Dose schedules are being continually revised and new side effects recognized. Oxford University Press makes no representation, express or implied, that the drug dosages in this book are correct. For these reasons the reader is strongly urged to consult the pharmaceutical company's printed instructions before administering any of the drugs recommended in this book.

Concise Oxford Textbook of Medicine

Concise Oxford Textbook of Medicine

Edited by

John G. G. Ledingham
Emeritus Professor of Medicine,
University of Oxford

David A. Warrell
Professor of Tropical Medicine
and Infectious Diseases; Director of
the Centre for Tropical Medicine,
University of Oxford

OXFORD
UNIVERSITY PRESS

OXFORD
UNIVERSITY PRESS

Great Clarendon Street, Oxford OX2 6DP

Oxford University Press is a department of the University of Oxford. It furthers the University's objective of excellence in research, scholarship, and education by publishing worldwide in

Oxford New York

Athens Auckland Bangkok Bogotá Buenos Aires Calcutta Cape Town Chennai Dar es Salaam Delhi Florence Hong Kong Istanbul Karachi Kuala Lumpur Madrid Melbourne Mexico City Mumbai Nairobi Paris São Paulo Singapore Taipei Tokyo Toronto Warsaw

with associated companies in Berlin Ibadan

Oxford is a registered trade mark of Oxford University Press in the UK and in certain other countries

Published in the United States by Oxford University Press, Inc., New York

First published 2000

A catalogue record for this title is available from the British Library

Library of Congress Cataloging in Publication Data
(Data available)

1 3 5 7 9 10 8 6 4 2

ISBN 0 19 262870 4

Typeset in Minion by Latimer Trend & Company Ltd, Plymouth
Printed in Italy on acid-free paper by
Vincenzo Bona s.r.l, Turin

Foreword
Professor Sir David Weatherall

This book is the lusty offspring of that ageing prima gravida, the *Oxford Textbook of Medicine* (OTM). Despite her advanced years, as evidenced by the fact that she is about to enter her fourth edition, she appears to have borne the long period of gestation of her offspring in reasonably good shape.

But why bring another infant of this type into an already overcrowded world? This question was very much in the mind of the editors of the first edition of the OTM. The omens were not good. Its predecessor, the last edition of *Price's Textbook of Medicine*, was not greeted with universal approval by the critics. An eminent professor of medicine had written that, like the dinosaurs, it was so large that it would collapse under its own weight and become extinct. While this criticism seemed to reflect a rather outmoded view of evolutionary biology, we could see his point.

Though a little discouraged by these comments, and not helped by one of our predecessors in Oxford who wrote that textbooks are only written by people with unhappy private lives, we decided to embark on the OTM. The reason was very simple. The three of us who became its founding editors were all striving to retain some competence in general internal medicine. The field had become vast and highly specialized and hence we found that we needed an up-to-date bird's eye view of the whole speciality which would give us an entré to any disease that we encountered and, even more importantly, point us in the right direction when we wished to analyse our patients in more detail. In addition, we felt the need for a book that would offer a reasonable grounding in both the scientific and pastoral aspects of internal medicine and which would present a more global picture of disease than standard western textbooks.

It appears that succeeding editions of the OTM have gone at least some way to meet these objectives. However, it is now a three-volume reference book, too daunting for medical students or young doctors to use as their companion and guide throughout their training. For this reason two of the original editors, John Ledingham and David Warrell, have condensed the OTM into a shorter version designed to fulfil these requirements.

As we move into the new millennium medical practice is going through an uneasy time. None of the richer western societies have come to grips with how to cope with the increasing expectations of medical care and its spiralling costs. Hospital-based practice has become increasingly compartmentalized and specialized. This has resulted in an increasing dearth of teachers who can provide students and young trainees with the kind of balanced picture of medical practice that they require. Furthermore, with the increasing age of the population, many patients have diseases in several different systems and present increasingly complex diagnostic and therapeutic problems. It is difficult to see how medicine will advance unless some of its practitioners maintain the old skills of the generalist, combined with a special interest. The editors of this book are two of the best general physicians that it has been my privilege and pleasure to work with over the years. This smaller version of the OTM seems to have inherited some of the better genes from its parent, and, in particular, carries the generalist stamp of its editors. I feel sure that it will be an invaluable guide and friend for students and young doctors during their early training and I wish it all the success that it undoubtedly deserves.

Oxford
April 2000

Section Editors

Disorders of the blood
Paul Moss, Institute of Molecular Immunology

Haemostasis and thrombosis
David Keeling, Consultant Haematologist, Oxford Radcliffe Hospitals; Honorary Senior Clinical Lecturer, University of Oxford

Neurology; Disorders of voluntary muscle
Peter Rothwell, MRC Senior Clinical Fellow; Honorary Consultant Neurologist, Radcliffe Infirmary, Oxford

Psychiatry
Eleanor Feldman, Consultant Psychiatrist, University of Oxford

Oxford University Press

Project Editor: Dr Irene Butcher

Development Editor: Kate Martin

Production Controller: Gill Watts

Design Manager: Claire Walker

Typographer: Jonathan Coleclough

Publisher: Alison Langton

Illustrations: Technical Graphics Department, Oxford University Press

Indexer: Caroline Sheard

Types of men 5

The physician

Hygiene is the corruption of medicine by morality. It is impossible to find a hygienist who does not debase his theory of the healthful with a theory of the virtuous. The whole hygienic art, indeed, resolves itself into an ethical exhortation, and, in the department of sex, into a puerile and belated advocacy of asceticism. This bring it, at the end, into diametrical conflict with medicine proper. *The aim of medicine is surely not to make men virtuous; it is to safeguard and rescue them from the consequences of their vices. The true physician does not preach repentance; he offers absolution.* (Editor's italics.)

H. L. Mencken (1923)

Preface

'Compendium: an abridgement of a larger work or treatise, giving the sense and substance, within smaller compass' (*Oxford English Dictionary*)

Concise versions of longer textbooks have been a successful part of Oxford publications for many years. Although shorter (and some, like this one are still quite large), they have been remarkably comprehensive and have often been preferred to the parent volumes for everyday use. An early example was the appearance in 1932 of *The Shorter Oxford English Dictionary*, a work which, with its successors, provides more than adequately for most readers, and is certainly more often consulted than is the full *OED*. The third edition of the *Oxford Textbook of Medicine* runs to over 5000 pages in three bulky volumes, compared to the first edition of some 2500 pages. It seemed to us, and to many colleagues whose advice we sought, ripe for a concise version. The substantial growth of the full Textbook reflected the increase of medical knowledge, the sometimes untrammelled enthusiasm of our authors for their appointed subjects, the indulgence of the editors and the provision of new sections on medical ethics, clinical trials, forensic medicine and clinical oncology. But much was also attributable to the editors decision to include chapters that were somewhat tangential to the essentials of clinical medicine. The editors also decided, in the full Textbook, to make each contribution complete in its own right, rather than to cross refer to a single account in the many areas in which overlap was inevitable.

The decision to produce this concise textbook, an epitome of the full *OTM*, was much influenced by the realization that, with tight editing, we could abridge the original text without loss of clinical information. This is important since most readers consult medical textbooks about particular clinical problems outside their own regular experience, be they students, general practitioners, or hospital physicians. The need, therefore, has been to produce a single volume, distilling from the original text an authoritative account of the essentials of clinical practice, while preserving an emphasis on the scientific basis of medicine. This was a much more difficult task than we had anticipated. But although it also took longer than we had thought it would, we did complete it in less than the 30 years (1902–32) needed to derive the Shorter from the full Oxford English Dictionary! Even so we echo the view of the editor of the *Concise Dictionary of National Biography* (1882–1930) who wrote of his work: 'The labour involved in condensing so massive a work ... has been great. No one without practical experience of a similar undertaking is likely to realise the vast amount of time and trouble which the preparation of this volume has entailed.'

The initial editing of the sections on psychiatry, haematology and neurology was done by Drs Eleanor Feldman, Paul Moss, and Peter Rothwell respectively and we are particularly grateful to them. Professor Julian Hopkin was kind enough to review (critically, but most helpfully) the respiratory section. We thank, too, the many authors for their help and tolerance of editorial decisions, especially when these seemed cruelly and capriciously procrustean. Perhaps our greatest debt is to Kate Martin and Irene Butcher from OUP, both of whom undertook an immense amount of expert work, while always preserving remarkable good humour in managing the editors, even when they were being unusually obtuse. Eunice Berry, who has been involved in all three editions of *OTM* was, yet again with this concise edition, an enormous help to DAW and to the Press.

We regret that we were not able to continue the partnership with David Weatherall that yielded three editions of *OTM*, but we are more than grateful for his advice and support as well as the nice things that he has said in the Foreword to this book. We hope that this offspring of the original Textbook, with which he was so closely involved, will not disappoint him or our other readers.

Oxford D.A.W.
June 2000 J.G.G.L.

Contents

Contributors

P. Aaby Professor, Danish Epidemiology Science Centre, Copenhagen, Denmark
16.20 Measles

J. P. Ackers Teaching Programme Director, London School of Hygiene and Tropical Medicine, UK
16.95 Trichomoniasis

M. W. Adler Professor of Genito-Urinary Medicine, University College London Medical School, UK
17.1 Sexually-transmitted diseases: epidemiology and control

D. Adu Consultant Physician and Nephrologist, Queen Elizabeth Hospital, Birmingham,UK
12.7 Idiopathic glomerulonephritis
12.11 Infections and associated nephropathies

P. Anderson Consultant, World Health Organization Regional Office for Europe, Copenhagen, Denmark
14.10 Assessing drug abuse and use of brief interventions

M. Asif Research Fellow in Cardiothoracic Transplantation, Department of Respiratory Medicine, University of Sheffield, UK
4.45 Lung and heart-lung transplantation

Tar-Ching Aw Consulting Occupational Toxicologist, National Poisons Information Service (Birmingham Centre), City Hospital, Birmingham, UK
18.13 Vibration

***R. R. Bailey** Nephrologist, Christchurch Hospital, New Zealand
12.18 Urinary tract infection
12.19 Vesicoureteric reflux and reflux nephropathy

M. J. Baines Consultant Physician, St Christopher's Hospice, London, UK
15 Palliative medicine

L. R. I. Baker Consultant Physician and Nephrologist, St Bartholomew's Hospital, London, UK
12.22 Urinary tract obstruction
12.27 Genitourinary tuberculosis

C. R. M. Bangham Professor, Department of Immunology, Imperial College School of Medicine, St Mary's Campus, London, UK
16.36 HTLV-1 and -II and associated diseases

K. M. Bannister Head of Renal Unit, Royal Adelaide Hospital, South Australia
12.1 Clinical physiology of the kidney: tests of renal function and structure

R. Bannister Honorary Consultant Neurologist, The National Hospital for Neurology and Neurosurgery, London and Oxford Regional and District Health Authority, UK
13.7 The autonomic nervous system

D. Barlow Consultant Physician, Department of Genitourinary Medicine, St Thomas's Hospital, London, UK
16.42 *Neisseria gonorrhoeae*

*It is with regret that we report the death of Dr R. R. Bailey.

A. J. Barrett Chief, Bone Marrow Transplantation Unit, National Heart, Blood, and Lung Institute, National Institutes of Health, Bethesda, Maryland, USA
3.4 Acute myeloblastic leukaemia

M. F. Bassendine Professor of Hepatology, University of Newcastle upon Tyne, UK
5.33 Primary biliary cirrhosis

P. H. Baylis Professor and Dean of Medicine, University of Newcastle upon Tyne, UK
7.2 The posterior pituitary
12.2 Water and sodium homeostasis and their disorders

J. I. Bell Nuffield Professor of Medicine, University of Oxford, UK
6.13 Diabetes mellitus

M. K. Benson Consultant Chest Physician, Osler Chest Unit, The Churchill Hospital, Oxford, UK
4.36 Pleural disease
4.40 Pleural tumours
4.41 Mediastinal tumours and cysts

V. Beral Director, Imperial Cancer Research Fund's Cancer Epidemiology Unit, Oxford, UK
17.6 Cervical cancer and other cancers caused by sexually transmitted diseases

R. J. Berry Visiting Professor, University of Lancaster, UK
18.11 Ionizing radiation

D. B. Bethell Specialist Registrar in Paediatrics, John Radcliffe Hospital, Oxford, UK
16.37 Dipththeria

C. M. Black Professor of Rheumatology, Royal Free Hospital, London, UK
10.9 Connective tissue disorders and vasculitis: an introduction
10.12 Systemic sclerosis

S. R. Bloom Professor of Medicine, Hammersmith Hospital, London, UK
5.5 Hormones and the gastrointestinal tract
7.15 Non-diabetic pancreatic endocrine disorders and multiple endocrine neoplasia

N. A. Boon Consultant Cardiologist, Royal Infirmary of Edinburgh, UK
2.20 HIV-related muscle disease
2.34 Coarctation of the aorta as a cause of secondary hypertension in the adult

I. C. J. W. Bowler Consultant Microbiologist and Infection Control Doctor to the Oxford Group of Hospitals and Honorary Senior Clinical Lecturer, University of Oxford, UK
16.8 Nosocomial infections

D. J. Bradley Professor of Tropical Hygiene, University of London and Director, Ross Institute, London School of Hygiene and Tropical Medicine, UK
16.84 Malaria

D. P. Brenton Professor, Director of Medical Education, University College London Hospitals Trust, UK
6.5 Inborn errors of amino acid and organic acid metabolism

R. Brettle Consultant Physician, Infectious Disease Unit, Western General Hospital, Edinburgh, UK
14.12 Physical complications of drug abuse

V. Broadbent Consultant Paediatric Oncologist, Addenbrooke's Hospital, Cambridge, UK
3.31 The histiocytoses

M. J. Brown Professor of Clinical Pharmacology, University of Cambridge, UK
2.33 Phaeochromocytoma

A. D. M. Bryceson Consultant Physician, Hospital for Tropical Diseases, London, UK
16.94 Leishmaniasis

C. Bunch Consultant Physician and Medical Director, Oxford Radcliffe Hospital NHS Trust, UK
3.28 Introduction to the lymphoproliferative disorders
3.29 The lymphomas

Danai Bunnag Professor Emeritus, Clinical Tropical Medicine, Mahidol University, Bangkok, Thailand
16.110 Liver fluke diseases of humans

W. Burgdorfer Rocky Mountain Laboratories, National Institute of Allergy and Infectious Diseases, National Institutes of Health, Hamilton, Montana, USA
16.65 Lyme disease

A. K. Burroughs Consultant Physician and Hepatologist, Royal Free Hospital, London, UK
5.36 Cirrhosis, portal hypertension, and ascites

T. Butler Professor and Chief, Division of Infectious Diseases, Department of Internal Medicine, School of Medicine, Texas Technical University Health Sciences Center, Lubbock, USA
16.51 Plague

A. E. Butterworth Formerly MRC External Scientific Staff and Honorary Professor in Medical Parasitology, University of Cambridge, UK
16.109 Schistosomiasis

F. I. Caird Formerly David Cargill Professor of Geriatric Medicine, University of Glasgow, UK
19.1 Medicine in old age

J. S. Cameron Emeritus Professor of Medicine, Guy's Hospital, London, UK
12.5 Common presentations of renal disease
12.15 Rheumatological disorders and the kidney: systemic lupus erythematosus, mixed connective tissue disease, scleroderma, Sjögren's syndrome, and rheumatoid arthritis
12.21 Gout, purines, and interstitial nephritis

D. J. S. Carmichael Consultant Nephrologist, Southend Hospital, Essex, UK
12.26 Prescription drugs and renal function

C. C. J. Carpenter Professor of Medicine, Brown University School of Medicine, Providence, Rhode Island, USA
16.46 Cholera

R. W. Carrell Professor and Head of Department of Haematology, Addenbrooke's Hospital and University of Cambridge, UK
4.17 Chronic obstructive pulmonary disease

D. P. Casemore Clinical Scientist, PHLS Cryptosporidium Reference Unit, Glan Clwyd District General Hospital, Bodelwyddan, Clwyd, UK
16.87 Cryptosporidium and cryptosporidiosis
16.88 Cyclospora

D. Catovsky Professor of Haematology, Institute of Cancer Research and Royal Marsden Hospital, London, UK
3.3 The classification of leukaemia
3.7 Chronic lymphocytic leukaemia and other leukaemias of mature B and T cells
3.8 Myelodysplastic syndromes

D. A. Chamberlain Consultant Cardiologist, Royal Sussex County Hospital, Brighton, UK
2.2 The syndrome of heart failure

L. E. Chapman Chief, Epidemiology Activity, HIV and Retrovirology Branch, Division of AIDS, STD, and TB Laboratory Research, National Center for Infectious Diseases, Centers for Disease Control, Atlanta, Georgia, USA
16.13 Human infections caused by simian herpesviruses

R. W. Chapman Consultant Gastroenterologist, John Radcliffe Hospital, Oxford, UK
5.34 Primary sclerosing cholangitis

Seung-Yull Cho Professor, Department of Molecular Parasitology, Sungkyunkwan University College of Medicine, Suwon, Korea
16.108 Diphyllobothriasis and sparganosis

***A. B. Christie** Honorary Consultant, Fazakerly Hospital, Liverpool, UK
16.19 Mumps: epidemic parotitis
16.37 Dipththeria
16.55 Anthrax

M. L. Clark Senior Lecturer, St Bartholomew's Hospital, London, UK
5.20 Tumours of the gastrointestinal tract

A. R. Clarkson Associate Professor of Medicine, University of Adelaide, Australia
12.6 Immunoglobulin A nephropathy, Henoch-Schönlein purpura, and thin membrane nephropathy

A. J. S. Coats Professor and Honorary Consultant Cardiologist, Royal Brompton and Harefield NHS Trust, Harefield Site, Middlesex, UK
2.2 The syndrome of heart failure

S. M. Cobbe Walton Professor of Medical Cardiology, University of Glasgow, UK
2.5 Cardiac arrhythmias

B. J. Cohen Clinical Scientist, Public Health Laboratory Service, London, UK
16.33 Parvoviruses

J. Cohen Professor and Chairman of Department of Infectious Diseases and Microbiology, Imperial College School of Medicine, Hammersmith Hospital Campus, London, UK

R. D. Cohen Professor of Medicine, St Bartholomew's and the Royal London Hospital Medical School of Medicine and Dentistry, London, UK
6.17 Disturbances of acid-base homeostasis
12.32 The renal tubular acidoses
16.117 Infection in the immunocompromised host

J. Collinge Professor and Director, MRC Prion Unit and Head, Department of Neurogenetics, Imperial College School of Medicine at St Mary's Hospital, London, UK
13.17 Prion diseases

D. A. S. Compston Professor of Neurology, University of Cambridge, UK
13.19 Demyelinating disorders of the central nervous system

C. P. Conlon Consultant Physician in Infectious Diseases, John Radcliffe Hospital, Oxford, UK
5.22 Gastrointestinal infections
16.7 Travel and expedition medicine
16.35 HIV infection and AIDS

M. Contreras Professor of Transfusion Medicine, Royal Free and University College Medical School, London, UK
3.25 Acquired haemolytic anaemia

M. R. Cooper CAB International, Wallingford, Oxfordshire, UK
18.3 Poisonous plants and fungi

J. Couvreur Professor of Paediatrics, Hôpital d'Enfants Armand Trousseau, Paris, France
16.86 Toxoplasmosis

P. J. Cowen Professor, University Department of Psychiatry, Oxford, UK
14.6 Psychopharmacology in medical practice

T. M. Cox Professor of Medicine, University of Cambridge, UK
5.10 Disaccharidase deficiency
6.2 Glycogen storage diseases
6.3 Inborn errors of fructose metabolism
6.4 Disorders of galactose and pyruvate metabolism and pentosuria

W. I. Cranston Emeritus Professor of Medicine, United Medical Schools of Guy's and St Thomas' Hospitals, London, UK
18.5 Drug-induced increases of body temperature

D. H. Crawford Professor of Medical Microbiology, University of Edinburgh, UK
16.12 The Epstein-Barr virus

I. Crome Professor of Addiction Studies, University of Wolverhampton, UK
14.10 Assessing drug abuse and use of brief interventions

D. W. M. Crook Consultant Microbiologist/Infectious Disease, University of Oxford (John Radcliffe Hospital), UK
2.25 Infective endocarditis
4.4 Microbiological methods in the diagnosis of respiratory infections
13.25 Bacterial meningitis
16.8 Nosocomial infections

G. W. Csonka Honorary Consultant in Venereology, St Mary's, St Stephen's, and Charing Cross Hospitals, London, UK
16.69 Syphilis

J. Cunningham Consultant Nephrologist and Physician, Royal London Hospital and Honorary Senior Lecturer St Bartholomew's and The Royal London School of Medicine, UK
12.31 Renal tubular disorders

J. V. Dacie Emeritus Professor of Haematology, Imperial College School of Medicine, London, UK
3.13 Paroxysmal nocturnal haemoglobinuria

D. A. B. Dance Consultant Microbiologist/Director, Public Health Laboratory, Derriford Hospital, Plymouth, Devon, UK
16.50 Melioidosis and glanders

H. J. Dargie Consultant Cardiologist, Western Infirmary, Glasgow, UK
2.2 The syndrome of heart failure

J. H. Dark Consultant Cardiothoracic Surgeon and Director, Cardiopulmonary Transplantation, Freeman Hospital, Newcastle upon Tyne, UK
2.3 Cardiac transplantation

P. G. Davey Professor of Pharmacoeconomics, University of Dundee and Honorary Consultant Physician in Infectious Diseases, Dundee Teaching Hospitals Trust, UK
16.5 Antimicrobial therapy

M. J. Davies BHF Professor of Cardiovascular Pathology, St George's Hospital Medical School, University of London, UK
2.8 The pathophysiology of ischaemic heart disease

P. D. O. Davies Consultant Respiratory Physician, Aintree Hospital NHS Trust, Liverpool, UK
16.59 Tuberculosis
16.60 Disease caused by environmental mycobacteria

A. M. Davison Professor of Renal Medicine, St James's University Hospital, Leeds, UK
12.13 Renal manifestations of malignant disease
12.14 Sarcoidosis and the kidney

P. T. Dawes Consultant Rheumatologist, Staffordshire Rheumatology Centre, Burslem, Stoke-on-Trent, Staffordshire, UK
10.1 Rheumatology: Introduction

K. Dawkins Consultant Cardiologist and Clinical Services Manager, Wessex Cardiothoracic Centre, Southampton General Hospital, UK
2.12 Exercise testing

***D. P. de Bono** British Heart Foundation Professor of Cardiology, University of Leicester Medical School, UK
2.14 Coronary angioplasty

D. M. Denison Professor of Clinical Physiology, Cardiothoracic Institute, University of London, UK
18.8 Aerospace medicine
18.9 Diving medicine

J. Dent Clinical Professor of Medicine and Director, Department of Gastroenterology, Royal Adelaide Hospital, South Australia
5.1 Symptomatology of gastrointestinal diseases
5.3 Diseases of the oesophagus

P. Dieppe Professor and Director, MRC Health Services Research Collaboration, University of Bristol, UK
10.1 Rheumatology: Introduction

M. Doherty Professor of Rheumatology, University of Nottingham Medical School, UK
10.5 Crystal-related arthropathies

M. Donaghy Reader in Clinical Neurology, University of Oxford, UK
13.1 Neurology: Introduction
13.29 The motor neurone diseases

S. Dover Consultant Physician and Gastroenterologist, West Glasgow Hospitals University NHS Trust, UK
6.7 Porphyrin metabolism and the porphyrias

R. H. Dowling Professor of Gastroenterology, Guy's Hospital, London, UK
5.7 Small-bowel bacterial overgrowth

R. M. du Bois Consultant Physician, Royal Brompton Hospital and Honorary Senior Lecturer, National Heart and Lung Institute, London, UK
4.18 Parenchymal lung disease: Introduction
4.19 Cryptogenic fibrosing alveolitis

*It is with regret that we report the deaths of Dr A. B. Christie and Professor D. P. de Bono.

C. R. K. Dudley Consultant Nephrologist, The Richard Bright Renal Unit, Southmead Hospital, Bristol, UK
2.18 Cholesterol embolism

B. O. L. Duke River Blindness Foundation, Lancaster, UK
16.96 Filariasis
16.97 Lymphatic filariasis

D. T. Durack Consulting Professor of Medicine, Duke University Medical Center, Durham, North Carolina, USA
16.115 Fever of unknown origin

S. R. Durham Upper Respiratory Medicine, Imperial College School of Medicine at the National Heart and Lung Institute, London, UK
4.11 Allergic rhinitis ('hay fever')

B. G. M. Durie Division of Hematology/ Oncology, Department of Medicine, Cedars-Sinai Comprehensive Cancer Center, Los Angeles, California, USA
3.30 Myeloma and other paraproteinaemias

P. N. Durrington Professor of Medicine, Department of Medicine, Manchester Royal Infirmary, UK
6.11 Lipid and lipoprotein disorders

G. M. Dusheiko Professor of Medicine, Royal Free Hospital, London, UK
5.40 Hepatic granulomas

C. J. Eastmond Consultant Rheumatologist, Aberdeen Royal Infirmary, UK
10.3 Seronegative spondylarthropathies

S. W. Eber Professor of Paediatrics, Universitäts-Kinderklinik, Göttingen, Germany
3.22 Genetic disorders of the red-cell membrane

A. L. W. F. Eddleston Professor of Liver Immunology and Dean, Guy's, King's and St Thomas' School of Medicine, London, UK
5.32 Autoimmune hepatitis

C. R. W. Edwards Professor of Medicine, University of London and Principal, Imperial College School of Medicine, UK
7.6 Adrenocortical diseases

A. M. El Nahas Professor of Nephrology, University of Sheffield, UK
12.29 Chronic renal failure

M. Elia Head of Clinical Nutrition Group, MRC, Dunn Clinical Nutrition Centre; Honorary Consultant Physician, Addenbrooke's Hospital, Cambridge, UK
8.4 The use of enteral and parenteral nutrition

M. Eliakim Professor of Internal Medicine; Chairman, Department of Medicine, Bikur Cholim Hospital, Jerusalem, Israel
6.16 Recurrent polyserositis (familial Mediterranean fever, periodic disease)

E. Elias Professor and Consultant Liver Physician, Queen Elizabeth Hospital, Birmingham, UK
5.30 Jaundice

B. T. Emmerson Emeritus Professor and Honorary Research Consultant, University of Queensland and Princess Alexandra Hospital, Brisbane, Australia
12.25 Toxic nephropathy

M. A. Epstein Fellow of Wolfson College, Oxford and Emeritus Professor of Pathology, University of Bristol, UK
16.12 The Epstein-Barr virus

S. J. Eykyn Professor and Honorary Consultant in Clinical Microbiology, St Thomas's Hospital, London, UK
16.38 Streptococci and enterococci
16.40 Staphyloccoci
16.45 Anaerobic bacteria

C. G. Fairburn Wellcome Principal Research Fellow and Professor of Psychiatry, University of Oxford, UK
14.20 Eating disorders

M. Farrell Senior Lecturer/Consultant Psychiatrist, Addiction Resource Centre, The Maudsley Hospital, London, UK
14.9 Substance abuse: Introduction
14.10 Assessing drug abuse and use of brief interventions
14.12 Physical complications of drug abuse
14.16 Strategies for managing drug and alcohol problems
14.18 Particular problems in special settings

M. J. G. Farthing Professor and Director, Digestive Diseases Research Centre, St Bartholomew's Hospital, London, UK
5.13 Malabsorption in the tropics

E. J. Feldman Consultant Liaison Psychiatrist and Honorary Senior Clinical Lecturer in Psychiatry, John Radcliffe Hospital, Oxford, UK
14.3 Schizophrenia
14.19 The use of the Mental Health Act and common law in mentally disordered general hospital patients

M. J. Field Associate Professor of Medicine, University of Sydney, Australia
12.1 Clinical physiology of the kidney: tests of renal function and structure

J. D. Firth Professor of Medicine, University of Cambridge, UK
12.28 Acute renal failure

S. P. Fisher-Hoch Director, Fondation Marcel Merieux, Laboratoire Jean Merieux P4, Lyon, France
16.26 Alphaviruses
16.30 Arenaviruses
16.31 Filoviruses: Marburg and Ebola fevers

E. Fitzsimons Consultant Haematologist, Monklands District General Hospital, Airdrie, UK
6.7 Porphyrin metabolism and the porphyrias

D. Fliser Assistant Professor of Internal Medicine, Medical School Hannover, Germany
12.9 Diabetic nephropathy

P. Föex Nuffield Professor of Anaesthetics, University of Oxford, UK
4.35 Adult respiratory distress syndrome

J. C. Forfar Consultant Cardiologist, John Radcliffe Hospital and Honorary Senior Lecturer in Medicine, University of Oxford, UK
2.2 The syndrome of heart failure

P. Frith Consultant Ophthalmic Physician, Radcliffe Infirmary, Oxford, UK
The eye and disease

C. S. Garrard Consultant Physician in Intensive Care, John Radcliffe Hospital, Oxford, UK
4.35 Adult respiratory distress syndrome
4.44 Management of chronic respiratory failure

J. S. Garrow Professor of Human Nutrition, St Bartholomew's Hospital, London, UK
8.3 Obesity

D. H. Gath Clinical Reader in Psychiatry, University Department of Psychiatry, Warneford Hospital, Oxford, UK
14.2 Mood disorders

K. C. Gatter Professor of Pathology and Head of Department of Clinical Biochemistry and Cellular Science, John Radcliffe Hospital, Oxford, UK
3.28 Introduction to the lymphoproliferative disorders
3.29 The lymphomas

M. G. Gelder Emeritus Professor of Psychiatry, University of Oxford, UK
14.1 Psychiatry in medicine
14.3 Schizophrenia
14.5 Non-pharmacological management of mental disorders

C. Gerada Principal in General Practice, Hurley Clinic, Kennington, London, UK
14.17 Drug dependency in pregnancy

H. Ghodse Professor of Psychiatry, St George's Hospital Medical School, University of London, UK
14.18 Particular problems in special settings

D. G. Gibson Consultant Cardiologist, Royal Brompton Hospital and Harefield NHS Trust, London, UK
2.23 Valve disease
2.26 Pericardial disease

G. J. Gibson Professor of Respiratory Medicine, University of Newcastle upon Tyne, UK
4.34 Drug-induced lung disease

F. J. Giles Assistant Professor, University of California at Los Angeles, USA
3.30 Myeloma and other paraproteinaemias

D. J. Girling Senior Scientific Staff, MRC Cancer Trials Office, Cambridge, UK
16.59 Tuberculosis
16.60 Disease caused by environmental mycobacteria

F. V. Gleeson Consultant Radiologist, Churchill Hospital, Oxford, UK
4.2 Thoracic imaging

R. Gokal Consultant Nephrologist and Physician, Manchester Royal Infirmary, UK
12.29 Chronic renal failure

M. H. N. Golden Professor of Medicine (Nutrition), University of Aberdeen, UK
8.2 Severe malnutrition

J. Goldman Professor of Leukaemia Biology and Chairman of Department of Haematology, Imperial College School of Medicine, Hammersmith Hospital, London, UK
3.6 Chronic myeloid leukaemia

E. C. Gordon-Smith Professor of Haematology, St George's Hospital Medical School, University of London, UK
3.12 Aplastic anaemia and other causes of bone marrow failure
3.23 Haemolysis due to red-cell enzyme deficiencies
3.25 Acquired haemolytic anaemia

J. M. Grange Reader in Clinical Microbiology, Imperial College School of Medicine; Visiting Professor, Royal Free and University College Medical School, London, UK
16.59 Tuberculosis
16.60 Disease caused by environmental mycobacteria

D. W. R. Gray Lecturer and Honorary Consultant in Transplantation, Nuffield

Department of Surgery, John Radcliffe Hospital and Oxford Transplant Centre, Churchill Hospital, Oxford, UK
12.29 Chronic renal failure

M. Greaves Professor of Haematology, University of Aberdeen, UK
3.39 Thrombotic disease

B. M. Greenwood Manson Professor of Tropical Medicine, London School of Hygiene and Tropical Medicine, UK
16.2 The host's response to infection
16.39 Pneumococcal infection
16.41 Meningococcal infection

R. J. Greenwood Consultant Neurologist, Homerton Hospital and the National Hospital for Neurology and Neurosurgery, London, UK
13.28 Neurosyphilis

B. Gribbin Consultant Cardiologist, John Radcliffe Hospital, Oxford, UK
2.25 Infective endocarditis

J. Grimley Evans Professor of Clinical Geratology, University of Oxford, UK
19.1 Medicine in old age

N. R. Grist Emeritus Professor of Infectious Diseases, University of Glasgow, UK
16.22 Enteroviruses

D. I. Grove Director of Clinical Microbiology and Infectious Diseases, The Queen Elizabeth Hospital, Woodville, South Australia
16.100 Nematode infections of lesser importance

D. J. Grundy Honorary Consultant in Spinal Injuries,The Duke of Cornwall Spinal Treatment Centre, Salisbury District Hospital, Wiltshire, UK
13.9 The management of spinal cord injury

J. P. Grünfeld Professor of Nephrology, Hôpital Necker, Paris, France
12.12 Renal amyloidosis, cryoglobulinaemia, light-chain deposition disease, and fibrillary glomerulonephritis
12.17 Clinical aspects of inherited renal disorders

A. G. Guevara Director, Laboratory of Clinical Investigations, Community Services Hospital Vozandes, Quito, Ecuador
16.93 American trypanosomiasis

M. R. Haeney Consultant Immunologist, Hope Hospital, Salford, UK
5.23 Immune disorders of the gastrointestinal tract

P. J. Hammond Consultant Physician/ Endocrinologist, Harrogate District Hospital, Harrogate, UK
5.5 Hormones and the gastrointestinal tract
7.15 Non-diabetic pancreatic endocrine disorders and multiple endocrine neoplasia

***A. E. Harding** Professor of Clinical Neurology, Institute of Neurology, University of London, UK
13.40 Mitochondrial myopathies and encephalomyopathies

Tranakchit Harinasuta Professor of Tropical Medicine, Faculty of Tropical Medicine, Mahidol University, Bangkok, Thailand
16.112 Intestinal trematodiasis

M. J. G. Harrison Emeritus Professor in Clinical Neurology, University College London, UK
13.13 Coma

I. Haslock Consultant Rheumatologist, South Cleveland Hospital and Visiting Professor in Clinical Bioengineering, University of Durham, UK
10.6 Back pain and periarticular disease

D. Hawkins Consultant Physician (Genitourinary Medicine), St Stephen's Centre, Chelsea and Westminster Hospital, London, UK
14.12 Physical complications of drug abuse

P. N. Hawkins Professor and Clinical Director, National Amyloidosis Centre, Department of Medicine, Royal Free and University College Medical School, Royal Free Campus, London, UK
6.15 Amyloidosis

K. E. Hawton Professor of Psychiatry and Consultant Psychiatrist, University Department of Psychiatry and Warneford Hospital, Oxford, UK
7.11 Disorders of sexual function

R. J. Hay Professor of Cutaneous Medicine, Guy's, King's, and St Thomas' School of Medicine, London, UK
16.63 Nocardiosis
16.81 Fungal infections (mycoses)

B. Hazleman Consultant Rheumatologist, Addenbrooke's Hospital, Cambridge, UK
10.8 Miscellaneous conditions

D. J. Hendrick Consultant Physician and Honorary Senior Lecturer, University of Newcastle upon Tyne, UK
4.25 Lymphocytic infiltrations of the lung
4.26 Extrinsic allergic alveolitis
4.29 Pulmonary alveolar proteinosis
4.30 Pulmonary amyloidosis
4.31 Lipoid (lipid) pneumonia
4.32 Pulmonary alveolar microlithiasis

M. F. Heyworth Chief of Staff, VA Medical Center and Professor, Department of Medicine, University of Pennsylvania, Philadelphia, USA
16.90 Giardiasis, balantidiasis, isosporiasis, and microsporidiosis

Tran Tinh Hien Vice Director, Centre for Tropical Diseases (Cho Quan Hospital), Ho Chi Minh City, Vietnam
16.37 Dipththeria

T. W. Higenbottam Consultant Physician and Respiratory Physiologist, Papworth and Addenbrooke's Hospitals, Cambridge, UK
4.45 Lung and heart-lung transplantation

S. L. Hillier Research Associate Professor of Obstetrics and Gynecology, University of Washington, Seattle, USA
17.3 Vaginal discharge

D. Hilton-Jones Clinical Director, Oxford Muscular Dystrophy Muscle and Nerve Centre, Department of Clinical Neurology, Radcliffe Infirmary, Oxford, UK
13.39 Metabolic and endocrine myopathies

T. D. R. Hockaday Honorary Consultant Physician, Radcliffe Infirmary, Oxford, UK
6.13 Diabetes mellitus

J. R. Hodges Professor of Behavioural Neurology, MRC Cognition and Brain Sciences Unit, Cambridge, UK
13.16 Dementia

H. J. F. Hodgson Professor of Medicine, Imperial College School of Medicine, Hammersmith Campus, London, UK
5.11 Whipple's disease (*Tropheryma whippelii* infection)
5.12 Short gut syndrome

A. V. Hoffbrand Professor of Haematology, Royal Free Hospital, London, UK
3.18 Megaloblastic anaemia and miscellaneous deficiency anaemias

J. M. Hopkin Professor of Medicine, University of Swansea, UK
4.6 Upper respiratory tract infection
4.8 Suppurative pulmonary and pleural infections
4.9 Chronic specific infections
4.10 Respiratory infection in the immunosuppressed
4.20 Bronchiolitis obliterans
4.23 Pulmonary vasculitis and granulomatosis
16.82 *Pneumocystis carinii*

***A. P. Hopkins** Director of the Research Unit, Royal College of Physicians, London, UK
13.11 Epilepsy in later childhood and adult life

I. A. Hughes Professor of Paediatrics, University of Cambridge, UK
7.7 Congenital adrenal hyperplasia

B. J. Hunt Consultant, Departments of Haematology and Rheumatology, Guy's and St Thomas' Trust, London, UK
3.38 Acquired coagulation disorders

C. W. Hutton Consultant Rheumatologist, Derriford Hospital, Plymouth, Devon, UK
10.4 Osteoarthritis

C. W. Imrie Consultant Surgeon, University of Glasgow, UK
5.26 Acute pancreatitis

M. Irving Professor of Surgery, University of Manchester, UK
5.24 The peritoneum, omentum, and appendix

D. Isaacs Head of Department of Immunology and Infectious Diseases, Royal Alexandra Hospital for Children, Sydney, Australia
16.6 Immunization
16.9 Respiratory tract viruses

P. G. Isaacson Professor of Morbid Anatomy, University College London Medical School, UK
5.9 Enteropathy-associated T-cell lymphoma

D. A. Isenberg Professor of Rheumatology, University College London, UK
10.11 Systemic lupus erythematosus and related disorders

K. Ishikawa Director, Department of Internal Medicine, Higashi Nagahara Hospital, Osaka, Japan
2.35 Takayasu's disease

H. S. Jacobs Professor of Reproductive Endocrinology, University College London Medical School, UK
7.8 Ovarian disorders
7.9 The breast

R. Jacoby Professor of Old Age Psychiatry, University of Oxford, UK
19.2 Abuse of elderly people

O. F. W. James Professor of Geriatric Medicine, University of Newcastle upon Tyne, UK
5.35 Alcoholic liver disease and non-alcoholic steatosis hepatitis

W. P. T. James Professor and Director, The Rowett Research Institute, Aberdeen, UK
8.1 Nutritional requirements

B. Jennett Emeritus Professor of Neurosurgery, Institute of Neurological Sciences, Glasgow, UK
13.14 Brainstem death

D. P. Jewell Professor of Gastroenterology, John Radcliffe Hospital, Oxford, UK
5.1 Symptomatology of gastrointestinal diseases
5.8 Coeliac disease

*It is with regret that we report the deaths of Professor A. E. Harding and Dr A. P. Hopkins.

5.14 Crohn's disease
5.15 Ulcerative colitis
5.42 Miscellaneous disorders of the gastrointestinal tract and liver

A. R. Johns Consultant Forensic Psychiatrist and Lead Clinician, Denis Hill Unit, Bethlem Royal Hospital, Beckenham, London, UK
14.14 Management of withdrawal syndromes

A. M. Johnson Reader in Epidemiology, Department of Genito-Urinary Medicine, University College London Medical School, UK
17.2 Sexual behaviour

A. W. Johnson CAB International, Wallingford, Oxfordshire, UK
18.3 Poisonous plants and fungi

E. A. Jones Chief of Hepatology, Department of Gastrointestinal and Liver Diseases, Academic Medical Centre, Amsterdam, The Netherlands
5.37 Hepatocellular failure

N. Jones Department of Virology, John Radcliffe Hospital, Oxford, UK
16.17 Orf
16.18 Molluscum contagiosum

M. Joy Consultant Cardiologist, St Peter's Hospital, Chertsey, Surrey, UK
2.16 Vocational aspects of coronary artery disease

J. A. Kanis Professor in Human Metabolism and Clinical Biochemistry, University of Sheffield Medical School, UK
7.5 Disorders of calcium metabolism
12.30 Renal bone disease

T. Kawasaki Director, Japan Kawasaki Disease Research Center, Tokyo, Japan
10.17 Kawasaki disease

W. R. Keatinge Emeritus Professor of Physiology, Queen Mary and Westfield College, London, UK
18.4 Heat
18.6 Cold, drowning, and seasonal mortality

P. G. E. Kennedy Burton Professor of Neurology, University of Glasgow, UK
13.26 Viral infections of the central nervous system

M. G. W. Kettlewell Consultant Surgeon, Oxford Radcliffe Trust, UK
5.18 Colonic diverticular disease

M. M. Kliks President, CTS Foundation, Honolulu, Hawaii
16.98 Guinea-worm disease: human dracunculiasis

B. Knight Emeritus Professor of Forensic Pathology, University of Wales College of Medicine, Cardiff, UK
20 Forensic medicine (medical jurisprudence: legal medicine)

R. Knight Associate Specialist in General Medicine, Royal Sussex County Hospital, Brighton, UK. Formerly Professor of Parasitology, Department of Microbiology, University of Nairobi, Kenya
16.83 Amoebiasis
16.99 Ancylostomiasis, strongyloidiasis, and other gut strongyloid nematodes
16.106 Other gut cestodes

J. B. Kurtz Consultant Virologist, PHLS Birmingham Heartlands Hospital, Birmingham UK
16.10 Herpes simplex virus infections
16.71 Legionellosis and legionnaires' disease

D. G. Lalloo Senior Lecturer, Liverpool School of Tropical Medicine and Honorary Consultant Physician, Royal Liverpool University Hospitals, UK
16.52 Yersiniosis
16.53 Pasteurellosis
16.54 Tularaemia

H. P. Lambert Emeritus Professor of Microbial Diseases, St George's Hospital Medical School, University of London, UK
16.1 An approach to the patient with suspected infection

D. J. Lane Consultant Chest Physician, Oxford Radcliffe Hospital, UK
4.1 The clinical presentation of chest diseases
4.13 Asthma
4.15 Cystic fibrosis
4.22 Pulmonary vasculitis and granulomatosis
4.23 Pulmonary haemorrhagic disorders
4.24 Pulmonary eosinophilia

H. E. Larson Private Practice, Internal Medicine and Infectious Diseases; Attending Physician Marlborough Hospital and Metrowest Medical Center, Framingham, Massachusetts, USA
16.58 Botulism, gas gangrene, and clostridian gastrointestinal infections

N. F. Lawton Consultant Neurologist, Wessex Neurological Centre, Southampton General Hospital, UK
13.23 Benign intracranial hypertension

J. G. G. Ledingham Emeritus Professor of Clinical Medicine, University of Oxford, UK
2.2 The syndrome of heart failure
2.30 Pulmonary embolism
2.32 Secondary hypertension
2.36 Lymphoedema
12.3 Idiopathic oedema of women
12.4 Disorders of potassium metabolism
13.31 The POEMS syndrome

J. W. LeDuc Medical Officer, Division of Communicable Diseases, World Health Organization, Geneva, Switzerland
16.29 Bunyaviridae

P. J. Lee Consultant in Metabolic Medicine, University College London Hospitals Trust, UK
6.5 Inborn errors of amino acid and organic acid metabolism

T. Lehner Professor, Guy's, King's, and St Thomas' Schools of Medicine, Dentistry and Biomedical Sciences, Guy's Campus, London, UK
5.2 The mouth and salivary glands
10.16 Behçet's disease

C. C. Linnemann, Jr Professor, Departments of Medicine and Pathology and Laboratory Medicine, University of Cincinnati, Ohio, USA
16.49 Bordetella

***C. M. Lockwood** Reader in Therapeutic Immunology and Honorary Consultant Physician, Addenbrooke's Hospital, Cambridge, UK
10.10 Vasculitis

S. Logan Senior Lecturer in Paediatric Epidemiology, Institute of Child Health, London, UK
16.27 Rubella

D. A. Lomas Lecturer in Medicine and Honorary Consultant Physician, Addenbrooke's Hospital and University of Cambridge, UK
4.17 Chronic obstructive pulmonary disease

M. S. Losowsky Emeritus Professor of Medicine, University of Leeds, UK
5.6 Investigation and differential diagnosis of malabsorption

S. E. Lux Professor of Pediatrics, Harvard Medical School, Boston, Massachusetts, USA
3.22 Genetic disorders of the red-cell membrane

L. Luzzatto Cancer Centre, Memorial Sloan Kettering Hospital, New York, USA
3.13 Paroxysmal nocturnal haemoglobinuria
3.24 Glucose 6-phosphate dehydrogenase (G6PD) deficiency

G. A. Luzzi Consultant in Genitourinary/HIV Medicine, South Buckinghamshire NHS Trust, Wycombe Hospital, High Wycombe, UK
16.35 HIV infection and AIDS

D. C. W. Mabey Professor of Communicable Disease, London School of Hygiene and Tropical Medicine and Consultant Physician, Hospital for Tropical Diseases, London, UK
16.76 Chlamydial infections

J. T. Macfarlane Consultant Physician in General and Respiratory Medicine, City Hospital, Nottingham, UK
4.7 Acute lower respiratory tract infections
16.71 Legionellosis and legionnaires' disease

S. J. Machin Professor of Haematology, University College and Middlesex School of Medicine, London, UK
3.34 Introduction to disorders of haemostasis and coagulation
3.35 Purpura

I. J. Mackie Non-Clinical Lecturer in Haematology, University College London, UK
3.33 The biology of haemostasis and thrombosis
3.34 Introduction to disorders of haemostasis and coagulation

C. R. Madeley Emeritus Professor of Clinical Virology, University of Newcastle upon Tyne, UK
16.23 Viruses causing diarrhoea and vomiting

A. Maden Consultant Forensic Psychiatrist, Bethlem Royal and Maudsley Hospital and Senior Lecturer, Institute of Psychiatry, London, UK
14.18 Particular problems in special settings

M. M. Madkour Consultant Physician, Military Hospital, Riyadh, Saudi Arabia
16.56 Brucellosis

J. I. Mann Professor, Department of Human Nutrition, University of Otago, Dunedin, New Zealand
2.10 Epidemiology and prevention of ischaemic heart disease

M. J. Marmot Professor, Department of Epidemiology and Public Health, Royal Free and University College Medical School, London, UK
2.10 Epidemiology and prevention of ischaemic heart disease

T. J. Marrie Professor of Medicine and Associate Professor of Microbiology, Dalhousie University, Halifax, Nova Scotia, Canada
16.74 *Coxiella burnetii* infections (Q fever)

***C. D. Marsden** Professor of Neurology, National Hospital for Neurology and Neurosurgery, London, UK
13.12 Narcolepsy and related sleep disorders
13.20 Movement disorders

***P. D. Marsden** Professor of Medicine, University of Brasilia, Brazil
16.93 American trypanosomiasis

V. J. Martlew Consultant Haematologist, Royal Liverpool Hospital, UK
3.41 Transfusion of blood and blood components

*It is with regret that we report the deaths of Dr. C. M. Lockwood, Professor C. D. Marsden, and Professor P. D. Marsden.

A. D. Mason Chief, Laboratory Division, US Army Institute of Medical Research, Fort Sam Houston, Texas, USA
18.10 Lightning and electric shock

W. B. Matthews Professor Emeritus of Clinical Neurology, University of Oxford, UK
13.3 The motor and sensory systems, midbrain, and brainstem
13.8 Spinal cord

R. S. Maurice-Williams Consultant Neurosurgeon, Royal Free Hospital, London, UK
13.10 Disorders of the spinal nerve roots

R. T. Mayon-White Consultant Public Health Physician, Public Health Directorate, Oxfordshire Health Authority, Oxford, UK
16.3 Epidemiology and public health

R. A. Mayou Professor of Psychiatry, University of Oxford, UK
14.4 Organic (cognitive) mental disorders
14.7 Psychiatric emergencies and problems arising in accident and emergency departments

K. E. L. McColl Professor of Gastroenterology, Western Infirmary, Glasgow, UK
6.7 Porphyrin metabolism and the porphyrias

J. B. McCormick Center for Bacterial and Mycotic Diseases, Centers for Disease Control, Atlanta, Georgia, USA
16.26 Alphaviruses
16.30 Arenaviruses
16.31 Filoviruses: Marburg and Ebola fevers

I. G. McFarlane Consultant Biochemist, Institute of Liver Studies, King's College School of Medicine and Dentistry, London, UK
5.32 Autoimmune hepatitis

A. M. McGregor Professor of Medicine, King's College School of Medicine and Dentistry, London, UK
7.3 The thyroid gland and disorders of thyroid function

N. McIntyre Professor of Medicine, Royal Free Hospital, London, UK
5.36 Cirrhosis, portal hypertension, and ascites

W. J. McKenna Professor of Cardiac Medicine, St George's Hospital Medical School, University of London, UK
2.19 Myocarditis, the cardiomyopathies, and specific heart muscle disorders

A. McMillan Consultant Physician, Department of Genito-urinary Medicine, Edinburgh Royal Infirmary, UK
17.5 Infections and other medical problems in homosexual men

T. W. Meade Professor and Director, MRC Epidemiology and Medical Care Unit, Wolfson Institute of Preventive Medicine, London, UK
2.10 Epidemiology and prevention of ischaemic heart disease

A. Meheus Professor and Chairman, Department of Epidemiology and Community Medicine, University of Antwerp, Belgium
17.1 Sexually-transmitted diseases: epidemiology and control

S. A. Misbah Consultant Clinical Immunologist, Leeds General Infirmary, UK
10.18 Cryoglobulinaemia

J. J. Misiewicz Honorary Consultant Gastroenterologist and Joint Director (Gastroenterology), Central Middlesex Hospital, London, UK
5.4 Peptic ulceration

T. P. Monath Vice-President, Vaccines Research and Medical Affairs, OraVax Inc./Peptide Therapeutics p.l.c., Cambridge, Massachusetts, USA
16.28 Flaviviruses

M. R. Moore Professor of Medicine, National Research Centre for Environmental Toxicology, University of Queensland, Australia
6.7 Porphyrin metabolism and the porphyrias

H. G. Morgan Emeritus Professor of Mental Health, University of Bristol, UK
14.8 The patient who has attempted suicide

P. J. Morris Nuffield Professor of Surgery, University of Oxford, UK
2.17 Peripheral arterial disease

N. J. McC. Mortensen Consultant Surgeon and Clinical Reader in Colorectal Surgery, John Radcliffe Hospital, Oxford, UK
5.18 Colonic diverticular disease

A. G. Mowat Senior Clinical Lecturer in Rheumatology, University of Oxford, UK
10.15 Polymyalgia rheumatica and giant-cell arteritis

J. Moxham Professor of Respiratory Medicine, Guy's, King's and St Thomas' School of Medicine, London, UK
4.42 Definition and causes
4.44 Management of chronic respiratory failure

E. R. Moxon Action Research Professor of Paediatrics, University of Oxford, UK
16.6 Immunization
16.47 *Haemophilus influenzae*

M. F. Muers Consultant Physician, Department of Respiratory Medicine, Leeds General Infirmary, UK
4.5 Diagnostic bronchoscopy and tissue biopsy

P. A. Murphy Professor of Medicine, Johns Hopkins University School of Medicine, Baltimore, Maryland, USA
16.4 Physiological changes in infected patients
16.116 Septicaemia

I. M. Murray-Lyon Consultant Physician and Gastroenterologist to Charing Cross Hospital and Chelsea & Westminster Hospital, London, UK
5.38 Primary liver tumours

R. Naoumova MRC Clinical Scientist, MRC Molecular Medicine Group, Hammersmith Hospital, London, UK
2.7 The pathogenesis of atherosclerosis

D. G. Nathan President, Dana-Farber Cancer Institute, Boston, Massachusetts, USA
3.2 Stem cells and haematopoiesis

G. Neale Consultant Physician, Addenbrooke's Hospital, Cambridge, UK
5.21 Vascular and collagen disorders

G. H. Neild Professor of Nephrology, University College London Medical School, UK
12.10 Haemolytic uraemic syndrome

J. Neuberger Consultant Physician, Queen Elizabeth Hospital, Birmingham, UK
5.41 Drugs and liver damage

J. M. Neutze Professor of Medicine and Cardiologist, Green Lane Hospital, Auckland, New Zealand
2.22 Cardiac aspects of rheumatic fever

C. I. Newbold Professor of Tropical Medicine, University of Oxford, UK
16.84 Malaria

A. J. Newman Taylor Professor of Occupational and Environmental Medicine, National Heart and Lung Institute, London, UK
4.14 Occupational asthma

J. Newsom-Davis Professor Emeritus, University of Oxford, UK
13.1 Neurology: Introduction
13.38 Disorders of neuromuscular transmission

P. Newton Wellcome-Mahidol University Oxford Tropical Medicine Research Programme, Faculty of Tropical Medicine, Mahidol University, Bangkok, Thailand
16.67 Leptospirosis

S. Nightingale Consultant Neurologist, Royal Shrewsbury Hospital, UK
16.36 HTLV-1 and -II and associated diseases

G. Nuki Professor of Rheumatology, University of Edinburgh, UK
6.6 Disorders of purine and pyrimidine metabolism

J. G. Olson Epidemiologist–Laboratory Manager, US Navy Medical Research Unit No. 2 (NAMRU-2) National Institute of Public Health (NIPH) Laboratory, Phnom Penh, Cambodia
16.75 Bartonellosis, cat scratch disease, bacillary angiomatosis-peliosis, and trench fever

D. Overbosch Consultant Physician, Department of Tropical Medicine, Havenziekenhuis and Institute of Tropical Medicine, Rotterdam, The Netherlands
16.107 Cysticercosis

J. M. Oxbury Consultant Neurologist, Radcliffe Infirmary, Oxford, UK
13.2 Disturbances of higher cerebral function

S. M. Oxbury Consultant Clinical Neuropsychologist, Radcliffe Infirmary, Oxford, UK
13.2 Disturbances of higher cerebral function

J. Paul Consultant Medical Microbiologist, Brighton Public Health Laboratory, Sussex, UK
16.80 'Newer' and lesser known bacteria causing infection in humans
16.113 Non-venomous arthropods

I. Peake Professor of Molecular Medicine, University of Sheffield, UK
3.36 The pathogenesis of genetic disorders of coagulation

J. M. S. Pearce Honorary Consultant Neurologist, Hull Royal Infirmary, UK
13.21 Headache

P. E. Pellett Chief, Herpesvirus Section, Centers for Disease Control and Prevention, Atlanta, Georgia, USA
16.15 Human herpesviruses 6, 7, and 8

M. B. Pepys Professor of Medicine and Head of Department of Medicine, Royal Free and University College Medical School, Royal Free Campus, London, UK
6.15 Amyloidosis

S. P. Pereira Senior Registrar in Gastroenterology/General Medicine, Guy's Hospital, London, UK
5.7 Small-bowel bacterial overgrowth

P. L. Perine Professor of Epidemiology, School of Public and Community Medicine, University of Washington, Seattle, USA
16.68 Non-venereal endemic treponematoses: yaws, endemic syphilis (bejel), and pinta

C. J. Peters Chief, Special Viral Pathogens Branch, Division of Viral and Rickettsial Diseases, Centers for Disease Control and Prevention, Atlanta, Georgia, USA
16.13 Human infections caused by simian herpesviruses

T. J. Peters Professor of Clinical Biochemistry, King's College School of Medicine and Dentistry, London, UK
14.13 Nutritional deficiency syndromes complicating alcohol abuse

T. E.A. Peto Professor and Consultant Physician in Infectious Diseases, Oxford Radcliffe Hospital NHS Trust, UK
4.5 Microbiological methods in the diagnosis of respiratory infections

***Prida Phuapradit** Professor of Neurology, Mahidol University, Bangkok, Thailand
13.25 Bacterial meningitis

M. J. Pippard Professor of Haematology and Head of Department of Molecular and Cellular Pathology, Ninewells Medical School, University of Dundee, UK
3.16 Iron metabolism and its disorders

J. M. Polak Professor of Endocrine Pathology, Imperial College School of Medicine, Hammersith Campus, London, UK
5.5 Hormones and the gastrointestinal tract

P. A. Poole-Wilson Professor of Cardiology, Imperial College School of Medicine, National Heart and Lung Institute, London, UK
2.2 The syndrome of heart failure

J. S. Porterfield Formerly Reader in Bacteriology, Sir William Dunn School of Pathology, University of Oxford, UK
16.29 Bunyaviridae

R. E. Pounder Professor of Medicine, Royal Free and University College Medical School, Royal Free Campus, London, UK
5.4 Peptic ulceration

M. A. Preece Professor of Child Health and Growth, Institute of Child Health, University College London, UK
7.13 Disorders of growth

***J. S. Prichard** Professor of Medicine, St James's Hospital, Dublin, Eire
2.27 Pulmonary oedema
2.28 Pulmonary hypertension
2.29 Cor pulmonale

N. B. Pride Professor of Respiratory Medicine, Imperial College School of Medicine, Hammersmith Hospital Campus, London, UK
4.3 Lung function testing
4.17 Chronic obstructive pulmonary disease

J. Pritchard Senior Lecturer in Paediatric Oncology, Institute of Child Health and Consultant, Hospital for Sick Children, London, UK
3.31 The histiocytoses

A. T. Proudfoot Director, National Poisons Information Service (Edinburgh Centre), Royal Infirmary, Edinburgh, UK
18.1 Poisoning with drugs and chemicals

B. A. Pruitt Professor of Surgery, University of Texas Health Science Center at San Antonio, USA
18.10 Lightning and electric shock

*It is with regret that we report the deaths of Professor Prida Phuapradit, Professor J. S. Prichard, and Professor A. E. G. Raine.

Swanjai Pungpak Associate Professor of Clinical Tropical Medicine, Mahidol University, Bangkok, Thailand
16.110 Liver fluke diseases of humans

Sompone Punyagupta President and Chairman, Department of Medicine, Vichaiyut Hospital, Bangkok, Thailand
16.103 Angiostrongyliasis

C. D. Pusey Professor of Renal Medicine, Imperial College School of Medicine, Hammersmith Hospital Campus, London, UK
12.8 Rapidly progressive glomerulonephritis and antiglomerular basement membrane disease

N. P. Quinn Professor of Clinical Neurology, Institute of Neurology, University College London, UK
13.4 Subcortical structures—the cerebellum, thalamus, and basal ganglia

A. J. Radford Emeritus Professor, Flinders University of South Australia
16.105 Hydatid disease

Prayong Radomyos Professor, Faculty of Tropical Medicine, Mahidol University, Thailand
16.112 Intestinal trematodiasis

***A. E. G. Raine** Professor of Renal Medicine, St Bartholomew's Hospital, London, UK
2.32 Secondary hypertension
12.24 Hypertension: its effects on the kidney

A. C. Rankin Senior Lecturer in Medical Cardiology, Royal Infirmary, Glasgow, UK
2.5 Cardiac arrhythmias

P. J. Ratcliffe Professor of Renal Medicine, Institute of Molecular Medicine, University of Oxford, UK
12.29 Chronic renal failure

A. J. Rees Regius Professor of Medicine, University of Aberdeen, UK
12.8 Rapidly progressive glomerulonephritis and antiglomerular basement membrane disease

D. Rennie Professor of Medicine, University of California, San Francisco, USA
18.7 Diseases of high terrestrial altitudes

J. Richens Clinical Lecturer, Academic Department of Sexually Transmitted Diseases, Royal Free and University College Medical School, London, UK
16.44 Typhoid and paratyphoid fevers
16.78 Donovanosis (granuloma inguinale)
16.79 Rhinoscleroma

B. K. Rima Professor of Molecular Biology, The Queen's University of Belfast, UK
16.19 Mumps: epidemic parotitis

E. Ritz Professor of Medicine, Ruperto Carola University of Heidelberg, Germany
12.9 Diabetic nephropathy

I. A. G. Roberts Senior Lecturer and Consultant in Haematology, Imperial College School of Medicine, Hammersmith Hospital Campus, London, UK
3.5 Acute lymphoblastic leukaemia

A. Ronald Associate Dean, Research; Distinguished Professor, Medicine, Medical Microbiology, and Community Health Sciences, University of Manitoba, Winnipeg, Canada
16.48 *Haemophilus ducreyi* and chancroid

R. J. M. Ross Reader in Endocrinology and Honorary Consultant Physician, University of Sheffield and Northern General Hospital, Sheffield, UK
7.14 Puberty

R. W. Ross Russell Consultant Physician, St Thomas's Hospital, National Hospital for Neurology and Neurosurgery, and Moorfields Eye Hospital, London, UK
13.5 Visual pathways

D. J. Rowlands Consultant Cardiologist, Manchester Heart Centre, UK
2.4 The electrocardiogram

P. Rudge Consultant Neurologist, National Hospital for Nervous Diseases, London, UK
13.6 The cranial nerves

T. K. Ruebush II Chief, Malaria Section, Division of Parasitic Diseases, Centers for Disease Control, Atlanta, Georgia, USA
16.85 Babesia

R. C. G. Russell Consultant Surgeon, The Middlesex Hospital, London, UK
5.28 Tumours of the pancreas

T. J. Ryan Clinical Professor of Dermatology, University of Oxford, UK
11 Diseases of the skin

M. O. Savage Professor of Paediatric Endocrinology, St Bartholomew's and the Royal London School of Medicine and Dentistry, St Bartholomew's Campus, London, UK
7.12 Normal and abnormal sexual differentiation
7.14 Puberty

G. F. Savidge Professor and Clinical Director, Haemophilia Reference Centre, St Thomas's Hospital, London, UK
3.37 Clinical features and management of the hereditary disorders of haemostasis

J. W. Scadding Consultant Neurologist, The National Hospital for Neurology and Neurosurgery, London, UK
1 Pain management

K. P. Schaal Professor and Director, Institute for Medical Microbiology and Immunology, University of Bonn, Germany
16.62 Actinomycoses

R. B. H. Schutgens Professor, Free University of Amsterdam, The Netherlands
6.9 Peroxisomal disorders

T. G. Schwan Head, Arthropod-borne Diseases Section, Laboratory of Vectors and Pathogens, Rocky Mountain Laboratories, National Institute of Allergy and Infectious Diseases, National Institutes of Health, Hamilton, Montana, USA
16.65 Lyme disease

J. Schwebke Associate Professor of Medicine, University of Alabama at Birmingham, USA
17.3 Vaginal discharge

D. G. I. Scott Consultant Rheumatologist, Norfolk and Norwich Healthcare NHS Trust, UK
10.9 Connective tissue disorders and vasculitis: an introduction

J. Scott Professor of Medicine, National Heart and Lung Institute, Imperial College School of Medicine, Hammersmith Hospital, London, UK
2.7 The pathogenesis of atherosclerosis

A. Seaton Professor of Environmental and Occupational Medicine, University of Aberdeen, UK
4.33 Pneumoconioses

A. W. Segal Professor of Medicine, University College and Middlesex School of Medicine, London, UK
3.27 Leucocytes in health and disease

M. H. Seifert Consultant Rheumatologist, St Mary's Hospital, London, UK
10.7 Septic arthritis

G. R. Serjeant Director, MRC Laboratories (Jamaica), University of the West Indies, Kingston, Jamaica
12.16 Sickle-cell disease and the kidney

C. A. Seymour Professor of Clinical Biology and Metabolism, St George's Hospital Medical School, University of London, UK
5.25 Congenital and hereditary disorders of the liver, biliary tract, and pancreas
6.10 Trace metal disorders

K. V. Shah Professor of Immunology and Infectious Diseases, Johns Hopkins University School of Hygiene and Public Health, Baltimore, Maryland, USA
16.32 Papovaviruses

M. Sharpe Senior Lecturer and Honorary Consultant in Psychological Medicine, University of Edinburgh, Royal Edinburgh Hospital, UK
16.118 Chronic fatigue syndrome (postviral fatigue syndrome and myalgic encephalomyelitis)

R. J. Shaw Medical Director and Professor of Respiratory Medicine, Imperial College London Medical School, Hammersmith Hospital Campus, London, UK
4.21 The lung in collagen-vascular diseases
4.28 Eosinophilic granuloma of the lung and lymphangioleimyomatosis

M. C. Sheppard Professor of Medicine and Head, Department of Medicine, University of Birmingham, UK
7.4 Thyroid cancer

J. M. Shneerson Director, Respiratory Support and Sleep Centre, Papworth Hospital, Cambridge, UK
4.37 Disorders of the thoracic cage and diaphragm

M. Siebels Department of Internal Medicine, Division of Nephrology, University of Heidelberg, Germany
12.9 Diabetic nephropathy

C. A. Sieff Associate Professor of Pediatrics, Harvard Medical School, Boston, Massachusetts, USA
3.2 Stem cells and haematopoiesis

H. A. Simmonds Senior Lecturer, United Medical and Dental Schools of Guy's and St Thomas' Hospitals, London
12.21 Gout, purines, and interstitial nephritis

D. I. H. Simpson Professor of Microbiology and Immunobiology, Queen's University, Belfast, UK
16.26 Alphaviruses

V. Sitprija Professor of Medicine, Department of Medicine, Chulalongkorn Hospital Medical School, Bangkok, Thailand
16.67 Leptospirosis

M. B. Skirrow Honorary Emeritus Consultant Microbiologist, Public Health Laboratory, Gloucester Royal Hospital, UK
16.43 Enterobacteria, Campylobacter, and miscellaneous enteropathogenic food-poisoning bacteria

P. Sleight Professor Emeritus of Cardiovascular Medicine, University of Oxford, UK
2.13 Myocardial infarction

D. H. Smith Senior Lecturer and Honorary Consultant Physician in Tropical Medicine, Liverpool School of Tropical Medicine, UK
16.92 Human African trypanosomiasis

G. L. Smith Professor of Virology, Sir William Dunn School of Pathology, University of Oxford, UK
16.16 Poxviruses

R. Smith Consultant Physician and Consultant in Metabolic Medicine, John Radcliffe Hospital and Nuffield Orthopaedic Centre, Oxford, UK
6.18 Metabolic effects of accidental injury and surgery
8.1 Nutritional requirements
9 Disorders of the skeleton

M. L. Snaith Senior Lecturer in Rheumatology, University of Sheffield, UK
10.11 Systemic lupus erythematosus and related disorders

J. Somerville Consultant Physician for Congenital Diseases, Royal Brompton Hospital and National Heart Hospital, London, UK
2.21 Congenital heart disease in adolescents and adults

S. G. Spiro Professor and Clinical Director of Medicine, University College Hospitals London Trust, UK
4.38 Lung cancer
4.39 Pulmonary metastases

C. J. F. Spry Professor of Cardiovascular Immunology, St George's Hospital and Medical School, London, UK
3.32 The hypereosinophilic syndrome

S. Stagno Katharine Reynolds Ireland Professor and Chairman, Department of Pediatrics, University of Alabama at Birmingham, USA
16.14 Cytomegalovirus

J. A. Stewart Chief, Clinical Virology Section, Public Health Service, Centers for Disease Control, Atlanta, Georgia, USA
16.15 Human herpesviruses 6, 7, and 8

J. H. Stewart Professor of Medicine, Western Clinical School, University of Sydney, Australia
12.20 Kidney disease from analgesics and non-steroidal anti-inflammatory drugs

R. A. Stockley Professor in Respiratory Medicine, Queen Elizabeth Hospital, Birmingham, UK
4.16 Bronchiectasis
4.17 Chronic obstructive pulmonary disease

J. R. Stradling Consultant Physician, Churchill Hospital, Oxford, UK
4.12 Upper airways obstruction
4.43 Sleep-related disorders of breathing

J. Strang Professor and Director, Addiction Research Unit, National Addiction Centre, The Maudsley/Institute of Psychiatry, London, UK
14.9 Substance abuse: Introduction
14.10 Assessing drug abuse and use of brief interventions
14.11 Reducing the harm resulting from drug abuse
14.15 The legal aspects of controlled drug prescribing
14.16 Strategies for managing drug and alcohol problems
14.18 Particular problems in special settings

P. R. Studdy Consultant Physician, Harefield, Mount Vernon, and Watford Hospitals, UK
4.27 Sarcoidosis

J. A. Summerfield Professor, Division of Medicine, Imperial College School of Medicine, St Mary's Campus, London, UK
5.25 Congenital and hereditary disorders of the liver, biliary tract, and pancreas
5.29 Diseases of the gallbladder and biliary tree

Pravan Suntharasamai Associate Professor, Department of Clinical Tropical Medicine, Mahidol University, Bangkok, Thailand
16.104 Gnathostomiasis

R. Sutton Consultant Cardiologist, Royal Brompton Hospital, London, UK
2.1 Syncope and palpitation
2.6 Pacemakers

J. D. Swales Professor of Medicine, University of Leicester, UK
2.31 Essential hypertension

R. H. Swanton Consultant Cardiologist, Cardiac Services Directorate, The Middlesex Hospital, London, UK
2.11 Angina and unstable angina

N. Sykes Consultant Physician, St Christopher's Hospice, London, UK
15 Palliative medicine

D. A. Taberner Consultant in Haematology, Withington Hospital, Manchester, UK
3.39 Thrombotic disease

I. C. Talbot Professor of Histopathology, St Mark's Hospital, Harrow, Middlesex, UK
5.20 Tumours of the gastrointestinal tract

D. Taylor-Robinson Professor of Genitourinary Microbiology and Medicine, Imperial College School of Medicine, St Mary's Hospital, London, UK
16.76 Chlamydial infections
16.77 Mycoplasmas

G. M. Teasdale Professor of Neurosurgery, University of Glasgow, UK
13.24 Head injuries

P. J. Teddy Consultant Neurosurgeon, Radcliffe Infirmary, Oxford, UK
13.22 Intracranial tumours
13.27 Intracranial abscess

A. C. Thomas Senior Specialist and Consultant in Tissue Pathology, Institute of Medical and Veterinary Science, Adelaide, Australia
12.6 Immunoglobulin A nephropathy, Henoch-Schönlein purpura and thin membrane nephropathy

H. C. Thomas Professor of Medicine, Imperial College School of Medicine, St Mary's Hospital Campus, London, UK
5.31 Clinical features of viral hepatitis

H. J. W. Thomas Consultant Gastroenterologist, St Mary's Hospital, London and Senior Lecturer, ICRF Colorectal Cancer Unit, St Mark's Hospital, Harrow, Middlesex, UK
5.20 Tumours of the gastrointestinal tract

J. E. P. Thomas Medical Consultant, Anglo American Corporation Services Ltd., Harare, Zimbabwe
16.109 Schistosomiasis

P. K. Thomas Emeritus Professor of Neurology, Royal Free Hospital, London, UK
13.6 The cranial nerves
13.18 Inherited disorders of the nervous system
13.30 Peripheral neuropathy

D. G. Thompson Professor of Gastroenterology, Hope Hospital, Salford, Lancashire, UK
5.1 Symptomatology of gastrointestinal diseases
5.17 Functional bowel disease and irritable bowel syndrome

M. O. Thorner Henry B. Mulholland Professor and Chair, Department of Medicine, University of Virginia Health Sciences Center, Charlottesville, USA
7.1 Anterior pituitary disorders

A. J. Thrasher Wellcome Clinical Research Scientist Fellow and Lecturer, Institute of Child Health, London, UK
3.27 Leucocytes in health and disease

Ph. Thulliez Head, Laboratoire de la Toxoplasmose, Institut de Puériculture de Paris, France
16.86 Toxoplasmosis

P. Tookey Research Fellow, Institute of Child Health, London, UK
16.27 Rubella

P. P. Toskes Professor and Director, Division of Gastroenterology, Hepatology, and Nutrition, Department of Medicine, University of Florida College of Medicine, Gainsville, USA
5.27 Chronic pancreatitis

T. A. Traill Professor of Medicine, Johns Hopkins University, Baltimore, Maryland, USA
2.24 Cardiac myxoma

T. Treasure Professor of Cardiothoracic Surgery, St George's Hospital, London, UK
2.15 Coronary artery bypass grafting

***J. D. Treharne** Reader in Virology, Institute of Ophthalmology, University of London, UK
16.76 Chlamydial infections

L. A. Turnberg Professor of Medicine, University of Manchester, UK
5.1 Symptomatology of gastrointestinal diseases

P. C. B. Turnbull Head, Anthrax Section, Centre for Applied Microbiology and Research, Porton Down, Salisbury, Wiltshire, UK
16.55 Anthrax

***R. C. Turner** Professor of Medicine, Radcliffe Infirmary, Oxford, UK
6.14 Hypoglycaemia

F. E. Udwadia Emeritus Professor of Medicine, Grant Medical College and J.J. Group of Hospitals, Bombay, India
16.57 Tetanus

J. A. Vale Director, National Poisons Information Service (Birmingham Centre) and Clinical Lecturer, University of Birmingham, UK
18.1 Poisoning with drugs and chemicals

P. Vallance Professor and Director, Centre for Clinical Pharmacology, University College London Medical School, UK
2.9 Vascular endothelium, its physiology and pathophysiology

Sirivan Vanijanonta Associate Professor, Faculty of Tropical Medicine, Mahidol University, Bangkok, Thailand
16.111 Lung flukes (paragonimiasis)

P. J. W. Venables Reader in Immunorheumatology and Consultant Physician, The Kennedy Institute of Rheumatology, London, UK
10.13 Sjögren's syndrome

D. H. Walker Professor and Chairman, Department of Pathology; Director, WHO Collaborating Center for Tropical Diseases, University of Texas Medical Branch at Galveston, USA
16.72 Rickettsial diseases including ehrlichioses

J. A. Walker-Smith Professor of Paediatric Gastroenterology, Royal Free Hospital, London, UK
5.19 Congenital abnormalities of the gastrointestinal tract

J. Walton Honorary Consultant in Neurology, Oxford, UK
10.14 Polymyositis and dermatomyositis
13.32 An introduction
13.33 The muscular dystrophies
13.34 The floppy infant syndrome
13.35 Myotonic disorders
13.36 Inflammatory myopathies
13.37 Miscellaneous disorders

R. J. A. Wanders Professor, Academic Medical Center, University Hospital of Amsterdam, The Netherlands
6.9 Peroxisomal disorders

C. P. Warlow Professor of Medical Neurology, University of Edinburgh, UK
13.15 Cerebrovascular disease

D. A. Warrell Professor of Tropical Medicine and Infectious Diseases and Director of the Centre for Tropical Medicine, University of Oxford, UK
13.25 Bacterial meningitis
13.26 Viral infections of the central nervous system
13.41 Pyomyositis, tropical pyomyositis, or tropical myositis
16.7 Travel and expedition medicine
16.24 Rhabdoviruses: rabies and rabies-related viruses
16.25 Colorado tick fever and other arthropod-borne reoviruses
16.64 Rat bite fevers
16.66 Other Borrelia infections
16.84 Malaria
16.114 Pentastomiasis (porocephalosis)
18.2 Injuries, envenoming, poisoning, and allergic reactions caused by animals

M. J. Warrell Centre for Tropical Medicine and Infectious Diseases, John Radcliffe Hospital, Oxford, UK
16.11 Varicella-zoster virus infections: chickenpox and zoster
16.21 Nipah virus
16.24 Rhabdoviruses: rabies and rabies-related viruses
16.25 Colorado tick fever and other arthropod-borne reoviruses

J. A. H. Wass Professor of Endocrinology, University of Oxford, UK
7.16 Endocrine manifestations of non-endocrine disease

M. F. R. Waters Honorary Consultant in Bacteriology, Middlesex Hospital, London, UK
16.61 Leprosy (Hansen's disease, hanseniasis)

G. Watt Chief, HIV Interaction Section, Retrovirology Department, Armed Forces Research Institute of Medical Sciences (AFRIMS), Bangkok, Thailand
16.73 Scrub typhus

R. W.E. Watts Visiting Professor, Department of Medicine, Imperial College School of Medicine and Honorary Consultant Physician, Hammersmith Hospital, London, UK
6.1 The inborn errors of metabolism: general aspects
6.8 Lysosomal storage diseases
6.12 Disorders of oxalate metabolism
12.23 Urinary stone disease (urolithiasis)

D. J. Weatherall Regius Professor of Medicine, University of Oxford, UK
2.30 Pulmonary embolism
3.1 Haematology: Introduction
3.9 Polycythaemia vera
3.10 Myelosclerosis
3.11 Primary thrombocythaemia
3.14 Erythropoiesis and the normal red cell
3.15 Anaemia: pathophysiology, classification, and clinical features
3.17 Normochromic, normocytic anaemia
3.19 Disorders of the synthesis or function of haemoglobin
3.20 Other anaemias resulting from defective red-cell maturation
3.21 Haemolytic anaemia: the mechanisms and consequences of a shortened red-cell survival time
3.23 Haemolysis due to red-cell enzyme deficiencies
3.26 The relative and secondary polycythaemias
3.40 The blood in systemic disease

R. A. Weiss Professor of Viral Oncology, Wohl Virion Centre, Windeyer Institute of Medical Sciences, University College London, UK
16.35 HIV infection and AIDS

L. Westrom Associate Professor of Obstetrics and Gynaecology, University of Lund, Sweden
17.4 Pelvic inflammatory disease

H. C. Whittle Deputy Director, MRC Laboratories, Fajara, The Gambia
16.20 Measles

P. J. Wilkinson Consultant Medical Microbiologist and Group Director, Public Health Laboratory, University Hospital, Nottingham, UK
16.70 Listeria and listeriosis

C. B. Williams Consultant Physician in Gastrointestinal Endoscopy, St Mark's Hospital, Harrow, Middlesex, UK
5.20 Tumours of the gastrointestinal tract

D. G. Williams Professor of Medicine, Guy's, King's College and St Thomas' Hospitals Medical and Dental School, Guy's Campus, London, UK
12.11 Infections and associated nephropathies
12.15 Rheumatological disorders and the kidney: systemic lupus erythematosus, mixed connective tissue disease, scleroderma, Sjögren's syndrome, and rheumatoid arthritis

R. Williams Professor and Director, Institute of Hepatology, University College London Medical School, UK
5.39 Liver transplantation

R. C. Williams Chief Medical Officer, GKN plc, Redditch, Worcestershire, UK
18.12 Noise

C. G. Winearls Consultant Nephrologist/Clinical Director, Oxford Kidney Unit, The Churchill Hospital, Oxford, UK
12.28 Acute renal failure
12.29 Chronic renal failure

D. L. Wingate Professor of Gastrointestinal Science, St Bartholomew's and the Royal London Hospital School of Medicine and Dentistry, London, UK
5.16 Disorders of motility

A. A. Woodcock Professor of Respiratory Medicine, Northwest Lung Centre, Wythenshawe Hospital, Manchester, UK
4.18 Parenchymal lung disease: Introduction
4.19 Cryptogenic fibrosing alveolitis

*It is with regret that we report the deaths of Dr J. D. Treharne and Professor R. C. Turner.

A. J. Woodroffe Renal Physician, Royal Adelaide Hospital, Australia
12.6 Immunoglobulin A nephropathy, Henoch-Schönlein purpura and thin membrane nephropathy

H. F. Woods Professor of Medicine, University of Sheffield, UK
6.17 Disturbances of acid-base homeostasis

B. P. Wordsworth Professor of Rheumatology, University of Oxford, UK
10.2 Rheumatoid arthritis

D. J. M. Wright Consultant Microbiologist, Imperial College School of Medicine, Charing Cross Hospital, London, UK
16.69 Syphilis

V. M. Wright Consultant Paediatric Surgeon, Royal London Hospital, UK
5.19 Congenital abnormalities of the gastrointestinal tract

F. C. W. Wu Senior Lecturer (Endocrinology), Royal Infirmary and University of Manchester, UK
7.10 Disorders of male reproduction

V. Zaman Professor of Microbiology, The Aga Khan University, Karachi, Pakistan
16.89 Sarcocystosis
16.91 Blastocystis hominis
16.101 Other gut nematodes
16.102 Toxocariasis and visceral larval migrans

A. J. Zuckerman Professor of Medical Microbiology; Principal and Dean, Royal Free and University College Medical School, London, UK
16.34 Hepatitis viruses and TT virus

J. N. Zuckerman Senior Lecturer and Elective Tutor, Royal Free Hospital Medical School, London, UK
16.34 Hepatitis viruses and TT virus

Plate section

The eye and disease *P. Frith*

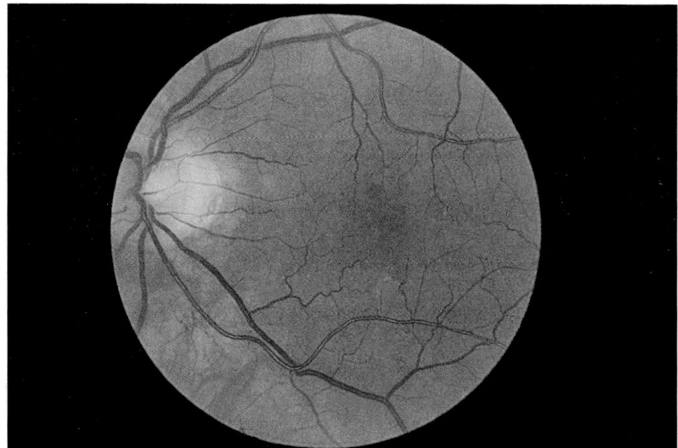

Plate 1 **Normal optic disc and macula.** The optic disc lies nasal to the fovea and is the visible head of the optic nerve where nerve fibres bend through a right angle within its pink outer rim. The disc margin should be definable, at least in part; if not, disc swelling may be present. The central paler cup is devoid of nerve fibres; it enlarges in chronic glaucoma as nerve fibres are destroyed and the rim shrinks or notches progressively, and becomes obliterated with disc swelling. Central and branch retinal vessels emerge from and return to the disc; the arteries are usually thinner and more shiny than the veins. The disc may become swollen, cupped, atrophic, or the site of neovascularization. As a congenital abnormality the disc may be tilted, have a pigmented rim or pale halo of surrounding atrophy, or come to contain pearly drusen. The fovea, lying temporal to the disc, is used for detailed vision as in reading; it is best visualized by dilating the pupil and asking the patient to fixate the ophthalmoscope light.

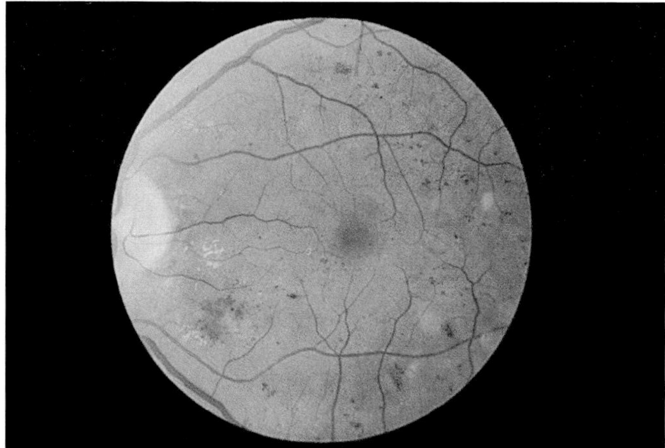

Plate 2 **Background diabetic retinopathy.** 'Background' is a term applied to diabetic retinopathy which is not an imminent threat to sight. 'Dot and blot' describes a mixture of red lesions, including microaneurysms and haemorrhages of different sizes, which often occur together with hard exudate though this does not extend to within one disc diameter distance of the fovea. In this plate the macula is the area of retina shown, temporal to the optic disc and enclosed by the arching major branch vessels; the darker fovea lies at its centre.

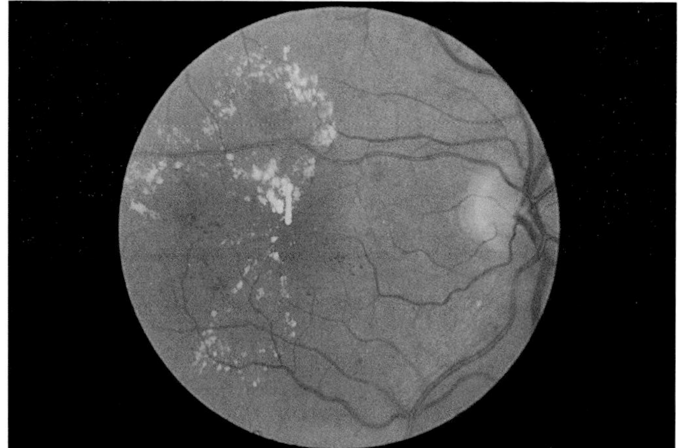

Plate 3 **Diabetic maculopathy.** Areas of focal leakage from capillaries within the diabetic retina form characteristic circular-shaped, (circinate), hard exudate containing protein and lipid which has leaked into and become trapped within the extracellular spaces. If exudate extends closer than one disc diameter towards the fovea, sight may be threatened. Red lesions at the centre of circinate exudates can be targeted by focal laser therapy which seals the leakage, hopefully causing regression of visible exudate over the following months. Such maculopathy must be detected by screening the retinal appearance, as treatment is preferably given before vision falls irretrievably. Note that as here, a characteristic site for exudation is temporal to the fovea.

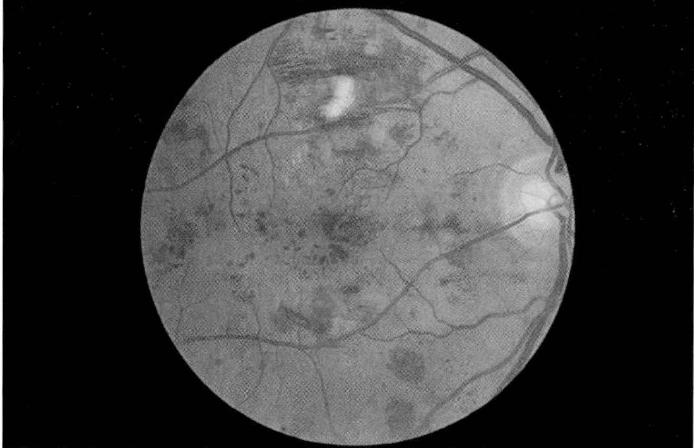

Plate 4 **Preproliferative diabetic retinopathy.** Some diabetics develop retinal capillary ischaemia, particularly of the peripheral retina, which may become severe enough to stimulate retinal neovascularization. Ominous signs include multiple blot haemorrhages, numerous cotton wool spots (microinfarcts), and dilatation or beading of larger retinal veins. Risk of neovascularization increases particularly with poor diabetic control and in pregnancy. Paradoxically, acute tightening of diabetic control may also precipitate transient ischaemic retinal changes. Fluorescein angiography will demonstrate the extent of capillary closure at this stage and so may help to predict the likelihood of neovascularization.

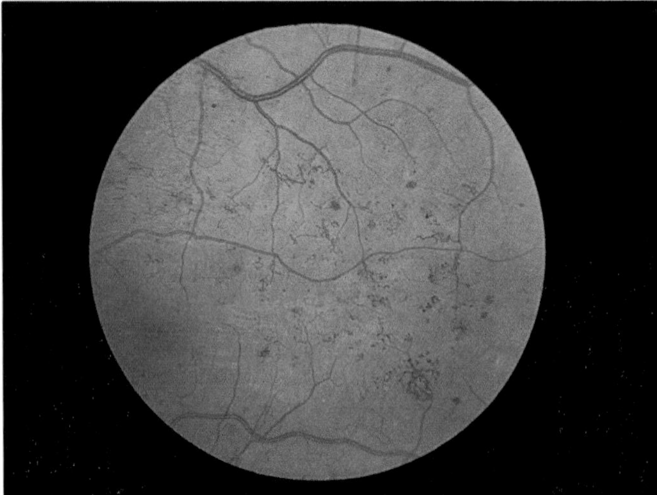

Plate 5 Proliferative diabetic retinopathy. In the peripheral retina or on the optic disc, sites of neovascularization become visible first as dilated capillary loops (intraretinal microvascular abnormalities or IRMA) which can then bud into frankly aberrant branching and looping tufts which leak profusely on angiography. At this stage, panretinal photocoagulation (PRP) laser treatment, using thousands of burns, destroys ischaemic areas which are providing the neovascular stimulus. With successful photocoagulation, the rate of new vessel formation slows and established new vessels eventually regress. Vision is usually normal in the early stages of neovascularization, unless vitreous haemorrhage occurs or maculopathy is also present.

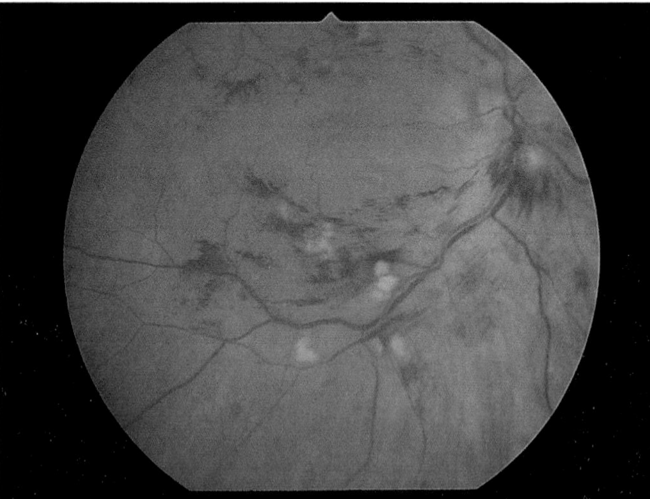

Plate 7 Accelerated hypertension retinopathy. Flame haemorrhages, multiple cotton wool spots (microinfarcts), and swelling of the optic disc are characteristic of hypertension sufficient to disrupt capillary integrity. Hard exudate is less common, and lacks the focal circinate pattern common in diabetes, though a macular 'star' may form with regression of acute ischaemic features as diffuse macular oedema resolves. Vision often remains normal until macular oedema occurs. These retinal changes are a warning for mandatory urgent control of blood pressure. Proteinuria is almost invariable and renal function may already be impaired The diastolic blood pressure is usually greater than 110 mmHg if associated with accelerated retinopathy.

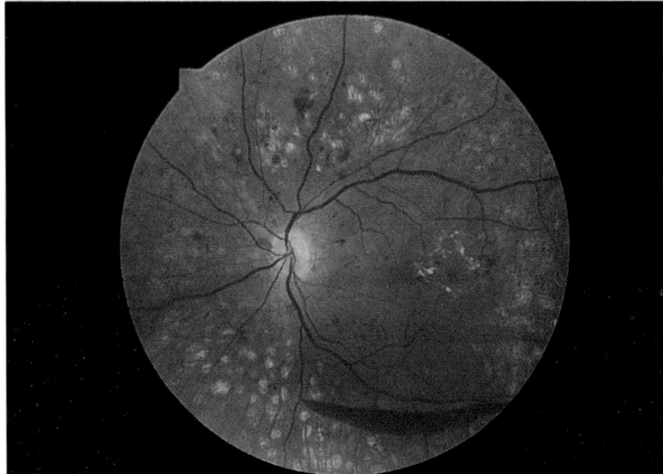

Plate 6 Treated proliferative diabetic retinopathy. Laser burns appear as numerous focal chorioretinal scars (whose size and density depend on the laser technique used) lying outside the macula and optic disc. This patient also has a recent haemorrhage of meniscal shape settling between the retina and vitreous which indicates that new vessels are still present and actively bleeding despite treatment, so more photocoagulation is necessary. This patient has also been treated using focal laser applied temporal to the fovea for macular exudates which have resolved and so is doubly at risk of eventual visual loss if treatment fails.

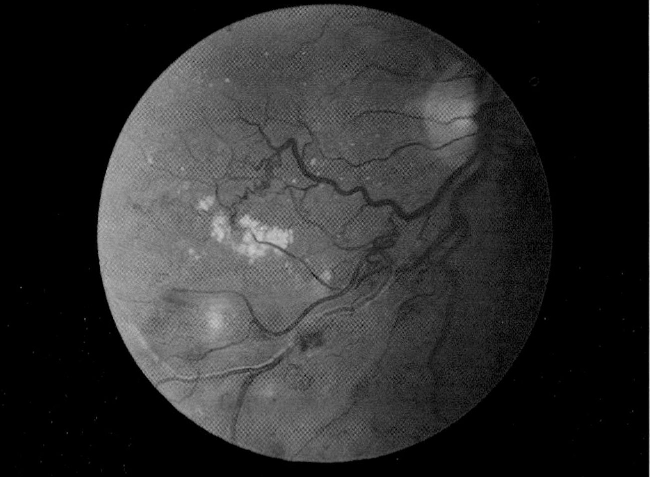

Plate 8 Occlusion of branch retinal vein. Haemorrhage and oedema, often with microinfarcts, occur in a wedge-shaped area drained by the branch vein which itself becomes distended. The vein often occludes at an arteriovenous crossing. In the example shown, inferior hemivein occlusion causes a monocular superior central visual field defect of acute onset. Retinal vein occlusion is usually an *in-situ* thrombotic event and should prompt a search for vascular risk factors incuding hypertension, hyperlipidaemia, diabetes, haematological abnormality, or glaucoma.

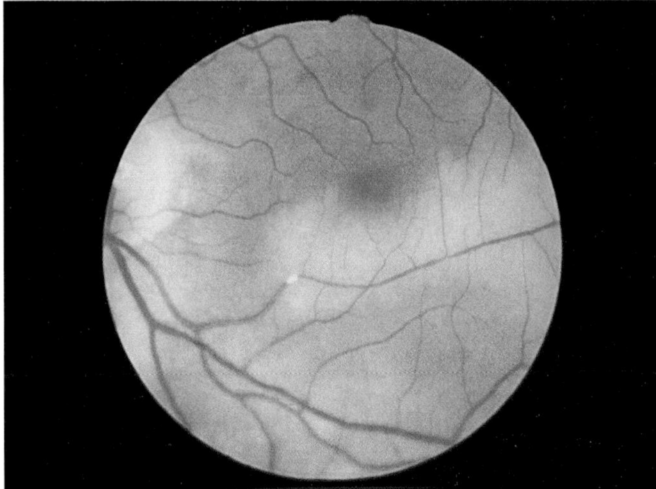

Plate 9 **Occlusion of branch retinal artery.** Retinal artery occlusion is usually an acute embolic event. Here, a bright embolic fragment is lodged in an inferior branch arteriole, with death and pallor of the section of retina it supplies. The acute field defect produced is similar to, but more complete than that of a branch venous occlusion, and usually persists. Search should be made for proximal sites of emboli – frequently the ipsilateral carotid bifurcation (atheroma) or the heart (mural thrombus, endocarditis, atrial myxoma).

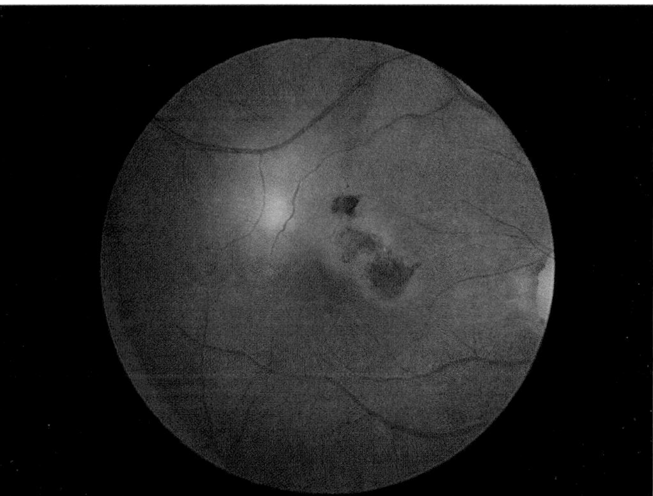

Plate 11 **Toxoplasmosis.** The combination of an inactive pigmented chorioretinal scar and a fresh, acutely active 'fluffy' focus is characteristic of *Toxoplasma gondii* infection of the choroid and retina. This is usually acquired congenitally from a primary infection in the mother. Retinal cysts remain dormant until reactivation occurs later in life, causing attacks of blurring of vision with floaters due to inflammatory cells in the vitreous. Systemic treatment is sometimes necessary, using a combination of oral antimicrobial with corticosteroid, especially if vision may be irretrievably damaged by involvement of the optic nerve head or fovea. Recurrent attacks may be expected.

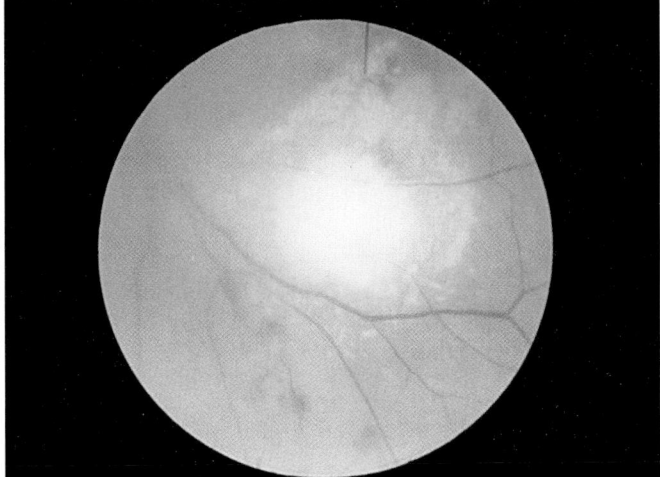

Plate 10 **Staphylococcal endophthalmitis.** Bloodborne organisms may settle in the choroid or retina, causing focal infection. The patient may describe recent onset of disturbance of vision, perhaps with the 'floaters' characteristic of inflammmatory cells in the vitreous. Vitreous aspirate may yield diagnostic material. Response to appropriate treatment can be observed, with resolution of the acute 'colony' into an inactive scar. Here, the infection was staphylococcal, and occurred in a diabetic with skin sepsis. Endophthalmitis is an unusual cause of intraocular inflammation but it is important to diagnose so that treatment may be tailored to the organism responsible. The eye finding may also prove a clue to the systemic infection.

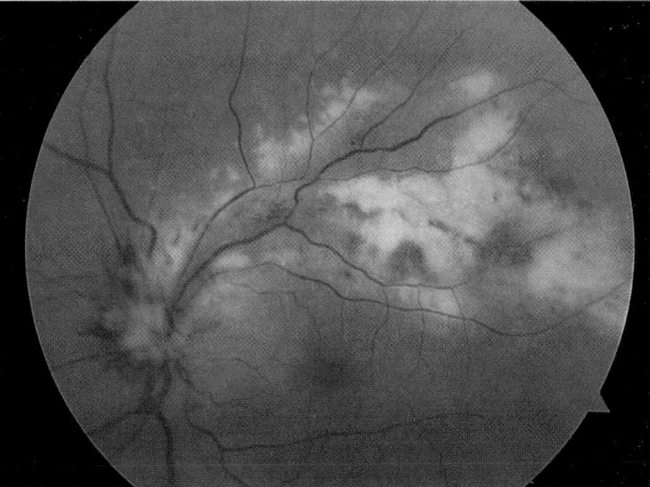

Plate 12 **Cytomegalovirus (CMV) retinitis.** The 'pizza' appearance is characteristic of cytomegalovirus infection of the retina, with pale areas of retinal necrosis associated with haemorrhage. This retinitis affects about one-third of patients with AIDS in whom the T4 lymphocyte count falls below 0.10×10^9/l.Treatment with virustatic agents such as ganciclovir, foscarnet, or cidofovir will control expansion of the lesions and forestall blindness, but treatment should be maintained for the duration of relative lymphopenia. Life expectancy of patients with CMV retinitis used to be several months, but has improved considerably since the use of combination antiretroviral regimes to reduce the immunosuppressive effects of HIV infection.

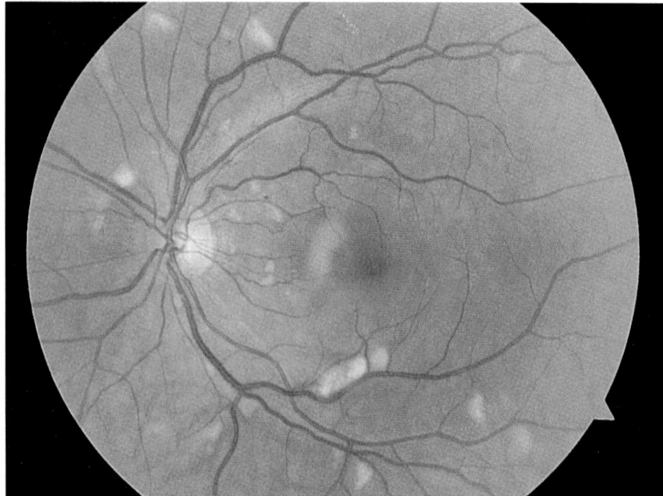

Plate 13 Cotton wool spots in HIV infection. Retinal microinfarcts must be distinguished from retinitis. They are characteristically multiple, often bilateral, associated with little or no haemorrhage, and occur between the branches of retinal vessels rather than tracking along them. With magnification they can be seen to have a striated, feathery appearance due to focal swelling of nerve fibres in the superficial retina. The patient is usually asymptomatic, so floaters due to inflammatory cells in the vitreous are absent. Cotton wool spots are frequent at all stages of AIDS, particularly after pneumonia. Other associations apart from HIV infection, include acute pancreatitis, cardiac bypass surgery, multiple fractures with fat microemboli, and systemic vasculitis especially dermatomyositis.

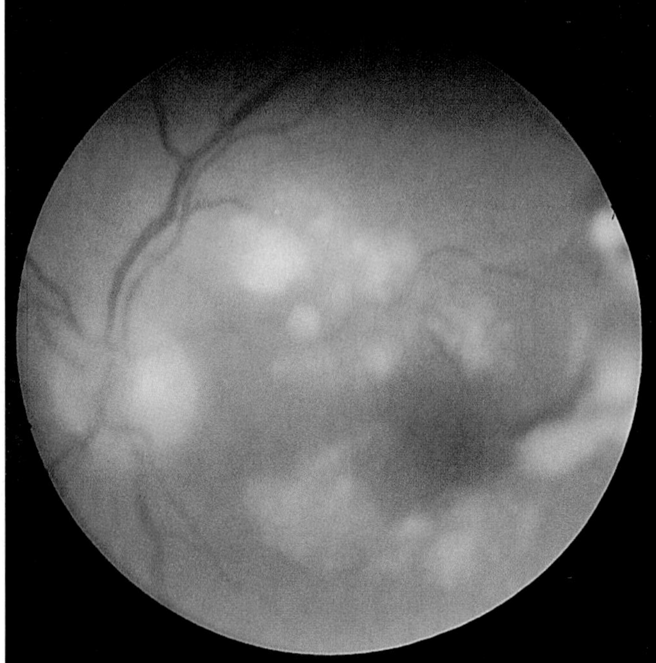

Plate 14 Candida endophthalmitis. Collections of fluffy rounded colonies of fungal hyphae within the vitreous are typical of an indolent Candida infection of the interior eye. The organisms seed from the circulation, often entering via intravenous lines, illicit drug injections, or dental drilling, though some patients have no such history. Characteristically there are also pale foci of chorioretinal infection without associated haemorrhage. The patient usually notices floaters due to the vitreous opacities. Vitreous aspiration may demonstrate hyphae or yield positive culture. Treatment with amphotericin or flucytosine may be appropriately initiated by intravitreal injection and continued systemically.

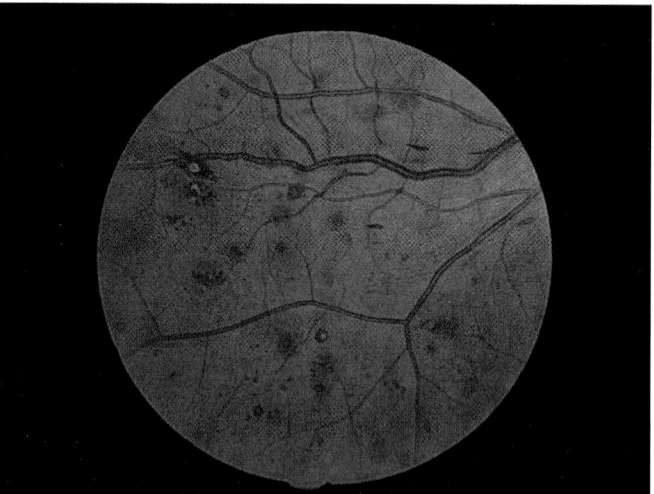

Plate 15 Retinal haemorrhages in leukaemia. Multiple and bilateral retinal haemorrhages in the absence of diabetes or hypertension always raise a suspicion of haematological disorder, acute or chronic. Haemorrhages are related to the degree of anaemia, hyperviscosity, and thrombocytopenia. Here an elderly man presented to his optometrist with acute fall in vision and multiple bilateral retinal haemorrhages were easily visible. Some have white centres due to a central microinfarct and so resemble Roth spots. Larger retinal veins are also dilated. His lymphocyte count was greatly elevated, consistent with chronic lymphocytic leukaemia. The retinal haemorrhages resolve with treatment of the underlying condition and prognosis for vision is usually good.

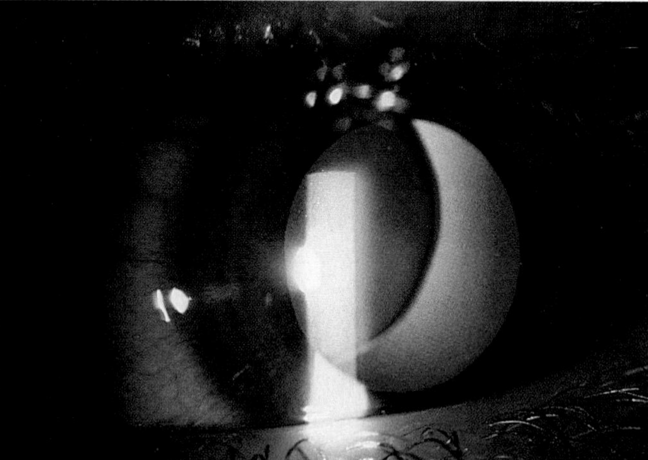

Plate 16 Marfan's syndrome with dislocated lens. Dislocation of the lens in Marfan's syndrome is due to weakness in the suspensory fibres because of fibrillin abnormality. The lens characteristically displaces upwards and to either side but may be asymmetrical in extent and direction. The mildest degree of abnormality results in a central but unstable lens and manifests as fluttering of the iris on eye movement (iridodonesis) detectable using the slitlamp. Here, the lens is clearly displaced to the left hand side in an 18-month-old child who came for screening after her father died from aortic rupture. This appearance would be visible using the ophthalmoscope, showing against the red reflex after dilating the pupil with 1 per cent trocaimide drops. Lens instability strongly suggests Marfan's syndrome if there are other consistent features; other possible diagnoses are homocystinuria (usually downward displacement) or isolated ectopia lentis.

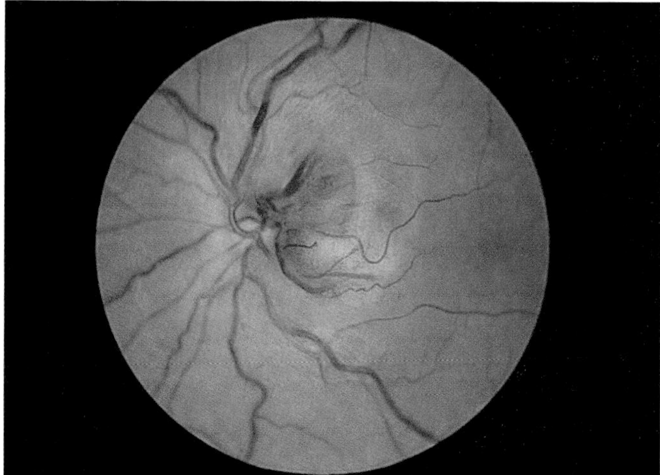

Plate 17 Angioma of von Hippel-Lindau disease. Retinal angiomas in von Hippel-Lindau disease can be single or multiple, large or small, central or peripheral, and may remain asymptomatic. Here a large raised vascularized lesion arising from the optic nerve head presented with acute loss of vision and a central scotoma. The lesion had the typical appearance of an angioma, fluorescing early and profusely on fluorescein angiography. Some lesions, particularly the smaller and more peripheral, are amenable to laser photocoagulation. There were others in the posterior fossa, causing unsteadiness of gait, and in the cervical spine, causing paraesthesiae in the hands. The patient will require regular screening for the development of new angiomas at several sites and also for phaeochromocytoma and malignant renal tumour. Other family members should also be screened as this is a dominant gene.

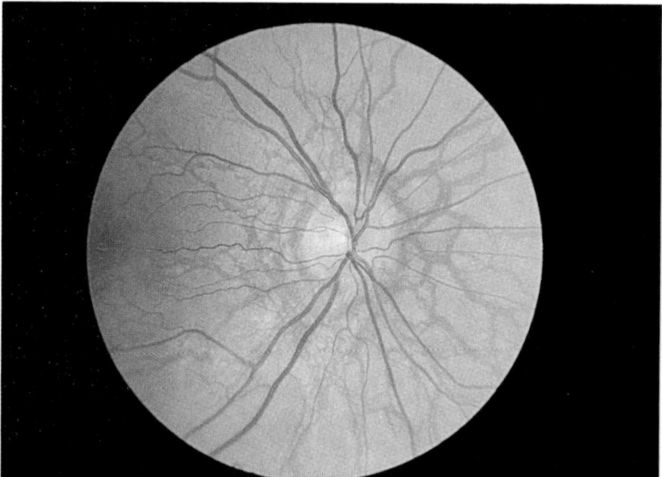

Plate 19 Angioid streaks of pseudoxanthoma elasticum. Cracks appearing in the elastic Bruch's membrane which supports the retina look like dark blood vessels (hence 'angioid') which cross beneath the retinal branch vessels. Such streaks are often most prominent around the optic nerve head, radiating from it to extend into the more peripheral retina. Streaks underlying the fovea carry a worse prognosis for vision as the patient may develop a neovascular tuft which may bleed and scar the fovea with irretrievable loss of central vision. Such defects are rarely amenable to laser treatment, but fortunately in many patients the streaks remain stable for long periods. Pseudoxanthoma elasticum is the most common abnormality associated with angioid streaks; the skin signs are often obvious, usually in the neck, axillae, or groins, but biopsy may be necessary to demonstrate more subtle microscopic abnormalities of the elastic structure in skin.

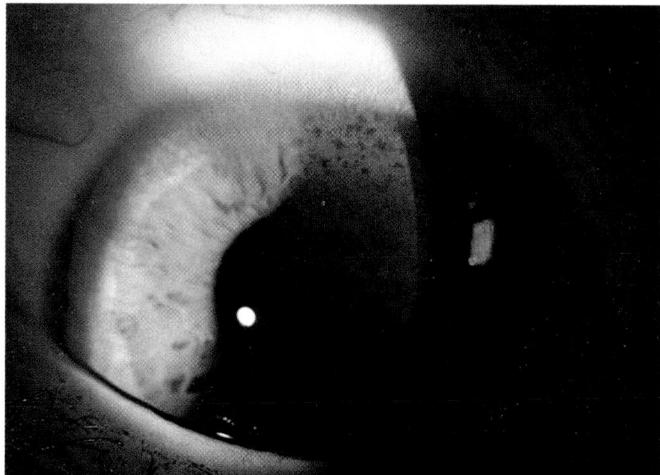

Plate 18 Kayser-Fleischer ring in Wilson's disease. The appearance of copper deposited deep in the peripheral cornea, within Descemet's membrane, is an extremely important sign virtually diagnostic of Wilson's disease. The ring should be carefully sought by slitlamp and can go unnoticed in the earlier stages when it is faint and partial, appearing first above and below before extending laterally to make a full ring. The typical colour is greenish, brown, or orange, and the texture at first delicate. Here the beam of the slitlamp shines from the right side and the deposit is visible at the top of the cornea with a freckled texture, extending from the periphery and fading towards the centre – looking very similar to the underlying iris, but in a different plane. The deposit disappears if treatment succeeds in de-coppering the patient's tissues.

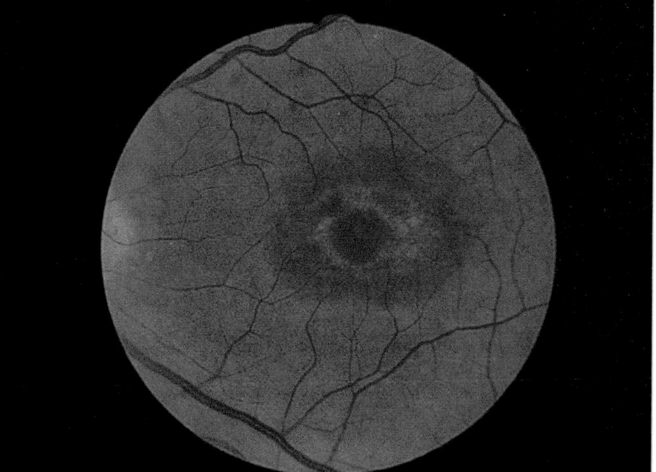

Plate 20 Bull's eye maculopathy associated with chloroquine use. The antimalarial chloroquine may cause retinal toxicity, especially if used in high dose and for the long periods typically necessary to control inflammatory skin or joint manifestations, as in SLE or rheumatoid arthritis. Formulary equations allow total dose of base to be calculated for each patient, and screening for retinal abnormality should be undertaken above the stated threshold. The characteristic appearance is an increase in pigmentation around the fovea to form a concentric, target-like zone. Macular sensitivity is also reduced and may progress to become symptomatic with blurring and loss of central vision which becomes irreversible. The optimum method of screening is controversial. Hydroxychloroquine appears to carry a negligible risk and is often a prudent substitute.

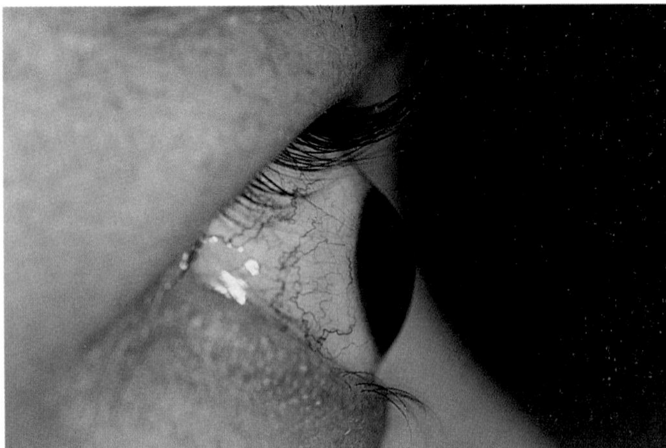

Plate 21 Thyroid ophthalmopathy. The immunological disorder which associates autoimmune thyroid disease with pathology in the orbit is still poorly understood. Characteristic clinical signs are due to increased pressure in the orbital tissues such as muscle and fat which produces exophthalmos (also termed proptosis), double vision, and congestion of the exterior eye and optic nerve. Here there is protrusion of the eye with swelling of both eyelids and chemosis of the conjunctiva as oedema fluid collects beneath it. Retraction of the upper lid suggests current thyrotoxicosis, though patients may also be euthyroid or hypothyroid when the eye problem presents. The appearance may be asymmetrical and it is wise to remember that thyroid ophthalmopathy is the most common cause of orbital disease and exophthalmos in European populations. MR imaging may be helpful in reaching a diagnosis, characteristically showing smooth swelling of the extraocular muscles, especially inferior and medial recti.

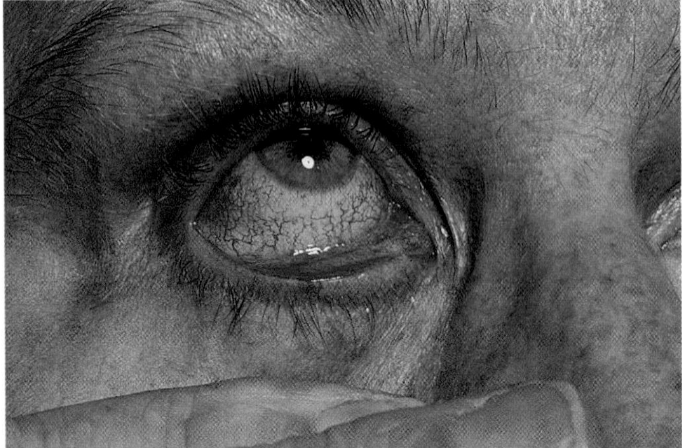

Plate 22 Episcleritis. Episcleritis is quite common, not a threat to sight, and is only occasionally associated with systemic disease such as vasculitis or infection. It manifests as redness and bogginess of the eye surface, sometimes only over a sector of the visible sclera, and the eye is uncomfortable but not painful, with normal vision. The attack of inflammation is self-limiting. Many patients are treated topically with corticosteroid drops which may hasten recovery though the condition tends to recur. If scleritis is unlikely, the patient should be reassured and treatment minimized; further investigation is not warranted.

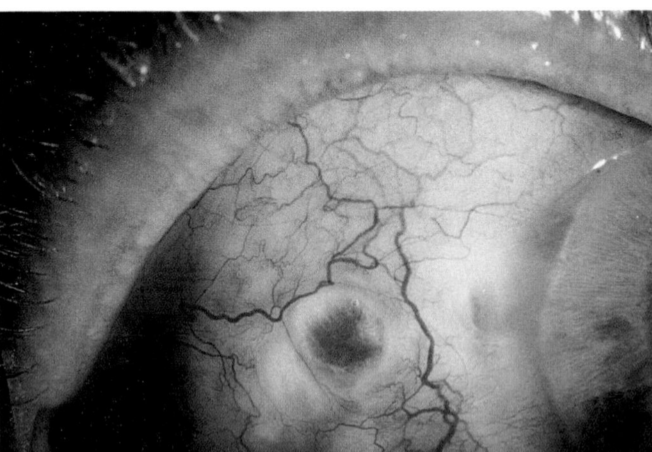

Plate 23 Scleral perforation in rheumatoid arthritis. Systemic vasculitis often underlies the serious condition of scleritis in which the eye surface becomes not only inflamed but also ischaemic, due to closure of blood supply within the superficial episclera.The characteristic pain may be severe enough to prevent sleep and is worsened by eye movement, though in a minority of patients pain is absent. If the process extends to the posterior part of the globe there may be double vision, and sight may be affected if the optic nerve is involved. Rheumatoid arthritis is the most common association; occasionally Wegener's granulomatosis or polyarteritis. Local treatments usually fail and systemic treatment is necessary to control pain and possible destruction of the eye coat. Thinning of sclera may even result in perforation, as shown here. To treat or pre-empt such an emergency requires specialist advice and tailored immunosuppression, sometimes with immediate or pulsed corticosteroid and cyclophosphamide.

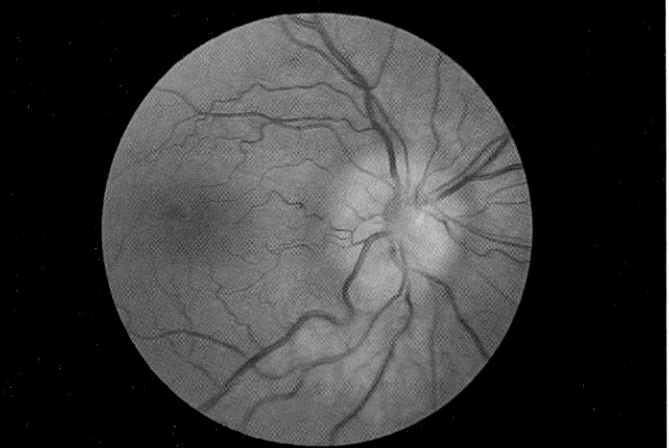

Plate 24 Papilloedema. 'Papilloedema' by convention refers to disc swelling resulting from raised pressure within the optic nerve sheath, usually secondary to transmission of raised intracranial pressure. The pink rim enlarges sideways and forwards with loss of definition of the disc margin and cup with congestion of capillaries on the rim and of retinal veins. The blind spot will be found to be enlarged but other tests of optic nerve function remain normal unless there are chronic sequelae due to compromise of a sufficient proportion of nerve fibres within the disc. On the other hand, an intrinsic optic nerve pathology such as inflammation (optic neuritis), ischaemia (as in giant cell arteritis – see below), compression (for example, by meningioma), or intrinsic tumour (glioma) tends to compromise function early, may cause optic disc swelling in the acute stages if the lesion is anterior and will lead to optic atrophy in the longer term.

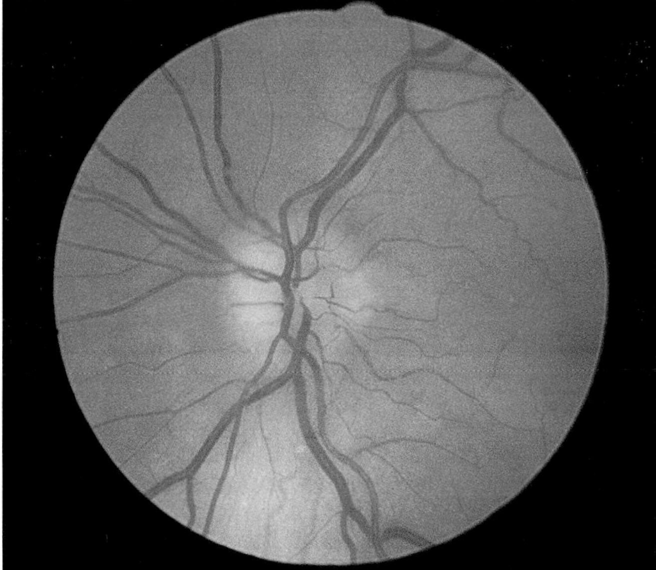

Plate 25 Ischaemic optic neuropathy of giant cell arteritis. The pale swollen optic disc associated with sudden loss of vision is entirely characteristic of acute ischaemic optic neuropathy. In older patients temporal ('giant cell' or 'cranial' – all synonymous) arteritis must be suspected and investigated promptly by measuring systemic inflammatory indices (ESR and CRP) and usually by temporal artery biopsy. The striking feature may be associated haemorrhage around the disc, but the critical feature is pallor. This is associated with impaired visual acuity, visual field defect (central, altitudinal, or total) and a relative afferent pupil deficit (RAPD). The central and branch retinal vessels are usually normal, though cotton wool spots which represent retinal microinfarcts may occur in the acute stages and the retinal veins may be mildly congested due to pressure within the optic disc . Optic atrophy will follow. The acute condition requires immediate and urgent suppression of inflammation using systemic corticosteroid.

Plates for Section 5 Gastroenterology

5.2 The mouth and salivary glands

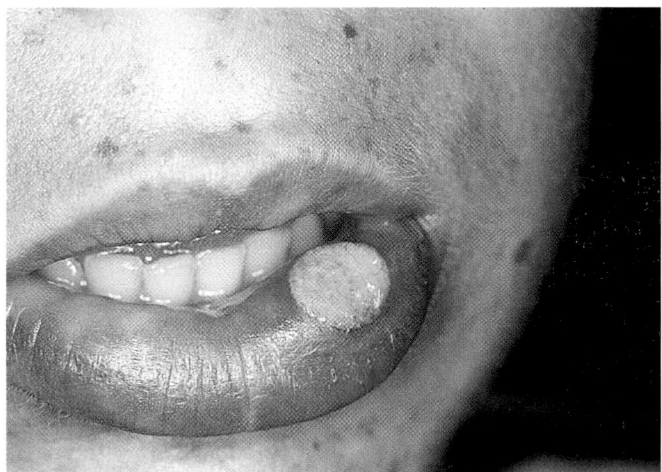

Plate 1 Aphthous ulcer.

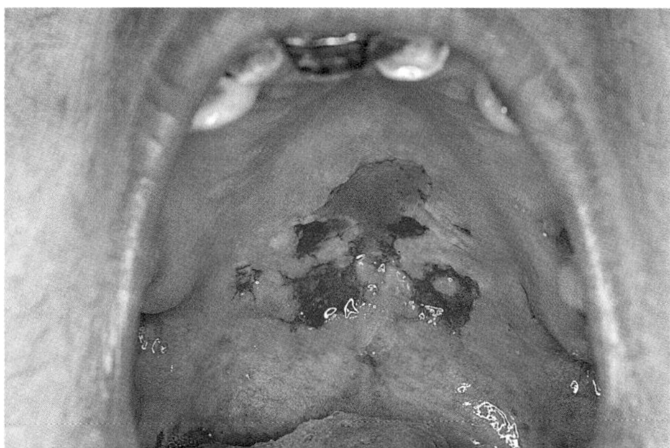

Plate 2 Pemphigus.

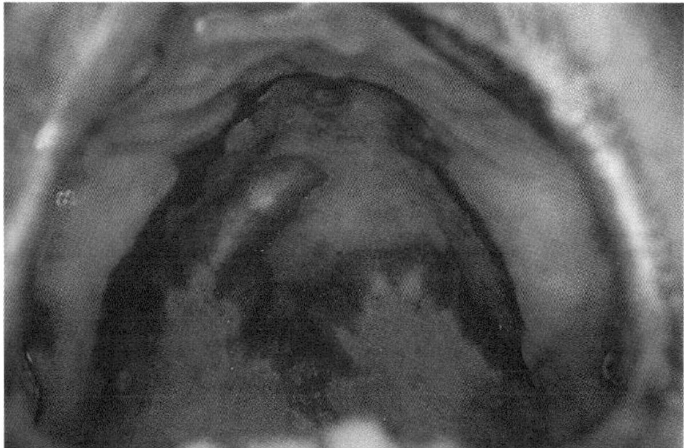

Plate 3 Erythema multiforme.

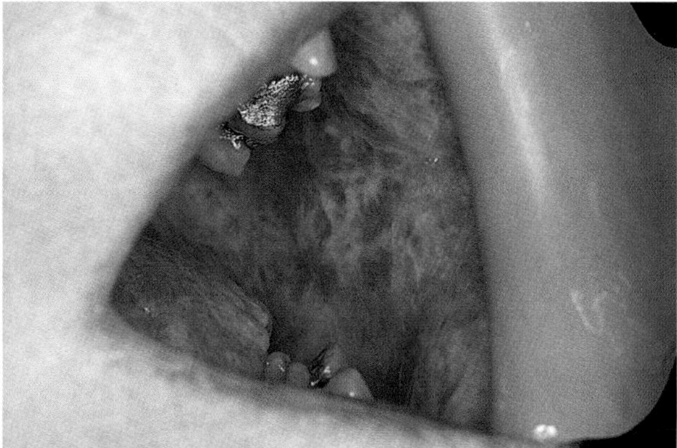

Plate 4 Lichen planus.

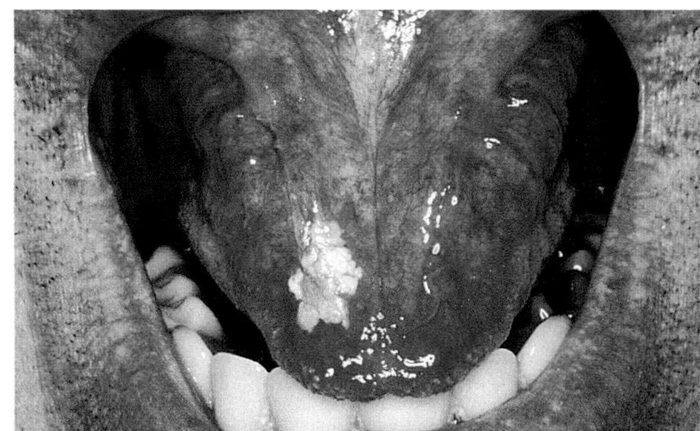

Plate 5 Leukoplakia.

5.20 Tumours of the gastrointestinal tract

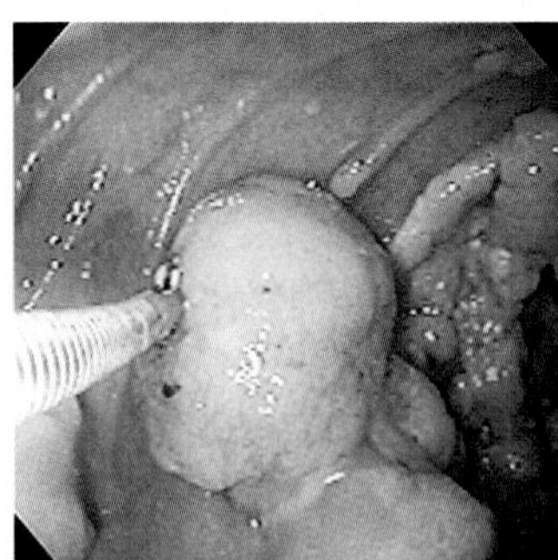

Plate 1 Duodenal adenomatous polyps in familial adenomatous polyposis.

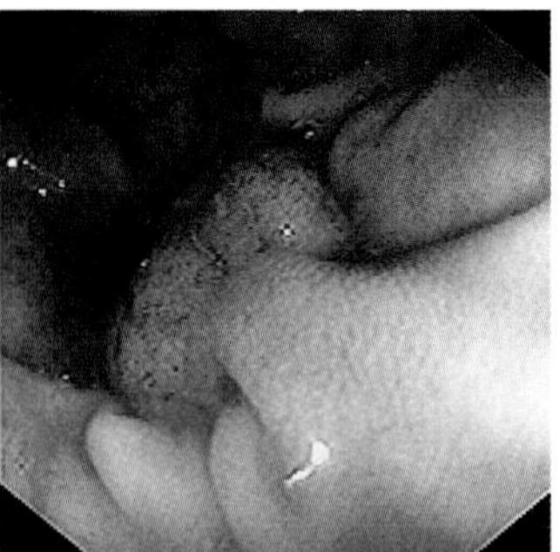

Plate 2 Stalked (pedunculated) benign adenoma in the colon.

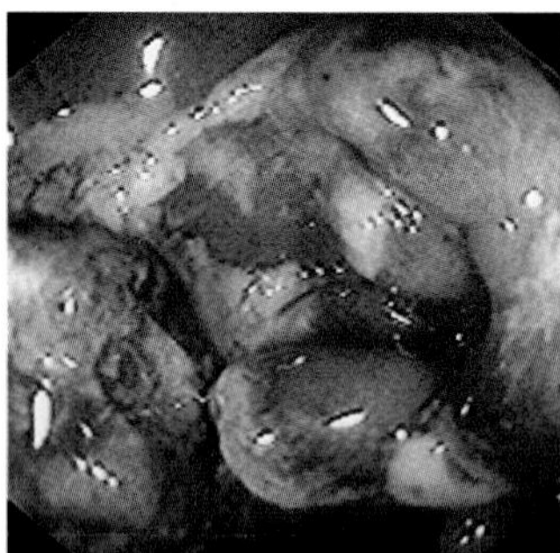

Plate 3 Multiple inflamed-looking polyps in 'cap polyposis' of the distal sigmoid colon.

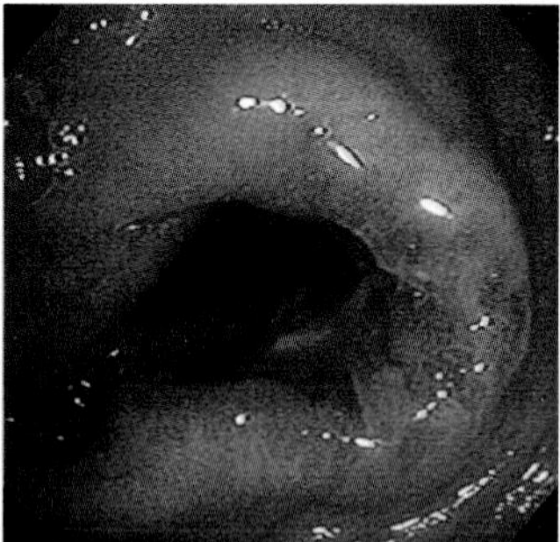

Plate 4 Tell-tale ulceration at the distal margin of a malignant stricture of the colon; note the raised edge of normal undermined mucosa.

Plates for Section 6 Metabolic disorders

6.10 Trace metal disorders

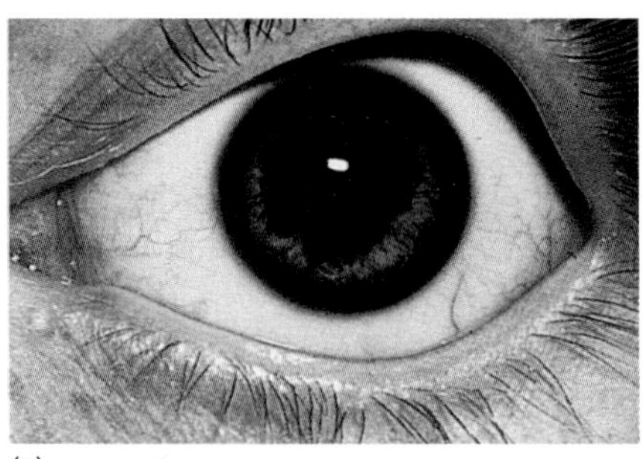

(a)

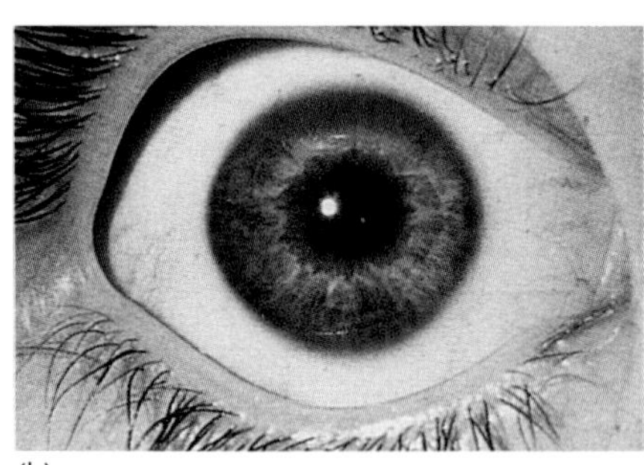

(b)

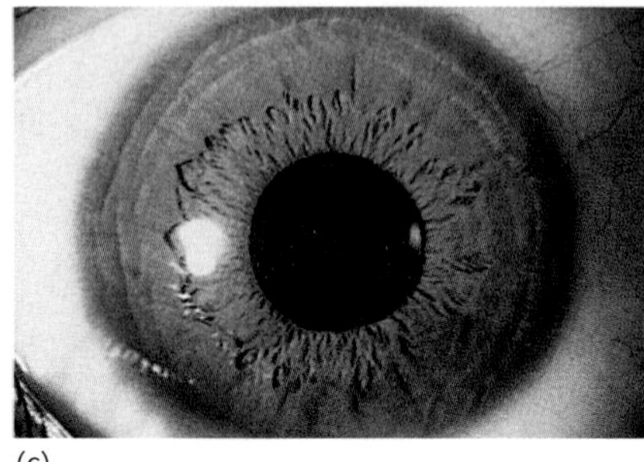

(c)

Plate 1 Kayser–Fleischer rings

6.11 Lipid and lipoprotein disorders

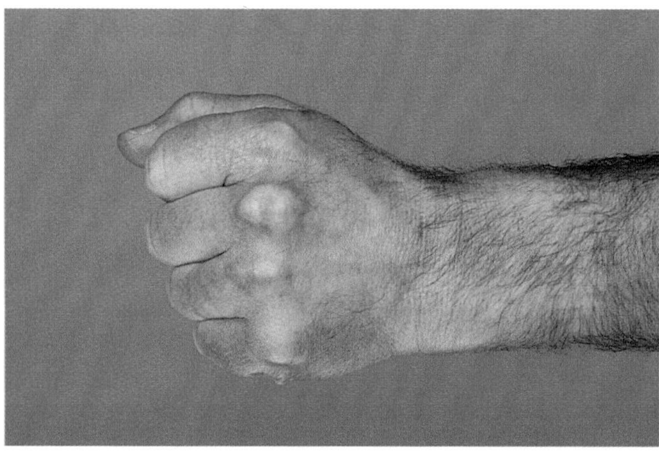

Plate 1 Tendon xanthomata on the dorsum of a hand (heterozygous familial hypercholesterolaemia).

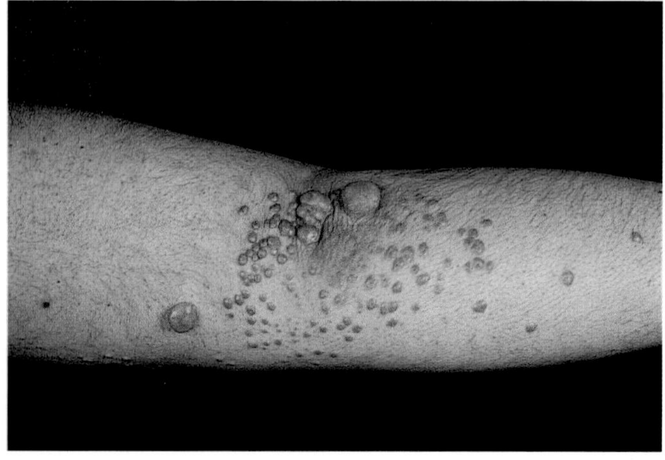

Plate 2 Eruptive and tuberose xanthomata on an arm (type III hyperlipoproteinaemia with marked hypertriglyceridaemia).

Plates for Section 7 Endocrine disease

7.6 Adrenocortical diseases

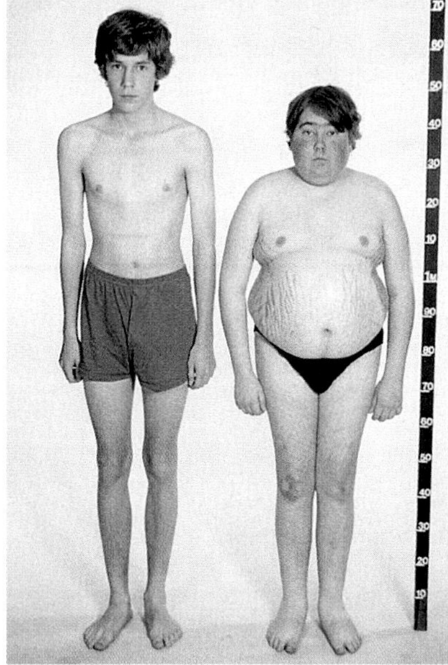

Plate 1 Cushing's disease.

Plates for Section 10 Rheumatology

10.5 Crystal-related arthropathies

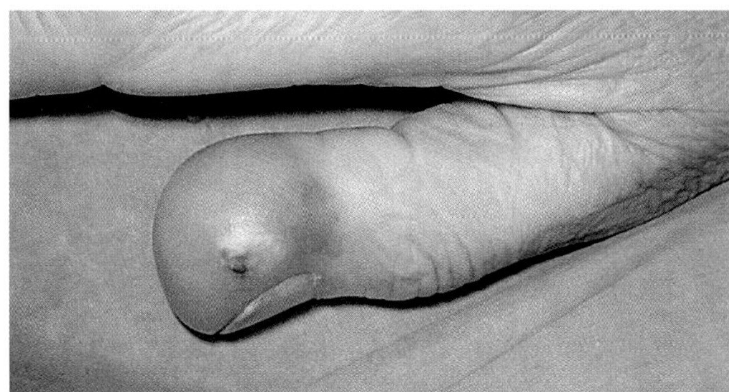

Plate 1 Gout in right thumb.

10.10 Small-vessel vasculitis

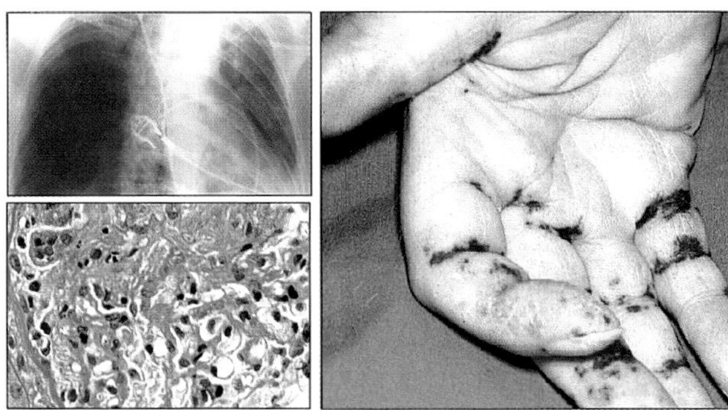

Plate 1 Microscopic polyangiitis in a 50-year-old woman affecting predominantly left lung (radiograph), kidneys (biopsy showing a high power view of the glomerulus with segmental fibrinoid necrosis—staining orange with Martius Scarlet Blue) and skin (hand). (Pathology kindly provided by Dr D. Peat.)

10.11 Systemic lupus erythematosus and related disorders

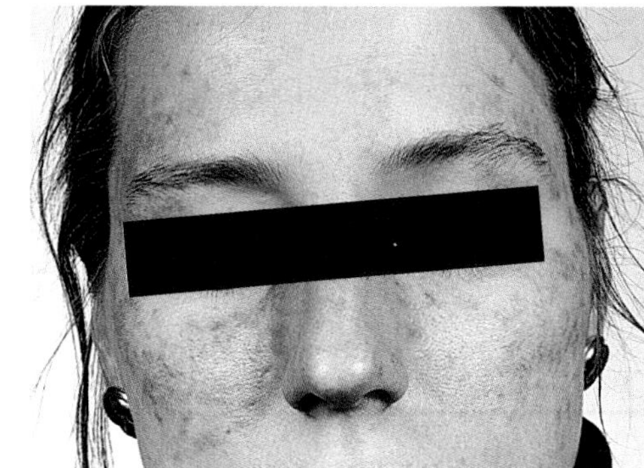

Plate 1 Butterfly (malar) rash: subacute malar rash, with erythema, vasculopathy, and early scarring.

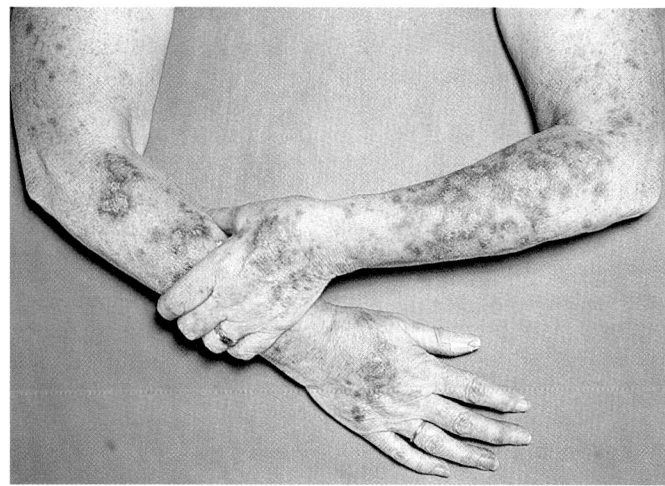

Plate 2 Subacute cutaneous lupus erythematosus in a patient with anti-La antibodies.

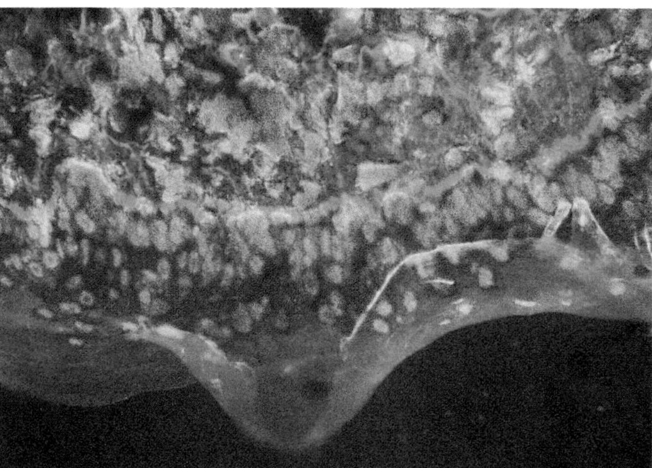

Plate 3 Lupus band test: deposition of IgG and complement at the dermoepidermal junction in the clinically normal skin of a lupus patient.

10.12 Systemic sclerosis

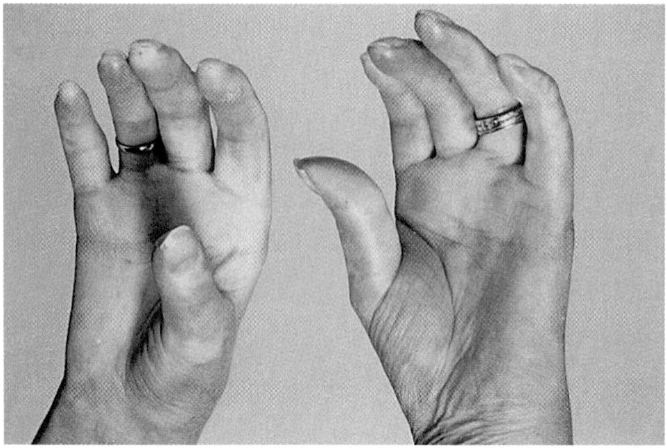

Plate 1 Scleroderma.

Plates for Section 11 Common diseases of the skin

(a)

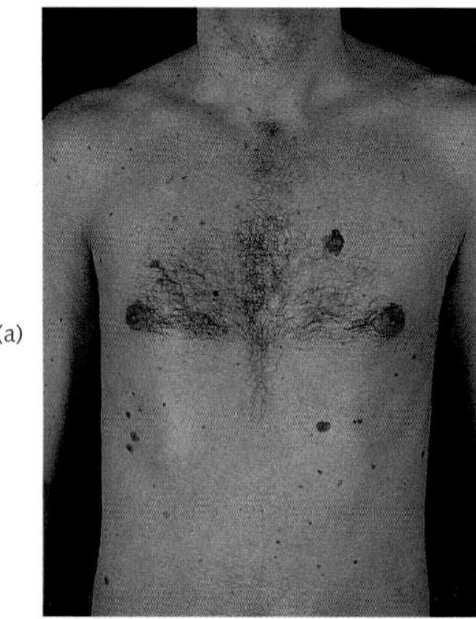

(b)

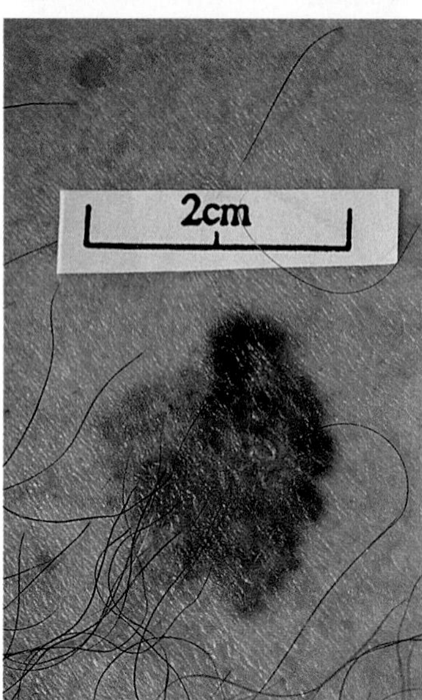

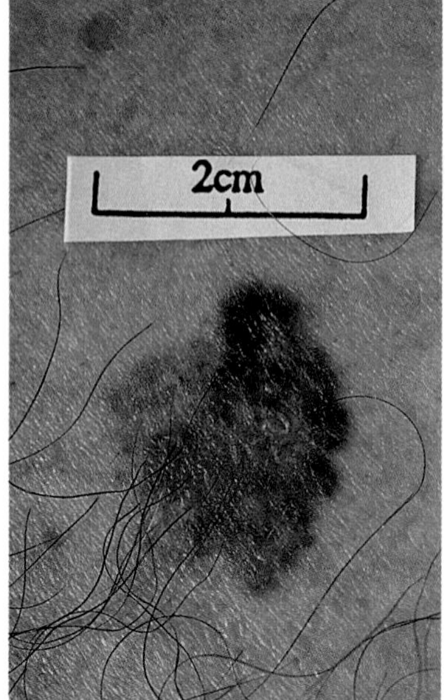

Plate 1 (a) In a patient with multiple atypical naevii, one may stand out as different from the others and can be seen to be a melanoma. (b) It has an irregular outline and contains numerous different shades of brown pigmentation.

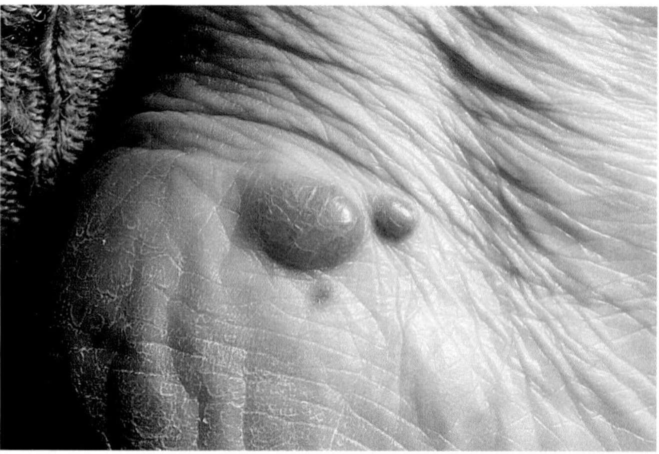

(a)

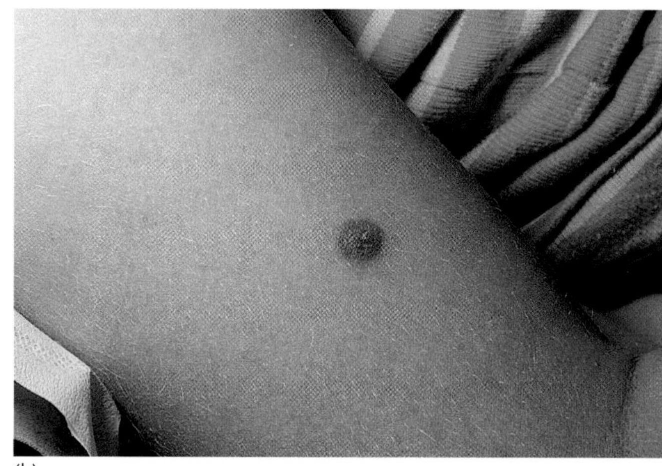

(b)

Plate 2 (a) Most primary melanomas will have some pigmentation even so-called amelanotic melanoma. (b) Spitz naevii were formerly called juvenile melanoma because of their histological resemblance to melanoma, but their biological behavior is benign.

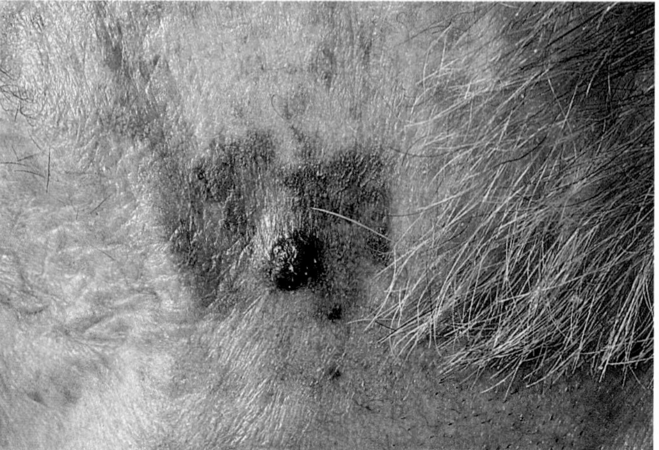

Plate 3 Nodular melanoma arising in a macular lentigo maligna (lentigo maligna melanoma).

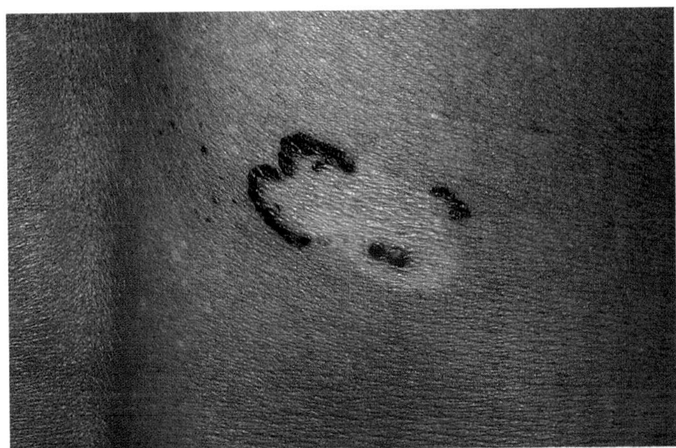

Plate 4 Regression in a melanoma making histological assessment of prognosis impossible.

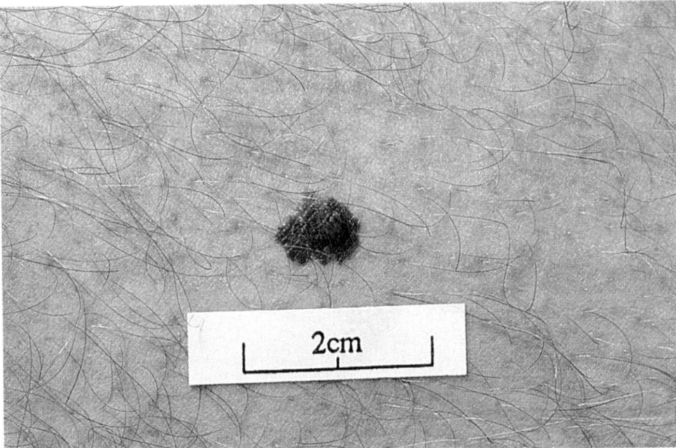

Plate 5 Melanoma most often arises *de novo* on normal skin and grows radially as well as vertically. Early detection requires identification of atypical morphology of smaller lesions.

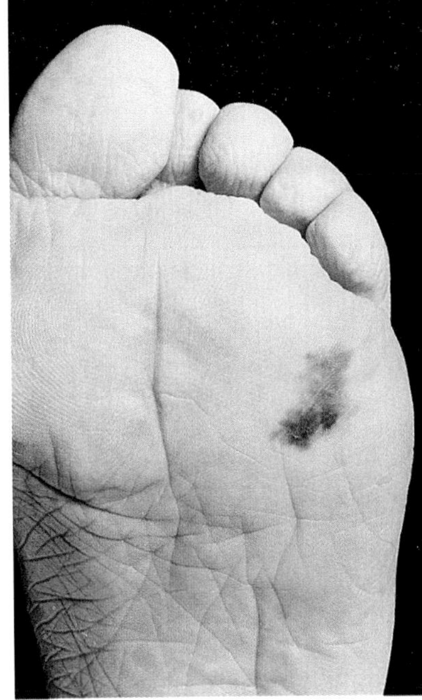

Plate 6 Acral lentigenous melanoma can be difficult to distinguish from benign junctional naevii on the palms and soles.

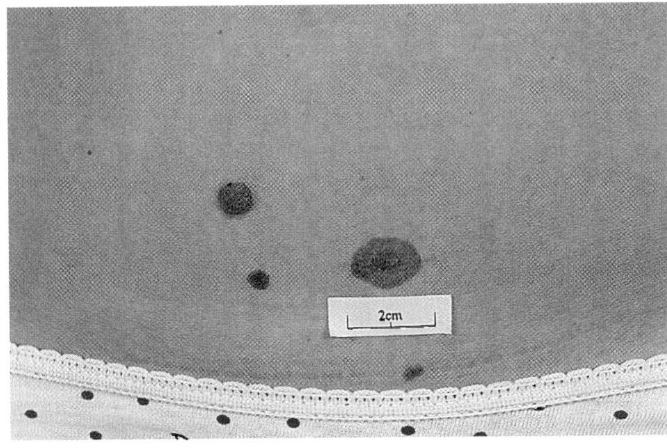

(a)

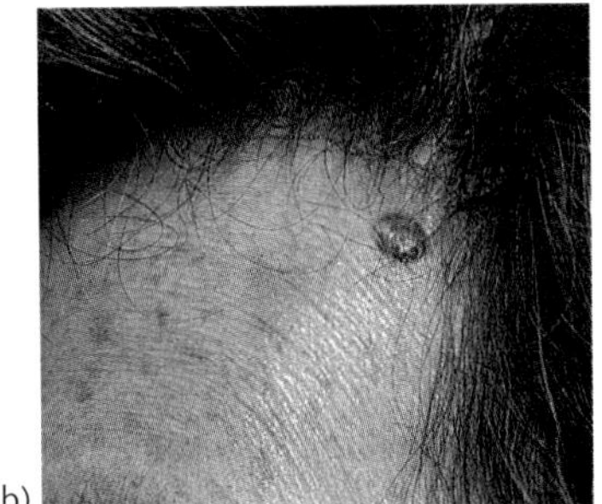

(b)

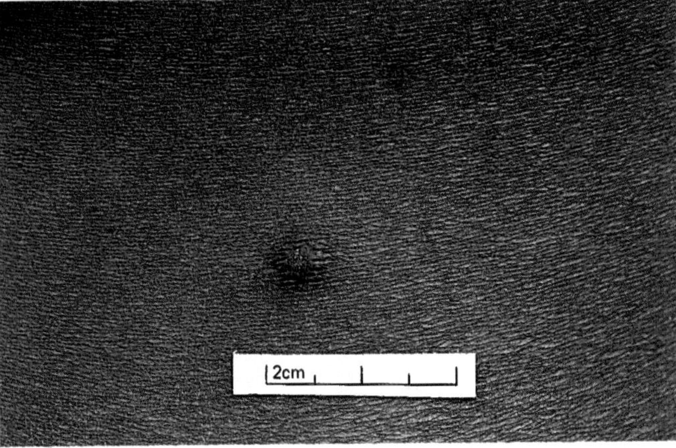

(c)

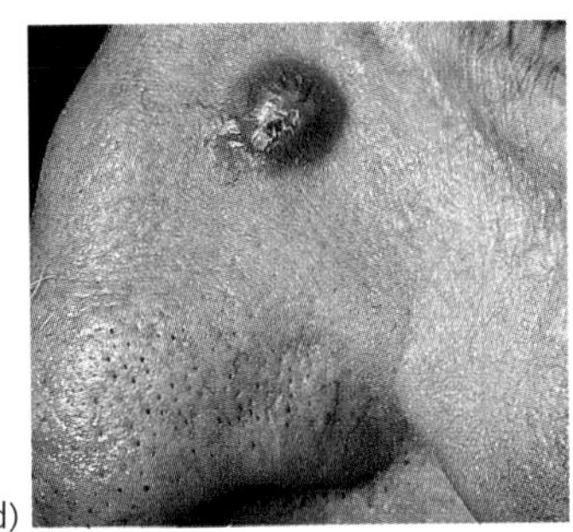

(d)

Plate 7 Lesions commonly confused with melanoma include (a) naevus en cocarde, which are central compound naevii with a surrounding macular junctional component, giving the appearance of a fried egg. Blue naevii (b) are often deeply pigmented, but the pigmentation is uniform and a blue tinge is discernible. Dermatofibromas (c) are sometimes easier to diagnose on palpation as they are hard and tethered to the skin. They may feel like a split pea. Pigmented basal cell epitheliomas (d) often have a rolled edge; however sometimes biopsy provides this unexpected diagnosis.

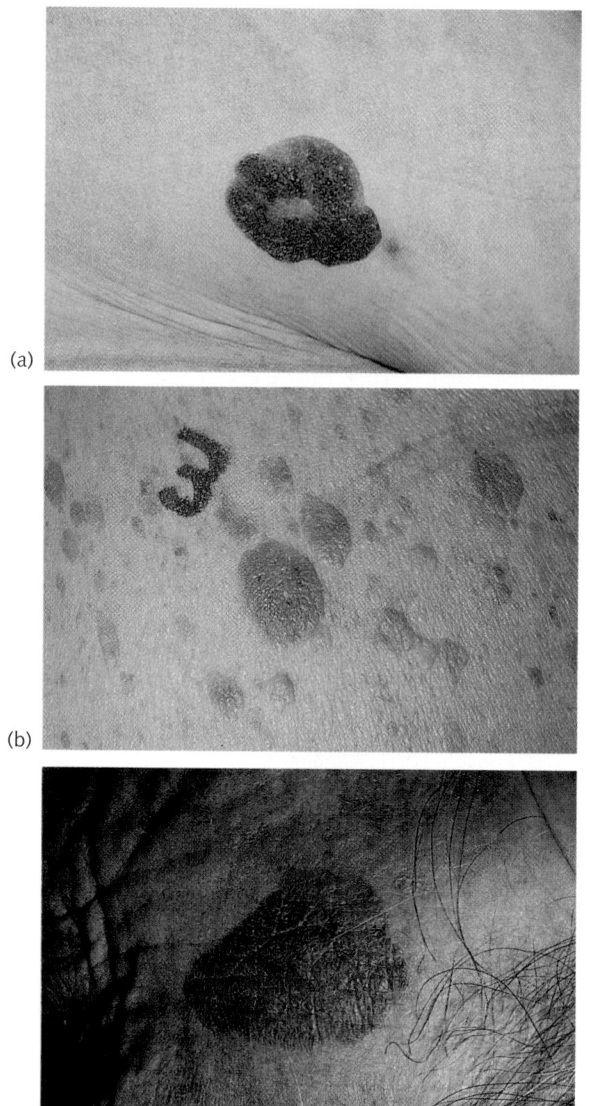

Plate 8 Seborrhoeic warts are often numerous and come in a variety of shapes and sizes. They may be deeply pigmented and elevated (a) or pale (b). They may also be macular (c). Characteristically they have a waxy surface and a 'stuck on' appearance.

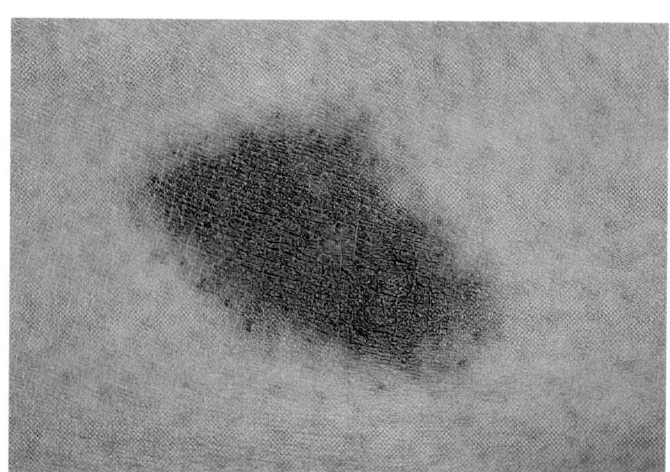

Plate 9 Congenital naevii are often larger than acquired naevii, but are usually evenly pigmented. They have a greater risk of malignant change.

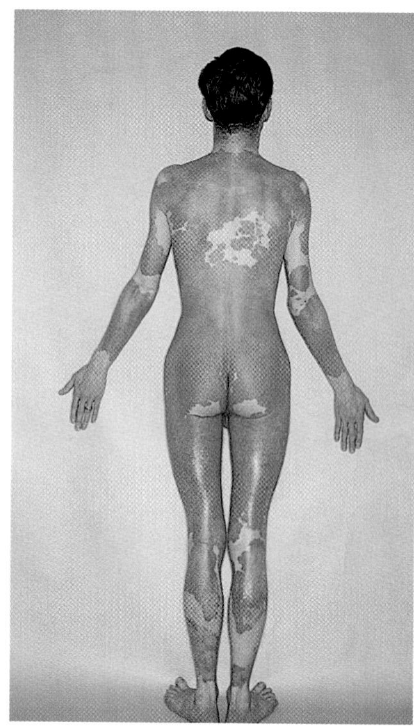

Plate 10 Erythroderma of psoriasis.

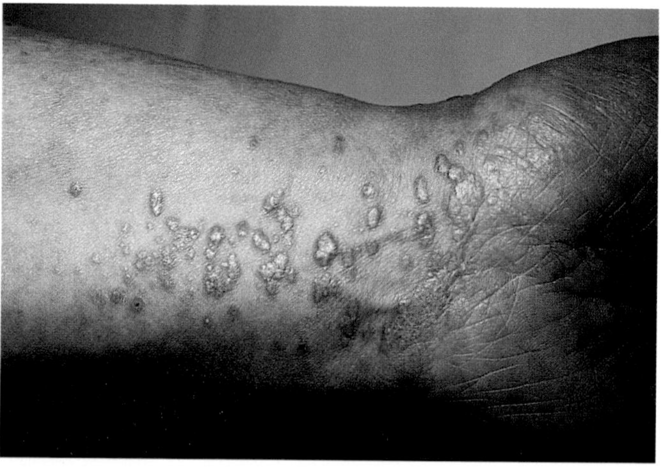

Plate 11 Distribution of the rash of lichen planus is symmetrical favouring the wrists. The lesion is flat topped, violaceous, and shiny.

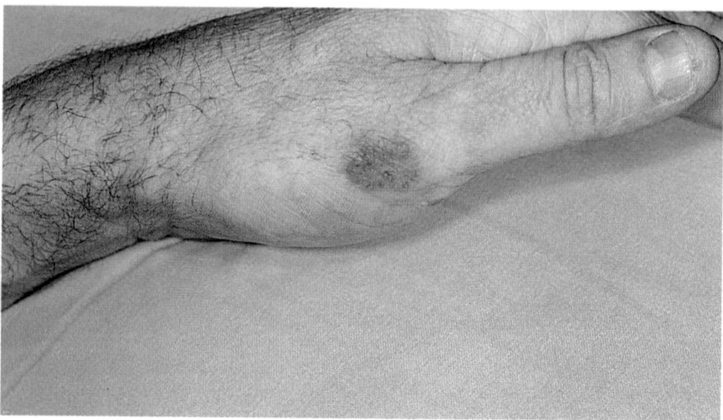

Plate 12 *Mycobacterium marinum*, a fish tank infection.

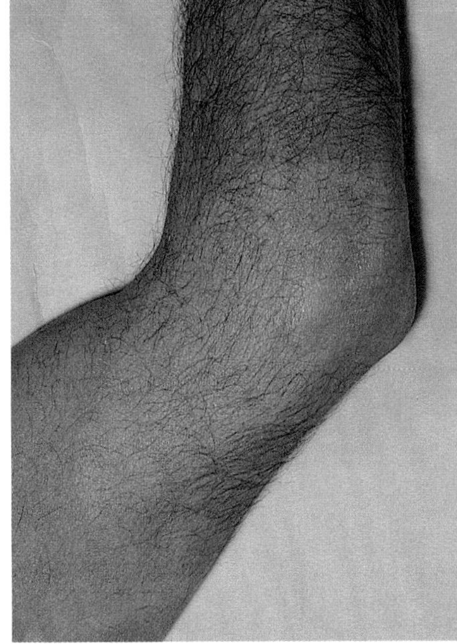

Plate 13 Hyperpigmented anaesthetic lesion of leprosy.

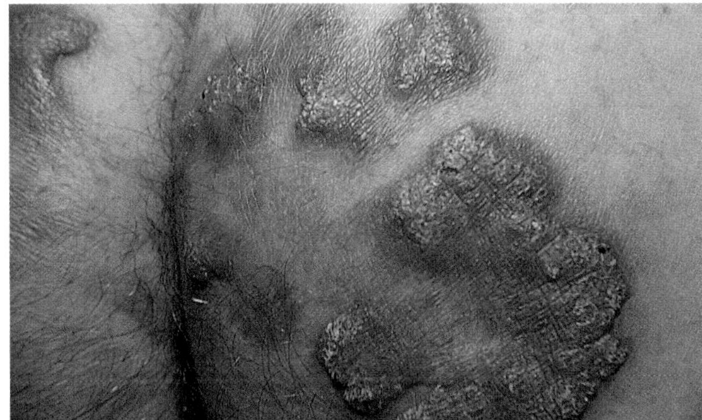

Plate 15 Lupus verrucosa.

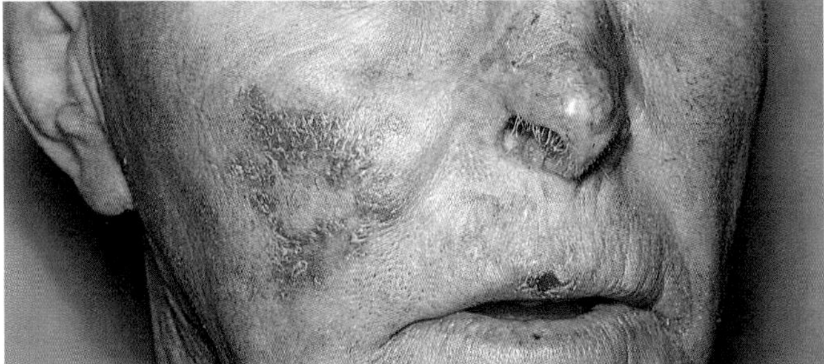

Plate 14 Lupus vulgaris.

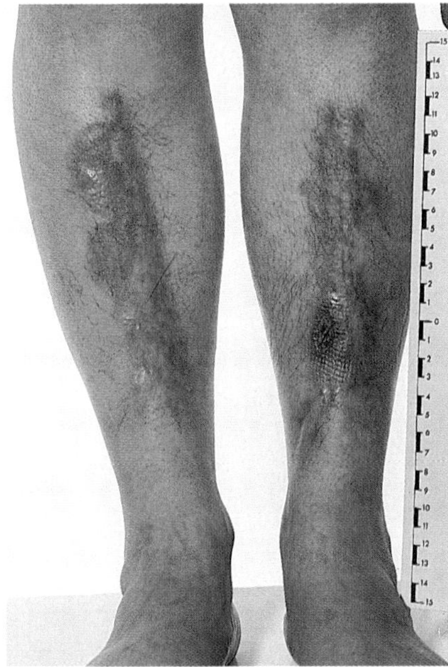

Plate 16 Necrobiosis lipoidica diabeticorum.

Plates for Section 16 Infectious disease

16.10 Herpes simplex virus infections

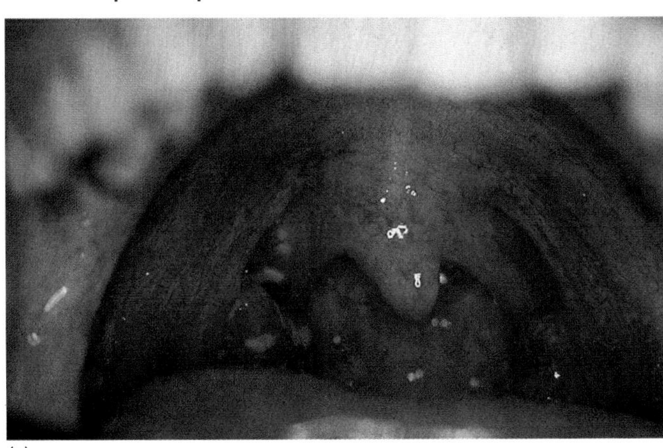

(a)

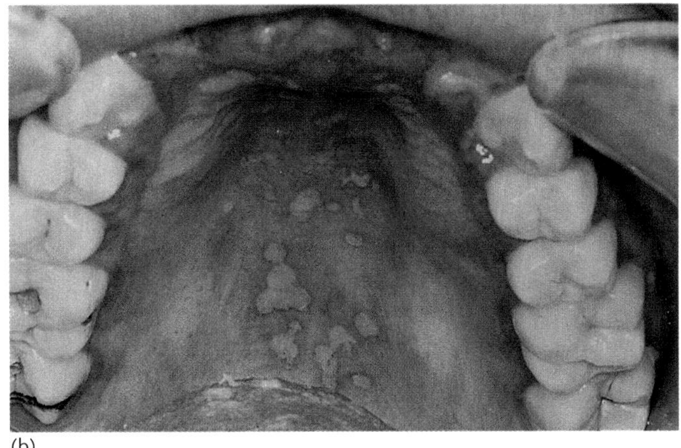

(b)

Plate 1 (a) Primary herpetic gingivostomatitis, part of generalized HSV-2 infection. The lesions on the soft palate are indistinguishable from the 'herpangina' in certain coxsackievirus infections. (b) Primary herpetic gingivostomatitis.

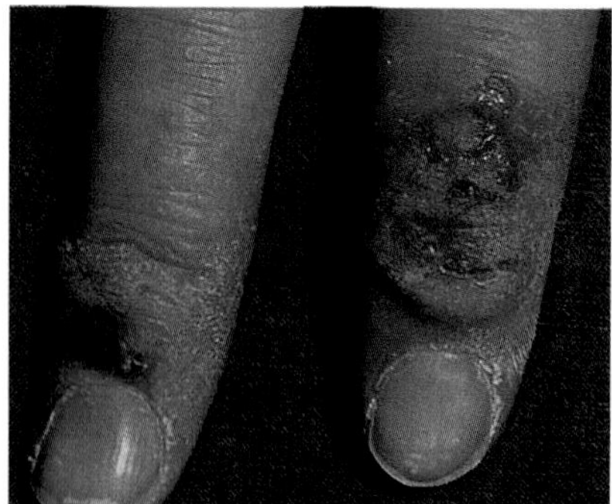

Plate 2 Herpetic whitlow with spread to an adjoining finger.

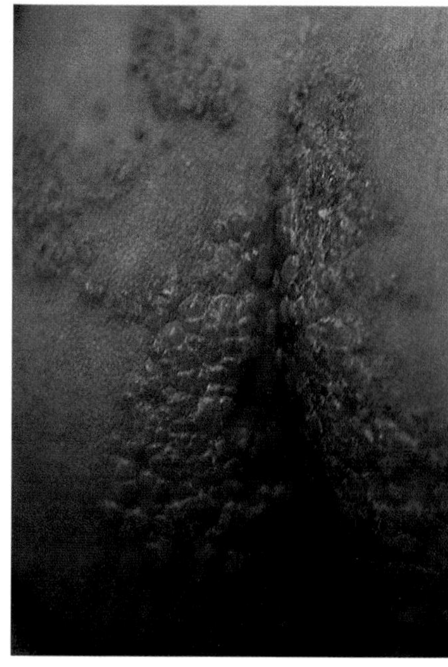

Plate 3 Primary HSV-2 of the buttocks.

16.11 Varicella zoster

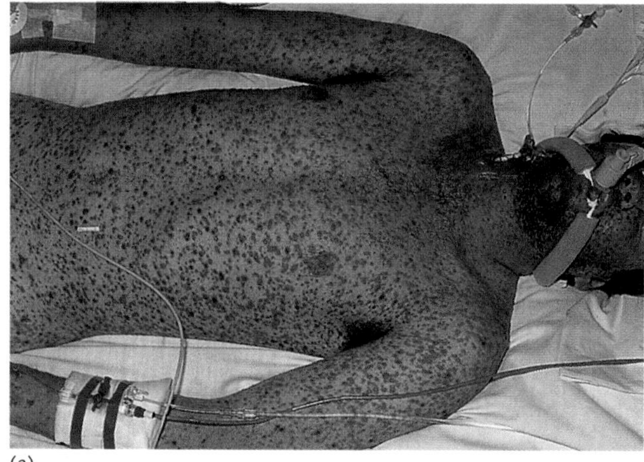

(a)

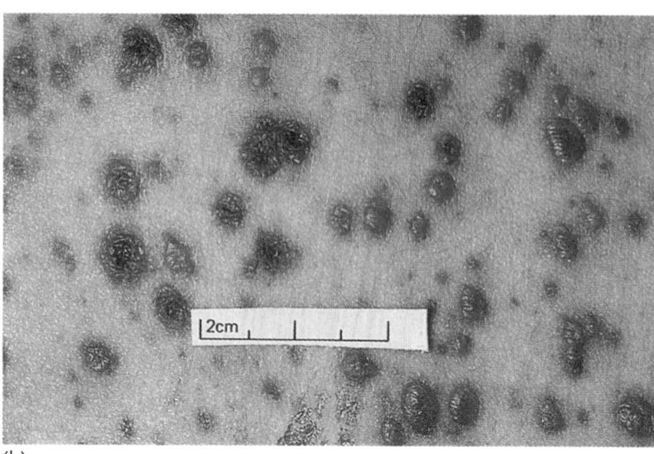

(b)

Plate 1 (a) Dense chickenpox eruption in a young man with severe infection also involving the lungs. (b) Details of the rash.

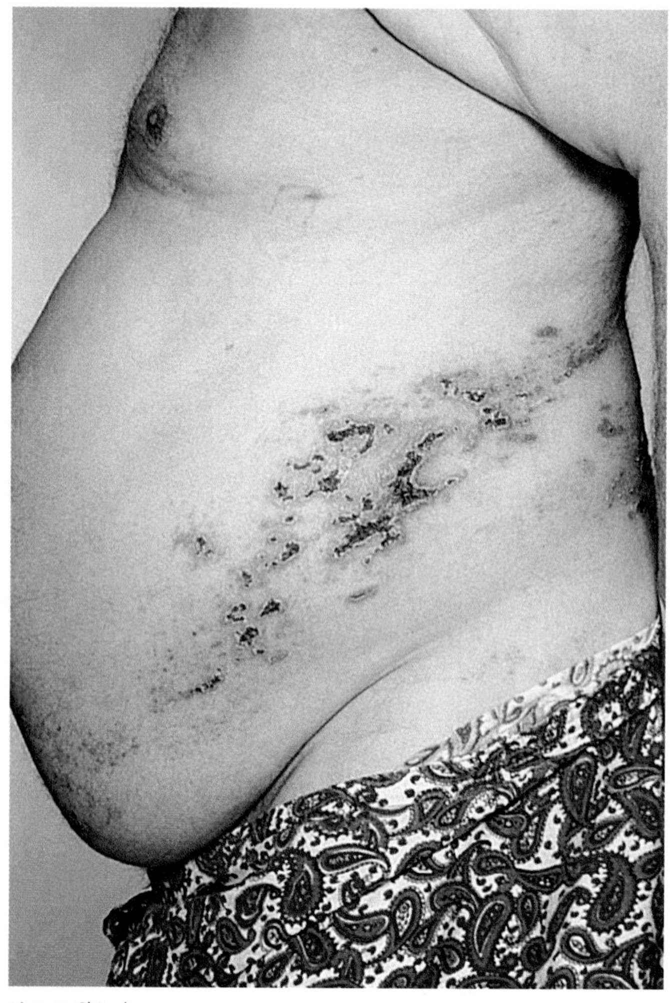

Plate 2 Shingles.

16.15 Human herpesviruses 6, 7, and 8

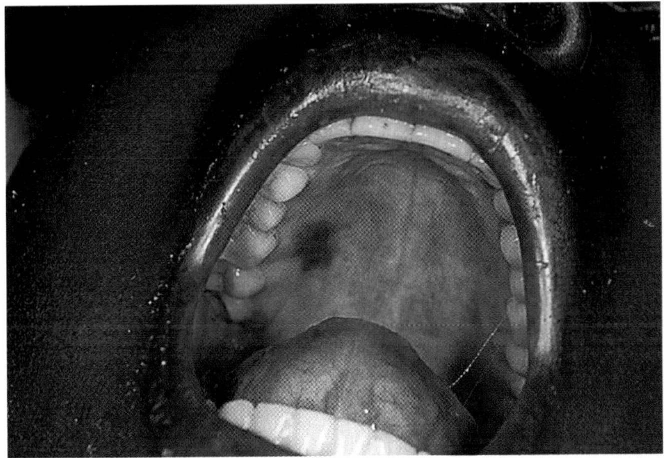

Plate 1 Kaposi's sarcoma of the palate in a seropositive patient.

(a)

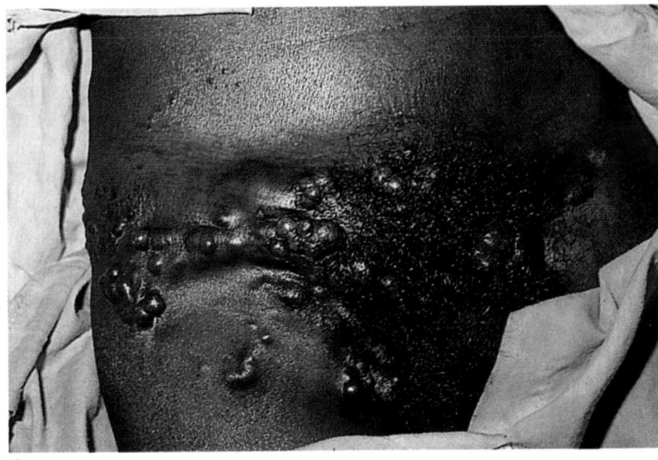

(b)

Plate 2 (a) and (b) Extensive invasive Kaposi's sarcomas in an HIV-seropositive man.

16.17 Orf

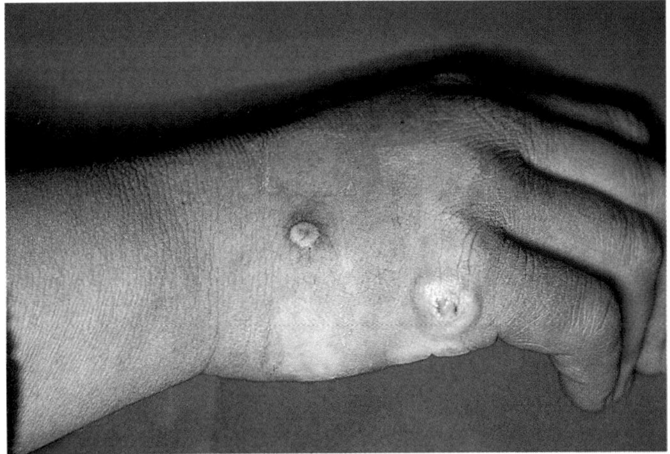

Plate 1 Orf, a sheep pox virus, is a common zoonosis in agriculture.

16.33 Parvoviruses

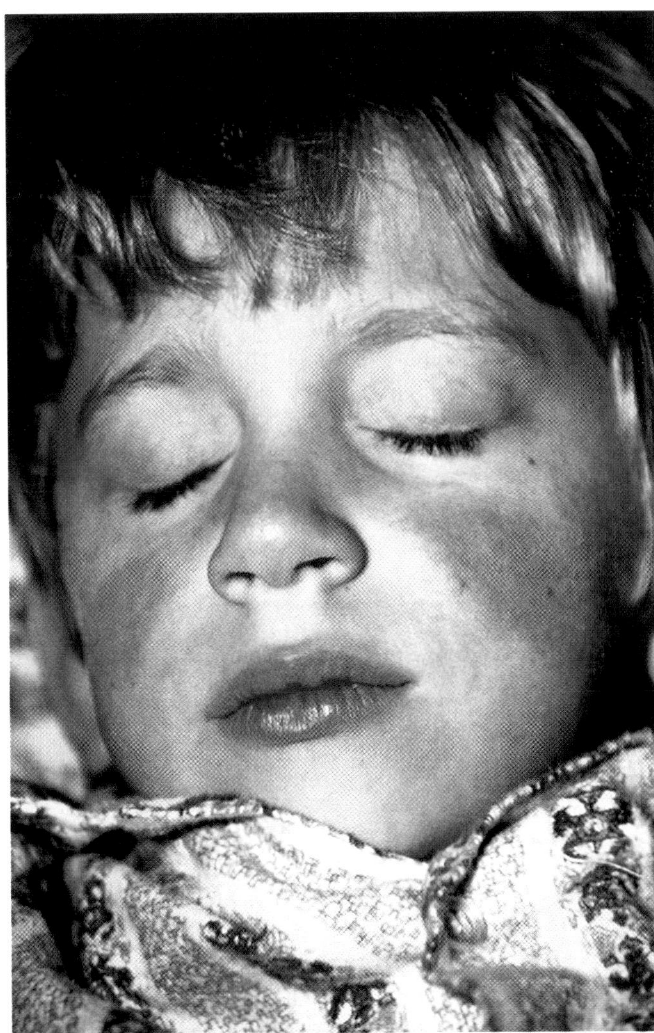

Plate 1 'Slapped cheek' rash of erythema infectiosum: note circumoral pallor (by courtesy of Dr Ken Mutton).

16.35 HIV infection and AIDS

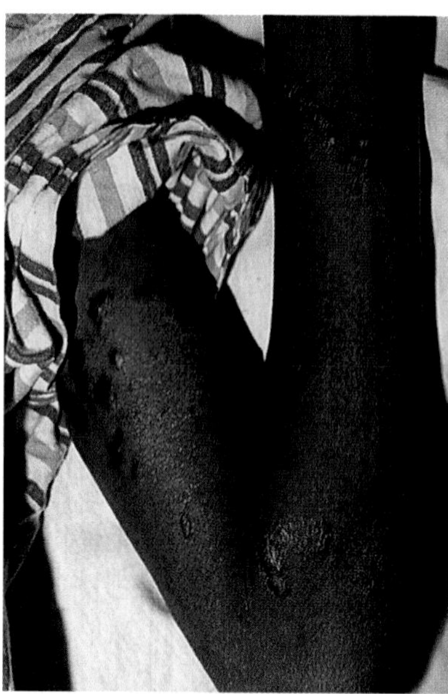

Plate 1 Multiple cutaneous Kaposi's sarcomas in an HIV-seropositive woman.

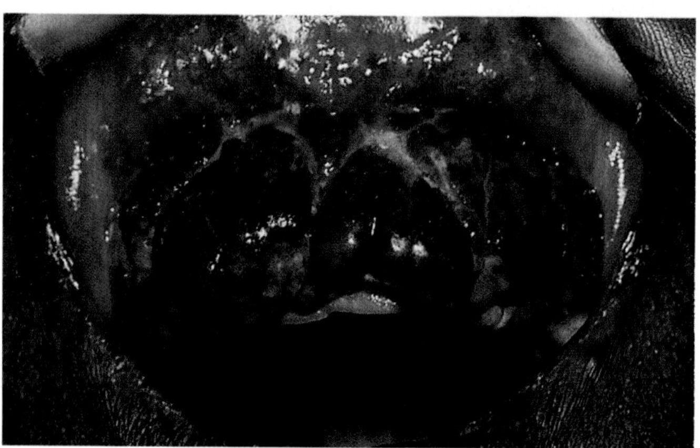

Plate 2 AIDS-associated Kaposi's sarcoma of the gum (copyright M.A. Ansary and C. Conlon, Lusaka).

16.38 Pathogenic streptococci

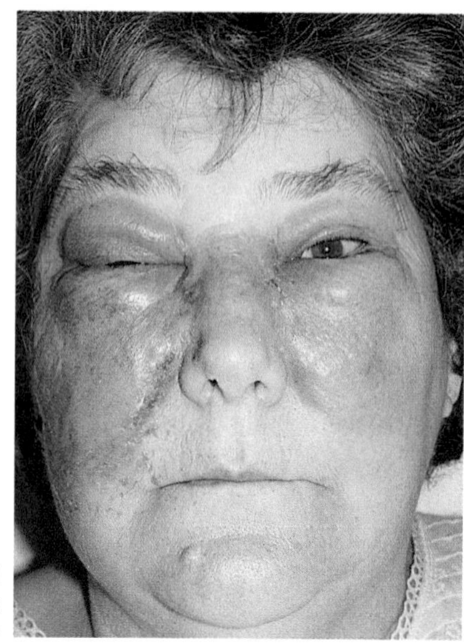

Plate 1 Bilateral facial erysipelas. (Copyright S. Eykyn.)

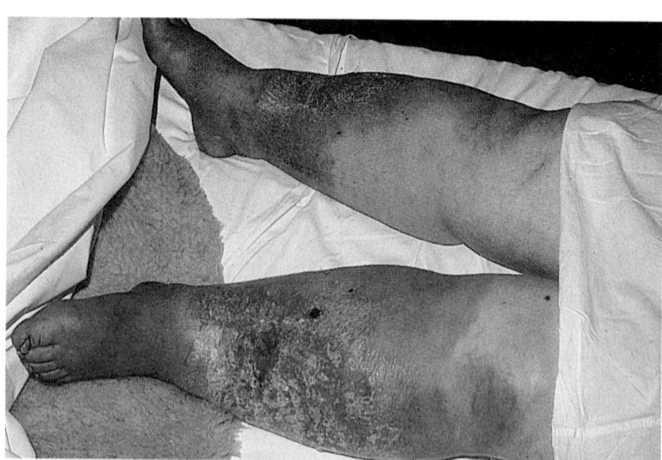

Plate 2 Cellulitis. (Copyright S. Eykyn.)

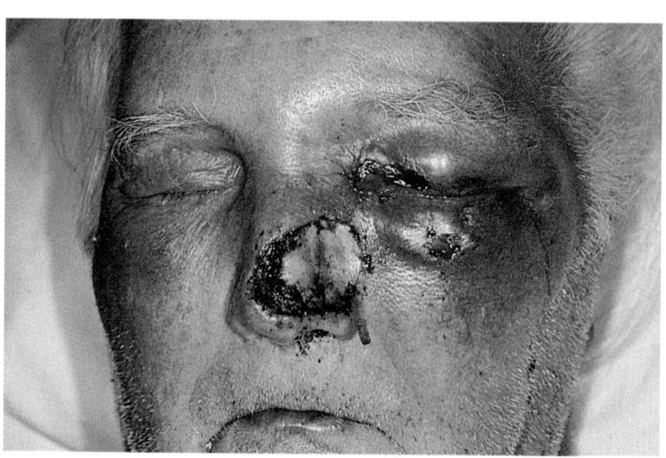

Plate 3 *Streptococcus pyogenes* bacteraemia 3 days after a skin graft. (Copyright S. Eykyn.)

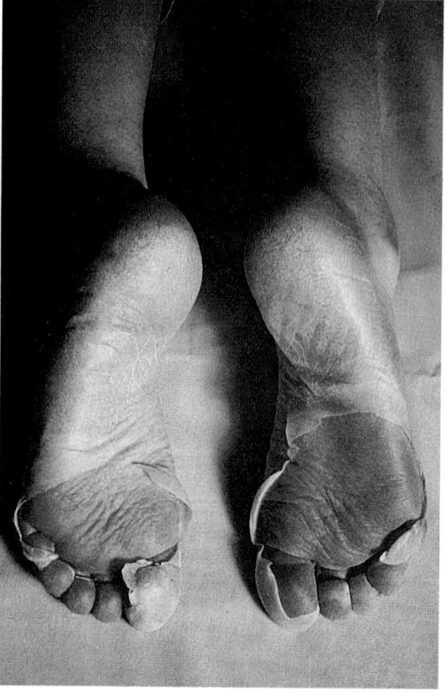

Plate 4 Peeling of the skin of the soles of the feet in a patient with *Streptococcus pyogenes* pericarditis. (Copyright S. Eykyn.)

16.41 Meningococcal infection

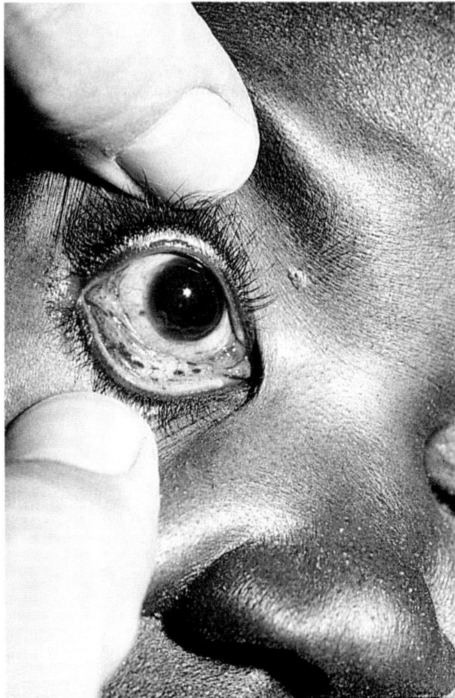

Plate 1 Petechiae in the conjunctiva of a patient with meningococcal disease. (Copyright D.A. Warrell.).

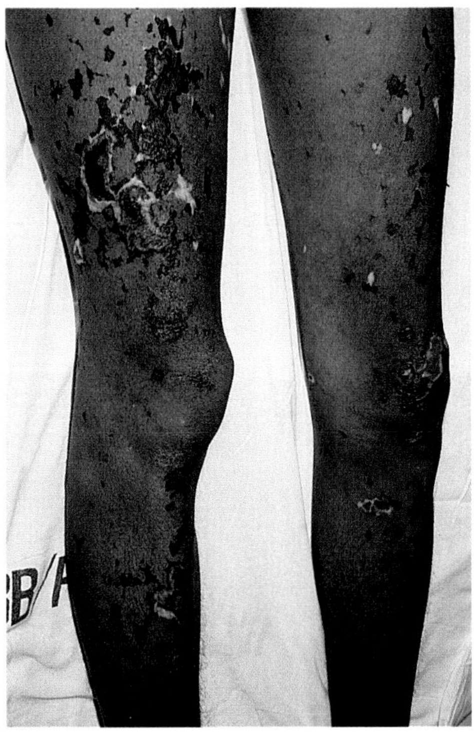

Plate 2 Cutaneous vasculitis as a complication of meningococcal disease.

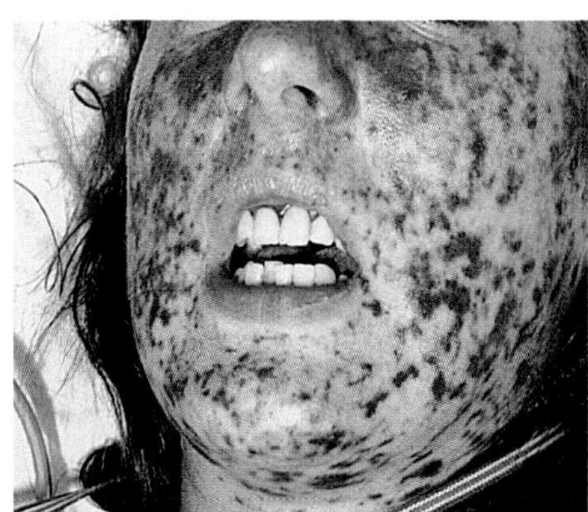

Plate 3 Meningococcal septicaemia.

16.54 Tularaemia

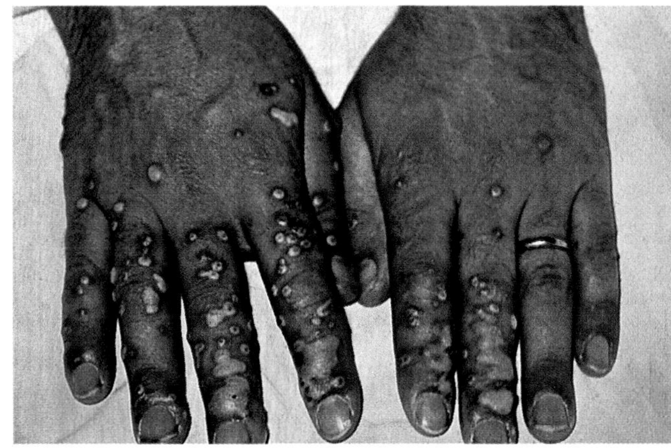

Plate 1 Hands in a case of ulcero-(cutano)-glandular tularaemia (by courtesy of A. Berglund, Falund, Sweden).

16.60 Disease caused by environmental mycobacteria

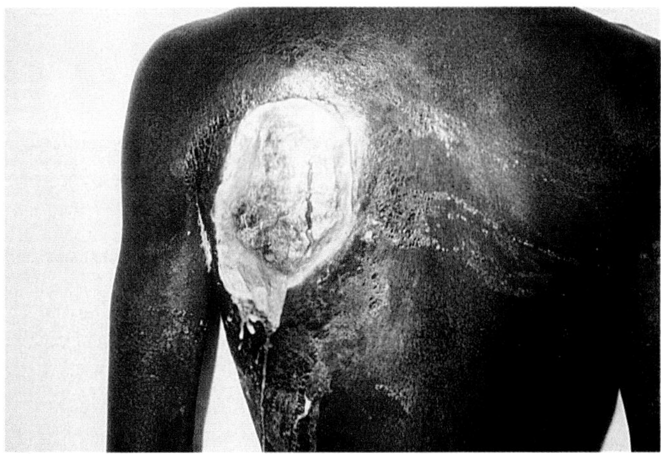

Plate 1 *Mycobacterium ulcerans* infection (Buruli ulcer). Large ulcer overlying the left scapula, showing discharge of liquefied necrotic subcutaneous fat.

16.72 Rickettsial diseases including the ehrlichioses

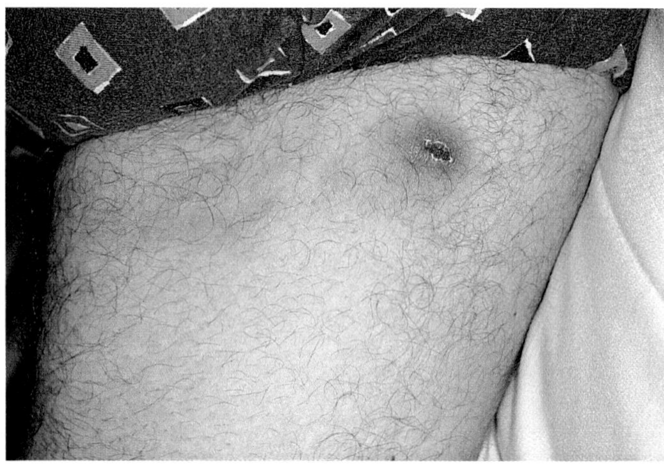

Plate 1 Boutonneuse fever (South African tick typhus). Eschar with lymphangitic lines spreading towards the femoral lymph nodes in a patient who had visited the Kruger National Park, South Africa, 7 days earlier. (Copyright D.A. Warrell.)

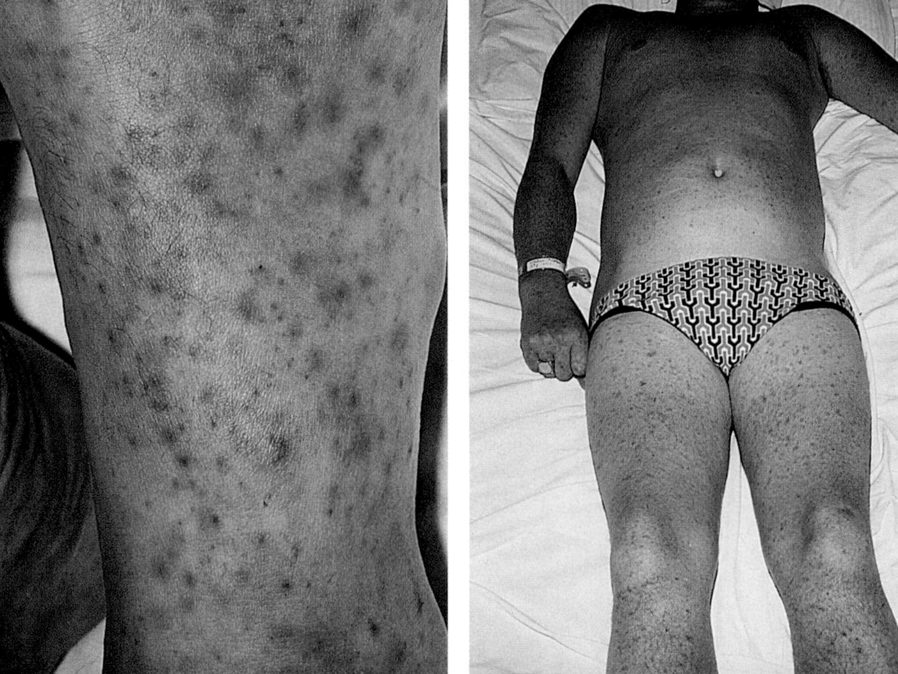

Plate 2 and 3 Boutonneuse fever (South African tick typhus) in a British traveller (Copyright E. Dunbar.)

16.73 Scrub typhus

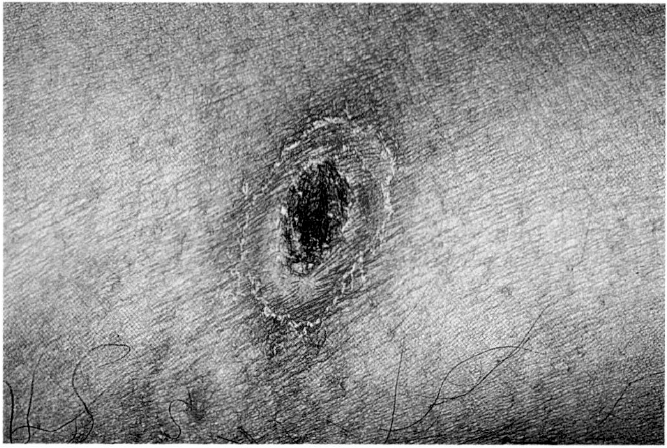

Plate 1 Eschar at site of a mite bite 10 days previously on the lower abdomen of a Thai patient. (Copyright D.A. Warrell.)

16.75 Bartonellosis, cat scratch disease, bacillary angiomatosis-peliosis, and trench fever

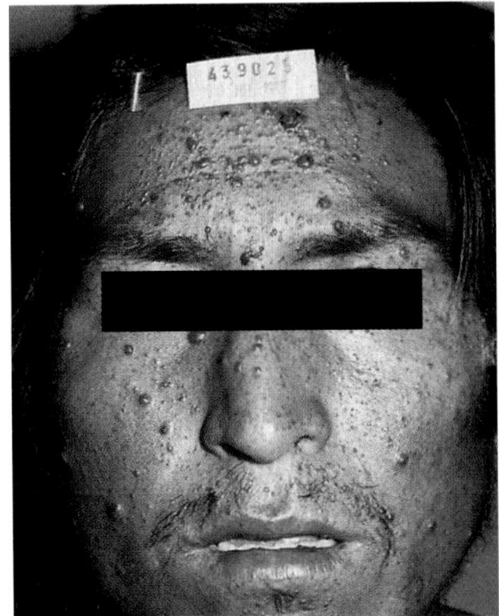

Plate 1 Miliary haemangioma-like lesions of 'verruga peruana'.

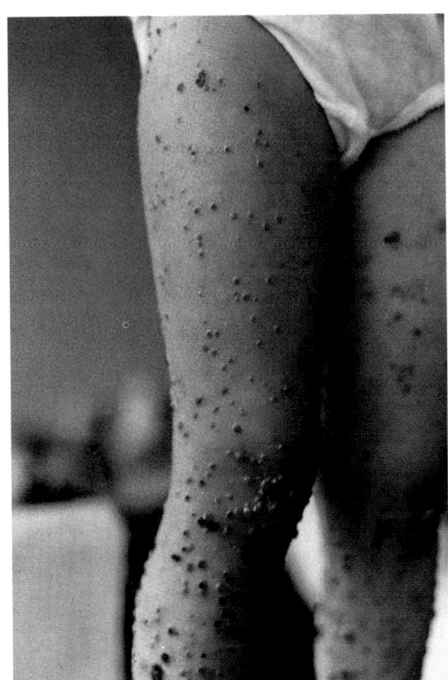

(a)

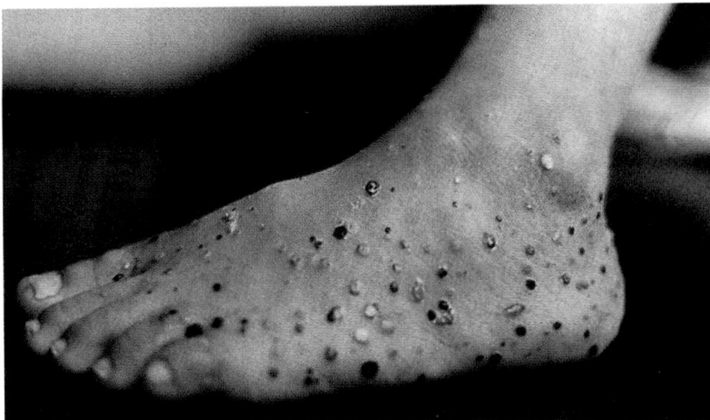

(b)

Plate 2 (a, b) Nodular lesions of 'verruga peruana'.

16.76 Chlamydial infections

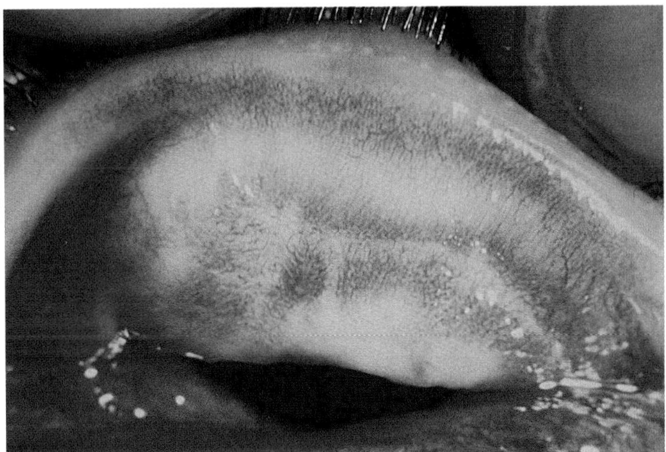

Plate 1 Everted upper eyelid showing trachomatous scarring.

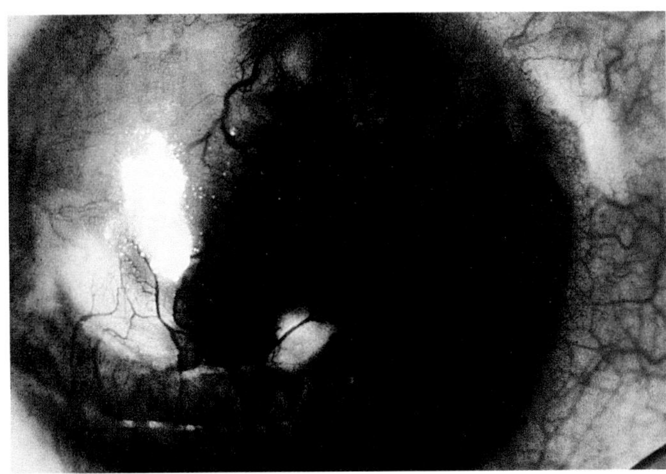

Plate 2 Extensive neovascularization of the cornea (pannus) due to trachoma.

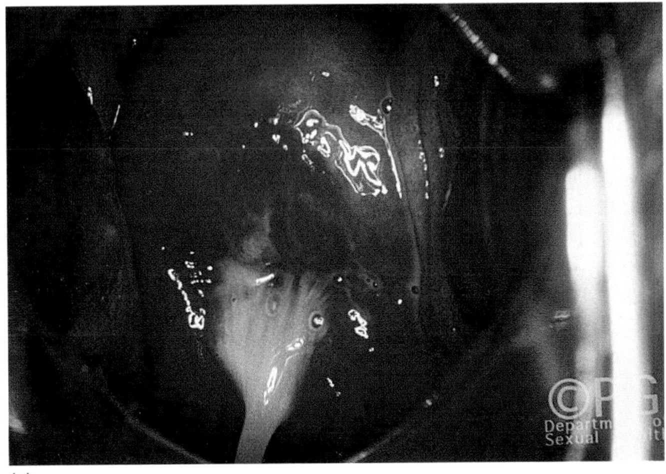

(a)

Plate 3 *See caption overleaf.*

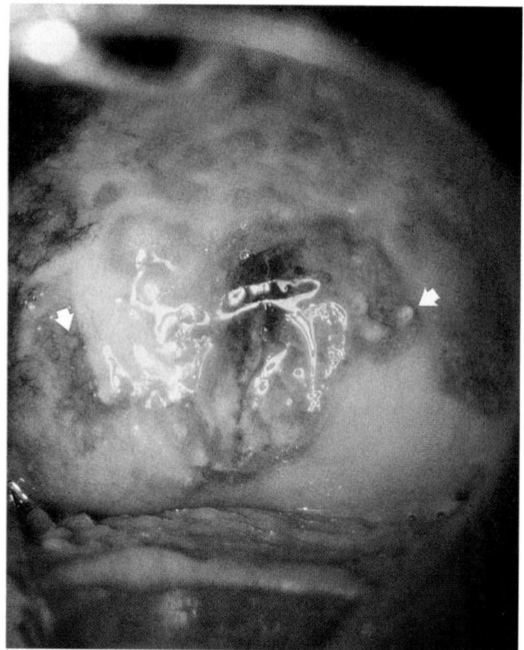

(b)

Plate 3 (a) Mucopurulent cervicitis; (b) follicular cervicitis.

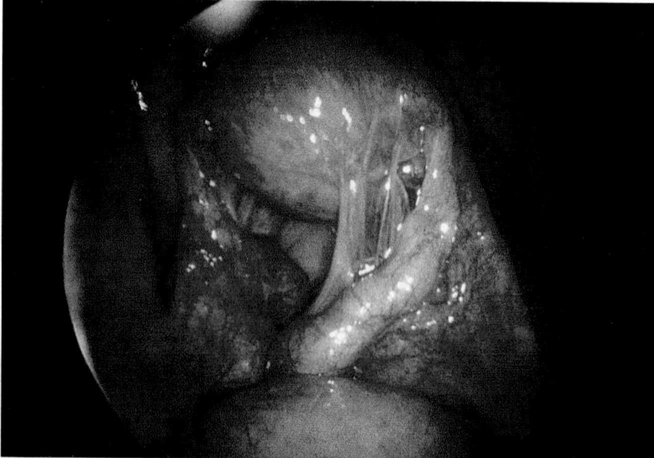

Plate 4 Laparoscopic view of inflamed fallopian tube due to *C. trachoma*. (By courtesy of P. Greenhouse.)

16.81 Fungal infections (mycoses)

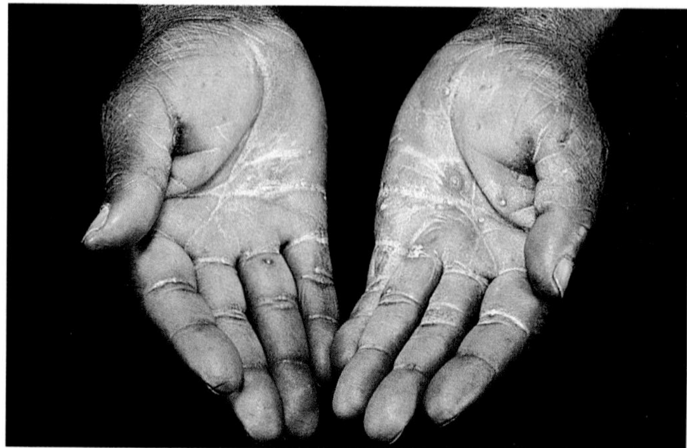

Plate 1 Palmar scaling due to *Trichophyton rubrum*.

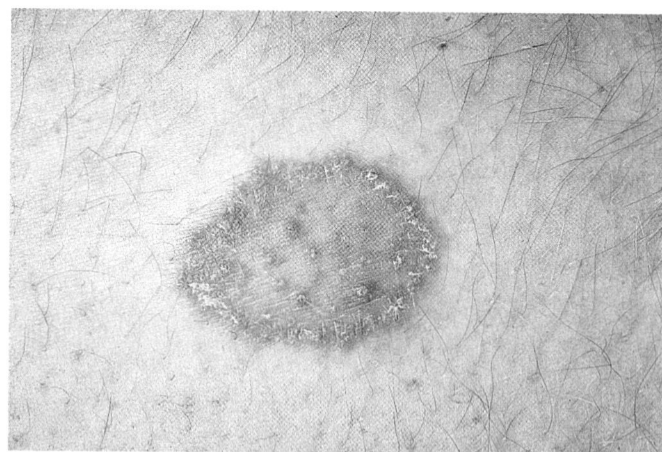

Plate 2 Tinea corporis due to *Microsporum gypseum*.

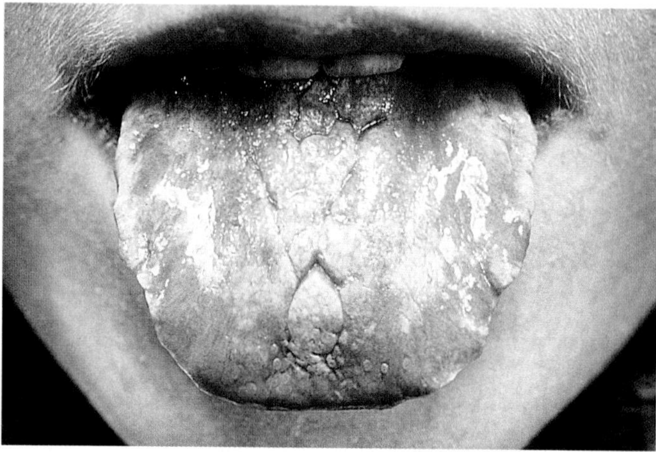

Plate 3 Oral candidosis in a patient with chronic mucocutaneous candidosis.

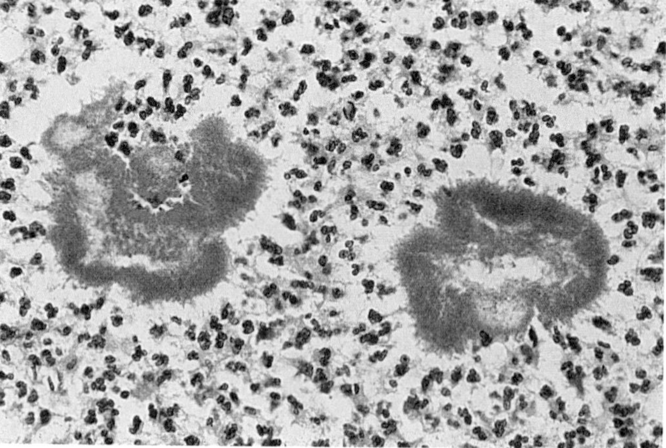

Plate 4 Grains in abscess in actinomycetoma (*Nocardia brasiliensis*) (H & E).

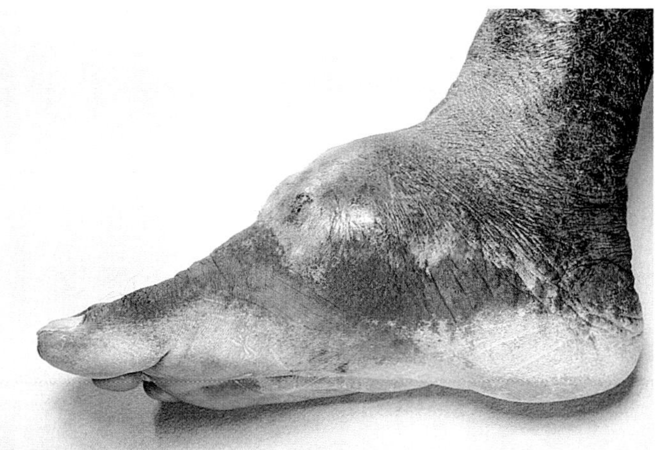

Plate 5 A mycetoma caused by *Madurella grisea.*

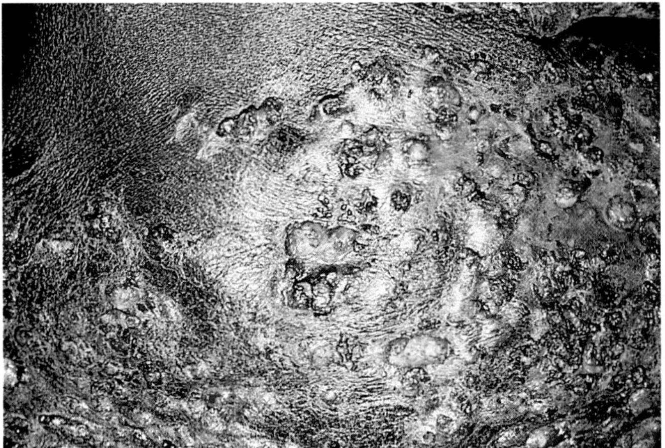

Plate 6 *Nocardia brasiliensis* actinomycetoma draining sinus.

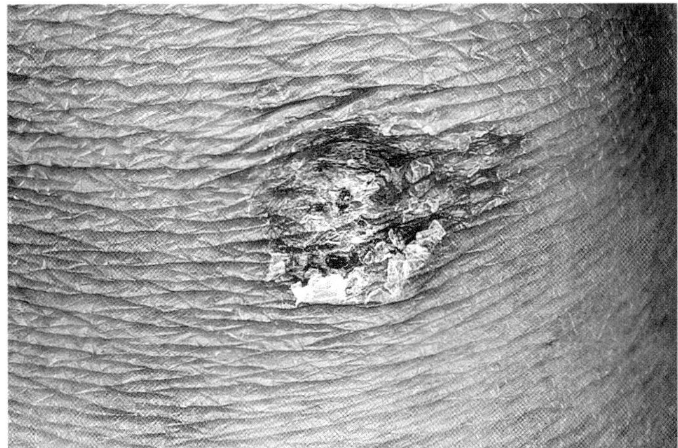

Plate 7 An early lesion of chromoblastomycosis.

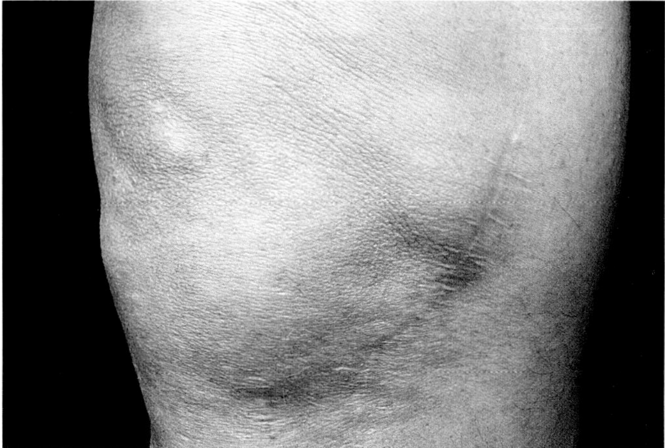

Plate 8 Arthritis due to disseminated coccidioidomycosis.

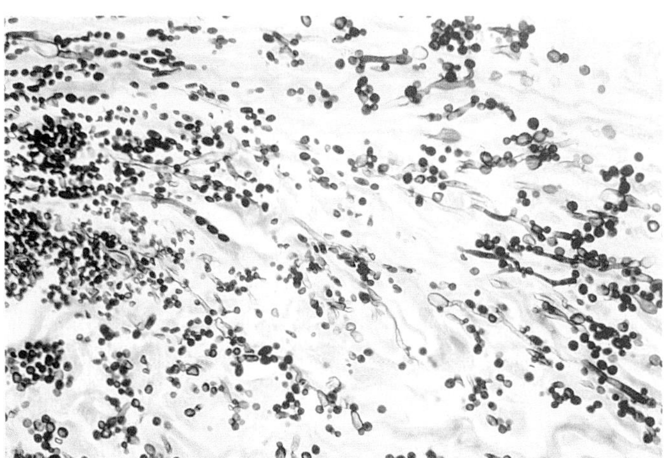

Plate 9 Candidosis disseminated to skin (methenamine silver × 516).

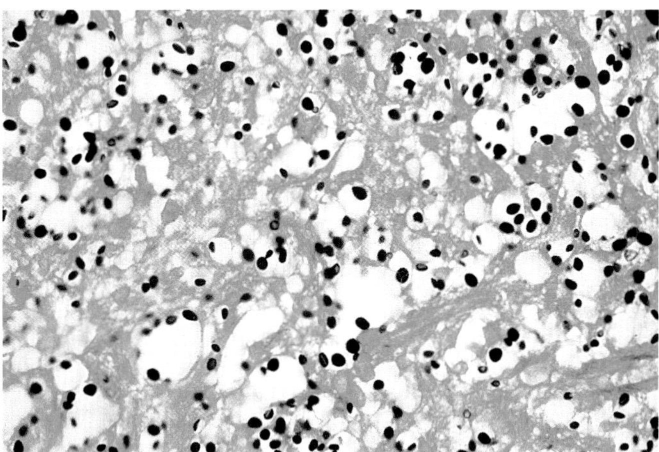

Plate 10 Disseminated cryptococcosis (methenamine silver × 52).

16.83 Amoebiasis

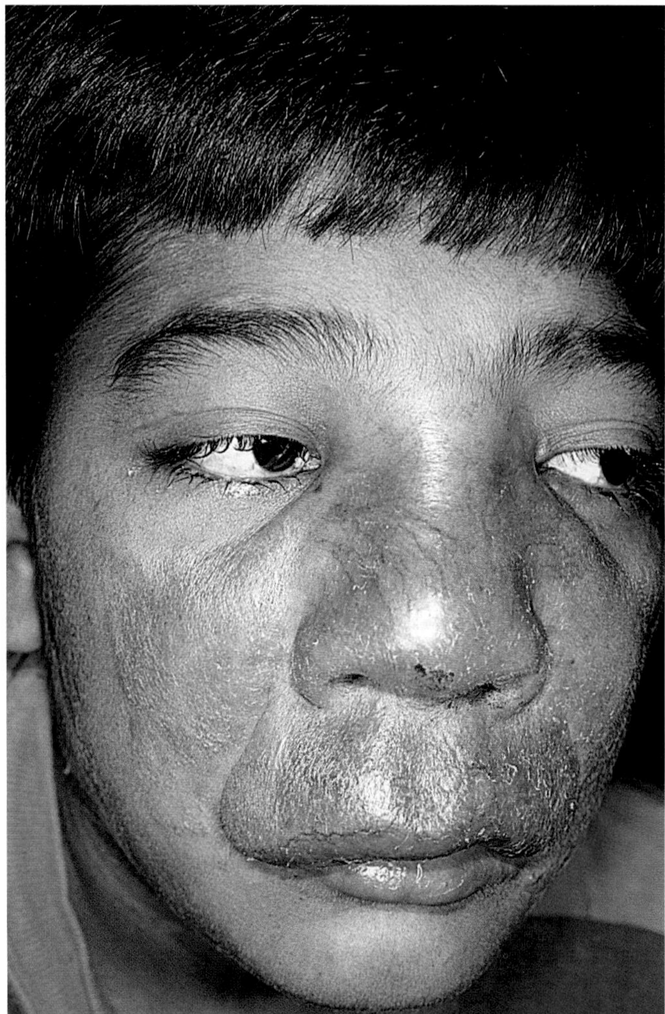

(a)

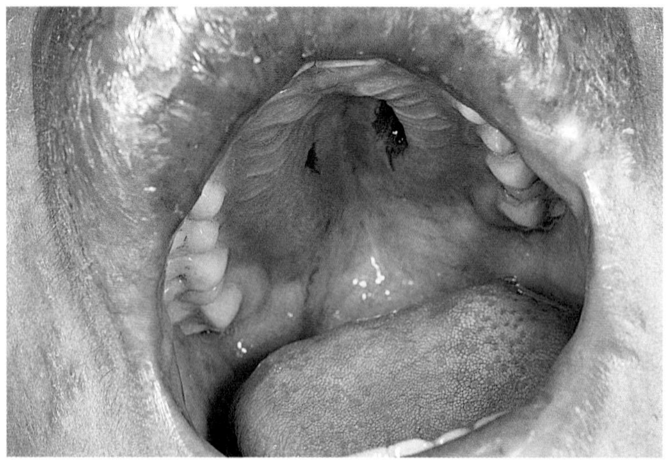

(b)

Plate 1 Sixteen-year-old Peruvian boy with a chronic facial lesion that had been present for 3 years (a), perforating lesion of the palate (b), and intracranial space-occupying lesions caused by *Balamuthia mandrillaris*. (Copyright D.A. Warrell.)

16.84 Malaria

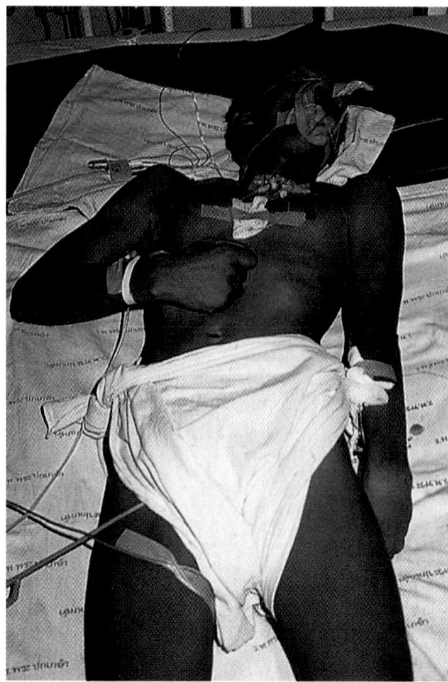

Plate 1 Decorticate rigidity in a Thai man with cerebral malaria. (Copyright D.A. Warrell.)

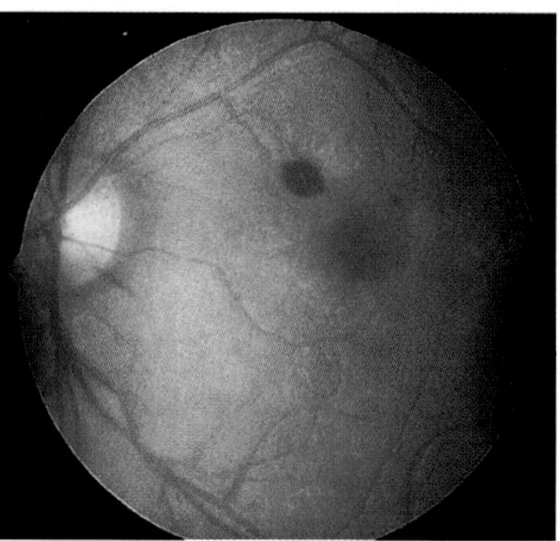

Plate 2 Retinal haemorrhages close to the macula in a Thai patient with cerebral malaria. (Copyright D.A. Warrell.)

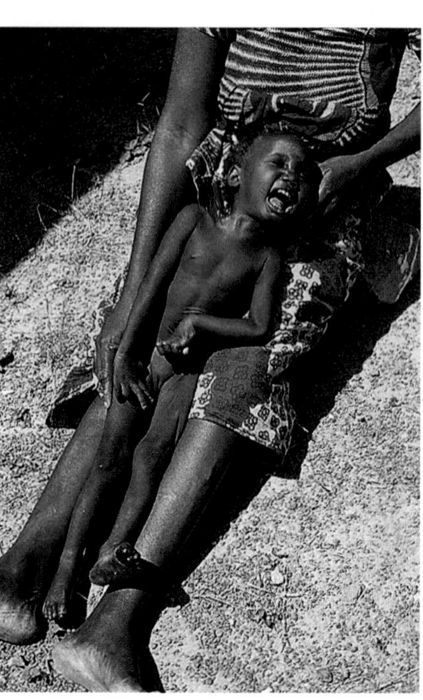

Plate 3 Hemiplegia and other severe residual neurological sequelae in a Nigerian child who survived an attack of cerebral malaria. (Copyright D.A. Warrell.)

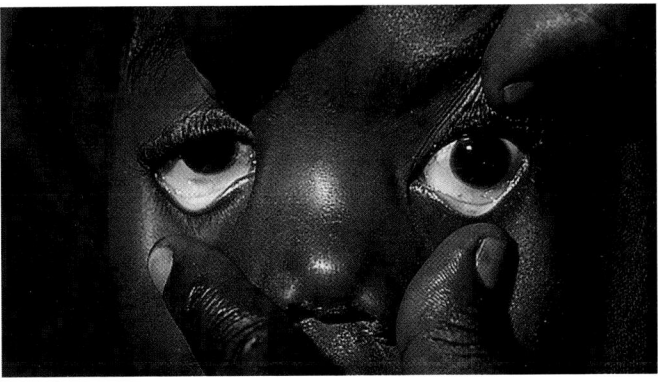

Plate 4 Profound anaemia (haemoglobin 1.2 g/dl) in a Kenyan child with *P. falciparum* parasitaemia. (Copyright D.A. Warrell.)

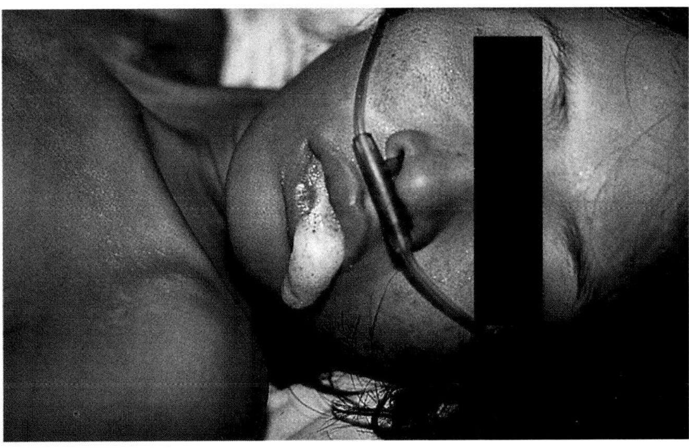

Plate 6 Fatal pulmonary oedema developing 3 h postpartum in a Thai woman with cerebral malaria; the fetus was stillborn (by courtesy of Professor Sornchai Looareesuwan, Bangkok).

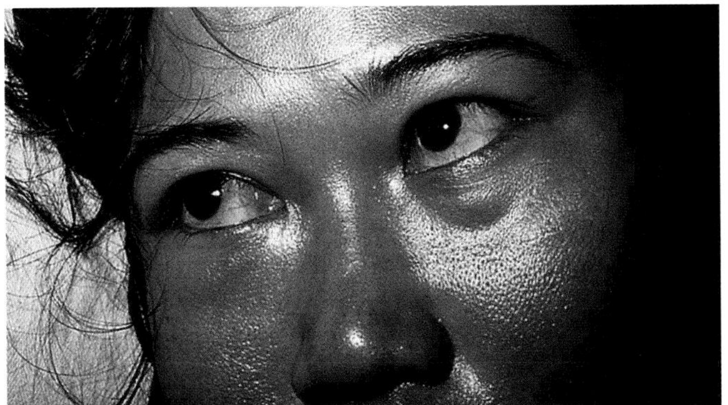

Plate 5 Deep jaundice in a Thai woman with severe falciparum malaria. (Copyright D.A. Warrell.)

Gametocytes		Schizonts		Trophozoites		
Female	Male	Mature	Immature	Old	Young	
						P. falciparum
						P. vivax
						P. malariae
						P. ovale

Plate 7 Malaria parasites developing in erythrocytes (by courtesy of the Wellcome Trust, London).

16.86 Toxoplasmosis

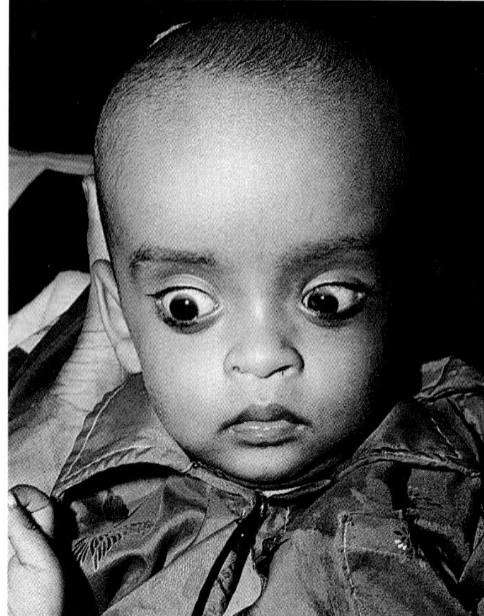

Plate 1 Hydrocephalus complicating congenital toxoplasmosis. (Copyright Professor Viqat Zaman.)

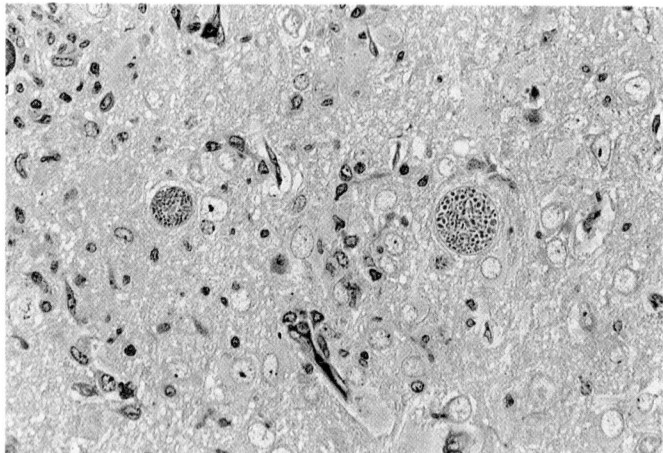

Plate 2 Encysted toxoplasmosis in brain. (Copyright Professor Viqat Zaman.)

16.87 Cryptosporidium and cryptosporidiosis

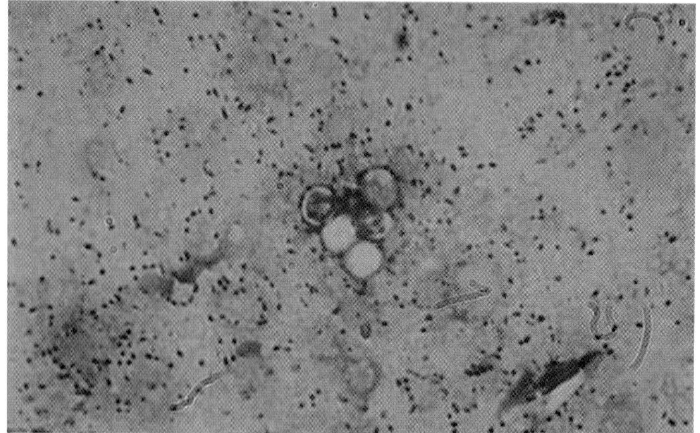

Plate 1 Modified Giemsa-stained faecal smear showing oocysts of *C. parvum*, examined with × 100 oil-immersion objective lens. The uniformity of size (4.5–5 μm) but variability of staining of oocysts can be seen. The eosinophilic nuclei and basophilic bodies of the sporozoites can be clearly seen within the oocysts that have taken up the stain. (Plates 1 to 3 of Chapter 16.87 provided from photographs by A. Curry and D.P. Casemore.)

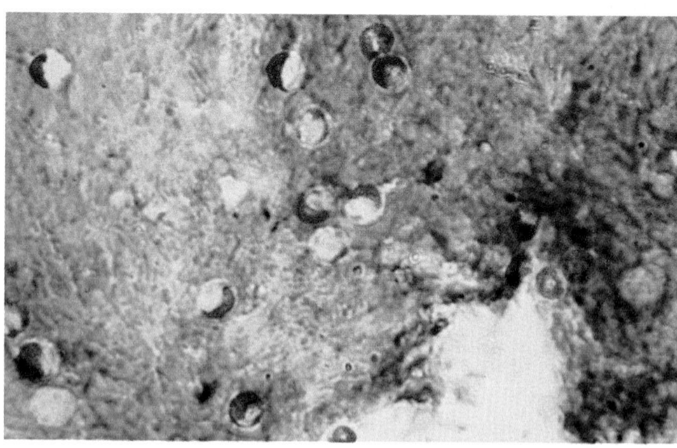

Plate 2 Modified Ziehl–Neelsen-stained faecal smear showing oocysts of *C. parvum* examined with × 100 oil-immersion objective lens. The uniformity of size (4.5–5 μm) but variability os staining of oocysts can be seen.

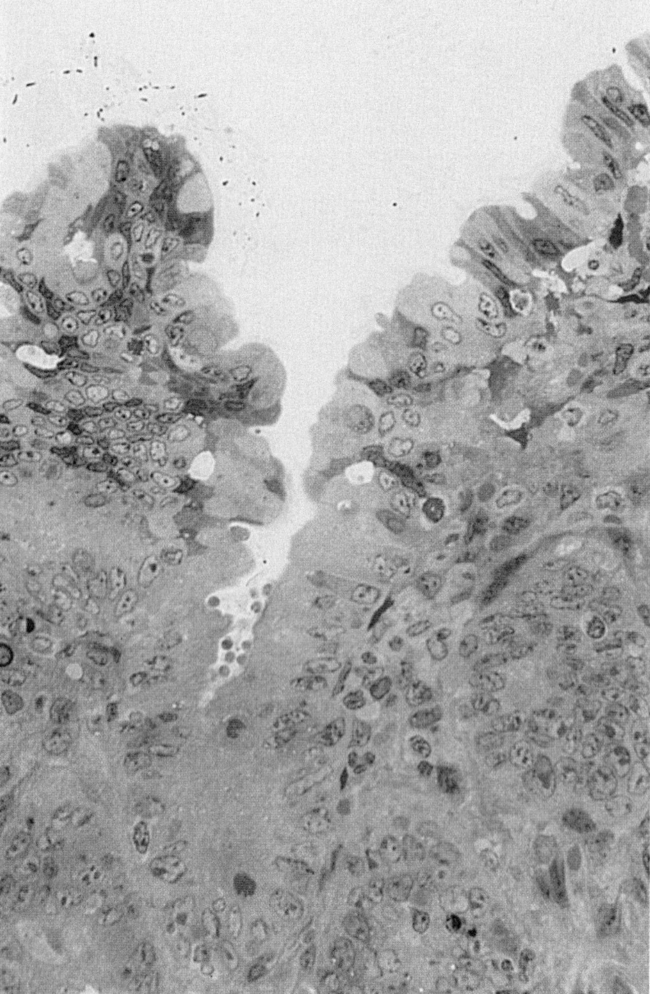

Plate 3 Toluidine blue-stained, semithin section of human rectal biopsy tissue of an AIDS patient with cryptosporidiosis. The apparently pseudo-external location of the parasite can be seen, the true location being intracellular but extracytoplasmic.

16.88 Cyclospora

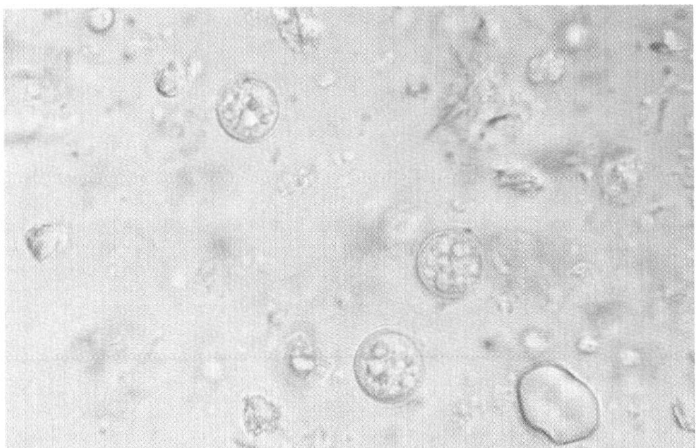

Plate 1 Unstained wet preparation of human faecal material showing oocysts of *Cyclospora* sp., examined with × 100 water-immersion objective lens by phase-contrast microscopy. The uniformity of size (8–10 μm) and the morular (mulberry) internal structure of the oocysts can be seen.

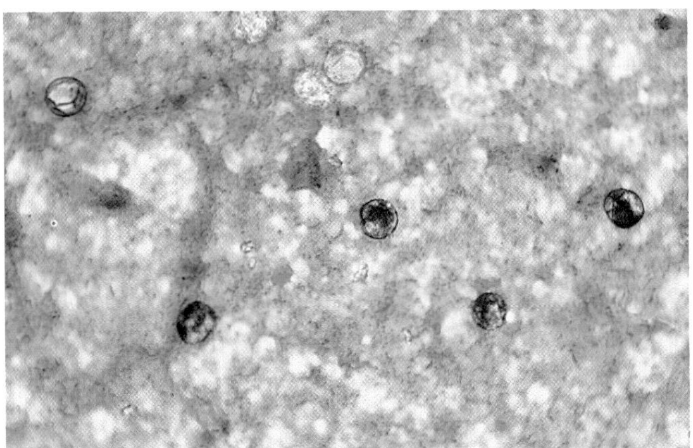

Plate 2 Modified Ziehl–Neelsen-stained faecal smear showing oocysts of *Cyclospora* sp. examined with × 50 oil-immersion objective lens. The uniformity of size (8–10 μm) but variability of staining of the oocysts can be seen. Apart from the greater size, the oocysts can be distinguished from those of *Cryptosporidium parvum* by the different pattern of acid-fast staining. Unstained oocysts within the smear sometimes show the morular structure apparent in wet preparations.

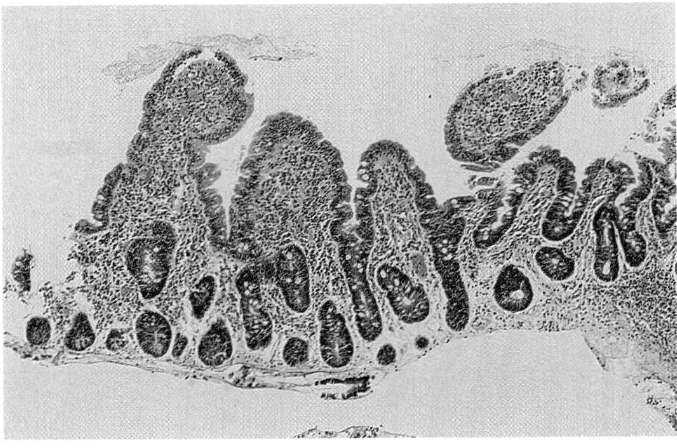

Plate 3 Jejunal biopsy from a patient with cyclosporiasis showing jejunitis with blunting of villi (low power H&E stain). (By courtesy of Dr Sebastian Lucus, London.)

16.95 Trichomoniasis

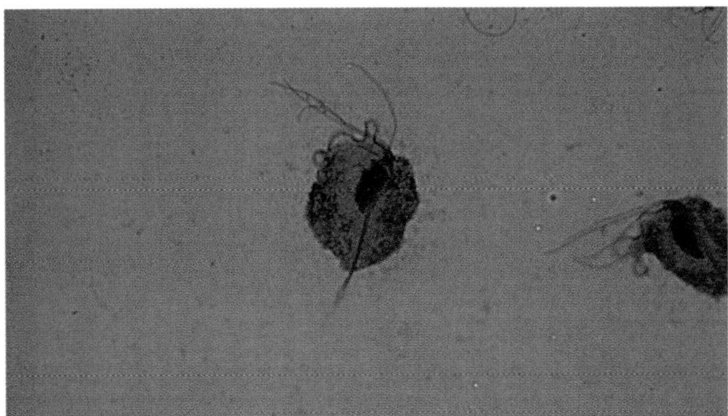

Plate 1 Trichomonads, Giemsa stain, in vaginal secretions. (Copyright J.P. Ackers.)

16.97 Lymphatic filiariasis

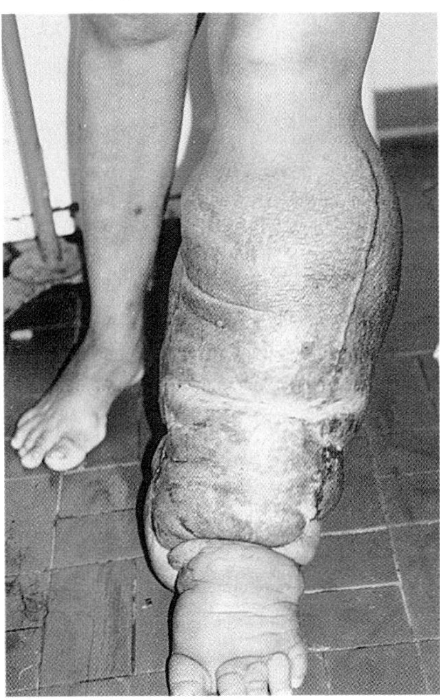

Plate 1 Man from north-eastern Brazil with severe lymphatic oedema (elephantiasis) of the left leg. (Copyright Pedro Pardal.)

16.99 Ancylostomiasis, strongyloidiasis, and other gut strongyloid nematodes

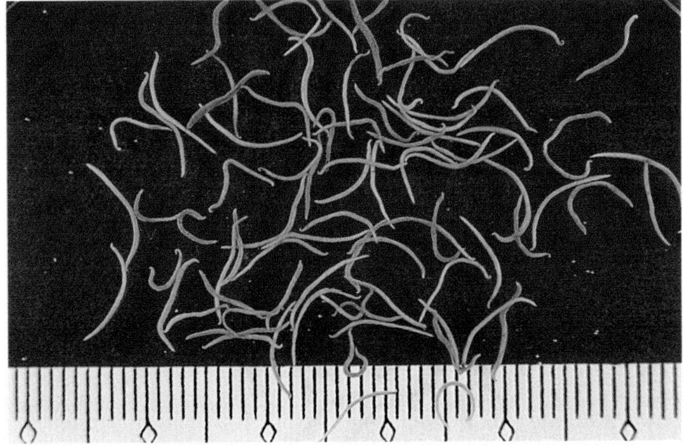

Plate 1 Ancylostoma.

16.101 Other gut nematodes

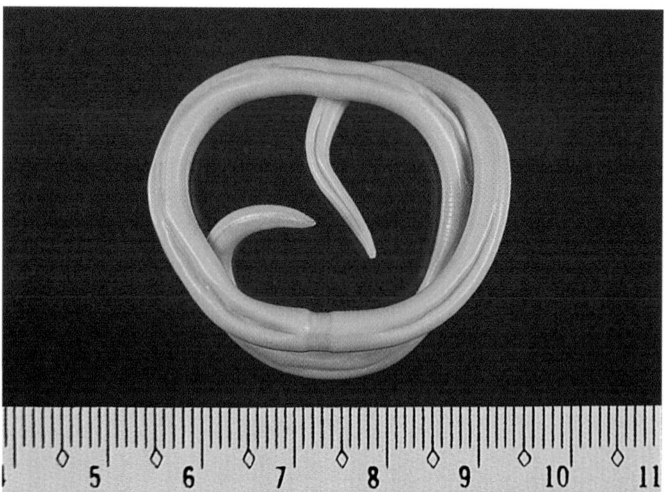

Plate 1 Ascaris.

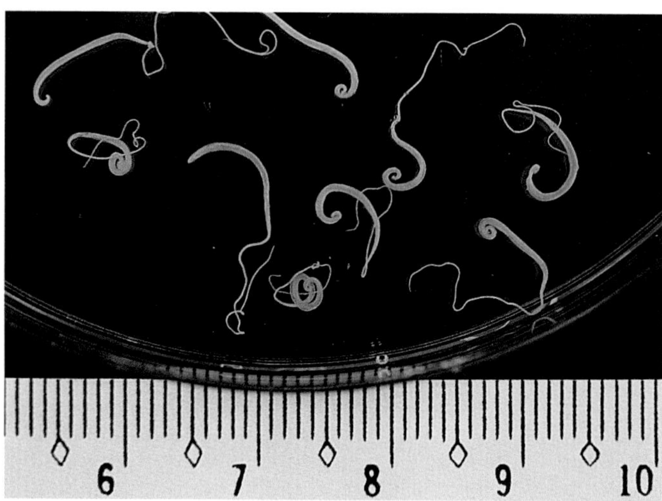

Plate 2 Trichuris.

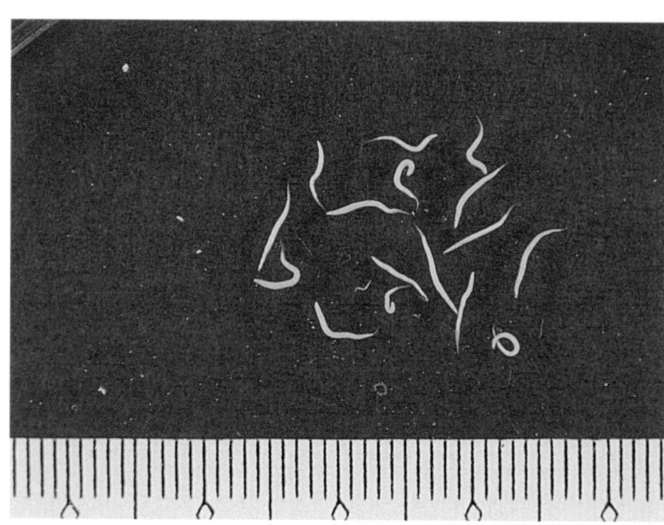

Plate 3 Enterobius.

Plates for Section 18

Chemical and physical injuries and environmental factors and disease

18.2 Injuries, envenoming, poisoning, and allergic reactions caused by animals

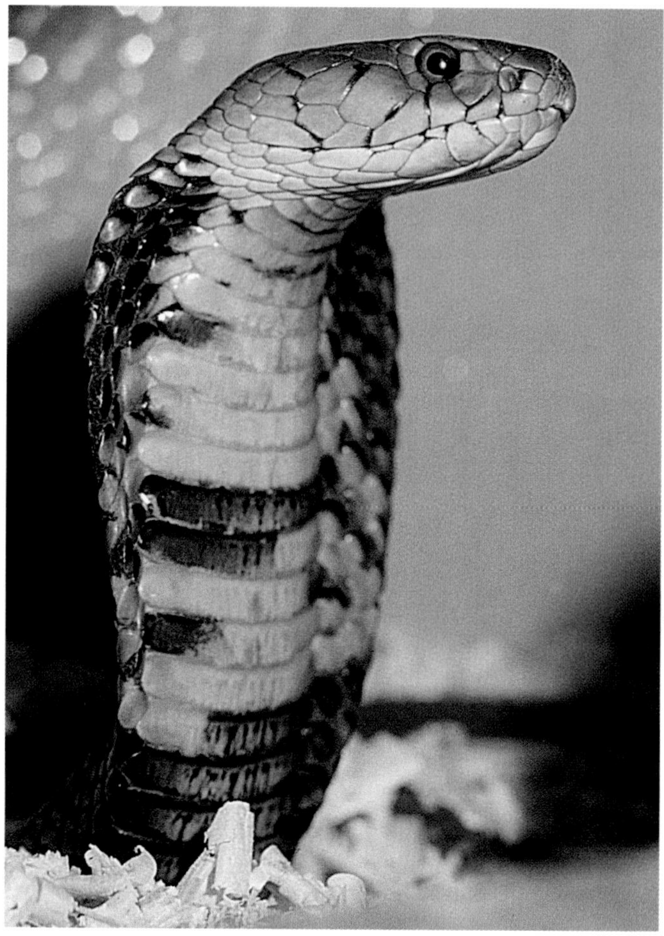

Plate 1 Mozambique spitting cobra (*Naja mossambica*). (Copyright D.A. Warrell.)

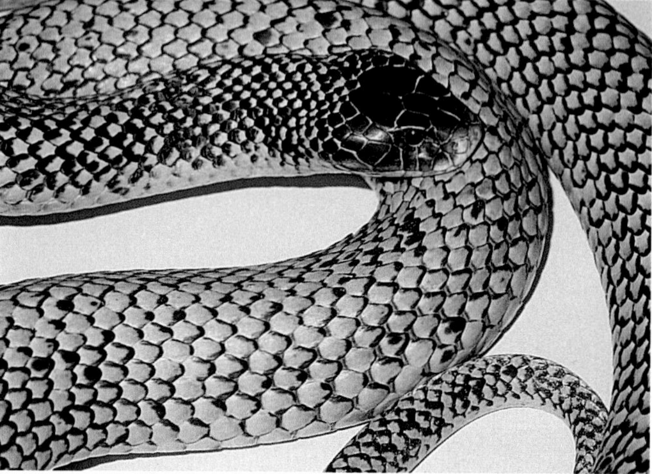

Plate 2 Australasian elapid: king brown or Mulga snake *(Pseudechis australis)*. (Copyright D.A. Warrell.)

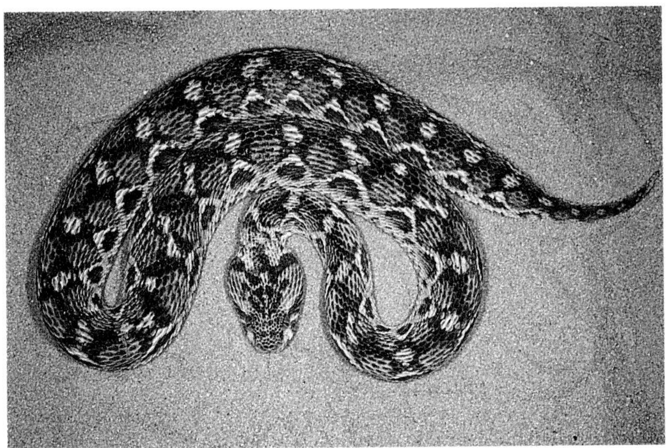

Plate 3 Saw-scaled or carpet viper from Saudi Arabia (*Echis pyramidum*).

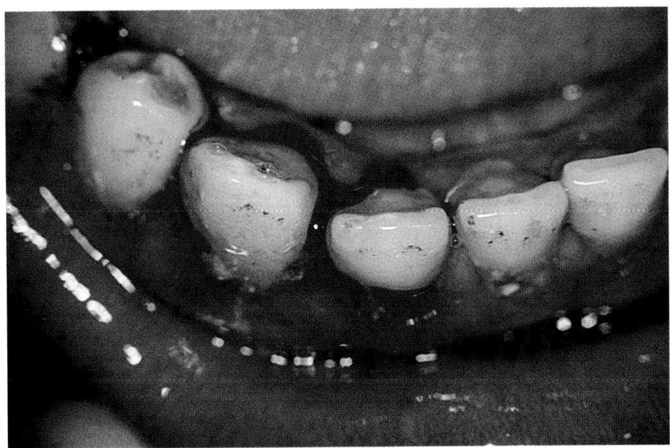

Plate 6 Bleeding from gingival sulci in victim of the West African saw-scaled or carpet viper (*Echis ocellatus*).

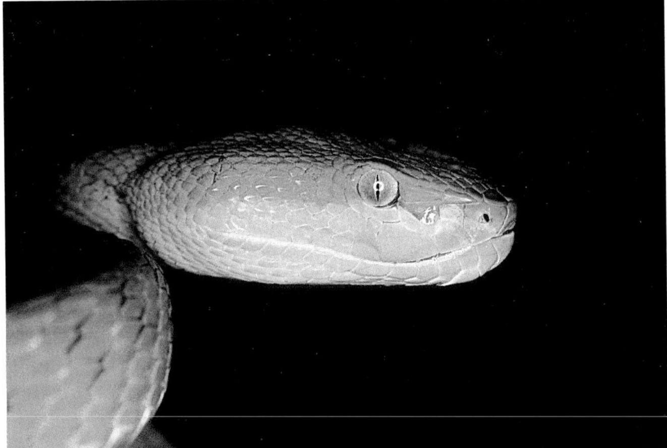

Plate 4 White-lipped pit viper (*Trimeresurus albolabris*) showing heat-sensitive pit between eye and nostril. (Copyright D.A. Warrell.)

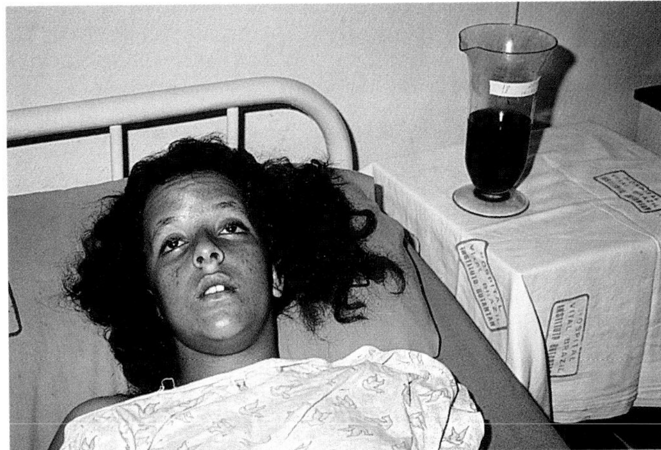

Plate 7 Brazilian girl bitten 24 hours previously by a tropical rattlesnake (*Crotalus durissus terrificus*). She has bilateral ptosis, paralysis of the facial muscles, and gross myoglobinuria resulting from generalized rhabdomyolysis. (Copyright D.A. Warrell.)

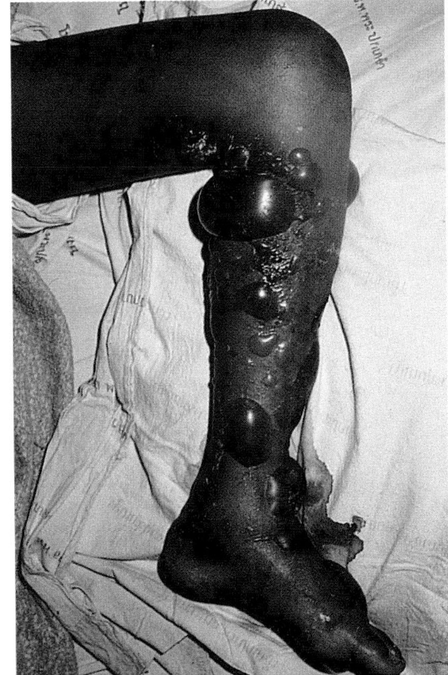

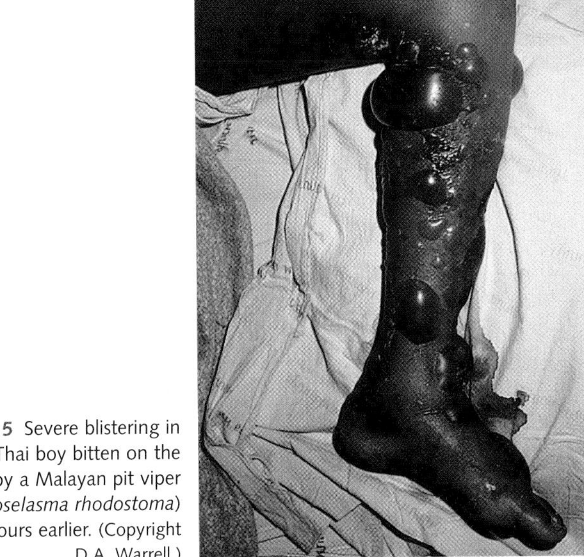

Plate 5 Severe blistering in a Thai boy bitten on the leg by a Malayan pit viper (*Calloselasma rhodostoma*) 48 hours earlier. (Copyright D.A. Warrell.)

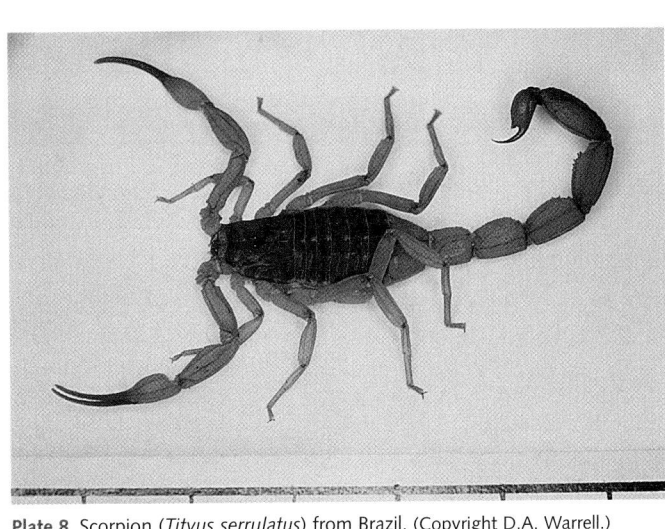

Plate 8 Scorpion (*Tityus serrulatus*) from Brazil. (Copyright D.A. Warrell.)

18.3 Poisonous plants and fungi

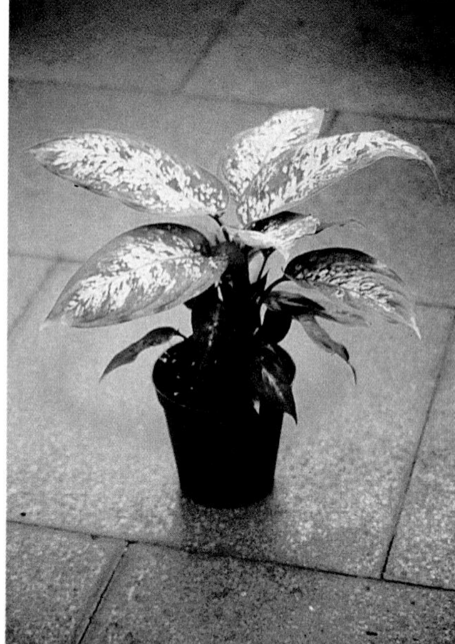
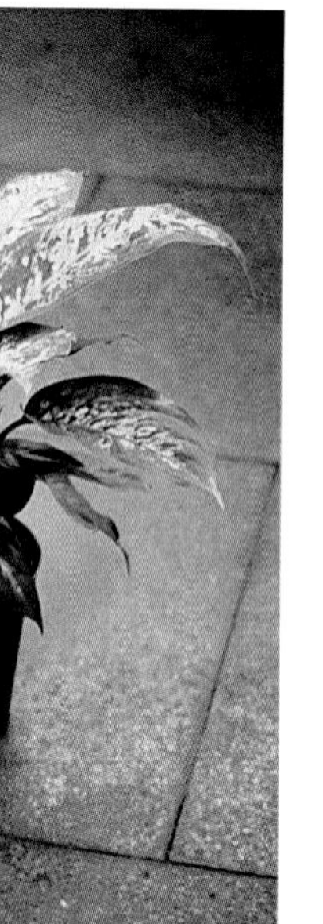

Plate 1 Dumb cane, *Dieffenbachia* sp. (GTC).

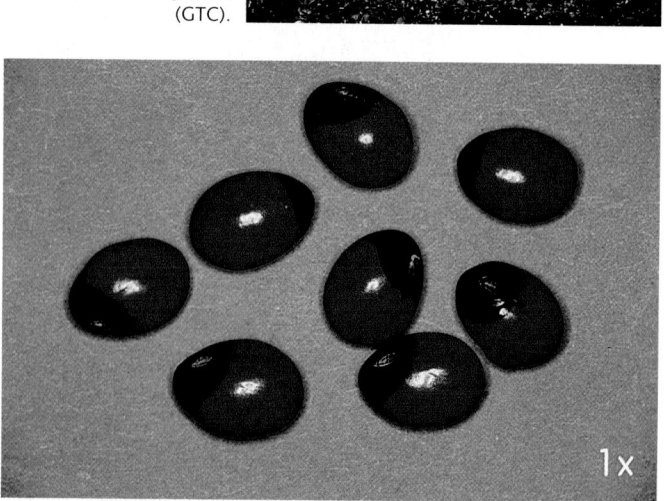

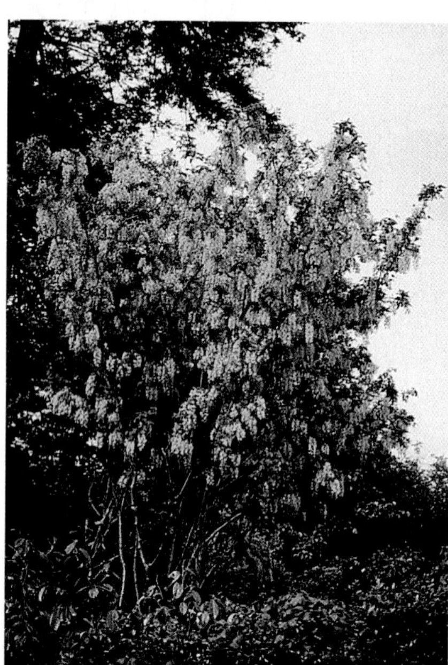
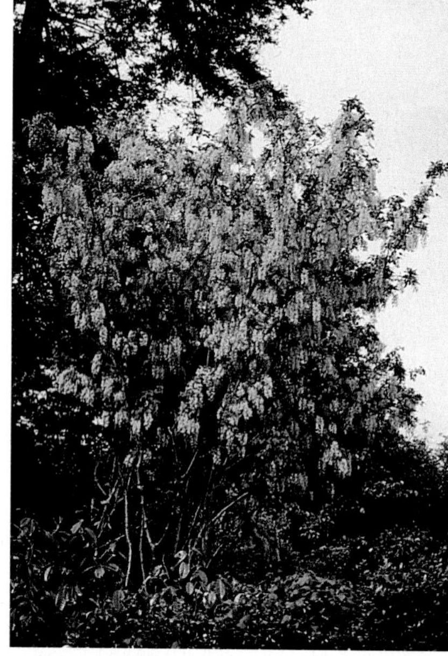

Plate 2 Laburnum, *Laburnum anagroides* (GTC).

Plate 3 Jequirity beans, *Abrus precatorius* (RBG, Kew).

Plate 4 Castor beans, *Ricinus communis* (GTC).

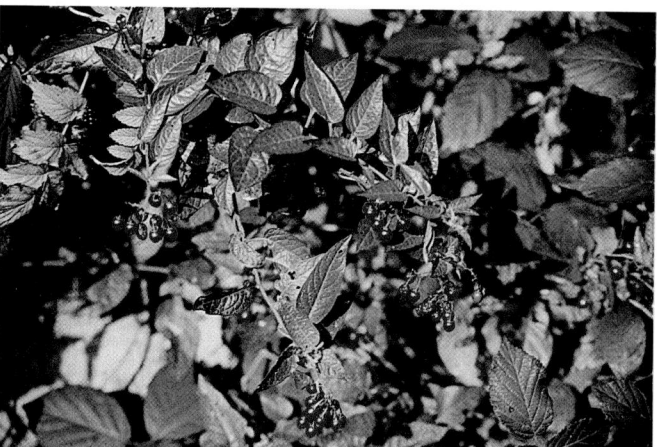

Plate 5 Woody nightshade, *Solanum dulcamara* (GTC).

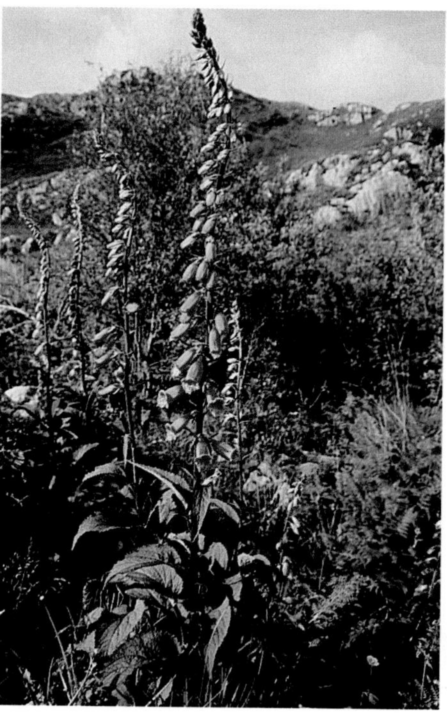

Plate 6 Foxglove, *Digitalis purpurea* (GTC).

Plate 7 Oleander, *Nerium oleander* (GTC).

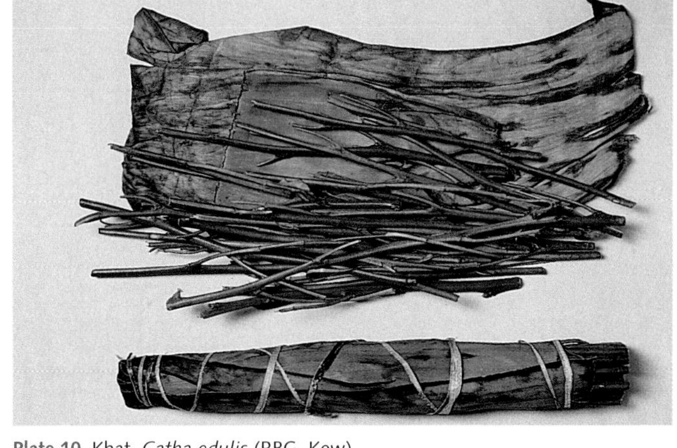

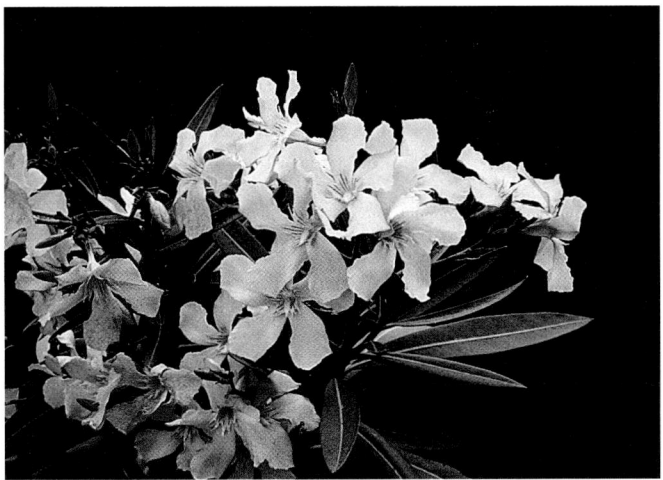

Plate 10 Khat, *Catha edulis* (RBG, Kew).

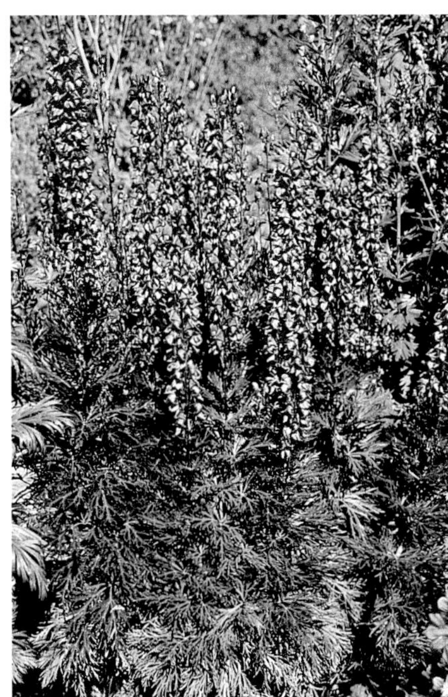

Plate 8 Monkshood, *Aconitum* sp. (GTC).

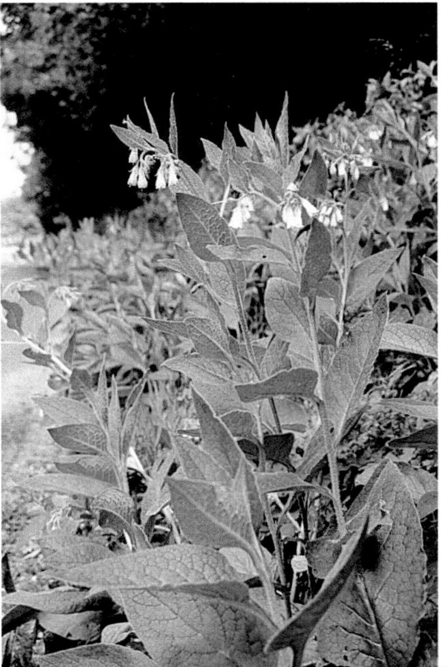

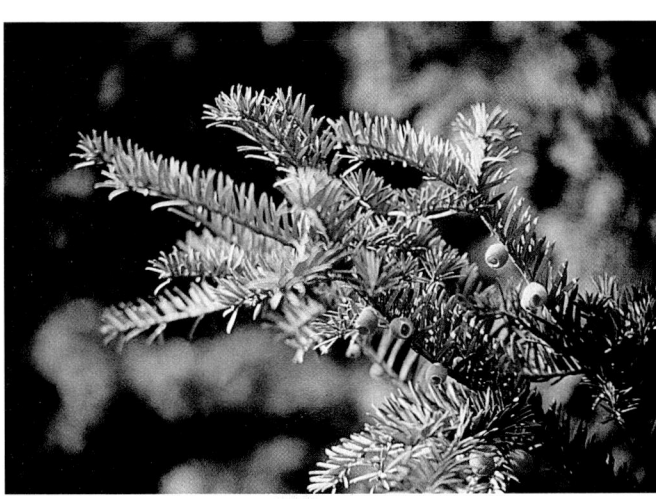

Plate 11 Comfrey, *Symphytum officinale* (GTC).

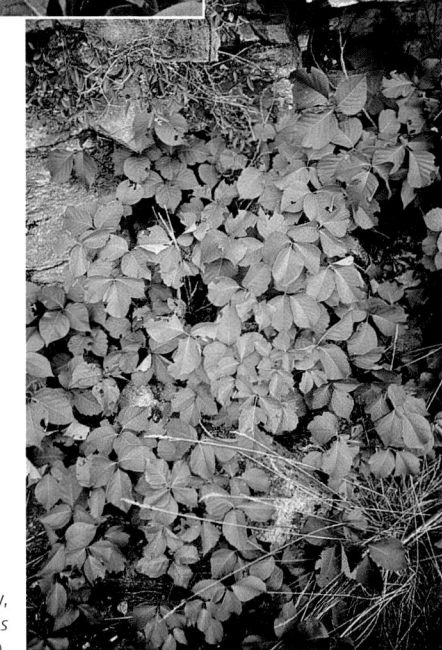

Plate 9 Yew, *Taxus baccata* (GTC).

Plate 12 Poison ivy, *Toxicodendron radicans* (MCC).

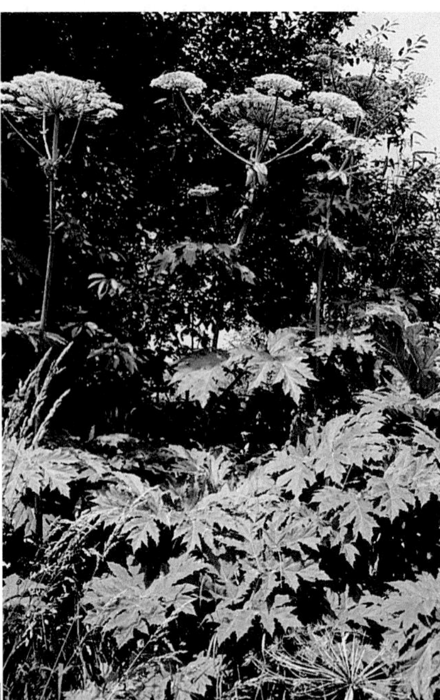

Plate 13 Giant hogweed, *Heracleum mantegazzianum* (GTC).

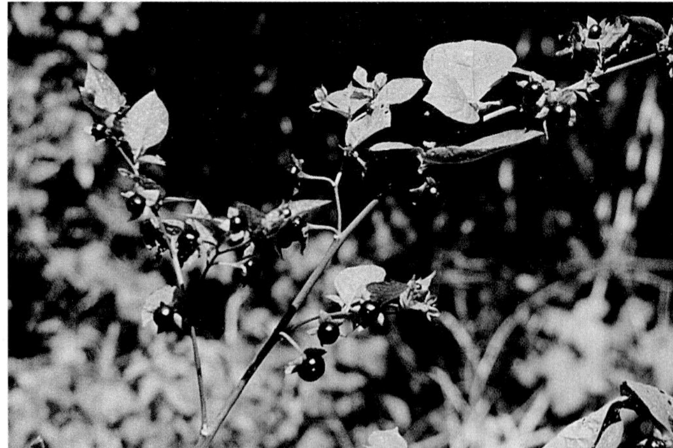

Plate 16 Deadly nightshade, *Atropa belladonna* (GTC).

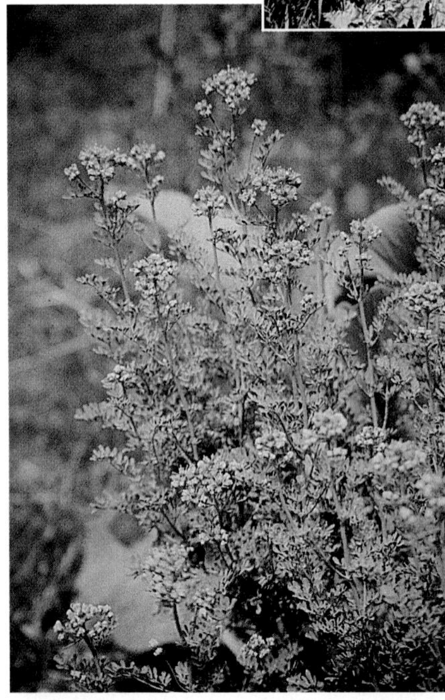

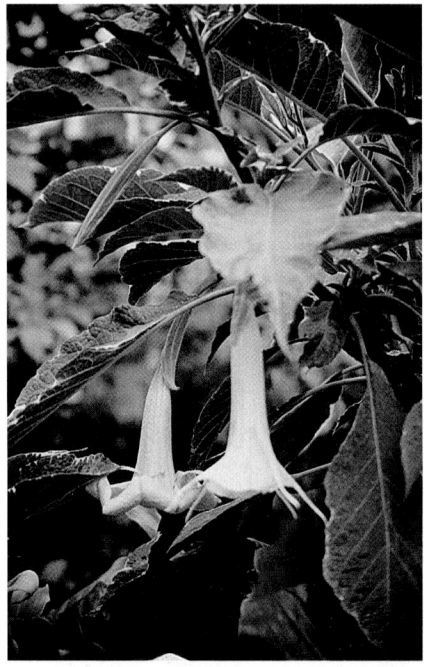

Plate 14 Rue, *Ruta graveolens* (GTC).

Plate 17 Angel's trumpets, *Brugmansia* sp. (GTC)

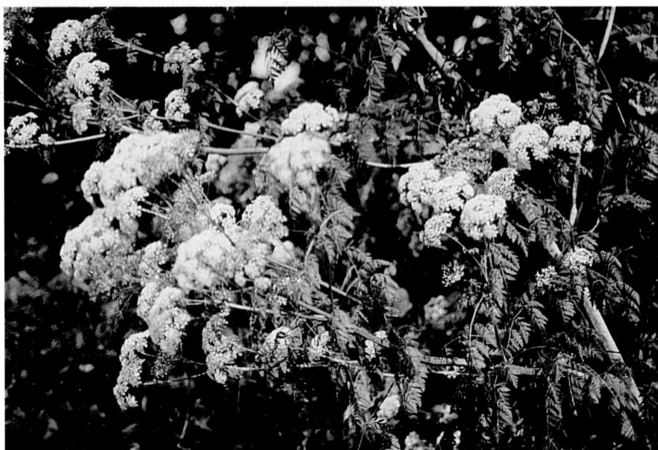

Plate 15 Hemlock, *Conium maculatum* (GTC).

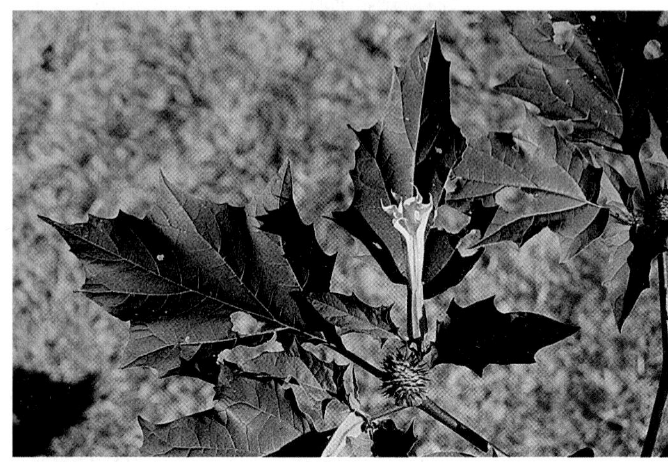

Plate 18 Thorn apple, *Datura stramonium* (GTC).

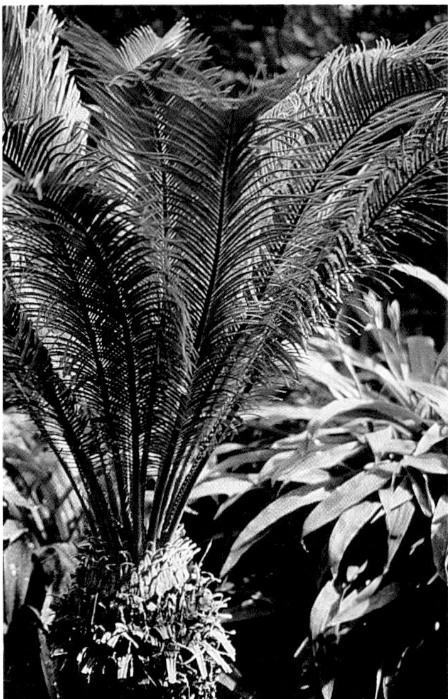
Plate 19 Cycad, *Zamia* sp. (GTC).

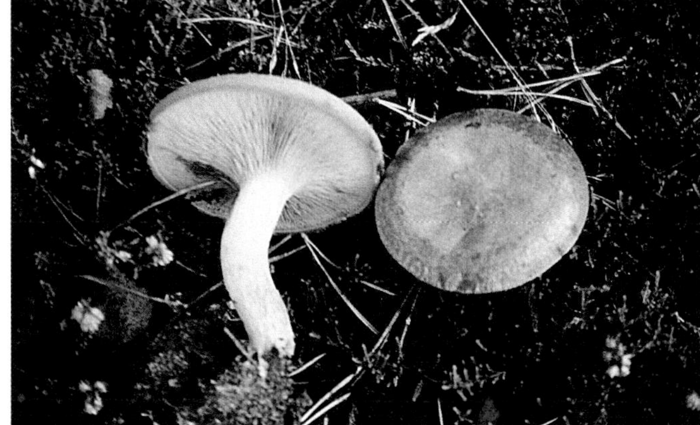
Plate 22 Roll-rim cap, *Paxillus involutus* (GTC).

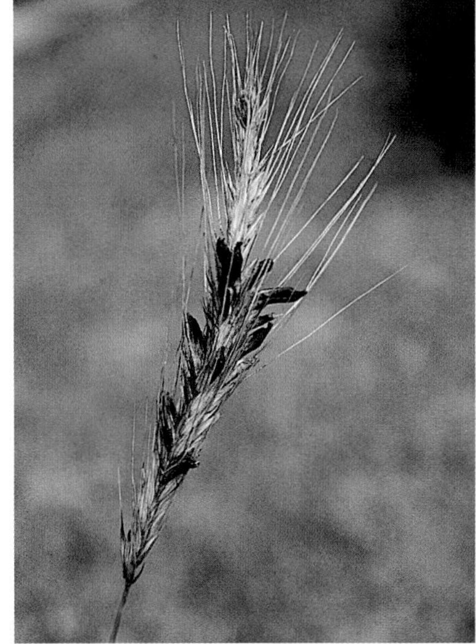
Plate 23 Ergot, *Claviceps purpurea* (JW).

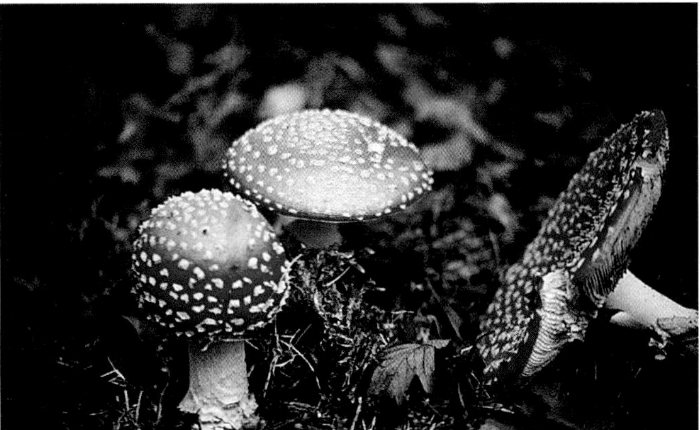
Plate 20 Fly agaric, *Amanita muscaria* (GTC).

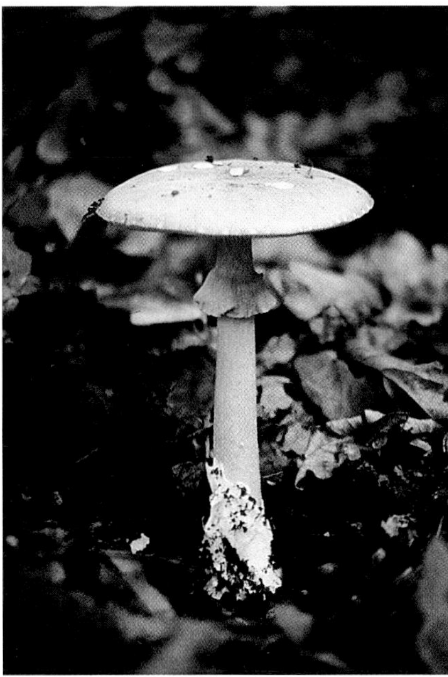
Plate 21 Death cap, *Amanita phalloides* (GTC).

We should like to thank the following for permission to reproduce their photographs: The Trustees, The Royal Botanic Gardens, Kew (RBG, Kew), G.T. Cooper (GTC), M.C. Cooper (MCC), and Professor J. Webster (JW).

Section 1
Pain management

Contents

Section 1

Pain management

J. W. Scadding

It is particularly important that junior doctors, especially house officers (interns) should feel confident about the assessment and management of pain.

Definition

Nociceptive pain is common and arises from damaged tissues, the pain then mediated by an intact nervous system. *Neuropathic* pain, due to damage to the nervous system itself, is less common, and much more difficult to treat, partly because many of its causes are irreversible and partly because its mechanisms are different and less well understood.

The pathophysiology of pain is described in OTM3, pp. 3936–9. Here the account is limited to clinical manifestations and management.

Neuropathic pain

This term embraces all pain due to lesions of the sensory pathways, both peripheral and central. The many causes include damage to peripheral nerves, nerve root and spinal cord lesions, and damage to the thalamic and critical areas in brainstem and cerebral cortex and subcortex. Conditions affecting the primary sensory neurone (including the dorsal root ganglion and dorsal root) are much more common than the central causes.

Deafferentation

The amount of sensory loss with neuropathic pain is variable, even within a single diagnostic category and shows no direct relationship to the severity of the pain. However, the greater the deafferentation the more likely it is that central nervous system mechanisms are important in generating the pain. Secondly, methods of counter-stimulation, such as transcutaneous electrical nerve stimulation (TENS), are less likely to be effective if there is significant deafferentation, and thirdly, any treatment that is likely to increase already severe deafferentation may make the pain worse.

Clinical features of neuropathic pain

The major ones are given in Table 1. A focus of damage in peripheral tissues often cannot be demonstrated. The quality of the pain is outside the patient's previous experience, making it difficult to describe. There are often paroxysmal shooting or shock-like pains in addition to continuous background. Changes in emotional state and fatigue may cause intensity to vary over short periods. The onset of neuropathic pain is often delayed. For example, it is characteristic for thalamic pain to develop at an interval of 2 or 3 months following thalamic infarction, and myelopathic pain may take many months to develop following spinal cord trauma. Neuropathic pain and associated hyperalgesia, allodynia (the perception of pain from a normally non-painful stimulus), and hyperpathia are not necessarily confined to the territory of an affected nerve or root but may radiate widely, indicating secondary central involvement; this can cause diagnostic difficulty.

Table 1 Clinical features of neuropathic pain

Quality of pain: often burning, raw, aching, gnawing
Additional paroxysmal, shock-like pains
Pain associated with some sensory impairment
Associated allodynia, hyperalgesia, and hyperpathia are common
Sympathetic dysfunction is common, particularly with peripheral nerve lesions
Sometimes associated with changes of reflex sympathetic dystrophy
The onset of pain may be immediate or delayed
Pain intensity is often markedly altered by fatigue and emotion

However, there is often a clear anatomical correlation of pain and sensory abnormality, and the presence of sensory loss is particularly helpful in distinguishing neuropathic from nociceptive pain.

Associated abnormalities of local or regional sympathetic activity are common, particularly with peripheral nerve lesions, but may also occur with root, cord, or thalamic lesions. The possible role of abnormal sympathetic outflow in producing or maintaining neuropathic pains, and the therapeutic implications, are discussed below.

Pain in peripheral neuropathy

Pain seems to be related to the acuteness of degenerative change and preferential involvement of small fibres by the underlying disease, particularly when there is also marked regenerative activity in the nerves. In some mononeuropathies there is tenderness at the site of the nerve lesion which is due to local inflammation and structural abnormality in the nerve. This is pain signalled by the nervi nervorum and is thus nociceptive rather than neuropathic in type.

Ischaemia can be shown to provoke pain and paraesthesiae in certain situations, for example carpal tunnel syndrome, and it is likely that ischaemia is a contributory factor in some neuropathies, for example diabetic mononeuropathy and the mononeuropathies associated with connective tissue disease which have a microangiopathic basis.

Abnormal sympathetic activity is important in maintaining causalgia. Sympathetic block may relieve pain and associated allodynia and hyperpathia in patients with causalgia and other types of post-traumatic neuralgia, whether or not there are signs of abnormal sympathetic function in the affected limb.

Some symptoms and signs associated with peripheral nerve injury implicate secondary changes in the central nervous system, particularly in dorsal horn cells and their funtions. These include the almost immediate onset of pain and associated sensory abnormalities in some patients (for example, causalgia following gunshot wounds) which develop before the peripheral abnormalities have had time to develop. Allodynia, hyperpathia, and reflex sympathetic changes may all extend beyond the territory of the affected nerve and indicate central factors.

These secondary central changes may become irreversible so that any therapeutic interventions, particularly peripheral, are bound to have, at best, a limited effect.

Table 2 Causes of reflex sympathetic dystrophy

Peripheral tissues	Peripheral nerve and dorsal root
Soft-tissue injury, including infection	Peripheral nerve trauma
Fasciitis, tendinitis, bursitis, ligamentous strain	Brachial plexus lesions
Fractures and dislocations	Post-herpetic neuralgia
Arthritis	Root lesions, particularly trauma
Deep venous thrombosis	*Central nervous systems*
Arterial thrombosis	Spinal cord lesions, particularly trauma
Immobilization	Head injury
	Cerebral infarction
	Cerebral tumours Idiopathic

Reflex sympathetic dystrophy and causalgia

Clinical features

Reflex sympathetic dystrophy describes a group of conditions, the common features of which include pain, allodynia, hyperpathia, sudomotor and vasomotor changes, and dystrophic changes which may affect both soft tissues and bone, leading to major loss of function in the affected limb. When dystrophic changes are marked, it is sometimes called Sudeck's atrophy. This diagnosis embraces a number of disorders such as algodystrophy, post-traumatic osteoporosis, acute atrophy of bone, and neurovascular dystrophy. There are many causes, but little is known as to why the condition develops in only a tiny minority of patients with the various lesions listed in Table 2. The diagnosis is a clinical one. The condition may be self-limiting and mild, but in some cases it is relentlessly progressive, leading to a painful, very sensitive, useless limb.

Causalgia means burning pain, a term commonly used to describe such pain associated with partial lesions of major limb nerves, when there is nearly always accompanying allodynia, hyperpathia, and vasomotor and sudomotor abnormalities, thus fulfilling the criteria for reflex sympathetic dystrophy.

Pathogenesis

This is uncertain. The often widely radiating allodynia and hyperpathia are mediated by large afferent myelinated fibres and, in many patients, can be temporarily relieved by sympathetic blockade. According to the most popular explanation, the initiating painful cause leads to noxious input to the spinal cord, which, by an unknown mechanism, leads to reflex sympathetic activation via sympathetic, preganglionic neurones in the intermediolateral column of the spinal cord. This increases sympathetic efferent postganglionic activity which, again by some undetermined mechanism, is capable of sensitizing the terminals of undamaged primary afferent fibres in the periphery, lowering their threshold to stimulation, leading to an increased afferent barrage, in this way completing a vicious circle. Sympathetic block would break the vicious circle by removing the peripheral sensitization of primary afferent terminals.

Treatment

Simple analgesia is rarely effective. Strong analgesics, including opiates, often have only marginal effect. Sympathetic block may sometimes dramatically relieve symptoms. If so, a series of blocks combined with physiotherapy may be sufficient gradually to reverse the condition. In refractory cases, prolonged analgesia by epidural local anaesthetic infusions together with physiotherapy may be successful. There have been no adequately controlled trials of any treatment of reflex sympathetic dystrophy, but there are reports of improvement with systemic corticosteroids, NSAIDs, calcitonin, antiepileptic drugs, calcium-channel blockers, and tricyclic antidepressants; in severe cases none of these may be effective.

Requests for amputation by patients should be resisted because of the high risk of the development of phantom limb pain, although there is some evidence that the incidence of stump and phantom pain may be reduced if good analgesia can be produced prior to amputation for 2 or 3 days by spinal block and maintained pre-operatively and for a period postoperatively.

All patients suspected of having or developing reflex sympathetic dystrophy should be urgently referred to a pain clinic since there is evidence that early treatment may prevent the development of severe consequences.

Pain due to central nervous system lesions

The lesions that lead to central neuropathic pain usually involve the spinothalamic tract or its rostral thalamoparietal projection. Within the thalamus, lesions involve the main sensory nuclei, which receive both the medial lemniscal pathway and part of the spinothalamic tract.

There is usually accompanying sensory impairment although loss may be subtle and is often of dissociated spinothalamic type. There is no clear correlation between the severity of the pain and the degree of sensory loss. Pain from *spinal cord lesions* may be localized, unilateral, or bilateral, but is often diffuse and widespread below the level of the lesion. It is sometimes particularly severe in the perineum. The pain is usually continuous and may have an aching, stinging, burning, cramping, or vice-like quality. Superimposed focal or diffuse paroxysmal pains are common. Pain is usually unprovoked but may be exacerbated by movement, fatigue, or emotion.

Vascular lesions in the pons and medulla are the commonest *brainstem lesions* leading to pain. Multiple sclerosis, tumours, syrinx, and tuberculoma are occasional causes.

Thalamic pain is almost always caused by infarction; haemorrhage and arteriovenous malformation are occasional causes and, very rarely, tumours. Therapeutic surgical lesions in the main thalamic sensory nuclei may lead to thalamic pain and the naturally occurring lesions causing pain always produce damage predominantly in these nuclei, with sparing of the medial and posterior nuclei.

Cortical and subcortical lesions leading to pain are extremely rare but vascular lesions, trauma, and tumours are recorded causes. Pain has also been observed after hemispherectomy for severe epilepsy with infantile hemiplegia, or for the treatment of tumour.

Therapeutic considerations

How the many pathophysiological changes to central nervous system damage interact is uncertain, but the multiplicity of possible abnormalities may help explain the great variations between patients in the development of pain with either peripheral or central nervous system lesions. Neuroablative treatments advocated in the past have been unsuccessful and emphasis has now moved towards stimulation procedures.

Psychological aspects of pain

Psychological factors are often of great importance in chronic pain. Individual responses to pain vary enormously for many reasons, including importantly personality, domestic and employment considerations, cultural influences, and all too often the problem of secondary gain from medical attention or medicolegal considerations.

Psychiatric factors and chronic pain

Depression is common in patients with chronic pain and may be an aggressive or even causative factor. Pain is a common symptom too in patients who present with numerous somatic symptoms associated with unshakeable conviction that they have a serious disease (somatization disorder). Others may be frankly hypochondriacal. Psychogenic pain may be one manifestation of a number of underlying problems. Clinicians in pain clinics see many such patients whose management may need the help of a psychiatrist.

Multidisciplinary pain clinics best comprise an anaesthetist, physiotherapist, occupational therapist, and psychologist, but the availability of others, particularly a neurologist and a psychiatrist, is important.

Local measures

Counterstimulation

Regardless of the type of pain, whether nociceptive or neuropathic, counterstimulation techniques may be helpful. These simple and effective methods are all too often neglected in favour of systemic drug treatment.

Some musculoskeletal pains respond to heat, delivered by a heat pad or radiant heat. Neuropathic pains tend to be exacerbated by cold but an exception is post-herpetic neuralgia in which regular application of cold packs for 20 minutes may reduce troublesome allodynia for up to several hours.

Both nociceptive and neuropathic pains may respond to vibration and ultrasound, of which vibration is the more practical long term since it can be used regularly by the patient at home.

Transcutaneous electrical stimulation (TENS), acting by segmental inhibition, has been shown to be effective in a wide range of different chronic pains, but is probably more effective for neuropathic than nociceptive pains. A trial period of 2–3 weeks, with the patient experimenting with different electrode placements, is essential before concluding that TENS is unhelpful.

Acupuncture probably works by segmental inhibition and by diffuse noxious inhibitory control. Cerebrospinal fluid endorphin levels are raised by acupuncture but not by TENS, and TENS-induced analgesia is not reversed by naloxone.

Simple lignocaine ointment, although poorly absorbed, is sometimes helpful in areas of severe allodynia and hyperpathia, particularly in patients with painful scar syndromes, tender amputation stumps, and post-herpetic neuralgia. Local capsaicin (0.075 per cent) may also be effective in these situations.

Local anaesthetic blocks to peripheral tissues, peripheral nerves, or roots may be useful in three ways. First, the origin of a particular pain may be more accurately defined. Secondly, injection into a peripheral trigger point, for example in muscle, may reduce widely radiating pain and offer effective treatment with one or a series of injections; and thirdly, in the case of neuropathic pain due to peripheral nerve or root lesions, failure to relieve all the pain with an adequate peripheral nerve or root block indicates an element of secondary central pain, which will be less amenable to peripheral measures. There is some evidence that lesions including trigger points in muscle, painful scars, and peripheral nerve lesions such as neuromas may respond better to a combination of local anaesthetic and corticosteroid.

Epidural injection of a local anaesthetic, with or without an opiate, can produce analgesia over a wide area. In relief of chronic pain, single or repeated epidural injections may have a partial, lasting effect in some patients. The use of highly lipid-soluble opiates such as fentanyl ensures rapid local absorption into neural tissue in the region, producing good analgesia, with less risk of drug spread. Low back pain with root pain not amenable to surgery, arachnoiditis, and brachalgia with neck pain may respond well to such treatment.

A further treatment of pain of non-malignant origin is the epidural infusion of a local anaesthetic and an opiate over periods of 2–3 weeks. In some patients this may produce a degree of long-lasting or even permanent pain relief.

A variable degree of motor block is produced by epidural analgesia, together with loss of bladder and bowel control, although it is usually possible to titrate the amount of drug used to produce localized unilateral sensory blockade which causes minimal motor deficit and spares sphincter function. Epidural or intrathecal infusion of opiate over long periods has proved useful in the management of pelvic pain due to cancer.

Injection of very low concentrations of morphine into the third ventricle may produce profound analgesia, associated with a low risk of respiratory depression. This procedure has been advocated for the relief of bilateral pain due to cancer affecting the neck and skull base.

Sympathetic blocks

Intravenous injection of phentolamine has some value in indicating which patients have sympathetically maintained pain and in predicting the response to other types of sympathetic block, either local anaesthetic block of cervical and lumbar sympathetic ganglia or intravenous regional guanethidine block. For sympathetically maintained pain associated with peripheral nerve lesions, there is sometimes a cumulative analgesic effect from a series of such blocks. The results of permanent sympathectomy, produced either surgically or chemically with phenol, are often disappointing. For these reasons, repeated temporary sympathetic blocks are preferable.

Systemic drugs (for further details see Section 15)

Analgesics are the mainstay of drug treatment. They should be given regularly, if possible by mouth. Paracetamol, aspirin, NSAIDs, weak opiates (e.g. codeine, dihydrocodeine, dextropropoxyphene) partial opiate agents (e.g. buprenophine) mixed agonist/antagonist drugs (e.g. pentazocrine) and strong opiates may be very efficacious in nociceptive pain, but less so for those of neuropathic origin. In pain due to cancer recourse to opiates is often necessary.

Psychotropic drugs: antidepressants, minor tranquillizers, and neuroleptic drugs

In addition to true antidepressive effects which may be useful, tricyclic agents enhance the bulbospinal 5-HT mediated analgesic pathway to the dorsal horn. An analgesic effect of amitriptyline has been shown in some neuropathic pains, notably post-herpetic neuralgia, but zimoldine, which has greater serotoninergic effect than amitriptyline, is less effective, and the newer, serotonin re-uptake inhibitor drugs have not been shown to be superior to amitriptyline in their analgesic effect.

Benzodiazepines may be helpful for short-term relief of anxiety and of muscle spasm, but sedation, dysphoria, dependence, and severe withdrawal effects in some patients limit their use.

Neuroleptic drugs have often been advocated for the treatment of neuropathic pains but, in the absence of clear evidence of useful effect in controlled studies, these drugs are best avoided. An exception is chlorprothixene, which is occasionally helpful in a variety of neuropathic pains and which does not produce extrapyramidal effects at the doses used (up to 45 mg/day).

Antiepileptic drugs have no effect in nociceptive pains. With the exception of the specific effect of carbamazepine in trigeminal neuralgia, antiepileptic drugs are also disappointingly ineffective in neuropathic pains. Although claims have been made for carbamazepine, phenytoin, valproate, and clonazepam in a variety of neuropathic pains, positive results have only emerged from poorly controlled short-term trials.

Membrane-stabilizing drugs

Intravenous infusions of lignocaine at doses as small as 1 mg/kg have been shown to reduce neuropathic pain and associated allodynia and hyperpathia, but this is not a practical long-term treatment. Mexiletine, which can be taken orally has been shown to have a short-term analgesic effect in painful diabetic peripheral neuropathy, but long-term treatment in this and other neuropathies has no demonstrable analgesic effect.

Role of surgery in the treatment of chronic pain

The indications for surgical treatment for chronic pain are now few. A variety of approaches have limited application. These include peripheral neurolysis, rhizotomy, specific lesions to the dorsal root-entry zone, antrolateral cordotomy, thalamotomy, or even leucotomy. These and techniques of stimulation in the central nervous system are described in OTM3, pp. 3945–6.

Rehabilitation

The importance of rehabilitation for patients with chronic pain cannot be overemphasized. For many, their pain has been the major focus of their lives for long periods and the effects far reaching in terms of limitation of work and other activities and impact on personal relationships. Detailed discussion of rehabilitation is beyond the scope of this chapter, but one point is worth emphasizing. When any pain-relieving procedure, however temporary, is successful, it is essential that the use of the affected painful part begins immediately. Thus, with sensory or sympathetic blocks, the physiotherapist should be present to start passive and active movements straight away. Analgesia alone is insufficient to regain function and unless strenuous immediate efforts are made, rehabilitation is likely to fail.

Further reading

Wall, P.D. and Melzack, R. (eds). (1994). *Textbook of pain* (3rd edn). Churchill Livingstone, Edinburgh.

Section 2
Cardiology

Contents

Symptoms of heart disease

Chapter 2.1

Syncope and palpitation

R. Sutton

Chest pain in ischaemic heart disease and the breathlessness and oedema of heart failure are dealt with in later chapters, but syncope and palpitation are also common and important problems.

Syncope

There are many causes of syncope; those due to cardiovascular diseases are shown in Table 1 and those of neuroendocrine origin in Table 2. There are many other causes of repeated episodic events, often described by the patient as 'blackouts'. The history is vital here and, apart from epilepsy, an important diagnosis to consider is hyperventilation in Da Costa's syndrome comprising the triad or left submammary stabbing pain, palpitation, and worrying awareness of breathing.

Electrical disturbances of cardiac function cause syncope either by reduction of the mechanical efficiency of the heart, or by complete interruption of cardiac activity due to asystole complicating atrioventricular block. Ventricular tachyarrhythmia, most commonly seen in coronary heart disease, can also cause syncope. Technical faults in pacing systems can result in asystole, due to sudden complete lack of pacing or, occasionally, very rapid pacing may occur. Inappropriate choice of pacing mode, mostly ventricular, may be associated with retrograde conduction to the atria causing them to contract during ventricular systole with regurgitation of blood into pulmonary veins. This has the effect of ventricular under filling and resultant low cardiac output known as pacemaker syndrome.

The neuroendocrine causes of syncope largely comprise cardioinhibition and vasodepression. Vasovagal syncope is the most frequent and in many ways the best understood. Upright posture is an almost invariable feature, leading critically to the pooling of 500–1000 ml of blood in the lower limbs and to reduction in central blood volume. Susceptible people show higher than normal plasma concentrations of adrenaline and vasopressin prior to the attack. These cause vigorous left ventricular contraction and sensitization of left ventricular baroreceptors, respectively. Reduced cardiac filling on standing then triggers the sensitized baroreceptors to manifest a reflex that is appropriate in left ventricular dilatation—bradycardia and vasodilatation. In the context of low central blood volume this reflex is disastrous for the maintenance of blood pressure. In addition to the increased sensitivity of left ventricular baroreceptors, there is some evidence in sufferers of recurrent vasovagal attacks of an abnormal positive gain in the reflex at brainstem level. In the autonomic neuropathies the mechanism is different and results from a failure of the normal adaptations to the erect posture.

Table 1 Cardiovascular causes of recurrent syncope

Cardiac—electrical	Vascular
• Tachyarrythmias	• Dissection of the aorta
• supraventricular tachycardias	• Takayasu's disease
• ventricular tachyarrhythmias	• Carotid stenosis
• Bradyarrhythmias	• Vertebrobasilar disease
• sinoatrial node disease	• Subclavian steel
• atrioventricular block	• Pulmonary embolism
• Pacemaker malfunction	• Pulmonary hypertension
• technical faults	• Migraine
• pacemaker syndrome	• Transient ischaemic attack
Cardiac—structural	
• Aortic stenosis	
• Hypertrophic cardiomyopathy	
• Pulmonary stenosis, including	
• tetralogy of Fallot	
• Myocardial infarction	
• Obstruction of a prosthetic valve	
• Atrial ball thrombus	
• Cardiac tumour	
• Cardiac tamponade	

Table 2 Neuroendocrine causes of syncope

• Carotid sinus syndrome	• Other central nervous diseases, e.g. Shy–Drager syndrome
• Vasovagal syndrome	• Drug-induced
• Glossopharyngeal syndrome	• α-adrenoceptor blockade
• Cough	• methyldopa and levodopa
• Micturition	• tricyclic antidepressants
• Defecation	• thiazide diuretics
• Deglutition	• phenothiazines
• Postural or orthostatic	• benzodiazepines
• hypotension	
• Autonomic neuropathies	
• Diabetes mellitus	
• Alcohol	
• Idiopathic	
• Prolonged bed rest	
• Sympathectomy	

Presentation

True syncope is of sudden onset and brief duration, typically lasting less than 1 min. When it has been caused by structural cardiac or vascular causes, other symptoms may emerge; for instance in obstructive cardiac disease (classically aortic stenosis) it tends to occur on exertion. When the cause is a bradyarrhythmia, and in some of the neuroendocrine disturbances, sudden loss of consciousness tends to be devoid of warning, whereas, syncope due to tachyarrythmia is often heralded by palpitation and the vasovagal syndrome typically is preceded by tiredness, yawning, air hunger, boredom, nausea, and occasionally palpitation, which lead to dizziness and a rather gradual greying into syncope. Only a minority of vasovagal sufferers, usually older patients, give no history of prodrome.

Observers report striking pallor in syncope and often wonder if the patient is dead. Cyanosis supervenes in the second half of the first minute. There may be epileptiform movements and incontinence of urine (but rarely faeces). Recovery from cardiac causes is associated with a bright flush; episodes that are due to neuroendocrine causes do not end with a flush because of the longer time course of vasodepression.

Sequelae of syncope

Syncopal attacks may result in injury. They are also occasionally followed by a transient neurological defect which may lead to diagnosis of a transient ischaemic attack but unconsciousness is rarely associated

Table 3 Differential diagnosis of syncope

	Syncope	Epilepsy
Warning	Cardiac minimal or none rushing noise in head falling backwards Vasovagal definite prodrome	Minimal typical prodrome
Colour changes	Cardiac White, blue, red Vasovagal White, blue, white	Red, blue
Timing of convulsion and incontinence	After 30 s	Before 30 s
Injury	Trauma on falling	Trauma on falling plus that self-inflicted
Recovery	Usually rapid	Slow
Pre-ictal amnesia	None	Present
Physical examination	No pulse	Pulse present

with transient ischaemic attacks. The cause of neurological sequelae may be either systemic embolism from the left atrium in sinoatrial node disease or focal cerebrovascular disease giving a more persistent and severe perfusion defect than that experienced by the brain overall.

Incidence and mortality

It has been estimated that as many as 30 per cent of the population experience at least one episode in a lifetime and perhaps every individual is capable of fainting given unfavourable circumstances. More than 1 per cent of all emergency room attendance is reported to have been for syncope. The most common cause of these is vasovagal syncope, but in some 50 per cent of cases the cause remains undiagnosed. Unexplained syncope carries a much better prognosis for survival than cardiac syncope; one series has given the respective mortalities as 6 versus 30 per cent. Recurrent syncope, despite investigation and treatment of a probable cause, seems to carry an appreciable mortality and justifies detailed investigation including tilt testing and cardiac electrophysiological studies with ventricular extrastimulation to reveal a tendency to ventricular tachyarrhythmias.

Differential diagnosis

A challenge to the clinician is separation of syncope and epilepsy (Table 3). The value of the history from patient and observer cannot be overstated. The type or lack of warning, the sequence and timing of colour changes, the timing of convulsions and incontinence, the type of injury, the speed of recovery and the existence of pre-ictal amnesia are most important.

Palpitation

When palpitation is severe or frequent enough for medical consultation, careful analysis of the patient's description can often reveal the type of arrhythmia underlying the symptoms. Extrasystoles, often reported as missed beats, typically have a compensatory pause and potentiation of the post-pause beat. Such extrasystoles are usually of no pathological significance but cause worry, which is likely then to be self-propagating, because anxiety is the most prominent cause of awareness of perhaps long-standing and previously asymptomatic extrasystoles. The history should include questions about alcohol consumption, caffeine, nicotine, and other drugs, as all of these agents favour extrasystolic activity.

Tachyarrhythmias will be given different descriptions by the patient and it is usually possible to ascertain whether the arrhythmia is regular or irregular and approximately how fast. Symptoms of impending or actual syncope are often features associated with palpitation and, in general, the most important rhythm disturbances are those associated with dizziness and syncope. The clinician will also want to know about onset and its timing, duration and mode of termination, including the effect on the attack of any spontaneous Valsalva-type manoeuvres, for example, vomiting. The other symptoms which coincide with arrhythmias are also of importance: dyspnoea, sweating, chest pain, polyuria. Polyuria tends to occur only in arrhythmias where atrial and ventricular systole are simultaneous, resulting in atrial wall stretch and release of large quantities of atrial natriuretic peptide.

Palpitation may also accompany bradyarrhythmias, with symptoms resembling those of missed beats. Unpleasant awareness of the heart beat may also be experienced in relation to its forcefulness, for instance with impending vasovagal syncope, in the postprandial state, and in hypertrophic cardiomyopathy.

Da Costa's syndrome (effort syndrome, soldiers heart, cardiac neurosis) most commonly reflects anxiety about the heart. It responds well to confident diagnosis and firm reassurance without more than a minimum of investigation.

Because palpitation is such a ubiquitous symptom it does not lend itself to the detailed and exhaustive descriptions of all its associations. The management of both syncope and palpitation is discussed in other sections of the book in the context of the underlying associated conditions.

Further reading

Kapoor, W.N., Karpf, M., Maher, Y., *et al.* (1982). Syncope of unknown origin: the need for a more cost-effective approach to its diagnostic evaluation. *Journal of the American Medical Association*, **247**, 2687.

Kenny, R.A., Ingram, A., Bayliss, J., and Sutton, R. (1986). Head-up tilt; a useful test for investigating unexplained syncope. *Lancet*, **i**, 1352–5.

Wayne, H.H. (1961). Syncope: physiological considerations and an analysis of the clinical characteristics in 510 patients. *American Journal of Medicine*, **30**, 418.

Chapter 2.2

The syndrome of heart failure

A. J. S. Coats and P. A. Poole-Wilson with contributions from J. G. G. Ledingham, D. A. Chamberlain, J. H. Dargie, and J. C. Forfar

Definitions

'Heart failure' is an unfortunate term. It has negative connotations for the patient and describes imprecisely several different clinical situations. Left and right heart failure are quite distinct clinical syndromes, although they frequently coexist. Subdivisions into forward, backward, and high output failure have not proved to be particularly useful. A more useful classification is dependent on the predominant pattern of left ventricular dysfunction, be it systolic, diastolic, or mixed. Whatever the complexities of the ventricular pathophysiology, a well-recognized clinical pattern is identifiable as 'heart failure', one which has proved a useful description of a complex syndrome for many years.

The pertinent features of any definition of heart failure are that the clinical picture is: (1) initiated by a reduction in effective cardiovascular (usually left ventricular) functional reserve; (2) associated with symptoms either at rest or at an unexpectedly low level of exertion; and (3) associated with characteristic pathophysiological changes in many disparate organ systems. In simple terms heart failure is a syndrome in which a reduction in left ventricular function causes pathophysiology which produces symptoms and exercise limitation.

A clinical picture similar to that of heart failure can develop when ventricular function is normal. These include volume overload conditions such as endotoxic high-output shock, severe anaemia, arteriovenous fistulae or shunts, and pressure overload conditions such as acute hypertensive crisis or prosthetic heart valve occlusion. Acute, chronic, or acute on chronic are also useful subdivisions. The acute syndrome usually presents dramatically with dyspnoea, tachycardia, pulmonary or peripheral oedema and underperfusion of systemic organs. Exercise intolerance is the prominent feature of chronic failure, and when it is severe there may also be chronic pulmonary and peripheral oedema with breathlessness at rest. Acute exacerbations are then common.

Epidemiology

Heart failure is common with an estimated incidence of 20–30 per 1000 per year and a prevalence overall of about 1 per cent. The prevalence increases with age, reaching 30 per cent in the over-80 year olds. Paradoxically, improvements in the management of acute myocardial infarction and chronic heart disease has led to more heart failure, as more people survive to develop it later in life.

Aetiologies

In Western societies the most common causes are ischaemic heart disease, hypertension, and idiopathic dilated cardiomyopathy. Some hypertensives may develop a dilated poorly functioning heart with an eventual normalization in arterial pressure; such cases may be diagnosed as idiopathic dilated cardiomyopathy. Previously common causes such as nutritional disorders or complications of rheumatic valvular disease are now rare. In less developed societies, infective causes still underlie the majority of cases. Particular disorders may be common in individual societies. These include Chagas' disease in Central and Southern America, iron overload in certain tribes in southern Africa, and nutritional deficiency states in the world's poorest countries. More than one cause of heart failure can coexist, such as hypertension and ischaemic heart disease.

Pathophysiology

Cardiac structural changes

Structural changes in the heart are common. There is usually enlargement of the left ventricular cavity (except in diastolic dysfunction and restrictive or constrictive cardiomyopathies). The shape of the ventricle also becomes more spherical. This can occur quickly after a myocardial infarction via stretching of the infarcted territory or more slowly in a process termed 'remodelling'. A similar change in shape is seen in dilated cardiomyopathies but not in the restrictive cardiomyopathies. The more spherical shape of the 'remodelled' and enlarged ventricle increases the stress of the myocardial wall and may thereby worsen myocardial ischaemia. Change in shape may also disrupt the conformational changes which normally occur during the isovolumic contraction phase in which the apex of the ventricle constricts in a twisting motion and pushes the blood into the base of the ventricle. When the ventricle is spherical at rest this intraventricular redistribution of blood is not possible and the net effect is a reduction in the efficiency with which the blood is ejected. Cardiac enlargement has long been known to be an adverse prognostic sign.

At the microscopic level there is an increase in the collagen content of the extracellular matrix, in part related to increased wall stress and in part to neurohormonal activation. This change reduces ventricular wall distensibility and may affect the efficiency with which active restorative forces can assist the diastolic filling process. It may also help explain the frequent coexistence of systolic and diastolic functional deterioration in an enlarging ventricle in chronic heart failure.

Enlargement of the ventricle is associated with a thinning of the ventricular wall with resultant realignment of the intercellular attachments between individual myocytes ('cell slippage'). There are also a reduced number of tight junctions between myocytes in the failing ventricle.

Functional abnormalities

Overall circulatory function

Cardiac power output is defined as cardiac output times the pressure drop across the systemic circulation. It is well-preserved at rest, even in severe heart failure, but its maximal reserve is reduced progressively as failure progresses. However, the measurement of cardiac power output tells us little of the underlying mechanisms. Attempts have been made, therefore, to define the components of ventricular function to assist in monitoring the patient's clinical course and the response to treatments.

Systolic dysfunction

Systolic dysfunction is most easily recognized by direct haemodynamic measurements showing a reduced peak rate of pressure rise within the ventricle (positive dP/dt maximum), an increased filling pressure (left ventricular end-diastolic pressure) or by indirect measurement of ventricular volumes. If there is a reduction in myocardial contractile function, an enlargement of the ventricle and a greater preload will enhance ventricular emptying via the Frank–Starling mechanism. The ventricle will operate at an increased end-diastolic and end-systolic volume. This can be measured by pressure and volume estimations by ventriculography (either radiographic or radionuclear) or echocardiography. The ejection fraction carries information about ventricular volumes and global ventricular function and is an important predictor of longevity, but it is a poor predictor of the severity of symptoms.

Diastolic dysfunction

Diastole is a complex process affected by many factors including heart rate, atrioventricular delay, atrial contractility, active myocardial recoil, passive ventricular wall stiffness, and the efficacy of ventricular systole and the residual end-diastolic volume and pressure within the ventricle. It is therefore not surprising that no simple measure of 'diastolic function' has been developed, and those measures that have been used are affected profoundly by systolic function and heart rate. Diastolic functional disturbance is, however, important, as there are cases of heart failure with a small heart and normal or even increased left ventricular ejection fraction. Abnormalities of diastolic filling may include increased filling pressures, delayed pressure fall within the ventricle and a greater than normal dependence on the effects of atrial contraction for ventricular filling. Such cases form the minority of cases of heart failure but are seen increasingly in older patients in whom senile myocardial fibrosis occurs more frequently. Other, rarer, causes include hypertrophic cardiomyopathy, infiltrative conditions such as amyloid heart disease, and the acute effects of ischaemia or the chronic effects of advanced hypertrophy in response to hypertension. Differentiation from systolic dysfunction is important because of differing effects of treatment; for instance, vasodilators may be less useful in diastolic dysfunction because of the requirement for high ventricular filling pressures in this condition.

Diastolic dysfunction can be quantified by a variety of measurements. The most commonly employed are the rate constant of isovolumic relaxation of the ventricle during early diastole (tau), the early to late peak filling velocity ratio (E/A) across the mitral valve on Doppler echocardiography, and the peak rate of ventricular filling on radionuclear gated acquisition (MUGA) scans in end-diastolic volumes per second. None of these is independent of the loading conditions of the ventricle, nor of atrioventricular delay and heart rate, nor of the effect of systolic dysfunction.

Non-cardiac features

Peripheral vascular changes

There is a reduction in large arterial compliance leading to an increase in impedance to ventricular outflow. Thus impaired ventricular reserve is further stressed and there is an increase in myocardial wall stress. The causes probably relate to sympathetic and possibly local renin–angiotensin activation.

There have been few reports of structural changes in the microvasculature but the endothelial-dependent vasomotor control systems are disordered; the vasodilator system is impaired both in the myocardial vessels and in the periphery. Tumour necrosis factor is elevated in some cases of chronic heart failure, and there have been reports of enhanced activity of the endothelin vasoconstrictor system.

Respiratory

The lungs

An acute reduction in left ventricular performance causes a rapid increase in left ventricular filling pressures and hence pulmonary venous pressures leading to fluid accumulation in the lungs. This decreases the compliance of the lung, thereby reducing vital capacity and increasing the work of breathing. It may also, via oedematous swelling of the bronchial mucosa, cause a non-asthmatic bronchial constriction which can mimic asthma and further increase respiratory muscle work. With more severe pulmonary venous hypertension the alveolar membrane becomes thickened and oedematous and this may impair gas exchange leading to an increase in the alveolar–arterial oxygen gradient and eventually arterial hypoxaemia. Frank pulmonary oedema leads to the clinical picture of gross dyspnoea, hypoxaemia, lung crepitations, and the production of copious quantities of pink frothy sputum.

In chronic heart failure, the patent remains dyspnoeic but the changes in the lungs are far less marked. Pulmonary venous pressures may even be normal if diuretic treatment is effective. Subtle changes in lung function include a reduction in gas diffusing capacity, intermittent non-asthmatic bronchial constriction and a purported increase in dead space ventilation. Alterations in the volume, strength, and fatiguability of the respiratory musculature have also been described, similar to those seen in limb musculature.

Respiratory control

Patients with heart failure, even in the absence of pulmonary oedema, have an increased ventilatory response to exercise, while maintaining normal arterial blood gas tensions. They show a reduced maximal oxygen consumption, an early dependence on anaerobic metabolism and an increased ventilatory equivalent for carbon dioxide even at low work levels. Why this occurs is not certain. There may be a primary increase in dead-space ventilation due to a reduction in the ability of the right ventricle to perfuse adequately all lung regions, or the development of ventilation/perfusion mismatching. An alternative is that something other than the rate of carbon dioxide production causes the increased exertional ventilation. There are several candidate stimuli such as lactate, arterial potassium, or adenosine. There is also a neural pathway in the control of ventilation utilizing group III and IV afferents from skeletal muscle. These are sensitive to the metabolic state of exercising muscle and transmit signals to mediate reflex increases in ventilation as well as peripheral vasoconstriction and sympatho-excitation. Mild alterations in gas exchange could reduce the rate of delivery of oxygen to the metabolizing tissues and act as a stimulus to increased ventilation. This could explain the beneficial effects of oxygen supplementation on exercise tolerance. In addition sensitivity of the arterial and central chemoreceptors has recently been shown to be elevated. It is not certain, however, that a reduction in diffusing capacity is quantitatively important nor that oxygen supplementation works via increasing net oxygen delivery to the tissues. The effect of high inspired oxygen is non-specific in reducing peripheral chemoreflex drive and thereby relieving the sensation of dyspnoea.

The sleep-apnoea syndrome

Episodes of apnoea may cause nocturnal oxygen saturation to fall episodically to below 80–85 per cent. The pattern is reminiscent of Cheyne–Stokes respiration well recognized in severe heart failure. The mechanisms of both abnormalities are incompletely understood. In some cases of sleep apnoea there is an obstructive element with obesity and pharyngeal occlusion. In others there appears to be an alteration in the central sensitivity to carbon dioxide so that oscillating levels of respiratory drive and hence arterial oxygen saturations develop. Sleep apnoea, as well as Cheyne–Stokes breathing and alterations in low frequency heart rate variability, may all reflect harmonic oscillations of chemoreflex/baroreflex interaction (see OTM3, pp. 2232–3).

Musculoskeletal

Structure

Fibre atrophy, changes in the distribution frequency of type IIa and IIb fibres, reduced mitochondrial density, volume, and number of cristae have all been described in skeletal muscle in moderate or severe heart failure. There is also a substantial reduction in muscle bulk, sometimes amounting to cachexia, but it is not possible to be sure of a specific skeletal myopathy of heart failure. Even so, these changes probably reflect a deficiency of oxygen delivery rather than the effects of primary reduction in the amount of exercise performed.

Function

In chronic heart failure there is a reduction in the strength of both small and large muscle groups, probably because of inherent defects in the quality of the muscle itself. There is also early fatiguability resulting in reduced physical activity, which leads to further muscle wasting and dysfunction.

Metabolism

Abnormalities of skeletal muscle metabolism in heart failure include early depletion of phosphocreatine, early acidification, accumulations of inorganic phosphate, reductions in the rate of resynthesis of phosphocreatine and of rate of removal of adenosine diphosphate. These changes are not the result of impaired blood flow, but probably reflect changes in oxidative enzymes in skeletal muscle.

Autonomic and neuroendocrine systems

Activation of the neuroendocrine system helps to support the circulation but in the long term is harmful. Adverse consequences include hypoperfusion of organs, myocardial toxicity, increased susceptibility to ventricular arrhythmias and progression of the underlying disease, be it ischaemia or cardiomyopathy.

The renin–angiotensin–aldosterone system

In untreated heart failure there is a mild activation of the systemic renin system, augmented by the use of diuretics. In addition, there is probably activation of the local systems in heart, kidney, brain, and blood vessel walls. The beneficial effects of inhibition show how important these systems may be. In the kidney, increased local angiotensin II may contribute to reductions in renal blood flow and glomerular filtration rate (**GFR**), especially on exercise. In very severe failure, angiotensin-mediated efferent arteriolar constriction maintains transcapillary hydraulic pressure (and therefore filtration) when overall perfusion pressure is unduly low.

The autonomic nervous system

There is activation of the sympathetic nervous system early in heart failure and a concomitant reduction in resting vagal tone. There is no clearly understood mechanism for this, particularly in mild cases.

Investigation of sympathovagal balance is limited by the lack of precise and quantifiable methods, but analysis of variations of heart rate variability shows promise in this context. The pattern in heart failure is very abnormal with a dramatic reduction in total heart rate variability and a selective loss of the higher frequency rhythm characteristic of respiratory sinus arrhythmia, and a relative preservation of low and very low frequency rhythms. This pattern is associated with high risk for the development of unstable ventricular arrhythmias and cardiac sudden death. Plasma noradrenaline levels correlate both with the degree of left ventricular failure, and with prognosis.

β-Receptor function

Chronic sympathetic activation leads to a depletion in myocardial catecholamine stores and a downregulation of β-1 receptors on the myocardium. There is also a decoupling of receptors from the post-receptor response, all of which lead to a loss of myocardial response to increased sympathetic drive. Clinically this manifests as chronotropic incompetence, loss of response to sympathomimetic stimulation and impaired exercise tolerance.

The natriuretic peptide systems

These peptides are natriuretic and also relax peripheral vasculature. Their release is increased in chronic heart failure associated with cardiac enlargement, but the significance of the increased plasma levels is uncertain; their natriuretic effects appear blunted in heart failure. There is increasing interest in the ability of elevated natriuretic peptide levels to become a biochemical marker of left ventricular systolic dysfunction.

The vasopressin system

Vasopressin concentrations are increased in chronic heart failure to levels that induce marked effects. Its actions are a combination of arteriolar vasoconstriction as well as renal water retention.

The kidney—oedema in heart failure

Oedema in heart failure is the consequence of retention of salt and water by the kidneys which behave in a way that resembles their response to haemorrhage. Yet blood volume is expanded rather than reduced leading to the concept of reduced 'effective' blood volume. Where this 'ineffectiveness' might be sensed is not certain, but candidates are arterial baroceptors and the low pressure receptors in atrial, ventricular, and juxtapulmonary capillaries. Those on the arterial side are more likely to be responsible, sensing in some way inadequate filling of the arterial tree by the sick heart. This concept of reduced 'effective' blood volume is also invoked to explain renal salt and water retention when cardiac output is much increased—as in hyperthyroidism, arteriovenous fistula, anaemia, or beriberi—so-called 'high output cardiac failure'.

Increased sympathetic tone, activation systemically and locally of the renin-angiotensin system could all plausibly be involved to explain the renal inability to excrete sodium and water normally, but, sodium retention in particular is likely to result from the summation of many influences on the kidney.

How does the kidney retain sodium in heart failure?

In moderate or severe heart failure, there is striking reduction in renal blood flow with relative preservation of GFR particularly during exercise. These haemodynamic changes, probably mediated by increased efferent arteriolar tone favour sodium reabsorption by increasing oncotic and reducing hydrostatic pressures in the peritubular capillaries. The effects of 'loop' diuretics suggest that there must also be increased sodium reabsorption in the loop of Henle and/or distal nephron mediated by factors which are unknown. Animal studies support an intrarenal redistribution of blood flow with juxtamedullary sodium-retaining nephrons better perfused than cortical nephrons, but there remains considerable doubt as to whether this occurs in humans.

Venous pressure and oedema

Cardiac oedema was once attributed to a primary rise in central venous pressure leading to a parallel increase in tissue capillary pressure and via Starling forces to increased filtration and decreased reabsorption of fluid, resulting in oedema and a reduction in plasma volume. This concept is untenable. In many patients sodium retention clearly precedes any rise in central venous pressure. At no stage in the development of clinical or experimental heart failure has blood volume been shown to be reduced. A reduction in lymphatic fluid return because of an increased central venous pressure is certainly a possible factor, but oedema must ultimately result from primary renal retention of salt and water.

Renal dysfunction

Low arterial pressure and the effects of the circulating and intrarenal neurohormonal systems described above contribute to impair renal excretory function in heart failure. Mild increases in blood urea, with lesser ones of plasma creatinine are common and overenthusiastic diuretic therapy can provoke significant renal failure. In very severe heart failure, when glomerular filtration is dependent on angiotensin-mediated efferent arteriolar tone, angiotensin-converting enzyme (ACE) inhibitors can induce significant oliguria or even anuria, readily reversed when the drug is withdrawn.

Electrolyte disturbances

These occur largely as a result of diuretic therapy, favouring hyponatraemia, hypokalaemia, alkalosis, and magnesium depletion.

Other organ systems

The liver

Hepatic congestion is due to venous engorgement of the liver and can result in an increase in size, local tenderness, and minor derangements in liver function. In severe cases nausea and right hypochondrial discomfort develop, and rarely jaundice. Impaired albumin and clotting factor production (important for those taking warfarin), and malabsorption may result.

Gastrointestinal tract

Intestinal mucosal oedema can contribute to malabsorption and a higher rate of intestinal angiodysplasia can lead to recurrent blood loss, another problem for patients who require anticoagulation.

Clinical assessment

History and clinical examination are aided by chest radiography, echocardiography and, in selected cases, by cardiac catheterization, radionuclide techniques and imaging modalities. Exercise testing with respiratory gas analysis can help establish the cause of symptoms in patients with coexisting heart and lung disease.

Treatment (Table 1)

Salt and water retention—diuretics

Conservative measures

The value of bed rest and moderate sodium restriction has been known for years, but these simple approaches have been neglected since the advent of potent diuretics. Supine bed rest enhances venous return, increases cardiac output and the secretion of atrial natriuretic peptide and increases the proportion of the output reaching the kidneys, thus facilitating natriuresis and diuresis and enhancing the efficacy of diuretic therapy. In the stabilized patient, however, there is evidence of the benefit of regular physical exercise improving symptoms and exercise tolerance. Strict sodium restriction to an intake of 20–30 mmol/day is an unpleasant treatment, found impractical or unacceptable by most patients, but more modest restriction may reduce the need for drugs and thus reduce risks of toxicity.

Fluid restriction (intake confined to 500–1000 ml/24 h) was once commonly prescribed for heart failure and there are still good reasons for this approach in advanced failure, as a number of factors combine to reduce the ability of the kidneys to excrete free water.

Table 1 Treatment of chronic heart failure

Mild to moderate	Severe
No added salt	Increase loop diuretic
ACE inhibitor	?Metolazone
Low-dose β-blocker (bisoprolol, metoprolol, carvedilol)	Add spironoloactone 25-50 mg/day
Digoxin for atrial fibrillation	ACE inhibitor
	Nitrate
	Anticoagulate
	Consider digoxin, inotropes
	Cardiac transplantation

Diuretics

By increasing urinary excretion of salt and water, diuretics reduce cardiac preload and thereby relieve congestion. Most, with the exception of spironolactone, influence renal tubular reabsorptive mechanisms in relation to their concentration in the tubular fluid which they reach largely by the organic ion transport mechanisms in the proximal convoluted tubule. Because of strong protein binding, loop agents and thiazides do not enter tubular fluid by glomerular filtration in significant amounts. The efficacy of a diuretic in individual cases depends therefore not only on inherent potency and site of action, but also critically on renal perfusion and tubular function as well as the antinatriuretic neurohumoral factors associated with heart failure. In the presence of heavy proteinuria, protein binding of diuretics in tubular fluid may also limit their efficacy.

Thiazide diuretics

The hazards of extreme hypovolaemia, and of serious electrolyte disturbance are less with thiazides. In maximal doses, these agents are capable of inhibiting reabsorption of some 5 per cent of the filtered load of sodium, quite enough for many patients with cardiac oedema. The dose–response curve of thiazides is flat, with little difference between small and large doses. Most thiazides affect urinary salt excretion for some 8–10 h but some, like chlorthalidone, last for as long as 24–36 h.

Potassium supplements

All thiazides tend to increase urinary potassium losses to a degree dependent on tubular flow rate, the delivery of sodium to the distal nephron, and the extent of secondary aldosteronism present. Chloruresis and potassium loss both tend to produce alkalosis, which further inhibits renal potassium conservation. The rate at which potassium may be lost is, therefore, variable and the need to provide supplements or not, equally variable. There is no doubt that severe potassium depletion can be provoked by thiazide treatment, especially by chlorthalidone, and that such depletion can potentiate cardiotoxic effects of digitalis analogues. When in doubt the wisest course is to prescribe supplements, or to combine treatment with one of the distally acting agents which promote potassium retention. Preparations providing thiazide diuretics and potassium in the same tablet are often prescribed, but the amounts of potassium incorporated may not suffice to prevent hypokalaemia; separate preparations of the diuretic and of potassium supplements are preferable.

Potassium-sparing diuretics

Spironolactone, amiloride, and triamterene all act on the distal nephron, promoting modest increases in sodium excretion and significant inhibition of potassium secretion. Spironolactone is a true antagonist of aldosterone. Effective doses range from 25 to 400 mg daily and depend on the degree of aldosteronism present. Side-effects of nausea and abdominal discomfort complicate higher dosage and prolonged use is commonly complicated by the development of gynaecomastia. The onset of action is delayed for a full 24–72 h. There is recent evidence of particular benefit from low dose (25–50 mg) spironolactone in severe (grade IV) heart failure.

Triamterene and amiloride block luminal sodium channels directly. Triamterene is rather less potent and less well tolerated than amiloride, which is as effective in conserving potassium and excreting sodium as is spironolactone, but free of the side-effect of gynaecomastia. Effective doses range between 5 and 20 mg daily.

The addition of any of these agents to thiazides or 'loop' diuretics augments sodium excretion and reduces potassium loss, but to a variable degree depending on haemodynamic factors and the activity of the renin–aldosterone system. It is *not* safe to assume potassium homeostasis without regular checks of plasma levels, particularly in the first 1–2 weeks after their introduction.

'Loop' diuretics

Loop agents all act principally by inhibiting sodium chloride cotransport in the ascending limb of the loop of Henle, which is critical to the mechanisms of urinary concentration and dilution. They are all extremely potent, and promote a considerably greater excretion of chloride than of sodium. They tend to increase urinary potassium losses in an amount dependent on the extent of secondary hyperaldosteronism present and the degree of alkalosis induced by chloride deficiency or any pre-existing potassium depletion.

These drugs are potentially dangerous particularly in the elderly. Their remarkable potency results in a risk of extreme hypovolaemia, postural hypotension, circulatory failure, and uraemia when they are given without proper supervision, particularly to patients whose disease could well be controlled by less drastic agents. Weight loss from diuretic therapy should be achieved ideally at a rate not exceeding 1–2 kg/day. These caveats apart, 'loop' diuretics properly prescribed provide a major advance in the care of patients whose oedema cannot be controlled by less powerful drugs. Given by mouth, all begin to induce natriuresis and diuresis within 1–2 h and have a peak effect at about 4 h, which is complete at about 6 h. The relatively short period of action can be used to tailor treatment for individual patients. The threshold dose required to produce a natriuresis in any given case may be increased for a number of reasons, including slow gastrointestinal absorption, reduced renal perfusion, impaired secretory function of the proximal tubule, as well as the sodium-retaining consequences of increased activity of the renin–angiotensin system and other neurohumoral mechanisms. In this situation, larger individual doses are required as a first step, with increased frequency of administration as the second.

Resistant oedema

Combinations of loop agents, thiazides, and distal acting drugs may fail to control fluid retention, particularly when cardiac failure coexists with impaired renal function. In such cases, metolazone has been shown to be remarkably effective when combined with a loop agent. Indeed its addition may produce an excessive natriuresis and it is often wise to begin with a small dose, e.g. 2.5–5 mg on alternate days, increasing if necessary to a maximum dose of 20 mg/day.

In extreme cases ACE inhibitors may cause an acute fall in GFR, oliguria, and uraemia secondary to inhibition of angiotensin-mediated efferent arteriolar tone.

When fluid retention persists despite therapy, there is a need to decide whether to increase the dose of ACE inhibitor or of a diuretic first. Cold extremities and a rise in blood urea above 20 mmol/litre (BUN over 60 mg/100 ml) indicates predominance of poor cardiac output, best treated by an increase in ACE inhibition, together with a reduction in diuretic dose. When blood urea concentrations are below some 12–18 mmol/l (BUN 36–54 mg/100 ml) and the extremities are warm, it may be more effective to increase the dose of diuretic first.

In cases with delayed, or inadequate absorption of loop agents due to intestinal oedema, higher blood levels can be achieved by the use of bolus doses given intramuscularly or intravenously. More effective and more comfortable for the patient is a slow infusion given by a low pump delivering the total 24-h dose in 100 ml or less of 5 per cent dextrose.

Contraindications and complications during diuretic therapy

There are some cardiac conditions in which removal of fluid from the circulation is quite inappropriate, despite clear evidence of an elevation in central venous pressure. These include constrictive pericarditis, pericardial tamponade, right ventricular infarction, pulmonary embolism, or mitral valve disease when cardiac output is severely compromised.

Prolonged treatment with loop agents or thiazides induce hyperuricaemia and may cause gout. Hyperglycaemia can be provoked by thiazides particularly, and the risk appears greatest in the elderly. Hypercalcaemia is increasingly recognized as a consequence of thiazide treatment. Hyponatraemia represents more of a problem and, hypomagnesaemia is often not sufficiently recognized (see below).

Diuretic-induced hyponatraemia

This complication is never, or almost never, due to sodium depletion, but almost always due to a relative water overload. A number of factors contribute. Increased tubular reabsorption of sodium in the proximal tubule results in less sodium and chloride delivered to the diluting sites. Excretion free water is thereby decreased. It is decreased further by the use of diuretics which inhibit electrolyte transport at these diluting sites. In addition, patients with cardiac insufficiency are often thirsty. Finally, plasma levels of antidiuretic hormone are increased in severe heart failure. Mild hyponatraemia needs no treatment, although it is a sign of a guarded prognosis. More severe hyponatraemia accompanied by symptoms requires treatment. If diuretics cannot be reduced, the addition of an ACE inhibitor may increase cardiac performance and renal perfusion, but on occasion hyponatraemia follows ACE inhibition. Water restriction is then only moderately effective and is rarely tolerated by patients. Demethylchlortetracycline has been tried in this situation but usually without great benefit.

Magnesium depletion

Both 'loop' diuretics and thiazides can provoke magnesium depletion. Symptoms and signs are rare but can include depression, muscle weakness, refractory hypokalaemia, hypertension, and ventricular or atrial dysrhythmias resistant to treatment. Treatment with magnesium glycerophosphate is quite well accepted in doses of 3–6 g daily providing 12–24 mmol of magnesium per 24 h. Other possible preparations include magnesium hydroxide which gives approximately 20 mmol in 15 ml but at the risk of diarrhoea and less efficient absorption.

Acute pulmonary oedema (see Chapter 15.23)

Apart from morphine, the most effective treatment is intravenous injections of 'loop' diuretics. Frusemide 20–40 mg increases urinary salt and water excretion within 2 min, reaching a peak at 5–10 min and complete within 25 or 35 min. There is some evidence that the beneficial effects can be attributed not only to natriuresis and diuresis but also to falls in left atrial pressure the result of dilatation of venous capacitance vessels.

Digitalis—maintenance therapy: indications and regimens

Maintenance therapy may be indicated for the management of heart failure due to systolic ventricular dysfunction. Much debate has centred around the value of digitalis long-term use in patients in sinus rhythm. The situation has been clarified by 14 studies using digoxin. Significant benefits included one or more of the following: subjective measures, heart failure scores, haemodynamic measures, exercise capacity, and frequency of hospital admission. One of the trials showed that the benefits of digoxin were additive to those of ACE inhibitors. A subsequent randomized study showed that withdrawal of it in patients treated with diuretics and ACE inhibitors led to worsening heart failure. Against the evidence of benefit must be set the possibility of harm. Some consider that cardiac glycosides should be used with particular caution in patients with severe coronary heart disease because the threshold to ventricular fibrillation may be lowered. Evidence is inconclusive that digitalis is an independent risk factor for death, but it cannot be pronounced innocent in this regard. The case at present is 'not proven'. The DIG study, involving over 7500 patients found no significant effect of digoxin on mortality, although there was a reduction in the rate of admission to hospital.

Assessment of ventricular rate during exercise should be made before deciding the dose to control atrial fibrillation, but in the presence of good renal function up to 250 µg digoxin twice daily may be required. Higher doses are very rarely needed. More commonly, smaller doses are dictated by impaired renal function or by unwanted effects. For most patients with sinus rhythm and good renal function, a dose of digoxin of 250 µg daily is usually appropriate but, with impaired renal function, smaller doses are necessary. Digitoxin may be better in this situation because accumulation is less likely. The usual dose is 100 µg daily or rarely 200 µg daily. Lower doses should be given in the presence of impaired liver function.

Measurement of plasma concentrations

Blood samples should be drawn when plasma concentrations after oral dosage have passed the absorption peak and fallen to a plateau, which then decays at a rate corresponding to the elimination half-life of the drug. In practice this requires sampling after an interval of about 8 h from the last oral dose. Exercise affects interpretation of results, by increasing the binding of digoxin to skeletal muscle. Plasma concentrations after a period of rest can be increased by as much as 75 per cent compared with those during exercise. Pregnancy and renal impairment can produce falsely elevated plasma glycoside concentrations in some assays.

Therapeutic plasma concentrations of digoxin are in the range of 1–2 µg/litre. Those for digitoxin are approximately 10–15 times higher, due chiefly to greater protein binding.

Digitalis toxicity

There is considerable variation in the plasma and tissue concentrations at which toxicity occurs. Serious toxicity is unusual with plasma concentrations below 2 µg/litre, and are likely to be present with concentrations more than 3 µg/litre. Between these figures some patients have a satisfactory therapeutic response while others have troublesome adverse effects.

The extracardiac toxic effects include fatigue with profound muscular weakness, severe visual disturbances, nausea and anorexia, abdominal pain, vomiting, diarrhoea, headache, restlessness, and agitation.

In the absence of heart disease or very large overdose, the cardiac manifestations are usually relatively benign. First-, second-, and third-degree atrioventricular block may occur, but severe bradycardia or long pauses are unlikely because the rate of subsidiary junctional pacemakers tends to be accelerated by the glycosides. In patients with heart disease the manifestations are usually more serious. While almost any rhythm disturbance can occur, the following may be regarded as characteristic: frequent ventricular extrasystoles, junctional and ventricular rhythms or tachycardias; atrial tachycardias with varying degrees of atrioventricular block, bradycardia due to sinoatrial block; an unduly slow ventricular response in atrial fibrillation, progressive regularization of ventricular response in atrial fibrillation due to the emergence of accelerated junctional beats, and ventricular fibrillation. Some digitalis-induced arrhythmias are very complex and difficult to analyse. With very high plasma levels, asystole may occur. This may be associated with refractory hyperkalaemia.

Treatment of digitalis toxicity

In most patients it is sufficient to withhold the drug, and especially in the presence of hypokalaemia, to give potassium. Potassium may be contraindicated when atrioventricular block is present because the conduction defect may be exacerbated. Atropine and pervenous pacing have an occasional role in the management of bradyarrhythmias.

A specific antidote (Digibind, Ovine) is valuable because of the risk to life in severe toxicity. The antibody fragments rapidly bind intravascular and interstitial digoxin. Their small size permits rapid diffusion into the interstitial space where binding of free digoxin sets up a concentration gradient leading to the egress of tissue stores of the glycoside. An initial clinical response can usually be expected within 60 min, and complete reversal of toxicity within about 4 h. If renal function is normal, the bound digoxin is excreted with a half-life of approximately 16 h. The dose is based on body weight and plasma digoxin concentration for patients toxic from excessive maintenance therapy or on the amount ingested after a single dose. Allergic reactions have occurred in less than 1 per cent of patients. Recrudescence of toxicity is rare, but caution is needed if renal

Table 2 Vasodilators in common clinical use

Drug	Mechanism	Arterial	Venous
Nitrates	Cyclic GMP	+	++
Hydralazine	Unknown	++	–
ACE inhibition	Angiotensin II	++	+
Calcium antagonists	Calcium entry	++	–
Angiotensin receptor antagonist	AT1 receptor	++	+

failure is severe enough to prolong greatly the elimination of the digoxin–antibody complex, which may eventually release free digoxin.

Lidocaine or phenytoin may be effective for serious arrhythmias, even if they are of supraventricular origin. β-adrenoceptor-blocking agents are useful for ectopic ventricular arrhythmias but may precipitate heart failure or bradyarrhythmias in susceptible patients. Electrical cardioversion may precipitate ventricular fibrillation and should be considered only for the most pressing indications. The lowest effective energy should be used. Dialysis and haemoperfusion are ineffective for both digoxin and digitoxin toxicity because the large tissue stores equilibrate relatively slowly with the much lower concentrations in plasma.

β-Blockers

Recent controlled trials (undertaken largely in relatively young men) have shown major benefit from the use of selective β-blockers (bisoprolol, metoprolol, carvedilol) in stable mild and moderate heart failure due to left ventricular systolic dysfunction. Overall mortality was reduced by some 30 per cent and that due to sudden death by 44 per cent. Initial doses should be small (e.g. metoprolol 5 mg) and increased only slowly over weeks or months. The position with regard to symptomless heart failure, diastolic heart failure, heart failure in the elderly, and severe heart failure (grade IV) is uncertain and these drugs should be avoided in these groups until further evidence is available.

Vasodilators

In most cases of heart failure, balanced vasodilatation with agents that reduce both preload and afterload leads to the greatest haemodynamic improvement and clinical benefit. A simple classification based on whether the major site of action is on arteries or veins is widely adopted (Table 2). The way in which reduction in venous (preload) or arterial (afterload) tone or both affect the cardiac output is illustrated in Fig. 1.

Nitroprusside

Nitroprusside is a balanced vasodilator which can only be given intravenously and whose rapid onset and offset of action renders it only suitable, but eminently so, for the acute situation; close haemodynamic monitoring both of systemic arterial and right heart pressures are essential during its use. As light degrades the parent compound, the delivery system must be shielded. The dose ranges from 10 μg/kg per min up to 30 μg/kg per min depending on response. A typical indication for its use would be a patient with low cardiac output and high filling pressures due to poor systolic left ventricular function resulting from dilated cardiomyopathy, acute myocardial infarction, chronic coronary heart disease, acute or chronic aortic or mitral incompetence, or acute ventricular septal defect following

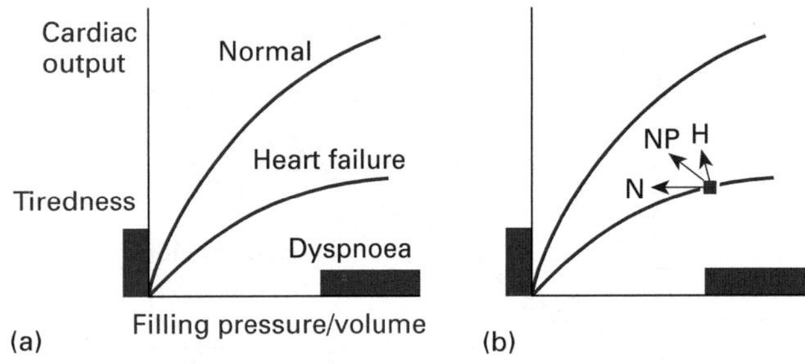

Fig. 1 (a) Schematic diagram of normal and depressed left ventricular function curves relating filling pressure and cardiac output. (b) Effects of vasodilatation. (i) arteriolar vasodilatation with hydralazine (H); cardiac output rises more than filling pressure falls. Tiredness expected to improve; (ii) venous dilatation with nitrates (N); filling pressure falls more than cardiac output rises. Dyspnoea expected to improve; (iii) 'balanced' vasodilation with nitroprusside (NP); both cardiac output and filling pressure improve. Dyspnoea and tiredness expected to improve.

acute myocardial infarction. Two main problems complicate its use. Hypotension is best avoided by starting at a very low dose and by close continuous monitoring of systemic arterial and pulmonary capillary wedge pressures. Second, toxic metabolites of cyanide or cyanate accumulate in patients with liver or renal dysfunction. These problems make many prefer nitrates which are safer, and as effective.

Nitrates

Glyceryl trinitrate is prepared in intravenous, sublingual, and transcutaneous formulations, while the mainstays of oral therapy are isosorbide mono- or dinitrate. They all cause vascular smooth muscle relaxation, particularly in veins, by increasing intracellular cyclic guanine monophosphate. Though some decrease in arteriolar tone also occurs, this effect is seen predominantly in the capacitance and pulmonary vessels resulting, acutely, in a reduction in preload. Frequently repeated doses of nitrate lead to the development of tolerance.

Hydralazine

This drug is an arteriolar smooth muscle relaxant. Its acute haemodynamic profile is shown in Fig. 1, but these effects do not translate into long-term benefit in controlled trials. The contribution of hydralazine with isosorbide dinitrate is more effective and is now the only way in which hydralazine is used in heart failure. The value of the combination was shown in the two Veterans Heart Failure trials (V-HeFTI and II—see Fig. 2). But ACE inhibitors are superior in controlling symptoms, in exercise capacity and in reducing mortality. Moreover, some one-third of patients cannot tolerate the combination because of headache, palpitation, or nasal congestion. Overall, hydralazine plus isosorbide is a second line approach, although a trial has shown benefit from adding this combination to ACE inhibition. Doses of hydralazine begin at 37.5 mg four times a day, and of isosorbide 20 mg four times daily, increasing to a maximum tolerated dose averaging 400 and 150 mg/day respectively.

Calcium channel blockers

These agents are arteriolar vasodilators acting by decreasing the slow inward calcium current that promotes arterial smooth muscle contraction. The main concern in their use in heart failure is that they also decrease calcium availability within cardiac myocytes, which decreases contractility. Interest in heart failure is therefore centred on those agents with relatively greater effects on the peripheral vascular calcium channels, such as nifedipine, felodipine, and amlodipine.

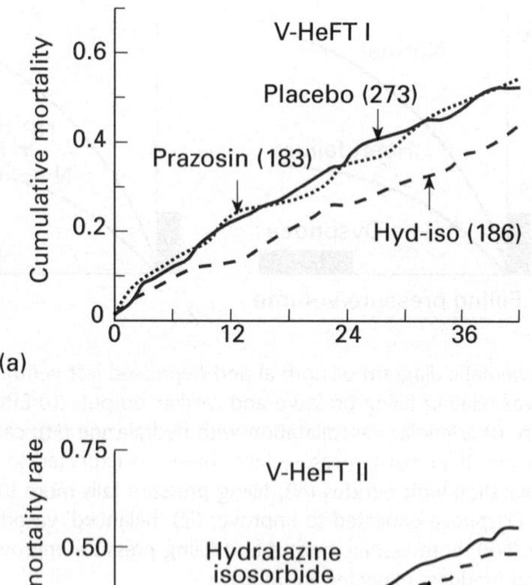

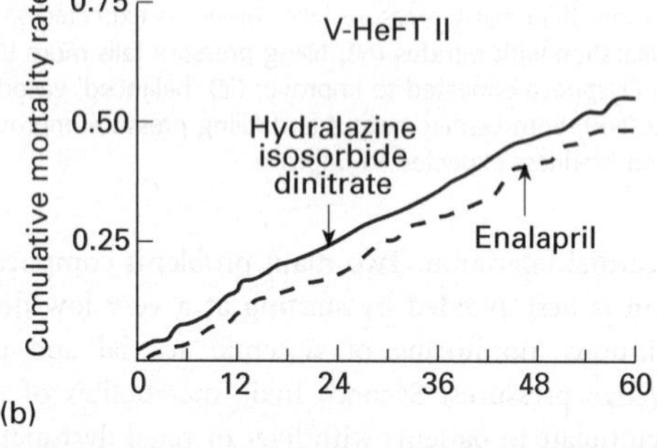

Fig. 2 (a) Cumulative mortality rates with time (months) in V-HeFT I. Hydralazine/isosorbide dinitrate (Hyd-iso) group has a lower mortality trend than prazosin and placebo. (b) Cumulative mortality rate with time in V-HeFT II. Enalapril group has a significantly lower mortality ($P = 0.08$) than hydralazine/isosorbide dinitrate.

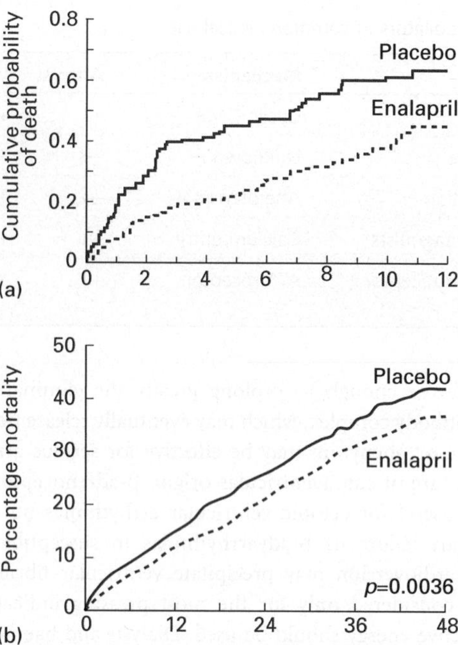

Fig. 3 (a) Cumulative mortality in CONSENSUS I. Clear survival advantage of enalapril is obvious as is the overall poor prognosis of severe heart failure. (b) Cumulative mortality in SOLVD treatment trial (T). Significant survival advantage of enalapril is noted.

There are few long-term studies on their value in heart failure but several reports have shown that nifedipine may lead to deterioration, probably reflecting its negative inotropic effects and, in some cases, the ill effects of secondary reflex neuroendocrine activation.

Angiotensin-converting enzymes inhibitors

ACE inhibitors are superior to other vasodilators. Their effects depend mainly on the inhibition of conversion of angiotensin I to II, both systemically and locally, although their action in inhibiting destruction of bradykinin may also be important.

The major benefits of their use probably derives from arterial and venous dilatation, reducing cardiac filling pressures, wall stress, chamber size, and myocardial hypertrophy and increasing left ventricular ejection fraction. Adverse effects are few. In advanced renal failure, any tendency towards hyperkalaemia may be aggravated and in very severe heart failure with low renal perfusion pressure, inhibition of angiotensin-mediated efferent arteriolar vasoconstriction may so reduce glomerular transcapillary hydraulic pressure as to cause acute but reversible renal failure.

Clinical efficacy

Heart failure is a progressive disorder and deterioration depends, at least in part, on a vicious cycle of increasing neurohumoral activation leading to increased vascular resistance and escalating cardiac work and dysfunction. ACE inhibitors and β-blockers are well placed to disturb this cycle and a number of studies have confirmed that the former reduce the rate of progression of heart failure and delay the onset of symptoms in patients with asymptomatic left ventricular dysfunction. They also reduce mortality in all grades of heart failure, including that after myocardial infarction (Fig. 3).

Table 3 Guidelines for starting ACE inhibitors

Confirm left ventricular systolic dysfunction (e.g. by echocardiography)
Check routine blood chemistry
Temporarily omit diuretic for 24–36 h
Stop potassium supplements or potassium-sparing diuretics
Initiate therapy under supervision
Consider admission if:
>80 mg frusemide/equivalent
systolic blood pressure <100 mmHg
serum creatinine >200 μmol/litre
serum potassium >5.0 mmol/litre
History of CVA or TIA
Peripheral vascular disease

Place in management

The effects of ACE inhibitors on survival, disease progression and the development of myocardial infarction make them mandatory treatment in all grades of symptomatic heart failure, although certain precautions should be taken before treatment is started (Table 3). In most studies they have been combined with diuretics and, when used alone have proved inadequate. In mild to moderate left ventricular function they are now also combined with β-blockers.

Treatment can be begun in most patients with mild or moderate heart failure without admission to hospital, but in those with severe heart failure on high doses of diuretics admission is essential.

A low dose should be given initially (e.g. 2–6.25 mg captopril, 2.5 mg enalapril). The patient should remain seated or supine until the peak haemodynamic effect of the drug has been observed (1–2 h with captopril, 2–6 h with other ACE inhibitors). Head-down tilt of the bed and intravenous saline will usually correct symptomatic hypotension. Once treatment has been successfully introduced, the dose can be increased to achieve maximum symptomatic benefit, though this may be delayed for weeks or months.

Adverse effects

First dose hypotension

A precipitous fall in blood pressure, occasionally accompanied by a bradycardia can occur in response to the first dose of an ACE inhibitor. This is usually only seen in volume depleted patients, and those on large doses of diuretic. In patients at risk a small test dose of a short-acting inhibitor is advisable, e.g. captopril 2 mg or perhaps 6.25 mg, with close observation of the blood pressure response over the subsequent 1–2 h. Correction of fluid-volume status may permit subsequent uncomplicated reintroduction of ACE inhibitors in patients who have shown this phenomenon. It is also important to ensure that significant pulmonary or obstructive valve disease has not been missed and that the patient does not have an unusual type of heart muscle disease causing diastolic dysfunction, for example, amyloid.

Renal dysfunction

Small increases in plasma creatinine (i.e. $\leq$ 10 per cent increase) are common when ACE inhibitions are used to treat advanced heart failure, but serious renal dysfunction is rare. Even so, frequent monitoring of blood urea, serum creatinine and urine output are essential when ACE inhibitors are introduced in patients with severe left ventricular dysfunction.

Hyperkalaemia

Modest hyperkalaemia (plasma potassium 4.6–5.8 mmol/l) is to be expected when ACE inhibitors are given to patients whose GFR is less than 20–30 ml/min. Volume depletion and extrarenal uraemia increase the likelihood of hyperkalaemia and co-prescription of a non-steroidal anti-inflammatory or potassium-conserving diuretic much increases the risk.

Cough

There is a small but significant increase in its incidence during ACE inhibitor therapy but, in trials, this has not led to more withdrawals in the actively treated patients. Cough should not be attributed immediately to ACE inhibition, and pulmonary congestion or airways obstruction must be excluded; even if it is due to the ACE inhibitor, the patient may be able to tolerate it and in some it may, on occasion, resolve spontaneously.

Other adverse effects

Taste disturbance, skin rash, proteinuria, and leucopenia have been rare in recent trials. Angio-oedema is another rare but troublesome complication.

Catecholamines

Haemodynamic profiles and usage of catecholamines

In contrast to the use of β-blockers in stable mild to moderate heart failure catecholamines can be used intravenously to provide short-term circulatory support in acute severe failure. They enhance the inotropic state of the heart, although both salbutamol and low-dose dopamine have the useful actions of peripheral, splanchnic, or renal vasodilatation and noradrenaline may cause vasoconstriction.

Table 4 Adrenergic receptor subtypes

Receptor	Action on circulation
α-1	Vasoconstriction (increase in contractility)
α-2	Vasoconstriction. Presynaptic sympathetic inhibition.
β-1	Increase in heart rate (sinus node)
	Increase in contractility (atrium, and ventricle)
	Increase in conduction (atrioventricular node)
β-2	Vasodilatation (bronchodilatation).
Dopaminergic-1	Renal and mesenteric vasodilatation.
Dopaminergic-2	Vasodilatation

Table 5 Adrenergic receptor activity of endogenous and synthetic catecholamines

Catecholamine	Receptor subtypes					
	α-1	α-2	β-1	β-2	DA-1	DA-2
Dopamine	++	+	++	0	+++	++
Noradrenaline	+++	++	+++	+−	0	
Adrenaline	++	++	+++	++	0	
Isoprenaline	0	0	+++	+++	0	
Dobutamine	+	+ −	+++	++	0	
Salbutamol	0	0	+	+++	0	
Dopexamine	0	0	+	++	++	+

Any increase in the inotropic state of the heart, also increases myocardial oxygen consumption to a greater or lesser extent. An increase in heart rate will further augment oxygen demand as will the development of tachyarrhythmias. Catecholamine usage in an individual patient requires careful consideration of the balance between augmented short-term cardiac performance and longer-term adverse effects on myocardial oxygen demands.

Adrenergic pharmacology

Classification of adrenergic receptors into α and β subtypes has been considerably refined (Table 4) and now includes α-1, α-2, β-1, β-2, and dopamine receptor subtypes. In chronic heart failure, cardiac efferent sympathetic activity is increased coupled with impairment of neuronal reuptake further increasing intrasynaptic noradrenaline concentration. However, tolerance to the action of both endogenous and exogenous catecholamines arises through β-adrenoceptor down-regulation.

Noradrenaline, adrenaline, and dopamine and their synthetic derivatives interact with the six adrenoceptor subtypes shown in Table 4 according to their specificity and affinity for these receptors (Table 5). Human ventricular muscle contains predominantly β-1-adrenoceptor subtypes in close proximity to the adrenergic synapse, mediating an inotropic response. The sinoatrial node, however, may respond preferentially to β-2-adrenoceptors distributed throughout the specialized tissue and responsive to circulating catecholamines (adrenaline/noradrenaline) as well as neuronally released noradrenaline.

Table 6 Catecholamine dosage

Drug	Infusion rate (μg/kg/min)
Dopamine dopaminergic	1–5
β-1	5–10
β-1/α	10–40
Noradrenaline	0.01–0.07
Adrenaline	0.06–0.18
Isoprenaline	0.01–0.15
Dobutamine	2.5–10

Dopamine

Effects are dose-dependent; the renal and mesenteric circulation, and to a lesser extent the coronary and cerebrovascular vessels dilate at low-dose (Table 6). The most important clinical effect is on the kidney with increased renal blood flow, glomerular filtration, and natriuresis. This action is especially useful in the management of persistent heart failure associated with reversible reduction in myocardial contractility or with impaired diuretic responsiveness as a result of renal artery vasoconstriction. Dopaminergic vasodilatation is antagonized by phenothiazines and by butyrophenones. Higher doses activate β-1-adrenoceptors leading to an increase in myocardial contractility and heart rate and an increase in myocardial oxygen demand. Yet they may augment coronary perfusion pressure. High-dose dopamine infusion leads to dominant α-1-adrenoceptor actions and peripheral vasoconstriction.

Noradrenaline

The main actions of noradrenaline are α-receptor-mediated vasoconstriction and β-1-adrenoceptor-mediated enhancement of contractility. Arteriolar vasoconstriction significantly increases blood pressure and cardiac output usually decreases. Heart rate usually falls because of baroreceptor mediated vagal stimulation and sympathetic withdrawal (as a result of elevated blood pressure) of β-1-adrenoceptor stimulation. Vasoconstriction is most intense in muscle, skin, liver, and kidney. Actions on the myocardium result from increased afterload, increased preload, and increased contractility. Myocardial oxygen demand will increase. Noradrenaline is useful in the short term to improve cerebral and coronary perfusions in shock, during resuscitation and may be used to counteract hypotension as a result of vasodilator therapy. It has little role in the longer term when adverse effects on oxygen demand are likely to be hazardous.

Adrenaline

Action on α- and β-adrenoceptors (most notably the β-1-adrenoceptors) in the heart augments cardiac contractility and increases heart rate, automaticity, and conduction. Vasoconstriction and increase in blood pressure are less pronounced than with noradrenaline. At low dose, systemic vascular resistance may fall while at higher doses vasoconstriction is evident. Myocardial oxygen demand is substantially and progressively increased and tachycardia and cardiac arrhythmias may limit usefulness particularly with acute circulatory failure. The main use is in short-term acute inotropic support, for example during cardiopulmonary resuscitation.

Isoprenaline

Isoprenaline has powerful β-adrenoceptor stimulatory actions, producing increases in heart rate, inotropic state and atrioventricular conduction and automaticity. Peripheral vascular and pulmonary vascular resistance fall from β-2-adrenoceptor stimulation. Systolic blood pressure may rise from cardiac effects, although diastolic pressure normally falls. Myocardial oxygen consumption increases greatly and arrhythmias and myocardial ischaemia frequently limit dose.

Isoprenaline is most frequently used for its chronotropic action as a short-term intravenous infusion in patients with symptomatic bradycardia, for example heart block. The infusion rate may be adjusted to achieve a heart rate alleviating acute symptoms, pending longer-term management such as cardiac pacing. Rarely, oral medication (30–60 mg 6-hourly) is necessary if other chronotropic measures are not available.

Dobutamine

This drug has some β-1-adrenoceptor selectivity and hence has less effect on the sinus node and on heart rate. Enhancement of left ventricular contractile activity provides a useful short-term role for it in shock states with primary or secondary ventricular disease. Effects on heart rate and arrhythmogenesis, however, are not infrequently limiting.

Salbutamol

This β-2-adrenoceptor agonist causes peripheral vasodilatation and hence afterload reduction. Increases in heart rate limit clinical usefulness and alternative vasodilator agents are usually to be preferred.

Dopexamine

Dopexamine is a dopamine analogue acting on β-2-adrenoceptors and some dopamine receptors. The combined effects of renal, hepatic, and splanchnic vasodilatation with peripheral vasodilatation offer a haemodynamic profile that may be of value, although increases in heart rate, as with dobutamine, can restrict its use.

Phosphodiesterase inhibitors

Emoximone and milrinone are selective phosphodiesterase inhibitors with primary myocardial effects. These drugs increase cardiac contractility, promote ventricular relaxation and cause modest peripheral vasodilatation. Improvements in myocardial performance are short lived, and both atrial and ventricular arrhythmias may be increased.

Prognosis

In severe heart failure where patients are symptomatic at rest (NYHA class IV) the prognosis is very poor, with a survival rate of 1 year or less. Even in mild heart failure (class II–III), the mortality rate is 8–10 per cent per year.

Many parameters have prognostic value in patients with heart failure (Table 2). The most important are: (1) the extent of left ventricular dysfunction; (2) the degree of functional limitation; (3) the electrolyte disturbance; (4) the degree of neurohumoral dysfunction; and (5) electrophysiological or electrocardiographic indicators of ventricular arrhythmogenesis.

Non-sustained ventricular tachycardia on Holter monitoring is a sign of an increased probability of mortality from sudden death. Class I antiarrhythmic agents can reduce the frequency of ventricular tachycardia, but the Cardiac Arrhythmia Suppression Trial, of three such agents, showed that, despite reducing the frequency of ventricular arrhythmias, there was an increased rate of sudden death, presumably due to some proarrhythmic effects. Similarly a low ejection fraction is an adverse prognostic sign, and it was expected that agents which improve ejection fraction should increase survival. Positive inotropic oral agents, such as milrinone, in controlled studies increase ejection fraction but with a reduced survival. Thus the only justifications for treatment are to slow the progression of the underlying disease, to relieve symptoms, or to use agents proven to improve survival.

Further reading

Benedict, C.R., Shelton, B., Johnstone, D.E., *et al.* (1996). Prognostic significance of plasma norepinephrine in patients with asymptomatic left ventricular dysfunction. *Circulation*, **94**, 690–7.

Clark, A.L., Poole Wilson, P.A., and Coats, A.J.S. (1997). Exercise limitation in chronic heart failure: the central role of the periphery. *Journal of the American College of Cardiology*, **28**, 1092–102.

Cleland J.G.F., Swedberg, K., and Poole-Wilson, P.A. (1998). Successes and failures of current treatment of heart failure. *Lancet*, **352** (suppl.1), 19–28.

Cohn, J. (1996). The management of chronic heart failure. *New England Journal of Medicine*, **335**, 490–8.

Richards, A.M. and Nicholls, M.G. (1999). Aldosterone antagonism in heart failure. *Lancet*, **354**, 789–90.

Sharpe, N. (1999). Benefit of β-blockers for heart failure: proven in 1999. *Lancet*, **353**, 1988–9.

The Digitalis Investigation Group. (1997). The effect of digoxin on mortality and morbidity in patients with heart failure. *New England Journal of Medicine*, **336**, 525–33.digoxin therapy in patients with chronic heart failure. *American Journal*

Chapter 2.3

Cardiac transplantation

J. H. Dark

Patient selection

Heart failure will be due either to idiopathic dilated cardiomyopathy or ischaemic heart disease in more than 90 per cent of recipients. Other presenting diagnoses are shown in Table 1. Patients with congenital heart disease are often excluded because of a high pulmonary vascular resistance secondary to uncorrected shunts, but, an increasing number who had palliative procedures as children are now presenting with irreversible ventricular failure in early adulthood.

Transplantation for an active myocarditis has a poor outcome and when the heart is involved in a systemic disease; compromise of other organs will often determine survival.

Referral for transplantation should only be made when conventional treatment has failed, and the anticipated prognosis is clearly worse than that offered by transplantation. If there is any suggestion of reversible ischaemic damage, coronary artery surgery should be seriously considered before transplantation.

Table 1 Indications for transplantation

Ischaemic cardiomyopathy
Idiopathic dilated cardiomyopathy
Congenital heart disease
Valvular heart disease
Restrictive/obstructive cardiomyopathy
Anthracycline toxicity

Table 2 Contraindications to transplantation

Absolute	Relative
Coexistent systemic illness with poor prognosis	Insulin-dependent diabetes Obesity
Active infection	Recent pulmonary embolism
Malignancy	Peptic ulcer disease
Elevated PVR > 8 Wood units	Elevated PVR > 4 Wood units
Severe peripheral or cerebrovascular disease	Psychosocial instability

PVR, pulmonary vascular resistance.

A list of standard exclusions is shown in Table 2. The number of patients who could benefit from cardiac transplantation is estimated to be 20–60 per million of population. The number of cardiac donors is approximately 6 per million in the UK, although a little higher in the USA, and up to 10 per million in some countries.

The cardiac donor

Most donors will have died from intracerebral or subarachnoid haemorrhage or head trauma. Positive serology for human immunodeficiency virus and hepatitis B, previous cardiac surgery, or a history of ischaemic heart disease are contraindications, as is prolonged ante-mortem hypotension. Donors into their fifties and sixties are acceptable if they have normal coronary arteries. Intravenous drug abuse, addiction to cocaine, and death due to tricyclic antidepressants or carbon monoxide poisoning are also contraindications. Management of the donor, matching between donor and recipient and perioperative management are described in OTM3, p. 2256.

Immunosuppression

Immunosuppression is achieved principally by corticosteroids, cyclosporin, and azathioprine. All are given in maximum tolerable doses for the first 4–6 weeks. Cyclosporin is monitored by measuring trough levels: doses of 5–10 mg/kg per day are required for levels of about 400 ng/litre, but deteriorating renal function often dictates a reduction in dose. For azathioprine a target leucocyte count of below 5000/mm^3 usually requires a dose of 1.5–3 mg/kg per day. Prednisolone is typically given in a dose of 1 mg/kg per day, reducing to 0.2 mg/kg per day after a few weeks. Steroids may be successfully stopped after 3 months in a proportion of patients.

Monitoring for rejection episodes

Acute rejection causes diastolic dysfunction of the ventricle with preservation of systolic function. Clinical clues are often sparse, with perhaps a third sound, elevated filling pressures, and occasionally atrial flutter. Non-invasive tests are not generally helpful. Monitoring of the adequacy of immunosuppression is achieved by regular transvenous endomyocardial biopsy.

Complications

Infection after transplantation remains a substantial risk, particularly in the early postoperative months. Later, despite excellent survival and functional rehabilitation there remains the problem of continuous immunosuppression and chronic rejection, usually manifested as accelerated coronary artery disease in the transplanted heart (see below). Almost all cardiac transplant recipients develop significant hypertension that in the past has been related to the use of cyclosporin. However, recipients of other organs, such as liver or lungs also given cyclosporin have a lower incidence of hypertension and there seems little doubt that a combination of pre-operative disease, denervation of the heart, and inappropriate fluid retention puts these patients at particular risk. Chronic immunosuppression increases the risk of malignancy. Apart from skin cancer, related to exposure to sunlight, there is an increased incidence of non-Hodgkin's lymphoma, nearly always of B-cell type and an uncontrolled response to latent Epstein–Barr virus (EBV) infection. Cyclosporin, and probably the other immunosuppressants, inhibit the suppressor T cells which usually exert control on EBV-infected lymphocytes. With loss of control these lymphocytes proliferate, usually at extranodal sites and often in association with the transplanted organ. Reduction of the immunosuppression together with high-dose intravenous acyclovir will usually result in shrinkage and disappearance of these lesions.

Coronary disease in the transplanted heart

Even in the absence of overt rejection there is probably continued immunological damage to the endothelium of the coronary arteries of the transplanted heart, which is the zone of contact with the recipient. This leads to subintimal hyperplasia and thickening of the wall of the artery, which can be detected as early as 6 weeks after transplantation and is progressive. By 5 years, 40–50 per cent of recipients will have developed angiographic evidence of this disease, and it will go on to be the most common late cause of death after transplantation.

This accelerated coronary disease differs substantially from typical atherosclerosis. It comprises a diffuse, symmetrical, and proliferating process resulting in cylindrical narrowing and involving intramuscular as well as epicardial vessels. It is not associated with pretransplant diagnosis, age of donor, blood pressure, lipids, or smoking. It does seem to be more severe in patients with a history of frequent early rejection episodes, lending credence to the immunological hypothesis of its origin. Because the transplanted heart undergoes complete denervation, angina seldom occurs and the usual presentation is either with sudden death or a silent myocardial infarction. Surveillance angiography remains the only effective means of diagnosis. Angioplasty for focal lesions has been described, but restenosis is frequent and the long-term benefit is questionable. The only effective treatment is retransplantation.

Results of transplantation

Most centres report a 1-year survival of 85–90 per cent and a 5-year survival of 75 per cent. Long-term experience is scanty but extrapolation of survival curves suggests that 50 per cent of patients will live 10 or 12 years after their transplant.

Further reading

Goldstein, D.J., Oz, M.C., and Rose, E.A. (1998). Implantable left ventricular assist devices. *New England Journal of Medicine*, **339**, 1522–33.

Hunt, S.A. (1998). Current status of cardiac transplantation. *Journal of the American Medical Association*, **280**, 1692–8.

Kobashigawa, J.A., Leaf, D.A., Lee, N., *et al.* (1999). A controlled trial of exercise rehabilitation after heart transplantation. *New England Journal of Medicine*, **340**, 272–7.

Chapter 2.4

The electrocardiogram

D. J. Rowlands

Normal electrocardiographic appearances

The basic electrocardiographic waveform

The basic electrocardiographic (ECG) waveform consists of three recognizable deflections termed 'P wave', 'QRS complex', and 'T wave' (Fig. 1). The P wave is the manifestation of atrial myocardial depolarization. Depolarization of the sinoatrial node is not recognizable and can only be inferred from the shape and direction of the P wave. The QRS complex is the manifestation of ventricular myocardial depolarization. The S–T segment and T wave represent ventricular myocardial repolarization. Atrial myocardial repolarization is indicated by the Ta wave, which is a small, asymmetrical negative wave following the P wave. The Ta wave is usually obscured by the QRS complex, which occurs at the same time. The Ta wave usually becomes easily recognizable during sinus tachycardia (especially during exercise) as it then increases in size and becomes a rounded negative wave beginning before the QRS complex and extending into the S–T segment. A prominent atrial repolarization wave occurring during an exercise stress test is frequently wrongly interpreted as S–T segment depression. The key to avoiding this error is to recognize that the negativity begins before the QRS complex.

QRS waveform nomenclature

The QRS complexes usually have the largest voltages and virtually always the highest frequency components of the various ECG deflections and usually consist of 'sharp', pointed deflections. The presence and relative size of the several possible components of the QRS complex may be indicated by a convention using combinations of the letters q, r, s, Q, R, and S (Fig. 2). If a given component is considered to be large, an UPPER CASE letter is used, if it is considered to be small a lower case letter is used.

The twelve conventional electrocardiogram leads

Unipolar, bipolar, and augmented leads

Leads I, II, and III are the bipolar limb leads. The remaining three limb leads and the six precordial leads are the unipolar V leads. All

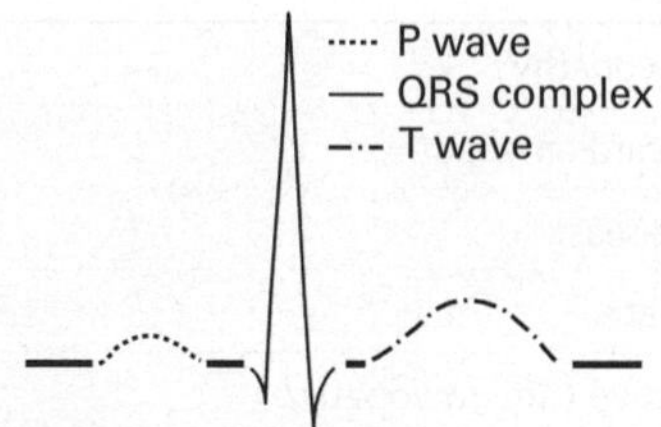

Fig. 1 The basic ECG waveform.

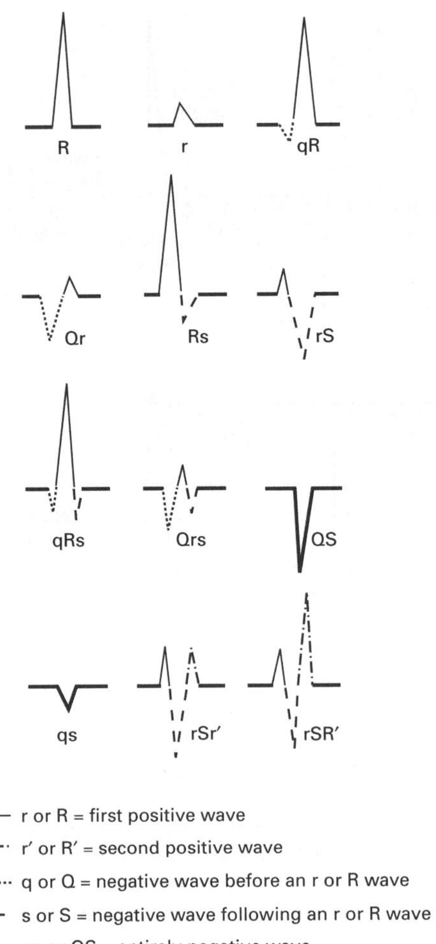

Fig. 2 QRS waveform nomenclature.

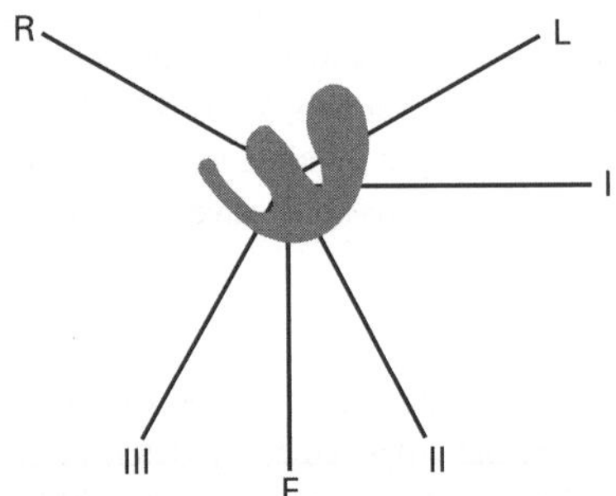

Fig. 3 The arrangement of the frontal plane leads. Note that leads II, III, and F are inferior to the heart, I and L are anterolateral to the heart, and R looks into the cavity of the heart
(reproduced, with permission, from Rowlands, 1991).

currently available ECG machines use augmented limb leads (i.e. they record aVR, aVL, and aVF as opposed to VR, VL, and VF).

The six limb leads (frontal plane leads)

The limb leads consist of the three bipolar leads (leads I, II, and III) and the three augmented, unipolar leads aVR, aVL, and aVF. Their orientation around the heart is illustrated in Fig. 3. The orientation of leads aVR, aVL, and aVF with respect to the heart is intuitively obvious because the limbs act as linear conductors (like wires). The left arm connection is therefore effectively 'looking at the heart' from the left shoulder, the right arm connection from the right shoulder, and the foot lead connection from the pelvic area. One practical consequence of this is that it does not matter whereabouts on any given limb the electrode is attached. The orientation of the bipolar leads with respect to the heart is not so obvious (because they are bipolar leads) but may be worked out from the known polarities of the conventional connections used in the bipolar leads. Thus, for example, because lead I is recorded with the left arm connected to the positive and the right arm to the negative terminal of the recorder, the position of lead I is effectively that obtained by subtracting the right arm vector from the left arm vector. To subtract vector R from vector L one reverses the direction of vector R and adds it to vector L. Inspection of Fig. 3 reveals that if this is done the resulting 'direction' of lead I is effectively horizontally to the left of the heart. In a similar manner it can be shown that the effective orientations of leads II and III with respect to the heart are as shown in Fig. 3.

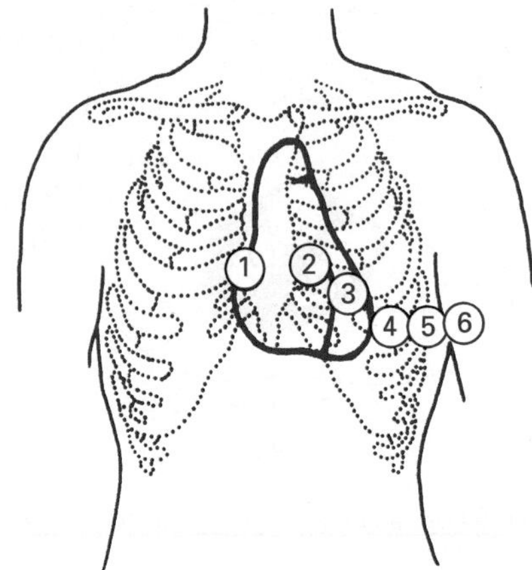

Fig. 4 The positions of the precordial leads. V_1, is located at the right sternal margin in the fourth intercostal space, V_2 at the left sternal margin at the fourth intercostal space, V_4 at the intersection of the left midclavicular line and left fifth intercostal space, V_3 mid-way between V_2 and V_4, V_5 at the intersection of the left anterior axillary line with a horizontal line through V_4, and V_6 at the intersection of the left midaxillary line with a horizontal line through V_4 and V_5
(reproduced, with permission, from Rowlands, 1991).

The six precordial leads (chest leads)

For each precordial lead, the positive (recording) terminal is connected to an electrode at an agreed site on the chest wall. As the connection to the negative terminal of the recorder is the 'indifferent' one formed by joining together leads R, L, and F, the chest leads are 'V' leads and are designated $V_{1'}$′, $V_{2'}$′, $V_{3'}$′, $V_{4'}$′, $V_{5'}$′, and $V_{6'}$′. As the torso, unlike the limbs, acts as a volume conductor, the waveform obtained depends critically on the siting of the recording electrode. The standard siting is shown in Fig. 4. The important relationships of the precordial leads to the cardiac chambers are shown in Fig. 5.

The normal electrocardiogram

Precordial leads—normal QRS appearances

QRS morphology

The QRS complex in V_1 typically shows a small initial positive wave followed by a larger negative wave and in V_6 a small initial negative wave followed by a large positive wave. In general the size of the initial positive wave (r or R) increases progressively from V_1 to V_6 (Fig. 6(a)). The direction of the initial part of the QRS is generally

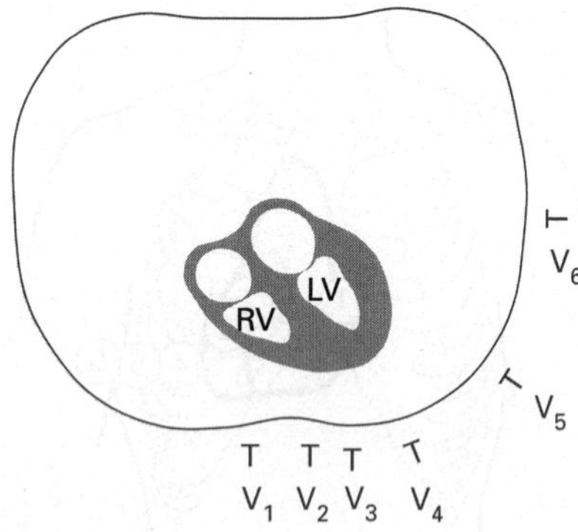

Fig. 5 The precordial leads and their important anatomical relationship to the main cardiac chambers
(reproduced, with permission, from Rowlands, 1991).

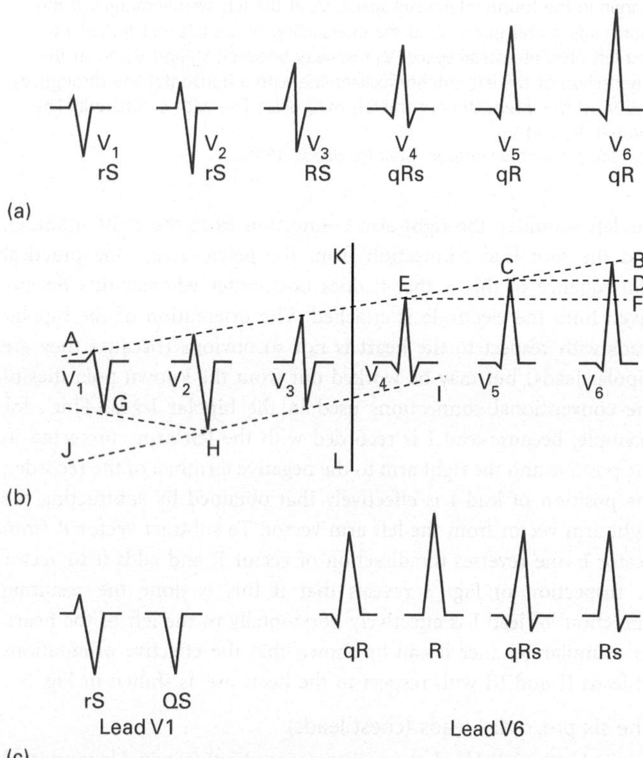

Fig. 6 Morphology of the precordial QRS complexes. (a) Typical normal morphology. (b) Normal variation in R wave amplitude and S wave depth. The R wave in each lead is usually larger than in the preceding lead from V1–V6 (line AB)—but it is quite normal for the R wave in V6 to be smaller than that in V5 (line CD) or for the R wave in V5 to be smaller than in V4, provided that the R wave in V6 is also smaller than that in V5 (line EF). The size of the S wave diminishes progressively across the leads (line JI), although that in V2 is often greater than that in V1 (line GHI). Leads before the line KL have an initial positive deflection and those after it a negative one, KL marking the transition zone between right and left ventricular configurations (reproduced, with permission, from Rowlands 1991). (c) Possible normal QRS configurations in V1 and V6.

upward (i.e. positive) in V_1–V_3 and downward (i.e. negative) in V_4–V_6. That is, V_1–V_3 show initial r waves and V_4–V_6 initial q waves. Leads showing an rS complex are being primarily influenced by right ventricular myocardium and leads showing a qR complex by left ventricular myocardium. The transition zone between right and left is normally between V_2 and V_4 (Fig. 6(b)). If the transition zone

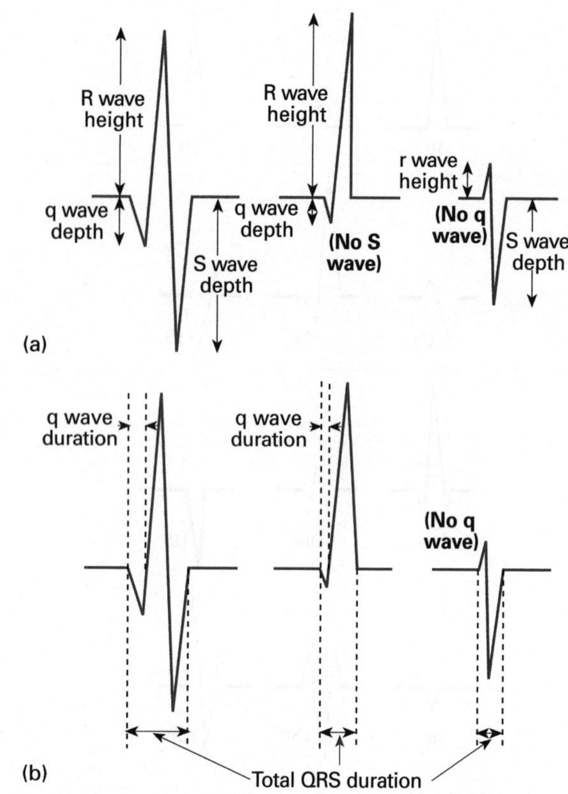

Fig. 7 The dimensions of constituent waves within QRS complexes. (a) Wave voltage measurements. (b) Wave duration measurements
(reproduced, with permission, from Rowlands, 1991).

occurs further to the left in the precordial series (for example between V_5 and V_6) the heart is said to be clockwise rotated. Conversely, if it is moved to the right, the heart is said to be counter-clockwise rotated. Clockwise and counter-clockwise rotation refer to a normal state of variability between one subject and another and are not in themselves indicative of abnormality. Although, V_1 usually shows an rS complex and V_6 a qR complex, it is also possible for V_1 to show a QS complex and for V_6 to show a monophasic R wave, a QRS complex or an Rs complex (Fig. 6(c)).

QRS dimensions

The dimensions of the individual waves of the precordial QRS complexes are of crucial importance in determining normality or otherwise. Figure 7 shows how measurements within the QRS complexes are obtained. The criteria for normality are:

1. *Minimum voltage*: at least one R wave in the precordial leads must exceed 8 mm in height.
2. *Maximum voltage*: (a) the tallest R wave in the left precordial leads must not exceed 27 mm; (b) the deepest S wave in the right precordial leads must not exceed 30 mm; (c) the sum of the tallest R wave in the left precordial leads and the deepest S wave in the right precordial leads must not exceed 40 mm.
3. *Maximum duration*: the total QRS duration in any one precordial lead must not exceed 0.10 s (two and a half small squares).
4. *q wave criteria*: (a) no precordial q wave must equal or exceed 0.04 (one small square); (b) precordial q waves must not have a depth greater than a quarter of the height of the R wave in the same lead and

5. *The ventricular activation time*, also known as 'intrinsic deflection time', in leads facing the left ventricle (i.e. showing qR complexes) must not exceed 0.04 (one small square).

Normal precordial T waves (adults only)

Lead V_1

In this lead 80 per cent of normal adults have upright T waves and 20 per cent have flat or inverted T waves. Inverted T waves in V_1 are only abnormal if they were known to be upright in a previous ECG.

Lead V_2

About 95 per cent of normal adults show upright T waves and 5 per cent have flat or inverted T waves in V_2. However, if the T wave in V_2 is inverted when it was formerly upright, it is abnormal. Further, if there is T wave inversion in V_2 with an upright T wave in V_1 the T wave in V_2 is abnormal.

Leads V_3–V_6

The T wave is normally upright in these leads. T wave inversion in V_4, V_5, or V_6 is always abnormal. Inversion in V_3 as well as in V_1 and V_2 may (rarely) be found in healthy young adults.

T wave size

There are no strict criteria for T wave size. In general the tallest precordial T wave is found in V_3 or V_4 and the smallest in V_1 and V_2 and the T wave should not be less than one-eighth and not more than two-thirds of the height of the preceding R wave in each of the leads V_3–V_6.

Normal precordial S–T segments

The S–T segment must not deviate by more than 1 mm above or below the isoelectric line in any precordial lead.

Normal precordial P waves

The P waves are usually upright from V_4 to V_6. Upright or biphasic P waves may occur in V_1 and V_2. If the P waves are biphasic, the negative (terminal) component of the P wave should have an area no greater than the positive (initial) component.

Limb leads—normal QRS appearances

Only three criteria determine the normality or otherwise of the QRS complexes in the limb leads:

(1) the size of any q waves in aVL, I, II, or aVF;

(2) the size of the R waves in aVL and aVF;

(3) the electrical axis of the heart.

Q wave size

Any q wave in leads I, II, or aVF must not exceed one-quarter the height of the ensuing R wave and must not equal or exceed 0.04 s in duration. Any q wave present in aVR or lead III should be ignored irrespective of its size. Q waves present in aVL should fulfil the same criteria as those in leads I, II, or aVF unless the frontal plane QRS axis is more positive than +60 degrees in which case large q waves in aVL are acceptable, as aVL is then a cavity lead.

R wave size

The R wave in aVL must not exceed 13 mm and that in aVF must not exceed 20 mm.

The frontal plane axis

The electrical axis of the heart must not lie outside the limits of –30 to +90 degrees (travelling clockwise). The significance and technique of determination of the electrical axis are described in larger texts.

Limb leads—normal S–T segments

Normal S–T segments do not deviate above or below the isoelectric line by more than 1 mm.

Limb leads—normal T waves

In general, the T waves and QRS complexes in the limb leads are concordant, i.e. when the QRS complexes are upright, the T waves are upright and vice versa. A normal T wave will always be negative in aVR and positive in I and II. T waves can be positive or negative in aVL, aVF, and II without necessarily indicating abnormality. A rough guide to assess normality of the T waves in the limb leads is:

(1) in any lead in which the QRS is predominantly upright, the T wave must be clearly upright and vice versa;

(2) in any lead in which the algebraic sum of QRS deflections is close to zero, the T wave may be positive or negative (though small in either case) or isoelectric (flat);

(3) the normal T wave is always upright in leads I and II.

Limb leads—normal P waves

Lead II normally shows the best P wave. In it, the normal P wave duration does not exceed 0.12 s and its height does not exceed 2.5 mm.

Electrocardiographic changes in myocardial hypertrophy

Left ventricular hypertrophy

Increased bulk of the left ventricle increases the voltage induced during left ventricular depolarization. This results in taller R waves in the left precordial leads and deeper S waves in the right precordial leads and in prolongation of the time taken to for the depolarization wave to travel from the endocardium to epicardium, i.e. it increases the ventricular activation time. In addition, secondary changes in depolarization alter the S–T segments and T waves. The ECG criteria for left ventricular hypertrophy are:

(1) at least one R wave in the left precordial leads exceeds 27 mm;

(2) at least one S wave in the right precordial leads exceeds 30 mm;

(3) the sum of the tallest R wave and the deepest S wave in the precordial leads exceeds 40 mm;

(4) the largest positive or negative deflection in the limb leads exceeds 20 mm;

(5) the intrinsic deflection time (ventricular activation time) exceeds 0.04 s;

(6) S–T segment depression and T wave inversion may occur in the left precordial leads and in those limb leads which face the left ventricle.

The presence of one or more of the above abnormalities indicates the presence of left ventricular hypertrophy only provided that the total QRS duration does not exceed 0.10 s. Left ventricular hypertrophy is a graded, rather than an all-or-none diagnosis. The greater the number of criteria fulfilled, the more confident one can be of the diagnosis. The voltage criteria have the greatest sensitivity and the intrinsic deflection time the greatest specificity. Caution should be exercised when diagnosing left ventricular hypertrophy on the basis of voltage criteria alone, especially if the patient is slim. An example of clear-cut ECG changes of left ventricular hypertrophy is shown (Fig. 8).

Right ventricular hypertrophy

Increased bulk of the right ventricle gives rise to higher voltages during right ventricular depolarization, increasing the size of the positive deflection in the right precordial leads. In addition, it shifts the electrical axis towards the right and changes the S–T segments and T waves, in leads facing the right ventricle, because of secondary changes in the repolarization process. The ECG criteria for right ventricular hypertrophy are:

(1) a positive deflection equal to or greater than the negative deflection in V_1 (RS, Rs, qR, rR′) in the presence of a normal total QRS duration;

(2) a mean frontal plane QRS axis more positive than +90 degrees;

(3) S–T segment depression and T wave inversion in right precordial leads.

The more features present, the more convincing is the ECG evidence for right ventricular hypertrophy but, in general, the combination of a dominant positive deflection of the QRS in V_1 and an abnormal degree of right axis deviation (axis more positive than +90 degrees) establishes the diagnosis. An example is shown in Fig. 9.

Atrial hypertrophy

The ECG changes in left atrial hypertrophy reflect an increase in the voltage and duration of the left atrial depolarization wave. As the terminal part of the normal P wave is produced by left atrial depolarization, the total P wave duration is prolonged. In addition, the P wave tends to be bifid in lead II and biphasic in V_1. In V_1 the area of the (terminal) negative component exceeds the area of the (initial) positive component (see Fig. 10). Right atrial hypertrophy increases the peak voltage of the P wave, usually best seen in lead II, where P wave voltage is abnormal when it equals or exceeds 3 mm.

Bundle branch block

Total failure of conduction in the right or left branches of the bundle of His can only be diagnosed with confidence from the appearances in the precordial leads, although there are also changes in the appearances of the limb leads.

Right bundle branch block

The primary change is a delay in depolarization in the right ventricular free wall. This results in the development of a second positive wave in right ventricular leads (and a second negative wave in left ventricular leads), and prolongs the total QRS duration. The essential ECG features of right bundle branch block are:

(1) a total QRS duration of 0.12 s or more; and

(2) the presence of a secondary positive wave in V_1 (rsR′, rR′).

In addition, secondary changes occur, but these are not in themselves essential for the definitive diagnosis. These include:

(3) deep and slurred S waves in lead I, aVL, and V_4–V_6; and

(4) secondary S–T, T changes in leads V_1–V_3.

An example of the appearance of right bundle branch block is shown in Fig. 11.

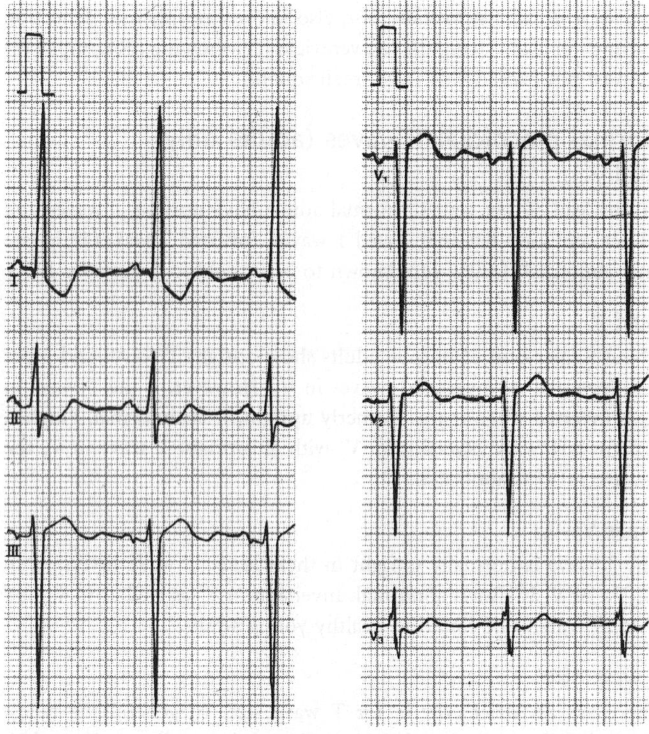

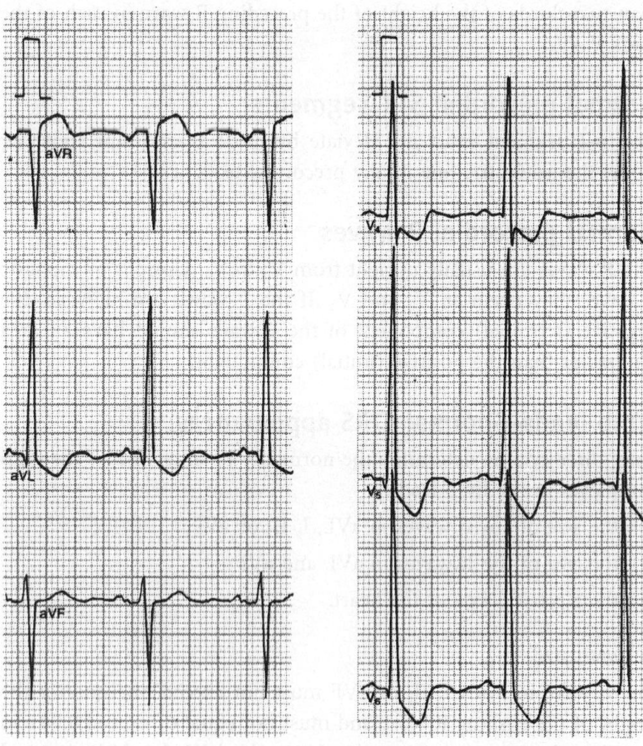

Fig. 8 Left ventricular hypertrophy. There is evidence also of left atrial hypertrophy
(reproduced, with permission, from Rowlands, 1991).

Left bundle branch block

This induces more extensive change in the ECG appearance. Not only is depolarization of the free wall of the left ventricle delayed,

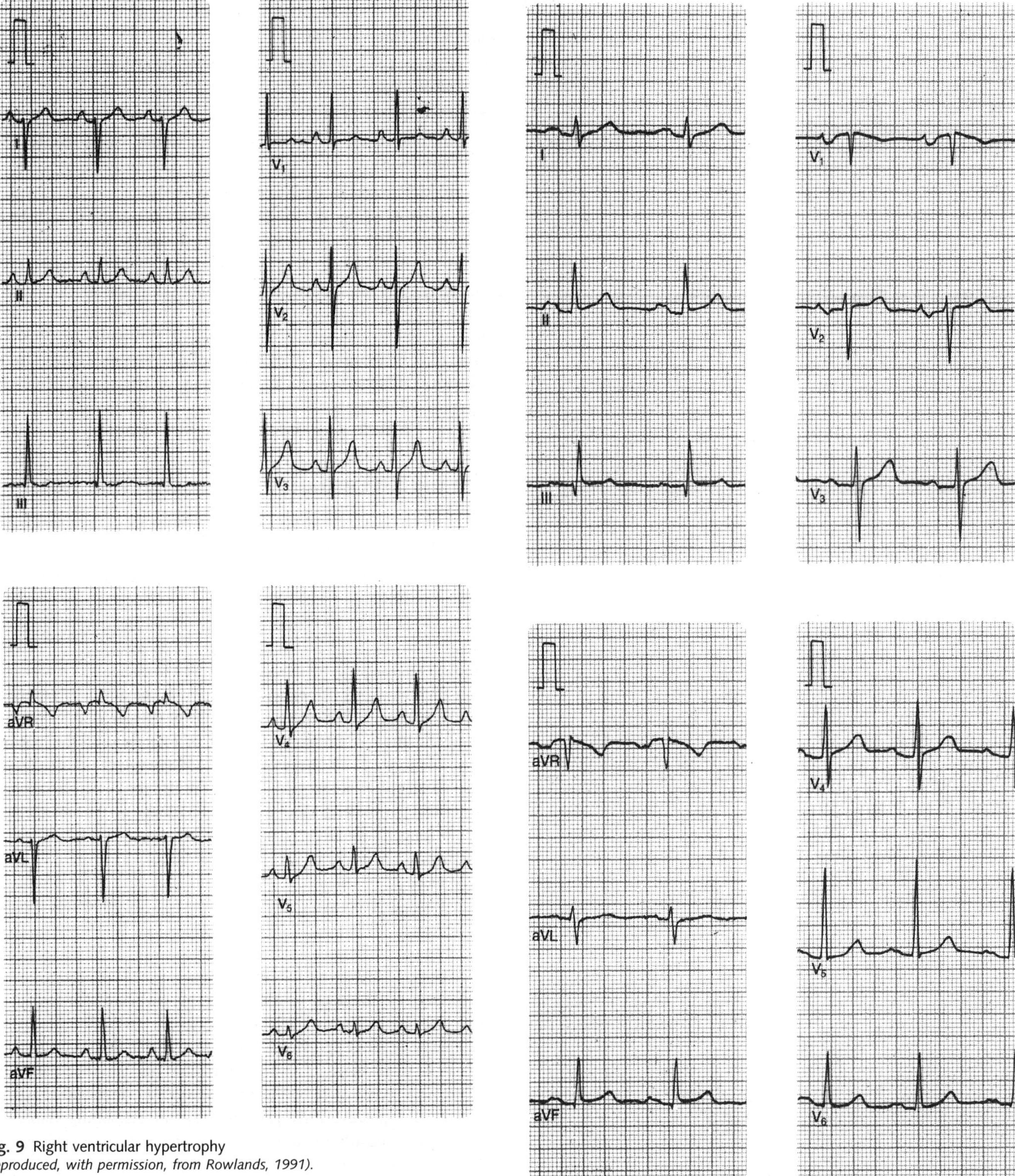

Fig. 9 Right ventricular hypertrophy
(reproduced, with permission, from Rowlands, 1991).

Fig. 10 Left atrial hypertrophy. Broad, bifid P waves in lead II. Biphasic P waves in V_1, with dominant negative component
(reproduced, with permission, from Rowlands, 1991).

but also the direction of depolarization of the interventricular septum is from right to left instead of from left to right as in the normal ECG. This reversal gives rise to widespread and major alterations in the QRS complexes in every lead. The diagnostic criteria for left bundle branch block are:

(1) a total QRS duration equal to or in excess of 0.12 s;

(2) absence of the normal (septal) q waves in lead I, aVL, and V_4–V_6;

(3) the absence of a secondary r wave in V_1.

This last criterion is necessary to prevent confusion in cases of right bundle branch block, which gives a QRS deviation of 0.12 s or

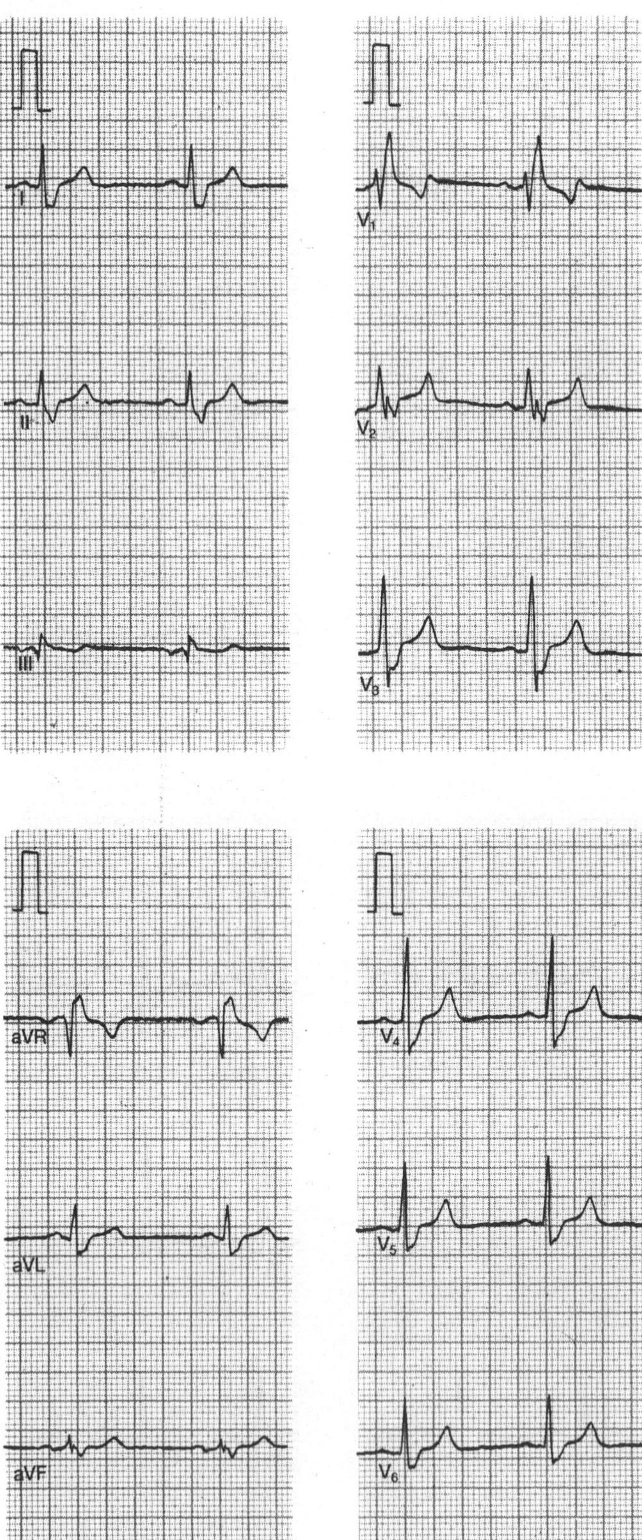

Fig. 11 Right bundle branch block
(reproduced, with permission, from Rowlands, 1991).

more, occurring in the presence of pronounced clockwise cardiac rotation, which gives loss of q waves in left ventricular leads. The finding of a secondary r wave in V_1 in the presence of an abnormally wide QRS complex indicates the presence of right bundle branch block. Secondary changes also inevitably occur but these are not diagnostic. These include:

(4) secondary S–T depression and T wave inversion in leads I, aVL, and V_4–V_6;

(5) broad QS waves in V_1–V_3;

(6) notching of the R waves giving rise to rsR′ or M-shaped QRS complexes;

(7) broad, R waves in leads I, aVL, and V_4–V_6.

An example of the ECG appearances in left bundle branch block is shown in Fig. 12. The changes in left bundle branch block so disturb the normal pattern of the ECG that none of the usual criteria can be applied for determining any other abnormality of the QRS complexes, S–T segments, or P waves. When left bundle branch block is present, a diagnosis of right or left ventricular hypertrophy, myocardial ischaemia or infarction, or of non-specific changes in the S–T segments and T waves cannot easily or reliably be made (see under Diagnosis of acute myocardial infarction in the presence of left bundle branch block (below) for further discussion).

The electrocardiogram in ischaemic heart disease

QRS changes in myocardial infarction

Inappropriate low R wave voltage and abnormal q waves indicate infarction. These two changes represent parts of the same process. The development of increased negativity (abnormal q waves) and the reduction in the normal positivity (loss of R wave height) of QRS complexes in the precordial leads each result from a loss of underlying viable muscle, with a consequent reduction in the normally generated positive voltage. When there is full thickness infarction in an area underlying the precordial leads there is total loss of the positive deflection and a totally negative wave (QS complex) occurs. This is a result of depolarization of the posterior wall of the ventricle travelling (posteriorly) from endocardium to epicardium in the normal way and no longer swamped by the usual simultaneous and dominant depolarization towards the exploring electrode of the anterior wall of the ventricle.

The normal precordial QRS complexes show a progressive increase in the R wave height from V_1 to V_6 (Fig. 13). In the presence of infarction of part of the left ventricle, the positive waves overlying the necrotic area will be reduced in size (Fig. 14). Loss in R wave height can only be used as a criterion for myocardial infarction if either: (1) larger, normal R waves are visible on both sides of the infarcted zone, or (2) previous ECGs are available demonstrating the normal R wave height for that particular lead in that particular subject. If a major part of the thickness of the myocardial wall is infarcted, the positive wave generated by any remaining viable left ventricular myocardium underlying the electrode is insufficient to overcome the negative deflection induced by the normal depolarization of the interventricular septum from left to right and of the free wall of the right ventricle (or the posterior wall of the left ventricle) from endocardium to epicardium. In this situation an abnormal q wave will develop. In the precordial leads, a q wave is abnormal if its duration is equal to or in excess of 0.04 s or if its depth is greater than one-quarter the height of the ensuing R wave in that lead. In Fig. 14, the q wave in V_4 satisfies this criterion. If the infarction involves the full thickness of the ventricular wall, no R wave is generated and an entirely negative (QS) wave develops (Fig.

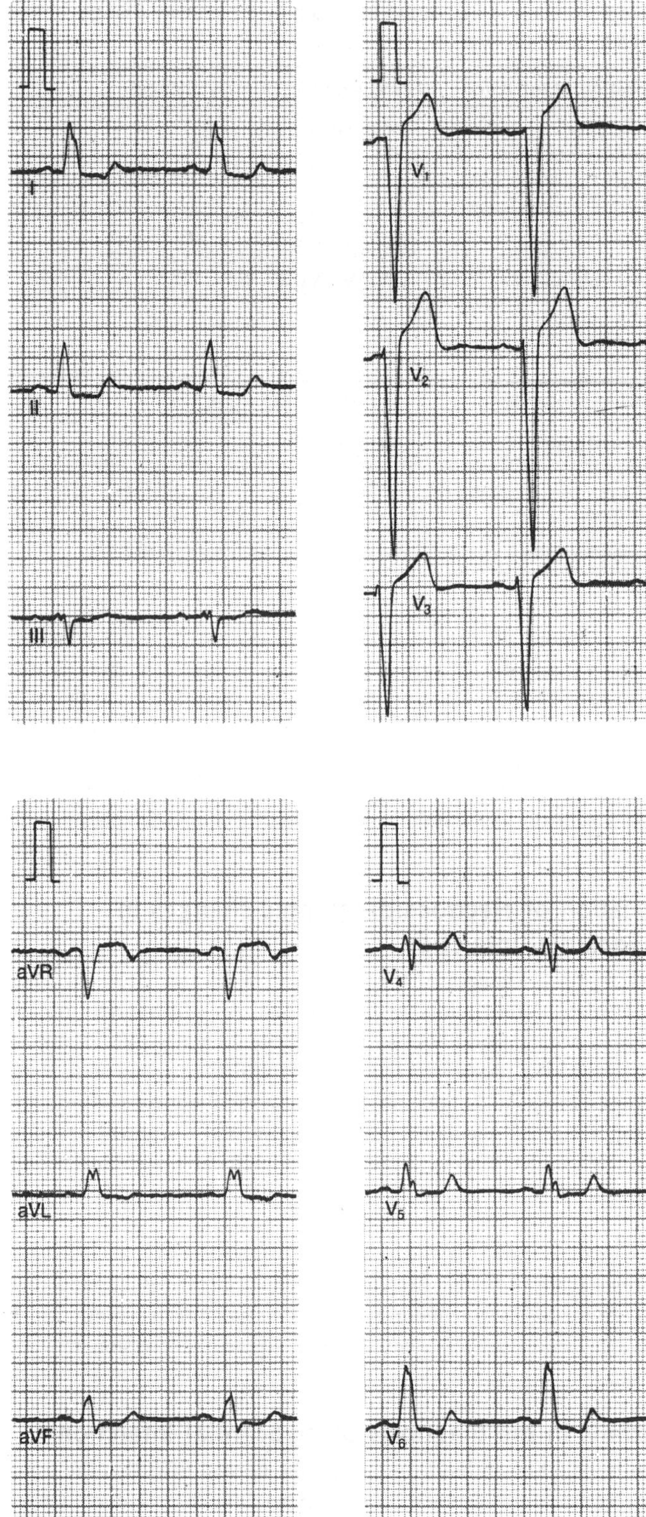

Fig. 12 Left bundle branch block
(reproduced, with permission, from Rowlands, 1991).

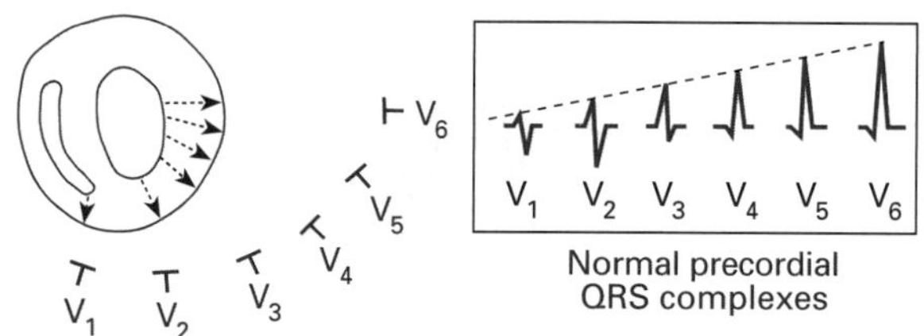

Fig. 13 Normal R wave progression in the precordial series
(reproduced, with permission, from Rowlands, 1991).

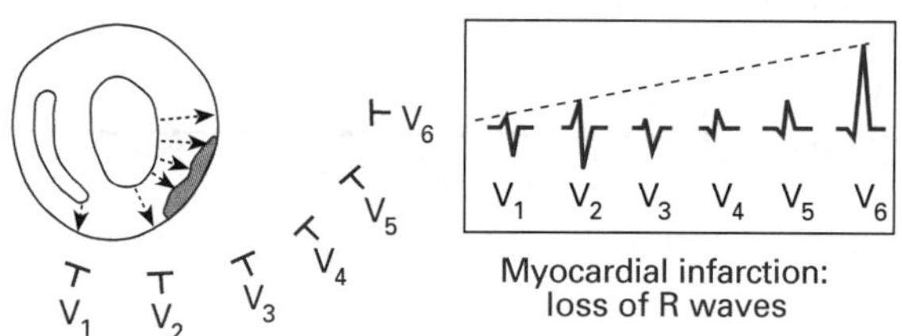

Fig. 14 Loss of R wave height in myocardial infarction. The R wave height is reduced in leads V_3–V_5
(reproduced, with permission, from Rowlands, 1991).

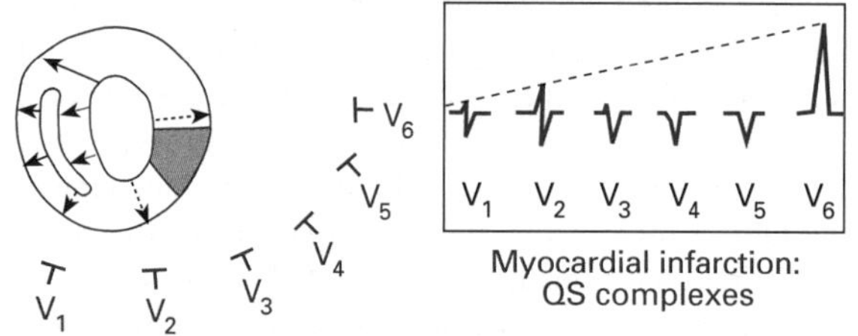

Fig. 15 Transmural myocardial infarction. QS complexes are seen from V_3 to V_5
(reproduced, with permission, from Rowlands, 1991).

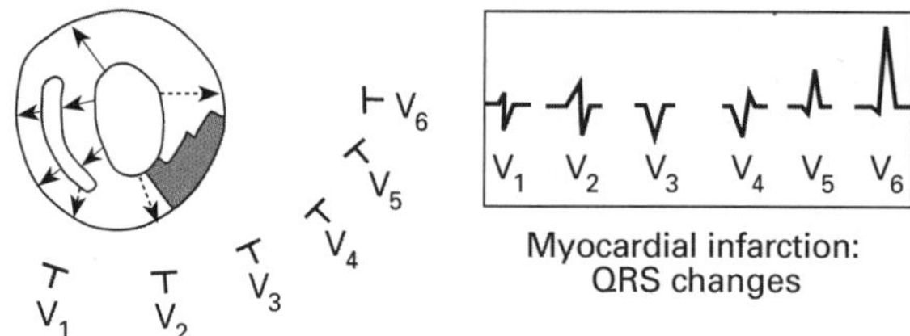

Fig. 16 Varying thickness infarction
(reproduced, with permission, from Rowlands, 1991).

15). Figure 16 shows the appearances produced in the precordial leads when infarcts of varying thickness occur under each of three precordial electrodes. The QRS complex in V3 is of QS type and indicates transmural infarction at this site. The appearances in V_4 indicate a substantial loss of myocardium underlying that electrode. The q wave is abnormal in duration and depth. The appearances in V_5 indicate a thinner zone of infarction. The q wave is not, in itself, abnormal but the R wave height is less than would be predicted from the height of the R waves present in V_2 and V_6.

The diagnosis of myocardial infarction in the limb leads depends entirely on the presence of abnormal q waves. q waves of any size may be seen in the normal ECG in aVR and in lead III. In leads I, II, and aVF, q waves equal to or greater than 0.04 s in duration or with a depth in excess of 1/4 the height of the ensuing R wave are abnormal and, unless ventricular pre-excitation or a defect of intraventricular conduction is known to be present, indicate myocardial infarction. The same is also true of abnormal q waves in aVL, except when the mean frontal plane QRS axis is equal to or more positive than +60 degrees; in this situation aVL becomes a cavity lead like aVR.

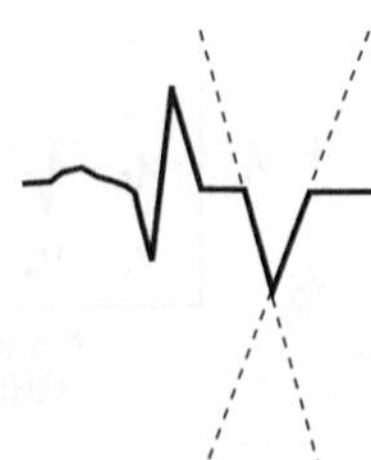

Fig. 17 Deep symmetrical T wave inversion. This is not truly specific but is typically found in association with myocardial ischaemia or infarction *(reproduced, with permission, from Rowlands, 1991).*

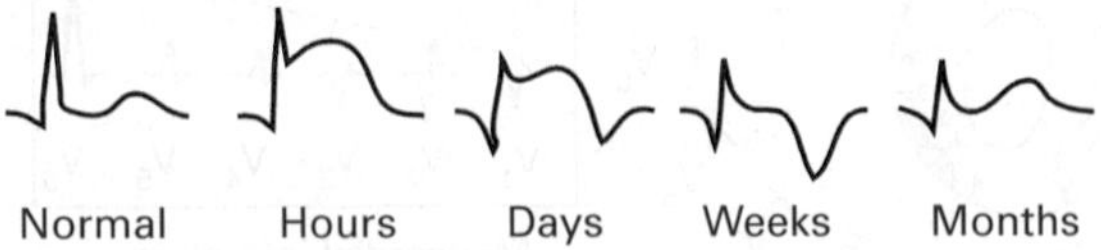

Fig. 18 Sequential changes in acute myocardial infarction *(reproduced, with permission, from Rowlands, 1991).*

S–T segment changes of infarction

Only changes in the QRS complexes provide definitive evidence of infarction, but in the acute stages S–T segment shift occurs. This is evidence of injury to, rather than infarction of, the myocardium. Thus, although in the vast majority of cases the development of typical S–T segment elevation is followed by the development of definitive QRS changes, occasionally S–T segment changes will revert to normal within hours or days. The essential change of myocardial injury is deviation of the S–T segment above the isoelectric line which must be in excess of 1 mm to be significant. Minor degrees of S–T segment elevation in the right precordial leads are very common in normal ECGs and up to 2 mm may be accepted as normal in V_1 and V_2. Significant S–T segment elevation occurs in transmural and subepicardial infarction in leads facing the infarct. S–T segment depression occurs in leads facing the infarct when it is subendocardial. S–T segment depression also occurs as a reciprocal change (see below) in leads opposite to those showing the primary changes of acute infarction.

T wave changes of infarction

These include flattened, diphasic, and inverted (negative) T waves. None of these is specific. While they are always abnormal in leads V_4–V_6 and in those limb leads showing clearly upright QRS complexes, they may be caused by factors other than infarction or ischaemia, including electrolyte changes, digitalis effect, pericarditis, myocarditis, changes in body position, and changes in oesophageal temperature. T wave changes are never, in themselves, reliable indicators of infarction, although characteristic T wave changes do occur, the most typical of which is the development of deep, symmetrically inverted T waves (Fig. 17).

The sequence of electrocardiographic changes in infarction

Any combination of the QRS, S–T segment, and T wave changes described above may occur in relation to acute infarction but commonly a typical sequence of changes can be recognized (Fig. 18). Typically, S–T segment elevation (which is convex upwards) appears within hours of the onset. At this stage no change in the QRS complex can be recognized. Within 1–3 days, reduction in the R wave height occurs, abnormally deep and broad q waves develop, some reduction in the extent of S–T segment elevation occurs, and there is development of T wave inversion. After the first few days the S–T segment elevation disappears completely. The deep, symmetrical T wave inversion typically persists for weeks before reverting to normal. The changes in the QRS complex are usually permanent but may occasionally disappear if the infarct is small and the scar subsequently shrinks.

Table 1 Location of myocardial infarction by the primary changes in the 12-lead electrocardiogram

Location of infarction	Leads showing primary changes
	Typical changes
Anteroseptal	V_1, V_2, V_3
Anterior	V_2, V_3, V_4
Anterolateral	V_4, V_5, V_6, I, aVL
Extensive anterior	V_1, V_2, V_3, V_4, V_5, V_6, I, aVL
High lateral	aVl (plus high precordial leads)
Inferior	II, III, aVF
Inferolateral (apical)	II, III, aVF, V_5, V_6, I, aVL
Inferoseptal	II, III, aVF, V_1, V_2, V_3
	Other changes
Posterior	V_1, V_2
Subendocardial	Any lead (usually multiple leads)

Location of electrocardiographic changes in myocardial infarction

Primary ECG changes of the type described above occur in leads facing the infarct. It follows that the leads in which such primary changes occur indicate the location of the infarct (Table 1), but in addition to the primary changes, 'reciprocal' changes occur in leads opposite those facing the infarction. These are the inverse of primary changes (e.g. S–T segment depression instead of S–T segment elevation and tall, pointed T waves instead of symmetrical T wave inversion). The inferior limb leads (II, III, and aVF) are reciprocal to the anterior leads (the precordial leads, lead I, and aVL) and vice versa.

Subendocardial infarction does not always produce recognizable changes in the ECG and such changes as do occur are usually apparent only in the S–T segments or T waves. Persistent deep symmetrical T wave inversion or persistent flat S–T segment depression may be found.

Pitfalls in the diagnosis of myocardial infarction

Left bundle branch block so distorts the normal ECG that the usual criteria for the diagnosis of myocardial infarction are no longer applicable. In the presence of ventricular pre-excitation neither left branch bundle block nor myocardial infarction should be diagnosed by the non-expert.

Diagnosis of acute myocardial infarction in the presence of left bundle branch block

The three most reliable criteria for the diagnosis of acute myocardial infarction in the presence of pre-existing left bundle branch block are:

(i) at least one lead shows 1 mm or more of ST segment elevation concordant with the QRS complex (i.e. in the same direction as the dominant direction of the QRS);

(ii) ST segment of at least 4 mm and discordant with the QRS;

(iii) ST depression of 1 mm or more in V_1, V_2, or V_3.

Ambulatory electrocardiography (Holter monitoring)

This technique permits long-term ECG recording in patients during their normal, everyday activity. It is useful in the detection, diagnosis, and quantification of arrhythmias, the evaluation of anti-arrhythmic therapy, and in detecting pacemaker malfunction. It may also be useful in the recognition of the intermittent myocardial ischaemia from changes in the configuration of the S–T segments and T waves.

The most common equipment used records over 24 h the record then being analysed by a variety of techniques much helped by the computer programs. There are also systems available for brief recording of the ECG following recognition by the patient of any possible significant symptom. Such intermittent devices are particularly useful when it is difficult to detect otherwise an arrhythmia causing paroxysmal symptoms.

Patient diary

An important part of ambulatory monitoring is the daily log kept by patients of all relevant activities and symptoms and the times when various medications (especially anti-arrhythmic drugs) are taken. Most recorders are equipped with an event marker which the patient is instructed to press when any relevant symptoms occur. Events coincidental with these symptoms and the timing of these symptoms should be logged in the diary.

Normal database and artefacts

Normal, healthy subjects at rest (and especially during sleep) not uncommonly demonstrate profound sinus bradycardia (35–40 per min), sinus arrhythmia with R–R intervals of up to 2 s, the Wenckebach phenomenon (Mobitz type I second-degree atrioventricular block), junctional escape beats, and occasional atrial and ventricular premature beats. However, some arrhythmias are not known to occur in normal subjects and are always significant. These include Mobitz type II second degree atrioventricular block, ventricular tachycardia, and complete heart block. Brief episodes of atrial fibrillation not uncommonly occur without any patient awareness. S–T segment shifts may be artefactual unless the low frequency response of the recording equipment is of the highest calibre, but with top class equipment primary, spontaneous (commonly 'silent', i.e. painless) ischaemic S–T segment shift can be recognized.

Artefactual arrhythmias' may occur from inadequate skin preparation, poor electrode localization or securement or from inadequate recorder or playback quality. A transient loss of signal (as a result of electrode movement) can mimic asystole and sinus pauses and intermittent heartblock can be mimicked by transient slowing or sticking of the tape during playback. Pseudotachycardia can occur because of slowing of the tape speed during recording in cases of battery depletion, recognized because the heart rate progressively increases towards the end of the recording and because the P waves, QRS complexes, and T waves all become progressively narrower at the same rate as the R–R interval appears to shorten.

Although a 24-h ambulatory record represents a considerable advance in the magnitude of data collection compared with a 12-lead ECG it still represents a very small time window and has, for example, only a 1 in 30 chance of catching an event which occurs monthly.

Further reading

MacFarlane, P.W. and Lawrie, T.D.V. (1989). *Comprehensive electrocardiology.* Pergamon Press, Oxford.

Rowlands, D.J. (1991). *Clinical electrocardiography.* Gower Medical Publishing, London.

Sgarbossa, E.B. and Galen, W. (1998). Electrocardiology. In *Textbook of cardiovascular medicine,* (ed. E.J. Topol). Lippincott-Raven.

Cardiac arrhythmias

Chapter 2.5

Cardiac arrhythmias

S. M. Cobbe and A. C. Rankin

Arrhythmias may occur in the absence of cardiac disease, but are more commonly associated with structural heart disease or external provocative factors.

Disorders of impulse formation and conduction

Bradyarrhythmias may result from impairment of impulse formation or conduction in the sinoatrial node or of conduction in the atrioventricular (AV) node due to factors such as sympathetic withdrawal, vagal stimulation, or drugs. Intrinsic degenerative disease of the sinus node may also result in failure of normal sinus rhythm. Idiopathic conducting system disease results in impairment of AV conduction, which may also be affected by myocardial ischaemia, infarction, infiltration, or surgical trauma.

Mechanisms of arrhythmogenesis

The exact mechanism responsible for cardiac tachyarrhythmias is not known in all cases. There is commonly a complex interaction between an underlying substrate such as previous myocardial infarction, a triggering event such as an extrasystole and modulating influences of which sympathetic stimulation and myocardial ischaemia are the most important. The principal mechanisms responsible for tachyarrhythmias are those of abnormal automaticity, triggered activity, and re-entry (Fig. 1).

Automaticity

Abnormal automaticity is defined as an inappropriate increase in the rate of discharge of a tissue having pacemaker properties (Fig. 1(a)), most commonly seen in the presence of ischaemia, sympathetic stimulation, or drug toxicity, especially digoxin. Automatic tachycardias are not inducible by extrasystoles.

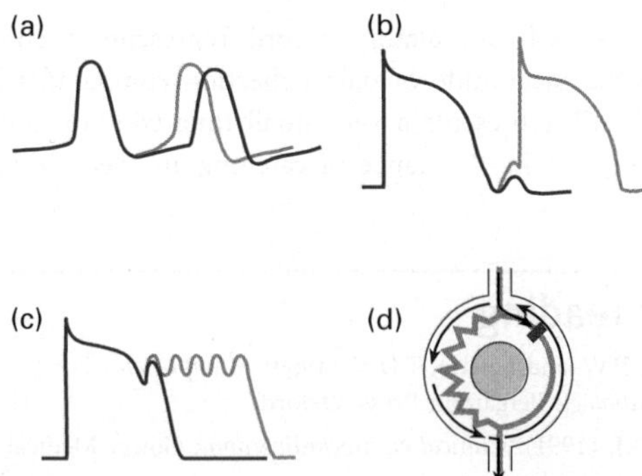

Fig. 1 Mechanisms of arrhythmias. (a) Increased automaticity; (b) triggered activity due to delayed after-depolarizations; (c) triggered activity due to early after depolarizations; (d) re-entry circuit. See text for details.

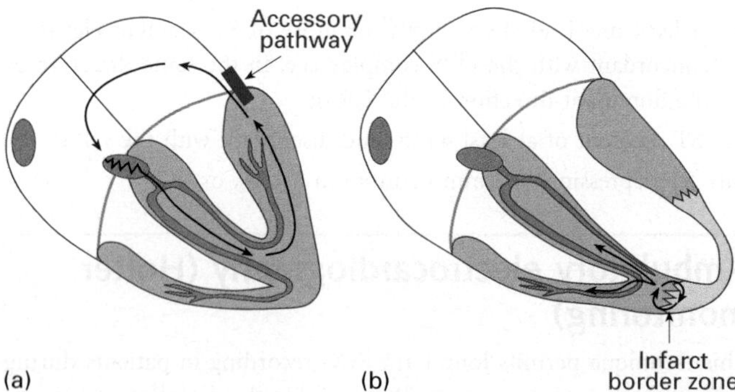

Fig. 2 Clinical examples of re-entry tachycardias. (a) Macro re-entry circuit involving an accessory pathway, which results in atrioventricular re-entry tachycardia; (b) micro re-entry circuit at the border zone of a myocardial infarction.

Triggered activity

This refers to automaticity resulting from external stimulation, and may arise in tissues which do not demonstrate physiological automaticity. Its relevance to clinical arrhythmias is uncertain, but some do behave in a manner consistent with triggered activity. Two forms of depolarization cause triggered activity *in vitro*. Delayed after-depolarizations are seen as small, subthreshold depolarizations after full repolarization of the action potential 1 (Fig. 1(b)). Their amplitude is increased by tachycardia or intracellular calcium overload, and may reach a level at which a spontaneous action potential is generated, potentially initiating a sustained tachycardia. Delayed after depolarizations are the likely mechanism of digitoxic arrhythmias. Early after-depolarizations, in contrast, are seen during the plateau phase of the action potential, prior to repolarization (Fig. 1(c)), and are more evident at slow heart rates, particularly in the presence of hypokalaemia and hypomagnesaemia. Drugs that prolong myocardial repolarization (class IA and class III antiarrhythmics, tricyclic antidepressants, organophosphorus insecticides, and many others) predispose to the appearance of early after-depolarizations *in vitro*. These agents are associated with the acquired long QT syndrome and the arrhythmia of torsades de pointes (see below).

Re-entry

The majority of sustained tachycardias, atrial, junctional or ventricular, arise by re-entry. The establishment of a re-entry tachycardia requires the presence of a potential circuit comprising two limbs with different refractoriness and conduction properties (Fig. 1(d)). A premature beat may result in the development of block in one limb of the circuit, while the activity is conducted by the other. If this conduction is sufficiently slow, the tissue distal to the site of block in the other limb is no longer refractory on the arrival of the depolarizing wavefront and conducts the activity retrogradely. This, in turn, results in re-activation of the slowly conducting pathway and thus a circus movement tachycardia is established. Macro re-entry describes a re-entry circuit over a large area, such as in the presence of an accessory pathway (Fig. 2(a)). In contrast, micro re-entry may occur in a relatively small area, for example, when normal myocardium is adjacent to the border zone of an old infarction in which conduction velocity is slowed (Fig. 2(b)).

Symptoms of arrhythmias

Symptoms of tachyarrhythmias depend on a variety of factors including the rate, its difference from the patient's sinus rate, the degree of irregularity of the rhythm, and the presence or absence of underlying cardiac disease. A low cardiac output may cause syncope. Other symptoms include a feeling of rapid palpitation, angina, or dyspnoea. Paroxysmal supraventricular tachycardia may be associated with polyuria due to release of atrial natriuretic peptide. Ectopic beats are commonly asymptomatic, but may produce a sensation of the heart 'missing a beat' often followed by a bump in the chest due to the more powerful post-ectopic beat.

Bradyarrhythmias may cause sudden death, syncope (Stokes–Adams attacks) or dizziness. Continuous bradycardia without asystolic pauses may produce fatigue, lethargy, dyspnoea, or mental impairment.

Table 1 Principles of ECG diagnosis of arrhythmias

Obtain 12-lead or multichannel recordings if possible	
Atrial activity	P waves visible? Normal P wave morphology and axis? Flutter/fibrillation waves? Atrial rate?
Ventricular activity	Ventricular rate? Regular or irregular? Normal QRS morphology and duration? Bundle branch block or bizarre QRS morphology? Variation in QRS morphology/axis?
Atrioventricular relationship	PR interval—fixed or varied? Retrograde P waves? Atrial versus ventricular rate?

Investigation of arrhythmias

Clinical assessment must include a detailed description of symptoms, precipitating factors (e.g. exercise, alcohol), and a search for underlying heart disease.

Electrocardiography

The key to diagnosis is to record a high-quality electrocardiogram (ECG) during the arrhythmia (Table 1). Holter monitoring (see Chapter 2.4) can provide records over 24–48 h and also allows analysis of heart rate variability, a reduction in which appears to be predictive of sudden death. Infrequent arrhythmias can be documented using

Table 2 Classification of antiarrhythmic drug activity

	ECG effect				Tissue effect			
	HR	PR	QRS	QT	SA node	Atrium	AV node	Ventricle
Class Ia	0	0/–	+	++	0	++	–	++/– –
Ib	0	0	0	0/–	0	0	0	++/–
Ic	0	+	++	+	0	++	0/+	++/– –
Class II	–	+	0	0	++	++	++	+/0
Class III	0/–	0/+	0	++	0/+	++	0/+	++/– –
Class IV	0/–	+	0	0	0/+	0/–	++	0/+
Digoxin	0/–	+	0	0	0/+	0/–	++	0/–
Adenosine	–	+	0	0	++	0/–	++	0/+

ECG effect: +, increases; –, decreases; 0, no effect; HR, heart rate.

Tissue effect: +, antiarrhythmic activity; –, potential adverse or proarrhythmic effect; 0, no effect.

patient activated recorders. High resolution ECG, using signal averaging to reduce background noise, may reveal areas of slow conduction which might allow re-entrant-ventricular arrhythmias.

Cardiac electrophysiological study

More detailed investigation requires invasive methods. Multipolar electrodes are inserted to record from the atrium, ventricle, His bundle, and from the coronary sinus if accessory pathways are suspected. The site of conduction delays may be identified, but the principal indication is the evaluation of tachyarrhythmias. Sustained arrhythmias may be initiated and terminated by extrastimuli, and their pattern of activation can be studied in detail. Programmed stimulation of tachycardias can be used to assess the efficiency of antiarrhythmic drugs.

Management of arrhythmias

Antiarrhythmic drug therapy

All antiarrhythmic drugs have potentially serious side-effects. They may worsen arrhythmias or produce new ones, possibly life-threatening. Prediction of the efficacy of a given drug for a given arrhythmia is imprecise and therapy is begun on the basis of trial and error, supported if necessary by more detailed investigation.

The Vaughan Williams classification of antiarrhythmic drug action is based on effects on the cardiac action potential, but many agents have multiple actions, the net result of which cannot be predicted easily. Furthermore, the classification is based on drug effects in isolated tissue, and does not predict effects mediated indirectly via the autonomic nervous system. The ECG features of the major classes of antiarrhythmic drug activity and the principal sites of action are listed in Table 2. Individual drugs are described in Table 3.

Class I activity

Class I drugs act by inhibition of the rapid inward sodium current and have local anaesthetic activity. Ia agents cause lengthening of action potential duration, and have intermediate effects on the onset and recovery kinetics of the sodium channel and hence on intracardiac conduction. Ib agents shorten the cardiac action potential duration, and have very rapid offset kinetics which result in minimal slowing of normal intracardiac conduction. Ic drugs have no major effect on action potential duration, but produce the most long-lasting effect on cardiac sodium channel kinetics, and the most marked slowing of intracardiac conduction.

Class II activity

Class II drugs antagonize the arrhythmogenic effects of catecholamines.

Class III activity

Drugs of this class lengthen the cardiac action potential duration and hence effective refractory period. They have a broad spectrum of activity against atrial, supraventricular, and ventricular arrhythmias. Several pure class III drugs are under clinical evaluation and are likely to be licensed in the near future. Amiodarone is a complex agent which has class I, II, III, and IV antiarrhythmic actions. Sotalol is a non-selective β-adrenoceptor antagonist which also possesses class III activity. Bretylium is a sympathetic neuronal blocker which acts by initial release of noradrenaline from the sympathetic nerve terminal. It has moderate class III activity.

Class IV activity

Class IV drugs reduce the inward calcium current in sinoatrial and AV nodal tissues. The effects are almost exclusively on AV nodal conduction, where slowing may interrupt a re-entry tachycardia involving the AV node, or slow the ventricular response in atrial fibrillation (**AF**).

Digoxin

The antiarrhythmic activity appears to be mediated predominantly via vagal stimulation. There is slowing of AV nodal conduction which may terminate or prevent the initiation of tachycardias involving the AV node, or slow the ventricular rate in AF. As vagal tone is withdrawn during exercise, the effect in slowing the ventricular rate in AF is less evident on effort than at rest.

Adenosine

Adenosine produces transient slowing of the sinus node and AV nodal block, and is thus effective for the termination of arrhythmias involving the AV node. It is of particular value in view of its extremely short plasma half-life (approximately 2 s), which confers safety. It must be administered by rapid intravenous injection, using incremental bolus doses from 3 to 12 mg.

Non-pharmacological therapy

Physical manoeuvres

Tachycardias involving the AV node may be terminated by manoeuvres which produce transient vagal stimulation. Although carotid sinus massage is the time-honoured technique the Valsalva manoeuvre, particularly performed in the supine position, is more effective.

Pacing

Re-entry tachycardias may be terminated by the delivery of appropriately timed extrastimuli which depolarize part of the re-entry circuit prior to the arrival of the wave front. Simple overdrive pacing may be effective in the termination of atrial flutter, AV nodal re-entry, AV re-entry tachycardia, or sustained ventricular tachycardia (**VT**) (Fig. 3). The cardiac chamber in question is paced at a rate just above that of the tachycardia for periods of 10–15 beats. Repeated attempts may be necessary at gradually increasing rates. Overdrive atrial or ventricular pacing may result in atrial and ventricular fibrillation (**VF**) respectively, and facilities for cardioversion must be

Table 3 Commonly used antiarrhythmic drugs

	Principal indication	Dose IV	Oral	Adverse effects
Class Ia				
Quinidine	AF cardioversion VT prophylaxis	–	1–2 g/day	Hypersensitivity, gastrointestinal symptoms, QT prolongation, hypotension
Disopyramide	VT prophylaxis VT termination	2 mg/kg	300–600 mg/day	Negative inotropy, QT prolongation, parasympathetic blockade, (urinary retention, dry mouth, blurred vision)
Procaineamide	AF cardioversion VT termination VT prophylaxis	100 mg/5 min up to 1000 mg 1–6 mg/min	2–6 g/day	Hypotension, QT prolongation, gastrointestinal upset, lupus syndrome
Class Ib				
Lignocaine	VT termination VT/VF prophylaxis	100 mg bolus 1–4 mg/min	Ineffective	CNS–confusion, dysarthria, fits
Mexiletine	VT prophylaxis	–	600–1000 mg/day	CNS–dizziness, ataxia, gastrointestinal symptoms
Class Ic				
Flecainide	AF cardioversion AF prophylaxis WPW prophylaxis VT prophylaxis	2 mg/kg	100–300 mg/day	Proarrhythmia, negative inotropy, CNS disturbance
Class II				
Atenolol	AF prophylaxis AF rate control SVT prophylaxis	–	50–100 mg/day	Bradycardia, negative inotropy, Cold extremities, bronchoconstriction, lethargy
Class III				
Sotalol	AF termination AF prophylaxis WPW prophylaxis VT prophylaxis	2 mg/kg	160–480 mg/day	Bradycardia, negative inotropy, cold extremities, bronchoconstriction, lethargy, QT prolongation
Amiodarone	AF termination AF prophylaxis WPW prophylaxis VT prophylaxis	300 mg in 30 min then 1200 mg/24h	600–1200 mg/day loading first 2 weeks then 100–400 mg/day	Photosensitivity, skin pigmentation, hypo- or hyperthyroidism, alveolitis, hepatitis, peripheral neuropathy, epididymitis
Class IV				
Verapamil	SVT termination SVT prophylaxis AF rate control	5–10 mg	240–480 mg/day	Negative inotropy, AV block, flushing, constipation
Other				
Digoxin	AF rate control	0.5–1 mg	0.0625–0.5 mg/day	Anorexia, nausea, vomiting, AV block, atrial and ventricular arrhythmias, toxicity
Adenosine	SVT termination	3–12 mg by incremental bolus	Ineffective	Flushing, chest pain, bronchospasm, transient AV block

AF, atrial fibrillation; SVT, supraventricular tachycardia (atrioventricular nodal and atrioventricular re-entrant tachycardia); VT, ventricular tachycardia; WPW, Wolff–Parkinson–White syndrome.

available. Implantable antitachycardia pacemakers have been used in patients with recurrent, drug refractory tachycardias.

External cardioversion/defibrillation

Direct current cardioversion remains the most effective and immediate means of terminating sustained tachycardias. R-wave synchronized cardioversion using low energies may be effective in terminating atrial flutter or AF, although in the latter case, higher energies may be necessary. Sustained VT may be terminated by synchronized direct current shock, normally requiring energies of 100–360 J. The most important use of D/C counter-shock is in the termination of VF (Fig. 4). Advisory external defibrillators, which analyse the cardiac rhythm automatically and advise as to whether a shock should be delivered have allowed individuals such as ambulance crew to defibrillate successfully.

Implantable cardiovertor defibrillators

Patients at high risk of sudden cardiac death as a result of previous sustained ventricular arrhythmias or out-of-hospital cardiac arrest may be treated with an implantable cardiovertor defibrillator.

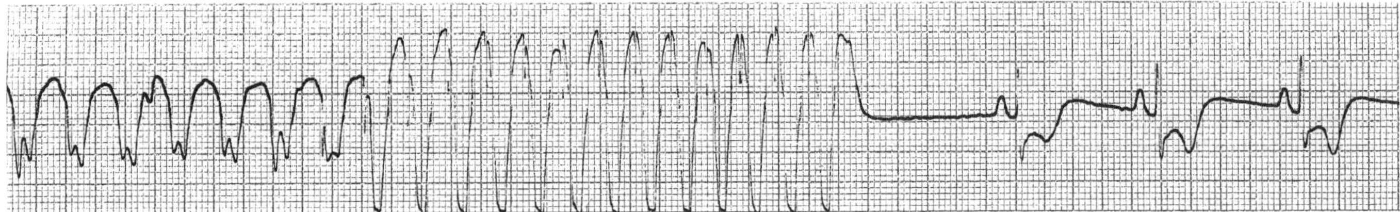

Fig. 3 Termination of ventricular tachycardia by overdrive ventricular pacing.

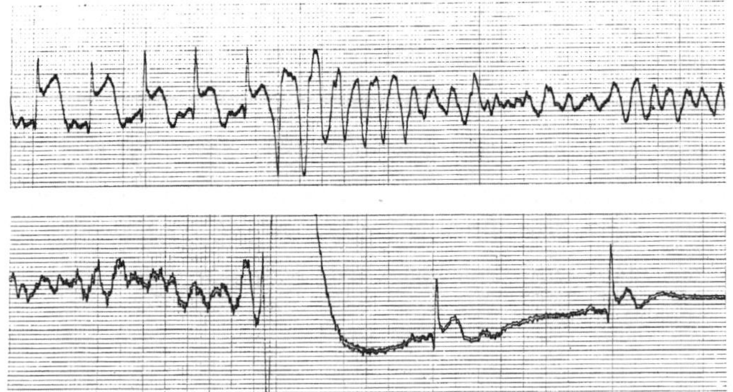

Fig. 4 Ventricular fibrillation is initiated by an 'R-on-T' ventricular extrasystole (above). Defibrillation (200 J direct current shock) terminated the ventricular fibrillation and restored sinus rhythm.

Ablation

Selective ablation of part of a re-entry circuit or of the bundle of His is increasingly used in the management of troublesome arrhythmias. Radiofrequency ablation of accessory pathways is the treatment of choice in the Wolff–Parkinson–White syndrome, and is indicated in drug refractory AV nodal re-entry tachycardia, atrial tachycardia, or atrial flutter. Ablation is feasible in a proportion of patients with VT. His bundle ablation with permanent pacemaker implantation is indicated in medically intractable paroxysmal AF or where the ventricular rate cannot be controlled by pharmacological means in permanent AF.

Surgery

The role of surgery is diminishing with the development of other techniques for ablation. Surgical management of recurrent VT is suitable for selected patients with adequate left ventricular function in whom the site of a micro re-entry circuit can be mapped. This commonly arises in the subendocardial area at the border zone between normal and aneurysmal tissue (see Fig. 2(b)). Subendocardial resection will result in permanent suppression of the tachycardia.

Individual arrhythmias

Sinoatrial disease

This is most commonly caused by degeneration of the sinus nodal cells particularly in the elderly, and is associated in about 20 per cent of cases with bundle branch fibrosis (see below). It may also be associated with coronary artery disease, particularly involving the right coronary artery. Conduction block may occur between the sinus node and the atrium (sinoatrial block), resulting in 'dropped' P waves (Fig. 5). More prolonged suppression of sinus node activity results in periods of sinus arrest, which may be terminated by an escape beat from the sinus node, AV junction or ventricle. Where the sinus rate is permanently slower than the junctional rate, continuous AV junctional rhythm will be present (Fig. 6).

Patients with sinus node disease can be asymptomatic, or may present with dizziness, or syncope. If the correlation between bradycardia or sinus pauses and symptoms can be demonstrated, permanent pacemaker implantation is indicated but such treatment in asymptomatic patients is not necessary. These patients also have an increased predisposition to atrial tachyarrhythmias (bradycardia/tachycardia syndrome).

Carotid sinus hypersensitivity

A hypersensitive carotid sinus reflex leads to reflex bradycardia or cardiac standstill resulting in dizziness or syncope. The condition is diagnosed by the demonstration of a sinus pause greater than 3 s or the appearance of AV block in response to 5 s carotid sinus massage. When a clear association between bradycardia and symptoms can be documented, implantation of a permanent pacemaker is indicated.

Vasovagal syndrome

Vasovagal syncope is common, particularly among young people. A malignant vasovagal syndrome occurs in older patients who are subject to episodes of dizziness and syncope, particularly when upright. There is no evidence of conventional sinoatrial disease, but provocation by tilt table testing will provoke bradycardia and hypotension. Effective treatment is uncertain, but vagally mediated bradycardia can be prevented by a pacemaker.

Atrioventricular conduction disturbances

Impairment may be intranodal or infranodal. The site cannot be identified with certainty from the surface ECG, but can be by intracardiac recording. Intranodal block is not associated with QRS abnormalities, but infranodal block is commonly associated with bundle branch block.

Electrocardiographic features

The normal upper limit of PR interval is 0.20 s and, if the value exceeds this, first-degree AV block is present (Fig. 7). In second-degree block, there is intermittent failure of conduction from atrium to ventricle. In type I (Wenckebach) second-degree block, a characteristic pattern of increasing PR interval duration followed by a non-conducted P wave is seen (Fig. 8). The QRS morphology is commonly normal. In type II second-degree block there is sudden failure of conduction, without preceding increase in PR interval (Fig. 9). This is commonly associated with bundle branch block. Regular non-conducted P waves may result in 2:1, 3:1 of conduction. In complete heart block there is complete dissociation between atrial and ventricular activity. The ventricular rate is then slower than the atrial rate, regular and with a QRS morphology dependent on the site of the escape rhythm.

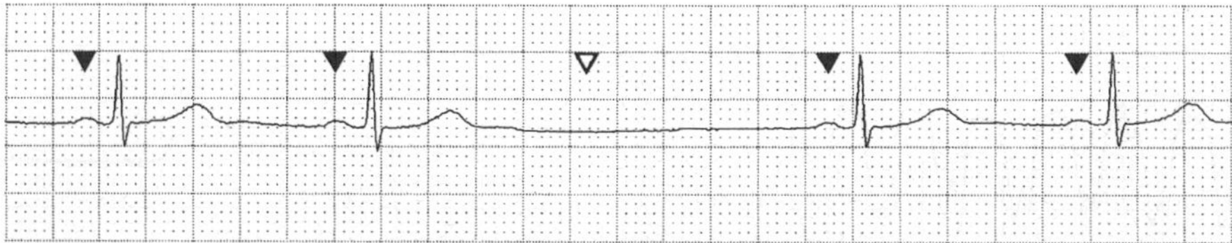

Fig. 5 Sinoatrial exit block. A pause occurred because of the absence of a P wave (open arrow). The timing of the sinus beats, however, is not interrupted, indicating that the sinus node discharged but the impulse failed to excite the atria.

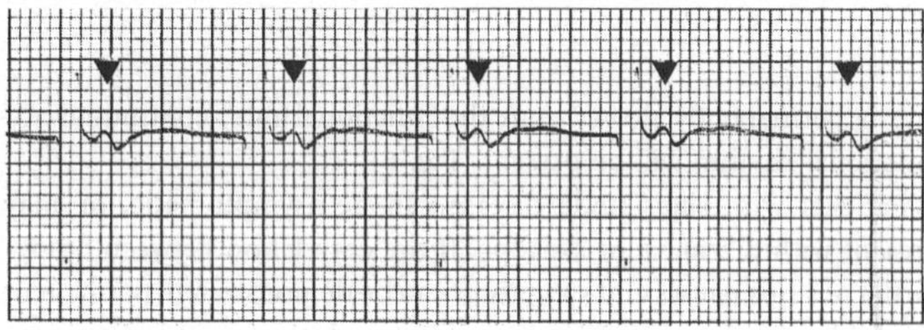

Fig. 6 Junctional rhythm. No P wave precedes the QRS complexes, but P waves are seen following them (arrows).

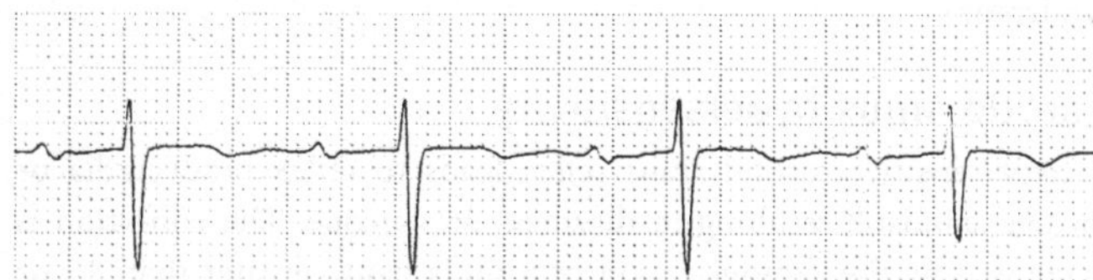

Fig. 7 First-degree heart block. The PR interval is prolonged (0.32 s).

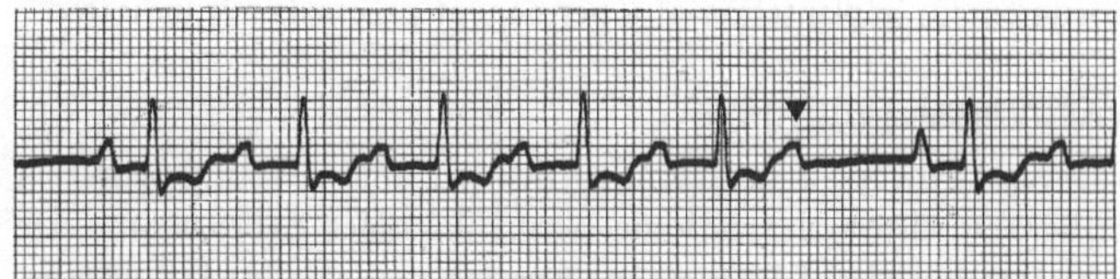

Fig. 8 Second-degree heart block, type I (Wenckebach). The PR interval progressively prolongs until there is failure of conduction following a P wave (arrow).

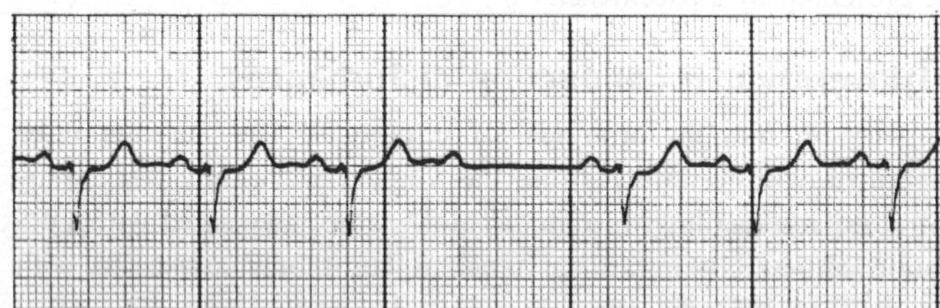

Fig. 9 Second-degree heart block, type II. A non-conducted P wave occurs without preceding prolongation of the PR interval.

Patients may present with symptoms of bradycardia (see above). When the ECG is normal or shows only mild disturbance, ambulatory recording may be required to detect intermittent high-degree AV block. AV conduction disturbances may be preceded by or associated with various degrees of bundle branch block.

Aetiology

The causes of AV block are listed in Table 4. The most common is idiopathic fibrosis of the conducting system, which occurs with increasing frequency from the seventh decade of life. AV block may occur acutely in myocardial infarction. Inferior infarction predominantly affects AV nodal conduction by vagal overactivity, and possibly adenosine release from ischaemic myocardium. First-degree, Wenckebach second-degree block, or third-degree block may occur, but these are usually transient. In contrast, AV conduction disturbance secondary to anterior myocardial infarction is normally due to extensive infarction of the interventricular septum involving the left and right bundle branches after the division of the bundle of His. This may result in type II second-degree block or complete AV block, with a lower probability of recovery of normal conduction. AV nodal blocking drugs may produce conduction disturbance. The combination of intravenous verapamil in patients already receiving β-adrenoceptor blockers is particularly hazardous. Vagally mediated conduction disturbances may occur in highly trained athletes, or in conjunction with carotid sinus syndrome or vasovagal syndrome. AV conduction disturbances can arise in structural congenital heart disease such as endocardial cushion defects, but also as an isolated congenital abnormality, commonly in association with maternal systemic lupus erythematosus in the presence of the Ro/La antibody.

Table 4 Causes of AV block

Causes
Drugs—digoxin, verapamil, β-blockers, class I antiarrhythmics
Idiopathic conducting system fibrosis
Acute myocardial ischaemia/infarction
Infiltration—calcific aortic stenosis, sarcoid, scleroderma, syphilis, tumour
Infection—diphtheria, rheumatic fever, endocarditis, Lyme disease
Vagal—athletic heart, carotid sinus, and vasovagal syndrome
Dystrophia myotonica

Management

First-degree AV block produces no symptoms and does not require treatment. Wenckebach-type second-degree block is normally associated with a reliable subsidiary pacemaker and a low risk of progression to complete heart block. In the majority of instances, treatment is not necessary. Type II second-degree block is generally indicative of a high risk of progression, suggesting the need for a permanent pacemaker even in the absence of symptoms. Complete block, except in an acutely reversible condition, is an indication for a permanent pacemaker, urgent with Stokes–Adams attacks. One exception is in congenital complete heart block, when the escape rhythm is often relatively fast (50–60 per min) with a narrow QRS morphology.

The risk of progression from chronic bifascicular block to complete heart block is low, and patients without symptoms do not require a pacemaker. Trifascicular block (first-degree AV block plus left or right bundle branch block with left or right axis deviation) implies advanced conduction system disease, and permanent pacing is usually advised.

Asystole

Asystole is usually the end-point of all arrhythmias resulting in cardiac arrest. It may also occur as the initiating reason for arrest, sometimes

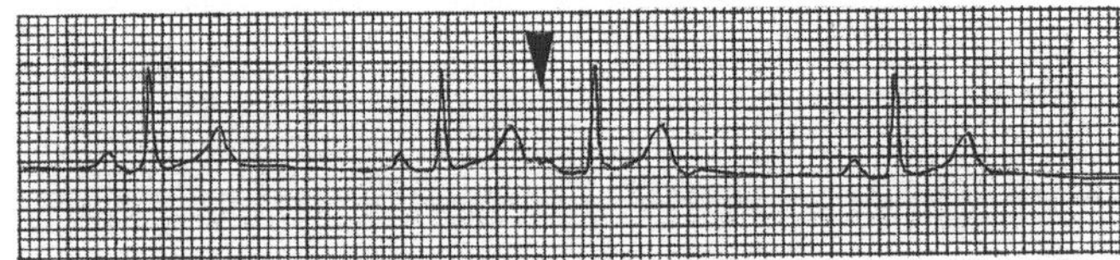

Fig. 10 Atrial extrasystole (arrow).

the result of profound vagal discharge, and is the likely cause of cardiac arrest in strangulation or hypoxia. Persistence of P waves without ventricular activity is normally termed ventricular standstill rather than asystole. The management of asystole is discussed below.

Extrasystoles

Atrial extrasystoles

Atrial extrasystoles are recognized by a premature P wave of different morphology from the sinus P wave and which may be hidden within the ST segment or T wave of the preceding sinus beat. If AV and bundle branch conduction have recovered following the previous sinus beat, the atrial extrasystole will be followed by a normal QRS complex (Fig. 10). If not, the PR interval may be prolonged or the impulse may not be conducted at all. It is important to distinguish non-conducted atrial extrasystoles from second-degree AV block or sinus arrest. Sometimes, atrial extrasystoles are conducted through the AV node but encounter bundle branch refractoriness in which case a bundle branch block pattern of the QRS complex will be identified.

Atrial extrasystoles are common in healthy people, particularly with increasing age. Their frequency is increased by alcohol or caffeine and by increased atrial pressure or stretch, as in cardiac failure or chronic mitral valve disease, when they may be harbingers of AF.

Drug treatment is rarely necessary, although β-adrenergic blockers may be used; class I drugs should be avoided in view of their proarrhythmic risk.

Atrioventricular junctional extrasystoles

Junctional extrasystoles produce a premature, normal QRS complex in the absence of a preceding atrial extrasystole. The atria as well as the ventricles may be activated, resulting an inverted P wave which may be simultaneous with the QRS complex, or inscribed within the ST segment. The significance and management of junctional extrasystoles are similar to those of atrial extrasystoles.

Ventricular extrasystoles

Ventricular extrasystoles are identified by bizarre wide QRS complexes not preceded by a P wave. There is often ST segment depression and T wave inversion. Ventricular extrasystoles commonly bear a constant coupling interval to the previous QRS complex. Retrograde activation through the AV node may occasionally produce an inverted P wave. Ventricular extrasystoles may be intermittent, or occur with a fixed association to the preceding normal beats, i.e. 1:2, 1:3 (bigeminy or trigeminy). Where extrasystoles are of differing morphologies the term multifocal is used. Two extrasystoles in a row are described as a couplet, and three or more in succession as a salvo. Occasionally, a focus may arise which discharges at its own intrinsic rate, independent of the preceding QRS complex, with variable myocardial capture. This arrhythmia, termed parasystole, results in extrasystolic beats which bear no consistent relationship to the preceding QRS complex.

Ventricular extrasystoles can occur in otherwise normal hearts, but are found particularly in the presence of structural heart disease. They occur commonly in the acute phase of myocardial infarction, but also in the postinfarction phase, in the presence of severe left ventricular hypertrophy, hypertrophic cardiomyopathy, or congestive heart failure. Symptoms require treatment in a minority of cases. The major controversy in management centres on their prognostic significance. Frequent ventricular extrasystoles (>10/h) are an independent risk factor for mortality, particularly sudden death, after myocardial infarction. Frequent extrasystoles also confer an adverse prognosis in congestive cardiac failure. Trials to improve prognosis by suppression of extrasystoles with class I agents have not shown a significant reduction in mortality, and meta-analysis suggests an increased mortality. The Cardiac Arrhythmia Suppression Trial, was terminated prematurely following the demonstration of a significant increase in sudden death and all-cause mortality in patients treated with flecainide or encainide. These results contrast with evidence that β-blockade will reduce sudden death and all-cause mortality in postinfarction patients. There is at present no convincing evidence that suppression of asymptomatic extrasystoles in any clinical context is associated with an improvement in prognosis, with the possible exception of the use of amiodarone in dilated cardiomyopathy. If extrasystoles require suppression on symptomatic grounds, the safest option is β-blockade.

Supraventricular tachycardias

Differential diagnosis of narrow QRS complex tachycardias

Most supraventricular tachycardias have normal AV conduction and QRS morphology, but sometimes rate-related bundle branch block may widen the QRS complex making it difficult to distinguish from ventricular tachyarrhythmias. The characteristic ECG features of the principal supraventricular arrhythmias are listed in Table 5. Careful study of all leads is necessary to identify retrograde P waves. Flutter waves are most commonly evident in the inferior limb leads or in lead V1. Transient interruption of AV nodal conduction by vagal stimulation or intravenous adenosine is of particular value in revealing the mechanism of tachycardia. Atrial tachycardias (including flutter and fibrillation) will not be terminated, but an increase in AV block will reveal the underlying atrial tachycardia (Fig. 11), while tachycardias utilizing the AV junction as part of the re-entry circuit will be terminated.

Atrial fibrillation (AF)

The prevalence of AF increases with age and may be as high as 5 per cent in the very elderly. The mechanism is thought to be macro re-entry in most instances. The ECG findings in AF of recent onset are of rapid, irregular 'f' waves at a rate of 350–600/min, associated with an irregular ventricular response. With increasing duration of AF, the amplitude of the 'f' waves diminishes until they are no longer visible, when diagnosis depends on the absence of P waves and the irregular ventricular response.

Clinical features

Paroxysmal attacks may last anything from a few s to a few days. At this stage, the ventricular rate is often rapid and the patient may have severe symptoms. After a variable period which may be as much as several years, AF typically becomes chronic, when the ventricular rate is often slower and the patient is commonly unaware of the irregular pulse. There are numerous causes of AF (Table 6), but sometimes

Table 5 Diagnosis of narrow QRS tachycardias

Arrhythmia	P waves Rate/min	Morphology/axis	P–R relationship	Other
Sinus tachycardia	100–150	Normal	1:1 normal PR	Rarely >150 except exercise
Sinus re-entry	100–140	Normal	1:1 normal PR	Abrupt ↑ HR
Atrial tachycardia	150–200	Abnormal	1:1 with prolonged PR or 2:1	
Atrial flutter	300	Flutter waves Negative II, III and a VF	Variable 1:1 to 4:1 or Wenckebach	Ventricular response regular or irregular
Atrial fibrillation	450–600	'f' waves or isolectric	–	Irregular ventricular response
AVNRT	140–220	Retrograde	Usually synchronous	Normal resting ECG
AVNRT fast/slow	120–150	Retrograde	R–P′ > P′R	Frequent/incessant
AVRT	150–220	Retrograde	RP′ < P′R Inverted P′ in ST segment	WPW or concealed accessory pathway

P—, retrograde P wave; AVNRT, atrioventricular nodal re-entry tachycardia; AVRT, atrioventricular (orthodromic) re-entry tachycardia; WPW, Wolff–Parkinson–White syndrome.

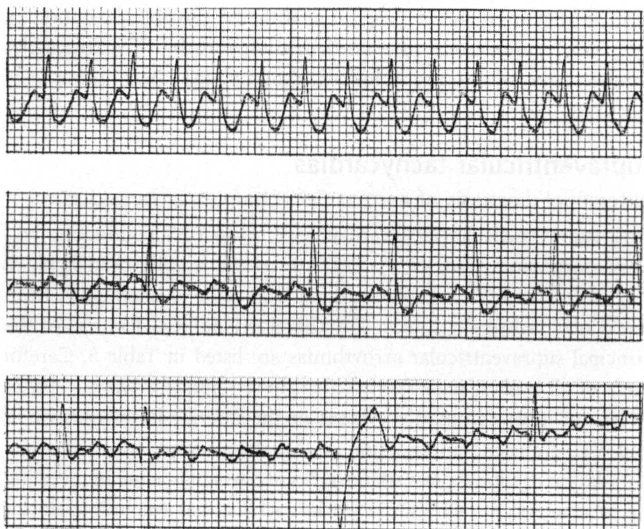

Fig. 11 Atrial flutter with 1 : 1 atrioventricular conduction (above), 2 : 1 conduction (middle) and following adenosine administration (below) (6 mg intravenous injection 10 s previously).

Table 6 Aetiology of atrial fibrillation

Increased atrial pressure/wall tension—mitral valve disease, congestive heart failure, left ventricular hypertrophy, restrictive cardiomyopathy, hypertrophic cardiomyopathy, pulmonary embolism, atrial septal defect
Myocardia ischaemia/infarction
Thyrotoxicosis
Alcohol
Sinoatrial disease
Infiltration—constrictive pericarditis, tumour
Infection—myo/pericarditis, pneumonia
Retrograde activation–WPW syndrome, ventricular pacing
Cardiac or thoracic surgery
Idiopathic—'lone' atrial fibrillation

WPW, Wolff–Parkinson–White.

none can be identified ('lone' AF). The adverse prognostic significance of AF is due in part to its association with organic heart disease and in part because of the risk of stroke. The risk is small in paroxysmal AF in the absence of organic heart disease, but is increased fivefold in chronic fibrillation, and as much as 17-fold in patients with mitral stenosis.

Loss of the atrial contribution to left ventricular filling may result in a modest reduction in cardiac output, which can be important in the presence of impaired ventricular function. More commonly, symptoms arise as a result of a rapid uncontrolled ventricular rate.

Management

Management depends on the duration of an episode, the presence of organic heart disease and any precipitating factors. An attempt to restore sinus rhythm should be made unless fibrillation is obviously of long-standing or associated with advanced heart disease. Underlying precipitating factors such as thyrotoxicosis should be corrected before attempting cardioversion. Synchronized direct current cardioversion under general anaesthesia is commonly effective. Drug cardioversion may be achieved with class Ia, Ic, or III agents. Class Ia agents accelerate the ventricular rate by their anticholinergic action on the AV node, and must be used in combination with digoxin. The original agent used was quinidine (1–2 g/day), but satisfactory results have been reported with flecainide given intravenously (2 mg/kg over 30 min), sotalol (1.5 mg/kg intravenously over 30 min), or amiodarone (300 mg intravenously over 30 min followed by 1200 mg per 24 h until cardioversion).

Prophylactic therapy is commonly necessary in paroxysmal AF or to maintain sinus rhythm following successful cardioversion. No drug is entirely satisfactory. Quinidine appears to increase mortality and is best avoided. Class IC agents and sotalol have been shown to be of benefit. β-Blockers are probably the safest option but are of relatively low efficacy. Amiodarone is effective and may be used at low dosage (100–200 mg daily) but its side-effects are such that it is only indicated when the arrhythmia fails to respond to other drugs.

If drug therapy failed completely, His bundle ablation and permanent pacemaker implantation may be indicated (see above). However, the natural history of paroxysmal AF is to revert into chronic fibrillation where the ventricular rate is often well controlled and symptoms improved.

Management of chronic AF is concerned with control of ventricular rate. Although digoxin is effective in achieving control of the ventricular rate at rest in most patients, the heart rate is poorly controlled on exercise. Additional agents to slow the ventricular rate, such as verapamil, diltiazem, and β-blockers, are commonly prescribed. They do not improve exercise tolerance acutely, but long-standing poorly controlled AF may result in impairment of ventricular function (tachycardiomyopathy) which can be avoided by adequate rate control.

Prophylaxis against thromboembolism should be considered in all patients. Cardioversion may be associated with embolism, and patients should ideally be treated with warfarin for a minimum of 3 weeks. When the arrhythmia is of less than 48 h origin, intravenous heparin prior to cardioversion is acceptable. Chronic anticoagulation is indicated in patients with mitral valve disease and in patients with non-rheumatic AF possessing risk factors for thromboembolism (age over 75 years, left ventricular dysfunction, hypertension, diabetes). Aspirin is less effective than warfarin but may be acceptable in lower risk subjects.

Atrial flutter

Atrial flutter produces a typical 'sawtooth' pattern of atrial activity on the ECG with a rate close to 300/min. Flutter waves are commonly negative in the inferior limb leads and positive in lead V1. Atrial flutter may be associated with either a regular or irregular ventricular response. Two to one AV conduction producing a regular tachycardia of 150/min is common, but occasionally, 1:1 conduction produces a rate approaching 300/min. Flutter waves are not seen easily with faster ventricular rates, and transient slowing of AV conduction may be necessary to make the diagnosis (Fig. 11).

The causes of atrial flutter are similar to those of AF. It carries a lower risk of thromboembolism. Termination of atrial flutter may be achieved by drug or electrical cardioversion as described above for AF. An additional method is by rapid atrial pacing at a rate approximately 10 per cent above the flutter rate. Bursts of such pacing may restore sinus rhythm, or precipitate AF. Prophylaxis involves the same agents as in paroxysmal AF.

Atrial tachycardia

The term describes a tachycardia with an atrial rate slower than in atrial flutter, usually between 120 and 250/min. There may be a degree of AV block, although 1:1 AV conduction may occur. The ECG shows regular P waves which do not show the same 'sawtooth' appearance as in atrial flutter.

When the cause is sinus node re-entry, P wave morphology is normal. Automatic atrial tachycardia shows a different P wave morphology, commonly with a longer PR interval. The rate characteristically accelerates before reaching a rate of 125–200/min; this arrhythmia is not started or terminated by atrial extrasystoles. Atrial tachycardia with block is a manifestation of digitalis toxicity when the ventricular rate may be relatively slow and careful evaluation of the ECG is necessary to identify the problem. Multifocal atrial tachycardia, in which rapid irregular, discrete P waves of three or four different morphologies are seen, occurs in severely ill, elderly patients or in association with acute exacerbation of pulmonary disease. It is rarely responsive to digoxin, but success with intravenous verapamil, or magnesium, has suggested triggered activity as the underlying mechanism.

The clinical context of atrial tachycardia is commonly the same as for AF and flutter, except for the association with digitalis toxicity. The approach to management is identical to that of AF.

Junctional re-entry tachycardias

All regular, paroxysmal tachycardias with narrow QRS complexes were previously grouped together 'supraventricular tachycardias', or as 'paroxysmal atrial tachycardias'. These terms are obsolete because it is now possible to identify the exact mechanisms in most instances. When atrial arrhythmias are excluded, the vast majority are junctional re-entry tachycardias, either AV nodal re-entry or AV re-entry (see below). Correct recognition of these arrhythmias is important in the context of effective curative measures, such as ablative techniques.

Atrioventricular nodal re-entry tachycardia

The basis of the arrhythmia is the presence of two functionally distinct AV nodal pathways (Fig. 12). One conducts more rapidly but with a longer refractory period; the other has slow conduction but a shorter refractory period. In sinus rhythm, AV nodal conduction occurs via the fast route and the PR interval is normal. A sufficiently premature atrial extrasystole blocks the fast pathway, but slow pathway conduction may continue and be sufficiently slow as to allow the fast pathway to recover excitability prior to activation reaching the distal end of the pathways. The stage is then set for a re-entry circuit with antegrade conduction via the slow pathway and retrograde via the fast pathway. Characteristically, antegrade activation of the ventricles and retrograde activation of the atria occur virtually simultaneously, resulting in the P wave being 'buried' within the QRS complex, or producing a very small distortion of the terminal QRS, which cannot be recognized easily without careful comparison with the ECG during sinus rhythm. The tachycardia is readily terminated by appropriately timed extra stimuli or by overdrive pacing. A less common variant of AV nodal tachycardia may arise when antegrade conduction in the tachycardia is via the fast pathway with retrograde conduction via the slow pathway. The atrium is then activated well after the QRS complex, characteristically producing an inverted P′ wave with the R–P′ interval greater than the P′–R interval during tachycardia (Fig. 13). Occasionally, slow/fast and fast/slow tachycardias coexist in the same patient.

AV nodal re-entry tachycardia commonly presents in childhood or adolescence, although it can appear at any age. Attacks happen at random intervals, although clustering may occur. There is no specific association with other organic heart disease. Palpitation is normally well tolerated.

Termination of an attack is achieved by producing transient AV nodal block. This is achieved by vagotonic manoeuvres, by intravenous verapamil (5–10 mg) or by intravenous adenosine (3–12 mg). Intravenous β-blockade is less effective. β-blockers, sotalol, verapamil, or digoxin can all be useful in prophylaxis. Atrial pacemakers have been used successfully in patients refractory to drugs or intolerant of side-effects. These do not prevent attacks, but can usually terminate them by overdrive pacing salvoes within a minute or so. Radiofrequency ablation of the slow pathway is increasingly used as curative treatment. There is a low risk of inducing complete AV block and results are excellent.

Fig. 12 Atrioventricular nodal re-entry tachycardia. Mechanism of initiation by atrial extrasystole. See text for details.

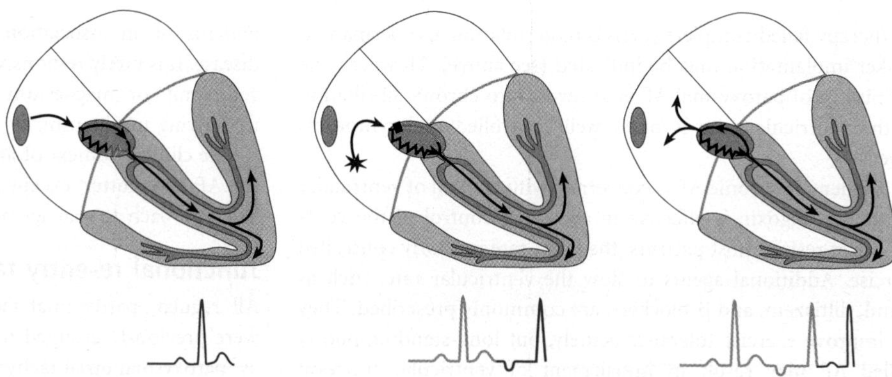

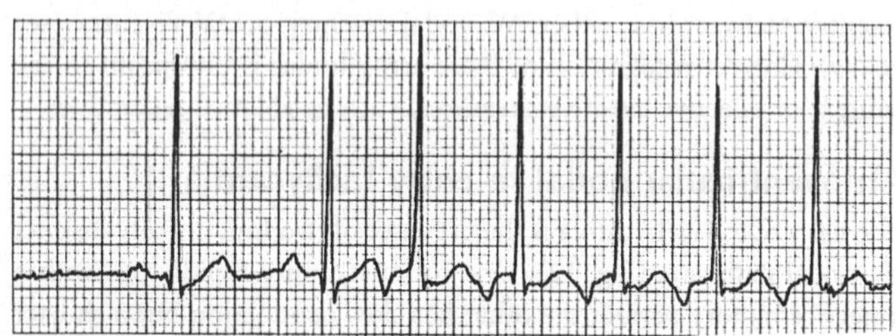

Fig. 13 Atypical atrioventricular nodal re-entry tachycardia ('long RP'). Inverted P' waves precede the QRS complex during tachycardia (compare with preceding sinus beats).

Atrioventricular re-entry tachycardia

The re-entry circuit in this tachycardia also involves the AV node but, in addition, uses an accessory pathway. The mechanism of the common form, orthodromic tachycardia, is illustrated in Fig. 14. The refractory period of the accessory pathway is commonly longer than that of the AV node; hence a premature atrial extrasystole may find the accessory pathway refractory, but be conducted through the AV node. If sufficient delay has occurred, the accessory pathway will have recovered excitability sufficiently to allow retrograde activation from the ventricle to atrium, with the establishment of a re-entry circuit. As the circuit involves activation of the ventricles via the His–Purkinje system, the QRS morphology will be normal, unless rate-related bundle branch block develops. Retrograde atrial activation is identified by the presence of an inverted P wave inscribed early in the ST segment. In sinus rhythm, the presence of an accessory pathway may be revealed by the characteristic features on the ECG of 'pre-excitation' (Fig. 15).

Pre-excitation syndromes (Wolff–Parkinson–White syndrome)

The most common of the pre-excitation syndromes is the Wolff–Parkinson–White syndrome in which one or more accessory pathways are present. Although these can lie at any point in the AV ring, the commonest sites are in the left free wall and the posteroseptal region.

The ECG appearances of the syndrome arise from early activation of the myocardium adjacent to the ventricular insertion of the accessory pathway (Fig. 14). There is no AV delay, hence the PR interval is shortened but slow intraventricular conduction results in a slurred initiation of the QRS complex (the delta wave) (see Fig. 16). The remainder of the ventricle is excited via the normal His–Purkinje system. The degree of pre-excitation during sinus rhythm is variable. It may be intermittent, if the refractory period of the accessory pathway is close to the sinus cycle length, or latent, if the delta wave is obscured due to rapid AV nodal conduction. Agents which enhance AV nodal conduction increase the proportion of ventricular tissue activated via the His–Purkinje system and will lessen the appearances of pre-excitation. In contrast, transient slowing of AV nodal conduction enhances the proportion of the ventricle excited by the accessory pathway. This phenomenon is used to diagnose latent pre-excitation by the administration of adenosine or verapamil during sinus rhythm.

AV (orthodromic) re-entry tachycardia is the characteristic arrhythmia in the Wolff-Parkinson-White syndrome. Rarely, the refractory period of the AV node exceeds that of the accessory pathway. A tachycardia can then arise which has antegrade conduction via the accessory pathway and retrograde conduction via the AV node (antidromic tachycardia). The QRS morphology is grossly abnormal and

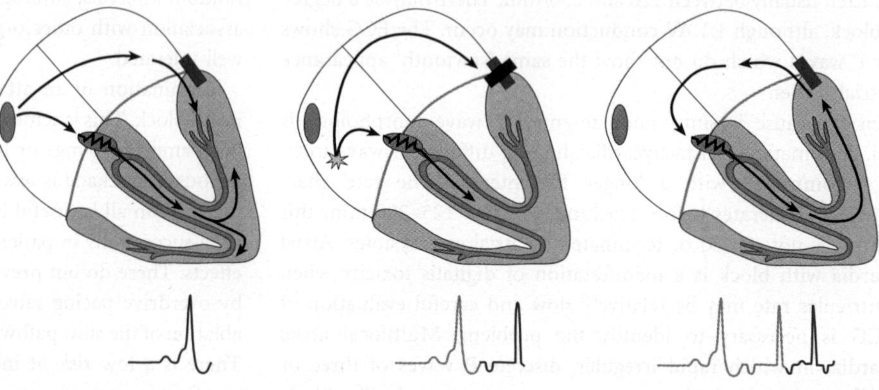

Fig. 14 Atrioventricular re-entry tachycardia. Mechanism of initiation by atrial extrasystole. See text for details.

its appearance is dependent upon the site of insertion of the accessory pathway.

Some accessory pathways conduct only retrogradely (concealed accessory pathway), hence the resting ECG is normal. These patients are not at risk of pre-excited AF (see below) but are still prone to orthodromic re-entry tachycardia.

Other forms of pre-excitation include the Mahaim pathways, usually direct AV connections with slow conduction properties typical of AV nodal tissue. Evidence for atrionodal pathways associated with a short PR interval but no delta wave and susceptibility to supraventricular tachycardias (Lown–Ganong–Levine syndrome) remains controversial.

The major concern in Wolff–Parkinson–White syndrome is pre-excited AF because conduction via a fast accessory pathway, bypassing the normal AV nodal slowing, results in AF being conducted at a rapid rate to the ventricles. If the refractory period of the accessory pathway is sufficiently short, the very rapid ventricular conduction may degenerate into VF. The degree of pre-excitation during AF varies, giving a characteristic pattern of an irregular ventricular response with QRS morphology ranging from normal to fully pre-excited. The exact QRS morphology will depend on the site of insertion of the accessory pathway.

Clinical features

ECG delta waves occur in approximately 1.5 per 1000 of the population but many who have them never experience paroxysmal tachycardia. The risk of sudden death due to rapid pre-excited AF appears to be very low among patients who have not had any symptomatic tachycardias, but increases in symptomatic patients. Analysis of spontaneous or induced episodes is important in assessing risk. The identification of consecutive pre-excited RR intervals of less than 250 ms identifies a higher risk group, although even in them, the absolute risk remains low. Accessory pathway conduction tends to become slower with increasing age. Patients who have experienced AF with relatively slow ventricular rates are unlikely to develop faster ventricular responses subsequently. Spontaneous disappearance of antegrade accessory pathway conduction is well documented in patients with low risk pathways. Wolff-Parkinson-White syndrome may be associated with Ebstein's anomaly but has no other clinical associations.

Management

Orthodromic re-entry tachycardia is terminated by AV nodal blocking manoeuvres such as vagal stimulation, verapamil, or adenosine. The management of pre-excited AF requires particular care, as digoxin or verapamil paradoxically accelerate ventricular rate and are contraindicated. In the presence of severe haemodynamic disturbance, direct current cardioversion is the treatment of choice. When patients are more stable, agents which slow antegrade conduction through the accessory pathway, such as intravenous flecainide, sotalol, or amiodarone are all effective.

Symptomatic patients with Wolff-Parkinson-White syndrome should be evaluated for the risk of pre-excited AF. Intermittent pre-excitation is commonly associated with a long accessory pathway refractory period and a low risk of life-threatening tachycardias. Disappearance of the delta wave in response to a class Ia or Ic antiarrhythmic drug also suggests a low risk. The safety and efficacy of radiofrequency ablation of accessory pathways is such that this is now the treatment of choice in symptomatic patients with ventricular pre-excitation, and for patients with concealed accessory pathways whose symptoms are not controlled by medical therapy, or who do not wish to consider long-term antiarrhythmic drug therapy. The site of the accessory pathway is mapped and ablation is undertaken at the same session (Fig. 16). If radiofrequency ablation fails or is not available, medical therapy may be used.

Flecainide or sotalol are the best choice for prophylaxis of orthodromic re-entry tachycardia. Amiodarone is also effective but less advisable in young people because of its potential adverse effects.

Diagnosis of wide QRS complex tachycardias

While it is safe to assume that virtually all narrow complex tachycardias have a supraventricular origin, wide complex tachycardias may arise either from the ventricle, or from supraventricular mechanisms when associated with pre-excitation or bundle branch block (Table 7). Misdiagnosis and mismanagement most commonly arise when VT is not recognized and is misdiagnosed as 'SVT with aberration'. This can arise as a result of a number of factors:

1. The clinical context is not considered. Middle-aged or elderly patients presenting with a recent history of wide complex tachycardia and who give a history of myocardial infarction or congestive heart failure are more likely to have ventricular than supraventricular tachycardia.
2. VT is assumed to cause haemodynamic collapse. This is not necessarily the case, if the rate is not excessively fast or if underlying cardiac function is good. Conversely, supraventricular tachycardias may cause syncope, hypotension, or shock if sufficiently rapid.
3. VT can present with a typical history of paroxysmal self-terminating tachycardia, just as in the case of supraventricular tachycardia.
4. Lack of detailed analysis of the ECG during tachycardia may lead to misdiagnosis.

The response to transient AV nodal blockade will assist considerably in diagnosis. The response to adenosine (Table 8) will permit distinction between atrial, junctional, and VT in many patients (Fig. 17).

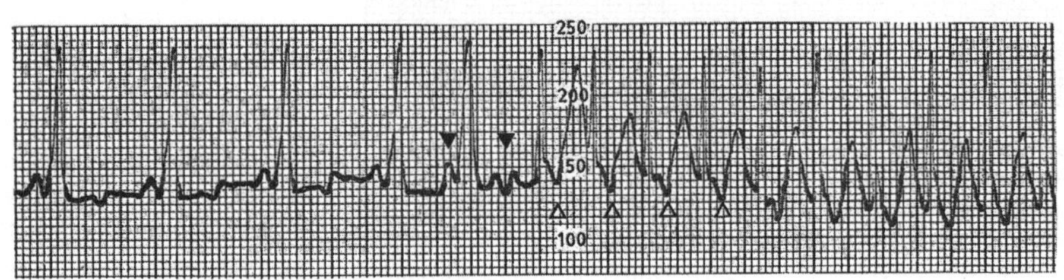

Fig. 15 Initiation of atrioventricular re-entrant tachycardia by atrial extrasystoles (arrows). Note the presence of short PR interval and delta wave during sinus rhythm, with normalization of QRS complex and appearance of retrograde P′ waves (open arrows) during tachycardia.

Table 7 ECG features of wide complex tachycardia

	Atrial rhythm	Atrioventricular relationship	ECG morphology: Tachycardia	ECG morphology: Sinus rhythm
Irregular ventricular response				
AF/AFL with previous BBB	'f' or flutter waves	Irregular	Typical BBB	BBB
AF/AFL with functional BBB	'f' or flutter waves	Irregular	Typical BBB	Normal
Pre-excited AF	'f' waves	Irregular	Varying normal/pre-excited	WPW
Torsades de pointes	Obscured	–	Varying QRS axis	Long QT
Regular ventricular response				
Ventricular tachycardia	Sinus or retrograde	AV dissociation or 1:1/2:1 VA conduction	Abnormal wide complexes	?Old MI
	VA conduction		QRS > 0.14 s Extreme axis deviation Fusion/capture beats Concordance RBBB tachycardia with Rsr— in V1 or qS in V6	
AFL with BBB	Flutter waves	2:1	Typical BBB	WPW or normal
AVRT with functional BBB	Retrograde atrial activation	1:1		
AVNRT with functional BBB	Synchronous with QRS	1:1	Typical BBB	Normal
Antidromic tachycardia	Obscured in QRS	1:1	Pre-excited	WPW

AF, atrial fibrillation; AFL, atrial flutter; AV, atrioventricular; AVNRT, atrioventricular nodal re-entry tachycardia; AVRT, atrioventricular (orthodromic) re-entry tachycardia; BBB, bundle branch block; MI, myocardial infarction; RBBB, right bundle branch block; VA, ventriculoatrial; WPW, Wolff–Parkinson–White syndrome.

Ventricular tachyarrhythmias

Definitions

VT is defined as the presence of five or more consecutive ventricular beats at a rate of 120 per min or greater. Sustained VT comprises a salvo lasting for 30 s or more. Non-sustained episodes last between five beats and 30 s. Monomorphic VT demonstrates a consistent QRS morphology during each paroxysm, while in polymorphic VT the QRS morphology is constantly changing. Polymorphic VT may degenerate into VF and the ECG distinction between the two is difficult. Torsades de pointes is a characteristic type of polymorphic VT with an undulating variation in QRS morphology as a result of variation in axis. The term is best reserved for the arrhythmias arising in association with QT interval prolongation.

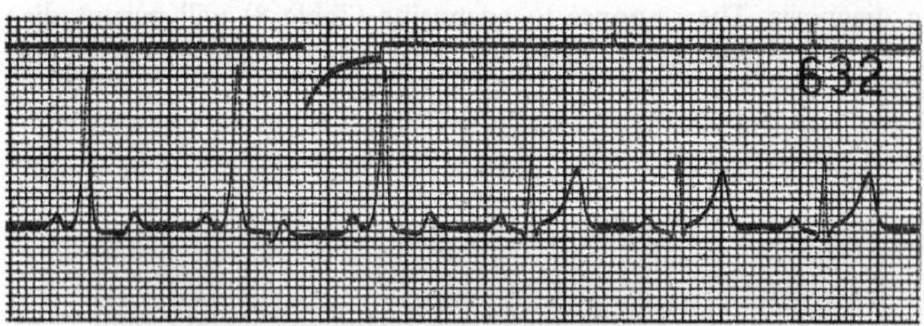

Fig. 16 Radiofrequency ablation of an accessory pathway. The patient had Wolff-Parkinson-White syndrome with evidence of ventricular pre-excitation on the surface electrocardiogram during sinus rhythm (short PR interval, delta wave). One beat after switching on the current (indicated by deflection in marker channel, above) the QRS becomes normal, indicating successful ablation of the accessory pathway.

Table 8 Diagnostic use of intravenous adenosine

Arrhythmia	Response
Atrial tachycardia Atrial flutter Atrial fibriliation	Transient AV block reveals atrial arrhythmia. Rarely terminated
AVNRT AVRT	Terminates tachycardia by antegrade (AV) block)
Ventricular tachycardia	Not terminated 1:1 VA conduction may be blocked, revealing AV dissociation

AV, atrioventricular; AVNRT, atrioventricular nodal re-entry tachycardia; AVRT, atrioventricular (orthodromic) re-entry tachycardia; VA, ventriculoatrial.

Sustained monomorphic ventricular tachycardia

This arrhythmia occurs most commonly in the presence of heart disease, particularly recent or remote myocardial infarction. The usual mechanism is one of micro re-entry with slow conduction occurring at the border of the infarcted area where surviving muscle fibres are interdigitated with fibrous tissue (see Fig. 2(b)). Less common mechanisms include macro re-entry involving the bundle branches, or triggered activity.

Electrocardiographic characteristics (see Table 7)

The presence of AV dissociation is a particularly important feature to seek in a wide complex tachycardia as it makes the diagnosis of VT virtually certain (Fig. 17). Careful search for P waves perturbing the QRS complex or T waves is necessary, ideally using multichannel recordings. Fusion and capture beats are diagnostic of VT and should

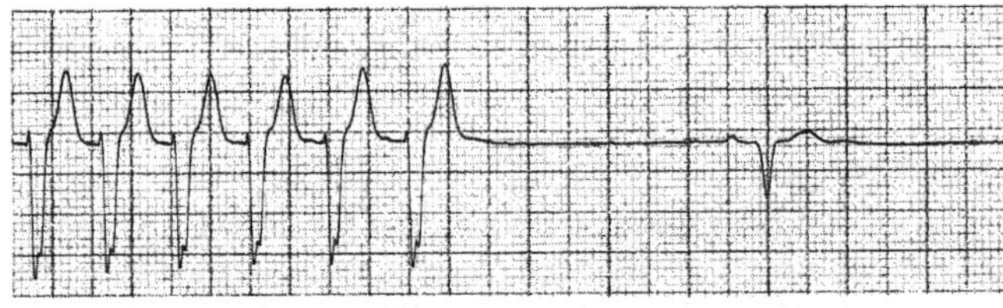

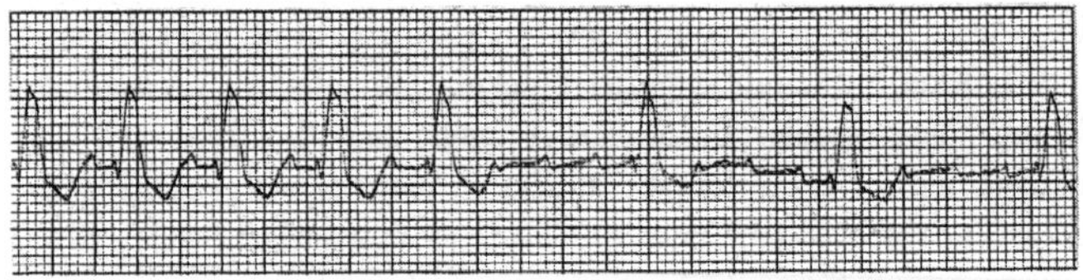

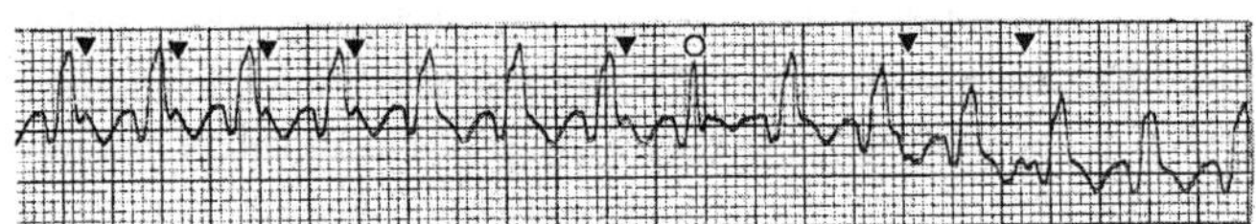

Fig. 17 Responses of broad complex tachycardias to intravenous adenosine. Supraventricular tachycardia is terminated (above), atrial flutter is revealed (middle) and ventricular tachycardia is not terminated (below), although retrograde ventriculoatrial block results in atrioventricular dissociation (P waves are arrowed) and a fusion beat (open circle).

be carefully sought. A fusion beat appears when activation of the ventricle is partly via the normal system and partly from the tachycardia focus. Occasionally, a fortuitously timed P wave allows the development of a capture beat of normal QRS morphology without interrupting the tachycardia. When dissociated P waves cannot be recognized with certainty, direct recording of atrial activity by an oesophageal or right atrial ECG may help. AV dissociation in VT is not invariable; retrograde ventriculoatrial conduction may give either 1:1 ventriculoatrial conduction or higher degrees of ventriculoatrial block. If 1:1 ventriculoatrial conduction is interrupted temporarily by adenosine, AV dissociation or the appearance of a fusion or capture beat may be identified (Fig. 17). The QRS duration in VT is commonly greater than 0.12 s, and values greater than 0.14 s are particularly suggestive. Specific morphological patterns may be identified (Table 7). Concordant positive or negative QRS complexes across the chest leads suggest VT, as does extreme axis deviation. Different abnormal QRS morphologies during tachycardia on different occasions are highly suggestive of VT.

Aetiology

Sustained VT in acute myocardial infarction is commonly of an unstable, polymorphic type, which either terminates spontaneously or degenerates into VF. Sustained monomorphic episodes occur in the subacute phase, or at any time after myocardial infarction, even many years later, particularly in association with left ventricular dilatation and aneurysm formation. Sustained VT may complicate any condition associated with ventricular dilatation or fibrosis such as dilated cardiomyopathy, hypertrophic cardiomyopathy, or previous ventriculotomy. Attacks in younger patients may arise in association with arrhythmogenic right ventricular cardiomyopathy; these patients may have no other symptoms or signs of cardiac disease, but dilatation of the right ventricle can be demonstrated on echocardiography or angiography (see Chapter 2.19). VT has been associated with mitral valve prolapse. Sustained monomorphic tachycardia may occur as a proarrhythmic response to antiarrhythmic drugs, particularly class Ic agents, which produce a characteristic slow, incessant tachycardia at a rate of 120–150 per min, especially after intravenous administration. There remains a minority of patients with ventricular tachycardia who have no evidence of structural heart disease. In some the arrhythmia originates from the right ventricular outflow tract, while in others the tachycardia arises from the anterior or posterior fascicle of the left bundle branch.

Clinical features

These will depend on the rate and duration of the arrhythmia and the underlying cardiac reserve. Rapid VT may present as cardiac arrest, syncope, or left ventricular failure. Slower tachycardias in patients with good cardiac function may present only as palpitation, or may be asymptomatic. Physical examination will reveal a rapid regular pulse rate and possibly signs of shock or left ventricular failure. If AV dissociation is present, intermittent cannon waves may be seen in the jugular veins and variations in the intensity of the first heart sound may be heard. In the presence of ventriculoatrial conduction there may be regular cannon waves with 1:1 or 1:2 relationship with the arterial pulse.

Management

Ventricular tachycardia is a medical emergency. If there is cardiac arrest, or the patient is unconscious, immediate direct current cardioversion is necessary. If the patient is conscious but hypotensive, urgent synchronized direct current cardioversion under general anaesthesia or diazepam sedation is used. Tachycardias which are better tolerated may be terminated by intravenous lignocaine 100 mg, repeated if necessary after 5 min. Second-line drugs include procainamide, disopyramide, and amiodarone. Amiodarone normally has a slow onset of action but may be effective if the tachycardia is well tolerated. Flecainide is not advised in view of the risk of developing incessant tachycardia. All antiarrhythmic drugs have significant negative inotropic actions which may further impair the haemodynamic status of the patient if sinus rhythm is not restored. For this reason, no more than two antiarrhythmic drugs should be given before recourse to alternative therapy. Pacemaker termination of VT may be very effective (see Fig. 3), particularly if the tachycardia is relatively slow, or has been slowed by drug therapy but facilities for cardioversion must be available in view of the risk of acceleration of the tachycardia or degeneration into VF.

After recovery, clinical assessment for evidence of underlying heart disease should be supported by ECG, echocardiography, and/or radionuclide ventriculography. Particular attention should be paid to the possibility of arrhythmogenic right ventricular cardiomyopathy in young patients. In those with ischaemic heart disease, exercise testing is important to identify any reversible ischaemia. Coronary arteriography is needed for those with ischaemia-related tachycardia and evidence of a left ventricular aneurysm sought. Signal averaged ECG may be needed to detect the mechanisms of the tachycardia.

The risk of recurrence or sudden death is 40 per cent in the first year after the initial event.

Unless there is a clear precipitating factor, patients require antiarrhythmic drug prophylaxis but the efficacy of any given choice cannot be predicted; thus it is necessary to demonstrate efficacy and to exclude proarrhythmic responses. If episodes of VT, sustained or non-sustained, are occurring frequently, it is sufficient to administer antiarrhythmic drugs under continuous ECG monitoring, and to demonstrate that salvoes of tachycardia have been suppressed completely. Unfortunately, many episodes of sustained VT are infrequent, and suppression of brief salvoes of non-sustained attacks may not correlate with protection from recurrence of sustained events. Under these circumstances, electrophysiological testing is indicated. If a sustained monomorphic tachycardia can be induced, a drug is given and the study repeated once stable plasma levels have been achieved. Suppression of inducibility of the tachycardia is associated with a substantially reduced risk of recurrence and an improved prognosis.

Class I drugs have been the traditional agents in the treatment of VT. However, clinical trials have shown them to be inferior to sotalol and amiodarone in the prevention of recurrence and sudden death, and Class I agents are no longer recommended for routine use. Recent randomized trials comparing soltalol and amiodarone with the implantable cardioverter defibrillator in patients with inducible sustained VT or spontaneous life-threatening ventricular arrhythmias have shown superior survival in patients receiving the defibrillator. Thus defibrillator therapy is becoming first-line treatment in a large proportion of these patients. Modern devices are implanted into the pectoral region with an endocardial electrode in the right ventricular apex. These devices combine antitachycardia pacing (Fig. 3) with 'back-up' defibrillation.

In patients for whom defibrillator therapy is inappropriate or unavailable, treatment with sotalol or amiodarone is commonly used. Patients in whom VT is rendered non-inducible or haemodynamically well tolerated on amiodarone therapy have a good prognosis. Adjuvant β-blockade, if haemodynamically well tolerated, appears to improve survival in patients at high risk of sudden death treated with amiodarone.

Prognosis

Three-year survival varies from 80 per cent in patients in whom arrhythmia induction is suppressed by antiarrhythmic drug therapy to 40 per cent in those in whom no effective suppression is achieved and empirical therapy is used. The 3-year survival in patients treated with an implantable cardioverter defibrillator following life-threatening ventricular arrhythmias in a recent trial was 75 per cent versus 64 per cent in drug treated controls.

Accelerated idioventricular rhythm

The term is used to describe a continuous ventricular rhythm with a rate less than 120/min, commonly occurs in acute myocardial infarction, and appears to be a marker of successful thrombolytic therapy. No treatment is necessary.

Non-sustained ventricular tachycardia

Salvoes of non-sustained VT occur in association with acute myocardial infarction, left ventricular dysfunction, or left ventricular hypertrophy due to hypertension, aortic stenosis, or hypertrophic cardiomyopathy. They may also be an incidental finding in patients with no evidence of organic heart disease.

Clinical features

If salvoes are short and not particularly rapid, they may be asymptomatic. More prolonged episodes may result in dizziness or presyncope, and occasionally in syncope. This arrhythmia carries no proven risk of sudden death in those without evidence of underlying heart disease. After myocardial infarction it is an independent risk factor for sudden cardiac death, particularly if associated with impaired left ventricular function. It is also an adverse prognostic factor in hypertrophic cardiomyopathy, but its significance in hypertensive left ventricular hypertrophy is uncertain. In advanced cardiac failure, it is associated with an increased risk of cardiac death, not selectively of sudden death.

Management

If no significant heart disease is present, and the patient is asymptomatic, no treatment is indicated. Symptomatic treatment in the absence of significant heart disease should be with antiarrhythmic drugs least likely to be complicated by proarrhythmic reactions such as β-blockers; calcium channel blockers are effective occasionally. Failing these, sotalol or a class I agent may be necessary. The management of asymptomatic attacks in patients with organic heart disease is controversial. There is no evidence that antiarrhythmic drugs improve survival in postinfarction patients. Low-dose amiodarone has been recommended in the management of hypertrophic cardiomyopathy with non-sustained VT, and has been shown to improve survival in one study of patients with congestive heart failure. Because of the risk of sustained VT, patients with symptoms and underlying heart disease should be investigated by signal averaged ECG. Those with good ventricular function and normal signal averaged ECG are at low risk and suitable for treatment by β-blockers. Those in whom ventricular function is impaired and the signal averaged cardiogram abnormal need programmed ventricular stimulation and management as described above for sustained VT.

Torsades de pointes and the long QT syndromes

Torsades de pointes (twisting of points) is an atypical VT characterized by a continuously varying QRS axis (Fig. 18). Paroxysms are commonly repetitive and normally self-terminating, although they may degenerate into VF. They are associated in the preceding beats with evidence of marked QT prolongation, and frequently with morphological abnormalities of the T waves such as T–U fusion, gross increases in T wave amplitude or T wave alternans. In the congenital syndromes, they are often associated with increases in sinus rate, while in the acquired syndromes a slowing of the heart rate, and in particular a postextrasystolic pause often initiates the arrhythmia. This produces a characteristic 'short–long–short' sequence of initiation.

The combination of QT interval prolongation during sinus rhythm with intermittent torsades de pointes is described as the long QT syndrome. This may be congenital or acquired. Specific mutations in genes encoding for the sodium or potassium channels in the cardiac cell have been identified in patients with congenital long QT syndromes. Delayed closure of the sodium channel results in prolongation of inward current, while potassium channel mutations result in delayed repolarization. Both mechanisms result in prolongation of the QT interval and increased predisposition to early after-depolarizations. In the acquired syndrome, predisposing factors are Q–T prolongation, bradycardia, hypokalaemia, and hypomagnesaemia, all of which predispose to early after-depolarizations.

A variety of congenital long QT syndromes has been identified. The Jervell–Lange–Nielsen syndrome is an autosomal recessive condition associated with neural deafness. The Romano–Ward syndrome is an autosomal dominant condition without deafness. Sporadic idiopathic cases have been reported. Attacks of torsades de pointes in the congenital syndromes are commonly associated with sympathetic stimulation such as exercise, wakening, or fright. Paroxysms may produce syncope which if prolonged may be complicated by convulsion. For this reason, the syndrome may often may be misdiagnosed

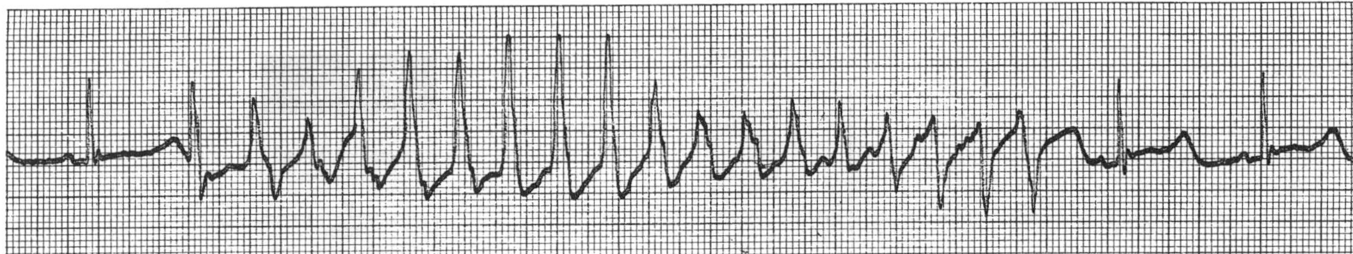

Fig. 18 Torsades de pointes. Note the marked QT interval prolongation in the sinus beats.

Table 9 Acquired (pause dependent) long QT syndromes

Drug-induced
• Antiarrhythmic drugs—classes Ia, III
• Vasodilators—prenylamine, ketanserin, lidoflazine
• Psychotropics
Electrolyte disturbances
• Hypokalaemia, hypomagnesaemia, hypocalcaemia
Metabolic
• Hypothyroidism, starvation, anorexia nervosa, liquid protein diet
Bradycardia
• Sinoatrial disease, atrioventricular block
Toxins
• Organophosphorus insecticides, heavy metal poisoning

as epilepsy. A family history of recurrent syncope or sudden death may be obtained.

Many factors may predispose to the development of the acquired long QT syndrome (Table 9). The clinical presentation is of recurrent dizziness and syncope, and the condition may easily be misdiagnosed as self-terminating polymorphic VT or VF unless the characteristic morphology of torsades de pointes and the associated QT interval prolongation is recognized.

Management

Individual paroxysms of are normally self-limiting but, if they are persistent, cardiac arrest will occur and emergency defibrillation is necessary. Accurate diagnosis is essential in order to avoid empirical antiarrhythmic drug therapy which may worsen the arrhythmia. Indeed, antiarrhythmic drug therapy is one of the commonest causes of torsades de pointes. Attacks of syncope in the congenital long QT syndrome are effectively treated with high-dose β-blockade. If this is unsuccessful, selective high left stellate ganglionectomy has been employed successfully. Occasionally, pacemaker or defibrillator implantation is necessary for resistant cases.

Prevention of recurrent attacks in the acquired long QT syndrome involves discontinuation of predisposing drugs or other agents. Intravenous magnesium sulphate (1–4 g) appears to be a safe and effective emergency measure. In view of the association of paroxysms of tachycardia with bradycardia and pauses, an attempt to increase heart rate should be made, for example by atrial or ventricular overdrive pacing at a rate of 90–100/min. Alternatively, isoprenaline infusion may be utilized given caution in cases of acute ischaemia.

The prognosis of untreated congenital long QT syndrome is poor, with a high incidence of sudden death in childhood. Retrospective data indicate the 15-year survival in patients following their first episode of torsades de pointes improved from 50 per cent in untreated cases to 90 per cent following treatment with β-blockade and/or left stellate ganglionectomy. The prognosis of acquired long QT syndrome is excellent provided the underlying predisposing factors are identified and avoided.

Ventricular fibrillation (VF)

VF is defined as a chaotic, disorganized arrhythmia with no identifiable QRS complexes (Fig. 4). The mechanism is of multiple, unstable reentry circuits. The ECG pattern depends on the duration. Recent-onset fibrillation is described as 'coarse', with a peak-to-peak amplitude of about 1 mV (1 cm). With increasing duration, the amplitude diminishes and 'fine' VF is less likely to be amenable to successful electrical defibrillation.

VF may represent the end-point of cardiac disease of many aetiologies. It may occur during acute myocardial ischaemia, and is the principal cause of death in the first 2 h following acute myocardial infarction. VF during myocardial infarction is subdivided into primary, occurring without warning in an otherwise stable patient, and secondary, where it occurs in the context of left ventricular failure and cardiogenic shock. In acute myocardial infarction, VF is often initiated by an R on T extrasystole. That occurring in chronic heart disease is most commonly a result of degeneration of rapid VT. VF is rarely self-terminating, and normally causes cardiac arrest, the management of which is discussed below.

Cardiac arrest

Cardiac arrest may arise as a result of a ventricular tachyarrhythmia, asystole, or ventricular standstill, or to electromechanical dissociation, where cardiac output is absent despite continuing ECG evidence of cardiac electrical activity (Table 10).

The initial signs are pulselessness and rapid loss of consciousness, associated with pallor or a grey appearance. The diagnosis of pulselessness should be based on an attempt to feel a large pulse such as the carotid. Respiratory activity may persist for some time after cessation of circulation, and the presence of agonal respiratory efforts in no way excludes the diagnosis of cardiac arrest. Pupillary dilatation is a relatively late occurrence. The majority of successful resuscitations occur within the first 5 min, and long-term success is rare if resuscitation is delayed more than 15 min.

Management

Basic life support

All medical and paramedical staff should be capable of performing basic life support. The first rescuer should shout or telephone for

Table 10 Causes of cardiac arrest

Electrical
- Ventricular fibrillation
- Rapid ventricular tachycardia
- Pre-excited atrial fibrillation
- Asystole
- Complete atrioventricular block with ventricular standstill

Hypoxia/acidosis
- Respiratory arrest

Metabolic
- Hyperkalaemia

Electromechanical dissociation
- Massive haemorrhage/hypovolaemia
- Circulatory obstruction – massive pulmonary embolism, myxoma, prosthetic valve obstruction, air embolism
- Cardiac tamponade
- Tension pneumothorax
- Massive infarction – 'dying heart'
- Drug overdose/intoxication
- Hypothermia

assistance. The vital steps are as simple as ABC. A is for *airways*, indicating that airways obstruction should always be excluded by passing a finger to the back of the tongue. The airways should be cleared by extending the cervical spine and pulling the jaw forwards. B is for *breathing*, using expired air by a mouth-to-mouth or mouth-to-mask approach, pinching the nose to avoid leakage. C is for *circulation*. External cardiac massage should be initiated by chest compression of the lower sternum at a rate of 60 per min. The ratio of chest compressions to lung inflations should be 5:1 if two rescuers are present or 15:2 if the rescuer is single-handed.

Advanced cardiac life support

This involves application of a defibrillator or ECG monitor to identify the cardiac rhythm, with appropriate therapy as determined by the findings. Protection of the airways and avoidance of aspiration requires endotracheal intubation. A large vein should be cannulated for drug administration, although endotracheal administration is an alternative. The guidelines recommended by the European Resuscitation Council are shown in Fig. 19. The probability of survival is greatest in VF. Advisory external defibrillators allows more rapid provision of defibrillation by individuals without detailed training in ECG recognition.

Management of initially successful resuscitation

If the patient remains unconscious, artificial ventilation may be necessary and abnormalities of arterial blood gasses or serum potassium will need correction. If multiple episodes of VF have occurred, lignocaine by bolus and continued infusion should be given. Persistent bradycardia may require atropine or temporary pacing. Persistent hypotension is best treated by dobutamine 2.5–10 μg/kg/min with dopamine 2.5–5 μg/kg/min. Urine output should be carefully monitored. Severe anoxic cerebral damage may cause convulsions which may require treatment by anticonvulsant drugs.

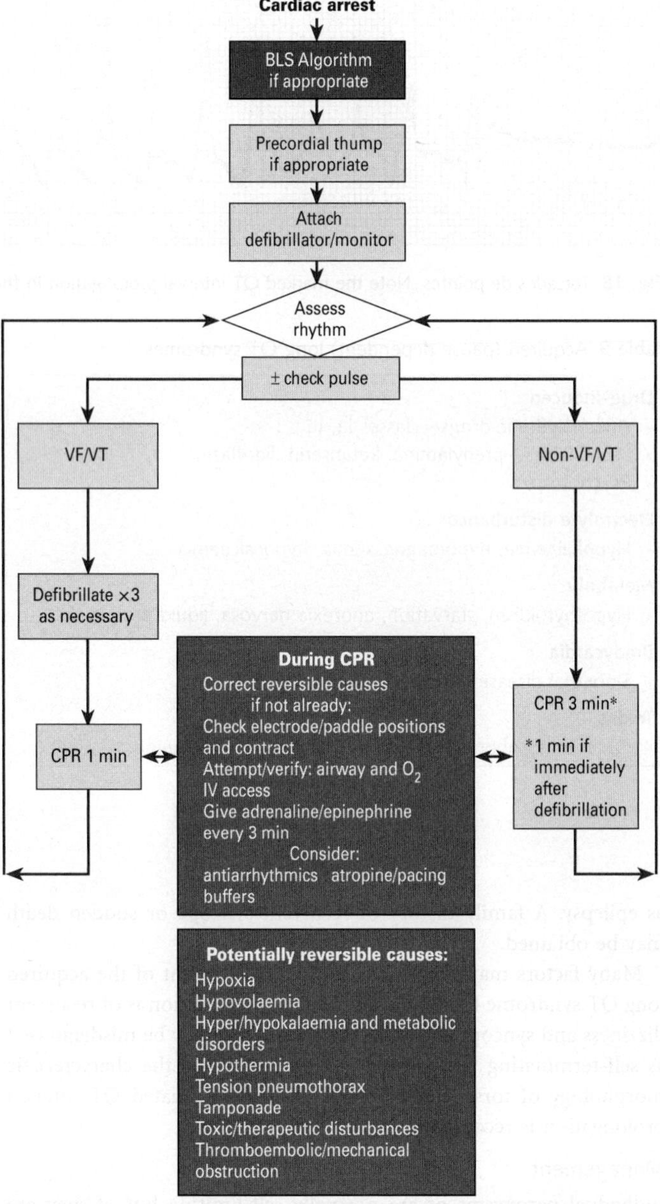

Fig. 19 Guidelines for advanced life support from the European Resuscitation Council. DC, direct current; BLS, basic life support; CPR, cardiopulmonary resuscitation.

Prognosis

The majority in whom a successful outcome occurs will have regained consciousness within 24–48 h, although they may remain confused with memory loss for more prolonged periods. There is no evidence that elective hyperventilation, dexamethasone, or mannitol will improve cerebral recovery.

Successful resuscitation after VF which occurs as a complication of electrophysiological studies is almost 100 per cent, and that occurring during exercise stress testing is 90 per cent. Survival after primary fibrillation in cardiac care units after acute myocardial infarction is good, whereas that of secondary fibrillation in patients with left ventricular failure or cardiogenic shock is very poor. The outcome of cardiac arrest in general wards is generally poorer, as a result of slower response times, greater average age, and differing underlying pathology. The survival rate in episodes occurring out of hospital varies between 15 and 25 per cent. The low survival following asystole is a feature of both in hospital and out of hospital series and reflects the nature of cardiac pathology. Similarly, electromechanical dissociation is normally caused by a catastrophic cardiovascular event which is rarely amenable to immediate correction, thus survival is unusual.

Survivors should be assessed to determine the risk of recurrence. If VF has occurred in the first few hours of a typical Q wave myocardial infarction, the risk of recurrence is low, and no prophylactic therapy other than conventional postinfarction β-blockade is indicated. Patients with VF arising as a result of acute ischaemia with known, extensive heart disease who have not sustained an acute infarction remain at high risk, and should be evaluated by exercise testing and coronary arteriography with a view to revascularization. When the cardiac arrest occurs after a previous myocardial infarction, VF will usually have been the result of degeneration of a preceding rapid VT. These patients are at risk of recurrent arrest and require full electrophysiological evaluation. Most of them will require drug prophylaxis or implantation of a cardioverter defibrillation.

Overall, survival of those surviving to be discharged from hospital following cardiac arrest is in the order of 50–60 per cent at 5 years.

Further reading

Cannom, D.S. and Prystowsky, E.N. (1999). Management of ventricular arrhythmias: detection, drugs, and devices. *Journal of the American Medical Association*, **281**, 172–9.

Morady, F. (1999). Radio-frequency ablation as treatment for cardiac arrhythmias. *New England Journal of Medicine*, **340**, 534–44.

Tresch, D.D. and Thakur, R.K. (1998). Ventricular arrhythmias in the elderly. *Emergency Medicine Clinics of North America*, **16**, 627–48.

Chapter 2.6

Pacemakers

R. Sutton

Pacemakers are most often used to control bradycardia but there are now increasing indications for their use in tachycardias.

Bradycardias requiring pacing comprise: (1) diseases of the ventricular conduction system and of the atrioventricular node; (2) pathology of the sinoatrial node and atria; and (3) disturbances of the neuroendocrine heart rate control mechanisms. The most common pathology in the His–Purkinje system in Western countries is patchy fibrosis perhaps autoimmune in origin; similar fibrotic damage is found in sinoatrial node disease. The aetiology of the neuroendocrine disturbances is unknown. In South America the most common conduction system lesion is that caused by Chagas' disease. Other conditions and therapies affecting ventricular conduction include coronary artery disease, cardiomyopathy, calcific aortic valve disease, surgical correction of some congenital defects, and congenital atrioventricular block.

Tachycardias arising from the ventricles when pacing may be considered are mostly related to coronary artery disease or cardiomyopathy, whereas atrial tachyarrhythmias share their aetiology with that of sinoatrial node disease.

Indications for pacing

Symptoms provide the major indication for cardiac pacing: syncope, dizziness, and heart failure. When complete or second-degree atrioventricular block exist, a pacemaker is advisable, even in the absence of symptoms, as asystole is common and mortality is significantly reduced by pacing. In sinoatrial node disease it has been conventional, hitherto, to pace only to obviate symptoms without expected benefit in mortality, but in more recent studies using atrial and dual chamber pacing, survival is improved and systemic embolism may be avoided. This evidence is now sufficient to consider these types of pacing in patients with asymptomatic sinoatrial node disease.

In carotid sinus syndrome, pacing has been shown to have symptomatic benefit but its place in vasovagal syndrome is not yet defined. In other conditions prophylactic pacing is controversial; these include evidence of conduction tissue disease without symptoms following myocardial infarction or cardiac surgery. Temporary pacing controls many transient arrhythmias but these do not usually require such treatment for longer than 72 h.

Techniques

The implantation of a pacemaker is usually performed under local anaesthesia. The central cephalic approach by incision or the subclavian percutaneously are the veins of choice for the lead, which is passed to the right atrium through the tricuspid valve, and positioned in the apex (anterior) of the right ventricle, or if an atrial lead is used to the right atrium. Prophylactic antibiotics are recommended for a few days after surgery.

Technology

The unit, now weighing 15–35 g, contains a lithium-iodine cell battery giving up to 10 years life. All pacemakers have 'sensing' capability where an amplifier picks up spontaneous cardiac activity and uses this to recycle the pacemaker's output. Thus, if the patient returns to normal sinus rhythm, the pacemaker output is inhibited; as soon as the rate of the spontaneous rhythm falls below the set rate of the pacemaker, stimulation of the heart recommences (demand function). It can be excluded by placing a magnet over the pacemaker, excluding the sensing amplifier from the circuit, rendering the unit asynchronous or fixed rate.

Pacemakers now have an external programmer which can communicate bidirectionally by radiofrequency. It can receive the present settings of rate, output, sensitivity, and refractory periods as well as information on lead and battery function or pacemaker settings can be adjusted to suit the patient's need.

Physiological pacemakers

Pacing the heart at a single rate is not physiological. New technology now allows the patient's physiological state to determine the pacing rate. Two approaches have been followed. First, use of the atria which often function normally in atrioventricular block. Atrial activity is detected via an atrial lead and ventricular pacing via a ventricular lead follows after a suitable interval. The second approach has been to determine the need for a given heart rate by means of a piezoelectric crystal sensor, which acts as a vibration sensor or accelerometer, but other more physiological systems are in use or development. These, when combined with dual chamber systems, allow paced cardiac function to resemble sinus rhythm much more closely.

Results

Permanent pacing results in abolition of symptoms and a marked prolongation in life expectancy in atrioventricular block. Dual chamber pacing gives improved life expectancy over ventricular pacing when heart failure is a presenting feature and atrial or dual chamber pacing also offers benefits in life expectancy in sick sinus syndrome. No such benefits have yet been demonstrated in the case of neuroendocrine disturbances of heart rate.

Complications

The incidence of infection should be less than 1 per cent. Erosion of the pacemaker through the skin has now been almost eliminated with modern lightweight units. Thromboembolism is extremely rare. Local problems such as pain and haematoma are rarely severe.

Perforation of heart or venous system is usually benign: and is now rare. If a lead becomes displaced from the endocardium, loss of capture results. This tends to occur in the first few weeks after implant and may be fatal in those who are pacemaker dependant. Modern tined leads have reduced this incidence to less than 2 per cent. Fracture of the wire, insulation, or both occurs rarely and may be anticipated by alterations in the electronic analysis of the pacemaker pulse. Infection may result in endocarditis at the lead tip and, may necessitate removal, and the use of temporary endocardial pacing. The power required to capture the heart may rise progressively, requiring a higher pacemaker output or a new lead.

Most pacemaker circuit faults occur either as a result of ingress of body fluids or failure of connections between the discrete components and the silicon chip.

The environment provides most hazards to the pacemaker patient. Electromagnetic interference may arise from many sources, including weapon and theft detectors. Most pacemakers revert to asynchronous mode under these conditions without risk to the patient. Some new software-based highly complex pacemakers may dump their programs in the face of surgical diathermy. Special care is required in these cases. Halothane and related anaesthetic gases raise the energy required for capture of the heart and should be avoided. Close contact with leaky microwave ovens and working with special apparatus, such as arc-welders, are contraindicated for pacemaker patients because of possible inappropriate inhibition or acceleration.

Ventricular extrasystoles are not uncommon immediately following lead implant. Occasionally ventricular pacing may be associated with retrograde A-V conduction. This may be asymptomatic or may cause syncope, dizziness, or heart failure. Treatment is by use of an atrioventricular sequential pacemaker.

Further reading

Andersen, H.R., Nielsen J.C., Thomsen, P., *et al.* (1997). Long-term follow-up of patients from a randomised trial of atrial versus ventricular pacing in sick sinus syndrome. *Lancet*, **350**, 1210–16.

Sutton, R., Rydén, L., and Bourgeois I. (1999). *An illustrated practical guide to rate variable pacing. Foundations of cardiac pacing*, Vol. 2. Futura Publishing Co. Inc., Armonk, New York.

Ischaemic heart disease

Chapter 2.7

The pathogenesis of atherosclerosis

R. Naoumova and J. Scott

Atherosclerosis is the underlying cause of heart attacks, strokes, and peripheral vascular disease. It is a focal arterial disease which affects the innermost layer of large and medium-sized arteries and represents a protective inflammatory–fibroproliferative response against different agents that can cause the disease and is characterized by deposition of lipids. Atherosclerosis develops slowly over many years and does not usually become clinically manifest before the fourth or fifth decade. The earliest lesions are fatty streaks. These consist of an accumulation of lipid-engorged macrophages (foam cells), and T lymphocytes in the arterial intima. The fatty streaks progress to intermediate lesions, composed mainly of foam cells and smooth muscle cells. With time smooth muscle cells lay down relatively large amounts of connective tissue and form a fibrous cap which covers the advanced lesion of atherosclerosis (or fibrous plaque), the deeper portion of which consist of macrophages, T lymphocytes, smooth muscle cells, connective tissue, necrotic debris and varying amounts of lipid material, predominantly extracellular cholesterol and its esters, some in a crystalline form.

Plaques may impede the blood flow, giving rise to ischaemic symptoms for example angina, intermittent claudication; or they can undergo denuding injury with limited thrombosis and unstable angina, or deep fissuring with sudden complete occlusion of coronary arteries and myocardial infarction. In the cerebral circulation the same process causes transient ischaemic attacks and completed stroke. Plaques that are at high risk of thrombosis or rupture are called vulnerable or unstable plaques. They are characterized by a large lipid-rich core with surrounding inflammation, a thin cap which is varying in stiffness and thickness, a disorganized pattern of collagen fibrils in the cap, a high macrophage density and a reduced smooth muscle cell content. Plaques with these characteristics are distributed across the whole range of stenosis from angiographically invisible to high degree obstructive ones.

The pathogenesis of atherosclerosis (Fig. 1)

Atherosclerosis develops as a response to repeated vascular-wall injury promoted by several risk factors (Table 1). Oxidatively damaged low-density lipoproteins (**LDL**), the toxins in tobacco smoke, the sheer stress of hypertension, homocysteine, and infectious agents (viral and bacterial) can all cause endothelial dysfunction. The dysfunctional endothelium undergoes a protective response, with the expression of adhesion molecules, growth-promoting substances, and activation of the blood coagulation cascade. Monocytes and T lymphocytes adhere to the activated endothelium and themselves become activated and produce growth factors, cytokines and chemoattractants. The adherent white blood cells migrate into the arterial intima and smooth muscle cells are recruited from the intima and media. With the repeated rounds of injury and repair, palisades of smooth muscle cells, matrix

Table 1 Risk factors for atherosclerosis

Risk factor
Male gender
Race
Diet high in saturated fat and cholesterol, low in fruit, grain, and vegetables
Family history of premature coronary heart disease in first degree relative (men <55 years, women <65 years)
Hypercholesterolaemia (total cholesterol >5.0 mmol/l (190 mg/dl))
Cigarette smoking
Hypertension
Low high-density cholesterol (<1 mmol/l (40 mg/dl))
Diabetes mellitus
Obesity
High lipoprotein (a)
High fibrinogen
High homocysteine

proteins, lipid-laden macrophages, and T lymphocytes accumulate to form the atherosclerotic plaque.

LDL has a central role in the pathogenesis of atherosclerosis. It may enter the intima by transcytosis or through the damaged endothelium, where it undergoes low grade modification by oxidative free-radicals to form minimally modified LDL. This adheres to the matrix proteins of the arterial wall, where it undergoes further oxidation. Free radicals are produced from macrophages and from nitric oxide (**NO**) derived from endothelial cells. This is compounded by the products of tobacco smoke and by homocysteine. Oxidation of the lipid or protein moieties or both renders the lipoprotein atherogenic. Analysis of lipid and protein oxidation products isolated from human atherosclerotic tissue implicate lipoxygenases and the phagocytic enzyme myeloperoxidase as playing a major part at different stages of plaque development.

Oxidized LDLs are not internalized via the LDL receptor but through so-called scavenger receptors, such as SR-AI, SR-AII, CD36, and others, which are expressed in the macrophages accumulating at the site of the vessel wall injury. The accumulation of cholesteryl esters in the cells gives the cytoplasm it characteristic foamy appearance and initiates the atherogenesis. Lipid and cholesterol peroxidation products, minimally oxidized LDL can regulate expression of several pro- and antiatherogenic genes. Oxidized LDL and fatty acid oxidation products regulate several transcription factors such as nuclear factor κB (**NF-κB**) and peroxisome proliferator-activated receptor γ (**PPARγ**).

The cells of the atherosclerotic plaque

Endothelial cells

In the earliest stages of atherogenesis, damaged endothelial cells become dysfunctional. They start producing growth factors, cytokines, chemoattractants, clotting factors, and adhesion molecules. The result is the recruitment and transformation of monocytes into macrophages, and the recruitment and proliferation of smooth muscle cells. Thrombotic processes are activated. There is chronic alteration of vascular tone as a result of disordered NO production and signalling. Sloughing of the endothelium occurs at a later stage, when plaques become complicated and split or fissure.

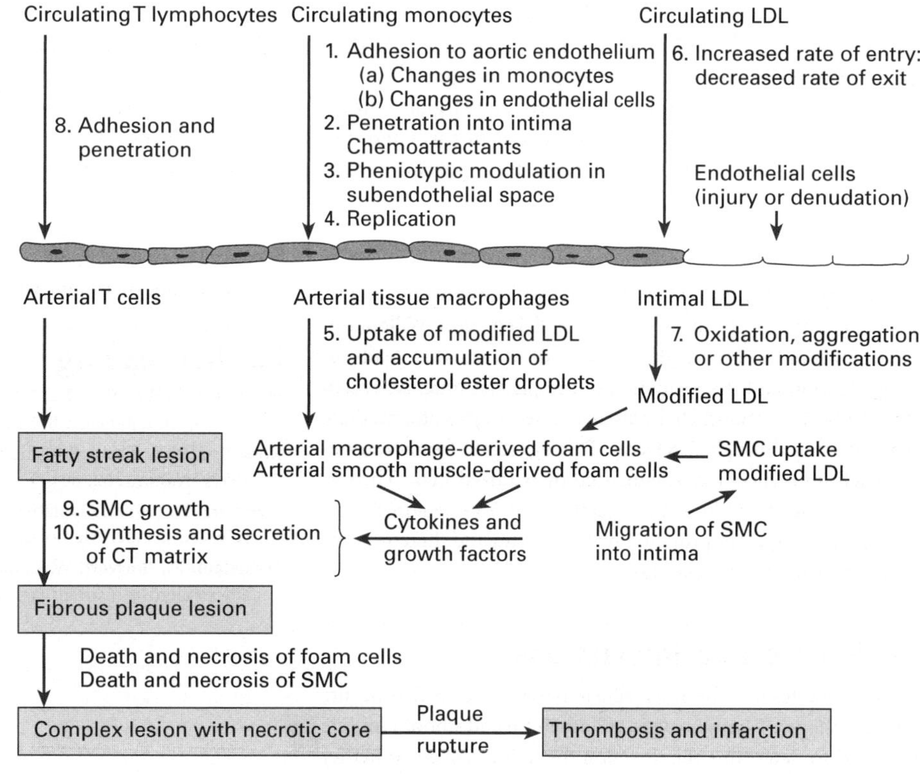

Fig. 1 Schema outlining a current consensus regarding the sequence of events in atherogenesis. SMC, smooth muscle cell.
Reproduced with permission from Rifkind, B.M. (ed.). (1995). Lowering cholesterol in high-risk individuals and populations, p.340. Marcel Dekker Inc., New York.

Monocyte/macrophages

The conversion of monocytes into phagocytically active macrophage is associated with the expression of scavenger receptors. These are cell surface proteins which can bind and internalize not only oxidized LDL but also conformationally modified albumins, oxidatively damaged cells, apoptotic cells as well as wide variety of pathogens (including viral and bacterial). PPARγ is involved in the conversion of macrophages into foam cells by exposure to oxidized LDL and especially oxidation products of linoleic acid.

The activated macrophages secrete a wide variety of growth-modulating substances and chemoattractants. Phagocytic macrophages produce free radicals and are induced to produce NO. This itself generates free radicals and promotes further oxidative damage to LDL. Macrophages also secrete proteolytic enzymes, which contribute to the necrosis and liquefacation of the core of advanced plaques and render it prone to rupture.

Vascular smooth muscle cell

Under the influence of proinflammatory cytokines and growth factors, smooth muscle cells in the plaque switch from contractile to a secretory phenotype to produce extracellular matrix. In addition they increase the cell surface adhesion molecules and the expression of cytokines, growth factors, and molecules involved in extracellular matrix remodelling. NF-κB is an important regulator of the expression of some of these proteins.

T lymphocytes

Immunocompetent cells accompany atherosclerotic plaques at all stages of development. T lymphocytes infiltrating the plaque recognize oxidized LDL and heat shock proteins and this triggers antibody responses. Activated T lymphocytes secrete cytokines which control macrophage activation, scavenger receptor expression and metalloproteinase secretion. Cytokines secreted by both T lymphocytes and macrophages modulate smooth muscle cell proliferation, NO production, and apoptosis, and induce endothelial activation.

Organ transplantation is associated with accelerated graft atherosclerosis. Immunosuppressive drugs are beneficial in this condition suggesting that T-lymphocyte activation plays an important part in transplant atherosclerosis (see Chapter 2.3).

Platelets

Platelets undergo activation when exposed to thrombogenic agents at the site of damage. Agonists such as collagen, von Willebrand factor and fibrinogen initiate the cascade of events that leads to platelet aggregation and the formation of the platelet plug. Activated platelets bind both to endothelial cells and to leucocytes and mediate leucocyte tethering through P-selectin. This aggregate formation between platelets and leucocytes is enhanced by oxidized LDL. Thrombin-activated platelets induce the secretion of interleukin-8 and monocyte-chemoattractant protein-1 by monocytes and thereby stimulate their adhesion by extravasation.

Cell and molecular interactions

In atherosclerotic lesions the intercellular networking, which occurs among macrophages, T lymphocytes, endothelium and smooth muscle cells, is critical to determine the direction the lesion will go. Whether or not a lesion will progress, remain static or undergo regression may be in part a reflection of which genes will be expressed in the different cell types during their interaction.

Growth factors generally promote mitosis or cellular hyperplasia, but can, in certain circumstances, block cell growth. Cytokines play a part in the inflammatory response, and may also act as mitogens and chemoattractants and can inhibit cellular processes. Some growth factors can also act as chemoattractants. Many of these substances are controlled by transcription factors responding to inflammation and promoter elements that respond to shear stress such as NF-κB. Activated NF-κB is found in atherosclerotic lesions but not in normal vessels. Molecular interactions are often local having both autocrine and paracrine effects. An account of the many growth factors, cytokines, adhesion molecules, matrix proteins, and coagulation factors thought to be involved in atherogenesis can be found in OTM3, pp. 2293–4 as well as in recent review articles.

Treatment of atherosclerosis

The treatment of atherosclerosis aims to prevent ischaemic attacks. Lipid lowering especially with statins (HMG-CoA-reductase inhibitors) has been shown to increase plaque stability. The beneficial effects of statins on clinical events may involve additional non-lipid mechanisms that modify endothelial function, inflammatory responses, plaque stability, and thrombus formation. The stable plaque is characterized by reduced lipid core, increased thickness of the cap, decreased number of activated macrophages and T lymphocytes and increased number of smooth muscle cells. The lipid core fills in with fibrous tissue leading to solid plaque which does not disrupt. Several large clinical trials showed a reduction in acute coronary events and strokes as well as in overall mortality following long-term treatment with statins. The prophylactic use of low-dose aspirin also helps to prevent thrombosis in those with atherosclerosis.

Early intervention on the major risk factors for atherosclerosis can lead to marked decrease in its prevalence. The reduction in the death rates from coronary heart disease in western Europe and USA in the recent decades can be attributed to improvement in life style (diet, exercise, smoking) and adequate treatment of the major risk factors (hyperlipidaemia, hypertension, diabetes). In addition to patients with genetically determined hyperlipidaemia and those with clinically manifested atherosclerosis, patients with diabetes mellitus, hypertension, and also individuals with two or more major risk factors for atherosclerosis are appropriate candidates for early and aggressive lipid-lowering treatment with statins.

Further reading

Holvoet, P. and Collen, D. (1997). Thrombosis and atherosclerosis. *Current Opinion in Lipidology*, **8**, 320–8.

Ross, R. (1993). The pathogenesis of atherosclerosis: a perspective for the 1990s. *Nature*, **362**, 801–9.

Steinberg, D. (1997). Oxidative modification of LDL and atherogenesis. Lewis A. Conner Memorial Lecture. *Circulation*, **95**, 1062–71.

Terkeltaub R., Boisvert, W.A., and Curtiss, L.K. (1998). Chemokines and atherosclerosis. *Current Opinion in Lipidology*, **9**, 397–405.

Chapter 2.8

The pathophysiology of ischaemic heart disease

M. J. Davies

Atherosclerosis and ischaemic heart disease

The critical lesions of atherosclerosis in relation to ischaemic heart disease is the initial plaque. Examination of coronary arteries of young people who had died from accidents have shown that the earliest lesions (fatty streaks) are flat yellow dots or streaks on the intima. Each comprises lipid filled modified monocytic (foam) cells which have accumulated beneath intact endothelium. Next appears extracellular lipid, followed by smooth muscle cells and increasing amounts of collagen. The final lesion is a raised fibro-lipid plaque, the basis of clinical symptoms and events. Many plaques are situated eccentrically, with a residual arc of normal vessel wall opposite the plaque. The typical advanced plaque has a core of extracellular lipid (Fig. 1), which is encapsulated by fibrous tissue produced by smooth muscle cells, and a fibrous cap separating the core from the lumen. The cap has considerable tensile strength due to high concentrations of collagen and elastin and is covered by endothelium on its luminal surface.

Advanced plaques and clinical symptoms

Many advanced plaques cause no symptoms and are angiographically invisible. The artery in this situation has responded to the plaque by increasing its external diameter, thus accommodating the plaque without compromising the lumen. Larger plaques overcome the remodelling process and cause focal narrowing of the lumen. and when it is reduced by more than 50 per cent in diameter, flow is limited when myocardial oxygen demand rises. The result is stable exertional angina.

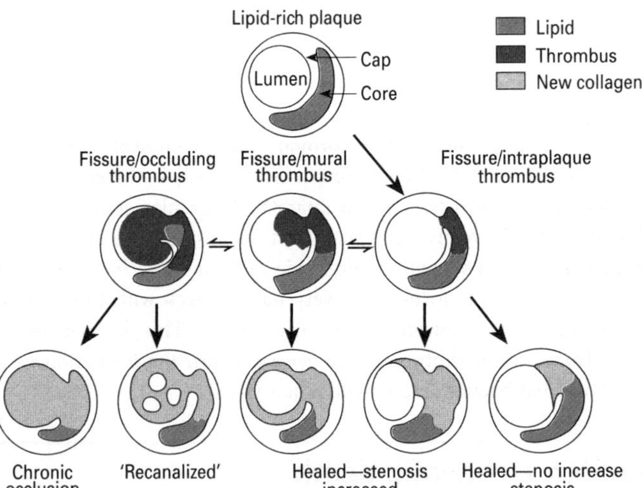

Fig. 1 Potential outcome of an episode of plaque disruption. A healing process is initiated with fibrinolysis and followed by smooth muscle proliferation. This proliferation restabilizes the plaque and may often lead to an increase in the degree of stenosis.

A second mechanism for the production of symptoms is thrombosis on an advanced plaque, producing an acute reduction of blood flow and acute myocardial infarction or unstable angina. The third process is altered vascular tone. Normal coronary arteries dilate in response to an increase in blood flow; in atherosclerosis the arteries undergo paradoxical vasoconstriction. This abnormal response is characteristic both of areas with angiographic lesions, and adjacent segments which ostensibly look normal.

Progression of coronary atherosclerosis

Data on progression are derived from serial angiography. Individual patients vary widely in the overall rate of progression; the rate of progression of individual stenoses is also variable. In general, progression is episodic; lesions that appear between two angiograms often develop at points where the vessel previously appeared normal or minimally diseased. A significant proportion of these 'new' lesions are very high grade or even totally obstructive and may appear without any overt signs of acute ischaemia.

Thrombosis in atherosclerosis

Two processes cause thrombosis on plaques. In the first (superficial injury) there is endothelial denudation over the plaque. Subendothelial collagen is exposed and a platelet-rich thrombus forms over the surface. Approximately one in four of larger thrombi that occlude coronary vessels are due to severe superficial injury of this kind. In the second (deep intimal injury) the plaque splits or tears through the cap. Blood enters the lipid core to meet a thrombogenic mixture of tissue factor, collagen and lipid. A platelet-rich thrombus forms within the plaque which may then extend into the lumen. Plaque fissuring covers a wide spectrum of severity; at one extreme there are microfissures no more than a few hundred microns across; at the other, the whole cap may be torn over a centimetre of the artery. When blood enters the core, thrombosis is inevitable but does not always lead to luminal obstruction.

Pathogenesis of plaque fissuring

Plaque cap tearing reflects the imposition of increased mechanical stress on an area weakened in its ability to withstand such stress. Circumferential wall stress is normally distributed evenly across the vessel wall but the soft core cannot carry its share which is carried by the cap. The larger the core, the greater the angle that the core subtends; the thinner the cap, the greater is the concentration of force on the cap in systole. The cap tissue itself may also undergo physical changes reducing its mechanical strength.

Evolution of thrombi

The initial response to a thrombus is lysis but thrombus which is not removed invokes local smooth muscle proliferation and replacement by collagenous tissue (organization). Combinations of lysis and organization mean that following coronary thrombosis a wide range of putative outcomes exist (see Fig. 1). These range from chronic total occlusion to restoration of a normal lumen. Minor plaque fissures and intraplaque thrombosis are found in people who have died from accidents but who have not had clinical evidence of ischaemic heart disease. Such subclinical events are important in episodic progression to coronary atherosclerosis.

The concept of stable and unstable plaques

Vulnerable plaques are those with a high risk of thrombosis; unstable plaques are those actually undergoing thrombosis. Vulnerability is a reflection both of the amount of lipid present and the degree of inflammatory activity in the plaque. Regression of atherosclerosis following the lowering of plasma lipid levels may reduce plaque lipid and lead to a more solid fibrous plaque, so reducing the frequency of new acute ischaemic events.

The pathology of angina

Stable angina

Stable angina is caused by segments of stenosis of more than 50 per cent in diameter in one, two, or three of the major coronary arteries. The smooth regular stenoses often remain unchanged for long periods. Plaques may then be concentric involving the whole circumferences or eccentric with a normal vessel wall opposite the plaque, when vascular tone in the normal segment can alter lumen size. Some subjects with stable angina have entirely fibrous concentric plaques; perhaps whose disease remains stable for years. Others have a high proportion of lipid-rich plaques, and therefore a higher risk of an acute event. Most subjects with stable angina have a mixture.

Autopsy studies show that up to 40 per cent of subjects with stable angina, even when there is no previous infarction, have a totally occluded artery at some point. At such a point the lumen may be occluded by fibrous tissue with extensive bridging collaterals in the adjacent adventitia, or there may be a number of new vascular channels within the original lumen.

Unstable angina

In crescendo angina there is a non-occluding thrombus projecting into the lumen from an underlying plaque fissure. Angiography then reveals stenosis characterized by an irregular outline, eccentric indentation, overhanging edge, and intraluminal radiotransluscent thrombus. The surface of such a plaque at autopsy is covered by platelet-rich thrombus, and distal embolization of small clumps of platelets occurs. These microemboli are associated with focal microscopic myocardial necrosis. In less severe cases, the association with thrombosis becomes less certain. Altered or enhanced vascular tone at segments of eccentric stenosis is a substantiated alternative mechanism.

Acute myocardial infarction

Infarction in heart muscle may be regional or diffuse. Regional infarction is further subdivided into transmural and non-transmural (subendocardial). Diffuse infarction usually consists of a circumferential necrosis of the subendocardial zone and the papillary muscle of the left ventricle. In regional infarction the cause lies in occlusion of the subtending artery, in the vast majority of cases by thrombosis. Rare exceptions include coronary spasm, dissection, and embolism. Three-quarters of all thrombi are due to a plaque disruption, the remainder being due to superficial intimal injury. Diffuse infarction is due to a more general failure of myocardial perfusion, often following prolonged hypotension and is exacerbated by ventricular hypertrophy and high left ventricular diastolic pressure.

Structure of human infarction

Regional transmural infarction usually results in the changes of coagulative necrosis with uniform appearances throughout the infarcted zone. In contrast, many non-transmural infarcts appear to be built up by the coalescence of smaller focal areas of necrosis of different ages and contraction band necrosis indicating reperfusion. In the healed phase, when fibrosis has replaced the dead tissue, strands and islands of surviving myocytes embedded in the scar are common.

The pathology of complications of human infarction

Sudden death due to ventricular arrhythmias during acute infarction is not directly related to infarct size and has a maximal risk in the first 24 h, when there are islands of ischaemic, but still viable, myocardium with the potential to cause re-entry circuits.

Cardiogenic shock is directly related to the proportion of the left ventricular muscle mass that has been lost.

Cardiac rupture, responsible for 5–8 per cent of the mortality of acute infarction comes in two forms. In the first, rupture occurs within 24 h and appears as a ragged tear at the margin of dead and viable myocardium. In the second, rupture occurs later, and is through an infarct that has thinned and become aneurysmal. Ventricular septal defects complicating infarction have similar pathology, and may be anteroseptal due to left anterior descending coronary occlusions or posteroseptal due to right coronary occlusion. Papillary muscle rupture may involve one or several heads of either the anterolateral or posteromedial papillary muscle. While many such ruptures are associated with extensive free wall infarction, older people may have a very localized infarct of papillary muscle with resultant rupture caused by occlusion of the left marginal coronary artery.

Infarct expansion and remodelling

Following infarction, the ventricular shape may undergo very drastic changes. In the first 24 h the dead area may thin and stretch due to slipping and tearing of bundles of myocytes. When organization and repair by fibrosis occurs, the expanded shape of the infarct zone is retained permanently. Left ventricular cavity size is increased and the residual surviving myocardium may also undergo compensatory hypertrophy.

Infarct thinning and expansion is a complication of transmural and large regional infarcts; its predominant cause is proximal occlusion of the left anterior descending coronary artery. Survival of a rim of subpericardial muscle prevents expansion, which is therefore not a complication of non-transmural infarcts. Ventricular aneurysms are closely related in many cases to infarct expansion. The aneurysmal bulge may be diffuse, with a very wide neck or more localized with a narrow neck. One form has a very narrow neck with the bulk of the aneurysm sac outside the ventricle itself. This is thought to result from partial rupture of the ventricle with the formation of a subpericardial haematoma (pseudoaneurysms).

Sudden ischaemic death

Two mechanisms appear to be involved in sudden cardiac death. One is by way of a new acute event due to coronary thrombosis or spasm; the other is of a fatal arrhythmia arising in a scarred and/or hypertrophied left ventricle. There is no agreement on the relative frequency of these two mechanisms.

Further reading

Coronary heart disease. (1996). *Lancet*, **348** (Suppl. 1), 1–31.

Detry, J.M. (1996). The pathophysiology of myocardial ischaemia. *European Heart Journal*, **173** (Suppl. G), 48–52.

Chapter 2.9

Vascular endothelium, its physiology and pathophysiology

P. Vallance

Endothelial cells are metabolically highly active and exert a profound influence on vascular reactivity, thrombogenesis, and the behaviour of circulating cells (Fig. 1). Abnormalities of endothelial function have been implicated in a wide variety of diseases ranging from atheroma and hypertension to acute inflammation and septic shock. The properties of endothelial cells vary between arterial and venous beds, between micro- and macrovasculature, between organs and between different parts of individual organs. This heterogeneity has implications for physiology, pathophysiology, and therapeutics, and some examples are discussed below.

Anatomy of endothelium

Endothelial cells lie with their long axis aligned in the direction of the blood flow. The underlying smooth muscle cells lie radially so that a single endothelial cell comes into contact with many smooth muscle cells and vice versa (Fig. 2). The total area of the luminal surface of endothelium is in excess of 500 m^2. These highly specialized cells are ideally placed to mediate communication between blood and the vessel wall, they detect signals in the lumen of the vessel and translate them into messages understood by underlying smooth muscle or passing blood cells.

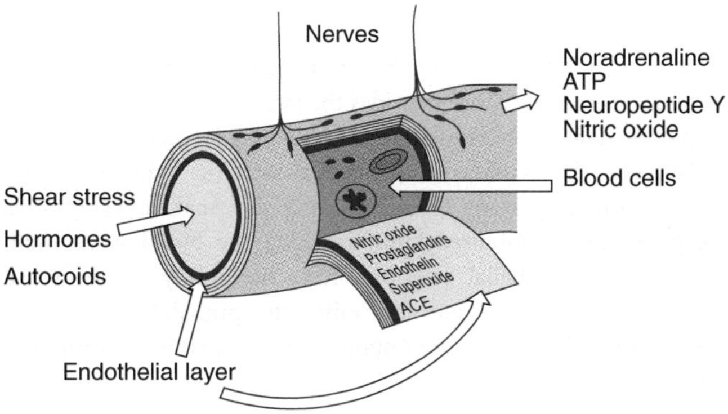

Fig. 1 The vascular endothelium detects chemical (e.g. hormonal), physical (e.g. shear stress or intraluminal pressure), and cellular signals in the lumen of the vessel and adjusts its output of vasoactive mediators accordingly. Nerves lying in the adventitia exert a predominant constrictor influence whereas the endothelium exerts a predominant dilator influence. Together these systems provide mechanisms for the rapid adjustment of vascular tone in response to central (nervous) and local (endothelial) activation.

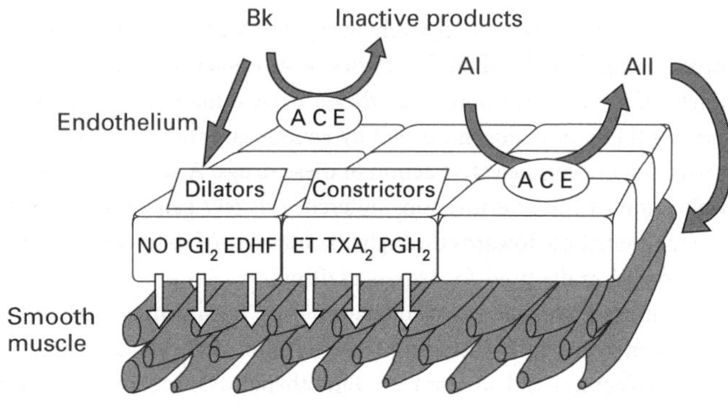

Fig. 2 Vasoactive mediators produced by endothelial cells. Dilator and constrictor mediators are synthesized and released. ACE is located on the cell surface and converts angiotensin I into angiotensin II and metabolizes bradykinin to inactive products. Bradykinin stimulates the release of dilator mediators. Abbreviations: NO, nitric oxide; PGI_2, prostacyclin; EDHF, endothelium-derived hyperpolarizing factor; ET, endothelin; TXA_2, thromboxane A2; PGH_2, prostaglandin H_2; Bk, bradykinin; AI, angiotensin I; ACE, angiotensin-converting enzyme

Control of vascular tone

Endothelium extracts and inactivates circulating hormones, converts inactive precursors into active products, and synthesizes and releases a variety of vasoactive mediators which allow the vessel to respond to changes in the local milieu (Figs 1 and 2).

Vasodilators

Nitric oxide

Nitric oxide (NO) is responsible for basal arterial endothelium-dependent dilator tone. It is synthesized from l-arginine and has a half-life of only a few seconds. It diffuses from endothelium into underlying smooth muscle, where it binds to the haem moiety of guanylate cyclase and produces a conformational change that leads to enzyme activation. The subsequent increase in cyclic guanosine monophosphate (**cGMP**) relaxes the smooth muscle. NO is also released on the luminal surface where it inhibits platelet activation. Contact with haemoglobin rapidly inactivates NO to prevent any downstream effect. In addition to activation of guanylate cyclase, NO also inhibits cytochrome *c* oxidase and may act as a regulator of mitochondrial function and tissue oxygen consumption.

Inhibition of NO synthesis leads to rapid vasoconstriction and hypertension. The basal generation of NO in resistance vessels appears to offer a counterbalance to the basal constrictor effects of the sympathetic nervous system. The precise physiological stimuli for the production of NO are not yet known, but probably include shear stress and platelet-derived mediators. The response to increased shear stress accounts for flow-dependent vasodilatation while that to aggregating platelets may protect against adverse effects of intravascular platelet activation. NO synthesis is also stimulated by acetylcholine, bradykinin, and substance P. In many vessels its release contributes to the vasodilator actions of these mediators, which are known as 'endothelium-dependent vasodilators'.

Venous endothelium releases NO when stimulated by acetylcholine or bradykinin, but not under basal conditions. Nor do human veins release much NO in response to platelet-derived mediators. Indeed, aggregating platelets constrict veins, due to the unopposed action of the mediators on vascular smooth muscle. One consequence of the difference between arteries and veins is that the guanylate cyclase in venous smooth muscle is relatively upregulated and veins respond to lower amounts of NO than do arteries or arterioles. NO is the active moiety of glyceryl trinitrate and other nitrovasodilators, and the low basal synthesis of endogenous NO by venous endothelium accounts, in part, for the venoselective action of these drugs. A second potential implication of the arteriovenous difference in NO generation is that it might contribute towards the higher failure rate of venous compared with arterial grafts used for bypass grafting.

Diminished NO-mediated dilatation has been implicated in a number of conditions including hypertension, diabetes, and hypercholesterolaemia, and in smokers. Endothelial dysfunction precedes the development of overt atheroma and there is a relationship between risk factors for ischaemic heart disease and impaired responsiveness of coronary arteries to endothelium-dependent vasodilators. Hypercholesterolaemia, even in the absence of atheroma or in children, is associated with abnormal endothelium-dependent vasodilatation in coronary and peripheral arterioles, and modified low-density lipoproteins (**LDLs**) appear to inhibit NO synthesis or speed its destruction. NO is also destroyed by oxygen free radicals (e.g. superoxide anion which is also generated by endothelial cells) and this might be an important mechanism linking oxidant stress to cardiovascular disease. Certain common genetic polymorphic variants of the endothelial NO synthase gene appear to be associated with enhanced coronary artery disease, possibly due to deficient endothelial NO generation. In experimental models, loss of NO enhances atherogenesis and predisposes to vasospasm and vessel occlusion, and in patients flow-dependent dilatation is lost and the response to sympathetic stimulation in the coronary circulation is converted from dilatation to unopposed constriction.

Overproduction of NO is also associated with disease and mediates the vasodilatation of certain types of inflammation. Bacterial endotoxin, and certain cytokines, including interleukin-1, may lead to expression of a second NO synthesizing enzyme in the endothelium, the vascular smooth muscle itself, and inflammatory cells infiltrating the vessel wall. This inducible NO synthase can produce large amounts of NO over long periods, contributing to tissue damage and causing profound vasodilatation and hypotension (septic shock).

Prostanoids

The endothelium is a rich source of prostanoids, including the vasodilators prostacyclin and prostaglandin (**PG**) E_2 and PGD_2. However, whereas inhibition of NO leads to profound and widespread changes in vascular tone, inhibition of prostanoid synthesis does not. Renal vasculature is an exception; aspirin and other non-steroidal anti-inflammatories vasoconstrict the kidney. In the fetus and newborn, indomethacin leads to closure of the ductus arteriosus and a fall in cerebral blood flow suggesting a significant contribution of endothelium-derived prostanoids to cardiovascular control at this stage of development. Vasodilator prostanoids are also important in the vascular changes of inflammation and expression of the pro-inflammatory isoform of cyclo-oxygenase (COX II) can be induced within endothelial cells.

Endothelium-derived hyperpolarizing factor

The endothelium mediates hyperpolarization of underlying smooth muscle and this causes relaxation. The identity of a putative diffusible factor mediating such an effect is not yet known.

Vasoconstrictors

Endothelins

The endothelins are a family of potent vasoconstrictor 21-amino-acid peptides related to the sarafatoxin snake venoms. Three endothelins have been described; endothelin 1, 2, and 3, and there are at least two endothelin receptors in human blood vessels: ET_A and ET_B.

Endothelin-1, synthesized from 'big endothelin' within human endothelial cells, is a potent and long-lasting constrictor of human blood vessels. Endothelin receptor antagonists cause vasodilatation and reduce blood pressure suggesting that basal generation of endothelin contributes to a slowly modulating vasoconstrictor tone in humans. Low concentrations of endothelins also appear to enhance responses to certain other constrictor agents and this might be important in determining the overall reactivity of blood vessels *in vivo*. While it is clear that activation of the ETA receptor subtypes mediates vasoconstriction, activation of the ETB subtype may mediate either constriction, dilatation, or both, depending on the blood vessel and the concentration of endothelin. Physiological stimuli for the release of endothelins remain unclear, but might include hypoxia, thrombin, and transforming growth factor β.

Elevated circulating levels of endothelin-1 occur in patients with myocardial infarction, diabetes, and renal failure, and local increases are seen in the venous blood draining the hand of patients with Raynaud's disease and in coronary sinus blood of patients with coronary vasospasm. A role for endothelin in the pathogenesis of vasospasm associated with subarachnoid haemorrhage and some types of renal ischaemia is suggested by animal experiments, and endothelin antagonists are in clinical trial for the treatment of hypertension, heart failure, and renal disease.

Increased production endothelin has been directly implicated in the pathogenesis of a very rare form of secondary hypertension caused by malignant haemangioendothelioma, in which there is proliferation of atypical endothelial cells. In this condition the degree of hypertension correlates with plasma levels of endothelin and when the tumour is removed blood pressure and plasma endothelin levels fall.

Angiotensin-converting enzyme

Angiotensin-converting enzyme (**ACE**) is located primarily on the luminal surface of the endothelium. It converts angiotensin I to angiotensin II and also metabolizes bradykinin to inactive products. The pulmonary vasculature provides the largest area of endothelium, and is important in the regulation of circulating levels of angiotensin II. However, the activity of endothelial ACE in systemic vessels may be more important in determining the final concentrations of angiotensin II and bradykinin reaching the blood vessel wall. Furthermore, endothelial cells also have the ability to synthesize renin and its substrate and this raises the probability that local renin–angiotensin systems are important in local control of vascular tone.

Prostanoids

The endothelium synthesizes thromboxane (**TXA_2**) and the unstable prostaglandin endoperoxides PGG_2 and PGH_2. Overproduction of constrictor prostanoids by the endothelium has been implicated in animal models of diabetes and hypertension but the significance of these findings in human disease remains uncertain.

Regulation of platelet function and haemostasis

The endothelium synthesizes and releases prothrombotic and antithrombotic factors, with the antithrombotic ones predominating under basal conditions.

Platelets

Endothelial cells inhibit platelet aggregation and adhesion, and disaggregate aggregating platelets. Two mediators are of particular importance: NO and prostacyclin (or PGE_2 in microvascular endothelium). They act through different second messenger systems—cGMP for NO and cyclic adenosine monophosphate for prostacyclin. Thiols and sulphydryl-containing molecules may react with NO to produce more stable adducts, including nitrosocysteine and nitrosoglutathione which may form *in vivo* and enhance the antiplatelet effects of the L-arginine/NO pathway. Loss of NO and prostacyclin at sites of endothelial damage or dysfunction promotes the formation of platelet aggregates and may contribute to thrombosis and vessel occlusion. Inflammatory mediators or repeated endothelial injury lead to the formation of unstable prostaglandin endoperoxides, platelet-activating factors, and von Willebrand factor, and further increase platelet adhesion and activation.

Coagulation

Heparan sulphates are found on the surface of endothelial cells and antithrombin III is expressed on the endothelial cell surface. Together these provide a mechanism for binding and inactivating thrombin. In addition, endothelial cells participate in the activation of protein C; protein S is secreted and thrombomodulin is found on the cell surface. In the quiescent state, expression of these anticoagulant factors predominates; however, once activated, the endothelium may promote coagulation: receptors for clotting factors appear on the endothelial surface, von Willebrand factor is secreted, and tissue factor is expressed. Bacterial endotoxin, inflammatory cytokines, and glycosylated proteins activate the endothelium and shift the balance in favour of coagulation.

Thrombolysis

The endothelial cell surface has a fibrinolytic pathway. Urokinase and tissue plasminogen activator are secreted and there are specific binding sites for plasminogen activators and plasminogen. Thrombin, adrenaline, vasopressin, and stasis of blood may be stimuli for tissue plasminogen activator release from human endothelium.

Plasminogen activator inhibitor I (PAI) is also synthesized and bound by endothelium, providing a pathway for local inhibition of the fibrinolytic system. Under basal conditions fibrinolysis is dominant, but the balance may be altered by a variety of local and circulating factors, including inflammatory cytokines and lipoprotein (a), which inhibits plasminogen binding and hence plasmin generation. In the presence of atherosclerosis the fibrinolytic properties of endothelium appear to be diminished.

Cellular adhesion

The resting endothelium prevents cells from adhering fully to the vessel wall but allows leucocytes to roll along its surface. The regulation of 'rolling', adhesion, and migration is governed largely by cell adhesion molecules, which are expressed in varying amounts on the endothelial cell surface and interact with complementary adhesion molecules on circulating cells. The degree of expression and the type of adhesion molecules expressed determines the 'stickiness' of the endothelium for different cell types. Expression of adhesion molecules is an important mechanism of cellular adhesion during inflammation but is also important in the recruitment of monocytes in atherosclerosis. NO and prostacyclin inhibit the adhesion of white cells to endothelium, an effect mediated by changes in the expression or configuration of adhesion molecules.

Cell growth

Healthy 'quiescent' endothelium inhibits proliferation of the underlying smooth muscle. Endothelium-derived vasodilator, antiplatelet, and antithrombotic mediators tend to inhibit cell growth whereas vasoconstrictor prothrombotic mediators tend to promote it. The basal antiproliferative effects of the endothelium may retard the development of atherosclerosis and intimal proliferation and in experimental models endothelial damage is associated with smooth muscle cell growth and neointima formation. A number of important endothelium-derived growth factors have been described. Vascular endothelial growth factor (**VEGF**) appears to be particularly important and can initiate re-vascularization and affect vascular re-modelling. Early trials of gene transfer of VEGF for peripheral vascular disease have been reported.

Cytokines

Interleukins-1, -6, and -8, and colony-stimulating factors are synthesized by endotoxin-stimulated endothelial cells, and tumour necrosis factor (**TNF**) -α by smooth muscle cells. A large number of cytokines alter endothelial functions, upsetting the balance of vasoactive mediators, and altering thrombotic activity and expression of adhesion molecules. Interleukin-1β increases the synthesis of NO and a variety of prostaglandins whereas TNF appears to initiate endothelial damage and dysfunction and may impair the ability of the endothelium to respond to hormonal and physical signals. Pro-inflammatory cytokines enhance the endothelial generation of thrombin, platelet-activating factor, von Willebrand factor, and plasminogen activator inhibitor; alter endothelial permeability; increase expression of some adhesion molecules; and may also cause endothelial cell damage and death. The ultimate effect of any cytokine will depend on the local concentration achieved, kinetics of its release, and the local environment of other cytokines and mediators into which it is released. Enhanced generation of certain cytokines might be important in mediating endothelial dysfunction in systemic inflammatory conditions and also in cardiovascular disorders, including heart failure and acute coronary syndromes.

Transport and metabolism

Transfer of molecules from the bloodstream into the vessel wall occurs by transport through the endothelial cells or between them. Transport between cells occurs when endothelial cells contract to leave intercellular gaps, an important mechanism of localized oedema formation. Transport through cells is an important mechanism for the passage of certain macromolecules, including insulin.

Lipoprotein lipase is located on the endothelial cell surface and receptors for LDLs are present in varying amounts. In quiescent endothelium lipoprotein lipase is active but there are few LDL

Table 1 Therapies for acute cardiovascular events and their effects on endothelial function

Drug	Effect on endothelium
Nitrovasodilators	Mimics endogenous nitric oxide
Low-dose aspirin	Restores balance of endothelial/platelet prostanoid synthesis in favour of endothelium
Thrombolytics	Enhances usual endothelial thrombolytic capacity
Heparin	Mimics usual anticoagulant effect of heparan sulphates on endothelium
Balloon angioplasty	Acutely disrupts endothelial integrity

receptors, indicating that healthy endothelium provides a barrier for entry of LDL into the vessel wall. Under conditions in which LDL is taken into the endothelium, modification by oxidation occurs and this step may stimulate atherogenesis.

Signal detection by endothelial cells

Endothelial cell membranes express a large number of receptors for circulating hormones, local mediators, and vasoactive factors released from blood cells, and express specialized ion channels and other cell surface proteins that can sense local changes in pressure and flow.

Therapeutic implications

Certain therapeutic interventions result in endothelial damage. Antibodies directed against the endothelium are found after heart transplantation and endothelial dysfunction may contribute to the rapid development of coronary disease seen in transplant recipients. Balloon angioplasty damages the endothelium and this has been implicated in the development of postangioplasty vasospasm, thrombosis, and restenosis. Venous coronary artery bypass grafts are more prone to occlusion than arterial grafts, and this may reflect differences between arterial and venous endothelium. Acute disruption of endothelial function may promote vasospasm, thrombosis, and occlusion and chronic changes enhance atherogenesis. Many existing therapies for acute cardiovascular disorders have significant effects to replace or restore endothelial function (Table 1). New drugs or therapeutic approaches targeted towards endothelial biology which are in clinical trials include endothelin receptor antagonists, novel NO donors with antiplatelet or other effects, antioxidants, inhibitors of NO synthases as anti-inflammatory agents, drugs affecting adhesion molecule expression or function, and gene transfer of NO synthase genes and vascular endothelial growth factor.

Further reading

Noll, G. and Luscher, T.F. (1998). The endothelium in acute coronary syndromes. *European Heart Journal*, **Suppl. C**, C30–8.

Wu, K.K. and Thiagarajan, P. (1996). Role of endothelium in thrombosis and hemostasis. *Annual Revue of Medicine*, 47, 315–31.

Chapter 2.10

Epidemiology and prevention of ischaemic heart disease

M. G. Marmot, J. I. Mann, and T. W. Meade

Occurrence of ischaemic heart disease

In England and Wales 30 per cent of all deaths among men and 22 per cent among women are the result of ischaemic heart disease (IHD), which is also the commonest cause of death in most industrialized countries. Although death rates from IHD in the UK have been falling since the 1970s they are still uncomfortably high (Table 1).

In recent years, in addition to the approximately 156 000 deaths every year in England and Wales, there have been, on average, 115 000 hospital discharges with the diagnosis IHD. In 60 per cent of all fatal myocardial infarctions, death occurs in the first hours after the attack. Most IHD deaths, therefore, occur too rapidly for treatment to influence prognosis, hence the importance of prevention.

Regional and ethnic differences in the UK

Death rates from IHD are higher in Northern Ireland, Scotland, and the north of England than in Wales or southern England and South Asians living in the UK have a higher rate of premature death from IHD than have the indigenous population.

International differences

There are marked international differences in the rate of occurrence of IHD. In one study among men aged 40–59 years initially free of IHD, the annual occurrence of new cases varied from 15 per 10 000 in Japan to 198 per 10 000 in Finland. Mortality statistics show a similar picture (Table 1). Some of the variation is undoubtedly due to differences in diagnostic practice and in coding of death certificates, but numerous studies using comparable methods have confirmed that real differences exist.

The experience of migrants suggests that these variations are likely to be the result chiefly of environmental or behavioural differences. People who have migrated from a low-risk country (e.g. Japan) to a high-risk country (e.g. the United States) tend to have rates of IHD approaching that of the host country.

The current international picture is one of marked contrasts (Fig. 1). Many countries with traditionally high rates of IHD have now experienced declines: among these are the United States, Finland, and other countries of western and northern Europe. By contrast, countries of central and eastern Europe and Singapore have shown marked increases over the last two decades. That an epidemic of IHD is not the inevitable consequence of wealth is shown by Japan, which has experienced a 40 per cent decline over a 20-year period.

Risk factors for ischaemic heart disease

Age and gender

The incidence of IHD increases exponentially with age, and in middle age the rate in men is three to four times that in women. After the menopause, the male/female ratio narrows. This could be due to loss

Table 1 Age-standardized death rates per 100 000 population aged 35–74 from IHD; selected countries

Country	Year	Men	Women
Latvia	1994	919	303
Russian Federation	1994	812	280
Estonia	1994	707	252
Belarus	1993	664	256
Lithuania	1994	663	223
Czechoslovakian Republic	1993	460	166
Hungary	1994	452	173
Ireland	1992	380	136
Romania	1993	367	166
Bulgaria	1994	352	132
Finland	1994	346	98
UK	1994	325	120
New Zealand	1993	308	120
Denmark	1993	306	120
Poland	1994	281	84
Norway	1993	276	81
Croatia	1994	269	132
Sweden	1993	252	77
USA	1993	248	100
Austria	1994	241	80
Germany	1994	237	79
Australia	1994	217	79
Canada	1994	212	75
Israel	1994	199	93
The Netherlands	1994	196	67
Greece	1994	168	48
Italy	1992	153	43
Spain	1993	130	36
Portugal	1994	128	47
France	1994	94	24
Japan	1994	49	18

Data from British Heart Foundation Database 1998, with permission.

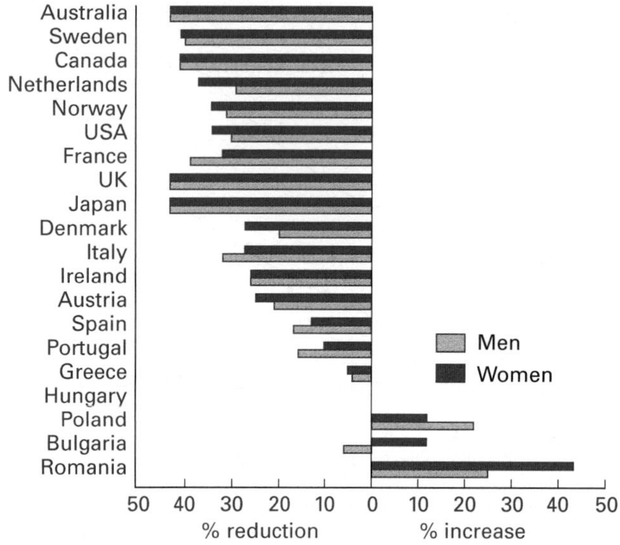

Fig. 1 Changes in death rates from IHD, men and women aged 35–74 (1983–1993), selected countries
(taken, with permission, from the British Heart Foundation database, Fig. 1.5(b), p. 21)

of a protective effect in women, loss of a harmful effect in men, or even killing off of male susceptibles.

Most of the studies on risk factors have been in middle-aged men, so that there have been doubts as to whether those identified in men could properly be accepted for women. It is now clear that they can, although the magnitude of the association may vary. It is important to distinguish between relative and absolute risk. For a number of factors, the relative risk declines with age, but *pari passu* the absolute risk may increase so that detection of risk factors in the elderly continues to be useful.

Physiological risk factors

Lipids and lipoproteins

Total cholesterol and low-density lipoprotein

No other blood constituent varies so much between different populations as serum cholesterol. From New Guinea to east Finland the mean serum cholesterol ranges from 2.6 to 7.02 mmol/litre (100–270 mg/100 ml) when estimated by the same method in the same age and sex group. The extent to which total cholesterol correlates with the geographic variation of IHD varies in different studies. In the Seven Countries Study, mean cholesterol values were highly correlated with IHD death rates ($r = 0.8$), accounting for 64 per cent of the variance between cohorts. In the MONICA study the classic risk factors (cholesterol, blood pressure, and smoking) accounted for a much smaller proportion of such variance. More important is the fact that among individuals within populations the association is exceptionally strong. In over 20 prospective studies in different countries, total serum cholesterol has been shown to be related to the rate of development of IHD, the association being 'dose' related, occurring in both sexes and independent of all other measured risk factors. The association in the Multiple Risk Factor Intervention Trial (**MRFIT**) study is shown in Fig. 2. Risk of IHD varies over a fivefold range in relation to serum cholesterol levels found in an average American population. There is no discernible critical value, the risk tending to increase throughout the range. While the absolute risk associated with any given cholesterol value varies in different parts of the world, within almost every population sampled, the risk is greater in people with higher than lower levels and the association is apparent in older as well as younger people. Multiple measurements in an individual improve the accuracy of appraisal of risk, the extent of which is magnified by the presence of other risk factors.

The association of total cholesterol with IHD derives chiefly from the low-density lipoprotein (**LDL**) fraction and to some extent also intermediate density lipoprotein. LDL particle size may be a particularly important determinant of premature IHD; small particles

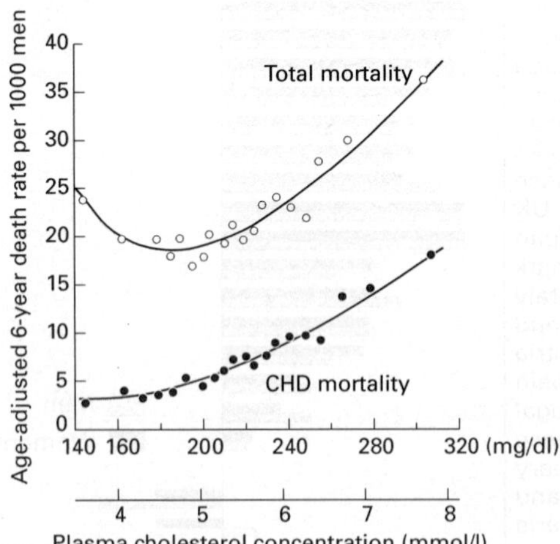

Fig. 2 Within-population relationship between plasma cholesterol and ischaemic heart disease and total mortality. From the study of >360 000 men screened at entry to the MRFIT study.

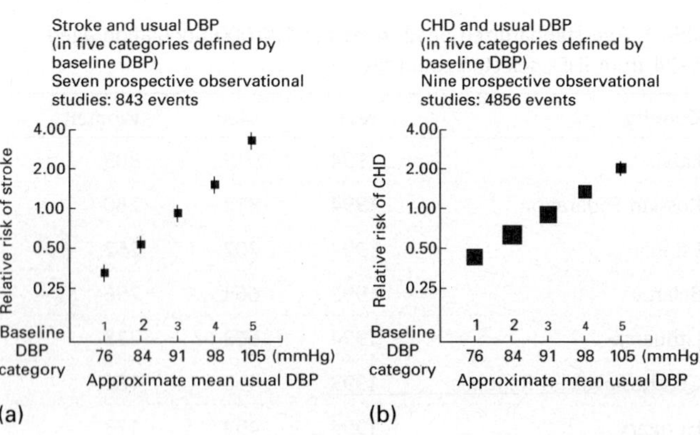

Fig. 3 Relative risks of stroke and ischaemic heart disease (IHD) estimated from combining the results of several studies. The solid squares represent disease risks in each category relative to risk in the whole study population. The sizes of the squares are proportional to the number of events in each diastolic blood pressure (DBP) category. The vertical lines represent 95 per cent confidence intervals.

(less than 225 Å) have been associated with a threefold increase in risk of myocardial infarction.

Triglycerides and very low-density lipoprotein (VLDL)

Increases in total triglycerides and VLDL are usually associated with increased IHD rates in prospective studies, although without the clear graded increase in risk seen for cholesterol. The extent to which the increased risk is independent of other measures of lipid metabolism has not been clearly established. The Framingham study data suggest a causal association only in the presence of reduced levels of high-density lipoprotein (**HDL**). Other studies support this; 'abnormal' VLDLs (i.e. relative cholesterol-enriched VLDLs) may be important predictors. Further studies which include measurement of VLDL are required to settle the point.

High-density lipoprotein

HDL is a protective factor against IHD. Women have higher levels than men and there is little change with age. The protective effect seems more marked in women than men. Low HDL may be associated with obesity, cigarette smoking, lack of physical activity, impaired glucose tolerance, or non-insulin-dependent diabetes, as well as a genetic predisposition. Some studies have found that the protective effect is not sustained when controlling for the effects of other risk factors, but an analysis of four large American prospective studies suggests than an increment of 1 mg/100 ml (0.026 mmol/1itre) is associated with a 2–3 per cent reduction in IHD. The protective effect appears to be mediated via the HDL 2 subfraction.

Plasma apolipoproteins

Atherosclerotic disease has also been associated with reduced levels of apolipoprotein A1, and high ones of apolipoprotein B. These two apolipoproteins form the major protein components of HDL and LDL, respectively, so that these observations are hardly surprising. However, because the association appears to be independent of plasma lipid levels, and has sometimes been noted in the absence of any elevation of them, it may be that such measurements, as well as those of apolipoprotein A2 and apolipoprotein E, may be better predictors of the risk of IHD than measurements of total lipids. More information is required from large prospective trials.

Lipoprotein (a) (Lp (a))

Concentrations are not normally distributed and vary from near zero to more than 100 mg/100 ml. Higher levels have been associated with various manifestations of atherosclerosis, and may help to differentiate those subjects with familial hypercholesterolaemia who develop IHD, from those who remain relatively free of it. Lp (a) appears to remain an independent risk factor after adjusting for the effects of LDL-C, but data from prospective studies are not available. Lp (a) may have thrombogenic as well as atherogenic effects. It is structurally similar to plasminogen and may compete with plasminogen for binding sites on endothelial cells and monocytes thus inhibiting fibrinolysis and promoting thrombus formation.

Total homocysteine

Raised levels of total homocysteine (**tHcy**) have been confirmed as a risk factor of IHD in case–control and cohort studies. The risk appears to be as great as that conveyed by the classical risk factors. tHcy levels may be lowered by increasing dietary, or providing supplementary, folate in the form of tablets or fortified foods. Trials to establish the clinical value of such approaches are under way.

Arterial pressure

Raised arterial pressure appeared to be responsible for about 40 per cent of the variance in the 10-year follow-up of IHD mortality in the Seven Country Study. Within populations increased blood pressure has been shown consistently to be associated with a subsequent increase in IHD risk (Fig. 3). The relationship is linear and graded; no cut-off dividing 'hypertension' from normal pressure. Systolic blood pressure is as good a predictor as is diastolic. In middle-aged men, it is estimated that 20 mmHg higher systolic blood pressure is associated with 60 per cent higher cardiovascular mortality and 40 per cent higher mortality from all causes combined.

Overweight

Obese men and women develop cardiovascular disease more frequently than non-obese. The lowest risk occurs at a body mass index (weight/height^2 in kg/m^2) of 23. Not all prospective studies support an association between overweight and IHD, in part perhaps because they have 'adjusted' for the effects of associated factors, such as hypertension and hyperlipidaemia. Central adiposity, measured by increased waist/hip ratio, is particularly related to IHD risk. The mechanism may be via a pattern of metabolic disturbance (see below).

Glucose intolerance and insulin resistance

Impaired glucose tolerance and diabetes, both insulin dependent and non-insulin dependent, all increase the risk of IHD. The risk correlates with fasting insulin levels and levels 2 h after a glucose load. Whether insulin contributes to risk directly or by association with central obesity, hypertriglyceridaemia low HDL cholesterol and hypertension (syndrome X—the insulin resistance syndrome) is difficult to assess. There is also a strong association between plasma insulin levels and concentrations of plasminogen activator inhibitor (PAI-1). PAI-1 is itself an independent risk factor for myocardial infarction.

Haemostatic variables

Fibrinogen

There is now consistent evidence that fibrinogen levels play a central part in the onset and progression of arterial disease in the heart, brain, and peripheral circulation and they almost certainly influence the outcome of such interventions as coronary and peripheral artery bypass grafting. The independent association of fibrinogen concentrations with the incidence of IHD is of the same magnitude as that for cholesterol. Fibrinogen is an acute phase protein. High levels might therefore reflect the underlying degree of arterial wall damage, which has many of the characteristics of an inflammatory reaction. However, a high fibrinogen level, whatever its origins, is likely to predispose to thrombosis through a variety of mechanisms including increasing blood viscosity, the amount of fibrin formed when coagulation is initiated, impaired clot deformity and its cofactor function in platelet aggregation. Fibrinogen also contributes to the atheromatous process.

The recent availability of a WHO standard for fibrinogen and the relative ease of measuring it mean that it can now be introduced into routine clinical practice.

Factors VII, VIII, and antithrombin III

High factor VII activity levels may also contribute to IHD, although the evidence from prospective studies is not consistent. Impaired fibrinolytic activity, which can be assayed either by 'global' tests such as the lysis time or through individual components including tissue plasminogen activator and PAI-1, is also involved as are high levels of factor VIII activity and low antithrombin III levels. However, measurements of none of these components are yet easy for widespread clinical use.

Platelets

While there is no doubt about the involvement of platelets in thrombosis, there are at present no tests that have been convincingly associated with later clinical events.

Nutrition and ischaemic heart disease

Fats

The major dietary fatty acids and food sources from which they are derived are shown in Table 2.

Table 2 The major dietary fatty acids and food sources from which they are derived

	Common name	Food source(s)
Saturated fatty acids		
C12:0	Lauric	Coconut oil
C14:0	Myristic	Butter, high fat dairy products, coconut oil
C16:0	Palmitic	Palm oil, lard, beef dripping, suet, butter
C18:0	Stearic	Occurs in meat and many other foods
Monounsaturated fatty acids		
C16:1	Palmitoleic	Present in small amounts in a wide variety of foods
C18:1	Oleic	Olive oil, avocado, peanut oil, cashew nuts, almonds, hazelnuts, rapeseed oil (with low erucic acid content), sardines, tuna
C22:1	Erucic	Rapeseed
Polyunsaturated fatty acids		
n-6 C18:2	Linoleic	Safflower oil, corn oil, wheatgerm oil, cottonseed oil, sunflower oils and seeds
n-3 C18:3	Linolenic	Widely distributed in foods but usually associated with C18:2
n-6 and n-3 C18:2 and C18:3		Walnuts and walnut oil, soy-bean oil, wheatgerm oil, rape-seed oil (with low erucic acid)
n-3 C20:5	Eicosa-pentaenoic acid	Salmon oil, cod liver oil
n-3 C22:6	Docosa-hexaenoic acid	Mackerel oil

Chemical notation: C12:0= 12 carbon atoms, no double bonds; C22:1= 22 carbon atoms, one double bond; C18:2 (ω6) = 18 carbon atoms, two double bonds; first double bond occurs at C6–C7.

Intake of saturated fatty acids (**SFA**) has been shown to correlate with IHD rates in cross cultural comparisons and in studies which have examined changing IHD rates within countries. Prospective studies of individuals within a population have not shown an association between intake and IHD, but were based on a single point estimate of dietary intake, related to the occurrence of IHD many years later. Several intervention studies have shown that the reduction of dietary SFA can reduce the incidence of IHD events to an extent correlating to the fall in plasma cholesterol, but even these findings do not provide conclusive evidence for a causal role, as dietary intervention aimed at reducing SFA, results in other potentially contributory changes. Nevertheless, the effect of SFA on atherogenic lipoproteins provides strong corroborative evidence. LDL levels may be appreciably increased or decreased by raising or reducing dietary intake of SFA, especially myristic acid (C14:0) or palmitic (C16:0) acids.

Low rates of heart disease in Mediterranean countries suggest that some aspect of the local diet might be protective. Olive oil, consisting largely of oleic acid (C18:1), has been a prime candidate. In the Seven Countries Study, intake of monounsaturated fatty acid was negatively correlated with IHD rates. When olive oil replaces a proportion of dietary SFA, LDL levels fall without a concomitant decrease in HDL. Naturally occurring monounsaturated fatty acid can also increase the resistance of LDL to oxidative modification. These benefits are seen only with naturally occurring monounsaturated fatty acid with a *cis* configuration. This may be modified in some manufacturing processes (e.g. in certain margarines) to a *trans* configuration, which also occur naturally in small quantities. *Trans* monounsaturated fatty acid increase LDL and lower HDL.

Polyunsaturated fatty acids (**PUFA**) may have an n-6 or an n-3 configuration. The former are derived chiefly from plant and seed oils, the latter from fish oils and various nuts. Several prospective studies have linked low intakes of n-6 compounds with increased risk of subsequent IHD and the Seven Countries Study suggested that n-6 compounds might protect against it. A reduced risk of IHD has coincided with advice to increase these n-6 fatty acids. Their beneficial effect could be mediated by lowered LDL or by reduced platelet aggregation. In contrast, very high levels of intake of n-6 PUFA have been associated with an increased risk of gallstones, reduced levels of HDL-C, a possible increase in oxidation of LDL and, in experimental animals, an increased risk of neoplasms.

The possibility that n-3 PUFA might reduce the risk of IHD started with the realization that Greenland Eskimos have low rates of such disease despite consuming a diet high in cholesterol and total fat. This fat is derived almost exclusively from marine foods rich in n-3 fatty acids (eicosapentaenoate, C20:5 and decosahexaenoate, C22:6). In a large cross-sectional study in which levels of adipose tissue fatty acid were related to undiagnosed IHD, higher levels of C20:5 were associated with a reduced level of such disease. In one secondary prevention study, regular fish intake has also been shown to reduce the risk of subsequent total mortality.

The protective effect might be attributable to anti-thrombogenic effects in inhibiting conversion of arachidonic acid to thromboxane A_2 and by facilitating the production of prostaglandin I_3. The n-3 fatty acids also lower plasma triglycerides, but may on occasion increase LDL. This group of fatty acids may also reduce the risk of IHD by reducing insulin resistance. The precise balance between n-3 and n-6 PUFA remains to be determined and may prove to be an important aspect of reducing the risk of IHD by dietary change.

Increased intake of dietary cholesterol can be associated with elevation in LDL, but perhaps only with very high intakes. Some individuals may hyper-respond to dietary cholesterol, while others show little change in LDL response, which is influenced by the coincident intake of SFA, a low intake, much reducing any adverse effect.

Carbohydrate and dietary fibre

Diets high in complex carbohydrate and dietary fibre (non-starch polysaccharide, **NSP**) are associated with a reduced risk of IHD. Such diets, which are associated with low levels of LDL, are invariably low in SFA and it is impossible to disentangle separate effects. Soluble forms of NSP, found in barley, oat and rye products, lentils, chick peas, fruits high in pectin, and cooked dried beans, have a small effect on LDL independent of the associated reduction in SFA. Insoluble forms of NSP do not influence lipid metabolism. There is no convincing evidence that sucrose or other simple sugars are associated with an increased cardiovascular risk.

Proteins

Vegetarians and vegans have been shown in prospective studies to have a decreased risk of IHD when compared with meat eaters, and have lower levels of LDL and factor VII suggesting that the atherogenic as well as the thrombogenic risk might be decreased. It has not been clearly established whether it is vegetable protein or some other attribute of the vegetarian diet which confers the protection.

Fruit, vegetables, and vitamins

Although antioxidants have been suggested to protect LDL lipids and apolipoprotein B against peroxidation, recent data suggest no benefit from taking supplements of vitamins A, C, and E. There is however, clear benefit from taking liberal amounts of fruit and vegetables. Recommended intake of these is five portions per day, amounting to some 14 oz. Such an intake has been associated with a fall, not only in death rates from IHD, but also in death rates overall. It may be that the mechanism of protection is not dependent on vitamins A, C, and E in the diet, but due to some other effect. Other antioxidant nutrients, for instance flavonoids, may be as important, or more so than these vitamins.

Sodium intake

Excess dietary salt might influence risk of ischaemic disease by way of raising arterial pressure, but this is not proven. The effect of dietary salt on blood pressure is discussed in Chapter 2.31.

Other nutritional issues relevant to diet and ischaemic heart disease

The public has been bombarded with nutritional advice, some of which is valid, some without any justification, and some based on half truths. Oatbran may reduce LDL and nicotinic acid can certainly lower LDL and VLDL, but only in pharmacological doses, and benefit must be very small. Similarly n-3 PUFA do have an effect on thrombogenesis and on VLDL but have inconsistent effects on LDL and total cholesterol except in pharmacological quantities. The safety of such preparations taken in large amounts has not been established and while it seems reasonable to recommend an increased intake of fish, it is inappropriate to advise large amounts of these fatty acids in concentrated form until such safety has been established. On the other hand, it now seems that garlic can favourably influence a whole range of cardiovascular risk factors.

Data on any association between coffee drinking, cholesterol levels and IHD are not consistent but any hypercholesterolaemic effect may be related to method of preparation. Boiled coffee may be more hypercholesterolaemic than that prepared in other ways.

Environmental influences in early life

Environmental influences in early life may influence the risk of later IHD. Weights at birth and 1 year of males born between 1911 and 1930 have been related to subsequent mortality. Those with the lowest early weights had the highest death rates from IHD; the standardized mortality ratio fell from 111 in men who weighed 8.2 kg or less at 1 year to 42 in those who weighed 12.3 kg or more. Subsequent levels of blood cholesterol and risk of developing diabetes have also been related to impaired growth and development in early life.

Smoking

A higher incidence of and risk of dying from IHD is found in smokers of cigarettes in northern Europe, North America and Australia. The more cigarettes smoked, the greater is the risk. In countries where other risk factors are lacking and the overall level of IHD is low (e.g. in Japan and China) smoking does increase the risk of ischaemic disease but to a much lesser degree. The risk of smoking cigars and pipes is lower than that for cigarettes.

The case that smoking is a cause of rather than an association with IHD is strengthened by: (1) the consistency of the relationship; (2) its strength (a risk approximately threefold greater among heavy smokers than among non-smokers); (3) its independence of other

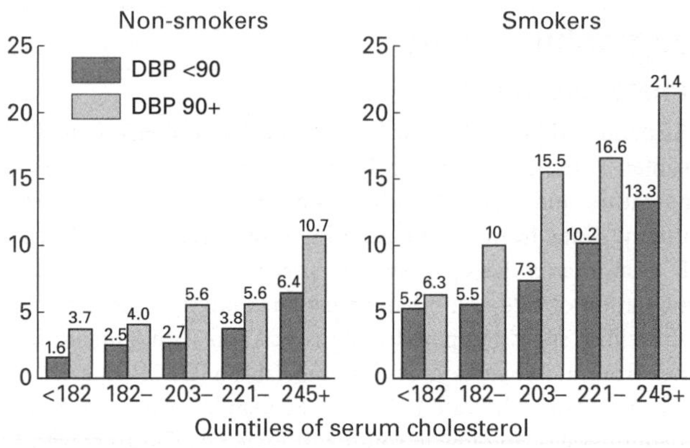

Fig. 4 Ischaemic heart disease death rate/1000 according to blood pressure, serum cholesterol level and smoking in males aged 35–57 screened for entry into the MRFIT study.

factors; (4) the lower risk of IHD among ex-smokers; (5) the time relationship (for example, in England and Wales over the last 20 years, IHD has become more common in working class men than in middle and upper class men, and at the same time smoking has decreased in middle and upper class men to a greater extent than in working class men).

Multiplication of effect of risk factors

Plasma cholesterol level, blood pressure, and smoking each have independent and additive effects on IHD risk (Fig. 4). At each level of blood pressure and plasma cholesterol, smokers have a higher risk than non-smokers. Similarly, the effects of each of the other two risk factors are independent. Smoking leads to an approximate doubling of risk, but the absolute death rate from IHD in a smoker with diastolic pressure greater than 90 mmHg and in the highest quintile of plasma cholesterol is about 13 times that of men in the lowest risk category.

Physical activity

Several prospective studies have shown vigorous exercise to protect against IHD. HDLs, triglycerides, insulin sensitivity, blood pressure, obesity, and fibrinolytic activity are all influenced favourably by physical activity. It is, however, not clear how much exercise is enough. In studies of sedentary executive grade civil servants, the protective effect was limited to vigorous aerobic exercise. Vigorous was defined as activity liable to reach peaks of energy expenditure of 7.5 kcal/min (31.5 kJ/min). Other studies find no threshold of vigorous activity, but a graded effect: the more exercise, the greater the apparent protection.

Alcohol

Heavy drinking is associated with higher levels of blood pressure and possibly with stroke, but several reports show that non-drinkers have a higher mortality from IHD than people who consume a moderate amount of alcohol (up to three drinks per day). Data combining results from a large number of prospective studies are shown in Fig. 5. The consistency of this finding in different population groups from different cultures makes it likely that a moderate intake of alcohol is truly protective against IHD. Although there has been much speculation that there is something specially protective about wine, the evidence does not at this stage suggest that one form of alcoholic drink is more protective than another. Regular alcohol raises the level of plasma HDL cholesterol and is associated with lower levels of plasma fibrinogen.

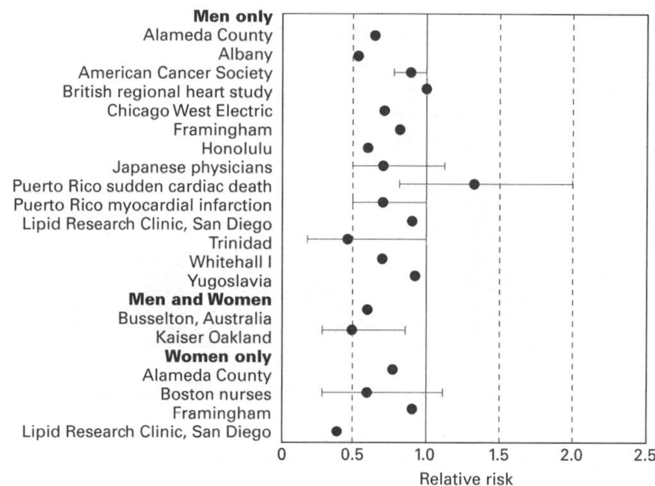

Fig. 5 Relative risk of ischaemic heart disease in moderate drinkers compared with non-drinkers in longitudinal studies. A relative risk of less than one means that moderate drinkers have a lower ischaemic heart disease risk than non-drinkers. The horizontal lines are 95 per cent confidence intervals, where available.

Steroid hormones

The excess of IHD rates in men compared with women has fuelled speculation that female hormones may be protective against ischaemic disease. It was shown in the 1970s and 1980s that women who used oral contraceptives were at increased risk. If they also smoked, the risk was further increased. Studies are in progress to determine if newer low-dose preparations give the same risk; and what the risk might be in women in Africa, Asia, and Latin America. Hormone replacement therapy decreases the relative risk by about 0.5. Progestogens are now prescribed with oestrogens because of the problem of endometrial cancer with sole use of oestrogens. It is not known what this change will do to the cardioprotective effect of oestrogens.

Ethnic differences

In the UK, black immigrants from the Caribbean have low IHD rates compared with the average; by contrast immigrants from the Indian subcontinent have higher rates than average. Similarly, South Asians have higher rates than the local population in Trinidad, Fiji, Singapore, and South Africa. In the UK, South Asians have a high frequency of the syndrome of insulin resistance, low levels of HDL cholesterol, high levels of plasma triglycerides, and central adiposity. This may underlie both their high rate of diabetes and of IHD. How much of this is genetic and how much environmental is not yet certain, although the observations suggest a strong genetic influence.

Socio-economic differences

Ischaemic heart disease is more common in wealthy countries than in poor ones. Paradoxically, in wealthy countries it is the poorer groups who are most at risk. In England and Wales this is a change; since the 1950s mortality from IHD in working class men has risen more steeply than in middle and upper class men, overtaking the latter by the 1960s. Figure 6 shows data from the Whitehall study of British civil servants: the lower the job grade the higher the mortality

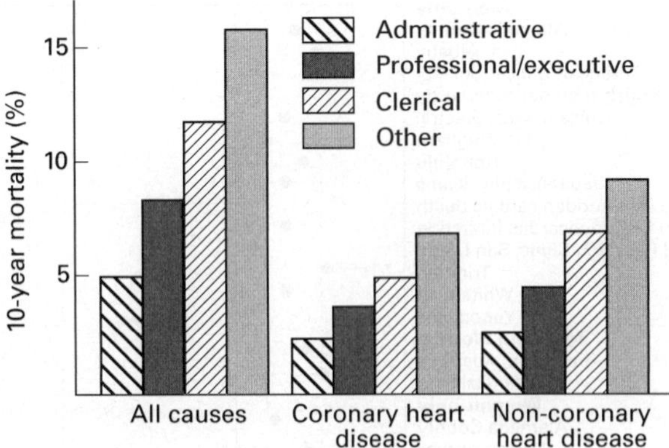

Fig. 6 Mortality in 10 years according to grade of employment in the Whitehall study of British civil servants. Administrators are the highest, 'other' the lowest grade.

from IHD and other causes of death. In addition, more than one report shows a rise in unemployment to be followed by a rise in IHD mortality.

The reasons for the change are not completely understood. Smoking has become relatively more common in working class men and women; they eat somewhat different diets including lesser amounts of fruit and vegetables (but not more fat); they tend to be more overweight; they have higher mean blood pressures; they report less leisuretime physical activity. Although these life-style factors contribute to the marked social variations in IHD incidence, they do not fully explain the differences seen. Psychosocial factors play an important part.

Psychosocial effects

Psychosocial factors have long been thought to cause IHD. The difficulty has been to demonstrate this scientifically. Two main approaches have been taken: (1) to identify potentially stressful situations which may increase the risk, and (2) to identify a particular 'ischaemic prone' behaviour pattern.

Stressful situations

Widowers have a higher mortality from IHD in the 6 months following bereavement than married men of the same age. There is some other evidence that stressful life events may precipitate myocardial infarction. Evidence from Scandinavia, the United States, and Britain support the hypothesis that jobs characterized by high demand and low perceived control are associated with an increase in risk of IHD. Other studies have also shown that low levels of social support outside work are associated with higher IHD death rates.

Coronary-prone behaviour patterns

The type A individual is aggressive, striving, ambitious, restless, and excessively concerned with time and deadlines. Type A individuals had been shown to have greater than twice the risk of developing IHD than type Bs independent of the other known coronary risk factors. More recent data fail to support the link between the full type A behaviour pattern and IHD. The focus has shifted to hostility. Both hostility and depression have been linked to IHD risk.

Geographic factors

Climate and season

In England and Wales, the mortality from IHD is consistently higher in winter. Throughout the year there is an inverse association between temperature and IHD; the lower the temperature the higher the mortality. Data from North America show that there is a rise in IHD deaths after heavy snowfalls; perhaps the consequence of a combination of cold and the unaccustomed physical activity entailed in shovelling snow. Support for an association with climatic factors comes from a comparison of IHD mortality rates in different parts of Great Britain. The rate is high in Scotland, north-west England, and South Wales, and low in south-east England. The areas with high mortality rates in general have lower average temperatures than the low mortality areas. The regional differences in mortality are also negatively correlated with socio-economic factors and water hardness, making it difficult to disentangle specific effects.

Water hardness

Studies in many countries have shown a negative association between water hardness and IHD mortality. Adjustment for climatic and socio-economic differences between towns reduces but does not abolish the association; however, to date there is no evidence that artificial softening of water increases the mortality from heart disease.

Prevention

Strategies of prevention

The high-risk approach seeks to identify people at high risk of IHD and modify their risk by treatment or other means. The population approach seeks to modify population levels of risk and, *pari passu*, to prevent high-risk states from occurring. These two are complementary, but the population approach has the potential for delivering greater gains. In the case of hypertension, for example, a high risk approach seeking to treat those with systolic pressures over 170 mmHg would save only a relatively small number of deaths. The majority of deaths 'attributable' to hypertension occur in those many more people with a more modest elevations of arterial pressure. Any approach therefore which would lower the average blood pressure of the population would be the most effective way to reduce fatalities associated with hypertension—the population approach.

Evaluating prevention

Trials to assess the potential of various approaches to prevention have had limitations, first, because many have addressed the modification of only one risk factor in a multifactorial disease; second, as atheroma starts early in life, trials involving the middle-aged and elderly might be expected to have a limited effect; third, most of the trials have not been designed specifically to assess effects on overall mortality and *post hoc* attempts to do so have caused confusion. More recently, a multifactorial approach has evolved.

Single factor intervention studies

Cholesterol reduction by means of diet and drugs

Recent trials in secondary prevention (Symvastatin Survival Study—4S; and Cholesterol and Recurrent Events—CARE) leave no doubt of the benefits of lowering cholesterol in established IHD and perhaps also in patients with other evidence of clinical atherosclerotic disease. The debate now centres around what level of plasma cholesterol should be the threshold for treatment. In secondary prevention the CARE study showed benefit from Pravastatin in patients with 'average' serum concentrations (total cholesterol less than 6.2 mmol/l, and LDL cholesterol between 2.9 and 3.6 mmol/l) It is reasonable therefore to recommend dietary or drug treatment in all who have had a myocardial infarct with initial LDL cholesterol concentrations at or above 2.5 mmol/l.

The position in primary prevention is less clear, although the WOSCOPS study in men with initial LDL cholesterol between 4 and 6 mmol/l showed a reduction in subsequent coronary events of 33 per cent over 5 years of follow-up (see OTM3, p. 1814). The debate concerns which group, from a cost–benefit point of view, should be treated by drugs. Most would agree that, in primary prevention, drugs should be used only in those seen to be at high risk.

Blood pressure reduction

Epidemiological data suggest that successful treatments of hypertension should reduce the incidence of IHD by some 20–25 per cent. In the event meta-analyses have shown a reduction nearer 14 per cent, but perhaps more in elderly patients at greater risk.

Pharmacological approaches to haemostatic factors in primary prevention

Even low-dose aspirin may lead to serious bleeding so that the general use of aspirin is not indicated. However, for those at increased risk, aspirin leads to a substantial reduction in non-fatal myocardial infarction but considerably less, if at all, in fatal events. This reduction can be achieved with 75 mg aspirin daily, a dose which appears to avoid the risk of cerebral haemorrhage observed in primary prevention with higher doses. Low-intensity oral anticoagulation with warfarin to an international standardized ratio of about 1.5 reduces the incidence of IHD events, particularly fatal ones, and causes no more serious bleeding than low dose aspirin. Concurrent low-dose aspirin and low (dose-adjusted) dose warfarin reduce all events, non-fatal or fatal, by about 33 per cent and also leads to no more serious bleeding than aspirin or warfarin alone, provided blood pressure is not raised. In the presence of hypertension, such combined therapy does increase the rate of cerebral haemorrhage.

So far, there are no selective fibrinogen-lowering agents and the value of newer fibrates, e.g. bezafibrate, for their fibrinogen-lowering as well as lipid-modifying properties, are currently under investigation.

Multiple risk factor intervention trials

In the Oslo trial, half the men at high risk as a result of smoking or cholesterol levels of 7.5–9.8 mmol/l received dietary education and advice to stop smoking with the other half controls. An impressive reduction in total coronary events was observed (Table 3) in association with a 13 per cent fall in cholesterol and a 65 per cent reduction in tobacco consumption.

The MRFIT study in which men at high risk were randomized to special care or usual care showed a reduction of 10 per cent IHD over 10 years in the special care group despite rather similar reductions in risk factors in each group. In the European Collaborative Study, people working in factories in several European countries were randomized to either receive advice aimed to modify a range of risk factors or to act as controls. The reduction in IHD was related to the degree of alteration in risk factors achieved but in Britain there were only minimal changes in the intervention group and no reduction of IHD.

Table 3 Major clinical events and mortality in the Oslo study

Event	Intervention group (n=604)	Control group (n=626)
Coronary deaths (including sudden death)	7	17
Non-fatal myocardial infarction	18	28
Stroke	4	4
Total cardiovascular disease	29	49
Coronary bypass surgery	1	8
Total deaths	19	31

Practical application of these findings

Recent declines in the incidence of IHD in countries with traditionally high rates, together with marked geographical and social variations in incidence show that IHD is in principle a preventable disease. An approach involving attention to many potential adverse factors in life-style appears to confer benefit even when started in middle age. Prevention should aim to include the whole population, rather than focusing solely on high-risk individuals. Strategies for prevention need to reach beyond the life-style interventions to encompass the social and economic factors that influence IHD through individual behaviours and psychosocial effects.

Further reading

Antiplatelet Trialists Collaboration (1994). Collaborative overview of randomised trials of antiplatelet therapy-1. Prevention of death, myocardial infarction and stroke by prolonged antiplatelet therapy in various categories of patients. *British Medical Journal*, **308**, 81–106.

British Heart Foundation (1998). *Coronary heart disease statistics.* British Heart Foundation, London.

Garber, A.M. and Browner, W.S. (1997). Cholesterol screening guidelines: Consensus, Evidence and Common Sense. *Circulation*, **95**, 1642–45.

Grundy, S.M., Balady, G.J., Criqui, M.H. *et al.* (1997). When to start cholesterol lowering therapy in patients with coronary heart disease—A statement for healthcare professionals from the American Heart Association Task Force on risk reduction. *Circulation*, **95**, 1683–85.

Meade, T.W. (1996). Oral anticoagulants in the secondary and primary prevention of myocardial infarction and coronary death. In: *Oval anticoagulants* (ed. L. Poller and J. Hirsh), pp. 132–42. Arnold, Hodder Headline Group, London.

Chapter 2.11

Stable and unstable angina

R. H. Swanton

Stable angina

Angina is characterized by a heaviness in the centre of the chest induced by effort or emotional upset. The sensation has been variously described as squeezing, crushing, gripping, band-like, choking, throttling, or a vice-like grip. Patients describe it as a great weight on their chest. It is typically central and symmetrical. In its early stages it is a discomfort rather than a pain. The sensation may radiate up the neck and throat into the jaws and ears and down both arms to the wrists. It does not usually reach the fingers. It may spread round to the back and into the epigastrium and both subcostal regions. Occasionally it may present only as an ache in the jaw or the wrist and forearm, without chest symptoms but always the relation to effort is the clue. It is usually worse if exercise is taken after meals, in the cold weather, or against a strong wind. It is more troublesome at high altitude. Patients may find that they can walk through their angina and continue to exercise without getting it again. Emotional triggers include arguments, watching exciting television, waiting in traffic jams, or sexual intercourse. Stable angina is predictable and is always relieved by rest.

Nocturnal or decubitus angina is as a more serious symptom precipitated by cold sheets, by tachycardia induced by dreaming, by alterations in coronary tone, or by the increase in wall stress of the left ventricle caused by an increase in end-diastolic volume when lying down. It may be partly related to the diurnal variation in blood pressure which starts to rise from about 4 to 5 a.m. It is relieved by sitting or standing up.

Unstable angina

This term has taken over from crescendo angina, pre-infarction angina, acute coronary insufficiency, and intermediate coronary syndrome. Angina is said to be unstable when it occurs with increasing frequency and severity. The pain is more prolonged and is not quickly relieved by nitrates. It is no longer predictable and comes on at rest. It is associated with ST segment depression and T wave inversion on the electrocardiograph (ECG). Transient bundle branch block or ventricular arrhythmias may also occur. It may be the prelude to an acute myocardial infarction and is an indication for urgent hospital admission.

Variant angina (Prinzmetal angina)

This term refers to a rare form of angina induced by coronary spasm. The pain comes on at rest unpredictably and is associated with ST segment elevation on the ECG. It may cluster in the early morning. Spasm may not always be relieved by nitrates and can cause arrhythmias or myocardial infarction. In many cases coronary spasm is associated with atherosclerotic lesions. Spasm in the presence of angiographically normal arteries is rare. The stimulus to spasm is unknown. Very occasionally patients have a history of migraine or Raynaud's phenomenon.

Differential diagnosis

Myocarditis commonly causes chest pain, reflecting associated myocardial ischaemia or pericarditis.

Pericarditis. The site of the pain is similar to that of angina but it is sharper, commonly exacerbated by inspiration. It may be relieved by sitting up and leaning forward and exacerbated by swallowing, twisting, or sternal pressure.

Aortic dissection can cause extremely severe pain, which is generally abrupt in onset, prolonged, and commonly felt in the back as well as in the chest.

Mitral stenosis. Angina can occur in mitral stenosis, either because of incidental or embolic coronary artery disease or, it has been suggested, from right ventricular ischaemia attributable to excessive systolic load with severe pulmonary hypertension.

Pulmonary embolism. Angina-like pain or chest discomfort (as well as pleuritic pain) can occur with major pulmonary embolism and may similarly reflect right ventricular overload and ischaemia.

Mitral valve prolapse may cause atypical chest pain. Traction on elongated chordae or kinking of the circumflex coronary artery has been implicated as a cause, but evidence is unconvincing.

Oesophageal pain other than heartburn due to acid regurgitation may be angina-like due to oesophageal dysmotility (spasm). The site, character, and radiation of this pain may be indistinguishable from those of cardiac pain, reflecting common root innervation. Acid reflux into the oesophagus may reduce coronary flow reserve to the point of inducing true angina (linked angina). A neurogenic cardio-oesophageal reflux has been incriminated affecting the coronary microvasculature. This has been shown in syndrome X patients (see below). These patients are often female with a hiatus hernia and this may confuse the diagnosis. Acid regurgitation often induces oesophageal dysmotility, but each can occur without the other, while either or both can be associated with chest pain or cause no symptoms. Oesophageal dysmotility may, like angina be induced by exercise, but unlike angina, it tends to follow rather than coincide with exertion. Oesophageal pain characteristically wakes the patient in the early hours of the morning, without the background of critically severe effort angina that is characteristic of nocturnal decubitus angina. Another potentially misleading feature is that the pain of oesophageal dysmotility can, like angina, be relieved by nitrites or calcium antagonists. The pain of oesophageal spasm can be severe with associated pallor, tachycardia, sweating, and dyspnoea attributable to activation of the sympathetic nervous system. It may then be indistinguishable from acute coronary syndromes and frequently causes admission to coronary care units. A useful test is that the swallowing of a bolus of saliva will often transiently relieve the pain of oesophageal spasm but not that of angina.

Oesophageal pain can reduce coronary flow to the point possibly of inducing true angina when the coronary reserve is already compromised.

Confirmation that chest pain is oesophageal demands rigorous criteria and temporal correlation of valid evidence of dysmotility (manometry) and of pH changes with the symptoms in question, but trials of omeprazole can be diagnostically useful and have practical and economic advantages over more sophisticated investigations.

Musculoskeletal and neurological causes. Bone pain from neoplasm, trauma, vertebral crush fracture, or rib stress fracture is associated with local tenderness and the diagnosis is confirmed by radiology. Intercostal muscle pain is similarly associated with local tenderness. Pain with local tenderness over the costo-chondral junctions, known as Tietze's syndrome, is a self-limiting condition.

Band-like, often unilateral thoracic root pains due, for instance to herpes zoster, diabetic mononeuritis, or tabes can also confuse. More common are ill-defined muscular pains without local tenderness, which may be recurrent. A useful clue to their origin is association with movement or position.

Psychological chest pain. Anxiety, attention-seeking, or pending legislation provide an overlay to the presentation of pain of any cause, amplifying symptoms whose cause must still be sought and managed.

Da Costa's syndrome. The triad of hyperventilation (awareness of breathing or a sensation of difficulty in getting enough air into the lungs), left submammary pain (often described as knife-like or stabbing) and palpitation is a common complaint given a number of names including circulatory neurasthenia, effort syndrome, soldiers heart, and cardiac neurosis as well as Da Costa' syndrome. It is a manifestation of anxiety ultimately about the presence of heart disease, although the symptoms often start spontaneously in a potentially anxious patient. It responds best to a confident diagnosis and firm reassurance and can be aggravated by unnecessary investigation which tends to increase concern rather than ameliorate it.

Pathophysiology of angina

Oxygen supply to cardiac muscle is normally increased by increasing coronary flow rather than oxygen extraction and coronary AVo_2 difference remains relatively constant at about 11 ml per 100 ml of blood. When myocardial oxygen demand exceeds supply ischaemia first results in breakdown of phosphocreatinine and adenosine triphosphate. Intracellular acidosis follows rapidly with release from ischaemic cells of potassium, protons, and lactic acid. These changes precede ST segment depression on the ECG, which in turn precedes angina. ST segment depression may occur without pain—silent ischaemia.

The three prime determinants of myocardial oxygen demand are heart rate, contractility, and wall stress. Wall stress is directly proportional to ventricular volume and ventricular pressure, and inversely to wall thickness. An increase in heart rate, contractility, ventricular volume or pressure will increase myocardial oxygen demand. The signal for coronary vasodilatation is probably locally released adenosine—an ideal messenger with a very short 2–10-s half-life. Adenosine deaminase on the surface of red cells rapidly converts adenosine to inosine. Adenosine is thought to be the cause of anginal pain when released from the ischaemic cell. Other metabolites released from the ischaemic cell cause vasodilatation, e.g. prostaglandin E series, lactate, bradykinin, hydrogen ions, and carbon dioxide.

Coronary flow depends on a pressure gradient between the aorta and intramyocardial coronary arterioles. Systole compresses the intramyocardial coronary arteries and during its ejection phase aortic and ventricular pressures are identical. Coronary flow is thus almost entirely diastolic. There are a number of conditions in which angina may occur despite normal coronary arteries. In aortic stenosis the gradient between aortic and left ventricular diastolic pressure may be insufficient for normal coronary flow. In extreme paroxysmal tachycardia diastole is much shortened compared with systole. High left ventricular pressure causing wall stress occurs in severe hypertension and hypertrophic obstructive cardiomyopathy as well as in aortic stenosis. High right ventricular wall stress in severe pulmonary hypertension is another cause as is anaemia when haemoglobin falls below 7–8 g/100 ml.

The common cause of angina is obstruction of coronary arteries whether atheromatous, thrombotic, or embolic. Large epicardial vessels are most commonly involved, although disease of tiny intramural vessels may be the cause of angina with a positive exercise test but normal coronary arteriograms (syndrome X) (see below).

Coronary tone is particularly important in determining flow in the presence of obstructive atherosclerotic lesions. The epicardial coronary arteries contain sympathetic ($\alpha > \beta1 > \beta2$), glucagon and histamine receptors. Endothelial factors regulating tone include nitric oxide, prostacyclin, thromboxane, and endothelin. The finely regulated balance between constriction and dilatation depends more on humoral and paracrine than neurogenic mechanisms.

Table 1 Causes of angina with normal coronary arteries

Angiogram misinterpretation, e.g. ostial lesion lesion right at origin of a branch lesion masked by vessel overlap
Coronary arteritis
Coronary spasm
Small vessel disease
Coronary emboli, e.g. from: atrial myxoma mural thrombus valve vegetation
Aortic valve stenosis
Hypertrophic obstructive cardiomyopathy
Syndrome X
Procoagulable state

Silent ischaemia

Silent ischaemia, recognized by ST depression on the ECG or reduced perfusion on thallium scanning in the absence of symptoms has been shown in 2.5 per cent of a normal male population and in stable angina up to 75 per cent of episodes of ST depression may be silent on Holter monitoring. Silent ischaemia is common in the morning and is found in 10 per cent of patients following myocardial infarction. Episodes of profound ST depression without symptoms should be investigated and treated as if they had been painful. Conventional treatment for stable angina reduces episodes of silent ischaemia. β-Blockade reduces the early morning peak of ST depression. Surprisingly silent ischaemia is of no prognostic value in stable angina, but carries an adverse prognosis in unstable angina or following myocardial infarction. These patients need coronary angiography.

Angina with angiographically normal coronary arteries

A few of these patients have non-cardiac pain but many have genuine angina and respond to anti-anginal therapy. A caveat is that repeated history taking by different doctors will educate the patient particularly when leading questions have indicated appropriate symptoms.

In addition a small number of patients who have had a myocardial infarction appear to have normal coronary arteries angiographically. These are often young patients and may be heavy smokers; they may be women on the contraceptive pill. Some of these cases may have a thrombotic or procoagulable state. Spontaneous lysis of previous thrombosis may then have occurred. Conditions which need to be excluded are polycythaemia, thrombocythaemia, antithrombin III deficiency, protein C or protein S deficiency, and the presence of the lupus anticoagulant. However, even after a procoagulable state has been excluded no cause may be apparent. Table 1 summarizes the more common causes of angina with normal coronary arteries.

Syndrome X

This term describes a group of patients with angina, a positive exercise test, and a normal coronary arteriogram. The patients are often middle-aged women. They probably represent a heterogeneous group but the cause of their angina is unknown. The problem may lie with the microvasculature (arterioles less than 100 μm in diameter). Vessels of this size cannot be seen on the coronary angiogram. There seems to be an abnormality of coronary flow reserve on effort: possibly due to a failure of dilatation or a diffuse fixed obstruction. Biopsies have shown abnormal intramural arteries and abnormalities in cellular ultrastructure with mitochondrial swelling. Ischaemia has been shown in some studies with atrial pacing and coronary sinus lactate measurements. Perfusion abnormalities have been seen on thallium scanning. On angiography, abnormally slow flow down the large epicardial coronary arteries is often seen. Abnormalities of both systolic function and diastolic function have been described with abnormal left ventricular filling rates and high end-diastolic pressures.

Patients with syndrome X must not be dismissed. Their angina is genuine and merits treatment. Patients can be reassured that the prognosis is good.

Assessment of the patient with stable angina

It is important to exclude anaemia, thyrotoxicosis, myxoedema, or rarely a high output state. Signs of hyperlipidaemia may include: arcus senilis or xanthelasma in a young patient, tendon xanthomas, ear lobe crease, or orange palmar crease. It is important to exclude aortic stenosis, hypertrophic cardiomyopathy, hypertension with a vigorous ventricle, and paroxysmal tachycardia.

The carotid, femoral, and iliac arteries should be auscultated for bruits. Absent, weak, or delayed peripheral pulses are noted. An attempt should be made to feel the abdominal aorta and, if there is doubt about its size, ultrasound performed to check its transverse dimension.

Diabetes may be detected by measurement of urine or blood sugar and careful examination of the optic fundi.

Myocardial perfusion scanning

In younger patients with a low likelihood of coronary disease and no risk factors, thallium scanning may be the only investigation needed. A normal stress thallium scan makes it extremely unlikely that a patient has coronary disease, whatever the history and treadmill exercise test show. It may confirm that a patient has reversible ischaemia or has had an infarct when this cannot be shown on the ECG (e.g. in left bundle branch block, or with pre-excitation). In patients who have had coronary arteriography it may identify which lesion or lesions is likely to be the cause of the patients symptoms. The size of the defect(s) has prognostic implications: large defects or high lung uptake of thallium indicating a poor prognosis. Reinjection of thallium may help to identify stunned myocardium which was initially thought to be dead scar tissue, but which may merit bypass grafting.

Unfortunately, thallium defects are not 100 per cent specific for coronary disease. They can occur in patients with normal coronary arteries. Small defects may occur in left ventricular hypertrophy, hypertrophic cardiomyopathy, syndrome X, myocardial infiltration, and even in left bundle branch block itself at high heart rates.

Treadmill exercise testing (see Chapter 2.12)

Thallium scanning has greater sensitivity and specificity than treadmill exercise testing but a gamma camera is more expensive than a treadmill and radiation is involved. Treadmill testing is part of the evaluation of patients with stable angina, but false positive tests are common in patients with a low pre-test prevalence of coronary disease (e.g. young women). The treadmill test is most useful in evaluating the severity of symptoms, the prognosis following myocardial infarction, the effect of drug treatment for angina or as a means of assessing the benefits of rehabilitation. Its use in diagnosis needs careful interpretation.

Stress echocardiography

Two-dimensional echocardiography can be used to identify ischaemic areas in the left ventricle by inducing hypokinesia on exercise or by infusing i.v. dobutamine. It is as sensitive as thallium scanning in the diagnosis of coronary disease but perfusion imaging may be more useful in assessing prognosis.

Coronary angiography

This remains the gold standard in diagnosis and has not yet been surpassed by magnetic resonance angiography. It provides anatomical detail and together with left ventriculography is useful in determining prognosis. It is performed on a day case basis and the overall mortality risk is less than 0.1 per cent. Higher risk cases require admission: e.g. the elderly, those with strongly positive exercise tests at low work load, insulin requiring diabetics, patients with renal failure or known poor left ventricular function.

Management of stable angina

The first stage involves alteration of the patient's life-style, coupled with drug therapy. If, then, angina is still unsatisfactorily controlled, coronary angiography with a view to coronary angioplasty or surgery is the next step.

Life-style changes

The patient must be strongly advised to give up smoking completely. Patients often complain about weight gain on giving up smoking but the adverse effects of obesity are trivial in comparison with the benefits from giving up smoking. Even so, every attempt should be made to control weight. Even modest elevations of cholesterol should be treated by diet or drugs in the light of the results of the 4-S and CARE studies. Plentiful fruit, vegetables, and oily fish are sensible recommendations but there is now no case for supplements of vitamins A, C, or E.

Alcohol should be allowed in moderation but intake should not exceed more than 2–3 units/day, as excess contributes to weight gain and large amounts may increase arterial pressure and can cause a dilated cardiomyopathy.

Some jobs will have to be given up at least temporarily by law: airline pilots, air traffic controllers, and heavy goods vehicle drivers. Coronary angiography is necessary for patients with these jobs, however mild their symptoms. Other jobs are clearly unsuitable: e.g. furniture removers, scaffolders, and miners. In some cases early retirement is necessary but it may be a mistake to encourage it for a patient whose angina may subsequently be relieved by angioplasty or surgery.

Driving in a private car may be continued unless traffic induces angina. Flight as an airline passenger is not contraindicated provided the angina is only mild and stable. The airline medical personnel should be informed, the patient should carry very little luggage and should be well insured for medical treatment abroad. An adequate supply of medication should be taken, with a reserve for any travel delays.

Vigorous competitive sports should stop. Regular daily exercise within the angina threshold should be encouraged with daily walks taking GTN prophylactically. On cold or very windy days the walks should be postponed. Swimming is allowed if the angina is stable. The patient should not dive, never swim alone, and swim only in heated pools. Scuba diving is prohibited. Sexual intercourse should be discussed, as the subject is often avoided by an anxious patient. It should be encouraged provided that the angina is stable and exercise tolerance reasonable. Glyceryl trinitrate (GTN) prophylaxis may be helpful but both anxiety and/or β-blockade may cause impotence.

Drug treatment

Nitrates

Nitrates reduce the preload by dilating the venous capacitance vessels in both systemic and pulmonary circuits. This reduces the ventricular diastolic pressure and volume, reducing diastolic wall stress in both ventricles. The arteriolar dilatation reduces afterload, which in turn reduces systolic wall stress. and myocardial oxygen demand. In addition there is an improvement in subendocardial coronary flow partly due to the fall in intracavity pressure and partly due to direct action. Two effects, however, may be disadvantageous. The first is a reflex tachycardia due to a fall in arterial pressure, and the second is a reduction in coronary perfusion pressure as the aortic pressure falls slightly, but the reduction in myocardial oxygen demand usually greatly outweighs these disadvantages.

Sublingual glyceryl trinitrate

The effect of an 0.5 mg tablet lasts about 30 min and often produces a transient headache and facial flushing, side-effects which often deter patients from using it. Some patients also feel nauseated. Patients should spit the tablet out as soon as their angina is relieved, as this will help curtail the headache; swallowing the tablet also inactivates it, as sublingual GTN is rapidly converted to inactive inorganic nitrite in the liver. Taken before exercise, one tablet can often prevent anginal pain. Postural hypotension and syncope can occur in unaccustomed heat.

In aortic valve stenosis peripheral vasodilatation may provoke hypotension and syncope, and in muscular subaortic stenosis nitrates increase the outflow tract gradient; similarly, nitrates will provoke hypotension in patients with severe mitral stenosis.

Many patients prefer a spray to tablets. It is quicker and easier to use.

Transdermal nitrates

Five or 10 mg patches are available. A patch applied once daily, provides a continuous low plasma nitrate level. Patches should be removed before going to bed to avoid nitrate tolerance (see below); alternatively, the patch can be used only at night to help prevent decubitus angina

Buccal nitrates

Buccal tablets placed between the gum and the upper lip are particularly useful for preventing nocturnal angina.

Oral nitrates

Isosorbide preparations are available in the mononitrate or dinitrate form. First-pass metabolism in the liver of the dinitrate preparation produces the active mononitrate, but a clear advantage in using mononitrate has not been proved. The drugs can be given up to three times a day but patients should be told to try and take their last dose by 6.00p.m. (provided they do not have decubitus angina) to allow for a nitrate-free period at night to avoid nitrate tolerance. Long-acting preparations are popular and may extend the drugs' action to 12 h. Patients who get decubitus angina or angina on waking in the morning should take their long-acting nitration on going to bed at night. The long-acting nitrate tablet must be taken only once during the 24 h period (e.g. isosorbide mononitrate slow release 60 mg once a day).

Intravenous nitrates

These are useful for the management of unstable angina. There is little to choose between isosorbide dinitrate (dose 2–10 mg/h IV) and GTN (dose 10–400 μg/min). Both will cause hypotension, tachycardia, and headache. Restlessness, nausea, and retching may also occur. Both are incompatible with polyvinyl chloride infusion bags or giving sets as the drug is adsorbed and up to 30 per cent of the potency may be lost. Polyethylene tubing is not a problem and a rigid plastic syringe with an infusion pump and a polyethylene tube is satisfactory.

Nitrate tolerance

This remains one of the chief drawbacks of oral nitrate therapy, but is not a problem with short-acting sublingual preparations. It is probably due to a depletion of sulphydryl groups needed for the production of nitrite ions. It occurs quickly on starting oral therapy (within a few days) and is best avoided by omitting nitrates for some point of the day (see above).

β-Adrenoceptor antagonists

β-blockers are the mainstay of treatment for angina and achieve their effect by reducing heart rate and myocardial contractility. They also reduce systolic wall stress by reducing afterload and arterial pressure.

Contraindications to β-blockade in relation to angina

Asthma of any degree, severe left ventricular dysfunction and second- or third-degree heart block or sinoatrial disease are strong contradictions. Prinzmetal's angina may be worsened by β-blockade leaving coronary α receptors unimpeded. Less important are considerations of masking hypoglycaemia symptoms in diabetes and worsening Raynaud's phenomenon or intermittent claudication. Cardioselective β-blockers appear to have little if any advantage in Raynaud's or claudication and should only be used in the presence of even very mild asthma and then only under very close supervision.

Side-effects

The most common side-effect is fatigue most apparent in the first few weeks of therapy. Fat-soluble drugs can produce nightmares, a lack of concentration, and some patients feel a fall in intellect. Limitation of exercise tolerance is to be expected. Cold peripheries are common even with cardioselective drugs. Impotence is common and one of the principal reasons for non-compliance. The elderly tolerate β-blockade poorly and small doses must be chosen initially, e.g. metoprolol 25 mg thrice daily. Asymptomatic resting bradycardia is not an indication to reduce the dose and patients may need reassurance in this context. β-blockade is used only with great care in patients on verapamil as the combined negative inotropic effect of the two drugs may provoke left ventricular failure.

Calcium antagonists

There are numerous calcium antagonist drugs with remarkably different structures. The three most common are the dihydropyridine group (e.g. nifedipine, nitrendipine, nicardipine), the phenylalkylamines (e.g. verapamil, prenylamine, gallopamil), and the benzothiazepines (e.g. diltiazem). Modification of these drugs has produced longer-acting agents (e.g. amlodipine, felodipine, nisoldipine).

Calcium antagonists can be used as monotherapy for angina and are particularly useful where β-blockade is contraindicated. They can be used in combination with β-blockade and synergize usefully with them. The exception is verapamil, which is best avoided with β-blockade. They are the drugs of choice in variant angina (Prinzmetal's angina) and in angina due to syndrome X (see above).

Verapamil, with its potent negative inotropic effect, is useful in patients whose angina is due to hypertrophic obstructive cardiomyopathy or hypertension, but has potent effects on delaying conduction in the atrioventricular node. There is little to choose between nifedipine, diltiazem, or verapamil in the treatment of angina; delayed release of preparations are available for all three. Agents with longer half-lives, equally effective are amlodipine, nisoldipine, and felodipine. Diltiazem is the most cardio-specific.

Side-effects

Calcium antagonists often produce a facial flush, and sometimes headache and dizziness, symptoms which tend to decrease within the first few weeks of therapy. Postural hypotension is possible. Gravitational peripheral ankle and shin oedema is common and does not respond well to diuretics. Gum hyperplasia is a less common side-effect. All calcium antagonists cause constipation. Pruritus can occur with any of the agents. Palpitation due to reflex tachycardia is to be expected in those patients on dihydropyridines unless they are also on β-blockade. Left ventricular failure may be precipitated by any calcium antagonist (particularly verapamil) if used in patients with poor left ventricular function. Diltiazem may cause marked sinus bradycardia in the elderly and should be used in low doses in this age group, especially if the patient is already on β-blockade.

Contraindications to calcium antagonists

They should be avoided in pregnancy and in women of child-bearing age unless reliable contraception is being used. All calcium antagonists are excreted in breast milk and the drugs are best avoided in lactating mothers. They are avoided also in patients with poor left ventricular function but in difficult cases amlodipine can be tried with care. Other contra-indications are: second- or third-degree atrioventricular block, digoxin toxicity, and sino-atrial disease unless covered by a pacemaker. Nifedipine and other dihydropyridines should be avoided in patients with aortic stenosis at sub-value or valve level as vasodilatation will increase the outflow tract or valve gradient. Calcium antagonists increase plasma digoxin levels and digoxin dosage may need to be reduced. Grapefruit juice should be avoided in patients taking dihydropyridines.

Potassium channel openers

Opening the potassium channel leads to relaxation of vascular smooth muscle. Nicorandil reduces preload and afterload in a similar way to nitrates, but without the problem of tolerance. It can be used in combination with other antianginal agents or as monotherapy. It is well absorbed, only slightly protein bound, with a half life of 1 h. The starting dose is 10 mg twice daily to a maximum of 30 mg twice daily. Headache is a common early side-effect; flushing, dizziness, and a reflex tachycardia may occur, and the drug should be avoided in patients with poor left ventricular function.

Management of unstable angina

Hospital admission is necessary. The patient should be nursed in a calm and quiet environment, with light sedation and restricted visitors. ECG monitoring, oxygen, and finger tip oximetry are established. Blood is taken on arrival for CPK MB level and for the myocyte proteins Troponin T or Troponin I. Troponins have been shown to have a better predictive value of future cardiac events than CPK MB. Levels of Troponin T (cTnT) of >0.1 ng/ml indicate a high-risk group. Raised levels of cTnT are thought to indicate continuing distal embolization of platelet microthrombi from the proximal thrombotic lesion in the coronary artery.

Basic treatment

Diamorphine 2.5–5.0 mg is the analgesic of choice. Additional cyclizine or metoclopramide may be needed as an anti-emetic. A combination of soluble aspirin 150 mg daily, and a β-blocker without sympathomimetic activity are prescribed. A long-acting nitrate is given orally and this is switched to the intravenous route if the angina does not settle quickly (e.g. i.v isosorbide dinitrate 2–10 mg/h).

Low molecular weight heparin

Low molecular weight heparin is started twice daily by subcutaneous injection (e.g. dalteparin 120 iu/kg,) or enoxaprin (1 mg/kg). Dalteparin has been shown to be superior to aspirin alone in the FRISC study and in addition enoxaparin superior to unfractionated intravenous heparin in the ESSENCE study in unstable angina in reducing the incidence of death, myocardial infarction, or recurrent angina as a combined end-point. The low molecular weight heparin is also easier to manage clinically as no monitoring of anticoagulation (such as the activated partial thromboplastin time or thrombin time) are needed. Anti-factor Xa activity is higher and the low molecular weight heparins are also less likely to cause thrombocytopenia, and are more resistant to the effects of activated platelets. Finally, unfractionated heparin may cause a rebound effect when it is discontinued.

Calcium antagonists

Calcium antagonists have not been shown to reduce mortality in unstable angina and nifedipine should be avoided unless the patient is on a β-blocker. Slow release diltiazem may be added to β-blockade.

Platelet glycoprotein IIb/IIIa antagonists

This group of drugs has been shown to be valuable in unstable angina in reducing Q wave infarcts and mortality. They have also been shown to reduce complications of coronary angioplasty in patients with unstable angina (EPIC trial), and to improve the results of coronary stenting (EPISTENT trial). Present evidence is largely based on intravenous agents (abciximab, tirofiban, and eptifibatide). The drugs are very expensive (approximately £750 per course) and are given with aspirin and heparin. The drugs are not identical and abciximab is known to possess longer antiplatelet activity as well as the ability to block other receptors (e.g. vitronectin and MAC 1), not possessed by other agents. Oral agents are now in production but their long-term effects still need assessing, particularly regarding long-term bleeding problems.

At present a bolus dose and infusion of abciximab is used prior to coronary angioplasty in unstable angina, and also if possible prior to the transfer of unstable cases from an admitting hospital to an interventional centre. In unstable angina patients in the CAPTURE trial abciximab was shown to be particularly beneficial in those patients who have a troponin T level of >0.1 ng/ml. It is also used during an angioplasty procedure in a more stable case if thrombotic complications develop.

Thrombolytic agents

In spite of the fact that coronary microthrombi have been seen at coronary angioscopy in patients with unstable angina, thrombolytic agents are not indicated and have not proved of value in unstable angina on their own. There is, however, increasing interest in the use of a reduced dose of a thrombolytic agent with abciximab with patients having a primary angioplasty for myocardial infarction.

Coronary angioplasty

This is best performed when the patient's symptoms have settled. Several trials have shown no long-term advantage in routine early investigation which can prove more dangerous than initial conservative medical treatment (TIMI IIIB trial and the VANQWISH trial). At angiography significant coronary disease will be found in 90 per cent of cases of whom about 10 per cent will have left main stem stenosis.

Aims of medical treatment

Angina must be kept stable and patients should be able to complete stage 2 of the Bruce protocol on the exercise treadmill. Failure to achieve these goals means that medical treatment has failed; these patients require coronary angiography with a view to either percutaneous transluminal coronary angioplasty (**PTCA**) or coronary artery bypass surgery (**CABG**).

Angioplasty versus medical treatment

The prognosis for medically treated patients is improving and the annual mortality for single vessel disease managed medically is approximately 2 per cent, and 4 per cent for two-vessel disease. The ACME trial compared angioplasty and medical treatment in patients with stable angina due to single vessel disease. Patients had a better exercise tolerance following angioplasty, but there was no difference in survival in the short 6-month follow-up. The cost of angioplasty was greater and there were more cardiac events in the angioplasty group. This trend was confirmed in the larger RITA 2 trial with a greater symptomatic improvement in the PTCA group over a median 2.7-year follow up, particularly in those patients with severe angina. There was a very slight excess hazard in the PTCA group due to the procedure itself.

Angioplasty versus coronary artery bypass surgery

Eight trials have compared PTCA with CABG and all have similar conclusions. Both strategies are effective at relieving angina, with PTCA initially cheaper and with the patient returning to work quicker than with CABG. There is no difference in prognosis with either option, but patients in the PTCA group have a much higher incidence of the need for revascularization in the first year of follow up than patients in the CABG group (33.7 per cent vs 3.3 per cent respectively). These trials were conducted in the pre-stent era, and coronary stenting has made a considerable difference to restenosis and the need for reintervention.

Choice of treatment

Patients with single- or two-vessel disease are usually managed with PTCA if the anatomy is favourable, or medically if symptoms are not severe and the lesions are not threatening. For patients with three-vessel disease surgery is more likely to carry a long-term prognostic benefit and symptom relief especially if left ventricular function is poor or if the patient is diabetic. Even clearer is the prognostic advance of CABG over medical treatment in patients with significant left main stem stenosis.

In the lifetime of a patient with coronary disease three coronary artery-bypass procedures would be considered an absolute limit. In patients who have already had coronary bypass grafting angioplasty has an additional role in delaying or obviating the need for 'redo' surgery in patients of all age groups in patients with multivessel disease or degenerative graft disease.

Further reading

Boden, W.E., O'Rourke, R.A., Crawford, M.H., Blaustein, A.S., Deedwania, P.C., Zoble, R.G., *et al.* (1998). For the Veterans Affairs Non-Q-Wave Infarction Strategies in Hospital (VANQWISH) trial investigators. *New England Journal of Medicine*, **338**, 1785–92.

Cohen, M., Demers, C., Gurfinkel, E.P., Turpie, A.G.G., Fromell, G., Goodman, S., *et al.* for the ESSENCE Study Group. (1997). Enoxaparin (low molecular weight heparin) versus unfractionated heparin for unstable angina and non-Q-wave myocardial infarction: primary endpoint results from the ESSENCE trial. *New England Journal of Medicine*, **337**, 447–52.

Pocock, S.J., Henderson, R.A., Rickards, A.F., Hampton, J.R., King, S.B. III, Hamm, C.W., *et al.* (1995). Meta-analysis of randomised trials comparing coronary angioplasty with by-pass surgery. *Lancet*, **346**, 1184–9.

RITA 2 Trial Participants. (1997). Coronary angioplasty versus medical therapy for angina: the second Randomised Intervention Treatment of Angina (RITA 2). *Lancet*, **350**, 461–8.

The CAPTURE Study. (1997). Randomised placebo controlled trial of abciximab before and during coronary intervention in refractory unstable angina. *Lancet*, **349** 1429–35.

The EPIC Investigators. (1994). Use of monoclonal antibody directed against the platelet glycoprotein IIb/IIIa receptor in high risk coronary angioplasty. *New England Journal of Medicine*, **330** 956–61.

The EPISTENT Investigators. (1998). Randomised placebo-controlled and balloon-angioplasty controlled trial to assess safety of coronary stenting with use of platelet glycoprotein IIb/IIIa blockade. *Lancet*, **352**, 87–92.

The FRISC Study Group. (1996). Low molecular weight heparin during instability in coronary disease. *Lancet*, **347**, 561–8.

Chapter 2.12

Exercise testing

K. Dawkins

Exercise testing is a pivotal investigation in the assessment of the patient with possible coronary heart disease. Correct interpretation requires a knowledge of the protocol used, the exercise duration

Table 1 Bruce protocol

Stage	Speed (mph)	Gradient (%)	Time (min)	Cumulative time (min)
1	1.7	10	3	3
2	2.5	12	3	6
3	3.4	14	3	9
4	4.2	16	3	12
5	5.0	18	3	15
6	5.5	20	3	18

achieved, the symptom(s) limiting exercise, the haemodynamic response observed, together with any electrocardiographic changes provoked by the test.

Physiological changes with exercise

During upright dynamic exercise there is an increase in oxygen intake in relation to raised metabolic demands up to a maximum (Vo_2max) above which oxygen uptake reaches a plateau. Vo_2max for an individual depends on age, gender, weight, muscle mass, and fitness. The normal cardiovascular response to dynamic exercise includes an increase in heart rate, blood pressure, venous return, stroke volume, and oxygen extraction. Peak heart rate correlates well with Vo_2max, but declines with increasing age. The maximum predicted heart rate for patients can be calculated from the equation, heart rate max $=$ $0.65 \times$ age (years). In untrained individuals, changes in stroke volume are secondary to alterations in heart rate as a means of increasing cardiac output with exercise. Systemic blood pressure increases linearly with increasing work until Vo_2max is reached, at which point there may be a slight decrease in diastolic pressure due to a fall in systemic vascular resistance secondary to both arterial and venous dilatation. Alterations in oxygen extraction with increasing levels of exercise are particularly important as a method of increasing oxygen delivery in patients with a low cardiac output.

Protocols and equipment

A number of protocols provide satisfactory results, but a maximum symptom-limited one increases sensitivity. A test carried out to 85 per cent of the maximum predicted heart rate may miss 50 per cent of the ischaemic responses that could have been identified had the test been continued to maximal effort. A protocol should be chosen that can be applied to a wide variety of individuals; an aggressive one should not be applied to the elderly, or the infirm, whereas too gentle a protocol may result in failure to reach the maximum heart rate (and therefore Vo_2max) because of the prior onset of muscle fatigue. The standard or modified Bruce protocol is in common use (Table 1).

Many of the current exercise testing systems consist of an integrated treadmill and electrocardiograph machine with pre-programmed protocols which can be selected by the operator. During the test the speed and gradient increase automatically and a full 12-lead electrocardiograph is recorded after each stage.

Indications

The majority are undertaken to determine the presence or severity of coronary disease, to stratify patients for risk following acute myocardial infarction, or to evaluate the effect of therapy in a patient with known coronary artery disease. Less frequent indications include the provocation of arrhythmias and the assessment of heart rate response prior to permanent pacing. Exercise testing in asymptomatic individuals is more contentious (see below).

Contraindications

These include patients who have suffered a very recent myocardial infarction, with unstable angina, or who are known to have high-risk coronary anatomy (e.g. left mainstem stenosis). Patients with infections including myocarditis, pericarditis, infective endocarditis should not undergo exercise testing. It is unlikely to be of value and may be dangerous in patients with arrhythmias with a rapid ventricular response at rest (e.g. atrial fibrillation, supraventricular, or ventricular tachycardia). Patients with aortic stenosis, or dilated or hypertrophic cardiomyopathy, can undergo exercise testing with care, but it is wise to use a submaximal protocol.

Risks

Mortality related to exercise testing in patients with coronary disease varies from 0.25 to 0.10 per 10 000 and the incidence of ventricular tachycardia or ventricular fibrillation requiring DC cardioversion is some 1 in 5000. Other documented complications of exercise testing include acute myocardial infarction, stroke, and retinal detachment.

Probability theory

As in any test there is a trade-off in exercise testing between sensitivity and specificity such that any increase in sensitivity is achieved at the cost of reducing specificity. For example, if the magnitude of the exercise-induced ST segment depression used to define positivity is increased from 1.0 to 1.5 mm, the specificity increases from 89 to 100 per cent but the sensitivity decreases from 62 to 48 per cent.

The usefulness of the test is dependent on the pretest likelihood of coronary disease; in a population with a low prevalence there may be more false-positive responders than true-positive responders, thereby rendering the test clinically useless.

False-positive and false-negative responders

Numerous causes of false-positive response have been reported (Table 2). Many protocols specify a resting ECG in both the lying and standing position before beginning exercise to exclude patients with repolarization changes provoked by changes in posture. False-negative tests occur in subjects taking β-blocking drugs, which should therefore be withdrawn 24 h before testing. Most commonly a false-negative result occurs because the test is discontinued prematurely.

Exercise test interpretation

The provocation of symptoms is an important part of the exercise test. Angina occurring at a low workload, either *de novo* or following a myocardial infarct is associated with a poor prognosis.

The timing, distribution, and severity of ST segment depression, together with the speed of normalization during recovery are all important factors in identifying the presence, severity, and prognosis of coronary artery disease. ST segment depression is recognized in three patterns (upsloping, horizontal, and downsloping) measured in

Table 2 Causes of a false-positive exercise test response

Causes
Changes in posture
Hyperventilation
Left or right ventricular hypertrophy (e.g. systemic hypertension, aortic stenosis)
Pre-excitation (e.g. Wolff–Parkinson–White syndrome)
Left or right bundle branch block
Mitral valve prolapse syndrome
Dilated cardiomyopathy
Elevated right ventricular end-diastolic pressure (e.g. pulmonary embolism, pulmonary stenosis)
Vasoregulatory asthenia
Drug therapy (e.g. digoxin, lithium, phenothiazines)
Hypokalaemia
Food or glucose ingestion

Table 3 Reasons to terminate an exercise test

Symptoms (severe/progressive chest pain, breathlessness, dizziness/ syncope)
Profound ST segment depression (>5mm)
Change of rhythm (e.g. ventricular tachycardia)
Progressive fall in blood pressure or heart rate
Patient appears unwell (pale,vasoconstricted, etc.)
Elevated blood pressure (>200 mmHg systolic)
Patient unable to continue

millimetres of depression 80 ms after the J point. Other features of myocardial ischaemia include inability to increase the heart rate, a fall in blood pressure, an increase in R-wave amplitude (indicative of ventricular cavity dilatation), exercise-induced ventricular arrhythmias, and a flat blood pressure response to exercise. Isolated T wave changes are unreliable indices of myocardial ischaemia.

There is a tendency to over-report ST segment changes; a convention of 2 mm (or more) depression 80 ms after the J point should be regarded as a 'positive' response offering an acceptable compromise between sensitivity and specificity.

Reasons for terminating an exercise test

Too often a test is terminated prematurely such that no useful clinical data are obtained. Similarly, an arbitrary cut-off at some heart rate below maximum (e.g. 150 beats/min or 75 per cent maximum) limits usefulness. Good reasons for terminating an exercise test are shown in Table 3.

Radionuclide exercise testing

The sensitivity and specificity of exercise testing for coronary artery disease can be enhanced by the addition of radionuclide myocardial imaging. Stress and rest images are compared thereby identifying 'fixed' defects indicative of myocardial infarction and 'reversible' defects as a consequence of myocardial ischaemia. The addition of single photon emission tomography allows the identification of abnormalities of regional myocardial perfusion. Exercise perfusion scintigraphy is indicated in four groups of patients.

1. Patients performing an inadequate amount of exercise (due to fatigue, arrhythmias, β-blocking drugs, etc.).
2. Patients with a resting electrocardiographic abnormality (e.g. left bundle branch block).
3. When exercise precipitates chest pain without associated electrocardiographic abnormalities).
4. If an 'ischaemic' electrocardiographic response occurs in the absence of symptoms.

Further reading

Fletcher, G.F., Flipse, T.R., Kligfield, P., and Malouf, J.R. (1998). Current status of ECG stress testing. *Current Problems in Cardiology,* **23**, 353–423.

Lim, P.O., MacFadyen, R.J., Clarkson, P.B., and MacDonald, T.M. (1996). Impaired exercise tolerance in hypertensive patients. *Annals Internal Medicine,* **124**, 41–55.

Lindahl, B., Andren, B., Ohisson, J., Venge, P., and Wallentin, L. (1997). Noninvasive risk stratification in unstable coronary artery disease: exercise test and biochemical markers. FRISC Study Group. *American Journal Cardiology,* **80** (5A), 40–4E.

Chapter 2.13

Myocardial infarction

P. Sleight

This chapter might better be titled 'suspected acute myocardial infarction' as the distinction between a definite myocardial infarction and an episode of unstable angina is often only possible retrospectively, based on the development of new Q waves on the electrocardiograph (ECG), and/or serum cardiac enzymes raised to more than twice the normal level. This distinction is somewhat arbitrary as the detection of raised enzymes has been shown to be dependent on the frequency of blood sampling. Nevertheless, it has some merit in that the mortality of unstable angina (including some small and undetected myocardial infarctions) is much less than that of acute myocardial infarction.

Coronary heart disease accounted for 26 per cent of all deaths in the UK in 1991, 1 in 3 men and 1 in 4 women (Fig. 1). More than 1 in 15 men die of coronary heart disease before the age of

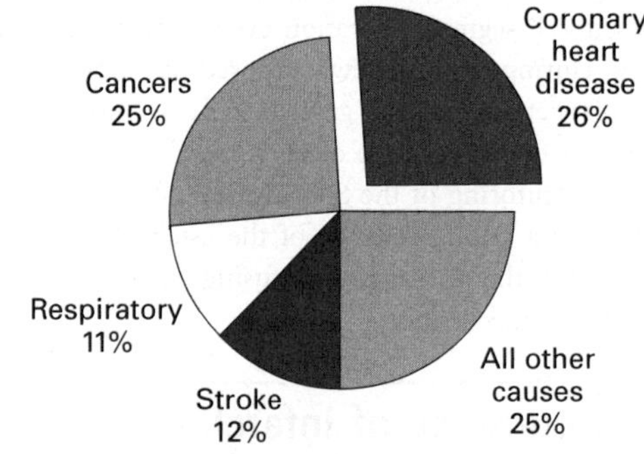

Fig. 1 Causes of death, UK 1991. Sources: OPCS and Government Statistics *(from Coronary Prevention Group/British Heart Foundation database 1992, with permission—see OTM3, p.2349 for full details).*

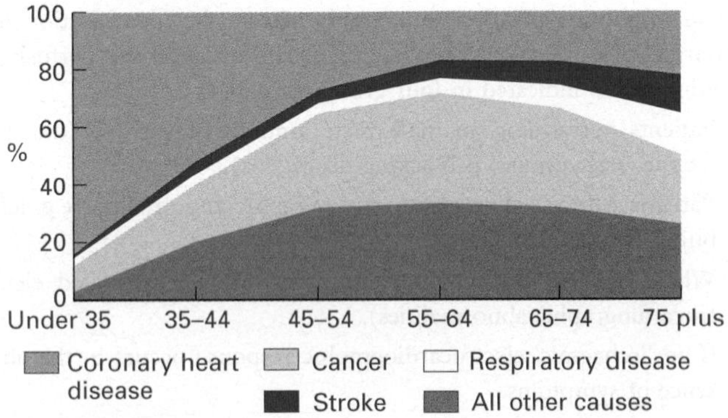

Fig. 2 Age related causes of death, UK 1991, men. Sources: OPCS and Government Statistics
(from Coronary Prevention/Group/British Heart Foundation database 1992, with permission—see OTM3, p.2349 for full details).

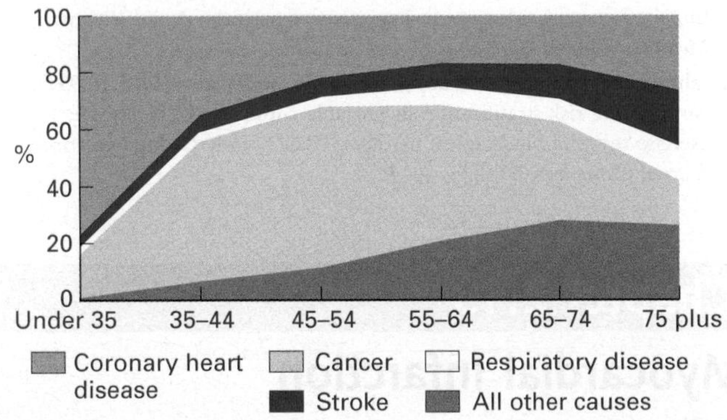

Fig. 3 Age related causes of death, UK 1991, women. Sources: OPCS and Government Statistics
(from Coronary Prevention Group/British Heart Foundation database 1992, with permission—see OTM3, p.2349 for full details).

65—accounting for more than one-quarter of all premature deaths. Women follow the same trend, but lag men by about 10 years (Figs 2 and 3).

Variation in coronary disease mortality within and between countries is marked and the reasons for this are discussed in Chapter 2.10.

Coronary artery thrombosis is now known to be the cause of myocardial infarction in some 90 per cent of cases (see Chapter 2.8). It is also now clear that the process of thrombosis and lysis is a dynamic balance. Serial angiography during evolving infarction and during treatment with intracoronary streptokinase has shown a repeated opening and closing of the artery with accompanying rapid ECG changes in ST segment elevation even during the infusion of the lytic agent. During lysis the newly exposed thrombus is extremely attractive to platelets, hence the great benefit of antiplatelet agents such as aspirin in the early phase of myocardial infarction.

Continuous monitoring of the S–T segment shift during lysis has been shown to be a good predictor of the establishment or not of reperfusion, despite the potentially confusing effects of the presence or absence of collateral vessels.

Time of occurrence of infarction

The time of onset of myocardial infarction shows a marked circadian rhythm with a peak onset in the early hours of the day, after waking, and a second peak after 5 p.m. In addition, there is an increasing incidence during the week to a peak on Friday and a weekend decline. It is likely that these peaks are related factors caused by the increase in sympathetic tone on arousal and with excitement. These include platelet activation, rise in blood pressure with subsequent liability to plaque rupture, and increased susceptibility to arrhythmia.

Presentation

About 70 per cent of deaths occur outside hospital and many are sudden and arrhythmic, emphasizing the importance of prevention together with public education in closed chest cardiac massage and mouth-to-mouth resuscitation.

The earlier the patient is seen during a myocardial infarction, the more difficult it may be to make the diagnosis correctly. This may be particularly so in older patients in whom the symptoms or signs may be atypical. Lack of pain may be partly because of increasing autonomic neuropathy with age (especially in diabetics) and partly because of increasing numbers of collateral vessels. In epidemiological surveys, Q wave infarction on the ECG could not be linked with a clinical episode of myocardial infarction in about 30 per cent of the population screened.

Thus the presentation of acute myocardial infarction varies widely and is influenced mainly by the amount of pain or arrhythmia produced by the infarction. Large infarcts, due to the proximal occlusion of one of the main coronary arteries with few protective collateral vessels, present either as sudden death or severe chest pain which demands immediate attention. Smaller infarcts due to occlusion of more peripheral vessels or of proximal vessels which have been bypassed by collateral vessels may be less painful and hence present later, say 4–12 h from the onset of pain or chest discomfort. Such smaller infarcts may present with arrhythmia, syncope, or heart failure.

Symptoms and signs of myocardial infarction

The attack may be completely unheralded, the first manifestation being sudden death. However, when such patients have been resuscitated about three-quarters reveal that they have experienced some premonitory chest discomfort and may even have consulted a physician about this. Many patients describe a non-specific prodromal phase of undue fatigue or shortness of breath, probably caused by a growing but subtotal thrombus which limits cardiac reserve. New onset of angina, or a sudden deterioration of angina often indicates an evolving thrombus.

The pain of a typical myocardial infarction is usually central, felt deep behind the sternum as a tightness, crushing, or bursting sensation. It is generally perceived to be serious or life-threatening. The pain may also be felt in the back, between the scapulae, and sometimes only there; it may radiate down the arms to the wrists, most often in the left arm. Radiation to the jaws is also characteristic; this may be the only site of pain. Jaw pain is unusual in oesophageal syndromes and should always arouse suspicion.

The pain is often accompanied by nausea and sometimes vomiting, particularly with large transmural infarction. This has been attributed to stimulation of the Bezold–Jarisch reflex, which arises from receptors in the left ventricle, and gives rise to hypotension, bradycardia, and vomiting due to acute neurogenic gastric dilatation. The efferent arm is vagal, hence the bradycardia. The vagus also has a powerful negative inotropic effect on the left ventricle and this, together with the reflex bradycardia, causes a dramatic fall in blood pressure which is rapidly reversed by intravenous atropine.

Because the ischaemic left ventricle becomes immediately stiff, patients may become short of breath due to raised pulmonary venous pressure. This stiffness is also responsible for pulmonary oedema, resulting in arterial desaturation for up to 48 h.

Physical signs may be remarkably few at first so the diagnosis depends largely on the history. A third heart sound may be present, together with signs of autonomic dysfunction due to vagal reflexes as above, or due to sympathetic reflexes causing tachycardia and sweating. A frequent sign is a raised venous pressure. Most commonly this results from increased sympathetic tone to the venous system from baroreceptor sensing of the lowered arterial pressure. It may also be the result of right ventricular infarction. In more severe infarctions there may be circulatory collapse, hypotension, and shock. Because of the vasovagal reflex disturbances outlined above it is best to reserve the term shock to patients whose hypotension, clammy sweating, pallor, oliguria, and mental obfuscation does not respond to atropine. True shock carries a very high mortality of about 80 per cent, whereas the transient shock-like state from vagal dysfunction is not particularly dangerous.

Differential diagnosis

The differential diagnosis of chest pain mimicking angina or myocardial infarction is discussed in Chapter 2.11. Particularly important in the context of a suspected myocardial infarct are aortic dissection and unstable angina.

Aortic dissection

Distinction from dissection of the aorta is of prime importance in view of the dangers for this of lytic treatment. Equally or even more painful than myocardial infarction, the pain is usually tearing, reaches an immediate peak and may travel outside the usual boundaries of true cardiac pain, e.g. into the abdomen. The patient can frequently describe the exact moment of onset, which may be precipitated by some sudden movement. Dissection may be suspected when the patient appears shocked but with a blood pressure at relatively normal levels. It is important to look for extravasation of blood, into the pleura. Absent or unequal pulses are quoted in most books but are noted in fewer than 5 per cent of dissections. When seen later in its course aortic dissection usually gives rise to fever due to extravasation of large quantities of blood; this together with an aortic diastolic murmur (when the aortic root is involved) may lead to a mistaken diagnosis of bacterial endocarditis.

Unstable angina

Usually the pain of myocardial infarction lasts longer than 20–30 min. If it is accompanied by significant ST elevation (say >1–2 mm in each of two limb leads or >2 mm in two chest leads), infarction is much more likely than unstable angina (where the occluding thrombus is usually subtotal). When the ECG shows only T wave inversion or ST depression, the distinction is more difficult and is best made by the duration of an episode of constant pain. Right ventricular chest leads should be done in all such cases (particularly if the ST depression is inferior) in order to rule out right ventricular infarction, which may easily be missed on a routine ECG. This carries a prognosis as grave as left ventricular infarction. Prinzmetal angina is uncommon; the ECG may show such extreme ST elevation that the QRS may appear bizarre and wide and be mistaken for extreme BBB. This diagnosis is often clinched by a rapid response to intravenous or oral nitrates.

Management of suspected myocardial infarction

Home or hospital? Initial assessment

A few years ago, it was reasonable to consider treatment at home, particularly for patients seen late after the onset and when the condition appeared stable. Indeed when other factors are present, such as other illness, poor quality of life, or clear contraindications to lytic treatment, home treatment may still be sensible; but the combination of thrombolytic treatment and aspirin has now transformed management. This therapy can halve mortality and may even abort the infarction if begun within the first 60–90 min. Because it carries a small risk of bleeding, particularly cerebral haemorrhage, it is important to assess the balance of risks, and to do so quickly—ideally within 20–30 min of arrival in casualty. Other investigations should be carried out later except where there are compelling reasons, e.g. suspicion of aortic dissection.

In the majority of cases the decision has to be clinical and depends on the history, a rapid examination, and an ECG. Three types of ST segment elevation may cause confusion. First, where there has been a prior myocardial infarction with aneurysm formation, ST elevation may persist over the dyskinetic area. It is usually accompanied by Q waves, which may help distinguish this from a recent myocardial infarction. Second, ST segment elevation in leads V1 and V2 may follow a deep S wave as a normal variant and does not necessarily indicate infarction. Third, pericarditis may cause ST elevation, but this is usually widespread and is often dome-shaped, i.e. convex upwards. An effusion on the echo together with a history of upper respiratory infection or malignancy may be helpful.

The most immediate need is to relieve pain with an adequate dose of intravenous morphine or diamorphine (5–10 mg), often given with an antiemetic. Relief of pain reduces sympathetic discharge and hence reduces cardiac work. Doses are often inadequate and overcautious. Oxygen will have been given routinely in the ambulance and emergency room and should be continued for 24–48 h.

Aspirin (160–320 mg) should be chewed immediately the diagnosis is clear. Thrombolysis should also be started quickly, in the emergency room unless a coronary care bed is available immediately; time is crucial. Treatment within 1 h of onset of symptoms saves about 30–35 lives per thousand patients treated. By 2–3 h from onset this has dropped to 23/1000, at 4–6 h to 20/1000 and from 7 to 12 h to 17/1000 fewer deaths at 5 weeks, compared with treatment without thrombolysis (Fig. 4).

Causes of delay in treatment and how to lessen these

The longest delay is the time it takes for a patient to decide to call medical help. Educational campaigns have had very limited impact on this, but, individual counselling may help. It is important to warn patients with angina, who have experienced a previous myocardial infarction, or who are at high risk of myocardial infarction, that they should not delay calling for help if pain persists for 20 to 30min and has not responded to trinitrin therapy. They should of course already be taking prophylactic aspirin (75 to 325 mg daily).

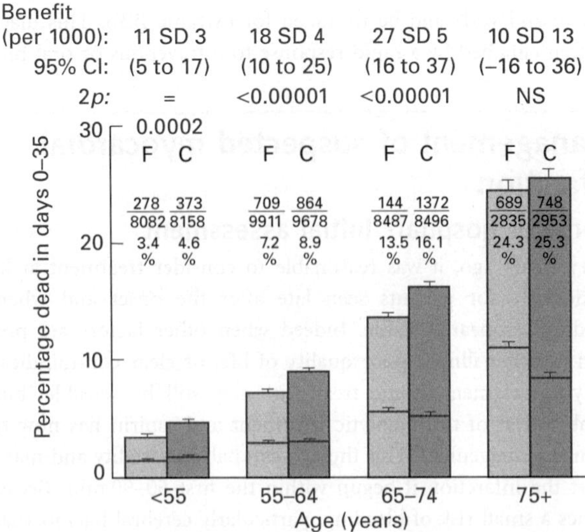

Fig. 4 Absolute effects on fibrinolytic therapy on mortality during days 0–35 subdivided by age. The unstratified percentage dead during days 0–35 among all those allocated fibrinolytic therapy and all those allocated control in these trials. Fibrinolytic (F) and Control (C). The absolute numbers and percentage are given above the respective columns and the absolute benefit per thousand at the top. The horizontal lines divide deaths in days 0–1 (below) and 2–35 (above)
(from Fibrinolytic Trialists Collaboration (1993), Lancet, with permission—see OTM3, p.2349 for full details).

Community practice delays: prehospital care

Delays by general practitioners are generally surprisingly small. Ambulance delays are also generally small in Western urban society, but may be more in rural areas. In such cases initiation of thrombolytic treatment at the patient's home has proven beneficial and safe. Where paramedics initiate domiciliary treatment this has usually been in conjunction with a hospital physician, who has received a transmitted ECG by phone or fax from the home or ambulance. Paramedics may also insert an intravenous line and administer pain relief and aspirin.

Some general practitioners resent being bypassed, and important medical and/or social data may not accompany the patient. Perhaps the best plan is for the general practitioner to be called first. He or she can assess the probability of myocardial infarction on the phone and, if in doubt, call an ambulance before leaving base.

Hospital delays

These remain a problem in busy emergency departments. They can be overcome by proper co-ordination between cardiologists, and admitting medical and nursing staff.

Risk assessment early in myocardial infarction

Lytic treatment carries a risk of serious adverse effects approaching 0.5 per cent, so it is not sensible to use it if immediate short-term risk of death is about 1 or 2 per cent only as in a small inferior myocardial infarct in a patient aged 45–50 with a stable circulation and no further pain. Overall, the mortality of acute myocardial infarction is about 8 per cent at 4–5 weeks but with wide variation depending on a number of factors.

Age

Age is by far the most important predictor of risk. Infarction is not only much more common with increasing age but the case fatality increases greatly so that by 5 weeks after onset it is over 25 per cent for those over 75 years, over 15 per cent for 65 or older, about 10 per cent for 55 and less than 5 per cent for those under 45 years (see Fig. 4).

Sex

Even after matching for age, women have a case fatality more than 50 per cent higher than for males. The reasons for this are not entirely clear. They appear to have more advanced disease at presentation, in smaller coronary arteries, and with a worse response to many treatments, including lytic therapy.

Size and site of infarction

Anterior carries about twice the risk of inferior myocardial infarction (5-week fatality 13 per cent versus 7 per cent). The number of leads showing ST elevation and the sum of the ST segments is also a powerful indicator of risk. ST segment depression also carries a poor prognosis (fatality approximately 15 per cent at 5 weeks), probably because it is often associated with multivessel disease and a history of prior infarction. The index infarction is often subendocardial and not localized, which may explain why benefit from lysis is less clear.

Bundle branch block (**BBB**) may disguise the site of infarction and also make the assessment of the ST segment unreliable. Even if the age of the BBB is uncertain, the presence of right or left BBB together with a suspicious history generally indicates a large myocardial infarction, and a poorer prognosis. On the other hand, an initially normal ECG carries a 5-week mortality risk of less than 2–3 per cent. Patients with a prior history of myocardial infarction, diabetes, or hypertension have an increase in risk about 50 per cent greater than those without.

Finally, patients who present with circulatory problems particularly a blood pressure below 100 mmHg and/or a tachycardia above 100/min have a poor prognosis. The risk of death approaches 60 per cent when both are present. If true shock is diagnosed (see above) the risk is over 80 per cent.

Heart failure

Evidence of pulmonary oedema is a highly important predictor of future mortality. This is true regardless of the measured ejection fraction.

Further investigations

Echocardiogram

An echocardiogram can assess left ventricular wall motion in cases of diagnostic difficulty where the ECG is equivocal or where there is old infarction. A reduced ejection fraction is a powerful index of prognosis, but is not exactly concordant with clinical heart failure (Fig. 5); together with signs of failure this identifies patients with poor prognosis.

Chest radiograph

Only if there is a real suspicion of aortic dissection should it be done before treatment. Dissection may be suspected if the upper mediastinal shadow is wide, although an unfolded aorta may also cause this. Irregularity of the outline of the knuckle, with a linear silhouette with angles, is particularly suspicious. Magnetic resonance imaging is the most sensitive investigation to confirm dissection.

Blood tests

Cholesterol concentrations fall rapidly after infarction and it may be weeks or months before the patients normal level is reached. The

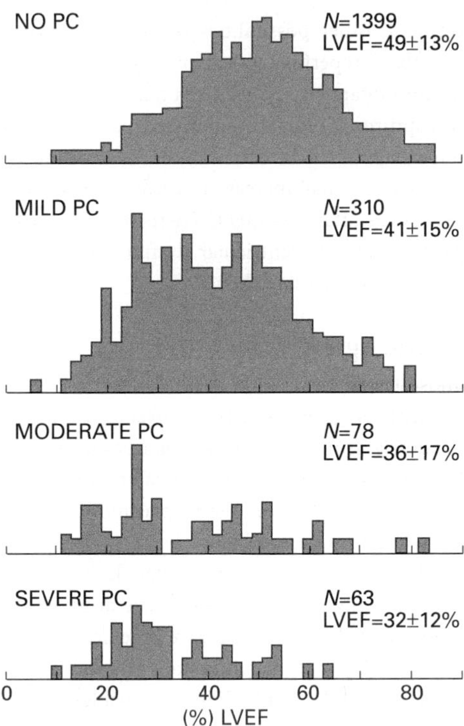

Fig. 5 Data from 1850 surviving AMI patients from the MPIP and MDPIT studies. Note the considerable overlap between different ejection fractions (LVEF) and the presence or absence of failure (PC = pulmonary congestion). Patients can still experience failure (and a poor prognosis) and yet have an ejection fraction which is relatively normal
(from Gottleib et al. (1992), American Journal of Cardiology, with permission—see OTM3, p.2349 for full details).

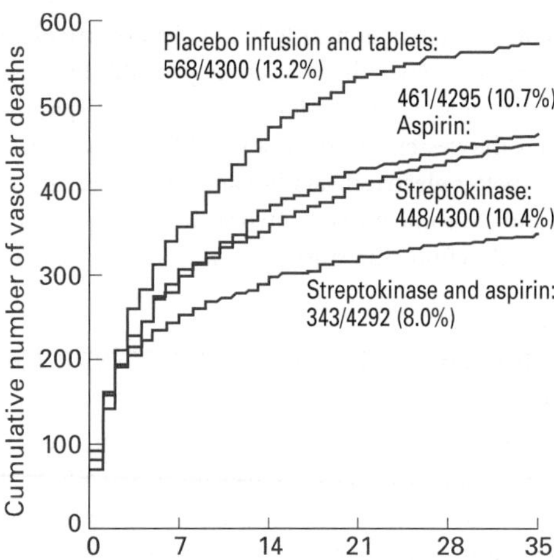

Fig. 6 Cumulative vascular mortality in days 0–35 in patients allocated to double-placebo, aspirin alone (160 mg daily for 1 month), streptokinase alone (1.5 million units intravenously over 1 h), or the combination. Note that aspirin has a similar effect on mortality whether or not streptokinase is present, but that the combination of streptokinase and aspirin is additive
(from ISIS-2 Trial (1988), Lancet with permission—see OTM3, p.2349 for full details).

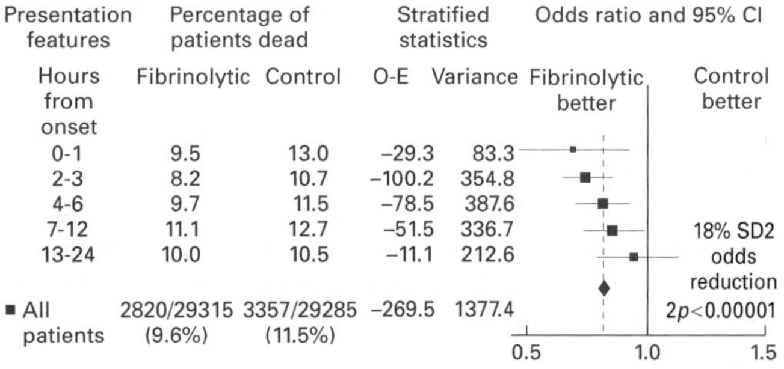

Presentation features	Percentage of patients dead		Stratified statistics		Odds ratio and 95% CI
Hours from onset	Fibrinolytic	Control	O-E	Variance	Fibrinolytic better / Control better
0-1	9.5	13.0	−29.3	83.3	
2-3	8.2	10.7	−100.2	354.8	
4-6	9.7	11.5	−78.5	387.6	
7-12	11.1	12.7	−51.5	336.7	18% SD2
13-24	10.0	10.5	−11.1	212.6	odds reduction
▪ All patients	2820/29315 (9.6%)	3357/29285 (11.5%)	−269.5	1377.4	$2p<0.00001$
					0.5 1.0 1.5

Fig. 7 Benefit of thrombolysis versus control divided by hours from onset of myocardial infarction. Note that statistical benefit is clear up to 12 h from onset, but earlier treatment is more effective. The filled squares are proportional in size to the number of events for that particular comparison. The horizontal lines are the 95 per cent confidence limits
(from FTT Collaboration, (1993), Lancet, with permission—see OTM3, p.2349 for full details).

level taken early after infarction is a good guide and should always be checked.

Most laboratories record the SGOT or AST and the serum creatinine kinase. Myocardial creatinine kinase is specific to heart muscle and therefore more useful. A rise in concentration of these enzymes usually occurs by 6 h from the onset, peaks at 24 h and falls to normal by 3–4 days. The height of the peak is a good guide to the amount of myocardial necrosis. LDH is released more slowly and persists longer (2–4 days). It is non-specific and may (like non-specific creatinine kinase) come from other sites of damage or injury. The creatinine kinase enzymes can be fractionated further so that by comparing the ratio of MM and MB subforms it is possible to date the time of onset of infarction. Other tests measure serum myoglobin or troponin. These smaller molecules are released much earlier and may therefore be used early to identify infarction when the ECG is equivocal.

Management of the subsequent course

The patient is usually nursed in the semi-sitting position at about 45 degrees. Uncomplicated cases are mobilized progressively from the second day. An average length of stay in hospital is usually 5–7 days, but may be shorter when successful reperfusion by drugs or percutaneous transluminal coronary angioplasty (**PTCA**) or surgery has limited the severity of the infarction. Early mobilization has been shown to be beneficial both physically and psychologically. The uncomplicated patient may spend 1–2 days in the coronary care unit and then transfer to an intermediate care unit or to a general ward.

Thrombolytic treatment

Two large trials—GISSI-1 and International Study of Infarct Survival (ISIS-2)—have confirmed the value of lytic treatment. In the ISIS-2 trial, aspirin alone reduced mortality by 23 per cent, streptokinase alone by 25 per cent and the combination by 45 per cent (Fig. 6). In both trials the best results were seen when treatment was given within 4 h, but there was evidence of benefit from treatment even as late as 24 h in ISIS, although not in GISSI. The GUSTO trials comparing streptokinase with an accelerated regimen of tissue plasminogen activator has similarly confirmed that patients treated within 2 h of onset had approximately half the early mortality of those treated within 2–6 h.

How long after infarction is lytic therapy still useful?

An overview of over 130 000 patients confirms that treatment can give benefit up to 12 h from onset (Fig. 7), a view confirmed by LATE (plasminogen activator) and EMERAS (streptokinase) trials. The mechanisms of late benefit appear to be: (1) less ventricular dilatation in the months after a myocardial infarction, probably by a combination of better scar formation and additionally, better 'splinting' of the ventricle when the vessels are open and stiffened by higher pressure perfusion; (2) better electrical stability and protection against serious arrhythmia; and (3) some possible myocardial salvage when the initial course of the infarction was stuttering, with subsequent myocardial 'stunning'.

What are the electrocardiographic criteria for treatment?

The most benefit from lysis occurs in those patients with suspected myocardial infarction who have ST elevation or BBB on the initial ECG. Patients with other changes such as ST depression, T wave inversion, or a normal ECG may even be harmed by lysis as hazards may balance benefits in smaller infarcts. It is difficult to understand the apparent lack of benefit in patients with ST depression, as they are at high risk and certainly are mostly experiencing a myocardial infarction.

When the ECG does not show ST elevation it is reasonable to repeat it at intervals and only use thrombolytics if ST elevation develops; some would treat immediately with lytics as the risk is high. At present there are insufficient trial data to be sure what is the correct procedure.

Age

Although the proportional benefit of lysis is less for older patients, their risk is much higher and so the absolute benefit is the same or greater than in young patients. Although the risk of haemorrhagic stroke is greater in older patients, particularly with tissue plasminogen activator (see below), there is a shortfall of thrombotic and embolic stroke with streptokinase. So fear of stroke should not deter one from using thrombolysis in the old.

Blood pressure

Hypertension is a relative contraindication to lysis because of the increased risk of cerebral haemorrhage, but this risk should be assessed in comparison with the risk from the myocardial infarction. In the Fibrinolytic Therapy Trialists' (FTT) overview patients with a history of hypertension benefited from lysis. Patients presenting with systolic pressures below 100 mmHg also benefit and that streptokinase itself causes hypotension is not a good reason to withhold it in such patients.

Diabetes

Diabetics appear to benefit as much as non-diabetics. Although retinal haemorrhage from retinopathy is sometimes listed as a contra-indication to thrombolysis, it is very little reported and must be extremely rare.

Previous infarction

Patients who have had a prior myocardial infarction benefit somewhat less than those experiencing a first attack, but should still be treated.

Hazards of thrombolysis

The hazards of lysis are very uncommon—a total of about 5–10/1000 patients treated. The most obvious risk is haemorrhage, particularly cerebral haemorrhage, which is strongly related to increasing age and blood pressure. Other hazards include a small excess of deaths associated with impaired left ventricular function, perhaps due to haemorrhage into necrotic myocardium as the risk increases with delay in treatment; other possibilities include excess calcium entry into damaged cells at reperfusion or damage to the collagen skeleton. Haemorrhage into infarcted myocardium may also be responsible for early cardiac rupture; in non-thrombolysed patients ruptures recur over the first few days but after thrombolysis it occurs most commonly in the first 12–24 h. A small increase in cardiac arrest can also occur in the first few hours after treatment. Thereafter, this early risk from haemorrhage, rupture, left ventricular dysfunction, and reperfusion arrhythmia is overcome by later benefit.

Choice of lytic agent

The three most tested drugs are streptokinase; a derivative of it, anistreplase, which is given as a bolus over 3–5 min and releases streptokinase slowly from the plasminogen streptokinase complex; and recombinant tissue plasminogen activator, which has the same amino acid sequence as human tissue plasminogen activator, but differs in its coating of sugars.

Both streptokinase and anistreplase suffer derive from the streptococcus—so that many patients already have antibodies as a result of previous infections. This necessitates a large dose. Both are highly allergenic and so a big rise in antibodies follows after a few days and persists for years. The antibodies are capable of neutralizing a subsequent dose, so for second use it is preferable to use tissue plasminogen activator, which is not antigenic. However, in countries which cannot afford this, a higher dose of streptokinase is an alternative. There is no advantage from the use of hydrocortisone as prophylaxis against anaphylactic shock which, after streptokinase is extremely rare.

Effects of different agents on recanalization

Two trials (TIMI-1 and ECSG) compared streptokinase or tissue plasminogen activator for efficacy in recanalizing blocked coronary arteries. Both showed patency at 90 min, better with plasminogen activation. Fatality was least when full patency was restored.

The GUSTO trial included a substudy of patients in whom angiography was performed at 90 min, 3 h, 24 h, and 7 days. Four regimens were compared—streptokinase with subcutaneous heparin; streptokinase with intravenous heparin; accelerated tissue plasminogen 100 mg given in 90 min rather than the previous standard of 3 h and a combination of less than 90 mg tissue plasminogen activator + 1 million units of streptokinase given over 1 h. Ninety-minute patency was slightly better with accelerated tissue plasminogen activator than the combination arm; both were better than the two streptokinase regimens, but all regimens showed similar effectiveness at 3 h, with patency slightly better with the combination arm than the others. More than half the patients were entered in less than 2 h. More rapid lysis with accelerated tissue plasminogen activator was associated with a small reduction in mortality, but a significant 3/1000 increase in stroke.

Mortality comparisons by lytic agent

A recent overview (which includes GUSTO) compared the results of streptokinase versus tissue plasminogen activator ('accelerated' regimen) and found no difference in mortality overall, or in patients divided by age, by blood pressure or by time to treatment. As in the GUSTO trial there was a significant excess of stroke with tissue plasminogen activator of 4/1000 treated. (Fig. 8)

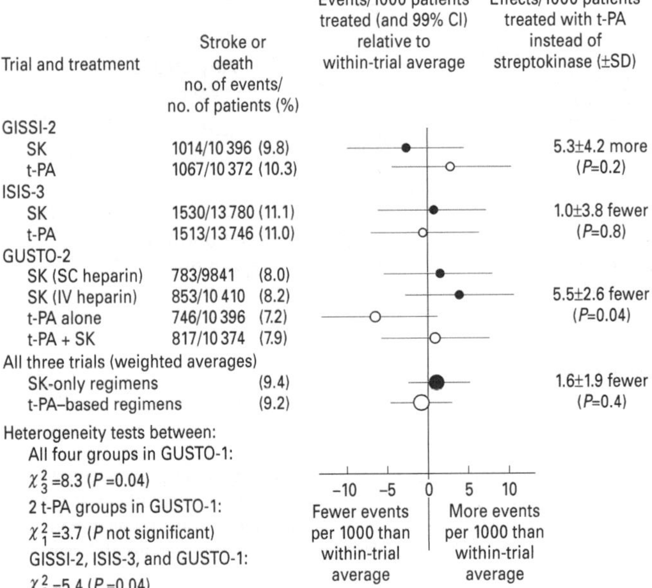

Trial and treatment
Stroke or death no. of events/ no. of patients (%)
Events/1000 patients treated (and 99% CI) relative to within-trial average
Effects/1000 patients treated with t-PA instead of streptokinase (±SD)
GISSI-2
SK 1014/10 396 (9.8)
t-PA 1067/10 372 (10.3)
5.3±4.2 more (P=0.2)
ISIS-3
SK 1530/13 780 (11.1)
t-PA 1513/13 746 (11.0)
1.0±3.8 fewer (P=0.8)
GUSTO-2
SK (SC heparin) 783/9841 (8.0)
SK (IV heparin) 853/10 410 (8.2)
t-PA alone 746/10 396 (7.2)
t-PA + SK 817/10 374 (7.9)
5.5±2.6 fewer (P=0.04)
All three trials (weighted averages)
SK-only regimens (9.4)
t-PA-based regimens (9.2)
1.6±1.9 fewer (P=0.4)
Heterogeneity tests between:
All four groups in GUSTO-1:
χ^2_3=8.3 (P=0.04)
2 t-PA groups in GUSTO-1:
χ^2_1=3.7 (P not significant)
GISSI-2, ISIS-3, and GUSTO-1:
χ^2_2=5.4 (P=0.04)
−10 −5 0 5 10
Fewer events per 1000 than within-trial average
More events per 1000 than within-trial average

Fig. 8 Stroke or death in the three large, directly randomized comparisons (GISSI-2, ISIS-3, and GUSTO-1) of the standard streptokinase regimen with more intensive tissue plasminogen activator-based fibrinolytic regimens. For each treatment group the number of events per 1000 patients treated (with its 99 per cent confidence interval [CI] is plotted, after subtraction of the overall average number of events per 1000 patients treated in that trial. Solid circles denote streptokinase-only regimens; open symbols denote tissue plasminogen activator-based regimens. (Subtraction of the overall within-trial risk does not affect the difference between the different groups in one trial, but merely centres the results for each trial on the same vertical line.) The weighted average of the results from the three trials has weights proportional to the number of patients in those trials. (SK denotes streptokinase, SC subcutaneous, and IV intravenous).
(From New England Journal of Medicine, 1997; **336***: 847–860 with permission.)*

Risk differences: excess stroke with tissue plasminogen activator and anistreplase

The reason why tissue plasminogen activator (100 mg) given over 1 h produces better patency at 90 min than streptokinase (1.5 million units) given over 1 h, yet produces no greater benefit in mortality may be because any small advantage of earlier recanalization is offset by a greater risk of cerebral haemorrhage with the more aggressive agent (Fig. 9). With tissue plasminogen activator, this excess risk is strongly related to systolic pressure, and to age. This excess with age was not seen with streptokinase and the gradient related to pressure was much shallower. One reason for these differences may be because streptokinase-associated hypotension may be protective; streptokinase may also be less likely to lyse old clots in Charcot–Bouchard aneurysms in the cerebral white matter.

The FTT overview shows that below a systolic pressure of 125 mmHg and an age of 55 the risk of cerebral haemorrhage is extremely low with either agent.

A reasonable conclusion is that there may be some marginal benefit for accelerated tissue plasminogen activator for the very early patient (seen within 2–3 h) with a severe myocardial infarction, who is not at risk of haemorrhagic stroke by reason of hypertension or age (under about 60 years), but tissue plasminogen activator is at least 10-fold more expensive than streptokinase, and becomes very expensive per life saved in such low risk patients.

Anistreplase

Anistreplase was first tested in the AIMS study in patients with ST elevation less than 6 h from onset of symptoms. The resulting 42 per cent reduction in 30-day mortality was, at that time, the most promising of all agents tested. However, compared with tissue plasminogen activator and streptokinase in the ISIS-3 study, anistreplase showed no mortality difference and was intermediate between streptokinase and tissue plasminogen activator with regard to safety, resulting in two fewer strokes/1000 than tissue plasminogen activator, and 2/1000 more than streptokinase.

The advantage of easier administration as a 30-mg bolus given over 3–5 min is somewhat reduced by the need to keep it refrigerated. It is more expensive than streptokinase but less than tissue plasminogen activator.

Other thrombolytic agents

Urokinase is similar to streptokinase, but is not allergenic. It is inexpensive and therefore a viable alternative to tissue plasminogen activator for second-time use. Other agents which appear promising are r-PA, a derivative of tissue plasminogen activator with a longer half-life, and staphylokinase.

Does heparin add significant advantage to aspirin in patients receiving thrombolysis?

The FTT overview, together with GUSTO, show no advantage for the routine use of any form of heparin added to streptokinase. It may be justifiable when there is high risk of, or existing, ventricular mural thrombus, or continuing arrhythmia, or poor left ventricular function. For tissue plasminogen activator the evidence is inadequate to allow judgement, but most physicians still use intravenous heparin added to aspirin after tissue plasminogen activator. Heparin may induce a state of thrombocytopenia; less commonly there may be associated agglutination of platelets and paradoxical thrombosis, which can be arterial or venous. Platelet counts should be carried out during longer term (>5 days) heparin therapy.

Other methods of acute revascularization in myocardial infarction

Coronary angioplasty (PTCA) without thrombolytic therapy, has become increasingly popular. It has the advantage of avoiding the risks of bleeding from the lytic agent, but not those of intensive heparinization, which leads particularly to bleeding from the catheter entry site. Trials of PTCA in myocardial infarction have shown that the time to open the artery can be very comparable with lytic agents. Other advantages of PTCA are that the resultant stenosis is generally less than with lysis, with better flow and hospital discharge may be more rapid. A recent trial of conservative versus aggressive therapy with PTCA in non-Q wave myocardial infarction and unstable angina (VANQWISH) shows the hazards of the latter, with lower mortality in the conservative arm.

PTCA may be a viable option in well supplied communities, but it is not an option in most countries. Nor do we have enough information about the later restenosis rate, or about its safety in settings with less experienced operators. Immediate coronary bypass surgery can also be a safe option but again has major resource implications.

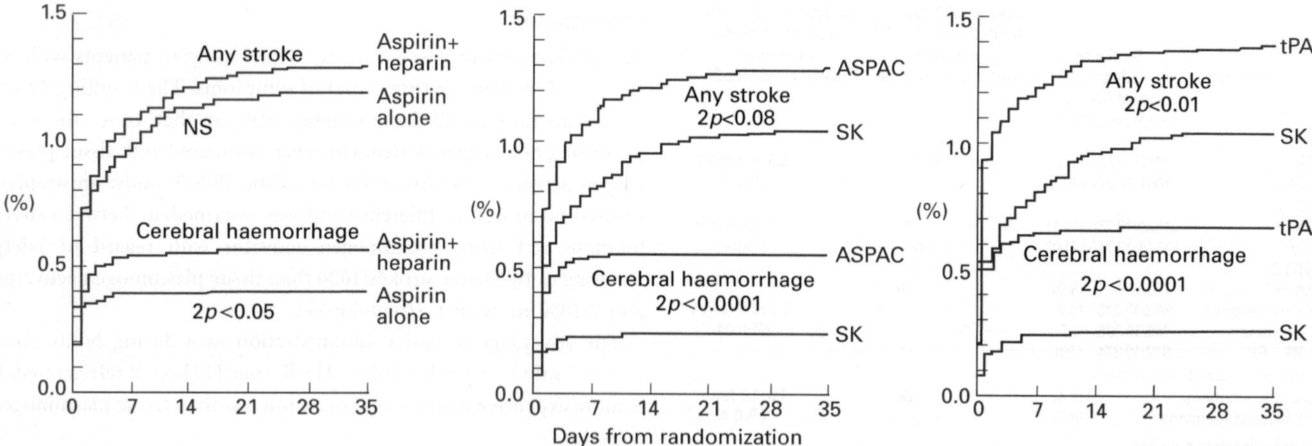

Fig. 9 Cumulative percentage with any stroke (upper lines) and with definite or probable cerebral haemorrhage in hospital up to day 35 or prior discharge, from the ISIS-3 Trial of the Comparison of streptokinase, conventional 3 h/100 mg tissue plasminogen activator regimen, and APSAC. (a) All patients allocated aspirin plus heparin (thicker line) versus all allocated aspirin alone; (b) all patients allocated streptokinase (thicker line) vs all allocated APSAC; (c) all patients allocated streptokinase versus all allocated tissue plasminogen activator. The same excess risk of stroke with tissue plasminogen activator over streptokinase was also seen in GISSI-2 and in the GUSTO-1 trial
(from ISIS-3, (1992), Lancet, with permission—see OTM3, p.2349 for full details).

Other agents for the acute stage of myocardial infarction

Nitrates

Sublingual trinitrin (0.4 mg) may help distinguish unstable angina or a prolonged attack of stable angina from an incipient myocardial infarction. It can be safely repeated on recumbent patients. Intravenous nitrate therapy is similarly in widespread use (5–10 mg/min initially). It is safe and helpful in suppressing pain in unstable angina; it relieves cardiac work by peripheral venodilation and reduction of venous return, and by reducing cardiac afterload. Nitrates may also have effects on platelets, reducing aggregation.

Small-scale trials suggest that nitrates may have beneficial long-term effects by reduction of ventricular dilation after myocardial infarction. ISIS-4 and GISSI-3 have respectively tested oral isosorbide mononitrate, and intravenous nitrate followed by a skin patch. In neither was there any significant reduction in mortality. The problems of side-effects and tolerance are addressed in Chapter 2.11.

Angiotensin-converting enzyme inhibitors

They are of great importance in the convalescent phase of myocardial infarction, where they have been shown to be particularly effective in patients who have had heart failure, or evidence of impaired left ventricular function in the acute phase. Their place as *routine* treatment in the acute phase is growing. Although there was no benefit in the CONSENSUS II trial, ISIS-4 (captopril), and GISSI-3 (lisinopril) showed a small but significant reduction of about 5–6/1000 in 5-week mortality. This benefit doubles with larger infarcts, prior infarcts, or left ventricular dysfunction; in GISSI-3. The majority of avoided deaths were due to prevention of cardiac rupture and arrhythmic deaths.

Magnesium

Magnesium has been tested because of potential anti-arrythmic effects. The LIMIT study did show benefit in left ventricular function and not in relation to arrhythmias. ISIS-4 showed a slightly higher mortality in those given magnesium, and an increase in asystole, shock, and heart failure. Hence use of intravenous magnesium should be confined to those few patients in whom deficiency is suspected (e.g. long-term diuretics or hyponatraemia).

β-Adrenoceptor blockade

The ISIS-1 and MIAMI trials have tested intravenous followed by oral β-blockade in the acute phase of myocardial infarction. Both showed a 13–15 per cent reduction in hospital deaths, although only ISIS-1 (16 000 patients compared with about 5500 in MIAMI), reached statistical significance. Almost all of the effect on mortality was in the first 24–36 h with a particular reduction in cardiac rupture.

Despite the trial results, use of intravenous β-blockers was rare in Europe, but is now increasing. Concern about hypotension and anti-inotopic effects means that in practice, this approach can only be used in good to moderate risk patients.

Calcium channel blocking agents

These are used commonly despite considerable evidence for harm, and certainly no evidence for good in the early phase of myocardial infarction. Verapamil, or diltiazem, are useful in the convalescent and later phase provided the patient has not experienced heart failure or has poor left ventricular function. The dihydropyridines, such as nifedipine, have no place in the acute or later phase of myocardial infarction except in the rather rare cases of coronary spasm, or in conjunction with β-blockade.

Inotropic agents, shock, and surgical treatments

Despite the risk of increasing cardiac work inotropes can be useful in temporary support in shock and in left ventricular failure (see Chapter 2.2). There is anecdotal evidence that acute angioplasty may be effective in shock, often requiring temporary use of an intra-aortic balloon pump. In some cases, shock may be the consequence of papillary or chordal rupture when prompt surgery may be life-saving.

Antiarrhythmic therapy

Ventricular fibrillation and tachycardia

Lignocaine

Present policy is to avoid the prophylactic use of anti-arrhythmic agents which generally have negative inotropic effects and may be importantly proarrhythmic. An overview of all randomized trials of the prophylactic use of lignocaine showed that, although ventricular fibrillation was reduced significantly, asystole was similarly increased; the balance was an increase in mortality.

Ventricular fibrillation is satisfactorily treated by DC shock. Lignocaine is used only after a patient has experienced ventricular fibrillation. For recurrent ventricular arrhythmia an implanted defibrillator or amiodarone is a useful agent (see below).

Atrial fibrillation

DC shock is not usually advised as there is a high likelihood of recurrence. Digitalis given intravenously may be toxic and oral digitalization is rather slow to control the rate. If the patient is not distressed it is often possible to wait a few hours for spontaneous reversion. Otherwise treatment is a matter for individual choice, as there are no good trials to guide one. There are potential proarrhythmic problems in the use of quinidine, flecainide, and procainamide. Some would use a small intravenous dose of a β-blocker or intravenous verapamil despite negative inotropic effects. Intravenous amiodarone 600 mg/day by a central venous line is probably the most effective agent, is non-toxic in short-term use and is not noticeably depressant of left ventricular function. Occasional instances of torsades de pointes have been described. Amiodarone has been tested after myocardial infarction in randomized trials, and found to be safe and probably effective. It may be continued intravenously for the initial few days and then orally, aiming at a long-term dose of about 200 mg/day but only in those patients in whom arrhythmia recurs.

Heart block

Heart block is more common with inferior than anterior infarction because the right coronary artery supplies the atrioventricular node and because vagal reflexes are more likely from this area. It is then often transient and does not necessarily imply a very large myocardial infarction. When heart block occurs with an anterior infarction it generally is associated with a very large lesion and the prognosis is grave. Pacing is only required when a low heart rate is compromising the circulation. Prophylactic pacing for first- and second-degree block is not advised and may compromise lytic therapy.

Pericarditis

This is a common complication especially of anterior infarction. It rarely causes tamponade unless anticoagulant therapy leads to pericardial bleeding. The associated pain causes anxiety, but responds well to non-steroidal anti-inflammatory drugs (**NSAIDs**). Pericarditis occurring 3–6 weeks after infarction is likely to be part of Dressler's syndrome. It is then often accompanied by fever, a raised erythrocyte sedimentation rate and pleuritic pain. This (probably) autoimmune syndrome also responds to NSAIDs or aspirin, but in some cases a short course of prednisolone is required.

Shoulder–hand syndrome

Pain in the left shoulder, with restricted movement, may occur in the weeks after myocardial infarction. It usually subsides with symptomatic treatment and physiotherapy.

Risk assessment and treatment after myocardial infarction

Patients with left main stenosis and multiple vessel stenosis have the highest risk, particularly if there has been substantial ventricular damage and a reduced ejection fraction (<40 per cent). Revascularization helps such patients and may do so in many others. Patients who have recovered from a small infarct, with an uncomplicated course, free of angina, and who are young may have a 1 year mortality less than 1–3 per cent. Such good risk patients must be distinguished from those who may have a 1-year risk of mortality of 20–40 per cent. Overall, the first-year risk after myocardial infarction is about 10 per cent. Thereafter it flattens rapidly to 3–5 per cent depending on age and left ventricular function.

There is a huge variation worldwide in the extent of investigation and treatment of patients who have survived a myocardial infarction, but with little evidence of much mortality benefit from more aggressive therapy.

Routine angiography or not after myocardial infarction

There are several reasons to doubt the wisdom of routine post-infarct angiography. First, the next event may recur on an innocent-looking plaque and not the one that caused the infarct. Although a severe lesion may go on to occlusion, such an event might not be as dangerous as anticipated—for instance when there is a good supply of collateral vessels or the subtended myocardium is already infarcted. Second, residual stenosis may include thrombus which may reabsorb. Third, too many physicians find it difficult to resist revascularization after angiography even if the procedure would not be helpful.

A final and compelling reason for caution is that prognosis is more dominated by the state of the left ventricle, than by the number of anatomically narrowed vessels seen. A classic study has shown that if the left ventricular ejection fraction is normal the 5-year survival is excellent.

Other methods of risk assessment

A number of non-invasive tests may be used to select patients with a poor prognosis from those who have a low risk but simple clinical markers should dominate any scheme of risk assessment. These are age, the presence of definite heart failure in the acute stage (however transient), continuing chest pain in the acute stage despite therapy with nitrates, heparin, β-blockade, and aspirin, a poor exercise ability, a clinically large infarction and the presence of serious arrhythmia,. Knowledge of the ejection fraction adds a little more. Exercise testing adds some further, but small, discrimination but can show patients what they can do safely, and so raises damaged morale. Radionuclide or echo assessment or left ventricular function during exercise or dipyridamole may identify ischaemic, but viable myocardium.

Holter monitoring and electrophysiological testing

Sudden death from ventricular fibrillation or asystole can to some extent be predicted by these techniques, but not with any great sensitivity or specificity. There is now more emphasis on newer analyses such as heart rate variability to identify autonomic imbalance, measurement of late potentials on the signal averaged ECG, and measurement of QT dispersion. These complex investigations should be used only when the above clinical indications suggest high immediate risk, or when the patient continues to have rest pain while on full medical therapy in hospital.

Conclusion

In high-risk patients after a large infarction, or equally in patients who have settled down after a period of unstable angina or a small myocardial infarction, it is sensible to proceed directly to coronary angiography or after an abnormal low level exercise test carried out before discharge.

For the others, a full symptom-limited exercise test can be performed at about 4 weeks after myocardial infarction. Angiography with a view to revascularization should be considered if the test shows definite early and prolonged ischaemia, or if the patient can only manage a low level of exercise (less than 5 min on the Bruce protocol).

Complications and consequences of myocardial infarction: prophylaxis

Prevention of reinfarction

β-Blockade

Large trials have shown that β-blockade given for 2–3 years after myocardial infarction reduces the risk of reinfarction and of sudden death by 20–30 per cent, as well as being highly effective against arrhythmia and angina. A varying proportion of patients (about 50 per cent) cannot tolerate these agents. Verapamil or diltiazem may then be useful and equally effective substitutes.

Calcium entry blockade

No calcium channel blocker has been shown to be beneficial in the first 48 h after myocardial infarction. Later, verapamil reduces the risk of reinfarction and sudden death by about 20–25 per cent but has no overall beneficial effect on patients who have had heart failure in the acute phase. The results of diltiazem treatment have been less impressive.

Further reading

ACE-Inhibitor Myocardial Infarction Collaborative Group. (1998). Indications for ACE-inhibitors in the early treatment of acute myocardial infarction: systemic overview of individual data from 10 000 patients in randomized trials. *Circulation*, 97, 2192–4.

Baigent, C., Collins, R., Appleby, P., Parish, S., Sleight, P., and Peto, R. on behalf of ISIS-2 (Second International Study of Infarct Survival) Collaborative Group. (1998). ISIS-2: 10-year survival among patients with suspected acute myocardial infarction in randomised comparison of intravenous streptokinase, oral aspirin, both, or neither. *British Medical Journal*, **316**, 1337–43.

Collins, R., Peto, R., Baigent, C., and Sleight, P. (1997). Aspirin, heparin and fibrinolytic therapy in suspected acute myocardial infarction. *New England Journal of Medicine*, 336, 847–60.

Fibrinolytic Therapy Trialists' (FTT) Collaborative Group. (1994). Indications for fibrinolytic therapy in suspected acute myocardial infarction: collaborative overview of early mortality and major morbidity results from all randomised trials of more than 1000 patients. *Lancet*, 343, 311–22.

ISIS-4 (Fourth International Study of Infarct Survival) Collaborative Group. (1995). ISIS-4: a randomised factorial trial comparing oral captopril versus placebo, oral mononitrate versus placebo, and intravenous magnesium sulphate versus control among 58 050 patients with suspected acute myocardial infarction. *Lancet*, 345, 669–87.

Chapter 2.14

Coronary angioplasty

*D. P. de Bono**

Percutaneous transluminal coronary angioplasty (PTCA) comprises inflation of a balloon to compress an atheromatous lesion, creating one or more tears within the plaque or in the normal vessel wall opposite. Arterial pressure then distends the vessel and subsequent remodelling usually preserves the new lumen (Fig. 1). In most cases, an expanding metal scaffold, or stent, is also implanted to stabilize the vessel wall and prevent recoil.

Complications of angioplasty

The most important immediate complication is abrupt vessel closure, and the most important long-term one is restenosis.

Abrupt closure

This may be due to thromboembolism, coronary spasm, thrombosis *in situ*, or dissection of the vessel wall. Thromboembolism is prevented by aspirin pretreatment (150–300 mg daily), high-dose intravenous heparin, (typically 10 000 units) during angioplasty, and careful attention to catheter flushing. Coronary spasm usually responds to nitrates or calcium antagonists given by direct intracoronary injection. Thrombosis *in situ*, either at the time of or within the next 12 h, is commonest in the presence of pre-existing thrombus, as in unstable angina or after myocardial infection. The risk of thrombosis in these patients is reduced by giving the platelet Gp IIb/IIIa blocker abciximab. Stent thrombosis is prevented by careful stent placement, monitored if necessary using intravascular ultrasound, and by a 1-month course of ticlopidine or clopidogrel. Coronary dissection is usually readily dealt with by stent implantation. Average procedure-related mortality rates for PTCA are 0.5–0.8 per cent and emergency bypass surgery may be needed in 1–2 per cent.

Restenosis

Restenosis can be defined angiographically as relative or absolute loss of gain following dilatation, and clinically as recurrent symptoms and a positive exercise test within 6 months. Symptoms developing later than 6 months are more likely to be due to a new lesion.

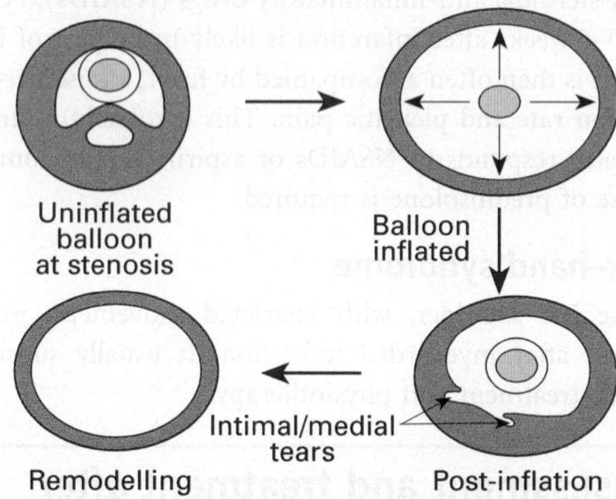

Fig. 1 Changes in the vessel wall during angioplasty.

*It is with regret that we report the death of Professor D. P. de Bono.

Restenosis is more common in males, smokers, diabetics and in left anterior descending lesions. No medication has consistently been shown to affect it. Stent implantation reduces clinical restenosis from 25–30 per cent to 15–20 per cent, partly by decreasing elastic recoil, partly because stented vessels have a larger post-procedure diameter. The restenosed vessel may be redilated, with a risk of further restenosis of about 30 per cent. In-stent restenosis is harder to redilate and may need special techniques (atherectomy, rotablation) or bypass grafting. It is currently uncertain whether elective stent implantation can be justified for all patients.

Indications and clinical results

Stable angina

PTCA is usually the intervention of choice for patients with single or two-vessel coronary disease who have angina not adequately controlled by medical treatment. The RITA-2 (Randomized Intervention Treatment of Angina) trial compared results of angioplasty with continuing medical treatment. Symptom relief was better with PTCA, at the cost of a slightly increased risk of death or myocardial infarction. The RITA I trial had earlier compared angioplasty with bypass grafting. After 2 years of follow-up, mortality, non-fatal infarction, and angina status were similar in the two groups. Patients given angioplasty were more likely to return to work early, but needed more subsequent interventions and were more likely to continue taking medical treatment. The initial cost of angioplasty was about half that of bypass surgery, but after 2 years this increased to about 80 per cent. Relative contraindications include diabetes, continued smoking, long occluded segments, diffuse coronary disease, and vessel diameter <2.5 mm. The primary success rate of angioplasty is >98 per cent in experienced centres but is lower when segments are completely occluded rather than stenosed (80–90 per cent).

Unstable angina

The success rate is high when lesions are suitable for angioplasty but the risk of abrupt closure is greater than in stable angina. Results of angioplasty are better in patients who can be stabilized with medical treatment and undergo PTCA as an elective procedure.

Myocardial infarction

Angioplasty as a primary treatment results in patency rates at least as good as those for thrombolysis, with the additional advantages of more rapid reperfusion and less bleeding complications, but resources for such an approach are rarely available. The role of 'rescue' angioplasty in patients who fail to reperfuse following thrombolytic therapy is being evaluated. Angioplasty may be indicated in patients with recurrent ischaemia presenting as unstable angina or reinfarction after initially successful thrombolysis or in patients who develop stable angina following infarction.

Angioplasty as a salvage procedure after coronary bypass surgery

Angioplasty is frequently the treatment of choice for patients developing recurrent angina after coronary bypass surgery. Vein graft stenoses are readily dilated, but tend to recur, and usually require stent implantation. Old vein grafts sometimes have a very friable intima, and dilatation may cause distal embolism of atheromatous material. This can be avoided by putting in a long stent after minimal predilatation. Thrombosed vein grafts should be treated initially with a thrombolytic agent, to prevent distal displacement of thrombus. Internal thoracic artery grafts seldom stenose but PTCA may be needed for anastomotic stenosis or new lesions in the native vessel.

Management of the pre- and post-angioplasty patient

Patients should be warned prior to angioplasty that in the event of abrupt vessel closure emergency surgery will be required, and that restenosis may occur.

Previous treatment with aspirin (300 mg immediately, then 150 mg daily) reduces the risk of abrupt vessel closure and supplements the heparin given at the time of the procedure. There is no evidence that nitrates or calcium antagonists given prior to angioplasty are any more effective than those given during the procedure. Use of ticlopidine/clopidogrel and abciximab is discussed above. Post-PTCA aspirin is usually continued indefinitely for its beneficial effect on outcome in coronary disease; there is no evidence that it reduces restenosis. High cholesterol, diabetes, and hypertension are vigorously treated for the same reason.

Patients with sedentary occupations may return to work within a few days. Regular exercise (walking, cycling, swimming) should be increased progressively within the limits of comfort. In the UK, licensing to drive a heavy goods or passenger carrying vehicle may be permitted 3 or more months after successful angioplasty provided the driver can safely complete at least the first three stages of the standard Bruce protocol exercise test without symptoms or signs of cardiac dysfunction, having been off cardioactive medication for at least 48 h.

Further reading

Goy, J.J. and Eeckhout, E. (1998). Intracoronary stenting. *Lancet*, **351**, 1943–9.

RITA-2 Trial Participants. (1997). Coronary angioplasty versus medical therapy for angina: the second Randomised Intervention Treatment of Angina (RITA-2) trial. *Lancet*, **350**, 461–8.

Chapter 2.15

Coronary artery bypass grafting

T. Treasure

Indications for surgery to relieve symptoms

Coronary artery bypass grafting is a highly effective means of relieving angina. Currently, over 90 per cent of patients are free of angina a year after surgery and this benefit is maintained in 80 per cent at 5 years and 60 per cent at 10 years.

Grafting should be considered to relieve angina in any patient in whom activity or enjoyment of life is curtailed by angina despite medical treatment. On average the likelihood of leaving hospital alive is 97 per cent, a figure that will apply to the typical male, aged 55–65, with triple vessel disease and no worse than moderate impairment of left ventricular function. This estimate should be adjusted up or down according to individual risk factors.

Indications for surgery to improve prognosis

Factors associated with a poor prognosis and improvable by surgery include left main stem stenosis, disease involving all three vessels with poor left ventricular function, disease in the proximal segment of the left anterior descending vessel and evidence of ischaemia at a low workload. Factors adversely affecting the risk of surgery include older age, female gender, obesity, renal impairment, diabetes, hypertension, and chronic respiratory disease.

Overall, the more severe and extensive the coronary artery disease, the greater is the comparative benefit of operation over medical treatment, while the outlook is very similar for the two managements if the disease is less severe. The worse the left ventricular function, the greater the comparative benefit of surgical over medical management.

The coronary bypass operation

Over 75 per cent of patients in contemporary UK practice receive three or more grafts.

Vascular conduits

Internal mammary artery

Eighty-five per cent of patients have at least one arterial graft, usually an internal mammary artery to the left anterior descending coronary artery. Intercostal branches are divided and the origin from the subclavian artery is left intact whenever possible, but the artery itself can be divided and used as a free graft to extend its range when its advantages still obtain. Both arteries can be used, but sternal healing may be compromised and increased operating time and increased risk of haemorrhage add to morbidity, outweighing any potential advantage . Double internal mammary artery grafting is an attractive option in younger patients but is unproven.

Patients with a pedicled left internal mammary artery graft to the left anterior descending coronary artery are more likely to be alive, free from myocardial infarction, and of angina at 10 years than those with a vein graft. Patency rate at 10 years can be as good as 95 per cent.

Vein grafts

In over 90 per cent of patients, vein grafts still make up the total of two to five grafts. The long saphenous is most commonly used but it may be unusable or unavailable due to varicose disease or its surgical treatment. Alternatives are the short saphenous, which is a technically satisfactory conduit but surgically less accessible, and arm veins, which are fragile and more difficult to use.

There are no good data to suggest there is any difference in the results between these veins but all vein grafts deteriorate with time. There is an early phase of thickening over the first few months, when a new layer, derived from platelets, fibrin, and circulating cells, is formed concentrically on the intimal surface. The attrition rate for vein grafts is about 2 per cent per annum with a high incidence of disease in the wall and occlusion from 7 years onwards. Patency at 10 years is only about 50 per cent.

Other arterial grafts and artificial conducts

The right gastroepiploic artery and inferior epigastric artery have also been used, the former requiring opening of the peritoneum with each limited to the inferior surface of the heart. Synthetic grafts or glutaraldehyde fixed arterial tissue grafts have proved rather unsatisfactory. In an attempt to increase the proportion of arterial grafts an increasing number of surgeons use the radial artery particularly since 1997 and 1998. The results remain to be seen.

Risk factors for perioperative death

In the UK during the early 1980s the death rate for coronary surgery levelled out to between 2.5 and 2.7 per cent, but in the 1990s with higher-risk cases being put forward, it has risen again to over 3 per cent. This figure is comparable with worldwide data and is applicable to the typical, patient who is male, aged 60–70, has surgery for chronic stable angina, has had some previous ischaemic damage to the myocardium, has triple vessel disease, and has four grafts at an elective operation, including a mammary graft to the left anterior descending coronary artery. Factors that increase the perioperative risk are greater age, emergency operation, unstable angina, recent myocardial infarction, left main stem disease, worse distal vessels, worse left ventricular function, other disease, small stature, and female gender, in approximate order of importance. Elderly women undergoing emergency surgery for multivessel disease face a risk of 10 per cent or more. Conversely, the factors that are associated with lower risk are an undamaged left ventricle and fewer vessels diseased. A 50-year-old having a single graft has a risk of less than 1 per cent.

Perioperative morbidity

Cardiac morbidity

Perioperative infarction

Localized myocardial infarction, occurs in about 2 per cent of cases. It results from occlusion of the grafted vessels or side branches of an artery where endarterectomy has been performed. More diffuse myocardial damage is more common but is less easy to define, and the wide range of estimates of its frequency reflect this.

Low output state

This is usually seen in patients with poor pre-operative left ventricular function, or those brought to theatre with evolving infarction. Treatment is supportive with intra-aortic balloon counterpulsation, afterload reduction with nitrates, and judicious use of inotropes. Techniques of myocardial reperfusion with substrate enhancement have something to offer in these cases and some will be supported temporarily with mechanical assistance of the left ventricle in the hope that there will be recovery of 'stunned myocardium'.

Cardiac arrhythmia

Atrial fibrillation and supraventricular tachycardia occur in 20–30 per cent of patients undergoing coronary surgery at about 2–5 days after operation. A wide range of prophylactic therapies have been suggested but the incidence is essentially unchanged. The important aetiological factors seem to be age and obesity, perhaps with hypoxia and left atrial distension being the proximate mechanisms. These arrythmias are almost without exception benign, and do not recur after the perioperative period. Heart block is seen immediately after surgery in about 5–10 per cent but persisting conduction abnormalities requiring permanent pacing are rare.

Acute ventricular arrhythmias, including ventricular fibrillation, are relatively uncommon.

Central nervous system damage

Stroke

Discrete central nervous system damage is seen consistently after coronary surgery with an incidence of about 2 per cent. It is age related, increasing from 0.5 per cent for patients in their fifties, to 5 per cent in patients over 70 years of age. The most common cause is embolism of atherosclerotic debris from the ascending aorta. Most cases are relatively mild and recover, but a minority have persisting severe disability. Stroke is sufficiently common, and the consequences so serious that the risk should be specifically mentioned prior to surgery.

Global cortical damage

Diffuse cerebral injury causing alteration in short-term memory and concentration is common but is only discernible by comparison of carefully performed neuropsychological tests before and after surgery. It can then be identified in one-third of patients at 2 months after surgery, and persists at 1 year.

Damage to other organs

Damage to other organs including the lung, kidney, and gastro-intestinal tract are more common with increasing bypass time, more severe disease and older age. They are rare in the routine elective case.

The outlook after coronary surgery

The probability of being alive 1 year after surgery is 95 per cent. Survival at 5 years is 88 per cent, and remains good at 10 years when 75 per cent can expect to be alive. At least half of the deaths are cardiac. Infarction, and the return of angina are more likely with incomplete revascularization and correlate with subsequent graft occlusion. Progression of disease in the native system is a major contributory factor and it is probable that thorough attention to risk factors will reduce the rate of progression of both graft and native vessel disease. Secondary prevention with low-dose aspirin improves graft patency.

Further reading

Hirsch, W.S., Ledley, G.S., and Kotler, M.N. (1998). Acute ischaemic syndromes following coronary artery bypass graft surgery. *Clinical Cardiology*, 21, 625–32.

Katz, M.M., Gersh, B.J., and Cox, J.L. (1998). Changing practice of coronary bypass surgery and its impact on early risk and long-term survival. *Current Opinion in Cardiology*, 13, 465–75.

Schussheim, A.E. and Fuster, V. (1998). Antithrombotic therapy and venous graft disease. *Current Opinion in Cardiology*, 13, 459–64.

Chapter 2.16

Vocational aspects of coronary artery disease

M. Joy

Almost 800 000 patients in the USA and at least 180 000 in the UK survive myocardial infarction each year. Nearly half of these will not have reached the age of retirement. In the US about 330 000 coronary artery bypass grafts are carried out each year and half of these are performed on people under the age of 65; some 300 000 American patients undergo percutaneous transluminal coronary angioplasty of whom two-thirds have not reached retiring age. The figures for Europe in general, and for the UK in particular are more modest; in the UK a total of some 18 000 coronary artery bypass procedures and 7300 percutaneous transluminal coronary angioplasty procedures were carried out in 1991. After myocardial infarction only about three-quarters of those eligible to return to work do so and only half will still be in employment 5 years later. A 10-year renew by the Coronary Artery Surgery Study has shown no difference in the work status between those treated surgically and those managed medically. After uncomplicated percutaneous transluminal coronary angioplasty the majority of those in work remain in it, but recrudescence of angina is associated with loss of employment.

Table 1 Canadian Cardiovascular Society classification of angina pectoris

Class I	Symptom-free for all normal activities; angina with strenuous or prolonged effort
Class II	Minor limitation. Symptoms with brisk effort on stairs, in the cold, or after meals
Class III	Significant limitation of ordinary activity. Symptoms with one flight of stairs or walking on the flat at a normal pace
Class IV	Any physical activity may provoke symptoms. Angina at rest

Data from Campeau, L. (1976). Grading of angina pectoris. *Circulation*, **55**, 522–3.

Recovery versus rehabilitation

In the last 10 years increasing attention has been paid to rehabilitation which starts in hospital and involves education with regard to risk factors, counselling, and emotional and psychological support. Exercise training has psychological value and helps the physiological deficit; it may also reduce the risk of further coronary events or mortality.

A number of factors influence return to work apart from the input of rehabilitation programmes. Adverse factors include age, the presence of significant symptoms, lower socio-economic status, poor motivation, a perception of 'illness', and inadequate social support. Other considerations include the availability of welfare payment, preferment of governments to pay sickness rather than unemployment benefit, and a raft of other problems, which include a desire on the part of the employer to retire an individual on account of concern about his/her ongoing suitability to perform at an appropriate level. Finally, there is failure to meet the medical fitness requirements laid down for certain occupations.

Fitness to work

Advice on fitness for work in the presence of coronary artery disease requires two considerations. The first is the level of symptoms, if any; the second is the predicted outcome and any deleterious effect of continued employment. The severity of angina is best described using the Canadian Cardiovascular Society's classification (Table 1). Breathlessness may conveniently be described using the New York Heart Association classification (Table 2).

There is no reason why the majority of patients who are class I from the symptomatic point of view, and who have been satisfactorily assessed, cannot continue to work.

Table 2 New York Heart Association functional classification of symptoms

Class I	Cardiac disease without symptoms on ordinary effort
Class II	Minor limitation of activity by symptoms
Class III	Marked limitation of activity by symptoms
Class IV	Symptoms at rest or on minimal exertion

Reproduced from the Criteria Committee of the New York Heart Association (1973). *Nomenclature and criteria for diagnosis for diseases of the heart and great vessels.* (7th edn) New York Heart Association/Little, Brown Co., Boston, with permission.

Some occupations, however, have statutory or non-statutory fitness requirements. Employment under hazardous circumstances, such as in the offshore oil industry, fire fighting, or the lifeboat services, are examples of this. The transportation industries (road, marine, aviation) and some recreational pursuits such as diving and flying are covered by statutory fitness requirements. Professional diving medical standards are the responsibility of the Health and Safety Executive in the UK while the railways have no statutory fitness standards in common with gliding, hang gliding, and amateur diving. The associated problems bear further consideration.

Coronary artery disease and transportation

Road

There are about one million holders of vocational driving licences in the UK. Three-quarters of a million hold large goods vehicle (**LGV**) licences and some 200 000 have passenger carrying vehicle (**PCV**) licences. These two groups of (vocational) licences are now called group II while the ordinary driving licence is now called the group I licence.

Although taxis carry passengers for hire and reward, only a group I licence is usually required. This also applies to emergency vehicles (of less than 7.5 tonnes). Their regulation, however, is the responsibility of individual municipal authorities, who may add additional medical standards up to and including those of the group II holders.

European legislature has not yet achieved consensus with regard to cardiological limits for driving licences. In the UK, the driver and vehicle licensing agency (**DVLC**) has produced a standard for both group I and group II licences. These have appeared in two publications—DVLA CLE1111 and in the *At a glance* guide to current medical standards.

Motor vehicle licensing

Group I licences

Group I drivers are legally required to notify the DVLA of any 'relevant' or prospective disability. Their doctors are also required to inform the patient if any bar to driving is thought to be present. This implies any condition which may lead to sudden impairment of consciousness or to sudden physical disability. The cardiological standards for group I are pragmatic and appropriate. Angina disbars only if particularly frequent or if it occurs at the wheel. Following myocardial infarction the subject should not drive for a month; after which a return to driving depends on the absence of other disqualifying conditions. Successfully treated heart failure does not disbar. Following coronary artery surgery the subject should not drive for at least a month while after coronary angioplasty a delay of only 1 week is required, provided that symptoms have not recurred.

Group II licences

Group II licence holders also require group I licences and are required to submit themselves to medical, but not electrocardiographic examination at entry, at age 45, 5-yearly until age 65, and then annually. Angina disbars whether or not freedom from the symptom can be achieved by medication. Likewise heart failure disbars. Following myocardial infarction, coronary angioplasty and coronary artery surgery the requirements are broadly similar and rely upon the generally favourable prognosis that is associated with normal or near normal left ventricular function in the absence of demonstrable myocardial ischaemia. In practice this depends on the symptom limited exercise electrocardiogram, and in the duration of the walking time. The subject who, 3 months after the index event, can complete at least three stages of the standard Bruce protocol or equivalent, off all cardioactive treatment for 24 h, without electrocardiographic change representing myocardial ischaemia, may, at the discretion of the Driver and Vehicle Licensing Agency, be considered for relicensing. Further, annual review may be demanded. Failure to increase blood pressure or the emergence of significant rhythm disturbance during the exercise test is likely to disbar.

Coronary angiography *per se* is not required, but if it has been carried out there should be no reduction of the left ventricular ejection fraction below 40 per cent, overall: nor should there be reduction of the intraluminal diameter of greater than 50 per cent in the proximal part of the left anterior descending coronary artery or in two or more major coronary vessels (greater than 30 per cent of the left main coronary artery). The group II licence holder is legally required to inform the Driver and Vehicle Licensing Agency of any relevant or prospective disability.

Motor racing

A competition licence is required for all competitive driving and this contains a medical declaration. The regulatory body in the UK is the Royal Automobile Club Motor Sports Association. For further details see OTM3, p. 2359.

Flying

Standards of operation and of personnel licensing, including medical certification, are agreed by international statute. The responsible agency is the International Civil Aviation Organization. The European Civil Aviation Convention will eventually become the European regional regulatory agency. At present, the Civil Aviation Authority (CAA) is the responsible certificatory agency in the UK. A number of reviews of cardiological problems in professional aircrew have been carried out to define with as much precision as possible acceptable latitude in standard fitness requirements (see e.g. Proceedings of the First European Workshops on Aviation Cardiology).

The 1 per cent rule in aviation

Any demonstrated abnormality should not carry a risk of 1 per cent or greater of any sudden adverse event/year. An 'event' in this context refers not only to sudden and total incapacitation, but also to symptoms which may cause subtle, rather than complete, impairment of function, for instance angina or rhythm disturbances. Professional aircrew with less than 1 per cent risk of event are given an 'as/with co-pilot' endorsed licence and those with a risk greater than 1 per cent are not licensed. The medical standards required of recreational licence holders are less rigorous.

Symptomatic coronary artery disease disbars from all forms of certification to fly. In the UK, recertification following myocardial infarction is possible subject to left ventricular function being normal or near normal, to there being no demonstrable obstruction of the coronary circulation remote from the artery subtending the infarcted area greater than 30 per cent, and no evidence of myocardial ischaemia on symptom-limited exercise electrocardiography/scintigraphy. Class I (i.e. professional) certification in such a circumstance is subject to restriction to fly 'as/with or with a co-pilot'. No such restriction applies to a private pilot who may be in sole command of an aircraft. No pilot, following a myocardial infarction, can expect unrestricted class I certification to fly an aircraft carrying passengers. Annual cardiological follow up with exercise electrocardiography is required.

Nine months after coronary artery bypass or successful percutaneous transluminal coronary angiography, an asymptomatic airman who has no demonstrable evidence of myocardial ischaemia (exercise electrocardiography), and who has demonstrably patent coronary bypass grafts with satisfactory run-off, or, who has maintained the dilatation of a treated vessel (residual stenosis less than 30 per cent) at angiography immediately before recertification, may be considered for recertification on an annual basis. Further coronary angiography is required not later than 5 years later.

Sea

Individual nations are responsible for standards of craft flying their national flag. In the UK medical standards for those going to sea are laid down in the Merchant Shipping (Medical Examination) Regulations (1983). These have statutory authority. Below the age of 18 all have an annual medical examination. Between the ages of 18 and 40 examination should be not exceed intervals of 5 years. After 40 the frequency is increased to 2 years. Those working on bulk chemical carriers may require more frequent examination and blood tests. Most cardiovascular problems including angina and myocardial infarction disbar from service at sea. There are no explicit standards for recertification following coronary artery surgery or percutaneous transluminal coronary angiography but the potential for a favourable decision may be present through a medical referee appointed by the Department of Transport.

The lifeboat service

In the UK there are two categories of operation, inshore (rivers and estuaries) and offshore. Inshore craft carry a crew of two to three. Offshore may operate for several hours at a time in extremes of cold and wet and in high seas, with crews of five to six.

Medical examinations are carried out on entry and 5-yearly thereafter. Age limits for service are 45 years for inshore operation and 55 years for offshore operation. A recent advisory committee has concluded that no lifeboatman in whom the diagnosis of coronary artery disease has been made, or is suspected, can serve, irrespective of treatment but the possibility of expert review, following appeal, exists.

Railways

The responsibility for application of medical standards of railwaymen in the UK is vested in the Department of Transport. Footplatemen require a class F certificate. The frequency for medical examination for class F holders is at entry, 5-yearly until age 55, again at $57\frac{1}{2}$ and 60, and 2-yearly thereafter. For class A, examination is carried out at entry, at age 30, 40, 45, and 5-yearly thereafter until 60, following which there is a further examination at age 63. The presence of overt or suspected coronary artery disease denies certification to operate a locomotive on a main line. There is the possibility of recertification following a myocardial infarction or following revascularization of the myocardium; an individual, having been excluded from mainline operations, might then find employment on a branch line. The operation of locomotives in marshalling yards and sheds is possible by railwaymen who are symptom-free on or off treatment for cardiovascular diseases.

Diving

Most divers are covered by the Diving Operations at Work Regulations (1981). Medical examinations are carried out annually. Any history of ischaemic heart disease, whether symptomatic or not, debars from diving. This applies whether or not there has been myocardial infarction or revascularization of the myocardium but divers have the statutory right of appeal to the Health and Safety Executive.

Fire service

Standards for firemen in the UK are laid down by the Home Office and medical examinations are carried out annually. Applicants have to be at least 18 years and under 31 years old and fit for any manual work. Coronary artery disease, whether or not there has been myocardial infarction and/or revascularization of the myocardium disbars from active duties.

Other

The armed forces in the UK, and the police force, have their own medical standards, which are similar to those of the civilian agencies.

Microlight flying and ballooning require a Civil Aviation Authority class D certificate embodying a short medical declaration and medical examination by a general practitioner. Microlight (and glider) instructors require a Civil Aviation Authority class III certificate with a medical examination carried out by an authorized medical examiner.

Regulatory agencies

A number of these exist. Their names and addresses can be found in OTM3, pp. 2361–2.

Further reading

Joy, M. (1992). First European Workshop in Aviation Cardiology. *European Heart Journal*, **13** (Suppl. H), 1–175.

Joy, M. and Bennett, G. (1984). First United Kingdom Workshop in Aviation Cardiology. *European Heart Journal*, **5** (Suppl. A), 1–163.

Joy, M. and Bennett, G. (1988). Second United Kingdom Workshop in Aviation Cardiology. *European Heart Journal*, **9** (Suppl. G), 1–179.

Chapter 2.17

Peripheral arterial disease

P. J. Morris

Most arterial disease is due to atherosclerosis, but embolism, trauma, and vasospastic disorders are also important. Atherosclerosis is found in all major arteries beyond middle age, and, indeed, if the fatty streak represents the first stage, it is widespread even in childhood. In addition to narrowing of vascular lumen, the destruction of the media by the atheromatous process may lead to dilatation of the

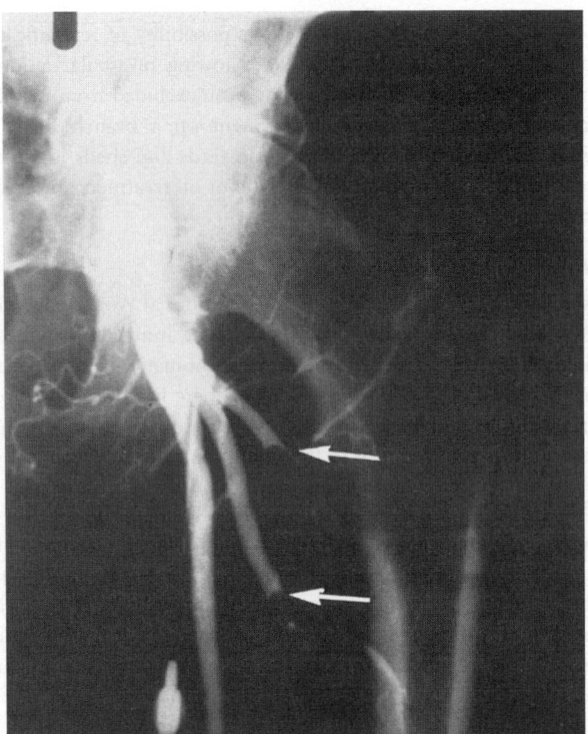

Fig. 1 A femoral angiogram showing the typical appearance of an embolus. Two emboli (arrows) can be seen in branches of the profunda femoris artery.

affected artery rather than occlusion. Occlusive arterial disease is often considered a different entity to aneurysmal disease, but whether they represent different manifestations of the same process or different processes of degeneration remains uncertain.

The distribution of atherosclerosis is peculiarly consistent in that plaques occur in large arteries with a high pressure, and at their bifurcations, or where there is kinking or external pressure on the artery, as in the adductor canal.

Risk factors for atherosclerosis and the underlying pathophysiology are discussed elsewhere (Chapters 2.8 and 2.10).

Clinical presentation

Acute ischaemia of a limb

The patient presents with a painful, pale, pulseless limb. Most commonly this is due either to acute thrombosis on an atheromatous stenosis or plaque, or to lodging of an embolus in a major artery. There is no difference on clinical examination of the acutely ischaemic limb whatever the cause. A previous history of claudication suggests that it may be due to thrombosis, while a history of a previous myocardial infarction, the presence of atrial fibrillation, rheumatic heart disease, or an abdominal aortic aneurysm would favour embolism. However, only an angiogram will enable an accurate diagnosis (Fig. 1). Arterial trauma is becoming increasingly common. A rare cause of acute ischaemia in the lower limb is phlegmasia cerulea dolens, in which massive thrombosis of all the major veins of the limb occurs with gross swelling causing obstruction of the arterial supply.

Chronic ischaemia of a limb

The manifestations of chronic ischaemia range from muscle pain on exercise relieved by rest (intermittent claudication), through rest pain and/or non-healing ulceration, to frank gangrene of the distal part of the limb. A relatively rare form of ischaemia in the Western world, but more common in South-east Asia, is Buerger's disease (thromboangiitis obliterans), which describes a syndrome of vasculitic disease in the medium-sized arteries of the lower limb, and less commonly in the upper limb, occurring almost always in young males who are heavy smokers and often associated with episodes of thrombophlebitis.

Clinical examination will reveal the absence of the appropriate pulses. Although the diagnosis of a severely ischaemic limb is usually quite apparent, that of intermittent claudication may present difficulties. Classically, the patient will complain of a cramp-like pain, for example in the calf after walking at a constant pace, which disappears within minutes of resting, only to reappear again at the same distance as the patient walks again. Failure of the pain to disappear on resting or its reappearance at a shorter distance after each rest should suggest a possible musculoskeletal cause, especially if distal pulses are present on examination. Pulses can be present in a limb distal to proximal disease, albeit weaker than the normal side, if there is good collateral flow, but then exercise to the point of claudication will lead to their disappearance. Doppler pressures at the ankle at rest will be lower than the brachial pressure and will fall markedly after exercising for 1 min on a treadmill. Angiography is performed if reconstructive surgery is to be considered, but is not used as a diagnostic tool. A variety of conditions may mimic intermittent claudication. These include such disorders as spinal stenosis, and arthritis of the knee and hip.

Aneurysms

Abdominal aortic aneurysm

This is the most common aneurysm encountered in clinical practice and may present in one of three ways.

1. *Ruptured or leaking aneurysm*: the patient classically presents with the triad of pain, hypotension, and a pulsatile mass in the abdomen, but only 50 per cent of patients will present with all three features. The pain tends to be epigastric radiating through to the back, but may be situated in the loin or even in the testicle. Indeed, one of the most common misdiagnoses is renal colic. A pulsatile mass may be overlooked, especially in the obese patient, if an attempt is not made specifically to feel for it in a patient with an acute abdomen or shock. In general, femoral pulses will be present and the femoral arteries tend to be ectatic.
2. *Symptomatic or expanding aneurysm*: the patient presents with abdominal pain, usually epigastric, or with pain in the back of relatively recent onset, and is found to have a pulsatile mass. Occasionally, the presenting features are of ureteric obstruction when a fibrotic inflammatory reaction similar to retroperitoneal fibrosis has occurred around the aneurysm, or of an embolus of the lower limbs causing acute ischaemia.
3. *Asymptomatic aneurysm*: the patient is found to have a pulsatile mass on examination for some other condition, or an aneurysm is detected on a plain radiograph or ultrasound of the abdomen.

Thoracic aortic aneurysm

Syphilis was once the commonest cause, but the vast majority of cases today are due to atheroma, with a small number resulting from previous trauma. Syphilitic aneurysms usually involve the ascending aorta, whereas atheromatous aneurysms are evenly distributed between the ascending aorta, arch, and descending aorta. Most thoracic aorta aneurysms are asymptomatic, and detected by chance on chest radiography. The first presentation is often death due to sudden rupture. Very large aneurysms may cause anterior chest pain, or pressure-related phenomena, such as superior vena caval obstruction, dysphagia, or stridor. Involvement of the aortic valve or sinus of Valsalva in lesions of the ascending aorta cause aortic regurgitation and angina even if coronary vessels are healthy.

Dissecting aortic aneurysm

Dissection is associated with degeneration of the media of the aorta and most patients are hypertensive. In about 50 per cent of cases the dissection starts in the ascending aorta, the next most common site being just distal to the origin of the left subclavian artery. The arch and the abdominal aorta are uncommon sites of origin. Pain, either substernal or in the upper back, is the most striking presenting feature, often with radiation to the neck or arms. An aortic diastolic murmur or a pericardial friction rub may be heard with a dissection of the ascending aorta, and there may be a significant diminution in the pulse and blood pressure in the right arm. A dissection of the descending thoracic aorta may extend into the abdominal aorta and involve all its major branches, thus being associated with acute renal failure, mesenteric ischaemia, or ischaemia of the lower limbs.

Popliteal aneurysms

These are not uncommon and are often associated with aneurysmal disease elsewhere. Although sometimes causing pain due to pressure on surrounding structures, they most commonly present as a pulsatile mass behind the knee or with ischaemia of the distal limb due to thrombosis or embolism.

Other aneurysms

Less commonly, aneurysms may occur in the iliac, femoral, carotid, splenic, renal, or one of the splanchnic arteries. With the exception of carotid or femoral artery aneurysms, which will usually present as a pulsatile mass, those elsewhere tend to be asymptomatic until they cause a major intra-abdominal bleed, more often fatal than not. Splenic artery aneurysms are the most common intra-abdominal ones apart from those of the aorta or iliac vessels, and are seen more frequently in younger women, in which case there is a marked tendency to rupture during pregnancy. Mycotic aneurysms are rare, and usually are seen today as a complication of bacterial endocarditis (Fig. 2).

Vasospastic syndromes

Raynaud's syndrome is the commonest of these and is described in Chapter 10.13.

Acrocyanosis virtually only occurs in women and is characterized by cold blue extremities, worse in cold weather. The symptoms are not episodic, and all peripheral pulses are present.

Livedo reticularis is characterized by persistent patchy reddish-blue mottling of skin which tends to be worse in cold weather. It may sometimes be associated with chronic ulceration. It is due to random spasm of cutaneous arterioles, with secondary dilation of capillaries and venules. There may be underlying systematic lupus erythematosus or other vasculitis in some cases.

Reflex sympathetic algodystrophy (Sudek's atrophy) describes a number of related conditions in which causalgic pain and vasomotor instability are common features—see OTM3, p. 3941.

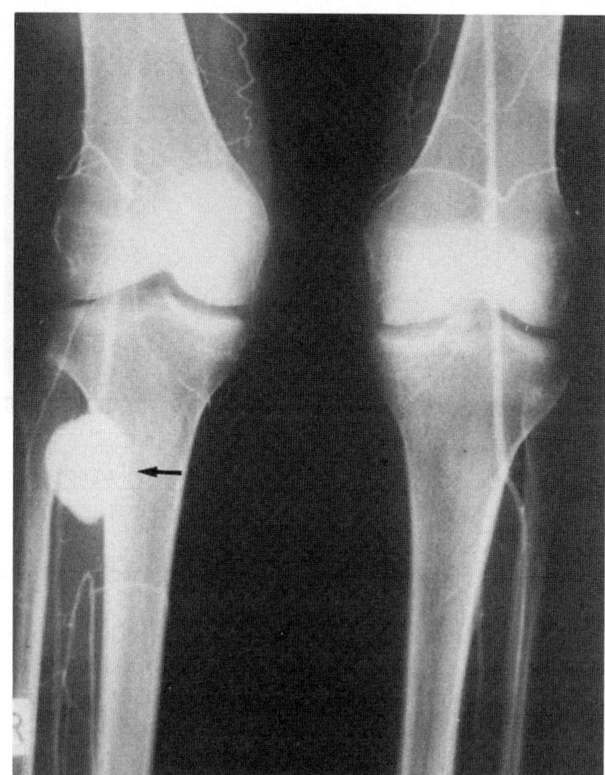

Fig. 2 A mycotic aneurysm (arrow) at the bifurcation of the distal popliteal artery in a young woman with subacute bacterial endocarditis. Other aneurysms were present in the left iliac artery and the right profunda femoris artery.

Thoracic outlet compression

Compression of any one of the subclavian vein, subclavian artery, or the lower trunk of the brachial plexus, or all three structures, may occur due to a variety of anatomical abnormalities at the thoracic outlet. A cervical rib is the most common recognized cause, but compression can occur despite normal anatomy as the structures cross the first rib into the axilla. Symptoms tend to occur for the first time in early middle age, particularly in women. Neurological symptoms predominate, such as pain which is usually poorly defined, paraesthesia in the C8–T1 distribution and loss of small muscle function in the hand. Vascular symptoms are due to either arterial or venous obstruction. Arterial obstruction may present as a unilateral Raynaud's phenomenon or pallor and pain in the hand when using the arm above the head, or at a later stage with distal emboli to the fingers from a post-stenotic aneurysm. Venous obstruction often presents in the younger person as a spontaneous axillary vein thrombosis.

Intestinal ischaemia

Acute

Patients presenting with acute intestinal ischaemia are usually elderly, with evidence of generalized atheromatous disease. Atrial fibrillation or a mural thrombus after myocardial infarction may be the source of emboli. Acute intestinal ischaemia may also be due to venous thrombosis, which is associated with portal hypertension, peritonitis, or a blood dyscrasia. Furthermore, in a significant number of patients with acute intestinal ischaemia, no major arterial or venous obstruction is found at laparotomy or autopsy, the ischaemia being

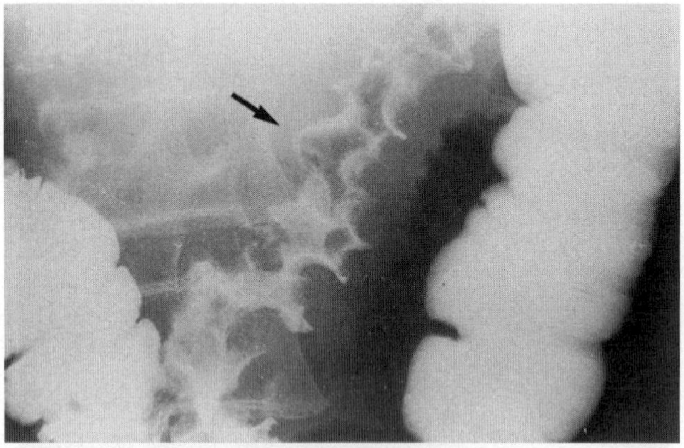

Fig. 3 Barium enema in a 68-year-old man with left-sided abdominal pain and positive occult bloods showing the typical appearance of an ischaemic colitis (arrow).

presumed to be due to low flow associated with cardiac failure or shock.

The patient presents with an acute abdomen, colicky abdominal pain, nausea, and vomiting, associated with tenderness in the early stages but later with the signs of peritonitis. Diarrhoea is common, and is often bloody, especially with acute ischaemia of the large bowel. A peritoneal tap will reveal a serosanguineous aspirate containing leucocytes and, at a later stage, bacteria. A plain radiograph of the abdomen may show complete absence of gas shadows at an early stage, or fluid levels, sometimes localized to the ischaemic segment of small bowel, while a typical scalloped or fingerprinting appearance in the large bowel may be apparent on barium enema (Fig. 3). However, only an angiogram will confirm the obstruction of a major mesenteric artery with either an embolus or thrombus. Whether this is justified in the investigation of possible intestinal ischaemia is debatable. Unless there is obstruction of at least one other major mesenteric artery, severe ischaemia of the intestine is unlikely to occur. The mortality of acute intestinal ischaemia is of the order of 75 per cent, and only early diagnosis and surgical exploration offers the patient a chance of survival.

Chronic

Patients with chronic intestinal ischaemia present with postprandial, central, colicky abdominal pain, and weight loss. Usually two of the three main arteries supplying the bowel have to be obstructed for symptoms to result. Angiography defines the vascular lesions but cannot confirm that they are responsible for symptoms. True chronic intestinal ischaemia of this cause is rare enough, but even rarer, if ever, must be the concept of compression of the coeliac artery by an unusually low median arcuate ligament of the diaphragm.

Extracerebral vascular disease

Carotid artery ischaemia

Atheromatous disease of the origin of the internal carotid artery commonly presents as a transient ischaemic attack (TIA), or amaurosis fugax. The majority of TIAs are embolic, arising from an ulcerated and/or stenosed origin of the internal carotid artery, but emboli may also arise from the heart. TIAs, especially in the presence of severe bilateral carotid artery disease, may be haemodynamic in nature, rather than embolic. Disease of the internal carotid artery may present as a full-blown stroke, without preceding warning. Amaurosis fugax

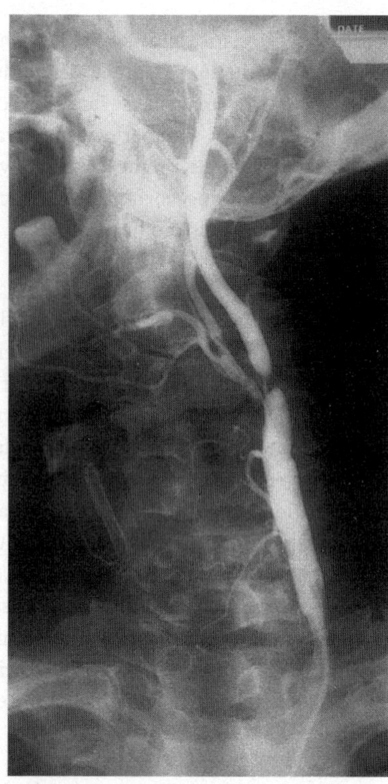

Fig. 4 A carotid angiogram showing a severe stenosis of the internal carotid artery.

describes a unilateral loss of vision lasting only minutes, often resembling the sensation of a blind being pulled down over the eye. A bruit may be heard over the carotid bifurcation, but its absence does not exclude internal carotid artery disease. Examination of the fundus may reveal a platelet or cholesterol embolus in the retinal arterial circulation.

A duplex scan of the carotids allows imaging of the carotid bifurcation and measurement of the degree of stenosis. The gold standard no longer remains carotid angiography (Fig. 4), as there is a 1–4 per cent risk of a stroke following it. For this reason it is appropriate to proceed with surgery on the basis of a satisfactory duplex scan without an angiogram, which is only performed if the duplex scan is unsatisfactory. A computed tomography scan or magnetic resonance image of the brain should always be performed to exclude other pathology and ascertain the presence of cerebral infarcts. Magnetic resonance angiography can also be valuable where the duplex scan is unsatisfactory.

Vertebrobasilar ischaemia

Symptoms of vertigo, ataxia, diplopia, dysarthria, and drop attacks suggest this diagnosis. Tingling and numbness of face and mouth in half of the body may also occur as may transient hemiparesis. Episodes of visual impairment are common, varying from reduced vision in one half-field to impairment of vision on both sides.

Vertebrobasilar ischaemia is haemodynamic rather than embolic in origin. Bilateral disease of the vertebral artery may be responsible, but usually only in the presence of carotid artery disease or a non-intact circle of Willis. Uncommon causes are the subclavian and innominate artery steal syndromes. In the former the steal is from the vertebral artery on the side of the occlusion, particularly while using that arm. In the latter there is a steal down both the vertebral and carotid arteries on the right side, again often associated with use of the right arm.

Renovascular disease

The most common form is renal artery stenosis, but also included are renal artery aneurysm, arteriovenous fistula, and trauma to the renal artery. The majority of stenoses are atheromatous in origin (over 70 per cent), a much smaller proportion being due to one of several types of fibromuscular dysplasia, and rarely associated with non-atheromatous aortic aortitis, e.g. mid aortic syndrome.

The presentation and diagnosis of renovascular hypertension are discussed in Chapter 2.32.

Investigation of patients with arterial disease

Detection of risk factors

Hypertension and smoking are most important. Hyperlipidaemia should also be treated. Polycythaemia should not be overlooked, but although there is some evidence that hyperfibrinogenaemia may be associated with peripheral vascular disease, the evidence is not sufficiently strong to warrant this investigation in most patients. Urine examination for glucose and a random blood glucose should be performed in all patients.

Non-invasive assessment of arterial disease

Physiological measurements

The physiological dysfunction of arterial obstruction requires correction rather than the anatomical lesion. Most commonly, Doppler ultrasound is used to measure pressure in peripheral vessels. Measurement at the ankle before and after exercise, provides an objective assessment of the degree of arterial obstruction. The ankle pressure is expressed as a pressure index which is the ratio of the systolic pressure at the ankle to that in the brachial artery. Normal indices at rest range from 0.9 to 1.2, while those in patients with intermittent claudication range from 0.4 to 0.9. In patients with severe ischaemia and rest pain the indices are below 0.4. After exercise the pressure, and hence the index, falls in the presence of significant arterial obstruction, the rate of recovery giving further information about the degree of ischaemia.

Non-invasive imaging techniques

Ultrasound imaging of large arteries allows the size of aneurysms and the presence of thrombus within the lumen to be determined, and is an ideal way of following small asymptomatic abdominal aortic aneurysms where surgery is not indicated. Colour duplex ultrasound has increased the utility of this technique further is now the method of choice for investigating patients with putative carotid artery disease. It is also used to demonstrate peripheral arterial disease in the legs, avoiding the need for angiography in many instances. Magnetic resonance angiography may replace conventional angiography in selected situations.

Invasive assessment of arterial disease

Angiography remains most valuable, although being replaced by duplex scanning in many instances. Complications such as thrombosis due to intimal damage, clot embolism, or cholesterol embolism, are uncommon. The resolution of digital subtraction angiography is inferior to that of a conventional angiogram, but can be enhanced by the intra-arterial injection of contrast. This technique has proven valuable in certain areas, such as the carotid bifurcation, the renal arteries, abdominal aortic, and peripheral arterial aneurysms, and in the sequential evaluation of known arterial lesions or of reconstructive surgery.

Management of the ischaemic limb

General management

Attention must be paid to the cleanliness of ischaemic feet or hands, and particular care must be given to the cutting of toe nails. Walking to the point of claudication several times during each day may improve collateral circulation, ultimately increasing the walking distance. Reconstructive surgery should not be considered in patients presenting with intermittent claudication until the symptoms have been present for at least 3 months, for it is possible that the claudication distance will improve significantly over the succeeding months as collateral circulation develops.

Drugs

A variety of vasodilator drugs have been tried but they have no place in management. Prostacyclin has not been shown to be of value in the ischaemic limb. Anticoagulants again have no place in the management of occlusive arterial disease, other than during reconstructive surgery. Recent evidence from controlled trials suggests that patency of infrainguinal grafts is prolonged by the prophylactic use of low-dose aspirin after reconstructive surgery.

Reconstructive arterial surgery

Aortoiliac reconstruction

Occlusive disease of the aortoiliac segment may be treated either by endarterectomy or the insertion of a prosthetic graft. Either procedure may give satisfactory results, but endarterectomy is best restricted to relatively localized disease. The long-term patency of bypass grafts appears superior to endarterectomy in the aortoiliac area, but endarterectomy does not preclude a subsequent graft.

Reconstruction below the inguinal ligament

Femoropopliteal grafts are performed for occlusion of the superficial femoral artery, usually running from the common femoral artery to either the proximal popliteal artery above the knee or the distal popliteal artery below the knee. Autologous saphenous veins are the preferred material. Prosthetic grafts do as well for above-knee procedures, but are markedly inferior when below-knee surgery is required.

Femorotibial grafts: where no popliteal artery is present but one of the three distal arteries is patent (anterior tibial, posterior tibial, or peroneal), it is possible to use one of these for insertion of a graft arising from the common femoral artery. This type of procedure is only performed for limb salvage, and vein is always used if possible. The salvage rate in critically ischaemic limbs has been impressive, at least in the short term.

Profundaplasty: when a stenosis at the origin of the profunda femoris artery exists together with a block of the superficial femoral artery, profundaplasty, with or without a local endarterectomy, may significantly improve the circulation to the limb. This is a simple procedure which can be performed under local anaesthetic and is ideal as a limb-salvage procedure in a poor-risk patient.

Extra-anatomical bypass grafts

In aortoiliac disease in patients considered not well enough to undergo aortoiliac reconstruction, a prosthetic graft can be brought subcutaneously from the axillary artery to the femoral artery on the same side, with another graft taken off this in the region of the iliac fossa to the opposite femoral artery.

Where one iliac artery only is obstructed, a prosthetic graft can be brought subcutaneously from the femoral artery on the side with a normal flow, to the common femoral or profunda femoris artery on the obstructed side. This technique is now preferred even in younger patients with unilateral iliac obstruction.

Factors influencing graft patency

The site of the graft is important, for prosthetic grafts have a very high patency rate above the inguinal ligament, approaching that of vein grafts, whereas below the inguinal ligament they are to be avoided if at all possible. Both the inflow and outflow from a graft are also important. Continued smoking decreases the likelihood of long-term patency in reconstructed arteries some fourfold. Management of hypertension, diabetes, and hyperlipidaemia, is just as important.

Complications of reconstructive surgery

The major complications are graft thrombosis, haemorrhage, and infection. Infection in the vicinity of an arterial anastomosis or a prosthetic graft represents the most serious, for it can lead to erosion of anastomoses and life-threatening haemorrhage. Prosthetic graft infection generally can be eradicated only by excising the graft, and replacing it with a new one, well away from the infected site but aggressive long-term antibiotic therapy and more conservative surgical management may be an appropriate alternative approach to this dreadful problem.

Embolectomy

There is no case for procrastination with anticoagulants when acute ischaemia is caused by an embolus; the only treatment is embolectomy which can be performed under local anaesthesia using a Fogarty balloon catheter. It can be successful even after 4 weeks, provided the limb is still viable.

Thrombolysis

Acute ischaemia due to embolism or thrombosis can sometimes be treated by thrombolysis. This has now become relatively common practice for the initial management of the acutely ischaemic, but viable, limb, although haemorrhage is a significant complication.

Sympathectomy

In severe limb ischaemia due to occlusive arterial disease when reconstruction is not possible, a lumbar sympathectomy may be performed. Although chemical sympathectomy by the paravertebral injection of phenol into the vicinity of the sympathetic chain is a simple procedure, it is not as effective as an operative sympathectomy in which the chain and the second and third ganglion are removed. However, the results of sympathectomy are not overly impressive.

Percutaneous transluminal angioplasty (see Chapter 2.14)

The lesion for this treatment par excellence is the localized iliac artery lesion, not greater than 2.5 cm long, where over 90 per cent of dilatations are immediately successful with 2-year patency rates of about 80 per cent. Successful dilatation of localized stenoses or occlusions of the superficial femoral artery have been achieved with lesions of less than 10 cm, the immediate success rate being of the order of about 70 per cent. The use of dilatation is now being explored for limb salvage in blocks of the superficial femoral artery in patients considered at high risk for reconstructive surgery. In functional renal artery stenoses percutaneous transluminal angioplasty is becoming the first line of attack for most lesions, and the use of a stent for ostial lesions has allowed these lesions to be treated by interventional radiology. The complication rate for this procedure is small in experienced hands and certainly less than for reconstructive surgery. Complications include distal embolization, significant groin haematomas, thrombosis, false aneurysm, and even death.

Amputation

The rate of amputation in hospitals with a specialist vascular unit has not declined, presumably due to the increasing age of the population. The level of amputation is dictated both by the limb-fitter's requirements and the likelihood of obtaining primary healing. In occlusive arterial disease there is no place for local amputations of gangrenous toes or even part of the foot, unless this is preceded by a successful graft restoring distal circulation. If possible, a below-knee amputation should be performed rather than above knee. No satisfactory method exists for determining whether the flaps of a below-knee amputation, have an adequate blood supply to achieve primary healing. Nevertheless with care some 75 per cent of below-knee amputations will heal primarily or with a modest delay.

Rehabilitation of a patient after an amputation must start as soon as there is recovery from the anaesthetic and continue until the patient is mobile on an artificial limb. Nevertheless the number of patients who become fully rehabilitated with an artificial limb remains depressingly low.

The diabetic foot (see also Chapter 6.13)

The diabetic with peripheral arterial disease not only has small artery disease but is likely to have large artery disease as well. If large artery disease exists, this should be dealt with, as reconstruction of an obstructed major artery will improve healing of the distal lesion even in the presence of small vessel disease. After local amputations of gangrenous toes healing is slow. If infection is present, the lesion must be laid open extensively with excision of any necrotic tissue or involved tendons.

Management of aneurysms

Abdominal aorta

Ruptured

This is a true surgical emergency, and the patient should be taken immediately to the operating room where placement of a clamp on the aorta above the aneurysm should take preference over resuscitation, radiography, or the cross-matching of blood. The results of surgery are poor; at best, about 50 per cent of patients survive. Not all patients should be operated on, but the decision not to operate may be difficult. As a general guideline, patients over 80 years of age who have been hypotensive for over 1 h have a poor prognosis.

Symptomatic aneurysm

A symptomatic aneurysm should be operated on whatever its size, for if the symptoms are truly due to the aneurysm then rupture within weeks to months is very likely. Severe cardiac or respiratory disease is sometimes a contraindication to surgery. There may be a place for aortic stenting (discussed below). Tacking of a sheet of Dacron over the aneurysm, in the hope that this will be incorporated in a thick fibrous reaction around it, hence preventing further dilatation, has sometimes appeared protective.

Asymptomatic aneurysm

If the aneurysm is large (greater than 6 cm), there is little doubt that it should be dealt with surgically, for there is good evidence that the likelihood of subsequent rupture is high. In the case of the smaller aneurysms, two courses are available. Either the patient is followed regularly and the size of the aneurysm monitored by ultrasound, or surgery is advised provided that the patient's general health is reasonably sound. The latter course can only be advised provided that a competent vascular surgeon is available, for in the best hands, the hospital mortality associated with an elective replacement of an abdominal aortic aneurysm is about 2 per cent. Even patients with a small aneurysm show a decreased survival compared with an age- and sex-matched population without an aneurysm. This difference is due only in part to subsequent rupture of the aneurysm, but also to death from cardiac and cerebral vascular disease. The insertion of intraluminal stents within the aortic aneurysmal lumen, although promising initially is proving to be beset with immediate and longer-term problems, and its place in the treatment of aortic aneurysms remains to be established.

Popliteal artery

These should always be bypassed or replaced, even though asymptomatic, for if a popliteal aneurysm presents with a severely ischaemic leg due to thrombosis or distal embolization, limb salvage is usually not possible.

Thoracic aorta

Rupture of thoracic aortic aneurysms is nearly always fatal, and in these few who reach the operating room, the chances of survival are remote.

Elective resection of aneurysms of the ascending thoracic aorta or aortic arch presents a formidable challenge because of the necessity to interrupt the cerebral circulation. Furthermore, the aortic valve may have to be replaced and coronary arteries reimplanted in lesions of the ascending aorta, while the innominate, left common carotid, and subclavian arteries need to be reimplanted after replacement of the aortic arch. These procedures are performed under cardiopulmonary bypass together with bypass to the cerebral circulation.

Elective replacement of descending thoracic aortic aneurysms carries the risk of spinal cord ischaemia and renal ischaemia during the period of clamping, and for this reason many surgeons employ extracorporeal bypass to perfuse the lower half of the body while the reconstruction is performed.

Hospital mortality is still high, especially in the case of aneurysms of the ascending aorta or arch, and is at least 10 per cent even in the most experienced hands.

Dissecting aneurysm

The results of treatment of dissecting aneurysms of the thoracic aorta are poor. There are advocates of both surgical and medical treatment, and perhaps a combination of both provides the best chances of survival. Medical treatment is directed at reducing the blood pressure to normal or below normal levels, while surgical treatment is directed at resection of the aorta at the origin of the dissection, closure of the dissection proximally and distally, and replacement of the defect in the aorta by a Dacron prosthetic graft. Mortality remains high.

Thoracoabdominal aorta

An aneurysm involving the thoracic as well as the abdominal aorta presents major problems as the coeliac, superior mesenteric, and renal arteries arise from it. Virtually no patients have survived an emergency resection of such aneurysms, and the mortality of elective resections is still about 30 per cent. The most satisfactory approach is to insert a Dacron prosthetic graft from the thoracic aorta to the distal abdominal aorta, followed by implantation of the major intra-abdominal arteries before disconnecting the aneurysm. This inevitably results in prolonged ischaemia of the kidneys and bowel, which is largely responsible for the high mortality.

Other arteries

Aneurysms of other arteries, such as the femoral, splenic, and renal arteries, should be excised and replaced with a graft if greater than 1.5–2.0 cm in diameter or if symptomatic.

Extracerebral vascular disease

Carotid artery ischaemia

Management of symptomatic internal carotid artery stenosis depends on the degree of stenosis. Patients with tight internal carotid artery stenosis (greater than 70 per cent) have been shown in two large trials to have had fewer strokes after endarterectomy than with medical treatment. The perioperative rate of major stroke or death was 2.1 per cent, in the American trial and 3.5 per cent in the European.

For stenoses of 30–70 per cent, the data do not support a role for carotid endarterectomy and patients in this category continue to be entered into both trials.

In patients with transient ischaemic attacks associated with mild or moderate stenosis, treatment should comprise aspirin 300 mg daily and attention to hypertension, hyperlipidaemia, and smoking. If aspirin is not tolerated, dipyridamole may be used. Continuing transient ischaemic attacks despite therapy may justify carotid endarterectomy. Patients undergoing carotid endarterectomy should continue on aspirin through surgery and thereafter.

Vertebrobasilar ischaemia

Surgical reconstruction of diseased vertebral arteries is now rarely performed, unless there is associated significant internal carotid artery disease when carotid endarterectomy may increase intracerebral circulation in general.

The subclavian steal syndrome is managed by an extra-anatomical bypass either from the axillary artery on the non-affected side to the axillary artery on the affected side, or a graft between the common carotid and the subclavian artery. The innominate steal syndrome is usually dealt with by inserting a graft from the aortic arch to the distal innominate artery via a median sternotomy. In both instances treatment is possible by angioplasty, especially in the case of the subclavian artery stenosis, where the risk of distal cerebral embolization is low.

Renovascular disease

Renal artery stenosis believed to be the cause of hypertension, with or without associated renal dysfunction, may be treated by transluminal angioplasty or open reconstructive surgery.

Renal artery aneurysms, if greater than 1 cm in diameter, are best treated surgically. This usually requires removal and cooling of the

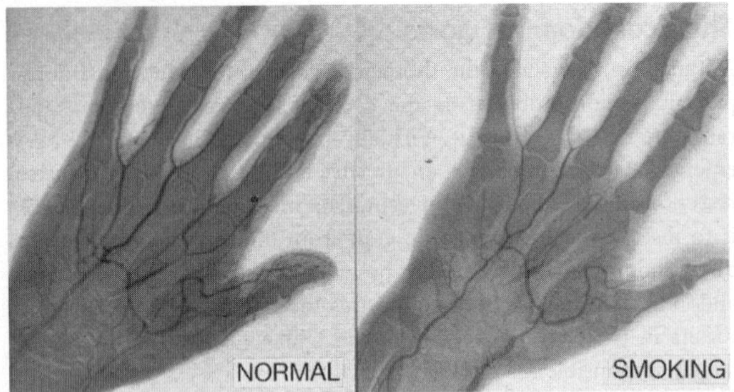

Fig. 5 An angiogram of the hand of a patient with Raynaud's disease, before and after smoking half a cigarette, showing the induced vasospasm of the small arteries of the hand.

kidney, with resection of the aneurysm and reconstruction of the vasculature on the bench, followed by reimplantation of the kidney in the iliac fossa.

Management of vasospastic disorders

General measures

The basis of all treatment initially should be advice on keeping warm and firm encouragement to stop smoking (Fig. 5). Battery-warmed gloves are of value in severe cases.

Drugs

Reserpine is sometimes useful, and some striking claims for benefits of intra-arterial reserpine, at least in the short term, for patients with severe Raynaud's syndrome have been made. Nifedipine is the most commonly used drug for this condition at present. Another approach to severe Raynaud's syndrome, which does result in short-term beneficial effect, is a guanethidine block, the guanethidine being injected intravenously with a tourniquet on the proximal part of the limb. Plasmapheresis has also been used in some cases, with benefit. The use of prostacyclin infusion is discussed in Chapter 10.13.

Sympathectomy

This should be reserved for the patient with severe symptoms despite general measures and drug treatment. Although most patients get an excellent result from sympathectomy in the early months after the operation, relapse after 6 months to 2 years, occurs in about one-third of patients with Raynaud's disease, and in two-thirds of patients with Raynaud's phenomenon. The results of sympathectomy are not so good once significant trophic changes have occurred.

Management of intestinal ischaemia

Acute intestinal ischaemia

Often the patient presents late and with irreversible ischaemia of part of the bowel, requiring immediate laparotomy and resection. If any patients are to benefit by embolectomy or reconstruction, the possibility of this diagnosis must always be borne in mind in the patient with generalized atheromatous disease or a source of embolism who presents with an acute abdomen. The diagnosis can only be established by angiography or, less reliably, at surgery.

If embolectomy or thrombectomy can be performed successfully, it not only reduces the length of bowel that has to be resected but also enhances the healing of the anastomosis. If there is the slightest doubt about the viability of any bowel not resected, the abdominal wall should be loosely closed in a single layer and a second laparotomy performed after 24 h. Unfortunately, in at least 50 per cent of cases of small- and large-bowel ischaemia an obvious blockage of a main artery or venous thrombosis is not demonstrable.

Ischaemia of the large bowel presents with a spectrum of clinical features ranging from mild abdominal pain to frank necrosis of the colon. The more severe examples will be managed by laparotomy and excision of the ischaemic bowel; preservation of large bowel is not nearly so critical as of small bowel. The less severe examples can be watched, but with immediate laparotomy if any signs of peritonitis develop. These patients often present months to years later with an ischaemic stenosis and obstruction requiring resection of the stenosed segments.

Chronic intestinal ischaemia

If this diagnosis can be established, restoration of arterial flow beyond a stenosis can be achieved by a bypass graft from the aorta to the involved mesenteric artery, endarterectomy and patch plasty or transaortic endarterectomy for a lesion at the origin of the artery. In patients in whom a median arcuate ligament syndrome is defined, division of the ligament will result in cure.

Management of thoracic outlet compression

When a clearly defined anatomical abnormality accounts for the clinical features, surgical treatment is indicated, as for instance by excision of a cervical rib. When no apparent abnormality exists, exercises directed at strengthening the shoulder girdle muscles may be of benefit. If no improvement follows, the most appropriate procedure is excision of the first rib, which relieves most cases whatever the cause. If damage to the subclavian artery has occurred as a result of long-standing compression, a post-stenotic aneurysm may be present, when resection of the artery and replacement with a graft is necessary.

Further reading

Girolami, B., Bernardi, E., Prins, M.H., *et al.* (1999). Treatment of intermittent claudication with physical training, smoking cessation, pentoxifylline, or nafronyl: a meta-analysis. *Archives of Internal Medicine*, **159**, 337–45.

Golledge, J. (1997). Lower-limb arterial disease. *Lancet*, **350**, 1459–65.

Jackson, M.R. and Clagett, G.P. (1998). Antithrombotic therapy in peripheral arterial occlusive disease. *Chest*, **114** (Suppl. 5), s666–82.

Chapter 2.18

Cholesterol embolism

C. R. K. Dudley

When atheromatous plaques ulcerate, the matrix may embolize. If the dislodged material is sufficiently large, occlusion of a major artery results in infarction of the organ or ischaemia of the limb supplied.

This has been termed atheroembolism to distinguish it from cholesterol crystal embolism where more numerous smaller particles, composed principally of cholesterol crystals, lodge in a number of small arteries simultaneously. The presence of a collateral circulation usually prevents infarction, and the event frequently runs a subclinical course. However, with multiple showers of cholesterol emboli, tissue damage results. Cholesterol embolism commonly affects the lower limbs, gastrointestinal tract, and kidneys. The clinical features are those of a systemic disorder with renal failure which can mimic vasculitis.

Epidemiology

The incidence of cholesterol crystal embolism found at post mortem is high: 77 per cent after aortic surgery, and 30 per cent and 25.5 per cent respectively when autopsies were performed within 6 months of aortography or cardiac catheterization. In contrast, the clinical syndrome is rare complicating less than 2 per cent of cardiac catheterizations. The condition is most frequently seen in older male patients with overt vascular disease. Although spontaneous cholesterol embolism may occur, it is much more common after vascular surgery or invasive radiology including aortography, angiography, and angioplasty. It has also been proposed that, by preventing thrombosis of ulcerating atheromatous plaques, anticoagulants favour the dissemination of atheromatous material from the plaques, and cholesterol embolism following the use of thrombolytic agents has been reported on rare occasions.

Clinical features

Symptoms are often non-specific with fever, weight loss, and myalgia. Other features are determined by the pattern of organ involvement, and are usually referable to the gastrointestinal tract, kidneys, and lower limbs. Bilateral skin changes over the lower extremities are the most common physical finding, and include livedo reticularis, 'trash feet', blue toes (acral cyanosis), and focal digital necrosis. Ulceration, nodules, purpura, and petechiae have also been described. Despite these skin changes and the presence of calf claudication (or frank myositis), pedal pulses may be felt easily, as only small vessels are occluded in this disorder. Carotid and femoral bruits are frequently heard, reflecting widespread atherosclerosis.

Abdominal pain, gastrointestinal bleeding, and pancreatitis may occur, and embolism to the stomach, small bowel, colon, gallbladder, and spleen have all been reported.

Renal involvement is common and usually manifests as a subacute stepwise deterioration in renal function over 2–6 weeks, invariably accompanied by a worsening of pre-existing hypertension. Acute renal failure with necrotizing glomerulonephritis and crescent formation has been described, but is rare. Transient ischaemic attacks, amaurosis fugax, and strokes can occur, and spinal cord infarction has also been reported. Thus a typical case is an elderly man presenting after angiography with progressive renal failure accompanied by livedo reticularis of the lower body and focal digital ischaemia of the toes.

Investigations

Laboratory findings frequently include a raised erythrocyte sedimentation rate and leucocytosis. Transient eosinophilia is common and may be pronounced. In rare cases thrombocytopenia and disseminated intravascular coagulation result. Depending on the tissue involved, elevated levels of creatine phosphokinase, amylase, lactate dehydrogenase, serum aspartate aminotransferase, and alkaline phosphatase may all be observed. Hypocomplementaemia has been described by only one group in the last decade, and other factors including the use of contrast media may have accounted for any complement activation. Mild proteinuria is generally present and urine microscopy may be bland or reveal red cells, white cells (particularly eosinophils), hyaline, and granular casts.

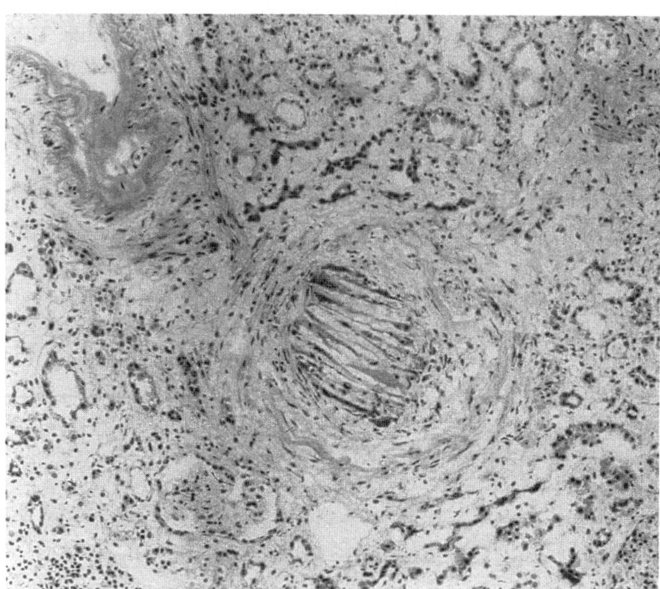

Fig. 1 Renal biopsy demonstrating the characteristic needle-shaped cholesterol clefts occluding a medium-sized renal arteriole with surrounding inflammatory cell infiltration, intimal proliferation, thickening, and concentric fibrosis. There is extensive autolysis (post-mortem sample).

Histology

The definitive diagnosis can usually be made from biopsies of kidney, skin, or muscle, although sampling error may miss the lesion. Diagnoses have also been made from gastric biopsy, prostatic curettage, and bone marrow. The demonstration of characteristic biconvex needle-shaped cholesterol clefts within the lumen of arteries or arterioles, which remain after the crystals have dissolved during histological preparation, is diagnostic (Fig. 1). In fresh samples the crystals can be identified by birefringence under polarized light, and specific histochemical stains.

Pathophysiology

Cholesterol crystals in the vascular lumen are believed to trigger a localized inflammatory and endothelial vascular reaction. An inflammatory cell infiltration occurs, and multinucleated giant cells engulf the cholesterol crystals which are resistant to the scavenger effects of macrophages and may remain in place for many months. The inflammatory phase is followed by intimal thickening with concentric fibrosis and occlusion of the vessel, resulting in ischaemia, infarction, or rarely necrosis of the distal tissue.

In the kidneys, small arteries and arterioles of diameter 150–200 μm are occluded, resulting in patchy areas of ischaemia and small areas of infarction. Crystals may also be seen within the glomeruli. In chronic cases, ischaemia produces a wedge-shaped lesion involving all components of the renal cortex radiating towards the capsule. The glomeruli appear ischaemic and hyalinized and the tubules become atrophic and separated by interstitial fibrosis (Fig. 1). Grossly, the kidneys may be reduced in size with a rough granular surface and wedge-shaped scars.

Differential diagnosis

Spontaneous cholesterol crystal embolism associated with renal failure, fever, rash, and eosinophilia may not unreasonably be misdiagnosed as a vasculitic illness such as polyarteritis nodosa, Churg–Strauss syndrome, microscopic polyarteritis, Wegener's granulomatosis, or bacterial endocarditis. Under these circumstances a renal biopsy is required to make the diagnosis. Cholesterol embolism should be considered in the differential diagnosis of a multisystem disease in elderly patients.

Clinical course and management

Mortality is high owing to the occurrence of coexisting cardiac and vascular disease together with renal failure in elderly patients. Renal impairment frequently progresses and may require dialysis, but partial recovery or stabilization has been reported even after several months of dialysis.

There is no effective therapy. Steroids, aspirin, dipyridamole, low-molecular-weight dextran, anticoagulants, and sympathetic blockade have all been tried but without benefit. Occasionally, the source of cholesterol emboli can be identified in a young and otherwise fit patient. In this limited circumstance there may be a role for surgical replacement of the diseased vessel with a graft.

Prevention is important. In patients with diffuse atherosclerosis, angiography should be strictly limited and careful attention must be paid to angiographic techniques including arterial approach (brachial instead of femoral for cardiac catheterization), use of softer and more flexible catheters, and reduced catheter manipulation.

Further reading

Lye, W.C., Cheah, J.S., and Sinniah, R. (1993). Renal cholesterol embolic disease. Case report and review of the literature. *American Journal of Nephrology*, 12, 489–93.

Mannesse, C.K., Blankestijn, P. J., Man In 'T Veld, A.J., and Schalekamp, M.A.D.H.' (1991). Renal failure and cholesterol crystal embolization: a report of 4 surviving cases and a review of the literature. *Clinical Nephrology*, 36, 240–5.

The cardiomyopathies

Chapter 2.19

Myocarditis, the cardiomyopathies, and specific heart muscle disorders

W. J. McKenna

Myocarditis

Definition

Clinicians may make a diagnosis of myocarditis following the acute onset of heart failure, arrhythmia, or electrocardiographic (ECG) changes, often in temporal association with viral infection in otherwise healthy, usually young, individuals. Pathologists have provided definitions based on varying criteria for myocyte necrosis and cellular infiltration, but the lack of accepted criteria for the histological diagnosis has hampered assessment of the incidence, natural history, treatment, and prognosis of myocarditis. In 1987 the Dallas criteria for histological diagnosis were developed to test the hypothesis that immunosuppression would modify left ventricular dysfunction and prognosis of patients with idiopathic myocarditis. A major multicentre trial failed to provide conclusive results, in large part because only 200 of over 2000 patients with 'clinical suspected myocarditis' fulfilled the criteria and could be randomized. The finding of diagnostic histological changes in less than 10 per cent of patients with 'clinical myocarditis' is a function of several factors including variable clinical diagnostic criteria, restrictive histological criteria, endomyocardial biopsy sampling error, and reliance on histology alone for the assessment of inflammation.

Aetiology and pathogenesis

Myocarditis is usually idiopathic, with a probable infective cause documented in less than 20 per cent of cases. Different agents have regional predominance, for example *T. cruzi* in South America or Coxsackie B in North America and Europe. Most viral infections in humans have multisystem involvement, and there is evidence to suggest that the heart is usually involved, although without symptomatic or significant clinical abnormalities. The determinants of severity in humans are uncertain, although the young (aged less than 1 year) are prone to more severe illness.

In myocardial involvement in Chagas' disease (*T. cruzi*), the acute phase is usually subclinical; but, a minority develop an acute febrile illness with myocarditis or pancarditis including endocardial thrombus formation and pericardial effusion. The disease then enters a long latency period; 20 years after the initial infestation, about 30 per cent of patients will have developed chronic Chagas' disease, but less than a third of these have parasitaemia. Present evidence suggests postinfectious autoimmune pathogenesis. Macroscopic and histological changes are similar to dilated cardiomyopathy with atrial and ventricular dilatation, myocyte hypertrophy, extensive fibrosis, and chronic lymphomononuclear cell infiltrates.

Clinical presentation and management

Myocarditis is usually a subclinical illness but may cause palpitation, atypical chest pain, ECG abnormalities, or arrhythmias without demonstrable change in global or regional left or right ventricular function. Cardiac failure or arrhythmias are usually associated with cardiac chamber dilatation and/or impaired systolic performance. Cardiac failure may be fulminant and fatal. Myocarditis and pericarditis often coexist .

There is no specific therapy for the management of either idiopathic or viral myocarditis. Heart failure and arrhythmias should be treated as appropriate. The role of antiviral and immunosuppressive therapy remains uncertain.

With the exception of the very young and the very old, prognosis is usually good. The determinants of acute myocarditis progressing to a chronic illness are discussed in dilated cardiomyopathy below.

The cardiac presentation of Chagas' disease resembles that of myocarditis and dilated cardiomyopathy. Conduction defects and arrhythmias are particularly common and may precede chamber dilatation and cardiac failure. The echo findings are of increased chamber dimensions, often with distinctive left ventricular posterior wall hypokinesis and relatively normal interventricular septal motion. In advanced disease an apical aneurysm is common, and in asymptomatic patients 10–15 per cent have apical dyskinesis. Diagnostic confirmation requires previous geographical exposure and either a positive complement fixation test for the antigens of *T. cruzi* or demonstration of parasites in the blood by xenodiagnosis. Treatment with antiparasitic drugs (e.g. nifurtimox, benzimidazole) may reduce parasitaemia, but does not cure the disease or prevent progression.

Table 1 Systemic diseases associated with specific heart muscle disorders

Metabolic/endocrine	**Malignancy**
• Diabetes mellitus	• Metastatic
• Gout	• Carcinoid
• Thyroid disease	**Infections**
• Acromegaly	• Rheumatic fever
• Phaeochromocytoma	• Tuberculosis
• Morbid obesity	• Syphilis
Infiltrating disorders	• Infective endocarditis
• Sarcoidosis	**Neuromuscular**
• Amyloidosis	• Duchenne dystrophy
• Haemochromatosis	• Becker
Systemic vasculitis	• Fascioscapulohumeral
• Systemic lupus erythematosus	• Emery–Dreifuss
• Scleroderma	• Limb-girdle
• Polyarteritis nodosa	• Distal myopathy
• Rheumatoid arthritis	• Mitochondrial myopathies
• Wegener's granulomatosis	• Oculopharyngeal
• Seronegative arthropathies	• Myotonic dystrophy
• Ankylosing spondylitis	**Drug use/dependence**
• Reiter's disease	• Alcohol
• Psoriatic arthritis	• Cocaine
• Ulcerative colitis	• 'Ecstasy' (MDMA)
• Crohn's disease	• Amphetamines

Cardiomyopathies

The cardiomyopathies are classified as hypertrophic, dilated, or restrictive; a classification which is useful in relation to natural history, treatment, and prognosis. Discovery of mutations in genes encoding sarcomeric contractile proteins in familial hypertrophic cardiomyopathy and a probable autoimmune pathogenesis of dilated cardiomyopathy indicates that knowledge of aetiology and pathogenesis will ultimately require a new classification.

Dilated cardiomyopathy

Definition

Dilated cardiomyopathy is characterized by unexplained dilatation and impaired contractile performance of the left ventricle. Potential causes of ventricular dysfunction, particularly coronary artery disease and systemic hypertension, must be excluded. Calcific aortic stenosis may be overlooked as a cause, particularly when the murmur is soft or absent. Specific heart muscle disorders should also be considered (Table 1). A primary cardiac presentation of diabetes mellitus, connective tissue disorders, and neuromuscular disease is rare, but arrhythmias or progressive conduction disturbance with mild left ventricular dysfunction may provide the earliest evidence of cardiac sarcoidosis. Dilated cardiomyopathy is a diagnosis of exclusion.

In North America and Europe symptomatic dilated cardiomyopathy has an incidence and prevalence of 20 per 100 000 and 38 per 100 000 respectively and remains the commonest indication for cardiac transplantation. Pedigree analysis reveals familial disease in at least 25 per cent of cases and an additional cohort (10–20 per cent) with mild abnormalities of left ventricular performance who may have early presymptomatic dilated cardiomyopathy. Inheritance is most consistent with autosomal dominant and incomplete penetrance, although X-linked families have been reported.

Pathology and pathogenesis

Macroscopic examination reveals dilated cardiac chambers, mural thrombi, and platelet aggregates with normal coronary arteries. Histology shows patchy perimyocyte and interstitial fibrosis and various stages of myocyte death, as well as myocyte hypertrophy and rare isolated inflammatory cells. These findings are non-specific. Alcohol, like pregnancy, may precipitate cardiac failure in predisposed individuals, but an additional specific aetiological or pathogenetic role remains uncertain. Viral involvement is supported by animal models and by rare patients, with an association with abnormal Coxsackie serology, or by hybridization studies which show non-replicating enteroviral genome in a variable proportion (10–50 per cent) of myocarditis-dilated cardiomyopathy hearts. An autoimmune pathogenesis is supported by animal experiments and the findings of a cardiac and disease-specific autoantibody in over 30 per cent of patients and their first-degree relatives, as well as inappropriate major histocompatibility complex class II expression on endothelial cells from cardiac tissue, and a weak HLA DR4 association.

Diagnosis

Initial presentation is usually with symptoms of cardiac failure but an arrhythmia, a systemic embolus, or the finding of an ECG or radiographic abnormality during routine screening may prompt earlier diagnosis. The familial nature of dilated cardiomyopathy indicates that a correct diagnosis is of importance as there is now the potential to identify the disease at an early or preclinical stage. Systolic blood pressure is usually low with a narrow pulse pressure and a low volume arterial pulse. Pulsus alternans may be present and the jugular veins may be distended with a prominent V-wave reflecting tricuspid regurgitation, with liver engorgement, peripheral oedema, and ascites.

The precordium often reveals a diffuse and dyskinetic left ventricular and occasionally right ventricular impulse. The apical impulse is usually displaced laterally. Paradoxical splitting of the second heart sound may reflect left bundle branch block, which occurs in approximately 15 per cent of patients. With the development of pulmonary hypertension, the pulmonary component of the second heart sound may be accentuated. Characteristically, a presystolic gallop or fourth heart sound is present before the development of overt cardiac failure, and, once cardiac decompensation has occurred, a third heart sound is often heard. Systolic murmurs are common, reflecting mitral and, less commonly, tricuspid regurgitation.

Unexplained cardiac failure during pregnancy or within the 3 months following birth is often labelled as peripartum cardiomyopathy. Unrecognized pre-eclamptic heart disease should be excluded, as this has a different prognosis and recurs with increasing severity during subsequent pregnancies unless prevented by aspirin treatment. In those with peripartum cardiomyopathy, there is often uncertainty whether the cardiac failure is acute (potentially myocarditis) or chronic and exacerbated by the haemodynamic stress of pregnancy and labour (dilated cardiomyopathy). When there is persistence of left ventricular chamber dilatation or impaired systolic performance, the diagnosis of peripartum cardiomyopathy can legitimately be made. The natural history is uncertain, although it is probable that the adverse effect of subsequent pregnancy is less adverse than the literature would suggest, particularly in those with only mild residual abnormalities of left ventricular structure and function.

Investigations

By the time of diagnosis, a normal ECG is rare and most patients show features consistent with diffuse myocardial abnormalities. Twenty per cent are in established atrial fibrillation, and paroxysmal supraventricular and ventricular arrhythmias are common.

Maximal exercise testing, ideally with respiratory gas analysis, provides a simple reproducible measure of functional capacity and is also useful to exclude ischaemia and assess risk of arrhythmia. Two-dimensional echocardiography, provides a repeatable measure of cardiac cavity dimensions and systolic performance, and assessment of regional wall motion as well as mural and intracavitary thrombi.

Coronary arteriography should be performed if doubt remains regarding a potential ischaemic aetiology. Cardiac catheterization is only necessary for measurement of pulmonary vascular resistance in those with very severe or rapidly progressive disease in whom cardiac transplantation may be required. Endomyocardial biopsy can help to exclude myocarditis and specific heart muscle disorders and to detect the presence of viral genome and markers of immune activation. Many of the systemic diseases which are associated with heart muscle disorders have typical clinical, immunological, and biochemical features. In their absence, a routine screen is probably not cost effective. However, investigation should include serum phosphorus (hypophosphataemia), serum calcium (hypocalcaemia), serum creatinine and urea (uraemia), thyroid function tests (hypothyroidism), and serum iron/ferritin (haemochromatosis).

Natural history and prognosis

The true natural history is uncertain because the diagnosis is usually not made until clinical features, which are late manifestations, become obvious. Then the prognosis is poor and related to the degree of left ventricular dilatation and impaired contractile performance; only a minority of patients (less than 25 per cent) will either stabilize or improve. Data from 1970s and 1980s indicate 50 per cent mortality from progressive heart failure or its complications in the 2 years following diagnosis. Survival should be improved by recognition of asymptomatic family members and by management including the early introduction of angiotensin-converting enzyme (ACE) inhibitors, aggressive treatment of arrhythmias, and the availability of cardiac transplantation.

Treatment

Heart failure is treated with digoxin, diuretics, and the early introduction of ACE inhibitors. Vigorous exercise and significant alcohol intake are proscribed. Low dose β-blockade with gradual dosage augmentation as tolerated over 3–6 months is often beneficial, but, rapid administration of β-blockers or their withdrawal after chronic administration may precipitate rapid deterioration and they should be used cautiously. If sustained or symptomatic arrhythmias are documented, amiodarone (100–400 mg daily) is effective in both supraventricular and ventricular disturbances.

Systemic and pulmonary emboli are common; but precise guidelines for anticoagulation are not established. Patients with mural or intracavitary thrombi or with established or paroxysmal atrial fibrillation should be fully anticoagulated. Those with severe left ventricular dysfunction (ejection fraction below 20 per cent) or atrial dilatation (more than 40 mm) should be at least partially anticoagulated.

The other major complication is sudden death. The mechanism is probably a ventricular arrhythmia, although bradyarrhythmias may be more likely in patients with severe disease such as those awaiting cardiac transplantation. ECG monitoring and electrophysiological studies do not identify patients at risk. The role of low-dose amiodarone (200–300 mg daily) in the prevention of sudden death is being examined in several multicentre studies. The practical, although unproven, approach is to treat those with frequent episodes of asymptomatic non-sustained ventricular tachycardia during ECG monitoring, as well as those with symptomatic or documented ventricular arrhythmia.

Cardiac transplantation provides a lifeline in those with progressive deterioration. Results are best when surgery is performed as an elective procedure; it should be considered in all patients with moderate to severe left ventricular impairment.

Hypertrophic cardiomyopathy

Definition

Hypertrophic cardiomyopathy is characterized by a hypertrophied and non-dilated left and/or right ventricle in the absence of a cardiac or systemic cause. Such a diagnosis of exclusion presents problems. Does the patient with moderate systemic hypertension and 2 cm left ventricular hypertrophy have one or two diseases? Is 2 cm hypertrophy a physiological response in a highly trained athlete? The presence of other causes of left ventricular hypertrophy highlights a major limitation of the current definition.

Pathology

The left, the right, or both ventricles may be involved. Hypertrophy on the left is usually asymmetric, involving the anterior and posterior septum and the free wall more than the posterior wall. Right ventricular hypertrophy, which is usually symmetric, is seen in over 30 per cent of patients; isolated right ventricular hypertrophy is rare. Over 60 per cent of patients will have structural abnormalities of the mitral valve, including increased leaflet area, elongation of the leaflets, or anomalous papillary muscle insertion into the anterior mitral leaflet. Another common finding is a patch of endocardial thickening just below the aortic valve which results from contact of the septum with the anterior mitral leaflet in patients with mitral leaflet abnormalities and/or reduced left ventricular outflow tract dimensions.

Histologically, affected myocardium shows interstitial fibrosis with gross disorganization of the muscle bundles resulting in a whorled pattern. The cell-to-cell orientation of muscle cells is lost and there is disorganization of the myofibrillar architecture within a given cell. Myocardial cells are wide, short, and often bizarre in shape. Foci of disorganized cells are often interspersed among areas of hypertrophied cells that are otherwise normal in appearance. Such changes are not completely specific: congenitally abnormal hearts may also show fibre disarray, and some disarrangement is found at the junction of the septum with the anterior and posterior walls of the left ventricle in normal subjects. However, the extent of myocyte disarray in normal subjects rarely exceeds 5 per cent, while in hypertrophic cardiomyopathy up to 40 per cent of the myocardium may be involved. Occasionally, extensive myocyte disarray is found in macroscopically normal hearts in patients who experience typical clinical features. Such patients highlight the broader phenotype and suggest that hypertrophy may be a secondary rather than a primary abnormality.

Genetics

Hypertrophic cardiomyopathy is usually familial with autosomal dominant transmission and a high degree of penetrance. Morphological and clinical features typically present during childhood or adolescence, but may not be apparent until growth has been completed. Variable expression of the disease is common, even within families bearing the same gene defect. Mutations in the DNA encoding β cardiac myosin heavy chain (chromosome 14), α tropomyosin (chromosome 15), and cardiac troponin T (chromosome 1) have been identified in over 50 per cent of pedigrees evaluated. Hypertrophic cardiomyopathy is emerging as a disease of sarcomeric contractile proteins. The majority of the mutations involve a single base pair change, which results in an amino acid substitution in exons encoding highly conserved regions of these contractile protein genes. Many of these mis-sense mutations alter the charge of the amino acid, which would be predicted to have a significant effect on the function of the encoded polypeptide, and preliminary observations suggest a worse prognosis in those so affected. However, marked heterogeneity of phenotypic expression and prognosis within a family indicates that other factors are important.

Pathophysiology

Disarray

It is probable that the disorganized architecture provides a substrate for electrical instability and contributes to diastolic abnormalities.

Systole

Most young and some old patients have evidence of hyperdynamic systolic function with rapid, early, and near complete ventricular emptying. Approximately 30 per cent of patients with such function have recordable gradients at rest between the body and outflow tract of the left ventricle; an additional 20–25 per cent develop such a gradient following manoeuvres that increase myocardial contractility or result in a decrease in ventricular volume. The presence and magnitude of a gradient are not only determined by systolic contractile performance, but are also a function of left ventricular outflow tract size and geometry. The most plausible mechanism is that venturi forces from increased ejection velocity in the narrowed outflow tract draw the anterior and posterior mitral leaflets towards the septum. In the majority of patients with resting left ventricular gradients, at least 70 per cent of stroke volume has already been ejected by the onset of the gradient.

Table 2 Potential causes of ischaemia in hypertrophic cardiomyopathy

Increased muscle mass	Systolic compression of arteries
Elevated diastolic filling pressures	Adequate capillary density
Enhanced myocardial oxygen demand (increased wall stress)	Impaired vasodilatory reserve

Diastole

Diastolic abnormalities are common, although variable. The isovolumic phase is prolonged, filling is slow, and the proportion of filling volume that results from atrial contraction may be increased. Occasionally, there is rapid early filling with restrictive physiology which resembles the situation in constrictive pericarditis or endocardial fibrosis.

Ischaemia

Despite normal epicardial coronary arteries, myocardial ischaemia is common and is caused by several mechanisms (Table 2).

Prevalence and diagnosis

Prevalence is estimated to be between 1 per 1000 and 1 per 5000. Diagnosis is based upon the demonstration of unexplained myocardial hypertrophy, with wall thickness exceeding two standard deviations for gender-, age-, and size-matched populations. A left ventricular myocardial segment of thickness 1.5 cm or more in an adult of normal size in the absence of a recognized cause is also considered diagnostic. Isolated right ventricular hypertrophic cardiomyopathy is extremely rare. Less stringent criteria, should be applied to first-degree relatives of an affected individual where the probability of carrying the disease gene increases from less than 1 per 1000 to 1 in 2. A negative diagnosis made before adolescent growth has been completed must require subsequent reassessment, but development *de novo* has not been reported in adults.

Problems in diagnosis arise in highly trained athletes and patients with hypertension in whom the hypertrophic response appears greater than expected. Athletes can increase myocardial mass to a maximum increase of 2–3 mm in the left ventricular wall. The determinants of the hypertrophy in hypertension are in part racially determined; the African response is clearly greater than that of white subjects. In athletes and hypertensives, the diagnosis is dependent on the total clinical picture. An athlete who has 1.7 cm left ventricular hypertrophy with either a small left ventricular cavity or a family history of hypertrophic cardiomyopathy probably does have the condition, whereas one with negative family history and a normal left ventricular cavity probably does not. There is the potential for molecular genetics to provide a 'gold standard' but at present the finding of a relevant mutation confirms disease but its absence does not exclude it.

Clinical features

History

Some 50 per cent of adult patients present with breathlessness on exertion, chest pains, sustained palpitation, or sudden death. The remainder are picked up during screening of affected families (as are most children and adolescents), or by physical signs or ECG changes. Some 15–25 per cent of patients have experienced syncopal episodes but in only a minority are there findings suggestive of an arrhythmia or conduction disease. Rarely, patients present with paroxysmal nocturnal dyspnoea, cough, ascites, or peripheral oedema.

Physical examination

In the majority of patients abnormal signs are subtle. Most patients have a rapid upstroke arterial pulse, best felt in the carotid area, which reflects dynamic left ventricular emptying. Most also have a forceful left ventricular cardiac impulse. In about a third of patients the jugular venous pulse may demonstrate a prominent 'a' wave reflecting diminished right ventricular compliance. The first and second heart sounds are usually normal but, unless patients are in atrial fibrillation, there is either a loud fourth sound, reflecting increased atrial systolic flow into a non-compliant ventricle, or a palpable atrial beat reflecting forceful atrial systolic contraction. An ejection systolic murmur is present only in those patients (one-third) who have a resting left ventricular outflow tract gradient. This murmur starts well after the first heart sound and ends well before the second. It is best heard at the left sternal border radiating towards the aortic and mitral areas but not into the neck or the axilla. The intensity varies with changes in ventricular volume: it can be increased by manoeuvres that decrease afterload or venous return (amyl nitrate, standing, Valsalva) and decreased by those that increase afterload and venous return (squatting, phenylephrine). The majority of patients with a gradient also have mild mitral regurgitation which may be difficult to distinguish by auscultation; Radiation to the axilla is often the best clue. A mid-diastolic rumble may occasionally result from increased transmitral flow in patients with severe mitral regurgitation; more commonly, it occurs in isolation, presumably reflecting inflow tract turbulence. Murmurs of aortic incompetence may develop following myotomy or myectomy or infective endocarditis. A pulmonary systolic murmur reflecting right ventricular outflow tract obstruction, is rare; usually associated with severe biventricular hypertrophy and more common in the young.

Investigations

Electrocardiography

The ECG is normal in 5 per cent of symptomatic and 25 per cent of asymptomatic patients, particularly the young. At the time of diagnosis, 10 per cent are in atrial fibrillation. The majority of patients have an intraventricular conduction delay, 20 per cent left axis deviation, and 5 per cent right bundle branch block; complete left bundle branch block is uncommon. ST-segment depression and T-wave changes are the most common abnormalities, usually associated with voltage changes of left ventricular hypertrophy and/or deep S waves in V1–V3. Occasionally, giant negative T waves are seen. Repolarization changes alone or isolated voltage criteria for left ventricular hypertrophy are unusual. Approximately 20 per cent of patients have abnormal Q waves either inferiorly (2, 3, and aVF) or, less commonly, in leads V1–V3. P-wave abnormalities of left and/or right atrial overload are common. Occasionally, a short PR interval may be associated with a slurred upstroke to the QRS complex, similar to that seen in Wolff–Parkinson–White syndrome, although usually not associated with pre-excitation.

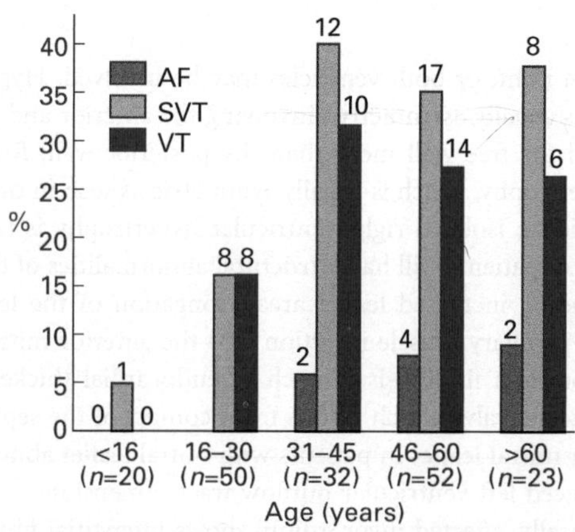

Fig. 1 The relation between arrhythmias and age in hypertrophic cardiomyopathy. SVT, supraventricular tachycardia; VT, ventricular tachycardia; AF, atrial fibrillation.

The incidence of arrhythmias during 48-h ambulatory ECG monitoring increases with age (Fig. 1). Non-sustained ventricular tachycardia is detected in 25–30 per cent of adults, and although asymptomatic, represents an approximately sevenfold increased risk of sudden death. Sustained supraventricular arrhythmias (more than 30 s) are poorly tolerated unless the ventricular response is controlled, and carry a risk of embolism.

Imaging

The extent and severity of myocardial hypertrophy is best evaluated with two-dimensional echocardiography and Doppler studies. Typically, left ventricular end-systolic and end-diastolic dimensions are reduced, and the left atrial dimension is increased. Ejection fraction and velocity of fibre shortening, are increased. Colour Doppler detects left ventricular outflow tract turbulence and, combined with continuous-wave Doppler measures, the peak velocity of left ventricular blood flow and outflow tract gradients. Early closure or fluttering of the aortic valve leaflets and Doppler evidence of mitral regurgitation are often seen in association with systolic anterior motion of the mitral valve.

Cardiac catheterization

Cardiac catheterization is not necessary for diagnosis but coronary arteriography may be necessary in patients in whom there is suspicion of coincident ischaemic heart disease.

Exercise testing

Maximal exercise testing may show the VO_2 max to be moderately reduced even in patients who claim that their exercise tolerance is not limited. Approximately one-third of younger patients have an abnormal blood pressure response with drops of 25–150 mmHg from peak recordings despite an appropriate increase in cardiac output. Preliminary observations suggest that these changes are likely to be of prognostic significance. ST-segment changes associated with symptoms of angina, are found in 25 per cent of patients, but their prognostic significance is uncertain.

Electrophysiological studies

These may occasionally be necessary to identify accessory pathways or to aid management of sustained monomorphic ventricular tachycardia.

Natural history

A gradual deterioration of left ventricular function is characteristic with a significant incidence of sudden death. The annual mortality from sudden death is 2–3 per cent in adults and 4–6 per cent in children and adolescents attending a referral centre. It is even greater in young patients with recurrent syncope or a family history of 'malignant' hypertrophic cardiomyopathy. The figures from non-referral hospitals are lower.

Left ventricular hypertrophy is not progressive once growth is completed, but symptoms of left ventricular dysfunction may continue to develop. Endocarditis is a rare complication of left ventricular outflow tract turbulence and/or mitral regurgitation. Antibiotic prophylaxis is important in appropriate patients.

Prognosis

In adults, the finding of non-sustained ventricular tachycardia during ECG monitoring is associated with a sevenfold to eightfold increased risk of sudden death. It is the best single marker of the high-risk adult, with a sensitivity of at least 70 per cent and a specificity of 80 per cent. However, the positive predictive accuracy of ventricular tachycardia is low (22 per cent), reflecting the fact that most patients with this condition do not die suddenly. In adults, no other clinical or investigative feature is associated with or predictive of sudden death. Children and adolescents with recurrent syncope and those who have two or more affected siblings who have died suddenly are at increased risk. The young pose problems of both identification and therapy. Most are asymptomatic, many are athletic, and even those at apparently low risk have an annual mortality from sudden death of 3–4 per cent.

Possible initiating mechanisms of sudden death include haemodynamic deterioration with reduced stroke volume following a physiological tachycardia or an arrhythmia as well as hypotension developing in the presence of a normal stroke volume but altered baroreflex control of vasomotor tone.

Management

β-Adrenoceptor blockers, particularly propranolol, and calcium antagonists, especially verapamil, are the mainstay of therapy. Both decrease myocardial oxygen consumption and blunt the heart rate response on exercise, allowing more time for ventricular filling. Both exert a negative inotropic effect, reducing hyperdynamic systolic function and left ventricular gradients; they may also improve diastolic filling.

Surgery is another option. The conventional indication has been a resting left ventricular outflow tract gradient of more than 50 mmHg in patients refractory to medical therapy. The commonest operation has been to remove a segment of the upper anterior septum The operation carries a perioperative mortality of 3–10 per cent, but successful surgery confers symptomatic and haemodynamic improvement. Mitral valve replacement produces excellent results.

Arrhythmias

Most patients who develop atrial fibrillation do well with digoxin and anticoagulant treatment but in a few the loss of the atrial systolic contribution to ventricular filling may be critical. In them, amiodarone 300 mg for 4–6 weeks may result in a return to sinus rhythm or facilitate electrical cardioversion. Sustained episodes of paroxysmal atrial fibrillation or supraventricular tachycardia represent a risk of haemodynamic collapse and emboli. Amiodarone in low doses (1000–1400 mg weekly) is effective in suppression and controls the ventricular response should breakthrough occur. The threshold for anticoagulation should be low as embolic complications are common. Episodes of non-sustained ventricular tachycardia are common but are rarely symptomatic, and therapy is warranted only if prognosis can be shown to be improved (see below).

Table 3 Identifiable and treatable mechanisms of sudden death in hypertrophic cardiomyopathy

Paroxysmal atrial fibrillation	Amiodarone
Sustained monomorphic ventricular tachycardia	Amiodarone ± an implantable cardioverter defibrillator
Ischaemia	High-dose verapamil
Conduction disease	Pacemaker
Accessory pathway	Ablation

Prevention of sudden death

The problem is to identify those at high risk and provide appropriate therapy (Table 3). The risk associated with non-sustained ventricular tachycardia is reduced by amiodarone 100–1400 mg/week. In the young, management is compromised by the lack of sensitive non-invasive prognostic indicators, although those with established markers (adverse family history or syncope for instance) may benefit from amiodarone, myectomy or the provision of an implantable cardioverter defibrillator, the choice dependent on suspected mechanisms.

Restrictive cardiomyopathy

Restrictive cardiomyopathy, with impaired filling of one or both ventricles is usually caused by endomyocardial fibrosis. Two variants are recognized. Tropical endomyocardial fibrosis accounts for 10–20 per cent of deaths from heart disease in Africa. In temperate countries the condition is typically associated with hypereosinophilia (see Chapter 3.31 and OTM3, pp. 2396–8). The pathology is similar in advanced cases with or without hypereosinophilia and each variant is considered to be a different manifestation of the same disease process. Idiopathic myocardial restrictive cardiomyopathy with and without myocardial fibrosis, is rare. Infiltrative diseases (amyloidosis, sarcoidosis, Gaucher's disease), storage diseases (haemochromatosis, glycogen storage disease, Fabry's disease), and endomyocardial disease associated with malignancies (metastases, carcinoid, radiation, anthracycline toxicity) may also have a restrictive pattern of physiology and mimic restrictive cardiomyopathy.

Pathology

In endomyocardial fibrosis, the fibrosis and overlying thrombosis involves the inflow tracts and apices of one or both ventricles, but spares the outflow tracts. Necrotic, thrombotic, and fibrotic stages have been defined in patients' hypereosinophilia. In the necrotic stage there is an acute inflammatory reaction characterized by eosinophilic abscesses in the myocardium with associated necrosis and arteritis. The endocardium is often thickened and mural thrombi may develop. Release from eosinophil granules of ribonucleases and other proteins is the mechanism whereby hypereosinophilia can damage the myocardium, but it is not known why cardiac lesions occur in only a few patients with very high eosinophil counts. Nor is it known why the myocardium is specifically affected. Endocardial thrombus formation may be severe with massive intracavitary thrombosis causing restriction to ventricular filling and a low output state with high filling pressures. During the necrotic and thrombotic stages the disease may mimic hyperacute rheumatic carditis. If the patient survives, healing by fibrosis results in adverse effects on ventricular filling volume and atrioventricular valve function which underlie the cardiac dysfunction.

Clinical features and management

Cardiac diagnosis and assessment

Left-sided disease may present with symptoms of pulmonary congestion and/or mitral regurgitation, and right-sided with raised jugular venous pressure, hepatomegaly, ascites, and tricuspid regurgitation.

Echocardiography provides the best non-invasive means of confirming the diagnosis. There may be intracavitary thrombus with apical cavity obliteration or bright echoes from the endocardium of the right or left ventricle with tethering of the chordae and reduced excursion of the posterior mitral valve leaflet. Typically, ventricular dimensions and wall thickness are normal whereas the atria are grossly enlarged. Left ventricular filling terminates early and is followed by a plateau phase coincident with the third heart sound.

Impairment of ventricular filling is reflected by the rapid rise of pressure in mid-diastole (square root sign). Systolic function is normal. Mitral and tricuspid regurgitation may be severe, and both ventricles appear abnormal in shape on angiography owing to obliteration of the apices. These changes result from the thrombotic and fibrotic stages of the disease. During the early acute phase the appearances of the left and right ventricle are far less abnormal; and the diagnosis can best be confirmed by endomyocardial biopsy.

Management

Most hypereosinophilic cases are idiopathic but some are associated with malignant disease. Investigation and management of hypereosinophilia *per se* is addressed in Chapter 3.31. Cases with cardiac involvement are usually given prednisolone 7.5–15 mg/day to reduce the release of granule proteins into the myocardium, but medical management of advanced cardiac disease is not very effective and there is a 2-year mortality of 35–50 per cent. Congestive symptoms can be improved with diuretics, although too great a reduction in ventricular filling pressure will lead to a reduction in cardiac output. Arrhythmias should not be treated unless they are sustained or associated with symptoms. Drugs which significantly slow the heart rate may be deleterious because of the small stroke volume. Given the risk of venous thrombosis and systemic emboli, both warfarin and antiplatelet drugs are advised.

Surgery with mitral and/or tricuspid valve replacement with or without decortication of the endocardium can give good long-term symptomatic results although there is a significant perioperative mortality (15–20 per cent).

Arrhythmogenic right ventricular dysplasia

This is characterized pathologically by fibrofatty replacement of the right ventricular myocardium and clinically by arrhythmia and sudden death. The disease is often familial with autosomal dominant inheritance and incomplete penetrance. The incidence is unknown. It occurs worldwide, but with a high incidence in the Veneto region of northern Italy.

Aetiology and pathogenesis

The fibrofatty replacement of the myocardium may be focal or widespread, usually involves the subepicardial layer of the right ventricular free wall, and when severe may appear transmural. It is unclear whether the genetic basis predisposes to a degenerative disease with atrophy and fibrofatty replacement of right ventricular myocardium or whether there is an infectious or genetically determined immune pathogenesis.

Clinical presentation and management

Clinical features include manifestations of abnormalities of the right ventricle, ECG changes, sudden death or arrhythmias of right ventricular origin. Imaging usually reveals segmental dilatation or localized aneurysm(s) of the right ventricular free wall. The typical ECG shows inverted T waves in right ventricular precordial leads and ventricular postexcitation 'epsilon waves', as a consequence of inhomogenous and delayed right ventricular depolarization.

Palpitation and/or syncope result from sustained ventricular arrhythmia. Sudden death related to exercise may be the initial manifestation, particularly in young athletes.

Diagnosis based on right ventricular endomyocardial biopsy is difficult because of the segmental nature of the disease, and relies on the clinical demonstration of characteristic structural, functional, and electrophysiological abnormalities.

In the absence of sustained ventricular arrhythmia most patients will be asymptomatic. Progression from localized to more diffuse right ventricular involvement with ventricular arrhythmia or right ventricular failure has been reported. In long-standing disease, the left ventricle may be involved.

Asymptomatic patients should have exercise testing and Holter monitoring to detect occult arrhythmias. Antiarrhythmic treatment is warranted in patients with palpitation, syncope, or sustained ventricular arrhythmia.

Specific heart muscle disorders

Cardiac manifestations of systemic vasculitis

Systemic lupus erythematosus

Clinical cardiac involvement is observed in 50–60 per cent of patients, while evidence of microvasculitis is found in almost all patients at autopsy. Pericarditis is the commonest cardiac lesion (60–75 per cent at autopsy) and is symptomatic in the majority. Other manifestations, particularly myocarditis and non-infective endocarditis of the mitral valve (Libman–Sachs endocarditis) are common but usually subclinical. Antiphospholipid syndrome can be associated with cardiac, particularly valvular, involvement. Management is discussed in Chapter 10.11. Prophylaxis against infective endocarditis should be considered in the presence of valvular disease.

Systemic sclerosis

Cardiac involvement is characterized by patchy myocardial fibrosis from gradual obliteration of small vessels. Pericarditis is common and congestive cardiac failure, in advanced disease, is progressive and carries a poor prognosis. Echocardiography typically shows features of dilated or restrictive cardiomyopathy. No therapy has been proved to alter these cardiac manifestations.

Rheumatoid arthritis

This is often associated with pericarditis and tends to correlate with the severity of the joint disease and the presence of rheumatoid

Table 4 Cardiovascular abnormalities in neuromuscular disorders

Condition	Transmission	CM	CD	TA	SD	CHF	Cardiovascular pathology	Genetic defect
Duchenne	XLR	+ Uncommon Common	–	–	–	+	Replacement fibrosis (posterobasal and lateral LV wall)	Xp21 absence of dystrophin
Becker	XLR	Common	–	–	–	+	Replacement fibrosis (posterobasal and lateral LV wall)	Xp21 altered size and/or quantity of dystrophin
Facioscapulo-humeral	AD	–	+	–	–	–	Replacement fibrosis (conduction system)	Chr 4q35
Emery–Dreifuss	XLR	+	+	+	+	+	?	Xq28
Limb-girdle	AR/AD	+	–	+	–	+	?	Chr 15 (AR)
Distal myopathy	AD	–	+	–	–	–	?	None known
Mitochondrial myopathies	Cytoplasmic	+	+	–	–	–	?	Mitochondrial
Oculopharyngeal	AD	–	+	–	–	–	?	?
Myotonic dystrophy	AD	+ Uncommon	+	–	+	+ Uncommon	Fibrosis, fatty infiltration and atrophy of the conduction system	Chr 19 myotonin kinase

AD, autosomal dominant; AR, autosomal recessive; CD, cardiac disease; TA, tachyarrhythmia; CHF, congestive heart failure; Chr, chromosome; CM, cardiomyopathy; LV, left ventricular; SD, sudden death; XLR, X-linked recessive; + present; – absent.

*Allelic forms of the same genetic defect.

Up-to-date clinical and molecular references can be accessed from the online *Mendelian inheritance in man.*

nodules. A pericardial rub can be heard in up to 30 per cent of patients, and a pericardial effusion can be identified echocardiographically in up to 50 per cent. Rheumatoid pericarditis has a good prognosis and usually responds to corticosteroid therapy although this treatment cannot prevent the rare development of constrictive pericarditis. Myocarditis has been reported in up to 20 per cent post mortem and is associated with severe vasculitis or joint disease; however, such patients are not usually symptomatic and overt congestive cardiac failure is rare.

Seronegative arthropathies

Ankylosing spondylitis, Reiter's syndrome, psoriatic arthritis, and the gastrointestinal arthropathies, are associated with a combination of pancarditis, proximal aortitis, or aortic regurgitation (which may be clinically silent) and varying degrees of conduction disease including complete heart block; long-standing disease may result in amyloid deposition.

Muscular disorders

Cardiomyopathy may be associated with evidence of a skeletal myopathy, although this may be subclinical. Conversely, many muscular disorders (Table 4) show varying degrees of cardiac involvement.

Miscellaneous heart muscle disorders

Cardiac involvement in sarcoidosis, amyloidosis, and thyroid dysfunction is described elsewhere. These diagnoses are not always obvious and the disease may present with predominant cardiac manifestations.

Further reading

Braunwald, E. (ed). (1992). *Heart disease. A textbook of cardiovascular medicine.* W.B. Saunders, Philadelphia.

Nava, A., Rossi, L., and Thiene, G. (ed.) (1997). *Arrhythmogenic right ventricular cardiomyopathy/dysplasia.* Elsevier, Amsterdam.

Keeling, P.J., Gang, Y., Smith, G., *et al.* (1995). Familial dilated cardiomyopathy in the United Kingdom. *British Heart Journal*, **73**, 417–21.

Spirito, P., Seidman, C.E., McKenna, W.J., and Maron, B.J. (1997). The management of hypertrophic cardiomyopathy [Review]. *New England Journal of Medicine*, **336**, 775–85.

Woodroof, J.F. (1980). Viral myocarditis: a review. *American Journal of Pathology*, **101**, 427–79.

Chapter 2.20

HIV-related heart muscle disease

N. A. Boon

The heart is involved in approximately 50 per cent of patients with acquired immune deficiency syndrome (**AIDS**) (see also Chapter 16.35) but this cause significant symptoms in less than 10 per cent, and death in no more than 5 per cent. The common lesions are listed in Table 1. Although tuberculous pericardial effusion is a major problem in Africa, left ventricular dysfunction due to myocarditis or dilated cardiomyopathy is the most important cardiac manifestation in the Western world.

Myocarditis and dilated cardiomyopathy

Postmortem studies have demonstrated some form of myocarditis in approximately 40 per cent of patients with AIDS and this is thought to be the substrate for the global left ventricle systolic dysfunction that is evident on echocardiography in up to 20 per cent of patients with advanced human immunodeficiency virus (**HIV**) infection. Specific forms of myocarditis (e.g. *Toxoplasma gondii*) occur but these are rare and heart muscle disease is usually due to an idiopathic focal

Table 1 Cardiac lesions in AIDS

Myocardial disease	*Pericardial effusion*
• Myocarditis • non-specific • infectious • Dilated cardiomyopathy • Isolated right ventricular dilation • Neoplastic infiltration • Kaposi's sarcoma • Lymphoma	• Sterile • Infectious • Neoplastic ***Endocarditis*** • Marantic endocarditis (non-bacterial thrombotic endocarditis) • Infective endocarditis

lymphocytic myocarditis. The inflammatory infiltrates are composed mainly of CD8 + lymphocytes with increased major histocompatibility complex class I antigen expression in keeping with an autoimmune reaction. HIV 1 has been found in the heart of some patients. Co-infection with cardiotropic viruses (e.g. cytomegalovirus), oxidative stress due to micronutrient deficiency, and direct cytokine-mediated injury may also contribute to myocardial damage.

Zidovudine damages cardiac muscle in rats and there are reports of improved cardiac function following its withdrawal in AIDS patients with heart failure. Other potentially cardiotoxic drugs used in HIV infection include pentamidine (which may cause ventricular tachycardia), gancyclovir, and interferon-α2a.

Clinical features

HIV-related heart muscle disease tends to occur in the late stages of AIDS and presents with heart failure or otherwise unexplained cardiomegaly. The symptoms and signs of heart failure can be subtle and are sometimes mistakenly attributed to anaemia or chest infection.

Treatment

Unless there is a myocardial infection that may respond to specific antimicrobial therapy treatment is palliative. The prognosis is very poor (particularly among patients with lymphatic myocarditis) with few patients surviving more than 12 months. Conventional treatments for heart failure are worthwhile but vasodilators are often tolerated poorly. In patients with severe heart failure zidovudine should be withdrawn but can be restarted if there is no demonstrable improvement in cardiac function within 4–6 weeks.

Isolated right ventricular dilatation

Dilatation of the right ventricle without any other demonstrable heart disease is a common finding in HIV patients and is usually due to pulmonary hypertension associated with repeated respiratory infections, thromboembolic disease, emboli acquired through intravenous drug use, or a variant of primary pulmonary hypertension.

Neoplastic infiltration

Disseminated Kaposi's sarcoma may involve the heart, particularly the epicardium and subepicardial fat, but seldom causes significant cardiac morbidity or mortality. Cardiac malignant lymphomas are usually derived from B cells, may be focal or diffuse, and may cause pericardial effusion and tamponade, ventricular arrhythmias, heart block, and sudden death.

Further reading

Barbaro, G., Di Lorenzo, G.D., Grisorio, B., and Barbarini, G. (1998). Incidence of dilated cardiomyopathy and detection of HIV in myocardial cells of HIV positive patients. *New England Journal of Medicine*, 339, 1093–9.

Currie, P.F., Jacob, A.J., Foreman, A.R., Elton, R.A., Brettle, R.P., and Boon, N.A. (1994). Heart muscle disease related to HIV infection: prognostic implications. *British Medical Journal*, 309, 1605–7.

Chapter 2.21

Congenital heart disease in adolescents and adults

J. Somerville

Introduction

The population of adolescents and adults with congenital heart disease in the UK increases each year by some 7 per cent because of the growing success of cardiac surgery in infants and children. Natural survivors (without surgery) comprise those with mild lesions that do not produce problems until after the second decade and others with more serious complex anomalies, inoperable, or who escaped surgery during infancy and childhood, but whose circulatory physiology is compatible with survival. The majority, amounting to about 75 per cent of the whole, are patients who have had cardiac surgery in infancy and childhood.

Congenital abnormalities of the heart and cardiovascular system are reported in about 7–11/1000 live births. It is doubtful if all the trivial lesions are recognized in childhood and so the true incidence may be higher. During infancy, 50–60 per cent of these patients need medical and surgical help. In the first decade after infancy, a further 25–30 per cent require the cardiac surgery to maintain or improve life. Some 80 per cent of patients with congenital cardiac lesions now reach adolescence or older age.

Natural survivors

These include those with bicuspid or mild aortic valve stenosis, subaortic stenosis, mitral valve abnormalities, small ventricular septal defects (VSDs), atrial septal defects (ASDs) (more commonly secundum than primum), pulmonary valve stenosis, persistent duct or fistulae, Ebstein's anomaly, and mild coarctation of the aorta. Symptoms develop later in life because of calcification in valves, progressive myocardial dysfunction, infective endocarditis, or the onset of arrhythmias. Survival with more serious lesions will have resulted from the development of postnatal adaptive changes in the heart or pulmonary circulation. Such changes may be ultimately destructive, protective, or beneficial.

Unnatural (post-surgery) survivors

These patients require continued medical care; many have residual dysfunction, the result of the evolution of the original lesion.

Postnatal adaptive changes

Adaptive mechanisms change the form and function of the heart and pulmonary circulation over time. Among the problems which may arise are:

1. Progressive hypertrophy of abnormally placed muscular bands may lead to obstruction to pulmonary blood flow as in acquired 'infundibular stenosis' bipartite right ventricle.
2. Deposition of endocardial fibrosis/elastic tissue may develop in architecturally abnormal outflows—for example, fixed subaortic stenosis or fixed infundibular stenosis. These lesions may calcify after 20 years; the same process occurs as a result of endocardial jet lesions.
3. Compensatory hypertrophy of ventricular myocardium in response to obstructive and/or regurgitant valvular lesions progresses with time to fibrosis and irreversible dysfunction.
4. Increasing pulmonary arteriolar disease, by raising pulmonary vascular resistance, reduces or reverses shunts through associated defects.
5. Spontaneous closure or diminution in size of VSDs and ducts can occur, through different pathological mechanisms.
6. Valves or outflow tracts may calcify, particularly abnormal semilunar valves or a right ventricular outflow tract that is narrowed. The tricuspid valve in severe pulmonary stenosis is often the site of annular calcification. Simple congenital valve lesions that have not caused sufficient haemodynamic disturbance to require surgical intervention before the age of 20 years are prone to develop calcification later. The most trivial obstruction caused by a bicuspid aortic valve may not declare itself until the seventh or eighth decades as calcific aortic stenosis. Atrioventricular valves also calcify when subjected to pressure loads imposed by distal obstructive lesions. The time taken for calcification to cause rigidity and increased obstruction depends on the initial degree of obstruction and generally occurs earlier in males.
7. Chordae tendinae of malformed, abnormally attached atrioventricular valves and valves subjected to unusual stresses may rupture. This complication tends to occur late in such anomalies as univentricular hearts, tricuspid atresia, double-outflow right ventricle, classic transposition of the great arteries, and even with such simple lesions as bicuspid aortic valve stenosis.
8. Aortic valve cusps may prolapse into subarterial VSDs causing aortic regurgitation and signs of spontaneous diminution or closure of the defect.
9. Myocardial dysplasia may be extensive in the presence of structural congenital cardiac anomalies. When dysplastic myocardium is subjected to abnormal pressure, the consequent increases in muscle mass may then itself contribute to obstructions to flow as well as disturb the normal contractile pattern of the ventricle. In congenital aortic stenosis, for example, disproportionate septal bulging and late mitral valve prolapse may occur.

Changes in cardiac form that develop in response to disordered anatomy and physiology may be initially beneficial but later the effects are excessive, leading to death. It is likely that if structural lesions can be corrected early, many of these adverse adaptive changes will be prevented.

Morphological changes within the heart and vessels continue in patients who have had extracardiac palliative surgery, a factor to consider when deciding the timing of more definitive surgery.

Lesions are here separated into cyanotic and acyanotic.

Cyanotic congenital heart disease

Central cyanosis is seen when the arterial oxygen saturation is below 85 per cent. When the patient is anaemic, cyanosis may not be obvious despite reduced arterial oxygen saturation. If the presence of central cyanosis is doubtful at rest, exercise or warmth should make it obvious. It is associated with clubbing of the fingers and toes unless arterial desaturation has been established recently. Extracardiac problems are found in adolescents and adults with cyanotic congenital heart disease:

Polycythaemia

In adults with cyanotic congenital heart disease, the haemoglobin and haematocrit are often extremely high causing increased blood viscosity and secondary symptoms: muzziness, headaches, and a tendency to spontaneous thromboses. Venesection, 500–750 ml, relieves such symptoms. The ideal haemoglobin concentration is 17–18 g/dl but in patients in whom concentrations regularly reach levels of 23–25 g/dl it is dangerous to reduce the level acutely to below 20 g/dl. In patients with values exceeding 20 g/dl there is a place for venesection and replacement before surgery to prevent thromboses during or soon after the procedure.

Venesections should be done with the patient at rest for a period of hours. The volume removed must be replaced by dextran or plasma; More than 1000 ml of blood should not be removed at one session, and if this order of venesection is needed, it should be done on two separate occasions separated by at least 24 h. The practice of venesection without fluid replacement is dangerous, particularly in patients with the Eisenmenger reaction. Patients feel weak for 5–10 days after excessive venesection, particularly if volume has not been replaced.

Gout

An elevated blood uric acid is common in adult cyanotic heart disease in both sexes, perhaps because of increased red-cell turnover and associated impaired renal function. There may be attacks of acute gout in classical sites, and thiazide diuretics may precipitate the problem.

Renal problems

The first signs of renal dysfunction are albuminuria and sometimes microscopic haematuria with a few casts. Later, creatinine clearance is reduced and oliguria, even anuria, may follow dehydration from any cause. This can be prevented by awareness and provision of adequate fluid intake. Patients with long-standing polycythaemia and reduced circulating plasma volume are at risk of an acute deterioration in renal function in relation to surgical procedures. Large doses of contrast media can provoke renal failure and hypertonic media may cause cerebral or pulmonary oedema in patients with impaired renal function.

Skin sepsis

Adolescents and young adults with cyanotic congenital heart disease frequently have widespread, pustular acne. Spontaneous systemic sepsis from this is unusual but wounds heal poorly and systemic infection following surgery is common.

Gums

Patients frequently have troublesome, bleeding, 'spongy' gums. Periodontitis and tooth loss occur prematurely, sometimes hastened by an associated enamel defect. Early and constant attention to oral hygiene is necessary.

Thrombosis and bleeding

Spontaneous venous and, less commonly, arterial thromboses are consequences of increased blood viscosity. Their occurrence is reduced by regular venesection and the avoidance of dehydration, prolonged immobilization, and oestrogen contraceptive pills. Low-oestrogen preparations have been associated with thromboembolism in patients with haemoglobin levels over 16 g/dl but can be prescribed with minimal risk in the mildly cyanosed with lower haemoglobin levels.

Any invasive procedure, including venepuncture or intravenous infusion, may precipitate venous thrombosis. This is dangerous because of the risk of paradoxical emboli causing strokes and cerebral abscess. Attacks of spontaneous cortical and cerebral venous thrombosis occur in those with very high haematocrits and mimic the symptoms of cerebral abscess.

In thrombotic lesions outside the brain, anticoagulants may be used, but the danger of haemorrhage is then always present because control is difficult, particularly in patients with the Eisenmenger reaction. Long-term anticoagulation is best avoided, but if the clinical situation requires it small intravenous injections of heparin sufficient to prolong the bleeding time slightly above normal or aspirin to reduce platelet stickiness are recommended. Conventional doses of heparin are contraindicated because of the danger of catastrophic haemorrhage. Subcutaneous and intramuscular injections of heparin may cause large haematomas and should be avoided. If bleeding complicates anticoagulation, caution is required in reversing the anticoagulant effects, as thrombotic incidents develop readily.

Spontaneous bleeding, except from the gums, is uncommon. Patients with long-standing, severe polycythaemia often have multifactorial clotting defects and defective thromboplastin generation. Assessment of clotting function is needed before surgery and fresh blood, plasma, and sometimes platelet transfusion should be available.

Relative anaemia

Apparently healthy haemoglobin concentrations may not be high enough for tissue oxygenation when cardiac function is impaired. In a very cyanosed patient a haemoglobin of 16–17 g/dl may represent important anaemia. Anaemia in cyanotic heart disease is uncommon but is one of the causes of malaise in cyanotic patients and is usually missed when the haemoglobin is above 14 g/dl.

Cerebral abscess

This diagnosis should be excluded in any cyanotic patient with congenital heart disease who presents with stroke, new headache and vomiting, personality change, transient weakness or paraesthesiae, or unexplained low-grade fever and apathy.

Pregnancy

Women with all forms of cyanotic congenital heart disease have difficulty in carrying a fetus to term. The main problem is the high incidence of spontaneous abortions between weeks 10 and 20. Those with moderate cyanosis (excluding Eisenmenger), and arterial saturation above 85 per cent, and with haemoglobin below 17 g/dl may carry to term without a problem, but there is a high incidence of premature and low birth-weight infants. Such patients need short labour, prevention of dehydration, and immediate attention to sepsis and to thrombotic or haemorrhagic complications. Pregnancy in patients with the Eisenmenger reaction only exceptionally results in a live, normal child. It is a risk to the mother's life, may accelerate deterioration, and should be discouraged. Termination carries risks but if done early these are less than those of pregnancy.

Contraception

High-oestrogen contraceptive pills are absolutely contraindicated, and there is a small but definite risk of thrombosis and embolic complications in cyanotics taking low-oestrogen preparations. Progesterone-only pills have fewer risks but are not completely protective. Sterilization may be the best solution, but even this operation has risks in patients with the Eisenmenger reaction and should be done only in optimal circumstances.

Arthritis

Adolescents and adults with chronic cyanotic congenital heart disease often complain of painful knees, ankles, and sometimes wrists. The periarticular tissues become thickened with severe long-standing clubbing. The ends of the long bones may become tender, as part of hypertrophic osteoarthropathy. Occasionally the joint pains become acute, involving all joints including the spine. Non-steroidal anti-inflammatory drugs may help but may provoke gastric bleeding or fluid retention precipitating right heart failure.

Causes of cyanosis in congenital heart disease

The haemodynamic disturbances that lead to central cyanosis are:

1. *Right-to-left shunt* Systemic venous blood can pass from the right side of the heart to the left at atrial, ventricular, or aortopulmonary level when defects or a patent foramen ovale are present. The abnormalities allowing a shunt are: (a) pulmonary vascular disease (Eisenmenger reaction); (b) pulmonary arterial stenosis or banding; (c) pulmonary valve stenosis or atresia; (d) abnormal right ventricular function without a, b or c; (e) tricuspid stenosis/atresia; (f) large Eustachian valve with ASD or patent foramen ovale.
2. *Complete mixing of systemic and pulmonary circulations* This occurs in single atrium, univentricular heart, and common trunk. The severity of central cyanosis depends on complications such as the degree of right ventricular obstruction or of pulmonary vascular disease present; the more severe, the lower is the systemic arterial oxygen saturation.
3. *Abnormalities of connection* (a) classic transposition of the great arteries when right ventricular blood is ejected directly into ascending aorta and left ventricular blood to the pulmonary artery; (b) inferior or superior vena caval drainage to the left atrium; and (c) total anomalous pulmonary venous drainage.
4. '*Pulmonary*' *cyanosis* in pulmonary arteriovenous fistula and late after anastomosis of the superior vena cava to the pulmonary artery for treatment of tricuspid atresia (Glenn's operation).

Note that (1), (2), and (3) often coexist in various combinations.

Specific disorders

Fallot's tetralogy

This anomaly comprises: (a) a large, subaortic, VSD with cephalad borders formed by aortic valve cusps, and (b) abnormal, rotated infundibular bands, which can form infundibular stenosis. The pulmonary valve may be mildly stenosed, bicuspid, or normal. Occasionally a suprapulmonary valve stenosis coexists and may be the main obstruction in patients who survive to adult life. Pulmonary arterial anatomy is variable. It depends on the size of pulmonary blood flow, which in turn relates to severity, form of the obstruction, changes in the peripheral pulmonary arterioles, and any earlier attempts to improve pulmonary blood flow by 'shunts'. The other two features of the 'tetralogy', right ventricular hypertrophy and overriding aorta, are secondary to (a) and (b).

In adult natural survivors the pulmonary arteries are usually well developed. Added problems in adults include calcification of the pulmonary valve (after 25 years), aortic regurgitation, and right ventricular failure after 40 years with extensive fibrosis of the myocardium.

Symptoms and presentation

Effort dyspnoea is usual and there may be symptoms from polycythaemia. Rhythm disturbances include atrial fibrillation (after 40 years), supraventricular tachycardia, and spontaneous ventricular ectopics from the right ventricle. Right heart failure is uncommon below 40 years, but may be precipitated by pregnancy, rhythm disturbances, or chronic anaemia. Infective endocarditis tends to involve the aortic valve and less often the tricuspid secondary to the jet lesions from the contiguous aortic valve cusp. Mitral valve endocarditis is rare.

Signs

Clubbing and cyanosis are variable. Pulses are full and carotid pulsation is prominent. The aortic pulsation may be palpable in the suprasternal notch, and often visible; 'a' and 'v' waves are easily seen in the jugular venous pulse, which may be elevated with rapid 'x' descent if there is right heart failure. The right ventricular impulse is palpable but not the left unless there is an additional lesion. The second sound is single (aortic) and there is a pulmonary systolic murmur whose length and intensity is related to the severity of the pulmonary stenosis. The milder the stenosis the more the pulmonary flow and the longer and louder is the murmur associated with thrill in the mildest cases.

The term 'acyanotic Fallot', refers to the condition of a large, subaortic, VSD and moderate infundibular stenosis, which permits a normal or increased pulmonary blood flow initially; cyanosis appears later or after effort but is not always present at rest. The murmur is then so loud and long that it sounds like that of a VSD. It diminishes with fever, hot weather, and inhalation of amyl nitrite or any other cause of vasodilation. No murmur arises from the VSD because it is so large.

Variable added signs include an ejection click from the dilated aorta, and a late, delayed, diastolic murmur when the pulmonary valve is calcified. Aortic regurgitation when present causes an immediate diastolic murmur that may be associated with right heart failure and widening of pulse pressure. The venous pressure increases when regurgitation is severe because of reflux into the right as well as the left ventricle. When right heart failure develops, a pansystolic murmur appears low at the left sternal edge from tricuspid regurgitation. The left ventricle enlarges if there has been a previous functioning shunt or aortic regurgitation.

Investigations

Electrocardiographic (**ECG**) features include P pulmonale, right axis deviation, right ventricular hypertrophy, and right bundle-branch block (only in older patients). The P–R interval is lengthened in some patients over 40 years. The characteristic findings on chest radiographs, and at catheterization and angiography are described in OTM3, p. 2403.

Table 1 Differential diagnosis of Fallot

1. Single ventricle and pulmonary stenosis
2. Corrected transposition
3. Double outlet right ventricle with VSD and pulmonary stenosis
4. Transposition of the great arteries
5. Atrioventricular defect with pulmonary stenosis
6. Multiple VSDs or defects not in the Fallot position
7. Bipartite right ventricle with VSD

See OTM3, pp. 2404–5.

Treatment

Complete repair is the ideal. If the haemoglobin exceeds 21 g/dl and there is severe pulmonary atresia, there may be a place for a preliminary shunt procedure to reduce the red-cell mass and the early complications of polycythaemia; in cases so managed, complete repair should be done 6–12 months later. Adults with Fallot's may have symptomatic benefit from late repair but may also require pulmonary valve replacement and have a higher surgical morbidity than children.

Associated congenital cardiac anomalies

A number of congenital cardiovascular abnormalities may coincide with Fallot's (see OTM3, pp. 2403–4). The differential diagnosis of the classical tetralogy includes a number of conditions with similar clinical signs (Table 1).

Fallot's tetralogy after surgery

Patients mostly survive because of earlier palliative shunts or radical repair with closure of the VSD and removal of pulmonary stenosis. Only a few reach adult life without earlier surgery. Systemic-to-pulmonary arterial shunts increase pulmonary blood flow, and this reduces cyanosis at the cost of volume overload on the left side of the heart. Aortic regurgitation is common when shunts have been *in situ* for many years. A number of shunt procedures have been used:

Blalock–Taussig

The subclavian artery is anastomosed to the right or left pulmonary artery.

Subclavian autograft

A subclavian is joined to a pulmonary artery after transection at its origin and reimplantation lower in the descending aorta.

Modified Blalock

This involves the interposition of a tube prosthesis between the subclavian artery and ipsilateral pulmonary artery.

Waterston

A window is made between the ascending aorta and the right pulmonary artery.

Potts

An anastomosis is made between the descending aorta and the left pulmonary artery. The complications which occur after palliative shunts are listed in Table 2.

After radical repair

Patients who have had radical repair have dramatic relief of symptoms and of hypoxia. Residual signs and problems depend on the completeness of the repair, and the duration of follow-up. Clubbing and

Table 2 Complications of palliative shunts

1. Closure or diminution of size of shunt
2. Acquired atresia of infundibulum and/or pulmonary valve
3. Development of bronchopulmonary collaterals
4. Subclavian steel after Blalock
5. Cerebral abscess
6. Infective arteritis (aortic valve or shunt)
7. Aortic regurgitation
8. Biventricular failure
9. Shortening of ipsilateral arm after Blalock
10. Pulmonary vascular disease

Table 3 Complications after radical repairs of Fallots

1. Residual VSD
2. Residual pulmonary stenosis
3. Patent foramen ovale and shunt reversal on exercise
4. Rhythm disturbance
5. Infective endocarditis
6. Right ventricular aneurysm
7. Pulmonary hypertension
8. Pulmonary regurgitation
9. Aortic regurgitation
10. Heart failure

See OTM3, pp. 2406–7.

cyanosis should disappear, but the jugular venous 'a' wave is still larger than normal and the right ventricle may remain overactive. A systolic ejection murmur is expected, with wide splitting of the second heart sound (related to complete right bundle-branch block in 85–90 per cent) and a diminished pulmonary component preceding a short diastolic rumble of pulmonary regurgitation. Exceptionally, the patient has no murmurs and a normal second sound. The ECG should show sinus rhythm, variable patterns of right bundle-branch block, and variable electrical axis. T inversion may persist and extend to V5.

Complications after radical repair vary according to the surgery performed (Table 3). Those with well-repaired lesions mostly live normal lives. They may safely take the contraceptive pill, and have a low risk of infective endocarditis. They are also safe to undertake pregnancy, but there is an increased risk of producing a child affected by congenital heart disease, particularly when the mother has had Fallot's tetralogy.

Defects with pulmonary hypertension

The Eisenmenger reaction (syndrome)

The Eisenmenger complex—pulmonary hypertension with reversed or bidirectional shunt from right to left sides of the heart—can occur as a result of a number of defects associated with pulmonary hypertension and pulmonary vascular disease (Table 4).

Table 4 Eisenmenger complex: associated defects

Ventricular septal defect (VSD)*
Double outflow right ventricle (DORV)*
A–V canal
Truncus
Aortopulmonary defect
Duct (patent ductus arteriosus)*
Transposition of the great arteries (TGA) with VSD, duct, after shunts, rare with ASD
Double inlet ventricle (single, common, uni) ± mitral atresia*
Tricuspid atresia with large VSD
Atrial septal defect (ASD)
Ostium primum
Common atrium
Hemi-anomalous pulmonary venous damage
Total anomalous pulmonary drainage (TAPVD)
Pulmonary atresia (complex) with large congenital systematic collaterals

*Rarely associated with coarctation which should *not* be operated on in adolescents/adults in this situation.

Certain factors predispose to the establishment of early pulmonary vascular disease. These are Down syndrome, birth at high altitude, associated left-sided lesions with other defects such as mitral stenosis or regurgitation, coarctation, congenitally abnormal lung arteries, multiple chest infections, chronic upper-airways obstruction, diaphragmatic hernia, and perinatal asphyxia. Patients with ASD generally acquire pulmonary vascular disease later in adolescence or adult life than in the case of other defects when it usually dates from early infancy or childhood (below 2 years).

The prognosis is partly related to the site of the defect. Those with an Eisenmenger duct have the best prognosis and survival to the sixth or even seventh decade, has been documented.

Symptoms

Dyspnoea is related to the degree of hypoxia. In patent ductus, symptoms appear when desaturated blood reaches the head, usually in adolescence; with the other defects, dyspnoea occurs earlier.

Effort syncope is a frequent symptom of primary pulmonary hypertension and is associated with a low fixed cardiac output. Sometimes there is angina of effort.

Excess sinus tachycardia with palpitation occurs with exercise, heat, or fright. After 35–40 years, paroxysmal supraventricular tachycardia is common, particularly with ASD. The onset of atrial fibrillation produces a rapid downhill course.

There may be massive haemoptysis (pulmonary apoplexy), which is usually terminal when it is associated with the rupture of capillaries or occasionally a pulmonary artery itself. Smaller haemoptyses may occur as the result of infarction and thromboses *in situ*. The incidence of haemoptysis increases with age, starting late in the second decade. It is always a sinister symptom and often heralds the end. If there is evidence of pulmonary infarction, small doses of intravenous heparin by infusion can be given with caution. With persistent fever and the development of a line of air around the pulmonary shadow, a mycetoma should be suspected and a search made for fungi in sputum and antibodies.

Right heart failure develops after the age of 40 years in sinus rhythm or is precipitated by supraventricular arrhythmias.

Physical signs

Pulmonary hypertension produces right ventricular hypertrophy, a pulmonary systolic click, and loud pulmonary valve closure. The patient may not be cyanosed at rest. With a duct, the toes are clubbed and more cyanosed than the hands. The behaviour of the second sound reveals the site of the defect, single with VSD or single ventricle, normally split with aortopulmonary shunts, fixed with ASDs. As the right ventricle fails, the second sound becomes delayed and fixed. Murmurs do not arise from the defects themselves as they are too large to offer any turbulence, but a pansystolic murmur may appear from tricuspid regurgitation when the right ventricle fails. An immediate diastolic murmur of pulmonary regurgitation is frequent and age related. The ECG shows varying degrees of right ventricular hypertrophy and axis shift.

Differential diagnosis

Patients with the Eisenmenger syndrome must be distinguished from those with acyanotic Fallot and transposition with pulmonary stenosis. An abnormal right ventricle with reversed interatrial shunt may also be confused with the Eisenmenger syndrome; a large 'a' wave, quiet right ventricle without murmurs, and a normal P2 with normal or small pulmonary arteries on the chest radiograph should confirm this diagnosis.

Management

The general advice for care of adult patients with cyanotic heart disease should be followed (see above). Any sudden change in volume may lead to death and should be prevented when possible. Patients should not go to an altitude above 1000 m. Flying is permissible, but oxygen should be available and used. Long flights are a risk and it is important to avoid dehydration, alcohol consumption, and sitting for long periods. Ordinary driving licences can be issued provided there is no syncope. Appropriate drug management of arrhythmias and heart failure should be instituted when indicated but it is important to remember that all drugs which may lower blood pressure should be avoided. Any change in cerebral state, new headaches, or transient cerebral signs require exclusion of cerebral abscess. Indwelling intravenous lines are a potential source of systemic embolism and even expert nurses require special warning about the avoidance of air bubbles, which carry a particular risk in the presence of right-to-left shunts. A cerebral embolism may result from a local peripheral vein thrombosis or a cerebral abscess may be the consequence of a minor skin infection.

Heart/lung transplantation offers hope for some of these patients when they become severely disabled with hypoxia but without other organ dysfunction.

Pregnancy carries risks to mother and fetus. Maternal risk of death may still be of the order of 20 per cent but, it is possible to bring a patient with Eisenmenger through pregnancy to a satisfactory outcome, provided the oxygen saturation is above 85 per cent and she is young. There is a high incidence of spontaneous abortion and still births, premature births, low birth weight, and increased incidence of congenital heart disease in the fetus. Early induction of labour or elective caesarean section are advised. Oxygen, as much as can be tolerated, will help raise oxygen saturation and the patient's well-being.

The progesterone-only contraceptive pill can be used, but an intrauterine device, with antibiotic prophylaxis at the time of insertion may be better, or the use of a diaphragm and condom.

Table 5 Other causes of cyanotic congenital heart disease (see OTM, pp. 2407–19)

Pulmonary atresia with VSD
Pulmonary valve stenosis with reversed interatrial shunt
Pulmonary arterial stenoses
Tricuspid atresia
Ebstein's anomaly
Abnormal right ventricle with reversed inter atrial shunt
Abnormal connections of systemic and pulmonary veins
(a) Interior vena cava to left atrium
(b) Superior vena cava to left atrium
(c) Total anomalous venous drainage
(d) Hemianomalous venous drainage
(e) Partial anomalous pulmonary veins
Transposition of great arteries (arterioventricular concordance; ventricular arterial discordance)
Corrected transposition (arterioventricular discordance; ventricular arterial discordance; anterior aorta to the left)
Corrected malposition (arterioventricular; ventricular arterial concordance; mitral/aortic discontinuity, anterior aorta)
Double outflow right ventricle
Double outlet left ventricle
Double inlet ventricle
Univentricular heart with mitral atresia
Pulmonary arteriovenous fistula

Other causes of cyanotic congenital heart

These are many (Table 5) and are described in OTM3, pp. 2407–19.

Acyanotic congenital heart disease in adults

Right-sided obstructive lesions and other anomalies of the right side of the heart

The main anomalies are pulmonary valve stenosis, 'lone' infundibular stenosis, bipartite right ventricle, pulmonary arterial stenoses, idiopathic dilatation of the pulmonary artery, and Ebstein's anomaly.

Pulmonary valve stenosis

Severe pulmonary valve stenosis is uncommon in adults unless there has been previous surgery. Patients with severe lesions may be cyanosed, depending on an association with ASD or patent foramen ovale. There is evidence that in some patients the disease is not limited to the pulmonary valve. There may be associated left ventricular disease, hypertrophic or dilated.

Table 6 Physical signs in pulmonary valve stenosis (PVS)

	Mild	Moderate	Severe
Pulse	Normal	Normal	Small
Jugular venous pressure	Normal	Dominant 'a' wave on inspiration or exercise	Giant 'a' wave
Apex beat	RV palpable	RV+ +	RV + +
Auscultation	Loud pulmonary ejection click, increases on expiration	Clock close to S_1 (absent if valve thick)	No click
	A_2/P_2 interval wide, increases on inspiration	A_2/P_2 interval wider, increases on inspiration	P_2 often very late, soft or not heard
	P_2 audible but late Grade 2 ejection murmur increases on inspiration, maximal 2nd left interspace	P_2 audible but late Grade 3 murmur + thrill	Loud murmur + thrill—late crescendo over A_2
Other			Mild clubbing (variable)
			Peripheral cyanosis Malar flush

Anatomy and physiology

The stenosed pulmonary valve may be bicuspid or tricuspid, a pliable dome, or the thick lumpy valve that is usual in patients with Noonan's syndrome and related syndromes. After 35–40 years of age, the valve calcifies and may become regurgitant. When right ventricular pressure is high, calcification develops in the tricuspid valve ring, sometimes involving a cusp. The effects of pulmonary valve stenosis are to disturb right ventricular function. Right ventricular hypertrophy occurs when resting right ventricular pressure exceeds 50 mmHg. Later fibrosis causes dilatation, tricuspid regurgitation and failure worsened or precipitated by atrial flutter or fibrillation.

Symptoms

Fatigue, slight dyspnoea, and effort syncope are features of severe pulmonary valve stenosis. Dyspnoea is more pronounced when there is cyanosis from a reversed intra-atrial shunt. Acyanotic patients are usually symptom-free until the onset of atrial fibrillation or flutter and right heart failure. Adult patients with mild-to-moderate pulmonary valve stenosis (right ventricular pressures 40–60 mmHg) may appear after the age of 50 years in right heart failure in sinus rhythm. Infective endocarditis on lone pulmonary valve stenosis is unknown unless part of the generalized septic process; routine prophylaxis is thus unnecessary.

Signs

These depend on the severity of the obstruction and secondary effects on the right ventricular myocardium (Table 6). Pulmonary regurgitation occurs when the valve calcifies.

In right heart failure, the pulse is small and irregular, the jugular venous pressure high with huge 'v' waves of tricuspid regurgitation, and there is a third sound that increases on inspiration. A loud pansystolic murmur, difficult to distinguish from the pulmonary ejection murmur, often occurs at the left lower sternal edge. In such cases, the ejection murmur at the pulmonary area is short.

The ECG reflects the severity of right ventricular hypertrophy, ranging from right axis deviation in the mildest cases to increased R wave voltage and S–T wave changes over the right ventricular leads. P pulmonale is usual and no true left ventricular complexes are recorded in V_6. With increasing age and/or failure, complete right bundle-branch block can develop.

Differential diagnosis

When stenosis is trivial it may be confused with mild aortic valve stenosis or ASD. To differentiate mild pulmonary valve stenosis from modest ASD may be difficult. Other causes of a long systolic murmur at the left sternal edge include VSD, infundibular stenosis, subaortic stenosis, and pulmonary artery stenosis. Severe pulmonary valve stenosis in failure with right ventricular dilation may be confused with Ebstein, pericardial effusion (no murmurs), or even VSD with atrial fibrillation.

Treatment

The late results of pulmonary valvotomy are excellent; 95 per cent of patients are relieved of any symptoms and endocarditis is not a risk. Murmurs persist and pulmonary regurgitation is common. Patients with lumpy, dysplastic valves can be left with serious pulmonary incompetence, which can lead, 15–20 years later, to progressive right ventricular dilatation, and failure with atrial flutter, and fibrillation. Pulmonary valve replacement has been helpful in a few but the heart diminishes little in size once extreme dilatation has occurred and the tricuspid valve may also require surgery. Provided pulmonary valve and annulus obstruction is relieved, infundibular stenosis should regress. Cyanosis and dyspnoea on effort may appear if the foramen ovale remains open and can be helped by closure.

'Lone' infundibular stenosis

Anatomy and physiology

Fixed, right ventricular outflow-tract obstruction below the pulmonary valve is caused by muscle bands that are abnormally placed, at first causing slight obstruction and then slowly hypertrophying in postnatal life; the pulmonary valve may be normal, bicuspid, or minimally stenosed. The infundibular stenosis can appear as the only anomaly but careful searches should show evidence of a VSD (subtricuspid or muscular) that has earlier closed spontaneously leaving only a scar. The speed with which infundibular obstruction develops relates to the stimulus from right ventricular hypertension, initially determined by the size of the VSD, the degree of abnormal rotation, and size of the bands; probably also the amount of abnormal muscle within the displaced band. Slow enlargement/hypertrophy of bands may cause obstruction to become critical in adults and, by then, thickened endocardium in the outflow of the right ventricle covers the bands and contributes to the obstruction.

Symptoms and signs

Murmurs may have been documented since early childhood. A click never precedes the long, pulmonary ejection systolic murmur, which is maximal in the third left interspace, and is conducted into the pulmonary area; it increases on inspiration. P_2, when audible, is delayed and diminished.

Left-sided obstructive lesions and other anomalies affecting the left side of the heart

The main anomalies causing left ventricular-outflow obstruction are aortic valve stenosis, bicuspid aortic valve, aortic regurgitation, fixed subaortic stenosis, supra-aortic stenosis, and coarctation of the aorta. Kinked aorta (at isthmus), aorto-left ventricular tunnel, mitral anomalies, and left atrial obstruction may present exceptionally after childhood.

Aortic valve stenosis

Minor congenital abnormality of the aortic valve (bicuspid, slight tricuspid fusion) is said to be the most common congenital lesion of the cardiovascular system.

Congenital stenosis can be critical at any age. When it has been moderate to mild, with gradients of 20–40 mmHg in childhood, it may become more significant around puberty during or after the period of rapid growth; less commonly, serious problems arise in the third and fourth decades. Isolated calcific aortic stenosis in patients over 60 years of age results from the deposition of calcium on a congenitally abnormal valve. Valve calcification is less in the female. In patients under 30 years with critical obstruction the valve remains pliable, with flecks of calcium in small myxomatous masses attached to the cusps. Severe calcification under 30 years seems only to occur after previous valvotomy, infection, or with a metabolic upset such as hypercholesterolaemic or hypercalcaemic states. The mildly deformed aortic valve (bicuspid, tricuspid, or rarely quadricuspid) may be regurgitant.

The physical signs depend on severity and pliability. The condition should be differentiated from fixed subaortic stenosis as the surgical treatment is different. The pathology may not be limited to the aortic valve. Patients can have an unusually thick (>2 cm) ventricular septum, secondary mitral valve dysfunction, and aortic disease with systemic hypertension unmasked after aortic valvotomy or valve replacement.

Fixed subaortic stenosis

The lesion is an accumulation of fibroelastic tissue in the form of a crescent or a complete ring. It may be close to the aortic valve, eccentric, and oblique or 1–2 cm beneath. It is never 'membranous' and is attached to a sheet of fibroelastic tissue overlying the bulging and usually excessively hypertrophic ventricular septum, depending on the age of the patient. It causes left-ventricular outflow obstruction, which is often only mild or moderate; when severe, the septal hypertrophy contributes rather than the narrowing of the outflow tract. It can present in childhood at the age of 2–3 years but more commonly in adolescence and sometimes in an adult. Secondary aortic regurgitation occurs from jet lesions or associated congenital abnormalities; mitral regurgitation may also be an acquired complication.

There is increasing evidence that this is a lesion acquired in postnatal life. Other congenital anomalies of the heart or cardiovascular system occur in 60 per cent, for instance duct, VSD, aortic valve stenosis (bicuspid or tricuspid), and coarctation. There is an interrelation between fixed subaortic stenosis and obstructive hypertrophic myopathy.

Symptoms and presentation

These are as for other forms of aortic stenosis. Left ventricular failure occurs after the age of 40 years. Infective endocarditis is a lifelong risk.

Signs

Pulses are full and often slightly jerky, but they may be small and sharp when obstruction is severe. There is a prominent 'a' wave in the jugular venous pulse if the ventricular septum is thick and encroaching on the right ventricular cavity, and a carotid thrill. The apex is left ventricular, powerful, and displaced to the left. There is an ejection systolic murmur not preceded by a click and maximal in the third left intercostal space, conducted to the apex and neck. The aortic second sound is usually audible but often delayed and splitting may be difficult to detect, or may be reversed. In adults a short, immediate diastolic murmur of aortic regurgitation is present.

Echocardiography may show premature closure of the aortic valve and a thick, abnormal ventricular septum. Cross-sectional echocardiography reveals the shelf protruding beneath the aortic valve, which may extend on to the anterior cusp of the mitral valve. A very thick, abnormal ventricular septum is commonly seen and abnormal movements of the mitral cusps are frequent. It can be difficult to differentiate from hypertrophic obstructive myopathy. The aortic valve is thickened, regurgitant, and opens abnormally.

Treatment

The lesion should be resected when producing obstruction. Ventricular muscle often behaves as in hypertrophic obstructive cardiomyopathy following operation. A picture of congestive myopathy with progressive fibrosis may appear after age of 40–50 years.

The aortic valve has a lifetime risk of endocarditis, as jet lesions remain after resection.

The mortality of early resection is low but problems can return. Reoperation may be hazardous. Total aortic-root/valve replacement may be necessary to provide real relief of obstruction.

Supra-aortic stenosis

Supra-aortic stenosis describes a narrowing above the aortic valve contiguous with the commissural attachments. It may be mild, without causing a gradient, or there may be severe fibrous constriction above the coronary orifices. Surgical attention is focused on the stenosis and removal may be thought to cure the condition. Unfortunately, this is not so as the disease is not localized to the supra-aortic area. The central aorta beyond is grossly abnormal, often diffusely hypoplastic. This is most severe in those with obvious aortic hypoplasia, where intimal changes may be found even in childhood. The same changes in the medial layers occur in those without apparent diffuse narrowing of the aorta and irrespective of whether the supra-aortic stenosis is part of the 'hypercalcaemic' syndrome with its characteristic facies and other features, familial with normal physical features, or sporadic with none of the known associations. This disorder, which extends throughout the major conducting arteries, appears in severely affected patients to fade out in the region of the common iliac arteries. The actual supra-aortic stenosis is probably

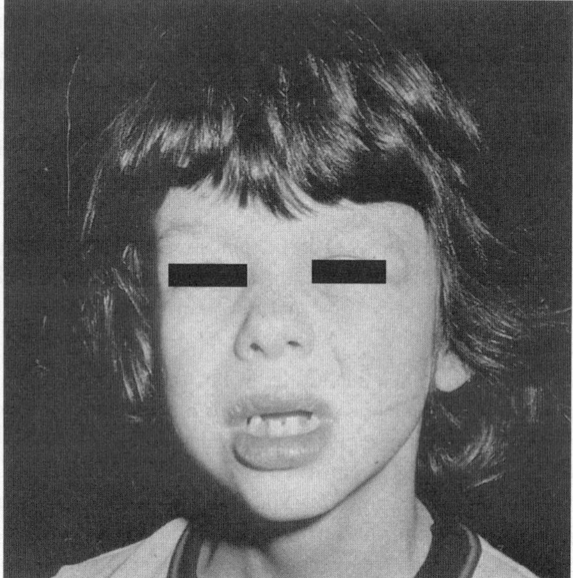

Fig. 1 Classic face associated with supra-aortic stenosis (William's syndrome). Large ridged teeth, prominent jaw, and supraorbital ridges.

the result of more extensive damage at a vulnerable site in the conducting arteries, as are the other stenoses at origins of major arteries.

Important supra-aortic stenosis has not been found at birth or infancy and so it is doubtful if the lesion is truly congenital. It should, like subaortic stenosis, be regarded as acquired in postnatal life, occurring as part of a congenital arteriopathy. Stenoses occur at other sites, for instance carotid, innominate, mesenteric, sometimes renal, and peripherally in the pulmonary arteries in about 50 per cent of patients.

Another abnormality is the degree and form of the left ventricular hypertrophy that often coexists; this appears to be disproportionate to the degree of outflow obstruction and is often associated with severe, irregular hypertrophy involving the septum, resembling the appearance in hypertrophic cardiomyopathy. Occasionally, the problem complicates other structural congenital heart anomalies such as pulmonary and aortic valve stenosis, duct, or VSD.

Symptoms

When supra-aortic stenosis occurs with the 'hypercalcaemic' facies, a history of early illness in infancy with failure to thrive, repeated infections, and constipation is characteristic. Cardiac symptoms are not present early. Angina occurs late when the arteries are often pathologically thick and abnormal. Sometimes a stenosis at the origin of a coronary artery causes angina. Syncope may occur if there is marked septal hypertrophy or atrial rhythm disturbances in older patients. Fits in adolescence are associated with severe hypertension and carotid or innominate obstruction.

Dyspnoea occurs when the myocardium is grossly hypertrophied, with secondary mitral regurgitation. Infective endocarditis on the aortic valve is a risk and leads to aortic regurgitation. Antibiotic prophylaxis is therefore essential. Supraventricular tachycardia may cause problems after the age of 30 years.

If the arteriopathy is part of the 'burnt-out' hypercalcaemic syndrome, the face is characteristic (Fig. 1), with prominent jaw and supraorbital ridges, large teeth, mental retardation, and exuberant

Table 7 Causes of ostium secundum ASD

1. Oval fossa defects (75%)
2. Inferior vena caval defects (7%)
3. Superior vena caval defects (11%)
4. Coronary sinus defects (rare)
5. Hemianomalous pulmonary venous drainage

personality. Familial cases look normal, and siblings and parents should then be examined.

Treatment

A gradient of over 50–60 mmHg should be relieved, particularly if there is evidence of left-ventricular and septal hypertrophy. This may be done by 'gusseting' but this can disturb aortic valve function with resultant aortic regurgitation. The systolic blood pressure can reach 250 mmHg and requires therapy. Total aortic root and valve replacement with homograft and reimplantation of coronary arteries may be needed.

Coarctation of the aorta

This subject is addressed in Chapter 2.34.

Communications between systemic and pulmonary circulation (septal defects)

Atrial septal defect

Defects in the atrial septum are often not detected until they cause symptoms in adult life. There are two anatomical groups, atrioventricular defects (see later) and ostium secundum defects.

Ostium secundum defects

These do not border the atrioventricular valves and are named according to the site in the atrial septum. They may be in the sinus venosus or secundum septum, but are grouped together because of clinical similarity (Table 7).

Physiology

The effects of an interatrial left-to-right shunt are increased volume load and dilatation of the right atrium and right ventricle, increased pulmonary blood flow and enlarged pulmonary arteries, increase in size of pulmonary veins, and reduced flow to the left ventricle and aorta, which becomes smaller than normal with time.

The factors that influence the blood flow across the defect are compliance of the right ventricle, compliance of the left ventricle, the size of the defect, and atrioventricular valve function. In sinus rhythm the left-to-right flow across the defect is mainly during diastole, but when atrial fibrillation occurs the shunt becomes systolic. Increased blood flow across the defect is caused by left-sided lesions or by increased systemic resistance. The shunt is decreased by tricuspid valve disease, impaired right ventricular filling, by pulmonary stenosis, and pulmonary hypertension. Central cyanosis results from reversal of the shunt.

Symptoms/natural history

Symptoms from secundum defects usually arise in adult life: in 10–20 per cent in the third decade, a few more in the fourth, and in the majority of those over the age of 40. By 50 years, 75 per cent have disability and heart failure, precipitated by atrial fibrillation. Dyspnoea, bronchitis, palpitation, cyanosis, and chronic progressive failure, with haemoptysis follow. Patients over 60 years who remain

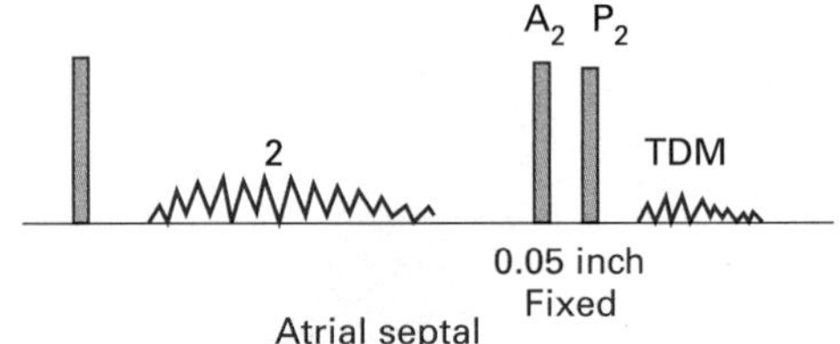

Fig. 2 Auscultation in atrial septal defect. TDM = tricuspid diastolic murmur.
(Reproduced by courtesy of Dr P. Wood.)

in sinus rhythm may slip into right heart failure from chronic fibrosis in the stretched ventricle. Paradoxical emboli are rare but do occur, particularly with extracardiac surgery or trauma. Pulmonary hypertension complicates about 8 per cent, producing massive cardiac enlargement, cyanosis, and severe failure. It is acquired in relation to thromboembolism, pregnancy, and life at high altitude. When atrial fibrillation complicates a small ASD, this lesion may be missed as the heart may not be enlarged and the signs are subtle.

Signs and investigations

Girls with an ASD are said to be slender ('gracile habitus'). Pulses are normal or small when complicated by mitral disease, or an unusually large shunt. Jugular venous pulsations are exaggerated, with easily distinguished 'a' and 'v' waves. Central cyanosis can be seen in association with a right-to-left shunt through the defect.

The right ventricle is overactive and dilated with gentle parasternal pulsation and the left ventricular impulse should be impalpable at the apex. On auscultation the first sound is loud (tricuspid valve closure) and often split, sometimes widely. The second heart sound is widely split in inspiration and expiration. The time interval between A_2 and P_2 is characteristically fixed to the ear but may widen on inspiration and not close on expiration when the defect is small. It becomes unusually wide with bradycardia, right ventricular failure, mild pulmonary stenosis, complete right bundle-branch block, and severe mitral regurgitation, which favours earlier closure of the aortic valve. Pulmonary valve closure (P_2) is loud in adults with ASD irrespective of pulmonary artery pressure. A pulmonary systolic click is common in adults over 40 years.

The classic auscultatory features of ASD are shown in Fig. 2. The diastolic murmur is not present in very small defects and in very large hearts with tricuspid regurgitation as the ring is too large to offer any resistance to the torrential flow. A pansystolic murmur occurs in patients in failure from tricuspid regurgitation. Apical murmurs from added mitral valve dysfunction appear with advancing years and a pulmonary diastolic murmur is common over the age of 50 or in younger patients with pulmonary hypertension.

The chest radiograph of patients in sinus rhythm is typical (Fig. 3)

The ECG typically shows right axis deviation, sharp right atrial P waves, slight prolongation of the P–R interval, partial right bundle-branch block, and absent QR in V_5–V_6. With increasing age there is, an increase in the height of secondary R waves, increasing width of the QRS, and progressive T inversion across RV leads. Left axis deviation may be present in 7 per cent with secundum defects or can be acquired in middle life. P mitrale may develop when the P–R interval is greater than 0.20 s. Prolongation of the P–R interval above 0.20 s occurs in huge defects, and in patients over 40 years.

Cross-sectional echocardiography should show the defect but sometimes in adults it is difficult to find a clear window to profile the atrial septum unless the transoesophageal route is used.

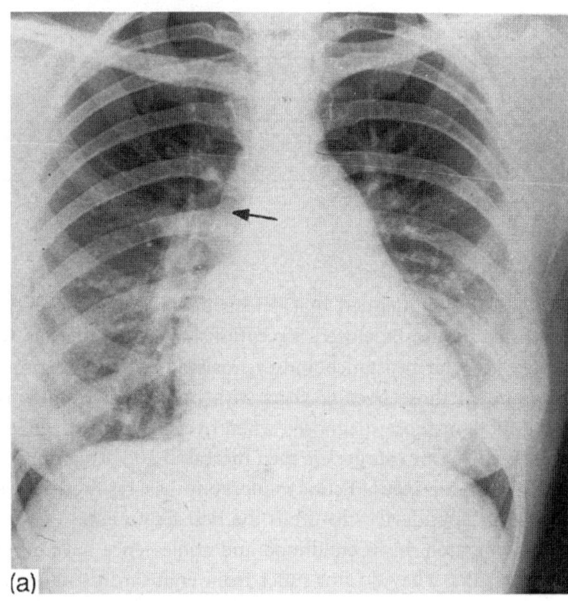

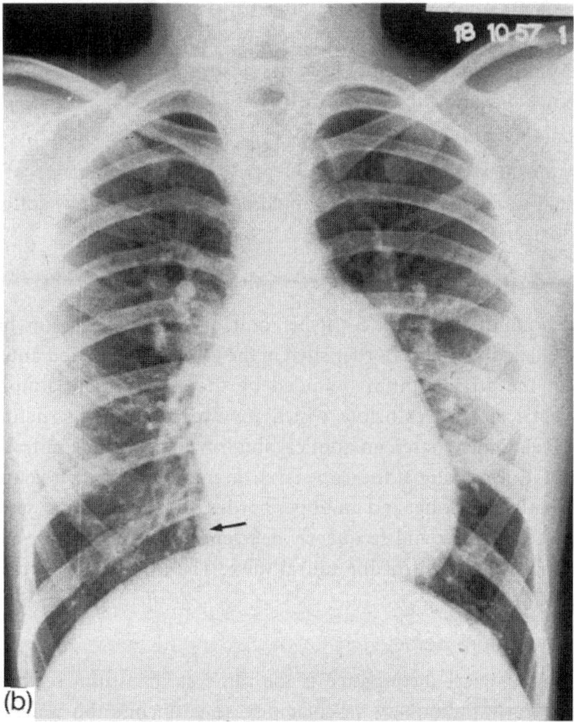

Fig. 3 (a) Chest radiograph from a patient with 'secundum' atrial septal defect showing cardiomegaly, pulmonary plethora, and small aorta. Special features are dilated superior vena cava (arrow) because there is anomalous right upper lobe pulmonary vein entering it in association with superior vena cava defect. (b) Chest radiograph from a patient with 'secundum' atrial septal defect showing cardiomegaly, pulmonary plethora, and small aorta. Special features are dilation of inferior vena cava opposite the uncommon inferior vena cava defect.

Differential diagnosis

This includes particularly mild pulmonary stenosis. In elderly patients with cardiomegaly and atrial fibrillation, ASD may mimic cor pulmonale, rheumatic mitral disease, or cardiomyopathy.

Table 8 The three main forms of atrioventricular defects

1. Ostium primum (75%)
2. Common atrioventricular canal (20%)
3. Common atrium (5%)

See OTM pp. 2426–7.

Treatment

It is generally recommended that defects large enough to give clear physical signs should be closed. Exceptions are when there is raised pulmonary vascular resistance and cyanosis due to the Eisenmenger reaction, and in those over 65 years with only small shunts. There are also doubts in those diagnosed when over 50 years of age, as the risk of morbidity from surgery is then increased and atrial fibrillation tends to persist or recur. Echocardiography has resulted in earlier diagnosis. In these, device closure is the best treatment.

Patients operated on in childhood and adolescence have excellent long-term results. They do not suffer from endocarditis unless there are left-sided valve problems. Mitral regurgitation occasionally appears. Some adults 15–25 years after surgery suffer supraventricular rhythm disorders. Pre-operative rhythm disorders should not prevent surgery in young patients because closure reduces not only the incidence but also the effects of rhythm disturbances.

The patent foramen ovale

Many normal adults (possibly 50 per cent) retain patency of the foramen ovale. Device closure should be done in those few suffering paradoxical emboli.

Atrioventricular defects

These account for about 5–10 per cent of ASDs. The lesion has a sickle-shaped cephalad border sited in the lower (caudal) and anterior part of the atrial septum bounded by the anatomically abnormal atrioventricular valves below, which are also commonly structurally abnormal. Other shared anatomical abnormalities include mitral and tricuspid valves lying at the same level, an outflow of the left ventricle that is unusually long, and an upper border of the ventricular septum depressed caudally and frequently deficient. These features result in abnormal attachment of the mitral valve. The three main forms are listed in Table 8.

Ostium primum defect

The physiological disturbance is the same as in ostium secundum defects. Early pulmonary vascular disease is uncommon unless the defect is large, mitral regurgitation is severe, or there are added lesions such as supramitral valve membrane, coarctation, or duct. Mitral regurgitation increases the left-to-right shunt and in many there is a left ventricular/right atrial shunt through the apex of the cleft. The natural history is worse than in ostium secundum ASD because of associated mitral regurgitation and the disturbance of conducting tissue. Behind the posterior edge of the defect is the atrioventricular node and beneath is the bundle of His, which may be stretched or damaged. Some patients can be symptomatic in childhood, but many reach adolescence and adult life without problems, particularly if mitral regurgitation is mild or absent. Symptoms arise from nodal bradycardia or tachycardia, complete block, and later atrial fibrillation or flutter. Infective endocarditis occurs uncommonly. Pulmonary vascular disease develops in about 8 per cent. Patients with ostium primum defect can survive to the eighth decade but most die before 30 years. The symptoms are as in other ASDs but with the addition of infective endocarditis and syncope from heart block. Signs are also similar to those of secundum patients but with the addition of a pansystolic murmur from an incompetent mitral valve in 75 per cent.

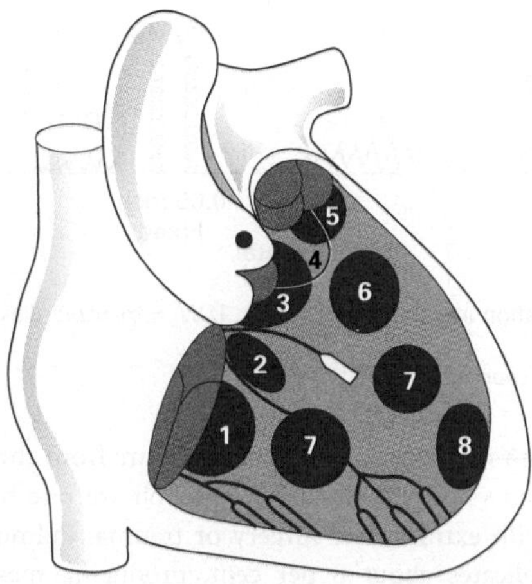

Fig. 4 Diagram to show simple classification of types of ventricular septal defect as seen from the right ventricle. 1–5, subvalvar; 1, inlet; 2, subtricuspid; 3, subaortic; 4, subarterial doubly committed; 5, subpulmonary; 6–8, muscular; 6, outlet; 7, central; 8, apical; MPM, medial papillary muscle.

Diagnosis

The diagnosis of ostium primum should be made in a patient with the signs of ASD and mitral regurgitation, and an ECG showing left axis deviation or abnormal initial activation. Two-dimensional echocardiography shows the lesion clearly, as does left ventricular angiography.

The ECG distinguishes the atrioventricular defects from ostium secundum by the presence of left axis deviation in the standard leads associated with an rSR in V_1, and other features typical of ASD. When severe right ventricular hypertrophy coexists, the axis may be shifted to the right shoulder and the pattern of ventricular activation may be less easily recognized from the standard leads, which show SI, II, and III dominance. Fifty per cent have prolongation of the P–R interval, and P mitrale is common.

Treatment and prognosis

Closure of ostium primum defects and repair of mitral clefts causing regurgitation is recommended in all patients unless there is pulmonary vascular disease, a small shunt below 1.5:1, or very abnormal mitral valve anatomy. Device closure is contraindicated because of the proximity of atrioventricular valves. Despite good anatomical 'correction' there may be late problems. Morbidity and mortality are caused by arrhythmias, and mitral regurgitation, which progresses if originally moderate or severe. Endocarditis may develop on mitral valves and rarely subaortic stenosis may progress.

Common atrioventricular canal and common atrium

These rarer forms of atrioventricular defects are described in OTM3, pp. 2427–8.

Ventricular septal defects

The natural history is dependent not only on the size of the defect but also on its site, which may be subvalvar or muscular related (either apical central or posterior in the muscular septum). Defects may be single or multiple (Fig. 4). Subaortic VSDs do not close spontaneously as the cephalad border is the aortic valve. In contrast, defects beneath the tricuspid valve close spontaneously or become small and are the defects seen most frequently in adults; small, single, muscular defects also behave like this. Large subaortic or subarterial defects in adults manifest as the Eisenmenger syndrome or mild Fallot. Small subpulmonary or doubly committed subarterial defects in adults present with aortic regurgitation. Subtricuspid and submitral defects associated with left axis deviation are rare in adults except in those with the Eisenmenger reaction.

Adults and adolescents with VSDs present as follows: (a) small defects, without elevation of right ventricular pressure and a shunt below 2:1; (b) moderate-sized defects with slight elevation of right ventricular pressure and infundibular gradient, and shunts between 2 and 2.5:1; and (c) large defects in association with advanced pulmonary vascular disease or infundibular and/or mild pulmonary valve stenosis.

Symptoms

These relate to the size of the defect and complications. Patients present as follows:

1. Infective endocarditis, most commonly caused by *Streptococcus viridans*, tends to take an insidious course. It is an indication for surgical closure of the defect and there is a place for removal of a large vegetation during the illness.
2. Atrial fibrillation after 30 years of age can precipitate right-sided congestion with tricuspid regurgitation and a left ventricular to right atrial shunt. The patient should be converted to sinus rhythm as soon as possible. It may be worthwhile closing the defect, however small, as the left ventricular to right atrial shunt can be surprisingly large.
3. Aortic regurgitation may develop with a small VSD or complicate larger subaortic defects. The differential diagnosis of VSD with aortic reflux is from causes of a continuous murmur, which include duct, fistulae, and ruptured sinus of Valsalva aneurysm.
4. Aneurysm of the ventricular septum is an acquired abnormality from spontaneous closure of a VSD beneath the septal cusp of the tricuspid valve. It normally produces no clinical problems.
5. Large left ventricle disproportionate to the expected size for a small VSD; prolapse of the mitral cusp may be found in these patients.
6. Spontaneous closure can occur in adolescents and in adults.

Diagnosis of small/moderate ventricular septal defect

Pulses, venous pressure, and apex beat are normal. There is a pansystolic murmur, associated with a thrill, maximal at the left sternal edge in the third or fourth interspace. With larger defects the left ventricle is prominent and overactive, and a delayed diastolic murmur is present at the apex.

The ECG may be normal. The axis may be leftward or there may be true left-axis deviation. A mild form of rSr is frequent in V_1 with features of left ventricular dominance and upright T waves in V_5 and V_6. Diagnosis is confirmed by two-dimensional echocardiography or left ventricular angiography.

Treatment

Treatment (surgical closure) depends upon symptoms and complications. Without them none is necessary. The prognosis of a small VSD is generally excellent if aortic regurgitation and endocarditis are excluded.

Complications

Most patients reaching adult life after earlier surgical closure of a VSD are well, but problems that may arise include: early and late heart block, ventricular ectopics and ventricular tachycardia, late sinoatrial problems, myocardial damage and dysfunction manifesting as failure, tricuspid mitral regurgitation and aortic regurgitation, and progressive pulmonary hypertension. Pulmonary vascular disease is uncommon when surgery has been done in infancy, but some with large defects closed after the age of 2 years are left with pulmonary artery pressures of 40–60 mmHg. If there is doubt about the normality of the pulmonary arterioles, patients should be discouraged from mountaineering, living at high altitude, taking the contraceptive pill or slimming drugs, or indulging in athletics. The question of pregnancy requires careful judgement.

Residual defects despite surgery is common in patients operated on before 1974–75. They should be protected from infective endocarditis and the defect closed early.

Coronary artery anomalies

Congenital anomalies of the coronary arteries are often symptomless but may cause premature angina, sudden death, persistent ventricular ectopics, or even underlie a cardiomyopathy. A left coronary artery arising from the pulmonary artery may be detected first in adult life but death is more usual in infancy or childhood. This may present with a continuous murmur with evidence of infarction on the ECG, or with a left ventricular aneurysm or mitral regurgitation, chronic failure, or as sudden death. Treatment is surgical—grafting of the left coronary artery into the aorta.

Single coronary arteries may be discovered in young patients with angina or a dilated left ventricle appearing as congestive myopathy or sudden death.

Coronary artery fistulae may cause a continuous murmur at the left sternal edge and enter the right ventricular outflow, the right atrium, or exceptionally the left ventricle. They may 'steal' from the other coronary arteries and the myocardium, causing angina.

Aberrant course of coronary arteries, such as when the right arises from the left sinus or the left from a right sinus may lead to compression between aorta and pulmonary artery, particularly during circumstances that provoke systolic hypertension. This may cause angina, ischaemic signs on the ECG, and even sudden death. Rerouting may be needed.

Aortopulmonary shunts

Persistent duct (ductus arteriosus)

When the duct remains open into the second decade and thereafter, a left-to-right shunt from just proximal to the aortic isthmus to the bifurcation of the pulmonary arteries occurs. The main pulmonary artery and branches dilate and may cause pulmonary regurgitation. The pulmonary veins, left atrium, left ventricle, and aorta are dilated. The pulmonary arterial systolic pressure may be moderately elevated and the diastolic pressure is low. The pulmonary and systemic pressures may be equal with a balanced or reversed shunt.

Symptoms include breathlessness if there is ventricular dysfunction. Atrial fibrillation may result in heart failure. Infective endocarditis may cause the first symptoms.

Signs

The pulse is jerky and the carotids prominent. The left ventricle is overactive and dilated. The pulmonary arterial pulsation maybe palpable. A continuous murmur, enhanced on expiration, is best heard in the second left intercostal space. The second heart sound is normally split with a loud pulmonary component. A delayed diastolic murmur may be heard at the apex. With large ducts there may be no continuous murmur; instead there is a variable-length systolic murmur in the pulmonary area. A pulmonary ejection click is common and the signs of pulmonary regurgitation may be obvious.

The main differential diagnoses are from conditions such as VSD with aortic regurgitation, aortic stenosis with regurgitation, or absent pulmonary valve with pulmonary regurgitation.

Treatment

Closure of all ducts that allow a left-to-right shunt is recommended. Many can now be closed by a device instead of surgery.

Further reading

Somerville, J. (1996). Congenital heart disease in adolescents and adults. In: *Oxford textbook of medicine*, (3rd edn) (ed. D.J. Weatherall, J.G.G. Ledingham, and D.A. Warrell), pp. 2398–431. Oxford University Press, Oxford.

Chapter 2.22

Cardiac aspects of rheumatic fever

J. M. Neutze

A detailed description of rheumatic fever is given in Chapter 2.26 (and see also Chapter 16.38). Here the account is confined to the cardiac aspects of the disease which result from an abnormal reaction to infection with group A beta haemolytic streptococci.

Although rheumatic fever was the major cause of acquired heart disease in children in Western countries before the 1940s, the incidence has since declined dramatically. In underdeveloped countries it remains a major problem, with annual incidence of 100 per 100 000 in childhood, compared with fewer than 5 per 100 000 in most Western countries.

Pathology

The classic histological feature is the Aschoff nodule which has a widespread distribution and can be found in myocardial tissue, although most valvular lesions consist of less organized collections of chronic inflammatory cells. The nodules heal by fibrosis, sometimes leading to extensive myocardial scarring.

The mitral valve leaflets become thickened with impairment of closure, exacerbated by dilatation of the annulus. Progressive distortion of the leaflets and sub-valvar apparatus may lead to severe regurgitation. Leaflet and chordal fusion may lead to mitral stenosis, the structure of the valve becoming severely distorted by progressive fibrosis and eventually calcification. This process usually progresses slowly over many years, but proceeds rapidly in some children in developing countries. Thickening of the cusps of the aortic valve is also seen, the edges developing a characteristic rolled appearance. The dominant functional abnormality is aortic regurgitation.

Clinical features of cardiac disease

Rheumatic carditis

Symptoms usually present 1–3 weeks after the streptococcal infection. When carditis occurs in the course of an acute illness (mostly in the 6–15-year age group), signs become obvious in the first week in three-quarters of the patients. In patients with a subacute course, carditis may become manifest later in an illness featuring low-grade fever, pallor, and joint aches. The most common manifestation is the development of mitral regurgitation, consisting of a modest apical systolic murmur but sometimes progressing to a severe leak with an overactive and dilating heart, dyspnoea, and an increasing murmur. The appearance of an early diastolic murmur of aortic regurgitation may clinch the diagnosis of rheumatic fever. Aortic regurgitation may also progress rapidly to a severe leak. Echo Doppler studies have shown clear evidence of valve involvement when cardiac signs are restricted to a modest, innocent-sounding murmur. Although some myocardial involvement probably occurs almost universally, severe impairment of ventricular function is uncommon. When pulmonary venous congestion and heart failure develop, severe mitral (and/or aortic) regurgitation are usually present with a modest reduction in myocardial contractility. As the heart dilates, stretching of the mitral valve ring exacerbates the leak, and dilation of the right heart may produce severe tricuspid regurgitation.

Pericarditis may accompany myocarditis, and a moderate pericardial effusion may develop. A third heart sound is common, sinus tachycardia is usual, and supraventricular and ventricular ectopic beats may occur. The P–R and Q–T intervals may be prolonged on the ECG. Carditis is thus diagnosed by the presence of new or changing murmurs, pericarditis, or heart failure.

Diagnosis of the cardiac lesions

There is no single diagnostic test for rheumatic fever and many factors cause problems in diagnosis (see Chapter 2.26). Cardiac murmurs heard in an appropriate clinical context may reflect a minor congenital cardiac lesion first noticed during a viral infection. Changing murmurs, evidence of involvement of mitral and aortic valves and evidence of myocarditis, and/or pericarditis favour rheumatic fever. Echocardiography can provide valuable information in experienced hands.

Treatment of acute rheumatic fever

Overall management is discussed in Chapter 2.26. Rest remains a cornerstone in treatment, based on repeated clinical observations and supported by a single clinical controlled trial in the pre-penicillin era. Once the acute phase reactants have settled, modest restriction of exercise is recommended for 2 weeks only. Measurement of phase reactants should be continued at 2-weekly intervals for 2 months. With this regimen a rebound is unlikely in patients with arthritis alone, but may occur in patients with carditis.

Anti-inflammatory drugs

Joint pains and fever usually settle rapidly with aspirin or steroids. However, over 170 papers failed to show that aspirin has any effect on the duration of the illness or the extent of valve damage after the illness. Meta-analysis of controlled trials of steroids also failed to show either effect. Although steroid is often given to patients with moderate carditis, covering withdrawal with aspirin because of the rather common rebound in symptoms, there is no scientific basis for routine use of either drug except for the control of joint pains and fever. On the other hand prednisone sometimes appears to help progressive heart failure. The required dose is usually not more than 40–60 mg daily, and gradual reduction can usually start within 1 week. Three points should be noted:

1. Treatment should not be started until the diagnosis is secure.
2. When there is evidence of deteriorating cardiac function, a severe valve lesion is present and valve repair or replacement may give the only chance of survival.
3. Aspirin and prednisone depress acute-phase reactants. The bout cannot be considered settled until the erythrocyte sedimentation rate and C-reactive protein have been normal in successive weeks, the first measurements being taken 2 weeks after stopping suppressive treatment.

Recurrence of rheumatic carditis

The risk of recurrence is highest in the first 3 years after the first attack, in young patients, and in patients with rheumatic heart disease. Carditis with a recurrence is more common in those patients in whom it was present in the first attack but it may occur in any patient. Recurrent attacks frequently lead to progressive deterioration in valvular and myocardial function.

Prophylaxis

The group A streptococcus remains uniquely sensitive to long-term, low-dose penicillin, which may be administered orally or parenterally. Regrettably, non-compliance can reach astonishing levels with oral prophylaxis. The minimum treatment period for patients without carditis is often given as 5 years, or to 18 years of age, but recurrences beyond 5 years are by no means uncommon. Annual recurrence rates above 5 per cent were recorded in years 10–15 in the pre-penicillin era. A minimum treatment period of 10 years is desirable. For patients with established heart disease more prolonged prophylaxis is mandatory and treatment is recommended to at least the age of 40 years.

Recommended treatment programme

Benzathine penicillin. Under 9 years or 27 kg: 0.9 megaunits every 4 weeks (not monthly). Over 9 years or 27 kg: 1.2 megaunits every 4 weeks. Penicillin VK or penicillin G 250 mg: 1–2 mg daily may be given in special cases.

OR *sulphadiazine.* Under 9 or 27 kg: 0.5 g. Over 9 years or 27 kg: 1.0 g daily

OR *erythromycin.* 250 mg twice daily for the patient allergic to both benzathine penicillin and sulphadiazine.

Blood levels 2 weeks after benzathine injections are extremely low and recurrences have been reported in a small percentage of compliant patients receiving 4-weekly injections; 3-weekly injections are then recommended.

Anaphylaxis to penicillin occurs in approximately 1/10 000 with death in about 1/30 000–50 000 injections. The risk is greatest in patients with advanced heart disease. Adrenaline and a resuscitation protocol must always be available. The risks are very much lower than the risks of recurrent attacks of rheumatic fever.

Further reading

Albert, D. A., Harel, L. and Karrison, T. (1995). The treatment of rheumatic carditis: A review and meta analysis: *Medicine, Baltimore*, 74, 1–12.

Taranta, L.M. (1947). Treatment of acute rheumatic fever and acute rheumatic heart disease. *American Journal of Medicine*, 285.

Wilson, N.J. and Neutze J.M. (1995). Echocardiographic diagnosis of subclinical carditis in acute rheumatic fever. *International Journal of Cardiology*, 50, 1–6.

Chapter 2.23

Valve disease

D. G. Gibson

Mitral stenosis

Aetiology

Chronic rheumatic heart disease is by far the most common cause of mitral stenosis, although a number of other pathological processes exist. It may be congenital, when it is frequently associated with other lesions including aortic or subaortic stenosis or coarctation of the aorta. In such cases, the chordae are usually short, and the spaces between them obliterated. The leaflets are thick, with rolled edges. The insertion of the papillary muscles may be abnormal. In parachute mitral valve, there is only a single papillary muscle. Congenital mitral stenosis may be associated with hypoplasia of the left ventricular cavity and the aorta, and also with endocardial fibroelastosis. Causes of acquired mitral stenosis, other than rheumatic, are rare, but include patients with calcified mitral valve ring, infective endocarditis, when bulky vegetations may cause obstruction or granulomatous infiltration in association with eosinophilia. In nodular rheumatoid arthritis, thickening of the valve cusps does not cause true mitral stenosis, but in systemic lupus erythematosus, treatment of Libman–Sachs endocarditis with steroids may lead to fibrosis of the cusps with commissural fusion. The combination of ostium secundum atrial septal defect and mitral stenosis (Lutembacher's syndrome) is probably fortuitous.

Rheumatic mitral stenosis

Incidence

The incidence of mitral stenosis approximately parallels that of acute rheumatic fever. It is commonest in the Middle East, the Indian subcontinent and the Far East, with an approximate incidence of chronic rheumatic heart disease of the order of 10 per 100 000.

Pathology

The valve becomes distorted with fusion of the commissures. The cusps are thickened, and frequently develop thrombus on their atrial surfaces. The subvalvar apparatus may also be affected, with thickening, fusion and contraction of the chordae tendineae. Finally, the valve cusps or ring may become calcified. The left ventricle is usually normal or small in pure mitral stenosis. The left atrium is enlarged: its wall may be histologically normal, but sometimes, muscle fibres are disrupted. Mural thrombosis may be present, most commonly on the free wall just above the posterior mitral valve cusp (McCallum's patch). In long-standing cases, calcification of the left atrial wall may develop in plaques on its endocardial surface. Changes of pulmonary venous congestion, pulmonary hypertension, and haemosiderosis may develop in the lungs, with dilation and hypertrophy of the right ventricle and functional tricuspid regurgitation.

Pathophysiology

The main disturbance in mitral stenosis is to left ventricular filling. When the valve area is reduced to about 2.5 cm^2, ventricular filling rate falls. This does not matter at rest when heart rate is slow and filling period relatively long, but during exercise as the heart rate increases, flow can only be maintained by increasing the pressure difference between the atrium and ventricle. If the valve area is smaller, the pressure difference is present at rest, and mean left atrial pressure rises. Patients with symptomatic mitral stenosis have a valve area of 0.75–1.25 cm^2, and a pressure drop as high as 20–30 mmHg across the valve during diastole. Cardiac output then falls and pulmonary vascular resistance usually increases. Left ventricular cavity size may be increased in the middle aged or elderly with mitral stenosis and the end-diastolic pressure may rise. A number of factors contribute including restriction of filling, coronary emboli, and distortion of the septum by right ventricular hypertrophy and overload. Chronic left atrial hypertension causes a corresponding rise in pulmonary capillary pressure; clinical evidence of pulmonary congestion appears when it reaches about 25 mmHg. Reactive pulmonary hypertension is a further problem.

Clinical picture

Symptoms

These usually appear insidiously. Less frequently, the onset is abrupt with an attack of acute pulmonary oedema, systemic embolism, or the onset of atrial fibrillation. The most common symptom is breathlessness and, less frequently, fatigue, or palpitation. Anginal pain may result from previous coronary embolism, or possibly from pulmonary hypertension and right ventricular hypertrophy. Recurrent chest infection or winter bronchitis are very characteristic. Haemoptysis is common, and caused by chest infections, pulmonary infarction, acute pulmonary oedema, or 'pulmonary apoplexy' (the rupture of a small blood vessel within the lung). Systemic embolism from the left atrium is common, particularly when atrial fibrillation is present. Pulmonary emboli may originate in the right atrium. Salt and water retention is common.

Physical examination

In pure mitral stenosis, the character of the pulse is normal, although its amplitude may be decreased and the rhythm irregular due to atrial fibrillation. All arterial pulses should be checked in view of the possibility of previous arterial emboli. Palpation at the apex may reveal a palpable first sound (a 'tapping apex') and, less frequently, a palpable opening snap. It may also be possible to feel pulmonary valve closure if severe pulmonary hypertension is present. A left parasternal heave is usually due to right ventricular hypertrophy caused by pulmonary hypertension. On auscultation the classical findings are a loud first sound, preceded by a presystolic murmur if the patient is in sinus rhythm, an opening snap and a delayed diastolic murmur. The opening snap is characteristic, usually loudest at the lower left sternal edge, less commonly the apex or the base, and is absent if the valve structure is severely disorganized. The delayed diastolic murmur starts after the opening snap, separated from it by an appreciable interval. If the stenosis is mild, the murmur is short, but if the murmur lasts throughout diastole at a normal ventricular rate, the degree of stenosis is likely to be at least moderately severe.

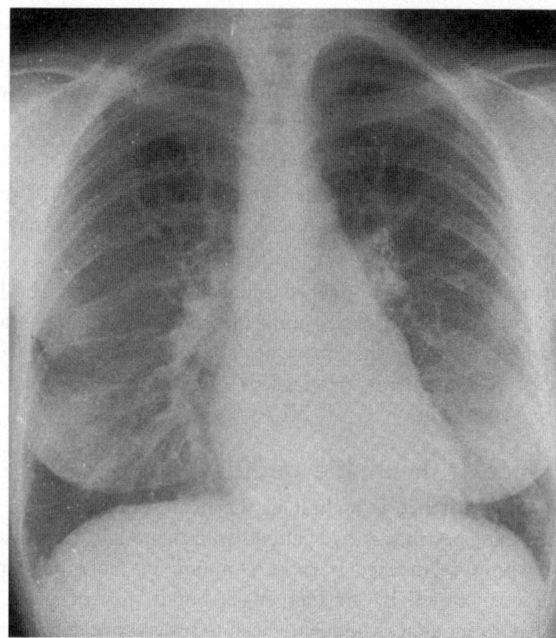

Fig. 1 Chest radiograph from a patient with pure mitral stenosis. Heart size is normal, but the left atrial appendage is enlarged. The upper lobe vessels are dilated and there are Kerley lines at both bases.

In some patients no diastolic murmur can be heard even at slow heart rates (silent mitral stenosis). These patients often have pulmonary hypertension, but the reason for the absence of a murmur is not clear.

Chest radiograph

The appearance of mitral stenosis are characteristic (Fig. 1). The most frequent abnormality is selective enlargement of the left atrium. Mitral valve calcification may be visible on the posteroanterior film just to the left of the spine. The upper lobe veins may be dilated with the patient in the erect position, indicating that left atrial pressure is raised, and the main pulmonary artery may be enlarged due to pulmonary hypertension. Pulmonary oedema may develop, with lymphatic lines, basal pleural effusions, generalized hazy shadowing, and finally obvious interstitial oedema. Long-standing left atrial hypertension may cause pulmonary haemosiderosis.

The electrocardiograph (ECG) is not generally very informative but in sinus rhythm may show bifid P waves in lead II and a dominant negative deflection in V1 reflecting left atrial hypertrophy, together with evidence of right ventricular hypertrophy.

Echocardiography has greatly improved diagnosis and management of mitral valve disease and has rendered cardiac catheterization unnecessary other than to assess the coronary circulation or as a prelude to balloon valvuloplasty.

Differential diagnosis

Left atrial myxoma may mimic all the physical signs of mitral stenosis including delayed diastolic and presystolic murmurs, loud first sound, and opening snap ('tumour plop', actually a modified third sound) (see Chapter 2.24).

Cor triatriatum may mimic mitral stenosis, particularly in childhood.

Pulmonary veno-occlusive disease may also present as silent mitral stenosis, often with a raised pulmonary wedge but a normal left atrial pressure.

Ostium secundum atrial septal defects (see Chapter 2.21) can resemble mitral stenosis because of a tricuspid flow murmur but the distinction is easily made by echocardiography.

In the *Austin Flint murmur* of severe aortic regurgitation the delayed diastolic murmur is due to the effects of the regurgitant stream of blood impinging on the anterior cusp or the mitral valve and is easily demonstrated by echocardiography.

Treatment

Medical

1. Patients below the age of 21 require penicillin prophylaxis against further attacks of acute rheumatic fever
2. Atrial fibrillation should be treated with a digitalis preparation to control the ventricular rate. Anticoagulant therapy should be given to all patients with atrial fibrillation, unless there are very strong contraindications, and perhaps also in middle aged and elderly patients in sinus rhythm in whom the incidence of embolism is not negligible.
3. Fluid retention responds well to treatment with diuretics.
4. Chest infections should be treated promptly with appropriate antimicrobials.
5. In all patients with valvular heart disease, prophylactic antimicrobial should be given for all dental manipulations and potentially septic hazards.

Mitral valvuloplasty

Fusion of the mitral commissures is susceptible to rupture by inflating a catheter-mounted balloon across the valve orifice but not all patients are suitable for valvuloplasty. There should be no more than minimal regurgitation. Ideally, the cusps should be pliable, with no calcification in the commissures. The subvalve apparatus should not be scarred or contracted, and clot in the left atrial appendix should have been excluded by transoesophageal echocardiography. Using this procedure, a satisfactory fall in transmitral pressure difference is usually achieved, and maintained in the short and medium term. Mitral regurgitation may be provoked, sometimes severe enough to require valve replacement.

Surgery

Available surgical procedures include mitral valvotomy, open or closed, and mitral valve replacement. The choice depends on the anatomy of the mitral valve, the age of the patient, and the surgical resources available. Closed mitral valvotomy is a relatively simple procedure. It is appropriate in a young patient, in sinus rhythm, with evidence of a mobile anterior cusp. Symptom-free follow-up of 30 years or more occurs regularly after this procedure. Open valvotomy allows a more complete procedure to be undertaken and the subvalvular apparatus can be inspected and adherent chordae divided. Valve replacement will be required if the cusps are greatly thickened or calcified but should not be considered in patients in whom the haemodynamic disturbance is mild, as the prosthesis causes a resting diastolic pressure drop across it, as well as interfering with systolic and diastolic left ventricular function.

Prognosis

Mitral stenosis is usually a progressive disease, although the rate is unpredictable. Surgical treatment has improved the prognosis considerably. Although mitral valvotomy does not prevent progression of the rheumatic process, or reduce the risk of infective endocarditis, it is not unusual to see a patient several decades after surgery still with effectively normal flow velocities across the mitral valve. It is still premature to assess the long-term prognosis of patients who have been treated by valvuloplasty. The life of biological mitral valve substitutes, particularly the porcine xenograft, is limited to no more than 10 years in the majority of patients above the age of 21, and considerably less than this in children. The use of biological valves should thus be confined to the very elderly, and to young women who wish to undertake pregnancy knowing that repeat surgery will be needed.

Mixed mitral valve disease

Mitral stenosis with regurgitation is almost invariably rheumatic in origin. The regurgitation is not usually severe in terms of the volume load that it imposes on the left ventricle, but the increased stroke volume is associated with an increased mitral diastolic pressure drop and the presence of mitral regurgitation implies a more damaged mitral valve.

Symptoms

The main complaint is of progressive reduction in exercise tolerance, although dyspnoea is frequently less prominent than fatigue or palpitation on exertion. Exacerbation of symptoms may result from chest infection or fluid retention, and systemic embolism remains a possibility.

Physical examination

Patients are usually in atrial fibrillation. The pulse character is normal. The venous pressure may be raised due to increased right ventricular end-diastolic pressure, to tricuspid valve disease, or to obstruction to right heart filling due to massive enlargement of the left atrium. A left parasternal heave is often present. The first sound is not usually palpable and a sustained apex beat suggests the presence of additional aortic valve disease or impaired left ventricular function. The first heart sound is soft, reflecting thickening or calcification of the anterior cusp, rather than the degree of mitral regurgitation, and the opening snap either soft or absent. The pansystolic murmur, loudest towards the axilla, reflects fibrosis and retraction of the posterior cusp. The delayed diastolic murmur is not usually of full length, but may be loud. Ankle oedema or ascites are unusual in the absence of tricuspid regurgitation.

The chest radiograph shows an enlarged heart with selective enlargement of the left atrium which may increase to a volume of up to 3 litres ('giant left atrium'—Fig. 2). There may be calcification in its wall as well as in the mitral valve cusps. The lung fields show similar changes to those of pure mitral stenosis.

The ECG confirms atrial fibrillation and may show voltage changes of left ventricular hypertrophy.

Echocardiography shows characteristic changes and again renders cardiac catheterization unnecessary unless to assess the coronary circulation.

Diagnosis and treatment

This is not usually in doubt. The severity of the overall lesion is best determined from the symptoms. Attempts to determine the relative importance of the stenosis and regurgitation are unhelpful, as the mitral regurgitation is seldom severe. It is more important to establish the presence or absence of other valvular lesions, particularly of the aortic and tricuspid valves. A giant left atrium is not necessarily

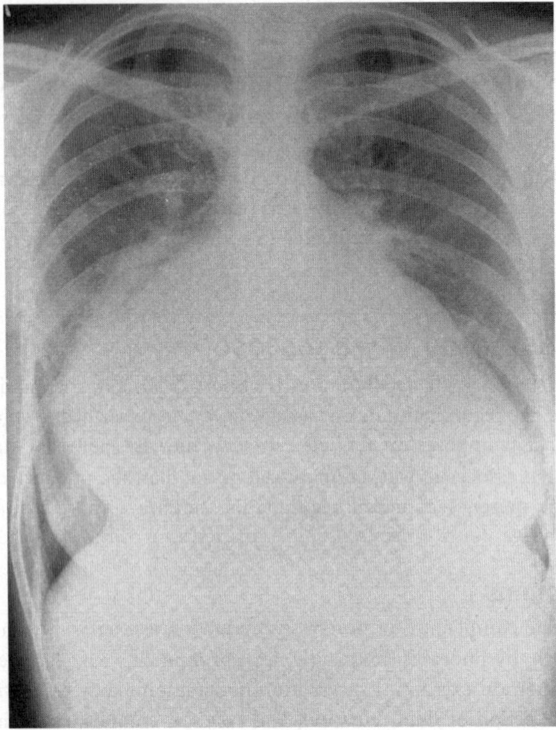

Fig. 2 Chest radiograph from a patient with mixed mitral valve disease, showing gross cardiac enlargement, due mainly to dilation of the left atrium.

evidence that the disease is severe, and its presence may actually improve the prognosis by damping the oscillations of the left atrial pressure. Similarly, the presence and severity of any pulmonary hypertension is not of major importance in determining the severity of the symptoms, or in assessing the timing or risk of operation. Treatment is on the same lines as for pure mitral stenosis, except that valvuloplasty is likely to be inappropriate, and operation will almost certainly involve mitral valve replacement.

Mitral regurgitation

Aetiology

There are a number of causes of pure mitral regurgitation (Table 1). The most common of these is the floppy mitral valve (also called mucinous or myxomatous degeneration, or ballooning or billowing mitral valve). It is relatively common above the age of 50, and is a non-inflammatory process which may affect either cusp, partially or completely. The most striking abnormality is an increase in cusp area, causing folding and upward doming into the left atrium during systole. The chordae may become elongated, tortuous, and thinned, predisposing to chordal rupture. The abnormal chordae can undergo fibrosis, as can the cusps, leading to an erroneous diagnosis of chronic rheumatic involvement. Ulceration of the cusps may also occur, predisposing to thrombosis on their surface, and also to infective endocarditis. The ring circumference may be normal or increased. The papillary muscles are normal.

The cause of sporadic cases of floppy mitral valve is unknown. However, similar appearances may complicate Marfan's syndrome, pseudoxanthoma elasticum, Ehlers–Danlos syndrome, and osteogenesis imperfecta.

Infective endocarditis is an important cause of mitral regurgitation. It may occur on an otherwise normal valve particularly in the old or

Table 1 Common causes of pure mitral regurgitation

Structure affected	Anatomical fault	Pathogenesis
Valve cusps	Congenital cleft	Primary atrial septal defect
		Isolated
	Redundant cusps	Floppy valve
		Marfan's syndrome
	Perforation	Infective endocarditis
	Scarring	Rheumatic
	Iatrogenic	Fenfluramine
Chordae	Redundant	Floppy valve
		Marfan's syndrome
		Other CT diseases
	Rupture	Floppy valve
		Marfan's syndrome
		Other CT diseases
		Infective endocarditis
		Rheumatic
	Shortening	Rheumatic
		EMF
Papillary muscle	Dysfunction	Ischaemic heart disease
		Cardiomyopathy
	Prolapsing cusp	Various
	Rupture	Acute myocardial infarction
Valve ring	Dilatation	Severe LV disease
	Calcification	Various

CT, connective tissue; EMF, endomyocardial fibrosis, LV, left ventricular.

debilitated, but more commonly there are minor congenital abnormalities such as floppy mitral valve, hypertrophic cardiomyopathy, valve calcification, or previous rheumatic disease.

Pathophysiology of mitral regurgitation

There is a large increase in left ventricular output. Ejection begins almost immediately after the start of left ventricular contraction, and at the time of aortic valve opening, up to one-quarter of the stroke volume may already have entered the left atrium. Left atrial pressures are increased, with the V wave sometimes reaching 50–60 mmHg. These high pressures shorten the phase of isovolumic relaxation and greatly increase the velocity of early diastolic left ventricular filling. Left ventricular end-diastolic cavity size is not greatly increased but end-systolic size is considerably smaller than normal due to the low force opposing ejection. Left ventricular output is maintained by a sinus tachycardia.

Clinical picture

The clinical picture is very variable, depending on the underlying pathology, the severity of the regurgitation, and whether or not the left ventricle is diseased. Tachycardia is frequent, and the pulse is 'jerky'. The venous pressure is usually normal. The apex beat is prominent and sustained, and may be double due to a palpable third sound. A systolic thrill may also be present. A left parasternal heave reflects the presence of systolic expansion of the left atrium or of left ventricular disease, rather than right ventricular hypertrophy. The first sound is normal or reduced in intensity and the most prominent features are a loud pansystolic murmur and a third heart sound. If the mitral regurgitation is very severe, left atrial and left ventricular pressures equalize before the end of systole, so that the murmur stops early. In cases presenting with acute pulmonary oedema and shock, the mitral valve is effectively absent, and there is no murmur at all. The position at which the amplitude of the murmur appears maximal varies between patients.

Diagnosis

This is made from the clinical picture and is best confirmed by echocardiography.

Ruptured chordae tendineae

The onset of symptoms is usually gradual but may be so sudden that patients are able to describe exactly what they were doing at the onset. In these latter cases, the symptoms are most severe at their onset, and improve over the next few weeks, as the ventricle adapts to the volume load. Even in this compensated phase, exercise tolerance may be severely limited. The most severe cases may present in intractable pulmonary oedema but, when the regurgitation is only moderately severe, it is remarkably well tolerated for many years with minimal symptoms.

Papillary muscle dysfunction

Function of the papillary muscles may be disturbed in a number of ways. They may be affected by ischaemic or other left ventricular disease, so that their ability to contract is impaired. If left ventricular cavity size is greatly increased, the relation between wall movement and papillary muscle shortening becomes abnormal. In hypertrophic cardiomyopathy, the greatly hypertrophied papillary muscles and abnormal cavity shape may contribute to the characteristic forward movement of the whole mitral valve during systole.

Mitral regurgitation attributed to papillary muscle dysfunction is usually mild. The clinical picture is usually dominated by the left ventricular disease. A late or pansystolic murmur often varies in its intensity and timing from day to day, and becomes softer with successful treatment of the underlying condition. Echocardiography demonstrates a large cavity with poor wall movement.

Ruptured papillary muscle

This is a rare complication of acute myocardial infarction. Complete rupture may occur, or less commonly, only a single head may be involved. Complete rupture usually occurs 2–5 days after the infarct, and is rarely associated with survival for more than 24 or 48 h without very prompt surgical intervention. Death is due to cardiogenic shock and pulmonary oedema. A pansystolic murmur may sometimes be audible at the apex. Partial rupture occurs rather later after the infarct and causes a striking deterioration in clinical state, along with the development of a pansystolic murmur. It can be diagnosed by echocardiography and treated by early mitral valve replacement.

Mitral prolapse

This has been a confused subject as assessment and definition have varied between observations made by operation, angiography, or echocardiography. As demonstrated by echocardiography, it does not represent a single entity (see OTM3, p. 2460). Many patients have floppy mitral valves, with varying degrees of regurgitation. In others, the primary abnormality may be cardiomyopathy. However, identical echocardiographic findings have been documented in up to 21 per cent of presumably normal females of college age. In addition, it may not be possible to demonstrate prolapse by echocardiography in patients with clear-cut mid-systolic click and late systolic murmur. Although these findings are non-specific, they do have a number of important clinical associations.

1. Non-rheumatic mitral valve disease, with evidence of mitral prolapse, is a significant cause of infective endocarditis. All patients in whom minor mitral valve abnormalities are suspected should have antimicrobial prophylaxis.
2. Young people with clear-cut mitral prolapse have a significantly increased risk of cerebral embolism from non-bacterial thrombotic vegetations. This is unusual, and there is no indication to treat all patients with long-term anticoagulants.
3. A minority of patients develop chest pain, characteristic of angina, or more commonly 'atypical' but often associated with inferior T wave changes on the resting ECG. Coronary arteriography is normal.
4. Ventricular ectopic beats are common. Much less frequently, recurrent ventricular arrhythmias may occur; very rarely these may be life threatening. It is these unusual cases that form the basis of reports of sudden death in this condition. Approximately half of such cases had a history of syncopal or presyncopal episodes. A late systolic murmur was common, but a mid-systolic click was unusual. The resting ECG almost invariably showed T wave abnormalities and ectopic beats. The autopsy appearances were those of floppy mitral valve.

Endomyocardial fibrosis (see Chapter 2.19)

The clinical picture is of progressive mitral or tricuspid insufficiency of insidious onset, together with restriction of ventricular filling by subendocardial scarring. When the tricuspid valve is mainly involved, there is gross fluid retention, whereas mitral or combined involvement leads to pulmonary oedema. Emboli from the right or left ventricle are common.

Mitral ring calcification

Heavy calcification of the mitral valve ring is a disease of the elderly, and is more common in females, and is associated with aortic stenosis or hypertension. It usually causes no symptoms, but is a potential source of systemic emboli, and a focus for infective endocarditis. Approximately half the patients have abnormalities of conduction, including atrioventricular block, sinus node disease or bundle branch block. Mild mitral regurgitation is common. In the absence of complications, no treatment is required other than prophylaxis against infective endocarditis.

Differential diagnosis of mitral regurgitation

This includes ventricular septal defect, aortic stenosis, and tricuspid regurgitation. Physical signs usually differentiate and the true diagnosis is confirmed by echocardiography.

Treatment

Mild or moderately severe mitral regurgitation does not require treatment apart from prophylaxis for endocarditis. When regurgitation is due to papillary muscle dysfunction, treatment is that of the

Table 2 Types of aortic stenosis

Valvular	***Fixed subaortic***
• Congenital	• Membrane
• Fused commissure 'bicuspid'	• Tunnel
• Rheumatic	***Supravalvular***
• 'Senile' (calcified tricuspid valve)	
• Infective endocarditis (rare)	
• Hyperlipidaemia (rare)	

underlying condition. Severe mitral regurgitation, which causes significant symptoms in spite of medical treatment, is best managed by mitral valve surgery either repair or replacement. After acute chordal rupture, it is often possible to treat patients medically with rest, diuretics, and vasodilators for 1–2 weeks, while the left ventricle enlarges to compensate for the increased volume load. Clinical improvement may be striking, so that surgery then becomes a less hazardous procedure than an emergency operation in the acute stage would have been.

Aortic stenosis

The obstruction is most commonly at the level of the valve itself, but may also be immediately above the sinuses or within the left ventricle (Table 2).

Valvar aortic stenosis

This is most common in the elderly, but may present at any age. Congenital aortic stenosis presents most frequently in infancy or childhood. A much more common abnormality, the congenital bicuspid valve, may be detected as an incidental finding early in life, but does not usually give rise to significant haemodynamic abnormality unless it becomes calcified or involved by infective endocarditis. Rheumatic aortic stenosis may result in calcification. Senile or degenerative aortic stenosis which results from deposition of calcium in a tricuspid valve in the absence of any inflammatory process, is becoming increasingly common in an ageing population.

Pathophysiology

The systolic pressure drop between the left ventricular cavity and the aorta in symptomatic cases, may be greater than 50–70 mmHg at rest, and reach over 200 mmHg on exertion. As a result left ventricular hypertrophy develops, although the cavity size remains normal or reduced. This hypertrophy and associated fibrosis causes the stiffness of the myocardium to increase so that the end-diastolic pressure may rise causing pulmonary congestion and predisposes to ventricular arrhythmias. Late in the disease the cavity becomes dilated and more spherical in shape. In the majority of cases, calcification is confined to the aortic valve, but in a minority it may spread to involve the anterior cusp of the mitral valve or the atrioventricular node, giving rise to a prolonged P–R interval or even to complete heart block. Obstructive coronary artery disease may contribute to symptoms or the impairment of left ventricular function.

Clinical picture

Symptoms

The three characteristic clinical features of aortic stenosis are breathlessness, chest pain, and syncope. Breathlessness occurs at first on exercise, but later at rest. Paroxysmal nocturnal dyspnoea is common in late stages of the disease. Typical anginal pain can occur in patients in whom the coronary arteries are normal. The mechanism for this may represent the effect of abnormal myocardial relaxation in left ventricular hypertrophy on coronary flow. Syncope probably reflects a number of different types of disturbance. In some patients, it is related to exertion and appears to be due to hypotension resulting from the combination of exercise-induced vasodilation and a fixed cardiac output. In others, it results from transient complete atrioventricular block due to involvement of the atrioventricular node by calcification, carotid sinus hypersensitivity, or even from short periods of ventricular tachycardia or fibrillation. Similar mechanisms may underlie the increased incidence of sudden death in these patients. Patients with long-standing aortic stenosis may present with severe breathlessness, a large heart on radiography, a small volume pulse with a normal upstroke, a third heart sound, and pansystolic murmur due to papillary muscle dysfunction suggesting dilated cardiomyopathy. Investigation to exclude aortic stenosis which might be suitable for surgical treatment is essential in such a presentation.

Clinical examination

The carotid pulse is slow rising with a reduced amplitude and an early notch on the upstroke, followed by a thrill. The venous pressure is usually normal until late in the disease, but a small 'a' wave may relate to the presence of left ventricular hypertrophy (Bernheim 'a' wave). The apex beat is sustained and often double, due to the presence of an additional left atrial impulse. The first sound is normal or soft, and may be preceded by a fourth heart sound. The second sound is single when the valve is calcified. When left ventricular disease is severe, pulmonary valve closure is accentuated. The characteristic ejection systolic murmur is maximal at the base of the heart, and is also audible over the right common carotid artery. An additional short, soft early diastolic murmur is nearly always present, although this does not imply haemodynamically significant aortic regurgitation.

ECG characteristically shows changes of left ventricular hypertrophy, although it may be entirely normal, even in the presence of severe aortic stenosis. Left atrial hypertrophy is shown by a bifid P wave in lead II or a dominant negative deflection in V1. Conduction disturbances may be present. Poor progression of R waves across the chest leads is common, and may be caused by septal hypertrophy rather than anterior myocardial infarction.

Echocardiography is the best technique to confirming the diagnosis and assessing functions (Fig. 3) but cardiac catheterization may be needed to confirm the pressure gradient across the valve in the minority of cases in whom continuous wave Doppler is difficult for technical reasons.

Treatment

Medical treatment has little to offer in aortic stenosis; in mild cases it is unnecessary, and in severe ones ineffective, but all patients with aortic stenosis, should have prophylactic antimicrobials for any potentially septic hazard. Patients with severe left ventricular disease and fluid retention will benefit from a period of bed rest and treatment with a diuretic before operation is contemplated, but the primary abnormality cannot be significantly modified by diuretic agents. Severe aortic stenosis requires intervention. Aortic balloon valvuloplasty is almost uniformly ineffective in adults in whom the cusps are calcified. Aortic valve replacement, however, is an extremely effective operation. In uncomplicated cases, it can be carried out with low mortality and morbidity, and thus should be considered in all patients in whom

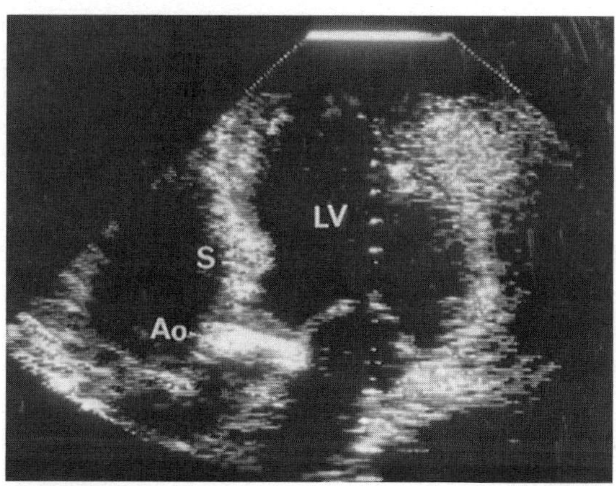

Fig. 3 Aortic stenosis, two-dimensional echocardiogram from apical four-chamber view, showing left ventricle (LV) and heavily calcified aortic valve (Ao). Se, septum.

the disease causes significant symptoms. Associated coronary artery disease is usually treated with bypass grafting at the same operation. Aortic valve replacement is also effective when significant aortic stenosis is complicated by severe left ventricular enlargement, although the risks of surgery are naturally somewhat greater.

Aortic stenosis and incompetence

Aetiology

The combination usually results from chronic rheumatic heart disease, but may also be caused by infective endocarditis on a previously stenotic valve.

Clinical picture

The clinical features do not differ significantly from those of pure aortic stenosis, except that breathlessness is usually the most prominent symptom. The character of the carotid pulse is modified, being bisferiens, a term that describes the presence of a notch half way up the upstroke. Left ventricular hypertrophy is shown by a sustained apical impulse, with or without a palpable left atrial contraction. The diagnosis is confirmed by aortic systolic and diastolic murmurs, maximal down the left sternal edge. If the patient is in atrial fibrillation, evidence of additional rheumatic mitral valve disease should be sought.

Chest radiography shows moderate cardiac enlargement and, in older patients, evidence of aortic valve calcification. Echocardiography can be used to measure left ventricular cavity size and thus to gain some idea of the severity of the regurgitation from the stroke volume. The pressure drop across the aortic valve is estimated by continuous wave Doppler, and colour flow mapping can give some idea of the extent of regurgitation. The main differential diagnosis is from pure aortic stenosis, or regurgitation. The indications for surgery are similar to those for pure stenosis or regurgitation.

Aortic regurgitation

Aortic regurgitation may result from a number of pathological mechanisms (Table 3).

Table 3 Causes of aortic regurgitation

Cusp	*Ring*
• Distortion	• Dilatation
• Rheumatic	• Dissecting aneurysm
• Rheumatoid	• Marfan's syndrome
• Fenfluramine	• Syphilis
• Perforation	• Ankylosing spondylitis
• Infective endocarditis	• Reiter's syndrome, ulcerative colitis
• Traumatic	***Loss of support***
	• Subaortic ventricular septal defect

Pathology

Rheumatic involvement leads to cusp thickening, with rolled edges, and fused commissures. There may be superimposed calcification or thrombosis. Infective endocarditis may lead to cusp destruction or perforation and may spread to involve the sinus of Valsalva, the atrioventricular node and the interventricular septum, where abscess formation may occur. Dilatation of the aortic ring may cause aortic regurgitation with normal cusps as in Marfan's syndrome, isolated medionecrosis, ankylosing spondylitis, rheumatoid arthritis, Reiter's syndrome, or relapsing polychondritis. Syphilitic aortitis causes dilatation of the valve ring, with aneurysm formation of the ascending aorta and involvement of the coronary ostia. Dissecting aneurysm involving the aortic root may separate the cusps from the valve ring; and the presence of a high ventricular septal defect or Fallot's tetralogy may leave the cusps unsupported from below.

Pathophysiology

There is an increase in left ventricular stroke volume with a corresponding increase in left ventricular cavity size, but wall thickness is usually within normal limits. In moderately severe cases, the stroke volume is twice normal, and when it is severe, up to three or even four times normal. The end-diastolic pressure in the aorta is low, so that the resistance to ejection of blood by the left ventricle is reduced. This, together with the large stroke volume, explains the characteristic rapid upstroke and large volume pulse. In long-standing cases, left ventricular cavity size increases out of proportion to the stroke volume, with loss of the normal myocardial architecture, so that the cavity becomes more spherical in shape, the walls stiffer, and the end-diastolic pressure increased.

Clinical picture

Patients may remain asymptomatic for many years. Ultimately breathlessness begins, usually on exercise, but the presenting symptom may be nocturnal dyspnoea, or an attack of acute pulmonary oedema precipitated by severe exertion. Chest pain may result from a low coronary perfusion pressure during diastole, coexistent coronary artery disease, or ostial involvement in syphilitic aortitis. A similar retrosternal pain, aggravated by exertion, may develop in patients with aneurysms of the ascending aorta, which seems to originate from the aortic root itself.

The carotid pulse has a large amplitude and a rapid upstroke, (collapsing). There may be visible arterial pulsation in the neck (Corrigan's sign). Other signs which depend on a large pulse volume and peripheral vasodilation include capillary pulsation in the nail beds. Durosiez's sign is elicited by compression of the femoral artery and listening proximally with the stethoscope for a diastolic murmur. It implies retrograde flow in the femoral artery due to aortic regurgitation that is at least moderately severe. The peripheral pulses

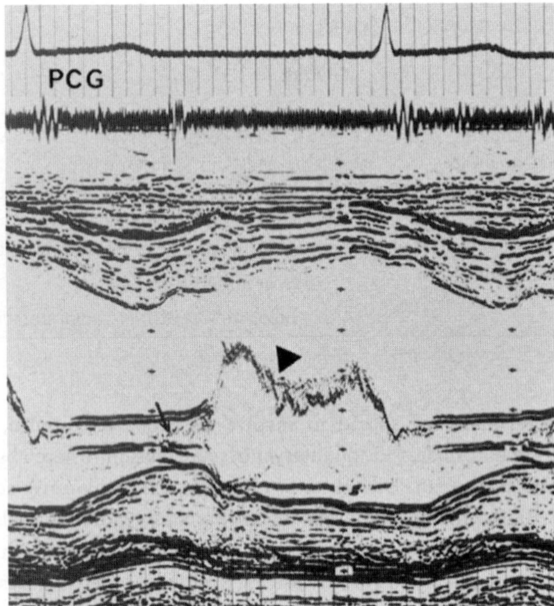

Fig. 4 Chronic aortic regurgitation, M-mode echocardiogram, showing 'flutter' on the anterior cusp of the mitral valve, marked by the arrow. PCG, phonocardiogram.

should always be checked to exclude the presence of coarctation of the aorta. The venous pressure is normal until late in the course of the disease. The left ventricular impulse is sustained. The early diastolic murmur, usually maximal down the left sternal edge, may be loudest at the apex or even in the left axilla. An ejection systolic murmur is nearly always present, due to increased flow across the valve. Aortic valve closure is not usually audible, but pulmonary hypertension may increase the pulmonary second sound. A third heart sound may be present, if the left ventricular cavity is dilated but, more commonly, a delayed diastolic murmur may be audible, indistinguishable from that of mitral stenosis (Austin Flint murmur). In addition, there may be a mitral pansystolic murmur due to dilatation of the valve ring.

The ECG shows left ventricular hypertrophy. Left bundle branch block may develop, and a long P–R is suggestive of disease of the aortic root.

Echocardiography confirms the diagnosis and allows calculation of the stroke volume and defines the anatomy of the aortic valve and root (Fig. 4).

Assessment

It is not enough to establish the presence of aortic regurgitation; its severity must be estimated and the state of the left ventricle assessed. In uncomplicated cases, the severity can be judged indirectly from the carotid pulse and from the heart size on chest radiography, but direct measurement of left ventricular cavity size and stroke volume by echocardiography or angiography is much more satisfactory. It is usually unnecessary to establish the exact aetiology, although it is important to exclude infection and investigate the presence of disease of the aortic root.

Treatment

Mild aortic regurgitation is well tolerated and requires no treatment other than prophylactic antimicrobial to prevent infective endocarditis. Patients with moderately severe regurgitation should receive prophylactic angiotensin-converting enzyme inhibitor, which delays

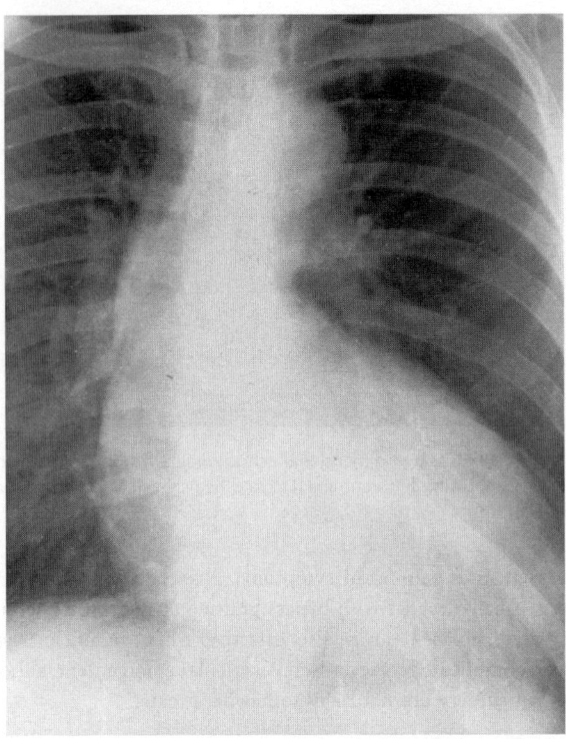

Fig. 5 Chest radiograph from a patient with chronic aortic regurgitation showing cardiac enlargement and dilation of the ascending aorta.

surgery by 3–4 years. Severe regurgitation should be treated by valve replacement. Evidence of left ventricular disease, aortic root disease, increasing heart size on chest radiography (Fig. 5), or cavity size on echocardiography, or a history of infective endocarditis, are all indications for early operation. Those not selected for surgery require regular review as left ventricular disease may develop over as short a period as 1–2 years in the absence of symptoms.

Acquired tricuspid valve disease

Tricuspid stenosis

Organic tricuspid stenosis is almost invariably due to chronic rheumatic heart disease, and usually coexists with mitral valve disease, although its incidence is about one-tenth. The two conditions are similar both with respect to their pathology and to the functional disturbance that they cause. The primary functional abnormality is obstruction to right ventricular filling associated with a diastolic pressure drop across the valve. This causes an increase in right atrial pressure, which leads to ascites and peripheral oedema

Clinical picture

The problem is to recognize the presence of additional tricuspid stenosis in a patient known to have mitral and possibly also aortic valve disease. A number of indications may be sought. Tricuspid stenosis is often associated with an 'a' wave in the venous pulse and with evidence of right atrial hypertrophy on ECG. A separate tricuspid delayed diastolic murmur may be audible, maximal down the left sternal edge or in the epigastrium. Echocardiography confirms the diagnosis, and the diastolic pressure drop can be estimated by continuous wave Doppler. Previously undiagnosed tricuspid stenosis may be unmasked by successful mitral valve surgery.

Table 4 Causes of tricuspid regurgitation

Organic	*Functional*
• Rheumatic	• Fenfluramine
• Infective endocarditis	• Cirrhosis of the liver
• Ebstein's anomaly	• Endomyocardial fibrosis
• Atrioventricular defect	• Prolapsing cusp
• Carcinoid syndrome	

Treatment with diuretics is not very satisfactory. Definitive treatment is either valvotomy or repair. Isolated tricuspid stenosis, developing after mitral valve surgery can be dealt with by balloon valvuloplasty if the anatomy is suitable. Tricuspid valve replacement is avoided whenever possible, because of the pressure drop in diastole across all prostheses.

Tricuspid regurgitation

A number of different pathological processes may cause tricuspid regurgitation (Table 4). It is frequently functional, occurring in association with dilatation of the right ventricular cavity.

Organic tricuspid regurgitation may be congenital, as an isolated abnormality, or associated with Ebstein's anomaly. A cleft right-sided atrioventricular valve may also occur in ostrium primum atrial septal defect. Acquired organic tricuspid regurgitation may be rheumatic in origin, or result from infective endocarditis of a previously normal valve, which occurs particularly commonly in intravenous drug users. Right-sided endomyocardial fibrosis causes scarring and distortion of the tricuspid subvalvular apparatus. The carcinoid syndrome is associated with severe tricuspid regurgitation, and similar findings may occur after methysergide therapy, and in long-standing hepatic cirrhosis. Mid-systolic prolapse of the tricuspid valve can occur in exactly the same way as that of the mitral valve, and is common in Marfan's syndrome. Organic tricuspid regurgitation has been described as a long-term consequence of radiotherapy to the thorax, when it may be associated with features of pericardial constriction or restrictive myocardial disease, making its diagnosis difficult.

The *clinical features* are those of severe and chronic elevation of the venous pressure, often in association with disease on the left side of the heart. The symptoms are non-specific, but are often related to the development of oedema or ascites: hepatic enlargement may be associated with nausea and upper abdominal or epigastric pain aggravated by exercise. The mean venous pressure may be very high, greater than 15 cm, with pulsations visible in the retinal vessels or palpable in the femoral veins. The high venous pressure is also responsible for occasional protein-losing enteropathy. In approximately two-thirds of patients, there is associated systolic expansile pulsation of the liver. In long-standing cases, hepatic fibrosis develops, associated with mild jaundice. In approximately one-third of cases, a tricuspid pansystolic murmur is present, which is audible down the left sternal edge. Echocardiography is the best way of making the diagnosis.

Treatment with diuretics deals with fluid retention, and may even allow right ventricular cavity size to decrease restoring competence to the tricuspid valve. Surgical treatment is avoided if possible, but if the regurgitation is very severe, and the fluid retention requires doses of diuretics large enough to cause significant metabolic consequences, intervention may be considered, but postoperative jaundice is very common.

Pulmonary valve disease

Acquired pulmonary valve disease is unusual. The most common form is associated with severe pulmonary hypertension and dilatation of the pulmonary valve ring, causing mild regurgitation and a soft early diastolic murmur (the Graham–Steell murmur). Rheumatic pulmonary regurgitation is extremely rare, and when present contributes little to overall disability. Pulmonary regurgitation may also form part of the carcinoid syndrome, or follow pulmonary valvotomy for pulmonary stenosis.

Management of patients with valve prostheses

Valve prostheses may be mechanical or biological. Mechanical prostheses are likely to be the ball and cage type (e.g. Starr–Edwards), the tilting disc, or the bileaflet. Biological prostheses consist of a plastic stent on which cusps made from some biological material are mounted. The cusps may be derived from porcine aortic valve or pericardium. The main factors guiding choice is the durability of the prosthesis and the likely incidence of thrombotic complications. Present operative mortality is in the region of 3–5 per cent for single valve replacement and approximately 10 per cent for double valve replacement. Ten-year survival after single valve replacement is approximately 50–55 per cent, and after double valve replacement 35–45 per cent.

Late complications of valve replacement

Thromboembolism is a problem with all mechanical prostheses. Long-term anticoagulant therapy is essential but even with satisfactory control an incidence of significant events, of 1–2 per cent per annum can be expected. Anticoagulant therapy itself also causes bleeding complications severe enough to require admission to hospital with an incidence of approximately 1 per cent per annum. Frequent embolization may be associated with thrombosis of the prosthesis, and reoperation and replacement with a biological prosthesis may be necessary. The incidence of thromboembolic complications is much lower with biological prostheses, so that long-term anticoagulant therapy can be dispensed with in patients in sinus rhythm after aortic or mitral valve replacement.

Infection: Patients with prostheses—mechanical or biological—are at greatly increased risk of infective endocarditis. All patients should receive full antimicrobial prophylaxis for dental manipulations and other potentially septic hazards in a course lasting for at least 48 h, rather than in a single dose. Established infective endocarditis in this situation rarely responds to antimicrobial therapy alone. A second valve replacement is nearly always required.

Prosthetic dysfunction is also an important cause of morbidity. Malfunction is much more common with biological prostheses, when cusps may become calcified, perforated, or detached. Calcification of porcine bioprostheses in an aortic homograft, usually takes some 10–15 years. Mechanical prostheses are subject to thrombosis. Deterioration in function may be insidious over a period of several months or years due to ingrowth of organized clot. Alternatively, the prosthesis may clot acutely; the patient presenting with pulmonary oedema or in a low cardiac output state, and the closing click of the prosthesis no longer audible. Operation is then required as soon as possible. If the condition of the patient precludes anaesthesia, intravenous streptokinase should be given, at a dose of 500 units immediately, followed by 100 000 units hourly, although a risk of systemic embolism must be accepted. Such treatment may be associated with improvement within a few hours; the streptokinase is then neutralized, and surgery undertaken.

Paraprosthetic regurgitation in the aortic position may have been present since the original operation, but regurgitation suddenly appearing always raises the possibility that the prosthesis might have become infected.

Recognizing prosthetic dysfunction: Stenosis or regurgitation associated with a prosthesis does not have the same physical signs as the corresponding lesion of the native valve. In general, it presents as deterioration in cardiac state, whose progress may be acute or chronic. When a mitral prosthesis is involved, there are characteristically no murmurs, other than those of tricuspid regurgitation; a systolic murmur may be present in aortic valve dysfunction, but its intensity and timing differs little from that of a normally functioning prosthesis. The clinical picture may thus be indistinguishable from that of heart failure, when the possibility of prosthesis must be considered. This requires echocardiography, Doppler, and possibly cardiac catheterization.

Haemolysis: All mechanical prostheses are associated with increased intravascular haemolysis but this rarely gives rise to clinical problems. It may become significant with a normally functioning prosthesis when the patient has a compensated haemolytic state of some different aetiology. Mild paraprosthetic regurgitation, whose severity is insufficient to give rise to any haemodynamic complications, may cause clinically significant haemolysis. Provided that haemolysis is not severe, such cases can usually be treated with iron and folic acid, but a requirement for repeated transfusion, is a strong indication for reoperation.

Left ventricular disease is now a major cause of morbidity and mortality after valve replacement. Contributing factors include preoperative disease, myocardial damage during bypass, the effects of the prosthesis, and coexisting coronary disease. The earliest clinical evidence, apart from breathlessness, may relate to right rather than left ventricular disease, with elevated venous pressure, fluid retention, and hepatic congestion. The differential diagnosis of ventricular disease after valve replacement is with prosthetic dysfunction best distinguished by echocardiography.

Further reading

Carabello, B. and Crawford, Jr. R.A. (1997). Medical progress: Valvular heart disease. *New England Journal of Medicine*, **337**, 32–41.

Cohen, D.J., Kuntz, R.E., Gordon, S.P.F., *et al.* (1992). Predictors of long-term outcome after percutaneous balloon mitral valvuloplasty. *New England Journal of Medicine*, **337**, 1329–35.

Devereux, R.B. (1998). Appetite suppressants and valvular heart disease. *New England Journal of Medicine*, **339**, 765–6.

Groves, P.H. and Hall, R.J.C. (1992). Late tricuspid regurgitation following mitral valve surgery. *Journal of Heart Valve Disease*, **1**, 80–6.

Leatham, A. and Brigden, W. (1990). Mild mitral regurgitation and the mitral prolapse fiasco. *American Heart Journal*, **99**, 659–64.

Oakley, C.M. and Burkhardt, D. (1993). Optimal timing of surgery for chronic mitral or aortic regurgitation. *Journal of Heart Valve Disease*, **2**, 223–9.

Ruttley, M.S.T. (1992). The chest radiograph in adult heart valve disease. *Journal of Heart Valve Disease*, **2**, 205–17.

Schon, H.R. (1994). Hemodynamic and morphologic changes after long term angiotensin converting enzyme inhibition in patients with chronic valvular regurgitation. *Journal of Hypertension* **12** (Suppl. 4), S95–104.

Selzer, A. (1987). Changing aspects of the natural history of aortic stenosis. *New England Journal of Medicine*, **317**, 91–8.

Vonpatanasin, W., Hillis, D., and Lange, R.A. (1996). Medical progress: Valvular heart disease. *New England Journal of Medicine*, **336**, 407–16.

Chapter 2.24

Cardiac myxoma

T. A. Traill

Cardiac myxomas are not common, but are important because they can present in a number of ways, and because the majority are easily and permanently removed by surgery. Estimates of the prevalence range from 1 to 5 per 10 000 in autopsy series, or 2 per 100 000 in the general population, with a sex ratio of 2 : 1 in favour of women. The majority of patients are between 30 and 60 years. Most cases are sporadic, but in Carney's syndrome (LAMB syndrome; NAME syndrome; Swiss syndrome) there is lentiginosis, multiple myxomas (most of them cardiac), and various kinds of endocrine overactivity or tumour, including Cushing's syndrome, acromegaly, and Sertoli cell tumour. Myxomas in Carney's syndrome may arise anywhere in the heart, are commonly multiple, and frequently recur. Inheritance is as an autosomal dominant, with centrofacial freckling as the most obvious marker of the phenotype.

Other benign cardiac tumours are the papillary fibroelastoma, usually attached to the leaflet of one of the left-sided valves, and lipoma. Malignant cardiac tumours include angiosarcoma, fibrosarcoma, malignant fibrous histiocytoma, leiomyosarcoma, and secondary deposits.

Pathology

Cardiac myxomas are benign polypoid masses arising from a stalk, ranging in size from 3 cm to as much as 10 cm or more, with a smooth or lobulated surface and gelatinous consistency. They are frequently covered with adherent thrombus. More than 75 per cent occur within the left atrium, with the base of the pedicle arising from the fossa ovalis or its rim. Occasionally they arise from the base of the mitral valve leaflets, from the posterior part of the left atrium, or from within the right atrium. Sometimes they grow in both atria, in the form of a dumb-bell.

The histology is that of a loosely woven, sparsely cellular connective tissue tumour, with very infrequent mitotic figures. Several cell types are identifiable. It is suggested that the source is a primitive multipotential mesenchymal cell, and that the predilection of these tumours for the atrial septum reflects the abundance of such cells in this region.

Clinical features

Presentation

Left atrial myxomas may mimic mitral stenosis, and cause left atrial obstruction. They may be the source of emboli to the systemic

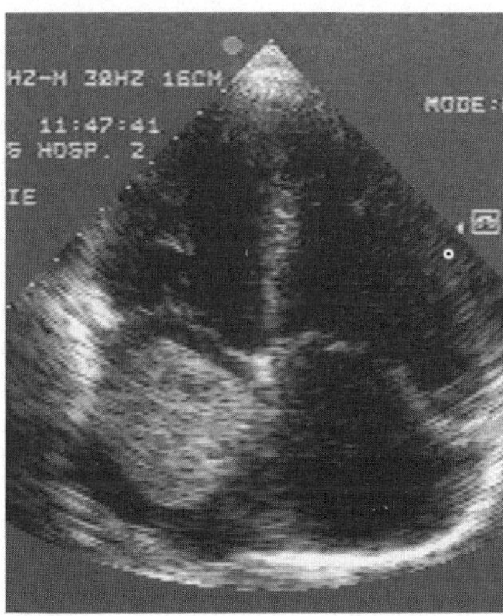

Fig. 1 Echocardiograph in the four-chamber view showing a myxoma occupying much of the left atrium.

circulation, and occasionally may present as a constitutional illness with fever. Right atrial myxomas seldom cause symptoms until they are very large, when they cause right atrial obstruction with elevated systemic venous pressure, splanchnic congestion, and oedema.

Left atrial obstruction: The presenting symptoms include progressive breathlessness, orthopnoea, paroxysmal nocturnal dyspnoea, fluid retention, and atrial arrhythmias. Examination suggests rheumatic heart disease.

Systemic emboli occur in about 40 per cent of patients and are frequently the first manifestation. Such emboli often occur while patients are in sinus rhythm. They may be sizeable, for example large enough to occlude the aortic bifurcation, and besides thrombus they frequently contain tumour material, so that histological examination may be diagnostic.

Constitutional effects predominate in about one-quarter of patients. These include fever, weight loss, Raynaud's phenomenon, finger clubbing, a raised erythrocyte sedimentation rate, and elevated immunoglobulin levels. Other abnormalities include anaemia, polycythaemia (associated particularly with right atrial tumours), leucocytosis, and thrombocytopenia. Such changes may lead to an initial diagnosis of infective endocarditis in patients who have heart murmurs, or to the suspicion of collagen vascular disease or occult malignancy.

Physical signs: Specific signs of myxoma are inconspicuous or absent in many patients. In others they vary from a prominent first heart sound to changes suggestive of mitral valve disease. Apical systolic murmurs are somewhat more common than diastolic rumbles, and occasionally there are signs of pulmonary hypertension with accentuated pulmonary closure and tricuspid regurgitation. Some patients have an audible 'tumour plop' in early diastole, analogous to a mitral opening snap. It is often recognized only after echocardiographic diagnosis. A rare but specific feature of the condition is variation of the auscultatory findings with change in posture.

Echocardiography has proved reliable for recognizing these tumours (Fig. 1). Transoesophageal echocardiography affords the opportunity to examine the tumour and its attachment with great precision.

Differential diagnosis after echocardiography is seldom difficult. Large masses may occasionally be difficult to distinguish from left atrial ball thrombus. Smaller left atrial masses may be papillary fibroelastomas, atrial septal aneurysms, or infective vegetations caused by endocarditis. Masses in the right atrium may also represent thrombus, sometimes propagated from the inferior vena cava, or occasionally venous extension of abdominal cancers, for example hypernephroma.

Treatment and prognosis

Atrial myxoma is treated by surgical removal. Except in patients with severe pulmonary hypertension, or those with profound debility, the risk is low, comparable with that of surgery for mitral valve disease. The results of surgery are good. Some patients are left with mitral regurgitation but this is seldom severe. Recurrence is uncommon except in Carney's syndrome. In these patients regular echocardiographic follow-up is required, at intervals of 6 months.

Further reading

St. John Sutton, M.G., Mercier, L.-A., Giuliani, E.R., and Lie, J.T. (1980). Atrial myxomas: a review of clinical experience in 40 patients. *Mayo Clinical Proceedings*, 55, 371–6.

Chapter 2.25

Infective endocarditis

B. Gribbin and D. W. M. Crook

Definition and classification

Infective endocarditis is characterized by a microbiological inflammation of the lining of the heart chambers, heart valves, and great vessels. Classically, the fulminant form is likely to be caused by virulent organisms such as *Staphylococcus aureus*, often attacking normal heart valves, whereas a more indolent form may present as chronic ill health of weeks or months duration, usually in patients with a pre-existing cardiac abnormality involving less virulent organisms such as the *Streptococcus viridans* group of organisms. However, the clinical effect of a given organism cannot be predicted and is modified by several other influences such as whether it has been community or hospital acquired, previous use of antibiotics, the presence of prosthetic heart valves, and a history of intravenous drug abuse. It is therefore best to classify infective endocarditis by the organism involved, the valves affected, whether native or prosthetic and with identification of other relevant clinical features.

Incidence

Infective endocarditis is uncommon, with an estimated annual incidence of 22 cases per million population in England and Wales giving rather more than 1000 cases each year, although this is almost certainly a considerable underestimation.

The pattern of the disease has changed since the advent of antibiotics. There is now an increasing incidence in the over 60s, who are more likely to have degenerative valve disease such as aortic sclerosis or calcification of the mitral annulus and to be exposed to invasive investigation and therapy. Overall, mitral valve prolapse is the most common underlying abnormality, with the aortic valve affected more often in elderly people. Endocarditis has also emerged as a serious complication of valve surgery and intravenous drug abuse.

Microbiology (see also Section 16)

Infective endocarditis can be caused by many species of bacteria and some fungi, but streptococci and staphylococci are responsible for 60 and 25 per cent of cases, respectively. The majority of causative organisms reside either in the mouth or on the skin. Chewing and tooth brushing result in a transient bacteraemia. The source of staphylococci is mainly the skin. A range of species-specific characteristics determine which organisms cause endocarditis, relating to tropism of organisms for heart valves and the type and course of the disease.

'*Streptococcus viridans*' is a group of α-haemolytic streptococci responsible for most cases of streptococcal endocarditis. They include *S. mitis*, *S. sanguis*, *S. angiosis*, (milleri), *S. salivarius*, *S. mutans*, and a distinct group of nutritionally variant streptococci. They usually inhabit the oropharynx, but *S. bovis* usually inhabits the bowel, and endocarditis caused by this organism is associated with an underlying gastrointestinal lesion, usually an adenoma or carcinoma of the large bowel. Viridans streptococci are of low pathogenicity and produce a subacute clinical picture, although *S. milleri*, frequently causes metastatic septic foci.

β-Haemolytic streptococci rarely cause infective endocarditis, but group A organisms can be responsible for fulminant disease and group C, G, and B streptococci may affect normal heart valves in adults, producing an acute form of infective endocarditis.

Enterococcus faecalis and *E. faecium* are the enterococci most commonly encountered. They form part of the normal faecal flora and are of low pathogenicity, characteristically producing subacute disease comprising between 5 and 15 per cent of infective endocarditis in most series. These organisms are resistant to most classes of antimicrobials. Cure depends on killing the organisms with a combination of gentamicin or streptomycin and a penicillin or a glycopeptide (e.g. vancomycin).

Staphylococci are the second most common cause of endocarditis. Coagulase negative staphylococci comprise many species, the most important in endocarditis being *S. epidermidis*. These organisms are associated with prosthetic valve endocarditis and infection on native valves in the elderly. The resulting disease is usually subacute.

Staphylococcus aureus endocarditis usually presents in one of four settings. First, community acquired fulminant disease affecting mainly the left sided native valves with multiple systemic emboli, rapid valve destruction, central nervous system involvement (including meningitis) and carrying a mortality of some 30 per cent. The source of such an infection is often obscure. Second, an acute febrile illness originating from an intravenous line which is untreated may evolve into the fulminating disease described above. Third, fulminant disease on prosthetic valves. Lastly, right sided endocarditis in intravenous drug abusers; these cases are relatively protected from the serious complications of multiple septic emboli, which instead lodge in the lung and produce impressive pulmonary infiltrates.

Gram-negative bacteria account for just under 10 per cent of all cases of endocarditis and a higher proportion of cases affecting prosthetic valves or related to intravenous drug abuse. *Pseudomonas* spp. and *P. aeruginosa* are leading causes in this group. Intravenous drug abusers present with right-sided disease indistinguishable from right-sided *Staphylococcus aureus* endocarditis. Left-sided disease caused by these organisms presents acutely and has a fulminant course characterized by multiple systemic emboli.

The oropharyngeal **HACEK** group of organisms (*Haemophilus* spp., *Actinobacillus actinomycetemcomitans*, *Cardiobacterium hominis*, *Eikenella corrodens*, *Kingella kingae*) can cause an endocarditis with insidious symptoms and very large vegetations.

Coxiella burnetti can also cause endocarditis. The organism both lacks a cell wall and is an obligate intracellular parasite and so is not culturable in standard media; recognition of this infection depends on serological tests. Many other organisms are rare causes of endocarditis (see OTM3, pp. 2437–8).

Fungal endocarditis accounts for approximately 1 per cent of all cases of endocarditis, but causes a greater proportion of the intravenous drug-abuse cases and prosthetic valve-associated endocarditis. *Candida* spp. and *Aspergillus* spp. account for the majority of cases. Large vegetations and the poor recovery of fungi (other than *Candida* spp.) from blood cultures often delays recognition. Histological examination and culture of emboli may be helpful in demonstrating a fungal aetiology.

Culture-negative endocarditis. Approximately 5 per cent of cases of endocarditis will fail to yield a positive blood culture. Some organisms such as obligate intracellular pathogens (e.g. *Coxiella burnetti*), filamentous fungi (e.g. *Aspergillus* spp.), fastidious organisms (e.g. HACEK), or nutritionally defective streptococci may not produce recognizable growth with standard culture techniques. In some cases, serological tests or histological examination of samples of vegetations may reveal the causative agent.

Pathogenesis

The ideal haemodynamic conditions for producing infective endocarditis consist of a high-pressure source forcing blood through a narrow orifice into a low-pressure chamber. High velocity jets of blood damage endothelial cells explaining why satellite lesions may form on the left atrial wall in mitral reflux, on chordae tendineae in aortic reflux, and on the tricuspid valve and free right ventricular wall in ventricular septal defect; also why low-pressure haemodynamic forces such as exist in mitral stenosis, large ventricular septal defects, and atrial septal defects are unlikely to result in endocarditis. A sterile vegetation is thought to be the initial lesion and is composed of platelets, fibrin, and macrophages. Organisms adhere to this and multiply, and endocarditis ensues. Vegetations are more common on the left side of the heart and on the free margins of incompetent valves, particularly on the atrial aspect in mitral reflux and the ventricular side in aortic reflux. They are also found on the right side of the ventricular septum in ventricular septal defects and distal to the constriction in coarctation of the aorta.

Immunology

Persistent bacteraemia produces a sustained stimulation of the host's immune system, resulting in, high-level antibody production by B lymphocytes. The non-specific antibodies are associated with rheumatoid factor (present in 20–50 per cent of cases), antinuclear factor, and cryoglobulins, and produce a generalized hypergammaglobulinaemia. Specific antibodies may be involved in a number of systemic effects. Circulating immune complexes may pass through capillary walls and be deposited in subendothelial tissues. Complexes may also form *in situ* but, in either case, complement factors are then activated and acute inflammatory injury ensues. Peripheral manifestations of infective endocarditis may not be due solely to immune-complex deposition. Roth spots in the fundi, Osler's nodes, and petechial haemorrhages may have more than one cause, including immune-complex deposition, microembolization, and increased capillary permeability.

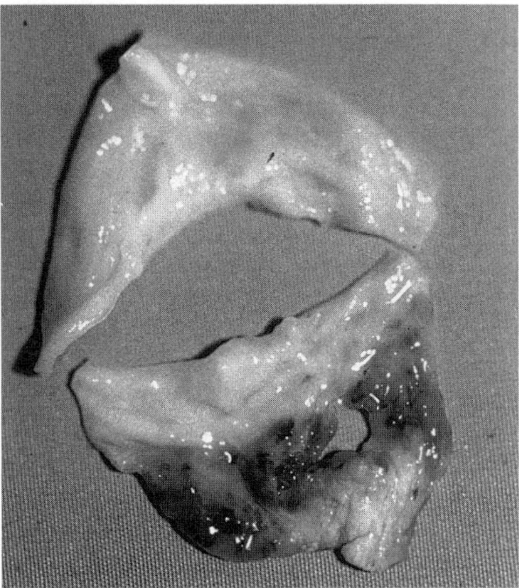

Fig. 1 Endocarditis on a bicuspid aortic valve showing vegetations and a perforation of one cusp.

Vasculitic skin lesions are likely to be manifestations of immune-complex deposition, as are the main renal manifestations of the condition, focal glomerulonephritis, diffuse proliferative glomerulonephritis and, rarely, membranoproliferative glomerulonephritis (see Chapter12.7).

Pathology

Underlying heart disease

This may be rheumatic, congenital, degenerative (aortic sclerosis or stenosis, mitral annulus calcification), related to mitral valve prolapse, or absent. In the UK, underlying heart disease will not previously have been detected in some 40 per cent of patients with infective endocarditis.

Congenital heart disease is present in most children with endocarditis and in approximately 10 per cent of adults.

The presence of any foreign material in the heart increases the risk of infective endocarditis, although this is extremely rare for pacemakers.

Pathology of complications

Some vegetations for example in fungal and HACEK endocarditis (see above) can be very large, even sufficient to obstruct a valve orifice.

In some patients, erosive rather than proliferative lesions are prominent, leading to perforation of cusps, ruptured chordae, and severe valve reflux (Fig. 1). Local necrosis with abscess formation burrowing into adjacent tissue may occur. Around the aortic valve, this process can damage the conducting pathways of the heart and can weaken the aortic root so causing an aneurysm of a sinus of Valsalva. The area of continuity between the aortic and mitral valves may also be involved in aneurysm formation and fistulae, leading to shunting of blood into the pericardial sac, the left atrium or other adjacent chamber.

Multiple myocardial abscesses are another complication, and evidence of myocarditis can be found in nearly all patients studied at autopsy.

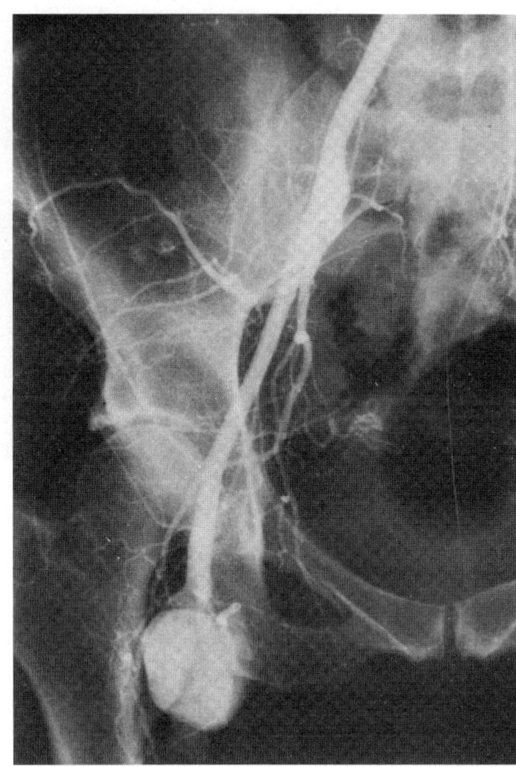

Fig. 2 A mycotic aneurysm of the right femoral artery.

Pericarditis can follow the direct spread of infection from a valve ring or myocardial abscess, and can also occur as a complication of coronary embolism and myocardial infarction. A sterile pericardial effusion can also occur, presumably as an immunological phenomenon.

Systemic emboli occur more commonly than can be detected clinically. Risk of a first embolism is related to the organism involved, with the greatest incidence found in patients with *Staphylococcus aureus* infection whether or not vegetations can be shown on echocardiography, whereas in *Streptococcus viridans* infection the risk is increased sevenfold if vegetations are found. There is no consistent evidence that unequivocally relates risk of embolism to the size of vegetations- at least for bacterial endocarditis. The threat from emboli falls quickly after starting antibiotic treatment. In ventricular septal defects and other forms of right-sided endocarditis, emboli pass into the pulmonary circulation and present clinically as pneumonia or pulmonary infarction.

Microemboli may be one of the causes of the peripheral stigmata of the condition such as Osler's nodes and the small petechial haemorrhages found in the skin and mucous membranes. They may also be responsible for an inflammatory myocarditis.

Mycotic aneurysms, from septic emboli, can be multiple (Fig. 2).

Symptoms and signs of infective endocarditis

The clinical presentation is less likely nowadays to fall easily into acute or subacute types. It may be atypical, especially in elderly individuals; the first symptoms may be neurological or psychiatric or

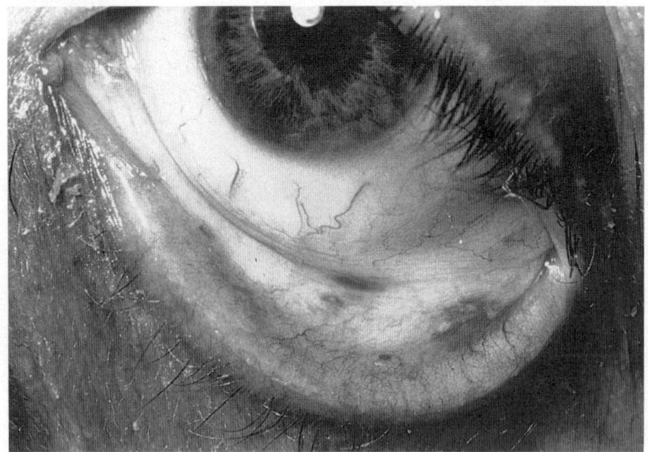

Fig. 3 Conjunctival haemorrhages from a case of endocarditis.

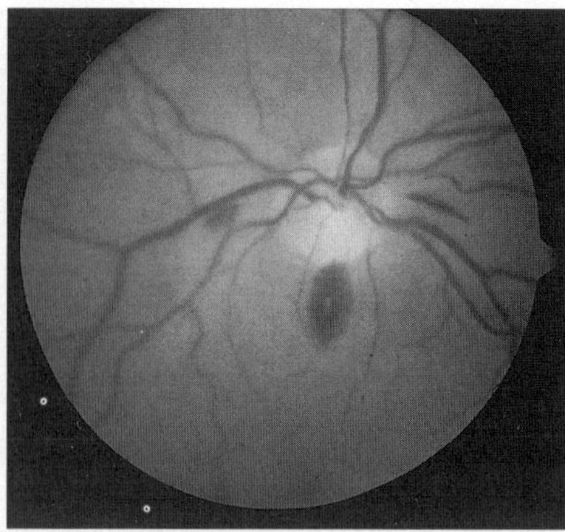

Fig. 4 Roth spot in the fundus of a patient with endocarditis.

perhaps follow sudden loss of vision due to occlusion of the central retinal artery. More commonly the clinical features are characteristic, with fever, marked constitutional symptoms, and evidence of heart disease. The clinical course then is governed by four main elements: the extent of cardiac damage, the risk and effect of systemic emboli, the degree of metastatic septic seeding, and the immunological response.

Fever occurs at some time in nearly all patients and in most it is prominent and associated with sweats, chills, and occasionally rigors. It may be low grade, falling to normal some time during a 24-h period, but spikes over 40°C may occur. Elderly patients, those in congestive cardiac failure, and those in renal failure may have a blunted pyrexial response.

Constitutional symptoms consist of malaise, with aches and pains, and are often summed up as 'flu-like'. In some, anorexia and weight loss are prominent, and in others, exhaustion. Headaches and arthritis are less common and rarely severe. Pleuritic chest pain and cough may be prominent in patients with right-sided endocarditis, the former also occurring in patients who develop a splenic infarct.

New cardiac symptoms and signs are uncommon at the time of presentation although, if endocarditis complicates a cardiac abnormality severe enough to cause effort dyspnoea or anginal pain, the infection with its concomitant fever and anaemia is likely to cause further deterioration. Cardiac failure is the most sinister complication and most common cause of death often reflecting acute aortic or mitral reflux or myocardial infarction from a coronary embolism.

Heart murmurs are detected in nearly all with a subacute presentation and in the majority of acute ones. Some day-to-day variation in the intensity of murmurs is not uncommon and the importance of changing murmurs in infective endocarditis lies in the detection of progressive valve damage. A pericardial friction rub indicates the need to investigate the possibility of infection tracking from a valve-ring abscess.

In *extracardiac manifestations* only petechial haemorrhages are common. These are not specific but in the appropriate clinical context support the diagnosis. Particular care should be taken when examining the eyes because small conjunctival haemorrhages are more significant than isolated splinter haemorrhages (Fig. 3). In this regard, lesions in the proximal portion of the nail bed are more likely to be due to endocarditis. Haemorrhages may be found in the fundi and some with central, pale areas have come to be called Roth spots (Fig. 4). Osler's nodes are circumscribed, indurated, red, tender lesions that occur most frequently in the pulps of the fingers and toes but may also be found in the thenar and hypothenar eminences and on the sides of the fingers. They may be multiple and usually disappear after a few days. Janeway lesions are rare, thought to be due to septic embolization, and are described as transient, non-tender, macular patches on the palms of the hands or soles of the feet, and occasionally the fingers and toes. Clubbing of the fingers is usually seen in patients with long-standing disease. Splenomegaly is variable and, although most likely to be prominent in those with a chronic illness, may not be detected in patients with infection of considerable duration and yet be obvious in someone presenting with a 2-week history.

Renal infarction may present with loin pain and haematuria. *Glomerulonephritis* (see Chapter 12.7 and OTM3, p. 3174) is seldom severe enough to cause endstage renal failure but more often function may be compromised sufficiently to justify close monitoring of potentially nephrotoxic drugs such as gentamicin. Haematuria and proteinuria are not uncommon. These renal abnormalities usually disappear with effective antibiotic treatment. Rarely, a progressive rise in serum creatinine with haematuria and proteinuria can be caused by an acute interstitial nephritis, itself caused by penicillin or other antimicrobial, in which case the fever persists and there may be a coincident skin rash. Renal abscesses are rare.

Neurological abnormalities are common and may be the mode of presentation, especially in elderly people. A fluctuating confusional state with short-term memory impairment, disorientation, and behavioural changes may be prominent. Cerebral emboli, mainly in the distribution of the middle cerebral artery, have been reported to occur in 17 per cent of cases of endocarditis and can lead to hemiplegia, sensory loss, and other focal abnormalities. Haemorrhagic transformation of an ischaemic infarct caused by septic embolization is the most common cause of intracerebral haemorrhage. Similar features may follow rupture of a mycotic aneurysm, which tragically may occur up to 2 years after apparent cure of the infection.

Meningoencephalitis characteristically produces headache and neck stiffness. The cerebrospinal fluid is usually sterile but may show an increase in white cells. In *Staphylococcus aureus* endocarditis, purulent meningitis may be demonstrated, with the organism grown from the spinal fluid. Multiple cerebral abscesses are then the rule, whereas a single, large collection of pus is more typically a complication of endocarditis in children with cyanotic congenital heart disease.

Investigations

Blood culture

This should be done as soon as possible in any patient suspected of having endocarditis. Normally three samples from different venepuncture sites are taken over a 24-h period. Seriously ill patients should be started on antibiotics after two or three samples have been taken over 1–2 h. Conversely, it may be best to continue culturing for a few days in less severe cases, particularly when the patient has already had a short course of antibiotic treatment or if initial cultures are negative at 48 h. Blood cultures are positive in about 90 per cent of cases; in nearly all of these the organism will be grown from the first sample, and negative cultures should occur in less than 5 per cent of cases. Some negative results can be explained by poor culture techniques or by previous antibiotic treatment. Furthermore, some organisms, for example the HACEK group, may require several weeks to grow in culture and advice should be sought about special culture techniques for anaerobes, microaerophilic organisms, nutritionally variant streptococci, and fungi. *Coxiella burneti* and *Bartonella quintana* should always be considered in culture-negative cases, as should fungi.

Blood tests

The haemoglobin concentration is likely to be well maintained in acute cases, whereas in subacute infections values below 10.5 g/dl occur in the majority; the anaemia is normochromic and normocytic. The white-cell count is variable, usually high with an acute presentation, and usually normal with the more subacute presentation of *Streptococcus viridans*. The erythrocyte sedimentation rate is elevated in 90 per cent of cases, as is the C-reactive protein. In subacute cases the concentration of immunoglobulins rises and the presence of autoantibodies can be inferred from a high titre of rheumatoid factors.

The *ECG* should be recorded early in the course of the illness. Serial records can show changes that imply extension of infection, myocardial damage, and haemodynamic deterioration. New prolongation of the P–R interval in cases of aortic valve endocarditis signifies likely extension of the infection from the aortic ring into the conducting tissue at the top of the intraventricular septum, and a similar suspicion can be raised if left bundle-branch block develops. Prominent supraventricular or ventricular arrhythmias may be the only indication of an extravalvular abscess or myocarditis. Changes of acute myocardial infarction due to embolization may provide an explanation for sudden clinical deterioration, and marked ST segment depression in someone with acute aortic reflux indicates poor subendocardial perfusion and unlikely survival with medical treatment alone.

Echocardiography provides serial records of chamber dimensions and ventricular function as well as detecting evidence of pre-existing rheumatic or degenerative valve disease. Detection of vegetations can support a clinical suspicion of endocarditis (Fig. 5). Two-dimensional echocardiography can detect vegetations as small as 2–3 mm. Transoesophageal echocardiography can detect vegetations as small as 1–1.5 mm with a sensitivity and specificity of over 90 per cent and with colour-flow Doppler can show perforations of valve leaflets, abscesses, fistulae, and aneurysms. Transoesophageal echocardiography should be considered for patients thought to have aortic

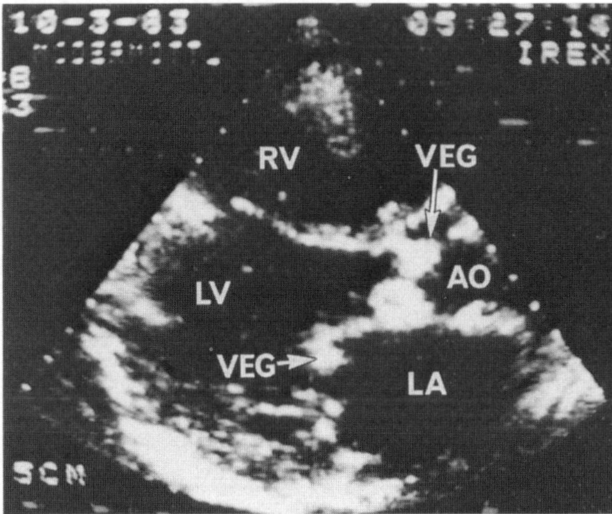

Fig. 5 Two-dimensional echocardiogram showing vegetations (veg) on the aortic valve and the anterior leaflet of the mitral valve. LA, left atrium; AO, aorta; RV, right ventricle; LV, left ventricle.

root infection, those with prosthetic valve endocarditis, those who have persisting fever or other features of continuing infection despite appropriate antibiotic treatment, and those with negative blood cultures.

Diagnosis of infective endocarditis

Criteria for the diagnosis, which is often difficult, are shown in Table 1. Definite endocarditis requires the presence of two major criteria or one major and three minor, or five minor criteria.

Special clinical problems

Aortic root infection

Severe damage to the aortic valve leading to reflux and cardiac failure may be accompanied by electrocardiographic evidence of prolonged atrioventricular conduction and/or a pericardial rub, indicating the possibility of an aortic ring abscess, best confirmed by transoesophageal echocardiography. If present, the subsequent course is likely to be one of sudden catastrophic cardiac failure.

The combination of the clinical features of an aortic root abscess with valve reflux is generally accepted as an indication for surgery. The results then are largely determined by pre-operative left ventricular function and are likely to be better in those patients referred before the onset of severe cardiac failure.

Infective endocarditis in children and elderly people

In most instances the presentation in children is similar to that in adults but peripheral stigmata, such as Osler's nodes and petechial haemorrhages, are less common and severe constitutional symptoms with joint pains and splenomegaly more common. Right-sided endocarditis complicating tetralogy of Fallot or ventricular septal defect may present with pneumonia, pleuritic chest pain, and haemoptysis.

Elderly people are particularly at risk of developing endocarditis. Enterococcal infection occurs in elderly men who have had instrumentation of the urinary tract. The clinical presentation is often atypical, with confusion and lethargy. Fever may not be evident and the physical signs unimpressive, although careful scrutiny may detect

Table 1 Diagnosis of infective endocarditis

(a) Criteria for diagnosis of infective endocarditis
Definite infective endocarditis
(1) Pathological criteria
Micro-organisms; demonstrated by culture or histology in a vegetation, *or* in a vegetation that has embolized, *or* in an intracardiac abscess, *or*
Pathological lesions: vegetation or intracardiac abscess present, confirmed by histology showing active endocarditis
(2) Clinical criteria, using specific definitions listed below
Two major criteria, *or*
One major and three minor criteria, *or*
Five minor criteria
Possible infective endocarditis
Findings consistent with infective endocarditis that fall short of 'Definite' but not 'rejected'
Rejected
Firm alternate diagnosis
Resolution of manifestations, with antibiotic therapy for 4 days or less, *or*
No pathological evidence of infective endocarditis at surgery or autopsy, after antibiotic therapy for 4 days or less.

Table 1 *continued*

(b) Definitions of terminology used in criteria
Major criteria
(1) Positive blood culture for infective endocarditis
Typical micro-organism for infective endocarditis from two separate blood cultures.
Viridans streptococci, *Streptococcus bovis*, HACEK group, *or*
Community-acquired *Staphylococcus aureus* or enterococci, in the absence of a primary focus, *or*
(2) Persistently positive blood culture, defined as recovery of a micro-organism consistent with infective endocarditis from:
(i) Blood cultures drawn more than 12 h apart, *or*
(ii) All of three or a majority of four or more separate blood cultures, with first and last drawn at least 1 h apart
(3) Evidence of endocardial involvement
(a) Positive echocardiogram for infective endocarditis
(i) Oscillating intracardiac mass, on valve or supporting structures, *or* in the path of regurgitant jets, *or* on implanted material, in the absence of an alternative anatomic explanation, *or*
(ii) Abscess, *or*
(iii) New partial dehiscence of prosthetic valve, *or*
(b) New valvular regurgitation (increase or change in pre-existing murmur not sufficient)
Minor criteria
Predisposition: predisposing heart condition *or* intravenous drug use
Fever: ≥38.0°C (100.4°F)
Vascular phenomena: major arterial emboli, septic pulmonary infarcts, mycotic aneurysm, intracranial haemorrhage, conjunctival haemorrhages, Janeway lesions
Immunological phenomena: glomerulonephritis, Osler's nodes, Roth spots, rheumatoid factor
Microbiological evidence: positive blood culture but not meeting major criterion as noted previously† *or* serological evidence of active infection with organism consistent with infective endocarditis
Echocardiogram: consistent with infective endocarditis but not meeting major criterion as noted previously

HACEK = *Haemophilus* spp., *Actinobacillus actinomycetemcomitans*, *Cardiobacterium hominis*, *Eikenella* spp., and *Kingella kingae*.

*Including nutritional variant strains.

†Excluding single positive cultures for coagulase-negative staphylococci and organisms that do not cause endocarditis.

peripheral stigmata such as haemorrhages in the conjunctivae, the fundi, or the mucous membranes of the mouth.

Prosthetic valve endocarditis

The cumulative risk of this complication is now considered to be about 2–4 per cent over the life-span of the valve. The first few months are the main danger period. When infection occurs early (within 2 months of surgery) the assumption is that organisms have gained entry during the perioperative period. Coagulase-negative staphylococci, predominantly *Staphylococcus epidermidis*, are the most common organisms isolated; approximately half of the early cases can be attributed to this and *Staphylococcus aureus*, with Gram-negative bacilli, diphtheroids, and *Candida* spp. causing most of the remainder. The disease tends to produce circumferential necrosis of the valve annulus, which leads to separation of the sewing ring and the development of a periprosthetic leak. Abscesses may track into adjacent myocardium, particularly if staphylococci are involved. Less common, and mainly affecting the mitral valve, is functional stenosis caused by ingrowth of vegetations. The clinical picture may be one of persisting postoperative fever, although in time valve malfunction will be recognized. Other causes of persisting postoperative fever include lung infections, the postperfusion syndrome, cytomegalovirus infection from transfused blood or the postpericardiotomy syndrome. The mortality of *early* prosthetic valve endocarditis is high. Persisting fever on treatment, evidence of annular abscess formation, non-streptococcal aetiology, and heart failure are predictors of a high mortality.

The microbiological profile of *late-onset* prosthetic valve endocarditis is similar to that of native valve involvement, with streptococci assuming the predominant role. The clinical presentation is also similar. The mortality of late prosthetic valve endocarditis is now about 20–30 per cent, although recent evidence suggests this figure is reduced by early surgery.

Infective endocarditis in drug addicts

The annual risk of endocarditis for intravenous drug users is estimated at 2–5 per cent, with this being the main diagnosis in 5–8 per cent of drug addicts admitted to some hospitals in the US.

Typically, the patient is a young male addict without previously recognized heart disease and with a relatively short history of illness. Skin colonization with *Staphylococcus aureus* is common and this organism accounts for more than half of cases. Enterococci and streptococci are more commonly isolated in left-sided disease and together make up about 20 per cent of cases, with fungal endocarditis, usually left sided, occurring more often in the addict population. Double and even multiple infections are also more common in addicts.

The clinical presentation of tricuspid valve endocarditis owes much to the shedding of emboli into the pulmonary circulation. Apart from fever, chills and myalgias, dyspnoea, cough, haemoptysis, and pleuritic chest pain make up the typical features. Abnormal physical signs in the heart may be few, particularly if the patient presents early. The venous pressure is likely to be elevated but the absence of a large 'V' wave should not rule out the possibility of tricuspid reflux. One should always consider right-sided endocarditis in mainline addicts who present with pneumonia. The chest radiograph can show pleural effusions and nodular densities, which may cavitate.

Staphylococcal infection of the tricuspid valve has a good prognosis if adequately treated with antibiotics, but if surgery is necessary valvulectomy may be the preferred option, with valve replacement deferred until after microbiological cure. Gram-negative or fungal infections may only be controlled after surgical excision of the valve.

The presentation of left-sided endocarditis in addicts is usually acute, with rapid valve damage and early development of heart failure. Valve replacement may be required and the risks of surgery are no greater than in non-addicts.

Management

In most instances adequate antibiotic treatment is all that is required but in selected cases, usually patients in cardiac failure, surgery has an important part to play, sometimes early in the clinical course.

In general the consensus is that bactericidal drugs should be used in preference to bacteriostatic, that parenteral treatment is indicated, and that bolus intravenous injections are preferable and possibly more effective than intravenous infusions or intramuscular administration. If indwelling intravenous needles are used, they should be changed every 2 days or at the first sign of local inflammation. In most cases a subcutaneous line tunnelled into the subclavian vein should be used and will allow drug administration over a 4–6-week period with very little risk of secondary infection. The best drug to give depends on the species as well as the results of sensitivity tests. For example, ampicillin is the preferred treatment of susceptible enterococci, whereas penicillin is preferred for susceptible *Streptococcus viridans*. Tests such as minimum inhibitory concentration (MIC) and minimum bactericidal concentration (MBC) are no longer considered necessary in the routine management of patients with endocarditis.

Initial therapy

In patients judged to be too ill to allow awaiting the results of blood cultures, the choice of empirical agent depends on clinical features. For native valve endocarditis with a subacute onset, the likely cause is *Streptococcus* spp., and ampicillin 2 g 6-hourly or penicillin 2.4 g 4-hourly, together with, gentamicin 1 mg/kg 8-hourly should be given. If the presentation is acute, a penicillinase-resistant antistaphylococcal penicillin such as flucloxicillin or nafcillin should be given in a dose of 2–3 g 6-hourly. Empirical treatment of endocarditis of prosthetic valves should cover *Streptococcus* spp., *Enterococcus* spp., *Staphylococcus aureus*, and methicillin-resistant coagulase-negative staphylococci. Vancomycin or teicoplanin and gentamicin are a good choice. Treatment of intravenous drug-abuse cases should include cover for *Staphylococcus aureus* and Gram-negative bacilli, requiring an aminoglycoside, a penicillinase-resistant penicillin (e.g. flucloxacillin), and an antipseudomonal β-lactam (e.g. piperacillin).

Treatment for specific agents

Table 2 outlines suitable regimens for various infective agents. Further details can be found in OTM3, pp. 2446–8.

Q fever and chlamydial and mycoplasmal endocarditis are relatively resistant to antimicrobial therapy. The mainstay is a tetracycline hydrochloroquine combination, usually with rifampicin. This regimen is bacteriostatic and prolonged or even indefinite treatment is need to control this form of endocarditis. Antimicrobial treatment combined with surgery may produce cure in some patients.

Culture-negative endocarditis should initially be treated with a combination of ampicillin and an aminoglycoside for 4–6 weeks. If the patient fails to respond, a further exhaustive search must be made for an aetiological agent or an alternative diagnosis.

The treatment of *fungal infective endocarditis* requires combined surgical and medical treatment. Amphotericin B is the drug of choice and should be given for a prolonged course and in a total dose of 2–3 g. Two new triazole drugs, fluconazole and itraconazole, offer some promise, but remain to be evaluated adequately. As itraconazole inhibits *Aspergillus* spp. it may offer a therapeutic option for endocarditis caused by this organism.

Surgical treatment

It is now accepted that surgery should be done in the presence of active infection if otherwise warranted. The main indications are presented in Table 3.

Postoperative survival is largely determined by pre-operative left ventricular function. Those at risk include those with *Staphylococcus aureus* endocarditis characterized by rapid tissue destruction, those with evidence of aortic root infection, and those with changing heart murmurs indicating further valve damage. The presence of valvular vegetations visualized by echocardiography is not by itself an indication for surgical referral but complications including emboli and heart failure appear more common in this group. Any patient with progressive cardiac failure should be referred early for a surgical opinion and even those with mild to moderate failure on medical treatment are best served by referral to a cardiac centre, where surgery can be done if necessary.

Although valve replacement is the usual surgical procedure, abscess formation around the aortic root may have to be dealt with by means of root replacement with a conduit and valve. Excision of the tricuspid valve may be the surgical treatment of choice in intravenous drug addicts, and attempts are being made to conserve heart valves by means of debridement of large vegetations and repair—again mainly of the tricuspid valve.

Persisting fever in a medically treated patient

Fever lasting for more than a week, or recurring after a period of defervescence, identifies a high-risk group with an increased mortality. There is an association with *Staphylococcus aureus* infection, peripheral stigmata such as petechial haemorrhages and Osler's nodes, and embolization of major vessels. Vigorous attempts should be made to

Table 2 Antibiotic regimens used to treat infective endocarditis in adults

Organisms[1]	Drug[2]/dose	Duration (weeks)
***Streptococcus* spp. *and Enterococcus* spp.**		
Penicillin MIC < 0.1 μg/ml (highly susceptible streptococci)	Penicillin G 1.2–2.4 g i.v. 4-hourly *or* Penicillin G 1.2–2.4 g i.v. 4-hourly *and* gentamicin 1 mg/kg i.v. 8-hourly (measure levels) *or* streptomycin 7.5 mg/kg i.m. 12-hourly	4 2
Penicillin allergy (highly susceptible streptococci) Non-anaphylactic type	Cephalothin 2 g i.v. 4-hourly *or* cefazolin 1 g i.v. 8-hourly	4
All types of allergy	Vancomycin 30 mg/kg divided i.v. 12-hourly (measure levels)	4
Penicillin MIC ≥0.1 and <0.5 μg/ml (relatively resistant streptococci)	Penicillin G 2.4 g i.v. 4-hourly *and* gentamicin 1 mg/kg i.v. 8-hourly (measure levels) *or* streptomycin 7.5 mg/kg intramuscular 12-hourly	2
Penicillin MIC >0.5 μg/ml (resistant streptococci) and *Enterococcus* spp.	Ampicillin 3 g i.v. 6-hourly *or* 2 g i.v. 4-hourly *or* penicillin G 2.4 g i.v. 4-hourly *and* gentamicin 1 mg/kg i.v. 8-hourly (measure levels) *or* streptomycin 7.5 mg/kg intramuscular 12-hourly	4–6
Penicillin allergy (applies to resistant and relatively resistant streptococci)	Vancomycin 30 mg/kg divided i.v. 12-hourly *and* gentamicin 1 mg/kg i.v. 8-hourly (measure levels) *or* streptomycin 7.5 mg/kg intramuscular 12-hourly	4–6
Staphylococcus spp.		
Penicillin susceptible *S. aureus* coagulase-negative staphylococci	Penicillin G∗ 2.4 g i.v. 4-hourly	4–6
Penicillin-resistant and methicillin susceptible *S. aureus*	Flucloxacillin∗ / Nafcillin∗ / Oxacillin } 2 g.i.v. 4-hourly	4–6
Penicillin allergy: non-anaphylactic type	Cephalothin∗ 2 g i.v. 4-hourly *or* cefazolin∗ 1 g i.v. 8 hourly	4–6
All types Methicillin-resistant *S. aureus* (MRSA) Penicillin- or methicillin resistant coagulase-negative staphylococci	Vancomycin∗ 30 mg/kg divided i.v. 12-hourly (measure levels)	4–6
Prosthetic-valve coagulase-negative staphylococci infection (Give appropriate antimicrobial listed above) If susceptible add	Aminoglycoside (e.g. gentamicin 1 mg/kg i.v. 8-hourly) *and* rifampicin 300 mg p.o. 8-hourly	2 4–6
HACEK[3]	Ampicillin 2 g i.v. 4-hourly *or* third-generation cephalosporin (e.g. ceftriaxone) i.v. *and* gentamicin 1.5 mg/kg i.v. 8-hourly (measure levels)	4
Pseudomonas aeruginosa	Aminoglycoside (e.g. gentamicin) i.v. 8-hourly (measure levels) *and* ceftazidime 2 g i.v. 8-hourly *or* piperacillin 3 g i.v. 4-hourly *or* imipenem 1 g i.v. 6-hourly	6
Enterobacteriacae	Aminoglycoside (e.g. gentamicin) i.v. 8-hourly (measure levels) *and* third-generation cephalosporin (e.g. ceftriaxone) i.v. *or* imipenem 1 g i.v. 6-hourly	4–6
Other penicillin susceptible Gram-positive organisms[5]	Penicillin 2.4 g i.v. 4-hourly *or* Ampicillin 2 g i.v. 4-hourly *and* gentamicin 1 mg/kg i.v. 8-hourly (measure levels)	4
Other penicillin resistant Gram-positive organisms and/or penicillin allergy[5]	Vancomycin 30 mg/kg divided i.v. 12-hourly (measure levels) *or* cephalosporin i.v. (test MIC) *and* gentamicin 1 mg/kg i.v. 8-hourly (measure levels)	4
Neisseria spp.	Penicillin 2.4 g i.v. 4-hourly *or* third-generation cephalosporin (e.g. ceftriaxone) i.v.	4
Fungal	Amphotericin B 1 mg/kg i.v. daily 2–3 g total dose	4

[1] In cases of infective endocarditis caused by unusual organisms, further reference should be made to specialist literature.

[2] Organisms must be susceptible by MIC to the drugs used.

[3] HACEK, *Haemophilus* spp., *Actinobacillus actinomycetemcomitans, Cardiobacterium hominis, Eikenella corrodens, Kingella* spp.

∗Other Gram-positive organisms, *Corynebacteria* spp., *Listeria* spp., *Propionibacteria* spp.,

∗Combined with gentamicin (or other aminoglycoside to which the isolate is susceptible) i.v. for 3–5 days.

Table 3 Main indications for surgery in infective endocarditis

• Cardiac failure due to valvular disease—moderate or severe
• Aortic reflux with progressive annular infection-abscess, aneurysm, fistulae
• Persisting infection despite optimal medical treatment
• Prosthetic valve endocarditis caused by staphylococci or organisms relatively resistant to antibiotic
• An unstable or stenosed prosthetic valve
• Fungal endocarditis

detect the presence of abscesses of the valve-ring or splenic, renal or cerebral. Otherwise the temptation to alter appropriate antibiotic treatment should be resisted, unless drug hypersensitivity is thought to be present, a diagnosis based on exclusion. A low-grade fever with skin rashes and possibly eosinophilia are suggestive of the latter.

Prognosis

The most common cause of death is heart failure. Prognosis is worse in cases of prosthetic valve endocarditis, especially of the aortic valve, and in elderly patients, and if diagnosis and treatment have been much delayed. Major emboli can occur even after completion of antibiotic treatment, and late rupture of a mycotic aneurysm can tragically maim a patient who has apparently made a complete recovery. Overall mortality is quoted at about 20 per cent for native valve endocarditis and a survey of endocarditis in the British Isles during 1981 and 1982 gave a mortality of 30 per cent for staphylococcal infections, 14 per cent for bowel organisms, and 6 per cent when sensitive streptococci were involved. Fungal infection carries a worse prognosis.

The prognosis for patients undergoing surgery is largely determined by pre-operative left ventricular function.

Prevention

It has not been possible to prove that antibiotic prophylaxis in humans prevents infective endocarditis. Despite this, prophylactic antibiotics should be used because animal endocarditis can be prevented by prior administration of antibiotics and evidence has linked endocarditis with previous dental and other forms of instrumentation. Nevertheless, dental and medical procedures account for only a very small proportion of cases. Poor oral hygiene may be a more important predisposing factor. Even so, dental procedures do cause a transient bacteraemia and prophylactic antibiotics can provide a protective efficacy of about 50 per cent for first-attack endocarditis occurring within 30 days of a procedure. In susceptible patients, antistreptococcal antibiotic prophylaxis is given for any dental procedure causing gingival bleeding. Instrumentation and surgery of the alimentary and genitourinary tracts may also cause bacteraemia with group D streptococci and Gram-negative organisms and requires prophylactic treatment (Table 4).

A vexed question is how to identify patients at risk. Patients with known valvular disease should have antibiotic cover, as should those with a past history of rheumatic fever and those with a heart murmur, unless judged to be normal. Mitral valve prolapse is associated with an increased risk and should be covered in the presence of a murmur of mitral reflux. Patients with congenital defects should be offered prophylaxis, as should postoperative patients if prosthetic materials have been used or if residual valve or septal defects persist. It is not

Table 4 Recommendation for endocarditis prophylaxis in adults

1. **Dental extractions, scaling, or periodontal surgery. Surgery or instrumentation of the upper respiratory tract**
UNDER LOCAL OR NO ANAESTHESIA
(a) *For patients not allergic to penicillin and not prescribed penicillin more than once in the previous month.*
Amoxycillin 3 g as a single oral dose 1 h before the procedure
(b) *For patients allergic to penicillin*:
Clindamycin 600 mg as a single oral dose 1 h before the procedure
UNDER GENERAL ANAESTHESIA
(c) *For patients not allergic to penicillin and not given penicillin more than once in the previous month:*
Amoxycillin 1 g i.v. or 1 g i.m. in 2.5 ml of 1 per cent lignocaine hydrochloride just before induction plus amoxycillin 0.5 g p.o. 6 h later
or Amoxycillin 3 g oral dose 4 h before anaesthesia followed by a further 3 g dose by mouth as soon as possible after the procedure
or Amoxycillin 3 g together with probenecid 1 g orally 4 h before the procedure
PATIENTS WHO SHOULD BE REFERRED TO HOSPITAL
(i) Patients with prosthetic valves for a general anaesthetic
(ii) Patients for a general anaesthetic who are allergic to penicillin or have had penicillin more than once in the previous month
(iii) Patients who have had a previous attack of endocarditis
(d) *For those patients not allergic to penicillin and who have not had penicillin more than once in the previous month.*
Amoxycillin 1 g i.v. or 1 g i.m. in 2.5 ml of 1 per cent lignocaine hydrochloride plus 120 mg gentamicin i.v. or i.m. at induction, then 0.5 g amoxycillin orally 6 h later
(e) *For patients allergic to penicillin or who have had penicillin more than once in the previous month*
(i) Vancomycin 1 g by slow i.v. infusion over at least 100 min followed by gentamicin 120 mg i.v. at induction or 15 min before the surgical procedure
or (ii) Teicoplanin 400 mg i.v. plus gentamicin 120 mg i.v. at induction or 15 min before the surgical procedure
or (iii) Clindamycin 300 mg i.v. in 50 ml dilutent over 10 min at induction or 15 min before the surgical procedure, followed by 150 mg orally or i.v. in 25 ml dilutent over 10 min 6 h later
2. **Genitourinary surgery or instrumentation**
As for 1(d) or 1(e) above, directed against faecal streptococci
3. **Obstetric, gynaecology, or gastrointestinal procedures**
Cover is suggested only for patients with prosthetic valves or a previous attack of endocarditis and is as for 1(d), 1(e)(i), or 1(e)(ii), directed against faecal streptococci

Copies of these recommendations are available from the British Heart Foundation, 14 Fitzhardinge Street, London W1H 4DH.

necessary for patients with an isolated secundum atrial septal defect, ligated persistent ductus arteriosus, permanent pacemaker, or after coronary bypass surgery.

In patients with prosthetic valves and those with a previous history of endocarditis, parenteral antibiotic cover should be given for any procedure that could conceivably cause a bacteraemia. This includes uncomplicated childbirth, which is otherwise not an indication for prophylactic treatment.

Further reading

Danjani, A.S. *et al.* (1997). Prevention of bacterial endocarditis. Recommendations of the American Heart Association. *Circulation*, **96**, 358–66.

Moon, M.R., Stinson, E.B., and Craig Miller, D. Surgical treatment of endocarditis. *Progress in Cardiovascular Diseases*, **40** (3), 239–64.

Sandre, R.M. and Shafran, S.D. (1996). Infective endocarditis: review of 135 cases over 9 years. *Clinical Infectious Diseases*, **22**, 276–86.

Chapter 2.26

Pericardial disease

D. G. Gibson

Causes

Diseases affecting the pericardium are given in Table 1.

Acute idiopathic pericarditis, most commonly affecting young adults, is usually sporadic. A viral cause can be found in about half. Coxsackie B virus is most common, but others, including ECHO type 8, rubella, hepatitis B, mumps, and influenza may also be identified. Epidemics may occur, with approximately equal numbers of patients developing pericarditis and myocarditis. The most common feature is chest pain, but 'flu-like symptoms, palpitations, orchitis, encephalitis, and radiographic appearances of pneumonitis or pleural effusion have all been reported. The condition is usually self-limiting, but a minority of cases follow a relapsing course over the succeeding 6–12 months.

Table 1 Diseases affecting the pericardium

Acute idiopathic pericarditis	*In association with systemic disease:*
Infections:	• connective tissue disorders
• viral	• (rheumatoid arthritis, systemic
• bacterial (including tuberculosis)	• lupus erythematosus, systemic
• toxoplasmosis	• sclerosis, rheumatic fever,
• amoebiasis	• polyarteritis nodosa, Churg–
• histoplasmosis	• Strauss syndrome, giant cell
• actinomycosis	• arteritis)
• nocardiosis	• uraemia
• echinococcal	• hypothyroidism
Other inflammatory:	*Neoplastic:*
• postcardiotomy	• primary or secondary
• Dressler's syndrome	*Physical agents:*
Haemorrhage:	• radiotherapy
• trauma	• blunt trauma
• aortic dissection	
Drug-induced chylopericardium	

Pyogenic infection of the pericardium is much less common. It is usually due to blood-borne infection of a previously sterile pericardial effusion, or the result of direct spread from the lungs or pleural space. Occurring more commonly in an immunologically compromised patient, the organisms most commonly involved are staphylococci, pneumococci, or streptococci.

Tuberculous infection is an important cause of pericardial disease, particularly in the Third World (see Chapter 16.59).

Fungal pericarditis caused by actinomycosis, coccidioidomycosis, and histoplasmosis have all been recorded, the last leading to constriction and calcification. Pericardial calcification by *hydatid disease* may require surgical treatment if cardiac compression occurs.

Evidence of acute pericarditis may be found in up to 15 per cent of patients in the first 24–72 h after acute *myocardial infarction*. Pericardial involvement is also characteristic of the *post-cardiotomy* and *Dressler syndromes*. Small pericardial effusions are common in *acute rheumatic fever* and are rarely followed by constriction.

Pericardial involvement may be a major manifestation of *rheumatoid disease*, particularly in male patients with positive serology. Transient pericardial pain, symptomatic pericardial effusion, and particularly pericardial constriction may all occur. Pericardial involvement is also common in *systemic lupus erythematosus*. Pericardial pain, asymptomatic effusion, and chronic constriction have also been reported. Pericardial effusion may also be seen in association with *systemic sclerosis*, and the vasculitic syndromes.

The pericardium is often involved in untreated or inadequately treated *chronic renal failure*. The most common manifestation is fibrinous pericarditis, associated with bloody pericardial effusion. Tamponade is common in untreated cases. Collagenous thickening of the epicardium is less common, but may give rise to myocardial constriction.

Pericardial effusion occurs in untreated *hypothyroidism*, although clinically silent. It subsides when thyroid replacement therapy is given.

Malignant involvement of the pericardium may be due to a primary tumour, or more commonly to secondary involvement. Clinical manifestations include supraventricular arrhythmias as well as pericardial tamponade or constriction.

Pericarditis caused by *irradiation* is usually asymptomatic. It may occur at the time of irradiation or at any time over the succeeding years, and effusion may be large enough to require drainage. In a small minority of patients, pericardial constriction may develop up to 40 years after the original irradiation.

Haemorrhage into the pericardium may occur with aortic dissection involving the ascending aorta. If the leak is large, it causes pericardial tamponade and death, but a small volume of blood is not uncommon. Pericardial haemorrhage may also result from stab wounds or blunt injury, cardiac surgery, or be induced by excessive anticoagulant therapy. It may follow invasive procedures such as myocardial biopsy or pacemaker insertion. Delayed tamponade causes a characteristic syndrome of elevated venous pressure, fluid retention, and a low cardiac output, which resembles myocardial disease. Haemorrhage may also be the basis of delayed pericardial constriction which can occur up to 10 years after open heart surgery.

Acute pericarditis

Clinical findings

There are three main components to the clinical syndrome of acute pericarditis: chest pain, pericardial rub, and electrocardiogram (**ECG**) changes. The pain is usually retrosternal, continuous, and sharp in character. It is frequently aggravated by sudden movements or deep inspiration, and is relieved by sitting up. Less commonly it may resemble angina, or may be mild and 'atypical'. The onset of the pain is usually sudden, but in idiopathic pericarditis, it may have been preceded by several days' malaise or other non-specific symptoms.

On examination, the main abnormality is a pericardial rub. In patients in sinus rhythm it has two components, corresponding to atrial and ventricular systole. Rubs are frequently evanescent, and may vary with posture. They are often louder in inspiration. An irregular pulse may reflect supraventricular ectopic beats, atrial fibrillation, or flutter.

The ECG shows symmetrical elevation of the ST segments by 1 mm or more in all leads other than aVr in over 90 per cent. Early in the illness, the T waves are upright, but over the next 2–3 weeks they become flattened and inverted as the ST segment changes regress. These T wave changes are variable in incidence, direction, and extent. They usually resolve completely, but a minority of patients may be left with minor non-specific abnormalities.

Echocardiography is the method of choice for detecting pericardial effusion.

Idiopathic acute pericarditis is usually self-limiting, requiring simple analgesics only. Pericarditis due to Dressler's or the postcardiotomy syndrome responds well to aspirin, or if more severe, to a non-steroidal anti-inflammatory drug, or moderate doses of steroids. Associated pericardial effusion is treated on its own merits: only rarely does it need to be drained. Supraventricular arrhythmias are treated in the standard way.

Pericardial tamponade

Pericardial tamponade is the result of the effusion increasing pericardial pressure enough to interfere with ventricular filling. The volume of fluid needed varies considerably; if it has collected slowly, 1–2 litres may be present, but if rapidly, or the pericardium is rigid, much less may cause tamponade.

When pericardial pressure is raised, right and left atrial pressures rise to maintain a normal transmural pressure across the ventricular walls during filling which occurs only in early diastole. Stroke volume is small and fixed, and an adequate cardiac output depends on a rapid heart rate. Peripheral resistance increases to maintain arterial pressure. Pulsus paradoxus is an important sign in which there is an exaggerated fall in arterial pressure on inspiration, a sign also present in acute asthma and obstructive lung disease. In the absence of these, the upper limit of the fall on inspiration is 10 mmHg. In severe tamponade, the reduction in pulse pressure can readily be palpated at the radial artery, and, with critical circulatory embarrassment, the pulse may disappear altogether with inspiration. In milder cases, arterial paradox is sought using the sphygmomanometer. The mechanism of pulsus paradoxus is still uncertain (see OTM3, p. 2477).

Abnormal right ventricular filling is reflected in the venous pulse. The pressure is always raised: if it is not the diagnosis of tamponade must be questioned. Usually, it is very high, and it may be difficult to see the top. A further increase occurs with inspiration (Kussmaul's

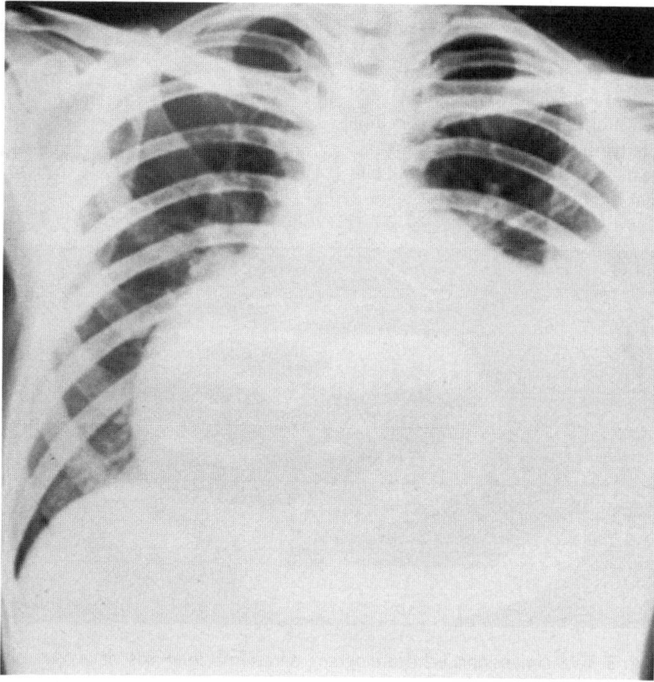

Fig. 1 Posteroanterior chest radiograph of a patient with a large pericardial effusion. The heart shadow is greatly enlarged and globular in configuration. The lung fields are normal.

sign) which may require a central venous line for detection. This is a non-specific finding and merely reflects the inability of the right heart to deal with an increase in stroke volume, so is seen in a variety of conditions including right ventricular disease and pulmonary hypertension. Although '*x*' and '*y*' descents are visible, their amplitude is small, reflecting the main disturbance of elevation of the mean venous pressure. Unlike pericardial constriction, therefore, abnormalities of the venous pulse are not particularly helpful in making the diagnosis. The precordium is quiet, and added heart sounds are absent.

Chest radiography shows a large globular heart (Fig. 1). Pulmonary oedema is most unusual.

The ECG shows tachycardia, often with low-voltage QRS complexes. If the effusion is large, electrical alternans is present. The alternate QRS complexes may show differing morphology (Fig. 2), with the heart swinging to and fro in a large effusion.

Echocardiography allows rapid and unequivocal diagnosis (Fig. 3). Evidence for circulatory embarrassment is diastolic collapse of the right ventricle or right atrium and a striking increase in the amplitude of septal motion with respiration.

The condition must be distinguished from severe ventricular disease, massive pulmonary embolism, hypovolaemia, or overwhelming sepsis. Hypovolaemia is ruled out by a high venous pressure, while the absence of added heart sounds and pulmonary congestion makes severe ventricular disease unlikely. Massive pulmonary embolism is accompanied by a right ventricular third sound and characteristic ECG abnormalities. An echocardiogram should settle the matter.

Treatment

Pericardial tamponade needs urgent treatment, particularly if there is obvious arterial paradox, or if the effusion is of recent onset and

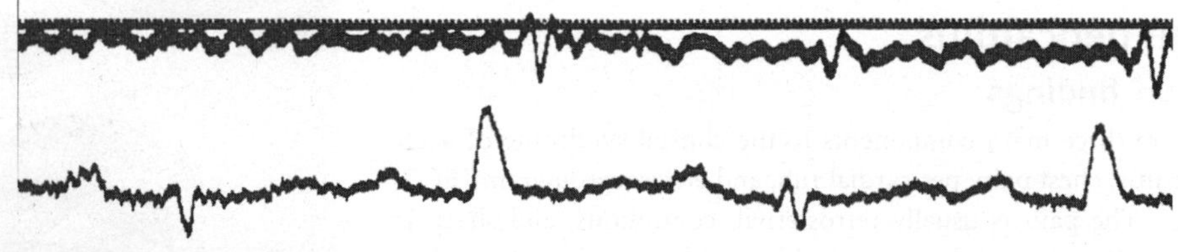

Fig. 2 Electrocardiogram from a patient with massive malignant pericardial effusion showing electrical alternans. Note that all are sinus beats with the same PR interval, but that the QRS axis alternates.

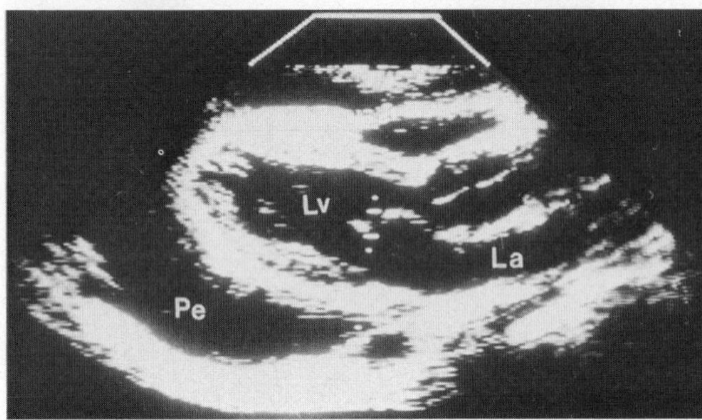

Fig. 3 Two-dimensional echocardiogram, parasternal long axis view, showing a large pericardial effusion (Pe) posterior to the left ventricle (LV). La, left atrium.

fluid is collecting rapidly. In a shocked patient cardiac output can be improved or maintained by infusion of saline or colloid to increase right ventricular filling pending urgent aspiration of the effusion which should preferably be done in an area where resuscitation facilities are available. It is helpful to perform an echocardiogram immediately before the start of the procedure to determine the safest spot to insert the needle, and to get some idea of the best direction to aim it. The subcostal or apical routes may be used. The former is more satisfactory if the heart is accessible in this way, as damage to the anterior descending coronary artery is possible from the apex. The depth of the pericardial fluid can usually be confirmed when the local anaesthetic is inserted. A larger needle or a polythene cannula should then be inserted, and up to 500 ml of fluid removed. Continuous drainage should then be instituted. Many pericardial effusions, particularly malignant ones, are heavily blood-stained, and may be indistinguishable from blood when they are withdrawn. These can be distinguished from puncture of a chamber by their colour, because they are very desaturated, and by their failure to clot, because they are defibrinated.

Aspiration is not the best way of managing pericardial effusion definitively. It does not always prevent recurrence, and it is often not possible to make a diagnosis from analysis of the pericardial fluid alone. A limited thoracotomy allows an adequate specimen of pericardium to be removed for histology, and assures drainage of the pericardial space by making a window to the pleura. It also deals with a loculated effusion and allows removal of blood clots which can give rise to delayed tamponade.

Pericardial constriction

Pericardial constriction seriously limits ventricular filling. The myocardium may also be involved, particularly in its subepicardial layers. Constriction usually affects both ventricles symmetrically, but in rare cases it may be more localized.

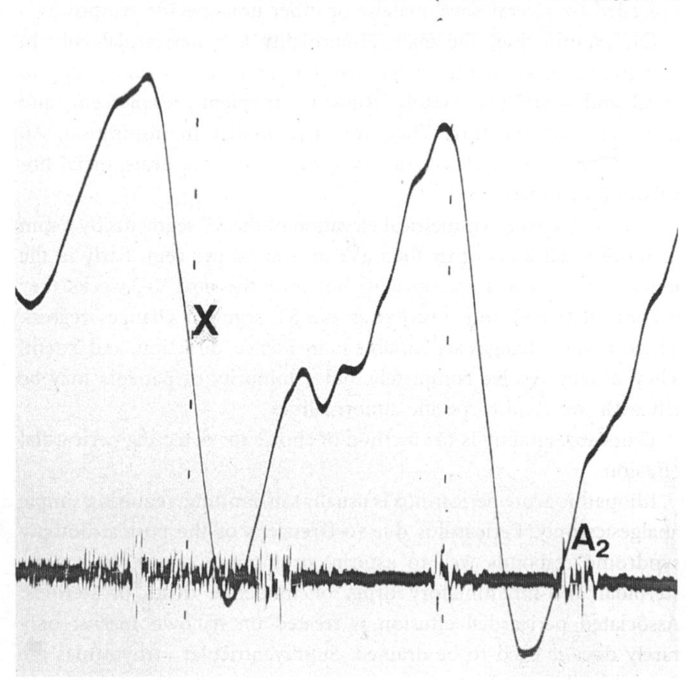

Fig. 4 Jugular venous pulse recording showing a dominant X descent in a patient with pericardial constriction. A2, aortic valve closure (time marker = 500 ms.

Pathophysiology

Pericardial constriction prevents cardiac filling in late diastole. As the pericardium is indistensible, a normal or reduced stroke volume causes a striking increase in filling pressure. Right and left atrial filling are usually equally compromised. End-diastolic pressures are thus equal to within 1–2 mmHg in all four cardiac chambers. This persists with respiration and even with fluid loading, and is the main criterion on which the invasive diagnosis of constriction is based. The ventricular pressure trace during filling is characteristic. It rises rapidly in early diastole, then stops abruptly, often with a slight rebound, it then remains constant for the remainder of diastole (the 'square root sign'). Abnormal early diastolic filling is also reflected in the transmitral Doppler trace. The jugular venous pulse is characteristic. Overall pressure is raised, with the dominant descent during systole, the X descent (Fig. 4). This systolic descent is independent of right atrial systole, occurring later in the cardiac cycle than the 'a' wave. Flow in the superior cava is also systolic, reflecting the increase in right atrial volume at this time. This combination of an increase in right atrial volume with a fall in right atrial pressure is caused by the increase in right atrial capacity as the tricuspid ring moves towards the apex of the right ventricle as it ejects. In all cases of constriction of clinical significance, the mean venous pressure is raised, and the inferior cava dilated. Stroke volume is reduced, so that tachycardia or atrial fibrillation are common. Fluid is retained leading to peripheral oedema and ascites.

Clinical findings

These are dominated by obstruction to right ventricular filling. Venous pressure is raised by 15 cm or more, showing abrupt systolic and, to a lesser extent, early diastolic descents. The precordial impulse is not usually palpable and the heart sounds are soft. There may be an early diastolic sound, sometimes referred to as a ventricular 'knock'. The liver is enlarged and, in patients with long-standing disease, there may be wasting and jaundice. Ascites is often more prominent than peripheral oedema, particularly when the patient has been treated with large doses of diuretics.

In rarer presentations, localized constriction may compress the outflow tract of the right ventricle or may mimic mitral or tricuspid stenosis, or a greatly raised venous pressure may lead to a protein-losing enteropathy, or to a classic nephrotic syndrome.

The heart may be normal in size or enlarged on chest radiograph, but the lung fields are clear. Pericardial calcification may be present as multiple plaques or more frequently, as a rim covering the diaphragmatic and anterior surfaces of the heart.

The ECG often shows atrial fibrillation, low voltage QRS complexes and non-specific T wave abnormalities but there are no diagnostic features. Computed tomography scanning or magnetic resonance imaging can demonstrate the extent and distribution of pericardial thickening. Echocardiography is unhelpful so that unless the diagnosis is very obvious, cardiac catheterization is still usually performed. The diagnostic finding is equal end-diastolic pressures in the two ventricles, persisting with respiration and fluid challenge.

The main *differential diagnosis* is from restrictive myocardial disease, usually as the result of fibrosis or infiltration. It may be very difficult to distinguish between these two conditions or even severe tricuspid regurgitation. However, there are a number of approaches:

1. *Anatomical.* A thickened or calcified pericardium makes a diagnosis of constriction very likely. Similarly, if echocardiography shows the appearances of amyloid it is very likely that restrictive myocardial disease is present. Tricuspid regurgitation can readily be diagnosed by echocardiography.
2. *Haemodynamic.* Raised ventricular filling pressures, with a square root sign on the pressure pulse, increased early diastolic filling velocities and shortened early filling periods do not distinguish. The most useful haemodynamic feature is equalization of diastolic pressures within the heart, persisting with fluid challenge. A dominant systolic (X) rather than (Y) descent on the jugular venous pulse is also very characteristic.
3. *Clinical progress.* The venous pressure in patients with restrictive myocardial disease usually drops with diuretic treatment, but it is very rare to be able to bring the venous pressure down to normal in a patient with constriction.

In a minority of cases, it is necessary to perform an exploratory thoracotomy in order to make the diagnosis.

Pericardial constriction must also be distinguished from other causes of raised venous pressure. Superior caval obstruction is excluded by the presence of venous pulsation. Right ventricular inflow may be obstructed by tricuspid stenosis or, very rarely, by a right ventricular tumour. These possibilities can be easily excluded by echocardiography or recording the venous pulse.

Treatment

Mild pericardial constriction can often be managed by diuretics. If this fails, surgery should be considered, but the operation is often difficult and is not always successful, particularly when the pericardium is calcified, and when there is fibrosis of the myocardium.

Postoperative pericardial disease

A modified type of pericardial tamponade occurs after open heart surgery due to blood clots within the pericardium, but may also occur with trauma or uraemia. It presents as a fall in urine flow and cardiac output, a reduction in skin temperature, and hypotension. The atrial pressures may be normal or raised, and the classic arterial and venous pulse abnormalities are absent. Clot may also compress the right atrium. This characteristically occurs towards the end of the first postoperative week. The main clinical features are fluid retention and elevation of the venous pressure.

Pericardial constriction as a long-term complication of open heart surgery may occur in 1–2 per cent of patients. It presents as chronic elevation of the venous pressure, and is often diagnosed as postoperative 'heart failure'. The diagnosis is made from a recording of the venous pulse, which shows a dominant X descent on the pressure and Doppler records. It can usually be controlled by a small dose of diuretic, but in a minority of cases, pericardial surgery may be needed.

Recurrent acute pericarditis

This is uncommon, but can occur any time up to 10 years after an episode of acute pericarditis of any aetiology. Its most common manifestation is chest pain, although occasionally it may present as recurrent pericardial effusion. Constriction appears to be a most uncommon complication, as does the development of significant myocardial disease and the overall prognosis is good.

Tuberculous pericardial constriction

In the Third World, tuberculous pericardial constriction runs a very different course from that seen in developed countries. It occurs early in the disease and may be the presenting feature. Patients present with sinus tachycardia, a very high venous pressure, ascites, and weight loss. The venous pressure often does not show the characteristic pattern of systolic dip. A third heart sound is present in about half the patients. There is no pericardial calcification. Treatment is by antituberculous chemotherapy. Added steroids make clinical improvement significantly more rapid, with heart rate and venous pressure returning more rapidly to normal.

Further reading

Baldwin, J.J. and Edwards, J.E. (1976). Uremic pericarditis as a cause of tamponade. *Circulation*, 53, 896–901.

Fowler, N.O. and Harbin, III A.D. (1986). Recurrent acute pericarditis: follow-up study of 31 patients. *Journal of American College of Cardiology*, 7, 300–5.

Strang, J.I.G. (1984). Tuberculous pericarditis in Transkei. *Clinical Cardiology*, 7, 667–70.

Vaitkus, P.T. and Kussmaul, W.G. (1991). Constrictive pericarditis versus restrictive cardiomyopathy: a reappraisal and update of diagnostic criteria. *American Heart Journal* 122, 1431–41.

Chapter 2.27

Pulmonary oedema

*J. S. Prichard**

Acute fulminant pulmonary oedema is a terrifying but uncommon event in which patients literally drown in their own body fluids. Much more commonly it is less acute, for breathlessness disturbs the patient long before serious alveolar flooding has begun. Because pulmonary oedema is so commonly seen as a manifestation of left-sided heart disease the wide range of other causes are too often forgotten (Table 1).

Physiological considerations

Fluid balance between the capillaries and the interstitial space

The movement of water from the lung capillaries into the interstitium is regulated by the permeability of the endothelium to water and protein and by the imbalance of hydrostatic and osmotic forces across the membrane. The Starling hypothesis suggests that perturbation of any one of five factors could lead to oedema (Figs 1 and 2). These are capillary hydrostatic pressure (P_{cap}), interstitial tissue pressure (P_{int}), plasma colloid osmotic (oncotic) pressure (π_{cap}), endothelial permeability (expressed by κ and σ), and lymphatic function. Abnormalities in the first four will cause oedema by increasing water entry to the interstitial space, while impaired function of the last will diminish drainage.

The development of pulmonary oedema is characterized by the relationship between tissue water and microvascular hydrostatic pressure. In the normal lung, water content rises only slowly until capillary pressure reaches 25–30 mmHg. Thereafter, rise is rapid. The curve is shifted leftwards by decreased interstitial pressure, increased endothelial permeability, decreased plasma oncotic pressure, or impaired lymphatic drainage (Fig. 3). Toleration of pulmonary capillary pressures as high as 25–30 mmHg without oedema is determined primarily by the protective effects of the lining lymphatics which can increase removal of water some three- to 10-fold before they are overwhelmed.

Hydrostatic pulmonary oedema

[illegible]crease in capillary hydrostatic pressure speeds the rate of water flo[illegible]interstitium. As long as lymphatic pumping can keep pace, th[illegible]ill expand only slightly, but once its capacity is exceeded, accu[illegible]an oedema fluid with a low protein content begins. This sta[illegible]wer parts of the lung and is associated with a characteristic [illegible] of blood flow away from the bases.

In conditions where pulmonary vascular p[illegible] are chronically elevated, the lymphatics undergo hypertrophy so tha[illegible]e elevations of pulmonary vascular pressure will produce acute life-threatening oedema at levels that, when reached chronically, cause little distress.

High permeability pulmonary oedema

Endothelial damage speeds the flux of both water and proteins into the intestinal space, so that the oedema fluid has a high protein

Table 1 Causes of pulmonary oedema

Hydrostatic pulmonary oedema

- Pulmonary venous hypertension—cardiogenic. Left ventricular failure; mitral stenosis and regurgitation; left atrial thrombosis; left atrial myxoma; cor triatriatum; loculated pericarditis
- Pulmonary venous hypertension—non-cardiogenic. Veno-occlusive disease; congenital pulmonary venous stenosis; mediastinal granulomas, fibrosis, masses; neurogenic
- Pulmonary arterial hypertension. Hyperkinetic states (extreme exercise, left–right shunts, hypoxia, anaemia, thyrotoxicosis); pulmonary emboli; high altitude

Permeability oedema

- *Drugs and circulating toxic substances*. Hydrochlorthiazide; phenylbutazone; aspirin; methylsalicylate; nitrofurantoin; hydralazine; bleomycin; heroin; morphine; methadone; dextropropoxyphene; paraquat; alloxan; α-naphthylthiourea; coral snake venom; silver nitrate; ammonium chloride; ammonium sulphate; chelating agents; oleic acid (fat embolus); diltiazem; iodine containing contrast media; interleukin-2
- *Immunological*. Goodpasture's syndrome; antilung serum; Stevens–Johnson syndrome
- *Radiation*.
- *Viral infection*.
- *Aspirated toxic substances*. Fresh water; salt water; stomach contents
- *Inhaled toxic substances*. Smoke; nitrogen oxides; ozone; chlorine; cadmium oxide; oxides of sulphur; carbonyl chloride; phosgene; lewisite; oxygen
- *Metabolic*. Hepatic failure; renal failure
- *Mechanical endothelial disruption*. ?Neurogenic pulmonary oedema
- *Mechanical epithelial disruption*. ?Pulmonary hyperinflation
- *Other causes of permeability oedema*: adult respiratory distress syndrome. Particularly: shock lung; septicaemia; pancreatitis; burns; fat embolism; cardiopulmonary bypass; banked unfiltered blood; amniotic fluid embolism

Reduced alveolar septal tissue interstitial pressure

- *Upper airways obstruction, acute*. Laryngospasm; epiglottitis; laryngotracheobronchitis; spasmodic croup; foreign body; tumour; upper airways trauma, strangulation, peritonsillar abscess, Ludwig's angina; angio-oedema; near drowning; ?asthma
- *Upper airways obstruction, chronic*. Obstructive sleep apnoea; adenoidal, tonsillar, or nasopharyngeal mass; thyroid goitre; acromegaly

Reduced plasma colloid osmotic pressure

- Rare as sole cause. Contributes to oedemas of adult respiratory distress syndrome, hepatic and renal failure, fluid overload, myocardial infarction. Important when hypoproteinaemia occurs with other oedemogenic conditions

Failure of lymphatic clearance

- Lymphangitis carcinomatosa; mediastinal obstruction; lung transplant; contributes to oedema in adult respiratory distress syndrome, malaria, silicosis

*It is with regret that we report the death of Professor J. S. Prichard.

Fig. 1 (a) The lung endothelial membrane is permeable to water and electrolytes but less permeable to macromolecules. (b) The Starling equation: $Q_1 = K(P_{cap} - P_{int}) - K\sigma(\pi_{cap} - \pi_{in})$ where Q_1 is the net fluid filtration rate, K is the filtration coefficient, σ is the reflection coefficient, $(P_{cap} - P_{int})$ is the hydrostatic pressure gradient from the capillary lumen to interstitial space and $(\pi_{cap} - \pi_{in})$ is the oncotic pressure difference across the capillary membrane.

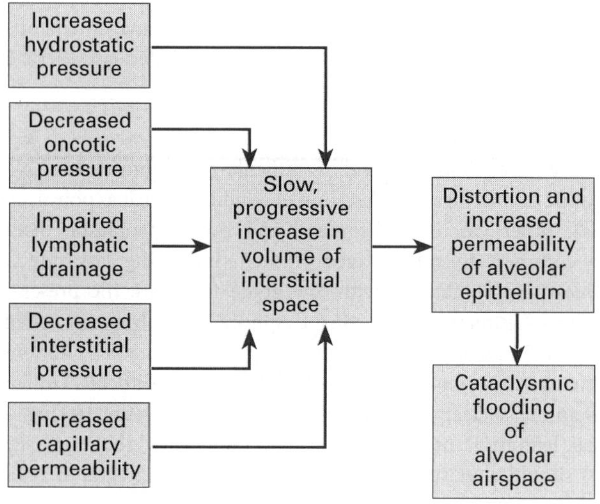

Fig. 2 The initiation of pulmonary oedema and the sequence of development.

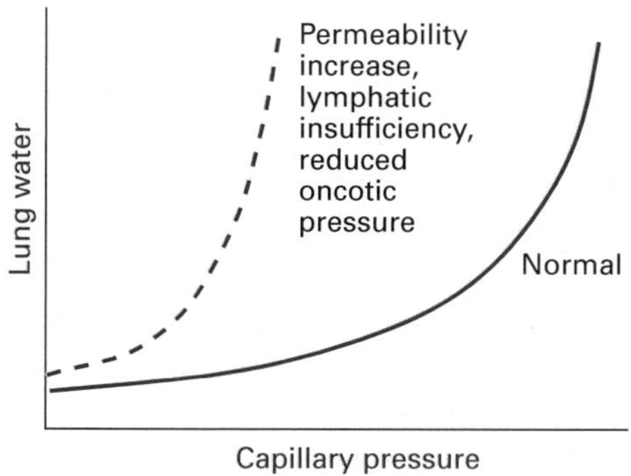

Fig. 3 Lung water content and capillary pressure. In the normal lung tissue, the water content does not begin to increase until capillary pressure is approximately 30 mmHg. Where colloid osmotic pressure (e.g. plasma protein concentration) is reduced, endothelial permeability is increased or the lymphatic pump is impaired, the whole curve is shifted to the left. *(Reproduced from Prichard, J.S. (1982). Edema of the lung. Charles C. Thomas, Springfield, Illinois, with permission.)*

content. Fibrinogen in it tends to coagulate and the residual coagulum impairs lymphatic drainage and becomes the skeleton in which lung fibrosis may develop.

The causes of permeability oedema (Table 1) broadly fall into two major groups—those in which damage appears to result from a perturbation of the normal defence mechanisms and those in which it is caused directly by toxic substances.

The first group is exemplified by septic shock when the mechanisms relate to those of the acute inflammatory response. The inflammatory cascades are of particular importance in relation to pulmonary oedema because they result, when inappropriately or uncontrollably activated, in the syndrome of adult respiratory distress syndrome (**ARDS**), in which pulmonary oedema is the consequence of changes in permeability.

Lung oedema may also result from damage to the airspace epithelium from inhaled and aspirated liquids and gases or from mechanical trauma such as stretching. The mechanisms of these causes of oedema are commonly assumed to relate to direct physical tissue damage, but alveolar macrophages may often be important initiators.

Reduced plasma oncotic pressure

A reduction in plasma oncotic pressure increases fluid transudation into the lung and leads to pulmonary oedema at lower hydrostatic pressures than would otherwise be expected. This possibility is frequently overlooked in clinical practice, where it may be of importance after transfusion of crystalloids, and in ARDS. A useful clinical guide to the danger is the difference between pulmonary wedge pressure and colloid osmotic pressure. The normal lower limit of this index is about −12 mmHg, but at levels below −9 mmHg the risk of oedema is considerably enhanced.

Lymphatic oedema and the lung lymphatics

The lymphatic system is capable of increasing the tissue clearance rate of tissue fluid at least 10-fold before becoming overwhelmed. In chronic venous and capillary hypertension even larger lymph flows occur because of lymphatic hypertrophy.

Oedema soon develops when lymphatic drainage is occluded experimentally. This has clinical relevance for patients with lung transplants, in whom initial alveolar flooding is common. Lymphatic oedema also plays a part in lymphangitis carcinomatosa and in facilitating oedema in patients with silicosis and malaria.

Reduced interstitial pressure

Tissue pressure within the interstitial space can be altered independently of intravascular events by changes in intrapleural pressure. Thus when extreme negative intrapleural pressures occur, the interstitial perialveolar tissue pressure can fall considerably below its normal subatmospheric level and accelerate the rate of fluid movement into the interstitium.

The sequence of oedema accumulation

When oedema fluid begins to accumulate in lung tissue it does so first around fissures, blood vessels, and airways. When this 'sump' has become near maximally dilated, swelling and thickening of the alveolar wall begin. Finally, fluid begins to accumulate in the alveoli at a point where total lung water has increased by about 30 per cent (Fig. 4), at first confined to the alveolar angles, with later complete flooding of individual alveoli.

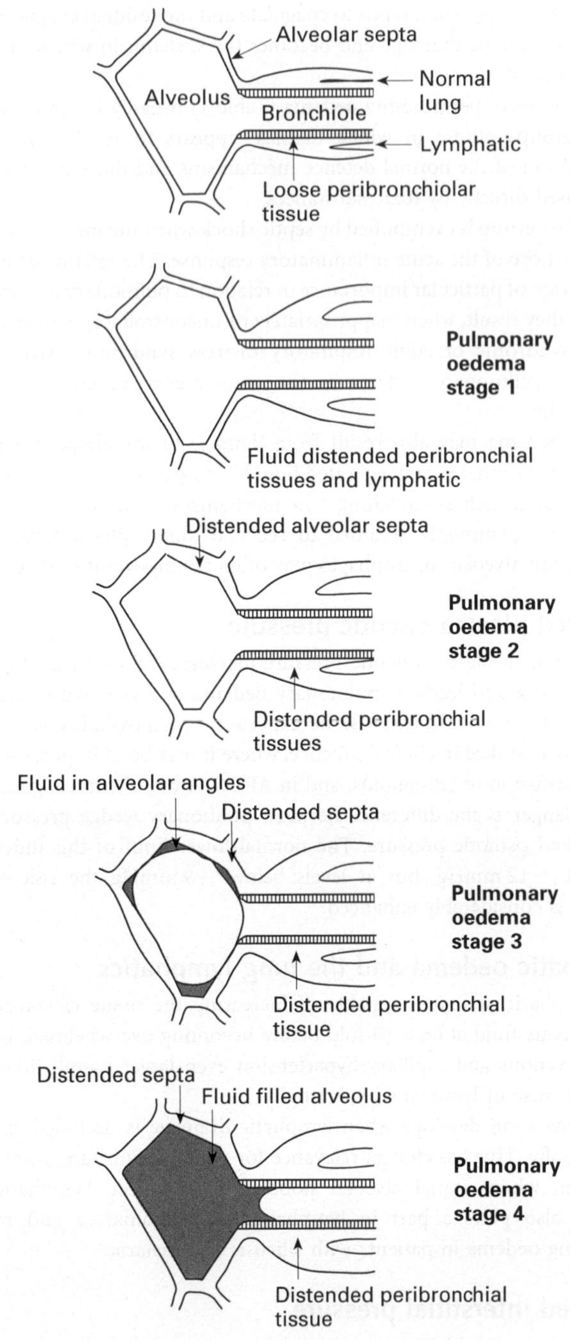

Fig. 4 Stages in the development of pulmonary oedema. Stage 1: peribronchial swelling; stage 2: distended alveolar septa; stage 3: limited accumulation of fluid in alveolar angles; stage 4: alveolar flooding. *(Reproduced from Prichard, J.S. (1982). Edema of the lung. Charles C. Thomas, Springfield, Illinois, with permission.)*

The resolution of pulmonary oedema

Hydrostatic and oncotic oedema can resolve completely and rapidly but this is rarely the case with permeability oedema, where slow disappearance and permanent lung damage are the rule.

Resolution of hydrostatic oedema occurs in two phases—return of the capillary pressure towards normal and then lymphatic and osmotic resorption of tissue and alveolar fluid. In cardiac failure, the shift of blood from the pulmonary circulation to the systemic by sitting up is the most powerful method of reducing capillary pressure, but other mechanisms have also been suggested, including:

1. Progressive hypovolaemia (from fluid extravasation into the lung).
2. Increasing plasma oncotic pressure from the relatively greater transendothelial loss of water than of plasma protein.
3. Hypoxic vasoconstriction of the muscular pulmonary arteries causing a fall in capillary pressure.

The clearance mechanisms in permeability oedema are considerably less efficient because fibrin has coagulated in the interstitium, lymphatics, and alveoli and because the endothelium and epithelium have been damaged. The problem in the alveoli is compounded by the inactivation of surfactant by fibrin and continuing high permeability of the alveolar epithelium. The incompletely removed coagulum acts as a skeleton for fibrosis.

Reconstruction of epithelium and endothelium may occur. In the case of the alveolar epithelium, cell replacement is by trans-differentiation from type II pneumocytes but this is rarely complete.

Clinical aspects

Causes of pulmonary oedema

Descriptions of the clinical manifestations and management of the more common diseases listed in Table 1 are provided elsewhere. But certain rarer conditions need comment here.

Pulmonary venous thrombosis

This is a rare condition and is difficult to diagnose. It may be idiopathic or may be a manifestation of conditions such as polyarteritis nodosa, other vasculitic disorders, and occult neoplastic disease. More common in middle-aged women, increasing lassitude and breathlessness, sometimes with low grade fever, are the presenting symptoms. Ultimately, gross effort dyspnoea and pulmonary oedema, usually with pleural effusions, develop. The signs of pulmonary hypertension are present but proof of diagnosis is difficult. Difficulty in obtaining a clear pulmonary artery wedge pressure tracing and normal left atrial pressure (measured directly by the trans-septal route) should alert suspicion. Pulmonary artery angiography should demonstrate poor segmental drainage in the regions affected by thrombosis. Open lung biopsy will confirm the diagnosis but is dangerous.

High-altitude oedema

Some apparently normal people who ascend rapidly to high altitudes experience acute pulmonary oedema. The condition is a particular instance of the oedema that occurs in severe hypoxia and develops only in that minority of individuals who have an exaggerated acute pulmonary arterial pressor response to hypoxia and who develop pulmonary hypertension at high altitude (see Chapter 18.7).

Pulmonary oedema with pulmonary arterial hypertension

Occasionally, pulmonary arterial hypertension secondary to high output states, such as large shunts, can be associated with pulmonary oedema especially following exercise.

Pulmonary oedema following acute intracranial lesions

A large variety of intracranial lesions may occasionally be associated with acute pulmonary oedema. It is probable that damage to the nucleus of the tractus solitarus and the hypothalamus lead to severe systemic vasoconstriction, which shifts blood to the pulmonary circulation, causing an extreme paroxysm of pulmonary hypertension—

reaching 410/200 in one recorded case. In addition, pulmonary venoconstriction increases pulmonary capillary pressure even in excess of that which would have been predicted from the pulmonary arterial pressure.

Pulmonary thromboembolism

This may occasionally lead to florid pulmonary oedema and two hypotheses have been proposed: (1) local overperfusion caused by the diversion of blood flow away from the occluded site, and (2) humoral alteration of permeability.

Expansion pulmonary oedema

The incidence of pulmonary oedema after expansion of a collapsed lung is low, but more likely when the area has been collapsed for some time. The occurrence may be reduced by ensuring that the negative pressures in the pleural space during re-expansion do not exceed 10 cmH_2O, that the procedure is terminated if cough develops and that not more than 1500 ml are aspirated at any one time when collapse is related to an effusion. The mechanism is uncertain.

Postobstructive pulmonary oedema

The initiating event is a markedly negative pulmonary intestinal space pressure generated by forceful inspiratory effort against obstructed upper airways. Postobstructive oedema should be suspected wherever there is the rapid onset of dyspnoea, cyanosis, frothy pink sputum production, and radiological pulmonary infiltrates after the rapid relief of upper airways obstruction. The onset is usually immediate but, occasionally, delays of up to 2 h have been reported.

Unilateral oedema

Unilateral oedema may arise from posture (lying on one side during oedema development), increased perfusion of one lung secondary to a systemic to pulmonary shunt, unilateral venous occlusion (either from unilateral veno-occlusive disease or from extrinsic compression), or unilateral lymphatic pathology such as lymphangitis carcinomatosa.

The diagnosis of pulmonary oedema

The characteristic symptom is breathlessness—probably generated by an inappropriate awareness of respiratory effort and by firing of 'J' (juxta-alveolar) receptors. Breath sounds are diminished at the bases and fine lung crepitations found, the latter probably caused by the sudden opening of a succession of small airways. The ronchi (musical sounds) that are sometimes heard, and that may cause diagnostic confusion, can arise either from bronchiolar wall oedema or from vagally mediated reflex bronchospasm. The chest radiograph is a sensitive tool for spotting early pulmonary oedema (Fig. 5).

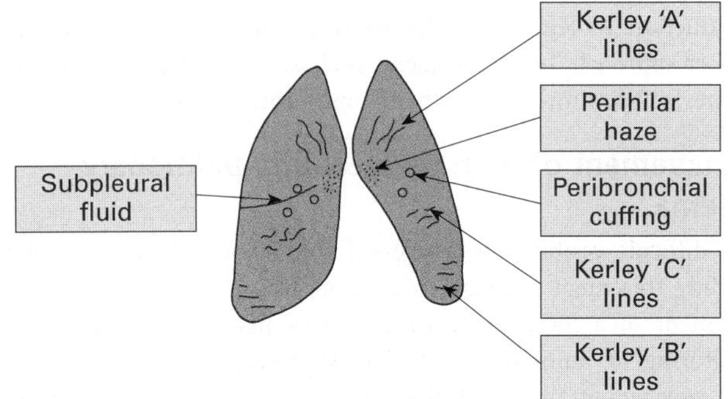

Fig. 5 Characteristic radiological appearances in interstitial oedema (see text).
(Reproduced from Prichard, J.S. (1982). Edema of the lung. Charles C. Thomas, Springfield, Illinois, with permission.)

Pulmonary function in oedema of the lung

The oedematous lung shows a mixture of restrictive and obstructive defects, although the former dominate. Sometimes, airflow resistance may cause a reduction in forced expiratory volume in 1 s and forced vital capacity.

Tachypnoea (mechanism uncertain) is a prominent feature of all forms of pulmonary oedema. Total ventilation (V_E) is high relative to the prevailing level of carbon dioxide consumption, but is expended mainly in dead-space ventilation and this normally maintains normocapnoea.

In acute, severe cases the usual blood gas abnormalities are hypocapnia and hypoxia. The hypoxia is a result of ventilation/perfusion mismatching. The hypocapnia is accounted for by tachypnoea, but, in about 20 per cent of severe cases, hypercapnia is seen, even when no chronic airflow disease coexists.

In the more chronic permeability oedemas—as in ARDS—the overwhelming problem is continuing severe hypoxaemia. Three mechanisms have been proposed: (1) diffusion impairment; (2) low ventilation/perfusion (V_A/Q) values; and (3) shunt ($V_A/Q < 0.005$).

Treatment of pulmonary oedema

Acute cardiogenic and fluid overload pulmonary oedema

By far the most common causes are acute and chronic left-sided heart disease, although overenthusiastic use of intravenous normal saline is often an additional factor. The patient is most comfortable in the 'trunk up, legs down' position which helps pool blood in the dependent parts and reduce central venous pressure. Morphine, diuretics, and oxygen are the fundamentals of current treatment. Thigh cuffs inflated to occlude venous return can help as a form of a bloodless phlebotomy and venesection with removal of 200–500 ml of blood is still an effective treatment when other measures are not available.

Morphine acts centrally to relieve the distress of dyspnoea. It also vasodilates the systemic venous system, shifting blood from the lesser to the major circulation. It is best administered by slow intravenous injection in a total dose of 2–10 mg at a rate of 2 mg/min.

A bolus dose of frusemide (or other loop diuretic), administered intravenously, acts both by 'pharmacological phlebotomy' and as a diuretic. If the patient is *in extremis* or heavily sedated, it is wise to catheterize the bladder for, as a result of the diuresis, bladder distension may induce intense reflex systemic vasoconstriction leading, on occasion, to disastrous cardiac overload.

Hypoxia is relieved with a standard face mask or nasal prongs delivering oxygen at relatively high flow rates—up to 10 litres/min—providing an inspired concentration of about 60 per cent. If the patient's arterial oxygen tension continues to fall, and/or hypercapnia develops, tracheal intubation and intermittent positive pressure ventilation will be needed.

The use of digoxin needs thought. If the patient is already receiving this it may best to discontinue it, at least temporarily, to avoid digitalis toxicity, particularly when diuretics may cause hypokalaemia. Otherwise digoxin is helpful, of course in the presence of uncontrolled atrial fibrillation, but also when the patient is in sinus rhythm.

Reduction in left ventricular overload by use of vasodilators is another approach. Inotropic agents such as dopamine or dobutamine require facilities for haemodynamic monitoring.

Management of high permeability pulmonary oedema

This difficult problem is addressed in Chapter 4.36. In essence, the only treatment available is to limit transendothelial fluid flow. Placement of a Swan–Ganz catheter is a first step for this allows monitoring of pulmonary vascular pressures in order to optimize fluid replacement and control the reduction of pulmonary capillary pressure, using diuretics.

The role of oncotic pressure management is uncertain. Low plasma oncotic pressures are a feature of many cases of ARDS and permeability oedema but, as the endothelium is damaged, any supplementally administered colloid will not only enter the interstitial space but will also be unable to exert oncotic pressure.

Oxygen is given at as high a fractional inspired oxygen concentration as is necessary to keep the arterial partial pressure of oxygen near to the normal level—and no more—because, in permeability oedema: (1) high oxygen levels may lead to absorption atelectasis in areas of low ventilation/perfusion, and (2) oxygen toxicity may become a problem where prolonged administration is necessary. Continuous positive pressure during spontaneous breathing may be tried and may obviate the need for intubation and mechanical ventilation. The latter buys time for healing or improvement of underlying disease. Extracorporeal membrane oxygenation with carbon dioxide removal has not yet been shown to promote lung healing or improve prognosis.

Further reading

Simon, R.D. (1993). Neurogenic pulmonary edema. *Neurologic Clinics*, 11(2), 309–23.

Chapter 2.28

Pulmonary hypertension

*J. S. Prichard**

Pulmonary hypertension is said to be present when the systolic pulmonary arterial pressure at rest exceeds 30 mmHg or the mean pressure 20 mmHg. Sustained pulmonary hypertension is usually a result of chronic hypoxia from lung disease or high blood flow through the lung generated by cardiac shunts, when the pulmonary hypertension is a secondary phenomenon. Occasionally the immediate problem is in the pulmonary vasculature itself (primary pulmonary hypertension).

Probably in every case two changes are present simultaneously. The first is constrictive vascular disease, in which the rise in resistance is a consequence of smooth muscular contraction. The second is restrictive vascular disease, in which structural, non-contractile remodelling of the pulmonary vascular system has reduced the capacity and increased the resistance to blood flow in the system. The balance between these varies greatly from case to case but generally, the milder the hypertension, the less the restrictive component.

*It is with regret that we report the death of Professor J. S. Prichard.

Table 1 Pulmonary hypertension—aetiology

Idiopathic
- Primary pulmonary hypertension
- Pulmonary veno-occlusive disease
- Pulmonary haemangioendotheliomatosis

Secondary to:
- Persistently increased pulmonary blood flow (pre-tricuspid and post-tricuspid shunts)
- Left atrial hypertension
- Chronic hypoxia*
    - chronic lung disease
    - thoracic musculoskeletal disease
    - dwellers at high altitudes
- Pulmonary embolism
    - thromboembolism
    - foreign body embolism from intravenous drugs
    - amniotic fluid embolism
- Collagen and autoimmune diseases
- Pulmonary vascular toxins—including:
    - drugs (aminorex, ?oral contraceptives, ?phenformin), plants (*Crotolaria* and *Senecio* spp.), denatured rapeseed oil (oleoanilide)
- Parasitic lung disease
- Hepatic cirrhosis
- Altered blood rheology (sickle-cell disease)

*Causes of cor pulmonale are set out in more detail in Chapter 2.29.

Classification of pulmonary hypertension

Classification by aetiology is shown in Table 1. In the West, the most common causes of secondary hypertension are persistent hypoxia from chest disease and high pulmonary blood flow from cardiac shunts; other causes are quite uncommon.

Classification by histopathological changes produces a slightly different pattern. All forms of chronic pulmonary hypertension show medial hypertrophy of the muscular arteries and proliferative intimal lesions but, in addition, certain characteristic patterns are recognized.

1. *Plexogenic pulmonary vasculopathy.* Primary pulmonary hypertension, hypertension from increased pulmonary blood flow, hepatic cirrhosis, and certain types of toxic pulmonary hypertension share the characteristic abnormality of plexogenic arteriopathy.
2. *Hypoxic pulmonary vasculopathy.* Characteristic vascular changes emerge in long-term hypoxia, irrespective of whether there are associated parenchymal lung changes or not (e.g. in high-altitude dwellers, thoracic deformity).
3. *Congestive pulmonary vasculopathy.* Venous outflow obstruction and pulmonary oedema lead to distinctive parenchymal changes and pulmonary haemosiderosis in addition to non-plexogenic vascular changes.

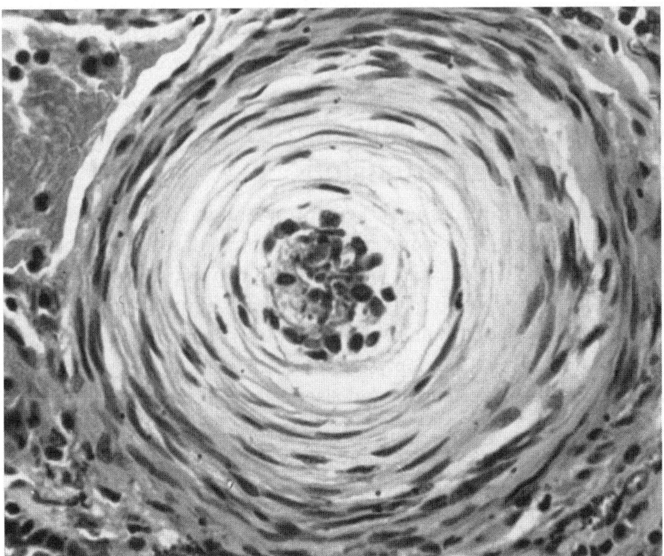

Fig. 1 Transverse section of a small muscular pulmonary artery from a woman of 26 years with a aortopulmonary septal defect and pulmonary hypertension. There is pronounced concentric intimal proliferation ('onion skin proliferation').
(Reproduced from Harris P. and Heath D. (1986). The Human pulmonary Circulation, p. 252 Livingstone, Edinburgh, with permission. Micrograph kindly supplied by Professor D. Heath.)

4. *Embolic pulmonary arteriopathy.* The presence of eccentric intimal fibrosis of muscular arteries in early primary pulmonary hypertension can occasionally make the distinction between primary disease and microthromboembolic disease extraordinarily difficult, if the embolus itself is not identified.
5. In *parasitic disease* (such as pulmonary schistosomiasis or hydatid disease), tumour, amniotic fluid embolus, collagen disease and foreign body embolism, morphological changes are closely associated with the particular aetiology.

Necrotizing vasculitis is a terminal feature of all types of pulmonary hypertension and is not particular to any. Similarly, dilatation, atherosclerotic change, and aneurysm in the larger elastic arteries are secondary results common to all syndromes where high pressure has been persistent and severe.

Pulmonary hypertension associated with high pulmonary blood flow

Histological changes

Congenital cardiac septal defects subject the pulmonary circulation to continuous haemodynamic stress. Six stages of histological change are recognized:

1. *Muscularization.* Arterioles are prominent with loss of elastic tissue and the appearance of circularly oriented muscle in the media. Muscular arteries hypertrophy.
2. *Cellular intimal proliferation.* The newly muscularized arterioles show proliferation of intimal cells progressively reducing the size of the lumen.
3. *Progressive fibrous vascular occlusion.* Fibroblasts then appear and lay down collagen fibres to produce an 'onion skin proliferation' (Fig. 1). Progressive fibroelastosis eventually causes complete occlusion.
4. *Appearance of complex 'dilation lesions'.* Three 'dilatation lesions' then develop:
   (a) Plexiform lesions consist of distensions of the smallest pulmonary arteries to form thin wall sacs with connections to the alveolar capillaries. Endothelial proliferation and thrombosis often occur within them.
   (b) Vein-like branches of hypertrophied muscular arteries emerge from parent arteries proximal to a point of obstruction. They act as collateral channels to the alveolar capillaries.
   (c) Angiomatoid lesions (seen in association with ventricular septal defect) arise in small pulmonary arteries just proximal to points of fibrotic occlusion.
5. *Chronic vascular dilation with haemosiderosis.* The dilation lesions allow diapedesis of erythrocytes and rupture easily. Foci of haemosiderin laden macrophages appear.
6. *Necrotizing arteritis of the muscular arteries* is found only in extreme cases. Disruption of the endothelium and intima allows fibrinogen into the media producing fibrinoid necrosis, as in malignant systemic hypertension.

Pathophysiology of high-flow pulmonary hypertension

Pulmonary arterial pressure and vascular resistance rise in parallel with severity of histological changes. A number of studies have tried to distinguish contributions to increased resistance by vasoconstriction or by fixed stenosis and suggest that in the lowest grades of abnormality the dominant effect is vasoconstriction, but as the disease progresses the relative contribution of restrictive, fixed stenosis becomes progressively greater.

Pulmonary hypertension associated with pulmonary venous hypertension

Pathological changes

The lung is engorged with blood and veins and capillaries are distended. In the veins there is intimal fibrosis and medial hypertrophy of the smooth muscle. An increase in the basement membrane of the alveolar capillary wall ranges from a thickness of 8–10 nm to between 15 and 30 nm. Frequently, there is a subendothelial infiltration of hyaline mucopolysaccharide. The endothelial cells may become oedematous and membranous type 1 pneumocytes are lost and replaced by granular type 2 pneumocytes.

Interstitial oedema causes wide separation of cells and fibrils. With persistence of oedema there is proliferation of reticular and elastic fibrils so that the alveolar capillaries become embedded in connective tissue. Red blood cells pass through capillary walls, split the basement membranes and subsequently disintegrate. They are ingested by macrophages which group together to give pulmonary haemosiderosis. Mast cells appear as a secondary response to the haemosiderosis. Occasionally, microlith—and even bone—formation may occur.

The arterial changes are the first three stages of plexogenic arteriopathy. But, dilatation and plexiform lesions do not develop. The distribution of changes in the lung follows a gradation from base to apex.

Pathophysiological changes

Pulmonary arterial pressure increases more rapidly than wedge pressure. This increase in resistance may protect the capillaries and delay the onset of oedema. Under normal circumstances perfusion increases progressively from the apex of the lung towards the base in the upright position at rest. When pulmonary venous hypertension is present the upper portions of the lungs become more perfused than the bases. This reversal may be caused partly by structural changes in the vessels, but there is an additional component from vasoconstriction.

Pulmonary hypertension following long-term hypoxia

Chronic hypoxia from any cause stimulates the formation of smooth muscle bundles, arranged longitudinally within the intima and media of the muscular pulmonary arteries, extending proximally. Muscularization of the arterioles between their internal and external elastic laminae also occurs. In addition, there is destructive loss of lung parenchyma if chronic lung disease is present.

Tropical disease and pulmonary arterial hypertension

Red cell sequestration in the lungs in sickle cell disease leads to local areas of infarction and acute pulmonary hypertension. Recurrent episodes can lead to microvascular destruction, fibrosis, and chronic hypertensive changes.

Granulomas may form in the lungs—in schistosomiasis from *Schistosoma mansoni* but less commonly from *Schistosoma japonica.* The early symptoms are allergic with attacks of asthma and mild fever. Severe pulmonary hypertension develops slowly, leading to chronic right heart failure within a few years.

Filariasis and tropical eosinophilia associated with helminth infestations other than filariasis produce both an allergic and granulomatous response to the larvae with scattered lesions in the lungs. Again, attacks of asthma, often with purulent blood-streaked sputum, are the presenting symptoms. Gradually the insidious symptoms of fatigue and breathlessness herald the development of pulmonary hypertension.

Pulmonary hypertension associated with hepatic disease

Pulmonary hypertension of the plexogenic form is a rare association of liver disease, most commonly cirrhosis or portal hypertension. The mechanism is obscure. The slightly increased pulmonary vascular flow seems too mild to be of significance. Thromboemboli in the lung via portopulmonary anastomoses are an unproven explanation. Dietary factors in association with portopulmonary venous anastomoses may also contribute.

Pulmonary hypertension and collagen vascular diseases

In systemic lupus erythematosus, polymyositis, dermatositis, systemic sclerosis, rheumatoid arthritis, and juvenile rheumatoid arthritis, pulmonary hypertension has been reported where there was no apparent pulmonary parenchymal disease. Histological examination has revealed an obliterative vascular disease which has on occasions shown a plexogenic pattern. The situation is further confused by the fact that positive antinuclear antibody serology (titre >1 : 80) occurs in about 50 per cent of patients with primary pulmonary hypertension, suggestive of a link between that condition and the collaganoses.

Clinical features common to secondary pulmonary hypertension

Intense fatigue, breathlessness even at rest, and faintness on exertion, often culminating in syncope, are all symptoms of severe pulmonary hypertension. Chest pain resembling angina may occur. As the disease progresses symptoms and signs of right heart failure develop.

Episodes of pleural pain with haemoptysis suggest recurrent pulmonary embolism. Haemoptyses without pain occur in severe pulmonary venous hypertension and also in the late states of plexogenic arteriopathy.

On examination, a small volume pulse, peripheral vasoconstriction, cool extremities, and peripheral cyanosis all reflect the low cardiac output. Except in hypoxic pulmonary hypertension, central cyanosis is not a notable feature unless there has been reversal of a previous left-to-right intracardiac shunt or recurrent pulmonary emboli. Right ventricular hypertrophy underlies a palpable right ventricular heave and the 'a' wave in the neck veins becomes prominent. Atrial fibrillation is often a late manifestation.

As pressure rises further, the pulmonary component of the second heart sound is accentuated. A third heart sound heralds the onset of right heart failure when the central venous pressure rises, with fluid retention and peripheral oedema. Dilatation of the right ventricle and stretching of the valve ring leads to the systolic murmur of tricuspid incompetence which increases during inspiration and to a 'v' wave in the jugular venous pulse. Tricuspid incompetence accelerates right heart failure and to the peripheral oedema may be added pulsatile swelling of the liver and eventual cardiac cirrhosis and ascites. The pulmonary valve may become incompetent, leading to a basal early diastolic murmur. An early pulmonary systolic ejection sound or even a short murmur may be heard when there is significant dilation of the main pulmonary trunk.

When pulmonary arterial hypertension has developed secondary to obstruction of the pulmonary venous outflow, basal lung crepitations may indicate significant pulmonary venous hypertension.

Functional investigations in secondary pulmonary hypertension

The chest radiograph is frequently dominated by primary pathology, but various features that result from pulmonary hypertension itself will frequently be detectable. Enlargement of the main pulmonary trunk is usual but variable. The left and right main pulmonary arteries and their proximal branches are also enlarged, and the peripheral pulmonary arteries may appear pruned. Patients with large septal defects show plethoric lung fields with engorged peripheral vessels.

Radioisotope lung scans can help in distinguishing thromboembolic disease from primary pulmonary hypertension.

The electrocardiogram (ECG) is likely to show the pattern of right ventricular hypertrophy with right axis deviation. Right atrial hypertrophy is shown by tall, often peaked P waves in right precordial leads and in the inferior leads. The pattern may be modified when both pulmonary venous and pulmonary arterial hypertension are present (as in mitral stenosis). Other changes depend on the primary pathology but right bundle branch block is common in all forms of pulmonary hypertension.

The echocardiograph assists in assessing the severity of the pulmonary hypertension. In venous pulmonary hypertension, it helps to verify the presence and severity of mitral stenosis and to exclude rarer conditions such as left atrial myxoma and cor triatriatum.

Cardiac catheterization and pulmonary angiography give direct evidence of the presence and severity of pulmonary hypertension, allowing assessment of whether arterial, venous, or mixed hypertension is present. Pressures and flows can be related and pulmonary vascular resistance calculated.

Arterial blood gas analysis is useful in the differential diagnosis of intracardiac shunts, in assessing the likelihood of hypoxic cor pulmonale and in detecting ventilation–perfusion abnormalities.

Primary pulmonary hypertension

Clinical features

This rare disease most often presents between 20 and 45 years and is twice as common in women as in men. Occasionally (in about 7 per cent), it may be familial and due to an autosomal dominant inheritance with incomplete penetrance.

The initial clinical manifestations are diverse and include dyspnoea (60 per cent), fatigue (20 per cent), chest pain (10 per cent), palpitations, syncope, and swollen ankles. Often diagnosis is delayed for between 1 and 2 years both because of the ill-defined nature of symptoms and because of the paucity of physical signs in the early stages.

On examination, the major features are the presence of third and fourth right heart sounds with, less frequently, pulmonary ejection and regurgitant murmurs. Tricuspid incompetence is often present and right ventricular hypertrophy may be detected. Raynaud's phenomenon is only slightly more common than in an age- and sex-matched population. A degree of arterial hypoxia is found but this is rarely sufficient to cause cyanosis at the time of diagnosis.

Histopathology

The features are those of plexogenic pulmonary arteriopathy and, both in the larger and smaller vessels, are indistinguishable from those in pre- and post-tricuspid shunts.

Investigations

In about 30–50 per cent of cases antinuclear antibodies can be detected despite the absence other features—immunological or clinical—of collagen disease. Abnormalities in one or more of various tests are present in about 90 per cent of patients but none is diagnostic:

1. *The radiograph* almost invariably shows enlargement of the main and hilar pulmonary arteries with pruning of the peripheral vasculature.
2. *Perfusion scans* are almost equally distributed between those that show segmental abnormalities and those in which the perfusion remains homogeneous.
3. *The ECG* shows right axis deviation, right ventricular hypertrophy and right ventricular strain to a degree corresponding to the hypertension.
4. *Echocardiography* demonstrates a small or sometimes normal-sized left ventricle but, at diagnosis, right ventricular enlargement is present in 75 per cent of patients.
5. *Pulmonary function* shows a mild restrictive disease with reduced diffusing capacity and mild arterial hypoxaemia.
6. *Cardiac catheterization.* Mean pulmonary arterial pressure is usually increased about threefold (to approximately 60 mmHg), although right atrial pressures are not greatly elevated. Wedge pressure is normal and cardiac index is marginally reduced. Resistance is usually in the range 15–25 mmHg/litre per min per m.

The diagnosis of primary pulmonary hypertension is by exclusion. By far the most difficult alternative to exclude is progressive thromboembolic disease.

Prognosis and natural history

The outlook, if untreated, is very poor. The median survival is slightly less than 3 years from diagnosis and death results from progressive right heart failure, pulmonary thromboembolism, pneumonia, or may be sudden. Survival is negatively correlated with pulmonary artery pressure and with right atrial pressure, and positively with cardiac index. Other factors indicating poor prognosis include dyspnoea, the presence of Raynaud's phenomenon and decreased lung diffusing capacity for carbon monoxide.

Treatment

Worthwhile treatment includes the reduction of pulmonary vascular resistance by vasodilators and the use of anticoagulants.

Calcium channel blockers, when used in high dosage can not only produce sustained haemodynamic improvement but also have a dramatic effect on survival. Continuous prostacyclin infusion by portable pump has also been shown to reduce pulmonary vascular resistance and the effects are sustained for up to 18 months. Inhalation of nitric oxide and use of thromboxane A synthesis inhibitors are newer approaches. Two lines of evidence point to the use of anticoagulation:

1. In 1984 a retrospective Mayo Clinic study suggested that, in 120 patients who had unexplained pulmonary hypertension, survival was significantly better if anticoagulants had been given irrespective of whether subsequent pathology was plexogenic or thromboembolic. A similar result appeared in a recent extensive study of the long-term benefit of high-dose calcium channel antagonists.
2. There have been reports in the 1950s of primary pulmonary hypertension regressing during anticoagulant treatment.

These data fit with evidence of raised fibronectin levels in primary hypertension and the inability of clinical (and occasionally even pathological) methods to distinguish between primary and microthromboembolic disease, suggesting an important role for deranged local thrombotic mechanisms amenable to anticoagulant treatment.

A plan for assessment and for evolving a treatment strategy is shown in Fig. 2.

The breathlessness is not particularly relieved by oxygen, although its effect in relieving vasoconstriction makes long term use theoretically sensible.

Experience of combined heart–lung transplantation is as yet small but in selected patients has had success.

Rare causes of apparently primary pulmonary hypertension

The slimming drugs aminorex fumarate and fenfluramine have been associated with pulmonary hypertension as has adulterated rape seed oil. Phenformin has been suggested as a rare cause, as have some early oral contraceptives. Herbs such as *Crotolaria* and *Senecio* (ragweed), which contain pyrrolizidine alkaloids, are suspect and can

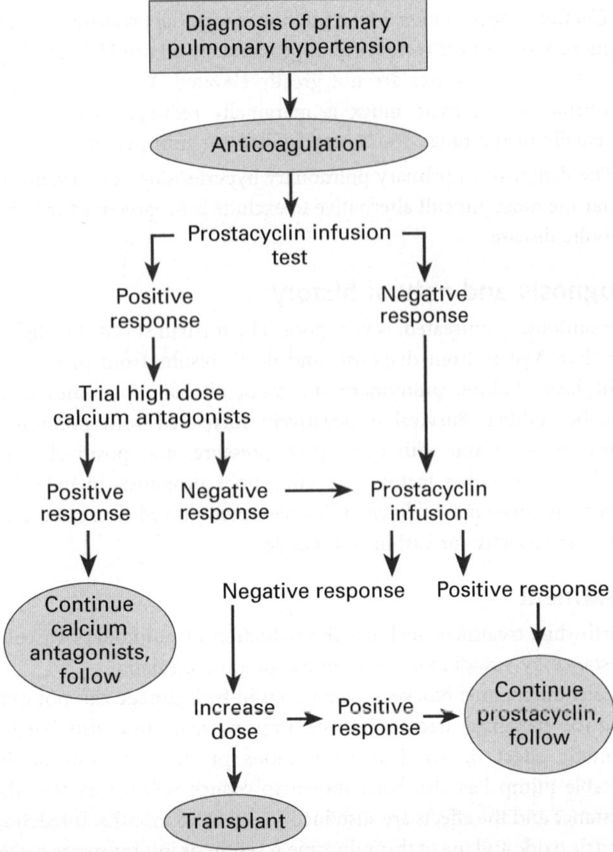

Fig. 2 Assessment and treatment of the patient with primary pulmonary hypertension
(Dr L. Rubin, personal communication).

occasionally be found in health stores. Foreign body emboli in intravenous drug users are another rare, but increasing, cause.

Recurrent systemic venous thromboembolism maybe difficult to exclude and pulmonary angiography or even lung biopsy may be necessary. Even then, the diagnosis may be in doubt but, as thrombosis may contribute to primary pulmonary hypertension, and as anticoagulation may be used in its treatment of this disease, the distinction may not be as important as was once thought. Open biopsy, from several different sites, is needed for accuracy; this inevitably imposes risks. It should be reserved for those cases where there is deep doubt about aetiology and serious apprehension that a remediable cause is being missed.

Further reading

D'Alonzo, G.E. *et al.* (1997) Survival in patients with primary pulmonary hypertension. *Annals of Internal Medicine*, 115, 343–9.

Rich, S., Kaufmann, E., and Levy, P.S. (1992). The effects of high doses of calcium channel-blocker on survival in primary pulmonary hypertension. *New England Journal of Medicine*, 327, 77–81.

Chapter 2.29

Cor pulmonale

*J. S. Prichard**

The term cor pulmonale describes structural or functional right heart changes caused by diseases of the lung, thoracic cage, or respiratory control mechanisms. Right heart hypertrophy and eventual failure are consequences of a high afterload produced by pulmonary hypertension, itself a result of physiological and anatomical changes in the lung caused by the primary disease. Cor pulmonale may be secondary to many diseases (Table 1) and the features of one or more of these will be present. A common pattern of abnormalities of the smaller pulmonary blood vessels can be found wherever cor pulmonale has developed. There is development of longitudinal muscle in the intima

Table 1 Diseases associated with cor pulmonale

Diseases of the lung parenchyma and intrathoracic airways
• Chronic obstructive lung disease
• Asthma (severe, recurrent, or chronic)
• Bronchiectasis (including cystic fibrosis)
• Pulmonary interstitial fibrosing and granulomatous diseases
Occlusive pulmonary vascular disease*
• Multiple pulmonary emboli
• Schistosomiasis
• Filariasis, tropical eosinophilia
• Sickle-cell disease
Disorders of the thoracic cage
• Kyphosis (particularly when deformity angle >100°)
• Scoliosis (particularly when deformity angle >120°)
• Thoracoplasty
• Pleural fibrosis
Neuromuscular disease
• Poliomyelitis
• Myasthenia gravis
• Amyotrophic lateral sclerosis
• Myopathies and muscular dynstrophy
Disturbance of respiratory control
• Idiopathic hypoventilation syndrome
• Obesity–hypoventilation syndrome
• Cerebrovascular disease
Obstruction of extrathoracic airways*
• Tonsils and adenoids in children

*These causes of cor pulmonale are not discussed in this chapter.

*It is with regret that we report the death of Professor J. S. Prichard.

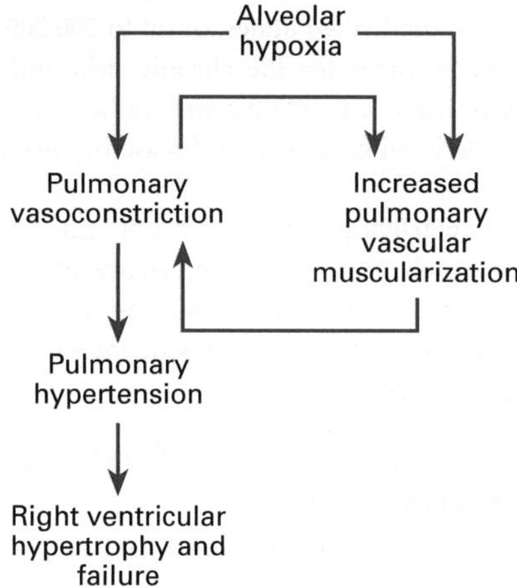

Fig. 1 The pathogenesis of cor pulmonale.

of pulmonary arterioles and muscular pulmonary arteries together with a distinct media of circular muscle in the pulmonary arterioles. Medial hypertrophy in the muscular pulmonary arteries is less pronounced. The extent of right ventricular hypertrophy varies greatly. Increases in weight range from slightly above normal (60 g) to as high as 200 g, and the right ventricular wall thickness may become greater than 0.5 cm. The left ventricle may also hypertrophy, perhaps a response to hypoxia and/or erythrocytosis and the carotid body is enlarged by an increased number of chief cells.

Pathophysiology

Hypoxia is the initiating event common to all forms of cor pulmonale. This leads to pulmonary vasoconstriction and pulmonary hypertension. The hypoxia acts synergistically with vasoconstriction and raised intravascular pressures to induce smooth muscle hypertrophy. Constriction of the hypertrophied muscle and subsequent intimal fibrosis produce sustained hypertension and right heart failure follows (Fig. 1). Oedema is most marked when hypercapnoea coexists with hypoxaemia.

Sodium and water retention may not be the only cause of oedema; much of it may be due to a shift of fluid from the intracellular to the extracellular compartment.

Clinical course

The period of hypoxia and pulmonary arterial hypertension that precedes the onset of cor pulmonale may vary greatly from months to years. The first attack of right heart failure is frequently triggered by an episode of pulmonary infection. It is usually treated satisfactorily at first but relapses occur with increasing frequency and with less response to treatment until eventually death results.

In the West, the most common cause is chronic obstructive airways disease, usually in men in their late 50s. The disease is more common among the hypoxic 'blue bloaters' than among the emphysematous 'pink puffers'.

The prognosis remains poor. In the 1960s and 1970s between 50 and 60 per cent of patients with chronic obstructive airways disease and cor pulmonale died within 3 years of the onset of cardiac failure, but survival now is probably somewhat longer.

Clinical signs

The enlarged right ventricle may produce a sternal heave, while cardiac pulsation may also be felt in the epigastrium. An increased pulmonary component of the second heart sound, a pulmonary valvular click, and (unless bundle branch block is present) shortening of the interval between the components of the second heart sound all denote pulmonary hypertension. Frequently, when frank right heart failure is present, the systolic murmur of tricuspid incompetence can be heard and a right ventricular third heart sound develops. More rarely, the diastolic murmur of pulmonary incompetence may occur.

When the right heart begins to fail, the central venous pressure becomes raised and, if tricuspid incompetence has developed, a 'v' wave can be seen. An enlarged and often tender liver becomes palpable and, in the presence of tricuspid incompetence, may be pulsatile. Oedema commonly forms in the legs and/or sacrum. Ascites and pleural effusion are relatively rare.

Blood gas tensions

$Pa\text{O}_2$ is usually in the range 6–7 kPa (45–53 mmHg) or lower. If the primary disease is associated with alveolar hypoventilation, $Pa\text{O}_2$ tensions rise to between 8 and 9 kPa (60–68 mmHg) (or higher). On the other hand the interstitial lung diseases are associated with hyperventilation and carbon dioxide tensions are below normal.

Diagnosis

The diagnosis of cor pulmonale requires that the respiratory disease is sufficiently severe to generate the necessary degree of hypoxia; and that no other cause of pulmonary hypertension is present. The minimal degree of hypoxia required is an arterial partial pressure of oxygen ($Pa\text{O}_2$) below 9.0 kPa (approximately 68 mmHg) but this is only a very rough guide. Studies of oxygen tension during sleep may be necessary to establish the diagnosis in patients when waking oxygen tensions are only mildly lowered.

Management

The cornerstones of management are to treat this primary disease, to provide oxygen to reduce pulmonary vascular resistance and to treat oedema with diuretics. Other approaches include venesection and the use of digoxin and pulmonary vasodilators.

Supplemental oxygen

For long-term therapy oxygen must be given in low dose (2 l/min) or low concentration (24 per cent) continuously for at least 12–15 h each day; continuous use for 24 h has a greater benefit than for the shorter period. Mortality, morbidity, and frequency of hospital admissions are reduced and pulmonary arterial pressure and haematocrit may fall. Selection of patients for such treatment is important. They should be stable when assessed and have on two occasions an arterial oxygen pressure ($Pa\text{O}_2$)< 7.3 kPa (55 mmHg), an arterial carbon dioxide pressure ($Pa\text{CO}_2$) >6.0 kPa (45 mmHg), and a forced expiratory volume of <1.5 litres. Delivery is by mask, nasal prongs, or transtracheal catheters.

Early results suggested that long-term oxygen therapy would confer up to 5 years additional survival in hypoxic chronic obstructive airways disease. However, recent evaluations show that this is not being achieved. Many patients comply poorly with the regimen.

Diuretics

Diuretics reduce oedema, improve peripheral circulation, allow improved ventricular contractile efficiency by reducing intravascular volume, and may improve gas exchange in the lung if pulmonary extravascular water has increased.

Venesection

An increase in haematocrit in chronic hypoxia is an adaptive response to reduced oxygen saturation. As the haematocrit rises progressively above 50 per cent, blood viscosity increases significantly and this, together with thrombosis and sludging in the pulmonary circulation, adds to right ventricular strain. These disadvantages begin to outweigh the advantages of the increased oxygen-carrying capacity and venesection has been advocated. Optimal benefit is obtained by reduction of haematocrits above 60 per cent to values in the mid or low 50s. This should be achieved by exchange transfusion with low molecular weight dextran solutions.

Pulmonary vasodilators

A large number of drugs including hydralazine, the nitrates, nifedipine, verapamil, uradabil, captopril, and prostaglandins I_2 and F_2, have been shown to act as vasodilators in the hypoxic pulmonary circulation, but clinical benefit is not proven. Adverse effects include systemic hypotension and diminished arterial oxygen saturation The latter arises from an increased intrapulmonary ventilation/perfusion imbalance. In general, pulmonary vasodilators cannot yet be recommended.

The effects on inhaled nitric oxide have been encouraging and pulmonary haemodynamics have improved without any deleterious effect upon ventilation/perfusion balance and shunt.

Lung transplantation

A limited number of severe lung diseases that cause hypoxia and cor pulmonale may be treated satisfactorily by lung transplantation.

Further reading

Baudoin, S.V., Waterhouse, J.C., Tahtamouni, T., Smith, J.A., Baster, J., and Howard, P. (1990). Long term domiciliary oxygen treatment for chronic respiratory failure reviewed. *Thorax*, 45, 195–8.

Palevsky, H.I. and Fishman A.P. (1990). Chronic cor pulmonale. *Journal of the American Medical Association*, 263, 2347–51.

Chapter 2.30

Pulmonary embolism

J. G. G. Ledingham and D. J. Weatherall

The vast majority of pulmonary emboli consist of thrombi which have originated in the deep veins of the legs and pelvis, although the embolic material may on rare occasions arise from malignant tumours, from amniotic tissue, from fat and even from aggregations of parasites that have invaded the venous system.

Incidence

Precise figures are difficult to come by, but those quoted for pulmonary embolism as a cause of *death* in hospital range from 20 000 to 50 000 per annum in the United States, or up to 200 000 when deaths in nursing homes, hospitals for the chronic sick, and at home are taken into account. Many patients die *with* rather than *from* emboli, particularly the elderly with malignant disease or chronic cardiac or lung disease.

Some 300 000 to 600 000 patients suffer a pulmonary embolism in the United States each year, with a mortality of 30 per cent, if untreated, and some 3–8 per cent dying despite treatment, either from recurrent embolism or more often with embolism complicating an underlying fatal disorder.

Deep vein thrombosis (see also Chapters 3.32–38 and OTM3, Section 22.6)

The occurrence of a pulmonary embolus may be the first and often the only indication of venous thrombosis which occurs postoperatively in some 50 per cent of major orthopaedic operations, in some 20–30 per cent after other major surgery and in 30 per cent of medical patients and 60 per cent of surgical ones at postmortem.

The major risk factors, apart from recent surgery, are immobility for more than 3 or 4 days, age over 40 years, previous venous thrombosis and/or embolism, presence or suspicion of malignant disease, sepsis, obesity, and varicose veins. The risk is increased in pregnancy, in the puerperium, in young women taking the oral contraceptive pill, and in the nephrotic syndrome. Rarer conditions include paroxysmal nocturnal haemoglobinuria, homocystinuria, and Behçet's disease. It is important to screen for a lupus anticoagulant, for a deficiency of antithrombin III or proteins C and S and for resistance to activated protein C, especially in younger patients who have sustained deep venous thrombosis and/or pulmonary embolism without a precipitating cause and in those who have recurrent episodes, or where there is a family history. Deficiencies of antithrombin III or proteins C and S are rare, but resistance to activated protein C is probably much more common and has been reported in between 20 and 60 per cent of patients in some series. These conditions are described further in Chapters 3.32–38.

It is not uncommon to encounter patients with deep venous thrombosis in the legs who have recently completed a long journey by air, but apart from anecdotal reports there is no evidence that air travel is a major risk factor for venous thrombotic disease. There are similar gaps in our knowledge about the risk of long car journeys or cigarette smoking.

Clinical features

Venous thrombosis of the legs and pelvis

The cardinal features are pain and swelling. There may also be muscle tenderness and pain on extending the foot, Homan's sign; both are non-specific. Additional signs include an increased temperature on the affected side, cyanotic discoloration of the limb, and engorgement of the superficial veins.

The clinical diagnosis of venous disease is not easy. Conditions which may mimic it include simple muscle strain, infection involving the skin or muscle, a ruptured Baker's cyst or plantaris muscle, and many other traumatic conditions. Streptococcal infections of the skin of the lower limbs are very common in old people, and may closely mimic venous disease. It is essential, therefore, to confirm the diagnosis by venography or, by Duplex Doppler ultrasound. The latter is particularly useful for identifying a ruptured Baker's cyst or a muscle haematoma.

Axillary vein thrombosis

This is a rare condition, which may be due to obstructive lesions in the axilla but, more often, occurs without any apparent cause. Although embolic disease is said to be rare, it does occur. The physical signs are characterized by swelling of the arm, dilatation of the superficial veins over the arm and anterior chest wall, and a cyanotic hue.

Superficial thrombophlebitis

This is usually seen in patients with varicose veins of the legs but may accompany some of the prethrombotic states including malignant disease. It is characterized by a painful swelling along the course of the superficial veins. The pain gradually subsides and leaves hard thrombotic cords, which can be felt along the course of the veins. It does not seem to be a risk factor for pulmonary emboli.

Management

In most cases, heparin should be administered and warfarin started at the same time. If there are no remaining risk factors it is current practice, based on the results of several trials, to continue with oral anticoagulants for 6–12 weeks after the episode. If there is extensive above-knee or pelvic vein involvement, or gross swelling of the arm due to an axillary vein thrombosis, and provided there are no contraindications, fibrinolytic therapy should be used to try to reduce the severity of the post-thrombotic syndrome.

There is still considerable controversy about whether it is necessary to anticoagulate every patient with venous thrombotic disease which is confined to below the knees. Pulmonary embolic episodes seem to be extremely rare and anticoagulant therapy has important side-effects. More information is required on this question.

Full details of the ways of administering anticoagulants, monitoring progress, and the management of complications, are given in Chapters 3.32–38.

The syndrome of pulmonary embolism

Symptoms and signs vary from none (perhaps the most common) to the life-threatening collapse which follows an acute, massive blockage of the pulmonary circulation. Diagnosis is most difficult when the clinical setting does not raise suspicion and when symptoms and signs are minimal. A chronic syndrome of repeated small pulmonary emboli may be particularly difficult, but equally important to detect.

Acute minor pulmonary embolism

When emboli are small and have impacted in terminal pulmonary arteries or arterioles it is likely that there will be no symptoms or signs. Small emboli give rise to only very minimal local inflammatory response, because the dual blood supply to the lungs from both the pulmonary and bronchial arteries protects against infarction. Involvement of tissue immediately adjacent to the pleura may, however, cause pleuritic chest pain with or without an audible rub. In most cases there are no visible changes on the chest radiograph but some 24 h after the event there may develop an initial area of non-specific pulmonary shadowing, followed sometimes by a characteristic linear scar, but more often resolving without trace. There may also be a small effusion at the base of the lung, which is often bloodstained.

Haemoptysis is uncommon. When it does occur it does so some 3–7 days after the initiating event.

Massive pulmonary embolism

This life-threatening condition is much rarer. When preceding cardio-pulmonary function has been normal the syndrome requires acute obstruction of at least 50 per cent of the pulmonary vascular tree, but lesser degrees of obstruction produce the same effects in the presence of previous cardiac dysfunction. The immediate haemodynamic consequences of impaction of these large emboli follow only partly from the direct anatomical effects of the occlusion of the major vessels. More important are a number of secondary effects arising from neurogenic reflexes and local release of vasoactive substances, 5-hydroxytryptamine and thromboxane from accumulated activated platelets, for example. Reflex effects include vasoconstriction of both pulmonary and coronary arteries and, on occasion, marked vasodilatation of peripheral systemic vessels.

The acutely increased right ventricular afterload results in a sudden rise in end-diastolic pressure, consequent elevation of the jugular venous pressure, considerable dilatation of the right ventricle often with tricuspid regurgitation and a rise in pulmonary artery pressure. The latter does not exceed 40–50 mmHg unless there has been preceding right ventricular hypertrophy. The delayed emptying of the right ventricle and coincident fall in left ventricular stroke volume may be detectable in widening of the interval separating the sounds of aortic and pulmonary valve closure but the pulmonary component is not increased in volume. Third and fourth heart sounds are commonly heard and may summate to produce a true gallop rhythm because of the associated increase in heart rate. A combination of a reversed Bernheim effect (displacement of the interventricular septum into the left ventricular cavity) and the reduced pulmonary blood flow result in a substantial fall in systemic stroke volume. This and peripheral arterial vasodilatation combine to cause a substantial fall in systemic arterial pressure.

Clinical features

Clinical features of a massive pulmonary embolism are collapse associated with an acute onset of severe breathlessness. In addition, there may be central chest pain resembling angina.

Patients are equally dyspnoeic in the prone and upright positions and are not relieved by sitting up. There is usually marked jugular venous engorgement but there are no abnormal breath sounds. There is marked hypotension, often some degree of pulsus paradoxus and perhaps a gallop rhythm. If the embolus breaks up and moves to the periphery there may be pleuritic chest pain, a pleural rub, and, later a blood-stained pleural effusion.

Chronic repeated pulmonary emboli

Repeated episodes of pulmonary embolism, silent, and producing trivial symptoms may result ultimately in pulmonary hypertension and the clinical manifestations of cor pulmonale. This condition is usually insidious in its clinical course and when established has a very poor prognosis (see Chapter 2.29. The source of emboli is usually the veins of the legs or pelvis but renal vein thrombosis complicating chronic nephrotic states may be an occult source. Pulmonary artery pressures may be very high and even exceed systemic pressures in this condition with associated gross right ventricular hypertrophy. The major symptoms are breathlessness and syncope on exertion.

Signs are those of right ventricular hypertrophy, and a loud pulmonary second sound. Right ventricular failure develops later.

Diagnosis

The diagnosis of a minor embolism may be made on clinical grounds alone when circumstances render it highly probable; for instance, when pleuritic pain or transient acute breathlessness have occurred 10–14 days after major surgery or injury. It is sometimes justified to treat by anticoagulation without investigation, especially if the perceived risks of potential ill effects of such treatment appear minimal. Most commonly, however, it is important to seek a source of embolism in the legs, pelvis, or renal veins by venography or ultrasound techniques and evidence of occlusion of pulmonary vessels by ventilation perfusion scanning or angiography.

The most accurate method of proving pulmonary embolism is angiography, but less direct methods are used unless massive embolism is suspected when this technique is obligatory if surgery is envisaged. Less definitive investigations may also be used to aid diagnosis.

Arterial blood gases

Hypoxaemia and hypocapnoea are common after major pulmonary embolism and may also be found after more minor events. Absence of these phenomena, on the other hand, by no means excludes embolism and their presence is non-specific. The precise stimulus to hyperventilation is unknown and there is also difficulty in understanding the reasons for hypoxaemia when it is present.

Chest radiographs

These are nearly always normal in acute minor pulmonary embolism. In more major cases vascular shadows may be reduced in the oligaemic area. Other signs of major embolism include prominence of the hilar shadow of the affected main pulmonary artery at the site of enlargement of a large clot. Inflammatory changes resulting from moderate-sized emboli may also be visible, or there may be a small pleural effusion.

Electrocardiographic changes

These do not occur as a result of minor pulmonary embolism and for practical purposes are confined to those who have suffered a major acute event or who have 'packed' multiple small emboli chronically, resulting in pulmonary hypertension and right ventricular hypertrophy. Even after major pulmonary emboli with obvious haemodynamic disturbance, changes on the electrocardiograph occur in only 80 per cent of cases. These include the classic S1, Q3, T3 pattern in the limb leads, T wave inversion in the right ventricular chest leads, and, on occasion, right bundle branch block.

D-DIMER/concentrations

D-DIMER/concentrations in plasma may be raised for some 2–3 days after pulmonary embolism, but also after venous thrombosis without embolism, after myocardial infarction and indeed in any event in which fibrin deposits in the circulation. In one series of 171 patients with possible pulmonary embolism the diagnosis was confirmed in 55 and in 54 of these plasma levels of D-dimer were in excess of 500 µg/l. In this series the sensitivity of the test was 98 per cent but the specificity only 39 per cent. In general clinical practice neither this, nor estimation of concentrations of fibrin degradation products are much used.

Ventilation perfusion scanning

A perfusion scan is the most commonly used screening test for the investigation of a suspected acute minor pulmonary embolism. Indeed a normal scan makes any but the smallest embolism unlikely. Abnormal scans are reported to show a low, moderate, or high probability of embolism, an approach which reflects the lack of certainty with which this investigation can be interpreted.

Low probability scans are reported when perfusion scans without ventilation images have revealed subsegmental defects, or when larger defects have been matched with coincident ventilation defects.

Moderate probability is suggested by segmental or larger perfusion defects without any information about ventilation; or by scans revealing many subsegmental defects with normal ventilation patterns.

High probability exists when segmental or larger defects are accompanied by normal ventilation of the unperfused areas of lung.

The presence of pre-existing lung disease makes for difficulty when mismatched areas coincide with areas of previously existing abnormality on the chest radiograph.

Studies correlating the results of lung scans with those of pulmonary angiography have demonstrated angiographic evidence of embolism in some 60–85 per cent of those whose scans were designated 'high probability', in some 15 per cent of those with 'low probability' and intermediate numbers in the other categories. The Prospective Investigation of Pulmonary Embolism Diagnosis (**PIOPED**) study showed a sensitivity of scintigraphy alone of 98 per cent, but a specificity of only 10 per cent. Eighty-eight per cent of patients with high probability scans had angiographic lesions, whilst only 32 per cent of those with low probability reports had had an embolism demonstrable by angiography; the figures for low probability was only 12 per cent. Even when the clinical setting was taken into account a number of emboli detected by angiography were missed by scanning and results were particularly difficult to interpret in the presence of pneumonia, bronchospasm, or when there had been a previous episode of pulmonary embolism. While only 2 per cent of subjects with high probability scans had not suffered an embolism, 59 per cent of all angiographically detected emboli were 'missed' if a report of high probability was taken as the only diagnostic criterion.

This study, then, confirms pulmonary angiography as the gold standard of investigation but the data also demonstrate that the combination of a low probability scan and an unconvincing clinical case makes embolism unlikely and a completely normal scan very unlikely indeed.

Pulmonary angiography

In the PIOPED study in which 1111 patients underwent angiography, the mortality was 0.5 per cent, there were major complications in 1 per cent and minor in 5 per cent. Thirteen subjects developed renal dysfunction, requiring dialysis in some, a complication more common in the elderly. The deaths occurred only in very ill patients many of whom had not had an embolism. High pulmonary artery pressures, a large volume of injected contrast and the presence of an embolism were not factors thought to have affected outcome but allergy to contrast material is a potential hazard and there are dangers in performing angiography with conventional contrast media when right ventricular end-diastolic pressure exceeds 20 mmHg.

Indications for pulmonary angiography

An angiogram has most to offer when clinical evidence is uncertain and the scan shows only moderate probability. In this situation the value of the procedure must be weighed against its ill effects. Often the decision will be made to anticoagulate without angiography, but if there are seen to be hazards of such treatment to be weighed against the risks of a further more serious event, the finding that 30 per cent of positive angiograms in the PIOPED series occurred in those whose scans showed only moderate probability strengthens the case for an angiogram.

Treatment

Acute minor pulmonary embolism

Unless there are serious concerns about ill effects of anticoagulation it is common and sensible practice to begin treatment with intravenous heparin with the intention of withdrawing anticoagulation if subsequent investigations indicate that an embolism has not occurred. A reasonable regimen is to give a loading dose of 5000 units, followed by a total of 30 000–40 000 per 24 h, the precise amount dictated by regular measurements of the activated partial thromboplastin time which should be kept between 1.5 and 2.5 times the control value. The risk of significant haemorrhage complicating this approach has been assessed at about 7 per cent. There may be advantage in those judged to be at particular risk in using one of the low molecular weight heparin products. Anticoagulant efficacy appears to be no less good, with perhaps a lesser risk of haemorrhagic complication.

Heparin therapy, however given, is generally required for an initial 4–5 days before being replaced by oral anticoagulants. Coumarin anticoagulant drugs are the ones most commonly used and they are introduced at least 48 h before it is planned to withdraw heparin.

Fibrinolytic drugs in acute minor to moderate embolism

The Urokinase Pulmonary Embolism Trial comparing treatment by heparin alone with heparin plus urokinase provided evidence for more rapid improvement in lung scans among patients given urokinase, but there was no difference in the occurrence of repeated emboli or in mortality between the two groups. There have been a number of studies of the efficacy of recombinant tissue plasminogen activators given with heparin compared with standard therapy. There is some evidence from these that right ventricular function and lung perfusion improves more rapidly after thrombolysis. Whether or not this approach truly reduces the risks of further embolism, reduces mortality, or reduces the already minimal risk of later morbidity related to long-term pulmonary hypertension is uncertain.

Acute major pulmonary embolism

Immediate resuscitation and the application of measures to maintain cardiac output and reduce hypoxaemia to a minimum are the first steps. It is essential to maintain right ventricular filling pressure to a level that maximizes cardiac output and maintains arterial pressure. Plasma expanding solutions should be infused to maintain blood pressure and organ perfusion, even when central venous pressure is already raised substantially. Vasodilatory drugs and diuretics are particularly to be avoided.

The difficult question is then to decide between medical and surgical treatment and in the medical option whether to give heparin alone or thrombolytic drugs followed by heparin.

When haemodynamic disturbances are controlled by the above measures, heparin treatment is commonly effective, even though it does not lyse emboli, so that occluding lesions cannot be cleared by natural fibrinolysis for 7–10 days. When the circulatory state remains precarious, or worsens, it is a moot point whether to continue heparin and await improvement or to proceed to surgery or thrombolysis (Fig. 1). Much will depend on the local availability or otherwise of an experienced surgical team. In a centre regularly accustomed to embolectomy the results of surgery appear very similar to those of thrombolysis. But there is no case for the occasional pulmonary embolectomy when thrombolytic therapy is feasible. A determining factor may be the presence of a major contraindication to thrombolysis (Table 1). A compromise approach is to break up emboli which have lodged in major pulmonary vessels, dispersing the fragments to more distal sites using the guide wire and/or catheter itself introduced in the course of pulmonary angiography. Pulmonary embolectomy should only be undertaken when thrombolysis is contraindicated and shock and hypotension cannot be relieved by plasma volume expansion and other conservative measures for maintaining arterial pressure. In one series of 139 patients treated in a specialist unit between 1964 and 1986 the mortality of embolectomy was about 30 per cent.

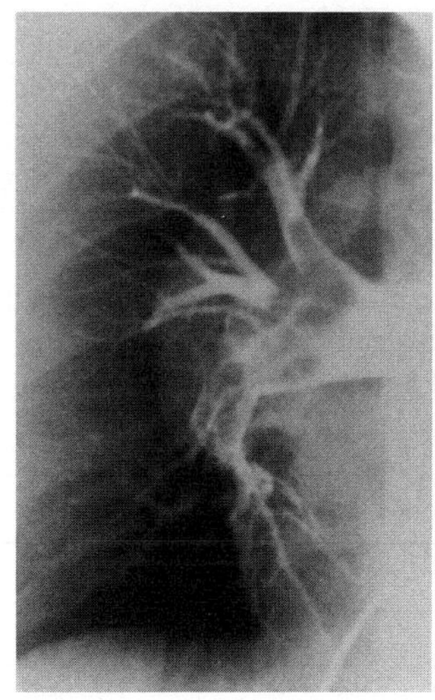

(a)

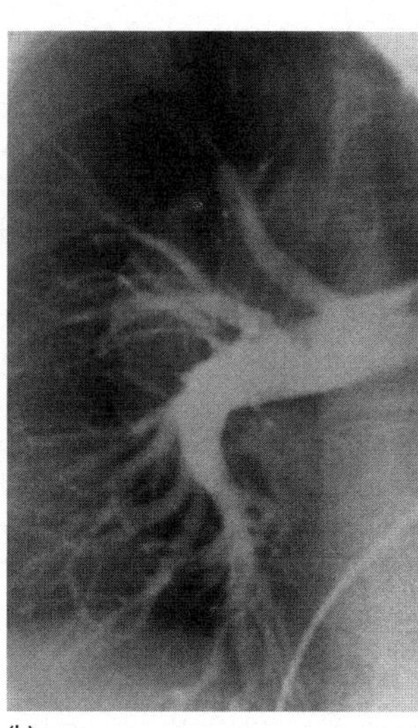

(b)

Fig. 1 (a) Angiogram of the pulmonary artery demonstrated clot at its bifurcation. (b) Pulmonary artery shown in (a) but 2 h after clot lysis by tissue-type plasminogen activator.
(By courtesy of Drs E.W.L. Fletcher and B. Gribbin.)

Table 1 Contraindications to thrombolytic treatment

Preceding stroke
Recent (7–14 days) head injury or neurosurgery
Active bleeding from the gastrointestinal tract
Severe diabetic retinopathy
Major surgery
Cardiopulmonary resuscitation
Postpartum

Duration of treatment

When there has been a readily recognized precipitating event such as recent surgery or injury, a 3-month period is commonly advocated after venous thrombosis, and 6 months or more if there has been an embolism in addition. However, it has also been suggested that a period of 3 weeks might suffice in such cases, and the British Thoracic

Society currently recommends 4 weeks in this situation. These recommendations do not apply to patients with persistent risk factors for further thromboembolism nor to those whose emboli were sufficiently large to result in thrombolytic or surgical treatment. In them the choice lies between anticoagulation for 3–6 months or treatment for life.

An analysis of 171 studies of long-term anticoagulants for a variety of causes, reveals a total incidence of haemorrhagic complication of 23 per cent and of major bleeding of 8 per cent in those treated for thromboembolism, although no fatal cases were reported in these series. The risk was substantially higher when the internationally normalized ratio was kept between 3 and 4.5 rather than between 2 and 3.

Further reading

Bauer, K.A. (1994). Hypercoagulability—a new co-factor in the protein C anticoagulant pathway. *New England Journal of Medicine*, **330**, 566–7.

Bradey, A.J.B., Crake, T., and Oakley, C. (1991). Percutaneous catheter fragmentation and distal dispersion of proximal pulmonary embolus. *Lancet*, **338**, 1186–9.

Carson, J.L., Kelly, M.A., Duff, A., *et al.* (1992). The clinical course of pulmonary embolism. *New England Journal of Medicine*, **326**, 1240–5.

Maternal and Neonatal Haemostasis Working Party of the Haemostasis and Thrombosis Task Force (1993). Guidelines on the Prevention, investigation and management of thrombosis associated with pregnancy. *Journal of Clinical Pathology*, **46**, 489–96.

Stein, P.D., Athanasoulis, C., Alavi, A., *et al.* (1992). Complications and validity of pulmonary angiography in acute pulmonary embolism. *Circulation*, **85**, 462–8.

The PIOPED Investigators (1990). Value of the ventilation-perfusion scan in acute pulmonary embolism. Results of the prospective investigation of pulmonary embolism diagnosis (PIOPED). *Journal of the American Medical Association*, **263**, 2753–9.

Thromboembolic Risk Factors (THRIFT) Consensus Group (1992). Risk of and prophylaxis for venous thromboembolism in hospital patients. *British Medical Journal*, **305**, 567–74.

Chapter 2.31

Essential hypertension

J. D. Swales

Definition and prevalence

Blood pressure, like height and weight, is a biological characteristic of the individual, depending on many genetic and environmental factors. Distribution curves in Western populations are smooth and unimodal, slightly asymmetrical, and with a tail to the right which becomes more pronounced with age. As there is no cut-off point in these curves separating 'normotension' from 'hypertension' the definition of hypertension (a quantitative deviation from the mean) becomes an arbitrary one, variably selected according to expected adverse effects of a given pressure against the adverse effects of diagnosis and treatment. The lower the selected criterion, the higher the apparent prevalence. Further, blood pressure normally falls with repeated measurement, so that definition using a single reading will yield a much higher apparent prevalence than with an average value taken on several occasions (Fig. 1). More than 95 per cent of those designated hypertensive will have no primary cause; the diagnosis of essential hypertension is one of exclusion. A variety of measures have been suggested as the threshold for the diagnosis, ranging from 140/90 mmHg or more (multiple readings—USA) to 160/95 mmHg or more (1975 WHO definition) Such definitions and prevalence figures are of little clinical or scientific value. Much more relevant are the blood pressure levels at which treatment is initiated. As this threshold varies in different countries even this figure has only limited practical value.

Ethnic and population differences in blood pressure

Adult black people in the US have higher blood pressures than white people. This difference has not been consistently observed in the UK, where black people of Caribbean origin and Asians have similar blood pressures to white people of similar social background. Social factors are very important in these comparisons. Thus, there is an inverse relationship between educational achievement and blood pressure in both black and white people. Some rural populations (in Africa, South America, India, and Australia) have lower pressures at all ages and show very little rise in pressures with age. Environmental factors account for these differences because in several cases it has been shown that when individuals migrate to an urban environment blood pressure rises. Diet and social stress are the major candidates. While most of the rural populations have a low salt intake (see below) other dietary factors may be important. The clinical importance of population differences in blood pressure lies in demonstration of the feasibility of modifying environmental factors to produce a reduction in population blood pressure which could have substantial public health benefits.

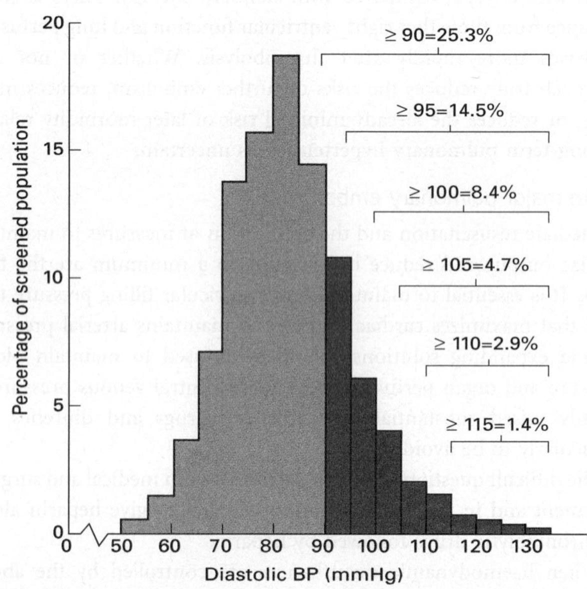

Fig. 1 Effect of different cut-off points on apparent prevalence of blood pressure, based upon single blood pressure measurements in a healthy population
(reproduced from Swales et al. 1991, with permission).

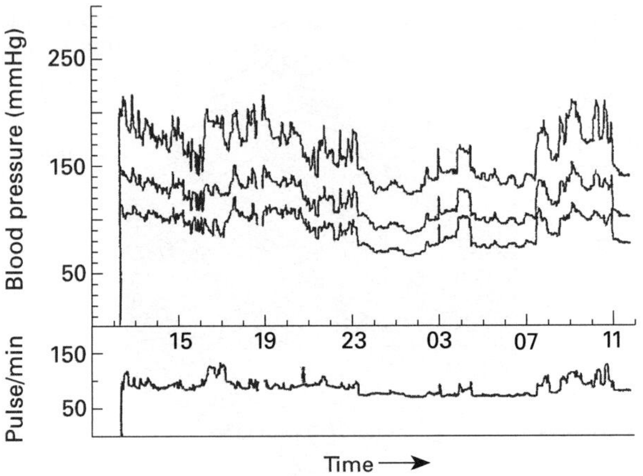

Fig. 2 Changes in blood pressure (measured by intra-arterial cannula) over 24 h
(reproduced from Swales et al. 1991, with permission).

Intraindividual blood pressure variation

Blood pressure shows great variability. Exposure to pain, mental stress, exercise, or sexual intercourse give rise to rapid elevation of pressure. Blood pressure also changes over the 24-h period, reaching its nadir during the early hours of the morning and reaching a maximum on rising (Fig. 2).

Genetic factors

The correlation between blood pressures in blood relatives of hypertensives is relatively weak and of little clinical value in screening programmes. Thus, the average correlation coefficient when blood pressures are corrected for age and sex is only of the order of 0.2. This suggests that the influence of the underlying genetic mechanisms is diluted by environmental factors and blood pressure variability. Adoption studies have shown a correlation between parents and natural children approximately twice as great as the correlation between parents and adoptive children and a similar relationship was observed for the correlation between siblings. The importance of environmental influences was illustrated by a correlation of blood pressure between adoptive siblings approximately twice as great as that between parent and adoptive child. Twin studies suggest a rather higher genetic contribution. Overall, these studies suggest that genetic factors contribute about 30 per cent to blood pressure variance.

The genes (probably more than five) that contribute to human essential hypertension have not been identified. There is a family linkage with the angiotensinogen gene, however, and there are, phenotypic associations with hypertension such as high body mass index, insulin resistance, and hyperlipidaemia. Some rare forms of secondary hypertension are due to mutations in a single gene. These include Liddle's syndrome (epithelial sodium channel gene) and glucocorticoid suppressible hyperaldosteronism (11-β-hydroxy-steroid dehydrogenase gene).

Environmental factors

Nutrition

Some studies have shown that subjects with lower birth weight and higher placental weight have higher blood pressure in middle age. It has been suggested on these grounds that maternal malnutrition may be an important determinant of the risk of subsequent hypertension (and other cardiovascular disease). However, birth weight reflects the influence of many factors and the processes responsible for this association have not been clarified. 'Central' obesity measured by waist to hip circumference correlates better with blood pressure than overall body mass, perhaps associated with genetic or humoral factors, but intervention trials have shown that reduction in body weight is associated with reduction in blood pressure. The mechanism is unknown.

High alcohol intake

More than 6 units/day, where 1 unit equals half a pint of beer, one measure of spirits, or a glass of wine has been shown to be associated with elevated blood pressure, independent of body mass index, age, or social class. The relationship between alcohol intake and blood pressure is causal, as reduction in intake in heavy drinkers lowers blood pressure.

Electrolyte intake

A number of studies, where different cultures are compared, have shown a positive association between sodium intake and blood pressure and a negative association between potassium intake and blood pressure. By combining the two into a sodium–potassium ratio a closer correlation has been observed. By contrast, analysis of electrolyte intake and blood pressure within a single culture has failed in most cases to show a significant association. Intervention studies in which sodium intake is restricted or potassium intake increased have shown modest effect in hypertensive subjects but only minimal or no effects in normotensives. Only if sodium intake is restricted to extremely low levels (less than 10 mmol/day), has blood pressure been lowered substantially. On current evidence the contribution of excessive sodium intake or inadequate potassium intake to hypertension in Western society is small. Some population studies have suggested that subjects with a low calcium or magnesium intake have higher blood pressures but intervention trials have either failed to show any effect or shown minimal effects when dietary intake of these electrolytes was increased.

Vegetarian diet

Vegetarians have lower blood pressures at all ages than omnivores. When omnivores change to a vegetarian diet blood pressure falls in both normotensives and hypertensives by a few mmHg. Increased intake of fruit and vegetables has been shown to lower blood pressure in omnivore hypertensives. One possibility is that unsaturated vegetable fats lower blood pressure. Saturated (ω-3) fish oils have been shown to lower blood pressure in several studies.

Stress

An acute major rise in blood pressure can be produced by acute pain, tension, or mental stress but it is much more difficult to show that chronic stress produces sustained elevation of blood pressure. Stress is difficult to measure and stressful circumstances have different effects on individuals. While there are clear social differences in human blood pressure these are not necessarily related to occupation or stress, although, it has been possible to demonstrate an association between 'job strain' and blood pressure.

Mechanisms of hypertension

The final common pathway in the genesis of hypertension appears to be in the vessels that maintain peripheral resistance, as cardiac output is normal in chronic hypertension. The resistance vessels in patients with hypertension show a reduction in luminal diameter associated with an increase in wall thickness. The close relationship between resistance vessel wall to lumen ratio and blood pressure appears to be secondary to the increased pressure but this does not entirely exclude a role for genetic factors modulating resistance vessel structure. Some of the rat genetic models of hypertension show enhanced smooth muscle growth and proliferation in tissue culture but so far there is no evidence for a primary abnormality of smooth muscle growth in humans. A reduction in the total number of resistance vessels is another genetically mediated possibility.

Autonomic nervous system

Essential hypertension in young subjects is associated with slightly elevated circulating noradrenaline and increased pulse rate and cardiac output. Genetically preconditioned autonomic over activity and social stress probably play important complementary roles.

Although baroreceptor sensitivity is reduced in hypertensive patients this is probably the result of structural changes in the walls of the large arteries in which the baroreceptors are situated causing them to become more inelastic. Rendering baroreceptors totally insensitive by denervation increases blood pressure variability but does not cause sustained increases in blood pressure.

Sodium

Blood pressure is remarkably sodium dependent in most patients with chronic renal failure, but sodium restriction produces only a modest fall in blood pressure in patients with essential hypertension (see above). This response is variable and it has been claimed that there is a discrete group of subjects with essential hypertension who are 'sodium sensitive' but the reproducibility of this phenomenon is poor. Essential hypertensives as a group show no increased sodium intake, no impairment of sodium excretion, and no increased body sodium content. At most, dietary sodium may amplify other blood pressure raising mechanisms and contribute secondarily to the rise in blood pressure with age.

Humoral mechanisms

The renin–angiotensin–aldosterone system, kallikrein–kinin, atrial natriuretic peptide, endothelin prostaglandin, and renomedullary lipid systems have all been implicated at one time or another, but there is no persuasive evidence to implicate any of these systems as a primary cause of essential hypertension, although they may respond to the rise in blood pressure.

Natural history

Mortality

Insurance company data show progressive increases in mortality with increasing systolic and diastolic blood pressures (Fig. 3). This relationship is continuous, with no break in the curve below which blood pressure ceases to be a risk factor. Indeed, those individuals with blood pressure below the population mean have a relative mortality less than the population average. Systolic and diastolic blood pressures are independent risk factors. Cardiac deaths are increased two- to threefold in patients with isolated systolic hypertension (i.e. systolic blood pressure over 160 mmHg, diastolic blood pressure below 95 mmHg).

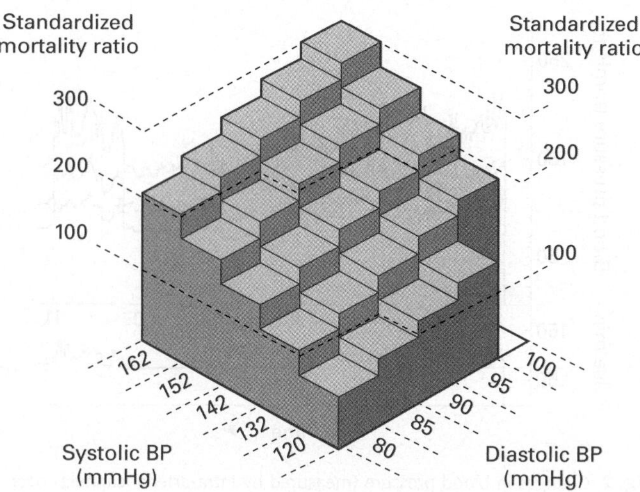

Fig. 3 Standardized mortality ratios in a healthy population. Note that systolic and diastolic pressures are independent risk factors. Risk progressively increases throughout the 'normal blood pressure range' *(reproduced from Swales et al. 1991, with permission).*

Mild hypertension and prognosis

Mild hypertension is a much more common problem than moderate or severe hypertension in unselected clinical practice. Even modest elevation of blood pressure impairs prognosis substantially. Thus, the life expectancy of a 35-year-old man with a casual blood pressure of 150/100 is reduced from 41.5 to 35 years; at 55 the relevant figures are 23.5 years and 17.5 years. Approximately half the hypertensive deaths in the Framingham population occurred in patients with blood pressures of 140 to 160/90 to 95 mmHg.

Prognosis in malignant hypertension (see also Chapter 12.24)

The presence of malignant hypertension greatly worsens prognosis. Before effective antihypertensive medication was available malignant hypertension was associated with a 1-year life expectancy of only 10–20 per cent. This has now been radically altered, particularly when effective treatment is begun early. Current 5-year survival rates are in excess of 80 per cent among patients who were free of significant renal impairment at presentation. Malignant hypertension is now much less common as a result of earlier detection and effective treatment.

Specific morbidity of hypertension

Cerebrovascular disease

In the Framingham study hypertensive patients were six times more likely to develop a stroke than normotensive controls. Although it seems probable that the risk of cerebral haemorrhage is more closely related to blood pressure than the risk of cerebral infarction, a high proportion of strokes (70–80 per cent) in unselected populations are due to cerebral infarction and there is no doubt that hypertension is a risk factor for cerebral infarction as well as cerebral haemorrhage.

Cardiac disease

In the Framingham study patients with hypertension were three times more likely to develop coronary heart disease and chronic heart failure than normotensive people. Heart failure as a result of hypertension becomes progressively more common with advancing age. Other studies have shown a smooth relationship between diastolic and systolic blood pressure and cardiac mortality.

Peripheral arterial disease

This is twice as common in hypertensive patients as normotensive controls. Smoking as a risk factor greatly outweighs blood pressure, although the two risks are additive.

Renal failure

Renal failure as a result of essential hypertension is almost always the consequence of the malignant phase. Although hypertension has been reported as the cause of renal failure in as many as 25 per cent of patients entering replacement programmes, the diagnosis in many such patients must be uncertain. In many cases renal failure is the result of renal arterial disease due to hypertension (ischaemic nephropathy). There is no doubt, however, that uncontrolled hypertension exacerbates renal failure in patients with primary renal diseases.

Pathology

Blood vessel changes

Large arteries

Hypertension produces medial thickening in the aorta and large arteries associated with disruption and uncoiling of elastic fibres and increase in the relatively inelastic collagen. Calcium is deposited secondarily. These changes are associated with ageing as well: the two processes are additive so that loss of elastic reservoir function of these vessels (the Windkessel vessels) occurs at an earlier age in hypertensive than in normotensive subjects. The decrease in arterial compliance allows the pressure wave generated during systole to be transmitted throughout the arterial tree in a less dampened form thereby increasing pulse pressure. The shape of the arterial wave form is also altered as a result of early return of the reflection wave from the periphery. This boosts the arterial pressure wave in late systole and so increases the stress on the arterial wall. This accounts for the association between pulse pressure and cardiovascular mortality.

Decreased compliance of the large arteries also has an important effect on the carotid and aortic baroreceptors which become less sensitive.

Atheroma in hypertension

There is a close association between the development of atheroma and blood pressure. The key process in atherogenesis in the hypertensive patient is probably increased endothelial permeability arising as a result of local stress. This allows exposure of the subendothelial arterial wall to growth factors derived from endothelium, macrophages, and platelets (see Chapter 2.7).

Resistance vessel changes

The increase of the wall to lumen ratio results in an increased reactivity to pressor agonists. The major histological change is growth and remodelling of the medial smooth muscle cells.

The heart

Angina and myocardial infarction in the hypertensive patient are usually due to coronary atheroma. The stimulus to left ventricular hypertrophy is unquestionably left ventricular load but the response to pressure may be amplified by activation of the renin–angiotensin–aldosterone system or increased sympathetic nerve activity. The bad prognosis carried by left ventricular hypertrophy in the hypertensive patient could reflect integrated exposure of the circulation to raised pressure. This is, however, not a sufficient explanation. The increased risk is also probably due to ischaemia produced by the increased muscle mass or the increased prevalence of simple and complex ventricular arrhythmias. The decrease in ventricular compliance also probably predisposes patients to left ventricular failure.

Cerebral blood vessels

Cerebral infarction in a hypertensive patient is usually attributable to atheroma of one of the larger cerebral arteries (usually the middle cerebral). Intracerebral haemorrhage is usually the result of rupture of a small intracerebral degenerative aneurysm (Charcot–Bouchard aneurysm). These lesions develop in the small perforating arteries in the region of the basal ganglia, thalamus, and the internal capsule. The incidence of Charcot–Bouchard aneurysms is closely correlated with age and blood pressure.

Hypertensive encephalopathy

When blood pressure rises above the autoregulatory range, focal areas of vasodilatation and oedema occur; haemorrhages, localized ischaemia, and infarction may result, giving rise to the clinical picture of encephalopathy.

The kidney in essential hypertension

In non-malignant hypertension renal blood flow is reduced, but glomerular filtration rate is preserved with an increase filtration fraction. Intracapillary glomerular pressure is increased. Hyaline degeneration is particularly observed in the afferent arterioles. Progressive hyalinization of nephrons accounts for the slow decline in glomerular filtration rate with age. The rate of this loss is increased in essential hypertension.

Blood vessels in malignant hypertension

The malignant phase occurs when blood pressure rises rapidly. In more long-standing hypertension arteriolar hypertrophy is protective. The characteristic pathological change is fibrinoid necrosis. The normal structure of the vessel wall is replaced with fibrin-like material. Fibrinoid necrosis is usually associated with focal areas of vasodilatation and increased permeability, primarily a mechanical effect. The endothelium of the dilated segments is disrupted and the vessel wall becomes permeable, allowing exudation of plasma into the media. The intima may become massively thickened by concentric collagenous rings until the lumen is almost obliterated. Changes in the glomerular vessels lead to rapidly progressively renal failure associated with increased glomerular permeability, proteinuria, and haematuria. Encephalopathy is caused by pressure-induced dilation of cerebral vessels and resultant oedema. Cerebral haemorrhage may occur. Death without treatment is largely due to rapidly progressive renal failure.

The clinical features of essential hypertension

Symptoms

Elevated blood pressure is usually asymptomatic. In some cases the knowledge that a patient has high blood pressure creates a fertile soil for the growth of functional symptoms particularly headache. 'Labelling' a patient as hypertensive may lead to increased absenteeism from work. Epistaxis is not particularly associated with mild hypertension but is more common in moderate to severe cases. Where patients present with epistaxis and high blood pressure it is important to dissociate hypertension as a cause of epistaxis from a pressor response to the episode.

When target organs are damaged, secondary symptoms arise. Other than stroke, angina, or myocardial infarcation, the commonest will be those of left ventricular dysfunction. The malignant phase is a cause of headache and may present with visual disturbance caused by retinal haemorrhage.

Measurement of blood pressure

Using the conventional sphygmomanometer, systolic pressure is taken to be that at which sounds return (Korokoff phase I). As the pressure is further lowered the sounds suddenly become muffled (Korotkoff phase IV) and shortly afterwards disappear (Korotkoff phase V). Both phase IV and phase V sounds have been used as estimates of diastolic pressure. Phase V is now recommended. Auscultatory measurement of blood pressure is often carried out badly: interobserver and even intraobserver variability is often unacceptably high. There are a number of important precautions which have to be taken.

Bladder and cuff

The bladder has to be long enough and wide enough to achieve adequate occlusion of the brachial artery when the pressure within the cuff equals arterial pressure. If the cuff is too small inadequate pressure will be applied and blood pressure will be overestimated. The length of the bladder should be at least 80 per cent and the width of the bladder at least 40 per cent of the circumference of the arm. Mercury manometers should be vertical and should read zero when no pressure is applied to the cuff. Aneroid manometers require regular calibration (at least yearly) by comparison with a mercury manometer.

Technique

Patients should be comfortable seated or supine. The arm should be held horizontal and supported at mid-sternal level. Tight or restrictive clothing should be removed from the arm. An appropriate sized cuff should be applied so that its mid-point lies over the position of maximal pulsation of the brachial artery. Blood pressure should be recorded in both arms on initial examination and the arm found to have the higher pressures subsequently used. Systolic blood pressure is initially determined by palpation and then the stethoscope is lightly placed over the brachial artery and the cuff pressure raised to approximately 30 mm above the point at which the radial pulse disappears and then released at the rate of 2–3 mm/s. Both systolic and diastolic blood pressure should be read to the nearest 2 mm mark. The point of disappearance of sounds (phase V Korotkoff) is preferable to the point of muffling (phase IV). In some situations sounds can be detected down to zero cuff pressure. This is often the case in pregnancy. Under these circumstances the fourth phase has to be used.

Semi-automatic (electronic) devices are now extensively used and, with concerns about the use of mercury, likely to replace the mercury sphygmomanometer. Reliability is variable and validation and regular calibration are essential.

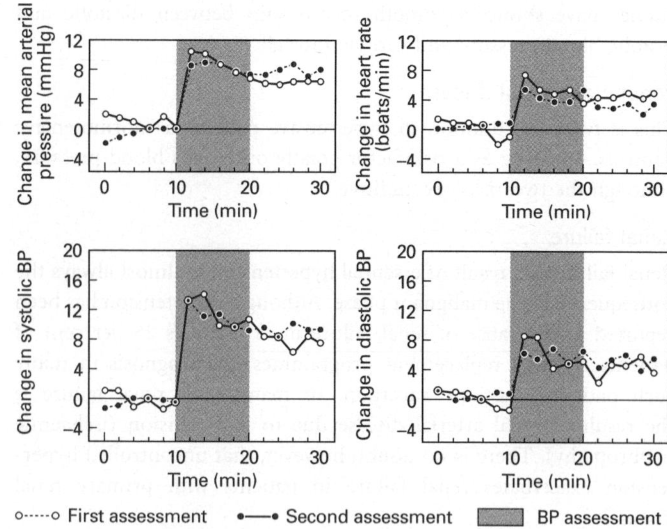

Fig. 4 White coat hypertension measured by an intra-arterial cannula on two occasions. Note the rise in blood pressure when a doctor approached the patient
(reproduced from Swales et al. 1991, with permission).

Indirect ambulatory blood pressure monitoring

Indirect monitoring can be carried out either by patient-triggered measurement or automatic measurement with cuff inflation at regular intervals. Ambulatory monitoring has demonstrated major divergences between casual blood pressure in the clinic and blood pressure levels outside it. In most cases clinic measurements are higher. In some cases dramatic elevations of blood pressure occur when measurements are carried out by a doctor (white coat hypertension) (Fig. 4). Although the evidence is not conclusive, it seems probable that average blood pressures measured by ambulatory monitoring are better predictors of cardiovascular risk than clinic measurements. Epidemiological and trial data are all based on clinic measurements. Increasingly, however ambulatory monitoring is being used in initial patient assessment to evaluate patients whose blood pressure is only elevated when measured in a clinic. Patients who show absence or attenuation of the normal fall in blood pressure at night are at increased cardiovascular risk ('non-dippers').

Fundal examination

Fundal appearances provide vital information on vascular pathology and prognosis in hypertension. The Keith Wagener classification is still used. In *grade I* the light reflex from the arterial wall is increased as a result of thickening, and in *grade II* the arterial light reflex is wider still and gives rise to a homogeneous silver wire appearance. Nipping of the retinal vein occurs largely as a result of the optical effect of the thickened arterial wall preventing visualization of the column of blood within the vein. These changes are produced by ageing as well as hypertension. Generalized reduction in arterial diameter with a consequent reduction in arterial-to-venous ratio is probably the most sensitive retinal sign of elevated blood pressure. In *grade III*, lesions may occur singly or in combination. Flame-shaped haemorrhages owe their character to constraints imposed by nerve fibres. Dot and blot haemorrhages are deep to the nerve fibres and so are not limited in the same way. Hard or waxy exudates represent the end results of fluid leakage into of the retina from damaged vessels often with associated nerve vessel damage. Soft exudates or cotton-wool patches are aetiologically and ophthalmoscopically quite different. They are usually larger and have a woolly, ill-defined edge. They are not true exudates but nerve fibre infarcts caused by hypertensive vascular occlusion. In *grade IV* severe arteriolar damage leads to papilloedema. The surrounding retina is often oedematous and small radial haemorrhages and cotton wool exudates are common. Grade III and IV changes are diagnostic of the malignant phase, requiring urgent assessment and treatment.

Management of essential hypertension

Establishing the diagnosis

When there is no clinical suspicion of secondary hypertension (see Chapter 2.32), extensive investigation for a primary cause is unnecessary. Measurement of serum urea, sodium, potassium, and creatinine, urinary microscopy, and dip stick measurement of protein are sufficient.

Assessment of the effects of hypertension

Examination of the fundi and detection of left ventricular hypertrophy provide the best evidence of severity of hypertension. When changes are detected, the possibility of white coat hypertension can be discounted, but in many patients with high arterial pressure there are no other abnormal signs. In them, and in ambulatory monitoring, white coat hypertension may be revealed. Echocardiography is the best way to detect early left ventricular hypertrophy. Heart failure and grade III or IV fundal changes indicate the need for urgent treatment.

Concurrent disease and risk factors

A history of smoking, the presence of glucose intolerance or diabetes, and hyperlipidaemia increase the cardiovascular risks of hypertension and may tip the balance in favour of active treatment, as well as requiring management in their own right. A history of obstructive airways disease contraindicates the use of β-blockers and gout usually contraindicates thiazide diuretics.

Advice and non-pharmacological treatment

Drug treatment of hypertension often creates unpleasant symptoms in an individual who previously felt perfectly well. It is essential therefore to explain the significance of high blood pressure. Many patients find difficulty in grasping the concept of blood pressure variability. Often they are alarmed at single high readings. Discussion of a simple plan for assessment, which involves evaluation of blood pressure on repeated measurement and explanation that treatment will not necessarily improve subjective symptoms, encourages a realistic approach by patients. Except for those who present with severe hypertension, repeated measurements of blood pressure should be carried out before drug therapy is considered.

This period of assessment can be combined with advice and non-pharmacological treatment. The duration of the period of observation and the number of blood pressure measurements that need to be carried out before a decision about drug therapy is made depend upon the severity of hypertension. A period of 3–6 months observation with measurements every 2–4 weeks is often appropriate for mild hypertension (diastolic blood pressure less than 110 mmHg) without advanced retinopathy. This period should probably be curtailed for diastolic blood pressures of 110 mHg or more unless a marked 'white coat' response is demonstrated with ambulatory monitoring.

Non-pharmacological treatment

Dietary methods include weight reduction, alcohol withdrawal, sodium restriction, and potassium supplementation. Behavioural methods include physical training, biofeedback, and relaxation.

Weight reduction

Dietary weight reduction in obese subjects produces a useful fall in arterial pressure. Even a weight loss of 3 kg on average produces a fall in blood pressure of 7/4 mmHg.

Alcohol withdrawal

The elevated blood pressures in heavy drinkers (more than 6 units of alcohol per day) are lowered by withdrawal. This is not related to changes in weight or electrolyte intake.

Sodium restriction

The average intake of sodium in Westernized cultures is 120–180 mmol/day. Severe sodium restriction (to less than 10 mmol/day) produces substantial blood pressure lowering but is not feasible. Moderate sodium restriction (to 70–80 mmol/day) can be achieved by abstaining from adding salt at the table, avoiding salt in cooking, and avoiding heavily salted processed foods. Such moderate salt restriction enhances the effects of angiotensin-converting enzyme (ACE) inhibitors, β-blockers, and diuretics. Curiously, it seems to be ineffective in patients treated with calcium antagonists. As sole therapy, moderate salt restriction has a modest blood pressure lowering action in some patients (particularly in the older age groups). The individual response to moderate salt restriction is variable and it is worth a therapeutic trial during the period of assessment if patients are willing.

Potassium supplementation

Doubling potassium intake (i.e. supplementing it by about 80 mmol/day) has a modest blood pressure lowering action of the same order of magnitude as moderate sodium restriction. Indeed, the natriuresis produced by potassium loading may contribute to the blood pressure reduction observed. There is no justification for potassium supplementation as an independent form of treatment for essential hypertension. Advising patients to consume liberal quantities of fruit and vegetables may be justified on general grounds.

Other dietary manoeuvres

Fish-oils (ω-3 fatty acids) lower blood pressure in hypertensive patients. The effect only appears to be seen in those whose consumption of fish is low. Olive oil has been shown to have a very small blood pressure lowering effect in some studies, but there is little evidence to support a therapeutic effect of other unsaturated fatty acids. Claims have been made for calcium and magnesium supplementation, but these are not persuasive and have no place in clinical practice.

A diet high in fruit and vegetables has been shown to have a blood pressure lowering effect approaching that of monotherapy. The specific dietary component is uncertain, although potassium probably plays a part.

Physical exercise

Repetitive isotonic exercise produces a useful fall in blood pressure independently of any fall in weight. Moderate exercise in the form of daily jogging or brisk walking is probably sufficient to have a useful effect in lowering blood pressure, as well as improving well-being.

Behavioural therapy

There is some evidence that biofeedback and relaxation exercise can lower blood pressure in some hypertensive patients, but training is costly in terms of labour and, unless regularly reinforced, the effects of behavioural treatment tend to diminish with the passage of time.

Antihypertensive drug treatment

The British Hypertension Society recommend that drug therapy should be given if diastolic blood pressure averages 100 mmHg or more over the assessment period. In the USA a lower threshold (over 90 mmHg) is suggested, and WHO recommends treatment for those whose diastolic pressures remain over 95 mmHg at 3 months of observation. Although the differences between these varying recommendations seem small they have important implications for the number of patients treated. For instance, 25.3 per cent of patients at the Hypertension, Detection and Follow-up Program Screening Study had a blood pressure equal to or more than 90 mmHg, 14.5 per cent had a value equal to or more than 95 mmHg, and only 8.4 per cent had diastolic blood pressures equal to or more than 100 mmHg. It is probable therefore that reducing the threshold of treatment from 100 to 95 mmHg increases the number of patients eligible by 73 per cent. At some point the costs of treatment and the potential adverse effects outweigh the benefits. This balance differs substantially from patient to patient, and also depends upon the treatment employed. Ideally we should attempt to identify the patients at high risk so that we can avoid unnecessary treatment of those at low risk. Other factors (smoking, hyperlipidaemia, left ventricular hypertrophy, glucose intolerance) should reduce the threshold for treatment to 95 or even to 90 mmHg. Two major trials have demonstrated that the benefits of lowering systolic blood pressure are as great (or, in the elderly probably greater) than lowering diastolic blood pressure. The British guidelines suggest a threshold of 160 mmHg, while the USA guidelines recommend 140 mmHg.

The effect of drug treatment

Trials of efficacy have required large numbers of patients, as the incidence of overt cardiac or cerebrovascular disease is relatively low in those with moderately elevated blood pressures. The conclusions have shown an impressive degree of concordance. Meta-analysis of the data has demonstrated that for a drug-induced fall in diastolic blood pressure of only 5–6 mmHg, the incidence of strokes was reduced by 38 per cent and coronary heart disease by 16 per cent in patients with mild hypertension (Fig. 5). Epidemiological observations indicate an excess risk for stroke of 40 per cent for an increase of 5–6 mmHg, so that at least over the period of the trial the risk of stroke attributable to hypertension was totally reversed. The impact of treatment on coronary events is more difficult to interpret. Although pooling of trials does indicate a significant impact, this probably falls short of complete reversibility of the risk attributable to hypertension. The reasons for this are still controversial (see below).

Selection of therapy

Treatment is normally begun with a single agent (Table 1). Combination tablets are, however, becoming more popular as individual doses can be lowered and the risk of adverse events therefore reduced. Examples are the combination of thiazide and potassium sparing diuretic, which is widely employed, and the combination of an ACE inhibitor and thiazide diuretic. An exception is hypertension in pregnancy where methlydopa is widely used.

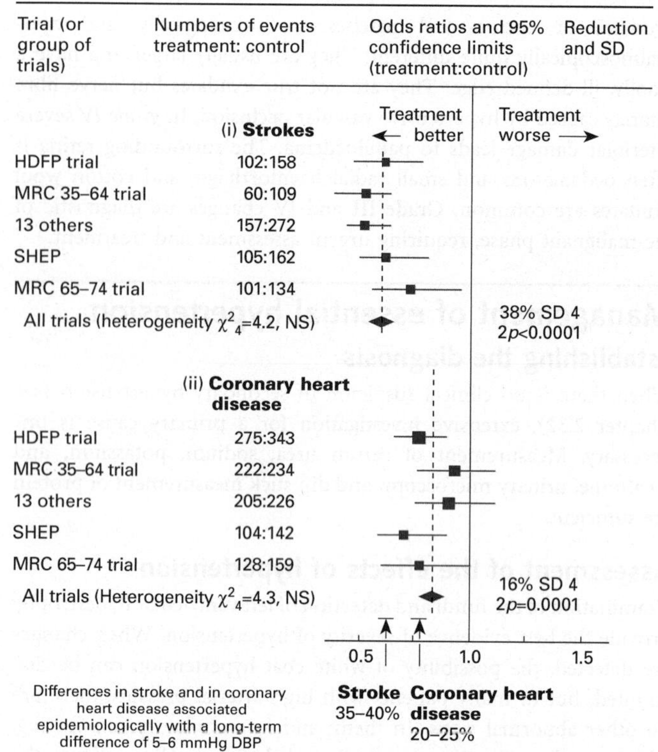

Fig. 5 Meta-analysis of end-point trials in the treatment of mild hypertension. Results from the 13 smaller trials are pooled together and the larger trials listed separately.
(Reproduced from Collins, R. and Peto, R. (1994). In Textbook of Hypertension (ed. J.D. Swales) Blackwell Scientific Publications, Oxford with permission.)

Six classes of agent are widely used. A seventh class, i.e. the centrally acting agents (methyldopa and clonidine) are not now recommended as first-line therapy because of the relatively high incidence of central side-effects (particularly sleepiness and depression).

Thiazide diuretics

These are effective and cheap. The major concern in their use has been metabolic adverse effects. These include increased total cholesterol, impairment of glucose tolerance, and hypokalaemia. It has been suggested that these undesirable effects may oppose the beneficial consequences of lowering blood pressure, and thus account for the failure of therapy to have a greater effect on the incidence of myocardial infarction. This is certainly not the case in elderly subjects, among whom diuretics have been associated with a greater reduction in cardiac events than β-blockers in endpoint trials (Fig. 6). Comparison of β-blockers and diuretics in younger subjects has given rise to more equivocal findings. The Medical Research Council (MRC) and HAPPHY trials failed to show any difference in outcome between diuretics and β-blockers. However, total infarction in the MRC trial (i.e. silent plus clinical myocardial infarction) was decreased by β-blocker treatment only and the HAPPHY trial showed a better cardiac outcome in the β-blocker-treated group. The dose of diuretic used may be an important factor. The earlier trials used high doses. Metabolic disturbances are minimal or non-existent at low doses (e.g. bendrofluazide 2.5 mg/day). There is no justification for exceeding this, or an equivalent dose.

Table 1 Drugs and dosages in the treatment of hypertension

Drug class	Drug	Dosage and regime
Diuretics	Bendrofluazide	2.5 mg o.d.
	Chlorthalidone	12.5 mg o.d.
	Amiloride	5 mg o.d.
	Triamterene	150–250 mg o.d.
β-Blockers	Propranolol*	80–160 mg b.d.
	Oxprenolol*	40–160 mg t.d.s.
	Pindolol	15–30 mg o.d.
	Sotalol	80–200 mg o.d.
	Timolol	10–30 mg o.d. or b.d.
	Acebutolol	200–400 mg o.d. or b.d.
	Atenolol	25–100 mg o.d.
	Bisoprolol	5–20 mg o.d.
	Metoprolol	100–200 mg o.d. or b.d.
	Celiprolol	200–400 mg o.d.
Calcium-channel blockers	Nifedipine (Retard)	10–40 mg b.d.
	Nicardipine	20–40 mg twice daily to t.d.s.
	Isradipine	2.5–10 mg b.d.
	Felodipine	5–20 mg o.d.
	Diltiazem SR	90–180 mg b.d
	Amlodipine	5–10 mg o.d.
	Verapamil	120–240 mg b.d.
Angiotensin-converting enzyme inhibitors	Benazepil	2.5–20 mg b.d.
	Captopril	12.5–50 mg twice daily or t.d.s.
	Enalapril	2.5–40 mg o.d.
	Fosinopril	10–40 mg o.d.
	Lisinopril	2.5–40 mg o.d.
	Perindopril	2–8 mg o.d.
	Quinapril	5–40 mg o.d.
	Ramipril	1.25–10 mg o.d.
	Trandolapril	1–4 mg o.d.
Angiotensin receptor blockers	Losartan	25–50 mg b.d.
	Valsartan	80–320 mg o.d
	Irbesartan	150–300 mg o.d.
α-Blockers	Prazosin	0.5–10 mg b.d.
	Doxazosin	1–16 mg o.d.
	Terazosin	1–20 mg o.d.
	Indoramin	25–100 mg twice daily or t.d.s.
Combined α–β	Labetalol	100–400 mg b.d.
Central	α-methyldopa	250 mg–1 g twice daily or t.d.s.
	Clonidine	0.05–0.4 mg t.d.s.
Vasodilators	Hydralazine	25–100 mg b.d.
	Minoxidil	2.5–25 mg b.d.
	Diazoxide	50–500 mg b.d.

Low-dose thiazide diuretics are preferred first-line treatment in elderly hypertensive subjects.

β-Blockers

These too have potentially adverse metabolic effects, producing an increase in serum triglycerides and a decrease in high-density lipoprotein (HDL) cholesterol. These effects are seen less with cardioselective agents and not at all in agents with intrinsic sympathomimetic activity. β-Blockers have the additional advantage of efficacy in reducing the incidence of a second myocardial infarction. They probably remain first-line therapy in younger patients (i.e. below the age of 65) who do not suffer from obstructive airways disease, peripheral vascular disease, or cardiac failure.

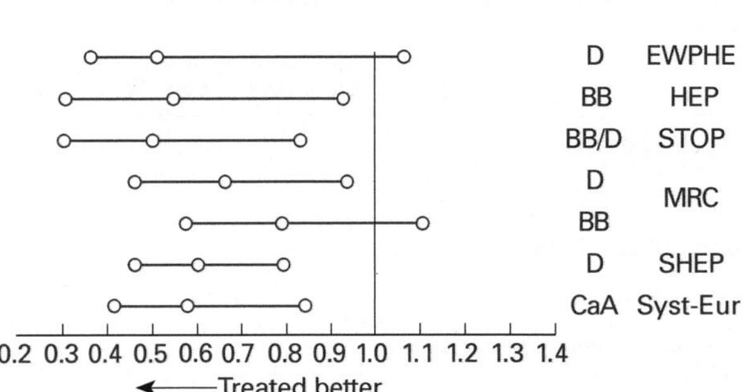

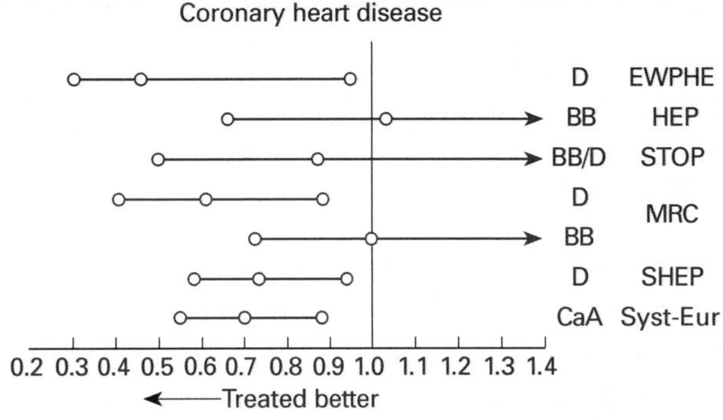

Fig. 6 Meta-analysis of the five trials of treatment in the elderly. While the impact upon stroke was significant in most cases, the impact on coronary heart disease appeared to be better with diuretics ('D') and calcium antagonists (CaA) than with β-blockers (B.B), where data on the two were presented separately.

Angiotensin-converting enzyme inhibitors

These are well tolerated, apart from the relatively high incidence of chronic dry cough (15 per cent). There are two serious side-effects, but these are rare in carefully screened patients.

Hypotension following the first dose is occasionally observed in patients with high levels of renin in plasma, usually as a result of previous intensive diuretic therapy or in severe and malignant hypertension. In any of these circumstances it is essential to start with the lowest available dose and to monitor blood pressure closely for several hours. In most patients it is probably sufficient to instruct them to take the first dose before retiring at night.

Acute renal failure may follow the use of ACE inhibitors in patients with critically reduced renal blood flow, i.e. bilateral tight renal artery stenosis or renal artery stenosis to a single kidney. Under these circumstances, and when cardiac output is low enough to produce comparably poor renal perfusion, angiotensin II causes arteriolar vasoconstriction in the efferent glomerular vessels, therefore maintaining intraglomerular filtration pressure. Blocking its formation removes this effect, resulting in a drastic fall in glomerular filtration caused by the fall in transglomerular capillary hydraulic pressure.

There are no completed comparative end-point trials of the use of ACE inhibitors in uncomplicated essential hypertension. Claims have been made that their usage might have a greater impact than those of other agents on coronary events as a result of beneficial effects upon cardiac mass, insulin resistance, and the absence of effect on serum lipids. These arguments are theoretical; as yet, ACE inhibitors cannot be considered routine first-line treatment of uncomplicated hypertension. Their major role is in those patients in whom the

Table 2 Selection of different classes of drugs in different clinical situations

	D	β-B	ACE	ARB	CaB	α-B
< 60 years healthy		+				
> 60 years healthy	+					
Ischaemic heart disease		+				
Previous infarction		+				
Cardiac failure/dilatation	+	−	+	+		
Black subjects	+				+	+
Diabetics			+	+	+	+
Contraindications to or poor tolerance of other therapy	+	+	+	+	+	+

D = diuretics; β-B = β-blockers; ACE = ACE inhibitors; ARB = angiotensin receptor blockers; CaB = calcium blockers; α-B = α-blockers.

preferred first-line agents cannot be used or have proved unacceptable and in specific situations (Table 2).

Calcium antagonists

Suggestions that these agents might increase the incidence of coronary artery disease are controversial and most physicians continue to use them. The major disadvantage of earlier dihydropyridine agents was activation of the sympathetic system with headache, sweating, palpitation, and burning sensations in the skin. Oedema is another adverse effect. Longer-acting agents and slow release preparations have reduced these problems.

Case–control studies and systemic reviews of clinical trials have suggested that short-acting dihydropyridine calcium channel blockers are associated with increased mortality from coronary heart disease. Although this finding has been challenged there is no indication for these agents in treating hypertension.

Angiotensin receptor (AT_1) blockers

These agents specifically inhibit the renin–angiotensin system at the angiotensin receptor level. Their main pharmacological difference from ACE inhibitors is therefore the absence of kinin potentiation. This probably accounts for the absence of cough as a side-effect. They are particularly useful in patients who have ACE-inhibitor induced cough, or sensitivity the incidence of adverse effects is low.

α-Adrenoreceptor blockers

These are less extensively used as first-line therapy. The longer acting α-blockers (doxazosin and terozasin) are well tolerated, although occasional postural hypotension is seen. α-Blockers have a beneficial action upon plasma lipids producing a slight increase in HDL cholesterol and a reduction in low-density lipoprotein cholesterol. How far this can be translated into reduced incidence of ischaemic heart disease is unknown. α-Blockers provide a reasonable alternative treatment to the preferred first-line agents (Table 2).

Vasodilators

Hydralazine was once extensively used. The main disadvantages were autonomic activation and the development of a lupus-like syndrome in patients with the slow acetylator genotype.

Minoxidil and diazoxide are extremely potent vasodilators reserved for patients whose blood pressure is resistant to other medication. The major disadvantages with both are severe oedema and hair growth. In addition, T wave changes in the electrocardiogram may be due to an increase in cardiac work as a result of generalized vasodilatation. Diazoxide has the added disadvantage of causing glucose intolerance and diabetes in over half of patients treated long term and is very little used now.

Combination therapy

When a single drug does not control blood pressure there is a choice between substituting another drug or adding a second agent. The latter is more generally favoured because it is more likely to produce early effective blood pressure control. Certain combinations are logical and effective. These include adding a β-blocker or an ACE inhibitor to a diuretic or adding a calcium channel blocker to a β-blocker. α-Blockers can be combined with any other class of agent. Some combinations are less effective, e.g. ACE inhibitor and β-blocker or calcium channel blocker and diuretic. These combinations are not contraindicated, however, and there may be other indications in the form of coexistent morbidity for using them.

Target blood pressure

The objective of treatment should be to maintain diastolic blood pressure in the range 80–90 and systolic blood pressure below 160. The Hypertension Optimal Treatment (**HOT**) study reported the lowest incidence of cardiovascular events when patients achieved a systolic blood pressure of 138 mmHg and a diastolic blood pressure of 83 mmHg. However, the gains from further reductions below 140/90 were marginal. There is evidence from HOT and the UK Prospective Diabetes Study that tight blood pressure control is important in preventing diabetic vascular complications. In diabetics therefore blood pressures of 130–140 mmHg systolic and 80–85 mmHg diastolic should be targeted.

Resistant hypertension

Poor compliance is a common cause and is often difficult to detect. In some cases it may be necessary to admit a patient to hospital and supervise administration of treatment.

White coat hypertension

Diagnosis requires ambulatory monitoring, although the absence of target organ damage and left ventricular hypertrophy despite apparent poor control provide a clue.

Genuine refractory hypertension

This occurs in a minority of patients. On occasions, previously well controlled blood pressure may escape from control. Under these circumstances enquiries should be made about other pharmacological agents which may be inhibiting the response such as sodium retaining drugs (particularly non-steroidal anti-inflammatory agents), sympathomimetics, antidepressants, and adrenal steroids. In other cases alcohol excess may be the reason. Where none of these explanations can be demonstrated more potent regimens may be required. The combination of calcium channel blocker, ACE inhibitor, and diuretic is particularly effective. Alternatively, a combination of minoxidil with a β-blocker and diuretic will control blood pressure in the large majority of cases. Probably the most potent combination of all is minoxidil, an ACE inhibitor and diuretic.

Malignant hypertension

This requires immediate treatment, but parenteral therapy is normally contraindicated because of the risk that an over-rapid reduction in pressure at a time when autoregulation of cerebral blood flow is compromised carries the risk of acute cerebral or retinal infarction. Oral therapy producing a gradual fall in blood pressure over 3–4 days is normally sufficient. Parenteral treatment is required in the presence of encephalopathy and, on occasion, when there is associated left ventricular failure.

Hypertensive encephalopathy

This is manifest by fluctuating neurological signs associated with high blood pressure and usually advanced retinopathy. The critical feature is the fluctuation of signs. Encephalopathy is more common in patients whose hypertension has developed over a relatively short period of time and who have not therefore had the opportunity to develop protective vascular hypertrophy. It is particularly seen in hypertension of pregnancy, in association with renovascular hypertension, in scleroderma renal crisis, or in acute nephritic syndromes.

Blood pressure must be reduced immediately. The agent of choice is sodium nitroprusside although other vasodilators such as diazoxide, hydralazine, or nitroglycerine can be given parenterally. The major danger is precipitation of cerebral infarction through an excessive fall in blood pressure. 'Excessive' in this situation may include restoration of blood pressure to apparently normal levels. It is, therefore, inadvisable to lower diastolic blood pressure in the first 24–48 h below 100 to 115 mmHg.

Further reading

Joint National Committee on Prevention, Detection, Evaluation and Treatment of High Blood Pressure (1997). Sixth Report. *Archives of Internal Medicine*, **157**, 2413–45.

Sever, P., Beevers, G., Bulpitt, C., Lever, A., Ramsay, L., Reid, J., and Swales, J.D. (1993). Management guidelines in essential hypertension: report of the Second Working Party of the British Hypertension Society. *British Medical Journal*, **306**, 983–7.

Swales, J.D. (1995). *Manual of hypertension*. Blackwell Science, Oxford.

Taubes, G. (1998). The (political) science of salt. *Science*, **281**, 898–907.

Chapter 2.32

Secondary hypertension

A. E. G. Raine and J. G. G. Ledingham*

An underlying cause is unlikely to exist in more than 10 per cent of unselected hypertensives. Even so there are a number of conditions in which appropriate treatment may cure hypertension. These include Cushing's syndrome, primary aldosteronism and liquorice addiction (see Section 7), phaeochromocytoma, renin secreting tumour, and hypertension associated with the contraceptive pill, but the commonest underlying causes are renal and renovascular disorders.

*It is with regret that we report the death of Professor A. E. G. Raine.

Renal and renovascular hypertension

Frequency

Different series have indicated a prevalence of renal parenchymal disease of 3–4 per cent in unselected hypertensive populations and of renovascular disease between 1 and 5 per cent.

Hypertension in renal disease

Most patients with severe renal impairment become hypertensive and raised arterial pressure is an early feature of all glomerular diseases and of adult polycystic disease. Salt and water retention in advanced renal failure is an important mechanism and in some cases plasma renin levels may be inappropriately high in relation to sodium balance. These are not the only mechanisms, however, as many uraemic patients have no relationship between blood pressure and blood volume, plasma renin activity, or the product of the two. Sympathetic activity is increased in hypertensive dialysis patients and abnormalities of the vasdilator nitric oxide pathway may also contribute, a possibility supported by observations of up to ninefold increases of circulating levels of endogenous inhibitors of nitric oxide synthesis in uraemic patients.

Renovascular hypertension

The two most common causes are atheromatous disease and fibromuscular hyperplasia. Other much rarer causes include dissecting aneurysm of the aorta, renal arterial thrombosis or embolism, abdominal trauma, neurofibromatosis, post-irradiation fibrosis, and Takayasu's arteritis.

Hypertension arises at least in part because underperfusion of the kidney leads to activation of the renin–angiotensin system which may cause the initial rise in pressure. When there is stenosis of a sole functioning kidney or of both kidneys, hypertension subsequently becomes dependent on volume and sodium retention and plasma renin may then return to normal levels. When there is moderate unilateral stenosis, plasma renin may be normal, but is more inclined to rise when stenosis is severe. Peripheral plasma renin assays are therefore not of value in the diagnosis of renovascular hypertension.

Clinical diagnosis of renal and renovascular hypertension

History

A family history of adult polycystic disease, Alport's syndrome, or other hereditary nephropathy should be sort. Symptoms such as gross haematuria, frothy urine (proteinuria), or dysuria may have been noticed. Polyuria and nocturia are only evident when renal function has declined to less than 50 per cent of normal. Malignant hypertension or hypertension in the adolescent or young adult (under 30 years) should always raise suspicion of renal, renovascular, or other form of secondary hypertension. Equally, hypertension arising over a short space of months in late middle age in a patient known to have been previously normotensive suggests acquired atheromatous renovascular disease as should exacerbation of hypertension in a previously well controlled patient. Angiotensin-converting enzyme (**ACE**) inhibitors may cause an acute deterioration in renal function when severe renovascular disease is present; a significant (>50 mol/l) increase of plasma creatinine within 7–10 days of starting an ACE inhibitor should always raise the possibility of renovascular disease.

Physical examination

Occasionally large kidneys can be felt, suggesting polycystic disease or hydronephrosis. More rarely, a palpable bladder may indicate obstructive uropathy or pallor, foetor and uraemic pigmentation may indicate advanced renal failure.

Renovascular disease is frequently associated with coronary artery disease and peripheral vascular disease; palpation of peripheral pulses and auscultation of bruits over femoral and carotid vessels as well as over the abdomen is particularly important. An abdominal or epigastric bruit has a low predictive value for renovascular disease, but a continuous or systolic–diastolic one is much more suggestive.

Investigations

The presence of haematuria or proteinuria either makes it essential to perform urine microscopy. Blood biochemistry may show elevation of urea and creatinine concentrations.

Twenty-four-hour urine collection gives reasonably accurate quantitation of protein excretion. Proteinuria in moderate and severe essential hypertension rarely exceeds a total of 1 g in 24 h. In bilateral renovascular disease up to 3 or 4 g in 24 h may be found, but heavy proteinuria, greater than this level, usually indicates underlying glomerular disease.

Renal ultrasound should be performed in any patient with suspected renal hypertension. It may reveal polycystic kidney disease or obstructive uropathy. It will show whether the kidneys are reduced in size or have parenchymal thinning, suggesting established chronic renal disease. In addition, it will show whether the kidneys are of unequal length, increasing the likelihood of renovascular disease. If an inequality of more than 1.5 cm in length is found, further investigations for renovascular disease are indicated.

The intravenous urogram remains useful in the diagnosis of chronic pyelonephritis with renal scarring, which is the most common cause of hypertension in patients aged under 20.

Renal biopsy may be valuable in determining whether renal impairment in patients with malignant hypertension is a consequence of hypertension itself, or whether an underlying primary renal disease is the precipitant. This distinction has a major bearing on outcome; in a Japanese survey of 69 patients presenting with accelerated hypertension and renal impairment, renal survival was 60 per cent after 5 years in patients with underlying essential hypertension, and only 4 per cent over 18 months in patients with chronic glomerulonephritis.

Treatment of hypertension in chronic renal disease

Early and effective treatment is essential, both because hypertension will accelerate progressive renal disease and because of the high risk of later cardiac and vascular complications in these patients (see Chapter 2.29).

Hypertension in acute renal disease

The increase in blood pressure may be rapid and severe, sufficient to cause the malignant phase or the neurological manifestations of hypertensive encephalopathy.

Renin-secreting tumours

Benign haemangiopericytomas in the kidney may contain cells resembling those of the juxtaglomerular apparatus which secrete renin, and are a very rare cause of potentially curable hypertension, associated with hypokalaemic alkalosis. Hypertension is often severe, and most frequently arises in the second to fourth decade, affecting males and females equally. The tumours are usually small, and are easily missed on angiography. Diagnosis may be supported by demonstration of elevated renin activity in the renal venous blood on the affected side. The response to surgical removal of the tumour is excellent.

A similar syndrome may result from hypersecretion of renin from Wilms' tumour, from renal cell carcinoma or from extrarenal tissues such as pancreatic, pulmonary, hepatic, or Fallopian tube carcinoma. The incidence of hypertension in patients with renal cell carcinoma ranges from less than 10 per cent to 50 per cent.

Renovascular disease

Atheromatous disease or fibromuscular dysplasia?

Renal angiography detects renovascular disease and determines whether it is due to atheroma or to fibrous dysplasia. In the former, which comprise 65–75 per cent of all cases of renovascular hypertension, patients are generally over 50 years old and are often smokers. There is usually extensive aortic atheromatous disease, together with atheromatous narrowing of one or both renal arteries. The lesions are usually located at or near the junction of the renal artery and the aorta, and quite frequently there is total occlusion of one renal artery as a result of the atheromatous process (Fig. 1).

The aorta appears normal in fibromuscular dysplasia and the lesions occur in the distal two-thirds of the renal arteries, often extending into the intrarenal branches. The radiological appearance resembles a string of beads (Fig. 2), and is caused by alternating areas of stenosis (due to medial fibrosis) and aneurysmal dilatation in areas where the internal elastic lamina and vascular smooth muscle are deficient. These lesions may affect one or both renal arteries, and may also occur in the carotid, coeliac axis, mesenteric, and iliac vessels, although involvement of these sites rarely leads to symptoms or to complications. Fibromuscular dysplasia is much more common in women, and occurs predominantly in the third and fourth decade.

Although demonstration of these anatomical abnormalities is straightforward, that they are the cause of hypertension and that correction will lower blood pressure is more difficult to ascertain. Even when moderate or severe renal arterial stenosis is present, it may not be relevant. As many as 20 per cent of patients with demonstrated renal artery stenosis by angiography may be normotensive. Proof that a stenotic lesion is functionally important requires demonstration of an improvement in hypertension or in renal function after correction of the stenosis by angioplasty or surgery.

Investigation of renovascular disease

Rapid sequence intravenous urography

This was once the screening test for renovascular hypertension. Pictures taken at 1-min intervals for 5 min show a delay in first appearance of the nephrogram, and subsequent increased density of the pyelogram, together with asymmetry of kidney size. The sensitivity and specificity of the test are imperfect, being 80 per cent and 85 per cent, respectively, for unilateral renovascular disease and less if bilateral disease is present. For these reasons it is largely replaced by isotope renography.

Renal vein renin ratio

Renal vein renin concentration has been measured both to aid diagnosis and to attempt to predict the outcome of surgery. The technique is invasive, involving bilateral catheterization and sampling from each renal vein, and the adjacent vena cava above and below the origin of the vein. A renal vein renin ratio of 1.6 or greater is

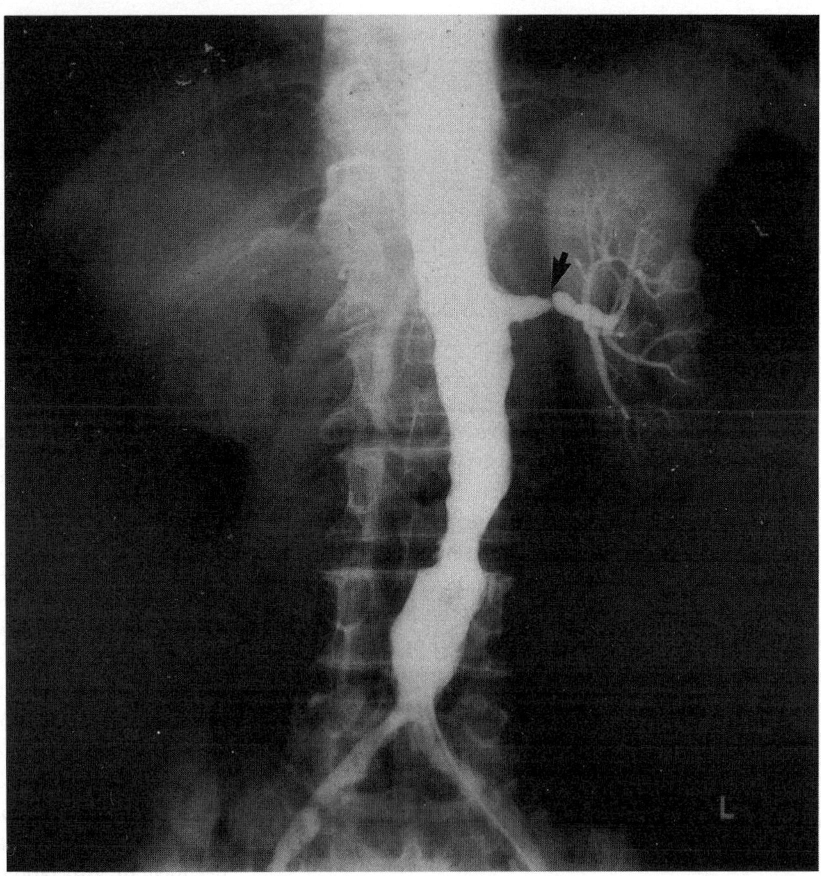

Fig. 1 Aortography in a 65-year-old man with severe atheromatous disease, with extensive aortic atheroma, total occlusion of the right renal artery, and a tight stenosis of the left renal artery (arrow).

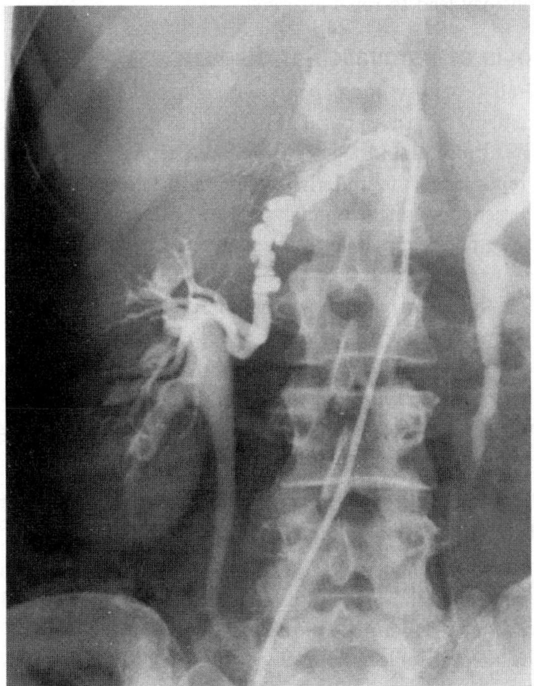

Fig. 2 Selective right renal angiography in a patient with hypertension due to fibromuscular dysplasia.

taken to be indicative, and diagnostic accuracy may be improved by sodium restriction or captopril administration. Although this test has shown a specificity of 90–95 per cent in different series, it has poor sensitivity, as between 30 and 60 per cent of patients with renal vein renin ratios below 1.6 have been found to benefit from surgical treatment. Further difficulties arise when the disease is bilateral, or when segmental areas of renal ischaemia are present. This approach has now fallen into relative disfavour.

Captopril challenge test

The test is simple, involving measurement of plasma renin activity before and 60 min after oral administration of 50 mg captopril. Initial retrospective data claimed remarkable sensitivity of 100 per cent and specificity of 98 per cent. Subsequent prospective evaluations have had mixed success, confirming a high sensitivity, but a limited specificity of 80–90 per cent. *Captopril renography* is an alternative and widely used approach to diagnosis of renovascular hypertension (see Chapter 12.1). The predictive value of this test is improved considerably if it is reserved for patients with clinical clues suggesting renovascular disease; even so, it may be argued that in such cases the only means of obtaining an unequivocal diagnosis is to perform angiography.

Renal angiography

Renal angiography showing renal arterial disease cannot predict whether there will be improvement after intervention. It carries a risk of radiocontrast-induced acute renal failure, those at most risk being patients who are volume-depleted or have diabetic nephropathy. There is also a significant morbidity from local haemorrhage from cholesterol embolism, and mortality may approach 0.1 per cent.

Table 1 Progression of untreated atherosclerotic renovascular disease

No. of patients	Initial degree of luminal narrowing (%)	Stenosis unchanged (%)	Progression without occlusion (%)	Progression to total occlusion (%)
78	<50	69	26	5
30	50–75	53	37	10
18	75–99	61	0	39

Adapted from Schreiber *et al.* (1984).

Treatment of renovascular disease

Progression of untreated renovascular disease

In the majority of patients with a renal arterial stenosis of 75 per cent or greater, hypertension is improved by correction of the stenosis, although not necessarily cured. Minor stenoses of less than 50 per cent are usually treated conservatively, but the practice of preventative correction of even these lesions is increasing to minimize the future risk of ischaemic renal failure. This risk is significant, as the natural history of untreated atherosclerotic disease is one of continuing progression. The Cleveland clinic series (Table 1) showed that nearly 40 per cent of patients with a 75–99 per cent stenosis developed complete occlusion within a mean period of 2 years of follow-up. Progressive disease was even found in a third of patients who had stenosis of less than 50 per cent. Progression of this degree of severity is much less of a problem in fibromuscular disease, although it has been observed in half or more of patients in some series, with occasional total occlusion.

Indications for surgery or angioplasty

No prospective trials comparing medical and surgical treatment, or angioplasty have been completed.

Renal vascular surgery should be undertaken only in specialized centres, and even in these the overall expectation of cure of hypertension by surgery is unlikely to be more than 50 per cent. Features favouring a corrective approach include the presence of fibromuscular disease, relative youth, absence of severe extra renal vascular disease, a positive result on tests such as captopril renography, a good long-term blood pressure response to converting enzyme inhibition, and, especially, a lesion or lesions which appear suitable for intervention, together with a relative absence of distal small vessel intrarenal atherosclerosis.

Nephrectomy is rarely appropriate and is only indicated when the affected kidney contributes less than 10 per cent to overall renal function. A number of reconstructive techniques are used, including endarterectomy, bypass grafting, 'bench' repair and auto-transplantation of the iliac fossa. All are hazardous in advanced atheromatous disease.

Percutaneous transluminal renal angioplasty is now established as an effective and relatively safe method of correction of renal vascular stenosis. Ostial lesions, which occur frequently in atheromatous disease, are usually least suitable for angioplasty. Complications occur in up to 15 per cent of patients, the most severe being renal artery dissection, occlusion or perforation, and cholesterol embolism to the renal or lower limb vasculature.

The results of angioplasty vary widely. The procedure is technically successful in 70–100 per cent of cases reported, and rates for improvement of hypertension range from 10–75 per cent. Restenosis is common, occurring in 20 per cent or more of patients at up to 2 years follow-up. The results for fibromuscular disease are better than those for atherosclerotic disease.

Medical treatment

Diuretics should be used with caution, as in unilateral disease volume depletion with accompanying hyponatraemia and hypokalaemia is not uncommon, as a consequence of pressure natriuresis in the unaffected kidney. Calcium entry blockers have been established to be safe and reasonably effective; β-blockers are an acceptable alternative. *Converting enzyme inhibitors should be used with caution in patients with renovascular disease.* They are very effective in reducing blood pressure but they carry the risk of causing a marked fall in glomerular filtration rate (see Chapter 2.31 and OTM3, p. 2541). The risk of this complication is increased by volume depletion or excessive diuretic therapy, and irreversible loss of renal function has been described in 15 per cent of a group of patients with hypertension or congestive cardiac failure and intrarenal arteriosclerosis in whom renal function declined in association with converting enzyme inhibitor therapy. Animal studies have also suggested that long-term converting enzyme inhibition may lead to renal atrophy.

Prognosis of renovascular disease

The overall prognosis for patients with atheromatous renovascular disease remains relatively poor. The detected frequency of renovascular disease as a cause of endstage renal failure has increased, and it is at present reported as the underlying disease in between 8 and 14 per cent of patients commencing dialysis. The outlook for these patients is especially poor, and in one series 5-year survival was less than 10 per cent, half that of dialysis patients with diabetic nephropathy and one-sixth that of patients with glomerulonephritis. These figures undoubtedly reflect attrition due to severe generalized atherosclerosis. Patients with atheromatous bilateral renovascular hypertension are also at high risk of recurrent severe pulmonary oedema. This complication is probably related to sodium retention, and may be effectively eliminated by successful renal revascularization.

Unilateral renal parenchymal disease

The unilateral parenchymal diseases which may give rise to hypertension are shown in Table 2. Pyelonephritic scarring from reflux or dysplasia of a single kidney are the most common.

Improvement in blood pressure after nephrectomy can occur, although there are no tests which will predict outcome. Nephrectomy without benefit in blood pressure is to be avoided. If there is appreciable remaining function in the affected kidney, surgery specifically designed to relieve hypertension should only be undertaken when blood pressure is uncontrolled, despite maximal tolerated doses of combinations of antihypertensive drugs, including converting enzyme inhibitors, minoxidil, and calcium channel blockers.

Table 2 Unilateral renal parenchymal disease causing hypertension

Chronic pyelonephritis	Tuberculosis
Reflux nephropathy	Trauma
Dysplastic kidney	Radiation fibrosis
Segmental hypoplasia (Ask–Upmark kidney)	Simple renal cysts
Obstructive uropathy	

Oral contraceptives and hypertension

Hypertension has been reported to occur in as many as 15 per cent of women taking the pill or as few as 1 per cent. A figure of 5 per cent is commonly quoted. Although the rise in pressure is usually mild, rare patients have developed severe or even malignant hypertension reversed by withdrawal of oral contraceptives. The mechanism of the rise in pressure is not known and evidence that the oestrogen content, rather than progestogen, is the cause is not well supported by the available data. Even so a pill containing 30 g of oestrogen is less likely to cause hypertension than is one containing 50 g. There have been reports of hypertension occurring in women taking norethisterone alone, reversed by withdrawal of the drug, but most reports record no increase in arterial pressure when normotensive women are given progestogens alone.

In most patients with hypertension induced by oral contraceptives, withdrawal of the pill corrects blood pressure within 3 months, although a longer period (up to 18 months) may be needed in a few cases.

Whether or not women with established hypertension should be denied oral contraception is less easy to decide. Much will depend on individual circumstances, but most doctors will at least discourage patients in this category as both elevated blood pressure and regular consumption of oral contraceptives carry an increased risk of coronary artery and cerebrovascular disease.

Further reading

Isles, C. G., Robertson, S., and Hill, D. (1999). Management of renovascular disease: a review of renal artery stenting in ten studies. *Quarterly Journal of Medicine*, **92**, 159–67.

Schreiber, M.J., Pohl, M.A., and Novick, A.C. (1984). The natural history of atherosclerotic and fibrous renal artery disease. *Urology Clinics of North America*, **11**, 383–92.

Weidmann, P., Benelta-Piccoli, C., Stetten, F., *et al.* (1976). Hypertension in renal failure. *Kidney International*, **9**, 294–301.

Wilcox, C.S. (1993) Use of angiotensin-converting enzyme inhibitors for diagnosing renovascular hypertension. *Kidney International*, **44**, 1379–90.

Chapter 2.33

Phaeochromocytoma

M. J. Brown

Incidence and importance

Phaeochromocytoma is a rare tumour. *In vivo* estimates of incidence are unreliable because none has been undertaken in an unselected group of patients. It is safe to say that the incidence is less than 1 per cent and more than 0.1 per cent of hypertensives. Despite its rarity, phaeochromocytoma justifies consideration because it combines the potential for being lethal if not diagnosed and treated, and for cure in most patients if diagnosed.

Catecholamine biochemistry

An understanding of the tests used to diagnose phaeochromocytoma requires reference to an outline of both the synthetic and degradative pathways of catecholamine metabolism. The precursor amino acid is phenylalanine; tyrosine is the substrate for the rate-limiting step in the biosynthetic pathway, by which tyrosine hydroxylase yields L-dopa. Decarboxylation of L-dopa yields the first catecholamine in the pathway, dopamine. Occasionally this can be the principal catecholamine secreted by phaeochromocytomas, or more often by childhood neuroblastomas. But usually dopamine is further hydroxylated to noradrenaline. This *N*-methylation usually occurs in only two sites: the adrenal medulla and certain hindbrain nuclei involved in blood pressure control. The enzyme, phenylethanolamine-*N*-methyltransferase, outside the central nervous system is dependent for induction on glucocorticoids, which are provided in the adrenal through the portocapillary circulation. The clinical importance of this is threefold. First, extra-adrenal phaeochromocytomas rarely produce adrenaline. Second, the normal adrenal produces mainly adrenaline, and accounts for less than 2 per cent of circulating noradrenaline. Third, when a tumour is present in the adrenal, the disruption of the portocapillary circulation causes a reversal of the normal adrenaline to noradrenaline ratio. The relevance of these to the clinical features and diagnosis of phaeochromocytoma will become apparent.

The metabolic breakdown of catecholamines is due to two principal enzymes, monoamine oxidase and catechol-*O*-methyltransferase (COMT). In phaeochromocytoma, adrenaline and noradrenaline are liberated directly into the bloodstream, rather than mainly into the synaptic gap around sympathetic nerve endings. Noradrenaline released from these is largely recaptured by neuronal and extraneuronal uptake, and metabolized before any free amine escapes into the bloodstream. Consequently, the proportion of parent amine to metabolite is usually higher in blood and urine in the presence of a phaeochromocytoma than in any other cause of elevated catecholamine production.

The most abundant product of breakdown is vanillylmandelic acid (VMA). Normetanephrine and metanephrine are produced by COMT from noradrenaline and adrenaline, respectively.

Analyses

Most routine laboratories screen 24-h urines measuring metabolites because they offer an integrated measure of total catecholamine release over this period; VMA is the product least prone to interference, L-dopa being the only drug which can cross-react in measurement through its equivalent metabolite, homovanillic acid. Quantitation of VMA is less sensitive than other measures, but it is very rare that a patient with a secreting phaeochromocytoma has a 24-h VMA result that is entirely normal. The problem is more that of distinguishing a true positive among the relatively large number of hypertensive patients with results in the grey zone. Metanephrines are arguably more sensitive than VMA, but their assay is more prone to interference by drugs, especially by β-blockers.

The measurement of free catecholamines is a more specialized procedure.

Most phaeochromocytomas also secrete one or more neuropeptides, especially neuropeptide Y. Much rarer, but essential to detect preoperatively, is adrenocorticotrophic hormone which may cause a coexisting ectopic adrenocorticotrophic hormone syndrome.

Pathology

The anatomical distribution of phaeochromocytomas closely parallels the sites where chromaffin tissue is present at the time of birth. Pathological differences between extra-adrenal phaeochromocytomas at various sites are not relevant to clinical practice except as a possible explanation for the failure of some head and neck phaeochromocytomas to accumulate the noradrenaline analogue used in radionuclide scanning.

In some patients, mainly those with associated abnormalities such as the multiple endocrine neoplasia (**MEN**) type 2 syndrome or in von Hippel Lindau syndrome (**VHL**), the tumour is familial. The genes for both these disorders have been identified.

Most phaeochromocytomas are benign but the pathologist can rarely provide a clear distinction between benign and malignant. On the one hand, benign tumours can appear to be invading the capsule of the tumour, which is often ill-defined, while on the other, malignant tumours may show no mitoses because of their slow rate of division.

Clinical features

Hypertension is the most common form of presentation but others include unexplained heart failure or as part of multiple endocrine neoplasia, or other rarer associated genetic diseases. In the last groups, the diagnosis is made by screening patients with or without specific clinical features of a phaeochromocytoma. In hypertensive patients, a spontaneous history or direct enquiry will usually reveal at least one of a group of characteristic symptoms. The most common are headache, sweating, and palpitations. Less frequent are episodes of pallor, a feeling of 'impending doom' and paraesthesiae. Examination rarely reveals useful signs, but an exception is a Raynaud's type of discoloration over the extremities and the larger joints in the limbs.

Occasionally phaeochromocytomas can present with a dangerous syndrome, due to acute haemorrhage and infarction of the tumour. This gives rise to a unique combination of the features of retroperitoneal haemorrhage and intermittent hypertension, which is pathognomonic but even prompt recognition of the diagnosis is not always sufficient to save patients presenting with this particular crisis. At the other extreme, not all patients with a phaeochromocytoma, causing severe hypertension, have any specific symptoms.

Many of the symptoms of phaeochromocytoma can be ascribed to the effects of the catecholamine excess, and disappear rapidly on initiation of appropriate treatment. Some remain more difficult to explain, including the sweating whose control in healthy subjects is usually ascribed to cholinergic sympathetic innervation. Because large tumours secrete principally noradrenaline, even when arising within the adrenal, tachycardia is usually only modest, and can be replaced altogether by reflex bradycardia when episodes of hypertension are triggered by the release of noradrenaline alone. In a few patients, catecholamine excess can cause myocardial necrosis. These are rare presentations and clinical features are usually less impressive than expected, possibly because the adrenoceptors have been downregulated by years of exposure before the diagnosis.

Diagnosis

There are two distinct questions to ask when considering the diagnosis. The first is, 'Does the patient have a phaeochromocytoma?' the second is, 'Where is it?'. The tests required to answer the first question are mainly biochemical, whereas the second is answered by radiological investigation. A golden rule is that the first question should be answered before proceeding to the second. No single radiological investigation is sufficiently accurate to detect more than 80–90 per cent of phaeochromocytomas, whilst computed tomography scanning is sufficiently sensitive to detect small non-functional adenomas in the adrenal that should not lead to further investigation in the absence of biochemical abnormalities.

The symptoms of a functioning phaeochromocytoma may be absent; to avoid missing the diagnosis, therefore, it is reasonable to screen some patients presenting only with hypertension, a few with unexplained heart failure, and even fewer, those with the MEN or VHL syndromes. Although the diagnosis is often postulated in other patients without hypertension but complaining of palpitation, headaches, sweating, or panic attacks, the chance of such patients having a phaeochromocytoma is very small.

There is no single perfect or 'best' test for screening. Twenty-four-hour urine VMA is a good initial screen in most patients, supplemented when necessary with the specialized catecholamine analyses. A single plasma measurement can miss the very occasional phaeochromocytoma with truly episodic secretion. An entirely normal 24-h urine VMA measured in a good laboratory is most unlikely in the presence of a phaeochromocytoma; Patients are asked to avoid vanilla containing foods during the collection and to undertake three collections, but a vanilla-free diet is unnecessary because the dietary contribution to VMA excretion is small.

VMA results which are less than twofold above the upper limit of normal cannot usually be considered pathognomonic of tumour. Most patients whose urine contains more than this will prove to have a phaeochromocytoma, and a threefold elevation is almost always diagnostic. The patients who need further analyses are those with less than twofold elevation, of whom only a very small proportion (less than 5 per cent) will have a phaeochromocytoma. Here, the single most helpful measurement is of the plasma catecholamines. In most patients with a phaeochromocytoma, the plasma noradrenaline will be at least twofold elevated.

Suppression tests

If the urinary VMA measurement or resting plasma noradrenaline does not resolve the diagnosis, there are two further useful investigations. The most widely used is a pharmacological suppression test, in which physiological elevations of noradrenaline release are temporarily suppressed by administration of either the ganglion-blocking drug, pentolinium, or centrally acting α2-agonist, clonidine. The former has three advantages: (1) it is most effective at suppressing noradrenaline release in patients with elevated sympathetic nervous activity but without a phaeochromocytoma; (2) it suppresses release of adrenaline from the adrenal medulla; and (3) it has a short half-life (approximately 20 min) so that the test can be completed in the outpatient clinic. Clonidine has the advantage of suppressing release of noradrenaline even when the basal level is normal, but in practice, when this is the case a suppression test is rarely necessary; as pentolinium is entirely excreted by the kidneys it should not be given if plasma creatinine exceeds 150 μmol/litre.

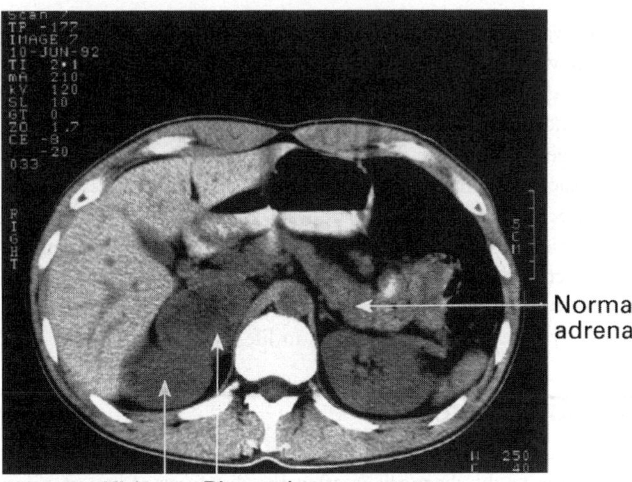

Fig. 1 CT scan of right adrenal phaeochromocytoma. The phaeochromocytoma has the typical non-homogeneous appearance due to areas of haemorrhage and infarction. The normal left adrenal has the typical tricornuate appearance with concave borders.

Patients should rest supine for 15–30 min before the test. Plasma catecholamines are measured in two samples taken 5 min apart from an intravenous cannula, and in two further samples taken 10 and 20 min after an intravenous bolus of pentolinium 2.5 mg. They should remain supine for a further 60 min, and their erect arterial pressure should be checked before they are allowed to leave the clinic. A normal response to pentolinium is a fall of both plasma noradrenaline and adrenaline concentrations into the normal range or by 50 per cent from baseline but there may be little fall in plasma catecholamine values when the basal levels are already within the normal range.

Measurement of plasma adrenaline is a useful clue to the location of a phaeochromocytoma; it is exceptional for extra-adrenal phaeochromocytomas to secrete adrenaline (because of the lack of cortisol stimulation). Most adrenal phaeochromocytomas do secrete adrenaline, although the proportion of noradrenaline to adrenaline is reversed from that in normal subjects.

Localization of phaeochromocytomas

Computed tomography (**CT**) scanning is the method of choice, as 90 per cent of phaeochromocytomas arise in the adrenal (Fig. 1). The adrenal is easy to visualize and cortical tumours can be distinguished from those of the medulla. Phaeochromocytomas are usually larger than Conn's tumours, and may appear non-homogeneous because of areas of haemorrhage and infarction. Even so diagnostic mistakes will be made if the differentiation between tumours is attempted radiologically rather than biochemically as the majority of adrenal cortical tumours are non-functional.

It is preferable to withhold CT for extra-adrenal phaeochromocytomas until the radiologist can be given some clue as to where to concentrate. In about 85 per cent of patients, this can be achieved by radioisotope scanning, using the iodinated analogue of noradrenaline, *m*- iodobenzylguanidine (**MIBG**). This may carry either an [^{123}I] or [^{131}I] label. The former is more sensitive but also more expensive, and may be misinterpreted if users are unaware that normal adrenal glands also accumulate MIBG. There is a case for undertaking MIBG scanning in addition to CT, even for patients found to have an adrenal phaeochromocytoma, to identify extra-adrenal secondary deposits when tumours are malignant, and because there may be coexisting adrenal and extra-adrenal phaeochromocytomas.

If these investigations fail to localize a phaeochromocytoma diagnosed by biochemical assays, the next step is to undertake selective venous sampling from various sites in the vena cava and the veins which drain into it. An arterial sample taken at the end of the procedure enables sites with a positive veno-arterial difference to be readily detected.

The place of angiography has not been entirely removed by CT scanning. As phaeochromocytomas are vascular tumours, they provide a good tumour blush, and angiography should resolve equivocal CT scans. This procedure can provoke an outpouring of catechols. Patients must be fully α-blocked and preferably also β-blocked prior to angiography, and their blood pressure pulse rate and electrocardiogram monitored during the procedure with phentolamine and practolol readily available to treat rises of arterial pressure or tachycardia.

Other investigations

It is important to check blood glucose and all patients should be screened for an associated medullary carcinoma of the thyroid by a plasma calcitonin estimation (see Chapter 7.15). Unusual symptoms may indicate the need for a gut peptide screen. The other monogenic syndrome—VHL—should be suspected when there is a personal or family history of tumours or when small adrenal tumours secrete only nonadrenaline. The finding of a retinal angioma on direct ophthalmoscopy makes the diagnosis.

The very rare patient who cosecretes adrenocorticotrophic hormone will be detected by the gross hypokalaemia of the ectopic adrenocorticotrophic hormone syndrome; because adrenocorticotrophic hormone release may be inhibited by noradrenaline prior to initiation of α-blockade, it is important to re-check the electrolytes after a few days of α-blocking treatment.

Treatment

The definitive treatment is surgical removal. Even the small number of phaeochromocytomas which can be recognized to be malignant preoperatively may still benefit from resection of the primary tumour. The task for the physician is to make the surgery safe. The mainstay of medical treatment is α-blockade, but not all patients require β-blockade. The objective of this treatment is not solely control of blood pressure but also to expand blood volume, which is always reduced in phaeochromocytoma patients. The α-blocker of choice is phenoxybenzamine, an irreversible agent, which destroys the α-receptor by alkylation. Prazosin, doxazosin, and labetalol, cause competitive blockade, which can be overcome by a surge of noradrenaline release from the tumour.

The starting dose of phenoxybenzamine is 10 mg daily. The effect is cumulative, and takes several days to reach maximum. It is reasonable to aim for a diastolic blood pressure between 90 and 100 mmHg during treatment, and to admit patients for 5 days preoperatively, during which time the dose is increased until there is at least a 10 mmHg postural fall in blood pressure and little if any variability in arterial pressure.

The need for β-blockade is indicated by tachycardia, which may become apparent only after treatment with phenoxybenzamine. It is usually better to use a β1-selective agent so that the peripheral vasodilatation mediated by β2-receptors is not affected. The lowest dose possible should be used as there may be a period of hypotension upon removal of the tumour, normally offset by the ability to mount a tachycardia. If hypotension does occur, it should not be treated with pressor agents, but by volume replacement, supplemented if necessary by β1-agonists.

The treatment of malignant phaeochromocytomas remains unsatisfactory. The rate of growth is usually slow but the prognosis can vary between the extremes of local recurrence at intervals of many years, and rapid demise sometimes precipitated by surgery. These tumours are not particularly sensitive either to chemotherapy or to radiotherapy. There has been interest in the use of therapeutic doses of MIBG, as a means of targeting high doses of radioactivity to the tumour, and some patients show considerable regression after such treatment. Long-term results are less certain. If pharmacological effects of the tumour remain a problem despite debulking, high doses of phenoxybenzamine are usually preferable to α-methyltyrosine. The latter is an inhibition of noradrenaline synthesis; its effects on noradrenaline production in the brain causes sedation and depression.

Prognosis

Ninety per cent of phaeochromocytomas are benign but because of the difficulties in ascertaining malignancy, all patients should be followed indefinitely with at least an annual measurement of arterial pressure and analysis of one of the indices of catecholamine secretion. The removal of a phaeochromocytoma in the majority cures hypertension, especially in younger patients.

Further reading

Manger, W.M. and Gifford, R.W. (1996). *Clinical and experimental pheochromocytoma.* (2nd edn). Blackwell.

Chapter 2.34

Coarctation of the aorta as a cause of secondary hypertension in the adult

N. A. Boon

Most coarctations are found beyond the left subclavian artery and either above or just below the ductus arteriosus. Preductal coarctation usually presents with heart failure in infancy and is commonly associated with a patent ductus arteriosus and a variety of other cardiac defects. Postductal coarctation tends to be less severe and approximately 20 per cent of cases are diagnosed for the first time in adolescents or adults.

Coarctation is more common in males and is sometimes a feature of Noonan's and Turner's syndromes. There is a bicuspid aortic valve in at least 50 per cent of patients and this may lead to aortic valve disease in later life. The condition is also associated with cerebral artery (berry) aneurysm.

Partial obstruction of the aorta has several important consequences. First, there is progressive elevation of the arterial pressure in the proximal vasculature. Second, a collateral circulation develops from the subclavian and axillary arteries through the internal mammary, scapular, and intercostal arteries. Collateral vessels may eventually become enormous. Third, there may be aneurysmal dilatation of the aorta immediately before or after the stenosis.

The exact mechanism of hypertension is disputed but resetting of the baroreceptors, decreased aortic wall compliance and generalized vasoconstriction due to increased renin–angiotensin or sympathetic nervous activity have all been implicated. This may explain why the blood pressure sometimes remains high following surgical correction, particularly if this is carried out late in life.

Clinical features

In young adults coarctation of the aorta is usually asymptomatic and the first clue to the diagnosis is often the discovery of hypertension or an abnormality on a routine chest radiograph. Occasionally the condition presents with infective endocarditis, which may occur at the site of the coarctation or, more commonly, on an associated bicuspid aortic valve. Cerebral haemorrhage may be due to rupture of a cerebral artery aneurysm or uncontrolled hypertension.

Older patients may present with heart failure attributable to aortic valve disease, hypertension, or premature coronary disease. Aortic dissection and aortic aneurysm are also recognized features. These complications account for the substantial reduction in life expectancy observed in untreated coarctation of the aorta (Fig. 1).

Physical signs

Hypertension in the upper limbs is almost invariable and there is often a greatly exaggerated rise in blood pressure during exercise. The lower limbs are sometimes underdeveloped and the femoral pulses are absent or weak and delayed. Collateral vessels in the back muscles are often palpable and may be visible. The apex beat is forceful and there may be a systolic thrill in the suprasternal area. Auscultation may reveal an ejection systolic click if there is an associated bicuspid aortic valve, accentuation of the aortic component of the second heart, and an atrial or fourth heart sound due to left ventricular hypertrophy. Murmurs may arise from the aortic valve, the coarctation itself, or arterial collaterals and it may be difficult to distinguish one from another. There is often an ejection systolic murmur over the base of the heart and occasionally aortic regurgitation gives rise to an early diastolic murmur at the left sternal edge.

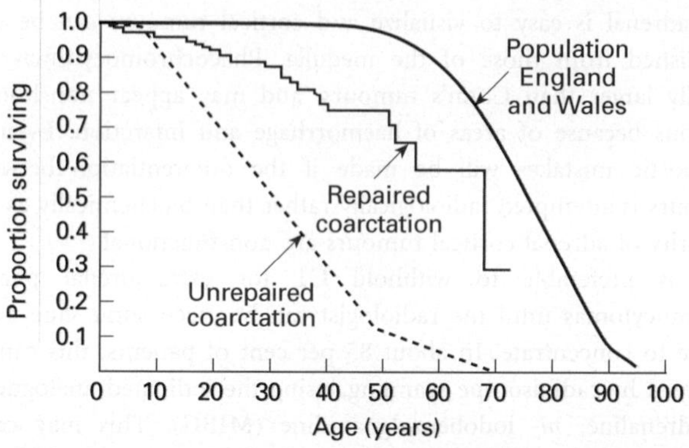

Fig. 1 Comparative survival, excluding deaths in the first year of life, of the general population and patients with repaired and unrepaired coarctation of the aorta *(redrawn, with permission, from Bobby et al. (1991)).*

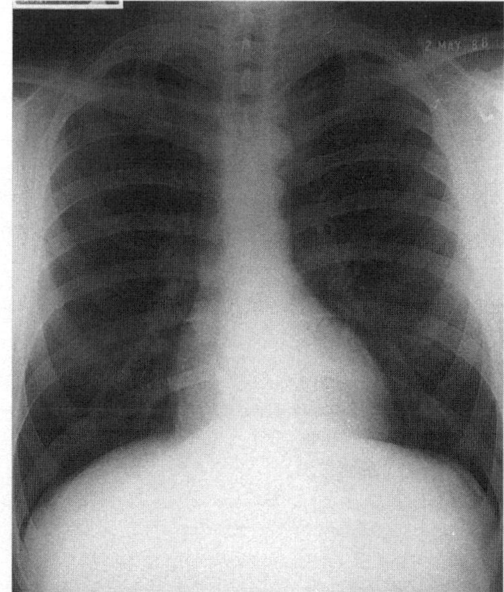

(a)

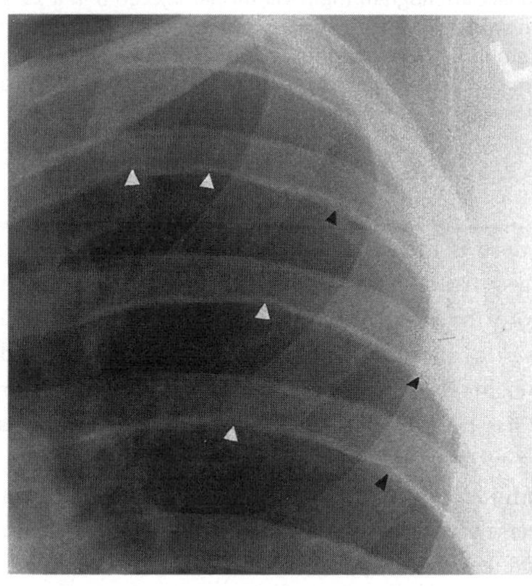

(b)

Fig. 2 (a) Chest radiograph from a patient with hypertension and coarctation of the aorta showing an abnormal aortic knuckle (the '3' sign). (b) Chest radiograph from a patient with hypertension and coarctation of the aorta showing bilateral rib notching (arrowheads).

Turbulence at the coarctation produces a widespread systolic murmur that is often best heard over the back, where there may also be systolic or continuous bruits arising from the collateral vessels.

Investigations

The chest radiograph usually shows subtle but pathognomonic changes (Fig. 2). The coarctation and associated pre- or post-stenotic dilatation of the aorta may be visualized by two-dimensional echocardiography, angiography, computed tomography scanning, or magnetic resonance imaging. The pressure gradient across the stenosis can be measured by Doppler echocardiography or catheterization but is critically dependent on the degree of collateral flow into the lower aorta and must therefore be interpreted in conjunction with the relevant clinical and anatomical information.

Treatment

Surgical repair improves life expectancy and reduces blood pressure. Early postoperative complications include paradoxical hypertension, mesenteric ischaemia and paraplegia due to infarction of the spinal cord. The perioperative mortality for elective surgery in adults is less than 1 or 2 per cent in most centres. Balloon angioplasty is a safe and effective treatment for recurrent coarctation following surgery and has also been used to treat native coarctation. However, long-term results of balloon dilatation are unknown and there is concern that angioplasty may be followed by a high incidence of recoarctation and aneurysm formation. The long-term prognosis appears to be inversely related to the extent and duration of pre-operative hypertension; hence early repair is usually advisable. Residual or recurrent hypertension is common after repair; relapse is due occasionally to recoarctation. Premature death is frequently due to rupture of an aortic or cerebral aneurysm, or heart failure.

All patients with coarctation remain at risk of developing infective endocarditis and therefore require appropriate antibiotic prophylaxis.

Further reading

Bobby, J.J., Emami, J.M., Farmer, R.D.T., and Newman, C.G.H. (1991). Operative survival and 40 year follow up of surgical repair of aortic coarctation. *British Heart Journal*, **65**, 271–6.

Fawzy, M.E., Sivanandam, V., Galal, O., Dunn, B., Patel, A., Rifai, A., *et al.* (1997). One- to ten-year follow-up results of balloon angioplasty of native coarctation of the aorta in adolescents and adults. *Journal of the American College of Cardiology*, **30**, 1542–6.

Swan, L., Wilson, N., Houston, A.B., Doig, W., Pollock, J.C.S., and Hillis, W.S. (1998). The long-term management of the patient with an aortic coarctation repair. *European Heart Journal*, **19**, 382–6.

Chapter 2.35

Takayasu's disease

K. Ishikawa

Takayasu's disease, a chronic inflammatory arteriopathy, occurs the world over but is most frequently diagnosed in young Oriental women. The main site of occurrence is the aorta and/or its main branches but the pulmonary artery is also often involved. Inflammatory changes in the affected vessels lead to occlusive changes in the lumina, often combined with dilation and secondary thrombus formation. Major complications are Takayasu's retinopathy, secondary hypertension, aortic regurgitation, and aortic or arterial aneurysm. The disease may also be called occlusive thromboaortopathy, aortitis syndrome, and non-specific aortoarteritis.

Aetiology

The cause remains unknown. An autoimmune mechanism is possible and there can be a good response to corticosteroid therapy during the inflammatory stage. Attempts to demonstrate circulating antibodies against antigens of the arterial wall, have given both positive and negative results. Group A streptococcal infection, association with tuberculosis, hormonal imbalance, ethnic susceptibility, and genetic predisposition may be pathogenetic factors.

Pathology

There is a panarteritis of the aorta and its main branches and of the pulmonary artery. The lesions begin with a mesoperiarteritis with subsequent fibrosis, followed by fibrotic thickening of the adventitia and the vasa vasorum, leading to intimal fibrosis, which progresses to marked thickening, often with thrombi. The destruction of the arterial wall leads to both stenotic and ectatic changes of the lumen, especially occlusion. These affected portions are clearly demarcated from the adjacent normal sites and segmental 'skipped' lesions are observed.

Clinical features and diagnosis

Clinical features are protean. There is often a long interval between the onset, and the establishment of the diagnosis, which is usually made when patients are between the ages of 20 and 40 years. The disease is much more frequent in women.

Patients in the early phase show evidence of inflammation with an elevated erythrocyte sedimentation rate (ESR), increased levels of C-reactive protein, increased α2-globulin and gammaglobulin, and slight normochromic anaemia. During this phase, most patients have symptoms of malaise, headache, fever, easy fatiguability, dizziness, transient visual disturbance, neck pain, mild palpitation and dyspnoea, arthralgia, stiffness of shoulders, and nausea. Syncopal attacks are not uncommon. Haemoptysis occurs rarely. Some patients, however, never suffer these symptoms. In them, the disease may present with its complications, for example pulselessness or hypertension. Some cases are picked up solely on investigation of a raised ESR. When the degree of narrowing of the involved arteries is advanced, cardiovascular symptoms and signs predominate. These include moderate or severe dyspnoea and palpitation on exertion, chest and back pain, recurrent syncopal attacks, intermittent claudication of the arms or legs, asymmetric pulses or pulselessness, bruits over the affected arteries, and high blood pressure.

It is vital, in making the diagnosis, to think of it in the first place. The extent of the disease can be assessed clinically by a 'pulse-bruit-pressure' diagram which records pulse volume, bruits, tenderness over vessels, and local arterial pressure (including retinal) at various regions. Plain radiographs will often show widening of the aortic knuckle, aortic calcification, irregularity of the contour of the left lateral margin of the descending thoracic aorta, and focal areas of decreased pulmonary vascular shadowing. Perfusion lung scanning or pulmonary arteriography aid diagnosis; pulmonary hypertension is not uncommon (Fig. 1). Total aortography is indispensable for the confirmation and differential diagnosis from congenital aortic coarctation at unusual sites, the aortitis of giant cell arteritis, and atherosclerosis alone. Coronary arterial lesions attributed to this disease are rare.

Treatment and prognosis

Medical

Patients in the inflammatory stage respond moderately well to corticosteroid therapy. Not only are non-specific symptoms reduced, but progression of arterial involvement can be retarded or prevented. Arteriographic stenoses often improve. The recommended initial daily dose is usually 30–50 mg of prednisolone per day, more often the

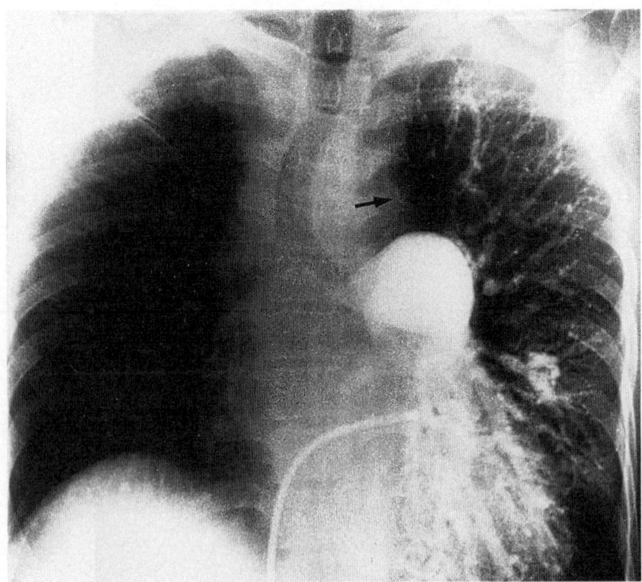

Fig. 1 Pulmonary arteriogram (right ventricular injection) in a 25-year old Japanese man with Takayasu's disease in the active stage, the extensive type, and in group III. Note occlusion of the right pulmonary artery, and elevation of the ipsilateral diaphragm. There is calcification of the aortic knob (arrow).

latter. The dose is then reduced gradually, depending on response, but prolonged treatment (an average period of 9 years) is usually needed before the drug can be withdrawn completely. In patients unresponsive to steroid therapy alone, cyclophosphamide (2 mg/kg body weight) is sometimes added. Percutaneous transluminal angioplasty has been used when the inflammatory stage has settled, but the long-term results are as yet unknown.

The inflammatory activity does not worsen during pregnancy, but various adverse cardiovascular events, including intrapartum cerebral haemorrhage, can occur. An evaluation of the disease before pregnancy, planning the mode of delivery, and intrapartum and anaesthetic considerations, are particularly important.

Surgical

Surgical treatments include reconstructive surgery of the aorta and its main branches, endarterectomy, aneurysmectomy, aortic valve replacement, and, rarely, coronary artery bypass grafting. Some results are excellent, for instance in hypertension secondary to coarctation of the aorta or to renal artery stenosis, but are not so good for those in the advanced phase. If inflammation is active, the possibility of suture failure or aneurysm formation, as well as occlusion of the graft, is higher than is the case of arterial disease of other causes; a healthy area of the arterial wall must be available and selected for the site of graft anastomosis. An increased ESR should be lowered by steroid therapy to a normal level before surgical treatment. In a series of 120 patients, the 20-year overall survival rate after diagnosis was nearly 83 per cent.

Further reading

Ishikawa, K. (1978). Natural history and classification of occlusive thromboaortopathy (Takayasu's disease). *Circulation*, 57, 27–35.

Ishikawa, K. (1988). Diagnostic approach and proposed criteria for the clinical diagnosis of Takayasu's arteriopathy. *Journal of American College of Cardiology*, **12**, 964–72.

Ishikawa, K. and Maetani, S. (1994). Long-term outcome for 120 Japanese patients with Takayasu's disease: clinical and statistical analyses of related prognostic factors. *Circulation*, **90**, 1855–60.

Chapter 2.36

Lymphoedema

J. G. G. Ledingham

Local oedema can be caused predominantly by inadequacy of lymphatic drainage of extracellular fluid. Such inadequacy may be related to hypoplasia of lymphatic vessels or to structural change related to trauma, surgery, inflammation, fibrosis, or neoplasm.

Anatomical considerations

Lymphatic capillaries are thin-walled, blind-ended structures lined by endothelial cells with a discontinuous basement membrane. Anchoring filaments, attached laterally, probably alter the size of intercellular clefts. Vesicles within the endothelial cells probably undertake pinocytosis of proteins, macromolecules, and cell debris taken up by the highly permeable lymphatic vessels. Lymphatic capillaries join to form the collecting lymphatics of larger dimension, lined also by endothelium, but now with a continuous basement membrane, a layer of smooth-muscle cells, valves retarding retrograde flow, and adrenergic innervation. Collecting lymphatics merge to form larger vessels, which tend then to aggregate along veins. The largest lymphatic trunks ultimately join either the right lymphatic duct or the thoracic duct.

Normal physiology

The formation of interstitial fluid is determined by Starling forces and by the coefficient of ultrafiltration of the relevant capillary wall. Filtration pressure on the arteriolar side is regulated by the precapillary arteriolar sphincter as well as by gravitational forces, whereas on the venous side there is no such sphincter to 'protect' from high venous pressures. On passive standing, arterial and venous pressures in the legs increase in parallel, so that the arteriovenous gradient is not altered; but absolute hydrostatic pressure increases according to the vertical distance of the capillary in question below the heart. The capillary pressure in the feet on quiet standing is some 125 cm of water. The normal plasma oncotic pressure is some 33 cm of water. Not surprisingly, the volume of the feet increases rapidly over 2–3 min on quiet standing, and after 10–15 min, swelling continues steadily at a rate of some 20–30 ml/h. The mechanisms preventing more rapid capillary transudation and oedema in such a situation are threefold. The most important is precapillary vasoconstriction. Extreme ultrafiltration of the much reduced blood flow results in only modest changes in hydrostatic and oncotic pressure in the extracellular fluid, but a marked increase in intracapillary oncotic pressure. Venous blood draining a foot passively dependent for some 30–40 min may contain protein up to a concentration of over 9 g/l with a haematocrit as high as 52 per cent. This rise in oncotic pressure is critical to the limitation of the formation of tissue fluid.

Lymphatic flow

Local fluid accumulation results in considerable dilatation of the lymphatic vessels, mediated in part by the physical action of the attached fibrils such that distension of the extracellular fluid space pulls on the walls to increase the lumen. Although tissue-fluid formation is increased in dependent limbs, there is no corresponding increase in lymphatic flow in the absence of muscular activity. Passive or active exercise does, however, increase lymphatic flow very considerably. The lymphatic vessels normally return some 2–4 litres of extracellular fluid to the circulating blood volume each 24 h. Capillaries leak protein, some of which is returned to the circulation by the lymphatics which at rest, contain proteins in the concentration some 15–20 per cent of that in blood.

Lymphatic oedema

Congenital lymphatic hypoplasia may induce local oedema from earliest infancy. Familial oedema (Milroy's disease), coming on at any age in either sex but mostly at puberty and in girls, is also due to lymphatic hypoplasia. Sporadic as well as familial cases are well recognized.

Structural damage to the lymphatic systems may be the consequence of neoplastic infiltration, of scarring from trauma or irradiation, or chronic lymphangitis from such infective organisms as *Wucheria bancrofti*, *Brugia malayi*, *Br. timori*, or lymphogranuloma venereum.

Obstructed lymphatic vessels dilate, rendering valves incompetent, and the walls become thickened. Stagnation of tissue fluid stimulates local interstitial inflammation and ultimately fibrosis. The swelling of lymphatic oedema is usually asymmetrical, painless, pits readily initially, and subsides at night. With time, however, fibrosis develops in the interstitial tissues, such that the oedema resolves much less easily with posture and becomes 'brawny' (firm and non-pitting). The skin may then become considerably thickened and pigmented. Indolent ulcers tend to develop at sites of pressure. The skin of a chronically oedematous area is abnormally susceptible to bacterial infection, particularly with the streptococcus.

Treatment is unsatisfactory. The affected part should be elevated above the heart whenever possible, and at other times supported externally by firm elastic bandage or appropriate graded elastic stockings, applied after a period of postural drainage. Devices designed to massage the affected part through the night or at other times of rest can be helpful. Prevention of skin sepsis, or its prompt treatment, are important.

Further reading

Michel, C.C. (1979). Fluid movement through capillary walls. In *Handbook of physiology: the cardiovascular system*, (2nd edn), Vol. IV, pp. 375–409. American Physiological Society, Washington DC.

Mortimer, P. and Regnard, C.F.B. (1986). Lymphostatic disorders. *British Medical Journal*, **293**, 347–8.

Section 3
Haematology

Contents

Chapter 3.1

Introduction

D. J. Weatherall

The study of blood is one of the most fascinating branches of clinical medicine. There are very few diseases that do not produce changes in the blood at some time during the course of the illness. Furthermore, the primary disorders of the blood and blood-forming tissues can give rise to extremely diverse clinical manifestations, which may involve any of the organ systems. In addition, haematological abnormalities are frequently encountered in patients in whom the primary problem is non-haematological.

An approach to patients with haematological disorders

The diagnosis of blood diseases follows the same process as any other condition; expertise in the laboratory will never make up for an inadequate history and clinical examination.

History

In taking a history from a patient who is suspected of having a haematological disorder, certain factors are of particular importance. The symptoms of anaemia are described in detail later in this section. However, it should be remembered that a slowly developing anaemia may be completely asymptomatic, even when the haemoglobin level is extremely low. Other general symptoms are of great importance, particularly weight loss, night sweats, bone pain, and pruritis. While moderate nocturnal sweating is common in anxiety states, drenching sweats requiring several changes of nightclothes and sheets are a more ominous symptom, often associated with infection or lymphoproliferative disease. Pruritus occurs with many disorders of the blood. When associated with lymphoma it is non-specific, but when it accompanies the myeloproliferative disorders it is often precipitated by warmth such as getting into bed or a hot bath. A detailed drug history is also essential; there are very few drugs that do not produce haematological side-effects.

When investigating anaemia a detailed dietetic history is essential and it is important to ask specifically about symptoms such as a sore tongue, bleeding gums, dysphagia, dyspepsia, disturbance of bowel habit suggestive of malabsorption, and rectal bleeding. Patients are often referred to haematological departments for investigation of easy bruising. Many people, particularly women, bruise easily and the key question is whether the bruising is unusual for them. Is it spontaneous or related to only mild trauma? It is also extremely helpful to enquire into certain key episodes in a patient's life that may provide a clue as to whether there is an inborn bleeding tendency. These include circumcision, dental extraction (was a return to the dentist for stitching or packing ever required?), menstruation, surgical procedures, and so on.

Assessment of menstrual blood loss is an important part of the history in women with iron deficiency, as well as for assessing haemostatic function.

Family histories are particularly important for the diagnosis of blood diseases. It is not only essential to ask for a family history of anaemia or bleeding disorders; the racial origin of the patient's ancestors may also give valuable clues for the cause of anaemia. A detailed personal history is also essential. Cigarette or cigar smoking is probably the most common cause of mild polycythaemia, and alcohol can produce remarkably diverse haematological changes. A detailed occupational history may reveal exposure to industrial solvents or other agents responsible for bone marrow depression; unusual hobbies may also result in contact with toxic agents.

Physical examination

The examination of a patient with a haematological disorder follows the same pattern as any physical examination but there are certain aspects of particular importance. On general inspection it is essential to examine the skin carefully for evidence of bruising, purpura, infiltration, or ulceration. The distribution and pattern of bruising or petechiae may be diagnostic, particularly in disorders such as Henoch–Schönlein purpura, senile purpura, scurvy, purpura due to venous obstruction, and the painful bruising syndrome. Thrombŏcytopenic purpura is often seen most easily over pressure areas; a few lesions in these regions are easily overlooked. Cutaneous lymphoma may mimic a variety of skin diseases. Chronic leg ulceration is a common finding in sickle-cell anaemia; it also occurs occasionally with other genetic haemolytic anaemias. The perianal region and perineum should be carefully inspected. There may be perianal infiltration, particularly in the monocytic leukaemias, and it is very important to recognize perianal infection early in neutropenic patients. Rectal examination should be avoided in neutropenia for fear of disseminating infection. Potential sites of infection in compromised patients must be examined daily. They include the skin, intravenous infusion sites, the mouth and throat, and the perineum. Mild jaundice may be a useful indicator of haemolysis, while a greyish pigmentation of the skin is common in patients with iron overload, both primary and secondary to repeated transfusion. There is an association between vitiligo and pernicious anaemia. In patients with polycythaemia there may be suffusion of the conjunctivae, a high colour, and prominence of the vessels over the face, neck, and upper part of the chest. The nails should be examined for unusual fragility; flattened, spoon-shaped nails, koilonychia, which are supposed to be diagnostic of chronic iron deficiency, are now rarely seen.

An assessment of the size of the lymph nodes and an inspection of other lymphatic tissue are a major part of the examination of patients with haematological disorders. It is most important to develop a systematic approach to lymph-node examination. Each group of nodes in the head and neck, axillae, and groins, together with the epitrochlear nodes, must be examined in detail. In the head and neck it is useful to start with the occipital nodes, then move to the preauricular and postauricular nodes, and, finally, to examine systematically the anterior and posterior triangles and supraclavicular regions. The scalp should be inspected for signs of infestation and secondary infection due to scratching in children with enlarged occipital or posterior cervical nodes. Soft, tender nodes usually indicate infection. Large, firm nodes are characteristic of lymphoma. Hard nodes occur in secondary carcinoma, although calcified nodes, matted together and attached to skin, are still encountered in patients with tuberculous adenitis. The approximate size of the nodes should be recorded, together with whether they are mobile, attached deep or superficially, and discrete or matted together. It is also very important to examine the tonsils and adenoids, particularly in a patient suspected of having a lymphoproliferative disease.

A detailed examination of the mouth should include the state of the tongue, mucous membranes, gums, teeth, and fauces. Glossitis, as evidenced by a smooth, depapillated tongue, occurs in iron-deficiency and megaloblastic anaemia. Small, black bullae (blood blisters) on the tongue or mucous membranes, which burst and leave superficial ulcers, are characteristic of thrombocytopenic purpura. Gingival hypertrophy is sometimes found in patients with acute leukaemia, particularly the monocytic type, and in some individuals with megaloblastic anaemia due to phenytoin therapy. Ulcers of the mouth and fauces occur in all forms of acute leukaemia. Oral infection, often associated with ulceration, is very common in neutropenic patients. Candidosis may be seen on the fauces, tongue, or mucous membranes. The teeth may be badly formed and the bite may be abnormal in patients with severe forms of thalassaemia. Dental abscesses are common in patients with neutropenia; suspect teeth should be gently percussed for evidence of apical infection. Telangiectases may be found on the lips and oral mucous membranes of patients with hereditary telangiectasia.

On abdominal examination the most important questions are the size of the liver, whether there is splenomegaly, and if there are any palpable para-aortic lymph nodes. It is not possible to learn how to examine the spleen from a textbook, but a few hints may be helpful. Very large spleens tend to move downwards and medially towards the right iliac fossa and can be missed if the examiner does not start palpating from this region, moving upwards and medially towards the left subcostal region. The secret of success is to persuade the patient to breathe just deeply enough to move the spleen down without contracting the abdominal muscles. The examiner should wait for the spleen tip to meet their fingers rather than to try to find it by deep palpation. Once defined, the position of the lower border of the spleen should be recorded in centimetres, vertically below the costal margin. Be gentle! The author has seen enlarged spleens ruptured by overenthusiastic medical students.

The eyes are a mine of information in patients with haematological disorders. The conjunctivae may show mild icterus not obvious in the skin, and there may be haemorrhages in bleeding disorders. Pingueculae of the conjunctivae are seen in Gaucher's disease. Retinal haemorrhages are common in patients who have had a sudden fall in haemoglobin level and the combination of anaemia and thrombocytopenia is particularly likely to lead to severe retinal bleeding. Proliferative abnormalities of the retinal vessels are often seen in patients with sickling disorders, particularly haemoglobin sub-cutaneous disease. The hyperviscosity syndrome associated with macroglobulinaemia and some forms of myeloma is characterized by fullness of the retinal veins, which are sometimes broken up into segments like a string of sausages. These changes are often associated with widespread retinal haemorrhages. Optic atrophy may occur in patients with severe vitamin B_{12} deficiency.

Examination of the musculoskeletal system may be particularly rewarding in patients suspected of having genetic disorders of blood. In patients with coagulation defects such as haemophilia, recurrent bleeding into joints may produce a chronic deforming arthritis. Muscle haematomata are also common and are easily missed. A mild refractory anaemia is a very common accompaniment of rheumatoid arthritis. Painful arthritis of the large joints may be the presenting symptom of primary haemochromatosis. Gout is a common complication of all the myeloproliferative diseases. Bone tenderness or local swelling are found in patients with myeloma or sickle-cell anaemia. In children with thalassaemia or other hereditary haemolytic anaemias there may be reduced growth, bossing of the skull, and facial deformities. A wide variety of skeletal changes may occur with congenital hypoplastic anaemia.

The use of the laboratory

Finally, the diagnosis and management of blood disease requires an examination of the blood and, if appropriate, the bone marrow. It is essential to ask for an examination of the blood film in any patient who is suspected of having a haematological disorder. More can be learnt from the help of an experienced morphologist than any other investigation in clinical haematology.

In the section that follows we shall describe briefly the normal blood count and what can be learnt from a peripheral blood film and bone marrow examination. It cannot be emphasized too strongly that the most useful information is obtained by very close liaison between the laboratory and the ward.

Examination of the blood

Constituents of normal blood

Blood consists of several different types of cells suspended in plasma. The formed elements of the blood, or blood cells, consist of the red cells, white cells, and platelets. The red cells are biconcave discs approximately 7 to 8 mm in diameter and consist of a membrane that contains a concentrated solution of haemoglobin and a variety of other proteins, salts, and vitamins. Normally they are of a uniform shape and size, and contain similar amounts of haemoglobin. On supravital staining, approximately 1 per cent of the red cells show a reticular appearance. These are newly released cells and because of their staining characteristics are called reticulocytes.

The white cells are classified according to their morphological appearances into granulocytes (polymorphonuclear leucocytes), monocytes, and lymphocytes. The granulocytes and monocytes are phagocytic cells while the lymphocytes are involved in a variety of immune mechanisms. The granulocytes can be further classified according to their maturity. In the newly produced forms, band cells or juvenile polymorphonuclear leucocytes, the nucleus is horseshoe-shaped but single. In a normal blood film the majority of the granulocytes have matured beyond this stage and their nuclei consist of two or more lobes separated by thin, filamentous chromatin strands. These cells are about 12 to 15 mm in diameter. The granulocyte series is further classified according to the staining characteristics of the granules into neutrophils, eosinophils, and basophils. The monocytes are of similar size to the granulocytes but have oval nuclei with a slate-coloured cytoplasm, which may contain some fine granules. There are two morphologically distinct forms of lymphocyte: a large cell with a diameter of 8 to 16 mm and a smaller one measuring 7 to 9 mm. Both forms are round and have a light-blue cytoplasm. The platelets are disc-shaped cells measuring approximately 2 to 3 mm in diameter. In normal blood they are relatively homogeneous in structure.

A more detailed description of the structure and function of these different blood cells and their precursors appears later in this chapter.

Investigation of the blood—the normal blood count

A full blood count can be carried out on a 5-ml anticoagulated blood sample. A stained blood film is prepared for morphological examination of the different cells. Using cell counters, the relative volume of packed red cells and white cells, the haemoglobin level, and the red-cell, white-cell, and platelet counts can be determined. From a series of calculations relating the volume of packed cells, haemoglobin level, and red-cell count, it is possible to derive a series of absolute indices that provide useful information about the size and degree of haemoglobinization of the red cells. Finally, the relative numbers of reticulocytes and the erythrocyte sedimentation rate can be determined.

The stained blood film

An examination of the stained blood film is the most important investigation in haematology. Each of the cell types is studied separately.

The red cells are examined to assess their degree of haemoglobinization and their shape; if both are normal, they are described as normochromic and normocytic. Disorders of the red cell are frequently associated with changes in their morphology or staining properties. These include variation in size or anisocytosis; an increase in size or macrocytosis; a reduction in size or microcytosis; variability in shape or poikilocytosis; pale staining or hypochromia, which suggests underhaemoglobinization; and variation in the degree of staining from cell to cell, which is called anisochromia. In addition to these changes there may be more specific alterations in the morphology of the red cells. Some of these, together with the different clinical disorders with which they are associated, are summarized in Table 1 and illustrated in Fig. 1.

The white cells may be abnormal in number or morphology. An increased white-cell count is called a leucocytosis. If this involves the polymorphonuclear series, it is called a polymorphonuclear leucocytosis. An elevated eosinophil, basophil, monocyte, or lymphocyte count is called an eosinophilia, basophilia, monocytosis, or lymphocytosis, respectively. A reduced white count is called a neutropenia or lymphopenia, depending on the cell type involved. An absence of granulocytes in the blood is called agranulocytosis. As is the case for the red-cell series, much can be learned by morphological examination of the white cells. A blood film is said to show a 'shift to the left' if there are relatively more 'young' polymorphonuclear leucocytes present than normal. This is reflected by an increased proportion of band forms and, in more extreme cases, by a variable number of myelocytes or metamyelocytes. In acute bacterial infections, vacuoles may appear in the cytoplasm of polymorphonuclear leucocytes. In addition, the granules may become morphologically abnormal; heavy granulation of this type is called toxic granulation. A variety of genetic changes of nuclear configuration or of the granules of the polymorphonuclear leucocytes has been described; these are discussed later in this section.

Table 1 Significance of morphological and staining variations of the red cells

Change	Clinical significance
Hypochromia	Defective haemoglobinization; usually iron deficiency or defective haemoglobin synthesis
Microcytosis	As above
Macrocytosis	Dyserythropoiesis or premature release; may indicate megaloblastic erythropoiesis or haemolysis
Anisochromia	Variability of haemoglobinization or presence of young red-cell populations, e.g. in haemolysis
Spherocytosis	Usually indicates damage to membrane; may result from a genetic disorder of the membrane or an acquired defect often due to antibody or other damage to the cell
Target cells	Large 'floppy' cells that occur with deficient haemoglobinization or in liver disease; also occur in hypoplenism
Elliptocytes	May result from a genetic defect in the red-cell membrane but also occur in a variety of acquired conditions including iron deficiency
Poikilocytes: include burr cells, helmet cells, schistocytes, fragmented forms etc.	Usually indicates trauma to red cells in microcirculation or severe oxidant damage
Sickle cells	Occur in sickling disorders
Acanthocytes	Occur in genetic disorders of lipid metabolism
Inclusions: iron granules (siderocytes), Howell-Jolly bodies and Cabot's rings (nuclear remnants), basophilic stippling, and Heinz bodies	Iron granules and nuclear remnants are often seen after splenectomy. Basophilic stippling indicates accelerated erythropoiesis or defective haemoglobin synthesis
	Heinz bodies are precipitated haemoglobin or globin subunits

The packed-cell volume, haemoglobin level, and red-cell indices

A great deal can be learnt about the character of an anaemia from a few simple haematological tests. The volume of packed red cells (**PCV** or haematocrit) can be estimated either by centrifugation of a blood sample or by a conductivity method in which it is derived from measurement of the red-cell volume and the number of red cells using an electronic counting system. The haemoglobin concentration is usually determined spectrophotometrically by comparing a test sample with a stable standard, usually of the cyanmethaemoglobin derivative. Although for many years red-cell counting fell into disrepute, it has now become part of a standard blood count because of the accuracy of electronic cell counters.

Normal values for the PCV, haemoglobin level, and red-cell count are shown in Table 2. It is important to become familiar with the variability of these figures at different stages of development and between the sexes (Table 3). By combining information obtained from these measurements the red-cell indices can be estimated. The mean cell haemoglobin (**MCH**), which is derived from the haemoglobin value and the red-cell count and is expressed in picograms (pg), gives a reliable indication of the amount of haemoglobin per cell. The mean cell haemoglobin concentration (**MCHC**) represents the concentration of haemoglobin in g/dl of erythrocytes. The mean cell volume (**MCV**), calculated in femtolitres (fl), gives an indication of the size of the erythrocytes. Hence it is elevated in patients with macrocytic disorders and reduced in the presence of microcytic red cells. The normal values at different stages of development are summarized in Table 3.

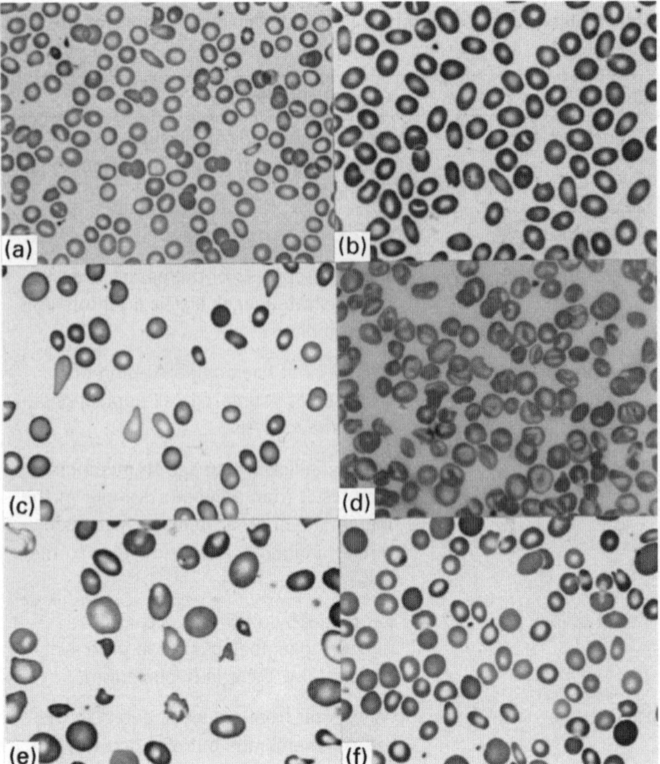

Fig. 1 Morphological changes of the red cells (600–800 ×). (a) Hypochromia and microcytosis. (b) Elliptocytosis. (c) Poikilocytosis (myelosclerosis). (d) Target cells and intracellular crystals (haemoglobin C disease). (e) Macrocytosis and anisocytosis (pernicious anaemia). (f) Dimorphic picture—normochromic and hypochromic (sideroblastic anaemia).

The total and differential leucocyte count

It should be remembered that the total white-cell count shows remarkable variability even in the same individual at different times. There are variations during the menstrual cycle and a marked diurnal rhythm, with minimum counts in the morning with subjects at rest. Activity may increase the white-cell count slightly, as may emotional stress and eating. Furthermore, the differential white-cell count varies considerably during normal human development. There is a preponderance of lymphocytes during the first few years of life and of polymorphonuclear leucocytes during later development and in adult life. These normal variations are shown in Table 3.

The platelet count

This is most accurately determined with an electronic cell counter, although a rough approximation can be obtained by using a counting chamber. There is marked variation in the normal platelet count and the range in health is approximately 130 to 400 × 10^9/l.

Blood volume, red-cell mass, and plasma volume

Because the haemoglobin level or PCV may vary due to expansion or contraction of the plasma volume, it is sometimes necessary to measure the red-cell mass and plasma volume directly. This is usually done by radioisotope dilution. The red-cell volume (**RCV**) is measured by labelling the red cells with ^{51}Cr and the plasma volume (**PV**) by the use of isotope-labelled albumin. In practice it is usual to calculate the RCV or PV in ml/kg. The wide range of normal values is summarized in Table 2.

The erythrocyte sedimentation rate (**ESR**)

The ESR is a measure of the suspension stability of red cells in blood. It is usually expressed in mm and is obtained by measuring the distance from the surface meniscus to the upper limit of the red-cell layer in a column of blood after 60 min. The ESR depends on the difference in specific gravity between the red cells and plasma but is influenced by many other factors, particularly the rate at which the red cells clump or form rouleaux. The increased sedimentation rate of clusters of cells reflects reduced fluid friction resulting from a decreased surface:volume ratio. Rouleaux formation is related to the concentration of fibrinogen and, to a lesser extent, of α_2- and γ-globulins in the plasma.

The ESR is still widely used as a non-specific index of organic disease. It is elevated in many acute or chronic infections, neoplastic diseases, collagen diseases, renal insufficiency, and any disorder associated with a significant change in the plasma proteins. Anaemia may cause an increased rate of sedimentation, and although many attempts have been made to develop correction factors to allow for this variable, none is satisfactory. Like all haematological measurements, the ESR changes in certain physiological states, particularly in pregnancy and with increasing age. In men and women over the age of 60 a slightly elevated ESR is often found without an obvious cause (Table 2).

Other haematological investigations

The simple tests that have been outlined in this section form the general screening investigations for all haematological disorders. In later sections we will describe the more specialized investigations that are often required to diagnose specific disorders of the red cells, white cells, and platelets, or of haemostasis and coagulation. Normal values for some of these investigations are given in Table 2.

Examination of the marrow

Bone marrow can be examined by needle aspiration, closed needle biopsy, or open surgical biopsy. In adults the sites most easily available are the sternum and the anterior or posterior iliac crests. In children of less than a year old the anterior surface of the tibia is the site of choice, but in older children the iliac crest is suitable. After aspiration of the marrow, films are made and stained with a Romanowsky stain. Needle or surgical biopsy samples are fixed and sectioned by standard methods.

The marrow films are examined initially under low-power microscopy to assess the overall cellularity and for the presence of abnormal cells. It is sometimes useful to obtain a differential count and from this the myeloid/erythroid (M/E) ratio can be determined. This is approximately 3:1 in health, although, if there is increased erythroid activity, it may fall to unity or less. It should be remembered that differential counts may be quite inaccurate because the precursors may not be distributed homogeneously. This is a particular problem in disorders in which there are abnormal cells in the marrow. Having determined the overall cellularity, the morphology of the individual cells is examined. The degree of maturation of the red cells, white cells, and megakaryocyte series is assessed and the marrow is examined carefully for the presence of any abnormal cells.

A biopsy (trephine) specimen is particularly useful for looking at overall cellularity and relating the amount of haemopoiesis to the amount of fatty tissue. It is of particular value if an aspiration yields a 'dry tap' when it may show replacement by fibrous or tumour tissue, which may not aspirate readily. Using appropriate

Table 2 Haematological values for normal adults

Red-cell count		*β-Thromboglobulin*	<50 ng/ml
Men	$5.0 \pm 0.5 \times 10^{12}$/l	*Platelet factor 4*	<10 ng/ml
Women	$4.3 \pm 0.5 \times 10^{12}$/l	*Protein C*	<10ng/ml
Haemoglobin		Function	0.70–1.40 u/ml
Men	150±20 g/l	Antigen	0.61–1.32 u/ml
Women	140±20 g/l	*Protein S*	
Packed-cell volume (PCV; haematocrit value)		Total	0.78–1.37 u/ml
Men	0.45±0.05 (l/l)	Free	0.68–1.52 u/ml
Women	0.41±0.04 (l/l)	*Heparin cofactor II*	55–145%
Mean cell volume (MCV)		*Autohaemolysis (37°C)*	
Men and women	92±10 fl	48 h without added glucose	0.2–2.0
Mean cell haemoglobin (MCH)		48 h, with added glucose	0–0.9%
Men and women	29.5±2.5 pg	*Cold agglutinin titre (4°C)*	<64
Mean cell haemoglobin concentration (MCHC)		*Serum iron*	13–32 μmol/l (0.7–1.8 mg/l)
Men and women	330±15 g/l	*Total iron-binding capacity*	45–70 μmol/l (2.5–4.0 mg/l)
Red-cell distribution width (RDW)		*Transferrin*	1.2–2.0 g/l
As CV	13.2±1.6%	*Ferritin*	
As SD	42.5±3.5 fl	Men	20–300 median 100 μg/l
Red-cell diameter (mean values)		Women	15–150 median 30 μg/l
Dry films	6.7–7.7 μm	*Serum vitamin B12*	160–760 ng/l
Red-cell density	1092–1100 g/l	*Serum folate*	3–20 μg/l
Reticulocyte count	0.5–2.0% (25–85×10^9/l	*Red-cell folate*	160–640 μg/l
Blood volume		*Plasma haemoglobin*	10–40 mg/l
Red-cell volume		*Serum haptoglobin*	0.6–2.7 mg/l
Men	30±5 ml/kg	*HbA2*	2.2–3.5%
Women	25±5 ml/kg	*HbF*	<1.0%
Plasma volume	45±5 ml/kg	*Methaemoglobin*	<2.0%
Total blood volume	70±10 ml/kg	*Sedimentation rate*	
Red cell lifespan	120±30 days	(1 h at 20±3°C) (upper limits)	
Leucocyte count	7.0± 3.0 × 10^9/l	Men:	
Differential leucocyte count		17–50 years	10 mm
Neutrophils	2.0–7.0×10^9/l (40–80%)	50–60 years	12 mm
Lymphocytes	1.0–3.0×10^9/l (20–40%)	61–70 years	14 mm
Monocytes	0.2–1.0×10^9/l (2–10%)	>70 years	30 mm
Eosinophils	0.04–0.4×10^9/l (1–6%)	Women:	
Basophils	0.02–0.1×10^9/l (<1–2%)	17–50 years	19 mm
Platelet count	130–400 × 10^9/l	50–60 years	19 mm
Bleeding time		61–70 years	20 mm
(Ivy's method)	2–7 min	>70 years	35 mm
(Template method)	2.5–9.5 min	*Plasma viscosity*	
Prothrombin time	12–16 s	25°C	1.50–1.72 mPa/s
Partial thromboplastin time (PTT)	30–46 s	37°C	1.16–1.33 mPa/s
Thrombin time	15–19 s	*Heterophile (anti-sheep red cell) agglutinin titre*	<80
Plasma fibrinogen	2.0–4.0 g/l		
Fibrinogen titre	≥128	After absorption with guinea-pig kidney	<10
Plasminogen			
Function	0.75–1.35 u/ml		
Antigen	0.76–1.36 u/ml		
Euglobulin lysis time	90–240 min		
Antithrombin III			
Function	0.86–13.2 u/ml		
Antigen	0.79–1.11 u/ml		

Expressed as mean±SD (95% range).

After Dacie and Lewis (1994).

Table 3 Haematological values for normal infants and children

	At birth (full term)	Day 3	1 month	2–6 months	2–6 years	6–12 years
Red-cell count ($\times 10^{12}$/l)	6.0±1.0	5.3±1.3	4.2±1.2	3.8±0.8	4.6±0.7	4.6±0.6
Haemoglobin (g/l)	165±30	185±40	140±30	115±20	125±15	135±20
Packed-cell volume/haematocrit	0.54±0.10	0.56±0.11	0.43±0.12	0.35±0.07	0.37±0.03	0.40±0.05
Mean cell volume (MCV) (fl)	110±10	108±13	104±19	91±17	81±6	86±8
Mean cell haemoglobin (MCH) (pg)	34±3	34±3	34±6	30±5	27±3	29±4
Mean cell haemoglobin concentration (MCHC) (g/l)	330±30	330±40	330±40	330±30	340±30	340±30
Reticulocytes (%)	2–5	1–4.5	0.3–1	0.4–1	0.2–2	0.2–2
Leucocyte count ($\times 10^{9}$/l)	18±8	15±8	12±7	12±6	10±5	9±4
Neutrophils ($\times 10^{9}$/l)	5–13	3–5	3–9	1.5–9	1.5–8	2–8
Lymphocytes ($\times 10^{9}$/l)	3–10	2–8	3–16	4–10	6–9	1–5
Monocytes ($\times 10^{9}$/l)	0.7–1.5	0.5–1	0.3–1	0.1–1	0.1–1	0.1–1
Eosinophils ($\times 10^{9}$/l)	0.2–1	0.1–2.5	0.2–1	0.2–1	0.2–1	0.1–1

Expressed as mean±2 SD or 95% range.

After Dacie and Lewis (1994).

stains it is possible to estimate the amount of iron and reticulin in the marrow.

Assessment of bone marrow activity and distribution

Some indication of marrow function is obtained from its morphological appearances and from the M/E ratio. It is also possible to measure the rates of production and turnover of the red-cell series using radioactive iron (see Chapter 3.16). It is sometimes necessary to attempt to estimate the distribution of the haemopoietic marrow, and this is usually done by using isotopes to produce scintograms that show the distribution of erythropoietic or reticuloendothelial marrow throughout the body. Erythropoietic marrow can be visualized using the short-lived, positron-emitting isotope ^{52}Fe with a scintillation camera. In health this shows erythropoietic marrow in the ribs, spine, pelvis, scapula, and clavicle, with a variable amount in the skull. The reticuloendothelial portion of the marrow can be labelled with a radiocolloid with an appropriate particle size; the most effective and commonly used is ^{99}Tc^{m}-sulphurcolloid.

Further reading

Beutler, E., Lichtman, M.A., Coller, B.S., and Kipps, T.J. (ed.) (1994). *Williams hematology*, 5th edn. McGraw-Hill, New York.

Dacie, J.V. and Lewis, S.M. (1994). *Practical haematology*, 8th edn. Churchill Livingstone, Edinburgh.

Nathan, D.G. and Oski, F.A. (1993). *Hematology of infancy and childhood*, 4th edn. Saunders, Philadelphia.

Chapter 3.2

Stem cells and haemopoiesis

C. A. Sieff and D. G. Nathan

Normal haemopoiesis in the adult is sustained by the production of blood cells from their recognizable precursors in the bone marrow, their survival in the vasculature, and their demise in the reticuloendothelial system, predominantly in the spleen, the liver, the lung, and the marrow itself. Though the concentration of cells in the blood varies widely, it is notable that the values observed in normal individuals are remarkably consistent, particularly considering the vast differences in the lifespans of these cells. For example, the mean lifespan of granulocytes in the peripheral blood may be measured in hours. In contrast, platelets survive for 7–10 days. Though platelets are removed from the blood in part by random forces, most of their lifespan is dictated by metabolic changes within them that lead to predetermined death in about 7–10 days. Normally, red cells are almost entirely lost by a process of metabolic decay that begins after the erythrocyte has attained an age of approximately 100 days. Lymphocytes have very dramatic differences in lifespan. Some are removed from the circulation in 2 or 3 weeks by a process that is not well understood. Others, particularly certain T lymphocytes, are thought to survive for the entire lifespan of the individual, carrying within them the programmes embossed upon them by the thymus.

Though steady-state concentrations of the blood cells vary from each other by three logs or more, the actual marrow production rates that maintain them are very similar. Approximately 5×10^4 red cells, 2×10^4 platelets, and 2×10^4 granulocytes must be produced per microlitre of blood per day to maintain a normal blood count. Lymphocyte production must be considerably lower because the bulk of lymphocytes in the peripheral blood are the long-lived T lymphocytes described above.

These relatively constant production rates of blood cells are regulated by a highly complex marrow tissue characterized morphologically by recognizable, differentiating precursor cells. These cells are renewed by a population of morphologically unrecognizable progenitor cells, some of which are in turn derived from stem cells. The differentiating precursor cells and their progenitors are packed together into fronds surrounded by endothelial cells that separate the marrow cells from the venous sinuses. The mature blood cells find apertures through the endothelial cells and migrate between them to fall into the sinuses, the currents of which carry them into the peripheral blood.

In this chapter, the physiology of haemopoiesis in the marrow is described. To understand this process, its ontogeny and comparative development must first be reviewed.

Phylogeny and ontogeny

In the developing human being, haemopoiesis moves through several overlapping anatomical and functional stages, beginning in the yolk sac, entering the hepatic phase at 6 weeks', and the marrow phase at 20 weeks' gestation. Transfer to the bone marrow phase is generally complete at birth. These anatomical shifts in sites of haemopoiesis are associated with marked alterations in functional properties, particularly of globin synthesis in the red cell.

Marrow anatomy

The relative red (active) marrow space of a child is much greater than that of an adult, presumably because the high requirements for red-cell production during neonatal life demand the resources of the entire production potential of the marrow. During postnatal life the demands for red-cell production ebb, and much of the marrow space is slowly and progressively filled with fat (Fig. 1). In certain diseases that are usually associated with anaemia, such as myeloid metaplasia, haemopoiesis may return to its former sites in the liver, spleen, and lymph nodes.

The microenvironment of the marrow cavity is a vast network of endothelial cell-lined vascular channels or sinusoids that separate clumps of haemopoietic cells. The haemopoietic cells are found in close association in the intrasinusoidal spaces with a stromal network that includes fibroblastoid cells and fat cells. Stromal cells, endothelial cells, and macrophages produce many of the haemopoietic growth factors necessary for the survival, proliferation, and differentiation of progenitor cells.

Function of stem cells and progenitors

The progenitors of the recognizable precursor cells are mononuclear 'blast' cells with large nuclei, prominent nucleoli, and basophilic cytoplasm devoid of granules. These primitive progenitor cells are present at extremely low frequencies, approximately 1 in 10^4 to 10^5 marrow cells for the stem-cell population and 1 in 10^3 for their committed progenitor progeny. A single pluripotent stem cell is capable of giving rise to increasingly committed progenitor cells according to the schema outlined in Fig. 2. These committed progenitors are destined to form differentiated recognizable precursors of the specific types of blood cells.

Pluripotent stem cells are defined most stringently as cells capable of reconstituting haemopoiesis after transplantation. They are capable of both self-renewal and differentiation, perhaps under the influence

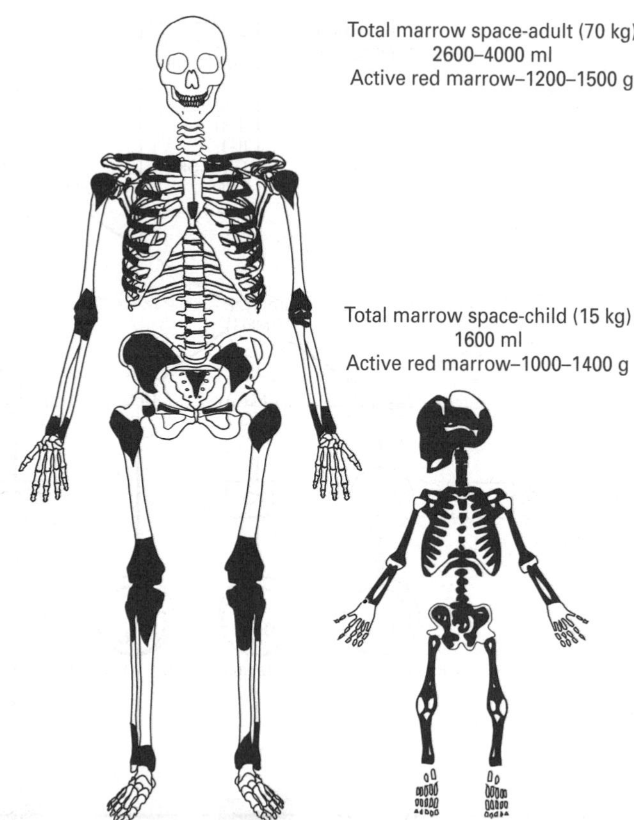

Fig. 1 A comparison of active red marrow-bearing areas in a child and adult. Note the almost identical amount of active red marrow in the child and adult despite a fivefold discrepancy in body weight.
(Reproduced with permission from MacFarlane, R.G. and Robb-Smith, A.H.T. (ed.) (1961). Functions of the blood, p. 357. Blackwell Scientific, Oxford.)

of certain non-lineage-specific growth factors such as the interleukins IL-1, IL-3, IL-6, IL-11, and Steel factor (SF), or unidentified stromal interactions. Their commitment to the various differentiation programmes appears to be random, and leads to a broad array of more mature lineage-committed progenitors that are themselves responsive to lineage-restricted growth factors, including erythropoietin and the granulocyte and macrophage colony-stimulating factors (G-CSF and M-CSF, respectively). Some of the lineage-restricted growth factors, particularly erythropoietin, are produced in response to the circulating levels of differentiated blood cells.

The lineage-committed progenitors are characterized by limited proliferative potential that depends upon the presence of specific growth factors. The latter interact with specific receptors on progenitor surfaces; therefore, they are not capable of indefinite self-renewal. In fact, they 'die by differentiation' to mature precursors of the blood cells. The maintenance of their numbers ultimately depends upon the presence of lineage-specific growth factor and on random influx into their pool from the pluripotent stem-cell pool.

Therefore, amplification of blood-cell production occurs at the level of the committed progenitor pool, while maintenance of the progenitors depends upon the capacity of members of the pluripotent stem-cell pool to differentiate into the committed progenitor pool.

Progenitors can exist outside the marrow. A number of early haemopoietic cells, including the pluripotent stem cells and certain committed progenitor cells, have been demonstrated in the circulation

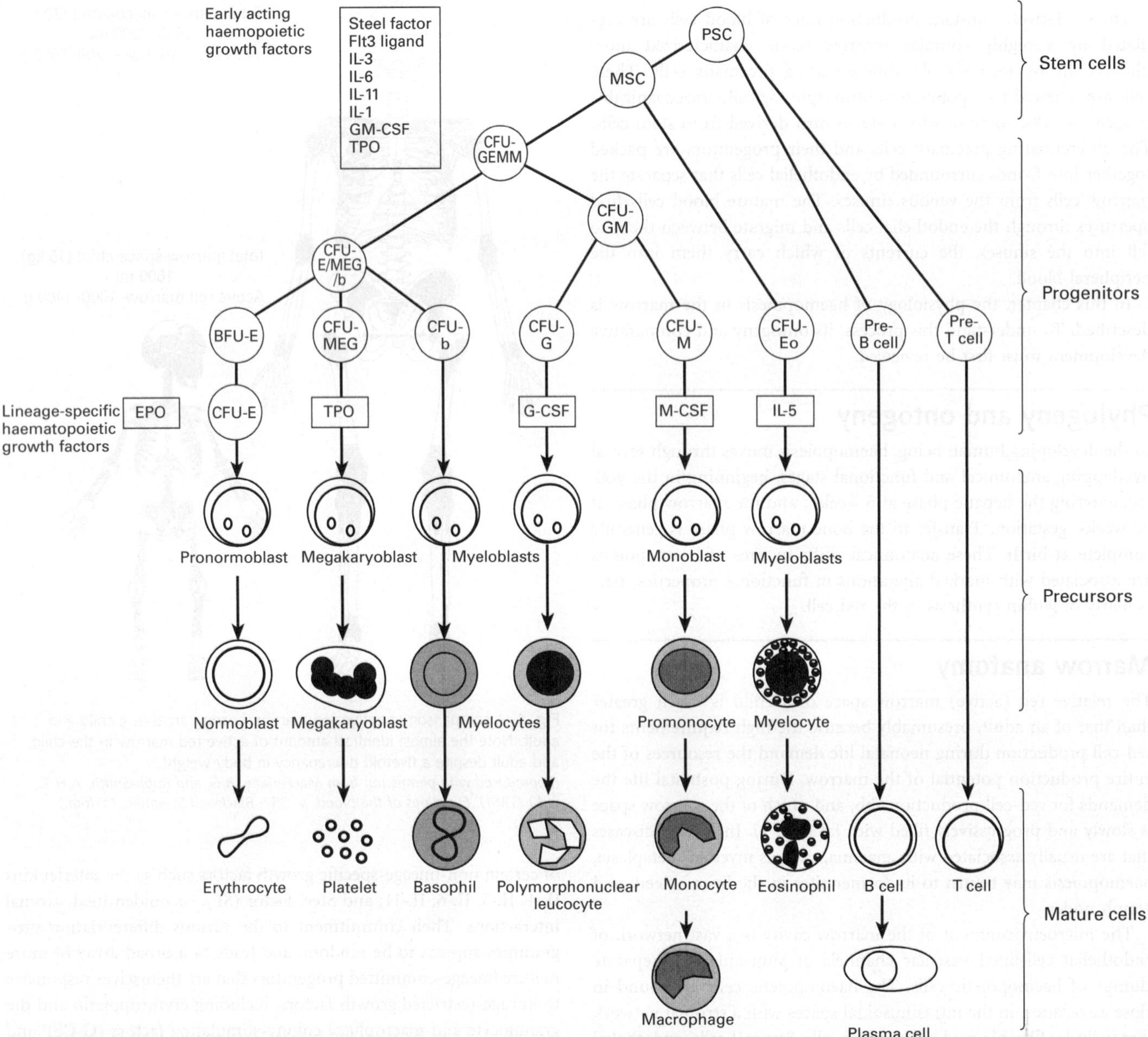

Fig. 2 The maturation sequence of progenitor cells. The sequence is characterized by a progressive approach to single-lineage commitment. The term 'stem cell' connotes a high capacity for self-renewal, but all progenitors have some self-renewal capacity.

of normal individuals and experimental animals. The capacity of haemopoietic stem cells to negotiate the circulation is especially significant in relation to bone marrow transplantation, which is carried out by an infusion of bone marrow cells from the donor into the circulation of the recipient. Murine transplantation studies with highly purified stem cells demonstrate that B and T lymphocytes are derived from the same population of stem cells as the other cellular elements of blood (Fig. 2).

Erythropoiesis

The rate of erythropoiesis is driven by anaemia or hypoxia, both of which stimulate a class of peritubular kidney cells through what is likely to be a haem-containing oxygen sensor to transcribe the erythropoietin (EPO) gene and release the hormone into the blood. The hormone acts via the erythropoietin receptor found on erythroblasts and erythroid progenitors to stimulate their division and differentiation. The least-mature committed erythroid progenitor is known as an erythroid burst-forming unit or BFU-E. When it differentiates *in vitro* under the influence of lineage non-specific factors such as SF, IL-3, or GM-CSF and EPO it forms large colonies of erythroblasts and reticulocytes that may contain as many as 50 000 cells. The colonies, derived from single cells, have a burst-like appearance because they are composed of multiple subcolonies. BFU-Es progressively mature during their sojourn in the marrow and in doing so gain in sensitivity to erythropoietin until they reach the stage at which they are known as erythroid colony-forming units (CFU-E).

Phagocytopoiesis

The development of a clonal assay for granulocyte and macrophage progenitors preceded the development of erythroid progenitor assays by nearly a decade, yet a clear understanding of the regulation of myeloid differentiation remains elusive. Figure 2 illustrates the development of granulocyte, monocyte, and macrophage production from the pluripotent stem cell. The colony-forming unit—granulocyte–macrophage (**CFU-GM**) derived from the pluripotent progenitor gives rise to separate granulocyte and monocyte progenitors (**CFU-G** and **CFU-M**), which, under the influence of unique colony-stimulating factors, G-CSF and M-CSF, differentiate to mature granulocytes and/or monocytes, respectively. Both IL-3 and GM-CSF affect a similar broad spectrum of human myeloid progenitor cells. This includes colonies that contain granulocytes, erythrocytes, monocytes, and megakaryocytes (**CFU-GEMM**), eosinophils (**CFU-Eo**), CFU-GM, CFU-G, and CFU-M.

Monocytes leave the circulation and differentiate further to become fixed tissue macrophages. These tissue macrophages include alveolar macrophages and hepatic Kupffer cells, dermal Langerhans cells, osteoclasts, peritoneal macrophages, pleural macrophages, and possibly brain microglial cells though the origin of these is still uncertain.

The granulocyte compartment itself is more complex than either the erythroid or megakaryocyte compartments. The circulating half-life of the newly rapidly deployed granulocyte is only 6.5 h. In order to meet sudden demands, an additional non-circulating granulocyte pool exists in the spleen, marginated around blood vessels, and in a readily releasable bone marrow pool. The rate at which new myeloblasts or monoblasts are produced by progenitors *in vivo* is not known, but exhaustion of progenitors in infection, particularly in the neonatal period, is associated with a fatal outcome due to a failure of granulocyte production.

Megakaryocytopoiesis

The regulation of megakaryocyte progenitors, their development into megakaryoblasts and their subsequent progressive maturation into platelet-shedding, multinucleated cells are all influenced by growth factors. The most important appears to be thrombopoietin which has recently been cloned and is now being used in clinical trials.

Clinical studies with haemopoietic growth factors

Several recombinant haemopoietic growth factors are currently under evaluation. The initial studies focused on erythropoietin in the anaemia of chronic renal failure (see also Chapter 12.29) and GM-CSF or G-CSF in both transient and long-standing, bone marrow-failure syndromes. More recently, other haemopoietic growth factors such as M-CSF, IL-3, SF, and thrombopoietin are coming under scrutiny. Erythropoietin has found a useful role in the treatment of anaemia associated with a variety of chronic diseases and in haematological disease such as myeloma. GM-CSF and G-CSF can shorten the period of neutropenia following myelosuppressive chemotherapy and their influence on survival is now being studied in trials. Most patients with Kostmann's syndrome, a rare inherited severe failure of neutrophil production, respond dramatically to G-CSF treatment, and patients with other defects of neutrophil production such as cyclic neutropenia and chronic idiopathic neutropenia may also benefit.

Further reading

Bunn, H.F., Gu, J., Huang, L.E., Park, J.W., and Zhu, H. (1998). Erythropoietin: a model system for studying oxygen-dependent gene regulation. *Journal of Experimental Biology*, **210**, 1197.

Clark, S., Nathan, D.G., and Sieff, C.A. (1997). The anatomy and physiology of hematopoiesis. In *Hematology of infancy and childhood* (ed. D.G. Nathan and S.H. Orkin). W.B. Saunders, Philadelphia, PA.

Enver, T., Heyworth, C.M., and Dexter, T.M. (1998). Do stem cells play dice? *Blood*, **92**, 348; discussion 352.

Metcalf, D. (1998). Lineage commitment and maturation in hematopoietic cells: the case for extrinsic regulation. *Blood*, **92**, 345; discussion 352.

Metcalf, D. (1998). The molecular control of hematopoiesis: progress and problems with gene manipulation. *Stem Cells*, **16**, 314.

The leukaemias and other disorders of haemapoietic stem cells

Chapter 3.3

The classification of leukaemia

D. Catovsky

The classification of leukaemia has evolved over the years from a purely morphological approach, based on the appearances of the leukaemic cells in peripheral blood and bone marrow films, through cytochemical techniques and, lately, to a greater reliance on monoclonal antibodies against cellular antigens. The next decade will see a major input from cytogenetic and molecular methods. The object of any classification is to define disease entities with distinct biological and clinical features.

A broad classification includes two large groups historically designated acute and chronic (Table 1). Acute leukaemias are malignancies with little evidence of differentiation; the characteristic cells are immature blasts. It is in this group that techniques other than

Table 1 The classification of leukaemia

Acute leukaemias	*Chronic leukaemias*
Myeloid (AML):	Myeloid:[1]
M0–M7 (see Table 3)	Chronic granulocytic (CGL)[1]
Lymphoblastic (ALL):	Atypical chronic myeloid (aCML)[1]
B-lineage—common ALL	Chronic neutrophilic
etc. (see Table 5)	Chronic myelomonocytic (CMML)[1]
T-lineage—T-ALL	Juvenile CMML
Biphenotypic:	Chronic eosinophilic
Myeloid and lymphoid	Lymphoid:
Hypocellular	B-lineage—CLL and others[2]
	T-lineage—T-PLL and others[2]

[1] French, American, British (FAB) group classification (see OTM3, p. 3399 for source).

[2] See Chapter 3.7.

Table 2 Immunological classification of acute leukaemia

Marker	Lymphoblastic (ALL)[1] B-lineage	Lymphoblastic (ALL)[1] T-lineage	AML (MO–M7)
CD2	–	+	–
CD3(c)	–	+	–
CD7	–	+	–
CD10	+	–	–
CD19	+	–	–
CD22(c)	+	–	–
CD13	–	–	+
CD33	–	–	+
MPO(c)	–	–	+[2]

(c) Cytoplasmic expression.

[1] Classification of ALL subtypes, see Table 4.

[2] MPO (myeloperoxidase) is negative in erythroid precursors (M6) and megakaryoblasts (M7).

Table 3 The classification of acute myeloid leukaemia

Myeloblastic leukaemia	*Myelomonocytic*
M0: minimal differentiation	M4: granulocytic–monocytic
M1: poorly differentiated	M4Eo: with bone marrow eosinophilia
M2: differentiated	
Promyelocytic	*Monocytic*
M3: hypergraunlar	M5a: monoblastic
M3V: microgranular variant	M5b: monocytic
	M6: Erythroleukaemia
	M7: Megakaryoblastic

French, American, British (FAB) group classification:; Bennett *et al.* (1976, 1985*a*, 1985*b*, 1991).

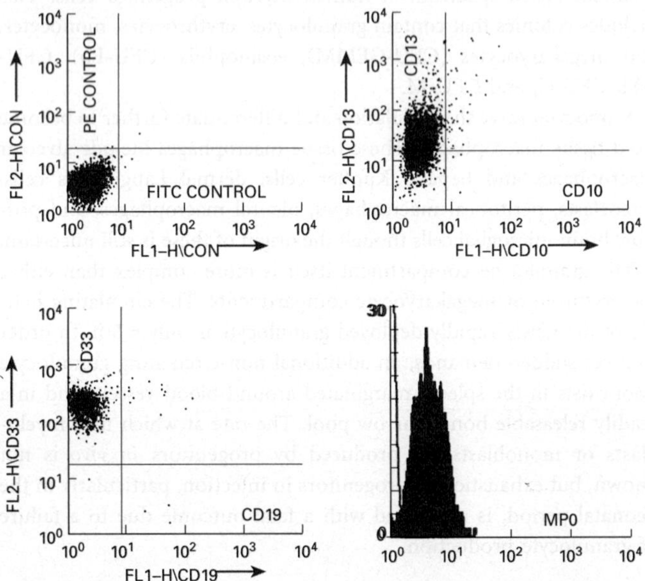

Fig. 1 Flow cytometric analysis of a case of acute myeloid leukaemia using double monoclonal antibodies conjugated with two different fluorescent dyes: phycoerythrin (PE) and fluorescein isothiocyanate (**FITC**) shown in the control panel (top left). The blast cells are CD13+ and CD10– (top right), CD33+ and CD19– (bottom left) and anti-MPO+ (bottom right).

morphological tests are essential for classification. The chronic leukaemias show maturation, which is more easily recognized by morphology, although in the diseases of lymphocytes the various subtypes can only be accurately defined by means of monoclonal antibodies.

Acute leukaemias

There are two major groups of acute leukaemia, lymphoblastic (**ALL**) and myeloid (**AML**). Both affect children and adults but with different frequency: 80 per cent of patients with AML are adults (over the age of 15 years) and 20 per cent children, including infants; in contrast, 85 per cent of those with ALL are children (under 15 years) and 15 per cent adults. In AML there are few differences in most disease features between children and adults; conversely, the differences between childhood and adult ALL are significant.

For a diagnosis of acute leukaemia it is necessary to identify blasts as the main cellular component. With a few cytochemical reactions it is possible to distinguish the two main forms, ALL and AML. However, because these cytochemical methods are largely negative in ALL, it is now essential to apply a battery of monoclonal antibodies, which can be used as markers for the two ALL cell lineages, B and T, and of AML blasts (Table 2). These monoclonals define the immunophenotype of the disease. In immature cells, some antigens are expressed first in the cytoplasm (c), then in the cell membrane.

In addition to the monoclonal antibodies listed in Table 2, other markers can be used to distinguish ALL from AML. One is the DNA polymerase terminal deoxynucleotidyl transferase (**TdT**), which is demonstrated by an antibody in all cases of ALL, both B and T. A proportion of AML (25 to 30 per cent) also expresses TdT, although not in all cells and, if a quantitative procedure is applied, with less intensity. The routine use of monoclonals and TdT has also disclosed the existence of acute leukaemias that express antigens of more than one lineage, usually lymphoid and myeloid. These cases are designated mixed lineage or biphenotypic (see below).

Bone-marrow trephine biopsies are useful for the diagnosis of cases that yield a 'dry tap' or a hypocellular specimen in aspirates. This is the case in two forms of acute leukaemia: megakaryoblastic or AML-M7 (Table 3) and hypocellular acute leukaemia; the blasts in the latter are nearly always myeloid.

Acute myeloid leukaemia

The French, American, British (**FAB**) group aimed to standardize the diagnostic criteria for the different forms of AML (Table 3) that reflect all the lines of myeloid differentiation. Although most types can be recognized by morphology and cytochemistry (see Fig. 1), there are two types, M0 and M7, which require positive evidence by monoclonal antibodies. The biological significance of the FAB classification of AML was emphasized by the correlation of several of the defined subtypes with non-random chromosome translocations (Table 4). The latter are more reliable for identifying patients with a good or bad prognosis.

AML-M0

This is the most immature form of myeloblastic leukaemia. The blasts are negative by cytochemistry but positive with one or more of the AML markers. The incidence of M0 is around 5 per cent of all AML and there is evidence that this disease has a poor prognosis.

Table 4 Chromosome translocations in acute myeloid leukaemia (AML)

AML type	Chromosome translocation	Genes involved[1]
M2	t(8;21)(q22;q22)	*ETO-AML1*
M3 and M3V	t(15;17)(q24;q21)	*PML-RARa*
M4Eo	inv(16)(p13;q32)	*CBFB-MYH11*
M5	t(11;19)(q23;p13)	*MLL-ENL*
AML with basophilia	t(6;9)(p23;q34)	*DEK-CAN*

[1] Detected by molecular methods: Southern blots, polymerase chain reaction or *in situ* hybridization.

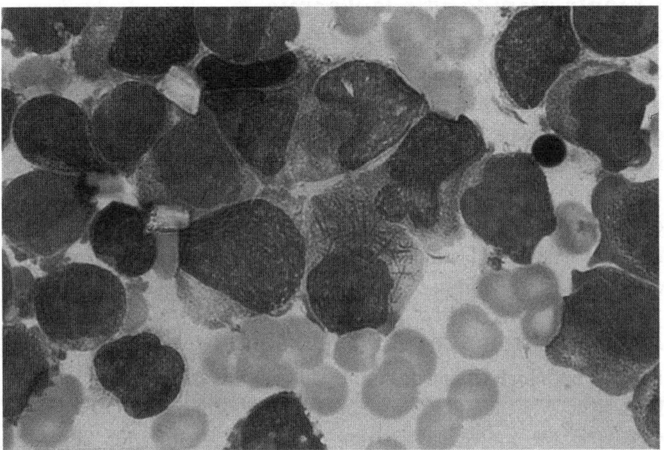

Fig. 2 Bone marrow aspirate from a case of acute myeloid leukaemia M3 (hypergranular promyelocytic) showing a cell with multiple Auer rods ('faggots').

AML-M1

This form of AML is also poorly differentiated; it differs from M0 in the demonstration of myeloid features by the cytochemical reactions of myeloperoxidase and Sudan black B.

AML-M2

This is AML with differentiation beyond promyelocytes. In 15 per cent of M2 cases the cells show the translocation t(8;21) (Table 4).

AML-M3

This comprises 7 to 8 per cent of all AMLs. Typical cases can be recognized by morphology: the blasts are bilobed, heavily granular, and show bundles of Auer rods or 'faggots' (Fig. 2). M3 affects young adults, who present with a low white blood-cell count and a bleeding tendency. M3 variant cases have a high white blood-cell count, the blasts are deceptively hypogranular and may resemble monocytes, but the nucleus is bilobed rather than reniform (kidney-shaped). A unique feature of both typical and variant M3 is the translocation t(15;17) (Table 4) and the important role of all-*trans* retinoic acid in treatment.

AML-M4

These cases show evidence of granulocytic and monocytic differentiation. The latter is confirmed by the ANAE reaction in more than 20 per cent of the blasts, a raised serum and/or urine lysozyme, and peripheral blood monocytosis. M4Eo is a variant form defined by the presence of bone marrow eosinophilia, with these cells showing prominent basophilic granules in addition to the eosinophil granules.

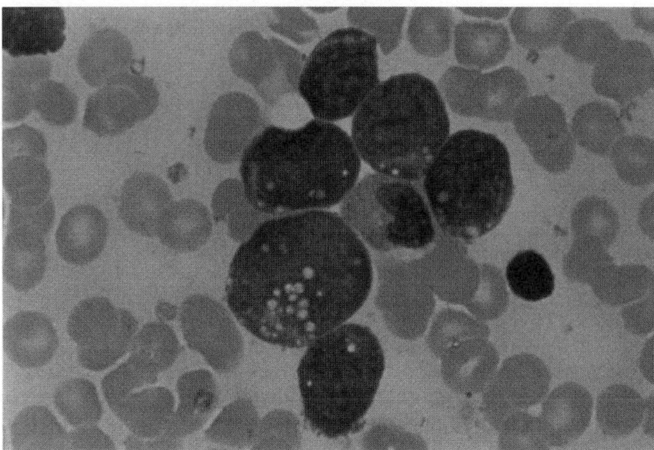

Fig. 3 Bone marrow film from a case of acute lymphoblastic leukaemia (ALL) L3 (Burkitt type) that corresponded immunologically to B-ALL (Table 4). The blasts have a deep basophilic cytoplasm with vacuoles.

M4Eo cases are associated with a unique chromosome abnormality (Table 4).

AML-M5

Two forms of monocytic leukaemia can be identified by morphology. M5a is immature and common in infants. In M5b the cells are more mature and lysozyme levels are raised. M5 is associated with a high white-cell count, lymphadenopathy, and gingival hypertrophy.

AML-M6

Because these cases always show features of trilineage myelodysplasia it is necessary to distinguish them from primary myelodysplasia. The blasts in M6 are nearly always myeloblasts, but in rare cases they may be erythroid precursors.

AML-M7

This form of AML includes most cases with features of 'acute myelofibrosis', that is a fibrotic bone marrow with blasts, abnormal megakaryocytes, and circulating blasts shown to be megakaryoblasts by their reactivity with monoclonal antibodies against platelet glycoproteins.

Acute lymphoblastic leukaemia

ALL represents the clonal proliferation of immature lymphoid precursors. The characteristic cell is the lymphoblast, which has a high nuclear:cytoplasmic ratio and lacks cytoplasmic granules. Myeloperoxidase, Sudan black B, and ANAE are negative.

The FAB group described three morphological types of ALL: L1, seen in 80 per cent of childhood cases, L2, seen in 20 per cent, and L3 or Burkitt type (Fig. 3), seen in 1 to 3 per cent.

The diagnosis and classification of ALL subtypes now relies mainly on the immunophenotype (Table 2). Based on the sequential appearance of certain antigens during B- and T-cell differentiation, a subclassification of ALL can be delineated (Table 5). The most important marker of the B lineage is the common-ALL antigen, which is recognized by monoclonal antibodies of the CD10 cluster. CD10 is expressed in the blasts of 75 per cent of childhood ALL cases, hence the designation common ALL. Less mature lymphoblasts (early or pro B-ALL) do not express CD10, and this is seen in 10 per cent of childhood cases and in 30 per cent of adult ALL. Pre-B-ALL blasts express cytoplasmic μ-chains (without light chains).

Table 5 Immunological classification of acute lymphoblastic leukaemia (ALL)

B-lineage	*T-lineage*
Early-B (CD10–)	Pre-T (CD2–)
Common ALL (CD10+)	T-ALL (CD2+)
Pre-B ALL (cyt. μ+)	
B-ALL (membrane Ig)	

The various forms of ALL have distinct prognostic features that are related to the associated chromosome abnormalities.

Clinical classification

A practical classification of ALL is to divide the cases according to age into adult and childhood ALL. Adult ALL has many biological and clinical differences from childhood ALL: more cases of L2 morphology and a Philadelphia (Ph)-positive karyotype and fewer with hyperdiploidy, which is a good prognostic feature in children. The classification in Table 5 could be adapted to this division of childhood and adult cases.

Common ALL

This is the most frequent form of ALL in children and includes the cases with a better prognosis. The main diagnostic criterion is the demonstration of the common-ALL antigen (CD10+).

Early or pro B-ALL

This was formerly described as null ALL, but has now been redefined by the presence of the early B-cell antigens CD19 and CD22 (cytoplasmic) and negative CD10.

Pre-B-ALL

This is defined by the expression of μ-chain in the cytoplasm and persistence of CD10.

B-ALL

This is defined by evidence of membrane immunoglobulin (heavy and light chains) and is associated with L3 morphology (Fig. 3) and the translocation t(8;14). B-ALL probably represents the leukaemic presentation of non-endemic Burkitt lymphoma. In adults it may also represent the transformation of a pre-existing follicular lymphoma; in such cases t(8;14) coexists with t(14;18). The prognosis of B-ALL is very poor with conventional therapy, but has improved dramatically with newer and more intensive regimens.

T-ALL

These cases evolve with a thymic mass and high white-cell count. There is overlap with T-lymphoblastic lymphoma, a condition in which, by convention, the bone marrow contains less than 25 per cent lymphoblasts.

Biphenotypic acute leukaemia

These are cases in which markers of different cell lineages (usually B and myeloid) are coexpressed on the same blast cells. Biphenotypic leukaemia comprises 5 per cent of all acute leukaemias and frequently shows rearrangement of immunoglobulin and/or T-cell receptor genes, even in cases presenting as AML. Because of the distinct biological and molecular changes and poor prognosis associated with these cases, it is of clinical value to recognize biphenotypic leukaemia as a distinct type using well-defined diagnostic criteria.

Hypocellular acute leukaemia

These are rare AML cases that present with pancytopenia and a 'dry tap' bone marrow, which are shown on adequate bone-marrow trephine biopsies to be hypocellular (in contrast to the expected hypercellularity). The biopsies may resemble aplastic anaemia but show distinct clusters of blasts as well as a number of these cells in the circulation.

Chronic leukaemias

These are malignancies in which mature leucocytes are the predominant cell. As for the acute leukaemias, there are two main groups, myeloid and lymphoid, with two representative disorders, chronic granulocytic (CGL) and chronic lymphocytic (CLL) (see Chapter 3.7).

Chronic granulocytic leukaemia

CGL is also known as chronic myeloid leukaemia (CML), although the former term describes more closely the haematological features of the disease. CML may be used as a generic term for the whole group. CGL has a distinct chromosome marker, the Ph chromosome, resulting from the reciprocal translocation t(9;22), and cases which are Ph-negative often have the same molecular rearrangement. The diagnosis of CGL can be established by the morphological appearance of peripheral blood and bone marrow films, and is confirmed by cytogenetic and/or molecular analysis.

Atypical chronic myeloid leukaemia

Patients with high leucocyte counts who are Ph chromosome-negative form a heterogeneous group. Some have morphological features of CGL and the molecular rearrangement *BCR-ABL*, and should be considered together with the Ph-positive cases as CGL because of their treatment response and natural history. Another group has atypical morphological features by comparison with CGL and do not show *BCR-ABL* rearrangement. This subgroup should be regarded as a separate group and has a worse prognosis than classical CGL.

Chronic myelomonocytic leukaemia (CMML)

Cases of CMML with high leucocyte counts (e.g. 10–30 × 10^9/1) could be considered together with other forms of CML rather than with the myelodysplastic syndromes. The major feature is monocytosis, but there may also be moderate to high levels of serum and urinary lysozyme and myelodysplastic changes in the bone marrow.

Rare forms of chronic myeloid leukaemia

Other types of chronic myeloid leukaemia that occur infrequently are chronic neutrophilic, juvenile CMML, and chronic eosinophilic leukaemia.

Chronic neutrophilic leukaemia

This occurs in adults over 50 years of age, who have normal haemoglobin and platelet counts. The blood film shows predominantly neutrophils without immature forms.

Juvenile CMML

This comprises 2 per cent of childhood leukaemias. Patients are under 5 years of age and have systemic symptoms. In contrast to CGL, there is monocytosis without basophilia or eosinophilia. Characteristically, the levels of fetal haemoglobin are high.

Chronic eosinophilic leukaemia

It is difficult to distinguish this from the hypereosinophilic syndrome. In favour of the latter is the absence of chromosome abnormalities and immature forms, whilst their presence suggests eosinophilic leukaemia.

Chapter 3.4

Acute myeloblastic leukaemia

A. J. Barrett

Acute myeloid leukaemia (AML) affects adults and children but has an increased incidence with advancing age. Over 80 per cent of patients are over 60 years of age and there is a worldwide distribution. The prospects for cure of younger adults and children with AML are improving due to new treatment concepts derived from a better understanding of the disease process, intensive therapies such as bone marrow transplantation, and better supportive care. The cause of AML is unknown. Over 50 per cent of cases arise *de novo* but some appear secondary to an underlying problem (Table 1).

The proliferation of leukaemic blast cells leads to crowding of the bone marrow and results in bone marrow failure. Patients become anaemic, thrombocytopenic, and neutropenic. The leukaemia cells spill into the blood and spread to the spleen, liver, and to a lesser extent the lymph nodes and other organs (Fig. 1).

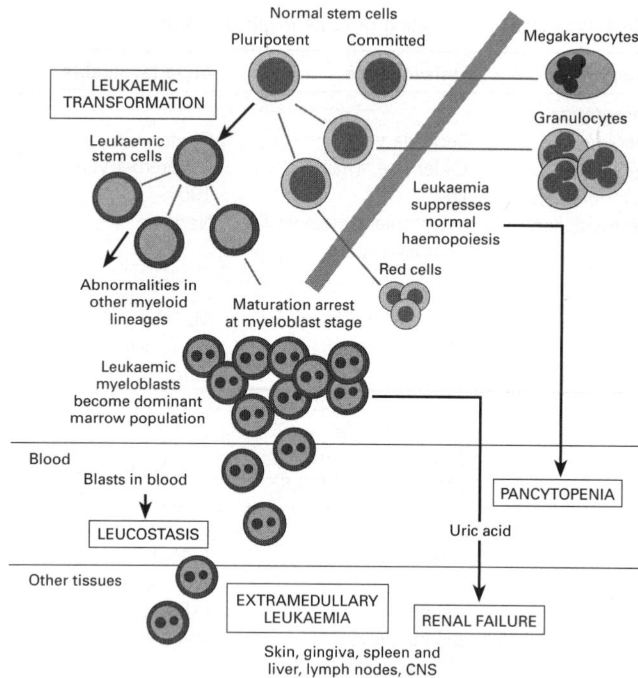

Fig. 1 Pathophysiology of acute myeloblastic leukaemia.

Presentation

In *de novo* AML the onset is typically abrupt, usually with a history of less than 6 weeks. The symptoms are often vague. Patients may complain of lassitude and headaches. Many of these symptoms are related to the development of anaemia. Sometimes they may notice an increased tendency to bleed. Nosebleeds, menorrhagia, gum bleeding, bruising, or a petechial rash may prompt the patient to visit their doctor. Presentation with infection is less common: patients may develop bacterial infection causing mouth ulcers and septic skin lesions especially in the perianal area. Sometimes the presence of extramedullary disease such as leukaemic skin deposits, gum hypertrophy, or neurological involvement may be the reason for presentation. The clinical signs of AML are often subtle. Careful observation may reveal the presence of a poorly healing injury, petechial haemorrhage, modest hepatosplenomegaly, and lymphadenopathy.

Table 1 Aetiology of acute myeloid leukaemia

Primary (de novo)	*Secondary (cont.)*
Cause unknown	Acquired marrow disorders:
Secondary	Myelodysplastic syndromes
Congenital disorders:	Chronic myeloid leukaemia
Fanconi anaemia	Other myeloproliferative disorders
Trisomy 21	(myelofibrosis, polycythaemia vera,
Chediak–Higashi disease	essential thrombocythaemia)
Wiskott–Aldrich	Severe aplastic anaemia
syndrome	
	Therapeutic agents:
	Fractionated radiotherapy
	Cytotoxics (alkylating agents,
	nitrosoureas, procarbazine, razoxane,
	others)
	Environmental factors:
	Accidental irradiation, nuclear
	weapons, benzene, toluene

Particular features are associated with certain AML subtypes. Acute promyelocytic leukaemia (AML M3) is associated with a consumption coagulopathy and may present with catastrophic haemorrhage. Gum hypertrophy and skin deposits are a feature of AML M4 and M5. These conditions, and an explanation of their classification are considered in Chapter 3.8.

Diagnosis

The diagnosis of AML can only be confirmed by examination of the blood and bone marrow.

The blood count is variable. There is usually a mild to moderate anaemia and the platelet count is usually low—below 100×10^9/l. Almost any leucocyte count may be encountered, from below 1×10^9/l to over 200×10^9/l. In most cases, examination of the blood film reveals the presence of blast cells. The hallmark of AML is the presence of Auer rods in the cytoplasm of blast cells. This feature is diagnostic of AML but occurs in less than 25 per cent of patients.

Examination of a bone marrow aspirate is essential. The marrow is usually hypercellular and crowded with blast cells, which usually constitute over 90 per cent of the cells in the aspirate. It is not always possible on morphological grounds alone to determine whether the leukaemia is of myeloid or lymphoid origin; cytochemical staining, immunophenotyping, and cytogenetic analysis are standard diagnostic tools.

Subclassification of AML

The first distinction is between primary (*de novo*) AML and secondary AML. Many patients developing secondary AML will already have been treated for defined myeloid disorders such as myeloproliferative diseases, myelodysplastic syndromes, or congenital disorders such as

Table 2 Prognostic classification of acute myeloid leukaemia

Category	Unfavourable	More favourable
Presentation		
Aetiology	Secondary	*De novo*
Age	Older age, infants	Children>1 year
Performance score	Low	100%
Extramedullary disease	Involvement of central nervous system	None
Morphological		
	M0 Undifferentiated M1 Undifferentiated myeloid M4 Myelomonocytic M5 Monocytic M6 Erythroleukaemia M7 Megakaryoblastic	M2 Myeloid with granulocytic differentiation M3 Promyelocytic
Karyotype		
	t (9;22) CML	t (15;17) promyelocytic
	del 5q)	t (8;21)
	del 7q) MDS	Inversion 16
	Chromosome breaks (Fanconi)	
	Deletion 11(q23)	

CML, chronic myeloid leukaemia; MDS, myelodysplastic syndrome.

Fanconi aplasia. In some instances, however, AML is the first indication of another underlying disorder.

The morphological classification is described in Chapter 3.3. Morphology quite accurately predicts the presence of the specific chromosome translocations: t(15;17) in acute promyelocytic leukaemia or abnormalities of chromosome 16 associated with M4 with eosinophilia. Together these have prognostic significance identifying favourable or less favourable outcomes with treatment (Table 2). It is essential to identify acute promyelocytic leukaemia (AML M3) because of the severe coagulopathy associated with this form of AML, and its specific responsiveness to all-*trans*-retinoic acid.

Management

Aims of treatment

The wide age range of presentation of AML and different prognoses associated with particular varieties demand different approaches to management. For example, the aim of treatment in a child or young adult newly presenting with AML is to achieve a cure of the leukaemia with as intensive a treatment programme as necessary. On the other hand, a palliative approach would be appropriate in an elderly patient presenting with a secondary AML. The patient's choice in selecting the treatment approach is of paramount importance. This implies the need for a frank discussion with the patient and relatives outlining the nature of the leukaemic process, its natural history, and an honest assessment of the likely outcome with the various treatment options. The first decision to make for a patient presenting for the first time with AML is whether or not to attempt to induce remission. No definite rules can be made, but there is a growing tendency to offer intensive treatments to older patients with AML. Once remission has been induced, further treatment is directed towards achieving a cure of the disease. Currently there is no consensus on the optimum postremission therapy.

Relapse of the leukaemia presents a fresh treatment dilemma. Sadly, as more patients die with AML than are cured, it is important to emphasize the continuing responsibility the haematologist has beyond the stage of active treatment.

Table 3 Supportive care for acute myeloblastic leukaemia

Monitoring
Daily or alternate daily: Blood count, electrolytes, liver function
Weekly: Bacteriological screen, chest radiograph
When indicated: Blood cultures, bone marrow aspirate
Anaemia
Transfusions of packed red cells to maintain haemoglobin above 10 g/dl
Haemorrhage
Transfusions of 3–12 donor units of platelets to maintain count above 10–20 × 10/l
Regular coagulation screens: replacement of coagulation factors with fresh frozen plasma, cryoprecipitate as required
Infection prevention
Protective isolation: single room, reverse-barrier isolation, clean food
Oral antibiotics: septrin/ciprofloxacin/colistin/neomycin
Oral antifungals: amphotericin/nystatin/fluconazole
Pulmonary aspergillosis: amphotericin aerosol
Herpes simplex labialis: oral acyclovir
Infection treatment
Fever regimen: initiated if temperature rises above 38°C
First line: aminoglycoside+broad-spectrum penicillin IV
Second line: (no response after 48 h, or deterioration) ceftazidime and vancomycin IV
Third line: (no response after 48 h, no organism isolated) amphotericin IV
Nutritional
Parenteral feeding if >10% loss of body weight
Intravenous analgesia for painful stomatitis
Psychological
Frank discussions, optimistic attitude, regular daily visits and progress updates, family support, early discharge as soon as haematological recovery permits

Supportive care (Table 3)

Proper care of the cytopenic patient is a prerequisite to giving treatment of sufficient intensity to achieve remission and cure of AML. Patients require almost constant venous access and installation of a semi-permanent, indwelling, right atrial catheter greatly facilitates their management.

Infections during the neutropenic period are derived from endogenous commensals, from bacteria and fungi present in the immediate environment, in food and drink, or acquired by direct human contact. Three approaches are employed to reduce the risk of infective death during treatment, as follows.

Prevention of autoinfection

Autoinfection is reduced by the administration of non-absorbable oral antibiotics. Alternatively, patients are given oral septrin, or ciprofloxacin. Candida infection can be prevented by using an antifungal agent.

Protective isolation

In the past this approach was taken to extremes but most AML treatment units now adopt a more relaxed approach to protective isolation, nursing the patient in a single room with restricted access to visitors and provision of 'clean' food.

Prompt treatment of suspected infection

The practice of taking blood for culture and giving intravenous antibiotics to patients with fever is the key to the successful management of neutropenia. A range of potent bactericidal broad-spectrum antibiotics is now available. Each hospital has its own particular treatment policy. In principle, first-line agents should cover Gram-positive and Gram-negative organisms including *Pseudomonas* spp. This can be achieved with a combination of an aminoglycoside with a broad-spectrum penicillin. Failure to obtain a response of the fever requires a change to second-line treatment with a different antibiotic combination (for example, vancomycin and ceftazidime). In patients not responding to antibacterial treatment an invasive fungal infection should be suspected and intravenous amphotericin should be commenced even in the absence of any localizing features of infection.

Lastly, the importance of the psychological support of the patient by the care team cannot be overemphasized. Step-by-step explanation of treatment details and regular progress reports are essential aspects of the management of patients with life-threatening disorders who have to remain in hospital for considerable periods during their treatment.

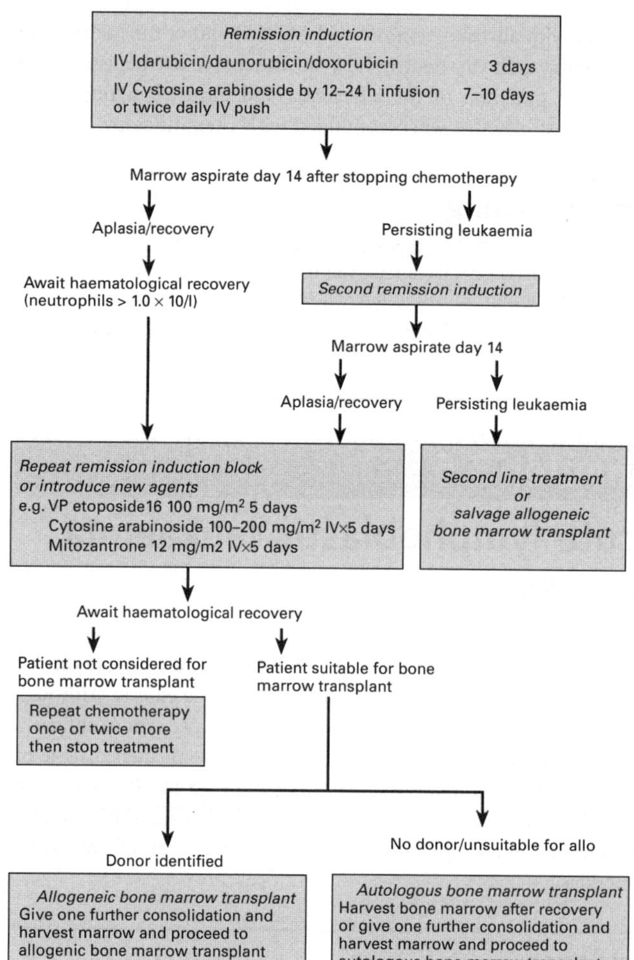

Fig. 2 Treatment response in acute myeloblastic leukaemia.

Remission induction (Fig. 2)

The goal of remission induction treatment is to give chemotherapy to reduce the leukaemic load to a point at which the bone marrow becomes temporarily aplastic. This permits the recovery of normal haemopoiesis. Most remission induction schedules employ the combination of cystosine arabinoside and an anthracycline administered in a treatment block of 7–10 days. Many schedules also include a third agent such as thioguanine or etoposide. In responding patients the blood count falls, blasts disappear from the blood, and the bone marrow becomes hypocellular. At 2 to 3 weeks a marrow aspirate is taken to assess progress. Complete remission is defined as the presence of a normal blood count, and a cellular marrow containing fewer than 5 per cent blasts.

Modern treatments achieve remission in up to 90 per cent of patients. However, there are clear prognostic differences in the likelihood of achieving remission. Increasing age is a major negative prognostic factor.

Postinduction treatment

The majority of patients achieving remission relapse unless further treatment is given. Generally, most patients receive one to four postremission treatment cycles. The strategy is to use different combinations of agents than those employed in remission induction in order to protect against relapse from drug-resistant cells. Agents such as mitozantrone, 5-azacytidine, etoposide, and cytosine arabinoside are used in combination in treatment blocks of 5 to 10 days, with intervals of about a month between courses to allow for haematological recovery.

Bone marrow transplantation (Fig. 2)

The place of stem-cell transplantation is still under evaluation. Although both autologous and allogeneic transplantation reduce the rate of leukaemia relapse, they carry a significant treatment-related mortality—in the region of 25 per cent for allografts up to 10 per cent for autografts. Their role is being studied in multi-centre trials.

Relapse rates for patients achieving remission vary widely according to the disease type. In general, *de novo* AML has a much greater chance of sustained remission than secondary AML. Younger patients and children especially have a lower chance of relapse. Recent series report disease-free survivals for children of over 50 per cent, but for adults this figure falls to around 25 per cent and decreases markedly in patients over the age of 65 years.

Treatment of acute promyelocytic leukaemia with all-*trans*-retinoic acid

The t(15;17) chromosome translocation specific for acute promyelocytic leukaemia (**APML**) is believed to cause an alteration in the signalling properties of the retinoic acid receptor–ligand complex.

Treatment with all-*trans*-retinoic acid (**ATRA**) allows the maturation of leukaemia cells to neutrophils, in the process exhausting the proliferative potential of the leukaemia and inducing a remission. ATRA is most effective when combined with chemotherapy.

Further reading

Bennett, J.M. *et al.* (1985). Proposed revised criteria for the classification of acute myeloid leukaemia: a report of the French–American–British cooperative group. *Annals of Internal Medicine*, **103**, 620–5.

Burnett, A.K. and Eden, O.B. (1997). The treatment of acute leukaemia. *Lancet*, 349, 270–5.

Chapter 3.5

Acute lymphoblastic leukaemia

I. A. G. Roberts

Acute lymphoblastic leukaemia (**ALL**) is a biologically diverse disease that can affect any age group from neonates to the elderly. Although modern therapeutic strategies can cure around 70 per cent of children, over 70 per cent of adults with ALL ultimately die of their disease or complications of its treatment. Approximately 30 to 40 per cent of paediatric cancers are acute leukaemias, of which around 80 per cent are ALL. In adults, ALL forms about 20 per cent of the acute leukaemias.

Incidence

Recent data from the United States show an age-adjusted incidence of ALL of around 1.0 to 1.3 cases per 100 000. This varies with age, sex and, possibly, race. There is a well-recognized peak at the age of 2 to 5 years, then a drop which holds steady until the age of 60 years when the rate begins to increase again; this hints at the existence of two distinct diseases with independent risk factors. ALL in children is approximately 30 per cent more common in boys overall; this effect is more marked in T-ALL in which the ratio of affected boys: girls is 4:1.

Aetiology

A number of risk factors for the development of ALL have been identified (Table 1). Some single-gene defects associated with an increased risk of ALL are fairly well characterized. Chromosomal disorders, which may involve several genes, such as Fanconi anaemia and Down's syndrome, are also important predisposing risk factors for the development of ALL, although acute myeloid leukaemia (**AML**) is much more common in the former than ALL. Familial cases of ALL are well described and there is an approximately fourfold risk that a sibling of a child with ALL will also develop the disease. In the vast majority of cases of ALL, however, an underlying hereditary cause cannot be identified. ALL results from a clonal expansion of immature lymphoblastic cells that are already committed to the B- or T-cell lineage. At the molecular level, several specific karyotypic abnormalities are associated with particular subtypes of ALL and appear to be of prognostic value.

Table 1 Risk factors for acute lymphoblastic leukaemia

Hereditary	*Environmental*
Single-gene diseases:	Radiation
Bloom's syndrome	Diagnostic radiographs
Ataxia telangiectasia	Radiotherapy
Schwachman's syndrome	Nuclear accidents/warfare
Achondroplasia	? Radiation from nuclear
Xeroderma pigmentosum	power installations
Primary immunodeficiency diseases,	Viruses
e.g. congenital X-linked	HTLV-1
agammaglobulinaemia	*Others**
Chromosomal disorders	Smoking
Fanconi anaemia	Electromagnetic fields
Down's syndrome	Pesticides
Other familial associations	Chloramphenicol
Siblings, especially twins	

*Causal association not proven.

Table 2 Clinical features of acute lymphoblastic leukaemia at presentation

Common signs and symptoms	*Unusual presentations*
Lethargy and irritability	Aplastic anaemia
Pallor	Eosinophilia
Fever	Isolated renal failure
Bone and joint pain	Pulmonary nodules
Bleeding, bruising, and petechiae	Pericardial effusion
Hepatosplenomegaly	Skin nodules
Lymphadenopathy: usually generalized and painless	
Central nervous disease (5% of children, 15% of adults)	
Mediastinal mass (especially in T-ALL)	

Clinical features

Presentation

Patients may present acutely or insidiously with symptoms present for several weeks or even months. Symptoms reflect the uncontrolled growth of leukaemic cells in bone marrow and extramedullary sites, particularly the lymphoid system. The most common presentations and some of the more unusual ones are shown in Table 2. The differential diagnosis may include immune thrombocytopenia, neuroblastoma, rheumatoid or other forms of acute arthritis, infectious mononucleosis and related viral infections, tuberculosis, aplastic anaemia, lymphoma, and myeloproliferative disorders, including chronic myeloid leukaemia.

Central nervous system disease is uncommon at presentation, but if prophylactic treatment is not given (see later) it has been shown to occur in the majority of patients. The presenting symptoms and signs are due to raised intracranial pressure and include headache, nausea, vomiting, lethargy, irritability, papilloedema, and nuchal rigidity. Occasional patients present with cranial nerve palsies, particularly of the IIIrd, IVth, VIth, or facial nerves. The diagnosis of central nervous disease is made by examination of the cerebrospinal fluid; the pressure, protein, and leucocyte count are usually elevated, with a normal or reduced glucose. Where ALL relapse presents in the CNS the peripheral blood count may be normal. However, relapse of ALL in the bone marrow is usually noted concurrently or within weeks.

Table 3 The FAB classification of acute lymphoblastic leukaemia

FAB class	Cytological appearance	Incidence (%)
L1	Small lymphoblasts with scanty cytoplasm	85
L2	Larger, more heterogeneous lymphoblasts with more cytoplasm	10–15
L3	Large lymphoblasts with deeply basophilic vacuolated, cytoplasm	1–3

Although hepatosplenomegaly is common, liver function tests are usually normal or only mildly deranged. In boys the testis is a fairly common site of relapse of ALL, occurring in 10 to 15 per cent. It presents as painless, usually unilateral, testicular enlargement. Testicular relapse may be isolated but is often followed by relapse in the bone marrow.

Diagnosis

In most cases the diagnosis is straightforward. The majority of patients are anaemic, neutropenic, and thrombocytopenic due to leukaemic infiltration of the bone marrow. The total leucocyte count is usually in the range of 5000 to 25 000 × 10^9/l. However, leucocyte counts of in excess of 100 000 × 10^9/l and under 5000 × 10^9/l are not uncommon. All patients should have a bone marrow aspirate and trephine biopsy. This is essential to confirm the diagnosis of ALL, in particular distinguishing it from AML which is treated in an entirely different way, and allows an accurate diagnosis of the subtype of ALL to be made. This is based on the morphology of the leukaemic cells assessed by standard and special cytochemical stains, their immunophenotype, and their karyotype. The diagnosis may be particularly difficult in patients who present with pancytopenia: in such patients it may be necessary to repeat the bone marrow aspirate and biopsy after a few weeks.

Classification of the subtypes of ALL

Morphology

The leukaemic blast cells in ALL can be quite heterogeneous in their appearance under the light microscope. As for AML, the French–American–British (**FAB**) Co-operative Working Group devised a classification scheme based on particular morphological characteristics. The FAB classification of ALL (Table 3) is widely used and appears to have some prognostic value, although, with the exception of L3, it does not correlate with the immunophenotype or karyotype of the ALL cells.

Immunophenotyping

Most haematology laboratories now use a panel of monoclonal antibodies that allow ALL cells to be classified into five main groups: **B cell;** early B, common, pre-B, and mature B; and **T cell.** Useful monoclonal antibodies for identifying T cells are CD7, CD2, and CD3; antibodies for B cells include CD19 and CD22; in most cases of ALL the leukaemic cells are also positive with CD10, which is known as the **CALLA** or common ALL antigen.

Cytogenetics

Karyotypic abnormalities can be identified in leukaemic blast cells from around 80 per cent of patients with ALL. These abnormalities are either numerical, that is chromosome loss (hypodiploidy) or gain (hyperdiploidy), or structural, usually translocations. Many of the structural karyotypic abnormalities can be related to specific immunophenotypes—t(8;14) with B-ALL, t(1;19) with pre-B ALL and t(1;7) with T-ALL for example. Both types of abnormalities have prognostic significance. The best prognosis is associated with hyperdiploidy with a modal number of chromosomes in excess of 50.

Management

Long-term survival in childhood ALL currently approaches 70 per cent and efforts are now directed towards minimizing the long-term side-effects of chemoradiotherapy by not overtreating children with a low probability of relapsing. In adults, however, long-term disease-free survival is 30 per cent at best and attempts to intensify treatment are continuing.

Current concepts of treatment

There are four main components to our current approach to treating ALL in any age group:

(1) remission induction;

(2) intensification chemotherapy;

(3) prophylaxis of central nervous system involvement;

(4) maintenance treatment.

During all these phases of treatment the importance of good supportive care cannot be overemphasized.

Remission induction

The most useful drugs for achieving remission have been shown to be oral prednisolone, intravenous vincristine, and intramuscular or subcutaneous L-asparaginase. These three drugs given in combination over 3 to 4 weeks are sufficient to induce complete remission in more than 95 per cent of children and around 80 per cent of adults.

Intensification chemotherapy

This aims to further reduce minimal residual leukaemia. The nature of the intensification used has been varied in different studies in order to try and target the patients at highest risk of relapse. The addition of drugs such as cytosine arabinoside and daunorubicin at this stage of treatment has been successful in improving survival.

Prophylaxis in the central nervous system

Current treatment schedules are based on risk factors and use either intrathecal or intravenous methotrexate and/or cranial irradiation.

Maintenance treatment

The addition of 2 to 3 years of maintenance treatment has been shown to be of definite value in ALL. The drugs used are continuous oral 6-mercaptopurine and weekly methotrexate together with monthly vincristine and prednisolone. During maintenance treatment all patients should be treated with continuous, low-dose co-trimoxazole to prevent infection with *Pneumocystis carinii.*

Treatment of central nervous leukaemia

A small proportion of patients present with disease in the central nervous system. This is treated by intrathecal chemotherapy, craniospinal irradiation, and systemic chemotherapy as for marrow disease, including intensification and maintenance therapy. Some 10 per cent of patients without evidence of central nervous disease at diagnosis will experience a central nervous relapse despite appropriate prophylaxis. The choice of treatment is difficult, particularly for those who have previously received cranial irradiation, as the toxicity of further irradiation may be considerable. Nevertheless, reinduction with systemic chemotherapy and intrathecal therapy is successful in a proportion of patients and long-term cure is still possible.

Treatment of relapsed ALL

The most common site of relapse of ALL, in patients who have received central nervous prophylaxis, is the bone marrow. In most children and in 50 to 60 per cent of adults a second remission can be induced. The treatment for relapsed ALL usually consists of the same chemotherapy as employed to induce remission at the initial presentation, although in patients with early relapse alternative agents, such as high-dose cytosine arabinoside or methotrexate, may be used. Following this, most centres now offer allogeneic bone marrow transplantation. Overall, the role of marrow transplantation in ALL is still controversial.

Late effects of treatment for ALL

The increasing number of patients surviving long-term after treatment for ALL, particularly childhood ALL, has highlighted the importance of lifelong follow-up of such patients to assess the late effects of high-dose chemoradiotherapy. The most common late effects are those due to structural damage in the central nervous system, endocrine abnormalities, and second malignancies. Cognitive defects appear to be mild but common and include reduction in Intelligence Quotient, impaired memory, and difficulty with mathematical problems and concentration. The most common endocrine abnormality is growth hormone deficiency, but this is rarely a clinical problem. Primary hypothyroidism occurs in around 3 per cent of children. There are now many examples of successful parenthood after treatment for ALL in childhood and no excess of malignancies or congenital abnormalities have been reported in the offspring. Second malignancies occur in around 8 per cent of long-term survivors, the most common being intracranial tumours and haematological malignancies, including AML and non-Hodgkin's lymphomas.

Prognosis

Prognostic factors and risk groups

Currently, those factors that appear to be useful prognostically fall into two categories: pretreatment variables (for example, age) and treatment-dependent variables.

The important pretreatment variables are age, the leucocyte count at diagnosis, the immunophenotype, and the karyotype of the ALL cells. For age, the poorest prognosis is in infants and in patients over 60 years. It is clear that patients who present with a leucocyte count in excess of 100 000 × 109/l fare worst. T- and B-ALL phenotype and certain karyotypes, for instance t(8;14) and t(9;22), also have a poor prognosis.

The important treatment-dependent variables are the initial response to a single cytostatic drug and the time taken to achieve complete remission. Patients with a good initial response and a short time to remission are twice as likely to achieve long-term disease-free survival.

The prognostic information from all these studies has been used by several groups to stratify patients into different risk groups and should result in more rational therapy for all patients with ALL. In addition, the application of molecular techniques to the detection of minimal residual disease or early relapse may yield data critical for tailoring therapy to individual patients.

Survival

In childhood, 60 to 70 per cent of patients can now be cured using chemotherapy and central nervous prophylaxis. For those that relapse, allogeneic bone-marrow transplantation will cure around 25 to 35 per cent, chemotherapy possibly rather fewer. In adulthood, long-term disease-free survival with chemotherapy alone varies from 5 per cent in high-risk ALL to around 50 per cent in low-risk disease. Novel therapeutic strategies, perhaps based on the exciting new information becoming available from studying the molecular and biological basis of ALL, are an important goal for the future.

Further reading

Burnett, A.K. and Eden, O.B. (1997). The treatment of acute leukaemia. *Lancet*, **349**, 270–5.

Chessells, J.M. (1998). Relapsed acute lymphoblastic leukaemia in children: a continuing challenge. *British Journal of Haematology*, **102**, 423–38.

Greaves, M.F. (1997). The aetiology of acute leukaemia. *Lancet*, **349**, 344–9.

Roberts, W.M., Estror, Z., Ouspenskaia, M.V., Johnston, D.A., McClain, K.L., Zipf, T.F. (1997). Measurement of residual leukaemia during remission in childhood acute lymphoblastic leukaemia. *New England Journal of Medicine*, **336**, 317–23.

Weisforf, D.J., Woods, W.G., Nesbit, M.E., *et al.* (1994). Allogeneic bone marrow transplantation for acute lymphoblastic leukaemia: risk factors and clinical outcome. *British Journal of Haematology*, **86**, 62–9.

Chapter 3.6

Chronic myeloid leukaemia

J. Goldman

Chronic myeloid leukaemia is a clonal disease of the pluripotential haemopoietic stem cell, whose progeny proliferates and eventually usurps all normal marrow function. One landmark in our understanding of the pathogenesis of chronic myeloid leukaemia was the discovery of the Philadelphia (**Ph**) chromosome in 1960; another was the characterization of the *BCR-ABL* chimeric gene. Until the 1980s, chronic myeloid leukaemia was assumed to be incurable but it has become apparent in the last 10 years that it can be cured by bone marrow transplantation. Unfortunately the proportion of patients eligible for this is still relatively small.

Natural history

Most patients have a relatively homogeneous disease characterized by the presence of a Ph chromosome in marrow metaphases. There are several rare variants in which the *BCR-ABL* chimeric gene is absent (see Chapter 3.3).

The incidence of chronic myeloid leukaemia appears to be constant worldwide and occurs in about 1 per 100 000 of the population. Chronic myeloid leukaemia is rare below the age of 20 years but occurs in all decades, with a median age of onset of 40 to 50 years. The risk of developing the disease is slightly but significantly increased by exposure to high doses of irradiation but, in general, all cases are 'sporadic' and no predisposing factors are identifiable.

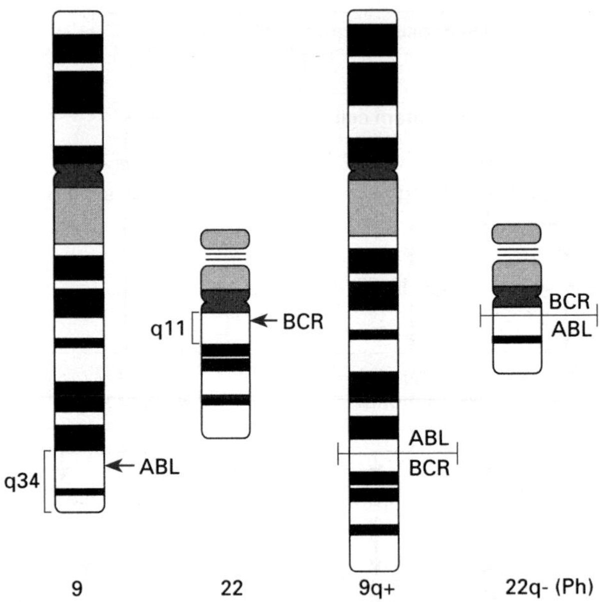

Fig. 1 A schematic representation of the Philadelphia chromosome showing the mechanism of formation of the chimeric *BCR-ABL* gene. Note that the positions of the normal ABL and BCR genes on chromosomes 9q34 and 22q11, respectively, are shown to the left; to the right are the Ph (22q–) chromosome bearing the *BCR-ABL* fusion gene and the 9q+ (which bears the reciprocal chimeric gene designated *ABL-BCR*).

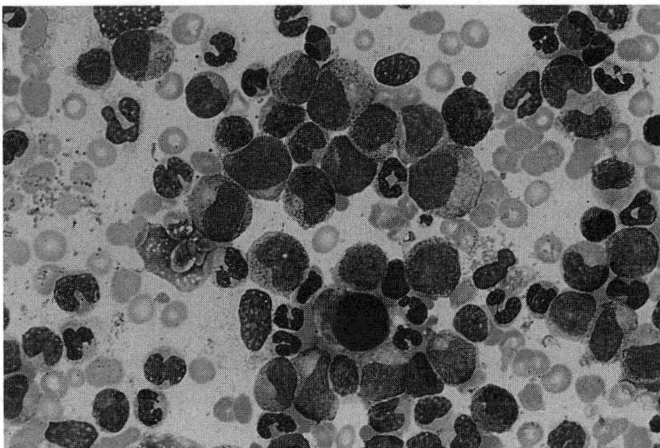

Fig. 2 Peripheral-blood appearances of a patient with chronic myeloid leukaemia at diagnosis. Note increased numbers of leucocytes including immature granulocytes and occasional blast cells.

Chronic myeloid leukaemia is a biphasic or triphasic disease that is usually diagnosed in the initial 'chronic' or stable phase. The chronic phase typically lasts for 2 to 6 years, but it may on occasion last more than 10 or even 15 years. Unpredictably it transforms to a more aggressive phase, described as acute or blastic transformation. In the majority of cases the diseases evolves somewhat more gradually through an intermediate phase described as 'accelerated' disease, which may last for months or occasionally years, before frank transformation. The duration of survival after the onset of transformation is usually 2 to 6 months so the median survival from diagnosis is 4 to 5 years.

Cytogenetics and molecular biology

The Ph chromosome is an acquired cytogenetic abnormality that characterizes all leukaemic cells in chronic myeloid leukaemia. The Ph chromosome is formed as a result of a reciprocal translocation of genetic material between the long arms of one number 22 chromosome and one number 9 chromosome, an event described as t(9;22)(q34; q11) (Fig. 1). In patients with chronic myeloid leukaemia the Ph chromosome is present in all myeloid cell lineages, in some B cells, and in a very small proportion of T cells. The translocation results in juxtaposition of 5′ sequences from the *BCR* gene with 3′ *ABL* sequences derived from chromosome 9. Thus the Ph chromosome carries a chimeric gene, designated *BCR-ABL* (Fig. 1), that encodes a protein of 210 kDa and has tyrosine kinase activity.

Clinical features

Approximately half of patients present with symptoms and the rest as a result of 'routine' blood tests. Symptoms include lethargy, loss of energy, shortness of breath on exertion, or weight loss. Increased sweating is characteristic. Spontaneous bruising or unexplained bleeding from the gums and/or the intestinal or urinary tract are relatively common. Visual disturbances may occur. The patient may have pain or discomfort in the splenic area or may have noticed a lump or mass in the right upper abdomen.

Between 60 and 80 per cent of patients have splenomegaly at diagnosis. The spleen varies from just palpable to being so large that it occupies all the left side of the abdomen. The liver is frequently also enlarged. Patients with very high leucocyte counts may have features of leucostasis with retinal-vein engorgement and pulmonary insufficiency.

In established transformation the spleen is frequently enlarged and may be painful. The liver may become very large. Patients may develop fever, lymphadenopathy, or, very rarely, lytic lesions of bone.

Haematology

Patients with splenomegaly are usually anaemic, while the haemoglobin concentration may be normal in those with 'early' disease. The leucocyte count at diagnosis is usually between 50 and 200×10^9/l. The film shows a full spectrum of cells in the granulocyte series, ranging from blast forms to mature polymorphs (Fig. 2). Blast cell percentages higher than 12 suggest that the patient is already in acceleration or transformation. The percentage of eosinophils and basophils is increased. Platelet numbers are usually increased in the range 300 to 600×10^9/l. The alkaline phosphatase content of the neutrophil cytoplasm is characteristically diminished or absent.

The bone marrow is usually examined to assess the degree of marrow fibrosis, to make cytogenetic analyses, and to exclude transformation. The marrow aspirate shows hypercellular fragments and chronic-phase blast cells number 2 to 10 per cent. The marrow biopsy shows dense hypercellularity and the reticulin content may be normal or modestly increased.

The haematological picture in acceleration may show anaemia and either greatly increased or reduced platelet numbers in a manner not accounted for by treatment.

Blastic transformation is defined by the presence of more than 30 per cent blasts or blasts plus promyelocytes in the blood or marrow. Cytochemical stains and immunophenotyping reveal a myeloid transformation in 70 per cent of patients, lymphoid blast cells in 20 per cent of patients, the remaining10 per cent having mixed myeloid and lymphoid characteristics.

Biochemical changes are non-specific. Patients diagnosed in chronic phase may have a slightly raised serum uric acid or serum alkaline phosphatase. The lactic dehydogenase level is usually raised. In transformation the serum uric acid may be raised, sometimes substantially, and tests of liver function are usually moderately abnormal.

Management

Chronic phase

There is no immediate urgency to start treatment in asymptomatic patients with leucocyte counts below 100×10^9/l. Most patients will, however, prefer to be treated once the diagnosis is confirmed. If the possibility of treatment by bone marrow transplantation is excluded or uncertain, treatment should be initiated with hydroxyurea or interferon-α. Hydroxyurea is usually started with 1.0 to 2.0 g daily by mouth and continued indefinitely. The leucocyte count starts to fall within days and the spleen gets smaller. It is usually possible to reverse all features of chronic myeloid leukaemia within 4 to 8 weeks of starting treatment. The dosage can then be titrated against the leucocyte count, the usual maintenance dose being between 1.0 and 1.5 g daily. The drug has relatively few side-effects. Busulphan was formerly used to treat all new patients but is now infrequently used. However, the drug is useful in older patients whose compliance is uncertain.

Interferon-α is a member of a large family of glycoproteins of biological origin with antiviral and antiproliferative properties. Treatment with interferon-α probably prolongs survival by perhaps 1 or 2 years in the majority of patients. It seems reasonable to offer interferon-α to all newly diagnosed patients who are not candidates for allogeneic bone marrow transplantation and to continue treatment for as long as the drug is tolerated. Interferon-α must be administered by subcutaneous injection and is not without side-effects. Almost all patients experience fevers, shivers, muscle aches, and general influenza-like features on starting the drug; these last 1 to 2 weeks but may be alleviated by paracetamol. They recur when the dosage is increased. A significant minority of patients cannot tolerate the drug because of lethargy, malaise, anorexia, weight loss, depression and other affective disorders, or alopecia.

Younger patients with HLA-identical sibling donors should be offered the opportunity of treatment by allogeneic bone marrow transplantation. Most specialist centres exclude from consideration patients over the age of 50 or 55 years. In general, patients are 'conditioned' for transplant with cyclophosphamide followed by total-body irradiation or with the combination of busulphan and cyclophosphamide. Bone marrow collected from the donor is infused intravenously on day 0. If all goes well, reasonable marrow function is achieved in 3 to 4 weeks and the patient leaves the hospital. For patients with chronic myeloid leukaemia treated by transplantation with marrow from HLA-identical siblings, the overall leukaemia-free survival at 5 years is now 60 to 70 per cent. There is a 20 per cent chance of transplant-related death and a 15 per cent chance of relapse. The use of 'donor leucocytes' obtained from the transplant donor and infused into the patient has proven of great value in curing patients with leukaemic relapse. For this reason patients surviving without haematological evidence of disease can be monitored by the polymerase chain reaction which can detect very low numbers of *BCR-ABL* transcripts in the blood or marrow. Such assays can be predictive of relapse and may therefore direct the early use of donor leucocyte infusions.

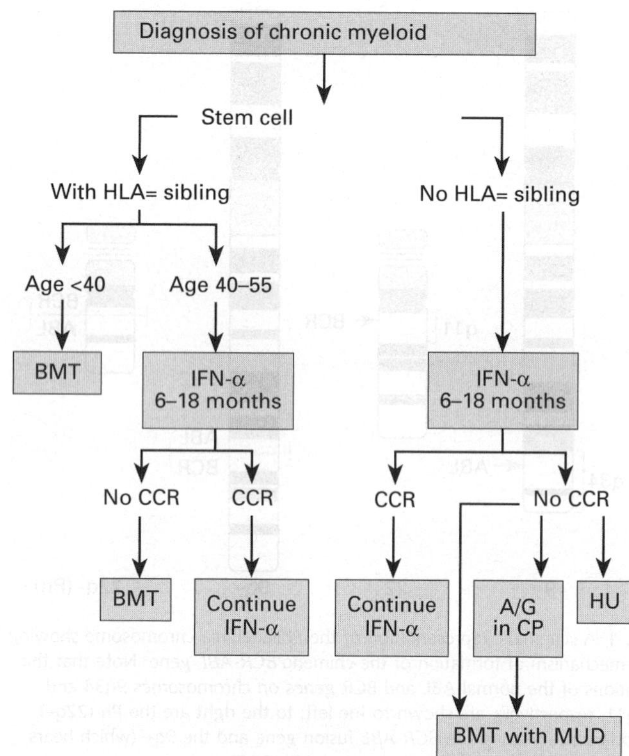

Fig. 3 An algorithm showing a possible approach to the management of a newly diagnosed patient aged 55 years or less. Blood- or marrow-derived stem cells can be cryopreserved at diagnosis. Patients with HLA-identical siblings may be allografted or treated first with interferon-α (**IFN-a**). In the latter case, those who achieve continuing cytogenetic responses (**CCR**) may have their bone marrow transplant (**BMT**) delayed. Patients without HLA-identical siblings may be treated initially with IFN-α. Non-responders may be treated with hydroxyurea (**HU**), by autografting (**A/G**) in chronic phase (**CP**), or by transplant with a 'matched' unrelated donor (**MUD**).

This qualified success with bone marrow transplants from matched siblings has led to the increasing use of 'matched' unrelated donors for transplantation in patients with chronic myeloid leukaemia, although the results are less good than with sibling transplants.

Autologous bone marrow transplantation with stem cells collected during recovery from high-dose chemotherapy are currently being evaluated in clinical trials. An integrated approach to the management of the 'younger' patient with chronic myeloid leukaemia is shown in Fig. 3.

Advanced-phase disease

Patients in blastic transformation may be treated with combinations of cytotoxic drugs in the hope of prolonging life, but cure can no longer be a realistic objective. Patients in lymphoid transformation may be treated with a little more optimism than those with a myeloid transformation, and are frequently returned to a second chronic phase. Allogeneic bone marrow transplantation from HLA-matched sibling donors can be done in the accelerated phase and blast transformation, but the results are currently poor.

Further reading

Goldman, J.M. (1994). Management of chronic myeloid leukaemia. *Blood Reviews*, **8**, 21–9.

Gratwohl, A., *et al.* (1998). Risk assessment for patients with chronic myeloid leukaemia before allogeneic blood or marrow transplantation. *Lancet*, 352, 1087–92.

Sawyers, C.L. (1999). Chronic myeloid leukemia. *New England Journal of Medicine*, 340, 1330–40.

The Italian Cooperative Study Group on Chronic Myeloid Leukemia (1994). Interferon alfa-2a as compared with conventional chemotherapy for the treatment of chronic myeloid leukemia. *New England Journal of Medicine*, 330, 820–5.

Chapter 3.7

Chronic lymphocytic leukaemia and other leukaemias of mature B and T cells

D. Catovsky

The principal methods used for diagnosis and classification of the chronic lymphoid leukaemias include peripheral blood and bone marrow films, bone marrow trephine biopsies, immunophenotyping, and histological evaluation of involved organs. Physical examination should include palpation of lymph nodes, liver, and spleen, and details noted of any skin infiltration. Results of cytogenetic and DNA analysis help to elucidate pathogenesis and may acquire a role in disease classification in the near future.

There are two broad disease categories to be considered: primary lymphoid leukaemias and leukaemia/lymphoma syndromes. Both can be subdivided, according to their cell derivation, into B- and T-cell types (Tables 1 and 2).

Chronic lymphocytic leukaemia

This is the most common form of lymphocytic leukaemia, accounting for 70 per cent of cases. In Western countries, chronic lymphocytic leukaemia (**CLL**) accounts for 25 per cent of all cases of leukaemia. It is less common in the Far East, comprising 2 per cent of cases.

Table 1 Primary lymphoid leukaemias

B-cell type	*T-cell type*
Chronic lymphocytic leukaemia (CLL)	Large granular lymphocyte leukaemia
Prolymphocytic leukaemia (B-PLL)	Prolymphocytic leukaemia (T-PLL)
Hairy-cell leukaemia (HCL)	Sezary-cell leukaemia
HCL variant	

Table 2 Leukaemia/lymphoma syndromes*

B-cell type	*T-cell type*
Follicular lymphoma	Adult T-cell leukaemia/lymphoma (ATLL)
Mantle-cell lymphoma	
Splenic lymphoma with circulating villous lymphocytes (SLVL)	Sezary syndrome
	Peripheral T-cell lymphoma
Lymphoplasmacytic lymphoma	Large-cell lymphoma (T)
Large-cell lymphoma (B)	

*Primary non-Hodgkin's lymphoma evolving with leukaemia.

Chronic lymphocytic leukaemia generally affects people over the age of 50 years and has a male to female ratio of 1.8:1.

Diagnostic criteria include a lymphocytosis of greater than 10×10^9/l and more than 30 per cent lymphocytes in bone marrow aspirates. The lymphocytes in chronic lymphocytic leukaemia have a distinct morphology: small size, round nucleus, clumped nuclear chromatin, and scanty cytoplasm; smear cells are common. A minority of cells are larger, with a prominent nucleolus, and have been designated prolymphocytes. Cases with more than 10 per cent prolymphocytes have been designated **CLL/PL,** PL standing for prolymphocytes.

Clinical features

Almost one-third of patients are diagnosed by chance, with lymphocytosis and no specific symptoms or physical signs. Others present with lymphadenopathy or symptoms of anaemia. The lymphadenopathy is usually symmetrical and of moderate size, involving the neck, axillae, and inguinal regions. Other nodal areas involved can be ascertained by chest radiographs and abdominal computed tomographic (**CT**) scan. Splenomegaly of variable size is found in 50 per cent of cases; hepatomegaly is less common.

Systemic symptoms such as weight loss or night sweating are not common but, when present, correlate with bulky abdominal disease. Fever usually indicates infection or transformation.

Membrane markers

The immunophenotype of chronic lymphocytic leukaemia is unique within the B-cell disorders: CD5 and CD23 positive, FMC7 negative, CD79b negative, and weak or negative CD22. These five markers and the weak SmIg expression represent the typical phenotype of chronic lymphocytic leukaemia.

In early chronic lymphocytic leukaemia the bone marrow shows minimal interstitial or nodular involvement, but with disease progression the normal, bone marrow fat spaces are replaced by lymphocytes. There is a mixed interstitial and nodular pattern, and in advanced disease the involvement is diffuse or 'packed'.

Staging

The course of CLL is very variable. Some patients may never require treatment and others have a progressive course with short survival. An important advance in management was the development of two staging systems (Rai and Binet) that can predict prognosis. Both systems use simple information: blood counts and physical signs, namely lymphadenopathy and hepatosplenomegaly.

In the Binet system stages A and B have no anaemia (Hb >10 g/dl) or thrombocytopenia (platelets $>100 \times 10^9$/l), and have a different degree of organ enlargement. Stage A patients have either no palpable nodes (including liver and spleen as nodal areas) or have one or two involved areas. Stage B patients have three, four, or all five involved nodal areas, which include nodes in cervical, axillary, and inguinal regions, spleen, and liver. Stage C patients have anaemia (Hb <10 g/dl) and/or thrombocytopenia (platelets $<100 \times 10^9$/l), and correspond to stages III and IV of the Rai system. The relative distribution of stages at presentation is: stage A, 45 to 50 per cent; stage B, 25 to 30 per cent; stage C, 20 to 25 per cent.

Complications

Infections, particularly of the upper respiratory tract, are the chief cause of morbidity in chronic lymphocytic leukaemia. Pneumonia is the main cause of death in 30 per cent of cases, usually in patients with advanced disease. The main predisposing factor for the infections is hypogammaglobulinaemia.

Autoimmune phenomena, chiefly haemolytic anaemia with a positive direct antiglobulin test due to warm autoantibodies, are a feature in 5 per cent of cases. The proportion of cases with a positive Coombs' test is higher than the number with frank haemolysis. Not infrequently, the haemolytic anaemia is precipitated by the initiation of therapy with alkylating agents or fludarabine in advanced CLL. Immune thrombocytopenia is seen in 2 per cent of cases.

Other malignancies are not uncommon in chronic lymphocytic leukaemia and it is unclear whether this relatively high incidence reflects age or a greater predisposition due to the disease itself or its associated immunodeficiency.

The most consistent chromosome abnormalities in chronic lymphocytic leukaemia are trisomy of chromosome 12 and deletions of the long arm of chromosome 13 (13q14).

Prognostic factors

The main prognostic factors in CLL are stage followed by age, sex, and response to therapy. The median survival of stage A patients is over 10 years, of stage B 6 years, and stage C 4 years. The lymphocyte doubling time and the degree of bone marrow infiltration are also independent prognostic variables

Treatment

Because of the variable outlook it is important to consider treatment for those with early and stable disease separately from patients with progressive, symptomatic, and/or advanced disease. For this purpose, staging is the first criterion to take into account.

The majority of stage A patients have no symptoms and may be observed for a while to determine whether the disease has a stable pattern, before deciding whether treatment is necessary.

Treatment is indicated for patients with stages B and C or stage A with clear evidence of disease progression. Disease progression is defined as a downward trend in haemoglobin or platelets, rising lymphocyte counts (doubling times less than 1 year), development of lymphadenopathy, and systemic symptoms.

Traditionally the first line of treatment has been with oral alkylating agents, particularly chlorambucil. This may be used at low dose daily for several weeks or as 'pulses' of higher dose therapy. However, a new generation of drugs, the nucleoside analogues (Table 3), are proving of great value in the treatment of chronic lymphocytic leukaemia and other low-grade lymphoid malignancies. The two with the greatest activity in chronic lymphocytic leukaemia are fludarabine and 2-chlorodeoxyadenosine. Trials are currently addressing the question of whether or not fludarabine should be used as the first-line treatment in CLL, but the drug appears to be the agent of choice for second-line therapy. So far there is no evidence that it provides any survival advantage when compared with chlorambucil, but durations of remissions are longer. Fludarabine can potentiate the effect of cyclophosphamide when used in combination because it inhibits DNA repair.

Splenectomy

The indications for splenectomy are therapy-resistant disease with significant residual splenomegaly, hypersplenism, and drug-resistant autoimmune complications. Because of the poor humoral immunity in chronic lymphocytic leukaemia the prophylaxis after splenectomy should rely mainly on long-term oral penicillin and less on antipneumococcal vaccines.

Table 3 Treatments used in chronic lymphocytic leukaemia

Alkylating agents
- Chlorambucil intermittently (10 mg/m²/day×6 days, monthly)
- Chlorambucil continuously (4–5 mg/day)

Combinations
- COP: cyclophosphamide, oncovin, prednisolone (5-day monthly courses)
- Chlorambucil plus epirubicin (chlorambucil intermittently as above; epirubicin: 50 mg/m² IV day 1; both monthly)
- CHOP: COP plus doxorubicin (doxorubicin 50 mg/m² IV day 1) monthly

Splenic irradiation
- (1 Gy once or twice/week to 10 Gy)

Corticosteroids
- Prednisolone 30 mg/m² for 3 weeks plus 1 week tailing off for stage C patients before other drugs. High dose methyl prednisolone IV, 1 g/m² (5-day monthly courses)

Nucleoside analogues
- Fludarabine IV push 25 mg/m² daily (5-day monthly courses)
- Fludarabine (as above) plus cyclophosphamide IV, 250 mg/m², both for 3 days
- 2'-Deoxycoformycin IV push 4 mg/m² (once a week or every 2 weeks)
- 2-Chlorodeoxyadenosine IV infusion (0.1 mg/kg per day × 7 days every 4–5 weeks)

Supportive care

This includes long-term antibiotic prophylaxis and/or their availability for use as soon as signs or symptoms of infections appear, and intravenous immunoglobulin replacement therapy to prevent serious bacterial infections in selected patients. Other measures include blood transfusions and vitamin supplements to correct deficiencies.

Transformation

There are two well-known forms of transformation in chronic lymphocytic leukaemia: a subtle one with an increased proportion of prolymphocytes, seen in some patients from presentation and known as CLL/PL, and a more dramatic change to a high-grade non-Hodgkin's lymphoma with diffuse large-cell/immunoblastic histology, known as Richter's syndrome. CLL/PL is seen in 10 per cent of patients, and is associated with trisomy of chromosome 12 and p53 deletions in 50 per cent of cases. Richter's syndrome is seen in at least 5 per cent.

The large-cell transformation may be localized or generalized and the classical Richter's syndrome is associated with deteriorating clinical status and systemic symptoms such as fever, weight loss, and sweating. The prognosis is poor, with a median survival of less than 6 months. Alkylating agents are not effective and probably nor is fludarabine. Combinations of the type used in high-grade, non-Hodgkin's lymphoma (for example, CHOP; Table 3) may induce remissions.

Patients with CLL/PL have progressive disease that may respond to first-line therapy as for chronic lymphocytic leukaemia, but the

Table 4 Membrane phenotype in leukaemias of mature B cells

Marker	CLL	B-PLL	HCL	NHL[1]
SmIg	Weak	Strong	Strong	Strong
CD22	Weak	Strong	Strong	Strong
CD5	+	+/−	−	−/+
CD23	+	−	−	−/+
FMC7	−	+	+	+
CD79b	−	+	+	+

[1] Non-Hodgkin's lymphoma (follicular, mantle-cell lymphoma, and SLVL); all other abbreviations as in Tables 1 and 2.

overall response rate is close to half that of patients with typical chronic lymphocytic leukaemia. Fludarabine may be effective too, but in a lower percentage of cases.

B-cell prolymphocytic leukaemia

The main features are splenomegaly without peripheral lymphadenopathy, anaemia, thrombocytopenia, and a high white-cell count, usually over 100×10^9/l. The diagnosis is made by examination of peripheral blood films in which the predominant cells are prolymphocytes. Small lymphocytes, as in chronic lymphocytic leukaemia, are rarely seen.

The immunophenotype of B-cell prolymphocytic leukaemia (Table 4) is different from that of chronic lymphocytic leukaemia and the differential diagnosis should be with CLL/PL, mantle-cell non-Hodgkin's lymphoma, and the hairy-cell leukaemia variant. In contrast to CLL, the evolution of B-cell prolymphocytic leukaemia is always progressive, with a median survival of 3 years. Several forms of treatment have been used in the past with moderate success: splenic irradiation, combination chemotherapy, and splenectomy. Fludarabine and 2-chlorodeoxyadenosine (CdA) have been shown to induce remission in 50 per cent of patients.

Hairy-cell leukaemia

Hairy-cell leukaemia is characterized by cytopenia and splenomegaly in two-thirds of cases; monocytopenia is a consistent finding. Most patients have circulating hairy cells but leucocyte counts rarely exceed 10×10^9/l. Hairy cells are larger than lymphocytes, their nucleus has a homogeneous, loose chromatin pattern without a visible nucleolus (except in the hairy-cell leukaemia variant), and they have an abundant cytoplasm with broad-based projections or villi. The nuclear outline is often kidney-shaped. The bone marrow trephine biopsy shows a unique pattern of infiltration with characteristic clear zones in between the cells. Bone marrow aspirates are, as a rule, unsuccessful.

The immunophenotype is different from CLL but similar to other B-cell disorders. Four other monoclonal antibodies have shown specificity for hairy cells, CD103, CD11c, CD25, and HC2, and are positive in most cases. Two of these, CD25 and HC2, are negative in the hairy-cell leukaemia variant. A well-known cytochemical property of hairy cells is the presence of tartaric acid-resistant acid phosphatase, which is still useful for diagnostic purposes.

Treatment and prognosis

The prognosis of patients with hairy-cell leukaemia has improved dramatically with the advent of three forms of treatment: interferon-α, 2′-deoxycoformycin (**DCF**), and 2-chlorodeoxyadenosine (**CdA**). Splenectomy, which was the mainstay of treatment in the past, is now reserved for patients presenting with very large spleens that are disproportionate to the degree of bone marrow involvement. Interferon-α improves the blood counts and the bone marrow but rarely induces prolonged complete remissions; treatment always needs to continue to maintain a response. CdA and DCF induce complete remissions in over 75 per cent of patients with few (3 per cent) non-responders. Once treatment is discontinued the majority of complete responders remain in remission for more than 5 years.

B-cell lymphomas in leukaemic phase

Several types of low- or intermediate-grade non-Hodgkin's lymphomas of B-cell type present or evolve with a leukaemic blood picture of more than 5×10^9/l circulating lymphoid cells (Table 2). The two types of non-Hodgkin's lymphoma that most commonly develop a leukaemic phase are follicular lymphoma and splenic lymphoma with villous lymphocytes (**SLVL**).

The circulating cells in follicular lymphoma are small, have no visible cytoplasm, the nuclear chromatin has a smooth pattern, and they show regularly deep nuclear clefts. Leukaemia in follicular lymphoma is associated with widespread disease, tends to run a more aggressive course, and requires more intensive treatment.

SLVL is a distinct, low-grade non-Hodgkin's lymphoma (splenic marginal zone lymphoma) characterized by splenomegaly, moderate lymphocytosis ($10–30 \times 10^9$/l), and a small monoclonal band, and/or free light chains in the urine in 50 per cent of cases. The circulating lymphocytes have a small nucleolus and a cytoplasm with conspicuous villous projections that are often seen polarized in one end of the cell. The bone marrow is minimally involved early in the disease and splenectomy is a useful treatment for SLVL. Leukaemia is also common in mantle-cell lymphoma. The circulating cells in mantle-cell lymphoma are of medium to large size with an irregular nuclear outline.

Large granular lymphocytic leukaemia

Most cases with a persistent T-cell lymphocytosis of greater than 5×10^9/l lasting for more than 6 months without an identifiable cause are likely to represent clonal proliferation of large granular lymphocytes. Large granular lymphocytes have abundant cytoplasm with prominent azurophil granules. Half of the patients have splenomegaly without lymphadenopathy and are neutropenic or, less frequently, suffer from other cytopenias. The membrane phenotype shows mature T cells that are typically CD4−, CD8+ and, characteristically, express one or more antigens associated with natural killer cells, for example CD11b, CD16, CD56, or CD57. Although many patients do not require active treatment, a significant minority present a therapeutic problem. Treatments that have been effective in some patients are cyclosporin A, prednisolone plus an alkylating agent, and 2-deoxycoformycin (DCF).

T-cell prolymphocytic leukaemia

This disease is characterized by splenomegaly, lymphadenopathy, and high leucocyte counts, usually rising rather rapidly above 100×10^9/l. The membrane phenotype is typically that of a CD4+ T lymphocyte but one-third of cases coexpress CD4 and CD8 or are CD4−, CD8+. The median survival of T-cell prolymphocytic leukaemia in our series has been 7 months. Complete and partial responses can be obtained with DCF and the 'humanized' monoclonal antibody CAMPATH-1H.

T-cell lymphomas in leukaemic phase

T-cell non-Hodgkin's lymphomas develop leukaemia more frequently than do B-cell lymphomas. Two diseases in particular regularly evolve with circulating lymphoma cells in the peripheral blood: adult T-cell leukaemia/lymphoma (ATLL) and Sezary syndrome.

ATLL

ATLL has a distinct geographical distribution affecting mainly the south-west islands of Japan, the Caribbean basin, and some parts of South America (Brazil and Chile). The demonstration of antibodies to human T-cell leukaemia lymphoma virus (HTLV)-I, the causative agent of ATLL, is one of the tests necessary for diagnosis. Diagnosis is made by the demonstration of ATLL cells in peripheral blood films. These cells have an irregular nucleus with poly-lobed configuration and many atypical forms. Patients with ATLL have generalized lymph-adenopathy, splenomegaly, and skin rashes. Leucocyte counts are variable but are often less than 50×10^9/l. Hypercalcaemia is present in two-thirds of patients and tends to be difficult to control. The median survival of ATLL is 6 months. Patients are treated as having high-grade non-Hodgkin's lymphoma, but remissions are transient and opportunistic infections are common. Interferon and anti-retroviral drugs are proving of some value.

Sezary syndrome

This is a form of cutaneous T-cell lymphoma characterized by erythroderma and circulating Sezary cells. Sezary cells are mature T cells with a CD4+, CD8– immunophenotype. Treatment is as for high-grade non-Hodgkin's lymphoma.

Further reading

Bennett, J.M. *et al.* (1989). Proposals for the classification of chronic (mature) B and T lymphoid leukaemias. *Journal of Clinical Pathology*, **42**, 567–84.

Catovsky, D. and Foa, R. (1990). *The lymphoid leukaemias.* Butterworths, London.

Moreau, E.J., Matutes, E., A'Hern, R.P., *et al.* (1997). Improvement of the chronic lymphocytic leukemia scoring system with the monoclonal antibody SN8 (CD79b) *American Journal of Clinical Pathology*, **108**, 378–82.

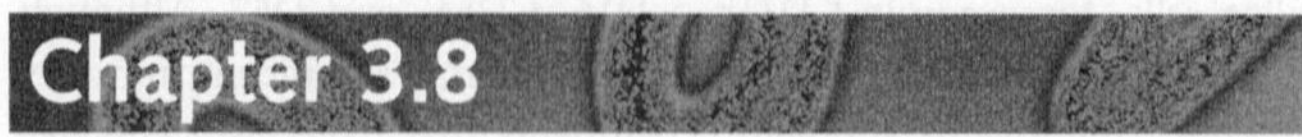

Chapter 3.8

Myelodysplastic syndromes

D. Catovsky

Definition

Myelodysplastic syndromes are acquired, clonal, and progressive cytopenias associated with a hypercellular bone marrow and ineffective haemopoiesis. As a rule, two or three of the bone marrow cell lineages are involved in myelodysplastic syndromes but, rarely, only one may be affected

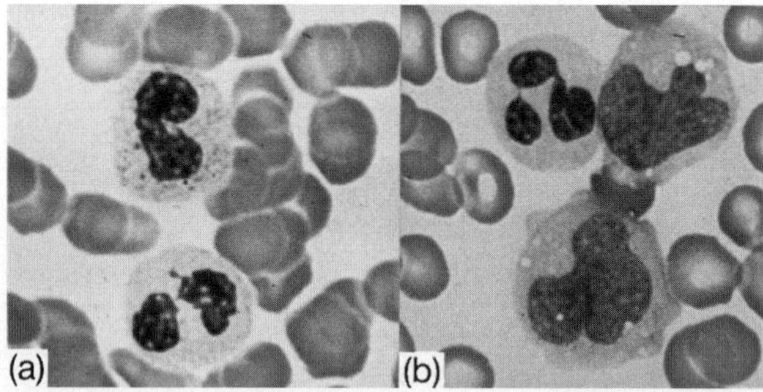

Fig. 1 Peripheral blood cells of myelodysplastic syndrome: (a) neutrophils with the Pelger anomaly; (b) monocytes and a neutrophil from a case of chronic myelomonocytic leukaemia. 900 ×.

Two major types of myelodysplastic syndrome can be recognized, both carrying an increased risk of transformation to acute myeloid leukaemia: (i) primary myelodysplastic syndrome, the most common, has no known cause, and (ii) secondary myelodysplastic syndrome, which results from the use of chemotherapeutic agents.

Clinical and laboratory features

Myelodysplastic syndromes almost always affect adults over the age of 50 years. Secondary myelodysplastic syndrome affects, as a rule, younger patients. The disease is rare but well documented in children. Anaemia, fever, or bleeding manifestations are the most common presenting symptoms. There are usually few, if any, significant physical signs. Splenomegaly is found in 20 per cent of cases, more often associated with one of the forms of myelodysplastic syndrome, namely chronic myelomonocytic leukaemia.

The key elements for diagnosis, in the presence of persistent anaemia or pancytopenia, are the examination of peripheral blood and bone marrow films.

Haematological findings

Anaemia is the most constant feature and is usually normocytic and normochromic, or moderately macrocytic. The red cells may show anisopoikilocytosis and nucleated forms. Reticulocyte counts are usually low. The white-cell count is variable but often low. Leucocytosis with a monocytosis is only a feature of chronic myelomonocytic leukaemia. Neutropenia is seen in one-third of cases. A common finding is the presence of abnormal hypogranular neutrophils (Fig. 1). Thrombocytopenia is less frequent than anaemia and neutropenia but the blood film may show large or even giant platelets and, rarely, megakaryocyte fragments.

Bone marrow

The marrow aspirate is always normocellular or hypercellular, displaying quantitative and qualitative changes with maturation defects in two or three of the cell lineages. These features are summarized in Table 1 (Figs 2 and 3). The presence of more than 15 per cent of ringed sideroblasts is a feature of acquired idiopathic sideroblastic anaemia. The trephine biopsy is usually hypercellular, with few remaining fat spaces. The abnormal localization of immature precursors (ALIP), clusters of blasts in the central spaces of the marrow and not along the endosteal spaces where they are normally found, has been considered a distinct feature of myelodysplastic syndromes. Myelofibrosis is not a feature of primary myelodysplastic syndrome

Table 1 Features of myelodysplasia in the bone marrow-cell lineages

Dyserythropoiesis: ringed sideroblasts; nuclear fragments; multinuclearity; abnormal nuclear shape; karyorrhexis; cytoplasmic vacuolation; megaloblastic changes (Fig. 2)
Dysgranulopoiesis: agranular or hypogranular neutrophils and myelocytes; hyposegmented nucleus (Pelger anomaly); abnormal chromatin clumping; hypersegmented neutrophils, occasionally with bizarre shapes; blasts with few or no granules; irregular distribution of cytoplasmic basophilia
Dysmegakaryopoiesis: micromegakaryocytes; large or small mononuclear forms; megakaryocytes with multiple, small, round nuclei; small cells with bilobed nuclei (Fig. 3)

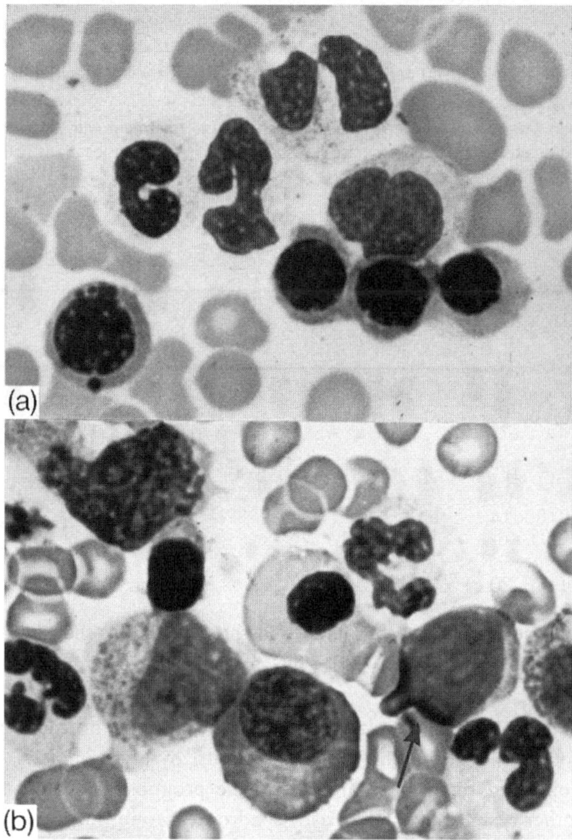

Fig. 2 Bone marrow appearances in myelodysplastic syndrome. (a) Erythroblasts from a case of refractory anaemia; one of them shows nuclear fragments. (b) Cells from a case of refractory anaemia with excess of blasts. Note a blast cell (arrow), hypogranular neutrophils, and a late erythroblast with megaloblastic features. 900 ×.

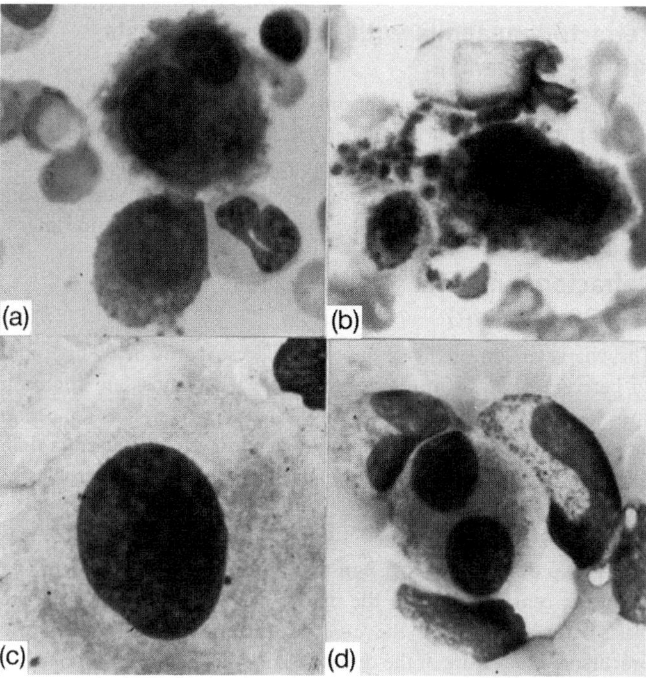

Fig. 3 Qualitative abnormalities of megakaryocytes: (a, b, d) binucleated or trinucleated micromegakaryocytes; (c) large mononuclear form. 900 ×.

Table 2 FAB classification of myelodysplastic syndromes

Disease (abbreviation)	Percentage of blasts	
	BM	PB
Refractory anaemia (RA) RA with ringed sideroblasts (RAS)	<5	<5
RA with excess of blasts (RAEB) Chronic myelomonocytic leukaemia (CMML)*	5–20**	<5
RAEB in transformation (RAEB-t)	21–30**	>5

After Bennett *et al.* (1982).

BM, bone marrow; PB, peripheral blood.

*Absolute monocytosis (>1 × 10^9/l; frequently >5 × 10^9/l).

**This percentage takes into account all BM cells; in cases with >50% erythroblasts the percentage of blasts is calculated by excluding the erythroid cells. If this percentage is >30% in any of the assessments the diagnosis is acute myeloid leukaemia.

but it is not rare in secondary myelodysplastic syndrome. The megakaryocytic abnormalities can be appreciated in biopsy sections as well as films obtained from aspirates.

Classification

The FAB classification (Table 2) has been found to be reproducible and a basis for comparisons between different series. The main features considered for the classification, in the presence of dysmyelopoiesis, are: (i) the proportion of marrow blasts (fewer than 5 per cent, 5–20 per cent, and between 21 and 30 per cent); (ii) the presence of ringed sideroblasts; (iii) blood monocytosis; and (iv) the presence of blasts and/or Auer rods in blood films.

The five categories of myelodysplastic syndrome should not be considered as rigid entities. Progression from one to another, usually from refractory anaemia to refractory anaemia with an excess of blasts (**RAEB**), and from RAEB to RAEB in transformation (**RAEB-t**) (see Table 2) is frequently seen. In addition, all of them can progress to acute myeloid leukaemia, although with different frequency.

Refractory anaemia (20–30 per cent)

Patients with refractory anaemia often have a macrocytic anaemia which may be associated with neutropenia and thrombocytopenia. Blast cells are not seen in blood films and are not prominent in the marrow (less than 5 per cent). Infections and bleeding are the main clinical problems.

Refractory anaemia with ringed sideroblasts (10–15 per cent)

This is characterized by anaemia and the presence of ringed sideroblasts in the marrow. There is typically a dimorphic blood picture; platelet and white-cell counts are often normal. It has a chronic course with a significantly lower risk of evolution to acute myeloid leukaemia than other types of myelodysplastic syndrome.

Refractory anaemia with an excess of blasts (20–30 per cent)

The characteristic of this group is the presence of between 5 and 20 per cent of blasts in the bone marrow. Cytopenias are common and are associated with marked dysplastic changes. This condition has a higher incidence of evolution to acute myeloid leukaemia than refractory anaemia and refractory anaemia with ringed sideroblasts.

RAEB in transformation (10–15 per cent)

This group differs from RAEB in that there are over 20 per cent (up to 30 per cent) of blasts in the marrow and/or 5 per cent or more blasts in the blood. Rarely, the presence of Auer rods in the granulocyte precursors is a feature of the disease. RAEB-t defines a group of cases with intermediate features between myelodysplastic syndrome and acute myeloid leukaemia.

Chronic myelomonocytic leukaemia (5–15 per cent)

The peripheral blood is characterized by neutrophilia and monocytosis (in excess of 1×10^9/l) and the only consistent cytopenia is thrombocytopenia, which is often responsible for bleeding manifestations. In contrast to other types of myelodysplastic syndrome, 30 per cent of patients with chronic myelomonocytic leukaemia have moderate splenomegaly. Patients with chronic myelomonocytic leukaemia are often elderly, and in some the disease runs a chronic course. However, overall median survivals are short (1–2 years), with one-third of cases evolving to acute myeloid leukaemia.

Differential diagnosis

Other causes of anaemia, for example renal or liver disease and nutritional deficiencies, should be excluded. The blast count can be used to exclude acute myeloid leukaemia. The bone marrow trephine will help to exclude aplastic anaemia and hypoplastic acute myeloid leukaemia (foci of blasts in a hypocellular bone marrow). Chromosome analysis is useful, particularly in cases of refractory anaemia if one of the typical clonal abnormalities of a myelodysplastic syndrome is demonstrated (see Table 3).

Chromosome and cellular abnormalities

Clonal karyotypic abnormalities can be demonstrated in the marrows of 50 to 70 per cent of patients with myelodysplastic syndromes. The incidence of chromosome abnormalities in secondary myelodysplastic syndrome is between 90 and 100 per cent. The most frequent abnormalities in myelodysplastic syndromes are listed in Table 3 (Fig. 4)

Some abnormalities have been described in association with particular types of myelodysplastic syndrome. For example, 5q–, when found in refractory anaemia or, less frequently, in RAEB, constitutes a distinct syndrome, 'the 5q– syndrome'. This is found more often

Table 3 Chromosome abnormalities in myelodysplastic syndromes (MDS)

Monosomy or deletion of chromosome 5 [–5; del(5q)]*
Monosomy or deletion of chromosome 7 [–7; del(7q)]*
Translocation t(1;7)
Trisomy 8 (+8)
Abnormal 11q23**
Deletion 12p [del(12p)]
Isochromosome 17q
Trisomy 19 or 21 (+19,+21)
Deletion 20q [del(20q)]
Abnormal 21q22**

*These are seen in 30–40 per cent of primary and secondary MDS; del(7q) is illustrated in Fig. 4.

**Seen in MDS/acute myeloid leukaemia secondary to treatment with drugs targeted against DNA-topoisomerase II, usually as balanced translocations with other chromosomes

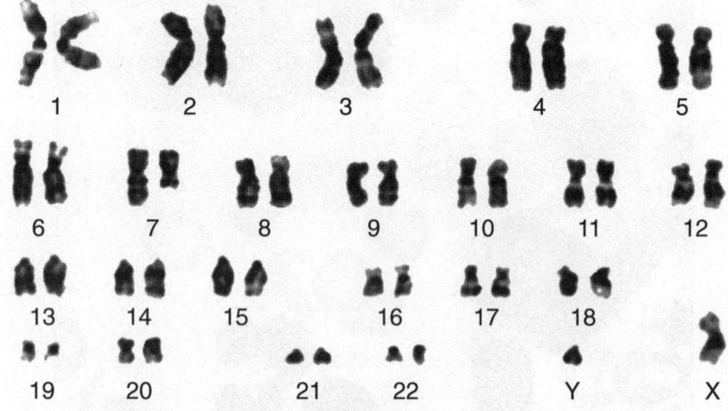

Fig. 4 Karyotype of a patient with myelodysplastic syndrome showing deletion on the long arm of chromosome 7, del(7q).

in women and is characterized by macrocytic anaemia, normal white-cell counts, normal or high platelet counts, dyserythropoiesis, and hypolobulated micromegakaryocytes. The prognosis is better than with other types of myelodysplastic syndrome. Monosomy 7 (–7), on the other hand, has been associated with abnormal neutrophil function and childhood cases of myelodysplastic syndrome.

The evolution to acute myeloid leukaemia is high (75 per cent) in cases with complex karyotype abnormalities, and twice as high in cases of myelodysplastic syndrome with chromosome abnormalities than in those without them.

Changes observed in therapy-related myelodysplastic syndromes seem to bear a relationship to the type of agent(s) used to treat the primary malignancy. In cases treated with alkylating agents the most common abnormalities are of chromosomes 5 and 7. In patients treated with etoposide and teniposide the most common abnormalities involve balanced translocations of chromosomes 11 and 21 with breakpoints at 11q23 and 21q22 (Table 3).

Prognosis

The median survival of patients with myelodysplastic syndrome ranges from 12 to 28 months. The main causes of death are complications resulting from the cytopenias and evolution to acute myeloid leukaemia.

A number of prognostic factors have been identified. The FAB classification (Table 2) has been shown to correlate with prognosis, the worst groups being RAEB and RAEB-t, both of which have the highest rate of evolution to acute myeloid leukaemia. An increase in blast cells is one of the bad prognostic features. Patients with fewer than 5 per cent of marrow blasts, for example in refractory anaemia and refractory anaemia with ringed sideroblasts, have median survivals of 3 to 5 years in some series.

An international scoring system for evaluating prognosis based on the results of cytogenetic analysis and the percentage of bone marrow blasts was proposed recently. This allows the separation of patients into four distinct risk subgroups: good, intermediate 1 and 2, and high, which predicts the timespan to evolve into acute myeloid leukaemia and the median survival.

Complications

Infections due to neutropenia and bleeding due to thrombocytopenia are the most common causes of death in patients with refractory anaemia, with or without ringed sideroblasts. Neutrophil function is depressed in myelodysplastic syndromes and infections may be a feature in patients with normal neutrophil counts.

An evolution towards acute myeloid leukaemia is the inevitable outcome in 30 to 50 per cent of patients with RAEB and with chronic myelomonocytic leukaemia, and in greater than 50 per cent of those with RAEB-t. This course is less common in refractory anaemia with or without ringed sideroblasts.

Secondary myelodysplastic syndrome

This condition is now seen with increasing frequency in younger patients who have been treated intensively or for prolonged periods with cytotoxic drugs. Many cases of secondary acute myeloid leukaemia evolve through a phase of myelodysplastic syndrome. Several factors may help to distinguish secondary from primary myelodysplastic syndromes. Secondary myelodysplastic syndromes show early macrocytosis, a hypocellular marrow, or an increase in reticulin fibres leading, sometimes, to myelofibrosis.

Treatment

Because of the life-threatening nature of myelodysplastic syndromes, the choice of active treatment to induce a remission or provide simple supportive care must be made with extreme care. Anaemia without other evidence of marrow failure could always be supported by blood transfusions to keep haemoglobin levels above 8 g/dl. A therapeutic trial of folic acid, pyridoxine, and/or vitamin B_{12} should be considered to identify responsive anaemias. For moderate neutropenias, antibiotics or antifungal agents should be given at the first sign of infection. For patients with more than 5 per cent blasts, or with marked cytopenia, supportive measures may not be enough to prolong survival.

A number of agents that induce differentiation and maturation of leukaemic cells have been used to treat patients with myelodysplastic syndrome. One of them, *cis*-retinoic acid, can improve the anaemia in some patients with refractory anaemia or refractory anaemia with ringed sideroblasts. Another, cytosine arabinoside (**Ara-C**), has been used at low doses, 10 mg/m^2 subcutaneously twice a day for 2 or 3 weeks, in order to induce haematological remissions. High-dose Ara-C in combination with anthracyclines is indicated in RAEB-t, where response rates can approach those obtained in acute myeloid leukaemia. Oral etoposide and hydroxyurea may be beneficial in chronic myelomonocytic leukaemia, particularly in cases with leucocytosis and involvement of, for example, spleen, lymph nodes, skin, and pleura.

Intensive combination chemotherapy, as used in acute myeloid leukaemia, should be considered for younger patients with myelodysplastic syndrome but remissions with this approach are generally short. Supralethal therapy with drugs and total-body irradiation, followed by a bone marrow transplantation from an HLA-identical sibling, have been tried with some success in younger patients with primary and secondary myelodysplastic syndromes. This is the only treatment that can achieve cure.

Haemopoietic growth factors may correct cytopenias in some patients with myelodysplasia. The two most commonly used growth factors, GM-CSF and granulocyte (G)-CSF, may both increase the levels of neutrophils in up to 70 per cent of patients. At present it is unclear whether this therapy can have a significant impact on survival. Recombinant erythropoietin has been used to improve anaemia and responses have been noted in 20 per cent of cases. Combinations of erythropoietin with other growth factors may be particularly valuable.

The choice of treatment in a myelodysplastic syndrome depends on a number of factors, of which the patient's age and prognostic features are the most important. Even if a decision for active treatment is considered, it is unclear at present which are the best agents or drug combinations.

Further reading

Bennett, J.M., *et al.* (1982). Proposals for the classification of the myelodysplastic syndromes. *British Journal of Haematology*, **51**, 189–99.

Greenberg, P., *et al.* (1997). International scoring system for evaluating prognosis in myelodysplastic syndromes. *Blood*, **89**, 2079–88.

Hirst, W.J.R. and Mufti, G.J. (1993). Management of myelodysplastic syndromes. *British Journal of Haematology*, **84**, 191–6.

Chapter 3.9

Polycythaemia vera

D. J. Weatherall

The term 'polycythaemia' is used to describe an increased red-cell count, packed-cell volume, or haemoglobin level. Two main types are recognized: (i) relative, in which there is a reduction in plasma volume with a normal red-cell mass; and (ii) absolute, in which there is a genuine increase in the red-cell mass. The absolute polycythaemias are divided into primary polycythaemia or polycythaemia rubra vera which is a myeloproliferative disorder of unknown aetiology, and the secondary polycythaemias, which result from a variety of different pathological mechanisms.

Here we shall consider polycythaemia vera because there is good evidence that this condition results from the neoplastic proliferation of a multipotent haemopoietic progenitor cell. The relative and secondary polycythaemias, and the differential diagnosis of an increased haemoglobin level, are considered in Chapter 3.26.

Aetiology

Polycythaemia vera results from the abnormal proliferation of red-cell precursors derived from a single haemopoietic progenitor cell with the capacity for differentiation down red-cell, white-cell, and platelet lines. The tendency to develop myelosclerosis in the later stages of the illness may be the result of the production of growth factors, such as platelet-derived growth factor, by the abnormal megakaryocyte line. Erythropoietin levels are normal or low, and on *in vitro* culture the red-cell precursors from patients with this disorder show unstimulated erythropoiesis. It thus appears that the basic defect in polycythaemia vera is a proliferation of precursors that behave quite independently of the normal erythropoietin regulation system.

There is a considerable incidence of acute leukaemic transformation in patients with polycythaemia vera, and, in this sense, polycythaemia vera can be looked upon as a preleukaemic condition.

Haemodynamics and oxygen transport

Optimum oxygen transport occurs at packed-cell volumes (PCVs) of between 40 and 50 per cent. If no compensatory mechanisms occurred, there would be a reduced rate of oxygen transport even with a moderate increase in the PCV. In fact, even at relatively high PCVs, oxygen transport is adequate because there is an increase in the total blood volume, an increased cardiac output, and a fall in peripheral resistance. Indeed, at a PCV of 60 per cent there may be some increase in oxygen delivery. Unfortunately, however, polycythaemia vera is a disease of middle and old age and is frequently associated with cardiovascular disorders such as hypertension and coronary artery and cerebrovascular disease. Hence, these compensatory mechanisms tend to break down, and this is particularly likely to occur at PCVs in excess of 60 to 65 per cent. In addition, there may be a marked reduction in the cerebral blood flow at high PCV levels, and this, together with associated cerebrovascular disease and a high platelet count, makes the cerebral circulation particularly vulnerable to occlusive episodes.

While many of the complications of polycythaemia vera are related to the haemodynamic changes secondary to increased blood viscosity, there is the added factor of the abnormal function of the aberrant cell line. Thrombotic episodes probably result from the reduced flow of thick, viscous blood together with the high platelet count that commonly accompanies the disorder. There is also defective haemostasis, probably due to abnormal platelet function. Hence, polycythaemia vera is characterized by the bizarre association of both thrombotic and bleeding tendencies, associated with cardiovascular complications.

Symptoms

The disorder sometimes starts insidiously. On the other hand, patients may first present with an acute, dramatic complication such as a cerebrovascular accident or major thrombotic episode.

Non-specific complaints, probably related to circulatory disturbances in the nervous system, are most common and include headache, dizziness, vertigo, tinnitus, and visual disturbances including blurring and diplopia. There may be a cardiovascular presentation with angina, intermittent claudication, or recurrent venous thrombosis or embolic disease. Other symptoms include an increased bruising tendency, bleeding, and abdominal pain due to a peptic ulceration or splenomegaly. The condition may be first recognized during the course of investigation for gout. A particularly common symptom is severe and intractable pruritus. This has a very characteristic relation to warmth and frequently occurs after getting into bed at night or bathing.

Physical findings

Many patients with polycythaemia vera are plethoric and show a cyanotic tinge to the nose, ears, and lips. Typically there is injection of the conjunctivae and a flush over the neck and upper half of the trunk. At least 75 per cent of patients have splenomegaly sometime during their illness. The size of the spleen varies greatly and radiological investigation may be necessary to demonstrate that it is enlarged. A moderate degree of hepatomegaly is present in up to one-half of patients. Although arterial hypertension has been thought to be a common accompaniment of polycythaemia vera, it is difficult to be sure about this because polycythaemia vera occurs at an age when hypertension is extremely common.

Haematological changes

Typically there is an increase in the haemoglobin and in the PCV, which may be over 70 per cent. These findings are associated with an absolute increase in the red-cell mass. In the majority of patients there is an elevation of either the white-cell or platelet count, or both. Bone marrow examination shows an active marrow, but erythropoiesis is normoblastic and there are no diagnostic features. A variety of abnormalities of platelet function have been demonstrated.

Many patients are hyperuricaemic, and secondary gout is quite common. The arterial oxygen saturation is usually normal, although, interestingly, mild degrees of unsaturation may occur occasionally in patients with otherwise well-documented polycythaemia vera. The leucocyte alkaline phosphatase is usually increased, which helps to distinguish cases with very high white-cell counts from chronic myeloid leukaemia, in which the level is reduced. The serum vitamin B_{12} content and the capacity of the serum to bind vitamin B_{12} are often markedly increased. Cytogenetic abnormalities occur in many cases and 20q+ translocations are particularly common.

Differential diagnosis

Usually there is little difficulty in diagnosing polycythaemia vera. The finding of an increased haemoglobin level and PCV, an increased red-cell mass, splenomegaly, and an associated elevation in the white-cell and/or platelet count is diagnostic. Provided that an absolute polycythaemia has been demonstrated by red-cell mass estimation, the only difficulty is ruling out the various causes of secondary polycythaemia; this problem is considered in Chapter 3.26. Where there is diagnostic uncertainty individuals should be followed carefully and their polycythaemia managed by venesection. Some will develop the typical features of polycythaemia vera after several months or years, while in others a cause of secondary polycythaemia such as a tumour may show itself after an equally long period.

Course and prognosis

It is extremely difficult to give an accurate prognosis in this disorder. It appears that younger patients survive longer and that the prognosis for those who present with a major complication at the onset is considerably worse than those who present with minimal symptoms.

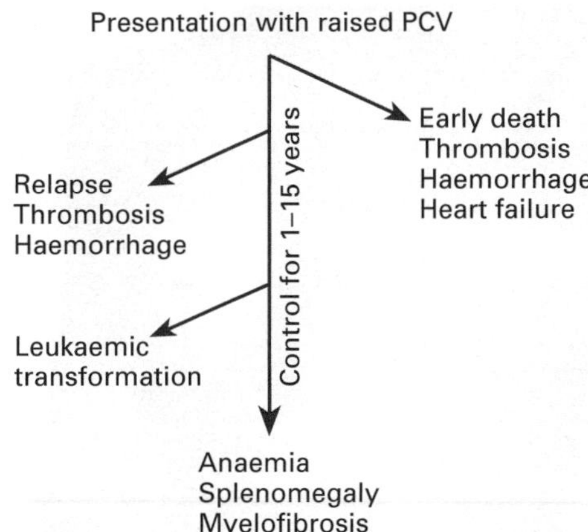

Fig. 1 Schematic representation of the natural history of polycythaemia vera.

The median survival time varies from 9 to 14 years, with some variation depending on the form of therapy (see below).

During the course of the illness (Fig. 1) there may be vascular or thrombotic complications, particularly if the PCV is allowed to remain in excess of 55 per cent or more; a very high platelet count is also associated with an increased incidence of thrombotic and haemorrhagic complications. In many of those patients who do not die of vascular complications, the polycythaemia gradually 'burns out' and is replaced by anaemia, massive splenomegaly, and progressive fibrosis of the bone marrow. At this stage the illness is indistinguishable from primary myelosclerosis (see Chapter 3.10). The other form of termination of polycythaemia vera is acute leukaemia. It is now clear that the frequency of this complication is, at least in part, related to the form of treatment (see below) and it may occur either acutely or insidiously.

Management

Currently, polycythaemia vera is not curable and hence the objectives of management are to maintain well being and to diminish the likelihood of complications for as long as possible. This is achieved by reducing a dangerously high PCV into a safer range by venesection and then by maintaining this level, either by regular venesection or the use of myelosuppressive agents, or both. At the same time an attempt is made to maintain the platelet count at a safe level and to control other complications such as hyperuricaemia and secondary folate deficiency with appropriate drugs.

Because patients with high PCVs are at great risk of thrombotic episodes it is important to initiate a venesection regimen as soon as the diagnosis is clear. It is usually possible to remove 350 to 500 ml of blood every other day until the PCV is reduced to the normal range. In emergencies, preoperatively for example, more blood may be removed and replaced by an equal volume of plasma.

Once a normal PCV has been attained, maintenance therapy should be started. In young patients in whom the platelet count is not dangerously high, it is better to try to maintain the PCV at a normal level by regular venesection to keep the PCV below 50 per cent, and ideally below 45 per cent. After a while changes of iron deficiency will be observed although this is rarely a problem.

In older patients who cannot tolerate regular venesection, or in younger patients in whom there is a very high platelet count, myelosuppressive therapy is indicated. The type of myelosuppressive treatment has been a major controversy for many years, mainly because of the fear that the use of these agents might provoke leukaemic transformation. The use of chlorambucil is associated with a significantly higher frequency of leukaemic transformation. The use of ^{32}P also seems to increase the likelihood of the development of leukaemia, although because of the time interval involved this does not seem to preclude its use in older patients. Several studies have shown that it is possible to control high platelet counts and the other features of polycythaemia vera by the use of continuous hydroxyurea.

So which form of myelosuppressive therapy should be used in polycythaemia vera? In older patients it seems reasonable to use ^{32}P. Following venesection to a normal PCV, a dose of ^{32}P, 3 to 5 mCi (2.5 mCi/m^2), should be given intravenously. Sometimes a second, smaller dose, 2 to 3 mCi of ^{32}P, is required 3 to 4 months after the initial injection in order to bring the disease under complete control. The condition then often remains quiescent for months or even years. It is most unusual to produce severe marrow hypoplasia with this regimen. In younger patients hydroxyurea can be used. It should be started at a dose of 500 mg to 1 g daily and the dose tapered down as control is achieved

A variety of agents reportedly improve the pruritus of polycythaemia vera, none of which has been uniformly successful. This distressing symptom seems to respond best to myelosuppressive treatment. Additional relief may be obtained from the use of H_1- or H_2-blockers. Hyperuricaemia should be managed with allopurinol.

In the later, 'burnt out' stages of the illness, when there is massive splenomegaly and myelofibrosis, the management is similar to that for primary myelosclerosis (Chapter 3.10). It consists of blood transfusion, iron and folate replacement, and, occasionally, splenectomy if there is gross hypersplenism. In patients who develop an acute leukaemic transformation the management is as described for acute leukaemia, although acute leukaemia superimposed on polycythaemia vera is usually very refractory to treatment.

Further reading

Beutler, E. (1994). Polycythaemia vera. In *Williams haematology* (ed. E. Beutler, M.A. Lichtmann, B.S. Coller, and T.J. Kipps). McGraw-Hill, New York.

Chapter 3.10

Myelosclerosis

D. J. Weatherall

The term 'myelosclerosis' is used to describe progressive fibrous replacement of the bone marrow and is used synonymously with myelofibrosis. The condition may be part of the myeloproliferative syndrome or may be secondary to the effects of other neoplastic disorders of the bone marrow, metabolic changes involving vitamin D or its metabolites, and a variety of other conditions that provoke a fibrous reaction by an unknown mechanism.

Primary myelosclerosis

Primary myelosclerosis is a myeloproliferative disorder, which is characterized by anaemia and abnormal proliferation of haemopoietic precursors associated with a variable degree of fibrosis of the bone marrow and myeloid metaplasia in the spleen, liver, and other organs.

Aetiology

The cause of myelosclerosis and myeloid metaplasia is unknown. It seems likely that the abnormal haemopoietic elements which constitute the myeloid metaplasia of the spleen, liver, and other organs result from the neoplastic proliferation of an abnormal stem-cell population. It is currently believed that the fibrotic reaction results from the release of platelet-derived growth factor for fibroblasts, or related factors from the abnormal line of megakaryocytes.

The fibrous tissue in the bone marrow is demonstrated with the silver stain for reticulin which identifies mainly collagen and fibronectin.

During the evolution of myelosclerosis the two major pathological processes, progressive fibrosis of the bone marrow and myeloid metaplasia of the liver, spleen, and lymph nodes, seem to occur simultaneously, although there is remarkable variability between patients in the rate and extent of these changes. The fibrosis of the marrow is extremely patchy and there may be areas of hyperplasia that can cause diagnostic difficulties. The hyperplasia involves all the precursor cells, particularly megakaryocytes. Major factors in producing the clinical picture of myelosclerosis are progressive bone marrow failure and hypersplenism.

Clinical features

The presenting symptoms in myelosclerosis are extremely variable. The disorder may first be recognized because an enlarged spleen is discovered accidentally. Sometimes it is large enough to cause abdominal distension or a dragging sensation in the left upper quadrant. On the other hand, the first symptoms may be progressive anaemia, weight loss or general ill health, bone pain, or acute abdominal pain due to a splenic infarct. Some patients are first referred to dermatologists with pruritus, which has the same distinctive relation to warmth as occurs in polycythaemia vera. Occasionally, the early clinical picture reflects abnormal platelet function and there may be increased bruising, unexplained gastrointestinal blood loss, or bleeding after minor trauma (Fig. 1).

The only physical finding that is almost invariably present is splenomegaly which may be massive. There is usually some degree of hepatomegaly.

Finally, since about one-third of patients with myelosclerosis have a patchy osteosclerosis, the condition may first be recognized by the finding of an unusual bone radiograph in a patient who is having a radiological examination for another cause.

Haematological changes

Anaemia may be quite mild in the early stage of the illness but usually becomes more severe as the disorder progresses. The red cells are characteristically misshapen, with many tear-drop-shaped forms (Fig. 2). These changes are the real hallmark of myelosclerosis. Quite often there are nucleated red cells in the peripheral blood.

The white-cell count is often elevated and consists mainly of mature neutrophils, but there are usually some immature forms (Fig. 2). These changes, together with the presence of nucleated red cells, constitute a leucoerythroblastic reaction. The platelet count is variable. In the earlier stages of the illness there is often a moderate thrombocytosis. As the disease progresses and the spleen enlarges, the platelet count tends to fall and severe thrombocytopenia may be a troublesome feature. The platelet morphology is abnormal; the changes are characterized by giant forms and occasional shreds of megakaryocyte cytoplasm in the peripheral blood (Fig. 2).

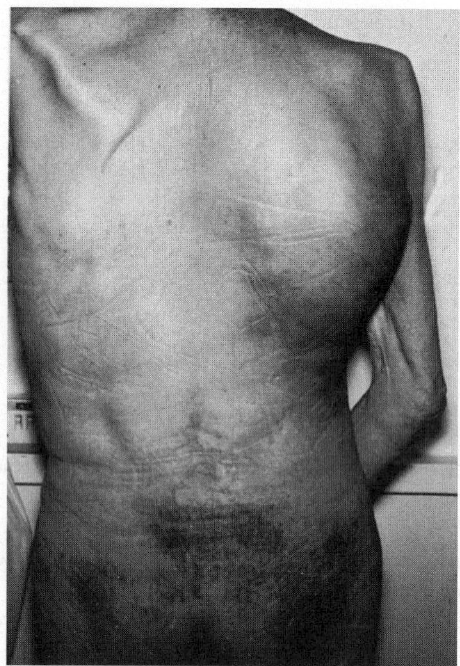

Fig. 1 A massive haematoma over the scapula region with tracking down in the tissue planes of the back in an 81-year-old patient with myelosclerosis and abnormal platelet function.

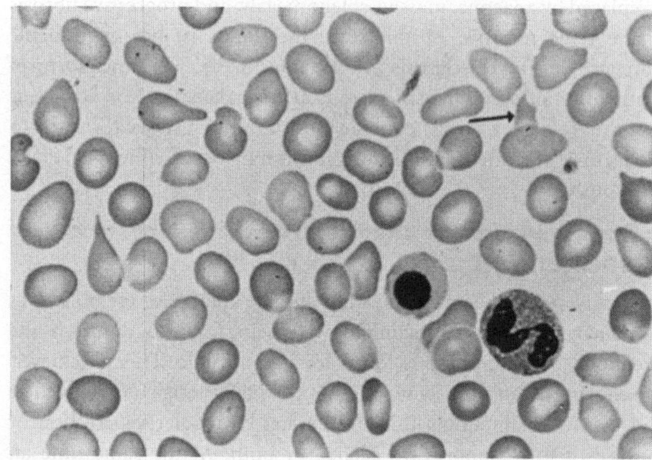

Fig. 2 Haematological changes in myelosclerosis. A peripheral blood film showing tear-drop cells, a nucleated red cell, and a grossly distorted cell marked by the arrow.
*(From Liebold, P.F. and Weed, R.I. (1975). Clinical Haematology, **4**, 353, with permission.)*

Bone marrow aspiration usually yields a 'dry' tap but the biopsy will show extensive fibrosis with islands of haemopoietic cells, and megakaryocytic hyperplasia (Fig. 3).

Although many cytogenetic abnormalities have been reported in this disorder, there are no specific chromosomal changes that are of diagnostic help.

There is usually an elevated uric acid level and the neutrophil alkaline phosphatase is variable. In addition, abnormalities of haemostasis and coagulation are common.

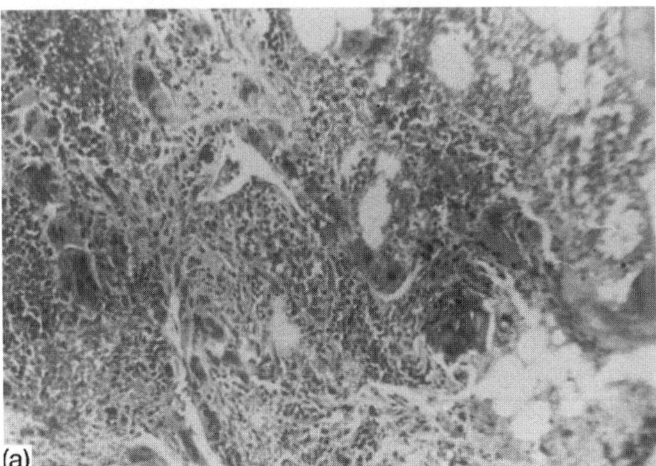

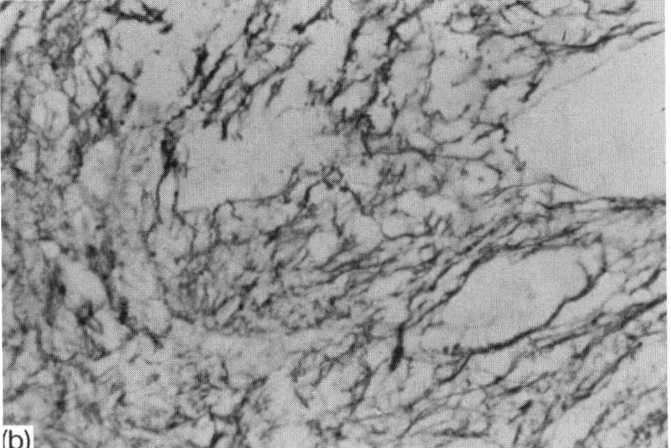

Fig. 3 (a) Bone marrow appearances in myelosclerosis. A biopsy showing a hyperplastic fragment with marked megakaryocytic hyperplasia. (b) Silver stain showing the marked increase in reticulin.

Differential diagnosis

The typical picture of myelosclerosis with a massive spleen and fibrosed bone marrow usually produces no diagnostic difficulty. Nevertheless, the disorder must be distinguished from the other myeloproliferative diseases and other causes of secondary marrow fibrosis.

Complications

The major complications of myelosclerosis relate to the massive splenomegaly. Splenic infarction with associated pain over the spleen or in the left shoulder tip is relatively common. Trauma to the large spleen may cause it to rupture, either into the abdominal cavity or with the production of a perisplenic haematoma. Secondary gout is common. Secondary folate deficiency is also common and may cause a sudden worsening of the anaemia. Presumably because of abnormal platelet function or peptic ulceration, chronic gastrointestinal blood loss occurs and the anaemia of myelosclerosis may be made worse by coexistent iron deficiency. Serious bruising and haematoma formation may result from mild trauma (see Fig. 1). There is also an association between myelosclerosis and portal hypertension, which may be accompanied by bleeding from oesophageal varices.

Course and prognosis

The course of myelosclerosis is variable. Some patients retain a relatively normal haemoglobin level and have a minimal splenomegaly for many years. More commonly there is a gradual decline in the patient's general condition with a progressive worsening of the anaemia, and increasing splenomegaly, which may reach enormous proportions. Although the median survival is usually given as approximately 5 years there is a very broad scatter and it is not at all uncommon for patients to live 10 to 20 years after myelosclerosis has been diagnosed. Approximately 20 per cent of cases terminate in acute myeloblastic leukaemia.

Treatment

There is no definitive treatment for patients with myelosclerosis. They should be followed carefully and complications such as iron or folate deficiency corrected. If they become symptomatic due to progressive anaemia, they should be started on a blood transfusion programme, although particular care is required when transfusing patients with this disorder. Although splenic irradiation and chemotherapy have been used in an attempt to reduce the size of the spleen, the results are equivocal. Some benefit may be obtained from a judicious use of busulphan or hydroxyurea. It is wise to start with a low dose of hydroxyurea, 500 mg daily for example, and gradually to increase it keeping a careful watch on spleen size and white-cell and platelet counts.

The place of splenectomy is controversial. It is impossible to anticipate how long patients will take to develop symptoms referable to splenomegaly. Postoperative thrombocytosis can still be extremely difficult to manage. Furthermore, some patients develop progressive hepatomegaly after splenectomy. For these reasons it is better to manage myelosclerosis conservatively and to reserve splenectomy for those rare cases in which splenic pain and severe hypersplenism become a major feature of the illness.

Acute myelosclerosis and acute megakaryoblastic leukaemia

Acute myelosclerosis is probably a myeloproliferative disorder that involves primarily the megakaryocyte or its precursor, and for this reason it is preferable to call the condition acute megakaryoblastic leukaemia. It is characterized by the rapid onset of anaemia, low-grade fever, bleeding, increased disposition to infection, and, sometimes, generalized bone pain. The spleen is either impalpable or only slightly enlarged. There may be marked bone tenderness.

The blood picture is characterized by pancytopenia with a leucoerythroblastic reaction. The disease has an extremely poor prognosis and does not respond well to conventional treatments, although some patients have been treated successfully by bone marrow transplantation.

Secondary myelosclerosis

There is a wide variety of disorders that may be associated with increased reticulin formation in the bone marrow. Secondary myelosclerosis is frequently associated with a leucoerythroblastic anaemia. Some of these conditions are summarized in Table 1 and include all forms of leukaemia, lymphomas, and myeloproliferative disorders.

The malignant form of systemic mastocytosis may develop *de novo* or superimposed on urticaria pigmentosa. It is a disease of the sixth and seventh decades and is more common in males. The symptoms are very varied and include general malaise, recurrent diarrhoea,

Table 1 Disorders associated with myelofibrosis (full references are given in McCarthy 1985)

Malignant	*Non-malignant*
Idiopathic myelosclerosis	Renal osteodystrophy
Acute myelosclerosis (acute megakaryoblastic leukaemia)	Vitamin D deficiency
	Hypoparathyroidism
Chronic myeloid leukaemia	Hyperparathyroidism
Acute lymphoblastic leukaemia	Grey platelet syndrome
Hairy-cell leukaemia	Systemic lupus erythematosus
Polycythaemia vera	Systemic sclerosis
Systemic mastocytosis	Thorium dioxide administration
Hodgkin's disease	
Myeloma	
Secondary carcinoma	

paroxysmal hypertension or hypotension, pruritus, the skin manifestations of urticaria pigmentosa, hepatosplenomegaly, dense sclerotic bone changes, and an increased number of mast cells in the skin, liver, lymph nodes, and bone marrow. Rarely, mast cells spill into the peripheral blood in large numbers giving rise to the picture of mast-cell leukaemia. The condition is diagnosed by demonstrating mast-cell infiltration of a lymph node or bone marrow using special staining techniques. Symptoms can sometimes be controlled by the use of H_1- or H_2-receptor antagonists. The prognosis from the time of diagnosis is variable. Many patients run a long course, terminating, in some cases, in leukaemia.

Other causes of marrow fibrosis include vitamin D deficiency, renal failure, and tuberculosis.

Further reading

McCarthy, D.M. (1985). Fibrosis of the bone marrow: content and causes. *British Journal of Haematology*, 59, 1–7.

Chapter 3.11

Primary thrombocythaemia

D. J. Weatherall

Primary thrombocythaemia is a myeloproliferative disorder characterized by hyperplasia of the megakaryocytes and a marked increase in the platelet count. There may be an associated increase in the white-cell count or even in the red-cell count, and the dividing line between this disorder and polycythaemia vera may be indistinct.

Aetiology and pathogenesis

Primary thrombocythaemia has a similar pathogenesis to the other myeloproliferative disorders and results from the abnormal proliferation of a stem-cell line, which, in this case, differentiates mainly towards the megakaryocyte/platelet compartments.

The platelets are morphologically abnormal and the platelet count is usually higher than that observed in thrombocytosis, that is, an increased production of normal platelets. The clinical features of this disorder are the result of the high platelet count and the functional abnormalities of the platelets produced by the abnormal cell line. As expected, the very high platelet count is associated with a thrombotic

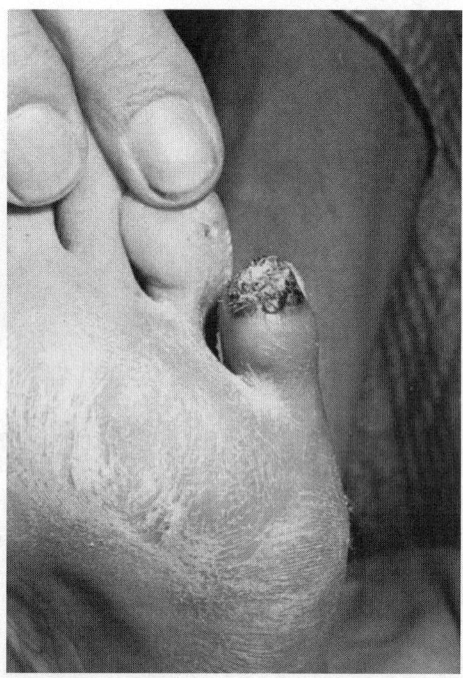

Fig. 1 A thrombotic lesion with infarction of the end of the toe in a patient with primary thrombocythaemia.

tendency but, because of abnormal platelet function, bleeding is often a major feature of the disease.

Clinical features

The most common symptom is abnormal bleeding, usually spontaneous. The most usual site is the gastrointestinal tract but haematuria and spontaneous bruising occur commonly. Interestingly, the disorder is not associated with genuine purpuric lesions. Thromboembolic phenomena are less frequent than bleeding and include thrombosis of the splenic vein and the superficial or deep veins of the legs, pulmonary emboli, thrombotic lesions of the vessels of fingers and toes (Fig. 1), and erythromelalgia. These bizarre peripheral vascular complications may be present for many years without a marked elevation in the platelet count. The spleen is often enlarged, at least in the early stages of the illness.

Laboratory findings

The main finding is a greatly elevated platelet count, which is often in excess of 800 to 1000 × 10^9/l. The platelet morphology is abnormal, with many large and bizarre forms, and aggregates in the peripheral blood. The bone marrow shows marked megakaryocytic hyperplasia. There is usually a mild polymorphonuclear leucocytosis and occasionally a slight elevation in the packed-cell volume. Tests of platelet function are often abnormal.

Thrombocythaemia must be distinguished from other causes of an elevated platelet count (Table 1), although in these disorders it is very unusual to find platelet counts in excess of 800 × 10^9/l.

Course and prognosis

The natural history is very variable. Although many patients run a course punctuated by episodes of bleeding, thrombosis, embolism, and other complications, the condition can also be surprisingly mild.

Table 1 Causes of a raised platelet count

Myeloproliferative disorders	*Secondary thrombocytosis (cont.)*
Primary thrombocythaemia	Malignant disease
Polycythaemia vera	Post-splenectomy
Myelosclerosis	Splenic atrophy; sickle-cell disease, coeliac disease
Chronic myeloid leukaemia	Drugs: vincoids, adrenaline
Secondary thrombocytosis	Post-thrombocytopenia
Bleeding	Haemolytic anaemia
Inflammatory disorders	
Rheumatoid arthritis	

Indeed, young patients who present without symptoms may live for many years without suffering any ill effects. There have been occasional reports of acute leukaemic transformation.

Treatment

Because this condition is rare trials to assess the available treatments are only just beginning. The thrombotic risk appears to be related to the underlying risk factors for thrombosis in the patient, such as age and hypertension. As young patients often remain asymptomatic for many years, it seems reasonable to leave them untreated under regular surveillance, and to initiate therapy only if symptoms occur or if the platelet count is progressively rising. In older patients the platelet count should probably be reduced to below 500×10^9/l. Hydroxyurea is the best tried agent. It is given as a dose sufficient to reduce the platelet counts to a safe level, reducing to a maintenance dose. Treatment options include hydroxyurea, interferon-α, busulphan, ^{32}P, and anagrelide, although busulphan and ^{32}P are generally only used in older patients. Aspirin may also be added in those patients who do not appear to be at risk of haemorrhage. In emergencies the platelet count can be lowered rapidly by plateletpheresis.

Further reading

Schafer, A.I. (1994). Primary thrombocythaemia. In *Williams haematology* (ed. E. Beutler, M.A. Lichtmann, B.S. Coller, and T.J. Kipps). McGraw-Hill, New York.

Chapter 3.12

Aplastic anaemia and other causes of bone marrow failure

E. C. Gordon-Smith

Bone marrow failure is a relatively common cause of peripheral blood cytopenia. The pathogenesis of most of these disorders is unknown but they can be classified according to the assumed mechanism of failure (Table 1).

Acquired aplastic anaemia

Definition

Acquired aplastic anaemia is a syndrome of haemopoietic stem-cell failure, characterized by peripheral blood pancytopenia associated

Table 1 Classification of bone marrow failure

Diseases	
Acquired	**Congenital**
Haemopoietic stem-cell failure	
Acquired aplastic anaemia	Fanconi anaemia Dyskeratosis congenita
Haemopoietic failure during differentiation	
Pure red-cell aplasia	Diamond–Blackfan anaemia
Amegakaryocytic thrombocytopenia	Thrombocytopenia with absent radii (TAR)
Chronic acquired neutropenia	Kostmann's syndrome
Proliferative dysplasias with abnormal differentiation	
Myelodysplastic syndromes	Congenital dyserythropoietic anaemias
Refractory anaemia (RA)	
RA with ringed sideroblasts	
RA with excess blasts	
Chronic myelomonocytic leukaemia	
Abnormal environment	
Proliferative dysplasias with fibrosis	Osteoporosis
Myelofibrosis	
Infiltrations	
Leukaemias/lymphomas	
Lipid-storage disease (e.g. Gaucher's disease)	
Amyloid	
Infections	
HIV	
Dengue fever	
Parvovirus B19	
Bone marrow necrosis	

with hypoplasia of the bone marrow in which there is neither fibrosis nor infiltration by malignant cells. Vitamin B_{12} and folate levels are normal, and the disorder is not associated with other dietary deficiencies. A classification is shown in Table 2.

- *Inevitable aplastic anaemia*: This occurs following exposure to cytotoxic drugs or irradiation. The severity and duration of aplasia is dose-related and recovery usually occurs 1 to 6 weeks after the cytotoxic agent is discontinued. With very high-dose radiation, stem-cell killing is complete and recovery does not occur.
- *Idiosyncratic acquired aplastic anaemia*: This is the disease to which the term 'aplastic anaemia' is usually applied without further qualification. The disease arises spontaneously or may follow exposure to normal doses of a variety of drugs that do not usually cause haematological disturbances. The nature of these agents is discussed in greater detail below.
- *Immune aplastic anaemia*: This is an uncommon disorder, which, again, may follow exposure to certain drugs or some virus infections, particularly infectious mononucleosis. It may also be associated with other autoimmune disorders. Unlike the idiosyncratic aplastic anaemias, recovery usually occurs 2 to 3 weeks after withdrawal of the offending agent, or spontaneously. In some instances it is possible to demonstrate inhibitors of granulopoiesis or erythropoiesis *in vitro*.

Table 2 Classification of aplastic anaemia (AA)

Disease	Causes	Characterization
Inevitable AA	Cytotoxic drugs Radiation	Dose-dependent Predictable recovery
Idiosyncratic AA	Drugs/chemicals Viruses (e.g. hepatitis) Idiopathic	Not dose-dependent Prolonged course Recovery unpredictable
Immune AA	Autoimmune disease Viruses (e.g. Epstein–Barr)	Usually short duration Antibodies may be detectable
Inherited AA	Autosomal recessive disease Sex-linked (usually)	Fanconi anaemia Dyskeratosis congenita
Malignant AA	Acute leukaemias (usually ALL*) Myelodysplastic aplasia	Transient: leukaemia develops later Prolonged or preleukaemic Cytogenetic abnormalities common

*ALL, acute lymphoblastic leukaemia.

- *Inherited aplastic anaemia (Fanconi anaemia)*: This is an autosomal recessive inherited disorder in which hypocellularity of the bone marrow and pancytopenia develop, usually during childhood. It is associated with skeleton and skin abnormalities, described in greater detail below.
- *'Malignant' aplastic anaemia*: This occurs in association with acute leukaemia or myelodysplastic syndrome. The aplastic presentation of acute leukaemia is more common in childhood, particularly with acute lymphoblastic leukaemia.

Idiosyncratic acquired aplastic anaemia

Aetiology

In about two-thirds of cases of aplastic anaemia it is not possible to identify any likely cause. Amongst the rest, drugs, viruses, and environmental toxins may be identified as probable causes. Drugs have been implicated in the aetiology of aplastic anaemia for 50 years or more and the list of implicated drugs is long (Table 3). However, in many cases the association with the disease is weak. The agents most commonly implicated are chloramphenicol and phenylbutazone. Aplastic anaemia is more likely to occur after a second or subsequent exposure to the drug than after the first exposure.

Viruses are also implicated in the aetiology of aplastic anaemia, particularly hepatitis viruses. Up to 10 per cent of patients in Western series of aplastic anaemia, particularly in the younger age group, give a history of jaundice and/or hepatitic symptoms some 6 weeks before the pancytopenia develops. In many instances, disturbances of hepatocellular function have been demonstrated. The hepatitis is usually hepatitis B surface-antigen negative, but the precise aetiology of the hepatitis is normally unidentified. Hepatitis A and C are not clearly associated with the disease.

Various domestic and recreational drugs and chemicals have been implicated in the cause of aplastic anaemia. 3,4-Methylenedioxymethamphetamine ('Ecstasy') has been associated with transient aplastic anaemia. DDT and other insecticides, particularly lindane and pentachlorophenol, have been linked to aplastic anaemia, although the evidence is not strong.

Table 3 Drugs strongly associated with an increased risk of aplastic anaemia

Antibiotics	*Anticonvulsant*
Chloramphenicol	Hydantoins:
Sulphonamides:	Phenytoin
Salazopyrine	Mephenytoin
Co-trimoxazole	Carbamazepine
	Phenacemide
Anti-inflammatory agents	Ethosuximide
Phenylbutazone	
Oxyphenbutazone	*Psychotropic*
Indomethacin	Phenothiazines
Sulindac	Remoxipride
Diclofenac	
Piroxicam	*Antimalarial*
Penicillamine	Quinacrine (Mepacrine)
Gold salts	Maloprim
Thyrostatic	*Antidiabetic*
Carbimazole	Chlorpropamide
Thiouracils	Carbutamide
Potassium perchlorate	Tolbutamide

Note: Many of these drugs have also been associated with a variety of other blood dyscrasias, particularly neutropenia or agranulocytosis.

Incidence and epidemiology

Aplastic anaemia is a rare disease. In Europe and the United States the incidence is probably between 2 and 5 per million of the population per year. All age groups may be affected, possibly with peaks between 20 and 30 years, and again in older patients. There is a slight preponderance of males, possibly reflecting the greater risk amongst men of exposure to toxic substances at work. In the Far East the incidence of aplastic anaemia is much higher and the male preponderance much more obvious. This may be related to the greater use of chloramphenicol and the increased risk of hepatitis. The risk factors seem to be environmental rather than genetic, as people of the same ethnic groups in the West have a lower incidence.

Pathogenesis

The way in which the various agents bring about aplastic anaemia is unknown. The main defect is a failure of the pluripotent, haemopoietic stem cells in the bone marrow to proliferate and differentiate into mature blood cells. *In vitro* experiments with long-term bone marrow culture show that aplastic marrow stromal cells are able to support haemopoiesis from normal stem cells, but aplastic stem cells continue to grow abnormally on normal stroma. In addition, the effectiveness of immunosuppression as a primary treatment modality implies that an autoimmune process may contribute to stem-cell damage.

Diagnosis and pathology

The diagnosis of aplastic anaemia is made on the basis of findings in the peripheral blood and bone marrow. In the blood there is pancytopenia with no abnormal cells present. The anaemia is usually normocytic at presentation but may be macrocytic, even strikingly so, particularly in chronic cases. The reticulocyte count is low. Neutrophils are invariably reduced and the count may be very low. Circulating neutrophils may have rather heavy granulation, so-called 'toxic' granulation, and a high alkaline phosphatase content. The eosinophils and basophils are usually also depleted and monocytopenia is usual. The reduction in the lymphocyte count is more

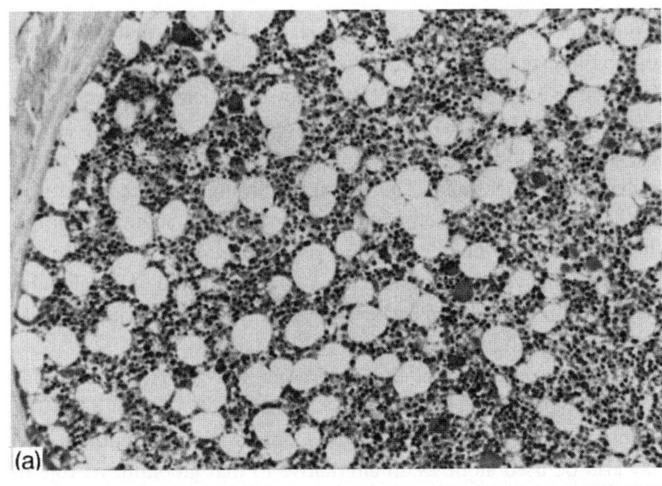

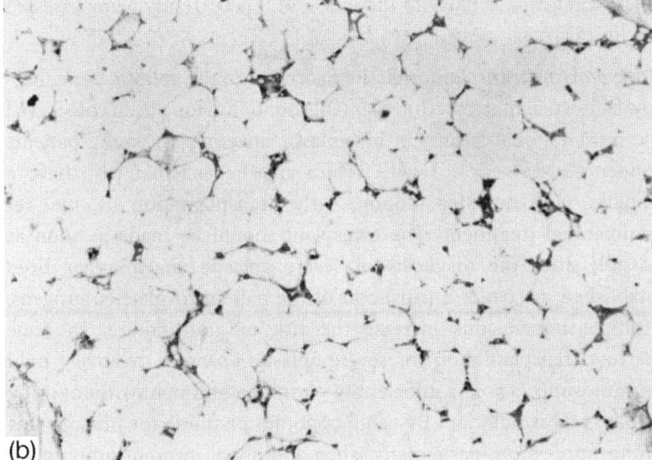

Fig. 1 Trephine biopsies of adult posterior iliac crest. (a) Normal marrow. (b) Severe aplastic anaemia.

variable; in children particularly it may be relatively high so that the total white-cell count may be normal. It is only when the differential white-cell count is done that the severe neutropenia is recognized. The platelet count is reduced and the relatively uniform smallness of the platelets is an indication that production has failed.

Bone marrow aspiration is usually easy; fragments are obtained which are fatty, and there is a reduction of haemopoietic cells in the trails. In aplastic anaemia there may be a patchy loss of cellularity throughout the marrow so that one aspirate may yield relatively normal-looking marrow. The diagnosis of aplastic anaemia should therefore not be made on a bone marrow aspirate alone, and assessment of cellularity should be made on a trephine biopsy, which shows replacement of the normal cellular marrow by fatty marrow. The reticulin network of the marrow is reduced commensurately with the reduction in the overall cellularity. Focal areas of preserved cellularity may be seen in the trephine, and it is one of the mysteries of aplastic anaemia that these foci do not repopulate the remainder of the marrow (Fig. 1). Residual cells also include normal lymphocytes, plasma cells, and macrophages. Malignant cells are not seen. Where haemopoiesis has not been completely abolished, the remaining areas may demonstrate abnormalities of differentiation, particularly in the red-cell series (dyserythropoiesis). In the early stages of aplastic anaemia, erythrophagocytosis by macrophages may be quite prominent.

Table 4 Criteria of severe aplastic anaemia*

Neutrophils	$<0.4 \times 10^9$/l
Platelets	$<10 \times 10^9$/l
Reticulocytes	$<10 \times 10^9$/l
Bone marrow	>80 per cent of remaining cells are non-myeloid

*Any three of the above four present for at least 2 weeks.

Clinical features

The clinical features of aplastic anaemia arise from the results of deficiencies of the cellular elements of the blood. Bleeding manifestations are often the first that take the patient to seek help from the doctor. Minor signs of the bleeding tendency present first—excessive bruising or a petechial rash may be noticed. Commonly, there is bleeding from the gums or nose. Haemorrhages in the buccal mucosa may occur, and retinal haemorrhages may be a portent of serious bleeding. The anaemia also develops slowly and the patient may complain only of mild fatigue or shortness of breath on marked exertion. Infections may be a presenting feature. Infections anywhere aggravate the effect of thrombocytopenia, particularly in the mouth. There are no specific physical findings in aplastic anaemia.

The progression of the disease is variable and depends upon the severity and completeness of the marrow damage. This has led to the establishment of criteria for severe aplastic anaemia (Table 4), which have proved to be very useful in stratifying patients when different treatments have been compared.

The identification of the group with severe aplastic anaemia is important because, for these patients, early bone marrow transplantation is the treatment of choice if a suitable donor is available. The subsequent course for patients who survive is variable. Spontaneous recovery, apparently to complete normality, may occur even after several years of pancytopenia. Other patients may remain stable for many years, and then gradually haemopoietic activity decreases further and they become anaemic, eventually dying of infection or bleeding. Abnormal clones of cells may develop with a greater frequency in these patients than in a normal population. Paroxysmal nocturnal haemoglobinuria is the most frequent clonal abnormality to evolve in aplastic anaemia (see Chapter 3.13). Myelodysplastic syndromes and acute myeloid leukaemia may also develop following aplastic anaemia.

Treatment

The treatment of aplastic anaemia has two main components. The first is to protect and support the patient from the consequences of pancytopenia and to keep him alive so that there may be a chance of spontaneous recovery. The second is to try to accelerate the recovery of the bone marrow by whatever means, without eradicating the chance of spontaneous recovery.

Support and protection

For the aplastic patient this depends upon reducing potential sources of infection to a minimum and replacing deficient cells by transfusion (see Chapter 16.117). Infections may arise from the environment or from sources of bacteria and other agents within the patient. As with all immunosuppressed patients, significant and lethal infections may arise from contamination with organisms that are not normally pathogenic. Exogenous infections are more likely in a hospital environment than at home, so any patient with aplastic anaemia admitted to hospital must be nursed in a clean and preferably sterile area.

Wearing an apron and hand washing by staff are important measures.

Endogenous infection arises from organisms carried within the patient, particularly in the upper respiratory passages and the gastrointestinal tract. Scrupulous skin and oral hygiene is essential. Repeated mouth washing with an antiseptic such as chlorhexidine or with hydrogen peroxide should be done regularly and after eating. The skin should be cleaned regularly with antiseptic. The role of bowel decontamination remains unclear.

Once an infection is established it is essential to treat it as soon as possible. Systemic antimicrobials must be given as soon as fever or signs of infection occur and appropriate samples have been sent to the laboratory. If an organism is isolated the antibiotics should be changed, according to the sensitivities of the organism. Because the most common exogenous infections arise from *Pseudomonas* or *Klebsiella* spp., and the endogenous ones from aerobic organisms of the gastrointestinal tract, the antimicrobials used in the first instance must be appropriate to those organisms. Most centres use a combination of aminoglycoside with a second antimicrobial likely to have activity against *Pseudomonas* spp. or a third-generation cephalosporin (suitable regimens are described in Section 16). Localized skin infections carry a particularly grave prognosis because it is difficult to achieve adequate antimicrobial concentrations in the oedematous lesion. A major problem in aplastic anaemia is to decide when to discontinue the antimicrobials. The patient may become afebrile and apparently well, but when the antimicrobials are stopped, infection by the original organism is all too likely to return unless the neutropenia recovers. Growth factors may play a role but there is little place for granulocyte transfusions (see Section 16).

Transfusion of red cells and platelets is the other main standby in the management of aplasia. Red-cell transfusions usually present few problems, but it must be remembered that the platelet count will fall and catastrophic haemorrhage may occur during transfusion. Platelets should always be given before starting a red-cell transfusion in the pancytopenic patient and preferably also at the end in order to avoid this complication. Repeated platelet transfusions usually lead to the development of antibodies and resistance to platelet concentrates. The antibodies may be anti-HLA or antiplatelet-specific antigens. Resistance is indicated by an inability to raise the platelet count by platelet transfusion. It may then become impossible to control bleeding manifestations without the use of appropriately matched platelet donations. White-cell filtration is valuable in patients with aplastic anaemia and appears to reduce the chances of sensitization. Platelets may be given either regularly or only when required to control bleeding episodes.

Further details of the management of patients with marrow failure are given in Section 16.

Specific measures

Immunosuppression A somewhat serendipitous series of observations led to the introduction of immunosuppressive treatment using antilymphocyte globulin. The rate of recovery after such treatment is usually slow, with few patients showing a response before about 3 months, and in some instances much later. Many patients treated in this way still require some transfusion support even a year or more after treatment, and may indeed continue with neutropenia and/or thrombocytopenia for many years, though independent of transfusion or hospital care. It is worth achieving even a modest improvement in blood count because, with neutrophil counts above 0.5×10^9/l and platelets above 30×10^9/l, an independent and relatively safe existence is possible. If the patient fails to respond to the first course of antilymphocyte globulin (usually prepared in a horse), a second course may be given. Some 50 per cent of patients respond to the first course with partial or complete remission, and about 40 per cent of non-responders will achieve some improvement with rabbit antilymphocyte globulin. The optimum timing of a second course still has to be determined but most groups wait about 4 months. There seems to be no advantage in giving more than a 5-day course of antilymphocyte globulin. Reactions during infusion of the globulin are common and serum sickness occurs in some 75 per cent of patients, requiring treatment with corticosteroids.

Steroids appear to offer little additional benefit. However, cyclosporin, 5 mg/kg per day, does appear to increase the rate of remission of aplastic anaemia when given after antilymphocyte globulin and may also be used alone as an alternative to that globulin. Its role in aplastic anaemia is likely to increase and it is currently being assessed in clinical trials.

Bone marrow transplantation Replacement of the aplastic bone marrow by normal marrow from a suitable donor has long been considered the most rational treatment for aplastic anaemia. In young patients (under 40 years or so) with severe aplastic anaemia who have a suitable HLA-matched donor, early transplantation is the recommended treatment. The transplant should be made as soon as possible after the diagnosis of severe aplastic anaemia has been established, to avoid sensitization of the patient to platelet antigens. Multiple transfusions increase the risk of graft failure. In bone marrow transplantation for severe aplastic anaemia, relatively mild immunosuppression is sufficient to permit engraftment without using whole-body irradiation. By using cyclophosphamide for pregraft immunosuppression, particularly when additional immunosuppression is given through antilymphocyte globulin, the risk of graft failure has been reduced to less than 10 per cent. Cyclosporin is given after bone marrow infusion to protect against rejection and to modify graft-versus-host disease. The success of HLA-matched, sibling transplants is now about 70 per cent, rising to better than 90 per cent for untransfused patients.

Other treatments

Androgens were the first drugs used in the treatment of aplastic anaemia that had any degree of success. High-dose anabolic (androgenic) steroids are given by mouth, but their usefulness is limited by hepatotoxicity (including the development of hepatocellular carcinoma and the formation of multiple venous lakes called peliosis hepatis) and virilization (Fig. 2). In patients who do respond it takes about 3 months before effects are seen and recovery of the blood count is thereafter slow. Occasionally, patients become androgen-dependent and stopping therapy leads to a relapse. For this reason, androgens should be tailed off slowly and the dose adjusted to response.

Congenital aplastic anaemia (Fanconi anaemia)

The most common of the inherited disorders which produce aplastic anaemia is that described by Fanconi in 1927. The disorder is inherited as an autosomal recessive and is associated with multiple developmental abnormalities, particularly of the skin and skeleton.

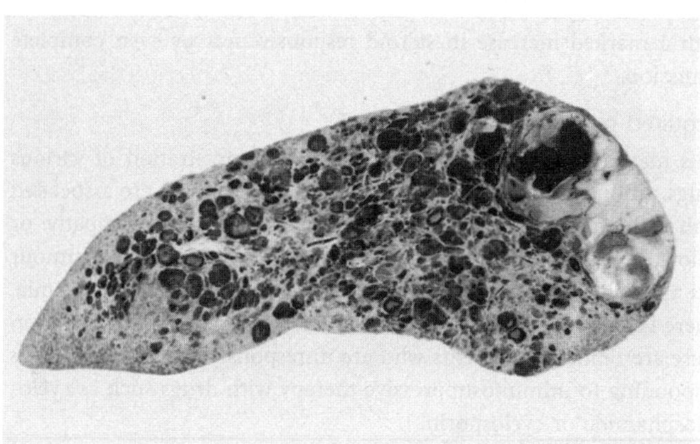

Fig. 2 Hepatocellular carcinoma in the liver of a patient with Fanconi anaemia treated for 4 years with anabolic steroids; the liver also shows multiple venous lakes (peliosis hepatis), another side-effect of anabolic steroids.

Haematological features

Patients with Fanconi anaemia usually have a normal or nearly normal blood count at birth and during infancy. The disease presents with the effects of pancytopenia, usually about the age of 5 years or later. Bleeding due to thrombocytopenia is the most common presentation, with anaemia second. The neutrophil count is often relatively well preserved for some years after severe thrombocytopenia and anaemia develop. The bone marrow becomes progressively hypocellular over the years.

Cytogenetic findings

The characteristic finding in Fanconi anaemia is multiple, non-specific abnormalities in the chromosomes, particularly when cells are stressed by exposure to DNA crosslinking agents. These consist mainly of chromatid breaks and aberrations. It appears that these lesions arise as a result of the failure of one of the DNA repair systems.

Clinical features

The features of the full-blown Fanconi anaemia are characteristic. In some cases, diagnosis may be difficult because of absence of the characteristic skeletal and skin features, and *formes frustes* probably exist. Infants are of low birth weight and remain small for age after birth. The skin is often mildly pigmented with areas of deeper pigmentation producing *café-au-lait* spots, sometimes with areas of depigmentation. Skeletal abnormalities occur in two-thirds of patients, particularly involving the bones of the forearm and thumbs. Abnormalities of the kidneys are also common. Mental development is usually normal.

Prognosis and treatment

The outlook in Fanconi anaemia is poor. Untreated, the disease is usually relentless. Treatment with anabolic steroids may bring about a remission of variable duration. The development of acute leukaemia is common and may be the presenting feature. Fanconi anaemia should be suspected in all children presenting with acute myeloid leukaemia under the age of 10 years. Its detection is important, at least for identifying the familial nature of the disease for the purpose of genetic counselling.

There are well-documented reports of patients with Fanconi anaemia going into spontaneous remission at the time of puberty, but this does not happen often and there is no way of predicting who will recover.

Bone marrow transplantation is the only curative form of treatment for these patients, but it carries special risks. The cells in Fanconi anaemia are very sensitive to the cyclophosphamide and irradiation used to immunosuppress patients before transplantation, and the doses given have to be greatly reduced to prevent severe skin and bowel toxicity. With these modifications the success of bone marrow transplants from HLA-matched donors is similar to that for acquired aplastic anaemia.

Aplastic presentation of malignant disease

There are a number of syndromes in which aplasia and acute leukaemia seem to be linked.

Acute lymphoblastic leukaemia of childhood

This may present in a form indistinguishable from aplastic anaemia. Blasts are not seen in the peripheral blood, and the bone marrow aspirate and trephine are hypocellular without any obvious infiltration by malignant cells. The aplasia in these children usually recovers rapidly, sometimes in response to corticosteroids. Some 6 to 8 weeks later leukaemic cells emerge in the peripheral blood. It is suggested that the aplasia is an early result of the leukaemia or possibly part of the body's reaction against leukaemia. It has also been suggested that corticosteroids should be given to all young children with aplastic anaemia as a diagnostic test for acute leukaemia. Whilst acute lymphoblastic leukaemia in childhood is the most common association, aplasia preceding acute myeloid leukaemia in this way has been described and adults are occasionally affected.

Hypoplastic myelodysplasia (see also Chapter 3.8)

Myelodysplasia may present with a hypocellular bone marrow.

Clonal disorders following aplastic anaemia

Some patients who survive for several years with aplastic anaemia may eventually develop acute leukaemia, though this is relatively rare (1–3 per cent). There may indeed be a period of apparent remission before the acute leukaemia develops, usually after a period of myelodysplasia. The emergence of clones associated with paroxysmal nocturnal haematuria has already been mentioned. Relapse or the emergence of an abnormal clone occurs in 25 to 40 per cent of patients with aplastic anaemia who have been treated with immunosuppression only.

Bone marrow failure affecting single cell lines

There are a number of conditions in which anaemia, neutropenia, or thrombocytopenia develop in isolation as a result of the failure to produce these cells by the bone marrow. The conditions may be inherited or acquired and the main disorders are listed in Table 5.

Pure red-cell aplasia (PRCA)

Pure red-cell aplasia is characterized by an anaemia with a marked reduction or absence of reticulocytes in which the neutrophils and platelet count are normal. The bone marrow is cellular, with normal granulopoiesis and megakaryocytes. There may be a complete absence of red-cell precursors or there may be precursors present up to a

Table 5 Bone marrow failure affecting single cell lines

Cause	Example
Red cell aplasia	
Inherited	Diamond-Blackfan syndrome
Idiopathic, acquired (?autoimmune)	With or without thymoma With other autoimmune disorders
Drug induced	Penicillamine Diphenylhydantoin Chlorpropamide Chloramphenicol
Virus induced	Aplastic crisis in haemolytic anaemia (Parvovirus) Transient erythroblastopenia in childhood
Riboflavin deficiency	Experimental
Neutropenia	
Inherited	Infantile genetic agranulocytosis (Kostmann syndrome) With pancreatic insufficiency (Schwachman–Diamond syndrome) Others
Idiopathic, acquired (? autoimmune)	?Cyclical
Drug induced	Thiazides Semisynthetic penicillins
Virus induced	Rubella
Amegakaryocytosis	
Congenital	With total absence of radii Isolated
Acquired	Variant of aplastic anaemia

certain stage of development but not beyond, so-called 'maturation arrest'. Both congenital and acquired forms exist.

Congenital pure red-cell aplasia (Diamond–Blackfan anaemia)

In most instances, anaemia is present at birth or is detected shortly afterwards. There is a profound reticulocytopenia, often with no reticulocytes present in the peripheral blood. There is no hepatosplenomegaly. The white-cell count and platelet counts are normal. Skeletal abnormalities may be present, of which triphalangeal thumb is the most common, but many children have no dysmorphic features. There are no disturbances of growth, of the skin, or other organs as are seen in Fanconi anaemia. The disorder is mainly sporadic or has an autosomal recessive inheritance. There is no chromosomal instability.

Treatment presents many problems. Most of these children, if treated early enough with corticosteroids, will respond and the haemoglobin level can be brought back to normal or maintained at normal levels after transfusion. However, if the condition is steroid-dependent, major problems may result from the continued use of corticosteroids in the doses necessary to maintain remission. Some of the side-effects may be reduced by using an intermittent regimen of corticosteroids on alternate days or even alternate weeks. Transfusion of the patients will permit normal growth but will produce all the other problems of iron overload, so that chelation therapy is required from an early stage.

During the course of the disease the spleen may enlarge and transfusion requirements increase. In these patients, splenectomy may reduce transfusion requirements and occasionally is associated with a marked increase in steroid responsiveness or even complete remission.

Acquired pure red-cell aplasia

This may occur *de novo* or following the administration of various drugs. About 10 to 15 per cent of the idiopathic cases are associated with a thymoma. The red-cell aplasia may precede, accompany, or follow the development of the thymoma, but excision of the tumour has a variable effect with no guarantee of recovery from the anaemia. There is an unpredictable responsiveness to corticosteroids; however, there are reports of patients who are unresponsive to corticosteroids responding to immunosuppressive therapy with drugs such as cyclophosphamide or cyclosporin.

Pure red-cell aplasia may also occur in association with acquired idiopathic hypogammaglobulinaemia and other autoimmune diseases. Occasionally, the direct antiglobulin test (Coombs' test) may be weakly positive, usually with complement on the surface of the red cell. There may be a severe thrombocytopenia in some cases. The presence of such autoimmune phenomena suggests that the patient has a better chance of responding to corticosteroids than in their absence. Pure red-cell aplasia may be associated with lymphomas, and evidence of an underlying lymphoma may be obtained by finding evidence of immunoglobulin or T-cell-receptor gene rearrangement in the marrow even when histological proof is lacking.

Erythroblastopenic anaemia in childhood

The 'aplastic crises' that occur in patients with haemolytic anaemia are usually due to infection with parvovirus and are covered in Chapter 3.19. Transient erythroblastopenia of childhood may also have a viral aetiology, though this is not so clearly demonstrated. The anaemia, with reticulocytopenia, usually occurs in children from 18 to 26 months of age (range 1–72 months). There is usually a history of preceding viral or bacterial illness. Recovery occurs within a few weeks of diagnosis, although the patient may need transfusion in the mean time.

Isolated defects in white-cell or platelet production

These conditions are described in Chapter 3.27 and are summarized in Table 5.

Further reading

Clarke, A.A., *et al.* (1998). Molecular genetics and Fanconi anaemia: new insights into old problems. *British Journal of Haematology*, **103**, 287-96.

Gordon-Smith, E. (1992). Bone marrow transplantation for acquired aplastic anaemia. In *Bone marrow transplantation in practice* (ed. J. Treleaven and J. Barrett), pp. 137–49. Churchill Livingstone, Edinburgh.

Marsh, J.C. (1998). Treatment options in severe aplastic anaemia. *Lancet*, **351**, 1830-1.

Chapter 3.13

Paroxysmal nocturnal haemoglobinuria

J. V. Dacie and L. Luzzatto

Paroxysmal nocturnal haemoglobinuria (**PNH**) is an uncommon acquired disorder, bearing some relation to aplastic anaemia, and characterized by the production of an abnormal line of blood cells that are unusually prone to lysis by complement. It affects both sexes and individuals of all racial groups. It is essentially a disease of adults, the majority of patients presenting between 20 and 40 years of age; it is rare, but not unknown, in childhood.

Aetiology and pathogenesis

Paroxysmal nocturnal haemoglobinuria is an acquired, clonal disease originating in a haemopoietic stem cell. It is possible to demonstrate that not only the patient's red cells, but also the granulocytes, the platelets, and usually the lymphocytes are abnormal. Although at one time in the evolution of the disease the abnormal red-cell progenitors largely replace normal red-cell progenitors—as happens in leukaemia—in PNH the abnormal clone gradually disappears in some patients, and if the patient has sufficient surviving normal stem cells he or she will eventually recover.

The relationship between PNH and aplastic anaemia is intriguing and uncertain. It is possible that marrow aplasia facilitates the growth of the PNH clone by reducing competition by normal stem cells. It may be that the PNH clone is able to escape from the pathogenetic mechanism, possibly immunological, that is suppressing normal stem-cell growth.

Biochemical basis of paroxysmal nocturnal haemoglobinuria

PNH is a beautiful example of biochemical research leading to an explanation of clinical observations. The most obvious abnormality of blood cells in PNH is the increased sensitivity of the red cells to complement-mediated lysis. However, it has become apparent that numerous surface proteins are either much reduced or completely lacking from PNH cells, and that all these proteins share the fact that they are attached to the cell membrane through the same chemical structure: a glucosylphosphatidylinositol (**GPI**) anchor. The somatic mutations in PNH are now known to affect the *PIG-A* gene that transfers *N*-acetylglucosamine to phosphatidylinositol, and thus cells belonging to the PNH clone are deficient in GPI-linked molecules.

Mechanism of haemolysis

The increased haemolysis in PNH is primarily intravascular and is thought to derive from continuous activation of the alternative pathway of complement activation. Why haemolysis should increase during sleep or intercurrent illness is unknown

Clinical findings

The onset of the disease is usually insidious, with gradually increasing symptoms of anaemia and perhaps slight jaundice, with or without the intermittent passage of dark urine (haemoglobinuria). In some cases, by contrast, an episode of massive haemoglobinuria, typically noticed first thing in the morning, may first bring the patient to the doctor. Some patients present simply with anaemia, or with attacks of abdominal pain, in which cases the diagnosis may be delayed considerably. Haemolysis may be exacerbated by infection, even a minor one such as the common cold, a blood transfusion, a surgical procedure, menstruation, exposure to cold, vaccine inoculations, and possibly 'stress'.

The physical signs are not distinctive. There is usually slight to moderate jaundice. The spleen is sometimes palpable a few centimetres below the costal margin and the liver may be slightly enlarged too.

The urine is red-brown to almost black in colour if it contains haemoglobin, methaemoglobin, or both. A constant finding, even in the absence of free haemoglobin, is haemosiderinuria—the presence in the urine deposit of numerous small granules giving a positive Prussian-blue reaction for free iron. The granules are derived from renal tubular cells that have taken in haemoglobin from the glomerular filtrate and, after the haemoglobin molecule has been broken down, retain the iron derived from haem in the form of haemosiderin. Despite the retention of iron, renal function is usually, although not invariably, well preserved.

Associated symptoms, signs, and complications

Many patients suffer from attacks of abdominal pain due to thrombosis occurring within small veins in the portal system. This varies from a feeling of vague discomfort to severe colic or cramp and may be accompanied by vomiting, which may persist for hours. Headaches are less common

Thrombosis and thromboembolism are in fact the most frequent cause of death in PNH. Veins almost anywhere in the body may be involved; particularly serious is major thrombosis within the portal system and intrahepatic venous thrombosis leading to the Budd–Chiari syndrome.

Some patients seem to be unusually susceptible to bacterial infections. This generally correlates with granulocytopenia, but there is no clear evidence of defective neutrophil function.

Pigment gallstones may form in patients with PNH and may lead to cholecystitis or obstructive jaundice. This seems to be less common than in other types of haemolytic anaemia, probably because most of the haemoglobin is excreted through the urine.

Patients may also present with iron deficiency due to haemosiderinuria.

Many patients suffering from PNH have a history of pancytopenia and may have been diagnosed originally as suffering from aplastic anaemia. However, this association takes several forms and the hypoplasia may precede or follow the development of the appearance of the PNH clone.

Leukaemia may develop in PNH but it is not common, the risk of transformation being around 1 per cent.

Course of the disease and chances of recovery

PNH is a very chronic disorder. The median survival is around 10 years. Interestingly, an appreciable proportion of PNH patients (perhaps 10–15 per cent) recover completely.

Blood picture

The characteristic finding is anaemia, neutropenia, and thrombocytopenia, accompanied by reticulocytosis. All these features are highly variable depending on the form and severity of the disease.

The blood film is usually unremarkable. Plasma haptoglobins are typically absent.

Diagnosis

The 'classical' test is the acidified serum test, often referred to as the Ham test, which demonstrates that a proportion of the patient's red cells are unusually sensitive to lysis by human complement. In the last few years flow cytometry has become a valuable diagnostic aid in PNH, by demonstrating the presence of two cell populations when either red cells or white cells are stained with antibodies having specificity for one of the GPI-linked proteins characteristically lacking from the surface of the abnormal cells.

From the clinical point of view it is important not to forget that PNH is a possible diagnosis in any patient presenting with anaemia of obscure origin.

Treatment

The only definitive treatment for PNH is bone marrow transplantation. In cases in which bone marrow failure has progressed to the stage of qualifying for a diagnosis of severe aplastic anaemia, and if an HLA-identical sibling is available, transplantation must therefore be regarded as the treatment of choice. For patients with haemolytic PNH, and for all those who do not have a potential donor, treatment must be supportive. Blood transfusion is imperative when exacerbation of haemolysis threatens life, but it should not be scheduled regularly. It is imperative to use on-line white-cell filters for all transfusions. Iron deficiency is common and should be treated.

Any patient with PNH who has experienced venous thrombosis, whether peripheral or hepatic, should be placed on prophylactic warfarin for as long as he or she has evidence of the disease, because there is serious risk of recurrence, and venous thrombosis is one of the main causes of death. There is no clear consensus on the use of anticoagulants in patients who have not suffered a clear venous thrombosis. For the treatment of hepatic venous thrombosis (Budd–Chiari), there is an immediate indication for thrombolytic therapy with tissue plasminogen activator.

Further reading

Hillmen, P., Lewis, S.M., Bessler, M., Luzzatto, L., and Dacie, J.V. (1995). *New England Journal of Medicine*, 333, 1253–8.

Packman, C.H. (1998). Pathogenesis and management of paroxysmal nocturnal haemoglobinuria. *Blood Reviews*, 1, 1–11.

The red cell

Chapter 3.14

Erythropoiesis and the normal red cell

D. J. Weatherall

The circulating red cells and their nucleated precursors in the bone marrow comprise a functional unit called the erythron.

The early stages of erythropoiesis

The red-cell precursors are derived from pluripotential stem cells. Using *in vitro* culture techniques with plasma clots or methylcellulose as supporting media and erythropoietin, it is possible to culture two populations of erythroid precursors from blood and bone marrow: colony-forming units, erythroid (CFU-E); and erythropoietin-dependent burst-forming units, or BFU-E. It is believed that the BFU-E form an amplification compartment, which can respond to the requirements for erythropoiesis by rapid contraction or expansion. The CFU-E mature directly into pronormoblasts, which are the first cells in the erythroid maturation pathway that can be recognized morphologically.

Morphological and biochemical development of the red cell

The total maturation time of the identifiable red-cell precursors in the bone marrow is approximately 7 days. The first 4 days are spent in cell division and the remaining 3 days are devoted to maturation and haemoglobin synthesis, during which the nucleus is extruded. The red-cell precursor, now called a reticulocyte, remains in the marrow for a further 24 h and then moves into the peripheral circulation where it matures into a red cell in approximately 1 day. The 1 per cent of the total red-cell mass destroyed every 24 h are replaced, in normal individuals, by a comparable number of reticulocytes.

The immediate precursors of the reticulocyte are the normoblasts, which gradually accumulate haemoglobin during their differentiation. Once they lose their nucleus the reticulocyte is formed. It is estimated that between 5 and 10 per cent of the red-cell precursors are lost during their passage through the marrow. In certain disorders of red-cell maturation this level of 'ineffective erythropoiesis' is considerably elevated above the normal baseline.

During red-cell development, DNA and RNA synthesis ceases, the mitochondria and RNA are lost, and the cell is then able to metabolize glucose only through the anaerobic Embden–Meyerhof pathway. In addition, the mature cell has a hexose monophosphate shunt that normally provides little energy but is of great importance in protecting the cell against oxidative damage.

Regulation of erythropoiesis

Erythropoiesis is stimulated by the hormone erythropoietin, which is produced in response to hypoxia by interstitial cells in the kidney. In fetal life it appears to be produced mainly in the liver. During the

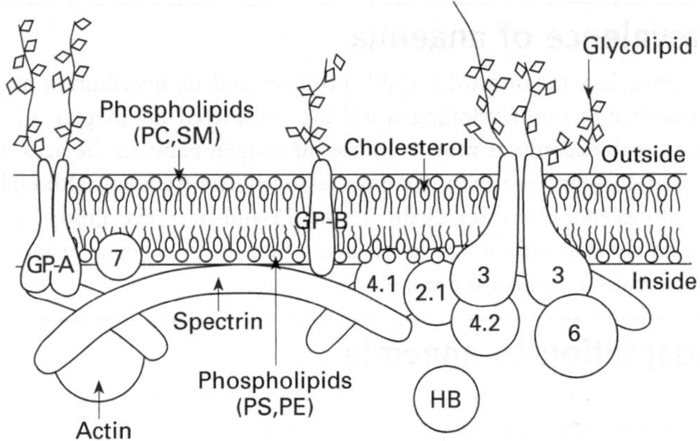

Fig. 1 Diagram of the red-cell membrane showing the relation of integral and internal membrane proteins to the lipid bilayer. The numbers refer to individual membrane proteins. GPA and GPB are glycophorins A and B, respectively; PC, phosphatidylcholine; SM, sphingomyelin; PS, phosphatidylserine; PE, phosphatidylethanolamine.
(Reproduced with permission from Brain, M.C. (1982). Blood and its disorders, 2nd edn (ed. R.M. Hardisty and D.J. Weatherall), p. 45. Blackwell Scientific, Oxford.)

transition from BFU-E to CFU-E the red-cell progenitors become increasingly sensitive to erythropoietin, the major physiological regulator of red-cell production.

The fact that erythropoiesis is regulated by a hormone produced by the kidney has important clinical implications. For example, the anaemia of renal disease is partly due to defective production of erythropoietin. Some renal tumours synthesize erythropoietin and cause polycythaemia. Severe hypoxia, as occurs in chronic lung disease or congenital heart disease, is associated with a marked drive to erythropoietin production and hence a variable increase in red-cell output. Recombinant erythropoietin has proved to be of great value in patients with a variety of haematological disorders and also in chronic renal failure.

Several factors are essential for the normal function of the bone marrow including iron, vitamin B_{12}, folate, and probably certain other vitamins including pyridoxine, ascorbic acid, riboflavin, and vitamin E.

The red cell

The mature red cell is a biconcave disc, 7.5 μm in diameter, 2.5 μm thick at the periphery, and 1 μm thick at the centre. This shape provides an optimal surface area for respiratory exchange. The cell is composed of about 70 per cent water, the remainder consisting of haemoglobin and small amounts of lipid, sugar, and enzyme proteins.

The red cell maintains itself in the circulation for about 120 days and keeps its haemoglobin in a state suitable for oxygen transport during this time. Its three major components are membrane, haemoglobin, and metabolic pathways.

Membrane (see also Chapter 3.22)

The red-cell membrane is a lipid bilayer with intercollated proteins (Fig. 1). There are two main classes of membrane proteins: the peripheral proteins and the integral membrane proteins. The former make up an extensive submembranous reticulum called the red-cell cytoskeleton, which is responsible for the shape, integrity, and flexibility of the cell membrane. The proteins of the cytoskeleton are described in Chapter 3.22. The integral membrane proteins consist of an anion transport protein, a glucose transport protein, and the sialoglycoproteins, glycophorins A, B, and C.

The critical functions of maintaining red-cell shape and deformability are mediated by these different components of the membrane and depend on a constant supply of energy. In later sections we shall see how primary or secondary abnormalities of the membrane lead to changes in function and hence to premature destruction of red cells.

Haemoglobin

The major haemoglobin of adult red cells, haemoglobin A, is a tetramer of two α- and two β-chains consisting of 141 and 146 amino acids, respectively. The heterogeneity and genetic control of haemoglobin is considered in Chapter 3.19. Each globin chain is attached to a haem molecule, a protoporphyrin ring that contains an iron atom and which can reversibly bind oxygen. The oxygen binding of whole blood is ideally suited for oxygen transport. The sigmoid shape of the curve, which reflects the allosteric properties of haemoglobin, is beautifully adapted to oxygen transport.

The position of the oxygen dissociation curve can be modified in several ways. One major influence is that oxygen affinity is decreased with increasing CO_2 tensions (the Bohr effect). Increasing concentrations of 2,3-diphosphoglycerate (**2,3-DPG**), a constituent of the red cell, shift the oxygen dissociation curve to the right, that is, cause a state of reduced oxygen affinity, while diminishing concentrations have the opposite effect.

Red-cell metabolism

The mature red cell has no nucleus or mitochondria and no tricarboxylic acid cycle. Its major source of energy is the glycolytic Embden–Meyerhof pathway. Glucose is metabolized via this pathway with the production of lactate, with a net gain of 2 mol of ATP and the reduction of 2 mol of NAD to NADH per mol of glucose. The other energy pathway is the hexose monophosphate shunt in which there is a reduction of 2 mol of NADP to NADPH per mol of glucose. In addition, there is a 'metabolic siding' in the Embden–Meyerhof pathway that is regulated by diphosphoglycerate mutase and generates 2,3 DPG.

The metabolic functions of the red cell can be summarized as follows. First, it must maintain its osmotic stability through the activity of its membrane pumps. This critical transport function is driven by ATP. Second, it must maintain the iron of haemoglobin in the reduced state, by reducing Fe^{3+} to Fe^{2+}. The enzyme system involved, methaemoglobin reductase, is driven by NADH. Third, 2, 3-DPG must be generated to act as a modulator of haemoglobin function (see below). Fourth, the sulphydryl groups of haemoglobin and membrane proteins must be protected by maintaining adequate amounts of reduced glutathione. This system is dependent on NADPH generated from NADP via the pentose pathway. Finally, NAD must be synthesized from nicotinic acid, glutamine, glucose, and inorganic phosphate, and NADP formed by the reaction of NAD and ADP. A breakdown of any of these critical metabolic functions causes shortening of the red-cell survival and/or abnormal oxygen transport.

The lifespan of red cells

The lifespan of red cells, normally about 120 days, can be assessed by several methods. In clinical practice, labelling a sample of circulating cells with ^{51}Cr is the most convenient technique. The normal $t_{1/2}$ of

^{51}Cr-labelled cells is 25 to 36 days. By the use of suitable external counters it is possible to determine the sites of red-cell destruction.

Red-cell destruction and the fate of haemoglobin

In health, erythrocytes are phagocytosed by the reticuloendothelial cells of the spleen, liver, and elsewhere. The changes of the ageing red cell that allow them to be identified and removed from the circulation are still not fully understood.

Once in reticuloendothelial cells, the haemoglobin liberated from the phagocytosed red cells is degraded. The first stage is the splitting up of haem and globin. The iron is split off from the haem molecule and reutilized for haemoglobin synthesis. Similarly, the globin fraction is broken down and the amino acids reutilized. Haem is converted to biliverdin by the enzyme haem oxygenase. One molecule of carbon monoxide is produced with each biliverdin molecule. The subsequent degradation of biliverdin via the action of biliverdin reductase, and the chemistry of the production and excretion of bilirubin is considered in detail in Section 5.

Further reading

Bull, B.S. (1994). Morphology of the erythron. In *Williams hematology* (ed. E. Beutler, M.A. Lichtman, B.S. Coller, and T.J. Kipps). McGraw-Hill, New York.

Erslev, A.J. (1994). Production and destruction of erythrocytes. In *Williams hematology* (ed. E. Beutler, M.A. Lichtman, B.S. Coller, and T.J. Kipps). McGraw-Hill, New York.

Testa, N.G. and Molineux, G. (1993). *Haemopoiesis: a practical approach.* IRL Press/Oxford University Press, Oxford.

Chapter 3.15

Anaemia: pathophysiology, classification, and clinical features

D. J. Weatherall

Anaemia is usually defined as a reduction of the haemoglobin concentration, red-cell count, or packed-cell volume (PCV) to below normal levels.

The definition of anaemia

The World Health Organization recommends that anaemia should be considered to exist in adults whose haemoglobin levels are lower than 13 g/dl (males) or 12 g/dl (females). Children aged 6 months to 6 years are considered anaemic who have haemoglobin levels below 11 g/dl and those aged 6 to 14 years below 12 g/dl. These guidelines are rather arbitrary, and a major problem is that there may be many apparently normal individuals whose haemoglobin concentration is below their optimal level.

Prevalence of anaemia

Anaemia is a major world health problem and its distribution and prevalence in the developing world are considered in Chapter 3.15. In general, anaemia is most common in women between the ages of 15 and 44 years and then becomes relatively less frequent, although the prevalence increases again in the 75-and-over age group. Interestingly, it is only in the latter group that the prevalence in males and females is almost the same.

Adaptation to anaemia

The function of the red cell is to carry oxygen between the lungs and the tissues. However, tissue oxygenation is the result of a complex series of interactions of different organ systems of which the red cell is only one. Obviously the cardiac output, ventilatory function, and state of the capillaries are of great importance as well. A decreased capacity of any of these components may be compensated for by increased activity of the others in an attempt to maintain tissue oxygenation.

By reducing the oxygen-carrying capacity of blood, anaemia tends to reduce the arteriovenous oxygen difference and this may be compensated for by the following mechanisms: (i) modulation of oxygen affinity; (ii) redistribution of flow between different organs; (iii) increase in cardiac output; and (iv) reduction of mixed venous oxygen tension to increase the arteriovenous oxygen difference.

Intrinsic red-cell adaptation

Anaemia, by lowering the haemoglobin concentration, proportionately reduces the oxygen-carrying capacity of the blood. As a response to this there is an increase in 2,3-diphosphoglycerate (2,3-DPG) concentration in the red cell, shifting the dissociation curve to the right, thereby enhancing tissue oxygen delivery by up to 40 per cent.

Local changes in tissue perfusion

In anaemia there is vasoconstriction of the vessels of the skin and kidney; this mechanism has little effect on renal function. The organs that gain from the redistribution seem to be mainly the myocardium, brain, and muscle.

Cardiovascular and pulmonary changes

When the haemoglobin level falls below 7 to 8 g/dl there is an increase in cardiac output, both at rest and after exercise. Vasodilatation plays the dominant role in this response, but the reduction in blood viscosity produced by a relatively low red-cell mass may contribute.

In extreme cases or in those with cardiac disease, symptoms of heart failure may develop. At this stage the plasma volume is almost always increased.

Theoretically, an increase in respiratory rate should not improve the oxygenation of the tissues. Curiously, however, severe anaemia is associated with dyspnoea. Although in some patients this may be related to incipient cardiac failure, in most cases it appears to be an inappropriate response to hypoxia which is centrally mediated.

Clinical manifestations and classification of anaemia

Clinical effects of anaemia

Because anaemia reduces tissue oxygenation it is not surprising that it is associated with widespread organ dysfunction and hence an extremely varied clinical picture. The picture depends, of course, on whether the anaemia is of rapid or more insidious onset.

After acute blood loss the red-cell mass and plasma volume are reduced proportionately and the symptoms are mainly of volume depletion. Hence the picture of rapid blood loss is characterized by the typical syndrome of shock, with collapse, dyspnoea, tachycardia, a poor volume pulse, reduced blood pressure, and marked peripheral vasoconstriction.

With anaemia of a more insidious onset, the compensatory mechanisms outlined above have time to come into play. In mild anaemia there may be no symptoms or simply increased fatigue and slight pallor. As the anaemia becomes more marked the symptoms and signs gradually appear. Pallor is best discerned in the mucous membranes; the nailbeds and palmar creases, although often said to be useful sites for detecting anaemia, are relatively insensitive for this purpose. Cardiorespiratory symptoms and signs include exertional dyspnoea, tachycardia, palpitations, angina or claudication, night cramps, increased arterial pulsation, capillary pulsation, a variety of cardiac murmurs, reversible cardiac enlargement, and, if cardiac failure occurs, basal crepitations, peripheral oedema, and ascites. Neuromuscular involvement is reflected by headache, vertigo, light-headedness, faintness, tinnitus, roaring in the ears, cramps, increased cold sensitivity, and haemorrhages in the retina. Acute anaemia may occasionally give rise to papilloedema. Gastrointestinal symptoms include loss of appetite, nausea, constipation, and diarrhoea. Genito-urinary involvement causes menstrual irregularities, urinary frequency, and loss of libido. There may be a low-grade fever.

In the elderly, in whom associated degenerative arterial disease is common, anaemia may present with the onset of cardiac failure. Alternatively, previously undiagnosed coronary narrowing may be unmasked by the onset of angina. Other symptoms of arterial degenerative disease may be also exacerbated or unmasked; intermittent claudication and a variety of neurological pictures associated with cerebral arteriosclerosis for example. It is important that anaemia is recognized as a contributing factor to the symptoms of these degenerative diseases as its correction may frequently bring about considerable symptomatic improvement.

Table 1 The main groups of anaemias classified according to the underlying cause

Reduced red-cell production:	*Increased rate of red-cell destruction:*
Defective precursor proliferation	Haemolysis
Defective precursor maturation	Loss of red cells from the circulation:
Defective proliferation and maturation	Bleeding

Table 2 Main causes of anaemia due to defective production of red cells

Reduced proliferation of precursors	*Defective maturation of precursors*
Iron deficiency anaemia	Nuclear maturation:
Anaemia of chronic disorders:	Vitamin B_{12} deficiency
Infections, malignancy, collagen	Folate deficiency
disease, etc	Erythroleukaemia
Reduced erythropoietin production:	Cytoplasmic maturation:
Renal disease	Iron deficiency
Reduced oxygen requirements:	Disorders of globin synthesis
Hypothyroidism	Disorders of haem and/or iron metabolism
Hypopituitarism	Disorders of porphyrin metabolism
Reduced O_2 affinity of haemoglobin	Unknown mechanism:
Primary disease of the bone marrow:	Congenital dyserythropoietic anaemias
Aplastic anaemia:	Infection
primary	Toxins and chemicals
secondary to drugs, irradiation, chemicals, toxins, etc.	
Pure red-cell hypoplasia	
Infiltrative disorders:	
leukaemia	
lymphoma	
secondary carcinoma	
myelofibrosis	

Causes and classification of anaemia

A reduction in the red-cell mass can result from either defective production of red cells or an increased rate of cell loss, either by premature destruction or bleeding. Decreased production of red cells may result from a reduced rate of precursor proliferation in the bone marrow or from failure of maturation leading to their intramedullary destruction, namely ineffective erythropoiesis. Based on this approach a very simple pathophysiological classification of anaemia can be derived (Table 1) in which the causes are divided into failure of red-cell proliferation, defective maturation, haemolysis, and blood loss.

Anaemia due to defective proliferation of red-cell precursors

The major causes of this group of anaemias are an inadequate supply of iron, primary diseases of the bone marrow that involve stem cells or later erythroid precursors, or a reduction in the amount of erythropoietin reaching the red-cell precursors (Table 2).

Iron deficiency results in defective erythroid proliferation and also in abnormal maturation of the red-cell precursors due to defective haemoglobin synthesis. Chronic inflammatory disorders and related conditions also interfere with the iron supply to precursors, probably by blocking the release of catabolized red-cell iron from reticulo-endothelial cells. The basic defect in iron-deficiency anaemia and that due to inflammation is similar, therefore, in that the supply of iron is inadequate to meet the requirements for erythropoiesis. Defective proliferation of red-cell precursors can also result from any of the causes of bone marrow failure (Table 2).

Finally, decreased proliferation of the red-cell precursors may result from erythropoietin deficiency. The most common cause is chronic renal failure. A similar mechanism may be involved in conditions in which the tissue requirement for oxygen is reduced. These include various endocrine disorders such as hypothyroidism and hypopituitarism. It may also explain the mild anaemia associated with haemoglobin variants with decreased oxygen affinity.

As a group, the hypoproliferative anaemias are associated with a low reticulocyte count and defective proliferation of the bone marrow precursors. The red cells are usually normochromic and normocytic, although there may be a mild macrocytosis. If the anaemia is due to iron deficiency, the cells are hypochromic. If granulopoiesis is normal, the defect in red-cell proliferation is reflected by an increase in the myeloid:erythroid (M/E) ratio.

Defective red-cell maturation

Defects of red-cell maturation may involve primarily nuclear or cytoplasmic maturation (Table 2). Those involving nuclear maturation include vitamin B_{12} and folic acid deficiency and other causes of megaloblastic anaemia, and some of the primary marrow disorders including erythroleukaemia. The important causes of defective cytoplasmic maturation include the inherited disorders of globin synthesis, the thalassaemia syndromes, and the genetic and acquired defects of iron metabolism that characterize the sideroblastic anaemias. There are other genetic defects of red-cell maturation, the congenital dyserythropoietic anaemias, in which the aetiology is unknown.

The main pathological mechanism common to all the anaemias that result from maturation abnormalities is ineffective erythropoiesis. There is marked erythroid proliferation, but many of the precursors are destroyed in the bone marrow before they enter the circulation. Hence, the characteristic finding is marked erythroid hyperplasia with a reduction in the M/E ratio, associated with a low reticulocyte count. Because of the significant intramedullary destruction of precursors there is usually an elevated level of bilirubin and lactate dehydrogenase and there are nearly always morphological abnormalities of the red-cell precursors. The anaemias that are associated with abnormal nuclear maturation, such as those due to vitamin B_{12} and folic acid deficiency, are characterized by megaloblastic erythropoiesis and macrocytic red cells, while those caused by abnormal cytoplasmic maturation are characterized by normoblastic hyperplasia and hypochromic and microcytic red cells.

Blood loss

The clinical picture associated with an acute loss of a large volume of blood is that of hypovolaemic shock.

Anaemias due to chronic blood loss may develop very insidiously and cause considerable diagnostic problems. Chronic blood loss from the gastrointestinal tract or uterus of more than 15 to 20 ml per day produces a state of negative iron balance (see Chapter 3.16). Assuming that the patient starts with a normal body store of iron, which is usually in the region of 1 g, the bone marrow will be able to maintain a normal haemoglobin level until the iron stores are totally depleted. At this stage there is no demonstrable iron in the bone marrow, the plasma iron level starts to fall, and then later the haemoglobin level starts to fall. The typical red cell changes may only develop later.

Haemolytic anaemia

When the lifespan of red cells is shortened there is a compensatory increased rate of red-cell production. This is reflected by a raised reticulocyte count and a macrocytosis due to the presence of young cells in the peripheral circulation. Because of the increased rate of red-cell destruction, there is an increased production of bilirubin, which leads to mild icterus and the presence of increased amounts of urobilinogen in the urine and stool. Thus the haemolytic anaemias are characterized by a variable degree of anaemia, a reticulocytosis, and hyperbilirubinaemia. Their causes and pathophysiology are considered in detail in Chapter 3.21.

It should be remembered that many anaemias associated with abnormal proliferation or maturation of red cells have a haemolytic component. For example, there may be a slightly shortened red-cell survival time in patients with pernicious anaemia or thalassaemia and yet there may be a very poor reticulocyte response. Similarly, there is a haemolytic component in the anaemia due to inflammation or malignancy, but again the marrow response is poor. In such cases it may be necessary to measure the lifespan of the red cells directly in order to determine the magnitude of the haemolytic component as compared to defective proliferation or maturation.

General approach to the anaemic patient

Clinical assessment

The clinical assessment of patients with anaemia has two main objectives. First, it is essential to determine the degree of disability caused by the anaemia and hence how quickly treatment must be started. Second, as much information as possible about the likely cause of the anaemia must be obtained from a detailed clinical history and physical examination. There is no place for the 'blind' treatment of anaemia without first establishing the cause.

In assessing the severity of the anaemia and how urgently treatment should be instituted, a detailed history of the patient's exercise tolerance must be obtained. Similarly, a full cardiac and respiratory examination should be made. The finding of profound anaemia with signs of cardiac failure indicates that urgent treatment is required. If the anaemia is associated with marked splenomegaly there will almost certainly be an increased blood volume and, particularly if there are already signs of cardiac failure, the patient may well go into acute left ventricular failure if transfused. Severely ill patients with profound anaemia require immediate treatment in an environment where they can be under constant observation, have regular measurements of the central venous pressure, and where they can be managed by experienced clinical and nursing staff.

An account of history-taking and clinical examination in patients with haematological disorders was given in Chapter 3.1. It cannot be emphasized too strongly that in many cases the anaemia is a symptom of a non-haematological disorder.

Haematological investigation

A preliminary blood count and blood film examination should classify anaemia into hypochromic–microcytic, and macrocytic or normochromic, normocytic varieties (Table 3). In middle-aged women with a history of several pregnancies or heavy menstrual loss it is reasonable to assume that a hypochromic anaemia is due to iron deficiency and treat them with iron without further investigation. However, hypochromic anaemia in males or young or postmenopausal women always suggests blood loss and should be investigated accordingly. If there is any doubt about a hypochromic anaemia being due to iron deficiency, the serum iron level and total iron-binding capacity should be established. Hypochromic anaemia with a normal serum iron suggests a genetic or acquired defect in haemoglobin synthesis, common causes being thalassaemia and sideroblastic anaemia. The diagnosis of a macrocytic anaemia always requires further investigation and should be followed up with a bone marrow examination. A macrocytosis with a normoblastic bone marrow may result from alcohol abuse, haemolysis, or, occasionally, one of the refractory anaemias with hyperplastic bone marrow (see Chapter 3.20). Macrocytic anaemias with megaloblastic bone marrows are usually due to vitamin B_{12} or folate deficiency and should be investigated accordingly. If there is macrocytosis with a reticulocytosis, hyperbilirubinaemia, and a normoblastic marrow, a haemolytic anaemia is likely.

The normochromic, normocytic anaemias often cause more diagnostic difficulty. Some help can be gained from a determination of whether the white-cell and platelet counts are normal. If there is

Table 3 The main causes of anaemia classified according to the associated red-cell changes

Hypochromic–microcytic (reduced MCV, MCH, and MCHC)
Genetic:
Thalassaemia
Sideroblastic anaemia
Acquired:
Iron deficiency
Sideroblastic anaemia
Chronic disorders (mildly hypochromic, occasionally)
Normochromic–macrocytic (increased MCV)
With megaloblastic marrow:
Vitamin B_{12} or folate deficiency
With normoblastic marrow:
Alcohol, myelodysplasia
Polychromatophilic–macrocytic (increased MCV)
Haemolysis
Normochromic–normocytic (normal indices)
Chronic disorders:
Infection, malignancy, collagen disease, rheumatoid arthritis
Renal failure
Hypothyroidism, hypopituitarism
Aplastic anaemia or primary red-cell hypoplasia
Primary disease of bone marrow, leukaemia, myelosclerosis, infiltration with other tumours
Leucoerythroblastic (indices usually normal)
Myelosclerosis
Leukaemia
Metastatic carcinoma

associated neutropenia and thrombocytopenia, a primary disease of the bone marrow is likely and bone marrow examination should be made to determine whether there is hypoplasia of the various precursor forms, hypoplastic or aplastic anaemia, or whether the pancytopenia results from infiltration of the bone marrow as occurs in the various forms of leukaemia. If there are nucleated red cells or young white cells on the peripheral film (that is, a leucoerythroblastic picture), a bone marrow examination is essential as this type of reaction usually indicates infiltration of the bone marrow with abnormal cells, either as part of a primary marrow disease such as leukaemia, or metastatic carcinoma. In the normochromic–normocytic anaemias in which the white-cell count and platelet count are normal, it is also helpful to make a bone marrow analysis. The most common cause is anaemia of chronic disorders. Another particularly common cause is chronic renal failure. After these conditions have been excluded, there remain the chronic anaemias associated with endocrine deficiencies (see Chapter 3.40) or the primary red-cell hypoplasias.

The management of anaemia

The management of specific forms of anaemia is described in detail in subsequent chapters. However, a few principles can be outlined here. In general, a cause should always be sought before treatment is instituted. As mentioned above, most cases of iron-deficiency anaemia require further investigation for a source of blood loss. If there is a clear-cut history of poor diet, multiple pregnancies, or obvious uterine bleeding, it is reasonable to start iron therapy and observe the haemoglobin level both during the period of treatment and for some months after iron therapy has been stopped. A rise in the haemoglobin level of approximately 1 g/dl per week indicates a full haematological response. In the megaloblastic anaemias it is quite reasonable to start treatment with vitamin B_{12} and folic acid once a diagnosis has been established and blood samples have been obtained for determining serum folate and B_{12} levels. The precise cause of the megaloblastic anaemia can be established at leisure once these samples have been obtained. A brisk reticulocyte response 5 to 7 days after initiating therapy suggests that there will be a full restoration of the haemoglobin level to normal. Failure of response of a hypochromic anaemia to adequate iron therapy should be managed by first finding out whether the iron is being taken and, if so, by determining the serum iron level. If it is normal, causes of hypochromic anaemia that are not associated with iron deficiency, thalassaemia and sideroblastic anaemia for example, should be sought. Similarly, refractory macrocytic anaemias require detailed analysis of the bone marrow morphology as there may be an underlying preleukaemic state.

Blood transfusion should always be avoided unless the haemoglobin level is dangerously low, when it is reasonable to transfuse the patient up to a safe level and then allow the haemoglobin to return to normal following appropriate treatment of the underlying cause. The decision whether to transfuse an anaemic patient depends mainly on the severity of the anaemia and its cause. For example, a young patient with a haemoglobin of 5 g/dl who is shown to have an active duodenal ulcer should probably be transfused because they would be at severe risk from a further brisk bleed from the ulcer. On the other hand, a patient of similar age with a similar haemoglobin level due to chronic nutritional iron deficiency might well be allowed to restore their haemoglobin level on oral iron therapy.

Occasionally, patients present in gross congestive cardiac failure with profound anaemia. This picture is usually seen in elderly patients with long-standing pernicious anaemia or iron deficiency. This type of condition still carries a high mortality and requires urgent treatment. Such profoundly anaemic patients require transfusing up to a safe level, namely a haemoglobin value of 6 to 8 g/dl. This can usually be achieved by the slow transfusion of two or three units of red cells with the intravenous administration of a potent diuretic such as frusemide with each unit. Ideally a central venous-pressure line should be inserted before the transfusion is started. In extreme cases an exchange transfusion may be needed.

Further reading

Oski, F.A. (1993). Differential diagnosis of anemia. In *Hematology of infancy and childhood* (ed. D.G. Nathan and F.A. Oski), pp. 346–53. Saunders, Philadelphia, PA.

Chapter 3.16

Iron metabolism and its disorders

M. J. Pippard

Iron is required by all cells, yet the chemical reactivity that underlies its requirement in many biological oxidation–reduction reactions carries with it the potential, when present in excess, for causing life-threatening tissue damage. It is thus not surprising that both iron

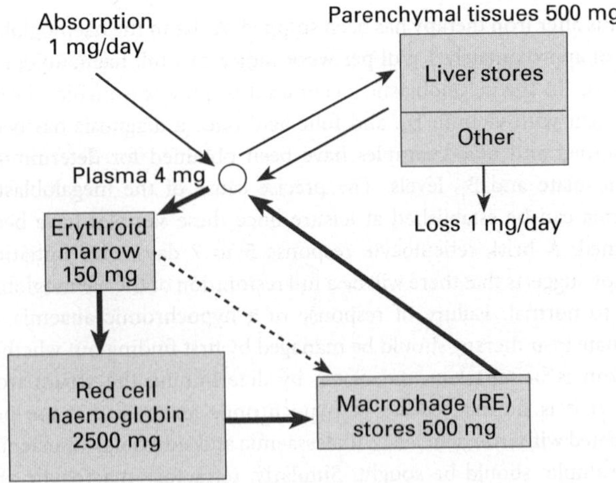

Fig. 1 The principal metabolic pathways of iron. These are dominated by iron supply for erythropoiesis and turnover of iron from senescent red cells (heavy arrows). The normal minor component of ineffective marrow erythropoiesis is shown by the broken line.

deficiency and iron overload affect many body systems, with a wide range of clinical manifestations.

Distribution of body iron

Iron-containing compounds may be separated into those in which iron has a vital functional role, and those that maintain body iron homeostasis through iron transport and iron storage. All three groups need to be considered when assessing disturbances of iron status.

Functional iron-containing compounds

Ferrous iron is an essential component of haem, allowing haemoglobin and myoglobin to bind oxygen reversibly as it is transported to, and stored in, the tissues. Of the 3 to 4 g of iron normally present in adults, 60–70 per cent is in the haemoglobin of circulating red cells and bone-marrow erythroid precursors, with another 10 per cent in the myoglobin of muscle cells. Other functional haem- or iron–sulphur-containing proteins account for less than 5 per cent of body iron.

Proteins of iron transport and storage

The redox activity of iron, upon which oxidative metabolism depends, is potentially toxic through its capacity to catalyse the production of damaging oxygen free radicals. In addition, any 'free' iron risks conversion to highly insoluble, and biologically unavailable, ferric hydroxide. These chemical constraints have been met by the evolution of specialized proteins for plasma iron transport (transferrin), cellular uptake of transferrin-bound iron (transferrin receptors), and iron storage (ferritin). Transferrin and ferritin hold ferric iron in a soluble, relatively non-toxic, and available form. As iron stores accumulate, there is an increasing tendency for cytoplasmic ferritin to undergo partial lysosomal degradation to form insoluble haemosiderin. This second form of storage iron is responsible for the Prussian-blue staining of iron-rich tissues with Perls' reagent. Only a tiny fraction of the total body iron (less than 0.1 per cent) is bound to plasma transferrin. By contrast, storage iron may normally be up to 1 g, but the amount is variable and it may be much lower or absent. It is found mainly in macrophages and hepatocytes, as shown in Fig. 1, which also illustrates the principal pathways of iron exchange.

Iron exchange

Body iron is normally rigorously conserved and reutilized (Fig. 1) and there is no active iron-excretion mechanism. Iron absorption must therefore be regulated to balance small, unavoidable losses (approximately 1 mg each day in exfoliated mucosal and skin cells, and insensible blood losses from the gut), and increased physiological requirements associated with growth, menstruation, and pregnancy.

Iron absorption

Dietary iron is approximately 6 mg/1000 kcal. However, the overall bioavailability of the iron (about 15 per cent in 'Western' diets) is more critical than the absolute amount, and is dependent upon the dietary make-up and gut luminal factors. Non-haem iron, which predominates in vegetable foods, forms the majority in most diets. Its absorption is enhanced by vitamin C and decreased by tea, bran, and phytates. By contrast, small amounts of dietary haem iron, derived from foods of animal origin, are relatively well absorbed. Iron balance is thus more precarious, and iron deficiency more likely, in people eating a diet low in animal foods.

Internal iron exchange

Iron movements around the body are normally dominated by the need to supply adequate iron for haemoglobin synthesis in developing erythroblasts (Fig. 1). Up to 90 per cent of plasma iron is taken up by these cells. At the end of their lifespan, red cells are broken down within macrophages, the iron being either released back to circulating transferrin or stored as macrophage ferritin and haemosiderin. The hepatocytes, with a two-way exchange of iron with plasma iron, act as a buffer, taking up and storing excess iron when the transferrin iron saturation is increased, and releasing it at times of increased iron need. As a result the liver is a principal target for iron accumulation in chronic iron overload.

Iron transport and cellular iron uptake

Transferrin iron binds to transferrin receptors before being taken into cells by receptor-mediated endocytosis. Transferrin synthesis occurs mainly in the liver and is transcriptionally regulated, the level of synthesis being inversely related to iron stores. Serum transferrin concentrations (measured by immunological assay or as a total iron binding capacity, TIBC) are thus increased in iron deficiency and decreased in iron overload (Table 1). After cellular uptake the transferrin is separated from its iron in the acid environment of the endosome.

Ferritin iron

Ferritin is a spherical protein capable of binding up to 4500 iron atoms in its core. All cells possess the capacity to synthesize ferritin in response to iron excess. Immunological assay of serum ferritin concentration thus provides an indirect assessment of overall cellular iron status and body iron stores.

Regulation of cellular iron homeostasis

Recent work has revealed the importance to iron homeostasis of a cytosolic iron regulatory protein (**IRP**). Depending upon the amount of available iron within the cell, the IRP undergoes a reversible conversion between iron-poor and iron-rich forms. Iron-poor IRP binds to regulatory iron-responsive elements (**IREs**) in mRNA, inhibiting the translation of ferritin protein, but stabilizing transferrin

Table 1 Factors influencing serum iron, total iron binding capacity (TIBC), and ferritin measurements

Measurement	Increase	Decrease
Serum iron (normal 10–30 μmol/1)	Iron overload Liver disease Decreased erythropoiesis (e.g. aplastic anaemia) Haemolysis/ dyserythropoiesis (e.g. pernicious anaemia)	Iron deficiency Infection/inflammation
Serum TIBC (normal 45–70 μmol/1)	Iron deficiency Pregnancy Oral contraceptive	Iron overload Infection/inflammation Protein loss/ malnutrition
Serum ferritin (normal 15–300 μg/l but age and sex dependent)	Iron overload Liver disease[1] Infection/inflammation Malignancy Haemolytic anaemia Hyperthyroidism Spleen or bone marrow infarction	Iron deficiency

[1] May be massive increase with severe hepatocellular damage.

receptor mRNA and thus increasing transferrin receptor synthesis. The reverse effects occur with iron-rich IRP, which functions as a cytoplasmic aconitase and can no longer bind to the IRE. This coordinated regulation of the two iron proteins acts to maintain a constant intracellular iron content.

Measurement of iron status

Unfortunately there is no one test, or combination of tests, that is optimal for all circumstances. This is because abnormalities may affect only one iron compartment or may develop sequentially. In addition, factors other than iron status affect many of the measurements (Tables 1, 2).

Storage iron

Measurement of the serum ferritin concentration is reproducible and well correlated with iron stores in normal people. In the neonate, values increase as the high haemoglobin present at birth declines and its iron is moved into stores, and then falls to a nadir at 6–12 months of age as the growing infant exhausts the iron reserve. After puberty, the serum ferritin increases through adult life, except in premenopausal women, who have lower mean concentrations (approximately 30 μg/1) than men (approximately 100 μg/l). These values correspond to iron stores of around 300 and 1000 mg, respectively. Concentrations below 15 μg/l are specific for storage-iron depletion but values above 300 μg/l do not necessarily indicate iron overload. This is because ferritin synthesis is increased by factors other than iron, and because damage to ferritin-rich tissues can release large amounts into the circulation. Where doubt remains, it may be necessary to look for Prussian blue-stainable iron in bone marrow macrophages (in the differential diagnosis of iron deficiency) or in a liver biopsy (in the diagnosis of parenchymal iron overload). Non-invasive approaches to determining tissue iron content include dual-energy computed tomography and magnetic resonance imaging.

Transport iron

Serum iron concentration in association with TIBC is useful in diagnosing iron deficiency, where a reduced saturation of TIBC indicates impaired iron supply to the tissues. An increase in transferrin saturation is the first change in the development of parenchymal iron loading, and its measurement remains an essential part of screening for iron overload.

Disturbances in iron status

With much of the world's population eating a predominantly vegetarian diet containing poorly available iron, only slight increases in physiological iron requirements or pathological blood loss (for example, related to hookworm infestation) may lead to a failure to maintain iron balance and hence to the development of progressive iron depletion. Much less commonly, patients with disorders in which iron absorption is upregulated, or in whom parenteral iron is given in the form of regular blood transfusions, are at risk of slowly progressive, and potentially fatal, accumulation of storage iron.

Iron deficiency

Prevalence

It has been estimated that 30 per cent of the world's population are anaemic. In developed regions the figure may be nearer 8 per cent. Prevalence is particularly high in preschool children (51 per cent in less-developed, and 13 per cent in more-developed regions). Approximately 500 million people are estimated to be affected by anaemia due to iron deficiency.

Pathophysiology

Haematological effects

In the early stages of iron-deficient erythropoiesis the haemoglobin concentration and red-cell indices may still be in the normal range. However, a transferrin saturation below 16 per cent is insufficient to maintain normal erythropoiesis. Further iron depletion leads to increasingly severe dyserythropoiesis and anaemia. The bone marrow shows moderately increased numbers of red-cell precursors with 'ragged' cytoplasm but there is no increase in circulating reticulocytes. Small, poorly haemoglobinized red cells are produced, some of which are distorted (Fig. 2) and have a shortened lifespan. The platelet count is commonly increased.

Effects on other tissues

These are less well-defined but include atrophy of buccal and gastric mucosal surfaces and the formation of oesophageal postcricoid mucosal webs. Conflicting roles for iron in protecting against or exacerbating the risk of infection have been proposed. Iron-deficiency anaemia seems to be accompanied by impaired mental development and function in children; this deficit may not be restored by treatment with iron.

Clinical features

Features of iron-deficiency anaemia are non-specific. Up to 50 per cent of patients show glossitis, which may proceed to almost complete loss of lingual papillae. Angular stomatitis is less specific. Nails may be brittle and flattened, though the almost diagnostic spoon-shaped deformity of koilonychia (Fig. 3) is now rare in UK practice. Dysphagia may be due to an oesophageal web (Patterson–Kelly or Plummer–Vinson syndrome). This is a premalignant condition that may occur in the absence of anaemia, usually in middle-aged women. Pica may

Table 2 Development of iron deficiency with gradual depletion of body iron content

	Normal	Storage-iron depletion	Iron-deficient erythropoiesis	Iron-deficiency anaemia
Iron stores				
RE marrow iron	Present	Trace/absent	Absent	Absent
Serum ferritin (μg/l)	15–300	20	10	<10
Serum TIBC (μmol/1)	45–70	70	75	>75
Iron supply to tissues				
Transport iron:				
Serum iron (μmol/l)	10–30	20	<10	<7
Saturation of TIBC (%)	16–60	30	<16	<10
Tissue iron needs:				
Serum transferrin receptor (mg/l)	2.8–8.5[1]	<8.5	>8.5	>8.5
Marrow sideroblasts (%)	30–50	30–50	<10	<10
Red-cell protoporphyrin (μmol/mol Hb)	<80	<80	>80	>80
Red-cell production				
Haemoglobin (g/dl)	>13(♂) >12(♀)	>13(♂) >12(♀)	>13(♂) <12(♀)	<13(♂) <12(♀)
Mean red-cell volume (MCV) (fl)	80–92	80–92	80	<80
Mean red-cell haemoglobin, MCH (pg)	27–32	27–32	27	<27
Morphology	Normal	Normal	Normal	Microcytic/hypochromic

[1] Kansas City monoclonal antibody ELISA.

The boxes indicate the stages in development of iron deficiency at which abnormalities in the tests first appear.

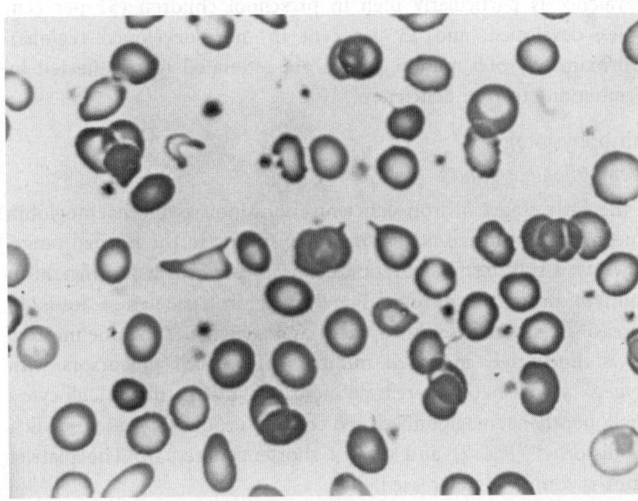

Fig. 2 The peripheral blood film in iron-deficiency anaemia showing pale and distorted red cells. 970 ×.

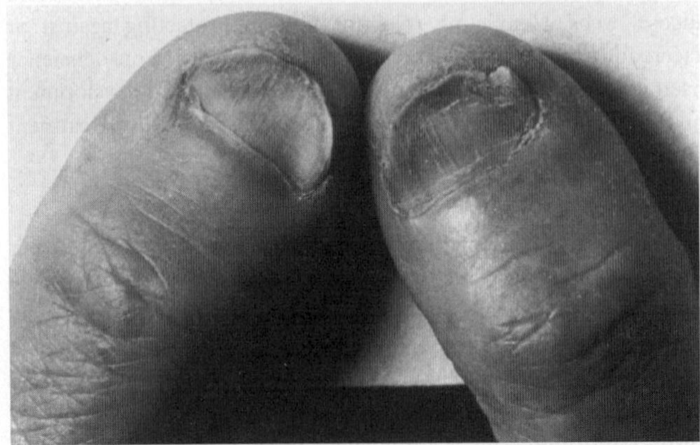

Fig. 3 Koilonychia in chronic iron-deficiency anaemia.

occur in both children and adults, with ingestion of ice, clay, soap, or other unusual materials.

Diagnosis

In a microcytic anaemia with an obvious cause for a negative iron balance, measurement of either serum ferritin or transferrin saturation and the subsequent haematological response to iron therapy will confirm the diagnosis. These measurements of iron status will also help to distinguish iron deficiency from other causes of impaired haemoglobin synthesis and microcytic anaemia (for instance, thalassaemia trait, sideroblastic anaemia). In hospital patients the chief differential diagnosis is the anaemia of chronic disorders. This is typically a normocytic or mildly microcytic anaemia, which has to be distinguished from the early stages of iron deficiency. Distinction depends upon demonstrating normal or increased iron stores, associated with reduced serum iron and TIBC if the anaemia is due solely to inflammatory disease. Unfortunately, the serum ferritin is an acute-phase reactant and in inflammatory disease its values may be in the normal range despite coexistent iron deficiency. Nevertheless, a serum ferritin level below 50 mg/l is usually associated with iron deficiency in rheumatoid arthritis, chronic renal disease, and inflammatory bowel disease. A bone marrow biopsy stained for iron is often the quickest way to be certain of iron status. The recent introduction of an immunological measurement of serum transferrin receptors (increased in iron deficiency) may eventually prove useful in these circumstances.

A diagnostic problem may be seen in patients with chronic renal failure who are receiving treatment with recombinant human erythropoietin. Here, demand for iron by the stimulated erythroid marrow may be greater than the rate at which it can be mobilized from macrophage iron stores, giving rise to a 'functional' iron deficiency and failure to sustain a rising haemoglobin concentration, despite apparently adequate iron stores.

Aetiology

It is vital that the underlying cause of negative iron balance should be identified, and where possible treated. The most likely cause depends on the age and sex of the patient. Dietary insufficiency is likely to play a part only at times of increased physiological demands for iron. These occur during rapid growth in infants between the age of 6 and 24 months (particularly if birth weight, and thus initial body iron content, was low), adolescents (particularly girls), and in premenopausal women (particularly with heavy menstrual blood loss or multiple pregnancies). In the UK there is a high incidence of iron deficiency among Asian women of childbearing age who eat a vegetarian diet containing poorly available iron. The 30 per cent increase in red-cell mass in pregnancy imposes a requirement for an extra 500 mg of iron in addition to the 200–300 mg of iron transferred to the fetus, mainly during the second half of pregnancy. The iron in the increased red-cell mass will be reclaimed after delivery, but after allowance for blood loss at the time of birth, the total iron cost of pregnancy is around 500 mg. There is a case for continued use of prophylactic iron supplements, at least during the second half of pregnancy, though a daily dose of 30 mg of elemental iron, rather than the customary 100 mg, is likely to be adequate and better tolerated. In older children, men, and postmenopausal women there is likely to be a pathological cause for iron deficiency, usually increased blood loss from the gut. Malabsorption of iron may occasionally be responsible.

Increased blood loss

Gastrointestinal bleeding is usually clinically inapparent and often intermittent. It may therefore be difficult to detect. Faecal occult blood tests may help, but even if they are negative endoscopic and/or barium studies should be done in males and postmenopausal women. Small-bowel barium studies may occasionally help. Typical causes are peptic ulceration, colonic carcinoma, oesophagitis, gastritis, polyps, and angiodysplasia. In children there may be bleeding from a Meckel's diverticulum. Oesophageal varices and haemorrhoids usually cause overt gastrointestinal blood loss. In the tropics the principal cause of gastrointestinal blood loss is hookworm infestation, where the blood loss is proportional to the number of parasites. In premenopausal women, before embarking on gastrointestinal studies, menstrual blood losses should first be assessed. These are notoriously difficult to estimate, though some idea can be obtained from the number of towels used and the duration of each period. The mean menstrual loss is about 40 ml, but over 10 per cent of women have menorrhagia with losses greater than 80 ml (equivalent to over 1 mg daily) and a high risk of developing iron deficiency.

In patients in whom these investigations show no cause for gastrointestinal bleeding the development of serious underlying disease is rare but careful follow up is required.

Bleeding into the urinary tract is uncommon and is usually clinically obvious, in schistosomal infestation for example. Occult loss, as haemosiderin, may occur in chronic haemolysis due to a prosthetic heart valve or paroxysmal nocturnal haemoglobinuria. Regular blood donation should also be recognized as a drain on iron reserves.

Malabsorption

Iron deficiency is occasionally the sole manifestation of coeliac disease, and though this may be diagnosed in childhood it may present for the first time at any age. Evidence of hyposplenism may be detected by red-cell changes on a blood film and should lead to consideration of a jejunal biopsy. Partial gastrectomy is also a potential cause of iron deficiency.

Treatment

The essential search for the underlying cause of iron deficiency should not delay the start of iron treatment. Where iron deficiency has been attributed to increased physiological demands for iron, without extensive investigation, patients should be followed regularly to avoid missing a source of blood loss.

Oral iron should be used, except in special circumstances, as parenteral iron can have serious adverse effects and does not increase the speed of resolution of the anaemia. In adults, 120–180 mg of elemental iron per day in divided doses should be given. Probably the most commonly used treatment is ferrous sulphate which contains 60 mg of elemental iron per 200 mg. Adverse effects include nausea, abdominal pain, diarrhoea, and constipation. They are related to the amount of available iron in the gut lumen.

The maximum response to treatment is a daily increase of 0.1–0.2 g/dl in haemoglobin concentration. Treatment is arbitrarily continued for about 3 months after resolution of the anaemia to provide a small reserve iron store.

Parenteral iron should be used only in those completely unable or unwilling to take oral iron, or where this cannot keep pace with continuing blood loss. Intramuscular injections or intravenous infusions are available but there is a risk of anaphylaxis.

Refractory hypochromic anaemia

Failure of treatment is commonly due to the patient not taking oral iron. Continuing severe blood loss, associated inflammatory disease, or malabsorption may also limit the response. It is essential to reassess the diagnosis of iron deficiency, as other causes of hypochromic anaemias include many of the iron-loading anaemias (see below and Chapters 3.19, 3.20).

Iron overload

The absence of a physiological pathway for the excretion of excess iron means that patients with an increased iron intake (Table 3) are at risk of progressive accumulation of iron and potentially lethal tissue damage. A primary inherited disorder of iron metabolism (hereditary haemochromatosis) may be responsible, or iron overload may be secondary, usually to disordered erythropoiesis. Where excess iron is derived from regular blood transfusions it is easy to recognize and to quantify (each unit of 450 ml of whole blood contains approximately 200 mg of iron). Where the iron is from inappropriate absorption in a normal diet, the risk may be concealed until the patient presents with established tissue damage.

Iron and tissue damage

The term 'haemochromatosis' is usually employed to describe the association of iron loading in parenchymal cells (especially in liver, heart, and endocrine glands) with tissue damage and fibrosis. As it is generally used in association with hereditary haemochromatosis it is useful to refer to other iron-loading disorders as secondary iron overload, with or without tissue damage. The mechanism by which iron produces cellular damage remains uncertain but is likely to involve the generation of oxygen free radicals.

Hereditary haemochromatosis (see also Chapter 6.10)

Aetiology and pathology

Hereditary haemochromatosis results from an inborn error of iron metabolism. The gene involved appears to be member of the human

Table 3 Causes of iron overload

Causes of severe iron overload
Repeated blood transfusions:
Congenital anaemias (e.g. β-thalassaemia major, sideroblastic anaemia, red-cell aplasia)
Acquired refractory anaemias (e.g. myelodysplasia, chronic renal failure, aplastic and myelodysplastic syndromes)
Excess iron absorption:
Hereditary haemochromatosis
Massive ineffective erythropoiesis (e.g. β-thalassaemia intermedia, sideroblastic anaemia, congenital dyserythropoietic anaemia)
Excess iron uptake:
SubSaharan dietary iron overload (Bantu siderosis) from traditional beer of high iron content (plus additional genetic determinant of increased iron absorption)
Excess parenteral iron therapy
Causes of modest iron overload
Chronic liver disease:
Alcoholic cirrhosis
Portacaval anastomosis
Porphyria cutanea tarda
Causes of focal iron overload[1]
Pulmonary haemorrhage:
Idiopathic pulmonary haemosiderosis
Chronic haemoglobinuria:
Renal tubular haemosiderosis (e.g. paroxysmal nocturnal haemoglobinuria, sickle-cell disease)

Conditions in the upper part of the table may potentially give rise to severe iron overload (>5 g excess in adults) with a risk of tissue damage. In conditions shown below the line any increase in total iron burden is small, redistribution of body iron may play a major part, and a localized increase in tissue iron may then have more specific clinical effects than those of generalized iron overload.

[1] In these circumstances local iron sequestration may occur in the presence of a generalized iron deficiency.

leucocyte antigen family (**HLA**) and has been termed *HFE*. Certain forms of this gene lead an increased absorption of iron from the gut. In established disease concentrations of iron in the liver and pancreas may be 50–100 times normal, and in the heart 10–15 times normal. Both the liver and heart are usually enlarged, with cirrhosis and myocardial fibrosis. When cirrhosis is marked, less iron is found in regenerating liver nodules, and hepatocellular carcinoma develops in 25–30 per cent of established cases. The anterior pituitary, thyroid, parathyroid, and adrenal glands also show heavy iron deposition.

Inheritance

Only homozygotes show full expression of the disease, though clinically insignificant increases in liver iron may occur in a minority of heterozygotes. Hereditary haemochromatosis is rare before adult life, but in juvenile cases males and females have been equally affected.

Clinical features

Around 70 per cent of patients first develop symptoms between the ages of 40 and 60 years, with a male to female incidence of 9:1. Excessive dietary iron intake or blood loss (including menstruation and regular donation of blood) will accelerate or delay manifestation of the disease; blood loss presumably accounts for the lower incidence in women. The clinical features (Table 4) extend far beyond the classical triad of diabetes, hepatomegaly, and slate-grey skin pigmentation (associated with increased deposits of melanin). Symptoms

Table 4 Clinical features of hereditary haemochromatosis

Symptoms	%	Signs	%
Weakness, lethargy	74	Skin pigmentation	82
Loss of libido	56	Hepatomegaly	76
Impotence	56	Testicular atrophy	50
Weight loss	53	Splenomegaly	38
Abdominal pain	50	Cardiac disease	35
Arthritis	47	Loss of body hair	32
Confusion, stupor	12	Ascites	15
Peripheral neuritis	9	Gynaecomastia	12
Vertigo	6		
Vomiting	6		

For source see OTM3, p. 3478.

of diabetes, gonadal failure, and arthritis may be present for several years before the diagnosis becomes otherwise obvious. Nearly all patients develop some degree of glucose intolerance and many require insulin therapy. Hypogonadism is commonly hypogonadotrophic in origin. Arthritis is more frequent in older patients and is characterized by articular chondrocalcinosis. Cardiac failure and arrhythmias may occur at any age but are a more common presenting feature in younger patients; rapid clinical deterioration and death may result.

Diagnosis

A high degree of clinical suspicion is needed, given the variety of clinical manifestation. Laboratory tests are centred on the demonstration of parenchymal iron loading and assessment of the function of the main 'target' organs. Liver biopsy is important both to confirm iron overload and to assess tissue damage. Genetic typing of *HFE* is valuable since a mutation (*C282Y*) is found to be homozygous in most patients of north European origin. Causes of secondary iron overload should be excluded. Liver disease, particularly when due to alcohol, may cause problems in differential diagnosis. It shares a number of clinical features with hereditary haemochromatosis as well as having a serum transferrin saturation and ferritin concentration that may be increased out of proportion to iron stores. The high iron content of some alcoholic drinks and enhancement of iron absorption by alcohol probably increase the likelihood of homozygous disease reaching full clinical expression. Liver biopsy usually distinguishes these conditions.

Treatment and prognosis

Regular phlebotomy has dramatically altered the causes of death in hereditary haemochromatosis. Phlebotomy greatly reduces mortality from cardiac and hepatic failure, but hepatocellular carcinoma now accounts for a large proportion of deaths in established disease. Earlier diagnosis may reduce this risk. Arthritis and hormonal function may not improve after phlebotomy.

Most patients tolerate weekly phlebotomy of 450 ml (200 mg iron), maintaining a haemoglobin concentration above 12.0 g/dl. Serum ferritin concentrations decline during treatment, which may need to be continued for 2–3 years as total iron load is usually around 20 g and may be as much as 40 g. As iron depletion approaches, serum iron and haemoglobin concentration fall. The frequency of phlebotomy should then be decreased, with maintenance treatment at around 2–6 units removed each year for the rest of the patient's life. The aim should be to maintain a normal transferrin saturation and a serum ferritin in the low normal range.

Screening and early diagnosis

First-degree relatives of patients with hereditary haemochromatosis are at risk for the disease. All those over the age of 10 years should be tested for any increase in serum transferrin saturation and ferritin concentration as well as *HFE* genotyping. Careful monitoring and institution of phlebotomy before there is tissue damage will avoid morbidity and gives the prospect of a normal life expectancy.

Iron-loading anaemias

In chronic refractory anaemias, iron overload may result from the need for regular blood transfusions or from excessive absorption of dietary iron (see Table 4). In the spectrum of thalassaemia disorders (Chapter 3.19) both mechanisms are found. The problems of assessing iron overload are somewhat different in these two groups of patients.

Transfusion iron loading

Cardiac iron toxicity frequently occurs in patients who have received more than 100 units of blood (20 g iron), and other parenchymal tissues are damaged in a pattern similar to that seen in hereditary haemochromatosis. The rate of iron loading is predictable. The serum ferritin may be much higher than is usually seen in hereditary haemochromatosis and is a poor guide to precise amounts of iron overload. Levels in excess of 4000 μg/l may reflect additional factors such as haemolysis, liver damage from iron, or transfusion-associated hepatitis. Liver biopsy is not justified as a routine, as the presence of iron overload is not in doubt. Other investigations to assess tissue damage may be needed.

Gastrointestinal iron loading

The degree of anaemia is not helpful in predicting the risk of iron loading in patients with dyserythropoiesis who do not require blood transfusions. A much better guide is the degree of erythroid marrow expansion, which can be measured by morphological or ferrokinetic techniques in presymptomatic patients. Such patients should be followed up regularly, as described for the screening and early diagnosis of hereditary haemochromatosis.

Treatment

Where possible the rate of iron loading should be reduced. In β-thalassaemia major, splenectomy may reduce transfusion requirements if there is hypersplenism.

Iron-chelation therapy

The only iron-chelating agent in widespread current clinical use is desferrioxamine (Desferal®). While highly specific for iron, this drug has to be given by injection, with slow infusions (intravenous or subcutaneous) being most effective. Ascorbic acid can be used to enhance desferrioxamine treatment but the dose of ascorbate should not exceed 100 mg/day.

Planning chelation therapy

Standard chelation treatment now consists of subcutaneous infusions of desferrioxamine given over 10–12 h, usually on six nights each week, using a small infusion pump (Fig. 4). Initially, 24-h urine collections for iron measurements should be made after increasing

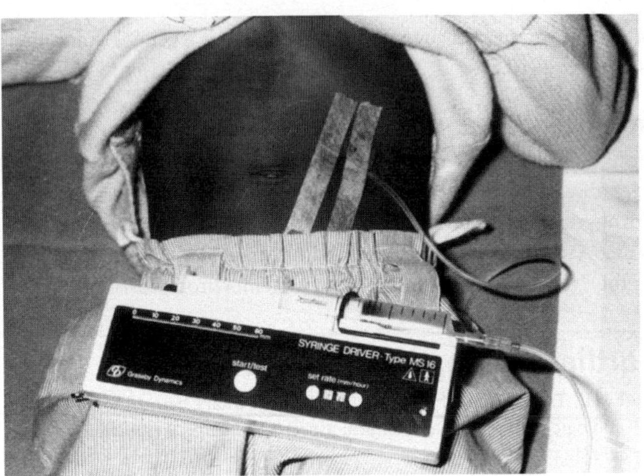

Fig. 4 Subcutaneous infusion of desferrioxamine in a thalassaemic child using a portable, battery-driven pump. The syringe is connected via narrow-bore tubing to a fine-gauge butterfly needle inserted deeply into the subcutaneous fat of the anterior abdominal wall.

doses (0.5–3.0 g as 12-h subcutaneous infusions) on successive days. In all but the most heavily iron-loaded patient the urine iron excretion tends to level off at higher doses, and the optimal dose may be selected as that giving maximal iron chelation before the plateau is reached. In most cases this will be around 50 mg/kg body weight by 12-h subcutaneous infusion each night. It is also worthwhile giving a single, larger, intravenous infusion (for example, 150 mg/kg) at the time of each regular blood transfusion. Annual testing of sight and hearing should be performed, but overall desferrioxamine has been remarkably non-toxic given the need for large continuous doses over many years.

Response to treatment

Thalassaemic patients complying with therapy have improved cardiac function. Prevention of pubertal growth failure due to iron loading in thalassaemia is dependent on starting chelation early in life, and treatment should ideally begin before there is a serious iron burden, usually by around the age of 3 years. The dose should be reassessed at annual intervals as patients grow, and in relation to the serum ferritin concentration.

Oral iron chelation

A number of potential oral iron-chelating agents have been examined over the last few years but none are ideal at present.

Non-transfused patients

Iron overload due to excess iron absorption may be treated with subcutaneous desferrioxamine or, if tolerated, by phlebotomy.

Excess iron intake

Oral iron

Prolonged oral iron ingestion in normal people does not usually produce significant iron loading. However, in patients with hereditary haemochromatosis or dyserythropoietic anaemias the rate of iron loading may be considerably increased.

Sub-Saharan dietary iron overload

A high prevalence of iron overload in Black Africans has been reported in sub-Saharan Africa. This iron loading is associated with a high intake of iron in beer prepared in iron pots but a genetic component is also required.

Iron overload and liver disease

Iron stores can be mildly increased in many forms of chronic liver disease, this tendency being exacerbated by portacaval shunt. Porphyria cutanea tarda (Chapter 11.5), a photosensitive dermatitis, is associated with mild increases in iron stores and with the mutation of the *HFE* gene found in hereditary haemochromatosis.

Further reading

Bothwell, T.H. and MacPhail, A.P. (1998). Hereditary hemochromatosis: etiologic, pathologic, and clinical aspects. *Seminars in Hematology*, 35, 55–71.

Brock, J.H., Halliday, J.W., Pippard, M.J., and Powell, L.W. (ed.) (1994). *Iron metabolism in health and disease*. Saunders, London.

Cook, J.D. (1994). Iron deficiency anaemia. *Baillière's Clinical Haematology*, 7, 787–804.

Chapter 3.17

Normochromic, normocytic anaemia

D. J. Weatherall

The finding of a mild normochromic anaemia is one of the most common problems in every branch of clinical practice. It is important to decide whether the anaemia is important and how far it should be investigated.

The first decision to be made is whether the blood findings represent 'anaemia' for the particular patient. There is a wide range of 'normal' values for any particular age and knowledge of any previous blood count can be useful. Most of the normochromic, normocytic anaemias are secondary to other diseases; a minority reflect a primary disorder of the blood. Some of the more common causes are summarized in Table 1.

Anaemia of chronic disorders (ACD)

This is the most common of the normochromic, normocytic anaemias and is found in association with chronic infection, all forms of inflammatory diseases, and in malignant disease. Although it may be extremely mild and asymptomatic, the presence of this blood picture should always alert the clinician to the possibility of there being a serious underlying disease.

Table 1 Some normochromic, normocytic anaemias

Anaemia of chronic disorders	*Marrow failure*
Inflammation	Pure red-cell aplasia
Neoplasia	Aplastic anaemia
Renal failure	Infiltration
Endocrine failure	*Acute blood loss*
Hypothyroidism	*Polymyalgia rheumatica*
Hypopituitarism	

Pathogenesis

The precise mechanism of the ACD is still not understood, but the most constant feature is a low serum iron level despite adequate iron stores in the reticuloendothelial elements of the bone marrow. This suggests that there is a block in the release of iron to the developing red-cell precursors. There may also be a degree of haemolysis.

Clinical and laboratory findings

The ACD is usually mild, although in patients with severe inflammation the haemoglobin may fall to levels at which symptoms are experienced. Although the anaemia is usually normocytic and normochromic there may be mild hypochromia with a slight reduction in the mean cell haemoglobin and mean cell volume, particularly in children. The reticulocyte count is in the normal range.

The most important findings are a reduction in the serum iron concentration and a concurrent reduction in the level of transferrin. This means that the percentage saturation of the iron-binding capacity is usually normal or only slightly reduced. This observation clearly distinguishes ACD from true iron-deficiency anaemia. This distinction can also be confirmed by measuring the serum ferritin level, which is usually in the normal range in patients with ACD while it is low in those who are iron deficient.

In the bone marrow, iron staining shows a paucity of iron in the red-cell precursors and an accumulation of iron in the storage elements of the marrow. Again, this distinguishes ACD from true iron deficiency. The abnormal distribution of iron in an adequately stained sample, together with the low serum iron, is the true hallmark of ACD and a finding that should always be followed up by a search for an underlying inflammatory or neoplastic condition.

Other forms of normochromic, normocytic anaemia

Other causes of this type of blood picture include renal disease, endocrine disease, and early iron deficiency. Polymyalgia rheumatica and giant-cell arteritis are nearly always associated with a moderate normochromic, normocytic anaemia together with a marked increase in the erythrocyte sedimentation rate. However, particularly in elderly patients, anaemia may be the presenting feature and the symptoms of polymyalgia or cranial arteritis may be minimal or even absent. This is quite a common variant of the polymyalgia syndrome and should always be considered in old people with anaemia and a very high sedimentation rate who do not have a paraprotein in the blood. The anaemia responds quite dramatically to corticosteroids.

Management

Mild, non-specific anaemias should always be investigated because they may be the first indication of a serious underlying disease. It is important to try to distinguish between ACD and iron deficiency or other non-specific normochromic, normocytic anaemias. The most common causes of ACD that lead to diagnostic problems are low-grade urinary-tract infections, chronic sinus infection, and occult malignancy.

The treatment of anaemias of this type is essentially that of the underlying disease. No haematinic will produce a rise in the haemoglobin level, although erythropoietin may help. As mentioned above, a trial of steroids may be valuable to recognize the polymyalgia syndromes.

Further reading

Erslev, A.J. (1994). Anemia in chronic disease. In *Williams hematology* (ed. E. Beutler, M.A. Lichtman, B.S. Coller, and T.J. Kipps). McGraw-Hill, New York.

Chapter 3.18

Megaloblastic anaemia and miscellaneous deficiency anaemias

A. V. Hoffbrand

The megaloblastic anaemias are a group of disorders characterized by a macrocytic anaemia and distinctive morphological abnormalities of the developing haemopoietic cells in the bone marrow. In severe cases, the anaemia may be associated with leucopenia and thrombocytopenia. Megaloblastic anaemia arises because of inhibition of DNA synthesis in the bone marrow, and this is usually due to the deficiency of one or other of two water-soluble B vitamins: vitamin B_{12} (cobalamin) or folate. B_{12} deficiency may also cause a severe neuropathy, but whether this occurs with folate deficiency is controversial. In a minority of cases, megaloblastic anaemia arises because of a disturbance of DNA synthesis due to a drug or to a congenital or acquired biochemical defect that causes a disturbance of B_{12} or folate metabolism, or that affects DNA synthesis independent of B_{12} or folate. B_{12} and folate are discussed first and the other rare megaloblastic anaemias are mentioned at the end of this chapter.

Biochemical and nutritional aspects of vitamin B_{12} and folate

Vitamin B_{12}

Biochemistry

There are four major forms of this vitamin known to exist in man. 5′-Deoxyadenosylcobalamin (**ado-B12**) accounts for about 80 per cent of the total, while methylcobalamin (methyl-B_{12}) is the other active coenzyme form. Hydroxo- and cyanocobalamin are therapeutic forms present in only trace amounts in human tissues. B_{12} is known to be involved in only three reactions in human tissues: as ado-B_{12} in the isomerization of methylmalonyl CoA to succinyl CoA and of α-leucine to β-leucine, and as methyl-B_{12} in the methylation of homocysteine to methionine, a reaction that also requires methyltetrahydrofolate (Fig. 1).

Nutrition

Vitamin B_{12} is synthesized by micro-organisms; animals obtain it by eating parts of other animals or animal produce (milk, cheese, eggs, etc.), or vegetables foods contaminated by bacteria. A normal mixed diet contains between 5 and 30 μg daily and total B_{12} in man is about 3–5 mg. To maintain normal body stores, daily requirements are of the order of 2 μg. It takes 3–4 years for deficiency to develop if supplies are totally cut off.

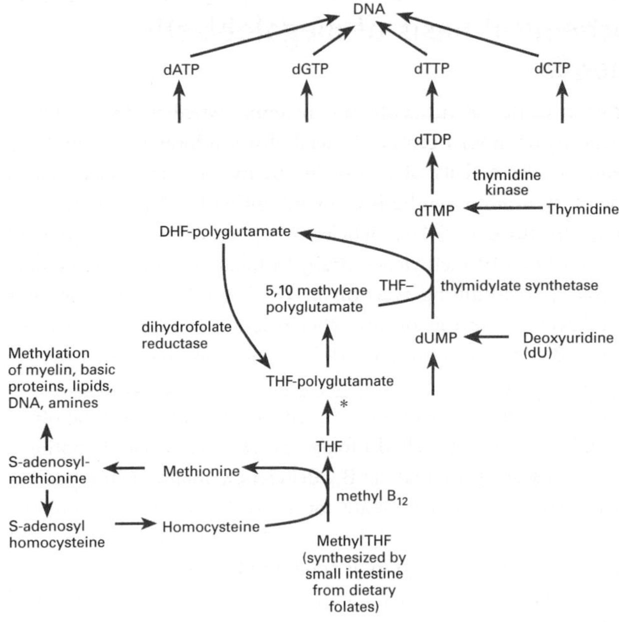

Fig. 1 Suggested mechanisms by which B_{12} deficiency affects folate metabolism and interferes with DNA synthesis. Indirect involvement of B_{12}, as methyl B_{12}, in DNA synthesis is suggested by the 'methylfolate' trap ('tetrahydrofolate starvation') hypothesis. Methyl-B_{12} is involved in the formation of intracellular THF from plasma methyl-THF*. THF and/or its formyl derivative are the 'ground substances' from which all folate coenzymes are made by glutamate addition and single carbon unit transfer (see text). 5,10-Methylene-THF polyglutamate is involved in thymidylate synthesis. D, deoxyribose; A, adenine; G, guanine; T, thymine; C, cytosine; TP, triphosphate; DP, diphosphate; U, uridine; THF, tetrahydrofolate.

Absorption and transport

Vitamin B_{12}, whether dietary or in bile, needs to bind to intrinsic factor (**IF**) for absorption. IF is a glycoprotein produced by the gastric parietal cells. The B_{12}–IF complex attaches passively to specific IF receptors (cubulin) on the terminal ileum where the B_{12} is absorbed. B_{12} in plasma is 80 per cent attached to a glycoprotein, transcobalamin (**TC**) I, which does not enhance cellular uptake of B_{12}. A closely related molecule, TC III, carries only 0 to 10 per cent of plasma B_{12}. The most important plasma B_{12}-binding protein is TC II, which actively enhances the uptake of B_{12} by tissues.

Folate

Biochemistry

This vitamin exists in nature in over 100 forms, all of which are derivatives of folic (pteroyl glutamic acid) acid. The biochemical reactions of folates involve the transfer of a single carbon group from one compound to another. Of these reactions, three are involved in the synthesis of DNA precursors.

Nutrition

Folate occurs in most foods, the highest concentrations being found in liver. People eating Western diets have an average normal daily intake of 250 μg and body stores are about 10–12 mg. Normal adult requirements are about 100 μg daily. Folic acid itself is not present in food but is used therapeutically. Folates are absorbed rapidly, mainly through the duodenum and jejunum, and transported in plasma—two-thirds unbound and about one-third loosely bound to albumin. As for B_{12}, there is an enterohepatic circulation of folate.

Biochemical basis of megaloblastic anaemia

All known causes of megaloblastic anaemia, whether due to drugs, deficiencies, or inborn errors of metabolism, inhibit DNA synthesis by reducing the activity of one of the many enzymes concerned in purine or pyrimidine synthesis or by inhibiting DNA polymerization from its precursors. Folate deficiency, by reducing the supply of the coenzyme, 5,10-methylene-tetrahydrofolate, inhibits thymidylate synthesis, a rate-limiting reaction in DNA synthesis. B_{12} does not have a direct role in this or any other reaction in mammalian DNA synthesis. B_{12} deficiency inhibits DNA synthesis indirectly by its effect on folate metabolism.

An explanation for the effect of B_{12} deficiency on folate metabolism is provided by the tetrahydrofolate (**THF**) starvation hypothesis (Fig. 1). This suggests that in B_{12} deficiency, folate is 'trapped' as methyl-THF, the monoglutamate form which enters cells from the plasma, because of the need for methyl-B_{12} in the conversion of methyl-THF to THF. The 'trap' is supposed to lower the intracellular supply of THF, from which, after glutamate addition, all folate coenzymes are made. The result is that B_{12} deficiency or inactivation puts a block between methyl-THF entering cells from plasma and the formation of intracellular folate polyglutamate coenzymes (Fig. 1). This causes a rise in plasma folate, a low level of intracellular folates, and reduced activity of all reactions requiring folate coenzymes, including those involved in DNA synthesis.

Clinical features and causes of megaloblastic anaemia

Although pernicious anaemia is only one of the many causes of megaloblastic anaemia (Tables 1, 2, and 3), it is convenient to describe the general clinical features of the anaemia under this heading because it is the most frequent cause of megaloblastic anaemia in Western countries. The laboratory findings and treatment of pernicious anaemia and other megaloblastic anaemias are discussed later.

Acquired pernicious anaemia

Definition

A disease of unknown origin in which there is atrophy of the stomach leading to severely reduced or absent IF secretion with consequent severe malabsorption of B_{12}, and B_{12} deficiency.

Aetiology and associated diseases

Although a disease of the stomach, pernicious anaemia is considered with blood diseases because it usually presents with anaemia; indeed, it is the most common cause of megaloblastic anaemia in many countries. It is a disease of older persons with an incidence of 127/100 000 in Caucasians—less than 10 per cent of patients are under 40 years of age; there is a female:male ratio of about 1.6:1. There is a higher incidence (about 44 per cent compared to 40 per cent) in people with blood group A compared with controls in Britain. It occurs in all races and there is a higher incidence in close relatives of either sex, with a positive family history in about 30 per cent of cases. Carcinoma of the stomach occurs in about 4 per cent of patients with pernicious anaemia, about three times the control rate. Pernicious anaemia may also be associated with other 'autoimmune' diseases, particularly primary myxoedema, thyrotoxicosis, Hashimoto's disease, Addison's disease, and vitiligo. About 55 per cent of patients show thyroid antibodies and 33 per cent with primary myxoedema have parietal-cell antibody. Close relatives may also show these diseases or their associated antibodies. Antibodies are present in serum and gastric juice directed against parietal cells and IF. Parietal-cell antibody is present in the serum of 85 to 90 per cent of patients. Two antibodies to IF exist in serum: type I ('blocking') occurs in about 50 per cent and is directed against the B_{12}-binding site; type II (to the ileal binding site) occurs in 30 to 35 per cent but only if type I antibody is also present. The antibodies to IF are virtually specific for pernicious anaemia, but parietal-cell antibody occurs in many subjects with atrophic gastritis without pernicious anaemia. Histopathology reveals a gastritis in which all layers of the body and fundus of the stomach are atrophied.

Table 1 Causes of B_{12} deficiency and malabsorption of B_{12}

1. *Causes of severe B_{12} deficiency*

(a) Nutritional:
- vegans
- long-continued extremely poor diet (rarely)

(b) Malabsorption:
- Gastric causes
  - acquired (addisonian) pernicious anaemia
  - congenital intrinsic-factor deficiency or abnormality
  - total and partial gastrectomy
  - destructive lesions of stomach
- Intestinal causes
  - gut, flora associated with (jejunal diverticulosis, ileocolic, fistula, anatomical blind loop, stricture, Whipple's disease, scleroderma, HIV disease)
  - ileal resection and Crohn's disease
  - chronic tropical sprue
  - selective malabsorption with proteinuria
  - irradiation to cervix
  - HIV disease
  - fish tapeworm
  - transcobalamin II deficiency

2. *Causes of malabsorption of B_{12} usually without severe B_{12} deficiency*

- Simple atrophic gastritis, gastric bypass, severe chronic pancreatitis
- Zollinger–Ellison syndrome, adult coeliac disease, giardiasis
- Drugs: PAS, colchicine, neomycin, slow K, ethanol, metformin, phenformin, anticonvulsants
- Deficiencies of folate, B_{12}, protein

Clinical features

The general features of megaloblastic anaemia are similar, whatever the underlying cause. Particular clinical features may point to the underlying disease. In pernicious anaemia, the anaemia usually develops gradually, perhaps over several years, and symptoms may not occur until it is severe. The most common complaints are due to the anaemia, while loss of mental and physical drive, numbness, or difficulty in walking suggest neuropathy. Psychiatric disturbances are common and range from mild neurosis to severe organic dementia. It is possible that they occur in the absence of anaemia or macrocytosis. Mild jaundice is frequent. Loss of appetite and weight, indigestion, and episodic diarrhoea are frequent. Older patients may present with congestive heart failure. In a few patients, bruising due to thrombocytopenia is marked. On the other hand, many patients are diagnosed because a routine blood test is performed.

Table 2 Causes of folate deficiency

1. Poor diet

- Especially poverty, psychiatric disturbance, alcoholism, dietary fads, scurvy, kwashiorkor, goat's milk anaemia, partial gastrectomy, other gastrointestinal disease

2. *Malabsorption*

- Gluten-sensitive enteropathy (child or adult or associated with dermatitis herpetiformis)
- Tropical sprue
- Congenital specific malabsorption
- Minor factor: partial gastrectomy, jejunal resection, inflammatory bowel disease, lymphoma, systemic infections
- Drugs: cholestyramine, sulphasalazine, methotrexate, ? others (see (5) below).

3. Excessive requirements

- Physiological
- Pregnancy
- Prematurity and infancy
- Pathological:
  - (a) Malignancies—leukaemia, carcinoma, lymphoma, myeloma, sarcoma, etc.
  - (b) Blood disorders—haemolytic anaemia (especially sickle-cell anaemia, thalassaemia major), chronic myelosclerosis
  - (c) Inflammatory—tuberculosis, malaria, Crohn's disease, psoriasis, exfoliative dermatitis, rheumatoid arthritis, etc.
  - (d) Metabolic—homocystinuria (some cases)

4. *Excess urinary excretion*

- Congestive heart failure, acute liver damage, chronic dialysis

5. *Drugs*

- Mechanism uncertain
- Anticonvulsants (diphenylhydantoin, primidone, barbiturates)
- ? nitrofurantoin
- ? alcohol
- Also drugs causing malabsorption of folate (see (2) above)

6. *Liver disease*

- Mixed causes above, and poor storage.

Physical signs, if present, are those of anaemia, perhaps with mild jaundice, giving the patient a so-called lemon-yellow tint. A few patients with either B_{12} or folate deficiency develop a widespread brown pigmentation that is reversible with the appropriate therapy. The tongue may be red, smooth, and shiny, occasionally with ulcers. A mild pyrexia up to 38 °C is common in patients with moderate to severe anaemia. The liver may be enlarged, while the cardiovascular system shows changes due to anaemia. Patients with pernicious anaemia may also have features of an associated disorder on presentation—most commonly myxoedema, but other thyroid disorders, vitiligo, carcinoma of the stomach, Addison's disease, and hypoparathyroidism, may precede, occur simultaneously with, or follow the onset of the anaemia.

Vitamin B_{12} neuropathy

B_{12} deficiency (but not folate deficiency) may cause a symmetrical neuropathy affecting the lower limbs more than the upper (Section 13), which usually presents with paraesthesiae or with ataxia, particularly in the dark. In some cases, loss of cutaneous sensation, muscle weakness, urinary or faecal incontinence, an optic neuropathy, or psychiatric disturbance dominates. The neuropathy is due to severe B_{12} deficiency

Table 3 Megaloblastic anaemia not due to vitamin B_{12} or folate deficiency

1. ***Abnormalities of B_{12} or folate metabolism***

- Congenital:
  - Transcobalamin II deficiency or functional abnormality
  - Inborn errors of folate metabolism e.g. methylfolate transferase deficiency
  - Homocystinuria and methylmalonic aciduria (some cases)
  - Acquired:
  - Nitrous oxide
  - Dihydrofolate reductase inhibitors: methotrexate, pyrimethamine, trimethoprim, ?pentamidine, triamterene

2. ***Independent of B_{12}* or folate**

- Congenital:
  - Orotic aciduria, (responds to uridine)
  - Lesch–Nyhan syndrome, ? responds to adenine
  - Thiamine-responsive
  - Some cases of congenital dyserythropoietic anaemia
- Acquired:
  - AML FAB M_6, other myeloid leukaemias (some cases)
  - Myelodysplasia
  - Drugs:
  - Antimetabolites: 6-mercaptopurine, cytosine arabinoside, hydroxyurea, 5-fluorouracil, azathioprine, etc.
  - Alcohol

but may occur with mild or no anaemia. It may be due to any cause of severe B_{12} deficiency, most commonly pernicious anaemia. The biochemical explanation for the neuropathy is unclear, but impaired methylation of myelin due to a reduced ratio of *S*-methionine to *S*-adenosyl homocysteine has been suggested.

General tissue effects of B_{12} and folate deficiencies

Both deficiencies cause macrocytosis and other abnormal features including glossitis and angular cheilosis and a mild malabsorption syndrome. In both sexes, sterility (reversible with B_{12} or folate therapy) may result from effects on the gonads.

It is now established that folic acid supplements at the time of conception and in early (first 12 weeks) pregnancy reduce the incidence of neural-tube defects (anencephaly, encephalocele, and spina bifida). The incidence of neural-tube defects is higher, the lower the maternal serum and red-cell folate and serum B_{12} levels, even when they are in the conventional normal range. There is considerable evidence that raised serum homocysteine levels are associated with a higher incidence of neural-tube defects, and with an increased incidence of peripheral vascular disease, coronary vascular disease and myocardial infarction, cerebral vascular disease, and deep-vein thrombosis. Raised serum homocysteine levels are associated with low levels of serum and red-cell folate and of serum B_{12} and vitamin B_6 ($\mathbf{B_6}$), and of low dietary intake of folate or B_6. A frequent polymorphism (G ® mutation at nucleotide 677 (alanine 225 ® valine)) in the gene coding for the enzyme 5,10-methylenetetrahydrofolate reductase (MTHFR) leads to a thermolabile enzyme, lower serum and red-cell folate levels than in a control population, and is associated with a higher incidence of neural-tube defects and with arterial disease. Congenital homocysteinaemia due to a homozygous defect in one of three enzymes concerned in homocysteine metabolism (cystathionine synthase, methionine synthase, or MTHFR) is associated with the development of cardiovascular disease in teenage years or early adulthood.

Increased folate intake or folic acid therapy can lower homocysteine levels, particularly in those with the highest initial levels. As yet, however, there are no published data that folic acid administration can reduce the incidence of arterial disease or thrombosis, although this seems likely.

Other causes of B_{12} deficiency

Juvenile pernicious anaemia

A few cases of typical pernicious anaemia have occurred in children.

Congenital deficiency or structural abnormality of intrinsic factor

About 40 cases have been reported of a child being born with absent or non-functioning IF but an otherwise normal stomach on biopsy and normal secretion studies (for example, of acid). Inheritance is autosomal recessive.

Total gastrectomy

All patients who have this operation will develop B_{12} deficiency, which usually presents between 2 and 6 years' postoperatively, and they should be treated with prophylactic B_{12} injections from the time of the operation.

Partial gastrectomy

Up to 6 per cent of these patients may develop megaloblastic anaemia, but usually the cause is malabsorption due to an abnormal jejunal flora.

Small-intestinal lesions

Colonization of the upper small intestine with colonic bacteria may lead to malabsorption of B_{12}. It appears that the bacteria destroy IF. Infestation with the fish tapeworm (*Diphyllobothrium latum*) has a similar effect.

Resection of a metre or more of terminal ileum

This causes severe malabsorption of B_{12}. Other diseases that affect ileal structure rarely cause severe B_{12} deficiency.

Selective malabsorption of B_{12} with proteinuria (Imerslund's disease, Imerslund–Gräsbeck syndrome)

This congenital disorder with autosomal recessive inheritance is the most common cause of megaloblastic anaemia due to B_{12} deficiency in childhood. The child secretes IF normally but is unable to transport B_{12} across the ileum to portal blood. The proteinuria, present in over 90 per cent of cases, is benign, non-specific, and persists after B_{12} therapy. The clinical presentation of the disease is identical to that of congenital IF deficiency.

Impaired synthesis, processing, or ligand biding of cubulin due to an inherited mutation within the gene most probably underlies the disease. Cubulin is also expressed on proximal renal tubules.

Dietary B_{12} deficiency

This occurs most commonly in Hindus who omit all animal produce from their diet. The incidence of overt megaloblastic anaemia is much lower than the incidence of subclinical deficiency assessed by the serum B_{12} assay. These individuals have low B_{12} stores. In India, babies have been born B_{12}-deficient with megaloblastic anaemia caused by severe B_{12} deficiency (due to poor diet or sprue) in the mother. Dietary deficiency of B_{12} also occurs in non-Hindu vegans, and rarely in non-vegetarian people living on inadequate diets because of poverty.

Folate deficiency

Clinical features

The main clinical features of megaloblastic anaemia due to folate deficiency are similar to those when the anaemia is due to B_{12} deficiency, except that a severe neuropathy does not occur and the underlying disease tends to be different. Less severe folate deficiency may nevertheless be associated with an increased risk of cardiovascular disease and, if present at conception and in early pregnancy, with neural-tube defects in the offspring (see above).

Nutritional folate deficiency

Minor degrees of nutritional folate deficiency are frequent in most countries, but severe folate deficiency may account for about 17 per cent of all cases of megaloblastic anaemias in Britain. It occurs mainly in the old and poor and psychiatrically disturbed living alone on an inadequate diet. In some countries, nutritional folate deficiency may be the main cause of megaloblastic anaemia, often presenting in pregnancy (for example, in Burma, Malaysia, Africa, or India).

Malabsorption (see Chapters 5.6–5.13)

Gluten-induced enteropathy

Folate deficiency occurs in virtually all untreated patients, the serum folate being subnormal whether or not megaloblastic anaemia is present; red-cell folate is subnormal in 80 per cent or more. Anaemia occurs in about 90 per cent of adult cases, owing to folate deficiency alone in 30 to 50 per cent and to mixed iron and folate deficiency in the remainder. Virtually all children show subnormal serum and red-cell folate levels; anaemia is most often due to combined iron and folate deficiency, but 'pure' megaloblastic anaemia also occurs.

Tropical sprue (see Chapter 5.13)

Malabsorption of folate occurs in all severe untreated patients; however, in the first year of the disease up to 60 per cent of patients appear to be cured by folic acid alone.

Congenital specific malabsorption of folate

This is a rare, autosomal recessive abnormality. Affected children all show features of damage to the central nervous system (mental retardation, fits, athetotic movements) and present with megaloblastic anaemia responding to physiological doses of folic acid given parenterally but not orally.

Increased folate utilization

Pregnancy

This, associated with poor nutrition, is probably the most common cause of megaloblastic anaemia worldwide, if folic acid supplements are not taken. The frequency of the anaemia was about 0.5 per cent in most Western cities and up to 50 per cent in some areas of Asia and Africa until the introduction of prophylactic folic acid. The incidence increases with parity and is higher in twin pregnancies. Folate requirements in a normal pregnancy are thought to be increased to about 300 to 400 μg daily, some 200 to 300 μg above normal. Lactation may also precipitate megaloblastic anaemia postpartum.

Prematurity

In premature infants, the expected fall in folate levels after birth is particularly steep and a number of such infants have developed megaloblastic anaemia, particularly if infections, feeding difficulties, or haemolytic disease with exchange transfusion have occurred. Prophylactic folic acid (for example, 1 mg weekly for the first 3–4 weeks of life) may be given, particularly to those babies weighing less than 1.5 kg at birth.

Malignant diseases

Mild folate deficiency is frequent but treatment is rarely indicated.

Blood disorders

Chronic haemolytic anaemia Requirements for folate are raised in patients with increased erythropoiesis, particularly when there is ineffective erythropoiesis. Folic acid is usually given in sickle-cell anaemia, thalassaemia major, hereditary spherocytosis, and warm-type autoimmune haemolytic anaemia.

Chronic myelofibrosis Circulating megaloblasts, increased transfusion requirements, severe thrombocytopenia, or pancytopenia may be the first indication that folate deficiency has developed. Polycythaemia vera is not a cause of folate deficiency.

Sideroblastic anaemia Folate deficiency, usually mild, may occur in about half of acquired cases.

Excess urinary loss of folate

Haemodialysis and peritoneal dialysis remove folate from plasma. Folic acid (for instance, 5 mg weekly) is now usually given prophylactically to patients with renal failure who require long-term dialysis.

Drugs

Alcohol

Folate deficiency may occur in spirit-drinking alcoholics. The main factor is poor nutrition. Beer drinkers seem relatively immune to folate deficiency because of the high folate content of beer. The usual macrocytosis in less severe, non-anaemic alcoholics is not related to folate deficiency.

Anticonvulsants, barbiturates

Diphenylhydantoin, primidone, and barbiturate therapy may be associated with some degree of folate deficiency. The mechanism for the deficiency is undetermined.

Laboratory investigation of megaloblastic anaemia

This consists of three stages: (i) recognition that megaloblastic anaemia is present; (ii) distinction between B_{12} or folate deficiency (or rarely some other factor) as the cause of the anaemia; (iii) diagnosis of the underlying disease causing the deficiency (Table 4). It should be noted, however, that more minor degrees of B_{12} or folate deficiency may exist which may not cause haematological changes yet may be associated with cardiovascular disease or with, in pregnancy, neural-tube defects in the offspring.

Recognition of megaloblastic anaemia

The peripheral blood

There is a raised mean corpuscle volume (MCV) to between 100 fl and 140 fl, and oval macrocytes are seen in the blood film. In mild cases, macrocytosis is present before anaemia has developed. The MCV may be normal if there is associated iron deficiency, when the blood film appears dimorphic, or if the anaemia develops acutely over the course of a few weeks. The reticulocyte count is low for the degree of anaemia, usually of the order of 1 to 3 per cent. The peripheral blood film also shows hypersegmented neutrophils (which have nuclei with more than five lobes) and the leucocyte count is often moderately reduced in both neutrophils and lymphocytes. The platelet count may be moderately reduced.

Table 4 Laboratory diagnosis of megaloblastic anaemia

1. *General tests*
- Peripheral blood film and count
- Bone marrow
- Serum bilirubin, iron, LDH

2. *Tests for B_{12} or folate deficiency*
- Serum B_{12} and folate; red-cell folate
- Serum homocysteine and methylmalonic acid levels
- Deoxyuridine suppression test

3. *Tests for cause of B_{12} or folate deficiency*
- B_{12} deficiency:
  - Serum antibodies to parietal cell, intrinsic factor
  - Serum immunoglobulins
  - Gastric secretion; intrinsic factor, acid,
  - Endoscopy, gastric biopsy
  - Barium meal + follow-through
  - Radioactive B_{12} absorption tests (alone, with intrinsic factor, after antibiotics, with food)
  - Proteinuria, fish tapeworm ova, intestinal flora, etc.
- Folate deficiency:
  - Small-intestinal function
  - Xylose, glucose, vitamin A, fat, B_{12} absorption
  - Duodenal or jejunal biopsy
  - Barium follow-through
  - Tests for many underlying conditions

Biochemical changes

These include a slight rise in serum bilirubin (up to 50 μmol/l), mainly unconjugated, and a rise in serum lactic dehydrogenase. Both are due to ineffective haemopoiesis

Bone marrow

The bone marrow is hypercellular in moderate or severely anaemic cases. The myeloid–erythroid ratio is often reduced or reversed. The erythroblasts are larger than normal and show asynchronous maturation of the nucleus and cytoplasm, nuclear chromatin remaining primitive with an open, lacy, fine granular pattern despite normal maturation and haemoglobinization of the cytoplasm. Excessive numbers of dying cells may be present. Giant and abnormally shaped metamyelocytes and megakaryocytes with hypersegmented nuclear lobes are also usually present.

Deoxyuridine suppression test

This is an *in vitro* biochemical test for B_{12} or folate deficiency based on the presence of a block in thymidylate synthesis. Normally deoxyuridine reduces the incorporation of radioactive thymidine into DNA by inhibiting thymidine kinase. In patients with B_{12} or folate deficiency there is a block in the conversion of dUMP (uridine monophosphate) to dTMP (thymidine monophosphate) and therefore less inhibition. Correction of the test *in vitro* with B_{12} or methyl-THF can be used to differentiate the two deficiencies.

Differential diagnosis

Other causes of macrocytosis include a high reticulocytosis, aplastic anaemia, red-cell aplasia, liver disease, alcoholism and myxoedema, the myelodysplastic syndromes, myeloid leukaemias, cytotoxic drug therapy, chronic respiratory failure, myelomatosis, and other causes of a leucoerythroblastic anaemia or paraproteinaemia. Once a bone marrow biopsy has been done, the principal differentiation is from other causes of megaloblastosis, particularly myelodysplasia. Other causes of megaloblastic anaemia not due to B_{12} or folate deficiency are listed in Table 3.

Diagnosis of B_{12} or folate deficiency

The peripheral blood and bone marrow appearances are identical in folate or B_{12} deficiency. Special tests are, therefore, needed to distinguish between the two deficiencies. The deoxyuridine suppression test has been described already (see above), and is used for a reliable and rapid diagnosis in some laboratories.

Subnormal serum B_{12} levels are found in cases of megaloblastic anaemia due to B_{12} deficiency, being extremely low in B_{12} neuropathy. Subnormal serum B_{12} concentrations in the absence of tissue B_{12} deficiency occur in pregnancy and in severe nutritional folate deficiency. Raised serum B_{12} levels may be seen in myeloproliferative diseases (chronic myeloid leukaemia, polycythaemia rubra vera, or in eosinophilic leukaemia for example).

A third and less widely used test for B_{12} deficiency is the measurement of the serum concentration of methylmalonic acid (MMA) or 24-h urine excretion of MMA. Serum MMA levels and excretion of MMA are raised in B_{12} deficiency but not in folate deficiency. Serum homocysteine levels are raised in B_{12} or folate deficiency and have been suggested as more sensitive tests than haematological changes or even vitamin assays. However, homocysteine levels are also affected by age, sex, dietary methionine and vitamin B_6 intake, renal function, alcohol consumption, and drugs (for example, corticosteroids and cyclosporin).

Folate deficiency

Direct tests include the serum and red-cell folate assay. The serum folate level is always low in folate deficiency (and is normal or raised in B_{12} deficiency unless folate deficiency is also present). Red-cell folate is a better guide than the serum folate to tissue folate stores.

Diagnosis of the cause of B_{12} deficiency

Although the clinical and family history and the clinical findings may point to pernicious anaemia or some other cause of B_{12} deficiency, it is important to establish this for certain. A brief dietary history will rapidly establish whether or not the patient is a vegan or takes a very inadequate diet. Radioactive B_{12} absorption tests are valuable to demonstrate B_{12} malabsorption and to differentiate gastric from small-intestinal lesions as the cause. The patient, after an overnight fast, is fed an oral radioactively labelled dose of cyanocobalamin, usually 1 μg of ^{57}Co-labelled B_{12}. Absorption can be measured by whole-body counting, liver uptake, faecal excretion, by plasma radioactivity, or by 24-h urinary excretion after a non-radioactive, parenteral flushing dose of 1 mg of B_{12} (Schilling test). Hydroxocobalamin instead of cyanocobalamin, as originally described, can be used to flush absorbed, labelled B_{12} into urine.

Normal subjects absorb more than 30 per cent of the 1-μg dose. In patients with a gastric cause, malabsorption is corrected when the labelled B_{12} is given with IF, whereas if the lesion is in the small intestine, the absorption does not improve with IF. Treatment with broad-spectrum antibiotics may improve the absorption in the stagnant-loop syndrome. In some patients with pernicious anaemia the absorption with IF only improves substantially after weeks of B_{12} therapy, possibly due to slow recovery of ileal function from the effects of B_{12} deficiency.

Gastric secretion studies in pernicious anaemia reveal achlorhydria. Endoscopy gastric biopsy will show features of gastric atrophy and helps to exclude gastric carcinoma. Serum should be tested for antibodies to IF and parietal cells.

Diagnosis of the cause of folate deficiency

An inadequate diet is usually, at least partly, implicated, but an exact estimate of dietary intake from the clinical history is impossible. Often it is the general social circumstances that suggest a poor intake. Drug intake, particularly of barbiturates, is important. Many underlying inflammatory or malignant diseases may exaggerate the tendency to folate deficiency in patients with inadequate diets. The main cause of folate malabsorption is gluten-induced enteropathy; in patients with severe folate deficiency, a jejunal biopsy is usually necessary. In certain tropical countries sprue may cause a generalized malabsorption syndrome in which folate deficiency commonly occurs.

Treatment of megaloblastic anaemia

Therapy is aimed at correcting the anaemia, completely replenishing the body with the deficient vitamin, treating the underlying disorder, and preventing relapse. In most cases, it is possible to diagnose which deficiency is present before starting therapy.

Vitamin B_{12} deficiency

Hydroxocobalamin, 1000 μg intramuscularly given six times at several days' interval over the first few weeks, will restore normal B_{12} stores.

Response to therapy

The patient feels better within 24–48 h, and the mild fever, if not due to infection, falls to normal. A painful tongue and uncooperative, disorientated state may also be improved in 48 h. The reticulocyte count peaks after 5–7 days. The white-cell count becomes normal by the third to seventh day and the platelet count rises and may reach levels of $500–1000 \times 10^9$/l before falling to normal at about 10–14 days. The bone marrow reverts to normoblastic by 36–48 h, although giant metamyelocytes persist for 10–12 days. The neuropathy always improves with therapy but residual deficits remain in some patients, particularly in those with symptoms of over 3 months' duration before the institution of therapy.

Maintenance

Hydroxocobalamin, 1000 μg intramuscularly, is given once every 3 months for life in pernicious anaemia and most other causes of B_{12} deficiency to prevent relapse. In a few patients with B_{12} deficiency, the underlying cause can be reversed; for example, expulsion of the fish tapeworm, improvement of a vegan diet, surgical correction of an intestinal stagnant loop. A few micrograms of B_{12} can be absorbed each day in pernicious anaemia from oral doses of 1000 μg or more by passive diffusion, but this maintenance therapy is reserved for those who cannot have injections—for example those with a bleeding disorder or who refuse them. Vegans may be maintained on much smaller oral doses of B_{12} each day, such as 50 μg as a tablet or syrup.

Prophylactic B_{12}

B_{12} therapy should be given from the time of operation after total gastrectomy or after ileal resection if a B_{12} absorption test post-operatively reveals malabsorption of the vitamin.

Folate deficiency

This is corrected by giving 5 mg folic acid by mouth daily. It is essential to exclude B_{12} deficiency so that precipitation of a neuropathy is avoided. It is usual to continue for at least 4 months until there is a completely new set of red cells, although body stores will theoretically be normal within a few days of therapy. The response to therapy is as described for B_{12}. The decision whether or not to continue folic acid beyond 4 months depends on whether or not the cause can be corrected. In practice, long-term folic acid is usually needed only in patients with severe haemolytic anaemias (for example, sickle-cell anaemia and thalassaemia major), myelofibrosis, and in gluten-induced enteropathy when a gluten-free diet is either unsuccessful or not feasible. In patients on a gluten-free diet, assessment of folate status is one simple way of following the improvement in absorption.

Prophylactic folic acid

This should be given to all pregnant women (doses of 400 μg daily are used, often combined with an iron preparation) and, if the diet is poor, to all women likely to become pregnant. Larger (for example, 5 mg daily) doses are given if there has been a previous infant with a neural tube-deficit. Folic acid is given to patients undergoing regular haemodialysis or peritoneal dialysis, and to premature infants weighing less than 1.5 kg at birth, and to selected patients in intensive care units or those receiving parenteral nutrition.

Fortification of the diet with folic acid (in flour) in now carried out in the USA and is being considered in Britain to reduce the occurrence of neural-tube deficits in children.

Folinic acid (5-formyl-THF)

This reduced folate is used to prevent or treat toxicity due to methotrexate or other dihydrofolate reductase inhibitors.

Severely ill patients

Some patients, usually elderly, are admitted to hospital severely ill with megaloblastic anaemia, perhaps in congestive heart failure, or with pneumonia. In this case, it is necessary to commence therapy immediately after obtaining blood for B_{12} and folate assay and aspirating bone marrow, before it is known which deficiency is present. Both vitamins should be given simultaneously in large doses. Heart failure and infection should be treated in conventional fashion. However, blood transfusion should be avoided, except in cases of extreme anaemia when 1–2 units of packed cells may be given slowly, accompanied by removal of a similar volume of blood from the other arm, and diuretic therapy.

Other therapy

Hypokalaemia may occur during the response to therapy and oral potassium supplements should be given to those with initial heart failure or if severe hypokalaemia is demonstrated. Iron deficiency commonly develops in the first few weeks of therapy.

Megaloblastic anaemia due to inborn errors of folate or B_{12} metabolism

Folate

A number of babies have been described with congenital deficiency of one or other enzyme concerned in folate metabolism. Nearly all showed impaired mental development.

Vitamin B_{12}

Congenital deficiency of transcobalamin II (TC II) may occur and is variable in severity. The serum B_{12} level is usually normal, B_{12} being bound to TC I. Absorption of B_{12} is impaired. Treatment is with massive doses of B_{12} (for example, 1000 μg intramuscularly three times each week). In contrast, in subjects with rare, inherited, low levels of TC I, low serum B_{12} levels occur, but haemopoiesis is normal. Abnormalities of enzymes concerned in the synthesis of ado-B_{12} cause methylmalonic aciduria with or without megaloblastic anaemia.

Megaloblastic anaemia due to acquired disturbances of folate or B_{12} metabolism

Folate

Therapy with dihydrofolate reductase inhibitors (for example, methotrexate) may cause megaloblastic anaemia.

Vitamin B_{12}

Nitrous oxide (N_2O)

This anaesthetic gas oxidizes B_{12} to an inactive form. Megaloblastosis develops within hours and recovers over several days when exposure to N_2O is discontinued. Neuropathies have been described in people (for example, dentists and anaesthetists) repeatedly exposed to the gas. When N_2O is used as an anaesthetic for patients with low B_{12} stores, megaloblastic anaemia or neuropathy may be precipitated months later, due to failure to replenish B_{12} stores by absorption.

Megaloblastic anaemia not due to folate or B_{12} deficiency or to a metabolic defect

Congenital

Orotic aciduria

This is a rare recessive disorder involving two enzymes in pyrimidine synthetase and presents with megaloblastic anaemia in the first few months of life. The diagnosis is made if needle-shaped, colourless crystals of orotic acid are found in the urine. Treatment is with uridine (1 to 1.5 g daily).

Thiamine-responsive anaemia

This may be associated with sideroblastic change. There is a fault in thiamine phosphorylation.

Congenital dyserythropoietic anaemia

Some cases of congenital dyserythropoietic anaemia show megaloblastic changes not due to B_{12} or folate deficiency.

Acquired

Megaloblastic changes are often marked in acute myeloid leukaemia (AML)/M6 and less commonly in other forms of AML. They also occur in about 50 per cent of patients with primary acquired sideroblastic anaemia and in other myelodysplastic syndromes. The exact site of the block in DNA synthesis in these syndromes is unknown.

Drugs that directly inhibit purine or pyrimidine synthesis (for instance, cytosine arabinoside, 5-fluorouracil, hydroxyurea, 6-mercaptopurine, or azathioprine) may cause megaloblastic anaemia.

Other deficiency anaemias

Vitamin C

Anaemia is usual in scurvy but the pathogenesis is complicated. It is likely that vitamin C has a direct effect on erythropoiesis, but folate and iron deficiencies, haemorrhage, or haemolysis often complicate the picture. Minimum adult daily requirements for vitamin C are about 10 mg but 30–70 mg is recommended. The anaemia of scurvy is typically normochromic, normocytic with a slightly raised reticulocyte count to 5–10 per cent and a normoblastic marrow with erythroid hyperplasia. Extravascular haemolysis occurs in many of the patients.

Protein deficiency (see Section 8)

Anaemia is usual in both 'pure' protein deficiency, kwashiorkor, and in protein-calorie malnutrition (marasmus). The anaemia also occurs in patients with gastrointestinal disease and severe malabsorption. The anaemia is typically normochromic, normocytic, and of the order of 8.0–9.0 g/dl. Typically erythropoietin levels are low and in many patients, the anaemia is complicated by infection, folate or iron.

Further reading

Boushey, C., Beresford, S., Omenn, G., *et al.* (1995). A quantitative assessment of plasma homocysteine as a risk factor for vascular disease. Probable benefits of increasing folic acid intakes. *Journal of the American Medical Association*, 274, 1049–57.

Daly, S., Mills, J.L., Molloy, A.M., *et al.* (1997). Minimum effective dose of folic acid for food fortification to prevent neural-tube defects. *Lancet*, 350, 1666–9.

Graham, I.M., Daly, L.E., Refsum, H.M., *et al.* (1997). Plasma homocysteine as a risk factor for vascular disease: the European concerted action project. *Journal of the American Medical Association*, 277, 1775–81.

Kozyraki, R., Kristiansen, M., Silahtaroglu, A., *et al.* (1998). The human intrinsic factor—vitamin B12 receptor: molecular characterization and chromosomal mapping of the gene to 10p within the autosomal megaloblastic anemia (MGAI) region. *Blood*, 91, 3593–600.

Molloy, A.M., Daly, S., Mills, J.L., *et al.* (1997). Thermolabile variant 5,10-methylenetetrahydrofolate reductase associated with low red-cell folates: implications for folate intake recommendations. *Lancet*, 349, 1591–3.

Wald, N.J., Watt, H.C., Law, M.R., *et al.* (1998). Homocysteine and ischaemic heart disease: results of a prospective study with implications regarding prevention. *Archives of Internal Medicine*, 158, 862–7.

Wickramasinghe, S.N. (ed). (1995). Megaloblastic anaemia. *Baillière's Clinical Haematology*, 8, 441–699.

Chapter 3.19

Disorders of the synthesis or function of haemoglobin

D. J. Weatherall

Disorders of the synthesis or structure of haemoglobin may be either inherited or acquired. The inherited disorders of haemoglobin are the most common single-gene disorders in the world's population. The World Health Organization has estimated that approximately 7 per cent of the world's population are carriers for important haemoglobin disorders. In many of the developing countries, where there is still a very high mortality from infection and malnutrition in the first year of life, these conditions are not yet recognized as an important public health problem. However, once economic conditions improve and infant death rates fall, the genetic disorders of haemoglobin start to place a major burden on the health services. This phenomenon has already been observed in parts of the Mediterranean region and South-East Asia.

Table 1 Disorders of haemoglobin

Genetic	*Acquired*
• Thalassaemia	• Methaemoglobin
• Structural variants	• Carbonmonoxyhaemoglobin
• Hereditary persistence of fetal haemoglobin	• Sulphaemoglobin
	• Defective synthesis:
	• Haemoglobin H/leukaemia
	• Other neoplastic disorders

As a result of mass migrations of populations from high incidence areas these conditions are being seen with increasing frequency in parts of the world where they have not been recognized previously. Because some of them, particularly sickle-cell anaemia and the more severe forms of thalassaemia, can produce life-threatening medical emergencies, it is important for clinicians to have at least a working knowledge of their clinical features, management, and prevention.

The structure, genetic control, and synthesis of haemoglobin

Structure

Human haemoglobin is heterogeneous at all stages of development; different haemoglobins are synthesized in the embryo, fetus, and adult, each adapted to the particular oxygen requirements of these changing environments.

The human haemoglobins all have a tetrameric structure made up of two different pairs of globin chains, each attached to one haem molecule. Adult and fetal haemoglobins have α-chains combined with β-chains (Hb A, $\alpha_2\beta_2$), δ-chains (Hb A_2, $\alpha_2\delta_2$), or γ-chains (Hb F, $\alpha_2\gamma_2$). In embryos, α-like chains called zeta (ζ)-chains combine with γ-chains to produce Hb Portland ($\zeta_2\gamma_2$), or with ε-chains to make Hb Gower 1 ($\zeta_2\varepsilon_2$), and α- and ε-chains combine to form Hb Gower 2 ($\alpha_2\varepsilon_2$). Fetal haemoglobin is itself heterogeneous; there are two kinds of γ-chains, which differ in their amino acid composition at position 136, where they have either a glycine or an alanine residue; those with glycine are called $^G\gamma$ chains, those with alanine $^A\gamma$. The $^G\gamma$ and $^A\gamma$ chains are the product of separate ($^G\gamma$ and $^A\gamma$) loci.

Classification of the disorders of haemoglobin

The main groups of haemoglobin disorders are shown in Table 1. The genetic disorders are divided into those in which there is a reduced rate of production of one or more of the globin chains, the thalassaemias, and those in which there is a structural change in a globin chain leading to instability or abnormal oxygen transport. In addition, there is a harmless group of mutations that interfere with the normal switching of fetal to adult haemoglobin production; these conditions are known collectively as hereditary persistence of fetal haemoglobin. The acquired disorders of haemoglobin can be subdivided into those characterized by defective synthesis of the globin chain and those in which the structure of the haem molecules is altered, leading to inefficient oxygen transport.

The thalassaemias

Introduction

Definition and classification

The thalassaemias are a heterogeneous group of genetic disorders of haemoglobin synthesis, all of which result from a reduced rate of

Table 2 The thalassaemias

α-Thalassaemia	δβ-Thalassaemia
α°	(δβ)°
α^+	Haemoglobin Lepore $(\delta\beta)^+$
β-Thalassaemia	(εγδβ)°-Thalassaemia
β°	δ-Thalassaemia
β^+	

Table 3 The β-, δβ-, and γδβ-thalassaemias

Type of thalassaemia	Findings in homozygote	Findings in heterozygote
β°	Thalassaemia major[1,2]	Thalassaemia minor
	Hbs F and A_2	Raised Hb A_2
β^+	Thalassaemia major[1,2]	Thalassaemia minor
	Hbs F, A and A_2	Raised Hb A_2
δβ	Thalassaemia intermedia	Thalassaemia minor
	Hb F only	Hb F 5–15%; Hb A_2 normal
$(\delta\beta)^+$	Thalassaemia major	Thalassaemia minor
(Lepore)	or intermedia Hbs F and Lepore	Hb Lepore 5–15%; Hb A_2 normal
εγδβ	Not viable	Neonatal haemolysis
		Thalassaemia minor in adults, with normal Hbs F and A_2

[1] Occasionally have thalassaemia intermedia phenotype.

[2] Many patients with thalassaemia are compound heterozygotes for different molecular forms of β° or β^+ thalassaemia.

production of one or more of the globin chain(s) of haemoglobin. They are divided into the α-, β-, δβ- or γδβ-thalassaemias according to which globin chain(s) is produced in reduced amounts (Table 2 and see Table 3). In some thalassaemias no globin chain is synthesized at all, and hence they are called α°-or β°-thalassaemias, whereas in others some globin chain is produced but at a reduced rate; the latter conditions are called α^+- or β^+-thalassaemias. The δβ- and γδβ-thalassaemias are always characterized by an absence of chain synthesis; thus they are (δβ)°- and (γδβ)°-thalassaemias. Because thalassaemia occurs in populations in which structural haemoglobin variants are common, it is not at all unusual for an individual to receive a thalassaemia gene from one parent and a gene for a structural haemoglobin variant from the other. Furthermore, both α- and β-thalassaemia occur commonly in some countries and hence individuals may receive genes for both types. These different interactions produce an extremely complex and clinically diverse series of genetic disorders, which range in severity from death *in utero* to extremely mild, symptomless, hypochromic anaemias.

The thalassaemias are inherited in a simple Mendelian codominant fashion. Heterozygotes are usually symptomless, although they can be easily recognized by simple haematological analysis. More severely affected patients are either homozygotes for α- or β-thalassaemia, compound heterozygotes for different molecular forms of α- or β-thalassaemia, or compound heterozygotes for one or other form of thalassaemia and a gene for a structural haemoglobin variant. Clinically, the thalassaemias are classified according to their severity into major, intermediate, and minor forms. Thalassaemia major is a severe transfusion-dependent disorder. Thalassaemia intermedia is characterized by anaemia and splenomegaly, though not of such severity as to require regular transfusion. Thalassaemia minor is the symptomless carrier state. While these descriptive terms do not have a precise genetic meaning, they remain useful in clinical practice.

The β-thalassaemias

The β-thalassaemias are the most important types of thalassaemia because they are so common and produce severe anaemia in their homozygous and compound heterozygous states.

Distribution

The β-thalassaemias occur widely in a broad belt ranging from the Mediterranean and parts of North and West Africa through the Middle East and Indian subcontinent to South-East Asia. In some populations carrier frequencies for the various forms of β-thalassaemia range between 2 and 30 per cent. It should be remembered that β-thalassaemia is not entirely confined to these high incidence regions; it occurs sporadically in every racial group.

Molecular pathology

Nearly 200 different molecular lesions responsible for the defective synthesis of the β-globin chains have been determined in β-thalassaemia. Some of these lesions completely inactivate the β-globin genes leading to the phenotype of β°-thalassaemia; others cause a reduced output from the genes and hence the picture of β^+-thalassaemia. Most mutations are single-base changes, or small deletions or insertions of one or two bases at various points in the genes. They can affect the coding sequence, RNA splicing, or gene regulation.

Pathophysiology

The molecular defects in the β-thalassaemias result in absent or reduced β-chain production. Synthesis of the α-chain proceeds at a normal rate and hence there is imbalanced globin-chain synthesis with the production of an excess of α-chains (Fig. 1). In the absence of their partner chains the α-chains are unstable and precipitate in the red-cell precursors, giving rise to large intracellular inclusions. These interfere with red-cell maturation, and hence there is a variable degree of intramedullary destruction of red-cell precursors, that is to say ineffective erythropoiesis. Those red cells that do mature and enter the circulation contain α-chain inclusions which interfere with their passage through the microcirculation, particularly in the spleen. These cells are prematurely destroyed and thus the anaemia of β-thalassaemia results from both ineffective erythropoiesis and a shortened red-cell survival. The anaemia is a stimulus to increased erythropoietin production from the kidneys and this causes massive expansion of the bone marrow, which may lead to serious deformities of the skull and long bones. Because the spleen is being constantly bombarded with abnormal red cells, it hypertrophies and the resulting splenomegaly causes red-cell pooling and an increase of the plasma volume, which contribute to the anaemia.

As mentioned previously, fetal haemoglobin production largely ceases after birth. However, some adult red-cell precursors (F cells) retain the ability to produce a small number of γ-chains. Because the latter can combine with excess α-chains to form haemoglobin F, cells

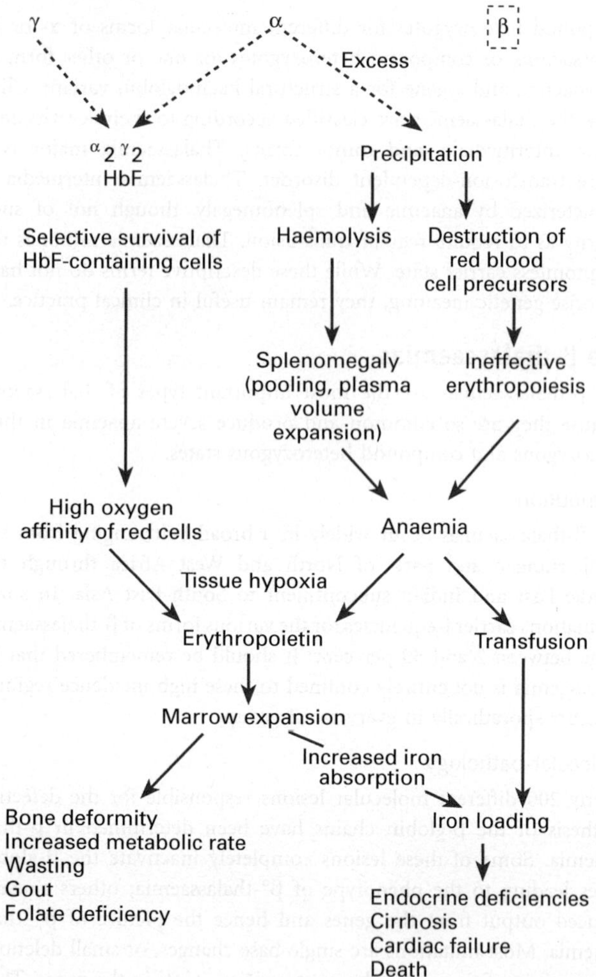

Fig. 1 The pathophysiology of β-thalassaemia.

that make relatively more γ-chains in the bone marrow of people with β-thalassaemia are partly protected against the deleterious effect of α-chain precipitation. Because these cells have a selective survival advantage they appear in the blood, and hence a raised fetal haemoglobin level is characteristic of all the β-thalassaemias. Furthermore, because δ-chain synthesis is unaffected, the disorder is characterized by a relative or absolute increase in haemoglobin A_2 ($\alpha_2\delta_2$) production. These interactions are summarized in Fig. 1.

It follows that if the anaemia is corrected with blood transfusion the erythropoietic drive is shut off, growth and development are improved, and bone deformities do not occur. On the other hand, each unit of blood contains 200 mg of iron; with regular transfusion there is a steady accumulation of iron in the liver, endocrine glands, and myocardium. Thus, although well-transfused thalassaemic children grow and develop well, they die of iron overload unless steps are taken to remove iron.

The severe homozygous or compound heterozygous forms of β-thalassaemia

These are the most common and most important forms of thalassaemia and give rise to a major public health problem in many parts of the world.

Clinical features

Most severe forms of β-thalassaemia present within the first year of life with failure to thrive, poor feeding, intermittent bouts of fever, or failure to improve after an intercurrent infection. At this stage the affected infant looks pale, and in many cases splenomegaly is already present. There are no other specific clinical signs and the diagnosis depends on the haematological changes outlined below. If the infant is put on a regular blood-transfusion regimen at this stage, early development is normal. However, if iron chelation is not instigated further symptoms occur at puberty, when the effects of iron loading due to repeated blood transfusion start to appear. If, on the other hand, the infant is not adequately transfused, the typical clinical picture of severe β-thalassaemia develops. Thus the clinical manifestations of the severe forms of β-thalassaemia have to be described in two contexts: the well-transfused child, and the child with chronic anaemia throughout early life.

In the well-transfused thalassaemic child growth and development are improved. However, if iron chelation is not introduced with the transfusion regime there is a gradual accumulation of iron and the effects of tissue siderosis start to appear by the end of the first decade. The normal adolescent growth spurt fails to occur and hepatic, endocrine, and cardiac complications of iron overloading produce a variety of problems including diabetes, hypoparathyroidism, adrenal insufficiency, and liver failure. Secondary sexual development is delayed, or does not occur at all. By far the most common cause of death, which usually occurs toward the end of the second or early in the third decade, is progressive cardiac damage. The use of intensive chelation therapy is able to prevent or delay this distressing termination.

The clinical picture in children who are inadequately transfused is quite different. There is progressive splenomegaly, and hypersplenism may cause a worsening of the anaemia, sometimes associated with thrombocytopenia and a bleeding tendency. Because of the bone marrow expansion there may be hideous deformities of the skull, with marked bossing and overgrowth of the zygomata giving rise to the classical facies of β-thalassaemia (Fig. 2(a)). These changes are reflected by striking radiological changes, which include a lacy, trabecular pattern of the long bones and phalanges and a typical 'hair on end' appearance of the skull. Because of the massive marrow expansion resulting from the chronic anaemia, these children are hypermetabolic, run intermittent fevers, lose weight (Fig. 2(b)), and may become acutely folate-depleted with worsening of their anaemia. Further complications include infections, bone fractures, gout, and a bleeding tendency. Iron loading occurs from both transfusions and increased intestinal absorption.

Haematological changes

There is severe anaemia and the haemoglobin values on presentation range from 2 to 8 g/dl. Although the red cells are hypochromic and microcytic, the red-cell indices, as derived from an electronic cell counter, may give surprisingly normal results, although usually the mean corpuscular haemoglobin and volume (MCH, MCV) are reduced. The appearance of the stained peripheral blood film is grossly abnormal (Fig. 3). The red cells show marked hypochromia and variation in shape and size. There are many hypochromic macrocytes and misshapen microcytes, some of which are mere fragments of cells. There is a moderate degree of anisochromia and basophilic stippling. There are always some nucleated red cells in the peripheral blood and, after splenectomy, these are found in large numbers. There is usually a slight elevation in the reticulocyte count. The white-cell and platelet counts are normal unless there is hypersplenism when they are reduced. The bone marrow shows marked erythroid hyperplasia.

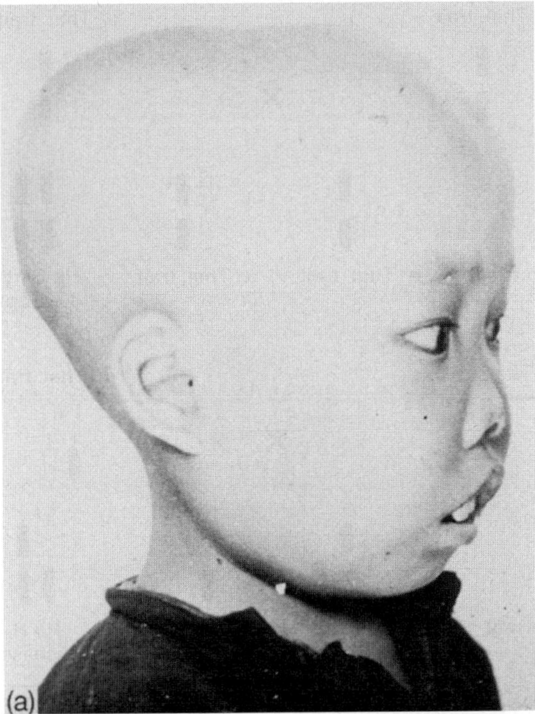

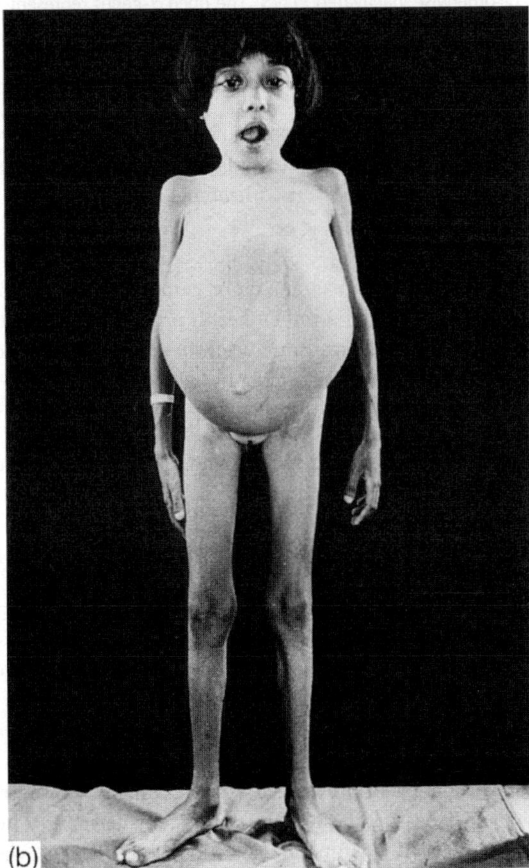

Fig. 2 Homozygous β-thalassaemia: (a) Skull and facial deformity due to bone marrow expansion. (b) Gross wasting of the limbs and hepatomegaly in an undertransfused child.

The bilirubin level is usually elevated and haptoglobins are absent. The ^{51}Cr red-cell survival is shortened. Without adequate chelation the serum iron and ferritin levels rise progressively.

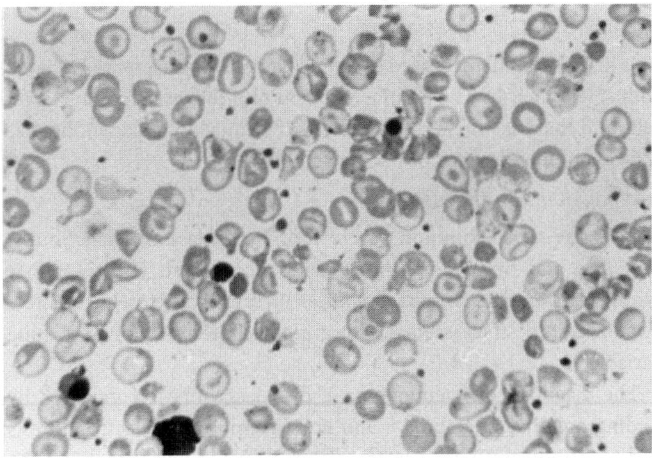

Fig. 3 Peripheral blood film in homozygous β-thalassaemia (630 ×, Leishman stain).

The haemoglobin F level is always elevated. In β°-thalassaemia there is no haemoglobin A and the haemoglobin consists of F and A_2 only. In β^+-thalassaemia the level of haemoglobin F ranges from 30 to 90 per cent of the total haemoglobin. The haemoglobin A_2 level is usually normal and is of no diagnostic value.

Heterozygous β-thalassaemia

Carriers for β-thalassaemia are usually symptom-free except during periods of stress such as pregnancy when they may become anaemic. Splenomegaly is rarely present.

Haematological changes

There is mild anaemia with haemoglobin values in the 9 to 11 g/dl range. The red cells show hypochromia and microcytosis with characteristically low MCH and MCV values. The reticulocyte count is usually normal. The bone marrow shows moderate erythroid hyperplasia.

Haemoglobin changes

The characteristic finding is an elevated haemoglobin A_2 level in the 4 to 6 per cent range. There is a slight elevation of haemoglobin F in the 1 to 3 per cent range in about 50 per cent of cases. A less common form occurs in which the haemoglobin A_2 is not elevated.

β-Thalassaemia in association with haemoglobin variants

It is quite common for an individual to inherit a β-thalassaemia gene from one parent and a gene for a structural haemoglobin variant from the other. Only three are of real importance—sickle-cell β-thalassaemia, haemoglobin C β-thalassaemia, and haemoglobin E β-thalassaemia.

Sickle-cell β-thalassaemia

The clinical manifestations vary considerably from race to race. In African populations the condition is usually characterized by mild anaemia and few sickling crises. On the other hand, in Mediterranean populations sickle-cell β°-thalassaemia occurs and is often associated with a clinical picture indistinguishable from that of sickle-cell anaemia.

Diagnosis rests on the clinical features of a sickling disorder found in association with a peripheral blood picture with typical thalassaemic red-cell changes, namely a low MCH and MCV. The diagnosis can be confirmed by haemoglobin electrophoresis and a family study.

Haemoglobin C β-thalassaemia

This disorder is characterized by a mild haemolytic anaemia associated with splenomegaly. The peripheral blood film shows numerous target cells and thalassaemic red-cell changes. Haemoglobin electrophoresis shows a preponderance of haemoglobin C.

Haemoglobin E β-thalassaemia

This is the most common severe form of thalassaemia in South-East Asia and throughout the Indian subcontinent. HbE is poorly synthesized and the resulting clinical picture may closely resemble homozygous β°-thalassaemia. However the clinical phenotype is quite variable.

The diagnosis of haemoglobin E β-thalassaemia is confirmed by finding only haemoglobins E and F on haemoglobin electrophoresis and by demonstrating the haemoglobin E trait in one parent and the β-thalassaemia trait in the other.

The δβ-thalassaemias (see Table 3)

Molecular genetics and classification

Disorders due to reduced β- and δ-chain synthesis are much less common than those due to defective β-chain production alone. It is usual to classify this group of conditions into the δβ-thalassaemias and the haemoglobin Lepore thalassaemias (in which the δ and β genes are fused and produce a δβ-fusion protein).

Clinical and haematological changes

In the homozygous state for δ β-thalassaemia there is a mild degree of anaemia with haemoglobin values of 8 to 10 g/dl. There is often a moderate degree of splenomegaly but these patients are usually symptomless except during periods of stress such as infection or pregnancy. Haemoglobin analysis shows 100 per cent haemoglobin F. Carriers have thalassaemic blood pictures, elevated levels of haemoglobin F of 5 to 20 per cent, and normal levels of haemoglobin A_2.

The homozygous state for haemoglobin Lepore is similar to that of homozygous β-thalassaemia, although in some cases it may be milder. The haemoglobin consists of F and Lepore only. Carriers have thalassaemic blood pictures associated with about 5 to 15 per cent haemoglobin Lepore.

There is a group of genetic disorders of haemoglobin production, encountered most commonly in Black-African populations, called collectively 'hereditary persistence of fetal haemoglobin'. Homozygotes have a mild thalassaemia-like blood picture but are not anaemic. They have 100 per cent haemoglobin F. Heterozygotes show no haematological abnormalities and carry 20 to 30 per cent haemoglobin F. These disorders are due to gene deletions involving the δ- and β-globin genes, and therefore appear to be extremely mild forms of δβ-thalassaemia in which the lack of δ- and β-chain production is almost entirely compensated for by the synthesis of the γ-chains of haemoglobin F.

The γδβ-thalassaemias

Heterozygotes with this rare phenotype have severe haemolytic disease of the newborn. If they survive the neonatal period they develop normally; in adult life they have the haematological picture of heterozygous β-thalassaemia and a haemoglobin pattern consisting of haemoglobin A, no elevation of haemoglobin F, and a normal level of haemoglobin A_2. The homozygous state is not compatible with survival.

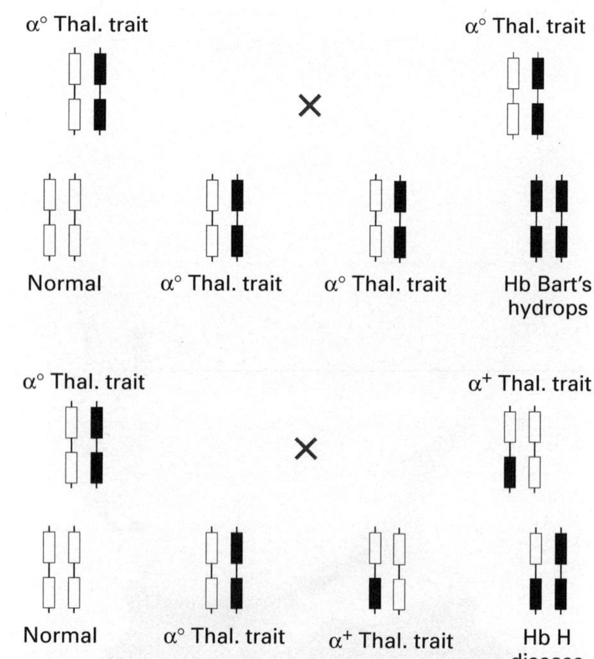

Fig. 4 The genetics of α-thalassaemia. The black α-genes represent gene deletions or otherwise inactivated genes. The open α-genes represent normal genes. α°-Thalassaemia and α^+-thalassaemia are defined in the text.

Other β-thalassaemia variants

Several rare variants have been described including forms that produce significant disease in heterozygotes, 'silent' heterozygote states, and heterozygous disease without raised haemoglobin A_2.

The α-thalassaemias

Although the α-thalassaemias are more common than the β-thalassaemias they pose less of a public health problem. This is because the severe homozygous forms cause death *in utero* or in the neonatal period and the milder forms do not produce major disability.

Distribution

The α-thalassaemias occur widely through the Mediterranean region, parts of West Africa, the Middle East, isolated parts of the Indian subcontinent, and throughout South-East Asia. The serious forms of α-thalassaemia are restricted to some of the Mediterranean island populations and South-East Asia.

Definition and inheritance

There are two α-globin genes on each chromosome and a normal individual therefore has four functional genes. If both genes on a chromosome are non-functional the heterozygote carrier has two functional α-globin genes and the resulting condition, with mild hypochromic anaemia, is known as α°-thalassaemia. If, however, only one of the genes on the affected chromosome is defective a heterozygote would have three functional α-globin genes. This virtually silent phenotype is termed α^+-thalassaemia. To put it another way, the terms α°- and α^+-thalassaemia describe haplotypes—the products of two linked α-chains on one of a pair of homologous chromosomes 16. The complexity arises when these different genetic lesions are inherited together (Fig. 4). If two α°-thalassaemia chromosomes are inherited there are no functional α-globin genes left and this is incompatible with life (Table 4). On the other hand, co-inheritence

Table 4 The α-thalassaemias

Type	Homozygotes	Heterozygotes
α°	Hb Bart's hydrops	Thalassaemia minor
α^{+}(deletion)	Thalassaemia minor	Normal blood picture[2]
α^{+}(non-deletion)	Hb H disease[1]	Normal blood picture[2]

[1] Haemoglobin H disease more commonly results from the compound heterozygous inheritance of α° and either variety of α^{+}-thalassaemia.

[2] There may be very mild red-cell hypochromia.

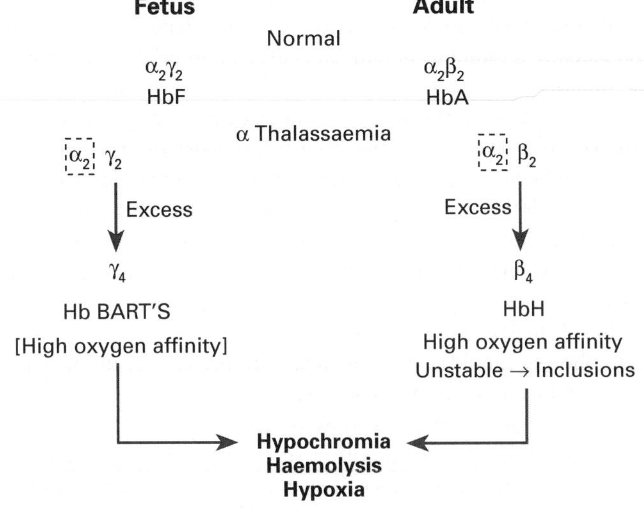

Fig. 5 The pathophysiology of α-thalassaemia.

of α°-thalassaemia and α^{+}-thalassaemia leaves one intact α-globin gene and results in the syndrome of haemoglobin H disease.

The α°-thalassaemias result from the deletion of both linked α-globin genes. The molecular basis of the α^{+}-thalassaemias is more variable; in most cases one of the α-globins is deleted, while less commonly one is inactivated by a mutation.

Because α°-thalassaemia is largely confined to South-East Asia and the Mediterranean islands it is in these populations that the haemoglobin Bart's hydrops syndrome and haemoglobin H disease cause public health problems. In contrast, α^{+}-thalassaemia occurs very commonly throughout parts of West Africa, the Indian subcontinent, and the Pacific island populations but is not a significant clinical problem, even in the homozygous state.

Pathophysiology

Unlike β-thalassaemia, the excess globin chains that are produced do not precipitate immediately, but form soluble homotetramers, γ4 (Hb Bart's) in infancy, and β4 (Hb H) in adults. Hence the pathophysiology of α-thalassaemia is different to that of β-thalassaemia (Fig. 5). Erythropoiesis is more effective but there is a shortened red-cell survival due to haemoglobin H precipitation in older red cells. Haemoglobins Bart's and H have excess γ-chains or β-chains, respectively, resulting from deficiency in α-chains. These haemoglobins have a very high oxygen affinity and are physiologically useless.

The haemoglobin Bart's hydrops syndrome

This results from the homozygous state for α°-thalassaemia and is a common cause of fetal loss throughout South-East Asia and in Greece and Cyprus. Affected infants produce no α-chains at all and hence can make neither fetal nor adult haemoglobin.

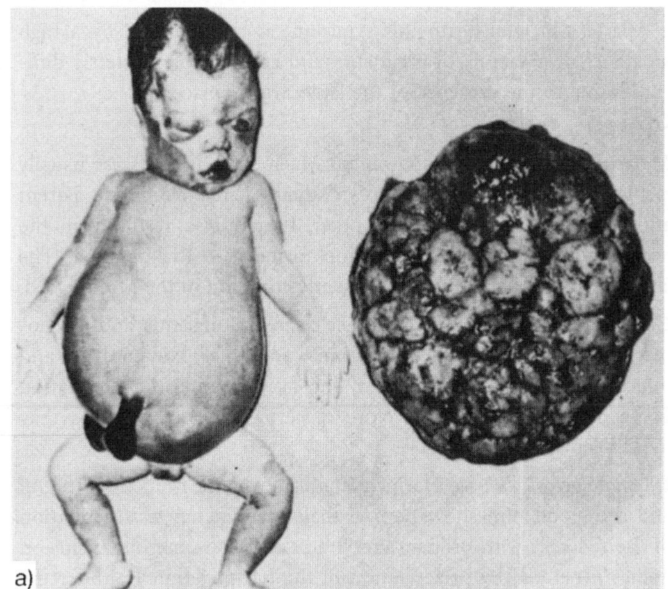

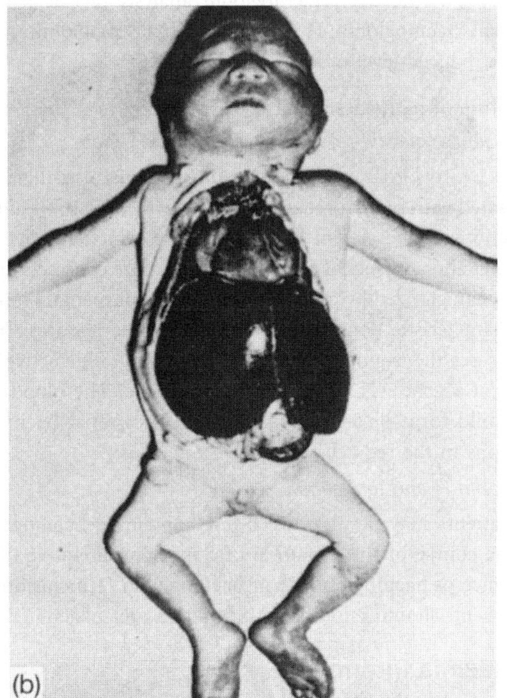

Fig. 6(a, b) The haemoglobin Bart's hydrops syndrome: (a) a hydropic infant with massively enlarged placenta; (b) autopsy findings with an enlarged liver.
(Both reproduced by permission of Professor P. Wasi.)

The clinical picture is very characteristic (Fig. 6). These infants are usually stillborn between 28 and 40 weeks, or if they are live-born take a few gasping breaths and then expire within the first hours after birth. They show the typical picture of hydrops fetalis with gross pallor, generalized oedema, and massive hepatosplenomegaly. There is a very large, friable placenta. All these findings are due to severe intrauterine anaemia. The haemoglobin values are in the 6 to 8 g/dl range and gross thalassaemic changes are seen on the peripheral blood film with many nucleated red cells. The haemoglobin consists of approximately 80 per cent haemoglobin Bart's and 20 per cent of the embryonic haemoglobin, Portland ($\zeta_2\gamma_2$).

Apart from fetal death this syndrome is characterized by a high incidence of toxaemia of pregnancy and considerable obstetric difficulties due to the presence of the large, friable placenta.

Haemoglobin H disease

Molecular genetics and pathogenesis Haemoglobin H disease usually results from the inheritance of α°-thalassaemia from one parent and α^{+}-thalassaemia from the other. It may also result from the homozygous state for non-deletion forms of α-thalassaemia. The latter form of inheritance is particularly common in the Middle East.

Clinical features There is a variable degree of anaemia and splenomegaly but patients usually survive into adult life. Oxidant drugs and infection and hypersplenism may increase the rate of precipitation of haemoglobin H and therefore exacerbate the anaemia, as may hypersplenism.

Haematological changes Haemoglobin values range from 7 to 10 g/dl and the blood film shows typical thalassaemic changes. Incubation of the red cells with brilliant cresyl blue reveals numerous inclusion bodies generated by precipitation of the haemoglobin H under the redox action of the dye. Haemoglobin analysis reveals from 5 to 40 per cent haemoglobin H together with haemoglobin A and a normal or reduced level of haemoglobin A_2.

Other forms of α-thalassaemia

*α-Thalassaemia/mental retardation (**ATR**) syndromes*

There are two disorders in which acquired forms of α-thalassaemia are associated with mental retardation. The first, ATR 16, results from long deletions at the end of chromosome 16 which remove the α-globin genes and a variety of other genes. The more common disorder, ATRX, is characterized by a more severe degree of mental retardation with a characteristic constellation of dysmorphic features. In these X-linked cases the α-globin genes are intact but are defective due to mutation of a gene *XH2* on the X chromosome. The blood picture shows a mild form of α-thalassaemia with occasional haemoglobin H inclusions in the red cells.

Haemoglobin H and leukaemia

Elderly patients may develop a cell line containing haemoglobin H during the course of the evolution of a myeloproliferative disorder. The presence of haemoglobin H or haemoglobin H inclusions in an elderly patients should raise the suspicion of a preleukaemic disorder.

Thalassaemia intermedia

Definition and pathogenesis

The term thalassaemia intermedia is used to describe patients with the clinical picture of thalassaemia, which, although not transfusion-dependent, is associated with a much more severe degree of anaemia than that found in heterozygous carriers for α- or β-thalassaemia. Many of the conditions described earlier in this section follow this clinical course—haemoglobin C or E thalassaemia, the various δβ-thalassaemias and haemoglobin Lepore disorders, and the wide variety of conditions that can result from the interactions of the different β- and δβ-thalassaemia determinants, for example. However, some children appear to be homozygous for β-thalassaemia yet run a much milder course than is usually the case. Sometimes this is due to co-inheritence of α-thalassaemia or less severe β-thalassaemia mutations.

Clinical and haematological changes

The clinical features are extremely variable. At one end of the spectrum are individuals who are virtually symptom-free, and, except for moderate anaemia, are completely normal. At the other there are patients who have haemoglobin values in the 5–7 g/dl range and who develop marked splenomegaly, severe skeletal deformities due to expansion of bone marrow, and, as they get older, become heavily iron-loaded because of increased intestinal absorption of iron. Recurrent leg ulceration, folate deficiency, symptoms due to extramedullary haemopoietic tumour masses in the chest and skull, gallstones, and a marked proneness to infection are particularly characteristic of this group of thalassaemias.

The laboratory diagnosis of thalassaemia

The thalassaemias should be suspected when a typical thalassaemic blood picture is found in an individual of an appropriate racial group. The homozygous states for the severe forms of β-thalassaemia are easily recognized by the typical haematological changes associated with very high levels of haemoglobin F. The heterozygous states are recognized by microcytic hypochromic red cells and an elevated level of haemoglobin A_2. The δβ-thalassaemias are characterized by the finding of 100 per cent haemoglobin F in homozygotes, and 5–15 per cent haemoglobin F together with a normal level of haemoglobin A_2 in heterozygotes (see Table 3).

When β-thalassaemia is diagnosed, a quantitative haemoglobin electrophoresis should be done to exclude the presence of an abnormal haemoglobin variant such as haemoglobin E or Lepore.

The haemoglobin Bart's hydrops syndrome is recognized by the finding of a hydropic infant with a severe anaemia, a thalassaemic blood picture, and the presence of 80 per cent or more haemoglobin Bart's on haemoglobin electrophoresis. Haemoglobin H disease is identified by the finding of a typical thalassaemic blood picture with an elevated reticulocyte count, generation of multiple inclusion bodies in the red cells after incubation with brilliant cresyl blue, and the finding of variable amounts of haemoglobin H on haemoglobin electrophoresis. There are no really useful diagnostic tests for the different α-thalassaemic carrier states, although α°-thalassaemia heterozygotes usually have typical thalassaemic red-cell changes with a normal haemoglobin A_2 value.

Prevention and treatment

Because there is no definitive treatment, most countries in which the disease is common are putting a major effort into its prevention.

Prevention

There are two major approaches to the prevention of the thalassaemias-population: screening with genetic counselling or prenatal diagnosis. Prenatal diagnosis can be made by globin-chain synthesis studies of fetal blood samples obtained by fetoscopy at 18 to 20 weeks' gestation, or fetal DNA analysis on amniotic fluid cells after chorion biopsy.

Because prenatal diagnosis of thalassaemia is available it is very important to discuss the genetic implications of the condition when carriers are detected by chance, regardless of the individual's racial background.

Symptomatic treatment

This is based upon regular blood transfusion, the judicious use of splenectomy if hypersplenism develops, and the administration of chelating agents to attempt to deal with the problem of iron overload from regular blood transfusion. The object should be to maintain the haemoglobin level between 9 and 14 g/dl. If there is a marked

Table 5 Clinical disorders due to structural haemoglobin variants

Disorder	Variants
Haemolysis and tissue damage	Haemoglobin S
Drug-induced haemolysis	Haemoglobin Zürich and other unstable haemoglobins
Chronic haemolysis	Unstable haemoglobin variants
	Haemoglobin C
Congenital polycythaemia	High-affinity variants
Congenital cyanosis	Haemoglobin(s) M
	Low-affinity variants
Hypochromia: thalassaemic phenotype	Haemoglobin E
	Haemoglobin Constant Spring

increase in transfusion requirements hypersplenism should be suspected. Splenectomy should be done as late as is feasible and, if possible, not in the first 5 years.

The only useful chelating agent for the prevention or treatment of iron overload in thalassaemia is desferrioxamine. Therapy should be started as early as possible, but for practical purposes this usually means somewhere between the second or third year or later.

The role of bone marrow transplantation is still controversial. Recent results suggest that if it is done early in life, with marrow donated from an HLA-compatible sibling, there is over an 80 per cent chance of curing the disease. These results need confirmation by larger series, but, at the time of writing, there seems to be a genuine place for marrow transplantation, particularly in families who find regular transfusion and chelating agents difficult to manage.

If well looked after, these children can have a relatively normal childhood, and the recent advances in the use of chelating drugs may mean that some of the distressing side-effects of iron loading that occur at puberty may at least be delayed, and possibly prevented indefinitely.

Structural haemoglobin variants

Over 400 structural haemoglobin variants have been described, most of which result from single amino acid substitutions. A classification of the diseases that result from structural abnormalities of haemoglobin is shown in Table 5.

Nomenclature

Originally, the structural haemoglobin variants were named by letters of the alphabet, but later it was decided to designate new haemoglobin variants by the place of origin of the first patient in whom they were characterized. It is customary to call the heterozygous (carrier) state the 'trait' and the homozygous condition the 'disease'. For example, haemoglobin S heterozygotes (genotype *AS*) are said to have the sickle-cell trait, while individuals homozygous for the sickle-cell mutation (genotype *SS*) are said to have sickle-cell disease.

The sickling disorders

Sickling disorders (Table 6) consist of the heterozygous state for haemoglobin S, or the sickle-cell trait (AS), the homozygous state, or sickle-cell disease (SS), and the compound heterozygous state for haemoglobin S together with haemoglobins C, D, E, or other structural variants. In addition, there are several disorders that result from the inheritance of the sickle-cell gene, together with different forms of thalassaemia.

Table 6 The major sickling disorders

Disorder	Genotype (normal= $\alpha\alpha/\alpha\alpha.\beta/\beta$)
SS disease (sickle-cell anaemia)	$\alpha\alpha/\alpha\alpha\ \beta^S/\beta^S$
SC disease	$\alpha\alpha/\alpha\alpha\ \beta^S/\beta^C$
SD disease	$\alpha\alpha/\alpha\alpha\ \beta^S/\beta^D$
S–β thalassaemia	$\alpha\alpha/\alpha\alpha\ \beta^S\beta^\circ$ or β^S/β^+
S–hereditary persistence of fetal Hb	$\alpha\alpha/\alpha\alpha\ \beta^S/-*$
S–α thalassaemia	α-/$\alpha\alpha$ or α-/α-β^S/β^S

*Indicates β-gene deletion.

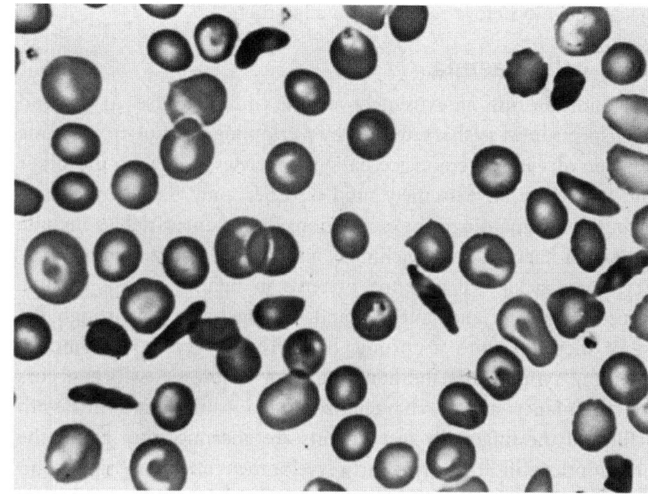

Fig. 7 Irreversibly sickled cells in the peripheral blood (1000 ×, Leishman stain).

Pathogenesis

Haemoglobin S differs from haemoglobin A by the substitution of valine for glutamic acid at position 6 in the β-chain. During their passage through the circulation, red cells containing haemoglobin S at a high concentration go through a series of cycles of sickling and desickling, and finally the cells become irreversibly sickled (Fig. 7). Sickling has two main effects: a chronic haemolytic anaemia and vascular blockage with tissue infarction.

Distribution

The sickling disorders occur very frequently in African and some Indian populations and, sporadically, throughout the Mediterranean region and the Middle East. There are extensive pockets in India but the disease has not been seen in South-East Asia. It is thought that the high frequency of the sickle-cell gene occurs because carriers are more resistant than normal individuals to *Plasmodium falciparum* malaria.

Clinical features

Except in conditions of extreme anoxia such as flying in unpressurized aircraft, the sickle-cell trait causes no clinical disability. However, it is possible for individuals to suffer vaso-occlusive episodes if they

Table 7 Acute exacerbations ('crises') in sickle-cell (SS) disease

1. Thrombotic: • Generalized or localized bone pain • Abdominal • Pulmonary • Neurological	**3. Haemolytic**
	4. Sequestration: • Spleen • Liver • ?lung
2. Aplastic	**5. Various combinations of above**

become unusually hypoxic under anaesthesia, and therefore all individuals of the appropriate racial background should have a sickling test (see below) before receiving an anaesthetic.

Sickle-cell anaemia

This condition runs an extremely variable clinical course. At one end of the spectrum it is characterized by a crippling haemolytic anaemia interspersed with severe exacerbations or crises, while on the other hand it may be an extremely mild disorder, only found by chance on routine haematological examination. Important variables include the level of haemoglobin F, climate, and socioeconomic factors.

Typically, sickle-cell anaemia presents in infancy with a variable degree of anaemia and jaundice and most patients go through the rest of their life with a chronic haemolytic anaemia. A common presenting symptom is the hand-and-foot syndrome, which occurs early in infancy and is characterized by a painful dactylitis with swelling of the fingers or feet. Infants are anaemic from about the third month of life and during early development often have significant splenomegaly. In most cases this gradually resolves due to repeated infarction of the spleen, a condition called autosplenectomy. Typically, the haemoglobin is in the 6 to 8 g/dl range with a reticulocyte count of 10 to 20 per cent. There is chronic, mild icterus with an elevated bilirubin level. Examination of the peripheral blood film shows anisochromia and poikilocytosis with a variable number of sickled erythrocytes (Fig. 7). As the children grow older the haematological changes of hyposplenism develop.

In some studies, children have tended to be short for their age, while postadolescents were usually tall. The only other physical sign that is frequently present is chronic leg ulceration; this is discussed in a later section.

Complications

The chronic haemolysis of sickle-cell disease is interspersed with acute exacerbations of the illness called sickling crises. Furthermore, a series of serious and life-threatening long-term complications develops in many patients with symptomatic sickle-cell anaemia.

The different forms of sickle-cell crises are summarized in Table 7. The most common is the painful crisis. This is sometimes precipitated by infection, dehydration, or exposure to cold. The episode starts with vague pain, often in the back or bones of the limbs. The pain is almost certainly due to blockage of small vessels with sickled erythrocytes. Occasionally, abdominal pain is the major symptom and this may be associated with distension, rigidity, and quiet bowel sounds, a picture very similar to an acute abdominal emergency.

Two other serious forms of thrombotic crises occur, which are known as the 'lung' and 'brain' syndromes. The 'lung' syndrome is characterized by acute dyspnoea and pleuritic pain and is due to infarction of major pulmonary vessels. It is often preceded by a rapid fall in the packed cell volume, which may reflect sequestration of sickled cells in the pulmonary vessels. Neurological complications usually present in childhood, either as fits, transient neurological symptoms resembling ischaemic attacks, or with a fully developed stroke. There is a tendency for recurrent episodes. Recent evidence suggests that strokes may be predicted by regular transcranial Doppler ultrasonography to detect stenosis of cerebral vessels.

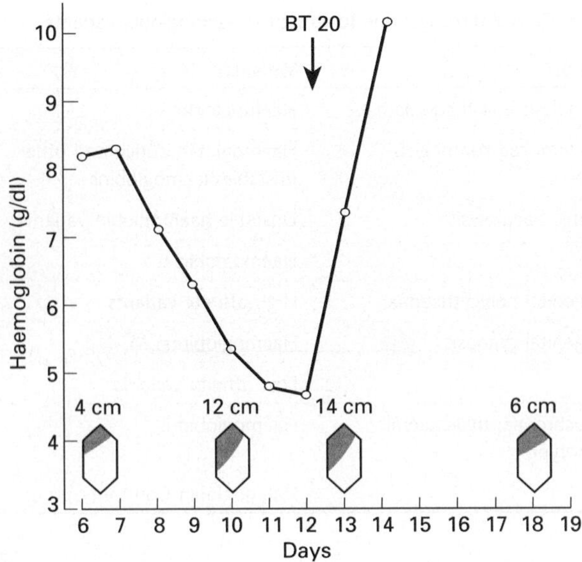

Fig. 8 Hepatic sequestration crisis in sickle-cell anaemia. BT, blood transfusion.

During painful crises there may be a marked increase in the rate of haemolysis with a fall in the haemoglobin level. Such haemolytic episodes are relatively uncommon. Much more serious are periods of transient bone marrow aplasia called aplastic crises. These seem to result from intercurrent infection, particularly due to parvoviruses, and frequently affect more than one sibling in the same family.

Finally, and most serious, are the sequestration crises. These occur mainly in babies and young children and are characterized by a rapid enlargement of the spleen or liver, which become engorged with sickled erythrocytes. As the crisis progresses a large proportion of the total red-cell mass may be trapped in the spleen or liver, and death may occur due to gross anaemia. These episodes show a tendency to recur in the same individual. Hepatic sequestration, which may occur in adults, is easily overlooked if the liver size is not monitored carefully (Fig. 8).

The most common cause of death in sickle-cell anaemia appears to be a sequestration crisis or acute infection, or both. A variety of organisms is involved, particularly *Pneumococcus* spp., and in some tropical countries typhoid infection of bone infarcts leads to typhoid osteomyelitis.

Pregnancy may be uneventful, or associated with an increased incidence of painful crises. There is a slightly increased incidence of maternal mortality and a definite increase in the rate of fetal loss.

Chronic complications

The chronic complications of sickle-cell anaemia result largely from repeated episodes of vascular occlusion. Almost any organ can be involved. The bones are particularly prone to infarction. Aseptic necrosis of the humeral or femoral heads may lead to their destruction, and bone infarcts may become secondarily infected to produce osteomyelitis.

Progressive renal dysfunction and failure is of particular importance (see Chapter 12.16). There is a progressive inability to concentrate the urine, leading to polyuria, nocturia, and enuresis. Chronic glomerular damage leads to chronic renal failure, which is a major contributor to or cause of death, particularly in patients over the age of 40 years.

There is increasing evidence that chronic lung disease may be an important determinant of complications and death. Chronic leg ulceration is also an important problem and may run a relapsing course for 10 or 20 years. Recurrent attacks of priapism may lead to chronic deformity of the penis. Vaso-occlusion in the eye due to ischaemia of the retinal vasculature is reflected by proliferative retinopathy with progressive visual loss. This complication occurs more frequently in haemoglobin subcutaneous disease.

Because of the chronic haemolysis, gallstones are very common and are seen in over 30 per cent of children by the age of 15 years.

Course and prognosis

Some patients with sickle-cell anaemia go through life with few complications, but there is a subset who undergo repeated crises, strokes, and incapacitating bone disease.

There is a marked difference in course and prognosis between populations. There are very few good data about the overall survival, although it seems likely that it is shortened. The most common cause of death at all ages is acute infection, while it appears that renal failure is becoming a more frequent cause of death in older sickling populations.

Laboratory diagnosis

The sickle-cell trait causes no haematological changes and is diagnosed by the finding of a positive sickling test together with haemoglobins A and S on electrophoresis (Fig. 9). Sickle-cell anaemia is diagnosed by the finding of anaemia, an elevated reticulocyte count, sickled erythrocytes on the peripheral blood film, a positive sickling test, and a haemoglobin electrophoretic pattern characterized by the absence of haemoglobin A and a preponderance of haemoglobin S with a variable amount of haemoglobin F (Fig. 9). The diagnosis is confirmed by finding the sickle-cell trait in both parents.

Management

Like all genetic diseases the first priority should be prevention. Prospective genetic counselling has not proven to be very successful. Prenatal diagnosis is undertaken in some centres.

It is important to identify patients with sickle-cell anaemia as early as possible. In high-risk populations neonatal screening programmes should be established. As soon as the disease is identified babies should receive daily oral penicillin and a pneumococcal vaccine.

Most patients with sickle-cell anaemia manage well with relatively low haemoglobin levels, and regular blood transfusion is generally not required. Adaptation to anaemia is particularly successful because of the low oxygen affinity of haemoglobin S. Episodes of infection should be treated early, and in populations in which the diet is low in folate, regular folate supplements should be added. Patients should be given access to a unit that is used to managing the disorder and advised to come early at the first sign of a painful crisis.

All but the mildest painful crises should be managed in hospital. The patient should be fully examined for evidence of underlying infection and then given adequate intravenous fluids, oxygen, antibiotics, and analgesia. It should be remembered that the pain may

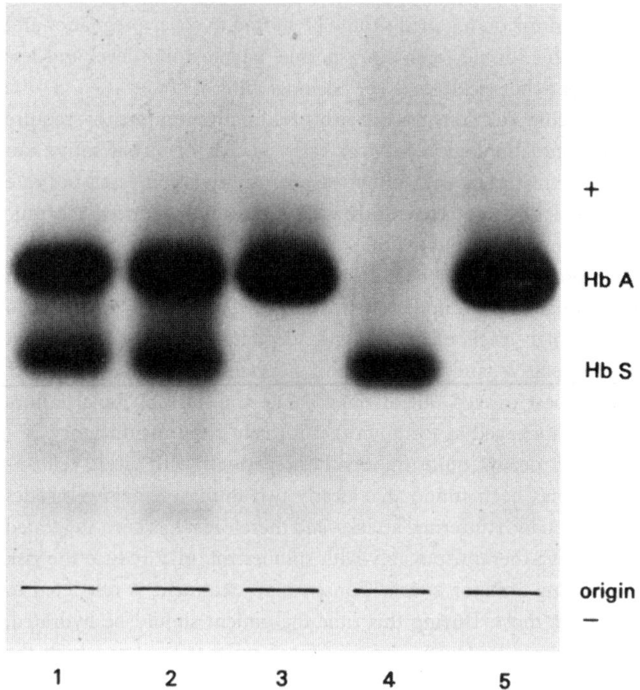

Fig. 9 The haemoglobin pattern in the sickling disorders (starch gel electrophoresis, protein stain, pH 8.5). The following are shown (left to right): (1 and 2) the sickle-cell trait; (3) normal; (4) sickle-cell anaemia; (5) normal.

be excruciating. It may be necessary to administer strong analgesics, but because of the danger of respiratory depression, this should only be done in an environment in which patients are under close observation, with regular monitoring of blood gases.

The packed cell volume or haemoglobin level, and reticulocyte count should be estimated at least daily, and perhaps twice daily. But unless there is a fall in the haemoglobin level or evidence of an impending aplastic crisis, as evidenced by a drop in the reticulocyte count, transfusion is not required. If the haemoglobin level falls due to increased haemolysis or bone marrow failure, a blood transfusion should be given to restore the haemoglobin level to normal or slightly higher. A sequestration crisis is an indication for urgent transfusion and very close surveillance because profound anaemia may develop over a period of hours. Hence, patients with a sickling crisis should have regular abdominal examinations to assess spleen and liver size to try and anticipate impending episodes of sequestration. Complications such as the brain or lung syndrome should be treated by partial exchange transfusion. The level of sickle cells should be reduced to below 30 per cent. If the initial haemoglobin level is lower than 5 to 6 g/dl, this can be achieved by transfusion up to 13 g/dl followed by regular 'top-up' transfusions to reduce endogenous erythropoiesis. If the initial haemoglobin value is unusually high (for example, in excess of 9 g/dl) it is better to carry out a partial exchange transfusion.

Hypertransfusion or exchange transfusion can be used to cover major surgical procedures or in patients who are having recurrent crises. Splenectomy may be indicated in cases with hypersplenism. Similarly, because sequestration crises seem to recur in the same infant, this may also be an indication for splenectomy.

There is no special treatment required during pregnancy except for regular surveillance and folate supplementation. If the haemoglobin level drops significantly, or if there are recurrent crises, a regular transfusion regimen should be started to cover pregnancy and delivery. This should maintain a normal haemoglobin level and less than 30 per cent sickle cells (or haemoglobin S).

Ocular complications, particularly proliferative retinopathy, require expert ophthalmological advice; early results of proliferative retinopathy treatment with either xenon arc or argon laser indicate that the risk of vitreous haemorrhage is significantly reduced. Chronic hip pain and difficulty with walking due to aseptic necrosis of the femoral heads may require total hip replacement. Any surgical procedure should be undertaken with great caution. It is critical to maintain high levels of oxygen and adequate hydration throughout the preoperative and postoperative period. Major procedures are probably best carried out after exchange transfusion. Renal failure should be managed as for any other form of renal insufficiency.

Priapism occurs quite frequently in patients with sickle-cell anaemia. It has been found that nearly two-thirds of major episodes are preceded by 'stuttering' attacks, and therefore it has been suggested that effective therapy, possibly with stilboestrol, may reduce the risk of sustaining a major attack. Conservative treatment is restricted to 24 h at the most. During this time the patient should be hydrated, given adequate analgesia, and transfused up to a level at which the number of sickleable cells is below about 30 to 40 per cent. If there is no improvement by these simple measures, a cavernosus–spongiosum shunt should be considered.

Recent trials suggest that daily hydroxyurea is effective at raising Hb F levels and reducing the frequency of crises. Such therapy is now widely used in selected patients. Allogeneic bone marrow transplantation can cure the disease but has the risk of causing significant morbidity and mortality. Its role is being assessed in prospective trials.

Other sickling disorders

The other sickling disorders include the interaction of haemoglobin S with haemoglobins C, D, β-thalassaemia, and some of the rarer haemoglobin variants. In many of these conditions the clinical manifestations are little different from the sickle-cell trait, but haemoglobin subcutaneous disease and SD disease more closely resemble sickle-cell anaemia.

Haemoglobin SC disease

This disease is relatively common in West Africans and is characterized by a milder anaemia than sickle-cell disease. Aseptic necrosis of the femoral or humeral heads or unexplained haematuria are common complications. A serious complication is the damage that may follow repeated blockage of the retinal vessels, which leads to retinitis proliferans, retinal detachment, and permanent blindness.

Haemoglobin SC disease is diagnosed by finding a mild anaemia with splenomegaly and characteristic morphological changes of the red cells including many target forms. The sickling test is positive and haemoglobin electrophoresis shows haemoglobins S and C in about equal proportions. One parent shows the sickle-cell trait and the other the haemoglobin C trait.

In severe thrombotic episodes, patients with haemoglobin SC disease should be well hydrated and treated with anticoagulants. Severe retinal disease is treated by coagulation therapy. In the life-threatening thrombotic episodes of pregnancy a partial exchange transfusion should be carried out.

Haemolysis due to other common haemoglobin variants

After haemoglobin S the second most common variant in West Africa is haemoglobin C. The homozygous state for haemoglobin C, haemoglobin C disease, is characterized by a mild haemolytic anaemia with splenomegaly. The blood film shows 100 per cent target cells, and haemoglobin analysis shows C with small amounts of F. This is a mild disorder and no specific treatment is required.

The most common haemoglobin variant throughout south-east Asia and the Indian subcontinent is haemoglobin E. The homozygous state for this variant, haemoglobin E disease, is characterized by a very mild degree of anaemia with a slight reticulocytosis. The blood film shows mild morphological changes of the red cells, which are hypochromic and microcytic, resembling the changes seen in some forms of thalassaemia. Again, no treatment is required for this mild anaemia.

Haemoglobin variants that migrate in the position of haemoglobin S but do not sickle have been given the general title of haemoglobin D. The compound heterozygous state for haemoglobins S and D produces a disorder very similar to sickle-cell anaemia.

The unstable haemoglobin disorders

The unstable haemoglobin disorders are a rare group of inherited haemolytic anaemias that result from structural changes in the haemoglobin molecule, which cause its intracellular precipitation with the formation of Heinz bodies. These make the cells more rigid and hence cause their premature destruction in the microcirculation. Most of the unstable haemoglobins result from single amino-acid substitutions or deletions.

Clinical features

All these conditions are characterized by a haemolytic anaemia of varying severity and splenomegaly. There may be a history of the passage of dark urine, particularly during episodes of infection. Like all chronic haemolytic anaemias, there is an increased incidence of pigment gallstones. The condition may become worse during periods of intercurrent infection and, in the more severe forms, such episodes are associated with life-threatening anaemia. Patients with unstable haemoglobins are at particular risk of haemolytic episodes following the administration of oxidant drugs such as sulphonamides.

Laboratory diagnosis

This condition should be thought of in any familial haemolytic anaemia, particularly if a red-cell enzyme deficiency cannot be demonstrated. The peripheral blood film shows the typical features of haemolysis but the red-cell morphology may be relatively normal. Occasionally there is a mild degree of hypochromia and microcytosis. Unless splenectomy has been carried out, Heinz bodies are not seen in the peripheral blood.

The most characteristic feature of the unstable haemoglobins is their heat instability, and some of the variants can be characterized by haemoglobin electrophoresis.

Treatment

There is surprisingly little experience of the effects of splenectomy. If the symptoms and signs are severe, for instance impairing development or well being, splenectomy should be considered.

Haemoglobin variants that cause abnormal oxygen binding

Aetiology

The high oxygen-affinity haemoglobin variants result from single amino-acid substitutions at critical parts of the haemoglobin molecule. These substitutions are involved in the configurational changes that underlie haem/haem interaction and the production of a sigmoid oxygen dissociation curve (see Chapter 3.14). All the high oxygen-affinity variants have a left-shifted oxygen dissociation curve with a reduced P_{50}. Thus the variant haemoglobin holds on to oxygen more avidly than normal haemoglobin and this leads to tissue hypoxia. This in turn causes an increased output of erythropoietin and an elevated red-cell mass.

Clinical features

Most patients are completely healthy and are only found to carry the variant when a routine haematological examination shows an unusually high haemoglobin level or packed cell volume. The condition should be suspected in any patient with a pure red-cell polycythaemia associated with a left-shifted oxygen dissociation curve. The diagnosis can be confirmed by haemoglobin analysis. In asymptomatic patients no treatment is necessary. If the patient has associated vascular disease with symptoms of coronary or cerebral artery insufficiency the haematocrit should be reduced by regular venesection.

Low oxygen-affinity variants

This condition should be thought of in any patient with an unexplained congenital cyanosis.

Methaemoglobinaemia and carboxyhaemoglobinaemia (carbonmonoxy- haemoglobinaemia)

Methaemoglobinaemia is a condition characterized by increased quantities of haemoglobin in which the iron of haem is oxidized to the ferric (Fe^{3+}) form. Carboxyhaemoglobinaemia (carbonmonoxy-haemoglobinaemia) results from the binding of carbon monoxide to the haem molecules.

Pathogenesis

If a single haem is oxidized it alters the conformation of the haemoglobin molecule so that the oxygen affinity of the other three haems is increased. Thus methaemoglobin, carboxyhaemoglobin, and cyanmethaemoglobin all have very high oxygen affinities with 'left-shifted' oxygen dissociation curves, and hence are associated with impaired unloading of oxygen to the tissues.

Methaemoglobinaemia

Methaemoglobinaemia causes a variable degree of cyanosis and should be thought of in any patient with significant central cyanosis in whom there is no evidence of cardiorespiratory disease. Methaemoglobin concentrations of 10 to 20 per cent are tolerated quite well but, because it is useless as an oxygen carrier, levels above this are often associated with dyspnoea and headache. Surprisingly, it is unusual for patients with chronic methaemoglobinaemia to have an increased haemoglobin level or red-cell count.

Methaemoglobinaemia may arise as a result of a genetic defect in red-cell metabolism or haemoglobin structure, or may be acquired following the ingestion of various oxidant drugs and toxic agents.

Genetic methaemoglobinaemia. There are two forms of inherited methaemoglobinaemia. The first results from a deficiency in red-cell NADH-diaphorase and is inherited as an autosomal recessive. Homozygotes have elevated levels of methaemoglobin and are cyanosed from birth. Heterozygotes seem to be unusually susceptible to the oxidant action of drugs. The second results from a structural alteration in either the α- or β-globin chains of haemoglobin. These haemoglobin variants are associated with cyanosis that is present from early life and have a dominant form of inheritance.

The diagnosis is confirmed by spectroscopic examination of the blood and by determination of methaemoglobin levels. Genetic methaemoglobinaemia due to NADH-diaphorase deficiency is readily treated by the administration of ascorbic acid, 300 to 600 mg daily by mouth in divided doses, or by the administration of methylene blue. Genetic methaemoglobinaemias due to structural haemoglobin variants do not respond to treatment.

Acquired methaemoglobinaemia. Acquired methaemoglobinaemia usually results from the administration of drugs or exposure to chemicals that cause oxidation of haemoglobin, including chromate, chlorate, and quinones. Nitrite, often used as a preservative, is one of the most common methaemoglobin-forming agents; nitrates, after conversion to nitrites in the gut, may cause serious methaemoglobinaemia in infants. Other agents that commonly cause methaemoglobinaemia include phenacetin, primiquin, sulphonamides, and various aniline-dye derivatives.

Chronic ingestion may lead to chronic methaemoglobinaemia with or without a haemolytic anaemia. Exposure to a large amount of these agents, and the development of in excess of 50 to 60 per cent methaemoglobin, can cause vascular collapse, coma, and death.

Methaemoglobinaemia with haemolytic anaemia. The haemolytic action of oxidant drugs is described later (Chapter 3.25). Chronic methaemoglobinaemia with haemolytic anaemia characterized by Heinz body formation and fragmented red cells occurs commonly in patients receiving dapsone, salazopyrine, or phenacetin. This condition is usually innocuous and can be modified by adjusting the dose of the drug.

Treatment

In cases of chronic acquired methaemoglobinaemia, the drug or chemical agent should be removed where possible. If continued therapy is required, it should be at a lower dose. Acute toxic methaemoglobinaemia may present as a serious medical emergency. Methylene blue should be given intravenously unless the methaemoglobinaemia is due to chlorate poisoning.

Carboxyhaemoglobinaemia

Carbon monoxide has an affinity for haemoglobin approximately 210 times that of oxygen. At levels of 5 to 10 per cent there may be no symptoms, but above 20 per cent there is usually headache and weakness. Levels of 40 to 60 per cent or more lead to unconsciousness and death. Carbon monoxide poisoning is discussed in Chapter 18.1 and secondary polycythaemia due to chronic exposure is considered in Chapter 3.26.

Further reading

Cao, A. and Rosatelli, M.C. (1993). Screening and prenatal diagnosis of the hemoglobinopathies. *Baillière's Clinical Haematology*, 6, 263–98.

Higgs, D.R. (1993). α-Thalassaemia. *Baillière's Clinical Haematology*, 6, 117–50.

Mansouri, A. and Lurie, A.A. (1993). Concise review: methemoglobinemia. *American Journal of Hematology*, 42, 7–12.

Serjeant, G.R. (1992). *Sickle cell disease*, 2nd edn. Oxford University Press.

Stamatoyannopoulos, G., Nienheis, A.W., Majerus, P.W., and Varmus, H. (1994). *The molecular basis of blood disease*, 2nd edn. Saunders, Philadelphia, PA.

Thein, S.L. (1993). β-Thalassaemia. *Baillière's Clinical Haematology*, 6, 151–76.

Chapter 3.20

Other anaemias resulting from defective red-cell maturation

D. J. Weatherall

In some dyserythropoietic anaemias the precise defect is not yet known (Table 1). They are characterized by erythroid hyperplasia of the bone marrow associated with a low and inappropriate reticulocyte response, together indicating ineffective erythropoiesis.

The sideroblastic anaemias

These genetic or acquired disorders are characterized by severe dyserythropoiesis, marked iron loading of the red-cell precursors and, in some cases, widespread haemosiderosis (Table 2).

Definition

There is an abnormal accumulation of iron in the mitochondria of erythroblasts. Staining with Prussian blue or other iron stains reveals a ring of iron granules in the perinuclear region (Fig. 1). Such red-cell precursors are called 'ring' sideroblasts, characteristic of all the sideroblastic anaemias.

Table 1 Anaemias in which defective red-cell maturation and increased ineffective erythropoiesis is a major factor

Abnormality of DNA synthesis	• Congenital dyserythropoietic anaemias
• Vitamin B_{12} deficiency	• Myelodysplastic syndrome (see Chapter 3.8)
• Folate deficiency	• Infection
• Drugs (antipurines, antipyrimidines)	• Chemicals and toxins
Defective cytoplasmic maturation	
• Disorders of globin synthesis:	
• Thalassaemia	
• Disorders of haem and/or iron metabolism:	
• Sideroblastic anaemia	

Table 2 The sideroblastic anaemias

Congenital	***Acquired (cont.)***
• X-linked	• Secondary:
• ? others	• Drugs—INAH, chloramphenicol, etc.
Acquired	• Alcohol
• Primary or idiopathic (myelodysplastic syndrome)	• Lead
	• Malabsorption
	• Secondary carcinoma
	• Other systemic disorders

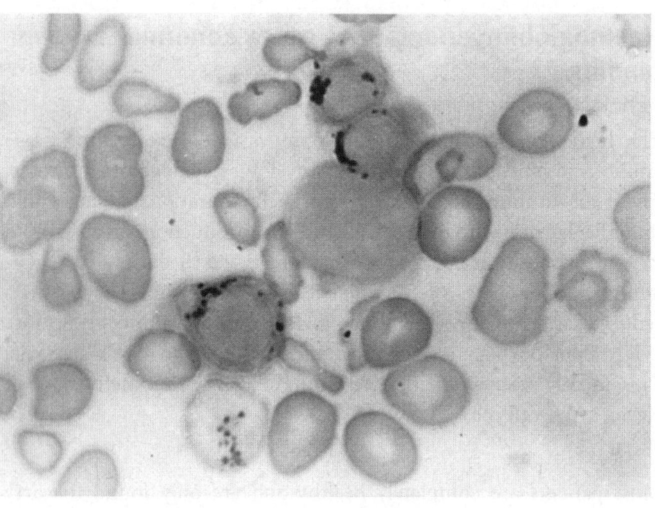

Fig. 1 Bone marrow treated with a stain specific for iron showing typical ring sideroblasts (800 ×).

Aetiology and pathogenesis

All the sideroblastic anaemias are characterized by hypochromic red cells together with iron loading of their precursors. Some are believed to result from defective haem production. The genetic sideroblastic anaemias are probably heterogeneous at the molecular level but some patients have enzyme mutations in the haem synthesis pathway.

The primary, acquired form of sideroblastic anaemia is a neoplastic condition of the bone marrow that forms part of the myelodysplastic syndrome. In some types of sideroblastic anaemia, specific mitochondrial toxins such as chloramphenicol, phenacetin, and paracetamol can be implicated. The sideroblastic anaemia of lead poisoning probably results from inhibition of δ-aminolaevulinic acid synthase and haem synthase. Alcohol and the antituberculous drugs may interfere with pyridoxine metabolism and hence with the early steps of haem synthesis.

As in other causes of ineffective erythropoiesis, there is an increased rate of gastrointestinal iron absorption leading to generalized haemosiderosis.

The genetic sideroblastic anaemias

These are extremely rare, sex-linked conditions. They usually appear in early childhood and are characterized by a mild to moderate anaemia with haemoglobin values in the 6 to 9 g/dl range and some degree of splenomegaly. The peripheral blood film shows hypochromic and normochromic cells (Fig. 2). The bone marrow shows erythroid hyperplasia and the presence of a large proportion of ring sideroblasts. Haemosiderosis may develop.

Acquired sideroblastic anaemia

Primary

The primary idiopathic type is the most common. No underlying cause can be identified. It is now considered a myelodysplastic condition (see Chapter 3.8). Typically there is a mild macrocytic anaemia with dimorphic morphology.

Secondary

In these anaemias, there is demonstrable exposure to toxins or drugs, such as alcohol, antituberculosis drugs (isoniazid, cycloserine, and pyrazinamide), and lead or an association with a variety of systemic diseases such as infections, endocrine abnormalities, and collagen-vascular diseases.

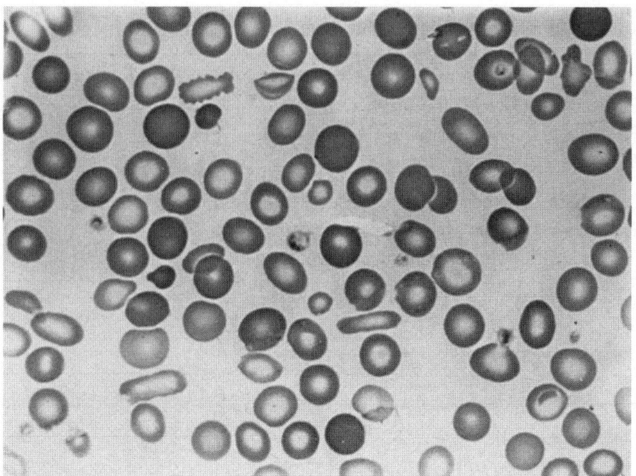

Fig. 2 Genetically determined sideroblastic anaemia. The peripheral blood film shows a dimorphic population with both normochromic and misshapen hypochromic microcytic red cells (800 ×. Leishman stain).

Diagnosis and treatment

Examination of the blood film and marrow is essential. The genetic sideroblastic anaemias usually require no treatment. Pyridoxine should be given (see below), although in most cases there is no response. Secondary folate deficiency should be excluded and the patient should be carefully followed up with regular serum iron and ferritin estimations, using venesection or chelation as appropriate.

In the acquired sideroblastic anaemias a careful search for an underlying cause should be made. Pyridoxine should be given; a high dose in the order of 25–100 mg, or even more, thrice daily may be required to obtain a haematological response. However, in most cases this will produce either no response or a short-lived reticulocytosis with no increase in the haemoglobin level. If patients become symptomatic they should receive regular blood transfusions. Serum iron and ferritin levels should be monitored.

Other dyserythropoietic anaemias

Congenital dyserythropoietic anaemias (CDA)

These disorders are defined by their bizarre red-cell precursor morphology and associated serological findings. These conditions usually, although not always, present early in life with anaemia and unusual red-cell changes. Bone marrow examination shows marked erythroid hyperplasia, the most striking feature being the presence of multinucleated red-cell precursors. Several types of CDA are recognized. In type 1 there are megaloblastoid erythroblasts with internuclear chromatin-bridge formation, that is to say the cell nuclei are incompletely separated from each other. Type 2 is characterized by erythroblastic multinuclearity and a positive acid-serum lysis test using the sera of some, but not all, individuals. This disorder has been called HEMPAS—*h*ereditary *e*rythroblastic *m*ultinuclearity with *p*ositive *a*cid *s*erum lysis. Type 3 is characterized by erythroblast multinuclearity with large, abnormal erythroblasts which have been called gigantoblasts. There have been case reports of clinical responses to interferon treatment.

Dyserythropoiesis and infection

Dyserythropoiesis may occur in association with a variety of infections, particularly of viral and parasitic origin. The most extreme example is virus haemophagocytic syndrome. This disorder is usually seen in immunosuppressed patients and is characterized by a rapidly progressive anaemia together with marked erythroid hyperplasia, dyserythropoiesis, and erythrophagocytosis of red-cell precursors by bone marrow macrophages. Although little is known about the natural history of this disorder it seems to carry an extremely poor prognosis. Dyserythropoiesis is also a feature of *Plasmodium falciparum* malaria infection (see Chapter 16.84). In any severely ill patient with progressive anaemia in whom the marrow shows dyserythropoietic changes, an underlying infection should be suspected.

Further reading

Mollin, D.L. (1965). A symposium on sideroblastic anaemia. Introduction: sideroblasts and sideroblastic anaemia. *British Journal of haematology*, **11**, 41–8.

Chapter 3.21

Haemolytic anaemia: the mechanisms and consequences of a shortened red-cell survival time

D. J. Weatherall

The normal red cell survives for approximately 120 days in the circulation. If the bone marrow is healthy and can compensate, red-cell survival can be reduced by as much as eight times without the development of significant anaemia. However, if the red-cell survival time is less than 15 days anaemia is inevitable.

Haemolytic mechanisms

Premature destruction of red cells occurs either because the red-cell membrane is abnormal in structure or function, the cells are subjected to excessive physical trauma in the circulation, or because they have become unusually rigid due to the precipitation or abnormal molecular configuration of haemoglobin.

The site of red-cell destruction depends on the type and degree of damage to the cells. For example, complement-damaged cells develop large holes in their membrane and are destroyed in the circulation, whereas IgG-coated cells are removed by interaction with macrophages in the reticuloendothelial elements of the spleen and liver.

Constant bombardment of the spleen by abnormal red cells results in splenomegaly and many haemolytic anaemias are associated with progressive splenomegaly and secondary hypersplenism.

Compensatory mechanisms

The haematological and biochemical changes which result from haemolysis reflect both compensatory mechanisms aimed at restoring the circulating red-cell mass to normal, and the results of an increased rate of haemoglobin breakdown from the prematurely destroyed red-cell population.

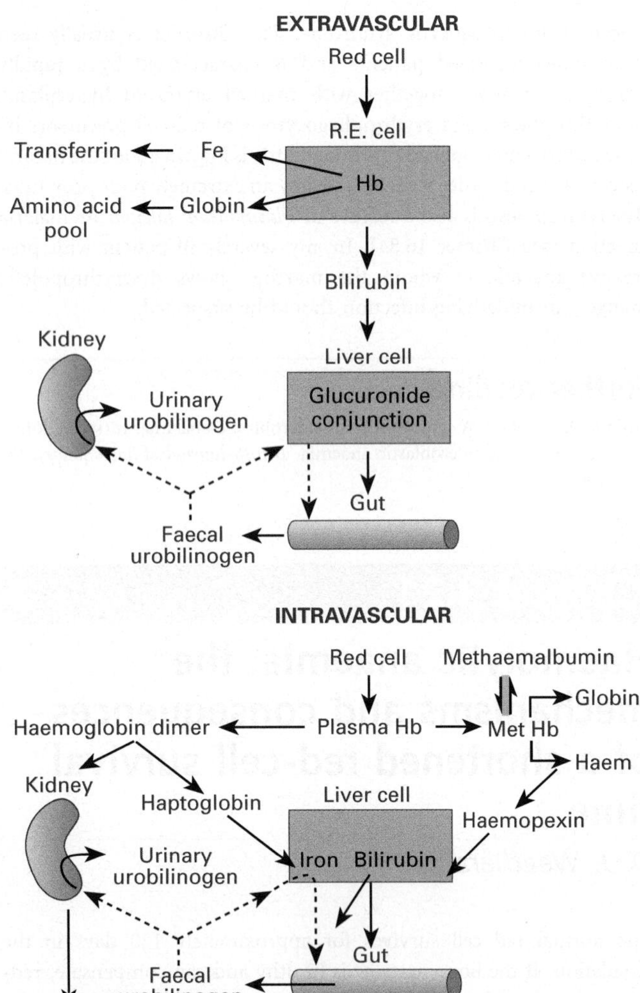

Fig. 1 Pathways of haemoglobin catabolism in haemolytic anaemia.

Within a few days of the onset of haemolysis, the reticulocyte count increases and erythroid hyperplasia of the bone marrow becomes apparent. There is increased demand for iron and folate. The spread of erythroid marrow down the long bones may lead to bone deformities similar to those observed in the severe dyserythropoietic anaemias. If the haemolysis has been present from early life, there is often extramedullary haemopoiesis in the spleen, liver, and lymph nodes.

Haemoglobin catabolism

After haemoglobin is liberated into the circulation it is bound to haptoglobin, this haptoglobin–haemoglobin complex is then rapidly removed into the reticuloendothelial system (Fig. 1). A reduction in the serum haptoglobin level provides an extremely sensitive index of intravascular haemolysis. If the binding capacity of haptoglobin is exceeded, haemoglobin appears in the plasma where it is degraded to haem which binds to a β-glycoprotein called haemopexin. When both haptoglobin and haemopexin are saturated, free haemoglobin appears in the plasma where it is rapidly oxidized to methaemoglobin, dissociated, and the haem bound to albumin to form methaemalbumin. The latter produces a dirty-brown discoloration of the plasma. If there is severe intravascular haemolysis, free haemoglobin may appear in the urine where much of the liberated iron is converted into haemosiderin. Renal tubular cells containing haemosiderin are cast off and appear in the urine; haemosiderinuria is the most reliable indication of chronic intravascular haemolysis. Due to increased red-cell breakdown all haemolytic anaemias show an increased production of faecal and urinary urobilinogen.

Table 1 General approach to the diagnosis of haemolytic anaemia

1. Is there evidence of an increased rate of red cell production?
Blood film—polychromasia, macrocytosis
Reticulocyte count—elevated
Marrow–erythroid hyperplasia
2. Is there evidence of an increased rate of red cell destruction?
Bilirubin level—elevated
Faecal and urinary urobilinogen—elevated
Plasma haptoglobin and haemopexin—reduced
^{51}Cr $t_{\frac{1}{2}}$—reduced
3. Is the haemolysis mainly intravascular?
Plasma haemoglobin—elevated
Methaemalbumin—present
Haemoglobinuria—present
Haemosiderin in urine—present (if chronic)
4. Where are the red cells being destroyed?
^{51}Cr labelling and external counting
5. Why are the red cells being destroyed?
Genetically determined
Morphology–spherocytes, ovalocytes, etc.
Haemoglobin analysis
Enzyme assay
Acquired
Immune—Coombs' test
Non-immune—red cell morphology
Associated disease
Ham's test, etc.

Recognition of haemolysis

There is variable reticulocytosis and the bone marrow shows erythroid hyperplasia. The serum bilirubin level is raised and serum haptoglobins are either reduced or absent. In the presence of severe intravascular haemolysis there may be free haemoglobin in the plasma and urine, and in all states of chronic intravascular haemolysis there is a variable degree of haemosiderinuria. Usually there are also specific features to identify the exact cause of the haemolytic anaemia.

In the majority of haemolytic anaemias there is some enlargement of the spleen. In some cases it is useful to measure the red-cell survival time directly and to try to determine the site of red-cell destruction (Chapter 3.14). An approach to the clinical and laboratory diagnosis of haemolysis is summarized in Table 1.

Classification of the haemolytic anaemias

The haemolytic anaemias are usually classified into two main groups: (i) genetically determined, and (ii) acquired (Table 2). The commonest inherited haemolytic anaemias in the world's population, the genetic disorders of haemoglobin structure and synthesis, are described in Chapter 3.19. The other common inherited and acquired forms of haemolytic anaemia are described in the following chapters.

Table 2 Main groups of haemolytic anaemias

Genetic disorders of the red cell	*Acquired disorders of the red cell*
• Membrane	• Immune
• Hereditary spherocytosis	• Isoimmune; Rh or ABO
• Hereditary ovalocytosis	• incompatibility
• Stomatocytosis	• Autoimmune; warm or cold
• Pyropoikilocytosis	• antibodies
• Other 'leaky' membrane disorders	• Non-immune
• ?March haemoglobinuria	• Trauma
• Acanthocytosis	Valve prosthesis
	Body surface
• Haemoglobin	• Membrane defects; PNH, liver
• Sickling disorders	
• Haemoglobins C, D, and E	• disease
• Unstable haemoglobins	• Parasitic disorders
• Thalassaemia syndromes	• Bacterial infection
• Energy pathways	• Physical agents, drugs, and
• Hexose-monophosphate shunt	• chemicals
• Embden—Meyerhof pathway	• Hypersplenism
• Others	• Defective red cell maturation

Further reading

Williams, W.J., Beutler, E., Erslev, A.J., and Lichtman, M.A. (1994). *Haematology*, (5th edn). McGraw Hill, New York.

Chapter 3.22

Genetic disorders of the red-cell membrane

S. W. Eber and S. E. Lux

Structure of the red-cell membrane

The red blood-cell membrane consists of an external lipid plasma membrane and an inner, membrane-bound, proteinaceous membrane skeleton (Fig. 1). Mutations in genes that encode proteins of the membrane skeleton often cause haemolytic anaemias.

Spectrin is the major skeletal protein and is commonly mutated in hereditary elliptocytosis and pyropoikilocytosis. Spectrin forms tetramers that are crosslinked by actin and protein 4.1. The membrane skeleton is attached to proteins in the lipid bilayer by ankyrin and protein 4.1.

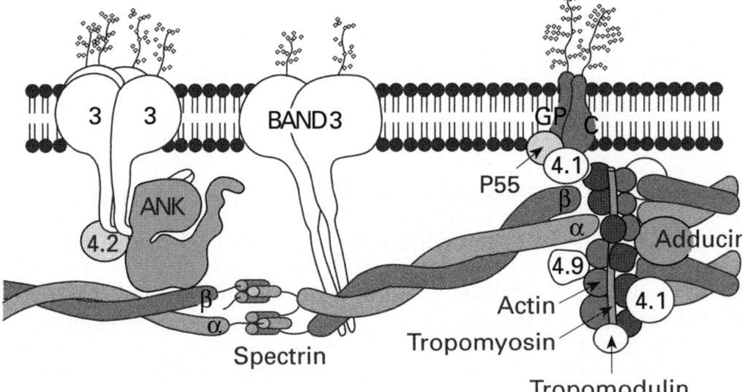

Fig. 1 Schematic illustration of the major components of the red-cell membrane and membrane skeleton.

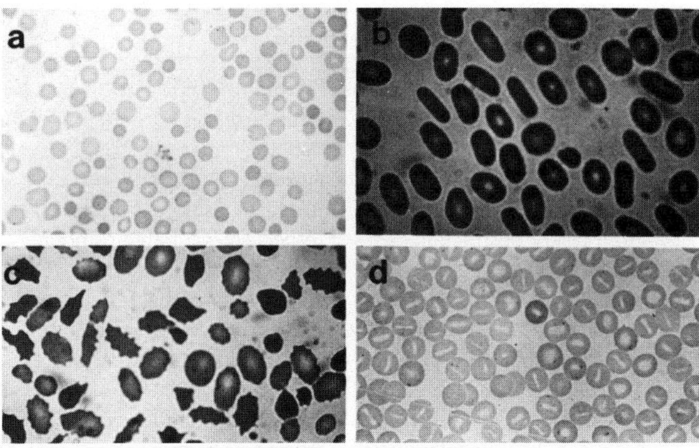

Fig. 2 Altered red-cell morphology: (a) spherocytes; (b) elliptocytes; (c) poikilocytes; (d) stomatocytes.

Congenital membrane defects

Red blood-cell morphology and osmotic fragility are the most useful tests for detecting membrane defects. The blood film may show spherocytes, elliptocytes, membrane fragments, poikilocytes, stomatocytes, acanthocytes, or target cells (Fig. 2). The osmotic fragility test measures the ability of red cells to resist lysis in hypotonic solutions. Spherocytes and stomatocytes have a reduced surface-to-volume ratio and can tolerate less osmotic swelling than normal cells before they lyse. Membrane protein analysis or DNA sequencing may be valuable.

Hereditary spherocytosis

Hereditary spherocytosis is an inherited haemolytic anaemia, characterized by osmotically fragile, partially spherical cells that are selectively trapped by the spleen. The disease occurs in all races, but is particularly common in northern Europeans, in whom the prevalence is about 1:5000. There are at least two patterns of inheritance: 75 per cent of the families show a classic autosomal dominant pattern. Most of the remainder are sporadic cases due to *de novo* mutations or autosomal recessive forms.

Pathogenesis

The molecular lesion mostly resides in the genes for ankyrin, band 3, or protein 4.2—in effect the proteins that bind the membrane skeleton to the lipid bilayer rather than the proteins involved in the 'horizontal' interactions (spectrin, actin, and protein 4.1) that hold the skeleton together.

Clinical features

The clinical characteristics of hereditary spherocytosis are listed in Table 1. The severity is variable (Table 2). Patients with mild hereditary spherocytosis (about 25 per cent of cases) have 'compensated' haemolysis—that is a normal or near-normal haemoglobin concentration combined with an elevated reticulocyte count. The moderate form of hereditary spherocytosis accounts for roughly two-thirds of cases and these patients have a chronic haemolytic anaemia. They may require exchange transfusions for hyperbilirubinaemia in the neonatal period and additional transfusions may be required during the first months of life, due to sluggish marrow erythropoiesis. However, by 1 year of age, patients with moderate hereditary spherocytosis reach a steady state, with haemoglobin values of 7–11 g/dl and reticulocyte counts over 10 per cent. About 10 per cent of patients have moderately

Table 1 Characteristics of hereditary spherocytosis

Clinical manifestations	*Laboratory features*

• Anaemia
• Splenomegaly
• Intermittent jaundice:
  • From haemolysis
  • From biliary obstruction
• Aplastic crises
• Inheritance:
  • Dominant—75 per cent
  • Non-dominant —25 per cent
• Rare manifestations:
  • Leg ulcers
  • Extramedullary haemopoietic
  • tumours
  • Excellent response to splenectomy
	• Reticulocytosis
	• Spherocytosis
	• Elevated MCHC
	• Increased osmotic fragility (especially incubated osmotic fragility test)
	• Negative Coombs' test
	• Decreased red-cell spectrin, or spectrin and ankyrin, or protein 3, or protein 4.2c
	• Frameshift mutations of ankyrin,or band 3, or b-spectrin, frequent *de novo* mutations

severe or severe disease. Those with severe disease require regular transfusions to keep the haemoglobin level above 6 g/dl. The inheritance is nearly always autosomal recessive, and both parents show minimal signs of increased haemolysis.

Complications

Most patients with moderate hereditary spherocytosis experience one or more haemolytic crises, usually associated with viral infections. These are characterized by increasing jaundice and haemolysis, but transfusions are rarely required. Aplastic crises due to parvovirus B19 may occur. Untreated older children and adults with hereditary spherocytosis often develop bilirubinate gallstones secondary to increased bilirubin production, but the frequency after the age of 30 parallels the frequency in the general population.

Other complications include gout, indolent ankle ulcers, or a chronic erythematous dermatitis on the legs. All these complications disappear after splenectomy. A rare severe complication occurring mostly in elderly adults with otherwise mild hereditary spherocytosis is extramedullary haemopoietic tumours, often located in the thorax.

Diagnosis

The hallmarks are anaemia, jaundice, and splenomegaly. The morphology and osmotic fragility test are typical. Membrane analysis is occasionally warranted. There are only a few disorders that can be confused with hereditary spherocytosis. ABO incompatibility may be difficult to distinguish from hereditary spherocytosis in the neonatal period. In later life, autoimmune haemolytic anaemias must be excluded. Spherocytes occur as a secondary phenomenon in burns, snake bites, and clostridial sepsis and may be seen in microangiopathic haemolytic anaemias, oxidant haemolysis, unstable haemoglobins, and haemoglobin C disease.

Treatment

Splenectomy cures almost all patients with spherocytosis, eliminating anaemia and reducing the reticulocyte count to near-normal levels (1–3 per cent). However, the indications for splenectomy should be weighted carefully as there is a risk of postsplenectomy infections. Splenectomy should be delayed until the age of 5 years or more if possible and to at least 2–3 years of age in all cases, even if chronic transfusions are required in the interim. All patients with moderately severe and severe spherocytosis should be splenectomized. Patients with moderate spherocytosis should be splenectomized if they suffer from reduced vitality or physical stamina due to anaemia, or if, later in life, anaemia compromises vascular perfusion of vital organs or extramedullary haemopoietic tumours develop. We defer splenectomy in patients with mild, compensated haemolysis. Whether patients with moderate, asymptomatic anaemia should have a splenectomy remains controversial. All splenectomized patients should receive appropriate vaccinations and antibiotic prophylaxis.

Hereditary elliptocytosis

Although hereditary elliptocytosis is quite frequent (approx. 1 in 2500 in the Caucasian North European population), it is less important clinically than hereditary spherocytosis. Only about 10 per cent of patients have significant haemolysis, mostly as newborns and during early infancy (transient infantile poikilocytosis). In some cases this can be life threatening. Four clinical phenotypes can be distinguished.

Table 2 Clinical classification of hereditary spherocytosis (HS)

	Mild HS	Moderate HS	Moderate to severe HS	Severe HS[1]
Haemoglobin (g/dl)	11–15	8–12	6–8	< 6
Reticulocytes (%)	3–8	≥8	≥10	≥10
Bilirubin (mg/dl)	1–2	≥2	2–3	≥3
Spectrin[2] (% of normal value)	80–100	50–80	40–80[3]	20–50
Osmotic fragility Fresh blood	Normal or slightly increased	Distinctly increased	Distinctly increased	Distinctly increased
Incubated blood	Increased	Distinctly increased	Distinctly increased	Markedly increased
Splenectomy	In general not necessary	If transfusions are needed, if decreased vitality	Necessary, not under the age of 5 years	Necessary, not under the age of 5 years

[1] Patients are in need of regular transfusions.

[2] Normal: 245±27∗ 10^3 copies per cell.

[3] Caused by different primary defects the spectrin concentration of the RBCs varies.

1. *Mild hereditary elliptocytosis*: This is usually very mild in heterozygous carriers; there is no anaemia and only mild haemolysis (reticulocyte counts of less than 4 per cent). However, moderate to severe haemolytic anaemia does occur in homozygous or combined heterozygous offspring. The defect is usually in the 'horizontal' interactions that hold the membrane skeleton together, particularly spectrin or protein 4.1.
2. *Hereditary pyropoikilocytosis*: This moderately severe to life-threatening haemolytic anaemia is characterized by remarkable red-cell fragmentation and microcytosis, bizarre poikilocytosis, and heat-sensitive red cells that fragment at 45 to 46 °C instead of the normal 49 °C. It typically results from homozygosity or compound heterozygosity for spectrin mutations.
3. *Spherocytic hereditary elliptocytosis*: This rare, autosomal dominant condition has features of both hereditary spherocytosis and hereditary elliptocytosis. Patients have a mild to moderate haemolytic anaemia characterized by rounded elliptocytes, occasional spherocytes, and a positive osmotic fragility test. The indications for splenectomy, which is curative, are the same as for hereditary spherocytosis. The molecular cause of the disease is unknown.
4. *South-East Asian ovalocytosis (Band 3 defect)*: This curious autosomal dominant polymorphism is very prevalent (up to 30 per cent) among Melanesian, Indonesian, and Malaysian aborigines, but is rarely seen in other populations. It is characterized by rounded elliptocytes, some with a unique morphology (a transverse bar that divides the central clear space), which are extraordinarily rigid and resist invasion by a variety of malarial parasites. Surprisingly there is little or no associated haemolysis.

Treatment

Splenectomy is indicated only in moderately severe and severe cases of hereditary elliptocytosis or hereditary pyropoikilocytosis and, especially as spontaneous regression occurs in some infants, should be postponed to at least the third year of life and preferably the fifth year or later.

Hereditary defects in membrane cation permeability

Conditions

Hereditary stomatocytosis

In this rare, autosomal dominant disease an inherited defect in membrane permeability causes a massive Na^+ influx and may result in severe haemolysis. Red cells show a mouth-like band of pallor (i.e. 'stoma') across the centre of the red cell.

Hereditary xerocytosis

In this rare, autosomal dominant disorder, the permeability of K^+ is altered and red cells are dehydrated. Patients have a mild to moderate haemolytic anaemia and the osmotic fragility is decreased.

Treatment

In both stomatocytosis and xerocytosis splenectomy bears a high, lifelong risk of thromboembolisms and can no longer be recommended.

Further reading

Eber, S.W., Gonzalez, J.M., Lux, M.L., *et al.* (1996). Ankyrin-1 mutations are a major cause of dominant and recessive hereditary spherocytosis. *Nature Genetics*, **13**, 214–18.

Handin, R.I., Lux, S.E., and Stossel, T.P. (1995). *Blood, principles and practice of hematology*, pp. 1701–1818. Lippincott, Philadelphia, PA.

Stewart, G.W., Amess, J.A.L., Eber, S.W., *et al.* (1996). Thrombo-embolic disease after splenectomy for hereditary stomatocytosis. *British Journal of Haematology*, **93**, 303–10.

Chapter 3.23

Haemolysis due to red-cell enzyme deficiencies

E. C. Gordon-Smith and D. J. Weatherall

These haemolytic anaemias are usually non-spherocytic, and may dominate the clinical picture or be part of a more generalized disorder, depending on whether or not the enzyme deficiency is expressed only in the red blood cells. Deficiencies of the enzymes of the glycolytic pathway produce a relatively constant degree of haemolysis; those of the hexose monophosphate shunt, which provides reducing power, produce haemolysis in the presence of oxidative stress.

Normal red-cell metabolism

Glucose is metabolized mainly through the anaerobic, glycolytic, Embden–Meyerhof pathway, with lactate as the end-product (Fig. 1). There is a net production of 2 mol of ATP and the reduction of 2 mol of NAD^+ to NADH per mol of glucose (Chapter 3.14). The other principal energy pathway is the hexose monophosphate shunt (also known as the pentose phosphate pathway), in which there is reduction of $NADP^+$ to NADPH. Under 'normal' conditions about 10 per cent of glucose is metabolized via the shunt, but flux through the pathway can increase markedly in the face of oxidant stress.

There is a 'metabolic siding' in the Embden–Meyerhof pathway called the Rapoport–Luebering shunt, which is controlled by diphosphoglycerate mutase and which generates 2,3-diphosphoglycerate (**2,3-DPG**). The latter plays an important part in controlling oxygen transport. Enzyme defects vary considerably in their effects on 2,3-diphosphoglycerate production, and hence on oxygen transport and the degree of compensation for anaemia.

Inherited enzyme deficiencies

Deficiencies of many of the enzymes of the glycolytic and reducing pathways have been described but most are rare (Table 1). However, two are relatively common: glucose-6-phosphate dehydrogenase (G6PD) deficiency in the reducing pathway and pyruvate kinase deficiency in the glycolytic. The various G6PD deficiency disorders are described in Chapter 3.24.

Pyruvate kinase deficiency

Pyruvate kinase catalyses the last step in the glycolytic pathway that produces the net gain in ATP from the metabolism of glucose (Fig. 1).

Deficiency of pyruvate kinase is the most common of the inherited red-cell enzyme defects after G6PD deficiency. It has been reported in many different races, and both sexes are affected equally. The most commonly described form is inherited as an autosomal recessive. Homozygotes have haemolytic anaemia, mild to moderate splenomegaly, and a gross deficiency of red-cell pyruvate kinase activity, while heterozygotes are clinically and haematologically normal and have about half the usual amount of pyruvate kinase activity in their red cells.

Aetiology and pathogenesis

There is a deficiency of ATP and the accumulation of glycolytic intermediates, particularly 2,3-diphosphoglycerate and phosphoenol pyruvate. In the absence of efficient glycolysis the red cell must obtain its energy requirements by other means. In the severe pyruvate kinase-deficient patient there is a marked reticulocytosis, and probably most of the red cells' energy is derived by oxidative pathways related to the residual mitochondria in the younger cell population. After splenectomy the reticulocyte count rises markedly, often up to 70 per cent or more of circulating cells. Pyruvate kinase deficiency shows a remarkable degree of molecular heterogeneity.

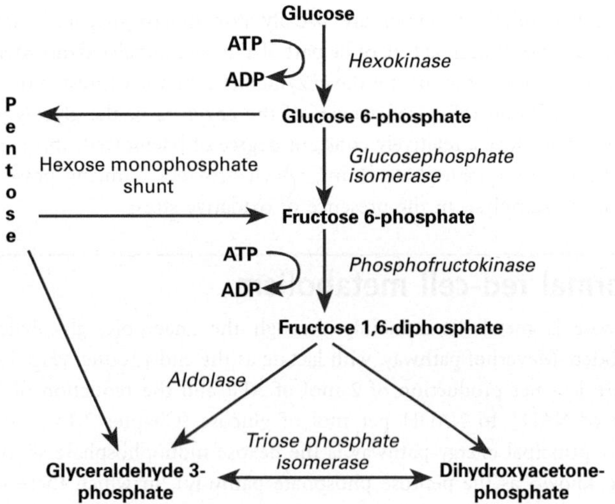

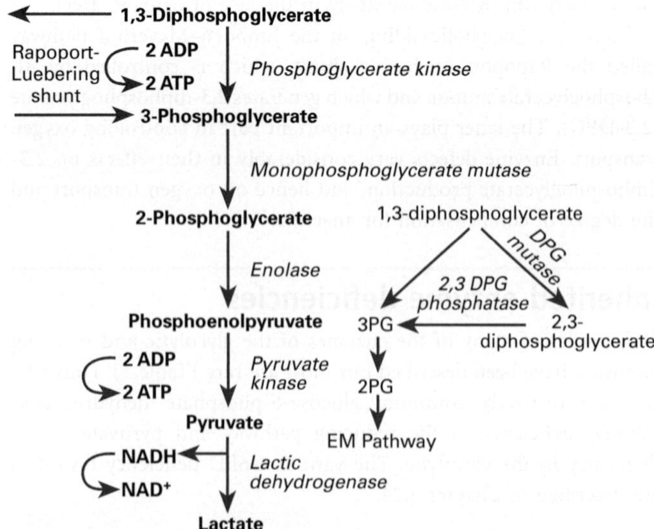

Fig. 1 The relationship between the main red-cell glycolytic pathway (Embden–Meyerhof) and the other metabolic pathways. The insert shows the production of 2,3-DPG in the Rapoport–Luebering shunt.

Table 1 Some red-cell enzyme deficiencies

Pathway and enzyme	Clinical features
Embden–Meyerhof	
• Hexokinase	• Rare; haemolytic anaemia (HA) mild to severe
• Glucose phosphate isomerase	• HA mild to severe
• Phosphofructokinase	• Mild HA ± myopathy (Tariu's disease)
• Aldolase	• Rare; mild HA ± mental retardation
• Triosephosphate isomerase	• Neuromuscular anomalies+moderate HA
• Phosphoglycerate kinase	• Rare; HA ± mental and phagocytic deficiencies; X-linked
• Pyruvate kinase	• Common; mild to severe HA
Hexose monophosphate shunt and glutathione (GSH) metabolism	
• Glucose-6-phosphate dehydrogenase	• Very common, X-linked (see Chapter 3.24)
• GSH peroxidase or reductase	• Rare; variable oxidant-sensitive HA
• GSH synthetase and α-glutamyl cysteine synthetase	
Nucleotide metabolism	
• Pyrimidine-5'-nucleotidase	• Mild to moderate HA • Basophilic stippling
• Adenylate kinase	• Rare; mild HA
Methaemoglobin reduction	
• NADH: methaemoglobin reductase	• 10–35% methaemoglobin
	• Heterozygotes cyanosed with oxidant drugs
• NADPH: methaemoglobin reductase	• Methaemoglobinaemia only after oxidant stress
Nucleotide synthesis	
• Orotidine 5'-phosphate pyrophosphorylase	• Megaloblastic anaemia
• Orotidine 5'-phosphate decarboxylase	• ± Mental retardation
• 5'-phosphoribosyl 1-pyrophosphate synthetase	

Clinical features

Severe pyruvate kinase deficiency may present at birth with neonatal jaundice and haemolysis, sometimes requiring exchange transfusions. There is a variable degree of chronic haemolysis throughout life, with jaundice, anaemia, splenomegaly, and even bone changes similar to those seen in thalassaemia in the most severe cases. There is often a marked exacerbation of the anaemia during periods of stress such as infection or pregnancy. Interestingly, however, the anaemia is very well tolerated, probably because high levels of red-cell 2,3-diphosphoglycerate cause a right shift in the oxygen dissociation curve. Aplastic crises may occur.

Laboratory diagnosis

The blood picture shows all the hallmarks of chronic haemolysis and the stained blood film shows polychromasia and macrocytosis with a varying number of irregularly contracted red cells. The diagnosis is confirmed by an assay for pyruvate kinase.

Therapy

There is no specific therapy but patients normally improve after splenectomy. Postsplenectomy, the platelet count may be greatly elevated ($600–1000 \times 10^9/l$) and patients may need long-term, low-dose aspirin to reduce the risk of deep-vein thrombosis. Standard postsplenectomy prophylaxis should be given. Transfusion is required during periods of exacerbation of the haemolysis. Folic acid is required to prevent deficiency.

Other enzyme deficiencies

Pyrimidine 5′-nucleotidase deficiency is an autosomal recessive trait, causing a variable haemolytic anaemia characterized by marked basophilic stippling of the red cells. An acquired form of this enzyme deficiency occurs in severe lead poisoning. Splenectomy does not appear to be effective. Several rare red-cell enzyme deficiencies are associated with multisystem disease, usually neurological (Table 1).

A general approach to congenital non-spherocytic haemolytic anaemia

When young children present with haemolysis, the first step is to look for one of the acquired causes of haemolytic anaemia. Once these have been excluded, and abnormalities of the red-cell membrane and haemoglobin have been ruled out, the level of red-cell G6PD and pyruvate kinase should be determined. This will leave a number of patients in whom no diagnosis can be made, and they should then be referred to centres capable of analysing all the red-cell enzymes and glycolytic intermediates. In practice, only a small proportion of cases of this type can be ascribed to a particular enzyme deficiency, and in the majority no specific abnormality can be found.

Further reading

Beutler, E. (1990). Hereditary nonspherocytic haemolytic anemia: pyruvate kinase and other abnormalities. In *Hematology*, 4th edn (ed. W.J. Williams, E. Beutler, A.J. Erslev, and M.A. Lichtman), pp. 606–12. McGraw-Hill, New York.

Beutler, E. (1993). The molecular biology of enzymes of erythrocytic metabolism. In *The molecular basis of blood diseases*, 2nd edn (ed. G. Stamatoyannopoulos, A.W. Nienhuis, P.W. Majerus, and H. Varmus), pp. 331–50. Saunders, Philadelphia, PA.

Chapter 3.24

Glucose 6-phosphate dehydrogenase (G6PD) deficiency

L. Luzzatto

Definition

Glucose 6-phosphate dehydrogenase (**G6PD**) is a key enzyme in redox metabolism. G6PD deficiency is an inherited condition in which red cells have a markedly decreased activity of G6PD, which predisposes to haemolytic anaemia.

Biochemistry

Red cells are vulnerable to oxidative damage both from oxygen radicals that are generated continuously from within the red cell and from any oxidizing agent that may be present in the plasma. These oxygen radicals are converted into hydrogen peroxide which must be detoxified by glutathione peroxidase and catalase. G6PD, the first enzyme of the pentose phosphate pathway (see Fig. 1), catalyses the conversion of glucose 6-phosphate (**G6P**) and NADP to 6-phosphogluconolactone and NADPH. NADPH is crucial for the operation of both glutathione peroxidase (via glutathione reductase) and catalase (because it stabilizes this enzyme).

Genetics

The inheritance of G6PD deficiency has a mendelian X-linked pattern. Therefore males have only one G6PD gene and must be either normal or G6PD-deficient. By contrast, females, having two G6PD genes, can be normal or deficient (homozygous), or intermediate (heterozygous). Moreover, due to X-chromosome inactivation, heterozygous females are genetic mosaics and the abnormal cells of a woman heterozygous for G6PD deficiency are just as deficient as those of a hemizygous deficient man. At the genetic level all mutations in the G6PD gene are structural and affect the catalytic function or *in vivo* stability of the protein.

Epidemiology

G6PD deficiency is distributed worldwide but has a high prevalence in Africa, Southern Europe, the Middle East, South-East Asia, and

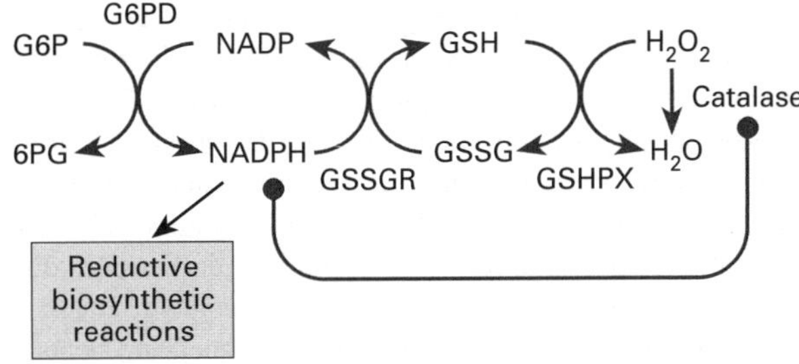

Fig. 1 The role of G6PD in red-cell metabolism: NADPH plays a dual role in the (i) regeneration of glutathione (**GSH**) and (ii) stabilization of catalase (see also Chapter 3.23).

Table 1 Drugs and other agents that can cause haemolysis in G6PD-deficient people

Drugs	Definite association	Possible of doubtful association[1]
Antimalarials	Primaquine Pamaquine Pentaquine	Chloroquine Quinacrine Quinine
Sulphonamides	Sulphanilamide Sulphacetamide Sulphapyridine Sulphamethoxazole	Sulphamethoxypyridazine Sulphoxone Sulphamerizine Sulphadiazine Sulphadimidine Sulphisoxazole
Sulphones	Thiazolesulphone Dapsone	
Nitrofurans	Nitrofurantoin	
Antipyretic/ analgesic	Acetanilide	Aspirin Aminopyrine Acetominophen Phenacetin
Other drugs	Nalidixic acid	Ciprofloxacin PAS Norfloxacin L-DOPA
	Niridazole	Chloramphenicol Doxorubicin
	Methylene blue	Vitamin K analogues Probenecid
	Phenazopyridine	Ascorbic acid Dimercaprol
Other chemicals	Naphthalene Trinitrotoluene Toluidine blue	

[1] These drugs can probably cause haemolysis only when given at high doses.

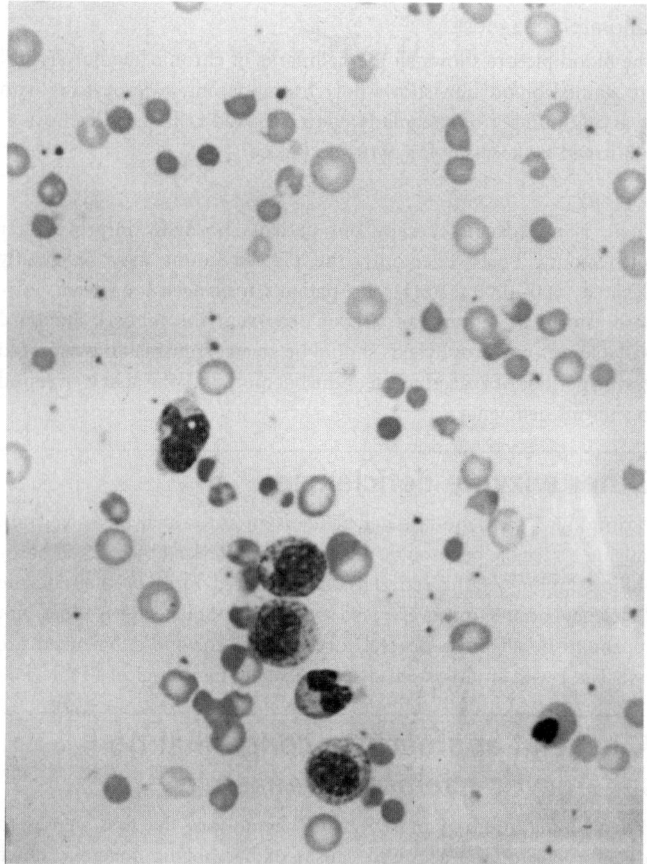

(a)

(a)

Fig. 2(a, b) Blood film in a case of acute haemolytic anaemia in a G6PD-deficient patient (favism). (a) Romanovsky stain, showing marked poikilocytosis, polychromatic macrocytes, bite cells, nucleated red cells, and a shift to the left in the granulocytic series. (b) Supravital stain with methyl violet, showing the characteristic Heinz bodies.

Oceania. The frequency of G6PD deficiency in males may be up to 20 per cent or more in some of these areas. Different G6PD variants underlie G6PD deficiency in different parts of the world. The overall geographical distribution of G6PD deficiency and its heterogeneity is strongly influenced by the relative resistance of heterozygous G6PD red cells to the effects of *Plasmodium falciparum* malaria.

Clinical manifestations

Acute haemolytic anaemia

The vast majority of individuals remain clinically asymptomatic throughout their lifetime. However, they are all at risk of developing acute haemolytic anaemia in response to three types of triggers: (i) drugs (see Table 1), (ii) infections, and (iii) fava beans. Typically, a haemolytic attack starts with malaise, weakness, and abdominal or lumbar pain. After an interval of between several hours and 2–3 days the patient develops jaundice and produces a dark urine, due to haemoglobinuria. In the majority of cases the haemolytic attack, even if severe, is self-limiting and tends to resolve spontaneously. Depending on the severity of the anaemia, the haemoglobin level may be back to normal in 3 to 6 weeks. The most serious threat in adults is the development of acute renal failure. An important feature of haemolysis in G6PD-deficient patients is the fact that G6PD gradually decays during red-cell ageing, and thus a haemolytic attack selectively destroys older red cells because they have a more severe shortage of G6PD.

The anaemia varies from moderate to extremely severe and is due largely to intravascular haemolysis. The blood film shows anisocytosis, polychromasia, and other features associated with acute haemolysis, including spherocytes (Fig. 2); in severe cases numerous red cells may appear to have unevenly distributed haemoglobin ('hemighosts'), or to have had parts of them bitten away ('bite cells'). Staining with methyl violet reveals the presence of 'Heinz bodies', consisting of precipitates of denatured haemoglobin (Fig. 2).

Favism

This is one of the more spectacular forms of acute haemolytic anaemia associated with G6PD deficiency; it can occur at any age, but is more common in children. Haemoglobinuria develops within 6 to 24 h and is associated with the child becoming first very fractious and then lethargic, and often with fever, abdominal pain, diarrhoea, and sometimes vomiting. Physical examination reveals pallor, tachycardia, jaundice, and an enlarged spleen; in severe cases there may be evidence of hypovolaemic shock or, more rarely, of high-output heart failure. The cause of favism is the ingestion of fava beans, although favism does not follow their ingestion in every case.

Neonatal jaundice

The clinical picture of neonatal jaundice related to G6PD deficiency differs from the 'classical' Rhesus-related neonatal jaundice in two main respects: (i) it is very rarely present at birth, and the peak incidence of clinical onset is between day 2 and day 3; (ii) there is more jaundice than anaemia, and the anaemia is very rarely severe. The severity of G6PD-related neonatal jaundice varies enormously.

Chronic non-spherocytic haemolytic anaemia

A small minority of patients has a chronic anaemia of variable severity. The patient is practically always a male, and in general he presents because of unexplained jaundice. Frequently the onset is at birth, and a diagnosis is made of neonatal jaundice which may be severe enough to require exchange transfusion. Subsequently the anaemia recurs and the jaundice fails to clear completely; or the patient is only reinvestigated much later in life, perhaps because of gallstones in a child or in a young adult. Usually the spleen is moderately enlarged in small children, and subsequently it may increase in size sufficiently to cause mechanical discomfort, or hypersplenism, or both. The red-cell morphology is not characteristic, and for this reason it is referred to in the negative as being 'non-spherocytic'. In this condition, unlike in the acute haemolytic anaemia described above, haemolysis is mainly extravascular.

Laboratory diagnosis

The final diagnosis must rely on the direct demonstration of decreased activity of the enzyme in red cells. Most screening tests are adequate for diagnostic purposes in patients who are in the steady state, but not those in the posthaemolytic period or with other complications; also, the tests cannot be expected to identify all heterozygotes. Ideally, every patient found to be G6PD-deficient by screening should then be retested for confirmation by a quantitative assay. For practical purposes it is most unlikely that a woman will have clinical manifestations if her G6PD level is more than 70 per cent of normal.

Treatment

Prevention and management

Favism is entirely preventable by not eating fava beans. Prevention of drug-induced haemolysis is possible in most cases by choosing alternative drugs. A common problem is the need to give primaquine for the eradication of malaria due to *Plasmodium vivax* or *P. malariae*; in these cases the administration of a lower dosage for a longer time is the recommended approach, which will still cause haemolysis, but of an acceptably mild degree.

In acute cases the anaemia may vary from being mild to one requiring blood transfusion. Recovery is the rule. The management of neonatal jaundice does not differ from that of neonatal jaundice due to other causes. In chronic non-spherocytic haemolytic anaemia, folic-acid supplements and regular haematological surveillance may suffice. Rarely the anaemia is so severe that it is transfusion-dependent. Splenectomy has proven beneficial in severe cases. Genetic counselling should be offered.

Further reading

Beutler, E. (1991). Glucose 6-phosphate dehydrogenase deficiency. *New England Journal of Medicine*, **324**, 169–74.

Chapter 3.25

Acquired haemolytic anaemia

E. C. Gordon-Smith and M. Contreras

The acquired haemolytic anaemias are caused by many different agents but the pathogenesis may be divided into immune and non-immune causes.

The immune haemolytic anaemias

Introduction

Pathogenesis

Immune haemolysis may occur when antibody or complement are attached to the red-cell surface. Antibodies bound to the red-cell membrane cause binding to macrophages (by the Fc receptors on the latter), with subsequent phagocytosis of the red cell. The antibodies may be IgG, IgA, or IgM, depending upon the aetiology. When IgG is bound, destruction of red cells tends to occur in the spleen. IgM antibodies are bound most avidly at low temperatures and give rise to the cold autoimmune disorders (see below). IgM antibodies also fix complement to receptors on the red cell so that haemolysis occurs through complement activation. Destruction of cells takes place throughout the macrophage system and spleen, but direct intravascular lysis occurs if sufficient complement is bound.

Antibody directed against the red-cell membrane may be provoked in a number of ways, which will be discussed below in more detail under the particular disorders.

The presence of antibody or complement on the surface of the red cell is detected by the direct antiglobulin test, the Coombs' test. Antibody that reacts against normal red cells of a similar blood group may be detected in the serum by the indirect antiglobulin test, and eluates may be prepared from the antibody-coated cells to test the specificity of the antibody. The temperature at which the antibody is most active and the class of immunoglobulin involved are also required for reaching a diagnosis.

Table 1 Drug-induced immune haemolytic anaemia

Mechanism	Drugs	Dosage of drug which produces haemolysis	Coombs' test	Reaction of eluate	Haemolysis
Hapten-membrane association	Penicillin, cephalosporins, insulin	High; exposure for some weeks	Mainly IgG	Reacts against drug-coated cells only	Extravascular
Immune complex	Stibophen, quinidine and quinine, p-aminosalicylic acid, isoniazid, phenacetin, anatzoline, sulphonamides, sulphonylureas, amidopyrine, dipyrone, rifampicin, insecticides	Low; second or subsequent exposure produces immediate haemolysis	Usually complement only	Reacts against drug-coated cells and sometimes against free drug	Intravascular acute
Autoimmune	α-Methyldopa, mefenamic acid, levodopa	Prolonged normal dosage	IgG	Reacts against normal red cells in the absence of the drug	Extravascular (usually slight)

Drug-induced immune haemolytic anaemia

There are three principal ways in which drugs cause the development of antibodies that bind to the red cells' surface (Table 1).

Hapten-membrane association

Some drugs, of which penicillin is the best-understood example, are bound to red cell-membrane proteins by covalent bonds. The drug–protein complex then acts as an antigenic determinant that binds specific antibody, which is mainly IgG in type. The haemolysis is gradual in onset but may be profound. The direct antiglobulin test is strongly positive, but antibodies in the serum will not react with normal red cells of the same type unless penicillin is also present. When the drug is withdrawn, haemolysis ceases fairly promptly, though the direct antiglobulin test may remain positive for 60 to 80 days.

Immune-complex formation

Many drugs have been incriminated in acute haemolytic anaemia (Table 1) but the number of case reports for each individual drug is small. The antibodies are usually IgM, which activates complement components and produces profound intravascular haemolysis with haemoglobinaemia and haemoglobinuria. The direct antiglobulin test is positive due to complement. Antibodies that are lytic for normal red cells only in the presence of the drug are found in the serum. Once the drug is withdrawn the haemolysis stops and the haemoglobin level rapidly returns to normal.

'Autoimmune' drug-induced haemolytic anaemia

Three drugs, α-methyldopa, mefenamic acid, and levodopa have been found to provoke the development of autoantibodies directed against red cell-membrane constituents, occasionally producing haemolytic anaemia. Haemolysis is usually moderate and spherocytes may be seen in the blood film. Haemolysis stops fairly rapidly after withdrawal of the drug, and steroid therapy is rarely indicated.

Autoimmune haemolytic anaemia

Haemolytic anaemia due to antibodies directed against normal red cell-membrane constituents may arise as a 'primary' event in otherwise healthy individuals, or may be associated with a number of other diseases. Table 2 shows that most secondary cases are associated with either malignancy of the lymphoid system or with more generalized autoimmune disorders. Autoimmune haemolytic anaemia may be further classified according to the temperature in which the antibodies are most active against normal red cells *in vitro*. In warm autoimmune haemolytic anaemia, the antibodies are most active at 37 °C, while in cold autoimmune haemolytic anaemia they are most active at low temperatures, 4 °C for example.

Table 2 Autoimmune haemolytic anaemias (AHAs)

	Warm	Cold
Primary	Idiopathic AHA Evans' syndrome (AHA and thrombocytopenia)	Idiopathic, chronic cold haemagglutinin disease (CHAD)
Secondary	Systemic lupus erythematosus, other autoimmune disorders Lymphomas (particularly chronic lymphocytic leukaemia and Hodgkin's disease) Drugs Ovarian teratoma, other cancers	Lymphomas (particularly histiocytic), paroxysmal cold haemoglobinuria, infectious mononucleosis Mycoplasma pneumonia Other virus infections (rare)

Warm autoimmune haemolytic anaemia

This is an uncommon disorder that may arise at any age and affects females slightly more than males (in a ratio of about 3:2). It is more common in older age groups because of its association with lymphoid neoplasms.

Clinical features

The onset and severity are variable. Most patients present with a progressive anaemia or mild jaundice, although rarely there is a fulminant illness with intravascular haemolysis. At the other extreme, the direct antiglobulin test may be positive but insufficient antibody is present to produce a shortening of the red-cell lifespan. Sometimes the symptoms and signs of the associated disorder dominate the clinical picture; however, the autoimmune haemolytic anaemia equally commonly precedes the discovery of the primary disease, sometimes by months or years. The spleen is usually palpable but rarely attains a great size.

Haematological features

Anaemia and reticulocytosis are the most marked features of the blood count. Nucleated red cells may be seen in the peripheral blood.

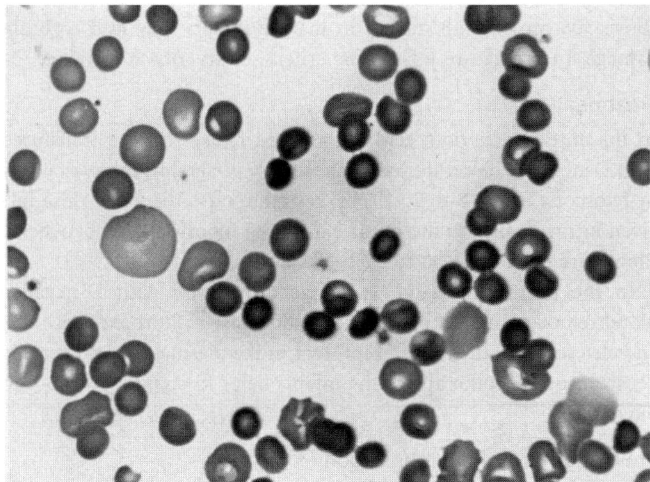

Fig. 1 The peripheral blood changes in autoimmune haemolytic anaemia. There is marked anisocytosis and anisochromia with many macrocytes and microspherocytes. The macrocytes reflect the reticulocytosis (1000 ×, Leishman stain).

In uncomplicated autoimmune haemolytic anaemia the platelet count is normal or high, again a reflection of general marrow drive, but in some patients the platelets are also destroyed by antibody and the haemolysis is accompanied by thrombocytopenia (Evans' syndrome). Autoimmune haemolytic anaemia and immune thrombocytopenia may also occur at different times in the same person.

The peripheral blood film may suggest the diagnosis (Fig. 1). Spherocytosis occurs in many but not all cases, and the cells may show autoagglutination. The direct antiglobulin test is positive in virtually all cases of warm autoimmune haemolytic anaemia.

The site of destruction of red cells depends upon whether sufficient complement is fixed to cause intravascular haemolysis or whether the antibody coating promotes phagocytosis by macrophages. When only IgG is bound to the red cell, destruction takes place mainly in the spleen.

Treatment

The aim of treatment in autoimmune haemolytic anaemia is to keep the patient in the best possible health with the minimum of iatrogenic problems until the autoantibody disappears and haemolysis stops. In many patients the antibodies disappear after a period varying from a few months to more than 10 years. Transfusion may be life-saving in the acute phase and should not be delayed because of an apparent incompatibility of crossmatch; ABO-matched blood that appears least incompatible should be used.

Corticosteroids are the first measure used to control haemolysis. Prednisolone, 80 mg daily, is effective in most patients and there is rarely any benefit in using higher doses. This dose may usually be reduced to 20 mg daily over a period of 2 to 3 weeks but thereafter a more cautious reduction should be used to find the minimum controlling dose. A maintenance dose of 10 mg prednisolone daily is acceptable in adults and side-effects may be reduced further if the drug is given on alternate days. Azathioprine may exert a steroid-sparing effect, allowing a reduction in steroid dose.

Splenectomy should done only when an adequate trial of corticosteroids has proved ineffective. The type of antibody present and the results of ^{51}Cr-survival studies with surface counting may sometimes provide some help in deciding whether to remove the spleen.

Cold autoantibody syndromes

Disorders due to autoantibodies that react most strongly at low temperatures may arise as primary (idiopathic) conditions or may be secondary to a variety of diseases (Table 2).

Chronic cold haemagglutinin disease

Cold haemagglutinin disease in a chronic form is a disease of elderly patients, usually of unknown cause but occasionally associated with lymphoma. Episodes of painful acrocyanosis and numbness (Raynaud's phenomenon) with a variable degree of intravascular haemolysis are the main features.

The blood film made at room temperature shows gross autoagglutination, which is absent if the blood is taken at 37 °C and the films prepared at this temperature. The direct antiglobulin test is positive, with complement bound to the red-cell surface. Antibodies in the serum are monoclonal, IgMk, and nearly all have anti-I specificity. The disease progresses slowly, with a gradual rise in titre and thermal range of the cold antibody, and may end with a malignant lymphoma after 10 years or more.

The main treatment is to keep the patient warm, but intermittent treatment with chlorambucil or fludarabine may reduce the antibody level and lead to temporary improvement. Steroids and splenectomy are of no benefit. Blood transfusion should be avoided if possible; if absolutely necessary, it should be given slowly and via a warming coil.

Acute cold haemagglutinin disease

An acute intravascular haemolysis due to a rise in titre of anti-I antibodies may occur following *Mycoplasma pneumoniae* infection. The haemolysis appears about 10 to 14 days after the onset of respiratory symptoms and is usually transient, but occasionally patients require transfusion. A rise in anti-I IgM antibodies is also found in infectious mononucleosis but acute haemolytic anaemia is rare.

Paroxysmal cold haemoglobinuria

Paroxysmal cold haemoglobinuria is a rare disorder caused by a complement-fixing antibody, the Donath–Landsteiner antibody, with anti-P activity. The condition used to arise most commonly in congenital syphilis but most cases are now associated with virus infections such as mumps, measles, or chickenpox. Acute intravascular haemolysis, accompanied by abdominal pain, peripheral cyanosis, and vascular symptoms of Raynaud type, occurs a few minutes after exposure to cold. The diagnosis is confirmed by identification of the Donath–Landsteiner antibody, which fixes itself to the red cell in the cold and binds on complement; this causes lysis as the cells are warmed.

Episodes are self-limiting and no specific treatment is required.

Haemolytic anaemia of the fetus and the newborn

Haemolytic disease of the fetus and newborn (**HDN**) is a condition in which the lifespan of the infant's red cells is shortened by the action of specific IgG red-cell alloantibodies derived from the mother by active transfer across the placenta. The disease begins in intrauterine life and may result in death *in utero*. In liveborn infants, the haemolytic process is maximal at the time of birth; however, jaundice and anaemia become more severe after birth.

The most common cause of HDN in the Western world is still anti-D, followed by anti-c, anti-K and anti-E. Although anti-A, and/

or -B are the most common IgG antibodies in women with blood group O, they very rarely cause clinically significant HDN.

The amount of red-cell destruction that follows the binding of IgG antibodies in HDN can be variable; hence a positive Coombs' test in a newborn infant is not synonymous with haemolytic disease. It is often difficult to decide whether there is any increased red-cell destruction because, in almost all newborn infants, the serum bilirubin concentration rises during the first 2 to 3 days of life and there is a fall in haemoglobin concentration, which continues for about 2 months.

Clinical manifestations of RhD haemolytic disease

The disease due to anti-RhD shows a wide spectrum of severity. Not all D-positive infants born to mothers with anti-D in their serum are affected by HDN. Some infants are only mildly affected, with jaundice and anaemia developing in the first week of life. More severely affected infants develop profound hyperbilirubinaemia. The most severe manifestation of HDN is profound anaemia, developing *in utero* as early as the eighteenth week of gestation and leading to hydrops fetalis with a high mortality.

RhD immunization may occur in 10 per cent of pregnancies in RhD-negative Caucasian women who have a D-positive infant. Immunization is due mainly to transplacental haemorrhage from the fetus to the mother, which occurs at delivery in over 50 per cent of cases. Spontaneous transplacental haemorrhage may occur in the third trimester and its volume can be quantitated by the acid-elution technique of Kleihauer. The chance of transplacental haemorrhage is increased in ectopic pregnancy and with obstetric interventions.

In approximately 1 per cent of RhD-negative women who deliver a first D-positive child, anti-D is detectable at the end of pregnancy; it is detectable 6 months' postpartum in 7 to 9 per cent of D-negative women with a D-positive child, and in a further 9 per cent (17 per cent altogether) at delivery of the second D-positive infant.

Antenatal assessment of severity

All pregnant women should be grouped for ABO and D at least twice: at the first visit and at delivery. The serum should be tested for alloantibodies at the first visit and if found positive, followed-up monthly up to the twentieth week and at 2-weekly intervals thereafter. Unimmunized D-negative women should be retested at 20 weeks and, if negative, retested at 28 weeks, when antenatal prophylaxis should be considered. All women should have their serum retested at delivery and if D-negative, unimmunized, and carrying a D-positive child they should be given RhD immunoglobulin (see below). Amniocentesis can be performed from 28 weeks' gestation onwards, if HDN is expected, to estimate the amount of bile pigment in the amniotic fluid. Ultrasonography also helps in the diagnosis of severe HDN from 18 weeks' gestation onwards, but measuring the haemoglobin and packed cell volume in a fetal blood sample is the best method to assess the severity of haemolytic disease *in utero* reliably.

Postnatal assessment of severity

If the direct antiglobulin test on cord red cells is positive, the cord haemoglobin level is the best indicator of severity in infants who may need exchange transfusion; 13.6 g/dl is the lower limit of normal in full-term infants. A cord plasma bilirubin concentration of 68 mmol/l (4 mg/dl) or more may also be an indication for exchange transfusion. If exchange transfusion is not indicated immediately, the plasma bilirubin concentration should be monitored every few hours; levels above 306 mmol/l (18 mg/dl) in mature infants may lead to brain damage. In premature infants the criteria of severity are stricter.

Treatment

In the antenatal period, severely affected fetuses can be transfused with D-negative blood intraperitoneally or, preferably, intravascularly by fetoscopy from 18 to 20 weeks' gestation onwards. High-dose IgG given intravenously to the mother has been reported to be beneficial. Premature delivery at 30 to 32 weeks also helps.

In the postnatal period, exchange transfusion with D-negative blood removes anti-D-coated cells, which have a short survival time, and also removes the bilirubin present in the plasma, thus preventing kernicterus. Phototherapy of the infants helps to convert bilirubin to biliverdin.

Prevention of RhD immunization

Some 20 μg of anti-D immunoglobulin are able to suppress maternal immunization by 1 ml of D-positive red cells (2 ml of blood). The standard dose of anti-D immunoglobulin varies in different countries between 100 and 300 mg given within 72 h of the delivery of an RhD-positive child. Transplacental haemorrhages not covered by the standard dose should be quantitated and additional anti-D given as necessary. About 1 to 2 per cent of RhD-negative women are immunized earlier, during pregnancy. This can be prevented by giving anti-D immunoglobulin antenatally, either with 100 μg anti-D at 28 and 34 weeks' gestation or with a single dose of 300 μg at 28 weeks.

Non-immune acquired haemolytic anaemias

Damage to the red-cell membrane leading to haemolysis may occur in certain infections, through oxidative damage brought about by various drugs and chemicals, or through physical damage to the red cell. Except in infection, where immune mechanisms probably play some part in the destruction of red cells, intravascular haemolysis is the usual result.

Infections causing haemolytic anaemia

These include malaria (see Chapters 3.40 and 16.84) and toxoplasmosis. With the latter, fetal infection *in utero* may give rise to a very severe disease resembling HDN. Stillbirth and premature delivery are common, and the infant may be hydropic and severely anaemic with erythroblasts in the peripheral blood. Rarely, acquired toxoplasmosis produces a haemolytic anaemia in adults.

Severe bacterial infections may lead to disseminated intravascular coagulation and a microangiopathic haemolytic anaemia (see below). *Clostridium perfringens* septicaemia is associated with an intense intravascular haemolysis, microspherocytosis, and fragmentation of the red cells.

Chemically induced haemolysis

Haemolysis may be caused by a number of drugs and chemicals that are oxidative or produce oxidative metabolites.

Pathogenesis

Some drugs and chemicals are strong oxidants and may overcome the reducing power of red cells. Individuals with glucose 6-phosphate dehydrogenase (**G6PD**) deficiency and newborn infants are more prone to develop haemolysis due to the administration of oxidants.

Two distinct syndromes occur as a result of oxidant stress. Some strongly oxidizing chemicals such as arsine or chlorate, which may be encountered in industry or used for self-poisoning, produce an intense haemolysis together with disseminated intravascular coagulation and acute renal failure. Constitutional symptoms occur and there may be cyanosis due to associated methaemoglobinaemia. The blood film is bizarre, with red-cell ghosts, fragments, and microspherocytes. The platelet count may fall. Blood transfusion, haemodialysis, and exchange transfusion may be needed. The management of acute methaemoglobinaemia is discussed in Chapter 3.19.

In contrast, the usual result of normal individuals taking oxidant drugs such as dapsone or sulphasalazine for long periods is a chronic intravascular haemolysis. Cyanosis due to the presence of methaemoglobin and sulphaemoglobin may be prominent. The peripheral blood film shows red cells that are irregular and contracted, often with only a segment of the membrane apparently normal. Heinz bodies (precipitated haemoglobin) may be seen but are uncommon unless the spleen has been removed. Withdrawal of the drug will terminate the haemolysis but it is not always possible to stop treatment, particularly with dapsone or sulphasalazine. Provided the haemolysis is well compensated it is reasonable to continue the treatment together with iron and folate supplements. If anaemia is a problem, it may be necessary to reduce the dose of the drug.

Mechanical haemolytic anaemias

Fragmentation of red cells by mechanical trauma occurs either when foreign material has been inserted into large blood vessels at surgery or where small blood vessels have been partially blocked by fibrin strands. The former has been called cardiac haemolysis and the latter microangiopathic haemolytic anaemia.

Cardiac haemolysis

The insertion of prosthetic valves or patches into the heart or aorta usually leads to some destruction of circulating red cells. Under certain circumstances this process can be sufficient to produce severe haemolytic anaemia. Mitral-valve prostheses produce severe haemolysis less commonly than aortic, but when they do the anaemia is often profound. Cardiac haemolysis is aggravated by an increase in cardiac output so that exercise and anaemia itself may increase the rate of cell destruction. The acuteness of the haemolysis may give some indication as to its cause. Severe haemolysis occurring immediately postoperatively suggests a surgical cause. Gradually increasing haemolysis after the patient has left hospital suggests that exercise is promoting turbulence or possibly that iron deficiency is aggravating the anaemia and increasing the turbulence. A delayed onset of haemolysis, particularly after some years in patients with ball-valve prostheses, suggests distortion of the ball or other abnormalities of the prosthesis and reoperation may be necessary. The peripheral blood film shows fragmented red cells with microspherocytes in most cases.

Oral iron should be given so that iron deficiency does not develop as a result of haemosiderinuria. Intractable haemolysis may be an indication for surgical re-exploration.

Microangiopathic haemolytic anaemia

Microangiopathic haemolytic anaemia is a term used to describe intravascular haemolysis due to the mechanical destruction of red cells as a result of a variety of pathological changes in small blood vessels. The condition has been described in association with a variety of systemic disorders, some of which are summarized in Table 3.

Pathogenesis

Microangiopathic haemolytic anaemia develops in many different disorders associated with pathological changes in small vessels, of which microthrombi in capillaries and arterioles, fibrinoid necrosis, necrotizing arteritis, and invasion of capillary walls by malignant cells are the most common.

Table 3 Causes of microangiopathic haemolytic anaemia

Disease	Microangiopathy
Haemolytic-uraemic syndrome	Microthrombi in renal arteries and capillaries
Thrombotic thrombocytopenic purpura	Disseminated intravascular coagulation (DIC)
Renal cortical necrosis	Necrotizing arteritis
Acute glomerular nephritis	Necrotizing arteritis
Pre-eclampsia	Fibrinoid necrosis, DIC (?)
Malignant hypertension	Fibrinoid necrosis. Intimal proliferation in renal vessels
Disseminated carcinomatosis (especially mucinous types)	DIC, tumour emboli (?)
Polyarteritis nodosa	Arteritis
Wegener's granulomatosis	Arteritis
Systemic lupus erythematosus	Arteritis
Homograft rejection	Microthrombi in transplanted organ
Meningococcaemia and other septicaemias	DIC
Cavernous haemangioma	?Local vascular anomalies or thrombosis
Purpura fulminans	?Microthrombi in skin vessels
Polycarboxylate interferon induction	DIC

Some of the disorders that produce microangiopathic haemolytic anaemia are associated with disseminated intravascular coagulation, and it has been suggested that microthrombi cause haemolysis because the red cells are fragmented during their passage through the fibrin clots in the small vessels. While this is certainly true in some cases, the relationship between intravascular coagulation and microangiopathic haemolytic anaemia is far from clear-cut.

Clinical features

Microangiopathic haemolytic anaemia is characterized by a haemolytic anaemia of varying severity. It is usually seen in a clinical setting of one of the disorders summarized in Table 3.

The haemolytic–uraemic syndrome and thrombotic thrombocytopenic purpura are considered separately below. The presence of renal disease, pre-eclampsia, or septicaemia usually presents no diagnostic difficulty. If a patient presents with microangiopathic haemolytic anaemia with no obvious associated disease, it is important to rule out an underlying carcinoma or collagen-vascular disease. The most common tumours associated with this condition are mucus-secreting carcinoma of the stomach, lung, breast, or large bowel. These are nearly always widely disseminated and it is often possible to demonstrate tumour cells in the bone marrow. If disseminated carcinomatosis can be excluded, it is necessary to proceed to investigation for collagen-vascular disorders.

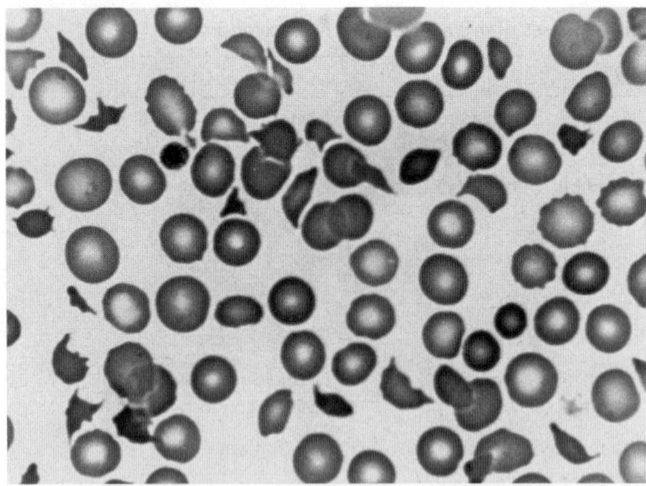

Fig. 2 The peripheral blood changes in microangiopathic haemolytic anaemia. This patient had recurrent thrombotic thrombocytopenic purpura and the marked fragmentation of the red cells together with microspherocytosis is evident on the blood film (1000 ×, Leishman stain).

The diagnosis is made largely on the basis of a haemolytic anaemia in the presence of certain morphological appearances of the red cells, which show marked fragmentation and some microspherocytes (Fig. 2); the Coombs' test is negative. A reduced platelet count suggests that there may be an associated disseminated intravascular coagulation.

The only really successful approach to the treatment of microangiopathic haemolytic anaemia is to find and eradicate the underlying cause. Severe anaemia requires blood transfusion.

Haemolytic–uraemic syndrome (see Chapter 12.10)

Pathogenesis

Haemolytic–uraemic syndrome is most often a disease of infancy, although the peak incidence is variable. There is a seasonal variation and it is more common in the northern hemisphere in the late spring and early summer.

There is widespread damage to the vascular endothelium with secondary fibrin deposition particularly involving renal arterioles and glomerular capillaries. These changes are also widely found throughout all the organ systems. It is presumed that the red-cell changes are secondary to damage during their passage through these small vessels.

Clinical and haematological features

The syndrome usually develops after a febrile illness accompanied by diarrhoea, often bloody, and vomiting in a previously healthy child. There may be marked gastrointestinal symptoms, including bloody diarrhoea and abdominal pain. A virulent strain of verotoxin-producing *Escherichia coli*, 0157, has been responsible for a number of epidemics.

Evidence of acute intravascular haemolysis with rapidly developing anaemia develops during or shortly after the prodromal illness and may precede the onset of oliguria. Purpura and bleeding may also occur during the acute phase. Drowsiness, convulsions, and coma may develop, and death may occur during the acute phase from uncontrollable anaemia, haemorrhage, or hypertension.

About one-third of patients do not develop oliguria at all, about one-third have oliguria for up to 10 days, and the remainder up to 4 weeks or longer. The majority of patients without oliguria recover completely without treatment. The longer the period of oliguria, the more likely it is that the condition will go on to a chronic renal failure. The overall death rate from haemolytic–uraemic syndrome varies from about 2 to 10 per cent.

The blood film shows fragmentation of red cells with occasional spherocytes. In contrast to cardiac haemolytic anaemia, thrombocytopenia is common, although not invariable. There is often a moderate leucocytosis. Usually there is laboratory evidence of intravascular haemolysis with a raised plasma haemoglobin level, methaemalbumin, low or absent serum haptoglobins, and, sometimes, haemoglobinuria. Coagulation studies give equivocal and often conflicting results, although in some cases there is evidence for a consumptive coagulopathy.

Management

The mainstay of treatment is supportive care, transfusion, hydration, control of hypertension, and, if necessary, dialysis.

Thrombotic thrombocytopenic purpura

Thrombotic thrombocytopenic purpura (TTP) is a disorder that has some similarities to the haemolytic–uraemic syndrome, but it occurs mainly in adults. The classical pentad of clinical features is thrombocytopenia, microangiopathic haemolytic anaemia, fluctuating neurological signs and symptoms, fever, and renal impairment. The renal aspects are considered in greater detail in Chapter 12.10.

Aetiology and pathogenesis

Both sporadic and familial forms of TTP are described; in either form a common pathway seems to be the deficient function of a protease which cleaves von Willebrand factor (vWF), thus reducing its multimeric size. Many of the sporadic cases appear to follow the development of an IgG autoantibody that inhibits protease function, whereas in constitutional forms the protease is deficient for other reasons.

Clinical features

The disorder affects females more commonly than males (about 2:1) and may occur at any age, but with a peak incidence around 35 years of age. The onset is often sudden, with the development of fever and signs of neurological damage, including convulsions, coma, transient or permanent paralyses, and bizarre psychiatric disturbances, sometimes with hallucinations; the neurological features often fluctuate widely. Purpura may accompany or follow the neurological signs and there may be severe bleeding, particularly from the gastrointestinal tract. Anaemia is not usually severe, although occasionally there may be dramatic intravascular haemolysis with haemoglobinuria.

The illness may run a fluctuating course of days or weeks and some patients may have a series of acute episodes with apparent recovery in between. The most common causes of death are sudden cardiac arrest, bleeding, cerebrovascular accident, or renal failure.

Haematological and biochemical changes

There is a mild to severe haemolytic anaemia with fragmentation and contraction of the red cells. This is associated with a variable degree of thrombocytopenia; in some cases the platelets may almost disappear from the peripheral blood. In some cases, coagulation studies show evidence of a consumption coagulopathy but this is not often marked.

Examination of the plasma by gel electrophoresis and immunostaining may demonstrate the presence of high molecular-weight von Willebrand multimers, though these may disappear during the acute phase.

Proteinuria is usual, often with other evidence of renal damage in the form of casts and red cells, together with a raised blood urea and reduced creatinine clearance. In some cases there may be serological findings suggestive of systemic lupus erythematosus. Hypertension is common.

There appears to be a subgroup of patients with a thrombotic thrombocytopenic purpura-like illness who give a long history of relapses going back to childhood, often initiated by a disorder resembling the haemolytic–uraemic syndrome. Also, thrombotic thrombocytopenic purpura seems to be particularly prone to occur during pregnancy or in the postpartum period and this may account for the slight excess of young women affected by this disease. It is often associated with miscarriage. Removal of the fetus does not always lead to remission.

Plasma exchange is the most effective form of treatment and the use of cryosupernatant seems especially valuable. Up to 12 consecutive, daily exchanges may be required to produce a response and relapse is not uncommon. A proportion of patients may respond to infusion of fresh frozen plasma without exchange.

March haemoglobinuria

Haemoglobinuria follows walking or running on a hard surface and lasts for a few hours. Other sports such as karate may produce the same effect. There may be some systemic symptoms, such as nausea and abdominal pain, but usually the haemoglobinuria is symptomless. The blood film is normal in appearance and fragments are not seen.

Treatment is not usually necessary, but the insertion of a springy sole into running shoes will usually prevent haemolysis.

Haemolytic anaemia of burns

Extensive burns produce intravascular haemolysis with microspherocytosis and fragmentation in the peripheral blood. The direct action of heat is probably important in the pathogenesis but intravascular coagulation in the postinjury period may play some part.

Acquired disorders of the cell membrane

Paroxysmal nocturnal haemoglobinuria is the most common acquired disorder of the red-cell membrane (see Chapter 3.13).

Lipid disorders

Changes in the lipid content of plasma may induce red cell-membrane changes that lead to some shortening of the cell's survival. Abnormalities of membrane lipid metabolism may contribute to the haemolysis of liver disease and disorders associated with hyperlipidaemia.

Liver disease

There is a shortening of the red-cell lifespan in most patients with acute hepatitis, cirrhosis, and Gilbert's disease (see Section 5). In Gilbert's disease the decreased red-cell survival and slight reticulocytosis suggest that haemolysis may contribute to the increased unconjugated bilirubin, but it seems probable that it is only a minor factor and that deficiency of the enzyme UDP-glucoronyl transferase is mainly responsible. In biliary obstruction and mild liver disease, target cells are seen in the peripheral blood. In more severe disorders, acanthocytosis is prominent. Zieve's syndrome is the association of haemolytic anaemia with abdominal pain, cirrhosis, hyperlipidaemia, and jaundice in chronic alcoholics. The peripheral blood contains spherocytes and the osmotic fragility is increased, unlike most liver disorders in which it is reduced.

Wilson's disease (see Chapter 6.10)

Acute haemolysis, usually intravascular, may be a presenting feature in Wilson's disease. It may be caused by the presence of free copper in the plasma.

Hypersplenism

A significant enlargement of the spleen is frequently associated with a slightly shortened red-cell survival even though the red cells are intrinsically normal.

Anaemia of chronic disorders and renal disease

The haemolytic component of the anaemia of chronic disorders is described in Chapter 3.17.

Further reading

Dacie, J.V. (1992). *The haemolytic anaemias*, Vol. 3, *The autoimmune haemolytic anaemias*, 3rd edn. Churchill Livingstone, Edinburgh.

Moake, J.L. and McPherson, P.D. (1990). von Willebrand factor in thrombotic thrombocytopenic purpura and the hemolytic–uremic syndrome. *Transfusion Medicine Reviews*, 4, 163.

Mollison, P. L. *et al.* (1993). *Blood transfusion in clinical medicine*, 9th edn, Chapters 3, 5, and 12. Blackwell Scientific, Oxford.

Chapter 3.26

The relative and secondary polycythaemias

D. J. Weatherall

The word 'polycythaemia' means an increased red-cell count, packed cell volume (PCV), or haemoglobin level. This chapter reviews the diagnostic approach to this condition as well as the common causes and their management. It is important to remember that polycythaemia rubra vera (Chapter 3.9) is responsible only for a minority of cases.

Classification and pathogenesis

A high haemoglobin level can occur for two main reasons (Table 1). First, there may be a reduction in the plasma volume with a normal red-cell mass (relative polycythaemia). Second, there may be a genuine increase in the red-cell mass (absolute polycythaemia).

An increased red-cell mass may occur due to neoplastic proliferation of haemopoietic progenitors (polycythaemia rubra vera) or from increased levels of erythropoietin. Raised erythropoietin may be appropriate due to hypoxia or there may be inappropriate secretion of high levels of erythropoietin, usually from an erythropoietin-secreting tumour.

An approach to the patient with polycythaemia

Apparent polycythaemia is a common clinical problem and it is useful to develop a logical approach to diagnosis (Fig. 1).

The first rule is that, unless the haemoglobin level is extremely high, never diagnose polycythaemia on a single blood count. Care must be taken to ensure that a count is obtained when the patient is well hydrated, is not receiving large doses of diuretics, and has not had a heavy night's alcohol intake the day before the blood sample is taken. Heavy smokers who have a mild polycythaemia should be asked to stop smoking and their blood counts repeated several weeks later. Also, it should be remembered that the haemoglobin level and PCV have a large standard deviation; many referrals for the investigation of polycythaemia stem from an ignorance of normal haematological values.

The next step is to decide whether it is a true or relative polycythaemia by performing a plasma volume and red-cell mass determination. If there is an absolute polycythaemia it is necessary to decide whether this is polycythaemia rubra vera (Chapter 3.9) or a secondary cause.

The causes of secondary polycythaemia are summarized in Table 2. Hypoxia due to chronic obstructive airways disease is by far the most common, and blood-gas analysis, either at rest or after exercise, is advisable. Cyanotic heart disease usually presents no diagnostic problems, but occasionally patients are encountered who have arteriovenous malformations that may not be obvious clinically. Again, analysis of the arterial oxygen saturation will provide a clue to the diagnosis. If available a P_{50} estimation is useful—if reduced, indicating a left shift in the oxygen dissociation curve, the carboxyhaemoglobin level should be estimated; patients are often unreliable about their smoking habits! If this is normal and the P_{50} is low, there must be an intrinsic abnormality of the red cells, either of the haemoglobin or of the red-cell enzymes. If the P_{50} is normal, a source of inappropriate erythropoietin production should be looked for. The most likely site is the kidney, either a hypernephroma or a renal cyst. An erythropoietin assay is a valuable confirmatory investigation.

Table 1 Mechanisms for the production of polycythaemia

Relative
Reduced plasma volume
Absolute
• Normal or low erythropoietin levels; abnormal proliferation polycythaemia vera
• Increased erythropoietin levels:
• Appropriate: lung disease, cyanotic heart disease, altitude, abnormal haemoglobin, hypoventilation, decreased 2,3-diphosphoglycerate production
• Inappropriate: renal tumour; other erythropoietin-secreting tumours; after renal transplant; genetic defect in erythropoietin regulation

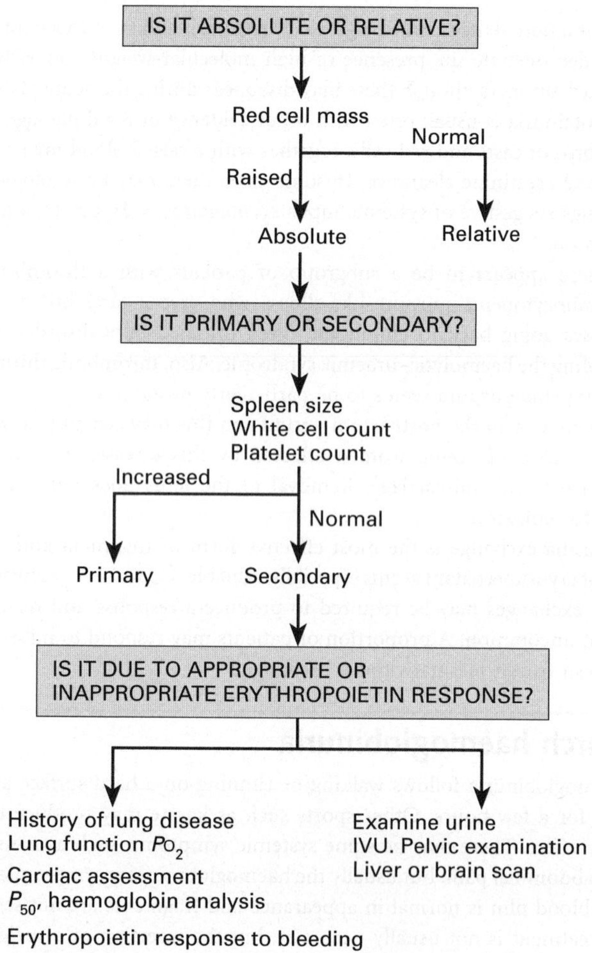

Fig. 1 Flow chart of investigations for polycythaemia.

Table 2 Clinical classification of polycythaemia

Relative or *pseudopolycythaemia* ('stress' polycythaemia)
True polycythaemia
Primary
Polycythaemia rubra vera
Secondary
Altitude
Chronic lung disease
Cyanotic congenital heart disease
Renal disease:
tumours, cysts, hydronephrosis, post-transplant
Non-renal tumours:
hepatoma, cerebellar haemangioma, uterine fibromata
Endocrine:
Cushing's disease, phaeochromocytoma
Genetic:
abnormal haemoglobin
abnormal erythropoietin response
abnormal 2,3-diphosphoglycerate metabolism
Obesity:
Pickwickian syndrome
other causes of hypoventilation

In a number of patients no cause can be found ('idiopathic erythrocytosis') and it is worthwhile keeping them under regular surveillance.

Relative polycythaemia

The term describes an elevated haemoglobin level or PCV that results from a contraction of the plasma volume and is not associated with an absolute increase in red-cell mass. Some patients have a clear disturbance of fluid balance leading to diminished plasma volume such as may occur in severe dehydration, following diuretic therapy, and in various endocrine disorders such as Addison's or Cushing's diseases. Others seem simply to have red-cell masses at the upper limit of normal and a slightly contracted plasma volume.

The typical clinical picture of relative polycythaemia is the overweight middle-aged male who is slightly hypertensive and has a haemoglobin value in the 18 to 20 g/dl range and a PCV of 49 to 55 per cent. There are no specific symptoms or signs that can be attributed to this 'disorder' and usually the presenting feature is an associated medical condition, most often cardiovascular disease or hypertension. With the exception of an elevated haemoglobin and PCV the rest of the haematological findings are completely normal.

In the past it was thought sufficient, once the diagnosis of relative polycythaemia was made, to reassure the patient strongly and to stop examining his or her blood. Suitable advice was given about weight reduction, the control of hypertension, and stopping smoking. Although this is still the case, there is some evidence that the mild elevation of blood viscosity that occurs in patients with PCVs in the 50 to 55 per cent range may predispose towards coronary artery and cerebrovascular disease. It may be reasonable to venesect patients who have had episodes of coronary artery or cerebrovascular disease and who have persistently elevated PCVs, or those who have a particularly bad family history of cardiovascular disease. It is much more difficult to make a case for venesection in asymptomatic patients.

Secondary polycythaemia

Some of the causes of secondary polycythaemia are listed in Table 2. Chronic obstructive airways disease is probably the most common and the therapeutic value of venesection in such patients remains controversial. In any congenital heart disease with a right-to-left shunt there may be arterial oxygen unsaturation and extreme secondary polycythaemia (see Chapter 2.21). Some children with severe congenital heart disease of this type may have PCVs in excess of 80 per cent. There is a genuine risk of thrombotic episodes, particularly if these children become dehydrated due to an intercurrent illness. There may be an indication for venesection, particularly before surgery, although the precise value of reducing the haematocrit is not clear. Carboxyhaemoglobin due to smoking is one of the most common causes of secondary polycythaemia. Heavy smokers may have carboxyhaemoglobin levels as high as 15 per cent of. A variable degree of polycythaemia is found in patients and their affected family members with high oxygen-affinity haemoglobin variants (Chapter 3.19).

A variety of disorders can cause inappropriate erythropoietin production including renal, cerebellar, or hepatic tumours. Mild polycythaemia has also been reported in patients with other forms of renal pathology including hydronephrosis and polycystic disease.

Although the most common form of hereditary polycythaemia is due to abnormal haemoglobins with a high oxygen affinity, there remain families in which this is not the cause. Abnormalities of the erythropoietin receptor are responsible in some cases.

Further reading

Erslev, A.J. (1994). Secondary polycythemia. In *Williams hematology* (ed. E. Beutler, M.A. Lichtman, B.S. Coller, and T.J. Kipps). McGraw-Hill, New York.

The white cells and lymphoproliferative disorders

Chapter 3.27

Leucocytes in health and disease

A. J. Thrasher and A. W. Segal

Leucocytes form the cellular basis of host defence against pathogens. They can be divided into phagocytic cells (which include neutrophils, monocytes, dendritic cells, and eosinophils) and non-phagocytic cells (the basophils and lymphocytes). Phagocytic cells and basophils are primary effector cells in acute inflammation, they modulate cellular and humoral immunity through the release of immunoregulatory cytokines, and are responsible for the ingestion and digestion of cellular and non-cellular debris.

Morphology and composition

Granulocytes are classified into neutrophils, eosinophils, and basophils on the basis of the staining characteristics of granules in their cytoplasm. They have irregularly shaped, lobed nuclei, and are also referred to as polymorphonuclear leucocytes.

Neutrophils

A mature neutrophil contains about 5000 granules, of which one-third are known as primary (or azurophil) granules which contain myeloperoxidase, lysozyme, and most of the antimicrobial molecules. The secondary (or specific) granules are smaller and contain membrane components that are stored and transferred to the plasma membrane when the cell is activated. The main function of these cells is in providing immunity against bacterial and fungal infections and in the removal of exogenous and endogenous debris.

Eosinophils

Eosinophils are much less numerous than neutrophils, making up only 1 to 6 per cent of blood leucocytes. They contain high concentrations of basic proteins, such as major basic protein and eosinophilic cationic protein, and are attracted to sites of inflammation by products released from T lymphocytes, mast cells, and basophils. The eosinophil has both proinflammatory and cytotoxic activity and is believed to play a primary part in host defence mechanisms against metazoan parasitic infection.

Basophils

Basophils make up less than 0.2 per cent of blood leucocytes, and unlike other members of the granulocyte family, are non-phagocytic.

Basophils release preformed mediators from granules including heparin, histamine, and platelet-activating factor. Degranulation is initiated by antigens that crosslink specific IgE to the surface of the cell by high-affinity Fc receptors. They are thought to be important in parasitic disease and immunoregulation.

Monocytes/macrophages

The functional status of monocytes depends on their degree of activation, which is determined by both macrophage-activating factors and physical contact with tumour cells or micro-organisms. Phagocytosis of micro-organisms and digestion of ingested cellular debris are the most prominent effector functions of monocytes/macrophages. In addition, activated cells produce many immunomodulatory molecules including interferon-β, interleukin-1 (IL-1), tumour necrosis factor-α, and IL-6, as well as reactive oxygen intermediates. Cytokines released from macrophages not only act locally, but exert hormonal effects throughout the body, resulting in fever, synthesis of acute-phase proteins, and tissue catabolism. Related specialized cells, known as dendritic cells, play a crucial role in antigen presentation.

Lymphocytes

Lymphocytes undergo maturation in lymphoid tissues of the body and constitute about 20 per cent of blood leucocytes. They can be separated into two main types, B cells and T cells. B lymphocytes develop predominantly in the bone marrow, while T lymphocytes develop in the thymus. Natural killer (NK) cells are the third population of lymphocytes and can kill cells expressing low levels of HLA molecules. Further details on lymphocyte biology can be found in OTM3, pp. 141–53.

Distribution and regulation of leucocytes

Granulocytes and monocytes have short lifespans—the development of mature neutrophils in the bone marrow takes about 7 days. Before their release from the bone marrow, mature cells remain in a storage pool for a variable length of time. In normal states this pool contains 10–15 times the number of granulocytes found in peripheral blood, but they can be released prematurely from marrow should the need arise. In the circulation, leucocytes are either in the circulating pool or the marginating pool adherent to microvascular endothelium, each with roughly equal numbers of cells. Mature neutrophils remain in the circulation for up to 12 h, and then migrate into the tissues to perform their biological function where they survive for 1–3 days.

Unlike granulocytes, which are terminally differentiated, monocytes can differentiate further into macrophages and related specialized cells, such as dendritic cells. After 24–48 h in the circulation, they enter tissues and differentiate into large macrophages that are widely spread throughout every tissue and organ of the body, where they may persist for months or years.

Haemopoietic growth factors control the proliferation and maturation of progenitor cells by interacting with specific cell-surface receptors. The most important are the colony-stimulating factors, which include granulocyte–macrophage colony-stimulating factor (GM-CSF) and granulocyte colony-stimulating factor (G-CSF). These have been shown to accelerate myeloid recovery after high-dose chemotherapy and stem-cell transplantation and are used widely in clinical practice. They are also valuable for releasing donor progenitor cells into the circulation prior to the collection of peripheral blood for use in stem-cell transplantation.

Overall, 50–70 per cent of leucocytes circulating in blood are granulocytes. During infancy there is a predominance of lymphocytes. In some areas of Africa, the adult neutrophil to lymphocyte ratio may be reversed.

Leucocyte dysregulation

Neutrophilia

An increase in the numbers of neutrophils in the circulating compartment (for example, above 10 × 109/l) is described as neutrophilia or neutrophil leucocytosis. Neutrophilia commonly accompanies bacterial infection and tissue injury, where there is an early release of cells from the bone marrow. Consequently, immature band cells and metamyelocytes may be found in the circulation, giving rise to a blood picture described as 'left shifted'. Other causes of neutrophilia include corticosteroids, an acute stress response, intense muscular activity, hyposplenism, and malignant disease. Extreme neutrophilia, often greater than 30×10^9/l, may occur in disseminated malignancy, disseminated tuberculosis, and severe infection, particularly in splenectomized individuals, and needs to be differentiated from chronic granulocytic leukaemia and other myeloproliferative diseases. The neutrophil alkaline phosphatase score is characteristically low in leukaemic disorders and high in most other neutrophilic states.

Neutropenia

A circulating neutrophil count below 1.5×10^9/l is usually abnormal, although lower counts may be normal for certain non-White genetic groups. Patients with neutrophil counts less than 0.5×10^9/l are at increased risk of infection.

Inherited neutropenia

Congenital agranulocytosis (Kostmann's syndrome) This is characterized by persistent severe neutropenia and bone marrow morphology suggestive of maturational arrest at the promyelocyte stage. Children develop frequent and severe infections starting in infancy.

Cyclic neutropenia A rare condition characterized by cyclic fluctuations in numbers of neutrophils, monocytes, eosinophils, lymphocytes, platelets, and reticulocytes with a periodicity of 3–4 weeks. Patients suffer from fever, mouth ulceration, and serious infections at times when the neutrophil count is low. The defect appears to be at the level of stem-cell regulation, but may improve spontaneously with time.

In both these conditions, regular treatment with G-CSF has been shown to augment neutrophil counts, and to decrease the frequency of serious infection.

Acquired neutropenia

The most common causes are viral or bacterial infection, radiotherapy, and cytotoxic drug therapy. Many drugs may produce idiosyncratic cytopenia and antithyroid drugs present a particularly high risk. Miscellaneous causes include hypersplenism, megaloblastic anaemia, autoimmune and isoimmune destruction, marrow infiltration by malignant cells, idiopathic aplasia, and drug-induced immune destruction. Felty's syndrome is a rare condition in which splenomegaly and neutropenia occur together with rheumatoid arthritis.

Eosinophilia (see also Chapter 3.32)

An elevated eosinophil count above 0.5×10^9/l is seen in a number of clinical conditions. It is most frequently associated with atopic disease, invasive parasitic infection, and drug hypersensitivity, but may also be a feature of malignancy, hypoadrenalism, and vasculitis.

Basophilia

The regulation of basophil and mast-cell lineages appears to be disordered in myeloproliferative disorders and in systemic mastocytosis. Basophilia is a classic feature of chronic granulocytic leukaemia. In systemic mastocytosis and the related cutaneous disorder urticaria pigmentosa, proliferation of mast cells within tissues is common, but systemic elevations of mast-cell numbers occur only rarely in mast-cell leukaemia. Urticaria, anaphylaxis, and asthma may occur.

Monocytosis

Absolute monocytosis is an infrequent finding, but may occur in cases of chronic infection, chronic neutropenia, Hodgkin's disease, and monocytic leukaemia.

Lymphocytosis

A lymphocytosis is most frequently associated with viral infection, in particular infectious mononucleosis, acute human immunodeficiency virus (**HIV**) infection, rubella, cytomegalovirus, and infectious hepatitis. It may also occur during bacterial infection, particularly brucellosis and tuberculosis, and in toxoplasmosis.

Lymphopenia

Absolute lymphopenia is an uncommon finding, but may be associated with marrow failure, immunosuppressive therapy, corticosteroid therapy, autoimmune disease, HIV infection, and systemic lupus erythematosus.

Leucocyte biology

Human polymorphonuclear neutrophils are the primary effector cells in acute inflammation. They are rapidly recruited from the bloodstream to sites of infection or inflammation, initially by an increase in local blood flow and vascular permeability, and then by the processes of adhesion to endothelial cells, transendothelial migration, and chemotaxis. Once at these sites they ingest and phagocytose foreign particles, and release a range of biological mediators. The importance of adhesion processes is revealed by the syndrome of leucocyte adhesion deficiency, a rare inherited disease characterized in its severe form by recurrent life-threatening bacterial and fungal infections. Such patients have mutations in genes coding for adhesion molecules. In the Wiskett–Aldrich syndrome, mutations in a gene involved in the regulation of the cytoskeleton lead to severe defects in motility of dendritic cells, monocytes, and possibly lymphoid cells. Neutrophil mobility is also reduced in a number of acquired conditions, both idiopathic and in association with diabetes, infection, malnutrition, severe burns, and drug therapy. The clinical relevance of subtle abnormalities of mobility is questionable.

Phagocytosis and killing

Polymorphonuclear leucocytes kill bacteria and fungi by a combination of oxidative and non-oxidative mechanisms:

- *Oxidative killing*: activation of polymorphonuclear leucocytes and phagocytosis of opsonized particles is associated with a massive increase in oxygen consumption known as the respiratory burst. This generates hydrogen peroxide and free oxygen radicals.
- *Non-oxidative killing*: neutrophil cytoplasmic azurophil granules contain an abundance of antimicrobial proteins such as lysozyme and cathepsin G that are active even in anaerobic conditions.

Disorders of killing and digestion

Disorders of oxidative mechanisms

Chronic granulomatous disease This is a heterogeneous group of inherited conditions and occurs with a frequency of about 1 in 500 000 births. Approximately two-thirds of cases are X-linked and due to cytochrome mutations, whilst one-third are recessively inherited. There is marked susceptibility to pyogenic and fungal infection, and often considerable growth retardation. Onset of symptoms is usually in childhood, and the appearance of symptoms at an early age predicts greater likelihood of complications and death. Common sites of infection include the skin, lymph nodes, lung, liver, and bone. The most prevalent organisms cultured from these sites are *Staphylococcus aureus*, Gram-negative bacteria, and *Aspergillus fumigatus*, although many other organisms may participate. A characteristic sterile granulomatous reaction develops in the tissues of many patients, and may represent an attempt to eliminate indigestible material. Diagnosis is made on the basis of the clinical picture, and evidence of failure of superoxide production by neutrophils and monocytes

Disorders of granule constituents

Myeloperoxidase deficiency This is a relatively common, autosomal recessive disorder that occasionally results in impaired killing of bacteria and fungi *in vitro*. Most patients remain asymptomatic and free of infection. Rarer syndromes include Chediak–Higashi syndrome and specific granule deficiency (see OTM3, p. 3560).

Tissue damage by leucocytes

In addition to their essential role in host defence, human leucocytes are being increasingly implicated as mediators of tissue damage in inflammatory disorders such as adult respiratory distress syndrome, inflammatory bowel disease, emphysema, and asthma. In a physiological inflammatory response, release of mediators by leucocytes is carefully regulated and directed towards foreign particles. However, persistent or inappropriate activation of these cells releases potent proinflammatory molecules that can inactivate tissue protease inhibitors. α_1-Antitrypsin (α_1-protease inhibitor) deficiency is an example of an inherited disease in which the balance is in favour of tissue damage because of deficiency of a protective factor.

Leucocyte function tests

Any patient who has suffered from recurrent episodes of infection or infection by unusual organisms should be investigated for defects in host defence mechanisms. A careful history, family history, and clinical examination may suggest a specific diagnosis. As neutrophil functional defects are uncommon causes of increased susceptibility to infection, it is first necessary to exclude other more common conditions that involve complement, humoral, and cell-mediated mechanisms. Initial screening tests should include a full blood count and differential white-cell count, lymphocytic subset immunoglobulin levels, complement levels, and skin testing with purified protein derivative, and candida. HIV infection should be excluded in those individuals deemed to be at risk. If the patient is anergic, specific analysis of T-cell number, distribution, and function is indicated. Deficiency of one or more classes of immunoglobulin suggests a primary defect of B cells, or a secondary effect of T-cell dysfunction. Morphological evaluation of the leucocytes may also be useful. If this initial evaluation fails to identify the cause, then more specific tests of white-cell function can be performed. These include the assessment of cell mobility *in vitro* and measurement of the activity of the respiratory burst

Treatment of patients with a leucocyte disorder

All defects in leucocyte function require correct identification of the cause, and treatment or removal of precipitating factors. Routine management is supportive and relies on the avoidance of exposure to infectious material, prophylaxis with antibiotics, and, where appropriate, immunization. Leucocyte numbers may be augmented with colony-stimulating factors. Immunoglobulin deficiencies can be replaced with pooled human immunoglobulin when clinically indicated. In acute infection broad-spectrum intravenous antibiotics and white-cell transfusions form the mainstay of treatment. Inherited leucocyte disorders with a poor prognosis may be considered for allogeneic bone marrow transplantation, if a suitable donor is available.

Further reading

Kuly, J. (1997). *Immunology*, 3rd edn. W.H. Freeman, New York.

Chapter 3.28

Introduction to the lymphoproliferative disorders

C. Bunch and K. C. Gatter

Proliferation of lymphocytes in response to antigenic stimuli commonly leads to enlargement of lymph glands and other lymphoid tissues. Usually the antigenic stimulus is an infecting organism, the lymphadenopathy is short-lived, and the glands return to their normal size after successful control of the responsible infection. Occasionally, however, the proliferative response is more prolonged and may itself give rise to clinical problems.

Persistent lymphadenopathy may simply reflect repeated antigenic challenge—as commonly occurs in young children suffering upper respiratory infections during the winter months. Alternatively, it may be due to persistence of antigen, possibly because the immune response is inadequate or because an infecting organism is difficult to eliminate. In other instances, such as rheumatoid arthritis and other collagen-vascular disorders, lymphadenopathy is associated with an abnormal immune response directed against 'self' antigens. Finally, and much less commonly, autonomous proliferation of a neoplastic clone of lymphoid cells may occur—giving rise to one of the malignant lymphoproliferative disorders considered in Chapter 3.29.

Organization of the immune system

Many of the clinical features of lymphoproliferative disorders can be explained by the fact that, structurally, the immune system is represented by lymphoid tissue strategically placed throughout the body, networked together by a system of lymphatic vessels and the bloodstream. In addition to between 500 and 600 or so discrete lymph nodes, lymphoid tissue is found extensively in the oropharynx (Waldeyer's ring), bronchial tree, and gastrointestinal tract. Lymphocytes are also found in the bone marrow, where they tend to form small follicles, and of course in the spleen.

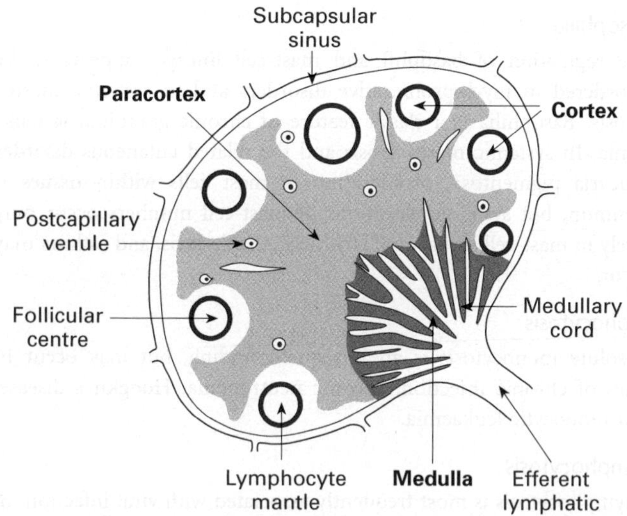

Fig. 1 Functional architecture of a normal lymph node.
(Reproduced from Arno (1980), with permission of the author and MTP Press.)

Lymph-node structure (Fig. 1)

Lymph nodes are arranged into outer cortical and inner medullary areas within a connective tissue capsule. Lymph enters the node via afferent lymphatics and percolates through radial sinusoids to the hilum, where it leaves the node via efferent lymphatics. Blood enters and leaves the node through hilar vessels: an extensive vascular network extends throughout the node, and specialized postcapillary venules allow extensive traffic of lymphocytes between the blood and lymphatic vessels.

Cells in the cortical areas are arranged into follicles with a pale centre known as the germinal centre. These comprise mainly B cells with a smaller number of T cells and non-lymphoid cells. The cuff surrounding the germinal centre consists of mature small lymphocytes. Within the centre itself, the most characteristic cell is a slightly larger lymphocyte known as a centrocyte. A number of larger cells can also be found, including macrophages (histiocytes), transformed lymphocytes or immunoblasts, and cells with a regular, centrally placed nucleus called centroblasts. Also within the germinal centre are follicular dendritic cells which act as antigen-presenting cells.

Following antigenic challenge, intense proliferative activity takes place in the germinal centre as B cells recognizing foreign antigens undergo clonal expansion and differentiation. The associated morphological changes follow the appearance of different types of cell within the germinal centre, and the various stages of B-cell differentiation are also reflected in the expression of different antigens. In part, this explains the diversity of lymphomas that can arise in the follicle centre, as malignantly transformed cells retain a limited but variable capacity for differentiation, which is reflected in their morphology, immunocytochemical phenotype, and behaviour.

The interfollicular and paracortical areas consist mainly of T cells. The medulla comprises cords of cells lining the sinusoids—the so-called medullary cords. These cells include fixed macrophages, plasma cells, lymphocytes, and connective tissue cells.

Table 1 Principal causes of lymphadenopathy

Inflammatory	*Granulomatous*
• Suppurating	• Infective
• Pyogenic infection	• Tuberculosis
• Non-suppurating	• Syphilis
• Infection—local or systemic	• Toxoplasmosis
• Immunologically-based	• Histoplasmosis etc.
Collagen disease	• Non-infective
Rheumatoid arthritis	• Sarcoidosis
Dermatopathic	*Malignant*
Drugs e.g. phenytoin	• Primary
Addison's disease	• Lymphoma
Thyrotoxicosis	• Leukaemia
Congenital	• Carcinoma
• Lymphangiomas	• Melanoma
• Cystic hygroma	• Sarcoma

Lymphoid tissue in other sites is arranged in a broadly similar fashion. The structure of the spleen is described in OTM3, pp. 3587–96.

Lymphocyte recirculation

Lymphocytes are not static, and there is extensive recirculation of cells throughout the immune system. Cells pass from the bloodstream to the lymphatic system through postcapillary venules within the lymph nodes, and return to the bloodstream by the thoracic duct.

Lymphadenopathy

Normal lymph nodes are impalpable, except in some very thin subjects. Palpable enlargement is commonly referred to as lymphadenopathy, even though the nodes may be simply reacting to antigenic stimulus in a normal fashion.

Causes

The main causes of lymphadenopathy are shown in Table 1. As indicated above, lymphadenopathy is most commonly due to infection, but other inflammatory disorders may be responsible. Lymphomas are relatively rare, and metastatic carcinoma is a more common cause of lymphadenopathy.

Clinical management

In many instances the underlying cause will be apparent after taking a careful history and performing a thorough clinical examination. The history should encompass the patient's general health and past illnesses, possible exposure to infection, including contact with animals or birds, foreign travel, and constitutional upsets such as fever, weight loss, sweats, or pruritus. Alcohol-induced pain at sites of affected nodes is characteristic of Hodgkin's disease.

Physical examination should take note of the location and extent of the lymphadenopathy, and the characteristics of the nodes themselves. Localized, tender lymphadenopathy should prompt a search for an infected lesion or portal of entry in the area drained by the node. Tender nodes are usually inflammatory or reactive, but rapid enlargement due to malignancy can stretch the capsule and produce pain and tenderness. Hard nodes, especially if fixed and matted together, suggest malignancy. When there is cervical lymphadenopathy, the throat and pharynx should be carefully examined. A full general examination should be performed, with particular attention to the size of the liver and spleen.

Investigations should include a full blood count, erythrocyte sedimentation rate, and examination of the blood film. These may be diagnostic in cases of leukaemia, or may point to a viral cause such as glandular fever. Additional investigations might include a chest radiograph, biochemical profile, and antibody screens for an infective cause, together with specific microbial cultures as appropriate.

Lymph-node biopsy

The cause of lymphadenopathy can be determined in the majority of instances by history, clinical examination, and the simple investigations outlined above. If this fails to yield a diagnosis, a lymph-node biopsy may be necessary. If the clinical suspicion of lymphoma is strong, and there are good reasons why treatment should not be delayed—perhaps because the patient's condition is deteriorating—a biopsy should be undertaken as soon as possible. If the suspicion is less strong, then one should wait at least until the results of preliminary investigations are to hand: during this time a number of infective and inflammatory conditions will resolve spontaneously.

The diagnostic yield is improved by careful selection of the node to be biopsied. Supraclavicular nodes are preferred, as axillary or inguinal nodes may be involved in reaction to coincident local trauma or infection in hands or feet. Similarly, enlarged nodes close to a malignant node may show only a reactive pattern and it is better to remove the largest node, even if this is technically more difficult. Occasionally, lymph-node enlargement is confined to internal lymph nodes (such as those in mediastinum, para-aortic, or mesenteric areas) not readily accessible to routine surgical biopsy. In these circumstances, material may be obtained by needle-core biopsy or fine-needle aspiration under radiological guidance. The biopsied specimen should not be put automatically into formalin: many of the techniques described below require fresh, unfixed tissue, and close liaison with the histopathologist is essential.

Fine-needle aspiration biopsy

Fine-needle aspiration biopsy done in consultation with the cytologist is gradually becoming more widely available as a simple, safe, and cheap investigation that often reveals a definitive diagnosis without recourse to surgery. However, in the case of suspected lymphoma it is not always possible to provide full diagnostic information with this material and biopsy is still considered to be an essential part of management.

Methods for the study of lymphoproliferative disorders

Conventional histological examination remains the cornerstone of diagnosis in a lymphoid biopsy, but the introduction of reliable immunoenzymatic staining techniques, coupled with the development of monoclonal antibodies, have added considerable refinement. Using these techniques and reagents the histologist can now readily identify the different cell types within lymphoid tissue and can accurately classify the immunological origin of most lymphoproliferative disorders (Fig. 2). Molecular biology techniques such as Southern blots and polymerase chain reaction (**PCR**) amplification to look for immunoglobulin and T-cell receptor gene rearrangements are increasingly used in routine practice.

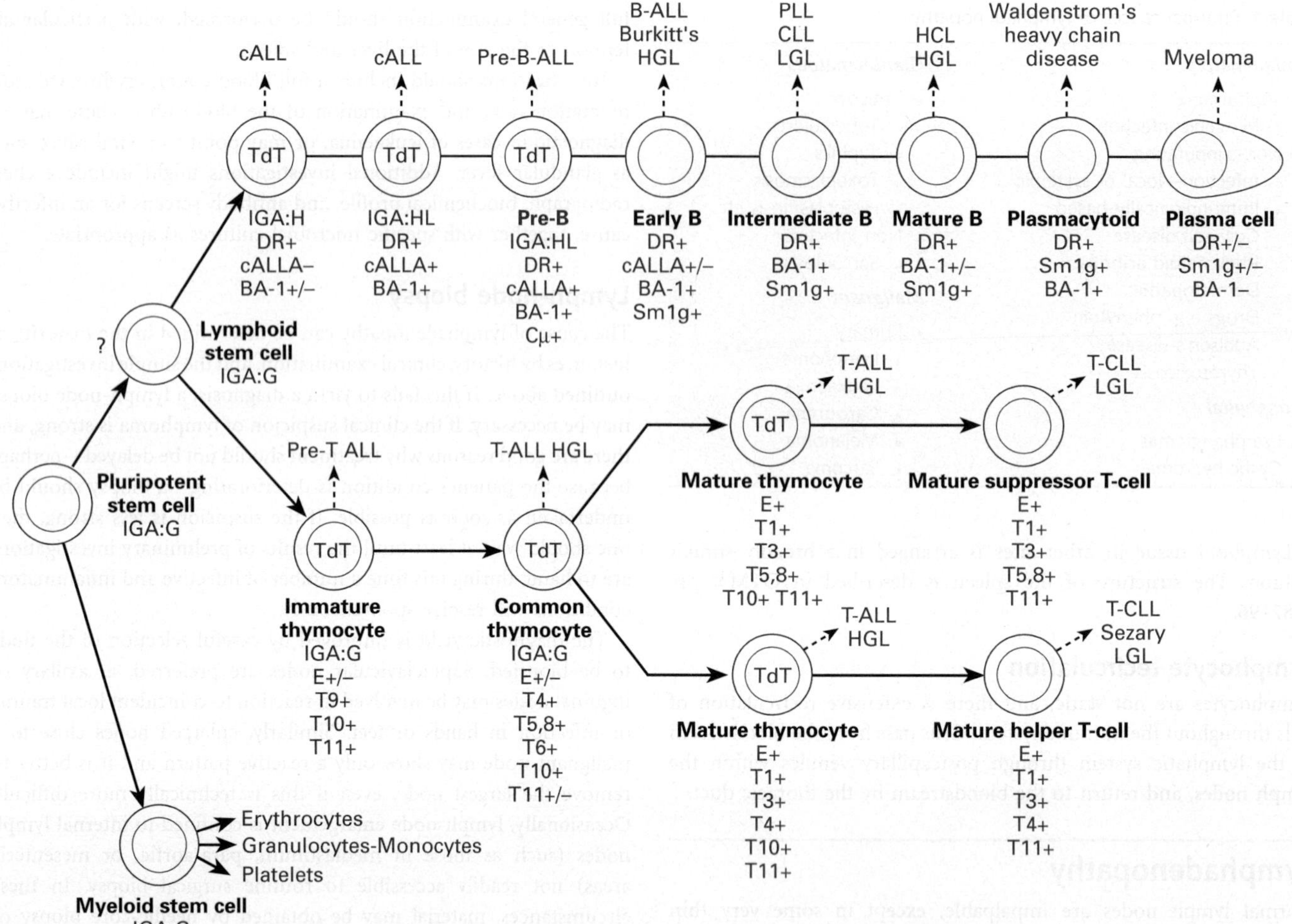

Fig. 2 A scheme of lymphocyte differentiation based on surface markers, enzyme, and molecular studies. Each 'cell' illustrated represents a phenotypically discrete stage in a continuum of differentiation. The pathways of differentiation are indicated by a solid arrow and the relationship of various developmental stages with lymphomas and leukaemias is indicated by a broken arrow. The phenotypic characteristics are indicated beneath each cell. IGA indicates the arrangement of immunoglobulin genes as follows: G, germline arrangement; H, heavy-chain genes rearranged; L, light-chain genes rearranged. T1, 3, 6, 8–11, and BA-1 represent reaction with monoclonal antibodies detecting various stages of T- and B-lymphocyte development, respectively. cALL, common acute lymphoblastic leukaemia antigen; TdT, terminal transferase; DR, HLA-DR expression; E, sheep erythrocyte, rosetting; Cμ, cytoplasmic μ heavy chain; SmIg, surface membrane Ig; CIg, cytoplasmic Ig (heavy and light chain); CLL, chronic lymphatic leukaemia; PLL, prolymphocytic leukaemia; HCL, hairy cell leukaemia; HGL, non-Hodgkin's lymphoma (high grade); LGL, non-Hodgkin's lymphoma (low grade).
(Modified from Foon, 1982.)

Patterns of lymph-node reactivity

Lymph nodes can be divided into three functional areas: the follicles, the paracortex, and the medullary sinuses. When lymph nodes respond to antigenic stimuli or invasion by infectious or neoplastic agents, changes often predominate in one of these areas, leading to one of three basic reactive patterns (Fig. 3).

1. *Follicular hyperplasia*: This occurs when either increases in the size or number of lymphoid follicles contribute to significant lymph-node enlargement. It is a common histological finding in enlarged lymph nodes during childhood and adolescence. The condition is self-limiting and an underlying cause is rarely discovered. Specific causes of marked follicular hyperplasia include rheumatoid arthritis, measles, and toxoplasmosis.
2. *Paracortical expansion*: This is characteristically seen in many viral infections, presumably due to a greatly increased stimulation of T lymphocytes. It may also occur after vaccination, granulomatous disease, and chronic skin diseases (dermatopathic lymphadenopathy).
3. *Sinus hyperplasia*: This is commonly seen in inflammatory or neoplastic conditions as well as lipidoses and Whipple's disease.

In conclusion, it should be emphasized that many conditions cause changes in each of the three areas of a lymph node, so that distinction between the three basic reactive patterns described above is not always clear.

Non-malignant lymphoproliferative disorders

Generalized lymphoproliferation is a feature of several infections, but the classic 'glandular fevers' are infectious mononucleosis, cytomegalovirus infections, and toxoplasmosis. Infectious mononucleosis is worthy of special mention as the virus responsible, the Epstein–Barr virus (EBV), preferentially infects B lymphocytes and most of the clinical features of the disease can be ascribed to an intense proliferation of T cells attempting to eliminate the infected B cells. In normal individuals the T cells keep infected B cells under permanent

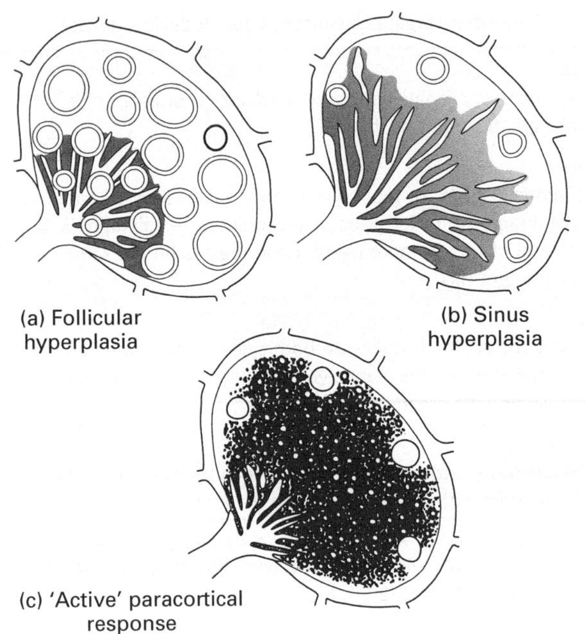

Fig. 3 Patterns of lymph-node reactivity. See text for description. *(Reproduced from Arno (1980), with permission of the author and MTP Press.)*

control, but in some immunodeficient patients B-cell clones can 'escape' the immune system producing a condition indistinguishable from an immunoblastic lymphoma.

A characteristic, generalized painless lymphadenopathy may develop in human immunodeficiency virus (**HIV**) infection, particularly in homosexual men. This is characterized by striking follicular hyperplasia.

Castleman's disease is a rare syndrome of hyperplasia of the lymph nodes that may be localized or generalized. It is characterized by nodules of small lymphocytes with a central vascular core replacing the germinal centre.

Further reading

Arno, J. (1980). *Atlas of lymph node pathology.* MTP Press, Lancaster.

Foon, K.A., *et al.* (1982). Surface markers on leukemia and lymphoma cells: recent advances. *Blood*, **60**, 1–19.

Stansfield, A.G. (1992). Non-neoplastic lymphoproliferative disorders. In *Oxford textbook of pathology*, Vol. 2b (ed. J.O. McGee, P.G. Isaacson, and N.A. Wright), pp. 1756–68. Oxford University Press, Oxford.

Chapter 3.29

The lymphomas

C. Bunch and K. C. Gatter

Lymphomas are neoplastic proliferations of cells of the immune system. The lymph nodes are the sites most frequently involved and progressive lymphadenopathy is the most common presentation. Involvement of other sites and organs may also occur and are sometimes the only manifestation. Lymphomas may be localized or widespread, and may or may not be associated with systemic symptoms. With modern treatment, many patients can be cured and a reasonable quality of life can be maintained in the remainder.

Classification

Lymphomas are classified by histology and immunophenotyping. The main division is into Hodgkin's disease and the non-Hodgkin's lymphomas. Most non-Hodgkin lymphomas are of B-cell origin, but 10–20 per cent express a T-cell phenotype.

Pathological grading of non-Hodgkin lymphoma generally correlates well with clinical behaviour.

Clinical features

The clinical features of the lymphomas are explained by the expansion of lymphoid tissue such as lymphadenopathy or splenomegaly together with the physical consequences of such expansion (e.g. superior vena caval obstruction or intestinal obstruction), secondary effects on the function of the immune system (immunodeficiency and autoimmune phenomena), and non-specific, systemic symptoms (fever, drenching night sweats, anorexia ,weight loss, and pruritus).

The most common manifestation of lymphoma is lymphadenopathy. Involvement of lymphoid tissue in other sites (extranodal involvement) is much more common in non-Hodgkin lymphomas than in Hodgkin's disease. Hodgkin's disease appears to spread from node to contiguous node via the lymphatics. It is thus more likely to be localized than widespread. Non-Hodgkin lymphomas spread via the bloodstream, and often involve cells that normally recirculate widely and continue to do so after malignant transformation; they are thus best considered as systemic disorders.

In general, the incidence of lymphomas increases with age, and most patients develop lymphoma are middle-aged or elderly. The principal exception is Hodgkin's disease, which has, in addition, a peak of incidence early in the third decade.

Diagnosis is made by history and clinical examination combined with a biopsy of a lymph node or other affected tissue.

Hodgkin's disease

Hodgkin's disease is about twice as common in males as in females, and shows two peaks of incidence—one in young adults, the other in the elderly. The hallmark of Hodgkin's disease is the Reed–Sternberg cell, a large cell with prominent nucleoli. It often shows monoclonal rearrangement of the immunoglobulin genes and is now thought to be derived from a B cell.

Aetiology

The aetiology of Hodgkin's disease remains unknown. An infectious agent has been postulated and Epstein-Barr virus (EBV) may be implicated in some cases.

Clinical features

Hodgkin's disease usually presents with painless enlargement of one or more groups of lymph nodes. The affected lymph nodes may already be quite large when first noticed, and subsequent growth may often be negligible, or the nodes may shrink or flutuate in size. The enlarged lymph nodes are firm, non-tender, and often feel rubbery.

Table 1 Common presenting sites for lymphadenopathy in Hodgkin's disease

Site	%	Site	%
Cervical	51	Abdominal	9
Mediastinal	24	Other	2
Axillary	18	Multiple sites	26
Inguinal	16		

For source see OTM3, p. 3570.

The neck and axillae are the sites most commonly involved at presentation (Table 1), although occasional cases present with disease confined to the mediastinum that is detected on routine chest radiograph. Presentations involving just infradiaphragmatic lymph nodes or extranodal sites are also relatively uncommon. Lymph node enlargement may occasionally give rise to local problems, such as superior vena caval obstruction from mediastinal lymphadenopathy. Splenomegaly may be present but does not always indicate involvement with Hodgkin's disease. Conversely, normal spleen size does not exclude involvement. Hepatomegaly is a feature of advanced disease. Bone involvement is rare early in the disease, but may be suggested by local areas of pain and tenderness. Local skin infiltration sometimes occurs, particularly in the thoracic wall as an extension from mediastinal or hilar node involvement, or in the region of massive lymph-node enlargement.

Systemic symptoms may affect about one-quarter of patients at presentation. Fever, drenching night sweats, and weight loss are especially significant and indicate a worse prognosis. Fever may occasionally show a clear cyclical variation; several days of fever may alternate with longer afebrile periods. Severe skin itching is a feature in some cases of Hodgkin's disease. Alcohol-induced pain in affected sites is a dramatic but rare feature.

Pathological features

The classical histological appearance of lymph nodes affected by Hodgkin's disease is proliferation of abnormal mononuclear cells and the diagnostic Reed–Sternberg binucleate or multinucleate cells. Four histological subtypes of Hodgkin's disease are recognized.

Nodular sclerosing (20–50 per cent of cases) The lymph node has a striking nodular appearance due to bands of collagenous connective tissue.

Mixed cellularity (20–40 per cent of cases) There is a mixed infiltrate with conspicuous granulocytes and plentiful Reed-Sternberg cells.

Lymphocyte predominant (10–15 per cent of cases) The infiltrate consists mainly of small lymphocytes.

Lymphocyte depleted (1–2 per cent of cases) This is characterized by large numbers of atypical mononuclear cells.

Management

Successful management is based on a full assessment of the extent of disease and the presence or absence of adverse prognostic features, followed by selection of appropriate therapy. Well over half of all patients with Hodgkin's disease can be cured, and many of the remainder can expect a survival measured in years rather than months. Careful consideration must be given to potential side-effects of any treatment protocol.

Table 2 Ann Arbor staging classification for Hodgkin's disease

Stage I Involvement of a single lymph-node region (I) or of a single extralymphatic organ or site (I_E)
Stage II Involvement of two or more lymph node regions on the same side of the diaphragm (II) or localized involvement of extralymphatic organ or site and of one or more lymph node regions on the same side of the diaphragm (II_E)
Stage III Involvement of lymph nodes on both sides of the diaphragm (III). There may also be splenic involvement (III_S), or localized involvement of extralymphatic organ or site (III_E)
Stage IV Involvement of extranodal sites, other than by direct invasion from an affected node, with or without lymph node involvement

For each stage, a qualifier 'A' or 'B' is used. 'A' denotes the absence and 'B' the presence of typical symptoms: weight loss, fever, drenching night sweats.
For source see OTM3, p. 3572.

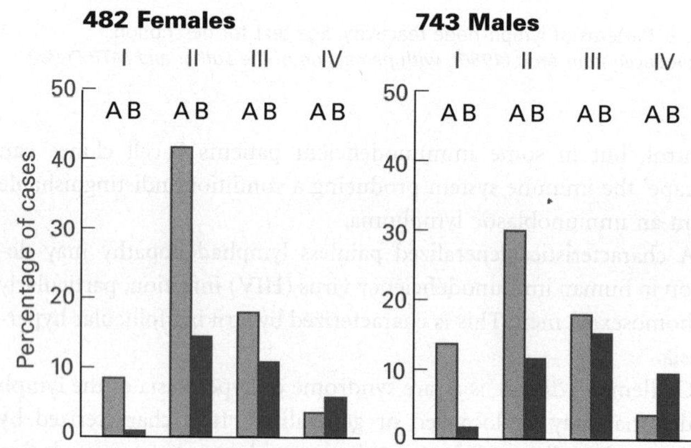

Fig. 1 Ann Arbor staging of Hodgkin's disease in relation to A or B symptom categories. Derived from data on 1225 consecutive untreated patients at Stanford University Medical Centre, 1961–77 *(reproduced by courtesy of Dr H.S. Kaplan).*

Staging

It is important to determine as accurately as possible the full extent of involvement with Hodgkin's disease, as this has an important bearing on prognosis and the selection of treatment. Truly localized disease can be effectively treated with radiotherapy with a very high chance of cure. Chemotherapy is appropriate for more widespread disease. A staging classification is in widespread use (Table 2 and Fig. 1). Involvement of lymph nodes in Hodgkin's disease has been shown to spread from one group to the next directly connected by lymphatics, and this has made it possible to predict certain patterns of disease.

The presence or absence of systemic symptoms of fever above 38 °C, drenching night sweats, and weight loss of more than 10 per cent of body weight in the 6 months before presentation has an adverse effect on prognosis and is taken into account in the staging classification. These so-called 'B' symptoms are rare in stage I disease, and if present in a patient with apparently localized disease a special effort should be made to exclude more widespread involvement, particularly of the mediastinal or para-aortic nodes.

Other investigations

The following investigations may further refine staging, or yield additional prognostic information.

Haematology

The blood count is usually normal in Hodgkin's disease, although patients with systemic symptoms or widespread disease frequently have anaemia and a raised ESR, both of which indicate a worse prognosis. A reactive leucocytosis may indicate very active disease or tissue necrosis. Lymphopenia is a poor prognostic sign. Moderate eosinophilia is occasionally found. Bone marrow involvement occurs in only a small percentage of cases but biopsy is often used in staging.

Radiology

In recent years computed tomography (CT) has largely replaced lymphangiography as the main radiological technique for assessing lymph node enlargement in the abdomen and pelvis. Plain chest radiography is also valuable. Magnetic resonance imaging (MRI) does not at present have a routine place in the investigation or staging of lymphomas but its use is likely to increase. The use of lymphangiography has declined since the introduction of CT scanning.

Treatment

The introduction of megavoltage radiotherapy and combination chemotherapy during the 1960s revolutionized the outlook for patients with Hodgkin's disease, and cure is now a realistic goal for the majority. While radiotherapy is appropriate for localized disease, in which it can be highly effective and relatively free of troublesome side-effects, widespread disease is best treated with chemotherapy initially, sometimes followed by radiotherapy.

Stages IA and IIA. The treatment of choice for most adult patients with stages IA and IIA is radiotherapy. Standard treatment involves extended-field, external-beam megavoltage irradiation designed to treat all the principal lymph node groups of the half of the body (upper or lower) in which the disease is localized.

Stages IB and IIB. Patients with clinically localized disease but clear-cut B symptoms probably have more widespread involvement than is apparent and are best treated with chemotherapy from the outset.

Stage IIIA. There has been considerable debate as to whether patients with stage IIIA disease are best treated with radiotherapy or chemotherapy but many centres now favour chemotherapy for all patients with clinical stage III disease.

Stages IIIB, IVA, and IVB. Patients with advanced disease (stages IIIB, IVA or IVB) should be treated with combination chemotherapy.

Management of chemotherapy

Various chemotherapy schedules have been employed in Hodgkin's disease. Combinations have been designed to include drugs with differing modes of action and toxicity, to exploit synergism, and allow effective doses to be used with acceptable toxicity.

The original combination of mustine, vincristine (Oncovin), procarbazine, and prednisolone (**MOPP**) was introduced in the late 1960s. Freedom from relapse is best achieved using full doses of drugs, but the chief drawback is toxicity. Mustine is powerfully emetogenic, induces sterility (especially in males), and may be associated with a higher risk of stem-cell damage leading to subsequent myelodysplasia or leukaemia. Vincristine causes peripheral neuropathy, especially in elderly patients. Variations of MOPP using chlorambucil in place of mustine and/or vinblastine in place of vincristine are thus widely used. They have a more acceptable toxicity and appear to be almost, or equally, as effective as MOPP. Combinations including the anthracycline adriamycin are also highly effective, and much less likely to cause infertility. A combination of adriamycin with bleomycin, vinblastine, and dacarbazine (**ABVD**) has been most widely employed. More recently, seven- or eight-drug combinations, such as MOPP/ABVD have appeared. Such intensive regimens may be better suited to patients with adverse prognostic features.

Maintenance chemotherapy is of no value and a total of three courses after complete resolution of the disease is adequate. In practice, this means that progress should be re-evaluated with a CT scan if appropriate after three courses, and again after a total of six, at which point the majority of patients will be in clinical remission. A dilemma arises in patients with initial bulky disease, especially in the mediastinum, which may not resolve completely after six (or even more) courses. Careful follow-up has shown that in most of these patients the residual abnormality is inactive residue or scarring. They can usually be followed up with one or two CT scans at 2-monthly intervals for reassurance. Alternatively, gallium scanning may help to distinguish active disease from inactive residue. If there is any doubt or evidence of progression, radiotherapy to the involved area is indicated.

Treatment of relapse

Patients who relapse after primary treatment with radiotherapy may be 'salvaged' with combination chemotherapy with a very good chance of cure. Alternatively, radiotherapy may produce excellent results in patients who relapse 8 or more years after initial therapy, or in the elderly.

Relapse in those treated initially with chemotherapy is more problematical. The prognosis appears to be especially poor in patients who initially received MOPP or similar regimens. Other possible approaches include the use of a different, non-cross-resistant, drug combination, or high-dose chemotherapy with haemopoietic stem-cell support (autologous bone-marrow transplantation or peripheral stem-cell transplantation (see OTM3, pp. 3696–701).

Complications of treatment

Since the majority of patients can expect to survive for many years after treatment, unwanted effects of therapy are very important.

Acute reactions to radiotherapy are usually self-limiting and include local skin reactions, mucositis and loss of taste. A widespread radiation pneumonitis may occasionally follow irradiation therapy, manifest by dyspnoea and a dry cough. Serious pulmonary fibrosis may be a later development, although it is very uncommon with properly planned irradiation. Cases of cardiomyopathy occurring several years after mediastinal irradiation have been reported. This complication is particularly associated with older age, concomitant administration of anthracycline drugs such as doxorubicin, and the use of single, anterior radiation fields, which give a very high pericardial dose. Radiotherapy may also be associated with hypothyroidism and growth retardation.

Vincristine may produce troublesome neurotoxicity. Most patients get some paraesthesiae and lose their ankle jerks, and occasional patients get severe pains, particularly in the legs and in the jaw, which may be quite intolerable. A change to vinblastine is indicated if this occurs. Ileus of the bowel may sometimes also be produced; constipation is common and should be avoided if possible in patients receiving vinca alkaloids. Myelosuppression is the most troublesome complication and limits the doses that may be given.

Infertility is a problem in patients receiving chemotherapy, especially with combinations that include mustine. Sperm and egg storage should be offered to all at risk. Chemotherapy is commonly associated with oligo- or amenorrhoea, but ultimate female fertility does not seem to be as frequently affected as male fertility. Early menopausal symptoms may be encountered, and may indicate the need for hormone replacement.

Patients successfully treated for Hodgkin's disease are at risk from second malignancies. A variety of malignancies has been encountered, but the most common are myelodysplasia and acute myeloid leukaemia. The risk is relatively small but appears to be proportional to the duration and intensity of treatment, being highest in those receiving both extended-field radiotherapy and chemotherapy.

Patients with Hodgkin's disease are particularly susceptible to infection because of the defects in cellular immunity and the myelosuppressive and immunosuppressive effects of treatment. Bacterial infections are common during chemotherapy, whilst herpes zoster is a frequent late complication.

Prognosis

Some 70–80 per cent of patients will survive to 5 years, most of whom can probably be considered cured. Prognosis depends on a number of factors including the extent of the disease, the presence of systemic (B) symptoms, histology (lymphocyte-predominant and nodular sclerotic histology having a better prognosis), age, and initial response to therapy.

Non-Hodgkin lymphomas

The non-Hodgkin lymphomas are by definition those lymphomas that lack the characteristic histopathological features of Hodgkin's disease; Reed–Sternberg cells are absent and the normal lymph-node architecture is not necessarily be disturbed. A rather loose definition of lymphoid tissue enables cells of the monocyte–macrophage lineage to be included: these cells are frequently described as histiocytes. Of 729 non-Hodgkin lymphomas immunophenotyped in Oxford during 1982–1992, 629 were of B-cell origin (88 per cent) and 99 were T cell (14 per cent). Only one case was unequivocally histiocytic.

The results of treatment for non-Hodgkin lymphomas have been much less satisfactory than in Hodgkin's disease, but are improving. Considerable effort has been made in recent years to characterize their aetiology, cellular and molecular biology, natural history, and response to treatment.

Aetiology and pathogenesis

There is now clear evidence that the majority, if not all, non-Hodgkin lymphomas arise from clones of a single mutant cell, and that in most cases the malignant cells show characteristics of B-cell differentiation, with most of the remainder being of T-cell origin.

Classification

Non-Hodgkin lymphomas vary greatly in their clinical and histopathological features leading to a plethora of classifications. In recent years our understanding of lymphoid differentiation has increased markedly, helped by immunological techniques that can pinpoint surface antigens on individual cells within suitable histological sections. This has led to a much clearer idea of the structure of normal lymph nodes, the traffic of cells through them, and the changes that occur after antigenic stimulation. More recent classifications of non-Hodgkin lymphomas have attempted to relate the nature of the malignant cell to its normal counterpart. Several such schemes have evolved, which vary mostly in their technical requirements and suitability for use with routine histopathological methods. All have prognostic significance, but it is not possible to make direct translations between the various classifications, and this makes comparisons of therapeutic trials difficult to interpret.

In an attempt to circumvent this problem, in 1981 an expert international panel reviewed clinical and histological material from 1175 patients. The result was a *Working Formulation of Non-Hodgkin's Lymphoma for Clinical Use*, which can be readily translated into any one of the standard classifications. This scheme (Table 3) was not intended to supplant any of those already in use, but to be a common language through which, for example, comparison of results of clinical trials might be made. One point to note is the category of 'intermediate' malignancy, which does not appear in any of the original six classifications on which this formulation was based. This distinction has not achieved any practical value, with most pathologists and clinicians continuing to apportion non-Hodgkin lymphomas to either a low- or high-grade category. These grades are based on the morphological features of lymphoma types, which are believed to correlate well with the natural progression of untreated disease.

Despite all the efforts put into the classification of non-Hodgkin lymphomas, accurate classification remains difficult or impossible in up to 10 per cent of cases.

The classification most widely used in Europe is that devised by Lennert's group in Kiel. This scheme was updated in 1988 (Table 4) to incorporate information gained from cell-marker studies, and when combined with a cytological/haematological approach enables a considerable consensus to be reached by non-specialist histopathologists working with routine biopsies. It has good prognostic correlations and successfully separates non-Hodgkin lymphomas into those with a relatively good prognosis (low-grade) and others with high-grade or poor prognostic features.

In the USA many other classifications is used. Many centres now use the Working Formulation as a classification, for which use it was not designed. To overcome this lack of harmony and to incorporate new information into lymphoma classification a group of international haematopathologists met in 1993 to discuss existing schemes. There was almost complete agreement between them on the entities that they were diagnosing. They have therefore put together a set of proposals as the REAL (Revised American European Lymphoma) classification in an attempt to simplify and co-ordinate diagnoses worldwide by emphasizing the recognition of disease entities (Table 5). The most radical aspect of this proposal is that for the first time it places emphasis on what pathologists really do rather than what a particular classification theory thinks they should do. If the concept of dealing with clinical and pathological entities is accepted, the artificial distinction of dividing lymphomas into low- and high-grade tumours can now be eliminated.

Clinical and pathological features

The non-Hodgkin lymphomas, with the exception of the lymphoblastic lymphomas, are relatively uncommon under the age of 40, and have a peak incidence in the 60–70-year-old age group. The presenting features may be similar to Hodgkin's disease with local or general lymph-node enlargement, with or without systemic symptoms, and a biopsy is always required to establish the diagnosis. The

Table 3 A working formulation of non-Hodgkin lymphomas for clinical usage (equivalent or related terms in the Kiel classification are shown)

Working formulation	Kiel equivalent or related terms
Low grade	
A. Malignant lymphoma	
Small lymphocytic	
consistent with CLL	ML lymphocytic, CLL
plasmacytoid	ML lymphoplasmacytic/lymphoplasmacytoid
B. Malignant lymphoma, folllicular	
Predominantly small cleaved cell; diffuse areas;	ML centroblastic-centrocytic (small), follicular±diffuse
sclerosis	
C. Malignant lymphoma, folllicular	
Mixed, small cleaved and large cell; diffuse areas;	
sclerosis	
Intermediate grade	
D. Malignant lymphoma, follicular	
Predominantly large cell	
diffuse areas	ML centroblastic-centrocytic (large), follicular±diffuse
sclerosis	
E. Malignant lymphoma, diffuse	
Small cleaved cell	
sclerosis	ML centrocytic (small)
F. Malignant lymphoma, diffuse	
Mixed, small and large cell	ML centroblastic-centrocytic (small), diffuse
sclerosis	ML lymphoplasmacytic/lymphoplasmacytoid, polymorphic
epithelioid cell component	
G. Malignant lymphoma, diffuse	
Large cell	ML centroblastic-centrocytic (large), diffuse
cleaved cell	ML centrocytic (large)
non-cleaved cell	ML centroblastic
sclerosis	
High grade	
H. Malignant lymphoma	
Large cell, immunoblastic plasmacytoid	ML immunoblastic
clear cell	
polymorphous	T zone lymphoma
epithelioid cell component	Lympyhoepithelioid cell lymphoma
I. Malignant lymphoma	
Lymphoblastic	
convoluted cell	ML lymphoblastic, convoluted cell type
non-convoluted cell	ML lymphoblastic, unclassified
J. Malignant lymphoma	
Small non-cleaved cell	
Burkitt's	ML lymphoblastic, Burkitt type and other B lymphoblastic
follicular areas	
Miscellaneous	
Composite	–
Mycosis fungoides	Mycosis fungoides
Histiocytic	
Extramedullary plasmacytoma	ML plasmacytic
Unclassifiable	–
Other	–

Reproduced with permission from the Non-Hodgkin's Lymphoma Pathologic Classification Project (1982).

spread of disease is, however, unlike Hodgkin's disease, with no clear anatomical spread from one area to a contiguous one and a much greater propensity to extranodal spread (Table 6).

B-cell lymphomas

B-cell lymphomas are those that express at least one of the pan-B-cell antigens CD19, 20, and 22, and usually demonstrate surface or cytoplasmic immunoglobulin. Genotypically, all B-cell malignancies show clonal immunoglobulin-gene rearrangement.

Low-grade B-cell lymphomas

Lymphocytic lymphoma

The common B-cell type of lymphocytic lymphoma is often arbitrarily separated from chronic lymphocytic leukaemia (CLL) on the basis of the degree of involvement of the blood and/or marrow. The disease is confined to lymph nodes at presentation in a small number of cases, but the bone marrow usually becomes involved as the disease progresses. As with CLL, the pace of progression is variable and, in some patients, proliferation may reach a plateau and remain stable

Table 4 Updated Kiel classification of non-Hodgkin's lymphoma

Low-grade B	Low-grade T
Lymphocytic—chronic lymphocytic and prolymphocytic leukaemia; hairy-cell leukaemia	Lymphocytic—chronic lymphocytic and prolymphocytic leukaemia
Lymphoplasmacytic/cytoid (LP immunocytoma)	Small cerebriform cell—mycosis fungoides, Sézary's syndrome
Plasmacytic	Lymphoepithelioid (Lennert's lymphoma)
Centroblastic/centrocytic:	Angioimmunoblastic (AILD, LgX)
• follicular ± diffuse	T zone
• diffuse	Pleomorphic, small-cell (HTLV-1 ±)
Centrocytic	
	High-grade T
High-grade B	Pleomorphic, medium and large cell (HTLV-1 ±)
Centroblastic	Immunoblastic (HTLV-1 ±)
Immunoblastic	Large cell anaplastic (Ki-1+)
Large-cell anaplastic (Ki-1+)	Lymphoblastic
Burkitt's lymphoma	**Rare types**
Lymphoblastic	
Rare types	

From: *Lancet* (1988), i, 292–3.

Table 5 The REAL classification of non-Hodgkin lymphomas (NHL)

Morphology	% NHL	Immunotype
B-cell neoplasms		
Lymphocytic: small lymphocytes	7	Surface Ig CD5+ CD10– CD23+
Immunocytoma: lymphoplasmacytic	3	Cytoplasmic Ig CD5– CD10– CD23–
Follicular centre: centroblastic/centrocytic	25	Surface Ig CD5– CD10+ bcl-2+
Mantle cell: centrocytic	2	Surface Ig CD5+ CD10– CD23–
MALToma: marginal zone (centrocyte-like)	3	Surface Ig CD5– CD10– CD23–
Large cell: centroblasts and immunoblasts	37	Surface Ig CD5– CD10–
Burkitt's: cohesive medium-sized blasts, 'starry sky' appearance	2	Surface Ig CD5– CD10+
Lymphoblastic: lymphoblasts	<1	Cytoplasmic Ig –/+ CD10+ Tdt+
T-cell neoplasms		
Lymphocytic: small lymphocytes	<1	CD4 or 8+
Cutaneous (mycosis fungoides/Sézary syndrome): small cerebriform cells	2	CD4+
Peripheral: extremely variable but usually includes medium and large pleomorphic cells with differing admixtures of reactive cells and blood vessels	8	May show marked heterogeneity of T-antigen expression CD4 or 8+
Lymphoblastic: lymphoblasts	1	CD7+ may be CD4 or CD8+ Tdt+
Anaplastic large cell: Large pleomorphic blast cells with prominent nucleoli	5	CD15– CD30+ EMA+ may be, T, B or null phenotype

EMA, epithelial membrane antigen.

Note: Rare entities and primary bone-marrow neoplasms, e.g., myeloma and hairy-cell leukaemia, have been omitted. The percentages given reflect USA and European practice but may be considerably different elsewhere (especially in Asia). Full details of this classification are given in Harris *et al.* (1994). *Blood*, **84**, 1361–92.

for many years. In general, the features are similar to those of CLL (see Chapter 3.7) including impaired humoral immunity in a significant proportion and paraprotein production in a few.

Immunocytic lymphomas

In this group there is an accumulation of cells that appear intermediate in morphology between lymphocytes and plasma cells, and which contain monoclonal intracellular immunoglobulin. Lymph nodes, gut, or spleen may be involved singly or in combination, or plasmacytomas may develop—often in association with the respiratory tract. The majority of these patients have an IgM paraprotein, when the condition is known as Waldenström's macroglobulinaemia. This may be associated with symptoms of hyperviscosity (see Chapter 3.30).

Myeloma is obviously related closely to this group of tumours but is traditionally considered separately as a primary haematological malignancy.

Follicular lymphoma

This is sometimes known as centroblastic/centrocytic lymphoma and is the most common type of non-Hodgkin lymphoma recognized in the West. It accounts for about 20 per cent of all non-Hodgkin lymphomas, and about one-third of all low-grade lymphomas It is

Table 6 Some general clinical differences between Hodgkin's disease and non-Hodgkin lymphomas (NHL)

Hodgkin's disease	Non-Hodgkin lymphomas
More often localized to one or more discrete groups or nodes	Commonly generalized (though not necessarily obvious clinically)
Waldeyer's ring and gut lymphatic tissue rarely affected	Waldeyer's ring and/or gut c commonly involved
Extranodal involvement (marrow, skin etc.) uncommon	Extranodal involvement common Primary extramodal lymphomas are usually non-Hodgkin lymphoma

characteristically a disorder of middle to old age, and most often presents with localized lymph-node enlargement. However, careful assessment will usually reveal more widespread involvement of other lymph nodes and the bone marrow.

Follicular lymphoma is believed to arise as a malignant transformation of germinal-centre cells and histologically comprises two cell types: the majority are small cleaved cells or centrocytes, together with scattered blast cells known as centroblasts. Most cases at presentation show a nodular pattern similar to reactive follicular hyperplasia, although mantle zones are poorly formed or absent and tingible-body macrophages are scarce. The demonstration of light-chain restriction by immunocytochemistry is useful in confirming the histological diagnosis.

Although the clinical course of this type of lymphoma is often initially benign or indolent, treatment at best produces a temporary clinical regression or remission, and cure is usually impossible, even with aggressive treatment. Ultimately the disease progresses, often over many years, and may end in frank transformation to a high-grade, diffuse, large-cell lymphoma. Such high-grade transformations imply clonal evolutions, and in some cases aggressive treatment can eliminate the high-grade clone, although the original, low-grade disease eventually returns.

A frequent cytogenetic abnormality in follicular lymphoma is the translocation of part of chromosome 14 to chromosome 18, bringing the *bcl-2* gene into apposition with immunoglobulin heavy-chain genes.

Mantle-cell lymphoma

This lymphoma was originally named centrocytic lymphoma. This subtype is much less common than follicular lymphoma and constitutes a replacement of the lymph node by a pure proliferation of small, cleaved cells indistinguishable morphologically from germinal-centre centrocytes. Initially it was believed to be a proliferation arising from the germinal centre, but immunophenotypic and genotypic studies have shown it to be quite distinct from germinal-centre cells. Currently, the evidence is much in favour of the tumours arising from cells in the mantle zone surrounding germinal centres, leading to the suggestion it should be renamed mantle-cell lymphoma. Although generally grouped with the low-grade lymphomas, the clinical course is more aggressive, and may need to be included in the intermediate category.

High-grade B-cell lymphomas

Large-cell lymphoma

These tumours comprise about 20 per cent of non-Hodgkin lymphomas and include two separate tumour types, centroblastic and immunoblastic. Centroblastic lymphomas are believed to arise from germinal centres, either primarily or as a secondary transformation from a low-grade lymphoma. In the case of immunoblastic lymphoma, it is unclear whether it arises exclusively from a plasmacytic course of differentiation or as a further stage of germinal-centre cell differentiation. Both tumours are composed of diffuse, uniform infiltrates of large blast cells and may be primary (arising *de novo*) or secondary (following transformation of a low-grade B-cell lymphoma). There is debate amongst pathologists as to whether or not these two categories can be separated reliably but even the most ardent subclassifiers agree that the therapy should be identical for both tumours. The small survival advantage for centroblastic lymphoma claimed by some sources depends crucially on the grounds for recognizing the tumour.

Burkitt's lymphoma

This lymphoma is the most common neoplasm in children in a wide equatorial belt of Africa and in New Guinea. It is known as endemic Burkitt's lymphoma to distinguish it from a small number of cases with a similar histological appearance seen in Europe and North America (so-called non-endemic Burkitt's lymphoma). The peak incidence is in the 4–7-year age group, and over 80 per cent of cases occur between the ages of 3 and 12 years.

Burkitt's lymphoma has a characteristic histological picture composed of a diffuse infiltrate of medium-sized blast cells. This tumour has a high proliferation rate, as evidenced by numerous mitotic figures, which is partially offset by the cell death demonstrated by the large number of apoptotic cells. This gives rise to large amounts of cellular debris, which is phagocytosed by macrophages giving the characteristic 'starry sky' pattern. Unlike lymphoblastic non-Hodgkin lymphoma, Burkitt's lymphoma has a tendency to grow in uneven clusters, giving a pattern of apparent cohesion between the cells. This can be the single most important feature in helping to distinguish Burkitt's lymphoma from either large-cell or lymphoblastic non-Hodgkin lymphoma.

The clinical picture of endemic Burkitt's varies somewhat with the age of the subject, the typical jaw tumours (Fig. 2) being most common in younger patients. These tumours usually arise in molar or premolar regions of the jaws, leading to loosening of the teeth. They may involve the mandible or maxilla, and in the maxilla may extend upward to involve the orbit.

Abdominal involvement is also present in the majority of cases, retroperitoneal masses, ovarian tumours, hepatic involvement, or gastrointestinal tumours being common. Involvement of the testes and breast may also occur. The masses may extend into the cranium or involve the spinal cord to give paraplegia. There may also be involvement of bones with tumour. Lymph-node involvement is relatively uncommon. A different pattern of disease is seen in non-endemic cases, which predominantly involve lymph node, bone marrow, and gastrointestinal tract.

One of the reasons that Burkitt's lymphoma has aroused such interest is the close association between the tumour and high titres of antibodies against EBV and the cellular antigens determined by it. Burkitt has drawn attention to the geographical distribution of the tumour and the importance of tumour-free gaps in tropical Africa, and has deduced that malarial infection may increase the tendency to neoplasia resulting from infection with a virus (EBV) that usually produces a non-malignant lymphoid proliferation. The connection with the presence of EBV is not clear, although the viral genome is

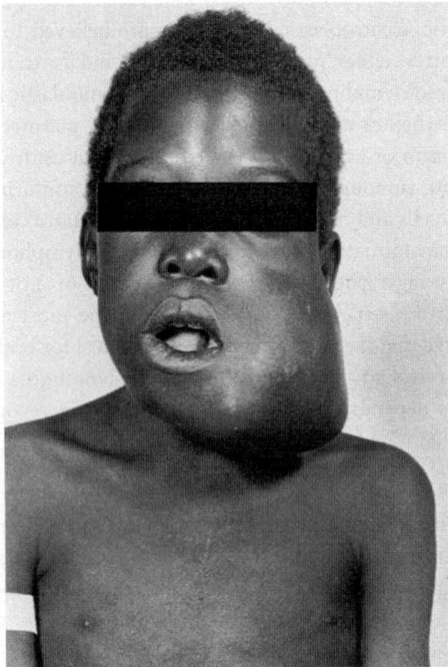

Fig. 2 Jaw tumour in a child with Burkitt's lymphoma *(reproduced by courtesy of Professor D.H. Wright).*

incorporated into the tumour-cell nuclei, a feature rarely seen in non-endemic Burkitt's or found in other conditions associated with the EBV such as nasopharyngeal carcinoma.

A translocation between chromosomes 8 and 14 (t[8;14][q24.13: q32.33]) is characteristic of Burkitt's lymphoma. The abnormalities involving chromosome 14 have been found in relation to a variety of other lymphomas, particularly of B-cell origin.

Burkitt's lymphoma is traditionally classified separately from other non-Hodgkin lymphomas. Although most research points to an origin from follicle-centre cells there are strong arguments for separating Burkitt's lymphoma from the common follicle-centre cell tumours. Burkitt's lymphoma shows no evidence of cytoplasmic immunoglobulin and no follicular pattern, and lymph node and spleen involvement, which is common in follicle-centre cell tumours, is relatively rare. Furthermore, the behaviour and response to therapy is quite different from that of centroblastic (large-cell) lymphoma in adults.

Lymphoblastic lymphoma

B-cell lymphoblastic lymphoma is an unusual condition occurring mostly in childhood, where it is almost always associated with acute lymphoblastic leukaemia. The tumour consists of a monotonous infiltrate of small to medium-sized blast cells with inconspicuous nuclear details. It can be difficult to distinguish morphologically from Burkitt's lymphoma, although the lack of nucleoli, phagocytic macrophages, and overcrowding and clumping of cells usually allows it to be recognized. Occasional adults with abdominal or mediastinal masses turn out to have B-cell lymphoblastic lymphoma that may not be associated with leukaemia.

T-cell lymphomas

A T-cell lymphoma expresses, at least partially, one or more of the following pan-T-cell antigens: CD2, CD3, CD4, CD7, and CD8. Genotypically, all T-cell malignancies show T-cell-receptor rearrangement, usually of the b-chain but occasionally only of the g/d-chain.

T-cell non-Hodgkin lymphoma is less common than the B-cell variety, comprising no more than 20 per cent in most series of Western patients. However, it comprises a much higher proportion in areas such as south Japan and the Caribbean where the human T-cell lymphotropic virus (HTLV-1) is endemic (see Chapter 16.36). Unlike most B-cell proliferations, T cells have a highly variable morphology, making the identity of neoplastic lesions and their classification extremely difficult. There are also no easily recognizable clonal markers, as both subtype antigens (CD4 or -8) may be absent or a reactive phenomenon. There is even debate over the reliability of T-cell-receptor gene rearrangements for this purpose.

Low-grade T-cell lymphomas

T-cell lymphocytic lymphoma

Morphologically these are similar to B-lymphocytic lymphomas and chronic lymphocytic leukaemias. A particular feature of the T-cell lymphocytic lymphomas is their predilection for the skin. This may be related to the known immunological functions of the skin and the fact that normal T cells interact dynamically with epidermal structures as part of the local immune response to invading antigen.

Primary cutaneous lymphoma

Primary lymphomas arising in the skin are almost always of T-cell origin and generally show a helper T-cell phenotype. Histologically, the epidermis is invaded by small cells with striking folded nuclei, often known as cerebriform or Lutzner cells. This infiltrate may form recognizable clusters in the epidermis known as Pautrier's microabscesses. As the lesion progresses, extension down into and beyond the dermis takes place. Two forms of primary cutaneous T-cell lymphoma are recognized (mycosis fungoides and Sézary syndrome) and are distinguished by their clinical features.

Mycosis fungoides is a progressive disorder that presents initially with a non-specific, scaly eruption, progressing eventually to the formation of multiple skin plaques and tumours, some of which may ulcerate. The disease tends to affect middle-aged men, and may be present for 20 years or more before systemic spread follows, with lymphadenopathy and visceral involvement. Death is often from unrelated causes, although internal organs may be found to be involved at autopsy.

Sézary syndrome may be considered as a generalized though insidious leukaemic variant of mycosis fungoides. It starts with a non-specific, eczematous, or licheniform skin eruption, which progresses to an intensely pruritic, generalized, exfoliating erythroderma, with a particular predilection for the face, palms, and soles. At this stage the condition bears a striking resemblance to acute graft-versus-host disease. Patchy hyperpigmentation and also some degree of lymphadenopathy are common. Plaque formation resembling that of mycosis fungoides is often found, and the histology of the two conditions at this stage is similar. Spontaneous remissions and exacerbations do occur, but the disease is ultimately fatal, with an average life expectancy of 5 years.

In both mycosis fungoides and the Sézary syndrome the malignant cell usually has a helper T-cell phenotype. When chromosomal studies have been done these have generally been abnormal, with marked aneuploidy. Occasionally, marker chromosomes have been detected, confirming a clonal origin.

Peripheral T-cell lymphoma

There are four T-cell lymphomas classified as low grade in the Kiel classification that have a similar neoplastic component. They differ mainly in the reactive elements surrounding them, presumably elicited by the lymphoma cells. These tumours are Lennert's lymphoma, angioimmunoblastic lymphoma, T-zone lymphoma, and small-cell pleomorphic lymphoma. Their common feature is a proliferation of small to medium-sized T cells, often with an associated vascular response. Eosinophils are a common component of the reactive lymphocytic infiltrate. Individual features of these disorders are discussed separately below. There is still no clear consensus on their behaviour, with many authorities believing them all to be high grade regardless of their morphology. In the REAL classification the T-cell tumours are treated as entities so that the concept of low- and high-grade categories has less relevance.

Lymphoepithelioid (Lennert's) lymphoma. This was originally described as a type of Hodgkin's disease but more detailed study has identified it as a T-cell lymphoma with a mixed population of malignant T cells interspersed with numerous small foci of epithelioid macrophages—that is, a granulomatous reaction. Its behaviour is that of a high-grade lymphoma.

Angioimmunoblastic lymphoma. This is a disease of older people, principally in their sixth or seventh decade, with only some 10 per cent being under 40 years of age. It presents with constitutional symptoms of fever, malaise, pruritus, polyarthralgia, anorexia, and weight loss. About half the patients have skin rashes, which may be maculopapular, purpuric, or urticarial. Lymphadenopathy is an almost invariable feature and it may involve both peripheral and internal lymph nodes. Hepatosplenomegaly is common, and lung involvement, arthritis, polyneuropathy, skin plaques and nodules, vasculitis, glomerulonephritis, oedema, and ascites have all been described in this condition. An autoimmune haemolytic anaemia is often found and a leucocytosis with eosinophilia is common. The ESR is usually raised, with a polyclonal hypergammaglobulinaemia.

The histological appearance of the glands is characterized by a proliferation of arborizing, postcapillary venules (the epithelioid venules) in the paracortex. In between the new vessels the interstitium is packed with a polymorphous selection of T cells with admixed polyclonal plasma cells. B-cell follicles are unrecognizable.

Initially, angioimmunoblastic lymphadenopathy with dysproteinaemia was believed to be non-neoplastic because, although virtually all patients died rapidly regardless of therapy, this seemed mostly to be due to the effects of immunodeficiency. However, the recognition that some developed obvious large-cell lymphomas, combined with careful molecular analysis, has identified the disease as a T-cell lymphoma.

Clinical behaviour and response to treatment is variable. Exposure to a known stimulus, for example, one which has produced an allergic drug reaction, should be avoided in future, and if the condition shows no tendency to regress spontaneously, treatment with prednisolone and possibly an immunosuppressive drug such as cyclophophamide is indicated. Once the condition has entered a clinically more obviously malignant phase, treatment appropriate to a high-grade lymphoma may be tried, but the prognosis is poor.

T-zone lymphoma In this lymphoma the B-cell areas are usually intact but surrounded by a polymorphic T-cell infiltrate, very similar to that seen in angioimmunoblastic lymphoma.

Pleomorphic small-cell lymphoma This lymphoma basically consists of the neoplastic infiltrate from the three tumours described above minus the granulomas, vascularity, or B-cell reaction. Like the high-grade pleomorphic T-cell lymphomas, with which it merges insidiously, it may be associated with HTLV-1 infection.

High-grade T-cell lymphoma

Pleomorphic lymphoma

This is a lymphoma composed of a mixture of pleomorphic cells of medium to large size. It can be extremely difficult to distinguish from the low-grade small-cell variant, and indeed the REAL classification recognizes this by putting all these tumours together as a single entity. Many cases, particularly in endemic areas, are associated with HTLV-1 infection. These cases are usually associated with an accompanying leukaemia and thus are known as adult T-cell leukaemia/lymphoma syndrome.

Adult T-cell leukaemia/lymphoma syndrome (ATL)

As might be expected from the association with the type C retrovirus HTLV-1, ATL tends to occur in clusters. It is an aggressive systemic disorder characterized by widespread lymphadenopathy, bone lesions, refractory hypercalcaemia, bone marrow, peripheral blood, central nervous, and skin involvement.

Angiocentric lymphomas

These are T-cell neoplasms characterized by invasion of vascular walls. This pathological entity encompasses a number of clinical syndromes such as polymorphic reticulosis, midline granuloma, and lymphomatoid granulomatosis. It is a rare disorder, though more common in Asia than in the West. The clinical course appears to depend on the proportion of large atypical cells.

Other forms of non-Hodgkin lymphoma

Anaplastic large-cell lymphoma

This is a recently recognized entity composed of large cells with abundant cytoplasm and pleomorphic nuclei. It has a characteristically cohesive growth pattern involving lymph nodes, often patchily, in the subcapsular sinuses and paracortex. Many cases were misdiagnosed as secondary cancer until antibodies against the activation antigen CD30 revealed the identity of this lesion as a malignancy of activated lymphocytes. Approximately 75 per cent of these lesions are T cell, 20 per cent B cell, and 5 per cent unidentifiable. Many have a characteristic t(2;5) chromosomal translocation.

This lymphoma occurs in two age peaks, one in older children and teenagers and one in elderly people. There is preliminary evidence in children that the tumour has a better prognosis than other high-grade large-cell lymphomas, whereas in adults there is no evidence yet that it is better or worse than other large-cell lesions.

Histiocytic lymphomas

Ever since the first description, in 1939, of a clinicopathological syndrome of hepatosplenomegaly, fever, and anaemia termed histiocytic medullary reticulosis, the literature has been full of case reports of macrophage-based neoplasms. Like the Loch Ness monster they are frequently cited but never caught. Most cases have been shown to be tissue deposits of monocytic leukaemia or T-cell lymphoma. If histiocytic lymphoma does exist it is so rare that for practical purposes it can be dismissed or lumped in with the high-grade large-cell lymphomas.

Table 7 Primary gastrointestinal non-Hodgkin's lymphoma

B-cell
Lymphomas of mucosa-associated lymphoid tissue (MALT):
(a) low-grade B-cell lymphoma of MALT
(b) high-grade B-cell lymphoma of MALT with or without a low-grade component
(c) immunoproliferative small-intestinal disease (IPSID) low-grade, mixed or high-grade
Mantle-cell lymphoma (lymphomatous polyposis)
Burkitt's or Burkitt-like lymphoma
Other types of lymphoma corresponding to peripheral lymph-node equivalents
T-cell
Enteropathy-associated T-cell lymphoma (EATL)
Other types unassociated with enteropathy

Primary extranodal lymphomas

Non-Hodgkin lymphomas have a tendency to involve structures other than lymph nodes, either by direct invasion (for example from mediastinal node into pleura, lung or pericardium) or more remotely. Extranodal spread occurs rarely in Hodgkin's disease. Primary extranodal presentations (without evidence of disease elsewhere) are less common and are almost exclusively confined to the non-Hodgkin group. A wide variety of tissues may be involved, most commonly the mucosa-associated lymphoid tissues (**MALT**) of gut, thyroid, lung, and salivary gland (the so-called MALTomas), the eye, and the skin.

MALTomas

These are a group of lymphomas showing common clinical and pathological features. They most commonly involve the stomach but other affected tissues are colon, thyroid, lung, and salivary gland. Maltomas may be low or high grade and are the most common primary gastrointestinal non-Hodgkin lymphomas, a classification of which is given in Table 7.

MALTomas are believed to arise from small centrocyte-like cells surrounding gut lymphoid follicles. These cells give rise to a low-grade malignancy with a marked propensity for invading epithelial glands but remain localized to the organ site, be it stomach or thyroid, for many years. It is assumed that high-grade MALTomas arise as a transformation of these low-grade tumours into large-cell lymphomas. Strikingly, even these high-grade lesions may remain localized for relatively long periods. This results in the important feature that fully resected MALTomas have a much better prognosis than their nodal counterparts.

Recent studies suggest that early gastric MALTomas may be driven by antigenic stimulation from *Helicobacter pylori* infection. Appropriate antibiotic therapy can result in dramatic regression of these lesions. It may well be that other antigens are stimulating MALTomas in other sites and might similarly respond to appropriate therapy.

Immunoproliferative small-intestinal disease (IPSID) (see also Section 5)

This condition is virtually confined to countries bordering the Mediterranean. It presents with malabsorption and consists of infiltration of small bowel by lymphoplasmacytic and plasma cells synthesizing only the heavy chain of IgA. Hence it is also known as α-chain disease. In the early stages, prolonged remission may be obtained with broad-spectrum antibiotics, indicating that these lesions may be preneoplastic and thus reversible. As the lymphoma progresses, it becomes virtually indistinguishable from other MALTomas and has a similar clinical and pathological course.

Other primary gastrointestinal lymphomas

See Section 5.

Lymphomatous polyposis

This presents with multiple small polyps in the small bowel infiltrated by a mantle-cell, non-Hodgkin lymphoma. These are true centrocytes and should be distinguished from the centrocyte-like cells of MALToma. Like nodal mantle-cell lymphoma it has a worse prognosis than its bland cytology might lead one to expect, and unlike MALToma it tends to spread rapidly to other sites.

Enteropathy-associated T-cell lymphoma (see Chapter 5.9)

This is similar or identical to nodal, high-grade, pleomorphic, T-cell non-Hodgkin lymphoma and usually arises as a complication of long-standing coeliac disease. There is some evidence that there are T cells that localize to the gastrointestinal tract and that enteropathy-associated T-cell lymphoma arises from these cells. This would make this lesion the T-cell equivalent of B-cell MALToma. Unlike the MALTomas, enteropathy-associated T-cell lymphoma has a grave prognosis.

Other extranodal non-Hodgkin lymphomas

Nervous system

Secondary involvement of the nervous system is a fairly common late complication of a variety of non-Hodgkin lymphomas. It usually affects the meninges, producing radicular or cranial-nerve symptoms, but may involve the brain in a focal or diffuse manner with headache, altered conciousness, and/or focal neurological signs. The prognosis is poor, but a combination of intrathecal chemotherapy and radiotherapy may relieve symptoms sufficient for consideration of high-dose salvage therapy.

Primary brain lymphomas are rare causes of intracranial neoplasia but are occasionally found on biopsy of intracranial lesions. Treatment outcome is highly unsatisfactory. Initial symptoms may be relieved by radiotherapy but recurrence either intracranially or systemically is usual. Intensive systemic chemotherapy may be a better alternative, but the rarity of the condition means that there are no large studies to guide rational therapy.

Primary B-cell non-Hodgkin lymphomas also arise in the orbit and the skin. Cytologically these have many similarities to MALTomas, although there are important differences such as a tendency to systemic dissemination (orbit) or lack of epithelial invasion (skin). In the skin the most common lymphoma is of T-cell origin and presents as mycosis fungoides or Sézary syndrome.

Management of non-Hodgkin lymphomas

The principles of management of patients with non-Hodgkin lymphoma are the same as for Hodgkin's disease described above. The same staging system is employed. It must be remembered, however, that non-Hodgkin lymphomas are frequently diseases of lymphocytes that may normally recirculate throughout the blood system and lymphatics. Non-Hodgkin lymphomas are thus more often widespread, and the pattern of spread is predominantly haematogenous rather than to contiguous lymph nodes via the lymphatics as in Hodgkin's disease. Extranodal involvement is thus also much more common, and special investigations such as endoscopy may be required in individual cases.

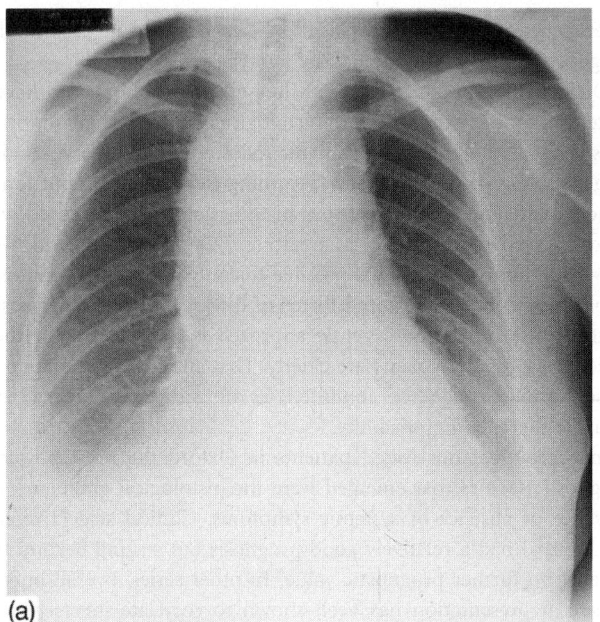

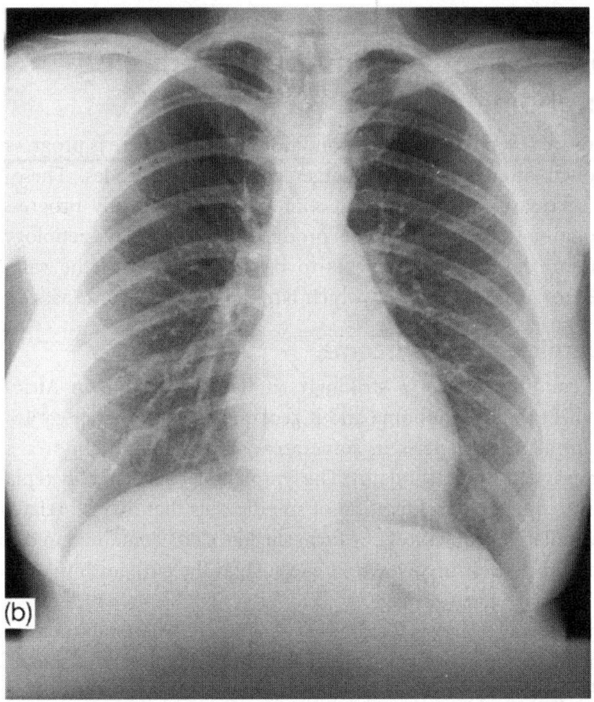

Fig. 3(a, b) A patient aged 31 at diagnosis, with malignant T-cell lymphoma associated with mediastinal obstruction, bilateral pleural effusions (which contained malignant T-cells), and involvement of the bone marrow but not of peripheral blood. Treated with aggressive chemotherapy on the lines of ALL, plus CNS prophylaxis with intrathecal methotrexate and 2 years maintenance chemotherapy. (a) Chest radiograph at presentation. (b) Six years later the patient remains well and in complete remission.

The most useful routine investigations are a full blood count and ESR, biochemical profiles (especially lactic dehydrogenase, which is elevated in some patients with high-grade tumours and may serve as a useful marker of disease activity), bone marrow examination, which should include aspirate and trephine, preferably from more than one site, chest radiograph (Fig. 3), and CT scan.

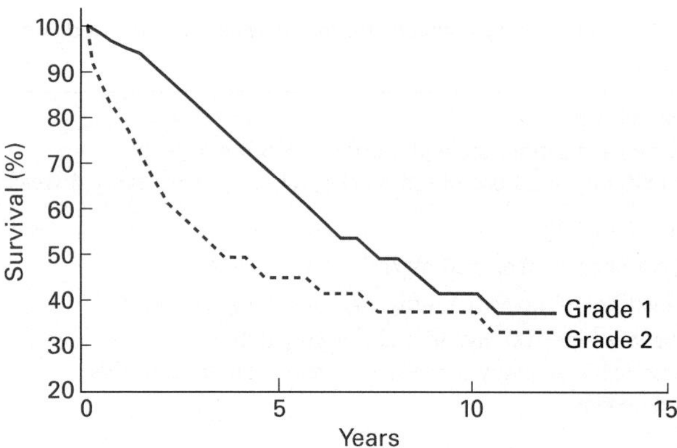

Fig. 4 Actuarial survival of patients with non-Hodgkin lymphoma. The graph is divided into low-grade (grade 1) and high-grade (grade 2) forms of the disease. Patients with high-grade lymphoma have an initial high death rate but the survival curve forms a plateau at 5 years, indicating that a significant proportion of patients are cured of their disease. Low-grade lymphomas, although having an indolent initial course, show a continuing death rate after 5 years and appear to be incurable with current therapies. By 10 years the survival rates of low- and high-grade lymphoma are similar. *(Data from the British National Lymphoma Investigation. (1988). Lancet,* **i***, 292–3.)*

Treatment

Over the years there has been less agreement about the optimal treatment for patients with non-Hodgkin lymphoma than with Hodgkin's disease, but recent improvements in classification, the introduction of less invasive investigations, and experience with different approaches to treatment have allowed a more rational approach to emerge. Many patients with non-Hodgkin lymphoma are elderly, their normal life expectancy may be limited, and attention to the quality of life is often at least as important as the duration of survival.

Low-grade tumours

Despite their more indolent course, few patients with low-grade non-Hodgkin lymphoma can be cured, even with aggressive cytotoxic therapy (Fig. 4). Exceptions are those in the minority with disease localized to one or two nodes, who may be cured by surgical removal and/or radiotherapy. Even so, long-term follow-up of such patients over 10 years or more will reveal a proportion with relapses at other sites. The aim of treatment in most patients with a low-grade non-Hodgkin lymphoma is therefore the control of symptoms and prolongation of good-quality survival rather than cure.

Some patients may not require therapy at first and can be treated only if symptoms occur, or can be anticipated from progression of the disease. Patients with stage I or II disease may be treated with radiotherapy to involved areas, particularly if node enlargement is producing local symptoms. Radiotherapy will generally produce good local control but the majority of patients will relapse in other sites sooner or later.

Various chemotherapeutic approaches for low-grade non-Hodgkin lymphoma have been suggested. Whilst the time required to achieve a remission is usually shorter with combination chemotherapy such as cyclophosphamide, vincristine, and prednisolone, randomized trials have shown that single-agent therapy with chlorambucil or cyclophosphamide may achieve just as good results with less toxicity, although taking longer to do so. Newer agents such as fludarabine, deoxycoformycin, and chlorodeoxyadenosine are currently under evaluation. Preliminary studies indicate that they may induce more

Table 8 Chemotherapy regimens for the treatment of non-Hodgkin lymphomas

Chlorambucil May be used continuously at a dose of 4–6 mg daily, or intermittently at a dose of 0.5 mg/kg daily for 3 days every 4 weeks
COP (CVP) • Cyclophosphamide 400 mg/m² orally, days 1–5 • Vincristine (Oncovin) 1.4 mg/m² (max 2 mg) IV, day 1 • Prednisolone 100 mg/m² orally, days 1 to 5 Course repeated every 3 weeks until remission or no further improvement
CHOP • Cyclophosphamide 750 mg/m² IV, day 1 • Vincristine (Oncovin) 1.4 mg/m² (max 2 mg) IV, day 1 • Adriamycin (hydroxydaunorubicin) 50 mg/m² IV, day 1 • Prednisolone 100 mg/m² orally, days 1–5 Course repeated every 3–4 weeks until remission + three further courses

complete responses than chlorambucil, but they are more difficult to administer, more toxic, and considerably more expensive, and do not at the moment appear to confer any long-term survival advantage.

Splenectomy may sometimes be helpful, either in patients whose disease is largely confined to the spleen or where hypersplenism is a feature. It may also be useful in the occasional patient with an autoimmune haemolytic anaemia where steroids or immunosuppressive treatment has failed or produced undesirable side-effects.

High-grade tumours

In high-grade non-Hodgkin lymphoma (lymphoblastic, large cell, and anaplastic large cell) the prognosis without treatment is extremely poor and aggressive combination chemotherapy is used. In contrast to low-grade non-Hodgkin lymphoma, the early mortality of high-grade disease is high but, paradoxically, patients who do go into remission may have prolonged disease-free survival and about one-third may be cured (Fig. 4).

Lymphoblastic lymphomas are best treated in a similar fashion to acute lymphoblastic leukaemia, including prophylaxis for the central nervous system.

Large-cell (centroblastic and immunoblastic) lymphomas are best treated with combination chemotherapy containing doxorubicin (Table 8). About one-half of all patients with large-cell lymphoma will have a complete response to CHOP, and about one-third overall will be cured. These somewhat disappointing results have led many to attempt more aggressive therapy with multiple (six, eight, or more) drug combinations. Whilst initial small series in selected patients were highly encouraging, recent large-scale randomized studies in less highly selected patients have shown no overall advantage over CHOP.

Attention is now being focused on the role of high-dose chemo/radiotherapy with haemopoietic stem-cell (marrow or peripheral blood) support. This is worth considering in relapsed patients or in those who have responded to CHOP but have adverse prognostic features, and randomized studies of its use in initial therapy are under way. However, it is currently an experimental approach, which should be confined to formal trials in specialist centres.

Prognosis

The prognosis of non-Hodgkin lymphoma is generally less good than that of Hodgkin's disease because this subset represents a much more heterogeneous group of neoplasms; this is reflected in the differing prognosis according to histological subtype.

One might expect patients with low-grade lymphomas to have a better prognosis than those with histologically more malignant forms. This generally holds true for patients followed for up to 5 years after diagnosis (Fig. 4), but it is now becoming clear that a proportion of patients with high-grade tumours histologically may be cured with more aggressive approaches to treatment. On the other hand, with low-grade tumours, a cure is possible for only a very small minority of patients with very localized forms of disease, even with aggressive treatment. A much more gentle approach is appropriate for these patients, especially as many are elderly. That antigenic stimulation by these tumours might be inhibited, as in gastric MALToma, is a valuable therapeutic possibility.

In a group of unselected patients in Oxford the most powerful prognostic factors that emerged were the histological grade and the presence or absence of systemic symptoms. Clinical stage I disease (all groups) had a relatively good prognosis but staging beyond this were of no further prognostic value. In other series, overall bulk of disease at presentation has been shown to correlate inversely with prognosis.

Miscellaneous conditions resembling lymphoma

There are several uncommon conditions in which there is progressive, although often non-fatal, enlargement of lymph nodes. These are not necessarily malignant, but some may subsequently progress to lymphoma, and may in time produce clues as to its aetiology. A common denominator appears to be an alteration of the vascular structure of nodes through which lymphoid cells have to pass.

Endemic Kaposi sarcoma

This condition shares a strikingly similar distribution in Africa to that of Burkitt's lymphoma and it accounts for approximately 16 per cent of all malignancies in some areas. It presents in children as a widespread lymphadenopathy. The lymph nodes are generally replaced by a sarcomatous proliferation of spindle cells that may be related to pericapillary fibroblasts. They form slit-like clefts containing red cells. When the process involves an organ such as the gut, death may occur from massive haemorrhage.

In Europe, Kaposi sarcoma is diagnosed when a much more indolent, vascular spindle-cell proliferation involves the skin, particularly of the extremities. Nodal and visceral involvement may supervene. It is uncertain to what extent the African childhood lymph-node disease and the adult Western skin tumour are identical.

A striking association between Kaposi sarcoma, human herpes virus 8, and AIDS has been recognized. This is described in Chapter 16.35.

Castleman's disease

This is a rare condition, also known as angiofollicular lymph-node hyperplasia. The original description was of a mediastinal mass, detected on chest radiograph, which on biopsy showed 'pseudo-follicles' with small lymphocytes surrounding capillaries, in the wall of which were concentric lamellae of plump, eosinophilic, endothelial cells, often resembling a Hassall's corpuscle in a normal thymus. Clinically, the condition may be asymptomatic, or associated with local symptoms such as cough and dyspnoea. Occasional patients may have constitutional symptoms such as fever and night sweats, and an associated anaemia and elevated ESR. In this form, the condition is generally benign, and asymptomatic patients may not require treatment, whilst surgical removal of the mass may relieve symptoms in those who are.

More recently, a histological form has been recognized (the 'plasma-cell variant') that is in contrast to the original description, which is now known as the 'hyaline vascular' variant. The plasma-cell variant is more often associated with systemic symptoms and a more generalized lymphadenopathy that may affect cervical, retroperitoneal or mesenteric lymph nodes. In some cases there may be one or more of *p*eripheral neuropathy, *o*rganomegaly (hepatomegaly and/or splenomegaly), *e*ndocrinopathy, a *m*onoclonal paraprotein, and *s*kin lesions—the so-called POEMS syndrome (Chapter 13.31). Occasional cases have been observed to progress to a frank non-Hodgkin lymphoma.

Lymphomatoid granulomatosis

This condition is characterized by a pleomorphic cellular infiltrate with atypical lymphocytoid and plasmacytoid cells, together with a granulomatous reaction. It affects adults between the third and sixth decades. The lungs are most commonly involved. Presenting features include cough, dyspnoea, pleuritic pain, fever, skin infiltrates, or neurological symptoms. A chest radiograph may show a nodular infiltrate. The diagnosis and distinction from Wegener's granulomatosis depends on biopsy (see Section 10).

The condition is now generally considered to be part of the angiocentric T-cell lymphomas and frequently progresses into an unequivocal florid lymphoma, often of a high-grade variety. The disorder is responsive to combined chemotherapy with cyclophosphamide and prednisone; long remissions can be obtained.

Histiocytic medullary reticulosis

This is a very rare disease of middle age, characterized by a fever, a rash, hepatosplenomegaly, and pancytopenia. Histiocytes in the splenic red pulp and hepatic sinusoidal cells show some erythrophagocytosis. As the disease progresses the architecture may be destroyed and tumour masses develop, especially in the skin and bones. Careful immunological review has shown that most of these cases are T-cell lymphomas.

Virus-induced haemophagocytic syndrome

This condition must be carefully distinguished from a purely reactive disorder that is seen occasionally in immunosuppressed patients. This has been termed the virus-induced haemophagocytic syndrome. There is often a history of a viral-like illness during the previous few weeks and laboratory investigation may reveal evidence of EBV or cytomegalovirus infection. Despite its reactive nature, this is a serious multisystem illness with a high mortality rate.

There is frequently an associated disseminated intravascular coagulation, and pancytopenia is invariable. The bone marrow shows increased numbers of histiocytes with prominent phagocytosis of red cells, platelets and nucleated cells. The histiocytes and cells are mature and morphologically normal.

Histiocytosis X (see Chapter 3.31)

Proliferation of cells with histiocytic features is evident in the histiocytosis X group of tumours, but although some of these have a malignant clinical course there is no good evidence that they are neoplastic.

Further reading

Armitage, J.O. (1993). Drug therapy: treatment of non-Hodgkin's lymphoma. *New England Journal of Medicine*, **328**, 1023–30.

Fisher, R.I. *et al.* (1993). Comparisons of standard regimen (CHOP) with three intensive chemotherapy regimens for advanced diffuse non-Hodgkin's lymphoma. *New England Journal of Medicine*, **328**, 1002–6.

Gordon, L.I., *et al.* (1992). Comparison of second-generation combination chemotherapeutic regimen (m-BACOD) with a standard regimen (CHOP) for advanced diffuse non-Hodgkin's lymphoma. *New England Journal of Medicine*, **327**, 1342–69.

Gray, G.M., Rosenberg, S.A., Cooper, A.D., Gregory, P.B. Stein, D.T., and Herzenberg, H. (1982). Lymphomas involving the gastrointestinal tract. *Gastroenterology*, **82**, 143–52.

Horning, S.J. (1994). Treatment approaches to the low-grade lymphomas. *Blood*, **83**, 881–4.

Linch, D.C. (1994). Management of histologically aggressive non-Hodgkin's lymphomas. *British Journal of Haematology*, **86**, 691–4.

Parsonnet, J., *et al.* (1994). *Helicobacter pylori* infection and gastric lymphoma. *New England Journal of Medicine*, **330**, 1267–71.

Safai, B. and Good, R.A. (1980). Lymphoproliferative disorders of the T-cell series. *Medicine (Baltimore)*, **59**, 335–51.

Shipp, M.A. *et al.* (1993). A predictive model for aggressive non-Hodgkin's lymphoma. The International Non-Hodgkin's Lymphoma Prognostic Factors Project. *New England Journal of Medicine*, **329**, 987–94.

Chapter 3.30

Myeloma and other paraproteinaemias

B. G. M. Durie and F. J. Giles

Pathological clonal expansion of plasma-cell populations results in a spectrum of disorders. This expansion may be overtly malignant, resulting in myelomatosis, Waldenström's macroglobulinaemia, a solitary plasmacytoma of bone, or an extramedullary plasmacytoma. A benign pattern of plasma-cell proliferation may result in monoclonal gammopathy of undetermined significance (**MGUS**), primary systemic amyloidosis, or comprise a component of the *p*olyneuropathy, *o*rganomegaly, *e*ndocrinopathy, *m*onoclonal gammopathy, *s*kin lesions (**POEMS**) syndrome (see Chapter 13.31).

Myelomatosis

Epidemiology and aetiology

Myelomatosis accounts for around 1.5 per cent of all malignancies and is rare below the age of 50 years. The most established risk factors for development of myelomatosis are old age and ionizing radiation. Many occupational hazards for myelomatosis have been noted and there appears to be a genetic component to susceptibility, although the size of this is not clear. While no specific chromosomal abnormality has been linked with myelomatosis, abnormalities of chromosome 14 occur in the majority of patients with cytogenetic abnormalities, and translocations involving the immunoglobulin heavy-chain gene are also commonly found.

Pathogenesis

The origin of malignant plasma cells is unknown but in 95 per cent of patients, malignant cells are widely disseminated to the axial skeleton, even at the earliest clinical stages of disease. Recent work has suggested that human herpesvirus 8 (**HHV-8**) infection of bone-marrow stromal cells is common in myeloma, and that this leads to the proliferation of plasma cells secondary to the production of a viral homologue of IL-6. The monoclonal (M) immunoglobulin protein reflects cell clonality, indicating that all the cells which are synthesizing it are descended from a single precursor. Bone-marrow plasma cells have a characteristic phenotype commonly expressing CD56 (NCAM), CD38 and lacking CD19. Serum IL-6 concentrations are elevated in patients with active myelomatosis, and this cytokine may play a role as an autocrine or paracrine growth factor. Lytic bone lesions with resultant hypercalcaemia commonly occur in myelomatosis and osteosclerotic lesions are occasionally seen.

Presentation

The clinical picture of myelomatosis is dictated by four main aspects: malignant plasma-cell proliferation, M-protein production, renal failure, and immunodeficiency.

Plasma-cell infiltration of the bone marrow results in impairment or failure of bone marrow function leading to anaemia, neutropenia, and thrombocytopenia. Anaemia, usually normochromic and normocytic, is common in myelomatosis and its symptoms may be dominant at the time of diagnosis in some 20 per cent of patients. Marrow invasion, the effect of tumour-related inhibitors of erythropoiesis, renal failure, and plasma-volume expansion secondary to M protein are the key factors in its pathogenesis. Erythropoietin is proving of some value in treatment.

At presentation, some 60 per cent of patients with myelomatosis have skeletal lytic lesions, with or without osteoporosis, wedging or collapse of vertebral bodies, or pathological fractures; some 20 per cent of patients have osteoporosis alone, and the remainder have no myelomatosis-related radiological abnormality. Because of the concentration of the disease in the axial skeleton, the main effects of osteoporosis and of lytic lesions are in the vertebrae, pelvis, ribs, and sternum. Bone pain, either diffuse or localized, is the predominant presenting symptom in 60 per cent of patients. Wedging and collapse of vertebral bodies, especially in the mid-dorsal, lower dorsal, and upper lumbar vertebrae, are common. With advanced disease, pathological fractures of the long bones, ribs, and sternum occur. There is no direct relation between severity of pain and the degree of skeletal involvement as assessed radiologically, apart from that associated with the wedging and collapse of vertebral bodies, or gross localized bone destruction. At presentation, some 25 per cent of patients have hypercalcaemia, in particular those with extensive lytic bone lesions. Characteristically the level of serum alkaline phosphatase remains normal except in the presence of healing fractures. Life-threatening episodes of acute hypercalcaemia leading to severe dehydration and uraemia may occur at any stage. In a small minority of patients with myelomatosis, plasma-cell infiltration of soft tissues is seen at presentation, and may be found in about 15 per cent of cases at autopsy.

The most serious clinical consequence of M-protein production, particularly that resulting from excessive synthesis of Bence-Jones protein, is the development of potentially irreversible renal damage. Of all patients with myelomatosis, 25 per cent are uraemic at presentation, with a further 25 per cent showing overt renal failure as the disease progresses. In a few cases the blood urea will fall to normal levels after rehydration.

Bence-Jones protein is the only M protein to be produced in approximately 15 per cent of patients with myelomatosis, while the cells of over 80 per cent of the remainder secrete Bence-Jones protein and complete immunoglobulin proteins. Bence-Jones protein consists of monoclonal light chains in a monomeric (molecular weight approx. 22 000 Da) or dimeric (approx. 44 000 Da) form, and enters the renal tubule with the glomerular filtrate. Bence-Jones protein is precipitated as a viscous mass in the collecting tubules and the distal convoluted tubules, causing obstruction. Proximal to the obstruction, the tubule dilates and epithelial cells atrophy. A number of other factors, such as hyperuricaemia, sepsis, disseminated intravascular coagulation, nephrotoxic drugs, renal-vein thrombosis, or direct infiltration by plasma cells or amyloid may contribute to the renal impairment (see Chapter 2.12).

Hyperviscosity syndrome associated with IgG myelomatosis occurs predominantly at very high M-protein concentrations. The hyperviscosity syndrome rarely occurs with a relative viscosity of less than 4, commonly at values of 6 or greater. Common components of the syndrome are ocular, haemostatic, and neurological disturbances accompanied by fatigue, malaise, or weight loss. Visual disturbances range in severity from mild impairment to abrupt loss of vision and are associated with characteristic retinal changes. A variety of neurological problems are also seen. Plasma volume increases with increasing viscosity, and may compromise cardiac function. A thrombotic tendency in patients with hyperviscosity syndrome may lead to presentation with deep venous thrombosis or pulmonary infarction.

Patients with myelomatosis have a much increased risk of bacterial infection, and some 10 per cent present in this way, often with pneumonia. Infections by both Gram-positive and Gram-negative organisms are increased. Infection is one of the most common causes of death in myelomatosis and early, intensive intervention is indicated where it is suspected. M-protein production is strongly associated with immunodeficiency, contributory factors being low serum concentrations of the normal immunoglobulins (immunoparesis) and suppression of the primary antibody response and cell-mediated immunity

Diagnosis, staging, and prognosis

The criteria for the diagnosis of myelomatosis (Table 1) include the presence of at least 10 per cent abnormal plasma cells in the bone marrow or histological proof of a plasmacytoma, and at least one of the following abnormalities: serum or urinary M protein or osteolytic lesions. Electrophoresis on a cellulose acetate membrane is satisfactory for screening the serum to detect M protein, while high-resolution agarose gel electrophoresis has the increased sensitivity necessary to detect smaller quantities of protein. Immunoelectrophoresis or immunofixation, or both, are confirmatory studies that can also define the immunoglobulin type and its light-chain class, which should be performed whenever myelomatosis, monoclonal gammopathy of undetermined significance, macroglobulinaemia, or amyloidosis are being considered, regardless of a normal-appearing or non-specific electrophoretic pattern. The recognition and quantitation of Bence-Jones protein in the urine depend on the demonstration of a

Table 1 Diagnostic criteria for multiple myeloma and monoclonal gammopathy of undetermined significance

Multiple myeloma *Major criteria* I. Plasmacytoma on tissue biopsy II. Bone marrow plasmacytosis with >30% plasma cells III. Monoclonal globulin spike on serum electrophoresis exceeding 35 g/l for IgG peaks or 20 g/l for IgA peaks, $\geq$1.0 g/24 h of κ or λ light-chain excretion on urine electrophoresis in the absence of amyloidosis *Minor criteria* (a) Bone-marrow plasmacytosis with 10–30% plasma cells (b) Monoclonal globulin spike present but less than levels in (III) above (c) Lytic bone lesions (d) Residual normal IgM <500 mg/l, IgA <1 g/l, or IgG <6 g/l Diagnosis is established when any of the following are documented in a symptomatic patient with clearly progressive disease. The diagnosis of myeloma requires a minimum of one major plus one minor criterion or three minor criteria that must include (a)+(b), thus: 1. (I)+(b), (I)+(c), (I)+(d) [I+(a) is *not* diagnostic] 2. (II)+(b), (II)+(c), (II)+(d) 3. (III)+(a), (III)+(c), III+(d) 4. (a)+(b)+(c), (a)+(b)+(d)
Indolent myeloma As per multiple myeloma except: I. No bone lesions or $\leq$3 lytic lesions, no compression fractures II. M-component levels IgA <50 g/l <70 g/l III. No symptoms or signs of disease, that is: (a) Karnofsky performance status >70% (b) Haemoglobin >100 g/l (c) Normal serum calcium (d) Serum creatinine <175 μmol/l (<20 mg/l) (e) No persistent or recurrent infection
Smouldering myeloma As per indolent myeloma with: No bone lesions Bone-marrow plasma cells 10–30%
Monoclonal gammopathy of undetermined significance I. Monoclonal gammopathy II. M-component levels IgA <20 g/l, IgG <35 g/l, <1.0 g/24 h of κ or λ light-chain excretion on urine electrophoresis III. Bone-marrow plasma cells <10% IV. No bony lesions V. No symptoms

monoclonal light chain by immunoelectrophoresis or immunofixation of an adequately concentrated sample from a 24-h urine collection.

A radiological survey of the entire skeleton is mandatory in the diagnosis of myelomatosis. The standard clinical staging system for myelomatosis is that of Durie and Salmon, with a stage I, II, and III differentiation as shown in Table 2.

The advent of computed tomographic (**CT**) scanning and magnetic resonance imaging (**MRI**) has greatly increased the sensitivity of detection of bone disease in myelomatosis. MRI is superior to CT scanning for screening large portions of the vertebral column and spinal canal, and for visualizing soft-tissue abnormalities. It clearly defines paraspinal or intraspinal tumour extension. It is of particular value in apparently solitary disease, where it may detect additional sites of involvement often missed by other imaging techniques.

Table 2 Myelomatosis: clinical staging system of Durie and Salmon

Stage I Low myeloma-cell mass (<0.6 $\times$ 10^{12} cells/m^2) *All* of the following: Hb >10 g/dl Serum calcium (corrected) $\leq$12 mg/dl* Radiographs are normal or show single lesion M-protein production value of: IgG <5 g/dl IgA <3 g/dl Urinary light-chain excretion <4 g/24 h
Stage II Intermediate myeloma-cell mass (0.6–1.2 $\times$ 10^{12} cells/m^2) Results fit neither stage I nor stage III
Stage III High myeloma-cell mass (>1.2 $\times$ 10^{12} cells/m^2) *Any* of the following: Hb $\leq$8.5 g/dl Serum calcium (corrected) >12 mg/dl* Radiographs show multiple lesions M-protein production value of: IgG >7 g/dl IgA >5 g/dl Urinary light-chain excretion >12 g/24 h

*Corrected calcium=calcium (mg/dl)–albumin (g/dl)+4.0.

Subclassification:

A=relatively normal renal function (serum creatinine value 2.0 mg/100 ml);

B=abnormal renal function (serum creatinine value 32.0 g/100 ml).

The prognosis for myelomatosis is dependent upon the stage and other prognostic factors including serum β_2-microglobulin and albumin levels at time of diagnosis. Of those patients diagnosed with myelomatosis, 75 per cent are reported to die 'directly' because of the disorder.

Therapy

It is important to consider both cytoreduction and ancillary treatment necessary to manage complications of the disease. Before proceeding to chemotherapy one must be sure of the diagnosis and need for therapy. This involves the exclusion of early forms of the disease or precursor states, such as monoclonal gammopathy of undetermined significance, which do not require treatment. Cytotoxic therapy has improved survival by reducing early deaths from complications and by slowing down tumour progression in some patients. Multidrug regimens consistently give higher response rates than the traditional melphalan/prednisone combination, but it is not clear that this translates into prolonged survival.

Induction therapy

In patients with stage I, smouldering or indolent myelomatosis, no specific antineoplastic or immunomodulatory therapy is currently indicated. Patients with stage I, II, or III disease that is symptomatic or progressive warrant systemic cytotoxic therapy. Commonly occurring indications for the institution of therapy are bone pain, hypercalcaemia, renal failure, marrow failure, or spinal-cord compression. All patients should be encouraged to drink 2 to 3 litres of fluid daily from the time of diagnosis.

Melphalan alone or in combination with prednisone (**MP**) has been the most widely used induction regimen for many years, but there is now debate as to whether or not more intensive regimes offer superior long-term survival. Certainly in those patients who are being considered for high-dose chemotherapy with stem-cell support, regimes such as vesicle-associated membrane protein (synaptobrevin, **VAMP**) or C-VAMP appear to allow better subsequent stem-cell harvests.

If MP is used, nadir absolute granulocyte counts should be monitored in patients on intermittent, oral alkylating-agent therapy. A typical induction regimen is melphalan 6 mg/m^2 and prednisone 100 mg/m^2 daily for 7 days each 28 days for six cycles.

Alternative induction regimens, for example vincristine, adriamycin, dexamethasone (**VAD**), may be of benefit to some patients with particularly aggressive tumours because these regimens may achieve higher overall or faster response rates. VAD is effective and relatively safe in patients with renal failure. Steroid pulses alone as induction therapy may be indicated where marrow function is suppressed. Conventional induction therapies are reported to result in median survival times of between 24 and 42 months, a clear improvement over the median survivals of 4 to 10 months achieved before the availability of suitable alkylating agents.

Numerous clinical studies with various α-interferons have demonstrated significant antitumour activity against myelomatosis, but its additive role in conventional induction regimens is still not clear.

Maintenance therapy

The majority of patients who achieve an objective response to induction therapy will enter a plateau phase of the disease, during which clinical assessments indicate a stable tumour burden. Continuing cytotoxic therapy beyond the time of objective response has repeatedly been shown not to prolong survival in myelomatosis. The addition of interferon-α appears to be able to prolong the plateau phase, although this has not been seen in all clinical trials.

Consolidation therapy

Autologous, bone marrow transplantation, using bone marrow and/or peripheral stem cells as rescue therapy, is an effective consolidation procedure in patients with myelomatosis. Most conditioning regimens incorporate high-dose melphalan and total-body irradiation. Complete remission occurs in 25 to 50 per cent of patients, but virtually all patients will relapse. Initial trial data suggests a survival benefit from autologous transplantation—some centres are performing double or even triple transplants. Allogeneic, bone marrow transplantation has also been tried. Although it uniquely offers a possibility of cure, morbidity and mortality rates remain high.

Relapse/refractory therapy

It is important to distinguish between two categories of patient covered by the term relapse/refractory. The first group is those who are truly refractory to first-line chemotherapy; it includes those who remain stable and are in a plateau phase at the time of diagnosis (and have a good prognosis) and a subgroup who actively progress while on induction therapy—the primarily resistant group. The second group comprises those who relapse after an initial response.

There are no satisfactory options for the treatment of refractory myelomatosis. A relatively effective approach is the use of simple, high-dose glucocorticoid (for instance, pulsed prednisolone, 100 mg on alternate days, reducing to 50 mg on alternate days when there is a response, or 28-day cycles of dexamethasone, 40 mg orally for 4-day blocks, starting on days 1, 9, and 17. The VAD regimen is also a useful regime in these circumstances.

The great majority of patients in the plateau phase will ultimately have evident overt progression of disease and patients stopping therapy must be closely monitored for the possibility of relapse.

Treatment of complications

Renal failure

The avoidance of dehydration has been shown to be one of the most important measures in the prevention of renal failure, and patients must maintain a minimal daily fluid intake of 3 litres. Aggressive therapy of hypercalcaemia, early control of disseminated intravascular coagulation, and care when using nephrotoxic drugs all decrease the risk of renal failure. It may be precipitated by the use of intravenous radiographic contrast media; the risk is reduced by ensuring adequate hydration and by using dyes of reduced osmolality.

Allopurinol should be prescribed for at least the first two courses of cytotoxic therapy. Moderate renal impairment can be completely reversed in many patients by rehydration. It is most likely to be effective when impairment is mild, and is independent of improvement in the underlying myelomatosis. Hypercalcaemia or urinary-tract sepsis need to be aggressively treated. VAD is probably the induction regimen of choice in the presence of severe renal failure. Despite initial concerns it is becoming clear that patients with myeloma can tolerate dialysis well.

Hypercalcaemia

Vigorous hydration and diuresis are the cornerstones of therapy whenever severe or symptomatic hypercalcaemia is diagnosed in myelomatous patients. Initial therapy of patients with severe hypercalcaemia should consist of rehydration with intravenous saline, the addition of a loop diuretic such as frusemide after expansion of the intravascular volume, and a bisphosphonate such as pamidronate. Corticosteroids are also effective.

Several trials have been performed to assess the ability of regular bisphosphonates (for example, oral clodronate or intravenous pamidronate) to reduce bone disease. Some studies have shown a reduction in the development of new lytic lesions and improved quality of life.

Anaemia

Transfusion-dependence in myelomatosis is an indication for specific therapy. Anaemia usually improves with response to chemotherapy, but it remains a significant problem in those patients with unresponsive or progressive disease. Erythropoietin is frequently successful in patients with myeloma.

Waldenström's macroglobulinaemia

Waldenström's macroglobulinaemia usually presents as a relatively indolent lymphoproliferative disorder with an IgM M protein and without bone lesions. Patients are usually in their sixties when first diagnosed. Fatigue, anaemia, hepatosplenomegaly, lymphadenopathy, and mucosal bleeding are common at diagnosis. Serum viscosity is increased in most patients and the hyperviscosity syndrome is evident in 70 per cent of patients at some stage of the disease; bleeding and visual disturbances are the most common manifestations. The M protein in Waldenström's macroglobulinaemia often behaves as a cryoglobulin. Typical signs and symptoms include peripheral vascular disease (Raynaud's phenomenon, acrocyanosis, ulceration and gangrene of the extremities), haemolytic anaemia, vascular purpura, and arthralgia. Waldenström's macroglobulinaemia may involve sites

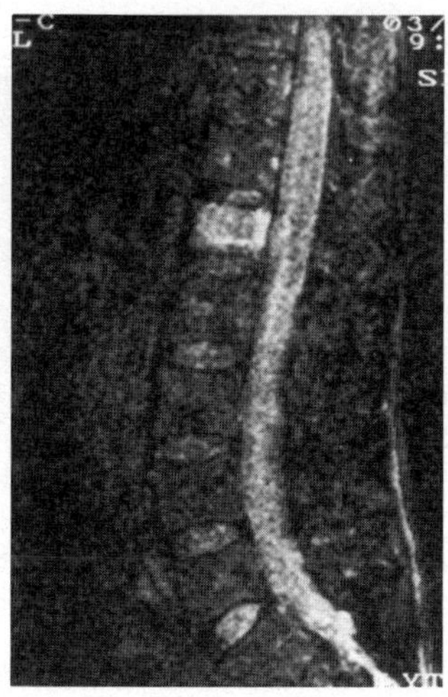

Fig. 1 (a) T_1-weighted MRI scan showing decreased signal intensity in L1 due to solitary plasmacytoma. (b) Short inversion time, inversion-recovery (STIR) MRI scan of the same lesion.

outside the marrow and reticuloendothelial system in some 10 per cent of patients, predominantly with infiltration of pulmonary tissue or the skin. Renal failure is relatively rare.

Anaemia due to plasma expansion, bleeding, and marrow suppression is almost universal at the time of presentation of Waldenström's macroglobulinaemia, and may be accompanied by neutropenia and thrombocytopenia. Peripheral lymphocytosis is usually a feature of late disease. The marrow is always involved, usually with a pleomorphic, diffuse infiltrate of lymphocytes, plasmacytoid lymphocytes, and plasma cells. Platelet function is usually abnormal due to defective platelet aggregation and adhesiveness following non-specific coating with M protein.

The IgM level required for the diagnosis of Waldenström's macroglobulinaemia has not been standardized and currently ranges from 10 to 30 g/l. The M-protein light chain is found in 75 per cent of patients and 70 per cent have Bence-Jones protein. In a Mayo clinic series of 430 patients with an IgM M protein, 56 per cent were associated with monoclonal gammopathy of undetermined significance, 17 per cent with Waldenström's macroglobulinaemia, 7 per cent with non-Hodgkin's lymphoma, 5 per cent with chronic lymphocytic leukaemia, 1 per cent with primary amyloidosis, and 14 per cent with lymphoproliferative disorders including patients with macroglobulinaemia-like features but having an IgM level of less than 30 g/l.

Median survival in Waldenström's macroglobulinaemia is approximately 6 years. Therapy is not curative and responses to chemotherapy are always transient. Chlorambucil, melphalan, or cyclophosphamide may control the disorder but rarely produce major remissions. It is not known whether combination cytotoxic therapy is more effective than single agents. The recent introduction of fludarabine and 2-chlorodeoxyadenine (2-CdA) therapy may improve the prognosis. In the hyperviscosity syndrome, plasmapheresis is the treatment of choice and may be dramatically effective, as 90 per cent of IgM is intravascular. It is usually necessary to remove 50 per cent of the total plasma volume and some four to six units of plasma may need to be removed daily until the relative serum viscosity is less than 4.

Solitary plasmacytoma of bone (Fig. 1)

Solitary plasmacytoma of bone may represent a very early stage of myelomatosis. Although any bone can be involved, it most frequently presents in the axial skeleton, with vertebral presentation in some 35 per cent of patients. Typical criteria for solitary plasmacytoma of bone include the presence of a single bone lesion predominantly consisting of plasma cells, negative skeletal survey, normal marrow aspirates and biopsies, and the absence of systemic signs or symptoms that could otherwise be attributed to myelomatosis. Immunoparesis is not a feature.

Definitive local radiotherapy relieves bone pain and eradicates the lesion in over 90 per cent of patients, with disappearance of M protein in 25–50 per cent. A generous margin of apparently uninvolved tissue should be included in the radiation fields. At least 10 per cent of irradiated patients have local recurrence and over 70 per cent go on to develop myelomatosis. The median time to the development of myeloma is 2 years, but there is no plateau. The median survival exceeds 10 years. Adjuvant or maintenance chemotherapy after initial radiotherapy has not been shown to slow progression to myelomatosis and poses the dual risks of drug resistance and secondary leukaemia.

Extramedullary plasmacytoma

Extramedullary plasmacytoma has a natural history distinct from those of myelomatosis and solitary plasmacytoma of bone. The median age at diagnosis is 59 years, with a predominance of males. The most common sites to be involved are the oronasopharynx and paranasal sinuses. In some 10 per cent of patients, extramedullary plasmacytomas are multiple or present in lymph nodes without evidence of a primary site. Treatment consists of local excision and wide-field radiation therapy, which should include regional nodes. Local recurrences occur in up to 30 per cent of cases, but dissemination does not necessarily follow and it has a lower rate of conversion to myelomatosis than has solitary plasmacytoma of bone.

Monoclonal gammopathy of uncertain (undetermined) significance (MGUS)

An M protein detected without concomitant evidence of an accompanying local or systemic disorder is designated an MGUS. It occurs in about 3 per cent of the normal population over the age of 70 years, and in 1 to 1.5 per cent of the normal population over 50 years. Out of patients presenting with an M protein, 65 per cent do not have an underlying neoplastic disease at diagnosis. In a Mayo Clinic series, 17 per cent of patients developed a lymphoplasmacytic disease at 10 years and 33 per cent at 20 years of follow-up. A serum M protein of more than 3 g/dl is more often associated with progression to neoplasia. The probability of progression is not affected by the heavy-chain isotype. The immunoglobulin levels other than the M protein are more commonly decreased in patients who will develop a lymphoproliferative disease. The presence of a monoclonal light chain is suggestive of a neoplastic process. It is mainly through the serial measurement of the M-protein level in the serum and urine, and intermittent clinical re-evaluation, that the character of disease can be assessed. The median survival of patients with MGUS is significantly reduced.

Further reading

Croucher, P.I., *et al.* (1998). Bone disease in multiple myeloma. *British Journal of Haematology*, 103, 902–10.

Smith, M.L., *et al.* (1999). Treatment of myeloma. *Quarterly Journal of Medicine*, 92, 11–4.

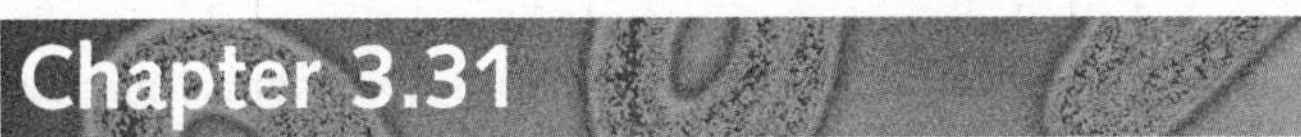

Chapter 3.31

The histiocytoses

V. Broadbent and J. Pritchard

The histiocytoses are a heterogeneous group of syndromes characterized by an abnormal proliferation of histiocytes. A classification of these is shown in Table 1 and may include both malignant and reactive conditions.

Class I disorder—Langerhans-cell histiocytosis ('histiocytosis X')

Definition and nomenclature

Langerhans-cell histiocytosis is a disorder in which cells with a phenotype similar to that of epidermal Langerhans cells cause tissue damage, possibly through excessive cytokine production. Formerly the disease was known as histiocytosis X, but the eponymous term

Table 1 Histiocytosis syndromes—a current working classification

Class I
Langerhans cell histiocytosis
Class II
Histiocytoses of mononuclear phagocytes other than Langerhans cells:
Haemophagocytic lymphohistiocytosis
Infection-associated haemophagocytic syndrome
Class III
Malignant histiocytic disorders:
Acute monocytic leukaemia (FAB M5)
Malignant histiocytosis
True histiocytic lymphoma
Class IV
Other histiocytosis syndromes:
Sinus histiocytosis with massive lymphadenopathy
Xanthogranuloma
Reticulohistiocytoma

See OTM3, p. 3606 for source.

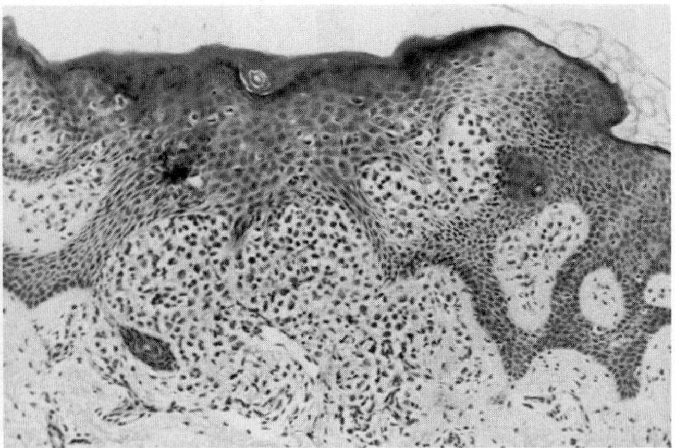

Fig. 1 Biopsy from skin involved in Langerhans cell histiocytosis. The infiltrate of histiocytes, eosinophils, and lymphocytes traverses the dermoepidermal junction. In this case, the rash resolved spontaneously (haematoxylin and eosin, 125 ×).

identifies the lesional cell more precisely and distinguishes the condition from other forms of histiocytosis. The terms eosinophilic granuloma, Hand–Schüller–Christian disease and Letterer–Siwe disease are outmoded and should no longer be used.

Pathogenesis

Langerhans cells are derived from haemopoietic stem cells in the bone marrow, which then migrate in the blood to the skin. They are powerful antigen-presenting cells, and an exaggerated cytokine response may explain most of the clinical and pathological features of Langerhans cell histiocytosis. Current ideas on pathogenesis implicate either an altered, dysfunctional population of Langerhans cells or an abnormal population of T cells producing trophic cytokines which attract normal Langerhans cells to sites of tissue involvement. There is still controversy as to whether or not the disease is a malignancy or a reactive process.

Histology

Early in the disease process, haematoxylin–eosin stained sections show infiltrates of pink-staining histiocytes (Langerhans cell histiocytosis cells (LCH cells)) surrounded by lymphocytes, eosinophils, and occasional giant cells (Fig. 1). A definitive diagnosis depends on the identification of Birbeck granules—tennis racket-shaped cytoplasmic inclusion bodies (Fig. 2) in lesional cells by electron microscopy, or positive CD1a surface-antigen staining.

Incidence

Peak age at presentation is 1–2 years, but with a range from birth to old age. Males are affected twice as commonly as females. Langerhans cell histiocytosis has been reported in twins and very rarely in other family members, although over 99 per cent of cases are sporadic.

Clinical manifestations

General features and prognosis

The clinical spectrum of the disease is wide. Single (organ)-system disease affects the skeleton, skin, lungs, or lymph nodes, in decreasing order of frequency; in most instances resolution is spontaneous and complete, though there may be residual lung fibrosis. By contrast, in 'multisystem' disease mortality can be as high as 50 per cent, despite intensive systemic therapy. Between these extremes are patients with

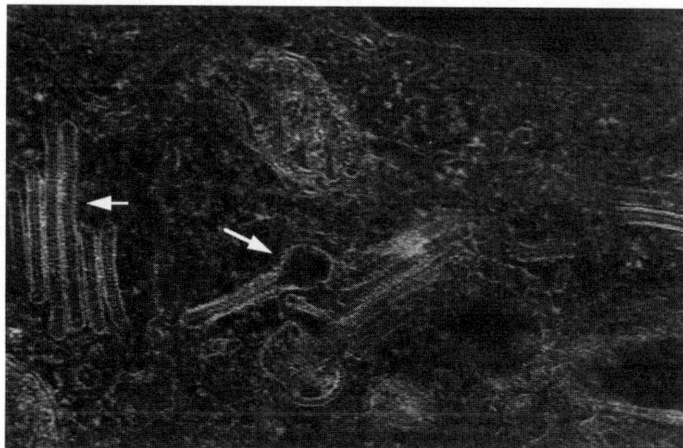

Fig. 2 Electron microphotograph showing Birbeck 'granules' (arrows) in Langerhans cells from a Langerhans cell histiocytosis skin infiltrate. The 'tennis racket' head and laminar structure of the racket 'handles' is clearly seen.

multisystem disease but without organ dysfunction; their disease usually responds to systemic therapy but runs a fluctuating course, eventually burning itself out, albeit with residual scarring in one or more organs.

Specific organs

Organs are listed in order of frequency of involvement.

Bone

Painful swelling of virtually any bone is the most common presenting feature and adjacent soft tissues or overlying skin or mucous membrane may be involved. Presentations include proptosis and cord compression. Skeletal radiographs are superior to bone scans in detecting bony lesions. Well-defined osteolytic lesions are typical (Fig. 3) (a sclerotic margin is regarded as evidence of healing), but periosteal reaction may be prominent and mimics the appearance of malignancy.

Skin

In infants, the typical skin rash occurs in the inguinal region and perineum, necklace area, axillary folds, and over the sacrum, and mimics seborrhoeic eczema. Scalp involvement resembles severe cradle cap. Brownish-pink papules with depigmented scars may be found on the trunk (Fig. 4). In neonates the lesions may resemble healing chickenpox with purplish, raised lesions scattered over the trunk, face, soles, and palms. The rash may be purpuric, especially if the platelet count is low.

Reticuloendothelial system

Cervical lymph nodes are most often affected but any group, including mediastinal and abdominal nodes, can be involved. A chronically discharging sinus may form if involved nodes erupt through the overlying skin. The spleen is often enlarged, and may reach an enormous size.

Ears

Aural discharge is common and may be caused by polypoid soft tissue extending from underlying bony disease or from extension of skin disease into the external auditory canal.

Peripheral blood and bone marrow

A mild anaemia of chronic disorders is relatively common. Blood eosinophilia does not occur. The CD4:CD8 ratio in blood is often inverted (2:1). Pancytopenia, usually found in infants presenting with pallor and petechiae or bleeding, and associated with hepatosplenomegaly, is an ominous finding. Bone marrow aspirates show infiltration with both phagocytic histiocytes and histiocytes typing as Langerhans cells.

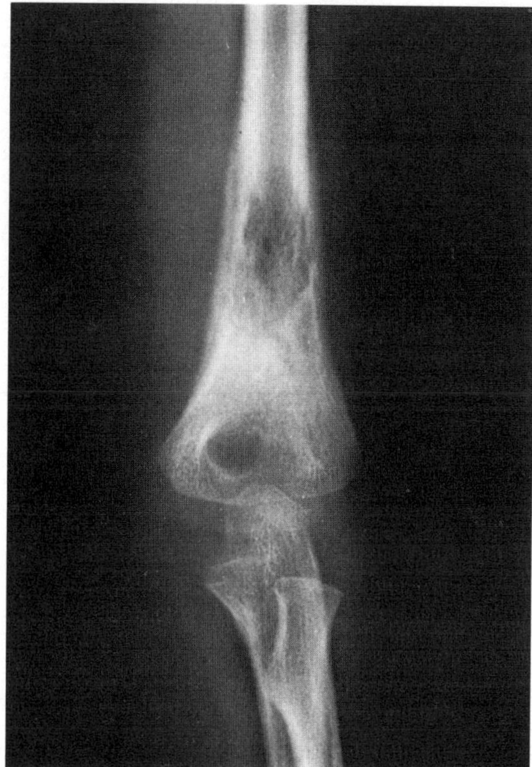

Fig. 3 Osteolytic lesion of the humerus in a 5-year-old boy presenting with a painful arm. When the periosteal reaction is as florid as this, the differential diagnosis includes osteomyelitis and malignancy, especially Ewing's sarcoma.

Liver

Liver involvement is often accompanied by a reduced hepatic synthesis of albumin and clotting factors (prolonged prothrombin time and/or partial thromboplastin time). Hepatomegaly and ascites are the most common clinical features. Rarely, obstructive jaundice, with a histological picture resembling sclerosing cholangitis, is the presenting feature. Solitary lesions in the liver parenchyma or porta hepatis may mimic a tumour or abscess.

Lungs

Lung disease may be the only manifestation of Langerhans cell histiocytosis in adults and is provoked by smoking. In young children, lung involvement may be symptomless but tachypnoea and rib recession are often seen. The earliest radiological abnormalities are interstitial shadows that cavitate, forming microcysts. As the cysts enlarge, bullae form and may rupture, causing pneumothorax. Pulmonary function tests show small, stiff lungs with reduced total lung volume and decreased compliance. Diagnosis is confirmed by finding LCH cells in bronchial washings or in a lung biopsy.

Central nervous system

The pituitary gland, stalk, and hypothalamus are most commonly involved and diabetes insipidus (see below) is the most common

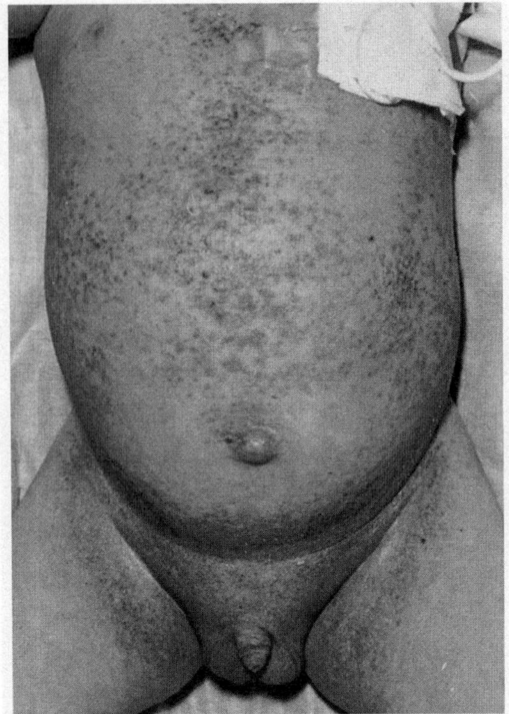

Fig. 4 Skin infiltration of characteristic distribution. Individual lesions are raised brownish-pink maculopapules. The rash is confluent in the groins and there are haemorrhagic areas on the anterior abdominal wall.

presentation. In chronic disease the cerebellar white matter may be involved, causing ataxia, incoordination, and nystagmus. Dural involvement and hydrocephalus can occur. A solitary intracerebral deposit may mimic a tumour. Enhanced computed tomography (CT) and magnetic resonance imaging (MRI) have led to detection of occult disease, especially in the cerebellar white matter. The natural history of cerebellar disease appears to be variable, some patients deteriorating rapidly and others having stable disease over many years.

Endocrine

Diabetes insipidus may pre-date the diagnosis of Langerhans cell histiocytosis. Thirst and polyuria developing within 4 years of diagnosis should be assumed to be due to diabetes insipidus. Growth failure is common.

Gastrointestinal tract

Involvement of oral mucosa, malabsorption, diarrhoea, failure to thrive, and mucus diarrhoea may all be seen.

Other organs

There are isolated reports of involvement of the thyroid, heart, and pancreas.

Diagnosis and evaluation

Definitive diagnosis of Langerhans cell histiocytosis requires the strict histopathological criteria outlined above—usually from skin or bone. Minimal investigations include full blood count, serum bilirubin and albumin, coagulation studies, skeletal survey, chest radiograph, and early-morning urine osmolality. Once evaluated the disease can be categorized into 'single system or multisystem, Langerhans cell histiocytosis, with or without organ dysfunction'. These variables have implications both for prognosis and treatment.

Differential diagnosis

Delay in diagnosis is usually due to failure to consider Langerhans cell histiocytosis as a possibility. Differentiation from familial or sporadic haemophagocytic lymphohistiocytosis is important. Sinus histiocytosis with massive lymphadenopathy (Rosai–Dorfman disease) should be considered if cervical glands are grossly enlarged. Malignant histiocytosis shares some clinical features with Langerhans cell histiocytosis.

Management

A rational approach is impossible because the cause is not understood. Now that the disease is not regarded as a malignancy, aggressive chemotherapy is no longer used. Current treatment approaches reflect the variation in severity and natural history of the disease.

Single-system disease

Spontaneous resolution of bony lesions is common and a period of observation is appropriate. Painful or unsightly lumps may require intervention and intralesional corticosteroids (20–80 mg methylprednisolone) is usually effective. Bony lesions that are inaccessible and might compromise vital organs (optic nerve, spinal cord) may require treatment with low-dose irradiation (7–10 Gy total dose); however, this form of treatment should be used only when there is no alternative, to reduce the risk of radiation-induced malignancy. Topical nitrogen mustard (mustine) in a 20 mg/dl solution, carefully painted on to active skin or aural lesions, is very effective. When the disease is confined, clinically, to a single lymph node that is removed for diagnosis, no further treatment is needed. Painful polyostotic disease or massive lymphadenopathy usually responds to a short course of corticosteroids. Indomethacin may be an effective analgesic.

Multisystem disease

Treatment of multisystem disease is more controversial. Symptomless patients may be managed by careful observation with a real chance of spontaneous resolution. When systemic treatment is required, cytotoxic drugs and corticosteroids, either alone or in combination, have been regarded as 'standard treatment', but no particular regimen has been shown to be superior. Vinblastine and etoposide are most often used, usually alone or with a corticosteroid. A variety of experimental treatments has been used for non-responders. These include cyclosporin, allogeneic bone marrow transplant, interferon-α, and 2-chlorodeoxyadenosine (2-CdA).

The management of diabetes insipidus is still controversial. There are reports of responses to pituitary irradiation given soon after symptoms (thirst and polyuria) develop. In most cases, however, lifelong replacement with 1-desamino-8-D-arginine vasopressin (DDAVP) is required.

Late sequelae

The outlook for patients with single-system disease is excellent, with minimal long-term sequelae. However, the majority of patients will have multisystem disease without organ dysfunction. Mortality in this group is low but about half are likely to have long-term morbidity. Problems include poor dentition, deafness, orthopaedic problems, small stature, diabetes insipidus, cerebellar ataxia, lung fibrosis, and cirrhosis.

Class II disorders

Haemophagocytic lymphohistiocytosis

Haemophagocytic lymphohistiocytosis is a multisystem disorder, more common in children but also seen in adults, in which there is activation or proliferation—or both—of phagocytic histiocytes, chiefly in the spleen, liver, bone marrow, skin, lymph nodes, and central nervous system. The infiltrate also contains many lymphocytes and haemophagocytosis is usually evident. The incidence (around 1:50 000) is similar in males and females, but this figure may be an underestimate because the disease is probably underdiagnosed. Haemophagocytic lymphohistiocytosis is considered to be a 'reactive' disorder, not a malignancy. Though the aetiology is unknown, between 30 and 50 per cent of all childhood cases have a genetic basis, with autosomal recessive inheritance. In other patients, including all adults, the disease is 'sporadic'—though often precipitated by infection, especially viral.

In decreasing order of frequency, presenting features are fever, splenohepatomegaly, lymphadenopathy, and neurological abnormalities. Etoposide (VP16) is often used for initial treatment and most patients respond. Corticosteroids are also used for their 'anti-inflammatory' action and intrathecal methotrexate often leads to remission of disease in the central nervous system. In a few patients, response to this 'triple therapy' is sustained, but in most cases the disease reappears between 3 and 24 months from diagnosis. Second and third remissions are usually brief, and most patients eventually die from 'organ failure' and complicating infection. Because there seems to be an underlying genetic defect manifest in bone-marrow stem cells, a number of centres have recently carried out bone marrow transplants.

Class III disorders

Malignant histiocytosis

Malignant histiocytosis must be differentiated histopathologically from the more common Ki 1-positive, anaplastic, large-cell lymphoma (usually of T-cell type), reactive 'haemophagocytic disorders', atypical Hodgkin's disease and 'sarcoma' of the interdigitating reticulum cell. Diagnosis requires positive staining of monoclonal macrophage-associated antigens.

Lymphadenopathy and hepatosplenomegaly are common and neurological involvement occurs. Cure can be achieved with combination chemotherapy.

Class IV

Rosai–Dorfman disease (sinus histiocytosis with massive lymphadenopathy)

In this rare disease lymph nodes are grossly distended by massive accumulations of bland, non-Langerhans cell histiocytes. Peak age is around 20 years. AfroCaribbean males are most commonly affected. Treatment may not be needed but can include steroids, radiotherapy, and chemotherapy.

Other class IV histiocytoses

A number of histiocytoses involving the skin, predominantly or exclusively, include juvenile xanthogranuloma, reticulohistiocytoma, and xanthoma disseminatum.

Further reading

Egeler, R.M. and D'Angio, G. (ed.) (1998). Langerhans cell histiocytosis. *Haematology/Oncology Clinics of North America*, **12**, 2.

Pritchard, J., Veverly, P., Chu, A., D'Angio, F., Davis, I., and Malpas, J. (ed.) (1994). The Proceedings of the Nikoras Symposia on the histiocytoses 1989–1993. *British Journal of Cancer*, **70** (Suppl. xxiii).

Chapter 3.32

The hypereosinophilic syndrome

C. J. F. Spry

The discovery that a person has marked eosinophilia is often unexpected. Nevertheless, in most such people there is a clear explanation, once the clinical features and results of investigations are known. Metazoan parasites are responsible in the majority of patients: hookworms, schistosomes, filariae, and roundworms are the main culprits in endemic areas. In other regions, asthma, hay fever, and drug reactions are frequent causes. Rarer causes include solid neoplasms, granulomatous and vasculitic diseases, and blood diseases. Even when an exhaustive range of investigations has been done, there remains a group of patients with no known cause for their marked eosinophilia and this diagnosis has been termed the idiopathic hypereosinophilic syndrome. The prognosis is usually excellent and this fact alone needs to be better known, as patients have died after receiving cytotoxic drugs in an attempt to put them 'into remission'.

Definition of the hypereosinophilic syndrome

Patients are considered to have the hypereosinophilic syndrome when they have: (i) persistent eosinophilia (blood eosinophil counts in excess of 1.5×10^9/l); (ii) no demonstrable cause for the eosinophilia; and (iii) one or more of a range of clinical problems. The diagnosis of the hypereosinophilic syndrome remains a provisional one and ought to be reviewed at intervals. This is because a small number of patients, who are considered initially to have no serious underlying cause for their disease, develop a lymphoma or lymphocytic leukaemia several months or years after presentation. In the hypereosinophilic syndrome, blood eosinophil counts rarely return to normal levels (less than 0.55×10^9/l), even when they are treated with steroids and other drugs that lower the counts in patients with reactive eosinophilia. The diagnosis should be reconsidered if blood eosinophil counts return to normal when steroids are first given.

Possible causes

By definition, the causes are unknown. However, there are two main ways by which eosinophilia could occur: an autonomous overproduction of eosinophils and their precursor cells in the bone marrow; or an appropriate response to excessive growth factors produced in other cells, for instance interleukin-5 (IL-5) from T lymphocytes. Other possibilities include alterations in receptors or signalling for the eosinophil-active peptide growth factors and abnormalities of feedback inhibition of growth-factor production.

Presentation and symptoms

The syndrome is most common in young and middle-aged men. The mean age of onset is 37 and it is rare after the age of 55 years. The sex ratio is 9:1 males:females.

Many of the symptoms at presentation are non-specific: generalized malaise, weight loss, sweating (especially at night), and itching of the lower legs. Other common features are respiratory symptoms (a severe dry cough, mainly at night, wheezing, and a blocked nose), gastrointestinal symptoms (indigestion, abdominal pain, alcohol intolerance, and diarrhoea), musculoskeletal symptoms (painful, swollen large joints, muscle aches, and pains), and neurological features ranging from focal peripheral nerve damage to diffuse cerebral lesions, retinal damage, and even strokes.

Physical findings are variable. The cardiological manifestations are described in OTM3, p. 2396–8. Splenomegaly is a common finding and in some cases may be marked. Dermatological changes include scratch marks, petechiae, and occasionally ulceration. There may be generalized lymphadenopathy, hepatomegaly, splinter or retinal haemorrhages, and neuropathy

Investigation

There should be a detailed assessment of possible exposure to parasites and travel to areas of endemic parasitic infection, as many of these (for example, filariasis, strongyloides, and trichinosis) can persist in asymptomatic forms for years. Current allergic diseases such as asthma and hay fever are usually obvious. Others require a range of studies to determine whether environmental antigens are causing reactions in the skin, respiratory tract, or gut. A total serum IgE assay can be particularly useful, as a normal level virtually excludes both parasitic infections and allergic diseases as a cause of persistent eosinophilia. Drug reactions producing eosinophilia may not be obvious when patients have been on treatment for months or years for other conditions.

Granulomatous and vasculitic diseases, including the Churg–Strauss syndrome and Wegener's granulomatosis, are particularly difficult to diagnose when the lesions do not produce focal symptoms and signs. Biopsies of involved sites should be obtained where possible. A range of solid tumours may produce eosinophilia even when they are small. The eosinophil count can then be used as a marker for disease recurrence after treatment.

Eosinophilia may be seen in a variety of blood diseases including chronic myeloid leukaemia, lymphomas, and acute lymphoblastic leukaemia. It is a notable feature in the M4EO subgroup of leukaemia where the increase in eosinophils with abnormal morphology may be confined to the bone marrow. Definite acute eosinophilic leukaemia is rare.

When other causes have been excluded and the patient is suspected of having the hypereosinophilic syndrome it is sensible to obtain baseline investigations from which to assess future change. In the blood, eosinophils often show a reduced number of granules. This is possibly the most useful single investigation in the hypereosinophilic syndrome, as there are few other diseases in which this occurs. Prominent vacuoles in eosinophils without loss of granules may point to an allergic cause for eosinophilia, such as a drug reaction. Blood neutrophil counts are also almost invariably increased in patients with the hypereosinophilic syndrome and neutrophils may show striking toxic granulation. Platelet counts are often low and if less than 80×10^9/l patients may also be anaemic, although a fall of haemoglobin levels to below 9 g/dl is unusual in this syndrome.

Marrow biopsies show an increase in all stages of eosinophil differentiation but there are no diagnostic characteristics. An abnormal karyotype is unusual but does suggest future development into a malignant process. Transformation of the hypereosinophilic syndrome to a leukaemic process does not occur unless there are features to suggest that the patient has a myeloproliferative disease at presentation. Biopsies of affected sites show eosinophil infiltration but no diagnostic features.

Treatment

Treatment should be directed at improving the patient's symptoms and remedying the complications, rather than returning blood eosinophil counts to the normal range.

Many fit patients in whom eosinophilia is a fortuitous finding require no treatment. There are no trials of treatment of the hypereosinophilic syndrome, but there are many case reports of treatment with a wide range of drugs. Patients with persistent systemic symptoms and/or signs of tissue damage should be treated initially with an oral corticosteroid. Many respond to 15–25 mg of prednisolone per day, and as symptoms improve it is possible to reduce the dose to a maintenance level of 7–15 mg/day. If steroids alone are unsuccessful, there are three other possibilities: hydroxyurea, 1–2 g daily; vincristine injections, 1.0–1.75 mg intravenously once every 2 weeks; or experimental forms of treatment such as interferon-α. Decisions about this should be strongly influenced by the fact that the syndrome is not cured by these drugs, although there may be weeks or months of relative improvement. It follows that treatment should always look to the long term; many of these patients will need treatment for over 15 years.

Prognosis

The prognosis of the hypereosinophilic syndrome is good, with approximately half of the patients alive 14 years after diagnosis. The main causes of death are thromboembolic disease, central nervous damage, and leukaemia. Generally, once an effective treatment regimen has been found, patients continue for many years with small fluctuations in their symptoms that are usually easily managed by temporary increases in steroid doses.

Further reading

Rothenberg, M.E. (1998). Eosinophilia. *New England Journal of Medicine*, **338**, 1592–600.

Haemostasis and thrombosis

Chapter 3.33

The biology of haemostasis and thrombosis

I. J. Mackie

The human organism has evolved complex mechanisms to ensure that no massive blood loss follows tissue damage and that circulating blood retains its fluidity. In response to vascular insult, blood around the site of damage is converted from a fluid to a solid state, with the formation of a primary haemostatic plug composed primarily of platelets and fibrin. This response is controlled so that the reaction remains localized and the entire vasculature is not blocked with thrombus. These responses and control mechanisms are known as haemostasis. Thrombosis may occur when there is a disorder or imbalance of the control mechanisms of haemostasis, or when there is an anatomical defect of the vessel wall or circulatory system.

Haemostasis involves the interaction of plasma proteins, platelets, endothelial cells, and blood flow. There is also an inter-relationship with leucocyte function, and haemostatic responses are closely linked with inflammation.

Platelet function

Platelet activation

Damage to the blood-vessel wall disrupts the layer of endothelial cells lining the luminal surface allowing platelets to adhere to the exposed subendothelial connective tissue. They secrete their granule contents which recruit more platelets to the site, leading to the formation of an aggregate of cells. Activated platelets also provide a procoagulant surface supporting the reactions leading to thrombin generation. Ultimately, fibrin is produced, which binds to the platelets and forms a network between them, adding mechanical strength to the platelet plug.

Platelet adhesion

Adhesion of platelets to areas denuded of endothelial cells requires specific structural components of the subendothelium, plasma proteins, and receptors on the platelet membrane. Platelets attach to extravascular matrices by surface receptors, most commonly from the integrin family. The integrins are heterodimeric proteins, each composed of an α- and a β-subunit, and platelets possess several types of integrin receptors as well as some non-integrin receptors that bind adhesive glycoproteins (Table 1).

The major platelet integrin receptor is glycoprotein (**Gp**)-IIb/IIIa, which can be activated by a variety of signals including exposure to extracellular matrix proteins such as collagen, and soluble activators such as ADP and thrombin. Gp-IIb/IIIa is responsible for much of the adhesion of platelets to the extracellular matrix proteins including fibrinogen, fibronectin, and von Willebrand factor (**vWF**). These proteins, have a common tripeptide sequence, Arg–Gly–Asp (**RGD**), which mediates their interaction with Gp-IIb/IIIa. Gp-IIb/IIIa is essential for normal platelet aggregation, allowing fibrinogen bridges to form between platelets.

Table 1 Platelet membrane receptors involved in adhesive-protein binding

Receptor	Subunit	Ligands
Integrins		
GpIIb/IIIa	$\alpha_{IIb}.\beta_3$	Fibrinogen, VWF, fibronectin, vitronectin (Vn), (?thrombospondin, collagen)
Vn receptor	$\alpha_v.\beta_3$	Vitronectin, fibrinogen, fibronectin, VWF, thrombospondin
GpIa/IIa	$\alpha_2.\beta_1$	Collagen
GpIc/IIa	$\alpha_5.\beta_1$	Fibronectin
GpIc′/IIa	$\alpha_6.\beta_1$	Laminin
Non-integrins		
GpIb/IX		VWF
GpIV(IIIb)		Thrombospondin

VWF, von Willebrand factor.

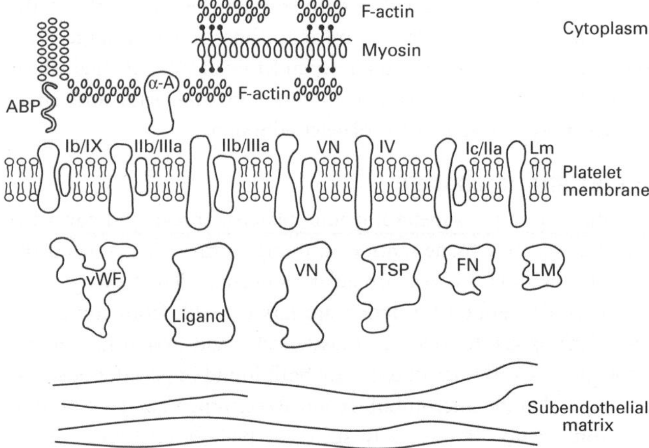

Fig. 1 Platelet adhesion. The platelet membrane phospholipid bilayer contains a variety of glycoprotein receptors to adhesive proteins (indicated by roman numerals, or VN for vitronectin and Lm for laminin receptor). At the cytoplasmic side of the membrane, some of these interact with cytoskeletal components. ABP, actin -binding protein; α-A, α-actinin; vWF, von Willebrand factor; VN, vitronectin; TSP, thrombospondin; FN, fibronectin; LM, laminin.

A number of adhesive glycoproteins are candidates as mediators of platelet adhesion to the subendothelium, among which are vWF, fibronectin, vitronectin, fibrinogen, and thrombospondin; vWF is clearly important in platelet adhesion, as congenital deficiency results in a mild-to-severe bleeding diathesis. The vascular endothelial cell synthesizes and secretes vWF directly into the subendothelial matrix as well as into plasma. It is also synthesized by megakaryocytes and stored in platelet α-granules. The protein is a macromolecule, existing as a series of multimers (1500–15 000 kDa); each of which is a polymer of dimers, themselves composed of two identical subunits (230 kDa) held together by disulphide bonds. There are discrete functional domains on the vWF molecule, with two separate sites responsible for platelet binding and a further site for binding to collagen. The platelet membrane has two classes of receptor for the factor, the Gp-Ib/IX complex, and the integrin receptor Gp-IIb/IIIa, which can also bind other adhesive proteins (Fig. 1; Table 1). Plasma

Table 2 Platelet α-granule proteins

β-Thromboglobulin	Fibrinogen
Platelet factor 4	Fibronectin
Platelet-derived growth factors	von Willebrand factor
Antiplasmin	Thrombospondin
α_2-Macroglobulin	Factor V
α_1-Antitrypsin	Albumin
Plasminogen activator inhibitor	Protein S

Table 3 Agents that cause platelet activation

ADP	Adrenaline
Collagen	Serotonin
Thrombin	Vasopressin
Thromboxane A_2	Cathepsin G
Arachidonic acid	Prostaglandins G_2 and H_2
Calcium ionophores	Phorbol myristate acetate

vWF does not interact with unstimulated circulating platelets, and for binding to occur either platelets have to be activated or plasma vWF must undergo a conformational change.

The receptor site for binding of vWF to the subendothelium probably involves collagen; collagen types I, II, and III have been shown to bind vWF. The contribution of this protein to platelet adhesion appears to be highly dependent on the shear rate at the vessel wall. At low shear rates, similar to those found in large veins and in arteries, adhesion occurs independently of vWF. At high shear rates in the vessel wall, similar to those in capillaries and small arterioles, vWF is essential for platelet adhesion.

Platelet shape change

After adhering to the subendothelium, platelets spread and cover the exposed connective tissue matrix. In doing so they change from the circulating discoid form to an irregular, elongated cell with cytoplasmic projections. Pseudopod formation appears to result from contractile activity analogous to that in muscle cells and requiring energy. Microfilaments and microtubules are both found in pseudopods, and it is thought that the microtubules control recruitment and dissolution of microfilaments. In the early stages of platelet activation, shape change is reversible, but strong stimuli cause the centralization of organelles, degranulation, and release accompanied by irreversible shape change and aggregation. The microtubules form a dense ring around the organelles, which liberate their contents into the channels of the surface connecting system.

Platelet-release reaction

Platelets possess two types of storage granules: dense granules that contain nucleotides and serotonin; and α-granules that contain a variety of proteins. Secretion of the platelet granules is thought to occur by fusion of the granule and surface connecting-system membranes in a process requiring calcium ions.

Adenine nucleotides are sequestered in the dense granules mainly as ADP and ATP, in a complex with calcium ions and pyrophosphate, and are not interchangeable with the nucleotides involved in general cell metabolism. A large amount of serotonin is also stored, it acts synergistically with other agents to activate platelets, and is a potent modulator of vascular tone and integrity.

α-Granules contain platelet-specific proteins, such as β-thromboglobulin and platelet factor 4 as well as fibrinogen and factor V (Table 2). Platelet factor 4 interacts with glycosaminoglycans such as heparan sulphate, dermatan sulphate, and chondroitin sulphate on the endothelial cell surface and neutralizes heparin.

β-Thromboglobulin is a potent stimulator of fibroblast chemotaxis, which may be important in wound healing, and it may inhibit prostaglandin I_2 production by endothelial cells.

Platelet aggregation

Platelet aggregation describes the property of platelets to cohere with one another in a specific process requiring energy, intracellular processes, and initiators. A large number of agents can act alone or together to stimulate platelets and cause their aggregation (Table 3). Aggregation is thought to proceed by at least three different pathways. The first is mediated by ADP released from the dense granules, the second requires the generation of prostaglandin endoperoxides and thromboxane A_2. The third pathway operates independently of ADP release or the generation of thromboxane A_2. One candidate as mediator of the third pathway is platelet-aggregating factor (**PAF-acether**).

In vivo, perturbed endothelial cells and erythrocytes are probably the main source of ADP, which is supplemented by ADP and serotonin from the platelet dense granules after the release reaction; but several other platelet activators would be present, such as collagen, thrombin, and platelet-derived thromboxane A_2, all of which can act in synergy. ADP probably plays an important part in the secondary aggregation response that follows the activation of adherent platelets at the wound site. There is a specific ADP receptor on the platelet membrane through which ADP downregulates adenylate cyclase, which thus reduces cAMP levels allowing a generalized activation of cytoplasmic enzymes favouring aggregation and secretion. ADP-binding to its receptor also leads to a conformational change in the Gp-IIb/IIIa receptor on the platelet membrane, so that fibrinogen can bind. Fibrinogen binding to Gp-IIb/IIIa along with the release of Ca^{2+} into the cytoplasm are essential for aggregation. Fibrinogen is the most likely candidate for the formation of interplatelet bridges during aggregation, and this interaction may well be stabilized by thrombospondin (Fig. 2).

Thromboxane A_2 binds to a specific receptor on the platelet membrane and lowers the threshold for release and aggregation. It can also act as a calcium ionophore, and liberates Ca^{2+} from the dense tubular system. It also inhibits prostaglandin E_1 and I_2 stimulation of cAMP production, although there is no effect on basal cAMP levels.

Collagen and thrombin at suitable concentrations cause platelet adhesion, phospholipase activation, and liberation of arachidonic acid from the membrane, as well as granular nucleotide release. The metabolism of arachidonate provides a series of compounds that influence platelet function.

Arachidonic acid metabolism

The rate-limiting step in prostaglandin and thromboxane synthesis is the liberation of arachidonate from the membrane phospholipids. This is brought about by the action of phospholipase C and diglyceride lipase on phosphatidyl inositides; and of calcium-activated phospholipase A_2 on phosphatidyl choline. Once liberated, arachidonate may be converted to a variety of possible products (Fig. 3) by the

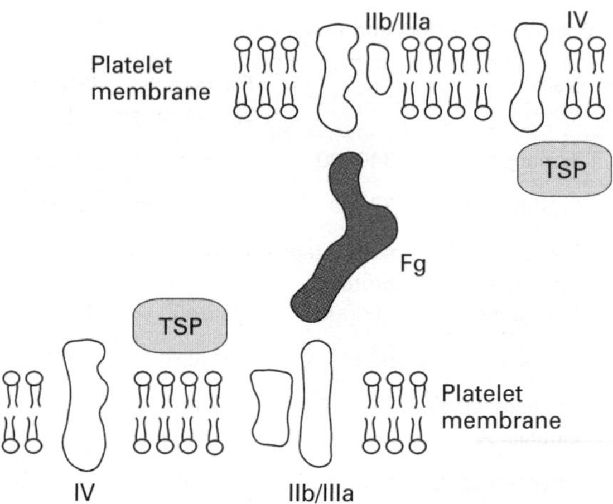

Fig. 2 Platelet aggregation. The terminal event in platelet aggregation is thought to be the binding of fibrinogen to glycoprotein-IIb/IIIa receptors on adjacent platelets. This fibrinogen bridge may be stabilized by thrombospondin bound to its receptor (Gp-IV).

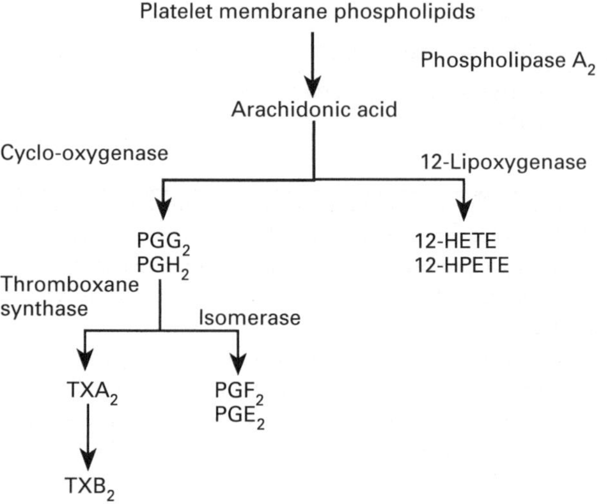

Fig. 3 Arachidonate metabolism.

cyclo-oxygenase and lipoxygenase pathways (ratio approximately 70: 30 per cent). Arachidonate is converted by cyclo-oxygenase to the prostaglandin endoperoxides, prostaglandins G_2 and H_2, and their main fate in platelets is rapid conversion to thromboxane A_2 by thromboxane synthetase. Thromboxane A_2 is an exceptionally potent constrictor of vascular smooth muscle and a strong platelet-aggregating agent.

Thrombin is the strongest of the physiological activators and causes shape change, secretion from dense and α-granules, and ultimately aggregation. It cleaves its own receptor forming a tethered ligand, and this results in the phosphorylation of G protein-coupled receptors and activation of phospholipase C.

Phosphatidyl inositol metabolism

There are three important messengers involved in the stimulus-response coupling that follows agonist binding at the platelet membrane—inositol triphosphate, calcium ions, and diglyceride. Diglyceride is produced as a result of the breakdown of phospholipids of the phosphoinositide class (Fig. 4), which are produced by the action of phospholipases when thrombin and other agents activate

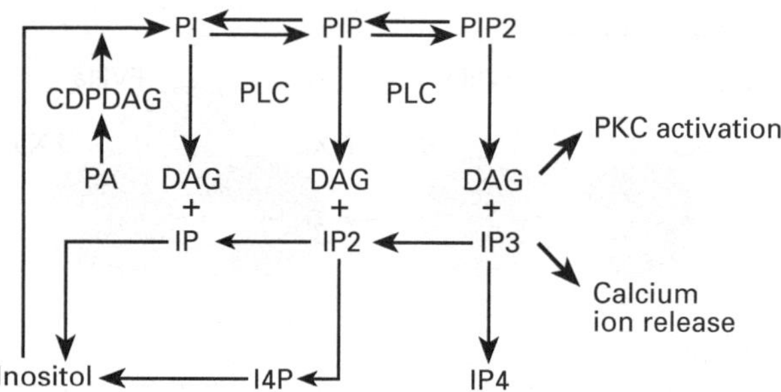

Fig. 4 The phosphatidyl inositol cycle. PLC, phospholipase C; PI, phosphatidyl inositol; PIP, phosphatidyl inositol 4-phosphate; PIP2, phosphatidyl inositol 4,5-bisphosphate; PA, phosphatidic acid; DAG, 1,2-diacylglycerol; CDPDAG, CDP-diacylglycerol; IP3, inositol 1,4,5-triphosphate; IP4, inositol 1,3,4,5-tetrabisphosphate; IP2, inositol 1,4-bisphosphate; IP, inositol 1-phosphate; I4P, inositol 4-phosphate.

platelets. Diglyceride is able to activate protein kinase C, and this enzyme phosphorylates a 40- to 47-kDa protein that appears to be associated with labilization of granules and calcium-ion secretion.

Inositol triphosphate has been implicated in the release of calcium from intracellular storage sites in cells and could function similarly with the dense tubular system of the platelet. An increase in the cytoplasmic, free calcium-ion concentration leads to the phosphorylation of the myosin light chain, with subsequent contraction and granule centralization, as well as several other calcium-mediated events associated with platelet activation.

Platelet calcium control

Platelets contain a high concentration of calcium; about 60 per cent is present in dense granules and can be secreted into plasma, but the cytoplasmic concentration is very low. A small amount of calcium is associated with the plasma membrane and most of the rest is located in the dense tubular system and may be released by thromboxane A_2-dependent and -independent pathways.

Platelet calmodulin regulates Ca^{2+} transport and appears to control the use and availability of Ca^{2+} in the cell. The major mechanism for downregulation of platelet function is the stimulation of adenylate cyclase, which increases the cAMP concentration. The effects of cAMP are probably exerted by inhibiting calcium flux and/or promoting calcium reuptake. Cyclic AMP is broken down by phosphodiesterase, which is stimulated by calcium-calmodulin.

Platelet coagulant activity

Platelets contribute to almost every stage of the coagulation system. They release calcium ions, factors V, XIII, and fibrinogen, as well as fibrinolytic substances and antithrombins. The platelet membrane provides a phospholipid surface on which reactions can occur, and has specific receptors for certain proteins, while others are non-specifically adsorbed to their surface, which results in the acceleration of coagulation reactions.

Platelet membranes have an asymmetrical distribution of phospholipids, with almost all the acidic (negatively charged) phospholipids such as phosphatidyl serine located in the inner leaflet of the plasma membrane. After platelet activation, the acidic phospholipids are translocated to the outer half of the membrane, while phosphatidylcholine moves to the inner half, in a phenomenon known as the 'flip-flop' reaction.

The exposed phosphatidyl serine and other negatively charged phospholipids account for the activity traditionally known as platelet

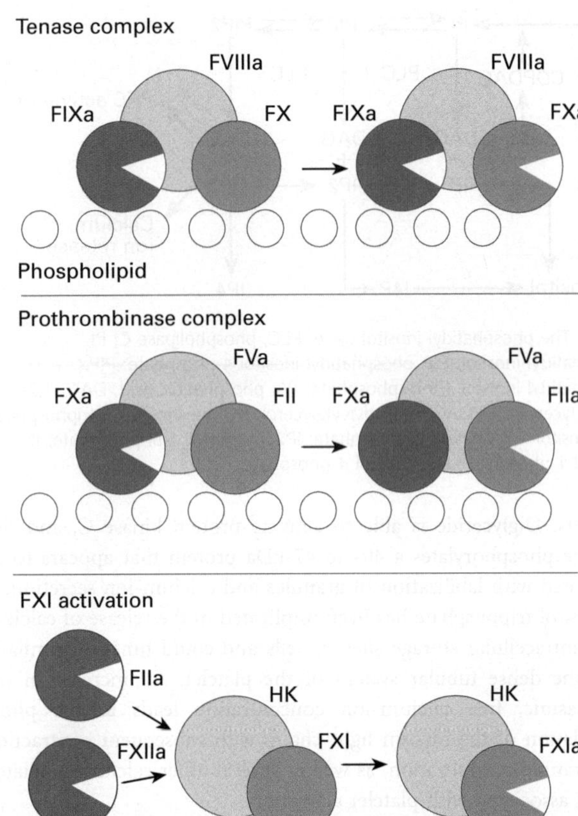

Fig. 5 Platelet coagulant activity. Pathways for the activation of prothrombin (prothrombinase complex), factor X (tenase complex), and factor XI, on platelet membrane phospholipids.

factor 3, by acting as a binding surface for the factor X and prothrombin activation complexes (Fig. 5). The vitamin K-dependent coagulation zymogens bind to the phospholipid surface by virtue of their γ-carboxyglutamic acid residues.

Activated platelets bind factor XI to their membranes in the presence of high molecular-weight kininogen. There is evidence that thrombin can activate factor XI at the platelet surface.

Inhibitors of platelet function

Increasing the level of platelet cAMP downregulates platelet function. Prostaglandins I_2 and E_1 bind to a membrane receptor, which results in the stimulation of adenylate cyclase and synthesis of cAMP from ATP. Adenosine and xanthines cause an increase in cAMP levels by inhibiting the enzyme responsible for cAMP degradation, phosphodiesterase.

Drugs such as aspirin cause the acetylation of cyclo-oxygenase, which results in irreversible inhibition of the enzyme.

Coagulation cascades

Coagulation factors

Coagulation factors were designated by roman numerals from I to XIII to avoid the confusion caused by various groups using different names for the same protein. Further numerals have not been assigned to the more recently discovered coagulation proteins, as it is clear that coagulation is a complex mechanism involving a large number

Table 4 Coagulation factors and Roman numerals

Factor	Names	M_r	Plasma concentration	Plasma half-life
I	Fibrinogen	340000	1.5–4 g/l	96–120 h
II	Prothrombin	72000	1–1.5 μg/ml	72 h
III	Tissue thromboplastin	43000 (apo-protein)	Tissue bound	
V	Proaccelerin	300000	10 mg/l	12–15 h
VII	Proconvertin	63000	500 μg/l	4–6 h
VIII	Antihaemophilic globulin A	200000	200 μg/l	10–18 h
IX	Antihaemophilic globulin B	55000	5–10 mg/l	18–30 h
X	Stuart–Prower factor	55000	10 mg/l	36 h
XI	Plasma thromboplastin antecedent	160000	5 mg/l	10–20 h
XII	Hageman factor	90000	40 mg/l	50–70 h
XIII	Fibrin stabilizing factor	320000	10 mg/l	100–120 h

of substances. The roman numerals are used for most of the factors (Table 4), except for factors I, II, and III, which are usually referred to as fibrinogen, prothrombin, and tissue factor, respectively; 'calcium ions' is used in preference to factor IV, and factor VI is redundant (it was found to be activated factor V).

The coagulation factors can be divided into enzymes, cofactors, and fibrinogen. The enzymatic coagulation factors generally circulate as an inactive, single-chain, zymogen form and become active after proteolytic cleavage, giving a two-chain form with the chains held together by disulphide bonds; this is usually accompanied by the release of a small activation peptide. The light chain, formed from the carboxy-terminal region, contains the active site, and the heavy chain from the amino terminal, contains the structural domains for binding to different cofactors and surfaces. The active forms are usually denoted by a lower case 'a' after the roman numeral. With the exception of factor XIII, which is a transglutaminase, they are all serine proteases related to trypsin. Some of the coagulation proteins are known as vitamin K-dependent factors (factors II, VII, IX, and X, protein C, protein S). The vitamin K-dependent proteins are synthesized in the hepatocyte and undergo post-translational modification in a carboxylase reaction. Certain glutamic acid residues in a specific structural domain of the protein undergo carboxylation of their γ carbon atom so that two carboxyl groups are attached, and γ-carboxyglutamic acid is formed. In this reaction vitamin K acts as a coenzyme,' the conversion of vitamin K to its epoxide form providing the energy for CO_2 fixation and γ-carboxylation (Fig. 6). The vitamin K epoxide is converted back into active vitamin K by a two-step reductase system. The reduction process is blocked by oral anticoagulants of the coumarin group, which interfere in the normal production of vitamin K-dependent factors. The γ-carboxyglutamic acid (Gla) residues are localized to a discrete region of vitamin K-dependent factors and facilitate the interaction of that region with phospholipids in the presence of calcium ions.

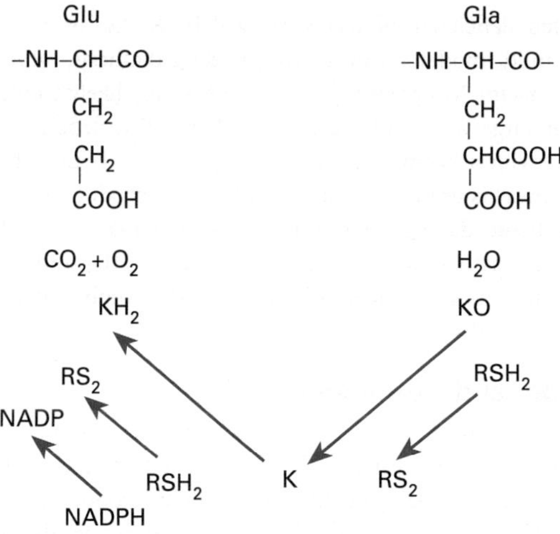

Fig. 6 Vitamin K-dependent carboxylation. Vitamin K (K) is first converted to a hydroquinone (KH_2) by either an NADPH-dependent or a dithiol (RSH_2)-dependent reductase enzyme. Specific glutamate residues (GLU) are γ-carboxylated (Gla) by a vitamin K-dependent carboxylase. During this reaction, the vitamin K hydroquinone is converted to vitamin K epoxide (KO). The latter is converted back to vitamin K.

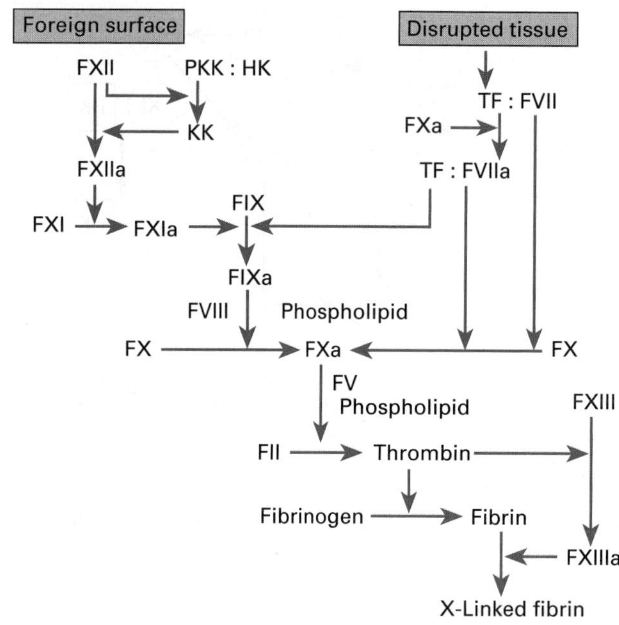

Fig. 7 The coagulation pathways. The coagulation cascade or pathways may be triggered by exposure of blood to foreign or extravascular surfaces, tissue rupture, and exposure of tissue factor, or platelet activation.

Factors V, VIII, high molecular-weight kininogen, tissue factor, as well as protein S, have no enzyme activity and act as cofactors in the activation of serine proteases.

The tissue factor-mediated pathway of coagulation

Tissue factor is exposed after trauma or cell damage, and usually remains localized at the site of injury. Thus when factor VII binds to tissue factor, the resulting factor X-activating complex remains localized at the cell surface. Factor VII is unusual because the zymogen form appears to have weak proteolytic activity on factor X. Tissue factor acts as a cofactor for the further activation of factor VII to factor VIIa by factor Xa and the activation of both factor IX and factor X by factor VIIa (Fig. 7). The resultant factor Xa exerts a positive feedback effect by cleaving factor VII to yield factor VIIa, which has enhanced activity on factor X, producing more factor Xa. The factor Xa remains phospholipid-bound, and forms a complex with factor V and prothrombin (the prothrombinase complex). Factor Xa cleaves prothrombin to produce thrombin, which is separated from its phospholipid-binding domain and can diffuse away from the phospholipid surface.

The interactions between these coagulation factors are dependent on the presence of calcium ions, which facilitate the binding of the vitamin K-dependent proteins to phospholipids. A constant theme in coagulation is the formation of reaction complexes composed of an enzyme, a substrate, a cofactor on an organizing surface (Fig. 8). In these reactions the surface is a phospholipid layer and the cofactor is tissue factor in the reactions involving factor VII, and factor V in the prothrombinase reaction. The cofactors act by increasing the reaction velocity, while the surface brings the reaction components together, so that a reaction is favoured (the K_m is lowered). The presence of both cofactors and phospholipid surfaces accelerates the reactions several thousand-fold.

A further action of factor VII is to activate factor IX to factor IXa, which itself can activate factor X—this may be the most important pathology *in vivo*.

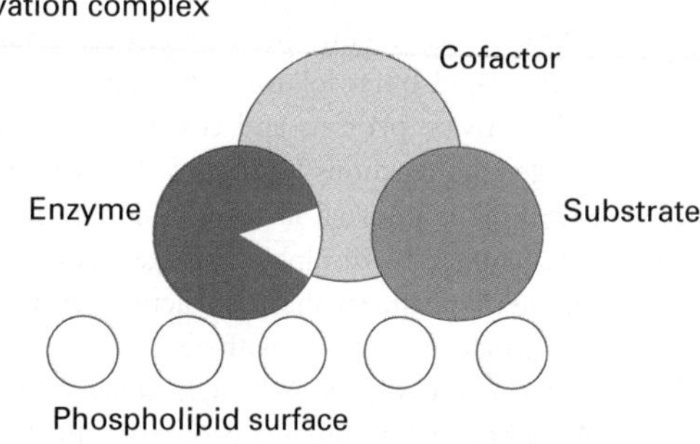

Fig. 8 Surface-mediated coagulation reactions. A constant theme in coagulation is the binding of an enzyme and its substrate to a surface, which is usually phospholipid. The conversion of substrate into product (an active protease) is catalysed by a cofactor which complexes with the other reaction components.

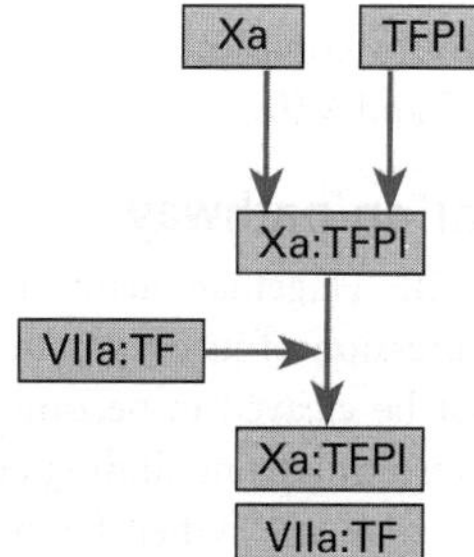

Fig. 9 Tissue-factor pathway inhibitor reactions. Tissue-factor pathway inhibitor (TFPI) binds to factor Xa and forms a quaternary complex with factor VIIa and tissue factor, resulting in inhibition of the extrinsic system.

When factor Xa accumulates, a complex is formed with a protein known as tissue-factor pathway inhibitor (**TFPI**) (Fig. 9). This complex can then form a tetramer with factor VIIa and tissue factor, resulting in the inhibition of factor VIIa and the tissue factor or extrinsic

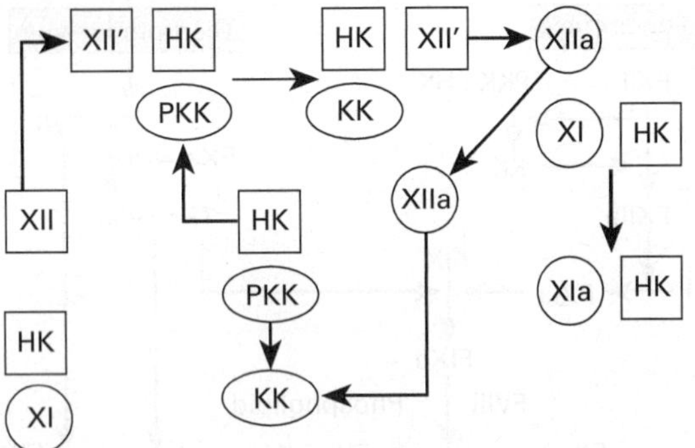

Fig. 10 Contact activation. Factor XII binds to charged foreign or extravascular surfaces and its active site becomes exposed, thus triggering the contact system. HK, high molecular-weight kininogen; PKK, prekallikrein; KK, kallikrein.

pathway of coagulation. However, activation of factor X by factor IXa (the tenase complex) is not affected.

The intrinsic system

There appear to be several mechanisms for the activation of factor XI. It can be cleaved by factor XIIa in the fluid phase, or at negatively charged surfaces; it can also be activated on platelet membranes in factor XIIa-dependent and -independent reactions. The latter may be due to several mechanisms, but the activation of factor XI by thrombin at the platelet surface has recently been described. Thus thrombin formed in an initial rapid burst following the exposure of blood to tissue factor could activate platelets and convert factor XI to factor XIa, and thus trigger the reactions leading to the further generation of thrombin. Factor XI is unusual in being a double molecule with two identical chains linked by disulphide bridges. This appears to be an amplification mechanism, so that two active serine centres are produced from a single interaction with factor XIIa or thrombin. Factor XI circulates as a complex with high molecular-weight kininogen (**HK**), which has surface-binding properties. Proteolytic cleavage of HK removes this binding function, and free factor XI does not readily bind to surfaces. Factor XIa acts on factor IX to produce factor IXa, which forms a complex with factor VIII, factor X, and phospholipid, in the presence of calcium ions, and liberates factor Xa. Thrombin cleaves factors V and VIII and makes them active as cofactors for the tenase and prothrombinase complexes. Prolonged exposure to high thrombin complexes causes further cleavage and inactivation of factors V and VIII.

The contact activation pathway

The exposure of factor XII (Hageman factor) to a variety of charged surfaces leads to the expression of its enzymatic activity. It is unclear whether factor XII must be cleaved to become active, or whether a confirmational change resulting from binding at a negatively charged surface can expose the active site. When factor XII becomes active, it is able to cleave prekallikrein (**PKK**) to yield kallikrein. PKK, like factor XI, circulates as a complex with HK, which acts as a cofactor and facilitates PKK binding at the surface. Kallikrein has a variety of substrates (Fig. 10) (including HK, which it cleaves with the loss of surface-binding capabilities) and liberates the vasoactive peptide bradykinin. Kallikrein acts in a positive feedback loop to activate further factor XII to factor XIIa, which can cause more generation of kallikrein. Kallikrein is able to activate complement by the alternative pathway.

Inherited deficiency of factor II, V, VII, X, IX, or VIII usually causes a mild, moderate, or severe bleeding diathesis, while in homozygous factor XI deficiency the patient is only likely to bleed after trauma or surgery. In contrast, factor XII and PKK deficiency are not associated with a haemorrhagic tendency. It is likely that the tissue-factor pathway is important for the early, rapid production of thrombin after tissue damage. The intrinsic system may then take over, initially with activation of factor IX by factor VIIa, and then with factor XI activation by the small amounts of thrombin generated by the extrinsic pathway.

Thrombin and fibrinogen

Fibrinogen is a large protein with a heterodimer subunit structure. It is composed of two each of three different polypeptide chains, α, β, and γ. They are held together by disulphide bonds near the N-terminal. Thrombin cleaves small peptides (fibrinopeptides A and B) from the α- and β-chains to form fibrin monomer. Fibrin monomer can interact with intact fibrinogen to give soluble complexes, but when sufficient fibrin monomers are formed, they undergo end-to-end polymerization to form long fibrin strands. When a sufficient molecular size is reached, these precipitate to give a solid fibrin clot. However, such a clot lacks tensile strength and would be easily washed away in flowing blood. A system for crosslinking the fibrin polymers to stabilize them therefore exists.

Fibrin-stabilizing factor (factor XIII or fibrinoligase) circulates in a zymogen form with a molecular weight of about 320 kDa, and is converted to an active transglutaminase by the action of thrombin. It is composed of two types of subunit, a and b, and possesses two of each type of chain (a2b2). The a-subunit contains the active, centre cysteine of the transglutaminase, while the b-subunit appears to act as a non-catalytic carrier protein. Factor XIII is synthesized in the liver and is present in plasma as well as in platelet α-granules. During the activation of factor XIII by thrombin, a small peptide is cleaved from subunit-a and a calcium-dependent dissociation of the b-subunits occurs, exposing the active centre. Factor XIIIa induces covalent-bond formation between fibrin strands to give dimers between the γ-chains of adjacent fibrin monomers. Then, at a much slower rate, polymers form between the α-chains of fibrin. Only when these inter-α-chain links are made does fibrin acquire its stable properties.

Thrombin inhibitors

As thrombin plays a pivotal role in the coagulation mechanism, it is not surprising that it has a number of inhibitors. The most important is antithrombin. A second heparin cofactor (heparin cofactor II, dermatan sulphate cofactor) has been more recently discovered and is discussed below. Antithrombin is also an important physiological inhibitor of factor Xa and can complex with most of the other serine protease coagulation factors. It is part of the serpin superfamily of proteins (Table 5), which show extensive sequence homology and have evolved from a primitive ancestral serine protease inhibitor. The serpins form a 1:1 irreversible complex with their target protease, and the complex is subsequently removed from the circulation and catabolized. Other examples of the serpin superfamily are given in Table 5.

The action of antithrombin is greatly potentiated by heparin, *in vitro* and *in vivo*, when used therapeutically or prophylactically. The physiological counterpart of heparin is probably heparan sulphate, which may be found on the endothelial cell surfaces. Heparin has a

Table 5 The serpin superfamily

Serpin	Target protease
AT-III	Thrombin, factor Xa, kallikrein
Heparin cofactor II	Thrombin, cathepsin G
α_2-Antiplasmin	Plasmin
PAI-1, PAI-2	t-PA, u-PA
PC inhibitor-1 (PAI-3)	APC, kallikrein, t-PA
α_1-Antitrypsin	Neutrophil elastase, factor XIa
Antichymotrypsin	Cathepsin G
C1 inhibitor	C1s, kallikrein, factor XIIa

Abbreviations as in text.

specific binding site for antithrombin and interacts with certain lysine residues in a particular domain of the antithrombin molecule. Heparin binding causes a conformational change that opens up the thrombin-binding site in antithrombin and greatly accelerates the inhibition of thrombin. Heparin is a highly acidic mucopolysaccharide composed of equal amounts of sulphated D-glucosamine and D-glucuronic acid, interlinked by sulphaminic bridges. Heparin is a mixture of molecules of varying chain length; longer chains, in addition to binding antithrombin, can also bind to and neutralize a positively charged site on thrombin. Factor Xa does not possess a similar positively charged site and shorter chains can give full anti-Xa activity. Antithrombin is synthesized mainly in the liver.

Heparin cofactor II is also a glycosaminoglycan-dependent thrombin inhibitor with many similarities in structure and function to antithrombin. However, it shows greater specificity for target proteases and, amongst the coagulation factors, only inhibits thrombin.

The protein C and S system

Protein C and protein S are involved in a pathway that leads to the degradation of the procoagulant cofactors Va and VIIIa. Both proteins are vitamin K-dependent, but protein S is unusual as it has no enzymatic activity. It is synthesized in the liver but is also released by platelets during activation.

Thrombin binds to several classes of receptor on the vascular endothelium: one of these is thrombomodulin, a transmembrane protein with an extensive hydrophobic region, which is synthesized and expressed by endothelial cells. Thrombin binds to thrombomodulin with high affinity and thrombomodulin blocks the procoagulant (fibrinogen clotting, factor V activation, and platelet activation) activities of thrombin. The thrombin–thrombomodulin complex binds protein C, which also binds to the membrane phospholipids. The protein C is cleaved by thrombin in a reaction catalysed by thrombomodulin (Fig. 11), to yield activated protein C.

Activated protein C binds to platelet and endothelial-cell membranes by interactions between its Gla residues and membrane phospholipids. The affinity of activated protein C for phospholipid membranes is increased by a cofactor protein S, which catalyses the inactivation of phospholipid-bound factors Va and VIIIa by activated protein C. Factors Va and VIIIa undergo proteolytic cleavage to yield a variety of fragments lacking procoagulant activity.

Protein S exists in two forms in plasma: 40 per cent of it is free protein and the remainder is complexed with a protein involved in regulating complement activation, C4b-binding protein (**C4BP**).

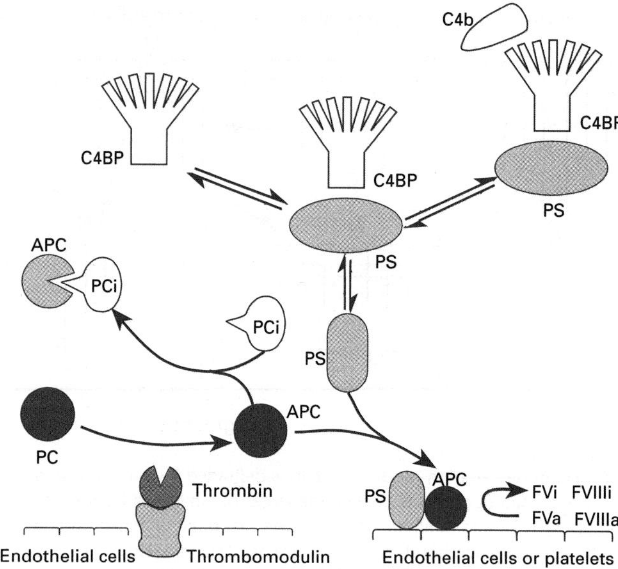

Fig. 11 The protein C anticoagulant system. PC, protein C; APC, activated protein C; PS, protein S; C4BP, C4b-binding protein; PCi, protein C inhibitor; FVi, inactivated factor V; FVIIIi, inactivated factor VIII.
(Modified from Hessing, M., et al. (1991). The interaction between complement component C4b-binding protein and the vitamin K-dependent protein S forms a link between blood coagulation and the complement system. Biochemical Journal, ***277****, 582, with permission.)*

Table 6 Fibrinolytic proteins

Protein	M_r	Concentration	Plasma half-life
Plasminogen	92000	0.2 mg/ml (2 μM)	2 days
t-PA	65000	5 ng/ml* (80pM)	5 min
u-PA (scu-PA)	54000	2 ng/ml (40pM)	8 min
PAI-1	48000	20 ng/ml (400pM)	7 min
PAI-2 PAI-3	60000 57000	0** 2 μg/ml (40nM)	
α_2-Antiplasmin	70000	70 μg/ml (1μM)	3 days

*Resting, unstimulated levels.
**250 ng/ml (4nmol) in late pregnancy.
Abbreviations as in text.

The free and complexed forms of protein S appear to be in equilibrium, but only the free form has activated protein C cofactor activity. C4BP is a multimeric protein composed of seven α-chains and one β-chain, linked by disulphide bridges. The protein S-binding site is located on the β-chain, but each α-chain of C4BP has a binding site for C4b, and both proteins can bind to the same molecule of C4BP.

Fibrinolysis (Table 6)

Fibrin degradation

Fibrin clots are broken down into small fragments and removed by the action of plasmin, which is generated by a variety of mechanisms within the fibrinolytic system. Plasmin is a serine protease produced by limited proteolysis from the zymogen plasminogen by the action of various plasminogen activator enzymes. Plasmin cleaves fibrin at a number of sites, so that progressively smaller fragments or fibrin

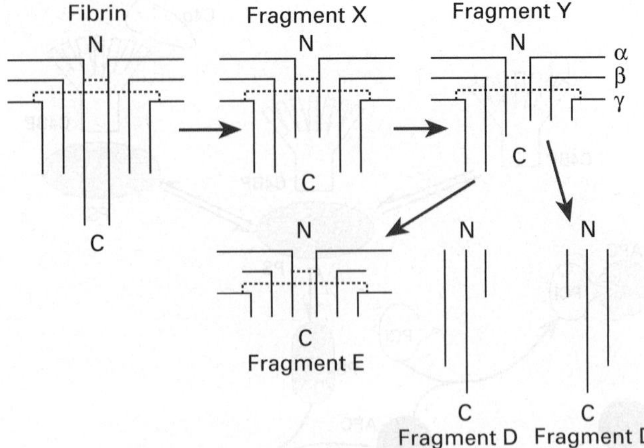

Fig. 12 Fibrin degradation products. Fibrin is degraded by plasmin into a series of degradation products (FDPs), the larger of which are known as fragments X, Y, D, and E. N, amino terminal; C, carboxy terminal; broken line indicates disulphide bonds of the N-terminal disulphide knot. *(Modified from Gaffney, P. (1987). In Haemostasis and thrombosis (ed. A.L. Bloom and D.P. Thomas), p. 233. Churchill Livingstone, Edinburgh, with permission.)*

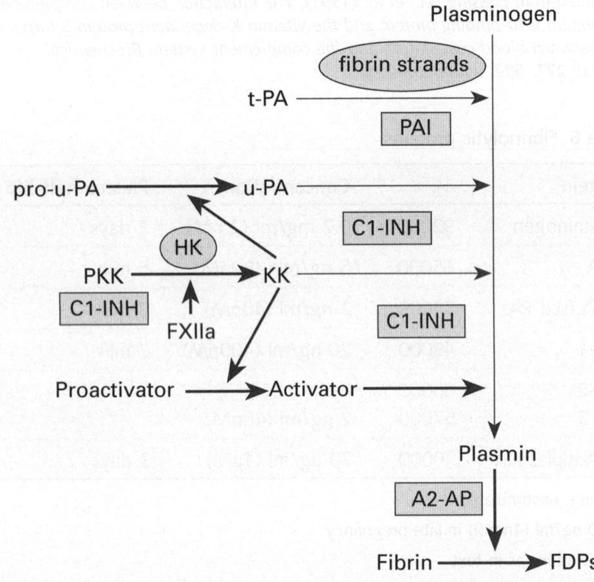

Fig. 13 Pathways of plasminogen activation. The various pathways leading to plasminogen activation are shown, as well as the inhibitors involved.

degradation products (**FDPs**) are formed (Fig. 12). The FDPs are able to bind to fibrin monomer and inhibit polymerization, thus interfering with fibrin clot formation. Plasmin also has the potential to cleave fibrinogen, but is usually prevented from doing so by the presence of a large molar excess of its fast-acting inhibitor α_2-antiplasmin. When crosslinked fibrin clots are lysed, X-oligomers and D-dimers are formed, and these have been used as clinical markers of increased lysis of fibrin, in contrast to non-specific lysis of fibrinogen.

Plasminogen activators and their inhibitors

There are a number of different plasminogen activators, including tissue plasminogen activator (**t-PA**), urokinase-type plasminogen activator (urokinase, **u-PA**), kallikrein, the kallikrein-activated proactivator, and neutrophil elastase (Fig. 13). In addition there are various exogenous activators such as the bacterial enzyme streptokinase, which binds to plasminogen to form an activator.

t-PA is synthesized by the vascular endothelial cell and released as a single-chain (**sc**) zymogen form, sct-PA. This zymogen is unusual because it has significant proteolytic activity; proteolytic cleavage to a two-chain (**tc**) form (t-PA, or tct-PA) enhances this activity. t-PA release can be stimulated by exercise and mental stress, venous occlusion, vasodilatation, adrenaline, thrombin, and cytokines. In plasma, t-PA is rapidly complexed by various forms of plasminogen-activator inhibitor (**PAI**).

The zymogen form of u-PA (scu-PA) is inactive and must be converted to the two-chain form (tcu-PA or u-PA) by kallikrein or plasmin to exert its activity, which, unlike t-PA, has no requirement for fibrin. u-PA is also found in large amounts in urine (urokinase), from which it was first isolated. u-PA secretion has been demonstrated from fibroblasts, epithelial cells, pneumocytes, and the decidual cells of placenta, but it can be secreted by endothelial cells under certain conditions.

PAI-1 is probably the predominant inhibitor in normal plasma; it is released by endothelial cells, but has a wide tissue distribution, and circulates in molar excess over t-PA. Platelets contain significant amounts of PAI-1, accounting for more than 90 per cent of the total blood PAI-1 concentration. However, the endothelium and liver are probably the main sources of plasma PAI-1.

PAI-2 is primarily a placental protein, and plasma levels are normally negligible, but increase during pregnancy and may be important for haemostasis at the placental interface, during pregnancy and parturition.

Plasminogen activation at fibrin surfaces

In normal blood, t-PA is unable to activate plasminogen because of the excess of PAI-1, and the rapid rate of complex formation. Furthermore, any plasmin that was formed would be rapidly inactivated by the excess α_2-antiplasmin. When a fibrin clot forms, t-PA released locally from the endothelial cells binds to the clot with a higher affinity than its interaction with PAI-1. The affinity of t-PA for plasminogen is increased about 400-fold when fibrin is present. Plasminogen has high- and low-affinity lysine-binding sites, which are responsible for binding to fibrin. Thus both t-PA and plasminogen are bound to fibrin and a cleavage occurs resulting in plasmin formation and fibrin degradation. Approximately 40 to 50 per cent of plasma plasminogen is reversibly bound to histidine-rich glycoprotein, which reduces the concentration of plasminogen available for activation.

The initial plasmin formed can clip the native plasminogen (Glu-plasminogen) to expose carboxy-terminal lysine residues (Lys-plasminogen) for which there are additional binding sites on the fibrin surface. Fibrin is also a cofactor for the conversion of Glu-plasminogen to Lys-plasminogen, and the activation of single-chain u-PA to the active two-chain molecule. Fibrin-bound plasmin is protected from its inhibitor α_2-antiplasmin and can cleave the fibrin clot. As the clot dissolves, the t-PA and plasmin become more accessible to their inhibitors and are complexed. Thus the system ensures that fibrinolysis is localized to the clot that needs to be removed, and native fibrinogen is not proteolysed.

Haemostatic reactions of the endothelial cell

The endothelial cell interacts with haemostasis at a variety of levels and influences all pathways. The luminal surface possesses anticoagulant and antithrombotic activities, and the endothelial cells synthesize and secrete a variety of substances.

The sulphated proteoglycans, including heparan and dermatan sulphates, are synthesized by endothelial cells and are incorporated into the extracellular matrix. Some of these glycosaminoglycans are also attached to the luminal surface of endothelial cells.

Thrombomodulin provides a specific high-affinity binding site for thrombin on the endothelial surface. It neutralizes the procoagulant activity of thrombin, and the complex may be regulated by internalization. When thrombin is bound to thrombomodulin, its activation of protein C is increased by 1000-fold. Activated protein C is able to diffuse away from the endothelium and bind to other phospholipid membranes, where it can cleave factors Va and VIIIa in reactions catalysed by protein S.

The vascular endothelium can synthesize and release t-PA, as well as releasing PAI-1.

Platelets do not adhere to the luminal surface of unperturbed endothelial cells, but will bind to damaged and thrombin-activated cells. The role of arachidonic acid metabolites and their exchange between platelets and endothelial cells in the maintenance of a thromboresistant surface has been relatively well studied. A major metabolite from endothelial cells is prostaglandin I_2 (**PGI_2**, prostacyclin). Cyclic prostaglandin endoperoxides (prostaglandins G_2 and H_2) released from platelets may be taken up by endothelial cells and rapidly converted to PGI_2. The latter is a potent inhibitor of platelet aggregation, adhesion, and secretion, which are mediated by the potentiation of adenylate cyclase after binding to a specific platelet-membrane PGI_2 receptor.

Endothelial cells synthesize tissue factor in response to a variety of agents, in a concentration- and time-dependent, reversible manner. At least 70 per cent of the synthesized tissue factor is expressed in the endothelial-cell membrane.

The endothelial cell is the principal site of synthesis of vWF and high molecular-weight multimers are packaged into structures known as Weible–Palade bodies, before their release into plasma.

Further reading

Bloom, A.L., Forbes C.D., Thomas, D.P., and Tuddenham E.G.D. (ed.) (1994). *Haemostasis and thrombosis*, 3rd edn. Churchill Livingstone, Edinburgh.

Coleman, R.W., Hirsh, J., Marder, V.J., and Salzman, E.W. (ed.) (1994). *Hemostasis and thrombosis—basic principles and clinical practice*, 3rd edn. Lippincott, Philadelphia, PA.

Chapter 3.34

Introduction to disorders of haemostasis and coagulation

S. J. Machin and I. J. Mackie

The normal haemostatic mechanism depends on several overlapping and sequential events including the vessel-wall response to injury, platelet adhesion and aggregation, and activation of the coagulation cascade leading to the generation of thrombin and the formation of fibrin. The haemostatic process is carefully balanced so that haemorrhage is promptly arrested and inappropriate thrombosis does not occur spontaneously. The causes of haemostatic abnormalities are numerous and it is essential to have a standardized initial approach to the clinical and laboratory diagnosis of any bleeding or thrombotic tendency.

Table 1 Screening tests for a bleeding tendency

For platelet disorders	*For coagulation disorders*
1. Bleeding time	1. Prothrombin time
2. Platelet count	2. Activated partial thromboplastin time
3. Fresh blood-film inspection	3. Thrombin time

General approach to the investigation of a bleeding tendency

The initial problem is usually to determine whether bleeding or bruising is due to a local factor, or to an underlying haemostatic abnormality. Often a mild abnormality only becomes apparent after trauma or a local precipitating lesion. Any bleeding disorder may be inherited or acquired and may result from one or more of five basic mechanisms:

(1) thrombocytopenia;

(2) functional platelet abnormality;

(3) blood vessel defect;

(4) coagulation factor(s) defect;

(5) excess fibrinolysis.

A careful clinical history, drug history, and physical examination should be undertaken. Generalized purpura usually reflects a failure of platelet function or number (thrombocytopenia) to maintain the integrity of the small blood vessels. Often the cause of the bleeding will be strongly suspected, but laboratory tests are always required to make a precise diagnosis and to define the severity of any abnormality.

Most patients with inherited disorders present in childhood, often with a family history of a bleeding tendency and excessive bleeding in response to minor operations, dental extractions, or trauma. However, mild defects may sometimes not present until adult life and occasionally in old age, often as a result of a minor trauma or operative procedure. If an inherited disorder is suspected, no effort should be spared to investigate other family members who might also be affected.

Generally, platelet bleeding starts immediately after the initiating event but once controlled it does not recur. By contrast, patients with coagulation-factor abnormalities do not bleed excessively after superficial cutaneous lacerations. However, they do produce internal bleeding or deep-muscle haematomas, and massive superficial bruising develops rather than purpura after minor trauma. Other episodes of internal bleeding, such as haematuria, epistaxis, gastrointestinal and retroperitoneal bleeding, are well-recognized manifestations of a primary coagulation-factor deficiency. This type of bleeding classically occurs up to several hours after the initial trauma and if untreated will, in severe cases, continue unabated for prolonged periods.

Initially a series of simple screening tests that are easy to do and give reliable results should be undertaken. The basic screening procedure outlined in Table 1 should be available in all routine haematology laboratories. If the screening tests suggest an abnormality, further specialized investigations should be performed, as outlined

Table 2 Sensitivity of coagulation screening tests to factor deficiency

Test	Detect abnormalities
Prothrombin time	VII, X, V (II, I)
Partial thromboplastin time	Prekallikrein, high molecular-weight kininogen, XII, XI, IX, VIII (X, V, II, I)
Thrombin time	I, raised FDPs, circulating heparin

FDPs, fibrin(-ogen) degradation products.

below. If the screening tests are all within normal limits it is unlikely that the bleeding tendency is related to a specific haemostatic disorder.

Screening tests for a coagulation-factor defect

This relies routinely on three simple screening tests: the prothrombin time; the activated partial thromboplastin time; and the thrombin time. The prothrombin time is measured by the addition of tissue thromboplastin and calcium ions; it gives an overall assessment of the extrinsic pathway. This test is relatively more sensitive to deficiencies of factors VII, X, and V than to defects of prothrombin or fibrinogen. To enable standardization of oral anticoagulant control, the results of the prothrombin time are often expressed as an international normalized ratio (**INR**). However, INR values should not be used to report prothrombin time tests for the investigation of a bleeding tendency or for patients not receiving oral anticoagulants.

The activated partial thromboplastin time (**APTT**) is measured by adding a platelet substitute reagent (usually a crude phospholipid extract), particulate material that is negatively charged to activate the contact system (such as kaolin, Celite, or ellagic acid), and calcium ions to a citrated plasma sample. This test detects abnormalities of all the coagulation factors except factor VII and XIII, but it is especially sensitive to defects of the early stage of the intrinsic system involving prekallikrein, high molecular-weight kininogen, and factors XII, XI, IX, and VIIIc. If a prolonged APTT is found the test should be repeated with a variable mixture of control normal plasma. This should indicate whether the abnormality is caused by a factor deficiency or an inhibitor, usually IgG in nature, that is inactivating part of the coagulation cascade. A simple factor deficiency will be significantly corrected by the addition of normal plasma, whereas very little correction of the prolonged time will occur if an inhibitor is present. An inhibitor pattern will be shown by inhibitors to a specific clotting factor, usually factor VIII, or non-specifically by a lupus anticoagulant or antiphospholipid antibody, which paradoxically may cause a thrombotic tendency.

The thrombin time is measured by simply adding thrombin and calcium ions to plasma. This test is prolonged by deficiency of fibrinogen (factor I), an abnormal fibrinogen molecule, or by the presence of inhibitors to the action of thrombin such as heparin or fibrin/fibrinogen degradation products. The significance of each of these screening tests is summarized in Table 2. Factor XIII deficiency will not be detected by these tests and if strongly suspected from clinical symptoms, particularly a delay in wound healing, a specific screening test based on the stability of preformed fibrin clots in the presence of acetate or urea should be done.

Whenever one of the screening tests is found to be prolonged the exact nature of the abnormality should be further defined by specific quantitative factor assays.

Screening tests for a platelet disorder

The peripheral platelet count, blood film examination, and the skin bleeding time are the first-line, basic laboratory tests of platelet involvement in haemostatic function. If the results of these tests are within normal limits it is unlikely that a platelet defect is responsible for excessive bleeding. Spurious or pseudothrombocytopenia may occur due to the presence of platelet agglutinins, which are often ethylenediaminetetraacetic acid (**EDTA**)-dependent. The stained blood film will show large clumps of platelets, and a repeat platelet count from a heparinized or citrated blood sample will reveal the true normal platelet count. Although a platelet count of 150×10^9/l is the lower limit of the normal range, spontaneous bleeding due to thrombocytopenia alone is unlikely to occur until the count has fallen below 50×10^9/l—and usually does not occur until it is below 20×10^9/l. Spontaneous bleeding usually occurs initially from the mucous membranes, especially the mouth and gums, often exacerbated by poor oral hygiene, or as skin purpura around areas of local pressure.

If the platelet count is normal or raised, a prolonged bleeding time is suggestive of one of the many congenital or acquired qualitative disorders of platelet function. Other non-platelet haemostatic disorders that may prolong the bleeding time are vascular abnormalities, particularly skin collagen defects, von Willebrand's disease, afibrinogenaemia, dysproteinaemias, severe anaemia, and chronic renal failure. The causes of a prolonged skin bleeding time are summarized in Table 3.

Table 3 Causes of a prolonged skin bleeding time

Thrombocytopenia due to:	Congenital qualitative platelet disorders	Congenital deficiency of coagulation factors	Hereditary connective tissue disorders	Acquired states
Marrow failure Platelet consumption or destruction	Bernard–Soulier syndrome Glazmann's thrombasthenia	von Willebrand's disease Afibrinogenaemia	Ehlers–Danlos syndrome (type III)	Liver failure Uraemia Dysproteinaemia
	Storage-pool disease Gray platelet syndrome	Factor V deficiency	Osteogenesis imperfecta	Myeloproliferative disease Acquired storage-pool disease
	Cyclo-oxygenase deficiency Thromboxane synthase deficiency Others unclassified			Drugs Diet Severe anaemia Polycythaemia (secondary)

When such screening procedures suggest a platelet functional disorder or if there is a high degree of clinical suspicion despite a normal bleeding time and platelet count, further platelet-function tests, particularly aggregation studies, should be planned in a systematic way. Unfortunately, as a preoperative screening test there is no evidence that the bleeding time is a predictor of the risk of haemorrhage. Drugs and certain dietary practices are the most common cause of a prolonged bleeding time and platelet dysfunction. Ideally, patients must refrain from taking drugs with known antiplatelet effects for at least 7 days before blood sampling. Because of the unreliability of the bleeding time in detecting mild degrees of platelet dysfunction, particularly storage-pool disease and some variants of von Willebrand's disease, many investigators will routinely perform platelet-aggregation studies with selective agonists such as ADP, collagen, arachidonic acid, and ristocetin as part of the initial screening test. von Willebrand factor activity should also be quantitated biologically by a ristocetin cofactor assay.

Further reading

Machin, S.J. and Mackie, I.J. (1989). Haemostasis. In *Laboratory haematology* (ed. I. Chanarin), pp. 263–399. Churchill Livingstone, Edinburgh.

Machin, S.J. and Preston, F.E. (1988). Platelet function testing. *Journal of Clinical Pathology*, **41**, 1322–30.

Chapter 3.35

Purpura

S. J. Machin

The term 'purpura' is used to describe small cutaneous extravasations of blood. More extensive cutaneous bleeding, which is often associated with purpura, is called 'ecchymosis', or bruising. Purpura is caused by thrombocytopenia, platelet dysfunction, or a primary cutaneous or vascular disease that may produce or mimic purpuric lesions. The causes of thrombocytopenia are numerous but can be broadly classified into decreased platelet production, diminished platelet survival, or abnormal distribution of the peripheral platelet mass due to hypersplenism. A pathogenic classification of thrombocytopenia is summarized in Table 1. Very often, several causes may be operative in the same patient. Defective platelet production is readily detected by a bone marrow aspirate. It is also possible to identify associated bone marrow disorders such as a haematological neoplasm, secondary carcinoma, alcoholism, or megaloblastic anaemia. These various conditions causing a primary bone marrow defect in platelet production are discussed in detail elsewhere.

Table 1 Pathogenic classification of thrombocytopenia

Defective bone marrow production
1. Megakaryocyte aplasia
2. Dysthrombopoiesis (a) infiltration (b) metabolic
B. *Diminished platelet survival*
1. Immune mediated
2. Excess platelet consumption
3. Structural platelet defects
C. *Loss from the systemic circulation*
1. Splenomegaly
2. Loss from the body—extracorporeal circulation

Table 2 Different types of immune-mediated thrombocytopenia

By autoimmunity
Autoimmune thrombocytopenia
Pseudothrombocytopenia
By alloimmunity
Neonatal alloimmune thrombocytopenia
Post-transfusion purpura
Refractoriness to platelet transfusion therapy
By drug-induced immune mechanisms
Drug-induced thrombocytopenia

Immune-mediated thrombocytopenia

Immune-mediated thrombocytopenia is one of the most commonly encountered haemostatic disorders. The different types are summarized in Table 2. In all these conditions thrombocytopenia is caused by circulating antibody binding to platelet-membrane surface antigen causing increased platelet destruction in the reticuloendothelial system, mainly in the spleen and liver. Antibody binding may also inhibit platelet function, particularly if this blocks the specific receptors of the platelet-activation pathway, usually glycoprotein (**Gp**)-Ib or the -IIb/IIIa complex.

Autoimmune thrombocytopenia

Autoimmune thrombocytopenia, or immune thrombocytopenia, usually presents without any obvious precipitating cause, and hence it is also referred to as 'idiopathic thrombocytopenic purpura', or **ITP**. In children, the disease is often preceded or accompanied by an acute viral infection and occurs equally between the sexes, whereas in adults it occurs more frequently in females and is rarely preceded by an infective illness.

The main objectives of the management of immune thrombocytopenia are to control the bleeding and, at the same time, determine whether the thrombocytopenia is secondary to a remedial cause.

Clinical findings

Immune thrombocytopenia may present with a few purpuric spots or bruises, or much more acutely with extensive purpura and bleeding from the mucous membranes. The skin lesions are widespread, although they tend to be more marked over pressure areas or below the site of a venous tourniquet. Oral lesions present typically as a dark 'blood blister' that bursts and leaves a small, pale, ulcerated region. The major danger is bleeding into the brain. Apart from the haemorrhagic findings there are no other characteristic physical signs; splenomegaly is not usually found and if present suggests that the thrombocytopenia is secondary to another disorder.

Particularly in children, ITP is usually a short, self-limiting illness that lasts up to 1 to 2 weeks and then resolves. A similar pattern may be seen in adults. However, in later life the disorder may follow a much more chronic, relapsing course, when it is referred to as chronic ITP. Chronic ITP may follow an acute episode or may be characterized by relapsing bouts of purpura, with or without bleeding, which may last for many years.

Haematological findings

The presenting platelet count is generally below 50×10^9/l and serious bleeding is unlikely unless the count is below 10×10^9/l. In acute ITP the platelets are larger than normal. Bone marrow aspirate shows increased numbers of megakaryocytes with immature cytoplasm, with evidence that they are producing platelets at an earlier stage of nuclear and cytoplasmic differentiation. Occasionally, normal or reduced numbers of megakaryocytes may be found. This is presumably because the antibody responsible for the thrombocytopenia is also recognizing an antigen expressed on the immature megakaryocyte surface. A bleeding-time test is not routinely done, although occasionally it may be significantly more prolonged than expected from the platelet count. Over the years several different tests have been developed to detect and quantitate the presence of platelet-associated immunoglobulin, but overall these tests have been disappointing and their significance remains uncertain.

Differential diagnosis

In a typical case the diagnosis is straightforward. However, in adults an associated disorder or drug-induced thrombocytopenia (see below) must be excluded.

The main disorders to be excluded are systemic lupus erythematosus (**SLE**), other autoimmune diseases, and lymphoproliferative disorders. Immune thrombocytopenia occurs in approximately 10 per cent of patients with SLE, and in some cases a diagnosis of ITP may precede the development of SLE by several years. The primary antiphospholipid syndrome, diagnosed by a positive lupus anticoagulant test and/or raised anticardiolipin antibodies, may also be associated with an immune thrombocytopenia. About 5 to 8 per cent of patients with immune thrombocytopenia also have a positive direct Coombs' test, which in some cases may be associated with an autoimmune haemolytic anaemia. This is known as Evans' syndrome.

Maternal ITP in pregnancy must be distinguished from incidental thrombocytopenia of pregnancy. This occurs in approximately 5 per cent of healthy women, with mild to moderate thrombocytopenia (usually a platelet count between 80 and 120×10^9/l). These women and their infants all remain well and no specific precautions or further investigations are necessary. Thrombocytopenia occurs frequently with human immunodeficiency virus (**HIV**) infections, with approximately 10 per cent of patients having platelet counts of less than 100×10^9/l due to an immune mechanism at some time during their disease.

Management

The treatment for immune thrombocytopenia depends on the degree of thrombocytopenia and the severity or risk of a major bleeding event. In the acute phase, with a platelet count of below 20×10^9/l, corticosteroids are still the mainstay of therapy. The results of several clinical trials have given rise to conflicting data. There would seem to be no difference between a high- or low-dosage regimen, and a dosage of between 0.25 to 0.5 mg/kg per day for 3 weeks in adults seems to be as effective as any higher dosage regimen. High doses of intravenous immunoglobulin (0.4 g/kg per day for 3 to 5 days) have also been shown to be effective. This response is usually transient and relapse usually occurs 10 to 20 days later. No superior response rates or efficacy have been demonstrated for the use of intravenous human gammaglobulin infusions, and because of the potential risks of viral transmission and high cost they should not be routinely used in the initial management of acute ITP. With a low-dose regimen of oral steroids approximately 60 to 70 per cent of patients achieve a response in their platelet count within 2 to 3 weeks, which in many adults may only be short term. In children, particularly for episodes following an acute viral illness, the acute phase is self-limiting and treatment is only required if the platelet count is dangerously low, or if there is bleeding.

Chronicity is defined as severe thrombocytopenia with platelet counts of less than 20 to 30 $\times$ 10^9/l for more than 6 months in adults and 12 months in children. For these patients splenectomy is the initial treatment of choice. A positive long-term response has been observed after splenectomy in 60 to 70 per cent of patients. There is a long-term risk after splenectomy of acute and chronic bacterial infections, particularly with pneumococcal and meningococcal organisms. As these infections may occasionally be fatal, patients should routinely be vaccinated against pneumococcal infections, preferably 2–3 weeks before splenectomy, and postoperatively they should receive long-term oral penicillin therapy. The 30 per cent or so of patients in whom splenectomy is ineffective pose a difficult long-term therapeutic problem. If the platelet count is above 40 to 50 $\times$ 10^9/l and the patient is asymptomatic, careful follow-up with no therapy is all that is required. Long-term, low-dose oral steroids may be necessary when spontaneous purpura or excessive bleeding occurs. If this is ineffective, or side-effects cause problems, a variety of secondary therapeutic options are available. These include long-term immunosuppression with cyclophosphamide or azathioprine, or the use of vincristine, vinblastine, vitamin C, anti-D infusions, and interferon-α therapy. The success rate with these agents is low.

Alloimmune thrombocytopenia

Alloimmunization against platelet-specific antigens occurs extremely rarely in neonates and after blood transfusion. Most cases are caused by immunization to the platelet antigen PLA1, part of the Gp-IIb/IIIa complex. Between 5 and 10 days after transfusion of a platelet-containing product there is a sudden fall in the platelet count associated with severe bleeding. The patient's own platelets are negative for the antigen involved but are also destroyed by the alloantibody.

Neonatal alloimmune thrombocytopenia results when the mother develops an antibody against a specific antigen on the fetal platelets. These alloantibodies cross the placenta and destroy the fetal platelets, which can result in severe intracerebral haemorrhage, either during fetal life or at the time of delivery. Usually these cases are unsuspected and about 50 per cent occur during the first pregnancy.

Thrombocytopenia due to excessive platelet consumption

Excessive peripheral platelet consumption occurs in acute and chronic disseminated intravascular coagulation (**DIC**) or in the thrombotic microangiopathic syndromes, thrombotic thrombocytopenic purpura, and the haemolytic–uraemic syndrome.

Thrombotic microangiopathies (see also Section 12)

Definition and clinical features

The thrombotic microangiopathies are a range of clinical syndromes characterized by microangiopathic haemolytic anaemia, thrombocytopenia, microvascular thrombosis, and multiple organ dysfunction and failure. Thrombotic thrombocytopenic purpura (TTP) is a rare, multiple system disease that occurs in approximately one per million of the population per year. TTP typically presents with fever, non-immune intravascular haemolytic anaemia associated with fragmented red cells, consumptive thrombocytopenia, renal failure, and various neurological deficits. Widespread microvascular thromboses consist of platelet aggregates and fibrin in capillaries and precapillary arterioles, predominantly involving the kidney, pancreas, adrenal, brain, and heart. The TTP syndrome has been associated with SLE, other connective tissue disorders, pregnancy, and oral contraceptive use. Rarely, there seems to be a familial association. In approximately 10 per cent of patients, multiple, recurrent relapses over prolonged periods have also been reported. However, in the majority of cases there is no known causal event or associated disease process. TTP is found in both sexes of all ages, with a slight predominance in females and a peak incidence between 30 and 40 years of age. It appears that the pathogenesis is the lack of a von Willebrand factor (**vWF**)-cleaving protease that results in unusually large vWF multimers in the circulation.

The haemolytic–uraemic syndrome (**HUS**) is usually defined as the association of thrombocytopenia and haemolytic anaemia with renal dysfunction, although occasional non-renal manifestations may also occur. HUS is more likely to occur in young children after a recent viral or acute gastrointestinal infection. The typical histological microvascular lesions are precipitated by vascular endothelial injury, which can be induced by a variety of infections and in particular those associated with endotoxin or verotoxin production. Occasionally childhood gastroenteritis caused by a verotoxin-producing serotype of *Escherichia coli* or shigellae has been reported to cause epidemic clustering of cases.

Diagnosis

This is suggested by the presence of a microangiopathic haemolytic anaemia, with fragmented red cells and thrombocytopenia, after excluding alternative diagnoses, particularly DIC. A clotting screen, including a thrombin time and fibrinogen level, is almost always within the normal range. There is often a mild increase in the reticulocyte count but the serum lactate dehydrogenase (**LDH**) level is often greatly elevated. Serial measurements of LDH along with haemoglobin levels and reticulocyte and platelet counts are the most valuable laboratory tests for assessing disease severity and response to therapy.

Treatment

The mainstay of treatment for acute TTP is plasma infusion or exchange with fresh frozen plasma. Recent multicentre clinical trials have shown that plasma exchange with approximately 3 litres of fresh frozen plasma daily gives a response rate of approximately 80 per cent, compared to approximately 60 per cent with fresh frozen plasma infusions alone. Although not as effective as plasma exchange, plasma infusion alone may be effective in mild cases and may also be useful as regular prophylaxis in patients with relapsing TTP. The unusually large multimers of vWF can be removed by plasma exchange, and the vWF cleaving protease is a component of normal fresh frozen plasma.

Unfortunately, despite an initial response to plasma exchange, some patients have an incomplete resolution and a prompt relapse. For refractory cases, high-dose steroids, vincristine, splenectomy, antiplatelet agents, or immunosuppressive therapy with a variety of drugs such as cyclophosphamide or azathioprine have occasionally been reported to be successful. Cases unresponsive to fresh frozen plasma infusions may respond to cryosupernatant. Cryosupernatant has processing activity for the unusually large multimers of vWF, but it lacks any actual vWF. Platelet transfusions are contraindicated because infusion of platelet concentrates may exacerbate the process and cause rapidly fatal, widespread microvascular thrombosis.

Table 3 Conditions in which acquired qualitative platelet disorders occur

• Uraemia	***Dysproteinaemias***
Myeloproliferative disorders	• Amyloid
• Essential thrombocythaemia	• Acquired von Willebrand syndrome
• Polycythaemia rubra vera	• Acquired storage-pool disease
• Chronic myeloid leukaemia	• Liver disease
• Myelofibrosis	• Autoimmune platelet disorders
Acute leukaemia	• Drugs
• Myelodysplasia	• Extracorporeal circulation

Excessive loss of platelets from the systemic circulation

Hypersplenism

Normally, approximately one-third of the total circulating platelet mass is in the spleen. Splenomegaly from any cause, particularly if the spleen is more than 4 cm enlarged, is often accompanied by thrombocytopenia. The principal cause is intrasplenic pooling of platelets, but occasionally accelerated destruction may also occur.

Acquired qualitative platelet defects

Abnormalities in platelet function with a normal or raised platelet count causing purpura and episodes of bleeding have been reported in a large number of acquired disorders. Frequently the specific biochemical defect in platelet function causing the abnormality is poorly understood. The conditions in which qualitative platelet disorders are recognized are listed in Table 3.

Uraemia

Many qualitative platelet defects have been recorded in renal failure, but the most important determinant of uraemic bleeding is low haematocrit, below 0.20, that frequently accompanies long-standing renal failure. The prolonged bleeding time in these patients is corrected by blood transfusion or the administration of recombinant erythropoietin to correct the anaemia. In addition, platelets show defective aggregation to adrenaline, collagen, and ADP; ristocetin-induced agglutination may also be impaired. An infusion of desmopressin (deamino-D-arginine vasopressin, **DDAVP**) may reduce the bleeding time in uraemia by promoting a rise of the circulating larger multimers of plasma vWF released from the vascular endothelial cells.

The precise uraemic retention product responsible for these platelet functional defects has not been identified, although it is believed to be the so-called middle molecules with molecular weights of between 500 and 5000.

Myeloproliferative disorders

Platelet defects associated with bleeding episodes as well as thromboembolic complications have been recognized in association with all the myeloproliferative disorders. Unfortunately, laboratory evidence of platelet dysfunction does not always correlate with bleeding. The most consistent defect of platelet aggregation is an impaired response to adrenaline.

Dysproteinaemias

Any cause of a raised paraprotein concentration may lead to a quantitative platelet defect. Paraproteins may bind to the platelet membrane and interfere with the normal function of specific receptors on the membrane surface. As platelets possess Fc receptors it has been proposed that paraproteins may specifically bind to them, and that inhibition of other activation receptors is merely mechanical. There is a high frequency of bleeding in IgA multiple myeloma and Waldenström's macroglobulinaemia in particular. Acute bleeding episodes can be controlled by plasma exchange and chronic bleeding by specific chemotherapy to reduce the paraprotein level.

Acquired von Willebrand's disease (see Chapter 3.37)

There are now several reports of von Willebrand's disease appearing in older people with no previous manifestations of a bleeding problem. The reported underlying mechanisms include an inhibitor, usually a paraprotein, against vWF, or accelerated clearance of that factor from the circulation by binding to abnormal lymphoid cells. Treatment of bleeding episodes with steroids, plasma exchange, and replacement with factor VIII concentrate containing significant quantities of vWF have been successful. Long-term immunosuppression and treatment of the primary underlying condition may lead to remission in the von Willebrand syndrome.

Acquired storage-pool disease

Deficiencies in both dense- and α-granule content, or a defect in their secretion, have been reported in several disorders as an acquired defect. These conditions include autoimmune disorders, particularly chronic idiopathic thrombocytopenia, DIC, TTP, chronic alcoholism, and various haematological malignancies. The depletion of platelet-granule contents has also been reported in patients with severe valvular disease, Dacron aortic grafts, and after cardiac–pulmonary bypass procedures.

Liver disease

Chronic liver disease is usually associated with excessive bleeding due to multiple deficiencies of blood coagulation factors, their inhibitors, and fibrinolysis. However, a variety of platelet functional abnormalities may significantly contribute to the increased bleeding tendency.

Drugs that inhibit platelet function

Many drugs have been shown to affect platelet function and these may occasionally precipitate bleeding. The most important are listed in OTM3, p.3629, Table 4 (and see also Further reading).

Non-thrombocytopenic vascular purpura

A variety of general medical conditions can result in widespread clinical purpura and must be distinguished from thrombocytopenia or platelet functional disorders. These include congenital or acquired primary disorders of blood vessels, connective tissue disorders, metabolic diseases, allergic diseases, or psychogenic bleeding disorders. The vascular defects that cause purpura are listed in Table 4.

Table 4 Vascular defects that may cause purpura

- Simple easy bruising
- Senile purpura
- Hereditary haemorrhagic telangiectasia
- Giant cavernous haemangioma

Hereditary connective tissue disorders

- Ehlers–Danlos syndrome
- Pseudoxanthoma elasticum
- Osteogenesis imperfecta
- Marfan's syndrome
- Scurvy
- Amyloid
- Dysproteinaemias
- Steroid therapy

Infections

- Streptococcal
- Viral
- Allergic vasculitis
- Psychogenic

Simple easy bruising

Purpuric lesions frequently occur in normal people, usually women. Single or multiple bruises appear spontaneously, mainly on the arms or legs, which rapidly resolve without any specific treatment. Those patients who consult physicians are usually exceedingly anxious or concerned for cosmetic reasons. No changes are found in the haemostatic screening tests and the patients should be reassured.

Senile purpura

Senile purpura is often found in older people, usually on areas exposed to mild but recurrent trauma such as the backs of the hands, the forearms, and the face. The purpura is caused by atrophy of the subcutaneous tissue with progressive loss of collagen and elastin fibres in the skin, which leads to inadequate support of the subcutaneous blood vessels. Mild shearing forces lead to rupture, and subcutaneous extravasation and spread of blood. There are no abnormalities in the haemostatic screening tests, although the skin bleeding time may be prolonged. The lesions retain their dark colour, often for several weeks, and unfortunately there is no specific therapy.

Hereditary haemorrhagic telangiectasia (Osler–Rendu–Weber syndrome)

This is a rare condition that is transmitted as an autosomal dominant trait. It presents with typical telangiectasiae that are found in the mucous membranes of the nose, lips, mouth, the whole of the gastrointestinal tract, urinary tract, vagina, and skin. The most common presentations are recurrent epistaxis or prolonged and progressive gastrointestinal bleeding from multiple sites, which lead to refractory chronic iron-deficiency anaemia. The standard coagulation screening tests are within normal limits. Repeated episodes of internal bleeding may have to be controlled by endoscopy or local cautery. Some patients respond to oral oestrogen therapy, which has been shown to convert columnar epithelium to stratified squamous epithelium.

Hereditary connective tissue disorders

There are several rare but readily recognized connective tissue disorders, including the Ehlers–Danlos syndrome, pseudoxanthoma elasticum, osteogenesis imperfecta, and Marfan's syndrome. All these can be present or be associated with recurrent purpura or skin bruising.

Metabolic causes of purpura

Severe scurvy, or vitamin C deficiency, typically presents with excessive bleeding from multiple sites including the gums, alimentary tract, joints, and brain. Perifollicular skin bleeding is also common. Although the bleeding time may be prolonged, the results of studies of platelet function are within normal limits. The diagnosis is confirmed by measuring leucocyte vitamin C concentrations and the bleeding rapidly responds to vitamin C supplements in the diet.

Primary and secondary amyloid can both cause skin purpura. Amyloid may be found infiltrating the small blood vessels and has also been shown to cause platelet functional abnormalities due to membrane coating by the amyloid fibrils.

Long-term administration of corticosteroids over several months causes atrophy of the collagen fibres that support the blood vessels in the skin. This causes widespread purpura and bruises, usually on the extensor surfaces on the hands, arms, and thighs. The purpura is similar in aetiology to the senile type. A similar distribution may also be seen in Cushing's syndrome.

Allergic purpuras

Various allergic vasculitic purpuras are caused by inflammation and infiltration of the blood-vessel wall as an anaphylactic reaction to a variety of agents including chemicals, toxins, infections, and physical stimuli. Henoch–Schönlein purpura is probably the most common and involves the skin, joints, alimentary tract, kidneys, heart, and central nervous system. There is often a preceding upper respiratory tract infection caused by a β-haemolytic streptococcus producing a rising antistreptolysin-O titre. Epidemics may occur in young children, with a fever followed by a purpuric rash that is often raised to the touch and classically affects the fronts of the legs, thighs, and buttocks. In addition, the patient may develop acute arthritis, gastrointestinal pain, and nephritis associated with proteinuria. The disease is usually self-limiting.

Psychogenic purpura

Most of these patients have a disturbed or overanxious personality. Very often the diagnosis is only suspected after numerous investigations have been made with all the results being within the normal range, despite continuing worrying and sometimes bizarre bleeding symptoms.

Further reading

McCrae, K.R. and Cines, D.B. (1994). Drug-induced thrombocytopenias. In *Thrombosis and hemorrhage* (ed. J. Loscalzo and A.I. Schafer), pp. 545–73. Blackwell Scientific, Cambridge, MA.

McMillan, R. and Imbach, P.A. (1994). Immune thrombocytopenic purpura. In *Thrombosis and hemorrhage* (ed. J. Loscalzo and A.I. Schafer), pp. 575–95. Blackwell Scientific, Cambridge, MA.

Moake, J.L. (1994). Thrombotic microangiopathies: thrombotic thrombocytopenic purpura and the hemolytic-uremic syndrome. In *Thrombosis and hemorrhage* (ed. J. Loscalzo and A.I. Schafer), pp. 517–27. Blackwell Scientific, Cambridge, MA.

Chapter 3.36

The pathogenesis of genetic disorders of coagulation

I. Peake

Qualitative or quantitative defects of the coagulation factors generally result in bleeding disorders. There are only three common and important genetic diseases of this type: factor VIII deficiency (haemophilia A), factor IX deficiency (haemophilia B), and von Willebrand's disease (von Willebrand factor deficiency). Although von Willebrand factor (**vWF**) is not strictly a coagulation factor, being involved in the primary haemostatic processes of platelet–subendothelium and platelet–platelet interactions, the disease is usually considered as a disorder of coagulation, particularly because, as discussed below, vWF and factor VIII have a physiological association.

The haemophilias are X-linked diseases that occur almost exclusively in males; female carriers are usually asymptomatic. Some 30 per cent of patients have no family history; that is, their disease results from new mutations. von Willebrand's disease shows a complex pattern of autosomal inheritance (usually dominant) and is the most common inherited human bleeding disorder, with up to 1 per cent of the population in some countries affected by a mild form. Haemophilias A and B show an incidence of 1 in 5000 and 1 in 30 000 males, respectively. Defects of other coagulation factors, such as factor V, VII, X, XI, are rare. They all follow an autosomal recessive pattern of inheritance.

Haemophilia A

Inheritance and diagnosis

Haemophilia A is due to a deficiency of coagulation factor VIII, which functions in the coagulation system as a cofactor with activated factor IX, phospholipid, and calcium in the activation of factor X. As discussed in Chapter 3.36, factor VIII deficiency can result in a life-threatening bleeding disorder and requires frequent and expensive treatment. Diagnosis is based on plasma factor VIII measurement using a variety of assays based either on procoagulant activity or, less commonly, on immunoassay. In general, levels of factor VIII correlate well with the frequency and severity of bleeding, and in most cases levels of biological activity correspond with immunological assay. Only in a few cases is functionally defective factor VIII seen; the so-called cross-reacting, material-positive (**crm+**) form, as factor VIII can be detected by an antibody reaction but not biologically.

Although carriers of haemophilia A will usually have reduced levels of factor VIII, on average to 50 per cent of the normal level, the wide normal range in plasma levels of that factor (50 to 200 per cent of normal) and the phenomenon of lyonization (random inactivation of one X-chromosome at an early stage of female embryogenesis), means that only some 80 per cent of carriers will have significantly reduced levels. Even when combined with the measurement of vWF (of value because the levels of factor VIII and vWF are linked in plasma), phenotypic assessment of carrier status carries only a 90 per cent probability. The advent of factor VIII gene analysis has significantly improved this assessment (see below).

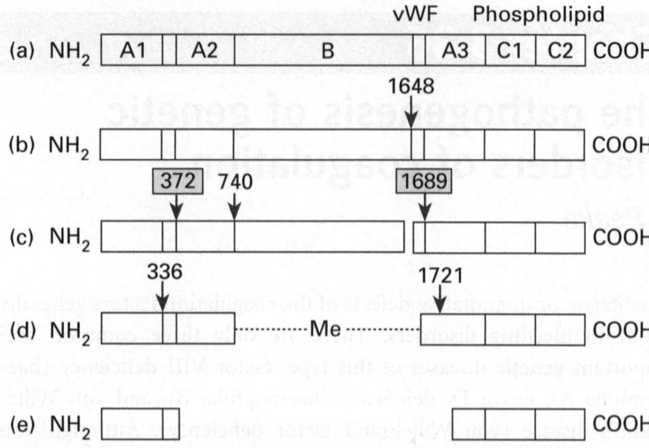

Fig. 1 A diagram showing the functional domains (von Willebrand factor (vWF) and phospholipid) and activation/inactivation of factor VIII (FVIII). (a) Full-length inert FVIII protein. (b) and (c) FVIII cleaved at residue 1648 by unknown protease to give heavy (A1, A2, B) and light chains (A3, C1, C2). (c) and (d) Activated FVIII after thrombin cleavage at residues 372, and 1689 and 740. (d) and (e) Inactivation of FVIII by cleavage at residues 336 by activated protein C and 1771 by factor Xa (and or thrombin).

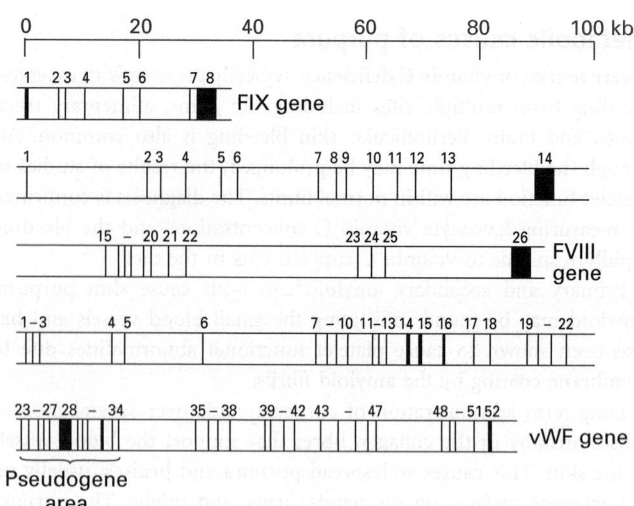

Fig. 2 Diagrammatic representation of the genes for factor (F) IX, VIII, and von Willebrand (vWF). Exons are numbered.

The molecular basis of haemophilia A

Factor VIII protein

Attempts to purify factor VIII from plasma were difficult, given the low plasma concentration and high instability of the protein. The cloning of the factor VIII gene and the sequencing of the cDNA, first reported in 1984, was therefore a major advance, and from the cDNA sequence, the amino acid sequence, size, and domain structure of the protein was deduced. Factor VIII is a glycoprotein (330 kDa) consisting in its native form in plasma of 2332 amino acids with three identifiable domain types in the sequence A1–A2–B–A3–C1–C2. Cleavage of an amino-terminal 19 amino-acid signal peptide occurs before release from the hepatocyte, where factor VIII is predominantly synthesized. Factor VIII circulates in plasma predominantly in a two-chain, metal-associated form (heavy (A1, A2, B) and light (A3, C1, C2)) in association with vWF. Thrombin activation of factor VIII by cleavage at two specific sites (Fig. 1) not only results in activation of the protein, but also dissociation of vWF.

Factor VIII gene

This is some 186 kb in length and is situated on the long arm of the X-chromosome. It encodes an mRNA of 9 kb and the gene itself comprises 26 exons (Fig. 2). Notable features of the gene are the large exon 14 (3.1 kb), which encodes the whole of domain B, and intron 22 (32 kb), which contains within itself the start points for two further genes, one entirely contained within the intron and apparently expressed in most tissues (*F8A*), and a second beginning within the intron and utilizing exons 23 to 26 of the factor VIII gene itself (*F8B*).

The genetic basis of haemophilia A

The majority of patients with haemophilia A have low or undetectable plasma levels of factor VIII protein. Only in crm+ patients can defective protein be identified, and even in these cases analysis of the small amount of protein obtained has proved to be extremely difficult. Our present knowledge concerning the defects causing haemophilia A is therefore almost entirely based on analysis of the factor VIII gene.

Since the factor VIII gene was cloned and DNA probes became available, a steady stream of mutations has been reported, and are now included on an Internet database that is updated annually (http://europium.mrc.rpms.ac.uk/).

No specific 'hot-spot' for mutations are apparent, although over 30 per cent of point mutations are at CpG dinucleotide sequences. Most missense mutations resulting in an amino acid change cause protein instability and only a few are associated with dysfunctional factor VIII molecules, explaining the relatively low proportion of crm+ patients alluded to above.

In almost 50 per cent of cases of severe haemophilia A, there is an apparent defect within intron 22, which leads to a failure in transcription across this intron. This has been shown to result from an inversion of a section of the X-chromosome at the tip of the long arm. This inversion results in separation of the factor VIII gene into two parts, separated by over 500 kb of DNA and is the cause of haemophilia A in almost half of severe cases.

Carrier detection and prenatal diagnosis of haemophilia A

Family studies in an X-linked disease such as haemophilia, resulting in precise assessment of carrier status and offering the option of prenatal diagnosis, can have a major impact on the medical, psychological, and social consequences of the disease. It has been estimated that for each patient an average of five to six potential carriers are present in the population. Obligate carriers (daughters of haemophiliacs or mothers of a haemophilic child with a maternal history of the disease) can be identified from the family tree. Possible carriers (daughters of carriers, female relatives of haemophiliacs on his maternal side, mothers with one haemophiliac son and no family history of the disease) require laboratory investigation to determine their carrier status.

Phenotypic assessment of carrier status in haemophilia A can be made by analysing plasma levels of factor VIII, because carriers will, on average, have 50 per cent of the normal female level. This method will only identify some 80 per cent of obligate carriers with certainty. The most precise method is to use gene analysis to identify the causative mutation within the patient's factor VIII gene, and to then analyse the potential carrier's gene for the same defect. This is now possible in some cases particularly where the chromosome inversion has occurred (see above), and with improving technology is becoming increasingly feasible. Where such techniques are unavailable, haemophilia gene tracking can be done by DNA polymorphism analysis.

Over 90 per cent of females are heterozygous (informative) for at least one of the FVIII gene polymorphisms, and therefore in haemophilia A families the affected gene can be tracked in the majority of cases.

Haemophilia B

Inheritance and diagnosis

Haemophilia B is an X-linked deficiency of factor IX and is clinically indistinguishable from haemophilia A. Factor IX functions at the same point in the coagulation system as factor VIII but as a serine protease, which, when activated, activates factor X (in the presence of activated factor VIII, calcium, and phospholipid). The diagnosis is made by measuring circulating levels of biologically active and/or immunologically detectable protein, the two measurements usually being in agreement, although crm+ haemophilia B is seen overall in about 25 per cent of patients. Carriers of haemophilia B have, on average, 50 per cent of the normal level of factor IX. However, as discussed earlier for haemophilia A, diagnosis of carrier status by factor IX assay is not optimal because only 70 to 80 per cent of obligate carriers have significantly reduced levels.

The molecular basis of haemophilia B

Factor IX protein

Factor IX is synthesized in the liver as one of the vitamin K-dependent serine proteases and is homologous to coagulation factors II (prothrombin), VII, X, and to protein C. The protein produced within the hepatocyte contains 454 amino acids. A short signal peptide and a propeptide, responsible for correct secretion from the cell and for γ-carboxylation (see below), respectively, are cleaved from the aminoterminal end before release from the cell, leaving a 415 amino-acid factor IX protein to circulate in the blood. This mature protein contains several, well-recognized functional domains (listed from amino- to carboxy-terminal): a γ-carboxylated glutamic acid (**Gla**) region containing 12 such residues and involved in phospholipid binding; two epidermal growth factor-like domains; an activation domain cleaved when factor IX is activated by factor XIa; and a serine protease or catalytic domain responsible for converting factor X to Xa.

Factor IX gene

This is on the long arm of the X-chromosome at Xq27 and contains eight exons encoding an mRNA of about 1.8 kb. The complete sequence of the gene (33 kb) has been determined.

The genetic basis of haemophilia B

The factor IX gene is a simple gene and has lent itself to detailed analysis using the polymerase chain reaction (**PCR**)-based procedures. As a result, in practically all cases of haemophilia B a genetic mutation can be found within the factor IX gene, or within its promoter regions.

The haemophilia B database (at http://www.umds.ac.uk/molgen/) contains details of many reported FIX gene mutations found in haemophilia B. Some 55 per cent of all entries and 32 per cent of unique mutations involve CpG dinucleotides. All nonsense mutations cause severe disease, and most missense mutations resulting in amino acid changes dramatically affect protein stability or release. Of the several unique mutations in the short 5' promoter region of the gene, almost all give rise to the 'Leyden' phenotype, characterized by the disappearance of the haemophilia after puberty.

Carrier detection and prenatal diagnosis of haemophilia B

To date, seven restriction fragment length polymorphisms (**RFLPs**) have been described within or directly flanking the factor IX gene, and, when all are used, over 90 per cent of females are heterozygous: in other words, informative for at least one. Because the complete DNA sequence of the gene is known, all are readily detected by PCR-based, DNA-amplification procedures.

von Willebrand's disease (vWD)

Inheritance and diagnosis

von Willebrand's disease is an autosomally transmitted bleeding disorder, usually inherited in a dominant fashion. Severe cases are rare though the incidence of mild vWD has been estimated to be as high as 1 per cent in some populations. It is caused by a qualitative and/or quantitative deficiency of von Willebrand factor—a multifunctional, multimeric plasma glycoprotein, of molecular weight from 5×10^5 to 20×10^7, synthesized within vascular endothelial cells and megakaryocytes. von Willebrand factor has two primary roles in haemostasis. First, it functions in primary haemostasis by binding both to platelets via the glycoprotein (**Gp**)-Ib, platelet-surface receptor and to exposed subendothelial matrix via collagen IV. This has the effect of bringing platelets into contact with exposed subendothelium and initiates the primary haemostatic process. It also mediates in platelet–platelet binding. Any defect in this process, such as defective von Willebrand factor in vWD, will result in poor primary haemostasis and a prolonged skin bleeding time. The second function of vWF is to bind to factor VIII and to protect it from destructive proteolysis after its release from the hepatocyte. Only after factor VIII has been activated by thrombin is vWF released. As a result of this close association, levels of factor VIII are often reduced in vWD in line with levels of vWF when compared to normal plasma levels, although there is a 50 times molar excess of vWF.

The diagnosis of vWD is often based initially on a prolonged skin bleeding time, reduced levels of plasma factor VIII, and autosomal inheritance. Qualitative and quantitative assessment of vWF is then made both immunologically (as vWF antigen) and by a functional test that relies on the ability of the factor to cause normal platelets to agglutinate (aggregate) in the presence of the antibiotic ristocetin. The ristocetin cofactor assay has been shown to be the best assessment of the biological activity of vWF in the disease when results are compared with the patient's skin bleeding time and history of bleeding.

In recent years, sophisticated tests have been established to assess the quality of von Willebrand factor in vWD. Of particular importance has been analysis of the multimer structure of vWF by gel electrophoretic separation of the multimers and their detection with specific labelled antibodies.

Classification of von Willebrand's disease (vWD)

A summary of the present classification of vWD as recommended by the vWD Sub-Committee of the ISTH is given in Table 1. This

Table 1 Diagnosis and molecular basis of von Willebrand disease

Type	Diagnostic criteria	Inheritance	Location of mutations
Type 1	Quantitative deficiency of VWF	Autosomal dominant or recessive	Generally unknown, no specific region
Type 2A	Qualitative defect of VWF Reduced platelet binding Lack of HMW VWF multimers	Autosomal dominant	A2 domain
Type 2B	Qualitative defect of VWF Decreased platelet binding	Autosomal dominant	A1 domain Cys509–Cys695 loop region
Type 2N	Qualitative defect	Autosomal recessive	FVIII binding domain D'–D3
Type 2M	Qualitative defect Reduced platelet binding Normal VWF multimer profile	Autosomal dominant	A1 domant
Type 3	Severe quantitative deficiency of VWF	Autosomal recessive	Throughout VWF gene e.g. deletion, terminal codon

classification is essentially based on vWF quantity, quality, and functionality (as observed by its ability to bind to platelets and FVIII in particular). Multimer profiles are of secondary importance but clearly reflect and, in part, can explain the properties of the vWF in each type of disease.

Types 1 and 3 VWD refer to partial or practically complete quantitative deficiency of plasma vWF, respectively. Type 1 represents over 70 per cent of all cases and may be present in up to 1 per cent of some populations. Type-3 VWD, however, is very rare with a reported incidence of approximately 1.5 per million population. Type 2 refers to qualitative vWF deficiency and is subdivided into four categories depending on the physiological properties of the vWF protein. Types 2A and 2M are variants having vWF with decreased platelet-binding ability, either with (type 2M) or without (type 2A) high molecular-weight vWF multimers. Type 2B refers to individuals with plasma vWF showing increased platelet-binding ability (to Gp-Ib/IX) and often shows loss of high molecular-weight multimers. Type-2N vWF has reduced FVIII-binding properties, often absent in the homozygous state. vWF multimer profiles are normal, as they are in type-1 disease.

Inheritance patterns are either dominant (type 1, 2A, 2B) or recessive (type-3 and type-2N families and some type-1 families). The overall picture is often complicated, particularly in type-1 families, where considerable variability in clinical symptoms and disease penetrance can be seen. Compound heterozygosity can be a confounding issue, and dominant negative effects (see below) can perhaps explain the patterns seen in some type-1 families.

The molecular basis of vWD

von Willebrand factor protein

von Willebrand factor (vWF) circulates in plasma as a series of multimers, each composed of a number of 230-kDa subunits joined initially at the carboxy terminal ends by disulphide bonds to give a dimer, and then at the amino terminal end of the dimers to form multimers of increasing length and size. The primary translation product of the vWF gene is a 2813 pre-pro-polypeptide, consisting of a 22 amino-acid signal peptide (necessary for the correct passage of vWF through the cell), a 741-residue propeptide, and the 2050-residue subunit found in all mature plasma and platelet vWF.

The vWF protein has four types of homologous domains (A, B, C, and D), all present in multiple copies, as indicated in Fig. 3. The

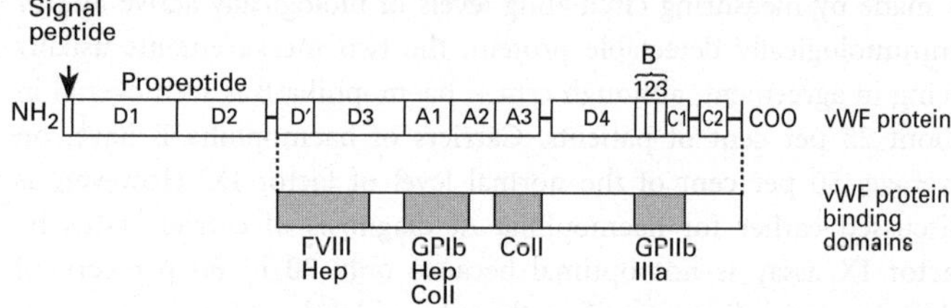

Fig. 3 A diagrammatic representation of pre-pro-vWF showing functional domains and regions of homology. FVIII, FVIII-binding domain; Hep, heparin-binding domain; Coll, collagen-binding domain; Gp-Ib-, platelet Gp Ib-binding domain; Gp-IIb -IIIa, platelet Gp IIb-, IIIa-binding domain.

functional domains of the protein have been identified using synthetic peptides and specific monoclonal antibodies and are also summarized in Fig. 3.

von Willebrand factor gene

The gene for vWF is found on human chromosome 12 (12p12-pter), although there is also a partial, non-translated pseudogene on chromosome 22, which shows only a 3.1 per cent divergence in sequence to the vWF gene. The gene is large and complex, spanning about 180 kb of DNA and containing 52 exons. The pseudogene is 21 to 29 kb in length, covering exons 23 to 34 of the complete gene (amino acids 227 to 1184).

The genetic basis of vWD

Analysis of von Willebrand factor from patients with vWD at a molecular level has not been possible and gene analysis, given its size and complexity, has proved difficult. A database of vWF mutations in patients with VWD can be found at http://mmg2.im.med.umich.edu/vwf. Southern blotting using complete and partial cDNA probes has identified a few complete or partial gene deletions in patients with severe type-3 vWD. However, PCR-based analysis of specific exons encoding known functional domains of the protein, and also reverse transcriptase (RT)-PCR of vWF mRNA from platelets, presumably originating from the parental megakaryocyte, have recently resulted in some interesting findings. To date, no defects have been identified in the vWF gene of patients with type-1 disease. Detailed analysis of exon 28, which encodes the A1 and A2 domains of the protein, has revealed missense mutations in almost all patients studied with type 2A and type 2B. The mutations in the type-2B patients are restricted to the loop region of the A1 domain, while those present in patients with type 2A are mainly in the A2 region between residues 742 and 875.

Type-2N VWD is now recognized to be more common than first thought, particularly as its resemblance to mild haemophilia A has led to the rediagnosis of several families. Point mutations are all within exons 18 to 23 encoding the first 272 residues of the mature vWF subunit. These cause missense mutations which result in reduced binding to factor VIII.

Carrier detection and prenatal diagnosis in vWD

von Willebrand's disease is usually inherited in a dominant fashion and thus carrier detection is unnecessary. Only in type 3 is recessive inheritance seen and in those rare cases, where the genetic basis of the disease is unknown, heterozygote diagnosis and prenatal diagnosis for a fetus at risk of severe disease can be made.

Other coagulation-factor deficiencies

Deficiencies of other factors involved in blood coagulation are rare and are inherited in an autosomal recessive manner. Deficiencies of prothrombin, factor X, factor VII, and factor V usually only result in clinical bleeding in the homozygous or compound heterozygous states. Heterozygotes, rather like carriers of haemophilia A or B, are usually asymptomatic. The genetic basis of the deficiencies has been revealed in a few cases, particularly in relation to factor XI deficiency, which, although rare, is found at a high frequency in Ashkenazim Jews, amongst whom 0.1 to 0.5 per cent are homozygous (9.5–13.5 per cent heterozygous). Heterozygotes are asymptomatic or have a very mild bleeding tendency, while homozygotes (or compound heterozygotes) show a considerable bleeding tendency. Two mutations within the factor XI gene (a change in the intron donor sequence in intron 14, and a nonsense mutation at codon Glu117) account for about half of the genetic changes in the abnormal factor XI genes.

Further reading

Antonarakis, S.E. and a consortium of more than 50 international authors (1995). Factor VIII gene inversions in severe haemophilia A: results of an international consortium study. *Blood*, **86**, 2206–12.

Forbes, C.D., Aledort, L., and Madhok, (ed.) (1998). *Haemophilia.* Chapman and Hall, London.

Sadler, J.E. (1998). Biochemistry and genetics of von Willebrand factor. *Annu. Rev. Biochem.*, **67**, 395–424.

Chapter 3.37

Clinical features and management of the hereditary disorders of haemostasis

G. F. Savidge

Hereditary disorders of primary haemostasis (Table 1)

Disorders characterized by platelet-adhesion defects

von Willebrand's disease (**vWD**) (Table 2)

This heterogeneous condition is the most common inherited bleeding disorder, with a prevalence of up to 125 per million of the world's population. It is characterized by quantitative and/or qualitative abnormalities in platelet, endothelial, and plasma von Willebrand factor (**vWF**) that prevent the binding of glycoprotein (**Gp**)-Ib to the subendothelial matrix, whereby the bleeding time becomes abnormally prolonged. Low levels of circulating factor VIII may occur due to the absence of vWF, which normally acts as a carrier protein and stabilizer for this factor.

The most common clinical symptoms are mucocutaneous haemorrhage, prolonged bleeding after minor trauma or surgical procedures, menorrhagia, and postpartum haemorrhage. Spontaneous bleeding into joints and muscles is unusual, but may occur with low levels of circulating factor VIII. Severe bleeding is unusual, and death from uncontrolled haemorrhage rare. In the common subtypes, symptoms decrease significantly after adolescence with normalization of plasma levels of vWF. vWD is subdivided into severe or mild disease, and treatment is determined by the nature of clinical symptoms and the specific subtype. The diagnosis is based upon the mode of inheritance, screening tests, platelet-function assays, plasma factor VIII levels, and measurements of plasma and platelet vWF (Table 2).

vWD types

Type-1 vWD. This 'classic' form of vWD, constituting some 75 per cent of all cases, is inherited as an autosomal dominant trait. Reduced levels of plasma vWF activity and antigenicity occur, with a concordant decrease in circulating factor VIII. The bleeding time is variably prolonged and related to clinical severity. Multimers of plasma vWF are fully identifiable, but in variably reduced concentrations. The therapeutic response to deamino-d-arginine vasopressin (**DDAVP**) is good, with an increase in plasma vWF activity and antigenicity, and in circulating factor VIII levels, with normalization of vWF multimers and the bleeding time

Type-2 vWD. This entity, comprising some 25 per cent of all cases vWD, is due to a qualitative defect in vWF. It is subdivided into types 2A, 2B, 2M, and 2N.

Type-2A vWD variant

In Type 2A, the mode of inheritance is autosomal dominant. Mutations have been reported, generally in the 134 amino-acid segment of the vWF-A2 homologous repeat. Large- and intermediate-sized multimers of vWF are absent from the plasma and platelets, while biologically

Table 1 Hereditary disorders of primary haemostasis

Disorder	Defined	Platelet count	Platelet size	Clot retraction	Aggregation studies: ADP	Aggregation studies: Collagen	Aggregation studies: Ristocetin	Serotonin release
von Willebrand's disease (vWD)	Abnormal von Willebrand factor	N but ↓ in type 2B and pseudo-vWD	Usually N	N	N	N	↓	N
Bernard-Soulier syndrome	GpIb, GpIX and GpV deficiency	↓	↑	N	N	N	Absent	N
Gray platelet syndrome	Absent α-granules	↓	N or ↑	N	↓	↓	N	↓
Storage pool deficiency	Reduced number of platelet dense bodies	N	N	N	N but ↓ 2 ° aggregation	↓	N	↓
Glanzmann's thrombasthenia	GpIIb-IIIa deficiency	N	N	Absent (type I) ↓ (type II)	Absent	Absent	N	N
Afibrinogenaemia	Plasma and platelet fibrinogen deficiency	N or ↓	N	N	Absent	Absent	Absent	N

↑ = increased values
↓ = decreased values
N= normal values
Gp = glycoprotein

inactive, smaller multimers are structurally abnormal. The bleeding time is prolonged, and both vWF reactivity to ristocetin and ristocetin-induced platelet aggregation (**RIPA**) are reduced. Therapeutic response to DDAVP is variable, although plasma levels of vWF antigen may increase.

Type-2B vWD variant

Unlike other forms of vWD, type 2B is characterized by increased reactivity between platelet Gp-Ib and the defective vWF. Type-2B mutations are clustered within a short segment of the homologous vWF-A I domain encoded entirely within exon 28, and the mode of inheritance is autosomal dominant. Platelets aggregate in response to lower concentrations of ristocetin than normal. Plasma multimers of vWF are usually of both low and intermediate size. The disorder presents with quite severe symptoms. DDAVP therapy is contra-indicated because the induced release of abnormal but highly reactive vWF from the endothelium may cause thrombocytopenia.

Type-2N vWD variant

This recently described variant is characterized by the inability of vWF to complex fully with circulating factor VIII. The genetic defect in the structure of the factor VIII-binding site on vWF is found exclusively in family members with an apparently phenotypic mild haemophilia, but with an autosomal recessive inheritance trait. Haemorrhagic symptoms are usually mild and are related to the circulating factor VIII deficiency. Platelet adhesion is normal because the binding-site defect on the vWF molecule does not participate in the platelet–subendothelial interaction.

Type-2M vWD variant

This variant resembles type 2A in phenotype, but unlike type 2A demonstrates high molecular-weight multimers and satellite bands relating to each multimeric form.

Type-3 vWD. Patients with type-3 vWD are relatively uncommon, but all exhibit very severe bleeding symptoms. Reported genetic defects include several mutations and gene deletions. Transmission is autosomal recessive. The activity and antigenicity of vWF are undetectable in plasma, platelets, and endothelial cells. Circulating levels of factor VIII (VIII:C) are low, with values approximating those seen in moderate haemophilia A. The clinical picture is one of a combined platelet-adhesion defect and a plasma coagulation-factor deficiency with mucocutaneous haemorrhage and muscle and joint bleeding. No increase in vWF is detected after DDAVP infusion, and treatment rests with replacement therapy.

Pseudo- or platelet-type vWD. This disorder, inherited as an autosomal dominant trait, is characterized by a lack of high molecular-weight multimers of vWF in the plasma. The abnormality is due to a mutation in the platelet Gp-Ib/IX complex, increasing its affinity for vWF. Bleeding symptoms are relatively mild and are commonly associated with thrombocytopenia. Replacement therapy or DDAVP infusions lead to rapid clearance of vWF with associated thrombocytopenia. Platelet infusions in conjunction with replacement therapy may secure haemostasis.

Therapy in vWD

The aim of treatment in vWD is to secure haemostasis by correcting the prolonged bleeding time through normalizing functional vWF levels. The cornerstone of treatment of severe vWD is replacement therapy with plasma-derived concentrates containing vWF and (and in some preparations factor VIII). In mild cases, DDAVP can be used, while antifibrinolytic and other adjunctive agents may be of value.

Replacement therapy. Cryoprecipitate is now no longer recommended due to the potential risks of viral transmission. Two factor VIII concentrates of intermediate purity (Haemate P and BPL 8Y), and one high-purity preparation (vWF concentrate LFB), have been shown to be reasonably effective. Plasma factor VIII levels (VIII:C) rise in proportion to the procoagulant factor VIII content of the concentrate administered, but subsequently they continue to be maintained for up to 72 h after a single infusion. This secondary transfusion-response is a unique feature of vWD, as the infused vWF acts as carrier protein for factor VIII, which is produced normally in this disorder. Replacement therapy is indicated in symptomatic patients with type-3 vWD, and in clinically severe and DDAVP-unresponsive type-1 and

Table 2 Clinical and laboratory features in common von Willebrand's disease (vWD) variants

Feature	Type 1	Type 2A	Type 2B	Type 3	Pseudo-vWD
Inheritance	Autosomal dominant	Autosomal dominant	Autosomal dominant	Autosomal recessive	Autosomal dominant
Bleeding time (BT)	Prolonged	Prolonged	Prolonged	Prolonged	Prolonged
Vwf: ristocetin cofactor (activity)	Reduced	Reduced	Normal/Reduced	Reduced	Reduced
Plasma vWf:Ag	Reduced	Normal/reduced	Normal/reduced (increased binding to platelets)	Reduced/absent	Normal/reduced
Plasma vWf multimers	Normal	Absent HMW multimers	Absent HMW multimers	Absent/only small multimer band	Absent HMW multimers (bound to platelets)
Platelet vWf:Ag	Normal/reduced	Absent HMW	Normal	Reduced/absent	Normal
Ristocetin induced platelet aggregation	Normal/reduced	Reduced	Increased at low restocetin concentrations	Absent	Hyperaggregation
Response to DDAVP	Increase in vWf and factor VIII BT correction	Variable but increase in factor VIII	Variable with intravascular platelet aggregation and thrombocytopenia	None	Intravascular platelet aggregation and thrombocytopenia
Response to vWf replacement therapy	Increase in vWf and factor VIII BT correction	Increase in vWf and factor VIII	Variable thrombocytopenia with increase in vWf and factor VIII	Increase in vWf and factor VIII	Intravascular platelet aggregation and thrombocytopenia

type-2 variants. In some cases of type-3 vWD, replacement therapy may induce the formation of alloantibodies to vWF, which complicates subsequent management. Concentrates are seldom justified in cases of mild vWD.

Therapy with DDAVP. DDAVP (0.3 μg/kg) as a slow intravenous infusion, or in some cases as a subcutaneous injection or intranasal insufflation, is the treatment of choice in mild type-1 vWD, and to a variable extent in type-2A vWD. DDAVP, which increases vWF by between 2 and 7 times can be given at 8- to 12-hourly intervals for 2 to 6 days, although in some cases tachyphylaxis may occur. As DDAVP also stimulates fibrinolysis, an antifibrinolytic agent (for example, tranexamic acid) is usually given concurrently. Adverse events are uncommon, but include facial flushing, hypotension, and water retention. The latter restricts its use in small infants. Benefits of DDAVP treatment in elderly patients with hypertension and cardiac failure should be assessed against possible thrombotic complications. DDAVP is contraindicated in type-2B and in pseudo-vWD because it may cause thrombocytopenia.

Adjunctive therapy. In mild vWD, antifibrinolytic preparations (for example, tranexamic acid) may be effective as the sole haemostatic agents for minor haemorrhage or minor surgery. In women of reproductive age with vWD, an oral contraceptive and tranexamic acid may control menorrhagia. As with other bleeding disorders, aspirin or related platelet-inhibitory agents and intramuscular injections should be avoided.

Bernard–Soulier syndrome

This rare, heterogeneous disorder, transmitted in an autosomal recessive fashion, is due to a deficiency of the platelet surface glycoproteins Gp-Ib, Gp-IX, and Gp-V, abolishing vWF-mediated platelet adhesion to the subendothelium. Homozygotes usually have a long history of excessive bleeding with frequent mucocutaneous haemorrhages. Menorrhagia is common. Most patients require blood transfusions at some time, and life-threatening bleeding frequently occurs.

Key diagnostic features include a mild to moderate thrombocytopenia with large, and occasionally giant, platelets. The bleeding time is prolonged and platelet aggregation to vWF and ristocetin, and to bovine vWF alone, are absent. Demonstration of absent or severely reduced platelet-surface Gp-Ib confirms the diagnosis.

No specific treatment exists, but platelet transfusion can be lifesaving, although high-titre alloantibodies can develop. Menorrhagia may respond to oral contraceptives and occasionally antifibrinolytic therapy can be helpful.

Disorders characterized by abnormal platelet activation

Grey-platelet syndrome

This rare syndrome is characterized by a mild to moderate thrombocytopenia with large platelets, and a moderate to severe bleeding disorder resembling a coagulation factor deficiency. The unusual name was derived from the grey colour of the platelets on Wright-stained blood smears, due to the almost total lack of α-granules in both platelets and megakaryocytes.

Storage-pool deficiency

This disorder, inherited as an autosomal dominant trait, is characterized by a moderate bleeding diathesis due to a deficiency in the granule-bound adenine nucleotides, ADP and ATP, associated with a decreased number of dense bodies in the platelets. Cystolic nucleotides involved in platelet metabolism are normal.

The bleeding time is moderately prolonged, and platelet-aggregation studies demonstrate a reduced response to ADP and collagen, with an ATP:ADP ratio greater than normal. Full platelet support, preferably with HLA-matched platelets, is recommended for severe haemorrhagic symptoms and for major surgical procedures. DDAVP infusions may correct the bleeding time and is useful for minor haemorrhages, while antifibrinolytic agents and oral contraceptives may be useful in menorrhagia.

Disorders characterized by defective platelet aggregation

Glanzmann's thrombasthenia

This rare disorder is characterized by moderate to severe mucocutaneous haemorrhages and menorrhagia. Symptoms usually begin in childhood, and pregnancy and delivery represent a severe haemorrhagic risk. Thrombasthenia is inherited as an autosomal recessive trait and a family history often reveals consanguinity, which may account for the remarkably uneven geographical distribution. The defect, which may involve either the *Gp-IIa* gene or the *Gp-IIIb* gene, results in a deficiency or an abnormality of the membrane glycoprotein complex Gp-IIb/IIIa at both platelet and megakaryocytic levels. As a result, fibrinogen cannot bind to the platelet membrane and platelet aggregation does not occur. The bleeding time is prolonged, and platelet-aggregation studies show an impaired-release reaction.

Treatment rests with the administration of HLA-matched platelet concentrates. Antifibrinolytic therapy or topical haemostatic agents may be of value in the treatment of minor bleeding, while oral contraceptives are effective for controlling menorrhagia.

Hereditary afibrinogenaemia

This rare disorder, normally included among the plasma coagulation-factor deficiencies, affects platelet function and makes the blood incoagulable. The condition is inherited as an autosomal recessive trait. In terms of primary haemostasis, afibrinogenaemia results in a grossly prolonged bleeding time and absent platelet aggregation involving the release reaction. The activated partial thromboplastin time (APTT), prothrombin time (PT), and thrombin times are profoundly abnormal.

Symptoms of mucocutaneous and joint or muscle bleeding, and fetal loss subsequent to implantation, occur, and haemorrhage from the umbilical stump is common. Treatment relies upon replacement therapy with fibrinogen concentrates and, where appropriate, antifibrinolytic therapy. Menorrhagia is well controlled by hormone therapy.

Hereditary disorders of secondary haemostasis

Disorders of the intrinsic coagulation cascade

Hereditary disorders of secondary haemostasis are usually the result of a single plasma-protein deficiency or abnormality, and are all associated with a similar clinical picture. In the following sections the clinical features of haemophilia A, the most common disorder of this kind, will be described in detail. The characteristics of the rarer disorders, and how they differ from haemophilia A, will be outlined for each individual disorder.

Haemophilia A

This X-linked recessive disorder is due to a deficiency or abnormality of factor VIII, which circulates in the plasma expressing both procoagulant activity (VIII:C) and antigenicity. It is bound to vWF (see Chapter 3.36). In most cases, factor VIII is quantitatively reduced with a proportional decrease in both VIII:C and VIII:AG levels. The incidence of haemophilia A in the population ranges from 1 in 10 000 to 20 000, but is rare in Chinese and uncommon in Black populations. Some 6000 patients are currently registered with haemophilia A in the UK. The fact that the mutation rate for the gene is high (up to 30 per cent) is important because a negative family history does not exclude haemophilia. In any one affected kindred, the expression of the genetic defect is consistent; all affected males demonstrate a similar level of factor VIII deficiency. A haemophiliac phenotype may occur in female heterozygous carriers due to skewed X-chromosome inactivation.

Clinical features of haemophilia A

The clinical severity is assessed by the frequency and nature of the bleeding, and the level of the factor VIII deficiency. Three degrees of clinical severity are recognized:

1. Severe haemophilia, with spontaneous haemorrhage into joints and muscles and severe bleeding after minor trauma. Factor VIII levels (VIII:C) are usually less than 1 IU/dl (1 per cent normal).
2. Moderate haemophilia, where bleeding occurs after minor trauma with few spontaneous symptoms. Factor VIII levels lie between 1 and 5 IU/dl.
3. Mild haemophilia when prolonged bleeding only occurs with trauma or following operative procedures. Basal factor VIII levels are between 5 and 40 IU/dl.

Infants with severe haemophilia have low levels of factor VIII at birth. It is unusual, however, for haemorrhagic symptoms to occur until the child becomes active.

Exceptionally, the first-born affected males may develop large cephalohaematomas and occasionally intracranial haemorrhage, particularly if labour is difficult or protracted, or with forceps delivery.

Haemarthroses. Episodic bleeding into joints is common in haemophilia. When inadequately treated, these haemarthroses lead to intra-articular pathology, secondary deformity, and eventual crippling. The knee, elbow, and ankle are most commonly affected. At the onset of joint haemorrhage, the patient may experience 'tingling' feelings, stiffness, or instability of the joint, evolving into a hot, swollen, and painful joint with restricted movement as blood fills the joint cavity. Clinical deterioration is directly related to the number of haemorrhages in any one joint. Bleeding occurs from the vascular synovium, and leads to synovial hyperplasia with hyperaemia and a tendency for further bleeding. With repeated haemorrhage, the synovium becomes fibrotic, with cartilage destruction, narrowing of the joint space, subchondral cyst formation, bone erosion, and osteophyte formation with eventual ankylosis. These features are referred to, collectively, as chronic haemophilic arthropathy. Haemorrhage into one specific joint more than twice a month, or more than three times in a 2-month period, produces a 'target joint'.

Haematomas and nerve-compression syndromes. Bleeding into muscles is common, and may lead to pressure necrosis of overlying skin or underlying bone, muscle contractures, and nerve-compression syndromes. The condition presents with pain on movement and later at rest, with swelling. Nerve compression may ensue, with pain, parasthesiae, numbness, motor impairment, and subsequent muscular atrophy. Volkmann's contracture is a consequence of bleeding into the muscular compartment of the forearm. Fibrosis following muscle haematomas is common, particularly in the calf, leading to shortening of the Achilles tendon and progressive walking difficulties. Retroperitoneal haemorrhage and bleeding into the ileopsoas muscle with femoral nerve compression are particularly important because they are common in severe haemophilia, and can be life-threatening.

Haemophilic cysts and pseudotumours. Inadequate treatment of haematomas may lead to cystic collections of blood that enlarge due to repeated haemorrhage. These pseudotumours infiltrate fascial planes, erode adjacent structures, and eventually rupture.

Haemorrhagic symptoms arising in other systems. Bleeding into the central nervous system and the renal and gastrointestinal tracts is common and may be life-threatening.

Next to acquired immune-deficiency syndrome (**AIDS**), intracranial haemorrhage is the most common cause of death with a reported incidence of up to 7.8 per cent. Although the mortality rate has dropped to some 30 per cent with modern treatment, over half the survivors suffer severe neurological sequelae, emphasizing the importance of prompt and adequate replacement therapy, even with trivial head injury.

Haemorrhage from the renal tract is common, and either frank or microscopic haematuria occurs in most patients. In many cases, haematuria is painless, transient, and clears spontaneously. In others, however, replacement therapy may be required. The indiscriminant use of antifibrinolytic agents in these cases may lead to disastrous consequences with ureteric-clot colic, obstruction, hydronephrosis, renal papillary necrosis, and renal failure.

Gastrointestinal bleeding is becoming more common, not so much as a symptom of the underlying factor deficiency, but as a manifestation of hepatic disease secondary to long-standing hepatitis C infection previously transmitted from blood products. Additionally, it may occur as a result of inappropriate use of non-steroidal anti-inflammatory agents for the management of haemophilic arthropathy. Bleeding from the mucous membranes of the mouth is common in children with haemophilia, and poses a specific problem because the mouth and tongue are moist and the haemostatic platelet plug is continually washed away. Treatment with replacement therapy and/or local haemostatic agents is mandatory in such cases because uncontrolled bleeding may lead to respiratory embarrassment.

Laboratory diagnosis

The laboratory diagnosis in haemophilia rests with the appropriate use of coagulation screening tests and the application of specific coagulation-factor assays. The APTT is usually prolonged, although in mild haemophilia with factor VIII levels in excess of 20 to 25 IU/dl the APTT may be normal, making specific assays of factor VIII mandatory for diagnosis.

Diagnosis of severe haemophilia is easy from the characteristic history, physical findings, and very low factor levels. Haemarthroses with progressive disability are rare in hereditary coagulation disorders other than haemophilia A or B. The diagnosis of mild haemophilia is more difficult as a characteristic clinical picture is lacking; therefore specific factor assays are essential to differentiate between deficiencies of other factors in the intrinsic coagulation cascade, and from vWD. In the vWD-2N variant, characterized by a defect in factor VIII-binding, the mode of inheritance is critical. In the initial assessment of patients with moderate and mild haemophilia A, the plasma factor VIII response to DDAVP is important, because an incremental rise in procoagulant factor VIII after DDAVP provides a safe and highly cost-effective therapeutic option for minor haemorrhagic symptoms, and obviates the use of expensive and potentially unsafe coagulation-factor concentrates.

Treatment of haemophilia A

Comprehensive care. The management of haemophilia and other bleeding disorders requires multidisciplinary expertise. The aim of comprehensive care is to offer specialist medical, surgical, and non-medical professional healthcare advice to affected individuals and their families.

Factor replacement therapy. Replacement therapy with factor VIII concentrates is the cornerstone of treatment for symptomatic severe, and DDAVP-unresponsive moderate haemophilia A. Adequate haemostasis is usually achieved when plasma factor VIII values exceed 30 to 40 IU/dl. Factor VIII concentrates can be given either as on-demand therapy for acute bleeding, or as prophylactic regimens to prevent haemorrhage. Treatment of haemorrhage is a medical emergency. Prompt replacement therapy is most cost-effective because bleeding is rapidly controlled, less concentrate is needed, and the progression of musculoskeletal deformities restricted.

Recombinant or virus-inactivated, plasma-derived, factor VIII concentrates should be used exclusively for replacement therapy. As hepatitis-B virus (**HBV**) and hepatitis-A virus (**HAV**) are known to be the more resistant viruses to current inactivation procedures, all patients who are seronegative should be immunized.

On-demand treatment and factor VIII dosage. Factor VIII dosage is based upon the observation that 1 international unit (IU) defined as that amount of factor VIII in 1 ml of fresh plasma per kg body weight increases the plasma factor VIII (VIII:C) level by 2 IU/dl (2 per cent). As the half-life of infused factor VIII is 8 to 12 h, and may be shorter with extensive haemorrhage or with febrile states, repeated doses are often necessary for haemostatic control.

Haemarthroses are adequately treated with 20 to 30 IU of factor VIII/kg repeated after 12 h, and possibly also at 24 and 36 h. Higher dosages and repeated infusions are necessary when there is pre-existing pathology in the affected joints or when initial treatment is delayed. Arthrocentesis is seldom indicated. Initial immobilization of the bleeding joint limits the need for analgesia, and isometric exercises followed by active movement, with hydrotherapy, or pulsed shortwave, should be started within 48 h. Night splints may be useful to prevent fixed–flexion deformities.

Intramuscular haemorrhage usually requires more intensive treatment, with doses of 20 to 40 IU/kg 12-hourly for several days. Complete bed-rest is recommended for ileopsoas bleeds.

For life-threatening bleeds, major surgery, or major trauma, a bolus infusion of 50 IU/kg of factor VIII followed by a continuous infusion at 2 to 4 IU/kg per hour is the most suitable management. Alternatively, after the bolus, 25 to 30 IU/kg (8- to 12-hourly) may be given with laboratory monitoring, to maintain the factor VIII level between 70 and 100 IU/dl.

Home infusion therapy is now a well-established form of treatment where the patient and his family are trained to infuse concentrates. This approach ensures the most prompt treatment for bleeding episodes and is highly cost-effective.

Prophylactic treatment with factor VIII

Intermittent prophylaxis. Intermittent prophylaxis in severe haemophilia is indicated during rehabilitation after major surgery, in 'target joint' management, and in chronic hypertrophic synovitis. In the treatment of 'target joints' and synovitis, 20–30 IU/kg of factor

VIII three times weekly for 3–6 months may induce improvement by promoting healing of the synovium.

Continuous prophylaxis. After adolescence haemophilic patients experience a more benign course of their disease. These observations have led to the introduction of continuous prophylactic programmes in children during the years of most frequent haemorrhage, with the objective of providing regular haemostatic cover and thus preventing spontaneous bleeding episodes. Children maintained on continuous prophylaxis with preinfusion levels of procoagulant factor VIII between 1 and 4 IU/dl achieve as normal a physical, educational, and social development as their unaffected peers.

Infective complications of replacement therapy

Millions of units of plasma-derived, coagulation-factor concentrates produced from hundreds of thousands of litres of plasma from as many individual blood donors may be used to control bleeding during the lifetime of a severe haemophiliac. It is not surprising that major safety issues in haemophilia care are related to the potential transmission of disease from plasma derivatives to the recipient.

The transmission of HIV-1, HCV, and HBV to patients receiving blood products is well recognized, and screening donated plasma for antibodies to these viruses and to viral components by the polymerase chain reaction (**PCR**) is mandatory. Virus-inactivation procedures of plasma-derived concentrates have been universally adopted and include dry-heating, pasteurization, steam and pressure treatment, solvent-detergent treatment, ultrafiltration, and the use of chaotropic agents. For HIV-1 and HCV all these methods seem to be effective, although concerns have been expressed on the transmission of non-lipid enveloped viruses. Recombinant factor VIII concentrates which are safe from viral infections are now available.

Factor VIII inhibitors (antibodies to factor VIII)

One of the most serious complications of blood-product therapy in haemophilia is the development of factor VIII antibodies (usually IgG1 or IgG4), since conventional replacement with factor VIII concentrate is rendered ineffective through antibody neutralization. Young children with severe haemophilia are at greatest cumulative risk (up to 32 per cent) of inhibitor development after relatively few exposure days (9–15 days). More than 80 per cent of inhibitors have developed before patients have reached the age of 9 years.

Factor VIII inhibitors are classified on the basis of the basal titre (assessed by the Bethesda assay in Bethesda units (**Bu**) per ml), and on their response to challenge with factor VIII concentrate *in vivo* (anamnestic response). Generally, two major types of factor VIII inhibitors are encountered: low-titre (less than 10 Bu/ml to human factor VIII), low responders (little, if any, anamnesis); and high-titre (more than 10 Bu/ml), high responders (inhibitor increase in excess of 10 times the basal level on factor VIII challenge). The correct classification of inhibitors is essential because it provides the rationale for effective clinical management.

Treatment of inhibitors can be directed at securing haemostasis alone or, additionally, eradicating the antibody. Low-titre, low-responding inhibitors are treated with either human or porcine factor VIII concentrates at a dosage and frequency of infusion high enough to swamp the antibody and achieve haemostatic levels of factor VIII.

In high-titre, high-responding inhibitors, depending on the inhibitor titre and the clinical status of the patient, porcine factor VIII or 'bypassing agents' may arrest haemorrhage. The 'bypassing agents' are human recombinant or plasma-derived concentrates containing activated coagulation factors, which trigger the coagulation cascades at levels below that at which the inhibitor is operative. The plasma-derived materials include FEIBA and Autoplex, which contain plasma-derived factors IXa, VIIa, and modified Xa. Recombinant factor VIIa concentrate is highly efficacious in securing haemostasis, with a success rate greater than 85 per cent. Immunodepletion of inhibitors with matrix-bound staphylococcal protein A using extracorporeal devices has been attempted with some success prior to high-dose factor VIII treatment.

Immune-tolerance induction programmes for inhibitor eradication in selected high-titre, high-responding antibody patients have met with considerable success, using dosages of factor VIII ranging from 100 IU/kg twice daily to 25 IU/kg three times weekly.

DDAVP and adjunctive therapy

As described for vWD, DDAVP (0.3 μg/kg) is the treatment of choice in mild and, in some cases, moderate haemophilia A—increasing factor VIII levels by 3.1–3.7-fold and peaking between 30 and 50 min after infusion. DDAVP with an antifibrinolytic agent is the treatment of choice in mild or moderate haemophiliacs undergoing dental surgery. It can also be given subcutaneously or by intranasal insufflation.

Haemophilia B (Christmas disease)

Haemophilia B (or Christmas disease) is less common than haemophilia A, with only 1200 patients registered in the UK. It is inherited as an X-linked recessive trait. Spontaneous mutations are uncommon. Several forms of haemophilia B have been defined with variable levels of factor IX antigenicity. One unique variant, haemophilia B Leiden is inherited as a factor IX antigen deficiency at birth and becomes progressively antigen-positive with age, and is associated with increasing factor IX functional levels.

Clinical features of haemophilia A and B are identical and diagnosis rests with the specific factor IX assay. Treatment of symptomatic haemophilia B, irrespective of clinical severity, rests with recombinant or virus-inactivated, plasma-derived, high-purity factor IX concentrates. The dosage of factor IX differs from factor VIII in that it has a longer half-life (14–20 h) and it is distributed into the extravascular space.

Factor XI deficiency

This disorder, which has a particularly high frequency in Ashkenazim Jewish populations is transmitted as an incompletely recessive autosomal trait, either as a major defect in homozygotes (factor XI less than 15 IU/dl) or as a minor defect in heterozygotes (factor XI, 15–45 IU/dl). Clinically, the deficiency presents as a mild bleeding disorder and may be associated with Noonan's syndrome. In homozygous patients the APTT is prolonged and factor XI levels of 3–15 IU/dl are seen. Therapy with factor XI concentrates and/or fresh frozen plasma is useful for severe haemorrhage and for surgery or trauma.

Disorders of the extrinsic coagulation cascade

Factor VII and factor X deficiencies

These disorders are transmitted as autosomal recessive traits, and clinically they are similar. Diagnosis rests with specific assays of the activity and antigenicity of factor VII or factor X. The haemostatic level of circulating factor VII is between 5 and 10 IU/dl and 10 to 20 IU/dl for factor X. Due to its short half-life (2–4 h), 4–6-hourly treatment with recombinant factor VIIa concentrates may be indicated for severe haemorrhage or surgical cover. In factor X deficiency, prothrombin-complex concentrate infusions are effective.

Disorders of the common pathway

Factor V deficiency

This uncommon, autosomal recessive disorder presents clinically with mild bleeding, particularly into mucocutaneous tissues, into the gastrointestinal and genitourinary tracts, and into the central nervous system. Low factor V levels by specific assay are diagnosed and the APTT and PT are prolonged. Some patients have a prolonged bleeding time. Fresh frozen plasma infusions usually control bleeding.

Prothrombin (factor II) deficiency

Hypoprothrombinaemia, an autosomal recessive disorder is rare, and usually presents as a mild bleeding disorder, although bleeding from the umbilicus is common. In inherited hypoprothrombinaemia, factor II levels are less than 10 IU/dl and the APTT and PT are abnormal. Treatment rests with prothrombin-complex concentrate infusions.

Disorders of fibrinogen

Afibrinogenaemia and hypofibrinogenaemia have been described under defects in primary haemostasis. Qualitative defects, the dysfibrinogenaemias, are inherited as autosomal dominant or codominant traits. Fibrinogen antigenicity is detectable, but dysfunctional abnormalities lead to impairment of one or more of the three stages involved in the conversion of fibrinogen to crosslinked fibrin, with abnormal fibrinopeptide A or B release, abnormal polymerization, or abnormal fibrin crosslinkage.

Most patients are asymptomatic, although in less than 30 per cent the disorder may present with a mild bleeding diathesis, thromboembolic symptoms, or impaired wound healing.

Prolonged thrombin and reptilase times, low clottable fibrinogen with normal fibrinogen antigen are characteristic of the disorders, and the APTT and PT are often abnormal. Haemorrhagic symptoms may require fibrinogen concentrates.

Factor XIII deficiency

Factor XIII deficiency is a rare, autosomal recessive condition.

Haemorrhage from the umbilicus is common and may be fatal. Cutaneous and muscular haematomas are usual, while haemorrhage after surgery or trauma may be severe. Wound healing is often impaired. Diagnosis rests upon clot solubility in 5 M urea and on specific functional assays for factor XIII. Virus-inactivated factor XIII concentrates are available and plasma factor XIII levels greater than 5 IU/dl will secure haemostasis. Due to the long half-life of factor XIII (72–96 h), prophylactic treatment on a 4-weekly basis is possible.

Disorders due to combined factor deficiencies

Disorders involving two or more separate factor deficiencies have been reported, many involving abnormal vitamin K-dependent proteins.

The most common is the combined deficiency of factors V and VIII. This is either transmitted as an autosomal recessive trait (type I) or as a dual abnormality of a combined gene (type II). Moderate to mild mucocutaneous haemorrhage is common, although severe bleeding may occur after surgery or trauma. Prolonged APTT and PT are common, and levels of 5–20 IU/dl of factor V and of factor VIII are diagnostic. Treatment rests with fresh frozen plasma or DDAVP, although factor VIII concentrates may be required for severe bleeding or for surgical cover.

Bleeding disorders due to hereditary antiprotease deficiencies

Severe bleeding is not uncommonly associated with hereditary α_2-antiplasmin deficiency, an autosomal recessive trait, attributed to premature lysis of fibrin clots. In homozygotes, α_2-antiplasmin levels are less than 10 U/dl. Treatment with antifibrinolytic agents or protease inhibitors may be beneficial.

Further reading

Colman, R.W., Hush, J., Mander, V.J., and Saltzman, E.W. (ed.) (1987). Basic principles and clinical practice. In *Haemostasis and thrombosis*, 2nd edn, p. 3621. Lippincott, Philadelphia, PA.

Lusher, J.M. and Kessler, C.M. (ed.) (1991). *Haemophilia and von Willebrand's disease in the 1990's. A new decade of hopes and challenges.* International Congress Series 943. Excerpta Medica, Amsterdam.

Seghatchian, M.J. and Savidge, G.F. (ed.) (1989). *Factor VIII—von Willebrand factor*, Vols I and II. CRC Press, Boca Raton, FL.

Chapter 3.38

Acquired coagulation disorders

B. J. Hunt

Acquired haemostatic disorders are secondary to an underlying disease. They may be due to either lack of production and/or excessive loss of haemostatic factors and/or the presence of inhibitory substances. In contrast to inherited coagulation disorders, they are usually associated with multiple haemostatic deficiencies (Table 1). A history and examination will indicate whether bleeding is due to local factors such ulceration, or whether an underlying acquired haemostatic defect such as that due to chronic liver disease is a contributory factor. Continued oozing from venepuncture and incision sites is a sign of haemostatic failure. Areas of cutaneous cyanosis and subsequent gangrene may also indicate disseminated intravascular coagulation before excessive bleeding becomes apparent. Acquired haemostatic defects that are not associated with active bleeding do not usually

Table 1 Changes in screening haemostatic assays in acquired coagulation disorders

	PT	PTT	Fibrinogen	Platelet count	FDPs
Liver disease	↑	↑	N/↑↓	↓	sl↑
Renal disease	↑/N	↑/N	↑	N/↓	sl↑/N
Disseminated intravascular coagulation	↑	↑	↓	↓	↑
Massive transfusions	↑	↑	N/↓	↓/N	↑/N
Fibrinolytic bleeding	sl↑	sl↑	↓	N	↑↑
Oral anticoagulants	↑↑	↑	N	N	N
Heparin	↑	↑↑↑	N	N	N
Idiopathic thrombocytopenic purpura	N	N	N	↓	N

N, normal; ↑, prolonged/elevated; ↓, decreased; sl, slight.

FDPs, fibrinogen degradation products; PT, prothrombin time; PTT, partial thromboplastin time.

Table 2 Haemostasis screening tests and factor assays in premature infants and term infants compared to the normal adult range

	Premature infants (28–34 weeks)	Term infants (38–41 weeks)	Normal adults
PT (s)	16–20	14–17	12–14
TT (s)	15–24	14–18	12–14
APTT (s)	50–65	40–50	30–40
Factor IX (%)	15–20	20–40	50–200
Factor VII (%)	20–60	35–70	50–200
AT-III (%)	25–35	45–75	80–120

PT, prothrombin time; TT, thrombin time; APTT, activated partial thromboplastin time; AT-III, antithrombin III.

need treatment and tend to correct themselves as the underlying disease process resolves.

Often a bleeding tendency is first suggested by screening tests: prothrombin time (PT); the partial thromboplastin time (PTT); thrombin time (TT); and fibrinogen levels and platelet count (other abbreviations used in this chapter are summarized in Table 2, and in Chapter 3.37).

Haemostasis in the newborn

The sites of bleeding in an infant include bleeding from the umbilicus, cephalohaematomas, circumcision, venepuncture sites, into the skin, and there is a particular risk of intracranial haemorrhage. Due to liver immaturity there is a fragile haemostatic balance with little reserve capacity to respond to haemorrhage, and multiple haemostatic deficiencies can easily develop in association with many disease states. The clinical spectrum of disseminated intravascular coagulation is wide in newborns; in some it is characterized by haemorrhage or thrombotic complications, whereas in others there may be few clinical signs. The management is similar to those of an adult with disseminated intravascular coagulation (see below).The constantly changing haemostatic mechanisms in newborns necessitate multiple reference ranges of normal values (Table 2).

Vitamin K deficiency bleeding in neonates

Presentation

The classical form of vitamin K deficiency bleeding has an incidence of about 1 in 200 to 400 in the absence of prophylactic therapy. It occurs in breast-fed, full-term infants, usually on the second or third day of life when concentrations of the K-dependent factors normally reach a nadir. It is due to the combination of lack of vitamin K in breast milk (less than 20 μg/l compared with 830 μg/l in formula milk), combined with poor vitamin K synthesis and stores.

The second form, or early-onset vitamin K deficiency bleeding, presents with bleeding in the first 24 h of life. Mothers of these infants have usually taken drugs that interfere with vitamin K metabolism, such as anticonvulsants or warfarin during the third trimester. A third type, that of late-onset, occurs after the first week of life in infants with malabsorptive diseases such as cystic fibrosis. Most respond to the administration of vitamin K except for the sick, very premature infants whose immature livers have poor synthetic ability.

Management

Prophylactic administration of 1 mg of vitamin K_1 intramuscularly within 24 h of birth was once standard practice. However, due to the possibility of an association between intramuscular vitamin K_1 in neonates and the later development of childhood cancer, oral vitamin K_1 is now widely used in the UK. It is given in doses of 2 mg, after birth, at 4–7 days, and in breast-fed infants at 1 month. Bottle-fed babies almost never suffer from vitamin K deficiency bleeding presumably, because they absorb enough of the 25 to 50 μg of vitamin K taken daily in supplemented milk formulas.

Certain risk groups, for example those with malabsorptive states or babies of women receiving anticonvulsants during pregnancy, require additional prophylaxis. Any woman receiving anticonvulsants during the third trimester should receive vitamin K supplements, 5 mg orally per day. Infants with haemorrhagic complications should receive vitamin K immediately, subcutaneously or intravenously rather than intramuscularly as this produces a large haematoma.

Vitamin K deficiency disorders

Vitamin K

Biochemistry

Vitamin K, a fat-soluble vitamin, is a cofactor for the post-translational carboxylation of specific glutamate residues of factors II, VII, IX, and X, as well as protein C and S within hepatocytes. γ-Carboxyglutamate residues bind via calcium ions to phospholipid templates and without them coagulation cannot proceed normally.

Sources

Vitamin K exists in two major chemical forms: vitamin K_1 (or phylloquinone), produced exclusively by plants; and vitamins K_2 (or menaquinones), the major dietary source, synthesized by microorganisms in the gut. Green, leafy vegetables are the richest source (100–500 μg/100 g) of K_1. Dietary contributions are made by other vegetables and fruit (1–50 μg/100 g); oils, fats, and margarine (1–100 μg/100 g); dairy products (0.5–5 μg/100 g); and bread and cereal products (0.1–10 μg/100 g).

The required daily intake of vitamin K is about 0.1–0.5 μg/kg. Most of the absorbed vitamin K passes to the hepatocytes, where liver stores are relatively low with a half-life of only a few days. Normal serum concentrations of vitamin K range from 150 to 800 pg/ml.

Vitamin K deficiency

Vitamin K deficiency in adults is due to poor dietary intake, malabsorption due to gut or pancreatic disease, hepatic immaturity or disease, or it may be iatrogenic due to oral anticoagulation. Clinical signs are uncommon unless the PT is more than 30 s.

Laboratory diagnosis

Baseline coagulation tests show prolonged PT and PTT but with normal TT and fibrinogen levels. Specific assays will show reduced amounts of factors II, VII, IX, and X. Correction of these values, and of the PT and APTT, follows vitamin K administration.

Management

The normal dose to prevent vitamin K deficiency is 10 mg intravenously a week. It should be given no faster than 5 mg/min because it can cause anaphylactoid reactions. Between 4 and 6 h are required before maximum benefit is obtained. Fresh frozen plasma or prothrombinase complexes will correct the coagulation abnormality immediately.

Coumarin anticoagulants

Oral anticoagulation is discussed in Chapter 3.39. Oral anticoagulants decrease the availability of vitamin K in the hepatocyte by acting as competitive inhibitors of vitamin K. Consequently, non-functional acarboxyl forms of factors II, VII, IX, X, protein C, and protein S are generated (proteins induced by vitamin K absence, **PIVKAs**).

The therapeutic range for oral anticoagulant control is based on the international normalized ratio (**INR**). This adjusts the PT so that it is expressed as if it had been measured using an international reference thromboplastin and consequently allows for uniform oral anticoagulant therapy. The most common complication of anticoagulant therapy is haemorrhage, which usually results from overdosage. If the INR is greater than 4.5 and there is little or no bleeding, treatment should be withdrawn and then resumed on a smaller maintenance dose once the INR has reached the normal range. If the INR is prolonged and associated with bleeding, a slow intravenous infusion of vitamin K, 1 mg, will reverse the prolongation, but the effect does not occur for 6 h, with a maximum at 24 to 36 h. A large dose such as 10 mg is not recommended unless there is life-threatening bleeding because it may prevent effective anticoagulation for up to 2 weeks. With serious haemorrhage, fresh frozen plasma or prothrombinase complexes (factors II, VII, IX, and X) will provide immediate correction.

Drug interactions

Drugs may potentiate the effects of oral anticoagulants or decrease the biological effects of anticoagulants by the induction of hepatic microsomal enzymes leading to increased warfarin metabolism.

Haemostasis and liver disease

Aetiology

Hepatocellular disease causes serious haemostatic defects, the severity of which is proportional to the extent of liver damage. In hepatic disease there is impaired synthesis of all coagulation factors and physiological anticoagulants, except for factor VIIIc, because it is produced at other sites including lymph nodes and spleen. Fibrinogen levels are usually normal unless the liver disease is severe. There is inadequate carboxylation of vitamin K-dependent coagulation factors in most patients, despite adequate vitamin K stores. This may be exacerbated by failed absorption of vitamin K due to biliary-tract disease. Liver disease can impair clearance of activated factors. Due to the diminished clearance of plasminogen activator and plasmin there is an enhanced fibrinolytic state. Platelet dysfunction is attributed mainly to increased levels of fibrin degradation products. Thrombocytopenia is common and related to a combination of reduced thrombopoietin production by the liver and hypersplenism.

Bleeding in liver disease is usually multifactorial in origin, for chronic liver failure induces non-haematological complications that contribute to bleeding. Portal hypertension causes varices that are fragile and easily ruptured, as well as splenomegaly and concomitant thrombocytopenia.

Laboratory investigation

The APTT and PT are prolonged, the latter being an excellent guide to hepatic function. The TT and fibrinogen levels are normal unless the liver disease is severe. An increase in plasma fibrinolytic activity is demonstrated by increased levels of fibrin degradation products.

Management

Abnormal coagulation results do not need treating unless the patient is not bleeding, although it is logical to give vitamin K_1, 10 mg intravenously if there is evidence of vitamin K deficiency, but this may not always improve the PT.

Local management of any local bleeding such as from a gastric or duodenal ulcer, or varices, is crucial. If a patient is bleeding the deficient proteins can be given in the form of fresh frozen plasma. If fibrinogen levels are very low, cryoprecipitate or fibrinogen concentrate can be given. Platelet transfusion is useful if there is thrombocytopenia and bleeding, and an infusion of deamino-D-arginine vasopressin (**DDAVP**) (see Chapter 3.37) may shorten the bleeding time by temporarily correcting platelet functional abnormalities.

Haemostasis and renal disease

In renal failure there is an increased likelihood of bleeding which parallels the degree of renal failure. The pathophysiology is only partly understood. Poor platelet function is the main defect, probably due to accumulation of toxic metabolites such as guanidinosuccinic acid and phenolic acid in the plasma and a deficiency of the larger multimers of von Willebrand factor, possibly due to increased proteolytic activity in uraemic blood. Anaemia contributes to the bleeding tendency by interfering with platelet–endothelial interactions. Coagulation factor deficiencies also occur. Deficiency of vitamin K-dependent factors results from malnutrition, antibiotic therapy, or uraemic enteritis. Rarely, isolated factor IX or factor XII deficiencies occur in the nephrotic syndrome, probably due to increased loss in the urine.

Laboratory investigations

The bleeding time is prolonged due to acquired platelet dysfunction, thrombocytopenia, and anaemia. The PT, APTT, and TT may be slightly or moderately prolonged. A disproportionately prolonged APTT may reflect factor IX deficiency, while prolongation of both PT and APTT may indicate vitamin K deficiency.

Management

Platelet transfusions have only a temporary effect because donor platelets acquire the uraemic defect within hours. Infusions of cryoprecipitate or DDAVP also temporarily shorten the bleeding time by increasing the levels of large multimers of von Willebrand factor. Transfusion of red cells or the administration of erythropoietin shortens the bleeding time in the long term. Correction of the platelet defects follows haemodialysis.

Disseminated intravascular coagulation

Disseminated intravascular coagulation (**DIC**) is defined as the widespread activation of haemostasis, with the formation of soluble or insoluble fibrin within the circulation. It is a pathological response to many underlying disorders. Initially the process is compensated for, but as the haemostatic factors are consumed in diffuse, small-vessel thrombosis, haemostatic failure may develop. In most cases bleeding is the major clinical problem; but in an important minority, about 10 per cent, widespread thrombosis is predominant.

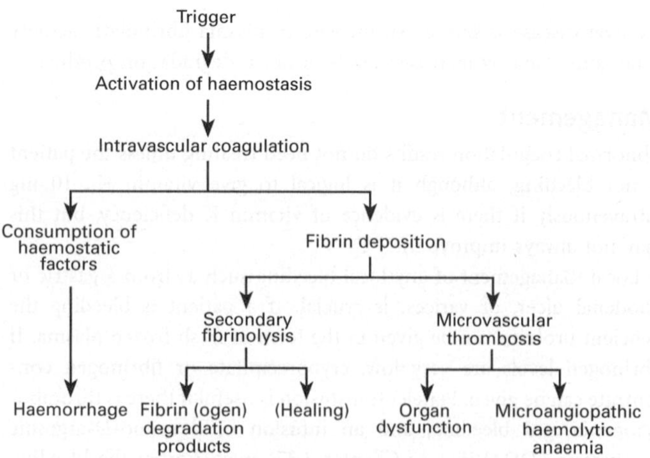

Fig. 1 The pathophysiology of disseminated intravascular coagulation.

The clinical syndrome is extremely variable in severity and rate of onset, and often occurs in desperately ill patients. Easy bruising and persistent oozing from venepuncture and intramuscular injection sites and around drainage tubes occurs and can progress to massive mucous-membrane bleeding and, rarely, to haemorrhage into the adrenal glands, which is known as the Waterhouse–Friderichsen syndrome.

If thrombosis is predominant, microthrombotic lesions are often found in the fingers and toes or there may be purpura fulminans and/or haemorrhagic bullae. The renal vasculature is usually involved at an early stage, while thrombi in the pulmonary vasculature can cause an acute respiratory distress syndrome and thrombi in the cerebral circulation will cause neurological abnormalities.

Pathogenesis (Fig. 1)

In DIC a powerful and/or persistent trigger activates the haemostatic mechanism. There are four potential, interactive mechanisms:

(1) activation of the extrinsic pathway by the expression of tissue factor on damaged tissues, and monocytes, especially due to surgery, burns, and heat stroke; infection; and some malignant tumours;

(2) intrinsic-pathway activation by immune complexes, bacterial lipopolysaccharide;

(3) platelet activation by bacterial endotoxin;

(4) pathological activation of haemostasis—for example, activation of factor X or prothrombin by proteolytic enzymes such as snake venoms.

Secondary activation of fibrinolysis follows the release of tissue plasminogen activator from the endothelium due to the effect of thrombin. The fibrinolytic system is capable of rapidly lysing large amounts of fibrin as it is formed, and thus maintaining vascular patency. Red cells are fragmented as they pass over the fibrin deposits in the microvasculature, leading to a microvascular haemolytic anaemia in 50 per cent of cases (see Chapter 3.25).

Aetiology (Table 3)

Within hospitals most cases of DIC are secondary to Gram-negative septicaemia or obstetric catastrophes which produce rapid and profuse bleeding problems. In contrast, intrauterine fetal death produces slow, progressive DIC with bleeding as a late complication.

Table 3 Clinical conditions complicated by disseminated intravascular coagulation

Infections	***Shock***
• Septicaemia	• Surgical trauma
• Viral	• Burns
• Protozoal (malaria)	• Heat stroke
• Rickettsial	***Immunological***
Obstetrics	• Immune-complex disorders
• Abruptio placentae	• Allograft reaction
• Amniotic fluid embolism	• Incompatible blood transfusion
• Placenta praevia	***Liver disease***
• Retained dead fetus	• Cirrhosis
• Eclampsia	• Acute hepatic necrosis
Malignancy	***Miscellaneous***
• Carcinoma of stomach, colon, pancreas, breast, lung, especially when metastatic	• Vascular malformations such as cavernous haemangioma
• Mucin-secreting adenocarcinomas	• Fat embolism
• Leukaemia, especially acute promyelocytic leukaemia	

Some neoplasms are associated with a low-grade DIC, especially adenocarcinomas, which may express tissue factor-like activity. In pancreatic carcinoma the release of trypsin may lyse and activate coagulation factors. Worldwide, the most common cause of death due to DIC is from snake-bite envenoming (see Chapter 18.2). Most venomous snakes belong to the Viperidae family, which includes vipers, rattlesnakes, and adders. For example, *Echis carinatus* (the saw-scaled viper) produces a venom that directly activates prothrombin, leading to complete defibrination, with death due to haemorrhage in 30 per cent of cases. The correct treatment of snake bites is to give the specific antivenom intravenously (see Chapter 18.2), if necessary in repeated doses.

Laboratory features

Initially, DIC produces few coagulation changes because the liver and bone marrow compensate for the consumption of haemostatic factors. However, if the trigger persists the haemostatic system will eventually fail. The main findings are thrombocytopenia (the platelet count is less than 100×10^9/l), increased levels of fibrin degradation products, and prolongation of PT, APTT, and TT due to factor deficiencies and the presence of fibrin degradation products. The fibrinogen level is usually reduced to between 0.5 and 1.5 g/l. The blood film may show red-cell fragmentation, evidence of microangiopathic haemolytic anaemia.

Management

If the patient is shocked they must be vigorously resuscitated to prevent exacerbation of DIC. It is imperative to treat the underlying cause, and appropriate broad-spectrum antibiotics should be given in septicaemia of unknown cause (see Chapter 16.116).

Serial laboratory assays of PT, APTT, fibrinogen level, platelet count, and fibrin degradation products are required as a guide to the replacement of blood components. The aim is to maintain the PT and PTT within a ratio of 1.5 of the control values, fibrinogen levels of greater than 1 g/l, and the haematocrit greater than 0.30. Fresh frozen plasma contains near-normal quantities of all the coagulation factors and inhibitors. Cryoprecipitate or fibrinogen concentrates can be given if fibrinogen levels are disproportionately low. Platelet concentrates should be given if the platelet count is less than 50×10^9/l.

The use of heparin and antithrombin concentrates in DIC remains controversial. They are given in an attempt to 'switch off' or inhibit the process that is activating coagulation, but this has only been shown to be clearly beneficial after an amniotic fluid embolism or incompatible blood transfusion. If thrombosis is predominant however, heparin is often used giving a continuous infusion of between 500 and 1000 U/h. An infusion of prostacyclin may be helpful in cases where pathological activation of platelets is a major factor. Antifibrinolytic agents should never be used as they may result in failure to remove fibrin thrombi and thus exacerbate multiorgan failure.

Hyperfibrinolytic bleeding or primary fibrinolysis

Bleeding may occur if there is excessive generation of plasmin with subsequent proteolytic degradation of plasma proteins and, in severe cases, large amounts of fibrin degradation products, hypofibrinogenaemia, and bleeding.

Aetiology

Some tissues, especially prostatic, are rich in plasminogen activator, excessive liberation of which may occur during prostatic surgery. It can occur during cardiopulmonary bypass, and especially during the reperfusion phase of liver transplantation. Iatrogenic fibrinolytic bleeding can occur through the use of exogenous fibrinolytic activators such as streptokinase or urokinase.

Acute promyelocytic leukaemia is associated with a bleeding diathesis that occurs against a background of bone marrow failure and thus thrombocytopenia. The usual finding of low levels of fibrinogen and increased titres of fibrin degradation products, minimally prolonged PT and PTT, and near-normal levels of antithrombin, suggest primary fibrinolytic bleeding rather than DIC as previously thought.

Laboratory investigation

Levels of fibrin degradation products (which include the D-dimer) assay are increased. More sophisticated tests will reveal decreased concentrations of plasminogen and α_2-antiplasmin, with increased amounts of tissue and/or urokinase plasminogen activators. The PT, PTT, and TT may be mildly prolonged due to fibrinogenolysis, with production of large quantities of fibrin degradation products.

Management

Tranexamic acid and aminocaproic acid, by [illegible] competitive inhibitors of plasminogen, are weak [illegible]nts and can be given intravenously or [illegible], given [illegible]00 000-KIU (kallikrein inactivat[illegible]enous bolus, is the most powerful antiplasmin ag[illegible]

In a[illegible]ytic leukaemia is controversial. Replacement th[illegible]sh frozen plasma and platelets should be instituted [illegible]ry.Trials of antifibrinolytics are promising. Transretinoic [illegible] by causing differentiation of the promyeloblasts may correct the haemostatic defect (see Chapter 3.5).

Perioperative bleeding

Excessive perioperative bleeding can be due to suture deficiency and/or derangement of haemostasis. The pathogenesis of non-surgical perioperative bleeding is not fully established. Cardiopulmonary bypass has been most comprehensively studied.

Cardiopulmonary bypass and bleeding

Haemorrhage remains an important complication of cardiac surgery, especially now that patients are requiring reoperation or complex procedures such as heart and lung transplantation, and have received antithrombotic therapy before surgery.

Pathogenesis

Cardiopulmonary bypass involves extensive contact between blood and the synthetic surfaces of the membrane oxygenator, which results in haemostatic activation. Large doses of heparin are given to the patient prior to bypass to prevent immediate clotting in the bypass circuit. During the bypass operation the activated clotting time (a variant of the whole-blood clotting time) is used to monitor anticoagulant therapy and is maintained above 400 s. At the end of the procedure the effect of heparin is reversed with protamine sulphate. Haemodilution is a consequence of extracorporeal circulation, but the fall in haematocrit and plasma proteins is about 30 per cent and thus not sufficient to cause a bleeding diathesis. Cardiopulmonary bypass through hypothermia and mechanical stresses produces platelet fragmentation with consequent thrombocytopenia (unusually less than 100×10^9/l) and platelet functional abnormalities. The latter tend to correct by about 3 h postoperatively. In the past the acquired haemostatic defect has been attributed to the acquired platelet defect; however, the efficacy of antifibrinolytic agents in reducing bleeding suggest that fibrinolytic activation is also a major cause of excessive bleeding.

Identification of those at risk of excessive bleeding

There is no assay to indicate which patients will suffer perioperative bleeding, unless screening reveals a previously undiagnosed congenital bleeding disorder. A history of previous or familial bleeding, together with a history of previous surgery and current drug therapy, are necessary before any surgical procedure. Before cardiac surgery, PT, PTT, and fibrinogen levels should be assayed. A bleeding time will give a guide to platelet function.

Prevention

Aprotinin is a basic polypeptide of bovine origin, and is a broad-spectrum serine protease inhibitor with a powerful antiplasmin effect. High-dose aprotinin reduces bleeding during repeat cardiac surgery by approximately 80 per cent. Lower doses of aprotinin have produced smaller reductions of blood loss. Shorter operating times have also resulted, probably due to a reduction of oozing; the operative fields remain 'bone dry'. Other antifibrinolytic agents such as tranexamic acid, given continuously during cardiopulmonary bypass, also reduce perioperative bleeding.

Immediate management of postcardiac surgical bleeding

Initially, the rate of filling of the chest drainage tubes should be checked to ensure that one is not filling more than the others, suggesting a bleeding vessel. A full blood count, PTT, PT, and fibrinogen are helpful, but rapid assays of platelet function and fibrinolytic activity (such as a thromboelastograph), which would be particularly useful, are not widely available. A bleeding time will give a guide to platelet function. It has been usual practice to give 6 units of platelets whatever the platelet count, in view of the acquired platelet abnormality. An antiplasmin dose of aprotinin (500 000 KIU) given intravenously may be useful.

Massive transfusion

This is defined as transfusion of stored blood of a volume equal to or greater than the patient's total blood volume in less than 24 h. The loss of haemostatic factors, consumption in clot formation, dilution with blood products and blood substitutes, and lack of replacement due to inadequate synthesis can result in bleeding diathesis.

Due to modern transfusion practice, dilutional reductions in coagulation factors are now more likely to occur than in the past. An increasing proportion of donor blood is collected for plasma retrieval (see Chapter 3.41), so that red-cell concentrates are produced that preserve red cells with minimal residual plasma and a lack of functioning platelets. However, it is important to appreciate that at least 1.5 blood volumes (that is, 7–8 l in adults) must be lost and replaced to produce a significant thrombocytopenia (less than 50×10^9/l) or clotting factor deficiencies. Platelets should be transfused to maintain a platelet count greater than 50×10^9/l or higher if there is also an acquired platelet function defect due to DIC. A bleeding time is supportive evidence of an acquired defect. It should be remembered that each platelet concentrate will also provide around 50 ml of fresh plasma. DIC may supervene, but cannot be predicted; delayed or inadequate treatment of shock is probably the common predisposing factor.

The use of blood substitutes may produce other haemostatic hazards. Dextrans, and to a lesser extent hydroxylethyl starch, have a fibrinoplastic effect: they accelerate the action of thrombin in converting fibrinogen to fibrin, which makes clots more amenable to fibrinolysis. Both are absorbed on to the platelet surfaces and von Willebrand factor, causing decreased platelet function and an acquired von Willebrand syndrome.

Management

It should be remembered that the major cause of death in massive transfusion is failure to maintain tissue oxygenation. It is imperative that the prime goal is the treatment of shock; haemostatic changes are a secondary issue and occur later. A transfusion of replacement blood components should be given as necessary according to screening coagulation tests, aiming to keep the platelet count greater than 50×10^9/l, PT and APTT less than 1.5 times the control value, and fibrinogen concentrations greater than 1.0 g/l.

Acquired inhibitors to coagulation factors

In the presence of coagulation factor inhibitors an abnormal APTT (or rarely an abnormal PT) cannot be corrected *in vitro* by a 30-min incubation of the patient's plasma plus an equal volume of normal plasma (called a 50:50 mix test). This test thus excludes a factor deficiency and implicates a circulating inhibitor. There are two main types: antibodies directed against coagulation proteins; and antiphospholipid antibodies.

An antibody may be directed against a specific coagulation protein, either in patients with congenital factor deficiencies or in previously haemostatically normal people. Specific autoantibodies have been reported against factor IX, von Willebrand factor, factors V, XII, XIII, and fibrinogen, but these are extremely rare. They may be associated with lymphoproliferative disorders or following recent blood transfusion. The most common target for inhibitors is factor VIIIc. Approximately 5 to 10 per cent of all patients with haemophilia A develop antibodies against factor VIIIc. Usually they occur after the administration of exogenous factor VIII, which, because of an alteration in the patients own factor VIII molecule, is recognized as a foreign protein (see Chapter 3.37).

Factor VIII inhibitors may rarely arise *de novo* in non-haemophiliacs, associated with conditions such as collagen disorders, penicillin sensitivity, cancer, and inflammatory bowel disease, or in the postpartum period, or in elderly people. The clinical course is variable but it is unusual for fatal haemorrhage to occur, and the antibodies may disappear within months or years. Most inhibitors are of the IgG class; rarely, IgA and IgM inhibitors are found in patients with paraproteinaemias.

The antiphospholipid antibodies are a heterogeneous group that bind to negatively charged phospholipid. *In vitro*, they prevent the interaction of coagulation factors with phospholipid that is a necessary part of the template for coagulation reactions. Thus phospholipid-dependent tests such as the PTT are prolonged. Paradoxically, *in vivo* however, these so-called anticoagulants produce an increased risk of both arterial and venous thrombosis (see Chapter 3.39).

Management

Considering management of the commonest acquired inhibitor—an acquired FVIII inhibitor—if there is serious bleeding, high doses of factor VIII can be given to overcome the inhibitor. Alternatively, plasma exchange may be used to remove the inhibitor, or blood products such as porcine factor VIII or factor IX concentrates or activated products can be administered to 'bypass' the need for factor VIII. Recombinant factor VIIa is proving to be particularly successful. Steroids and immunosuppressants may be beneficial in long-term management.

Isolated factor deficiencies

Factor X deficiency may occur rarely with amyloid disease due to the adsorption of factor X to amyloid fibrils. Some patients with amyloidosis also have increased fibrinolysis, probably due to amyloid deposits in the endothelium stimulating the release of tissue plasminogen activator.

Acquired von Willebrand's disease is found in hypothyroidism and is relieved by treatment with thyroxine.

Further reading

Aoki, N. (1989). Hemostasis associated with abnormalities of fibrinolysis. *Blood Reviews*, 3, 11–17.

Fielding, A., Machin, S.J., Goldstone, A.H., Solomon, E., and Gann, A. (1994). Acute promyelocytic leukaemia. *The Lancet*, **344**, 1615–18.

Hunt, B.J. (1991). Modifying perioperative blood loss. *Blood Reviews*, 5, 168–76.

Moia, M., *et al.* (1987). Improvement in haemostatic defect of uraemia after treatment with recombinant human erythropoietin. *Lancet*, ii, 1227–9.

Roberts, B. (ed.) (1991). Guidelines for transfusion for massive blood loss. In *Standard haematology practice* (The British Committee for Standards in Haematology). Blackwell Scientific, Edinburgh.

Shearer, M.J. (1995). Vitamin K. *Lancet*, **345**, 229–34.

Chapter 3.39

Thrombotic disease

M. Greaves and D. A. Taberner

Mechanisms of thrombus formation

Thrombosis arises from the interplay of many influences. Virchow's observation, made over 100 years ago, that the main influences in the pathogenesis of thrombosis are disturbances of the vessel wall, of the blood components, and of the dynamics of flow, have withstood the test of time (Fig. 1).

Pathogenesis of thrombosis

The role of the vessel wall

The healthy vascular endothelium has a range of antithrombotic properties (Table 1; Fig. 1).

Heparan sulphate, a glycosaminoglycan that is intimately associated with the luminal surface of vascular endothelial cells, greatly augments the thrombin-neutralizing activity of plasma antithrombin. In addition, the protein thrombomodulin, which is also a component of the endothelial cell wall, inhibits the procoagulant properties of thrombin and redirects its activity towards an anticoagulant role, in the activation of protein C and thus the neutralization of activated factors VIII and V.

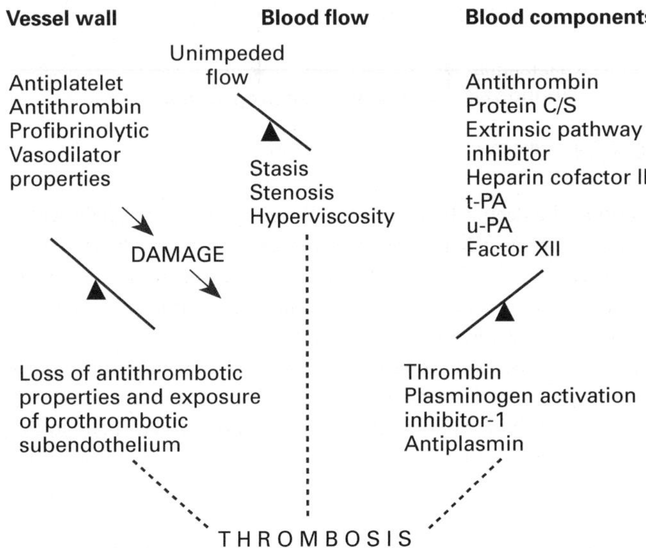

Fig. 1 Virchow's triad and the balance of pro- and antithrombotic factors.

Table 1 Antithrombotic properties of vascular endothelium

Modulation of thrombin activity
• Heparan sulphate
• Thrombomodulin
Modulation of platelet reactivity and release of vasodilators
• Products of arachidonic acid metabolism:
• Prostaglandin I_2
• 13-HODE
• Nitric oxide
Activation and localization of fibrinolytic activity
• Generation of tPA
• Affinity for tPA and plasminogen

13-HODE, 13-hydroxyoctadecadienoic acid; tPA, tissue plasminogen activator.

Tissue plasminogen activator, a central component of the fibrinolytic system, is synthesized by, and released from, vascular endothelial cells. It becomes bound on the endothelial surface, along with its substrate plasminogen. This serves to localize fibrinolytic activity for the rapid dissolution of any fibrin generated, whilst protecting against the risks of enhanced systemic fibrinolytic activity.

The metabolism of arachidonic acid, mobilized from membrane phospholipid by phospholipase, is central to one mechanism of platelet aggregation, through synthesis of prostaglandin endoperoxides and thromboxane A_2 within the platelet. In contrast, within the vascular endothelial cell the principal product of arachidonic acid is prostaglandin I_2, a potent inhibitor of platelet activation.

A potent, local, short-acting vasodilator previously known as endothelium-derived relaxing factor is now known to be nitric oxide. Acting through cGMP it is also capable of modulating platelet activation, and is also physiologically important in the inhibition of vascular occlusion.

The intact vascular endothelium thus possesses a comprehensive range of protective mechanisms that interact to maintain vascular patency. When the vessel wall is breached by trauma, the disruption of endothelial continuity allows platelet accumulation and fibrin generation to occur, thus effectively re-establishing vascular integrity. However, where the endothelium becomes damaged through disease, as in ulceration or rupture of an atheromatous plaque, the local loss of the antithrombotic properties of the vessel lining rapidly leads to thrombus formation and occlusion, with consequent tissue hypoxia and, often, infarction.

The role of blood components

The complex interactions between coagulation enzymes, their inhibitors, platelets, and fibrinolytic mechanisms are described in an earlier section.

The role of disturbed flow

Stasis promotes clot formation by allowing the local accumulation of platelets and activated clotting factors, especially thrombin. Endothelial hypoxia in areas of stasis may also contribute by impairing the antithrombotic functions of vascular endothelium.

In the venous system, stasis occurs as a result of immobility and a failure of the muscle pump necessary for forward flow in the deep veins of the lower limbs. In arteries, areas of relative stasis develop distal to the narrowed segments that are most commonly due to the luminal encroachment of atheromatous plaques.

The viscosity of blood is a major determinant of flow. The main contributors are the haematocrit and the concentration of fibrinogen, which determines the viscosity of plasma and also influences the tendency of erythrocytes to aggregate. Thrombotic complications are common in polycythaemia. It is also noteworthy that the plasma fibrinogen concentration is a potent risk factor for coronary and cerebrovascular thrombosis. It may contribute to this risk by its effect on blood viscosity and flow, as well as by its availability for conversion to insoluble fibrin by thrombin and by its cofactor activity in platelet aggregation.

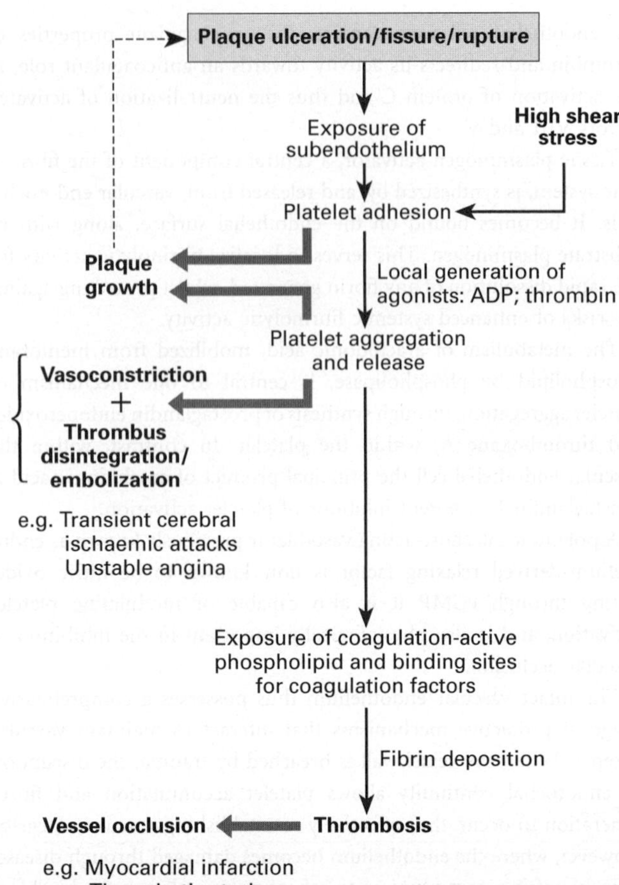

Fig. 2 The pathogenesis and consequences of arterial thrombosis.

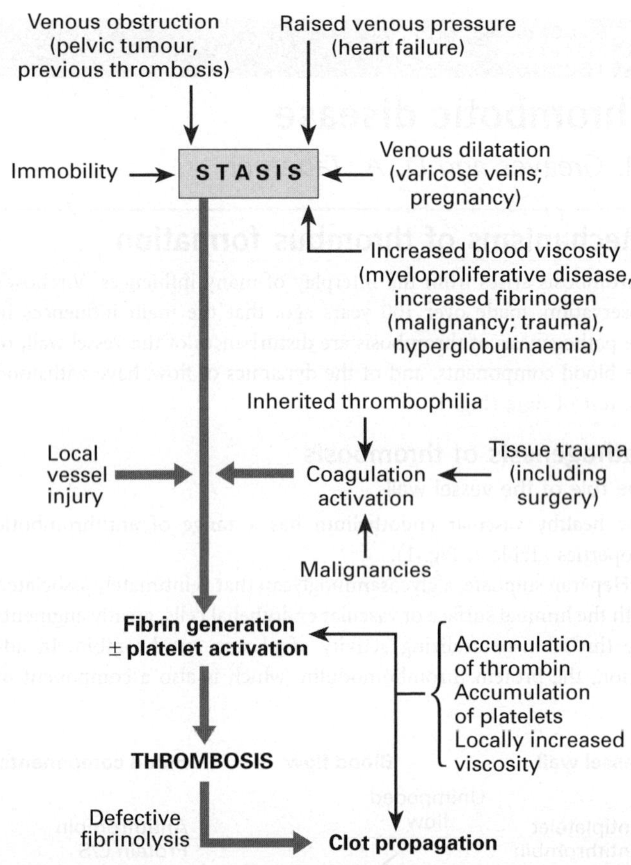

Fig. 3 The pathogenesis of venous thrombosis.

The pathogenesis of arterial thrombosis (Fig. 2)

The arterial system is one of high pressure and rapid flow. Arterial thrombosis almost invariably occurs in association with damage to the vessel wall caused by atherosclerosis. Whilst arterial disease results in ischaemic symptoms at times of increased oxygen demand, it is superadded thrombosis that produces acute ischaemia and infarction. Even if the antithrombotic control mechanisms are sufficient to prevent vascular occlusion and tissue damage, incorporation of platelets and fibrin into the plaque may none the less result in its growth and thus contribute to the pathogenesis of arteriosclerosis (Fig. 2). Platelets carry growth factors and mitogens in intracellular granules to sites of tissue injury. Their release from platelets incorporated into atheromatous lesions contributes to the accumulation of monocytes and the proliferation of smooth-muscle cells that are the hallmarks of the early vascular lesion.

The pathogenesis of venous thrombosis (Fig. 3)

Stasis is the predominant influence in venous thrombosis. This is supported by the clinical observations that the incidence of postoperative venous thrombosis is proportional to the duration of immobility and that, in hemiplegia, deep venous thrombosis most commonly affects the paralysed leg.

Imaging studies demonstrate that by far the commonest sites of origin are the deep veins of the calf. Isolated proximal-vein thrombosis is uncommon, unless there has been local vascular injury or compression.

Within the deep calf veins, many thrombi have their origin within the valve pockets, where venous flow is associated with the formation of vortices and local stasis. When the calf pump fails, due to immobility, venous dilatation, raised venous pressure, or venous obstruction (Fig. 3), further areas of stasis develop.

Although stasis is central to the pathogenesis of venous thrombosis, under experimental conditions blood within an isolated segment of vein remains fluid for some time. The addition of activated clotting factors rapidly results in clot formation, however. *In vivo*, activated clotting factors generated at sites of tissue trauma, including operative trauma, or in association with a malignant tumour, enter the circulation and result in fibrin generation in areas of stasis. Although platelets may become incorporated into the fibrin mesh, their role in thrombosis under conditions of low shear is a relatively minor one.

The consequences of deep venous thrombosis (see also Chapter 2.30)

The morbidity associated with acute thrombosis and the risk of pulmonary embolism are the immediate clinical consequences; the postphlebitic syndrome develops later in a proportion of cases. Thrombus confined to calf veins only rarely produces serious early or late morbidity and the risk of death from pulmonary embolism is low. However, at least 20 per cent of untreated calf-vein thromboses progress to the proximal veins of the lower limb and this carries a 50 per cent risk of pulmonary embolism. The postphlebitic syndrome eventually develops in over half of those afflicted by thrombosis in the ileofemoral veins, due to permanent damage to venous valves with or without residual occlusion of major veins, and consequent chronically increased venous pressure (Fig. 4).

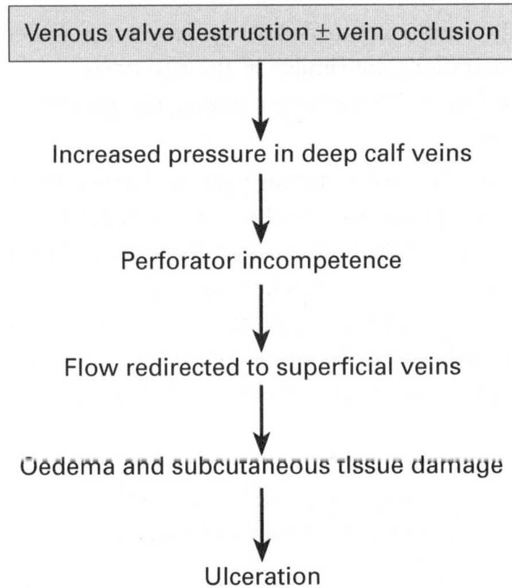

Fig. 4 The pathogenesis of the postphlebitic syndrome.

Table 2 Clinical risk factors for venous thromboembolism

Immobility	Malignancy
Tissue trauma, including surgery	Nephrotic syndrome
Myocardial infarction	Advancing age
Pregnancy and puerperium	Collagen vascular disorders, antiphospholipid syndrome
Oestrogens	Hyperviscosity states
Obesity	Congenital thrombophilia
Varicose veins	Therapy with coagulation-factor concentrate containing activated factors (II, IX, X concentrate)
Previous deep-venous thrombosis	
Congestive cardiac failure	

Hypercoagulable states

In many instances of thrombotic disease an underlying state of hypercoagulability appears to be a contributory factor. Occasionally this is due to an inherited defect in the natural anticoagulant mechanisms, the best characterized being deficiencies of antithrombin, protein C, or protein S. These disorders account for around 10 per cent of venous thrombosis in people under 45 years of age. More recently, resistance to activated protein C due to a mutation in the factor V gene has been described. Instances of a familial thrombotic tendency without deficiency of these anticoagulants are not uncommon, suggesting that there are other disorders of this type which remain to be identified. In homocystinuria, a genetic abnormality of cystathione synthetase is responsible for the development of arterial and venous complications, often at a young age.

More commonly, hypercoagulability is acquired. There is an increased tendency to thrombosis in a wide variety of disorders including malignancy, atherosclerosis, nephrotic syndrome, collagen-vascular disease, primary antiphospholipid syndrome, myeloproliferative disease, paroxysmal nocturnal haemoglobinuria, inflammatory bowel disease, and heparin-induced thrombocytopenia. Microvascular thrombosis is a central feature in disseminated intravascular coagulation, haemolytic–uraemic syndrome, and thrombotic thrombocytopenic purpura. Some additional clinical risk factors for thrombosis are listed in Table 2. These are all acquired hypercoagulable states. In none has a single abnormality of the coagulation or fibrinolytic mechanisms been identified, and in some the mechanisms underlying the prethrombotic state are not known.

Table 3 Familial thrombophilic conditions

Well-defined disorders	Uncommon disorders	Unproven
Antithrombin deficiency	Dysfibrinogenaemias	Factor XII deficiency
Protein C deficiency		Hypo (dys) plasminogenaemia
Protein S deficiency		tPA deficiency
Resistance to activated protein C		
Homocystinuria		

tPA, tissue plasminogen activator.

Inherited thrombotic disorders

The term familial thrombophilia has been applied to a group of disorders in which the increased tendency to venous thromboembolism is due to an inherited defect in, or deficiency of, a natural anticoagulant—antithrombin, protein C, or protein S—or to resistance to activated protein C. Some other familial abnormalities have also been identified, but they are either relatively uncommon or the association with a familial thrombotic tendency is unproven (Table 3).

Antithrombin deficiency

Antithrombin (formerly antithrombin III) is a member of the 'serpin' superfamily, being the major serine protease inhibitor, acting on thrombin, factor Xa, and also factors IXa and XIIa. It is a single-chain glycoprotein of 58 kDa and is synthesized by the liver. The inhibitory effect is through the formation of a 1:1 stoichiometric complex with the enzyme, which involves an active-site serine and a binding domain centred on Arg393 on antithrombin. The rate of enzyme inhibition is enhanced around 1000-fold by heparin, a sulphated polysaccharide, as well as by a heparin-like glycosaminoglycan heparan sulphate, which is present on the vascular endothelium. It is likely that a fraction of plasma antithrombin is bound to heparan sulphate at the luminal surface of the endothelial cell and is thus able to rapidly inactivate any locally generated serine protease.

The association between a familial deficiency of antithrombin and thromboembolism was first described in 1965. Inheritance is autosomal dominant. Estimates of the prevalence have been variable, in the range of 1 in 2000 to 1 in 40 000 of the population. The deficiency may be responsible for 2 to 5 per cent of the cases of venous thromboembolic disease presenting before the 45th year.

Molecular genetics. The human antithrombin gene has been localized to q23–25 of chromosome 1 and consists of seven exons over 19 kb of genomic DNA.

Individuals with antithrombin deficiency are usually heterozygous for the defect. The homozygous condition has been reported and is associated with a severe clinical course. The deficiency can be due to an overall reduction in both immunological and functional levels in plasma (type I) or to a dysfunctional variant (type II). The type- II variants are subclassified depending on the presence of altered reactivity with both heparin and thrombin (IIa), thrombin only (IIb), or heparin alone (IIc). This is of clinical significance as the incidence of thrombotic episodes is much lower in subjects heterozygous for a type-IIc variant than in other antithrombin-deficient subjects. Type-I defects account for 80 to 90 per cent of familial antithrombin deficiencies.

The advent of the polymerase chain reaction and direct sequencing techniques has allowed the description of over 30 mutations leading to type-I deficiency. Most cause frameshifts and the introduction of early stop codons into the coding sequence of the gene.

Over 20 dysfunctional variants (type II) with defective thrombin inhibitory activity and/or altered heparin affinity have been characterized. They arise from single-base mutations that alter the amino acid sequence of the mature protein. In some, a local structural change results, which affects the heparin -binding site. Variants with defective thrombin inhibitory activity usually involve mutations of the reactive centre of antithrombin.

Clinical features. Deep venous thrombosis of the lower limb and pulmonary embolism, often recurrent, are the most common presenting features. Thrombosis may also occur in other veins, including the mesenteric, cerebral, portal, and renal vessels, as well as the inferior vena cava. Presentation in pregnancy or during the puerperium is occasionally seen; surgery and immobilization are other precipitating factors. In one-third of cases no precipitating cause can be found for the presenting thrombotic event. Although there are reports of thrombotic stroke and other arterial events in subjects affected by antithrombin deficiency, the association with arterial thrombosis is weak.

Presentation before the age of 10 years is rare. However, it is estimated that an asymptomatic 15-year-old heterozygote has a 65 per cent risk of developing venous thrombosis by 30 years of age.

Protein C deficiency

Protein C is a glycoprotein that circulates as a covalently linked dimer of 62 kDa consisting of a 41-kDa heavy chain and a 21-kDa light chain. It is synthesized by the liver, and, having nine γ-carboxyglutamic acid residues, is dependent on vitamin K. Activation of the zymogen protein C is by cleavage of a 12-amino acid activation peptide from the amino-terminal end of the heavy chain by thrombin bound to an endothelial cell-surface receptor, thrombomodulin. When activated, protein C, a serine protease, has an anticoagulant function due to the inhibition of activated factors V and VIII, a process that requires protein S as cofactor, as well as phospholipid.

Familial protein C deficiency and its association with venous thromboembolism has been recognized since 1981. It is inherited as an autosomal dominant. The prevalence of the heterozygous state in the general population is a source of controversy. Studies based on subjects presenting with venous thrombosis suggest a prevalence of between 1 in 15 000 and 1 in 30 000. However, 1 in 200 to 300 healthy blood donors have been found to have levels consistent with a congenital deficiency of protein C. It may be that other, as yet unrecognized, factors play a part in the clinical expression of protein C deficiency. Clinical studies suggest that the disorder accounts for venous thromboembolic disease in around 4 per cent of individuals presenting before the 45th year.

Molecular genetics. The human protein C gene has been localized to chromosome 2 and nine exons have been identified.

Analogous to antithrombin deficiency, type-I and type-II deficiencies of protein C are recognized. Parallel reductions in functional and immunological levels are found in type-I deficiency and a relatively greater reduction in functional to immunological activity in type II. In contrast to antithrombin deficiency, in protein C deficiency the clinical manifestations are similar in the two types.

Over 30 different DNA changes within the protein C gene have been identified.

Clinical features Heterozygotes for protein C deficiency are prone to venous thromboembolic events, which may be recurrent (mainly deep venous thrombosis of the limbs), and pulmonary embolism. Cerebral venous thrombosis and splanchnic-vein thrombosis may occur. Superficial thrombophlebitis appears to be more common than in antithrombin deficiency. As discussed above, some heterozygotes remain asymptomatic despite plasma protein C levels of less than 50 per cent of normal.

Anecdotal reports suggest that there may be an increased risk of arterial thrombosis, especially stroke, but this has not yet been substantiated. If present, it is small compared to the risk of venous thrombosis.

In kindreds with protein C deficiency and thrombosis, 80 per cent of deficient individuals will be symptomatic before 40 years of age. An uncommon manifestation of protein C deficiency is warfarin-induced skin necrosis, where haemorrhagic infarction of the skin occurs, usually over an area of adiposity. It appears to be a thrombotic manifestation that is due to the relatively short half-life of protein C, such that, after administration of a vitamin K antagonist, the plasma level falls at a rate similar to that of factor VII, but in advance of II, IX, and X, resulting in a transient hypercoagulable state in the deficient subject.

Homozygous protein C deficiency is very rare. It is phenotypically variable. Most subjects have presented with a syndrome of 'purpura fulminans' within 12 h of birth. Large ecchymoses with purpuric and necrotic skin lesions, disseminated intravascular coagulation, and central nervous thrombosis are typical. Large-vessel thrombosis without skin necrosis may occur. In contrast, some homozygotes with a plasma protein C concentration of less than 10 per cent of normal have remained asymptomatic to adult life.

Protein S deficiency

Protein S is a glycoprotein that circulates as a single-chain species of 70 kDa. Approximately 35 to 50 per cent is bound, in plasma, to C4b-binding protein and only the unbound (free) form is functionally active. Protein S is synthesized by megakaryocytes and vascular endothelial cells, as well as in the liver, and is present in platelet granules. The mature protein has 11 γ-carboxyglutamic acid residues, and full synthesis is dependent on vitamin K. Free protein S forms a 1:1 stoichiometric complex with activated protein C on phospholipid surfaces in the presence of calcium, and thus has cofactor activity in the inhibition of activated factors V and VIII.

Familial protein S deficiency, with venous thromboembolism, was first described in 1984. It is inherited as an autosomal dominant trait and accounts for around 5 to 8 per cent of cases of venous thrombosis presenting before the age of 45 years.

Molecular genetics. The human protein S gene locus is on chromosome 3 and contains two genes, α and β. Only the α-gene is transcribed. It contains 15 exons and has not been fully sequenced. Polymorphisms have been described. The size and complexity of the protein S gene have rendered analysis of the molecular biology of the deficiency more difficult than that of protein C.

Based on the assay of free and bound protein S in plasma, three types of deficiency have been defined. In type-I deficiency there is a reduction in total protein S, most of which is bound to C4b-binding protein, resulting in reduced free protein S. The majority of these cases appear to result from silent alleles, that is a failure of mRNA production by the defective gene. In type-II deficiency, protein S function is impaired, although the total immunoreactive level is normal. Type-III deficiency is characterized by an alteration in the binding characteristics between protein S and C4b-binding protein that results in a reduced level of free protein S.

Clinical features. The manifestations are indistinguishable from those in heterozygotes for protein C deficiency, that is venous thromboembolism in various sites. Warfarin-induced skin necrosis has been reported. Again, although stroke, due to cerebral arterial thrombosis, has been recorded, an increased incidence in familial protein S deficiency has not been proven. It seems likely that, in congenital thrombophilia, there may be a minor increase in the incidence of arterial occlusive events in the presence of additional risk factors.

Activated protein C resistance

It has recently been noted that the anticoagulant response to protein C in its activated state is reduced in up to 50 per cent of selected subjects with a personal or family history of thrombosis. Furthermore, resistance to activated protein C is demonstrable in the plasma of up to 5 per cent of healthy individuals. This phenotype is related to a point mutation in the factor V gene (G→A at nucleotide 1691), affected individuals being heterozygous or homozygous for the mutation. This abnormality may therefore account for the tendency to venous thromboembolism in a very high proportion of subjects.

Dysfibrinogenaemia and thrombosis

Hereditary, functionally abnormal fibrinogen has been described in many kindreds but is not a common disorder. It is most usually detected by a prolongation of the thrombin time on screening tests. The majority of defects do not cause symptoms, but around 30 per cent result in a bleeding tendency, some with poor wound healing. Less than 10 per cent appear to be associated with a thrombotic tendency.

Other coagulation disorders and thrombosis

Several other abnormalities have been associated with a thrombotic tendency, but the relationship appears to be weak or is unproven. Homozygous deficiency of factor XII, a contact factor, produces no haemorrhagic risk, but, possibly due to failure of the contact activation of fibrinolysis, it may be associated with a thrombotic risk. Whether heterozygotes for factor XII deficiency suffer a thrombotic tendency is disputed.

Dysplasminogenaemia has been described in subjects with thrombosis but clinical problems have usually been restricted to the proband, other affected family members being clinically normal.

Reduced vascular release of tissue plasminogen activator has been reported as a familial disorder, but the vast majority of apparent defects in fibrinolysis in subjects with thrombosis are acquired and often transient. Increased production of plasminogen activation inhibitor-1 is the most frequent cause.

Heparin cofactor II is a plasma inhibitor of thrombin, but unlike antithrombin it does not inhibit factor Xa. Deficiency has been reported, with thrombotic disease, but the prevalence is similar in healthy subjects and those with a history of thrombosis, and heparin cofactor II deficiency is thus unproven as a risk factor.

Clinical management of inherited thrombophilia

Acute thrombotic events, almost always in the venous system, should be managed in the conventional way, using heparin and an oral anticoagulant drug (see below). In protein C deficiency, and probably protein S deficiency, because of the risk of warfarin-induced skin necrosis, oral anticoagulation should only be commenced after full heparinization and the use of a loading dose should be avoided. Predictably, deficiency of antithrombin results in a degree of heparin resistance so large doses may be required to achieve adequate prolongation of the clotting time. Antithrombin concentrates are available. Although antithrombin replacement therapy is unnecessary in most circumstances, it may be justified in life-threatening thrombosis or perhaps in thrombosis complicated by disseminated intravascular coagulation in antithrombin-deficient subjects.

The appropriate duration of oral anticoagulant therapy in familial thrombophilia is controversial. After an apparently spontaneous event, lifelong treatment must be considered. Other factors may influence this decision, including the teratogenic potential of warfarin in women of childbearing age, and the very variable clinical expression between kindreds in protein-C and protein-S deficiency states. Where venous thrombosis occurs after trauma or during pregnancy or the postpartum period, long-term anticoagulant therapy may not be justified; however, particular attention must be subsequently paid to prophylaxis at times of high risk.

Clinically unaffected family members with congenital thrombophilia require counselling, including advice to avoid additional risk factors such as oestrogen-containing oral contraceptives, and the need for prophylaxis perioperatively and during periods of immobilization. Management of pregnancy is especially difficult. As the risk appears to be greatest in antithrombin deficiency, prophylaxis should be considered throughout pregnancy and for 12 weeks' postpartum. Warfarin must not be given during the first trimester and around the time of delivery. Many obstetricians now elect to avoid warfarin before the postpartum phase, preferring subcutaneous heparin prophylaxis throughout pregnancy and accepting the, as yet, unquantified risk of symptomatic osteoporosis. In protein C or S deficiencies, decisions relating to prophylactic anticoagulant therapy in pregnancy will be influenced by the previous obstetric and thrombotic history. Prophylaxis for 12 weeks after delivery is a reasonable option in all cases.

Homocystinuria (see also Chapter 6.5)

Homocystinuria is an inborn error of metabolism in which a deficiency of cystathionine synthetase results in an accumulation of methionine and homocystine in the plasma and tissues, and increased excretion of homocystine in the urine. The prevalence is around 1 in 45 000 to 1 in 200 000. It is inherited in an autosomal recessive fashion.

The clinical phenotype is variable and includes mental retardation, ectopia lentis, skeletal abnormalities, and a high incidence of venous and premature arterial thrombotic disease.

Acquired prethrombotic states

The risk of thrombotic complications is variably increased in a range of disease states. In some, the pathogenesis has been at least partially determined, for example the possible role of antiphospholipid antibodies in thrombotic manifestations of autoimmune disease. More commonly, the underlying mechanism has not been determined and may be multifactorial.

Thromboembolism is a common complication of trauma, be it accidental or surgical. Pulmonary embolism is an important cause of postsurgical death and is underdiagnosed. Its prevalence is determined by a range of factors, especially the nature and duration of the surgical procedure, and the presence of preoperative risk factors including malignant disease, obesity, increasing age, varicose veins, and a prior venous thromboembolic event. The roles of thrombin generation and stasis in the pathogenesis of venous thrombosis were discussed earlier. Tissue trauma is followed, over a few days, by thrombocytosis and increased platelet reactivity, an increased concentration of plasma factor VIII, and a rise in plasma fibrinogen. Fibrinolysis is suppressed. These changes potentially contribute to the progression of the thrombotic process.

Thrombosis is a common complication of cardiac disease. Pulmonary embolism is frequent in subjects with congestive cardiac failure, and venous thromboembolism and stroke are recognized complications of myocardial infarction and arterial embolism of atrial fibrillation. Again, stasis and immobility are important contributors to the high risk of thrombosis. Furthermore, in the days following myocardial infarction, changes occur in platelets, factor VIII, fibrinogen (and hence blood viscosity), and fibrinolysis analogous to those after tissue trauma.

In patients with malignant disease, there is an increased risk of apparently spontaneous venous thromboembolism, an observation first made by Trousseau in 1868. Postoperative venous thrombosis is also more common, with an increased risk of two- to threefold. Cancer is two to three times more likely to become manifest in the 2 years after apparently idiopathic venous thrombosis than in the same period after thrombosis in which another recognized risk factor was apparent at diagnosis. Recurrent thrombosis is even more strongly associated with occult cancer. The risk is, however, not sufficient to warrant intensive invasive investigation of subjects presenting with idiopathic venous thromboembolism—providing the history and thorough clinical examination, and the results of simple investigations, do not suggest an underlying malignant disease. Whilst immobility, vessel involvement in tumour masses, and reactive increases in fibrinogen and other clotting factors may be contributory, other prothrombotic effects of cancer have been reported. Inappropriate intravascular coagulation may accompany cancer, particularly with a mucin-secreting adenocarcinoma. Tumour cells may express tissue factor or induce tissue-factor expression by monocytes. Factor X activators have been described in malignancy. Tumour cells may interact directly with platelets and endothelial cells, and may also secrete plasminogen-activator inhibitor.

In nephrotic syndrome in adults, arterial and venous thrombosis occurs. It is a rare complication of childhood nephrotic syndrome (see Chapter 12.5). Loss of anticoagulants, especially antithrombin, in the urine and platelet hyperactivity may contribute.

Whether there is a specific association between ulcerative colitis and venous thromboembolism is unclear, but thrombotic events may complicate the disease. Thrombotic complications are a major feature of Behçet's syndrome. Superficial thrombophlebitis, deep-vein thrombosis, caval thrombosis, cerebral venous thrombosis, and arterial occlusion, often with aneurysm formation, have been described. The thromboses probably occur in association with vasculitic lesions, but reactive increases in fibrinogen and factor VIII may contribute to the prethrombotic state. Antiphospholipid antibodies have been detected in Behçet's syndrome and may be prothrombotic.

Venous and arterial thrombosis, especially thrombotic stroke, are features of polycythaemia rubra vera and essential thrombocythaemia (Chapter 3.9 and 3.11). In paroxysmal nocturnal haemoglobinuria, death is frequently due to thrombotic complications (see Chapter 3.13). Venous thrombosis may affect the splanchnic circulation as well as limb vessels, hepatic and portal venous thrombosis being prominent features. The mechanisms have not been determined.

Although vascular occlusion in sickle-cell disease is due predominantly to the accumulation of non-deformable sickled erythrocytes in the microcirculation, venous thrombosis has been recorded.

Antibodies to phospholipid and thrombosis (see Chapter 10.11)

The association between circulating antibody reactive against (mainly negatively charged) phospholipid and thrombotic complications in systemic lupus erythematosus has been recognized for over 40 years. The antibodies may be detected as a 'lupus anticoagulant', as anticardiolipin, or as the 'biological false-positive' test for syphilis, depending upon the apparent phospholipid specificity of the antibodies and the physical presentation of the antigen in the tests. It is concluded that the lupus anticoagulant is present when there is a prolongation of a phospholipid-dependent test of coagulation, such as the activated partial thromboplastin time, without the presence of an inhibitor to an individual clotting factor or a factor deficiency. There is no specific test, but the kaolin clotting time or the dilute Russell's viper-venom time, with appropriate controls, reliably detect lupus anticoagulant. Paradoxically, the presence of the anticoagulant confers an increased thrombotic risk in systemic lupus, and there is no haemorrhagic tendency. Assays for anticardiolipin use purified cardiolipin, a phospholipid present in the inner leaflet of the mitochondrion, in a solid-phase system. Some antibodies react only in one type of assay—coagulation or solid phase—whilst others give positive results in both, with or without positivity in the Venereal Diseases Research Laboratory test.

Most individuals with serum that reacts positively for antiphospholipid do not have systemic lupus, but may have a history of thrombosis. However, the antibodies may also appear transiently after tissue trauma, in infections, and as a response to exposure to certain drugs (see OTM3, p. 3669, Table 4). Also, lupus anticoagulant is occasionally responsible for the finding of an unexpected prolongation of the activated partial thromboplastin time in a preoperative coagulation screen. Whether these transient and coincidental lupus anticoagulant/anticardiolipins are of pathogenic significance is open to some doubt, particularly as test positivity is often transient after tissue trauma or infection. The clinical significance of weakly positive tests for anticardiolipin is also open to question.

Antiphospholipids present in women of childbearing age have been associated with a strong tendency to pregnancy failure. Recurrent mid-trimester miscarriage, early pregnancy loss, fetal growth retardation, and the development of severe pre-eclampsia occurring unusually early in gestation have all been observed.

The primary antiphospholipid syndrome (PAPS)

PAPS refers to patients without systemic lupus erythematosus but with positive tests for antiphospholipid with a history of thrombosis and/or recurrent (three or more) miscarriages. Thrombocytopenia may also be present, and is presumably autoimmune. The risk of recurrent thrombosis, both arterial and venous, appears to be high. PAPS thus represents an acquired prethrombotic state with an autoimmune basis.

Thrombosis and antiphospholipid. The prevalence of thrombosis in people who test repeatedly positive for antiphospholipid is difficult to determine, owing to selection bias in published series. In systemic lupus the presence of lupus anticoagulant confers an approximately threefold increased risk of thrombotic complications.

In PAPS, thrombotic stroke is a particularly common manifestation and may be the presenting event. In these individuals, heart-valve abnormalities, sometimes with non-infective vegetations, may be present. The risk of recurrent thrombosis is high. Venous thromboembolism is also common and may occur in relatively unusual sites including the cerebral venous sinuses, portal and hepatic veins, and retinal veins. Small-vessel occlusion may occur. Involvement of dermal vessels may lead to livedo reticularis, first reported in association with thrombotic stroke. Whether they are of pathogenic significance, or merely an epiphenomenon, is not yet known.

Intervention is not usually indicated when antiphospholipid is detected incidentally, without thrombotic or obstetric complications. Aspirin, heparin, warfarin, and immunosuppressive agents have been used in the management of recurrent miscarriage and in thromboprophylaxis. Treatment failures are not uncommon and the optimal therapy has not been determined. The use of aspirin or warfarin in arterial thrombosis and warfarin in venous thrombosis is logical. In prophylaxis against recurrent miscarriage, aspirin is the usual initial treatment, with the introduction of prophylactic doses of heparin where aspirin fails. Corticosteroids have been used, but such treatment carries a high risk of maternal morbidity and their efficacy is unproven.

The pathogenesis of thrombosis in PAPS. Cause and effect have not been demonstrated, but various pathogenic mechanisms by which antiphospholipid could result in a prethrombotic state have been postulated. Binding to vascular endothelium, with inhibition of prostaglandin I_2 release, inhibition of fibrinolysis, and interference in phospholipid-dependent protein C activation, or in the anticoagulant effect of activated protein C have been demonstrated *in vitro*.

Recently, it has been shown that phospholipid may not be the target antigen for many of these antibodies, but rather a protein on which epitopes become exposed only when the protein itself becomes bound to negatively charged phospholipids. β_2-Glycoprotein I is such a phospholipid-binding protein that also has anticoagulant properties. It is a target antigen for many 'antiphospholipids'. Interaction with phospholipid-bound prothrombin has been demonstrated in some other sera apparently containing 'antiphospholipid'.

Clinical management of antiphospholipid syndrome. Anticoagulant therapy may not be indicated when the antibody is an incidental finding, although prophylaxis at times of additional risk is a wise precaution. Venous thromboembolism is treated with heparin and an oral anticoagulant; persistence of antiphospholipid may indicate an ongoing increased risk with the need for long-term treatment. Thrombotic stroke has a particularly strong association with antiphospholipid, and limited data suggest a high recurrence rate.

Numerous approaches have been recommended for preventing pregnancy failure in women with PAPS. There have been reports of success with aspirin, heparin, corticosteroids, and intravenous high-dose human immunoglobulin, as well as plasma exchange. Maternal morbidity from hypertension and gestational diabetes mellitus, as well as premature labour, appear to be significant risks of corticosteroid therapy. Subcutaneous heparin carries the risk of maternal osteopenia and the rare complication of severe thrombocytopenia. Until further information becomes available, one approach is to offer low-dose (75 mg daily) aspirin, together with close obstetric observation from confirmation of pregnancy, to women with three or more consecutive episodes of fetal loss and a positive test for antiphospholipid. In the event of failure, heparin prophylaxis (5000 U, twice daily, subcutaneously) may be added early in the next pregnancy, with close clinical observation.

Table 4 Indications for screening for thrombophilia

Tests for AT, protein C, protein S and activated protein C resistance	Tests for lupus anticoagulant and anticardiolipin
Venous thromboembolism presenting at <45 years of age	Venous thromboembolism presenting at <45 years of age
Recurrent venous thrombosis	Arterial thrombosis presenting at <45 years of age in the absence of risk factors
Venous thrombosis in an unusual anatomical site	
Positive family history of thrombophilia	Recurrent (≥3) abortion of unknown cause Early, severe pre-eclampsia For assessment of thrombotic risk in some cases of SLE

AT, antithrombin; SLE, systemic lupus erythematosus.

Atrial fibrillation

All patients in atrial fibrillation should be considered for prophylaxis against thromboembolism. Aspirin reduces the risk of stroke by 25 per cent and warfarin (INR 2–3) by 67 per cent. If the patient has any other risk factors for stroke (for example, previous stroke or transient ischaemic attack, heart failure, an enlarged left atrium, hypertension, diabetes) then warfarin is preferred.

Laboratory screening for thrombophilia

Thorough clinical assessment and simple laboratory investigations will suffice to detect most causes of the prethrombotic state. Screening for inherited thrombophilia is unlikely to be cost-effective if applied indiscriminately. However, it is indicated in younger people, particularly in the circumstances listed in Table 4. Identification of a deficiency allows rational decisions to be made about the duration of therapy for thrombotic events. It also leads to the identification of affected family members before clinical presentation. Although anticoagulant treatment will not necessarily be indicated, appropriate counselling and recommendations for prophylaxis during periods of high risk, pregnancy, and surgery for example, as well as avoidance of other risk factors, are important aspects of management. In screening it must be recognized that the plasma levels of antithrombin and protein C and S can be low in a variety of acquired states (Table 5), also that the results of samples taken during an acute event, and whilst on anticoagulant therapy, may be misleading. Currently it is recommended that, for antithrombin and protein C, both functional and antigenic assays are made; and, for protein S, both the levels of free and bound cofactor are measured.

Screening for antiphospholipid should also be done selectively and a comprehensive laboratory approach employed. This must include a coagulation screening test (activated partial thromboplastin time), as well as more specific tests (kaolin clotting time or dilute Russell's viper-venom time) and an assay for anticardiolipin (these investigations are defined in Chapter 3.34).

Anticoagulant and thrombolytic treatment

Fibrinolytic therapy

The fibrinolytic agents commonly used are plasminogen activators, which activate the proenzyme plasminogen to its active form, plasmin.

Table 5 Conditions in which acquired deficiency of antithrombin, protein C, or protein S may occur

Antithrombin	Protein C	Protein S
Liver disease	Liver disease and transplantation	Liver disease
Disseminated intravascular coagulation	Disseminated intravascular coagulation	Disseminated intravascular coagulation
Nephrotic syndrome	Cardiopulmonary bypass surgery	Pregnancy
Protein-losing enteropathy	Haemodialysis	Systemic lupus erythematosus
Major surgery		In association with antiphospholipid antibody
Acute thrombosis		
Drugs:	Drugs:	Drugs:
Heparin	Warfarin	Warfarin
Oestrogens	Asparaginase	Cancer chemotherapy
Asparaginase	Cancer chemotherapy	Oestrogens

Although they have the potential for generating plasmin action predominantly on the fibrin contained within a thrombus, they also induce a plasma proteolytic state. The resulting plasminaemia destroys fibrinogen and other circulating clotting factors and may induce serious haemorrhage.

Streptokinase and urokinase were the first lytic drugs to be used and they remain in widespread use. Streptokinase is cheaper but is antigenic. Both have low fibrin specificity.

The newer, more expensive agents—recombinant tissue plasminogen activator, acylated plasminogen streptokinase-activator complex (**APSAC**), and single-chain urokinase (pro-urokinase, scu-PA)—are more fibrin-specific. APSAC retains the allergic side-effects of streptokinase (rashes and, rarely, anaphylaxis). Dose-related side-effects, including hypotension, flushing, and nausea, are also seen with streptokinase, APSAC, and tissue plasminogen activator.

Fibrinolytic agents may be given locally or systemically. Local delivery via a catheter is particularly useful for peripheral arterial thrombolysis as it allows angiographic assessment of efficacy. For venous thromboembolism, local treatment has no advantages, while for myocardial infarction the number of patients requiring treatment and the degree of urgency makes intravenous systemic therapy a more practical choice.

Pulmonary embolectomy is reserved for life-threatening occlusion when the patients are deteriorating on medical management (see Chapter 2.30).

In myocardial infarction, prompt lytic treatment provides the most benefit. Intravenous streptokinase, APSAC, and recombinant tissue plasminogen activator all reduce mortality, with a 25 to 30 per cent reduction in the risk of death.

Antiplatelet drugs

Although there has been an interest in the role of antiplatelet agents in thrombotic disease for many years, only recently have clear indications for their use been formulated. Aspirin is of benefit in various groups of thrombotic patients such as survivors of myocardial infarction, and those with unstable angina, transient cerebral ischaemia, or ischaemic stroke. Using aspirin, the secondary prevention of myocardial infarction approaches 25 per cent, mortality from vascular accidents can be reduced by one-sixth, and non-fatal stroke by one-third. A recent meta-analysis indicates a beneficial effect of aspirin on mortality in all subjects with symptoms of arterial disease.

There is still controversy about the optimal dosage, but any dose between 30 and 300 mg appears to be effective; during initial therapy a loading dose of at least 120 mg is required for a full effect. There is a slightly increased risk of haemorrhagic stroke and minor bleeding, but the buffered or enteric-coated formulations provide good gastrointestinal tolerance. Of other antiplatelet drugs, dipyridamole is widely used but its efficacy is unproven. Ticlopidine is effective but causes reversible neutropenia and marrow aplasia and has been superseded by clopidogrel.

Anticoagulation

Heparin is the drug of choice for rapid anticoagulation. Unfractionated heparin (**UFH**) is usually given by bolus injection followed by continuous infusion, or by intermittent subcutaneous injection. Intermittent intravenous injection is associated with more bleeding than continuous infusion. In contrast, warfarin is given orally but takes 4 days to become fully effective.

When long-term anticoagulation is required, it is usual to start with heparin and then introduce warfarin, continuing heparin until warfarin has achieved a therapeutic level. For distal venous thrombosis, warfarin and heparin are normally started together; while for proximal venous thrombosis and pulmonary embolism, longer periods of heparin therapy may be helpful. Consequently, warfarin may be delayed until 3 to 7 days after starting heparin. A recent study has confirmed the need for heparinization in addition to oral anticoagulants in the treatment of venous thrombosis; if oral anticoagulants are used alone, recurrence is more likely.

Heparin

Heparin is a glycosaminoglycan composed of chains of alternating residues of d-glycosamine and uronic acid. Its major anticoagulant effect depends on a unique pentasaccharide with a high-affinity binding sequence to the endogenous coagulation inhibitor antithrombin. After its interaction with heparin, antithrombin undergoes a conformational change that markedly accelerates its ability to inactivate the serine proteases thrombin, factor Xa, and factor IXa. Thrombin is most sensitive to this interaction and a tertiary complex is formed during inactivation, heparin binding to both antithrombin and thrombin.

In contrast, the inactivation of factor Xa is achieved by binding to antithrombin without factor Xa interacting directly with heparin. Low molecular-weight heparin (**LMWH**) molecules containing fewer than 18 saccharides cannot bind antithrombin and thrombin simultaneously, and hence they have a relatively higher anti-Xa:anti-IIa ratio.

This makes potency and hence dosage comparisons between different LMWH formulations difficult. Furthermore, the altered pharmacological properties lead to longer half-lives after subcutaneous or intravenous injection. LMWH have some advantages over UFH: prophylaxis can be achieved with once-daily subcutaneous injections, and they provide better protection against postoperative venous thromboembolism in hip surgery. LMWHs produces a much more predictable anticoagulant response than standard heparin, and therefore they have become the treatment of choice for deep-vein thrombosis. The treatment dose can be calculated according to body weight and given subcutaneously once or twice a day without the need for monitoring or dose adjustment. This is at least as effective and at least as safe as treatment with UFH and clearly offers huge logistical advantages. If UFH is used, generally a loading dose of 5000 U is injected intravenously as a bolus when starting full heparinization. Subsequent heparinization is achieved by a continuous intravenous infusion of 24 000 to 32 000 U over 24 h (the lower dose is recommended for patients who have received recent thrombolytic therapy). Patients vary in their response to the anticoagulant effect of UFH, so that the dose is adjusted depending upon the degree of anticoagulation; the activated partial thromboplastin time (**APTT**) is the most popular method of monitoring therapy. Although APTT reagents differ in their response to UFH, treatment that aims at maintaining the APTT between 1.5 to 2.5 times the average laboratory control value is often used. However, current APTT reagents show increased sensitivity to UFH and higher ratios have recently been recommended. It is wise to seek advice from the local coagulation laboratory on the optimal APTT target range. Monitoring should be started 6 h after induction and continued daily, or more frequently, if the response is inadequate or excessive. Overdose responds within a few hours to a dose reduction or discontinuation; in underdosage a further intravenous bolus can be given, as well as increasing the infusion rate. Protamine is rarely required but is prompt and effective in neutralizing heparin. If bleeding is severe, protamine sulphate should be given in a dose of 1 mg for every 100 IU of heparin that have been infused over the previous hour.

Before heparinization a normal baseline prothrombin time and APTT help ensure that there is no important underlying coagulation defect. Delay in reaching a therapeutic concentration of heparin is associated with a higher incidence of recurrence and extension of venous thrombosis.

Haemorrhage is common with heparin therapy and can occur even when the APTT response is not excessive. Other major side-effects are thrombocytopenia and osteopenia. Thrombocytopenia may be associated with heparin-induced arterial thrombosis. Thrombocytopenia is a dangerous complication and is immune-mediated. It occurs more commonly with bovine than porcine heparin and usually 3 to 15 days after starting heparin, unless the patient was previously exposed. It is more common with higher doses and usually resolves within 4 days of stopping the drug. Heparin should be stopped immediately, and if alternative treatment is indicated, the drug of choice is danaparoid, which can be given until warfarin is effective. Re-exposure may be dangerous.

Osteopenia appears to be more likely after long exposure (usually in excess of 6 months). This is also a serious side-effect and can cause vertebral collapse. Urticaria and skin necrosis can occur with heparin. In the latter, the histological features suggest a hypersensitivity angiitis.

Oral anticoagulants

Oral drugs are generally used where anticoagulation is to be continued for more than 1 to 2 weeks. The preparation most widely used is warfarin, although the shorter acting agent nicoumalone, and the longer acting phenprocoumon, are also in regular use. Phenindione is not recommended because of the high incidence of skin rashes.

Oral anticoagulants compete with the action of vitamin K in the post-transcriptional carboxylation of glutamic-acid residues of clotting factors II, VII, IX, and X and the inhibitory proteins C and S. This takes place predominantly in the liver. Warfarin has a plasma half-life of 35 h and it takes about 1 week to achieve a steady anticoagulant effect. Hence, to optimize that effect, heparin and oral anticoagulants should be continued together for 7 days. In practice, heparin is often discontinued earlier when the prothrombin time is at an apparent therapeutic level. During the first few days of oral anticoagulation the defect is predominantly of factor VII, which is rate-limiting in the prothrombin time test. It is uncertain how effective this period of anticoagulation is in preventing thrombus extension. Therefore, for patients with pulmonary embolism or substantial proximal thrombosis, at least 5 days of combined oral anticoagulants and heparin are advisable. This will ensure adequate depression of all the coumarin-sensitive clotting factors before the heparin is discontinued.

The prothrombin time is used to monitor the effect of oral anticoagulants and guide dosage. In order to take into account the variation between laboratories the result is expressed on a common scale as an international normalized ratio (**INR**). The sensitivity of a local method is expressed as the international sensitivity index (**ISI**). This is the slope of prothrombin times obtained with the primary international reference preparation when plotted against local data for prothrombin time (**PT**) on a log scale: $INR = (PT\ ratio)^{ISI}$. For the majority of therapeutic indications the target range is 2 to 3, but in some instances higher ranges have been recommended. An INR of 3 to 4 is currently recommended to prevent systemic emboli in patients with mechanical prosthetic heart valves.

In patients with recurrent venous thromboembolism, in spite of an INR of 2 to 3, higher ranges have also been recommended. A full search for any underlying cause, particularly neoplasia, could be made.

In arterial disease, aspirin rather than oral anticoagulants is the first choice for therapy. However, oral anticoagulants may be used if transient cerebral ischaemic attacks continue in spite of aspirin therapy or endarterectomy. In view of the increased risk of cerebral haemorrhage with anticoagulation in cerebrovascular disease, a target INR of 2 to 3 is safer than higher ranges.

Warfarin is advised following myocardial infarction in certain patients who have a high risk of thromboembolism. Continuing anticoagulation, after 3 months, may be required where the left ventricle is diffusely dilated or poorly contracting.

Oral anticoagulants are sometimes used in an attempt to prevent further coronary thrombosis after myocardial infarction. However, the current view is that aspirin is preferred for secondary prophylaxis. If oral anticoagulants are used, INR values in the range 3 to 4 are usually advised.

The combination of warfarin and aspirin is potentially dangerous. For patients with a very high risk of further arterial thromboembolism, where such a combination may be justified, a high INR must be avoided and the target INR should be low (2–2.5) with very careful anticoagulant control.

During the induction phase of warfarin, daily monitoring is advised, at least for the first few days. This allows the response to be used as a guide to predicting the maintenance dose. Heparin, except in unusually high doses, does not substantially affect the INR. With a normal baseline INR a daily dose of warfarin of 10 mg is recommended for the first 2 days, with lower induction doses if there is an underlying coagulation defect, liver disease, cardiac failure, or in old or unusually small patients. The required maintenance dose varies considerably

Table 6 Drugs that interact with the effects of warfarin

Increase activity	May increase activity	Reduce activity
Alcohol abuse	*Antigout agents*	*Antibiotics*
Alcohol	Allopurinol	Rifampicin
Disulfiram	*Analgesics*	*Antiepileptics*
Anabolic steroids	Diflunisal	Carbamazepine
Oxymetholone	Flurbiprofen	Phenobarbitone
Stanozolol	Mefenamic acid	Primidone
Analgesics	Sulindac	Phenytoin
Azapropazone	Other NSAIDs	*Antifungals*
Phenylbutazone	*Anion-exchange resins*	Griseofulvin
Antiarrhythmics	Cholestyramine	*Barbiturates*
Amiodarone	*Antiarrhythmics*	*Hormone antagonists*
Propafenone	Quinidine	
Antibacterials	*Antibacterials*	Aminoglutethimide
Aztreonam	Enoxacin	*Oral contraceptives*
Cephamandole	Nalidixic acid	*Vitamins*
Chloramphenicol	Neomycin	Vitamin K
Ciprofloxacin	Norfloxacin	
Co-trimoxazole	Tetracyline	
Erythromycin	Other broad-spectrum antibiotics	
Metronidazole		
Sulphonamides	*Antidepressants*	
Trimethaprim	Fluvoxamine	
Antifungals	*Anticonvulsants*	
Fluconazole	Phenytoin	
Intraconazole	*Hypnotics*	
Ketoconazole	Chloral hydrate	
Micoconazole	*Lipid-lowering drugs*	
Clofibrates	Simvastatin	
Hormone antagonists	*Ulcer-healing drugs*	
Danazol	Sucralfate	
Tamoxifen		
Thyroid hormones		
Ulcer-healing agents		
Cimetidine		
Omeprazole		
Uricosurics		
Sulphinpyrazone		

between patients but is generally between 3 and 9 mg/day (mean 5 mg). Weekly testing is advised for the first few weeks, followed by 1–2-monthly if compliance and control are good. The hazards must be carefully explained to the patient, who should carry a dosage card that should be shown to all doctors, dentists, or pharmacists who deal with them. If there is any change in the patient's condition or medication, the physician should liaise with the anticoagulant clinic as more frequent INR testing may be required. For some patients, control is easy while in others the INR varies without explanation. Drug interaction is a major problem and prescribing requires care and vigilance in warfarinized patients (Table 6).

Haemorrhage is the main side-effect, and dosage omission with INR checking is essential if this occurs. If the INR is below 5.0, a search for a local cause of bleeding is necessary. For life-threatening haemorrhage, 5 mg of phytomenadione (vitamin K) should be given by slow intravenous injection, together with a prothrombin-complex concentrate (preparations usually contain factors II, IX, and X). One litre of fresh frozen plasma can be used instead of a prothrombin-complex concentrate, but may not be so effective. For less severe haemorrhage, when overdose is present (INR >5.0), 0.5 to 2 mg of vitamin K by slow intravenous injection or fresh frozen plasma may be required. For overdose without haemorrhage, and if the INR is below 7.0, missing 1 or 2 days' dosage with early review is sufficient. If the INR is above 7.0, even without haemorrhage, reversal with 0.5 mg of vitamin K_1 by slow intravenous injection or fresh frozen plasma should be considered. Caution is required to avoid complete reversal of anticoagulation in subjects with metal prosthetic heart valves.

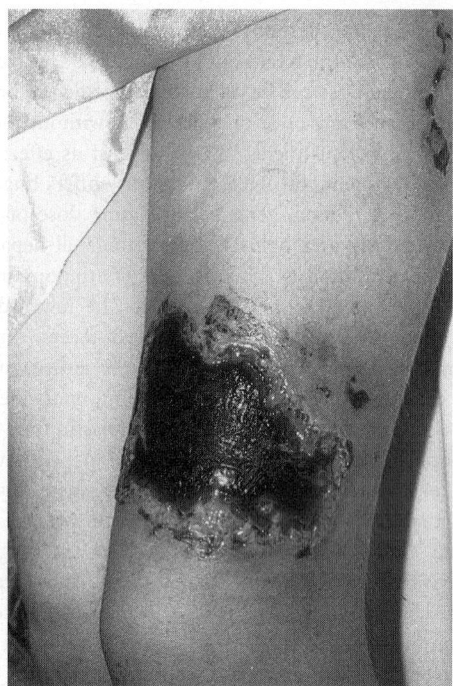

Fig. 5 Coumarin-induced skin necrosis in a patient heterozygous for protein S deficiency.

Other side-effects are very rare. Rashes and alopecia can occur. Skin necrosis is associated with oral anticoagulants, particularly during the induction phase; microscopy shows capillary thrombosis. An association between hereditary protein C or protein S deficiency and coumarin-induced skin necrosis is now recognized (see Fig. 5).

Warfarin is often given for 3 months for venous disease. For idiopathic, proximal deep-vein thrombosis (DVT) or pulmonary embolism 6 months is probably preferable, whilst for a distal DVT with a reversible precipitating factor (for example, surgery) 6 weeks may be adequate. Recurrent venous thrombosis is considered to be an indication for long-term oral anticoagulation. Long-term treatment may also be considered for patients with inherited thrombophilia after a single idiopathic event.

In patients on long-term warfarin, surgery is problematic. Minor surgery can be performed at an INR of less than 2.5. For more major surgery, the warfarin may have to be stopped and heparin substituted. The perceived risk of thromboembolism will dictate if prophylactic doses of heparin are felt to be adequate or if full-dose heparin is used perioperatively.

Warfarin causes a specific embryopathy and if possible should be avoided in pregnancy. The embryopathy is characterized by chondrodysplasia punctata, nasal hypoplasia, and neurological abnormalities, probably due to fetal haemorrhage. Anticoagulant regimens for pregnant patients reflect a balance between thrombotic and teratogenic effects. The warfarin effect on bone and connective-tissue development

Table 7 Incidence of venous thromboembolism in hospital patients according to risk group

	Deep-vein thrombosis (%)	Proximal-vein thrombosis (%)	Fatal pulmonary embolism (%)
Low-risk groups	<10	<1	0.01
Moderate-risk groups	10–40	1–10	0.1–1
High-risk groups	40–80	10–30	1–10

Low-risk groups
Minor surgery (<30 min) with no risk factors except age.
Major surgery (>30 min) with age <40 years and no other recognized risk factor.
Minor trauma or medical illness.

Moderate-risk groups
Major general, urological, gynaecological, cardio-thoracic, vascular or neurological surgery with age > 40 years or other recognized risk factor.
Major medical illness: heart or lung disease, cancer, inflammatory bowel disease.
Major trauma or burns.
Minor surgery, trauma, or illness in patients with previous deep-vein thrombosis, pulmonary embolism or thrombophilia.

High-risk groups
Fracture or major orthopaedic surgery of pelvis, hip, or lower limb.
Major pelvic or abdominal surgery for cancer.
Major surgery, trauma, or illness in patients with previous deep-vein thrombosis, pulmonary embolism, or thrombophilia.
Lower-limb paralysis (for example, hemiplegic stroke, paraplegia).
Major lower-limb amputation.

is maximal 6 to 9 weeks after conception, so subcutaneous heparin is often given for the first trimester. Moderate doses of heparin are required (for example, 10 000–12 000 U, twice daily) but even this may be insufficient to protect against thrombosis on mechanical heart valves. Some authorities therefore maintain such patients on warfarin throughout pregnancy. At delivery, the infant may itself be anticoagulated so that heparin is preferred during the last few weeks of pregnancy (for instance, at 36–40 weeks' gestation). Postpartum, warfarin can be safely used, even with breast feeding, as very little passes into the breast milk. If heparin is used throughout pregnancy there is a risk of oesteopenia.

Prophylaxis for venous thromboembolism (see also Section 2)

Anticoagulants

Pulmonary emboli continue to be a major cause of death in patients in hospital (Table 7). It is not solely a postoperative complication; only 1 in 4 of patients dying from pulmonary emboli in hospital has had recent surgery. In fatal embolism, preceding signs of thromboembolism are often present but not recognized. Serious notice must therefore be taken of any signs or symptoms suggesting venous thromboembolism in patients in hospital. Screening for embolism in asymptomatic individuals, though advocated, is not cost-effective. Routine prophylaxis for moderate- to high-risk patients is recommended, however (see Table 7). The relative merits of the various prophylactic measures available for use after major surgery can be judged from the data in a meta-analysis (shown in Table 8). Low-dose subcutaneous UFH (5000 U, 8 to 12 hourly) is widely used and

Table 8 Incidence of deep-vein thrombosis after major general surgery

	Mean incidence (%) by meta-analysis
No prophylaxis	25.1
Low-dose heparin	8.7
Graduated elastic compression stockings	9.3S
Intermittent pneumatic compression	9.9
Dextran	16.6
Aspirin	20.4

is suitable for moderate- and some high-risk groups. For hip and knee surgery, fixed-dose UFH is only moderately effective, and adjusted-dose or low molecular-weight heparin give better results. Adjusted-dose heparin requires careful laboratory monitoring and is less convenient than LMWH which can be given once daily.

General measures

In addition to the use of prophylactic anticoagulants there are a number of general measures that should be carefully instituted in an attempt to further reduce the frequency of venous thrombotic disease, both in hospital and general practice (see also Chapter 2.30).

In surgical practice there is now well-documented evidence that the use of elastic stockings in the perioperative period are of genuine value. Other simple measures such as early mobilization, the avoidance of dehydration, and the encouragement of leg exercises postoperatively are also useful. Particular attention should be paid to obesity and, where possible, major efforts at weight reduction should be instituted, particularly before 'cold' surgery. Many of these measures are also relevant to patients with serious diseases who may be immobile for prolonged periods.

It is also important to remember the dangers of venous thromboembolic disease in primary-care practice. There is increasing evidence that long journeys by aeroplane, particularly if associated with dehydration due to excessive alcohol intake, or any other form of prolonged immobilization, increase the likelihood of venous thrombosis. Similarly, patients who stay in bed at home for long periods are at increased risk, particularly those who are exposed to thrombogenic agents, the oral contraceptive pill for example, or who become dehydrated as part of an infective disorder.

Further reading

Anonymous (1992). How to anticoagulate. *Drug and Therapeutic Bulletin*, **30**, 7–80.

Bertina, R.M., Koelemann, B.P.C., Koster, T., *et al.* (1994). Mutation in blood coagulation factor V associated with resistance is activated protein C. *Nature*, **369**, 64–7.

Colvin, B.T. and Barrowcliffe, T.W. on behalf of BCSH Haemostasis and Thrombosis Task Force (1993). The British Society for Haematology guidelines on the use and monitoring of heparin 1992: second revision. *Journal of Clinical Pathology*, **46**, 97–103.

Gallus, A.S. (1992). Anticoagulant in the prevention and treatment of thromboembolic problems in pregnancy including cardiac problems. In *Haemostasis and thrombosis in obstetrics and gynaecology* (ed. I.A. Greer, A.G.G. Turpie, and C.D. Forbes), pp. 319–47. Chapman and Hall Medical, London.

Morris, G.K. (1992). Thrombolytic therapy and myocardial infarction. In *Thrombosis and its management* (ed. L. Poller and J.M. Thomson), pp. 231–44. Churchill Livingstone, Edinburgh.

Thromboembolic risk factors (THRIFT) Consensus Group (1992). Risk of prophylaxis for venous thromboembolism in hospital patients. *British Medical Journal*, **305**, 567–74.

Chapter 3.40

The blood in systemic disease

D. J. Weatherall

There are few diseases that do not produce some alteration in the blood. Here, some of the haematological changes that accompany and may be the presenting feature of general systemic diseases of patients of all ages will be summarized.

Malignant disease

By far the most common haematological finding in malignant disease (Table 1) is the anaemia of chronic disorders (Chapter 3.17). It may occur together with localized or widespread malignancy of any type and may respond to successful removal of the primary tumour. Remember that the anaemia may be complicated by chronic blood loss and superimposed iron deficiency.

Disseminated malignancy

Disseminated malignancy may be associated with a leucoerythroblastic picture characterized by the presence in the blood of immature myeloid cells together with some nucleated red cells and, sometimes, a mild reticulocytosis. This is very commonly accompanied by the presence of tumour cells in the bone marrow. Occasionally, widespread carcinoma leads to a leukaemoid reaction with white-cell counts in the range seen in chronic myeloid leukaemia (Chapter 3.27). The microangiopathic haemolytic anaemia of disseminated malignancy (Chapter 3.25) is most frequently found in association with mucin-secreting adenocarcinoma, particularly of the stomach, breast, and lung.

Less common forms of anaemia associated with cancer

Autoimmune haemolytic anaemia is sometimes found in patients with an underlying lymphoma and, rarely, with other forms of tumour. Pure red-cell aplasia may occasionally be the presenting feature in a patient with a tumour of the thymus. Finally, it should be remembered that there is an association between pernicious anaemia and carcinoma of the stomach and a patient may present with a megaloblastic anaemia associated with a malignancy of this type. Sideroblastic anaemias are occasionally found in patients with carcinoma.

Polycythaemia

The relationship between secondary polycythaemia and a wide variety of underlying neoplasms is discussed in Chapter 3.26.

Changes in the platelets and blood coagulation

An otherwise unexplained thrombocytosis may be the first indication of an underlying malignancy, even in the absence of chronic bleeding.

Table 1 Principal haematological changes in malignant disorders

Erythrocytes	
Anaemia of chronic disorders	All forms
Iron-deficiency anaemia	Gastrointestinal; cervix, uterus
Leucoerythroblastic anaemia	Stomach, breast, thyroid, prostate, bronchus, kidney
Microangiopathic haemolytic anaemia	Mucin-secreting tumours; stomach, bronchus, breast
Secondary myelosclerosis	As for leucoerythroblastic; also reticuloses
Selective red-cell aplasia	Thymus, lymphoma, bronchus
Immune haemolytic anaemia	Ovary; lymphoma; other carcinomas
Megaloblastic anaemia	Stomach; rarely others
Sideroblastic anaemia	Myelodysplastic syndrome
Polycythaemia	Kidney, liver, posterior fossa, uterus
Leucocytes	
Leucocytosis	All forms
Leukaemoid reactions	As for leucoerythroblastic anaemia
Eosinophilia	Miscellaneous carcinomas and reticuloses
Monocytosis	All forms
Basophilia	Myeloproliferative disease; mastocytosis
Lymphopenia	Carcinoma, reticuloses
Platelets	
Thrombocytosis	Gastrointestinal with bleeding; bronchus and others without bleeding
Thrombocytopenia	As for the microangiopathies
Acquired thrombocytopathy	Macroglobulinaemia; other paraproteinaemias
Coagulation	
Disseminated intravascular coagulation	Prostate, many others
Primary activation of fibrinolysis	Prostate
Selective impairment of coagulation	
Thrombophlebitis	All forms
Miscellaneous	
Abnormal proteins-cryofibrinogens	Prostate, others
Fetal proteins	Alpha-fetoprotein—liver and others
	Carcinoembryonic antigen (CEA)—gastrointestinal neoplasms
	Fetal haemoglobin—leukaemia, other tumours
Circulating tumour cells	All forms
Effects of cytotoxic drugs	All forms

Generalized haemostatic failure associated with disseminated carcinoma is considered in detail in Chapter 3.38 (Figs 1 and 2). A detailed analysis of the activities of the intrinsic and extrinsic pathways must be made as malignancies can be associated with a variety of specific coagulation disorders including factor inhibitors and deficiencies.

White-cell abnormalities

Apart from the leukaemoid reaction described above, persistent monocytosis or eosinophilia may be associated with Hodgkin's disease

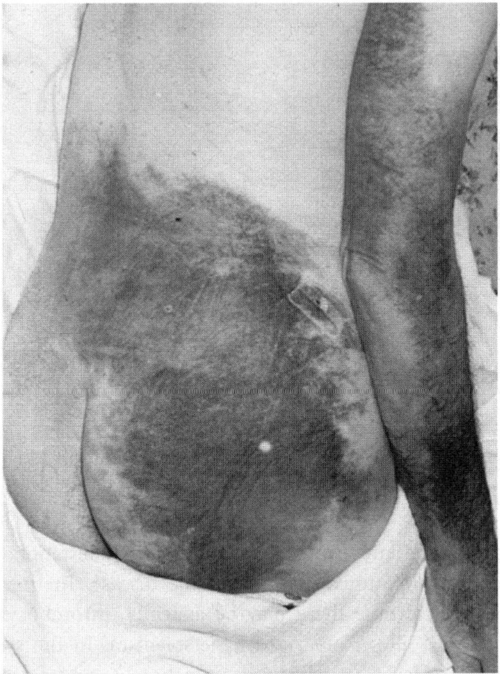

Fig. 1 Disseminated intravascular coagulation in association with carcinoma of the prostate. The patient started to bleed extensively from the iliac-crest marrow biopsy site and from venesection sites. Marrow biopsy showed widespread tumour metastases.
(Reproduced from Hardisty, R.M. and Weatherall, D.J. (ed.) (1982). Blood and its disorders, 2nd edn. Blackwell Scientific, Oxford, with permission.)

or with bronchial carcinoma. Persistent lymphopenia may occur in patients with Hodgkin's disease.

Infection

Acute bacterial infection

Most acute bacterial infections are associated with a neutrophil leucocytosis. This may be so marked, and associated with such a 'shift to the left' with production of myelocytes in the blood that the condition may present a leukaemoid type of reaction. Occasionally, however, the neutrophil response seems inadequate, or may be frankly neutropenic. This clinical picture is particularly common in newborn infants, especially those born prematurely. Monocytosis has been reported in patients with typhoid fever and sometimes in brucellosis or subacute bacterial endocarditis.

Some degree of anaemia is found almost invariably in patients with bacterial infection and usually presents a picture of the anaemia of chronic disorders. Haemolytic anaemia may occur in severe septicaemias and is usually associated with disseminated intravascular coagulation. Some organisms, *Clostridium welchii* for example, produce an α-toxin that acts as a lecithinase and causes fulminating intravascular haemolysis. Disseminated intravascular coagulation and thrombocytopenia is a relatively common accompaniment of severe bacterial infection.

Chronic bacterial infection

Chronic bacterial infection is usually associated with the anaemia of chronic disorders. Disseminated tuberculosis may be associated with leukaemoid reactions, pancytopenia, myelofibrosis, and even polycythaemia.

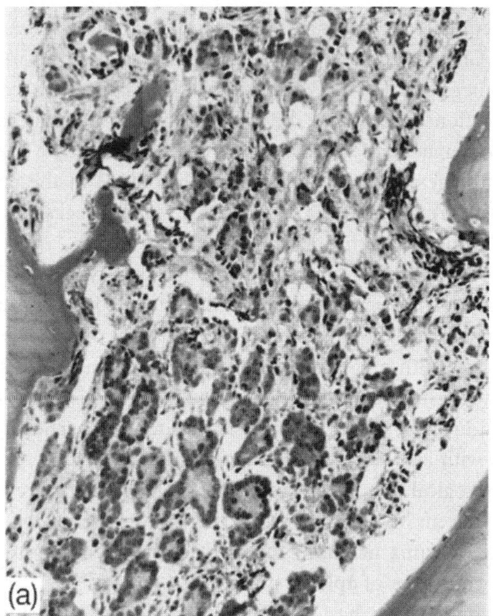

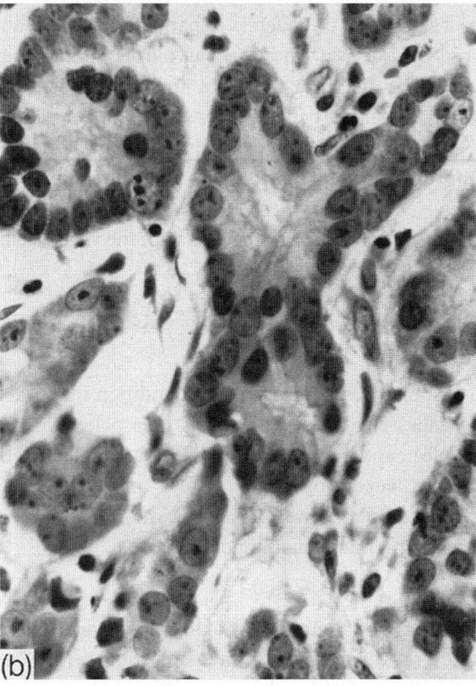

Fig. 2 Section prepared from Gardner-needle biopsies from bone marrow infiltrated with neoplastic cells; the primary tumour was in the prostate (haematoxylin and eosin stain). (a) 230 ×. (b) 920 ×.
(Reproduced from Hardisty, R.M. and Weatherall, D.J. (ed.) (1982). Blood and its disorders, (2nd edn). Blackwell Scientific, Oxford, with permission.)

Virus infections

Rubella, acquired in childhood or adult life, is often associated with a leucocytosis and an atypical lymphocytosis. A small proportion of patients develop an acute fulminating thrombocytopenic purpura approximately 4 days after the appearance of the rash. This is usually self-limiting but fatalities have been reported. Thrombocytopenia is also common in infants with congenital rubella, and this condition is also characterized by a non-immune haemolytic episode shortly after birth.

The haematological changes in infectious mononucleosis are described in Chapter 16.12. A very similar picture can occur in patients with cytomegalovirus (**CMV**) infection. In infants with congenital CMV infections there may be striking hepatosplenomegaly with purpura and anaemia. The anaemia is characterized by a haemolytic picture with the appearance of many normoblasts in the peripheral blood. This form of anaemia may last for several weeks and may be associated with severe thrombocytopenia.

Infections with human immunodeficiency virus type-1 (**HIV**-1) can cause lymphopenia, neutropenia, and thrombocytopenia. Anaemia is also common and bone marrow examination often reveals dyserythropoiesis with a variable degree of erythrophagocytosis. In addition to these haematological complications there is the added risk of drug-induced marrow hypoplasia, associated particularly with treatment with zidovudine (azidothymidine, AZT).

Haematological complications of infectious hepatitis are rare, but when they occur they may be extremely severe. Coombs' positive haemolytic anaemia has been reported, and there is an association with the occurrence of aplastic anaemia.

Human parvovirus has an affinity for red-cell progenitors and probably causes transient red-cell aplasia quite commonly. This only gives rise to a symptomatic anaemia in patients who have a markedly shortened red-cell survival, and thus parvovirus infection appears to be responsible for the aplastic crises in patients with sickle-cell anaemia, pyruvate kinase deficiency, or other congenital haemolytic anaemias. Viruses can cause acute damage to the bone marrow in immunosuppressed patients as part of the virus haemophagocytic syndrome.

The haematological changes associated with the virus haemorrhagic fevers are described in detail in Section 16.

Parasitic disease

Toxoplasmosis

Congenital toxoplasmosis can produce a condition identical to erythroblastosis fetalis. The clinical picture is of a pale, hydropic infant with a large spleen and liver associated with severe anaemia, thrombocytopenia, and a leucocytosis, often with a marked eosinophilia. In adult life the acquired forms of toxoplasmosis produce a clinical disorder resembling infectious mononucleosis.

Malaria

Malarial infection produces a variety of haematological abnormalities. The most severe changes occur in association with *Plasmodium falciparum* malaria infection. In acute infections in non-immune individuals there is usually minimal anaemia at the onset of the illness, but during the 2 to 3 weeks after treatment there may be a steady decline in haemoglobin level, the mechanism of which is not yet fully worked out. On the other hand, children or adults with chronic malaria, some degree of immunity, and low-level parasitaemias, may be severely anaemic at presentation with an inappropriately low reticulocyte count. The bone marrow is often hyperplastic and shows a marked degree of dyshaemopoiesis (Fig. 3) (see also Chapter 3.21). There may also be marked intravascular haemolysis and haemoglobinuria. Again, the mechanism is not certain, and although some of these patients may be glucose 6-phosphate dehydrogenase deficient, this is by no means the whole story. Thrombocytopenia is extremely common in patients with acute malaria. In addition, most forms of malarial infection are associated with neutropenia, and monocytosis has also been described.

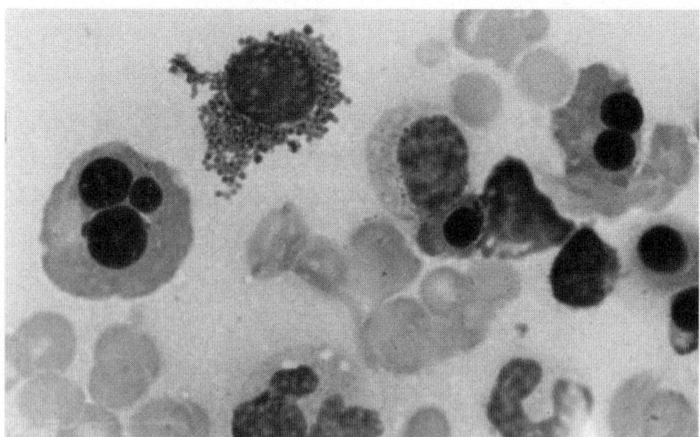

Fig. 3 Bone marrow appearances in *P. falciparum* malaria. There is marked dyserythropoiesis with several multinucleate red-cell precursors (Giemsa stain, 800 ×).

There are several interesting haematological manifestations of malaria associated with unusual forms of the disease. In the tropical splenomegaly syndrome there may be anaemia, thrombocytopenia, and neutropenia, all secondary to hypersplenism. In the syndrome of congenital malaria, in which the infection is contracted in intrauterine life from the mother, newborn babies have a febrile illness associated with profound anaemia that appears to result from the combination of haemolysis and bone marrow suppression.

Leishmaniasis

Particularly in young children, visceral leishmaniasis, or kala azar, is associated with hepatosplenomegaly, lymphadenopathy, and a pancytopenia. Early in the course of the disease there is often marked neutropenia and the marrow may be grossly infiltrated with parasitized macrophages. The anaemia is due mainly to a short red-cell survival; there is also an inappropriate marrow response and a variable degree of hypersplenism.

Hookworm

The haematological changes of hookworm infestation are described in Chapter 16.99. It is one of the most common causes of iron-deficiency anaemia in the world population. During the systemic phase of the illness, when the larvae invade the lungs, there may be a marked eosinophilia.

Visceral larva migrans

This condition is characterized by striking haematological changes including anaemia, a marked leucocytosis with eosinophilia, and changes in the titre of anti-A and anti-B blood-group antibodies.

Rheumatoid arthritis and related disorders

In patients with rheumatoid arthritis, anaemia is extremely common and usually follows the general pattern of anaemia of chronic disorders. It is occasionally complicated by genuine iron deficiency, which may result from a variety of causes including poor diet and chronic blood loss due to the effects of treatment, particularly ingestion of non-steroidal, anti-inflammatory agents. Ferritin estimation is useful in distinguishing chronic disease and iron deficiency. The platelet count is elevated in between 20 and 50 per cent of patients with rheumatoid arthritis and parallels the degree of activity of the illness. The haematological changes of Felty's syndrome (anaemia, thrombocytopenia, and marked neutropenia) are summarized in Section 10.

The management of the haematological manifestations of rheumatoid arthritis and Felty's syndrome is unsatisfactory. The anaemia generally reflects the activity of the disease. If there is genuine iron deficiency, iron replacement therapy is indicated. There is controversy about the best way to manage Felty's syndrome. After splenectomy there is sometimes a dramatic rise in the neutrophil and total leucocyte counts, but this is not always associated with a decreased incidence of infection. Furthermore, some patients show no change in the white-cell count after surgery.

There is also a variety of haematological changes secondary to drug therapy for rheumatoid arthritis and related disorders. Salicylates may produce chronic blood loss, while drugs containing phenacetin produce methaemoglobinaemia and Heinz body haemolytic anaemia that may sometimes be preceded by a marked eosinophilia. Oxyphenylbutazone and penicillamine may cause severe marrow depression. The administration of gold occasionally causes marked thrombocytopenia or pancytopenia.

Systemic lupus erythematosus and other collagen disorders

It is quite common for systemic lupus erythematosus (SLE) to present with a haematological disorder. This is not the case in the other collagen-vascular disorders. The most common blood change is anaemia, which occurs in nearly all patients at some stage of the illness. It is usually a mild anaemia of chronic disorders, which may be complicated by blood loss from analgesics or anti-inflammatory medication, renal impairment, or haemolysis. Acquired autoimmune haemolytic anaemia occurs in around 5 per cent of cases and may be the sole presenting feature. The Coombs' test is invariably positive with anticomplementary reagents and is positive with anti-IgG during episodes of acute haemolysis. Other forms of anaemia in SLE include hypersplenism and a hypocellular bone marrow.

The most consistent finding in the white-cell count in SLE is leucopenia which is often a combined neutropenia and lymphopenia. Mild eosinophilia occurs occasionally, particularly in association with skin involvement. A mild thrombocytopenia occurs in 10 to 25 per cent of all cases of SLE. More severe thrombocytopenia, producing a picture almost indistinguishable from idiopathic thrombocytopenic purpura, occurs in a small proportion of patients and may be the sole presenting feature in some.

An important abnormality of coagulation in SLE is the lupus anticoagulant. This is a circulating anticardiolipin which interferes with the binding of phospholipid to form prothrombin activator, and this affects the intrinsic and extrinsic clotting pathways (see Chapter 3.39). Although it causes a prolonged partial thromboplastin time, its presence in patients with SLE seems to produce a clotting rather than a bleeding tendency. A significant number of patients who have the lupus anticoagulant have recurrent thrombotic episodes including cerebral thromboses. It is also associated with recurrent spontaneous abortions and, possibly, with 'idiopathic' pulmonary hypertension.

The haematological changes in the other collagen-vascular diseases are much less impressive. They are all associated with the anaemia of chronic disorders. Polyarteritis nodosa may be characterized by an eosinophilia.

The interesting syndrome of polymyalgia rheumatica and temporal arteritis may present to the haematologist (Chapter 3.17 and Section 10). There are usually significant haematological changes characterized by a severe anaemia of chronic disorders with a marked elevation of the erythrocyte sedimentation rate (**ESR**). The leucocyte count is usually normal, although occasionally there may be a mild eosinophilia.

Renal disease

Almost all forms of renal disease are associated with haematological changes. However, by far the most important is the severe refractory anaemia that accompanies chronic renal failure. The anaemia has a complex aetiology including shortened red-cell survival, impaired red-cell production, or iron deficiency. Rarely, splenomegaly and hypersplenism or folate deficiency may develop.

The anaemia of chronic renal failure is normochromic and normocytic unless there is associated iron deficiency. The red cells show characteristic deformities with multiple tiny spicules and contracted poikilocytes. The total and differential white-cell count is usually normal in patients with chronic renal failure. However, neutrophil function and cell-mediated immunity are often depressed.

There is a variety of haemostatic defects in different forms of renal disease. Most forms of renal failure are associated with a bleeding tendency, which is seen in its most florid form in acute renal failure. The main features are purpura, and mucosal and gastrointestinal bleeding associated with abnormal platelet function and a prolonged bleeding time; these changes are reversible by dialysis. Many conditions that lead to renal failure are also associated with thrombocytopenia.

The nephrotic syndrome is characterized by a marked tendency to thrombosis. Platelet aggregation and release reactions are enhanced in this condition and protein loss in the urine may also play a part.

Polycythaemia

The polycythaemias associated with renal lesions and following renal transplantation are discussed in Chapter 3.26.

Treatment of the haematological complications of renal disease

The management of the anaemia of chronic renal failure has been revolutionized by the availability of recombinant erythropoietin (Chapter 12.29). The management of bleeding in patients with acute renal failure is based on correction of uraemia by dialysis and appropriate replacement therapy. If there is severe thrombocytopenia, platelet transfusions should be given.

Gastrointestinal and liver disease

Gastrointestinal blood loss

Blood loss in excess of 20 ml/day will always result in a negative iron balance and ultimately in iron-deficiency anaemia, the time taken depending on the body stores of iron when the bleeding started. The haematological picture shows the typical changes of iron-deficiency anaemia, and occasionally there are clues that this blood picture is associated with chronic blood loss. Quite frequently there is a mild to moderate thrombocytosis, and if iron is being taken there may be a dimorphic blood picture (Fig. 4), red-cell polychromasia, and a low-grade reticulocytosis. Target cells may indicate liver disease, whereas Howell–Jolly bodies suggest malabsorption due to adult coeliac disease complicated by hyposplenism.

The investigation of chronic gastrointestinal blood loss may be difficult (see Chapter 3.16). If gastrointestinal blood loss is suspected the first step is to confirm this by examining several stool specimens

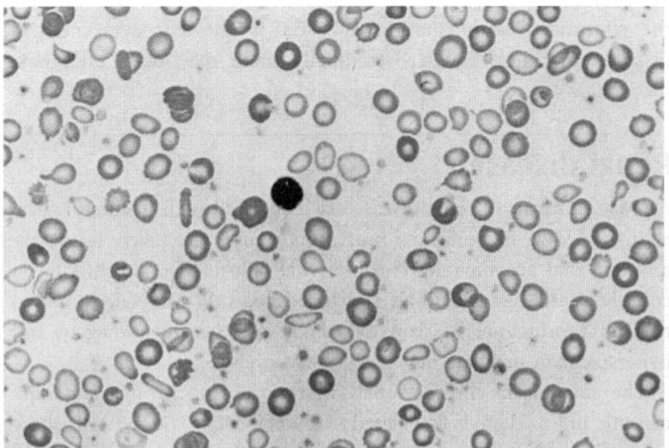

Fig. 4 Peripheral blood picture associated with gastrointestinal bleeding. The red cells show a dimorphic picture with hypochromic and normochromic forms. The platelet count is elevated, a typical finding in bleeding (Giemsa stain 600 ×).

for occult blood. If these are positive the next step is to determine the site of bleeding. This will usually require an upper gastrointestinal endoscopy and barium enema or colonoscopy. If these investigations do not provide a diagnosis, and there is persistent bleeding, the duodenum and small bowel should be studied radiologically. Occasionally it is necessary to resort to coeliac or superior mesenteric angiography.

Inflammatory diseases of the bowel

A mild anaemia of chronic disorders is a common accompaniment of inflammatory bowel disease and may be complicated by blood loss or dietary iron deficiency. In some cases of extensive Crohn's disease there may be an added factor of malabsorption. Anaemia occurs in about one-third of patients with this condition and occasionally it may be complicated by reduced vitamin B_{12} or folic acid absorption.

The anaemia of intestinal inflammatory disease may be made worse by drugs used in its management. Patients who receive salazopyrine for colitis occasionally develop an acute haemolytic anaemia associated with Heinz-body formation, and bone marrow depression may occur in patients receiving immunosuppressive treatment for colitis or Crohn's disease.

Whipple's disease may produce a clinical picture and blood changes that can mimic several primary haematological disorders. The typical clinical triad of diarrhoea, arthropathy, and enlarged lymph nodes is usually associated with a mild normochromic, normocytic anaemia, a raised ESR, and a polymorphonuclear leucocytosis. Quite often there is associated lymphopenia or eosinophilia.

Structural disease of the stomach and small and large bowel

The structural changes and resulting abnormalities of absorption associated with gastritis are described in detail in Section 5. Similarly, the various anatomical abnormalities of the small-gut and malabsorption syndromes that lead to vitamin B_{12} and folate deficiency are reviewed in Chapter 3.18. The relationship between gastric surgery and iron and vitamin B_{12} metabolism is discussed in Chapter 3.16 and Chapter 3.18.

Most anatomical lesions of the small bowel present to the haematologist as a macrocytic anaemia with a megaloblastic bone marrow due to vitamin B_{12} or folate deficiency, or as a refractory iron-deficiency anaemia. Several abnormalities of the small gut are associated with the production of a relatively profuse bacterial flora with subsequent utilization of vitamin B_{12}. These conditions include surgically produced blind loops, strictures, anastomoses between loops of small bowel, fistulae between various sections of the bowel, diverticula of the small bowel, malfunctioning gastroenterostomies, interference of gut motility in conditions such as scleroderma, Whipple's disease, post-vagotomy, and after extensive gut resection, where the disorder may also produce malabsorption. All these conditions are associated with defective vitamin B_{12} absorption, which can be partly corrected by the administration of broad-spectrum antibiotics but not by intrinsic factor.

Malabsorption syndromes may present to the haematologist in a variety of ways. In addition to classic megaloblastic anaemia there is a very high incidence of iron-deficiency anaemia, and in childhood this is the more common form of presentation. The peripheral blood changes of hyposplenism are quite frequently associated with an underlying malabsorption syndrome, which itself may also present with a bleeding disorder due to prothrombin deficiency following defective absorption of vitamin K.

Table 2 Haematological changes in liver disease

Virus hepatitis
Haemolytic anaemia, hypoplastic anaemia
Chronic active hepatitis
Immune haemolytic anaemia, hyperglobulinaemia
Chronic liver failure
Chronic anaemia is often complicated by: (a) blood loss and iron deficiency (b) alcohol, direct effect on marrow (c) folate deficiency (d) portal hypertension and hypersplenism (e) acute haemolytic episodes (e.g. Zieve's syndrome, spur-cell syndrome)
Thrombocytopenia, leucopenia, haemorrhagic diathesis due to: (a) deficiency of vitamin K-dependent factors (b) portal hypertension and hypersplenism (c) increased fibrinolysis (d) thrombocytopenia
Portal hypertension
Anaemia, leucopenia, thrombocytopenia, bleeding from varices
Obstructive jaundice
Mild anaemia, target-cell formation, masking of hereditary spherocytosis
Tumours
Polycythaemia, leukaemoid reactions, alpha-fetoprotein production
Liver transplantation
Haemorrhagic and hypercoagulable states

Liver disease

There is usually a moderate degree of anaemia in patients with chronic liver failure (Table 2). The red cells are normochromic or slightly macrocytic with mean corpuscular volume (MCV) values ranging from 100 to 115 fl. Target cells, variable polychromasia, and a slightly elevated reticulocyte count are often found. The degree of macrocytosis and target-cell formation corresponds reasonably well with the degree of liver failure. The actual mechanism of the anaemia is uncertain but includes nutritional folate deficiency and secondary iron deficiency.

A variety of different forms of haemolytic anaemia occur in patients with liver disease. In Zieve's syndrome there is jaundice, hyperlipidaemia, and haemolytic anaemia that follows an excessive alcohol intake (see Chapter 3.25). Acute haemolysis has been well documented in patients with viral hepatitis.

The haematological effects of alcohol

Anaemia is particularly common in chronic alcoholics. It has an extremely complex aetiology including a deficient diet, chronic blood loss, hepatic dysfunction, and the direct toxic effects of alcohol on the bone marrow. An unexplained macrocytic blood picture should always raise the possibility of alcoholism, although its absence does not rule out the diagnosis. Frank megaloblastic anaemia is usually seen in severe alcoholics who are poorly nourished, and is due to folate deficiency. Simple iron deficiency is also found commonly in alcoholics and probably reflects both a poor diet and chronic blood loss due to gastritis or bleeding varices. In addition, any of the haematological manifestations of liver disease may be found in alcoholics.

Alcohol also has deleterious effects on the white cells and severe alcoholics are prone to infection. The neutropenia of alcoholism may reflect both the toxic effect of alcohol on the marrow and folate deficiency. Thrombocytopenia is commonly seen in chronic alcoholics and may occur without accompanying folate deficiency or splenomegaly. Following withdrawal of alcohol the platelet count usually returns to normal, although it may become markedly elevated for a few days.

Chest disease

(See also carcinoma and tuberculosis, above, and secondary polycythaemia, Chapter 3.26).

Pneumonia

Most bacterial pneumonias are associated with a neutrophil leucocytosis. Two relatively common forms of pneumonia are associated with more specific haematological changes. In mycoplasma pneumonia, cold agglutinins can usually be detected in increased amounts towards the end of the first week in up to 80 per cent of cases. The cold antibodies are polyclonal IgM and to the red-cell I antigen. Although a positive Coombs' test has been described in these cases, and in most of them there is an increased reticulocyte count, serious haemolysis is rare. Occasionally, the condition is complicated by disseminated intravascular coagulation.

There is increasing evidence that in patients with pneumonia caused by *Legionella pneumophila* (Legionnaires' disease) there may be severe thrombocytopenia and, sometimes, lymphopenia. Several cases have been reported to be complicated by disseminated intravascular coagulation.

Pulmonary eosinophilia (see also Chapters 3.32 and 4.24)

This term refers to a group of disorders that have in common a raised eosinophil count in the peripheral blood in association with pulmonary infiltrates on the chest radiograph. The exact nature of many of the disorders that constitute this syndrome is uncertain. In its simplest form there may be a brief period of respiratory distress in association with eosinophilia. This condition is sometimes called Löffler's syndrome. At the other end of the spectrum there is a severe illness associated with widespread pulmonary infiltrates and eosinophilia, which may culminate with the features of polyarteritis nodosa.

The transient disorder described by Löffler probably represents a heterogeneous group of conditions including parasitic infection, hypersensitivity reaction to drugs, and allergic alveolitis (see Section 4). Another well-documented cause of pulmonary eosinophilia is hypersensitivity to fungi, particularly *Aspergillus fumigatus.*

Idiopathic pulmonary haemosiderosis and Goodpasture's syndrome (see Chapter 12.8)

These disorders occasionally present as a refractory anaemia with the characteristics of the anaemia of chronic disorders, although it may become markedly hypochromic and microcytic due to chronic blood loss.

Skin diseases

Megaloblastic anaemia and the skin

The relationship between skin disease and megaloblastic anaemia is controversial (see Chapter 3.18). There is no doubt that a proportion of patients with various dermatoses show evidence of folate depletion, at least biochemically, and in some cases, haematologically. This has been reported in patients with erythroderma, psoriasis, or extensive eczema. There is a well-documented association between malabsorption and dermatitis herpetiformis.

Endocrine disease

Pituitary and adrenal deficiency

A mild normochromic, normocytic anaemia is very common in patients with anterior pituitary deficiency. The mechanism is not absolutely clear, although the anaemia has many features in common with that of hypothyroidism and is fully responsive to appropriate replacement therapy. A similar pattern is seen in adrenal insufficiency.

Thyroid disease

Hypothyroidism is associated with a variety of haematological changes. The anaemia of uncomplicated myxoedema is normochromic and normocytic and, although macrocytic anaemia may be seen, it usually signifies coexistent megaloblastic anaemia.

Diabetes mellitus

Severe diabetic acidosis is often associated with a marked leucocytosis, even when there is no underlying infection. In addition, hyperosmolarity impairs neutrophil function, and reduced neutrophil migration has been observed in patients with diabetic ketoacidosis or poorly controlled hyperglycaemia.

Neuropsychiatric disease

Anorexia nervosa

About one-third of patients with severe anorexia nervosa have a mild normochromic, normocytic anaemia. There may also be mild neutropenia or thrombocytopenia.

Trauma

The brain is rich in thromboplastin activity and acute disseminated intravascular coagulation occurs quite commonly after severe head or brain injury.

Myasthenia gravis

The association between myasthenia gravis and pure red-cell aplasia is described in Chapter 3.6.

Abetalipoproteinaemia

This condition is characterized by an ataxic neurological disease, retinitis pigmentosa, fat malabsorption, and the absence of chylomicrons and low-density lipoproteins. It is caused by the failure to synthesize or secrete lipoprotein-containing products of the apolipoprotein B gene. It is characterized by the presence of from 50 to 90 per cent of acanthocytes in the peripheral blood. These are abnormal, spiky red cells, which have a moderately shortened survival. Despite these changes there is only a mild haemolytic anaemia.

Further reading

Stockman, J.A.I. and Ezekowitz, A. (1993). Hematologic manifestations of systemic diseases. In *Haematology of infancy and childhood* (ed. D.G. Nathan and F.A. Oski), pp. 1834–85. Saunders, Philadelphia, PA.

Weatherall, D.J. (1993). Hematologic manifestations of systemic diseases in children of the third world. In *Haematology of infancy and childhood* (ed. D.G. Nathan and F.A. Oski), pp. 1886–904. Saunders, Philadelphia, PA.

Chapter 3.41

Transfusion of blood and blood components

V. J. Martlew

The donor source

Homologous blood

Blood for transfusion in the UK is collected from healthy volunteers between the ages of 17 and 70 years. Each individual undergoes a standard interview with a healthcare professional at their first visit, and completes a tick-box questionnaire thereafter to ensure their continued fitness to donate. Particular emphasis is laid on risk activities which may be associated with transfusion-transmitted diseases.

Autologous blood

An individual who is likely to need blood transfusion to support forthcoming surgery and who is otherwise fit, may embark on a scheme to predeposit autologous blood to be returned during the perioperative period. Other methods of autologous transfusion include perioperative cell salvage and preoperative haemodilution for vascular procedures.

Preparation of blood components

Leucodepletion

In recent years component preparation has been changed to provide products leucodepleted at source by the Blood Centre to a specification requiring less than 5×10^6 leucocytes per donation. This has reduced the incidence of several previous side-effects of transfusion, including: non-haemolytic febrile transfusion reactions (NHFTR) attributed to cytokines released from leucocytes in stored blood; alloimmunization by human leucocyte antigens (HLA), which are found on white cells; and post-transfusion infections as a result of organisms transmitted in leucocytes (for example, cytomegalovirus (CMV) and human T-cell lymphoma leukaemia virus type-1 (HTLV-1)).

Apheresis

The requirement for leucodepletion has led to a marked increase in the direct procurement of platelet concentrate by thrombopheresis—red cells and plasma being returned to the donor during the procedure. A minimum of two adult doses of platelets are usually obtained in this way from a single donor, thereby minimizing antigen exposure to the patient. As no red cells are lost, donors may return more frequently at monthly or fortnightly intervals rather than the standard 16 weeks between whole blood donations.

Preparation of components from whole blood

The standard donation is 450 ml of whole blood, which is mixed with 63 ml of anticoagulant in a plastic container attached, in a sterile closed system, to a number of satellite packs, the choice of which is determined by the component requirement. Red cells, plasma, and platelets are separated by centrifugation, filtered to achieve a leucodepleted product and then transferred to containers for storage under conditions optimal for maintaining the viability of the specific component. Each component is labelled with a unique donation number, blood group, expiry date, production site, details of pack type, and anticoagulant solution. The storage and transport of all blood components is closely monitored and subjected to rigorous quality assurance.

Laboratory testing of donations

Donations are screened on every occasion the donor attends. Automated technology has been introduced in recent years to deal with samples, which are bar-code labelled with a unique donation number to minimize error in identification.

Microbiological screening

In the UK, donations are screened to exclude hepatitis C (HCV) and human immunodeficiency viruses-types 1 and 2 (HIV-1 + 2) by serological methods, and hepatitis B (HBV) by the surface-antigen test. Nucleic acid testing for transfusion-transmitted viruses is scheduled for introduction at the earliest opportunity to reduce the period between infection and laboratory identification of the donor. A proportion of donations are further screened to provide cytomegalovirus (CMV)-negative products for immunosuppressed recipients (for example, neonates and post-transplant patients).

Blood group determination

Almost 100 years after its first description, the ABO blood group system remains the most important consideration in the choice of

Table 1 Some examples of blood group systems

Blood group system	Symbols of common antigens
ABO	A_1 A_2 B H
Rhesus (Rh)	CDEce
MNS	MNSs
P	P_1 P_2
Kell	Kk
Lewis	Le^a Le^b
Lutheran	Lu^a Lu^b
Duffy	Fy^a Fy^b
Kidd	Jk^2 Jk^b
Ii	Ii

red cells for transfusion. Rhesus (D) typing is the other essential investigation to complete the grouping of donor blood.

Both donations and patient samples undergoing grouping require a confirmatory step before the blood group is formally reported. This may involve duplicate blood group determination in the laboratory for new cases or interrogation of the historical record for group on repeat samples. This recommendation of best practice in blood grouping emphasizes the importance of determining the correct ABO and rhesus (D) group for both donations and patients. Accurate identification of the individuals from whom the samples are collected—namely blood donors and hospital patients—is vital to ensure the integrity of this exercise.

Blood group antigens and antibodies

Red-cell antigens

Some antigens, for example rhesus (CcDEe), are found exclusively on red cells, while others may be present in tissue fluids or on the surface of other somatic cells (for instance, ABO and Lewis). The most common blood group systems of clinical significance are set out in Table 1. The physiological significance of their variable expression is largely unknown apart from a few recognized disease associations—for example: duodenal ulcer is more common in Group O individuals; carcinoma of the stomach is more frequently found in Group A patients; and Africans who lack expression of Duffy antigens (Fy^{a-b-}) are believed to have resistance to falciparum malaria.

Red-cell antibodies

Red-cell antibodies are immunoglobulins most commonly of classes IgG (dimers) and IgM (pentamers). The formation of such antibodies is usually dependent upon stimulation by the corresponding antigen. Where antigens are restricted to red cells (for example, rhesus), antibody formation may be induced either by blood transfusion or transplacental haemorrhage during pregnancy. By contrast, red-cell antibodies arising in the absence of any obvious stimulus are described as naturally occurring. The most common of these occur in the ABO system where antigens are not restricted to red cells. It is thought that antigens closely resembling those of the relevant blood group system, but present in bacteria and foods, may provide the appropriate stimulus to antibody formation.

Table 2 The ABO groups, corresponding naturally occurring antibodies and frequencies in the UK

Group of red cells	Antibody in serum	Approximate frequency (%)
A_1	anti-B	32
A_2	anti-B (+anti-A_1 in 10%)	1.0
B	anti-A	8
O	anti-A + anti-B	47
A_1B	None	2.3
A_2B	None or anti-A_1 (in 25%)	0.7

ABO blood group system

The commonly encountered groups in the ABO system and their associated antibodies are set out in Table 2. Their frequencies are expressed according to their distribution in the UK, although this varies considerably in different parts of the world.

Anti-A and anti-B antibodies combine with their corresponding antigens both *in vitro* and *in vivo* with associated complement fixation and, as naturally occurring antibodies, are present from an early age. The transfusion of ABO-incompatible red cells may cause the most serious complications for the recipient who may develop an acute intravascular haemolysis. Although Group O red cells do not bind anti-A or anti-B, ABO-matched red cells should be selected for the recipient wherever possible. Certain Group O individuals have high concentrations of anti-A (and occasionally anti-B) which may produce haemolysis in Group A or Group B recipients. The indiscriminate choice of Group O red cells for transfusion to patients with other ABO groups is to be avoided wherever possible.

The rhesus (Rh) blood group system

The five common antigens in the Rh system are CDEce. Anti-d has not been characterized. In the UK approximately 85 per cent of the population have Rh (D)-positive red cells, the remaining 15 per cent being Rh (D)-negative.

All Rh (D)-positive individuals have the D antigen expressed on their red cells, which is inherited as an autosomal dominant. A small proportion of these exhibit weaker expression of the D antigen, either as a result of a general reduction in the number of antigen sites per cell (D^{weak} and D^u) or as a result of the varied expression of D in the absence of one of the components of the D antigen itself ($D^{variant}$). Both D^{weak} and $D^{variant}$ individuals are Rh (D)-positive, but the $D^{variant}$ recipient is capable of making a variant anti-D directed against that portion of the D antigen site which is absent from their own red cells. They should therefore be recipients of Rh (D)-negative red cells.

Although Rh (D) is by far the strongest immunizing antigen of the Rh system, antibodies may also be stimulated by the other Rh antigens CcEe. Rh antibodies are IgG antibodies that readily cross the placenta and do not fix complement. Transfusion reactions arising from anti-Rh are usually extravascular, giving rise to delayed haemolysis over the next few days.

Compatibility testing

As donated blood is selected for transfusion on the basis of its ABO and Rh (D) groups, it is essential to check that the recipient has

Table 3 Specification of blood components

	Red cells	Platelet (adult concentrate dose)	Fresh frozen plasma	Cryoprecipitate
Storage temperature	4°C (2–6°C)	22°C (20–24°C)	≤ 30°C	≤ 30°C
Shelf life	35 days	5 days	1 year (frozen)	1 year (frozen)
Maximal time from storage to complete infusion	5 h		4 hour (post-thaw)	4 hour (post-thaw)
Compatibility requirements: ABO match	Yes	Yes	Yes	Yes
Rh (D)	All	Premenopausal females		
Further red cell phenotypes	Red antibodies present	No	No	No
Volume	280 ml (± 60 ml)	200 ml (± 40 ml)	225 ml (± 75 ml)	15 ml (± 5 ml)
Contents: Haematocrit	0.65 (± 0.10)	–	–	–
Platelets	–	2.4×10^{11}	–	–
White cells (all leucodepleted)	$< 5 \times 10^6$	$< 5 \times 10^6$	$< 5 \times 10^6$	$< 5 \times 10^6$
Fibrinogen	–	–	2–5 mg/ml	150–300 mg/pack
von Willebrand factor	–	–	–	80–120 IU/pack
Factor VIIIc	–	–	0.7 IU/ml	80–120 IU/pack
Anticoagulant: *CPD	Yes	Recovered whole blood	Yes	Yes
*ACD	–	Single donor apheresis	–	–

*CPD = citrate phosphate dextrose with adeninine
*ACD = acid citrate dextrose

no other red cell-antibodies, usually acquired as a consequence of pregnancy or previous transfusion, which might require extended testing of donor blood.

Both donation and patient samples are grouped and checked as described above to determine their ABO and Rh (D) type. Patient serum is then screened against a range of red cells using sensitive techniques including an indirect antiglobulin test at 37 °C to detect the presence of any other clinically significant antibodies. The addition of an antihuman globulin reagent, produced by injecting human antibodies into an animal of another species (for example, rabbit or sheep), enhances the detection of antibody in the patient. Donor red cells are then incubated with the patient's serum to exclude incompatibility, which would be indicated by agglutination. Laboratory techniques have been refined considerably over the years to enhance the sensitivity and specificity of antibody detection, while minimizing the delay in the provision of compatible blood to the patient. New technology associated with automated grouping and antibody screening may now permit the issue of ABO- and Rh (D)-matched red cells supported by an electronic crossmatch. Formal compatibility testing on the laboratory bench will continue to be required for patients found to have red-cell antibodies.

Some clinical applications of blood products

The basic specification of blood and plasma components in common use are set out in Tables 3 and 4.

Patient consent

In view of the hazards which may be associated with their transfusion, it is important to consider a risk–benefit analysis before prescribing such treatment. Wherever appropriate, patients must be offered alternatives to transfusion of homologous blood products. After full discussion with the patient and/or their family, as appropriate, the indication for blood transfusion must be clearly documented in the case notes.

Red-cell transfusion

There is no clinical evidence for a fixed haemoglobin value or haematocrit that should trigger a red-cell transfusion. Considerable anaemia will be tolerated by the young and fit, while frail older people with cardiac impairment will require red cells much earlier in situations of acute blood loss. Blood loss of up to 20 per cent of the blood volume can usually be satisfactorily restored by crystalloid and/or colloid solutions alone.

Additional, specific components may be required if bleeding continues after attempted surgical haemostasis and where the coagulation tests or platelet count are abnormal. Every effort should be made to establish a diagnosis before prescribing red cells for patients with chronic anaemia, since nutritional anaemias will respond to the appropriate haematinic supplements in time. A regular transfusion programme may be required for individuals with bone marrow failure or malignant infiltration.

Certain groups of patients with haemoglobinopathies (for example, thalassaemia major, sickle cell disease) may also require regular

Table 4 Plasma products fractionated from large donor pools

	Content	Volume(s) (ml)	Indications	Special hazards
Human albumin solution	5%	50; 100; 250; 500	(Colloid replacement) Burns	Concerns about safety after review intensive care use
	20%	5; 50; 100	Ascites (liver disease) Nephrotic syndrome	Sodium retention (20% only)
Human immunoglobulin	Variable			Anaphylaxis (anti-IgA)
Intravenous normal human			Deficiency antibody formation (congenital and acquired) Autoimmune disease	
Specific intramuscular: Anti-D			Prevention Rh(D) HDN	
Viral antibody			Passive immunity e.g. hepatitis A, B, Varicella zoster, Rubella, etc	
Coagulation* factor concentrates: Factor VIII			Haemophilia A	
Factor IX			Haemophilia B	
Factor VII			Factor VII deficiency	
Prothrombin complex			Anticoagulant overdose	
Antithrombin III			Antithrombin III deficiency	
Fibrin sealant			Local surgical	

*Recombinant products are now available to replace factor VII, VII and IX from a non-plasma source

transfusions of red-cells. Haematological guidance concerning red-cell phenotyping and the choice of product must be sought before the first transfusion. For example, potential recipients of stem-cell transplants may require CMV-negative red cells; red cells must be irradiated (25–30 Gy) to prevent graft-versus-host disease in recipients of stem-cell grafts. Red cells are no longer indicated in chronic renal failure—erythopoietin is now the treatment of choice.

Platelet transfusion

In adults, a platelet concentrate is prescribed for severe microvascular bleeding when the platelet count is less than $50 \times 10^9/1$, or rarely for patients with qualitative defects of platelet function in situations of acute blood loss.

In disorders of bone marrow function, platelets are transfused into thrombocytopenic patients with mucosal bleeding and/or acute infection to maintain a count in excess of $20 \times 10^9/1$. In the absence of such symptoms prophylactic platelets are prescribed to maintain a count in excess of $10 \times 10^9/1$.

Potential bone marrow recipients require CMV-negative platelets. All cellular blood products must be irradiated (25–30 Gy) before transfusion after the recipient has received a stem-cell graft.

Fresh frozen plasma

Fresh frozen plasma (15 ml/kg) is used to treat patients with microvascular bleeding who have abnormal results on coagulation screening.

In the absence of a prothrombin-complex concentrate it may be used in association with vitamin K to reverse severe bleeding associated with an anticoagulant overdose.

Cryoprecipitate

Cryoprecipitate is transfused as a source of fibrinogen in disseminated intravascular coagulopathy. It is no longer indicated in the management of von Willebrand's disease, as satisfactory virally inactivated sources of von Willebrand factor are now available for those patients who fail to respond to desmopressin (DDAVP).

Cryoprecipitate supernatant plasma

This frozen plasma is deficient in high molecular-weight, von Willebrand multimers. It is the replacement fluid of choice during plasma exchange in the treatment of thrombotic thrombocytopenic purpura.

Intravenous immunoglobulin

This is prescribed as a replacement to prevent bacterial infection in congenital hypogammaglobulinaemia and in acquired states often secondary to haematological malignancy (for example, myeloma, lymphoproliferative disorders) at a dose of 0.2 g/kg every 3 to 4 weeks.

Intravenous immunoglobulin may also be effective in suppressing inappropriate antibody production (for example, immune thrombocytopenia, Guillain-Barré syndrome) at a dose of 0.4 mg/kg daily for 5 days.

Special applications to the fetus and neonate

Red cells: haemolytic disease of the newborn (HDN)

Antenatal screening of the mother at booking and in the third trimester detects those with red-cell antibodies of clinical significance to the developing fetus. The routine administration of 500 IU of anti-D immunoglobulin to Rh (D)-negative mothers delivered of Rh (D)-positive infants has reduced the incidence of maternal anti-D sensitization to less than 1 per cent. As this dose will only deal with a leakage of 4 ml of fetal cells into the maternal circulation, the size of the remaining fetomaternal haemorrhage must be quantitated (for example, by Kleihauer or flow cytometry). The recent recommendation for routine antenatal prophylaxis with two doses during the third trimester as well as at times of increased risk of sensitization (for example, amniocentesis), will reduce this further.

When HDN does occur, regular ultrasound examination will detect early evidence of oedema as a sign of fetal anaemia which may require transfusion. Red cells for direct intrauterine transfusion to the fetus intravenously should be hyperconcentrated (haematocrit approximately 90 per cent) leucodepleted, CMV-negative, irradiated, and less than 5 days from collection. A similar product is required for the fetal anaemia that sometimes occurs in maternal infection with human parvovirus B19. Once the baby is born, exchange transfusion may be necessary in the early days of life using less-concentrated red cells (haematocrit < 65 per cent) but otherwise specially selected as for the fetus. Blood volume is higher in neonates (80 ml/kg) than in adults (70 ml/kg).

Platelets

Thrombocytopenia is associated with increased risk of bleeding in the very young ($< 50–100 \times 10^9$/l) and in the preterm infant ($<20–30 \times 10^9$/l in a full-term infant). Hyperconcentrated platelets, similarly CMV-negative and irradiated, should be ordered for such patients to minimize circulatory overload.

The thrombocytopenic infant of a mother with autoimmune thrombocytopenia may respond to intravenous immunoglobulin. In neonatal alloimmune thrombocytopenia caused by maternal IgG antibody to specific platelet antigens (usually human platelet antigen-1a, **HPA-1a**) inherited from the father, intrauterine transfusion with selected platelets may restore the platelet count to prevent bleeding during fetal life or at delivery.

Referral to specialists in fetal medicine is recommended for patients who may require intrauterine transfusion.

Table 5 Hazards of blood transfusion

Immunological
1. Haemolytic (a) Intravascular e.g. ABO; Lewis; P (b) Extravascular e.g. Rh; Kidd (Jk[a])
2. Leucocytic antibodies (a) Lymphocytoxic: HLA* (b) Specific, e.g. NA/system* (c) Transfusion associated lung injury (TRALI) (d) Donor T-cell—transfusion associated graft-versus-host disease (TA-GVHD)
3. Plasma antibodies (a) IgA (b) Gm (c) Drug induced, e.g. penicillin
4. Platelet antibodies (a) Lymphocytoxic HLA* (b) Specific e.g. HPA system
Non-immunological
1. Circulatory overload
2. Thrombophlebitis/phlebothrombosis
3 Embolism eg. air; catheter tip
4.** Non-immune haemolysis (a) Overheated red cells (b) Frozen red cells (c) Non-isotonic fluid addition (d) Bacterial infection
5.*** Iron overload (>20 g iron ~ 80 units red cells)
6. Massive transfusion (> blood volume in 24 h)
7. Transfusion transmitted infection (a) Protozoa, e.g. malaria; amoeba (b) Spirochaete, e.g. syphilis, yaws (c) Bacteria, e.g. Yersinia, Brucella (d) Viral, e.g. Hepatitis B, C; HIV 1+2; *CMV; *HTLVI; 1 Parvovirus B_{19}

*Leucodepletion minimizes risk.

**Prognosis as severe as immune cause.

***Occurs earliest in carriers of haemochromatosis gene.

Management of some complications of transfusion

Massive transfusion

When the total blood volume is exchanged within 24 h there is an associated dilution of platelets and coagulation factors in the recipient which must be monitored by serial coagulation screening. In the bleeding patient, replacement fluids should be prescribed on the basis of results of the coagulation profile, with administration of platelet concentrate in thrombocytopenia, fresh frozen plasma for coagulation factor deficiency, and cryoprecipitate as a source of fibrinogen. Associated metabolic problems may arise as citrate anticoagulant binds calcium to produce hypocalcaemia. Hyperkalaemia and rapid infusion of cold red cells reduce the pH so that both calcium and bicarbonate may be required.

Acute haemolytic transfusion reaction

The causes of this are set out in Table 5. The more serious cases involve acute intravascular haemolysis mediated by complement. The transfusion must be stopped immediately and good intravenous access established to maintain hydration and minimize renal damage. Renal function must be closely monitored and investigations set in train to confirm haemolysis (failing haemoglobin, rising bilirubin, haemoglobinaemia, methaemalbuminaemia) and determine its cause (blood culture recipient and all products transfused, repeat compatibility testing using stored pretransfusion and fresh post-transfusion sample). Specialist advice should be sought early about the management of deteriorating renal function. Coagulation screening should be arranged and component transfusion prescribed as indicated. If bacterial infection is suspected, intravenous antibiotics should be administered.

Delayed transfusion reactions

These reflect increased red-cell destruction by an extravascular mechanism leading to a fall in haemoglobin and rising bilirubin levels over about a week. In patients with impaired hepatic or renal function the consequences may be serious.

Iron overload

Those patients on long-term, red-cell transfusion programmes need to have their iron stores monitored, with a view to iron chelation therapy. A subcutaneous infusion of desferrioxamine at a dose of 2 g/20 ml of water over 12 h on several nights a week may prevent the organ damage associated with iron overload.

Post-transfusion purpura

Thrombocytopenia may occur, albeit rarely, 7–10 days after the transfusion of cellular products as a result of platelet-specific antibodies (anti-HPA). This is best treated by immunosuppression with high-dose steroids and intravenous immunoglobulin. Further transfusion should be avoided wherever possible.

Serious hazards of transfusion (SHOT)

In 1996, a national system was introduced for reporting serious hazards of transfusion centrally. The first annual reports have demonstrated that serious consequences occur more frequently as a result of failure to follow local procedures, particularly in patient identification, rather than following anticipated clinical hazards as listed in Table 5.

Post-transfusion infection must be reported to the local blood centre for urgent investigation of implicated donations. All other hazards should be reported directly to the SHOT office.

Prions

Over the last 10 years, an epidemic of bovine spongiform encephalopathy has been observed in cattle in the UK. Subsequently, a variant form of Creutzfeldt–Jakob disease has been recognized in humans, occurring in younger people. Both diseases have been linked to abnormal prion protein detected in the brain of affected cases. More recently, the pathological prion protein has been found in human appendix and tonsillar B lymphocytes. Although there is no reported incidence of transfusion-acquired prion disease, the preparation of blood components has been reorganized to supply exclusively leucodepleted products. An alternative plasma source has been procured as the current epidemic appears to be restricted to the UK.

Further reading

Consensus statement on red cell transfusion (1994). Proceedings of a consensus conference held by the Royal College of Physicians of Edinburgh (May 1994). *British Journal of Anaesthesia*, **74**, 857–9.

Daniels, G. (1995). *Human Blood Groups.* Blackwell Science, Oxford.

Hoffbrand, A.V., Lewis, S.M., and Tuddenham, E.D.G. (ed.) (1999). *Postgraduate haematology*, 4th edn, Chapters 9, 10, 11. Butterworth–Heinemann, Oxford

Lee, D., Contreras, M., Robson, S.C., Rodeck, C.H., and Whittle, M.K. (1999). Recommendations on the use of anti-D immunoglobulin for Rh (D) prophylaxis. *Transfusion Medicine*, **9**, 93–8.

McClelland, D.B.L. (ed.) (1996). *Handbook of transfusion medicine. Blood Transfusion Services of the United Kingdom*, 2nd edn. HMSO, London.

Norfolk, D., Ancliffe, P.J., Contreras, M., *et al.* (1998). Proceedings of the consensus conference on platelet transfusion organised by the Royal College of Physicians of Edinburgh in November 1997. *British Journal of Haematology*, **101**, 609–14.

UKBTS—NIBSC Liaison Group (1996). *Guidelines for the Blood Transfusion Service*, 3rd edn. HMSO, London.

Section 4
Respiratory disease

Contents

Chapter 4.1

The clinical presentation of chest diseases

D. J. Lane

The predominant symptoms of chest diseases are cough, breathlessness, chest pain and haemoptysis.

Cough

The cough reflex is initiated by stimulation of receptors in the larynx and major airways, by mechanical or chemical irritants. The afferent fibres run in branches of the superior laryngeal nerve and vagus.

A dry cough, short and repeated, is heard in tracheobronchitis and early pneumonia. In laryngitis the sound is hoarse and harsh. In abductor paralysis of the vocal cords it is prolonged and blowing. Weakness of thoracic muscles lessens the expulsive force and cough may be suppressed when there is severe thoracic or upper abdominal pain. Cough with expectoration in the morning is characteristic of chronic bronchitis and large volumes of yellow sputum throughout the day suggests bronchiectasis. Bouts of coughing when eating point to oesophageal or neuromuscular disease causing aspiration. A dry cough over many weeks can signify a neoplasm. A cough may be dry because there is nothing to produce, because secretions are swallowed, because of muscular weakness, or because secretions are too viscid.

Phlegm and sputum

Phlegm from the lower respiratory tract is often combined with secretions from the nose and pharynx and saliva to form sputum. In health, only about 100 ml of phlegm is produced each day and most of this is swallowed. Intrabronchial mucus exists in two layers, one of low viscosity and high elasticity touching the cilia and above this, a more viscous layer. Elasticity of phlegm depends on the rate of beating of the bronchial epithelial cilia. Airway mucus is 95 per cent water, the remainder being serous fluid and glycoprotein. There is a shift towards glycoprotein production in chronic bronchitis and greater transudate formation in asthma. Breakdown of leucocytes in infection increases the DNA content of sputum, making it less viscid and debris of cells and micro-organisms give it a yellow colour. Non-infected sputum is clear and often jelly-like (mucoid). Viscid mucoid sputum often with pellets or branching plugs is seen in asthma. City dwellers produce grey sputum. In lower respiratory tract infection, pus mixed with mucus produces mucopurulent sputum, but pure pus suggests a lung abscess or stagnant bronchiectatic cavity. Anaerobic organisms give sputum a particularly offensive odour. Large quantities of watery mucus may come from alveolar cell carcinoma.

Laboratory examination of sputum may be unrewarding in detecting infecting organisms, but cytology may reveal an underlying carcinoma and eosinophilia suggests airway allergy.

Table 1 Modified Borg Scale*

Number	Verbal description
10	Severe
9	
8	Moderately severe
7	
6	
5	Moderate
4	
3	
2	Slight
1	
0	None

*Modified from Borg, G.A.V. (1982). Psychological basis of perceived exertion. *Medical Science of Sports and Exercise*, **14**, 377–81.

Haemoptysis

A definite cause is only found in some 50 per cent of cases and it is important to be sure that the blood does truly come from the lungs and not from the nose or gastrointestinal tract. Haemoptysis is a classical presenting feature of tuberculosis, carcinoma, and bronchiectasis, but there are many other causes, for instance Goodpasture's syndrome, mitral valve disease, coagulation defects, or even endometriosis. It is rare in pulmonary embolism, when it reflects infarction of the lung.

Treatment of cough

Cough suppressants act centrally; most are opiate derivatives. They are invaluable in terminal bronchial carcinoma. Atropine can be useful to reduce the production of bronchial mucus and corticosteroids reduce secretion in alveolar cell carcinoma and in asthma. Aerosolized water is an effective expectorant. Volatile oils probably act as irritants. Mucociliary clearance increases under the influence of guiaphenesin, inhaled β-adrenergic agonists, or hypertonic saline. Mucolytic agents are ineffective. A source of life threatening haemoptysis is only rarely found at bronchoscopy, but topical adrenaline, balloon tamponade, or cold saline lavage may help, as may embolization of the appropriate bronchial artery.

Breathlessness

A complaint of breathlessness may reflect true dyspnoea, hyperpnoea, or hyperventilation. The history is critical in detecting the true nature of the complaint and the clinician must evaluate the quality of breathlessness, its timing, severity, and the circumstances which precipitate or relieve it.

Quality Asthmatics tend to recognize wheeze and usually find it more difficult to breathe in than out. A sense of suffocation is a feature of pulmonary oedema or massive pleural effusion. Phrases like I can't fill my lungs properly' suggest psychogenic breathlessness, but muscle weakness must be excluded.

Severity A simple visual analogue scale relating breathlessness to activity (Table 1) can be useful, but no scale deals with breathlessness which is significantly variable.

Table 2 Conditions causing breathlessness classified by rate of onset

1. Dramatically sudden: over minutes Pneumothorax Pulmonary embolism Pulmonary oedema 2. Acute: over hours Acute pulmonary infiltrations, e.g. allergic alveolitis Asthma Left ventricular failure Pneumonia 3. Subacute: over days Pleural effusion Bronchogenic carcinoma Subacute pulmonary infiltrations, e.g. sarcoidosis	4. Chronic: over months or years Chronic airflow obstruction Diffuse fibrosing conditions Chronic non-pulmonary causes, e.g. anaemia, hyperthyroidism 5. Intermittent: episodic breathlessness Asthma Left ventricular failure

Timing and occurrence The rate of onset can give a clue to diagnosis (Table 2), as can the circumstances precipitating breathlessness. Psychogenic breathlessness bears no relation to exertion. Breathlessness made worse by lying flat (orthopnoea) is characteristic of left ventricular failure or diaphragmatic paralysis. Nocturnal wakening with severe breathlessness (paroxysmal nocturnal dyspnoea) suggests left ventricular failure. The asthmatic wakes in the night with breathlessness, coughing, and wheezing. Postexertional breathlessness and the triggering of wheezing by irritants and allergic stimuli also suggest asthma.

Investigation of the breathless patient

If the clinical history points to chest disease simple lung function tests and radiology are the most useful investigations. Spirometry will define three groups; normal, an obstructive pattern, or a restrictive pattern (see Chapter 4.3). The chest radiograph is of most value in furthering the diagnosis of conditions giving a restrictive pattern. The farther investigation of a patient with airflow obstruction is dealt with in Chapters 4.14 and 4.17. Breathlessness in a patient with normal spirometry and a clear chest radiograph presents special problems. Asthmatics, when well may have normal lung function and cardiac conditions may be occult or intermittent. Neurological or muscular disorders affecting the muscles of respiration must always be considered and pulmonary hypertension is all too easily missed. Hyperthyroidism and anaemia should not be forgotten as causes of breathlessness.

Clues to psychogenic breathlessness include the sensation of inability to take a full breath, irregular breathing, paraesthesiae, and dizziness. Some patients with anxiety about their heart may also suffer palpitation and a stabbing left submammary pain.

Treatment

If management of the underlying condition does not relieve breathlessness, symptomatic treatment is unsatisfactory, but chronic bronchitics of the pink puffer' type can be helped by diazepam or promethazine. Opiates reduce breathlessness but can dangerously depress respiration; there has been a sad failure to find opiate derivatives with a more selective action on breathlessness.

Chest pain

The greater part of the lower respiratory tract is insensitive to pain. Most parenchymal lung disorders proceed to an advanced state without pain. However, the parietal pleura is exquisitely sensitive to painful stimuli and unpleasant sensations can arise from the tracheobronchial tree.

Pleurisy

Typical pleural pain is sharp and accentuated by respiratory movement. Afferent pain fibres from the central diaphragm run in the phrenic nerve to the cervical cord (C3/4), giving referred pain in the shoulder tip. The outer diaphragm is served by intercostal nerves (T7–12), causing referred pain to the upper abdomen.

Most conditions giving rise to pleuritic pain are acute and inflammatory in origin: either infection or infarction. Recurrent pleurisy should suggest bronchiectasis or embolism. In pleural effusion, the typical pleuritic pain largely disappears and is replaced by a dull ache. Pleural fibrotic disease is rarely painful, but pleural neoplasia frequently is. A superior sulcus tumour of bronchial origin (Pancoast's tumour) infiltrating the brachial plexus gives very severe pain in the shoulder and arm.

Pain from the chest wall

Chest-wall pain can mimic pleurisy. Epidemic myalgia or Bornholm disease (see Chapter 16.22) is a bothersome manifestation of Coxsackie B infection which can involve the intercostal muscles (pleurodynia). The pre-eruptive stage of thoracic herpes zoster gives a stabbing pain. Costal cartilage pain is generally not inflammatory, but can be troublesome. Rib fractures can present diagnostic problems. Metastatic disease of bone may be symptomatic before radiological change is evident.

Fleeting transient chest pains are often part of chronic, somatized anxiety states.

Central chest pain

Sensations arising from the major airways are unpleasant and referred to the anterior chest wall. Tracheal inflammation causes a raw, painful sensation retrosternally. Persistent coughing can itself lead to soreness in the upper airways and trachea.

The mediastinal structures of the thorax are responsible for a multitude of pains. Of central pulmonary lesions likely to give mediastinal pain, neoplasia is the most likely culprit.

Other pulmonary symptoms

A harsh inspiratory wheezing sound arising from obstruction in the larynx or major airways is termed stridor. Wheeze is the externally audible counterpart of the sounds heard with the stethoscope in asthma and obstructive bronchitis.

In response to changes in atmospheric conditions or to the inhalation of dusts or fumes, the patient with irritable airways will respond with cough, tightness in the chest, wheeze, or breathlessness.

General history in the patient with pulmonary disease

Emphasis in the history should be given to the cardiovascular system, fluid retention, deep venous thrombosis, the upper respiratory tract, the skin, and the locomotor and nervous systems. These may be pointers to metastatic spread or the non-metastatic manifestations of malignant disease. The past history may reveal atopy or tuberculosis. Previous chest radiographs may be obtainable for comparison.

A smoking history is essential. Alcohol, and steroid and immunosuppressive therapy will depress antibacterial defences, and a detailed drug history is essential because of toxic effects on the lungs (see Chapter 4.34).

A complete occupational and environmental history is of the utmost importance. Both inorganic and organic materials are hazards to the chest (see Chapter 4.33). Certain working environments may lead to exposure to organisms likely to cause pulmonary infection.

Finally, certain disorders have a familial predisposition. These include asthma and other atopic diseases (see Chapter 4.14) and cystic fibrosis (see Chapter 4.15).

Physical signs in pulmonary disease

Inspection of the chest

The normal respiratory rate is around 10 to 14 per min. A rate above 20 per min is seen in pneumonia, interstitial lung disorders, hypoxia, and anxiety. Painful conditions of the chest or upper abdomen cause an abrupt stop to inspiration. Deep sighs and an irregular breathing pattern are seen in psychogenic breathlessness. A regular alternation of apnoeic periods with increasing ventilation characterizes Cheyne–Stokes respiration, usually associated with cerebral lesions or severe heart failure.

Poor movement of the chest on one side only always indicates pathology on that side. Generally poor expansion is seen in severe airflow obstruction, with indrawing of intercostal spaces during inspiration.

An increased anteroposterior diameter to give a 'barrel chest' is as often a sign of osteoporotic kyphosis as it is of the hyperinflation of chronic airflow obstruction. Pectus carinatum (pigeon chest), an outward protuberance of the sternum, may reflect severe attacks of asthma in childhood. The opposite, pectus excavatum (depressed sternum), is a congenital anomaly. Scoliosis of skeletal origin is of importance because of the severe impairment of respiratory movement that it causes (see Chapter 4.37). Localized collapse and fibrosis may draw in the adjacent rib cage.

Palpation of the chest

The trachea should be localized in the suprasternal notch with the index finger. Deviation of the trachea to one side is either due to apical fibrosis pulling it to the affected side or a mass pushing the trachea across to the opposite side. The position of the apex beat can reflect pressure against or traction on mediastinal structures, or be due to intrinsic cardiac disease.

Percussion of the chest

In percussion the sides of the chest must be compared from identical sites. A dull note lacks resonance and is higher in pitch and softer than normal. It signifies the presence of solid tissue or fluid. It is important to delineate the surface markings of the dullness. Consolidation will follow the outline of the affected lobe, whereas the upper limit of a pleural effusion will be determined by gravity.

A hyper-resonant note occurs over hyperinflated lung as in emphysema or an air-filled space (bulla or pneumothorax).

Auscultation of the chest

Breath sounds

In the normal upright lung, breath sounds are loudest at the apex in early inspiration and at the bases in midinspiration. During expiration, normal breath sounds rapidly fade. Bronchial breathing, higher in pitch and more blowing in quality, is heard over airless lung as in consolidation, atelectasis, or dense fibrosis. Very quiet breath sounds are heard over hyperinflated lungs as in emphysema or when breath sounds are prevented from reaching the chest wall by a layer of air or fluid (pneumothorax, pleural effusion, malignancy).

Adventitious sounds

Crackles and interrupted non-musical sounds may be coarse or moist when they are due to the movement of sputum in large airways. Fine midinspiratory crackles are characteristic of pulmonary oedema and fibrosing alveolitis. Occasionally, a single mid to late inspiratory 'squawk' is heard in patients with a variety of pulmonary fibroses.

Wheezes signify obstruction in airways. A sound of single pitch (monophonic) which cannot be altered by coughing to shift mucus, signifies localized obstruction in a major airway. Several sounds of varying pitch (polyphonic) heard randomly in inspiration and expiration are typical of the widespread airways obstruction of asthma and chronic obstructive bronchitis.

A pleural rub, the diagnostic sound of pleurisy, is a superficial grating synchronous with late inspiration. Inflammation of the pleura close to the heart can give a friction rub that synchronises with the heart beat but will cease if the breath is held.

Voice sounds

A long sound such as 'ninety-nine' is transmitted by normal lung, but not by air space or fluid, and will pass through solid lung with undue clarity, even allowing whispered sounds to be heard (whispering pectoriloquy). Certain physical characteristics of solid lung allow low frequency sounds to be filtered out, leaving a sound of bleating or nasal quality (aegophony); this is particularly noticeable over collapsed lung adjacent to a pleural effusion.

The relevance of the general examination in respiratory disease

Overall appearance

Obesity places an added burden on the respiratory system, and can be an unfortunate complication of corticosteroid therapy. Weight loss is a feature of emphysematous obstructive lung disease, malignancy, and cystic fibrosis. Severe kyphoscoliosis can lead to hypoventilation, and Marfan's syndrome is associated with pneumothorax.

Table 1 Methods of investigation

CXR
Computed tomography (CT), including high resolution CT (HRCT)
Ultrasound
Magnetic Resonance Imaging (MRI)
Radionuclide imaging
Pulmonary and bronchial angiography
Superior vena cavography
Percutaneous lung biopsy

Cyanosis

Peripheral cyanosis in cold weather will leave the tongue still pink, whereas in central cyanosis the tongue will be blue. Most patients with a saturation of 90 per cent or less will appear cyanosed. Cyanosis is less marked in severe anaemia and more obvious in polycythaemia.

The skin and eyes

Eczema and urticaria point to an atopy. Erythema nodosum is a classical presentation of sarcoidosis. It may also be found in primary tuberculosis. Patients with diffuse neurofibromatosis and tuberous sclerosis can both develop a severe pulmonary fibrosis.

Clubbing of the fingers

Loss of the natural angle between the nail and the nail bed and a boggy fluctuation of the nail bed are cardinal signs of clubbing. Among chest disorders the causes include: (a) suppurative disease (bronchiectasis and empyema); (b) fibrosing alveolitis and asbestosis; (c) malignant disease of the bronchus and pleura. If finger clubbing is associated with hypertrophic pulmonary osteoarthropathy, malignancy is present in 95 per cent of cases.

Head and neck

Neurological disease of the pharynx or structural abnormalities of the larynx encourage aspiration and respiratory tract infection. A short thick neck, retrognathia, and a large uvula predispose to sleep apnoea. A goitre may be large enough to compress the trachea and cause stridor. Signs in the neck of intrathoracic malignancy are cervical lymphadenopathy and superior vena caval obstruction.

Investigation of respiratory disease

Chapter 4.2

Thoracic imaging

F. V. Gleeson

The mainstay of radiographic investigation of respiratory disease remains the chest radiograph (CXR) although there are now a multitude of additional imaging techniques to aid diagnosis (Table 1). Before submitting the patient to further investigation it is important that the CXR is technically adequate and correctly interpreted.

Techniques in thoracic imaging

Chest radiography

The standard view is a posteroanterior (PA) projection, taken with the patient erect and the anterior chest wall against the film cassette. This view may be supplemented by a lateral chest radiograph and, less often, oblique views of the ribs or a lordotic view to demonstrate more clearly the apices, although the advent of computed tomography (CT) has decreased their importance. The lateral view aids assessment of the retrocardiac and peridiaphragmatic areas and, with experience, the hila and major airways. The normal CXR and anatomy are shown in Fig. 1.

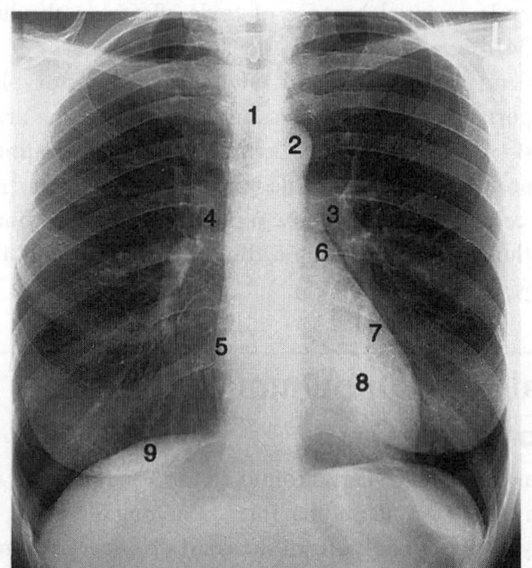

(a)

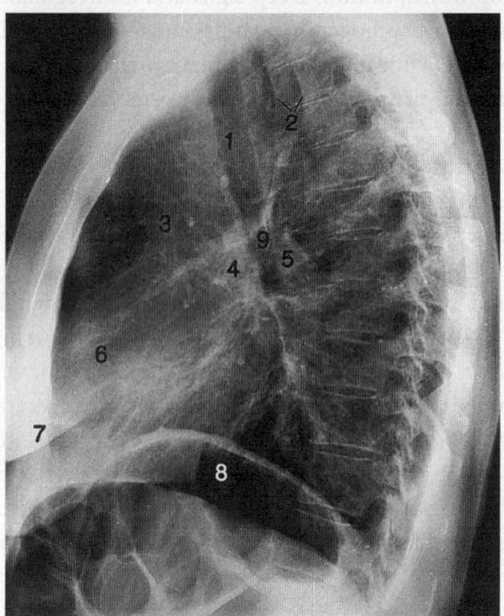

(b)

Fig. 1(a), (b) Normal radiographic anatomy. (a) posteroanterior chest radiograph: (1) trachea; (2) aortic arch; (3) left main pulmonary artery; (4) right main pulmonary artery; (5) right artial border; (6) left atrial appendage; (7) left ventricular border; (8) right ventricle; (9) right dome of diaphragm; (10) costophrenic angle; (11) breast shadow. (b) Lateral chest radiograph; (1) trachea; (2) scapulae; (3) anterior aortic arch; (4) right pulmonary artery; (5) left pulmonary artery; (6) right ventricle; (7) breast shadows; (8) gastric bubble under the left hemidiaphragm; (9) left main bronchus.

Table 2 Indications for CT of the thorax

Suspected or proven lung cancer. Confirms the presence of a mass, and is part of staging procedure (in conjunction with other investigations)
Elucidation of an abnormal mediastinal or hilar contour on CXR.
To aid diagnosis in patients with suspected diffuse lung disease.
Investigation of haemoptysis.
Investigation of pleural disease.
Investigation of suspected pulmonary emboli (spiral CT).
Investigation of patients with large airways disease (spiral CT).
To aid percutaneous needle biopsy or chest drain insertion.
As part of the staging procedures in patients with malignancies that metastasize to the lung or mediastinal lymph nodes.

Although most CXRs are performed using conventional radiographic equipment, more recently new techniques such as digital radiography have been introduced. Digital radiography enables the CXR to be viewed on a monitor as well as film, may be stored and retrieved in a similar fashion to other digital data, and has additional advantages such as data manipulation to aid diagnosis and improve image quality even from technically inadequate radiographic exposures.

Ultrasound

The main use of ultrasound is for the localization and characterization of pleural fluid collections prior to aspiration or drain insertion. Ultrasound may be used to differentiate pleural thickening from fluid in cases of uncertainty post CXR. It is also of value in assessing pleural invasion by cancers abutting the pleura and may be used to guide percutaneous needle biopsy in these cases.

Computed tomography

The ability of CT to delineate structures that are either not clearly defined or in some cases not visualized at all on CXR is responsible for its increased use in medicine (Table 2). The advent of Spiral CT has further expanded its role. Conventional CT produces cross-sectional images of varying thickness of the thorax. Section thickness ranges from 1 mm to 10 mm. Normal CT anatomy of the mediastinum is shown in Fig. 2. The use of thinner sections, high resolution CT (HRCT), has enabled more accurate diagnosis in patients with diffuse lung disease (Fig. 3). Conventional, 10 mm sections are of value in assessing the mediastinum, major airways, the pulmonary parenchyma for nodules, and the pleura. Spiral CT differs from conventional CT in acquiring a volume data set rather than cross-sectional data and also achieving this in a greatly reduced time. It is of value in assessing the vessels and major airways within the thorax. The ability to acquire a volume of data enables analysis and display of the images in multiplanar formats, further enhancing CT's diagnostic capabilities.

Magnetic resonance imaging (MRI)

Protons within the body become excited when placed in a strong magnetic field irradiated with a radiofrequency signal. Selective absorption of frequencies produces a magnetic resonance image. MRI is able to produce an image in any plane (Fig. 4) and has a number of advantages and disadvantages when compared to CT (Table 3).

Radionuclide imaging

Ventilation–perfusion imaging is, at present, the most frequently used method for diagnosing pulmonary emboli. Minute particles of technetium-99m labelled macroaggregates of albumin are injected intravenously and the patients thorax scanned in multiple projections. The gamma rays detected produce an image dependent on the degree of pulmonary perfusion, a significant defect representing an area of diminished or absent perfusion. These images are compared to the ventilation images produced when the patient inhales either of the inert gases xenon-133 or krypton-81m, or aerosolized technetium-99m. Perfusion defects not matched by ventilation defects are used to diagnose pulmonary embolic disease (Fig. 5). The scans must be interpreted in conjunction with a current CXR and clinical information. Due to the failure to directly visualize clot using isotope scanning, the diagnosis is given as a likelihood of embolic disease; unfortunately most patients' scans produce an indeterminate likelihood of emboli (see Chapter 2.30). Because of this, additional tests such as pulmonary angiography, spiral CT, and ultrasound of the peripheral veins are often performed.

Pulmonary and bronchial angiography: superior vena cavography

Pulmonary angiography is performed by injecting contrast into the pulmonary arteries catheterized via peripheral venous puncture (antecubital, jugular, or femoral vein). Thrombus if present is visualized as a filling defect within the pulmonary arteries. Bronchial angiography is performed with selective catheterization of the bronchial arteries arising from the aorta by a catheter introduced via puncture of the femoral artery. It is usually performed to enable embolization of hypertrophied bronchial arteries in patients with bronchiectasis and life-threatening haemoptysis. Superior vena cavography is performed by catheterization of the superior vena cava via peripheral venous puncture, most commonly in patients with suspected vena cava stenosis or obstruction. It is also now possible to insert a self-expanding metal stent at the site of narrowing at the same time and relieve the obstructive symptoms.

Percutaneous needle biopsy

Biopsy of pulmonary and mediastinal masses are most commonly performed to diagnose malignancy in patients with a mass seen on CXR. Lung needle biopsy is most commonly performed after sputum cytology and bronchoscopy have failed to produce a tissue diagnosis. The most common complications are pneumothorax and haemoptysis. The frequency of complications relates to needle size, number of biopsy attempts, depth of lesion from the chest wall, and lung function. Despite the relative safety of needle biopsy, it should only be performed after consideration of the risk to the patient and the benefit of obtaining a diagnosis.

Common radiological signs of disease

Pulmonary consolidation

This occurs when the normal air-filled spaces distal to the bronchi are filled with either fluid or solid material rather than air. This produces the characteristic radiological sign of an air bronchogram,

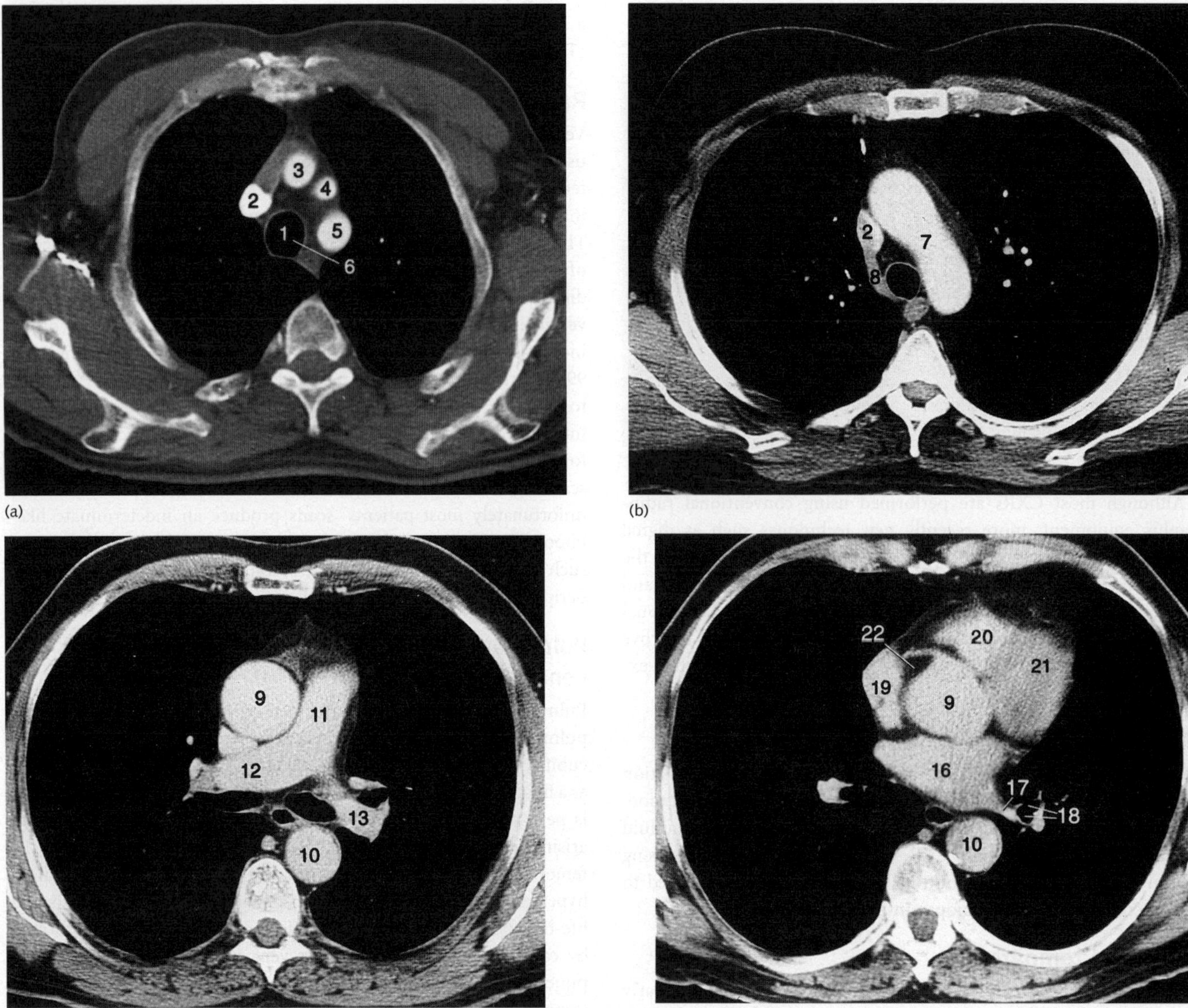

Fig. 2(a)–(d) CT with contrast enhancement to show the normal anatomy at four levels through the mediastinum: (1) trachea; (2) superior vena cava; (3) brachiocephalic artery; (4) left common carotid artery; (5) left subclavian artery; (6) oesophagus; (7) aortic arch; (8) azygos vein; (9) ascending aorta; (10) descending aorta; (11) main pulmonary artery; (12) right pulmonary artery; (13) left pulmonary artery; (14) right main bronchus; (15) left main bronchus; (16) left atrium; (17) left inferior pulmonary vein; (18) segmental bronchi of the left lower lobe; (19) right atrium; (20) right ventricular outflow; (21) left ventricle.

whereby the branching bronchi are clearly visualized against a background of increased radio-opacification. Consolidation may be focal or diffuse, and the most common causes are given in Table 4.

Pulmonary collapse

This may either involve a subsegment or segment of a lobe, a complete lobe, or an entire lung, dependent on the cause and the site of obstruction. Characteristic PA CXRs demonstrating lobar collapse are shown in Figs 6 to 10.

Septal lines

These represent thickening of the normal interlobular septa within the lung. Commonly called Kerley B lines, when seen on the CXR, these are 1 to 2 mm in thickness and 5 to 10 mm in length, lying perpendicular to the pleural surface. They are most frequently associated with pulmonary oedema and lymphangitis carcinomatosis, but may also occur in association with infection and other causes.

Reticular and reticular–nodular shadowing

This term is used to describe innumerable small linear opacities or linear and nodular opacities that produce the appearance of a net or a net that has small nodules superimposed upon it. These terms are usually used to describe pulmonary interstitial abnormalities such as pulmonary fibrosis.

Pulmonary masses and nodules

Masses represent lesions greater than 30 mm and nodules lesions 2 to 30 mm in size. Miliary nodules are 2 mm or smaller. The commonest cause of a pulmonary mass is carcinoma. The differential diagnosis

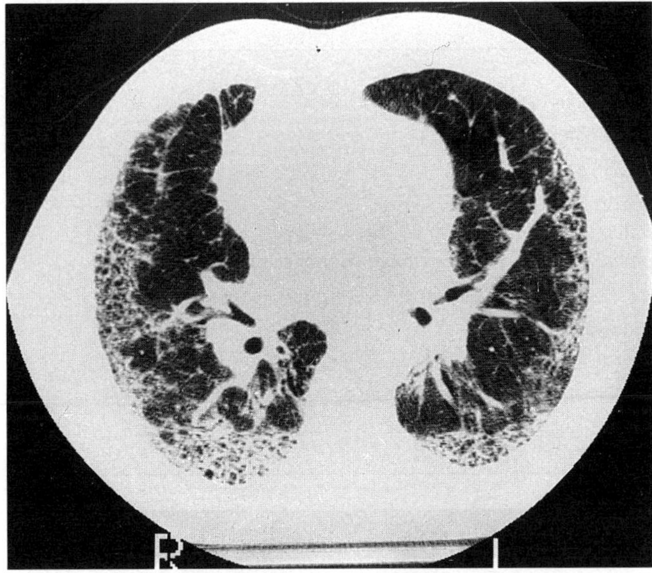

Fig. 3 High resolution CT of a patient with cryptogenic fibrosing alveolitis. The peripheral distribution of the disease and the fine detail of the small cystic air spaces in the destroyed fibrotic lung are clearly shown.

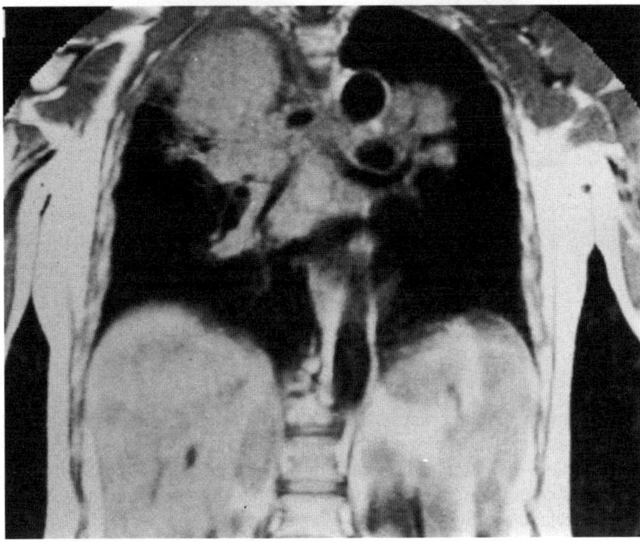

Fig. 4 Magnetic resonance image (coronal section) showing the relationship of an apical bronchial carcinoma to the chest wall and adjacent mediastinum. There are enlarged subcarinal lymph nodes and a metastatic deposit in the right adrenal gland
(by courtesy of Dr P. Goddard).

Table 3 Advantages and disadvantages of MRI compared to CT

Advantages	*Disadvantages*
• No ionizing radiation exposure required	• Poor spatial resolution
• Multiplanar capability	• Prolonged examination times
• Good contrast resolution	• Expensive
• Different image weighting allowing good soft tissue assessment	• Frequently not readily available
	• Poor visualisation of pulmonary parenchyma

in patients with pulmonary nodules and miliary nodules is given in Table 5.

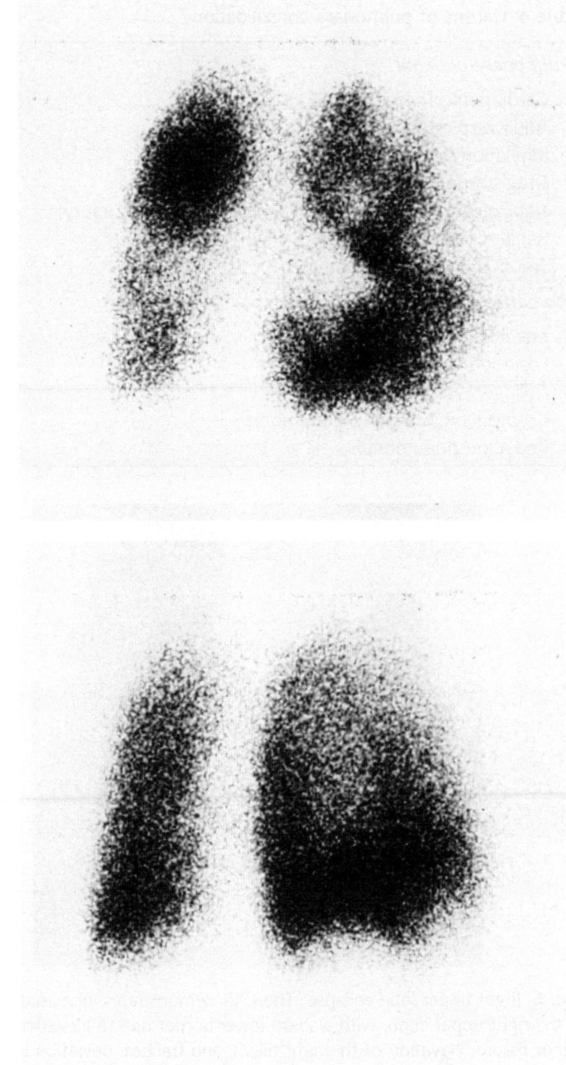

Fig. 5a, b A ventilation–perfusion radionuclide study (oblique views). The perfusion scan (a) shows a defect in the left mid-zone which is not matched on the corresponding view of the ventilation scan (b). The so-called mismatched defect is characteristic of a pulmonary embolus.

Radiological investigation of common clinicoradiological problems

Haemoptysis

Investigation is dependent on whether the CXR is normal or abnormal and whether there are other diagnostic markers of disease. Assuming that most patients are bronchoscoped, CT may be of value in staging tumour if detected by bronchoscopy or to provide a diagnosis such as bronchiectasis if the bronchoscopy is negative, and it is now thought that CT and bronchoscopy are complementary tests in patients with haemoptysis. Contrast enhanced CT may enable a diagnosis of pulmonary embolic disease to be made as the cause of haemoptysis when not expected clinically.

Suspected pulmonary embolic disease

Ventilation–perfusion scanning or contrast enhanced spiral CT are the accepted current methods of investigation. Isotope scans are readily available and their clinical utility has been confirmed by

Table 4 Causes of pulmonary consolidation

Pulmonary oedema	***Neoplasm***
• Cardiogenic/fluid overload	• Bronchoalveolar cell carcinoma
• Adult respiratory distress sydrome	• Lymphoproliferative disorders
• Inhalation injury (noxious gases)	***Blood***
• Drug abuse	• Contusion
• Neurogenic (raised intracranial pressure or head injury)	• Infarction
• Renal disease	• Idiopathic pulmonary haemorrhage (Goodpasture's syndrome)
• Traumatic (fat embolism)	***Other***
Exudative	• Sarcoidosis
• Infective consolidation	• Alveolar proteinosis
• Eosinophilic lung disease	
• Collagen vascular disease	
• Cryptogenic oranizing pneumonia	
• Radiation pneumonitis	

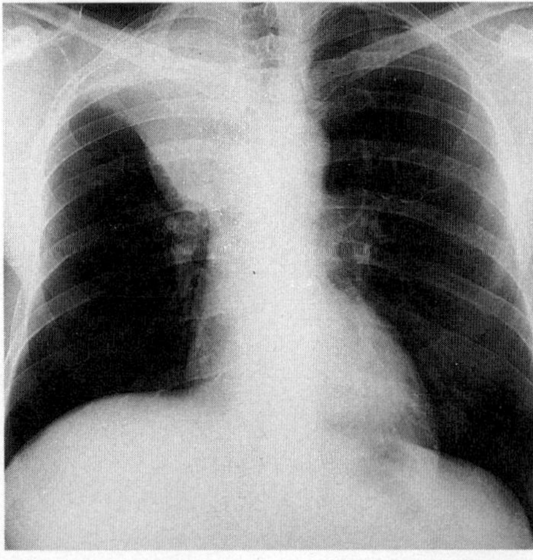

Fig. 6 Right upper lobe collapse. The CXR demonstrates increased opacity in the right upper zone, with a sharp lower border due to elevation of the minor fissure, elevation of the right hilum, and tracheal deviation to the right.

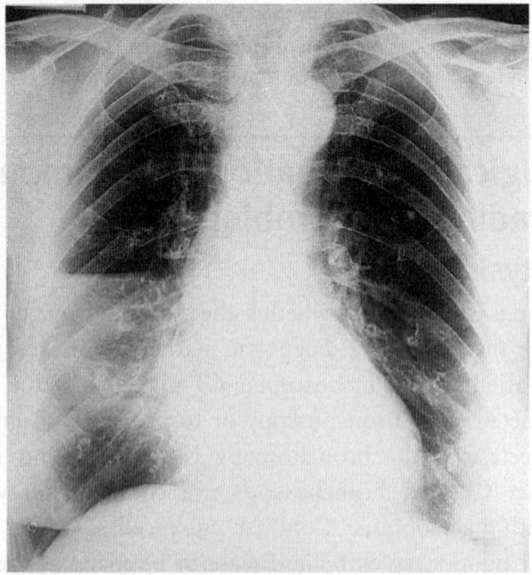

Fig. 7 Right middle lobe collapse. The CXR demonstrates increased right mid-zone opacification, and obliteration of the right heart border.

multiple studies. Spiral CT is less readily available and a much less well researched technique; despite this, the direct visualization of pulmonary artery thrombus and the studies available suggest that this technique is as useful as isotope studies, and may also be used to confirm or refute a diagnosis of emboli in patients with an indeterminate scan.

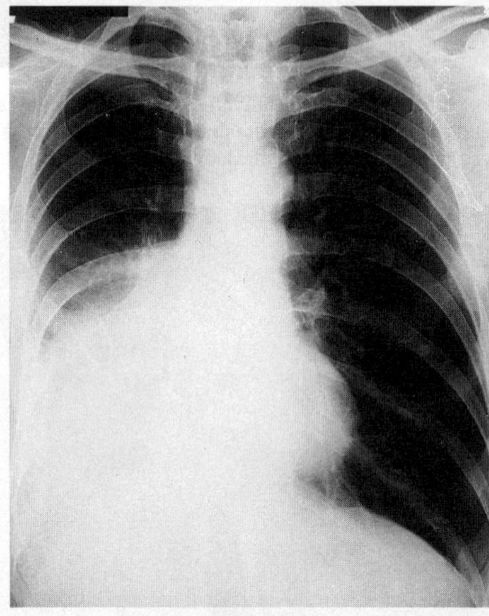

Fig. 8 Right lower lobe collapse. The CXR demonstrates increased density at the right base, elevation of the right hemidiaphragm with obscuration of its medial portion, and inferior displacement of the right hilum. (Although not seen in this case, the right heart border often remains clear, and there is tracheal deviation to the right).

Segmental/lobar/lung collapse

CT may be used to stage tumour diagnosed on bronchoscopy, but is also of value if extrinsic compression is suspected by demonstrating tumour or lymphadenopathy as the cause. If tumour or lymphadenopathy is confirmed on CT to be the cause of collapse and a tissue diagnosis has not been produced by bronchoscopy, percutaneous needle biopsy may be performed.

Opaque hemithorax

Ultrasound may be used to confirm a large pleural effusion or mass as the cause of an opaque hemithorax, particularly if a space-occupying cause rather than complete lung collapse is suspected from the CXR.

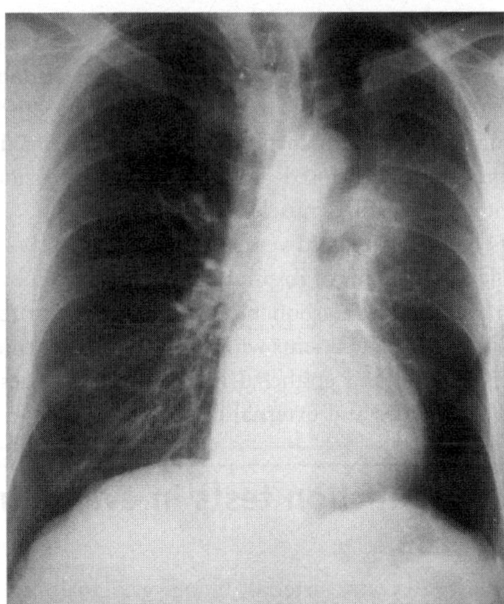

Fig. 9 Left upper lobe collapse. The CXR demonstrates a veil-like increase in density in the left upper zone, elevation of the left hilum, and tracheal deviation to the left.

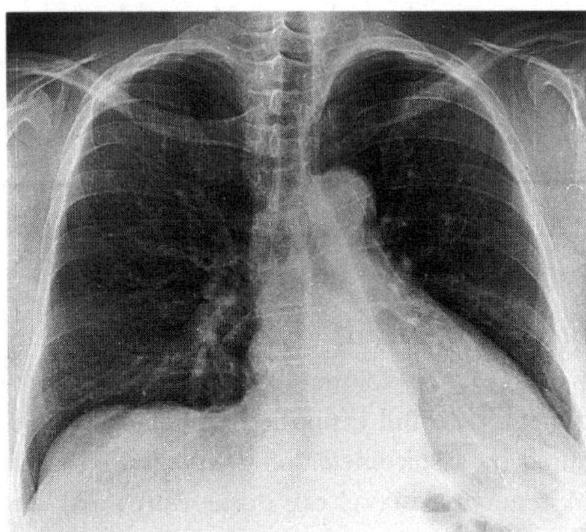

Fig. 10 Left lower lobe collapse. The CXR demonstrates a triangular density behind the heart, depression of the left hilum and loss of the medial border of the left hemidiaphragm.

Ultrasound may also be used to assist aspiration, drainage, or biopsy. CT may be helpful in assessing mediastinal involvement if a tumour is detected on bronchoscopy or ultrasound.

Pleural effusion

Ultrasound may confirm an effusion suspected on CXR, and demonstrate its nature. CT is of greater value than ultrasound in diagnosing a malignant cause for the effusion, and in targeting a site for biopsy if required.

Pulmonary mass

Retrieving previous CXRs is often the single most valuable act when a mass is revealed on CXR. A significant increase in size, greater than 25 per cent increase in diameter, is suggestive of malignancy. Other features such as calcification or spiculation are less reliable indicators of benign or malignant disease. If malignancy is suspected, CT may be used to confirm the size and site of the mass, whether it is solitary and whether associated with lymphadenopathy, and the presence or absence of metastatic disease. Percutaneous needle biopsy may be performed if a tissue diagnosis is required.

Table 5 Causes of pulmonary nodules

Solitary nodule	*Multiple nodules > 2mm in size*
• Granulomas	• Metastases
• Bronchial carcinoma	• Sarcoidosis
• Pulmonary metastasis	• Lymphoma
• Pulmonary adenoma	• Bronchoalveolar cell carcinoma
• Pulmonary hamartoma	• Multifocal pneumonia/abscesses
• Arteriovenous malformation	• Fungal disease
• Immunological disease (Wegener's granulomatosis, rheumatoid disease)	• Immunological disease
	• Multiple arteriovenous malformations
• Hydatid disease	• Hydatid disease
	• Fat emboli
Multiple nodules < 2mm in size	
• Miliary tuberculosis	
• Fungal disease	
• Pneumoconiosis	
• Sarcoidosis	
• Acute extrinsic allergic alveolitis	
• Metastases	

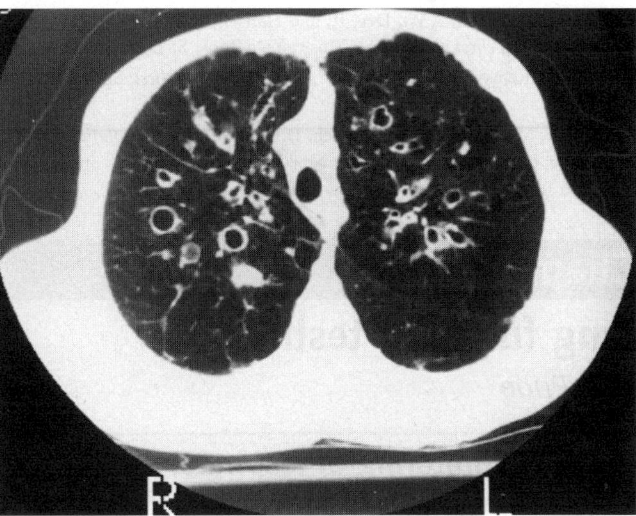

Fig. 11 High resolution CT showing thickened and dilated subsegmental airways characteristic of severe bronchiectasis.

Mediastinal mass

Computed tomography should be used in most instances to confirm the presence of and the position of the abnormality, and in a large number of cases will provide a specific diagnosis. MRI may be used as an alternative means of investigation, particularly in patients with suspected vascular abnormalities.

Bronchiectasis

Moderate or severe bronchiectasis may be apparent on CXR. However, significant numbers of patients with clinically-suspected bronchiectasis have a normal CXR, and these patients should now be investigated with HRCT (Fig. 11). The severity and extent of disease, that is the number of lobes involved, is readily assessed by HRCT.

Diffuse lung disease

In many instances the diagnosis may be apparent from the CXR, but HRCT has been shown to be more sensitive and specific in the diagnosis of diffuse lung disease. The success of this technique has been responsible for the decline in open lung biopsies performed in patients with diffuse lung disease. HRCT may also be used to target a site for open lung biopsy if a specific diagnosis may not be made, and in some cases to assess treatment response.

Pulmonary nodules

Combining clinical information, with the size, number, and distribution of nodules on CXR and other abnormalities such as hilar lymphadenopathy may enable a specific diagnosis to be made, although in the majority of patients without a leading clinical history or examination this is not possible. Further radiological investigation is usually with CT, when specific features such as calcification may be helpful. If there are no specific clinical or radiological pointers, percutaneous needle biopsy may be valuable in diagnosing a malignant or infectious cause.

Further reading

Armstrong, P., Wilson, A.W., Dee, P., and Hansell, D.M. (1994). *Imaging of diseases of the chest*, (2nd edn). Mosby Year Book, St Louis, MO.

Remy, J. and Remy-Jardin, M. (1996). *Spiral CT of the chest.* Springer-Verlag.

Webb, W.R., Muller, N.L., and Naidich, D.P. (1996). *High-resolution CT of the lung*, (2nd edn). Raven Press, New York.

Chapter 4.3

Lung function testing

N. B. Pride

Bedside monitoring of respiratory function in acute illness

Many tests of respiratory function depend on patient co-operation, limiting application in acute disease where they could be particularly useful. Current monitoring is usually confined to continuous measurement of oxygen saturation with oximetry, with frequent but intermittent measurements of arterial oxygen and carbon dioxide pressures (PaO_2, $PaCO_2$), pH, and of peak expiratory flow (PEF) to follow airway function. Transcutaneous electrodes can indicate trends in PCO_2 with a rather slow time constant; values are considerably higher than $PaCO_2$. Often it would be useful to follow minute ventilation, for instance in acute respiratory failure or severe asthma, but although chest wall movements (rib cage and abdomen) can be detected by pneumographs or magnetometers, these devices are very sensitive to changes in the position of the subject and therefore only provide qualitative information. The best solution at present is to place a portable pneumotachograph at the mouth for about 30 s. Fortunately, PEF remains a valid measurement in distressed patients with severe asthma as the expiratory effort to achieve true PEF is less in acute asthma than in the absence of airway obstruction; underestimates occur if PEF measurement is not preceded by a full inflation. In gross weakness of the respiratory muscles (crises of myasthenia gravis, Guillain–Barré syndrome), the vital capacity gives a better indication of respiratory reserve than PEF. Portable meters are now available for bedside measurement of mouth pressures developed during maximum inspiratory efforts and maximum expiratory efforts against a closed airway, and these provide a direct measurement of respiratory muscle strength.

In patients requiring assisted ventilation in the intensive care unit, a more detailed assessment of respiratory mechanics can be obtained with modern ventilators. Carbon monoxide transfer coefficient can be measured in intubated patients with a rebreathing technique. Lung water and endothelial and epithelial integrity can be assessed using radionuclide techniques and external counting.

Use of lung function tests in evaluating stable disease

During the last 20 years, arterial blood gas analysis, oximetry, regional ventilation and perfusion scans, and PEF monitoring have moved from the lung function laboratory to general hospital use. The standard tests widely available in lung function laboratories (Table 1) are most useful for assessing patients with airways obstruction and restrictive lung disease. More elaborate methods are needed to evaluate breathing problems during sleep (Chapter 4.43), function of the diaphragm, the central control of breathing, regional lung function, and the pulmonary circulation (Table 2), and these are not so widely available.

Tests of ventilatory mechanics

Static lung volumes (Fig. 1)

Vital capacity (VC) is the volume expired from full inflation (total lung capacity (TLC)) to full expiration (residual volume (RV)) and can be measured by a spirometer or by integrating expired flow at the mouth. A reduction in VC can occur with a reduction in TLC (as in lung fibrosis or inspiratory muscle weakness) or an increase in RV (as in emphysema, asthma, and other forms of intrapulmonary airway disease). In normal lungs resting end-tidal volume (functional residual capacity (FRC)) is about 50 per cent of the fully expanded volume of the lung (TLC).

FRC can be measured by:

1. Gas dilution: a known volume and concentration of a relatively insoluble foreign gas (usually helium) is allowed to mix with resident intrapulmonary gas, the volume of which is measured from the difference between the initial and final concentrations of marker gas. In normal lungs a single breath test provides a reasonable estimate of lung volume, but multibreath methods lasting more than 5 min may be required to achieve mixing and avoid underestimates in patients with intrapulmonary airway obstruction.
2. Whole-body plethysmograph method: the subject makes panting efforts against a closed shutter while seated in a large air-tight chamber. As mass movement of gas is prevented, changes in alveolar volume during this manoeuvre are due to compression and rarefaction of alveolar gas which are reflected by reciprocal changes in plethysmograph pressure, allowing absolute alveolar volume to be calculated using Boyle's law. The volume inspired during a maximum inspiration or expiration from FRC can then be measured with a spirometer to derive TLC or RV.

Table 1 Standard aspects of lung function assessed in lung function laboratories

Function	Available techniques	Applications
Airway function, including response to dilator and constrictor agents	Spirometry, peak expiratory flow Maximum flow–volume curves Body plethysmograph (airway resistance and flow–volume curves)	Airflow obstruction due to asthma, emphysema, chronic obstructive pulmonary disease, and extrathoracic airways obstruction Tests can all be repeated after bronchodilators or bronchoconstrictor challenges (such as histamine, methacholine, exercise, cold air, specific allergens, etc.) Constrictor tests are useful for diagnosis of asthma, when initial airway function is normal
Lung volumes and distensibility	Multibreath gas equilibration using helium Body plethysmography (thoracic gas volume) Lung compliance using oesophageal intubation	Hyperinflation in airflow obstruction Diagnosis of restrictive lung disease Distinguish cause of restrictive lung disease
Respiratory muscle function	Mouth pressures during maximum inspiratory and expiratory efforts	Systemic muscle disease Unexplained ventilatory failure or restrictive lung disease Severe hyperinflation
Pulmonary gas exchange	Single-breath CO transfer coefficient Pulse oximetry PaO_2 and $PaCO_2$ with simultaneous collection of expired gas: response to increasing inspired oxygen, etc.	Reduced with emphysema or interstitial lung disease Increased with intrapulmonary haemorrhage, asthma Detection of inefficiency in pulmonary gas exchange for O_2 or CO_2
Exercise capacity	Treadmill, cycle, step ergometry or progressive walk with measurement of work, O_2 consumption, heart rate, ventilation (O_2 saturation, PaO_2, $PaCO_2$) Simple tests of walking distance against time	Integrated performance of cardiorespiratory–muscular system Assessment of response to treatment or training programmes Assess disability in severe disease

Table 2 Additional aspects of respiratory function assessed in some lung function laboratories

Function	Available techniques	Applications
Disturbance of breathing, oxygenation, and upper airway occlusion during sleep	Monitoring oxygenation (oximeter) and chest wall movements during sleep Additional measurements to detect snoring, movement, blood pressure, EMG, EEG, heart rate, and transcutaneous PCO_2 may be used	Investigation of daytime somnolence, narcolepsy, unexplained respiratory failure or polycythaemia Adequacy of oxygen or other therapy in patients with COPD or respiratory muscle weakness
Diaphragm function	Transdiaphragmatic pressure, EMG of diaphragm and other muscles, electrical stimulation of phrenic nerves or magnetic stimulation of cervical nerve roots	Suspected diaphragm disease Further investigation of low mouth pressures with maximum voluntary efforts
Control of breathing	Ventilatory response to induced hypoxia or hypercapnia Non-invasive monitoring of chest-wall movements (pneumographs or magnetometers)	Investigation of unexplained hypoxia or hypercapnia Disorder of breathing rhythm
Pulmonary circulation Haemodynamics	Right-heart catheterization, echocardiogram–Doppler studies	Evaluation of pulmonary hypertension, resistance, and response to O_2 or vasodilator drugs
Epithelial/endothelial function	Clearance of injected or inhaled* (e.g. radio-aerosol of DTPA) markers	Progress of adult respiratory distress syndrome Lung damage after inhalation injury Interstitial lung disease
Regional lung function	Distribution of ventilation with radiolabelled gas or aerosols Distribution of blood flow with radiolabelled microspheres	Pulmonary embolism Assessment of suitability for pulmonary resection or bullectomy (plus tests of overall lung function)

*May also reflect airway epithelial function.

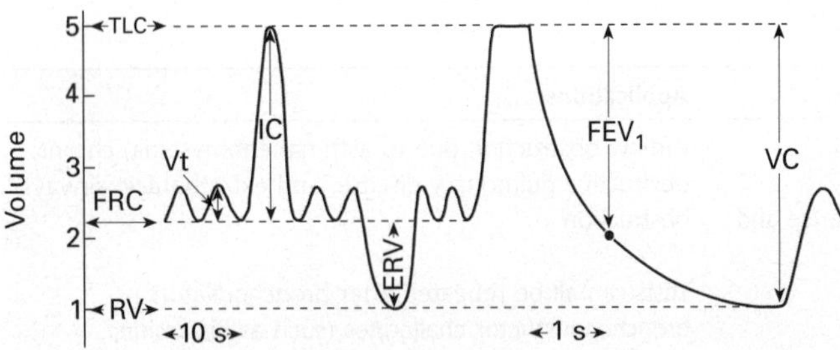

Fig. 1 Static and dynamic lung volumes indicated as a record of tidal breathing against time, followed by expiratory and inspiratory forced vital capacity manoeuvres for which the time scale has been expanded. TLC, total lung capacity; FRC, functional residual capacity; RV, residual volume; FEV_1, forced expiratory volume in 1 s; IC, inspiratory capacity; Vt, tidal volume; ERV, expiratory reserve volume; VC, vital capacity.

The plethysmographic method often gives higher values than the gas dilution method for FRC in severe intrapulmonary airway disease. Some of this difference occurs because plethysmography measures intrathoracic gas which barely communicates with the airway (bullae and other very poorly ventilated areas). An accurate estimate of thoracic volume can also be obtained from spinal CT or from planimetry of standard posteroanterior and lateral chest radiographs taken at full inflation. Corrections have to be made for tissue and vascular volumes of the lungs so as to estimate gas volume.

In normal subjects, FRC is passively determined by the balance between the inward recoil of the lungs and outward recoil of the chest wall. Reductions in VC in lung fibrosis, respiratory muscle weakness, heart failure, and chest wall deformity are accompanied by decreases in TLC and FRC. In obesity there is a reduced FRC. Intrapulmonary airway disease consistently leads to a rise in RV and FRC, while TLC is either normal or, in some subjects with emphysema, increased. When TLC is increased, the accompanying increase in RV is almost always greater so that there is still a decreased VC. When airway obstruction is severe, slowing of tidal expiratory flow results in FRC being considerably greater than the volume determined by lung and chest wall recoil. Alveolar pressure at the end of expiration, which is normally equal to atmospheric pressure, is then positive ('intrinsic' positive end-expired pressure (PEEP)) and provides a threshold load which has to be overcome by the inspiratory muscles before inspiratory flow can begin.

Lung recoil pressure and compliance

Lung recoil pressure (PL) is the difference between alveolar and pleural pressure. Pleural pressure is estimated from the pressure measured by a balloon-tipped catheter placed in midoesophagus. The relation between lung recoil pressure and volume is obtained by interrupting inspiration and expiration during vital capacity manoeuvres when mouth pressure will equal alveolar pressure. The change in volume (−V)for unit change in recoil pressure (−PL) is the static lung compliance (−V/−PL). Analysis of lung recoil and compliance helps in determining whether a reduction in TLC associated with low compliance is due to extrapulmonary (when there is a low LPl at TLC) or intrapulmonary (when there is an increased PL at TLC) disease. A low recoil pressure and a high static compliance are found in emphysema; the low PL reduces the driving pressure for expiratory flow and the distending forces on the airways, contributing to the airflow obstruction. Airway pressure during the end-inspiratory pause is often used to assess compliance in patients on assisted ventilation in the intensive care unit; this indicates the total compliance of lungs and chest wall which is normally about half that of the lungs alone. Dynamic lung compliance measured during ordinary or accelerated tidal breathing reflects the effects of airway disease as well as the static elastic properties of the lung and is reduced below static compliance when there is peripheral airway narrowing.

Tests of forced expiration and inspiration

The physiological basis of tests of forced expiration depends on the development of plateaux of expiratory flow at any particular lung volume once a certain minimum expiratory pressure is achieved. Provided that flow plateau conditions are achieved, the values obtained do not depend on the pressure applied but only on the mechanical characteristics of the lungs and airways. In contrast, tests of forced inspiration are much more dependent on the applied inspiratory pressures. Both forced expiration and inspiration can be analysed as change in volume versus time (by spirometry) (Fig. 1) or as change in instantaneous flow rate at the mouth (usually measured by a pneumotachograph) versus change in lung volume (maximum flow-volume curve) (Fig. 2). Standard spirometric measurements are the forced expiratory volume in 1 s (FEV_1) and the VC; the latter can be obtained from forced expiration (forced vital capacity (FVC)) or from a separate slower full expiration. In airway disease, FVC may be considerably less than the slow VC. Normally, FEV_1 is more than 70 per cent of VC. Two patterns of spirometric abnormality can be distinguished: 'obstructive' in which, although there is usually some reduction in FVC, FEV_1 is reduced even more so that the ratio FEV_1/FVC is low; and 'restrictive', in which a small FVC is associated with normal or even accelerated emptying on forced expiration and a normal or increased FEV_1/FVC ratio. The maximum flow-volume curve (Fig. 2) shows that, on expiration, flow normally rapidly rises to a peak value and then declines in an approximately linear fashion. Peak expiratory flow (PEF) can also be measured with a peak flow gauge. The most effort-dependent part of expiration is close to full inflation, and therefore in measuring PEF the subject must take a full inspiration and make a rapid and forceful start to the subsequent full expiration. Reduced PEF is most often due to airway disease, but is also found with expiratory muscle weakness and restrictive lung disease. For clinical assessment of ventilatory function, FEV_1 and VC (or FVC) are usually adequate, although these tests will not pick up mild airway disease. In asthma, the value of PEF is closely related to the value of FEV_1, and because PEF can be measured by simple meters which can be used by patients in the home or at work, this measurement is particularly useful for identifying asthmatic episodes and their response to treatment. The maximum flow-volume curve cannot be used to distinguish the site or mechanism of intrapulmonary airway narrowing, but distinctive curves are found when obstruction is extrathoracic (Fig. 2) (see also Chapter 4.12).

Airways resistance

Airways resistance is the ratio of driving pressure (difference between alveolar and mouth pressures) to instantaneous gas flow. Alveolar pressure can be obtained non-invasively with a body plethysmograph or derived from oesophageal pressure obtained via a balloon-catheter system. During quiet tidal breathing via the mouth in normal subjects about one-third of the total resistance is in the extrathoracic airway, about one-third is in the central intrathoracic conducting airways, and the remaining one-third is in the peripheral airways of less than

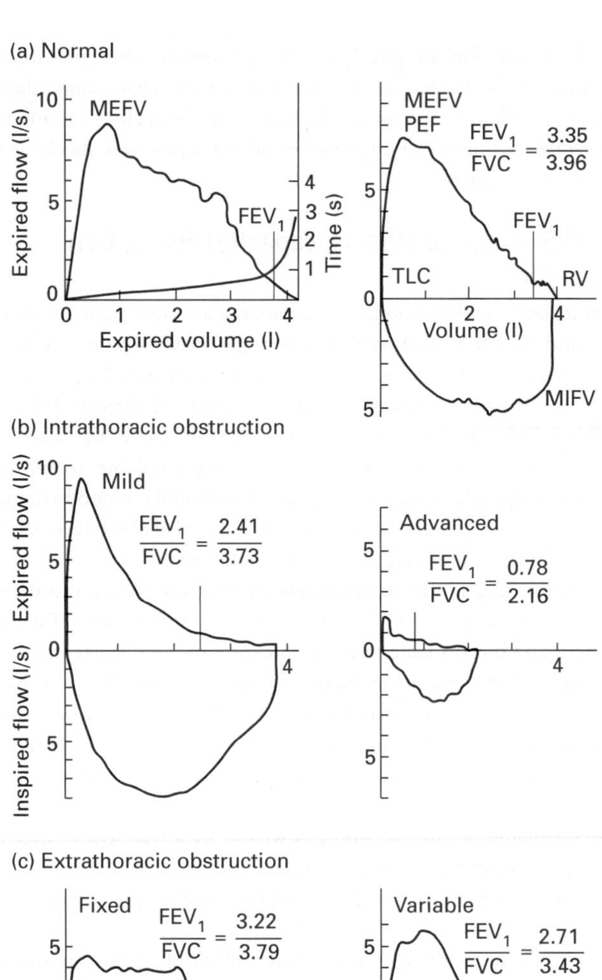

Fig. 2 Characteristic patterns of maximum flow-volume curves for normal subjects, and patients with intrathoracic and extrathoracic airway obstruction. (a) Normal subjects. Left: simultaneous record of maximum expiratory flow versus volume (MEFV, upper curve) and expired volume versus time (spirogram, lower curve) during a forced expiration in a healthy normal subject. The volume expired in first second (forced expiratory volume in 1 s, FEV_1) is indicated. Right: maximum expiratory and inspiratory flow-volume (MEFV, MIFV) curves in another normal subject. Note the different shape of the MEFV curve in the two normal subjects. PEF, peak expiratory flow; TLC, total lung capacity; RV, residual volume; FVC, forced vital capacity. (b) Intrathoracic airways obstruction. Left: mild obstruction. Despite preservation of a normal peak expiratory flow the MEFV curve shows marked convexity to the volume axis in contrast to the linearity or concavity to the volume axis in normal subjects. Right: severe obstruction with gross reduction on both the flow and volume axis and convexity to the volume axis. Reduction in flow on MEFV curve considerably greater than on MIFV curve. (c) Extrathoracic airways obstruction. Left: fixed obstruction pattern as seen in tracheal stenosis with reduction in flow on MEFV and MIFV curves and a distinctive plateau of flow on MEFV curve. Right: variable obstruction with inspiratory narrowing of the upper airway but preservation of a normal MEFV curve in a patient with severe obstructive sleep apnoea.

2 to 3 mm internal diameter. The precise value of resistance varies according to the lung volume at which it is measured, the phase of respiration (inspiration or expiration), the size of the laryngeal aperture, and the flow rate. In contrast, spirometry is more robust and less demanding technically. Consequently, at least in the UK, the measurement is used more for research into airway pharmacology than for routine clinical assessment.

Airway responsiveness

In subjects with asthma there is an increased tendency for airways narrowing to occur in response to a whole range of stimuli (e.g. exercise, hyperventilation, breathing cold air, hypo- or hyperosmolar aerosols, constrictor drugs such as histamine or cholinergic agonists, or mediators such as bradykinin or leukotrienes). This responsiveness can be quantified using an incremental dose–response technique. Histamine or methacholine is generally used as the stimulus and the dose is increased until a 20 per cent fall in FEV_1 is produced (Chapter 4.14). Airway responsiveness is often increased in smokers with chronic airflow obstruction, when it may reflect altered airway geometry and increased thickness of the airway wall.

Additional tests of airway function (see Table 3)

Respiratory muscle function

The simplest test of respiratory muscle function is to measure mouth pressure when maximum inspiratory or expiratory efforts are made against a closed valve. Inspiratory efforts are made at FRC or RV; expiratory efforts at full inflation (TLC). Portable meters for bedside use are now available. Properly performed, this test indicates the overall strength of inspiratory or expiratory muscles, but low values may be due to poor technique. Bilateral paralysis of the diaphragm can be suspected if there is orthopnoea and paradoxical inspiratory indrawing of the abdominal wall (particularly in the supine position). A reduction in VC in the sitting position is often found in respiratory muscle weakness; a further fall of >25 per cent in VC on adopting the supine position is characteristic of diaphragmatic weakness. Serial measurements of maximum effort mouth pressures (or, failing this, PEF or VC) may be useful in monitoring conditions where muscle strength varies rapidly (e.g. myasthenia gravis).

Respiratory muscle function is often impaired in generalized muscle disease and motor neurone disease and can then be the most important factor determining prognosis. Weakness is also common in polymyositis, some connective tissue disorders, notably systemic lupus erythematosus, and cachexia from whatever cause. Respiratory muscle function should be checked when there is unexplained restrictive lung disease or hypercapnia. Weakness of the respiratory muscles can be a limiting factor preventing weaning from assisted ventilation in the intensive care unit and is related to such factors as cachexia, muscle catabolism, electrolyte disturbance, and corticosteroid treatment, as well as the underlying lung disease.

An important factor compromising inspiratory muscle function is hyperinflation associated with severe airways obstruction. The raised FRC shortens the initial length of the inspiratory muscles so that they operate on a suboptimal part of their force-length curve and expend more energy to generate a given inspiratory pleural pressure, increasing their oxygen consumption, which may become a significant proportion of the total oxygen consumption.

Diaphragm function can be measured more directly by placing balloon-catheters in the oesophagus and stomach and obtaining transdiaphragmatic pressure from the difference between pressures in these two sites. Such measurements may be made during tidal breathing, maximum inspiratory efforts or in response to phrenic nerve stimulation. The phrenic nerves may be stimulated electrically directly in the neck or by magnetic stimulation, usually applied posteriorly over the cervical spine, which activates the relevant cervical nerve roots. Electromyography of the diaphragm may be used to assess phrenic nerve conduction and to detect changes suggestive of fatigue.

Tests of pulmonary gas exchange

Distribution and mixing of inspired gas

Inequalities of ventilation and inefficient gas mixing may be either between regions or within regions. The topographical distribution of ventilation can be examined by detecting the distribution of inhaled radionuclides such as xenon-133 or krypton-81m with external counters.

In normal subjects, much of the inequality in ventilation is on a regional basis; in the upright posture ventilation is greater in the dependent basal zones. In most diseases of the lung, however, inequalities within a region are of greater importance than inter-regional differences. This applies even in diseases such as asthma and emphysema, where obvious inequalities of ventilation are easily demonstrated by radioactive gas methods. Intraregional inequalities may be detected by a single breath test which measures the expired nitrogen concentration at the mouth after a preceding vital capacity breath of 100 per cent O_2. The rate of rise of expired nitrogen over the middle part of the expiration indicates the unevenness of ventilation: towards the end of the breath there may be a sharp rise in nitrogen concentration which indicates the beginning of closure of basal airways ('closing volume'). This test is a sensitive indicator of early lung damage as with smoking or occupational lung disease. Other techniques are based on the rate of equilibration when helium is washed in or nitrogen washed out of the lung to measure FRC.

Regional ventilation scans are most widely used in conjunction with regional perfusion scans to diagnose pulmonary embolism by the presence of 'unmatched' perfusion defects. They are also useful in assessment for lung volume reduction surgery or bullectomy, unilateral transradiancy, and suspected inhalation of foreign bodies. In bronchial carcinoma, defects in regional ventilation (and perfusion) are very often more severe than suspected from the chest radiograph. Using a combination of preoperative spirometry and regional ventilation scans quantifying the contribution of each lung, a reasonably accurate prediction of postoperative spirometry after pulmonary resection can be made. Because there is usually close concordance between ventilation and perfusion defects in bronchial carcinoma, the preoperative regional distribution of blood flow can also be used to make this prediction.

Transfer factor (diffusing capacity) for carbon monoxide

The transfer of carbon monoxide across the alveolar–capillary membrane and into combination with haemoglobin within the red blood corpuscle mimics the diffusive conductance of oxygen. By measuring carbon monoxide transfer at two or more levels of alveolar PO_2 it is possible to obtain separate values for transfer across the alveolar-capillary membrane and transfer into the haemoglobin within the red blood corpuscle and so derive pulmonary capillary blood volume. Values of carbon monoxide transfer are reduced if there is anaemia, but correction can be made for haemoglobin level.

In normal lungs, carbon monoxide transfer can be used to define a true diffusing capacity of the lungs, which depends on the diffusivity of the gas and the available area and thickness of the alveolar–capillary membrane. The standard technique is extremely simple: the subject inhales a full breath of a gas mixture containing a very low carbon monoxide concentration and the gas transferred during breath-holding for 10 s at TLC is measured. A rebreathing technique can be used also. In lung disease, carbon monoxide transfer is affected by inhomogeneities within the lungs as well as by a true loss of area or increase in thickness of the membrane, and for this reason the less precise term carbon monoxide transfer factor has been adopted in Europe.

Despite these theoretical limitations, values of carbon monoxide transfer (particularly when expressed per litre alveolar volume (transfer coefficient)) are useful in differential diagnosis (Table 4). Apart from the major reductions found in severe emphysema (which contrasts with a slight increase in asthma) and fibrosing alveolitis, smaller reductions are found in systemic sclerosis, chronic renal disease, graft-versus-host disease, pulmonary oedema, *P. carinii* pneumonia, pulmonary toxicity due to amiodarone, lymphangitis carcinomatosa, and a host of other conditions where the alveoli are involved with disease. However, the carbon monoxide transfer coefficient is also greatly influenced by pulmonary blood volume. An increase in blood volume per unit alveolar volume probably accounts for slightly increased values for the carbon monoxide transfer coefficient found

Table 3 Additional tests of airway function

Function	Available techniques	Applications
Cough responsiveness	Response to increasing doses of inhaled capsaicin or citric acid	Unexplained non-productive cough
Mucociliary transport	Clearance of radiolabelled inhaled particles from the lungs Ciliary beat frequency from bronchial or nasal brushings	Investigation of recurrent bronchopulmonary infections, Kartagener's syndrome, etc.
Detection of mild lung damage	Single-breath nitrogen test and 'closing volume'	Occupational and environmental lung disease
Exposure to cigarette smoke	Concentration of CO in expired air	Confirmation of smoking habit
Airway inflammation	Concentration of NO in expired air.	Assessing adequacy of anti-inflammatory treatment in asthma

Table 4 Examples of the value of carbon monoxide transfer coefficient in differential diagnosis

	Reduced	Normal or increased
Airway obstruction	Emphysema	Asthma
Chronic restrictive lung disease	Fibrosing alveolitis	Often remains normal in sarcoidosis; may be slightly increased when restriction is due to respiratory muscle weakness
Acute pulmonary infiltration	Pulmonary oedema	Intrapulmonary haemorrhage

Table 5 Determinants of arterial PO_2 and PCO_2

*Intrapulmonary abnormalities**
Impaired diffusion
Ventilation-perfusion mismatch
Alveolar shunt†
Extrapulmonary modifying factors
Inspired O_2 concentration/pressure
Total ventilation/breathing pattern (influence alveolar PO_2 and CO_2 excretion)
Cardiac output/whole body metabolism (influence mixed venous PO_2 and PCO_2)

*All characterized by an increased alveolar–arterial PO_2 difference.

†Extrapulmonary shunts (e.g. right-to-left intracardiac shunts) also lower arterial PO_2 and increase alveolar–arterial PO_2 difference.

with lung volume restriction in respiratory muscle weakness or after pneumonectomy. Values tend to be below normal in primary pulmonary hypertension, but increased when there is a right-to-left shunt in atrial septal defect. The avidity of carbon monoxide uptake by haemoglobin is utilized to make serial measurements of carbon monoxide transfer to monitor the number of haemoglobin binding sites (intra- and extravascular) accessible in the lungs in intrapulmonary haemorrhage.

Assessment of arterial hypoxaemia and hypercapnia (see Chapter 4.42)

Arterial PO_2 (PaO_2) and PCO_2 ($PaCO_2$) are determined by the interaction between the efficiency of the lungs as gas exchangers and extrapulmonary factors (oxygen in the inspired air, total ventilation, cardiac output, and oxygen consumption and carbon dioxide production).

The three types of abnormality in the lungs which impair pulmonary gas exchange (Table 5) are all characterized by an increased difference between mean alveolar and arterial PO_2 (Chapter 4.43).Most evidence suggests that, at least at rest, diffusion limitation is not important in the hypoxaemia of lung disease, and so resting alveolar–arterial PO_2 difference can be assumed to be due to either shunt (blood flow evading contact with alveolar gas) or to ventilation–perfusion imbalance chiefly due to units with very low ventilation-to-perfusion (V/Q) ratios. The distinction between ventilation–perfusion mismatch and shunt is of considerable practical importance, because the former can readily be corrected by modest increases in inspired oxygen concentration, while this is not the case with shunt. Increase in alveolar shunt is rare in chronic obstructive pulmonary disease (COPD) or asthma and even in patients with severe exacerbations of airway disease PaO_2 can almost always be raised to safe levels with modest rises in inspired oxygen concentration, thus minimizing the risk of worsening hypercapnia. In contrast, hypoxaemia due to shunt is difficult to correct with modest rises in inspired oxygen concentration. Shunt is found with permanent anatomical defects in the heart or with pulmonary arteriovenous malformations. However, effective alveolar shunts develop with acute lung diseases which lead to extensive fluid filling of alveoli, such as pulmonary oedema, severe pneumonia, and adult respiratory distress syndrome. Increases in inspired oxygen to levels which carry a risk of causing pulmonary toxicity are often required, but oxygenation can be assisted by applying positive end-expired pressure to expand the resting lung volume and recruiting additional alveolar surface area for gas exchange.

A reduced minute ventilation is an unusual cause of a low alveolar and arterial PO_2 and is accompanied by a rise in alveolar and arterial PCO_2. Apart from acute crises such as asphyxia due to obstruction of the upper airway or cardiorespiratory arrest, reduced total ventilation is only found with sedation induced by anaesthesia or drugs, with paralysis or gross weakness of the respiratory muscles, or with rare breathing disorders such as Ondine's curse where the central control of breathing is abnormal. In most patients with lung disease, including chronic obstructive pulmonary disease with hypercapnia, there is some increase in total ventilation above normal, which plays an important part in minimizing the effects of impaired pulmonary gas exchange.

The efficiency of carbon dioxide excretion can be assessed by measuring the difference between $PaCO_2$ and mixed expired PCO_2 to estimate the physiological dead space (Vd) for carbon dioxide as a proportion of tidal volume (Vt).

$$\frac{Vd}{Vt} = \frac{(PaCO_2\text{–mixed expired } PCO_2)}{PaCO_2}$$

Small increases in tidal ventilation, especially if associated with a larger tidal volume, are considerably more effective in reducing $PaCO_2$ than in raising PaO_2. Alterations in $PaCO_2$ have a profound effect on acid–base balance and arterial pH (see Chapter 4.43). Measurement of the difference between alveolar and arterial PO_2 and of physiological dead space for CO_2 provides simple, lumped estimates of the efficiency of pulmonary gas exchange in lung disease, which in fact is determined by large variations in ventilation–perfusion balance in different parts of the lungs.

Other constituents of expired air

Apart from oxygen and carbon dioxide, measurements of breath alcohol, carbon monoxide (usually to establish smoking status), and hydrogen (to detect bacterial overgrowth in the gut) have been used for many years. Recently, expired nitric oxide has been proposed as a simple marker of active airway inflammation in asthma and other potential makers of inflammation of oxidant stress are being investigated.

Control of ventilation

Measuring ventilation at rest has played a surprisingly small part in clinical assessment, except in the intensive care unit. Methods that require breathing via a mouth-piece with the nose clipped are not well tolerated by breathless patients—always add some dead space and generally increase minute ventilation. Less intrusive methods, in which surface pneumographs or magnetometers are used to measure expansion of rib cage and abdomen, have shown that minute ventilation in healthy subjects at rest is less than previously believed—commonly about 5 to 6 l/min. Unfortunately, absolute values with these methods are greatly influenced by postural changes but they are valuable for detecting irregularities in pattern of breathing, as during sleep.

Increased resting ventilation occurs in normal subjects during pregnancy, probably in response to increases in progesterone, and at altitude, when the effect is due to hypoxaemic stimulation of the carotid chemoreceptors. It also occurs with of aspirin poisoning and metabolic acidaemia, such as renal failure, diabetic ketosis, and lactic acidosis; acidaemia probably stimulates both peripheral and central chemoreceptors. Hyperventilation is a feature of many cardiorespiratory diseases, notably asthma, severe pneumonia, pulmonary embolism, and pulmonary oedema, and is associated with a respiratory alkalaemia; some of the increase in ventilation may be explained by hypoxaemic stimulation of the carotid chemoreceptors, but stimulation of vagal afferent receptors within the lungs also plays a part. Most of the conditions associated with hyperventilation are easily recognized; when there is no obvious cause the differential diagnosis often lies between pulmonary vascular disease and psychogenic hyperventilation. Psychogenic hyperventilation may be associated with dizziness, tetany, chest pain, paraesthesiae, and an erratic breathing pattern which settles during sleep (Chapter 4.1). Reduced total ventilation (hypoventilation) is much less common and is usually due to sedative drugs or neuromuscular disease, although occasionally it occurs with brainstem disease or severe metabolic alkalosis. In most patients with chronic obstructive pulmonary disease, minute ventilation is slightly above normal values; even in episodes of acute respiratory failure. Relatively small variations in the pattern of breathing can influence the development of hypercapnia in such patients.

Examining the ventilatory response to imposed hypoxia or hypercapnia is most useful when lung and respiratory muscle mechanics are normal, as in studies of the effects of drugs, anaesthesia, or sleep in normal subjects, Pickwickian patients with obesity, or unusual patients with abnormal central control of breathing due to brainstem pathology. Impaired responses to hypoxia and hypercapnia are also found in many patients with chronic airflow obstruction, but when there are abnormalities of ventilatory mechanics or respiratory muscle weakness, a given neurological output inevitably results in less ventilation than in a normal subject. A better idea of neurological output may be obtained by measuring oesophageal pressure throughout the breath or mouth pressure during a transitory 0.1 s occlusion at the start of a breath; these techniques have reduced the role of decreased central drive and emphasized the role of impairment of respiratory muscle and lung mechanics in limiting the ventilatory response in such patients.

Exercise capacity

Exercise tests play an important part in quantifying effort intolerance, investigating its cause, and monitoring progress and response to treatment and rehabilitation programmes. They are also used for confirming a diagnosis of exercise-induced asthma and ischaemic heart disease. An increased ventilation in relation to oxygen consumption is found at high work loads in normal subjects when blood lactate begins to rise (anaerobic threshold). In lung disease, increased ventilation is particularly found with fibrosing alveolitis and primary pulmonary hypertension; some of this increase may be due to stimulation of peripheral chemoreceptors by a fall in arterial PO_2 during exercise, but mechanoreceptor stimulation has also been implicated since increasing inspired oxygen does not restore exercise ventilation to normal values.

In chronic airflow obstruction and fibrosing alveolitis, exercise tolerance appears to be limited by the impaired ventilatory capacity and there is often a considerable fall in oxygen saturation, which in fibrosing alveolitis is due to impaired diffusion.

Quantitative exercise tests usually involve either a treadmill or a bicycle ergometer although progressive walk or step tests can be used in the absence of such equipment. Many clinical problems can be investigated by a simple progressive work load test on a bicycle ergometer measuring ventilation, heart rate, electrocardiogram, and oxygen consumption. This will often indicate whether exercise is limited by the cardiac response or by ventilation, and will give an objective measurement of maximum oxygen consumption. More elaborate measurements, including arterial blood gases and cardiac output, may occasionally be required. These tests indicate cardiopulmonary fitness and exercise capacity. Exercise tolerance (the amount of work a patient is prepared to achieve) can be assessed by the distance walked on the flat in 6 or 12 min in patients with more severe disability. In such patients, walking distance tests correlate well with disability in daily life; they evaluate motivation as well as cardiopulmonary status.

Further reading

Cotes, J.E. (1993). *Lung function*, (5th edn). Blackwell Scientific Publications, Oxford.

Gibson, G.J. (1995). *Clinical tests of respiratory function*, (2nd edn). Chapman and Hall, London.

West, J.B. (1995). *Respiratory physiology—the essentials*, (5th edn). Williams and Wilkins, Baltimore.

West, J.B. (1997). *Pulmonary pathophysiology*, (5th edn). Williams and Wilkins, Baltimore.

Chapter 4.4

Microbiological methods in the diagnosis of respiratory infections

D. W. M. Crook and T. E. A. Peto

A wide range of bacteria, viruses, fungi, and parasites colonize or infect the airways, lung, and pleura (Table 1). The diagnosis of a

Table 1 Bacterial, viral, and fungal respiratory pathogens

Colonizing organisms	Lung abscess
Hospital-acquired pneumonia	Mixed oropharyngeal flora, e.g. *Prevotella* spp. (anaerobes)
Pseudomonas aeruginosa	*Streptococcus* spp.
Escherichia coli	*Eikenella corrodens*
Klebsiella pneumoniae	**Non-colonizing organisms**
Staphylococcus aureus	*Legionella* spp.
Enterobacter spp.	*Nocardia* spp.
(many other *Enterobacteriacae* spp.)	*Chlamydia* spp.
Candida spp.	*Mycoplasma pneumoniae*
Aspergillus spp.	*Mycobacteria tuberculosis*
Cytomegalovirus (latent virus)	*Blastomyces braziliensis*
Community-acquired pneumonia	*Coccidioides immitis*
Streptococcus pneumoniae	*Histoplasma capsulatum*
Haemophilus influenzae	*Cryptococcus neoformans*
Moraxella catarrhalis	Respiratory syncytial virus
Staphylococcus aureus	Influenzae A and B
	Parainfluenza virus

respiratory tract infection can only be made clinically. The microbiology laboratory can only provide some clues as to the likely causative organism.

Some of the organisms that usually colonize the nasopharynx (e.g. *Streptococcus pneumonia*, *Haemophilus influenzae*) may spread to the lung and cause exacerbations of chronic bronchitis or pneumonia. Pathogens such as *Mycobacterium tuberculosis*, *Legionella pneumophila*, *Histoplasma capsulatum*, and the respiratory viruses do not colonize the nasopharynx but may infect the lung, after airborne or haematogenous spread, where they form an infected focus. The distinction between nasopharyngeal colonizers and non-colonizers is critical for the interpretation of microbiological tests of respiratory tract secretions, fluids, or tissues.

Samples for microbiological testing

1. Expectorated or induced sputum is liable to be contaminated with upper respiratory tract colonizers.
2. Respiratory secretions obtained by transtracheal aspiration are largely free from nasopharyngeal contamination. This procedure is useful when bronchoscopy is not available, but is unpleasant for the patient.
3. Bronchoscopy specimens (bronchoalveolar lavage, protected specimen brush, or lung biopsy) are relatively free of contaminating upper respiratory tract flora but there is a risk from bleeding and hypoxia which can sometimes require mechanical ventilation of a patient.
4. Fluid can be aspirated from the lung parenchyma through a fine needle introduced percutaneously in the case of peripherally located intrapulmonary cavities (abscesses) and in childhood and adult pneumonias. There are risks of pneumothorax, haemorrhage, and occasional sudden death.
5. Open-lung biopsy provides the most useful specimens, but this technique is too invasive for routine use.
6. Pleural fluid or pleural biopsy specimens obtained by percutaneous needle provide reliable samples free from contamination with nasopharyngeal-colonizing organisms.
7. Pleural fluid samples obtained from a chronically draining chest tube are not reliable, since chest drains rapidly become colonized with potential pathogens after insertion.
8. Blood cultures should be carried out in ill patients suspected of infection. Approximately 10 to 28 per cent of pneumococcal pneumonias are associated with bacteraemia. *H. influenzae*, *Staphylococcus aureus*, *Klebsiella pneumoniae*, and other organisms causing pneumonia can be cultured from the blood.

Microbiological examination of samples

Microscopy of unstained sputum

Hyphae of filamentous moulds (e.g. *Aspergillus* spp. in a patient with fever, neutropenia, and pulmonary infiltrates), yeasts (e.g. *Blastomyces* spp.), or ova of paragonomiasis may be seen in unstained sputum.

Direct examination of stained samples

Gram staining of expectorated sputum is useful only in diagnosing pneumococcal pneumonia. However, Gram staining of organisms in bronchoalveolar lavage fluid is highly predictive of pyogenic bacterial infection in patients with pneumonia. In community-acquired pneumonia, Gram-positive diplococci, pleomorphic Gram-negative coccobacilli, and Gram-positive cocci in clusters are likely to be pneumococci, *H. influenzae*, and *Staph. aureus* respectively. In nosocomial and ventilator-associated pneumonia, Gram staining of expectorated sputum or endotracheal aspirates is poorly predictive of the aetiology. However, when more than 7 per cent of cells in bronchoalveolar lavage fluid from a ventilated patient contain stainable intracellular organisms, the probability of pneumonia caused by these organisms is high (70–80 per cent). Gram staining of pleural fluid is useful; the presence of many neutrophils suggests an empyema, and organisms can be seen in up to 80 per cent of these cases.

In an appropriate clinical setting, detection of acid-fast organisms by Ziehl–Neelsen or rhodamine auramine staining of respiratory secretions or tissue is highly predictive of mycobacterial disease. Unfortunately, the sensitivity of the test is relatively low (20–78 per cent for sputum and less than 10 per cent for pleural fluid). Therefore a negative test result does not reliably exclude mycobacterial pulmonary or pleural disease.

Direct fluorescent antibody testing is a specific and sensitive test for detecting respiratory syncytial virus and *Legionella* spp. In children with suspected respiratory syncytial virus infection, the most accessible specimen is a nasopharyngeal aspirate. *Legionella* spp. can occasionally be detected in sputum or bronchoalveolar lavage fluid.

Pneumocystis carinii in respiratory secretions is highly predictive of pneumocystis pneumonia. In 80 per cent of AIDS patients with pneumocystis pneumonia, induced expectorated sputum samples are positive. Examination of bronchoalveolar lavage fluid or lung tissue stained with methenamine silver is highly sensitive (90 per cent) and is specific (more than 95 per cent) for *P. carinii.*

Histological examination of stained lung or pleural biopsy material may reveal tuberculous granulomas, schistosome ora, fungi (e.g. *Aspergillus* spp., *Rhizopus* spp., *Coccidioides immitis, H. capsulatum,* and *Blastomycosis braziliensis*), characteristic features of cytomegalovirus, or measles pneumonias.

Detection of antigens

Pneumococcal antigen detection by latex agglutination or countercurrent immunoelectrophoresis is highly specific with samples such as blood, pleural fluid, bronchoalveolar lavage fluid, or urine. The sensitivity is high (80 per cent) with pleural fluid but low with blood or urine.

Legionella antigen testing of urine is both sensitive and specific for serogroup 1 legionellosis. Cryptococcal antigen testing of serum is useful for diagnosing pulmonary cryptococcosis.

Culture

The isolation from sputum of respiratory pathogens that frequently colonize the upper respiratory tract does not reliably predict the aetiology of pneumonia or lung abscess. However, isolation of non-colonizing organisms is strongly associated with infection caused by these pathogens.

The isolation of organisms from a bronchoscopic protected specimen brush or bronchoalveolar lavage samples is useful in patients with suspected ventilation-associated pneumonia. Isolation of mixed aerobic/anaerobic oral flora from bronchoalveolar lavage specimens or lung aspirates suggests an aspiration or suppurative pneumonia. The culture of *Aspergillus* spp. in bronchoalveolar lavage fluid in neutropenic patients indicates invasive disease. Cytomegalovirus can be grown from respiratory secretions, but the sensitivity, specificity, and predictive value are uncertain. The growth of organisms from pleural fluid suggests a pleural infection and, if the organisms are pyognic, empyema.

Serological tests

Serodiagnosis is useful for viral, mycoplasma, chlamydial TWAR (which refers to the first two laboratory isolates of *Chlamydia pneumoniae,* TW-183 and AR-39), Q fever, and *Legionella* spp. infections. In histoplasmosis, coccidioidomycosis, filariasis, and echinococcus the presence of antibody suggests active infection.

Detection of specific DNA sequences

PCR is being assessed for the diagnosis of tuberculosis and pneumonia caused by *P. carinii, Mycoplasma pneumoniae,* and *L. pneumophila.*

The microbiological investigation of patients with pneumonia—one approach

The rational approach to making a microbiological diagnosis of a pulmonary infection rests on balancing the risk of the procedure to obtain reliable samples against the risk of treating empirically without defining the cause of a respiratory infection. There are empirical antibiotic regimens (e.g. cefuroxime and erythromcyin) that have negligible side-effects and adequately cover the majority of likely pathogens in community-acquired pneumonia (e.g. *Strep. pneumoniae, H. influenzae, Mycoplasma,* etc.). However, such an approach is inadequate if the patient is too ill to risk a poor response to a therapeutic trial. In such patients, bronchoscopic examination may be justified even if the patient subsequently requires mechanical ventilation. In less severely ill patients, bronchoscopy is justified if tuberculosis or rarer pathogens resistant to empiric treatment, such as fungi, parasite, or multiresistant bacterial infection, are suspected.

Further reading

Bartlett, J.G., Ryan, K.J., Smith, T.F., and Wilson, W.R. (1987). In *Cumitech 7A. Laboratory diagnosis of lower respiratory tract infections* (ed. J.A. Washington II). American Society for Microbiology, Washington, DC.

Pugin, J., Acukenthaler, R., Mili, N., Janssens, J.P., Lew, P.D., and Suter, P.M. (1991). Diagnosis of ventilator-associated pneumonia by bacteriological analysis of bronchoscopic and nonbronchoscopic 'blind' bronchoalveolar lavage fluid. *American Review of Respiratory Disease,* 143, 1121–9.

Research Committee of the British Thoracic Society and the Public Health Laboratory Service (1987). Community-acquired pneumonia in adults in British hospitals in 1982–1983: a survey of aetiology, morality, prognostic factors and outcome. *Quarterly Journal of Medicine,* 62, 195–220.

Wilson, S.M., McNerney, R., Nye, P.M., Godfrey-Faussett, P.D., Stoker, N.G., and Voller, A. (1993). Progress toward a simplified polymerase chain reaction and its application to diagnosis of tuberculosis. *Journal of Clinical Microbiology,* 31, 1007–8.

Chapter 4.5

Diagnostic bronchoscopy and tissue biopsy

M. F. Muers

Diagnostic bronchoscopy and tissue biopsy are an integral part of the investigation of respiratory disease, but should be regarded as complementary to, rather than substitutes for, simpler tests.

Bronchoscopy

Indications (Table 1)

Bronchoscopy is mainly used to investigate or confirm the possibility of carcinoma. The diagnosis does not depend just on tissue sampling, since many abnormal appearances are characteristic. Nor is it confined to visible lesions; the simultaneous use of flexible sampling instruments and fluoroscopy allows sampling from distal bronchi or lung parenchyma.

Techniques

Fibreoptic bronchoscopy

This is usually a day case procedure with local anaesthesia and light sedation. A posteroanterior and a lateral chest radiograph, and spirometry, are required beforehand. Any cardiac abnormalities need to be assessed, and arterial blood gases measured if spirometry is poor. Patients with coagulopathies or on anticoagulants need clotting studies.

Instruments should be carefully cleaned as a routine before every examination. They should be dismantled and all parts washed in neutral detergent before immersion for 20 min (routine) or 60 min (immunocompromised patients) in 2 per cent alkaline gluteraldehyde. Immediately before use they should be rinsed and wiped with sterile water or 70 per cent alcohol. Bronchoscopists and their assistants should be gowned and gloved, and should consider wearing masks and goggles to minimize the risk of HIV transmission, particularly in high incidence areas.

Patients are usually fasted for at least 2 h, and lightly sedated, usually by perioperative intravenous diazepam, midazolam, and/or fentanyl. Atropine, 0.6 mg intravenous is commonly given but is probably not necessary. The procedure can be undertaken without sedation, and this may be safer in patients with marked respiratory impairment, provided that local anaesthesia is adequate. Supplemental oxygen by nasal cannulae at 2 l/min usually maintains arterial saturation. Continuous oximetry is recommended.

The nares and oropharynx are sprayed with 4 per cent or 10 per cent lignocaine. The bronchoscope is best inserted through the nose. The mouth, with a mouth guard should be used only if access is difficult. The vocal cords are anaesthetized either by a previous transtracheal injection of 2–5 ml of 4 per cent lignocaine or 5 per cent cocaine, or by the injection of 2 ml aliquots of 2 per cent or 4 per cent lignocaine through the bronchoscope. Anaesthesia of the bronchial tree is obtained similarly.

A survey of 40 000 bronchoscopies in the UK during 1983 revealed a complication rate of 0.12 per cent and a mortality of 0.04 per cent.

Rigid bronchoscopy

This is useful if previous fibre-optic bronchoscopy has failed to make a diagnosis, if there is anxiety about uncontrolled bleeding, when operability is being assessed, when foreign body removal is being contemplated, in children, and for laser treatment, diathermy, and stent insertion. This is performed under general anaesthesia and oxygen Venturi ventilation.

Bronchoscopic biopsy techniques

Endobronchial sampling

The majority of endobronchial lesions are carcinomas, and these are best investigated by a combination of brushing or catheter samples from the surface for cytology, forceps biopsy for histology, and a bronchial 'wash' for cytology. Up to four or five forceps biopsies are advisable from a single lesion. For a bronchial 'wash' 20–40 ml of normal saline is injected over the lesion into the peripheral lung and the residual fluid aspirated into a trap. When this is done in addition to brush and forceps biopsy, the diagnostic yield is increased.

Table 1 Indications for bronchoscopy

Diagnosis

- Suspected malignancy
- Unexplained localized or diffuse radiographic opacity (e.g. 'persistent pneumonia')
- Unexplained respiratory symptoms (particularly haemoptysis, wheezing)
- Microbiological sampling (e.g. ? tuberculosis but no sputum; ? Pneumocystis carinii pneumonia in AIDS)
- Bronchoscopic bronchogram
- Multiple lung biopsies for post lung-transplant surveillance.

Therapy

- Removal of secretions or foreign body
- Palliation of carcinoma symptoms by laser, diathermy, cryotherapy, endobronchial radiotherapy, stents, photodynamic therapy.

Table 2 Bronchoalveolar lavage (a) Normal cellular constituents

Cells	Non-smoker	Smoker
Total ($\times 10^4$/ml)	13	42
PAM (%)	80–95	85–98
Lymphocytes (%)	<15	10
Neutrophils (%)	<3	<5
Eosinophils (%)	>0.5	<3

(b) Pathognomonic appearances

Cells	Diagnosis
Iron-laden PAMs	Haemosiderosis Pulmonary haemorrhage
PAS-positive PAMs Lamellar structures on EM	Alveolar proteinosis

PAM, pulmonary alveolar macrophage; PAS, periodic acid–Schiff stain.

Simple aspiration of natural secretions into a trap may also provide materials for cytology but in practice this technique is more useful for microbiological tests. It is not sensitive as a lone investigation for neoplasm.

Bronchoalveolar lavage (BAL)

This technique provides a sample of cells and fluid from the peripheral airways and alveoli of a lung segment or lobe. The naturally occurring cells are predominantly pulmonary alveolar macrophages, and include variable proportions of leucocytes. Changes in the proportions of these cells are rarely diagnostic, but can give support to a diagnosis, for example there is sometimes a high lymphocyte count in allergic alveolitis and active sarcoid. Some rarer findings are pathognomonic (Table 2). BAL is very useful in diagnosing infection in immunocompromised patients (see Chapter 4.10). The study of the chemicals in the supernatant is a widely used research procedure, but is not used in clinical practice.

For BAL, the bronchoscope is wedged into the chosen segment of lung and up to 300 ml of buffered normal saline at 37°C are instilled in 50 ml aliquots injected by syringe. Continuous suction is applied after each aliquot to aspirate the specimens into a trap. The fluid is spun down and the cell pellet examined.

Perioperative nasal oxygen is needed; caution is required if the FEV1 is less than 1.5 litres; transient pyrexia occurs after about 10 per cent of lavages.

Transbronchial biopsy

Usually under fluoroscopic screening, closed, flexible bronchial biopsy forceps are advanced to within 1 cm of the pleura and are then opened and moved gently backwards and forwards two or three times before being advanced more peripherally and closed. Specimens are put in formol saline for histology and others taken dry or in normal saline for culture.

A minimum of three or four biopsies should be taken from diffusely abnormal lung, and up to five or six from localized lesions, provided that no complications occur. These are more common in immunocompromised patients or in the presence of coagulopathies. Bleeding occurred in 0.5 per cent and pneumothoraces after 2.1 per cent of the 3500 procedures reported in the UK survey of 1983. Fluoroscopic screening significantly reduces the incidence of pneumothorax.

Transbronchial needle aspiration

A needle is advanced from its sheath in the bronchoscope through a bronchial wall and suction applied to obtain cytological specimens from tissue up to 1 cm from the surface. In this way subcarinal and paratracheal nodes can be sampled and when guided by CT; aspiration may avoid mediastinoscopy for the staging of lung cancer. Under fluoroscopy, peripheral coin lesions can be examined.

Bronchoscopic bronchography

This is an alternative to formal transcricoid or catheter bronchograms. Bronchographic contrast medium can be injected either directly through the suction channel or through a catheter. Segmental or lobar bronchograms or full unilateral or bilateral bronchograms of good quality can be obtained. However, the advent of high resolution CT has largely replaced bronchograms for the routine investigation of possible bronchiectasis, where it is available.

Percutaneous lung biopsy

Percutaneous fine-needle aspiration biopsy

This is used to sample peripheral lesions, particularly where malignancy is suspected. Large immediately subpleural lesions can be targeted using plain posteroanterior and lateral radiographs with skin markers, but all other lesions need to be examined under screening. This is usually either biplane or C-arm fluoroscopy, although now CT or real time ultrasonography is often preferred. A fine aspiration needle (0.5–1.0 mm, 25–17 gauge) is advanced perpendicular to the skin under local anaesthesia. Suction is applied and aspirated material is expressed on to slides for cytological examination or it may be cultured. Small needles, single passes, and lesions within 2–3 cm of the pleura cause a pneumothorax in less than 5 per cent of cases, but this rate rises substantially with larger needles, multiple passes, and deeper sampling. Slight haemorrhage may occur in 1–10 per cent of cases. Contraindications are untreated coagulopathies, severe coexisting lung disease, especially emphysema, and suspicion of a vascular malformation.

Percutaneous cutting-needle biopsy

The use of cutting needles allows histological examination of lung tissue. The Trucut biopsy needle is now favoured over the previous Silvermann needle, and spring loaded instruments such as the Biopty now make sampling easier. The technique is similar to fine-needle aspiration biopsy, but repeated biopsies are accompanied by a much higher complication rate. Pneumothorax is likely to occur in 20 per cent of cases with perhaps half of these requiring aspiration or tube drainage. Haemorrhage occurs in about 15 per cent. Theoretically, cutting needles can sample diffuse lung disease, but transbronchial biopsies are probably safer.

Open lung biopsy and video assisted thoracoscopic (VATS) biopsy

The sampling of lung tissue under direct vision is the final arbiter in obtaining a diagnosis of diffuse or focal lung disease. The indications are decreasing because of the increase in high resolution CT scanning (see Chapter 4.3) and transbronchial biopsies. These should be considered first in most cases. Video assisted thoracoscopic biopsy (VATS) is replacing formal mini thoracotomy in many centres because of the reduced morbidity and hospital stay. Sampling is best guided by CT, and the surgeon is advised to examine both visibly abnormal lung and nearby tissue where active disease, as opposed to fibrosis, is often found.

Mediastinal sampling

Mediastinal sampling is required when the clinical problem is either the diagnosis of a mediastinal mass or assessment of the operability of lung cancer.

Needle biopsy of the mediastinum

Mediastinal masses can be diagnosed by percutaneous needle biopsy. Screening is needed. Ultrasound allows sampling of anterior and posterior mediastinal masses which abut the chest wall; CT scanning allows any mediastinal mass to be sampled.

Surgical mediastinal sampling

This is required for assessment of operability, and for cases where needle biopsy has failed to produce an accurate diagnosis of a mediastinal mass. Mediastinoscopy is an endoscopic examination under general anaesthesia through a small cervical incision with a rigid instrument passing beneath the pretracheal fascia. It allows sampling of tissue or nodes within the superior mediastinum as far as the carina. Mediastinotomy involves a short transverse incision in the second intercostal space on either side. Exploration under direct vision is extrapleural, and is particularly useful in assessment of tumours arising in the left upper lobe. Complications, including bleeding and pneumothorax are less than 1 per cent if the surgeon is experienced. Mediastinal sampling under direct vision using VATS techniques is an alternative.

Pleura and pleural fluid sampling

Large pleural effusions can be sampled using the physical signs and the chest radiograph to direct the sampling 21-G venepuncture needle on a 20–50 ml syringe, into the intercostal space above the area of maximum dullness to percussion. Ultrasound guidance is better for small effusions. Diagnostic information is obtained from the appearance of the fluid (e.g. blood stained or chylous) and biochemical, cytological, and microbiological examination. Simple aspiration cytology has a diagnostic sensitivity of about 60 per cent for primary or secondary malignant pleural effusions, and about 75 per cent with repeated aspirations. Conventionally, exudates and transudates are separated using the criterion of a protein content (transudates contain <30 g/l. However, Light's criteria are probably more accurate for the diagnosis of exudates: pleural fluid/serum protein > 0.5, pleural fluid/serum LDH > 0.6; pleural fluid LDH > 200 IU/l.

Pleural biopsy

Percuataneous pleural biopsy using the Abram's needle should usually be done at the same time as the aspiration of pleural fluid if local pulmonary or pleural disease, as opposed to organ failure, is suspected as the cause. Strict asepsis and adequate local anaesthesia down to the pleural surface are mandatory, as is verification of the effusion by prebiopsy aspiration. Multiple samples should be taken for histology and in appropriate cases for culture, especially mycobacteria. If repeated fluid cytology is negative, routine biopsy increases the diagnostic yield for neoplasia by about 10 per cent. False negative biopsies are particularly common in mesothelioma. The Trucut needle is more appropriate when a pleural mass is present.

Thoracoscopy

Many pleural effusions remain undiagnosed even after aspiration and percutaneous biopsy. If further histological specimens are required, thoracoscopy is necessary. This involves the inspection and sampling of the visceral and parietal pleura, using a rigid 9 mm thoracoscope, usually under general anaesthesia. The technique which needs an experience operator, allows wide inspection of the pleural surface and multiple biopsies. Complications are rare. The technique has a sensitivity of greater than 90 per cent for pleural malignancy and tuberculosis, although mesothelioma may yield falsely negative samples.

Clinical applications

Perihilar lesions

In modern adult practice, the most common and important diagnosis is lung cancer. In nearly all cases where this is a possibility, fibreoptic bronchoscopy should be considered unless there are contraindications or good clinical reasons why further information is not required. The advantages of proceeding to bronchoscopy are that a tissue diagnosis may be obtained, operability can be assessed, and complications such as bronchial occlusion anticipated. More than 70 per cent of all primary lung neoplasms are within the field of view, with a diagnostic sensitivity of about 90 per cent for biopsy. It must be remembered however, that the differential diagnosis of primary lung cancer at bronchoscopy includes adenomas, metastatic deposits, and, more rarely, tuberculosis or sarcoidosis.

If a perihilar lesion is present on the radiograph, but bronchoscopy is entirely normal, further imaging, usually by CT, is needed, followed by a percutaneous needle biopsy, a mediastinotomy, or a VATS procedure. If endobronchial lesions are seen but biopsies are unhelpful, options are to rebiopsy, perform a transbronchial needle aspiration, or proceed to rigid bronchoscopy for bigger samples.

Circumscribed peripheral lung lesions (the 'coin' lesion) or solitary pulmonary nodule (SPN)

The first point to consider is whether such lesions need to be biopsied or whether, if the probability of a primary lung cancer is high, it is not better to proceed directly to thoracotomy with a frozen section before resection. In a few cases a policy of observation is justified but commonly even these eventually come to surgery. Algorithms are available to assist this decision. The possibility of a solitary metastasis, particularly from renal or adrenal primaries, must be carefully borne in mind.

For most cases, if biopsy is required, percutaneous fine-needle aspiration should be considered first. This is particularly so if the likely diagnosis is malignancy, since the specificity of this examination is nearly 100 per cent. However, cell typing is less accurate, perhaps 80 per cent. In cases where this fails to demonstrate malignancy, or a benign diagnosis is thought to be probable, a cutting needle biopsy should be done. Specificity for a benign diagnosis approaches 80 per cent. If the working clinical diagnosis is a vasculitis, even cutting needle biopsies are inappropriate, and open lung biopsy is recommended.

Diffuse parenchymal lung disease (pulmonary infiltrates and/or interstitial shadowing)

Widespread, bilateral, interstitial or alveolar shadows and also similar shadows confined to one lobe or segment of the lung, e.g. 'persistent pneumonia' are included under this heading.

Practical points are as follows:

1. Biopsy should not be considered until simpler non-invasive procedures such as a high resolution CT scan have been done.
2. Biopsy should not be considered if a tissue diagnosis will not result in any change of treatment, or will not allow a more accurate prognosis.
3. Biopsy should be performed by experienced operators or under their immediate supervision, and the safest technique should be preferred.
4. Biopsy should not be performed if the occurrence of a complication, particularly a pneumothorax, in the presence of reduced respiratory reserve, would endanger the patient.

Most physicians faced with this problem would first attempt a transbronchial biopsy under fluoroscopic control. Multiple biopsies provide alveolar tissue in 90 per cent of cases and diagnostically useful specimens in about 80 per cent. The disadvantage of these biopsies is their small size (1–2 mm^3) and crush artefact. Transbronchial biopsies are particularly indicated if the working diagnosis is sarcoidosis, allergic alveolitis, diffuse malignancy such as lymphangitis or alveolar cell carcinoma, or diffuse infection such as disseminated tuberculosis or pneumocystis. However, if the prior probability of these is low and rarer diseases such as leiomyomatosis, histiocytosis X, or a vasculitis are considered more likely, open lung biopsy is necessary.

If the probable diagnosis is a fibrosing alveolitis, the situation is even more complex. If all that is required is a confirmation of interstitial alveolar fibrosis and the exclusion of, for example, malignancy or granulomata, transbronchial biopsies may suffice although the proportion of negative or unsatisfactory specimens may be high. If a more detailed histological assessment is required, even after CT scanning, the physician should advise an open biopsy optimally by VATS. For the generality of other cases, the author would advise transbronchial biopsy first, proceeding to open biopsy if no diagnosis is achieved.

External masses and pleural disease

If the reason for enlarged supraclavicular nodes is thought to be carcinoma, the preferred investigation is fine needle aspiration biopsy. It is much harder to diagnose lymphoma or tuberculosis in this way and a cutting needle or excision biopsy is better. Subcutaneous masses thought to be due to tumour can be considered similarly.

Most pleural effusions can be diagnosed confidently with a combination of basic clinical information and needle aspiration with or without an Abram's needle biopsy. This should be the first approach. If it fails, repeat aspiration is often worthwhile and a repeat biopsy if the previous sample was poor. Ultrasound may usefully direct the biopsy to a localized area of pleural thickening. Failure to reach a diagnosis at this point is usually an indication for thoracoscopy. Bronchoscopy is usually unrewarding if the only radiographic abnormality is a small to moderate effusion.

Matters are different if a pleural effusion occurs in the presence of apparently diffuse pleural thickening. In industrialized countries, mesothelioma must be carefully considered alongside diffuse peripheral adenocarcinoma. The former is notoriously difficult to diagnose. Multiple pleural aspirations and punch pleural biopsies may be negative. Thoracoscopy occasionally helps in this situation. Whether to proceed to this or an open pleural biopsy is a difficult question since there is then a high incidence of tumour seeding in the skin—although this can be reduced by prophylactic postprocedure palliative radiotherapy. Biopsy solely for medicolegal purposes is usually not advisable.

Tuberculosis

Fibre-optic bronchoscopy with brush biopsies and a bronchoalveolar wash from the affected lung segments is recommended for cases where tuberculosis is suspected but sputum specimens are negative. Tuberculosis is an important differential diagnosis for large pleural effusions. Pleural fluid sampling is less satisfactory than pleural biopsies. Multiple biopsies need to be taken both for histological examination and for culture. In areas of high incidence, pleural adenosine deaminase (ADA) measurements may be helpful.

Mediastinal disease

Preoperative assessment in lung cancer

Mediastinal assessment is a prerequisite before surgery if a CT scan has shown possible inoperability due to mediastinal lymphadenopathy. Enlarged nodes need sampling because many are reactive and not malignant particularly if the primary is a squamous carcinoma. For this reason physicians should be very cautious in diagnosing inoperability just because mediastinal nodes are large on CT.

Mediastinal masses

If the prior working diagnosis is carcinoma, fine-needle aspiration biopsy is recommended. If this test is negative or there is an indication on the smear that the diagnosis may by thymoma or lymphoma, or if the prior working diagnosis is either of these or a benign lesion, then a cutting needle biopsy should be performed. It is unwise to diagnose thymoma or lymphoma on the results of fine-needle aspiration. In all other cases, open surgical biopsy is required.

Diagnosis in the immunocompromised host

Precise diagnosis, demanding invasive sampling, is required when pulmonary complications occur (Chapter 4.10).

Therapeutic bronchoscopy

Carcinoma

Bronchoscopic treatment of stenosing carcinomas, which often cause distressing stridor or breathlessness, can be performed using cryotherapy, diathermy, laser therapy, photodynamic therapy, or by placing intrabronchial stents. These provide immediate relief. Brachytherapy (endobronchial radiotherapy) utilizes a bronchoscopically-placed catheter to guide an intraluminal radioactive source which gives a locally high dose to the tumour, for example 10 Gy at 1 cm. A single procedure may produce good symptomatic and functional benefit and may supplement prior external beam treatment. These therapeutic techniques require considerably more practice than routine bronchoscopy, but are now becoming increasingly important in the palliation of lung cancer symptoms.

Further reading

Brewis, R. A. L., Corrin, B., Geddes, D. M., and Gibson, G. J. (eds) (1995). *Respiratory medicine*, (2nd edn). Diagnostic methods: Invasive techniques, Vol 1, pp 362–94. Balliere Tindall, London. [Three articles].

British Thoracic Society (1999). Guidelines on aspects of fibre optic bronchoscopy. *Thorax*, 54, in press.

Golden, J. A., Wang, K.-P., and Keith, F. M. (1994). Bronchoscopy, lung biopsy, and other diagnostic procedures. In *Textbook of respiratory medicine*, Vol 1, (2nd edn), (ed. J.F. Murray and J.A. Nadel), pp. 711–81. W B Saunders, Philadelphia.

Klech, H. and Pohl, W. (1989). Technical recommendations and guidelines for bronchoalveolar lavage [BAL]. Report of the European Society of Pneumonology Task Group on BAL. *European Respiratory Journal*, 2, 561–85.

Klech, H., Hutter, C. Macha, H.-N., and Loddenkemper, R. (1995). Interventional bronchoscopic procedures: Endobronchial radiotherapy, laser therapy and stent implantation. *European RespiratoryJournal*, 1, 332–60.

Respiratory infection

Chapter 4.6

Upper respiratory tract infection

J. M. Hopkin

Upper respiratory tract clinical syndromes include rhinitis (coryza, the common cold), pharyngitis, laryngitis, and laryngotracheal bronchitis. In any illness, these syndromes may occur in combination or may be accompanied by a lower respiratory tract infection (Chapter 16.9). Viruses (Table 1) are the principal cause of upper respiratory tract infection. The various respiratory DNA or RNA viruses may be transmitted by small droplet aerosol, as a result of sneezing or coughing; in this way adenovirus and influenza A and B (Section 16) are effectively transmitted, infecting many individuals to cause epidemics. In addition, respiratory syncytial virus and rhinoviruses can be spread by direct contact with infected secretions, hand to hand, or involving an intermediate fomite.

A specific diagnosis may be established by culture of the virus on suitable cell culture media, by direct detection of virus DNA from respiratory secretions, or by serology, retrospectively. The chief value

Table 1 Viruses causing respiratory infection by frequency

Upper respiratory infection	Lower respiratory infection
Rhinovirus	Respiratory syncytial virus
Coronavirus	Influenza A+B
Adenovirus	Parainfluenza
Parainfluenza	Measles
Echovirus	Adenovirus
Respiratory syncytial virus	Rhinovirus
Coxsackie A	Coronavirus
Influenza A and B	

of these techniques is in delineating the epidemiology of infections rather than clinical management.

Most upper respiratory illnesses are self-limiting, but may be complicated by significant secondary bacterial infection, usually *H. influenzae* or pneumococcus (see Chapter 16.47).

The common cold

The common cold syndrome is caused principally by rhinovirus and coronavirus infections. Respiratory syncytial virus and parainfluenza viruses may also cause the syndrome in adults, whereas they cause principally lower respiratory tract disease, either as bronchiolitis or pneumonia, in infants and toddlers (Table 1).

The array of virus subtypes, notably rhinovirus, ensures that no long-lasting immunity occurs, and adults continue to suffer between one and six coryzal illnesses annually. The familiar features of the common cold begin with nasal or nasopharyngeal stinging, progressing to variable nasal blockage and watery nasal discharge. In contrast with influenza, there is relatively little constitutional disturbance. Potential complications, due to secondary bacterial infection, include sinusitis (manifest as facial pain and nasal tenderness with purulent nasal discharge or retropharyngeal drip), middle-ear infection (with pain and deafness), or tracheobronchitis (with cough producing purulent sputum).

These secondary complications can be treated with antibiotic appropriate for *H. influenzae* or pneumococcal superinfection, such as amoxycillin or cotrimoxazole. Uncomplicated rhinitis requires no specific therapy, although large sums of money are spent by sufferers on 'over the counter' relief medications of marginal efficacy.

Croup

Croup represents one clinical form of laryngotracheal bronchitis in young children. It is characterized by a bark-like cough and respiratory stridor. Most episodes are caused by parainfluenza virus. The illness starts with cough, hoarseness, and fever. Croup symptoms follow and are typically worse at night. There may be accompanying signs of wheeze and there is usually hypoxaemia. Humidification of inspired air and oxygen supplementation are necessary supportive treatments. Nebulized epinephrine and systemic corticosteroids are used by many clinicians, and there is some trial evidence of efficacy.

Acute epiglottitis

Croup must be distinguished from acute infective epiglottitis, another febrile syndrome showing features of upper airflow obstruction. In this syndrome, often caused by *H. influenzae* infection, there is severe throat pain, painful dysphagia, and often the need to sit upright with jutted chin in an effort to maintain a patent airway. If the diagnosis is suspected, then expert laryngoscopy is essential when a nasally introduced endotracheal intubation may be required. Effective antimicrobial therapy, against local strains of *H. influenzae*, is essential.

Further reading

Geelhoed, G.C., Turner, J., and Macdonald, W.B. (1996). Efficacy of a small single dose of oral dexamethasone for outpatient croup. *British Medical Journal*, **313**, 140–2.

Kaiser, L., Lew., Hirschel, B. *et al.* (1996). Effects of antibiotic treatment in the common-cold. *Lancet*, **347**, 1507–10.

Wise, R. (1996). Antibiotics for the uncommon cold. *Lancet*, **347**, 1499.

Chapter 4.7

Acute lower respiratory tract infections

J. T. Macfarlane

Acute respiratory infections are one of the most common human illnesses.

Bronchial infections

Acute bronchitis in previously healthy people

This very common condition is usually believed to be caused by viral infections, particularly adenovirus, rhinovirus, or influenza virus in adults, and respiratory syncytial virus or parainfluenza virus in children and the elderly. Recent studies have suggested that secondary bacterial infections with *Streptococcus pneumoniae* and *Haemophilus influenzae* and atypical infections with *Mycoplasma pneumoniae* and *Chlamydia pneumoniae* may sometimes be present.

Symptoms include mild general malaise, retrosternal soreness, and initially a dry tickly cough. Sputum may be produced, initially mucoid but becoming mucopurulent. Associated upper respiratory tract symptoms, including sore throat and runny nose, are common. The patient does not look ill and the chest is clear. Investigations are not normally required; the white blood count will be normal and the chest radiograph clear.

Treatment is symptomatic. Controlled trials show no overall benefit from antibiotics. The decision to use antibiotics will be based on various considerations including duration of history, psychosocial factors, and pointers to bacterial infection such as purulent sputum and severity.

Patients who develop asthma often date their symptoms from an episode of acute bronchitis. It is important to identify and manage asthma appropriately in this situation. All too often patients receive multiple courses of antibiotics before the asthma is recognized.

Acute exacerbations of chronic bronchitis

Presentation

Patients with chronic bronchitis have a persistent production of excess bronchial mucus and are liable to repeated acute exacerbations, especially in the winter and characterized by an increase in sputum purulence and quantity, worsening cough and dyspnoea, sometimes associated with malaise and a mild fever.

Aetiology

H. Influenzae, Strep. pneumoniae, and *Moraxella catarrhalis* are the three commonest bacterial pathogens isolated from the sputum of patients with acute exacerbations of chronic bronchitis, in that order, but uncertainty surrounds their pathogenic role. Bacteria are rarely the causes of exacerbations of asthma. Viruses are important, particularly in the winter months, and *Mycoplasma pneumoniae* and

Chlamydia pneumoniae infections have also been implicated on occasions.

Clinical features

The clinical features reflect both the infection itself and the effect on the underlying cardiopulmonary disease. The cardinal symptoms include increasing dyspnoea and sputum volume and purulence. Variable wheezes and scattered coarse crepitations may be heard on auscultation. Radiographically the chest is usually clear, although some peribronchial thickening or subsegmental infiltration may be noted.

Management of acute exacerbation

Routine sputum culture is unnecessary during the exacerbation unless the patient is seriously ill, the presentation is unusual, or there is a known local problem with pathogens of altered antibiotic susceptibility. The role of antibiotics is controversial but they appear to hasten recovery in those with two or more symptoms, including increasing sputum volume or purulence, or dyspnoea. Studies have shown equally good response with numerous antibiotics, and the choice of antibiotic depends more on side-effect profile, local antibiotic susceptibilities, patient acceptability, and cost.

A popular first-line choice is amoxicillin for 5 to 7 days, with co-amoxiclav, quinolones, and newer oral cephalosporins being reserved as second-line therapy or if there is a high local prevalence of β-lactamase-producing *H. influenzae.* The associated problems of airflow obstruction, ventilatory failure, and cor pulmonale will require vigorous treatment when present.

Preventative measures

An influenza vaccination in the autumn is helpful, and pneumococcal vaccination is recommended. Antibiotic prophylaxis is rarely indicated or effective.

Pneumonia

Continuing importance of pneumonia and costs

Pneumonia is one of the leading causes of death in both the UK and North America and the most common cause of hospital attendance for both adults and children in developing countries. The impact on health service resources is also substantial. Respiratory infections are the commonest reason for general practitioner consultation. Pneumonia ranks as the third most common hospital-acquired infection, has a considerable mortality and morbidity, and considerably prolongs hospital stay.

Classification of pneumonia

A practical classification that helps to guide investigation, management, and therapy is outlined in Table 1. In this chapter we concentrate mainly on community-acquired pneumonia, hospital-acquired pneumonia, and recurrent pneumonia. Details of other pneumonia groups can be found in Section 16.

Table 1 Classification of pneumonia

Community-acquired pneumonia (CAP)
• Non-severe CAP. No unusual risk factors present
• Non-severe CAP. Risk factors present (related to host or environment)
• Severe CAP
Hospital-acquired pneumonia (HAP)
• Non-severe HAP. No unusual risk factors
• Non-severe HAP. Risk factors present
• Severe HAP. Early onset
• Severe HAP. Late onset
Immunocompromised associated pneumonia (IAP)
Georgraphically associated pneumonia (GAP)
Recurrent pneumonia

Community-acquired pneumonia

Introduction

Community-acquired pneumonia occurs twice as often in the winter months and is a common cause of acute hospital admission. The incidence in the community is probably around 4 adults per 1000 population and about three-quarters will be managed at home.

Types of community-acquired pneumonia

Community-acquired pneumonia can affect the previously healthy individual or the patient with underlying disease, particularly chronic lung disease.

Infection can result either from bacteria already colonizing the upper airways (e.g. *Strep. pneumoniae, H. influenzae*) or by direct droplet transmission from other infected individuals (e.g. respiratory viruses and mycoplasma), animals (e.g. Q fever, tularaemia, psittacosis), or infected water droplets (e.g. legionella infection).

The term 'atypical pneumonia' is used widely but can be confusing. It is best used to describe the community-acquired infections caused by intracellular respiratory pathogens, including *M. pneumoniae, Chlamydia* spp., *Legionella* spp., and *Coxiella burnetii,* which respond to macrolides or tetracycline but not to β-lactam antibiotics. *Legionella* spp. also cause hospital-acquired pneumonia.

Aetiology

There have been numerous, recent hospital studies of adults admitted from the community with pneumonia in the UK, Europe, and elsewhere which have produced a broad agreement on the current causes of community-acquired pneumonia (Table 2), although the relative frequency of some pathogens varies widely depending on where, how, and when the study was performed.

In some studies, no pathogen has been identified in over half the cases. Pneumococcal infection is probably the cause in many of these undiagnosed cases. However, antibiotics given before admission to hospital reduce the ability to culture common respiratory bacteria and some viral and atypical pneumonias are also underdiagnosed because both acute and follow-up serological samples are not taken.

The main conclusion from these studies is that community-acquired pneumonia is caused by a limited number of organisms which can be divided into (a) *Strep. pneumoniae* as the principal or 'core' pathogen and (b) other pathogens to be considered if additional host or environmental factors are present. Other bacteria include *H. influenzae* (particularly associated with chronic lung disease) and *Staphylococcus aureus* (particularly in association with influenza virus infection or steroid therapy). In some areas, legionella pneumonia is a significant problem, but in the UK it accounts for around 3 per cent of pneumonia cases overall. *Moraxella catarrhalis* pneumonia has been reported infrequently but is associated with severe chronic lung disease or lung cancer. Aspiration pneumonia in the community setting is usually caused by penicillin-sensitive anaerobic bacteria from the teeth crevices and oropharynx. Gram-negative enteric bacillary

Table 2 Causes of adult community-acquired pneumonia (CAP) found in 10 hospital-based studies performed in the last 10 years*

	CAP (%) (range (%)) (2679 patients)	Severe CAP (%) (233 patients)
No cause found	36 (3–50)	33
Strep. pneumoniae	25 (9–79)	27
Influenza virus	8 (5–8.5)	2
M. pneumoniae	7 (2–18)	2
Legionella spp.	7 (2–18)	17
H. influenzae	5 (2–11)	5
Other viruses	5 (1–10)	8†
Psittacosis/Q fever	3 (0–6)	1
Gram-negative enteric bacilli	3 (0–8)	2
Staph. aureus	2 (0–3)	5

*Severe CAP data from various studies based on intensive care units (overall mortality 39 per cent) are also included.

†Four of these patients had varicella pneumonia.

infections are very unusual as community pathogens unless there are particular risk factors such as severe comorbid disease or (for pseudomonal infections) bronchiectasis or cystic fibrosis.

Atypical pneumonias, particularly *M. pneumoniae* and *Chlamydia pneumoniae* infection, form a sizeable group, the former in younger patients of school or working age. Viral infections, of which influenza virus is the commonest followed by parainfluenza and respiratory syncytial virus infection, usually present in adults because of secondary bacterial pneumonia. Since influenza A was first isolated in 1933, a link between viral and subsequent bacterial infection has been recognized. Secondary bacterial pneumonia with *Strep. pneumoniae, H. influenzae,* or *Staph. aureus* is now the most common pulmonary complication of influenza and carries a poor prognosis. Rarely, the influenza virus itself causes pneumonia. Viral infection promotes bacterial adherence and colonization in the respiratory tract and reduces local defences by damaging mucociliary clearance and suppressing alveolar macrophages and lysozyme activity. Pregnant women and those with chronic cardiac or respiratory diseases are particularly at risk.

Some community-acquired pneumonia studies in the US more frequently report Gram-negative enteric bacillary, anaerobic, and staphylococcal infections, probably because of a larger proportion of debilitated patients, alcoholics, and drug abusers.

The few studies of community-acquired pneumonia not requiring hospital admission suggest a pattern very similar to hospital-based studies, except that legionella and staphylococcal infections are less common as they invariably cause a severe illness requiring hospital admission.

Epidemiology

Many respiratory pathogens have characteristic epidemiological features, a knowledge of which can be of value to the clinician (Fig. 1). Seasonal peaks vary from year to year, but bacterial infection are much commoner in the first quarter of the year at the time of increased influenza virus activity. In contrast, legionella infection is commoner in the summer months, sometimes related to foreign travel, hotel stays, and exposure to air conditioning and other water systems. Respiratory syncytial virus occurs in major epidemics in late autumn and early winter, affecting the very young and the very old.

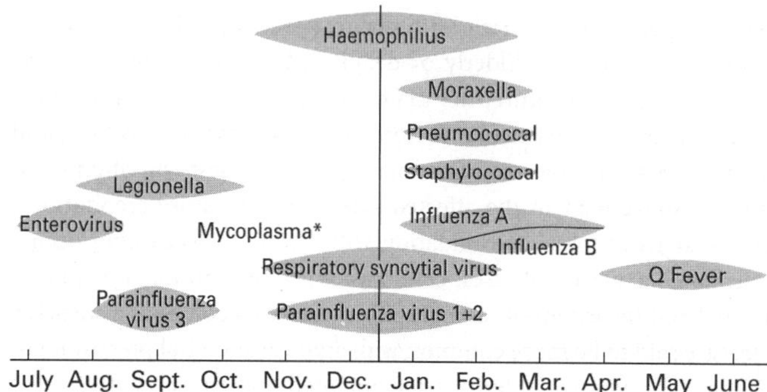

Fig. 1 Seasonal peaks in respiratory medicine. Respiratory pathogens usually occur throughout the year but many have seasonal peaks as well. *(Adapted from R. A. L. Blewis, J. Gibson, and D. M. Geddes, eds. (1990). Fig. 21.1.3. Balliere Tindall, London, with permission.)*

Whooping cough and mycoplasma have a much longer periodicity. Mycoplasma occurs in large epidemics every 3 to 4 years throughout the world, when suspicion will be heightened. The last epidemic was in 1994. Enquiry should be made about recent contact with pet birds or fowl at home or work (possible psittacosis), contact with farm animals (Q fever), recent foreign travel or stays in large hotels or hospitals (legionella pneumonia), or contact with others with pneumonia, influenza, or chicken pox.

Clinical features

It is not possible to guess the cause of pneumonia correctly from the history and signs on presentation as no pathogen produces an unique microbial pattern.

Symptoms

Males are affected twice as commonly as females. General symptoms include those of any febrile illness—malaise, anorexia, sweating, aches and pains, and headache. There may be a preceding history of upper respiratory tract symptoms, particularly with viral and mycoplasma infections. Respiratory symptoms are variable, but classically include cough, sputum, dyspnoea, pleural pain, and, less commonly, haemoptysis.

Sputum is usually mucoid, scanty, or absent early on in the illness, particularly with legionella and atypical pneumonias. Purulent sputum develops later, and can be pinkish coloured in classic pneumococcal infection.

Non-respiratory symptoms sometimes dominate the picture and mask the diagnosis. Lower-lobe pneumonia may present with an 'acute' abdomen. Marked confusion is seen in any patient with severe pneumonia, and is also a feature of legionella pneumonia in less seriously ill patients who may also have severe headache, cerebellar dysfunction, memory loss, and myalgia. Meningitis, hypoxia, and metabolic upset must also be considered in the confused patient.

With post-influenzal pneumonia the patient experiences the typical symptoms of influenza, starts to improve, and then 3 to 7 days later suddenly deteriorates with rigors, chest pain, dyspnoea, and cough with discoloured or blood-stained sputum. In approximately a third of cases, the pulmonary symptoms blend with the influenza.

Physical signs

The patient usually looks flushed and unwell with tachypnoea and a tachycardia. High temperatures (greater than 39.5°C) and rigors occur in young people, particularly with pneumococcal, staphylococcal, and legionella pneumonia. Elderly or debilitated patients may have little or no rise in temperature; the main sign is a raised respiratory rate. Herpes labialis is a particular feature of pneumococcal infection, and is found in a third of cases. Examination of the chest will often show reduced movement of the affected side and inspiratory crepitations. Classic signs of lobar consolidation with bronchial breathing occurs in less than a quarter of cases. On occasion, chest examination appears normal and the extent of radiographic shadowing comes as a surprise, a feature said to be more common with atypical and viral pneumonias.

The very young, elderly, or debilitated patient may have few respiratory symptoms and the diagnosis may be missed without careful chest examination and a chest radiograph.

Investigations

Investigations are performed to assess the severity and cause of the infection, to identify complications, and for epidemiological purposes.

General

The total white cell count is over 15.0 × 10^6/dl in the majority of patients with bacterial pneumonia, with the differential showing a neutrophila (Table 3). In legionella pneumonia it is usually less than 15.0 × 10^6/dl and sometimes there is a lymphopenia. In patients with uncomplicated atypical or viral pneumonia a near normal white cell count is usual. A low or very high white cell count is a poor prognostic sign. Cold agglutinins are present in over 50 per cent of cases with mycoplasma pneumonia.

Abnormal liver function tests, raised blood urea and creatinine, hyponatraemia, hypoalbuminaemia, proteinuria, and haematuria can be seen with any severe pneumonia (see later). Patients ill enough to require hospital admission will often be hypoxic. Hypercapnia denotes the onset of ventilatory failure. Signs of multisystem involvement are less usual with mycoplasma or viral pneumonia.

Specific

Many patients with mild pneumonia, treated successfully in the community, will not need any investigations, except for a chest radiograph after clinical recovery to confirm resolution. For patients who are ill enough to require hospital treatment, the aim is to identify the cause of the pneumonia and the severity of the infection as soon as possible. Blood, any pleural fluid, and sputum should be collected for culture, but positive rates are markedly reduced by prior antibiotics. However, antibiotic treatment should not be delayed if sputum cannot be obtained quickly, as occurs in a third of patients.

Gram staining of sputum (or respiratory secretions and pleural fluid) sometimes provides a quick and accurate indication of the pathogen in seriously ill patients if predominant numbers of one pathogen are seen. Although the specificity of the Gram stain is high, the sensitivity is low. Sputum culture is a relatively poor method of diagnosis for bacterial pneumonia, because the bacterial flora of sputum represents a mixture of organisms from the lower and upper respiratory tract, and potential respiratory pathogens such as staphylococci, meningococci, haemophilus, and streptococci can be part of the stable respiratory flora. The specificity may be improved by washing or diluting the sputum to remove upper respiratory bacteria. Isolation of a pathogen from blood (or pleural fluid) culture provides certain evidence of its importance and identifies those bacteraemic patients who have a worse prognosis.

The major limitation of diagnostic virology is the length of time required for isolating and identifying a particular virus. Direct antigen detection in respiratory secretions has been useful in the rapid diagnosis of respiratory syncytial virus bronchiolitis in children, and is being developed for other respiratory pathogens, including influenza, parainfluenza types 1 and 3, adenoviruses, mycoplasma, and chlamydia.

A four-fold or greater change in specific antibody titre is accepted as serological evidence of recent viral and atypical infection, but the result often arrives too late to influence management.

The majority of cases of legionella pneumonia are diagnosed serologically although seroconversion can be slow and a proportion of culture-proven cases never seroconvert. About a third of cases will have detectable antibody levels on admission. Only about 10 to 15 per cent are identified in the acute phase of the illness by culture or staining of the organism in respiratory secretions. Detection of legionella antigen in urine is a valuable early diagnostic tool and should be more widely available for clinical use.

Invasive techniques for investigating pneumonia (see Chapter 4.5)

They are usually considered for patients with severe infection, when it is considered important to sample uncontaminated lower respiratory secretions.

Induced sputum Although not strictly 'invasive', induced sputum using nebulized hypertonic saline has proved valuable in experienced hands for the early diagnosis of infection, particularly pneumocytis pneumonia in AIDS patients.

Percutaneous lung aspiration This technique has been used extensively to investigate pneumonia in children and adults and obtain samples of 'lung juice'. Pneumothorax can occur in up to 10 per cent but the need for drainage is unusual; significant haemoptysis is rare. The use of slim 25-gauge needles reduces complications and the technique can be performed at the bedside. It is contraindicated in patients on assisted ventilation.

Bronchoscopy Fibreoptic bronchoscopy will provide bronchial secretions, bronchoalveolar lavage fluid, and transbronchial biopsies from specified areas of the lung. The use of protected specimen brush catheters and quantitative culture largely overcomes the problem of contamination in the bronchoscope channel.

Transtracheal aspiration and injection Transtracheal aspiration is rarely used now owing to the availability and greater safety of bronchoscopy. However, a saline injection with a small 21-gauge needle and syringe through the cricothyroid membrane (without recourse to catheters etc.) will often be enough to produce a deep cough specimen of respiratory secretions, and this is a simple and safe technique.

Open-lung biopsy/video assisted thoracoscopic lung biopsy This acts as the 'gold standard' for diagnosing the cause of both infective and non-infective lung shadowing, particularly in the immunocompromised host. However, it is not used commonly as the risks of the procedure have to be weighed against the likelihood of discovering a diagnosis that would affect management or outcome.

Radiographic features

The initial radiographic pattern is not particularly helpful in differential diagnosis, as homogeneous shadows are also seen in over half the patients with atypical pneumonia. Pleural effusions and some degree of pulmonary collapse are seen in about a quarter of cases; sometimes the latter will be due to an endobronchial obstruction (e.g. tumour, foreign body, mucus plug). Lung cavitation is unusual except with anaerobic, staphylococcal, and pneumococcal serotype 3 pneumonia or in immunosuppressed patients. Pneumatoceles are only seen with staphylococcal infection.

The rate of radiographic resolution can be surprisingly slow, and lags considerably behind clinical recovery, particularly in older patients with chronic lung disease following bacterial infections. Atypical pneumonias clear more quickly than bacterial ones.

Differential diagnosis

The commonest diagnostic confusion is with pulmonary infarction or atypical pulmonary oedema. On occasions, the distinction is very difficult, and treatment may have to be given for more than one condition until the true diagnosis becomes clearer. Less common conditions that enter the differential diagnosis include alveolitis, pulmonary eosinophilia, cryptogenic organizing pneumonitis, bronchoalveolar lung tumours, and subdiaphragmatic conditions such as subphrenic abscess or acute pancreatitis.

Community-acquired pneumonia at extremes of age

The causes of pneumonia in the very young and the elderly show important differences. In neonates, infections are usually contracted from the mother's genital tract during delivery and include *Staph. aureus, H. influenzae* type B, streptococci, Gram-negative enteric bacilli, and *Chlamydia trachomatis.* In children under 2 years, the major respiratory pathogen is respiratory syncytial virus. At school age mycoplasma and pneumococcal infections are most usual, although *H. influenzae* infection is still occasionally seen.

Acute pneumonia in the elderly is common and carries a high mortality, ranging up to 30 per cent, often related to comorbid illness. The pattern of bacterial pathogens is very similar to that in younger adults, apart from a higher incidence of *H. influenzae,* associated with chronic lung disease. Anaerobic, staphylococcal, and Gram-negative enteric bacillary infections should be considered in increasingly elderly patients with increasingly severe comorbid diseases. Atypical infections such as mycoplasma and legionella are uncommon in the very young and the elderly, apart from reinfections with *Chlamydia pneumoniae,* which increase with age.

Management of community-acquired pneumonias

General measures

Patients with acute pneumonia should be in bed. Fever and pleuritic pain can often be relieved by regular analgesia. For patients managed at home, the severity of the illness and the need for hospital admission should be assessed regularly (see discussion of prognostic factors below). Pneumonia developing in even a previously well patient with influenza or chickenpox is particularly worrying. For patients ill enough to be in hospital, correction of fluid balance, hypoxia, and nutrition is very important. Patients with severe pneumonia should be admitted urgently to hospital and managed on a high dependency or intensive care unit. Early assisted ventilation can be life-saving. Chest physiotherapy and postural drainage are rarely helpful in the acute stage.

Specific measures

Antibiotics The cause of the pneumonia is not usually known when the patient is first seen and a logical 'best guess' antibiotic choice has to be made, depending on the type of patient, severity of infection, and any aetiological clues from the clinical picture. In all cases the 'core' pathogen *Streptococcus pneumoniae* must be adequately covered.

Non-severe pneumonia In most previously fit patients with non-severe pneumonia the most likely infecting agent is the pneumococcus or, less commonly, an atypical organism. An aminopenicillin such as oral amoxicillin is the commonest initial choice and is well tolerated, cheap, and mostly effective.

Table 3 Simple clinical features associated with severe pneumonia

Clinical features	Laboratory features
Confusion*	Blood urea > 7 mmol/l*
Respiratory rate < 30/min*	White cell count < 4 × 10^9/l or > 30 × 10^9/l
Diastolic blood pressure < 60 mmHg*	Arterial oxygen < 8 kPa
New atrial fibrillation	Serum albumin < 25 g/l
Multilobe involvement on chest radiograph	

*Three recent studies have found a large increase in chance of death if at least two of these features are present.

In younger, previously fit patients who do not respond to an aminopenicillin or in whom an atypical infection is suspected, particularly during a mycoplasma epidemic or in penicillin allergic individuals, erythromycin is an appropriate alternative choice. Gastrointestinal intolerance is less of a problem with the newer macrolides. Tetracycline is an alternative.

In those with chronic lung disease who fail to respond to amoxicillin or are moderately ill, β-lactamase-producing, ampicillin-resistant *H. influenzae* (7–20 per cent of isolates in the UK) and occasionally *M. catarrhalis,* must be considered. β-lactamase-stable alternatives include co-amoxiclav, quinolones, and newer generation cephalosporins. Concern about activity against the pneumococcus argues against the routine use of current quinolones as first line agents.

Severe pneumonia Severe pneumonia can evolve rapidly and antibiotics should be given parenterally without delay, and must cover all likely pathogens, especially pneumococcal infection. Penicillin-resistant pneumococci are a clinical problem in only a few countries so far. Other 'core' pathogens for severe community-acquired pneumonia include *L. pneumophila* and *Staph. aureus* (particularly during influenza epidemics). *H. influenzae* (particularly in those with chronic lung disease), and occasionally atypical, varicella and pneumocystis (in previously unrecognized patients with HIV infection) pneumonias are encountered (Table 2). High doses of intravenous ampicillin (500 mg–1 g, 6 hourly) or a cephalosporin such as cefuroxime (750 mg–1.5 g, 8 hourly) together with erythromycin (as erythromycin lactobionate 500–1000 mg, 6 hourly) or clarythromicin (500 mg, 12 hourly) provide good initial cover for all these pathogens. During a period of influenza, or where there is a chance of secondary staphylococcal pneumonia, flucloxacillin should be used as well. The antibiotics are adjusted appropriately as soon as investigations identify a specific pathogen.

Duration of antibiotic therapy Patients with uncomplicated pneumonia are usually treated with antibiotics for 5 to 10 days. The duration of therapy for those with more severe pneumonia is judged on clinical response. In the presence of lung cavitation, treatment may be needed for 3 to 4 weeks.

Identifying severe pneumonia and poor prognostic factors

Several studies have identified simple clinical and laboratory pointers that should be used for early identification of those with severe disease (Table 3). Prognosis is related to the pathogen, the host, and the

Table 4 Factors to consider when a patient with pneumonia is responding poorly to initial therapy

Factor	Action
Improvement expected too soon	Continue—review again (improvement slow in elderly and debilitated)
Diagnosis of pneumonia wrong (pulmonary infarction/oedema?)	Review history, examination, and data
Organism resistant to antibiotic/ unexpected organism involved	Review history: travel abroad? Avian contact? Review microbiological data Consider alternative or invasive investigations
Complicating pulmonary disease (e.g. bronchial obstruction, bronchiectasis)	Review chest radiograph; consider bronchoscopy
Local intrathoracic complications (e.g. empyema, lung abscess)	Repeat chest radiograph Aspirate any pleural fluid
Secondary complications (e.g. deep venous thrombosis, intravenous cannula infection)	Detailed clinical examination
Metastatic infective complication (e.g. arthritis, endocarditis, meningitis)	Detailed clinical examination
General factors (e.g. dehydration, hypoxia)	Treat appropriately
Allergic reaction to antibiotic (usually after several days therapy)	Take allergic history; look for rash; consider stopping/changing antibiotic

interplay between the two. A positive blood culture is a bad prognostic sign in bacterial pneumonias, as are pulmonary infections with *Staph. aureus* or Gram-negative enteric bacilli. Patients with atypical pneumonia generally do well. The mortality of community-acquired legionella pneumonia is 5 to 15 per cent. The mortality of post-influenzal bacterial pneumonia, especially staphylococcal, remains high. Mortality and morbidity rise with increasing age of the patient and the presence of coexisting chronic illness (such as cardiac or respiratory disease or diabetes).

Failure to improve

The majority of patients will improve quickly, a few days after starting treatment. If recovery is unsatisfactory the causes shown in Table 4 should be considered.

Intrathoracic complications

Pleural effusions are the commonest intrathoracic complication and a sample should always be aspirated to exclude an empyema. Usually these effusions are clear straw-coloured, sterile, sympathetic exudates which can still cause persisting fever and should be drained. Empyemas occur in up to 5 per cent of pneumonias; the incidence being higher with *Staph. aureus*, streptococci, and anaerobes.

Prevention of pneumonia

Pneumococcal vaccination is effective in reducing bacteraemic pneumococcal pneumonia in those who are particularly liable to severe infection (e.g. chronic respiratory and cardiac disease, sickle-cell disease, and splenectomy). Annual influenza vaccination gives some protection to patients who are debilitated and in whom an attack of influenza or its complications could be serious.

Hospital-acquired pneumonia

Introduction

Hospital-acquired pneumonia is a new episode of pneumonia developing more than 48 h after hospital admission. Such respiratory infections have been estimated to occur in 0.5 to 5 per cent of patients in hospital and to rank third behind urinary infections and wound infections in the frequency of hospital-acquired infections.

Pathogenesis

The infection usually arises from aspiration of nasopharyngeal contents, inhalation of bacteria from contaminated equipment such as ventilators, intubation and suction equipment, humidifiers and nasogastric tubes, or, rarely, by haematogenous spread from a distant site of infection.

Some aspiration of nasopharyngeal secretions is common even in healthy people, particularly during sleep. The normal lung defences copes easily with this, and the bacteria are relatively non-pathogenic. However, colonization of the nasopharynx with Gram-negative enteric bacilli from the hospital environment and from the patient's own gastrointestinal tract occurs in 30 to 40 per cent of patients in hospital. The frequency can be even higher in patients receiving broad-spectrum antibiotics or those who are seriously ill.

Patients who are ill, bed-bound, have impaired consciousness from their illness or from drugs, or who have neurological disease will be more likely to aspirate such pathogens. Reduced ability to clear bronchial secretions after a general anaesthetic and impaired coughing after thoracic or abdominal surgery are further risk factors, and occasionally impaired general antimicrobial defences contribute to the development of these infections. The presence of malignancy and the prior use of antibiotics, steroids, or cytotoxic drugs increase the risk.

The risk of postoperative pneumonia is associated with increasing age, smoking habit, obesity, the presence of chronic illness, long preoperative stay, prolonged anaesthesia, use of intubation, and thoracic and upper abdominal operations.

Pathogens implicated

The spectrum of pathogens encountered in hospital-acquired pneumonia is much wider and more varied than that for community-acquired pneumonia and it is helpful to consider firstly 'core' pathogens and then other pathogens. The likely pathogens can be categorized depending on the severity of the pneumonia, the presence of comorbid disease or prior antibiotic therapy, and the length of hospitalization. 'Core' pathogens which must be considered for all cases of hospital-acquired pneumonia include Gram-negative enteric bacilli (*Enterobacter* spp., *Escherichia coli*, *Klebsiella* spp., *Proteus* spp., and *Serratia marcescens*), *H. influenzae*, and Gram-positive organisms such as *S. pneumoniae* and methicillin-sensitive *Staph. aureus*. Other pathogens, in addition to the 'core' pathogens must be considered in certain circumstances.

In those with non-severe pneumonia, the 'core' pathogens are most likely. Additional risk factors will increase the risk of particular pathogens such as anaerobic infection after aspiration or *Staph. aureus* infection following multiple trauma, coma, or neurosurgery and legionella infection following steroid therapy or from a hospital environmental sources.

When severe hospital-acquired pneumonia occurs within 5 days of admission, the 'core' organisms are likely, in particular *H. influenzae* and Gram-positive pathogens. In severe pneumonia appearing later in the hospital stay, highly resistant Gram-negative organisms such as *Pseudomonas aeruginosa* and *Acinetobacter* spp. (especially for ventilator-associated pneumonia), and methicillin-resistant *Staph. aureus* (MRSA) (if prevalent locally) become more likely additional pathogens.

Clinical features and diagnosis

Pneumonia is usually identified by the development of fever, purulent respiratory secretions, elevated white cell count, and a new pulmonary infiltrate on the chest radiograph.

Identifying the pathogen is more difficult. Colonization of the oropharynx by a variety of hospital-acquired pathogens means that sputum examination is generally unhelpful. If blood, sputum, or pleural fluid cultures are negative, invasive techniques may be required to obtain lower respiratory secretions (see above). Bronchoscopy provides a convenient way of obtaining samples in ventilated patients. Serological tests for legionella infection should be considered.

Treatment

Logical empirical antibiotic therapy depends on time of onset of the pneumonia, the early assessment of severity, the appreciation of 'core' pathogens, and the identification of risk factors for other specific pathogens.

For non-severe hospital-acquired pneumonia, single antibiotic therapy is usually appropriate to cover the 'core' pathogens, unless additional risk factors are present. Options include a second or third generation cephalosporin such as cefuroxime, ceftriaxone, or cefotaxime, or a combination of a β-lactam antibiotic with a β-lactamase inhibitor (e.g. amoxycillin or ticarcillin, together with clavulanic acide) or a quinolone. The presence of specific risk factors will provide some guidance as to whether additional antibiotic therapy may be required to cover such pathogens as anaerobes, more resistant Gram-negative enteric bacilli, and legionella infection as well as the 'core' pathogens.

In a similar way to the empirical management of community acquired pneumonia, patients with severe infection must be identified early and started on combination antibiotic therapy to cover all likely pathogens. Severe hospital-acquired pneumonia occurring within 5 days of hospital admission is likely to be caused by the 'core' organisms and is treated like non-severe infection. For 'late' severe hospital-acquired pneumonia empirical therapy should also cover *P. aeruginosa* and *Acinetobacter* spp. in addition to the 'core' organisms. Combination antibiotics providing antipseudomonal cover are required, including an antipseudomonal β-lactam antibiotic together with one or both of an aminoglycoside and a fluorquinolone. MRSA may be a problem in some institutions. Despite therapy the mortality is high, ranging from 25 to 50 per cent, largely dictated by the underlying condition of the patient, and in survivors there is a considerable prolongation of hospital stay.

Prevention

Measures include prevention of smoking preoperatively, early post-operative mobilization, hospital staff hygiene, scrupulous care of respiratory equipment, and infection control in high risk areas such as intensive care units. Selective decontamination of the gastro-intestinal tract has been used with some success to prevent Gram-negative colonization of the lung in the intensive care unit.

Recurrent pneumonia

In patients with a history of three or more episodes of pneumonia, several possibilities need to be considered. Recurrent pneumonia in the same part of the lung raises the possibility of a localized bronchial or pulmonary abnormality, for example localized bronchiectasis or bronchial obstruction. When pneumonia recurs in different sites, a more generalized disorder is likely (e.g. chronic obstructive pulmonary disease, bronchiectasis, chronic sinusitis with aspiration of infected material, or, rarely, the immotile cilia syndrome). Non-respiratory problems include conditions that predispose to aspiration of pharyngeal or oesophageal contents and also the various causes of impaired immunity.

Further reading

American Thoracic Society (1993). Guidelines for the initial management of adults with community acquired pneumonia. *American Reviews of Respiratory Disease*, **148**, 1418–26.

American Thoracic Society (1996). Hospital acquired pneumonia in adults: diagnosis, assessment of severity, initial antimicrobial therapy, and preventive strategies. A consensus statement. *American Journal of Respiratory and Critical Care Medicine*, **153**, 1711–25.

Bartlett, J.G., Bretman, R.F., and File, T.M. (1988). Guidelines from the Infectious Disease Society of America. Community acquired pneumonia in adults: Guidelines for Management. *Clinical Infectious Diseases*, **26**, 811–38.

British Thoracic Society (1993). Guidelines for the management of community acquired pneumonia in adults admitted to hospital. *British Journal of Hospital Medicine*, **49**, 346–50.

Faitey, T. (1998). Antibiotics for respiratory tract symptoms in general practice. *British Journal of General Practice*, **48**, 1815–16.

Macfarlane, J.T. (1991). Community acquired pneumonia. In *Recent advances in respiratory medicine*, Vol. 5, (ed. D. M. Mitchell), pp. 109–24. Churchill Livingstone, London.

Macfarlane, J.T. (1994). An overview of community acquired pneumonia with lessons learned from the British Thoracic Society Study. *Seminars in Respiratory Infections*, **9**, 152–64.

Niederman, M.S. (1994). An approach to empiric therapy of nosocomial pneumonia. *Medical Clinics of North America*, **78**, 1123–41.

Chapter 4.8

Suppurative pulmonary and pleural infections

J. M. Hopkin

Lung abscess

Lung abscess describes suppurative, necrotic infection of lung (Table 1) seen typically as a cavitating opacity on chest radiography.

The commonest cause is pulmonary aspiration of material from the oropharynx which contains many anaerobes. Aspiration occurs to some small extent during sleep, but is cleared by mucociliary action and coughing. These defences are impaired during spells of impaired consciousness, as in general anaesthesia, alcoholism, drug overdosage, epilepsy, or cerebrovascular accident; other risk factors include oropharyngeal or periodontal sepsis. The dominant organisms are anaerobes; in hospital, colonization of the mouth and upper airways by aerobic Gram-negative bacteria and staphylococci make these organisms important. Aspiration lung abscesses occur at typical sites, influenced by gravity and bronchial geometry; aspiration in the supine position leads to disease in the apical segments of the lower lobes or posterior segments of the upper lobes.

Bronchial obstruction due to bronchial carcinoma or foreign body can also lead to infection of retained sputum and lung abscess. One or more lung abscesses may result from vascular embolization of infected material as in septicaemias of diverse origin, for example right-sided endocarditis, infected intravenous cannulae, and 'mainline' drug abuse; they often involve *Staphylococcus aureus* or less commonly *Streptococcus milleri*. Extension of a hepatic amoebic abscess can lead to formation of a secondary abscess in the right lower lobe. Necrosis of the lung can occur as a complication of severe pneumonia without significant aspiration or obstruction (e.g. *Staph. aureus* and *Klebsiella pneumoniae*).

Clinical features

The illness begins with shivers, fever, cough, and pleuritic chest pain. At some stage, the abscess discharges into a bronchus resulting in large amounts of bloodstained, purulent sputum. The patient appears toxic. There may be a local area of crepitation or bronchial breathing. Finger clubbing can develop rapidly. Empyema ensues in 20 to 30 per cent. A chronic course is recognized in which less severe symptoms progress over weeks or months. When one or more lung abscesses are secondary to a bacteraemic or septicaemic illness, the clinical picture may be dominated by the latter.

Diagnosis

When purulent sputum or fever imply infection, the diagnosis of abscess is suggested by the radiographic appearances of a pneumonic opacity with a cavity in which a fluid level may be seen. The differential diagnosis for a solitary cavitated lesion includes tuberculosis, fungal infection such as coccidioidomycosis, a cavitating squamous-cell carcinoma, pulmonary infarct, and pulmonary vasculitis. Blood cultures should be taken. Sputum should be examined by microscopy and culture for bacteria including anaerobes, mycobacteria, and fungi. Fibre-optic bronchoscopy is valuable in excluding bronchial obstruction or foreign body and may be useful in providing deep specimens for accurate microbiological assessment (Fig. 1) particularly in the immunosuppressed (Table 1).

Table 1 Causes of lung abscess

Condition	Micro-organisms
Pulmonary aspiration	Often anaerobes, *Actinomyces* species
Bronchial obstruction	Mixed organisms
Bacteraemia/septicaemia	*Staphylococcus aureus*, *Streptococcus milleri*, others
Spread from subphrenic or hepatic abscess	Coliforms, *Streptococcus faecalis*, *Amoeba histolytica*
Primary infection with cavitation	*Mycobacterium tuberculosis*
	Klebsiella pneumoniae, *Nocardia asteroides*
Immunosuppression (AIDS, leukaemia, chronic granulomatous disease)	Unusual organisms can be encountered, e.g. *Rhodococcus equi*, *Lactobacillus casei*

Management

The most important aspect of treatment is effective antimicrobial therapy. The organisms in aspirational disease are generally anaerobes, and unless aerobic Gram-negative organisms or staphylococci are recovered from early cultures, treatment can be based on benzylpenicillin, 2–3 MU, four times daily initially, changing to oral therapy once there has been clinical improvement. Treatment continues for 4 to 6 weeks. If there are doubts about the sensitivity of the anaerobe to penicillin, then metronidazole should be added. Postural drainage with vigorous percussion aids the clearance of pus.

If there is failure to resolve, bronchoscopy to allow the clearance of pus and assessment of malignant and other microbiological possibilities (Table 1) is required before considering surgical resection. Carcinoma requires definitive management and a distal abscess is no contraindication to surgery.

In lung abscess secondary to bacteraemia or septicaemia the antibiotic choice is dictated by blood culture results; pending these a broad spectrum combination of intravenous antibiotics is given.

Empyema

Thoracic empyema describes a purulent pleural effusion; the excess of white cells present denotes active intrapleural infection. A number of underlying causes are recognized (Table 2). Empyema usually follows a pulmonary infection in the form of pneumonia, lung abscess, or bronchiectasis, but may occur after septicaemia, thoracic surgery, or penetrating chest wounds, or following transdiaphragmatic extension from a subphrenic or hepatic abscess. Tuberculous empyema is a complication of advanced pulmonary disease. Lowered resistance to infection which is part of rheumatoid disease results in an increased risk of empyema.

Infection in the pleural space causes an inflammatory exudate and variable production of fibrinous adhesions between visceral and parietal pleura which may cause loculation of the fluid. Bronchopleural fistula may develop. Untreated there is sequential deposition of layers of fibrin with trapped cellular debris on both pleural surfaces, particularly the parietal.

The organisms involved depend on the underlying cause of the empyema, for example *Streptococcus pneumoniae* following simple pneumonia. Mixed growths are common otherwise involving anaerobes, staphylococci, and Gram-negative organisms; spread from an hepatic abscess may be due to amoebic disease (Chapter 16.83). *Aspergillus fumigatus* may produce an empyema years after surgery or artificial pneumothorax or pneumonectomy.

Clinical features and diagnosis

Empyema complicating acute pneumonia presents as failure of the pneumonia to resolve or as a recurrence of illness after an apparent recovery. The typical clinical features are malaise, fevers, and pleuritic pain. Careful examination reveals an area of stony dullness. The features of chronic empyema are continuing malaise, pain, sometimes purulent sputum, and progression to normochromic anaemia, weight loss, finger clubbing, and chest wall deformity. The chest radiograph (a lateral view needs to be included) shows

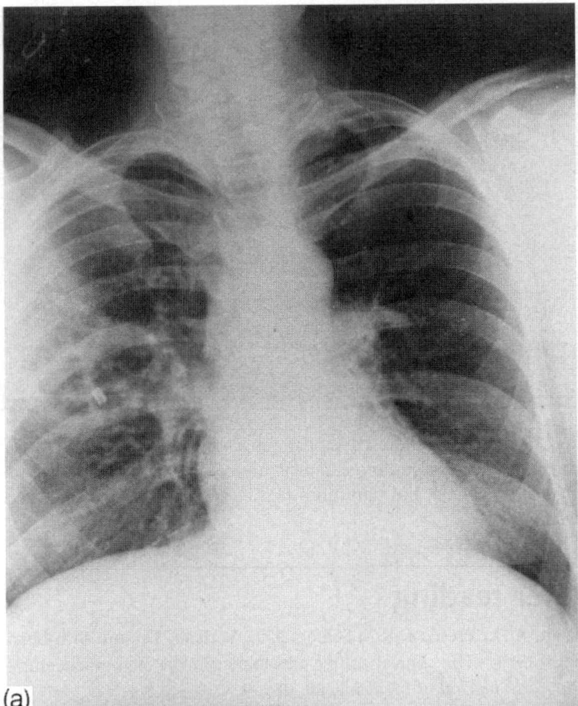

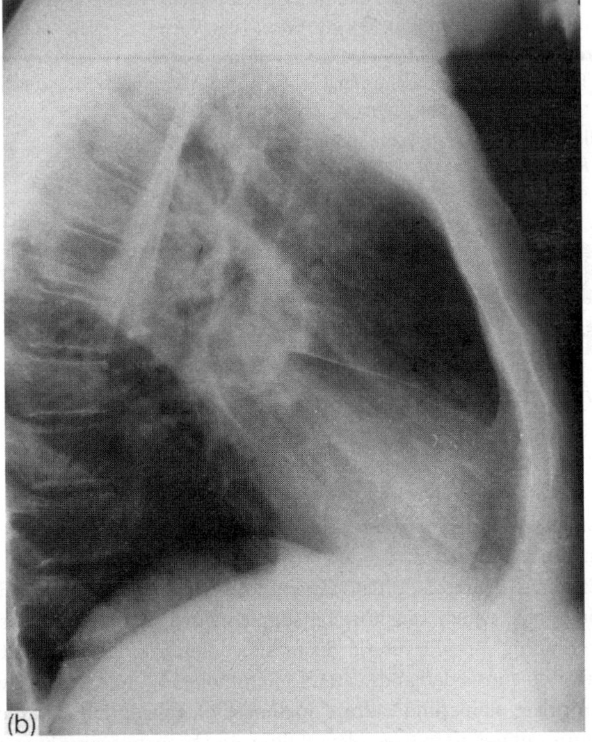

Fig. 1(a), (b) (a) Posteroanterior chest radiograph and (b) right lateral chest radiograph of a 50-year-old man with treated acute myeloid leukaemia, cough, and unremitting fever, showing an abscess in the right upper lobe. Microbiology on sputum was non-contributory, but specimens taken at bronchoscopy showed numerous Gram-negative rods which were found to be the anaerobe *Bacteroides bivius* on culture. An excellent clinical and radiological outcome followed treatment with metronidazole.

signs of effusion, which may be loculated, or a pleural mass (Fig. 2). A visible fluid level implies a leak of air from a previous

Table 2 Causes of empyema

Underlying condition	Micro-organism
Acute pneumonia	*Streptococcus pneumoniae*, others
Bronchiectasis, lung abscess	Mixed organisms, *Actinomyces* species
Post-thoracic surgery	Various organisms including late *Aspergillus fumigatus* infection
Bronchial obstruction, e.g. carcinoma	Mixed organisms
Penetrating injury	Various organisms including *Clostridium welchii*
Oesophageal perforation	Mixed organisms
Debility, e.g. rheumatoid disease	Mixed organisms
Spread from subphrenic abscess	Coliforms, *Streptococcus faecalis*, *Amoeba histolytica*
Primary infection	*Mycobacterium tuberculosis*, *Nocardia asteroides*

pleural aspiration, a bronchopleural fistula, or the presence of gas-forming organisms, for example *Clostridium welchii* in post-traumatic empyema.

The diagnosis of empyema is confirmed by the demonstration of purulent fluid on pleural aspiration; a wide-bore needle is used to ensure extraction of thick pus. The fluid aspirated needs careful microscopy and culture for aerobic and anaerobic bacteria, together with studies for tuberculosis and fungi.. Ultrasound or CT scan (Fig. 3) helps with assessment and the search for predisposing subphrenic or hepatic abscess, bronchiectasis, or obstructing bronchial tumour.

Treatment

Effective treatment of an empyema requires prompt drainage combined with appropriate antibiotics. The initial choice of antibiotics is usually made without microbiological guidance and should offer cover against a broad range of Gram-positive and Gram-negative organisms. The regimen should be revised in the light of clinical response and subsequent laboratory findings. Ampicillin (in high dosage) or cefuroxime will eliminate the more common anaerobic organism and can be combined with metronidazole if resistant species are suspected.

Pleural drainage can be attempted by repeated aspiration through a wide-bore needle, particularly if loculated collections can be identified with ultrasound guidance. A more conventional approach is to insert an intercostal drain, with regular saline flushes. Catheter drainage using a soft 12 French gauge catheter (e.g. Van Sonenberg) is more comfortable for the patient than the traditional large-bore tube. It is effective unless the pus is exceptionally thick and viscid, when a larger-bore catheter may be required. The use of intrapleural streptokinase can be used to help break down loculi and allow free drainage.

Empyema may fail to resolve because of unextractable thick pus, extensive loculation, the development of bronchopleural fistula, or the presence of gross fibrin and debris deposition on the pleura.

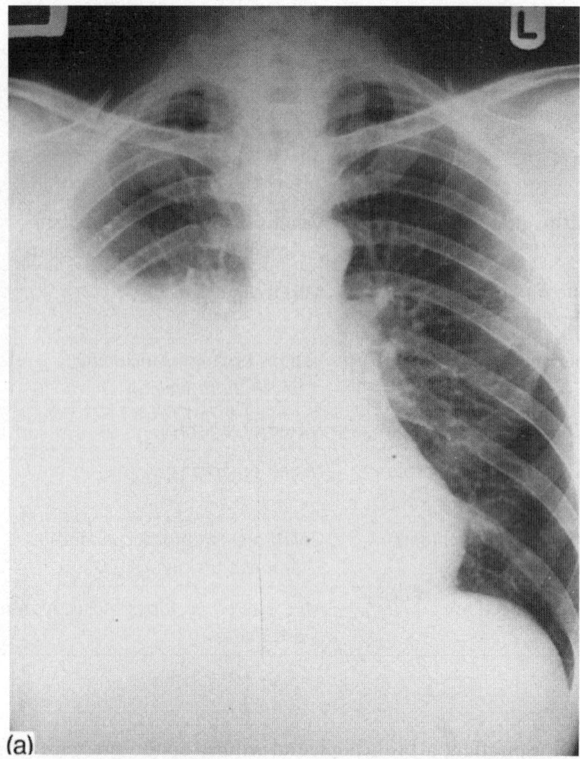

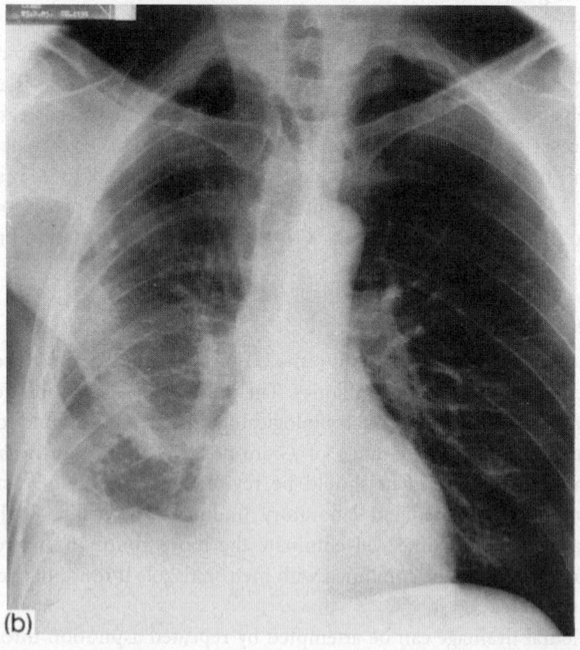

Fig. 2 Chest radiographs taken before (a) and after (b) treatment of a 51-year-old man with a chronic empyema and associated glomerulonephritis with renal impairment and the nephrotic syndrome. Microbiology on the pleural pus produced a growth of the Gram-negative *Morganella morgani*. Successful treatment of the empyema with surgery and appropriate systemic antibiotics also led to complete resolution of the renal lesion.

Thoracoscopy, if available, may allow breakdown of adhesions and placement of a fresh tube and resolution; otherwise formal surgery for the clearance of the pleural space and decortication of the lung or closure of a bronchopleural fistula is essential.

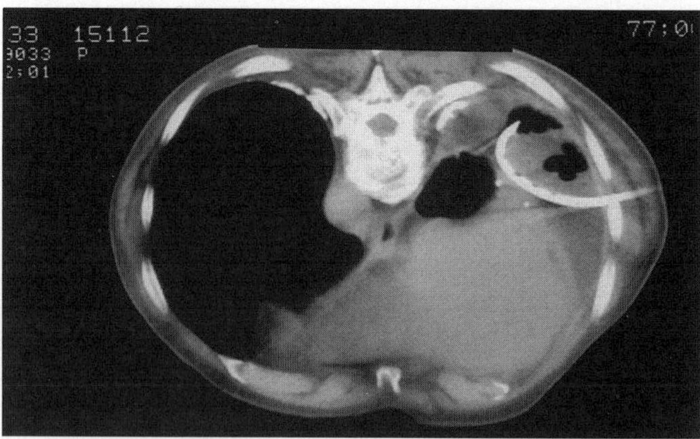

Fig. 3 CT scan of the thorax demonstrating empyema with an indwelling slim drainage tube. Large-bore cannulae are commonly used for the drainage of empyema, but slim tubes flushed regularly with saline can also be effective.

Further reading

Ferguson, A.D., Prescott, R.J., Selkon, J.D., Watson, D., and Swinburn, C.R. (1996). The clinical course and management of thoracic empyema. *Quarterly Journal of Medicine*, **89**, 285–9.

Hammond, J.M., Potgieter, P.D., Hanslo, D., Scott, H., and Roditi, D. (1995). The etiology and antimicrobial susceptibility patterns of microorganisms in lung abscess. *Chest*, **108**, 937–41.

Storm, H.K., Krasnik, M., Bang, K., and Frimodt-Moller, N. (1992). Treatment of pleural empyema secondary to pneumonia: thoracocentesis regimen versus tube drainage. *Thorax*, **47**, 821–4.

Wells, F.C. (1990). Empyema thoracis: what is the role of surgery? *Respiratory Medicine*, **84**, 97–9.

Chapter 4.9

Chronic specific infections

J. M. Hopkin

Bacteria, fungi, protozoans, and helminths can all cause pulmonary disease of slow evolution that results in chronic illness or death. Detailed accounts of these are given in Section 16. Geographical variation is significant.

Effective diagnosis often depends on clinical suspicion. Chest radiographs, which can now be supplemented in many centres by CT scanning, provide useful diagnostic pointers (Figs 1, 2, and 3). Formal diagnosis demands careful microbiological examination, with appropriate stains and culture methods, of appropriate samples—sputum, cutaneous masses, pleural fluid, and bronchoscopic broncho-alveolar samples if needed.

Tuberculosis is the leading cause of specific chronic respiratory infection world-wide. Notification rates are rising again in the wake of the AIDS epidemic and the increasing recognition of resistant strains is of great concern. Atypical mycobacteria cause cavitating apical disease, which is radiographically indistinguishable from *Mycobacterium tuberculosis*, in normal and debilitated hosts, such as the elderly or those with severe diabetes mellitus or rheumatoid disease.

Actinomyces species (true *Actinomyces* and *Arachnia* species) are oral cavity anaerobes which, after aspiration, produce indolent pulmonary

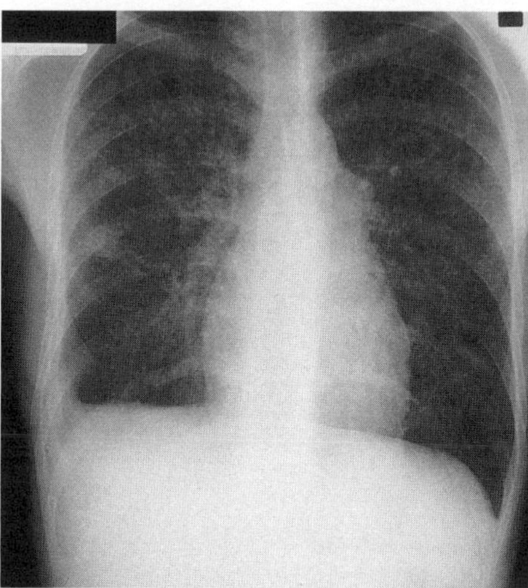

Fig. 2 Miliary tuberculosis (with small right pleural effusion) in a 20-year-old, HIV-negative Ugandan man.

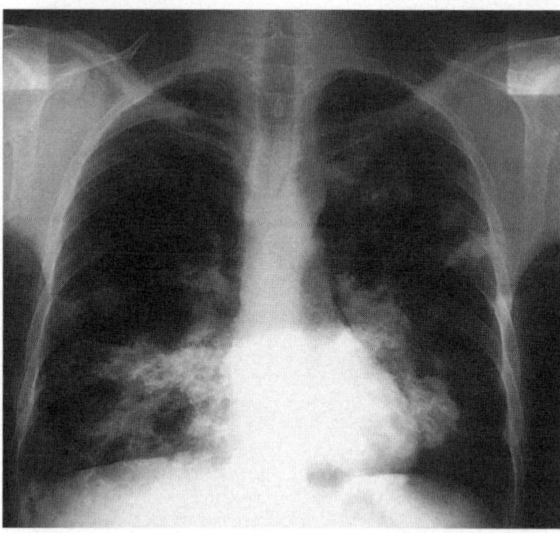

Fig. 3 Infiltrating and nodular shadows of South American blastomycosis scattered through the middle and lower zones in a 50-year-old Brazilian agricultural worker.
(By courtesy of Dr C.C. Fritscher.)

infection that can spread to mediastinum, pleura, and thoracic wall.

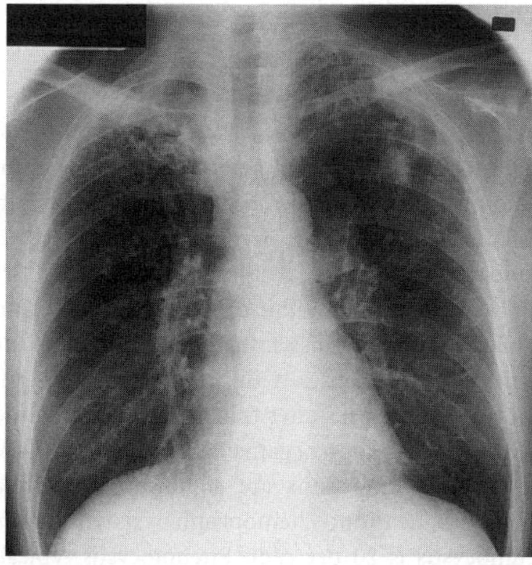

Fig. 1 Bilateral cavitating apical tuberculosis in a 60-year-old unemployed Briton who drank and smoked to excess.

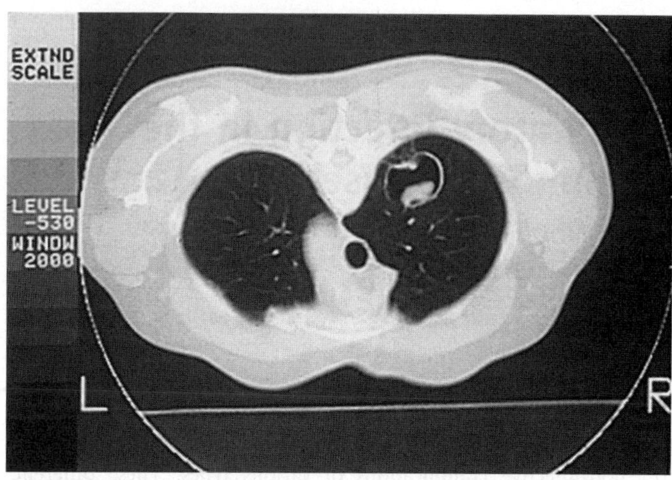

Fig. 4 CT scan showing an aspergillus mycetoma (or fungal ball) within a right apical lung cavity.

Nocardia asteroides, a saprophytic soil bacterium, causes chronic pulmonary infection that can disseminate in immunosuppressed and normal subjects.

Aspergillus fumigatus is a ubiquitous fungus that causes a range of respiratory syndromes: allergic bronchopulmonary aspergillosis, in which its antigens trigger intense bronchial inflammation in some atopic asthmatic individuals (Chapter 4.14); mycetoma (Fig. 4) in which the fungus colonizes a cavity within the lung, scarred by old tuberculosis or sarcoidosis for example, and cause variable haemoptysis; invasive pneumonitis in immunosuppressed subjects (e.g. on oncology or transplant programmes (Chapter 4.10); chronic empyema, often after surgery or trauma.

Other fungi, often of soil origin, are important causes of acute and chronic pulmonary infections in defined geographical regions: histoplasmosis, coccidioidomycosis, blastomycosis, paracoccidioidomycosis (or South American blastomycosis (Fig. 3)), and cryptococcosis.

Helminths cause pulmonary eosinophilia syndromes. Because of the deposition of larvae in the pulmonary circulation with ensuing intense inflammation and fibrosis, schistosomiasis can cause pulmonary hypertension and cor pulmonale. *Echinococcus granulosus* (hydatid disease) produces space-occupying rounded masses and cysts in the lung.

Amoebiasis of the liver can spread through the diaphragm, causing empyema or abscess/pneumonitis over or within the right lower lobe of the lung.

Further reading

Bergman, J.S. and Woods, G.L. (1996). Clinical evaluation of the Roche AMPLICOR PCR Mycobacterium tuberculosis. *Journal of Clinical Microbiology*, **34**, 1083–5.

Grzybowski, S. (1991). Tuberculosis in the third World. *Thorax*, **46**, 689–91.

Nolan, C.M. (1996). Multidrug-resistant tuberculosis in the USA: the end of the beginning. *Tubercle and Lung Disease* 77, 293–4.

Sudre, P., Hirschel, B.J., Gatell, J.M., *et al.* (1996). Tuberculosis among European patients with the acquired immune deficiency syndrome. *Tubercle and Lung Disease* 77, 322–8.

Chapter 4.10

Respiratory infection in the immunosuppressed

J. M. Hopkin

In the immunosuppressed, lung infections are particularly prominent (Chapter 16.117).

The pulmonary complications seen in the immunosuppressed may be due to: (a) infection with pathogenic organisms; (b) infection with opportunistic organisms of medium to low pathogenicity (Table 1); (c) non-infective complications of various types. These different entities often have overlapping clinical and radiographic features, and therefore pose diagnostic and therapeutic difficulties. Making a precise diagnosis, often with resort to invasive investigation, allows the use of highly specific and effective treatment, with the minimum of side-effects. This significantly improves the likelihood of survival.

An effective diagnostic approach requires knowledge of the potential pulmonary complications in the patient under care, a thorough clinical and radiographic assessment, and a strategy for further investigation.

Patterns of pulmonary complication

Cancer chemotherapy programmes

Profound neutropenia is a common occurrence during the early phases of treatment; therefore Gram-negative pneumonia is a special risk, and fungal pneumonia, particularly caused by *Aspergillus fumigatus*, is possible if the neutropenia is severe and prolonged. Later during the course of the illness, T-lymphocyte immune deficiency develops and with it the risk of pneumocystis pneumonia which, before the introduction of specific chemoprophylaxis, attacked annually 18 per cent of children with leukaemia.

Non-infectious complications include diffuse pneumonitis as a drug reaction to cytotoxic agents and leukagglutinin reaction of the lung in which diffuse radiographic change and hypoxaemia may follow white-cell transfusion.

Table 1 Opportunistic respiratory infection in the immunosuppressed

Defect	Infections
Neutropenia (e.g. treated leukaemia)	Bacteria (particularly Gram-negative and *Staphylococcus aureus*), (*Aspergillus fumigatus*, *Mucor* spp.)
Immunoglobulin deficiency (e.g. multiple myeloma, inherited defects)	Encapsulated bacteria (*Streptococcus pneumoniae*, *Haemophilus influenzae*)
T-lymphocyte deficiency (e.g. AIDS, organ transplant recipients, treated malignancy)	Fungi (particularly *Pneumocystis carinii*, *Cryptococcus neoformans*), cytomegalovirus, *Mycobacteria* (tuberculous and atypical), bacteria (including *Legionella pneumophila*, *Nocardia asteroides*)

(a)

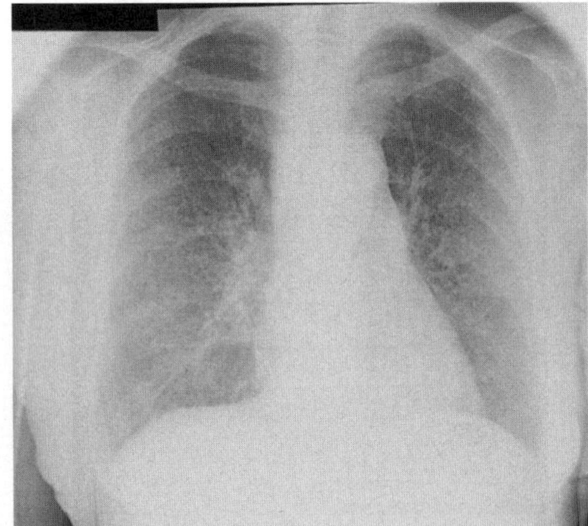

(b)

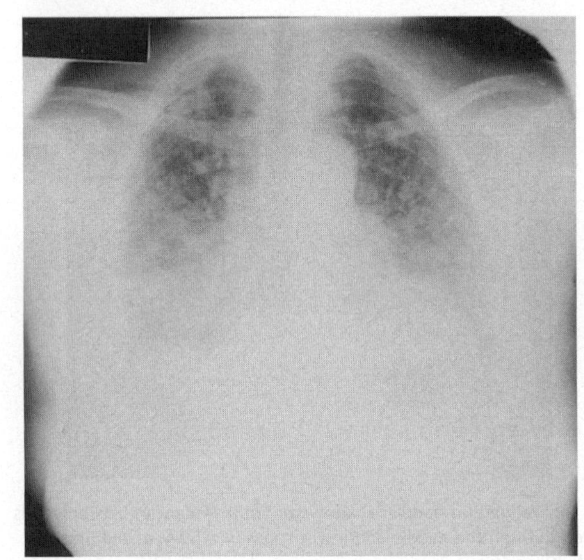

Fig. 1 Chest radiograph of a renal transplant recipient with tuberculosis showing (a) miliary changes and (b) nodular/confluent consolidative changes. The radiograph advanced to these appearances over 16–20 days. The diagnosis was established at alveolar lavage by Ziehl–Neelsen staining, and subsequently confirmed on culture as *Mycobacterium tuberculosis*.

Organ transplantation

Renal

Bacterial pneumonias, due to *S. pneumoniae* and Gram-negative bacteria including legionella, may occur at any stage after transplantation. Mycobacterial disease, particularly tuberculosis, is a high risk for individuals with a past history of tuberculosis or of likely past infection because of their ethnic origin or country of origin. The disease may take a rapid and disseminated pulmonary form (Fig. 1). Cytomegalovirus (CMV) causes a diffuse pneumonitis of mild to moderate severity 4 to 6 weeks after transplantation. The most severe form occurs in CMV-serology-negative recipients of a CMV-positive donor kidney. Fungal infections are significant, particularly with *Pneumocystis carinii*; without chemoprophylaxis the annual attack rate for pneumocystis is 20 per cent. Pneumocystis typically occurs 1 to 6 months after transplantation when immunosuppression is at its zenith, and causes a rapidly progressive diffuse pneumonitis that is fatal unless specific treatment is initiated quickly. Other fungal pneumonias can be caused by *A. fumigatus*, *Mucor* spp., *Fusarium* spp., and *Trichosporon* spp. and, in some parts of the world, by *Coccidioides immitis* and *Histoplasma capsulatum*. Non-infectious complications include pulmonary oedema (the result of impaired renal salt and water excretion, cardiac dysfunction, or fluid overload) and thromboembolism. The original renal-destroying disease may recur in the lung, for example in Wegener's granulomatosis or Goodpasture's syndrome.

Liver

The infective risks are similar to those listed for renal transplantation. Because of the prolonged surgery intubation, non-infectious complications include postoperative collapse and effusion, at the right lung base, and postoperative adult respiratory distress syndrome (Chapter 4.35).

Heart–lung

Infective complications are as for renal transplantation, but can also be due to *Nocardia asteroides* and *Toxoplasma gondii*, which may be transmitted with the donor heart. Non-infectious complications include collapse of the left lower lobe and paralysis of the left diaphragm (due to phrenic nerve cold injury) and pulmonary oedema, due to heart failure, and adult respiratory distress syndrome (post-pump syndrome). A common, late complication after lung transplantation is the development of obliterative bronchiolitis due to organ rejection (Chapter 4.20).

Bone marrow

Profound neutropenia makes Gram-negative pneumonia a special risk. Cytomegalovirus pneumonia, occurring at 6 to 12 weeks, is particularly common, is progressive, and carries a high mortality despite initiation of treatment (Chapter 16.14). Non-infectious complications include early pulmonary oedema due to large-volume donations of intravenous fluid or the cardiotoxicity of cytotoxic drugs. An often fatal interstitial pneumonitis, which is probably due to the direct pulmonary toxicity of the preparative irradiation and methotrexate therapy, is particularly common and fatal.

Acquired immunodeficiency syndrome (AIDS)

Bacterial pneumonia—due to pneumococcal infection, as well as *S. aureus*, coliforms, and legionella—occurs frequently. Chronic bronchial suppuration, associated with or without acquired bronchiectasis, occurs. Lung abscesses due to unusual organisms such as *Rhodococcus equi* occur.

Mycobacterial disease is important. Infection with *M. avium intracellulare* complex usually takes a systemic form, without pulmonary preponderance, and in the later stages of HIV disease. Tuberculosis occurs in the earlier phases of HIV infection as well as in AIDS. Multiple drug-resistant strains are documented in the US. Mantoux test negativity, accompanying extrapulmonary disease and atypical basal bilateral nodular radiographic features, are frequent.

Fungal infections are dominated by *P. carinii* pneumonia (Fig. 2) which had an annual attack rate of 70 per cent for AIDS subjects not receiving chemoprophylaxis. Pneumocystis pneumonia in AIDS is often of gradual onset and progression; if left untreated, the diffuse pneumonitis causes increasing hypoxaemia and death. Histoplasmosis and coccidioidomycosis pneumonias are increasingly documented. Cryptococcal infection generally presents with meningeal disease, but major pulmonary disease or pleural effusion also occurs.

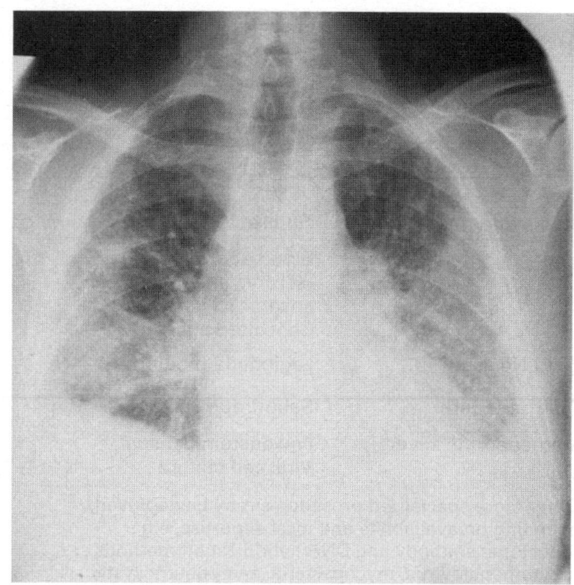

Fig. 2 Chest radiograph showing extensive bilateral consolidation radiating from both hila in pneumocystis pneumonia.

Non-infectious pulmonary complications of AIDS include a diffuse, usually non-aggressive, pneumonitis which in one form is characterized by CD8 lymphocytes infiltration. Some such reactions are due to drug reactions or, more rarely, alveolar proteinosis. Tumour occurs either as non-Hodgkin's lymphoma or Kaposi's sarcoma. Kaposi's sarcoma presents in the lung, usually after the development of extrapulmonary disease, and can cause focal bronchial disease, pulmonary change, hilar lymphadenopathy, or pleural effusion.

Hypogammaglobulinaemia

Hypogammaglobulinaemia may be due to a variety of congenital and acquired causes, and may be global or confined to subclass deficiency in IgA, IgG, or IgG_4. Pulmonary complications can take the form of recurring bronchial infection, the development of bronchiectasis, or bacterial pneumonias due to encapsulated pneumococci or *H. influenzae.*

The clinical picture

The respiratory illness may simply be an episode of acute bronchitis with cough and purulent sputum following a coryzal illness; in this there is little constitutional disturbance and no clinical or radiographic signs of pulmonary consolidation.

The more important clinical problem is the patient with breathlessness or radiographic consolidation accompanied by fever, for whom the differential diagnosis is broad and includes non-infectious disease. Fever itself, particularly when it is high and associated with chills, suggests infection, but can be due to non-infectious disease, for example drug reaction.

Tumour or bleeding at extrapulmonary sites may suggest the same process in the lung. Skin disease may be present in graft-versus-host disease, and cutaneous lesions may provide diagnostic clues to systemic vasculitis. Signs of intracerebral infection are a principal feature of cryptococcal disease and may complicate aspergillus and nocardial infections. Arthropathy and biochemical evidence of hepatitis occur frequently in cytomegalovirus disease. Haemoptysis may be part of an infective syndrome but also raises the possibility of pulmonary

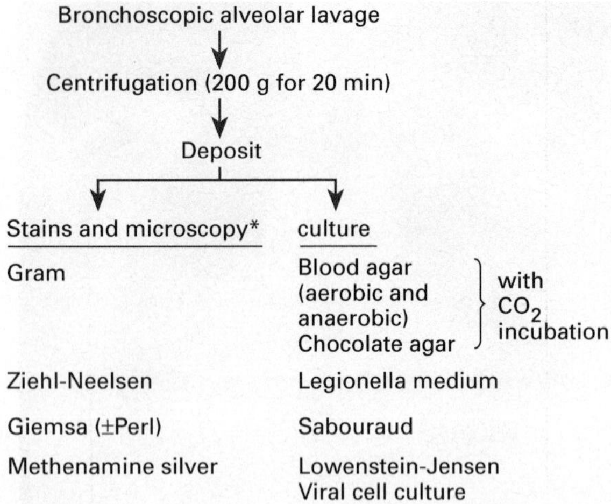

Fig. 3 Laboratory analysis of bronchoscopic alveolar lavage.

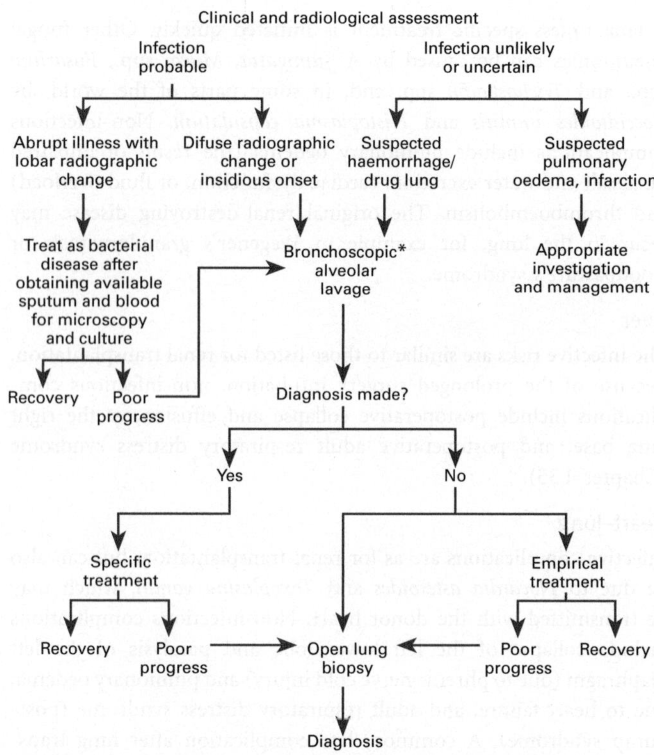

Fig. 4 An algorithm showing one approach to the investigation and management of pneumonia in the immunosuppressed. *Transbronchial biopsy should also be taken if drug-induced alveolitis is suspected. Percutaneous needle aspiration is an alternative diagnostic procedure for discrete pulmonary nodule(s).

embolism or haemorrhage. Pleurisy with pleural pain and pleural rub is not a feature of pneumocystis pneumonia, cardiogenic pulmonary oedema, or alveolar haemorrhage. In pneumocystis pneumonia, fever and breathlessness may precede definite radiographic changes; absence of auscultatory physical signs in the chest is characteristic.

Radiology

The chest radiograph provides evidence on the presence of pulmonary consolidation, its extent, distribution, and character, and the presence or absence of other features including those of cardiac failure (cardiomegaly, pulmonary venous congestion, and Kerley B lines) or pleural disease. The lateral chest radiograph is valuable in localizing lesions for further investigation by bronchoscopy. CT scanning provides more detailed anatomical information for targeting of sampling procedures. There are few microbe-specific radiographic changes; there can be a good deal of overlap between the radiographic features or Pneumocystis, mycobacterial, and cytomegalovirus infection. However, confluent segmental or lobar consolidation accompanying a very acute clinical illness strongly suggests bacterial pneumonia.

Lung sampling

Sputum, if expectorated, provides a valuable sample for preliminary microbiological assessment. It may be induced by the inhalation of nebulized hypertonic (3–6 per cent) saline; such samples have proved useful in the diagnosis of pneumocystis pneumonia in AIDS subjects.

Open-lung biopsy provides the best sample of pulmonary tissue but may precipitate the need for assisted ventilation or be complicated by pneumothorax or wound sepsis. Percutaneous lung biopsy or fine-needle aspiration, carrying the risk of bleeding or pneumothorax (proportionately related to the calibre of the needle), offers a useful method for sampling peripheral nodules. Bronchoscopic alveolar lavage but without transbronchial biopsy, is widely used in the immunosuppressed—producing diagnostic rates of 70 to 80 per cent. Alveolar lavage produces a large cellular sample from the alveolar space and is a good specimen for microbiological assessment by microscopy, the application of monoclonal antibodies and DNA probes, and culture (Fig. 3). Cytological examination of the fluid may help diagnose pulmonary haemorrhage and malignant infiltrates.

A practical approach to diagnosis and treatment (Fig. 4)

Episodes of bronchitis are typified by prominent cough producing purulent sputum but no clinical or radiographic evidence of consolidation. After sputum has been obtained for study, these episodes should be treated with an antibiotic effective against the likely pathogens *H. influenzae* and *Streptococcus pneumoniae.*

Pneumonia of abrupt onset and progress, with accompanying segmental or lobar radiographic shadowing, strongly suggests bacterial infection. Antibiotic treatment should start promptly after swift and simple microbiological investigation based on blood, urine, natural or induced sputum, and, if available, pleural fluid samplings. Treatment should be an intravenously-administered broad-spectrum antibacterial regimen.

When the pneumonia is less acute or when the chest radiograph shows more diffuse or nodular change the differential diagnosis enlarges and determined diagnostic methods are needed (see under Lung sampling above). Treatments are based ideally on the results obtained.

In pneumocystis pneumonia, the first-line treatments are high dosage cotrimoxazole or pentamidine. In the AIDS population, side-effects with these agents are common; reactions which include fever, rash, and renal impairment often demand change of therapy to the other agent or to other alternatives, including trimethoprim, dapsone, or naphthoquinone. Changing regimens because of failure of the pneumocystis pneumonia to respond is not useful, but the co-administration of corticosteroids is useful in accelerating recovery, particularly to AIDS patients. Despite the severity of the disease, aspergillus pneumonia can resolve when treated vigorously with amphotericin. Standard chemotherapeutic regimens are used for tuberculosis. Cytomegalovirus pneumonia is treated with the guanine analogue gancyclovir; addition of intravenous immunoglobulin should be considered in severe disease.

The severe hypoxaemia accompanying many of these pneumonias may demand a period of automatic ventilation, high concentrations of inspired oxygen, and the use of positive end-expiratory pressure. In transplant patients and oncology patients, immunosuppressive agents may need to be discontinued to allow recovery from pneumonia.

Prevention

Prevention of pneumocystis pneumonia depends on chemoprophylaxis with either thrice-weekly oral cotrimoxazole or monthly inhaled pentamidine; such prophylaxis is a routine part of certain leukaemia and organ transplantation programmes and the management of AIDS patients. Chemoprophylaxis against tuberculosis, with daily oral isoniazid over the first year, is appropriate in transplant recipients with a past history of tuberculous infection. Severe cytomegalovirus disease occurs in seronegative transplant recipients of seropositive blood products or transplant; avoidance of a positive organ is advised; live attenuated CMV vaccine can be given prospectively to seronegative transplant recipients. The risk of opportunistic pneumonia increases with the degree of induced immunosuppression; clinicians should define the lowest dosages of immunosuppressants capable of suppressing inflammatory vasculitis, maintaining an organ transplant, or eradicating tumour.

Further reading

Douglas, J.A., Shaw, R.J., and Hopkin, J.M. (1995). Respiratory disease in the immunocompromised host. In *Respiratory medicine* (ed. Brewis *et al.*), (2nd edn). Sanders, London.

Ettinger, N.A. and Trulock, E.P. (1991). Pulmonary considerations of organ transplantation. *American Review of Respiratory Diseases*, **143**, 1382–405; **144**, 213–23, 433–51.

Hopkin, J.M., Turney, J.H., Young, J.A., *et al.* (1983). Rapid diagnosis of obscure pneumonia in immunosuppressed renal patients by cytology of alveolar lavage fluid. *Lancet*, **ii**, 299–301.

Murray, J.F. and Mills, J. (1990). Pulmonary complications of human immunodeficiency virus infection. *American Review of Respiratory Disease*, **141**, 1356–72, 1582–98.

Wakefield, A.E., Millar, R.M., Guiver, L., and Hopkin, J.M. (1991). DNA amplification for the diagnosis of pneumocystis pneumonia from induced sputum. *Lancet*, **i**, 1378–80.

The upper respiratory tract

Chapter 4.11

Allergic rhinitis ('hay fever')

S. R. Durham

Introduction

Rhinitis, inflammation of the nasal mucosa, is defined as 'symptoms of nasal itching, sneezing, discharge, or nasal blocking which occur for more than 1 h on most days'. It is a common and increasing cause of morbidity and social embarrassment affecting 10 to 15 per cent of the population of the United Kingdom. The lining of the nose and paranasal sinuses is in continuity with the lower respiratory tract. Frequently, diseases of the upper and lower airways coexist.

Aetiology

Seasonal allergic rhinitis

Tree pollens are important in the spring and grass pollens during the summer. Weed pollens and mould spores predominate in the latter part of the summer and early autumn. Grass pollen counts above 50/mm^3 are considered high and represent the level at which most hay fever sufferers experience symptoms.

Perennial allergic rhinitis

The commonest cause of perennial allergic symptoms is the house dust mite (*Dermatophagoides pteronyssinus, Dermatophagoides farinae,* and *Euroglyphus maynei*) which is found in almost every home living in dust accumulated in carpets, bedding, fabrics, and furniture. Domestic pets, cats and dogs, are the second important cause of perennial allergy, identifiable in up to 40 per cent of children with asthma and/or rhinitis. Cockroach is a recently-identified perennial allergen in inner city areas.

Occupational rhinitis refers to rhinitis caused by an agent inhaled in the workplace. Occupations at risk include laboratory animal handlers (rats, guinea pigs, mice), bakers (flour), agricultural workers (cows, pollens, fungal spores), solderers (colophony), and users of rubber gloves, particularly surgeons (latex).

Pathophysiology

Immediate symptoms of allergic rhinitis result from the interaction between soluble allergen and IgE on the surface of mast cells in the nasal mucosa (Coombs classification type 1 immediate hypersensitivity) (Fig. 1). Mast-cell degranulation releases a wide range of mediators, including histamine and tryptase, and the generation of bradykinin. IgE-dependent activation of mast cells also results in the release of newly formed membrane-associated mediators derived from arachidonic acid. These include leukotrienes C4, D4, and E4, and prostaglandin D2.

Allergic inflammation is characterized by tissue eosinophilia and recruitment and actitivation of CD4+ T lymphocytes. Helper (CD4+) T lymphocytes may be subdivided according to their profile of cytokine release. 'TH_1-type' cells produce predominantly IL-2 and γ-interferon, whereas 'TH_2-type' cells produce mainly IL-4 and IL-5.

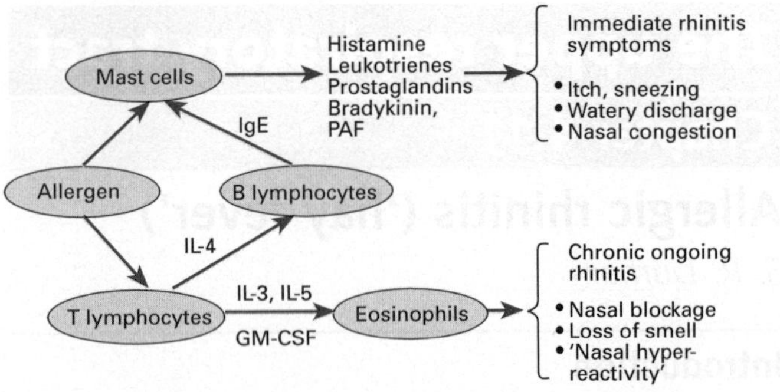

Mast cells → Histamine, Leukotrienes, Prostaglandins, Bradykinin, PAF → Immediate rhinitis symptoms
• Itch, sneezing
• Watery discharge
• Nasal congestion
Allergen → Mast cells; Allergen → T lymphocytes
T lymphocytes —IL-4→ B lymphocytes —IgE→ Mast cells
T lymphocytes —IL-3, IL-5, GM-CSF→ Eosinophils → Chronic ongoing rhinitis
• Nasal blockage
• Loss of smell
• 'Nasal hyper-reactivity'

Fig. 1 Hypothesis: pathogenesis of allergic rhinitis.

Both TH_1 and TH_2 cells produce IL-3 and granulocyte-macrophage colony-stimulating factor.

The biological properties of TH_2-type cytokines suggest their involvement in allergic rhinitis (Fig. 1). For example IL-4 is the major cytokine responsible for switching B-cell immunoglobulin production to IgE. IL-5 stimulates growth and activation of eosinophils and their selective adhesion to IL-4 upregulates VCAM-1 on the endolitheium which binds eosinophils via VCA-4.

Clinical diagnosis

History

Dominant itching, sneezing, and watery discharge suggests allergy as do associated eye or chest symptoms (asthma). A history of potential allergic triggers should be sought. As well as provoking immediate nasal symptoms, allergens may also result in late symptoms several hours after exposure which may not be recognized as being related to the previous exposure. Seasonality of symptoms and their relationship to work indicate the allergic trigger (i.e. occur at work or in the evening following work, with improvement at weekends and during holiday periods). The home environment, including the presence of domestic pets or birds, fitted carpets, etc. should be established. A personal or family history of atopy is extremely common in patients with allergic rhinitis. There are many other causes of rhinitic symptoms. Different causes may coexist. Therefore it is always important to consider the differential diagnosis (Fig. 2).

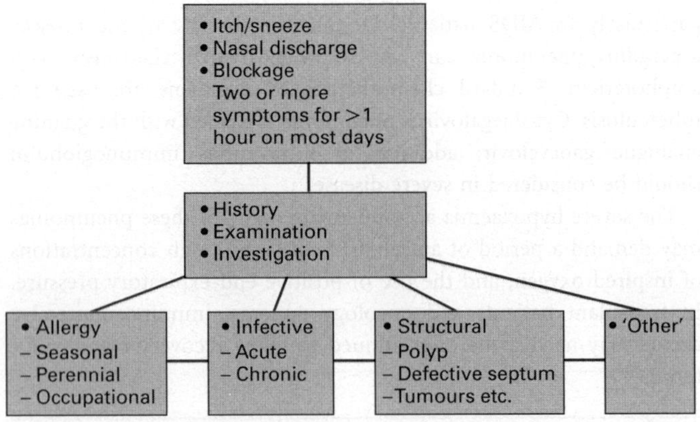

Fig. 2 Diagnosis of rhinitis. More than one cause may be present. 'Other' causes include hormonal (pregnancy, premenstrual), drugs (β-blockers, angiotensin converting enzyme inhibitors, cocaine abuse), idiopathic (nasal hyper-reactivity to persistent irritants, temperature changes, etc.), granulomatous conditions (Wegener's sarcoidosis), atrophic (old age, postsurgical), and, rarely, tumours (nose and sinuses).
(Based on Lund 1994.)

The presence of facial pain, fever, systemic upset, and mucopurulent discharge suggests an infective aetiology. Nasal obstruction which alternates with the nasal cycle is common to both allergic and infective causes. Nasal crusting and/or bleeding may occur in granulomatous disorders, atrophic rhinitis, or, rarely, tumour (particularly if associated with persistent unilateral symptoms). Impaired taste and/or smell is particularly common with nasal polyposis and may occasionally follow trauma (olfactory nerve damage). Enquiry regarding associated chest disease is important. Rhinitis and asthma coexist, and recognition and appropriate treatment of rhinitis may improve asthma control. The presence of infertility and recurrent respiratory infections (including bronchiectasis) should raise the possibility of abnormalities of mucus (Young's syndrome or cystic fibrosis) or ciliary dysfunction (primary ciliary dyskinesia, Kartagener's syndrome). Recurrent respiratory infections or a history of chronic rhinosinusitis should also raise the possibility of immune deficiency states including hypogammaglobulinaemia and acquired immune deficiency syndrome (AIDS). Hormonal imbalance (premenstrual symptoms, pregnancy, hypothyroidism, or acromegaly) may be associated with rhinitis. A history of trauma or previous nasal surgery should be sought. The efficacy, frequency, and regularity of previous treatments should also be established.

Examination

Local examination may be performed with a head mirror and speculum. Alternatively, an ophthalmoscope with an auroscope attachment may be used. Allergic rhinitis is accompanied by a pale bluish 'boggy' appearance of the nasal mucosa only if the patient has current symptoms. A red inflamed appearance with pus suggests an infective cause. A granular appearance with fine pale nodules is diagnostic of sarcoidosis. Enlarged turbinates may be confused with polyps by the unwary. If doubt exists, further examination with rigid and/or flexible endoscope should be performed. The identification of structural abnormalities such as polyps, deflected nasal septum, or enlarged turbinates is important since surgical treatment may be indicated. A major advance has been the development of techniques of minimally invasive endoscopic sinus surgery. Examination of the nose should also include tests of smell and examination of the ears, eyes, mouth, and throat. Examination of the chest and a general examination should also be performed in view of common associations with chest and systemic diseases.

Investigations

Skin-prick tests

In the presence of a clear history, particularly seasonal hay-fever symptoms, skin-prick testing is not essential.

Skin-prick tests should only be interpreted in conjunction with the clinical history. A useful basic skin-prick testing kit should include the following:

(1) a positive control (histamine 10 mg/ml);

(2) negative control (allergen diluent solution);

(3) house dust mite (*D. pteronyssinus*);

(4) grass pollen;

(5) cat fur;

(6) *Aspergillus fumigatus*.

Table 1 Treatment of allergic rhinitis

• Allergen avoidance (house dust mite, animal danders, occupational causes)
• Topical corticosteroids; check technique and place emphasis on regular use even when symptoms are absent
• Non-sedative antihistamines provide helpful combination treatment
• Sodium cromoglycate is useful for eye symptoms and is first choice in children
• Immunotherapy retains a place in pollen-sensitive patients unresponsive to the above measures
• If patient fails to respond, review diagnosis and treat any associated conditions (e.g. antibiotics for infection, surgery for structural problems).

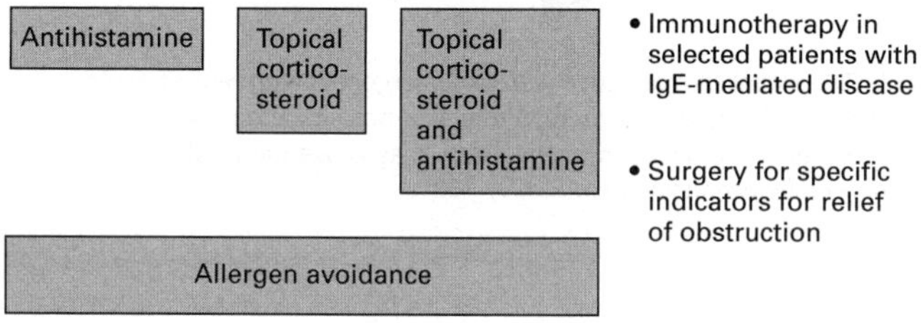

Antihistamine

Topical corticosteroid

Topical corticosteroid and antihistamine

Allergen avoidance

• Immunotherapy in selected patients with IgE-mediated disease

• Surgery for specific indicators for relief of obstruction

Fig. 3 Treatment of allergic rhinitis.
(Based on Lund 1994.)

Skin-prick tests should be performed with a sterile 23 gauge needle or lancet which is lightly inserted through the epidermis without inducing bleeding. Responses are recorded as mean weal diameter at 15 min. A positive prick test is defined as a weal diameter 3 mm or more greater than that of the negative control test. As an alternative to skin testing, allergen specific IgE concentrations in serum may be determined using radioallergosobent test (RAST).

Treatment

This involves the avoidance of provoking allergens where possible and the use of topical corticosteroids and oral H_1 selective antihistamines (Table 1 and Fig. 3).

Allergen avoidance

It is not possible to avoid pollens, although sensible advice includes wearing sunglasses and keeping windows tightly shut and avoid open grassy spaces. House dust mite avoidance measures include use of mite-proof bedding covers and removal of the bedroom carpet. A leaflet entitled *House dust mites: avoidance measures for allergy sufferers* is available from the British Allergy Foundation, Deepdene House, 30 Bellgrove Road, Welling, Kent DA16 3BY. Where animal exposure is relevant, there is frequent resistance to advice to remove a family pet. However, patients can be advised to avoid replacing animals, to confine them where possible, and to avoid contact with animals or contaminated clothing. Recent evidence suggests that washing the cat is extremely effective in reducing cat allergen exposure!

Pharmacotherapy

Topical corticosteroids are effective in 70 to 90 per cent of hay fever sufferers. Preparations include beclomethasone, budesonide, fluticasone, triamcinolone, and mometasone. Aqueous formulations are better tolerated and have a better local distribution in the nose. Side-effects are minor. The importance of regular treatment even when symptoms are absent should be emphasized. The drug should also be commenced before the hay fever season for maximal effect. Systemic effects are virtually absent at conventional doses.

A further advance has been the availability of potent specific histamine H_1 receptor antagonists with a low potential for anticholinergic side-effects and a low sedative profile. Antihistamines are particularly effective for sneezing, itching, and rhinorrhoea, although, unlike topical corticosteroids, they have little effect on nasal blockage. They are also effective for eye and throat symptoms. A rare but important complication of terfenadine is prolongation of the QT interval on the ECG. This only occurs when doses in excess of those recommended are employed, or in the presence of hepatic impairment or concomitant use of ketoconazole or erythromycin which modify the hepatic metabolism of terfenadine. Astemizole may have the same effect in overdose. Acrivastine, loratadine, cetirizine, ebastine, and fexofenadine are alternatives. All these drugs should be avoided during pregnancy.

Sodium cromoglycate is available as a topical nasal spray for use four times daily. It is less effective than topical corticosteroids. Topical cromoglycate eye drops (Opticrom) are effective for allergic eye symptoms in the majority of patients.

In a small proportion of patients whose symptoms are not controlled by the above measures, there is a place for a short course of prednisolone (20 mg daily for 5 days) which may also unblock the nose, thereby improving efficiency of topical corticosteroids. Topical decongestants should only be used for short periods (no more than 2 weeks) in view of the risk of tachyphylaxis and rebound persistent nasal blockage (rhinitis medicamentosa).

Immunotherapy

In patients with sole grass pollen allergy unresponsive to topical corticosteroids and antihistamines, immunotherapy (hyposensitization) retains a place in treatment. In view of the slight risk of anaphylaxis this treatment which involves injection subcutaneously of increasing concentrations of an allergen extract followed by monthly injections for 3–5 years should be confined to specialist clinics with immediate availability of adrenaline.

Further reading

Colloff, M.J., Ayres, J., Carwell, F., *et al.* (1992) The control of allergens of dust mites and domestic pets: a position paper. *Clinical Experimental Allergy*, **22** (Suppl. 2), 1–28.

Fleming, D.M. and Crombie, D.L. (1987). Prevalence of asthma and hayfever in England and Wales. *British Medical Journal*, **294**, 279–83.

Howarth, P.H. (1989). Allergic rhinitis: a rational choice of treatment. *Respiratory Medicine*, **83**, 179–88.

Lund, V. *et al.* (1994). International consensus report on the diagnosis and management of rhinitis. *Allergy*, **49** (Suppl. 19), 1–34.

Varney, V.A., Gaga, M., Aber, V.R., Kay, A.B., and Durham, S.R. (1991). Usefulness of immunotherapy in patients with severe summer hayfever uncontrolled by antiallergic drugs. *British Medical Journal*, **302**, 265–9.

Chapter 4.12

Upper airways obstruction

J. R. Stradling

Introduction

Above the larynx is conventionally regarded as the upper airway, but many of the conditions that can completely block off the main airway also affect the trachea, presenting in a similar way to those affecting the larynx and pharynx (Table 1).

Aetiology

Acute

Aspiration

Aspiration of an object sufficiently large to cause acute upper airway obstruction is usually due to its lodging in the larynx, since this is the narrowest portion of the upper airway. This is usually due to a piece of food and has been colourfully called the 'café coronary'. The patient will suddenly become distressed, be unable to talk and apparently unable to breath. Inspiration may not be possible to provide the air necessary for a good expulsive cough. The Heimlich manoeuvre was invented for this. If the patient is still upright then the helper stands behind with his arms clasped around the upper abdomen. A very forceful pull, backwards and upwards, will drive the diaphragm upwards, hopefully providing enough expired air to shift the aspirated food off the cords (Fig. 1). The principles of this manoeuvre can and should be taught to first aid workers. If the Heimlich manoeuvre fails, then it may be possible to dislodge the lump of food with a finger once the patient has become unconscious. The only alternative is an emergency cricothyrotomy which requires a hole to be made in the cricothyroid membrane just below the 'Adam's apple' of the thyroid cartilage and above the cricoid cartilage. Even a small hole (2 mm or so) will allow adequate ventilation and special large-bore curved needle kits are available for this purpose which are safer than an unskilled attempt at a tracheostomy.

Table 1 Causes of upper airway obstruction

Acute	Non-acute
Inhaled foreign body	Tumours
Oedema	Tracheal stenosis
Allergy	Post intubation
Angioneurotic oedema	Post tracheostomy
Smoke burns	Tracheal compression
Infections	Tumour
Pharyngitis	Thyroid
Tonsillitis	Aneurysm
Epiglottis	Tracheal abnormalities
Retropharyngeal abscess	Tracheomalacia
Croup	Scabbard trachea
	Tracheobronchiomegaly
	Tracheobronchopathia-osteochondroplastica
	Recurrent laryngeal nerve palsy
	Laryngeal dysfunction

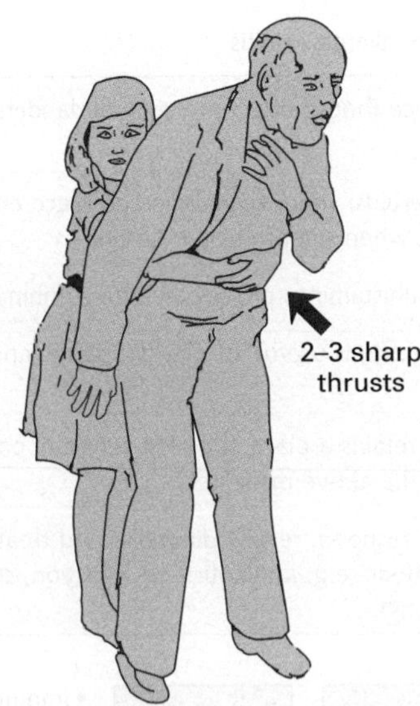

Fig. 1 The Heimlich manoeuvre for the emergency treatment of acute pharyngeal or laryngeal obstruction due to a bolus of food. Two or three sharp thrusts in the direction of the arrow may cause the food to be ejected. *(Reproduced by permission from Flenley 1990.)*

Oedema

Acute oedema of the larynx or pharynx is usually either due to allergy (atopic or non-atopic), a hereditary abnormality in the complement pathway, or inhalation of noxious gases.

Episodes of upper airway and facial oedema sometimes have no known cause and appear without warning. Often there will be an atopic history with a specific allergy, such as to insect stings. Some allergic reactions are not on the basis of atopy and IgE, but possibly through IgG or direct activation of other inflammatory pathways. Allergies to nuts, strawberries, etc. may involve this latter mechanism rather than IgE.

Treatment of these allergic causes of upper airway obstruction consists of subcutaneous (or intramuscular) adrenaline (1 ml of 1 in 1000) with antihistamines and steroids. Aerosolized adrenaline may also be useful, using 10 ml of 1 in 10000 in an ordinary nebulizer.

Hereditary angio-oedema is caused by a deficiency (true or functional) of plasma C1 esterase inhibitor due to one of several different mutations in the C1 inhibitor gene (autosomal dominant). There are also similar acquired forms of angio-oedema due to activation by a paraprotein. Absence of C1 esterase inhibitor allows greater activation of the whole complement pathway and its vasoactive products.

Diagnosis hinges on the clinical presentation, a positive family history, and low levels of C1 esterase inhibitor. In the form where normal amounts of inactive C1 esterase inhibitor are present, then it is necessary to demonstrate low C_4 levels during an attack. An episode of swelling is often precipitated by local trauma, such as a tooth extraction or a blow to the face, and lasts about 48 to 72 h. The skin manifestations do not itch in the way allergic oedema does. If adequate treatment is not available, 25–30 per cent of sufferers will eventually die from asphyxia. Treatment of the acute attack consists of adrenaline and steroids, although the response is much less satisfactory than in allergic oedema. Emergency tracheostomy or cricothyrotomy may be necessary. Purified C1 esterase inhibitor is available, but takes time to work. Danazol (or other androgenic steroid) raises C1 esterase inhibitor levels within a few weeks and is useful prophylaxis. Epsilon aminocaproic acid will prevent most attacks, mainly by inhibiting plasmin.

Hot smoke inhalation can burn the upper airway and contributes significantly to deaths due to fires. Upper airway obstruction due to heat injury and mucosal swelling usually develops within 24 h of exposure but stenosis due to scarring can develop later. A hoarse voice, stridor, severe conjunctivitis, burnt nasal hairs, and falling peak flow all suggest significant upper airway damage. Management usually consists of simple measures such as elevating the head of the bed and inhaling cool moist air with added oxygen. If peak flow continues to fall, then transfer to the ICU and bronchoscopy with the capability to intubate, guided by direct vision, is the correct approach.

Infections

Upper airway infections rarely cause obstruction in adults, but can do so in infants and young children; streptococcal pharyngitis, tonsillitis, and retropharyngeal abscesses being amongst the most important. Croup (due to parainfluenza and other viruses) is very common with narrowing of the subglottic trachea, sometimes with a thick purulent coating over the larynx and trachea: respiratory syncytial and parainfluenza viruses being the usual cause. Treatment consists of cool mist and supplemental oxygen, with careful monitoring of upper airway function.

Although again more common in children, acute epiglottitis, usually due to *Haemophilus influenzae*, can affect adults. A combination of pyrexia, drooling, hoarse voice, difficulty breathing, intense sore throat, and a stridor, are the usual presenting symptoms. The diagnosis may be missed initially but lateral neck radiographs show swelling of the epiglottis. Attempts to examine the back of the throat may precipitate further obstruction, particularly in children. Even tipping the head back for a lateral neck radiograph may be disastrous. Thus if there is evidence of difficulty breathing with stridor, and the clinical diagnosis is epiglottitis, then in children immediate transfer to intensive care and intubation for 48–72 h is the usual management whilst ampicillin or chloramphenicol control the infection. In adults, close monitoring on intensive care is probably adequate and prophylactic intubation is not routinely practised. General use of *Haemophilus influenzae* vaccines should make this problem increasingly rare.

Non-acute

Tumours

Laryngeal, and less commonly tracheal, malignant tumours are usually seen in smokers. The dominant cell type is squamous. Spread of a primary bronchial carcinoma into the base of the trachea is probably the commonest cause of upper airway obstruction in pulmonary practice.

Laryngeal tumours nearly always present with hoarseness, or voice change, and cough. Large airway tumours commonly go undiagnosed until far advanced. This is because they will mimic lower airways obstruction and chest radiography is often normal. Tumours may also respond to asthma therapy, showing temporary shrinkage with steroids which may further mask the real diagnosis.

If history, examination, and lung function tests suggest an upper airway obstruction, then some form of imaging is required. CT is the least invasive approach and therefore least likely to disturb the airway and make matters worse, but will of course provide no histology. Plain films (PA and lateral) may show tracheal narrowing but they can be very deceptive. Direct visualization by fibre-optic or rigid bronchoscopy is usually necessary for diagnosis and to aid future therapy, but care must be taken not to precipitate complete obstruction by taking biopsies.

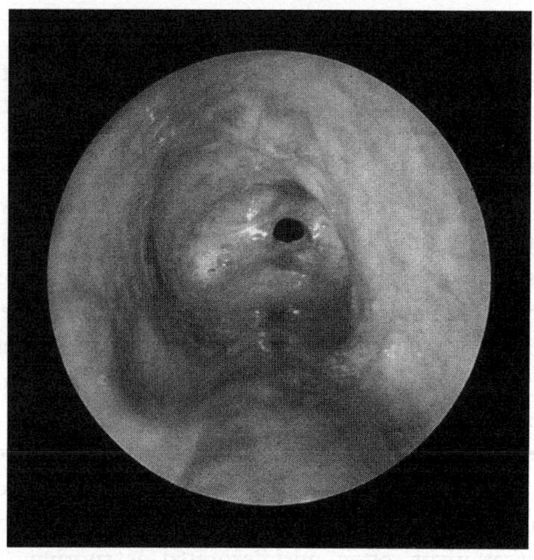

Fig. 2 Bronchoscopic view of a post-tracheostomy tracheal stricture. The remaining hole is about 2–3 mm diameter.
(By courtesy of Dr P. Stradling.)

Whilst waiting for other treatments to work or be organized, dexamethasone (12 mg a day), nebulized adrenaline (10 ml of 1:10000 up to six times a day), humidification of inspired air, and breathing Heliox (21 per cent O_2 in helium) are all that is really available. Improvement in the airway may be achieved by treatment of the tumour with chemotherapy or radiotherapy. Sometimes there is an initial swelling of the tumour so that steroids are usually prescribed first, with emergency treatments kept close to the patient (Heliox, adrenaline). If these therapies are not helping, then palliation can be achieved with the use of endobronchial silicone or metal stents, or bronchoscopically guided laser therapy and cryotherapy.

Unfortunately, in many cases upper airway obstruction from a tumour becomes a terminal event. Powerful sedation is indicated and the patient should be made unaware that he/she is asphyxiating and choking to death.

Tracheal stenosis

Tracheal stenosis usually develops some time after prolonged intubation or tracheostomy removal (Fig. 2). Radiology or bronchoscopy will usually confirm the diagnosis, already strongly suspected from the history. Temporary treatment may be possible by dilating the stricture at rigid bronchoscopy. Definitive treatment involves resection of the stenosed portion and reanastomosis.

Tracheal compression

External tracheal compression may be due to malignant or non-malignant conditions. Non-malignant causes include thyroid enlargement, aortic aneurysm, sclerosing mediastinitis, mediastinal neurofibroma, and Castleman's disease. If definitive treatment is not possible, then stenting the airway is the only treatment possible.

Tracheal abnormalities

Tracheomalacia may be secondary to prolonged external compression or a primary abnormality that presents in childhood. It is essentially a weakness or deficiency of the supporting cartilages, sometimes seen secondary to a long history of chronic airways obstruction. Symptoms are usually stridor, shortness of breath, and paroxysms of cough.

Tracheobronchiomegaly, relapsing polychondritis, and tracheobronchopathia osteochondroplastica are rare conditions that may lead to tracheal obstruction and are discussed in OTM3, pp. 2723–4.

Laryngeal dysfunction

Damage to one recurrent laryngeal nerve usually causes a weak voice that improves with time as the opposite cord 'learns' to compensate and move slightly across the midline to improve apposition. As one of the recurrent laryngeal nerves (carrying efferent and afferent traffic) is invaded or compressed (usually by tumour at the left hilum) differential effects on abductors and adductors of both cords may be seen. Because bilateral recurrent laryngeal nerve paralysis produces flaccid cords that lie passively midway between full abduction and adduction, rapid inspiration will draw the cords together and produce stridor, thus limiting exercise. The inspiratory stridor may be present initially just at night, often misinterpreted as snoring. The usual clinical history is of a voice change following thyroidectomy some years before, then over the following years nocturnal stridor develops with a reduction in exercise tolerance and even respiratory failure. Other causes include neurosyphilis, Arnold–Chiari type 1 malformation, and a proportion are idiopathic.

Laryngeal surgery can prevent inspiratory cord closure but at the expense of the voice, and thus a tracheostomy with speaking tube is the usual approach. If the night time obstruction is the main problem (with sleep disruption and daytime sleepiness) then nasal continuous positive airway pressure therapy will usually keep the cords apart during sleep.

Laryngeal destructive conditions such as rheumatoid arthritis can also lead to poor abduction with inspiratory stridor, particularly at night. In Shy-Drager syndrome (multisystem atrophy) there can be a fairly specific wasting of the laryngeal abductors, this also presents with inspiratory stridor (or apnoea) at night and can progress to respiratory failure.

Functional laryngeal abnormalities, with narrowing during either inspiration or expiration, can occur. This may occur due to psychological problems, but the syndrome blends with reflex laryngeal

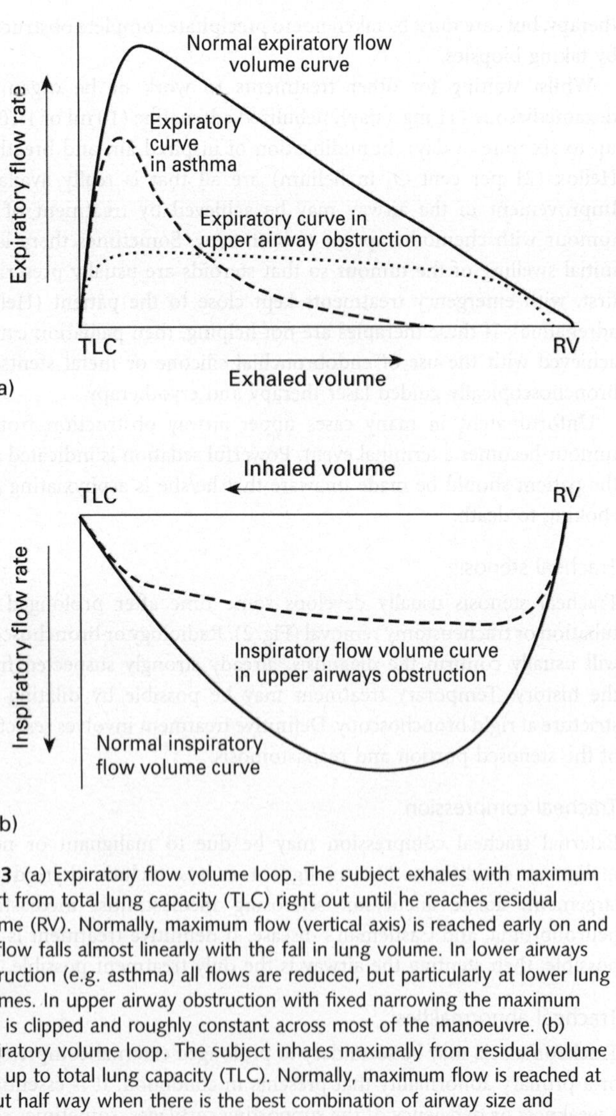

Fig. 3 (a) Expiratory flow volume loop. The subject exhales with maximum effort from total lung capacity (TLC) right out until he reaches residual volume (RV). Normally, maximum flow (vertical axis) is reached early on and the flow falls almost linearly with the fall in lung volume. In lower airways obstruction (e.g. asthma) all flows are reduced, but particularly at lower lung volumes. In upper airway obstruction with fixed narrowing the maximum flow is clipped and roughly constant across most of the manoeuvre. (b) Inspiratory volume loop. The subject inhales maximally from residual volume (RV) up to total lung capacity (TLC). Normally, maximum flow is reached at about half way when there is the best combination of airway size and muscle strength. In upper airway obstruction maximum flow is determined by the diameter of the fixed narrowing and roughly constant across the manoeuvre.

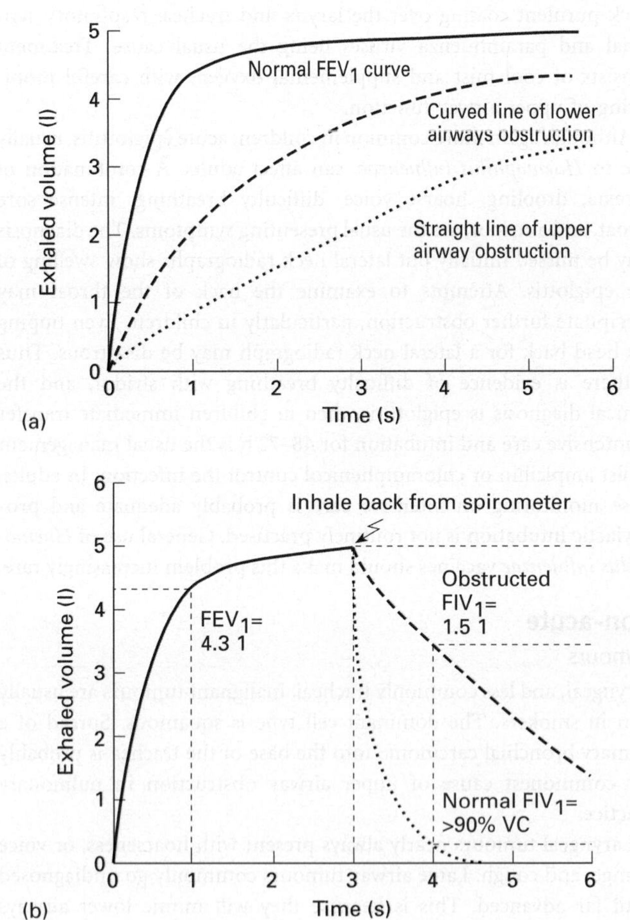

Fig. 4 (a) Curves of forced expiratory volume (FEV) against time. Normally exhalation is rapid and more than 75 per cent of the final volume (vital capacity—VC) is exhaled in 1 s (FEV_1). In lower airway obstruction, flows are slower and thus less air is exhaled at 1 s: the line is still curved because flows are falling. In upper airway obstruction, because flows are roughly constant at a low level set by the remaining orifice, the line is nearly straight and the FEV_1 also low. (b) Following a forced exhalation manoeuvre into a spirometer, a forced inhalation can be made. Normally inspiration is fast and the forced inspiratory volume in 1 s (FIV_1) is almost the vital capacity (VC). If there is upper airway obstruction, particularly extra thoracic such as at the vocal cords, then inspiration will be very limited and the FIV_1 small.

dysfunction in patients with asthma and following upper respiratory tract infections.

Clinical features

History

At rest the main airway can be reduced to 3 mm or so before respiratory distress and stridor occur. Thus, it takes little further obstruction to precipitate complete asphyxia. When upper airway obstruction is suspected, it is a medical emergency to assess severity, diagnose, and treat. If upper airway obstruction comes on slowly then it is most likely to be misdiagnosed as asthma or chronic airways obstruction. At first stridor or noisy breathing will only be heard on exercise but then begins to appear at lower and lower levels of activity. Sometimes the patient may be more symptomatic on lying down and is well aware that the blockage is 'somewhere in the neck', such complaints should be taken seriously, as should associated haemoptysis. A non-productive cough may be present and a change in the voice with shortness of breath should alert one to obstruction at the laryngeal level.

Examination

In pure upper airway obstruction the noisy breathing will localize to the upper airway and tend to be monophonic and stridulous. Harsh breathing rather than stridor may be present if there is a long segment of obstruction. On auscultation of the chest the only sound at the periphery will be the transmitted noise of the stridor. However there may be lower airway obstruction as well, which should not put one off further investigating a suggestive history.

If the upper airway obstruction is extrathoracic, the stridor will tend to be worse on inspiration and the converse may be true when the lesion is intrathoracic.

Investigation

Lung function

During a forced expiration from total lung volume down to residual volume there is a progressive fall in expiratory flow rates which is largely due to the airways getting smaller as the lungs get smaller. If, however, a fixed resistance is introduced (such as tracheal stenosis) then the maximal flow rate possible is almost independent of the lung volume. On a plot of airflow against lung volume (flow-volume loop, Fig. 3(a)), instead of the normal triangular appearance, there is more of a square appearance with the high flows (normally seen at larger lung volumes) severely clipped.

Even if the apparatus to do flow-volume plots or loops is not available, a peakflow meter and spirometry plot may be useful. Because the fixed extra expiratory resistance clips the high flow rates predominantly, then the peakflow rate (PEFR) will be reduced disproportionately to the FEV_1. This gives rise to a simple index of upper airway obstruction: FEV_1 in ml divided by the PEFR in l/min. Normally less than 10, this index usually (but not always) exceeds 10 when there is upper airway obstruction. For simple monitoring of progress, once the diagnosis is known (for example during treatment), the PEFR alone is probably adequate.

The other clue from simple spirometry is the shape of the FEV_1 curve. Normally this is a gentle, ever flattening curve because flow rates (the slope of the curve) are falling. Because of the fixed flow rate of upper airway obstruction this line will tend to be straighter (Fig. 4(a))

The normal inspiratory flow-volume loop is almost a half circle in shape (Fig. 3(b)). Again, if upper airway obstruction is present, this pattern may be replaced by a squarer shape due to the fixed resistance imposing a lower maximum inspiratory flow rate (Fig. 3(b)).

Vocal cord paresis due to bilateral recurrent laryngeal nerve damage is often very much worse on inspiration and simple spirometry can be particularly helpful here. The expiratory tracing will be normal as the cords are blown apart: if the patient then immediately inhales back from the spirometer (make sure a new in-line filter is present first) the inspiratory rate will be tortuously slow (Fig. 4(b)). The forced inspiratory volume in 1 s will often be much smaller than the FEV_1, whereas normally the reverse is true (Fig. 4(b)).

Further reading

Empey, D.W. (1972). Assessment of upper airways obstruction. *British Medical Journal*, **3**, 503–5.

Flenley, D.C. (1990). *Respiratory medicine*. Ballière Tindall, London.

Fraser, R.G., Paré, J.A.P., Paré, P.D., Fraser, F.S., and Genereux, G.P. (1990). *Diagnosis of diseases of the chest*, Vol. 3. W.B. Saunders, Philadelphia, PA.

Goldman, J. and Muers, M. (1991). Vocal cord dysfunction and wheezing. *Thorax*, **46**, 401–4.

Stradling, J.R. (1995). Commentary: upper airways dysfunction. *Thorax*, **50**, 696–7.

Airways disease

Chapter 4.13

Asthma*

D. J. Lane

Introduction

The clinical syndrome of asthma is defined as '... widespread narrowing of the intrapulmonary airways which varies either spontaneously or in response to treatment'. Such a definition allows informed investigation of the phenomenon, but suffers from a lack of precision in terms of 'how variable' (both degree and time-scale).

The introduction of the term 'inflammatory disease of the airways' has served to highlight an important aspect of the pathological anatomy of the condition, encouraged a shift in treatment, and offered some clarification of the nature of the asthmatic process. Yet there remains an underlying dilemma of how best to use the term asthma; whether it should signify a syndrome or a disease or diseases of which the syndrome is a part.

Causes of asthma

Asthma can arise at any age, with peaks of onset in childhood and middle life. Childhood asthma is usually associated with atopic allergy, whereas adult onset asthma often arises in non-atopic individuals. Both allergic and non-allergic asthma appear to have significant inherited components. Family and twin studies suggest that genetic

*Includes some text from Chapter 17.9.1(a) Asthma: basic mechanisms and management by A. J. Frew and S. T. Holgate (OTM3, pp. 2724–9).

and environmental components are required before asthma becomes evident. The ability to make large amounts of IgE directed against environmental allergens (atopy) is genetically controlled. Genetic studies reveal linkage to multiple chromosomal locations pointing to genetic heterogeneity for both atopy and asthma. Atopy is not sufficient alone to cause allergic asthma: environmental factors are equally important. Other individuals have allergic rhinitis or allergic conjunctivitis without clinical asthma. Respiratory tract viral infections have been linked with the development of asthma on both clinical and epidemiological grounds.

A wide range of organic and inorganic materials can sensitize occupationally-exposed individuals. With high molecular weight agents (e.g. rat urinary protein) IgE is usually demonstrable. In contrast, occupational asthma due to low molecular weight agents (isocyanates, acid anhydrides, plicatic acid, etc.) is less clearly linked to IgE and atopy is not a risk factor.

The pathology of asthma

Asthma is an inflammatory disorder of airways mucosa which causes bronchial hyper-responsiveness and small airway damage. In death from acute severe asthma, lungs show widespread obstruction of the small airways with mucus plugs containing fibrin and eosinophils. Death is due to asphyxiation secondary to endobronchial plugging. The bronchial epithelium may be shed into the airway. The basement membrane is thickened with subepithelial fibrosis and there is oedema and a mixed cellular infiltrate. Mild asthmatics show inflammatory changes similar to those in asthma deaths, with fragility of the bronchial epithelium, subepithelial fibrosis with deposition of types III and V collagen, and infiltration by activated eosinophils, mononuclear cells, and T lymphocytes. The extent of these changes parallels the degree of bronchial hyper-responsiveness. Histological studies of intrinsic non-allergic asthma and occupational asthma show very similar findings to the biopsy appearances of allergic asthma.

Inflammatory events in the bronchial mucosa

In patients with allergic asthma, exposure to a relevant allergen causes degranulation of mast cells in the airway lumen and mucosa. This leads to the release of histamine and a range of newly formed mediators which induce bronchoconstriction, oedema, mucus secretion, and vasodilatation. Acute bronchospasm usually resolves within 1 to 2 h but there may then follow renewed airway narrowing which is more persistent. This late-phase asthmatic response is associated with an inflammatory cell accumulation. Eosinophils are characteristic and cause damage to the bronchial epithelium. Growth factors induce proliferation of myofibroblasts which deposit collagens beneath the basement membrane. The production of IgE and the recruitment of eosinophils involves prominently the TH2 cytokines, IL-4, IL-5, and IL-15. Atopy can therefore be regarded as an immune disorder of TH2 predominance.

The recognition of asthma

Though the cardinal symptom of asthma is wheezing (see Chapter 4.1), a few asthmatics never wheeze, and many describe other airways symptoms such as cough, sputum production, chest tightness, or shortness of breath.

Asthmatic wheezing is polyphonic, present on inspiration and expiration, and often only heard on exercise or forced expiration. It

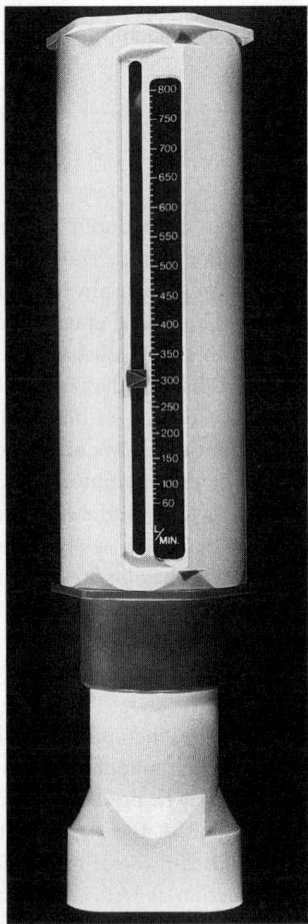

Fig. 1 The mini-Wright peak expiratory flow meter.

is produced by vibrations set up in small airways that are almost closed off. The sensation of tightness is not a pain and so should be distinguishable from angina pectoris and oesophageal spasm. Asthmatics generally find it more difficult to breathe in than out. Exertional shortness of breath for the asthmatic has both a variable component, which tallies with the waxing and waning of their airways narrowing, and a persistent, more fixed component.

Cough is one of the commonest symptoms of asthma in children and can be a lone symptom of the condition in adults. It is frequently accompanied by the expectoration of sticky, mucoid sputum.

The physical signs of asthma are those described for airways obstruction in Chapter 4.1 with special features (described below) that reflect severity in the acute severe attack. Objective confirmation of airways narrowing in asthma can be obtained using any of the tests of airways function described in Chapter 4.4. The test generally used in clinical practice is the peak expiratory flow (PEF) rate (Fig. 1). Results reflect changing levels of airflow obstruction with ease and accuracy and are more reliable than chest physical signs.

Features which suggest asthmatic airways narrowing are variability of pattern and timing. There is a classic diurnal pattern with symptoms disturbing sleep in the small hours of the morning (3–5 a.m.) with late afternoon the most trouble-free time. This diurnal pattern is disrupted by episodic attacks of asthma, some transient, lasting over minutes, others lasting for an hour or so, and yet others creating a more prolonged deterioration lasting for days on end. These patterns of symptoms are readily detected by a parallel variability in serial peak expiratory flow measurements (Fig. 2).

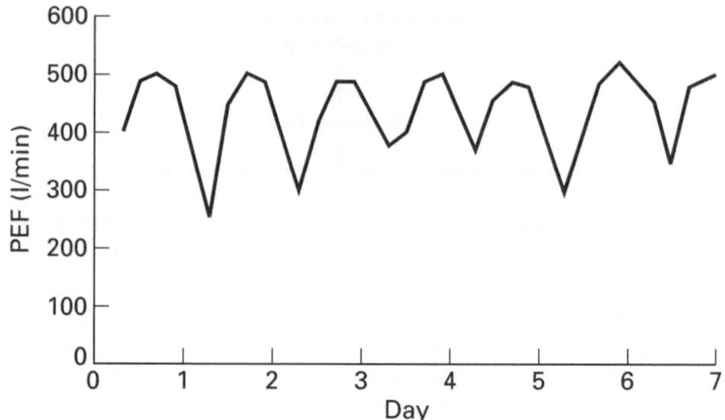

Fig. 2 Serial peak expiratory flow rates in a patient with nocturnal asthma.

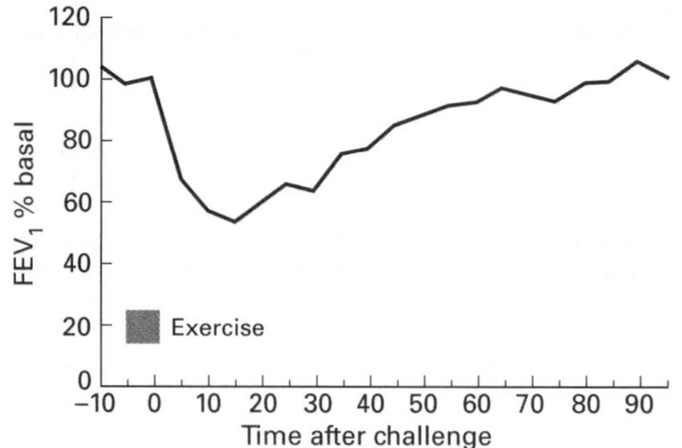

Fig. 3 Exercise-induced asthma: fall and recovery of FEV, as a percentage of basal value.

The clinical relevance of bronchial hyper-responsiveness

Asthmatic airways respond by narrowing to a whole variety of circumstances that leave healthy airways unaffected. This narrowing is caused by smooth muscle contraction, mucosal inflammation, and intraluminal mucus.

Deep inspiration

Following a deep inspiration to total lung capacity and a relaxed expiration, there is a transient increase in airways resistance that is over in 3 min. This type of reactivity may explain wheeziness after laughter or coughing, and can influence tests of forced expiration.

Environmental change

Temperature change, particularly to cold, smoke inhalation, perfumes, irritant gases, etc., can cause immediate tightness or coughing that settles over a space of a few minutes, provided that the provocation is not sustained.

Exercise-induced asthma

This is not a special and separate type of asthma, but an integral part of asthmatic symptomatology, especially in children and teenagers. Exercise-induced asthma does not only result in the curtailment of exercise because of shortness of breath or wheeziness but also is a highly characteristic worsening of symptoms after exercise has finished (Fig. 3).

The magnitude of the response is related to the level of ventilation achieved. Breathing moist humidified air will greatly reduce the degree of exercise-induced asthma, but conversely exercise in very cold weather when the air will also be very dry will enhance airways narrowing. Airways fluid osmolality is more important than temperature change in producing exercise-induced asthma.

Nocturnal asthma

This, too, is an integral part of asthmatic symptomatology. The subject awakes around 3 to 5 a.m. with cough, chest tightness, or wheezing. Objectively, there is increased airflow limitation reflected in reduced PEF. Even if sleep itself is not disturbed, lung function at the natural awakening time 2 or 3 h later will still be abnormal—the morning dip (see Fig. 2). This phenomenon, so dramatic in the asthmatic, is an exaggeration of a natural circadian rhythm detectable even in normal subjects if sufficiently sensitive tests of airways function are used. It is related to sleep itself and most closely parallels changes in circulating sympathomimetic amines, rather than corticosteroids.

The causes of bronchial hyper-responsiveness

The phenomena so far described are indicative of an existing state of bronchial hyper-responsiveness, but do not explain how that state was initiated in the first place. Three further triggers not only set off an attack of asthma, but can create that state *de novo*. They are allergic reactions, infections, and pollutants.

Allergic bronchial hyper-responsiveness

When individuals with an inherited allergic diathesis are exposed to allergens in appropriate concentrations and probably at appropriate times (in the evolution of their immune system), they will develop allergic disease. If these allergens are inhaled into the lungs, local IgE receptors will become sensitized and on further challenge the clinical result will be asthma.

Following allergen challenge, two time courses are defined: (1) an immediate reaction beginning within minutes of exposure and reaching a peak in 5 to 15 min; (2) a late reaction with its onset some 4 to 6 h after exposure which lasts for up to 24 h.

Immediate reactions can be prevented by the inhalation of disodium cromoglycate or a β_2-agonist prior to allergen exposure. Steroids have no obvious effect on the immediate reaction but abort the late reaction.

Several observations signify that allergic inflammation has created a state of bronchial hyper-responsiveness. First, histamine reactivity increases during the interval between the early and late reactions, and remains abnormal after the late reaction has recovered. Secondly, after a late reaction there can be a series of 'morning dips' in lung function on subsequent days (Fig. 4). Finally, pollen-sensitive asthmatics may complain of worsening exercise-induced asthma during the pollen season.

Bronchial hyper-responsiveness resulting from infection

In previously healthy individuals, an acute viral respiratory tract infection will create a state of bronchial hyper-reactivity for 3 to 6 weeks and this may sometimes evolve into persistent asthma. Mechanisms include epithelial damage, genetic predisposition, and type of infecting organism, for example respiratory syncytial virus infection in infancy.

Once bronchial hyper-responsiveness has been established, respiratory tract infection will trigger exacerbations of symptoms. About a

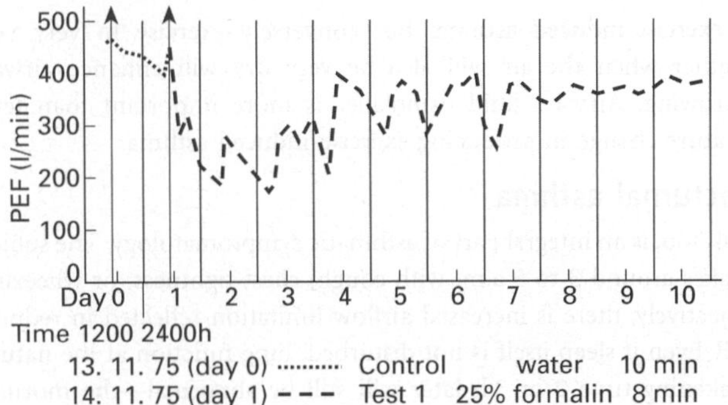

Fig. 4 A series of nocturnal dips following a single allergen challenge in a patient sensitive to formalin.
*(Reproduced from Hendrich, D.J. and Lane, D.J. (1977). Occupational formalin asthma. British Journal of Industrial Medicine, **34**, 11–18, with permission.)*

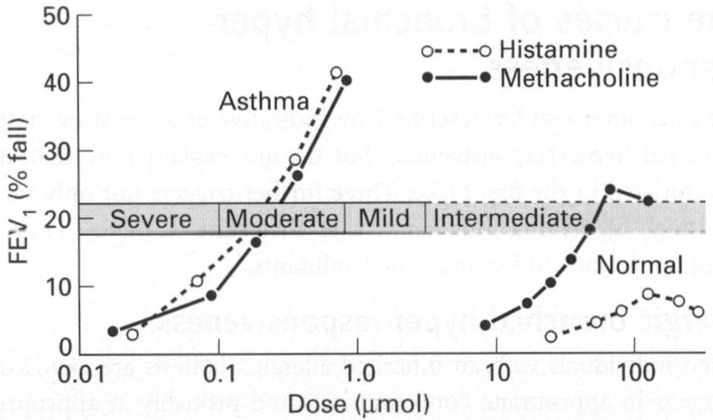

Fig. 5 Percentage fall in FEV_1 during challenge with histamine and methacholine in a normal subject and a moderately severe asthmatic.

half of asthmatics with an identified infection will have an exacerbation of symptoms. These can be amongst the most serious and prolonged of asthma attacks, with slow recovery.

Environmental pollution and bronchial hyper-responsiveness

Cigarette smoking creates hyper-reactive airways. However, in most smokers the fixed component is, or becomes, so dominant that it overwhelms the picture of reversible airways obstruction.

Other atmospheric pollutants, particularly nitrogen dioxide and ozone interact with allergens to increase reactivity. In an occupational setting certain pollutants (e.g. sulphur dioxide and chlorine) are capable of creating *de novo* a state of bronchial hyper-responsiveness.

Testing reactivity in clinical practice

Assessment of hyper-reactivity is most reliably carried out using inhalation challenges with histamine or methacholine. Testing involves the inhalation of logarithmically increasing doses of the challenge and measuring PEF or forced expiratory volume in 1 s (FEV_1) (Fig. 5). The dose of inhaled agent which produces a 20 per cent deterioration in function (PD_{20}) is the index of reactivity.

The clinical use of reactivity testing is confined to the diagnosis of the difficult or confusing case, research into mechanisms, and population epidemiological studies.

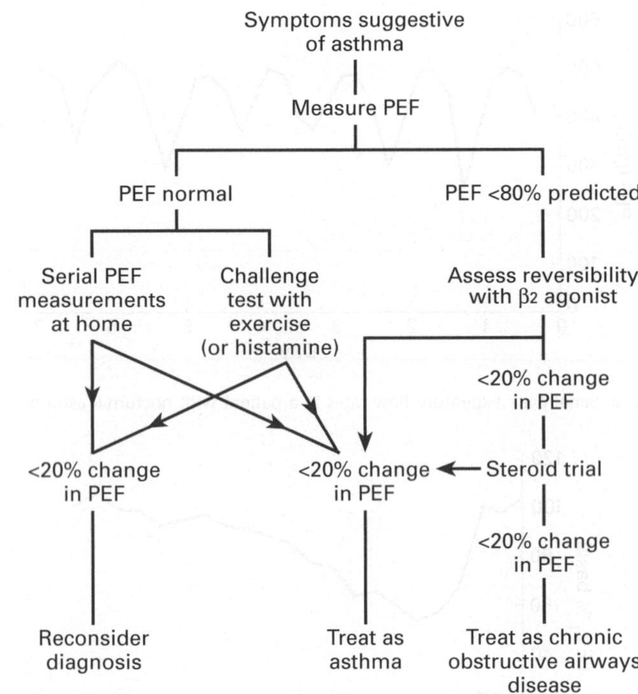

Fig. 6 A diagnostic algorithm for asthma.

A diagnostic algorithm for asthma

A clinical suspicion of asthma based on the symptoms described above in conjunction with variations in function under challenge or in response to therapy creates a diagnostic pathway suitable for most potential asthmatic subjects (Fig. 6).

The asthmatic disorders

If asthma is regarded as a syndrome of reversible airflow obstruction, then it becomes necessary to describe the disorders of which it is a clinical feature.

Extrinsic atopic (allergic) asthma

Atopic allergic individuals are generally young and often have other allergic disorders such as infantile eczema, urticaria, or allergic rhinitis. Such individuals have raised serum levels of IgE and positive skin-prick tests (a weal and flare reaction 15 min after the intradermal inoculation of a solution of allergen).

Intermittent exposure to allergens produces episodic attacks of asthma with or without rhinitis in appropriately sensitized individuals. In contrast, continuous exposure, for example to the house dust mite *Dermatophagoides pteronyssinus*, produces more continuous asthma.

In some individuals, asthmatic symptoms are confined to a particular pollen season. Sensitized individuals will have upper respiratory tract symptoms as well as wheezing. Hyper-responsiveness to histamine, exercise-induced asthma, and nocturnal awakening are all enhanced during the pollen season.

Inhaled allergens are far more important than ingested allergens in causing asthma in atopic individuals, but there are notable examples of the latter. The asthmatic response is then seldom exclusive; there is often associated urticaria, angio-oedema, gastrointestinal upset, and even full-blown anaphylaxis. Fruits, nuts, and shellfish are notorious for causing such symptoms in sensitized individuals.

Extrinsic non-atopic allergic asthma

This term describes individuals with asthma who show allergic airways responses often characterized by a late asthmatic reaction alone, but sometimes a dual reaction, yet who are not atopic. The best examples come from occupational asthma and are described in Chapter 4.14.

Allergic bronchopulmonary aspergillosis

Airways disease due to *Aspergillus fumigatus* spores has distinctive features. The allergen is found in garden compost. Spores are released in the autumn and early winter. Symptoms include exertional breathlessness and sputum production with bronchial casts and brown pellets. Chest radiographs can show transient infiltrates and collapse, due to mucus impaction. Repeated attacks lead to saccular bronchiectasis. Eosinophilia is marked, IgE is high, precipitating antibodies are present in the serum to Aspergillus antigens.

Oral and high dose aerosol steroids are needed for the acute episode. Antifungals, for example itraconazole, will reduce the fungal load.

Asthma with parasitic disorders

These disorders are discussed in Section 16.

Infective asthma

Many adult smokers with early chronic obstructive pulmonary disease suffer infections; there is often wheeze in these bronchitic illnesses. It is reversible to a degree with antibiotics and bronchodilators. Some of these individuals are atopic or have had asthma as children. Since both asthma and smoking are common, a concurrence of the two is quite frequent.

'Psychogenic' asthma

At one time it was thought that asthma was 'all in the mind'. Suggestion can certainly alter airways calibre. Panic, sufficient to produce acute hyperventilation, can initiate airways narrowing or worsen an evolving attack. Chronic stress can cause persistent asthma which can be quite resistant to therapy. However, it seems singularly unlikely that stress or emotional stimuli can initiate asthma in the absence of an underlying cause such as allergy or infection.

Asthma and gastro-oesophageal reflux

Acid reflux into the oesophagus and microaspiration both cause airways narrowing and symptoms of reflux are reported in up to 50 per cent of asthmatics. The association is not confined to adults or the non-atopic. Proton pump inhibitors will help in most instances.

Intrinsic asthma

In adult-onset asthma, infection, psychosocial stress, and occupational exposure can be responsible for wheezing, but there remain a group in whom no recognizable cause of asthma can be determined. These are intrinsic asthmatics.

By definition total IgE is normal and specific allergy tests are negative. However, eosinophilia is not absent from either sputum or blood. Histology of the airways epithelium is similar to that of asthma due to other causes. The clinical course is more likely to be progressive with persistent wheeze and eventual dependence on oral corticosteroids.

Drugs and asthma

Potentially dire consequences follow administering β-blockers, even in the form of eye drops, to asthmatics.

Some 2 per cent of asthmatics react adversely to aspirin and/or non-steroidal analgesics. Symptoms of streaming coryza followed by intense wheezing develop 10 to 20 min after ingesting. Nasal polyps grow after repeated attacks. The best policy is strict avoidance.

Asthma at different ages

Half of those who ever develop asthma will do so before the age of 10. The first onset of asthma in adults occurs evenly across the age bands. Once asthma has begun, it generally persists for some years. In children it will last for longer the earlier it begins. Many children have a remission of symptoms in the teens, but in at least 50 per cent there will be a recurrence at some time in adult life. Remission is less frequent if asthma begins later in life.

Boys predominate over girls early in life with sex ratios of three or four to one in infants. Later in life the sex ratio is around unity with females predominating in the elderly.

Most children who are asthmatic are also atopic, yet viral infections are a more likely trigger for attacks. Allergen-induced attacks occur with exposure to pets and pollens, and the ubiquitous house dust mite is undoubtedly responsible for much asthma in the young. During the school years exercise-induced asthma becomes troublesome. Despite the well-described symptoms of asthma in school children, only half those identified as asthmatic in epidemiological studies will have been formally diagnosed and appropriately treated.

By the teenage years many notice an easing of symptoms, although the highly atopic, particularly those with marked eczema, suffer persistent symptoms. Those foolish enough to smoke cigarettes lay down the foundations of subsequent decline into chronic airways obstruction.

Women may notice a distinct worsening of symptoms just before or during each menstrual cycle. The pattern of asthma in pregnancy is unpredictable. In many it remains stable, some feel much better, but others feel worse.

The worsening, or first appearance, of asthma in adults should prompt enquiry about occupation and any change of place of work. Asthma is inadequately recognized in the elderly but is worth diagnosing because it is treatable.

Acute severe asthma

The most dramatic attacks are very rapid in onset, the victim being transformed from a state of relative well being to one of life-threatening asthma in less than 30 min. These attacks may be brought on by a recognizable allergic trigger, and seem to differ from the infective attack which evolves over several days of worsening symptoms.

In the attack, the patient is desperately breathless, unable to move or complete more than a few words in one breath. Respiratory rate is rapid ($\geq$ 25/min) and there is a tachycardia ($\geq$ 110/min). Children attain much higher rates. Wheeze is usually readily audible, and a silent chest is a warning of extremely severe obstruction. Life-threatening features are bradycardia, hypotension, reduced respiratory effort, exhaustion, and coma.

A peak expiratory flow rate of 33 per cent or less of normal can be sufficient to be life threatening. Oximeter saturations below 90 per cent are likely in severe attacks. Hyperventilation usually lowers the $PaCO_2$, and any rise in $PaCO_2$ or a low pH are grave prognostic features.

Investigations in asthma

Lung function tests

These tests are mandatory and determine the degree of functional disturbance. Repeated tests are essential and therefore should be simple. Measurement of PEF using a portable meter satisfies these aims. Qualitative evaluation of peak flow charts (Figs 2 and 3) provides almost all the information required. There is little need for more complex tests. Plethysmographic lung volume and flow/volume loop measurements add sensitivity when lung function is only minimally disturbed.

Chest radiology

Chest radiology is frequently normal in asthma. Its use is confined to patients presenting diagnostic problems, usually for the exclusion of other disorders, such as pneumothorax, collapse, or consolidation.

Evaluating mechanisms

Atopic status is evaluated using skin-prick tests, total IgE, and specific IgE (radioallergosorbent tests), but does not influence therapeutic decisions. As an adjunct to influencing decisions on inhaled allergen avoidance, specific allergen tests can be valuable. In the difficult chronic asthmatic, there may be need for measurement of Aspergillus precipitins, gastro-oesophageal function, or quantitative immunoglobulins. A peripheral eosinophilia of the order of 5 to 10 per cent ($0.4–1.0 \times 10^9$/l) is not uncommon but counts higher than this range should alert to the possibility of vasculitis (see Chapter 4.28).

Differential diagnosis

It is rightly said that 'all that wheezes is not asthma'. In childhood the most worthwhile differential is inhaled foreign body. There is an increased prevalence of atopy in cystic fibrosis (Chapter 4.15), and in the early stages of the disease recurrent infection may present as wheezing episodes.

In older age groups single airway obstruction is more likely to be due to benign or malignant tumours. Diffuse airways obstruction in smokers and bronchiectatics is occasionally sufficiently reversible to deserve the label asthma.

Organic upper-airways obstruction (trachea, larynx, pharynx) can trap the unwary, as can functional upper-airways obstruction. This is a syndrome of variable, laryngeal obstruction due to tightly adducted vocal cords. Wheeze is intense. This is essentially a psychological disorder, though some have a history of mild genuine asthma, making the diagnosis difficult.

In the cardiovascular system, left-ventricular failure and very occasionally pulmonary emboli can present in a very similar manner to acute asthma.

Treatment

Allergen avoidance

When a recognized allergen is responsible for asthma it should be eliminated from the environment. The best examples come from occupational asthma (Chapter 4.14). Much effort has been expended in devising methods for reducing the load of *D. pteronyssinus* in household dust. Occlusive bedding covers are a key measure.

Domestic pets should be banished. Food that gives obvious allergic reactions is easy enough to exclude, but elaborate diets should be avoided. No asthmatic should take a β-blocker by any route. Aspirin and NSAIDs should be treated with caution. Asthmatics should not smoke tobacco actively or passively.

Table 1 Management guidelines for asthma

Avoidance of allergens and stopping smoking where appropriate
Step 1 Occasional use of relief bronchodilators
Step 2 For regular or persistent symptoms, night-time awakening or daily use of relief bronchodilators: low dose inhaled steroid, e.g. beclomethasone 100–400 μg twice daily[1]
Step 3 High dose inhaled steroid, e.g. beclomethasone 500–1000 μg twice daily OR[2] low dose inhaled steroid+additional bronchodilator, e.g. inhaled salmeterol 50 μg twice daily, inhaled ipratropium, or oral methylxanthine
Step 4 High dose inhaled steroids and regular bronchodilators
Step 5 Intermittent courses[3] or maintenance corticosteroids[4]
Step down: review progress regularly and reduce to minimum necessary to maintain control
[1] Alternative preventive therapy, e.g. DSCG 20 mg four times a day or nedocromil 8 mg twice daily suitable for young, atopic asthmatics
[2] The author favours this alternative using inhaled long-acting β_2 agonist
[3] One course may dampen airway inflammation sufficiently to allow other preventive therapy to work more effectively
[4] Seek specialist advice before taking this step

Prophylaxis

The foundation of present-day treatment of asthma is prophylactic, regular therapy to control symptoms. A scheme is outlined in Table 1. Treatment is built up until satisfactory control is achieved. This means freedom from symptoms, particularly nocturnal awakening, lung function within the normal range, and normal quality of life. The attainment of these aims is limited by treatment side-effects and patient compliance. Maintenance oral corticosteroids give well-recognized side-effects, but even aerosol corticosteroids are not free from toxicity (skin bruising, reduced bone density, and impaired hypothalamic–pituitary–adrenal axis function). Taking regular treatment is demanding and can appear unrewarding. Patients resent relying on medication, and may have fears about its safety. All these concerns must be met if prophylactic therapy is to be effective.

Aerosol corticosteroids are the corner stone of prophylactic therapy. The current standard steroid aerosols are beclomethasone, budesonide, and fluticasone.

In children, in young atopic adults, in those with mild disease, and in those with an aversion to steroids, disodium cromoglycate (Intal) or nedocromil (Tilade) can be tried.

Devices for inhaled therapy

The inhaled route is preferred whenever possible for asthma therapy. The device chosen should be that which the individual can use most effectively. The technique needs to be taught carefully and checked regularly. Large spacer devices (Fig. 7) reduce local side-effects in the mouth and systemic side-effects and deliver a greater percentage dose to the lungs. Dry powder devices are generally more expensive, more complex to use, and still suffer from problems of deposition in the oropharynx. Nebulizers should be reserved for patients who require

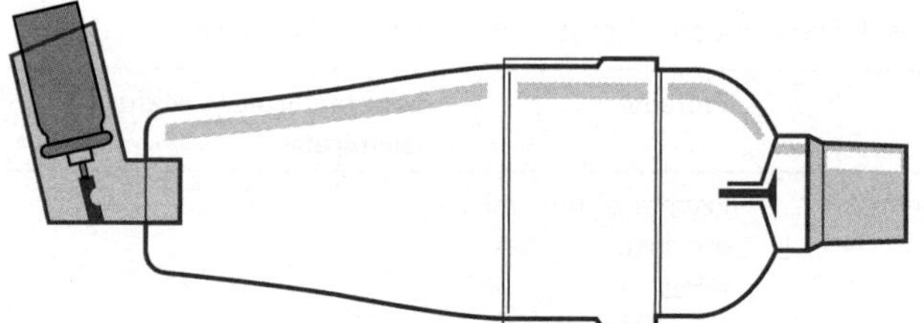

Fig. 7 A large-volume spacer (the Nebuhaler).

larger doses, cannot use any other device, or are likely to need unexpected emergency treatment for an acute attack.

Bronchodilators

Inhaled β_2-agonist bronchodilators give immediate relief in acute episodes. The dose can be repeated within 10 min if required or it can be increased. Long-acting inhaled β-agonists (salmeterol and eformoterol) given 12-hourly, improve function and symptom control and often obviate the need for high-dose inhaled steroids. Oral methylxanthine bronchodilators, such as theophylline and aminophylline, are occasionally helpful. Nausea and dyspepsia are limiting side-effects.

Oral corticosteroids

Short courses of oral corticosteroids are indicated in asthma as a diagnostic test, to gain good control when initiating treatment in more severe cases, when inhaled treatment proves unsatisfactory, and when intercurrent infection or allergen exposure produces a sharp decline in function. Prednisolone is prescribed from 20 mg/day in a child or small female to 40 mg/day in a heavy muscular male. The duration of the course depends on clinical and functional indices of recovery. Aerosol steroids should not be stopped during a course of prednisolone and should be continued after the oral drug has been stopped.

Maintenance oral corticosteroid therapy should be avoided whenever possible. Patients should be monitored for long-term side-effects, particularly diabetes and osteoporosis. In postmenopausal women on maintenance oral corticosteroids, cyclical diphosphonates and calcium supplements may halt the progress towards osteoporosis.

In those instances where prednisolone is required in a dose of more than 10 mg daily, consideration should be given to trials of other immunosuppressive agents, such as methotrexate or cyclosporin. These agents carry their own side-effects which must be balanced against those of the corticosteroid.

The acute attack

The approach to the acute attack is therapeutically simple but managerially complex. In essence, therapy consists of adequate doses of β_2-agonist bronchodilators, systemic steroids, and oxygen (Table 2). Only a few attacks will fail to respond to this scheme. For those that do, additional bronchodilators and ventilatory support will be required.

Attacks that include an element of anaphylaxis can benefit from subcutaneous adrenaline. Nebulized anticholinergics can speed recovery in the first 24 h if given with β_2-agonists. For the difficult attack, methylxanthines can be given as a slow intravenous infusion. Intravenous fluid replacement is important in severe attacks, to which potassium should be added to counteract the metabolic effects of high-dose β-agonist therapy.

Table 2 Treatment of a severe asthmatic attack

Immediate treatment in all patients
• Oxygen—highest concentration available (CO_2 retention is rarely a problem)
• Prednisolone 30–60 mg orally, or hydrocortisone 200 mg IV if $PaCO_2$ is raised or there is any doubt about tablet absorption, or both
• Salbutamol 2.5–5 mg or • Terbutaline 5–10 mg } via a nebulizer (driven by O_2 in hospital)

Table 3 Acute severe asthma—indications for intensive care

Patients with following features always require intensive care
• Hypoxia (PaO_2<8kPa) despite receiving 60% inspired oxygen
• Hypercapnia ($PaCO_2$>6kPa)
• Onset of exhaustion
• Confusion or drowsiness
• Unconsciousness
• Respiratory arrest

Ventilatory support is rarely needed, but the indications for its use (Table 3) should be clearly recognized by any physicians who handle acute asthma.

Failure to respond to therapy

Some asthmatics fail to respond as might be expected. It is always worth reconsidering the diagnosis. However, the fault often lies with therapy. The commonest is poor technique in using inhaled therapy. Secondly, the dose of the inhaled medication may be wrong—usually too low a dose of inhaled steroid. Equally, the patient may be neglecting to use correctly-prescribed therapy. Sometimes side-effects are real, and this issue also needs addressing.

Desensitization

In desensitization for allergic disease, the allergen is injected intramuscularly in increasing concentrations. Clinical trials support some benefit in allergic rhinitis, but very little in asthma.

Organization of care

Broader management strategies for asthma must recognize the need for planned care. There are some asthma deaths that no form of intervention could have avoided. However, there are others where errors of judgement on the part of the sufferer, the carers, or the medical attendants seem to have been at least partly responsible. In aiming to prevent these, the important issues are that the patient (carer) knows what to do and when to do it, and that the services that they contact are competent and skilled in handling acute asthma.

Steps can be taken when patients emerge from an attack to try to prevent further acute attacks. No patient should be discharged without prophylactic therapy or knowledge of how to proceed in the next acute attack.

Asthma is a condition where patients can take a leading role in managing their own illness. The asthmatic should have a clear action plan. This information can be provided by doctors, but increasingly it is being supplied by trained practice nurses running asthma clinics.

The National Asthma Campaign has taken a lead in patient education, providing literature, a telephone help line, and support groups.

Nationally-agreed guidelines for the treatment of asthma devised by a widely representative group show that there is resolve within the profession to set standards.

Death from asthma

Despite major innovations in the treatment of asthma, there has been no consistent improvement in mortality for many decades. There was a sharp increase in the late 1960s confined to young people (10–40 years) and there was a drift upwards, most marked in the elderly, from the mid 1980s, which has now begun to decline. Explanations for these trends, include changes in international classifications for disease and in physicians' habits in diagnostic labelling. An upsurge of asthma deaths in New Zealand in the 1980s has been linked with the use of the non-selective β_2-agonist fenoterol.

Epidemiological studies

There is a striking tendency for asthma to be more common in urban than in rural communities. In addition, when there is movement of a population group from a rural to an urban environment, the prevalence of asthma (and often of other atopic disorders) increases. These trends are partly due to changes in exposure to environmental allergens and partly to changes in immune responsiveness consequent upon an urban life style. Environmental pollution, especially from vehicle exhausts, is greater in cities, but there is no direct link between this and the rising prevalence of asthma.

Further reading

Anonymous (1993). Guidelines on the management of asthma. *Thorax*, 48, Supplements.

Hopkin, J.M. (1997). Mechanisms of enhanced prevalence of asthma and atopy in developed countries. *Current Opinion in Immunology*, 9, 788–92.

Platts-Mills, T.A.E., Tovey, U.R., Mitchell E.B., *et al.* (1982). Reduction of bronchial hyperreactivity during prolonged allergen avoidance. *Lancet*, ii, 675–8.

Rosenwaser, L.J. (1997). Interleukin 4 and the genetics of atopy. *New England Journal of Medicine*, 337, 1720–5.

Spitzer, W.O., Suissa, S., Ernst, P., *et al.* (1992). The use of beta-agonists and the risk of death and near death from asthma. *New England Journal of Medicine*, 326, 501–6.

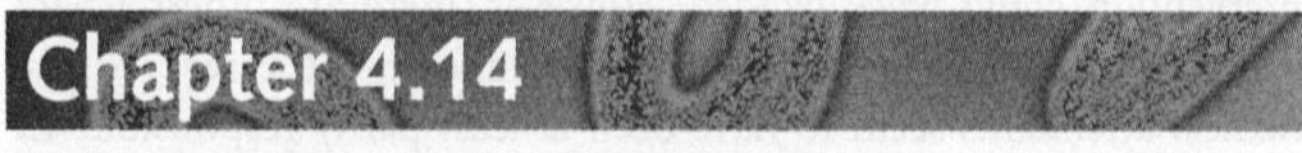

Occupational asthma

A. J. Newman Taylor

Introduction

Although agents inhaled at work can aggravate pre-existing asthma, the term occupational asthma is usually restricted to asthma initiated or induced by agents encountered at work.

Asthma may be initiated by respiratory irritants inhaled in toxic concentrations—'irritant'-induced asthma—or as the outcome of an acquired specific hypersensitivity response—'hypersensitivity'-induced asthma.

Table 1 Some important causes of occupational asthma

	Proteins	Low-molecular weight chemicals
Animal	Excreta of rats, mice etc; locusts, grain mites	
Vegetable	Grain/flour Castor bean Green coffee bean Ispaghula	Plicatic acid (Western red cedar) Colophony (pinewood resin)
Microbial	Harvest moulds *Bacillus subtilis* enzymes	Antibiotics,e.g. penicillins, cephalosporins
'Minerals'		Acid anhydrides Isocyanates Complex platinum salts Polyamines Reactive dyes

Hypersensitivity-induced occupational asthma is considerably the more frequent and it is important to recognize because in many cases asthma improves or resolves with avoidance of further exposure.

Causes

The described causes of 'irritant'-induced asthma are relatively few and include well-recognized respiratory irritants such as chlorine and ammonia. However, any respiratory irritant inhaled in concentrations toxic to airway epithelial cells is a potential cause.

In contrast, a considerable number of causes of hypersensitivity-induced occupational asthma have been identified. Some of the more important are listed in Table 1.

Importance of occupational causes of asthma

Occupational causes probably account for some 5 per cent of new cases of asthma in adult life. Occupational asthma is the single most frequent category of occupational lung disease reported in the UK. Some 1500 new cases are estimated to occur each year. The most frequently reported causes of asthma are isocyanates, grain and flour, wood dusts, colophony, and laboratory animals.

Pathology and pathogenesis

The airways of patients with asthma of occupational cause show a desquamative eosinophilic bronchitis with bronchial epithelial cell desquamation and infiltration of the airway wall by eosinophils and lymphocytes.

Hypersensitivity-induced occupational asthma caused by organic dusts and by some reactive chemicals is associated with specific IgE antibody production. It is probably the outcome of TH_2 lymphocyte stimulation, and the pathological changes observed are primarily the consequence of TH_2 lymphocyte–eosinophil interaction. In general, specific IgE has been identified to the protein causes of occupational asthma but to only a minority of the non-protein causes, such as acid anhydrides and reactive dyes which form stable conjugates with human serum albumin.

Clinical features

'Irritant'-induced asthma

Asthma caused by an inhalation accident is one manifestation of the general tissue injury to exposed mucosal surfaces—eyes, nose, throat, and bronchial airways—which follow an identifiable exposure to a toxic chemical. Running, swelling, and discomfort of the eyes, running and obstruction of the nose, and painful throat usually occur within minutes of the exposure and symptoms of asthma—shortness of breath, wheezing, chest tightness, and cough—develop within minutes or hours of the inhalation. In the majority of cases, asthmatic symptoms resolve spontaneously within a few weeks but occasionally can persist for several years.

Hypersensitivity-induced asthma

In hypersensitivity-induced occupational asthma, respiratory symptoms develop insidiously and do not usually follow a single identifiable exposure to the cause. Asthma develops after an initial symptom-free period of exposure, commonly within 1 year of starting a new job or changing jobs at work, although in some cases not until after several years of exposure. Characteristically, symptoms become increasingly severe during the working week and improve during absences from work at holidays and weekends. However, the relationship of respiratory symptoms to work may not always be appreciated by the patient. This is especially the case when symptoms develop during the second half of the day, and are most severe, as is characteristic of asthma, in the evenings, during the night, and on waking in the morning. Asthmatic symptoms can also persist for several days after avoidance of exposure and appreciable symptomatic improvement at weekends does not occur; improvement is usually sufficient to be appreciated by the end of a two-week holiday or deterioration recognized on return to work.

Diagnosis

The diagnosis of occupational asthma should be considered in any adult who develops asthma or whose asthma has deteriorated in working life. In 'irritant'-induced asthma, association of the onset with inhalation of a toxic chemical is usually clear. The association of asthma caused by a specific hypersensitivity reaction may be less apparent and the diagnosis is based on:

(1) exposure to a sensitizing agent at work;

(2) characteristic history of:

 (a) onset of asthma after an initial symptom-free period of exposure; and

 (b) deterioration in symptoms during periods at work and improvements during absence from work;

(3) results of objective investigations:

 (a) lung function tests;

 (b) immunological tests;

 (c) inhalation tests.

Investigations

Lung function tests

The most commonly used criterion for diagnosing asthma—improvement in airflow limitation (usually measured as forced expiratory volume in 1 s (FEV_1) or peak expiratory flow (PEF)) after inhalation of bronchodilator—may not be present in cases of occupational asthma because when seen away from work lung function may be normal and, if present, does not identify a work relationship. The measure of lung function most commonly used to identify work-related asthma is serial, self-recorded PEF made at 2 to 3-hourly intervals from waking to sleeping for 1 month during periods at and absences from work. The results can be summarized in a graphical display which records the best, worst, and average value for each day, allowing comparison of PEF during days at work with days off work (Fig. 1). When compared with the results of inhalation testing as the 'gold standard', serial, self-recorded PEF measurements have been found to be a sensitive and specific index of work-related asthma. The major diagnostic difficulties are patients who have evidence of asthma on peak flow records without a work relationship, of whom a proportion have occupational asthma; the commonest reason for this false negative response is insufficient time away from work for significant improvement to have occurred.

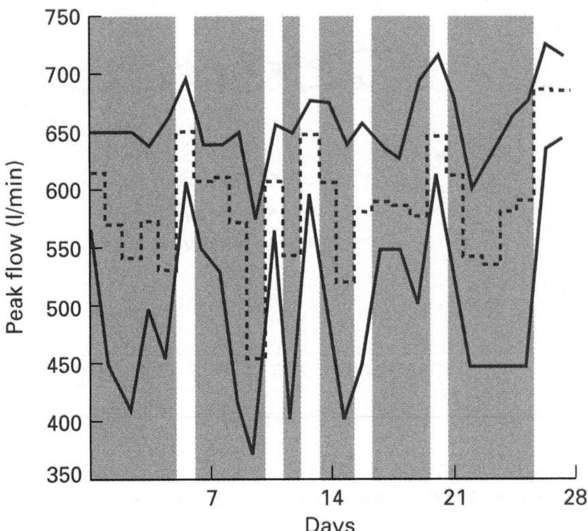

Fig. 1 Serial peak flow results in a baker sensitive to flour. The best, worst, and average value are plotted for each day. Shaded areas are periods at work, unshaded areas periods away from work. Peak flows are consistently worse in each work period and improved during each period away from work.

Immunological tests

The presence of specific IgE antibody, identified either by immediate skin test response or by immunoassay in serum to a soluble protein extract or a hapten protein conjugate, is evidence of sensitization to a specific agent. Specific IgE can be identified to most, if not all, protein causes of occupational asthma and to a small number of low molecular weight chemical causes of asthma—complex platinum salts, acid anhydrides, and reactive dyes.

Inhalation testing

The objective in an inhalation test is to expose the individual under single blind conditions to the putative cause of his asthma in circumstances which resemble as closely as possible the conditions of exposure at work. The patterns of airway response provoked by specific inhalation test have been distinguished by their time of onset and duration. Immediate asthmatic responses occur within minutes of the test exposure and usually resolve spontaneously within 1 to 2 h (Fig. 2). Late asthmatic responses develop one or more hours

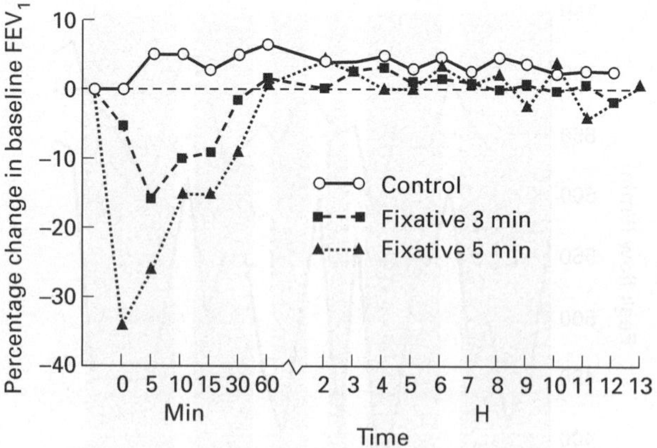

Fig. 2 Immediate asthmatic reactions in a radiographer provoked in inhalation tests of 3 and 5 min with radiographic fixative material, but not by control test.

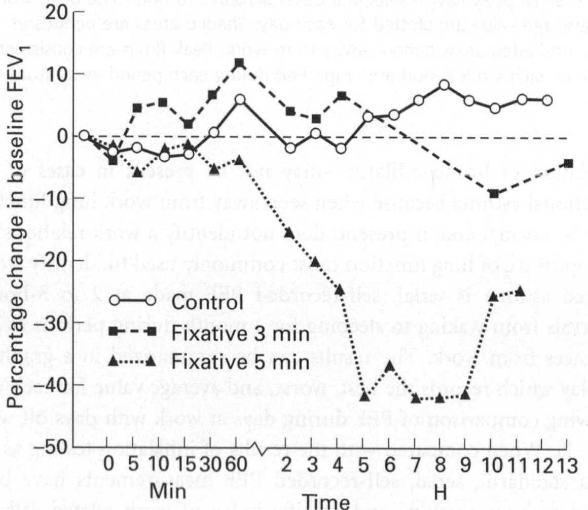

Fig. 3 Late asthmatic reaction in a platinum refiner provoked by exposure to the complex platinum salt ammonium hexachloroplatinate in a concentration of 10 mg but not 1 mg in 250 gm of lactose, the control material.

after the test exposure and can persist for 24 to 36 h (Fig. 3). Late asthmatic (but usually not immediate) responses are accompanied by an increase in non-specific airway responsiveness at 3 h and, less reliably, at 24 h after the test inhalation.

There are four major indications for inhalation tests with specific agents in the diagnosis of occupational asthma:

(1) where the agent considered responsible for causing asthma has not previously been reliably shown to do so;

(2) where an individual with occupational asthma is exposed at work to more than one potential cause which cannot be distinguished by other means;

(3) where asthma is of such severity that further uncontrolled exposure at work is unjustifiable;

(4) where the diagnosis or cause of occupational asthma remains in doubt after other investigations including serial PEF and immunological tests, where applicable, have been completed.

Inhalation tests should be undertaken only for clinical purposes, to inform future management decisions.

Differential diagnoses

The diagnosis of occupational asthma requires differentiation of asthma:

(1) from other causes of similar respiratory symptoms, in particular chronic airflow limitation and hyperventilation;

(2) of occupational from non-occupational cause;

(3) initiated by an agent inhaled at work from pre-existing or incidental asthma provided by non-specific stimuli encountered at work such as sulphur dioxide, exercise, and cold air.

Prognosis

Both 'irritant' and 'hypersensitivity'-induced asthma can persist for several years if not indefinitely, despite avoidance of exposure to the initiating cause. Isocyanates, colophony, plicatic acid from Western Red Cedar and acid anhydrides cause continuing asthmatic symptoms and airway hyper-responsiveness in more than 50 per cent of cases. Airway responsiveness and symptoms improve during the two first years of avoidance of exposure but subsequently plateau.

Those who remain exposed to the cause of their asthma are more likely to develop chronic asthma.

Management

Patients who develop occupational asthma in whom a specific cause is identified should be advised to avoid further exposure to the cause of their asthma.

Avoidance of further exposure may require a change or loss of job which, for social or financial reasons, may not be possible. Such individuals and others sensitized to biological dusts who are unable, at least in the short term, to change their job, should be advised to minimize exposure to the cause of their asthma and to wear adequate respiratory protection, most conveniently laminar flow equipment, when in contact with the organic dust. In addition, background prophylaxis such as sodium cromoglycate can minimize the risk of the provocation of asthma by indirect allergen contact, as from dust on colleagues' clothing. Nonetheless, it should be emphasized that such measures are temporary and in the long term, the means should be sought to avoid exposure to the cause of asthma.

When an individual does remain in employment exposed to the cause of his asthma, either directly or indirectly, the effectiveness of relocation or of respiratory protection needs to be monitored. This can be conveniently done by serial self-recordings of peak flow to determine whether or not asthma is continuing and, if so, if it is work related.

Prevention and control

Occupational asthma is one of the few situations in which application of current knowledge could reduce the incidence of asthma. The incidence of both 'irritant' and 'hypersensitivity'-induced occupational asthma can be decreased by improved control of exposure to their causes, the first by measures to prevent inhalation of irritant chemicals in toxic concentrations and the second by measures to minimize exposure in the workplace to airborne concentrations of the causes of the disease. Where this is not feasible (e.g. spray painting with isocyanates) protective equipment with airfed masks will be required.

Further reading

Bernstein, I.L., Chan Yeung, M., Malo, J.-L., and Bernstein, D.I. (eds) (1993). *Asthma in the workplace.* Marcel Dekker, New York.

Durham, S.R., Graneek, B.J., Hawkins, R., and Newman Taylor, A.J. (1987). The temporal relationship between increases in airway responsiveness to histamine and late asthmatic responses induced by occupational agents. *Journal of Allergy and Clinical Immunology,* 79, 398–406.

Malo, J.-L., Cartier, A., Ghezzo, J., Lafrance, M., McCante, M., and Lehrer, S.B. (1988). Patterns of improvement in spirometry, bronchial hyper-responsiveness and specific IgE antibody levels after cessation of exposure in occupational asthma caused by snow crab processing. *American Review of Respiratory Disease,* **138**, 807–12.

Meredith, S. K. and McDonald, J.C. (1994). Work-related occupational respiratory disease in the United Kingdom 1989–1992: A report of the SWORD project. *Occupational Medicine,* **44**, 183–9.

Venables, K.M., Topping, M.D., Nunn, A.J., Howe, W., and Newman Taylor, A.J. (1987). Immunologic and functional consequences of chemical (tetrachlorophthalic anhydride) induced asthma after 4 years of avoidance of exposure. *Journal of Allergy and Clinical Immunology,* **80**, 212–18.

Chapter 4.15

Cystic fibrosis

D. J. Lane

Introduction

Cystic fibrosis is a condition combining pancreatic insufficiency with repeated respiratory tract infections. It is the commonest potentially lethal, autosomal recessive disorder in Caucasians affecting one in 2000 live births.

Genetics and biochemistry

The gene in which mutations give rise to cystic fibrosis lies on the long arm of chromosome 7 and codes for the cystic fibrosis transmembrane conductance regulator (CFTR). The commonest abnormality (DeltaF508) involves a phenylalanine at amino acid 508. Some 54 per cent of north European and American cystic fibrosis patients are homozygous for DeltaF508 and another 20 per cent carry one copy. Over 200 other mutations have been identified, but there are still 18 per cent of cystic fibrosis patients in the UK with clinical disease but either just one or no identifiably abnormal gene. Across Europe there is a clear north-west to south-east gradient for the prevalence of DeltaF508 from 100 per cent in the Faroe Islands to 26 per cent in the southern former Yugoslavia and Turkey.

CFTR transports chloride ions across epithelial cell membranes. Defective chloride transport results in viscid, low water content secretions which clog the ducts of exocrine glands, particularly in the lungs and pancreas.

There appears to be no consistent correlation between the pulmonary disease and the presence of any genetic abnormality, though those homozygous for DeltaF508 are more likely to have pancreatic insufficiency.

CFTR is easily identified in the pancreas, intestine, and salivary glands, but little can be picked up in the lungs where an abundance might be expected. In contrast, CFTR is strongly expressed in renal tissue where the only clinical abnormality is unduly rapid excretion of certain antibiotics.

Pathology

Gastrointestinal tract (see Chapter 5.19)

In utero and in the neonatal period, proteinacious material within the pancreatic ducts leads to occlusion, inflammation, and fibrosis resulting in failure of enzyme secretion and steatorrhoea.

The lung

The neonate has normal lung histopathology. Early changes are mucous gland hyperplasia, pneumonitis, and mucus plugging leading to focal atelectasis and mucoceles. Cystic bronchiectasis and progressive lung destruction follows. Abnormal airway mucus encourages bacteria especially *Staph. aureus* and *Pseudomonas* spp.

Clinical features

Early life

Presentations which alert to the possibility of cystic fibrosis are meconium ileus, failure to gain weight, and respiratory tract infection. Meconium ileus is the commonest cause of neonatal death in cystic fibrosis. Fatty, offensive stools point to malabsorption and pancreatic insufficiency. Diagnosis of respiratory symptoms is the most difficult. Whooping cough or asthma may be suspected before cystic fibrosis. Salty sweat can be a useful guide.

The respiratory tract

Initial symptoms are cough, with vomiting of swallowed secretions but rarely expectoration. Repeated respiratory tract infections follow. The chest radiograph may show patchy areas of pneumonitis. Sputum is produced as the disease evolves. The mucopus is yellow–green in colour, excessive in quantity, and unpleasant in taste and smell. Blood-staining or frank haemoptysis are not infrequent.

Microbiology

Early colonizing bacteria are pneumococci and *Haemophilus influenzae.* Staphylococci seem to hasten bronchial wall damage. More serious is *Pseudomonas. Burkholdia cepacia* is particularly dangerous because of its antibiotic resistance and greater contagion.

Physiology

Small airways obstruction gives a raised residual volume/total lung capacity (RV/TLC) ratio, abnormal flow-volume loops, and increased $P(A\text{–}a)O_2$ gradient. As airways disease progresses, flow rates on forced expiration are reduced and vital capacity (VC) and TLC become smaller. Some patients have an asthmatic bronchial hyper-responsiveness.

Radiology

The plain chest radiograph reveals bronchiectasis (Fig. 1), with thickened airways, fibrosis, and emphysema emphasized on CT scans.

Respiratory complications

Haemoptysis can be massive, and even fatal. Pneumothorax occurs in 20 per cent. A persistent pneumothorax can become infected, leading to a pyohydropneumothorax.

Cicatrization between bronchiectatic areas leads to fixed airways obstruction.

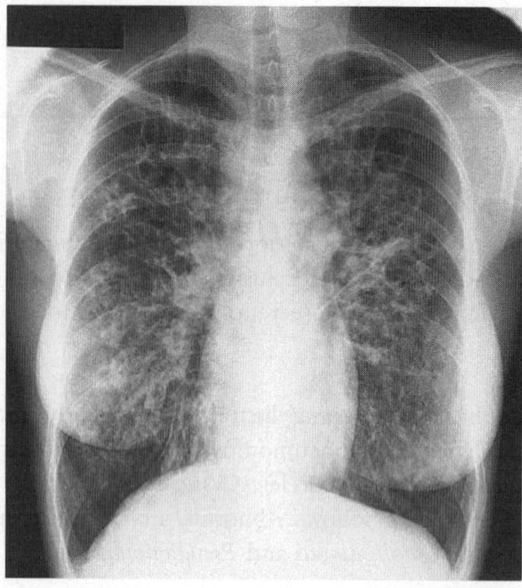

Fig. 1 Posteroanterior plain chest radiograph in an adult patient with cystic fibrosis.

Lung destruction and airways obstruction lead to ventilatory failure with hypoxaemia and carbon dioxide retention. Cor pulmonale ensues and in this state many cystic fibrosis patients will die.

Upper respiratory tract

Recurrent infections lead to chronic inflammatory damage and bacterial colonization. The nose is unduly susceptible to polyp formation

Abdominal manifestations

Steatorrhoea

Though pancreatic insufficiency is characteristic, up to 15 per cent, have no such problem. Classically the stools are pale, bulky, offensive, and difficult to flush away. Untreated, the malabsorption results in weight loss and cachexia. Loss of fat-soluble vitamins causes visual disturbance (vitamin A deficiency) and osteomalacic rickets (vitamin D deficiency). None of these complications need arise since pancreatic enzyme replacement is simple and effective (see below).

Rectal prolapse, volvulus, and intussusception

These bowel complications are only likely to occur in young children. Surgical intervention may be needed.

Distal intestinal obstruction syndrome

Small intestinal obstruction in adults presents with vomiting, abdominal pain, distension, and severe constipation. Subacute obstruction can be recurrent. Dilated loops of small bowel are visible on plain abdominal radiography. The pathogenesis is unclear.

Surgical treatment should be avoided, except as a life-saving measure. Intravenous hydration and parenteral feeding are needed with full doses of pancreatic enzymes, H_2 blockers, and acetylcysteine delivered directly to the bowel via a nasojejunal tube.

Liver and biliary tree

A fatty liver is common. In focal biliary fibrosis, a pathognomonic lesion leads to cirrhosis. Portal hypertension, resulting in splenomegaly, oesophageal varices, and ultimately hepatic encephalopathy, can follow. Older patients are liable to develop cholesterol gallstones.

Diabetes

Diabetes is increasingly common with the ageing cystic fibrosis population (one in 10, though 50 per cent may have abnormal glucose tolerance tests). Treatment is along conventional lines with oral hypoglycaemics or insulin.

Miscellaneous clinical manifestations

Arthropathy

An inflammatory arthropathy can occur in 10 per cent of older cystics. Spontaneous remission is usual. Non-steroidal anti-inflammatory drugs (NSAIDs) give symptomatic relief.

Vasculitis

Henoch–Schonlein-like phenomenon is uncommon. Antinuclear cytoplasmic antibody (cANCA) is positive in some 40 per cent. Oral corticosteroids are indicated.

Amyloidosis

As in other disorders where there is long-standing suppurative disease, secondary amyloidosis can develop.

Infertility

Over 90 per cent of males with cystic fibrosis are infertile. There is obstructive azoospermia. Women with cystic fibrosis can have children despite diminished fertility. Most women do not attempt pregnancy.

Psychological consequences of cystic fibrosis

Most children adapt well to their disease. Adolescents and adults can have problems coping with increasing disability. Cystics are often isolated and disadvantaged in employment. Close contact with family members, essential for their physical support, means that outside social contacts are few. Family dynamics can be seriously upset. Marriage is particularly stressful for adults, males realizing the significance of their infertility and women ill at ease with the consequences on their physical health of pregnancy. Despite this, adult patients with cystic fibrosis are generally remarkably robust.

Diagnosis

The sweat test

Two values of 70 mmol/l for sodium in apocrine gland secretions are diagnostic. Careful attention has to be paid to technique in performing the test. At least 100 mg of fluid is required for reliable analysis.

Neonatal screening

Low immunoreactive trypsin in serum and blood can detect the gastrointestinal effects of cystic fibrosis very early in life.

Prognosis

Until 1965 the median age at death of children with cystic fibrosis was 2 years. In 1993, 50 per cent of cystic fibrosis patients were still alive at 25 years. Those born with cystic fibrosis today are likely to survive beyond 40 years. Boys fare slightly better than girls. Survival is longer in children from social classes with non-manual occupations. The development of pseudomonas colonization is a poor prognostic feature.

There is no suggestion that the incidence of the disease is increasing, though the prolonged survival means a steady increase in prevalence.

Treatment

Nutrition

Diet

With effective pancreatic enzymes, restriction of dietary fat is no longer necessary. A full diet with high energy and calorie content is encouraged, aiming to keep body mass index within the normal range. Dietary supplements, and vitamins A and D should be given. The use of vitamins E and K, zinc, and selenium is more controversial.

Further nutritional support

With disability, decline in appetite and loss of weight necessitate nutritional support with high caloric supplements orally, via a nasogastric tube, or a gastrostomy. Exercise tolerance improves significantly when nutritional status is improved in these ways.

Pancreatic enzyme replacement

Pancreatic enzyme capsules of lipase, amylase, and protease in two strengths are available. A regimen is devised distributing capsules according to the probable intake at a given meal. Additional help with steatorrhoea can be obtained by adding an H_1 blocker

Diabetes, liver disease, and the other non-pulmonary complications are treated according to standard guidelines.

Treating bronchopulmonary disease in cystic fibrosis

Protection from infection

Avoiding contact with infectious respiratory tract illness in children and segregating patients with *B.cepacia* infection are sensible precautions. Cystic fibrosis patients should be immunized against the usual childhood illnesses, likewise influenza. Prophylactic flucoxacillin and nebulized colisitin probably improve prognosis.

Principles of the use of antimicrobial agents

Respiratory tract infection must always be taken seriously. Sputum culture and sensitivities warn of the emergence of bacterial resistance.

Antibiotics penetrate poorly into bronchiectatic cavities, and the alginate coating of *Pseudomonas* provides the microbe with protection. The rapid renal clearance of antibiotics in cystic fibrosis means that larger than usual doses have to be given. *Staphylococcus aureus*, *Pneumococcus*, and *H. influenzae* will respond to standard oral antibiotics.

Pseudomonas infection is serious. A vigorous attack when it is first isolated may sometimes eradicate it for months, even years. Regular treatment every 3 months is advocated by some, irrespective of clinical state.

Antimicrobials for *Pseudomonas*

Oral agents

The four quinolones are the only oral agents effective against *Pseudomonas* species but resistance emerges readily. Side-effects include gastrointestinal disturbance and cerebral dysfunction.

Inhaled agents

Three classes of antibiotic have been used by inhalation. The penicillins, particularly carbenicillin, cause sensitivity reactions in the airways. Aminoglycosides have been more successful and less trouble.

Colomycin (a polymyxin antibiotic) has been the most successful inhaled agent for the long-term treatment of pseudomonas infection. There is no evidence of absorption sufficient to give side-effects and the incidence of bacterial resistance is low.

Table 1 Antimicrobial agents for pseudomonas infection in cystic fibrosis

Oral	*Intravenous injection*
• Ciprofloxacin	• Azlocillin
• Ofloxacin	• Piperacillin†
*Inhaled**	• Ticarcillin†
• Colisitin	• Ceftazidime
• Tobramycin–under trial	• Aztreonam
• Meropenem	• Meropenem
	• Gentamicin*†
	• Netilimicin*†
	• Tobramycin*†

*The antipseudomonas penicillins have also been given by inhalation.

†Both also available with clavulanic acid.

*†High doses of aminoglycosides can be tolerated but check levels.

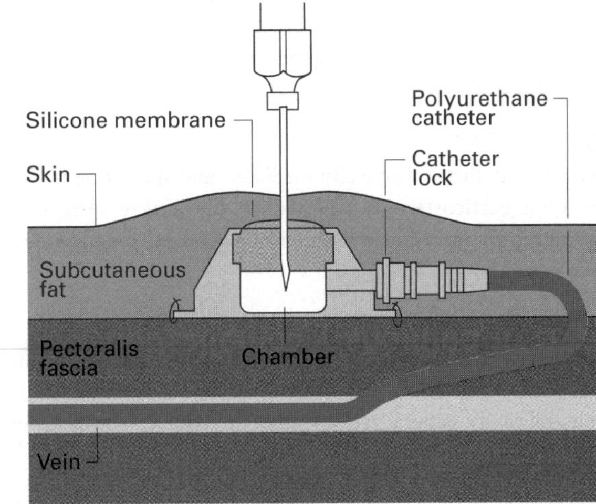

Fig. 2 Portacath venous access system.

Intravenous agents

There is an increasing trend towards intravenous therapy. The agents used and commonly recommended doses are listed in Table 1. A combination of two antibiotics is recommended. Chronic colonization leads to the need for almost continuous intravenous treatment and the increasing likelihood of development of resistance.

Venous access

Care must be taken to do as little damage as possible. Flushing after use is essential. Long lines are widely used. More permanent venous access through completely buried venous ports (Fig. 2) will eventually be necessary.

One of the greatest advances in the general management of cystic fibrosis patients has been self-management of venous lines. This has greatly decreased the number of inpatient days or hospital visits and has allowed cystic fibrosis patients to remain active and at work despite needing intravenous antibiotics. Newer devices contain preprepared antibiotic solutions which are automatically delivered slowly over a preset time. The device itself can be sited in a pocket.

Other therapeutic approaches

Reducing the viscosity of sputum

Acetylcysteine has been given by inhalation but frequently causes bronchospasm. DNA-ase can liquefy sputum, allow its more effective expectoration, and improve lung function.

Physiotherapy

Techniques which aid drainage of bronchial secretions are:

- postural drainage;
- percussion and vibration;
- forced expiration (huffing);
- controlled breathing.

The treatment of respiratory complications

Haemoptysis

Rest and adrenaline inhalations may help, and vasopressin or desmopressin have been used successfully. When bleeding is life-threatening, arterial embolization with metal coils has halted the bleeding.

Pneumothorax

This is treated along conventional lines with early recourse to surgery. Sclerosing agents are discouraged because the pleural damage may preclude later lung transplant. The best surgical approach is to use a thoracoscopic technique.

Airways obstruction

In some patients this is atopically mediated and should be treated as asthma. Oral corticosteroids will reduce the airway inflammation process caused by infection but should be reserved for patients with serious obstruction.

Aspergillus colonization

Colonization with *Aspergillus fumigatus* can cause allergic bronchopulmonary aspergillosis but also mycetomas, and if the fungus invades to the pleural cavity, generalized spread of infection can be devastating.

Respiratory failure

This is treated conservatively along the lines described elsewhere. Ventilatory support should be reserved for those patients who have a good prospect of benefiting from heart–lung transplant.

Heart-lung transplant

Combined heart and lung transplant is the favoured procedure for patients with cystic fibrosis. Their hearts can often be used for other patients.

There is a significant perioperative mortality, which is not surprising in view of the serious nature of the disease, but the subsequent attrition rate is slower. The 3-year survival is currently around 65 per cent and the 5-year survival is just over 50 per cent. When death is an imminent prospect these statistics represent a chance worth taking.

Patients are selected on the grounds of poor lung function (spirometric values less than one-third of the predicted value), arterial desaturation on exercise, and deteriorating quality of life. Patients need to have a stable background, a robust attitude, and strong home support. Prognosis is adversely affected by malnutrition, other organ failure, previous thoracic surgery, and preoperative intermittent positive-pressure ventilation. Rejection is dealt with along conventional lines. Obliterative bronchiolitis afflicts one in five patients after about the first year and is usually fatal.

Management strategies for cystic fibrosis

The highly specialized care necessary for the treatment of patients with cystic fibrosis has led to the creation of cystic fibrosis centres. Such centres need to be regionally based, and offer multidisciplinary care.

Prevention

Families with an affected child require genetic counselling. The risk of a further affected child is one in four; the risk of a carrier child is two in four. Accurate antenatal diagnosis is possible.

For female cystic fibrosis sufferers the risk of an affected child is relatively low, at one in 44, if the partner is not a carrier.

The future

One major hope for the future lies with gene therapy. In a mouse model of cystic fibrosis in which the murine CFTR gene has been ablated, inhalation of the gene restores the chloride channel function to normal and successful preliminary human studies have given hope for the future.

Further reading

Cheng, S.H., Gregory, R.J., Marshall, J., *et al.* (1990). Defective intracellular transport and processing of CFTR is the molecular basis of most cystic fibrosis. *Cell*, **63**, 827–34.

Cleghorn, G.J., Fortstner, G.G., Stringer, D.A., *et al.* (1986). Treatment of distal intestinal obstruction syndrome in cystic fibrosis with a balanced intestinal lavage solution. *Lancet*, **i**, 8–11.

Hyde, S.C., Gill, D.R., Higgins, *et al.* (1993). Correction of the ion transport defect in cystic fibrosis transgenic mice by gene therapy. *Nature*, London, **362**, 250–5.

Pinkerton, P., Duncan, F., Trauer, T., Hodson, M.E., and Batten, J.C. (1985). Cystic fibrosis in adult life: a study of coping patterns. *Lancet*, **ii**, 761–3.

Smyth, R.L., Higenbottam, T., Scott, J., and Wallwork, J. (1991). Cystic fibrosis 5—the current status of lung transplantation for cystic fibrosis. *Thorax*, **46**, 213–16.

Chapter 4.16

Bronchiectasis

R. A. Stockley

Introduction

Bronchiectasis is a condition in which there is chronic dilatation of the bronchi. It is usually suspected when patients present with a long history of persistent or intermittent sputum production in the absence of other known causes, such as asthma or smoking. In reality, the condition may coexist with these other causes.

There is a general impression that bronchiectasis is now less frequent or at least less severe than previously. This may reflect changes in socio-economic conditions, the introduction of immunizations, and the use of antibiotics.

Pathology

Gross inspection reveals the dilated bronchi that are pathognomonic of the disease (Fig. 1). The airways are inflamed, often tortuous and collapsible, and often contain secretions which may cause occlusion. There is a varying degree of parenchymal damage with scarring and fibrosis (Fig. 2). The condition is usually widespread but may be localized to the upper lobes if due to tuberculosis or related to an

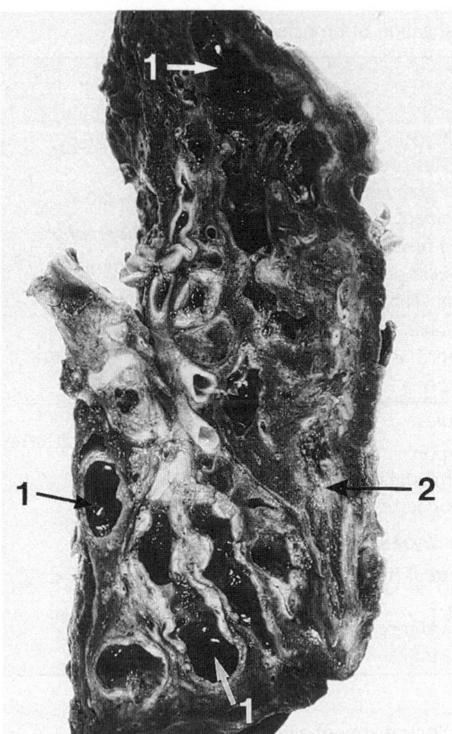

Fig. 1 Macroscopic appearance of extensive bronchiectasis of the lung. Dilated bronchi are arrowed (1). The remaining architecture is distorted and large white areas of fibrosis (arrow 2) are seen.

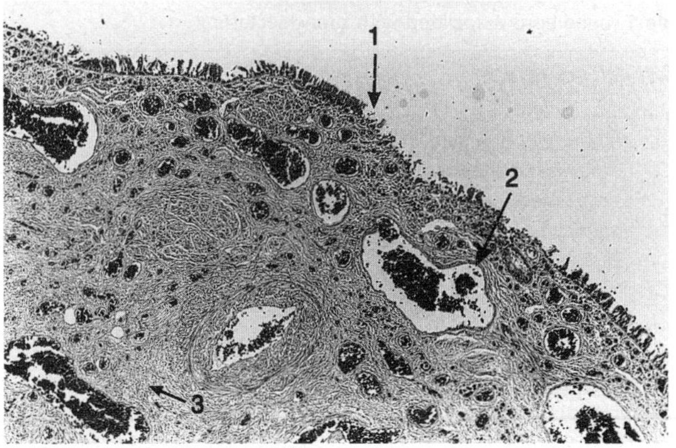

(a)

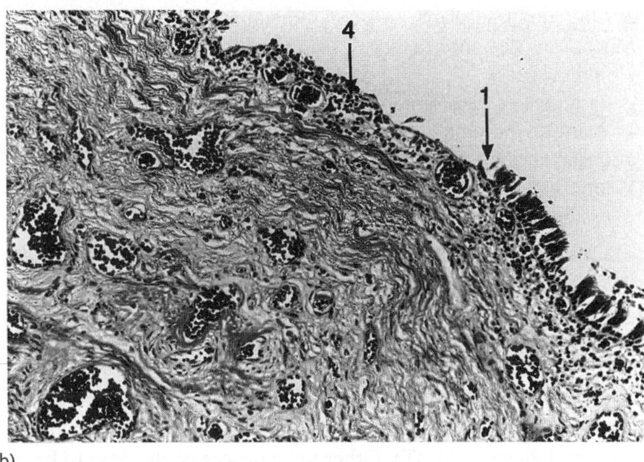

(b)

Fig. 2(a,b) Histological sections of bronchial wall in bronchiectasis highlighting some of the features (arrowed): (a) shows the epithelial damage with loss of ciliated epithelium (1), dilated submucosal blood vessels (2), and increased interstitial collagen (3). These features are seen at higher magnification (b) together with submucosal inflammatory cell infiltrate (4).

area distal to bronchial obstruction or the site of a previous lobar pneumonia.

Microscopically there is a varying degree of damage to the bronchial epithelium (Fig. 2). There may be areas of ulceration and the columnar ciliated epithelium is replaced patchily by squamous epithelium. There is goblet cell and mucus gland hyperplasia and the peribronchial connective tissue is often damaged or lost (leading to dilated but collapsible airways). There may be microabscesses in the bronchial wall and evidence of pulmonary vascular dilatation, occlusion, or hypertension. There is usually extensive inflammatory cell infiltration which consists of neutrophils (predominantly in the lumen) and mononuclear cells (in the bronchial wall). There is also a variable degree of tissue oedema and fibrosis.

Individual specimens show a wide range of severity which is in keeping with the wide range of clinical features (see later).

There are three major pathological types, although the distinctions are often unclear and different types may coexist:

1. Saccular bronchiectasis—this is less common today but is associated with the most severe damage and large saccular dilatation with loss of bronchial subdivisions.
2. Atelectatic bronchiectasis—this is usually lobar or segmental in distribution and occurs in the absence of other forms. It is usually related to proximal bronchial distortion or occlusion.
3. Follicular bronchiectasis—this is the most commonly encountered form of bronchiectasis. It is characterized by the formation of multiple lymphoid follicles which may distend and project into the bronchial tree. They are associated with extensive loss of the elastic tissue in the bronchial wall. The follicles themselves contain activated lymphocytes (predominantly CD8 positive cytotoxic/suppressor T cells). In addition, there is also an increase in B lymphocytes in the bronchial wall. At present it is known that many of these produce the IgA1 and IgA2 subclasses of immunoglobulins. It is unknown whether B lymphocytes producing the IgG subclasses are also increased in number but there is evidence of increased local production of the IgG subclasses 1 to 4.

Pathogenesis

The pathogenesis of bronchiectasis is only partly understood. Symptoms often date from childhood and are related (by the patient) to a single event described as 'pneumonia'. Several epidemiological studies have noted that bacterial pneumonia or more specified infections (whooping cough and measles pneumonia) may relate to the onset of symptoms in 30–60 per cent of patients. Unfortunately, most of the information is collected in retrospect and its validity has been questioned. Nevertheless, some infections have undoubtedly been linked to bronchiectasis including tuberculosis, whooping cough, adenovirus, and mycoplasma infections. Also the incidence and severity of bronchiectasis has probably decreased since the introduction of antibiotic therapy and immunization regimens providing circumstantial evidence that infection plays a role. The role of infection in the development of bronchiectasis is highlighted further by the association with identified defects in host defence (see Table 1).

Table 1 Conditions associated with bronchiectasis

Host defence defects	*Infection*
• Immune defects • Immunoglobulin deficiency • (primary and secondary) • Complement deficiency • Phagocyte defects • Chronic granulomatous disease • Chediak Higashi disease • Leucocyte adherence deficiency • Hyperimmune states • Allergic bronchopulmonary • aspergillosis • After lung transplant • Mucociliary clearance defects • Immotile cilia • Kartagener's syndrome • Young's syndrome • Cystic fibrosis • Bronchial obstruction (tumour or nodes)	• Tuberculosis • Measles pneumonia • whooping cough • Adenovirus 21, 3, and 7 *Mycoplasma pneumoniae* • Pneumococcal pneumonia • AIDS *Other inflammatory disease* • Gastric aspiration • Ammonia inhalation • Heroin • Inflammatory bowel disease • Rheumatoid arthritis • Vasculitis *Miscellaneous* • Inhalation of foreign body • Pulmonary fibrosis • Absence of bronchial cartilage • α_1-Antitrypsin deficiency • Yellow nail syndrome • Primary lymphoedema • Treated lymphoreticular malignancy

There may be a positive family history suggesting a genetic component as in cystic fibrosis and the immotile cilia syndrome and α_1 antitrypsin deficiency (α_1AT). Other toxic processes also lead to bronchiectasis including aspiration of gastric contents or inhalation of toxic chemicals such as ammonia. Table 2 summarizes the investigation of bronchiectasis and these investigations may reveal a cause.

Table 2 Investigation of bronchiectasis

Blood tests	*Radiology*
• Biochemistry • α_1-Antitrypsin • Aspergillus precipitins • Immunoglobulins (subclasses) • Complement components • Neutrophil function • Superoxide production • Bacterial killing • Chemotaxis • Adherence assays • Neutropenia *Genetic studies* • α_1-Antitrypsin • Cystic fibrosis gene and/or sweat chloride test *Mucociliary clearance* • Ultrastructural studies • Functional • nasal clearance • lung clearance	• Sinus radiograpy • Chest radiograpy • CT scan • Barium swallow *Electrocardiography* • Echocardiography • Right heart catheter *Lung function* • Arterial blood gases • Exercise capacity • Static lung volumes • Dynamic flow rates/reversibility • Sleep studies *Sputum culture* • Gram stain • Aerobic • Anaerobic • Selective medium

Table 3 Radiological abnormalities in bronchiectasis

Tramline shadows
Cystic lesions (often fluid filled)
Volume loss with crowding of vessels
Areas of atelectasis
Evidence of previous tuberculosis infection
Fibrosis
Evidence of previous heart surgery

Clinical features

The patients show a broad spectrum of clinical disease. Least affected subjects may have no symptoms or signs between clinical exacerbations. During these episodes they develop cough productive of purulent sputum associated with fever, occasional chest pain (localized to the area of the disease), a variable degree of breathlessness, and occasional haemoptysis. Clinical signs are non-specific but localized; medium to coarse crackles or wheeze may suggest the diagnosis particularly if symptoms date back to childhood or a severe acute respiratory illness (see later).

In more severely affected subjects sputum production becomes continuous (often large volumes) and varies from mucoid (clear) to frankly purulent, often changing during episodes of acute exacerbations. However, some patients continuously produce purulent secretions and these usually have the most extensive disease.

Patients often suffer from chronic or recurrent otitis and sinusitis (present in 30–40 per cent of patients). Indeed, postnasal drip, which occurs in approximately 75 per cent of patients, was thought to be important in the pathogenesis of bronchiectasis, although it may also reflect the same pathological processes in both the upper and lower respiratory tract.

Clinical signs

There are no specific signs for bronchiectasis. The patient may have a fruity, productive cough, signs of an associated disease (rheumatoid arthritis, lymphoedema, etc.), and finger clubbing (patients with persistent purulent bronchiectasis). The remaining signs may be minimal and confined to the chest, consisting of localized or widespread medium to coarse crackles, with or without wheeze. The most severely affected patients may have signs of cor pulmonale or respiratory failure.

Radiology

Plain radiographic examination of the chest may show many abnormalities (see Table 3). Collapse of the lung as indicated by atelectasis or 'crowding' of pulmonary vessels indicate an area of damage and consolidation that may become infected leading to bronchiectasis. On the other hand 'tram-line shadows' suggest bronchial wall oedema and cystic lesions (particularly if fluid filled) suggest saccular bronchiectasis.

The bronchogram (Fig. 3), once the 'gold standard' in the diagnosis of bronchiectasis, has been replaced by high resolution CAT scanning (Fig. 4). At present, all chest imaging should be regarded as complementary and used in conjunction with clinical features.

Secretion cultures

Bacteria are usually cultured from the secretions even at the end of successful antimicrobial therapy. Indeed it is often possible to identify and culture three or more different organisms from the same sample

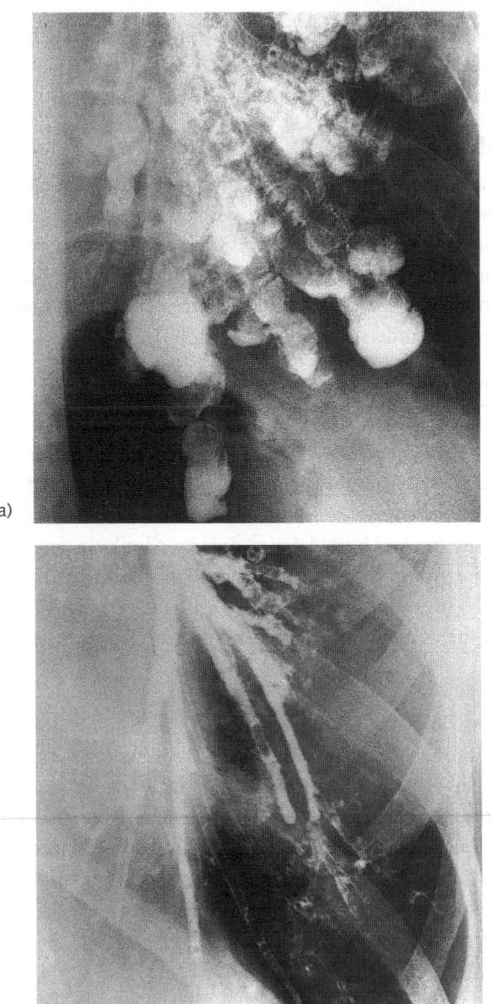

Fig. 3(a,b) Bronchograms of left lower lobe from two patients. (a) Demonstrates marked saccular dilatation usually seen as cystic lesions on plain chest radiograph. (b) Demonstrates long non-tapering bronchi characteristic of fusiform bronchiectasis that may demonstrate tram-line shadows on plain chest radiograph.

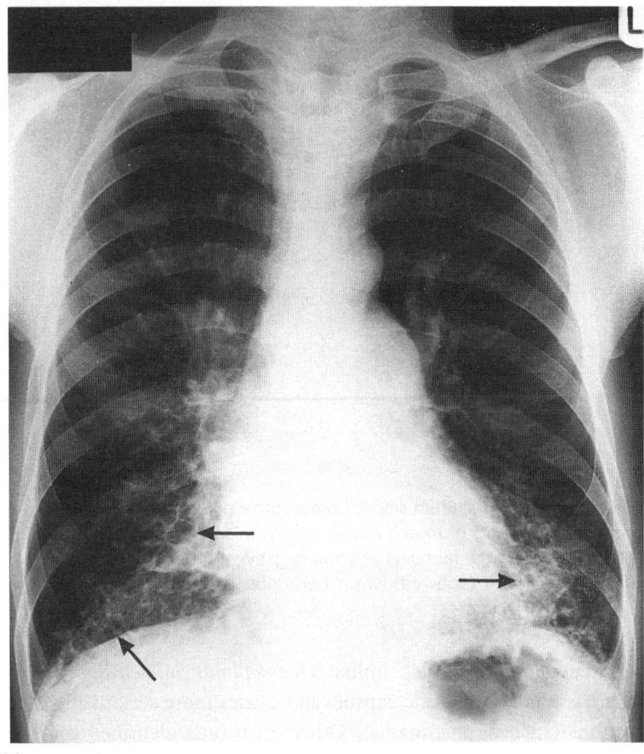

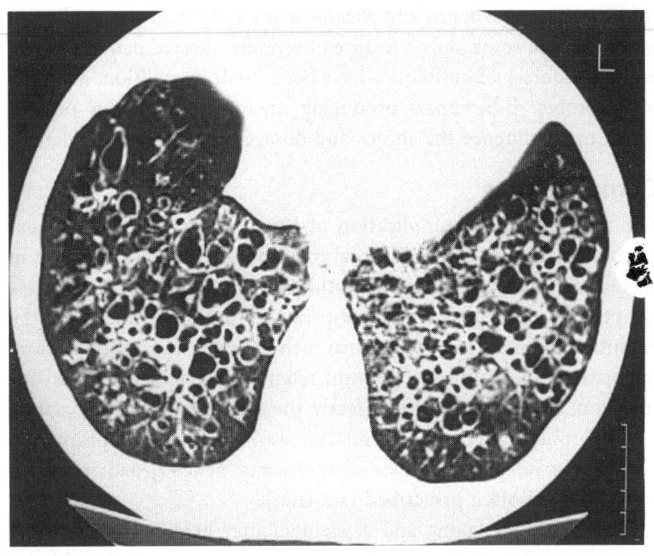

Fig. 4(a,b) Cystic lesions, arrowed on the chest radiograph, indicate the presence of saccular bronchiectasis demonstrated clearly on the corresponding CAT scan.

with aerobic and careful anaerobic techniques and the use of selective medium. Many of the organisms also colonize the mouth and hence can be reported as 'normal mouth commensals' in sputum samples that have been expectorated. Indeed, when there is concern over the infecting organism, direct aspiration of secretions using a transcricoid needle or fibre-optic bronchoscope has been recommended. However, the organisms isolated with these selective sampling techniques are usually the same ones seen in sputum and such invasive methods are rarely indicated.

Interpretation of sputum cultures requires collaboration between clinician, physiotherapist, and bacteriologist. It is important that the sample is sputum rather than saliva and this can be facilitated by the use of postural drainage. The sample should be analysed as soon as possible as standing or even cold storage may affect the culture of more fastidious organisms.

Gram stain is often useful to identify the presence of significant numbers of organisms (Fig. 5) and partially characterize them to help the initial choice of antibiotic. With careful culture techniques it is possible to identify most organisms present. Thereafter the significance of each isolate needs to be determined. It may be that all play a role by adding to the total bacterial load or that the appearance or an increase in the number of one of the organisms is the most important.

Some organisms are regularly identified and assumed to be important in determining the clinical status. Many of these organisms are rarely a problem in the normal lung. However, in the compromised lung (bronchitis, bronchiectasis, cystic fibrosis, etc.) they take on more significance. The organisms rarely cause invasive infections but colonize the airways and elicit an inflammatory response at this site. The organism most commonly isolated is *Haemophilus influenzae* (present in approximately 75 per cent of samples). It is unencapsulated

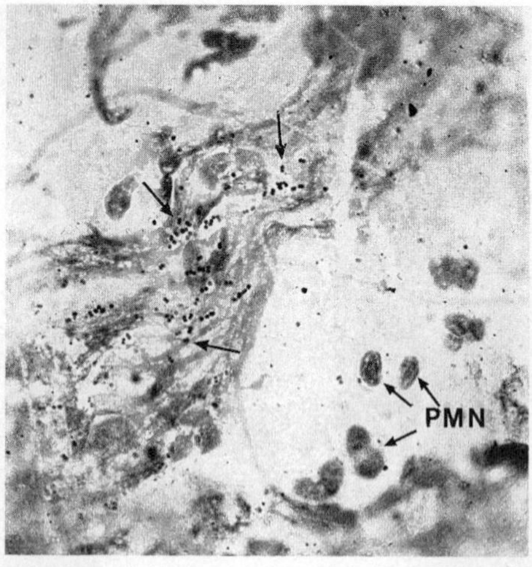

Fig. 5 Gram stain of sputum smear from a stable patient with bronchiectasis. Streaks of mucus can be seen with several neutrophils (PMN). There are large numbers of gram negative diplococci typical of *Moraxella catarrhalis* (arrowed) which were subsequently identified following primary culture.

(and hence non-typeable) unlike *Haemophilus influenzae* type B which has a polysaccharide capsule and causes more serious invasive infections (such as meningitis). Other organisms identified include *Streptococcus pneumoniae*, *Moraxella catarrhalis* (previous known as *Branhamella catarrhalis*), and *Pseudomonas aeruginosa* (mucoid type) which is more commonly a feature of severely-affected patients where multiple courses of antibiotics have been used. In addition, a variety of anaerobic, β-lactamase-producing organisms are often present which may influence the choice and dosage of antibiotic (see later).

Complications

The most common complication of bronchiectasis is an acute exacerbation. These vary from occasional to repetitive. An increase in symptoms (sputum volume, breathlessness, or chest pain) or new symptoms (haemoptysis and temperature) are all included in the definition of an exacerbation. Thus such episodes may reflect natural fluctuations in symptoms, sputum retention, increased airflow obstruction, as well as infection. Clearly, the regular presence of bacteria in the bronchial secretions tends to result in the assumption that they play a role in most exacerbations and hence broad spectrum antibiotics are often prescribed (see later).

Careful history taking and assessment may help clarify the exact cause. For instance, if the sputum is generally clear and remains so, it is unlikely that a bacterial infection is the cause of the deterioration and evidence of increased airflow obstruction with reversibility should be sought. Furthermore, even a change in sputum colour to purulent may indicate airflow obstruction as the cause if the cells in the sputum are eosinophils rather than neutrophils. The picture becomes more confusing when the sputum is usually purulent and symptoms worsen. A proportion of these episodes are also likely to represent increased airflow obstruction and evidence for this should still be sought and treated appropriately.

Nevertheless, many exacerbations are infective in origin. Features such as pyrexia, systemic symptoms (particularly if associated with a rise in ESR and/or acute phase proteins such as C reactive protein), and new changes on the chest radiograph are all suggestive. A proportion of these infective episodes (probably up to 30 per cent) are probably viral in origin and the remainder are presumed to be bacterial. Antimicrobial therapy is appropriate for such episodes whether presumed to be viral or bacterial since the former can result in a secondary bacterial 'infection'.

Haemoptysis

Mild transient haemoptysis occurs frequently in exacerbations of bronchiectasis and may vary from occasional streaks of blood to frank haemoptysis and from a single episode to recurrence with every exacerbation. The episodes are usually self-limiting but occasionally the haemoptysis can be severe and life-threatening and may require intervention (see under Management below).

Extrapulmonary spread of infection

Whereas brain abscesses used to occur as a result of vascular dissemination of organisms from the lung, this complication is rarely seen nowadays, presumably due to the prompt use of effective antibiotics. However, abscesses do not occur at other sites in the absence of any known host defence defects. Similarly, empyema has become less common in bronchiectasis in recent years although paradoxically empyema can occur in poorly treated lobar pneumonias resulting in the subsequent development of bronchiectasis.

Amyloidosis

Secondary amyloid has been recognized as a complication of bronchiectasis, although again it is now rare. It is assumed that most of the amyloidosis is caused by protein A deposition as with amyloidosis in other chronic disorders. However, it is possible that it may represent immunoglobulin light chain disease in some subjects receiving replacement therapy since many of the early IgG preparations were fragmented and hence contained free light chains.

Joint disease

A seronegative arthropathy has been described in bronchiectasis particularly during exacerbations of the disease. The symptoms can settle with appropriate antibacterial therapy suggesting it is directly related to the lung problem. The arthropathy may be the result of immune complexes formed between high levels of circulating immunoglobulins and bacterial antigens.

Vasculitis

Cutaneous vasculitis has been described in severe bronchiectasis with and without cystic fibrosis. Again the cause is thought to be circulating immune complexes.

Respiratory failure and cor pulmonale

A small proportion of the most severely affected patients deteriorate progressively and develop respiratory failure with clinical signs of hypoxia and CO_2 retention. In a proportion cor pulmonale will develop, eventually resulting in right heart failure. These complications are less common than previously, presumably as a result of improved management of the disease in its earlier stages.

Management

The majority of patients with bronchiectasis have minimal or undiagnosed disease. As such they have few symptoms most of the time and require or tolerate little or no medical intervention. Many of the symptoms (cough and sputum production) are often regarded as no more than a nuisance or a 'fact of life'. It is only when these symptoms become sufficient to interfere with 'normal' life that medical advice is sought and even then intervention may not alter the symptoms significantly.

Surgery

Surgery was once considered to be the main way to cure the disease but in most cases it proved ineffective. The disease was rarely localized to a single lobe or even lobes, although the severity in individual areas may have varied at the time of surgery. In addition, the underlying cause of the disease (immune deficiencies, etc.) still persisted in some patients. Furthermore, extensive chest surgery itself often led to atelectasis in the remaining lung during the postoperative phase, resulting in further lung damage. Many of the patients currently attending specialist clinics with bronchiectasis have had previous surgery aimed at 'curing' the disease. Thus, elective surgery is rarely undertaken except in a few limited cases including bronchiectasis following foreign body inhalation or severe lobar pneumonia in patients with persistent ill health.

However, surgery remains an option for persistent and extensive haemoptysis. Although most cases will settle spontaneously, this complication can be life-threatening. In such cases, localization of the bleeding to a single lobe or segment by bronchoscopy can result in a curative operation. More recently bronchial artery embolization has also proven effective and should be considered when lung function is poor.

Deficiency status

At present our understanding of deficiencies in the immune system is relatively superficial. Although gross deficiency states can be recognized (hypogammaglobulinaemia, IgA deficiency, complement deficiencies, neutrophil chemotactic defects) most cannot be treated. Furthermore, there may be many more subtle defects (epitope, specific IgG defects) that have yet to be identified. Thus, at present most patients with identified immune deficiencies have to be treated along conventional lines (see later).

However, replacement therapy is available for panhypogammaglobulinaemia, selective IgG and IgM deficiency, and IgG subclass (usually IgG2) deficiency. Treatment has been given as weekly intramuscular injections (often painful and ineffective) although now intravenous replacement is more effective and more acceptable to the patient. Selective IgA deficiency is not usually amenable to replacement therapy because the patient may have, or develop, IgA specific antibodies leading to anaphylaxis or immune complex deposition.

α_1-Antitrypsin (α_1AT) deficiency may be associated with bronchiectasis and this protein may also be involved in pathogenesis (see earlier). Replacement therapy is already approved in the US as a weekly infusion in patients with emphysema, and may prove useful in deficient subjects with bronchiectasis.

Other specific causes

Few of the other known causes of bronchiectasis respond to specific therapy. However, prompt therapy in allergic bronchopulmonary aspergillosis, relieving the obstruction, should modify the development of bronchiectasis. In addition, treatment of chronic rhinosinusitis and gastro-oesophageal reflux may improve respiratory symptoms. Finally, some cases of bronchiectasis associated with conditions such as rheumatoid arthritis may improve if the primary condition is treated adequately.

Physiotherapy

Postural drainage has long been considered a cornerstone of the management of bronchiectasis—because sputum accumulation might be harmful and clearance of damaged or obstructed areas might be beneficial. However, there is very little evidence to support this assumption.

With this reservation, many patients and doctors still advocate regular, twice-daily postural drainage, designed to allow the affected areas to be cleared at least temporarily. This does have the advantage of a marginal improvement in lung function (probably due to airways clearing) and a reduction in the frequency of cough and expectoration between episodes. Nevertheless, patient compliance (when assessed) has been shown to be poor.

More supervised physiotherapy during acute exacerbations, particularly when mucus expectoration becomes more difficult, appears helpful in relieving symptoms of chest discomfort and improving ventilation perfusion mismatching which may be critical in patients with respiratory failure. In addition, steam inhalations can also occasionally prove beneficial by facilitating expectoration whereas mucolytic therapy has largely fallen out of favour; treatment with human recombinant DNAse has proven ineffective in the absence of cystic fibrosis.

Drug therapy

At present, therapy is aimed predominantly at the airflow obstruction or infection that may be playing a critical role in the disease morbidity. However, as the pathogenesis of the condition becomes clarified alternative strategies are being considered and some have been assessed (see below).

Airflow obstruction

Many patients with bronchiectasis have relatively normal lung function but others develop progressive obstructive or restrictive lung disease. Indeed with the degree of inflammation, tissue damage, and repair (by fibrosis) it is surprising that lung function remains well preserved in many subjects. It is important to assess baseline lung function in all patients and review on a 6- to 12-monthly basis, particularly in those with most extensive and symptomatic disease.

Those with airflow obstruction should be investigated and treated for any reversibility, using a combination of inhaled β_2-agonists, anticholinergics, and steroids, as well as appropriate oral therapy.

The aetiology of any asthmatic component is uncertain (in the absence of allergic bronchopulmonary aspergillosis); independent asthma might simply coexist with bronchiectasis, or result from the airways inflammation due to bacterial colonization.

Airways infection

The airways of patients with bronchiectasis are usually colonized with bacteria. Though this may not represent 'infection' in the true sense, in many patients these organisms cause a host response leading to airways inflammation and persistent recruitment of neutrophils from the circulation resulting in purulent secretions (Fig. 5).

The precise role of these organisms in the pathology of bronchiectasis is uncertain but they are likely to contribute significantly. The mortality from bronchiectasis has changed following the introduction of antibiotics and complications such as amyloidosis, respiratory failure, and cor pulmonale have decreased. The Medical Research Council trial in 1957 demonstrated that prophylactic antibiotic therapy could prevent exacerbations and improve morbidity.

Indications for antibiotic therapy

Antibiotic therapy in bronchiectasis can be divided into short courses for exacerbations, prophylactic therapy to prevent or modify exacerbations, and continuous therapy. In general terms, management should go through each of these three stages with clinical response and observation determining introduction of the next step.

Acute exacerbation Although many acute infective exacerbations may be self-limiting or even viral in origin (up to 30 per cent) a course of antibiotic therapy appears helpful. Patients often develop an 'exacerbation' following an upper respiratory tract infection and it may be appropriate to start antibiotic therapy prior to the development of lower respiratory tract infection.

Recurrent exacerbations If a pattern of several 'exacerbations' each year develops, prophylactic therapy has to be considered dependent upon frequency or the morbidity associated with each episode. Prophylaxis may be confined to the winter months or given throughout the year, depending on the pattern. In general the threshold for the introduction of prophylactic therapy has been lowered as the potential pathogenic role of such episodes has become clearer.

Persistent infection Some patients with bronchiectasis persistently produce purulent secretions that contain numerous neutrophils—a state indicating a continuous host response in the lung to the organisms colonizing the airways. Such patients are more likely to show declining lung function.

The combination of bacterial colonization with an exuberant host response may lead to progressive deterioration through the release of proteinases, particularly elastase, from the neutrophils recruited to the lung. Neutrophil elastase has several potentially harmful effects: damage of ciliated epithelium and reduction of the cilia beat frequency; stimulation of mucus secretion and, together with its effect on cilia, reduction of mucociliary clearance; interference with other host defences by inactivating immunoglobulins and damaging the C3bi receptor on neutrophils, thus reducing bacterial phagocytosis and killing; degradation of lung connective tissues leading to further damage releasing fragments that are chemoattractant to neutrophils.

Bacterial toxins can also damage ciliated epithelia, and activated lung lymphocytes may damage host cells by antigen dependent cell cytotoxicity (ADCC). Figure 6 outlines the destructive, self-perpetuating sequence of these events. It is possible to break this sequence by successful antibiotic therapy.

Choice of antibiotic

Several factors influence the choice of the antibiotic used, including the sensitivity of the organisms involved and the need for the antibiotic to penetrate the scarred airways and secretions where the organisms reside.

The organism The predominant organism is *Haemophilus influenzae* (75 per cent) with *Streptococcus pneumoniae* and *Moraxella catarrhalis* making up most of the rest. These show good sensitivity to many orally-administered antibiotics although a degree of resistance is developing to some and in a small proportion of patients (particularly the most severely affected) *Pseudomonas aeruginosa* may become a persistent pathogen.

Haemophilus influenzae usually remains sensitive to amoxycillin although recent surveys show resistant rates ranging from 15–30 per cent across Europe. Resistance to erythromycin (19 per cent) is higher than that to ampicillin (15 per cent) in the UK, although resistance to tetracycline (1–2 per cent) and cephaclor (2 per cent) is lower and

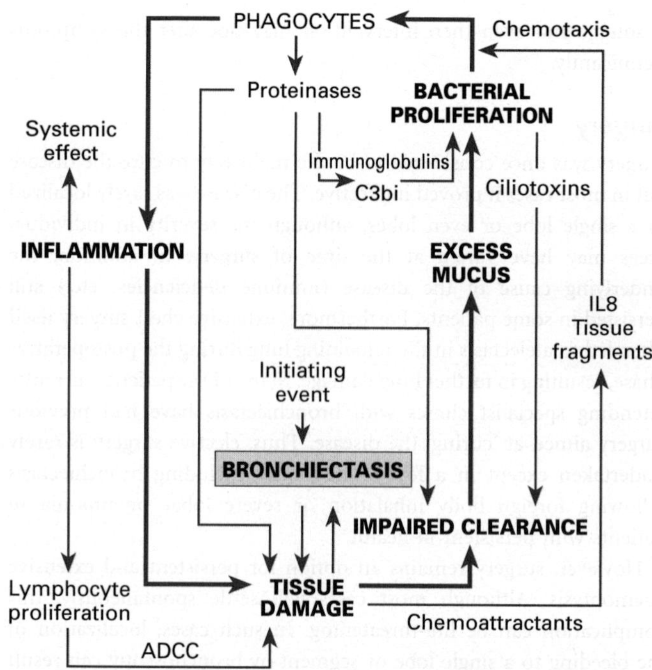

Fig. 6 Summary of the general concept of self perpetuation of lung damage in bronchiectasis. Following an initiating event that leads to the development of bronchiectasis, the tissue damage impairs mucociliary clearance resulting in sputum retention and bacterial proliferation. The subsequent recruitment of phagocytes may persist if the organisms are not cleared and a state of chronic inflammation is established. These various factors may amplify other steps in the sequence resulting in a failure of host defences and perpetuation of lung damage.

most organisms remain sensitive to co-trimoxazole and chloramphenicol. *Streptococcus pneumoniae* is still relatively sensitive to penicillin although erythromycin resistance is high whereas cephaclor resistance is negligible. *Moraxella catarrhalis* usually produces β-lactamase and is thus resistant to penicillins although macrolides and cephalosporins are still effective *in vitro*.

Antibiotics The initial choice usually rests between ampicillin/amoxycillin or cephaclor and clarithromycin (for penicillin-sensitive patients). Amoxycillin is easily tolerated, is fully absorbed from the gastrointestinal tract, and penetrates lung secretions well. However, as penicillin resistance of *Haemophilus influenzae* rises and the importance of *Moraxella catarrhalis* increases, the initial choice may alter to macrolides or cephalosporins. The role of newer antibiotics including the quinolones (e.g. Ciprofloxacin) is also becoming established although they should probably be reserved at present for specific indications such as penicillin resistance or *Pseudomonas* infection requiring oral therapy.

Acute exacerbation If the patient usually has no symptoms or their sputum is usually mucoid, an infective exacerbation is indicated by the production of purulent sputum and this usually responds to a short course (7–10 days) of amoxycillin or a similar alternative in conventional doses (e.g. 250–500 mg three times daily for amoxycillin).

In patients usually producing mucopurulent or purulent secretions management is more difficult. These patients have a significant bacterial load in the lung resulting in neutrophil recruitment during the stable state. If symptoms suggest an infective exacerbation it is still advisable to prescribe an antibiotic course. Mucopurulent sputum often becomes clear but may return to its pretreatment state within a few weeks although the symptoms of the exacerbation may not return. Patients with purulent sputum may notice no change in sputum colour unless high doses of antibiotics are used (amoxycillin 3 g twice daily; cephaclor 3–4 g daily), although symptoms may settle. If the sputum clears it may only be for 2–4 days, suggesting that the organisms responsible have only been suppressed temporarily. The failure of sputum colour to clear or the development of rapid relapse suggests long-term management may be required (see below).

For severe exacerbations where oral therapy has failed, or may not be appropriate, it is usual to embark upon broad spectrum intravenous therapy, especially to cover the less common organisms. In this instance initial Gram stain may help but often therapy remains empirical. Many agents can prove effective in individual cases including the aminoglycosides (when *Pseudomonas* is expected) or Imipenem with or without amoxycillin and metronidazole. Choice and dosage will depend upon individual hospital policy and local resistance patterns.

Prophylaxis Prophylactic therapy is indicated in patients who have frequent exacerbations and this can usually be achieved with oral therapy. In the original Medical Research Council trial (1957) the agent used successfully was tetracycline given twice a week and it should be achievable by other oral agents. Prophylactic therapy is also used for patients who persistently produce purulent secretions, in an attempt to 'break the vicious circle'. Although such patients appear clinically stable, studies have shown that continuous antibiotic therapy improves well being and reduces plasma acute phase proteins, suggesting that the presence of purulent sputum alone is associated with a low grade, systemic response.

The choice of regimen is influenced by the patient's clinical state prior to therapy. Those with mucopurulent secretions usually respond to conventional doses of antibiotic orally. However, patients whose secretions are usually deeply purulent (dark green) usually require high dosage orally (e.g. amoxycillin 3 g twice daily) or even nebulized (e.g. amoxycillin 500 mg twice daily). With such a regimen the response (clearance of secretions) can be maintained (Fig. 7). Clinical experience suggests that patients treated this way have few clinical exacerbations and, despite concern, the emergence of resistant organisms is unusual providing therapy is maintained.

Clinical exacerbations in patients treated prophylactically require careful sputum assessment and often short courses of parenteral therapy before returning to the usual regimen. Some patients treated successfully with prophylactic therapy may remain well (with mucoid sputum) even if treatment is stopped. Thus it seems sensible to attempt withdrawal of therapy after 4–6 months, but early relapse would indicate that prophylactic therapy should be long term.

A general summary of these principles and guidelines is indicated in Fig. 8.

Immunization

The role of immunization in bronchiectasis is uncertain. As with other forms of chronic obstructive pulmonary disease (COPD), regular immunization against influenza virus may be considered, but there are no formal studies of its efficacy. It is recommended in the most severely affected patients where severe influenza infection could precipitate respiratory failure and death.

Immunization with bacterial antigens is more contentious. The immunodominant antigens for *Haemophilus influenzae* and *Streptococcus pneumoniae* have yet to be characterized. Polyvalent vaccines are unlikely to benefit the patient since they are usually persistently exposed to the antigens of the bacteria that already colonize the airways and usually have excessive antibodies to bacterial antigens, both locally (in the lung) and systemically. The administration of extra bacterial antigen may thus be harmful. At present, immunization with polyvalent bacterial vaccines would be inappropriate for most patients with bronchiectasis.

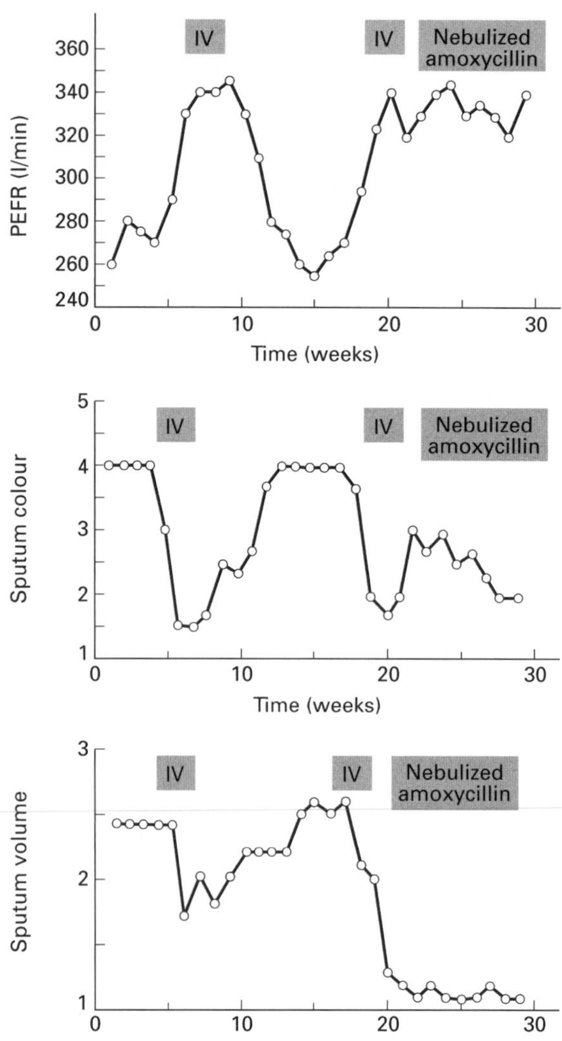

Fig. 7 Flow chart of PEFR and sputum characteristics of a patient with bronchiectasis. Sputum colour and volume are given as arbitrary units. High values for colour reflect the degree of purulent (1 = mucoid) and for volume (a value of 1 reflects little or not sputum/day). Following a 2-week course of intravenous therapy (IV), PEFR increases, sputum colour improves (becoming mucoid), and sputum volume decreases. However, there is a gradual return to the pretreatment state and a further course of IV therapy followed by regular nebulized antibiotic improves and maintains the lung function and sputum values.

Alternative therapy

As the inflammatory processes involved in bronchiectasis have become clarified, there has been interest in alternative ways of intervening.

Immunosuppressive therapy

The lung shows many features of an overexuberant immune response, some of which may be directed against autoantigens. Thus, immunosuppressive therapy may have a role in some patients. Corticosteroids

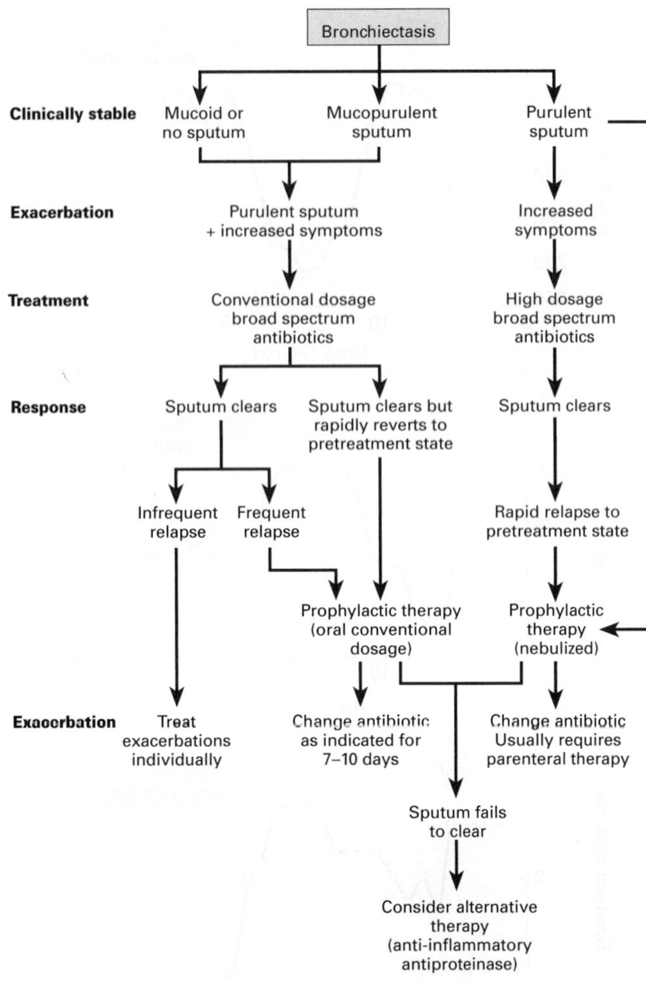

Fig. 8 Flow chart for the management of bronchiectasis, indicating treatment protocols. Note patients are assessed sequentially as indicated by symptoms with the exception of those who persistently expectorate purulent sputum where a strong case can be made for prophylactic therapy from the start.

have been used successfully in patients with severe endstage bronchiectasis related to cystic fibrosis. Furthermore, some patients with bronchiectasis associated with rheumatoid arthritis have shown dramatic improvement in their lung symptoms following aggressive immunosuppressive therapy for their joint disease.

At present, immunosuppressive treatment should be reserved for the most severely affected patients where conventional therapy has failed. Patients should be carefully monitored to ensure a positive clinical response with no detrimental effect occurs.

Neutrophil modulation

As recruitment of neutrophils to the lung results in release of harmful proteinases it may be possible to modulate their response. Non-steroidal anti-inflammatory agents can reduce neutrophil responses and may be considered in the management of severely affected patients.

Antiproteinases

Elastase activity is reduced or abolished and two of its effects—release of the chemoattractant IL-8 and damage to the C3bi phagocytic receptor on neutrophils—have been reversed during antiprotease therapy. It is unknown whether this approach affects the clinical features and progression of this disease.

Transplantation

Lung and heart/lung transplantation is being undertaken successfully in patients with severe endstage lung disease with or without cor pulmonale. Patients tend to be older than those with cystic fibrosis which affects their acceptance onto the programmes.

Further reading

Hill, S. L., Burnett, D., Hewetson, K. A., and Stockley, R. A. (1988). The response of patients with purulent bronchiectasis to antibiotics for 4 months. *Quarterly Journal of Medicine*, **66**, 163–73.

Medical Research Council (1957). Prolonged antibiotic treatment of severe bronchiectasis. *British Medical Journal*, **2**, 255–9.

Murphy, T. F. and Sethi, S. (1992). Bacterial infection in chronic obstructive pulmonary disease. *American Review of Respiratory Disease*, **146**, 1067–83.

Stockley, R. A. (1987). Bronchiectasis—new therapeutic approaches based on pathogenesis. *Clinics in Chest Medicine*, **8**, 481–94.

Whitwell, F. (1952). A study of the pathology and pathogenesis of bronchiectasis. *Thorax*, **7**, 213–39.

Chapter 4.17

Chronic obstructive pulmonary disease

N. B. Pride and R. A. Stockley with a contribution from R. W. Carrell and D. A. Lomas

Definitions and terminology

The term chronic obstructive pulmonary disease (**COPD**) has gradually displaced 'chronic bronchitis and emphysema' as a label for the type of airways obstruction seen predominantly in smokers and exsmokers. The emphasis on obstruction is useful, because the severity of obstruction is the major factor determining symptoms and prognosis. The non-specificity of the term reflects the difficulty in life of defining the respective roles of primary airways disease and emphysema in causing obstruction to airflow. Emphysema—defined as an 'increase beyond the normal in the size of air spaces distal to the terminal bronchiole accompanied by destruction of their walls and without obvious fibrosis'—is only detected reliably in life by imaging and lung function tests when it is relatively severe. In contrast 'chronic bronchitis', which is a synonym for chronic mucus hypersecretion, is easily diagnosed by the presence of chronic cough and expectoration not attributable to other lung disease. Thirty years ago, it was thought there was a direct connection between 'chronic bronchitis' and the development of airways narrowing. This has not proved to be the case; the pathological changes responsible for chronic mucus hypersecretion are predominantly in the central conducting airways which are not significantly narrowed by the accompanying gland hyperplasia and mucosal inflammation. The airways disease which contributes to the obstruction to airflow is in the smaller airways (Table 1). Both processes are strongly related to smoking, but many smokers have

Table 1 Serial distribution of airways resistance

	Normal (cmH_2O/l/s) (% of total)	Severe COPD (cmH_2O/l/s) (% of total)
Extrathoracic airway	0.5 (33)	0.5 (8)
Major intrathoracic conducting airways	0.5 (33)	1.0 (17)
Peripheral airways (<3 mm diameter)	0.5 (33)	4.5 (75)
Total	1.5 (100)	6.0 (100)

The values are for a typical patient with severe COPD during tidal breathing via the mouth. Extrathoracic resistance would be at least 1.0 cmH_2O/l/s when breathing through the nose.

chronic cough and expectoration without significant airways obstruction, while perhaps 25 per cent of smokers with obstruction of the peripheral airways do not have chronic expectoration. Hence, the term 'chronic bronchitis' has become a source of confusion in clinical practice.

Conventionally, other specific causes of diffuse, largely irreversible obstruction of the intrathoracic airways (Table 2), with the exception of α_1-antitrypsin deficiency, are excluded from the diagnosis of COPD.

The most troublesome diagnostic aspect of COPD is the overlap with chronic incompletely reversible asthma, a common alternative diagnosis in middle-aged and older patients. This distinction has never been clarified precisely; almost all patients with COPD show some short-term improvement after using bronchodilators, although this is usually less than 15 per cent of predicted forced expiratory volume in 1 s (FEV_1). Overlap terms such as 'chronic asthmatic bronchitis' are commonly used because of this difficulty. From the point of view of current therapy the distinction between COPD and chronic asthma is irrelevant (provided that a trial of corticosteroids is made in all severely obstructed patients) because the same drugs are used in asthma and COPD, but this may not be the case in future (specific treatments for α_1-antitrypsin deficiency and cystic fibrosis are already being developed). However, the two conditions have a very different prognosis for progression and mortality (much worse in COPD), and probably a different pathogenesis, so that the distinction is of critical importance for investigators and epidemiologists.

Aetiology (Table 3)

Clinically significant COPD arises following many years of a moderately accelerated decline in lung function in those smokers who are susceptible to the effects of cigarettes (Fig. 1). There is a wide variation in the susceptibility of individual smokers to develop progressive airflow obstruction, suggesting that other important risk factors remain to be identified. In the US, mortality rates for COPD in cigarette smokers are at least 10 times those in never-smokers; COPD causes about 15 per cent of all smoking-related deaths compared with 28 per cent attributed to lung cancer. Smoking promotes inflammation

Table 2 Some 'specific' causes of chronic airflow obstruction

Cystic fibrosis	Bronchiectasis
α_1-Antitrypsin deficiency	Bronchopulmonary dysplasia
Hypogammaglobulinaemia	Byssinosis
Obstructive bronchiolitis Irritant gas inhalation Virus infections Connective tissue disorders Following lung or bone marrow transplant Mineral dust inhalation	

Table 3 Risk factors for the development of chronic obstructive pulmonary disease

Increasing age	Ventilatory impairment reflects cumulative lifetime smoking history
Smoking habit	Some relation to number of cigarettes smoked per day; risk not reduced by reduction in tar content
Gender	Controversial, women may be more susceptible
Environmental pollution	Greater urban than rural death rates; linked to particulate pollution. Indoor pollution important in some societies
Socio-economic status	More common in individuals of low socio-economic status
Diet	High fish and antioxidant intake may reduce risk in smokers
Occupation	Cadmium workers probably have increased risk of emphysema, and coal and gold miners, and cotton and grain dust workers of chronic airways obstruction; many other inorganic dusts cause mucus hypersecretion but in most cases obstruction is mild or absent
Genetic factors	Severe serum α_1-antitrypsin deficiency is the strongest single risk, but is rare
Birthweight and childhood respiratory infections	Mortality related to weight at birth and at 1 year; chest infections in early life predict adult COPD

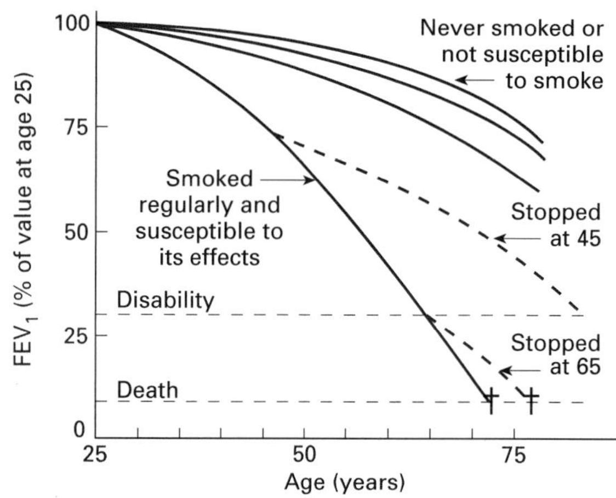

Fig. 1 Development of impairment of FEV_1 in a susceptible smoker as proposed by Fletcher and Peto. In practice there will be a range of rates of decline in FEV_1 in susceptible smokers. On stopping smoking there is no improvement in FEV_1 but the subsequent loss of FEV_1 is similar to that in healthy never-smokers.
(For source see OTM3, p. 2768.)

in the periphery of the lung either due to a direct toxic effect of tobacco smoke (e.g. oxidants) or by recruiting neutrophils and other inflammatory cells into the airways and airspaces. Occupational dust exposure undoubtedly plays a part. In some countries, domestic environmental factors may be of great importance; for instance in New Guinea household pollution due to heating and cooking within a small space is important, and COPD is more common in women than men. The established risk factors shown in Table 3 only account for a small part of the variability in the susceptibility of smokers to develop COPD. Two popular hypotheses have been that the susceptible smoker has a pre-existing asthmatic constitution with airways hyperresponsiveness which accentuates the effects of smoking (Dutch hypothesis) and that repeated bronchopulmonary infections lead to permanent airways damage and hence to COPD (British hypothesis). The role of repeated infections has not been proven in otherwise healthy smokers but may be important in young children; unidentified bronchiectasis may contribute to high reported rates of COPD in less developed countries.

Epidemiology

Prevalence

The high prevalence of chronic cough and expectoration in the UK was recognized long before cigarette smoking was widely adopted, but only became a subject for medical research after the smog disasters in London in the 1950s. At that time 20 to 30 per cent of middle-aged men had chronic cough and sputum; with the reduction in active smoking, environmental SO_2, and particulate pollution, this had dropped to about 15 to 20 per cent of middle-aged men and about 8 per cent of middle-aged women by the late 1980s.

COPD is the commonest cause of impaired spirometry in the population; by middle age about 18 per cent of male and 14 per cent of female smokers have FEV_1 values more than two standard deviations below the mean predicted values, in contrast to rates of about 7 per cent in men and women who have never smoked. These rates are probably somewhat higher than those observed in the USA. Although the rates for spirometric impairment are broadly similar to those for chronic cough, as already discussed, both changes are not necessarily found in the same individual smokers.

Mortality

Since about 1970, male mortality from COPD in the UK has steadily fallen in all except men aged more than 75 years. The total mortality in women is about one-third of that in men, but there is some upward trend over the same period, presumably reflecting increased smoking by women since the Second World War. Other countries, including the USA, report increasing mortality from COPD over the same period, mainly in elderly men. Because cigarette smoking has declined more dramatically in the US than in the UK, this is somewhat surprising; one factor may be that COPD was underdiagnosed in the US in the period before 1970. In many countries the expansion of cigarette smoking is relatively recent and, as with lung cancer, the peak of COPD mortality probably has not been reached. Reliable international comparisons are sparse, but it appears that death rates from COPD are particularly high in the UK and Eastern Europe and low in Southern Europe, Scandinavia, and Japan.

Within the UK mortality is higher in conurbations than in rural areas, and there are considerable regional variations with the lowest rates in south-east England. In part this may reflect the importance of poor socioeconomic status in determining mortality. Although cigarette smoking is now most prevalent in persons of low socioeconomic status, the mortality trend was evident at a time when cigarette smoking was relatively independent of this factor. Indeed, downward trends in overall mortality for chronic respiratory disease in the UK cannot all be explained by improvements in air pollution or reduction in cigarette smoking, and may reflect changes in social conditions and nutrition in early life.

Pathophysiology

Morbid anatomy

Changes are found throughout the tracheobronchial tree and lungs. In the central conducting airways, there is enlargement of submucosal glands and an increase in surface goblet cells which also extend into more peripheral airways than in normal subjects. There is often some evidence of persistent airway inflammation even during the interval between acute airway infections, but eosinophils and loss of surface epithelium are less prominent than in asthma although ciliary function is impaired. There may be some increase in airways smooth muscle.

In the smaller bronchi and bronchioles there are inflammatory changes, increased intraluminal mucus, thickening of all elements of the airway wall (although less marked than in asthma), fibrosis, and stenosis. These changes are the major source of the increased resistance to airflow in COPD (Table 1).

Emphysema is classified by its location: confined to the centre of a lobule (centrilobular, syn. centriacinar), diffuse throughout the lobule (panlobular, syn. panacinar) or paraseptal, a variety occurring around the periphery of lobes and associated with very little disturbance to lung function. Centrilobular emphysema is surrounded by macroscopically normal lung, tends to be more obvious in the upper lobes, and is not well identified by *in vivo* imaging. There is usually evidence of active inflammation in both centrilobular emphysema and in panlobular emphysema. Consequences of the emphysematous destruction of airspace walls are loss of pulmonary capillary bed and loss of attachments between alveolar and bronchiolar walls; these attachments are responsible for the normal increase in bronchiolar diameter as the lung expands, and so their loss may contribute to the airways obstruction. The relative contributions of airspace destruction and 'intrinsic' disease of the airway wall to the development of airways obstruction remain uncertain. The major effect of macroscopically visible emphysema (Fig. 2) is functionally to remove areas of the lung, because these areas receive little ventilation or blood flow. The importance of recognizing macroscopic emphysema may well be that it is associated with lesser degrees of airspace enlargement and loss of surface area in the remaining macroscopically normal and still functioning lung.

In advanced COPD there are also changes in the heart and pulmonary circulation (thickening of the walls of pulmonary arteries, particularly vascular smooth muscle in the media, and right ventricular hypertrophy) and enlargement of the carotid body. These changes are probably secondary to alveolar hypoxia. Loss of skeletal muscle mass, including the diaphragm, frequently occurs in advanced disease.

Cellular and molecular events

Our concepts of the molecular and cellular processes involved date back to the original identification of five subjects with a deficiency of the α_1 protein band seen on paper electrophoresis of serum. Three of these five subjects had severe emphysema (Fig. 2) at a relatively

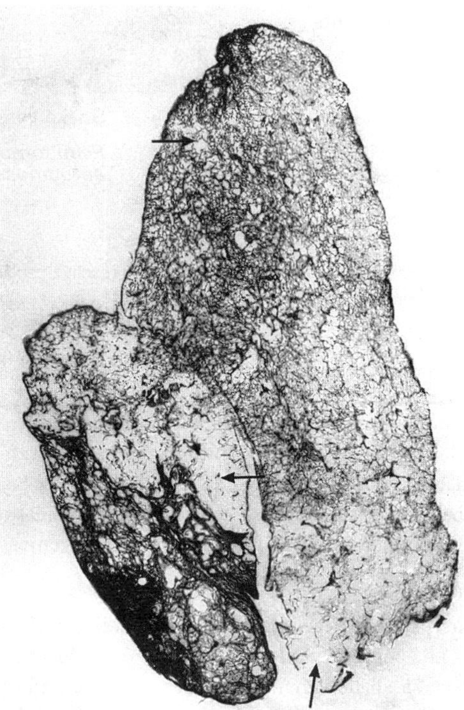

Fig. 2 Thin-layer section of whole lung of a patient with emphysema related to α_1-antitrypsin deficiency. Emphysematous 'holes' are seen throughout the lung parenchyma.

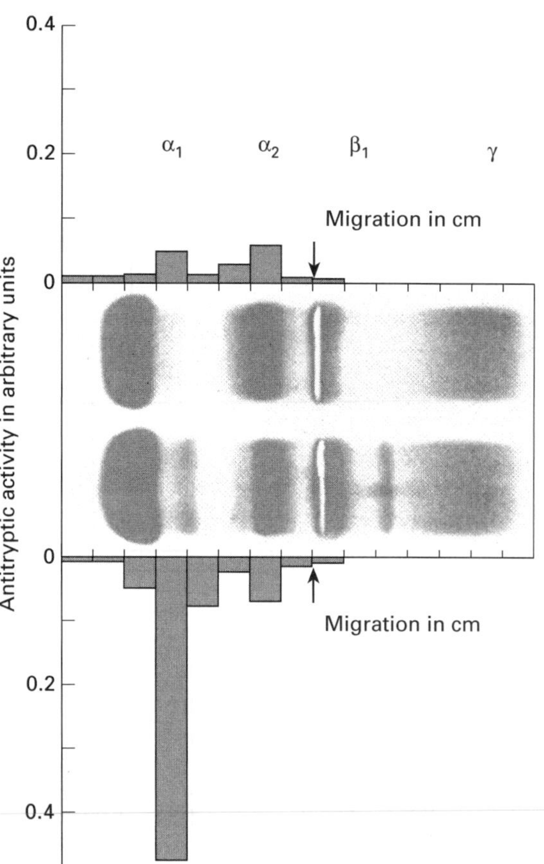

Fig. 3 Paper electrophoresis of plasma from a patient with α_1-antitrypsin deficiency (upper) is shown next to that of a normal subject (lower). The antitryptic activity of fractions from each protein band is shown, confirming that most of the activity is in the α_1 band.
(For source see OTM3, p. 2770.)

young age. Subsequent studies confirmed that the missing α_1 band was responsible for most of the antitryptic activity of the blood (Fig. 3) and contained a proteinase inhibitor which was called α_1-antitrypsin (also known more recently as α_1-proteinase inhibitor). Later it was shown that a proteolytic enzyme (papain) could produce airspace enlargement in animals. Thus, emphysema might occur in subjects with α_1-antitrypsin deficiency because an enzyme, normally controlled by the inhibitor, was able to digest lung tissues unopposed. Human neutrophil elastase was shown to produce emphysema in experimental animals. α_1-antitrypsin is the most potent inhibitor of this enzyme and hence neutrophil elastase became accepted as the most likely mediator of chronic lung damage. The enzyme is produced during neutrophil differentiation, and is packaged and stored in the azurophil granules prior to release of the cells from the bone marrow. Neutrophil elastase is a serine proteinase with a range of substrates. It degrades elastin; hence its ability to produce emphysema. It digests several other lung connective tissues including type IV collagen and fibronectin. Also it damages ciliated epithelium *in vitro*, reduces the beat frequency of cilia, induces mucus gland hyperplasia *in vivo*, and is an important secretagogue for mucus glands *in vitro* and may therefore mediate bronchial damage. Neutrophil elastase can also degrade immunoglobulins and the C3bi receptor on neutrophils that is responsible for phagocytosis and bacterial killing, and so reduce the efficiency of several other lung host defences. It also increases IL-8 production by bronchial epithelial cells, which is a potent neutrophil chemoattractant. These events are summarized in Fig. 4.

The proteinase–antiproteinase theory of COPD

Thus proteinases (particularly neutrophil elastase) damage many lung proteins and tissues. The lung and plasma contain inhibitors which can inactivate these enzymes and hence protect the lung. Inflammatory damage occurs when the enzyme activity exceeds the capacity of the inhibitors to inactivate them. Provided that the inhibitors dominate, lung damage is limited. This concept is the basis of the proteinase–antiproteinase theory of COPD. There are three ways that this balance may be disturbed: (1) decrease in protective inhibitor (as with α_1-antitrypsin deficiency); (2) increase in enzyme load (as with excess neutrophil recruitment); (3) a combination of (1) and (2).

Decreased inhibitor

This could be the result of either a primary or secondary defect, that is an absolute deficiency of the proteinase inhibitors or a relative deficiency due to inactivation of the protein present, thereby reducing its functional capacity. Evidence exists for both kinds of 'deficiency'.

α_1-Antitrypsin deficiency

People of European descent are particularly prone to disease arising from a genetic deficiency of the plasma protein α_1-antitrypsin. This is a 394-amino acid, 52 kDa, acute phase glycoprotein synthesized by the liver and by macrophages and present in the plasma at a concentration of 1.5 to 3.5 g/l. It functions as an inhibitor of a range of proteolytic enzymes but its primary role is to inhibit neutrophil elastase. Activated neutrophil leucocytes release elastase to break down connective tissue at sites of inflammation. This breakdown is limited by the antielastase activity of α_1-antitrypsin but if the plasma concentration of this protein falls below 40 per cent of normal, as in

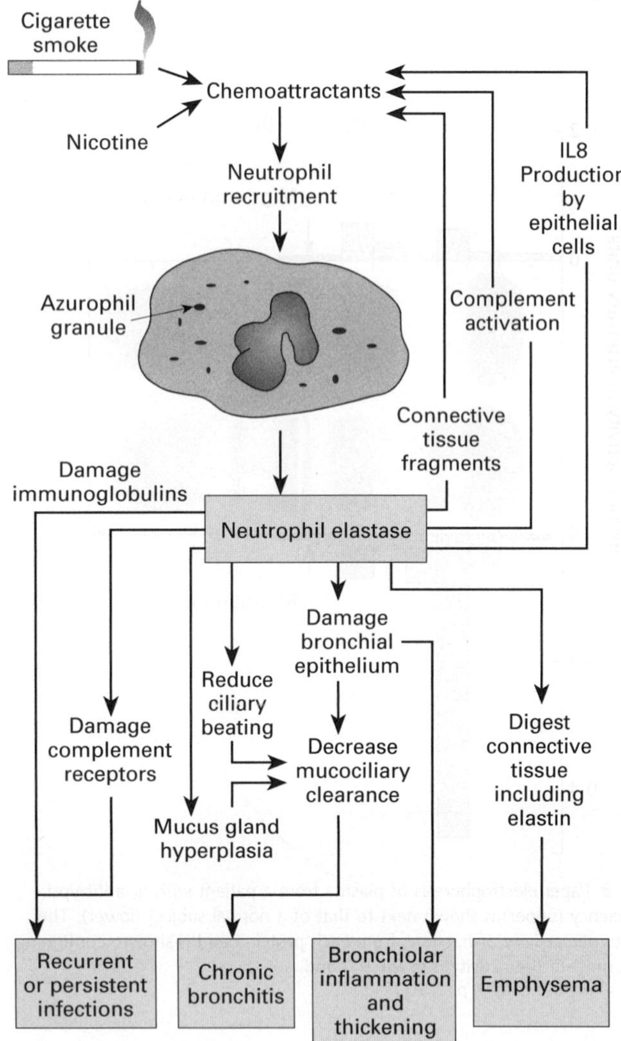

Fig. 4 Diagrammatic representation of some of the pathways involved in the perpetuation of features of COPD by neutrophil elastase. Development of lung damage alters lung defences, and destruction of tissues may perpetuate neutrophil recruitment leading to further damage.

genetic deficiency, then unimpeded tissue destruction may ensue. The most vulnerable tissue is the elastic connective tissue of the lung and the major consequence of α_1-antitrypsin deficiency is the premature onset of emphysema. This association between the deficiency of a protease inhibitor and the loss of lung elasticity has drawn attention to the way in which other factors, particularly cigarette smoking, contribute to the onset of emphysema.

Structure and function

α_1-Antitrypsin is the archetype of the serine protease inhibitor, or serpin, superfamily, members of which have closely related structures and functions. These inhibitors control the various inflammatory cascades, including coagulation (antithrombin), complement activation (C1-inhibitor), and fibrinolysis (α_2-antiplasmin). A surprising member of the family is angiotensinogen, which retains the same overall structure as the other members of the family but has lost its function as a protease inhibitor.

α_1-Antitrypsin functions by presenting its reactive centre methionine residue on an exposed loop of the molecule such that it

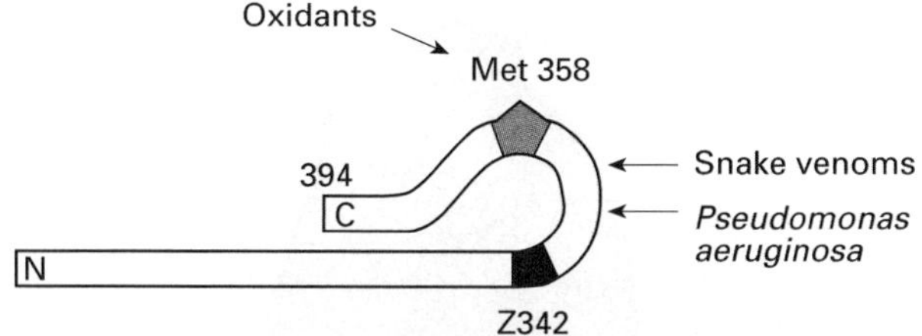

Fig. 5 α_1-Antitrypsin: inactivation by oxidation of the reactive centre methionine residue or by cleavage of the reactive centre loop.

forms an ideal substrate for the enzyme neutrophil elastase (Fig. 5). The exact fit between enzyme and inhibitor causes them to form a tightly bound 1:1 complex, which inhibits the enzyme and allows it to be eliminated from circulation. A reduction in the activity of antitrypsin may result from genetic deficiency, from oxidation of the methionine residue, or from cleavage of the reactive centre loop.

Genetic deficiency

α_1-Antitrypsin is subject to genetic variation resulting from mutations in the 12.2 kb, 7-exon gene at q31–31.2 on chromosome 14 (Table 4). Over 75 allelic variants have been reported and classified using the Pi (protease inhibitor) nomenclature, which assesses antitrypsin mobility in isoelectric focusing analysis. Mutations are inherited by simple Mendelian trait; the normal genotype is designated PiMM, a heterozygote for the Z gene is PiMZ, and a homozygote is PiZZ.

The medically interesting variants are those associated with deficiency: namely the S and Z mutants and the uncommon null (non-production) gene. Most important are the S and Z variants of α_1-antitrypsin, which are commonly found in Europeans. About 6 per cent of people of Northern European descent are heterozygotes for the S variant (PiMS) and 3 to 4 per cent for the Z variant (PiMZ).

Each of the deficiency genes results in a characteristic decrease in the plasma concentration of α_1-antitrypsin; the S variant forms 60 per cent of the normal M concentration and the Z variant 15 per cent. The critical level for health is a plasma concentration of at least 40 per cent of normal and therefore the common heterozygote states MZ (60 per cent) and MS (80 per cent) and the S homozygote (60 per cent) do not pose a threat to health. However the ZZ homozygote (15 per cent) and the SZ heterozygote (40 per cent) do predispose to emphysema.

One in 10 Northern Europeans is a carrier of a deficiency gene and 1 in 2500 has the PiZZ genotype which predisposes to disease. A greater number again are PiSZ heterozygotes which results in 'at risk' plasma levels of α_1-antitrypsin.

Molecular pathology of S and Z variants of α_1-antitrypsin

Z α_1-antitrypsin results from the substitution of a positively charged lysine for a negatively charged glutamic acid at position 342. The α_1-antitrypsin gene is normally translated but 85 per cent of the Z antitrypsin is retained within the endoplasmic reticulum, with only 15 per cent entering the circulation. The Z mutation distorts the relationship between the reactive centre loop and the β-pleated (A) sheet that forms the major feature of the molecule (Fig. 5). The consequent perturbation in structure allows the reactive centre loop of one antitrypsin molecule to lock into the A sheet of a second to form fibril-like loop–sheet polymers. The formation of these polymers is temperature and concentration dependent and localized to the endoplasmic reticulum of the hepatocyte (Fig. 6(a)). These chains of polymers become interwoven to form the insoluble aggregates which are the hallmark of antitrypsin liver disease (Fig. 6(b)). The S variant of α_1-antitrypsin is due to a valine→glutamic acid mutation at position 264. It also perturbs the structure of the protein to allow the formation of loop–sheet polymers which are retained within the hepatocyte. The rate of polymer formation is much slower than in the Z variant, which accounts for the absence of lung disease and the milder plasma deficiency.

Oxidation and inactivation

The need for an exact fit between enzyme and inhibitor provides a molecular explanation for the causative relationship between cigarette smoking and emphysema. The reactive centre of methionine of α_1-antitrypsin is readily oxidized to the much larger methionine sulphoxide, with a consequent loss of function as an inhibitor of elastase. Thus the oxidants released by stimulated neutrophils can oxidize the key methionine residue and switch off the activity of α_1-antitrypsin. Normally this switch mechanism is advantageous in allowing elastase activity to continue in the immediate vicinity of an inflammatory focus.

Cleavage and inactivation

The exposed molecular loop of antitrypsin renders it vulnerable to inactivation by other proteases such as those contained in snake venoms. The damaging effects of pulmonary infection with *Pseudomonas aeruginosa* is similarly explained by the secretion of a protease that specifically cleaves the exposed loop of α_1-antitrypsin allowing fulminant damage to lung connective tissue (Fig. 5).

Clinical features

α_1-Antitrypsin deficiency and emphysema

Patients usually present with increasing dyspnoea and weight loss, with cor pulmonale and polycythaemia occurring late in the course of the disease. Chest radiographs typically show bilateral basal emphysema with paucity and pruning of the basal pulmonary vessels. Upper lobe vascularization is relatively normal. Ventilation perfusion radioisotope scans and angiography also show abnormalities with a lower zone distribution. Lung function tests are typical for emphysema.

Decline in lung function in health and disease

After the age of 30 years in healthy non-smokers, the forced expiratory volume decreases by 35 ml/year, although there is considerable individual variation. By old age, most people will have an appreciable

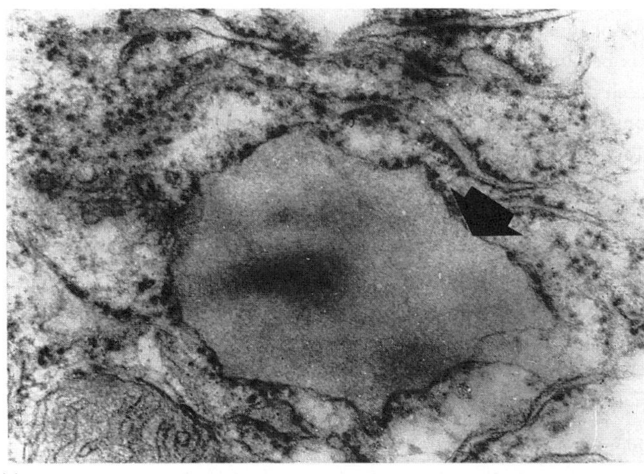

(a)

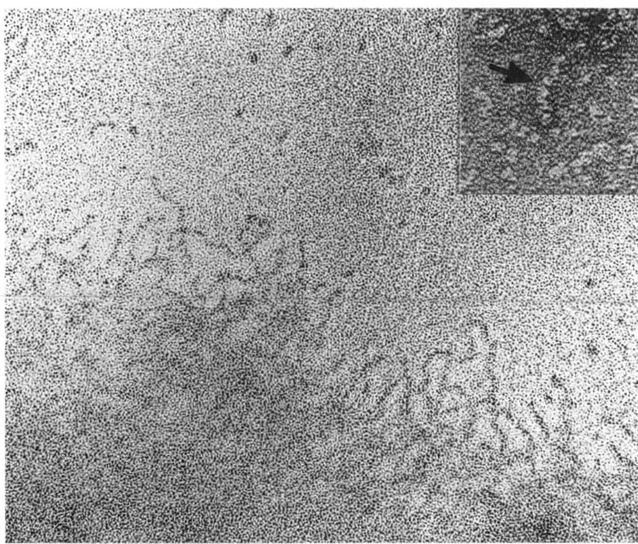

(b)

Fig. 6(a,b) (a) Electron microscopy (20 000 × magnification) of a hepatocyte from a Z homozygote showing a massive inclusion (arrow) in the endoplasmic reticulum. (b) Electron microscopy (222 000 × magnification) of Z antitrypsin loop-sheet polymers *in vitro* (inset and arrowed) and isolated from a patient undergoing liver transplantation for Z antitrypsin cirrhosis. The *in vitro* material is negatively stained with uranyl acetate whilst the hepatic inclusions are highlighted with platinum rotary shadowing.

Table 4 Summary of some of the mechanisms involved in α_1-antitrypsin deficiency

Allele	Genetic defect	Effect on α_1-antitrypsin
Z	Point mutation Glu^{342}GAG-Lys AAG	Spontaneous polymerization and reduced secretion
S	Point mutation Glu^{264} GAA-Val GTA	Increased intracellular catabolism
NULL$_{\text{isola de procida}}$	Gene deletion Deletion of 10 kb of the gene	No transcription
NULL$_{\text{Bellingham}}$	Point mutation Lys^{217}AAG-STOP TAG	mRNA degraded; no α_1-antitrypsin is made
NULL$_{\text{granite falls}}$	Frameshift nucleotide deletion Tyr^{160} TAC delete C-5′ shift STOP^{160} TAG	mRNA degraded; no α_1-antitrypsin is made
NULL$_{\text{mattawa}}$	Frameshift nucleotide insertion Leu^{353} TTA-insert T-Phe^{353} TTT-3′ shift-STOP^{376} TAG	No α_1-antitrypsin made
M$_{\text{mineral springs}}$	Point mutation Gly^{67} GGG-Glu GAG	Secretion of a non-functional protein

loss of lung elasticity but only occasionally in the non-smoker will this be clinically apparent. The loss of forced expiratory volume is accelerated to 80 ml/year in the ZZ antitrypsin homozygote. As a consequence, there is a hastened but still variable onset of emphysema. Most PiZZ non-smokers are free from dyspnoea up to the age of 50 years with an average age of death from respiratory disease being 67 years. Again there is considerable individual variation and, particularly in women, there is a good likelihood of a full life span without significant respiratory impairment. The outlook, however, is poor for the ZZ antitrypsin homozygote who is a heavy smoker as the loss in forced expiratory volume increases to as much as 300 ml/year. The onset of dyspnoea occurs around the age of 30 years with death from respiratory disease by the age of 50 years.

Liver disease

Z α_1-antitrypsin liver disease is characterized by the accumulation of the abnormal antitrypsin as diastase-resistant, periodic acid–Schiff-positive inclusions in the periportal cells. This insoluble material accumulates within the endoplasmic reticulum of hepatocytes (see Fig. 6), stimulating a massive increase in cellular degradative activity. The PiMZ and SZ individuals are able to degrade much of the abnormal antitrypsin, but not the Z homozygote, in whom aggregation overwhelms the degradative process resulting in antitrypsin accumulation, hepatocellular damage, and cell death. The accumulation of antitrypsin within hepatocytes is also seen with two other rare mutations, antitrypsin S_{iiyama} (53 phenylalanine → serine) and M_{malton} (52 phenylalanine deletion). Both of these point mutations result in perturbations of antitrypsin structure, which favour loop–sheet polymer formation. Polymer formation is temperature and concentration dependent, accounting for the variation in the number and density of liver inclusions between individuals. Antitrypsin is an acute phase protein and, as such, undergoes a manifold increase in production during even minor illnesses. At these times there may also be temperature increases of up to 41°C and the combined effects of the increase in protein concentration and temperature favour rapid polymerization, which leads to inclusion formation and liver disease.

Neonatal jaundice and juvenile cirrhosis

Eighty per cent of ZZ antitrypsin homozygote infants show biochemical evidence of hepatocellular damage in the first year of life. One in 10 develops neonatal hepatitis which presents as cholestatic jaundice and 6 per cent develop clinical evidence of liver disease without jaundice. These symptoms usually resolve by the second year but 10 to 15 per cent of patients with cholestatic jaundice progress to a juvenile cirrhosis. The reasons for this variable progression are not known; intercurrent illness will contribute but other hormonal and genetic factors may also be involved. Juvenile cirrhosis is three times more common in boys than girls and the likelihood of juvenile cirrhosis may be increased if there is a history of a Z homozygote sibling having developed liver disease. The overall risk of death from liver disease in PiZZ children during childhood is 2 to 3 per cent.

Adult liver disease

All PiZZ individuals have slowly progressive hepatic damage which is often subclinical and only evident as a minor degree of portal fibrosis. However, up to 50 per cent of ZZ antitrypsin homozygotes eventually present with clinically evident cirrhosis and occasionally with hepatocellular carcinoma. The presence of Z α_1-antitrypsin deficiency including the heterozygous PiMZ and PiSZ should always be considered before making the diagnosis of cryptogenic cirrhosis.

Associated conditions

α_1-Antitrypsin deficiency is associated with an increased incidence of bronchiectasis, glomerulonephritis, and panniculitis and probably also with inflammatory bowel disease. There is also a considerably increased incidence in both heterozygotes (PiMZ) and homozygotes (PiZZ) of antineutrophil cytoplasm antibodies (c-ANCA) with consequent risk of Wegener's granulomatosis.

Diagnosis

Severe genetic deficiency is readily diagnosed by the virtual absence of the α_1-antitrypsin band on protein electrophoresis. The deficiency is then assigned a Pi phenotype according to the migration of the protein on an isoelectric focusing gel. Most cases are detected in this way, as an incidental finding, but in some areas the systematic identification of homozygotes is achieved by neonatal blood-spot testing.

Treatment

Treatment depends largely on the avoidance of stimuli causing repeated pulmonary inflammation—primarily smoking. Patients with α_1-antitrypsin deficiency-related emphysema should receive conventional therapy with trials of bronchodilators and, where appropriate, assessment for long-term oxygen therapy and single lung transplantation. Some patients may benefit from resection of basal bullae to reduce lung volume and improve ventilatory mechanics but this has not been assessed in a controlled trial. Intravenous infusions of α_1-antitrypsin are feasible to replace the deficient protein. This approach has a sound physiological basis but the assessment of the protective effect of replacement therapy has been handicapped by the lack of a properly controlled trial. There is a good theoretical reason for short-term intravenous supplementation at times of stress, such as respiratory infections, but this too requires further evaluation.

All Z homozygotes have some liver damage and would be wise to avoid alcohol abuse. The deduction that loop–sheet polymerization of α_1-antitrypsin complicates the acute phase response highlights the importance of antipyretic agents in infants with PiZZ antitrypsin deficiency. Although this has yet to be proven by clinical trials, there is anecdotal evidence that these intercurrent illnesses account for the variation in progression of liver disease in infants. Moreover, there is good reason to believe that conservative treatments to lessen pyrexia and the inflammatory response will be of value in reducing α_1-antitrypsin aggregation within hepatocytes and hence liver disease. PiZZ homozygotes should be monitored for the persistence of hyperbilirubinaemia as this, along with deteriorating results of coagulation studies, indicate the need for liver transplantation. Parents with a child with severe Z α_1-antitrypsin liver disease require genetic counselling although the likelihood of similar severe liver damage in a subsequent Z homozygote sibling is less than 5 per cent.

The panniculitis associated with α_1-antitrypsin deficiency usually responds to dapsone 100 to 150 mg daily for 2 to 4 weeks but occasionally necessitates the administration of intravenous α_1-antitrypsin replacement therapy.

COPD in subjects with 'normal' α_1-antitrypsin

Most patients develop COPD against the background of normal concentrations of α_1-antitrypsin with the normal (PiM) phenotype. However, normal concentration does not necessarily mean normal function and there have been extensive studies of this possibility. α_1-Antitrypsin can be inactivated as an antielastase by previous complexing with enzymes, cleavage at or near the active site, and oxidation of the active site methionine leading to functional deficiency, although the relevance of these changes is uncertain.

Increased enzyme load

α_1-Antitrypsin–elastase balance often results from increased enzyme load. When neutrophils are in contact with connective tissues the cells are tightly adherent and release elastase at the interface, which produces high local concentrations of enzyme whilst partly excluding inhibitors such as α_1-antitrypsin. This privileged site enables a degree of connective tissue degradation to occur even in the presence of α_1-antitrypsin. Thus, factors which affect the number and activation of cells recruited to the lung will also influence the degree of connective tissue degradation. Studies with COPD patients have shown that polymorphonuclear leucocytes isolated from the blood are more responsive to chemotactic factors and so are recruited to the lungs in greater numbers and degrade more connective tissue than smoking- and age-matched healthy subjects. If this process were continuous, the net result would be more extensive lung destruction.

Other enzymes, inhibitors, and proteins

There are several other enzymes and inhibitors that may play a direct or indirect role in the development of COPD. Enzymes from the macrophages and bacteria have been shown to inactivate α_1-antitrypsin as an inhibitor of neutrophil elastase and may disturb the elastase–antielastase balance.

Proteinase 3, another serine protease from the neutrophil, also produces emphysematous lesions in an animal model. Cysteine proteinase (cathepsin B) also produces emphysema and bronchial damage when instilled into the lungs of hamsters. This enzyme is not inactivated by α_1-antitrypsin and causes damage independently of this inhibitor. Cathepsin B activity has been identified in the lung secretions of COPD patients.

A metalloproteinase (dependent upon metal ions for activity) with elastolytic activity (macrophage elastase) and other cysteine proteinases (cathepsin L and B) have been identified in the macrophage. Finally, bacteria may play a role, and a metalloelastase has been isolated from *Pseudomonas aeruginosa*.

More enzyme inhibitors are being identified in the lung, such as the secretory leucoprotease inhibitor which is made locally in the lung. This inhibitor is the dominant neutrophil elastase inhibitor in the bronchi and peripheral airways and has been identified in association with lung elastin. It is far more effective than α_1-antitrypsin in inhibiting neutrophil elastase that has become attached to elastin. An inhibitor of metalloproteinases (TIMP) has also been identified in lung secretions, as have cystatins which inhibit cysteine proteinases. These inhibitors will play a role in limiting lung damage by their respective enzyme classes.

Although there is uncertainty concerning the relative roles of these different enzymes and inhibitors in COPD, it is clear that emphysema is related mainly to the destruction of lung elastin. Lung tissue is subject to degradation and remodelling in health. In elastase-induced emphysema in animal models the initial loss of elastin leads to regeneration as the pathological changes evolve, and prevention of normal elastin fibre cross-linking during this regeneration phase worsens the pathological changes. Thus disorders of elastin may play a role in the development of emphysema, and emphysema is a recognized feature of cutis laxa.

Evolution of pathophysiology

Cough (associated with hypertrophy of mucous glands and mucus hypersecretion) and inflammatory changes in the respiratory bronchioles may develop in young adults early in their smoking history. In never-smokers spirometry shows little change in early adult life; age-related decline begins at about 30 years. In many smokers, however, some decline in FEV_1 occurs through the twenties. By middle age the FEV_1 may be significantly reduced (this is often associated with hyper-responsiveness of the airways to inhaled histamine and other agents) and the early changes of emphysema are developing, functionally revealed by reductions in lung recoil and carbon monoxide transfer coefficient. Because of the enormous total cross-sectional area of the peripheral airways, breathlessness on exertion does not develop until there is considerable pathological change and FEV_1 may be 50 per cent or less of the expected values. As the disease advances ventilation becomes uneven, reducing the efficiency of the lungs as gas exchangers and leading to falls in PaO_2 and increasing ventilatory requirements on exercise. Resting end-tidal volume (functional residual capacity, FRC) increases; although this widens the airways it increases the work of the inspiratory muscles, which are less able to generate inspiratory pressures because of their shorter length at the start of inspiration. Until FEV_1 drops below about one-third of predicted values there is hypoxaemia but not hypercapnia; this is because the inefficiency of the lungs as gas exchangers for carbon dioxide is overcome by a modest increase in resting ventilation. In advanced disease, this compensation is insufficient and hypercapnia often develops; this is related to a combination of the severity of airways obstruction and impaired ability of the inspiratory muscles to generate pressure. With advanced disease, moderate rises in pulmonary artery pressure are found; the precise contributions of loss of pulmonary vascular bed, hypoxaemia, structural changes in the pulmonary vessels, and increased blood viscosity associated with a high haematocrit are uncertain.

Airways obstruction and impaired gas exchange in patients with advanced COPD result from varying combinations of obstructive changes in the peripheral conducting airways (intrinsic airways disease) and destructive changes in respiratory bronchioles, alveolar ducts, and alveoli (emphysema). Many attempts have been made to characterize different patterns of clinical presentation or pulmonary function in COPD and to relate them to the presence and severity of emphysema. The best established contrast is between 'pink and puffing patients' (type A, 'fighters'), who are underweight with severe breathlessness, relatively normal blood gases, and without oedema, and 'blue and bloated' patients (type B, 'non-fighters') with severe hypoxaemia and hypercapnia, polycythaemia, and oedema, but without such severe breathlessness. Type A was originally thought to be associated with severe emphysema but this has not been confirmed in subsequent studies; retained ventilatory responsiveness to hypoxia is now thought to be a more important factor. There are distinct functional changes associated with emphysema which all reflect the airspace changes: an enlarged total lung capacity, a severely reduced carbon monoxide transfer coefficient, and loss of lung recoil. The enlargement in total lung capacity is responsible for the low, flat position of the diaphragm on full-inflation chest radiographs.

Clinical features

Symptoms

Patients may present either with chronic productive cough and recurrent bronchial infections, or with insidious breathlessness on exercise, or a combination of the two types of symptoms.

The tendency to bronchial infections is associated with impaired mucociliary clearance and chronic bacterial colonization of the normally sterile tracheobronchial tree. Diagnosis of chronic bronchitis requires a normal chest radiograph which effectively excludes tuberculosis, bronchiectasis, neoplasms, and many other lung diseases which cause cough. Other possibilities such as postnasal drip, aspiration, asthma, and immune deficiency may have to be excluded by appropriate investigations. Although lung function deteriorates during acute infections and takes several weeks to recover, there is no evidence that the progression of airways obstruction is related to the occurrence of recurrent infections in otherwise healthy smokers.

Airways obstruction leads to breathlessness on exertion and the insidious development of a reduced exercise capacity. A temporary exacerbation due to infection often triggers seeking medical advice. Some patients first present at a very advanced stage and give a short history, but prospective population studies have failed to identify subjects who show rapid and catastrophic falls in FEV_1.

Examination

There are no abnormalities on clinical examination in the earlier stages; diagnosis then depends on spirometry. With progression of the disease signs of hyperinflation (barrel-shaped chest, low position of the laryngeal prominence, loss of cardiac dullness, and lowering of hepatic dullness) develop and there may be increased frequency of breathing, use of accessory muscles, loss of the normal outward movement of the abdomen during inspiration, and wheeze, particularly in the second half of expiration. At the most advanced stage there is often pursed lip breathing, cyanosis, and indrawing of the lateral rib cage (Hoover's sign) on inspiration. Clubbing is not a feature. Ankle oedema may develop, often without any detectable abnormality of the heart or pulmonary circulation. A few patients develop gross cardiac enlargement, gallop rhythm, signs of tricuspid incompetence, raised jugular venous pressure, and hepatic engorgement. Signs of advancing respiratory failure (apart from cyanosis) are restlessness and confusion, a coarse tremor, and warm peripheries.

Investigations

Thoracic imaging

The chest radiograph is a relatively insensitive indicator of COPD; it is possible to die from COPD with a normal chest radiograph. The most striking changes are those due to enlargement of total lung capacity, which is found with emphysema but not usually when obstruction is due to intrinsic airway disease. The domes of the diaphragm are then low with loss of the normal curvature (often seen best on the lateral radiograph); with severe hyperinflation the insertions of the diaphragm into the ribs may be revealed due to loss of the normal area of apposition between diaphragm and rib cage at total lung capacity. A further sign of hyperinflation is an increased retrosternal airspace. Generalized emphysema is often difficult to diagnose with confidence; local differences in transradiancy and paucity of medium-size vascular markings, such as the characteristic bilateral basal transradiancy of α_1-antitrypsin deficiency, are more obvious. Bullae and panlobular emphysema are detected more easily than centrilobular emphysema. Signs of airway disease are few; airway wall thickening is not obvious, but a few patients with recurrent infections with COPD may have bronchiectatic changes.

Secondary effects on the circulation may develop with advanced disease, resulting in upper-zone prominence of medium-size pulmonary vessels, enlargement of the main branches of the pulmonary arteries (a standard measurement is right main descending artery more than 16 mm in diameter), and eventual enlargement of the heart.

Computed tomography has significantly improved the ability to diagnose generalized emphysema and bullae compared with conventional chest radiographs and is particularly useful to follow progression and for preoperative assessment when surgery to the lungs in considered.

Scans of regional ventilation and perfusion become patchily abnormal with the development of relatively mild airways obstruction. The coarse, moth-eaten defects seen are usually 'matched', affecting ventilation and blood flow similarly, but inevitably make it more difficult to detect additional vascular defects due to pulmonary embolism.

Heart (see also Chapter 2.29)

Electrocardiographic signs of right heart disease are usually modest, probably in part because they are masked by hyperinflated lung. Right-bundle branch block and P pulmonale in leads 2, 3, and aVf are common but do not bear a close relation to pulmonary artery and right-ventricular pressures. Evidence of right-ventricular hypertrophy is uncommon. Atrial fibrillation is the commonest arrhythmia. Echocardiographic assessment is also impeded by the hyperinflation, but some indirect estimate of pulmonary artery pressure and of the ejection fraction of the right ventricle can be achieved.

Blood examination

The major change is a raised haematocrit (secondary polycythaemia) in hypoxaemic patients. Smokers have about a 25 per cent rise in all elements of the white blood cell count; a rise in the percentage of eosinophils suggests an asthmatic component. Biochemical tests show a raised venous bicarbonate level in patients with established hypercapnia.

Sputum examination

In stable patients spontaneous and/or induced sputum contains more neutrophils and fewer eosinophils than in asthma and there are suggestions of differences in cytokine profile also. During infective exacerbations three main bacteria are cultured: *Haemophilus influenzae*, *Streptococcus pneumoniae*, and *Moraxella catarrhalis*. At present, most bacterial infections respond to a wide range of antibiotics so many physicians believe culture and tests of antibiotic sensitivity are only necessary if the patient fails to respond to the first course of antibiotics, but ampicillin-resistant *H. influenzae* is becoming increasingly common (15 per cent or more in some areas). So far, penicillin-resistant *Strep. pneumoniae* is very rare (less than 1 per cent) in many countries, including the UK, but isolated multiple-antibiotic-resistant organisms have been found in New Guinea, the Republic of South Africa, and Spain. After repeated courses of antibiotics *Pseudomonas* species may be predominant. *Staphylococcus aureus* is important during epidemics of influenza. The commonest organism causing a lobar pneumonia is *Strep. pneumoniae*, but smokers with COPD are at increased risk of *Legionella pneumophila* infections. Tuberculosis is relatively common in the elderly smoker, particularly if there is also alcohol abuse.

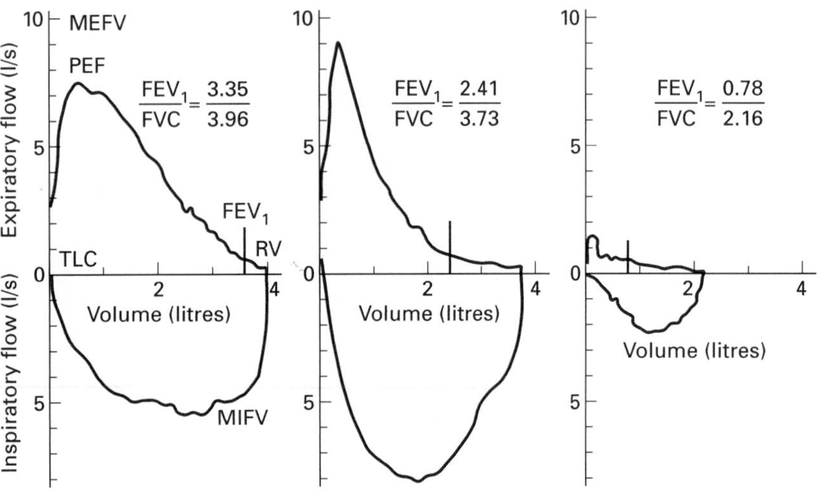

Fig. 7 Maximum expiratory and inspiratory flow-volume (MEFV and MIFV) curves in a normal subject (left), a smoker with mild intrathoracic airways obstruction (centre), and a patient with severe airways obstruction (right). PEF, peak expiratory flow; RV, residual volume; FVC, forced vital capacity; TLC, total lung capacity. With developing airways obstruction the earliest distinctive change is development of convexity of the flow signal to the volume axis (centre); in this subject, peak expiratory flow and the MIFV curve were normal. In severe obstruction there are gross reductions on both the flow and volume axes.

Respiratory function tests

Spirometry A low FEV_1 and FEV_1/vital capacity (VC) ratio are essential to the diagnosis; values of both depend on age, gender, and height. If the result is borderline, finding convexity to the volume axis of the expiratory limb of the maximum expiratory flow-volume curve is useful because this change occurs early in the development of obstruction (Fig. 7 centre).

The response to an inhaled β-adrenoceptor agonist and/or muscarinic antagonist should also be measured; a large increase immediately raises the prospect of a reversible ('asthmatic') component. Absence of an immediate bronchodilator response, while disappointing, should not prevent a full trial of corticosteroid treatment (see below).

Peak expiratory flow is better preserved than FEV_1 in COPD, so an initial assessment with full spirometric tests is necessary; once the diagnosis is established, peak expiratory flow can be used to monitor progress.

Carbon monoxide transfer coefficient Reduction in carbon monoxide transfer, particularly when expressed per litre of lung volume, indicates the extent of emphysema and contrasts with the normal or even increased transfer coefficient found in asthma.

Static lung volumes Residual volume (volume at the end of a full expiration) is increased and VC reduced. An increase in total lung capacity (TLC) indicates probable emphysema. However, the most important static lung volume is the volume at the end of a tidal expiration (functional residual capacity, FRC). In healthy subjects, FRC is about 0.5 TLC, rising slightly above this ratio beyond middle age. In severe COPD, the FRC/TLC ratio may be 0.7 or 0.8.

Respiratory muscle strength The maximum inspiratory pressure developed at FRC is reduced in severe COPD. The major factor is probably the muscle shortening due to the increased FRC but in advanced COPD there is often loss of weight and muscle bulk; the diaphragm and other respiratory muscles share in this loss of mass, reducing the pressures generated during both maximum inspiratory and maximum expiratory efforts.

Blood gases Resting PaO_2 falls as airways obstruction increases. Oximetry has made it easy to monitor oxygen saturation during outpatient visits and to assess the need for long-term oxygen at home. Hypercapnia can be suspected from elevation of venous blood bicarbonate. $PaCO_2$ is usually normal until FEV_1 is reduced below 1.2 litres. The chronicity of any elevated $PaCO_2$ can be judged from the pH, which tends to remain at about 7.40 in the steady state, particularly when the patient is on diuretics.

Exercise capacity Simple walking tests, such as the distance covered in 6 min, provide a useful summary of the patient's disability and can be supplemented by monitoring oxygen saturation with oximetry and by formal incremental exercise tests.

Management of chronic stable disease (Fig. 8)

Disability and prognosis in COPD are dominated by the severity of airways obstruction. While symptoms can be ameliorated by a large variety of treatments, radically improved prognosis is unlikely unless obstruction can be relieved or at least future decline slowed. Generally available options are to stop smoking and to be certain that the reversible component of airways obstruction is adequately recognized and treated. Removal from occupational dust exposure is desirable.

Stopping smoking

In smokers with minor airways obstruction there may be a slight improvement in FEV_1 on stopping smoking, but the major effect is to slow subsequent decline in FEV_1, nearly to that of healthy never-smokers (Fig. 9). In advanced COPD it is less certain that further decline in FEV_1 is slowed, so that there is a strong case for early intervention. Stopping smoking consistently results in a reduction in cough, expectoration, and acute respiratory infections, but patients should not expect improvement in breathlessness. Low tar cigarettes are associated with less cough but any slowing of decline in FEV_1 is slight. The benefits of stopping smoking on the subsequent development of cardiovascular disease and lung cancer (the incidence of which is increased, even allowing for smoking habit) apply equally to patients with COPD as to the rest of the population. Physician advice is important, particularly in encouraging repeated attempts to quit; nicotine replacement can assist addicted smokers.

Response to bronchodilator and corticosteroid treatment

Virtually all patients with chronic airways obstruction show some immediate response to treatment with β-adrenergic agonists, muscarinic antagonists, and theophylline, but these improvements are usually small. If the response is large, the possibility of further improvement with corticosteroids is evident. The patient at risk of undertreatment is the heavy smoker with a small immediate

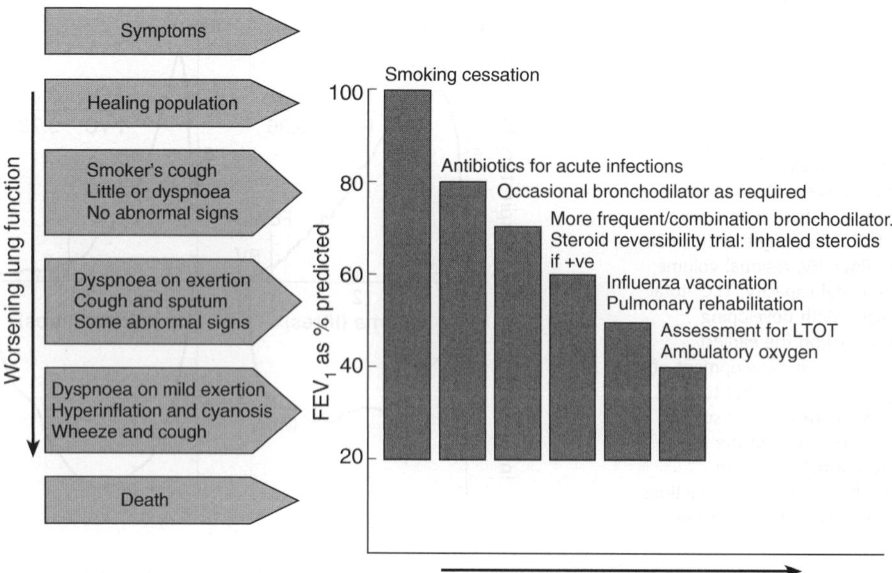

Fig. 8 Escalation of treatment of COPD as disability increases. *(Reproduced with permission from British Thoracic Society, 1997. Thorax,* **52** *(suppl. 5): S1–28.)*

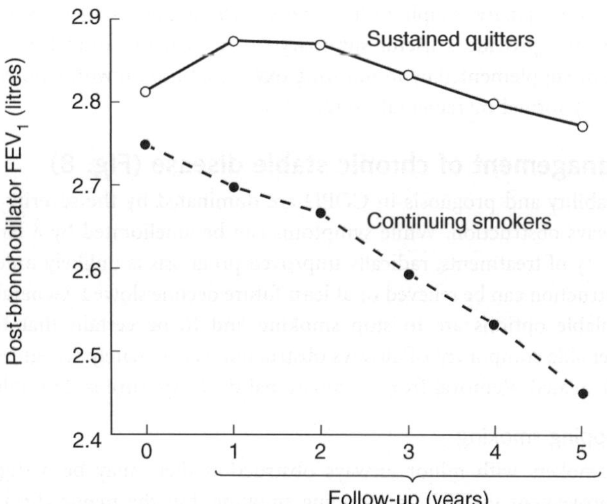

Fig. 9 Changes in postbronchodilator FEV_1 on quitting smoking compared to continuing smokers in subjects with mild airways obstruction. There was on average a small rise on quitting smoking but the important change is the slowing of subsequent decline in FEV_1. Data from Lung Health Study in North America. *(Reproduced with permission from Anthonisen et al., (1994), Journal of the American Medical Association,* **272**, *1497–1505.)*

bronchodilator response, particularly if there is evidence of emphysema. Conventional management is to make a 2 to 3-week trial of 30 to 40 mg of prednisolone daily, monitoring peak expiratory flow daily and spirometry at least at the beginning and end of a trial. In the great majority of 'responders', improvement can be sustained subsequently by inhaled corticosteroids. If there is a large improvement in airways obstruction, the prognosis should be dramatically improved. An alternative to oral corticosteroids is a trial of high-dose inhaled corticosteroids; this should be continued for 6 to 8 weeks.

A more difficult question is whether long-term treatment is beneficial even when the effects of such trials are negligible. Preliminary data from three large-scale studies of inhaled corticosteroids continued for 3 years in subjects with mild to moderate COPD suggest that inhaled corticosteroids may produce a small increase in lung function in the first few months but do not significantly alter subsequent long-term decline. The number of acute exacerbations may be reduced but further studies are required. In the meantime, it seems reasonable to decide their usage on the basis of short-term benefit.

In contrast with asthma, where β-agonists are clearly superior to muscarinic antagonists as inhaled bronchodilators, muscarinic antagonists are as effective overall as β-agonists in COPD. A combination of two or three types of bronchodilators is commonly used, but addition of effects is uncertain. Patients with severe COPD often claim more sustained relief from use of β-agonists and muscarinic antagonists via home nebulizers instead of conventional metered dose inhalers. Whether this is because of the increased dosage (there can be a 10-fold difference between the doses given by conventional inhalers and by nebulizers), the sequential inhalation, the more impressive mode of treatment, or the mimicry of crisis management in accident and emergency departments is uncertain, but several studies have suggested reduced hospital admissions in disabled patients.

The most commonly-used muscarinic antagonist, ipratropium, has to be taken three or four times a day, but longer acting alternatives are being developed. Longer-acting β-agonists, such as salmeterol or formeterol, may also be used for long-term therapy. As with corticosteroids, there has been interest in whether regular bronchodilator treatment, by diminishing airway hyper-responsiveness, might reduce annual decline in FEV_1 but 5 years of treatment with an inhaled muscarinic antagonist failed to attenuate decline in FEV_1 in a large North American study. At present, therefore, their use is also based on short-term benefit. When the effect is small there may be a divergence between subjective benefit and spirometric benefit.

Apart from relaxation of airways smooth muscle, β-agonists may have some anti-inflammatory effects, aid ciliary clearance, and increase mucus secretion; they are pulmonary vasodilators and modulate cholinergic neurotransmission. Theophyllines also have anti-inflammatory actions, increase ciliary clearance, and are mild ventilatory stimulants and diuretics; their ability to improve respiratory muscle performance is disputed.

Other drugs

Oral N-acetyl cysteine, a mucolytic and antioxidant drug, slightly reduces the number and length of bronchopulmonary infections. Trials of long-term antibiotics in the 1960s, admittedly with small doses and less effective drugs than now available, failed to attenuate decline in FEV_1. Preliminary studies of the replacement of α_1-antitrypsin in deficient individuals are in progress, aiming to keep plasma levels about 50 per cent of normal. Oral ventilatory stimulants (such as medroxyprogesterone, carbonic anhydrase inhibitors, or almitrine) can improve PaO_2 and $PaCO_2$ by 0.5 to 1.0 kPa but are not widely used.

Sedative drugs should almost always be avoided, although they may have a place under carefully monitored conditions in a few patients to control distressing dyspnoea. β-blocker drugs, even when relatively cardioselective or given as eye drops, can worsen airways obstruction.

Immunization

Immunization against influenza and pneumococcal infection seems sensible, although the protective effect of pneumococcal vaccination in patients with COPD may be less than in the general population.

Acute increases in breathlessness

It is not always easy to diagnose the cause of an acute increase in breathlessness in patients with more severe COPD, and often they are treated with a combination of increased bronchodilators (and possibly corticosteroids), antibiotics, and diuretics.

Acute respiratory infection

This is the most commonly diagnosed cause if there is an exacerbation associated with some evidence of infection (raised temperature, infected sputum, abnormal chest radiograph, and raised C-reactive protein) and wheeziness. The proportion of infections initiated by viruses is unknown and antibiotics are usually given empirically, the choice of antibiotics being determined by local sensitivity patterns to common bacteria such as *Strep. pneumoniae* and *Haemophilus influenzae*. Whereas in the stable outpatient state inhaled muscarinic antagonists (ipratropium, oxitropium) are as good as (and some would maintain better than) β-agonists for bronchodilatation, in acute exacerbations there is no evidence that muscarinic antagonists can add to the bronchodilatation produced by β-adrenergic agonists alone. There is evidence that initial improvement in airways function over the first few days is faster in patients given a course of systemic corticosteroids, but the effect is small.

Pneumothorax

COPD is the commonest cause of spontaneous pneumothorax in older patients. Detection by clinical examination may be difficult in the presence of hyperinflated lungs and because the degree of lung collapse is often modest. The threshold for inserting an intrapleural drain is lower than normal, both because of the greater significance of a small further loss in function when baseline function is compromised and because the abnormal lung does not readily collapse, so that the increase in pleural pressure cannot be estimated from the degree of collapse. Sustained re-expansion is often slow, requiring prolonged pleural intubation and the hazards of relative immobilization in elderly subjects.

Pulmonary embolism

This is also more difficult to detect in patients with COPD, but is common at autopsy. The usual presentation is with an unexplained increase in breathlessness. The most useful investigations are a rise in serum D-dimers and ventilation and perfusion scans; the common abnormality in stable COPD is matched ventilation and perfusion defects. Perfusion defects in areas that are still ventilated are more likely to be due to pulmonary embolism than to emphysema. Relative immobility, development of leg oedema, and high haematocrit all predispose to venous thrombosis in advanced COPD, but no studies provide useful guidance on whether anticoagulants should be routinely used long term in such patients in sinus rhythm.

Left ventricular failure

This is also common in COPD and is particularly dangerous because the ability of such patients to survive with low arterial PO_2 depends on maintaining at least a normal, and preferably a high normal, cardiac output. The coincidence of two common conditions may simply reflect that smoking is a major risk factor for both ischaemic heart disease and COPD, but other suggestions have been that left ventricular function may be compromised by arterial hypoxaemia or hypertrophy of the interventricular septum.

Advanced disease

Available medical treatments for advanced stable disease include long-term home oxygen, diuretics, venesection, nutritional supplementation, physiotherapy, and limb and respiratory muscle training. These treatments and the management of acute-on-chronic ventilatory failure are discussed in Chapters 4.44 and 4.45.

Surgical treatment

Some patients with large bullae can be improved by surgical obliteration. Lung transplantation, usually of a single lung, can provide dramatic relief of symptoms and improvement in lung function for patients with advanced COPD; shortage of donor organs effectively confines this option to a few patients who develop advanced disease at a relatively young age, often with bullous emphysema or α_1-antitrypsin deficiency. Consequently the development of lung volume reduction surgery for patients with advanced disease has aroused much interest, particularly in the USA. The goal of this operation is to reduce total lung capacity by about 20 to 25 per cent by removing the most emphysematous and poorly functioning areas in both lungs, which are identified by preoperative CT and ventilation scans and failure to collapse at operation. The obvious benefit is to improve chest wall mechanics and the resting length of the diaphragm and other inspiratory muscles, but early results suggest useful improvements in pulmonary elasticity and FEV_1 can be obtained. Currently, large trials are in progress to assess the precise indications for this operation and to examine how long any improvement is sustained. If a reduction in disability can be sustained for two or more years, this operation may provide worthwhile palliation.

Special categories of COPD

Bullous emphysema

Bullae (thin-walled airspaces more than 1 cm in diameter) may occur in otherwise normal lungs or in lungs where there is accompanying airways obstruction and generalized emphysema.

In the former case there are often no symptoms and the diagnosis may be fortuitous on a routine chest radiograph or with a spontaneous pneumothorax. If bullae occupy a third or more of a hemithorax, surgical obliteration improves lung function. However, the necessity for and timing of any surgical intervention is often difficult to assess in patients with no or few symptoms.

When bullae are associated with more severe airways obstruction the problem is to decide whether they are playing a significant part in a patient's breathlessness. This requires detailed anatomical and physiological assessment. Anatomical assessment is made by CT of the thorax. Functional assessment is more difficult. Uncommon patients who have significant ventilation of a bulla can be detected by scans of regional ventilation. In the remaining patients bullae act solely as space-occupying lesions and the problem is to assess the degree of interference with the surrounding lung and its ability to expand into the space provided in the hemithorax following surgical obliteration. There is no doubt that some patients with generalized airways obstruction can be helped by obliterative surgery, at least if bullae occupying one-third or more of a hemithorax can be obliterated but precise criteria for such surgery have not been developed. Indications for bullectomy should be clarified by the current interest in lung volume reduction surgery for generalized emphysema. Worthwhile palliation may last for some years; an alternative in younger patients is single-lung transplantation.

Bronchopulmonary dysplasia

This has become an important cause of mild chronic airways obstruction in childhood. It follows premature delivery and ventilation for respiratory distress of the newborn and may be associated with lack of full lung development during growth. Affected children may prove to be at particular risk of smoking-related damage in adult life.

Unilateral transradiancy of the lung (Swyer–James or Macleod's syndrome)

This is an uncommon condition in which there is unilateral airways obstruction, hyperinflation, and small central and medium-size pulmonary arteries. Because the contralateral lung is normal there may be few symptoms and the diagnosis may be made when a chest radiograph is taken for other reasons. The diagnosis can be confirmed by obtaining expiratory radiographs (the affected lung shows only a small decrease in volume and so may cause mediastinal shift), and scans of regional ventilation and perfusion. No treatment is required, but contraindications to smoking are amplified by the lower reserves of lung function.

Further reading

American Thoracic Society (1995). Standards for the diagnosis and care of patients with chronic obstructive pulmonary disease. *American Journal of Respiratory and Critical Care Medicine*, **152**, S77–120.

Anthonisen, N.R., Connett, J.E., Kiley, J.P., *et al.* (1994). Effects of smoking intervention and the use of an inhaled anticholinergic bronchodilator on the rate of decline of FEV1. The Lung Health Study. *Journal of the American Medical Association*, **272**, 1497–505.

Becklake, M.R. (1989). Occupational exposures: evidence for a causal association with chronic obstructive pulmonary disease. *American Review of Respiratory Disease*, **140**, S85–91.

British Thoracic Society and others (1997). Guidelines for management of chronic obstructive pulmonary disease. *Thorax*, **52** (suppl. 5), S1–28.

Eriksson, S., Carlson, J., and Velez, R. (1986). Risk of cirrhosis and primary liver cancer in alpha1-antitrypsin deficiency. *New England Journal of Medicine*, **314**, 736–9.

European Respiratory Society consensus statement (1995). Optimal assessment and management of chronic obstructive pulmonary disease (COPD). *European Respiratory Journal*, **8**, 1398–420.

Mahadeva, R. and Lomas, D.A. (1998). Alpha1-antitrypsin deficiency, cirrhosis and emphysema. *Thorax*, **53**, 505.

Murray, C.J.L. and Lopez, A.D. (1997). Alternative projections of mortality and disability by cause 1990–2020: global burden of disease study. *Lancet*, **349**, 1498–505.

Parenchymal lung disease

Chapter 4.18

Introduction

A. A. Woodcock and R. M. du Bois

Diseases of the parenchyma, or functioning gas exchanging regions, of the lung have conventionally been called interstitial lung diseases. However, histological examination demonstrates disease in the lung interstitium with coexistent disease, usually inflammatory or infiltrative, in the alveoli, terminal bronchioles, and/or the pulmonary capillary. Hence, this heterogenous group of diseases will be termed 'diffuse parenchymal lung diseases'.

Many diffuse parenchymal lung diseases are chronic and therefore have persistent radiographic abnormalities. Some, such as fibrosing alveolitis, asbestosis, and alveolar proteinosis, are often progressive in the absence of treatment, whereas others, such as sarcoidosis, extrinsic allergic alveolitis, and pulmonary eosinophilia run a more chronic relapsing–remitting course.The variable natural history mirrors the different disease mechanisms, the nature of the stimulus, the site at which it acts, and whether there is an immunological response or a non-immunogenic injury. To produce disease in the peripheral regions of the lung, inhaled dust must be of a size (1–3 μm) which can reach the periphery. Individual predisposition also helps determine disease (for example, not all budgerigar owners develop bird fancier's lung).

The clinician's role is to determine the nature of a diffuse lung disease before sufficient respiratory reserve has been lost and when treatment may still be effective.

An approach to patients with diffuse parenchymal lung disease

Producing a specific diagnosis may appear difficult because more than 180 causes of diffuse lung disease have been described (Table 1). This chapter aims to provide a logical diagnostic approach. Initially a full history, examination, lung function, chest radiograph, and usually a CT scan are carried out. Some patients can be satisfactorily managed on this information alone, but most patients need invasive investigations including fibreoptic bronchoscopy, bronchoalveolar lavage, and transbronchial or open lung biopsy. A diagnostic algorithm is described in Fig. 1. In diseases with such a variable natural history and response to treatment, it is important where possible to obtain a definitive diagnosis prior to treatment.

The history (especially the rate of onset of symptoms, occupations, hobbies, drugs) and examination are critical, and some differentiating features are described in Table 2.

Routine haematological and biochemical investigations are often unhelpful but specific tests can be valuable. A peripheral blood eosinophilia (above 1500/mm^3) suggests a pulmonary eosinophilia.

Table 1 Diffuse parenchymal lung diseases

Unknown causes	Known causes
With interstitial fibrosis	***Organic dusts***
• Cryptogenic fibrosing alveolitis	• Avian e.g. pigeon antigens
• Systemic sclerosis	• Fungal e.g. aspergillus
• Polymyositis	• Chemical e.g. diisocyanates
• Sjögren's syndrome	***Pneumoconiosis***
• Rheumatoid arthritis	• Fibrogenic inorganic dusts (e.g. asbestos, silica, hard metal alloy, beryllium, coal)
• SLE	• Inert inorganic dusts (e.g. iron, barium, tin)
• Ankylosing spondylitis	***Infection***
With granulomas	• Viruses (e.g. cytomegalovirus)
• Sarcoidosis	• Bacteria (e.g. tuberculosis)
• Wegener's granulomatosis	• Fungi (e.g. histoplasmosis)
• Langerhans' cell histiocytosis	• Protozoa (e.g. Toxoplasma, Pneumocystis)
• Eosinophilic granulomatosis (Churg–Strauss syndrome)	• Helminths (e.g. Ascaris, filaria)
• Lymphomatoid granulomatosis	***Drugs***
• Bronchocentric granulomatosis	• Producing lung injury (e.g. cytotoxic/chemotherapeutic, illegal opiates)
Inherited disorders	• Producing immunogenic lung injury (e.g. anti-inflammatory, cardiovascular)
• Tuberous sclerosis	• Causing eosinophilia (e.g. antibiotics, anti-inflammatory, anticonvulsant, cytotoxic)
• Neurofibromatosis	• SLE-like responses (e.g. hydrallazine)
• Hermansky–Pudlak syndrome	• Organizing pneumonia (e.g. acebutalol, gold, sulphasalazine)
• Lipid storage disorders	***Neoplasia***
• Familial fibrosing alveolitis	• Lymphangitis carcinomatosa
With vasculitis	• Lymphoma
• Wegener's granulomatosis	• Alveolar cell carcinoma
• Microscopic polyarteritis	***Miscellaneous***
• Rheumatic diseases (e.g. SLE, rheumatoid arthritis)	• Radiotherapy
• Hypersensitivity vasculitis (e.g. response to drugs)	• Gases (e.g. mercury vapour, high oxygen concentrations)
Individual pathology	• Chemical (e.g. paraquat)
• Cryptogenic pulmonary eosinophilia	• Associated with chronically elevated left atrial pressure, uraemia
• Idiopathic pulmonary haemosiderosis	• Multiple pulmonary emboli
• Pulmonary veno-occlusive disease	• Post-ARDS
• Lymphangio-leiomyomatosis	
• Lymphocytic interstitial pneumonia	
• COP (BOOP in the US)	
• Known causes: amiodarone, sulpha-salazine, acebutalol	
• Unknown cause: idiopathic	
• Alveolar proteinosis	
• Alveolar microlithiasis	
• Amyloidosis	

SLE, systemic lupus erythematosus; COP, cryptogenic organizing pneumonia; BOOP, bronchiolitis obliterans organizing pneumonia; ARDS, adult respiratory distress syndrome.

IgE levels are elevated in proportion to the eosinophilia in allergic causes such as helminthic infection and drug hypersensitivity, whereas disproportionately high eosinophil counts with a much more modest elevation in serum IgE are seen in cryptogenic pulmonary eosinophilia. Specific IgE measurements will confirm the identity of a suspected cause. Similarly, identification of precipitating antibodies to organic antigens will confirm exposure to suspected causes of extrinsic allergic alveolitis. If a vasculitis is suspected, cANCA positivity is highly suggestive of Wegener's granulomatosis. Rheumatoid factor and antinuclear antibody are often non-specific. Other more specific autoantibodies can be diagnostic, for example anticentromere antibody (limited systemic sclerosis); anti-DNA topoisomerase-1 (Scl-70) (diffuse systemic sclerosis); anti-aminoacyl t-RNA synthetase antibodies such as Jo1, PL-7, and PL-12 (polymyositis and other myositic diseases associated with fibrosing alveolitis); anti-SS-A and anti-SS-B (Sjögren's syndrome); anti-double-stranded DNA antibodies (systemic lupus erythematosus). It is important to look for autoantibodies in all patients with diffuse lung disease because the lung manifestation of the systemic disorder may antedate evidence of disease elsewhere. In rheumatoid arthritis, for example, the lung problem may occur 4 to 5 years before other abnormalities. Angiotensin-converting enzyme levels may be elevated in sarcoidosis, but this test is not specific and may be normal in progressive sarcoidosis.

Lung function tests

These usually show a restrictive ventilatory defect with reduced gas transfer (*DL*CO). They are non-discriminatory diagnostically but are essential for monitoring progression. Some patients have a combination of restriction combined with evidence of obstruction on the flow-volume loop, and have airways involvement (in e.g. sarcoidosis or Langerhans cell histiocytosis) or two diseases (e.g. alveolitis plus emphysema; usually with disproportionally low *DL*CO). In more subtle disease with normal gas transfer at rest, exercise tests can unmask

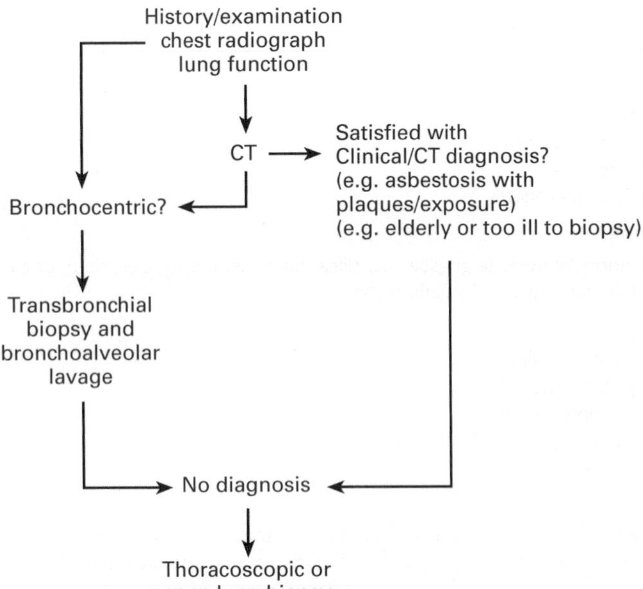

Fig. 1 Clinical approach to diffuse parenchymal lung disease.

abnormality; PaO_2 falls and the alveolar–arterial oxygen gradient (A–a gradient) widens, indicating abnormalities of gas exchange.

Radionuclide imaging

Gallium scanning may be helpful in determining the presence of lung disease when there is doubt. It is not specific, is time consuming, and has a considerable radiation burden. Other techniques of imaging, for example ^{99}Tc-DTPA scanning which measures epithelial permeability, ^{111}In-transferrin labelling which assesses microvascular leak, ^{111}In-neutrophil labelling to identify neutrophil traffic, and positron emission tomography in association with radiolabelled carbohydrate administration which indicates local increases in metabolic activity, are promising as specific indices of early inflammation, but their present role is still being defined.

Chest radiology

Chest radiography is one of the most important keys in differential diagnosis. Five important features should be noted:

(1) lung size;

(2) distribution of abnormalities;

(3) size and nature of nodular and reticular abnormalities;

(4) presence of confluent shadows;

(5) presence of pleural disease or lymphadenopathy.

The combination of these radiographic features and suggested diagnoses are seen schematically in Fig. 2.

Computed tomography

Fine-section CT (1–3 mm sections at 10–20 mm intervals) is more sensitive and specific than conventional chest radiography in differential diagnosis:

1. It gives a better perspective on distribution
2. It is abnormal earlier.
3. It can provide a high probability diagnosis (avoiding biopsy in the sick/elderly).
4. It guides the surgeon to the best biopsy site.

Table 2 Diffuse parenchymal lung disease: key points on history/examination

Wheeze	Airways involved (e.g. Langerhans cell histiocytosis/sarcoidosis)
Acute dyspnoea	? Heavy antigen exposure (e.g. farmers lung)
Cough	Common; non-discriminatory
Sputum	? Bronchiectasis
Haemoptysis	? Vasculitis e.g. Wegener's granulomatosis, microscopic polyarteritis
Smoking	Universal in Langerhans cell histiocytosis; increased in cryptogenic fibrosing alveolitis; reduced in sarcoidosis/extrinsic allergic alveolitis
Associated symptoms	e.g. arthritis (rheumatological diseases) dysphagia/Raynaud's (systemic sclerosis), muscle weakness (polymyositis)
Occupation	History from leaving school (critically important) e.g. asbestosis/siderosis
Hobbies	e.g. Avian exposure; mushroom growing
Drugs	? Immunosuppressed ? cytotoxics
Clubbing	Cryptogenic fibrosing alveolitis: 70%; rare in sarcoidosis/extrinsic allergic alveolitis/Langerhans cell histiocytosis
Crackles	Universal in cryptogenic fibrosing alveolitis; less common in other disorders

Bronchoalveolar lavage

Bronchoalveolar lavage has not fulfilled its promise as an alternative to lung biopsy as a diagnostic test in diffuse parenchymal lung disease, although useful information can be obtained from some patients. Specific examples are seen in Table 3. The differentiation of diffuse parenchymal diseases into those with a preponderance of either lymphocytes or granulocytes was initially promising, but further studies revealed that lymphocytes were not always present in granulomatous disorders; lymphocytes may be present at the earlier stages of fibrosing lung disorders and suggest a good response to therapy. Conversely neutrophils are present in the lungs of acute extrinsic allergic alveolitis and also in diseases such as sarcoidosis in a more fibrotic phase. The test can be of value where initial investigations have suggested one disease (e.g. fibrosing alveolitis) but a very high

Table 3 Bronchoalveolar lavage in diffuse parenchymal lung disease

Non-specific	
Lymphocytes:	Sarcoidosis/CFA (good prognosis)/very high in EAA
Neutrophils:	CFA/asbestosis/ARDS/bacterial infections
Specific	
Lipoproteinaceous material	Alveolar proteinosis
Giant cells	Hard metals
Langerhan's cells	Langerhan's cell histiocytosis
Infections	Immunosuppressed? e.g. *Pneumocystis carinii*

CFA, cryptogenic fibrosing alveolitis; EAA, extrinsic allergic alveolitis

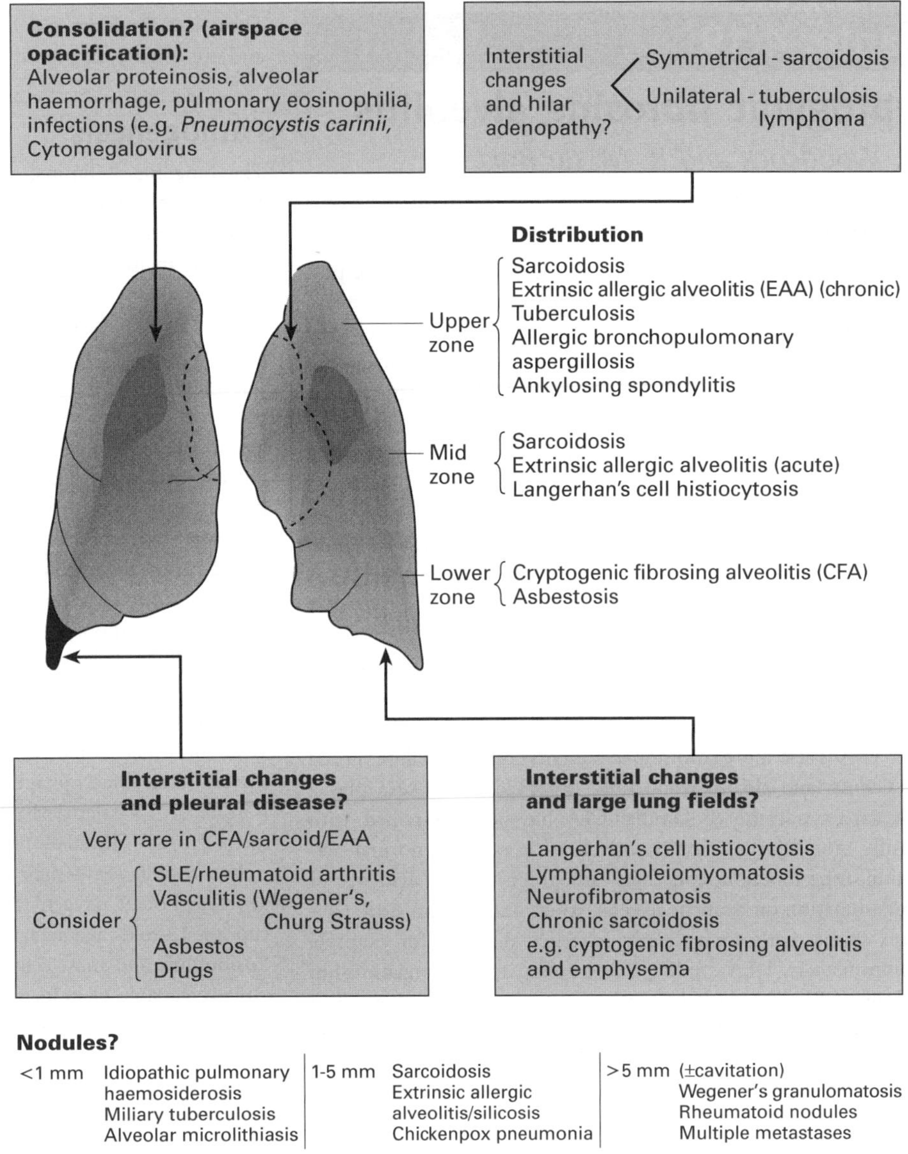

Fig. 2 Diffuse parenchymal lung disease: key points on chest radiograph.

percentage of one cell type (e.g. lymphocytes) would force the physician to reconsider the suspected diagnosis.

Lung biopsy

It is important to weigh up the relative risks of a biopsy procedure. In an elderly individual with poor respiratory reserve, particularly one in whom the other clinical features and high resolution CT have confirmed the diagnosis beyond reasonable doubt, biopsy is superfluous. However, in younger patients who may need to be treated for a prolonged period reasons should be sought for not performing a biopsy, rather than subject the patient to prolonged potent treatment with potentially major side-effects without the security of knowing precisely what process is being treated.

The type of biopsy procedure is determined by initial investigations. If bronchocentric or granulomatous disease is suspected (e.g. sarcoidosis, extrinsic allergic alveolitis, miliary tuberculosis, lymphangitis carcinomatosa) transbronchial biopsy together with bronchoalveolar lavage will provide diagnostic material in more than 80 per cent of instances. Transbronchial biopsy may result in pneumothorax or haemoptysis which are rarely serious (check clotting first).

For other suspected diseases, transbronchial biopsy is of little value and open or thoracoscopic biopsy are needed to provide adequate tissue for diagnosis and staging. Specialist pulmonary histopathological support is critical and experience concentrated in centres of expertise.

Further reading

Corrin, B. (1990). *Systemic pathology*, Vol. 5, *The lungs*. Churchill Livingstone, London.

Crystal, R.G. and West, J.B. (1991). *The lung. Scientific foundations*. Raven Press, New York

Chapter 4.19

Cryptogenic fibrosing alveolitis

A. A. Woodcock and R. M. du Bois

Definition

Cryptogenic fibrosing alveolitis (CFA; also known as idiopathic pulmonary fibrosis) is a clinical syndrome characterized by progressive dyspnoea, clubbing, late-inspiratory crackles, and a diffuse lower zone infiltrate on the chest radiograph. A rapidly progressive form has been termed the Hamman–Rich syndrome. CFA is characterized histologically by inflammation and fibrosis of the lung interstitium and alveoli. CFA usually occurs alone but can be associated with a number of other diseases especially systemic sclerosis and rheumatoid arthritis. It can occur at any age, but with increasing frequency over the age of 50. The male–female ratio is 1:1 and CFA is more common in smokers. Prevalence data is scarce, but the mortality in the UK is approximately 1500/annum and the disease prevalence is of the order of 5/100 000 and rising.

It is likely that CFA can result from a number of triggers. Recent data suggest that Epstein–Barr virus is present in the lungs of some patients with CFA and many patient histories suggest a viral illness at onset. CFA is also more common in patients occupationally exposed to metal dust, and also to wood fires. Inherited factors also play a role. A rare syndrome of familial CFA has been described with apparently non-affected family members (i.e. with normal examination, lung function, and chest radiograph) having evidence of lung inflammation on bronchoalveolar lavage and gallium scan. CFA can also coexist with some clearly inherited diseases, for example neurofibromatosis. HLA studies have shown no fixed relationship with 'lone' CFA, but in CFA with systemic sclerosis there is a relationship with DR3/DR52a. Drawing a parallel with asbestos exposure, not every exposed individual develops asbestosis and it is likely that trigger factors produce CFA only in genetically predisposed individuals.

Pathology

CFA is one of the 'interstitial pneumonias'. In this histological classification the two polar ends of the CFA spectrum, UIP (usual interstitial pneumonia) and DIP (desquamative interstitial pneumonia), are described separately. At one extreme is the rare DIP with a uniform infiltration of interstitium and alveolar spaces with mononuclear phagocytes with almost absent fibrosis, and at the other extreme is the 'honeycomb lung' form of UIP, with severe fibrosis. It is important to grade the cellularity and fibrosis components semiquantitatively in a lung biopsy as these predict prognosis. Other features, such as type 2 cell hyperplasia, loss of architecture, and vascular change, can also be scored.

The three other forms of interstitial pneumonia include:

(1) chronic organizing pneumonia (bronchiolitis obliterans organizing pneumonia in the US);

(2) lymphoid interstitial pneumonia (a lymphocytic pneumonia seen in Sjögren's syndrome, rheumatoid arthritis, lymphoma, and HIV);

(3) giant cell interstitial pneumonia (with bizarre giant cells in air spaces, seen in hard metal disease).

These last three are not forms of CFA but may mimic it clinically and are usually diagnosed at lung biopsy.

Pathogenesis

The lung has a limited repertoire of response to injury and the appearance at the endstage of any of the parenchymal lung diseases may be identical, that is 'honeycomb lung'. The initiating factors probably include environmental dusts and viruses, possibly acting in synergy.

In CFA, lung biopsies show the presence of secondary lymphoid follicles within the interstitium with abundant lymphocytes (predominantly CD4+ cells) and plasma cells, and macrophages. Many of the T cells express markers of activation, and have the surface phenotype of antigen-primed memory T cells (CD45RO+). In bronchoalveolar lavage fluid, an excess of lymphocytes seen in some patients may indicate a favourable response to corticosteroid therapy. Increases in one or more classes of immunoglobulins in the peripheral blood are usually seen in fibrosing alveolitis, and approximately 45 per cent of patients have non-organ-specific autoantibodies in their serum (antinuclear antibodies or rheumatoid factor).

Macrophages play a key role. They secrete chemotactic factors (e.g. LTB4, IL-8), tumour necrosis factor α, and IL-1 which increase the expression of the adhesion molecules ICAM-1, E-selectin, and VCAM-1, all of which enhance the traffic of other inflammatory cells to disease sites. Macrophages also synthesize growth factors such as fibronectin, platelet-derived growth factor, and insulin-like growth factor 1 which stimulate fibroblasts enhancing fibrosis.

Neutrophils (with their proteolytic enzymes and their capacity to generate potent oxygen radicals) are present in increased numbers (up to 15-fold, particularly in smokers) in lung lavage samples. Eosinophils and mast cells are also present in the lung interstitium and are capable of inducing lung injury.

There is an excess of collagen, with excess type III collagen (as opposed to type I) associated with a more active disease process which is more amenable to therapy. Transforming growth factor β is emerging as a potent fibroblast chemotactant and stimulator of fibrogenesis. Although injury and subsequent loss of lung tissue are irreversible, deposition of collagen is not an endstage process. In animal models, approximately 10 per cent of lung collagen is turned over every day.

Clinical features

History

Patients with CFA give a history of progressive breathlessness on exertion in the absence of wheeze. A cough is frequent but sputum is unusual. Haemoptysis is uncommon and should suggest the development of lung malignancy which occurs with a 14-fold excess frequency. Chest pain is uncommon. Weight loss, lethargy, and tremor may be present. (The implications of other associated symptoms and signs are given in Table 2 in Chapter 4.19.)

A full occupational history (from school leaving) is necessary to exclude inorganic dusts as the cause of fibrosing alveolitis. In particular, exposure to asbestos and hard metal can produce a disease which is clinically indistinguishable from cryptogenic fibrosing alveolitis. Causes of extrinsic allergic alveolitis due to avian or fungal antigens should be sought. It is important to obtain a history of other diseases, (e.g. systemic sclerosis, rheumatoid arthritis, polymyositis,

Table 1 Known causes of lung disease which may mimic fibrosing alveolitis

Extrinsic allergic alveolitis (chronic stage)
Occupational lung disease
Asbestosis
Hard metal disease
Drug therapy
Cytotoxic (e.g. bleomycin, busulphan, BCNU, methotrexate)
Antibacterial (e.g. nitrofurantoin, sulphasalazine)
Cardiological (e.g. amiodarone, tocainide)
Rheumatological (e.g. gold, D-penicillamine)
Analgesics (e.g. heroin)
Anticonvulsants (e.g. diphenylhydantoin)
Inhaled agents
Mercury vapour
Nitrogen dioxide
Ingested agents
Paraquat
Irradiation

Sjögren's syndrome, systemic lupus erythematosus, chronic active hepatitis, primary biliary cirrhosis, inflammatory bowel disease, renal tubular acidosis). Previous or current malignancy must be noted, particularly when cytotoxic therapy has been used. A full therapeutic drug history is required to exclude drug causes of fibrosis (Table 1).

Examination

Digital clubbing is present in approximately 70 to 80 per cent of patients. Fine crackles are universal, best heard at the lung bases. They occur at the end of inspiration in early cases but become paninspiratory in more advanced disease. At advanced stages of disease, central cyanosis may be evident, and the signs of right ventricular hypertrophy, pulmonary hypertension, and cor pulmonale with parasternal heave, gallop rhythm, loud pulmonary second heart sound, raised jugular venous pressure, and ankle oedema may be present.

Examination may reveal features that are consistent with other disease, such as arthropathy or the skin changes of systemic sclerosis or systemic lupus erythematosus. There may also be features to suggest an alternative diagnosis, for example mononeuritis multiplex or skin vasculitic lesions in necrotizing vasculitis; lupus pernio or erythema nodosum in sarcoidosis; or Kaposi's sarcoma with an opportunistic lung infection in AIDS.

Investigations

Imaging

A typical chest radiograph in CFA has small lung fields and reticulonodular shadowing at the periphery of the lung and at the bases, obscuring the right and left heart borders and making the diaphragmatic surfaces irregular (Fig. 1). In more advanced cases, all lung zones are involved, often with honeycomb shadowing. Rarely, the chest radiograph may be normal or present a diffuse 'ground-glass' pattern which is typical of desquamative interstitial pneumonia. Lymphadenopathy is rare on the chest radiograph, and pleural disease should suggest an alternative diagnosis, especially asbestosis.

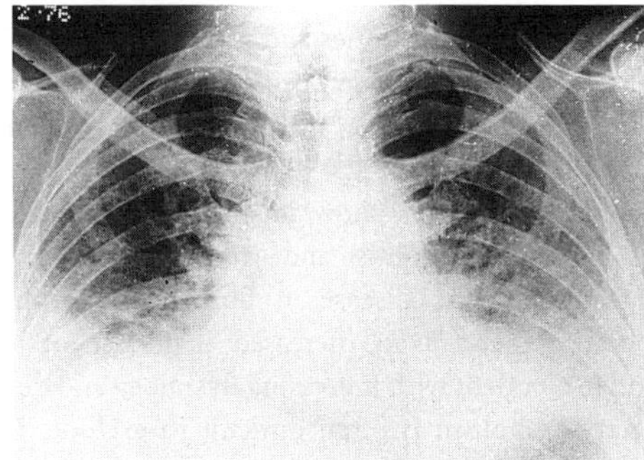

Fig. 1 Chest radiograph of a patient with advanced fibrosing alveolitis. The small lung fields with obscured right and left heart borders and both hemidiaphragms should be noted.

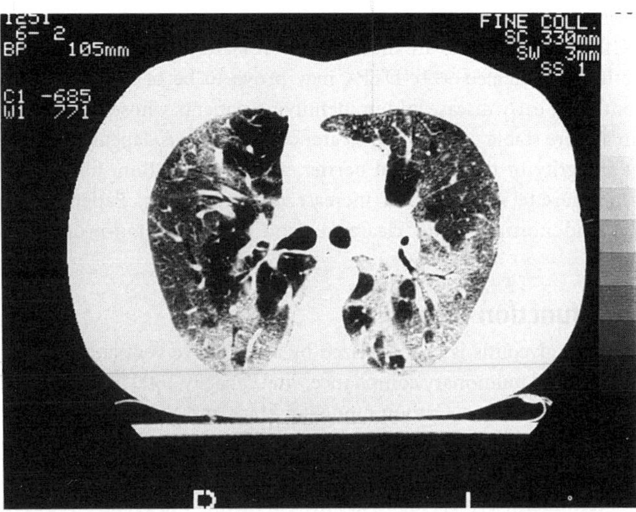

Fig. 2 High resolution CT of the lungs of a patient with fibrosing alveolitis. The widespread ground-glass opacification, denoting a more cellular histopathological pattern of disease, should be noted.

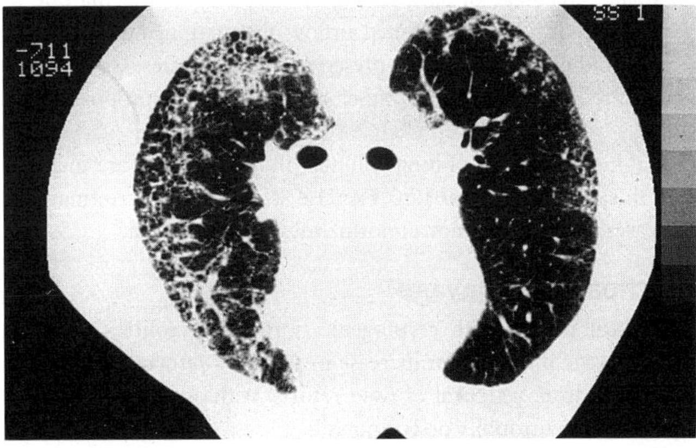

Fig. 3 High resolution CT of the lungs of a patient with fibrosing alveolitis. The predominantly peripheral abnormality should be noted. In the left lung the disease process is more extensive and has a reticular pattern indicative of a more fibrotic disease process.

High resolution computed tomography (HRCT) is virtually pathognomonic in cryptogenic fibrosing alveolitis. Typical early changes are of a peripheral rim of increased attenuation present posteriorly at the bases. In more cellular disease this assumes a ground-glass pattern (Fig. 2) but in more fibrotic, destroyed lung the pattern is reticular (Fig. 3). As disease becomes more extensive, these changes are observed in the other lung zones and more centrally. CT confirms that pleural disease is not present in fibrosing alveolitis but, in contrast with the plain chest radiograph, mediastinal lymphadenopathy is commonly present.

Ventilation–perfusion scans show mismatching of perfusion and ventilation in fibrosing alveolitis, and are completely unreliable in excluding thromboembolic disease in fibrosing alveolitis. This is important because there is an increased incidence of pulmonary embolism, and in a patient with increasing dyspnoea and deteriorating CFA, pulmonary embolism is often difficult to exclude. Pulmonary angiography may be necessary.

Gallium scanning is highly sensitive but not specific. It is expensive and needs two visits to hospital. It should be restricted to patients in whom other tests have failed to confirm a pulmonary problem but in whom disease is still suspected.

Other radionuclides are the subject of research. The clearance from the lung of inhaled 99Tc-DTPA may prove to be of value, both in identifying early disease and in identifying patients whose disease will run a more stable course. The clearance of isotope is dependent upon the integrity of the epithelial barrier, and inflammation, fibrosis, or even cigarette smoking will increase clearance rates, Patients with CFA and normal DTPA clearance tend to run a non-progressive course.

Lung function tests

Fibrosing alveolitis is characterized by a restrictive ventilatory defect with reduced pulmonary compliance, vital capacity, total lung capacity, and residual volume. Carbon monoxide transfer factor and coefficient are reduced .The blood gases may be normal initially but in progressive disease, PaO_2 is low due to V/Q mis-match. $PaCO_2$ is low early, but rises terminally. Typical blood gas measurements will reveal a reduced PaO_2 value with a normal or low $PaCO_2$ measurement. On exercise, hypoxaemia is exacerbated and the alveolar–arterial (A–a) gradient is widened.

A small percentage of patients have coexistent emphysema due to cigarette smoking. With combined airflow obstruction and restriction, the chest radiograph may have preserved lung volumes. Gas transfer (which is reduced by both emphysema and CFA) is disproportionally low.

Serial measurements of lung volumes and gas transfer are made to determine disease progression. Exercise is a useful discriminant in mild cases with only minor abnormalities of gas transfer.

Bronchoalveolar lavage

In a typical patient with cryptogenic fibrosing alveolitis, bronchoalveolar lavage produces an increase in total cell returns of three- to six-fold (up to 6 × 105/ml of fluid return) with an excess of (up to 20 per cent) neutrophils or eosinophils. Excess lymphocytes may be found and mast cells may be observed in a few patients. The prognostic value of bronchoalveolar lavage findings is uncertain. The presence of excess granulocytes, as opposed to lymphocytes, may be associated with a poorer response to treatment and prognosis. Very high lymphocytes suggest an alternative diagnosis (e.g. extrinsic allergic alveolitis).

Lung biopsy

Open-lung biopsy through either minithoracotomy or video-assisted thoracoscopic biopsy, with CT used to guide the surgeon, usually provides a definitive diagnosis and histological grading. Transbronchial biopsy is generally unhelpful, with adequate samples being obtained in only about 35 per cent of instances using this technique. Trephine drill biopsy and Trucut biopsy can be hazardous with unacceptable risk of haemorrhage and pneumothorax.

A decision to perform open-lung biopsy depends upon the individual case. A patient over the age of 65 with poor lung function, particularly with hypoxia at rest, is at high risk of any operative procedure. Under these circumstances, it is reasonable to make a clinical diagnosis, particularly with HRCT. However, with a younger patient, for whom prolonged treatment with potentially toxic drugs is being considered, it is important to establish a clear diagnosis before treatment is commenced.

Management

Detection of early disease at a time when symptoms are trivial or absent would provide the opportunity to prevent the disease advancing, but treatment at this stage would only be justifiable if reliable predictors of disease progression could be developed, and if potentially toxic treatments could reliably prevent progression. Treatment should be started if the patient is symptomatic or has deteriorating lung function. There have been few controlled clinical trials of treatment.

An objective response to oral corticosteroids (improvement in chest radiograph or lung function) occurs in a quarter of cases reported in the literature, with a subjective improvement in just over 50 per cent. The factors which predict a good response to corticosteroids include a patient with less dyspnoea, less radiographic abnormality, better PaO_2, an excess of lymphocytes on bronchoalveolar lavage, and a cellular open-lung biopsy. All these features would suggest early disease. Treatment generally commences at 1 mg/kg per d for 4–6 weeks. The dose is then reduced progressively but relapse is frequent and rapid, often at unacceptably high doses of steroids for long-term use. If the disease either stabilizes or improves, the patient should be maintained on prednisolone 20 mg every other day for a minimum of 1 year. If there is no response to corticosteroids or if deterioration occurs during dosage reduction, treatment should be replaced with a combination of prednisolone and an immunosuppressant.

A combination of prednisolone 20 mg on alternate days with cyclophosphamide (up to 125 mg/d) has been tested in a prospective controlled study comparing this regimen with high dosage corticosteroids. Objective response was found in approximately 20 per cent of patients and a small percentage of those who failed to respond to corticosteroids showed a response to the corticosteroid/cyclophosphamide regimen. The mortality at 5 years was not significantly different between the two treatment groups—approximately 50 per cent. A placebo group was not included. Maximum improvement may not be seen until after at least 6 months of treatment. Cyclophosphamide toxicity should be monitored by regular full blood counts and dipstick urine testing for haematuria.

An international trial of prednisolone/azathiaprine/cyclosporin is underway.

Single-lung transplantation is an option for younger patients with approximately 70 per cent of patients surviving 1 year and 45 per cent 5 years. At present, the shortfall in organs precludes many patients from being considered for transplantation, and with many patients with fibrosing alveolitis presenting over the age of 60 this reduces the numbers of patients for whom transplantation is an option.

When all treatment options have failed, supportive therapy is necessary. Supplemental oxygen may be required. Infection (especially opportunistic) should be investigated aggressively, treated promptly and often empirically. Differential diagnosis of deteriorating CFA, from for example *Pneumocystis carinii* pneumonia or even left ventricular failure is often very difficult. In the more terminal phases, opiates help to relieve the distressing breathlessness.

The most logical approach is to try and achieve disease stability, maintain that stability on a dosage of therapy which is acceptable for a period of a year, and then to discontinue treatment if disease stability is maintained. In practice, however, because of the high rate of relapse, low-dose maintenance therapy is continued indefinitely. Since prolonged use of immunosuppressant therapy has been associated with the development of malignancy, withdrawal of immunosuppression must be considered after 12–24 months of treatment and low-dose corticosteroids continued.

The potential for side-effects is of great importance when choosing a drug regimen. For example in an obese diabetic, high-dose prednisolone may provoke unacceptable side-effects, and a combination regimen would be preferable. In contrast, for an individual of child-bearing years, high-dosage prednisolone may be preferred in view of the risk of infertility. Prednisolone will produce a maximum improvement approximately 6 weeks after the start of therapy, whereas the combination therapy may require 3 to 6 months to see the maximum effect.

Prognosis

In all series, 50 per cent of all patients are dead within 5 years of presentation despite therapy. Improved survival is determined largely by those factors which predict good response to therapy. Detection and treatment of early disease is important. Real advances are only likely with a better understanding of pathogenesis and an increased awareness of early disease.

Further reading

See OTM3, pp. 2794–5.

Chapter 4.20

Bronchiolitis obliterans

J. M. Hopkin

Bronchiolitis obliterans is now recognized to occur in two distinct syndromes:

1. Bronchiolitis obliterans with organizing pneumonia (BOOP), otherwise known as cryptogenic organizing pneumonia (COP): in this, the bronchiolitis obliterans is part of a more major process affecting the alveoli and interstitium and the characteristic ventilatory defect is restrictive.
2. Constrictive bronchiolitis obliterans: in this, the histological changes are confined to the small airways and are associated with a progressive obstructive ventilatory defect.

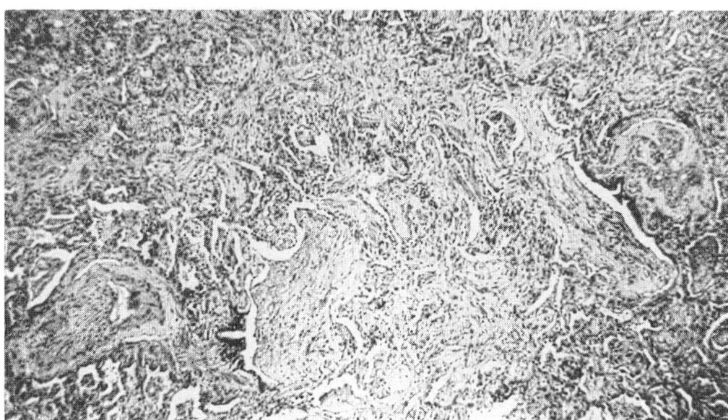

Fig. 1 Cryptogenic organizing pneumonia (or bronchiolitis obliterans with organizing pneumonia): photomicrograph of tissue from an open-lung biopsy shows fibrous tissue and inflammatory cell infiltration obliterating the bronchioles and extending to the alveoli.

Bronchiolitis obliterans with organizing pneumonia or cryptogenic organizing pneumonia

Buds or polyps of fibrous tissue, occurring patchily in the bronchioles and causing partial obstruction, extend into the alveolar sacs and are associated with a variable degree of interstitial inflammation and fibrosis (Fig. 1). Inflammatory cells, including lymphocytes, plasma cells, and also some neutrophils and eosinophils, aggregate within the fibrous tissue buds and tracts.

This pathology results from a variety of pulmonary insults including adult respiratory distress syndrome, organizing infections (e.g. *Pneumocystis carinii*, *Mycoplasma pneumoniae*, and viral infections), inhalation of toxic agents, and extrinsic allergic alveolitis. The distribution of the disease may be focal or diffuse, and in some instances the histological changes may be seen as a 'reaction' adjacent to a lung abscess, an area of pulmonary vasculitis, infarct, or other conditions.

Idiopathic BOOP is a syndrome that appears to follow a respiratory tract infection and presents as a subacute influenza-like illness with variable fever and malaise, cough, and dyspnoea. Crackles are usually audible on auscultation, and there is a restrictive pulmonary ventilatory defect with hypoxaemia. Chest radiograph abnormalities, best visualized on CT scanning, are typically multiple and strikingly peripheral in distribution (Fig. 2). Failure of an apparently infective illness to respond to antibiotics is often the first clinical clue to the diagnosis of idiopathic BOOP. Peripheral blood eosinophilia and autoantibodies are absent; there are no diagnostic 'blood test' abnormalities. Response to corticosteroids is good, and these can be slowly tapered over 6–12 months. The dilemma is whether to introduce corticosteroids in what initially appeared an infective illness. Fibre-optic bronchoscopic lavage, to allow culture of deep lung samples, is useful in excluding continuing bacterial infection, whilst many physicians proceed to a lung biopsy. The long-term outlook can be good, but over-rapid tapering of the corticosteroid dosage can lead to relapse.

Constrictive bronchiolitis obliterans

There is chronic bronchiolar inflammation with concentric bronchiolar luminal narrowing, submucosal fibrous thickening, and mucostasis. These features may also be seen in response to a range of

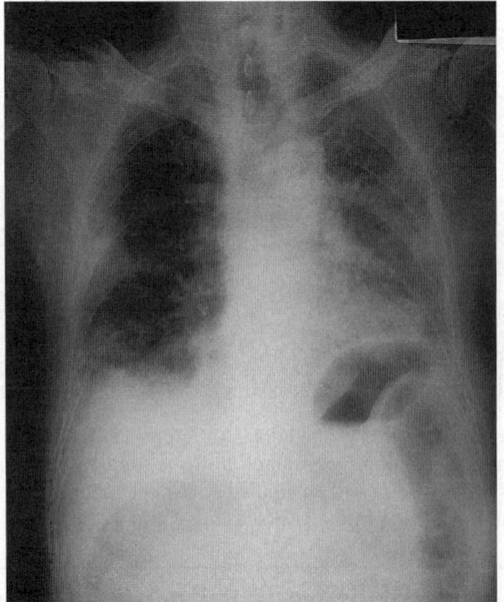

(a)

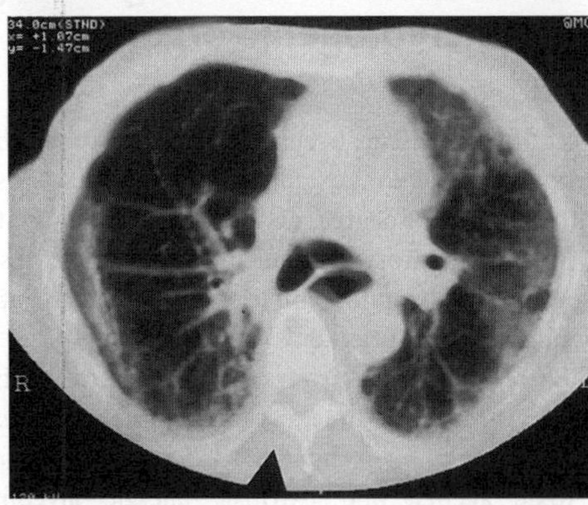

(b)

Fig. 2(a), (b) Cryptogenic organizing pneumonia (or bronchiolitis obliterans with organizing pneumonia): (a) plain chest radiograph and (b) CT of the thorax showing scattered peripheral pneumonic changes in an 80-year-old man who presented with influenza-like illness, cough, and dyspnoea. There were scattered crackles, a restrictive ventilatory defect, and hypoxaemia. No response followed antibiotic regimens over 1 month, but oral corticosteroids produced prompt, sustained improvement.

pulmonary insults—notably in rejection of a pulmonary allograft, as a complication of rheumatoid disease, as a result of viral infection in childhood (particularly by adenovirus), and following inhalation and injury from gases that include nitrogen dioxide, ammonia, and chlorine. In some cases there is no evident cause.

Bronchiolitis obliterans is an important complication of lung and heart-lung transplantation. Patients present with dyspnoea and progressive airflow obstruction; arterial oxygen haemoglobin saturations are reduced, but the chest radiograph is normal. The syndrome is thought to be due to chronic or repeated graft rejection; increased immunosuppression may occasionally result in improvement.

Constrictive bronchiolitis obliterans, as a rare complication of rheumatoid disease, presents with dyspnoea. Lung function tests show typical obstructive changes and the chest radiograph is normal except for hyperinflation. The disorder is usually progressive and not responsive to corticosteroids.

Postviral bronchiolitis obliterans in childhood may improve or remit, but the outlook is often poor. Progressive dyspnoea and airflow obstruction towards respiratory failure may develop with little or no useful response to corticosteroids.

Further reading

Davison, A.G., Heard, B.E., McAllister, W.A.C., and Turner-Warwick, M. (1983). Cryptogenic organizing pneumonitis. *Quarterly Journal of Medicine*, **52**, 382–94.

du Bois, R.M. and Geddes, G.M. (1991). Obliterative bronchiolitis, cryptogenic organizing pneumonitis, and bronchiolitis obliterans or bronchiolitis obliterans organizing pneumonia: three names for two different conditions. *European Respiratory Journal*, **4**, 774–5.

Epler, G.R., Colby, T.V., McLoud, T.C., Carrington, C.B., and Gaensler, E.A. (1985). Bronchiolitis obliterans organizing pneumonia. *New England Journal of Medicine*, **312**, 152–8.

Geddes, D.M. (1991). BOOP and COP. *Thorax*, **46**, 545–7.

Wright, J.L., Cagle, P., Churg, A., Colby, T.V., and Myers, J. (1992). Diseases of the small airways. *American Review of Respiratory Disease*, **146**, 240–62.

Chapter 4.21

The lung in collagen–vascular disease

R. J. Shaw

Rheumatoid arthritis

Rheumatoid arthritis is a symmetrical inflammatory polyarthropathy of unknown cause (see OTM3, pp. 2953–64). The different pulmonary manifestations of rheumatoid arthritis are listed in Table 1. These complications generally occur in the presence of well-established rheumatoid disease and are severe in less than 5 per cent of patients.

Pleural disease

Pleural disease is usually asymptomatic. Five per cent of patients have clinically evident pleural effusions with mild dyspnoea and pleuritic chest pain. The fluid is an exudate with high lactate dehydrogenase levels and shows mainly lymphocytes. Often the glucose and pH of the fluid are reduced, mimicking an infectious or malignant process. Excess of polymorphonuclear cells suggests a sterile or septic empyema. The pleural effusion either resolves spontaneously or remains for months or years without requiring any specific treatment. Empyema requires appropriate drainage.

Rheumatoid nodules

Rheumatoid nodules fall into two types; necrobiotic nodules and Caplan's syndrome, and are generally asymptomatic. The nodules

Table 1 Pleural/pulmonary manifestations of rheumatoid arthritis

Pleural disease.
Nodules (necrobiotic and Caplan's syndrome).
Interstitial lung disease.
Airways disease.
Others (infection including mycobacterial infection and bronchial sepsis, vascular disease, apical fibrobullous disease, thoracic cage immobility, drug-induced lung disease).

may cavitate, and thereby cause a spontaneous pneumothorax. Percutaneous needle aspiration of a necrobiotic nodule is rarely diagnostic. Radiographic surveillance is thus indicated since malignancy and tuberculosis are important differential diagnoses.

Caplan's syndrome represents development of either single or multiple nodules in coal miners with rheumatoid arthritis; but they can occur in other dust-exposed occupations. These nodules appear rapidly and often cavitate. Histologically, they are similar to necrobiotic nodules with the additional feature of dust-laden macrophages.

Interstitial lung disease

Histological evidence of interstitial inflammation and fibrosis is common in rheumatoid arthritis, but lung fibrosis is less commonly an important clinical problem. The clinical physiological radiographic manifestations resemble cryptogenic fibrosing alveolitis with progressive dyspnoea, tachypnoea, bibasilar fine crepitations, restrictive ventilatory defect and hypoxia on exertion. High resolution CT of early disease show bibasilar patchy alveolar infiltrates. In more severe disease, a fibrotic pattern supervenes with progression to radiographic honeycombing. There may be associated pleural disease. The lung histology is often non-specific, with evidence of inflammation and fibrosis or honeycomb lung. A predominant lymphocytic infiltration with germinal follicles adjacent to the airways of vessels (termed follicular bronchitis or bronchiolitis), rheumatoid nodules, pleural fibrosis, or adhesions suggest interstitial lung disease associated with rheumatoid arthritis, as opposed to lone cryptogenic fibrosing alveolitis.

The prognosis of lung fibrosis with rheumatoid arthritis is probably similar to that of cryptogenic fibrosing alveolitis, with conflicting evidence of the benefits of corticosteroid treatment and other immunosuppressants.

Airways disease in rheumatoid arthritis

Airways disease is uncommon in rheumatoid arthritis. Cricoarytenoid arthritis is manifest by ear pain, dysphagia, and the sensation of a foreign body in the throat although rarely with dyspnoea or stridor. Relapsing polychondritis in rheumatoid arthritis can affect the airways, causing upper airways obstruction. Airway infection in the form of bronchitis or bronchiectasis is twice as common in rheumatoid patients as in controls, possibly as a result in a debility or immunosuppression. Obliterative bronchiolitis where small airways (1–6 mm in diameter) are obliterated and replaced by scar tissue is a well-recognized but rare complication of rheumatoid arthritis.

Other pulmonary complications of rheumatoid arthritis

In addition to respiratory tract infection by conventional bacteria, infection with mycobacterium tuberculosis and non-tuberculosis mycobacteria may occur. Acute vasculitis as seen in systemic lupus erythematosus is only a rare complication of rheumatoid arthritis, although pulmonary hypertension in the absence of lung fibrosis is reported. Apical fibrobullous disease similar to that in ankylosing spondilitis is reported, and some patients experience problems associated with thoracic cage immobility. Differentiating rheumatoid arthritis from drug-induced lung disease can pose a problem since the drugs used for rheumatoid arthritis, namely gold salts, penicillamine, and methotrexate, are all associated with the development of pulmonary fibrosis. Withdrawal of any suspected drug is indicated.

Table 2 Pleuropulmonary manifestations of systemic lupus erythematosus

Pleuritis with or without effusion.
Acute lupus pneumonitis with or without pulmonary haemorrhage
Diaphragmatic dysfunction or shrinking lung.
Opportunistic infection in the setting of immunosuppressive drugs used in treatment.
Others

Systemic lupus erythematosus

Systemic lupus erythematosus is a common autoimmune disorder (see Chapter 10.11). The pleuropulmonary manifestations of systemic lupus erythematosus are listed in Table 2.

Pleural disease

Pleural disease is common in systemic lupus erythematosus. The pleural effusions may be bilateral, are usually small, and are exudates with a higher glucose and pH than that in rheumatoid arthritis. Antinuclear antibodies, anti-DNA antibodies, and LE cells may be found in the fluid; complement levels may be reduced.

Acute lupus pneumonitis with or without pulmonary haemorrhage

Acute lupus pneumonitis may be a transient lober or segmental event or a severe complication of systemic lupus erythematosus. It may accompany a generalized exacerbation of the disease. The severe syndrome consists of fever, dyspnoea, and hypoxaemia. Examination reveals tachypnoea, and fine or coarse crackles may be present. There are diffuse pulmonary infiltrates on the chest radiograph which may simulate adult respiratory distress syndrome. C-reactive protein is not usually elevated, complement levels may be low, and the ANF is usually strongly positive. An elevated carbon monoxide transfer suggest pulmonary haemorrhage. Bronchoalveolar lavage may help to identify infectious organisms, or in acute pulmonary haemorrhage it may show haemosiderin-laden macrophages. If serology is indecisive, open-lung biopsy is definitive, showing diffuse alveolar damage with inflammation, vasculitis, and pulmonary haemorrhage. Treatment of acute lupus pneumonitis requires large doses of corticosteroids or immunosuppressant agents.

Diaphragmatic dysfunction or shrinking lung

This syndrome presents with dyspnoea and loss of lung volume. Radiography shows small but clear lungs with high diaphragms bilaterally. The 'shrinking lungs' are probably due to diaphragm dysfunction, as these patients have a reduction in transdiaphragmatic pressures.

Systemic sclerosis and crest

Systemic sclerosis is a syndrome comprising inflammation and fibrosis of skin and internal organs. CREST (calcinosis, Raynaud's disease, oesophageal dismotility, sclerodactyly, and telangiectasia) is considered to be a more benign variant. There are three main pulmonary complications.

Recurrent bacterial infection

Poor oesophageal mortality predisposes to recurrent aspiration pneumonias which may contribute to lower-lobe fibrosis or bronchiectasis.

Pulmonary fibrosis

The majority of patients with systemic sclerosis will develop pulmonary fibrosis over time. This has similar symptoms, signs, lung physiology, chest radiograph, and high resolution CT changes to cryptogenic fibrosing alveolitis and responds poorly to treatment with corticosteroids or immunosuppresants.

Pulmonary hypertension

Pulmonary hypertension occurs in 25 to 50 per cent of patients with systemic sclerosis and two-thirds of those with CREST, where it may occur in the absence of pulmonary fibrosis. There is dyspnoea in the presence of a clear chest radiograph. The pathology of the vessels reveals intimal proliferation, medial hyperplasia, and perivascular hyperplasia.

Other reported pulmonary complications of systemic sclerosis include pleuritis, pneumothorax, pulmonary haemorrhage, and scar carcinoma.

Polymyositis and dermatomyositis

Polymyositis and dermatomyositis are characterized by muscle pain and weakness. The pleural and pulmonary complications include aspiration pneumonia (occurring due to diminished cough reflex or weak pharyngeal muscles), respiratory muscle weakness leading to loss of lung volumes, and basal atelectasis (which may progress to hypoventilation and respiratory failure). Fibrosing alveolitis is a rare, occasionally florid complication of both diseases. Lung cancer may be the promoter of the dermatomyositis.

Sjögren's syndrome

Sjögren's syndrome (commonly part of other collagen vascular diseases) may give rise to dryness and atrophic changes in the upper airways, leading to atrophic rhinitis, xerostomia (dry mouth), and xerotrachea. Xerotrachea or bronchitis sicca is perhaps the most common condition. It presents as an unremitting, non-productive cough. Patients may also have chronic bronchitis, recurrent infections, atelectasis, and obstructive airways disease. A proportion of patients develop one of a spectrum of diseases ranging from lymphocytic interstitial pneumonitis to pseudolymphoma (see OTM3, Chapter 17.10.8).

Mixed connective tissue disease

Mixed connective tissue disease combining features of systemic lupus erythematosus, systemic sclerosis, Sjögren's syndrome, and polymyositis. Patients with mixed connective tissue disease commonly have evidence of interstitial lung disease. As many as 80 per cent have impaired lung function, but most are asymptomatic, a proportion progress to fibrosing alveolitis and behave as patients with systemic sclerosis. Pulmonary hypertension may occur as in systemic sclerosis.

Ankylosing spondylitis

Pulmonary complications occur in under 2 per cent of patients with ankylosing spondylitis.

Apicofibrobullous disease has the radiographic features of bilateral progressive upper-zone fibrosis with cavitation. Patients may complain of cough, sputum production, and dyspnoea, or may be asymptomatic. The differential diagnosis includes tuberculosis. In advanced cases, the cavities can be infected by aspergillus or atypical mycobacteria.

The fusion of vertical bodies may reduce rib movement and thus lung volumes. However this usually causes little ventilatory impairment.

Behçet's disease

Behçet's disease (see Chapter 10.16) may have respiratory manifestations including haemoptysis, pleuritis, fleeting chest radiograph shadows, and pulmonary artery aneurysms. The Hughes–Stovin syndrome, which includes venous thrombosis and pulmonary aneurysms, may be a manifestation of Behçet's disease.

Further reading

Anaya, J.M., Diethelm, L., Ortiz, L.A., Gutierrez, M., Citera, G., Welsh, R.A., and Espinoza, L.R. (1995). Pulmonary involvement in rheumatoid arthritis. *Seminars in Arthritis and Rheumatism*, 24, 242–54.

Chapter 4.22

Pulmonary vasculitis and granulomatosis

D. J. Lane and J. M. Hopkin

Classification of these disorders is complicated by unclear aetiology, the wide variation in the size and distribution of vessels involved, and the variable clinical picture (see Chapter 10.10). Positive antineutrophil cytoplasmic bodies (ANCA) are present in Wegener's granulomatosis, most cases of Churg–Strauss syndrome, and microvasculitic polyarteritis nodosa, but are not present in systemic lupus and its allied disorders in which hypocomplementaemia and anti-DNA antibodies are typical (Table 1). The hypersensitivity vasculitides, in which the lungs are occasionally involved as part of a systemic disease, and the pulmonary vascular and granulomatous manifestations of the connective tissue disorders are described in Chapters 10.9–10.18. Modest HLA associations are known for certain connective tissue disorders. There are as yet no consistent associations with external agents.

Churg–Strauss syndrome: allergic granulomatosis

This occurs typically in young adults with a history of asthma; they develop evidence of systemic vasculitis in association with a marked peripheral eosinophilia, which may represent progression of allergic disease in response to an unusual, undetected antigen.

Clinical and laboratory features

There is a history of rhinitis and asthma, with onset usually in early adult life. Peripheral eosinophilia becomes marked and there are eosinophilic infiltrates in various organs, particularly the lungs. The appearance of vasculitis in the middle to late thirties suggests the diagnosis. The clinical course can be acute and rapidly fatal with heart failure, but it is more usually subacute and relapsing.

The diagnostic triad is thus asthma, eosinophilia, and systemic vasculitis. Pulmonary radiographic infiltrates accompanying the asthma are patchy and transient hilar lymphadenopathy, pleural effusion, and both fine small and large (non-cavitating) nodules are described. The eosinophilia is greater than 1.5×10^9/l—greater than seen in atopic asthma but less than in hypereosinophilic syndrome. Vascular lesions can affect the body widely, for example mononeuritis multiplex, painful lesions in the bowel, skin with a variety of maculopapular, urticarial, or purpuric rashes or granulomatous nodules, and a focal segmental glomerulonephritis. Skin-prick tests are often positive for common environmental allergens, with elevated serum IgE; antineutrophil cytoplasmic antibody are variably present. Necrotizing vasculitis can usually be demonstrated in vessels in and around the lesions, but granulomas occur in fewer than half the cases examined at autopsy.

Treatment

Oral corticosteroids are almost universally successful, transforming a previously poor prognosis; the treatment may need to be prolonged at low dosage to prevent relapse.

Wegener's granulomatosis

There is the classic triad of upper and lower respiratory tract granulomas combined with necrotizing focal glomerulonephritis in this, the best known and most easily identified of the pulmonary granulomatous vasculitides. It may occur with single organ involvement (limited Wegener's).

Clinical and laboratory features

Pulmonary involvement can cause haemoptysis and chest pain, but often the radiographic changes are more marked than symptoms or physical signs. The chest radiograph can show changing nodular pulmonary opacities, which frequently cavitate but may regress spontaneously (Fig. 1), more widespread 'pneumonic' shadows. Involvement of the trachea and bronchi may obstruct the airway and, occasionally an obliterative bronchiolitis may spread to bronchioles with atelectasis and pleural involvement.

Table 1 Classification of vasculitides

Granulomatous vasculitides
• Allergic granulomatosis and angiitis
• Classic Wegener's granulomatosis
• Limited Wegener's granulomatosis
• Lymphomatoid granulomatosis
• Necrotizing sarcoidal granulomatosis
• Bronchocentric granulomatosis
Hypersensitivity vasculitis
• Anaphylactoid purpura
• Mixed cryoglobulinaemia
• Vasculitis associated with malignancy, infection, drugs
Pulmonary vasculitis with connective tissue diseases
• Rheumatoid disease
• Systemic lupus erythematosus
• Systemic sclerosis
• Dermatopolymyositis
• Mixed connective tissue disease

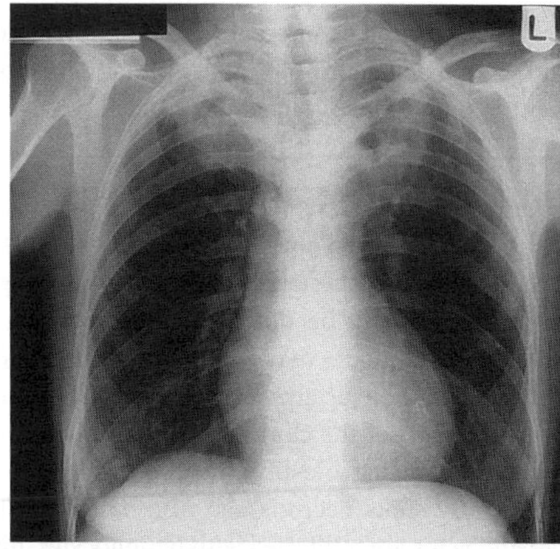

(a)

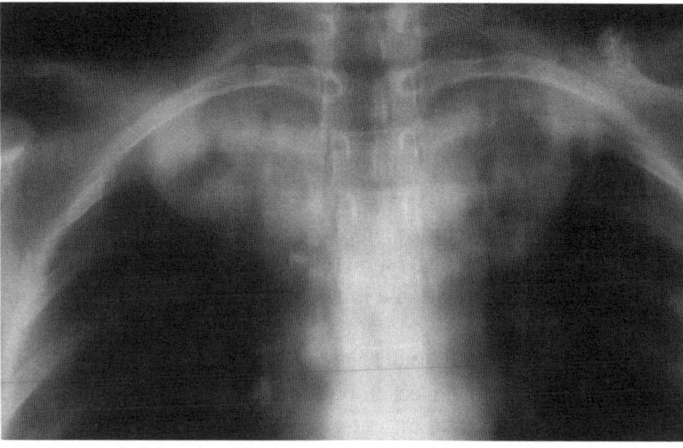
(b)

Fig. 1(a), (b) (a) Wegener's granulomatosis. (a) Radiograph showing bilateral cavitating apical masses in a woman with features of upper respiratory tract disease and glomerulonephritis. (b) Tomograms.

In the upper respiratory tract granulomas in the nose may produce little more than coryza with epistaxis and some nasal crusting, but extensive destruction is possible leading to nasal septal perforation and saddle nose, or there may be ulcerative lesions of the sinuses, palate, or pharynx.

The necrotizing glomerulonephritis is often asymptomatic but sometimes acute and fulminating.

There is often malaise, fever, and arthralgia—and there may also be vasculitic lesions in the skin, and the nervous and cardiovascular system.

Antineutrophilic cytoplasmic antibodies (directed at myeloperoxidase) are present; there is usually normochromic normocytic anaemia with elevated erythrocyte sedimentation rate. The lesions in the lung show granulomatous nodules built up from lymphocytes, plasma cells, and histiocytes; giant cells form, and the centre of the nodule is frequently necrotic and at a distance there is a necrotic vasculitis of both arteries and veins. The renal lesion is a focal necrotizing glomerulonephritis with frequent crescent formation.

Prognosis and treatment

Confusing symptoms and signs may lead to delayed diagnosis and thereby worsened prognosis because of progression of the renal lesion. Treatment of the disorder has been transformed by the use of cyclophosphamide therapy (2 mg/kg/day) continued for at least a year after remission. Corticosteroids are often added, certainly for an initial phase, and prescription on alternate days minimizes side-effects that can include opportunistic infection. An initial remission rate of over 90 per cent is now to be expected.

Necrotizing sarcoid granulomatosis

Presentation is usually with non-specific respiratory complaints such as cough or chest pain and chest radiology shows striking, usually multiple, nodules which may be down to miliary in size and are frequently confluent. Hilar nodes may be seen on the chest radiograph and are often found pathologically. Neither systemic vasculitis nor glomerulonephritis is part of the clinical picture; though rarely there is uveitis. The nodules are sarcoid-like, but the epithelioid giant-cell granulomas frequently show necrosis and also vasculitis. The walls of both arteries and veins are infiltrated with lymphocytes, histiocytes, and plasma cells, leading to vessel destruction and local infarction. Prognosis is good with untreated survivals of a decade or more. Oral corticosteroids, usually without cytotoxics, produce good remission; the occasional relapse responds equally well.

Bronchocentric granulomatosis

This morphological diagnosis lacks clear-cut immunological features, and there is increasing suggestion that this is a sustained bronchial inflammatory reaction to some inhaled antigen, for example fungus. It presents as localized pulmonary shadowing in a patient with persistent cough and dyspnoea; there is asthma in about half the cases and a high peripheral eosinophil count. Since there is an isolated mass or alveolar infiltrate on chest radiograph many are diagnosed histologically after thoracotomy. The lesions consist of necrotizing granulomas centred on an airway and surrounded by collapsed consolidated lung; epithelioid cells are arranged radially to form granulomas but there is no arteritis. The bronchial lumen is filled with inspissated mucus together with the ulcerated bronchial wall, and the peribronchial tissues is infiltrated by eosinophils and eosinophilic masses. Corticosteroids will clear the consolidation even though repeated courses may be needed.

Further reading

Hoffman, G.S. (1994). Emerging concepts in the management of vasculitic diseases. *Advances in Internal Medicine*, **39**, 277–303.

Hunder, G. (1996). Vasculitis: diagnosis and therapy. *American Journal of Medicine*, **100**(2A), 37S–45S

Liebow, A.A. (1973). Pulmonary angiitis and granulomatosis. *American Review of Respiratory Disease*, **108**, 1–18.

Niles, J.L. (1996). Antineutrophil cytoplasmic antibodies in the classification of vasculitis. *Annual Review of Medicine*, **47**, 303–13.

Chapter 4.23

Pulmonary haemorrhagic disorders

D. J. Lane

Pulmonary haemorrhage is suspected when haemoptysis is associated with radiographic alveolar shadowing (Fig. 1). The diagnosis is supported by the demonstration of a high transfer factor for carbon monoxide or multiple haemosiderin-laden macrophages in sputum, bronchoscopic alveolar lavage samples, or lung biopsy.

A range of different disorders can cause recurrent pulmonary bleeding and anaemia including chronic pulmonary venous congestion (mitral stenosis, left ventricular failure, pulmonary veno-occlusive disease), bleeding disorders, and thrombolysis which are discussed elsewhere in this book (see Sections 2 and 3).

Goodpasture's syndrome (see also Chapter 12.8)

This comprises pulmonary haemorrhage and glomerulonephritis. The syndrome is now usually considered as a triad of these two features together with the demonstration of autoantibodies to glomerular basement membrane. The basement antigen is now recognized to be the α-3 chain of type IV collagen. The majority of patients are smokers. It is thought that smoking or organic hydrocarbon exposure initiates endothelial damage and thus allows access of autoantibody to basement membrane in the kidney and lung.

In the lungs, there are red cells in the alveoli following acute bleeding and later haemosiderin-laden macrophages. The glomeruli show focal proliferative and necrotizing glomerulonephritis, usually with crescent formation. Presentation is with cough, breathlessness, and haemoptysis that is intermittent and ranges from occasional streaks to massive fatal bleeding. Renal disease may be missed at this stage because it is only evident as proteinuria or microscopic haematuria, but may progress rapidly to renal failure.

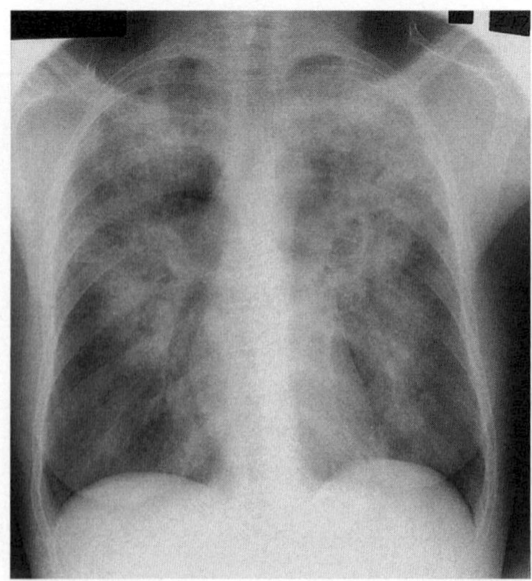

Fig. 1 Radiograph showing gross alveolar shadowing following major pulmonary haemorrhage in 60-year-old man with systemic vasculitis.

The chest radiograph shows single or multiple patchy shadows due to intra-alveolar blood. These resolve over the course of 2 weeks unless there is further bleeding. At the time of bleeding there may be arterial hypoxaemia and reduced lung volumes, but carbon monoxide gas transfer is increased as the inspired carbon monoxide is taken up by the blood within the lungs. This test can be used to monitor the progress of the pulmonary bleeding. Haemosiderin-laden macrophages are found in the sputum or at bronchoscopic alveolar lavage. Prolonged, severe bleeding leads to an iron-deficiency anaemia.

The diagnosis of Goodpasture's syndrome is confirmed by demonstrating circulating antibasement membrane antibodies (present in 90 per cent) or linear immunofluorescence on renal biopsy. The main treatment (see also Chapter 12.8) is plasma exchange, which must be started early before there is irreversible renal damage and continued until antibasement membrane antibodies are absent. Steroids and immunosuppressant drugs may be helpful temporarily to control the pulmonary haemorrhage, but probably have only a secondary role in controlling the renal disease. Patients should not smoke and should avoid hydrocarbon exposure. Pneumonectomy may be required for uncontrollable pulmonary haemorrhage.

Idiopathic pulmonary haemosiderosis

This is a rare disorder of children and young adults in which there is recurrent bleeding into the lungs. The extravasated blood is taken up by macrophages which become loaded with haemosiderin, and repeated bleeding may cause a marked iron-deficiency anaemia. Blood in the alveoli is in some way fibrogenic, and diffuse pulmonary fibrosis eventually develops. Other conditions which cause recurrent alveolar bleeding, such as mitral stenosis and chronic severe left ventricular failure (Section 2), can result in identical pathological changes.

Serum IgA is elevated in most cases and there are reports of associations with rheumatoid arthritis, antibodies to cow's milk, and exposure to gasoline products. Coeliac disease is another association, and this subgroup shows a high incidence of HLA B8 antigen. Idiopathic pulmonary haemosiderosis is probably a heterogeneous condition.

Patients present with either recurrent acute pulmonary bleeding, or progressive breathlessness with diffuse radiographic changes. Physical examination is unhelpful and the chest radiograph shows variable alveolar shadowing due to blood and, ultimately, fibrosis. These shadows clear completely over 1 to 3 weeks. Eventually a large bleed can be fatal. Lung function tests show progressive loss of volumes.

Supportive treatment is required during the acute bleeding, and artificial ventilation is occasionally required. There are case reports suggesting responses to avoidance of milk and gluten and to immunosuppressive agents including corticosteroids and cyclophosphamide.

Other causes of alveolar haemorrhage

Although the haemorrhage can be as dramatic as in Goodpasture's syndrome or as persistent as in idiopathic pulmonary haemosiderosis, it is generally overshadowed by other features of the underlying disease.

- Systemic vasculitides, particularly those such as Wegener's granulomatosis with prominent vascular necrosis, may present with alveolar haemorrhage; there may be a special association with those showing IgM antineutrophil cytoplasmic antibodies.
- Systemic lupus erythematosus can cause alveolar haemorrhage, which can be massive without evidence of pulmonary vasculitis.
- Rapidly progressive glomerulonephritis, whether immune complex mediated or not, may be accompanied by alveolar haemorrhage. In half of immunofluorescence-negative cases, haemoptysis and pulmonary infiltrates have been recorded although the pattern of the pulmonary disease is often mild.

Alveolar haemorrhage has been reported to result from various exogenous agents such as D-penicillamine, lymphangiography contrast media, and trimellitic anhydride fumes or powder.

Further reading

Leatherman, J.W., Davies, S.F., and Hoidal, J.R. (1984). Alveolar haemorrhage syndromes; diffuse and microvascular lung haemorrhage in immune and idiopathic disorders. *Medicine*, Baltimore, **63**, 343–61.

Chapter 4.24

Pulmonary eosinophilia

D. J. Lane

In this multicausal syndrome there is pulmonary radiographic shadowing and peripheral blood eosinophilia. These conditions can be broadly divided into three categories:

(1) pulmonary infiltrations due to an eosinophilic alveolar exudate without airways involvement, e.g. simple pulmonary eosinophilia, prolonged pulmonary eosinophilia, and eosinophilic pneumonia;
(2) pulmonary infiltration with eosinophilia but including a component of airways obstruction as well as parenchymal lung disease, e.g. allergic bronchopulmonary aspergillosis and tropical eosinophilia;
(3) pulmonary infiltrations with eosinophilia and with or without airways involvement but with systemic vascular or granulomatous pathology, e.g. polyarteritis nodosa, allergic granulomatosis, and the hypereosinophilic syndrome.

Conditions with eosinophilia as part of a well-defined disease and which may include pulmonary involvement (e.g. Hodgkin's disease) are excluded.

Löffler's syndrome (simple pulmonary eosinophilia)

Transitory, migratory pulmonary shadows with modest peripheral eosinophilia in patients with a mild self-limiting illness is typical. Most present with cough, sometimes with sputum discoloured by abundant eosinophils; a few have malaise and mild fever. The pulmonary shadows, simple or multiple, appear peripheral and sometimes rather nodular, and last a few days only. There is alveolar consolidation with an eosinophil-filled exudate. The eosinophil count usually ranges between 1×10^9 and 2×10^9/l. Patients are often atopic. The defined causes of the syndrome suggest an allergic reaction, and are various. Some are reactions to parasites, including *Ascaris lumbricoides* and occasionally *A. suum*, Ancylostoma, Trichuris, Trichinella, Taenia, and Strongyloides (see Section 16). Drugs are an important category, including *p*-amino salicylic acid, aspirin, sulfonamides (including the antimalarial combination sulfadiazine and pyrimethamine or Fansidar), penicillin, and imipramine, nitrofurantoin, toxic smoke, and lymphangiography contrast medium. A significant minority of cases of Löffler's syndrome remain unexplained. Drug withdrawal or treatment of a worm infestation is required.

Eosinophilic pneumonia and prolonged pulmonary eosinophilia

This syndrome is similar to simple pulmonary eosinophilia; indeed, the differences may simply lie in degree and duration. Prolonged pulmonary eosinophilia may last for several months, and is associated with more severe clinical symptoms than simple pulmonary eosinophilia. High fever is usual, weight loss and other systemic features may occur, for example skin and hepatic necrosis, hepatosplenomegaly, and atopic manifestations such as rhinitis, sinusitis, and angio-oedema. The pulmonary disease is usually extensive, causing dyspnoea and hypoxia with signs of consolidation on clinical examination and chest radiograph, in a peripheral distribution. Eosinophilic pleural effusion may occur. There are macrophages, lymphocytes, and eosinophils in the alveolar exudate and sometimes angiitis or granuloma formation reminiscent of the more sinister disorder of Wegener's granulomatosis. The eosinophil count is usually more than 1×10^9/ml. Causes, and hence treatment, cover the same range as for simple pulmonary eosinophilia, but often no cause is evident. These cryptogenic cases respond dramatically to oral corticosteroid therapy which is usually required for 6–12 months.

Pulmonary eosinophilia with bronchial involvement

Eosinophilia (counts of above 0.4×10^9/ml) is common in straightforward bronchial asthma. Figures greater than about 1.0×10^9/ml suggest that a specific cause should be sought. Two syndromes stand out:

1. Allergic bronchopulmonary aspergillosis (Chapter 4.13), which consists of asthma, fleeting pulmonary infiltrates with a tendency to mucus impaction, and bronchial wall damage which leads to proximal bronchiectasis. In many countries, Aspergillus sensitivity accounts for more than 90 per cent of such cases.
2. Tropical eosinophilia (see also Section 16) is a condition seen in the tropics and characterized by asthmatic airways obstruction, parenchymal lung damage, and a marked peripheral eosinophilia. The typical presentation is persistent dry cough, particularly at night, quickly followed by nocturnal wheezy breathlessness, fever, and haemoptysis. On auscultation, there may be both wheeze and crepitations. The typical radiographic appearance is of bilateral mottling. Untreated, persistent dyspnoea reflects irreversible airways obstruction and pulmonary fibrosis, and there can be terminal respiratory failure and cor pulmonale. Lung function tests show a mixed obstructive and restrictive defect. The peripheral white cell count is often greatly elevated with 20 per cent eosinophils. Microfilariae, notably *Wuchereria bancrofti* and *Brugia malayi*, are the cause. The pathological lesions (focal granulomata in an infiltrate of eosinophils, neutrophils, polymorphs, and macrophages) represent an allergic response to microfilariae transiently released into the circulation. High titres of IgE, IgG, and IgM to the parasite are present on serology. A good prognosis is possible if the condition is recognized and treated early with diethyl carbamazine in a daily dose of 6–8 mg/kg body weight orally, given for a week. Longer courses may occasionally be necessary.

Further reading

Crofton, J.W., Livingstone, J.L., Oswald, N.C., and Roberts, A.I.M. (1952). Pulmonary eosinophilia. *Thorax*, 7, 1–35.

Udwadia, F.E. (1993). Tropical eosinophilia: a review. *Respiratory Medicine*, 87, 17–21.

Chapter 4.25

Lymphocytic infiltrations of the lung

D. J. Hendrick

Introduction

A number of disorders are characterized by a prominent, even dominant, lymphocytic infiltration of the lung. Several are rare and poorly understood, while others are relatively common and have additional, more definitive characteristics. Classification of the latter group poses few problems, and individual diseases (for example sarcoidosis, extrinsic allergic alveolitis, cryptogenic organizing pneumonia, and some cases of cryptogenic fibrosing alveolitis) are satisfactorily distinguishable. They are described elsewhere.

For the first group classification poses an evolving challenge—largely because precise mechanisms and full natural histories are yet to be defined. These disorders are often considered to represent a spectrum of overlapping conditions from relatively benign infiltration of apparently normal lymphocytes without involvement of other cellular lines, through vasculitic and granulomatous inflammation, to frank malignancy. Apparent progression from disorder to disorder within the spectrum is not uncommon, but it is not always clear whether individuals affected in this way truly progress from one disease to another or have a single disease whose early manifestations are similar to (and mistaken for) those of less serious neighbours in the disease spectrum. This has given rise to an alternative view that one end of the spectrum comprises a group of inflammatory disorders whose vasculitic and granulomatous features link more appropriately with diseases such as Wegener's granulomatosis and sarcoidosis, while the other end comprises the various malignant lymphomas.

Nevertheless, dominant lymphocytic infiltration is a convenient, definitive feature from which to consider the small group of uncommon pulmonary diseases which are described in this chapter. There is often paraprotein production, implying that a lymphocyte clone is involved. Depending on severity, these disorders are characterized clinically by cough (usually dry) and progressive undue exertional breathlessness, although systemic features of fever, malaise, and weight loss may also be prominent. Clubbing is not common, but there are frequently inspiratory crackles at the lung bases. The chest radiograph shows a diffuse interstitial pattern or patchy 'pneumonic' infiltrates with the more benign disorders, but nodular shadows are more characteristic at the more malignant end of the disease spectrum.

Lung function tests show a non-specific pattern of ventilatory restriction with impaired parenchymal function.

Lymphocytic (and plasma-cell) interstitial pneumonitis

At the most benign end of the spectrum, lymphocytic (or lymphoid) interstitial pneumonitis is characterized by diffuse infiltration of the lung interstitium and alveolar walls with small mature lymphocytes, immunoblasts (activated lymphocytes), and plasma cells. Occasionally, plasma cells dominate the lymphoid cell infiltrate, and in these circumstances the term plasma-cell interstitial pneumonitis is preferred; and occasionally there is hypo- rather than hypergammaglobulinaemia. Lymphocytic pulmonary infiltration may occur in isolation without obvious cause or may be associated with HIV infection and a variety of autoimmune disorders, particularly Sjögren's syndrome or systemic lupus erythematosus. It may also be a consequence of a graft-versus-host reaction. When it occurs in children with AIDS, it is thought to be largely a consequence of Epstein–Barr infection.

The respiratory features are similar to those of cryptogenic fibrosing alveolitis, and open biopsy is generally required for definitive diagnosis. Slow progression is characteristic, although lymphocytic interstitial pneumonitis is rather more responsive to corticosteroid or other immunosuppressive therapy, and it sometimes remits spontaneously.

Benign lymphocytic angiitis

Lymphocytic infiltration is centred in small arteries and arterioles, although necrosis is characteristically absent. Not infrequently there is granuloma formation. Therefore it has vasculitic and granulomatous features. It is rare, relatively benign, and usually affects the lungs or the skin. Most often there is no obvious provoking cause, but there have been reports of it emerging as a consequence of drug administration (streptokinase), HIV infection, or intrathoracic malignancy (thymoma).

Pulmonary lesions are usually focal and most commonly present as asymptomatic nodules on a chance chest radiograph. The diagnosis is then made following biopsy or resection. However, there may be systemic symptoms, and treatment with corticosteroids or cytotoxic agents may be necessary. The disease may progress to produce the more characteristic features of lymphomatoid granulomatosis, but more typically there is spontaneous remission. This suggests that it is primarily a benign reactive vasculitis rather than a malignant lymphoma, and that lymphomatoid granulomatosis may initially behave similarly.

Angioimmunoblastic (immunoblastic) lymphadenopathy

This is a systemic, and often febrile, disorder characterized by widespread reactive lymphadenopathy and the infiltration of various organs by activated lymphoid cells, characteristically, but not uniformly, T lymphocytes. CD8+ cells, often clonal, are observed more commonly than CD4+ cells in affected organs, but in peripheral blood active disease is characterized by decreased numbers of T cells and an increase in B lymphocytes. The latter are possibly released from T-cell control and this might explain the frequency of paraprotein production. Blood vessels may be prominently infiltrated—hence the original term, angioimmunoblastic lymphadenopathy.

This disorder occurs most commonly in the elderly and frequently in isolation, but it is often a consequence of infection (prominently HIV infection in recent years in younger subjects) or drug administration (often antibiotics), and it may be associated with autoimmunity.

Respiratory involvement is not common. It usually comprises mediastinal or hilar lymphadenopathy, although diffuse interstitial infiltration and pleural effusion may occur.

Management requires treatment of any provoking cause and, if necessary, the use of corticosteroids or other immunosuppressive agents. Occasionally there is spontaneous remission, but more commonly a T-cell lymphoma evolves. Indeed, the view is strengthening that most cases are fundamentally peripheral (i.e. post-thymic) T-cell lymphomas.

Lymphomatoid granulomatosis

Cytochemical and immunogenetic investigations suggest that lymphomatoid granulomatosis is a low grade T-cell lymphoma, although the typical histological appearances of prominent infiltration of blood vessel walls (hence vasculitis) and granuloma formation have suggested a disease of more benign nature. The infiltrating cells comprise a mixture of lymphocytes, plasma cells, histiocytes, and atypical lymphoid cells, and their proliferation leads to luminal obstruction followed by ischaemic necrosis.

The disease is uncommon in childhood but occurs throughout adult life. The lungs are almost invariably affected, but skin, central nervous system, and renal involvement is frequently seen and there is often peripheral neuropathy. The disease is typically multifocal, affecting several organs, and may simulate disseminated carcinoma. Pulmonary lesions are usually discrete and nodular, whether single or multiple, but may vary in size from small nodules less than a centimetre in diameter to large masses several centimetres across. Occasionally outlines are irregular and indistinct, suggesting patchy consolidation, and cavitation may occur. An inflammatory cause may consequently be suspected.

Symptoms are commonly dominated by systemic upset (fever, malaise, weight loss), but respiratory involvement is likely to cause cough (sometimes with haemoptysis) or undue breathlessness. The involvement of other organs may provide valuable diagnostic insight, but biopsy is necessary for definitive diagnosis. Temporary improvement sometimes follows treatment with corticosteroids alone, but a realistic chance of complete remission requires cytotoxic therapy for lymphoma.

Lymphoma

At the malignant end of the disease spectrum lies lymphomatous infiltration of the lung. All lymphoma tumour types may involve the thorax, whether at presentation or during disease evolution, and lymph nodes, lymphatics, airways, and lung parenchyma may all become infiltrated.

A comprehensive review of lymphomas is beyond the scope of this chapter, and the reader is referred to Chapter 3.29 for full detail. In brief, lymphomas can be considered to be of the Hodgkin's type (a unique malignancy arising typically in lymphoid tissue, of uncertain cell origin, and characterized by the Reed–Sternberg cell) or the non-Hodgkin's type. The latter arise from B lymphocytes, T lymphocytes, or histiocytes (or their stem cells), and can be classified according to a variety of aetiological, histological, immunological, and clinical features. To the respiratory-physician the differentiation of Hodgkin's disease and high grade non-Hodgkin's lymphoma from low-grade non-Hodgkin's lymphoma is of particular value, since the first two are potentially curable with aggressive chemotherapy regimens.

When Hodgkin's disease involves the thorax it usually does so by infiltrating hilar or mediastinal lymph nodes, although localized, even diffuse, parenchymal infiltration occurs occasionally. Asymmetrical nodal enlargement favours lymphoma over sarcoidosis, but in endemic areas tuberculosis most frequently explains nodal asymmetry. Pleural effusion is not uncommon. Radiotherapy is normally curative for localized nodal disease and is invaluable as an adjunct in reducing local bulk when the disease is disseminated. It carries less risk than chemotherapy, which is required for parenchymal or disseminated disease and for the small proportion of patients with localized nodal disease who show features of poor prognostic significance.

Non-Hodgkin's lymphoma occurs more commonly than Hodgkin's disease, and tends to affect a rather older population. Its thoracic manifestations are similar to those of Hodgkin's disease, but it has a greater tendency to be disseminated at presentation, and to be less responsive to chemotherapy. Nevertheless, localized high grade tumours are often curable, and useful palliation is generally achieved for many years for low grade tumours.

Further reading

See OTM3, p. 2808.

Chapter 4.26

Extrinsic allergic alveolitis

D. J. Hendrick

The diffuse inflammatory disorder of the gas exchanging tissues which results from hypersensitivity to inhaled organic dusts is known as extrinsic allergic alveolitis (EAA) or hypersensitivity pneumonitis. For dust deposition to occur predominantly in the alveoli, particle size must be largely confined to the range 0.5–5 μm. This encompasses the diameters of many antigenic bacterial and fungal spores, and a large number of microbial species are now recognized causes. In addition, the disease has been noted to follow exposure to a variety of antigens derived from animal, vegetable, and even chemical sources, in both the workplace and the home.

Clinical features

Acute form

This is the most easily recognized because symptoms are often quickly distressing and incapacitating, and have a high degree of specificity. Recognition is particularly easy for groups such as farmers and pigeon fanciers for whom the risk of EAA is well known. Following a sensitizing period of exposure of weeks to years, the affected subject experiences repeated episodes of an influenza-like illness accompanied by cough and undue breathlessness some hours (usually 3–9) after commencing exposure to the relevant organic dust. The systemic influenza-like symptoms generally dominate those that are essentially respiratory in nature, and the subject complains most of malaise, fever, chills, widespread aches and pains (particularly headache), anorexia, and tiredness. He is unlikely to exercise himself and so may be less aware of undue shortness of breath, although he is likely to develop a dry cough without wheeze and some difficulty in taking deep satisfying breaths. Occasionally there is an asthmatic or bronchitic response in addition to that in the gas exchanging tissues, and wheezing or productive cough becomes a further feature.

The severity and duration of symptoms depend on exposure dose and the level of sensitivity. When occupation is responsible, the affected worker may feel unwell only at home during the following evening or night and be fully recovered by the next morning. Consequently the relevance of the workplace may be obscured. Following severe responses, however, complete remission may require days or even weeks, and in exceptionally severe cases, life-threatening respiratory failure may develop requiring intensive care.

Fever and gravity-dependent crackles comprise the major physical signs, with breathing being fast but shallow. Clubbing is very rarely seen. Hypoxia is typically accompanied by hypocapnia, but the chest radiograph is often normal unless the episode is severe. There is then a diffuse alveolar filling pattern. Spontaneous recovery can be expected to begin within 12–24 h, and can be accelerated with corticosteroids. It is generally complete.

Chronic and intermediate forms

In some subjects, EAA expresses itself in a much less dramatic, though potentially more serious, way. There is a slowly increasing loss of exercise tolerance due to shortness of breath but no systemic upset apart from an occasional prominent loss of weight. This is the result of diffuse pulmonary fibrosis which has often been progressing for years before the affected subject seeks advice. The slower the progression, the longer the delay, and the greater the likely degree of permanent fibrotic damage. Eventually hypoxia and pulmonary hypertension may supervene, and the right heart fails. There are no acute exacerbations, and the clinical features are similar to those of other varieties of pulmonary fibrosis. The chronic form of EAA is typically seen in the subject who keeps a single budgerigar/ parakeet in the home. The level of antigenic exposure to avian dust is relatively trivial but it is encountered almost continuously, particularly if the affected subject is a housewife or elderly pensioner largely confined to the home.

That the acute form of EAA can be produced by inhalation provocation tests in subjects with the chronic form of the disease emphasizes the major role that dose exerts in determining the clinical nature of the response, though differences in host responsiveness exert an important additional influence. Consequently, a range of intermediate forms will be recognized; there may be considerable variability in clinical features among individuals affected by the same source of antigenic exposure; and some subjects will experience different patterns of response at different times.

Causative agents

Table 1 lists the various agents reported to cause EAA. Most are micro-organisms that are found contaminating a variety of vegetable products. Although those associated with the most celebrated disorders—farmer's lung, mushroom worker's lung, and bagassosis—are

Table 1 Agents reported to cause extrinsic allergic alveolitis

Agent	Source	Appellation
Micro-organisms		
Alternaria	Paper mill wood pulp	Wood pulp worker's lung
Aspergillus clavatus	Whisky maltings	Malt worker's lung
Aspergillus fumigatus	Vegetable compost	Farmer's lung
Aspergillus versicolor	Dog bedding (straw)	Dog house disease
Aureobasidium pullulans	Redwood	Sequoiosis
Bacillus subtilis	Domestic wood	
Cephalosporium	Sewage	Sewage worker's lung
Cryptostroma corticale	Maple	Maple bark stripper's lung
Graphium	Redwood	Sequoiosis
Lycoperdon	Puffballs	Lycoperdonosis
Merulius lacrymans	Domestic wood	
Mucor stolonifer	Paprika	Paprika splitter's lung
Penicillium casei	Cheese	Cheese washer's lung
Penicillium chrysogenum/Penicillium cyclopium	Domestic wood	
Penicillium frequentens	Cork	Suberosis
Saccharomonspora viridis	Logging plant	
Sporobolomyces	Horse barn straw	
Streptomyces albus	Soil, peat	
Thermophilic actinomycetes (*Micropolyspora faeni, T. sacchari/vulgaris*)	Hay, straw, grain, mushroom compost, bagasse	Farmer's lung, mushroom worker's lung, bagassosis
Trichosporon cutaneum	Japanese summer air	Summer-type hypersensitivity pneumonitis
Miscellaneous: bacteria?, fungi?, amoebas?, nematode debris?	Air conditioners, humidifiers, tap water	Humidifier lung, ventilation pneumonitis, sauna taker's lung
Unknown	Roof thatch	New Guinea lung
Animals		
Arthropods (*S. granarius*)	Grain dust	Wheat weevil disease
Birds	Bloom?, excreta?	Bird fancier's lung
Fish	Fish meal	Fish meal worker's lung
Mammals		
Pituitary (cattle, pig)	Pituitary extracts	Pituitary snuff taker's lung
Hair	Fur	Furrier's lung
Urine (rodents)	Urinary protein	Rodent handler's lung
Vegetation		
Coffee	Coffee bean dust	Coffee worker's lung
Wood (*Gonystylus bacanus*)	Wood dust	Wood worker's lung
Chemicals		
Bordeaux mixture (fungicide)	Vineyards	Vineyard sprayer's lung
Cobalt dissolved in solvents	Tungsten carbide grinding	
Diphenylmethane diisocyanate	Plastics industry	
Formaldehyde*	Laboratory	
Pauli's reagent	Laboratory	
Pyrethrum	Insecticide spray	
Hexamethylene diisocyanate	Plastics industry	
Toluene diisocyanate	Plastics industry	
Trimellitic anhydride	Plastics industry	

*One subject, possibly toxic not allergic response

usually thermophilic, the majority are not. Some microbial contamination may occur during growth of the vegetable host, but most of the antigenic load is usually acquired after harvest. Therefore prolonged storage under damp conditions increases the risk of EAA substantially, while drying to reduce the water content below 30 per cent greatly reduces the risk.

Inevitably there are situations where contamination arises with a number of different microbes, and it is not possible to identify a single responsible agent. This is a characteristic feature with contaminated humidifiers and air conditioners, and a large variety of agents have been suggested as possible causes of humidifier lung, including bacteria, fungi, protozoa (amoebae), and metazoa (nematode debris). Some authors prefer to distinguish EAA attributable in such circumstances to micro-organisms growing in cool or cold water (humidifier lung) from EAA which arises from thermophilic organisms growing in heated water (ventilation pneumonitis).

Pathogenic mechanisms

Histology

Within 24–48 h of exposure the acute form of EAA is characterized by a non-specific, diffuse pneumonitis with inflammatory cellular infiltration of the bronchioles, alveoli, and interstitium accompanied by oedema and luminal exudation. With ongoing exposure, whether continuous or intermittent, the more familiar appearances of the subacute forms evolve. Epithelioid non-caseating granulomas are characteristic, but are generally less well formed and less profuse than in sarcoidosis, and are often evanescent. They can be recognized within 3 weeks of the initiating exposure, and generally resolve within 6–12 months. In parallel, fibrosis evolves alongside cellular infiltration of the interstitium with histiocytes, lymphocytes, and plasma cells. Macrophages with foamy cytoplasm may be prominent in the alveolar spaces, and organization of the inflammatory exudate may lead to intra-alveolar fibrosis. Obstruction or obliteration of bronchioles is common. Foreign-body giant cells may reflect the dependence of EAA on antigens derived from inhaled foreign material, as does a peribronchial predominance of the inflammatory response. Vasculitis is notably absent.

With continued exposure, progressive, widespread, and irreversible fibrosis may occur leading to disruption of the normal architecture of the lung. In advanced cases honeycombing may develop. Granulomas are no longer characteristic, and the overall appearance may differ little from other causes of progressive interstitial pulmonary fibrosis.

Immune mechanisms

An outline of the possible immunopathology through acute and subacute–chronic phases is illustrated in Fig. 1. The inflammatory reaction is dominantly lymphocytic or mononuclear rather than polymorphonuclear, though a transitory polymorphonuclear leucocyte response is typical immediately following exposure. The non-caseating granulomatous response during the subacute phases of the disease suggests cell-mediated hypersensitivity. The latter is thought to play a dominant role, and in animal models the disease is transferred from animal to animal only with sensitized T lymphocytes. This is not to say that other mechanisms play no role, nor that all inflammatory diseases of the gas exchanging tissues induced by organic dusts share a common mechanism.

Lymphopenia in peripheral blood within hours of the provoking exposure is a typical feature of acute exacerbations, with the T lymphocytes migrating from blood to lungs, but bronchoalveolar lavage in similarly exposed subjects has shown excess numbers of T lymphocytes whether they were clinically affected or not. Most investigators have detected a relative excess in the number of CD8+ T cells in exposed but asymptomatic subjects, thereby 'inverting' the normal ratio of CD4+ to CD8+. The balance appears to shift back towards CD4+ dominance in those with disease. These and other observations suggest that a relative impairment of suppressor-cell function, or of its activation following antigenic exposure, is fundamental to the development of EAA.

Cytokines, possibly together with anaphylotoxins from activated mast cells, are likely to be responsible for the systemic influenza-like symptoms that are so characteristic of the acute form of EAA. These symptoms are not specific, however, and are indistinguishable from those characterizing grain fever in grain workers, 'Monday fever' in cotton workers, humidifier fever in subjects exposed to microbially-contaminated humidifiers, and metal fume fever in welders.

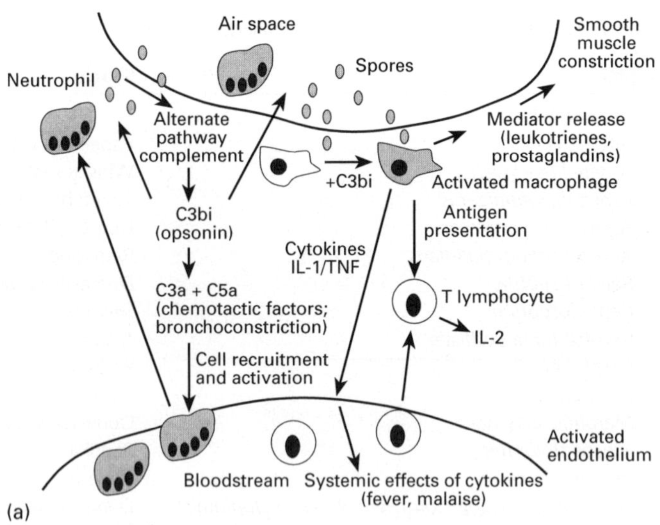

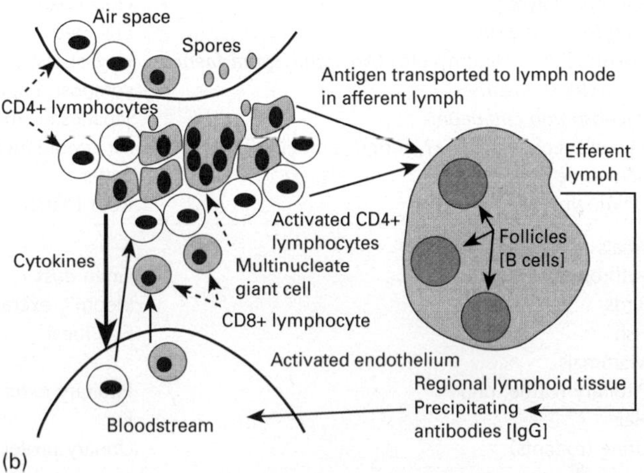

Fig. 1 (a) Possible immunopathogenesis: acute phase. (b) Possible immunopathogenesis: subacute–chronic phase.
(By courtesy of Dr G. Spickett.)

Relation to smoking and coeliac disease

Curiously, the disruptive effect of smoking on the alveolar membrane does not appear to augment the risk of EAA or to increase its severity. Rather, the reverse appears true. Although smoking enhances acute phase reactions and IgE production, it diminishes IgA, IgG, and IgM antibody responses, increases circulating CD8+ T-lymphocyte numbers, and probably reduces the incidence and severity of EAA.

Reports that cryptogenic fibrosing alveolitis and EAA (particularly bird fancier's lung) might be associated with coeliac disease led to the interesting hypothesis that in some cases absorbed food antigens from the disrupted bowel mucosa might play a role in the pathogenesis of the lung disorder. Alternatively, systemic hypersensitivity to a common inhaled and ingested avian antigen might give rise to similar immune reactions and diseases in the relevant target organs. However, the avian IgG antibody response seen in coeliac disease is distinct from that associated with bird fancier's lung and seems to be a response to dietary egg. It is not related to environmental exposure to birds but does correlate with the activity of the bowel disorder.

Investigation

Establishing a diagnosis of EAA involves three areas of investigation: lungs, exposure, and hypersensitivity.

Pulmonary

In the acute form the chest radiograph will commonly show no abnormality unless symptoms are severe. Normal radiographic appearances are particularly common with humidifier lung, possibly because antigen is presented in soluble aerosol form rather than particulate form. When the radiograph is abnormal, there is a widespread ground-glass appearance or an alveolar filling pattern, particularly in the lower and middle zones. This may resolve within a mere 24–48 h once exposure has ceased. In subacute forms, small irregular or nodular opacities are seen within the same distribution. These may persist for several weeks despite cessation of exposure. In contrast, the upper zones are predominantly affected by the irreversible fibrotic process that characterizes the chronic form of EAA. These radiographic appearances vary considerably from patient to patient, and correlate poorly with the clinical severity of the disease.

Computerized tomographic scans provide a much clearer picture of the radiographic abnormalities, particularly when thin section, high resolution techniques are used. No single feature or pattern has proved to be pathognomonic, but the abnormalities are seen to be distributed more uniformly than is apparent from the plain radiograph.

Lung function studies usually reveal little of note in the acute form of the disease unless there has been recent exposure. When impairment is seen, the pattern is one of reduced carbon monoxide gas transfer with restricted ventilation, decreased compliance, and (in the more severe examples) hypoxia of the arterial blood with hypocapnia, particularly on exercise. Although total lung capacity is reduced, residual volume is often increased, suggesting air trapping as a result of bronchiolar involvement. Occasionally there is also obstruction of the large airways, but this implies a coincidental asthmatic or bronchitic effect.

Transbronchial or open-lung biopsy may be indicated when other diagnostic procedures are not sufficiently definitive, but is not commonly needed and may not be definitive either. Biopsy may be particularly useful in suspected subacute or chronic forms of the disease when hypersensitivity is less obvious, or in the suspected acute form when there has been an unduly heavy exposure to microbial spores and there is the alternative (even additional) possibility of microbial invasion. Bronchoalveolar lavage, although more readily performed and less hazardous, has not proved to be as definitive as biopsy.

Environmental exposure

In many cases the history alone provides the evidence of relevant exposure, but this is not always reliable and independent measurements of environmental respirable contaminants, particularly microbial contaminants, may be invaluable. These are sophisticated investigations and are mostly indicated when EAA is first suspected in an environment, generally industrial, not previously associated with the disease.

Immunological

Laboratory demonstration of a serum IgG precipitating antibody response to the inducing organic dust is the most widely used method of 'confirming' hypersensitivity, but this is not fully satisfactory. Although affected subjects tend to have higher antibody levels than those who are exposed but unaffected, many investigators have found the antibody response to correlate more closely with exposure than disease. In practice, the absence of a precipitin response is extremely uncommon in subjects eventually proved to have EAA, provided that they are non-smokers. Cellular immune responses in blood (or skin) have not yet given rise to clinically useful diagnostic tests, though a T-lymphocyte response in bronchoalveolar fluid (lymphocytes represent 10 to 20 per cent or more of recovered cells) is characteristic. Again, lymphocytosis is seen also in asymptomatic although similarly exposed subjects, and during the hours immediately following exposure a polymorphonuclear leucocyte response may dominate, simulating cryptogenic fibrosing alveolitis.

When the diagnosis remains in doubt, some form of inhalation challenge test may be considered necessary. The simplest method involves comparison of experimental periods spent away from the suspected causal environment with similar periods of continuing exposure. The acute form of the disease is likely to be recognized in this way, although the procedure can be time consuming and there may be practical problems of compliance. When a definitive diagnosis is particularly important, laboratory-based inhalation challenge tests can be used. The influenza-like component of positive reactions tends to dominate the respiratory component, and objective evidence for positivity may be difficult to obtain. Thus, auscultation, chest radiography, measurement of gas transfer, and arterial blood gas analysis may all be too insensitive to provide useful diagnostic information, though changes in body temperature, circulating neutrophil and lymphocyte numbers, forced vital capacity, and exercise ventilation provide collectively high specificity and high sensitivity.

Differential diagnosis

Organic dust toxic syndrome is the term applied to a further disorder which occurs within hours of heavy respiratory exposure to dusts containing fungal toxins, particularly those released on decapping silos. It is the result of direct toxicity rather than hypersensitivity. Its effects are usually mild and self-limiting, but severe respiratory embarrassment may occur and there is a small risk of ongoing, and potentially fatal, fungal invasion of the lungs. This risk could be enhanced if corticosteroid treatment is given, and death has resulted in subjects who appear to have been fully immunocompetent. Not only does organic dust toxic syndrome occur in circumstances which favour the occurrence of EAA, but its clinical features have much in common with EAA, and to a lesser extent with nitrogen dioxide toxicity which also affects silo workers. Acute EAA may also simulate pulmonary infections, other immunological disorders of the lung, drug reactions, and even paraquat poisoning which sometimes occurs accidentally in farm workers.

When subacute or chronic forms of EAA are encountered, the differential diagnosis includes other diffuse infiltrative and fibrotic disorders of the lung. Most frequent are cryptogenic fibrosing alveolitis, sarcoidosis, pneumoconiosis, and tuberculosis.

Epidemiology

EAA is an uncommon but not rare disease. For every case there are 10 to 100 cases of asthma, but there is much greater geographic variation reflecting the much larger dependence of EAA on occupational causes. Its comparative scarcity limits epidemiological knowledge. Recent experience in Britain indicates that EAA accounts for only 2 per cent of occupational lung diseases. Almost 50 per cent of reported occupational cases affect farm workers, followed by 15 per cent affecting workers in material, metal, or electrical processing trades. Among farm workers, incidence varies from 40 to 100 cases per million per year. Contaminating micro-organisms underlie most reported cases, but in 20–30 per cent no causal agent is specified.

Figures for prevalence are more readily available than those for incidence, and demonstrate quite marked national differences. In developed countries, humidifier lung is recognized with increasing frequency in both the workplace and the home, and remarkable prevalences of 15–70 per cent have been suggested in populations from some contaminated offices in North America. Bird fancier's lung may be more prevalent in Britain, simply because of the great popularity of keeping budgerigars and pigeons, and the limited need for humidifiers. In areas of high rainfall where 'traditional' farming methods are used, the prevalence of farmer's lung may reach 10 per cent. This is likely to be the commonest cause of EAA in developing countries. Where modern farming methods are used, prevalences rarely exceed 2 to 3 per cent and may be much less. In the hot and humid regions of Japan, a seasonal summer growth of *Trichosporon cutaneum* in unsanitary and poorly ventilated homes is by far the commonest cause of EAA and accounts for about 75 per cent of all cases.

Management

Management of the individual

Management centres on reducing any further exposure to a minimum. There is no place for desensitization. Ideally, the affected individual changes or avoids the relevant environment completely, but this may mean a profound loss in income or great expense and is often unrealistic. Nor is it fully justified since continued exposure does not inevitably lead to progressive disease.

Occupational exposure can often be reduced substantially by changing the pattern of the affected individual's duties. A further option is the use of industrial respirators, which filter out 98–99 per cent of respirable dust from the ambient air. They are particularly valuable when exposures are intermittent and short-lived, but may be uncomfortably hot when worn for long periods or during heavy work.

Whatever course is followed, any continuing exposure should be accompanied by regular medical surveillance. If there is no progression, it is reasonable for some exposure to continue. When there is progressive disease, exposure should cease. This may involve a loss of earnings, and may entitle the affected worker to compensation. Rarely, the individual with progressive disease will refuse to change his occupation or hobby, and the physician must weigh the possible advantages of long-term corticosteroid therapy against the well-known risks.

Management of the environment

Once EAA is recognized in one individual, the environment concerned should be assessed for the risk it poses to others. In many circumstances this will be well known already. In others, the precise causal agent and its level of exposure will be unknown, and so the risk will not be quantifiable. In such unfamiliar circumstances there may be a need to survey the exposed population at risk, and investigate exposure levels in the occupational environment. Questionnaires and serological tests provide the most convenient tools for a clinical screening procedure. When large populations are involved, comprehensive investigation of a representative sample is sensible before major modifications to the working environment are contemplated.

Modifications can always be made to the environment to lessen the levels of exposure, but their extent will be limited by expense and should be justified by need. Dry storage and adequate ventilation are the two most important factors when vegetable produce is involved, and in some farming areas there is benefit in drying produce artificially after harvest. When ventilation and humidification systems are themselves responsible for EAA, major mechanical alterations may be necessary and the methods of humidification and temperature control may need to be changed. The crucial need is to reduce the ease with which normal airborne microbial contaminants are able to proliferate in water reservoir systems. For this there may be a role for 'biocide' sterilizing agents, but these are also likely to become airborne and respirable and so must have low intrinsic toxicity and sensitizing potency.

Outcome

No further exposure

With the acute form of EAA the 'sensitizing' period of exposure is often short and the disorder generally resolves without sequelae once the diagnosis is made and exposure ceases. However, one investigation has demonstrated continuing inflammation and alveolar membrane leakiness 2–15 years after exposure ceased. The significance of this is unclear, since all subjects were then asymptomatic and gave normal results to radiographic and lung function studies. With the chronic form of EAA there is little possibility for improvement following exposure cessation, but there is some risk of progression. Fortunately this is not common. Some affected subjects give clear accounts of increased responsiveness to a given level of exposure months or years after initial antigen exclusion, which suggests that protective mechanisms may be downgraded more quickly than those which are causal.

Continuing exposure

There is greater concern when exposure continues. This may lead not only to recurrent acute attacks but also to progressive and permanent fibrotic damage, though the latter course is followed by only a minority of affected subjects. A 2- to 40-year follow-up survey of 92 farm workers presenting with the acute form of farmer's lung showed that, while the majority continued to live on farms, only a minority developed radiographic evidence of pulmonary fibrosis (39 per cent) or impairment of carbon monoxide gas transfer (30 per cent). A similar 10-year outcome has been reported in pigeon fanciers with acute EAA; again, the majority elected to continue their antigenic exposures despite medical advice to the contrary. Important protective mechanisms must consequently emerge which lead to tolerance from the effects of further acute exposures or at least prevent the development of damaging fibrosis.

Whether the use of corticosteroids for acute episodes confers any long-term benefit is not yet clear, but one recent investigation failed to demonstrate any long-term functional differences between groups treated randomly with corticosteroids or placebo for the initial acute episode of farmer's lung.

Further reading

Braun, S.R., doPico, G.A., Tsiatis, A., *et al.* (1979). Farmer's lung disease: long-term clinical and physiologic outcome. *American Review of Respiratory Disease*, **119**, 185–91.

Hendrick, D.J., Marshall, R., Faux, J.A., and Krall, J.M. (1980). Positive 'alveolar' responses to antigen inhalation provocation tests: their validity and recognition. *Thorax*, **35**, 415–27.

Kokkarinen, J.I., Tukiainen, H.O., and Terho, E.O. (1992). Effect of corticosteroid treatment on the recovery of pulmonary function in farmer's lung. *American Review of Respiratory Disease*, **145**, 3–5.

Chapter 4.27

Sarcoidosis

P. R. Studdy

Sarcoidosis, a relatively common multisystem disease, is one of a large family of granulomatous disorders characterized by epithelioid cell granulomas. The presentation, duration of symptoms, and extent of tissue involvement is very variable. Although remarkably transient in most individuals, a proportion of whom are asymptomatic, it may uncommonly become a chronic problem with debilitating symptoms and premature death. Treatment remains controversial.

Aetiology

No cause has been discovered. Perhaps an unidentified agent interacts with the host to produce a disease in which immunological factors are important. If there is a transmissible agent, perhaps a virus or a protoplast form of *Mycobacterium tuberculosis*, it must have either an extremely low infectivity or an incubation period so protracted the initial contact goes unrecognized. The lungs and regional thoracic lymph nodes are most frequently involved, suggesting that the disease is caused by an inhaled agent provoking an initial alveolar injury followed by an influx of immune effector cells which maintain an inflammatory alveolitis.

There is a link between some manifestations of the disease and certain HLA patterns. The occasional occurrence of familial sarcoidosis and apparent excess concordance in monozygotic rather than dizygotic twins provides slight evidence that the susceptibility to sarcoidosis may be influenced by genetic factors.

Epidemiology

Sarcoidosis is recognized worldwide. The prevalence varies considerably (Table 1).

Most cases of sarcoidosis show characteristic chest radiograph abnormalities. Mass radiological surveys for England and Wales show a frequency of sarcoidosis of 13.8 men and 19.8 women per 100 000 population, with the highest prevalence in Irish women aged 25–34 years.

The incidence and course of sarcoidosis in different racial groups living in the same geographical area show considerable variation. In London, there is a 10-fold higher annual incidence in West Indian and Asians than in the indigenous white population. In the US and South Africa, sarcoidosis is more extensive and at least 10 times more common in the black than the white population.

Table 1 Reported prevalence of pulmonary sarcoidosis

Sweden (64)	Switzerland (16)
Denmark (48)	Yugoslavia (12)
West Germany (43)	France (10)
East Germany (4.1)	Italy (9)
Ireland (40)	Scotland (7)
United States (New York) (39)	Finland (5)
England (27)	Japan (2.5)
Norway (27)	Spain (1.2)
Holland (22)	

Numbers in parentheses are prevalence per 100 000

Based on data reported at international sarcoidosis conferences.

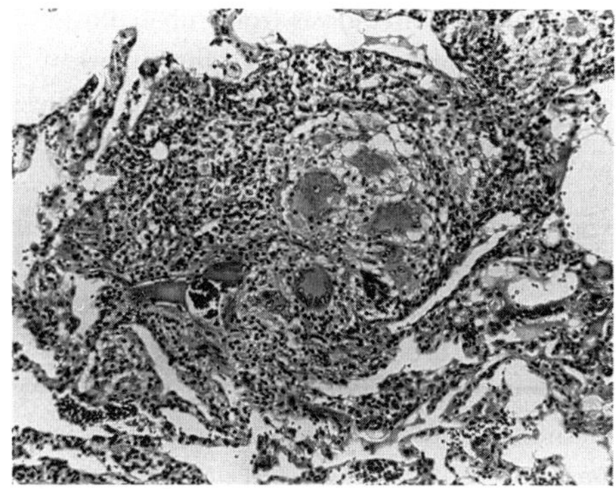

Fig. 1 Typical perivascular sarcoid granuloma in a lung biopsy containing many epithelioid cells, Langhans type giant cells, and lymphocytes. Haematoxylin and eosin. Magnification 40×.
(By courtesy of Dr Margaret Burke, Mount Vernon Hospital.)

Pathology

It is generally assumed the first step is the presentation of an unknown antigen by major histocompatibility complex class 11 macrophages to CD4 T cells of the TH1 subclass. This results in T-cell proliferation and release of immune mediators.

The increased CD4 helper T-lymphocyte response is maintained by the spontaneous release of interleukin 1 (IL-1) and interleukin 2 (IL-2) T-cell growth factors. Helper T lymphocytes accumulate at sites of disease activity, a fact readily demonstrated in the lungs by bronchoalveolar lavage studies. CD4 T-helper cells predominate over CD8 T-suppressor cells and in involved tissues the ratio of CD4 T-helper to CD8 T-suppressor cells may be as high as 10:1, compared to the ratio of 2:1 found in normal tissues. At uninvolved sites and in the peripheral blood, T lymphocytes are not 'activated' and are present in reduced numbers.

The characteristic non-caseating epithelioid-cell granulomas (Fig. 1) may occur in a variety of other conditions (Table 2). The earliest manifestation is an accumulation of mononuclear inflammatory cells and CD4 T-helper lymphocytes, soon followed by granuloma formation. In the early stages, the granulomas consist of focal, close-packed collections of macrophages and epithelioid cells surrounded by a peripheral ring of lymphocytes. CD4 helper cells and activated macrophages penetrate to the centre of the granulomata where the latter coalesce into epithelioid and multinucleate Langhans type giant cells. In the peripheral mantle, CD8 suppressor cells lie adjacent to

Table 2 Human pulmonary granulomatous diseases

Aetiology	Disorder
Known	Extrinsic allergic alveolitis. Chronic beryllium disease Infections. (mycobacteria, bacteria (brucellosis), fungi, protozoa, viruses, and worms) Foreign body (talc following IV drug abuse)
Unknown	Sarcoidosis. Wegener's granulomatosis. Churg-Strauss syndrome. Lymphomatoid granulomatosis. Langerhans' cell granulomatosis

numerous antigen-presenting macrophages. Central fibrinoid necrosis may occur in florid granulomas but true caseation is not seen, a finding that differentiates sarcoidosis from tuberculosis.

In the later stages of chronic sarcoidosis, three types of cytoplasmic inclusions may be present, particularly in the multinucleated giant cells: crystalline calcium carbonate, densely basophilic conchoidal (Schaumann's) bodies, and star-shaped asteroid bodies. These inclusions are not diagnostic of sarcoidosis and are present in many other granulomatous conditions.

When the disease remits, the granulomas may completely resolve, but those that remain are usually slowly replaced by featureless, hyaline scar tissue showing few, if any, diagnostic features (Fig. 2).

Humoral immunity is enhanced. B-cell activity is increased, probably in response to T-cell-derived B-cell growth factors, and results in non-specific polyclonal hyperglobulinaemia. Circulating immune complexes are frequently present in acute sarcoidosis at the stage of erythema nodosum, uveitis, and arthralgia.

Tuberculin sensitivity is reduced at the onset of sarcoidosis and a previously positive tuberculin test may become negative. About two-thirds fail to react to 100 IU of tuberculin (PPD). Normal reactivity to tuberculin is not necessarily restored when sarcoidosis remits. Low responsiveness or cutaneous anergy to other 'recall' antigens may be demonstrated.

Clinical features

Modes of presentation

Sarcoidosis may involve any organ (Fig. 3). Sarcoidosis occasionally presents in childhood and in the elderly, but usually between the ages of 20 and 35 years (Table 3). Onset may be:

- acute with erythema nodosum in a young adult usually indicates a self-limiting course with spontaneous resolution;
- insidious, in middle age, frequently associated with progressive fibrosis and permanent organ dysfunction.

Erythema nodosum and bilateral hilar lymphadenopathy (Lofgren's syndrome)

The combination of erythema nodosum immediately preceding bilateral hilar lymphadenopathy (BHL) sometimes with pulmonary mottling, is virtually diagnostic of acute sarcoidosis. The clinical picture is complete if there is anterior uveitis and superficial lymphadenopathy. Erythema nodosum, a pan nodular panniculitis, usually subsides within a month. The characteristic red hot, tender, shining, symmetrical lesions affect the shins, and infrequently the calves,

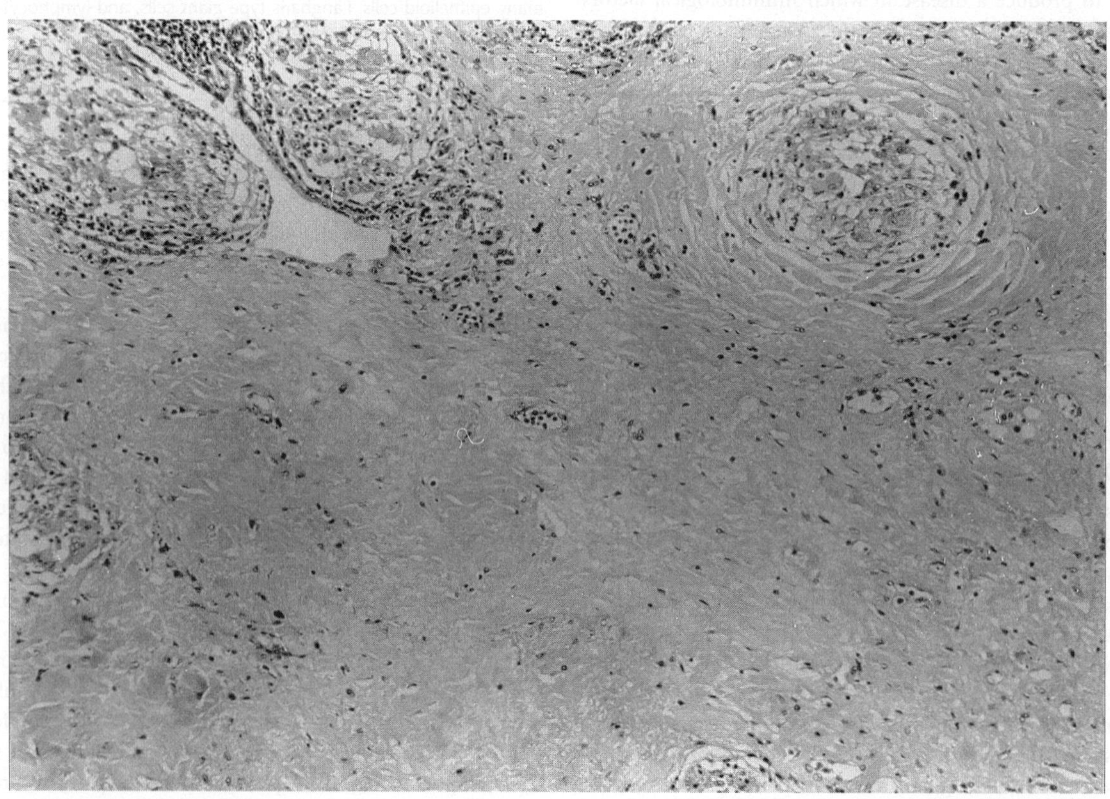

Fig. 2 Hyaline fibrosis with extensive replacement of lung tissue by fibrous tissue. The scattered, residual non-caseating granulomas in the interstitium should be noted. Haematoxylin and eosin. Magnification 10×.
(By courtesy of Dr Margaret Burke, Mount Vernon Hospital.)

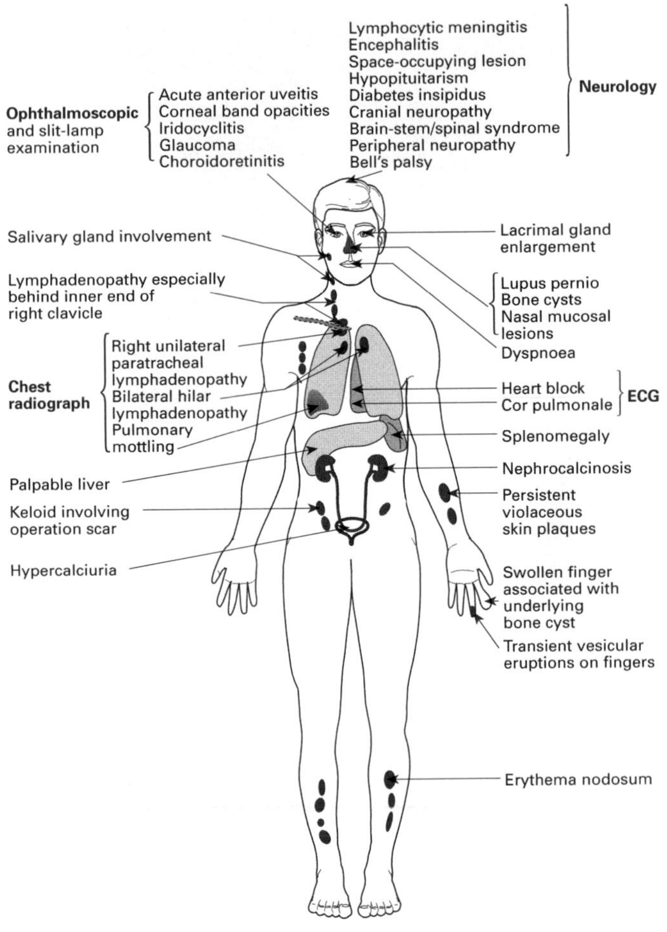

Fig. 3 Principal clinical features of sarcoidosis.

Table 3 First presenting symptoms of patients with sarcoidosis in the UK

Feature	White	Black	Asian
Abnormal chest radiograph	34	7	10
Respiratory symptoms	25	57	55
Constitutional symptoms	5	57	55
Erythema nodosum	20	8.5	17
Ocular symptoms	7	12	3
Superficial lymphadenopathy	3	34	17

Male and female data combined; figures expressed as a percentage.

For source of data see OTM3, p. 2820.

knees, buttocks, and upper outer aspect of the arms. Constitutional symptoms may occur, with abrupt onset of intermittent fever and troublesome polyarthralgia. Recurrence is unusual—in some 10 per cent, usually within 3 months but occasionally up to a year. Hilar adenopathy typically regresses within a year, and recurrence or late pulmonary sequelae are rare.

The proportion of cases of erythema nodosum attributed to sarcoidosis in the population depends upon the incidence not only of sarcoidosis but also of other infections including *M. tuberculosis*, haemolytic streptococci, and fungal infections such as coccidioidomycosis and histoplasmosis.

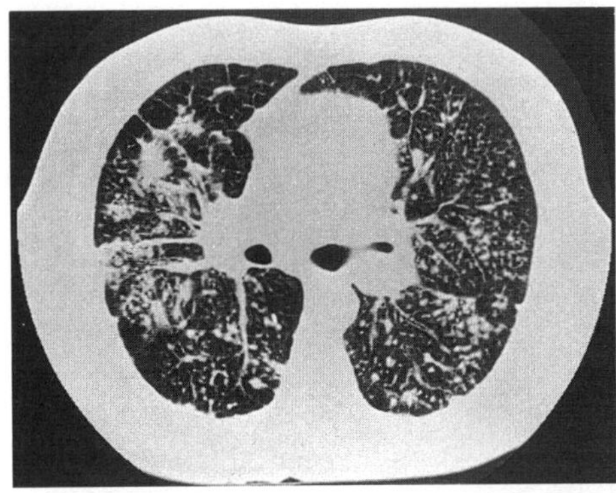

Fig. 4 Pulmonary sarcoidosis CT scan. Widespread nodules of varied size and shape are present throughout the lung fields. On the right side areas of irregular fibrosis are beginning to stretch and deform the lung parenchyma. *(By courtesy of Dr B. Strickland, Royal Brompton Hospital.)*

Uveoparotid fever (Heerfordt–Waldenstrom) syndrome

Uveoparotid fever is uncommon and presents acutely to run a chronic course with parotid gland enlargement uveitis, fever, and cranial nerve palsies (especially VII). Other components included bizarre neurological manifestations, lethargy, meningism, and cerebrospinal fluid pleocytosis.

Intrathoracic sarcoidosis

More than 90 per cent of patients show radiographic intrathoracic involvement. About a quarter are symptomless and about the same proportion present with trivial respiratory or systemic symptoms, which may include dyspnoea on exertion, usually gradual in onset, cough which is seldom productive, wheezing, and ill-defined constitutional symptoms. Individuals with extensive pulmonary infiltration may experience severe exertional dyspnoea, anterior chest discomfort, and persistent unproductive cough.

Auscultation of the chest is usually normal. Crackles and wheezes suggest other interstitial lung diseases, including fibrosing alveolitis and asbestosis. In advanced disease, the physical signs are compatible with fibrosis and airway obstruction from any cause. Finger-nail clubbing is rare. Slight haemoptysis may occur with endobronchial sarcoidosis. Marked haemoptysis in chronic sarcoidosis suggests complicating bronchiectasis or aspergilloma.

Chest radiology

Intrathoracic sarcoidosis can be radiographically staged as:

- stage 0—clear chest radiograph;
- stage 1—hilar and mediastinal lymphadenopathy;
- stage 2—hilar and mediastinal lymphadenopathy with pulmonary infiltration;
- stage 3—pulmonary infiltration without hilar adenopathy.

Thoracic CT scanning is more discriminating than conventional radiography, and often reveals widespread, multiple, ill-defined densities deployed along bronchovascular bundles, lymphatics, and interlobar septa when conventional posteroanterior chest radiography shows apparently clear lungs. CT is helpful in differentiating between equivocal glandular or vascular hilar enlargement (Fig. 4).

Bilateral hilar and mediastinal gland enlargement (Fig. 5) is not unique to sarcoidosis and may also occur in tuberculosis, coccidioidomycosis, histoplasmosis, lymphomas, and metastatic carcinoma.

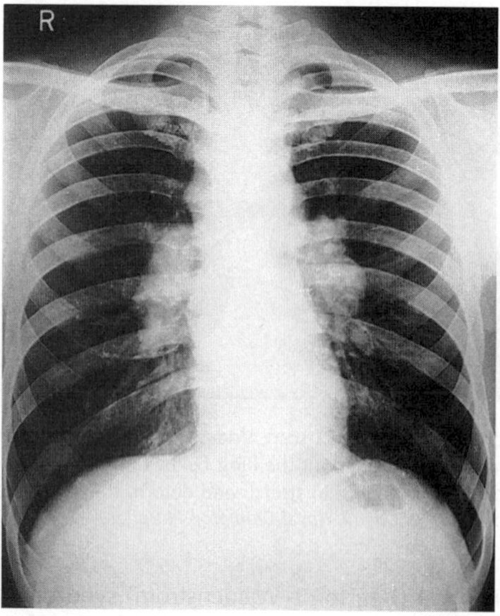

Fig. 5 Bilateral hilar gland enlargement. The right paratracheal lymph node is enlarged (stage 1 chest radiograph).

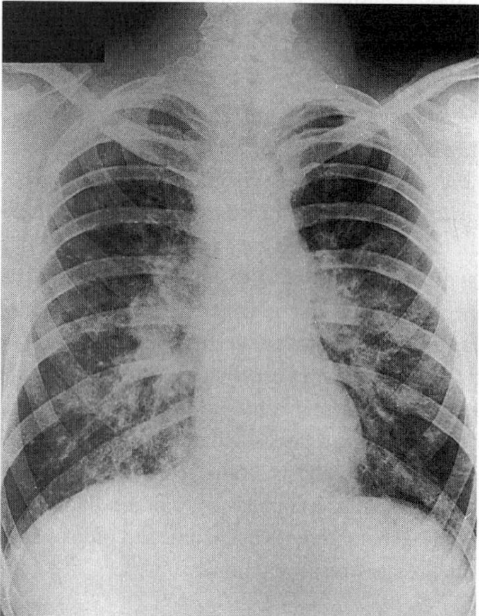

Fig. 6 Bilateral hilar gland enlargement and pulmonary infiltration (stage 2 chest radiograph).

The enlarged hilar nodes of sarcoidosis are roughly symmetrical, with clearly-defined outer borders and multiple, smooth contours suggesting discrete enlargement of individual lymph nodes. The right paratracheal nodes are involved in about half of patients. The anterior mediastinal nodes are seldom visibly enlarged in sarcoidosis, unlike lymphoma.

Pulmonary infiltration (Figs 6 and 7)

The most characteristic posteroanterior chest radiograph appearance is widespread symmetrical miliary, nodular, or confluent shadows ranging from 1–5 mm in diameter, densest in the middle zones or distributed more or less uniformly throughout the lungs. Less commonly, there are cloudy confluent shadows or nodular uniform opacities associated with widespread infiltration.

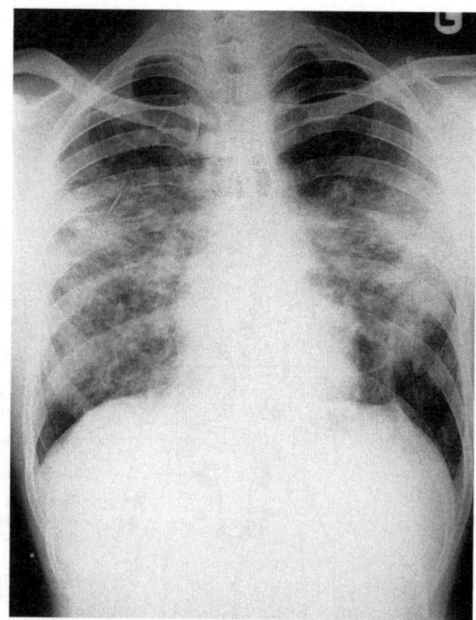

Fig. 7 Mid-zone pulmonary infiltration (stage 3 chest radiograph).

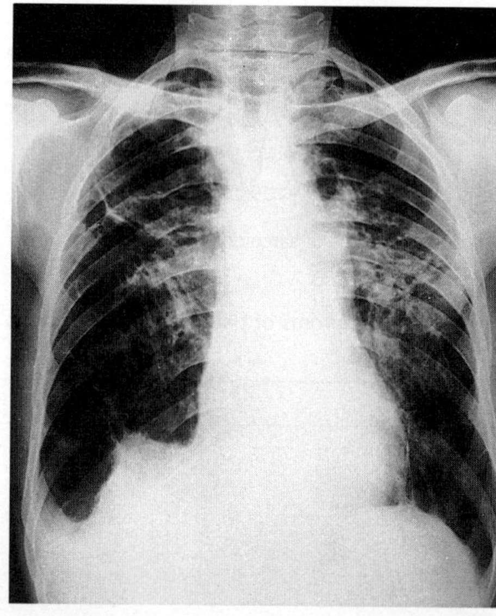

Fig. 8 Chronic fibrosis with upper lobe shrinkage characteristic of late stage sarcoidosis (stage 3 chest radiograph).

Mid-zone fibrosis is characteristic with coarse strands radiating from the hilum, often associated with loss of volume in the upper zones, elevation of the hilar shadows (Figs 8 and 9), and emphysematous hypertransradiant lower zones. Fibrosis occurs in those areas previously affected by the densest or most persistent infiltration. Thick-walled, small, moderate, or large-sized cavities are a feature of fibrotic pulmonary sarcoidosis, and may become colonized by *Aspergillus.* Large lung bullae are rare, and, even less commonly, patients with chronic fibrotic pulmonary sarcoidosis develop radiological features of generalized bullous emphysema. Lung fibrosis is irreversible and, when severe, may progress to gross functional impairment and terminal respiratory failure.

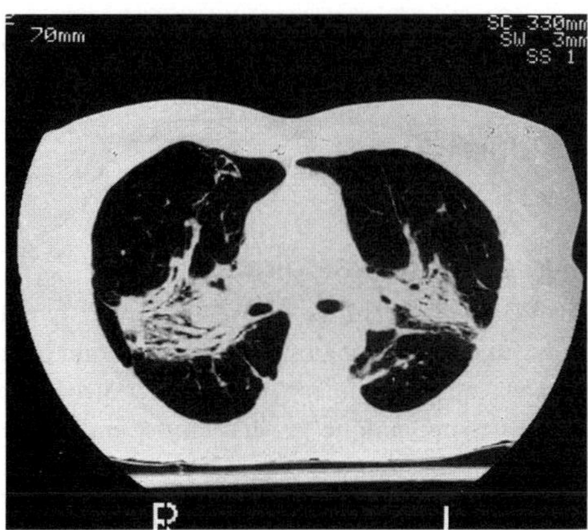

Fig. 9 Pulmonary sarcoidosis CT scan showing severe fibrosis in both mid-zones. Dilated bronchi are present with fibrotic masses surrounded by emphysematous lung.
(By courtesy of Dr B. Strickland, Royal Brompton Hospital.)

Calcification

The lungs and hilar lymph nodes can show scattered calcified foci in areas of hyaline fibrosis and plaque-like or 'eggshell' calcification may develop in persistently enlarged hilar or mediastinal glands.

Pleura

Symptoms are rare although CT scanning shows pleural involvement in up to one-third. A transient exudative lymphocytic pleural effusion may appear at any time. Pneumothorax is a rare complication.

Bronchial stenosis

This occurs as a late feature with distortion and narrowing of major bronchi by fibrosis and granulomas. A single lobar stenosis may improve with corticosteroids. Multiple segmental stenoses have a poor prognosis irrespective of treatment.

Prognostic significance of radiographic staging

Sarcoidosis resolves to leave radiographically clear lungs in half to two-thirds of patients:

- With Stage 1 radiography the prognosis is particularly good in white patients. Some 80 per cent resolve spontaneously and have a normal chest radiograph after a year and a further 10 per cent resolve during the second year. BHL persists in the remaining 10 per cent, with enlarged nodes and active disease. Only one-third of Afro-Caribbean and Asians achieve radiographic resolution.
- With Stage 2 chest radiography a quarter show radiographic pulmonary infiltration. Complete resolution eventually occurs in about half this group.
- With Stage 3 chest radiography complete radiological resolution occurs in only about a quarter. Many show moderate respiratory impairment and in some this may become critically severe.

Lymphoreticular involvement

Transient lymphadenopathy is common. Superficial glands are discrete and painless, with a firm, rubbery feel. The mediastinal nodes are most frequently affected and their enlargement is best demonstrated by thoracic CT scan. Peripheral lymphadenopathy is more frequent in black than white patients. The cervical and scalene nodes are often involved and may simulate Hodgkin's disease, which must be excluded by biopsy if there is any diagnostic doubt.

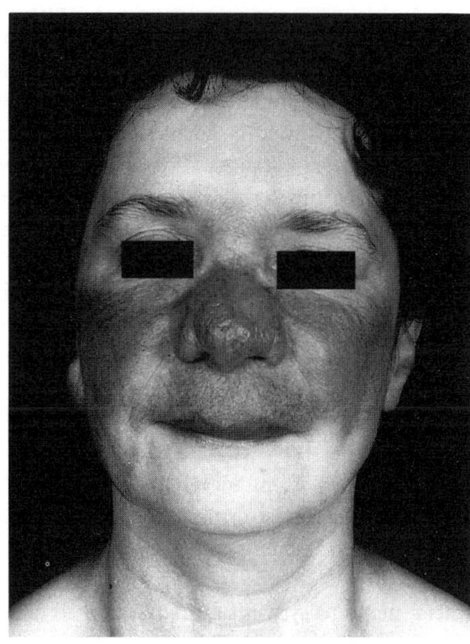

Fig. 10 Disfiguring facial skin lesion due to extensive lupus pernio.
(Reproduced with permission from James, D. G. and Studdy, P.R. (1993). Colour atlas of respiratory diseases, Mosby-Year Book, St Louis, 1993.)

The liver and spleen are often silently affected. Slight hepatosplenomegaly or transient biochemical 'cholestatic' abnormalities of liver function may be found in about a quarter. There may be discomfort when the spleen or liver are grossly enlarged. Cirrhosis, intrahepatic cholestasis, and gross splenic enlargement are rare, most frequent in black males, and associated with portal hypertension, oesophageal varices, and hepatic failure.

Skin

Skin involvement may be transient or chronic. Erythema nodosum and maculopapular eruptions are the commonest early lesions, frequently seen in white females, and often coincide with acute uveitis and BHL. Indolent violaceous skin plaques, subcutaneous nodules, and lupus pernio are features of late chronic fibrotic disease, particularly in Afro-Caribbean females. Lupus pernio is a chronic persistent violaceous skin infiltration with a predilection for the nose, cheeks, ears, scalp and terminal phalanges, (Fig. 10). Healing may leave unsightly telangiectatic facial scars and nasal deformity. Scars from surgery, trauma, or vaccination may be infiltrated by sarcoid granulomas and become raised, purple, and livid.

Sarcoidosis of the upper airways

Symptomatic upper respiratory tract sarcoidosis of the nose, nasopharyngeal mucosa, and larynx is uncommon. The inferior turbinates and septum are most commonly affected, with reddened granular hypertrophic polypoid nasal mucosa causing obstruction, crusting, discharge, and epistaxis. The nasal bridge may be widened due nasal bone involvement. Dyspnoea, wheezing, or stridor draw attention to laryngeal airway obstruction.

Ocular sarcoidosis

Uveitis occurs in about 25 per cent and, neglected, may lead to blindness. The uveal tract, iris, ciliary body, or choroid are frequently involved. Acute anterior uveitis (iridocyclitis) may be the first manifestation and presents abruptly with blurred vision, lacrimation, and photophobia. Clinically, the eyes are red with circumcorneal ciliary congestion and pupillary irregularity. Slit-lamp examination shows fine keratitic precipitates in the anterior chamber. Acute uveitis usually settles spontaneously or with local corticosteroids in a matter of weeks leaving no permanent damage. Chronic progressive sarcoid iridocyclitis with cataract and secondary glaucoma responds poorly to treatment. Conjunctival sarcoidosis results in phlyctenular conjunctivitis.

The lacrimal glands are rarely enlarged, but can be infiltrated by granulomas with reduced secretion of tears and dry eyes. Band keratopathy with deposits of calcium and exophthalmos due to sarcoid infiltration of the orbit are described.

Neurological sarcoidosis

Any part of the nervous system may be affected and 7 per cent show some evidence with cranial or peripheral neuropathies, or less commonly meningitis, encephalitis, pituitary involvement, or space occupying lesions.

Transient facial nerve palsy, with a predilection to affect the two sides of the face successively, is the most frequent acute neurological presentation. Full recovery should be expected with corticosteroids.

Acute or chronic meningitis may present with raised intracranial pressure, papilloedema, or obstructive hydrocephalus. Anterior pituitary granulomas seldom disturb function, but involvement of the posterior pituitary or hypothalamus may result in diabetes insipidus or, rarely, hypothalamic hypothyroidism, hypopituitarism, hyperprolactinaemia, somnolence, or alveolar hypoventilation. Space-occupying nodular cerebral lesions with symptoms and signs mimicking those of cerebral tumour, polyneuropathy with paraesthesiae and weakness in the limbs, transverse myelitis, or multiple lesions which mimic multiple sclerosis and amyotrophic lateral sclerosis may occur.

Cerebrospinal fluid raised pressure, elevated protein levels, pleocytosis, and low glucose level are common but of limited diagnostic value. Cranial CT scanning or magnetic resonance imaging are the most useful diagnostic investigations for cerebral sarcoidosis. Neurological sarcoidosis has a poor prognosis despite steroid treatment.

Cardiac sarcoidosis

Myocardial granulomas are found in 20 per cent of sarcoidosis autopsy cases, but cardiac involvement is usually localized and asymptomatic. The left ventricle, interventricular septum, and His–Purkinje conduction system are most frequently involved. The high frequency of sudden death reflects the risk of involvement of the conduction system by fortuitously-sited granulomata. Cardiac sarcoidosis may prove difficult to diagnose but is suspected when a patient with known sarcoidosis develops arrhythmias, bundle branch block, pericarditis, congestive cardiac failure, or dilated cardiomyopathy.

The prognosis is poor despite corticosteroids. A proportion require permanent pacemakers, and some in cardiac failure may be rescued by cardiac transplantation.

Locomotor system sarcoidosis

The bones, joints, and muscles can be involved. An acute, transient, migratory polyarthropathy accompanied by BHL and erythema nodosum is a common, early feature. Palpable tender muscle nodules, muscle wasting, and weakness occur in chronic sarcoidosis.

Bone involvement is uncommon and strongly associated with lupus pernio. The phalanges, metacarpals or metatarsals, and nasal bones are most frequently involved with cystic or destructive lesions. There are occasional reports of skull, rib, or vertebral body involvement.

Renal sarcoidosis

See Chapter 12.14.

Endocrine glands and sarcoidosis

Endocrine gland involvement is unusual. Rarely, hypothalamic–pituitary axis dysfunction due to posterior pituitary and hypothalamic involvement may cause secondary neurogenic diabetes insipidus. Diabetes insipidus is not unique to sarcoidosis, and the differential diagnosis includes chronic meningeal infection, metastatic malignancy (lung or breast), and histiocytosis X (eosinophilic granuloma), a rare condition which may mimic sarcoidosis.

Granulomas are occasionally detected in the anterior pituitary, pancreas, thyroid, and parathyroid glands, but very seldom disturb function.

Pregnancy and sarcoidosis

Sarcoidosis does not generally affect fertility or unfavourably influence the course and outcome of pregnancy. Active sarcoidosis tends to improve during pregnancy and may gradually worsen after delivery.

Diagnosis and investigations

Diagnosis is based on clinical presentation and radiographic, biochemical, and immunological findings. Some clinical presentations are so highly characteristic, for instance BHL with erythema nodosum, that histological confirmation is not required. With less characteristic presentations the diagnosis may only be accepted after positive tissue biopsies have been obtained.

Diagnostic histology

Fibreoptic bronchoscopy with multiple transbronchial biopsies is particularly useful, with low complication rate, high yield, and frequency of positive diagnosis greater than 80 per cent. Enlarged superficial lymph nodes or apparently involved skin may be biopsied. Mediastinoscopy gives access to the anterior mediastinal lymph nodes, has a high diagnostic yield, and helps to differentiate lymphoma from sarcoidosis. In obscure cases video-assisted transthoracoscopic (VATS) or open-lung biopsy provide a sufficiently large sample for diagnosis from precisely selected parts of the lung.

The Kveim–Siltzbach test, using human splenic tissue, is no longer recommended.

Lung function

Slight respiratory function impairment is common in early prefibrotic pulmonary sarcoidosis, but is seldom associated with symptoms. Routine tests may give results within the normal range. Abnormalities include a modest restrictive functional defect with reduction in lung volumes, slight impairment of gas exchange identified by a fall in PaO_2, widening of the alveolar–arterial difference ($P(A\text{–}a)O_2$) on exertion, and failure of the carbon monoxide transfer coefficient (K_{CO}) to rise with exercise. It is debatable whether small airway function is abnormal in early disease, although the widespread distribution of granulomata in the lung parenchyma implies small airway involvement.

As the disease progresses there is gradual loss of lung volume, more severe gas exchange abnormalities due to ventilation–perfusion inequalities, airflow obstruction caused by endobronchial sarcoidosis or bronchostenosis, and loss of compliance. A complaint of exertional dyspnoea is often associated with significant impairment of lung function. Resting hypoxaemia is a feature of severe pulmonary disease. Single measurements of lung function determine the extent of functional impairment, and serial measurements help in following progress and response to therapy.

Laboratory investigations

Hypercalcaemia and hypercalciuria occur in about 10 per cent. Disordered calcium homeostasis in chronic sarcoidosis may become persistent with nephrocalcinosis and renal calculi. Hypercalciuria is more common than hypercalcaemia. There may be a moderate or considerable elevation of serum calcium, normal serum phosphate, and normal or slightly raised alkaline phosphatase. The cause is an acquired increase in 1–25 dihydroxycholecalciferol (1,25-$(OH)_2$-D_3) synthesized by activated macrophages in the granulomas and independent of renal 1-hydroxylase, the normal physiological source of 1,25-$(OH)_2$-D_3. Patients with sarcoidosis are extremely sensitive to vitamin D and may suffer an exacerbation of hypercalcaemia or hypercalciuria when the skin is exposed to ultraviolet light during the summer. Hypercalcaemia due to sarcoidosis responds to corticosteroids which quickly lower 1,25-$(OH)_2$-D_3 levels and reduce intestinal hyperabsorption of calcium.

Total serum globulin and specific immunoglobulin levels are often raised; circulating immune complexes and raised IgM occasionally may be detected in the early acute sarcoidosis.

Monitoring disease activity

Activity is assessed by serial radiographs, serial measurements of pulmonary function, and clinical criteria, such as the presence or absence of weight loss, fatigue, malaise, fever, dyspnoea, or cutaneous lesions. Some two-thirds of patients with active sarcoidosis have raised serum angiotensin-converting enzyme (SACE) with the highest levels in clinically florid or radiographically extensive disease. SACE measurements can be helpful in monitoring disease activity, and broadly correlate with serial chest radiographs and lung function tests.

Course and prognosis

The outcome is usually good. Sarcoidosis remits without treatment in two-thirds of white and one-third of black patients, and is fatal in less than 3 per cent. Young, white, adult patients presenting with an abrupt onset of erythema nodosum and BHL have the best prognosis. Pulmonary resolution is much less likely when there is accompanying extrathoracic disease. The chest radiograph clears in only one-sixth with bone and skin lesions. Between the large proportion of transient benign cases and the very rare fatality lies a minority who are permanently disabled by tissue fibrosis in the lungs, eyes, kidneys, or other organs.

Treatment

There is no specific or curative therapy. Most aspects of sarcoidosis can be controlled by anti-inflammatory drugs. Corticosteroids improve local and constitutional symptoms and suppress granulomatous inflammation with, for instance, a fall in SACE activity, measurable increase in pulmonary function, or rapid clearing of radiographic infiltration. The dose and duration of corticosteroids treatment required to produce this effect varies considerably and the long-term benefit is uncertain.

Indications for corticosteroids in pulmonary or extrathoracic sarcoidosis are a matter of clinical judgement, balancing the relative risk of corticosteroid treatment against unpredictable long-term benefit. Indications are:

1. Progressive dyspnoea, deteriorating lung function, and worsening chest radiograph.
2. Hypercalcaemia and hypercalciuria.
3. Uveitis always requires corticosteroid treatment. Topical corticosteroid eyedrops and local atropine to maintain a dilated pupil may suffice. In all other cases the only safe course is to treat with systemic corticosteroids commencing with oral prednisolone.
4. Central nervous system involvement. High dose corticosteroids are advisable when symptoms are due to meningeal infiltration, local deposits in the brain, and spinal cord or cranial nerve involvement.
5. Myocardial sarcoidosis may respond to corticosteroids, particularly if there are arrhythmias due to active granulomas.
6. Corticosteroids should be considered for symptomatic muscle involvement, for disfiguring skin lesions, for glandular or significant splenic involvement, or when severe erythema nodosum persists or recurs.

The basic strategy is to start with a large enough dose of corticosteroids to suppress granuloma activity and favourably improve the clinical, radiographic, and physiological abnormalities. Prednisolone in a dose of 30–40 mg daily is normally sufficient. Corticosteroids should be discontinued in individuals showing no response after 4–6 weeks. In responders, the dose is slowly reduced over 6 months to a low maintenance level of 5–10 mg prednisolone per day. Occasional attempts should be made to withdraw treatment.

Non-steroidal anti-inflammatory drugs (e.g. aspirin, indomethacin) are of value in controlling musculoskeletal and cutaneous symptoms in subacute sarcoidosis.

Alternatives to corticosteroid treatment

The antimalarial drug chloroquine phosphate has a suppressive rather than curative effect upon progressive cutaneous, pulmonary, and extracutaneous sarcoidosis.

Cytotoxic or immunosuppressive drugs (chlorambucil, methotrexate, or azothiaprine) may be given exceptionally as single agents in the treatment of disfiguring chronic skin lesions or as a 'steroid-sparing' supplement to corticosteroid treatment.

Further reading

Du Bois, R-M., Holroyd, K.J., Saltini, C., and Crystal, R.G. (1991). Granulomatous processes. In: *The lung: scientific foundations* (ed. R.G. Crystal and J.B. West), pp. 1925–38. Raven Press, New York.

James, D.G. (ed.). (1994). *Sarcoidosis and other granulomatous disorders.* Vol. 73. Dekker, New York.

Scadding, J.G. and Mitchell, D.N. (1985). *Sarcoidosis* (2nd edn). Chapman and Hall, London.

Thomas, P.D. and Hunninghake, G.W. (1987). Current concepts of the pathogenesis of sarcoidosis. *American Review of Respiratory Disease*, **135**, 747–60.

Chapter 4.28

Eosinophilic granuloma of the lung and lymphangioleimyomatosis

R. J. Shaw

Eosinophilic granuloma

Eosinophilic granuloma is characterized by an abnormal proliferation of cells thought to arise from the dendritic cell lineage. These cells form granulomatous-like lesions within the lung and deform the alveolar walls. Lesions may cavitate and heal, resulting in foci of fibrosis giving a typical stellate scar. This process results in honeycombing with the formation of small cysts.

Eosinophilic granuloma affects men and women aged 20–40. It is almost confined to smokers. The main symptoms are cough and exertional dyspnoea. Spontaneous pneumothorax, presumably due to rupture of one of the small cysts, is a common complication and may give rise to pleuritic pain. The chest radiograph typically shows diffuse micronodular reticular changes which progress to cystic honeycombing. Pulmonary physiology reveals a mixed obstructive and restrictive pattern. Bronchoalveolar lavage may reveal atypical histiocytes or Langerhans' cells. The major identifying feature of these cells is an X body or Birbeck granule, which appears under the electron microscope as a tennis-racquet like structure in the cytoplasm. Lung biopsy is usually required to make the diagnosis. Eosinophilic granuloma may be complicated by manifestations of histiocytosis X in bone or by diabetes insipidus. Despite the confusing nomenclature, eosinophilic granuloma is not associated with peripheral eosinophilia. The clinical course is variable, with remission in 25 per cent, stable disease in 50 per cent, but a progressive deterioration in 25 per cent of patients. There are no accepted successful treatments, although some patients may respond to corticosteroids.

Lymphangioleimyomatosis

Lymphangioleimyomatosis is a rare disease occurring in premenopausal women which is characterized by proliferation of the smooth-muscle cells in the lymphatic vessels of the thorax and abdomen. The disease presents with dyspnoea due to the progressive interstitial lung disease, pneumothorax, chylous pleural effusion, or pulmonary haemorrhage. The chest radiograph changes are reticular shadowing including Kerley B lines due to dilated lymphatics, small nodules possibly due to hyperplastic smooth-muscle aggregates, and pleural effusions. Later in the disease honeycombing and cystic dilation occur, predisposing to pneumothorax. These changes are characteristic on CT scanning. The pulmonary physiology is similar to that of emphysema (decreased forced expiratory volume in 1 s (FEV_1), increased residual volume, and decreased *TLCO* and *KCO*). If untreated, most patients die within 10 years.

There are reports of response to antioestrogen therapy suggesting oestrogen dependence of the disease. A trial of treatment with medroxyprogesterone is appropriate and if no response is obtained, bilateral oophorectomy should be considered.

Further reading

Kitaichi, M., Nishimura, K., Itoh, H., and Izumi, T. (1995). Pulmonary lymphangioleimyomatosis: a report of 46 patients including a clinicopathologic study of prognostic factors. *American Journal of Respiratory and Critical Care Medicine*, **151**, 527–33.

Lieberman, P.H., Jones, C.R., Steinman, R.M., *et al.* (1996). Langerhans cell (eosinophilic) granulomatosis. A clinicopathologic study encompassing 50 years. *Journal of Surgical Pathology*, **20**, 519–52.

Chapter 4.29

Pulmonary alveolar proteinosis

D. J. Hendrick

First described in 1958, pulmonary alveolar proteinosis has proved to be a rare but interesting disorder that exerts its primary effects in the alveolar spaces. Over periods ranging from months to years, these become filled with an amorphous, largely cell-free, lipoproteinaceous material which is not readily expectorated. There are two major consequences. First, depending on the number of alveoli involved, the lungs become stiff, ventilatory function becomes restricted, shunting occurs at the alveolar/capillary level causing hypoxia, and in some cases there is death from respiratory failure. Second, there is complicating infection—generally with organisms associated with intracellular infection and impaired T-lymphocyte function.

Pathogenesis

Males appear to be affected more commonly than females, but all age groups may be involved. The cause in most cases is unknown, though an apparently identical (and relentlessly progressive) disorder can arise within months of massive exposure to respirable mineral dust, especially silica. This has been called acute silicoproteinosis or silicolipoproteinosis. A few cases have also been associated with haematological malignancies (usually after the use of cytotoxic agents) or immunodeficiency disorders.

The secreted material is rich in protein and phospholipid, and stains strongly with periodic acid Schiff (PAS) and eosin. It also contains structures resembling tubular myelin which are derived from lamellar bodies of surfactant-producing type II pneumocytes. The secretions themselves are chiefly the product of these cells, and the chief phospholipid (dipalmitoyl phosphatidylcholine) is a component of normal surfactant. It is unclear, however, whether the accumulation of these secretions results from excessive or abnormal production, or from impaired resorption by the type II pneumocytes or the alveolar macrophages. In most cases the PAS stain is taken up uniformly but in others, particularly those associated with haematological or immunological disorders, uptake is heterogeneous, and it has been suggested that fundamentally different processes underlie this 'secondary' form.

Clinical features

The affected subject usually presents with progressive shortness of breath or with a superimposed pneumonic illness. Occasionally, recognition follows an incidental chest radiograph. Cough is common and may be productive, particularly if there is infection. Low grade

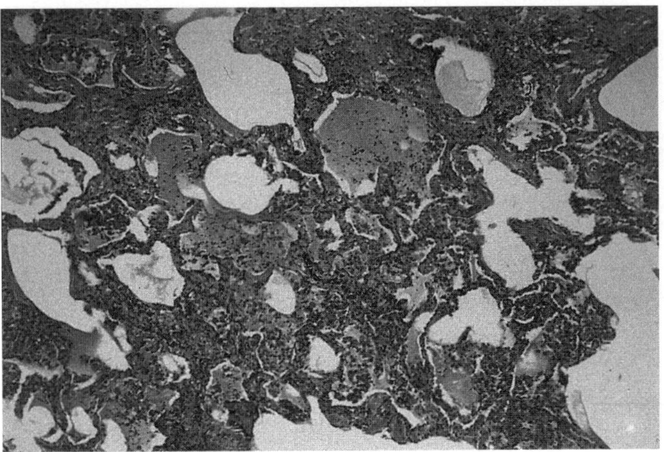

Fig. 1 Pulmonary alveolar proteinosis arising acutely following massive exposure to silica. (By courtesy of Dr D.E. Banks.) Some alveoli are filled with a characteristic non-inflammatory proteinaceous exudate. The lung interstitium shows fibrosis and inflammation which can be attributed to acute silicosis (haematoxylin and eosin, medium magnification).

fever, haemoptysis, and pleuritic pain occur infrequently. There may be crackles and clubbing in advanced stages, and fever becomes characteristic when infection supervenes. When nocardia is not responsible for this, aspergillus, candida, cryptococcus, cytomegalovirus, histoplasma, mucor, mycobacteria, pneumocystis, and viruses are the most common culprits.

Diagnosis

The chest radiograph characteristically shows an alveolar filling pattern, which radiates from the hila and simulates pulmonary oedema, but may be somewhat patchy and asymmetrical. A micronodular infiltration is occasionally seen, particularly in children. The key to diagnosis lies with the PAS-positive milky alveolar secretions, which contain no organisms and no excessive cellular response. Indeed macrophages may be deficient in numbers as well as function. Occasionally the sputum provides diagnostic material, identification of lamellar bodies or their debris by electron microscopy being particularly useful. These may be found within macrophages or pneumocytes, or may lie free within the secretions. More commonly, bronchoalveolar lavage or transbronchial lung biopsy (Fig. 1) is required.

Management

In perhaps a third of cases, no appreciable disability develops and the disease remits spontaneously or fails to progress. Corticosteroids are of no value and may increase the risk of infection. The most effective therapy has been physical removal of the secretions by bronchoalveolar lavage. This is usually performed under general anaesthesia using a double lumen endotracheal tube, one lung being repeatedly lavaged with a total of 20 to 50 litres of warm, sterile buffered saline while the other is mechanically ventilated. The procedure is then reversed. An alternative is sequential lobar lavage using a fibre-optic bronchoscope and a cuffed catheter. When severe respiratory failure has already supervened despite ventilatory support, cardiopulmonary bypass has been used successfully to maintain gas exchange during the lavage procedure. Further lavage is usually necessary every few weeks or months but the activity of the disease may then lessen. Sometimes there is relentless progression.

A considerable threat to life comes from complicating infection, and this should be quickly recognized and treated. An accelerated clinical course together with the development of fever, increased (and productive) cough, malaise, systemic illness, and the radiographic demonstration of cavitation or pleural effusion provide pointers to its development. Blood cultures together with smear and culture studies of sputum may identify the organism(s) responsible, but diagnostic bronchoscopy is often needed. When 'opportunistic' organisms are involved, their eradication may be difficult, perhaps reflecting an underlying impairment of macrophage function. It has consequently been argued that regular bronchoalveolar lavage, even in the absence of impaired exercise tolerance, may provide valuable prophylaxis.

Further reading

Claypool, W.D., Rogers, R.M., and Matuschak, G.M. (1984). Update on the clinical diagnosis, management and pathogenesis of pulmonary alveolar proteinosis (phospholipidosis). *Chest*, **85**, 550–8.

Hoffman, R.M., Dauber, J.H., and Rogers, R.M. (1989). Improvement in alveolar macrophage migration after therapeutic whole lung lavage in pulmonary alveolar proteinosis. *American Review of Respiratory Disease*, 139, 1030–2.

Chapter 4.30

Pulmonary amyloidosis (see also Chapter 6.15)

D. J. Hendrick

It is extremely rare for amyloidosis to exert a major effect in the lung, and only a few dozen cases (usually in the middle aged or elderly) have been reported over recent decades.

Pathogenesis

The material which is responsible for amyloid infiltration is composed of a fibrillar polypeptide and a non-fibrillar glycoprotein. They produce a unique α-pleated structure which may be deposited progressively and widely in the body's organs, eventually interfering with their function. The glycoprotein (amyloid P or AP protein) comprises a mere 10 per cent of amyloid tissue. It is derived from a parent serum protein (SAP) made in the liver and is common to all types of amyloid tissue. When radiolabelled, it can be used with whole body scintigraphy to assess the extent of the disease.

The fibrillar protein is of two distinct types:

1. AL protein, seen with 'primary' amyloidosis and amyloidosis associated with myeloma, is derived from immunoglobulin light chains and a plasma cell clone, whether benign or malignant. It may sometimes be detected in the serum as 'M-component' and in the urine as Bence Jones protein. When plasma cells and macrophages occur in focal aggregations within the lung and adjacent to localized deposits of amyloid tissue, it is likely that AL protein is generated locally. With systemic disease, it is more likely that the AP and AL proteins are manufactured at a distance and

then extracted from circulating blood for deposition in the target organ.

2. AA protein is seen with 'secondary' amyloidosis and most of the familial forms of amyloidosis and is derived from an acute phase serum component (SAA). The chronic inflammatory diseases associated with persistently raised levels of SAA (and C reactive protein) are those that are most commonly associated with secondary amyloidosis, but only a small minority of affected subjects show evidence of complicating amyloidosis. This implies derangement of the SAA protein in these subjects or of the SAA degrading process.

Although the patterns of organ dysfunction differ according to the type of amyloid protein, much overlap occurs and both become deposited widely with progressive systemic disease. It is unclear why deposition is a systemic process in some cases but a local one in others, but this is critical to the clinician and so is useful in classification (see Chapter 6.15).

Clinical features

Although the lungs may become infiltrated with both types of amyloid protein, this is particularly unusual for the AA protein. Even when the AL protein is involved, the kidneys and heart bear the brunt of systemic disease. The thoracic effects depend on deposition sites (which occasionally include hilar or mediastinal lymph nodes and pleura) and the following varieties, in descending order of epidemiological importance, are the most clearly recognized:

1. Laryngotracheobronchial: discrete and usually multiple masses of amyloid protein enlarge in the walls of the airways or the peribronchial tissues causing cough, obstruction, and sometimes bleeding. The obstructed airways may lead to wheeze, stridor, breathlessness, atelectasis, infection, and even bronchiectasis. A individual lesion may be polypoid, simulating the effects of a bronchial adenoma.
2. Parenchymal nodule(s): single or multiple masses, occasionally reaching the size of a tennis ball, develop within the lung parenchyma. They rarely cause symptoms or disrupt function, and may eventually calcify, cavitate, or even ossify. Fear of malignancy often leads to resection.
3. Alveolar–interstitial: amyloid tissue is deposited diffusely throughout the vasculature, alveolar walls, and interstitium, usually in association with systemic amyloidosis (Figs 1 and 2). There is progressive breathlessness and dry cough. Scattered crackles are characteristic and there may be pleural effusions. Eventually, respiratory failure may supervene as ventilation becomes increasingly restricted and gas transfer impaired, though death more commonly results from cardiac or renal involvement. Although amyloid infiltration of the pulmonary vasculature is usually of no clinical consequence, it has been reported to cause pulmonary hypertension and undue bleeding after biopsy.

Diagnosis

The diagnosis rests essentially on the demonstration of amyloid tissue in an affected organ. When the protein is derived from plasma cells or lymphocytes, it may be possible to demonstrate light chains in the urine or M-component in the serum, and a plasma cell or lymphocyte dyscrasia may be clinically evident. When systemic reactive amyloidosis is the diagnosis, a provoking chronic inflammatory disease should be obvious, and high levels of SAA and C reactive protein will be present in the serum. Histochemical studies in the laboratory should, in any event, identify the specific biochemical nature of the protein sampled at biopsy, as should the ultrastructural appearances at electron microscopy. When there is systemic disease from either cause, submucosal biopsy of the rectum usually provides a convenient source of diagnostic tissue.

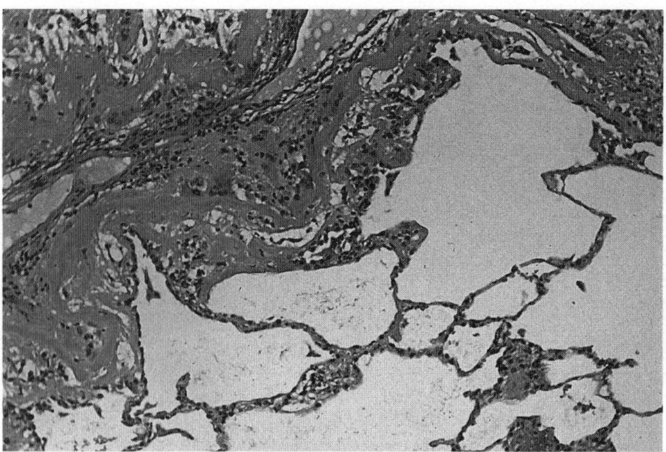

Fig. 1 Amyloidosis of the lung: alveolar–interstitial type [i] (by courtesy of Dr T. Ashcroft). The interstitial deposits of hyaline eosinophilic material with a foreign body type giant cell response in adjacent tissue are almost unique to amyloidosis affecting the lung (haematoxylin and eosin, medium magnification).

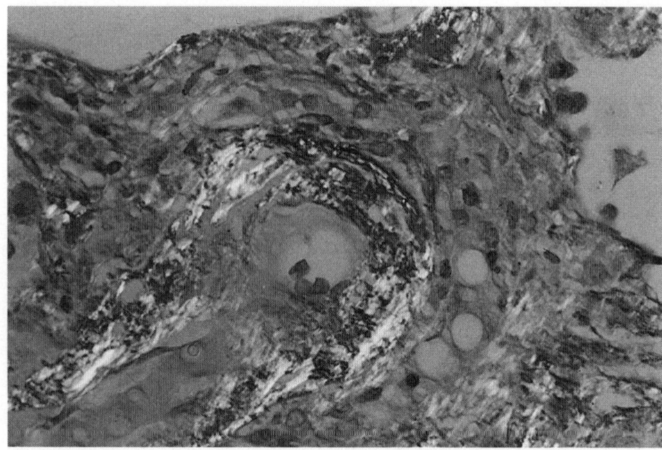

Fig. 2 Amyloidosis of the lung: alveolar–interstitial type [ii] (by courtesy of Dr T. Ashcroft). Amyloid gives a characteristic dichroic birefringence (Congo red stain under polarized light, high magnification).

Management

Treatment of the systemic disease associated with AL protein is usually unrewarding. There is an inexorable accumulation of amyloid tissue in the affected organs, and death occurs within 1 to 2 years. A response to cytotoxic agents (particularly alkylating agents) is encountered sporadically, but these agents are not often helpful unless survival in the short and medium term is ensured by organ transplantation. Corticosteroids may actually worsen deposition of protein in the kidneys. Ultimately, organ transplantation may become the only hope of survival, and when renal failure or cardiac failure is the only immediate threat to life, this is often carried out.

The outcome of systemic reactive amyloidosis is dependent on the accompanying inflammatory disease. If this can be controlled, the deposition of amyloid tissue may be halted. It may also be halted or lessened by the use of colchicine, which interferes with the metabolism of SAA. Nevertheless, systemic reactive amyloidosis usually ends fatally within a few years.

With the local forms of the disease, of whatever aetiology, the outlook is a good deal brighter. Progression is usually slow, and the disease may become quiescent.

Further reading

Kavaru, M.S., Adamo, J.P., Ahmad, M., Mehta, A.C., and Gephardt, G.N. (1990). Amyloidosis and pleural disease. *Chest*, **98**, 21–3.

Chapter 4.31

Lipoid (lipid) pneumonia

D. J. Hendrick

Exogenous

When mineral or vegetable lipids are deposited in the lung, they usually prove to be relatively inert but difficult to remove. Lung lipases have little effect, and the macrophages are slow to ingest and degrade the free or emulsified material. The result is often a chronic low grade inflammatory response that may lead to secondary infection and/or local fibrosis. It is known as lipoid (or lipid) pneumonia. It should be suspected whenever a 'pneumonic' illness is slow to resolve or is recurrent, especially if there is the possibility of impaired swallowing and recurrent aspiration. Some animal lipids are more readily degraded by lung lipases, thus releasing irritating fatty acids. In these circumstances a brisk pneumonitis may occur.

Pathogenesis

Aspiration of vegetable or mineral oil is not common in the population at large, but is seen not infrequently within certain subgroups—particularly those with impaired swallowing mechanisms. Most affected are the very young and the elderly, and among affected elderly subjects the use paraffin as an aperient is a common cause. The critical point is that paraffin and other oils are not irritating to the tracheal mucosa, and so coughing is rarely excited and aspiration readily occurs. Those fed by nasogastric tube are particularly vulnerable as are those fed regularly with high lipid diets. Adults with unimpaired swallowing are affected only sporadically, though shipwrecked sailors have occasionally aspirated diesel oil, and lipoid pneumonia has been recognized in workers exposed to oil mists and burning fats.

Clinical features

There may be no symptoms, the subject presenting by chance with an abnormal chest radiograph, but in about 50 per cent of cases there is productive cough with low grade fever. Often there is a cyclical course with intermittent symptoms. Repeated aspiration may lead to fibrotic shrinkage of the affected segment or segments, or to persistent consolidation. Either may closely simulate bronchial carcinoma, and many resections have been carried for this reason. When more substantial quantities are aspirated the radiographic abnormalities are necessarily more diffuse, and when dependent segments are involved the true nature of the disorder is more obvious.

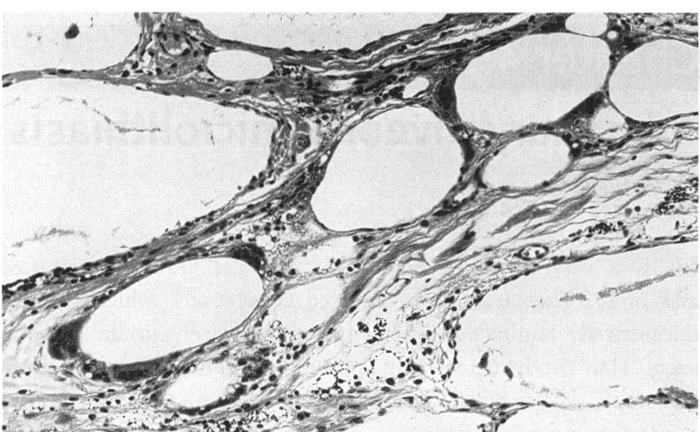

Fig. 1 Lipoid pneumonia due to aspirated paraffin (by courtesy of Dr T. Ashcroft). There is interstitial fibrosis containing oil vacuoles which are enclosed within multinucleated giant cells (haematoxylin and eosin stain, medium magnification).

Diagnosis

The key to diagnosis lies with the demonstration of lipid material within pulmonary secretions or alveolar macrophages, whether obtained from sputum or bronchoalveolar lavage. If lung tissue is resected or undergoes biopsy, there may be fibrosis, evidence of chronic inflammation, and foreign body granulomata/giant cells in addition to lipid material retained within alveoli and macrophages (Fig. 1). Computed tomography has recently identified excess deposits of lipid in lipoid pneumonia from its X-ray absorption characteristics, a technique which could offer a valuable alternative to biopsy or bronchoalveolar lavage in the diagnosis of 'atypical pneumonias'. Nuclear magnetic resonance scanning appears much less effective.

Management

Prophylactic management centres on minimizing any tendency to aspiration from impaired deglutition, on limiting the use of dietary lipids in such subjects, and on persuading the misuser of paraffin to adopt alternative habits. Once aspiration has occurred there may be a role for bronchoalveolar lavage since this may remove substantial quantities of lipid from the alveoli. During episodes of secondary bacterial infection, there is an obvious role for antibiotics.

Endogenous

The body may itself produce and retain lipid (mainly cholesterol) within the lungs, though this is not a common phenomenon. It occurs chiefly at sites of chronic inflammation, obstruction, or tissue necrosis and is derived from the necrotic cells. This lipid will also be ingested by macrophages and may be recovered in the sputum. Sputum macrophages laden with lipid are not therefore pathognomonic of aspiration from an exogenous source, though chemical tests can distinguish the two varieties and histological examination of affected lung does not show a granulomatous response to endogenous lipid. Endogenous lipid is most commonly deposited when chronic inflammation accompanies bronchiectasis, bronchial carcinoma, or some other cause of persisting localized bronchial obstruction, and appears to depend on cigarette smoking. The radiological appearances are of a persisting pneumonia.

Chapter 4.32

Pulmonary alveolar microlithiasis

D. J. Hendrick

This is a very rare and remarkable disorder (150–200 reported cases only). Tiny, 0.2–5 mm, calcified concretions, which may be concentrically laminated, are formed progressively in the alveolar spaces. They produce a striking and unique appearance on the chest radiograph. At present there are few clues to the cause and there is no effective means of therapy.

Pathogenesis

No abnormality of calcium metabolism has been demonstrated, and there has been no clear pattern of environmental, genetic, or gender dependence. An analytical study using X-ray energy spectroscopy and microscopic infrared spectroscopy showed no evidence of mineral dust deposition. It demonstrated that the calcified microliths were formed of calcium carboxyapatite. Formation did presumably occur within the alveolar spaces because some microliths were flushed out by bronchoalveolar lavage.

Clinical features

The disease usually presents in middle age, but the whole age spectrum may be involved. Almost invariably the affected subject is symptom-free when an initial film is taken for incidental reasons, and there may be wonder that this can be possible when the radiograph is so grossly abnormal. This is a consequence of there being no associated cellular, exudative, fibrotic, or vascular disruption of normal physiological processes. Physical signs are conspicuous by their absence for most of its long course, though crackles, clubbing (even hypertrophic pulmonary osteoarthropathy), and signs of respiratory failure may be observed ultimately.

In most cases, there is slow progression; eventually exercise limitation, dry cough, occasional haemoptysis, respiratory failure, and cor pulmonale supervene; the lungs becoming stiff, ventilation restricted, and gas transfer impaired. Survival of 10 to 20 years is characteristic. At death, extensive areas of the chest radiograph show a dense 'white-out' appearance due to the considerable accumulation of calcium, the lungs are difficult to cut, and they sink in water.

Diagnosis

The radiograph appearances of profuse small calcified nodules are specific, particularly in moderately advanced cases when the dense 'white-out' picture supervenes but symptoms are still absent or unimpressive. With less advanced disease biopsy or bronchoalveolar lavage should provide diagnostic tissue, but with transbronchial biopsy it may prove difficult to close the forceps and extract them through the fibre-optic bronchoscope. Initially, the chest radiograph shows a mere haziness of the lower zones, and computerized tomography may be useful in demonstrating the calcific nature of the nodular shadows. It may also confirm an early predominance for the basal and posterior segments. Measurement of lung function during the asymptomatic stage reveals little or no abnormality. As profusion and size of the calcified concretions increase, the lung fields become diffusely and densely opaque.

Management

In the absence of transplantation, treatment is merely supportive. A report of a 37-year-old man presenting in respiratory failure has recorded severe hypoxia and pulmonary hypertension. Considerable intrapulmonary shunting was demonstrated which was greatly improved by nasal continuous positive airway pressure, but not by conventional supplemental oxygen therapy.

Chapter 4.33

Pneumoconioses

A. Seaton

Most lung diseases are caused, at least in part, by inhalation of harmful material. A wide range of conditions, including lung cancer, pneumonia, asthma, alveolitis, pulmonary fibrosis, and toxic pneumonitis, may occur as a result of work-place exposure. Pneumoconiosis may be defined as fibrotic lung disease caused by inhalation of mineral dust.

In the West, dust control in mines and decline of the traditional extractive industries has reduced the incidence of pneumoconiosies, but increased use of asbestos through the 1960s to 1980s has caused a rise in mesothelioma. The industrialization of developing countries has stimulated the need for indigenous coal and minerals, and in China, South America, and India several million workers are employed in mining, often in conditions which ensure a high risk of pneumoconiosis. Fortunately, these problems are all potentially soluble by the application of preventive measures and these are emphasized in the sections that follow.

Coalworker's pneumoconiosis

Coalworker's pneumoconiosis is caused by inhalation of coal dust, a complex mixture of carbon, silicates, quartz, and other minerals. In Britain it is now uncommon, the annual incidence having declined from about 2000 in the 1960s to less than 100 today. New cases reflect mining conditions decades earlier, and a further fall is likely unless there is a relaxation of dust control in mines. In other Western countries there has also been a reduction in the incidence, but in China the disease is widespread.

Aetiology and pathology

The pathogenicity of coal dust depends on its inhalability to acinar level, respirable particles having an aerodynamic diameter equivalent to a sphere of unit density between 7 and 0.5 μm. Some coalmine dusts containing a high proportion of quartz (crystalline silicon dioxide) cause a reaction leading to the typical silicotic nodule (see section on silicosis). Most coal dust, however, contains little quartz and is not particularly toxic to macrophages *in vitro*. Studies in rats have shown that inhalation of relatively low concentrations of coal dust causes inhibition of macrophage migration and provokes an inflammatory response, mediated *inter alia* by interleukin-1 and tumour necrosis factor, resulting in the release of elastase and the

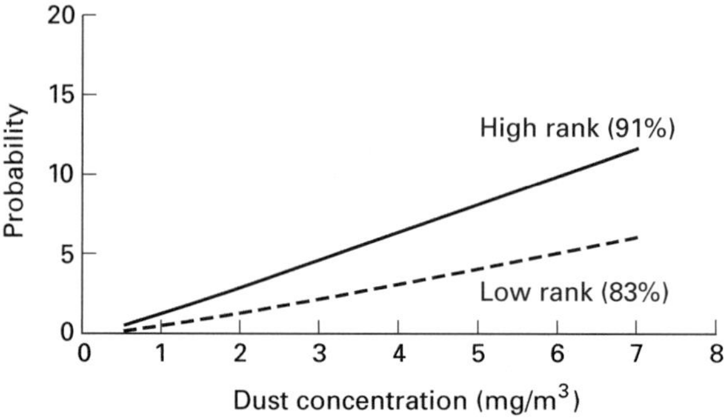

Fig. 1 Relationship between risk of category 2 or 3 radiological simple pneumoconiosis in relation to daily exposure over a working lifetime to different concentrations of coal dust. Note the greater risk in association with exposure to dust from coals of higher combustibility.

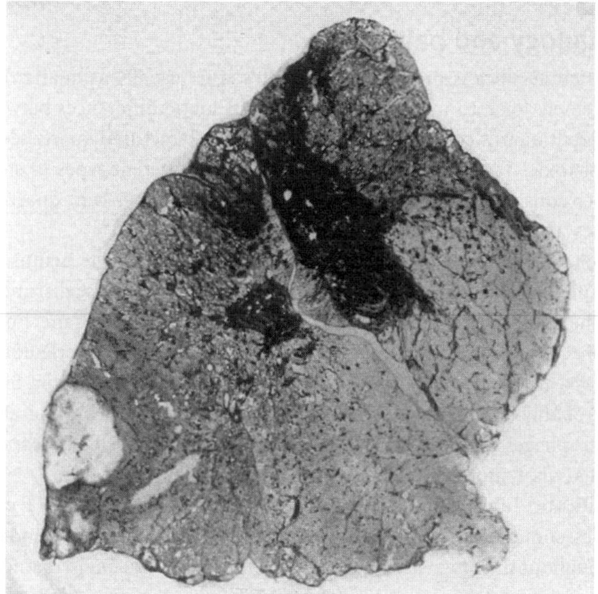

Fig. 2 Whole lung section of a coalminer whose radiograph is shown in Fig. 4, showing progressive, massive fibrosis.

degradation of fibronectin. It seems likely that these toxic effects are fundamental to the pathology of coalworker's pneumoconiosis, including the associated centriacinar emphysema.

The total amount of dust inhaled is a critical factor in the development of pneumoconiosis. Epidemiological studies have shown a relationship between cumulative dust exposure and radiological disease (Fig. 1). This is, however, not straightforward, some coal dusts being more toxic than others. As a general rule, the higher the combustibility (rank) of the coal, the more likely is its dust to cause pneumoconiosis.

Pathologically, coalworker's pneumoconiosis is characterized by multiple centriacinar and interlobular foci containing varying proportions of dust, inflammatory cells, macrophages, and reticulin or collagen, the coal macules. The presence of small discrete nodules is known as simple pneumoconiosis, and when sufficient numbers of these lesions are present they become visible on a radiograph. Progressive massive fibrosis (PMF) is present, by definition, when one or more of these lesions is more than 1 cm in diameter (Fig. 2). This occurs either by aggregation of several, usually collagenous, smaller nodules or by diffuse accumulation of dust associated with dead cells and ischaemic necrosis of lung tissue. The former, less common, mechanism occurs especially in relation to relatively high quartz exposures while the latter seems more frequent with exposure to high carbon dusts. There is a tendency for PMF to grow and be surrounded by bullous emphysema.

Clinical features

Miners most at risk are those working in the dustiest areas, face workers cutting coal, drilling for shot-firing, tunnelling, and drilling bolts into the roof. Opencast miners rarely work in such dusty circumstances, except in hot dry countries. Simple pneumoconiosis *per se* causes no symptoms, signs, or impairment. Radiological progression or regression occurs only very rarely after dust exposure ceases, occasional apparent regression being associated with the development of emphysema.

The threat from simple pneumoconiosis is that it predisposes to PMF, the risk being related to the profusion of opacities on the radiograph. PMF may occur during working life or appear for the first time years after dust exposure ceases, even when there is no apparent simple pneumoconiosis on the radiograph. In general, PMF progresses and causes a mixture of lung restriction and, due to associated emphysema, airways obstruction. Ultimately it may lead to cor pulmonale (see also Chapter 2.29). However, the rate of progression is very variable. In general, the earlier it develops, the more rapidly progressive and serious it is.

The patient with PMF may complain of shortness of breath and, later, symptoms of cor pulmonale. An unusual symptom is expectoration of the black contents of a cavitated lesion, melanoptysis. Finger clubbing is not a feature. Abnormal signs in the chest, if present, relate to the presence of bullae, though lobar collapse occurs rarely.

Coalworker's pneumoconiosis is not associated with an increased risk of tuberculosis or cancer. There is, however, evidence of a parallel association between dust exposure and two effects—pneumoconiosis and airways obstruction. The more dust a miner has been exposed to, the greater his risks of pneumoconiosis on the one hand and productive cough, reduction in forced expiratory volume in 1 s (FEV_1), and presence of centriacinar emphysema on the other. The effect of dust exposure is additional to that of smoking.

The radiological lesions in simple pneumoconiosis are predominantly rounded opacities between 1 and 5 mm in diameter, though small irregular and linear opacities and Kerley B lines are frequently present also (Fig. 3). The round opacities tend to be more profuse in the upper and mid zones whereas the irregular lesions predominate in the lower. PMF almost always starts in an upper zone, gradually increasing in size until it may occupy up to a third of the lung (Fig. 4). Such lesions are frequently multiple and often shaped like short fat sausages, their outer border curved with the chest wall and separated from the pleura by bullous emphysema. Calcification is not a feature, but cavitation may occur. Caplan's syndrome is the name given to the combination of rheumatoid disease and several round nodules (usually between 1 and 5 cm in diameter) in the lungs of a coalminer. The lesions have a rheumatoid histology and rarely cause any serious pulmonary impairment. They may cavitate and disappear. The radiological features of coalworker's and other pneumoconioses are described by a set of standard films produced by the International Labour Organization (ILO) for use in epidemiological studies.

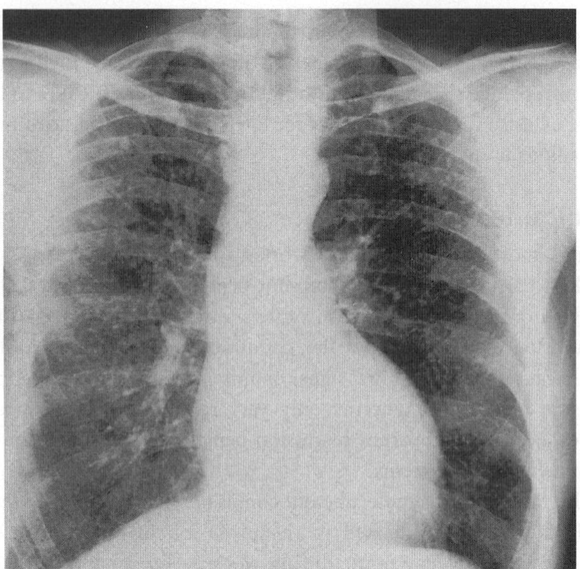

Fig. 3 Radiograph of a coalminer showing small round lesions of simple pneumoconiosis. Some irregular shadows are also present in the lower zones.

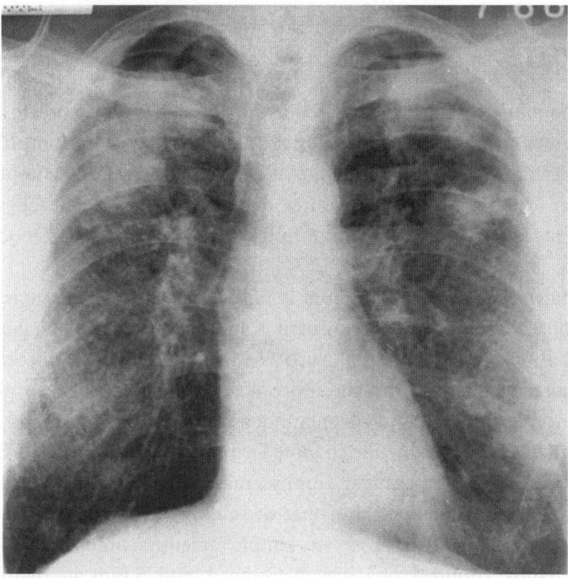

Fig. 4 Chest radiograph of the miner whose lung is shown in Fig. 2, showing progressive, massive fibrosis in upper zones and small round shadows through both lungs.

Prevention and management

Standards for coalmine dust levels have been based on the epidemiological relationship described above. Their success in preventing disease depends on regular monitoring of dust levels by gravimetric sampler, dust suppression by ventilation and the use of water at points of dust production, and regular radiography of the workforce. PMF is prevented by prevention of simple pneumoconiosis. This disease is now very rare indeed in Britain, where the standard is 7 mg/m^3, measured in the air returning from the coal face.

If a man develops simple pneumoconiosis late in his career, no action normally needs to be taken, apart from (in the UK) advising him to apply to the Department of Social Security (DSS) for assessment of disablement and possible benefit payments. A younger man, with years of dust exposure ahead, should be advised to work in an area of approved low dust conditions. Men with more than the earliest stages of radiological change are entitled to disablement benefits from the DSS, the value of these depending on the extent of disability. Benefits for airflow obstruction as an associated effect of coal dust exposure are also available in certain circumstances.

Silicosis

Silicosis is the fibrotic disease of the lungs due to inhalation of crystalline silicon dioxide. It is a risk of quarrying or carving almost any type of stone, mining or tunnelling, grinding, fettling in foundries, or sandblasting, if the dust generated contains quartz. In Britain, true silicosis is now quite rare, fewer than 100 cases being diagnosed each year, usually in men working in circumstances where the risks had been ignored.

Aetiology and pathology

Crystalline silica is present in the earth's crust usually as quartz. It is extremely toxic to macrophages, although subtle differences between different quartz-containing dusts exist. Freshly fractured quartz seems most toxic. The quartz content of dust from different types of stone varies considerably, from some sandstones of 100 per cent quartz to shales and slates with less than 10 per cent.

Inhaled particles of quartz small enough to reach the acinus are engulfed by alveolar and interstitial macrophages and cause disruption of the phagosome, probably by peroxidation of membrane lipids. There is release of inflammatory mediators, including interleukin-1, various growth factors, tumour necrosis factor, and fibronectin. Silica is probably transported across the alveolar epithelium by migrating macrophages and by endocytosis by type 1 alveolar cells. It is transported via lymphatics, much being deposited in hilar nodes.

Silicotic lungs show fibrous pleural adhesions, enlarged lymph nodes containing fibrotic, often calcified, nodules, and grey nodules throughout the lung varying from a few mm to several cm in diameter, more profuse in upper zones. They have a whorled appearance when cut across and may be calcified. The largest lesions consist of many nodules that have become confluent. Microscopically, the silicotic nodule consists of concentric layers of collagen surrounded by a zone of doubly refractile quartz particles, macrophages, and fibroblasts, and may contain remnants of the respiratory bronchiole and arteriole.

Acute silicosis macroscopically resembles pulmonary oedema. Microscopically, the alveoli are filled with macrophages and eosinophilic fluid, and the alveolar walls contain plasma cells, lymphocytes, fibroblasts, and quartz.

Clinical features

Silicosis presents a spectrum of clinical appearances. The most severe type, acute silicosis, results from very heavy exposure over only months, as in sandblasting without respiratory protection. Such patients become intensely breathless and die within a year or two. The radiograph shows apparent pulmonary oedema. Large hilar nodes are a recently described consequence of heavy short-term exposures. Less heavy exposure causes less dramatic disease, ranging from a progressive upper lobe fibrosis with slowly increasing exertional dyspnoea over several years (accelerated silicosis), to radiographic nodular change similar to coalworker's pneumoconiosis unassociated with symptoms or signs. The latter type is the most common and is usually associated with exposure to dust containing 10–30 per cent

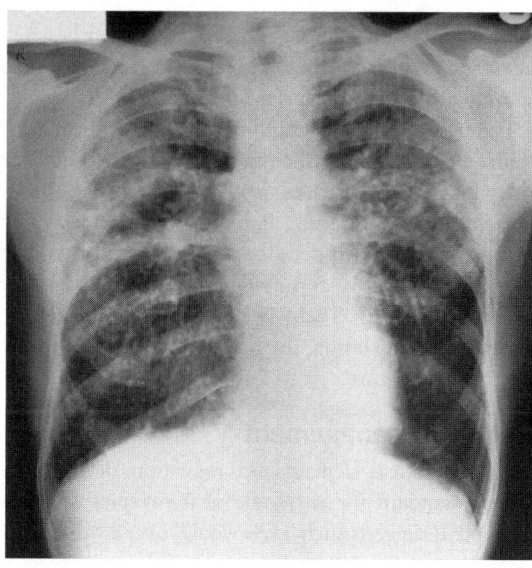

Fig. 5 Radiograph of slate miner, showing extensive simple silicosis in upper and mid-zones with early massive fibrosis and eggshell calcification of hilar nodes.

silica over a prolonged period. Simple nodular silicosis differs from coalworker's pneumoconiosis in that the lesions are larger (3–5 mm) and it progresses even after dust exposure ceases. Lesions increase both in size and profusion and PMF frequently develops (Fig. 5). Extensive simple silicosis may be associated with mild reduction of lung volumes but rarely with emphysema. PMF is, however, commonly associated with bullous disease. Accelerated silicosis and PMF cause lung restriction and may lead to cardiorespiratory failure.

Physical signs are usually absent and clubbing and crackles are not a feature. Diagnosis depends on a history of quartz exposure and the radiograph. The most characteristic feature is 3 to 5-mm nodules, predominantly in the upper zones and sometimes pathognomonic eggshell calcification in the hilar nodes. Silicosis may be complicated by tuberculosis, usually due to reactivation of a quiescent lesion, or other mycobacterial disease. There is some evidence of an association between silicosis and lung cancer, even when exposures to cigarette smoke and other occupational carcinogens have been accounted for, and lung cancer is now recognized as an occupational disease in patients with silicosis in Britain.

Subjects with silicosis, especially of the accelerated type, are at increased risk of the development of autoantibodies and of collagen diseases, which have been described in about 10 per cent of some series of silicotics. Focal glomerulonephritis has also been described probably as a direct toxic effect of quartz.

Prevention and management

Workers exposed to concentrations in excess of 1 mg/m^3 of respirable silica have a high risk of silicosis, and even at around 0.1 mg/m^3 a risk may still exist. The British Maximum Exposure Limit is 0.3 mg/m^3, and industry is obliged to keep exposures of workers below this level by appropriate dust suppression measures. If higher exposures are inevitable, the worker should wear respiratory protection though this is a second-best procedure. Once a worker has developed silicosis he should be prevented from further exposure. Sputum examination for tubercle bacilli is desirable in endemic areas. Workers with silicosis in UK should apply to the DSS for industrial injuries benefit.

Asbestosis

Asbestos is mined principally in Canada, South Africa, and the USSR. It is a generic term for a group of fibrous silicates, the most important being chrysotile (white), crocidolite (blue), and amosite (brown). Chrysotile, the most commonly used fibre, has a serpentine configuration and breaks up into microfibrils, while the other types are straight and less liable to dissolution. All are resistant to destruction which gives them their commercial value in fireproofing, insulation, reinforcement of cement, weaving into cloth, bonding in brake linings and plastics, and so on.

Asbestos causes pleural plaques, pleural effusion and diffuse pleural fibrosis, asbestosis, lung carcinoma, and mesothelioma, risks of the last three being related to the cumulative exposure to asbestos. Crocidolite and amosite are more dangerous than chrysotile, particularly with respect to mesothelioma.

The current incidence of asbestosis is about 100–150 cases annually in Britain, mostly in people working with asbestos in insulation, shipyards, or construction. Mesothelioma, the most important asbestos-related disease, occurs in about 1000 people in Britain each year, reflecting the increasing use of asbestos in construction and shipyards through the 1980s. It is likely to increase in incidence over the next two decades.

Aetiology and pathology

The harmful asbestos fibres are those less than 3 μm across and greater than 10 μm in length, sufficiently narrow to be inhaled to the acinus yet too long to be removed by macrophages. All types of asbestos are equally toxic to macrophages *in vitro* and all can cause fibrosis and carcinoma when inhaled by rats. Moreover, injection of any asbestos type (and indeed many fibrous non-asbestos minerals) into the peritoneum of rats causes mesothelioma. The weaker epidemiological association between mesothelioma and chrysotile may be due to the propensity of chrysotile to break up into short fibrils that can be removed from the lung by the action of macrophages. The fibrogenicity of asbestos is probably related, as with coal and silica, to damage to macrophages which are unable to remove fibres much longer than themselves and the liberation of substances that activate fibroblasts to produce collagen. Among those shown to result from experimental exposure of rats are tumour necrosis factor, and macrophage- and platelet-derived growth factors.

The asbestotic lung shows grey fibrosis, progressing to honeycombing, peripherally and in the lower zones. Yellow, shiny parietal pleural plaques are also usually present though these frequently occur also in the absence of pulmonary fibrosis. Microscopically there is diffuse fibrosis including asbestos bodies, asbestos fibres coated with a protein–ferritin complex. Pleural plaques have the appearance of basket-weave collagen.

Clinical features

Asbestosis occurs in people exposed regularly over years, as a result of the material being used or removed, and not as a result of occasional exposure. It is more likely to be seen in trades involving the application or removal of insulation than in asbestos production where control of fibre levels is nowadays more careful. It may first occur after exposure has ceased. The symptoms are shortness of breath and dry cough. Repetitive end-inspiratory basal crackles commonly precede symptoms, and finger clubbing occurs. The disease is usually progressive, resulting in increasing disability and cardiorespiratory failure.

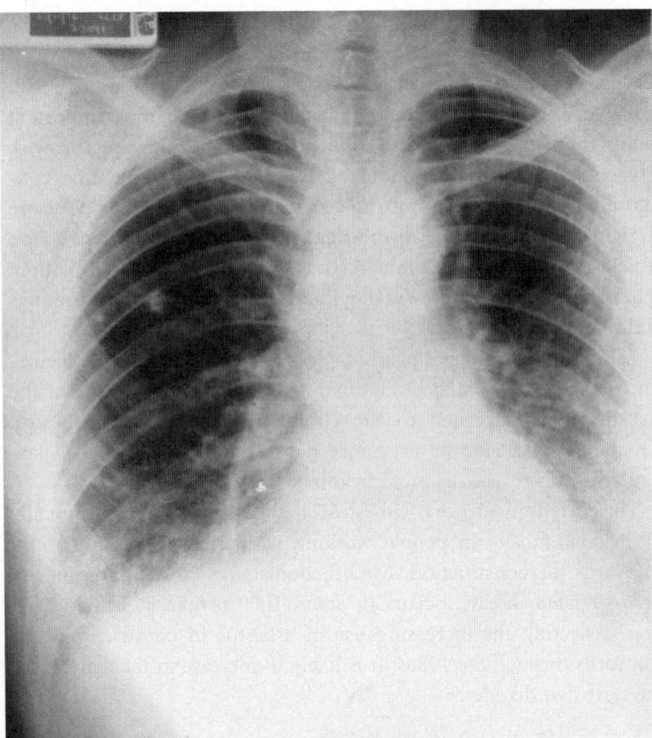

Fig. 6 Radiograph of lagger with asbestosis. Note irregular basal and mid-zone fibrosis.

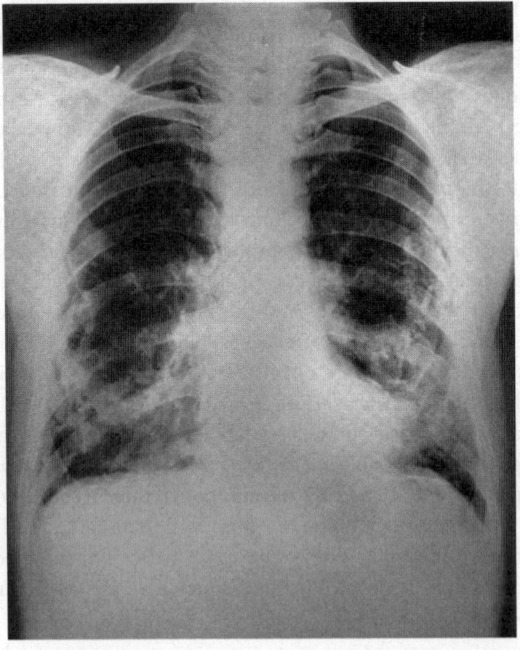

Fig. 7 Radiograph of lagger, showing extensive calcified pleural plaques.

Up to 50 per cent of smokers with asbestosis die of bronchial carcinoma and there is evidence of a multiplicative increase in risk with these two causes.

The radiological appearances are of predominantly basal, irregular shadowing progressing to honeycombing (Fig. 6). Pleural plaques, often calcified, indicate asbestos exposure and may help in the differential diagnosis (Fig. 7). In advanced asbestosis, the pulmonary fibrosis gives a shaggy appearance to the cardiac borders. As with other pneumoconioses, the radiological appearances are best described by the ILO standard films. Asbestosis causes a restrictive pattern of lung function, with reduced transfer factor.

Pleural plaques cause no symptoms. A diffuse form of pleural fibrosis, unilateral or bilateral which may restrict lung volumes, occurs infrequently. Inspiratory crackles may be heard over this in the absence of significant asbestosis. Rarely, a benign pleural effusion develops within the first two decades after exposure. It is diagnosed by the exclusion of infective and malignant causes and usually leads to diffuse pleural fibrosis. There is no evidence that any of these disorders causes mesothelioma, the risk of which relates to the prior extent of asbestos exposure.

Prevention and management

Prevention of asbestosis depends on reduction of exposure. The present British standard for chrysotile of 0.5 respirable fibres/ml is based on work that suggests such levels would, over a working lifetime, result in asbestosis in fewer than 1 per cent of those exposed. Stricter standards apply to crocidolite and amosite. Most industries are substituting other fibrous or crystalline minerals where possible. Some may be hazardous themselves and are under toxicological and epidemiological investigation.

Regular medical and radiological examination of asbestos workers is essential for the early detection of asbestosis and there is some evidence that removal of the worker from exposure at this stage is associated with slower progression. Workers should also be advised of the special dangers of smoking. Once asbestosis, bilateral pleural fibrosis, or mesothelioma is suspected, the UK worker should apply to the DSS for assessment for industrial injuries benefit.

Risks of asbestos-related disease in the non-occupationally exposed population

Much anxiety has been engendered in the general public by media interest in asbestos, and doctors may find themselves being asked about, for example, the risks to children of asbestos wall panelling in houses or asbestos inserts in ironing boards. It can be stated that asbestosis only occurs in people exposed to asbestos regularly, directly or indirectly, for years. Occasional or incidental exposure to asbestos can be dismissed as a cause of asbestosis. Lung cancer risks, similarly, seem to be increased only with exposures that lead to asbestosis, and individuals who don't smoke and who only have asbestos fittings in their houses can be reassured that their risks of this disease are negligible. Finally, the risk of mesothelioma is again dose-related, although it is well established that a sufficient dose of crocidolite or amosite can be inhaled in a period of intense exposure of a few months. Of the 1000 or so cases occurring in Britain each year, almost all give a history of having worked with asbestos and have large numbers of fibres in their lungs. Small and occasional exposures to asbestos are highly unlikely to entail an important risk.

Other pneumoconioses

Several silicates apart from asbestos are of commercial importance and some of these have been shown to cause pneumoconiosis. Talc, hydrated magnesium silicate, is mined as soapstone in the US, China, and the Pyrenees. It is milled and has many uses including cosmetics, the rubber industry, paints, ceramics, and pharmaceuticals. Kaolin, hydrated aluminium silicate, is quarried in south-western England, US, Japan, Egypt, Germany, and Czechoslovakia, and used mainly in ceramics, paper and paint manufacture and in pharmaceuticals. Fuller's earth, calcium montmorillonite, is an absorbent clay quarried in UK, US, and Germany. It is used in oil refining and bonding foundry moulds.

Talc is commonly contaminated with tremolite, a form of asbestos, and with silica. Talc pneumoconiosis resembles asbestosis, with finger clubbing and basal crackles, though radiological descriptions emphasize lesions predominantly in the mid-zones with nodular as well as reticular components. PMF has been described. Kaolin causes a pneumoconiosis similar to coalworker's pneumoconiosis, described in workers involved in drying and milling china clay. There is no evidence linking kaolin pneumoconiosis with carcinoma or tuberculosis. Fuller's earth has been described as causing a pneumoconiosis resembling that of coalworkers.

People in several villages in central Turkey have been exposed to erionite, a fibrous hydrated aluminium silicate, from use of local rock as stucco and whitewash in their homes. Pleural plaques, pulmonary fibrosis, lung cancer, and mesothelioma have been endemic in these villages. Erionite has no commercial use, but this illustrates the potential dangers of inhaling fine fibrous material, whether asbestos or some other mineral.

Two widely-used silicate materials are not established as causes of pulmonary disease: cement and vitreous fibres. Cement is often mixed with asbestos and asbestosis may occur in its production. Artificial vitreous fibres (glass wool and rock wool) have not so far been shown to cause pulmonary fibrosis or neoplasia in humans exposed to them.

Beryllium is a metal used in the nuclear industry, in alloys, and in the production of X-ray tubes. It is highly toxic when inhaled, and also causes granulomatous ulcers on contact with the skin. High concentrations cause an acute pneumonitis and tracheobronchitis, which may be fatal. Chronic berylliosis usually follows longer exposure to lower levels. No more than about 50 cases have been diagnosed in UK, but it has been recorded much more frequently in the US, in beryllium workers, wives exposed to dust from their husbands' clothes, and people living near the factories. The patient presents with cough and shortness of breath. Bilateral pulmonary mottling and diffuse irregular fibrosis are the usual radiographic features. The disease progresses, but the rate is very variable. There is restrictive lung function with low transfer factor. The pathology is identical to that of sarcoidosis.

The diagnosis is made on the exposure history, compatible clinical and histological features, and a negative Kveim test. An *in vitro* macrophage inhibition test is available in specialized centres. The progress of the disease can usually be controlled with corticosteroid therapy but this needs to be continued indefinitely in most cases. Berylliosis is prevented by keeping exposures below the threshold limit value (2 $\mu g/m^3$), and by use of respiratory protection.

Many other pneumoconioses have been described, though most are of very limited prevalence and relatively benign. Siderosis is a benign pneumoconiosis occurring in welders caused by iron oxide. The radiological lesions often regress after exposure ceases. Barium processing and tin refining may be associated with the development of dramatic radiological nodular shadowing, baritosis and stannosis respectively, also completely benign conditions, the appearances reflecting radio-opaque dust in macrophages. Work with hard metal (tungsten carbide) may cause asthma, allergic alveolitis, or pulmonary fibrosis, all probably due to cobalt in the metal and coolants used.

Further reading

Morgan, W.K.C. and Seaton, A. (1995). *Occupational lung diseases*, (3rd edn). WB Saunders, Philadelphia.

Mossman, B.T., Bignon, J., Corn, M., Seaton, A., and Gee, J.B.L. (1990). Asbestos: scientific developments and implications for public policy. *Science*, **247**, 294–301.

Peto, J., Hodgson, J.T., Matthews, F.E., and Jones, J.R. (1995). Continuing increase in mesothelioma mortality in Britain. *Lancet*, **345**, 535–9.

Chapter 4.34

Drug-induced lung disease

G. J. Gibson

Adverse effects of drugs on the lungs frequently present diagnostic problems. This account is limited to respiratory disease due to the direct effects of drugs in usual therapeutic doses. A detailed review is available and a comprehensive list of drugs which may injure the respiratory system has recently been published (see Further reading, below). This list is also available in updated form on the World Wide Web at: http://www.pneumotox.com/lungdrug.

Drug-induced asthma

Airway obstruction induced by drugs usually presents as an exacerbation of pre-existing asthma. In some cases, however, asthma is not recognized until 'uncovered' by the adverse effect of a drug. Less commonly, drug-induced asthma may develop *de novo*, usually in an occupational setting. The relevant drugs are classified as those which produce a predictable effect, related to their pharmacological properties, and those having an idiosyncratic effect (Table 1).

Pharmacological effects (Table 1)

Cholinergic drugs such as carbachol given systemically occasionally produce bronchoconstriction, and in very sensitive asthmatic patients exacerbations have occurred with pilocarpine eye drops. Prostaglandin $F_{2\alpha}$, if used to induce abortion, may be hazardous in asthmatic patients, while bronchoconstriction after thiopentone, opiates, and muscle relaxants (tubocurarine, suxamethonium, and pancuronium) is probably due to their capacity to release histamine.

More common is worsening of airway obstruction by β-adrenergic antagonist drugs, even the more selective agents. Of currently available drugs, propranolol is the least selective and most likely to provoke a reaction while atenolol and metoprolol are less likely to cause problems. Nevertheless, many patients with asthma will show reduction in forced expiratory volume in 1 s (FEV_1) or peak flow on therapeutic doses of these agents and considerable caution is necessary. The adverse effects of ophthalmic preparations are easily overlooked. Timolol, which is used commonly in eye drops for the treatment of glaucoma, is a potent, non-selective β-blocker which frequently has been associated with worsening asthma.

Idiosyncratic reactions (Table 1)

The most dramatic presentation of drug-induced asthma is as part of an acute anaphylactic reaction such as can occur with penicillin and intravenously-administered iron dextran. The drugs which most frequently exacerbate asthma are the non-steroidal anti-inflammatory

Table 1 Drugs which may exacerbate asthma

Pharmacological effects
Cholinergic agents (e.g. carbachol, pilocarpine)
Cholinesterase inhibitors (e.g. pyridostigmine)
Prostaglandin $F_{2\alpha}$
Histamine-releasing agents (e.g. curare derivatives)
β-Sympathetic antagonists
ACE inhibitors (cough without asthma more common)
Idiosyncratic effects
Oral
Aspirin and other NSAIDs
Nitrofurantoin (alveolar reaction more common)
Carbamazepine
Propafenone
Parenteral
Penicillin
Iron-dextran complex
Aminophylline
Hydrocortisone sodium succinate
N-acetylcysteine
Inhaled
Nebulized pentamidine
Occupational agents (e.g. antibiotics, methyldopa, cimetidine, piperazine)

agents (NSAIDs). Most patients who are sensitive to aspirin react also to other NSAIDs with widely differing chemical structures making an immunological reaction unlikely. All the anti-inflammatory agents incriminated are inhibitors of prostaglandin synthesis via the cyclo-oxygenase pathway, and it is presumed that their adverse effects are mediated by diversion of the metabolism of arachidonic acid towards production of bronchoconstrictor leukotrienes, but the precise mechanism of the idiosyncracy is unclear. Deaths have been reported with both aspirin and indomethacin. Of commonly used analgesic agents, paracetamol is least likely to provoke a significant response, although occasional adverse reactions are well documented.

Potential exacerbation of asthma by drugs used to treat it presents a particularly acute dilemma, as a drug effect may be difficult to dissociate from spontaneous deterioration. Worsening asthma after both intravenous aminophylline and hydrocortisone is rare but well documented. Steroid sensitivity relates mainly to hydrocortisone sodium succinate and appears to be particularly relevant to asthmatic patients who also show adverse reactions to aspirin and NSAIDs.

Drug-induced cough

Cough is a well-recognized side-effect of inhibitors of angiotensin-converting enzyme (ACE). It develops in 10 to 20 per cent of individuals so treated and is an effect of the class of drug rather than of specific agents. It is sometimes sufficiently troublesome to necessitate withdrawal of the drug. Exacerbation of asthma occurs much less commonly. ACE catalyses not only the conversion of angiotensin I to angiotensin II, but also the breakdown of bradykinin and substance P which are cough stimulants, offering a possible mechanism for this unusual adverse effect.

Table 2 Commoner drugs causing alveolar reactions

ARDS	
Hydrochlorothiazide	
Salicylates	
Tocolytic agents (e.g. isoxsuprine, ritodrine, terbutaline)	
Naloxone	
Cytosine arabinoside	
Low molecular weight dextran	
Diffuse lung injury (alveolitis) and/or fibrosis	
Oxygen	
Nitrofurantoin	
Amiodarone	
Tocainide	
Cytotoxic agents	
Bleomycin	Carmustine
Melphalan	6-Mercaptopurine
Mitomycin C	Azathiprine
Cyclophosphamide	Busulphan
Cytosine arabinoside	Chlorambucil, etc
Eosinophilic reactions	
Sulphonamides	Gold salts*
Nitrofurantoin*	Sulphasalazine
Penicillins	Penicillamine*
Tetracycline	Chlorpropamide
Methotrexate*	Chlorpromazine
Aspirin	Imipramine
Procarbazine	Carbamazepine
Naproxen	Phenytoin, etc

*Eosinophilia not consistent

Alveolar reactions

There is no generally agreed classification of alveolar reactions to drugs. They range from the adult respiratory distress syndrome (ARDS) at one extreme to insidiously developing pulmonary fibrosis at the other. The reactions are conveniently considered in three main groups (Table 2). Of the drugs which can produce ARDS, hydrochlorothiazide and salicylates are the commonest. With salicylates, reactions usually occur with frank overdose (as also occurs with opiates) but occasionally are seen in chronic ingesters with high serum levels. Infused β_2-adrenergic agonists used as uterine relaxants (tocolytics) to inhibit premature labour have also been associated with florid pulmonary oedema.

Numerous drugs produce widespread alveolar damage ('pneumonitis' or 'alveolitis') which may or may not be followed by fibrosis (Table 2). Patients may present acutely with cough, fever, shortness of breath, and occasionally systemic upset. Alternatively, slowly progressive fibrosis can develop, with gradually worsening dyspnoea and widespread radiographic shadowing. The mechanism(s) of such reactions are generally uncertain. With some drugs, including bleomycin, carmustine, amiodarone, and nitrofurantoin, there is a relation to dose or duration of treatment, while with others no dose-response effect is seen. Only the common causes are given in Table 2 and a comprehensive list is available (see Further reading below).

One of the commoner culprits is amiodarone. It has been estimated that approximately 6 per cent of patients taking 400 mg or more per day of the drug for 2 months or more will develop overt pulmonary toxicity. There have also been several well-documented cases taking smaller doses. The mechanism may include both immunologically-mediated and direct toxic effects. Histologically, the lung shows varying chronic inflammation, interstitial and intra-alveolar fibrosis, with characteristic 'foamy' macrophages. Occasionally, the histological picture is of 'bronchiolitis obliterans organizing pneumonia', also known as cryptogenic organizing pneumonia. Symptoms include progressive dyspnoea, cough, and occasionally pleuritic pain. Radiographic appearances are varied and include diffuse nodularity or alveolar 'filling', sometimes with upper lobe predominance and occasionally a pleural effusion. Differential diagnoses in the relevant patient population include left ventricular failure and pneumonia. If amiodarone lung toxicity is suspected, cessation of treatment is desirable, but the very long half-life implies that elimination is very slow. Corticosteroids probably suppress the reaction and sometimes allow continuation or retreatment in cases of 'malignant' dysrrhythmia unresponsive to other agents.

Cytotoxic and immunosuppressive drugs represent an increasing problem, with the majority reported to cause pulmonary complications. In most cases it is not clear whether the effect is due to direct toxicity or hypersensitivity. The recorded frequency of adverse reactions varies with the means by which they are detected with CT scanning showing a greater prevalence than plain radiography. The likelihood of overt lung involvement may be related to length of survival with the primary disease. Other factors which may increase toxicity include advanced age and synergistic effects with other drugs, pulmonary irradiation, or subsequent oxygen therapy.

Histologically, most cytotoxic drugs produce diffuse alveolar damage with destruction of pneumocytes, formation of hyaline membranes, and a variable inflammatory infiltrate and degree of fibrosis. Fibrosis is particularly common with busulphan and bleomycin and rare with methotrexate. With methotrexate and procarbazine (and very occasionally with bleomycin) there may be blood and tissue eosinophilia and correspondingly a good therapeutic response to steroids.

Eosinophilic reactions in the lung include conditions which may be classified as Löffler's syndrome, simple or prolonged pulmonary eosinophilia, and eosinophilic pneumonia. Tissue eosinophilia is a more consistent feature than peripheral blood eosinophilia. Historically, sulfonamides have been the drugs most frequently reported as causes of pulmonary eosinophilia and sulfonamide sensitivity may explain reactions to sulfasalazine and chlorpropamide. Nitrofurantoin can produce an acute eosinophilic reaction in addition to more insidious fibrosis. The roles of gold salts and penicillamine in this type of reaction have been a matter of some debate, but the evidence suggests that both can provoke a reaction. Penicillamine has been further incriminated in two rarer adverse pulmonary reactions: pulmonary haemorrhage and obliterative bronchiolitis.

The clinical severity of eosinophilic reactions is very variable, ranging from a transient and asymptomatic radiographic opacity to a severe illness with dyspnoea, cough, fever, and hypoxaemia due to widespread eosinophilic pneumonia. Concomitant asthma has been noted with carbamazepine, but is not otherwise a common feature. The chest radiograph shows fluffy opacities, frequently with peripheral or predominantly upper-lobe distribution. The reactions are often accompanied by a diffuse maculopapular skin eruption. The prognosis is usually good. Corticosteroids, if required for troublesome symptoms, usually produce rapid improvement.

Table 3 Drugs associated with pleural reactions

Drug-induced lupus	Isolated
Procainamide	Methysergide
Gold	Dantrolene
Hydralazine	Methotrexate
Isoniazid	Bromocriptine

Pulmonary vascular reactions

Pulmonary thromboembolism related to use of the contraceptive pill is well established; its frequency correlates with the oestrogen content and has been reduced with the use of low oestrogen preparations.

An association between pulmonary hypertension and the anorectic agent aminorex in the 1960s was of great theoretical interest. Although the epidemic of pulmonary hypertension subsided when the drug was withdrawn, recent evidence has confirmed that modern anorectic drugs such as fenfluramine are also associated with the condition.

Pleural disease

Drugs which have been associated with pleural reactions (fluid or thickening) are shown in Table 3. Several can produce a systemic-lupus-like syndrome. The main respiratory effects are on the pleura, but (as also with methysergide and bromocriptine) there is often some fibrosis of subjacent areas of the lung.

Methysergide may induce mediastinal or pleural fibrosis with or without retroperitoneal fibrosis. Improvement follows early withdrawal of the drug. Bromocriptine has structural similarities to methysergide and can also produce chronic pleural effusions and thickening. Methotrexate has been associated with pleurisy, independent of its alveolar effects. The smooth-muscle relaxant dantrolene produces an unusual type of pleurisy with effusion in which fluid and blood eosinophilia are prominent.

Further reading

Abenhaim, L., Moride, Y., Brenot, F., *et al.* (1996). Appetite-suppressant drugs and the risk of primary pulmonary hypertension. *New England Journal of Medicine*, **335**, 609–16.

Camus, P. and Gibson, G.J. (1995). Adverse pulmonary effects of drugs and radiation. In *Respiratory medicine*, (2nd edn), (ed. R.A.L. Brewis, B. Corrin, D.M. Geddes, and G.J. Gibson). Saunders, London.

Foucher, P., Biour, M., Blayac, J.P., *et al.* (1997). Drugs that may injure the respiratory system. *European Respiratory Journal*, **10**, 265–79.

Chapter 4.35

Adult respiratory distress syndrome

C. S. Garrard and P. Foëx

Introduction

The term adult respiratory distress syndrome (ARDS) is used to describe an acute, life-threatening respiratory failure which occurs in subjects with previously healthy lungs without primary left ventricular failure. It is associated with a large number of unrelated clinical disorders, yet has uniform physiological, radiological, and pathological features. There are morphological similarities to the neonatal respiratory distress syndrome.

Major trauma, acute hypovolaemic hypotensive Gram-negative septicaemia, and severe pulmonary infections are the most frequent precursors of ARDS (Table 1).

Clinical presentation

The development of ARDS varies in speed and intensity, but the morphological and symptomatic changes leads to a sequential progression of events:

- Phase 1—this is the period of initial resuscitation, with repletion of hypovolaemia. Excessive use of bicarbonate, loss of chloride in gastric contents, and oxidation of citrate in transfused blood may produce a metabolic alkalosis aggravated by a respiratory component following hyperventilation in response to pain. Unless there has been direct pulmonary damage, the lungs are clear to auscultation and the lung fields of the chest radiograph may be unremarkable.
- Phase 2—this is a period of 24–72 hours' duration when the patient is deceptively haemodynamically stable with no obvious respiratory distress except mild tachypnoea. Serial blood gas analyses at this time, however, might reveal subclinical hypoxaemia due to intrapulmonary shunting.
- Phase 3—during this period the hypoxaemia worsens. The patient becomes clinically cyanosed and dyspnoeic. The chest compliance falls, increasing the work of breathing and, if the patient is mechanically ventilated, requiring high inflation pressures. The chest radiograph may reveal the widespread bilateral intra-alveolar and interstitial infiltrates. Increasing hypoxaemia produces disturbed cerebral and renal function.
- Phase 4—refractory hypoxaemia develops with increasing pulmonary hypertension and right ventricular dysfunction in up to 50 per cent of patients. Hypercapnia and hypoperfusion contribute to a mixed respiratory and metabolic acidosis and multiorgan failure may follow.

Pathology

In the acute exudative phase, interstitial oedema is accompanied by damage to, and necrosis of, capillary endothelial and alveolar type I epithelial cells. Fibrin and platelet thrombi develop, and there is adherence of leucocytes to areas denuded of endothelium. Later, the oedema becomes perivascular, peribronchial, and intra-alveolar and accompanied by focal alveolar haemorrhages. Characteristic hyaline membrane lines the alveoli, alveolar ducts, and some respiratory bronchioles. In the chronic proliferative phase, there is regeneration of the capillary endothelium and alveolar epithelium accompanied by interstitial infiltration with lymphocytes, fibroblasts, and deposition of collagen which may proceed to fibrosis. The damaged type I alveolar cells are replaced by more granular type II alveolar cells with a thickening of the air–blood interface. The alveolar lining of surfactant, normally produced by these cells, is absent.

There is an increase in total lung water caused by a disturbance in the normal fluid flux between the intra- and extravascular compartments in the lung. Several factors contribute to the excess lung water:

1. Plasma protein osmotic pressure—in trauma and acute illness, there is a reduction in plasma protein concentration and oncotic pressure, which may be further reduced by crystalloid infusion. Reductions in plasma protein concentration lower the threshold at which pulmonary capillary hydrostatic changes become significant.
2. Lymph drainage—the normal lymph drainage is only 25–30 ml/h but this can increase 20-fold in response to relatively small changes in interstitial pressure from fluid accumulation. High intrathoracic pressures during intermittent positive-pressure ventilation (IPPV) or high levels of positive and expiratory pressure (PEEP) may impair this function.
3. Pulmonary capillary permeability and hydrostatic pressure—although stress-evoked sympathetic stimulation of the sympathetic nervous system in the critically ill will produce pulmonary venoconstriction and pulmonary hypertension, increased pulmonary vascular permeability with increased postcapillary resistance is largely responsible for the increase in lung water.

Table 1 Disorders associated with ARDS

1. *Hypovolaemic shock*	6. *Haematological*
2. *Infection*	(a) Disseminated intravascular coagulopathy
(a) Pulmonary (microbial, fungal, pneumocystis, malaria)	(b) Massive blood transfusion
(b) Extrapulmonary (septicaemia)	7. *Metabolic*
3. *Trauma*	(a) Diabetic ketosis
(a) Thoracic	(b) Uraemia
(b) Extrathoracic	8. *Neurogenic*
4. *Embolism*	(a) Cerebral oedema
(a) Fat	(b) Intracranial haemorrhage
(b) Amniotic fluid	9. *Drugs*
(c) Cellular aggregates	Including heroin, aspirin, propoxyphene, barbiturates, paraquat, protamine
5. *Inhalation*	10. *Other*
(a) Gas	*Inhalation*
(i) irritant (e.g. nitric oxide, smoke)	(a) Pancreatitis
(ii) Non-irritant (e.g. oxygen)	(b) High altitude
(b) Liquid	
(i) Gastric juice	
(ii) Fresh and salt water	

Pathogenesis

Neutrophils, complement activation, and cytokines

Neutrophils appear to play a key role in the pathogenesis of ARDS by sequestering in the lungs as a result of alternative pathway activation of complement with the release of neutrophil-aggregating components, particularly C5a. The neutrophils' intracellular granules release proteinases such as elastase, collagenase, and cathepsin which, by degrading structural components, lead to disorganization of the interstitium and damage the capillary endothelial and alveolar epithelial cells. Proteinases may also cleave fibrinogen, the Hageman factor, complement, and the other plasma proteins producing further embolization by blood constituents such as platelets, mast cells, fibrin, and fibrinogen degradation products. Histamine, platelet activated factor, serotonin, bradykinin, and other vasoactive substances may be released by these embolized blood products, contributing to the permeability and hydrostatic pressure changes in the pulmonary micro-circulation. The activated neutrophils may also be responsible for oxidant damage to the lung by the excessive generation of highly toxic oxygen radical molecules. The free radical superoxide ($O_2^{\cdot}$) can participate in several chemical reactions yielding hydrogen peroxide (H_2O_2) and the extremely cytotoxic hydroxyl radical (OH). These molecules are normally used in a protective role against bacteria but, by overwhelming the antioxidant defence mechanisms such as superoxide dismutase, they destroy intracellular enzyme systems and cell wall structure of both endothelial and alveolar epithelial cells. Free oxygen radicals cause the loss of the functional integrity of the cell membrane associated with an acute increase in alveolar–capillary permeability.

In septic ARDS, endotoxin may cause the release of tumour necrosis factor (TNF) from stimulated macrophages; this in turn activates neutrophils. In neutropenic states, there is not enough elastase to inhibit the action of TNF so that direct tissue injury may occur as well as injury mediated by neutrophil activation. Moreover, TNF induces the production of interleukin-1 (IL-1) by vascular endothelium, and stimulates macrophages to activate chemotaxis, and polymorphonuclear neutrophil leucocytes (PMNL) to degranulate.

Coagulation and fibrinolytic function

Increased procoagulant activity associated with depressed fibrinolytic activity in these patients encourages fibrin deposition in the lung while increased alveolar capillary permeability allows the fibrinogen substrate to enter the alveolar airspaces.

Arachidonic acid metabolism

There is increasing evidence that arachidonic acid metabolites might be involved in the pathogenesis of ARDS. They are released from cell membrane phospholipid, by activated neutrophils, mast cells, platelets, and complement-dependent mechanisms. Two functionally active groups of substances, the prostaglandins (PG) and the leukotrienes (LT), are produced by separate metabolic pathways (Fig. 1).

Oxidative metabolism of arachidonic acid by the cyclo-oxygenase pathway sequentially produces two cyclic endoperoxides (PGG_2 and PGH_2), which are converted by specific enzymes into vasoactive products, thromboxane A_2 (TXA_2), an intense pulmonary vasoconstrictor and platelet aggregator, and prostacyclin (PGI_2), an anti-aggregator and pulmonary vasodilator substance. While excess TXA_2 could result in pulmonary capillary hypertension (postcapillary vasoconstriction) and mechanical obstruction by microaggregates, increased prostacyclin production may increase intrapulmonary

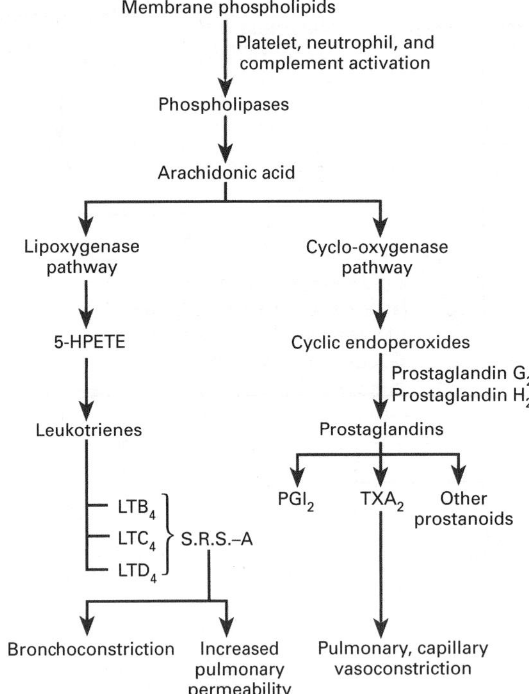

Fig. 1 Pathogenesis of ARDS: arachidonic acid metabolism.

shunting by preventing the normal hypoxic pulmonary vasoconstriction.

The alternative lipoxygenase pathway of arachidonic acid metabolism produces several groups of metabolites. Leucotriene B_4 is a potent neutrophil chemotaxin while leucotrienes C_4 and D_4 are the main constituents of the slow reacting substance of anaphylaxis (SRS-A) which, in the lung, can produce bronchoconstriction, microvascular vasoconstriction, and increased capillary permeability. A simplified sequence of the mechanisms involved is shown in Fig. 2.

Role of surfactant

Pulmonary surfactant is synthesized and secreted from alveolar type II cells. The major components of surfactant are phospholipids (85 per cent), neutral lipids, and at least three specific proteins (SP-A, SP-B, and SP-C). Saturated phosphatidylcholine (SatPC) is the main surface active component. SP-A is the major surfactant protein.

In ARDS patients, surfactant function is impaired early, and surfactant inactivation may also play a role. Proteins compete with surfactant for the surface of the alveoli and may interfere with the monolayer formation. This phenomenon may play a major role when surfactant concentration is low. In addition, lipid peroxidation products, including oxygen radicals, may interfere with the normal surface activity of surfactant. Surfactant increases macrophage migration and phagocytosis, enhancing the killing of bacteria, its deficiency in ARDS may decrease host defence. It also inhibits the migration of particulate matter from the alveoli.

While exogenous surfactant administration is effective in neonates with respiratory distress syndrome, there is only limited clinical experience in ARDS.

Physiological features

Abnormalities of pulmonary function correlate well with the pathological changes.

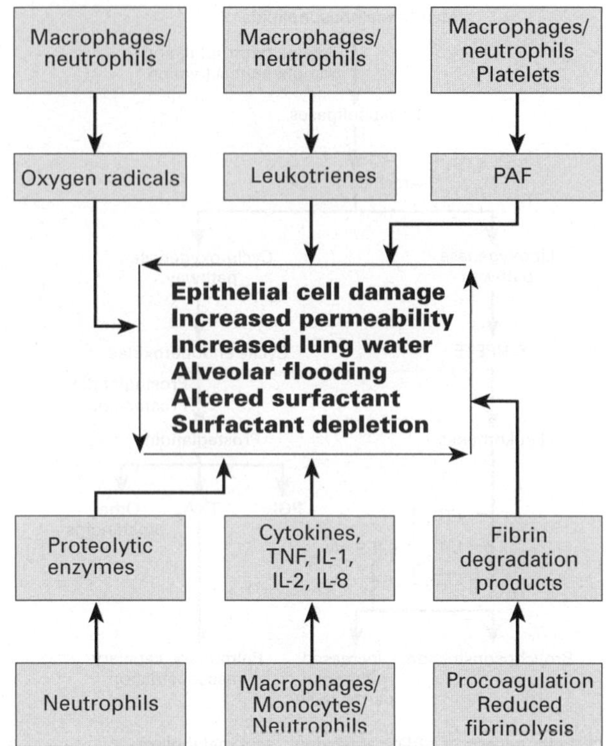

Fig. 2 A summary of the pathogenesis of ARDS.

Reduced compliance and lung volume

Altered surfactant production and function result in alveolar instability and diffuse microatelectasis. All lung volumes are reduced. Physiologically, the most important is the functional residual capacity (FRC) which, if greatly reduced, produces small airway closure during expiration, with air trapping in the distal alveoli. Subsequent absorption atelectasis produces more reduction in lung compliance and further impairs gas exchange. However, increased lung stiffness and reduced lung volume are not the result of homogenous mechanical abnormalities. The lungs of patients with ARDS can be divided into areas that are infiltrated, consolidated, or collapsed (poorly aerated and poorly compliant) and regions with near normal levels of compliance and ventilation.

Alterations in gas exchange

The most sinister feature of ARDS is an inability to maintain arterial oxygen tensions without toxic levels of inspired oxygen concentration (FiO_2). Three mechanisms operate in producing this hypoxaemia:

1. Perfusion of underventilated alveoli (*V*/*Q* mismatch). The fluid accumulation in the lung progresses from an interstitial to a peribronchial distribution before alveolar flooding occurs. Narrowing of the small airways results in a large number of alveoli, particularly in the dependent lung zones, having a reduced but finite V/Q ratio.
2. Perfusion of non-ventilated alveoli (true shunt). In ARDS the intrapulmonary shunt can increase to 60–70 per cent of cardiac output, mainly by perfusion of non-ventilated alveoli. This is caused by the loss of hypoxic vasoconstriction.
3. Impaired diffusion. In addition to thickening of the alveolar capillary septum, there is a reduced capillary blood volume with decreased transit time. The relative contributions of these three mechanisms are variable and not easily assessed. If true shunt rather than *V*/*Q* mismatch was the main contributor, increasing FiO_2 would not alter arterial oxygenation. In practice, however, increasing FiO_2 has a variable effect on the shunt, not only in different patients, but also in the same patient, during different phases of the disease. The usual response to very high FiO_2 is an increase in intrapulmonary shunt. In patients with ARDS, this active response is associated with a more favourable prognosis than a fixed shunt uninfluenced by increasing FiO_2.

Table 2 Criteria for diagnosis of ARDS

Characteristic chest radiograph
Hypoxaemia
Reduced lung compliance
Pumonary hypertension (>30/15 mm Hg)
Pulmonary capillary wedge pressure <18 mmHg
High protein pumonary oedema

Increased work of breathing

In spontaneously breathing patients, an increase in the dead space/tidal volume (V_D/V_T) ratio may be seen, particularly with microembolization of the pulmonary capillaries. Increased effort is required to keep the arterial carbon dioxide tension normal and reduced lung compliance can lead to respiratory failure unless respiration is mechanically assisted.

Pulmonary hypertension and right ventricular failure

The mediators of the inflammatory reaction are also responsible for pulmonary vasconstriction, platelet aggregation, microthrombosis, and direct tissue damage and pulmonary hypertension. Pulmonary vasoconstriction reduces blood flow to the ventilated areas of the lungs, and therefore contributes to the hypoxaemia.

Large increases in pulmonary artery pressure may cause right ventricular failure as the right ventricle is thin-walled and unable to withstand increases in afterload. Another mechanism is myocardial ischaemia. In the face of pulmonary hypertension, especially when aortic pressure is reduced, the pressure difference between aorta and right ventricle is reduced and systolic coronary flow to the wall of the right ventricle is decreased. Such a reduction in coronary blood flow may cause ischaemia even in the presence of normal coronary arteries. For this reason, administration of vasodilators may worsen the circulatory failure, while systemic vasconstrictors may improve cardiac output.

Diagnosis and management

ARDS should be suspected if acute respiratory failure ($PaO_2 < 6.7$ kPa breathing 60 per cent oxygen) occurs in association with a recognized precipitating cause and if the circulation is hyperdynamic with normal or slightly raised pulmonary capillary wedge (< 18 mmHg) and central venous pressures (Table 2).

The criteria by which ARDS is defined are reflected in the incidence, morbidity, and mortality reported in any particular series. Some recent reports do suggest a decline in mortality, possibly related to improved methods of conventional, mechanical ventilatory support.

Table 3 ARDS lung injury score

1. Chest roentgenogram score		
No alveolar consolidation		0
Aleolar consolidation confined to 1 quadrant		1
Aleolar consolidation confined to 2 quadrants		2
Aleolar consolidation confined to 3 quadrants		3
Aleolar consolidation in all 4 quadrants		4
2. Hypoxaemia score		
PaO_2/FiO_2	>300	0
PaO_2/FiO_2	225–299	1
PaO_2/FiO_2	175–224	2
PaO_2/FiO_2	100–174	3
PaO_2/FiO_2	<100	4
(PaO_2 in mmHg/unity for kPa/unity divide by 7.5)		
3. PEEP score (when ventilated)		
PEEP	$\leq$ 5 cm H_2O	0
PEEP	6–8 cm H_2O	1
PEEP	9–11 cm H_2O	2
PEEP	12–14 cm H_2O	3
PEEP	$\geq$15cm H_2O	4
4. Respiratory system compliance score (when available)		
Compliance	$\geq$80 ml/cm H_2O	0
Compliance	60–79 ml/cm H_2O	1
Compliance	40–59 ml/cm H_2O	2
Compliance	20–39 ml/cm H_2O	3
Compliance	$\leq$19ml/cm H_2O	4
The final value is obtained by dividing the aggregate sum by the number of components that were used		
No lung injury 0		
Mild to moderate lung injury 0.1–2.5		
Severe lung injury.>2.5		

(From: Murray, J.F., Matthay, M.A., Luce, J.M., and Flick, M.R. (1988). An expanded definition of the adult respiratory distress syndrome. *American Review of Respiratory Diseases*, **138**,720–3.)

Although ARDS severity scores are at best crude they do allow some comparison to be made between different groups of patients (Table 3). It is evident that patients do not usually die of hypoxaemia but from the complex disturbances that result from multiple organ system failure. The aim in the management of ARDS is to support all body systems until the integrity of the alveolar capillary membrane is restored.

Early recognition with appropriate pharmacological and supportive therapy favourably influences the prognosis, but, unfortunately, no simple laboratory test or bedside measurement accurately predicts the onset of this condition. The indices of pulmonary gas exchange and pulmonary compliance are not sufficiently sensitive to detect early interstitial oedema, becoming abnormal only when alveolar oedema occurs. Changes in lung volumes, particularly FRC, do occur earlier but are not applicable to bedside monitoring. Non-invasive methods of measuring lung water and permeability changes may prove to be useful in screening patients but perhaps the most useful method of identifying incipient acute respiratory failure is by C5a assays, high levels of which have been positively associated with the onset, but not the severity, of ARDS.

Ventilation and oxygenation

Intermittent positive-pressure ventilation (IPPV)

If the arterial oxygen tension cannot be maintained above 6.5 kPa with an FiO_2 of 0.5 in the spontaneously breathing patient, intubation and ventilatory support are generally indicated. A guide to indications for intubation and mechanical ventilation is shown in Table 4.

Table 4 Guidelines for the introduction of mechanical ventilation

1. *Inadequate ventilation*
Indicated by:
(a) Apnoea, upper airway obstruction, unprotected airway
(b) Respiratory rate > 35 breaths/min [normal range 10–20]
(c) Vital capacity < 15 ml/kg [normal range 65–75]
(d) Tidal volume < 5 ml/kg [normal range 5–7]
(e) Negative inspiratory force < 25 cmH_2O [normal range 75–100]
(f) $PaCO_2$ > 8 kPa (60 mmHg), [normal range 4.7–6.3 kPa (35–47 mmHg)]
(g) V_D/V_T ratio > 0.6 [normal range < 0.3]
2. *Inadequate gas exchange and oxygenation*
Indicated by:
(a) PaO_2 < 8 kPa, (60 mmHg) on $FiO_2 \geq$ 0.6
(b) (A-a)DO_2 on FiO_2 1.0 > 47 kPa (350 mmHg), [normal range 3.3–8.7 kPa (25–65 mmHg)]

After: Pontoppidan, H., Geffin, B., and Lowenstein, E. (1972). Acute respiratory failure in the adult. *New England Journal of Medicine*, **42**, 45–55.

The optimal mechanical ventilation strategy appears to be low volume, pressure limited ventilation with permissive hypercapnia. By limiting peak inspiratory pressures to less than 40 mmHg and accepting $PaCO_2$ values in the range 9 to 15 kPa the risks of barotrauma and the adverse circulatory effects of positive pressure ventilation can be largely avoided. Hypoxaemia will rarely be reversed by IPPV alone; other manoeuvres, designed to increase FRC and improve oxygenation, are usually required.

Positive and expiratory pressure (PEEP) and continuous positive airway pressure (CPAP)

The beneficial effects of PEEP/CPAP are produced by an increase in FRC, a decrease in intrapulmonary shunting, and an improvement of lung compliance. Its benefits are limited, however, by a reduction of cardiac output and the dangers of barotrauma (pneumothorax, pneumomediastinum, and surgical emphysema). While modest levels of PEEP (5–10 cm H_2O) are unlikely to reduce cardiac output, very high levels (up to 30 cm H_2O) impose the need to maintain the cardiac output by volume loading and inotropic support. The risk of barotrauma limits its use. More conventionally, a level of PEEP is selected which is compatible with an unchanged cardiac output or an unchanged static lung compliance.

A feature of the patient with ARDS is the extensive gravity dependent lung collapse resulting from nursing the patient for prolonged periods in the supine position. In the persistently hypoxic patient, significant improvement in oxygenation may be obtained by rolling the patient prone every 6–8 h.

Asynchronous independent lung ventilation (AILV)

This technique employs a double lumen endobronchial tube, each limb of which is connected to a separate ventilator, thus allowing optimum respiratory function to be obtained from each lung independently by varying ventilatory indices and inspired oxygen concentrations. AILV demands a high degree of nursing care to preserve accurate tube placement and the duration is limited by the risk of trauma to the bronchial tree.

High frequency ventilation (HFV)

Satisfactory gas exchange occurring at ventilatory 'frequencies' up to 40 Hz. HFV can be divided into high-frequency jet ventilation and high-frequency oscillation. HFV rests on enhancement of convection and accelerated diffusion of gas molecules. By delivering pulses of oxygen-enriched air, efficient alveolar ventilation and gas exchange is achieved with low transpulmonary pressures and reflex inhibition of spontaneous respiration. HFV minimizes the risk of barotrauma and minimal effects on pulmonary and systemic circulations. In clinical practice, humidification is difficult and its role in the management of ARDS has yet to be fully assessed.

Extracorporeal lung assist

Extracorporeal membrane oxygenation offered the hope that the lungs of patients with ARDS would have time to recover while oxygenation and perfusion of vital organs was maintained. However, the results of a randomized, prospective, multicentre trial in the US were disappointing in adults, yet favourable in a relatively high proportion of children with unrelenting pulmonary failure. Attention has been paid to extracorporeal CO_2 removal ($ECCO_2R$) using a large area membrane lung with low extracorporeal blood flows (1–1.5 l/min) to remove carbon dioxide. A low ventilatory rate (3 l/min) prevents atelectasis and oxygenation is maintained by using a carinal catheter delivering 300 ml oxygen/min. The low intra-alveolar tensions, low ventilatory rates, and low inflation pressures avoid the adverse effects of conventional IPPV. In a recent, randomized, rigorously controlled study, $ECCO_2R$ combined with low-frequency positive pressure ventilation offered no advantage over conventional ventilation.

An alternative approach uses an intracorporeal oxygenation device (IVOX®, Cardiopulmonics Inc., Salt Lake City, Utah, US). IVOX® is a polypropylene multifilament oxygenator which is heparin surface bonded. It is passed into the inferior vena cava via a femoral vein and oxygen is sucked through the hollow filaments. Although it has been used safely in patients, the potential benefit of IVOX® has not been established.

Liquid ventilation

Adequate and improved gas exchange has been achieved by ventilating the lungs of neonates and animal models with perfluorocarbon solutions saturated with oxygen. This technique exploits the phenomenon of the reduced surface forces between a liquid interface and the alveolus and the capacity of perfluorocarbons to carry up to 120 ml of oxygen per 100 ml of solution. The lung can be filled to FRC with the perfluorocarbon liquid and then slowly the liquid is topped up on a daily basis. This technique, although innovative and effective in early studies, needs further evaluation before it can be established in clinical practice.

Oxygen delivery

ARDS reduces the arterial oxygen content and cardiac output may be lowered by hypovolaemia or by PEEP. Inotropic support may therefore be required to restore effective oxygen delivery. The interdependence of biventricular function must be remembered. Right ventricular failure secondary to increased pulmonary vascular resistance impairs left ventricular forward flow and may also produce left ventricular compression by a leftward shift of the interventricular septum. In such instances the pharmacological reduction of the excessive pulmonary vascular resistance might be considered. Anaemia should be corrected.

Provided oxygen delivery is sufficient to meet demand, without evidence of tissue hypoxia (i.e. absence of lactic acidosis, cardiac arrhythmias, or mental obtundation), then arterial hypoxaemia should be well tolerated and is acceptable. This approach of 'acceptable' hypoxaemia together with permissive hypercapnia, if carefully monitored, should provide the best opportunity for recovery by avoiding the harmful effects of airway pressure and oxygen toxicity.

Oxygen demand

High oxygen requirements may be reduced by heavy sedation and, when indicated, muscle relaxation. Although hypothermia (30°C) reduces the oxygen demand, there is no firm evidence that it improves the prognosis in ARDS; oxygen availability is reduced by the leftward shift of the oxyhaemoglobin dissociation curve, thus lessening the benefits of hypothermia.

Oxygen supply dependency

The concept of oxygen supply dependency in ARDS remains controversial, and it is doubted that achieving 'supranormal' oxygen delivery targets offers any therapeutic benefit.

Oxygen toxicity

Histological changes of both early and late ARDS correlate with high inspired oxygen concentrations. Experimental evidence suggests that the elevated alveolar oxygen concentration, not the arterial oxygen tension, is responsible for the toxicity. The mechanism involves the reduction of molecular oxygen to highly reactive and potentially cytotoxic radicals, which overwhelm the antioxidant defence enzymes causing intracellular enzyme damage and loss of membrane integrity.

The severity of oxygen toxicity is dependent on both the FiO_2 and the duration of exposure. An FiO_2 of < 0.5 can be safely administered for prolonged periods, whereas an FiO_2 of > 0.8 can produce deleterious effects in the lung within 48 h. However, it is sometimes impossible to maintain adequate oxygenation unless potentially toxic inspired oxygen concentrations are used. In these circumstances, the full range of therapeutic manoeuvres should be employed in an attempt to lower the FiO_2.

Pulmonary haemodynamics

Infusions of vasodilator drugs such as glyceryl trinitrate, sodium nitroprusside, or prostacyclin all non-selectively reverse vasoconstriction throughout the whole pulmonary vascular bed reducing the pulmonary artery pressure, but at the expense of systemic arterial oxygenation as perfusion of poorly ventilated areas of the lung increases. Despite an increase in venous admixture, the increase in cardiac output associated with these agents may result in increased oxygen delivery, increased SvO_2 and thus increased SaO_2.

Selective vasodilation of pulmonary vessels in ventilated areas of the lungs can be obtained by inhalation of nitric oxide (NO), a powerful regulator of vascular smooth muscle tone. Low concentrations of nitric oxide (20–120 ppm) cause an immediate reduction in venous admixture as more blood flows through the well-aerated regions of the lung. Short half-life and rapid absorption by oxyhaemoglobin ensures that NO does not affect the systemic circulation. As a safeguard, NO levels in the inspired gas mixture can be monitored together with methaemoglobin levels in the patient's blood. At present, NO appears to offer an effective pharmacological method of improving gas exchange in ARDS.

Pulmonary hypertension in ARDS may also be caused by microembolization of the pulmonary circulation by particulate blood products. Neither the use of anticoagulants nor the infusion of streptokinase has been shown to be useful or safe. Cyclo-oxygenase inhibitors, such as the non-steroidal anti-inflammatory drugs, can reduce the pulmonary hypertension but without abatement of the increased permeability.

Fluid balance

Positive fluid balance may have a protective effect in preventing the development of ARDS and multiple organ failure. Once ARDS is established, adequate cardiac preload must be maintained to avoid hypoperfusion of other organ such as the kidneys. There is still debate about the effects of crystalloid and colloid infusions on the flux of water and solutes across the pulmonary endothelium when there is increased permeability as in ARDS. Careful monitoring of systemic and pulmonary perfusion pressures may be critical. By maintaining a pulmonary capillary wedge pressure (PCWP) between 8 and 12 mmHg a guide to the rate and volume of infused fluid can be obtained, while sequential measurements of plasma protein osmotic pressure and haematocrit enable the type of infused fluid to be more precisely selected. Note that high levels of PEEP may overestimate the PCWP and central venous pressure measurements. Relative or absolute fluid overload should be managed by diuretic therapy, but ultrafiltration may become a more efficient method of treating pulmonary oedema.

N-Acetylcysteine

N-Acetylcysteine is a free radical scavenger which may also counteract neurophil activation in the lung. It improves dynamic compliance, perhaps by reducing lung microvascular permeability, which would reduce interstitial oedema. *N*-Acetylcysteine may also increase surfactant secretion. In randomized studies of mild to moderate ARDS, acetylcysteine has not been shown to be of benefit but greater experience with the more severe forms of disease is desirable.

Prophylactic management

Steroids and non-steroidal anti-inflammatory agents

Although there are theoretical grounds to support their use, specific treatments to inhibit mediator cascades are largely experimental. Multicentre, randomized studies have failed to show significant benefit from corticosteroids, non-steroidal anti-inflammatory agents, or vasodilator prostaglandins.

Antibiotics

It is estimated that 85 per cent of patients with established ARDS have an infective focus, either intra- or extrapulmonary. Strict aseptic suctioning techniques must be used and the sterility of ventilators ensured. Intensive efforts must be made to identify the microorganism and appropriate antibiotics started. The changing bacterial pattern in patients on ventilators can be best determined by quantitative culture of bronchoscopic-protected specimen-brushings of the distal airways or bronchoalveolar lavage. When no organism can be isolated, the decision to start, and the selection of, empiric, combination broad-spectrum antibiotics should be based on clinical findings.

Parenteral nutrition

Patients with ARDS invariably suffer nutritional depletion which, if uncorrected, leads to muscle weakness, particularly of the respiratory muscles, and lessened cellular-mediated immunity, predisposing to infection. Hypophosphataemia and hypomagnesaemia can develop in long-term, critically ill patients and can contribute to muscle weakness and impaired ventilatory effort. Nutrition, ideally by the enteral route, should be started early in the management of ARDS patients.

Outcome

Provided multiple organ system support can be maintained, a positive attitude towards final recovery is justified. Even after periods of mechanical ventilation, high FiO_2s, and PEEP for up to 3–4 months a good functional outcome is possible. Biopsy-proven pulmonary fibrosis does not inevitably mean there is fixed, irreversible pathology. A mortality rate of over 50–60 per cent is generally quoted for the last decade although some recent reports have shown a fall in mortality to about 20 per cent. The chief determinants of the outcome relate not to the severity of the physiological defect, but to the presence of non-pulmonary organ system failure or sepsis syndrome. Pulmonary function testing 1 year following recovery from ARDS may show a reduction in vital capacity with a mild obstructive defect. In many patients the only abnormality may be a reduction in carbon monoxide transfer.

Further reading

Hickling, K.G., Henderson, S.J., and Jackson, R. (1990). Low mortality associated with low volume pressure limited ventilation with permissive hypercapnia in severe adult respiratory distress syndrome. *Intensive Care Medicine*, **16**, 372–7.

Hirschl, R.B., Pranikoff, T., Wise C, *et al.* (1996). Initial experience with partial liquid ventilation in adult patients with the acute respiratory distress syndrome. *Journal of the American Medical Association*, **275**, 383–9.

Ryan, D.P. and Doody, D.P. (1992). Treatment of acute pulmonary failure with extracorporeal support 100 per cent survival in a pediatric population. *Journal of Pediatric Surgery*, **27**, 1111–16.

Suchyta, M.R., Clemmer, T.P., Orme, J.J., Morris, A.H., and Elliott, C.G. (1991). Increased survival of ARDS patients with severe hypoxemia (ECMO criteria). *Chest*, **99**, 951–5.

Suter, P.M., Suter, S., Girardin, E., Roux-Lombard, P., Grau, G.E., and Dayer, J.-M. (1992). High bronchoalveolar levels of tumor necrosis factor and its inhibitors, interleukin-1, interferon, and elastase, in patients with adult respiratory distress syndrome after trauma, shock, or sepsis. *American Review of Respiratory Diseases*, **145**, 1016–22.

Chapter 4.36

Pleural disease

M. K. Benson

The pleural surfaces form the interface between the lung parenchyma and the chest wall. The parietal pleura is closely applied to the chest wall and the surfaces of the ribs. Medially it is adjacent to the pericardium and mediastinal structures. The visceral pleura covers the surface of the lungs and extends into the major fissures which separate the lobes of the lung. Between the two layers of pleura there is a potential space, the surfaces of which are lubricated by a thin layer of fluid. A number of pathological processes can affect the pleura. Inflammation results in characteristic pleuritic pain which is aggravated by deep inspiration, coughing, or sneezing. It is often accompanied by a pleural rub. The accumulation of fluid in the pleural space results in a pleural effusion. Air can also enter the

Table 1 Causes of pleural effusions

	Common	Less common
Transudates	Cardiac failure	Nephrotic syndrome Cirrhosis Peritoneal dialysis Myxoedema
Exudates		
Inflammatory (infective)	Parapneumonic	Subphrenic abscess
	Tuberculosis	Viral Fungal
Inflammatory (non-infective)	Pulmonary emboli	Collagen vascular disease Pancreatitis Drug reaction Asbestos exposure Dressler's syndrome Yellow nail syndrome
Neoplastic	Metastatic carcinoma Lymphoma	Mesothelioma Meigs' syndrome
Haemothorax	Trauma	Spontaneous Bleeding disorders
Chylothorax	Lymphoma Carcinoma Trauma	Lymphangio-leimyomatosis

pleural space resulting in a pneumothorax. Involvement of the pleura by metastatic malignant disease is common; primary tumours are rare.

Pleural effusion

A pleural effusion results from the accumulation of fluid in the pleural space. It is traditional to divide effusions into transudates and exudates, although blood, pus, or chyle may also present as collections of pleural fluid. Factors likely to result in excess fluid accumulation include the following:

(1) an imbalance between the hydrostatic and oncotic forces as defined in Starling's equation—such fluid is usually a transudate;
(2) an alteration in the permeability of pleural capillaries resulting in an exudate;
(3) impaired lymphatic drainage;
(4) abnormal sites of entry (e.g. transdiaphragmatic passage of fluid in patients with ascites).

The main causes are listed in Table 1.

Diagnostic approach to pleural effusion

Clinical features

Symptoms specifically related to pleural disease are pain and breathlessness. The extent to which these occur is likely to vary and clinical presentation will, at least in part, be determined by the underlying pathogenesis. Pleuritic pain which causes severe discomfort on coughing or deep inspiration is more typical of 'dry' pleurisy. It often improves as fluid accumulates, separating the inflamed pleural surfaces. The other major symptom is of breathlessness which only becomes apparent if there is a large effusion or in patients who already have impaired respiratory reserve. Abnormal physical signs may be absent if the effusion is relatively small but are often diagnostic if the effusion is large. The percussion note is very dull and breath sounds will be diminished or absent. Similarly, vocal resonance and tactile vocal fremitus will be absent. Compression of the lung above the effusion can result in signs of consolidation with bronchial breathing and increased vocal resonance. The position of the mediastinum will help in distinguishing between a large effusion and a collapsed lung. In the former, the mediastinum is central or displaced away from the side of the effusion, whereas in the latter deviation is towards the affected side.

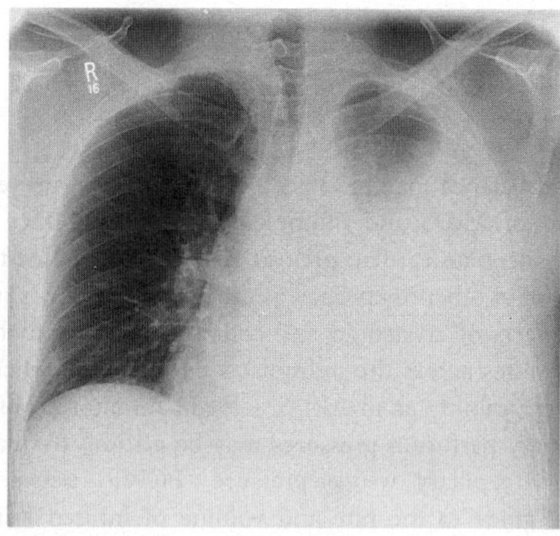

Fig. 1 Chest radiograph showing opacification of the left hemithorax and mediastinal shift indicating a large pleural effusion.

Investigation of pleural effusion

The presence of a pleural effusion should be suspected on clinical examination and can be confirmed by using radiographic imaging. Whilst clinical features play an important part in identifying the pathogenesis, examination of the pleural fluid or pleural biopsy material is most likely to lead to a definitive diagnosis.

Radiographic techniques

Radiography is helpful in identifying the presence of an effusion but is of limited value in determining the pathogenesis. A conventional posteroanterior chest radiograph is usually adequate. Small effusions, in the order of 500 ml, will result in blunting of the costophrenic angle. Larger effusions produce increased opacification and mediastinal shift (Fig. 1). Variations of the normal appearance will result if the fluid is loculated. Ultrasound can be helpful in confirming the presence and site of an effusion. It can also demonstrate the presence of septation and loculi. CT scans may complement ultrasound examination in demonstrating the site of a pleural collection and have the additional advantage of imaging the underlying lung (Fig. 2).

Thoracentesis

Percutaneous aspiration of pleural fluid is a relatively simple procedure which can be undertaken for diagnostic purposes and, in the case of larger effusions, can relieve breathlessness. For diagnostic purposes it is usually adequate to remove 50–100 ml of fluid. Unless the fluid is loculated, a conventional site for aspiration is posteriorly about 10 cm lateral to the spine and one intercostal space below the upper level of the fluid as detected by percussion. The skin and underlying tissues are infiltrated with local anaesthetic, care being taken to avoid the intercostal nerves and vessels which run immediately beneath the rib. Failure to obtain fluid can arise for a number of reasons including

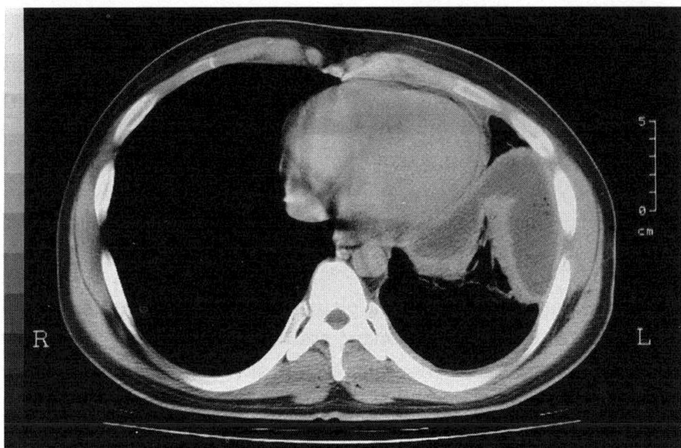

Fig. 2 CT scan demonstrating a loculated effusion due to empyema.

Table 2 Tests to evaluate cause of pleural effusion

Cell type		
Red blood cells	>100 000/mm^3	Trauma malignancy Pulmonary embolism
White blood cells	>10 000/mm^3	Pyogenic infection
Neutrophils	>50%	Pyogenic infection
Lymphocytes	>90%	Tuberculosis, lymphoma Malignancy
Eosinophils	>10%	No diagnostic, usually benign
Mesothelial cells	Absent	Tuberculosis
Malignant cells	Present	Malignancy
Biochemistry		
Protein concentration	>30 g/l	Exudate
Protein F:S ratio	>0.5	Exudate
LDH	>200 IU	Exudate
LDH F:S ratio	>0.6	Exudate
Glucose	>4 mmol/l	Rheumatoid arthritis, infection, malignancy
Amylase F:S ratio	>1	Pancreatitis
pH	>7.2	Malignancy, infection
Microbiology	Positive	Infection

F:S ratio, fluid-to-serum; LDH, lactic dehydrogenase.

misdiagnosis of the presence of fluid, incorrect site of aspiration, and the presence of viscid fluid. Ultrasound examination can be helpful in identifying the reason for a failed aspiration.

Examination of pleural fluid

Transudates are clear straw-coloured fluids which do not clot on standing. Many exudates are similar in appearance but can be somewhat turbid owing to the presence of cells. Blood-tinged fluid is of little diagnostic significance but a uniformly bloody effusion is likely to be associated with an underlying malignancy. Pus can sometimes be very viscid and difficult to aspirate. It is turbid in appearance, yellow in colour, and often foul smelling. Chyle is odourless and milky in appearance.

Biochemical, cytological, and microbiological examination of the pleural fluid can help to establish the underlying cause if this is not apparent on clinical grounds. The main features are listed in Table 2.

Pleural biopsy

Pleural biopsy may be indicated if initial analysis of pleural fluid fails to establish a diagnosis. It is of particular value if there is a suspicion of an underlying malignancy or tuberculosis.

Closed-needle biopsy is usually performed using an Abraham's or Cope's needle. The technique is similar to that used for pleural aspiration except that a small incision is made in the skin and subcutaneous tissues to enable ease of insertion of the needle.

Needle biopsy undoubtedly increases the diagnostic yield in patients with tuberculosis of the pleura. Aspiration alone gives positive results in approximately 25 per cent of cases and culture of biopsy material increases this to 50 per cent. The additional diagnostic yield in malignant disease is less dramatic with only a small percentage of biopsies being positive when cytology has been negative.

Thoracoscopy

Direct visualization of the pleura is technically possible using a thoracoscope. Diagnostic yield is increased to 90 per cent in patients with tuberculosis or pleural malignancy since biopsies can be taken from areas which are macroscopically abnormal.

Specific pleural effusions

Transudates

A transudate is characterized by low concentrations of protein and other large molecules. Excess fluid forms when there is an increase in capillary hydrostatic pressure or a reduction in colloid osmotic pressure. The former occurs predominantly in congestive cardiac failure and the latter when there is hypoalbuminaemia associated with nephrotic syndrome or hepatic disease.

Small effusions are common in congestive cardiac failure and the clinical features are usually sufficient to make a diagnosis. The effusions are frequently bilateral although unilateral effusions do occur and are more common on the right side. Resolution with treatment of the heart failure offers confirmation of the diagnosis.

Hypoalbuminaemia, which may occur in patients with chronic liver disease, is a major contributory factor to the development of generalized oedema. Ascites and pleural effusions are both common occurrences with effusions more often on the right than on the left.

Exudates

Neoplastic pleural effusions

Malignant involvement of the pleura is the commonest cause of a large pleural effusion. Most frequently this results from direct spread from a bronchogenic carcinoma. Breast cancer may spread via the lymphatic system whilst pleural involvement from primary disease in the ovary or gastrointestinal tract is usually by haematogenous spread. Extensive investigation for an asymptomatic primary is of limited value, although it may be appropriate to exclude disease originating in breast or ovary because of the potential response to hormonal treatment or chemotherapy. Lymphomas can occur at any age and account for approximately 10 per cent of malignant effusions.

Clinical features Symptoms directly attributable to the effusion are most commonly breathlessness or chest discomfort. Specific symptoms which can be attributed to the primary site are often absent although non-specific systemic symptoms are common.

Investigations Aspirated fluid is usually an exudate and may be blood-stained. Malignant cells can be identified in up to 60 per cent of cases. If the diagnosis remains in doubt, it may be appropriate to proceed to pleural biopsy, ideally obtaining material at thoracoscopy.

Table 3 Organisms resulting in emphysema thoracis

Single organisms (75%)	
Gram-positive aerobes	*Strep. milleri* +++
	Strep. pneumoniae ++
	Staph. aureus +
Gram-negative aerobes	*E. coli* +
	H. influenzae +
	Proteus +
Anaerobic bacteria	*B. melaninogenicus* ++
	Streptococci +
	Fusobacterium +
Fungi	*Candida* spp. +
Multiple organisms (25%)	*Strep. milleri* plus anaerobes

+++ -common; + -rare.

Treatment Palliative treatment is only necessary if the effusion is large and results in significant breathlessness. Percutaneous needle aspiration of 1 to 2 litres of fluid is a simple outpatient procedure and often results in considerable symptomatic benefit. The fluid is likely to recur and under these circumstances repeat aspiration may be an appropriate therapeutic option. An alternative approach is to attempt pleurodesis by draining the pleural space completely and using a sclerosant. The most effective approach is thoracoscopic insufflation of talc. An alternative is intercostal tube drainage and the use of tetracycline (500 mg in 100 ml saline). Adequate analgesia is necessary using both local anaesthetic into the pleural cavity and systemic analgesics.

Meigs' syndrome

This rare syndrome originally described an association between pleural effusions, ascites, and a benign ovarian tumour. Surgical removal of the tumour results in resolution of the pleural and peritoneal fluid. The cause of the pleural effusion is uncertain but there is no evidence of tumour spread and the syndrome should not be confused with effusions which can result from metastatic spread of ovarian cancers.

Endometriosis of the pleura

This rare condition is one in which endometrial tissue is implanted on visceral or parietal pleura. Catamenial pleuritic chest pain or a pneumothorax can be a presenting feature. Treatment is directed at suppressing ovulation using progesterones or androgens.

Infection

Inflammation or infection of the pleura is usually secondary to pneumonia or lung abscess. Other sources of infection can be subdiaphragmatic, associated with mediastinitis, or as a result of direct contamination following penetrating trauma or surgery. It can result in a dry pleurisy, a non-infected exudate (a parapneumonic effusion), or infected fluid (an empyema). The distinction between a parapneumonic effusion and an empyema is somewhat arbitrary since there can be a transition from one to the other. An empyema is frankly turbid, contains increased numbers of polymorphs, and has a low pH (usually less than 7). The spectrum of organisms most frequently encountered in the UK is listed in Table 3.

Tuberculous effusion

Pleural involvement with tuberculosis is a common manifestation of primary infection with direct extension from a subpleural focus. It is more common in younger patients and those of Asian origin. The presenting features are usually acute or subacute with fever, pleuritic pain, and breathlessness. The effusion is often large and tends to recur after initial aspiration. An excess of lymphocytes should alert the clinician to the possibility of tuberculosis. Isolation of organisms from the pleural fluid is difficult. A pleural biopsy is more likely to give a positive result showing granulomatous inflammation. Treatment involves the use of standard antituberculous chemotherapy together with adequate drainage, especially if there is frank pus.

Pulmonary emboli

Pleurisy, often associated with a pleural effusion, may be one of the presenting features of pulmonary emboli. The effusion is usually small and in itself does not require specific treatment. It is often blood-stained but the cellular content is variable and there are no diagnostic features. The diagnosis is based on clinical features supplemented by appropriate radiographic or isotopic imaging techniques.

Collagen vascular disease

Rheumatoid arthritis

Pleural effusions are the commonest pulmonary manifestation of rheumatoid arthritis occurring in about 3 per cent of patients with active disease. It is more common in men than women and may antedate the onset of joint symptoms in a small proportion of patients. Although usually unilateral, they may be bilateral in about 20 per cent of patients. The fluid is an exudate and may appear turbid due to cholesterol crystals. Polymorphonuclear cells usually predominate and although not specific to rheumatoid effusions, a diagnostic clue is the presence of a low glucose content. Pleural biopsy is non-specific although it may reveal the epithelioid cells and multinucleate giant cells found in rheumatoid nodules. Symptomatic treatment with anti-inflammatory analgesics is indicated if pleuritic pain is a feature. The majority of effusions resolve spontaneously within a few months.

Systemic lupus erythematosus

Pleural involvement is common in patients with this condition. Approximately 50 per cent of patients will have pleurisy at some stage and the majority of these will have an associated effusion although this is usually small.

Haemothorax

A haemothorax is a result of bleeding into the pleural space and is somewhat arbitrarily diagnosed on the basis of having a haematocrit more than half of peripheral blood. The majority are associated with penetrating or non-penetrating trauma. Spontaneous bleeding may occasionally occur in association with a pneumothorax and presumably result from tearing of pleural adhesions. Other rare causes include bleeding disorders and rupture of the thoracic aorta.

The treatment of choice is to insert an intercostal drain which permits evacuation of blood and then reduces the incidence of a subsequent fibrothorax. Continued bleeding will require thoracotomy.

Chylothorax

A chylothorax results from leakage of chylous fluid from the thoracic duct. The majority of cases are acquired either as a result of trauma or neoplastic invasion of the thoracic duct. A lymphoma accounts for the majority of malignancies. Other rare associations include pulmonary lymphangiolyomyomatosis, the yellow nail syndrome (the association of yellow nails, lymphoedema, pleural effusion, and bronchiectasis), and filariasis. Aspirated fluid is classically milky and opalescent due to the presence of fat globules. It needs to be distinguished from an empyema or pseudochyle. The latter occurs in chronic effusions and is due to the presence of cholesterol crystals which can usually be recognized on smears taken from the sediment.

Pneumothorax

A pneumothorax results from gas entering the potential space between visceral and parietal pleura. A spontaneous pneumothorax is the consequence of rupture of a bulla or cyst on the surface of the lung. Following penetrating trauma, atmospheric air may enter the pleural space through the wound or the visceral pleura may be punctured allowing entry of alveolar gas.

Pathophysiology

Because of the elastic recoil of the lung, pleural pressure is always less than alveolar pressure. Thus if there is a breach of the visceral pleura due to rupture of surface bullae, gas moves from lung to pleural space. As the lung collapses down, the pressures equilibrate and net flow of gas ceases. Occasionally the site of air leak acts as a one-way valve, allowing air to enter the pleural space during inspiration but preventing return flow during expiration. A tension pneumothorax results with mediastinal shift and compromised function of the opposite lung. Once the original leak has sealed, reabsorption of pleural gas occurs and re-expansion of the lung takes place.

Clinical syndromes

A spontaneous pneumothorax usually occurs without any warning or obvious precipitating factor. A primary pneumothorax occurs in individuals with apparently normal lungs. A secondary pneumothorax is a consequence of pre-existing lung disease.

Primary pneumothorax

This is a relatively common condition with an annual incidence of about 9 per 100 000. It is more common in young men with a male-to-female ratio of approximately 4:1. Patients often have a marfanoid appearance. About 20 per cent of patients who have had one pneumothorax are likely to have a recurrence. The frequency of recurrence increases with repeated pneumothoraces.

Secondary pneumothorax

Older patients presenting with a spontaneous pneumothorax are likely to have underlying lung disease as a predisposing factor. The commonest association is in patients with emphysema and obstructive airway disease or asthma. A secondary pneumothorax can also be associated with a lung malignancy and with pulmonary infection when necrotic lung may rupture into the pleural space. Rare associations include cystic fibrosis, histiocytosis X, lymphangiomyomatosis, pulmonary neurofibromatosis, Marfan's syndrome, and Ehlers–Danlos syndrome.

Iatrogenic pneumothorax

A number of diagnostic and therapeutic procedures have an associated risk of developing a pneumothorax. Percutaneous needle aspiration or lung biopsy carries the greatest risk with estimates ranging from 5 to 50 per cent. Attempted catheterization of subclavian veins can result in puncture of the lung.

Clinical features

A spontaneous pneumothorax will present with sudden onset chest pain and breathlessness. Inspiration is painful and breathing is shallow to minimize discomfort. Breathlessness is partly engendered by the difficulty in taking a deep breath, but is also dependent on the size of the pneumothorax and the presence of underlying lung disease.

Abnormal physical signs may be difficult to detect if the pneumothorax is small or the lungs are emphysematous. The most consistent finding is a reduction in breath sounds on the affected side. The percussion note will be resonant or hyper-resonant. A large pneumothorax under tension will result in mediastinal and tracheal shift away from the affected side. A left-sided pneumothorax may occasionally be associated with a clicking noise synchronous with the heart beat (Hamman's sign).

Table 4 Treatment options for a pneumothorax

Option	Indication
Natural resolution	Small primary pneumothorax
Aspiration	Large primary pneumothorax, particularly if the patient is breathless
Intercostal drain (± pleurodesis)	Failed aspiration Secondary pneumothorax
Thoracoscopy + pleuradesis	Recent pneumothorax Failed intercostal drainage
Thoracotomy	Recurrent pneumothorax
Limited pleurectomy	Failed intercostal drainage
Pleurodesis	
Ligation of bullae	

Investigations

Confirmation of a pneumothorax is best made by chest radiograph. The outer margin of the lung can be seen as a thin line with the space between it and the chest devoid of any lung markings. A large emphysematous bulla can occasionally be mistaken for a pneumothorax on both clinical and radiological grounds although the inner margins are usually concave.

Management

The diversity of therapeutic options listed in Table 4 is a manifestation of the uncertainty with respect to optimum treatment. Two principal therapeutic objectives are to achieve rapid resolution of the pneumothorax, particularly if there is evidence of respiratory distress, and to reduce the likelihood of recurrence.

Natural resolution

A small pneumothorax in an otherwise healthy patient may require no treatment other than reassurance and relief of pain. Non-steroidal anti-inflammatory drugs are usually effective in this respect. Admission to hospital is unnecessary provided that the patient has ready access to medical care and is advised to return if symptoms worsen.

Simple aspiration

This is the treatment of choice for a patient with a large, primary pneumothorax. If successful, it will not only speed resolution but relieve any associated breathlessness or chest discomfort. It is simple to perform and has negligible morbidity even in relatively inexperienced hands. An appropriate site for aspiration is the second intercostal space in the midclavicular line. Aspiration should stop if resistance is encountered or if a patient experiences undue discomfort. If more than 2 or 3 litres of air have been evacuated, it is likely that there is a persisting air leak. Simple aspiration is less painful and requires shorter duration of hospital stay than treatment with an intercostal drain.

Intercostal tube drainage

This approach is likely to be indicated if simple aspiration has failed although a decision should be influenced as much as by the patient's symptoms as by the size of the pneumothorax. It is more likely to be indicated in patients with underlying lung disease in whom even a small pneumothorax can result in severe respiratory failure. The preferred site is the fourth, fifth, or sixth intercostal space anterior to the midaxillary line. An adequate incision is made in the skin and underlying muscle such that a trocar and catheter can be advanced without force. Once in the pleural space, the catheter should be advanced towards the apex of the lung and connected to an underwater seal. Bubbling will cease once the air leak has sealed and the lung fully expanded. The value of additional suction is unproven and may simply serve to maintain the patency of the original air leak.

Pleurodesis

Pleurodesis is often undertaken in an attempt to obliterate the pleural space and reduce the likelihood of a recurrent pneumothorax. There are several potential techniques but the lack of any large comparative studies makes choice somewhat dependent on personal experience. Sclerosants can be introduced in conjunction with an intercostal drain or at thoracoscopy. Agents which have been used include silver nitrate, tetracycline, talc, fibrin 'glue', and blood. The lung needs to be fully inflated and a combination of local anaesthetic and systemic analgesic is required to minimize chest discomfort.

Surgical intervention

Thoracoscopic techniques have, to a considerable extent, superseded open thoracotomy. The main indications for surgery are a persisting air leak after prolonged intubation and recurrent pneumothoraces.

Pneumomediastinum

A pneumomediastinum can present in isolation or in association with a pneumothorax. Air tracks along the bronchovascular sheath to the hilum and mediastinum. It can be associated with sudden rises in alveolar pressure during sneezing or straining and in patients undergoing intermittent positive pressure ventilation. Precordial chest discomfort may be a presenting symptom and subcutaneous emphysema can be detected in the neck and supraclavicular fossae. No specific treatment is indicated since the condition is benign and self-limiting.

Further reading

Berger, H.W. and Magier, E. (1973). Tuberculous pleurisy. *Chest*, **63**, 88–92.

Fairfax, A.J., McNabb, W.R., and Spiro, S.G. (1986). Chylothorax: A review of 18 cases. *Thorax*, **41**, 880–5.

Getz, S.B. and Beasley, W.E. (1983). Spontaneous pneumothorax. *American Journal of Surgery*, **145**, 923–6.

Hunninghake, G.W. and Fauci, A.S. (1979). Pulmonary involvement in the collagen vascular diseases. *American Review of Respiratory Disease*, **119**, 471–503.

Jay, S.J. (1985). Diagnostic procedures for pleural disease. *Clinics in Chest Medicine*, **6**, 33–48.

Miller, A.C. and Harvey, J.E. (for Standards of Care Committee, British Thoracic Society) (1993). Guidelines for the management of spontaneous pneumothorax. *British Medical Journal*, **307**, 114–16.

Chapter 4.37

Disorders of the thoracic cage and diaphragm

J. M. Shneerson

Disorders of the spine

Scoliosis

Scoliosis is lateral curvature of the spine associated with rotation of the vertebral bodies.

Pathophysiology

A scoliosis reduces the compliance of the chest wall and to a lesser extent of the lungs because of their reduced volume. The distorted rib cage puts the inspiratory muscles at a mechanical disadvantage; those on the convexity are shortened and those on the concavity are lengthened. The maximum inspiratory and expiratory pressures are reduced and a restrictive defect develops. Exercise ability is linked to the degree of reduction of vital capacity (VC) and forced expiratory volume in 1 s (FEV_1). Cardiac output usually increases normally during exercise, but the pulmonary artery pressure rises rapidly. Its rate of increase is related to the oxygen uptake and inversely to the VC.

The arterial blood gases are normal in mild scoliosis, but a fall in the oxygen pressures (PO_2) is the first abnormality to be seen. This is due to suboptimal ventilation and perfusion matching, but there is usually less difference in function between the two lungs than might be expected from their anatomical distortion. Acute ventilatory failure may be precipitated by a chest infection or asthma, but chronic hypoventilation is seen initially during sleep, particularly in rapid eye movement (REM) sleep. Central apnoeas and hypopnoeas are frequent, particularly in REM sleep, and the severity of oxygen desaturation correlates with both the oxygen saturation during wakefulness and the VC. Chronic hypercapnia during the day develops particularly if the onset of the scoliosis is before 8 years of age, if it is high in the thoracic spine, more than around 100°, if there is respiratory muscle weakness, or if the VC is less than 1–1.5 litres.

Right ventricular failure often appears at the time that chronic hypercapnic respiratory failure develops and is associated with pulmonary hypertension due to hypoxic vasoconstriction, an anatomically restricted pulmonary vascular bed, and occasionally polycythaemia.

Symptoms and physical signs

The earliest feature is a change in the appearance of the patient, such as an asymmetry of the shoulders. Worsening breathlessness often signifies the development of complications such as respiratory failure. Fatigue and ankle swelling may coincide with this, and frequent awakenings from sleep, associated with excessive day-time sleepiness suggests that the subject is arousing from apnoeas and hypopnoeas.

Physical examination may reveal the cause of the scoliosis, such as neurofibromatosis, and any congenital abnormalities or associated muscle weakness.

Treatment

Spinal fusion or costectomy (in which parts of the ribs comprising the posterior hump are removed) may be of cosmetic value if scoliosis is severe. Spinal fusion may also prevent progression of the scoliosis, stabilize the spine, particularly in neuromuscular disorders, and in selected cases improve cardiac or respiratory function or prevent its deterioration. The latter is only of value in patients with muscle weakness, such as in Duchenne's muscular dystrophy or following poliomyelitis.

Acute ventilatory failure may require endotracheal intubation or non-invasive ventilatory support. Chronic ventilatory failure also responds to mechanical ventilation. Oxygen either at night or during the day, or both, is often dangerous because of the risk of hypercapnia. Nasal positive pressure ventilation is most commonly used, although negative pressure ventilation, usually with a cuirass or jacket, is also effective. The quality of life, arterial blood gases, and sleep structure can all improve with long-term, non-invasive ventilation. This also reduces the number of visits required by general practitioners and the number of drugs prescribed. Survival with treatment is around 75 per cent at 5 years, and 60 per cent at 10 years.

Kyphosis

Kyphosis is exaggeration of the normal thoracic anteroposterior curvature of the spine.

Pathophysiology

Kyphosis due to osteoporosis rarely causes any significant changes in respiratory function, but a sharp kyphosis (gibbus) caused by, for instance, tuberculous osteomyelitis of the spine (Pott's disease) causes it to become rigid. The costovertebral joints may also ankylose and limit rib cage expansion. This leads to a restrictive defect, but respiratory failure is uncommon unless the gibbus is high in the thoracic spine and appears in early childhood. The development of hypoxia, hypercapnia, pulmonary hypertension, and right heart failure are similar to scoliosis (see above).

Symptoms and physical signs

Slight breathlessness on exertion is common in the presence of a gibbus, but is rare in other types of kyphosis. Physical examination reveals the spinal deformity and limitation of rib cage expansion.

Investigations

The extent and severity of the kyphosis is usually well seen on a lateral chest radiograph. The changes in lung volumes are similar to scoliosis. The arterial PO_2 and PCO_2 are normal in most subjects, but the earliest abnormalities are revealed by sleep studies.

Treatment

Treatment of the acute tuberculous infection with chemotherapy is often effective in preventing a gibbus from developing. Once it has been established and respiratory failure has developed the only effective treatment is long-term respiratory support. This is best provided non-invasively by a nasal positive pressure ventilator rather than a negative pressure system since patients with a sharp kyphosis often find it difficult to lie in the supine position, which is required for negative pressure ventilation.

Ankylosing spondylitis (see also Chapter 10.3)

Pathophysiology

The rib cage becomes rigid once the affected joints become ankylosed. There is little spinal mobility, and a pronounced kyphosis often develops. Unlike other skeletal disorders affecting the thorax the functional residual capacity (FRC) increases because the rib cage becomes fixed at its own relaxation volume. This is greater than the normal FRC which is influenced by the inward pull of the elastic recoil of the lungs. Intercostal muscles often atrophy and the maximum inspiratory and expiratory pressures are reduced. Respiration depends increasingly on the diaphragm, but the ventilatory responses to exercise are virtually normal.

Chronic respiratory failure is very uncommon in ankylosing spondylitis unless another complication develops, such as airflow obstruction (which may be due to cricoarytenoid arthritis), pleural thickening or effusion, aspiration pneumonia related to impaired oesophageal motility, apical fibrobullous lung disease, which may be complicated by opportunist infections such as *Aspergillus fumigatus* or saprophytic Mycobacteria, or abdominal surgery, which restricts diaphragmatic function.

Symptoms and physical signs

Chest pain during sudden movements such as coughing and laughing is common when the active phase of the inflammation affects the thorax. Occasionally cricoarytenoid arthritis may present with hoarseness, stridor, or breathlessness, and extensive fibrobullous disease may cause breathlessness.

The most obvious physical sign is restriction of rib cage movement associated with prominent accessory muscle activity and abdominal respiratory movements.

Investigations

Chest radiography may show calcification of the paraspinal ligaments (bamboo spine) and complications of ankylosing spondylitis such as pleural thickening, aspiration pneumonia, and apical fibrobullous disease. The changes in lung volumes have been described above. Chest wall compliance is reduced but lung compliance is normal. The *K*CO is increased and arterial blood gases are normal both during rest and exertion.

Treatment

Physiotherapy and non-steroidal anti-inflammatory drugs may improve the vital capacity and chest expansion, particularly in the early phase of the disease or during acute exacerbations.

Disorders of the sternum and ribs

Congenital abnormalities

Congenital abnormalities of the ribs and sternum rarely cause any important respiratory problems. Occasionally, multiple congenital rib abnormalities may lead to paradoxical movement of the chest wall or impair diaphragm function. Agenesis and bifid sternum are rare but may require surgery in the neonatal period to stabilize the anterior chest wall.

Pectus excavatum

This depression deformity of the sternum may be seen at birth but often worsens during adolescent growth spurt, and may be associated with other abnormalities such as scoliosis. It is probably due to an increased inward pull on the sternum by the sternal diaphragmatic fibres or occasionally to an abnormally compliant chest wall. It rarely causes any symptoms. The lung volumes and arterial blood gases are virtually normal. Occasionally, right ventricular filling is impaired because of cardiac compression between the depressed sternum and the spine. Pulmonary outflow tract compression can cause a systolic murmur and atrial dysrhythmias may occur.

Surgery may be carried out for cosmetic reasons, but it has little or no effect on the mild restrictive defect or exercise ability, except in the rare situation where right ventricular filling is impaired or atrial dysrhythmias have developed.

Pectus carinatum

This protrusion deformity of the sternum usually develops during the adolescent growth spurt due to excessive and sometimes asymmetrical growth of the ribs or costal cartilages. Occasionally chest pain arises at the insertion of the intercostal muscles anteriorly or in the costal cartilages and anterior ribs. The lung volumes are normal and surgery is indicated only for cosmetic reasons and not to improve respiratory function or exercise ability.

Thoracoplasty

Introduction

The operation of thoracoplasty was developed for the treatment of pulmonary tuberculosis. Varying lengths of up to eleven ribs were removed in order to collapse the lung on the affected side. It has been superseded by antituberculous chemotherapy but is still occasionally required to treat chronic infections, particularly when there is a problem in obliterating the pleural space after pulmonary resection. As many as 30 000 operations were carried out in the UK between 1951 and 1960 and many patients still survive.

Pathophysiology

Resection of the ribs flattens the chest and reduces the volume of the thorax. Paradoxical rib cage movement may be seen and the chest wall compliance is reduced. A scoliosis is almost invariable and its severity is related to the number of ribs that are removed. Respiratory muscle function is also impaired, particularly on the side of the thoracoplasty. The restrictive defect that develops is proportional to the number of ribs that have been resected and exercise ability is limited by ventilatory factors. The ventilation and perfusion are both reduced almost equally on the side of the thoracoplasty so that the arterial PO_2 is often normal. The function of the contralateral lung is more important in determining the blood gases. Hypoxaemia usually appears during sleep before wakefulness and may be associated with hypercapnia. This may later persist during the day, particularly if the maximal inspiratory and transdiaphragmatic pressures are reduced.

Symptoms and physical signs

The symptoms of patients with a thoracoplasty are similar to those with a scoliosis, but if a productive cough develops a recurrence of pulmonary tuberculosis should be suspected. Right heart failure often develops insidiously either when respiratory failure appears or subsequently. Physical examination reveals a thoracotomy scar and a flattened area of chest in the region of the thoracoplasty which may move paradoxically. Accessory muscle activity is often marked, particularly on the side of the thoracoplasty.

Investigations

The chest radiograph shows the extent of the thoracoplasty, and of the previous tuberculous infection, and the results of other treatment for this. There is a restrictive defect, occasionally with airflow obstruction as well which may be either due to tuberculous endobronchitis or coincidental tobacco smoking. Maximum inspiratory and expiratory pressures are reduced and hypoxia with or without hypercapnia may be seen.

Treatment

Chronic ventilatory failure can be supported with non-invasive nocturnal mechanical ventilation with a nasal positive pressure ventilator, or alternatively with a negative pressure system such as a cuirass or jacket. Long-term oxygen therapy is dangerous if hypercapnia is present, but occasional patients have predominant hypoxaemia and benefit from oxygen.

Table 1 Main causes of diaphragm weakness

Unilateral	Bilateral
Congenital—e.g. agenesis, eventration	
Trauma	Trauma
Adjacent mass—e.g. neoplasm, aneurysm	High cervical cord lesions
Herpes zoster	Motor neurone disease
Poliomyelitis	Poliomyelitis
Peripheral neuropathy	Peripheral neuropathy
Neuralgic amyotrophy	Acute idiopathic polyneuropathy
Open heart surgery	Myopathies Muscular dystrophies

Disorders of the diaphragm

Aetiology

Diaphragmatic paralysis or paresis may be due to lesions affecting either the diaphragm itself or the phrenic nerve, its nucleus, or higher control centres or pathways (Table 1).

Pathophysiology

Unilateral weakness of the diaphragm causes it to move upwards (paradoxically) into the thorax during inspiration, particularly in the supine position when the weight of the abdominal contents pushes the diaphragm upwards. Recruitment of intercostal and accessory muscles partially compensates for loss of diaphragmatic activity, but the VC in the upright position is around 20–25 per cent less than normal and it falls a further 15 per cent in the supine position. Ventilation–perfusion matching is impaired, leading to hypoxia, but hypercapnia does not occur during wakefulness or sleep.

The physiological abnormality is much more marked in bilateral than unilateral diaphragm weakness. The whole diaphragm moves paradoxically during inspiration and expiration, and the intrapleural pressure changes are transmitted across it so that the abdominal pressure falls during inspiration and the anterior abdominal wall moves inward. The sitting VC is about 50 per cent predicted and may fall by a further 50 per cent when supine. Ventilation is particularly reduced at the bases in the supine position with relatively less change in perfusion, so that the arterial PO_2 falls. During sleep this effect together with the rapid respiratory rate, small tidal volume, and short inspiratory time contribute to hypoxia and hypercapnia.

Symptoms and physical signs

Unilateral diaphragm paralysis in adults rarely causes symptoms unless there is coexisting pulmonary disease or weakness of other respiratory muscles. In contrast, bilateral weakness can cause severe breathlessness. This may occur during exertion, but a specific feature is orthopnoea. This occurs within a few seconds of lying flat and is relieved promptly by sitting up, unlike left ventricular failure and nocturnal asthma.

There may be no definite abnormal physical signs in unilateral diaphragm weakness, but if this is bilateral orthopnoea is readily apparent and the abdomen moves paradoxically inwards as the diaphragm ascends during inspiration. Accessory muscle activity is present and bilateral basal dullness due to the high diaphragm is characteristic.

Investigations

The chest radiograph may show elevation of the diaphragm, either unilaterally or bilaterally, together with basal linear shadowing due to subsegmental lung collapse. Diaphragmatic screening or ultrasound examination will demonstrate whether the diaphragm is moving paradoxically, particularly during sniffing.

The low VC which falls further in the supine position is the hallmark of diaphragmatic weakness, but this can be confirmed by the finding of a low transdiaphragmatic pressure. Lung volumes are reduced except for the residual volume (RV) since the expiratory muscle strength is largely preserved. Phrenic nerve function can be estimated by measuring its conduction time which is normally less than about 9.5 ms. The arterial PO_2 is slightly reduced with a normal PCO_2 during the daytime. Similar features may be observed during sleep but hypercapnia may develop, particularly if other respiratory muscles are also weakened.

Treatment

Plication of the diaphragm may reduce breathlessness due to unilateral diaphragm weakness, but since this symptom is uncommon it is rarely indicated. Bilateral plication is not effective, and in the presence of bilateral weakness mechanical respiratory support may be needed. This is usually provided at night with a nasal positive pressure ventilator, although a negative pressure system using a cuirass or jacket may also be effective, and rocking beds have been used in the past.

Further reading

Gibson, G.J. (1989). Diaphragmatic paresis: pathophysiology, clinical features, and investigation. *Thorax*, **44**, 960–70.

Rochester, D.F. and Lindley, L.J. (1992). Neuromuscular and skeletal disease. In *Pulmonary complications of systemic disease*, (ed. J.F. Murray), pp. 303–84. Marcel Dekker, New York.

Shneerson, J.M. (1988). *Disorders of ventilation*. Blackwell Scientific Publications, Oxford.

Tobin, M.J. (ed.) (1990). The respiratory muscles. *Problems in respiratory care*, **3**, 257–546.

Neoplastic disorders

Chapter 4.38

Lung cancer

S. G. Spiro

General epidemiology

Lung cancer is the most common malignant disease in the Western world, and its incidence has increased rapidly in many countries. It has shown the greatest relative and absolute rise in mortality of any tumour this century in England and Wales, and particularly in Scotland. In the US it has been increasing in incidence by up to 10 per cent per year since the 1930s, but over the last decade there has been a levelling in the incidence, particularly in males.

Lung cancer causes 35 000 deaths per year in England and Wales, with 80 per cent of these occurring in men. In the European Community there were 1.35 million deaths per annum in men (the highest death rate from any tumour) and 229 000 deaths per annum in women during the period 1978–1982.

However, age-standardized mortality rates for cancer for 1985–1989 show that in the European Community lung cancer in men has by far the greatest mortality rate. Belgium has the greatest mortality (77.16 deaths per 100 000 population) with Scotland second, and England and Wales fifth.

Age-specific mortality data clearly show differences between age groups. While mortality continues to increase in the elderly, death rates among younger people are falling. Figure 1 analyses data in England and Wales relating the year of birth to death rate in age cohorts of 5 years for men and women. Each vertical set of points represents the mortality rate at different ages of persons born during a 10-year period surrounding a central year of birth. Male mortality at each age reaches the peak in the generation born between 1901 and 1916, but for women, whilst the pattern is similar, the peak death rates occur in those born during the 1920s. There is a cohort of elderly patients in the population with a high incidence of lung

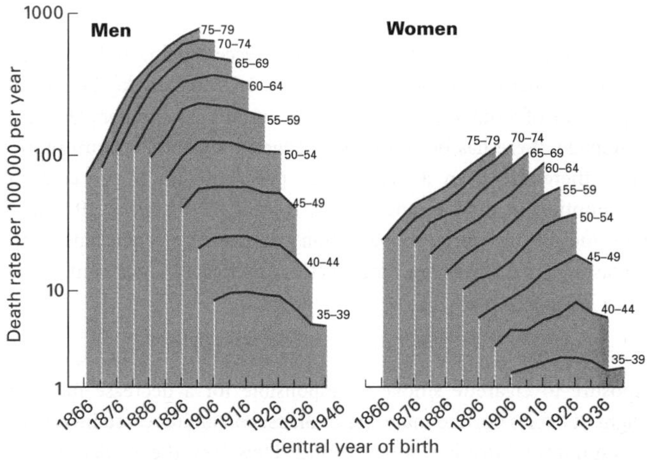

Fig. 1 Age-specific mortality from lung cancer in England and Wales during the period 1941–1980 plotted versus central year of birth. *(Reproduced with permission from Coggon and Acheson 1983.)*

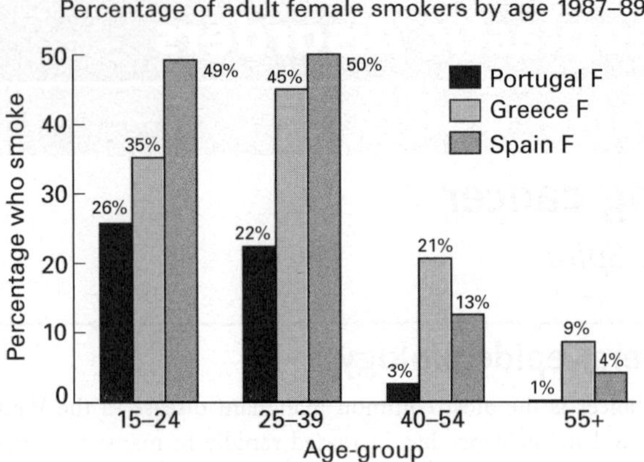

Fig. 2 Smoking by age in females in the European Community 1987–1989.

cancer; thus the average age of those presenting with lung cancer will slowly rise, at least for the next few years.

Aetiological factors

Tobacco

In every country, the increase in mortality from lung cancer coincided with tobacco usage, particularly cigarette smoking, after what seemed to be an appropriate latent interval. Prospective studies, amongst which the long-term study of British doctors is particularly informative, confirmed the increased risk of death from lung cancer from any tobacco use, but most specifically from usage of cigarettes; there was a strong dose-response relationship with the number of cigarettes smoked. The most important variable in smoking intensity is the number of cigarettes smoked; also the depth of inhalation, number of puffs, butt length, use of a filter, and the type of tobacco smoked. Wide differences in smoking habits are now seen between social classes, with 57 per cent of unskilled manual workers smoking compared with only 21 per cent of professional workers. However, during the last 5 years the number of adult men smoking in England and Wales has fallen from 64 to 36 per cent, but has remained at 35 per cent for adult women.

A recent European Community survey has shown that smoking is most prevalent among young people. The rates of smoking by age are even more striking for women. In Greece, Spain, and Portugal less than 10 per cent of women aged over 55 years smoke, but up to 50 per cent of women aged between 26 and 40 are smokers (Fig. 2).

Globally, there has been a huge change in cigarette consumption. While there has been a drop of 25 per cent and 9 per cent in consumption in the UK and the US respectively between 1970 and 1985, the overall world consumption has risen by 7 per cent, with increases in Asia (22 per cent), Latin America (24 per cent), and Africa (42 per cent).

Passive smoking

Exposure to cigarette smoke is responsible for a decrease in birth weight of babies born to maternal smokers, and an increased incidence of respiratory infection when young. However, the evidence that passive smoking predisposes to lung cancer is far from certain. Exposure histories may ignore the effect of the workplace, divorce, remarriage, and childhood exposure.

Table 1 Industrial products and processes known to cause or suspected of causing lung cancer

Fibre exposure (asbestos)	Chloromethyl ether
Nickel refining	Chromates
Aluminium industry	The electronics industry
Arsenic and arsenic compounds	Irradiation
Benzoyl chloride	Soots, tar, oils
Beryllium	Mustard gas
Cadmium	

Reproduced from Coggan and Acheson (1983), with permission.

Occupation

The association of asbestos with lung cancer is now firmly established. There is a much greater risk for the asbestos industry worker if he smokes cigarettes; one study identified the risk as 93 times that for non-smokers not exposed to asbestos. Exposure to radioactive isotopes, mainly radon daughters, occurs among various groups of miners, particularly those involved in the mining of pitchblende and uranium. Polycyclic aromatic hydrocarbons are responsible for the increased risk in workers in the gas and coke ovens and in foundry workers. Nickel refining, chromate manufacture, and arsenical industrial workers are also exposed to a higher risk of lung cancer. A summary of the important industrial products and processes involved appears in Table 1.

Pathology

A detailed understanding of the natural history, pathology, and pathogenesis of bronchial carcinoma is becoming increasingly important as the assessment, management, and prognosis of the disease depends largely upon the cell type and the presence or absence of metastasis at the time of presentation. It has been estimated that about seven-eighths of a tumour's life will have passed when it is diagnosed and that the vast majority will be disseminated at the time of diagnosis.

Bronchogenic carcinomas arise most commonly in segmental and subsegmental bronchi in response to repetitive carcinogenic stimuli or inflammation and irritation. The mucosal lining is most susceptible to injury at the bifurcation of bronchial structures. Dysplasia is followed by carcinoma *in situ* when the entire thickness of the mucosa may be replaced by proliferating neoplastic cells. These changes may be strictly localized or multicentric. A significant number of lung tumours arise in the periphery of the lung, perhaps three-quarters of adenocarcinomas and large-cell anaplastic malignancies, one-third of squamous (or epidermoid) carcinomas, and one-fifth of small-cell carcinomas.

The WHO classification of lung cancer according to cell type and the percentage distribution of each type of lung cancer is shown in Table 2. The squamous-cell tumour has a relatively slow growth rate (volume doubling time 90 days) and the lowest incidence of distant haematogenous metastasis. Small-cell tumours grow rapidly (volume doubling time 30 days) and there is very early dissemination with metastases being present in more than 90 per cent of patients at the time of diagnosis. Adenocarcinomas and anaplastic large-cell tumours occupy an intermediate position. Squamous-cell tumours, adenocarcinomas, and large-cell tumours are called non-small-cell lung

Table 2 Classification of epithelial tumours of the lung (based on revised WHO Classification)

	Frequency (%)		Frequency (%)
Main			
Epidermoid carcinoma (squamous cell)	35	Adenocarcinoma	21
		Acinar	
		Papillary	
		Bronchiolar alveolar	
Small-cell carcinoma	24	Large-cell carcinoma	19
Oatcell		With stratification	
Fusiform		With mucin-production	
Others		Giant-cell	
		Clear-cell	
Less common			
Tumours showing mixed differentiation		Bronchial gland	
		Adenoid cystic	
		Mucoepidermoid	
		Others	
Carcinoid tumours			
		Carcinoma *in situ*	

cancers, and the approach to their management differs from that for small-cell lung cancer.

Squamous (epidermoid) carcinoma

These tumours are composed predominantly of flattened neoplastic cells that stratify, form intercellular bridges, and elaborate keratin. About 60 per cent present as obstructive lesions in lobar and main-stem bronchi. As a result, distal pneumonia and abscess formation is common, and cavitation is seen in about 10 per cent. The cells are usually well differentiated, but in some cases differentiation is poor and the appearances are those of predominantly anaplastic cells, frequently arranged in the classical pattern of stratifying sheets.

Small-cell (oat-cell) anaplastic carcinoma

This is a pathologically and clinically distinct form of lung cancer, which may originate from the amine precursor uptake and decarboxylation (APUD) series of cells. The tumour is composed of neoplastic cells with dark, oval to round spindled nuclei and scanty, indistinct cytoplasm arranged in ribbons, nests, and sheets. This type of tumour presents as a proximal lesion in 75 per cent of cases and may arise anywhere in the tracheobronchial tree and rapidly invade vessels and lymph nodes. Extensive, advanced disease exists in more than half the patients on presentation. The cells secrete hormones which give rise to characteristic clinical syndromes in 10 per cent of cases.

Adenocarcinoma

This tumour forms acinar or granular structures, having prominent papillary processes, and may be mucin-provoking. About 70 per cent appear to originate peripherally in the lung and are frequently fairly circumscribed; in about 10 per cent the initial presentation is a pleural effusion.

Large-cell carcinoma

These tumours include all that show no evidence of maturation or differentiation. They are composed of pleomorphic cells with variable enlarged nuclei, prominent nucleoli and nuclear inclusions, and abundant cytoplasm; they are mucin-producing in many instances. Large-cell carcinoma is a smoking-related disease in over 90 per cent of patients.

Bronchioloalveolar cell carcinoma

The tumour tends to spread as cuboidal or columnar 'epithelium' along the lining of the alveoli, with single or multiple rows of cells and often papillary formation. There is production of a large amount of mucus in 20 per cent of cases and it is believed that malignant cells shed into the mucus may carry over into relevant anatomical sites in the contralateral lung. The tumour can spread within a lobe and occupy it fully. Sometimes, however, the tumour is multicentric in origin, and diffuse nodular lesions are to be found on radiographic examination in some patients. Invasion of neighbouring tissue and lymph nodes is common, but more distant spread is unusual.

Carcinoid tumours

Carcinoid tumours are described in Chapter 5.20.

Carcinoma *in situ*

Many investigators have suggested that cells undergoing malignant change do not necessarily invade the lungs at the onset of this biological mutation, but continue to exist at a particular location (cancer *in situ*). Exfoliated cancer cells sloughed from such a location may be seen fortuitously by the cytologist; even more rarely, such a site may be biopsied at bronchoscopy.

Genetics and biology

Genetic influences may play a role in the development of lung cancers, particularly in patients under 50. Individuals who extensively metabolize debrisoquine are at greater risk than those who are poor or intermediate metabolizers. The gene coding for this enzyme is located on chromosome 22.

Two major categories of cell lines have been established for small-cell lung cancer—classic and variant. Classic cell lines account for 70 per cent and are characterized by high expression of neuroendocrine markers such as L-dopa decarboxylase and bombesin/gastrin-releasing peptide, neurone-specific enolase, and creatine kinase-BB. The variant cell lines have selective loss of some of these neuroendocrine markers, and many variant small-cell lung cancer lines have substituted amplification of the c-*myc* oncogene. These neuroendocrine properties have important prognostic features—in most studies, survival in patients from whom a classic cell line is grown is better than those with variant cell lines.

Several monoclonal antibodies have been generated against lung-cancer-associated antigens. Thirty-six monoclonal antibodies raised against small-cell lung cancer have been grouped into eight clusters. No antigen is specific for small-cell lung cancer. Antibodies belonging to the major cluster (cluster 1) are directed against the neural-cell adhesion molecule (NCAM), whilst the nature of the other antigens remains unclear.

Lung cancer cells not only show mutations that activate dominant cellular proto-oncogenes, but also genetic mechanisms that inactivate recessive tumour suppressors. The commonest abnormality is a deletion in the short arm of chromosome 3, which is found in over 90 per cent of small-cell lung cancer and 50 per cent of non-small-cell lung cancer patients. Other sites of loss of heterozygosity include 11p, 13q, and 17p.

The dominant oncogene mutations in small-cell lung cancer are among the *myc* family. Amplification of c-*myc*, n-*myc*, and l-*myc* are late events in the pathogenesis of small-cell lung cancer, and are recognized mainly in patients who have relapsed after previous intensive chemotherapy.

Clinical features

The clinical abnormalities associated with lung cancer vary considerably. In about 5 per cent of patients the initial presentation is a radiographic abnormality found on routine examination and unassociated with symptoms; however, patients may present with extremely advanced disease from which death rapidly occurs.

The clinical features may be due to local development of the tumour in the lung, including bronchial obstruction, invasion of contiguous structures in the thorax and mediastinum, metastasis through blood or lymph vessels, and endocrine, metabolic, and neurological syndromes.

Cough is the most common initial presenting symptom. Patients who have a persistent cough should have a chest radiograph, particularly if they are 40 years or over and are smokers. A change in the cough habit is significant and also requires investigation. If cough is manifestly ineffective, involvement of the recurrent laryngeal nerve should be suspected.

Expectoration of sputum may be due to spread of the tumour itself or to infection occurring distal to partial bronchial obstruction.

Haemoptysis occurs as a sole presenting symptom in about 5 per cent of cases and at some stage in the disease in 50 per cent. Massive haemoptysis is rare except as a terminal event, and the common description is of coughing up blood every morning for successive days.

Localized, persistent wheeze even after coughing is a significant observation associated with obstruction of a larger or central airway.

Dyspnoea is a presenting symptom in only a small number of patients. As the disease progresses dyspnoea is inevitable, being proportional to the amount of lung involvement including collapse of the lung due to endobronchial disease causing airway narrowing or obstruction. Progressive breathlessness is also a salient feature of malignant pleural and, rarely, pericardial effusion, superior vena caval obstruction, and lymphangitis carcinomatosis.

Chest discomfort is a common symptom occurring in up to 40 per cent of patients at diagnosis and is often of an ill-defined nature. Pleural pain may occur in the presence of infection, but invasion of the pleura by tumour may be painless. However, invasion of the ribs or vertebrae causes continuous gnawing pain locally. A tumour in the superior pulmonary sulcus (Pancoast tumour) causes progressive constant pain in the shoulder, upper anterior chest, or interscapular region, spreading to the arm once the brachial plexus is invaded.

Lack of energy and, more particularly, loss of interest in normal pursuits are symptoms of great importance; a sensation of vague ill health commonly occurs.

Invasion of adjacent intrathoracic structures gives rise to certain specific clinical features. Involvement of the last cervical and first thoracic segment of the sympathetic trunk produces Horner's syndrome. Malignant infiltration of the recurrent laryngeal nerve—almost always the left branch because of its course adjacent to the left hilum—gives rise to vocal chord paralysis. Recurrent aspiration pneumonias may follow. Extension of the tumour with invasion or compression of the superior vena cava results in superior vena caval obstruction—awareness of tightness of the collar, fullness of the head, and suffusion of the face, particularly after bending down, blackouts, breathlessness, and engorgement of veins with a downward venous flow in the neck, the upper half of the thorax, and arms, often accompanied by oedema of the face.

Dysphagia is due to compression of the oesophagus from without by tumour masses and only rarely to direct invasion. Invasion of the phrenic nerve results in elevation and paralysis of the hemidiaphragm.

The clinical features associated with involvement of the ribs, spine, and pleura are described elsewhere. Very rarely bronchogenic carcinoma causes spontaneous pneumothorax. It must not be forgotten that spread of tumour to the other lung may occur or that synchronous primaries may coexist.

Metastatic lesions from lung cancer may occur in any organ of the body and produce symptoms which form the presenting complaint. Metastases to nodes, particularly those in the supraclavicular area are frequent. The side affected usually corresponds to the side of the lung lesion, the exception being that tumours from the left lower lobe may metastasize to the nodes in the right scalene area.

Bony metastases are common, particularly in small-cell tumours, and occur predominantly in the ribs, vertebrae, humeri, and femora. Early involvement may be detected by a rise in alkaline phosphatase of bony origin, isotope scanning, or biopsy. Liver secondaries are common and usually silent, although a rise in liver enzymes, particularly alkaline phosphatase, may be an early sign. CT scans and ultrasound may detect involvement in a liver which is not clinically enlarged. Metastases to the brain may account for the presenting symptom in lung cancer in 4 per cent of patients and may be encountered at some time in the illness in 30 per cent. The adrenal glands are involved in 15 to 20 per cent of patients, rarely producing symptoms. The skin should be examined for the presence of tumour spread and subcutaneous metastases may be found at almost any site.

Endocrine and metabolic manifestations (see also Chapter 7.16)

Cancer cells are able to synthesize polypeptides that mimic virtually all the hormones produced by conventional endocrine organs. From time to time the clinical features resulting from ectopic hormone secretion precede those of the pulmonary tumour, emphasizing the importance of a high index of suspicion in such circumstances.

Syndrome of inappropriate secretion of antidiuretic hormone (SIADH) (see also Chapter 7.2)

The continued secretion of vasopressin (ADH) in excess of the body's needs leads to overhydration in both the intracellular and extracellular compartments. The cerebral oedema resulting from water intoxication causes drowsiness, lethargy, irritability, mental confusion, and disorientation, with fits and coma being the most profound features. Peripheral oedema is remarkably rare. The patient is usually asymptomatic until the sodium falls below 120 mmol/l with a low serum osmolality. Urine osmolality usually exceeds 300 mosmol/kg. This syndrome is most commonly associated with small-cell cancer and may be obvious in 10 per cent of cases. Restriction of fluid to a daily intake of 700–1000 ml may redress the hyponatraemia, but demethylchlortetracycline (demeclocycline) 600–1200 mg daily is often highly effective, making water restriction unnecessary.

Ectopic ACTH syndrome (see also Chapter 7.6)

Secretion of an adrenocorticotrophic substance by a small-cell carcinoma leads to bilateral adrenal hyperplasia and to secretion of large amounts of cortisol. The onset of symptoms may be so acute that death may occur within a few weeks, and the typical features of Cushing's syndrome do not have time to develop. Chief clinical features are thirst and polyuria, oedema, pigmentation, and hypokalaemia. Hypertension and profound myopathy may also be present. Serum cortisol is often grossly elevated; the level is not suppressed by dexamethasone, loss of the diurnal rhythm of cortisol level occurs, and the hypokalaemic alkalosis can be severe.

Hypercalcaemia (see also Chapter 7.5)

Hypercalcaemia may be associated with ectopic secretion of parathormone or PTHrP by squamous-cell cancers but is also and more commonly due directly to the presence of multiple bone metastases. The main clinical features are nausea, vomiting, abdominal pain and constipation, polyuria, thirst and dehydration, muscular weakness, psychosis, drowsiness, and eventually coma. The associated dehydration requires replacement of 5 litres of fluid intravenously in 24 h. Corticosteroids (400 mg of hydrocortisone and 100 mg prednisolone in 24 h, initially) are effective in about half the cases. However, intravenous diphosphonates followed by oral maintenance therapy is now the treatment of choice.

Gynaecomastia

Swelling of the breasts, which may be painful, occurs mainly in the subareolar area, and there may be atrophy of the testes. Increased gonadatrophin production is the cause.

Other endocrine manifestations

Hyperthyroidism occurs rarely, but neither goitre nor eye signs are prominent features. Spontaneous hypoglycaemia, the masculinizing syndrome in young women, and hyperglycaemia are very rarely encountered. Pigmentation associated with α- and β-melanocyte-stimulating hormone may occur. The carcinoid syndromes are described in Chapter 5.20.

Neuromyopathies

The term carcinomatous neuropathy is used to describe those abnormalities of the central nervous system, the peripheral nerves, the muscles, and the autonomic nervous system occurring in association with malignancy. These disorders include myopathies (polymyositis, myasthenia, and dermatomyositis) and neuropathies (sensory and mixed sensorimotor, encephalopathy, and myelopathy).

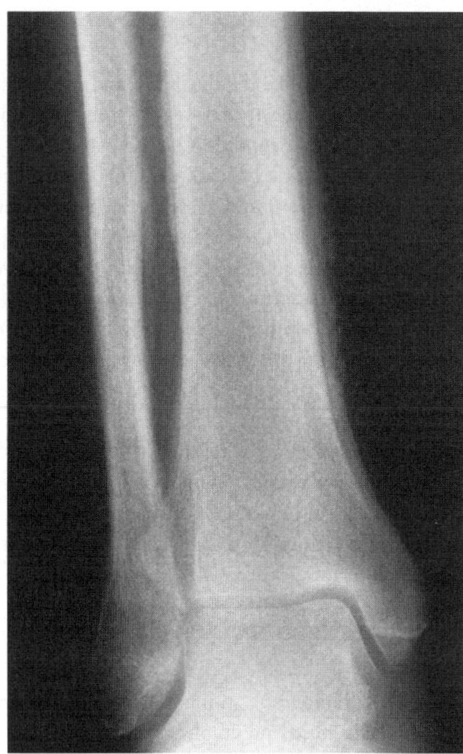

Fig. 3 Hypertrophic pulmonary osteoarthropathy showing persistent new bone formation.

Most neuromyopathies are not tumour-cell-type specific, except for the Lambert–Eaton syndrome seen in small-cell lung cancer patients, often preceding the appearance of a tumour by up to 15 months. It is characterized by proximal muscle weakness, depressed tendon reflexes, often returning following repetitive exercise, autonomic features, and difficulty with swallowing. There appears to be an association with the IgG heavy-chain allotypes GM2 and H LA-B8 for this condition which is currently treated with prednisolone and 3-4-amidopyridine 10–20 mg, four times daily.

Finger clubbing and hypertrophic pulmonary osteoarthropathy

Finger clubbing accompanies a variety of intrathoracic disorders. Gross clubbing is readily recognizable; its early presence may best be demonstrated by the ability to rock the nail on its abnormally spongy bed. Its incidence in lung cancer has been reported as being between 10 and 30 per cent. Clubbing may disappear after resection of tumour.

Hypertrophic pulmonary osteoarthropathy, which may be preceded by finger clubbing alone, consists of periostitis, arthropathy, and usually gross finger clubbing. It is most commonly associated with peripheral lesions and squamous tumours. The long bones of the extremities are affected by a periosteal reaction resembling elm bark; the changes are symmetrical and affect mainly ankles and wrists. The typical radiographic appearances are shown in Fig. 3. The affected areas are hot and painful and sometimes oedematous. Removal of the tumour is followed by immediate regression of hypertrophic pulmonary osteoarthropathy.

Staging and investigations

The investigations used to make the diagnosis and the assessment of lung cancer will vary according to the stage of presentation, the cell type, and the age and general condition of the patient.

The very rapid doubling time of small-cell lung cancer causes it to disseminate rapidly and widely, and at diagnosis is very rarely considered operable. However, the slower doubling times for squamous-cell cancers and adenocarcinomas, together with the relatively lesser tendency for the former to disseminate, makes surgery the best option whenever possible for the non-small-cell lung cancers. Anatomical staging classification demonstrates that the prognosis of non-small-cell lung cancer depends strongly on the extent (or stage) of the disease. The TNM staging system (T describing the primary tumour, N the extent of regional lymph node involvement, and M the absence or presence of metastases) allows an ordered assessment of investigations and selection of cases for surgery (Table 3).

The following investigations form the basis for the diagnosis and staging of patients with lung cancer.

Intrathoracic investigations

Radiological assessment

The value of the chest radiograph in the diagnosis and management of pulmonary neoplasm needs no emphasis.

The finding of a normal radiograph of the chest does not exclude bronchial carcinoma as patients presenting with haemoptysis and a normal chest radiograph are sometimes found to have a central tumour on bronchoscopy. The rounded or ovoid shadow of a peripheral tumour is described in greater detail below; these are sometimes cavitated (Fig. 4). The common appearance of a tumour arising from the main central airways (70 per cent of all cases) is enlargement of one or other hilum (Fig. 5); even experienced observers sometimes have difficulty in determining whether a hilar shadow is enlarged or not, and if there is any suspicion, investigation by bronchoscopy and/or CT should be pursued. Consolidation and collapse distal to the tumour may have occurred by the time that the patient presents, with the tumour itself often being obscured in the process. Collapse of the left lower lobe is often hard to identify (Fig. 6), as is a tumour situated behind the heart. Apically located masses or superior sulcus tumours (Pancoast tumours) may be misdiagnosed as pleural caps, and often have a long history of pain in the distribution of the brachial nerve roots. Loss of the head of the first, second, or third rib is not unusual (Fig. 7).

The mediastinum may be widened by enlarged nodes. Involvement of the phrenic nerve may lead to elevation of the hemidiaphragm. Tumour spreading to the pleura causes an effusion, which may be large. The ribs and spine should be carefully examined for the presence of metastasis. Spread of tumour from mediastinal nodes peripherally along the lymphatics gives the appearance characteristic of lymphangitis carcinomatosa—bilateral hilar enlargement with streaky shadows fanning out into the lung fields on either side.

Lung function

Evaluation of lung function is essential. Simple spirometry is usually adequate, but it may be necessary to evaluate exercise capability in a more sophisticated manner in some patients for whom surgery is being considered. Ventilation–perfusion lung scans give a good indication of the relative function of each lung in cases whose overall preoperative lung function appears to be borderline for resection.

Table 3 Definitions for staging bronchogenic carcinoma (American Joint Committee on Cancer Staging 1997)

T0	No evidence of primary tumour
TX	Tumour proven by the presence of malignant cells in bronchopulmonary secretions but not visualized radiographically or bronchoscopically, or any tumour that cannot be assessed
TIS	Carcinoma *in situ*
T1	A tumour that is 3.0 cm or less in greatest diameter, surrounded by lung or visceral pleura, and without evidence of invasion proximal to a lobar bronchus at bronchoscopy
T2	Tumour with any of the following features of size or extent: 3 cm in greatest dimension; Involves main bronchus ≥ 2cm distal to the carina; Invades the visceral pleura; Associated with atelectasis or obstructive pneumonitis that extends to the hilar region but does not involve the entire lung.
T3	Tumour of any size that directly invades any of the following: chest wall (including superior sulcus tumors), diaphragm, mediastinal pleura, parietal pericardium: or tumour in the main bronchus < 2cm distal to the carina, but without involvement of the carina: or associated atelectasis or obstructive pneumonitis of the entire lung
T4	Tumour of any size that invades any of the following: mediastinum, heart, great vessels, trachea, oesophagus, vertebral body, carina; or tumour with a malignant pleural or pericardial effusion, or with satellite tumour nodule(s) within the ipsilateral primary-tumour lobe of the lung
N0	No demonstrable metastasis to regional lymph nodes
N1	Metastasis to lymph nodes in the peribronchial or the ipsilateral hilar region, or both, including direct extension
N2	Metastasis to ipsilateral mediastinal lymph nodes and subcarinal lymph nodes
N3	Metastasis of contralateral mediastinal lymph nodes, contralateral hilar lymph nodes, ipsilateral or contralateral sclera, or supraclavicular lymph nodes
M0	No (known) distant metastasis
M1	Distant metastasis such as in scalene, cervical, or contralateral hilar lymph nodes, brain, bones, liver, or contralateral lung

Summary stage grouping		
Stage IA (operable)		
T1	N0	M0
Stage IB		
T2	N0	M0
Stage IIA (operable)		
T1	N1	M0
Stage IIB		
T2	N1	M0
Stage IIIa (sometimes operable)		
T3	N1	M0
T1	N2	M0
T2	N2	M0
T3	N2	M0
Stage IIIb (inoperable)		
Any T	N3	M0
T4	Any N	M0
Stage IV		
Any T	Any N	M1

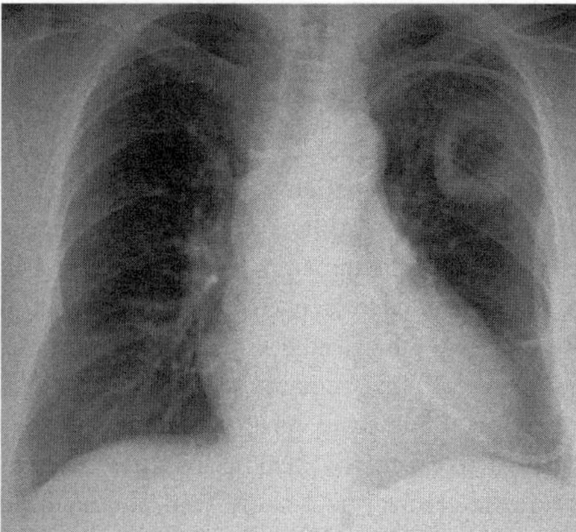

Fig. 4 Cavitating peripheral squamous-cell carcinoma.

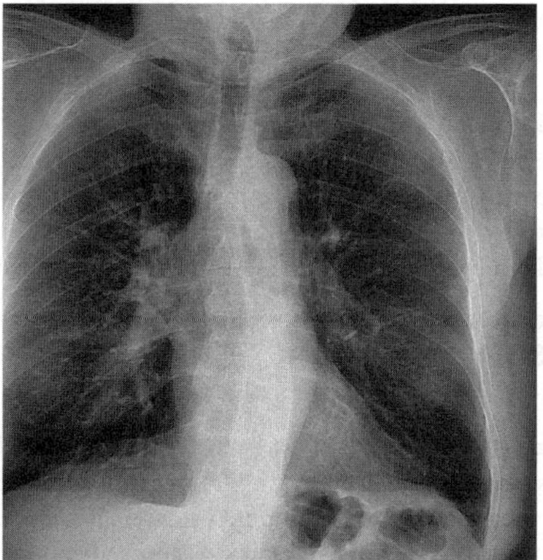

Fig. 5 Enlarged right hilum. Bronchoscopy revealed a tumour in right intermediate bronchus.

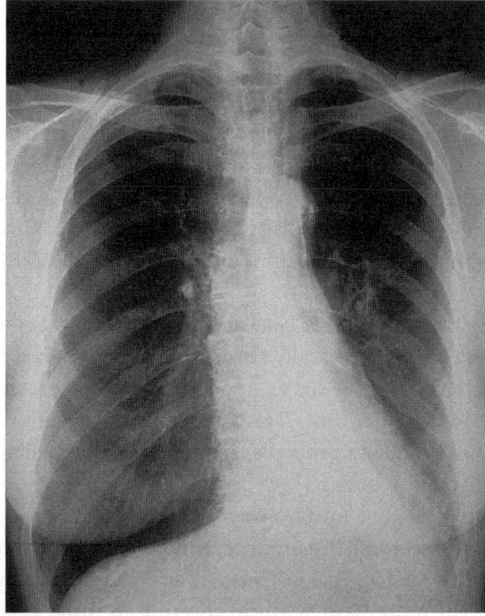

Fig. 6 Collapsed left lower lobe showing loss of the medial third of the left diaphragm.

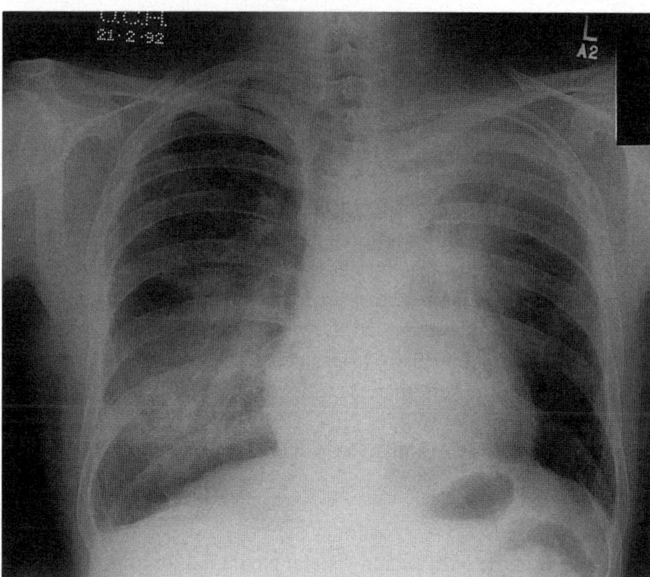

Fig. 7 Huge apical tumour with destruction of posterior parts of the second and third ribs.

Bronchoscopy

Bronchoscopy, which is described in detail in Chapter 4.5, is frequently the definitive diagnostic method in lung cancer. Tissue removed at bronchoscopy can establish the diagnosis and cell type. Most investigators perform a biopsy of a suspicious lesion, then brushings, and this can be followed by a small-volume lavage (50–150 ml). Whilst brushing cytology will add to the yield from biopsy, lavage only adds 1 to 2 per cent to the total diagnostic yield of lung tumours. Bronchoscopic examination also yields valuable information regarding suitability for surgical resection. Histological confirmation is now obtainable in 85 to 90 per cent of bronchoscopically visible lesions.

Transbronchial biopsy

Transbronchial biopsy via the fibreoptic bronchoscope can be useful in the diagnosis of circumscribed lesions beyond the range of direct vision or of more diffuse lesions such as may be seen in adenocarcinoma, bronchoalveolar-cell carcinoma, and lymphangitis carcinomatosis. It is advisable to manoeuvre the placement of the biopsy forceps under fluoroscopic control if a circumscribed lesion is to be biopsied. A positive yield of up to 60 per cent has been obtained from circumscribed lesions, and is greatest in those over 4 cm in diameter. Pneumothorax follows the procedure in about 5 per cent of cases and major haemorrhage in 1 to 2 per cent. Fatalities are extremely rare. However, trends are increasingly towards transthoracic percutaneous needle biopsy, often with CT guidance, for circumscribed lesions, and to use transbronchial biopsy for diffuse infiltrates.

Percutaneous needle biopsy

Percutaneous Trucut biopsy may be carried out on large lesions close to the pleura to obtain a core of tissue for histology, or with aspiration needle biopsy which only yields cytological smear preparations. These procedures should be performed under fluoroscopic, CT, or ultrasound control, and are best avoided in patients with poor respiratory function or with bleeding diatheses. Positive yields as high as 90 per cent have been reported. Cytological samples remain the least satisfactory for cell type specificity. Pneumothorax occurs in about

25 per cent of patients, with some 5 per cent requiring intubation. Haemoptysis may follow the procedure.

Sputum cytology

Cytological examination of sputum is a useful, non-invasive step in the diagnosis of malignant pulmonary disease. The yield increases according to the number of specimens examined, and three consecutive morning specimens should be submitted in the first instance. In one large study, in those in whom a diagnosis of lung cancer was made, the diagnosis came from a single specimen of sputum in 41 per cent; a second sample increased the yield to 56 per cent, a third to 69 per cent, and a fourth to 85 per cent. The positive incidence is lower with tumours less than 2 cm in diameter (40 per cent) and best with larger masses (60 per cent). Central tumour yields a higher proportion of positive results (60 per cent) than peripheral lesions (48 per cent).

Thoracoscopy

Visualization of the parietal and visceral pleura has an important part to play in the diagnosis of effusions and in pleural tumours as biopsy can be carried out under direct vision, and absence of pleural tumour is important in decisions about resectability of a lung tumour. Thoracoscopy is inadvisable in the absence of effusion or pneumothorax but, in otherwise operable tumours with a pleural effusion that is not bloodstained and without positive cytology or pleural biopsy, thoracoscopy may be a useful next step in determining operability.

Computed axial tomography (CT)

Thoracic CT scanning can identify the site, size, and extension of the primary tumour far more clearly than conventional radiology. It also identifies mediastinal lymphadenopathy which posteroanterior and lateral chest radiographs fail to show. Mediastinal lymphadenopathy on CT is arbitrarily taken to be pathological if the glands are greater than 1.0 cm in diameter. However, previous infective conditions, such as tuberculosis, and reactive hyperplasia to the tumour can cause appearances identical with that of malignant enlargement. Thus positive CT scans of the mediastinum may be falsely positive and mediastinal lymph node biopsy (mediastinoscopy) must be performed to confirm an abnormal finding.

Another potential advantage of CT is its ability to detect tumour invasion of the surrounding pleura and chest wall, in addition to the mediastinum itself. However, not all tumours with CT evidence of invasion prove unresectable, and if possible invasion of the mediastinum or chest wall is the only contraindication to resection then thoracotomy should be performed.

The predictive value of a negative CT is 90 to 95 per cent, and in such cases a mediastinoscopy can be omitted before thoracotomy. However, microscopic invasion of normal-sized mediastinal nodes is increasingly reported in patients with adenocarcinoma of the lung. Perhaps patients with this cell type should have a mediastinoscopy routinely prethoractomy, irrespective of whether the mediastinal lymph nodes appear normal in size on a staging CT scan.

Extrathoracic investigations

The ability to identify small metastatic deposits is as unsatisfactory for lung carcinomas as for other solid tumours. The techniques are relatively crude, and this partially explains the high extrathoracic relapse rate following so-called 'curative' resections for lung cancer. In patients with no symptoms other than those caused by their primary tumour, if there is no clinical evidence of neurological, hepatic, or bony disease and normal biochemistry, then imaging scans of brain, liver, and bones will be unhelpful. CT brain scans have a high accuracy in detailing cerebral metastases in patients with neurological symptoms. In patients with a palpable liver and/or abnormal liver function tests, a liver CT scan or ultrasound should be performed. CT scan of the upper abdomen identifies abnormalities of one or both adrenal glands in up to 10 per cent of patients considered for surgery. Fine-needle aspiration of the adrenal gland should be performed if this remains the only contraindication to pulmonary resection. Bone scans have a high false-positive rate due to Paget's disease, active arthritis, healing fractures, renal disease, and hyperparathyroidism. However, a bone scan should be ordered in patients with bone pain, local tenderness, or non-specific symptoms of weight loss or malaise.

Biopsy of enlarged lymph nodes and skin metastases should be carried out whenever indicated. If an isolated hepatic or bony lesion identified with isotope or CT scanning appears to be the only contraindication to surgery, this should be biopsied under radiological control.

The staging investigations for non-small-cell lung cancer are summarized in Fig. 8. The final procedure prethoracotomy is the assessment of the mediastinum. If CT scanning is normal, the surgeon can proceed directly to thoracotomy. If the CT scan is abnormal or is not available, mediastinal exploration should be performed first.

Treatment

Surgery

Surgery remains the modality most likely to cure non-small-cell lung cancer. In small-cell lung cancer the very occasional patient, usually presenting with a peripheral tumour, who remains operable after extensive staging investigations, is cured. These patients are rare, but have a 5-year survival rate in the region of 30 to 40 per cent.

Prior to surgery the patient should have been carefully staged (Fig. 8). All patients with stage IIIb disease (Table 3) should be rejected for thoracotomy, but those with stage I and II disease can be resected. Stage IIIa disease is technically resectable, but results are very poor if N2 (mediastinal node) involvement is macroscopically obvious at thoracotomy. In general, patients with squamous-cell carcinomas have higher 5- and 10-year survival rates than those with adenocarcinoma and large-cell carcinomas. Table 4 summarizes survival data at 5 years for preoperatively staged non-small-cell lung cancer. Clearly, small peripheral lesions with no nodal disease fare best (up to 70 per cent survival at 5 years), but the survival rate decreases with both size of tumour and presence of hilar node involvement.

In all, approximately 20 per cent of patients who present with non-small-cell lung cancer eventually come to thoracotomy. Of these, the overall survival rate at 5 years is approximately 25 per cent and at 10 years it is 16 to 18 per cent. Death from local or distant recurrence of the tumour is equally probable, highlighting the inadequacies of current staging techniques.

Pulmonary function must always be evaluated prior to consideration for resection. Pneumonectomy should probably not be undertaken if the patient cannot sustain a forced expiratory volume in 1 s (FEV_1) of more than 1.2 litres, bearing in mind that patients who have coexistent chronic obstructive airflow disease may not sustain the current value in exacerbations. In the middle range of

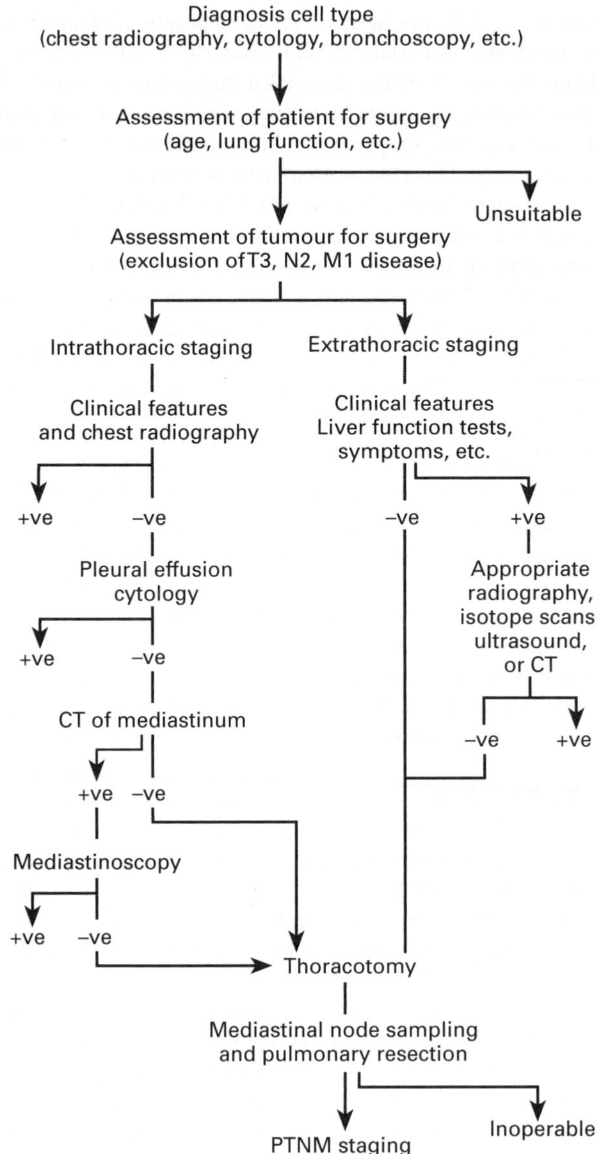

Fig. 8 Preoperative staging of non-small-cell lung cancer: +ve, positive; –ve, negative; PTNM staging, postsurgical pathological staging.
(See OTM3, p.2888 for source.)

ventilatory capacity the risk of resection is a matter of judgement based on the estimate of maximum tolerable resection and assessment of the functional integrity of the non-tumour-bearing lung. Combination of pulmonary function tests, including the 6 min walking test and regional function studies using 133-xenon, may be used in patients with borderline function.

Patients over 70 years of age appear to tolerate lobectomy as well as younger patients, although the mortality for pneumonectomy (8–10 per cent) is double that of those under 70. Hence resection should be encouraged in fit patients. Smokers should be persuaded to stop smoking before thoracotomy; continued smoking increases perioperative complications.

Radiotherapy

Patients who are excluded from surgery because of adverse prognostic factors, advanced stage of tumour, or other coincidental disease constitute the largest group treated with radiotherapy. Although the usual aim of radiotherapy will be palliative, there will be a small group of patients in whom more aggressive therapy will be used in the hope of cure, or at least long-term survival, particularly in those who have refused surgery. Radiotherapy for lung cancer is limited by the comparative radiosensitivity of three critical normal tissues likely to be included in the radiation beam: normal lung, spinal cord, and heart, each of which has a critical tolerance dose. There is no clear evidence for an optimum radical (curative) radiation dose, but doses of 5000 to 6000 rad (50–60 Gy) in 5 to 6 weeks are appropriate.

The role of radiotherapy

Alternative to surgery

In some patients with a technically resectable tumour, there may be medical contraindications for resection or the patient may refuse surgery. In general, the results of radical radiotherapy in these patients are inferior to the 5-year survival following surgery. The best result for radiotherapy was a 5-year survival rate of 22 per cent for peripheral squamous-cell cancers, but other series post a 5-year survival rate of 6 per cent.

Preoperative radiotherapy

Preoperative radiotherapy has been attempted in a few uncontrolled studies, but there is no evidence that this approach improves survival.

Postoperative radiotherapy

This has long been uncertain in value, but two recent, large, randomized studies and a meta-analysis showed no survival benefit for

Table 4 Cumulative percentage surviving 5 years and median survival by clinical and surgical TNM subsets (1986 Classification)

	Clinical			Surgical		
TNM subset	No.	Survival	Median survival	No.	Survival	Median survival
T1 N0 M0	591	61.9%	60 m	429	68.5%	60 m
T2 N0 M0	1012	35.8%	26 m	436	59.0%	60 m
T1 N1 M0	19	33.6%	20 m	67	54.1%	60 m
T2 N1 M0	176	22.7%	17 m	250	40.0%	29 m
T3 N0 M0	221	7.6%	8 m	57	44.2%	26 m
T3 N1 M0	71	7.7%	8 m	29	17.6%	16 m
Any N2 M0	497	4.9%	11m	168	28.8%	22 m

m = months.

Table 5 Objective average response to single-agent chemotherapy in lung cancer

Drug	Response (%)			
	Small-cell	Squamous-cell	Adeno-carcinoma	Large-cell
Ifosfamide	63	27	23	36
Vincristine	42	10	23	0
Epipodophyllotoxin	40	25	12	0
Cyclophosphamide	33	20	20	23
Methotrexate	30	25	30	12
Adriamycin	30	20	15	25
CCNU	15	30	20	17
Cisplatin	35	20	12	13

CCNU, chloroethyl-cyclohexyl-nitrosourea.

the addition of high-dose radiotherapy (50–60 Gy) to the mediastinal region following curative resection.

Radical radiotherapy for locally inoperable disease

In otherwise fit patients with small-volume intrathoracic disease which is not resectable, usually because of mediastinal involvement, it is common practice to attempt to cure with radiotherapy. Results are disappointing, even with doses of up to 60 Gy, with 5-year survival rates ranging from 5 to 17 per cent. Continuous hyperfractionated accelerated radiotherapy (CHART), when treatment is given as small fractions three times a day for 12 days has shown improved survival and better local disease control compared to daily fractionated dose radical radiotherapy. The results are particularly good in squamous cell cancers.

Palliation

The value of radiotherapy in palliating certain symptoms is beyond dispute. Haemoptysis and cough, can be controlled in up to 80 per cent of cases. Administration of two single fractions, each of 8.5 Gy, 1 week apart appears adequate. Dyspnoea from bronchial obstruction and dysphagia are also relieved in the majority of cases. Superior vena caval obstruction is relieved in about 80 per cent, but usually requires a more conventional course of five to ten fractions of radiotherapy. Pain from bone secondaries can be relieved in more than 50 per cent by a single fraction of 8 to 10 Gy, often given at the same time as a clinic visit. Brain metastases generally respond poorly to radiotherapy. A 48-h trial of dexamethasone, 4 mg orally four times daily, is recommended as initial management. If a worthwhile response follows the resolution of the oedema surrounding the metastases, then radiotherapy may consolidate this gain. Spinal cord compression is often preceded by pain and bony tenderness but responses to radiotherapy are disappointing.

Chemotherapy

Non-small-cell lung cancer

Although many cytotoxic drugs show modest activity against these tumours, there is no good evidence that they prolong survival in inoperable patients. Response rates (i.e. reduction in tumour volume by at least 50 per cent to single agents) of up to 30 per cent occur (Table 5), but there is no convincing evidence that chemotherapy prolongs survival. Newer agents such as etoposide, ifosfamide, cisplatin, navelbine, gemcytabine, and taxols have not conferred a significant survival advantage. Controlled studies incorporating combinations of cytotoxic agents in patients with advanced non-small-cell lung cancer, when compared with best supportive care, show little survival advantage. However, a recent meta-analysis of chemotherapy versus best supportive care in cases of advanced non-small-cell lung cancer reported a significant advantage for chemotherapy at 12 months after commencing treatment. Clearly more information is needed before the role of chemotherapy is defined with certainty. Clinical trials are also currently evaluating the possible use of chemotherapy as an adjuvant to surgery in locally inoperable tumours, and also before radical radiotherapy. These usually involve fit, relatively asymptomatic patients who tolerate chemotherapy well.

Small-cell lung cancer

This cell type has an explosive growth pattern so that the TNM staging makes no impact on prognosis or survival, almost certainly because staging puts most patients into the inoperable category and small metastases are not detected. However, simple staging has some prognostic impact, and those with limited disease (tumour confined to one hemithorax and the ipsilateral supraclavicular fossa) fare better than those with extensive disease (involvement of any site outside the hemithorax). The natural history of untreated small-cell lung cancer is about 3.5 months for limited disease and 6 weeks for extensive disease.

Small-cell lung cancer is much more sensitive to cytotoxic chemotherapy than the non-small-cell lung cancer tumours, with a much higher response rate to cytotoxic drugs (Table 5). Modern combination cytotoxic treatment, which is usually given every 3 weeks, has extended the median survival to 14–18 months for limited disease and to 9–12 months for extensive disease. Most combinations include cyclophosphamide, doxorubicin, etoposide, cisplatin, or vincristine, and give a complete response rate (i.e. disappearance of all measurable disease) of 40 to 50 per cent and a partial response rate (greater than 50 per cent reduction in tumour bulk) of 40 per cent, giving a total response rate of 80–85 per cent. Studies assessing the quality of life in patients presenting with small-cell lung cancer receiving chemotherapy have noted that over 70 per cent of patients have important symptoms such as weight loss, malaise, bone pain, dyspnoea, and haemoptysis at presentation. After 3 months of chemotherapy, relief of these symptoms occur in 60 to 70 per cent.

Intensifying the dosage or the frequency of administration of the cytotoxic agents has not shown benefit on median survival. Advantages are occasionally seen, but these have to be balanced by the increased toxicity resulting from this more aggressive approach.

Prognostic factors

Routine biochemical values such as serum sodium, albumin, and alkaline phosphatase allow separation of prognostic subgroups. Performance status and extent of disease are also important influences. For instance a good performance status and normal biochemical values (i.e. a good prognostic category) has a 2-year survival rate of 20 per cent, yet a correspondingly low performance status with one or more abnormal biochemical parameters (poor prognosis) has virtually no 2-year survivors (Fig. 9). Pretreatment weight loss of more than 3 kg indicates a worse prognosis.

Duration of treatment

Toxicity to chemotherapy increases with the number of courses given. Most of the tumour response occurs within the first three cycles.

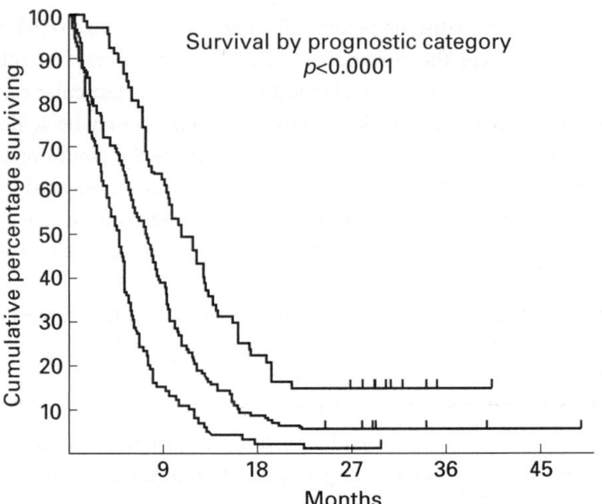

Fig. 9 The effect of prognostic grouping in survival in small-cell lung cancer. The upper curve represents good prognosis patients; the lower two curves are intermediate and poor prognosis groups respectively.

Studies attempting to minimize the duration of chemotherapy without adversely affecting survival have shown that six courses of combination chemotherapy, that is a course every 3 weeks, is optimal.

Long-term survival

Survival beyond 5 years is achieved in 5–7 per cent of patients with limited disease and <2 per cent with extensive disease. Most studies of long-term survival report late deaths due to other cancers, in particular non-small-cell lung cancers, in up to 30 per cent of these long-term survivors.

Radiotherapy

In addition to palliation of symptoms at relapse following chemotherapy, there is a small but definite benefit when thoracic irradiation is added to combination chemotherapy—a 5 per cent increase in survival at 3 years. Chest irradiation also significantly decreases the rate of recurrence at the primary tumour site and in the mediastinum. A total dose of 40 to 50 Gy is usually given.

Superior vena caval obstruction

Ten per cent of small-cell lung cancer patients present with this complication which responds as well as any presentation to chemotherapy. The onus is on the clinician to establish the diagnosis and the cell type of the tumour. Small-cell lung cancer should be treated with chemotherapy in the usual manner, whilst non-small-cell lung cancer should be treated with radiotherapy.

Cranial irradiation

Cranial metastases are common. Ten per cent of patients with an incomplete response develop brain metastases as their first site of relapse. Prophylactic cranial irradiation given at the end of chemotherapy will delay the presentation of cerebral metastases and also reduce their overall incidence. However, there is no evidence of prolonged survival.

General management

There are certain complications which require specific measures to alleviate symptoms.

Patients who seem likely to survive for 6 months or more and who have vocal chord paralysis find benefit from an injection of Teflon into the affected chord which may restore voice and reduces the risk of aspiration. Occurrence of upper airway obstruction causing stridor, or obstruction of the lower major airways, in non-small-cell lung cancer patients is usually initially treated with radiotherapy. Should this complication recur or be unsuitable for radiotherapy, it could be suitable for laser photocoagulation administered either via the fibre-optic bronchoscope or under general anaesthetic via a rigid instrument. Laser therapy for carcinoma of the bronchus is most suitable as a palliative treatment of tumours occluding large airways. Laser therapy is used predominantly for recurrence of tumour, usually after radiotherapy has failed. Trials are in progress assessing the additional benefits of endobronchial radiotherapy using irridium or caesium wires delivered via the fibre-optic bronchoscope. This procedure irradiates endobronchial tumour to a circumferential depth of about 1 cm, and will often produce a further remission. It is used where further external beam radiotherapy cannot be given because of the risk of exceeding normal tissue tolerance.

Infection distal to tumour requires antibiotic therapy and, where appropriate, oxygen therapy and bronchodilators. Severe recurrent haemoptysis may also be controlled by radiotherapy or laser.

Malignant pleural effusion recurs after aspiration unless the pleural space is obliterated. Chemical pleurodesis can be induced by intrapleural tetracycline and gives successful pleurodesis in 50 to 70 per cent of patients.

Prednisolone, 20 mg orally daily, is often used to improve the sense of well-being, as are blood transfusion or hyperalimentation.

Terminal care is described in Section 15, but the importance of the combined support to the patient and the family given by the family doctor, nursing and hospice organizations, and the hospital team cannot be emphasized too much.

Prevention

Lung cancer is almost totally preventable. The strategy of any preventive measures must be based on the observations that lung cancer is extremely rare in non-smokers. The risk increases proportionately to the amount smoked, the benefit from stopping smoking is evident within 5 years, and that the risk for an ex-smoker at any given time after stopping is determined by the length of time he or she had smoked before stopping. The promotion of cigarettes with low tar, nicotine, and carbon monoxide contents may have made a small contribution to prevention, but low-tar cigarettes are not a substitute for giving up smoking.

The identification of occupational hazards and implementation of appropriate measures to safeguard the health of employees are clearly important preventive measures, even although the number at risk is very small.

Prospective lung cancer screening programmes in males aged 45 years and above who smoke at least 20 cigarettes per day have been carried out using both chest radiography and pooled 3-day sputum analysis every 4 months. They are unlikely to form the basis of standard practice as there is no evidence that early detection is translated into increased cure rate.

Carcinoid tumours (see also Chapter 5.5)

The slow-growing, intrabronchial lesions previously grouped under the heading of bronchial adenoma have now been reclassified into bronchial carcinoids, adenoid cystic tumours, and mucoepidermoid tumours. They are not related to cigarette smoking, and tend to be diagnosed at a younger age than carcinoma of the bronchus. These tumours were once thought to be benign but they are potentially, and often frankly, malignant, being capable not only of destructive local growth but also of metastasis to regional lymph nodes in about one-third of patients and to distant organs in about 10 per cent. They are occasionally located in the trachea.

The most common symptoms are cough, haemoptysis, and recurrent pneumonia, although not infrequently the lesion is discovered on routine radiographic examination before symptoms develop. Carcinoids may produce the classical symptom pattern of intermittent cyanotic flushings, intestinal cramps and diarrhoea, bronchoconstriction, and cardiovascular lesions in a few cases when there are extensive liver secondaries. As the majority of the tumours occur in main stem or the proximal portions of lobar bronchi, bronchoscopy is usually the definitive diagnostic measure. The tumour appears as a white or pink polypid or lobulated mass, with the bronchial mucosa appearing to be intact. Biopsy may be followed by brisk haemoptysis.

Surgical resection is the treatment of choice. In the absence of regional spread or distant metastases 5-year survival prospects are excellent, but if there is involvement of regional nodes, survival rates fall to 70 per cent. The mechanism and management of the general symptoms of the carcinoid syndrome are described in Chapter 5.5.

Further reading

Carney, D.N. (1992). Biology of small-cell lung cancer. *Lancet*, **339**, 843–6.

Coggon, D. and Acheson, E.D. (1983). Trends in lung cancer mortality. *Thorax*, **38**, 721–3.

Goldstraw, P. (1992). The practice of cardiothoracic surgeons in the peri-operative staging of lung cancer. *Thorax*, **47**, 1–2.

Hansen, H.H. (1992). Management of small-cell lung cancer. *Lancet*, **339**, 846–9.

Izbicki, J.R., Thetter, O., Karg, O., *et al.* (1992). Accuracy of computed tomographic scan and surgical assessment for staging of bronchial carcinoma. A prospective study. *Journal of Thoracic and Cardiovascular Surgery*, **104**, 413–20.

Mountain, C.F. (1997). Revisions in the international system staging for lung cancer. *Chest*, **111**, 1710–17.

Saunders, M., Dische, S., Barrett, A., *et al.* (1997). Continuous hyperfractionated accelerated radiotherapy (CHART) versus conventional radiotherapy in non-small-cell lung cancer; a randomised multicentre trial. *Lancet*, **350**, 161–5.

Chapter 4.39

Pulmonary metastases

S. G. Spiro

Malignant metastasis to the lung may present as a solitary enlarging nodule, as multiple nodules, or with diffuse lymphatic involvement.

Solitary metastasis represents some 10 per cent of round lesions in general, but some 70 per cent in patients with a known malignancy. Colorectal cancer is the commonest tumour of origin. Diagnosis can usually be secured by percutaneous CT-guided biopsy. In rare cases, surgical excision may prolong survival or result in cure.

Multiple metastases range enormously in size and number from 'cannon balls' to miliary shadowing, and may be accompanied by hilar lymphadenopathy or pleural effusion. Breast, colon, renal, and lung primaries are the commonest underlying tumours, but others include tumours amenable to chemotherapy, such as testicular cancer and choriocarcinoma, and also sarcomas. Diagnosis may be achieved by cytology or histology on various samples from the pleura or lung and can occasionally be made from cytology on expectoration or induced sputum. Solitary or multiple Kaposi's sarcoma is a feature of AIDS, and can involve the bronchi and pleura as well as lung tissue.

Lymphangitis carcinomatosa is most commonly due to breast and primary lung tumours. The radiograph shows diffusely increased interstitial markings that may be accompanied by Kerley B lines, hilar lymphadenopathy, or pleural effusion. Diagnosis may be established by cytology from sputum or pleural fluid, but often requires bronchoscopic or transbronchial lung biopsy. Later, progressive and severe breathlessness with hypoxaemia often develops, and requires vigorous palliative relief with opiate and oxygen supplementation.

Occasionally metastasis, presenting as haemoptysis, may be confined to a bronchus and therefore is not visible on a plain chest radiograph. Renal carcinoma and malignant melanoma are recorded causes. Diagnosis requires bronchoscopy, and radiotherapy is usually effective in controlling the haemoptysis.

Further reading

Ishida, T., Kaneko, S., Yokoyama, H., *et al.* (1992). Metastatic lung tumours and extended indications for surgery. *International Surgery*, **77**, 173–7.

Lower, E.E. and Baughman, R.P. (1992). Pulmonary lymphangitis metastasis from breast cancer. Lymphocytic alveolitis is associated with favourable prognosis. *Chest*, **103**, 1113–17.

Stewart, J.R., Carey, J.A., Merrill, W.H., Frist, W.H., Hammon, J.W., Jr, and Bender, H.W., Jr. (1992). Twenty years' experience with pulmonary metastasectomy. *American Surgeon*, **58**, 100–3.

Chapter 4.40

Pleural tumours

M. K. Benson

Primary pleural tumours are relatively rare, although malignant mesothelioma has received much attention because of its increasing incidence and association with asbestos exposure. Pleural plaques are also associated with asbestos exposure but should not be regarded as true tumours since they represent local areas of fibrocollagenous thickening. The classic, benign tumour of the pleura is fibrous mesothelioma (pleural fibroma).

In contrast, pleural involvement by metastatic disease is very common. It can occur in association with most carcinomas but is particularly associated with primaries arising in the lung, breast, or colon. Malignant lymphomas may also present with pleural involvement. Tumours arising in adjacent structures, such as diaphragm and chest wall, may also invade the pleura. Both benign and malignant tumours can originate from muscle, adipose tissue, nerves, blood vessels, and bones. All are rare and the diversity of sites and types of tumour results in a variety of clinical presentations.

Benign tumours

Benign fibrous mesothelioma

These tumours are rare but can occur in virtually any age group. They bear no relationship to the development of malignant mesotheliomas and are not associated with exposure to asbestos or other industrial pollutants. They originate from a pedicle, usually from the visceral pleura. Macroscopically they are firm, lobulated, and well encapsulated. The cut surface is white or grey and can have a whorled appearance. They vary in size but can on occasions be very large with weights of 2 or 3 kg.

Clinical features

The tumours are often discovered on routine chest radiology in otherwise asymptomatic individuals. Large tumours can result in chest discomfort and breathlessness, presumably due to compression of adjacent lung. Spontaneous hypoglycaemia is an associated feature in a small proportion of patients.

Radiologically it may be difficult to decide whether a pleural-based nodule is arising from the pleura or within adjacent lung. The diagnosis is usually established after surgical excision. Although benign, with no potential for metastatic spread, there is a possibility of local recurrence if the pedicle has not been completely excised.

Malignant mesothelioma

A malignant mesothelioma derives from mesothelial cells and although most commonly arising in the pleura, can also occur in the peritoneum or rarely the pericardium. Malignant mesotheliomas were first recognised in the 1950s and during the next decade much evidence accumulated indicating a strong link between the exposure to asbestos and development of a mesothelioma. Asbestos is a collective term given to a group of silicate minerals commercially useful because of their heat resistant properties. Exposure to asbestos is greatest in those involved in mining or quarrying the material and in those who handle the raw fibres. Many workers engaged in the ship building industry in the 1940s and 50s were exposed to asbestos and it has also been widely used in the building industry. The incidence of asbestos-related diseases in the UK is still rising and this trend is set to continue well into the next century. This reflects the fact that there is a long interval, usually in excess of 20 years, between initial exposure and subsequent development of disease. Although most asbestos workers have been exposed to a mixture of fibres, there is good epidemiological evidence that crocidolite (blue asbestos) is more hazardous than chrysotile (white asbestos).

It is estimated that the annual incidence of developing a mesothelioma in subjects with no history of asbestos exposure is about one per million. The risk increases in those exposed to asbestos and is a function of a concentration of fibres and duration of exposure. Individuals exposed to low levels of environmental contamination also have a slightly increased risk. Endemic pleural mesothelioma has been reported from certain areas of central Turkey, Cyprus, and Greece and is related to local mining of zeolite and other asbestos minerals.

Pathology

A mesothelioma can arise from either visceral or parietal pleura, initially as a local mass associated with a pleural effusion. As it progresses, there is gradual encasement of the lung and extension into adjacent structures including chest wall and pericardium. Metastatic disease is relatively uncommon although involvement of the contralateral lung and pleura, liver, and bone are recognized sites for secondary spread.

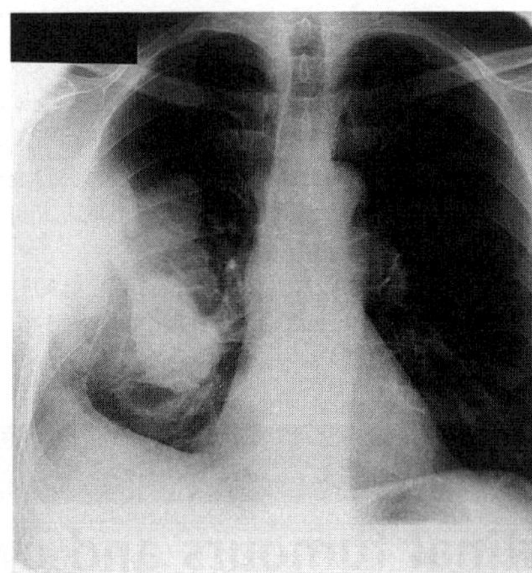

Fig. 1 Chest radiograph showing lobulated pleural thickening due to mesothelioma.

Histologically, the diagnosis can be difficult and there are a diversity of histological patterns ranging from well-differentiated epithelial or sarcomatous forms to more undifferentiated tumours. Even after biopsy, there may be difficulty in distinguishing between a malignant mesothelioma and benign pleural disease.

Clinical presentation

The age of presentation is usually between 50 and 70 and male predominance reflects occupational exposure. Symptoms due to local disease are mainly those of pain and breathlessness. Pain may be pleuritic in nature although is often a dull, continuous ache due to direct involvement of the chest wall.

Systemic symptoms include tiredness, anorexia, weight loss, fever, and sweats. Finger clubbing is rare. Physical findings are those of a pleural effusion but with advanced disease there is progressive reduction in chest wall movement.

Investigations

A chest radiograph often demonstrates a pleural effusion with a tumour being suspected if there is pleural thickening having a lobulated outline (Fig. 1). This can be more easily identified on a CT scan. Pleural aspiration with cytological examination of pleural fluid may reveal a definitive diagnosis in about one-third of patients. Biopsy may increase the diagnostic yield although even with samples obtained under direct vision at thoracoscopy or thoracotomy, there may be some diagnostic uncertainty.

Management

There is no effective curative treatment despite occasional enthusiastic reports of good results from radical surgery for limited disease. Response to radiotherapy is disappointing, although palliative relief of pain may be achieved if there is direct invasion of bone or nerve root. Regular analgesics or nerve blocks may also be helpful for localized pain. Pleural aspiration with pleurodesis is of benefit in the relief of breathlessness due to recurrent pleural effusions.

The prognosis is poor with a median survival of approximately 18 months. It is important to note that it is an industrially notifiable disease for which the patient and family can receive financial compensation.

Further reading

Hillerdal, G. (1983). Malignant mesothelioma in 1982: review of 4710 published cases. *British Journal of Diseases of the Chest,* 77, 321–43.

Jaurand, M.C., Bignong, J., and Brochard, P. (ed.) (1993). Mesothelial cell and mesothelioma. Past, present and future. *European Respiratory Review,* 3, review 11.

Peto, J., Hodgson, J.T., Matthews, F.E., and Jones, J.R. (1995). Continuing increase in mesothelioma mortality in Britain. *Lancet,* 345, 535–9.

Chapter 4.41

Mediastinal tumours and cysts

M. K. Benson

Anatomy

The mediastinum encompasses those structures within the thorax excluding the lungs. The superior boundary is the thoracic inlet represented by a plane at the level of the first rib. The inferior boundary is the diaphragm. Traditionally, the mediastinum has been subdivided into a number of compartments: classically a superior and inferior compartment with the latter being subdivided into anterior, middle, and posterior divisions. In fact, there are no true anatomical boundaries, and structures in the superior mediastinum are contiguous with those inferiorly. A more logical subdivision is simply into anterior, middle, and posterior compartments (Fig. 1). Such a division can help to compartmentalize what is a complex anatomy and to give some guidance as to the most likely pathology occurring in any particular area.

The anterior mediastinum is bounded by the sternum anteriorly and by pericardium and aorta posteriorly. It contains the remnant of the thymus gland, branches of the internal mammary artery, veins, and associated lymph nodes.

The middle mediastinum contains the pericardium, ascending aorta and aortic arch, the vena cavae, the brachiocephalic vessels, and the pulmonary arteries and veins. It also encompasses the trachea and major bronchi with their associated lymph nodes, the phrenic nerves, and, in its upper portion, the vagus nerve.

The posterior mediastinum is bounded anteriorly by the pericardium, laterally by the mediastinal pleura, and posteriorly by the vertebral bodies. It contains the descending thoracic aorta, oesophagus, azygos veins, thoracic duct, and autonomic nerves.

Lymph nodes are common to all three compartments and knowledge of their anatomical relationships together with their sites of drainage is helpful in interpreting an abnormal chest radiograph with mediastinal enlargement. The majority of the nodes lie in the middle mediastinum. Hilar nodes are located around bronchi and pulmonary vessels and receive afferent drainage from the lungs. Carinal nodes at the tracheal bifurcation surround the origin of right and left main bronchi. Paratracheal nodes are situated in front of and to either side of the trachea.

Posterior
Anterosuperior
Middle
(a)
Anterior
Middle
Posterior
(b)

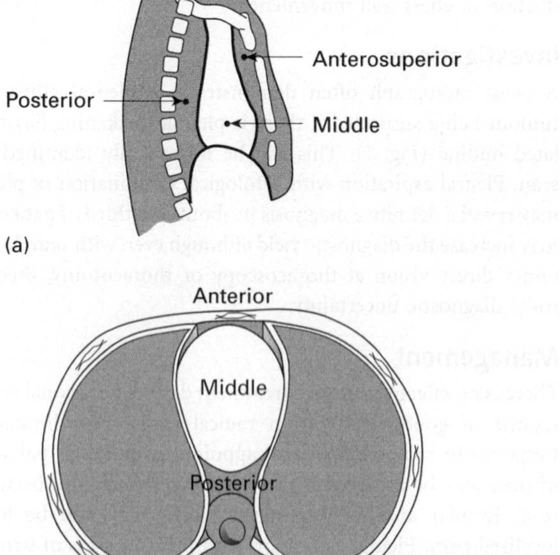

Fig. 1 A schematic representation of the mediastinal compartments: (a) lateral projection showing division into anterior (or anterosuperior), middle, and posterior compartments; (b) cross-sectional depiction.

Mediastinal masses

It is not surprising that the diversity of anatomical structures in the mediastinum is reflected by an equally diverse range of neoplastic, developmental, and inflammatory masses. Whilst clinical symptoms and signs may be of diagnostic value, a significant proportion of mediastinal masses, particularly those which are benign, tend to be asymptomatic and are usually detected on routine chest radiography. The advent of computed tomography and magnetic resonance imaging has provided accurate anatomical localization which can be of considerable diagnostic value, since most primary cysts and tumours of the mediastinum have characteristic compartments of origin (Table 1).

Table 1 Mediastinal masses

Anterior compartment	Middle compartment	Posterior compartment
←	Lymph nodes	→
	Sarcoidosis	
	Infections	
	(tuberculosis)	
	Lymphoma	
	Castleman's disease	
Thyroid	→	→
Retrosternal goitre		
Thyroid carcinoma		
Thymus	Vascular	→
Thymoma	Aneurysm of aorta	
Hyperplasia	Anomalous vessels	
Cyst		
Lymphoma	Pericardium	Neural tumours
	Cysts	Neurolemmoma
Germ-cell tumours	Fat pad	Neurofibroma
Teratoma		Ganglioneuroma
Seminoma	Bronchogenic cysts	Neuroblastoma
Other miscellaneous		Phaeochromocytoma
Parathyroid adenoma		

Lymph node masses and aneurysms of the aorta tend to be the exception and can be found in any of the mediastinal compartments.

General considerations: clinical features

Benign lesions tend to be asymptomatic and are most commonly detected on routine chest radiography. Patients presenting with symptoms are more likely to have malignant disease.

Non-specific symptoms of a constitutional nature, such as fever or weight loss, occur with certain types of tumour such as lymphomas or thymic tumours. The commonest symptoms are usually cough or chest discomfort and arise as a consequence of distortion of the normal mediastinal anatomy. Compression of vital structures can also result in specific symptoms such as stridor, dysphagia, or superior vena caval obstruction.

Diagnostic approach

The finding of a mediastinal abnormality on chest radiograph, whether or not accompanied by specific clinical features, is usually an indication for further investigation. Computed tomography can define the anatomy and relationship to normal structures. It is not ideal for determining the composition of any particular mass although it can demonstrate heterogenicity or the presence of calcification. Contrast enhancement can be used to identify vascular structures.

Fine needle aspiration is widely used in the investigation of mediastinal masses, particularly when performed in conjunction with CT scanning. The presence of a cyst can be confirmed by aspiration of clear fluid. Anterior mediastinal masses can easily be approached percutaneously although cytological examination alone is often insufficient and samples for histological examination are more likely to be of diagnostic value. Hence, there is still a place for open biopsy to be performed. Similarly, neural tumours arising in the posterior mediastinum usually require surgical resection and there is often little to be gained by preceding this with fine needle aspiration.

Anterior mediastinal masses

Thymus

The thymus is located in the superior portion of the anterior mediastinum. Radiographically, the normal thymus can only be seen in infancy. Regression occurs during childhood and there is fatty replacement of normal thymic tissue. Enlargement of the thymus is the commonest single cause of an anterior mediastinal mass. Possible causes include the development of a thymoma, thymic hyperplasia, thymic cyst, or involvement by lymphoma.

A thymoma derives from thymic epithelium and although these tumours are often benign, they can behave in a malignant fashion with invasion of adjacent structures. Distant metastases are rare. They occur mostly in middle-aged adults. Myasthenia gravis is an associated systemic disorder and, although reports vary, some 30 per cent of patients have an association between a thymic tumour and myasthenia. Rare associations include red cell aplasia, hypogammaglobulinaemia, systemic lupus erythematosis, and inflammatory bowel disease. The majority of thymomas are slowly growing, lobulated masses which are well encapsulated. Surgical resection can be expected to result in a cure. Local invasion is less common but often precludes complete resection and recurrence is the rule. Adjuvant radiotherapy can offer additional benefit to this group of patients.

Thymic hyperplasia is uncommon and presents as an enlargement of the thymus which retains normal morphology. Thymic cysts are also uncommon. They can contain straw-coloured fluid. They can arise in thymomas and also in Hodgkin's disease. Thus, thorough cytological examination of the cyst contents and wall must be carried out to exclude malignancy.

Thymic lymphoma is fairly frequent, particularly in patients with Hodgkin's disease. There are no specific diagnostic features although disease confined to the thymus is relatively uncommon.

Germ-cell tumours

This group of neoplasms includes tumours which are identical with certain testicular and ovarian neoplasms and are thought to be derived from primitive germ cells that have migrated to the mediastinum during oncogenesis. They include benign and malignant teratoma, seminoma, chorion carcinoma, and embryonal carcinoma. They usually present in early adult life. The benign tumours are more common in females and malignant tumours in males.

Mediastinal germ-cell tumours have a varied and often mixed histological appearance which can make pathological diagnosis difficult. Since malignant tumours may be very responsive to chemotherapy or radiotherapy, it is important to make a definitive diagnosis. This can be assisted by detection of elevated levels of α-fetoprotein, β-human chorionic gonadotrophin, and carcinoembryonic antigen.

Teratomas consist of a disorganized mixture of ectodermal, mesodermal, and endodermal tissues and can include skin, hair, cartilage, bone, and neural tissue. The majority are benign and often contained cystic areas. Unless there is a major contraindication to surgery, they should be excised to prevent further expansion and to exclude malignant change.

Seminomas are second in frequency to teratomas and occur almost exclusively in young men. They are radiosensitive and 5-year survival rates reach 75 per cent.

Thyroid masses

Retrosternal extension of an enlarged thyroid represents one of the more common causes of a mass in the superior mediastinum. The majority arise in the neck and extend into the anterior mediastinum through the thoracic inlet. They are usually multinodular and benign. The majority of patients are asymptomatic although compression of the trachea at the thoracic inlet can result in respiratory distress and is an absolute indication for surgical resection.

Middle mediastinal masses

Lymphadenopathy

Nodes in the middle mediastinum represent the most common site of intrathoracic lymphadenopathy. Reactive changes occur in association with many pulmonary infections although usually the nodes are not grossly enlarged and may be undetected on plain chest radiograph. Gross lymphadenopathy is a common manifestation of metastatic carcinoma, lymphoma, sarcoidosis, and primary tuberculosis. Less common causes can be due to drug toxicity, angioimmunoblastic lymphadenopathy, amyloidosis, and giant follicular lymph node hyperplasia (Castleman's disease (Fig. 2)). This latter syndrome, although rare, merits specific consideration. Its aetiology is unknown and it is not clear as to whether it represents a focus of lymphoid hyerplasia or has an infectious origin. The lesion consists of a vascular tumour with satellite lymphadenopathy. In addition to local symptoms due to compression, there may be systemic symptoms of fever, anaemia, and weight loss. There are no diagnostic radiographic features. The diagnosis is usually made after surgical resection or biopsy. The condition is regarded as benign although a small group

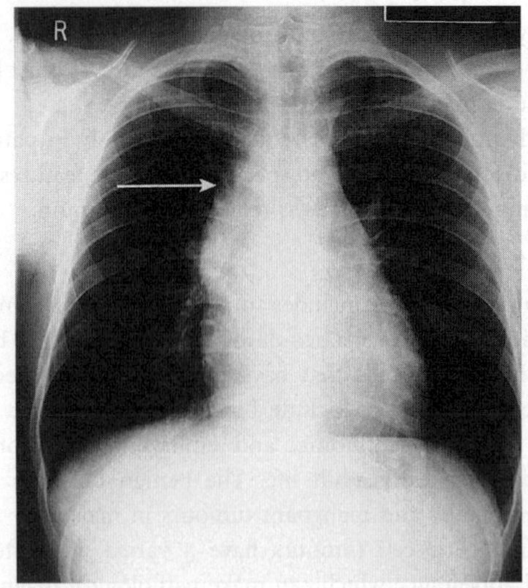

(a)

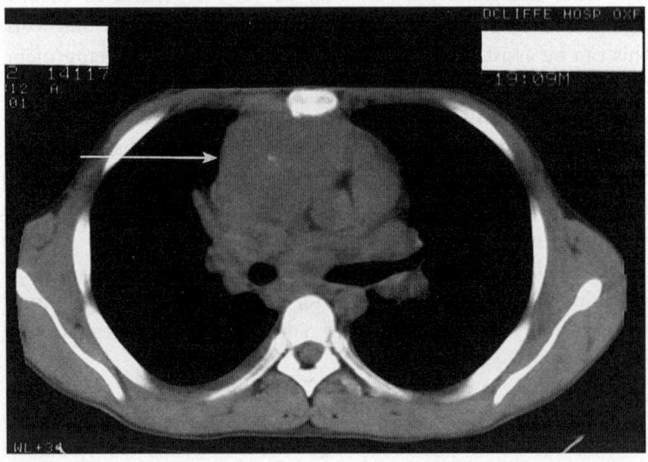

(b)

Fig. 2(a,b) Chest radiograph and CT scan showing large anterior mediastinal mass which on histology showed features of Castleman's disease.

of patients with multicentric disease have progressive hyperplasia, recurrent infections, and subsequent development of a frank lymphoma.

Mediastinal cysts

Cysts within the mediastinum represent a relatively common cause of a mediastinal mass. They can arise in association with the pericardium, bronchi, gut, or thoracic duct. The majority of patients are asymptomatic.

Pericardial cysts develop in relationship to the pericardium although rarely communicate directly with the pericardial sac. They are most commonly adjacent to the right heart border and can be mistaken for a pericardial fat pad or a hernia through the foramen of Morgagni. Surgical excision is unnecessary.

Bronchogenic cysts arise adjacent to the trachea or major bronchi (Fig. 3). They are lined by respiratory epithelium and can contain thick, inspissated mucus. Occasionally they communicate with the trachea resulting in an increased tendency to recurrent infection. Surgical excision is recommended if there are associated symptoms.

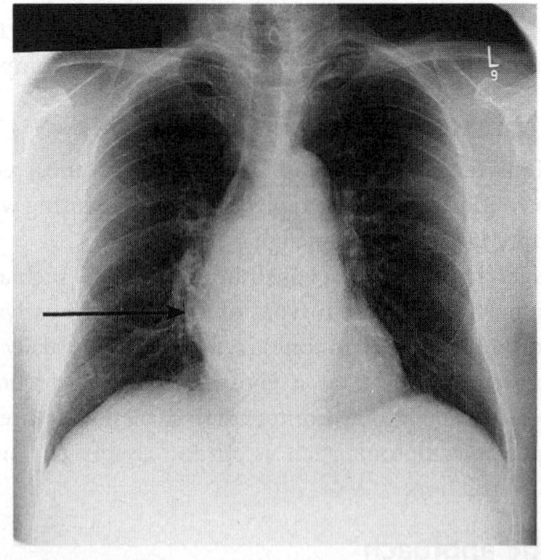

(a)

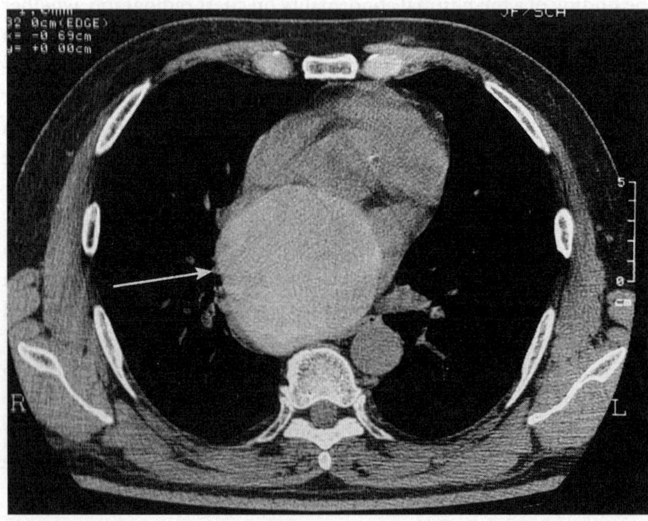

(b)

Fig. 3(a,b) Chest radiograph and CT scan showing a large mass in the mediastinum. This represents a large bronchogenic cyst which had been present for 20 years and was finally removed when compression of the oesophagus resulted in dysphagia.

Posterior mediastinal masses

Oesophageal lesions and aneurysms of the descending thoracic aorta can both result in abnormal shadows in the posterior mediastinum. Neural tumours comprise the vast majority of tumour masses. Overall figures suggest that some 25 per cent will be malignant, although this proportion is higher in children. Benign tumours tend to be asymptomatic, whilst malignant tumours cause pressure effects. Tumours arising from peripheral nerves include neurilemmoma (Schwannoma) and neurofibroma, together with their malignant counterparts. Tumours of the autonomic chain include ganglioneuroma and neuroblastoma.

A neurilemmoma is the commonest neural tumour arising in the mediastinum and usually presents in middle age. They can extend into the intravertebral foramen producing a dumb-bell appearance. CT scanning or magnetic resonance imaging should be undertaken prior to surgical excision.

Neurofibromata are also common and derive from the nerve sheath. They may be solitary although some 20 per cent of patients have a more generalized picture of neurofibromatosis. Surgical resection is recommended partly because of the small risk of developing a malignant neurosarcoma, which has a very poor prognosis.

Ganglioneuroma arise from the autonomic plexus and may have associated endocrine symptoms such as flushing, sweating, diarrhoea, and hypertension. They may be very large before becoming clinically apparent.

Ganglioneuroblastoma and neuroblastoma represent the malignant end of the spectrum and are predominantly tumours of infants and children. Neuroblastoma, in particular, is highly invasive and metastatic spread is often established by the time of presentation.

Further reading

Adkins, R.B., Maples M.D., and Hainsworth, J.D. (1984). Primary malignant mediastinal tumours. *Annals of Thoracic Surgery*, **38**, 648–59.

Childs, A.W., Goldstraw, P., Nicholls, J.E., Dearnaley, D.P., and Horwich, A. (1993). Primary malignant mediastinal germ cell tumours: improved prognosis with platinum based chemotherapy and surgery. *British Journal of Cancer*, **67**, 1091–100.

Davis, R.D., Oldham, H.N., and Sabesdon, D.C. (1987). Primary cysts and neoplasms of the mediastinum: recent changes in clinical presentation, methods of diagnosis, management and results. *Annals of Thoracic Surgery*, **44**, 229–37.

Lewis, B.D., Hurt, R.D., Payne, W.S., Farrow, G.M., Knapp, R.H., and Muhm, J.R. (1983). Benign teratomas of the mediastinum. *Journal of Thoracic and Cardiovascular Surgery*, **86**, 727–31.

Mullen, B. and Richardson, J.D. (1986). Primary anterior mediastinal tumours in children and adults. *Annals of Thoracic Surgery*, **42**, 338–45.

Respiratory failure

Chapter 4.42

Definition and causes

J. Moxham

Definition

Respiratory failure can be defined as specified degree of hyopoxia (arterial carbon dioxide pressure (PaO_2) less than 8 kPa or 60 mmHg) or hypercapnia ($PaCO_2$ more than 6.0 kPa or 45 mmHg).

Hypoxia

Failure of oxygenation is most commonly due to an imbalance between lung ventilation and perfusion. In pneumonia, for example, the consolidated lung is perfused but not ventilated. Although reflex reductions in perfusion of the non-ventilated area of lung do occur, this is not sufficient to avoid a large shunt of blood through the lung. Although impaired diffusion capacity can cause hypoxia (as in severe emphysema) and inadequate ventilation may also be responsible (as in obstructive sleep apnoea or sedative overdose), ventilation perfusion (V/Q) mismatches are the major mechanism of hypoxaemia in most patients with respiratory disease.

Hypoxia stimulates ventilation and when ventilatory capacity is adequate the response to hypoxia is hypocapnia. The capacity of hyperventilation to correct arterial hypoxia is limited by the full saturation of capillary blood in regions of the lung with normal V/Q ratios.

Effects of hypoxia

The ability to withstand hypoxia depends on whether it occurs acutely or is chronic, and it is tissue oxygen delivery and uptake that is vital. Thus, haemoglobin concentration and function, cardiac output and tissue perfusion, and peripheral tissue oxygen utilization are just as important as arterial oxygen tension and saturation.

Acute hypoxia

Minor hypoxia has few symptoms or signs, but acute severe hypoxia causes anxiety, restlessness, sweating, and, if sufficiently severe, confusion. Examination reveals central cyanosis, poor peripheral perfusion (blood flow is redistributed to more vital organs), and, importantly, tachycardia. Acute hypoxia is poorly tolerated if patients are anaemic or hypovolaemic, or have significant cardiac or vascular disease; thus severe hypoxia can precipitate angina in patients with anaemia, confusion in those with cardiac failure, or stroke in those with cerebrovascular disease.

Chronic hypoxia

When hypoxia develops slowly compensatory mechanisms come into play. The release of erythropoietin by the kidney, in response to chronic hypoxia, causes secondary polycythaemia which enhances the oxygen-carrying capacity of blood, but also increases blood viscosity which may eventually impair overall tissue oxygen delivery. Poor cerebral perfusion, secondary to high viscosity of blood, can contribute to lethargy, mental slowing, and confusion.

Acute hypoxia causes pulmonary hypertension due to pulmonary arterial vasoconstriction which reverses when hypoxia is corrected. Chronic hypoxia also causes pulmonary hypertension which, with time, becomes fixed as a consequence of secondary changes in the pulmonary vasculature, including muscular hypertrophy and intimal thickening.

Assessment of oxygenation

The clinical assessment of cyanosis is notoriously inaccurate. Though cyanosis can be detected at an SaO_2 of 90 per cent, it may not be obvious until the SaO_2 is approximately 80 per cent, given a normal haemoglobin concentration. Therefore cyanosis is a sign of severe hypoxaemia and a measurement of PaO_2 is essential for assessment.

Instantaneous, and if necessary continuous, non-invasive measurement by oximetry has greatly facilitated the assessment of oxygenation in patients with respiratory failure. Oximetry is least helpful when PaO_2 is near normal, in which case changes of 1–2 kPa cause little alteration in oxygen saturation. However, over the clinically important range of PaO_2, oxygen saturation monitoring provides accurate and useful information and is sensitive to small changes in PaO_2.

The effectiveness of oxygen uptake by the lung can only be accurately assessed by relating PaO_2 to the oxygen tension in inspired gas, that is the alveolar–arterial oxygen difference $P(A–a)O_2$ which is normally <2.5 kPa.

The alveolar–arterial oxygen gradient gives insight into the severity of impaired oxygenation by the lung and is particularly useful when assessing the progress of patients over days and weeks. During this period PIO_2, $PaCO_2$, and PaO_2 will all change, but sequential documentation of $P(A–a)O_2$ allows progress to be assessed accurately.

The alveolar–arterial oxygen gradient is a good measure of the oxygenating capacity of the lung, but it is equally important to assess the adequacy of tissue oxygenation. If tissue oxygen delivery is adequate, the oxygen saturation of venous blood returning to the heart from the peripheral tissues is normal (>75 per cent). If tissue oxygen delivery is inadequate, due for example to severe hypoxia, anaemia, or poor cardiac output, following the extraction of required oxygen by the peripheral tissues the venous oxygen saturation will be low. Measurements are best made using venous blood sampled from the pulmonary artery—mixed venous oxygen saturation.

Hypercapnia

The shape of the carbon dioxide dissociation curve is different from that for oxygen and over the relevant range the relationship between $PaCO_2$ and carbon dioxide concentration is almost linear compared with the sigmoid shape of the oxygen dissociation curve. Enhanced elimination of carbon dioxide from well-ventilated areas of the lung can compensate for the inadequate ventilation of abnormal areas. Thus many patients with pulmonary diseases which cause V/Q mismatch characteristically have hypoxaemia but a normal or low $PaCO_2$.

Overall, arterial PCO_2 is determined by the balance between carbon dioxide production and alveolar ventilation. When carbon dioxide production is constant $PaCO_2$ is determined solely by alveolar ventilation; hypercapnia is synonymous with hypoventilation.

Effects of hypercapnia

Acute hypercapnia causes restlessness, confusion, and flapping tremor. These central nervous effects are due to raised intracranial pressure and to increased cerebral blood flow; eventually cerebral oedema and papilloedema can occur. Peripherally, the acidosis caused by carbon dioxide promotes profound vasodilatation with bounding pulses and warm limbs. Chronic hypercapnia of gradual onset is better tolerated, but because hypoventilation is usually greatest at night patients often have poor sleep quality, tiredness, impaired intellectual performance, personality changes, and frequently report early-morning headaches which clear as ventilation improves upon wakefulness.

Assessment of hypercapnia

The symptoms and signs of hypercapnia are frequently both non-specific and insensitive.

Hypercapnia causes a respiratory acidosis. Carbon dioxide is in equilibrium with carbonic acid, and any increase in carbon dioxide increases this acid which dissociates into bicarbonate and hydrogen ions, thereby reducing pH. As a compensatory mechanism the kidney retains bicarbonate and pH is returned to normal (Fig. 1). Severe acidosis (pH less than 7.20) due to acute ventilatory failure carries a high mortality unless promptly reversed. However, well-compensated, chronic ventilatory failure, with a normal pH may persist for months or years, for example in patients with chronic obstructive lung disease. Other patients may only develop hypercapnia at night, for example some patients with kyphoscoliosis in whom a raised bicarbonate level and a significant base excess may be present by day even though $PaCO_2$ is normal.

Causes of respiratory failure

The causes of respiratory failure are given in Table 1. This table broadly divides the causes of respiratory failure into type 1 and type 2. In general terms this is useful, but the distinction must not be viewed as rigid since many of the conditions which give rise to type 1 failure can eventually progress to cause hypercapnia. Similarly, many of the causes of type 2 ventilatory failure cause hypoxaemia without hypercapnia early in their course.

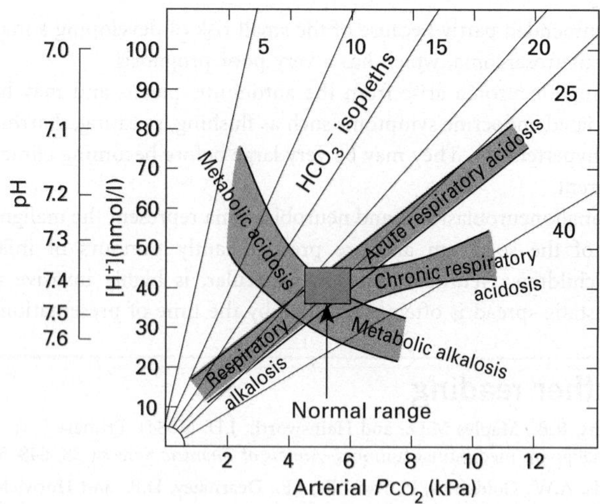

Fig. 1 Acid–base diagram: acute ventilatory failure causes hypercapnia and acidosis, renal retention of bicarbonate subsequently compensates the acidosis, and pH is restored to normal.

Table 1 Causes of types 1 and type 2 respiratory failure

Type 1 (oxygenation failure)
Acute asthma
Left heart failure
Adult respiratory distress syndrome
Pneumonia
Pulmonary fibrosis
Chronic bronchitis and emphysema
Bronchiectasis
Cystic fibrosis
Pulmonary vascular disease
Miscellaneous: lymphangitis, radiation pneumonitis, etc.
Type 2 (ventilatory failure)
Central nervous system abnormalities (e.g. trauma, drugs)
Neuromuscular diseases (e.g. Guillain–Barré syndrome, motor neurone disease)
Thoracic cage and pleural disorders (e.g. kyphoscoliosis, massive obesity)
Lung and airways diseases (e.g. severe acute asthma, upper airway obstruction, including obstructive sleep apnoea, severe chronic obstructive lung disease)

Further reading

Anthonisen, N.R. (1982). Hypoxaemia and oxygen therapy. *American Review of Respiratory Disease*, **126**, 729–33.

Warren, P.M., Flenley, D.C., Millar, J.S., and Avery, A. (1980). Respiratory failure revisited: acute exacerbations of chronic bronchitis between 1961–68 and 1970–76. *Lancet*, **i**, 467–71.

Chapter 4.43

Sleep-related disorders of breathing

J. R. Stradling

Introduction

There is a two-way interaction between sleep and breathing, such that alterations in the control of breathing with the onset of sleep lead to profound changes in ventilation, and these changes in ventilation can in turn greatly fragment sleep. Sleep-related obstruction of the upper airway (obstructive sleep apnoea syndrome, OSA) is a common disorder of variable severity (perhaps 0.5 to 1 per cent of the population) and presents across a range of disciplines. Central sleep apnoea, with loss of drive to breathe with sleep onset, is far less common and is associated with many different underlying causes.

Normal physiology of breathing during sleep

Table 1 shows the features of the two main stages of sleep, non rapid eye movement sleep (NREM, usually subdivided into stages 1 to 4, with stages 3 and 4 also known as slow wave sleep, SWS) and rapid eye movement sleep (REM, the stage during which we dream). During NREM sleep, the wakefulness drive to breath is lost (this is equivalent to a ventilation of about 5 l/min) and ventilation depends on the chemical drives to breathe (hypoxia and hypercapnia). There is also a general reduction in muscle tone that is greatest in REM sleep. During REM sleep other 'cortical' drives to breathe return and partially suppress chemical drives, similar to wakefulness. The body's defence mechanism against any failure of ventilation is arousal from sleep which restores compensatory mechanisms that seem to depend on wakefulness to function. There are various stimuli that alert and arouse the brain, an increase in inspiratory effort or ventilation being the most important (in normal subjects an inspiratory effort of −15 cmH_2O pleural pressure, or a ventilation of 15 l/min, is the approximate arousing level). However, hypoxia and hypercapnia alone can also provoke arousal, even in the absence of a ventilatory response.

Table 1 Sleep and breathing

	Non-rapid eye movement sleep	Rapid eye movement sleep
Electroencephalogram	Progressively slower frequency and higher amplitude	Similar to the awake pattern, irregular and high frequency
Eye movements	Initially slow and pendular, then none	Bursts of rapid binocular movements
Postural muscle tone	Reduced from wakefulness	Very much reduced or absent
Factors controlling breathing	Loss of 'wakefulness' input. Brainstem functions (and thus classical chemical stimuli) dominate, but are reduced compared to wakefulness	Cortical overriding and apparent reduction in responses to classical stimuli
Arousal response to asphyxia	For arousal to occur, a ventilatory response to small changes in PaO_2 and $PaCO_2$ are required (bigger changes in gases are required if there is no ventilatory response)	Larger changes in PaO_2 and $PaCO_2$ are required to produce a ventilatory response sufficient to provoke an arousal
Potential effects on breathing	Fall in min ventilation, rise in $PaCO_2$ and a fall in PaO_2 Reduction in compensatory mechanisms	Loss of use of accessory muscles of respiration
	Rise in pharyngeal resistance	Further rises in $PaCO_2$ and falls in PaO_2 are tolerated before rescue by arousal Further rise in pharyngeal resistance

Obstructive sleep apnoea

Definition

Sleep apnoea was first properly documented in neurophysiological sleep laboratories. Using simple oronasal airflow detectors it was realized that hundreds of episodes of cessation of breathing or apnoea, usually due to upper airway (pharyngeal) obstruction with associated snoring, produced marked sleep disturbance. Cessation of breathing for longer than 10 s is the arbitrary definition of apnoea in this context. Early work suggested that normal young people rarely had more than 30 or so apnoeas per night so that one definition of sleep apnoea syndrome was: more than 35 per night, or more than 5 per hour of sleep, of 10 s or longer apnoeas.

This definition is far too narrow and has been replaced with broader versions such as 'a sleep disruption syndrome, sufficient to cause daytime symptoms, that is due to a respiratory problem engendered by sleep itself'. Usually this is upper airway incompetence during sleep (mostly accompanied by snoring), but may also be due to primary problems of respiratory drive. The inclusion of symptoms in the definition emphasises the importance of defining a syndrome requiring treatment. As the pathophysiology of sleep apnoea is explained, the reasons for this shift in emphasis will become clear.

Aetiology (Table 2)

The pharyngeal airway serves two functions, swallowing and breathing, which require different design features. Swallowing requires a collapsible peristaltic tube and breathing requires a rigid open tube. These dual functions are achieved by having a floppy and collapsible muscular tube that is also capable of being held rigidly open by dilator muscles (such as genioglossus and palatopharyngeus). All these dilator muscles share in the reduced activation of skeletal muscle during sleep so that some pharyngeal narrowing occurs normally.

Table 2 Causes of obstructive sleep apnoea

Anatomical
Central (neck) obesity
Craniofacial abnormalities, e.g. micro- or retrognathia
Pharyngeal encroachment, e.g. tonsillar hypertrophy, tumours, mucopolysaccharidoses, oedema
Neuromuscular
Brainstem damage, e.g. Arnold-Chiari malformation
Neurological degenerative disorders, e.g. Shy-Drager syndrome
Myopathies, e.g. Duchenne dystrophy
Mechanism unclear
Hypothyroidism, acromegaly
Other provoking factors
Alcohol
Sedative drugs
Sleep deprivation
Increased nasal resistance

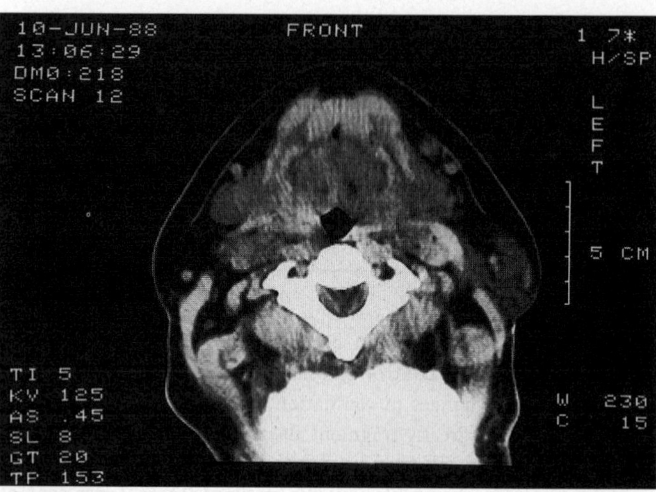

Fig. 1 CT slice at the level of the retroglossal space in a man with severe OSA. Note the considerable amount of subcutaneous fat and the circular airway which is normally wider side-to-side versus front-to-back.

There are many different abnormalities that can provoke excessive sleep-related upper airway narrowing, essentially either neuromuscular or anatomical.

Neuromuscular function

Early work looking at EMG activity in pharyngeal muscles during sleep found reductions of tone in patients with OSA. This was initially thought to explain the pharyngeal narrowing but it is now clear that this fall in inspiratory activity with sleep is normal. What is different in patients with OSA is that whilst awake they have increased inspiratory activity in the pharyngeal dilators, defending the airway in the face of narrowing influences, such as neck obesity and retrognathia. These anatomical abnormalities are discussed later.

In some primary neuromuscular problems (such as muscular dystrophy, brainstem lesions) there may be a specific loss of pharyngeal dilator activity worsened by sleep. This represents a very small proportion of cases of OSA and the larynx is sometimes the site of obstruction.

Instability of ventilatory control (e.g. in Cheyne–Stokes respiration of heart failure severe enough to produce recurrent central apnoeas) sometimes provokes a few obstructed breaths at the end of each central apnoea, when inspiratory drive returns to the diaphragm before the pharyngeal dilators are activated. This is only a secondary phenomenon, but may lead to misdiagnosis of the true underlying cause.

Anatomical causes

Simple encroachment of the pharyngeal lumen, for example by tonsillar hypertrophy, means that the normal fall in pharyngeal dilator tone with sleep can lead to critical narrowing and obstruction. There are many case reports of obvious anatomical abnormalities provoking OSA. For example tonsillar hypertrophy, pharyngeal oedema, tumours, acromegaly, mucopolysaccharidoses, and retro- or micrognathia. There are also abnormalities that 'load' the upper airway and require increased dilator muscle action that is then lost during sleep (e.g. high nasal resistance or increased external compression from neck obesity). Finally there may be mechanical problems of coupling the muscle activity so that it fails to dilate the pharyngeal lumen as effectively.

The majority of patients with OSA are overweight. In many clinics the average obesity index is well over 30 kg/m^2. This is equivalent to being about 30 per cent overweight, that is 95 kg (15 stone) at a height of 1.78 m (5'10"). Weight loss can certainly cure OSA and all studies looking at risk factors have found obesity to be dominant, accounting for at least 40 per cent of the variance in OSA severity. Neck circumference is a better predictor of OSA severity than obesity, suggesting that it is neck obesity and external pharyngeal loading that is important, rather than obesity per se. Neck imaging techniques have shown evidence of small amounts of extra fat directly around the pharynx, but the majority of the extra fat is subcutaneous (Fig. 1). Extra fat within the muscles may also interfere with their ability to dilate the airway, but this is speculative.

Although general obesity is of course related to neck obesity, the overall correlation is only about 0.75. Thus, a not particularly overweight man can have a big neck and vice versa. This is because fat distribution varies considerably between individuals. The 'female' distribution tends to be lower body and 'male' distribution more central.

Thus, the evidence is in favour of most OSA in adults being due to loading of the upper airway from obesity which can be fended off during wakefulness but, with the withdrawal of postural muscle tone with sleep, leads to excessive narrowing or collapse.

However, by no means all adult sleep apnoea can be explained by obesity or intrapharyngeal anatomical abnormalities. Careful cephalometric studies of facial and skull morphology have revealed that compared to control subjects some patients with OSA have longer faces, retropositioning of the mandible (measured as a more acute angle between the sella to nasion and nasion to supramentale planes), a downward movement of the hyoid, elongation of the soft palate, and a narrower anteroposterior distance behind the tongue. Some of these changes may be secondary to the years of sleep apnoea rather than part of the cause. However, the retropositioning of the mandible is likely to be truly contributory (Fig. 2), certainly surgery to advance the mandible can be curative. Inherited abnormalities of the lower craniofacial shape may also be the factor that explains familial clustering of sleep apnoea cases.

Retropositioning of the mandible may also be a legacy from childhood. There is evidence that nasal blockage and mouth breathing, very early in life, alters facial development (the so-called 'adenoidal

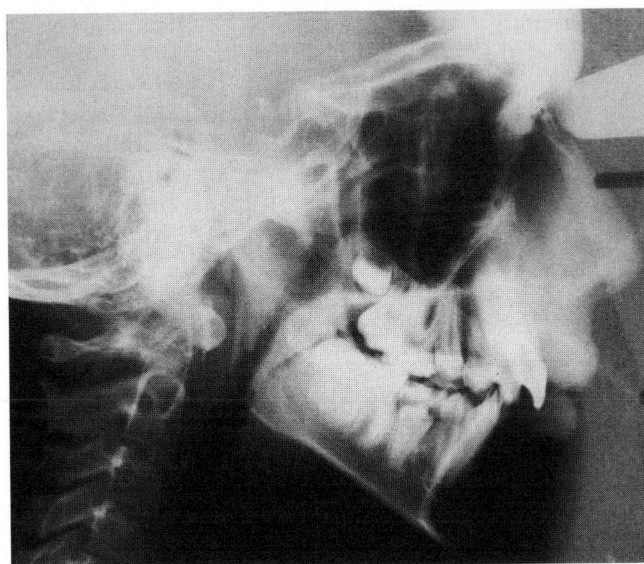

Fig. 2 Cephalostat (lateral view of skull for measurement purposes) from a patient with OSA caused by marked underdevelopment of the lower jaw.

facies'), one feature of which is abnormal development of the mandible. Following early adenoidectomy and resumption of nasal breathing, the mandible can remodel and return to its normal position and shape. Thus, one encompassing theory is that mandibular underdevelopment and obesity are two relatively common, independent risk factors for OSA which may be synergistic.

Other factors provoking OSA

Alcohol is a potent reducer of muscle tone and can further reduce pharyngeal dilator muscle tone during sleep, converting snoring to full apnoea. Other sedatives, such as the benzodiazepines, barbiturates, and opiates can do the same. Interestingly, sleep deprivation itself can reduce upper airway muscle tone during subsequent sleep and thus provoke a positive feed back of apnoea/sleep disruption/more apnoea.

Nasal blockage can contribute to the tendency of the pharynx to collapse by further lowering intrapharyngeal pressures during inspiration. This certainly leads to snoring, but may not be too important when there is full apnoea and flow ceases. Nasal obstruction may contribute to sleep apnoea over a long period by damage to the pharynx through years of snoring making it more collapsible, but improving nasal patency rarely cures OSA.

Hypothyroidism provokes OSA but the mechanism is not clear. It may partly be through weight gain or through tissue or fluid deposition in the pharynx. Alternatively there may be interference with muscle function directly. Replacement thyroxine only cures about half of the patients. Acromegaly causes sleep apnoea, probably through changes in pharyngeal shape.

Epidemiology

The prevalence of OSA depends very much on where the arbitrary cut off is drawn using sleep study derivatives for its definition, and whether symptoms are included. Some 0.3 per cent of men aged 35–65 years had severe, symptomatic OSA requiring nasal continuous positive airway pressure (CPAP) therapy and were responsive to such treatment; some 5 per cent had more than five dips per hour in SaO_2 of greater than 4 per cent SaO_2, but most of these subjects were not apparently symptomatic and did not have sleep apnoea syndrome. Sleepiness correlated best with snoring rather than OSA. Indeed more sleepiness seemed to be due to snoring more than to classical sleep apnoea.

Predictors of sleep apnoea in prevalence studies have been obesity (neck circumference in particular), snoring, age, self-reported sleepiness, and alcohol consumption. Snoring is more common in men than women, and clinical OSA itself is about five to ten times more common in men. After the menopause the prevalence in women probably increases.

Pathophysiology

Immediate consequences of sleep apnoea

Upper airway narrowing, sometimes with complete apnoea, usually starts on passing from awake to stages 1 and 2 of sleep. Once significant narrowing or obstruction occurs, increasing inspiratory effort occurs. The length of such events is highly variable, sometimes only a few seconds to well over a minute. At some point arousal occurs with a fall in upper airway resistance and increased ventilation with resolution of any asphyxia. With a return to sleep the cycle is repeated (Fig. 3). Hypoxaemia and mild hypercapnia usually (but not always) accompany these periods of obstructed breathing. The consequences of this are not clear, but because the blood gas derangements are so transient they may do little harm, unless there is already ischaemic heart disease, for example.

Hypoxaemia was thought to play a key role in provoking the arousal response that saves the patient from continuing asphyxia. Recent evidence shows that the main arousal stimulus is the actual inspiratory effort being made in response to asphyxia, rather than asphyxia per se. Normal subjects tend to wake when they have to make inspiratory efforts about three times larger than normal (10–20 cmH_2O pleural pressure swings). This degree of effort is easily reached in OSA when subatmospheric pressures of -80 cmH_2O can be recorded during the frustrated inspiratory efforts. In addition, such pressures can also be reached by heavy snorers, even if they do not develop hypoxaemia, and this will also lead to recurrent arousals with sleep fragmentation. This is because the greatly increased respiratory effort to overcome a partially obstructed pharynx (with loud snoring) can compensate fully and maintain gas exchange in some individuals, but at the expense of recurrent arousals. The importance of trying to measure these arousals has recently been appreciated, and technology to measure them automatically is being developed. Though there is a broad relationship between increasing sleep disruption and deteriorating daytime function, they are not particularly well correlated.

During the apnoea there is sometimes activation of the diving reflex that produces bradycardia, particularly when there is associated hypoxaemia. Upon arousal there is a sudden rise in blood pressure and usually a rise in pulse rate, due to activation of the sympathetic nervous system. During the actual frustrated inspiratory efforts the blood pressure falls with the reductions in intrathoracic pressure (pulsus paradoxus) and, in conjunction with the blood pressure rise on arousal, produces a very characteristic trace (Fig. 3). In addition to the increased nocturnal catecholamine secretion seen in patients with OSA, there is also a suppression of growth hormone and testosterone levels. There is marked polyuria during sleep (a reversal of the normal relative oliguria of sleep) but the mechanism is not clear although it may be related to the recurrent arousals or increased ANP production from right atrial distension (due to the large inspiratory efforts).

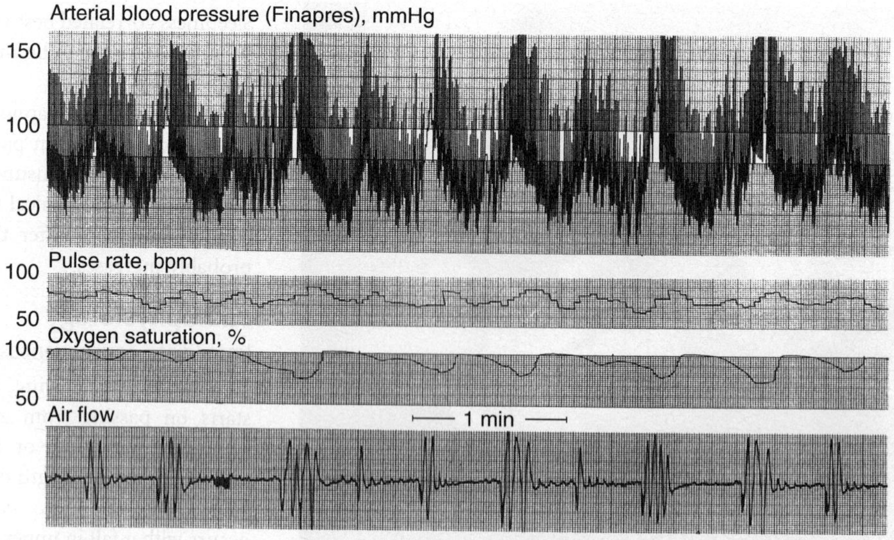

Fig. 3 Five minute tracing during sleep from a patient with obstructive sleep apnoea. The rises in blood pressure (top trace) and heart rate (second trace) coincide with the cessation of each apnoea and an arousal. During each apnoea (evident from the bottom airflow trace) frustrated inspiratory efforts are accompanied by falls in blood pressure (pulsus paradoxus).

Long-term consequences of obstructive sleep apnoea

The main reason for treating OSA is to relieve the daytime symptoms, mainly sleepiness. There is also a small amount of evidence that these patients have an increased, though unexplained, cardiovascular mortality due to myocardial infarction and stroke. Since several cardiovascular risk factors also contribute to the production of OSA (central obesity, smoking, alcohol), it is difficult to determine the contribution made independently by OSA to cardiovascular deaths. Possible mechanisms include sustained hypertension, intermittent nocturnal hypertension, increased catecholamine release, hypoxia-induced cardiac arrhythmias, insulin resistance, hyperlipidaemia, and left ventricular hypertrophy but as yet none of these are proven.

Clinical features

The main symptom of OSA is daytime hypersomnolence and this correlates broadly with the degree of sleep disruption. Early on in the development of the disorder the daytime sleepiness is little more than that often experienced by normal people after a few disturbed nights. Whilst occupied there is little difficulty concentrating and staying awake, but once activities become more boring then unwanted sleepiness intervenes. As the sleep disruption worsens then more and more activities will be interfered with. Particularly on long motorway journeys after dark, when sensory stimulation is low, sleepiness can be devastating. Initially there will be lane wandering with sudden arousal and correction. Accidents involving driving off the road, or driving into vehicles in front, are about seven times more common in patients with OSA. This sleepiness also impinges greatly on work performance and home life. It is important to ask the right questions to assess sleepiness and not be confused by tiredness, which is a lack of energy or desire to get up and do anything. Because of the insidious onset of OSA, the sleepiness may be regarded as normal by the patient and thus situational questions, such as contained in the Epworth Sleepiness Scale (Fig. 4), need to be asked.

A list of other symptoms seen in OSA is given in Table 3. There is usually a long history of gradually worsening snoring with apnoeas witnessed by the spouse, who may have long since moved out of the bedroom due to the snoring. There is likely to have been a weight gain over the last few years with an obesity index of greater than 30 kg/m^2 and a collar size of 17 inches or more. There is often a history of fairly high alcohol intake and smoking. On examination there may be nasal stuffiness, evidence of a small lower jaw (such as teeth crowding or several extractions for this problem), and a small pharynx with mucosal bogginess and wrinkling. It should be stressed, of course, that not all these features are likely to be present in one individual.

Part of the investigation of such patients should include an assessment for precipitating factors such as hypothyroidism and acromegaly. Other factors such as mucopolysaccharidosis, pharyngeal tumours, tonsillar hypertrophy, neurological disorders, and significant retrognathia will be more obvious.

Diagnosis

Following the history and examination, further tests may be appropriate, for example thyroxine or growth hormone estimations. Blood gases and simple lung function tests may be necessary if associated diurnal respiratory failure is suspected. A raised haemoglobin or venous [HCO_3^-] may also signify diurnal respiratory failure. A raised haemoglobin or venous [HCO_3^-] may also signify diurnal respiratory failure.

Unless the presenting problem is clearly not sleep-related, some form of sleep study will be required (Fig. 5). Simple systems can assess sleep fragmentation and arousals by looking for heart rate rises, body movements, or from the blood pressure rises using non-invasive beat-to-beat blood pressure monitors. Upper airway obstruction can be inferred from snoring, inspiratory flow limitation, and non-invasive measurements of pleural pressure. Failure of ventilation can be measured by finger oximetry, as long as supplemental oxygen is not being used. Accurate cut off points to define normality and abnormality are currently impossible, thus sleep studies remain qualitative aids to diagnosis and any possible or appropriate therapies.

In the past, the usual procedure was to employ full polysomnography that measured sleep state (with electroencephalography, EMG, and eye movement recordings) and respiratory variables (with ribcage/abdominal transducers, oronasal airflow thermistors, and oximetry). This investigation and its analysis are expensive, time consuming, and now unnecessary.

Treatment

Mild symptoms may resolve with simple treatments and advice (Table 4). Weight loss is undoubtedly effective but usually very difficult

How likely are you to **doze off or fall asleep** in the situations described in the box below, in contrast to feeling just tired?

This refers to your **usual way of life** in recent times.

Even if you haven't done some of these things recently try to work out how they would have affected you.

Use the following scale to choose the ***most appropriate number*** for each situation:-

0 = Would *never* doze
1 = *Slight* chance of dozing
2 = *Moderate* chance of dozing
3 = *High* chance of dozing

Situation	**Chance of dozing**
Sitting and reading	
Watching TV	
Sitting, inactive in a public place (eg. a theatre or a meeting)	
As a passenger in a car for an hour without a break	
Lying down to rest in the afternoon when circumstances permit	
Sitting and talking to someone	
Sitting quietly after lunch without alcohol	
In a car, while stopped for a few minutes in the traffic	

Fig. 4 This self administered scale for measuring sleepiness has a maximum total score of 24, up to 9 is considered normal.

Table 3 Symptoms of obstructive sleep apnoea

Most common (>60%)
Loud snoring
Excessive daytime sleepiness
Restless sleep
Unrefreshing sleep
Nocturia
Apparent personality changes
Witnessed apnoeas
Less common (10–60%)
Choking or shortness of breath sensations at night
Reduced libido
Nocturnal sweating
Morning headaches
Rare (<10%)
Nocturnal enuresis
Recurrent arousals/insomnia
Nocturnal cough
Symptomatic oesophageal reflux
Nocturnal angina

to achieve and sustain. Stopping sedatives and evening alcohol can help. No drug has shown any consistent effect.

If symptoms are severe then there is only one fully effective therapy, nasal continuous positive airway pressure (CPAP). This involves wearing a small mask over the nose whilst asleep that is kept at above atmospheric pressures by a low pressure pump (Fig. 6). Pressures in the region of 10 cmH_2O are enough to splint open the pharynx and resist collapse, thus allowing unobstructed breathing and undisturbed sleep (Fig. 7). The exact pressure required by the patient can either be established manually, or automatically by 'intelligent' CPAP machines that use snoring and other signals to adjust their pressure appropriately. The response to CPAP treatment is dramatic so that the daytime symptoms resolve rapidly, even after one night of treatment. The unpleasantness and unaesthetic appearance of this treatment repels patients initially but, with careful and thorough training, and once the benefits have been experienced, acceptance is over 80 per cent. Once established on nasal CPAP, a patient with OSA is likely to require it for life unless he can lose a significant amount of weight.

A less well established mechanical treatment for OSA is a mandibular advancement device worn at night. These are intraoral devices that hold the lower jaw forward and closed, thus enlarging the retroglossal space. In their simplest form they consist of two gum shields for the top and bottom teeth welded together to produce 75 per cent of maximum lower jaw protrusion when worn (Fig. 8). They clearly reduce snoring and mild to moderate OSA in some individuals, but their role in treatment is not yet established. Temporomandibular joint problems and lower jaw or teeth discomfort limit their acceptability.

A surgical treatment whose popularity is rapidly decreasing is uvulopalatopharyngoplasty (UPPP). This operation consists of removing part of the soft palate, any residual tonsils, and 'tightening

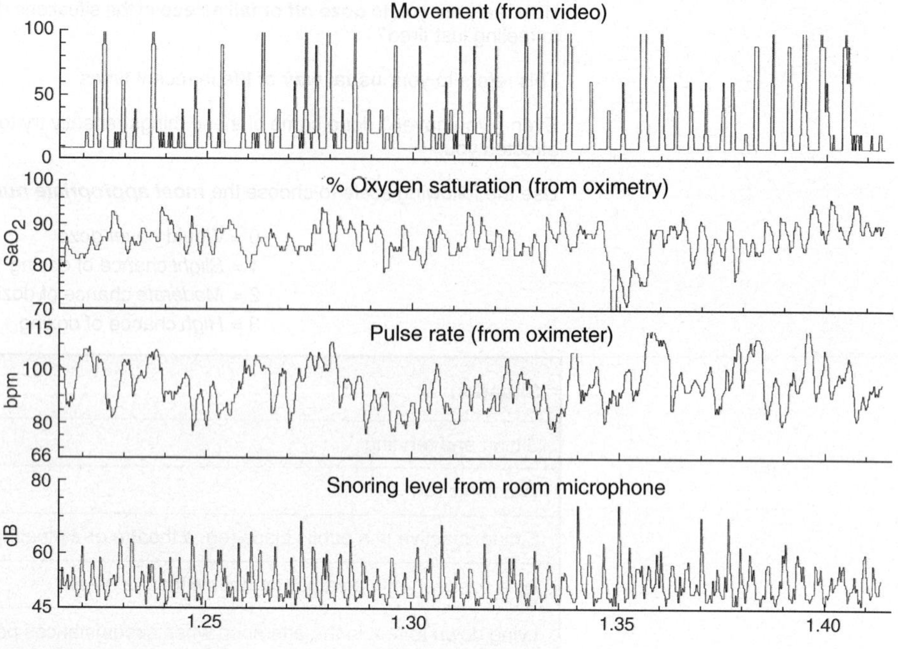

Fig. 5 Twenty minute tracing during sleep from a patient with obstructive sleep apnoea. Top trace is body movement (derived from digital processing of the video picture of the patient) and shows recurrent movement arousals throughout. The second tracing is oxygen saturation (pulse oximetry), the third line is heart rate (from the oximeter, showing again recurrent sleep disturbance), and the bottom trace is sound (room microphone) and shows the loud snoring associated with every resumption of ventilation after a apnoea. Normal sleep would be four straight lines.

Table 4 Advice for patients with mild to moderate OSA, usually worse when sleeping supine

(1)	Learn to sleep on your side and avoid sleeping on your back
(2)	No alcohol after 18.00 h
(3)	No sedatives
(4)	Lose weight
(5)	Stop smoking
(6)	Keep the nose as clear as possible

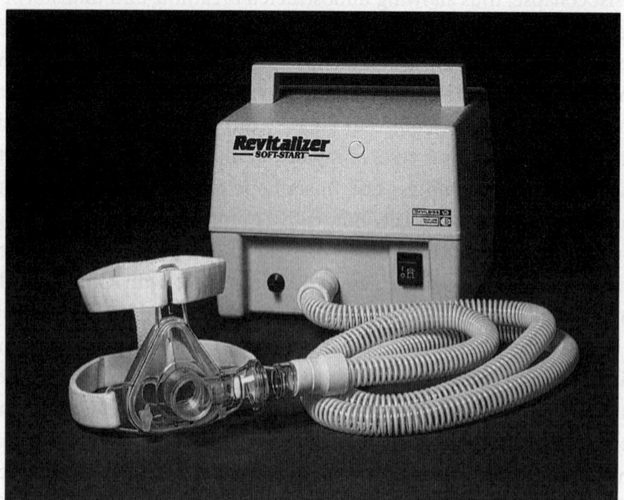

Fig. 6 Nasal continuous positive airway pressure system as used at home by patients with obstructive sleep apnoea.

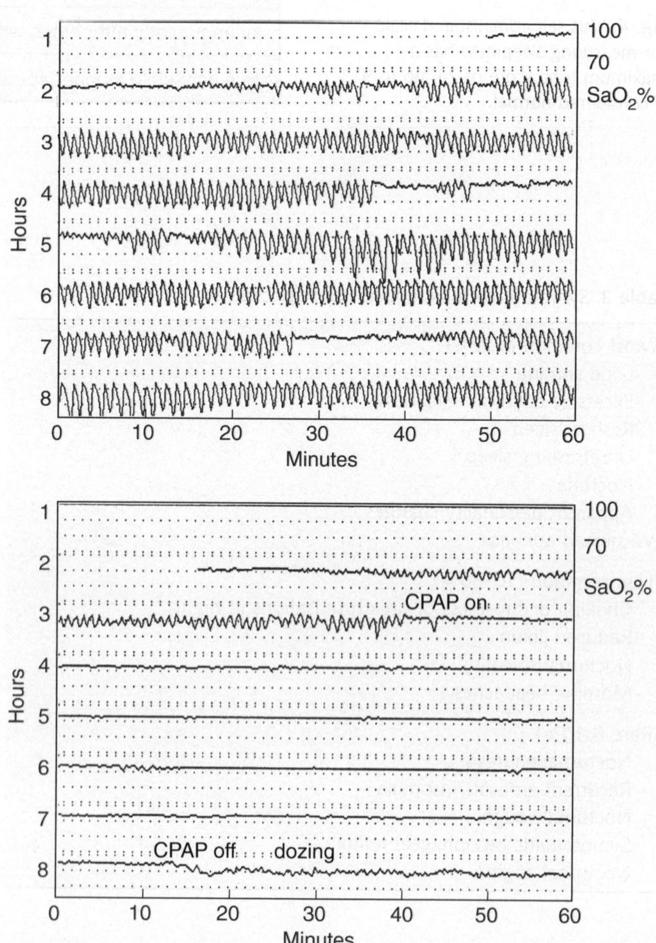

Fig. 7 Two all-night oximetry tracings from a patient with obstructive sleep apnoea, before treatment and during his first night on nasal continuous positive airway pressure (CPAP). Each tracing starts top left and finishes bottom right. Each tracing is eight continuous hours with the scale for each individual line scaled 70–100 per cent SaO_2.

up' the side walls of the pharynx. Although said to be good at reducing snoring, its success rate at treating OSA is not good: approximately 50 per cent of patients experience a 50 per cent improvement in the number of apnoeas per hour. Attempts to improve the selection of

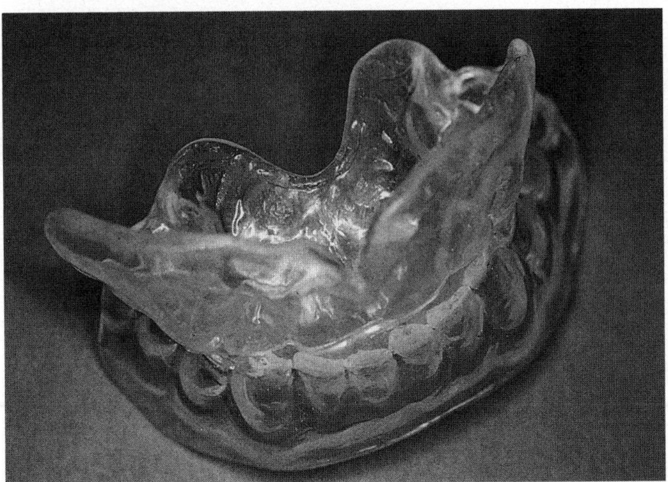

Fig. 8 Simple dental advancement device worn in the mouth at night to hold the lower jaw forward and closed during sleep. The resultant increase in retroglossal space can greatly improve snoring and mild to moderate sleep apnoea.

patients who might respond better to this operation have had very limited success, although thin patients with big soft palates, residual tonsils, and milder disease do the best. It is an extremely painful operation and very much a second option.

Surgical advancement of the mandible (and sometimes the maxilla) may be appropriate in highly selected cases. Tracheostomy was the first successful therapy and is very effective. Despite the subsequent problems of such surgery, it may still be appropriate in occasional patients.

Sleep-induced hypoventilation and central sleep apnoea

Breathing during sleep may also decrease not because of obstruction but because of a reduction in central output to the respiratory muscles, so called central (rather than obstructive) apnoea. There are many causes for central sleep apnoea, or hypoventilation, and the following is one way of classifying them (Table 5). In some situations the central apnoeas disturb sleep and present with daytime sleepiness, whereas in others presentation is more with symptoms of respiratory failure, such as morning headaches with cyanosis and confusion, ankle oedema, and shortness of breath on exertion.

Absent ventilatory drive

Brainstem abnormalities may damage the areas responsible for automatic, chemical control of ventilation. Whilst awake the wakefulness-related ventilatory drive (about 5 l/min) may remain adequate to maintain PaO_2 and $PaCO_2$ levels, but on falling asleep drive is reduced or even disappears with marked hypoventilation (or apnoea) and hypoxaemia: arousal in response to asphyxia is then necessary to restore the blood gases. This failure of brainstem automatic control can be congenital (so-called Ondine's curse) or acquired as the result of a stroke, infection, surgical damage, multiple sclerosis, or compression by tumour, syrinx, or Arnold–Chiari malformation.

Reduction of chemical drive can occur as a secondary problem when there is hypoventilation due to mechanical problems such as chronic airways obstruction or weak respiratory muscles. Chronic

Table 5 Suggested classification of causes of central apnoea

Type of central apnoea	Examples	Daytime arterial CO_2 level
1. Absent or reduced ventilatory drive	Brainstem damage or congenital abnormality Acquired blunting, e.g. secondary to lung disease	Raised
2. Unstable respiratory drive	Sleep onset, hypoxaemia, altitude, heart failure	Normal or low
3. REM related oscillations	Normal in REM sleep Due to neuromuscular disorders and respiratory muscle weakness	Normal or raised
4. Reflex central apnoea	Pharyngeal collapse inhibits inspiration	Normal
5. Apparent central apnoea (wrongly diagnosed)	Respiratory muscle weakness or gross obesity cause chest wall movement transducers to fail to demonstrate any ventilatory effort during *obstructive* apnoeas	Normal or raised

hypoventilation can lead to blunting of ventilatory drive, and this will lead to further, marked falls in ventilation on entering sleep.

Unstable ventilatory drive

The wakefulness-related ventilatory drive has a considerable stabilizing effect on ventilation by preventing it from falling below a certain level. If reasons for ventilatory instability exist then, by removing this stabilizing effect, sleep will allow periodic respiration to develop. The usual provoker of instability is an increased drive to breath; control theory shows that increasing the gain in a feedback system promotes instability through overshoot and undershoot. One of the best examples of increased drive is the hypoxaemia of altitude. The hypoxaemia steepens the CO_2 response line, promotes instability, and when sleep occurs there is the usual fall in ventilation. Both the resulting extra hypoxaemia and the return of ventilation due to the rise in CO_2 provoke arousal. This arousal provides yet more ventilatory drive which restores the blood gases with some overshoot and the cycle repeats. Thus periodic breathing with recurrent arousals is very common at altitude with the expected daytime consequences of both sleepiness and insomnia. Acetazolamide produces a metabolic acidosis and increases ventilation overall, the hypoxaemia is relieved and thus the ventilatory response to CO_2 becomes less steep. Both these factors restore stability and reduce the periodic respiration.

In left ventricular failure there is extra ventilatory drive from stimulation of interstitial lung receptors. This also provokes instability in conjunction with the longer circulation time seen in heart failure. This so called Cheyne–Stokes breathing is quite common in heart failure and through sleep disruption produces daytime sleepiness and complaints of nocturnal dyspnoea. The patient is usually aware that the dyspnoea disappears rapidly on arousal, unlike the paroxysmal nocturnal dyspnoea of pulmonary oedema. Treatment with either overnight oxygen or acetazolamide can sometimes greatly reduce the periodicity and improve both sleep quality and symptoms.

Rapid-eye-movement sleep apnoeas

During normal REM sleep the phasic bursts of eye movements are associated with transient falls in ventilation, with even apnoeas occurring. The ribcage muscles are affected most, but diaphragmatic excursion can also fall. Such periodicities are entirely normal.

The REM sleep inhibition of most muscles (apart from the diaphragm) can greatly reduce overall ventilation when accessory muscles of respiration are needed for breathing. Profound falls in ventilation and SaO_2 can occur on entering REM sleep in patients with neuromuscular diseases, chest wall abnormalities, and chronic airways obstruction. These periods of profound hypoventilation may accelerate the onset of diurnal respiratory failure.

Reflex apnoea

Central respiratory output can be modified by a number of reflexes from receptors in the upper airway. There appears to be a reflex from the pharynx that inhibits inspiratory flow when the pharynx is being sucked in and collapsed. This makes teleological sense as a slowing of inspiratory flow would reduce the collapsing tendency. There are some patients with pharyngeal collapse who, instead of struggling to inspire against the blocked airway, simply stop breathing (central apnoea) until they finally arouse, presumably in this case due to the fall in PaO_2 and rise in $PaCO_2$. These patients usually present with histories suggestive of OSA and do respond to nasal CPAP as one would expect.

Apparent central apnoea

The diagnosis of central apnoea depends on failing to detect evidence of respiratory effort during an apnoea. However in two circumstances, marked obesity and muscular weakness, the surface transducers may fail to register that inspiratory efforts are being made, leading to misclassification.

Overnight ventilation for central sleep apnoea or hypoventilation

The chronic respiratory failure associated with some neurological disorders (e.g. acid maltase deficiency, postpolio syndrome, motor neurone disease, Duchenne dystrophy) can progress to death even when quality of life may otherwise be very good. The same is true of the chest wall restrictive disorders, such as due to scoliosis and previous extensive thoracoplasty. However the respiratory failure can be reversed by supporting ventilation overnight. The response to this treatment can be dramatic with resolution of all symptoms and restoration of normal blood gases, even when off the ventilator during the day. The mechanism by which supporting ventilation at night corrects respiratory failure is not clear and there are three possibilities: resting of fatigued respiratory muscles, resetting of the respiratory centre back towards normal (a reversal of acquired blunting of drive), and improved lung and chest wall compliance following a period of greater lung expansion than the patients own inspiratory muscles can achieve. Tricyclic antidepressants such as protriptyline can virtually abolish the REM sleep periods (and thus the associated hypoxaemia) and have been shown to temporarily improve daytime blood gases. Whatever the explanation, there is no doubt that overnight ventilation is a life-saving therapy that in certain conditions can add decades of active life.

The recent development of comfortable nasal masks designed for CPAP therapy for OSA has revolutionized the overnight ventilation of these patients, who previously had to use cumbersome and inefficient negative pressure systems around the chest. Positive pressure ventilation can be given via a nose mask, although there are still many problems to be overcome when establishing patients on such equipment (particularly mask comfort and air leaks through the mouth).

Electrical pacing of the diaphragm is occasionally used for supporting ventilation in conditions where the phrenic nerve and diaphragm are intact and the problem is more central. This involves the implantation of bilateral phrenic electrodes and induction coils under the skin that are activated by external induction coils.

Further reading

Davies, R.J.O. and Stradling, J.R. (1996). The epidemiology of sleep apnoea. *Thorax*, **51** (suppl. 2), S65–70.

Ferguson, K.A. and Fleetham, J.A. (1995). Sleep-related breathing disorders: Consequences of sleep disordered breathing. *Thorax*, **50**, 998–1004.

Grunstein, R.R. (1995). Sleep-related breathing disorders: Nasal continuous positive airway pressure treatment for obstructive sleep apnoea. *Thorax*, **50**, 1106–13.

Stradling, J.R. (1993). *Handbook of sleep-related breathing disorders.* Oxford University Press, Oxford.

Stradling, J.R. (1997). Practical approach to sleep disordered breathing. In *Horizons in medicine*, (ed M. Farthing). Blackwell Scientific Publications, Oxford.

Chapter 4.44

Management of chronic respiratory failure

J. Moxham and C. S. Garrard

The most important causes of chronic respiratory failure and subsequent cor pulmonale are listed in Table 1. Pulmonary fibrosis and pulmonary vascular disease cause predominantly hypoxia (type 1 respiratory failure) and the development of hypercapnia only occurs late in these diseases. Obstructive sleep apnoea and central alveolar hypoventilation cause respiratory failure mainly during sleep. Chronic obstructive pulmonary disease (COPD) is by far the most common cause of hypercapnic (type 2) ventilatory failure.

Patients with chronic respiratory failure are hypoxic and breathless, particularly on exertion, and eventually develop hypercapnia and cor pulmonale. Any assessment of patients with chronic respiratory failure must address the mechanism, severity, and treatment of hypoxia, plus

Table 1 Important causes of chronic respiratory failure

Lung and airways	***Neuromuscular disorders***
• Pulmonary fibrosis	• Cervical cord lesions
• Pulmonary vascular disease	• Motor neurone disease
• Chronic bronchitis and emphysema	• Poliomyelitis
• Bronchiectasis and cystic fibrosis	• Muscular dystrophies and myopathies
• Obstructive sleep apnoea	
	Thoracic cage and pleural abnormalities
Central nervous system	• Kyphoscoliosis
• Central alveolar hypoventilation	• Thoracoplasty
	• Extreme obesity

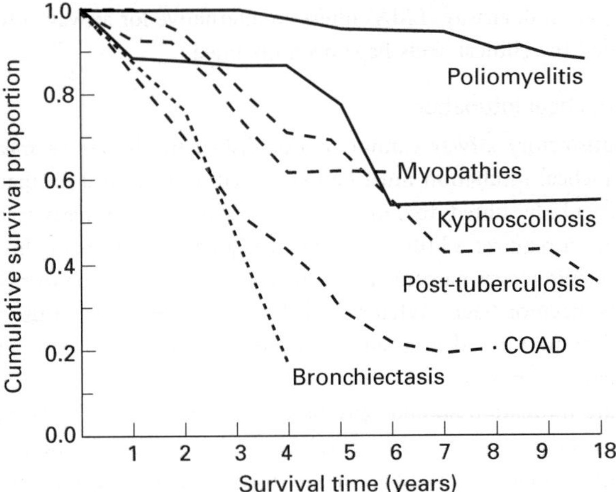

Fig. 1 Survival with long-term domiciliary ventilation in patients with neuromuscular and other disorders.
(See OTM3, p.2930 for source.)

the three crucial areas of central respiratory drive, respiratory muscle pump capacity, and the load imposed on the respiratory system by the disease (see Chapter 4.42). In different diseases the importance of each of these three components will vary. In patients with chronic respiratory failure, impairment of the central nervous system output is only rarely a problem and is most relevant in central alveolar hypoventilation syndromes. However, abnormalities of central ventilatory control are commonly part of the overall pathophysiology of ventilatory failure and, furthermore, a reduction of central nervous system output is an important component of respiratory failure in many patients during sleep. The increased load on the respiratory system imposed by disease processes is frequently self-evident, for example in pulmonary fibrosis, obstructive sleep apnoea, or obesity. Similarly, impairment of respiratory muscle pump capacity occurs in a wide variety of circumstances. Neuromuscular diseases, for example motor neurone disease or muscular dystrophy, are an obvious cause of reduced pump capacity. However, pump capacity is often impaired in less obvious ways: patients with COPD and hyperinflation have reduced inspiratory muscle capacity as a consequence of muscle shortening and patients with severe weight loss for whatever cause have respiratory muscle weakness.

On rare occasions chronic respiratory failure can be cured, for example when patients with cystic fibrosis are treated by lung transplantation, patients with severe obstructive sleep apnoea are managed with continuous positive airway pressure (CPAP), and patients with morbid obesity lose weight. Nevertheless, for most patients with chronic respiratory failure a cure is impossible, and an important aspect of management is careful assessment of the interrelated issues of central drive, respiratory load, and ventilatory capacity, as well as the management of chronic hypoxia.

Non-invasive ventilation

Long-term and domiciliary ventilation

Selected patients with chronic ventilatory failure are appropriately treated with long-term assisted ventilation, and many, particularly those with neuromuscular and chest wall disease, can do well (Fig. 1). A small number of patients, usually with advanced neurological disease or high cervical cord transection, are totally ventilator dependent and generally receive positive pressure ventilation via a tracheostomy. Some patients with high cervical lesions are managed by diaphragm pacing (see below). However, a much larger group of patients are capable of sustaining their own ventilation, albeit with hypoxia and hypercapnia, but require, or benefit from, intermittent ventilatory support, particularly at night. Intermittent ventilatory support can be provided via a tracheostomy, but most patients are treated non-invasively by either negative or positive pressure ventilatory devices.

The use of non-invasive ventilation has greatly increased in recent years, following the introduction of non-invasive positive pressure ventilation (NIPPV). Most commonly a nasal mask is used of the type employed in CPAP treatment of patients with obstructive sleep apnoea (see Chapter 4.43).

The usual indication for non-invasive ventilation (most commonly NIPPV) is chronic severe hypercapnic ventilatory failure due to chest-wall or neuromuscular disease. In general, NIPPV is only appropriate for neuromuscular patients with stable or slowly advancing disease. Kyphoscoliosis, when severe, eventually causes ventilatory failure and is ideally treated by nocturnal NIPPV, as is the ventilatory failure which can eventually develop in patients with thoracoplasty. The nocturnal hypoventilation and ventilatory failure of these patients is well controlled by NIPPV; supplemental oxygen is seldom needed, and daytime gases (off ventilation) gradually improve. Such patients report a large improvement in well-being, sleep quality, intellectual capacity, energy, and breathlessness. Cor pulmonale and pulmonary hypertension are reversed, and life expectancy is increased. The effectiveness and relative simplicity of NIPPV is such that all appropriate patients with severe chest wall or neuromuscular disease need careful supervision so that NIPPV can be considered at the correct time.

A number of patients with COPD and ventilatory failure have been treated by long-term nocturnal NIPPV. COPD patients are less easy to ventilate and less tolerant of the technique than patients with chest wall disease. NIPPV works best in COPD patients with hypercapnia and is not easily applied to the breathless patient with emphysema (the 'pink puffer'), in whom it can reduce breathlessness but with the danger that patients become ventilator dependent. When patients with COPD receive long-term domiciliary ventilation the outcome is less good than for neuromuscular disease (Fig. 1), and whether this treatment is superior to long-term oxygen therapy remains to be proved.

It is crucial to keep in mind that NIPPV is only feasible in patients who require intermittent ventilatory support. With prolonged periods of uninterrupted NIPPV the nasal mask can cause severe damage to skin and soft tissue.

Acute on chronic ventilatory failure

Many patients with severe neuromuscular or chest wall disease are precipitated into overt ventilatory failure by an intercurrent event, most commonly a respiratory infection. A period of NIPPV can control such ventilatory failure until the status quo is restored, and therefore intubation and mechanical ventilation, or death, is avoided. Similarly, many patients in ventilatory failure due to an acute exacerbation of COPD, who do not respond to conventional therapy and develop a worsening hypercapnic acidosis, can be managed successfully with NIPPV. Therefore non-invasive ventilation may become a powerful tool in the management of selected patients with acute on chronic ventilatory failure and may have the important economic advantage of not requiring intensive care unit facilities.

Weaning from mechanical ventilation

Patients who have difficulty in weaning from mechanical ventilation pose an important clinical management challenge. Many of these patients have pre-existing, chronic lung disease, and some have established ventilatory failure prior to their unavoidable admission to the intensive care unit. Recent clinical studies suggest that NIPPV may be a useful technique to facilitate weaning and achieve early discharge from the intensive care unit, thereby improving clinical outcome and saving scarce medical resources. Successful weaning from chronic ventilator dependency has been reported in patients with COPD as well as in those with neuromuscular and chest wall disorders. Prior to successful weaning, it is important that patients are able to co-operate with the NIPPV technique and that they are also independent of mechanical ventilation for short periods of time.

NIPPV and transplantation

NIPPV has been used as a 'bridge to transplantation' in patients with chronic lung disease, particularly those with cystic fibrosis. Patients with cystic fibrosis often become septic when intubated and ventilated, and have a poor prognosis; therefore NIPPV represents, in many ways, a preferred ventilation option.

Continuous positive airway pressure (CPAP)

Obstructive sleep apnoea is an important, even if unusual, cause of ventilatory failure for which the mainstay of treatment is CPAP. In other patients with chronic respiratory failure the role of CPAP is limited. CPAP can only be applied for relatively short time periods. Studies of patients with chronic airways obstruction suggest that in some patients the application of CPAP may reduce breathlessness and increase exercise capacity. However, not all patients report benefit and further studies are required.

Diaphragm pacing

The principal indication for diaphragm pacing is in the treatment of selected ventilator-dependent patients following high cervical cord injury. Pacing electrodes are implanted around the phrenic nerves. A radio receiver is implanted in the subcutaneous tissues, usually of the lower antrolateral rib cage. The advantage of diaphragm pacing is that it is possible to achieve adequate ventilation without application of any equipment to the airway. The best results are achieved in young adults with quadriplegia, and many of these have been satisfactorily paced for more than 10 years.

Management of acute respiratory failure

The treatment of acute respiratory failure consists of:

- establishing an airway;
- administering oxygen;
- maintaining adequate ventilation;
- identifying and treating the underlying cause;
- monitoring SaO_2 (pulse oximetry), ECG, and vital signs.

Establish an airway

Simple manoeuvres to re-establish and clear the airway must always be followed. These include positioning and maintaining the head and neck in the 'sniff position', inspection of the oropharynx, suctioning, and, if necessary, the insertion of an oral or pharyngeal airway. The laryngeal mask airway (LMA) offers an alternative for airway control provided the clinical skills have been obtained.

Endotracheal intubation

If a satisfactory airway cannot be established by the above means, endotracheal intubation must be performed. Orotracheal intubation is particularly suited to emergency intubation while nasotracheal intubation requires a little extra time. Coagulation defects or thrombocytopenia makes nasotracheal intubation inadvisable due to risk of serious haemorrhage. Whatever technique is selected, intubation should be performed in a safe and expeditious manner by the most experienced clinician available. Neuromuscular relaxant drugs to facilitate intubation should only be used by experienced personnel. The complications of endotracheal intubation are due to occlusion or displacement of the tube, and airway trauma. The appropriate endotracheal tube size for most adult males is 8–9 mm internal diameter; and for women, 7–8 mm. For children, a rough calculation using the child's age in years divided by 4, plus 4.0 will provide the tube internal diameter in mm. These smaller tubes are generally uncuffed.

It is essential that the endotracheal tube be securely anchored and the cuff inflation pressure restricted to less than 30 cm H_2O. High volume, low pressure cuffed tubes are generally recommended and cuff inflation pressures should be checked periodically using an anaeroid manometer and adjusted accordingly. Using higher cuff pressures does not improve airway protection against aspiration but only serves to damage the tracheal mucosa and risk later subglottic stenosis.

Difficulties with endotracheal intubation can be encountered in patients with a short 'bull' neck or receding lower jaw. Any patient with restricted neck and jaw movements (rheumatoid arthritis or cervical spine injury) or who have abnormal oropharyngeal anatomy (tumour or trauma) should also be considered to pose difficulties for intubation.

There are several options when a difficult intubation is anticipated. Inhalational anaesthesia by face mask can facilitate intubation but under no circumstances must muscle relaxants be given unless satisfactory airway access can be ensured. Awake intubation can be performed with topical anaesthesia. Blind nasal intubation or intubation using a fibreoptic bronchoscope or laryngoscope requires considerable skill and training but may be the safest option in establishing an airway.

Tracheostomy

Tracheostomy should only replace endotracheal intubation for specific indications and not merely after the elapse of a predefined time interval. Using modern endotracheal tubes and techniques, endotracheal intubation can be tolerated without permanent harm to the airway for months if necessary. It has been shown that the greater part of mucosal damage is done in the first week of intubation with little additional change thereafter.

However, much can be gained by the judicious selection of patients for tracheostomy either as the preferred primary route for airway access or as a replacement for endotracheal intubation. The common indications for replacement include the need for chronic or permanent ventilation, to help weaning after previously failed attempts at extubation, to facilitate oral nutrition, or the presence of upper airway complications of endotracheal intubation.

Table 2 Oxygen delivery systems

Method of delivery	FiO_2 achieved
Nasal cannula (1–2 l/min)	0.24 to 0.30
Venturi mask	0 24 to 0.50
Partial rebreathing mask	0.60 to 0.80
Non-rebreathing reservoir mask	Up to 0.90
Anaesthetic face mask or endotracheal tube	Up to 1.0

The same principles of cuff pressure management apply to tracheostomy tubes as do to endotracheal tubes. Tracheostomy is associated with fewer but more serious complications than endotracheal intubation. These include tube displacement, pneumothorax, severe haemorrhage, and wound infection.

Minitracheostomy

Minitracheostomy tubes are 3.5–4.0 mm diameter, cuffless tubes inserted percutaneously through the cricothyroid membrane, usually under local anaesthesia. A Seldinger technique for introduction of the minitracheostomy tube offers an alternative to the direct trochar method. Minitracheostomy allows suctioning lung secretions without the need for formal endotracheal intubation or tracheostomy. However, minitracheostomy tubes cannot be used for conventional ventilation, may result in local haemorrhagic complications, and may be source of infection.

Cricothyroidotomy

A cricothyroidotomy may be needed in life-threatening, upper airway obstructions where endotracheal intubation is not feasible and there is insufficient time to perform tracheostomy. Performed under local anaesthesia, a full sized tracheostomy tube can be inserted (6–8 mm internal diameter) to facilitate mechanical ventilation.

The administration of oxygen

Although there is limited safety information for oxygen therapy, the long-term administration of 50 per cent oxygen or 100 per cent oxygen for less than 24 h is usually considered acceptable. Nevertheless, hypoxia should never be tolerated through a concern over oxygen toxicity. Oxygen can be delivered by a variety of means depending upon the concentration desired and the patients minute ventilation. Details of some oxygen delivery systems are shown in Table 2.

Oxygen should be given in such concentrations as to prevent prolonged or even transient episodes of hypoxia. The well-recognized caveat that only controlled (limited) oxygen concentrations should be given to patients with chronic obstructive lung disease must be borne in mind. The response to oxygen therapy can best be measured continuously by pulse oximetry (SaO_2) or by intermittent arterial blood gas sampling.

Mechanical ventilation

The main indications for mechanical ventilation are ventilatory failure as indicated by a rising $PaCO_2$ or severe hypoxemia that cannot be corrected with high concentrations of inspired oxygen. The provision of efficient and safe mechanical ventilation is a skill that must be mastered by all physicians practising critical care. The basic principles still pertain despite the introduction of complex and sophisticated mechanical ventilators and the overabundance of studies claiming superiority of certain techniques over others. The application of common sense and sound physiological doctrine will serve better than devotion to an attractive technical innovation.

Indications for intubation and mechanical ventilation

Mechanical ventilation is not to be undertaken lightly since it is associated with much morbidity and some mortality. Yet, failure to intervene promptly can clearly have catastrophic consequences for the patient. The indications for mechanical ventilation fall into two broad categories:

(1) inadequate alveolar ventilation with increasing PCO_2; and

(2) inadequate gas exchange with increasing $(A–a)PO_2$ and arterial hypoxaemia.

Guidelines for mechanical ventilation in acute respiratory failure are shown in Table 3. The physician must always exercise judgement in the interpretation of these guidelines and anticipate problems before they arise. For example one of the simplest criteria for mechanical ventilation is a respiratory rate of 35 breaths per min or more. If, with a respiratory rate of 30 breaths per min, a patient is clearly fatiguing then an early elective intubation is preferred to an emergency procedure an hour or so later. Similarly, a progressive fall in vital capacity in a patient with myasthenia gravis receiving full medication may need ventilatory support though the critical value of less than 15 ml/kg is not broached.

The treatment of hypoventilatory respiratory failure consists of assisting ventilatory function usually by mechanical external means. Figure 2 shows a flow diagram outlining the decision process involved in the assessment of patients who may require mechanical ventilation.

Features and applications of a mechanical ventilator

The control mechanism that cycles the ventilator from inspiration to expiration may be electromechanical or electronic (utilizing microprocessor technology). Modern mechanical ventilators tend to fall into the latter category and offer a degree of sophistication that has greatly improved the safety and efficiency of mechanical ventilation.

Most adult patients are supported on volume/time cycled, pressure limited ventilators (volume ventilator or flow generator). The volume/time cycled ventilators deliver preset tidal volumes regardless of changes in lung compliance or impedance. The price paid for this desirable characteristic is that the inflation pressures must rise to overcome the mechanical load. To protect the patient against inadvertently high pressures, a pressure limit must be set. When this limit is reached the ventilator terminates inspiration regardless of the volume delivered and triggers an alarm.

Neonates and infants may be satisfactorily ventilated using time cycled, pressure limited devices (pressure ventilator or pressure generator). The pressure limited paediatric ventilator offers simplicity and reliable ventilation although the delivered tidal volume is difficult to measure. In the premature neonate these are not serious limitations and pressure limited ventilation is the preferred technique.

Specifically designed, compact, lightweight ventilators, driven by cylinder oxygen and utilizing fluid logic circuits are available for transporting ventilator dependent patients. They are pressure generators and can be used for both adults and children. By entraining air, a choice of either 60 per cent or 100 per cent oxygen is available.

Modes of ventilation

Depending upon the indications for ventilation, the clinician must select the mode of ventilation, choose the ventilation parameters, and adjust the ventilator alarms. The most commonly available ventilator modes include:

Table 3 Guidelines for introduction of mechanical ventilation

A. General indications in acute respiratory failure*
1. Inadequate ventilation Indicated by: (a) Apnoea, upper airway obstruction, unprotected airway (b) Respiratory rate >35 breaths/min [normal range 10–20] (c) Vital capacity < 15 ml/kg [normal range 65–75] (d) Tidal volume < 5 ml/ kg [normal range 5–7] (e) Negative inspiratory force <25 cmH_2O [normal range 75–100] (f) $Paco_2$>3 kPa (60 mmHg) [normal range 4.7–6.3kPa (35–47 mmHg)] (g) VDNT ratio > 0.6 [normal range < 0.3]
2. Inadequate gas exchange oxygenation Indicated by: (a) Pao_2 < 8 kPa (60 mmHg) on Fio_2 > 0.6 (b) (A-a)Do_2 on Fio_2 1.0 > 47 kPa (350 mmHg), [normal range 3.3–8.7 kPa (25–65 mmHg)]
B. Specific indications, with or without prevous respiratory pathology
3. Chronic obstructive lung disease (a) Failure of conservative measures (b) Inability to co-operate with care (c) Decreased consciousness (d) Cardiac instability (e) Apnoea (f) Severe respiratory acidosis (g) Acute management of nocturnal obstructive hypoventilation
4. Chronic restrictive lung disease (a) Severe hypoxaemia (b) Fatigue and impending exhaustion
5. Severe acute asthma (a) Failure of conservative measures (b) Obtundation (c) Cardiac instability (d) Increasing $PaCo_2$ (e) Fatigue and impending exhaustion.
6. Head trauma (a) Unconscious (b) Unprotected airway (c) Cerebral oedema (d) Apnoea or global hypoventilation.
7. Chest trauma (a) Flail chest with hypoventilation and hypoxaemia (b) Pulmonary contusion with hypoxaemia
8. Neuromuscular weakness (a) Apnoea or progressive hypoventilation (see above) (b) Airway protection, nocturnal hypoventilation/hypoxaemia (c) Organophosphate poisoning.
9. Other neurological disorders (a) Status epilepticus (b) Tetanus (c) High cervical spine injury
10. Upper airway protection (a) Loss of consciousness (b) Neck and oropharyngeal trauma (c) Epiglottitis (d) Acute neuromuscular event.
11. Drug overdose Apnoea, hypoventilation, airway protection, seizures

*For source see OTM3, p.2920.

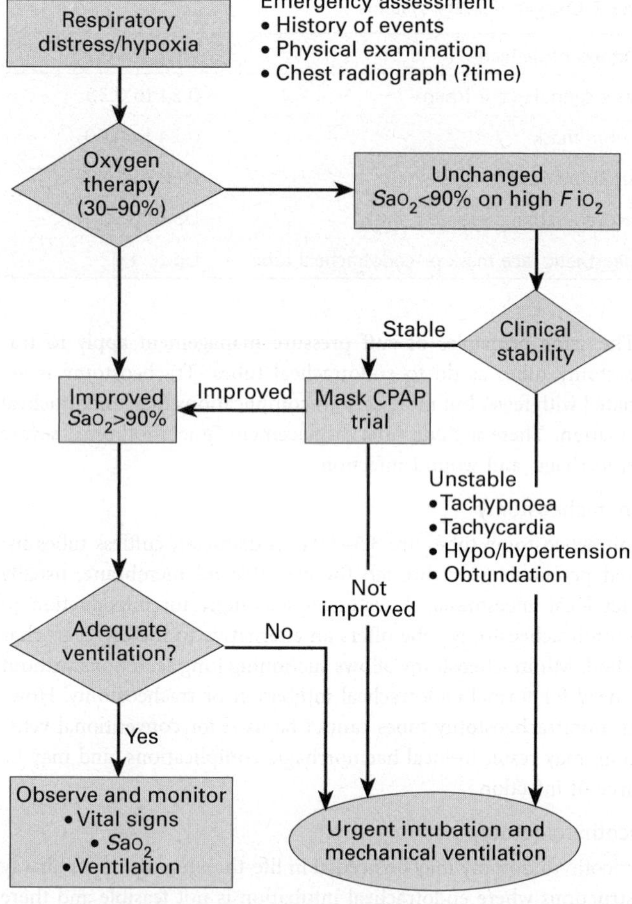

Fig. 2 Respiratory failure algorithm.

(1) control mechanical ventilation (CMV);

(2) assist control (triggered ventilation, volume cycled);

(3) intermittent mandatory ventilation (IMV or SIMV);

(4) pressure support (triggered ventilation, pressure cycled);

(5) others.

CMV provides time and volume cycled, pressure limited breaths at the preset rates but does not allow the patient to breathe spontaneously. This mode is suitable for the paralysed or heavily-sedated patient.

Assist control or triggered ventilation synchronizes the ventilator to the patient's own respiratory rhythm delivering a volume preset, pressure limited tidal volume. A trigger sensitivity must be selected (usually –0.5 to –2.0 cmH_2O) by which the patient can initiate volume preset breaths above the set rates. Patients have a tendency to hyperventilate on assist control. As a safety requirement, a high respiratory rate alarm is needed and a 'back up' ventilation rate must be set in the event of apnoea. Assist control is better tolerated than CMV and the patient requires less sedation.

IMV was originally devised for weaning but is now widely adopted as a maintenance mode. It provides the opportunity for the patient to breathe spontaneously and supplement the positive pressure minute ventilation. In the standard IMV mode there is a theoretical risk of stacking a ventilator breath on top of a spontaneous breath. However, this does not appear to be a significant problem and an appropriately set pressure limit should safeguard this causing inadvertent over-inflation of the lungs. More modern ventilators utilize the triggering or assist facility to synchronize the IMV breaths with the patient's own spontaneous breathing pattern (synchronized IMV, SIMV). The IMV mode is intended as partial ventilation support. With the patient taking spontaneous breaths, IMV is better tolerated than CMV. It results in lower mean airway pressures, has less effect on the cardiovascular system, and allows the patient to regulate their own PCO_2 to at least some degree.

Pressure support uses a triggering facility to deliver not a volume preset breath, as in assist control, but a pressure limited breath (i.e. as with paediatric pressure ventilation). The inspiratory flow rate is usually high so as to minimize phase lag and the work of breathing. Pressure support may be used alone or in conjunction with SIMV when it assists spontaneous breaths. Pressure support provides an efficient maintenance and weaning mode that is well tolerated by the patient. The trigger mechanism is usually a negative pressure threshold but some ventilators trigger on changes in circuit gas flow which potentially could be more sensitive and reduce the work of breathing.

Other modes of ventilation, such as pressure release, high frequency, inverse I:E ratio ventilation and bilevel constant airway pressure (biPAP), have their proponents. Evidence to indicate significant superiority of these modes over conventional methods of ventilation is not convincing. High frequency ventilation in its several forms has been recommended for use following reconstructive laryngeal, tracheal, or bronchial surgery or for patients with bronchopleural or bronchocutaneous fistulae. Even these applications may not offer much advantage, if any, over conventional modes. Mandatory minute ventilation (MMV) is an innovative mode whereby the combined spontaneous and mechanical ventilation must reach a minimum preset level. As the patient's spontaneous ventilation increases, the mechanically assisted breaths become fewer. Individual ventilators vary in their ability to achieve successful MMV.

Sighs

Before the advent of high tidal volume ventilation and positive end expiratory pressure/ constant positive airway pressure (PEEP/CPAP), sighs were added to the ventilation protocol to prevent progressive atelectasis. Each sigh was delivered two to six times per hour and was equivalent to about twice the conventional tidal volume. The risks of barotrauma probably outweigh the theoretical benefits.

Negative pressure ventilation

Negative pressure (tank) ventilators proved their worth during polio myelitis epidemics when large numbers of patients were supported for prolonged periods of time. Positive pressure ventilation has since largely replaced negative pressure ventilation except for specific indication. Like positive pressure ventilation, it is possible not only to generate enhanced tidal volumes but also to maintain lung inflation with the negative pressure equivalent of PEEP. In this context negative pressure ventilation has been successfully adopted in neonates with the respiratory distress syndrome. As an alternative to a large enclosure around the limbs and trunk (with the head and neck protruding) a curasse placed over the anterior thorax can facilitate the application of negative pressure to the chest. Recent developments of the curasse type of negative pressure ventilator (HayekS) permits high frequency oscillations to be used resulting in enhanced gas exchange.

Setting ventilator parameters

Once a ventilation mode has been selected (at least temporarily), ventilatory parameters must be set before attaching the patient to the ventilator. The ventilator parameters include:

(1) tidal volume
(2) ventilation rate
(3) inspiratory/expiratory (I:E) ratio
(4) flow waveform
(5) FiO_2 (0.21 to 1.0)
(6) pressure limit
(7) PEEP/CPAP (0 to 20 cmH_2O)

Tidal volume and ventilation rate

The delivered, inspiratory tidal volume may be set at 10–12 ml/kg body weight. This should be reduced if the patient has restrictive lung disease or has undergone lobectomy or pneumonectomy. Using respiratory rates of more than 10 breaths per min with such tidal volumes will provide full ventilatory support. If the patient is breathing spontaneously, an IMV mode will be preferred at rates of between 4 and 8 breaths per min. If assist control or pressure support is chosen the respiratory rate will be the patient's spontaneous rate and the tidal volumes achieved will depend upon lung compliance and the patient's inspiratory effort.

I:E ratio, inspiratory flow rate

The ratio of inspiratory to expiratory time (I:E ratio) will generally range from 1:2 to 1:4. This provides sufficient time for full passive exhalation. In patients with obstructive lung disease, failing to allow adequate time for exhalation results in hyperinflation (auto or intrinsic PEEP). The higher the set respiratory rate the shorter expiration becomes and the I:E ratio falls. This may lead to the paradoxical situation in the patient with COPD where the PCO_2 rises as the ventilator rate is increased!

The I:E ratio can be adjusted is several ways depending upon the make of ventilator. In some, a ratio can be selected directly, while in others, the inspiratory flow rate determines the duration of inspiration. An acceptable range for inspiratory flow rates is between 30 and 60 l/min (0.5 to 1.0 l/s).

Inspiratory waveforms

Many volume and time cycled (flow generator) ventilators allow the choice of several waveforms. Although there is little evidence to favour one over the other, a square waveform delivers the tidal volume in the least time and with higher peak pressures. A decelerating flow pattern results in lower peak pressures, longer inspiratory intervals, and lower I:E ratios.

Inspired oxygen concentration (FiO_2)

This should be constantly adjusted to provide adequate arterial oxygenation without hyperoxia. Too high a FiO_2 is frequently the cause of failure to wean COPD patients from a mechanical ventilator.

Pressure limit

Setting a pressure limit about 10 cmH_2O above the peak pressure reached during each ventilator cycle protects the patients against inadvertently high pressures experienced during coughing or straining. Hitting the pressure limit terminates inspiration and sounds an alarm.

PEEP/CPAP

Maintaining airway pressure above barometric pressure in a spontaneously breathing patient is called constant positive airway pressure (CPAP). The same pressure applied to a patient on intermittent

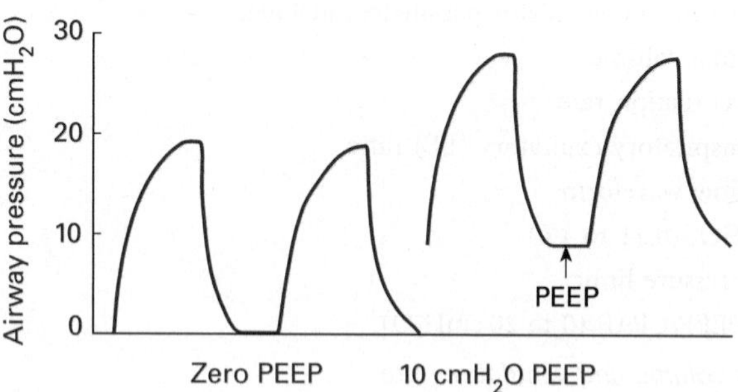

Fig. 3 Schematic of airway pressure measured without PEEP and following the addition of 10 cmH_2O PEEP. By preventing end-expiratory pressure from falling to zero, reinflation and recruitment of alveolar units is encouraged.

positive pressure ventilation is called positive end expiratory pressure (PEEP). PEEP/CPAP is used to correct lung volume (FRC) in conditions characterized by reduced lung volume such as ARDS or cardiogenic pulmonary oedema. It may also be of benefit in patients with flail chest segments by splinting the chest wall. The terms PEEP and CPAP can be used interchangeably provided that the differences regarding spontaneous and assisted ventilation are recognized (Fig. 3).

PEEP/CPAP is achieved by the inclusion of a resistance at the expiratory end of the breathing circuit. Ideally this resistance should be as close to a threshold resistor as possible, such as an under-water column. In practice, most of the valves produce some flow-dependent retardation of expiration that increases the work of breathing in spontaneously breathing patient. Continuous measurement of mixed venous SaO_2 with a suitable flow-directed pulmonary artery catheter is a particularly good method of evaluating the response to a change in PEEP/CPAP.

Trends in the application of PEEP/CPAP in patients with respiratory failure have changed over the years. The use of maximum tolerated levels of PEEP (super-PEEP) and 'best' PEEP have generally been replaced by concepts of 'least' or 'enough' PEEP to allow adequate arterial oxygenation with an FiO_2 less than 0.6. However, it is still not uncommon to have to consider levels of PEEP greater than 10 or 15 cmH_2O, particularly in patients with adult respiratory distress syndrome (ARDS). Care must be exercised to ensure that oxygen delivery is not impaired in the unbridled pursuit of improved arterial oxygenation.

Mask CPAP Continuous positive airway pressure (CPAP) can be applied without resorting to endotracheal intubation for the treatment of selected patients with acute respiratory failure. Close-fitting CPAP masks, which are very similar to standard anaesthetic masks, are widely available together with disposable circuitry and gas supply/pressure regulator mechanisms to ensure the safe delivery of air/oxygen mixtures. Suitable patients should be carefully selected and managed in a clinical area where appropriate observation and monitoring can be assured. This usually would be an intensive care, high dependency, or respiratory unit.

Ventilator monitors and alarms

The ventilation monitors and alarms that must be set and maintained include the following:

(1) exhaled tidal volume (VT), exhaled minute ventilation;

(2) spontaneous respiratory rate;

(3) airway pressure and circuit disconnect;

(4) peak airway pressure;

(5) FiO_2;

(6) inhaled gas temperature.

The importance of ventilator alarms cannot be overemphasized. The modern, microprocessor based ventilator is not only more efficient but is significantly safer than its earlier predecessors.

Clinical monitoring of mechanical ventilation

An essential aspect of monitoring is regular clinical examination of the patient, and inspection of the ventilator and ventilator circuit. Expansion of the chest should be symmetrical with each ventilator cycled breath (CMV, IMV), assisted breath (assist control or pressure support), or unassisted spontaneous breath (IMV). Auscultation should confirm air entry and detect any added sounds. The patient should be sat up or rolled side to side to allow inspection of the whole of the chest. The endotracheal tube should be secure and as comfortable as possible for the patient. The endotracheal cuff pressure should be adjusted to less than 30 mmHg or so that a small air leak becomes audible with a stethoscope on the side of the neck with each ventilator cycle. The ventilator circuit should feel warm but be free of significant amounts of condensed water. The humidifier temperature and water level should be checked.

The pulse oximeter has contributed significantly to the monitoring and safety of patients on mechanical ventilation. Not only does it provide a continuous measurement of oxygenation but also reduces the need for arterial blood gas sampling. Much can be appreciated from watching the ventilator pressure gauge with each cycle. In addition to evaluating peak inspiratory pressure, the clinician will be able to judge whether the patient is 'fighting' the ventilator. Comparing inspiratory and expiratory tidal volumes may indicate a leak in the circuit, either at circuit connections or at the endotracheal tube cuff. When peak pressures are high, the internal compliance of the ventilator and circuit (about 2–2.5 ml/cmH_2O) may account for much of the volume loss. A rough assessment of the compliance of the lung can be made by following the peak inflation pressures.

Weaning of mechanical ventilation

More than 80 per cent of patients who are ventilated postoperatively can be weaned simply by clinically evaluating their spontaneous ventilation on a 'T-piece' or similar circuit. The remainder require a progressive reduction in ventilatory support until measurement of ventilation parameters can be made. These parameters include the negative inspiratory force (NIF) and vital capacity (VC). A NIF greater than −25 cmH_2O or a VC greater than 10 ml/kg usually indicates sufficient ventilatory reserve for spontaneous ventilation. These parameters cannot be applied reliably to patients with severe COPD, instead blood gases have to be followed with each reduction in ventilation support. Modes of ventilation such as SIMV, IMV, and pressure support are very suitable for weaning since they allow gradual and progressive reduction in ventilation support. Regular clinical and physiological assessment after each reduction in ventilation support is essential. Failure to wean a patient successfully from mechanical ventilation should prompt the questions addressed in Table 4.

Complications of mechanical ventilation

Several complications of mechanical ventilation can be attributed to the local effects of the endotracheal tube upon the airway. These

Table 4 Questions to ask when weaning is difficult:

1. Is the endotracheal tube of optimal size? Small endotracheal tubes of <7mm internal diameter have a high resistance.
2. Has the patient been seated upright to aid lung mechanics?
3. Is there evidence of airway obstruction that would improve with bronchodilator or steroid therapy?
4. Are there respiratory depressant drugs being administered?
5. Is there evidence of occult neuromuscular disease? Exclude interactions with aminoglycosides.
6. Is there evidence of hypothyroidism, hypophosphataemia or hypomagnesaemia?
7. Is there a metabolic alkalosis? If so this should be corrected with potassium, chloride and volume as appropriate.
8. Is there evidence of malnourishment on history or simple laboratory test such as serum albumin.
9. Is tracheostomy indicated?
10. In COPD patients, are the target blood gases similar to the premorbid values?
11. Is there evidence of diaphragmatic dysfunction due to phrenic nerve injury ?

include airway obstruction due to endotracheal tube displacement and pressure necrosis leading to vocal cord injury and subglottic stenosis. The risk of nosocomial pneumonia is increased in the intubated patient. Many complications are the direct consequence of positive pressure ventilation. Haemodynamic effects such as reduced cardiac output, reduced renal perfusion, and salt and water retention are primarily the result of mechanical, neuroreflex, and humoral factors. Interstitial lung damage may occur due to positive pressure ventilation and this has prompted renewed interest in extracorporeal systems for the management of patients with ARDS.

The greatest concern relates to the risk of pneumothorax, pneumomediastinum, pneumopericardium, or subcutaneous emphysema. Pneumothorax is the most feared complication because it is associated with rapid deterioration unless dealt with quickly. Signs of barotrauma include arterial desaturation (pulse oximeter), sudden rise in peak airway pressure, hypotension and tachycardia, and finally circulatory collapse.

Tube thoracostomy is mandatory since progression to a tension pneumothorax is very likely. Emergency decompression with a 14 gauge cannula may produce temporary relief and may have a diagnostic role, but tube thoracostomy should be performed without delay and without radiographic confirmation if necessary. Blunt dissection through the parietal pleura with forceps and digital exploration of the pleural space prior to insertion of the thoracostomy tube is essential if lung damage is to be avoided.

Specific strategies in ventilator management

Restrictive lung disease

Patients with restrictive lung diseases such as sarcoidosis or fibrosing alveolitis should be ventilated with small tidal volumes of between 5 and 8 ml/kg at rates of 15 to 20 breaths per min. Oxygen need not be restricted in the manner recommended for patients with COPD.

Chronic obstructive pulmonary disease (COPD)

Most cases of acute on chronic respiratory failure can be managed successfully without mechanical ventilation. A small proportion of patients fail to respond to conservative measures and require ventilatory assistance. In many cases, the need for mechanical ventilation is the direct result of injudicious oxygen therapy. Low rate SIMV (6 to 8 breaths per min) or low pressure levels of pressure support are idea for COPD patients with acute on chronic respiratory failure. The $PaCO_2$ should be reduced very slowly towards but not to normal levels. The FiO_2 rarely needs to be higher than 0.35. High ventilator rates (<14 per min) are associated with high values of VDNT (>0.5). Paradoxically, as the ventilator rates are increased in an attempt to increase minute ventilation, the $PaCO_2$ may rise. To avoid intrinsic or autoPEEP, the I:E ratio should be maintained at 1:2 or more. Weaning can begin as soon as the precipitating cause of respiratory failure has been corrected. Weaning will be unsuccessful if there is any underlying metabolic alkalosis or the patient receives sedative or analgesic agents. The $PaCO_2$ can be allowed to rise slowly to above normal levels provided sufficient time is given for the blood pH to correct and the FiO_2 kept below 0.35. Carbon dioxide production can be minimized by providing balanced nutrition with calories being provided by both lipid and carbohydrate.

Asthma

Probably less than 1 per cent of acute severe asthma attacks require mechanical ventilation. However, it is apparent that some patients suffer cardiac arrest and die each year because intubation and mechanical ventilation was not performed in time. Hypercarbia alone is generally insufficient indication for ventilation but a combination of a rising $PaCO_2$, fatigue, failure of conservative measures, or arrhythmias does call for elective intubation and mechanical ventilation. Adequate oxygenation must be ensured by the administration of unrestricted and high concentrations of oxygen in contrast to the CO_2 retaining COPD patient for whom controlled oxygen (24–28 per cent) is generally indicated.

A philosophy of 'permissive hypercapnia' or 'controlled hypoventilation' should be adopted with the $PaCO_2$ remaining at elevated levels (7–8 kPa, 50–60 mmHg). Lower tidal volumes and respiratory rates are therefore possible. Deaths in ventilated asthmatic patients are rare but are usually the result of barotrauma, hypotension in volume depleted patients, arrhythmias, or lung infection.

Maximal bronchodilator therapy including corticosteroids are continued throughout the period of mechanical ventilation, supplemented if necessary with inhalational anaesthetics such as isoflurane or the intravenous anaesthetic ketamine. Both of these agents are potent bronchodilators. Rehydration and adequate humidification of inspired gases will ordinarily mobilize secretions and mucous plugs; if not, bronchoalveolar lavage may be indicated.

The use of extracorporeal membrane oxygenation and CO_2 removal has been reported in acute asthma. These must be considered exceptional cases and such techniques cannot be generally recommended.

Bronchopleural/bronchocutaneous fistulae

Although bronchopleural and bronchocutaneous fistulae can occur after trauma or lung infection, many arise during the postoperative period following lobectomy or pneumonectomy. To reduce the risk of this, low tidal volume, high respiratory rate ventilation should be adopted to minimize inflation pressures. High frequency ventilation would appear to be ideally suited to the prevention of bronchopleural fistula although evidence to prove superiority over conventional ventilation is lacking.

Compensation for the loss of tidal volume through the fistula is easily made by adjusting the ventilator but if the leak is large, endobronchial intubation may be necessary. Bronchopleural and bronchocutaneous fistulae are unlikely to close until the patient is weaned from the ventilator.

Further reading

Bott, J., Carroll, M.P., Conway, J.H., *et al.* (1993). Randomised controlled trial of nasal ventilation in acute ventilatory failure due to chronic obstructive airways disease. *Lancet*, **341**, 1555–7.

Brochard, L., Mancebo, J., Wysocki, M., *et al.* (1995). Non-invasive ventilation for acute exacerbations of chronic obstructive pulmonary disease. *New England Journal of Medicine*, **333**, 817–22.

Elliott, M. and Moxham, J. (1994). Non-invasive mechanical ventilation by nasal or face mask. In *Principles and practice of mechanical ventilation* (ed. M.J. Tobin), pp. 427–53. McGraw Hill, New York.

Garrard, C.S. (1992). Mechanical ventilation support in severe asthma. *Care of the Critically Ill*, **8**, 201–11.

Hershey, M.D. (1993). Ventilatory support of patients with respiratory failure. *International Anaesthesiolgy Clinics*, **31**, 149–68.

Hickling, K.G., Henderson, S.J., and Jackson, R. (1990). Low mortality associated with low volume pressure limited ventilation with permissive hypercapnia in severe adult respiratory distress syndrome. *Intensive Care Medicine*, **16**, 372–7.

Jubran, A. and Tobin, M.J. (1996). Monitoring during mechanical ventilation. *Clinics in Chest Medicine*, **17**, 453–73.

Leatherman, J.W. (1996). Mechanical ventilation in obstructive lung disease. *Clinics in Chest Medicine*, **17**, 577–90.

Lessard, M.R. and Brochard, L.J. (1996). Weaning from ventilatory support. *Clinics in Chest Medicine*, **17**, 475–89.

Moxham, J. and Shneerson, J.M. (1993). Diaphragmatic pacing. *American Review of Respiratory Disease*, **148**, 533–6.

Nava, S., Ambosino, N., Clini, E., *et al.* (1998). Non-invasive ventilation in the weaning of patients with respiratory failure due to chronic obstructive pulmonary disease: A randomised, controlled study. *Annals of Internal Medicine*, **128**, 721–8.

Sawicka, E.H., Loh, L., and Branthwaite, M.A. (1988). Domiciliary ventilatory support: an analysis of outcome. *Thorax*, **43**, 31–5.

Udwadia, Z.F., Santis, G.K., Steven, M.H., and Simonds, A.K. (1992). Nasal ventilation to facilitate weaning in patients with chronic respiratory insufficiency. *Thorax*, **47**, 715–18.

Chapter 4.45

Lung and heart–lung transplantation

M. Asif and T. W. Higenbottam

Introduction

In the last 18 years, lung and heart–lung transplantation have become established as treatments for a wide range of endstage lung and cardiopulmonary disease. The main advantage of transplant surgery is the replacement of lungs disrupted by chronic disease with normal lungs.

Postoperative medical care and immunosuppressive treatments continue to improve and as a result survival as well as the recipient's quality of life have been enhanced. Newer surgical techniques include the use of lungs from living, related donors. There remains the problem of too few organs to treat all potential recipients. Xenografts and 'cloned' organs remain for the future, but use of organs from non-heart-beating donors could offer the benefits of lung transplant surgery to a larger population by increasing the donor pool.

Obliterative bronchiolitis (OB), the main long-term complication, is often disabling and fatal. It results from chronic rejection and viral infections such as cytomegalovirus (CMV) and adenovirus. New and improved immunosuppressive therapies have proved less toxic and more effective in controlling rejection and so decreasing the incidence of OB. Prophylaxis and early therapy for CMV may also lessen the incidence. Specific therapies to impede the progressive obliteration of the airways are, however, still awaited.

Survival from lung and heart–lung transplantation

The International Society for Heart and Lung Transplantation (ISHLT) has registered 2428 heart–lung transplants, 4777 single lung, and 3278 bilateral/double lung transplants since 1981 at over 150 centres. Results are almost as good as those for other solid organ transplants.

Early deaths result from complications occurring during surgery and early postoperative care, late deaths from rejection, immunosuppressive treatment, and OB (Table 1).

Five-year survival according to the ISHLT registry is 40 per cent for heart–lung transplants, 40 per cent for single lung, and 48 per cent for bilateral/double lung transplants. Survival depends on the recipient's original disease. For unknown reasons, pulmonary arterial hypertension is associated with a poorer survival than emphysema.

Selection of the patients for referral for lung transplants

A working group for the American Thoracic Society, ISHLT, the European Respiratory Society, and the American Society of Transplant Physicians has recently provided guidelines for referral of potential lung transplant recipients.

The indications for lung and heart–lung transplant surgery

Physicians considering referral for transplant surgery should ensure that the patient has received optimal medical treatment but continues

Table 1 Causes of death after heart–lung transplantation ($n = 100$)

Death within 3 months	Death after 3 months
Rejection 1	Obliterative bronchiolitis 17
Infection 8	Infection 5
Tracheal dehiscence 2	Cerebrovascular event 1
Cerebrovascular event 2	Renal factors 1
Lung failure 2	Air traffic accident 1
Liver failure 1	
Graft-versus-host disease 1	

to deteriorate. Rarely, transplantation is offered for acute illness. Comorbid illness should be diagnosed and adequately treated.

Prognosis is worse in older than younger patients. The age limits are: 55 years for heart–lung transplants, 65 years for single lung transplants, and 60 years for bilateral lung transplants.

Chronic obstructive lung disease (COLD) (chronic bronchitis and emphysema)

Asthma must be excluded and patients should have received adequate rehabilitation and long-term oxygen therapy. Lung volume reduction surgery is an alternative for selected patients with extensive bilateral emphysema without respiratory failure.

Referral criteria are:

- $FEV_1 < 25$ per cent of the predicted value (without reversibility);
- and/or $PaO_2 \geq 7.3$ kPa with evidence of pulmonary hypertension;
- patients with elevated PaO_2 who continue to deteriorate despite long-term oxygen therapy.

Cryptogenic fibrosing alveolitis (CFA) or other forms of diffuse lung fibrosis

Single lung transplantation is effective for all forms of diffuse interstitial lung fibrosis, including sarcoidosis, the lung fibrosis of connective tissue diseases, and drug-induced diffuse lung disease. CFA is a rapidly progressive illness with high mortality and requires early referral as the medical treatment is usually ineffective.

Referral criteria are:

- symptomatic with deteriorating lung function despite maximal medical treatment with high-dose (daily dose > 20 mg prednisolone) corticosteroid:
- diffusing capacity (TLCO) and vital capacity less than 50–60 per cent of predicted values.

In systemic diseases with diffuse lung fibrosis, such as systemic sclerosis, it is important that the underlying disease is quiescent. Patients should be individually assessed.

Pulmonary arterial hypertension

All patients are anticoagulated to an INR of greater than 2.5. The development of right ventricular failure is the most important determinant of survival; this can be assessed by right heart catheterization.

- A cardiac index (CI) of more than 2.5 l/min per m^2, or mixed venous oxygen saturation (SvO_2) (pulmonary artery sample) of more than 60 per cent and a mean right atrial pressure (mRAP) of less than 12 mmHg indicates a good survival, of more than 60 per cent at 3 years.

If intravenous infusion of prostacyclin (PGI_2) during the right heart catheter study causes pulmonary vasodilation, an oral calcium channel blocker such as amlodopine can be used.

- In patients with advanced disease (CI < 2.5 l/min per m^2, or SvO_2 is < 65 per cent, or if the mRAP is > 12 mmHg) continuous intravenous PGI_2 or Iloprost (a prostacyclin analogue) can prolong life to beyond 3 years in over 80 per cent of patients.
- Only when these medical treatments have failed is lung transplantation considered.

In patients with thromboembolic pulmonary hypertension and evidence on pulmonary arteriography of central thrombi, obstructing lobar, and segmental pulmonary arteries, pulmonary thromboendarterectomy (PTEA) is effective. Referral of those patients not suitable for PTEA for transplantation again is after failure of medical treatment.

In selected patients, atrial septostomy can improve symptoms and may increase survival. Pulmonary venous hypertension, left ventricular failure induced veno-occlusive disease, and pulmonary capillary haemangiomatosis need early referral for transplantation as PGI_2 is contraindicated here.

Patients with pulmonary hypertension secondary to congenital heart disease (Eisenmenger's syndrome), should be considered for transplant surgery when they show evidence of right ventricular failure. Again CI < 2.5 l/min per m^2 and mRAP > 12 mmHg are appropriate indices for referral.

Criterion for referral is:

- failure of prostacyclin therapy to prevent decline in cardiovascular indices.

Cystic fibrosis

Lung transplantation is a particularly effective treatment when respiratory failure has developed. Usually FEV_1 is less than 20 per cent, $PaO_2 < 6.5$ kPa, and there is hypercapnia. It can also be used in patients with uncontrolled sepsis or haemoptysis.

Referral criteria are:

- $FEV_1 < 30$ per cent of the predicted value and/or frequent hospital admissions and developing cachexia;
- $PaO_2 < 7.3$ mmHg or $PaCO_2 > 6.7$ mmHg.

Paediatric lung transplantation

Indications include: pulmonary hypertension with and without structural cardiac disease, pulmonary vein stenosis and congenital abnormalities of lung development. All possible medical and surgical treatments should have been instituted and there must be evidence of progression and marked disability.

General medical conditions which influence the decision to refer for transplantation

1. Symptomatic osteoporosis requires treatment before a patient undergoes lung transplantation.
2. Severe musculoskeletal disease is a relative contraindication, progressive disease precludes surgery.
3. Corticosteroid therapy should be reduced to below 20 mg prednisolone per day.
4. Weight should be at least 70 per cent of ideal body weight.
5. Patients should be free of addiction, including to cigarette smoking.
6. Psychosocial disorders should have been resolved.
7. Invasive assisted ventilation precludes transplantation.
8. Colonization with fungi and atypical mycobacteria should be assessed individually. Pulmonary tuberculosis should have been fully treated before transplant surgery.
9. Systemic diseases should be quiescent or under medical control.

Patients are not considered for transplant surgery if they have any of the following:

- renal failure (creatinine clearance of < 50 mg/ml per min);
- HIV;
- active malignancy, 2 years for basal cell skin cancers, 5 years for solid tumours;
- hepatitis B antigen positivity, hepatitis C with biopsy-proven histological evidence of liver disease.

Table 2 Choice of lung and heart–lung transplants in the United Kingdom

Primary pulmonary hypertension	Bilateral lung transplant
Eisenmenger's syndrome	Heart–lung transplant
Chronic thromboembolic disease	Bilateral lung transplant
Cystic fibrosis	Bilateral lung transplant
Bronchiectasis	Bilateral lung transplant
Cryptogenic fibrosing alveolitis	Single-lung transplant
Emphysema	Single-lung transplant
Granulomatous and fibrotic lung disease	Single-lung transplant

Types of lung transplant operation (Table 2)

Single lung tranplantation

This is effective for diffuse lung fibrosis, including CFA, sarcoidosis, and histiocytosis X and emphysema. It is used in primary pulmonary hypertension but acute graft injury remains a common complication, and long-term complications such as OB markedly impair gas exchange. Long-term outcome is poorer than double lung and heart–lung transplantation.

Bronchiectasis should be excluded with high resolution CT in CFA and COLD as infection spreads from the native to the engrafted lung. If present, double lung transplantation is required.

Single lung transplantation allows treatment of two recipients. It does not require cardiopulmonary bypass, making it suitable for older patients.

Sequential bilateral lung transplantation

This is useful for suppurative lung diseases such as bronchiectasis, cystic fibrosis, and chronic obstructive bronchitis with or without emphysema and pulmonary hypertension. Since patients retain their own hearts they avoid chronic cardiac rejection. The operation does not necessarily require cardiopulmonary bypass.

Heart–lung transplantation

This was introduced for cystic fibrosis, primary pulmonary hypertension, and Eisenmenger's syndrome. Perfusion of the tracheal anastomosis is maintained through extensive collateral arteries from the mediastinum.

Two lungs and one heart are needed for a single recipient. The 'domino' operation was devised so that the recipients can donate their heart to another cardiac recipient. In many countries, sequential double-lung transplantation has replaced heart–lung transplantation for all except patients with Eisenmenger's syndrome.

Living related donors

Lobes from living family members can be grafted into children, mainly with cystic fibrosis. Survival and physiological improvement are good. There are only limited dangers to the donor.

Donor selection and organ procurement

Less than 20 per cent of some 1000 potential donors in the UK each year will be suitable. Brain death, prolonged assisted ventilation, and intensive care are associated with lower respiratory tract infection or acute lung injury that preclude lung donation (Table 3).

Table 3 Lung donor selection criteria

Age < 45 years
No past history of pulmonary disease including asthma
No thoracic trauma
No pulmonary or systemic infection
Normal chest radiograph
Short period of assisted ventilation
Normal lung compliance; peak respiratory airway pressure < 30 cmH_2O with tidal volume 15 ml/kg and respiratory rate 10–14 mm
Normal gas exchange; Pa_{O_2} > 13.5 kPa with Fi_{O_2} = 30%
HIV negative
For heart–lung transplantation
No heart disease
Normal electrocardiogram
Minimal inotropic requirements (dopamine or dobutamine < 10μg/kg/m)

Donor and recipient are matched according to ABO blood groups. The size match between donor and recipient lungs is currently based on their total lung capacity predicted from their sex, age, and height. Ideally, donors seropositive for cytomegalovirus are only used in cytomegalovirus-positive recipients. In many countries this is not possible and so prophylaxis is used with effective acute therapy of infections.

Prostacyclin, Iloprost, or PGE is infused into the pulmonary artery maximally vasodilating the pulmonary vasculature before the perfusate solution at 4° C is infused into the lung. This has enhanced graft function immediately after surgery and has extended ischaemic times to beyond 4 h, enabling the procurement operation to take place at a distant hospital.

Immediate postoperative care

The three main objectives are to establish effective immunosuppression, negative fluid balance, and extubation and mobilization.

Antilymphocytic globulin is no longer used after cardiac transplantation; the same may soon apply to lung transplantation. Instead, intravenous cyclosporine is used perioperatively. Thanks to better surgical and lung-preservation techniques, corticosteroids are no longer contraindicated in the postoperative period.

Despite improved preservation techniques, ischaemia can injure the lung. Hyaline membrane and alveolar capillary injury may be detectable soon after surgery, indicating the risk of non-cardiogenic pulmonary oedema. For this reason hypervolaemia is carefully avoided by fluid restriction and intense use of diuretics over the first 3 days.

Assisted ventilation is not usually required for prolonged periods after surgery if the lungs were satisfactorily preserved. The ideal is less than 24 h, allowing early mobilization. It is no longer necessary to isolate patients postoperatively to prevent infection during the induction of immunosuppression.

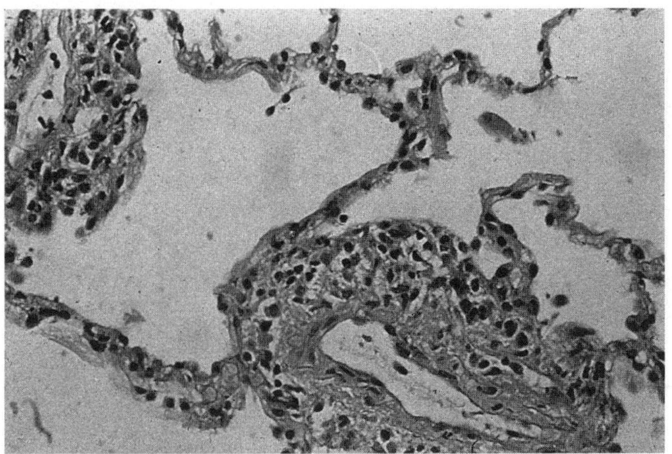

Fig. 1 A transbronchial lung biopsy showing a dense lymphocyte perivascular infiltrate type of acute rejection.
(See OTM3, p.2936 for source.)

Medical management after lung transplantation

This is directed to early diagnosis and treatment of rejection and infection, and the maintenance of adequate immunosuppression.

Acute rejection

Acute rejection is indistinguishable from pulmonary infection by clinical signs, radiology, or pulmonary function tests. Often the chest radiograph is normal in acute rejection. To distinguish between them it is necessary to perform fibre-optic bronchoscopy with bronchoalveolar lavage and transbronchial lung biopsy. Multiple biopsies, attempting to sample all lobes, are taken from one lung.

The biopsies are processed for histology, and specially stained to identify opportunistic infections. In acute lung rejection, perivascular lymphocyte infiltrates are seen (Fig. 1), as are lymphocytic infiltrates of bronchioles. Pneumonia can be diagnosed by identifying the pathogen with standard histological techniques. Rejection and infection can coexist. Examination of bronchoalveolar lavage specimens does not allow diagnosis of rejection.

Rejection is treated with daily intravenous methylprednisolone for 3 days. Doses between 125 and 1000 mg according to weight are required. Oral prednisolone is taken in decreasing doses for a further 10 days. Recurrent rejection is treated with continuous oral steroids; which are required in the long-term with cyclosporin and azathioprine by a third of patients.

A scheme of grading the severity of the histological appearances of acute rejection has been agreed internationally and so different transplant centres share the same treatment regimes and diagnostic procedures (Table 4).

Infection

Pulmonary infections include pneumonias, lower respiratory tract infections, and chronic suppurative lung disease such as bronchiectasis (Table 5). Diagnostic investigations include sputum cultures, blood, bronchoalveolar lavage, and transbronchial lung biopsy specimens for viral, bacterial, and fungal pathogens.

Recipients who are seronegative for cytomegalovirus before surgery are at high risk of developing cytomegalovirus pneumonia if they

Table 4 Histological classification of pulmonary rejection

Classification	Principal histological finding
Acute rejection	Perivascular mononuclear infiltrates with or without airway inflammation
Acute airway damage without fibrosis	Lymphocytic bronchitis or bronchiolitis without perivascular infiltrates
Chronic rejection of airways	Bronchiolitis obliterans
Chronic vascular rejection	Fibrointimal thickening of arteries and veins

Adapted from the working formulation of the Lung Rejection Study Group

Table 5 Early pulmonary infections after heart–lung transplantation

Site of infection	Number	Organism cultured		Deaths (%)
Pneumonia	7	*B. aeruginosa* *K. pneumonia*	6 1	43
Emphysema	3	*P. aeruginosa* *Staph. aureus*	2 1	66
Paratracheal abcess	2	*C. perfridens* *Staph. aureus* with *H. influenzae*	1 1	50
Acute bronchitis	3	*P. aeruginosa* *Staph. epidermidis*	2 1	0
Peritonitis	1	Enterococci	1	0
Septicaemia	1	*P. aeruginosa*	1	0

Infections which occurred in 17 of 100 heart–lung transplant patients within 30 days of surgery.

Table 6 International classification of the bronchiolitis obliterans syndrome (BOS)

Normal	FEV_1 > 80% baseline
Minimal BOS	79% > FEV_1 > 65% baseline
Moderate BOS	64% > FEV_1 > 50% baseline
Severe BOS	FEV_1 < 49%

Baseline FEV_1 is defined as the average of the best two values obtained at least 3 months after surgery.

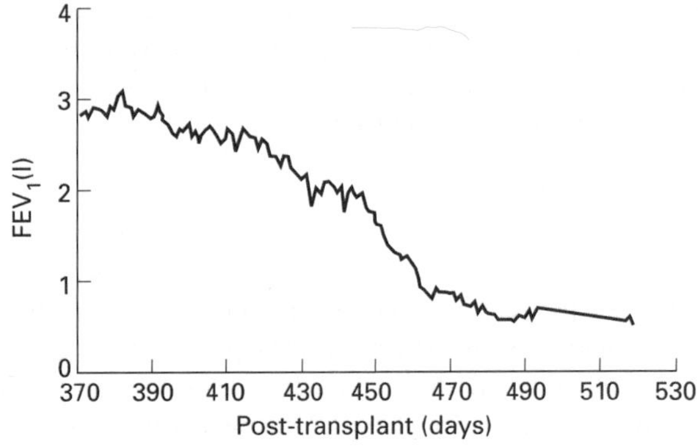

Fig. 2 An irreversible decline in FEV_1 is physiologically pathognomic of bronchiolitis obliterans.
(See OTM3, p. 2937 for source.)

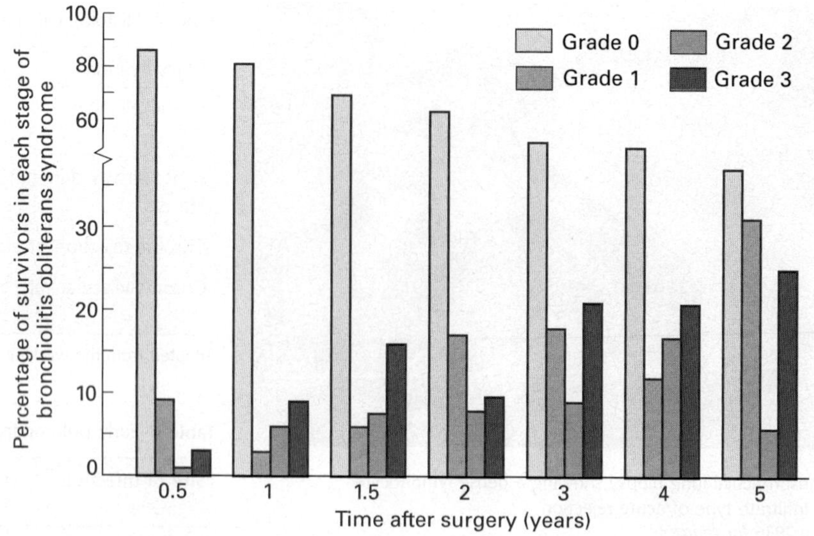

Fig. 3 The proportions of patients maintaining normal grade O (FEV_1 > 80 per cent), minimal grade 1 (80 per cent > FEV_1 > 65 per cent predicted), moderate grade 2 (65 per cent > FEV_1 > 50 per cent predicted), and severe grade 3 (FEV_1 < 50 per cent predicted) airflow obstruction.

receive organs from a seropositive donor. Treatment is with intravenous ganciclovir for 14 days. Latent herpes simplex virus infection can be reactivated in seropositive patients to cause pneumonia within the first 6 months of transplant surgery or when immunosuppression is increased. Seropositive recipients can be protected by prophylactic acyclovir for the first 6 months and when patients are treated for rejection. Epstein–Barr virus infections are usually reactivated and are also treated with acyclovir and may initiate lymphoproliferative disease.

Pneumocystis carinii pneumonia is precipitated by augmentation of immunosuppression. The organism is encountered in up to 30 per cent of bronchoalveolar lavage specimens from asymptomatic patients. Prophylaxis with oral trimethoprim (160 mg) and sulfamethoxazole (800 mg) each day has reduced the risk in heart–lung transplant patients. *Toxoplasma gondii* infection seldom affects the lung but causes a systemic illness, often with cardiac involvement. It is acquired when seropositive donor organs are used in a seronegative recipient. In these cases infection can be prevented by prophylactic pyrimethamine with folinic acid for the first 6 weeks after transplantation.

Yeast and fungal infections cause tracheobronchitis more commonly than pneumonia. Airway complications of single- and double-lung transplants are frequently associated with *Aspergillus fumigatus* infections. All infections with yeast or fungi, where quantitative counts of cultures or invasion are seen on biopsy, are treated with intravenous amphotericin. The liposomal preparation of amphotericin is effective and less likely to cause renal impairment.

Lymphoproliferative disease

Lymphoproliferative disease is caused by Epstein–Barr virus and occurs when immunosuppressive treatment is maximized. An incidence of 9.4 per cent has been reported in heart–lung transplant patients. Abnormal lymphoid tissue may be present within the lung, the mediastinum, or the small bowel. It is a B-cell expansion with features of a malignant lymphoma. Treatment with acyclovir and reduction of the level of immunosuppression may be effective. However, chemotherapy or radiotherapy may become necessary, particularly when lymph node involvement is found.

Nephrotoxicity and systemic hypertension

Cyclosporin can induce acute but reversible renal impairment as well as establish renal failure. This effect, together with systemic hypertension, is dependent on dose. Since higher doses are required in heart–lung and lung transplants than in other transplants, up to 44 per cent of patients require antihypertensive treatment.

Obliterative bronchiolitis

OB accounts for most late deaths after lung transplantation. There is submucosal fibrosis of the bronchioles which obstructs the lumen and extensive bronchiectasis of the central airways. Patients develop disabling severe airflow obstruction with an irreversible fall in FEV_1 (Table 6, Fig. 2). It is associated with frequent, acute rejection episodes. Patients with CMV infection are more prone to OB as are children who experience adenovirus infection. A common proliferative fibrosis of the airway is probably initiated by both infection and frequent rejection. There is no treatment, and patients ultimately die of respiratory failure.

With increasing time after surgery, more patients develop some degree of airflow obstruction. After 5 years, less than 50 per cent of heart–lung transplant patients will have a normal FEV_1 (Fig. 3). This condition has become the major limitation of lung and heart–lung transplantation.

Further reading

Akimine, S., Katayama, Y., Higenbottam, T., and Locke, T. (1998). Developments in inhaled immunosuppressive therapy for the prevention of pulmonary graft rejection. *Biodrugs*, 9, 49–59.

Cooper, J.D., Billingham, M., Egan, T., Hertz, M.I., and Higenbottam, T. A. working formulation for the standardisation of the nomenclature for clinical staging chronic dysfunction in lung allografts. *ISHLT Journal of Heart Lung Tranplantation*, 12, 713–16.

Higenbottam, T., Otulana, B., and Wallwork, J. (1990). The physiology of heart-lung transplantation in man. *News in Physiological Science*, 5, 71–4.

Wallwork, J. (1989). *Heart and heart-lung transplantation.* W.B. Saunders, Harcourt Brace Jovanovich, Philadelphia.

Section 5
Gastroenterology

Contents

Chapter 5.1

Symptomatology of gastrointestinal diseases

From contributions to OTM3 by J. Dent, D. P. Jewell, L. A. Turnberg, and D. G. Thompson

Dysphagia and other symptoms of oesophageal disease

Indigestion-like symptoms arising from the oesophagus

In the great majority of patients these symptoms arise from oesophageal mucosal irritation by refluxed gastric juice, ingested irritants or damage to the mucosa caused by infective agents. Reflux disease is overwhelmingly the most common cause (see Chapter 5.3 and OTM3, Chapter 14.6).

Heartburn is an episodic, lower retrosternal/epigastric burning pain that radiates upwards, sometimes to as high as the pharynx or jaw. Reflux may also induce lower retrosternal or epigastric burning without radiation, or a poorly localized lower chest/upper abdominal discomfort or unease. Pain tends to occur after food and is provoked by large, fatty, or highly spiced meals, by bending or stooping, or heavy physical exertion, and relieved by antacids.

Damage to the oesophageal mucosa from causes other than gastro-oesophageal reflux can lead to similar symptoms. Hypersensitivity of the oesophageal mucosa can be 'primary' (irritable oesophagus) or due to damage by infection, irradiation, or by injury induced by drugs or other substances.

Dysphagia

The term implies a sensation of mechanical difficulty with movement of food from the mouth to the stomach. High and low dysphagia should be distinguished, as their investigation and causes differ. With high dysphagia, oral, pharyngeal or upper oesophageal structural abnormalities or motor dysfunction are the causes. The patient has difficulty with ejection of boluses from the mouth, takes many swallows to clear a normal-sized bolus, and usually coughs and splutters due to aspiration. With low dysphagia, successful swallowing is followed by a sensation of food hold-up. The surface location of the sensation of obstruction is an unreliable indication of the site of obstruction.

Solid boluses are most likely to cause symptoms because they require more propulsive force than liquids. Association of dysphagia with swallowing of hard boluses above a particular size is strongly suggestive of a fixed narrowing, either due to extrinsic compression or oesophageal stricture. Oesophageal obstruction is confirmed by regurgitation of saliva and other oesophageal contents, and inability to swallow further boluses. Bolus impaction at an oesophageal stenosis can lead to secondary painful oesophageal spasm.

Duration, progression, and frequency

Typically, the dysphagia of motor disorders will have been present for many months or years at presentation. Non-specific motor disorders usually cause mild, intermittent dysphagia with solids. Steady progression of severity over a period of weeks is ominous, as it is usually due to malignant obstruction. The dysphagia of achalasia normally occurs with almost every meal and is frequently associated with regurgitation. Typically, the dysphagia of diffuse oesophageal spasm is associated with crushing retrosternal pain and occurs episodically and between episodes there is total freedom from dysphagia.

Regurgitation

Regurgitation is the effortless appearance of material in the pharynx without prior nausea, often misdiagnosed as vomiting. It is usually of small volume, but can be disabling. Symptoms should be evaluated critically to differentiate true vomiting from regurgitation. The regurgitation of reflux disease is typically episodic, but in severe cases it can occur after every meal. It changes little in pattern over months to years. Regurgitation is usually a prominent symptom in achalasia, occurring several times a week with gradual worsening over months to years.

Chest pain and pain on swallowing (odynophagia)

Oesophageal pain from both mucosa and muscle typically occurs retrosternally and may radiate into the arms or jaw. Not infrequently, the pain pattern is indistinguishable from cardiac pain if it is not clearly linked in time to swallowing.

Association of severe retrosternal pain with dysphagia points strongly towards diffuse oesophageal spasm or achalasia, but absence of this association does not rule out these diagnoses. Resolution of pain during high-level acid suppression suggests that the pain is reflux induced. Consistent lack of tight association of chronic chest pain with exertion makes an oesophageal more likely than a cardiac source.

Vomiting

Vomiting is a common symptom of many disorders. The clinical circumstances will often help in diagnosis of the cause. If it is in the morning soon after waking it is characteristic of pregnancy, alcoholism, and metabolic disturbances such as uraemia. Vomiting associated with psychological disorders usually occurs during or soon after a meal. Pyloric canal ulcers may also cause vomiting immediately after a meal. Delayed vomiting (more than 1 h after a meal) is the usual pattern associated with peptic ulcer, gastric carcinoma, gallbladder disease, and intestinal obstruction. Projectile vomiting is often seen in pyloric stenosis and is said to occur in patients with raised intracranial pressure.

The content of the vomitus may provide some diagnostic clues. 'Vomiting' of undigested food suggests that it is regurgitation secondary to achalasia, an oesophageal stricture, or a pharyngeal diverticulum. Intestinal contents in the vomitus suggest intestinal obstruction or ileus and the vomit usually has a faecal odour. Bilious vomiting characteristically occurs after gastric surgery. Altered blood ('coffee grounds') is of obvious significance.

Patients who are vomiting because of delayed gastric emptying may show gastric distension on physical examination and a succession splash may be present. Visible peristalsis may be seen in patients with gastric-outlet or intestinal obstruction.

Psychogenic vomiting is not uncommon and mainly affects women. There is often a long history (e.g. vomiting associated with school examinations). Vomiting normally occurs after a meal but can usually be suppressed until the patient reaches a bathroom or lavatory. It is frequently a feature of bulimia nervosa (see Chapter 14.8). The diagnosis should be recognized quickly and extensive investigation should be avoided.

Cyclical vomiting occurs in children and is characterized by recurrent attacks of severe vomiting, which may last for several days. The onset is sudden and may be associated with headache, abdominal pain, and, occasionally, fever. The syndrome usually starts before the age of 6 years and the frequency of the attacks varies from more than one a month to one or two each year. The cause is unknown. Organic disease, especially intracranial pathology, must be excluded. Most children gradually improve with increasing age and the attacks usually stop by the end of puberty.

Abdominal pain

Pain from specific viscera

Oesophageal disorders are unlikely to cause abdominal pain. Pain from the stomach and duodenum is usually midline in the epigastrium or in the right upper quadrant, but may be felt in the back. Small-intestinal pain is central and midline, usually colicky, and radiating into the back. Colonic pain can be felt centrally, along the line of the colon, or in the hypogastrium. It is often poorly localized but frequently radiates into the back or into the thighs. Pain from the gallbladder and bile duct is colicky and is felt in the right upper quadrant. Characteristically it is also felt in the back, between the scapulae or in the right shoulder tip. Pancreatic pain is epigastric and midline, radiates into the back, and is often made better by curling up and aggravated by lying flat.

Diagnosis

The major features of the pain to be determined are site, intensity, character, timing, and aggravating and relieving factors. Associated symptoms, such as bowel disturbance, vomiting, heartburn, and urinary and gynaecological symptoms must be elicited. Physical examination may reveal areas of abdominal tenderness, rebound tenderness, and rigidity. Abdominal distension or visible peristalsis must be looked for. Organ enlargement and the presence of masses must be excluded. A rectal examination is essential. The hernial orifices should be carefully examined and the abdomen should be auscultated for bruits. General examination may reveal the presence of fever, tachycardia, jaundice, weight loss, or anaemia.

Investigation of abdominal pain will be directed by the clinical findings. However, in cases of chronic pain it is not usually possible to make a firm clinical diagnosis as the symptom complexes of many diseases overlap, for example gastric ulcer, gastric carcinoma, duodenal ulcer, gallstones, or irritable bowel syndrome. Radiological and endoscopic investigations will therefore often be necessary. The diagnosis of specific disorders is dealt with in the appropriate sections.

Diarrhoea

Usually diarrhoea is thought of in terms of frequency of evacuation and consistency of stool, but it is not easy to set the limits beyond which diarrhoea may be said to occur. For example, a patient who is habitually constipated might complain of diarrhoea when his bowel frequency reaches twice per day and he would be right to do so as it might indicate serious bowel disease even though some arbitrarily defined frequency of bowel evacuation has not been reached. A clinical decision as to whether a given patient has diarrhoea or not usually depends, then, on that patient's normal bowel habit. A change to an increased frequency or looser consistency becomes suspicious without the need to define whether the patient has diarrhoea or not.

Another source of difficulty arises in the distinction between what patients and what doctors perceive as diarrhoea. Patients with carcinoma of the rectum, for example, may complain of diarrhoea when they pass blood and mucus, but may still pass normal formed stools. Faecal incontinence may also give rise to diagnostic difficulties. Many patients are reluctant to complain of incontinence, to which some social stigma is attached, and would rather complain of diarrhoea.

These observations emphasize that definitions of diarrhoea should not be slavishly adhered to and that a careful history is essential for accurate diagnosis.

Diagnosis

Diagnosis of acute infective diarrhoeal illnesses is usually straightforward and rests on a history of recent onset, perhaps with nausea, fever, and systemic upset. Staphylococcal 'food poisoning' will develop soon after ingestion of the offending food and may be severe but short lived. Viral gastroenteritis is usually milder, often without systemic upset and lasts 2–3 days. *Salmonella*, *Shigella*, and *Campylobacter* can cause more severe disease with fever and prostration. Abdominal pain is a more prominent feature of *Campylobacter* while the presence of blood and mucus in the stool suggests shigellosis or, occasionally, salmonellosis.

More difficulty is found with chronic, persistent, or intermittent diarrhoeal disease. In these cases an effort should be made to distinguish diarrhoea of large bowel and small bowel origin. Large bowel diarrhoea will tend to occur maximally on waking in the morning, be associated with pain relieved by defecation and perhaps accompanied by the passage of mucus. The presence of red blood in the stools of a patient with diarrhoea is a clear pointer towards a large bowel origin. Diarrhoea of small bowel origin does not occur at any particular time and pain is not usually relieved by defecation. A pale fatty stool, without fresh blood or mucus clearly indicates small bowel disease.

Associated symptoms such as anorexia and weight loss will suggest significant organic disease while long continued diarrhoea, perhaps for many years, without weight loss or systemic upset might indicate an irritable bowel syndrome. Intermittency of diarrhoea, precipitated by stress, would point towards a functional bowel disturbance while weight loss despite a good appetite should suggest thyrotoxicosis. A high proportion of patients with diarrhoea are being treated for another disease and many of the drugs used are found to be responsible for the diarrhoea. Particular culprits are antihypertensive agents including β-blockers, diuretics, antacids, and antibiotics. Patients who drink large volumes of beer should not be surprised if they have loose stools but some come to the doctor complaining of diarrhoea. The presence of skin rashes, mouth ulcers, 'conjunctivitis', or perianal disease, should alert one to the possibility of an underlying inflammatory bowel disease particularly Crohn's disease.

In addition to a full clinical examination a point should be made of inspecting the stool and performing a rectal examination.

Investigation

The investigation of a patient with persistent diarrhoea will depend on the history which may point towards a large or small bowel origin. Stool culture and sigmoidoscopy should be performed early, particularly in patients suspected of large bowel disease. Sigmoidoscopy with fibreoptic instruments is becoming increasingly used and it is often possible to examine the whole of the left side of the colon with little bowel preparation. The barium enema is less valuable

Where clinical features suggest small bowel disease evidence for deficiency of nutrients should be sought, and a faecal fat or xylose tolerance test may then be indicated. A radiological examination of the small bowel and a jejunal biopsy will provide indicators of underlying disease.

Persistent diarrhoea

There remains a difficult group of patients in whom diarrhoea persists but in whom all investigation has proved unhelpful. It is useful in such patients to admit them to hospital and make some simple measurements of stool output. Patients with stool outputs of less than about 400 g/day, and who complain of diarrhoea for which no cause has emerged on investigation, should be suspected of having an irritable bowel syndrome or anal incontinence. In others the complaint of diarrhoea is made because of frequency of defecation, although the amount of stool may be normal. The problem is then due to 'irritability' of the rectosigmoid or a defect in the reservoir function of the lower bowel.

In patients who have large volume of diarrhoea ($\geq$1 litre/day) the major differential diagnosis lies between an osmotic or a secretory cause.

Measurements of stool osmolality, and sodium and potassium concentrations are then useful. In a secretory diarrhoea the stool osmolality is close to the calculated total stool ionic concentration, $([Na^+] + [K^+]) \times 2$. On the other hand, in osmotic diarrhoeas, in which some other non-absorbed solute is causing the diarrhoea, the measured stool osmolality is considerably higher than the calculated total ionic concentration. A further test which helps differentiate these causes is to observe the effect on the diarrhoea of a 24–48-h fast. Osmotic diarrhoeas are markedly reduced by fasting but secretory diarrhoeas continue unabated.

Osmotic diarrhoea is most commonly caused by disaccharidase deficiency or occasionally by an osmotic purgative such as magnesium sulphate in a surreptitious purgative abuser. In chronic secretory diarrhoea a search may be made for very rare peptide-secreting tumours, such as the pancreatic islet adenoma of the Verner–Morrison syndrome which can be revealed by detecting raised plasma peptide concentrations. More common, but more difficult to detect, is the patient who is surreptitiously taking laxatives. The condition may be suspected when diarrhoea is severe and repeated investigation, often in several hospitals, has not revealed a cause. A previous psychiatric history, the presence of hypokalaemia, and the detection of melanosis coli are useful clues. Once suspected it is a simple matter to search for the offending purgative in the patient's locker and perform a screening test of urine and/or faeces for laxatives.

Constipation

Concepts of what constitutes constipation vary between societies and individuals. In western Europe, passage of stool by normal individuals ranges between two to three times per day to two to three per week. Three-quarters of the population pass approximately one stool per day. Constipation ranges in its presentation from an acute onset, which is usually taken to suggest organic obstruction, to a chronic lifelong disability, which usually indicates an intrinsic colonic neuromuscular disorder. The most common causes of constipation are shown in Table 1.

Table 1 Causes of constipation

Inadequate dietary fibre and fermentable carbohydrate
Immobility, disinclination to defaecate
Organic obstruction:
Neoplasm
Diverticular disease
Crohn's disease
Metabolic diseases:
Hypothyroidism
Hypercalcaemia
Extrinsic neurological diseases:
Spinal cord and sacral-nerve disease
Pudendal nerve damage
Parkinson's disease
Chronic intrinsic neuromuscular disease of the colon:
Hirschprung's disease
Chronic pseudo-obstruction
Systemic sclerosis
Diabetic neuropathy
Drug therapy:
Opiates
Anticholinergic agents including antidepressants
Iron therapy
Functional constipation

History

It is important to obtain a measure of the frequency, consistency, and volume of the stools. Infrequent desire to defecate suggests slow transit through the colon, while inability to expel faeces suggests obstructed defecation.

Sudden onset of constipation in a previously fit individual is a serious symptom and suggests intestinal obstruction, particularly if accompanied by increasing abdominal pain. Alternatively, constipation since childhood, with slow deterioration in function with time, almost certainly indicates a progressive neuromuscular degenerative disorder of the colon. Between these two extremes lie the most common modes of presentation. A dietary history is mandatory because the quantity of dietary fibre and fermentable carbohydrate ingested is the strongest determinant of faecal weight and defecatory frequency. The development of progressive obstruction of the colon must always be considered in adults, particularly those in whom the risk of colon cancer is high. A change in stool diameter together with the presence of blood in the stool can be indicators of malignant rectal obstruction. Metabolic diseases, in particular hypothyroidism, hypercalcaemia, and diabetes with autonomic neuropathy, should always be considered. Chronic constipation in young women who are otherwise well is characteristically worse during the latter phases of the menstrual cycle and also exacerbated by pregnancy.

Consumption of constipation-inducing medication such as opiates and anticholinergic agents, including antidepressants, must be excluded.

A family history of constipation suggests a chronic neuromuscular disease of the colon.

Clinical examination

The presence of hard faeces palpable in the colon is a useful confirmatory sign. Gross abdominal distension is unusual, except in individuals with severe megacolon due to colonic muscle disease or in those with psychiatric disorders and a severe disinclination to defecate.

Examination of the perineum and anus is mandatory. A rough guide to pelvic-floor dysfunction is obtained by examination of the perineum in the left lateral position while the patient either strains or coughs. Absence of normal pelvic descent suggests an abnormality of pelvic-floor relaxation. The visible descent of the perineum to the level of the ischial tuberosities after straining or coughing indicates damage to neuromuscular control of the pelvic floor, which is often accompanied by rectal mucosal prolapse. Inspection of the anus for fissures or fistulae, is also important, as local anal pain on attempted defecation is a powerful inhibitor of stool expulsion. A rectal examination and proctosigmoidoscopy should also be used to exclude organic disease of the rectum, to inspect the mucosa for melanosis coli, which is often an indicator of chronic laxative abuse, and to confirm the presence of solid faeces.

Management

In the vast majority of patients with simple constipation, the addition of poorly absorbed dietary carbohydrate is usually successful. Laxatives can be additionally prescribed if dietary modification fails, beginning with agents such as lactulose.

Specific stimulant laxatives can be tried in those individuals in whom defecation remains a problem despite bulking agents. These drugs act directly on the neuromuscular apparatus of the colon and stimulate faecal expulsion. They should only be used chronically with great reluctance. Enemas may be useful in obtaining colonic clearance of impacted faeces and as a prelude to longer-term laxative use. In intractable cases, regular, intermittent enemas may be the only way of managing the problem.

In young persons with severe symptoms and slow transit, where the life-style is severely impaired, subtotal colectomy can be of great benefit.

Acute gastrointestinal bleeding

The major causes of acute bleeding from the gastrointestinal tract are listed in Table 2.

Acute upper gastrointestinal bleeding

This presents as haematemesis and/or melaena. It is very rare for lesions distal to the ligament of Treitz to cause a haematemesis. However, brisk bleeding may occur from a proximal lesion, for example oesophageal varices, without haematemesis and present as melaena. Upper gastrointestinal bleeding can be severe enough to cause the passage of dark-red blood per rectum, which may cause diagnostic confusion. Table 3 shows the approximate frequency of lesions causing upper gastrointestinal bleeding. Rare causes include vascular abnormalities (telangiectasia, angiomas), leiomyoma, haemophilia, thrombocytopenia, Ehlers–Danlos syndrome, pseudoxanthoma elasticum, and rupture of the aorta into the duodenum. The role of aspirin in initiating bleeding from whatever cause is still controversial. All the anti-inflammatory drugs may be associated with bleeding.

Table 2 Causes of gastrointestinal bleeding

Inflammatory
Oesophagitis; gastritis; peptic ulcer; Crohn's disease; ulcerative colitis; enterocolitis—infective, ischaemic, radiation
Mechanical
Hiatus hernia; Mallory–Weiss tears; Meckel's diverticulum; diverticulosis coli
Neoplasms
Carcinoma; polyps—single, multiple; leiomyoma; carcinoid
Vascular
Varices; hereditary telangiectasia; angioma; aortointestinal fistula; mesenteric thrombosis or embolus; arteritis
Systemic
Chronic renal failure; thrombocytopenia; coagulation defects; connective tissue disorders; dysproteinaemia

Table 3 Causes of upper gastrointestinal bleeding and their frequency

Cause	Frequency (%)
Duodenal ulcer	35
Gastric ulcer	20
Acute gastric erosions/haemorrhagic gastritis	18
Mallory–Weiss tear	10
Gastric carcinoma	6
Oesophageal varices	5
Other	6

Assessment

When possible, the patient should be questioned about dyspepsia, vomiting, alcohol, drugs, previous episodes of bleeding, and jaundice. Pulse, respiratory rate, blood pressure, and the state of the peripheral circulation must be assessed. Specific signs to look for are those of chronic liver disease, iron deficiency, telangiectasia, and malignancy.

Blood should be taken for cross-matching and for determination of haemoglobin, haematocrit, platelet count, and prothrombin time.

Management

Intravenous saline should be given initially but, occasionally, uncrossmatched blood (blood group O, rhesus negative), albumin, or plasma expanders may be required. Central venous-pressure lines should be inserted into all patients over 65 years of age and into younger patients who show signs of a compromised blood volume (tachycardia in excess of 100/min; postural fall in systolic blood pressure of >20 mmHg). Transfusion should begin with whole blood in order to raise the haemoglobin to at least 10 g/dl. In general, 1 unit of blood raises the haemoglobin by 1 g/dl in an adult. Half-hourly observations of pulse, respiratory rate, and blood pressure are instituted, although these can be reduced in frequency once bleeding has stopped. The use of a nasogastric tube is controversial as it adds to the discomfort of the patient, it may cause fresh bleeding, and can cause erosions that may be confusing at subsequent endoscopy. Repeated nasogastric aspiration as a means of detecting a recurrent bleed is less sensitive than observing the pulse rate. The use of intravenous H_2-antagonists in the acute stage is common practice but there is little evidence to support this.

There may be some role for H_2-antagonists in patients in intensive care to prevent acute bleeding from stress ulcers or from gastric erosions but intragastric instillation of antacids may be a more effective measure.

For patients bleeding from oesophageal varices, further procedures may be necessary (see Chapter 5.3).

Diagnostic procedures

Once bleeding has stopped, and the patient is in a good haemodynamic state, the diagnosis of the cause of the bleeding can begin. Emergency endoscopy or barium meals while the patient is still bleeding often reveal little more than the fact that the stomach is full of blood. However, diagnostic procedures should be done within 24 h of bleeding because erosions and tears can heal rapidly.

The investigation of choice is upper gastrointestinal endoscopy as this will reveal tears and acute erosions of the stomach or duodenum that may frequently be missed radiologically and allows biopsies of a gastric ulcer or a tumour if found.

If a gastric or duodenal ulcer is found, the endoscopist should record whether there is active bleeding, whether a visible vessel can be seen in the base of the ulcer, or whether the ulcer crater is covered by a clot. These signs of recent bleeding have a very high predictive value for rebleeding.

Angiography should be reserved for patients with continuing bleeding in whom no cause has been found at endoscopy. It is useful in detecting angiomas, duodenal or ileal varices, bleeding from Meckel's diverticulum or non-specific ulcers of the ileum, and small-bowel tumours.

If emergency surgery is being considered, endoscopy may be indicated immediately, best performed under anaesthetic before surgery. The other possible indication for emergency endoscopy is when oesophageal varices are suspected, as the patients may be bleeding from mucosal lesions such as erosions or peptic ulcers. The subsequent management will obviously differ according to the endoscopic findings.

Indications for surgery

All patients presenting with acute upper gastrointestinal bleeding must be assessed by a physician and surgeon together. The indications for surgery will depend on the cause of bleeding; if from an erosive gastritis, surgery should be avoided if possible as the surgeon may have to do a total gastrectomy. Bleeding from a carcinoma is rarely severe and continuous enough to require emergency surgery. The management of bleeding varices is considered elsewhere (see Chapter 5.3 and OTM3, Chapter 14.6).

For peptic ulcers, early surgery can be recommended once initial resuscitation has been achieved. This is particularly so for elderly patients if there is continuous bleeding resulting in transfusion in excess of 6 pints. Bleeding to the point at which the central venous pressure cannot be maintained is a clear indication. Patients with recurrent bleeds should also be recommended for early surgery.

Endoscopic management

The methods used range from the injection of sclerosants, coagulation by diathermy or heater probes to Nd:YAG laser therapy and experimental methods of placing sutures or staples over the bleeding vessel. The most readily available technique is the injection of sclerosants.

Course and progress

The overall mortality of upper gastrointestinal bleeding is about 8–12 per cent and has remained constant since the 1960s. One of the major factors contributing to this apparent lack of progress is the increasing age of the population. So far, there is no evidence that early diagnosis by endoscopy or recourse to early surgery have greatly altered the overall prognosis, but it is now possible to predict which patients with gastric or duodenal ulcers are at particular risk from rebleeding. The presence of a clot or a visible vessel at the base of the ulcer has been shown to predict a high risk. It is possible that in this subgroup of patients, mortality may be reduced by an aggressive interventional approach.

Further reading

Langman, M.J.S. (1985). Upper gastrointestinal bleeding: the trials of trials. *Gut*, **26**, 217–20.

Rutgeerts, P., Gevers, A.M., Hiele, M., Broekaert, L., and Vantrappen, G. (1993). Endoscopic injection therapy to prevent rebleeding from peptic ulcers with a protruding vessel: a controlled comparative trial. *Gut*, **34**, 348–50.

Chapter 5.2

The mouth and salivary glands

T. Lehner

Dental caries and sequelae

Aetiology

Caries is an infection caused by aggregation of bacteria on the tooth surface. Prevalence is greatest in children and young adults affecting the occlusal surfaces and the enamel of the approximal surfaces of teeth. An increasing prevalence of root caries occurs later in life. The development of dental caries requires: (a) the presence of cariogenic bacteria capable of rapidly producing acid below the critical pH (4.1) for dissolving enamel, and (b) sugar in the diet that favours colonization of these bacteria and that can be metabolized by them to form acid. Among cariogenic organisms (*Streptococcus mutans*, *Streptococcus sanguis*, *Lactobacillus acidophilus*, *L. casei*, and *Actinomyces viscosus*) *S. mutans* is the most efficient. Sugar substrate for these organisms include starch, sucrose, glucose, fructose, and lactose. Of these the most important is sucrose. The major polysaccharide is dextran.

Pathology

The enamel becomes demineralized and plaque bacteria penetrate along the enamel prisms. Once the dentine is reached, destruction by decalcification and proteolysis of the dentine is rapid. The pulp reacts by an acute inflammatory response that results in necrosis.

Eventually, infection and toxic materials spread from the root-canal opening to the tissues around the apex of the tooth and induce periapical inflammatory changes, which may terminate in an acute or chronic abscess or a chronic granuloma. A dental abscess shows a mixed bacterial infection with a variety of streptococci, staphylococci, and other organisms.

There are two principal immunological mechanisms of protection against caries. One involves salivary IgA antibodies, the other involves all the humoral and cellular components elicited by systemic immunization. Antibodies, complement, polymorphonuclear leucocytes, lymphocytes, and macrophages pass from the gingival blood vessels to the gingival domain of the tooth.

Clinical features

Toothache is made worse by any hot or cold drink or food, affects the patient especially at night-time, and may radiate to the face and ear. If relief is not sought death of the dental pulp and the development of an acute swelling due to an abscess or cellulitis follows. With an acute abscess the inflammatory exudate may penetrate through the bone to the soft tissues; oedematous swelling of the face increases, and if the upper canine is involved may spread to the eyelid. The regional lymph nodes are tender and enlarged, there may be fever and some malaise.

Much less commonly a cellulitis may give rise to a spreading infection along the fascial planes, especially of the submaxillary and sublingual spaces. The inflammatory exudate may occasionally spread into the loose connective tissue of the glottis causing oedema and respiratory obstruction. The attendant brawny swelling of the neck and floor of the mouth, difficulty in swallowing, trismus, fever, and malaise is referred to as Ludwig's angina. An alternative chronic course is the development of a chronic pulpitis, granuloma, abscess, and eventually cyst around the apex of the offending tooth, and these may proceed without symptoms or only slight discomfort.

Treatment

The principles of treatment are to remove the caries, apply a non-irritant dressing to protect the pulp and restore the tooth with a filling. If the pulp is damaged irreversibly it will have to be extirpated and root-canal therapy instituted. The alternative is extraction of the offending tooth. A dental abscess is effectively dealt with by extraction, but if the tooth is to be saved, the pus is drained by an intraoral incision and/or establishing drainage through the root canal. Antibiotics are useful in acute abscesses and phenoxymethylpenicillin, 250 mg four times a day for about 7 days, is adequate. Cellulitis should first be treated by intramuscular benzylpenicillin, 1 MU four times a day. The swelling should then be incised and extraction of the tooth under general anaesthesia should take place as soon as the patient's condition permits it.

Prevention of dental caries is best practised by plaque removal, and by limiting the intake of sugar. The type of toothpaste used matters less than the method of tooth brushing, although fluoride in toothpaste decreases the incidence of caries in children by up to 40 per cent. Water fluoridation is the most effective public-health preventive measure.

Differential diagnosis

Toothache occasionally needs to be differentiated from sinusitis and neuralgia. An abscess or cellulitis caused by dental caries can be (rarely) confused with mumps.

Gingival and periodontal disease

Aetiology

A mild inflammation of the gingiva (gum) and slight destruction of the collagen of the periodontal membrane are found in most adults. Advanced destruction of the periodontal membrane, including the supporting bone, is found in about half of the middle-aged or older population. A close association has been found between accumulation of bacterial plaque and gingivitis. During this process a change occurs from a predominantly Gram-positive coccal form of plaque to a complex population of filamentous organisms, spirochaetes, vibrios, and Gram-negative cocci. Of the Gram-positive organisms, *Actinomyces viscosus* appears to be involved in the development of gingivitis. Gram-negative organisms, essential in the development of periodontal disease include *Porphyromonas gingivalis*, *Actinobacillus actinomycetemcomitans*, *Capnocytophaga* spp., and some spirochaetes.

Dental plaque may calcify, especially in adults and the elderly, to produce calculus, often found on the lingual surface of the lower incisors and the buccal surface of the upper molars. Chronic gingival inflammation may persist for many years and breakdown of the periodontal membrane, with loss of the supporting bone, may follow. This is known as periodontitis ('pyorrhoea'), and is the most important cause of loss of teeth after the age of 40.

Pathology

Periodontitis is a progressively destructive process leading to loss of teeth. The immunological processes are complex, with the protective–destructive mechanisms of lymphocyte and macrophage functions, antibodies, and complement activation. Repair, with collagen formation and destruction of the tissues, eventually leads to loss of support of the teeth.

Clinical features

The symptoms of chronic gingivitis or periodontitis are usually so mild that they often go unnoticed but there may be discomfort in teeth, bleeding of gums and associated halitosis, difficulty on eating, looseness of teeth, and occasionally abscess formation.

Differential diagnosis

Chronic gingivitis can be differentiated from acute ulcerative gingivitis by the sudden onset, malaise, characteristic halitosis, pain, and ulceration of the gingiva in the latter. Herpetic gingivostomatitis occurs predominantly in children and again the onset is acute, with fever, malaise, pain, and ulceration of the gingiva and oral mucosa (see below). Desquamative gingivitis may cause difficulties in differential diagnosis and the points to bear in mind are that the attached gingiva shows diffuse erosive areas and evidence of bullous lesions may be found in the oral mucosa.

Treatment

Plaque and calculi should be removed by regular scaling of the teeth. Prevention involves careful tooth brushing, with the aid of plaque-disclosing solutions and regular use of dental floss and wood points. Deep periodontal pockets can be treated by root planing, gingival curettage, or surgically.

Viral, bacterial, and fungal infections

Primary herpetic gingivostomatitis, recurrent herpetic infection (cold sores), Herpes zoster infection, herpangina, hand, foot, and mouth disease, oral manifestations of AIDS, and oral candidiasis are discussed in Section 16 of this textbook (see also OTM3, pp. 1846–65).

Bacterial infections

Acute (necrotizing) ulcerative gingivitis (Vincent's gingivitis; acute fusospirochaetal gingivitis)

Aetiology

It is caused by an infection, although the organisms responsible are disputed. Evidence is accumulating in favour of a mixed, bacterial pathogenesis of Gram-negative organisms (fusobacteria, veillonella, bacteroides, leptotrichia), which may be responsible for the lesions by their endotoxin activity. A number of predisposing factors are recognized; poor oral hygiene, accumulation of dental bacterial plaque, defective restorations, and pericoronitis are most important. The disease is seen more commonly in young adults and smokers.

Pathology and clinical features

The gum undergoes an acute inflammatory reaction, leading to necrosis of the epithelium and thrombosis of the small blood vessels. The clinical picture is the sudden onset of painful, bleeding gums and a characteristic foul breath. There is a rise in temperature, regional lymphadenitis, anorexia, and significant malaise. Oral examination reveals necrotic, punched-out ulcers, affecting predominantly the interdental gingiva. At times there are shallow necrotic ulcers affecting the oropharyngeal mucosa, which shows diffuse erythema (Vincent's angina).

Diagnosis

This disease is often confused with primary herpetic stomatitis, but in this patients are usually younger and their breath lacks the distinct foul quality of ulcerative gingivitis. Direct examination of a smear from the lesion reveals a large number of spirochaetal and fusiform organisms, with a decrease in the mixed bacterial flora.

Treatment

Metronidazole 200 mg by mouth three times daily for 3–4 days is very effective. Phenoxymethyl penicillin, 250 mg four times daily for a week is equally effective. Hydrogen peroxide mouthwash, and a variety of peroxyborate preparations are also useful.

Cancrum oris (noma)

This is a rapidly spreading gangrene of the lips and cheeks, mostly confined to children in parts of tropical Africa. It is thought to be an extension of acute ulcerative gingivitis when associated with other diseases, especially measles. Cancrum oris is very rare in the United Kingdom, but can be seen in terminal stages of leukaemia, especially when treated by cytotoxic, anti-inflammatory, and immunosuppressive drugs.

Tuberculosis

Oral tuberculosis is rare. Commonly, the presenting feature is a painful ulcer or a firm small swelling. Ulcers may be single or multiple, but they are usually large, with a depressed floor and some induration of the base. Diagnosis is based on microscopy and culture and a biopsy of the lesion. Oral tuberculosis responds readily to specific chemotherapy.

Syphilis

The chancre of the primary stage may present on the lip or tongue as a painless, small, firm nodule that breaks down and forms an ulcer with raised indurated edges. The regional lymph nodes then show discrete, rubbery enlargement. In the secondary stage, shallow, snail-track ulcers may affect the tonsils, tongue, or lips, and the saliva is highly infective. Gumma and leucoplakia are the typical oral manifestations of the tertiary stage. A gumma starts as a swelling of the palate, tongue, or tonsils; it undergoes necrosis and results in a painless, punched-out, deep ulcer, with a 'wash-leather' floor. The lesion may heal with scarring, or give rise to perforation. Leucoplakia usually affects the dorsum of the tongue as an irregular, diffuse white patch that cannot be rubbed off.

Table 1 Classification of oral ulcers

Recurrent oral ulcers
Minor, major aphthous, and herpetiform
Behçet's disease
Microbial infection
Primary and recurrent herpes simplex infection
Herpes zoster infection
Acute ulcerative gingivostomatitis
Tuberculosis
Syphilis
Neoplastic ulcers
Carcinoma
Leukaemia
Haematological disorders
Anaemia
Neutropenia, agranulocytosis
Dermatological disorders
Erosive lichen planus
Pemphigus
Benign mucous membrane pemphigoid
Erythema multiforme and Stevens–Johnson syndrome
Reiter's syndrome
Granulomatous disorders
Histiocytosis X
Wegener's granulomatosis
Iatrogenic agents
Drug allergy
Drug-induced agranulocytosis
Cytotoxic drugs
Radiotherapy
Trauma
Denture, teeth, or foreign body
Chemical

Oral ulceration

The main causes are listed in Table 1. Only some merit more description here.

Recurrent oral ulcers

Aphthous ulcers are common with a prevalence varying between 10 and 34 per cent (Plate 1). The aetiology is not known but there is recent evidence suggesting a T-cell response to a peptide within the sequence of heat shock protein. While emotional stress may influence the pattern of the disease, it is unlikely to be the direct cause. A family history is often present and the highest incidence of ulcers is recorded in siblings in whom both parents have recurrent aphthous ulcers. In some female patients there is a relationship between the ulcers and menstrual period; the onset of ulceration may coincide with puberty, or the ulcers may develop only after the menopause and often disappear during pregnancy.

Pathology

An early intense lymphomonocytic infiltration, especially with a perivascular distribution, is a constant histological finding. This is followed by a polymorphonuclear infiltration and a significant increase in the number of CD4 and CD8 subsets of T cells, Langerhans cells, and macrophages.

Clinical features

About 80 per cent of recurrent oral ulcers are of the minor type; and are found more frequently in women than men. Soreness 1–2 days before ulceration increases in severity especially on eating. The ulcers are round or oval, and enlarge in size, although they remain well under 1 cm. They have a yellow floor with a slightly raised margin and often marked surrounding erythema and oedema. The common sites of involvement are the mucosa of the lips and cheeks and margin of the tongue, and the ulcers last 4–14 days. The rate of recurrences varies from 1 to 4 months and is usually irregular.

Major aphthous ulcers are less common. Pain can be severe so that patients find it difficult to eat and often lose weight. Ulcers may enlarge to some 3 cm, may number as many as 10 and can mimic a carcinomatous lesion. In addition to the lips, cheeks, and tongue, the soft palate and tonsillar region are commonly involved. Healing may take 10–40 days and recurrences are so frequent that the patient suffers from continuous ulceration. The prevalence of major aphthous ulcers is raised in ulcerative colitis. A striking association has been found in smokers who give up the habit and develop recurrent aphthous ulcers.

Herpetiform ulcers may affect any part of the mouth. They account for less than 10 per cent of recurrent oral ulcers and are much more common in females. Patients present with pain on eating and talking, and often with dysphagia; malaise and loss of weight can be prominent. The lesions persist for 7–14 days and commonly new ulcers appear before the previous crop has healed.

It is important to differentiate both aphthous and herpetiform ulcers from those found in iron, folate or vitamin B_{12} deficiency. Ulcers relating to coeliac disease respond to a gluten-free diet. The shallow necrotic ulcers of agranulocytosis or neutropenia tend to persist at one site. Ulcers due to denture trauma are usually localized to the mucosa covering the mandibular and maxillary alveolus and the buccal and lingual sulci.

The differential diagnosis from pemphigus, benign mucous membrane pemphigoid, and erythema multiforme will be described below.

Treatment

Topical corticosteroids in aphthous ulceration are most effective if application is started during the prodromal phase, but later may reduce the severity and duration of ulceration. The most useful preparations are triamcinolone in orabase; hydrocortisone sodium succinate, 2.5 mg per tablet; and betamethasone, 0.5 mg per tablet. The tablets are kept in the mouth, or the ointment is applied to the ulcers, three to four times daily. Systemic prednisolone has to be resorted to occasionally in patients with major aphthous ulcers. Topical tetracycline is the drug of choice in suppressing herpetiform ulcers, but is also useful in controlling some major aphthous ulcers. The powder from a 250 mg capsule is dissolved in 10 ml of water and kept in the mouth four times daily.

Bullous lesions

Pemphigus vulgaris (see also Section 11)

This may present in the mouth, which is involved at some stage of the disease in most patients (Plate 2). Painful, fluid-filled blisters or bullae burst within a few hours, resulting in shallow ulcers. These persist for weeks or months, but new lesions recur. Oral manifestations may persist for many months, without overt ill-health but skin lesions, malaise, and loss of weight may occur at a later stage. The lesions can be differentiated from recurrent aphthous ulcers by the presence of bullae and when these ulcerate the edges lack the well-defined character of aphthous ulcers. The most important diagnostic test is the presence of acantholytic cells on microscopic examination of direct scrapings from the lesion and a biopsy must always be taken. Pemphigus must be differentiated from pemphigoid and dermatitis herpetiformis (see below). A less severe and rare variant of pemphigus vulgaris is pemphigus vegetans. Vegetation may be found on the oral mucosa and lips, and histological examination shows intraepithelial abscesses containing numerous eosinophils.

Treatment

Prednisolone is given initially in doses of 40–60 mg/day and gradually reduced to the minimal dose that will prevent formation of new lesions. The required dose may be reduced by adding azathioprine in a dose of 200 mg/day. Treatment with corticosteroids must be maintained for life and has completely changed the prognosis of the disease.

Benign mucous membrane pemphigoid (see also Section 11)

This rare disease affects women twice as often as men, usually over the age of 40 years.

Bullous lesions involve the oral mucosa, conjunctiva, and skin around the genitals and orifices, but in some patients only the mouth is involved. The bullae rupture within a day or two leaving erosions and ulcers. The gingiva is commonly involved, giving rise to persistent pain, bleeding, and a diffuse, raw, fiery red lesion. The oral lesions usually heal without scaring unlike those of the conjunctiva.

The disease persists, often with exacerbations and remissions, over many years. It is differentiated from pemphigus vulgaris on clinical grounds but only a biopsy examination will establish the diagnosis. There are no acantholytic cells and the bullae are subepithelial and not suprabasilar. Autoantibodies can be detected, in less than half the patients, binding to the basement membrane of epithelium and not to the interepithelial substance. The disease should be differentiated from linear IgA disease, and dermatitis herpetiformis.

Treatment

If the disease is confined to the mouth, topical corticosteroids are often adequate but with involvement of other sites, systemic corticosteroids are indicated.

Erythema multiforme (see Section 11)

The mouth can be affected without skin involvement. Painful, extensive erosions and ulcers have a predilection for the palate, tongue, and cheeks (Fig. 1 and Plate 3). The gum may show extensive erosions, which tend to bleed. Haemorrhagic crusting of the lips is often seen. The Stevens–Johnson syndrome is a rare variant.

If an offending agent is not found, the lesions may recur over many years. The diagnosis of oral lesions without skin manifestation

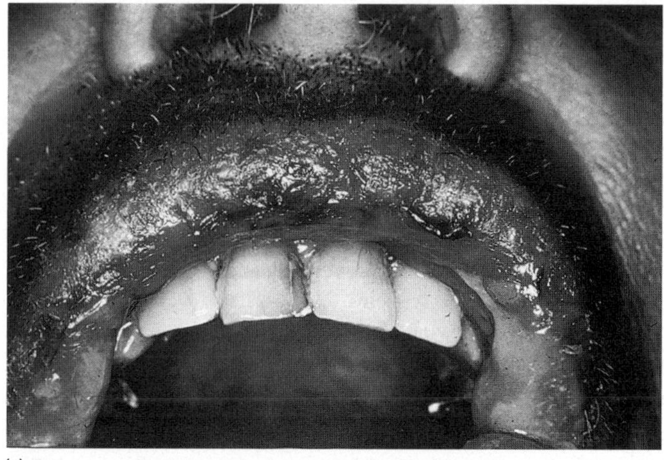

(a)

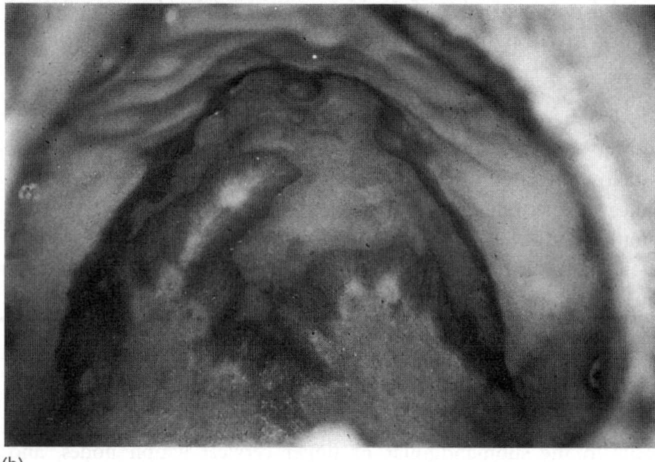

(b)

Fig. 1 Erythema multiforme: (a) haemorrhagic crusted upper lip; (b) diffuse erosion of the palate.

can be very difficult. The clinical features to note are the very extensive erosions affecting the palate, tongue, cheeks, and gingiva and the haemorrhagic crusting of the lips. An association with drugs or microbial infection is helpful. A biopsy can exclude pemphigus and erosive lichen planus. Behçet's disease is an important differential diagnosis.

Treatment

Any offending drug or infection should be eliminated. The oral lesions often respond to topical tetracycline.

Lichen planus (see Section 11)

Many patients with oral lichen planus do not have skin lesions. Mouth lesions may remain symptomless for years. Some patients complain of a furry thickening of the mucosa and others of pain or bleeding from the gums on eating. There are three types of oral lichen planus: hypertrophic, erosive, and bullous (Plate 4). The hypertrophic variety is most common and is usually seen in all three types. There are white striae and minute papules, most commonly affecting the posterior part of the buccal mucosa, lips, and dorsum of tongue, though the palate, gum, and floor of the mouth can also be involved. The striae criss-cross giving rise to a fine lacy or fern-like pattern, and less commonly a honeycomb or annular patter. The striae may fuse and result in a diffuse, somewhat smooth, shiny white plaque which may be difficult to differentiate from leucoplakia.

In bullous lichen planus a bulla is rarely seen, presumably because it bursts to produce ulcers. In erosive lichen planus there may be large shallow ulcers up to 3 cm in size, surrounded by white striae and papules. Except for discomfort, difficulties with eating, and occasionally loss of weight, there are no general manifestations and the regional lymph nodes are not enlarged, except with secondary infection. Lichen planus may affect only the gum, inducing a diffuse, fiery-red gingivitis and scattered erosions.

The striae and papules are sufficiently distinctive to differentiate lichen planus from other lesions, without the need for a biopsy, but the diffuse hypertrophic variety can be confused with leucoplakia. Erosive lichen planus may very occasionally lack the distinctive striae, and then erythema multiforme and benign mucous membrane pemphigoid should be excluded. Both systemic and discoid lupus erythematosus can present in the mouth as erosions, surrounded by a keratinized margin.

Treatment

In the absence of symptoms, hypertrophic lichen planus does not require treatment. Topical corticosteroids are usually effective in erosive lichen planus and suppress the striae and papules of the hypertrophic variety. Triamcinolone in orabase ointment applied four times a day is useful in localized lesions, but betamethasone 0.5 mg tablets are more effective, kept in the mouth three times daily. The lesions recur almost invariably, and corticosteroids may have to be applied with every relapse. In a very small number of patients, carcinomatous transformation, especially in the erosive type of lichen planus, can take place.

Leucoplakia

White patches of the oral mucosa that cannot be removed by scraping are referred to as leucoplakia (Plate 5). Among identified causes are physical and chemical agents, smoking, and microbial infections (*Candida*, syphilis, AIDS); some cases are congenital or hereditary. A cause cannot be found in about half the cases. The *microscopical features* show a spectrum of changes; at the benign end is epithelial keratosis alone, followed by hyperplasia and then epithelial atypia at the premalignant end. The lamina propria shows in parallel an increase in mononuclear cells, especially plasma cells. Carcinoma *in situ* is the least common histological finding.

Clinical features

The white patches vary from a soft, slightly thickened mucosa, involving a small or very large mucosal surface, to hard, irregular white plaques with intervening normal, erosive, or ulcerated sites. The latter (speckled leucoplakia) has a greater propensity to carcinomatous transformation. Any part of the oral mucosa or gum may be involved. Frictional keratosis is usually found along the occlusal line of buccal mucosa and presents as a linear white patch of even consistency. Smoker's keratosis shows a characteristic distribution of the soft and adjacent hard palate, as keratinized papules with central red dots. The distribution is due to involvement of the palatal mucous glands and the red dots are the openings of the ducts. It is usually caused by pipe smoking, but cigarettes may also cause diffuse keratosis, affecting most commonly the cheeks. Congenital and hereditary leucokeratosis shows diffuse, soft, white plaques, often with a folded surface. The lesions tend to be symmetrical; they affect the floor of the mouth.

All leucoplakias should be biopsied, except smoker's keratosis of the palate, as even small lesions have at times proved to be early carcinomas. It is also essential to find out the degree of epithelial atypia as this affects the prognosis. Direct examination of scrapings can be helpful in the presence of hyphae of candida; cultures should also be set up for candida. Serological tests are essential in the diagnosis of syphilitic leucoplakia.

Treatment

Smoker's keratosis is reversible in many instances. Frictional keratosis can also be cleared, if some local cause of irritation is removed. Candidal leucoplakia should be treated with topical antifungal drugs. Syphilis should be managed by a course of penicillin. Leucoplakia showing evidence of epithelial atypia should be excised and occasionally a skin graft may be required.

Most important is long-term follow-up, so as to detect in time the development of an incipient carcinoma. About 5 per cent of all leucoplakias undergo malignant changes and this figure increases to about 30 per cent in leucoplakias showing histological evidence of epithelial atypia. Malignancy is more commonly associated with speckled leucoplakia as well as syphilitic leucoplakia. Congenital or hereditary leukokeratosis were thought to be free of malignant changes, although recently a few cases with carcinomatous transformation have been reported.

Benign neoplasms, cysts, and developmental and inflammatory lesions of the soft tissues

There are numerous benign neoplasms and soft tissue lesions of the mouth. These include papilloma, fibroma, lipoma, neurofibroma, haematoma, pigmented naevus, lymphangioma, denture granuloma, fibrous polyp, pregnancy tumours, mucus retention, and extravasation cysts. Soft-tissue tumours present as painless, slow-growing swellings affecting any part of the mouth. Fibrous polyps are the most common and result from trauma or irritation from rough edges of carious teeth. Most of the tumours are sessile, some are pedunculated, and others flat and pigmented. They are usually symptomless except for bleeding from hamartomas and giant-cell reparative granulomas.

Definitive diagnosis depends on histological examination but a papilloma can be recognized by its firm, small, keratinized, finger-like processes. Lymphangiomas are soft swellings, which may cause considerable enlargement of the lip or tongue. Hamartomas are flat or nodular red lesions that may blanch when compressed; they are occasionally confused with pregnancy tumours, which are rather vascular granulomatous swellings of the gingiva. Giant-cell reparative granulomas are also very vascular, maroon-coloured lesions originating from the gingiva. Denture granulomas can be readily recognized from their relation to the flange of a denture. Mucous retention or extravasation cysts are small, often bluish swellings affecting the lips or cheeks.

Surgical excision, with a margin of normal tissue at the base of the lesion, is usually indicated. Pregnancy tumours, however, commonly regress spontaneously. Only the giant-cell reparative granuloma has a tendency to recur after excision.

Oral carcinoma

Carcinoma of the mouth accounts for about 2 per cent of all cancers in Britain. The prevalence increases after the age of 45 years and more than twice as many men as women are affected. The incidence has been decreasing over the last four decades. The cause is unknown, but smoking and alcohol have been implicated, and it is pipe or cigar smoking that have been associated with oral cancer. There is some evidence that *Treponema pallidum*, *Candida albicans*, human papilloma virus, and human immunodeficiency virus (**HIV**), may directly or indirectly influence the development of carcinoma. Among the predisposing lesions, leucoplakia is the best known. Submucous fibrosis is another precancerous condition and is found predominantly in India and Sri Lanka. It seems to be related to eating chillis and possibly betel-nut chewing, and affects the palate, buccal mucosa, and tongue.

Pathology

Squamous cell carcinoma in the mouth is usually a well-differentiated keratinizing neoplasm invading the surrounding tissue. Poorly differentiated and anaplastic oral carcinomas are much less frequent. Spread by local invasion and lymph node metastasis occurs at a late stage.

Clinical features

The lesion may comprise a lump or an ulcer that is resistant to healing and gradually enlarging in size. There may be little pain initially, but later discomfort and occasional bleeding may occur. Cancer of the tongue may give rise to local pain and earache. A dry mouth may be found in the early stages. Ulcers have a raised and often everted edge, and induration at the base. Any part of the mouth can be involved but the lips (usually the lower lip) and tongue are most common, each accounting for about 25 per cent of oral carcinomas. The floor of the mouth, gingiva, cheek, hard and soft palate, and oropharynx may account for about 10 per cent. Some patients may have two or even multiple carcinomas. Metastasis may occur to the submandibular or upper cervical lymph nodes, and occasionally to the submental nodes. A biopsy is essential for any long-standing or indurated lesion.

Adenocarcinoma of the small salivary glands may also present as a lump of the soft palate, lips, or cheeks and only a biopsy will establish the diagnosis. Carcinoma *in situ* is rare in the mouth, but it may present as a diffuse, erythematous, somewhat velvety lesion, affecting the mucosa of one-half of the soft palate or cheek.

Treatment

Surgical excision of the lesion and a margin of adjacent tissue may be extended if necessary to block dissection of the regional lymph nodes. Radiotherapy is an alternative, commonly used in primary treatment of cancer of the lip, in inoperable cases, or with recurrent carcinoma following surgery. Cytotoxic drugs have also been used with variable results.

Course and prognosis

The 5-year survival rates differ considerably with the anatomical site. Carcinoma of the lip has by far the best prognosis, and the 5-year survival rate is about 80 per cent. The figures for carcinoma of the tongue range from 25 to 35 per cent, floor of the mouth 20 to 40 per cent, cheek 30 to 50 per cent, and oropharynx, palate, and gingiva at about 25 per cent.

Salivary gland diseases

Xerostomia (dry mouth)

Dry mouth is common can be caused by anxiety and emotional stress. Antihistamines, phenothiazines, antihypertensive agents, diuretics, and preparations containing atropine are well recognized causes. Some diseases affect the salivary glands directly, e.g. Sjögren's syndrome and sialadenitis. It may be impossible to eliminate the cause. In such cases, palliative measures include frequent sips of water, meticulous oral hygiene, early treatment or preferably prevention of candidiasis by topical nystatin or amphotericin B. Some prefer glycerine, others carboxymethylcellulose as a lubricant, and the latter can be taken as a solution or aerosol (Glandosane). A mucin preparation can also be helpful as a spray or as a lozenge (Saliva Orthana).

Sialadenitis

Bacterial or viral infections and rarely allergic reactions may cause inflammation of the salivary glands, giving rise to acute, chronic, and allergic sialadenitis, and recurrent parotitis. Ascending acute infection of the parotid (*Staphylococcus aureus*, *Streptococcus viridans* or *S. pneumoniae*) used to be a common complication in elderly post-operative patients. Acute parotitis may also follow the use of drugs causing xerostomia. The most common cause of acute parotitis is mumps. Salivary glands are sometimes affected by HIV infection, with an enlargement of the parotid glands. Chronic sialadenitis is usually associated with duct obstruction and usually affects the submandibular gland. Recurrent sialadenitis may be associated with a decreased salivary flow causing retrograde infection.

Clinical features

The usual presenting symptom in acute cases is a painful swelling in one of the parotid glands of an elderly patient. Commonly the patient has a low-grade fever, oedema of the cheek, some trismus, and a purulent discharge may be expressed from the duct opening. In chronic sialadenitis there are usually features of duct obstruction of one of the submandibular glands. There is pain and swelling in the submandibular or retromandibular region, with a reddened duct orifice discharging pus. Recurrent parotitis presents as an acute pain and swelling of one or both parotid glands, with erythema of the duct orifices and pus discharging from them. There may be an associated fever and malaise. Recurrences vary from weeks to months and after repeated attacks the affected gland may remain enlarged.

There is little difficulty in the differential diagnosis between acute parotitis in the elderly and mumps in the healthy young subject. Discharging pus should be cultured. Recurrent parotitis can cause difficulties; sialography may show sialectasis and duct dilatation. In chronic sialadenitis there is usually clinical or radiological evidence of calculus and sialography may show duct dilatation.

A variety of granulomatous diseases may rarely affect the salivary glands, such as sarcoidosis, tuberculosis, syphilis, and actinomycosis. Allergic sialadenitis is also rare and to determine the allergic agent can be difficult.

Treatment

In acute, chronic, or recurrent sialadenitis, appropriate antibiotics should be used but surgical drainage may also be necessary. Oral hygiene is also important. There is no special treatment for mumps. In chronic sialadenitis the cause of obstruction, such as a calculus, should be removed. The treatment of recurrent parotitis is more difficult and if antibiotics do not control the disease, surgical intervention should be considered.

Salivary duct obstruction due to calculus

The presenting symptoms are a sudden unilateral swelling and pain of the gland related to eating. Examination reveals a soft swelling of the affected gland and careful digital palpation along the course of the salivary duct will localize the calculus. This may vary in size from a small grain to a concretion 10–20 mm in length. The localization of a stone in a duct should be confirmed by radiographs and the presence of calculi in the gland can be diagnosed only by radiography. If the calculus is near the orifice of the duct it can occasionally be teased out, otherwise surgical removal is indicated.

Salivary gland tumours

A variety of epithelial tumours affects the salivary glands. In the parotid, the commonest is the pleomorphic adenoma or mixed salivary tumour (74 per cent) followed by adenocarcinoma (12 per cent), adenoma (8 per cent), muco-epidermoid tumour (3 per cent), and acinic cell tumour (2 per cent). Only pleomorphic adenoma will be considered here.

Pleomorphic adenoma

This originates from epithelial cells of the ducts, acini, or myoepithelial cells which proliferate in duct-like structures, sheets, and cords, within a connective tissue stroma, which may show mucous, cartilaginous, or hyaline appearance. The lesion is encapsulated, although satellite tumours are often found outside the capsule. The tumour is usually found in adults and the parotid is most commonly affected, followed by the submandibular gland and rarely the sublingual. The minor glands can also be affected, most frequently in the glands of the palate, lips, and cheeks. The tumour presents as a small, painless swelling, which may take years to enlarge and is not attached to the overlying skin or mucosa. Adenocarcinoma, mucoepidermoid carcinoma, and adenoid cystic carcinoma may mimic pleomorphic adenoma in its slow growth, and can often be differentiated only on histopathological examination.

Treatment is by excision with a margin of normal tissue, as the tumour is radio-resistant. If left untreated the tumour may enlarge to a grotesque size. A small proportion may undergo carcinomatous transformation. The tumour has a bad record for recurrences after excision, thought to be due to residual satellite tumours outside the capsule.

Neoplasms, cysts, developmental lesions, and dystrophies of the bones and teeth

A number of such lesions can arise in the jaws including benign and malignant neoplasms, cysts and tumours of dental origin, dental malformations and various osteodystrophies. They are described briefly in OTM3 (pp. 862–3).

Halitosis

There are four possible sources of halitosis: the mouth, nasopharynx, lungs, and the gastrointestinal tract. Altered blood round the gum may be the most important oral cause, and this may be associated with debris or pus from gingivitis and periodontal pockets. A characteristic halitosis is found in acute ulcerative gingivitis. Chronic tonsillitis may be responsible for halitosis but atrophic rhinitis causing ozena is probably the most important cause to be excluded. Occasionally, respiratory tract infections may cause halitosis and a variety of gastrointestinal disorders have been associated with bad breath but with little evidence. Frequently all these sources of halitosis may be excluded without finding a cause.

Further reading

Bouquot, J.E., Weiland, L.H., and Kurland, L.T. (1988). Leukoplakia and carcinoma *in situ* synchronously associated with invasive oral/oropharyngeal carcinoma in Rochester Minn., 1935–1984. *Oral Surgery, Oral Medicine, Oral Pathology*, **65**, 199–207.

Greenspan, D. and Greenspan, J.S. (1996). HIV related oral disease. *Lancet*, **348**, 729–33.

Lehner, T. (1992). *Immunology of oral diseases*. Blackwell Scientific Publications, Oxford.

Lozada-Nur, F., Gorsky, M., and Silverman, S. (1989). Oral erythema multiforme: clinical observations and treatment of 95 patients. *Oral Surgery, Oral Medicine, Oral Surgery*, **67**, 36–40.

Williams, D.M. (1989). Vesiculobullous mucocutaneous disease: pemphigus vulgaris. *Journal of Oral Pathology and Medicine*, **18**, 544–53.

Williams, R.C. (1990). Periodontal disease. *New England Journal of Medicine*, **322**, 373–82.

Chapter 5.3

Diseases of the oesophagus

J. Dent

Gastro-oesophageal reflux disease

Gastro-oesophageal reflux occurs to some degree in everybody and should only be considered a disease when it gives rise to significant symptoms or complications. An abnormally high level of episodic exposure of the distal oesophagus to gastric contents is the most important functional defect. In most patients this is due to abnormal neural control of the sphincter and oesophageal body. In the majority of patients most reflux occurs during the day, predominantly after food, but in those with severe oesophagitis nocturnal reflux and its resultant acid exposure become important. Hiatus hernia is probably an important amplifier of defects of sphincter function and oesophageal clearance. In a small and ill-defined minority of patients, apparently normal levels of reflux induce typical symptoms, presumably because of oesophageal sensitization by a primary oesophageal mucosal sensory defect.

Oesophagitis

Excessive mucosal exposure to acid and pepsin leads to distal oesophageal ulceration in between one-third to one-half of patients with symptomatic reflux. The extent of ulceration varies from tiny patches of erosion to circumferential, extensive ulceration in a small minority. Peptic stricture and/or oesophageal columnar metaplasia (Barrett's oesophagus) are typically only associated with severe oesophagitis. Oesophageal adenocarcinoma is the main significance of columnar metaplasia and is dealt with later. Oesophageal columnar metaplasia also carries the risk of deep, benign oesophageal ulceration in the metaplastic segment. Occasionally, such ulcers erode into mediastinal structures or the pleural space often with a fatal outcome. Bleeding from oesophagitis is relatively common, but rarely life threatening.

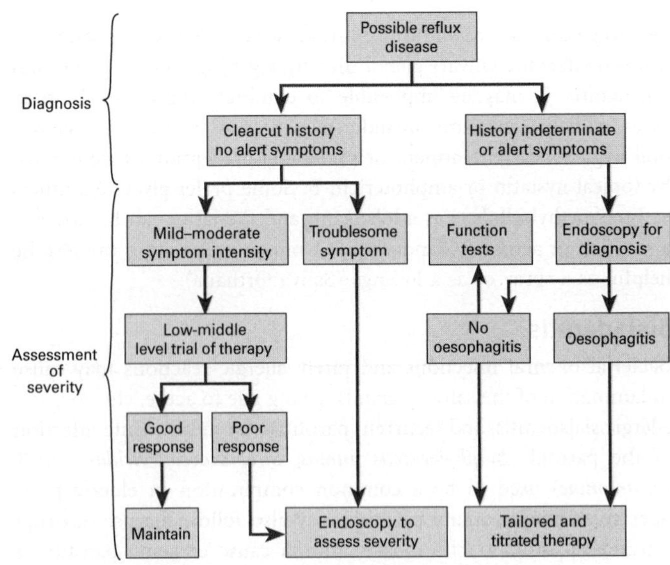

Fig. 1 Principal decision paths for management of reflux disease.

Symptoms

Heartburn is most important, but presentation may be with less-specific patterns of dyspepsia or with regurgitation, haematemesis, and dysphagia due either to stricture or oesophageal body motor dysfunction. Reflux-induced respiratory symptoms of hoarseness, persistent cough, and bronchospasm may predominate.

Diagnosis and assessment of severity

The history is pivotal for diagnosis because of the extremely high prevalence of reflux-induced symptoms and the lack of a definitive, inexpensive, diagnostic test for reflux disease. Endoscopy is the only test that can give sensitive recognition and grading of oesophagitis, and reliable diagnosis of oesophageal columnar metaplasia. Mechanically significant peptic stricture, gastric cancer, and chronic duodenal and gastric ulcer are also diagnosed with high sensitivity. The value of endoscopy is enhanced by the histological diagnosis of endoscopic biopsy and cytology brushings. Barium swallow and meal is insensitive for diagnosis of oesophagitis and cannot grade it, but other pathology such as gastric ulcer and oesophageal stricture is demonstrated with reasonable sensitivity. Barium swallow has an important role in the investigation of mechanisms of troublesome dysphagia, in recognizing extrinsic oesophageal compression, and in the assessment of anatomically complex hiatus hernia. Oesophageal function tests (pH monitoring, manometry, and radioisotope transit testing) may be helpful and are discussed in OTM3 (p. 1865). Steps needed for diagnosis are shown in Fig. 1).

Symptoms and the presence and severity of oesophagitis show poor correlation but the response of symptoms to low and medium levels of therapy (see Table 1 and below) gives an indirect approximation of severity and helps to determine further action.

Tailoring and grading therapy

Table 1 provides a framework. The lowest effective dose of any agent should be used in long-term therapy. Endoscopic findings allow the appropriate initial approach. Therapy is then graded upwards or downwards in order to find the lowest that is effective. Initial high-level medical therapy is likely to confirm the diagnosis, but is relatively expensive and uninformative about the best long-term approach.

Table 1 Levels of antireflux therapy

Low: antacids, non-drug measures
Middle: normal-dose H2-receptor antagonists, cisapride and sucralfate, ?bethanechol
Upper: 2–4 × normal ranitidine dose, × 2 normal famotidine dose omeprazole 10 mg, lanzoprazole 15 mg Combination of cisapride and standard-dose H_2-receptor antagonists
Highest: antireflux surgery, omeprazole 20 mg, lanzoprazole 30 mg

Initial low–medium-level therapy has the disadvantage of giving less useful diagnostic information and often, slow relief of symptoms, but it is relatively inexpensive and will usually identify patients with severe oesophagitis by their lack of response.

Non-drug measures and antacids

The efficacy of these approaches is often overrated. Most useful are avoidance of large meals and provocant foods, drinks, and physical activities. The benefits to reflux disease of stopping smoking, losing weight, and raising the bedhead are more debatable. Antacid may be effective in controlling heartburn.

Acid suppression

This treatment is highly efficacious. Proton-pump inhibitors have a special place, because of their overall efficacy in the control of acid secretion. Long-term acid suppression maintains patients free of symptoms and oesophagitis indefinitely, but withdrawal is usually associated with prompt relapse. The maintenance dose appears to be the same as the lowest effective healing dose. There have been concerns about the safety of long-term acid suppression but to date, follow-up of patients treated continuously for 5 or more years has shown no evidence of any important ill-effects.

Motility stimulants

Cisapride has a medium level of efficacy for both short- and long-term management. The principal effect appears to be on oesophageal acid clearance.

Other agents

Sucralfate, which is of medium-level efficacy, is believed to act by protecting the oesophageal mucosa from chemical injury. Bethanechol stimulates salivation and oesophageal contraction; at best it has only medium efficacy. Various formulations that include some mucosa coating or protective agent combined with antacid are probably no better than antacid alone.

Combination therapy

Cisapride and H_2-receptor antagonists in combination gives moderate results, but is a relatively unattractive option given the high efficacy of monotherapy with proton-pump inhibitors.

Antireflux surgery

In skilled hands, antireflux surgery is very effective with a small (about 0.5 per cent) mortality. Laparoscopic antireflux surgery is an important advance.

Management of complications

Dysphagia secondary to *peptic stricture* needs to be distinguished from the more common dysphagia due to defective triggering and control of oesophageal-body peristalsis (see below). Peptic stricturing is managed by a combination of peroral dilatation and healing of oesophagitis by either medical or surgical means.

Oesophageal columnar metaplasia (Barrett's oesophagus) is increasingly recognized as a consequence of oesophagitis (see below).

Respiratory disease may be the result of either direct aspiration of refluxed gastric contents, or from the reflex effects of gastro-oesophageal reflux. Proof of an association between coexistent reflux and respiratory disease is often difficult.

Regurgitation is the main problem in a small subgroup of patients who usually present complaining of 'vomiting'. Vigorous medical therapy sometimes controls the problem, but more often antireflux surgery is the only effective management.

Reflux is an important cause of *non-cardiac chest pain* (see below).

Idiopathic achalasia and achalasia-like states

These disorders are characterized by absent or incomplete relaxation of the lower oesophageal sphincter and impairment of oesophageal-body peristalsis. Idiopathic achalasia accounts for most cases and has an annual incidence of approximately 1–2/200 000; it affects all ages, but is most common in early to mid-adult life. The syndrome is also seen in Chagas' disease, occasionally in the intestinal pseudo-obstructive syndrome, as a manifestation of paraneoplastic neural dysfunction, and secondary to oesophageal amyloidosis. Impairment of inhibitory neural control of the distal oesophagus is the common abnormality, produced by neural damage at several sites; evidence of myenteric inhibitory neurone degeneration is probably most important.

Symptoms

Dysphagia with solids is the most common symptom. Regurgitation is also prominent. The regurgitated material tastes bland because it never enters the stomach. Cramping chest pain occurs in some patients during the early, hypercontracting phase of the disorder. Weight loss may occur. In some patients, symptoms remain static for many years, but in others there is a progression with increasing regurgitation, when respiratory problems secondary to aspiration can become a major feature.

Dilatation varies from a minor change to a grossly enlarged, colon-like oesophagus. Barium swallow shows a gastro-oesophageal junction that tapers smoothly to a closed sphincter, with occasional spurts of flow into the stomach (Fig. 2). In the absence of dilatation, a barium swallow is usually reported as normal. Oesophageal manometry is the only sensitive method for demonstration of the motor dysfunction, and is especially important in patients with no radiological abnormality. The important differential diagnosis is of malignancy of the gastric cardia. Endoscopy with biopsy and computed tomography scanning are helpful in this context.

Treatment

Calcium antagonists and β-adrenergic agonists compare poorly with mechanical disruption of the sphincter. Oesophagomyotomy (laparoscopic or thoracoscopic) is effective but associated with a 5–10 per cent risk of troublesome gastro-oesophageal reflux. Balloon dilatation often needs to be repeated, and in some hands fails in up to 40 per cent of patients, and carries a risk of perforation of about 5 per cent.

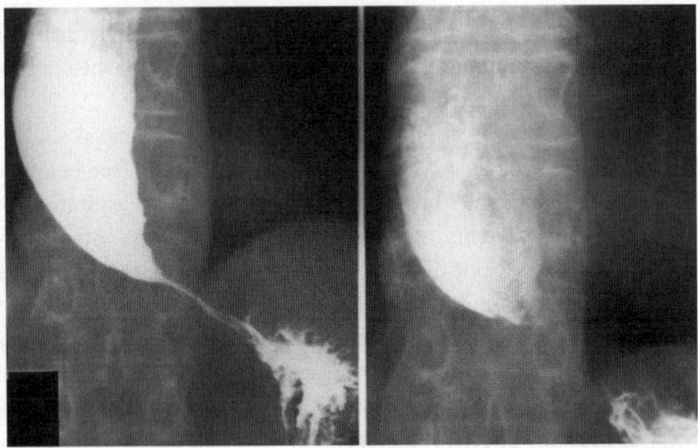

Fig. 2 Achalasia. Barium-filled dilated oesophagus; intact mucosa in distal achalasic segment.

Prognosis

If treatment is applied before the development of major dilatation, results are excellent, but achalasia carries an increased risk (ranging from 2 to 7 per cent) of oesophageal carcinoma. The average interval from diagnosis of achalasia to development of carcinoma has been estimated as 28 years. Some clinicians therefore recommend periodic screening endoscopy.

Diffuse oesophageal spasm

Episodic chest pain and/or dysphagia may result from spastic contractions of the distal half of the oesophagus in the absence of any precipitating structural stenosis. There may be an underlying disorder of neural control but evidence for this is lacking and the aetiology is unknown.

Symptoms

Virtually all patients have episodic, crushing, central retrosternal pain; cardiac ischaemia is often the first diagnosis. Intermittent dysphagia occurs in about two-thirds of patients and leads to temporary abandonment of eating until symptoms abate—usually over about 30 min, but episodes of oesophageal obstruction can last for several hours. In the majority, episodes occur less than once a month, but in severe cases these may occur several times a week, or each time food intake is attempted. Full-blown dysfunction is usually absent during investigation, but in a minority, there is asymptomatic motor dysfunction. Barium swallow then shows trapping of beads of contrast in the distal oesophagus—'the corkscrew oesophagus'—or sustained obliteration of the distal oesophageal lumen. Manometry may show intermittent, simultaneous, prolonged, and vigorous oesophageal contractions interspersed with normal swallow-induced peristalsis. Relaxation of the lower oesophageal sphincter is normal. The diagnosis is made from the history and the exclusion of other problems. Most important among these is Schatski ring (see below).

Treatment

There is no specific therapy. Nitrites, nitrates, and calcium antagonists may reduce symptoms; but reassurance is the most important measure. In the rare case of frequent, disabling spasm, long oesophagomyotomy can give good relief. There is no consistent progression of dysfunction and associated symptoms over time. Reports of progression to achalasia are probably explained by early spastic achalasia having been misdiagnosed.

Non-cardiac chest pain

Chest pain resembling cardiac pain may arise from oesophageal disorder such as reflux or spasm and may then respond well to appropriate therapy. Monitoring of oesophageal pH and mobility studies can be helpful but no clear diagnosis emerges in as many as 50 per cent of cases. In them, anxiolytics and antidepressants may be effective particularly in those in whom there is continuing anxiety about a cardiac origin of pain.

Miscellaneous motor disorders (see OTM3, Chapter 14.6)

Peristaltic pressure waves may exceed 250 mmHg (hypertensive peristalsis, nutcracker oesophagus) and can produce central cardiac pain. There are many other manometrically defined motor abnormalities associated or not with reflux, spasm, diabetes, or other autonomic dysfunction. 'Non-specific motor disorder' is characterized by multipeaked swallow-induced contractions in the distal oesophagus. Hypocontraction causes deranged transit and mild intermittent dysphagia particularly for solids. Prokinetic drugs may improve contractions but symptoms are rarely sufficient to warrant long-term treatment.

Oesophageal muscle diseases

Systemic sclerosis involves the smooth muscle of the oesophagus in as many as three-quarters of patients (see Chapter 10.13). Primary striated muscle disorders (such as dermatomyositis, polymyositis, inclusion body myositis, muscular dystrophy, and myasthenia gravis) may present with high dysphagia in association with oropharyngeal dysfunction.

Sliding hiatus hernia

About 90 per cent of hiatus hernias are of this type in which the gastro-oesophageal junction is displaced upwards into the thorax, giving a simple pouch of intrathoracic stomach. Symptoms of gastro-oesophageal reflux are the only ones of significance. These should be treated along conventional lines (see above). As many patients with hiatus hernia are asymptomatic, its demonstration should not be taken as diagnostic of reflux disease.

Rolling hiatus hernia

In this disorder, part of the stomach herniates through the hiatus alongside a normally situated gastro-oesophageal junction. This pattern of herniation may narrow the exit from the herniated pouch into the main stomach cavity. Some rolling hernias are also associated with displacement of the gastro-oesophageal junction above the hiatus (mixed hernias). Obstruction and distension of the pouch causes upper abdominal discomfort and can progress to strangulation. Gastric volvulus may obstruct the gastro-oesophageal junction. Both of these complications have a very high mortality and demand urgent surgery. Elective surgery is normally recommended to reduce and anchor rolling hiatus hernias in order to reduce these risks.

Schatski ring (B ring) and other rings and webs

The Schatski ring is a short luminal stenosis at the gastro-oesophageal junction (Fig. 3). The cause is unknown. With mechanically significant rings, intermittent dysphagia occurs on eating solids. Episodes of bolus obstruction are not unusual, with associated chest pain caused

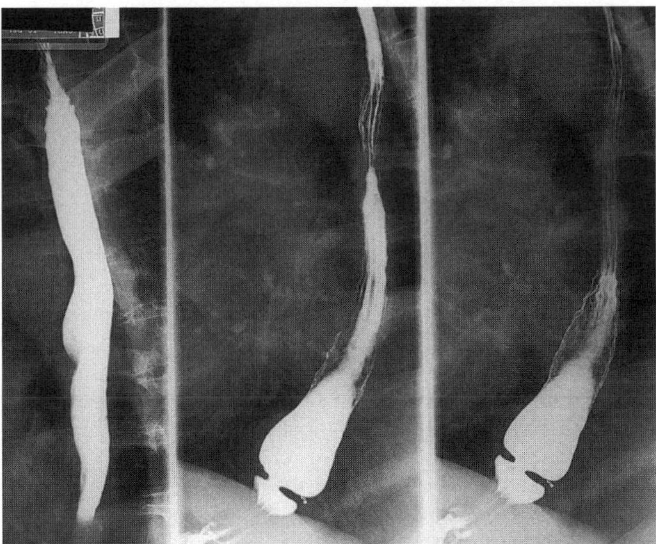

Fig. 3 Schatzki ring: thin, 2–4 mm in height, annular constriction at gastro-oesophageal junction; best shown on prone-oblique views.

by powerful oesophageal contractions. Failure to recognize a Schatski ring frequently leads to the incorrect diagnosis of oesophageal spasm. The diagnosis requires an expert radiologist. Disruption of the ring by peroral dilatation or endoscopic diathermy or laser is very rewarding. Other short oesophageal stenoses are due to peptic stricture, muscular rings, and cervical webs, with (Plummer–Vinson syndrome) or without iron-deficiency anaemia.

Oesophageal diverticula and pseudodiverticula

Wide-mouthed, multiple diverticula are characteristic of scleroderma oesophagus. In other cases, diverticula occur in the mid and distal parts, probably caused by 'blow-outs' secondary to hypercontraction motor disorders. It is rare for these to cause symptoms. They are best left undisturbed because leakage is common after surgical removal. Multiple intramural out-pouchings of barium are characteristic of intramural pseudodiverticulosis, which appears to be due to dilatation of submucosal gland ducts by an unknown process.

Extrinsic oesophageal compression

This is a relatively common cause of dysphagia, mainly from malignant mediastinal lymphadenopathy. Other causes include a grossly enlarged heart, aortic aneurysm, or congenital vascular abnormalities such as an aberrant right subclavian artery.

Mechanical, chemical, and radiation trauma

Mallory–Weiss tear

These mucosal tears extend across the gastro-oesophageal junction and are normally induced by vigorous straining associated with vomiting. Bleeding is the only consequence of significance. In 10 per cent of cases, bleeding is severe enough to cause hypovolaemia. The history is usually characteristic, but a definitive diagnosis requires endoscopy. Continued bleeding usually responds to endoscopic injection or electrocoagulation, vascular embolization, or vasopressin infusion. Very rarely, surgery is needed to underrun a persistently bleeding artery in the base of the tear.

Table 2 Common causes of medication-induced oesophageal injury

Severe injury—high risk	*Occasional injury*
Slow-release potassium chloride	Ascorbic acid
Non-steroidal anti-inflammatory agents	Mexiletine
Tetracycline	Slow-release theophylline
Quinidine	Captopril
	Phenytoin
Less severe injury—high risk	Zidovudine
Many antibiotics	
Iron supplements	

Boerhaave's syndrome

Straining and vomiting can cause oesophageal rupture, most often in the left lower third. Spillage of the gastric contents into the pleural space causes shock and chest and upper abdominal pain with radiation to the back, left chest, or shoulder. The chest radiograph becomes abnormal only some hours after rupture. Surgical repair and drainage are usually necessary, and if this is delayed beyond 24 h, mortality is very high.

Traumatic perforation

This may complicate oesophageal instrumentation. Perforation is suggested by the development of chest or epigastric pain directly after instrumentation, sometimes with dyspnoea. Pneumothorax and surgical emphysema are diagnostic. Broad-spectrum antimicrobials should be given on suspicion. The choice between conservative and surgical management should be based on the individual circumstances. Increasingly, instrumental perforation is being managed non-surgically with nasogastric suction, antimicrobials, and intravenous nutrition.

Caustic ingestion

This is addressed in OTM3, Chapters 8.3.1 and 8.3.5.

Medication-induced oesophagitis

Medications known to have an especially high risk for oesophageal damage are listed in Table 2. Symptoms are those of oesophagitis with stricturing. Such injury is the most likely cause of oesophagitis and/or benign stricture at the level of the aortic arch, where pills can lodge. Injury at the distal oesophagus, the other common site of hold-up, is often misdiagnosed as due to reflux disease.

Chemotherapy causes oesophageal disease in several ways. It may impair mucosal defences, reducing resistance to damage from other agents, and increase susceptibility to infective oesophagitis from immune suppression. Oesophageal transit and acid clearance may be impaired through neurotoxic effects of some agents. Fistulation or perforation may occur through cytotoxic effects on malignancy in the oesophageal wall.

Oesophageal neoplasms

Squamous cell carcinoma is the commonest oesophageal neoplasm. Adenocarcinoma usually arises in association with columnar metaplasia, or Barrett's oesophagus. Other oesophageal tumours are rare but include melanoma, lymphoma, carcinoid, leiomyosarcoma, small cell carcinoma, adenoid cystic carcinoma, and pseudosarcoma. Benign tumours include leiomyomas, lipomas, granular cell tumours, and squamous cell papillomas. The disorders are described in Chapter 5.20 and in OTM3 (pp. 1874–6 and Chapter 14.6).

Table 3 Major causes of infective oesophagitis

Pathogen	Management	Remarks
Immunocompetent patients		
Candida albicans	Topical/oral antifungals	By far most common
Herpes simplex	Acyclovir if severe	Unusual; may denude mucosa
Varicella zoster	Acyclovir if severe	In association with chickenpox/herpes zoster
Bacteria		Rare in well individuals
Immunocompromised patients		
Candida albicans	Systemic antifungals	Most common; oral disease almost diagnostic
Cytomegalovirus	Prophylaxis and treatment with ganciclovir or foscarnet	Part of systemic infection Sepiginous → giant ulcers distal half
Herpes simplex	Prophylaxis and treatment with acyclovir or foscarnet	Circumscribed ulcers, raised edges → coalescence Oral lesions.
Tuberculosis	Conventional	From miliary and local spread
Gram-positive cocci, Gram-negative bacilli	IV antibiotics	Often with systemic infection
Syphilis	Conventional	Associated with tertiary syphilis elsewhere → inflammatory stricture

Infective oesophagitis

Viral oesophagitis can cause major haemorrhage. Infective oesophagitis can damage the full thickness of the oesophageal wall and lead to stricturing. Diagnosis is often aided by the setting. Cutaneous or oral disease can suggest what is happening in the oesophagus. Endoscopy is the diagnostic method of choice. Mucosal appearances and the distribution of oesophageal lesions can be virtually diagnostic. In addition, biopsies and brushings allow histological diagnosis and identification of infectious agents. The more important causes are summarized in Table 3.

Other non-neoplastic mucosal diseases

Rarely, Crohn's disease can cause indolent, craggy ulceration and/or stricturing of the oesophagus. Oesophageal sarcoidosis can also mimic Crohn's disease. Other diseases affecting the oropharynx and oesophagus include epidermolysis bullosa, Behçet's disease, lichen planus, pemphigus vulgaris, bullous pemphigoid, benign mucous membrane (cicatricial) pemphigoid, and drug-induced disease (Stevens–Johnson syndrome and toxic epidermal necrolysis). Chronic, and less frequently, acute graft-versus-host disease may cause severe oesophageal problems through mucosal desquamation or mural damage. Resultant stricturing shows considerable variation in appearances.

Further reading

Quigley, E.M.M. (1997). Gastro-oesophageal reflux disease—spectrum or continuum? *Quarterly Journal of Medicine*, 90, 75–8.

Tytgat, G.N.J. (1995). Long term treatment for reflux oesophagitis. *New England Journal of Medicine*, 333, 1148–50.

Chapter 5.4

Peptic ulceration

J. J. Misiewicz and R. E. Pounder

Duodenal ulcer

Duodenal ulcer is a distinct break in the mucosa of the duodenum, almost invariably in the duodenal bulb, but occasionally more distal. The ulcer may be superficial, or may penetrate to the serosa.

Aetiology

It is not known why patients develop duodenal ulceration, nor why the clinical course is characterized by episodes of intermittent relapse. The characteristics of the disease appear to be changing towards a less severe form: why this should be so is not known. The strongest aetiological association is with infection of the gastroduodenal mucosa by *Helicobacter pylori*, which has important effects on gastric function. Eradication of the bacterium leads to healing and dramatic decrease in the incidence of relapse. *H. pylori* is an important aetiological factor in several other diseases of the foregut, including chronic gastritis, gastric ulceration, gastric cancer, mucosal associated lymphoid tissue lymphoma, and Ménétrier's disease.

Acid and pepsin

Although the presence of acid and pepsin is essential for the appearance of a duodenal ulcer it is probably only one of several aetiological factors operating in most patients. Ulceration is thought to be related to an imbalance between the damaging effects of acid and pepsin and mucosal defences. As a group, patients with duodenal ulcer secrete more acid than healthy people. Five factors may account for the tendency to hypersecrete acid and pepsin: (a) increased parietal cell mass; (b) increased stimulation of acid secretion; (c) increased parietal cell sensitivity to stimulants; (d) decreased inhibitory control of acid secretion; and (e) *Helicobacter pylori* induced hypergastrinaemia. Several of these abnormalities (hypergastrinaemia, raised basal and stimulated acid output, decreased inhibitory drive mediated by somatostatin, hyperpepsinogenaemia) disappear after eradication of *H. pylori*.

The abnormalities of acid output and gastrin release described above are subtle, difficult to investigate, and based on evidence collected from an intensive study of few subjects: it is uncertain whether they apply to all patients with duodenal ulcer. Much less is known about the importance of pepsin secretion, while knowledge of factors affecting mucosal defence and integrity is fragmentary.

Gastric emptying

The pH in the duodenal lumen is lower more frequently and for longer periods in patients with duodenal ulceration than in controls. These patients empty food from their stomachs faster so that after a meal there is less food available to buffer secreted acid as it passes into the duodenum, where acid is neutralized by bicarbonate. Patients with duodenal ulcer do not have a gross defect of pancreatic alkaline secretion, but the alkaline secretions of the duodenal mucosa are suboptimal.

Ulcerogenic drugs

Corticosteroids, aspirin, and non-steroidal anti-inflammatory drugs (**NSAIDs**) are commonly thought to be ulcerogenic, but the evidence that they cause chronic duodenal (or gastric ulcer) is not convincing. Anti-inflammatory agents can damage the gastric mucosa and are used to produce ulcer models in experimental animals for the testing of drugs. Extrapolation from these models to humans should be viewed with a certain amount of scepticism. However, the incidence of consumption of NSAIDs is high among patients with gastrointestinal bleeding, or perforation.

Psychological factors

Stress is often invoked as an important cause of duodenal ulcer. Chronic (as opposed to acute) stress is difficult to measure. Case–control studies suggest that patients with duodenal ulcer may be more stressed than controls exposed to similar events.

Epidemiological factors

Duodenal ulceration may affect 10–15 per cent of many populations. The prevalence is subject to marked geographic variation; for example, it is much more common in Scotland and northern England than in southern England; it is more common in the south of India than the north. Men are affected more than women, but the incidence is increasing in women, particularly after the menopause. In India and Africa the prevalence is higher in populations who eat a low-residue diet. There are weak associations with smoking, alcohol, and anti-inflammatory drugs. It is possible that there is a genetic predisposition; ulcers are more common in close family members, patients with blood group O and non-secretors of blood-group substances in the saliva.

Virtually all patients are infected with *H. pylori*, but there are many who are colonized by it but who do not develop an ulcer. The prevalence of this organism seems to be determined by socio-economic factors and the infection is usually acquired in childhood.

Clinical picture and natural history

The main symptom of duodenal ulceration is pain, classically epigastric, related to food, and occurring during the night, but there can be great individual variation. Indeed, severe ulceration to the point of perforation or haemorrhage can be virtually symptomless.

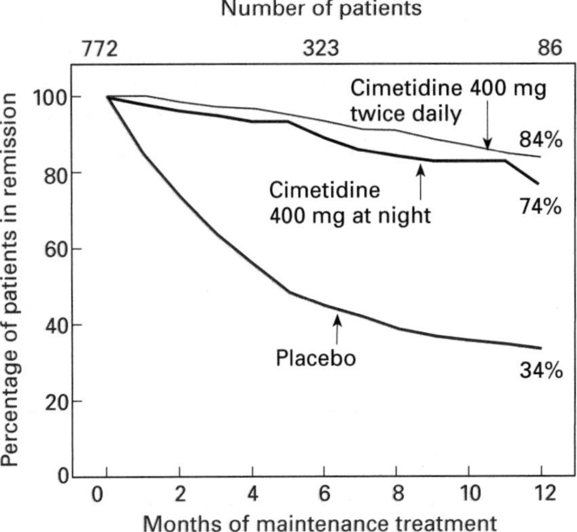

Fig. 1 Maintenance treatment of duodenal ulcer with cimetidine: results of double-blind trials from 22 centres (from the data of Burland, W., Hawkins, B., and Beresford, J. (1980). *Postgraduate Medical Journal*, **56**, *173)*.

Some 50 per cent of patients who die from a peptic ulcer are unaware of their ulcer at the time of their fatal admission. The cause of ulcer pain is not clear: it is not always directly related to intraduodenal acidity, but is rapidly relieved by antacids.

Nausea and vomiting are relatively unusual, unless there is severe pain or pyloric stenosis. Posterior penetration into the pancreas may cause mid-back pain, or pancreatitis. Major complications are rare; perhaps occurring in 1 per cent per year. Haemorrhage may cause haematemesis and/or melaena, or iron-deficiency anaemia. Perforation causes acute, severe pain, collapse, and peritonitis.

Duodenal ulceration is a condition of spontaneous relapses and remissions. The change in the clinical picture from relapse to remission can be remarkable. It is therefore unwise to make decisions about surgery during a relapse. Clinical trials show that within a year of treatment using a gastric acid antisecretory drug, 66 per cent of those receiving a placebo will have had a symptomatic relapse (Fig. 1), and approximately one-third of asymptomatic patients have recurrent ulcers when examined by endoscopy. Some patients suffer only a single episode of ulceration, while in others the illness is progressive, with rare remissions and severe complications. Spontaneous healing of duodenal ulcer may be delayed, and relapses are earlier and more frequent in patients who either continue to smoke cigarettes or take NSAIDs.

Diagnosis

Duodenal ulcer cannot be diagnosed by clinical history, because similar symptoms occur in other diseases (gastric ulcer, gastric cancer, or the irritable bowel syndrome). The patient often points to the epigastrium as the site of the pain, but this is not reliable. Physical examination may show epigastric tenderness, but is otherwise unhelpful, unless there is severe pyloric stenosis, when visible gastric peristalsis and a succussion splash are present.

The diagnosis is established by radiology or endoscopy. A barium meal, preferably air-contrast, will show deformity of the duodenal cap, but the differentiation between scarring, mucosal folds, and an active ulcer crater is less certain. Fibreoptic endoscopy is the best method of diagnosis. Even then, pyloric stenosis with retention of gastric contents, mucosal oedema, haemorrhage, or incomplete inspection of the base of duodenal cap can all cause the ulcer crater to be missed. Previous therapy may make the diagnosis more difficult or impossible. Duodenal ulcers are usually single, circular areas of discrete ulceration resembling oral aphthous ulcers, usually with a creamy yellow base.

The fasting plasma gastrin concentration should be measured in patients with severe or ectopic ulceration, or in those with continuing ulceration after adequate medical treatment or surgery, to exclude the Zollinger–Ellison syndrome. Serological and salivary tests for specific antibodies to *H. pylori* have been used to screen young dyspeptic patients. This approach needs further validation.

Chronic benign gastric ulcer

Ulcers can occur anywhere in the stomach, but most develop on the lesser curvature at the junction between the acid-secreting mucosa and that of the antrum. Special care must be taken to exclude malignancy in antral ulcers. Pre-pyloric ulcers resemble duodenal ulcers endoscopically and are best managed similarly.

Aetiology

Approximately 80 per cent of benign gastric ulcers are associated with *H. pylori* infection. There is also an association with NSAID medication. The gastric mucosa is probably injured by the combination of gastric acid, reflux of duodenal contents, and by *H. pylori* colonizing the antral epithelial cells. Patients with gastric ulcer tend to reflux their duodenal contents, a tendency that is aggravated by smoking cigarettes. Gastric-emptying time tends to be prolonged and retention of contents predisposes to ulceration.

Gastric ulceration was once a disease of young women but it is now common in both genders, in older age groups, and in patients of low socio-economic class.

Clinical picture and diagnosis

Patients typically present with epigastric pain. Although exacerbations of discomfort after meals, remitting pain, weight loss, and a long history are common, a confident diagnosis must not be made on clinical evidence alone. Many patients are asymptomatic until they present with a complication such as acute or occult gastrointestinal haemorrhage, or perforation. Up to a half of the patients develop recurrence. Diagnosis can be continued by double contrast barium meal (Fig. 2) or endoscopy. The latter allows biopsy and brush cytology, which is essential to exclude early carcinoma.

Acute erosive ulceration

Multiple superficial ulcers may develop in the oesophagus, stomach, or duodenum of acutely stressed patients, particularly after major trauma, extensive burns, or during shock or hypoxia. The main damage appears to be due to mucosal ischaemia and hypoxia. This type of ulceration usually presents with haemorrhage some days after the initial insult, which may be aggravated by coagulopathies associated with the primary disorder. H_2-receptor blockers can prevent the ulceration and haemorrhage. The recommended maximum doses are cimetidine (400 mg) or ranitidine (50 mg) intravenously 6-hourly, preferably as a continuous infusion. In the presence of renal insufficiency the dose should be decreased, as the drugs are mainly excreted by the kidney. Cimetidine very occasionally causes coma in severely ill people. Omeprazole is not generally available for intravenous use. Erosive ulcers can also develop in patients taking NSAIDs or excess alcohol.

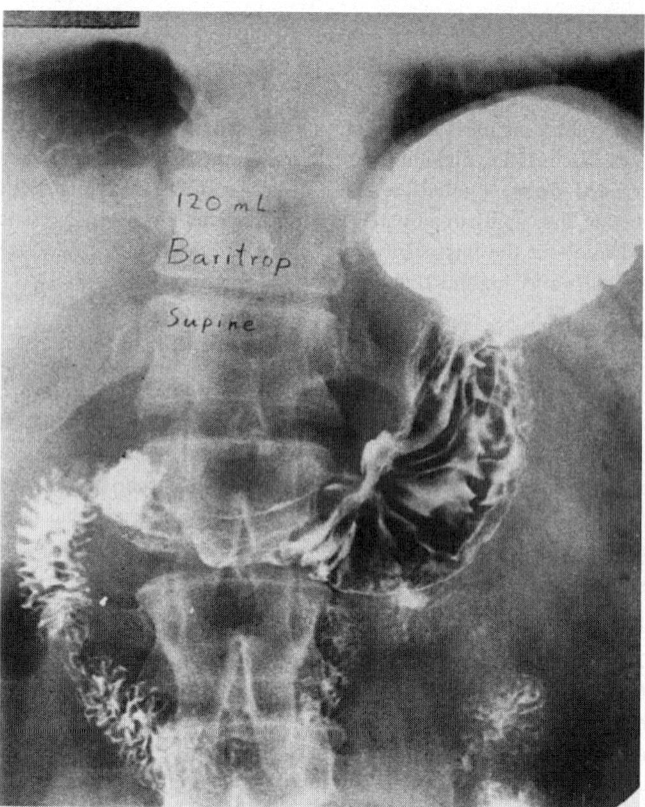

Fig. 2 Benign gastric ulcer demonstrated by air-contrast barium meal; mucosal folds reach the rim of the ulcer crater.

Non-ulcer dyspepsia (functional dyspepsia)

Dyspepsia is common, but only a small proportion of sufferers have organic disease. Ulcer-like symptoms, bloating with early satiety (dysmotility dyspepsia) or features suggesting reflux are common. Dysmotility dyspepsia may respond to motility-stimulating agents, such as cisapride. Reflux dyspepsia merges into gastro-oesophageal reflux disease. Medical treatment of ulcer-like dyspepsia is unsatisfactory in that response to gastric acid suppressants, or to eradication of *H. pylori*, is unpredictable. The prevalence of *H. pylori* in patients with functional dyspepsia is similar to that of the general population.

Duodenitis

This is an ill-defined condition, characterized at endoscopy by inflamed, haemorrhagic, and friable duodenal-cap mucosa; duodenal biopsies show acute inflammatory changes. Erosions may be present and symptoms then may be indistinguishable from those of duodenal ulcer and may be complicated by haemorrhage. Most patients are treated as if they have a duodenal ulcer; many will be colonized by *H. pylori*, but the effect of eradicating this organism on duodenitis has not been fully studied.

The Zollinger–Ellison syndrome Type II

This syndrome comprises severe peptic ulceration, hypersecretion of gastric acid, and an islet-cell tumour of the pancreas, secreting gastrin (gastrinoma). The tumours are usually found in the body or tail of the pancreas; may be multiple and can be malignant. The gastrin secreted is usually the G17 form (little gastrin), but smaller and larger molecular species have also been reported. Prolonged high plasma gastrin concentrations cause an increase of the parietal cell mass with consequent high basal and maximal acid secretion. Occasionally, a pancreatic gastrinoma is associated with hyperparathyroidism in Werner's syndrome (multiple endocrine adenomatosis I).

Most patients (95 per cent) have peptic ulcers in duodenum, stomach or oesophagus, often multiple, large, and penetrative. Ulceration often extends beyond the first part of the duodenum. Diarrhoea is present in 40 per cent and can be the only symptom. It is not due to hypergastrinaemia and may result from the low intestinal pH which denatures pancreatic enzymes causing steatorrhoea and precipitates bile salts.

Diagnosis

This initially depends on the detection of an elevated fasting plasma gastrin concentration, in the presence of acid in the stomach. Three conditions can cause marked hypergastrinaemia with increased acid output and aggressive peptic ulceration, but without the presence of a gastrinoma. First, hyperplasia of the gastrin-secreting cells of the antrum, called confusingly the Zollinger–Ellison syndrome type I (the classical condition is type II), which may represent the upper part of the normal range of gastrin and acid secretion. Secondly, a cuff of antral mucosa inadvertently retained at the end of the oversewn blind loop of a Polya partial gastrectomy results in the excluded antrum being bathed in alkaline duodenal and pancreatic secretion, thereby causing profound gastrin release. Thirdly, for a short time after massive small-intestinal resection, plasma gastrin concentrations rise markedly: possibly due to transient deficiency of an inhibitory gastrointestinal polypeptide.

Treatment with gastric-acid antisecreting drugs also results in a rise of plasma gastrin concentration. Excessive histamine release in patients with either systemic mastocytosis, or mast-cell leukaemia, may cause profound gastric hypersecretion, with normal or low plasma gastrin concentration.

The most reliable confirmatory investigation is the secretin test. Two units GIH secretin per kg are given by slow intravenous injection with the patient fasting. In normal individuals the plasma gastrin concentration drops, but in patients with the Zollinger–Ellison syndrome there is an immediate rise (within 1 or 2 min of the injection) to more than 50 per cent above the basal values. Patients with type I Zollinger–Ellison syndrome have a normal response to secretin, but those with an excluded antrum may still be confused with type II.

The pancreatic tumour may be small and difficult to find. Selective arteriography, ultrasound, or an abdominal computed tomographic scan may help to localize it.

Treatment

Until the mid-1970s the only possible treatment was total gastrectomy, combined with exploration and perhaps resection of the pancreas. Now most patients will respond to omeprazole, 40 mg twice daily. Failure is usually due to inadequate dosage. The optimal dose can be determined by measuring intragastric pH after breakfast and lunch: keeping the pH between 2.0 and 7.0. The H_2-antagonists now have no role in management, except as emergency intravenous treatment, using up to six times the normal dose. The role of surgery is now controversial. Some advise an attempt to remove the tumour together with selective vagotomy. Others would reserve surgery for those in whom omeprazole therapy has failed. Inoperable and progressive malignancy may respond to streptozotocin.

Complications of peptic ulcer

Perforation is more common in men and more frequent in duodenal than in gastric ulcers. A proportion of patients (approximately 50 per cent), perforate without any preceding history. The most common site is the anterior wall of the duodenal cap in duodenal ulcer or the lesser curve of the stomach in gastric ulcer. Rarely, ulcers may perforate into the biliary tract, filling it with air.

The *history* is of a sudden onset of abdominal pain. The abdomen is rigid, there is rebound tenderness, the abdominal respiratory movements and bowel sounds are absent, and liver dullness to percussion is diminished. A plain abdominal radiograph may show free air between the upper border of the liver and the diaphragm. Leucocytosis usually appears promptly. Difficulties in diagnosis arise in the elderly, or in the mentally ill, in patients in hospital for chronic illness, or in those on high doses of corticosteroids. In this group, 'silent' or painless perforations may occur; unexplained shock is the most common clinical finding.

Treatment is usually surgical. Medical management consists of continuous nasogastric suction, treatment of shock, electrolyte and fluid replacement, and antibiotic therapy with ampicillin, gentamicin, and metronidazole. Oversewing a perforated ulcer provides no long-term cure. The patient may need either maintenance treatment with an H_2-antagonist, eradication of *H. pylori*, or an elective, definitive reoperation.

The main causes of upper gastrointestinal *haemorrhage* are peptic ulceration or variceal bleeding. Variceal haemorrhage is relatively rare in the United Kingdom. Duodenal ulcer, gastric ulcer, erosive ulceration, and the Mallory–Weiss syndrome are all more common.

Diagnosis and management are described in Chapter 5.1 and in OTM3, Chapter 14.7.

Pyloric stenosis

More than 80 per cent of cases are due to duodenal ulcer. The diagnosis is suggested by a long history of peptic ulcer pain, with a more recent onset of vomiting. The vomitus contains food sometimes identified to have been eaten the previous day. Weight loss is usual. Visible gastric peristalsis and succussion splash are the physical signs. Dehydration, prerenal uraemia, or metabolic alkalosis may complicate the picture. A barium meal will show a dilated, often atonic stomach: food debris may be present in the lumen. Gastric emptying of barium will be grossly prolonged.

Pyloric stenosis caused by chronic duodenal ulcer must be differentiated from malignant tumours, the most common being antral carcinoma. Cancer of the head of the pancreas or lymphoma can also interfere with gastric emptying. Other causes are benign tumours (adenomatous polyp or annular pancreas), adult hypertrophic pyloric stenosis, and rarely, a pyloric or duodenal diaphragm. Treatment is surgical.

Medical treatment of duodenal and gastric ulcer

Patients should be treated medically in the first instance. Surgery is reserved for emergencies such as haemorrhage or perforation, complications such as pyloric stenosis or suspicion of malignancy, or failure of medical treatment.

Diet

Avoidance of fatty, fried, spicy, and rich meals is almost universal, but it is difficult to be certain how much of this is due to folklore, and how much to some undefined pathophysiological mechanism. Patients will almost invariably have excluded from the diet those foods that produce pain and distension. Detailed dietary advice is therefore unnecessary and can be summed up as 'avoid what upsets you, eat little and often, and go to bed with an empty stomach'.

Smoking and alcohol

There is little evidence to show that giving up smoking has an effect on the healing rate of duodenal ulcer, although faster healing rates of gastric ulcer have been reported, and relapse rates of duodenal ulcer have been shown to be significantly higher in smokers than in non-smokers. Excessive drinking must be discouraged, but total abstinence is not required for ulcer healing.

Rest, sedation, and psychotropic drugs

Rest and removal from stressful circumstances will act as a non-specific adjuvant to treatment, but sedation has no part to play. A small number of controlled trials suggest that tricyclic antidepressants accelerate the healing of duodenal ulcers in the short term, but there is insufficient evidence to recommend this as an established therapy.

Anticholinergics

There is no good evidence that conventional anticholinergics are useful in the short- or long-term healing of either gastric or duodenal ulcer. This picture has been modified by the introduction of pirenzepine, which is said to be more selective in blocking cholinergic receptors on or near gastric parietal cells. Data from controlled trials show that this drug (50 mg three times daily) does speed healing of duodenal ulcer.

Bismuth preparations

These have several modes of action, which include chelation with protein in the base of the ulcer, stimulation of local release of prostaglandins, and inhibition of secretion and activity of pepsin. However, probably the most important effect is the rapid and profound suppression of *H. pylori*. The main usefulness of bismuth salts is in their use in triple-therapy regimens for eradication of *H. pylori* (see below).

Helicobacter pylori

This organism is responsible for almost all cases of chronic, non-immune gastritis, which heals when the infection is eradicated. *H. pylori* is very strongly associated with duodenal ulcer, and also has associations with gastric ulcer and with gastric cancer. The factors that determine the occurrence of duodenal ulcer in a colonized individual are not understood. Some strains of *H. pylori* may be more pathogenic. These strains express a high molecular weight protein (about 120 kDa), associated with a cytotoxin (a product of the *CagA* gene), which has been shown to be cytopathic *in vitro*. In Western countries the prevalence of *H. pylori* increases with age, from some 20 per cent at 20 years to over 50 per cent at 50 years. The prevalence of *H. pylori* in developing countries is much higher, and may reach 80 per cent by the age of 5 years. The prevalence of *H. pylori* is inversely related to socio-economic status and to the sophistication of public health facilities; it is directly related to overcrowding. There is no evidence to show that *H. pylori* is itself carcinogenic; the link is probably through *H. pylori*-associated chronic gastritis proceeding to gastric atrophy.

H. pylori probably spreads through the oral/faecal route and the infection is acquired in early childhood. It grows only on the surface of gastric epithelial cells and below the protecting layer of adherent mucus. It also colonizes islands of gastric metaplasia in the duodenal cap; the damage to epithelial cells and the inflammatory reaction mounted by the host set the scene for the development of ulceration. *H. pylori* increases the release of gastrin from the antral G cells. The hypergastrinaemia is probably triggered by suppression of somatostatin release from antral D cells by *H. pylori*. Gastric acid output in response to GRF is about six times greater in *H. pylori*-positive duodenal ulcer patients, when compared with *H. pylori*-negative controls; *H. pylori*-positive controls secrete about three times the normal amount of acid when stimulated by GRP. Hyperpepsigenaemia is also present and all these changes are reversed by eradication of *H. pylori*.

Diagnosis of the presence of H. pylori

All diagnostic tests may be affected by previous medication with antibiotics, omeprazole, or bismuth-containing compounds. The most widely available diagnostic method is either one of the variants of the CLO test (see below), or the demonstration of *H. pylori* in an endoscopic biopsy. At least two biopsies need to be taken from the antrum. Biopsies from the gastric corpus are indicated, if the patient has been on proton-pump inhibitors.

The CLO test (on antrial biopsy material) and urea breath test depend on urease from hydrolysing urea to NH_4 and CO_2, the NH_4 producing a colour change in a pH-sensitive indicator. In the urea breath test, expired air is collected after ingestion of ^{13}C- or ^{14}C-labelled urea and the excreted, labelled CO_2 is measured by mass spectrometry, or scintillation counter, respectively. Both tests are highly specific and sensitive. Serological tests are available, and the fall in anti-*H. pylori* titre can be used to assess the results of treatment, but it takes several months for the antigen levels to decrease. Culture of *H. pylori* provides the diagnostic 'gold standard'. Specialized techniques are necessary and there is a proportion of failed cultures, even in experienced hands.

Treatment

H. pylori is difficult to eradicate. Its habitat is poorly penetrated by antimicrobial agents, and it can survive deep in the gastric pits, emerging later from these sanctuary sites. There is also ready development of resistant strains, principally to metronidazole, but also to other antimicrobials. Resistant strains are more prevalent in women (20 per cent) and in developing countries (80 per cent). The use of only one agent against infection is thus to be discouraged. Although resistance to tripotassium dicitrato bismuthate does not develop, and although the incidence of early relapse after a healing dose of bismuth is lower than after cimetidine, eradication rates on bismuth alone are negligible at less than 10 per cent.

A definitive treatment regimen for *H. pylori* infection has not yet been established. Large blinded trials, and direct comparisons of different therapies are generally lacking. Triple therapies usually comprise bismuth with two antimicrobials, but there have been encouraging results with the use of non-bismuth triple regimens—for example, ranitidine or omeprazole together with an imidazole (tinidazole or metronidazole), and an antimicrobial (amoxycillin or clarithromycin) given for 7–10 days. Eradication rates are very variable, but usually range between 70 and 80 per cent.

Microbial resistance, or non-compliance are the commonest causes of failure. Repeat endoscopy with bacterial culture of biopsies may help select an appropriate antibiotic regimen.

Indications for eradication

Eradication treatment should be offered to all *H. pylori*-positive, non-NSAID associated, duodenal and gastric ulcer patients, but not to patients with functional dyspepsia. Treatment will not work in all patients, so there is a need for counselling on the possible outcomes, especially in those in whom the treatment has changed.

Other treatments

Sucralfate is said to increase in viscosity on contact with gastric acid, forming a protective coating for damaged mucosa. It is also said to absorb pepsin and bile salts. It does not affect acid secretion, but does accelerate ulcer healing significantly. It is safe, the dose being 1 g four times daily before meals, but there is some systemic absorption of aluminium. Constipation is the only common side-effect.

The main limitation of *carbenoxolone sodium* therapy is unwanted aldosterone-like activity (sodium and water retention, hypertension, and hypokalaemia). It is used rarely because a range of safer medications is now available.

Histamine H2-receptor antagonists Histamine abundantly present in the gastric mucosa, is a powerful stimulant of gastric acid and pepsin secretion. Histamine, acetylcholine, and gastrin are all involved in the stimulation of the gastric parietal cell. There is a close interrelation between the three secretory stimulants, and the inhibition of one will markedly decrease the effects of the others. Histamine H_2-receptor antagonists inhibit gastric-acid secretion. H_2 receptor blockade by cimetidine ranitidine, or other similar agents inhibits gastric acid secretion by all known agonists. Basal and nocturnal acid secretion can be inhibited completely.

Short-term treatment of duodenal and gastric ulcer with H_2-receptor antagonists

Some 80–95 per cent of gastric or duodenal ulcers will heal after treatment for 4–8 weeks with H_2-receptor antagonists. Cimetidine 400 mg twice daily, or 800 mg at bedtime, are now the standard dose regimens. Ranitidine 300 mg at bedtime is equally effective (Fig. 3). Famotidine and nizatidine are given in bedtime doses of 40 and 300 mg, respectively. Administration is usually accompanied by rapid relief of symptoms.

If symptoms persist despite 8–12 weeks of therapy at a full dose, patients should be endoscoped, the remaining ulcer, if present, biopsied and the Zollinger–Ellison syndrome excluded. There may be a need for further therapy for *H. pylori*, but a change to omeprazole is indicated if after a further 8 weeks the ulcer has not healed. Long-term treatment with an H_2-blocker is used to prevent relapse or complications. The usual dose is half that used for acute ulcer healing.

Unwanted effects of H_2-receptor blockade

Mild hypergastrinaemia does occur during H_2-receptor blockade with the theoretical risk that prolonged hypergastrinaemia could lead to parietal-cell hyperplasia, and hypersecretion of acid once treatment is stopped leading to severe re-ulceration. Parietal cell hyperplasia has never been detected in humans, and the recurrence rate of duodenal ulcer is much the same in patients who have had 12 months' maintenance treatment as in those who have not.

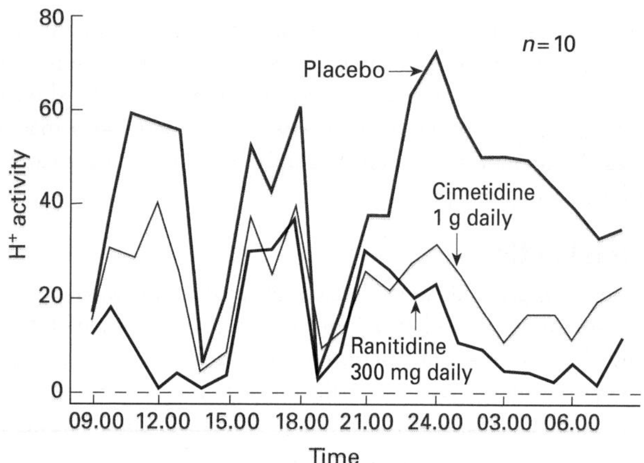

Fig. 3 Mean hourly H^+ activity (i.e. intragastric acidity) over 24 h in 10 patients with duodenal ulcer receiving placebo, cimetidine 1 g daily (four divided doses), or ranitidine 150 mg twice daily.
(Reproduced from Walt, R.P. et al. (1981). Gut, **22**, *49.)*

Sporadic instances of male erectile impotence have been reported in patients taking cimetidine, but this is not common. Prolactin concentrations increase after bolus intravenous cimetidine (but not after ranitidine), but oral treatment does not affect prolactin metabolism. Gynaecomastia in men and galactorrhoea in women has been occasionally reported: most commonly in patients treated with cimetidine for the Zollinger–Ellison syndrome. Blood concentrations of warfarin, labetolol, diazepam, and phenytoin are significantly higher in patients receiving cimetidine, so that smaller doses of these drugs may be necessary. Reversible mental confusion and coma have also been reported in elderly or severely ill patients receiving cimetidine. It may also cause a minor rise in creatinine or hepatic transaminases. The most common side-effect of cimetidine, mild sedation and tiredness, is rarely severe enough to interfere with treatment. There are no grounds for withholding long-term H_2-blockade because of possible carcinogenesis.

H^+, K^+-ATPase inhibitors

Omeprazole inhibits gastric-acid secretion by irreversible inhibition of the proton pump in the gastric parietal cells. Newer, similar drugs include lansoprazole and pantoprazole. Peak plasma concentrations of omeprazole occur 2–4 h after oral administration, but bioavailability increases during the first few days of treatment, probably because increasing inhibition of acid secretion results in less intragastric degradation. Individuals vary in their response to an oral dose of omeprazole, with approximately one-third of patients with duodenal ulcer demonstrating a profound decrease of intragastric acidity taking 20 mg every morning, and almost all patients responding to 40 mg every morning. There is a period of sustained hypoacidity when treatment is stopped abruptly, with normal intragastric acidity returning 3–7 days later.

Safety

The major concern is the theoretical possibility of increased susceptibility to enteric infection or infestation; also the proven development of bacterial overgrowth of the stomach and duodenum, and an unremitting rise of 24-h plasma gastrin concentration during treatment. Long-term treatment of rats with omeprazole results in the development of dose-dependent carcinoid tumours in the stomach. Similar carcinoids have occurred in patients with pernicious anaemia, but gastric carcinoids have not developed after prolonged treatment in humans using omeprazole.

Prostaglandins

Misoprostol is generally well tolerated, although a substantial minority of patients may notice either abdominal pain, or diarrhoea, particularly during the first few days of dosing. In addition, the drug has a uterotonic activity, which can induce abortion, and must therefore not be given to pregnant women, or to women of child-bearing age who may conceive during treatment. Misoprostol has not found a place in routine treatment of duodenal or gastric ulcer, because of unimpressive healing rates and fairly troublesome side-effects. It has been advocated as preventive therapy in patients receiving NSAIDs, and trials indicate a lower incidence of duodenal ulcer, or gastric ulcer, in those so treated.

Ulcers and NSAIDs

NSAID-associated duodenal ulcers and gastric ulcers occur largely in older patients, who are at risk of the potentially life-threatening complications of perforation or haemorrhage. The addition of H_2-receptor antagonists can prevent the development of duodenal ulcer, and added misoprostol prevents the formation of duodenal and gastric ulcer, but no trial has so far shown the incidence of ulcer complications to be lowered by these therapies. At present there is no indication for treating every patient on NSAIDs with either H_2-blockers or prostaglandin analogues; patients deemed at risk—those with a history of peptic ulcer, the very elderly, or frail individuals—should be selected for such treatment.

Antacids

Antacids are now mainly used for the symptomatic management of dyspepsia. Most regimens involve the use of a mixture of several alkalis—for example, sodium bicarbonate, aluminium hydroxide, calcium carbonate, and magnesium hydroxide. Aluminium–magnesium antacids are usually preferred to those containing sodium bicarbonate, because of the latter's high sodium content, short duration of action, and tendency to produce alkalosis. Calcium-containing antacids tend to stimulate gastric-acid secretion and may produce hypercalcaemia with impaired renal function.

Short-term management of peptic ulcer

It is mandatory to endoscope every patient with gastric ulcer when multiple biopsies and exfoliative cytology brushings must be taken. It is then ideal to repeat the endoscopy after 8–12 weeks of medical therapy to check that the ulcer has healed: if still present, histopathological evaluation must be repeated, because the diagnosis of early intramucosal carcinoma can be difficult to establish, and results of resection of early gastric cancer are good. By contrast, in duodenal ulcer, repeated endoscopy or radiology is unnecessary. Reinvestigation is only needed if complications occur, or before operation to provide the surgeon with up-to-date anatomical information.

Omeprazole produces the fastest healing and probably the best relief of daytime ulcer pain in the first days of treatment—but the shortest acceptable length of treatment with omeprazole is probably 4 weeks. Similar considerations apply to lansoprazole. Treatment to eradicate *H. pylori* could be offered to patients following remission of symptoms, but the present complicated drug regimens limit this strategy. Pirenzepine, misoprostol, or sucralfate may be useful in some patients and can be used if H_2-receptor antagonists or omeprazole are badly tolerated or unavailable.

Long-term management

A choice of strategies is available for the long-term management of duodenal ulcer: either intermittent therapy (giving full-dose H_2-blockade only at the time of ulcer relapse) or continuous therapy (giving low-dose bedtime H_2-blockade, with full-dose treatment only when there is rare symptomatic relapse). The best guide is the previous history of ulcer symptoms. The patient who has one or two relapses each year, but who remains well otherwise, does not need continuous medication, while the individual with continuous symptoms, or whose symptom-free periods are short, will tend to do better on continuous therapy. Despite reports to the contrary, there is no convincing evidence that 'rebound' ulceration is a serious problem in the post-treatment period. Some physicians prefer to tail off treatment. There are no experimental data to support this, but it is probably good practice. Maintenance therapy for gastric ulcer gives similar or better results.

Surgical treatment

In *duodenal ulcer*, absolute indications for surgical intervention are continuing or life-threatening haemorrhage, perforation, or pyloric stenosis. In the uncomplicated patient, frequent and severe recurrences, poor response to, or poor compliance with medication, residence in remote areas with limited access to medical facilities, and occupations where a sudden haematemesis or perforation may endanger the life of others all suggest the need for surgical intervention. Only rarely is the indication failed medical treatment.

Before an elective operation, the ulcer should be biopsied at endoscopy to exclude rare lymphoma, tuberculosis, Crohn's disease, or carcinoma. The patients' fasting plasma gastrin concentration should also be measured to exclude the Zollinger–Ellison syndrome.

In *gastric ulcer*, absolute indications for surgery are similar to those for duodenal ulcer, except that suspicion of carcinoma should lead to thorough re-evaluation: if neoplasm cannot be confidently excluded, it is safer to proceed to operation.

Choice of operation

Uncomplicated duodenal ulcer is now almost invariably treated by either a truncal vagotomy with a drainage procedure (pyloroplasty or gastroenterostomy), or by selective, or highly selective vagotomy. This latter operation denervates only the parietal cell mass, leaving the innervation of the antral pump, and thus control of gastric emptying, undisturbed. Gastric ulcers are usually dealt with by a Billroth-type partial gastrectomy: surgical texts can be consulted for details.

Outcome of surgery

Surgical treatment works well for properly selected patients with either type of ulcer. The main disadvantage of highly selective vagotomy for duodenal ulcer is a relatively high recurrence rate—some 5 to 15 per cent. Other types of vagotomy have a lower recurrence rate, but the incidence of unwanted effects such as postvagotomy diarrhoea, or dumping is higher. Vagotomy and antrectomy carries the lowest recurrence rate, but mortality is slightly higher than after vagotomy and drainage, where it is less than 1 per cent in good centres.

Recurrence is rare after elective partial gastrectomy for chronic gastric ulcer, but the mortality is about 3 per cent, mainly because gastric ulcer tends to be the disease of elderly patients from low socio-economic groups. Late or early dumping is an unwanted sequel. Later sequelae include weight loss, iron-deficiency anaemia, mild steatorrhoea, and occasional osteomalacia. There is also a slightly increased incidence of carcinoma in the gastric remnant.

Postsurgical recurrent ulcers

Duodenal ulcer may recur after vagotomy often in the duodenal cap, but after gastroenterostomy ulcers may form distal to the stoma in the jejunum. Most recurrences are due to the incomplete division of the vagal fibres: a few are previously undiagnosed cases of the Zollinger–Ellison syndrome. The diagnosis of recurrent duodenal ulcer is best established by endoscopy. Treatment is either by re-operation, at which undivided vagal trunks are identified, or a highly selective vagotomy is converted to another type, or a partial gastrectomy is performed. Results of re-operation are good, but repeated surgical procedures carry a higher morbidity and mortality. The alternative is aggressive medical treatment with an H_2-receptor antagonist or a proton pump inhibitor, and a further attempt to eradicate *H. pylori.*

Further reading

Blaser, M.J. (1998). *Helicobacter pylori* and gastric diseases. *British Medical Journal,* **316**, 1507–10.

El-Omar, E., Penman, I., Dorrian, C.A., Ardill, J.E.S., and McColl, K.E.L. (1993). Eradicating *Helicobacter pylori* infection lowers gastrin mediated acid secretion by two-thirds in patients with duodenal ulcer. *Gut,* **34**, 1060–5.

Laine, L. and Peterson, W.L. (1994). Medical progress: bleeding peptic ulcer. *New England Journal of Medicine,* **331**, 717–27.

Penston, J.G. and Wormsley, K.G. (1992). Maintenance treatment with H_2-receptor antagonists for peptic ulcer disease. *Alimentary Pharmacology and Therapeutics,* **6**, 3–29

Tytgat, G.N.J. (1994). Treatments that impact favourably upon the eradication of *Helicobacter pylori* and ulcer recurrence. *Alimentary Pharmacology and Therapeutics,* **8**, 359–99.

Chapter 5.5

Hormones and the gastrointestinal tract (see also Chapter 7.14 and OTM3, Chapter 12.10)

P. J. Hammond, S. R. Bloom, and J. M. Polak

Most of the gut peptides, such as cholecystokinin and substance P, have been identified within the central and peripheral nervous systems, playing a neuromodulatory part in many organs. They are synthesized in nerve cells in the gut and act locally as peptide neurotransmitters or neuromodulators. Their principal role is the integration of gastrointestinal function, by either autocrine or paracrine activity. The endocrine cells of the gastrointestinal tract are not grouped into anatomically distinct glands, like most endocrine cells, but are scattered through the length of the gastrointestinal tract. In addition to altering gastrointestinal function many peptides, such as gastrin, secretin, and enteroglucagon, probably play an important paracrine part in controlling the growth and development of the gastrointestinal tract.

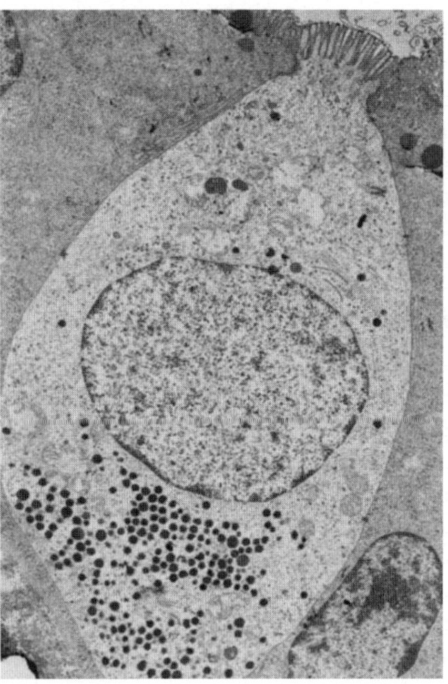

Fig. 1 Electron micrograph of mucosal endocrine cell showing well-developed microvilli and secretory granules grouped at the basal membrane (×5500).

Radioimmunoassay has allowed detection of gut peptides at very low concentrations in plasma and tissues. Furthermore, antibodies can be used in immunocytochemistry to demonstrate cellular and neuronal localization. Peptide localization is further defined by electron microscopy, which demonstrates specific storage granules (Fig. 1), and *in-situ* hybridization, which allows the sites of synthesis to be identified. The most recent advance has been the molecular characterization of hormone receptors by cloning techniques. This has demonstrated different receptors for the same ligand and provides an explanation for the diverse biological actions of many gut peptides in the same tissues.

Gastrin-cholecystokinin family

Gastrin occurs in a variety of molecular forms but all biological activity resides in the four carboxy-terminal amino acids. The major forms contain 17, 14, and 34 amino acids. Gastrin is particularly localized to the gastric antrum, where G17 is the predominant form, but is also found in the upper small intestine, mainly as G34; these are the predominant circulating forms. Gastrin release is particularly stimulated by protein ingestion and gastric distension. Its main physiological action is the stimulation of gastric acid secretion. Its other important part is its trophic effect on the gastric mucosa.

Cholecystokinin (CCK) has an identical terminal sequence to gastrin, but specificity is conferred by the adjacent three amino acids. It is found in the gut in 33, 39, or 58 amino acid molecular forms predominantly, and is produced by the I cells of the duodenal and jejunal mucosa. CCK secretion is stimulated by long-chain fatty acids and certain amino acids. There are two receptor subtypes, A and B. The CCK-A receptor appears to be involved in the stimulation of gallbladder contraction and trophic effects on the duodenum and pancreas.

The secretin family

The secretin family includes, in addition to secretin, glucose-dependent insulinotropic peptide, glucagon, enteroglucagon, vasoactive intestinal peptide, peptide histidine methionine, and growth hormone-releasing factor, which in addition to stimulating release of growth hormone, is also found in the small intestinal mucosa, where its function is unknown.

Secretin is a 27 amino acid peptide, produced by S cells throughout the duodenal and jejunal mucosa. The main stimulus to secretion is a duodenal pH of less than 4.5. It is probably also secreted late after a meal. The main role of secretin is stimulating production of watery, alkaline pancreatic juices in response to acid in the duodenum.

Glucose-dependent insulinotropic peptide (**GIP**) is a 42 amino acid peptide with considerable sequence homology at the N-terminal to secretin, glucagon, and vasoactive intestinal peptide. It is produced in the upper small intestinal mucosa but also in the gastric antrum and ileum. At pharmacological doses, GIP inhibits gastric secretions, and was originally named gastric inhibitory peptide. However, its physiological role appears to be as a component of the enteroinsular axis, being released in response to a mixed meal, particularly carbohydrates and long-chain fatty acids, and stimulating insulin release.

Vasoactive intestinal peptide (**VIP**) is a 28 amino acid peptide widely distributed through the central and peripheral nervous systems. The highest concentrations occur in the submucosa of the intestinal tract, where it is found in postganglionic intrinsic nerves. VIP is a potent stimulator of small intestinal and colonic enterocyte secretion of water and electrolytes. Other important actions include smooth muscle relaxation, stimulation of insulin release (counteracted by a direct glucagon-like effect), stimulation of pancreatic bicarbonate secretion, and relaxation of the gallbladder, pyloric sphincter, and circular muscle of the small intestine with contraction of the longitudinal muscle.

Peptide histidine methionine is a 27 amino acid neuropeptide with considerable sequence homology to VIP. It mimics the actions of VIP, but is less potent.

Pituitary adenylate cyclase-activating peptide has 27 and 38 amino acid forms and with considerable sequence homology to VIP, a similar tissue distribution and similar actions to VIP on intestinal secretion and motility.

Peptide products of preproglucagon

In the pancreas the major product of preproglucagon is glucagon, but in the intestine it is cleaved into *enteroglucagon*, and glucagon-like peptide (**GLP**) 1 and GLP2. *Enteroglucagon* is found in the mucosa of the ileum, colon, and rectum, and is released after a mixed meal. It is postulated that enteroglucagon has a trophic effect on the small intestinal mucosa and may be important in gut adaptation. GLP-1, a 36 amino acid peptide, is a more potent stimulus to insulin secretion than GIP, and inhibits secretion of glucagon and potentiates release of somatostatin.

Pancreatic polypeptide, neuropeptide Y, and peptide tyrosine

Pancreatic polypeptide has 36 amino acids and is produced by cells found at the periphery of the pancreatic islets. Concentrations rise dramatically after a meal, at least in part due to activation of the vagus. It inhibits pancreatic exocrine and biliary secretion.

Neuropeptide Y is a 36 amino acid peptide neurotransmitter, often colocalized with noradrenaline. It is found in both extrinsic adrenergic nerves to the myenteric plexus and in intrinsic nerves in the myenteric and submucosal plexi. It is a potent vasoconstrictor, inhibits intestinal secretion, and depresses colonic motility.

Peptide tyrosine tyrosine (**PYY**) is a 36 amino acid peptide found in endocrine cells of the ileum, colon, and rectum. It is released after a meal, and its main function appears to be to slow intestinal transit.

The gastrin-releasing peptides

The gastrin-releasing peptides are found in the gut in the intrinsic neurones of the myenteric and submucosal plexi, particularly in the stomach and pancreas. They are potent stimulators of gastrin and stimulate release of motilin and cholecystokinin, and pancreatic enzyme secretion.

Opioids

Leu-enkephalin, met-enkephalin, and dynorphin are widespread through the nerves of the myenteric and submucosal plexi of the gastrointestinal tract. Their principal actions appear to be inhibition of gastrointestinal secretion and increased smooth muscle contractility.

Tachykinins

Substance P is an 11 amino acid peptide causing smooth muscle contraction and vasodilatation. Substance P, neurokinase A, and preprotachykinin B are localized to neurones in the intestinal myenteric and submucosal plexi, collectively called tachykinins because of their rapid actions. Their principal effects are smooth muscle contraction, vasodilatation, and inhibition of intestinal absorption.

Other gut peptides

Motilin is a 22 amino acid peptide secreted by small intestinal M cells, whose density decreases from duodenum to ileum. Motilin appears to control the reflex motor activity of the small intestine, which occurs at approximately 2-hourly intervals in the fasted state, keeping the small intestine free of debris. The macrolide antibiotics, such as erythromycin, are motilin-receptor agonists, hence their side-effects of diarrhoea and abdominal cramps.

Neurotensin is a 13 amino acid peptide present in enteric neurones and N cells of the ileal mucosa. Plasma concentrations rise after a meal. Neurotensin inhibits gastric acid secretion and gastric emptying, and stimulates pancreatic exocrine and intestinal secretion.

Somatostatin is widely distributed throughout the central and peripheral nervous system, and is found in a variety of endocrine tissues. In the gastrointestinal tract it occurs in 14 and 28 amino acid forms. It is secreted by specific cells in the gastric and intestinal

Table 1 Inhibitory actions of somatostatin

Hormone release	Physiological function
Growth hormone	Lower oesophageal sphincter contraction
Thyroid-stimulating hormone	Gastric acid secretion
Insulin	Gastric emptying and secretions
Glucagon	Absorption of nutriments
Pancreatic polypeptide	Splanchnic blood flow
Gastrin	Gallbladder contraction and secretions
Secretin	Pancreatic enzyme and bicarbonate secretion
Gastric inhibitory polypeptide	
Motilin	
Enteroglucagon	

mucosa, by the D cells on the inner rim of the pancreatic islets, and is found in the enteric neural system. Five human somatostatin receptors have now been identified and cloned. Somatostatin inhibits hormone release and blocks the response of the effector tissue, and inhibits a wide range of gastrointestinal functions (Table 1). Its acts principally as a paracrine factor or neurotransmitter.

Calcitonin gene-related peptide, a 37 amino acid peptide, is a neurotransmitter and in the gut occurs in both extrinsic sensory nerves and intrinsic neurones. It inhibits gastric acid and pancreatic secretion and causes relaxation of vascular smooth muscle.

Galanin, a 29 amino acid peptide neurotransmitter, is found in the gut plexi and in nerves supplying the liver and pancreatic islets. Its main actions are inhibition of intestinal smooth muscle contraction and inhibition of postprandial insulin release.

Endothelin has been demonstrated in the plexi of the gastrointestinal tract and in mucosal epithelial cells, but its role in the regulation of gastrointestinal function is unknown.

Gut peptides in gastrointestinal disease

Gastric pathology

The most common cause of an elevated gastrin concentration is achlorhydria, a consequence of the loss of negative feedback on gastrin secretion by the low stomach pH, but very high concentrations are also found in the Zollinger–Ellison syndrome (see Chapter 5.4).

In peptic ulcer disease a decrease in somatostatin release in patients infected with *Helicobacter pylori* may influence the paracrine regulation of gastric function.

The dumping syndrome after gastrectomy or truncal vagotomy is associated with a marked increase in the postprandial rise of VIP, neurotensin, PYY, and enteroglucagon, and a decrease in the release of motilin. VIP and neurotensin may both contribute to the postprandial hypotension associated with dumping, but neurotensin may have a beneficial effect in slowing gastric transit. The long-acting somatostatin analogue octreotide, which inhibits release of these peptides and inhibits gastric emptying, is often a very effective treatment for this condition.

Malabsorptive conditions

These are associated with a decrease in the amount of peptides produced in the affected region, and a compensatory elevation of other peptides, particularly those implicated in adaptation to loss of absorptive surface, such as enteroglucagon. The postprandial peptide response in patients with untreated coeliac disease shows greatly reduced secretion of GIP and secretin, and a marked elevation of enteroglucagon, neurotensin, and PYY. The decrease in secretin and increase in PYY may be responsible for the reduced pancreatic exocrine and biliary secretion found in this condition. In tropical sprue, a different profile of postprandial peptide release is seen. There is marked elevation in enteroglucagon and PYY, but also in motilin secretion, while other peptides behave normally. Patients with chronic pancreatitis may have insulin-dependent diabetes, and basal, and meal and secretin-stimulated concentrations of pancreatic polypeptide are reduced if steatorrhoea is associated, probably reflecting the location of its secretory cells throughout the exocrine pancreas and on the periphery of the islets. The malabsorption associated with pancreatic exocrine insufficiency leads to an excess of nutriments in the colon, and as a result the concentrations of enteroglucagon, PYY, and neurotensin are raised. Cystic fibrosis is often associated with diabetes mellitus and pancreatic exocrine insufficiency. Fasting and milk-stimulated concentrations of pancreatic polypeptide are usually suppressed. GIP concentrations fail to rise after a milk stimulus, and this may contribute to the associated glucose intolerance.

Intestinal resection

Jejunoileal bypass (for massive obesity) results in glucose intolerance and hyperinsulinaemia, absence of line postprandial rise in GIP, and massive hypertrophy of remaining bowel, the last related to gross increases in secretion of enteroglucagon and neurotensin. After partial ileal resection, the concentrations of gastrin, enteroglucagon, pancreatic polypeptide, motilin, and PYY are elevated, but after colonic resection only gastrin and PP are raised.

Diarrhoea

In acute infective diarrhoea, the concentrations of enteroglucagon, PYY, and motilin are increased. Patients with Crohn's disease have an elevated pancreatic polypeptide, GIP, motilin, and enteroglucagon, while in ulcerative colitis there is a modest elevation in PP, GIP, motilin, and gastrin, the last in response to the associated hypochlorhydria.

Neuropathic disease

In conditions associated with destruction of intrinsic enteric nerves there is loss of the neurocrine peptides found in the affected region. Chagas' disease in the gastrointestinal tract can result in mega-oesophagus and megacolon. Concentrations of VIP and substance P are greatly reduced in biopsies from affected segments. Similar changes are seen in Hirschsprung's disease. Patients with the Shy–Drager syndrome have no abnormalities in neurocrine peptides. Acquired immune deficiency disease is frequently accompanied by diarrhoea without evidence of secondary infection, and reduced immunostaining for substance P, VIP, and somatostatin in biopsies suggests a neuropathic process may be responsible.

Carcinoid syndrome

The term carcinoid refers to tumours capable of producing serotonin (5-hydroxytryptamine; **5-HT**). Several different cell types either synthesize or take up 5-HT and so the term is applied to a variety of malignant tumours with different biological behaviour grouped by their similar histological appearances.

Primary gastrointestinal carcinoid tumours are derived from the embryonic foregut (thyroid, bronchus, stomach, common bile duct, and pancreas), midgut, or hindgut. The most common sites are the appendix and rectum, but these tumours are often found incidentally on histological examinations of appendicectomy and rectal biopsy specimens. These tumours are almost always benign. Rectal tumours are often multicentric and even when they metastasize are rarely associated with the carcinoid syndrome, which occurs in about 10 per cent of patients with carcinoid tumours. It does not develop when the tumour drains through a normal liver, and so midgut tumours have almost always metastasized, usually to the liver, before symptoms develop. The syndrome is most commonly due to a metastatic midgut tumour, about 50 per cent of which metastasize to the liver. Primary carcinoid tumours are bronchial in origin in about 10 per cent of cases, and rarely occur in the ovary and testis. Tumours in these sites may be associated with the syndrome in the absence of metastases. The annual incidence of the carcinoid syndrome is about 1 in 500 000.

Clinical manifestations

The cardinal feature of the classical syndrome is the flush, which predominantly involves the head and upper thorax, and is usually associated with a tachycardia, hypotension, and increased skin temperature. Patients may have a sensation of intense heat and wheezing may occur. Rarely, flushing extends to the trunk and limbs, and may be associated with lacrimation, facial oedema, and great distress. Attacks are paroxysmal, and usually unprovoked, although precipitating factors include alcohol or food ingestion, stress, emotion, or exertion. Flushing initially lasts for only a few minutes but as the disease progresses may become almost continuous, and such patients often develop a chronically reddened and cyanotic facial hue, with widespread telangiectasia, the leonine facies. This fixed flush is more commonly seen with bronchial carcinoids. Gastric carcinoids are often associated with raised, localized, weal-like areas of flushing, which are usually pruritic and may migrate.

The other characteristic feature is secretory diarrhoea, which may be profuse, and associated with cramping abdominal pain, nausea, and vomiting. Rarely these symptoms may result from small bowel obstruction from a large ileal tumour, but the majority of primary tumours are small. Hepatic metastases may cause right hypochondrial pain, and acute exacerbations may occur if metastases become ischaemic and undergo autonecrosis. Weight loss and, in the later stages, cachexia are common. Pellagra with dermatitis of sun-exposed areas may occur, the increased conversion of 5-hydroxytryptophan into 5-HT causing nicotinamide deficiency.

Cardiac valve abnormalities affect about 50 per cent of patients. They occur as a result of endocardial fibrosis, with plaques of smooth muscle in a collagenous stroma deposited on the valves. Lesions are almost always on the right-side, left-sided damage only occurring in association with bronchial carcinoids or atrioseptal defects with right to left shunting. The most common lesions are tricuspid incompetence and pulmonary stenosis. Bronchospasm may coincide with flushing attacks and arthritis occurs in a small number of patients. Sclerotic bone metastases may develop usually in association with foregut tumours.

Carcinoid tumours also have the potential to produce a variety of peptide products and may be associated with other syndromes, with or without the carcinoid syndrome. The most common of these is Cushing's, due to an ectopic adrenocorticotrophic hormone (**ACTH**)-secreting bronchial or pancreatic carcinoid. Carcinoid tumours may also be a feature of multiple endocrine neoplasia type 1.

Biochemistry

5-HT probably plays a part in the pathogenesis of some of the symptoms, particularly the diarrhoea and bronchoconstriction. It is metabolized to 5-hydroxyindole acetic acid (**5-HIAA**), which accounts for 95 per cent of the urinary excretion of 5-HT.

A variety of vasoactive substances may be secreted by carcinoid tumours, including bradykinin, histamine, substance P, and prostaglandins.

Investigations

The diagnosis is made on the basis of elevated concentrations of 5-HIAA in a 24-h urine collection. Various foods, including avocados, bananas, aubergines, pineapples, plums, and walnuts, should be avoided while collecting specimens to prevent false-positive results. A number of drugs and other substances interfere with the spectrophotometric assay; paracetamol, fluorouracil, methysergide, and caffeine give false-positive results, and ACTH, phenothiazines, methyldopa, monoamine oxidase inhibitors, and tricyclic antidepressants false-negatives.

Localization of tumours is rarely a problem, as most have gross hepatic metastases, visible on computed tomography (**CT**) scanning or abdominal ultrasonography. In those rare cases where the syndrome occurs in the absence of metastases, tumour localization may offer the prospect of cure, so chest radiographs and CT scans of the chest and pelvis should be taken. The indium-labelled somatostatin analogue, pentetreotide can help in localizing some of these tumours. 123-*m*-iodobenzylguanidine (**MIBG**) scanning is equally effective and can be useful in metastatic disease to demonstrate the extent of spread. Angiography may be of value in assessing suitability for hepatic embolization.

Treatment

Codeine phosphate, diphenoxylate, and loperamide may help to control the diarrhoea. Many of the symptoms can be controlled with 5-HT antagonists: cyproheptadine, a 5-HT type 2 receptor blocker, often helps the diarrhoea; ketanserin may be effective in reducing flushing; and the 5-HT type 3 receptor antagonist ondansetron can alleviate nausea and anorexia. H_1- and H_2-receptor blockade may be useful. These treatments have been largely superseded by the long-acting somatostatin analogue octreotide which inhibits the release of the mediators of the syndrome by the tumour and antagonizes their peripheral effects. It is effective in alleviating symptoms in over 90 per cent of patients. It may be life saving in the carcinoid crisis. The major drawback to octreotide is that patients develop resistance with time, and most become refractory to any form of treatment after about 4 years. Vitamin supplements containing nicotinamide are necessary when patients have pellagra. The treatment of cardiac manifestations is the same as for valve disease and cardiac failure of other causes. Patients with painful bony metastases may benefit from palliative radiotherapy.

Tumour debulking may provide palliative relief, and enucleation of large metastases may give some benefit. Rarely, patients with metastases localized to the liver and an identifiable primary tumour may be cured by resection of the primary and hepatic transplantation.

The most effective means of debulking is hepatic embolization. Octreotide should be given in high dose to cover this intervention.

Tumours respond rarely to chemotherapy with streptozotocin and 5-fluorouracil, or cyclophosphamide and doxorubicin. Interferon-α is more effective, with symptom relief and tumour stabilization or regression in up to 70 per cent of patients.

Tumour targeted radiotherapy, using ^{131}I-MIBG or ^{90}Y-DOTA-octreotide, is a novel technique for delivering local tumour irradiation and has proven effective in a few individuals.

Prognosis

The median survival from the time of diagnosis is about 5 years, with a range of up to 20 years. Thus palliation is very worthwhile in these patients, allowing them to lead a normal life until the terminal stages of the disease.

Further reading

Bloom, S.R. and O'Shea, D. (ed.) (1998). *Baillière's clinical gastroenterology: gastrointestinal endocrine tumours.* Baillière Tindall, London.

Malabsorption

Chapter 5.6

Investigation and differential diagnosis of malabsorption

M. S. Losowsky

Malabsorption can arise from defective digestion of foodstuffs within the lumen of the bowel, structural changes in its wall, or anatomical abnormalities in its lymphatic drainage. Although some degree of malabsorption has been demonstrated in a wide variety of systemic disorders, in many cases the gastrointestinal dysfunction plays a relatively minor part in the illness. The main causes are summarized in Table 1.

Clinical presentation of malabsorption

Some symptoms and signs are common to the syndrome of malabsorption whatever its cause. In the severe case the stools are typically loose, bulky, offensive, greasy, light coloured, and difficult to flush away. Stool frequency is usually increased, but not to the extent seen in colonic disease. The stools may, however, appear normal and even constipated, even though steatorrhoea is shown by faecal fat measurement. Steatorrhoea may be absent in any of the diseases of the small intestine. Abdominal symptoms include discomfort, borborygmi, and distension. The discomfort may follow food and mimic peptic ulcer, or it may be relieved by bowel action, thus mimicking the irritable bowel syndrome.

Nutritional deficiency may present with anaemia due to iron, folate, or vitamin B_{12} deficiency, bleeding due vitamin K deficiency, or bone disease secondary to vitamin D deficiency. Such deficiencies may be reflected by a variety of symptoms and signs including glossitis, pallor, pigmentation of the skin, petechiae or bruising, muscle pain, neurological abnormalities, a positive Chvostek or Trousseau sign, and skeletal abnormalities.

Features of general ill health include anorexia, weight loss, lethargy, tiredness on little effort, dyspnoea, and general irritability. In contrast to the usual anorexia, some patients have hyperphagia and a very high food intake. Finger clubbing occurs in some cases. In severe or prolonged disease, hypoalbuminaemia, oedema, electrolyte deficiencies, and dehydration may occur, as may amenorrhoea, infertility, and impotence.

Features related to the underlying cause include, for example, the finding of an abdominal mass in intestinal lymphoma or regional

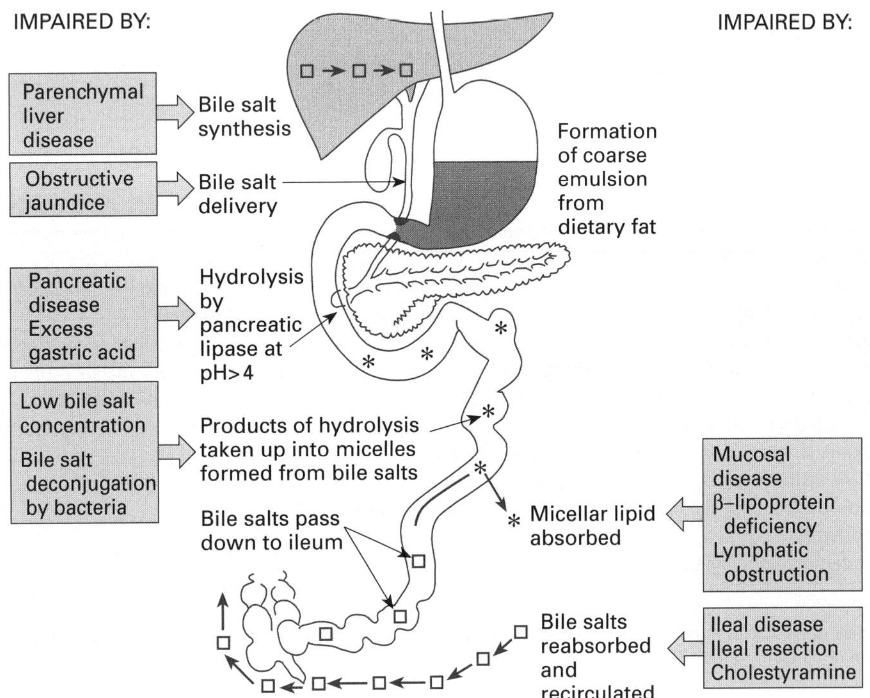

Fig. 1 Digestion and absorption of fat. Steatorrhoea may be caused by disease processes that impair different stages in the sequence of events.

Table 1 Classification of causes of malabsorption

Mucosal—definitive investigation: intestinal biopsy
Structure
- Food sensitivities:
  - gluten-sensitive enteropathy*
  - dermatitis herpetiformis
  - cows' milk sensitivity in infants
  - soya protein sensitivity
- Tropical sprue*
- Whipple's disease
- Intestinal lymphangiectasia
- Mast-cell disease

Function
- Alactasia
- Abetalipoproteinaemia

Structural—definitive investigation: usually small-bowel radiology
Crohn's disease*
Intestinal resection
Gastric surgery (see below)*
Radiation enteritis
Mesenteric arterial insufficiency
Small-intestine lymphoma or other malignancy
Blind loops, fistulae, diverticula, strictures
Idiopathic chronic ulcerative enteritis
Amyloidosis
Eosinophilic gastroenteropathy
Mechanisms of malabsorption after gastric surgery

- Poor mixing } not important
- Decreased gastric digestion } not important
- Lack of stimulus to bile and pancreatic secretion
- Rapid gastric emptying
- Intestinal hurry
- Afferent loop pooling of bile and pancreatic secretions
- Afferent loop bacterial overgrowth

- Pancreatic atrophy
- Unmasking of other disease: gluten sensitivity, alactasia, jejunal diverticula

- Inadvertent gastroileostomy } rare
- Gastrocolic fistula } rare

Infective—definitive investigation: usually microbiology
- Human immunodeficiency virus
- Acute enteritis
- Travellers' diarrhoea*
- Intestinal tuberculosis
- Parasitic disease of the intestine, especially giardiasis
- Whipple's disease
- Contaminated small bowel
  - Anatomical: blind loops, fistulae, diverticula, strictures
  - Motility disturbance: systemic sclerosis, intestinal pseudo-obstruction, diabetes mellitus, abdominal radiotherapy
  - Achlorhydria
  - Hypogammaglobulinaemia

Defective luminal digestion
Pancreatic
- Chronic pancreatitis*
- Carcinoma of the pancreas*
- Cystic fibrosis*
- Pancreatectomy
- Zollinger–Ellison syndrome
- Defective stimulation: intestinal disease, gastric surgery
- Malnutrition

Bile-salt mediated
- Parenchymal liver disease*
- Biliary obstruction*
- Bacterial degradation (in contaminated small bowel)
- Terminal-ileum disease*
- Terminal-ileum resection*
- Cholestyramine

Drugs
Neomycin
Cholestyramine
Colchicine
p-Aminosalicylic acid
Irritant purgative abuse
Phenindione
Metformin
Methyldopa
Methotrexate
Liquid paraffin
Ethyl alcohol
Antacids

Lymphatic obstruction
Congenital lymphangiectasia
Acquired lymphangiectasia: lymphoma, tuberculosis, cardiac disease

Disease outside the upper gastrointestinal tract
Endocrine disorders: hyperthyroidism, hypothyroidism, Addison's disease, hyperparathyroidism, hypoparathyroidism, diabetes mellitus, carcinoid syndrome
Collagen diseases
Ulcerative colitis

Widespread skin disease
Malnutrition

Specific biochemical defects
Pancreatic enzyme deficiencies, with normal structure
Enterokinase deficiency
Disaccharidase deficiency
Cystinuria
Congenital chloridorrhoea
Vitamin B_{12} malabsorption
Folate malabsorption
Acrodermatitis enteropathica

*Relatively common.

Some disorders cause malabsorption by more than one mechanism and are thus classified under more than one heading. This has the advantage of allowing consideration of different forms of treatment in the same patient.

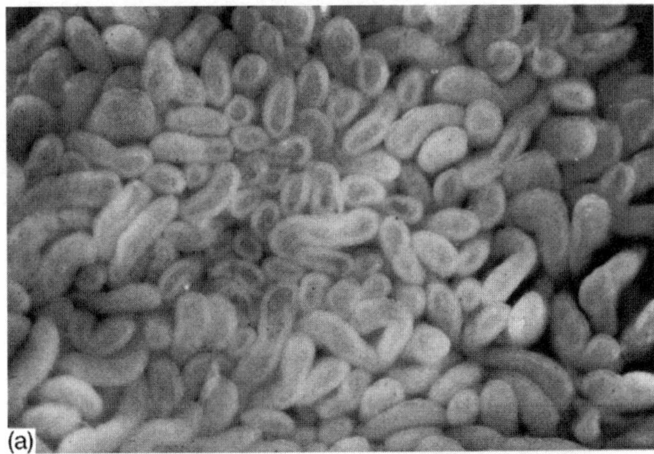

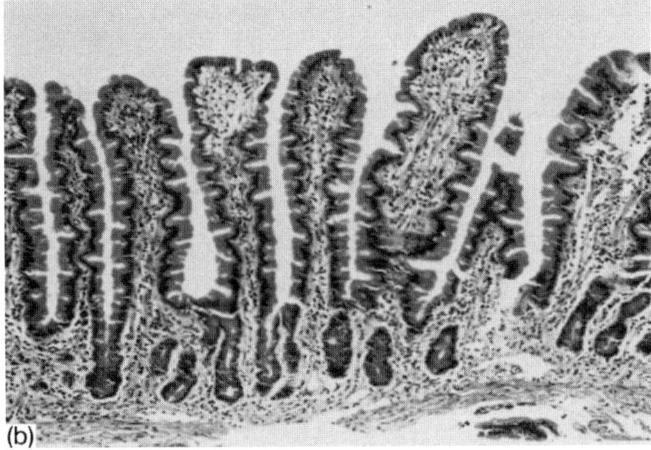

Fig. 2 (a) Dissecting microscopic appearance of normal jejunal mucosa showing finger-shaped and leaf-shaped villi. (b) Histological appearance of normal jejunal mucosa showing tall villi, several times as long as the crypts are deep. The epithelial cells are columnar with basal nuclei. There is a scattering of inflammatory cells deep into the mucosa.

enteritis, the dermatological changes of systemic sclerosis, facial flush and large liver suggestive of the carcinoid syndrome, signs of hypo- or hyperthyroidism, neurological impairment associated with abetalipoproteinaemia, ocular or neurological changes suggestive of diabetes mellitus, lymph node enlargement, arthritis and lung disease characteristic of Whipple's disease, or the dermatological changes characteristic of systemic mast-cell disease.

Investigation of suspected malabsorption

Demonstration of defective absorption

Fat malabsorption

The mechanisms of defective fat absorption are shown in Fig. 1. Estimation of faecal fat content is the standard investigation. Because the output of fat varies greatly from day to day faeces need to be collected for several days, preferably at least five, and the result expressed as average daily excretion. Faecal markers, intermittent or continuous, improve accuracy.

The quantity of fat in the stool depends on dietary intake which may vary by a factor of 4 to 5. Thus, the dietary intake must be known. Expressing the faecal fat as a percentage of dietary fat gives a meaningful basis of comparison between patients on different fat intakes and from time to time in the same patient if the fat intake varies. Ninety-three per cent absorption is the approximate lower limit of normal. Diarrhoea of any cause can lead to a modest increase in faecal fat. Faecal fat determined in this way gives an overall assessment of major physiological functions (Fig. 1). Repeated estimations are of value in assessing progress and the effects of treatment. In the case of the small intestine, adaptation may occur with compensatory increased function in non-diseased areas. Thus fat absorption may be normal with established disease, for example of the small intestine, the pancreas, or the liver. Many indirect methods of estimation of fat absorption have been devised. These include the use of radioactive fats, macroscopic or microscopic examination of faeces, and fat tolerance tests. Most correlate moderately well with faecal fat measurements.

Carbohydrate malabsorption

Xylose absorption test

An oral dose of xylose is given and the excretion in the urine measured for the ensuing 5 h. Excretion of greater than 22 per cent of a 5-g dose and greater than 17 per cent of a 25-g dose may be regarded as normal. This test rarely gives normal results in untreated coeliac disease or tropical sprue, and abnormal results rarely occur in patients with pancreatic disease. Abnormal results occur for reasons other than malabsorption. These include delayed gastric emptying, low urine flow, or poor renal function.

Lactose tolerance test

In patients with absent or low levels of lactase in the intestinal mucosa, either primary or secondary to intestinal mucosal disease, oral lactose is followed by little rise in the blood glucose. Diminished lactose digestion may also be due to resection of a major portion of the small intestine. The unabsorbed lactose reaching the colon is converted by bacteria to gas and lactic acid, which may cause inhibition of the absorption of salt and water by the colon and consequent abdominal discomfort and diarrhoea. These symptoms, following oral lactose, are presumptive evidence of alactasia. Direct measurement of lactase in mucosal biopsy specimens is a better test.

Protein malabsorption

Faecal nitrogen is a measure of protein malabsorption in severe pancreatic disease, and parallels faecal fat in some conditions. It is rarely used in diagnosis because much of the faecal nitrogen derives from sources other than dietary protein. Protein-losing enteropathy is assessed by measuring faecal radioactivity after intravenous injection of radioactive protein or other substance of similar molecular weight.

Vitamin B_{12} absorption (see also Section 3)

The absorption of vitamin B_{12} may be used as a test of function of the terminal ileum. The Schilling test consists of an oral dose of radioactive vitamin B_{12} followed by an intramuscular, large, 'flushing' dose of the non-radioactive vitamin B_{12} and measurement of urinary radioactivity, which reflects the amount absorbed. Confirmation that a low value is not due to pernicious anaemia or other gastric pathology can be obtained by repeating the test and giving intrinsic factor with the oral dose of vitamin B_{12}. If malabsorption is due to ileal disease, the result will remain abnormal.

Small bowel biopsy

There are remarkably few complications to this procedure. Bleeding is exceedingly rare provided that neither prothrombin time nor platelet count is grossly abnormal. Perforation of the intestine has occasionally been described in severely malnourished subjects. The

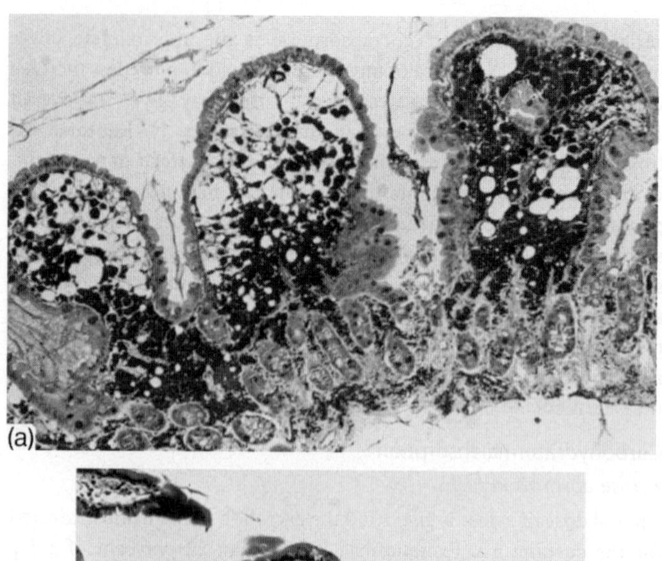

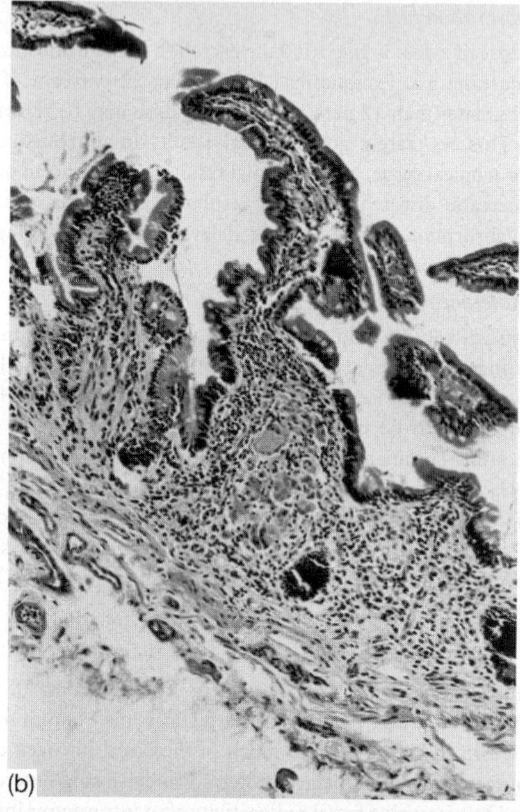

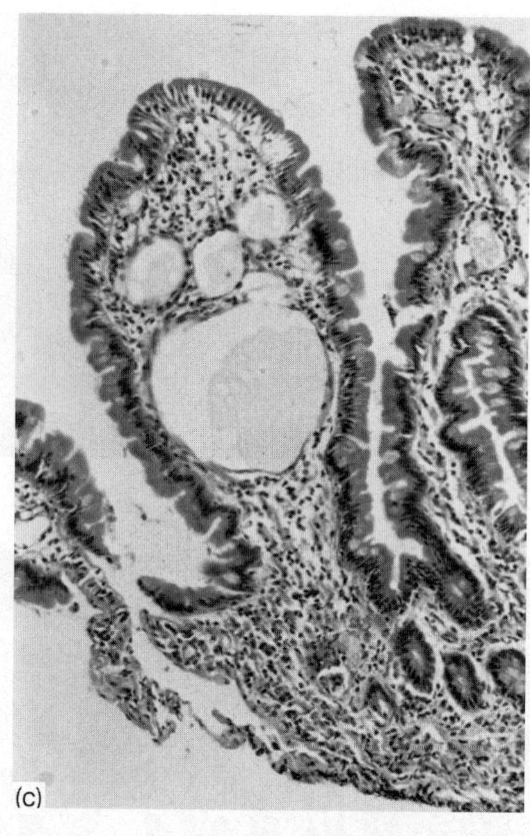

Fig. 3 (a) Whipple's disease: the villi are distended but the overlying epithelium is relatively normal. This periodic acid-Schiff stain demonstrates macrophages stuffed with deposits of glycoprotein, and distended lymphatic spaces within the villi. (b) Crohn's disease. At the base of a villus is a granuloma containing giant cells. (c) Intestinal lymphangiectasia. A villus is shown with grossly distended lymphatics in its core.

specimen can be examined and orientated on a plastic mesh, using the dissecting microscope. This enables an immediate rough assessment of the likelihood of pathology, certain recognition of severe villous loss, and an indication for sections at multiple levels if a patchy lesion is seen.

Histological interpretation

The normal upper small bowel in temperate zones shows a mixture of finger- and leaf-shaped villi (Fig. 2(a)). The epithelial cells are tall and columnar with basal, palisaded nuclei. There are a few lymphocytes between the epithelial cells. There is a scanty infiltrate of inflammatory cells in the lamina propria. The villi are several times as long as the depth of the crypts (Fig. 2(b)).

Duodenal samples overlying Brunner's glands may show villi that are rather flattened and this may apply in areas of jejunal samples that overlie lymphoid nodules. In tropical areas a wider range of appearances may be found in subjects with no evidence of disease.

The small intestine responds in a similar way to many different diseases. Milder lesions, consisting of (a) broadening of the villi, which may be branched or fused, (b) oedema and excess of inflammatory cells beneath the surface epithelium, and (c) sometimes reduction in the height of the epithelial cells and loss of their regular nuclear arrangement, are very non-specific. Causes include malignancy anywhere in the body, malnutrition, small bowel ischaemia, severe skin disease, bacterial overgrowth in the small intestine, various parasitic infestations of the small intestine, excess secretion of gastric acid as in the Zollinger–Ellison syndrome, and numerous other conditions. Total loss of villi and crypt hypertrophy is highly suggestive of coeliac disease but total or subtotal villous atrophy may be seen occasionally

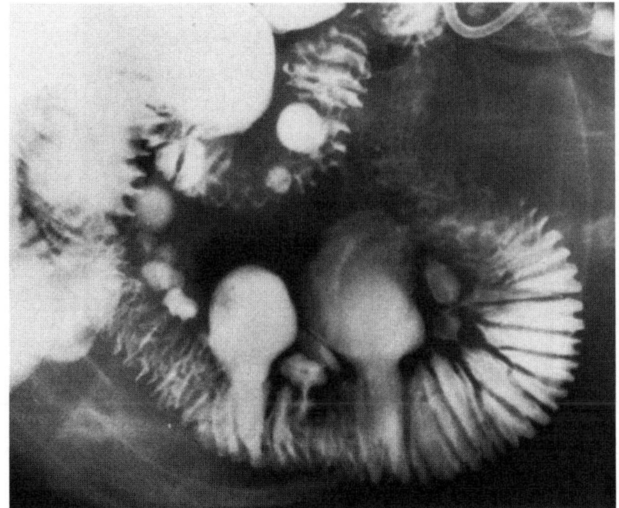

Fig. 4 Multiple diverticula of the small intestine shown by the technique of small bowel enema.

in other conditions, notably severe tropical sprue, cows' milk sensitivity and gastroenteritis in young children. Rarer causes of a severe villous lesion include soy protein intolerance, eosinophilic gastroenteropathy, immune deficiency syndromes, severe malnutrition, ischaemia of the small intestine, and damage due to drugs or irradiation.

Diseases with specific features (Fig. 3) include Whipple's disease, abetalipoproteinaemia, diffuse lymphoma, giardiasis and other infestations in which the parasites may be found, lymphangiectasia, and humoral immune deficiencies. *Mycobacterium avium intracellulare*, showing up acid-fast in the lamina propria and in inflammatory cells, may be found in immunocompromised patients, especially those with **AIDS**. Crohn's disease may show granulomas with giant cells (Fig. 3(b)). The lesion that follows radiotherapy may show villous loss without crypt hyperplasia. Specific stains may reveal amyloid infiltration.

Endoscopic biopsy of the duodenum

Coeliac disease may be strongly suspected from the endoscopic appearances of loss of folds in the duodenum, but there are pitfalls in interpreting duodenal biopsies. Villous flattening over Brunner's glands is a normal finding. Leaf-shaped villi are commoner in the duodenum and may appear as broadening. Duodenitis or an adjacent ulcer may cause inflammation. In some coeliac patients, the duodenal mucosa is much less affected than is the jejunal mucosa.

Enzyme measurements

Multiple deficiencies occur in any condition with gross histological change, but isolated deficiency of lactase is specific for primary alactasia.

Small-bowel radiology

The small bowel can be examined by a follow through after a barium meal, but a small bowel enema is better. Non-specific findings such as dilatation, thickened folds, and poor motility occur in many disorders of the small bowel that are accompanied by malabsorption. Flocculation of the contrast medium is a non-specific indication of excessive secretion. A definitive diagnosis of a cause for malabsorption may be obtained with diverticula, blind loops, strictures, or fistulas (Fig. 4).

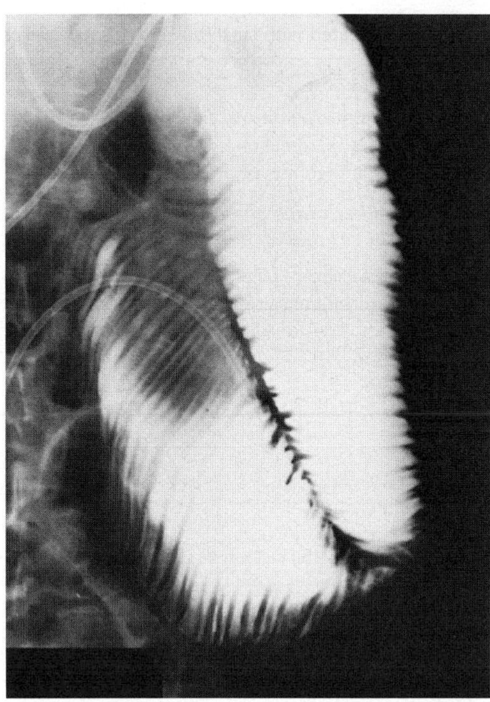

Fig. 5 Dilated small intestine with the transverse folds remaining very close together (the 'hidebound' bowel) diagnostic of systemic sclerosis of the small intestine.

In systemic sclerosis a severe motility disturbance may be accompanied by dilatation of the small bowel, but with the folds remaining close together (the 'hidebound' bowel) (Fig. 5). A diagnosis of Crohn's disease may be made if irregular, thickened folds, ulceration, narrowing of the lumen, and thickening of the wall are seen, particularly in the terminal ileum and more particularly if multiple, short segments of small bowel are affected ('skip lesions'). Differential diagnosis of such appearances includes tuberculosis, lymphoma, Henoch–Schönlein lesions, Behçet's disease, and mesenteric venous thrombosis which sometimes occurs in young females taking the contraceptive pill. Tumours of the small intestine, usually lymphomas, may appear as mass lesions or merely as rigidity or thickening of the wall. Strictures and ulcers may occur in coelic disease. In conditions of defective humoral immunity, multiple small lymphoid nodules may be found in the small intestine (nodular lymphoid hyperplasia) and should not be mistaken for lymphoma. Bacterial overgrowth is a cause of malabsorption, and is discussed in Chapter 5.7.

Further reading

W.S. Hanbrich, F. Schaffrer, and J.E. Berk (eds.). (1995). *Bockers gastroenterology*, (5th edn), pp. 996–1022. W.B. Saunders.

Chapter 5.7

Small bowel bacterial overgrowth

S. P. Pereira and R. H. Dowling

Small bowel bacterial overgrowth is a syndrome characterized, in its florid form, by weight loss, diarrhoea, malabsorption, and altered

Table 1 Conditions associated with small-bowel bacterial overgrowth

Gastric hypochlorhydria
• Chronic atrophic gastritis/pernicious anaemia
• Vagotomy and/or gastric resection
• Treatment with H_2; antagonists or proton-pump inhibitors
Anatomical abnormalities of the gut
• Postsurgical:
• Afferent loop of a Billroth II/Poly A partial gastrectomy
• Blind loop (side-to-end anastomosis)
• Recirculating loop (side-to-side anastomosis)
• Continent ileostomy
• Diverticula:
• Duodenal
• Jejunal
• Fistulae:
• Cologastric
• Ileogastric
• Colojejunal
• Ileojejunal
• Obstruction:
• Strictures
• Adhesions
Disordered intestinal motility
• Systemic sclerosis
• Diabetic autonomic neuropathy
• Intestinal pseudo-obstruction
• Amyloidosis
Miscellaneous
• Malabsorption in the elderly
• Hypo- or agammaglobulinaemia
• Cirrhosis
• Bacterial cholangitis

bile acid metabolism. It is due to proliferation of abnormal bacterial flora in the small intestine and is also known as the blind loop syndrome, the contaminated bowel syndrome and, in one specific example, the afferent loop syndrome.

Aetiology

Any situation in which gastric acid secretion is reduced, or intestinal motility is impaired, may lead to bacterial overgrowth. Anatomical disorders that result in stagnation of intestinal contents, or seeding of the proximal small intestine with colonic-type bacteria, also predispose to bacterial overgrowth (Table 1). In these situations, a small-intestinal flora develops which is predominantly anaerobic and closely resembles that of the colon with bacterial counts in the upper intestine rising to more than 10^5 colony-forming units per ml.

Decreased gastric acid secretion

Hypo- or achlorhydria, however caused, permits a larger than normal fraction of the bacteria ingested with food, or present in oropharyngeal secretions, to traverse the stomach and enter the small bowel.

Disorders of intestinal motility

Conditions associated with impaired peristalsis include systemic sclerosis, intestinal pseudo-obstruction, diabetic autonomic neuropathy, and, rarely, amyloidosis.

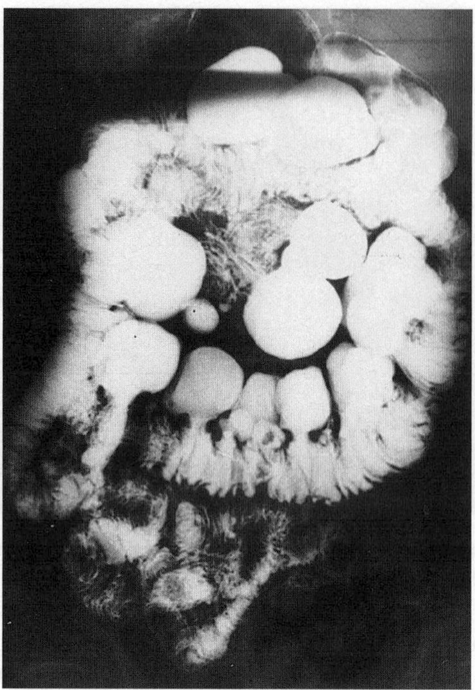

Fig. 1 Barium follow-through in a patient with small bowel bacterial overgrowth secondary to extensive jejunal diverticulosis: supine film. *(By courtesy of Dr D. MacIver.)*

Anatomical disorders

Stagnation of intestinal contents, with resultant proliferation of bacteria, may occur in the afferent limb of a Poly A or Billroth II gastrectomy, within duodenal or jejunal diverticula (Fig. 1), or as a result of chronic obstruction secondary to intestinal strictures or adhesions. Contamination of the proximal intestine with bacteria from the distal small bowel and/or colon—as a result of fistulas or distal small bowel resection—also predisposes to bacterial overgrowth.

Miscellaneous associations

These include malnutrition in some elderly patients, cirrhosis of the liver, and bacterial cholangitis (see OTM3, p.1912).

Pathogenesis

Malabsorption in bacterial overgrowth is due mainly to the metabolic consequences of the abnormal bacteria and, to a lesser extent, to patchy damage to small bowel enterocytes.

Fat malabsorption

In bacterial overgrowth, anaerobic species deconjugate the intraluminal bile acids, splitting the glycine or taurine conjugates from the steroid ring of the bile acid molecule to a variable degree. At the pH of the proximal small bowel (5.0–6.5), the deconjugated bile acids are largely protonated and partly solubilized. They are, therefore liable to premature absorption by passive non-ionic diffusion. Given their high pKa, deconjugated bile acids are also vulnerable to precipitation in the slightly acidic environment of the upper small bowel lumen, as inert crystals. These two factors result in intraluminal bile acid deficiency and, as a consequence, impaired micelle formation, fat malabsorption, and steatorrhoea.

Carbohydrate malabsorption

In patients with bacterial overgrowth, intraluminal fermentation of carbohydrates produces hydrogen, carbon dioxide, volatile short-chain fatty acids, and small amounts of alcohol. The generation of H_2 is the basis for both the glucose and lactulose breath H_2 tests for small bowel bacterial overgrowth.

Protein malabsorption

Hypoalbuminaemia has been reported in patients with bacterial overgrowth, but the mechanism for it is not completely understood. Contributing factors include deamidation of protein and amino acids by bacterial proteases, decreased hepatic protein synthesis, reduced mucosal uptake of peptides and amino acids and protein losing enteropathy.

Vitamin and mineral malabsorption

Partial vitamin B_{12} malabsorption is a common feature of small bowel bacterial overgrowth, and is probably due to bacterial uptake of the B_{12}-intrinsic factor complex in the contaminated proximal small bowel. Anaerobes also metabolize the complex to inactive analogues (cobamides), which act as competitive inhibitors of active B_{12} transport in the terminal ileum. These cobamides may also occupy vitamin B_{12} storage sites in the liver, at the expense of the normal storage form (B_{12} bound to transcobalamin II). Serum and red blood-cell folate levels are usually normal, and may even be high, due to bacterial synthesis of 5-methyl tetrahydrofolate.

The absorption of sterols and fat-soluble vitamins is even more dependent on intraluminal bile acids than that of ingested fat. In theory, therefore, luminal deficiency of conjugated bile acids should cause profound effects on the absorption of vitamins A, D, E, and K. In practice, however, fat-soluble vitamin deficiency has been described only rarely in patients with small bowel bacterial overgrowth. Iron deficiency is also unusual.

Water and electrolytes

Secretory and osmotic processes both contribute to the diarrhoea seen in bacterial overgrowth. Bacterial metabolites, such as hydroxylated fatty acids and deconjugated bile acids, stimulate secretion of water and electrolytes. Injury to the brush border of the enterocytes resulting in decreased absorption of fat, carbohydrate, and protein, may also contribute to diarrhoea by increasing the osmolality of small and large bowel contents.

Enterocyte damage

In patients whose small-intestinal mucosa is normal by light microscopy, subtle degenerative changes in the enterocyte can be seen on electron microscopy. Brush-border enzyme activity, and active transport of monosaccharides, fatty acids, and amino acids, are diminished. The causes of mucosal damage are unclear and there is still controversy about the overall importance of these changes.

Clinical features

Symptoms vary greatly, and many individuals with high bacterial counts, with or without haematological or biochemical evidence of malabsorption, may be asymptomatic. The clinical picture depends on: (a) the metabolic activity of the abnormal flora; (b) the resultant small bowel malabsorption; and (c) the predisposing condition. For example, patients may have duodenal or jejunal diverticulosis for years before the classical symptoms and signs of bacterial overgrowth—weight loss, diarrhoea, steatorrhoea, and vitamin B_{12} malabsorption—develop. Other symptoms, such as recurrent abdominal pain, early satiety, and bloating, are non-specific. In conditions such as Crohn's disease, systemic sclerosis, or intestinal pseudo-obstruction, the clinical features of the primary disease may be difficult to distinguish from those due to intraluminal bacterial proliferation. Less commonly, patients may present with isolated vitamin B_{12} deficiency, or evidence of fat-soluble vitamin malabsorption, such as night blindness (vitamin A deficiency), rickets osteomalacia, or proximal myopathy (vitamin D deficiency), or bleeding bruising secondary to vitamin K deficiency.

Diagnosis

The 'gold standard' for diagnosing overgrowth involves small-intestinal intubation and aspiration of duodenal or jejunal contents for quantitative culture of the small-intestinal flora. Cultured bacteria are often a mixture of anaerobes (Bacteroides, clostridia, enterococci) and aerobes such as coliforms (*Escherichia coli, Klebsiella*). Aspirated juice can also be examined for the proportion of deconjugated bile acids or the presence of short-chain fatty acids.

Indirect tests are based on the measurement of end-products of intraluminal bacterial metabolism of fat, carbohydrate, protein, vitamins or bile acids in the breath, urine, faeces, or serum. Although they have the advantage of being non-invasive, many do not adequately distinguish between bacterial overgrowth and other causes of malabsorption. These include measuring the urinary excretion of indican or phenols, or of xylose.

In contrast, increased fasting or postprandial serum unconjugated bile acids, or an increased ratio of serum unconjugated cholic acid to total cholic acid, have a sensitivity for bacterial overgrowth of 70–80 per cent. Serum unconjugated bile acids may also be increased in patients with ileal resection.

Breath tests (Fig. 2)

Breath tests rely on the pulmonary excretion of either labelled CO_2 following the administration of ^{14}C- or ^{13}C-labelled substrates, or of H_2 following the administration of glucose, lactulose, or a carbohydrate meal. The principle of the bile acid ([^{14}C]glycine-labelled glycocholate) breath test, is that anaerobic bacteria in the intestinal lumen deconjugate the labelled bile acid, liberating [^{14}C]glycine, which is then absorbed, transported to the liver and metabolized to release $^{14}CO_2$, which is then excreted in the breath. This test has a false-negative rate of up to 30 per cent, and it does not easily distinguish between small bowel bacterial overgrowth and other causes of bile-acid malabsorption, such as ileal dysfunction, unless faecal bile-acid excretion is also measured. In the presence of ileal dysfunction, [^{14}C]cholylglycine is malabsorbed and spills into the colon where it is metabolized by colonic bacteria, resulting in a delayed breath $^{14}CO_2$ peak and high faecal output of the label.

Bacterial fermentation of carbohydrate in the colon normally produces H_2, some 20 per cent of which is absorbed and excreted in the expired air. In small bowel bacterial overgrowth, H_2 is produced by anaerobic bacteria, thus leading to an early peak in H_2 excretion after 50 or 80 g glucose or 10–15 g lactulose by mouth. The specificity of this H_2 test is 80 per cent and its sensitivity ranges from 60 to 90 per cent.

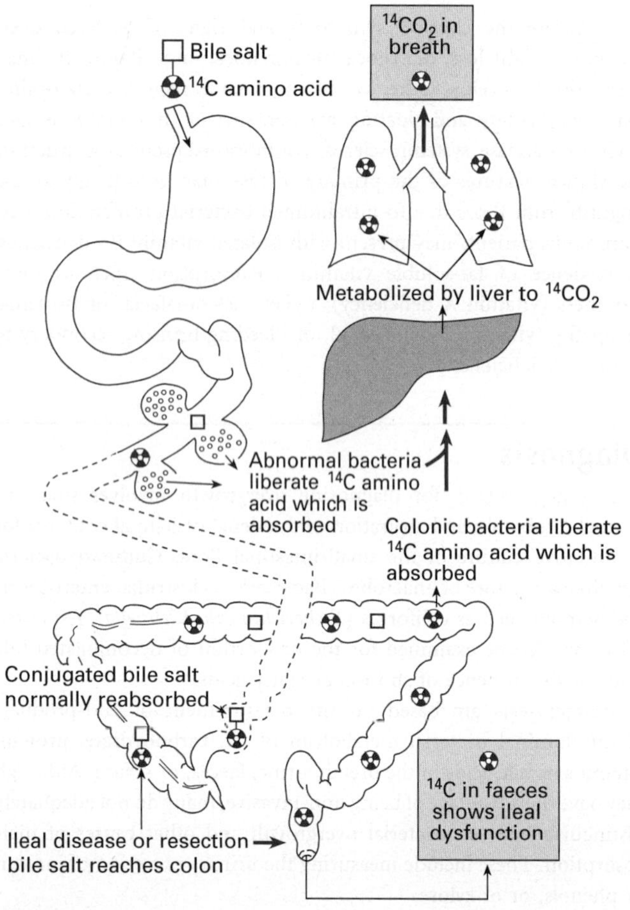

Fig. 2 The radioactive bile-acid breath test for detection of bacterial overgrowth in the small intestine. A false-positive result may be caused by ileal disease or resection, in which case there is also excess radioactivity in the faeces (see text).

Xylose is absorbed by the proximal small bowel and only minimally metabolized thereafter. In patients with terminal ileal disease or resection, virtually no xylose reaches the colon and $^{14}CO_2$ in expired air is not increased. In bacterial overgrowth, aerobic bacteria metabolizes the xylose producing $^{14}CO_2$ so that within 1 h there will be an increase in $^{14}CO_2$ in expired air in 65–85 per cent of patients.

Treatment

Management is divided into: (a) antimicrobial treatment; (b) nutritional support; (c) consideration of surgical correction of anatomical abnormalities; and (d) medical therapy of any underlying condition, such as diabetes mellitus or small bowel Crohn's disease.

Antimicrobials that have been shown to be effective include erythromycin, tetracycline, amoxycillin–clavulanic acid, trimethoprim–sulphamethoxazole, and the cephalosporins. Metronidazole is also effective. There have been few adequately controlled studies to guide the choice of antimicrobial, duration of treatment, or appropriate management of recurrent bacterial overgrowth. In general, after a 7–10-day course of antimicrobials chosen empirically, symptoms and absorptive abnormalities resolve and many patients remain well for months—despite the fact that small bowel bacterial counts may return to pretreatment values within a few weeks. If symptoms and/or absorptive abnormalities do not then resolve, duodenal aspiration and culture, together with antimicrobial sensitivity assays, are indicated. The results of uncontrolled trials suggest that, in patients who respond initially to antimicrobials but in whom symptoms recur within several weeks, cyclical antimicrobial therapy (for example, 1 week in 6), may be effective. Failure to respond may be due to antimicrobial resistance, antibiotic-associated diarrhoea, or an incorrect diagnosis.

Further reading

Kerlin, P. and Wong, L. (1988). Breath hydrogen testing in bacterial overgrowth in the small intestine. *Gastroenterology*, 95, 982.

King, C.E. and Toskes, P.P. (1983). The use of breath tests in the study of malabsorption. *Clinical Gastroenterology*, 12, 591–610.

Kirsch, M. (1990). Bacterial overgrowth. *American Journal of Gastroenterology*, 85, 231–7.

Chapter 5.8

Coeliac disease

D. P. Jewell

Coeliac disease is an inflammatory disorder of the small intestine induced by the gliadins of wheat, hordeins of barley, and secalins of rye. The inflammation is associated with loss of villous height and crypt hypertrophy that leads to malabsorption. The functional and histological abnormalities are reversed towards normal following exclusion of those cereals from the diet, but reappear on challenge.

Pathology

Mucosal inflammation can vary in severity and extent and can be patchy. The characteristic, but not specific, feature is loss of villous height so that, under a dissecting microscope, the mucosa appears completely flat (Fig. 1). This is confirmed on histological examination (Fig. 2). The mucosa may be completely flat or there may be very short, broad villi (subtotal villous atrophy). The total mucosal thickness is usually normal or only slightly reduced because the crypts become elongated (crypt hypertrophy). The surface epithelial cells become flattened, the basal polarity of their nuclei is lost, and the microvilli of the brush border become short and irregular.

Within the lamina propria, there is a marked infiltration of plasma cells, lymphocytes, n neutrophils, eosinophils, and mast cells. The proportion of intraepithelial lymphocytes is also increased in comparison with the number of enterocytes, although the absolute number is probably not increased.

There is an increase among plasma cells in those producing IgA, IgG, and IgM, although IgA cells still predominate. There is a marked increase in the crypt cell proliferation rate, shown by numerous mitoses at the base of the crypts, and mediated by cytokines released by the lymphocytes and macrophages. This leads to the elongation of the crypts and loss of villous height.

Three stages in the development of coeliac disease have been suggested—infiltrative, hyperplastic, and destructive. In the infiltrative stage, the epithelium becomes infiltrated with increased numbers of lymphocytes and this is the lesion frequently seen in patients with dermatitis herpetiformis. This leads on to some inflammation of the

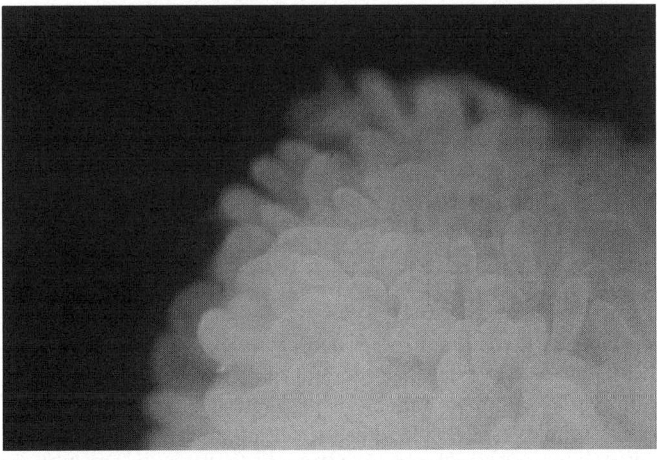

(a)

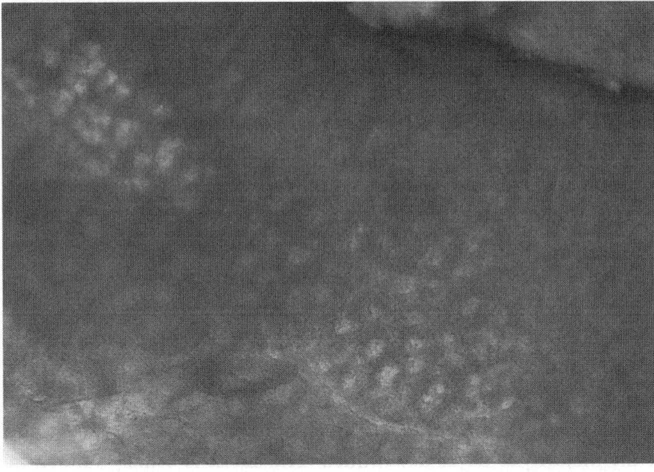

(b)

Fig. 1 (a) Dissecting microscopic appearance of a normal jejunal biopsy. (b) Dissecting microscopic appearance of coeliac disease.

lamina propria, with elongation of crypts. Both these stages are asymptomatic. The destructive stage is the full lesion with loss of villi and a marked inflammatory infiltrate. Whether this classification is representative of what actually happens, is not yet clear. There may also be a diffuse infiltration of other mucosal surfaces with lymphocytes and plasma cells. In particular, a proctitis has been recently recognized but this is only detected if a rectal biopsy is taken and is virtually never severe enough to cause symptoms.

Following a gluten-free diet, these changes return towards normal. In some 3 months the mucosa usually returns to normal in children but, in adults, minor changes may persist with a crypt/villous ratio of 1:2 rather than the normal ratio of 1:4. When patients in remission are challenged with gluten, histological changes may be seen within a few days. However, some patients may take much longer to relapse and there have been some individuals who have virtually no histological change for up to a year.

Epidemiology

Coeliac disease is primarily a disease of Caucasians and, is closely associated with the extended haplotype HLA-B8, -DR3, and -DQ2. The highest prevalence is seen in the west of Ireland, where it may be as high as 1 in 300. Throughout Europe, the prevalence ranges up to 1 in 6000, with the value in England being 1 in 1500. However, screening populations for endomysial antibody suggests a prevalence of 1 in 500. There is little sex difference, although some studies have shown a preponderance of women. There is a familial incidence, with about 10 per cent of first-degree relatives being affected, and studies of monozygotic twins have shown a concordance of 70 per cent.

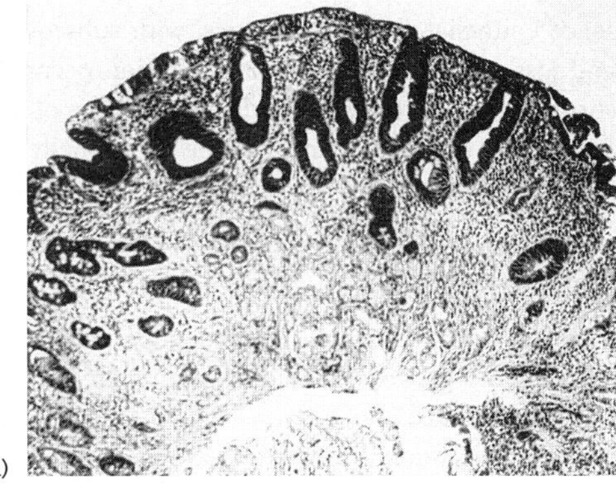

(a)

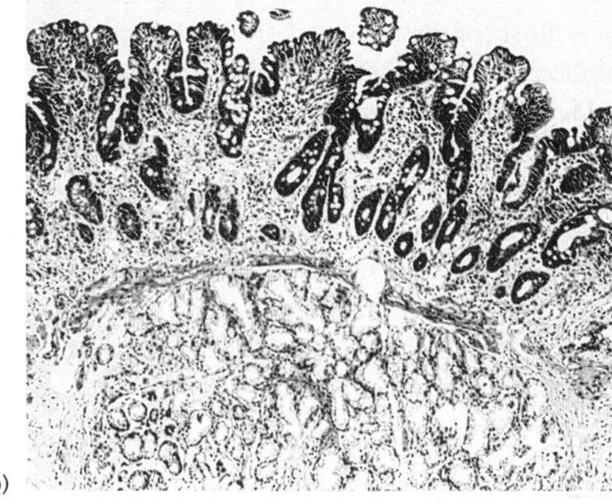

(b)

Fig. 2 Histological appearances of a distal duodenal biopsy in a patient with coeliac disease before (a) and after (b) a 3-month period on a gluten-free diet. Following treatment, there is much less inflammation and the villous pattern has begun to reappear.

Pathogenesis

The gliadin component of gluten and similar factors from rye and barley prolamins are the toxic dietary constituents, susceptibility being associated with HLA haplotypes B8, DR3, and DQ2 in north Europe and with B8, DR5/7, and DQ2 in south Europe. This difference is due to the fact that the same DRQ α–β heterodimer can be encoded on the same chromosome (*cis* position) in DR3 individuals or on opposite chromosomes (*trans* position) in DR5/DR7 individuals. It is not clear how this particular haplotype interacts with gluten to produce mucosal inflammation in one person whereas the majority of people with it are able to ingest gluten with impunity. The key may be previous infections with adenovirus 12. There is a dodecapeptide on the surface of A-gliadin which is similar to a peptide contained within an E1b protein of the virus. Many coeliac patients demonstrate cellular and humoral immune responses to the virus, and it is conceivable that the immune response to it cross-reacts with the gliadin peptide and thus induces intestinal inflammation. Another possibility is that other, non-HLA genes are involved.

The immunological reaction to the toxic peptides involves both humoral and cellular responses. The release of cytokines and inflammatory mediators is thought to amplify the immune response and to influence epithelial stem-cell kinetics, with subsequent crypt elongation and loss of villous height. Malabsorption occurs because of loss of absorptive area and the presence of a population of immature surface epithelial cells whose function may be additionally impaired by cytokines and inflammatory mediators.

Clinical features

In children, growth retardation and delayed puberty is a common presentation and if the gastrointestinal symptoms are minimal, the diagnosis can be overlooked.

In adults, the most common presentations are anaemia and variable abdominal symptoms of discomfort, bloating, excess wind, and an altered bowel habit. Mouth ulcers can be the presenting symptom. The anaemia is most commonly due to iron deficiency and frequently occurs in the absence of intestinal symptoms; but macrocytic anaemias also occur. Many patients presenting with diarrhoea, wind, and abdominal pain are wrongly diagnosed as having an irritable bowel syndrome. Less commonly steatorrhoea, weight loss, bruising, and other symptoms of nutritional deficiencies result from malabsorption.

There may be no physical signs but there may be those of iron deficiency, aphthous ulcers in the mouth, mild finger clubbing, and evidence of recent weight loss. Osteomalacia, bleeding, and ascites with hypoproteinaemic oedema are now very rare.

Diagnosis

The crucial test is a biopsy taken from the duodenal–jejunal junction using a Crosby capsule, or a distal duodenal biopsy taken at endoscopy.

Serological tests have been developed for screening but none has yet proved sufficiently reliable to replace the need for a small-intestinal biopsy. Endomysial antibodies have high specificity and sensitivity for the disease with a positive predictive value of over 95 per cent. IgA antibodies are measured hence patients with an associated IgA deficiency will have a false-negative result. Endomysial antibody titres fall as the disease goes into remission on a gluten-free diet. This antibody is directed towards intestinal transglutaminase. Endomysial antibodies are proving the most useful and are found in over 90 per cent of coeliacs of all ages. The titre of all three antibodies falls as the disease goes into remission on a gluten-free diet.

Assessment of malabsorption

Haematology

In addition to a blood count and film examination, measurements should be made of serum iron, iron binding capacity, red cell folate and vitamin B_{12} levels. B_{12} levels are low only in patients with extensive involvement of the small bowel. Mixed deficiencies of iron and folate are not uncommon.

Biochemistry

Faecal fat estimations are ideal but not always available. Malabsorption of vitamins A, D, E, and K is best assessed by measurement of serum β-carotene and plasma calcium, 25OHD3, alkaline phosphatase, and prothrombin time. Diarrhoea may cause hypokalaemia, hypomagnesaemia and hypoalbuminaemia can occur in severe cases, together with zinc deficiency.

Immunological tests

Serum immunoglobulin concentrations may be abnormal. The most common pattern is a raised IgA with a low IgM but virtually any pattern may be seen. Five per cent of patients have an associated IgA deficiency and loss of villous height and crypt hypertrophy frequently accompany common variable acquired immunodeficiency.

Radiology

Barium radiology cannot give a positive diagnosis of coeliac disease and is not usually necessary unless it is required to exclude other small-intestinal diseases.

Differential diagnosis

Few patients present with overt malabsorption, so the diagnosis of coeliac disease requires a high index of suspicion. In adults, infection with giardia, common variable hypogammaglobulinaemia, lymphoma, Crohn's disease, and other small-intestinal diseases such as radiation enteritis, amyloid, and Whipple's disease may all show villous flattening and mucosal inflammation. Tropical sprue is usually associated with partial villous atrophy—but has to be considered in patients who have spent time in endemic areas. Rarely, patients may be seen with a flat biopsy but with crypt hypoplasia—these do not respond to a gluten-free diet. Some patients with crypt hypoplasia also have a thickened band of subepithelial collagen, so-called collagenous sprue. Systemic diseases such as the vasculitides and systemic sclerosis may also be associated with an abnormal mucosal biopsy. Bacterial overgrowth of the small intestine may be associated with some mucosal inflammation and minor villous changes.

Dermatitis herpetiformis is commonly associated with an abnormal mucosal biopsy, and responds to gluten withdrawal. The skin lesions also respond to a gluten-free diet, albeit slowly.

Non-specific infections of the small intestine may lead to a degree of malabsorption and mucosal inflammation. The precise aetiology of the majority is never determined. The illness is usually sudden in onset and gets better spontaneously over several weeks ('temperate sprue'). Thus a patient presenting with a very short history and whose mucosal biopsy suggests coeliac disease must be considered carefully. HLA typing and the presence of serum endomysial antibodies may be helpful in making the correct diagnosis. If there is still doubt, the patient should be given a gluten-free diet but when the mucosa has recovered, a gluten challenge with subsequent biopsy should be undertaken.

Associated diseases

There is an increased prevalence of autoimmune diseases in patients with coeliac disease, especially those that are associated with HLA-B8 DR3 phenotype. These include diabetes, thyroid disease, and Addison's disease. Fibrosing alveolitis, systemic lupus erythematosus, and polyarteritis have also been reported. There may be an increase in epilepsy, especially temporal-lobe epilepsy, in coeliac patients. Also about 5 per cent of coeliacs have an isolated IgA deficiency.

Treatment

Once the diagnosis is confirmed, patients should be started on a gluten-free diet, which should also exclude barley and rye, but with oats the need is less clear. For all patients, the diet is a lifelong necessity. Nutritional supplements may be necessary at the start, but once a gluten-free diet has begun, mucosal recovery occurs rapidly so that long-term supplementation is rarely necessary. Patients with extensive mucosal damage may need a lactose-free as well as a gluten-free diet until there is histological recovery. Once patients have been on the diet for 3–4 months, a further small intestinal biopsy must be obtained to check for histological recovery. If the mucosa has not returned towards normal, a thorough review of the patient's diet is needed. Long-term follow-up is desirable but need only be on an annual basis once patients are stabilized. Patients should also be given details of the national Coeliac Society, if there is one.

Complications and prognosis

The two major complications of coeliac disease are an ulcerative jejunoileitis and a T-cell lymphoma, and some investigators consider the jejunoileitis to be a manifestation of a lymphoma. They usually occur in middle age and usually present with weight loss, anaemia, abdominal pain, and diarrhoea. For diagnosis, biopsies should be snap-frozen in liquid nitrogen to allow immunohistochemical analysis of T-cell markers and the detection of T-cell receptor rearrangements. The prognosis of a lymphoma complicating coeliac disease is poor (see below). In addition, there is a slight increase in the frequency of small-bowel carcinoma and of other gastrointestinal cancers, especially oesophageal tumours.

There is some evidence suggesting that the patients who develop malignant disease are those who have been poor compliers with the diet. For those who adhere to a strict diet, the prognosis is excellent.

Unresponsive disease

A rare group of patients with a flat small-intestinal biopsy fail to respond to a gluten-free diet despite meticulous attention to avoid even minute amounts of gluten over many months. Treatment of this group is difficult. Corticosteroids with or without azathioprine may help some, and oral cyclosporin may also be of benefit. Excluding dietary items such as soya can be tried, or an elemental diet that removes all dietary antigens. Some of these patients have a variety of central and peripheral neurological lesions of unknown cause. The neurological damage is slowly progressive and patients gradually lose weight despite full nutritional support. In some of these cases, the diagnosis of lymphoma and collagenous sprue may have been missed.

Further reading

Catassi, C., Ratsch, I.M., Fabiani, E., *et al.* (1994). Coeliac disease in the year 2000: exploring the iceberg. *Lancet*, **343**, 200–3.

Ferreira, M., Lloyd-Davies, S., Bulter, M., Scott, D., Clark., M., and Kumar, P. (1992). Endomysial antibody: Is it the best screening test for coeliac disease? *Gut*, **33**, 1633–7.

Halsted, C.H. (1996). The many faces of coeliac disease. *New England Journal of Medicine*, **334**, 1190–2.

Houlston, R.S. and Ford, D. (1996). Genetics of coeliac disease. *Quarterly Journal of Medicine*, **89**, 737–43.

Maki, M. and Collin, P. (1997). Coeliac disease. *Lancet*, **349**, 1755–9.

Chapter 5.9

Enteropathy-associated T-cell lymphoma

P. G. Isaacson

It was once thought that malabsorption in intestinal lymphoma was caused by the lymphoma. The reverse is true and there is now good evidence that enteropathy associated lymphoma is a consequent of coeliac disease.

Clinical features

The disease usually affects patients in their sixth or seventh decade who have previously shown evidence of coeliac disease or dermatitis herpetiformis. Presenting symptoms include weight loss, anaemia, abdominal pain, and diarrhoea. Some patients present with severe malabsorption unresponsive to gluten withdrawal. The lymphoma may also present as an abdominal emergency without any history of malabsorption but the features of coeliac disease are found in the uninvolved portion of the resected small intestine. There is sometimes a long latent interval during which inflammation with stricture formation is seen in the small intestine, overt lymphoma manifesting only later. In a small group of patients the lymphoma presents in secondary sites such as peripheral lymph nodes, skin, lungs, or elsewhere in the gastrointestinal tract, with only a minor focus in the small intestine that may be difficult to identify.

Jejunal biopsy usually shows villous atrophy with crypt hyperplasia but may only show minor changes that may be limited to an increase in intraepithelial lymphocytes, or may be normal, if the patient is already on a gluten-free diet. Barium studies usually show ulcers or strictures of the small intestine superimposed on a malabsorption pattern. Staging procedures may reveal evidence of disseminated lymphoma. The lymphoma may involve any segment of the small intestine but is more common in the jejunum where it occurs as multiple nodules, ulcers, and strictures or, less frequently, as a single large mass. The small intestine may appear normal, although there is usually considerable enlargement of mesenteric lymph nodes. In these circumstances, multiple lymph nodes, as well as the liver, should be biopsied.

The clinical course is very unfavourable except in a minority of patients in whom resection of a localized tumour has been followed by long remission.

Pathology

Histological features show great variation between cases and within any single case (Fig. 1). Intraepithelial tumour cells may be prominent. Interpretation is further complicated by the heavy inflammatory component, often containing many eosinophils, and extensive necrosis, which, together, may mask the neoplastic infiltrate. Granulomas may be present and cause confusion with Crohn's disease. The appearance of small bowel remote from the tumour are typically those of coeliac disease. Intra-epithelial lymphocytosis may be dense. The lymphocytes are small, without neoplastic features, but despite their innocuous appearance have, in at least two cases, been shown to be a part of the neoplastic clone. Episodes of ulceration followed

(a)

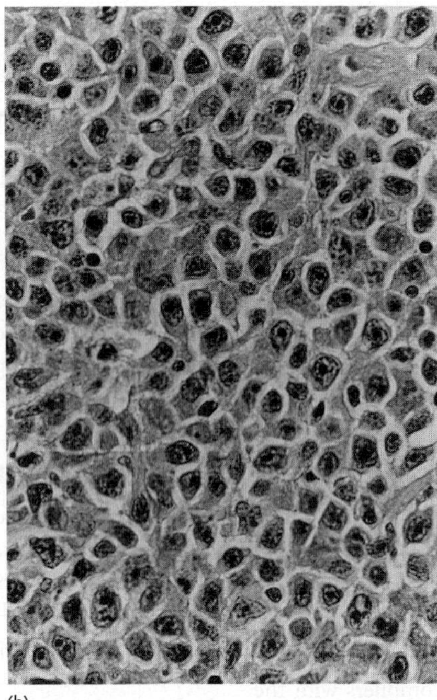

(b)

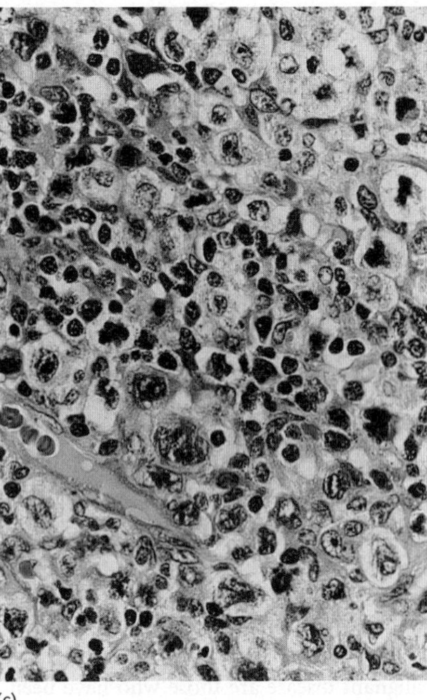

(c)

Fig. 1 Histological appearances of three different cases of enteropathy associated T-cell lymphoma showing the cytological variability. In (a) the tumour is composed of small to medium-sized lymphocytes; in (b) the tumour is composed of monomorphic, large immunoblasts; in (c) the tumour shows striking pleomorphism.

by remission (so-called ulcerative jejunitis; see below) can lead to a confusing appearance of the mucosa, with scarring and distortion, destruction of the muscularis mucosae, and the development of florid, pseudopyloric metaplasia. The mesenteric lymph nodes almost always show accompanying hyperplasia that may mask the malignant cells, which may be present in remarkably small numbers. Selective necrosis of lymph nodes, remote from the main lesion is a feature of some cases. The most commonly reported phenotype of the T cells is CD3+/–, CD7+, CD4–, and CD8–; the cells contain cytotoxic molecules and probably arise from intraepithelial T cells.

Chronic ulcerative jejunitis and enteropathy associated T-cell lymphoma

There is an overlap between enteropathic T-cell lymphoma and ulcerative jejunitis in which multiple ulcers may accompany the lymphoma and these may comprise the dominant feature. The relation between the two conditions is so close that some regard ulcerative jejunitis as a manifestation of enteropathy associated T-cell lymphoma. The opposite view, that the jejunitis is a disorder in its own right, is supported by those cases in which no evidence of lymphoma can be detected despite thorough investigation. Even in these cases, however, a monoclonal T-cell population may be present in the ulcers and prolonged follow-up is necessary to exclude malignancy in these cases.

Management

Excision of localized tumour may be followed by long remission or cure but most cases are multifocal or have already disseminated at diagnosis and require treatment appropriate for a high-grade non-Hodgkin's lymphoma. Some cases of ulcerative jejunitis, even when small foci of lymphoma are present, may respond to steroids.

Further reading

Holmes, G.K.T., Prior, P., Lane, M.R., Pope, D., and Allan, R.N. (1989). Malignancy in coelic disease—effect of a gluten-free diet. *Gut*, **30**, 333–8.

Swinson, C.M., Slavin, G., Coles, E.C., and Booth, C.C. (1983). Coelic disease and malignancy. *Lancet*, **i**, 111–15.

Chapter 5.10

Disaccharidase deficiency

T. M. Cox

Disaccharidases are enzymes required for the complete assimilation of all dietary carbohydrate with the exception of free monosaccharides—principally glucose and fructose. They are found on the luminal surface of the small gut; their activity may be reduced by genetically determined deficiencies of single disaccharidases or acquired by generalized disease of the intestinal mucosa. Deficiency causes a characteristic syndrome of carbohydrate intolerance.

Mucosal disaccharidases are optimally active at pH 6.0 and are present principally in the jejunum—but are also found in the ileum.

Colonic epithelial cells do not express appreciable disaccharidase activity and unabsorbed carbohydrate resulting from maldigestion of disaccharides proximally is fermented by bacteria in the colon to short-chain organic acids, hydrogen, and methane. In these circumstances, ingestion of carbohydrate may cause pain by distension of the bowel with fluid and gas, accompanied by irritant and watery diarrhoea.

Table 1 Carbohydrate intolerance syndromes due to deficiency of disaccharidases

Lactose intolerance
• Congenital (inherited) lactase deficiency • Lactase restriction (genetically determined) • Lactase deficiency secondary to intestinal disease
*Sucrose intolerance**
• Congenital asucrasia (inherited) • Sucrase deficiency secondary to intestinal disease
Trehalose intolerance
• Congenital atrehalasia

*Accompanied by reduced tolerance of starch.

Carbohydrate intolerance syndrome (Table 1)

Nausea, bloating accompanied by borborygmi and flatulence may be noticed within an hour of ingestion of food containing the offending sugars. Colicky pain precedes watery diarrhoea that is usually associated with flatus—and may be explosive. Diarrhoea can occur several hours after ingestion of the noxious food or drink. These symptoms may result from consumption of only a few grams of the offending sugar. Deficiency of particular disaccharidases is responsible for intolerance of specific foods and drinks: milk-containing products in the case of lactase deficiency; table sugar and starch in asucrasia; mushrooms (and probably shellfish) in the rare trehalase deficiency. Identification of a cause-and-effect relation is often impossible, given the ubiquity of sucrose and lactose in commercial foods.

Lactose intolerance

Most patients suffer either from lactase deficiency acquired as a result of intestinal disease, especially postinfective gastroenteritis in children, or as a result of genetically determined restriction of lactase expression.

Congenital lactase deficiency

This is caused by a severe inherited deficiency of mucosal lactase and is a life-long problem. In a few infants with the condition, diarrhoea may follow the first feed with breast milk. These patients respond well to exclusion of lactose in the diet. No such response is seen in patients with congenital glucose–galactose malabsorption.

Loss of lactase with age

In about 5 per cent of northern European adults as compared with more than 90 per cent in parts of Africa and Asia, there is a genetically determined decline in mucosal lactase activity after weaning, normally without consequence because consumption of dairy products is insignificant. Symptoms develop on exposure to excessive lactose-containing foods (Table 2) or medicines in late childhood or early adult life. With increasing migration of peoples and the adoption of Western-style diets, this physiological loss of lactase activity is a prevalent cause of abdominal distress. A significant proportion of patients considered to have irritable bowel disease, or other 'functional' disturbances may prove to have lactase deficiency. The lack of functional reserve of lactase activity also explains the frequency with which lactose malabsorption becomes manifest after partial gastrectomy and related procedures that enhance delivery of carbohydrate to the jejunum.

Table 2 Foods containing lactose

Fresh, dried, skimmed, non-fat, and condensed milks
Cream
Yoghurt
Cheese
Processed meats and sausages
Sauces, stuffings, salad dressings
Custard powder
Canned and dried soups
Biscuits, cakes, cookies, pancakes, waffles, dried cereals
Confectionery
Frozen and canned fruits
Instant coffee
Lactose is also frequently used as a filler in powdered medicines and tablets

Diagnosis of lactose malabsorption

This may be suspected in a patient with abdominal pain, flatulence, and diarrhoea after eating lactose-containing food or drink. Symptoms may occur for the first time after immigration from oriental or African countries to the West. The stool has an acidic pH (<6) and the osmolality of stool water is generally greater than 350 mosmol/kg due to the presence of lactate and other organic anions. Breath hydrogen analysis is a useful confirmatory test. The diagnosis may be confirmed by enzymatic assay of biopsied jejunal mucosa.

Secondary lactase deficiency

Lactase activity may be depressed by mucosal disease of the small intestine, classically infective gastroenteritis. Symptoms can persist for some days or even weeks before recovery, but resolve rapidly when dairy products are excluded from the diet. Decreased lactase activity also accompanies extensive and long-standing mucosal diseases—such as coeliac disease, intestinal giardiasis, and Crohn's disease. In secondary deficiencies of disaccharidases, intolerance of lactose predominates; but the use of high-calorie supplements containing maltose and sucrose may also cause the syndrome of carbohydrate maldigestion.

Sucrose-isomaltase (α-dextrinase) deficiency

This recessively inherited enzyme deficiency of the mucosal brush border is rare in all populations except Eskimos in whom the frequency of homozygotes is up to 10 per cent. Several genetic defects appear to be responsible; in some there is aberrant glycosylation and the enzyme is inefficiently transported to the brush border. Substantial degradation of the abnormal polypeptide occurs within the epithelial cell.

Intolerance of sucrose is responsible for most of the symptoms, which develop as sugar-containing foods are introduced during weaning. Intolerance of starch is less prominent, but ingestion of large, starchy meals may induce cramping discomfort, flatulence, and diarrhoea. While taking a normal diet, patients with deficiency of sucrase–isomaltase have persistent diarrhoea with the passage of acid and frothy stools containing increased concentrations of lactate.

The diagnosis may be suspected on the basis of the history of diarrhoea at weaning and on the character of the stools. Differentiation from coeliac disease, cow's milk allergy, infective or postinfective gastroenteritis, pancreatic failure, and disaccharide intolerance syndromes in relation to other inflammatory disease of the bowel is important, and biopsy of the jejunal mucosa for enzymatic assay and histological examination should be considered. Hydrogen breath tests after ingestion of sucrose and isomaltose may also prove to be useful in diagnosis.

Trehalase deficiency

A few patients have been reported with mushroom intolerance due to the absence of mucosal trehalase. Trehalose is found in the haemolymph of arthropods and in fungi, so that intolerance of crustacean shellfish as well as mushrooms in the diet might be expected.

Treatment

Dietary exclusion of the offending sugar is the best method of preventing symptoms. In hypolactasia, complete elimination is not usually required. An alternative treatment for lactose malabsorbers is the use of β-galactosidases obtained from yeast or other microorganisms. In the United States, β-galactosidase has been produced commercially from yeast 'LactAid' for hydrolysing lactose in milk and has been shown to reduce symptoms as well as breath hydrogen excretion in subjects with maldigestion of lactose. Similar studies have demonstrated the efficacy of β-galactosidase derived from *Aspergillus oryzae*, 'Lactrase'. The enzyme is taken in tablet form but the cost, compared with dietary exclusion, may not be justified.

Complete absence of sucrase–isomaltase activity in most patients with sucrose intolerance and the ubiquity of sucrose in modern diets complicates symptom management. Modest reduction of amylopectin-rich foods usually suffices but the necessary avoidance of sucrose-containing foods can be difficult. Ingestion of dried brewer's yeast after food may relieve the symptoms.

Further reading

Malagclada, J-R. Lactose intolerance. (Editorial.). *New England Journal of Medicine*, 333, 1–4,

Suarez, F.L., Savaiano, D.A., and Levitt, M.D. (1995). A comparison of symptoms after consumption of milk or lactose-hydrolysed milk by people with self-reported severe lactose intolerance. *New England Journal of Medicine*, 333, 53–4.

Chapter 5.11

Whipple's disease (*Tropheryma whippelii* infection)

H. J. F. Hodgson

Whipple's disease is a rare infection that may affect virtually any organ, but is usually dominated by small-intestinal involvement. This may be preceded or accompanied by arthralgia and fever and other systemic symptoms. Tissues are infected with a recently characterized Gram-positive, rod-shaped actinomycete, *Tropheryma whippelii*, and contain characteristic foamy macrophages. There is usually a good response to antibiotic therapy, which may have to be prolonged.

Pathology and aetiology

The small intestine and mesenteric lymph nodes usually show the most severe involvement (hence the synonym intestinal lipodystrophy). The small intestine is thick and oedematous, with stubby villi and dilated lacteals (secondary lymphangiectasia due to obstructed lymph flow through affected lymph nodes). The intestinal lamina propria is stuffed with macrophages, which stain brilliant magenta with periodic acid-Schiff (**PAS**) reagent (Fig. 1). Otherwise there is little inflammatory infiltrate, and the enterocytes are virtually normal. The mesenteric nodes contain fatty masses and foamy macrophages. There is often extraintestinal involvement, in spleen, lymph nodes, central nervous system (CNS), liver, lung, and heart, showing PAS-positive macrophages. Cardiac involvement may lead to endocarditis with vegetations.

The 1–2 μm long bacteria are the source of the PAS positive material. The organism (*Tropheryma whippelii*), a Gram-positive actinomycete, not closely related to any previously known species, was initially identified by amplification of bacterial 16S-ribosomal RNA from tissues, and culture of the organism was not achieved until some years later.

The rarity of the disease is unexplained. It is suggested that immune defects, in macrophage and T-cell function, may lead to colonization of the host by a low virulence organism. A weak association with the haplotype HLA-B27 has also been claimed.

Clinical features and diagnosis

Most patients are middle-aged men, but no group is exempt. Advanced disease presents with malaise, weight loss, diarrhoea, and arthralgias. Examination may show pigmentation, lymphadenopathy, anaemia,

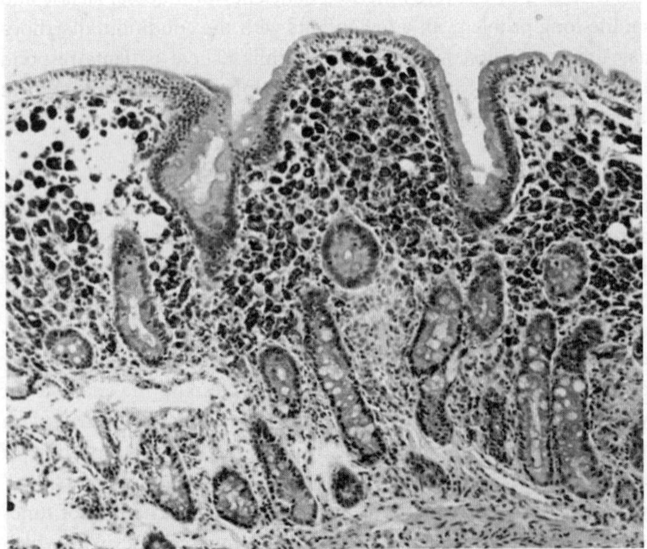

Fig. 1 Jejunal biopsy specimen from a 50-year-old male with Whipple's disease showing stunted villi and infiltration of lamina propria with densely staining macrophages (PAS × 150).

finger clubbing, hypotension, and oedema. Investigation of the gut quickly establishes the diagnosis in such cases. Diagnosis is more difficult if symptoms are limited to fever, arthritis, or other manifestations. Arthritis is peripheral, migratory, non-deforming, and seronegative, and may precede gut involvement by many years. Other clinical features include pleurisy, pulmonary infiltrates, pericarditis, chylous or serous ascites, endocarditis, cardiac conduction defects, coronary arteritis, and myopathy. Five to 10 per cent of patients may have CNS involvement—depression, apathy, fits, myoclonus, ophthalmoplegia, papilloedema, scotomas, pseudotumour, uveitis, meningitis, or a hypothalamic syndrome of insomnia, hyperphagia, and polydypsia.

Conventionally diagnosis is histological. Whether or not the intestine is involved clinically peroral duodenal or jejunal biopsy is usually an effective means of making the diagnosis. Endoscopically, flattened duodenal mucosa with lymphatic dilatation may be identified. Occasionally tissues outside the gut (such as lymph nodes) may be histologically abnormal despite normal intestinal histology. More recently polymerase chain reaction (**PCR**) analysis of tissue for bacterial RNA has been used to identify infection, and it is likely more cases without overt intestinal involvement will be recognized.

Other investigations are not diagnostic. Radiographs of affected small bowel characteristically show oedema and dilatation. Abnormal ultrasound and computed tomography (**CT**) scanning may show lymphatic masses, and brain CT demonstrate multiple ring-enhancing lesions. The erythrocyte sedimentation rate is elevated. Anaemia due to folate or iron deficiency, eosinophilia and thrombocytosis may be apparent, Steatorrhoea, hypocalcaemia, vitamin deficiencies, an elevated alkaline phosphatase, and hypoproteinaemia reflecting a protein-losing enteropathy occur with advanced gut disease.

Treatment and prognosis

Unrecognized and untreated the disease is eventually fatal. Antibiotic therapy is effective, although seriously ill and malnourished individuals require correction of their metabolic state, and occasionally short-term corticosteroid therapy is required. Many empirical antibiotic regimens are reportedly successful: penicillin alone, penicillin and streptomycin, tetracycline, co-trimoxazole, and cephalosporins. Clinical improvement occurs within a few days or weeks but long-term treatment is recommended. In particular the risk of a relapse with CNS manifestations is reduced if the regimen includes antibiotics that pass the blood–brain barrier. Parenteral penicillin and steroids for 2 weeks followed by doxycycline for a year is one recommended regimen, as is trimethoprim–sulphamethoxazole.

The gut mucosa returns to normal within a few months, although a few PAS-positive macrophages may persist. Even after initially effective treatment, relapse may occur, and there may be progressive CNS involvement in the absence of other systemic involvement. Early recognition of relapse can be made by return of bacteria in intestinal tissues, or by serial PCR analysis of tissues.

Further reading

von Herbay, A., Maiwald, M., Ditton, H.S., and Otto H.F. (1996). Histology of intestinal Whipple's disease revisited—a study of 48 patients. *Virchows Archiv*, **429**, 335–43.

Ramzan, N.N., Loftus, E., Burgart, L.J., *et al.* (1997). Diagnosis and monitoring of Whipple's disease by PCR. *Annals of Internal Medicine*, **126**, 520–7.

The SNFMI Research Group on Whipple's Disease. (1997). Whipple's disease. Clinical review of 52 cases. *Medicine*, **76**, 170–84.

Chapter 5.12

Short gut syndrome

H. J. F. Hodgson

Short gut syndrome is the result of substantial resections of the small intestine, and includes diarrhoea, malabsorption, and a number of longer-term metabolic sequelae. Severity and the range of metabolic consequences depend upon the site and extent of resection and the state of the remaining bowel.

Resections of more than half the intestine usually herald problems, and if less than 1 m remains, significant problems are inevitable. The outlook is worse if the remaining intestine is jejunum. When the remnant intestine is ileum, this can adapt to increase its absorptive capacity, food is slower in transit, and the specific transport mechanisms for vitamin B_{12} and bile salts are maintained. Outlook is also worse when (as in Crohn's disease) the remaining bowel is abnormal, when the ileocaecal valve has been removed or when there is additional loss of colon.

Mechanisms of diarrhoea

Diarrhoea occurs in response to eating. The mechanisms are complex and will vary between individuals. The main components include failure to absorb salt and water, failure to absorb nutrients and bile acids (an osmotic effect), and small bowel bacterial overgrowth. Gastric hypersecretion, perhaps related to high gastrin levels may also contribute.

Nutrient malabsorption and metabolic problems

Loss of surface area, interference with fat absorption, sequestration of solutes, and loss of specific binding sites all contribute to nutrient malabsorption.

Renal oxalate stones may result from hyperabsorption of dietary oxalate in the colon. Normally, oxalate is rendered insoluble by combining with calcium, but in the presence of excess fat, calcium is sequestered in calcium soaps. *Urate stones* may form with combined small- and large-intestinal resections, as the concentrated acid urine produced due to loss of bicarbonate-rich small-intestinal fluid encourages urate precipitation. *Gallstones* are also prevalent, reflecting the lithogenicity of bile associated with a depleted bile-salt pool.

D-Lactic acidosis appears to be the result of bacterial metabolism of unabsorbed carbohydrate to D-lactate. It is commonest after jejunal–ileal bypass, but can occur in the short gut syndrome too. Symptoms last 2–3 days and include lethargy, ataxia, double vision, and nausea. Antibiotic treatment for bacterial overgrowth and/or carbohydrate restriction are useful treatments.

Management

Management changes over time after massive small gut resection. Absorptive capacity increases over many months, reflecting adaptive changes, but enteral nutrition is required both for this to occur, and to prevent atrophy of the intestine, and should be therefore provided as soon as possible (see Chapter 8.4 and OTM3, Chapter 10.6).

Early postoperative management

Parenteral fluid and electrolyte replacement is likely to be mandatory. As adequate nutrient intake orally may only become feasible after a period of weeks or months, if at all, total parenteral nutrition is likely to be necessary and should be instituted early. Oral feeding should avoid the use of hyperosmolar high formulations, which tend to cause diarrhoea.

Subsequent dietary management

Some patients, usually those with between 1.25 and 1.5 m of small intestine or more remaining, can maintain a stable weight without a highly tailored diet, often by taking a greater than normal oral calorie intake, and tolerating diarrhoea. With more extensive resections, parenteral supplements are required. Meals should be small but frequent, based on solids, which are slowly released from the stomach. Lactose-containing preparations should be avoided and a low-fat diet, notably low in long-chain fats, prescribed. Restriction may need to be to less than 30 g of long-chain fats per day, with caloric requirements made up by medium-chain triglycerides, which are directly absorbed into the portal vein. Antimotility preparations such as loperamide should be prescribed. The combination of fat restriction and adequate hydration should prevent nephrolithiasis.

Supplementation

Parenteral vitamin B_{12} is mandatory if the ileum has been resected. Patients should be surveyed regularly for nutritional deficiencies, and oral vitamin supplements, and a metabolic mineral mixture prescribed. Oral calcium and magnesium supplements are advisable, although poorly absorbed; parenteral magnesium may be required.

Salt and water balance

Patients with less than 1 m of jejunum remaining always need parenteral salt and water supplements. 'Oral rehydration' mixtures may be necessary, best taken at an interval before breakfast and in the evening, to maximize absorption. If glucose–electrolyte mixtures are ineffective, glucose polymers provide increased amounts of glucose to aid salt absorption while maintaining isotonicity. The consumption of large volumes of water without salt may be counterproductive, causing an increased small-intestinal effluent containing effectively the same water volume now rendered isotonic with body salt. Some improvement in fluid losses may be obtained by decreasing gastric secretion by H_2-receptor antagonists or proton-pump inhibitors. Long-acting somatostatin, subcutaneously, has reduced intestinal fluid loss in patients with jejunostomies on oral feeding. Potassium balance is usually less disturbed than that of sodium.

Other approaches

Bacterial overgrowth should be suspected if diarrhoea worsens without other cause. Screening breath tests are not always definitive. Empirically prescribed antibiotics such as tetracycline, erythromycin, and metronidazole may often be helpful.

Long-term prospects

Adaptation of the remaining gut may allow discontinuation of parenteral supplementation. Many patients will require home total parenteral nutrition. Surgical reversal of a distal segment of the remaining small intestine, to provide an antiperistaltic break and increase absorption, has been advocated; this has obvious risks of further imperilling already limited small intestine and is doubtful value. Small-intestinal transplantation has been done in a very small number of individuals.

Further reading

Berger, D.L. and Malt, R.A. (1996). Management of the short-gut syndrome. *Advances in Surgery*, **29**, 43–57.

Chapter 5.13

Malabsorption in the tropics

M. J. G. Farthing

The common causes of malabsorption in the tropics differ from those in the industrialized world. Tropical malabsorption is not limited to the indigenous population but also affects travellers to these regions, who are susceptible to infective causes of malabsorption and also to less well-defined conditions such as tropical enteropathy and tropical sprue (Table 1).

Specific causes of tropical malabsorption

Intestinal infection

The majority of infections that produce malabsorption in the tropics cause an enteropathy in the small intestine with varying degrees of villous atrophy, crypt hyperplasia, and inflammatory infiltrates in the lamina propria and in some cases in the epithelium. Giardiasis is the most common protozoal infection causing chronic diarrhoea and intestinal malabsorption. *Cryptosporidium parvum* usually produces

Table 1 Tropical malabsorption

Specific		
Infection:		
	Protozoa	*G. intestinalis*
		C. parvum
		E. bieneusi
		I. belli
	Helminths	*C. philippinensis*
		S. stercoralis
	Bacteria	Enteropathogenic *E. coli, Mycobacterium tuberculosis*
	Viruses	Rotavirus
		Enteric adenoviruses (types 40 and 41)
		Norwalk viruses
		Measles virus
		HIV
Coeliac disease		
Lymphoma		
Severe undernutrition (kwashiorkor and marasmus)		
Primary hypolactasia		
Non-specific		
Tropical enteropathy		
Tropical sprue		

an acute, self-limiting, diarrhoeal illness but in the immunocompromised, chronic diarrhoea is common. The microsporidia, *Enterocytozoon bieneusi* and *Encephalitozoon itestinalis* and *Isospora belli* are also important infections causing malabsorption in **AIDS** patients. Heavy infection with *Strongyloides stercoralis*, including the hyperinfection syndrome, should be included in the differential diagnosis. *Capillaria philippinensis* is an important cause of intestinal malabsorption but in a highly restricted area in South-east Asia. The relation between human immunodeficiency virus and small-intestinal enteropathy is controversial, although there is some evidence to suggest that the virus itself may be responsible for small-intestinal damage.

Coeliac disease

Coeliac disease is rare in the tropics but may present for the first time there in expatriates. Confirmation of this diagnosis can be difficult in the tropical setting, particularly in distinguishing it from tropical sprue, but the morphological changes in the jejunum are usually more profound than those found in tropical sprue and will almost inevitably respond to gluten withdrawal but not to broad-spectrum antibiotics.

Lymphoma

Immunoproliferative small-intestinal disease (**IPSID**) and primary upper small-intestinal lymphoma (**PUSIL**) are found predominantly where socio-economic conditions are poor. Around the Mediterranean, the Middle East, South Africa, and South America these conditions may be related, with IPSID progressing to PUSIL. These disorders usually occur in a younger age group, in contrast to the primary intestinal lymphoma that occurs worldwide, most commonly in the elderly.

Severe undernutrition

The role of undernutrition in the pathogenesis of intestinal malabsorption and small-intestinal enteropathy remains controversial. Steatorrhoea complicating kwashiorkor and marasmus is reversed following restoration of nutrition and lesser degrees of malnutrition have no major impact on intestinal structure or function.

Primary hypolactasia

The practical importance of hypolactasia is small in Africa and Asia because adults avoid milk unless they wish to use it as a purgative. It does mean, however, that milk-based products cannot be used reliably in these regions as a nutritional supplement, given the frequency of reduced lactase activity in the indigenous population.

Non-specific tropical malabsorption

The aetiopathogenesis of tropical enteropathy and tropical sprue remains elusive and the relation between the two a matter for conjecture.

Tropical enteropathy

The jejunal morphology of people in many tropical regions is different from that of those living in temperate, industrialized areas, and broad leaf-shaped and/or tongue-shaped villi are the usual pattern, accompanied by increased crypt depth and an inflammatory infiltrate in the lamina propria and the epithelium. Tropical enteropathy has been detected in most tropical regions of Asia, Africa, the Middle East, the Caribbean, and Central and South America (Fig. 1). It can also be acquired by travellers from the developed world who reside and work in a tropical environment for a period of several months.

Aetiology

Climate alone does not appear to be a major factor, as in locations like Singapore where water quality, sanitation, and nutritional status are similar to industrialized countries, tropical enteropathy has not been found. The major contributors appear to be intestinal infection and nutritional insufficiency. The intestine is relatively resistant to nutritional insufficiency except when severe, and thus attention has focused on the microbiological milieu of the intestine. Two 'infective' factors may be important. Apparently healthy asymptomatic individuals (a) have a small intestine that is heavily colonized by aerobic and anaerobic organisms, and (b) excrete a range of established bacterial enteropathogens in their faeces. There is circumstantial evidence that it is the increased bacterial load of commensal and pathogenic micro-organisms which leads to the mucosal abnormalities in many parts of the developing world. There is also little to support a genetic basis for this condition.

Tropical sprue

Controversy continues to surround this disorder. Its aetiology is unknown. One of the problems has been the failure to establish an agreed definition of the syndrome, but 'malabsorption in deprived areas of the tropics when no bacterial, viral, or parasitic infection can be detected', probably serves best.

Epidemiology

Tropical sprue is predominantly a disease of southern and south-east Asia, the Caribbean islands and to a much lesser extent, of Central and South America. It virtually never occurs in expatriates in Africa, although there have been sporadic reports from South Africa, Zimbabwe, and Nigeria (Fig. 2). This suggests that the aetiological factor or factors are geographically restricted. Epidemics differ from other acute diarrhoeas in that they evolve over many months, with new cases continuing to appear after a year or more. In addition, the attack rates are higher in adults than children. Epidemics occur in south India around Vellore, in north India, Burma, and Puerto Rico.

Clinical features

The cardinal features are chronic diarrhoea, anorexia, abdominal bloating, and prominent bowel sounds. The illness in expatriates and in epidemics in the indigenous population often begins with an acute attack of diarrhoea associated with fever and malaise. The diarrhoea may then take on the features of steatorrhoea and be accompanied by weight loss. Lactose intolerance may develop as part of, and may be associated with, deficiencies of folic acid, vitamin B_{12}, and occasionally hypocalcaemia and hypomagnesaemia. Generally, the illness remits on returning home and after treatment with broad-spectrum antibiotics and folic acid, but in some individuals the disease becomes chronic. The clinical picture then becomes dominated by nutritional deficiencies producing anaemia, stomatitis, and glossitis, hyperpigmentation of the skin, and oedema as a result of hypoproteinaemia.

In a small number of patients the initial presentation involves only a mild or a subclinical illness and chronic diarrhoea and nutritional deficiencies develop months or even years after leaving a tropical

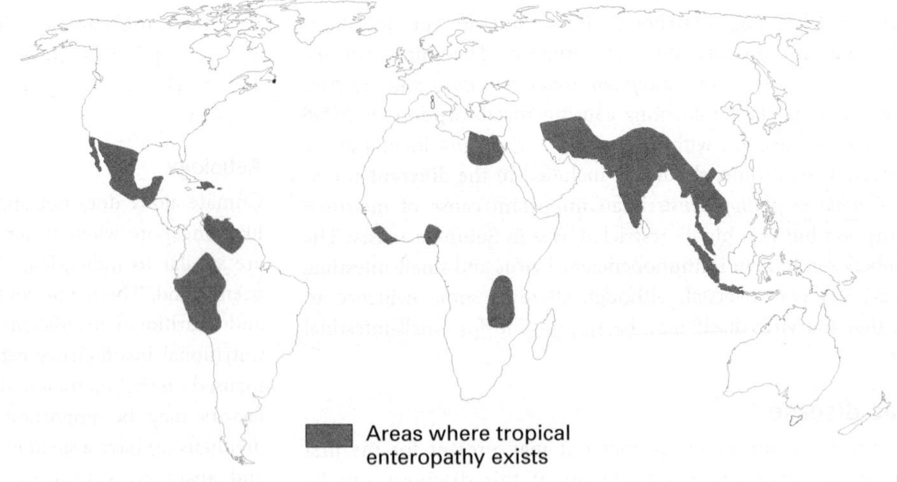

Fig. 1 Geographic distribution of tropical enteropathy.

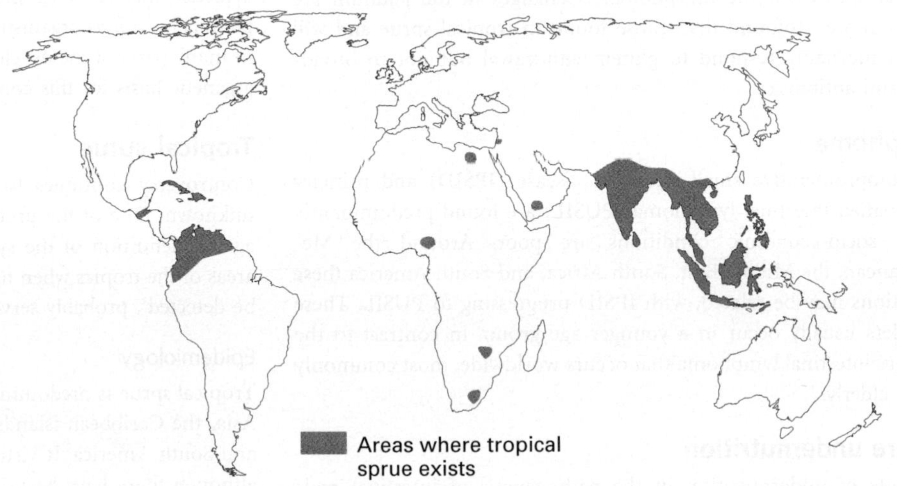

Fig. 2 Geographic distribution of tropical sprue.

environment ('latent sprue'). This has been described in Puerto Ricans living in New York and in Anglo-Indians in London.

Pathology

This is highly variable but generally relates to the duration and the severity of the clinical presentation.

Chronic atrophic gastritis

Many patients in southern India have reduced secretion of gastric acid and intrinsic factor as a result of chronic gastritis. This can result in vitamin B_{12} malabsorption, corrected by administration of intrinsic factor. The gastritis may persist after the enteropathy has recovered.

Enteropathy

The jejunal mucosal biopsy may be normal in the early stages, but there is usually a reduction in villous height, increase in crypt depth, and an inflammatory cell infiltrate in both the lamina propria and the epithelium. Electron-microscopic studies have suggested that the primary lesion is in the stem cells in the crypts.

Colonopathy

Colonic epithelial cells show structural abnormalities similar to those in the small intestine. Sodium and water absorption by the colon is impaired, related in part to the increased concentrations of unsaturated free fatty acids in the stool.

Pathophysiology

The major disturbances occur in the small intestine.

Intestinal absorption and secretion

Some patients have a net secretory state for water in the small intestine which can be dramatically improved by treatment with antibiotics. Malabsorption of amino acids, dipeptides, carbohydrates, fat, folic acid, and vitamin B_{12} is common as is lactose intolerance.

Intestinal motility

Mouth-to-caecum transit time is increased and in a small number may be reduced after treatment with tetracycline and folic acid. Fat malabsorption may be an important factor modulating small-intestinal transit.

Gut hormones

Fasting serum concentrations of motilin and enteroglucagon are increased in acute tropical sprue, with a further marked increment following administration of a standard test meal. The relation between the plasma enteroglucagon concentration and mouth-to-caecum transit time, suggests that enteroglucagon is a mediator of the increase in small-intestinal transit time.

Aetiopathogenesis of tropical sprue

Nutritional insufficiency, intestinal infection, and possibly toxins have all been implicated, but there is little evidence to suggest that undernutrition has any primary role. The bulk of the evidence suggests an infective aetiology. A variety of bacteria has been isolated from the jejunum in patients with tropical sprue (see OTM3, p.1934). In some areas there is bacterial colonization of the proximal small intestine with coliforms, but no single species has emerged that could explain tropical sprue in all locations. Viruses have been searched for as a cause without conclusive evidence of their involvement. It seems probable that the syndrome may have more than one cause.

Diagnosis

The first step is to exclude the specific causes of malabsorption, particularly intestinal infections. At least three stool specimens on separate days should be examined by microscopy, using appropriate stains to search for the parasites *Giardia intestinalis* and *C. parvum*, and in the immunocompromised *Isospora belli* and the microsporidia. If faecal microscopy is negative, and any of these infections strongly suspected, jejunal aspiration and jejunal biopsy may reveal the parasites. The jejunal biopsy will also be useful in diagnosing coeliac disease, as are the anti-endomysial and antireticulin antibodies. A barium follow-through examination and small-bowel biopsies will be necessary to exclude small-intestinal lymphoma or immunoproliferative small-intestinal disease. Once the specific aetiologies have been excluded, the presence of fat, vitamin B_{12}, and possibly D-xylose malabsorption, and a jejunal biopsy showing partial villous atrophy, allows the diagnosis of tropical sprue.

Treatment

Restoration of water and electrolyte balance and replacement of nutritional deficiencies are the priorities in the initial management. It is usually recommended that vitamin B_{12} be given parenterally, although iron and folic acid may be given orally. The question of broad-spectrum antibiotics remains controversial. Spontaneous recovery does occur. Symptomatic treatment with an antidiarrhoeal preparation such as loperamide is often advised.

Prevention

There are no specific preventive measures for tropical sprue. The incidence appears to be declining in overland travellers and expatriates. This may be related to the more liberal use of antibiotics for travellers' diarrhoea.

Further reading

Farthing, M.J.G., Kelly, M.P, and Veitch, A.M. (1996). Recently recognised microbial enteropathies and HIV infection. *Journal of Antimicrobial Chemotherapy*, 37 (suppl. B), 61–70.

Farthing, M.J.G. (1997). Tropical malabsorption and tropical diarrhea. In: *Gastrointestinal and liver disease* (B.F. Feltman, M.H. Scharschmidt, eds.), 6th edn, pp.1574–84. Sleisenger.

Chapter 5.14

Crohn's disease

D. P. Jewell

Crohn's disease is a chronic inflammatory disease of the gastrointestinal tract, the cause of which remains unknown. It is characterized by a granulomatous inflammation affecting any part of the tract, frequently in discontinuity, and by the tendency to form fistulae.

Epidemiology

Crohn's disease is well recognized in Europe, North America, and Australia but is rarely seen in India, tropical Africa, and South America. This may be largely due to the difficulty of diagnosing Crohn's disease in areas where intestinal tuberculosis is common. The disease is rare in Japan but its prevalence there appears to be increasing. There has been a striking increase in incidence and prevalence in Europe since 1950 (Table 1). Annual discharge rates for the disease in England and Wales rose from 2.8 per 100 000 in 1958 to 7.2 per 100 000 in 1971. The reasons for changing patterns of incidence are not clear. Crohn's disease occurs in all age groups but it is rare in early childhood and most commonly affects young adults. There is no marked sex difference, and no association with social class or occupation.

Genetics

Familial incidence varies from 6 to 15 per cent, and affected members of a family may have Crohn's disease or ulcerative colitis. Susceptibility genes have been located on chromosomes 3, 7, and 12, probably shared with ulcerative colitis, but a locus on chromosome 16 appears to confer specific susceptibility to Crohn's disease.

Aetiology

Environmental influences include smoking and intestinal luminal factors. There is a relative risk of 4–6 for Crohn's disease in smokers

Table 1 Incidence of Crohn's disease per 100 000 population

Aberdeen	1955–61	1.7
	1964–66	3.3
	1967–69	4.5
	1970–72	4.3
	1973–75	2.6
Cardiff	1934–70	1.1
	1971–77	4.6
Malmö	1958–65	3.5
	1966–73	6.0
Uppsala	1956–61	1.7
	1962–67	3.1
	1968–73	5.0
Stockholm	1955–59	1.5
	1960–64	2.2
	1965–69	3.6
	1970–74	4.5
	1975–79	4.1

compared with non-smokers, in striking contrast to the reverse association seen in ulcerative colitis. The role of luminal factors is suggested by the tendency of Crohn's colitis to heal if the colon is rendered non-functional by an ileostomy and by the effectiveness of an elemental diet for the treatment of active disease. Other mechanisms include diet, infective agents, ischaemia, and immune responses.

Diet

There is evidence of a higher intake of refined sugar and a lesser one of fibre in patients with Crohn's disease, but a controlled trial was unable to show that a low-sugar, high-fibre diet had any effect on the course of the disease over a 2-year period. Claims have been made that patients may benefit from dietary exclusion determined by a period on an elimination diet followed by challenge with individual foods, but the long-term benefit of dietary exclusion is by no means proven. Elemental diets of glucose and amino acids have been shown to have equal efficacy to prednisolone for treating active Crohn's disease but whether this effect is mediated by influencing bacterial populations, by removing dietary antigens, or by some other mechanism is unknown.

Infective agents

Most claims that viruses or cell wall deficient bacteria might cause Crohn's disease are discredited, but there is current interest in *Mycobacterium paratuberculosis* and measles virus. Evidence for either agent remains inconclusive (see OTM3, p. 1937).

Ischaemia

Abnormalities of mucosal arterioles have been detected in resected specimens of intestine affected by Crohn's disease. Many of the small vessels have been shown to be thrombosed, but in a rather patchy distribution, suggesting that much of the inflammation may rise from multifocal infarction. However, it is not possible to be sure whether these changes are primary or are secondary to inflammation.

Immune mechanisms

Serum concentrations of immunoglobulins and complement components are usually normal, although they may be raised in association with active disease. Neutrophil and monocyte functions, *in vitro*, show no defect. The number of peripheral blood T lymphocytes may be reduced but the proportion of phenotypic subsets (CD4, CD8) remains unchanged. Within the inflamed tissue, there is a marked increase of plasma cells, lymphocytes, macrophages, and neutrophils. Increased immunoglobulin production is predominantly of the IgG isotype but, with a greater proportional increase in the IgG2 subclass. T cells and macrophages in the lamina propria are activated. No consistent defect in immunoregulation has been found, although there may be an impaired facility to produce antigen-specific suppresser cells. Cellular activation results in the release of cytokines and inflammatory mediators, which may determine the course of the disease, whether fibrosing or fistulating.

Pathology

Crohn's disease may occur anywhere in the gastrointestinal tract, although the most common pattern is an ileocolitis. The disease is often discontinuous (skip lesions). Isolated involvement of the mouth, oesophagus, stomach, and anus is recognized but is extremely rare. The bowel is thickened and frequently stenosed. The serosal surface may be inflamed and the mesentery becomes oedematous. The regional mesenteric nodes are usually enlarged. The earliest lesion on the mucosal surface is an aphthoid ulcer. In areas of more severe disease, deep, fissuring ulcers occur in the oedematous and inflamed mucosa, giving rise to a cobblestone pattern. Long, serpiginous ulcers are a further characteristic feature. Strictures occur as a result of submucosal fibrosis and the affected intestine may become adherent to adjacent loops or other structures with the subsequent formation of fistulae.

Histologically, the inflammation is transmural and consists principally of lymphocytes, histiocytes, and plasma cells. Granulomas are found in only 65 per cent of patients. They are present in most cases with rectal disease but are much less common in ileal disease. The mucosal architecture is well preserved and, in the colon, goblet cells are usually present. Fissures, penetrating into the submucosa and lined with histiocytic cells, are frequently present.

Quantitative histological and enzyme studies have suggested that the whole of the gastrointestinal tract is abnormal in patients with Crohn's disease even though overt involvement is localized.

Clinical features

The majority of patients complain of diarrhoea (70–90 per cent), abdominal pain (45–66 per cent) and weight loss (65–75 per cent). Fever is also common (30–49 per cent). Obstructive symptoms (colic, vomiting) are much more commonly associated with ileal than colonic disease. Colonic disease causes rectal bleeding more commonly than ileal disease and is also associated with perianal disease and with extraintestinal manifestations, which are uncommon when the disease is confined to the ileum. Anaemia is common, and usually the result of iron deficiency or, less frequently, of vitamin B_{12} or folate deficiency. Other features of malabsorption are infrequent but with extensive small bowel disease, osteomalacia may occur and there may be a bleeding tendency secondary to vitamin K malabsorption. Deficiencies of magnesium, zinc, ascorbic acid, and the B vitamins are uncommon and usually due to inadequate intake.

A few patients present as acute appendicitis but have an acute terminal ileitis, only sometimes due to Crohn's disease. Diagnostic difficulties may also occur when patients present with fever, weight loss, and anaemia without diarrhoea or abdominal pain, or in ileocaecal disease with urinary frequency and dysuria due to ureteric involvement.

Physical examination may be normal but many patients will show evidence of anaemia. Glossitis and aphthous ulcers in the mouth, beaking or frank clubbing of the nails, evidence of weight loss, and a tachycardia are common. The affected bowel is usually tender and its thickening can sometimes be felt as an abdominal mass. Anal examination often shows the presence of fleshy skin tags, which have a characteristic violaceous hue. Anal fissures, perianal fistulae, and abscesses are particularly associated with colonic disease.

The extraintestinal manifestations are similar to those of ulcerative colitis. Table 2 lists those that are most frequently seen.

Complications

Intestinal obstruction due to strictures or fistulae between parts of the gut or between gut and bladder or vagina are more common than acute dilatation of the bowel (colonic diameter >5.5 cm)

Table 2 Extraintestinal manifestations of Crohn's disease

	Frequency (per cent)	Comment
Related to disease activity		
Aphthous ulceration	20	
Erythema nodosum	5–10	
Pyoderma gangrenosum	0.5	
Acute arthropathy	6–12	Large joints affected; transient, non-destructive
Eye complications:	3–10	
Conjunctivitis		
Episcleritis		
Uveitis		
Unrelated to disease activity		
Sacroiliitis	15–18	Usually asymptomatic; may be present in up to 50 per cent using isotope scanning; unrelated to HLA-B27.
Ankylosing spondylitis	2–6	75 per cent of patients have the HLA-B27 phenotype
Liver disease:	5–6	
Primary sclerosing cholangitis		Rare and poorly documented in Crohn's disease
Gallstones	Very common	Owing to malabsorption of bile salts from ileum
Chronic active hepatitis	2–3	
Cirrhosis	2–3	
Fatty change	6	Very common in ill patients requiring surgery
Amyloid, granulomas	Rare	

perforation or serious haemorrhage. The gross malabsorption that occurs with a gastrocolic or ileocolic fistulae is largely due to bacterial overgrowth of the small intestine. External fistulae to the skin also occur, but this is usually secondary to surgical intervention. Involvement of the ureter, can cause frequency with a sterile pyuria, a frank urinary tract infection, or a ureteric stricture with subsequent hydronephrosis. Hyperoxaluria and oxalate stones may be complications of ileal disease associated with steatorrhoea. Carcinoma of the colon may complicate Crohn's colitis in about 3–5 per cent of cases and small bowel carcinomas have been reported in association with ileal Crohn's disease. Amyloid may occur within the bowel or systemically.

Radiological appearances

A plain radiograph of the abdomen with decubitus films may show evidence of intestinal obstruction or suggest an inflammatory mass in the right iliac fossa. In acute Crohn's colitis, evidence of mucosal oedema and ulceration may be clearly seen and could obviate the need for barium studies, which should be avoided in the presence of severe, active disease. The plain film can also provide evidence of sacroiliitis or ankylosing spondylitis.

The small intestine is best examined by a small bowel enema. The earliest lesions are thickening of valvulae coniventes and small, discrete aphthoid ulcers. In more severe disease, cobblestoning, fissure ulcers, and thickening of the wall occur (Fig. 1). Areas of stenosis and dilatation may be present, and sinus tracts and fistulas may be demonstrated. The abnormal segment is usually well demarcated from the normal bowel.

Radiological examination of the colon is made with a double-contrast barium enema. Characteristic appearances of Crohn's colitis are similar to those described for the small intestine (Fig. 2). Table 3 lists the main features that differentiate the radiological appearances of Crohn's colitis from ulcerative colitis.

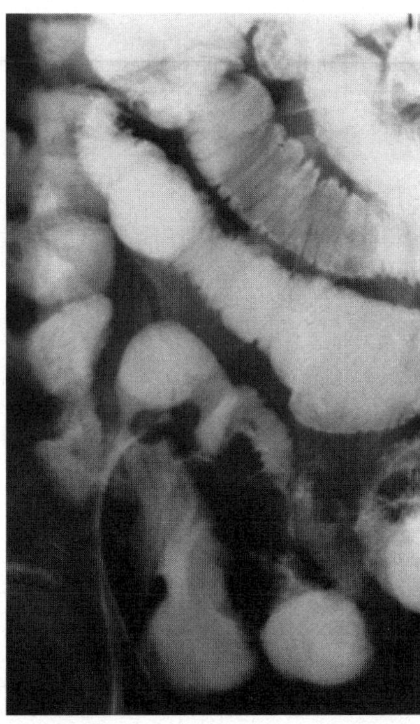

Fig. 1 Small bowel enema demonstrating Crohn's disease of the terminal ileum with fissure ulcers, ileocaecal fistulae, and partial obstruction. *(By courtesy of Dr D.J. Nolan.)*

Endoscopy

On sigmoidoscopy the rectal mucosa is frequently normal but may show a granular proctitis and occasionally the typical appearances of Crohn's disease. Histological examination of a rectal biopsy from a macroscopically normal rectum often shows an inflammatory infiltrate. Colonoscopy allows examination and biopsy of the whole colon and often terminal ileum.

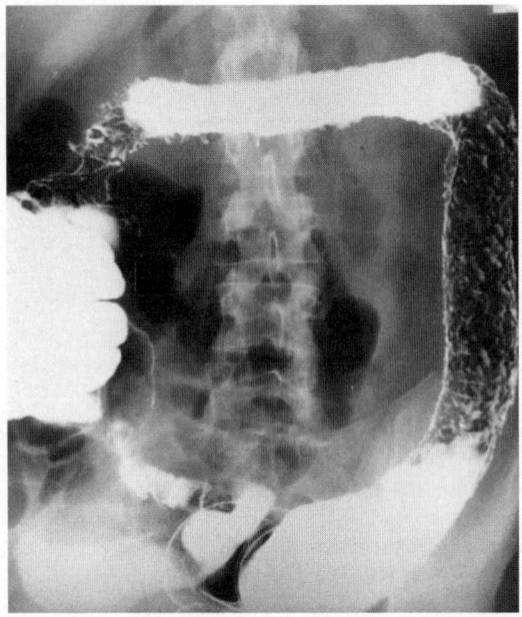

Fig. 2 Barium enema showing Crohn's disease of the colon and terminal ileum. Distal sigmoid, rectum, and a segment of ascending colon are normal. The diseased segments show loss of haustration, shortening, and fissure ulcers.
(By courtesy of Dr D.J. Nolan.)

Table 3 Differential diagnosis of Crohn's disease and ulcerative colitis

	Crohn's disease	Ulcerative colitis
Clinical features		
Bloody diarrhoea	Less common	Common
Abdominal mass	Common	Rare
Perianal disease	Common	Less common
Malabsorption	Frequent (ileal disease)	Never
Radiological features		
Rectal involvement	Frequently spared	Invariable
Distribution	Segmental, discontinuous	Continuous
Mucosa	Cobblestones, fissure ulcers	Fine ulceration
		'Double contour'
Strictures	Common	Rare
Fistulae	Frequent	Rare
Histological features		
Distribution	Transmural	Mucosal
Cellular infiltrate	Lymphocytes, plasma cells, macrophages	Polymorphs, plasma cells, eosinophils
Glands	Gland preservation	Mucus depletion, gland destruction, crypt abscesses
Special features	Aphthoid ulcers, granulomas, histiocyte-lined fissures	None

Endoscopically, the earliest lesion of Crohn's disease is a small aphthoid ulcer surrounded by normal mucosa with a normal vascular pattern. This contrasts with the erythema and loss of vascular pattern seen in ulcerative colitis. In more severe disease the mucosa becomes oedematous and is penetrated by fissuring ulcers to give a cobblestone appearance. A diffusely inflamed, granular, friable, and dark-red mucosa is more typical of ulcerative colitis. Pseudopolyps and mucosal bridges occur in both diseases.

Multiple biopsies should be taken, even from apparently normal areas, because granulomas may be present, which allow a precise diagnosis.

Upper gastrointestinal endoscopy is only indicated in the presence of appropriate symptoms or if abnormalities are noted on a barium meal. Deep, longitudinal ulcers may occur in the stomach together with rugal hypertrophy and a cobblestone appearance. In the duodenum the major differential diagnosis is duodenal ulcer but there is usually a 'cobblestone' mucosa surrounding the frank ulceration. Biopsies are usually helpful, although granulomas are found infrequently.

Laboratory data

Iron deficiency from intestinal blood loss is common but serum folate and vitamin B_{12} concentrations may also be low. Serum ferritin is the best indicator of iron stores in patients with chronic disease. A neutrophil leucocytosis is usually associated with active disease and there may be a thrombocytosis. The total lymphocyte count and number of circulating T lymphocytes may be reduced.

Hypokalaemia is associated with severe diarrhoea and the plasma urea concentration is often low, reflecting a poor dietary intake of nitrogen. Serum albumin is reduced in of active disease, largely due to down-regulation of albumin synthesis by cytokines such as interleukin (IL) -1, tumour necrosis factor, and IL-6, but sometimes it is also due to a protein-losing enteropathy. Serum immunoglobulins are normal or mildly elevated and there may be a rise in the α_2-globulins. A low serum calcium is unusual unless there is extensive small bowel disease, and a low urinary calcium is more likely to reflect a poor diet than osteomalacia. Mild elevations of the aspartate transaminase and alkaline phosphatase are more common, but persistence of abnormal liver tests suggests associated liver disease and should be investigated by liver biopsy and visualization of the biliary tree. Patients with extensive ileal disease or with ileal stricture may have increased faecal fat excretion, usually secondary to bacterial overgrowth, compounded by the low circulating pool and increased excretion of bile salts. Magnesium, zinc, and selenium deficiencies, are occasionally present.

Diagnosis

Intermittent abdominal symptoms and diarrhoea without systemic symptoms are often labelled as an irritable bowel syndrome. Weight loss, fever, and anaemia without gastrointestinal symptoms are another source of misdiagnosis. Even when the diagnosis seems sound, all patients must have: (a) stool examination to exclude pathogens; (b) sigmoidoscopy and rectal biopsy; (c) radiographs of the small and large intestine; and (d) colonoscopy with multiple biopsies is when the above investigations are equivocal and there are strong reasons for suspecting Crohn's disease, or if strictures are present.

Differential diagnosis

Few patients with an acute ileitis presenting as acute appendicitis subsequently develop Crohn's disease. Some cases are caused by *Yersinia*; the aetiology of the remainder is unknown. The main differential diagnosis of ileal Crohn's disease is tuberculosis. Laparoscopy may be helpful if serosal tubercles are present, as they can be biopsied and cultured. If doubt exists, corticosteroid therapy for Crohn's disease must be covered with antituberculous therapy. Other differential diagnoses include abdominal lymphoma, α-chain disease, actinomycosis, amyloid, Behçet's disease, and carcinoma of the small bowel.

The major differential diagnosis of Crohn's colitis is ulcerative colitis (Table 3). Thirty per cent of patients with ileal Crohn's disease may have a proctitis and may present in this way. In segmental colitis, ischaemia, tuberculosis, and lymphoma have to be excluded. Crohn's disease can be overlooked on the barium enema when it occurs in association with severe diverticular disease.

Assessment of activity

There is no satisfactory method of assessing activity of the disease. Fever or continuing weight loss are obvious indicators but severe disease can be present in the absence of any major symptom. Laboratory evidence of activity includes a reduced serum albumin, a rise in C-reactive protein and in the erythrocyte sedimentation rate. Another technique for the assessment of activity is the use of indium- or technetium-labelled neutrophils. The labelled cells preferentially migrate to inflamed mucosa and the increased uptake of isotope can be detected using a gamma-camera. Faecal excretion of the labelled cells can also be quantified and this has shown good correlation with a Crohn's disease activity index and albumin loss.

Management

Nutritional support

A low residue diet helps patients with strictures, a low fat diet those with steatorrhoea and a lactose free diet is required for those with hypolactosis. The value of elimination diets for the generality of patients is unproven. Iron and vitamin B_{12} deficiencies may need replacement and less commonly deficiencies of vitamins A, D, E, and K, and folic acid or B vitamins arise. Parenteral nutrition is often indicated for seriously ill patients.

Drug therapy

There is no indication for treatment in asymptomatic patients. Active disease can usually be controlled with corticosteroids. Severe disease requires intravenous prednisolone (60–80 mg daily) or hydrocortisone (400 mg daily), together with fluids and electrolytes. Most patients settle within 5–7 days and can then be changed to oral prednisolone (e.g. 40 mg daily). Patients with less severe disease can be treated with oral 20–40 mg prednisolone daily. Most patients will have made a good symptomatic response by 4–6 weeks; the dose can then be reduced over the next 3–6 weeks and finally stopped.

The role of 5-aminosalicylic acid-containing drugs is not so well defined for Crohn's disease as for ulcerative colitis. Sulphasalazine may have some beneficial effect on mildly active disease, especially affecting the colon. High-dose Pentasa (4 g daily) may be effective for active disease, and Claversal and Pentasa may have some benefits as maintenance treatment in order to prolong remission. Details of the new salicylate drugs are given in the next chapter.

For patients who continually relapse when steroids are withdrawn or when the prednisolone dose falls below 10–15 mg daily, azathioprine or 6-mercaptopurine will benefit some at a dose of 2.0–2.5 mg/kg but there is no way of predicting which patients will respond. These drugs usually take several weeks to exert their effects and, it may be worthwhile continuing therapy for 1–2 years. Controlled trials have shown that oral cyclosporin (5 mg/kg) is not effective but methotrexate (25 mg intramuscularly weekly) does have a steroid-sparing effect. Metronidazole, ciprofloxacin and augmentin are required for patients with small-intestinal bacterial overgrowth, perianal sepsis, and abscesses associated with fistulae.

Elemental diets have been shown to be as effective as prednisolone but the major problem is one of compliance. Polymeric diets may be as effective as elemental diets and are certainly more palatable.

Surgery

Indications include failure to respond to medical therapy, strictures causing mechanical obstruction, fistulae, and other complications such as abscess and perforation. Resection should be limited to removing the most severely affected segment and an end-to-end anastomosis should be made, even if there is some inflammation in the tissue being anastomosed. Bypass procedures should not be done. Fistulas are excised together with the segment of affected intestine and the subsequent anastomosis is usually best protected with a temporary ileostomy. For colonic disease, the choice is a split ileostomy or a proctocolectomy with terminal ileostomy. Colectomy with ileorectal anastomosis is associated with a high recurrence rate. Multiple short strictures should be dealt with by stricturoplasty rather than resection.

Management during pregnancy

The outcome of pregnancy is not influenced by the disease except in very severe cases where there may be an increased risk of abortion. Corticosteroids, sulphasalazine, and azathioprine are safe but methotrexate is teratogenic and must not be prescribed.

Course and prognosis

Patients are never cured of Crohn's disease. After a resection, the disease recurs in about 30 per cent of patients during the subsequent 5 years and in 50 per cent during the subsequent 10 years; of these, half will require further surgery. Recurrence rates, assessed by endoscopic appearance, are even higher than the rates quoted above, which are based on symptoms. Overall mortality varies from 10 to 15 per cent in different studies. Some reports suggest a worse prognosis for women, and for patients over the age of 50 years. Even so, the majority of patients will have a good prognosis with a mortality of only about twice that expected.

Further reading

Bickston, S.J. and Cominelli, F. (1998). Treatment of Crohn's disease at the turn of the century. *New England Journal of Medicine*, **339**, 401–2.

Fiochi, C. (1998). Inflammatory bowel disease: aetiology and pathogenesis. *Gastroenterology*, **115**, 182–205.

Hanauer, S.B. (1996). Drug therapy; inflammatory bowel disease. *New England Journal of Medicine*, **334**, 841–7.

Hodgson, H.J. (1996). Keeping Crohn's disease quiet. *New England Journal of Medicine*, **334**, 1599–1600.

Hodgson, H. (1999). Prospects of new therapeutic approaches for Crohn's disease. *Lancet*, **353**, 425–6.

Rhodes, J.M. (1997). Mucus and inflammatory bowel disease. *Quarterly Journal of Medicine*, **90**, 79–82.

Rutgeerts, P. and Vermeire, S. (1998). Clinical value of the detection of antibodies in the serum for the diagnosis of inflammatory bowel disease. *Gastroenterology*, 115, 1006–9.

Satsangi, J., Jewell, D.P., Rosenberg, W.M.C., and Bell, J.I. (1994). Genetics of inflammatory bowel disease. *Gut*, 35, 696–700.

Chapter 5.15

Ulcerative colitis

D. P. Jewell

Ulcerative colitis is a chronic inflammatory disease of the colon of unknown cause. It always affects the rectum and extends proximally to involve a variable extent of the colon. It is characterized by a relapsing and remitting course.

Epidemiology

Ulcerative colitis is a worldwide disease. Table 1 lists data for the high-incidence areas. In eastern Europe, Asia, Japan, and South America the incidence rates are at least 10-fold less. The age of onset peaks between 20 and 40 years but the disease may present at all ages from the first few months of life to the 80s. There is little difference between the sexes.

Genetics

Ten to 20 per cent of patients may have at least one other family member affected either with ulcerative colitis or with Crohn's disease. Most of the familial association is in first-degree relatives, with a preponderance of parent-sibling combinations in the US, whereas in the UK the disease is more commonly shared by siblings. Concordance rates in twins suggest that familial clustering reflects environmental rather than genetic influences, although the incidence of the disease in spouses of probands is very low. Susceptibility genes have been located to loci on chromosomes 3, 7, and 12. Disease phenotype and susceptibility to extra-intestinal manifestations are influenced by other genes, including HLA genes.

Table 1 Incidence of ulcerative colitis

	Period of study	Incidence (per 10^5)
USA		
Minnesota	1935–64	7.2
Baltimore	1960–63	4.6
UK		
Oxford	1951–60	6.5
Wales	1968–77	7.2
Aberdeen	1967–76	11.3
Denmark		
Copenhagen	1962–78	8.1
	1981–88	9.5
Holland		
Leiden	1979–83	6.8
Sweden		
Stockholm County	1975–79	4.3
Israel		
Tel-Aviv	1961–70	3.6

Aetiology

The main hypotheses that have been proposed include infection, allergy to dietary components, immune responses to bacterial or self antigens, an abnormality in epithelial cell integrity, and the psychosomatic theory.

Infection

No specific infective organism has been identified, but it has been suggested that strains of *Escherichia coli* by releasing enzymes or toxic products might damage the mucosa.

Food allergy

Allergic responses to milk proteins, eggs, and other dietary proteins have not been substantiated as an aetiological factor. The failure of ulcerative colitis to respond either to intravenous nutrition with nil by mouth or to colonic isolation by a split ileostomy are strong evidence that dietary factors play little part.

Environmental factors

Ulcerative colitis is more common in non-smokers than smokers, with a relative risk of 2–6. Ex-smokers have a particularly high incidence and this is highest for ex-heavy compared with ex-light smokers.

Immunopathogenesis

The intense infiltration of the inflamed mucosa with plasma cells, B and T lymphocytes, and macrophages suggests immunological activity. The predominant product of the plasma cells is IgG of the IgG1 and 3 subclasses which are synthesized in response to protein antigen and fix complement. As antibody to epithelial antigens, especially an 40-kDa protein, is a feature of ulcerative colitis, it is possible that autoimmunity plays a part. This concept is strengthened by the association with other autoimmune disorders and with circulating antibodies to neutrophils (pANCA).

CD4+, and CD8+ T cells are present in increased numbers but their proportions do not change significantly. There may be a failure of T cells to induce suppression to specific antigens, leading perhaps to some of the immunological overactivity characteristic of the disease. Certainly, T cells are activated and release cytokines.

The activated macrophages not only release inflammatory mediators but serine proteases, metalloproteinases, and cytokines. The release of interleukin (IL) -1, IL-6, and tumour necrosis factor will not only lead to tissue damage but will initiate an acute-phase response, down-regulate albumin synthesis, and induce fever. Changes in epithelial permeability induced by interferon-γ and inflammatory mediators, endothelial damage by a wide variety of cytokines and mediators leading to local ischaemia, and stimulation of collagen synthesis by transforming growth factor-β, IL-1, and IL-6 may all contribute to the inflammatory process.

Pathology

Ulcerative colitis always involves the rectum and in about 40 per cent of patients the disease is limited to the rectum and sigmoid. In adults, only about 20 per cent will have the whole colon involved. In mild disease, the mucosa is hyperaemic and granular but, as it becomes more severe, small punctate ulcers appear, which may then enlarge and extend deeply into the lamina propria. The mucosa can become intensely haemorrhagic. In patients with long-standing disease, inflammatory polyps may develop, usually in the colon and rarely in the rectum. In remission, the colonic appearances may return to normal. There is often narrowing and shortening of the bowel. Fibrous strictures complicating long-standing chronic disease are extremely rare. If an acute dilatation occurs, the bowel becomes thin and congested, and may perforate. Inflammation is largely confined to the mucosa. The lamina propria becomes oedematous, with dilated and congested capillaries, and extravasation of red blood cells. There is a cellular infiltrate of acute and chronic inflammatory cells.

Neutrophils invade the epithelium, usually in the crypts, giving rise to a cryptitis and eventually to a crypt abscess. Damage to the crypts leads to increased epithelial cell turnover and a discharge of mucus from goblet cells. With increasing inflammation, the surface epithelial cells become flattened, irregular, and eventually ulcerate. Deep ulcers may extend into the lamina propria, leading to inflammatory changes in the submucosa. Many of the acute changes may also be seen in infective colitides, but the diagnosis can be made with some accuracy if there are distorted crypt architecture, crypt atrophy, basal lymphoid aggregates, and a chronic inflammatory infiltrate.

In remission, the histological appearances may return to normal, but there is frequent evidence of bifid or shortened crypts, hyperplasia of the muscularis mucosae, neuronal hypertrophy, and Paneth-cell metaplasia at the base of the crypts.

Clinical features

Patients usually present with a gradual onset of symptoms, often intermittent, but which become progressively more severe, but the disease may mimic an infective colitis. The major symptoms include diarrhoea, rectal bleeding, the passage of mucus, and, less frequently, abdominal pain. The diarrhoea is often accompanied by urgency, tenesmus, and occasionally incontinence. With severe disease, patients are usually anorectic, nauseated, and have lost weight.

Patients may also complain of malaise, or of some of the extra-intestinal manifestations, especially recurrent aphthous ulcers of the mouth. When inflammation is confined to the rectum, patients often pass fresh blood, which is usually mixed with the stool but can be streaked on the surface. Those with mild attacks usually look well. Abdominal examination may reveal a tender colon but is often normal. Patients with a severe attack may be ill, with fever, salt and water depletion, anaemia, and evidence of weight loss. There may be oral candidiasis, aphthous ulceration, signs of iron deficiency, finger clubbing, and dependent oedema. The abdomen is often distended and tympanitic, with reduced bowel sounds and marked colonic tenderness.

Assessment of disease severity

In mild disease there are less than four stools daily, with or without blood, with no systemic disturbance and a normal erythrocyte sedimentation rate (**ESR**), but those with severe disease have at least six stools daily, with bleeding, and fever, tachycardia, a falling haemoglobin, hypoalbuminaemia, and raised ESR and C-reactive protein, and often a neutrophil leucocytosis and thrombocytosis.

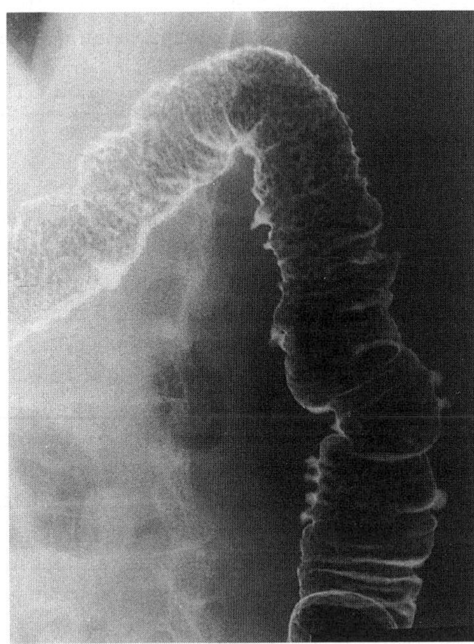

Fig. 1 A double-contrast barium enema in a patient with active ulcerative colitis. The figure is a close-up view of the splenic flexure to show extensive mucosal ulceration, loss of haustration, and narrowing of the colon. The patient also has diverticula in the descending colon.

Diagnosis

This is made on the history, the absence of faecal pathogens, and the endoscopic and histological appearances of the colon. Special culture conditions are required for *Campylobacter* spp., *Yersinia*, gonococci and *Clostridium difficile*. The possibility of an infection with *E. coli* 0157 must also be considered, especially in patients in whom bleeding and abdominal pain are predominant symptoms. An infective colitis with opportunistic organisms may occur in patients with immunodeficiency syndromes.

Sigmoidoscopy is safe, even in patients with a severe attack, and allows a biopsy to be taken and an assessment of severity to be obtained. Colonoscopy is best avoided in the acute stage. The earliest signs on sigmoidoscopy are blurring of the vascular pattern associated with hyperaemia and oedema, leading to blunting of the valves of Houston. With increasing severity, the mucosa becomes granular and then friable. With severe inflammation, the mucosa shows spontaneous bleeding and ulceration. Pseudopolyps tend to be in the colon rather than the rectum. Colonoscopy is useful for assessing the extent of disease and is mandatory for patients with a colonic stricture, and is also required for cancer surveillance. In severe attacks, a plain abdominal radiograph may detect a dilated colon or indicate the extent of disease by showing mucosal islands, or distended loops of small bowel, abnormal haustral pattern or mucosal oedema. Barium radiography is contraindicated in such cases but in less severe disease, a double-contrast barium enema can be safely given (Fig. 1) but the colon must not be overdistended and the procedure must be stopped if the patient complains of pain.

Biopsies help in grading severity as well as confirming the diagnosis. Biochemical abnormalities are rare in mild or moderate attacks but hypokalaemia, hypoalbuminaemia, and a rise in α_2-globulin frequently accompany a severe attack. Minor elevations of the aspartate transaminase or alkaline phosphatase seen in patients with a severe attack return to normal in remission. Persistent elevation, especially of alkaline phosphatase needs further investigation.

Differential diagnosis

The major differential diagnosis for those presenting with a slow onset is Crohn's disease, and in some 10 per cent of patients the diagnosis of indeterminate colitis has to be made. Collagenous colitis usually has only a mild inflammation on colonoscopy and is diagnosed on the basis of a thickened subepithelial collagen band (wider than 15 μm) seen in a rectal biopsy specimen. Lymphocytic colitis has a normal endoscopic appearance but shows a diffuse infiltration of the lamina propria with lymphocytes and eosinophils on histological examination. Ischaemic colitis may occur in the rectum, especially in the elderly, and can be diagnosed histologically. Radiation damage to the rectum may follow radiotherapy to the prostate. Rarely, colitis may be caused by non-steroidal anti-inflammatory drugs, gold, penicillamine, and 5-aminosalicylic acid, the latter a problem in those with known ulcerative colitis. Pseudomembranous colitis can occur without the use of antibiotics, especially in the elderly.

In acute cases, infective colitis must be excluded by stool culture. Sigmoidoscopic appearances are usually very similar to ulcerative colitis but a rectal biopsy can be useful in making the distinction. The common organisms causing an infective colitis are salmonellae, shigellae, and campylobacter. Yersinial infections may also cause a colitis and can pursue a chronic course over many months before resolving. *E. coli* 0157 often causes massive bleeding and may be associated with an haemolytic uraemic syndrome. For patients who have travelled in endemic areas, amoebic and schistosomal colitis must be considered. Causes of infective colitis in immunosuppressed patients include cytomegalovirus, herpes simplex, and *Mycobacterium avium intracellulare.* Sexually transmitted causes of proctitis do not usually cause diarrhoea and, especially with gonorrhoea, are associated with the passage of watery pus. Ulcerative colitis also has to be differentiated from irritable bowel syndrome, colonic polyps or carcinoma, diverticular disease, solitary rectal ulcer syndrome, and factitious diarrhoea.

Extraintestinal manifestations (Table 2)

Skin

A hypersensitivity rash to sulphasalazine (related to the sulphapyridine moiety), may be photosensitive. Erythema nodosum is mostly associated with active disease. Pyoderma gangrenosum is usually seen in active disease but occasionally persists despite inactive colitis (see OTM3, p. 3778).

Mouth

Aphthous ulcers are common in active disease. A sore tongue and angular stomatitis often accompany chronic iron deficiency.

Eyes

Episcleritis or an anterior uveitis occur in 5–8 per cent of patients. Local corticosteroids and treatment of active colitis usually lead to resolution.

Joints

An acute arthropathy occurs in 10–15 per cent of patients with active disease. It affects the larger joints and is usually asymmetrical, settling as the colitis goes into remission. Low back pain is usually due to a sacroiliitis unrelated to disease activity. It is not strongly associated with HLA-B27, and rarely progresses to ankylosing spondylitis, which occurs in only 1–2 per cent of patients.

Table 2 Extraintestinal manifestations of ulcerative colitis

Related to activity of colitis
- Aphthous ulceration of the mouth
- Fatty liver
- Erythema nodosum
- Peripheral arthropathy
- Episcleritis

Usually related to activity of colitis
- Pyoderma gangrenosum
- Anterior uveitis

Unrelated to colitis
- Sacroiliitis
- Ankylosing spondylitis
- Primary sclerosing cholangitis
- Cholangiocarcinoma

Liver disease

There may be persistent abnormalities in liver enzymes in about 3 per cent of patients, usually a rise in alkaline phosphatase. The overwhelming majority of these patients will have primary sclerosing cholangitis. Many patients with ulcerative colitis and sclerosing cholangitis remain well for many years. The colitis is often very mild, but the liver disease is progressive and ultimately leads to portal hypertension and liver failure. Sclerosing cholangitis is a premalignant condition and explains the association between ulcerative colitis and cholangiocarcinoma. Pathogenesis and treatment of the liver disease are discussed in Chapter 5.34.

Rare associations

Pericarditis has been described in association with an acute colitis but a true association is not yet proven. Amyloid occurs rarely. Rapidly progressing bronchiectasis has also been described.

Medical management

The most effective drugs for controlling active disease are the corticosteroids, systemically, topically, or in combination. Sulphasalazine, olsalazine, and mesalazine are often used to treat a mild colitis but prednisolone has been shown to be more effective and to control symptoms more rapidly. Corticosteroids are ineffective as maintenance therapy.

Proctitis can be remarkably difficult to treat. Initial therapy is usually a 5-aminosalicylic acid (5-ASA) drug by mouth in combination with topical therapy, with a corticosteroid or 5-ASA in the form of retention enemas, a foam preparation or a suppository. For patients who do not respond, oral prednisolone may be given. Some have sufficiently severe proctitis to warrant intravenous steroids, and occasionally colectomy may be necessary.

Patients with *mildly active disease* should be given oral prednisolone, 20 mg daily, together with topical steroids or 5-ASA. Treatment should be given for at least 4 weeks before being tailed off over the subsequent 3–4 weeks. Those with *moderately active disease* should be given 40 mg of prednisolone by mouth daily. The dose is reduced to 20 mg daily over 2–3 weeks and the regimen then follows that described for mild disease. In *severe disease* patients should be admitted to hospital and assessed by both physician and surgeon. Fluid and electrolyte losses are replaced; a blood transfusion should be given if the haemoglobin is less than 10 g/dl, and intravenous corticosteroids (e.g. hydrocortisone 100 mg, 6-hourly) given together with a twice daily rectal drip of hydrocortisone (100 mg in 100 ml water). Parenteral nutrition is indicated for patients who are malnourished. Provided there is improvement, treatment is continued for 5–7 days. At this time, a good response is one in which the patient feels well, there is no fever or tachycardia, the colon is not tender, and the diarrhoea has settled, to less than four motions daily. These patients can go on to oral prednisolone (e.g. 40 mg daily), a retention enema, an oral 5 ASA drug, and a light diet. Patients who deteriorate during the first few days or those who have not made a substantial improvement by the end of the first week should have urgent surgery. The difficult decision is when patients have made some improvement but are still not well. Continuing intravenous therapy for more than 7–10 days is rarely beneficial and surgery is usually required. In this group the introduction of a light diet towards the end of the first week of treatment often provides a guide to future management. If the pulse rises or a niggling fever develops, urgent colectomy is required. Intravenous cyclosporin given as a slow infusion (4 mg/kg) has shown promise in this group of patients but its precise role is still undergoing evaluation.

Approximately 25 per cent of patients with a severe attack will require an urgent colectomy. They can often be identified early using features, which have prognostic significance. These are the passage of more than nine stools, a pulse rate greater than 100/min, or a temperature greater than 38°C during the first 24 h of treatment. A serum albumin of less than 30 g/l or the failure of the C-reactive protein to fall are also poor prognostic signs. Seventy-five per cent of patients showing mucosal islands in the colon or having more than three loops of distended small bowel on a plain abdominal radiograph will come to urgent surgery.

In *chronic active disease* patients who relapse repeatedly when the dose of prednisolone falls below 10–15 mg/day may be helped by the addition of azathioprine 2.0–2.5 mg/kg per day, allowing the dose of steroid to be reduced or stopped. Beneficial effects usually need 4–6 weeks to be evident. High-dose prednisolone (40 mg) given on alternate days is another approach. Surgery must be considered when medical treatment has failed.

Maintenance of remission

Sulphasalazine 2 g daily may maintain remission for many years and reduces the rates of relapse some fourfold. Dose-related side-effects of nausea, anorexia, and headache are caused by the sulphapyridine component. Skin rashes, male infertility, agranulocytosis, and Heinz-body haemolytic anaemia are not dose dependent and are usually caused by the sulphonamide. Overall, some 10–15 per cent of patients cannot tolerate sulphasalazine. Other drugs containing the essential 5-ASA component are shown in Table 3. The newer drugs are more expensive but have equal therapeutic efficacy, and are associated with fewer side-effects.

Table 3 New salicylate drugs

	Characteristics
Mesalazine preparations	
Enteric coated:	
Asacol	Coated with Eudragit, S 5-ASA released at pH 7.0
Claversal, Salofalk	Coated with Eudragit, L 5-ASA released at pH 6.5
Controlled release:	
Pentasa	Tablets comprise 5-ASA granules coated with ethyl cellulose; released with time at pH greater than 6.5
Prodrugs	
Olsalazine (Dipentum®)	Two molecules of 5-ASA linked with an azo bond, which is split by colonic bacteria
Balsalazide (Colazide®)	5-ASA linked to an amino acid via an azo bond

5-ASA, 5-aminosalicylic acid.

Diet

A lactose-free diet is important for those developing hypolactasia. Individual patients may be intolerant of dairy products, wheat, or eggs, but the majority of patients should have a normal diet.

Local complications

Perianal lesions

Fissures, perianal abscesses, or haemorrhoids may occur but extensive lesions such as fistulas are exceptional and, if they occur, suggest Crohn's disease.

Massive haemorrhage

This occurs in association with severe attacks but is rare. Intravenous corticosteroids and transfusion are usually effective but urgent colectomy may occasionally be required.

Perforation

This carries a mortality of some 16 per cent. In patients receiving corticosteroids, the physical signs of peritonitis may not be obvious, and malaise, tachycardia, and reduced or absent bowel sounds may be the only clinical features. Plain abdominal films usually show free intra-abdominal gas. Perforation may complicate an acute dilatation but can occur in its absence. Management consists of immediate intravenous fluid, electrolytes, antibiotics, and hydrocortisone, followed by urgent colectomy.

Acute dilatation

This is defined as a transverse colon with a diameter of greater than 5.0–6.0 cm with loss of haustration seen on a plain radiograph, and occurs in about 5 per cent of patients with a severe attack and can be precipitated by hypokalaemia or the administration of opiates. Physical signs are often minimal but the patient is usually obtunded, the bowel sounds reduced, and the abdomen may become distended. If the colon is already dilated on presentation, intravenous steroids should be given. Approximately 50 per cent of patients will settle on medical therapy alone but urgent surgery is required for those who continue to deteriorate or do not improve within 24 h. If the colon dilates during the course of treating a severe attack, colectomy should be done.

Strictures

These occur very rarely in patients with long-standing disease. When they are present, colonoscopy with multiple biopsies must be done as there must be a high index of suspicion of carcinoma.

Pseudopolyps

These are common and may be filiform, sessile, or may form bridges. They are not premalignant and may occasionally regress.

Colonic carcinoma

This occurs mainly in patients who have had extensive disease for more than 10 years, especially if they have had recurrent attacks. The cumulative risk for patients with extensive disease is about 7–15 per cent at 20 years, with very little risk up to 15 years of disease. Carcinoma is usually, but not always, preceded by dysplasia. This can be detected histologically and has led to the use of colonoscopic surveillance programmes for patients with long-standing ulcerative colitis affecting most or all of the colon. Provided no dysplasia is found, the examination is repeated every 1–3 years. Prophylactic colectomy is indicated if dysplasia is present, especially if it is high grade.

Surgery

Surgery is required for severe inflammation unresponsive to medical therapy; for chronic active disease; and to prevent cancer. The choice of operation is partly determined by the expertise available and the activity of disease. Complete proctocolectomy was once the best approach but restorative proctocolectomy with an ileo-anal pouch is now often the treatment of choice.

Complications of the pouch, once the immediate surgery is over, include anal stenosis, adhesion obstruction, and pouchitis. Pouchitis occurs in 10–20 per cent of patients and consists of diarrhoea with blood and evidence of inflammation on endoscopy. It usually responds to metronidazole or ciprofloxacin but occasionally requires topical treatment with corticosteroids or 5-ASA. The causes of pouchitis include ischaemia, infection, and poor emptying but the majority of pouchitis attacks are unexplained.

Course and prognosis

The majority of patients have intermittent attacks, but the duration of remissions can vary from a few weeks to many years. About 10–15 per cent will have a chronic continuous course and a few (5 per cent) will have a severe first attack requiring surgery but fewer, if any, have one attack only and never relapse. Patients with extensive disease are more likely to have a severe attack within 1 year of diagnosis than patients with distal disease and are therefore at greater risk of colectomy. However, a year from diagnosis the risk of colectomy is similar in all groups with a cumulative rate of about 1 per cent per year. Only some 30 per cent of those with initial disease limited to the rectum will develop more extensive disease over 20 years. The development of patient self-help groups has been of value in providing education and an environment in which patients can regain confidence. The mortality rate for a severe attack, including urgent surgery, should now be less than 2 per cent. In the longer term, mortality differs hardly at all from that expected in a matched healthy population.

Ulcerative colitis in pregnancy

Women with ulcerative colitis have normal fertility, are not at increased risk of having a spontaneous abortion, and there is no evidence that pregnancy is a risk factor for relapse. If they do become pregnant, the chance of having a normal baby is the same as for healthy women, and there is no good evidence that corticosteroids, 5-ASA-containing drugs, or azathioprine are harmful.

Further reading

Fiochi, C. (1998). Inflammatory bowel disease: aetiology and pathogenesis. *Gastroenterology*, **115**, 182–205.

Hanauer, S.B. (1996). Drug therapy; inflammatory bowel disease. *New England Journal of Medicine*, **334**, 841–7.

Rhodes, J.M. (1997). Mucus and inflammatory bowel disease. *Quarterly Journal of Medicine*, **90**, 79–82.

Rutgeerts, P. and Vermeire, S. (1998). Clinical value of the detection of antibodies in the serum for the diagnosis of inflammatory bowel disease. *Gastroenterology*, **115**, 1006–9.

Satsangi, J., Jewell, D.P., Rosenberg, W.M.C., and Bell, J.I. (1994). Genetics of inflammatory bowel disease. *Gut*, **35**, 696–700.

Chapter 5.16

Disorders of motility

D. L. Wingate

The physiology of gastrointestinal motility is described in OTM3 (pp. 1951–55).

Abnormal motility

Disorders of motility become apparent because of the abnormal propulsion, or lack of propulsion, of ingesta and/or secretions rather than from symptoms arising from focal lesions of the neuromuscular apparatus of the digestive tract. As there is no agreed taxonomy for these disorders, it seems reasonable to divide them into primary disorders caused by specific nerve or muscle dysfunction, and secondary disorders where derangements of motility are incidental to systemic disease. Primary disorders have been classified according to the disturbance of transit—delayed, retrograde, or accelerated—while secondary disorders have been classified in terms of the underlying pathology.

Investigation

With the exception of oesophageal disorders, standard protocols of investigation have not been established, and some of the methods that are likely to become established—such as proximal small bowel manometry—are not yet widely available.

Radiology

Except in the oesophagus, where a barium swallow is often diagnostic of a motility disorder, conventional gastrointestinal radiology is often unhelpful in excluding a motility disorder. The transit of barium through the digestive tract is dissimilar from the transit of food, except in the oesophagus. Yet, barium radiology may yield some clues: a stomach that still contains significant residue after the normal period of fasting usually indicates delayed gastric emptying, and it is sometimes possible to suggest from the rate of transit of barium that the transit of food and secretions may be abnormal.

The admixture of contrast media with food is disliked by radiologists because the mucosal pattern is impaired, but this is the simplest technique for the study of motility disorders. Barium sulphate can be incorporated into food during preparation, as a 'bariumburger', or more simply, the patient can be asked to take sips of barium sulphate between mouthfuls of food.

Solid radio-opaque markers, usually small pieces of plastic into which barium sulphate has been incorporated, are valuable for studying colonic transit. In the presence of normal gastric emptying and small-intestinal transit, it is reasonable to assume that all the opaque markers eaten with a meal will have passed into the colon after 6–8 h. Subsequent radiological study of their distribution may give useful information about colonic stasis or accelerated transit. Similar information can be obtained by making radiographs of all stool samples subsequent to marker ingestion until all the markers have been recovered.

Manometry

Oesophageal manometry using multiple sensors is the 'gold standard' for the diagnosis of disordered oesophageal motility but is, in practice, rarely required because radiology has usually provided a diagnosis, and is readily available. *Gastric manometry* as an isolated procedure is rarely helpful, but observation of motility in a selected region together with that in the adjacent viscus may be of value. Gastro-oesophageal manometry will indicate whether the swallowing reflex in the oesophagus induces the appropriate receptive relaxation in the fundus. Antroduodenal manometry will indicate the integrity of the antral contractile mechanism, and also the integrity of gastro-duodenal co-ordination. *Duodenojejunal manometry* is a reliable method for confirming the integrity of the migrating complex (MMC) and its abolition by food. Absence of the MMC, or absence of the appropriate motor response to food, indicate enteric myopathy or neuropathy. *Colonic manometry* is neither practical nor useful as a routine procedure, but anorectal manometry is helpful in the investigation of faecal incontinence.

Radionuclides

Radionuclides can be incorporated in tracer quantities into palatable meals, and a γ-camera scan allows detailed observation over prolonged periods of time. The disadvantage of these techniques is the poor resolution of the image, and the difficulty of reconstructing continuous movements from serial scans. Radionuclides offer the best available method of studying gastric emptying. Scintiscanning is the current method of choice, and is now most often used for the detection of diabetic gastroparesis and for the study of postsurgical problems. Small bowel transit can also be studied using isotopes, but the length and convolution of the small bowel do not allow for anything less than major disturbances of transit to be studied; the same is true of the colon.

Breath tests

Breath tests are based upon the principle that transformation of ingested nutrients by colonic flora will release gases that can be detected in expired air, either as hydrogen from non-absorbed carbohydrates or labelled carbon dioxide from lipids or bile acids labelled with ^{13}C or ^{14}C. These tests are used to measure orocaecal transit; alternatively, the labelled substrate can be introduced by gavage at a selected level of the gut. They have proved useful in the assessment of small bowel transit time, but their value in clinical practice is limited, because when motility is disordered, invasion of the small bowel by colonic flora is common, and will result in spurious assumptions of rapid transit from the results of a breath test.

Endoscopy

Fibreoptic endoscopy has little to offer in the study of motility. Endoscopic visualization of bile reflux is not diagnostic, as a degree of bile reflux is physiological, but its appearance should prompt the endoscopist to biopsy the antral mucosa. Endoscopic diagnosis of hiatus hernia and pyloric stenosis is possible, but dynamic tests of function are required in order to determine whether the lesion is of functional importance. It is dangerous to rely on endoscopy in the diagnosis of oesophageal dysmotility; in particular, achalasia of the cardia is easily missed.

Ultrasonographic scanning

Ultrasound can now obtain clear rapid sequential images of the antrum and pylorus under physiological conditions.

Primary disorders of motility

Gastro-oesophageal reflux, oesophageal spasm, and achalasia are described elsewhere (see Chapter 5.1).

Gastric stasis (idiopathic gastroparesis)

Gastric stasis may be caused by mechanical obstruction, or more commonly may be a sequel of abdominal surgery; it can also be caused by autonomic neuropathy. Gastric stasis can, however, also occur as a primary motility disorder, when it is known as idiopathic gastroparesis. The cause, incidence, and nature of this disorder remain matters of controversy. Idiopathic gastroparesis presents with postprandial epigastric discomfort and distension, nausea, and vomiting. If, in such patients, investigation reveals: (a) delayed emptying of solids and liquids with scintigraphy; (b) hypomotility of the gastric antrum with manometry; (c) normal motor function in the rest of the digestive tract; or (c) absence of any associated systemic disease; then most physicians would concur with a diagnosis of idiopathic gastroparesis.

In the relatively few patients in whom the diagnosis can be made with confidence, therapy is often ineffective. 'Prokinetic' drugs such as metoclopramide and cisapride may produce some symptomatic improvement, and erythromycin (a motilin agonist as well as an antibacterial drug) is sometimes helpful. There are no reliable data on the natural history of this condition.

Adynamic ileus

Acute and reversible motor failure of the whole bowel is a normal occurrence after major abdominal surgery, and is considered below. It also occurs after major traumatic injury, and in some states of metabolic imbalance; the principles of diagnosis and management are as for the postsurgical state.

Chronic idiopathic intestinal pseudo-obstruction (CIIP)

This term includes a variety of rare disorders in which the patient presents, usually in childhood or early adult life, with the clinical features of subacute or acute intestinal obstruction, but in whom no actual obstruction can be found. The cause of CIIP is an intrinsic disorder of function of the bowel, which is usually due to myopathy of the smooth muscle or neuropathy of the enteric nerves, or a combination of both. The disorder may be familial, and some varieties are associated with disorders of other smooth muscle, usually in the urinary tract. One of the more common presentations of CIIP is that of megaduodenum, which appears to be due to a localized neuropathy of the duodenum; duodenojejunostomy is indicated.

In severely affected patients, drugs intended to stimulate motility are rarely effective. Surgery should be avoided unless life is threatened or the bypass of a segment of bowel is clearly indicated. Bacterial overgrowth secondary to stasis leads to chronic malnutrition; antibacterial therapy with metronidazole or tetracycline may lead to temporary improvement. When stasis is severe, the patient may be unable to eat enough to avoid malnutrition. Nutritional support, either enterally or parenterally, may be required. When CIIP is less severe, cisapride has been shown to produce short-term benefits in some patients.

There may be many more patients with symptoms of 'functional' disorders, often resembling the irritable bowel syndrome, who probably have neuropathy or myopathy of the bowel. In them, manometry of the upper small bowel can reveal abnormalities suggesting malfunction or damage to the enteric nervous system or to the smooth muscle. The increased use of manometry and the availability of laparoscopy to obtain full-thickness bowel biopsies that allow histopathological study of nerve and muscle will help to clarify this problem.

Hirschsprung's disease

This is a localized neuropathy of the colorectum, in which there is an aganglionic segment that acts as an obstruction to the transit of faeces; proximal to the segment, the bowel is dilated. Surgery is indicated.

Accelerated transit

Intestinal hurry

Intestinal hurry is an ill-defined disorder of motility, in which the transit of ingesta through the small intestine is excessively rapid. The result is the delivery to the colon of an excess fluid and nutrient load, the latter being then subject to bacterial fermentation, which causes osmotic dilution; the outcome is diarrhoea. Damage to the intrinsic innervation of the bowel as in diabetes, or to the extrinsic innervation as a sequel of vagotomy, are known factors. Another possibility is the persistence of powerful peristaltic activity, resembling the interdigestive migrating complex, in the postprandial phase. Too little is yet known about this condition; physicians continue to encounter occasional cases of chronic 'motor diarrhoea', in which the only abnormality is excessively rapid transit of the intestine, or intestinal hurry. Specific therapy does not exist, and the only form of management is conventional antidiarrhoeal medication.

Rectal incontinence

Chronic faecal incontinence may occur in the absence of anorectal disease. The primary disorder appears to be defective tonic contraction of the internal anal sphincter with defective compensation by the external sphincter. A number of surgical procedures have been attempted in this condition, and the results have been variable.

Secondary disorders of motility

Obstructed gastric outflow causes include congenital hypertrophic pyloric stenosis, duodenal bands or stenosis and adult pyloric stenosis complicating duodenal ulcer.

In *subacute intestinal obstruction* the usual causes are intrinsic, due to inflammatory disease of the bowel (Crohn's disease, tuberculosis) or extrinsic due to tumour or fibrous adhesions. The condition usually presents as episodes of colicky pain, sometimes associated with abdominal distension and vomiting. The diagnosis is not always simple; in the absence of any known predisposing cause, exploratory laparotomy is indicated, but it is important to prevent unnecessary exploration of patients with known enteric disease.

Postoperative ileus is a neurogenic condition in which the normal electrical slow wave is present in the smooth muscle, but either, as in the colon, does not excite any action potentials or, as in the stomach or small bowel, is not associated with normal patterns of motor activity. In humans, periodic activity starts shortly after wound closure with a rapid sequence of MMCs (migrating myoelectric complexes) that slows gradually over the next 60 h. The colon is inert after surgery, but motor activity returns to the stomach almost as rapidly as in the small bowel. But, although contractions are present, they are ineffective, and it is possible that a change in non-electrogenic tone is involved. The mechanism is thought to be adrenergic postsynaptic inhibition, triggered by a variety of stimuli including peritoneal inflammation, but much the most common cause is tactile stimulation of the bowel wall during surgery. It is an inevitable sequel of resection of the digestive tract, but is much diminished after procedures such as cholecystectomy in which the bowel remains intact. Bowel sounds are absent, flatus is not passed, and there is consequent gastric stasis, which may lead to vomiting of accumulated secretions. A plain radiograph of the abdomen in the upright posture shows dilated loops of bowel with multiple fluid levels (Fig. 1).

The condition is usually self-limiting. Recovery is hastened by the correction of any fluid or electrolyte imbalance, and by measures to 'defunction' the small bowel by aspirating gastric contents and administering fluid and nutrients by the parenteral route. Occasionally, the condition is prolonged, and many drugs have been tried in an attempt to terminate prolonged ileus, but with little success. Cisapride has so far shown the most promising results with the fewest unwanted side-effects.

Gastric stasis is an expected sequel of section of the vagus nerve, and consequently occurs during the early postoperative period after a vagotomy. It rarely persists.

Biliary gastritis may occur when the functional integrity of the pylorus is compromised by surgery. The diagnosis may reasonably be made when dyspeptic symptoms persist following vagotomy and pyloroplasty, provided that: (a) active ulcer disease is excluded and biliary reflux is confirmed at endoscopy; (b) antral gastritis is confirmed on biopsy; and (c) gastric aspiration repeatedly confirms the presence of bile. Medical treatment is a matter of trial and error: some cases will respond to antacids, some to carbenoxolone, and some to drugs such as metoclopramide or cisapride. A Roux-en-Y gastrojejunostomy is the operation of choice, and has shown to be an effective, if drastic treatment, if medical treatment has failed.

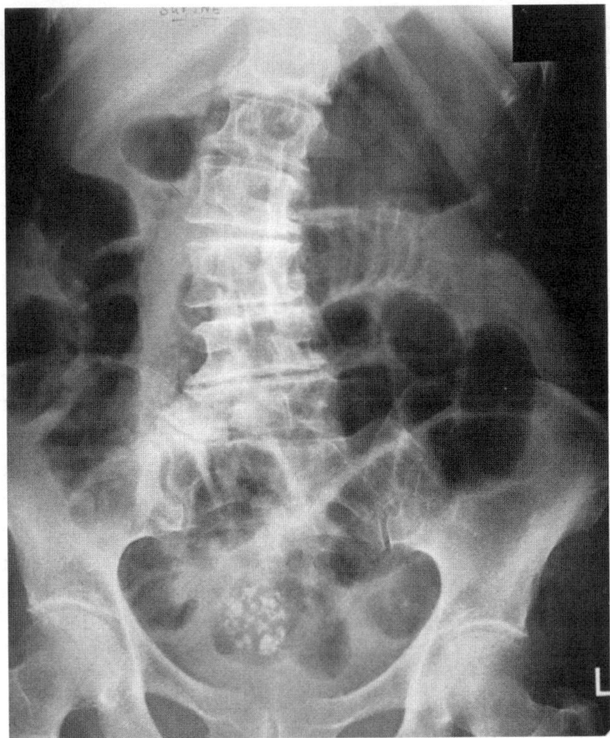

Fig. 1 Adynamic ileus of the small bowel, shown by dilated air-filled loops of bowel in this plain film taken in the supine posture. A few liquid levels were seen in an erect film taken at the same occasion. Severe degenerative changes in the spine and a calcified fibroid are also visible.
(Reproduced by courtesy of Dr Kreel.)

Gastric incontinence and the dumping syndrome

Gastric incontinence, or excessively rapid gastric emptying, is an uncommon sequel of gastric surgery that included a procedure to alter gastric drainage, usually pyloroplasty. Manifestations result from excessive input into the small bowel, of which the most common is the dumping syndrome. This includes postprandial weakness, sweating, flushing, and cramping abdominal pain. The mechanism is thought to be due to rapid delivery of hypertonic contents to the small intestine resulting in osmotic diminution of blood volume, and disturbances of carbohydrate metabolism leading to excessive insulin activity. Small, frequent meals should be substituted for large, infrequent meals and carbohydrate intake should be reduced. The addition of colloids, such as guar or pectin, is also helpful in reducing the rate of effective delivery of carbohydrate to the small intestine. If there is an associated motility disorder of the small bowel, as may occur after truncal vagotomy, gastric incontinence may lead to diarrhoea.

Where the problem cannot be managed by the adoption of a different pattern of eating, or the use of food additives, further surgery may be indicated. Reversal of a segment of proximal intestine, in combination with a Roux-en-Y procedure, may be helpful.

Diabetic gastroparesis and diarrhoea

Diabetic gastroparesis can be diagnosed by radiology, or on endoscopy after normal fasting. It may provoke vomiting in addition to abdominal distension and discomfort. Radionuclide imaging shows delayed emptying of solids rather than liquids. Manometry shows diminished or absent postprandial antral contractions, and absence of phase III of the MMC during fasting. The reported incidence depends upon whether impaired function or symptoms are used as the diagnostic criteria; functional impairment in diabetics is common, with only a relatively small proportion suffering from symptoms. Metoclopramide and cisapride have been shown to be beneficial in some cases, but the improvement is usually temporary. Erythromycin is more effective.

Diabetic diarrhoea is assumed to be due to autonomic denervation in the small bowel. It is characterized by intestinal atony, can be detected manometrically, and results in variable combinations of diarrhoea and steatorrhoea. There is no specific therapy, but as bacterial overgrowth of the small intestine may occur, antibacterial therapy sometimes affords a degree of relief.

Chagas' disease (see Chapters 16.92 and 16.93)

This is caused by *Trypanosoma cruzii.* The parasite has a predilection for smooth muscle, but it is the digestive tract that is particularly affected. T lymphocytes are sensitized by antigens from the parasite and cross-react with antigens on enteric neurones. The result is destruction of the myenteric plexuses with various manifestations; achalasia of the cardia, chronic pseudo-obstruction, and inertia of the colon may occur independently or in combination. The small bowel is relatively spared. Treatment consists of palliative surgery.

Systemic sclerosis

This may affect the digestive tract. The regions most commonly affected are the oesophagus and small intestine, where replacement of smooth muscle by collagen, and destruction of autonomic nerves may occur. These lesions may result in failure of oesophageal peristalsis, leading to dysphagia, and an adynamic small intestine in which bacterial overgrowth may occur. Manometry of the small intestine has shown diminished or absent MMC activity in affected areas.

Functional and psychomotor disturbances of motility

The classification of these conditions as motility disorders is not, for the greater part, based on scientific grounds. Their psychogenic nature is also, for the most part, an unverified assumption. Yet, of the major functions of the digestive tract—secretion, absorption, and motility—it is motility that is modulated from moment to moment by neural control. Successful management of these patients includes some common principles.

Many patients with functional disorders fear that they are suffering from some serious disease, usually malignancy. It is important that the physician make a positive diagnosis, and not a diagnosis by exclusion. Once sure that the problem is indeed functional, the physician should refrain from further investigations, and should explain to the patient that a positive diagnosis is now clear. An explanation of the problem, and any possible association with provocative factors in lifestyle, must be offered. The limitations of effective therapy must be explained, and patients must be firmly reassured that they are not suffering from the prodromal manifestations of serious organic disease. The prognosis of most functional complaints is that of little change, and this should not be concealed from the patient.

Although functional symptoms may present in a bewildering variety of permutations, certain syndromes predominate, and are more easily recognized. *Globus hystericus* presents with dysphagia at the level of the upper oesophageal sphincter usually accompanied by the persistent feeling of a lump in the throat. Investigation reveals no abnormality, but anxiety is a common feature. Because the syndrome is remarkably specific, it may be that this is a sensory disorder of motility, in which abnormal tension of voluntary muscle plays a part. As the principal fear of the patient is usually of oesophageal malignancy, adequate investigation followed by strong reassurance is required. *Rumination, or merycism*, comprises the effortless regurgitation of a meal into the mouth. Boluses of food are retropelled into the mouth at intervals during the first one or two postprandial hours, when the acidity of gastric contents is still insufficient to render them unpalatable. The retropulsion is due to a complex sequence of efforts that involve a rise in intra-abdominal pressure at the moment when the lower oesophageal sphincter opens during swallowing. Halitosis is one of the side-effects of the habit. It is important not to confuse this syndrome with normal gastro-oesophageal reflux. There is no known method of treatment beyond persuasion, which is rarely successful. *Psychogenic vomiting* which is self-induced, is a conversion symptom; that is, a symptom designed to draw attention to the patient as an invalid. Patients are commonly adolescent girls. There is usually a discrepancy between the alleged volume and frequency of vomiting, and an apparently adequate state of nutrition with unaltered body weight. *Irritable bowel syndrome* is discussed in Chapter 5.17 and *Constipation* in Chapter 5.1.

In *purgative abuse* some individuals surreptitiously take purgatives to the point where troublesome chronic diarrhoea prompts recourse to the physician. The psychopathology that leads such an individual to deny the use of purgatives is varied and the causes are often obscure. Suggestive features include hypokalaemia, finger clubbing, and persistence during abstention from food. Barium enema may reveal a colon lacking in haustrations, but the mucosal pattern is normal and this may be confirmed by endoscopic examination and biopsy. If anthracene purgatives are being used, pigmentation of the colonic mucosa may be present (melanosis coli). The abnormal outline of the colon together with the absence of mucosal damage suggests that disordered motility as well as disordered absorption may contribute to the diarrhoea.

The condition is only treatable when the purgatives are found and the patient is confronted with the evidence; this usually requires hospital admission. If the colonic innervation has been damaged by prolonged use of anthracene derivatives, such as senna, the diarrhoea may be replaced by troublesome constipation; this should be treated with osmotic purgatives. Psychiatric referral may be helpful in determining the cause of the habit.

Attacks of anorectal pain occur in some individuals without evidence of anorectal disease; the syndrome of *proctalgia fugax* is said to be more common among physicians. The cause of the attacks, which often occur at night and are sometimes associated with emotional stress, is disputed but spasm of the levator ani has been implicated. In some individuals, spasm of the anal sphincter may also play a part; in such cases, rectal examination may reveal a tight sphincter. Reassurance over the absence of organic disease is sometimes helpful, but there is no generally effective treatment.

Further reading

Kumar, D. and Wingate, D.L. (1993). *An illustrated guide to gastro-intestinal motility.* Churchill Livingstone, London.

Chapter 5.17

Functional bowel disease and irritable bowel syndrome

D. G. Thompson

Irritable bowel syndrome

This syndrome is characterized by abdominal pain associated with defecation, or a change in bowel habit together with disordered defecation and the sensation of abdominal distension. The diagnosis relies upon the presence of at least 3 months' abdominal pain that is relieved by defaecation and is associated with a change in frequency in defaecation and/or consistency of stool, together with two or more of the following symptoms: (a) altered stool frequency; (b) altered stool consistency; (c) altered ease of defaecation; (d) passage of mucus; (e) sensation of abdominal distension. The diagnosis is clinically based, and relies on history and examination. Identification of the syndrome is usually not difficult.

Clinical features

In addition to the elicitation of the above symptoms, many patients have food-related abdominal distension. Women may also complain of menstrual and bladder symptoms, and there is also an increased prevalence of psychosexual problems.

On examination palpation over the lower colon, particularly in the left iliac fossa, may produce discomfort, and a sigmoid colon containing faeces is often palpable. Similar tenderness may be present in the right iliac fossa. Rectal examination and sigmoidoscopy characteristically show pellety stools and a mucosa of normal appearance. On air insufflation during sigmoidoscopy, abdominal discomfort is often reproduced and relieved by its expulsion. Radiological and endoscopic examination of the colon is not mandatory unless there is suspicion of a structural colonic disorder, particularly neoplasia.

Pathophysiology

The hypothesis that many patients have a disorder of neuromuscular function of the gastrointestinal tract seems eminently plausible but incontrovertible evidence is lacking. Manometric studies of the colon show an increased contractile activity in patients with this syndrome, particularly after food, but the neurophysiological basis of this finding remains to be determined. Another hypothesis is that visceral sensation from the gastrointestinal tract is somehow enhanced.

There is also evidence that psychiatric disease and abnormal illness behaviour are more prevalent in patients with irritable bowel syndrome, but, the relation between the psychological problem and any neuromuscular abnormality remains uncertain.

Diet has been suggested as a pathogenic factor, because irritable bowel syndrome is uncommon in those parts of the world where a high-fibre diet is consumed. Faecal bulk can be increased by increasing fibre ingestion and some symptoms are improved, but studies of fibre intake and symptom development do not show a clear causal relation. True food allergy is readily distinguishable from irritable bowel by its extraintestinal symptoms and by a clear relation between ingestion of the food and symptom development. More subtle forms of intolerance (e.g. lactose intolerance, fructose intolerance) that produce gut symptoms without an accompanying immune response are much more difficult to recognize.

Functional bowel disease

Functional abdominal bloating

This is a disorder characterized by symptoms of abdominal fullness or distension, awareness of audible bowel sounds, and excessive flatus for at least 3 months without any evidence of either maldigestion and malabsorption or excessive consumption of poorly absorbed fermentable carbohydrate. This seems to be a variant of irritable bowel syndrome. As in irritable bowel syndrome, the prevalence of psychological disorders is high.

Functional constipation

This is defined as persistently difficult, infrequent defaecation, or the sensation of incomplete defaecation. The criteria required are two or more of the following for at least 3 months: straining at defaecation at least a quarter of the time; lumpy or hard stools at least a quarter of the time; the sensation of incomplete evacuation at least a quarter of the time; two or fewer bowel movements per week. Evidence of diabetes, hypothyroidism, and hypercalcaemia must also be sought.

The diagnosis is based on history and examination designed to exclude the possibility of more serious colonic disease, particularly cancer. It is important to enquire about immobility, concomitant drug therapy (particularly opiate analgesia), and a low roughage diet.

An abnormality of pelvic-floor relaxation on attempted defaecation is an unusual but important cause of constipation that should be suspected in those individuals who feel the need to defecate but cannot expel faeces despite severe straining. The absence of perineal descent on straining or coughing is a simple indicator of pelvic-floor dysfunction, while descent below the level of the ischial tuberosities indicates pelvic-floor weakness. Sigmoidoscopy identifies the presence of formed faeces, and excludes faecal impaction and obstruction of the lower colon.

A plain abdominal radiograph may confirm the presence of faecal material throughout the colon and indicate the diameter of the small intestine and colon, which helps exclude the rare cases of intestinal pseudo-obstruction and megacolon caused by intestinal myopathies and neuropathies. Electrophysiological and radiological assessment of anorectal function is indicated if there is evidence of abnormal perineal descent or rectal prolapse, as the accurate recognition of pelvic-floor dysfunction can influence the choice of therapy.

The cause of functional constipation is uncertain. In the mildest cases, dietary-fibre deficiency may be relevant; although, in the more severely affected patients, fibre supplementation does not abolish the problem and may even worsen it. An abnormality of colonic enteric nerves or muscle may be found, but for the great majority, no structural abnormality has been identified.

In a proportion of patients, almost invariably female, defaecatory dysfunction appears to be the major factor with a failure of relaxation in appropriate pelvic-floor muscles on attempted stool expulsion. This appears to be a 'learned' phenomenon with a psychophysiological aetiology. In other patients, low tone in the pelvic floor and rectal prolapse appear to be the result of damage to the pudendal nerve from straining at stool.

In some severely affected women, there is a relation between symptoms and the luteal phase of the menstrual cycle, which has led to the unproven suggestion of a sex-hormonal aetiology.

Functional diarrhoea

This is defined as the frequent passage of unformed stool without the presence of other features of irritable bowel syndrome. The diagnosis depends on the presence of two or more of the following findings for at least 3 months: unformed stool for more than three-quarters of the time; three or more bowel movements per day for more than half the time; increased stool weight of greater than 200 g/day. The diagnosis is achieved by exclusion of such conditions as inflammatory bowel disease, secretory diarrhoea, malabsorption, pancreatic insufficiency, gluten sensitivity, chronic infection, or laxative abuse.

Functional diarrhoea is assumed to be a disorder of neuroenteric function. In favour of this assertion are the findings of accelerated upper-intestinal transit following ingestion of a meal, and reduced rectal compliance.

Functional abdominal pain

The term refers to frequent, recurrent, or continuous abdominal pain for at least 6 months together, without relation between pain and recognizable events such as eating, defaecation, or menstruation, and in the absence of evidence of organic disease. Most of these patients exhibit chronic illness behaviour.

Management of functional bowel diseases

A review of 43 randomized, double-blind, placebo-controlled trials for the treatment of irritable bowel syndrome concluded that none offered evidence that any therapy was effective. In most trials the placebo responses were very high, usually up to 50 per cent.

What can be done to help patients with functional bowel disease? A principal task is explanation and reassurance. Attention to the patient's psychological state is important, as mood is a powerful modulator of symptom severity. In more severe cases, psychological treatment using a variety of methods, including 'dynamic psychotherapy', has been found to provide greater improvement than drug therapy alone.

In less severe cases, attention to treatment of symptoms is usually the approach taken. In patients with predominant constipation, supplementary dietary fibre and additional, poorly absorbed fermentable carbohydrates (e.g. pulses) increase faecal bulk, soften the stool, and may ease defaecatory difficulties. Wherever possible, long-term use of stimulant laxatives is best avoided because such drugs may themselves damage the colonic enteric–neural function. Osmotic laxatives and enemas are the mainstay of therapy.

For the patient who is unable to relax musculature of the pelvic floor on attempted defaecation, a variety of biofeedback techniques are now available. Success is high in those able to comply. Relaxation therapy, in particular hypnosis, also seems to provide benefit in those individuals who are prepared to participate.

For patients with diarrhoea-predominant symptoms, the size of and timing of meals may influence the frequency of the diarrhoea. Poorly absorbed foods such as fermentable carbohydrates are best taken in moderation. In the more persistent cases, symptoms can be improved by antidiarrhoeal agents, administered before the meal rather than after it.

In patients with pain-predominant symptoms, opiate-derivative analgesics are unlikely to help in the long term and may exacerbate symptoms because of their constipating effects. Antidepressants in low doses or 'antispasmodics' (e.g. hyoscine butyl bromide) are commonly prescribed, but a beneficial effect has yet to be proven.

On rare occasions, subtotal colectomy and ileorectal anastomosis will provide marked symptomatic benefit in severe, slow-transit constipation.

Further reading

Christensen, J. (1992). Pathophysiology of the irritable bowel syndrome. *Lancet*, **ii**, 1444–7.

Lynn, R.B. and Friedman, L.S. (1993). Irritable bowel syndrome. *New England Journal of Medicine*, **329**, 1940–5.

Schuster, M.N. (1993). Irritable bowel syndrome. In *Gastrointestinal disease* (ed. M.H. Sliesinger and Fordran), (5th edn), pp. 917–33. W.B. Saunders, Philadelphia.

Chapter 5.18

Colonic diverticular disease

N. J. McC. Mortensen and M. G. W. Kettlewell

Diverticula can be found throughout the gastrointestinal tract, but are seen most commonly in the sigmoid and descending colon.

Epidemiology

The prevalence of colonic diverticula increases with age in the UK and Australia, where they are rare in those under 30 years of age but occur in more than 50 per cent of those over 70; but colonic diverticulosis is very rare in African and Asian countries and right-sided disease predominates in Japan. Migration studies have shown that these differences are not genetic. Patients presenting with complicated diverticular disease have a low dietary-fibre intake, while vegetarians have a low incidence of the disease; but in spite of the introduction of high-fibre diets, there is no evidence that the incidence of acute diverticulitis is declining.

Aetiology

The development of diverticula can be ascribed to a lifelong diet deficient in dietary fibre. Modern, fibre-deficient diets give rise to stiff, viscous stools that need high intracolonic pressures to propel them. High luminal pressures cause a protrusion of the mucosa through vulnerable points in the sigmoid and descending colon, usually at the site where colonic blood vessels penetrate the wall.

Changes in the colon wall also play a part. With age, and following episodes of diverticulitis, the colonic wall becomes stiff and less distensible, aggravating the effects of raised intracolonic pressure. Diabetic patients are prone to diverticular disease at an earlier stage, suggesting a defect in glycolysation of colonic collagen with advancing age. In Ehlers–Danlos syndrome or Marfan's disease, diverticula are also seen at an unusually early age. It is not known why some diverticula and not others become symptomatic.

Pathology

The fully developed diverticulum consists of mucosa, connective tissue, and peritoneum. Thickening of the circular and longitudinal muscle narrows the colonic lumen and shortens the sigmoid like a concertina to give a saw-tooth appearance on barium enema. The diverticula occur as slit-like apertures between the muscle clefts.

Table 1 Indications for surgery

Sepsis	*Fistulae*
• Recurrent diverticulitis	• Colovesical
• Perforated diverticulitis	• Colovaginal
• Purulent peritonitis	• Ileocolic
• Faecal peritonitis	
• Pelvic or paracolic abscess	*Major haemorrhage*
Colonic obstruction	
• Inflammatory stricture	
• Fibrotic stricture	
• Suspected malignancy	

Inflammation in diverticular disease is the result of infection around diverticula, which spreads within the pericolic fat to form a dissecting abscess. Usually a single diverticulum is the cause of a pericolic abscess, perhaps initiated by the presence of a faecolith. Involvement of the peritoneum results in local peritonitis, which may become generalized in the event of a perforation. This may also give rise to intra-abdominal abscesses or fistulae to the bladder, small bowel, vagina, or uterus. Repeated episodes of diverticulitis lead to a contracted, narrowed sigmoid colon surrounded by fibrous tissue. Bleeding in diverticular disease can often be traced to an infected diverticulum, with erosion of a vessel in its wall or the formation of granulation tissue inside the diverticulum, which then bleeds.

Clinical features

Diverticula are usually discovered incidentally. Only some 10 per cent produce symptoms, and about 1 per cent require surgery.

Uncomplicated diverticular disease

Pain can be felt along the course of the colon, particularly over the sigmoid, and is often accompanied by a change in bowel habit with the passage of broken, pellety stools after considerable straining. The passage of blood with an unformed stool is unusual and should alert to the possibility of other pathology.

All patients should have sigmoidoscopy in addition to a barium enema to exclude a rectal or sigmoid carcinoma. A high-fibre diet should be recommended, including wholemeal bread, whole-wheat breakfast cereals, rough porridge or muesli, and fresh fruit and vegetables daily. A good clinical response is usually achieved by including two tablespoons of bran with the morning cereal, but about half the patients will experience gaseous distension or cramps on starting the high-fibre diet.

In patients with pain, antispasmodics such as mebeverine may be useful, and in a minority with repeated severe attacks an elective resection is indicated (Table 1). This is probably more effective than sigmoid myotomy but the latter may still be useful in some elderly or obese patients.

Complicated diverticular disease

Acute diverticulitis

Pain is felt over the left lower abdomen, and the patient may have a pyrexia, malaise, anorexia, and nausea. The white blood count is raised.

Treatment is with rest, antibiotics, usually cefuroxime 750 mg and metronidazole 500 mg 8-hourly, and analgesia. Most cases settle and the diagnosis can be confirmed after 2–3 weeks by barium enema. A narrow segment can sometimes be difficult to distinguish from a carcinoma and any doubtful cases can be clarified by subsequent colonoscopy. If symptoms fail to resolve, or recur, resection of the sigmoid colon may be necessary.

Diverticular abscess

Acute diverticulitis can lead to a local peritonitis with abscess formation, either in the paracolic or pelvic area. There may be a palpable mass and a swinging fever. When in doubt the diagnosis can be confirmed by ultrasound or computed tomography with rectal contrast.

It is wise to let an abscess localize while giving antibiotics, and analgesia. Some abscesses will be amenable to drainage by direct incision. More complicated collections are best drained by computed tomography guided aspiration or drain placement. There is rarely need for a proximal transverse colostomy. If drainage persists, an elective sigmoid colectomy with primary anastomosis can be done at a later time.

Perforated diverticulitis

The clinical picture is of severe intraperitoneal sepsis with toxaemia, ileus and abdominal pain, and septicaemia will often follow. Emergency laparotomy is almost always required, as well as antibiotic therapy—again cefuroxime and metronidazole. A Hartmann's procedure—removing the diseased sigmoid, oversewing the distal rectum, and bringing out an end colostomy, is now the most frequently used procedure (Fig. 1).

Faecal peritonitis is a catastrophic complication with a mortality of about 50 per cent particularly in the elderly. A diverticulum ruptures, liberating quantities of faeces into the peritoneal cavity. Rapid and severe shock with septicaemia ensues. Energetic resuscitation is necessary, followed promptly by Hartmann's operation.

Intestinal obstruction

Recurrent inflammation with fibrosis and muscular hypertrophy can lead to progressive stenosis and colonic obstruction, which is usually chronic but may present acutely. Conservative treatment is worth trying at first, provided a carcinoma has been excluded. With the aid of a stool softener the symptoms may resolve and the stricture gradually dilate. If these measures fail, a resection will be necessary.

Small-bowel obstruction

Sometimes a complication of acute diverticulitis, as the bowel may adhere to the inflammatory mass.

Colonic fistulae

A colovesical fistula usually presents with recurrent urinary-tract infections together with pneumaturia or faecuria. Carcinoma and Crohn's disease should be excluded. After removal of the affected sigmoid the fistula into the bladder is closed and urethral catheter drainage continued for a week.

Fistulae may also occur between the sigmoid and vagina, uterus, ureter, and ileum. They seldom heal spontaneously but do not always give rise to disabling symptoms. Sigmoid colectomy as a one-stage procedure is the best option, and colostomy is rarely required.

Haemorrhage

Major haemorrhage is uncommon. It is usually self-limiting, only requiring transfusion and supportive measures. It is vital to exclude other sources of bleeding by barium enema or colonoscopy. The source of a persistent major bleed must be sought urgently and selective angiography while the patient is bleeding is essential. Blind colonic resections have a particularly poor record and if the site of bleeding has still not been located, on-table colonic lavage via the appendix stump and intraoperative colonoscopy will usually target the bleeding segment.

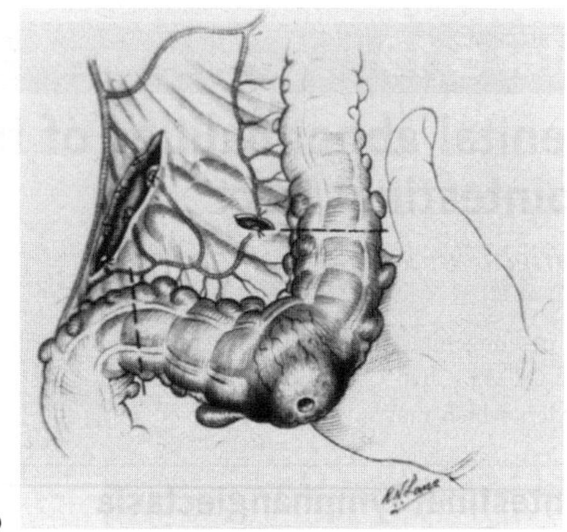

(a)

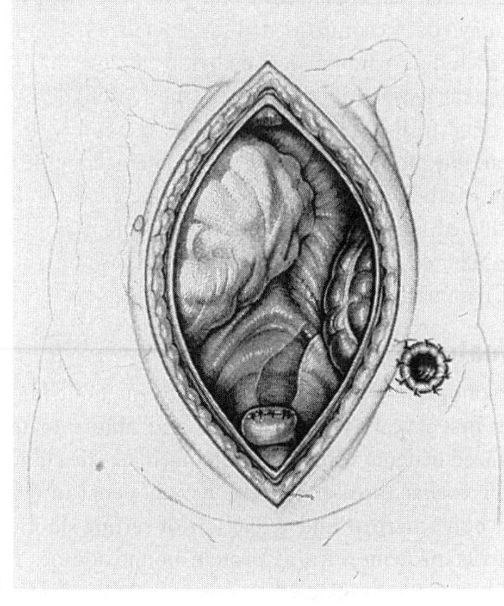

(b)

Fig. 1 (a) The area of sigmoid colon resected for perforated diverticular disease. (b) Hartmann's operation—the sigmoid colon has been resected, the rectum oversewn, and a left iliac-fossa colostomy fashioned.

Further reading

Cook, T.A. and Mortensen, N.J.McG. (1997). Diverticular disease of the colon. *Prescribers Journal*, 37, 213–29.

Chapter 5.19

Congenital abnormalities of the gastrointestinal tract

V. M. Wright and J. A. Walker-Smith

A number of congenital conditions present and are dealt with in infancy (see OTM3, Chapter 14.15). Here the account is confined to those disorders which may give rise to problems in adult life.

Small-intestinal lymphangiectasia

This can be a primary congenital abnormality or secondary to some other disease such as constrictive pericarditis. The primary abnormality may be accompanied by generalized lymphatic abnormalities including lymphoedema, chylous ascites, and hypoplasia of the peripheral lymphatic system, but the lymphatic abnormality may be confined to the small bowel and its mesentery. It is usually, but not invariably, accompanied by hypoproteinaemic oedema. The pathogenesis of the hypoproteinaemia has been attributed to the rupture of dilated lymphatic channels or to protein exudation from intestinal capillaries via an intact epithelium, where there is obstruction of lymphatic flow.

Clinical features

It is a rare condition, which may present throughout life but most often in the first 2 years with diarrhoea and failure to thrive and, later, generalized oedema with hypoproteinaemia. The clinical picture may resemble coeliac disease. There is lymphopenia in the presence of a normal bone marrow and reduction of serum albumin, serum IgG, and carrier proteins such as protein-bound iodine. The severe protein loss may be accompanied by enteric calcium loss, leading to hypocalcaemia. Steatorrhoea is common.

Diagnosis

Diagnosis is made by showing the characteristic lymphatic abnormality on small intestinal biopsy, but the lesion is patchy. One negative biopsy does not exclude the diagnosis. Barium studies in most cases show coarse mucosal folds.

Pathology

There is considerable variation in the distribution of the lymphatic abnormality along the length of the small intestine. Dilated lacteals may occur irregularly along the small bowel and there may be gross dilatation of lymphatics projecting into the lumen. Lymphatic proliferation and dilatation may also occur within the mesentery, as well as the serosal, muscular, and submucosal layers of the small-intestinal wall, and extend into the lymph nodes and occupy part of the nodal tissue.

Treatment

This is usually dietetic, as the lymphangiectasia is rarely localized enough to allow surgical excision to effect a permanent cure. Long-chain fat in the diet should be limited; this leads to a reduction in the volume of intestinal lymph and in the pressure in the dilated lymphatics. Albumin infusions are of little value in management as their benefit is so transitory. Steroids have been advocated but there is little evidence to justify their use. Continued adherence to a strict diet, at least through puberty, is recommended. Some dietetic management may usually need to be permanent.

Meckel's diverticulum

This diverticulum is the vestigial remnant of the vitellointestinal duct, and is located in the distal ileum within 100 cm of the ileocaecal valve. It is always antemesenteric. Although most people who have such a diverticulum are asymptomatic, complications may present in a variety of ways. In children these chiefly arise in association with the presence of ectopic gastric mucosa in the diverticulum. Other ectopic tissue, for example pancreatic tissue and colonic mucosa, may be found in some cases.

Clinical features

Rectal bleeding is the main symptom. This is usually the passage of bright blood rather than tarry melaena stools. Typically, the stool is at first dark in colour but later bright red. Bleeding may be acute, with shock requiring urgent blood transfusion, or it may be chronic. Most often bleeding from Meckel's diverticulum is associated with ulceration of the small bowel adjacent to ectopic gastric mucosa.

Small-intestinal obstruction may be due to a volvulus or an intussusception with the diverticulum as the leading part. Acute diverticulitis occurs and may produce a picture indistinguishable from acute appendicitis.

Diagnosis and management

When rectal bleeding occurs, other causes such as anal fissure, intussusception, peptic ulcer, oesophagitis, and colonic polyps must be considered.

Barium follow-through is usually unrewarding but a small bowel enema, may be more successful. A technetium scan is usually the most important investigation; technetium-99m concentrates in the gastric mucosa. When it is given intravenously, ectopic gastric mucosa appears as an abnormal localization on abdominal imaging with a gamma-camera. This technique should lead to earlier and more accurate diagnosis, but a negative result in a child with severe bleeding should not deter a surgeon from proceeding with a diagnostic laparotomy, which remains the final diagnostic test.

Congenital short intestine

There is a syndrome of congenital short intestine in association with malrotation and clinical features similar to those that follow massive intestinal resection. There is also another syndrome of congenital short intestine in association with pyloric hypertrophy and malrotation. This latter is due to an absence or diminution of argyrophil ganglion cells in the small-intestinal wall. These cells normally control peristalsis. In their absence, smooth muscle of the small-intestinal wall contracts spontaneously and rhythmically, but segmentation is not co-ordinated, the food bolus does not move forward, and there is work hypertrophy of smooth muscle.

Both syndromes are rare and often only diagnosed at laparotomy.

Hirschsprung's disease

In this condition, ganglion cells are absent in the bowel wall. The distal rectum is always aganglionic and the aganglionosis extends proximally for a variable distance. In 70 per cent the rectosigmoid is involved, in 20 per cent the aganglionosis extends proximal to the sigmoid for a variable distance up the colon, and in 10 per cent the aganglionosis extends into the small intestine. The aganglionic bowel is incapable of co-ordinated peristalsis and passively constricts, resulting in a mechanical obstruction. The incidence is approximately 1 in 5000 births.

Clinical features

The most important association is with Down syndrome. The diagnosis is aganglionic in infancy or soon after and initial treatment is to form a colostomy of the aganglionic bowel to allow the dilated hypertrophied proximal bowel to recover. Definitive surgery by excision of the aganglionic bowel follows, with anastomosis of ganglionic bowel to the anus. Long-term complications include faecal and urinary incontinence and impotence, but these are rare.

Further reading

See OTM3, Chapter 14.15.

Chapter 5.20

Tumours of the gastrointestinal tract

M. L. Clark, I. C. Talbot, H. J. W. Thomas, and C. B. Williams

Oesophageal tumours (see also Chapter 5.3)

Benign

Leiomyomas are the most common benign tumours of the oesophagus. They are often discovered incidentally or at autopsy. Mucosal ulceration is rare so that bleeding is uncommon. Only tumours that are large and cause dysphagia should be removed, by enucleation rather than resection. Rarely, fibrovascular polyps, lipomas, and other benign tumours are found.

Malignant

The majority of malignant tumours of the oesophagus have, until recently, been squamous carcinomas. However, in parallel with nutritional and other factors, the incidence of adenocarcinoma is now probably greater than of squamous carcinoma, at least in white men. The reasons for this recent change are complex and seem to be related to overnutrition, increasing gastro-oesophageal reflux, and Barrett's oesophagus, together with increased levels of gastric acidity associated with a falling incidence of *Helicobacter* infection.

Other malignant tumours—malignant melanomas, secondary tumours, plasmacytomas are rare. Gastrointestinal Kaposi's sarcoma is found in 50–60 per cent of patients dying with AIDS, but are particularly found in the mouth and hypopharynx. These tumours rarely lead to symptoms and do not require treatment.

Epidemiological and aetiological factors

Squamous carcinoma

In the UK the overall incidence of oesophageal carcinoma ranges from 5 to 10 cases per 100 000 people or 2.5 per cent of all malignant disease. The incidence varies considerably throughout the world, and there are sharp differences between regions only a few hundred miles apart.

Alcohol and tobacco consumption have been strongly implicated as aetiological factors. In Chinese populations there is an association with pickled vegetables which contain high concentrations of *N*-nitroso compounds.

There is an increased incidence of malignancy in patients with oesophageal strictures due to ingestion of corrosives as well as in patients who have been treated with radiation therapy. An increased incidence also occurs in patients with achalasia, or with coeliac disease, and the Patterson–Kelly (Plummer–Vinson) syndrome, is historically associated with carcinoma of the oesophagus.

There is no evidence of an inherited basis except in the rare skin disease tylosis palmae, which is characterized by hyperkeratosis of the palms and soles and in which oesophageal carcinomas affect up to 40 per cent of patients.

Adenocarcinoma

The large majority of these tumours arise in the columnar-lined epithelium of the lower oesophagus or occasionally in islands of columnar epithelium higher up (Barrett's oesophagus). This columnization arises from long-standing reflux, with an estimated 30–40 times increased risk of developing cancer. Adenocarcinoma of the gastric cardia with involvement of the lower oesophagus has become an increasing cause of malignant oesophageal obstruction. An unfortunate feature of columnar-lined oesophagus is that symptoms such as dysphagia are usually absent, even when there is severe and extensive Barrett's including dysplasia or even early carcinoma.

Clinical features

The median age of presentation is 68 years for both males and females. The dysphagia of malignancy is progressive and unrelenting; initially involving solids but eventually liquids too. Impact pain after eating may occur but more persistent pain in the front and back of the chest suggests infiltration and is a bad prognostic feature. Loss of appetite and weight loss are often present. Metastases are found at diagnosis in about 50 per cent of cases. The earliest spread is through the mediastinal tissues around the oesophagus but subsequently downwards to the gastric glands and to the liver. Direct spread involves the bronchi, lungs, and pleura, but also the aorta. Perforation and local sepsis, result in tracheo-oesophageal or other fistulae, or mediastinitis. Involvement of the recurrent laryngeal nerve causes hoarseness. By the time there is difficulty in swallowing saliva, cough, and other features of aspiration are common and may result in terminal bronchopneumonia. Anaemia may be present and palpable lymph nodes can be found in the neck.

Diagnosis

Barium swallow gives an accurate picture of the extent of any deformity, but endoscopy allows biopsies to be taken and, if appropriate, palliative dilatation or intubation performed. Combining brush cytological samples with biopsies will produce a diagnostic accuracy rate of 95 per cent. In tumours of the distal oesophagus it is important to differentiate between squamous or adenocarcinoma as the latter does not respond to radiotherapy.

A computed tomography (CT) scan will show the volume of the tumour and detect spread outside the oesophagus. Endoscopic ultrasound has an accuracy of nearly 90 per cent for assessing depth of infiltration and 80 per cent for staging lymph-node involvement.

Treatment

The overall results are poor. Surgery over the last 10 years has produced no improvement in long-term prognosis despite postoperative mortality having been reduced by half. Overall, of 100 patients presenting with an oesophageal cancer, approximately 50 per cent have resectable disease. Seven per cent of these will die postoperatively and of the remaining approximately 40 patients, 25 will survive 1 year, 10 will survive a second year, and 10 will survive into the fifth year.

It is important to differentiate between tumours that have not completely infiltrated the oesophageal wall and those that have spread; the latter are inoperable and patients should, if possible, be spared surgery.

Adjuvant chemo- or radiotherapy has not improved survival, but uncontrolled trials for radiotherapy alone have given results similar to those of surgery for squamous carcinoma.

Palliation can be achieved by stenting, laser photocoagulation, or ethanol injection to induce tumour necrosis with comparable results.

Stomach tumours

Benign tumours and polyps

The most common benign tumour is a leiomyoma. Most are asymptomatic but there can be superficial ulceration and gastrointestinal haemorrhage. Local removal is curative. Other benign gastric tumours include angiomas and gastric carcinoids.

Gastric polyps are uncommon and usually found by chance. The most common are cystic fundic gland polyps but regenerative or hyperplastic polyps are also frequent. None of these have malignant potential. They are often multiple and after biopsy can be safely left alone. Adenomatous polyps of the stomach are much less common and have a villous or tubulovillous architecture. There is no evidence to suggest that gastric cancers commonly arise from pre-existing adenomas, but these lesions should be removed endoscopically because of that possible risk. Large pedunculated polyps may bleed or obstruct outflow.

Carcinoma of the stomach

The occurrence of gastric carcinoma varies within and between countries. There is a high incidence in Japan, parts of Chile, and the mountainous regions of Costa Rica but a low one in the US. Gastric cancer is the sixth most common fatal malignancy in the UK and accounts for about 10 per cent of deaths from malignant disease. Data are accumulating that link *Helicobacter pylori* infection to an increased risk of carcinoma of the body and antrum of the stomach and WHO now accept *H. pylori* as a class I carcinogen. The relative risk in studies in the UK and USA is some two- to sixfold. Figure 1 outlines the pathological changes which may be involved.

Dietary factors that have been implicated include spiced or pickled foods, salt, and alcohol, as well as a diet low in fresh fish and vegetables. Levels of nitrate ingestion are high in areas of high incidence. Nitrates can be converted to nitrosamines by bacteria at neutral pH and nitrosamines are known to be carcinogenic in animals.

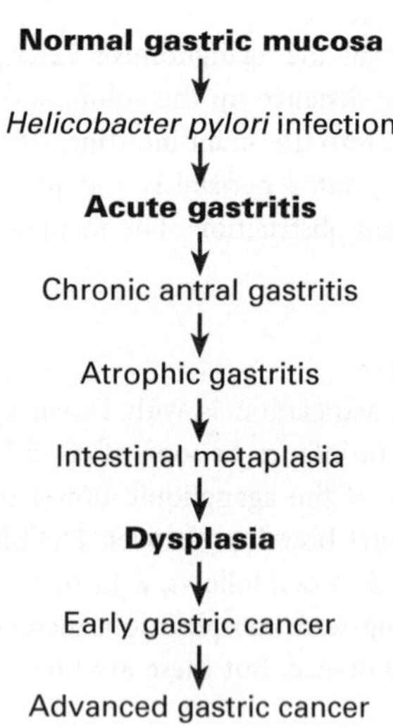

Fig. 1 Flow chart of pathogenesis of gastric cancer.

Nitrosamines are present in the stomach of patients with achylorhydria, who also have an increased risk. Smoking may account for the age-related increase in gastric cancer. Further evidence of genetic susceptibility is needed in view of the association of gastric carcinoma with blood group A.

Precancerous conditions

Patients with *pernicious anaemia* have a two to three times increased incidence of stomach cancer but surveillance programmes are unwarranted as the overall incidence is still low. *Benign gastric ulcers* are not premalignant, but it can be very difficult to differentiate between some benign and malignant ulcers, and malignant ulcers can heal on medical treatment. *Intestinal metaplasia* occurs more frequently in stomachs that contain a carcinoma, and in some early cases of carcinoma there appears to be a transition between metaplastic mucosa and carcinoma. Most cases of metaplasia develop after chronic, active gastritis, often secondary to infection with *H. pylori*. *Gastric resection* may result in metaplasia and chronic active gastritis and in most series there is an increased incidence of gastric carcinoma. Biliary reflux and/or *H. pylori* infection may be involved.

Screening

As resection of early gastric cancer results in 5-year survival rates of about 90 per cent, it has been suggested that mass screening might be introduced more widely, but on present evidence, screening is unwarranted, except possibly for individuals with the precancerous conditions discussed above. It seems doubtful, however, even in this group whether screening asymptomatic subjects can be justified.

Clinical features

There may be no symptoms in early cases, although weight loss may be a feature. The most common is epigastric pain, which may be relieved by food and antacids. In those with advanced diseases there is also nausea, anorexia, and weight loss with vomiting a problem in some half of the patients. Dysphagia can occur with tumours involving the fundus. Gross haematemesis is unusual but anaemia from occult blood loss is frequent. Patients can also present with abdominal swelling due to ascites or jaundice due to liver involvement. Metastases in bone, brain, and lungs produce appropriate symptoms.

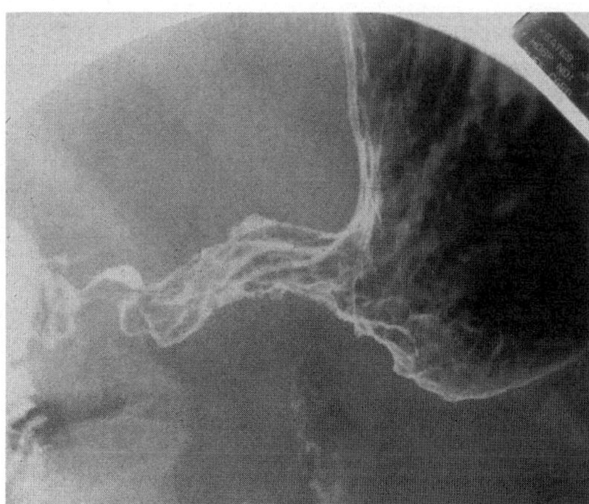

Fig. 2 Barium meal demonstrating circumferential narrowing and irregularity of the distal body and antrum of the stomach.

An epigastric mass is palpable in some 50 per cent of patients. A palpable lymph node is sometimes found in the left supraclavicular fossa (Virchow sign). Carcinoma of the stomach is the cancer most frequently associated with dermatomyositis and acanthosis nigricans.

Pathology

Gastric cancer is almost invariably adenocarcinoma. The antrum is the most frequent site but tumours arising in the cardia have increased in recent years, probably for reasons similar to those responsible for the increased incidence of oesophageal adenocarcinoma. A polypoid lesion is most common in the elderly and in high-frequency areas and may be associated with metaplasia and *H. pylori* infection. The diffuse type is composed of scattered or small clusters of cells, occurs in low-frequency areas, and in younger people; it is associated with extensive submucosal spread, which may result in the picture of 'linitis plastica' and has a worse prognosis.

Early gastric cancer is limited to the mucosa or submucosa. These cancers can be multifocal and they may spread superficially to cover a considerable area.

Diagnosis

Good-quality, double-contrast radiology (Fig. 2) is very accurate (90 per cent) but, because radiographic quality varies and because of the ability to obtain biopsy, endoscopy is the procedure of choice. However, one or more negative biopsies from the edge of an ulcer do not rule out malignancy, and it is recommended that eight to 10 biopsies be taken around the ulcer margin and from its base. Superficial brushing specimens for exfoliative cytology will further improve diagnostic accuracy. In assessing operability, CT has been disappointing and endoscopic ultrasound is probably better. Blood tests and ultrasound are used to detect secondary spread.

Treatment and prognosis

The 5-year survival rate after surgery for early gastric cancer in Japan is over 90 per cent. In more advanced cases, 5-year survival rates of 30–40 per cent have been obtained in Japan. Five-year survival rates after all resections published in English language journals from 1970 have increased from 21 to 28 per cent and after 'curative' resection from 38 to 55 per cent. More depressing is the 5-year survival rate of only 5 per cent in patients with carcinoma of the cardia.

Palliative surgery to relieve symptoms and to prevent obstruction and haemorrhage is helpful for the many patients found to be inoperable as far as a cure is concerned.

Adjuvant therapy with either chemotherapy or radiation does not produce significant improvement in survival. Chemotherapy alone for advanced disease involves new combinations of drugs introduced at regular intervals. The results show little improvement over the use of a single agent such as 5-fluorouracil and, although survival may be prolonged by a few months, the toxicity of the drugs limit their use. Cimetidine has been shown in a Danish study to improve survival and further trials with this agent are being conducted.

Other malignant tumours of the stomach

Primary lymphoma

Gastric lymphoma accounts for approximately 5 per cent of all gastric malignancies. It is usually a non-Hodgkin's lymphoma of the B-cell type arising from mucosa-associated lymphoid tissue (**MALT**). MALT tumours are associated with *H. pylori* gastritis. The clinical features are indistinguishable from those of other benign or malignant lesions of the stomach. Treatment is surgical combined with chemotherapy or radiotherapy; chemotherapy is used for widespread disease, although some MALT tumours respond to *H. pylori* eradication. The 5-year survival prognosis varies from 75 to 95 per cent, depending on whether the lymphoma is low or high grade.

Small-bowel tumours

Only 3–6 per cent of all gastrointestinal tumours and fewer than 1 per cent of all malignant lesions occur in the small bowel. Malignant tumours are more common than solitary benign lesions and 90 per cent of the former are symptomatic.

Benign adenomas, leiomyomas, and lipomas are the three most common solitary benign tumours. They are frequently asymptomatic, but pain can be due to intussusception. Insidious loss of blood leading to anaemia is another frequent manifestation. Haemangiomas are rare, occurring as small polyps found on angiography or by pre- or perioperative fibreoptic endoscopy of the small intestine.

Adenocarcinoma is the most common malignancy of the small intestine. It is found most often in the duodenum, especially the periampullary region, and jejunum. Carcinoid tumours form the next major group, while lymphoma and smooth-muscle tumours make up the remainder, the former two most often in the ileum. The small intestine may also be involved secondarily.

Lymphoma

Some 20–30 per cent of gastrointestinal non-Hodgkin's lymphomas occur in the small bowel in patients in the developed world, whereas in the Middle East over half of the lymphomas occur in the small bowel. Most tumours are of B-cell type, tending to form annular or polypoid masses in the distal ileum.

In coeliac disease and dermatitis herpetiformis there is an increased incidence of lymphoma, which is often T cell in origin (see Chapter 3.29). A tumour similar to Burkitt's lymphoma also occurs and commonly affects the terminal ileum of children in North Africa and the Middle East. Small-intestinal lymphoma is a frequent manifestation in patients with AIDS.

Immunoproliferative small-intestine disease (IPSID)

This is a B-cell lymphocyte disorder in which there is proliferation of plasma cells in the lamina propria of the upper small bowel, which produce truncated monoclonal heavy chains but lack associated light chains. IPSID occurs usually in countries surrounding the Mediterranean but it has also been found in other developing countries, and has recently been documented in the developed world. IPSID affects predominantly people in lower socio-economic groups in areas with poor hygiene. It presents as a malabsorptive syndrome, associated with diffuse lymphoid infiltration of the small bowel and neighbouring lymph nodes, and responds to tetracycline. This progresses in some cases to an immunoblastic lymphoma.

Adenocarcinoma

Patients with *familial adenomatous polyposis* may have polyps throughout their small gut, particularly in the periampullary region of the duodenum (Plate 1). About 12 per cent of such patients eventually develop an upper gastrointestinal malignancy, usually an adenocarcinoma of the ampulla of Vater. Screening by duodenoscopy has been suggested.

Coeliac disease is associated with an increased incidence of adenocarcinoma of the small bowel (as well as lymphoma) and an increase in incidence of all malignancies throughout the gastrointestinal tract and elsewhere in the body. There is some evidence that a gluten-free diet protects against the development of malignancy.

Crohn's disease of long duration is associated with an increased risk of adenocarcinoma of the small bowel.

Clinical features and diagnosis

Malignant tumours present with abdominal pain, anorexia, weight loss, anaemia, and diarrhoea. Most lesions can be detected on small-bowel follow-through but it is sometimes necessary to use a small bowel enema as the lesion can be extremely small. CT and ultrasound will demonstrate the bowel-wall thickening and the involvement of the mesentery and lymph nodes. Biopsy using a flexible enteroscope allows assessment of histology.

Treatment

Adenocarcinoma is treated surgically with wide excision. The 5-year survival is 10–20 per cent. Evidence for efficacy of radio- or chemotherapy is minimal. Lymphoma is also treated by surgical excision, with radiotherapy and/or chemotherapy. No universal treatment regimen for small-gut lymphoma has yet been agreed. The 5-year survival for T-cell lymphomas is only about 25 per cent; for B-cell tumours it varies from 75 to 50 per cent, depending on grade.

Colon polyps and polyposis syndromes

Colorectal polyps (Plate 2) may be single, occur together in small numbers, or may carpet the colon in hundreds or thousands as part of the polyposis syndromes. The majority prove to be adenomas with malignant potential. Histological examination is essential. Table 1 gives a general classification.

Table 1 Colonic polyps and polyposis: a classification

Pathogenesis	Polyps	Polyposis
Metaplastic	Hyperplastic	Hyperplastic polyposis
Inflammatory	Inflammatory	Inflammatory polyposis
Lymphatic	Benign lymphoid	Malignant lymphomatous polyposis
Traumatic	Mucosal prolapse syndrome	Inflammatory cap polyp polyposis (Plate 3)
Neoplastic	Adenoma	Familial adenomatous polyposis if >100
Hamartomatous	Juvenile Peutz–Jeghers	Juvenile polyposis Peutz–Jeghers syndrome Cronkhite–Canada syndrome
Stromal origin Type/neoplastic	Leiomyomatous polyp Lipomatous polyp	Cowden's syndrome
Hamartomatous	Vascular hamartoma Neurofibroma Ganglioneuroma	

Non-neoplastic polyps

Metaplastic (hyperplastic) polyps are the most common type seen on proctosigmoidoscopy, appearing as 2–4 mm pale shiny nodules in the rectum. They have a characteristic histological appearance with 'saw toothing' of the elongated mucosal crypts but normal-looking nuclei. These polyps have no clinical consequence, although 'mixed' polyps containing both adenomatous and hyperplastic tissue may occur. Multiple hyperplastic polyps proximal to the rectum may be associated with malignant potential and such patients need follow-up endoscopy.

Post-inflammatory polyps may be equally numerous and variable in size and shape, although classically thread-like. They are seen in the healed phase after one or more severe attacks of colitis (ulcerative colitis, Crohn's disease, schistosomiasis, etc.). Histologically, they are usually only tags covered by normal or mildly distorted epithelium.

Inflammatory polyps may be composed of granulation tissue and may cause bleeding or protein loss when large or numerous; they may require removal or biopsy for distinction from adenomas.

Hamartomatous polyps (principally juvenile or Peutz–Jeghers in type) are developmental malformations containing a disorganized mixture of normal intestinal tissues. Hamartomatous tissues have no malignant tendency but the polyps occasionally harbour a focus of dysplastic epithelium, which probably explains sporadic reports of malignancy in the stomach or colon in Peutz–Jeghers syndrome and the greater cancer risk in the colon in juvenile polyposis. Hamartomatous polyps are commonly large and stalked. Juvenile polyps show mucus-retention cysts and inflammation, whereas Peutz–Jeghers polyps have characteristic fibromuscular fronds radiating between the disorganized mucosal crypts. Juvenile polyps are a cause of bleeding in childhood. They can intussuscept and present at the anus or may be an incidental finding in middle age. Juvenile polyposis, defined as more than three to five colonic polyps (the small intestine and stomach are sometimes involved), requires endoscopic surveillance and polypectomy, and perhaps even colectomy and ileorectal anastomosis, as these patients have a considerably increased risk of colon cancer. Juvenile polyposis appears to be genetically heterogeneous, with germline mutations of the gene *SMAD4* (also know as *DPC4*) reported in some families. There is no evidence that solitary juvenile polyps have neoplastic potential and they do not require follow-up.

Hereditary mixed polyposis syndrome has been described, in which there are adenomatous, juvenile, and metaplastic polyps of the colon and an increased incidence of colorectal cancer; genetic studies have shown linkage to chromosome 6. Histologically, similar polyps occur throughout the gastrointestinal tract in the rare Cronkhite–Canada syndrome, resulting in diarrhoea and steatorrhoea associated with ectodermal abnormalities such as alopecia, nail dystrophy, and skin hyperpigmentation. Cowden's disease is an autosomal dominant predisposition to the development of multiple hamartomata. It is associated with breast and thyroid cancers and also colorectal cancer and has been shown to be caused by mutations of the *PTEN* gene.

Peutz–Jeghers syndrome of mucocutaneous pigmentation (Fig. 3) and gastrointestinal polyposis is inherited as a Mendelian dominant. The gene responsible has been identified as *LKB1*, a serine-threonine protein kinase, and presymptomatic molecular genetic diagnosis is now possible in these families. Polyps may occur anywhere in the intestine but associated malignancy is rarer in the colon than in the duodenal region and stomach. Operation may be advised if polyps over 1 cm in diameter are found in the small intestine, because there is a risk of intussusception and infarction. Gastroduodenal and colonic polyps may also bleed. They are best removed by 2-yearly snare polypectomy. It should also be noted that extragastrointestinal tumours occur with a prevalence approaching that of gastrointestinal malignancies in individuals affected by Peutz–Jeghers syndrome.

Neoplastic polyps

The majority of neoplastic polyps in the colon and rectum are adenomas. They range from the most frequent tubular adenomas, those with mixed or intermediate tubulovillous characteristics, to the rarer but larger and often sessile villous adenomas which have the greatest tendency to malignancy (Fig. 4).

Aetiological factors and pathology

Factors influencing the development of adenomas are genetic (e.g. familial adenomatous polyposis) and environmental, with dietary factors perhaps promoting the formation of carcinogens by way of changing bacterial flora and thereby their metabolic products. Adenomas are slow growing so that, although some 30 per cent of the elderly in the West have an adenoma, only 3–5 per cent develop carcinoma of the colon. All adenomas have epithelial dysplastic change of varying degree. Malignancy, more common the larger the tumour and the greater the degree of dysplasia, is diagnosed histologically, when dysplastic epithelium has crossed the muscularis mucosae (Fig. 5 and Table 2).

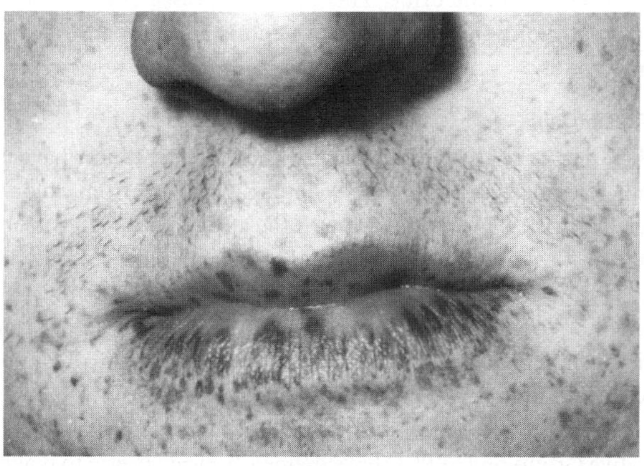

Fig. 3 Peutz–Jeghers patient showing characteristic lip pigmentation.

Tubular adenoma
Tubulovillous adenoma
Villous adenoma

Fig. 4 Diagrammatic representation of the histology of adenomatous polyps.

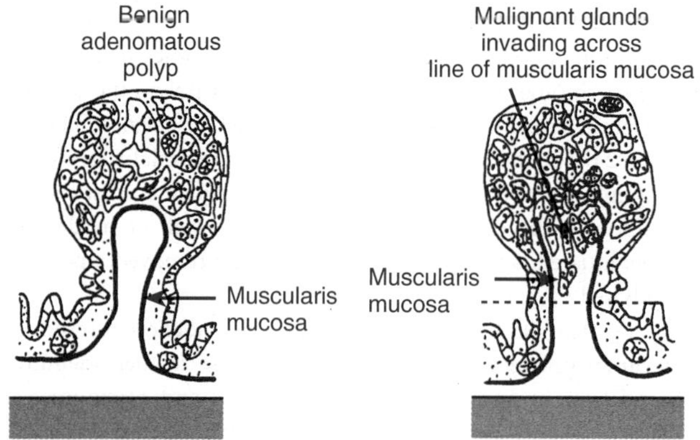

Fig. 5 Diagrammatic representation of the histology of a benign adenoma and a 'malignant polyp' showing adenoma and invasive adenocarcinoma (dotted line indicates snare transection line for complete removal).

Table 2 Frequency of invasive carcinoma in different types and sizes of adenomas in an endoscopic series

		Percentage with malignancy			
	Type as percentage of all adenomas	<1.1 cm	1–2 cm	>2 cm	All sizes
Tubular	75	1	3.0	10	2
Tubulovillus	20		5.0	11	6
Villous	5		6.0	38	18
All adenomas		1	5.5	16	5 (overall)

From Gillespie *et al.* (1979).

Most colon carcinomas originate from an adenoma; the average interval for a medium-sized adenoma to develop malignancy is thought to be about 5–7 years. Patients with adenomas have a higher risk of coexisting colon carcinomas or of developing one subsequently, the risk increasing with the number of adenomas found up to the almost 100 per cent lifetime risk in familial adenomatous polyposis.

Very small or intramucosal carcinomas are rarely found except in association with the unique flat pattern of dysplasia of chronic extensive colitis. The rare '*de novo*' carcinoma of about 1 cm in diameter probably arises from a non-polypoid ('*flat*') adenoma. Flat adenomas are rare in comparison with polypoid adenomas but may progress to adenocarcinoma and are easily missed at endoscopy.

Clinical features and management

Most colonic polyps are symptomless and are diagnosed on radiographs or by endoscopy. Larger ones may bleed intermittently. Mucus production, altered bowel habit, or abdominal pain are uncommon. Villous adenomas of the rectum can, rarely, present with profuse mucoid diarrhoea and hypokalaemic alkalosis.

Once found a polyp must be completely removed for histological assessment. Over 95 per cent are removable by endoscopic snare polypectomy or local electrocoagulation. Few are so large as to need surgical resection. Within 5 cm of the anus there is a likelihood of pain sensation and general anaesthesia may sometimes be advisable.

When carcinoma is identified in the removed polyp, the decision for or against resection of the bowel is a matter of balance. There is a less than 2 per cent chance of finding resectable metastatic carcinoma in the draining lymph nodes, which must be weighed against the risk of operation in the elderly. If the carcinoma is well or moderately well differentiated, and histologically completely removed, operation is not advised.

Once a patient has had one or more 'high-risk' adenomas removed, long-term surveillance is recommended, because further adenomas are found later in over 30 per cent of patients and carcinomas in 2–4 per cent. If only one or two 'low risk' (tubular adenomas <1 cm) are found no follow-up may be needed. For multiple, larger, or villous polyps the first colonoscopy check can usually be at 3 years. After a normal 3-year examination it may be safe to increase the subsequent intervals to 4–5 yearly. Follow-up stops at about 75 years of age.

Familial adenomatous polyposis

Familial adenomatous polyposis (**FAP**) is a dominantly inherited condition in which affected individuals develop hundreds to thousands of colonic adenomas, but also adenomas elsewhere in the gastrointestinal tract, particularly in the duodenal region. The prime reason for concern is the almost inevitable development of colorectal cancer. Carcinoma of the duodenum, ampulla, or bile duct occurs in a small but significant proportion of patients. Extraintestinal manifestations of FAP are now recognized and these include Gardner's syndrome with mesodermal tumours (desmoid tumours of the abdomen, osteomas of the mandible and skull, sebaceous cysts, and soft-tissue tumours of the skin), Turcot's syndrome with medulloblastomas of the brain, hepatoblastomas in children, and congenital hypertrophy of the retinal pigment epithelium (CHRPE).

It is unusual for adenomas to appear before adolescence and symptoms usually only occur when a carcinoma has developed. The mean age of symptomatic presentation is 36 years, whereas diagnosis can be made much earlier if members of FAP families are under surveillance from 12 to 14 years of age. Regular flexible sigmoidoscopy is necessary for all the first degree relatives of an FAP patient if presymptomatic genetic testing is not possible.

Colectomy with ileorectal anastomosis or proctocolectomy with ileoanal pouch is usually undertaken in FAP at the age of 17 to 18 years. If the rectum is retained any polyps are fulgrated at 6-monthly intervals, but 10 per cent will develop cancer of the rectal stump over a 30-year period. An ileorectal anastomosis may be converted to an ileoanal anastomosis with a pouch in those with an unmanageable number of rectal polyps. The role of non-steroidal anti-inflammatory drugs to reduce the incidence of adenomas and regular upper gastrointestinal endoscopy to remove duodenal adenomas is being assessed.

FAP is caused by inactivating/truncating mutations of the *APC* gene on chromosme 5. The *APC* gene product has a pivotal role in the control of cell division in the colonic epithelium and has been termed a 'gatekeeper'. Presymptomatic DNA diagnosis may be offered to families where their individual mutation has been identified. Up to 10 per cent of patients do not have a family history and their disease may be due to new mutations.

An attenuated from of FAP has been described with up to 100 colonic adenomas and a variable incidence of the extracolonic features. Attenuated polyposis is association with 3′ or 5′ germline mutations of the *APC* gene. Missense mutations of the *APC* gene have been described in families and may be associated with the presence of only a few adenomatous polyps but an increased risk of colorectal cancer.

Colorectal cancer

Adenocarcinomas of the colon and rectum are common. Other malignancies—lymphoma, sarcoma, and carcinoid—are very rare.

Epidemiology and aetiological factors

Colorectal carcinoma is the most common malignancy in the UK after lung cancer, and in the US after skin cancer. Men appear to be slightly more at risk for rectal cancer and women for colon cancer. The incidence of both increases with age, the average age at diagnosis being between 60 and 65 years.

Environmental (probably dietary) and genetic factors are both important in causation. The incidence is higher in northern Europe and North America than in southern Europe and South America or in Africa and Asia. Sporadic examples of colorectal cancer occur even in low-risk countries, unfortunately often in young people. There is some evidence that carcinogens or cocarcinogens may be produced by bacterial metabolism of bile salts or other sterols derived from animal fat. A contributory factor in populations eating a low-fibre diet may be explained by slow colonic transit, which gives more time for carcinogen production, concentration, and contact with the mucosa. Ethanol consumption, particularly beer drinking, has also been associated with colon carcinogenesis.

Ureterosigmoidostomy results, after 10–20 years, in a high incidence of colonic adenoma or carcinoma adjacent to the ureteric stoma, possibly due to carcinogen formation from bacterial action on nitrates/nitrites excreted in the urine. There is an increased risk of cancer in patients with long-standing ulcerative colitis and probably also with Crohn's colitis.

Genetic factors

The first degree relatives of a patient with colorectal cancer have two- to threefold increased risk of developing or dying from colorectal cancer. This risk is increased further if the affected individual is under the age of 45 years or if there is more than one affected individual in the family.

Hereditary non-polyposis colon cancer (HNPCC) is an autosomal dominant inherited predisposition to the development of colorectal cancer at a young age. Ther is no characteristic phenotype and the diagnosis is suggested by family history. The International Collaborative Group on HNPCC have defined clinical criteria to diagnose HNPCC (the 'Amsterdam Criteria'). These are: that colorectal cancer is present in three or more relatives, one of whom is a first degree relative of the other two, that colorectal cancer affects at least two generations, one case or more is diagnosed before the age of 50 years, and that FAP is excluded. HNPCC extracolonic tumours (see below) are now usually also included in the criteria. HNPCC may account for 1-2 per cent of cases of colorectal cancer.

In HNPCC colorectal cancer occures at a mean age of 45 years, two-thirds are in the right colon, and may be multiple. Extracolonic cancers also occur and these include endometrial, gastric, renal, small bowel, ovarian carcinomas, and astrocytomas. In women the lifetime risk of endometrial cancer is greater than that of colonic cancer. Rare familes with HNPCC develop benign keratoacanthomas of the skin, an association known as Muir-Torre syndrome.

HNPCC is caused by germline mutations of DNA mismatch repair genes. The two most commonly mutated are *MLH1* and *MSH2.* As a consequence of these mutations HNPCC cancers usually exhibit DNA microsatellite genetic instability as opposed to the chromosomal instability usually seen in sporadic colorectal cancer. Presymptomatic DNA genetic testing may be offered to families in whom the individual mutated gene has been identified.

Individuals with HNPCC and their first degree relatives should undergo 2-yearly, or even more frequent, coloscopic surveillance from the age of 25 as in HNPCC tumours may tend to rapid progression. HNPCC gene carrriers may elect to undergo a total colectomy rather than colonoscopic surveillance. The benefits of extracolonic surveillance are not proven but it has been recommmended that female patients should undergo annual pelvic ultrasound and endometrial aspirate and patients witha strong family history of gastric or renal tract tumours regular gastroscopy, renal ultrasound, or urine cytology.

The molecular genetic basis for colorectal carcinogenesis is increasingly understood, and involves a number of events, which cumulatively result in the progression from normal epithelium to adenoma and finally to invasive adenocarcinoma (see OTM3, pp. 1990–1).

The sequence of events is slow moving, making it possible to find and remove the lesion at its precancerous stage. Furthermore, colorectal neoplasms tend to grow into the lumen of the bowel, which makes them easier to diagnose and resect. Only the carcinoma of chronic ulcerative colitis is characteristically endophytic and even this appears usually to be preceded by a period of superficial dysplastic change, potentially allowing biopsy diagnosis and colon resection in the precancerous phase.

Pathology

The majority of bowel carcinomas occur distally in the rectosigmoid: 30 per cent occur in the rectum, 30 per cent in the sigmoid colon, and 30 per cent proximal to that.

The typical carcinoma is a polypoid mass with central ulceration and irregular, easily bleeding edges, which may spread to become a stricture. Infiltrating scirrhous colon carcinomas are rare. Spread is by local invasion rather than by venous or lymphatic routes, which accounts for a good prognosis when confined to the bowel wall. Invasion through to extramural tissues may involve adjacent organs such as the bladder. Involvement of larger veins results in early spread to the liver and poor prognosis, although occasionally liver metastases may be single and resectable. When lymphatics are invaded the spread is to nodes nearest to the growth. Dukes' staging classification (Fig. 6) allows assessment of likely 5-year survival (Table 3). The most frequent sites of metastases are liver (>60 per cent), lung (50 per cent), peritoneum (15 per cent), or skeleton (15 per cent).

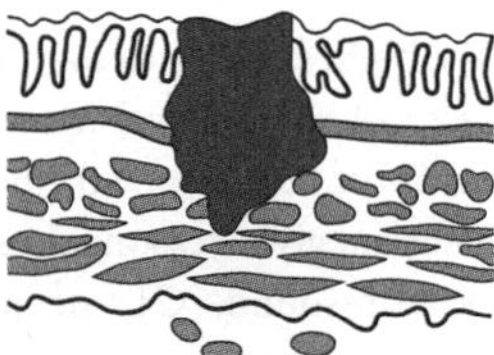
Dukes A
Tumour limited to bowel wall

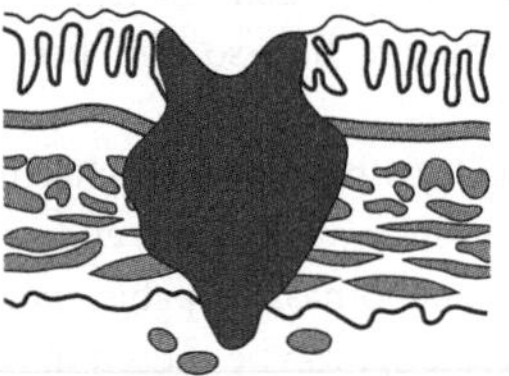
Dukes B
Tumour has penetrated through the bowel wall but lymph nodes are not involved

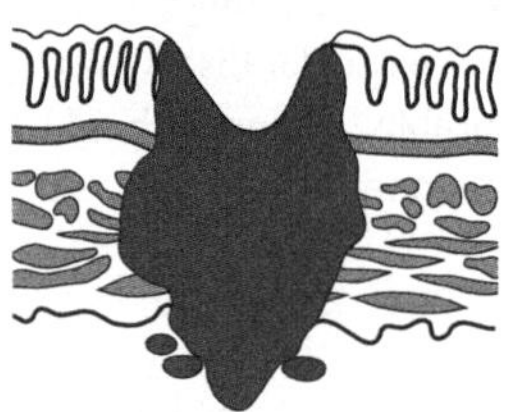
Dukes C
The lymph nodes are now involved

Fig. 6 Dukes' classification of colorectal carcinoma.

Table 3 Modified Dukes' classification and life prognosis for potentially curative colorectal cancer

Dukes' classification	Cases resected (per cent)	5-Year survival (corrected for other causes of mortality per cent)
A	15	95–100
B	40	65–75
C_1 (local nodes positive)	35	30–40
C_2 (apical node positive)	10	10–20

Clinical features and diagnosis (Plate 4)

Any large bowel cancer will bleed intermittently but rectal and sigmoid cancers are more likely to bleed overtly, the blood being mixed in with the stool. Alteration in previously regular bowel habit occurs if tumour obstructs the passage of stool in the narrow left colon. Flow through the capacious caecum or ascending colon is unaffected even by large tumours. For this reason the caecum is a 'silent area' in which large but symptomless carcinomas may occur, eventually presenting with iron-deficiency anaemia. Pain and weight loss are late symptoms, but even at this stage the slow-moving nature of colon cancer means that it may be resectable. A palpable mass does not invariably mean a bad prognosis, for the carcinoma may be small with faecal hold-up, or most of the mass may be due to surrounding inflammatory change or abscess formation.

The importance of early diagnosis is such that any new colonic symptoms should be taken seriously, especially in patients over 45 years of age. Faecal occult blood testing can be used to screen at-risk individuals but sensitivity and specificity are low. Flexible sigmoidoscopy allows examination of the distal colon (sometimes to the splenic flexure) and covers both the highest risk area for adenomas and carcinoma and the region where most radiological misses occur. Examination of the proximal colon is most accurate with the colonoscope. The double-contrast barium enema gives reasonable accuracy only for large lesions. Imaging by ultrasound, CT, or magnetic resonance imaging are disappointing except where spread of advanced cancer requires assessment. The lack of specificity of serological tests such as the carcinoembryonic antigen has so far been a disappointment.

Differential diagnosis must be made from localized ischaemic areas, solitary ulcer of the rectum, granulation-tissue masses, endometriosis, or inflammatory lesions such as amoebomas. Palpable masses with radiological features simulating carcinoma can be caused in the caecal area by an appendix abscess, tuberculosis, actinomycosis, or Crohn's disease, and in the sigmoid colon by diverticular disease with pericolic abscess formation. Whenever practicable, a biopsy should be taken before operating on an apparent carcinoma.

Screening and follow-up

Screening of asymptomatic populations for colorectal cancer has been undertaken using faecal occult blood testing followed by colonoscopy in those individuals with a positive test; this has been shown to reduce the mortality from colorectal cancer by between 15 and 33 per cent in large randomized controlled studies. Trials of one-off flexible sigmoidoscopy between the ages of 55 and 65 years are in progress.

In patients with colorectal cancer the entire colon should be imaged, if possible preoperatively, but, if not, postoperatively, to exclude synchronous tumours. As there is an increased risk of developing future polyps or carcinoma 3-yearly colonoscopic surveillance is recommended thereafter.

Treatment and results

The best treatment is excision, usually by surgical resection, except for snared polyps with invasion limited to the head, or occasional small and circumscribed rectal cancers suitable for local excision. Radiotherapy for rectal carcinoma may decrease the risk of local recurrence. Chemotherapy with 5-fluorouracil in combination with folinic acid agents has shown some improvement in survival time in disseminated disease and irinotechin to prolong survival in patients who have not responded to 5-fluorouracil. Adjuvant chemotherapy with 5-fluorouracil increases the cure rate in patients who have undergone a curative resection of Dukes' C stage colorectal cancer. Even in the 20 per cent of patients in whom metastases or extensive infiltration makes radical surgery impossible, resection of the primary tumour is usually desirable in order to prevent obstruction and the unpleasantness of bloody discharge. The operative mortality of colorectal resections is around 2 per cent overall.

The long-term results of surgery depend on the centre reporting as well as on the stage and grade of tumour. Specialist centres quote over 90 per cent of cases as suitable for radical or curative surgery, with corrected 5-year survival of 50–60 per cent overall and almost 95 per cent for Dukes' A cases. District general hospitals find only 50 per cent suitable for radical surgery and, have only 30 per cent corrected 5-year survival.

Carcinoma in ulcerative colitis

This subject is addressed in Chapter 5.15.

Other colonic and anal tumours

Carcinoid tumours of the large bowel are usually benign, do not produce the carcinoid syndrome, and can be locally resected. Kaposi's sarcoma may be found in the rectum in homosexuals and more generally in AIDS patients. Primary lymphoma of the colon is rare but polyposis-like involvement can occur either in primary malignant lymphomatous polyposis or as part of generalized lymphoma with multiple, umbilicated nodules present in the distribution of the lymphoid follicles in the colon and elsewhere in the gastrointestinal tract; diagnosis is made on biopsy, the polyps disappearing on chemotherapy. Localized lymphoma may be treated by resection or irradiation, depending on its site.

A number of anus-specific tumours may occur. They include variants of squamous carcinoma, condyloma, and malignant melanoma. Rarely, the anal region may be the site of precancerous skin conditions such as leucoplakia, Paget's disease, or Bowen's disease.

Further reading

Chow, W.H., Blot, W.J., Vaughan, T.L., *et al.* (1998). Body mass index and risk of adenocarcinomas of the esophagus and gastric cardia. *Journal of the National Cancer Institute*, **90**(2), 150–5.

Foulkes, W.D. (1995). A tale of four syndromes: familial adenomatous polyposis, Gardner syndrome, attenuated APC and Turcot syndrome. *Quarterly Journal of Medicine*, **88**, 853–63.

Sharma, V.K., Chockalingam, H., Hornung, C.A., Vasudeva, R., and Howden, C.W. (1998). Changing trends in esophageal cancer: a 15-year experience in a single center. *American Journal of Gastroenterology*, **93**(5), 702–5.

Spigelman, A.D., Murday, V., and Phillips, R.K. (1989). Cancer and the Peutz-Jeghers syndrome. *Gut*, **30**(11), 1588–90.

Vasen, H.F., Mecklin, J.P., Khan, P.M., and Lynch, H.T. (1994). The International Collaborative Group on HNPCC. *Anticancer Research*, **14**, 1661–4.

Chapter 5.21

Vascular and collagen disorders

G. Neale

Ischaemic disease of the gut

Ischaemic lesions may occur in the small or large intestine with or without evidence of gross vascular occlusion. The stomach is rarely affected. A list of causes is shown in Table 1.

Occlusion of major arteries

Atheromatous occlusion is the most common cause of mesenteric vascular insufficiency, often undiagnosed in life, probably because the slowness of the pathological process allows for the development of a compensatory collateral circulation. Intestinal infarction secondary to atheromatous occlusion of one major vessel is uncommon. Indeed, all three vessels may be occluded without visceral damage.

Thrombosis often develops on an ulcerated atheromatous plaque but may also occur spontaneously in polycythaemia, sickle cell disease, cryoglobulinaemia, and amyloidosis. Thromboangiitis obliterans (Buerger's disease, see Chapter 2.17) only rarely affects mesenteric vessels but in such cases the prognosis is poor.

Table 1 Causes of ischaemic disease of the gut

Major arterial occlusion
Thrombotic
Embolic
Inflammation (usually non-infective) of blood vessels (see Table 2)
Miscellaneous lesions damaging or compressing the arterial tree
Mesenteric venous thrombosis
Non-occlusive intestinal infarction (see Table 3)

Table 2 Vasculitides that may affect the gut

Involving vessels of all sizes
• Polyarteritis nodosa • (Churg–Strauss disease) • Giant-cell arteritis • Takayasu's arteritis • Transplant rejection
Involving predominantly medium and small vessels

• Wegener's granulomatosis
• Kawasaki disease
• Buerger's disease
• Malignant hypertension
• Vasculitis of collagen—vascular disorders:
  • Rheumatoid disease
  • Systemic lupus erythematosus
  • Progressive systemic sclerosis
  • Dermatomyositis

Involving predominantly small vessels
• Hypersensitivity angiitis (microscopic polyarteritis) • Henoch–Schönlein purpura • Serum sickness • Infective angiitis (e.g. typhoid, tuberculosis)

Systemic arterial embolism usually from the heart may account for up to one-third of cases of mesenteric vascular occlusion. Paradoxical embolism through a patent foramen ovale and embolism from aortic mural thrombi are uncommon causes.

Inflammation of blood vessels

Vasculitis may affect the splanchnic circulation in several multisystem disorders (Table 2), causing oedema, mucosal haemorrhages, focal ulceration, and focal necrosis with perforation. Occasionally healing leads to intestinal strictures. Secondary involvement of small vessels may also occur in inflammatory bowel disease, potassium-induced ulceration, eosinophilic granuloma, midline granuloma or irradiation.

Miscellaneous lesions

Vessels may be compressed by retroperitoneal haematomas, by neoplastic infiltration, and by proliferating fibrous tissue as in retroperitoneal fibrosis and around carcinoid tumours. Necrotizing arteritis in the splanchnic circulation may also occur a few days after surgical correction of coarctation of the aorta. Diffuse microthrombosis may result from disseminated intravascular coagulation and in the haemolytic–uraemic syndrome and thrombotic thrombocytopenic purpura. Renal failure often dominates the clinical picture but in most patients there is evidence of widespread involvement of the intestine.

Table 3 Intestinal infarction without vascular occlusion

Neonatal
• Necrotizing enterocolitis
Haemorrhagic enteritis or colitis
• Bacterial toxins (e.g. *E. coli* 0157:H7; *Clostridium perfringens*)
Necrotizing colitis
• Severe ileus often drug induced and rarely after surgery (intestinal pseudo-obstruction)
Focal ulceration
• Stress ulcers (especially stomach and duodenum) • Drug-induced ulcers (e.g. potassium, NSAIDs) • Radiation enteritis • Uraemic ulceration (especially in colon)
After prolonged period of poor perfusion
• Low-output cardiac failure (? digitalis predisposed) • Hyperviscosity syndromes • Polycythaemia and haemoconcentration

NSAIDs, non-steroidal anti-inflammatory drugs.

Mesenteric venous thrombosis

Thrombosis of mesenteric veins accounts for less than 10 per cent of cases of intestinal infarction. Causes include hypercoaguable states and complications of portal hypertension, peritoneal inflammation, and trauma. There is an association with pregnancy and oral contraceptives.

Non-occlusive intestinal infarction (Table 3)

Sporadic and epidemic cases of necrotizing enteritis without vascular occlusion have been described in all age groups and accounts for 25 per cent of cases of intestinal infarction. In adults, it is seen mainly in the elderly with severe, low-output cardiac failure and occasionally in the severely shocked.

Pathogenetic mechanisms

The hallmark of ischaemic bowel pathology is extensive coagulative necrosis, which commences in the mucosa and then spreads to deeper layers. The appearances are similar in both occlusive and non-occlusive forms. Non-occlusive focal ischaemia appears to underlie the pathogenesis of uraemic colitis, radiation enteritis, potassium-induced ulcers, and multiple stress ulcers of the upper gastrointestinal tract. The verotoxin of *Escherichia coli* 0157:H7 is another cause.

Clinical syndromes

Acute intestinal ischaemia

Acute intestinal ischaemia is primarily a condition of older people with cardiovascular disease, caused by necrosis, threatened or complete, of that part of the gut supplied by the superior mesenteric artery.

Clinical features

The onset is usually abrupt but may be insidious with colicky abdominal pain. Later the pain becomes constant. Diarrhoea is usual and frequently the motions contain blood. Vomiting occurs in some cases but haematemesis is rare. In the early stages the distress of the patient is out of all proportion to the physical signs. As the condition develops the abdomen becomes distended and silent with increasing tenderness, a positive rebound sign and signs of peripheral circulatory failure. Later, the patient becomes cyanosed and anuric. At this stage, intestinal necrosis has almost certainly gone beyond the point of recovery.

Prompt diagnosis depends on recognizing that the patient has suffered a potentially catastrophic event in the abdomen which needs urgent investigation and often laparotomy. Needling the peritoneal cavity usually produces blood-stained fluid. Plain radiograph of the abdomen may show non-specific dilatation of loops of intestine with multiple fluid levels. The presence of gas bubbles in the portal vein is diagnostic of intestinal necrosis at a stage when the patient is beyond recovery. Centres with appropriate facilities and experience should offer emergency mesenteric angiography. Papaverine should be infused into the superior mesenteric artery if vasoconstriction rather than vascular occlusion appears to be the cause.

Management

With or without angiography urgent laparotomy is necessary as soon as the patient is sufficiently fit. If a large vessel is occluded, the surgeon may be able to undertake embolectomy or reconstruct an occluded artery. In both occlusive and non-occlusive vascular disease it is necessary to decide how much intestine to resect. If there is doubt about the viability of the residual intestine the abdomen may be closed and, 24 h later, re-explored.

Many patients with acute intestinal ischaemia causing necrosis die. Those who recover have difficulty in maintaining their nutrition.

Chronic intestinal ischaemia

Atheroma of the visceral arteries commonly involves the coeliac axis and superior mesenteric artery. The inferior mesenteric artery is affected to a much lesser extent. Classically the patient suffers cramping abdominal pain 20–60 min after eating, sometimes relieved by analgesics or by vasodilator drugs. As the condition progresses the patient becomes afraid to eat and loses weight.

The finding of a systolic bruit is a doubtfully valid physical sign. Bruits may be detected in normal subjects, and may be absent in patients with severe visceral arterial disease. The diagnosis is made by excluding other conditions and correlating clinical symptoms with angiographic findings. Arterial reconstruction can be rewarding in selected cases.

Coeliac-axis compression

In occasional patients with chronic abdominal pain and an abdominal bruit, aortography shows apparent constriction of the coeliac axis by the median arcuate ligament. It has been claimed that 'intestinal angina' may be relieved by dividing ligament. Although patients claim to have been cured by surgery, the validity of the syndrome remains uncertain.

Focal ischaemia of the small intestine

Ischaemia of a segment of small intestine may cause local ulceration that on healing leads to stenosis. This may occur as a result of any of the vascular disorders described as above. More specific entities include ischaemic damage by a strangulated hernia, by an episode of blunt trauma to the abdomen, or by irradiation. A high concentration of potassium in the lumen of the intestine causes venous spasm and subsequently local arterial thrombosis, which may lead to ulceration and fibrosis. The patient presents with features of subacute obstruction of the small intestine. The stricture is located by radiological examination and requires surgery.

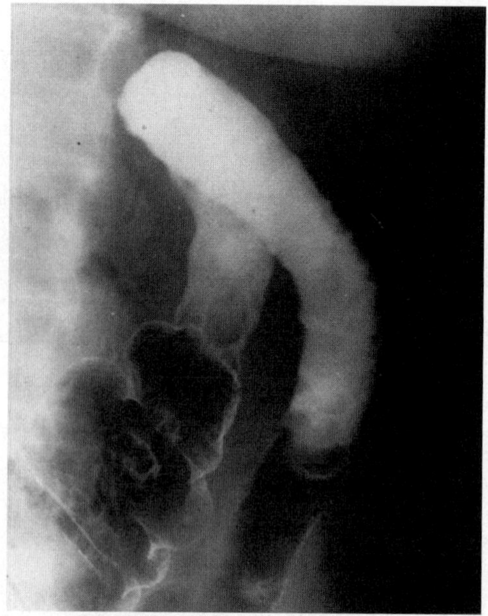

Fig. 1 Ischaemic colitis: barium enema showing thumb-printing at the splenic flexure.
(By courtesy of Dr A. Freeman, Addenbrooke's Hospital.)

Ischaemic colitis

The vascular anatomy of the colon makes it more prone to ischaemic damage than the small intestine. Also, damage may be more rapid and more severe than that occurring in the small intestine because of the effects of the high concentration of bacteria in the faecal stream. Blood flow to the colon may be impaired by any of the mechanisms described previously. In addition, colonic obstruction may reduce blood flow by increasing the intraluminal pressure.

Venous occlusion is also a possible cause of ischaemic colitis. The contraceptive pill has been incriminated but evidence remains suggestive rather than conclusive.

Clinical features

In the acute phase the clinician has to differentiate between mild disease, which responds quickly and effectively to supportive measures and treatment with appropriate antibiotics, and severe disease in which gangrene may develop. Most patients are between the ages of 50 and 70 years and often have a background history of atheromatous arterial disease, collagen disorder, or local colonic pathology. Typically the patient complains of pain in the left iliac fossa, nausea, and vomiting followed by the passage of a loose motion containing dark blood.

Marked tenderness in the left iliac fossa is the most constant physical sign. At colonoscopy the mucosa may be blue and swollen without contact bleeding. The rectum is invariably spared. Plain radiographs of the abdomen may show an abnormal segment of large intestine outlined with gas. Angiography is only occasionally helpful.

Contrast enema examination of the colon is a most useful way of demonstrating ischaemic damage. In the early phase, 'thumb printing' is the characteristic sign, which may persist for several days (Fig. 1). Subsequently, the mucosal appearances may return to normal or progress to mucosal ulceration, giving an appearance that may be indistinguishable from segmental ulcerative colitis or Crohn's disease, although the haustral pattern is usually not seriously disrupted and the ulcers are patchy and do not penetrate deeply. Again, these

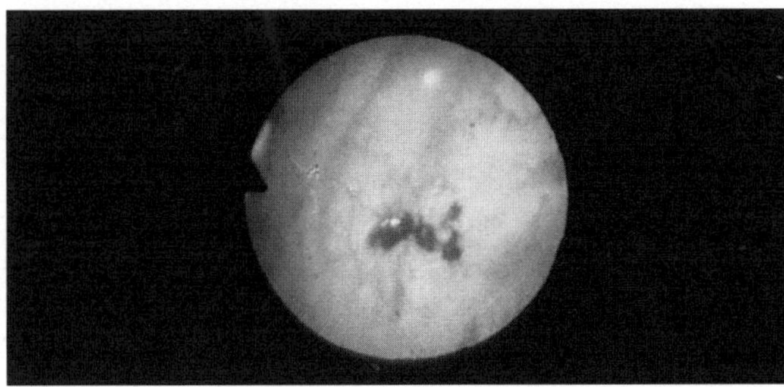

Fig. 2 Angiodysplastic lesion in the caecum, photographed through a colonoscope.
(By courtesy of Dr R. Hunt, RN Hospital, Haslar.)

changes may resolve spontaneously or progress to tubular narrowing with or without sacculation on the antimesenteric border.

Ischaemic colitis may be confused with dysenteric conditions, acute diverticular disease, acute inflammatory bowel disease, perforation of a hollow viscus, or left-sided peritonitis secondary to pancreatitis. The most important distinguishing features are the characteristic age range, the association with degenerative cardiovascular disease, and the distinctive, although not pathognomonic, radiographic and colonoscopic appearances.

Management

Treatment is initially with intravenous fluid and systemic broad-spectrum antibiotics. Well over 90 per cent of cases resolve spontaneously. A stricture may develop in up to a third of patients but this is usually asymptomatic and only rarely needs to be resected. Surgery is indicated if there is evidence of peritonitis, persistent bleeding, or of an underlying colonic disorder (such as carcinoma).

Other primary vascular disorders of the gut

Aneurysms of the aorta and its major branches (see Chapter 2.17)

Rarely, aneurysms fistulate into the stomach or duodenum, causing catastrophic bleeding and rapid death. Even more rarely intermittent bleeding may be difficult to diagnose.

Superior mesenteric artery syndrome

A syndrome of postprandial epigastric pain, distension, and vomiting may occur in asthenic young people, especially those who have lost weight or who are fixed in a position of hyperextension after spinal injury. Barium studies show a distended proximal duodenum with a sharp cut-off at the line where the superior mesenteric artery crosses the duodenum. Symptoms may be relieved if the patient adopts the prone position after meals and may disappear as the patient gains weight. Occasionally surgery is necessary. The condition must be distinguished from duodenal ileus caused by mesenteric bands, a condition that is associated with partial malrotation of the midgut.

Haemangioma

Haemangiomas are uncommon lesions of the gut but may cause painless bleeding, especially from the jejunum.

Intestinal telangiectasia

These lesions occur most commonly with Osler–Weber–Rendu disease and may lead to microscopic bleeding with anaemia, especially in adults.

Vascular dysplasia

This not uncommon disorder causes occult bleeding from the gut in older subjects. The lesions occur as small arteriovenous malformations or as foci of ectatic capillaries or veins with little supporting stroma; they are found predominantly in the caecum and ascending colon.

Patients give a history of recurrent anaemia or episodes of bleeding from the gut and usually have been investigated repeatedly without a firm diagnosis. The diagnosis may be made by direct visualization of the intestinal mucosa (Fig. 2) or by selective mesenteric arteriography (Fig. 3). Lesions may be multiple. Many patients can be treated successfully by fulguration of the lesion through an endoscope.

Intramural bleeding

Bleeding into the wall of the bowel may occur as a result of treatment with anticoagulants or from the inflammation of small vessels (as in Henoch–Schönlein purpura). The usual presentation is with colicky abdominal pain, with bleeding into the lumen of the gut. Appropriate barium examination may show the classical sign of 'thumb printing'.

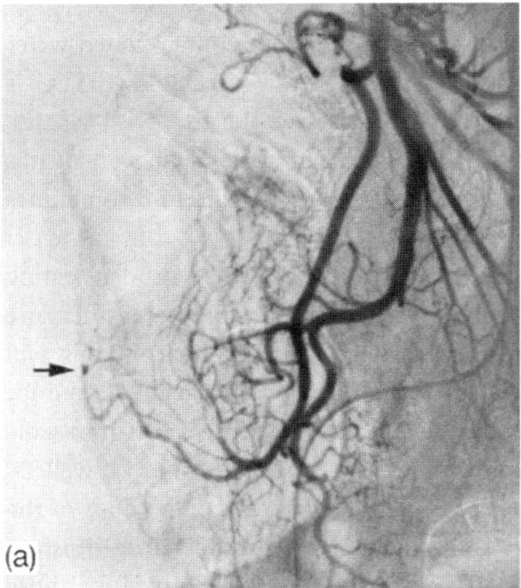

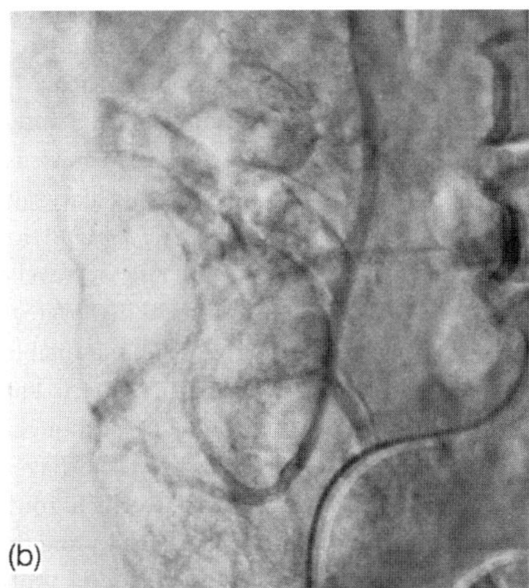

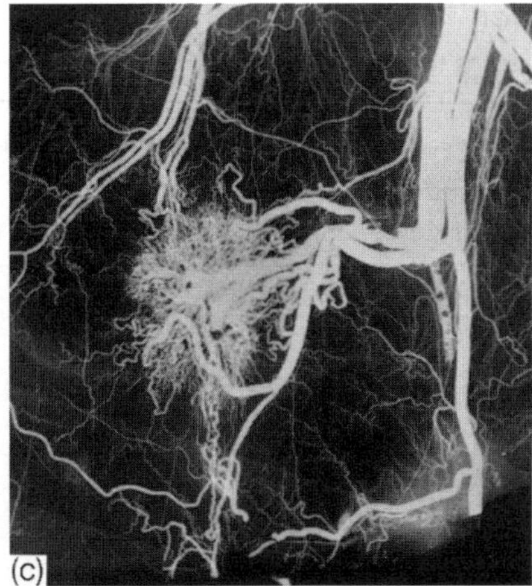

Fig. 3 Angiodysplastic lesion in the caecum: superior mesenteric angiogram in a 53-year-old man with anaemia for 20 years (no lesion found at previous operations). (a) Vascular lake in caecum (arrowed). (b) Capillary phase, showing early-filling vein arising from lesion. (c) Injected specimen magnified ×30).
(By courtesy of Dr D. J. Allison, Royal Postgraduate Medical School and reprinted with permission of the Editor of the British Journal of Medicine.)

Vasculitis and the collagen disorders

The gut may be involved in any of the systemic collagen and inflammatory vascular disorders. The manifestations may be due to vasculitis or to involvement of visceral muscle as in systemic sclerosis (see Chapters 10.11–10.17). Local vasculitis has been described involving individual intra-abdominal organs such as the appendix and gallbladder. The relationship to the systemic disorders is uncertain.

Further reading

Bradbury, A.W., Brittenden, J., McBride, K., and Ruckley, C.V. (1995). Mesenteric ischaemia: a multi-disciplinary approach. *British Journal of Surgery*, 82, 1446–59.

Chapter 5.22

Gastrointestinal infections

C. P. Conlon

Infections of the gastrointestinal tract produce a variety of symptoms and can be due to a large number of different infective agents. The most common symptom is diarrhoea, which leads to considerable morbidity and mortality worldwide, particularly among children in developing countries.

The types and severity of gastrointestinal infections are determined by a variety of epidemiological factors. Different age groups will have different risks, with the extremes of age being the most vulnerable. Overcrowding and poor sanitation predispose to epidemics. Most enteric infections in the tropics occur in the summer months, whereas in temperate regions, winter is the time of peak prevalence.

The organisms that cause the different gastrointestinal infections are considered in detail in Section 16. Here, the spectrum of different gastrointestinal disorders due to infection is summarized.

Clinical syndromes of gastrointestinal infection

Non-inflammatory diarrhoea

This is usually caused by viruses, bacterial enterotoxins, or protozoa (Table 1) affecting the proximal small bowel resulting in secretory diarrhoea, often associated with nausea and vomiting. There is very little bowel inflammation and no colonic involvement so pus cells are not found in faeces.

Table 1 Causes of non-inflammatory infective diarrhoea

Viruses	Bacteria	Parasites
Rotavirus	EPEC	Giardia
Norwalk	ETEC	Cryptosporidium
SRSV	*V. cholerae*	*Isospora belli*
Calicivirus	*V. parahaemolyticus*	
Astrovirus	*Staph. aureus*	
Adenovirus	*B. cereus* *C. perfringens*	

Abbreviations are explained in the text.

Viruses

Rotavirus most commonly affects those under the age of 5, disrupting cuboidal epithelium at the tips of villi producing severe watery diarrhoea. Older children and adults may be subject to attacks of severe nausea and vomiting due to viruses (sometimes called winter vomiting disease). This can be due to rotavirus, but usually other agents are involved. These include the Norwalk virus (identified in Norwalk, Ohio, USA) which also attacks the microvillus, but infections result more prominently with vomiting than with diarrhoea or fever. Other similar agents are small round structural viruses (SRSV), astroviruses, adenovriruses, and caliciviruses.

Bacteria

The most well-known bacterial cause of non-inflammatory diarrhoea is *Vibrio cholerae.* Adenyl cyclase activation by the 'A' subunit of the cholera toxin in intestinal mucosal cells can lead to a severe secretory diarrhoea, with depletion of water and salts from both intravascular and extracellular spaces, producing the classical clinical picture of cholera. *V. cholerae* can produce anything from asymptomatic excretion to mild watery diarrhoea through to fulminant disease and death. Many other bacteria can produce secretory diarrhoea via the elaboration of toxins. Cholera-like syndromes may result from infection with some strains of *Escherichia coli* (**ETEC**). These *E. coli* produce two types of enterotoxins, one heat labile (**LT**) and one heat stable (**ST**). LT is very similar to cholera toxin while ST is smaller and activates guanylate cyclase with an earlier onset of action than LT.

Food poisoning

This is described in detail in Section 16.

Travellers' diarrhoea

Symptoms usually arise within 2 weeks of arrival and normally only last for 3–5 days. Nausea and abdominal cramps are soon followed by the sudden onset of watery diarrhoea of mild to moderate severity. Vomiting may occur and, with some infections, there may be blood in the stool.

The organisms responsible are acquired from contaminated water or food, particularly unwashed fruit and raw vegetables. ETEC is responsible for about 50 per cent of cases worldwide, with viruses, particularly rotavirus, causing a significant minority. Other organisms include shigellae, salmonellae, campylobacter, giardia, and sometimes *Entamoeba histolytica.*

The risk of travellers' diarrhoea can be reduced by prudent eating and drinking. Water sterilization tablets and portable water filters are now readily available and simply boiling water for about 10 min will kill many enteric pathogens. Avoiding salads, raw vegetables, and ice also helps. Although prophylactic antibiotics, such as co-trimoxazole or doxycycline, have been shown to reduce the incidence of travellers' diarrhoea, their routine use cannot be recommended because of the risk of toxicity and the increasing emergence of multiply drug-resistant enteric bacteria. Antibiotic prophylaxis should be reserved for those at highest risk, such as patients with achlorhydria or those who are immunosuppressed. Pre-emptive treatment with a single dose of ciprofloxacin after the first loose stool has been shown to be effective.

Table 2 Infective causes of dysentery

Bacterial	Parasitic
Shigella spp.	*Entamoeba histolytica*
EHEC	*Balantidium coli*
Salmonella spp.	*Schistosoma mansoni*
Campylobacter jejuni	*S. japonicum*
V. parahaemolyticus	*Trichinella spiralis*
C. perfringens	
C. difficile	

EHEC, enterohaemorrhagic *E. coli*.

Chronic non-inflammatory diarrhoea

Giardiasis may cause chronic symptoms and eventually even lead to a malabsorptive state. In some children and in immunosuppressed adults, cryptosporidium may cause chronic diarrhoea. Viral, bacterial, and protozoal infections may all cause sufficient damage to small intestinal microvilli to lead to a secondary disaccharidase deficiency, so that if diarrhoea is prolonged, it is worth trying a lactose-free diet before embarking on more invasive investigations.

Other causes of chronic non-inflammatory diarrhoea include tropical sprue (Chapter 5.13) and bacterial overgrowth in the small intestine (Chapter 5.7).

Inflammatory diarrhoea

Acute inflammatory diarrhoea is usually bacterial and occasionally parasitic in origin, and may present with several distinct syndromes. Organisms commonly responsible include salmonellae, campylobacter, and shigella. In all cases, both the distal small bowel and the colon are involved and the inflammation leads to pus cells in the stool.

Acute dysentery

Patients may present with diarrhoea of sudden onset, often associated with abdominal cramps and a mild fever, when infected by some bacteria or parasites (Table 2). The frequent bowel movements often contain blood and mucus and there may be tenesmus. Microscopy reveals red cells and pus cells in the stool. Sigmoidoscopy may show an active proctitis, sometimes with ulceration; shallow and widespread with shigellae, deeper and more discrete with amoebiasis.

Bacteria

Shigella may produce symptoms after a very small inoculum ($<10^2$ organisms) and although *S. dysenteriae* and *S. flexneri* cause the most severe disease, *S. sonnei* and *S. boydii* are more common in the UK. Certain strains of *E. coli* (ETEC) may produce a very similar syndrome, but *Campylobacter jejuni* is emerging as one of the most common causes in developed countries, although the dysenteric symptoms tend to be milder than is seen with shigella infections. Salmonella infections are also an increasing problem with notable outbreaks of *Salmonella enteritidis* (phage type 4) gastroenteritis in the UK in the past few years. This particular species is associated with the consumption of undercooked eggs and poultry but many other *Salmonella* spp. can lead to inflammatory diarrhoea. Rarely, the abdominal pain may be severe enough with campylobacter or salmonella infections to mimic appendicitis and both infections have been known to cause toxic megacolon. All of the above organisms may be associated with a postdysenteric reactive arthropathy in patients with HLA-B27.

Both enteroinvasive *E. coli* (EIEC) and EHEC may cause bloody diarrhoea. *E. coli* 0157:H7 is responsible for a haemorrhagic colitis, associated with haemolytic–uraemic syndrome and presents in a manner similar to thrombotic thrombocytopenic purpura. *E. coli* 0157:H7 has caused large outbreaks of diarrhoea and haemolytic–uraemic syndrome in association with a variety of cooked meats.

Parasites

Entamoeba histolytica can cause a range of problems, but most adults with symptoms have a mild to moderately severe dysentery. The onset is gradual, with abdominal discomfort and flatulence followed by the frequent passage of watery, bloody stools. Fever is uncommon. Unlike amoebic abscesses, amoebomas are usually associated with an active dysentery. *Balantidium coli* may present in a manner indistinguishable from amoebic dysentery. Rarely, this parasite can cause acute appendicitis and sometimes chronic diarrhoea.

Acute schistosomiasis may cause bloody diarrhoea when the adult worms invade the gastrointestinal tract and start producing eggs. Sometimes these trematodes and their eggs are a cause of chronic, intermittent diarrhoea. Acute trichinosis may sometimes start with an inflammatory diarrhoea a week or two before the systemic features are manifest.

Pseudomembranous colitis after antibiotic treatment and necrotizing enteritis may produce similar symptoms.

Chronic inflammatory diarrhoea

This may occur with recurrent or relapsing bacterial infections, such as salmonellosis, or with protozoal infections, such as amoebiasis. Intestinal tuberculosis may lead to diarrhoea, although fever, abdominal pain, and weight loss are more common. Rarely, fungi like South American blastomycosis (*Paracoccidiodes brasiliensis*) or histoplasmosis may affect the gut, producing ulcerating or granulomatous lesions and causing abdominal discomfort and diarrhoea.

Invasive infections

Some intestinal infections present with a systemic illness in which fever and non-diarrhoeal abdominal symptoms predominate. Typhoid is the best example. Organisms causing a typhoid-like illness are: *Salmonella typhi*, *S. paratyphi* A and B, *Campylobacter fetus*, *Yersinia enterocolitica*, *Y. pseudotuberculosis*.

Many parasites can also cause abdominal symptoms and fever, often with eosinophilia. Infection with *Strongyloides stercoralis* can cause abdominal pain, diarrhoea, and abdominal distension. Many other nematodes, such as *Ascaris lumbricoides* or *Trichinella spiralis*, may present with gastrointestinal problems but may also be discovered during investigation of extraintestinal symptoms.

Schistosomal infection may present with bowel disturbance but may first present with 'swimmer's itch' or a more serious illness, Katayama fever, characterized by fever, urticaria, lymphadenopathy, diarrhoea, and eosinophilia. *Fasciola hepatica* or *Clonorchis sinensis*, may present with hepatomegaly or cholangitis.

The larval form of *Taenia solium* may cause cysticercosis in humans if excreted eggs are ingested.

Trypanosoma cruzi may damage the myenteric plexus anywhere in the gastrointestinal tract leading to motility problems. Other organisms infecting the gastrointestinal tract (for example, tuberculosis,

HIV, *Helicobacter pylori*) are described elsewhere. Whipple's disease (see Chapter 5.11) is caused by *Tropheryma whippelii.*

Diagnosis and management of gastrointestinal infections

Diagnosis

Particular note should be taken of foreign travel, the dietary history, the possibility of associated cases, and underlying medical problems. Vomiting in association with watery diarrhoea may indicate a non-inflammatory intestinal infection, while the presence of blood in the faeces points to an inflammatory enteritis. A history of current or recent antibiotic treatment may suggest *C. difficile* colitis. The clinical signs that should be noted are the presence and degree of dehydration, fever, evidence of toxaemia, and any extraintestinal manifestations.

Investigations should include culture of blood and stool, with light microscopy of stool to look for pus cells and parasites. If a viral cause is suspected, stool should be examined by electron microscopy. Rotavirus may be detected by an enzyme-linked immunosorbent assay, and other viruses may be found by tissue culture or radioimmunoassay.

Sigmoidoscopy and rectal biopsy may sometimes be helpful, particularly to identify parasites such as *Entamoeba histolytica* or *Schistosoma mansoni* and helps in the differential diagnosis of inflammatory bowel disease. Occasionally small-bowel biopsies and duodenal fluid aspirates may be needed to sort out chronic diarrhoea and in the differential diagnosis of conditions such as gluten enteropathy. Plain abdominal radiographs may be required to exclude a toxic megacolon and barium studies are useful in the work-up of bloody diarrhoea that is not settling or if intestinal tuberculosis is a consideration.

Differential diagnosis

Non-inflammatory diarrhoea is usually due to infective causes, but a variety of toxins can produce acute diarrhoea and vomiting, including heavy metals, such as cadmium and arsenic. Mushroom poisoning, for example with *Amanita phalloides*, may result in severe vomiting and sometimes diarrhoea along with other symptoms. Some fish contain toxins that may affect the gastrointestinal tract. Ciguatera poisoning has been associated with several hundred different species of fish in the Pacific and Caribbean. The toxin, derived from microalgae, produces neurological and gastrointestinal symptoms, the latter comprising nausea, vomiting, abdominal cramps, and diarrhoea. Scromboid poisoning results from the ingestion of poorly refrigerated fish in which bacteria have caused breakdown of histine in fish muscle to saurine, a histamine-like substance. The symptoms are like those of histamine poisoning, with diarrhoea in association with other reactions, such as flushing, generalized urticaria, myalgia, and swelling of the tongue and throat.

There are also endocrine causes of diarrhoea. These include carcinoid tumours, medullary carcinoma of the thyroid, and non-β-islet-cell tumours. Sometimes, diarrhoea is a major feature of thyrotoxicosis or hypoadrenalism. More chronic diarrhoea may result from coeliac disease or from disaccharidase deficiency.

Inflammatory diarrhoea of infective origin must be distinguished from inflammatory bowel disease. Although histological examination of the rectal biopsy may help, the diagnosis of inflammatory bowel disease may only be made with the passage of time in the absence of an infective cause being found. Sometimes acute diverticulitis or ischaemic colitis may present acutely with bloody diarrhoea and mimic infection. This occurs rarely with colonic cancers.

Table 3 Oral rehydration solutions

Constituents (mmol/l)	WHO	Dioralyte (Rorer)
Sodium	90	60
Potassium	20	20
Chloride	80	60
Base (citrate)	10	10
Glucose	110	90
Osmolality	310	240

Management

The mainstay of managing diarrhoeal diseases is the recognition and correction of water and electrolyte depletion. If vomiting is not a major feature then rehydration can usually be achieved using oral rehydration solutions (**ORS**) (Table 3). The **WHO** 'universal formula' takes the form of a powder containing 20 g glucose, 3.5 g sodium chloride, 1.5 g potassium chloride, and either 2.5 g sodium bicarbonate or 2.9 g trisodium citrate per litre of solution, usually packaged in aluminium foil in quantities appropriate to the volume of containers used for water in different tropical regions. However, in Western countries where faecal sodium losses are less, there are real fears of hypernatraemic dehydration. In these areas an ORS with a lower sodium content is preferable, for example Dioralyte (Rorer Pharmaceuticals). Clearly, fluids may need to be given intravenously or even subcutaneously.

Antidiarrhoeal agents such as diphenoxylate sodium and codeine phosphate, are used to relieve the symptom of diarrhoea. There are unsubstantiated fears that these drugs may increase the risk of toxic megacolon but there is some evidence to suggest that they may slow the clearance of organisms from the intestine. Loperamide may inhibit intestinal secretion but only in very large doses. Other agents like kaolin pectin have been promoted as absorbents of bacteria and their toxins but there is no evidence to suggest that they are any more effective than placebo and their use cannot be recommended. Solutions of bismuth salts may have an antiseptic role and have been shown to be useful in the prevention of travellers' diarrhoea.

Antibiotics are rarely indicated for diarrhoeal illnesses. In some instances, they may prolong carriage and excretion of the pathogen while at the same time increasing the chances of multiply resistant enteric pathogens emerging. However, in some circumstances specific therapy is indicated. Cholera symptoms will settle more quickly, and transmission in epidemics will be reduced, if tetracycline is given in addition to ORS. Typhoid and other enteric fevers need to be treated with an appropriate systemic antibiotic according to the sensitivity of the causative organism. Infections with non-typhoidal salmonellae or *Campylobacter jejuni* rarely require treatment unless the patient is ill and immunocompromised or there is a documented bacteraemia. Parasitic infections such as amoebiasis or giardiasis require specific chemotherapy.

Surgery has little role in the management of gastrointestinal infection unless there is a bowel perforation or torrential bleeding.

Public health

Patients admitted to hospital with presumed infectious diarrhoea should be nursed in side rooms to minimize the risk of nosocomial spread of the infection. Cases of food poisoning, typhoid, tuberculosis, etc. are notifiable in the UK.

Prevention

Most diarrhoeal illness can be prevented through good personal hygiene and the provision of adequate sanitation. Immunization against enteric pathogens is an ideal aim but progress has been slow. Current vaccines against *S. typhi* are relatively effective, those against *V. cholerae* very ineffective. New recombinant and cholera vaccines based on cholera toxin look promising and may also offer protection again ETEC. There are no effective vaccines against most bacteria, protozoa, or enteric viruses.

Further reading

Bell, B.P., Goldoft, M., Griffin, P.M., *et al.* (1994). A multistate outbreak of *Escherichia coli* 0157:H7-associated bloody diarrhoea and hemolytic uremic syndrome from hamburgers. *Journal of the American Medical Association*, **272**, 1349–53.

Bern, C., Martines, J., de Zoysa, I., and Glass, R.I. (1992). The magnitude of the global problem of diarrhoeal disease: a ten year update. *Bulletin of the World Health Organisation*, **70**, 705–14.

Blaser, M.J. (1998). *Helicobacter pylori* and gastric diseases. *British Medical Journal*, **316**, 1507–10.

Doyle, M.P. (1990). Pathogenic *Escherichia coli*, *Yersinia enterocolitica* and *Vibrio parahaemolyticus*. *Lancet*, **336**, 1111–15.

DuPont, H.L. and Ericsson, C.D. (1993). Prevention and treatment of traveler's diarrhea. *New England Journal of Medicine*, **328**, 1821–7.

Farthing, M., Feldman, R., Finch, R., *et al.* (1996). The management of infective gastroenteritis in adults. A consensus statement by an expert panel convened by the British Society for the Study of Infection. *Journal of Infection*, **33**, 143–52.

Goodgame, R.W. (1996). Understanding intestinal spore-forming protozoa: cryptosporidia, microsporidia, isospora and cyclospora. *Annals of Internal Medicine*, **124**, 429–41.

Gore, S.M., Fontaine, O., and Pierce, N.F. (1992). Impact of rice based oral rehydration solution on stool output and duration of diarrhoea: meta-analysis of 13 clinical trials. *British Medical Journal*, **304**, 287–91.

Sanchez, J.L. and Taylor, D.N. (1997). Cholera. *Lancet*, **349**, 1825–30.

Chapter 5.23

Immune disorders of the gastrointestinal tract

M. R. Haeney

Introduction

The gut is normally protected by several mechanisms. The acid pH of the stomach and the proteolytic enzyme content of the intestine are formidable barriers to many organisms, but a change in the normal microflora of the intestine or impaired gut motility may allow pathogenic bacteria to flourish. Microbial antigens that resist these defences and penetrate the epithelial surface encounter the mucosal immune system of gut-associated lymphoid tissues and the local and systemic activity of immunoglobulins described in OTM3, pp. 1836–7.

Table 1 Gastrointestinal disorders associated with common variable immunodeficiency and other forms of primary antibody deficiency

Infective	Other
Giardiasis	Pernicious anaemia-like syndrome
Campylobacter enteritis	Hypogammaglobulinaemic sprue
Cryptosporidiosis	Coeliac disease
Strongyloides stercoralis	Carcinoma of the stomach
Salmonella/shigella infection	Nodular lymphoid hyperplasia
Viral enteritis	Inflammatory bowel disease
Bacterial overgrowth	Non granulomatous jejunoileitis

Normally, the intestinal immune system steers a delicate course between the extremes of immunological incompetence, with resulting vulnerability to ingested pathogens and hypersensitivity to dietary antigens, with immunologically mediated reactions each time that antigen is eaten.

Primary immunodeficiency diseases

In the compromised host, most infections are due to common pathogens that are readily identified and controlled, but opportunistic infections (from agents not normally pathogenic) often elude isolation, may not respond to available drugs, and carry a high fatality.

The gastrointestinal complications of every known form of primary and secondary immunodeficiency are legion. Attention here will be focused on representative disorders.

Common variable immunodeficiency (CVI)

This group of heterogeneous disorders is characterized by low serum immunoglobulin levels, a normal or low proportion of circulating B lymphocytes and, in about one-third of patients, impaired cell-mediated immunity. Between 30 and 50 per cent of patients with CVI have gastrointestinal problems at some time. Virtually any part of the gastrointestinal tract may be affected (Table 1) but the most common complaints are diarrhoea and weight loss. Non-gastrointestinal manifestations are described elsewhere (see Chapter 5.3, OTM3).

Stomach in CVI

Achlorhydria is found in about 30 per cent of patients and the associated atrophic gastritis occasionally leads to a syndrome resembling pernicious anaemia. It differs from the classical disease in several respects: the atrophic gastritis involves the whole stomach without antral sparing; the serum gastrin concentrations remain normal; and autoantibodies to gastric parietal cells and intrinsic factor are absent. There is an increased incidence of carcinoma of the stomach, sufficiently common to warrant yearly gastroscopic examination in hypogammaglobulinaemic patients who have atrophic gastritis.

Small intestine in CVI

Infective complications

Although infestation with *Giardia lamblia* is the most common identifiable cause of malabsorption, in many patients the cause is never found. Giardiasis may also cause diarrhoea, villous abnormalities, vitamin B_{12} and folate malabsorption, steatorrhoea, disaccharidase deficiency, and protein-losing enteropathy but the pathogenetic mechanisms are poorly understood.

Cysts of *Giardia* may be found in fresh stool specimens, in duodenal aspirates or jejunal biopsies, but in difficult cases, it can be useful to give a therapeutic trial of metronidazole. Other parasitic infestations occur. *Cryptosporidium* infection occasionally causes self-limiting diarrhoea but has a much more sinister outcome in patients with human immunodeficiency virus (HIV) infection.

Bacterial infections also cause diarrhoea in patients with CVI and *Campylobacter jejuni* is frequently responsible. Rarely, *Campylobacter* causes an ascending cholangitis and hepatitis. Treatment is a 2-week course of erythromycin (500 mg, four times daily).

Shigella or salmonella diarrhoea do not occur more commonly than normal. Overgrowth of commensal bacteria is common, but bacterial counts rarely exceed 10^5 organisms/ml, compared with counts of more than 10^6/ml in the blind-loop syndrome. Nevertheless, it is common practice to treat these patients empirically with tetracycline and metronidazole, often with symptomatic improvement.

*Nodular lymphoid hyperplasia (**NLH**) in CVI*

Lymphoid nodules in the lamina propria of the gut are described in many disorders and occasionally in healthy individuals, but their presence should raise suspicion of common variable immunodeficiency. NLH occurs in 20–50 per cent of such patients but is not necessarily symptomatic. The nodules, 1–3 mm in diameter, appear as protrusions on fibreoptic endoscopy and as multiple filling defects on barium studies. When restricted to the rectum or colon NLH can present with rectal bleeding, abdominal pain, and features of intestinal obstruction.

The ultrastructure of these nodules is similar to that of Peyer's patches. The condition probably represents hypertrophy of the gut associated lymphoid tissue in response to antigens in the gut lumen. Although NLH is not premalignant in hypogammaglobulinaemia, intestinal lymphoma has been reported in apparently immunocompetent subjects with extensive small-bowel nodular lymphoid hyperplasia.

In a few patients with unexplained diarrhoea, the mucosal lesion resembles coeliac disease or tropical sprue but with reduced or undetectable plasma cells within the lamina propria. Indeed, in tropical regions, about 1 per cent of patients with 'sprue' may be suffering from a primary humoral immunodeficiency syndrome. Malabsorption in such patients can improve rapidly after replacement immunoglobulin therapy. Jejunoileitis is a rare feature of common variable immunodeficiency and has a poor prognosis.

Management

The cornerstone of treatment of antibody deficiency is immunoglobulin replacement (see OTM3, Chapter 5.3). Antibody-deficient patients respond as promptly as others to appropriate antibiotics but prolonged courses of treatment are usually needed.

Selective IgA deficiency (see also Section 5, OTM3)

Gastrointestinal manifestations are listed in Table 2.

Pernicious anaemia

The association with selective IgA deficiency conforms to the classical Addisonian type in that atrophic gastritis shows antral sparing and raised serum gastrin concentrations occur.

Table 2 Gastrointestinal disorders sometimes associated with selective IgA deficiency

Infections	Giardiasis; bacterial overgrowth
Autoimmune disease	Pernicious anaemia; antiepithelial-cell antibody
Hypersensitivity disorders	Coeliac disease; cows' milk protein intolerance; inflammatory bowel disease
Neoplasia	Carcinoma of oesophagus, stomach, colon
Other	Nodular lymphoid hyperplasia; disaccharidase deficiency.

Malabsorption and steatorrhoea

IgA deficiency occurs in about 1 in 40 of patients with coeliac disease, over 15 times more frequently than in the general population. Patients with selective IgA deficiency and a flat jejunal mucosa respond to dietary gluten withdrawal in a way typical of classical coeliac disease.

Antibodies to dietary antigens

Secretory IgA helps prevent absorption of food antigens through the intestinal mucosa and there is a high prevalence of serum antibodies to food proteins in patients with selective IgA deficiency. IgA-deficient subjects also tend to have autoantibodies to antigens such as collagen and IgA itself.

Gastrointestinal infection

With the exception of *G. lamblia* infestation, infections rarely persist. Even giardiasis is far less frequent than in CVI. Chronic diarrhoea and malabsorption have followed truncal vagotomy and gastroenterostomy for duodenal ulceration due to overgrowth of commensal bacteria in the upper intestinal tract.

Crohn's disease and ulcerative colitis

Crohn's disease and ulcerative colitis occur in patients with IgA deficiency but their frequency is difficult to judge from the widely varying published reports.

Malignant disease

Oesophageal, gastric, and colonic neoplasms have been reported but it is not certain whether the risk of malignancy is truly increased.

Management

Patients with selective IgA deficiency rarely warrant immunoglobulin replacement, unless IgG2 deficiency is also present. Antibodies to IgA develop in about a third of patients and high titres may cause severe reactions to plasma or blood transfusions or intravenous immunoglobulin preparations.

Other types of primary immunodeficiency

Gastrointestinal problems occur in other types of immunodeficiency affecting infants or children (see OTM3, p.1840, Table 3).

Secondary immunodeficiency

Secondary immunodeficiency is far more common than primary immunodeficiency. In many cases, it is of minor relevance but occasionally its severity may mask the underlying condition. AIDS is

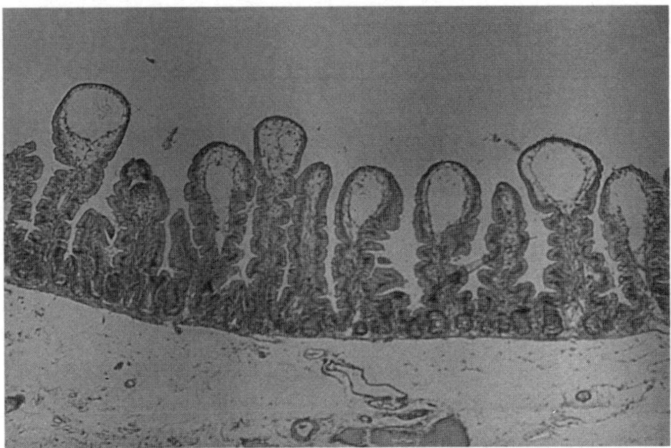

Fig. 1 A jejunal biopsy from a patient with intestinal lymphangiectasia showing dilated central lacteals.

a florid example of the gastrointestinal complications involving cell-mediated immunity predominantly. About half of the patients with HIV infection will have gastrointestinal involvement at some time and any level of the tract, from mouth to anus, can be involved.

The principal change in the small intestine is a partial villous atrophy, detectable early in the natural history. Enteropathogens causing intestinal infections are of the same types as in immunocompetent subjects but the infections are much more aggressive and invasive, and elicit little host immune response, so familiar symptoms and signs may be absent. Multiple infections and tumours may coexist.

The clinical features of HIV infection and AIDS are discussed in detail in Section 16.

Immunodeficiency secondary to gastrointestinal disease

Hypogammaglobulinaemia, particularly involving IgG, may be due to increased intestinal loss of immunoglobulin. A useful clue to this possibility is a low serum albumin. The main causes of protein losing enteropathy are discussed in Chapter 5.42).

Intestinal lymphangiectasia (see also Chapter 5.25) is an example of immunodeficiency resulting from increased loss of immunoglobulins and lymphocytes through the intestine. The basic defect is abnormal dilatation of the lymphatic vessels in the intestine. The condition may also occur secondarily to lymphatic obstruction, for example due to lymphomas in the intestine or constrictive pericarditis. The diagnosis should be suspected when there is T-cell lymphopenia, hypoalbuminaemia, and hypogammaglobulinaemia, and confirmed by finding dilated lymphatics in a jejunal biopsy (Fig. 1).

Food allergy and intolerance

Food allergy is one of the most controversial topics in medicine. It undoubtedly exists but extravagant claims that a staggering array of symptoms are due to food 'allergy' have confused the subject. The major cause of confusion lies in the lack of agreement on definitions and diagnostic criteria.

Definition

The term food allergy refers to a form of exaggerated reactivity (hypersensitivity) of the immune system to an ingested antigen. It should be used only when the abnormal reaction is proved to be immunologically mediated, either by IgE or some other immune mechanism (Table 3). The term food intolerance should be used to describe all abnormal, reproducible reactions to food when the causative mechanism is unknown or is non-immunological.

Aetiology

Food allergy

Up to 2 per cent of a protein meal can appear antigenically intact in the circulation. Non-IgE antibodies to proteins in cows' milk and eggs do occur in infants, but only if a large amount of the relevant protein is ingested. These antibodies gradually decline in the first few years of childhood. In contrast, relatively small amounts of protein are sufficient to induce relatively high antibody concentrations, including those of IgE type, in allergic children. Such infants tend to retain high concentrations of serum antibody during childhood.

Some forms of food allergy involve immune mechanisms other than IgE. For instance, in coeliac disease, there is strong evidence of exaggerated immunological reactivity to dietary gluten, but it is unclear whether local T-cell-mediated hypersensitivity, immune-complex formation, or other mechanisms cause the villous atrophy.

Food intolerance

This is much more common and includes irritant, toxic, pharmacological, or metabolic effects of foods, enzyme deficiencies, or even the release of substances produced by fermentation of food residues in the bowel. Some foods contain pharmacologically active substances (such as tyramine or phenylethylamine) that act directly on blood vessels in sensitive subjects to produce migraine. Traces of drugs, food additives (e.g. monosodium glutamate), colouring agents

Table 3 Classification of adverse reactions to foods

	Reproducible adverse reaction on food challenge		Immune mechanism		Non-immune mechanism	Examples
	Open	Blind	IgE	Other		
Food allergy	+	+	+	–	–	Immediate reactions to nuts, eggs, milk shellfish, fish
	+	+	–	+	–	Coeliac disease; cows' milk protein intolerance
Food intolerance	+	+	–	?	+	Irritable bowel syndrome (some); food-induced migraine; reactions to sulphites, nitrites, food additives
Food aversion	+	–	–	–	–	

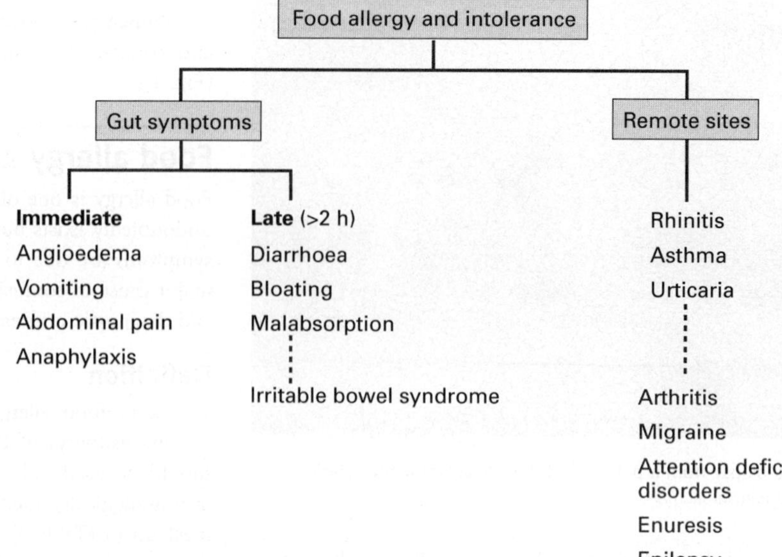

Fig. 2 Clinical spectrum of food allergy and intolerance. *(Redrawn from Chapel, H.M., Haeney, M.R., Misbah, S.A., and Snowden, H.N. (1999). Essentials of clinical immunology, (4th edn) by permission of the authors and Blackwell Scientific Ltd, Oxford.)*

(e.g. tartrazine), or preservatives (e.g. benzoic acid) can also cause symptoms in susceptible people by mechanisms that are ill understood, but are probably due to direct effects on mast cells.

Prevalence

There are no reliable data. Widely varying estimates are reported: between 0.3 per cent and 20 per cent of children suffer from, or have suffered from, symptoms caused by some form of dietary intolerance. Reactions to food additives are not as common as most people believe. In one study, 7.4 per cent of a survey population had symptoms suggestive of food additive intolerance; further clinical assessment and additive challenge showed a true prevalence of 0.01–0.23 per cent.

Clinical features

Food reactions can be early or late, confined to the gastrointestinal tract or occur at sites remote from the gut (Fig. 2).

Early reactions

These often occur within minutes or up to 2 h of ingestion, recur on challenge, and include, apart from gastrointestinal disturbances, such features as perioral rash, swelling of the lips, tingling of the throat, urticaria, angioedema, asthma, or even anaphylaxis. Such acute and severe allergic reactions are mostly due to IgE antibodies to foods and are the least controversial form of food allergy. They are fairly easy to diagnose and the offending food is readily identified, usually by the parent: the most common culprits are cows' milk (in infants), peanuts, eggs, fish, and shellfish. In some cases, anaphylaxis only occurs when the food is eaten immediately before exercise—food-induced, exercise-dependent anaphylaxis.

Late reactions

Symptoms occurring over 2 h after food ingestion, such as diarrhoea, bloating, or a fatty stool are suggestive of food intolerance, if not allergy. Features of the irritable bowel syndrome may be accompanied by allergic symptoms elsewhere but usually occur in isolation, without any evidence of an immunological reaction.

Remote symptoms

Some patients with acute, IgE-mediated reactions to foods also experience rhinitis, asthma, urticaria, angioedema, or eczema. However, eating the implicated foods does not always cause these remote systems. Sneezing bouts, blocked nose, or asthma can also occur after taking wine or other alcoholic drinks because of the irritant effect of sulphite preservatives or other components. This is not an immunological reaction. Many patients with atopic eczema find that certain foods provoke a transient red and blotchy rash but it is mainly in children that food makes eczema worse. Elimination diets rarely improve atopic eczema in adults. What is more debatable is whether food intolerance plays any part in remote symptoms such as migraine, attention deficit disorders, enuresis, or arthritis.

Specific syndromes of food allergy

Food allergy contributes to a number of common intestinal disorders. The immunological mechanisms are obscure but are not IgE mediated. In coeliac disease the intestinal damage is probably due to a local T-cell-mediated reaction to gluten.

Recognized syndromes of food intolerance

In a minority of patients, a relation to specific foods can be convincingly demonstrated. Sometimes, symptoms are provoked by the known irritant, pharmacological, or metabolic effects of food.

Most cases of *irrritable bowel syndrome* are unrelated to food intolerance but in a few—usually those with predominant diarrhoea, with some bloating and pain—a relation to specific foods can be demonstrated. Some patients are able to identify foods, such as cereals and dairy products, that provoke symptoms.

Lactose intolerance is not common in Europeans but affects up to 90 per cent of adult Africans and Orientals. It can occur as a transient result of gastroenteritis and even as a secondary effect of cows' milk protein intolerance.

Coffee and coffee withdrawal can provoke *migraine* in susceptible people. Certain cheeses cause headaches in many people, probably due to the tyramine content. Red wines, especially port, cause headaches in susceptible people because of their content of congeners.

Foods preserved by sulphites, particularly white wine, dried fruit, and fruit salads from supermarkets and restaurants sometimes provoke *asthma* by the release of sulphur dioxide.

Tartrazine and other coloured food dyes can sometimes trigger *urticaria* in sensitive subjects.

Chinese restaurant syndrome occurs when monosodium glutamate has been reported to cause a syndrome of chest pain, sweating, nausea, dizziness, and fainting in susceptible individuals.

Controversial issues

Behavioural problems in children

The belief that foods and food additives can induce *behavioural problems*, particularly attention deficit disorders is controversial.

Psychological distress in adults

Some patients with a multiplicity of vague and variable symptoms, such as fatigue and malaise, and disturbances of sleep, appetite, or libido turn to the diagnosis of food allergy as an explanation. Having made their own diagnosis, they have difficulty in accepting they are not allergic to foods, even though their food aversions may have resulted in a dangerously inadequate diet. Early diagnosis and sympathetic management is essential if unnecessary consultations and inappropriate allergy tests are to be avoided.

Diagnosis

Food allergy should not be diagnosed without clear evidence. Skin tests and radioallergosorbent tests are positive in about 75 per cent of patients who have IgE-mediated, acute, early reactions to foods such as nuts, egg, or fish. Usually, the offending antigen is obvious from the clinical history and confirmatory tests are needed only if there is doubt. In patients with late symptoms at sites remote from the gut (Fig. 2), skin and blood tests are notoriously unreliable. For most patients with suspected food intolerance, laboratory tests are of no diagnostic value.

Elimination diets and challenge tests form the basis of diagnosis. The relation between food and symptoms should be established by a placebo-controlled, double-blind challenge under medical supervision. In some cases it may be necessary to repeat the double-blind challenge several times before being convinced that the association between the food and the symptoms is not simply coincidental. Only about a quarter of reported 'adverse reactions' can be confirmed by double-blind challenge. Food challenges are not without risk: there is a danger of precipitating an anaphylactic reaction.

Treatment

Recognition of the offending food and its elimination from the diet is the cornerstone of treatment. In patients with acute, IgE-mediated reactions to a single food, such as shellfish, this is usually quite straightforward. Patients with violent anaphylactic reactions to foods need to be especially careful to avoid accidental exposure. A problem for such patients is the use of a food, most notably peanut, as an undeclared ingredient in manufactured foods or restaurant meals. Where there remains a risk of accidental ingestion it may be appropriate for some patients to carry a preloaded syringe of adrenaline for self-injection, after first being instructed in its use.

In less clear-cut situations, certain foods or food additives are eliminated empirically because they are frequently implicated in that form of food intolerance: for example, a diet free of azodyes, preservatives, and salicylates helps a proportion of patients with chronic intractable urticaria. Patients who seem intolerant of a wide range of foods may need a very restricted diet—sometimes called a 'few-food' diet. If symptoms are improved, then foods can be reintroduced one at a time. This is both diagnostic and therapeutic, but care is essential, as anaphylaxis can occur on reintroduction, especially in children.

Oral *sodium cromoglycate* has been used as an adjunct to diet in selected patients with food allergy, especially those with accompanying allergic reactions in the eyes, nose, and skin. Its effectiveness is still unproven.

Although *immunotherapy* (hyposensitization) is effective in wasp or bee venom anaphylaxis and in some forms of allergy to inhaled allergens, it is of no value in food intolerance.

Further reading

Bindslev-Jensen, C. (1998). Food allergy. *British Medical Journal*, **316**, 1299–302.

Teahon, K., Webster, A.D., Price, A.B., Weston, J., and Bjarnason, I. (1994). Studies on the enteropathy associated with primary hypogammaglobulinaemia. *Gut*, 35, 1244–9.

Strobel, S. and Mowat, A.M. (1998). Immune responses to dietary antigens: oral tolerance. *Immunology Today*, **19**, 173–81.

Chapter 5.24

The peritoneum, omentum, and appendix

M. Irving

Peritonitis

Most cases of infective peritonitis are secondary to diseases of intra-abdominal organs such as necrosis of the bowel, perforation of a neoplasm, appendicitis, Crohn's disease, colitis, diverticulitis, and perforation of peptic ulcer. Salpingitis may give rise to pelvic peritonitis. Less commonly, peritonitis may complicate ascites due to cirrhosis or the nephrotic syndrome. Common causative organisms are *Escherichia coli*, pneumococci, or streptococci. Pneumococcal peritonitis used to be encountered as a primary phenomenon but is not often seen now. Peritonitis may also complicate peritoneal dialysis. Tuberculous peritonitis is described elsewhere (see Section 16). 'Chemical peritonitis' may arise when acid, blood, talc, or glove powder are released into the peritoneal cavity.

Clinical signs and investigation

The characteristic picture of acute generalized peritonitis is one of agonizing abdominal pain in a patient who is pale and sweating, with shallow breathing, and who is lying absolutely still because every movement causes exacerbation of pain. Respiration is painful; the patient tends to breath with the thorax while holding the abdomen immobile, and will be unable to sit up. If asked to cough, those with generalized peritonitis will give an inadequate effort while those with localized disease will wince and immediately put a hand over the inflamed area. Another useful technique is for the examiner to place a hand 2 cm above the abdomen and ask the patient to raise the latter to touch the hand. This will prove impossible for one with acute generalized peritonitis.

Palpation will reveal widespread guarding, or rigidity in generalized cases, and similar signs over the inflamed organ in localized peritonitis. These signs may not be present in the very young or the very old, or may become less obvious when the disease is progressing or has been modified by analgesia, antibiotics, or corticosteroids. Most patients will be febrile with variable tachycardia, hypotension, oliguria, ileus, and vomiting.

Radiographs of chest and abdomen may show air under the diaphragm, distended loops of bowel, and fluid between loops. Aspiration of the peritoneal cavity through a fine needle may show leucocytes and organisms. Ultrasonography will reveal thickened bowel, and air and fluid in the peritoneal cavity and its recesses.

Treatment

The patient should be started on intravenous fluids to correct hypovolaemia. A nasogastric tube should be passed and the bladder catheterized. Cefuroxime and metronidazole should be given intravenously. Analgesic agents should also be given intravenously as absorption is unpredictable after intramuscular administration in such patients.

Intraperitoneal abscesses

Subphrenic and pelvic abscesses usually arise secondary to a perforated appendix or colonic diverticulum, or following a leak from an intestinal anastomosis. Occasionally, they may arise without obvious cause. The clinical picture is characterized by malaise, fever, and pain, often referred to the shoulder tip in the case of a subphrenic abscess. Physical signs are usually minimal, although in subphrenic abscess there may be a small, reactive pleural effusion on the affected side, and in pelvic abscess a boggy swelling may be felt on rectal examination. Plain radiographs of the abdomen may show gas and a fluid level under the diaphragm. The diagnosis may be facilitated by ultrasound examination and computed tomography (CT) scanning. Treatment is by percutaneous drainage under ultrasonographic or CT guidance. Open surgical drainage is virtually never required other than in thick, multilocular abscesses.

Most abscesses in other sites can also be readily detected by ultrasonography or CT scanning and drained percutaneously, but it is often difficult to detect an interloop abscess and therefore hard to ensure adequate drainage by this technique. In such patients, laparotomy may be the only way to ensure that the abscesses are detected and adequately drained.

Glove powder peritonitis

This condition has almost been eliminated by the use of starch-free gloves. Patients who develop it suffer abdominal pain, associated with an intermittent pyrexia, about a week to 10 days after operation. The abdomen is often swollen, with signs of free fluid and subacute intestinal obstruction. The condition can be treated conservatively but often the patient requires a further laparotomy.

Tumours of the peritoneum

The vast majority are the result of metastases from carcinomas arising in the gastrointestinal tract, the uterus, the ovary, the lung, and the breast. The only primary tumour of any significance arising from the peritoneum is the mesothelioma, commonly associated with exposure to asbestos.

Pseudomyxoma

In this rare condition the peritoneal cavity becomes distended with loculated masses of semitranslucent mucinous material. Although the usual cause is an ovarian cystic lesion, pseudomyxoma may arise from rupture of a mucocele of the appendix or from seeding throughout the peritoneum of a mucus-secreting neoplasm of the appendix or even *de novo*. Patients present with abdominal distension. Pseudomyxoma is difficult to treat because of its tendency to recur and of its lack of response to chemotherapy. The cystic masses can occasionally be excised but ultimately they accumulate, and eventually become inoperable. Debulking has a part to play and very vascular pseudomyxomas may occasionally be controlled by arterial embolization. Patients with chronic intestinal obstruction not amenable to operation may be successfully treated with home parenteral nutrition.

Adhesions

Adhesions following surgery or peritonitis may rarely give rise to pain relieved by laparoscopic division. Such adhesions tend to be small and may well give rise to pain by traction on a small area of parietal peritoneum.

Tuberculous peritonitis

Tuberculous peritonitis may be generalized or localized. The omentum is often extensively involved and forms a palpable mass in the upper abdomen. The diagnosis and management of this condition is described in Section 16. Symptoms are usually insidious and consist of fever, anorexia, and weight loss. In about 70 per cent of cases there is abdominal distension resulting from ascites.

Fungal and parasitic peritonitis

These rare forms of peritonitis present a similar clinical picture to that of tuberculosis. Fungal peritonitis usually occurs in patients who are immunosuppressed, or are being treated by chronic peritoneal dialysis. Cryptococcal infections affect immunosuppressed patients, and peritoneal schistosomiasis has been recorded, simulating malignant diseases.

Familial paroxysmal peritonitis

This condition is part of the syndrome of familial polyserositis or familial Mediterranean fever, described in Chapter 6.16.

Appendicitis and other appendiceal conditions

Incidence of appendicitis is now falling, possibly as the result of the more widespread use of high-residue diets.

Aetiology and diagnosis

The usual explanation attributes the inflammation to obstruction of the mouth of the lumen with a faecalith, but is challenged by some. Although there does not seem to be a sustainable pathological basis for a diagnosis of 'chronic appendicitis', the long-held belief in a 'grumbling appendix' could be explained by recurrent faecalithic obstruction. However, it is more likely that patients with such symptoms are afflicted by the irritable bowel syndrome.

Acute appendicitis can occur at any age. The incidence rises rapidly in children over the age of 5 years and reaches a peak during the second and third decades of life. The disease is not uncommon in elderly people and can occur in extreme old age.

Appendicitis can be a challenging diagnosis to make in children, elderly people, and pregnant women. The classical signs are seen most often in young and middle-aged individuals. The symptoms begin with colicky abdominal pain in the periumbilical region, perhaps caused by appendicular peristalsis to overcome the postulated faecalithic obstruction. Most patients vomit at this stage. If the faecalith is not expelled, venous congestion causes distension and bacterial growth occurs in the lumen. The wall of the appendix becomes inflamed and its arterial supply compromised. The great omentum wraps itself around the inflamed organ and the local peritonitis causes right iliac fossa pain and rebound tenderness.

In elderly people the incidence of perforation increases. These patients may have fewer of the classical physical signs and indeed may present with features of intestinal obstruction. They are less likely to have a leucocytosis than are younger patients.

In patients with retrocaecal appendicitis the ureter may be involved, leading to dysuria and inflammatory cells in the urine. An appendix in this position or one lying in the pelvis may also involve the psoas muscle, leading to psoas sign (flexion contracture of the hip).

Examination usually reveals tenderness and guarding in the right iliac fossa. Rectal examination rarely provides useful signs and indeed appendicitis should not be diagnosed just on a finding of rectal tenderness. If the appendix perforates, which it usually does at its base, localized peritonitis results and may be contained by the omentum and form an abscess. If not, then a spreading, generalized peritonitis ensues.

Differential diagnosis

Differential diagnosis from gynaecological causes may be difficult, especially in a woman, with pelvic peritonitis. In young adults, the presence of an element of small-bowel obstruction raises the possibility of Crohn's disease. Frank obstruction and dilated loops of bowel can be a feature of late appendicitis. Mesenteric adenitis, once a popular diagnosis, is probably only a rare cause of abdominal pain.

Investigations

The white-cell count is rarely of value unless a low one leads to a review of the diagnosis. Plain radiographs of the abdomen can reveal a large faecalith lying in the right iliac fossa or a dilated loop of small or large bowel caused by an associated ileus. Barium enema can show a filling defect at the base of the appendix or incomplete filling of the appendix. Ultrasonography is capable of showing the presence of the distended appendix. Peritoneal aspiration with a fine needle can show a cellular response suggestive of appendicitis. In confusing cases, a CT scan can occasionally be of value.

Treatment

The standard management is appendicectomy. The laparoscopic method is associated with less postoperative pain and wound infection.

Appendix abscess

When patients present with a 2–3-day history of appendicitis and a mass is found in the right iliac fossa, ultrasound should reveal any abscess. If found, it should be drained percutaneously. In the absence of persisting symptoms or recurrence of the abscess there is then no need for interval appendicectomy. However, any residual mass should be investigated with colonoscopic examination of the caecum to ensure there is no underlying neoplasia.

Non-acute inflammation of the appendix

Chronic inflammation of the appendix resulting from obstruction of its base with consequent accumulation of mucus in the lumen and the development of a globular swelling is an undoubted entity and can present as a mucocele. Such patients complain of discomfort in the right iliac fossa and occasionally a mass may be felt. The condition can be revealed by ultrasound examination.

Carcinoid tumour

Carcinoid tumour can be revealed histologically after appendicectomy. A small proportion will go on to metastasize to the liver and cause carcinoid syndrome (see Chapter 5.5).

Adenocarcinoma

Adenocarcinoma of the appendix is rare. It may present as acute appendicitis, may be an incidental finding at laparotomy, or can present as a mass in the right iliac fossa.

Other appendiceal tumours

Leiomyoma, fibroma, neuroma, neurofibroma, and ganglioneuroma have all been described but are curiosities. Similarly, occasional rare malignancies have been described, such as sarcoma and a condition called malignant mucocele. The treatment of these lesions follows the general principles outlined above.

Further reading

See OTM3, p.2011.

Chapter 5.25

Congenital and hereditary disorders of the liver, biliary tract, and pancreas

From contributions to OTM3 by J. A. Summerfield and C. A. Seymour

Congenital abnormalities of the biliary tree are described in OTM3, Chapter 14.21. They include congenital atresias and intrahepatic (Caroli's syndrome) and extrahepatic (choledochal cyst) dilatation of the bile ducts. Infantile polycystic liver disease is usually rapidly fatal because of associated renal disease. Adult polycystic liver disease may cause pain or discomfort in the right upper quadrant of the abdomen, usually in women in their fourth or fifth decade (see Chapter 12.12). Congenital hepatic fibrosis is an autosomal recessive condition usually diagnosed under the age of 10. The fibrosis causes portal hypertension and patients bleed repeatedly from oesophageal varices. Because liver function is well preserved, portocaval shunts can be successful, but liver transplantation is an alternative. The prognosis is determined also by associated renal abnormalities, which include dysplasia, medullary cystic disease, and adult-type polycystic kidneys.

Inherited metabolic disease affecting the liver

Haemochromatosis

This term refers to a group of conditions in which iron in the body is increased and is deposited in and damages the parenchyma of various organs. In the primary form, idiopathic haemochromatosis, iron overloading of liver is a major feature, determined by a gene situated on the long arm of chromosome 6 near the *A* locus of the human leucocyte antigen (**HLA**) system. Secondary forms of iron overload, such as occur with iron-loading anaemias, particularly thalassaemia major, present with similar features as far as the liver involvement is concerned.

Clinical features

Primary haemochromatosis is described in Section 3. Hepatomegaly in association with diabetes, skin pigmentation, cardiomyopathy, and joint disease is the typical presentation. In the early stages, it is rarely associated with clinical symptoms or signs of hepatic dysfunction, and liver enzyme tests are often normal when the patient first presents. A major complication is the development of hepatocellular carcinoma in association with cirrhosis and iron overload.

Hepatic pathology

In primary haemochromatosis parenchymal iron loading is found in conjunction with cirrhosis and is demonstrable by blue staining of iron granules with Perl's reagent. Any therapy that reduces or depletes the iron stores will often leave lipofuscin granules ('wear and tear' pigment), which do not stain for iron. In secondary haemochromatosis, iron granules may be more prominent in reticuloendothelial cells.

Investigations

Increased saturation of transferrin and increased serum ferritin concentrations correlate with the degree of iron overload in primary and secondary disease. Liver function tests may be normal or show slight increases in transaminases.

Genetic markers such as HLA (-A3, -B14) and DNA analysis have proved important in identifying genetic haemochromatosis. Direct methods of confirming the disease and monitoring treatment involve liver biopsy. Histological grading establishes the extent of overload and identifies the predominantly periportal and hepatocytic iron distribution. Genetic haemochromatosis has a more parenchymal distribution, whereas in secondary haemochromatosis, iron is localized to Kupffer cells and fibrotic areas. Measurement of the hepatic iron concentration by atomic absorption spectrophotometry correlates closely with measurement of iron stores by a desferrioxamine test.

Management of haemochromatosis

In the genetic type, iron depletion can be achieved by phlebotomy, with monitoring of liver iron concentrations by ferritin measurements and computed tomography or magnetic resonance imaging scanning. Screening of relatives by HLA typing and DNA studies is an essential prophylactic measure. In secondary forms of haemochromatosis, phlebotomy may be helpful. Iron overload in the iron-loading anaemias, thalassaemia for example, is best treated with prolonged subcutaneous desferrioxamine infusions or oral-chelating agents such as hydroxypyridones.

Other causes of secondary iron overload

Chronic alcoholic liver disease

Iron overload is found in some 30 per cent of alcoholics. The histological appearance of liver tissue shows Mallory bodies in addition to iron-induced damage to hepatocytes. Differentiation from genetic haemochromatosis heterozygotes can be difficult.

Porphyria cutanea tarda

This chronic condition results from a deficiency of uroporphyrinogen decarboxylase (see Chapter 6.7). The liver form is sporadic and the enzyme abnormality is restricted to the hepatocyte. Clinical expression is usually exacerbated by alcohol, oestrogens, iron, and other liver disease. The iron overload is of moderate order (less than four times the normal value) and responds, as does the porphyrin overload, to iron depletion by phlebotomy, which also resolves the skin lesions and reduces the light sensitivity of exposed areas of skin.

Copper toxicity

Wilson's disease

This inherited disorder of copper metabolism is characterized by increased body copper, predominantly in hepatocytes but also in the kidneys, cornea, and brain. It is described in detail in Chapter 6.10.

Chronic cholestatic syndromes

Intra- and extrahepatic disturbances in the secretion of bile, the major route of copper excretion from the body, can also lead to copper accumulation in the liver and elsewhere. These can arise with congenital abnormalities of the biliary tract (e.g. biliary atresia) or from secondary damage to the liver and biliary tract (e.g. primary biliary cirrhosis, Indian childhood cirrhosis). Unlike Wilson's disease, biliary-cell damage precedes the accumulation of copper, which increases with progressive cholestasis and exacerbates the destruction of hepatocytes and biliary cells.

The liver in cystic fibrosis

There is an increasing awareness of hepatic involvement in this disease, although pulmonary manifestations are still the main determinants of survival. This has become important now that lung transplantation is available for selected patients with the disease. To date, there is no mutation that identifies the patient at specific risk of developing liver disease. Liver involvement must be sought for in every patient.

Clinical features

Hepatic disease may occur at any age as focal biliary cirrhosis, as well as portal hypertension and liver failure in adolescents and young adults. Some patients have bile duct strictures, which may also contribute to liver damage. Cirrhosis is found in 10 to 15 per cent of adolescents, but hepatomegaly and portal hypertension is now found increasingly in patients with cystic fibrosis in their 20s. However, only 13 per cent of patients undergoing lung transplantation for severe cystic fibrosis have abnormal liver tests.

Investigations

Common abnormalities include increased alkaline phosphatase and γ-glutamyl transferase, but their levels do not correlate well with the degree of portal fibrosis and it is essential to make an ultrasonographic examination of the liver and gallbladder to exclude gallstones. Liver biopsy is the most informative investigation for suspected liver involvement and cholestasis.

Pathology

The liver in cystic fibrosis may vary in appearance from fatty change at birth to different degrees of bile duct obstruction. Mucous plugs in cholangioles are believed to be the cause of inflammation and proliferation, and predispose to chronic liver damage and cirrhosis. The parenchymal architecture and hepatocyte integrity are relatively well preserved. In most adult patients, focal biliary cirrhosis is the characteristic lesion. In older patients these fibrotic areas increase to involve the portal tracts and, later, the hepatic parenchyma. Established cirrhosis follows.

Up to 25 per cent of patients have abnormal liver function and extrahepatic lesions (such as strictures) of the common bile duct are present in nearly all patients suffering from liver disease.

Pathogenesis

The most reasonable explanation for liver involvement is that biliary-tract cells and hepatocytes may have the same impaired handling of electrolytes in affected patients that has been described for respiratory and secretory epithelia, (pancreas, salivary, and sweat glands) and that these cells are then more susceptible to injury and progressive fibrosis.

Management

There is, at present, no treatment for severe liver damage other than orthotopic liver transplantation. Treatment is directed towards portal hypertension (including sclerotherapy if varices bleed) and hypersplenism/splenic infarction (including splenectomy), and to the management of gallstones, biliary obstruction, and liver failure. In order to reduce the incidence of bile plugging, chenodeoxycholic acid is used in patients who have pancreatic, biliary, or liver problems.

Reye's syndrome

This syndrome of fulminant encephalopathy and acute hepatocyte dysfunction occurs in previously healthy children in the week following a viral infection. It is rare, acute, and can arise in children of any age. There are now increasing reports of Reye's syndrome in adults following flu-like illness.

Clinical features

A typical patient is usually between 6 and 14 years of age. Initial features are a trivial viral illness followed by persistent vomiting with increasingly severe encephalopathy, deepening confusion, and rapid progression to coma. In the latter stages, seizures occur in association with flaccidity, loss of deep tendon reflexes, and respiratory arrest. Typically, there are no clinical features of liver disease, and the diagnosis must be suspected in cases with transient increases in transaminases, an increased plasma ammonia, and hypoglycaemic episodes with prolonged prothrombin times, but tests of liver enzymes and function are often normal. Other abnormalities include a low plasma very low density lipoprotein, and increased serum concentrations of uric acid and creatine phosphokinase (CK-MM).

Diagnosis

Liver biopsy done under cover of fresh frozen plasma shows diagnostic features within a few days of onset of vomiting. Hepatocytes typically show a swollen, rounded contour with central nuclei, cytoplasmic fragmentation, and glycogen depletion. There is no hepatic necrosis or inflammation and the triglyceride found in hepatocytes is not the typical lipid droplets of chronic fatty liver. Ultrastructural changes include swollen, pleomorphic mitochondria; there is a reduction in mitochondrial enzyme activities with preservation of cytoplasmic enzymes. Progressive mitochondrial deformity occurs and is self-limiting over about 2–6 days after the onset of encephalopathy. Some evidence suggests a genetic predisposition.

Treatment

Early diagnosis and intensive care may improve the outcome. Maintenance of cerebral circulation and oxygenation is important, and mechanical ventilation is necessary to prevent hypoxia. Hypothermia should be avoided. Hypoglycaemia should be averted by dextrose infusions, and patients should be given appropriate therapy to reduce intracranial pressure.

Prognosis

Death rates vary from 10 to 50 per cent. Some survivors have permanent brain damage, which is probably related to the duration of the encephalopathic phase of the illness. The most effective way of preventing complications or death is to suspect the disease. There is a link with the use of aspirin and an increased predisposition to a Reye-like syndrome. Limiting the use of aspirin in children under 5 years has been associated with a significant reduction in the disease.

Inherited pancreatitis

Chronic pancreatitis may occur with autosomal dominant or more rarely autosomal recessive inheritance, often involving several generations of affected families. The major forms are idiopathic, and associated with cystic fibrosis, hereditary hyperlipoproteinaemia (types I and V), and hereditary hyperparathyroid disease.

Hereditary pancreatitis

This disease occurs in Caucasians as a rare autosomal dominant and presents in childhood. There is evidence for suppression of the gene for pancreatic structural protein (**PSP**) and its secretory form (**PSP-S**). There is also a possible association between this pancreatitis, expression of the *erb*-B2 receptor, and development of pancreatic carcinoma.

Clinical features

The condition usually presents in children, with recurrent episodes of acute abdominal pain lasting 1–2 days. Rarely, there are associated features of acute pancreatitis. After some years, steatorrhoea may develop; pancreatic calcification eventually occurs. Other complications include pancreatic pseudocysts, thrombosis of splenic and portal veins, and, in up to 25 per cent, the development of pancreatic carcinoma. Surprisingly, diabetes is rare.

Diagnosis

Increased serum amylase and lipase activities can be detected during attacks of abdominal pain,. Pancreatic calcification can be noted on plain abdominal radiographs. About half the patients have aminoaciduria, predominantly of cystine and lysine.

Differential diagnosis

Other causes of chronic pancreatitis associated with inherited disorders need to be excluded, such as cystic fibrosis, haemochromatosis, hereditary hyperlipoproteinaemias, and primary hyperparathyroidism.

Further reading

Desmet, V.J. (1992). Congenital diseases of the intrahepatic bile ducts, variations on the theme 'ductal plate malformation'. *Hepatology,* **16**, 1069–83.

Mastella, G. and Cipolli, M. (1999). The liver in cystic fibrosis. In *Oxford textbook of clinical hepatology,* 2nd edition (ed. J. Bircher, J.-P. Benhamou, N.McIntyre, M. Rizzetto, and J. Rodés), pp. 1403–19. Oxford University Press.

O'Brien, S., Keogan, N., Casey, M., *et al.* (1992). Biliary complications of cystic fibrosis. *Gut,* 33, 387–91.

Sherlock, S. and Dooley, J. (1997). *Diseases of the liver and biliary system.* Blackwell Science, Oxford.

Steindl, P., Ferenci, P., Dienes, H.P., *et al.* (1997). Wilson's disease presenting in patients with liver disease, 'a diagnostic challenge'. *Gastroenterology,* **113**, 212–18.

Walshe, J.M. and Yelland, M. (1993). Chelation treatment of neurological Wilson's disease. *Quarterly Journal of Medicine,* **86**, 197–204.

Diseases of the pancreas

Chapter 5.26

Acute pancreatitis

C. W. Imrie

Aetiological factors (Table 1)

Major factors

The two major aetiological factors, biliary disease and alcohol abuse, together account for over 80 per cent of cases. In those not obviously explained by these factors, endoscopic retrograde cholangiopancreatography (ERCP) often reveals very small stones in biliary sludge and bile crystals. The way in which the transient migration of small stones causes acute pancreatitis is not understood. But it is clear that the risk is much greater with small stones.

Alcohol abuse pancreatitis is usually found in young males who drink in excess of 80 g alcohol/day. Up to 10 per cent of patients may have both a biliary pathology and alcohol abuse. Alcohol may cause acute pancreatitis by acinar stimulation with ampullary spasm.

Table 1 Aetiological factors in acute pancreatitis

Major	Minor
Biliary disease	Post-ERCP
Alcohol abuse	Blunt trauma
	Coxsackie B
	Mumps virus
	Hyperlipoproteinaemia
	Ampullary tumour
	Hyperparathyroidism
	Worm infestation (SE Asia)
	Scorpion bites (Trinidad)
	Drugs

Table 2 Conditions that may occasionally be involved in the aetiology of acute pancreatitis

Hypothermia
Sclerosing cholangitis
α_1-Antitrypsin deficiency
Pancreatic cancer
Cancers metastatic to pancreas: Renal Stomach Breast Ovarian Lung
Virus infection: Hepatitis ECHO
Duodenal reduplication
Annular pancreas

Minor factors

Iatrogenic acute pancreatitis may be induced by surgical or endoscopic procedures involving the ampulla of Vater. ERCP carries a risk for acute pancreatitis of about 1 per cent. Following a therapeutic endoscopic sphincterotomy the risk of acute pancreatitis is approximately 3 per cent. Failure to clear the duct of stones and inadequate sphincterotomies are the two most common predisposing features.

Viral infection particularly mumps virus, Coxsackie B, and hepatitis can cause acute pancreatitis. One clinical feature that may prove useful is prodromal diarrhoea, which is rare in all other types of acute pancreatitis.

Drug-induced involvement with, e.g. valproic acid, azathioprine, L-asparaginase, and corticosteroids has (rarely) been associated with acute pancreatitis.

Hyperparathyroidism is now recognized to be an uncommon accompaniment of acute pancreatitis. The association is calculated at 0.1 per cent. Removal of the parathyroid adenoma usually relieves further attacks.

The association with types I and V *hyperlipoproteinaemia* is hard to validate. Most patients with the association have a high alcohol intake, but some with primary hyperlipoproteinaemia are prone to attacks of acute pancreatitis.

Hypothermia is a particularly important association in the elderly. In younger patients, alcohol abuse may be linked, particularly if patients fall asleep out of doors or in a cold, unheated house. Histologically, the acute pancreatitis is perilobular.

Blunt trauma from, e.g. sports injuries and traffic accidents may result in acute pancreatitis, usually from a crush injury to the body of the pancreas against the vertebral column.

Periampullary adenoma or cancer is an important association. Effective treatment of the tumour abolishes recurrent attacks.

Other rare causes are listed in Table 2.

Pathology

All patients with acute pancreatitis have microscopic evidence of necrosis, while macroscopic changes, particularly black discoloration, are confined to the most severe cases. Periductal necrosis is typical of biliary and alcohol causation. Less commonly, a perilobular necrosis is found, usually in patients with hypothermia or gross hypotension.

Clinical features

Sudden onset of severe upper abdominal pain with vomiting is the most common presentation. The pain may focus in the epigastrium, right or left upper quadrant, with penetration through to the back. Occasionally it encircles the upper abdomen. It tends to lessen in severity progressively over the first 72 h, and is unusually a significant factor beyond this time. Patients with stones in the common bile duct may be jaundiced, and cholangitis can supervene in a minority. Much milder degrees of jaundice may occur from compression of the lower bile duct in patients with alcohol-induced disease. Gross hypotension only occurs in the very severe cases. Bowel sounds are rarely present in the early phase and paralytic ileus may extend beyond 4 days. Indeed the duration of ileus is a useful marker of severity of disease.

In those with *mild attacks*, intravenous fluids and nasogastric suction may often be discontinued after 48 h. It is important to monitor the volume of nasogastric aspirate and urinary output to maintain adequate fluid replacement. Even in this category of patients it may occasionally be necessary to provide 4–5 litres of intravenous fluid in the first 24 h of the illness.

Patients with *severe attacks* may be pyrexial, hypotensive, markedly tachypnoeic, and suffer from acute ascites, pleural effusions, and prolonged paralytic ileus. Body-wall staining at the umbilical area (Cullen's sign) or in the flanks (Grey Turner's sign) can occur. Renal and respiratory compromise are common. The urine output and arterial oxygen saturation must be monitored, and arterial gas analysis may be needed three or four times in the first 24 h. These patients may often require intensive care for single or multi-organ failure, circulatory and ventilatory support.

Renal dysfunction may result not only from hypovolaemia, but also from renal arteriolar vasoconstriction and ultravascular coagulation in glomerular capillaries. In most cases, adequate fluid replacement and/or low-dose dopamine maintain adequate renal function, but acute tubular necrosis or even cortical necrosis may ensue.

Hypoxaemia is the hallmark of acute pancreatitis and reflects its severity. Shunting of blood in the pulmonary vascular bed may account for up to 30 per cent of cardiac output. Hypoxaemia can usually be reversed by the provision of humidified oxygen, but in severe cases, the pattern is similar to adult respiratory-distress syndrome. Hyaline membrane formation has been found in severe cases, when reversal of the respiratory insufficiency takes many weeks. Pleural effusions may be large enough to warrant aspiration.

Laboratory abnormalities

Levels of serum amylase over four times the upper limit of normal are usually taken as diagnostic, provided the clinical course corresponds. The lipase level is more specific; levels of twice the upper limit of normal are significant.

There are very high levels of circulating cytokines early in the disease. Tumour necrosis factor-α, platelet-activating factor, and interleukin 6 are present in greatest concentration in those with severe acute pancreatitis.

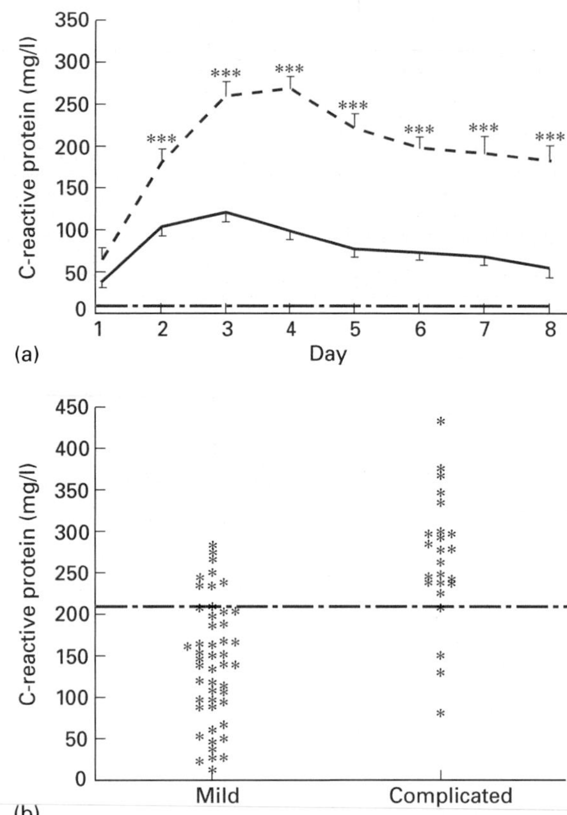

Fig. 1 (a) Sequential C-reactive protein concentrations in 47 patients with mild pancreatitis (—) and 25 with complicated attacks (- - -). Results are expressed as mean ± SEM; $*p < 0.05$; $**p < 0.01$; $***p < 0.001$ (mild versus complicated); (— - —), upper limit of normal for C-reactive protein. (b) Scattergram showing discrimination between mild and complicated attacks of pancreatitis based on the peak C-reactive protein concentration recorded on days 2–4. — - —. The peak concentration providing the best discrimination was ≥210 mg/litre.
(Reproduced with permission from British Journal of Surgery.)

Hypocalcaemia is a common feature, in some cases the result of loss of albumin, but in others reflecting a line fall in ionized calcium and an appropriate increase in concentrations of parathyroid hormone.

Disseminated intravascular coagulation is an uncommon complication. An increase in C-reactive protein is usual and is a useful marker of the severity of the disease and its progress (Fig. 1).

Pyrexia

This is a reflection of cell damage and necrosis and a low-grade fever is typical in the first 3–4 days. More severe or prolonged fever may result from ascending cholangitis especially in jaundiced cases. In severe disease, bacteria may reach the necrotic tissue around the pancreas, by transudation from the transverse colon.

Diagnosis

The diagnosis is usually made from the clinical presentation. Gross elevations of amylase and lipase in blood support it, while urinary amylase levels of greater than five times the upper limit of normal can be helpful in less typical cases. Peritoneal aspiration can be helpful

Table 3 Differential diagnosis of acute pancreatitis

Perforated duodenal ulcer	Ectopic pregnancy
Acute cholangitis	Renal failure
Acute cholecystitis	Macroamylasaemia
Mesenteric ischaemia/infarction	Ruptured aortic aneurysm
Small-bowel obstruction/perforation	Dissecting aortic aneurysm
Atypical myocardial infarction	Diabetic ketoacidosis

Table 4 Glasgow Prognostic Score

WBC	>15 000/mm^3
Glucose	>10 mmol/l (no diabetic history)
Urea	>16 mmol/l (despite IV infusion)
PO_2	<8 kPa (60 mmHg)
Albumin	<32 g/l
Calcium	<2.0 mmol/l
LDH	>600 international units/l
AST/ALT	>200 units/l

Any three or more factors = severe acute pancreatitis. The greater the number of factors, the poorer the prognosis.

WBC, white blood count; LDH, lactic dehydrogenase; AST, aspartate transferase; ALT, alanine transferase.

and the aspiration of more than 20 ml of free fluid without bacterial contamination is indicative of severe disease. Computed tomography (CT) may reveal pancreatic swelling, fluid collection, and change in density of the gland. Angiogram-enhanced CT scanning is mandatory to obtain the most useful information.

Differential diagnosis (Table 3)

High amylase levels not caused by pancreatitis may confuse. They are found in renal failure, in ectopic pregnancy, diabetic ketoacidosis, and after perforation of a duodenal ulcer. Similarly, mesenteric ischaemia or infarction can be associated with biochemical changes similar to those of acute pancreatitis, but in both these situations bacterial contamination of the peritoneal cavity will be detected by peritoneal aspiration. High levels in macroamylasaemia are due to failure of glomeruli to filter the larger molecules, so that urinary levels are very low.

Grading disease severity

The Glasgow scoring system of prognostic factors is shown in Table 4. CT scanning can also help assessment and regular monitoring of C-reactive protein provides a simple guide to severity and progress (Fig. 1).

Clinical management

Pain is treated with pethidine or buprenorphine; intravenous benzodiazepines may be required in severe cases. Morphine has a strong spastic effect on the sphincter of Oddi and is contraindicated. Rapid correction of hypovolaemia, monitored by measurement of the central venous pressure, and sufficient intravenous fluid to maintain a minimum urine flow of 30 ml/h are essential.

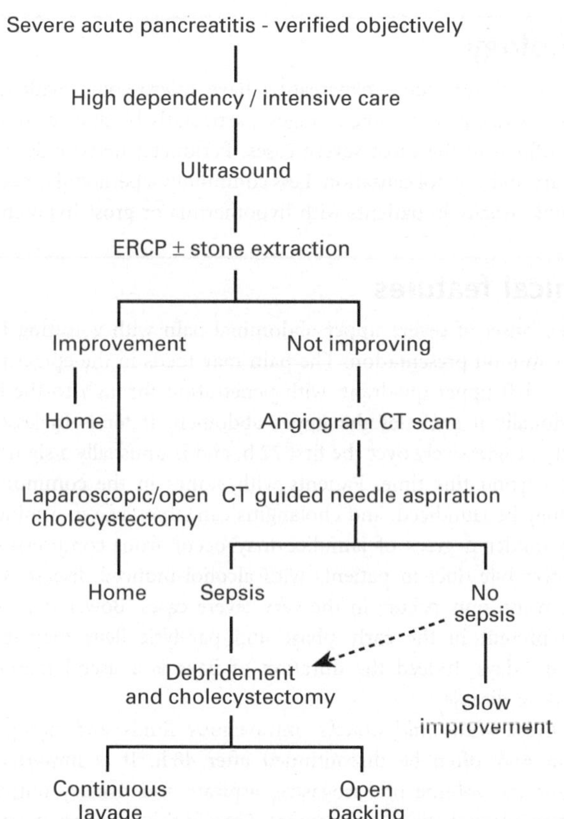

Fig. 2 Summary of management of acute pancreatitis.

If gallstones have been identified, laparoscopic or open cholecystectomy should be done in the same admission. In older and infirm patients, ERCP sphincterotomy alone is considered a satisfactory alternative.

The severely ill patient

An algorithm for the management of severe acute pancreatitis (Fig. 2) may prove valuable.

Two controlled studies and a large body of clinical data indicate that early endoscopic sphincterotomy in those with gallstone acute pancreatitis provides a significant therapeutic advantage. Intravenous antimicrobial therapy is recommended as a cover for ERCP sphincterotomy and the drugs most widely used include the third-generation cephalosporins and piperacillin. The administration of imipenem to patients with severe acute pancreatitis throughout the first 2 weeks of illness has been found to be of value in several studies. Fungal infection may be a problem in long-term management where broad-spectrum antimicrobials are given for more than 10 days.

Another approach has been to strive to lower the concentration of intestinal organisms by gut irrigation combined with antimicrobial therapy, in the belief that transudation of organisms from the transverse colon into the peripancreatic necrotic tissue may occur.

The role of surgery

Patients who develop infection in the necrotic tissue in and around the pancreas require open surgical debridement of the necrotic tissue. After the removal of the infected tissue there are two options. One is to establish a postoperative lavage system. Alternatively, if venous ooze is a particular problem, packing of the abdominal cavity with large cotton packs wrapped in non-adhesive paraffin gauze, together with limited or non-closure of the abdominal wall, has been advocated.

Debate continues as to whether only patients with infected necrosis warrant such surgical intervention. Some have strongly advocated that uninfected necrosis can be managed successfully without surgical intervention. The proportion of patients coming to surgery varies between 4 and 15 per cent rising to some 35 per cent in those with severe acute pancreatitis.

Nutrition and gallstone eradication

At the time of surgical debridement it is important to provide for postoperative nutrition by the insertion of a feeding jejunostomy. Cholecystectomy and common-duct clearance are indicated in patients with stones or biliary sludge. Indeed, all patients coming to surgery should have a cholecystectomy, as it is often impossible to identify small stones.

Pancreatic pseudocyst

This condition is probably overdiagnosed. It is recommended that the term 'acute fluid collections' be used at an early stage in the disease because these frequently disappear spontaneously. Even established pseudocysts can resolve spontaneously in about 50 per cent of patients. For those not resolving, synthetic somatostatin therapy (octreotide) given subcutaneously three times a day, can be helpful, either alone or combined with percutaneous drainage of the pseudocyst cavity. Percutaneous aspiration alone invariably results in recollection of the fluid quite rapidly, but infection is potentially associated with long-term percutaneous drainage.

Pancreatic ascites

This condition occurs either when a pancreatic pseudocyst spontaneously decompresses into the peritoneal cavity or a major pancreatic duct disrupts after trauma or pancreatitis, with escape of pancreatic juice into the peritoneal cavity. Treatment comprises either a combination of intravenous nutrition and octreotide therapy or surgical excision of the disconnected segment of pancreas.

Rare complications

Rarer complications of severe acute pancreatitis include splenic vein thrombosis and subcutaneous fat necrosis. The latter condition is sometimes referred to as Weber Christian disease—relapsing, nodular, non-suppurative panniculitis. Although some dispute that this is a true entity, it is reasonable to preserve the term when manifestations are classical. These comprise the occurrence of crops of tender nodules in the skin and subcutaneous fat on thighs, trunk, and buttocks, which may recur over several years, more commonly in middle-aged women. The lesions often ulcerate and, on healing, leave atrophic scars. Histological examination of biopsies shows inflammation involving fat lobules of the panniculus and small blood vessels show endothelial proliferation and oedema of the media, but not true vasculitis. The presence of the latter should suggest systemic lupus erythematosus or other vasculitic illness. Treatment of Weber Christian disease is difficult; prednisolone or immunosuppression may be tried but are often ineffective. There is an association in some cases with acute pancreatitis, pancreatic carcinoma and, in others, with α_1-antitrypsin deficiency. Panniculitis can also be a feature of lymphomas.

Further reading

Corfield, A.P., Cooper, M.J.C., and Williamson, R.C.N. (1985). Acute pancreatitis; lethal disease of increasing incidence. *Gut*, **26**, 724–9.

Larvin, M. and McMahon, M.J. (1989). APACHE II score for assessment and monitoring of acute pancreatitis. *Lancet*, **ii**, 201–4.

Ranson, J.H. (1982). Etiology and prognosis factors in acute pancreatitis, a review. *American Journal of Gastroenterology*, 77, 633–8.

Chapter 5.27

Chronic pancreatitis

P. P. Toskes

Patients with chronic pancreatitis come to medical attention largely due to two complaints—abdominal pain or maldigestion (diarrhoea, steatorrhoea, weight loss). The great variability in symptoms and the many causes of this disease have made its classification problematical. Three forms have been recognized: (a) chronic calcifying; (b) chronic obstructive; and (c) chronic inflammatory. Alcohol abuse and/or malnutrition are the most common causes of the calcifying type. Obstruction of the main pancreatic duct with secondary fibrosis in that part of the pancreas proximal to the obstruction leads to the obstructive type. Chronic inflammatory pancreatitis is not well characterized. Often irreversible changes occur in the gland, making a cure improbable.

Histologically, in advanced cases the gland may be fibrotic, calcified, and there may be marked dilation of the main duct. Inflammation and sclerosis with progressive damage to the acini and ducts are the histological hallmarks of chronic pancreatitis. Islet cells are usually lost more slowly than the exocrine part, thus preserving endocrine function relative to exocrine function.

Aetiology (Table 1)

Chronic alcoholism and cystic fibrosis are the most frequent causes in adults and children, respectively. Cholelithiasis rarely, if ever, causes chronic pancreatitis because a cholecystectomy is almost always done after the first or second attack of acute pancreatitis related to gallstones. Hypertriglyceridaemia may cause chronic as well as acute pancreatitis. Tropical pancreatitis (Africa and Asia) is characterized by calcific disease, glucose intolerance, and infrequent pain. Pancreatic exocrine impairment is not infrequent in patients with haemochromatosis and α-antitrypsin deficiency but this is usually not symptomatic. Secondary pancreatic exocrine insufficiency may occur after gastric surgery. The acid hypersecretion associated with gastrinoma may irreversibly inactivate lipase, causing steatorrhoea. Hereditary pancreatitis is described in Chapter 5.25. Developmental anomalies leading to pancreatitis will be discussed below.

Idiopathic chronic pancreatitis may account for up to 20 per cent of cases. These tend to present solely with unexplained abdominal pain, and have small-duct disease. A hormone stimulation test is necessary to detect them. Endoscopic retrograde cholangiopancreatography (**ERCP**) may miss up to 30 per cent of those with chronic pancreatitis who have abnormal hormone stimulation tests.

Pathophysiology

There remains controversy as to whether alcohol-induced disease is secondary to a primary reduced secretion of pancreatic-stone protein

Table 1 Conditions associated with chronic pancreatitis

Alcohol abuse
Cystic fibrosis
Malnutrition (tropical)
Pancreatic cancer
Gastrinoma
Trauma
Familial pancreatitis
Schwachmann's syndrome (pancreatic insufficiency and bone marrow dysfunction)
Trypsinogen deficiency
Enterokinase deficiency
Isolated deficiencies of amylase or lipase
Haemochromatosis
α_1-Antitrypsin deficiency
Postsurgery:
Pancreatic resection
Subtotal gastrectomy with Billroth I or II anastomosis
Truncal vagotomy and pyloroplasty
Idiopathic pancreatitis

or a direct toxic effect of alcohol. In tropical pancreatitis a combination of protein deficiency and a toxin in the diet, which is high in cassava or sorghum, may cause the disease. A primary defect in the electrolyte permeability of epithelium within the pancreatic ducts of patients with cystic fibrosis results in reduced fluid flow, producing hyperconcentrated proteinaceous secretions that precipitate and obstruct the ducts. The pathophysiology of the other causes of chronic pancreatitis is not understood.

Incidence

The prevalence in autopsy studies varies from 0.04 to 5.0 per cent. The only prospective study found a prevalence of 26.4 cases per 100 000 population and an incidence of 8.2 new cases per 100 000 per year, but this study was largely based on alcohol-induced pancreatitis.

Clinical features

The pattern, severity, and frequency of abdominal pain may vary considerably. It has no characteristic features and may be constant or intermittent. Eating may often increase its severity. Approximately 15 per cent of cases never suffer abdominal pain but present with steatorrhoea, diarrhoea, and weight loss.

Diagnosis

Computed tomography (CT) scans may reveal diffuse enlargement of the pancreas and, occasionally, a pseudocyst (Fig. 1). Ultrasonography may reveal calcification and dilatation of the pancreatic duct; calcification may also be seen on plain abdominal radiographs (Fig. 2). The levels amylase, lipase, or trypsin are usually not elevated except in patients who have a pseudocyst. There may be elevated

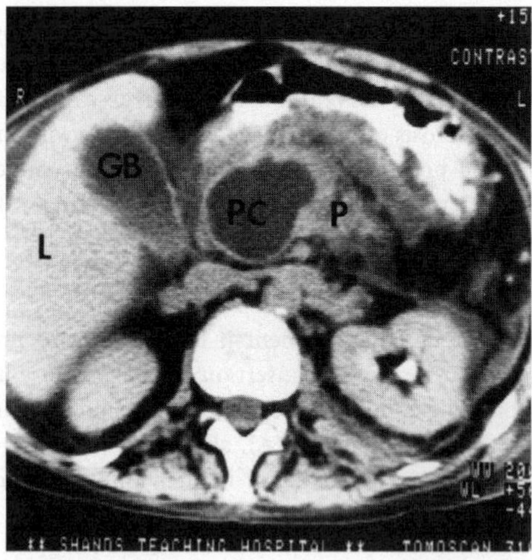

Fig. 1 CT scan demonstrating a pseudocyst (PC) in the head of the pancreas, diffuse enlargement of the pancreas (P) a normal liver (L), and normal gallbladder (GB).

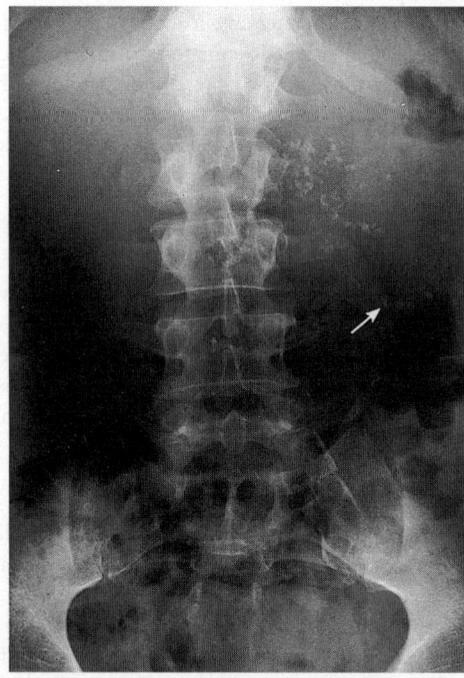
Fig. 2 Plain film of the abdomen showing diffuse pancreatic calcification; the arrow points to one of the calcified areas.

alkaline phosphatase secondary to an inflammatory reaction around the common bile duct. Some patients with severe disease may have elevated fasting blood-glucose levels.

A number of tests are available to assess structure and function of the pancreas (see OTM3, p. 2037). The most accurate means of detecting chronic pancreatitis is a combination of a hormone stimulation test and ERCP.

Management

The cornerstone of medical management is the use of pancreatic enzyme formulations. The principles of therapy are similar for treating pain or steatorrhoea. Pancreatic enzymes decrease abdominal pain in some patients. Those most likely to respond have small-duct disease;

Table 2 Frequently used pancreatic enzyme therapy

Pancrelipase
• Viokase (C), 8 tablets each time • Pancrease (E), 3 capsules each time
Pancreatin
• Creon (E), 3 capsules each time
Adjuvant
• Sodium bicarbonate, one 650-mg tablet before and after each meal and 1300 mg at bedtime for pain • H_2-receptor antagonists in usual acid-suppressive doses, twice a day • Omeprazole, 20 mg every day • The enzymes should be administered before meals; a bedtime dosage should be given if the enzymes are being used to treat pain

C, conventional preparation; E, enteric-coated preparation.

patients with large-duct disease do not respond well. Eight tablets or capsules of a potent, non-enteric-coated enzyme preparation should be given at mealtime and at bedtime, with appropriate adjuvant therapy (Table 2). Abstinence from alcohol is recommended and the diet should be moderate in fat (30 per cent), high in protein (24 per cent), and low in carbohydrate (40 per cent). Non-narcotic analgesics are the pain-relieving medications of choice.

Figure 3 outlines an approach to patients with abdominal pain thought to be secondary to chronic pancreatitis.

If there is large-duct disease, a lateral pancreaticojejunostomy should be done. Immediate pain relief occurs in 80 per cent of patients, sustained in about 50 per cent at 1–3 years. If the ducts are not significantly dilated, most patients can eventually have their pain controlled by adjusting enzyme and adjuvant therapy; for example, substitution of omeprazole for H_2-receptor antagonist, total parenteral nutrition with no food orally for several weeks, or performing a nerve block. It is now rare for a major pancreatic resection to be done for pain control. Octreotide in doses up to 200 μg three times daily given subcutaneously can be effective in lessening pain in severe disease.

Endoscopic therapy for pain has been disappointing. Only acute biliary decompression has been shown to be effective in controlled trials. Following stent placement, complications such as bleeding, sepsis, pancreatitis, and perforation have occurred, and stents can induce progressive ductal changes similar to the abnormalities seen in chronic pancreatitis.

Steatorrhoea is a late finding and does not occur until less than 10 per cent of lipase is secreted. Enzyme therapy (Table 2) controls steatorrhoea and diarrhoea effectively but formulations containing lipase in amounts of 25 000 units or higher have been associated with the occurrence of colonic strictures in patients with cystic fibrosis. No such problems have occurred in adult patients with chronic pancreatitis.

Decreasing the amount of long-chain triglyceride in the diet and/or adding medium-chain triglycerides may decrease the steatorrhoea and enhance weight gain and energy.

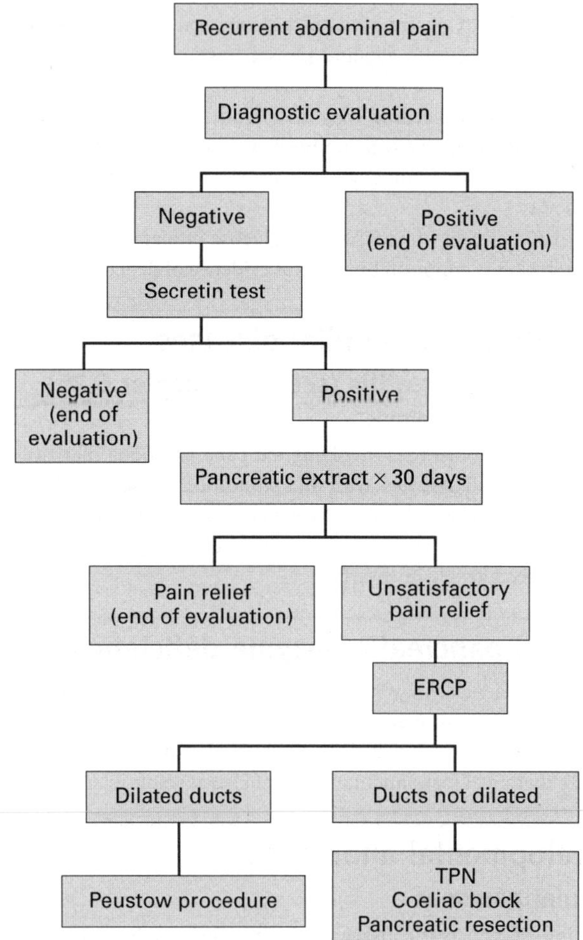

Fig. 3 Approach to management of chronic pancreatitis and abdominal pain.

Table 3 Complications of chronic pancreatitis

Structural	Metabolic
Phlegmon	Narcotic addiction
Pseudocyst	Diabetes mellitus
Abscess Ascites	Cobalamin (vitamin B_{12}) malabsorption
Common bile-duct obstruction	Subcutaneous fat necrosis
Duodenal obstruction	Bone pain
Splenic-vein thrombosis	Non-diabetic retinopathy
Gastrointestinal bleeding	Pancreatic cancer

Complications

Table 3 lists the structural and metabolic complications of chronic pancreatitis. Inflammatory masses are common. Ultrasonography and CT have helped in sorting out phlegmon from pseudocyst from abscess. The management of pseudocysts is currently being re-evaluated. Their ability to undergo late resolution may have been underestimated and the incidence of serious complications overestimated. In patients with minimal symptoms, no evidence of active alcohol abuse, and a mature pseudocyst not resembling a cystic neoplasm, non-intervention is appropriate.

True pancreatic ascites should be distinguished from 'reactive ascites' in which the ascitic amylase content is not nearly as high as in the pancreatic state. Patients with pancreatic ascites should have total parenteral nutrition and no food by mouth. Surgery may be needed if the ascites persists.

Management of obstruction to the common bile duct should be conservative unless the alkaline phosphatase remains very high or cholangitis develops.

Gastrointestinal bleeding may arise from portal hypertension associated with splenic-vein thrombosis or if a pseudocyst erodes into the duodenum or from a pseudoaneurysm within the wall of a pseudocyst.

Up to 30 per cent of patients have glucose intolerance. Vitamin B_{12} malabsorption is common but clinical evidence of deficiency is rare.

Hereditary and familial diseases

Hereditary pancreatitis (see also Chapter 5.25)

Schwachmann's syndrome

This is a familial disorder involving the pancreas, bone marrow, and skeletal system. Neonates with this condition present with severe steatorrhoea. The associated neutropenia leads to frequent infections. The steatorrhoea is well treated by pancreatic enzymes but severe skeletal defects result in dwarfism.

Isolated pancreatic enzyme deficiencies

Protease deficiencies may result from a deficiency of enterokinase or a deficiency in trypsinogen. The addition of exogenous enterokinase to duodenal secretions will distinguish. Both conditions respond to enzyme therapy. Lipase and colipase deficiency result in steatorrhoea.

Developmental anomalies

Annular pancreas

The ring of pancreatic tissue encircling the duodenum may lead to intestinal obstruction in the neonate or the adult. Non-specific symptoms of postprandial fullness, nausea, abdominal pain, and vomiting may be present for years before the diagnosis is made. The differential diagnosis should include duodenal webs, tumours of the pancreas or duodenum, postbulbar peptic ulcer, Crohn's disease of the proximal intestine, and adhesions. Patients with annular pancreas have an increased incidence of pancreatitis and peptic ulcer. Surgery may be necessary and retrocolic duodenojejunostomy is the procedure of choice.

Pancreas divisum

When the ventral and dorsal parts of the pancreas fail to fuse, pancreatic drainage is accomplished mainly through the accessory papilla. This anomaly is not often a predisposing factor to the development of pancreatitis, but the combination of pancreas divisum and a small accessory orifice may result in dorsal-duct obstruction. Patients with pancreatitis and pancreas divisum should be treated conservatively, including enzyme therapy. Endoscopic or surgical intervention is indicated only when these methods fail.

Further reading

Ammann, R.W., Heitz, P.U., and Kloppel, G. (1996). Course of alcoholic chronic pancreatitis; a prospective clinico-pathological long term study. *Gastroenterology*, 111, 224–31.

Forsmark, C.F. and Grendell, J.H. (1991). Complications of pancreatitis. *Seminars in Gastrointestinal Diseases*, 3, 165–76.

Toskes, P.P. (1993). Medical therapy of chronic pancreatitis. *Seminars in Gastrointestinal Diseases*, 3, 804–16.

Toskes, P.P. (1993). Chronic pancreatitis. *Current Opinion in Gastroenterology*, 9, 767–73.

Chapter 5.28

Tumours of the pancreas

R. C. G. Russell

Carcinoma

Carcinoma of the pancreas carries a particularly poor outlook. Fewer than 20 per cent of patients survive the first year and only 3 per cent are alive 5 years after the diagnosis.

Incidence

The disease is rare before the age of 45 years, but its occurrence rises sharply thereafter. Worldwide, there are large variations in incidence. In the United States, it was 9/100 000 in 1988, with a male/female ratio of 1.3:1. Afro-Caribbeans are more frequently affected, with an incidence of 15.2/100 000. In India, Kuwait, and Singapore the rate is less than 2.2/100 000; in Sweden it is 12.5 and in Japan the rate has risen sharply from 1.8 in 1960 to 5.2/100 000 in 1985. In the United Kingdom there were 5839 deaths from pancreatic carcinoma in 1995.

Risk factors

Cigarette smoking has the firmest link. Many studies have found that the relative risk in smokers is at least 1.5, and increases with the number of cigarettes smoked; the excess risk levels off 10–15 years after stopping smoking.

The second most important risk factor appears to be diet, notably a high intake of fat, meat, or both. A protective effect is ascribed to diet containing fresh fruits and vegetables. The suggestion that coffee consumption may contribute is controversial. A few of the 30 studies have suggested a possible increase in risk, but no prospective study has found a significant association.

There are families that develop hereditary pancreatitis and have a markedly increased risk of pancreatic cancer, suggesting that there may be a link between the two, but studies of non-hereditary chronic pancreatitis have also suggested a weak association. Diabetes mellitus is associated with pancreatic cancer, with a fourfold increase in the risk ratio.

Even after correction for smoking there appears to be a two- to fivefold increased risk of pancreatic cancer 15–20 years after partial gastrectomy. Increased formation of *N*-nitroso compounds by nitrate reductase-producing bacteria that proliferate in the hypoacidic stomach could be responsible for both the gastric and pancreatic cancers. Other possible carcinogenic influences include industrial toxins, socio-economic status, and viruses.

Pathology

Primary malignant epithelial neoplasms of the pancreas can occur either in the exocrine parenchyma or the endocrine cells of the islets of Langerhans but they are far more frequent in the former. Non-epithelial tumours are exceedingly rare. Ductal adenocarcinoma makes up between 75 and 92 per cent of pancreatic neoplasms and is twice as frequent in the head of the pancreas as in the body or tail. At the time of diagnosis, over 85 per cent of tumours have extended beyond the pancreas. Pancreatic adenocarcinoma has a proclivity for perineural invasion within and beyond the gland, although lymphatic spread also leads to early metastasis to adjacent and distant lymph nodes. The most common sites of extralymphatic involvement are the liver and peritoneum, and the lung is the most frequently affected extra-abdominal organ. Two histological pathological classifications are used commonly; the Armed Forces Institute of Pathology classification deals primarily with exocrine neoplasia. The other is from WHO, which combines endocrine and exocrine neoplasia as well as some non-neoplastic lesions (see OTM3, p. 2041).

Giant-cell carcinoma has no clinical distinguishing feature from ductal adenocarcinoma except for a tendency to a larger size at presentation and a shorter survival, with a median of only 2 months and few, if any, documented survivors at 1 year from diagnosis. The histopathological appearance is unmistakable, with large polypoid, often bizarre, giant mononucleated or multinucleated tumour cells that are obviously malignant.

Adenosquamous carcinoma presents in an identical manner to the ductal carcinoma. The ductal component is usually well differentiated but may be very small in quantity. Squamous metaplasia rather than squamous carcinoma may occur. The prognosis is poor.

Microadenocarcinoma is characterized by sheets of small oval or round cells with small or moderate amounts of cytoplasm and no neurosecretory granules. Necrosis is common but fibrosis is rare. These tumours have a particularly poor prognosis.

Mucinous adenocarcinoma is associated with a much longer survival. Histologically, the mucin-filled cystic spaces are separated by internal collagen septa. The mucin itself may produce biliary obstruction, and jaundice as a result of these tumours is not relieved by the insertion of a stent, which blocks with mucus.

Mucinous carcinoid features both mucin-producing ductal adenocarcinoma and carcinoid tumour. *Mucinous cystadenocarcinoma* is a variant that tends to occur in younger females and rarely involves the pancreatic head. The median size at presentation is large and the survival is generally better than for ductal adenocarcinoma. These tumours may show calcification on plain radiographs. The cysts are completely lined by columnar cells showing a wide range of histological appearance.

Pancreatoblastoma is a neoplasm of childhood and has a mixed cell type with ductal, acinar, epidermoid, and islet cells present. The prognosis is poor but rare long-term survivors have been recorded.

Papillary cystic tumour presents as a gradually enlarging, painful mass in the left upper quadrant in young women. It has a relatively good prognosis. The solid areas consist of sheets of small polyhedral cells with a moderate amount of eosinophilic cytoplasm.

Acinar-cell carcinoma is clinically associated with polyarthritis, skin lesions, and metastatic fat necrosis, possibly due to raised levels of serum pancreatic lipase. It consists of large, polyhedral acinar cells with basal, round nuclei and an abundant, dense, eosinophilic, granule-containing cytoplasm. It has a particularly poor prognosis.

Lymphoma can occasionally involve the pancreas and must be differentiated from other pancreatic masses.

Clinical features

Symptoms and signs

The early symptoms of non-hormone-producing pancreatic neoplasms are usually non-specific. Early symptoms are often ignored. Examples include epigastric bloating and flatulence (31 per cent), general fatigue and weakness (31 per cent), diarrhoea (25 per cent), vomiting (23 per cent), and constipation (13 per cent). Up to 90 per cent of patients will present with incurable advanced disease, with one or other of the classical triad of symptoms of pain, jaundice, or weight loss.

Painless jaundice carries the best prognosis if it is due to a tumour in the pancreatic head, as it need only be small and local to produce intrapancreatic bile-duct obstruction. If the jaundice is present when the tumour is in the body or tail of the pancreas, there is invariably metastasis to the lymph nodes in the porta hepatis. Pain is, overall, the most common symptom and is diffuse in the early stages, and may be posture related, similar to musculoskeletal disease, intermittent at onset, mimicking of biliary disease, and food related, suggestive of peptic ulcer. It is usually epigastric but one-quarter of patients also have back pain; some only have back pain. Pain in the left upper quadrant is suggestive of body and tail disease. Cramping abdominal pain may be secondary to fat malabsorption. Weight loss may be rapid despite normal appetite, due to steatorrhoea. There are other uncommon presenting symptoms: acute cholecystitis or acute pancreatitis; upper gastrointestinal haemorrhage; neuropsychiatric disturbance; diabetes mellitus; polyarthritis or painful skin nodules due to metastatic fat necrosis (especially with acinar-cell adenocarcinoma); pyrexia of unknown origin; clinical steatorrhoea; and, migratory thrombophlebitis or thromboembolic disease.

Important signs include an upper abdominal mass, icterus and scratch marks, hepatomegaly, palpable gallbladder (Courvoisier's sign), supraclavicular lymphadenopathy (usually left-sided), splenomegaly (due to portal or splenic vein compression, thrombosis or diffuse liver involvement), periumbilical mass (due to lymphatic spread along the line of the umbilical vein), ascites and/or peripheral oedema (including inferior vena caval obstruction), and thrombophlebitis.

Investigation

Blood tests

A number of non-specific abnormalities may be found including a raised erythrocyte sedimentation rate and C-reactive protein, a normochromic normocytic anaemia, and abnormal liver function tests. A number of tumour antigens can be assayed but no one of them can independently establish the diagnosis.

Ultrasonography, computed tomography, and magnetic resonance imaging

Each can detect pancreatic masses as small as 1–2 cm, dilatation of the pancreatic and bile ducts, hepatic metastases, and extrapancreatic spread. These techniques have shown that approximately 70 per cent of patients at presentation will have local extension, 40 per cent contiguous organ involvement, 40 per cent hepatic metastases, 30 per cent regional lymphadenopathy, and 85 per cent vascular involvement.

Endoscopic retrograde cholangiopancreatography (ERCP)

ERCP can define periampullary tumours with the possibility of biopsy and allows imaging and cytological sampling of both bile and pancreatic ducts, but in up to 12 per cent of patients the ductal system is normal.

Endoscopic and intraoperative ultrasonography

Endoscopic ultrasonography enables pancreatic tumours to be clearly evaluated, with clear views of the pancreas in over 90 per cent of studies. Peroperative ultrasonography has limited value except as a method of imaging the liver more accurately and defining the presence of metastases.

Percutaneous biopsy and cytology

Histological confirmation of the diagnosis is mandatory. The main disadvantage of the percutaneous technique is the small risk of tract seeding, which occurs only in patients with disseminated disease. The incidence of major complications is small (<2 per cent), with acute pancreatitis and haemorrhage being the most common.

Laparoscopy

This technique is useful in the determination of seedling deposits not visible by current imaging techniques. It also has a role as an independent predictor of operability and can be of great value when methods of imaging are unavailable.

Treatment

Surgery

A review of the results of resection in 4100 patients in 1987 showed that only 3.5 per cent survived 5 years. Later data suggest that a 5-year survival of 24 per cent can be achieved in a selected group with small tumours (2 cm or less in diameter) and no evidence of distant disease. Tumours of the ampulla of Vater have a much better (40 per cent) 5-year survival.

Radiotherapy

This may be useful in the treatment of tumours that are not resectable but are localized. Radiotherapy, combined with 5-fluouracil can improve median survival from 5 to 10 months. External beam treatment has a role as an adjuvant treatment after resection and can help palliation of pain.

Chemotherapy

5-Fluouracil can improve median survival and combinations with other agents such as doxorubicin and cisplatin can relieve pain.

ERCP and stenting

In cases in which the tumour has obstructed the bile duct, stent placement by ERCP can relieve jaundice and provide confirmation of the diagnosis by biopsy. The disadvantage of this approach is the risk of infection or pancreatitis which might delay the chance of curative surgery. Biliary drainage to reverse the ill-effects of cholestasis has not been of proven benefit in controlled trials.

Palliative care

The treatment of diabetes, steatorrhoea, and malnutrition improves the quality of life, and the management of pain by coeliac plexus block can be effective.

Further reading

Lillemoe, K.D. (1995). Current management of pancreatic carcinoma. *Annals of Surgery*, 221, 133–48.

Warshaw, A.L. and Del Castillo, F. (1992). Pancreatic carcinoma. *New England Journal of Medicine*, 326, 455–65.

Chapter 5.29

Diseases of the gallbladder and biliary tree

J. A. Summerfield

Disorders of the biliary system usually give rise to the symptoms and signs of biliary obstruction (cholestasis). Pain can range between abdominal discomfort to severe right hypochondrial colic caused by a sudden rise in biliary pressure. Jaundice, dark urine, and pale stools indicate obstruction of the bile duct. Itching is an important sign of biliary obstruction. Nausea and vomiting may be prominent in sudden obstruction of the bile duct, usually by a gallstone. The milder symptoms of flatulence and intolerance of fatty food are more common. Fever and rigors indicate bacterial infection of the biliary tract. In jaundiced patients, weight loss is usual and results from fat malabsorption due to the lack of bile acids reaching the gut. Prolonged biliary obstruction leads to skin changes: increased pigmentation and cholesterol deposits (xanthelasma and xanthoma). Finally, biliary cirrhosis may develop, causing the signs of portal venous hypertension and liver-cell failure.

Laboratory investigations

Most disorders of the biliary system give rise to the biochemical picture of cholestasis. A notable exception is gallstones in the gallbladder when the liver function tests are usually normal. In cholestasis, the serum bilirubin concentration may be normal or raised and most of the bilirubin is esterified (conjugated). Bilirubinuria is present. The disappearance of urobilinogen from the urine indicates complete biliary obstruction. Elevation of the serum alkaline phosphatase is an important but not invariable sign of biliary obstruction. Other biliary canalicular enzymes accumulate in the blood, including 5′-nucleotidase and γ-glutamyl transpeptidase. These enzymes are found only in the liver and are estimated if there is doubt as to whether the alkaline phosphatase is of bony or hepatic origin. Serum transaminases show only modest elevation in contrast to the rises that occur in hepatitis. The serum cholesterol concentration rises and may cause abnormalities of red-cell shape (target cells). A prolonged prothrombin time reflects intestinal malabsorption of fat-soluble vitamin K due to a lack of bile acids. Vitamin A and D deficiency may also develop. The serum albumin and γ-globulin concentrations are normal until biliary cirrhosis develops. A polymorphonuclear leucocytosis accompanies bacterial infections of the biliary system.

Imaging techniques

The preferred first investigation is ultrasonography (Fig. 1). Computed tomography (CT) and magnetic resonance imaging are used in complicated diagnostic problems. Hepatic scintiscanning with $^{99}Tc^{m}$-labelled HIDA (dimethyl acetanilide iminodiacetic acid) is an alternative and is of value in the diagnosis of acute cholecystitis. Oral cholecystograms are taken if ultrasound is not available and to determine whether the gallbladder functions in patients with gallstones being assessed for oral bile-acid dissolution therapy (see below). However, these investigations usually provide insufficient anatomical detail for planning of treatment. Then endoscopic retrograde

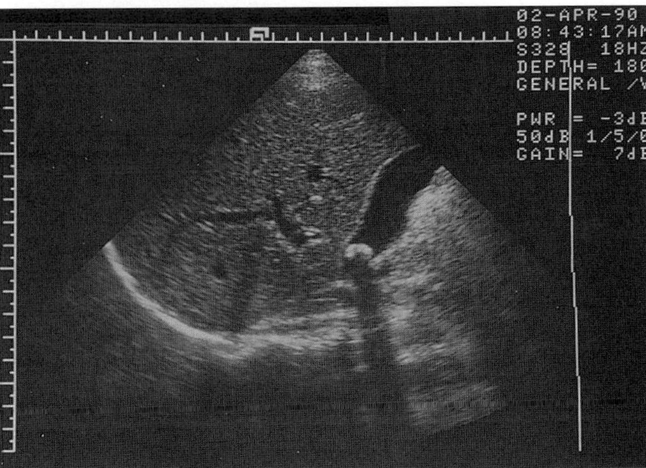

Fig. 1 Ultrasound scan of the gallbladder shows gallstones (arrowed) as bright round objects which cast acoustic shadows.

cholangiopancreatography (**ERCP**) or percutaneous transhepatic cholangiography (**PTC**) are used. Both these techniques carry small risks, including haemorrhage, biliary peritonitis, and cholangitis (PTC) and bowel perforation and cholangitis (ERCP).

Gallstone formation

Gallstone disease affects between 10 and 20 per cent of the world's population. Stones may be comprised largely of cholesterol (70 per cent) or of bile pigment. Cholesterol stones result from the secretion of cholesterol-saturated bile by the liver, but the precise reason for saturation is unclear. Pure cholesterol stones are usually solitary, but mixed cholesterol stones (cholesterol in a matrix of calcium bilirubinate, calcium phosphate, and proteins, Figs 2 and 3) are usually multiple and faceted. Pure bile pigment stones are black, hard, and brittle containing an insoluble black pigment, calcium bilirubinate, calcium carbonate and phosphate, calcium salts of fatty acids and bile acids. Brown pigment stones are soft and friable and comprise calcium bilirubinate cholesterol and calcium soaps. Cholesterol stones account for up to 70 per cent of gallstones in Europe and the USA. Brown pigment stones are common in the Far East and are associated with infection of the biliary tree with *Escherichia coli*, bacterioides, and clostridia. Black pigment stones are found in patients with cirrhosis, chronic obstruction of the bile duct, chronic haemolytic states, and malaria. About 50 per cent of all pigment stones are radio-opaque and they account for some 70 per cent of all opaque stones.

Natural history of gallstones

The majority of gallstones remain in the gallbladder and may give rise to no symptoms. Impaction of a stone in the neck of the gallbladder results in inflammation and the symptoms and signs of acute or chronic cholecystitis. Acute cholecystitis will subside if the stone spontaneously disimpacts or may progress to gangrene and perforation, or empyema, of the gallbladder. Gallstones may pass through the cystic duct into the bile duct, resulting in biliary obstruction and jaundice. Cholangitis is then a complication which can lead to a liver abscess. Gallstones may perforate through the inflamed gallbladder to form an internal fistula, usually to the small intestine or colon. A large gallstone passing into the small intestine may impact in the ileum, resulting in intestinal obstruction (gallstone ileus).

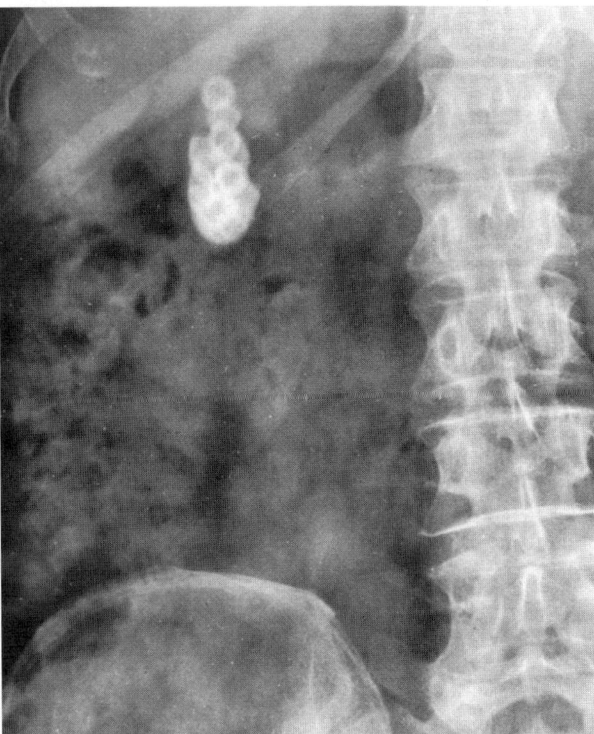

Fig. 2 Calcified gallstones. Gallstones contain sufficient calcium to be visible on a plain abdominal radiograph in about 10 per cent of patients. The gallbladder stones are surrounded by a ring of calcium salts.
(Reproduced from Sherlock, S. and Summerfield J.A. (1979). A colour atlas of liver disease, Wolfe Medical Publications, London, with permission.)

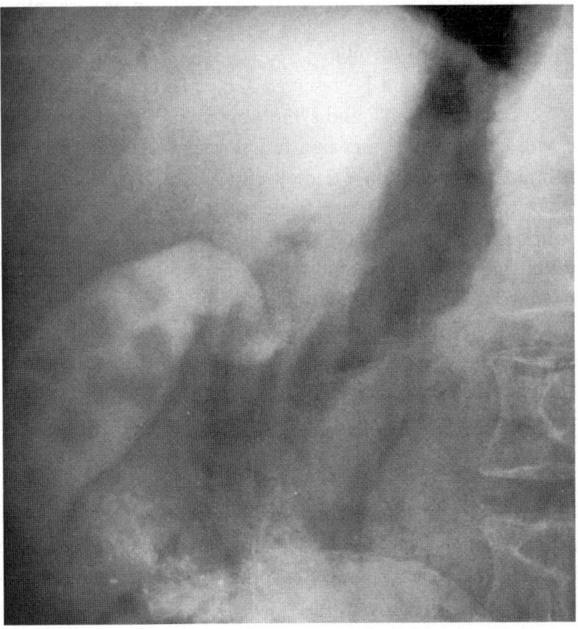

Fig. 3 Cholesterol gallstones. An intravenous cholangiogram has opacified the gallbladder showing multiple faceted radiolucent gallstones. These are typical features of cholesterol stones.

Treatment

The usual treatment for symptomatic gallstones is laparoscopic cholecystectomy, although medical treatments may be employed in selected patients (see below). In patients in whom 'silent' gallstones are discovered incidentally and in patients with minimal symptoms it is by no means clear that treatment is always the best solution. The problem revolves around the probability of serious complications in the future. It is appropriate to offer treatment to young patients and to advise against it in the elderly with other major medical problems. In fit, middle-aged patients with no or minimal symptoms it is reasonable to withhold surgery until it is warranted by symptoms or complications.

Gallstone dissolution and disruption

Chemical methods

Oral bile-acid therapy with chenodeoxycholic acid or ursodeoxycholic acid can dissolve cholesterol gallstones. These bile acids reduce the cholesterol saturation of bile and result in the leaching of cholesterol from gallstones. Ursodeoxycholic acid has advantages over chenodeoxycholic acid in that it does not cause diarrhoea or elevations of serum transaminases. The two dissolve gallstones better in combination than singly.

Contact dissolution of gallstones is a method whereby cholesterol stones in the gallbladder can be dissolved by the direct instillation of methyl tert-butyl ether (**MTBE**) into the gallbladder via a percutaneous catheter. MTBE is continually infused and aspirated with vigour until the stones have disappeared (which typically takes 5–7 h).

Physical methods

Extracorporeal shock-wave lithotripsy (**ESWL**) shatters gallstones into a coarse powder. The gallbladder must contain no more than three stones to allow accurate focusing of the shock waves.

In *endoscopic sphincterotomy* the bile duct is entered by a cannula passed via a duodenoscope and is opened by diathermy cutting of the ampulla of Vater. Stones are removed by balloon or wire catheters.

Patient selection and results

These treatments should be reserved for patients in whom the risk of cholecystectomy is high and symptoms mild. They are suitable for those with cholesterol stones in a functioning gallbladder (as judged by an oral cholecystogram). Radiolucent stones are usually, but not always, composed of cholesterol. Calcified stones do not dissolve (CT scans pick up low levels of calcification).

Oral bile-acid therapy should not be taken during pregnancy. The preferred treatment is a combination of chenodeoxycholic acid (7 mg/kg) and ursodeoxycholic acid (7 mg/kg). Gallstone dissolution usually requires 6–24 months of therapy, depending on stone size. Combining oral bile-acid therapy with ESWL speeds up the process greatly: gallstones will be cleared in more than 90 per cent of patients within 18 months. Furthermore, slightly calcified gallstones can be treated this way.

The most frequent side-effect of oral bile-acid therapy is diarrhoea, dose related, and usually mild and transient. Transient elevations of serum transaminase activity are also common. One year after gallstone dissolution about 30 per cent of patients will have had a recurrence. Unwanted effects of ESWL include biliary colic, skin petechiae, and haematuria.

Acute cholecystitis

Aetiology

Acute cholecystitis follows impaction of stone(s) in the cystic duct in over 90 per cent of patients. Continued secretion by the gallbladder leads to a rise in pressure. Inflammation of the wall results from the toxic effects of the retained bile and bacterial infection. The gallbladder bile is usually turbid but may become frank pus (empyema). Intestinal organisms, especially anaerobes, are commonly cultured from the gallbladder. Ischaemia in the distended wall may lead to infarction and perforation. Generalized peritonitis may follow but the leak is usually localized to form a chronic abscess. Some patients have repeated attacks of acute cholecystitis, which are probably exacerbations of chronic cholecystitis. Acute cholecystitis in the absence of gallstones (acalculous cholecystitis) is rare, but can be a problem in patients with **AIDS**, when cytomegalovirus and cryptosporidium are the most commonly associated organisms.

Symptoms and signs

The typical patient is an obese, middle-aged female, but there are many exceptions to this pattern. The principal symptom is pain, of fairly sudden onset, which is severe, continuous, or minimally fluctuating, and localized to the epigastrium or right hypochondrium, often radiating to the back. In uncomplicated cases the pain gradually subsides over 12–18 h. Flatulence and nausea are common but persistent vomiting suggests the presence of a stone in the common bile duct. Fever indicates a complicating bacterial cholangitis. Jaundice is usually a sign of a stone in the bile duct. The abdomen moves poorly with respiration. Right hypochondrial tenderness is present and is exacerbated by inspiration (Murphy's sign). Muscle guarding and rebound tenderness are common. The gallbladder is usually impalpable but occasionally a tender mass of omentum and gallbladder may be felt under the liver.

Investigations

There is usually a moderate polymorphonuclear leucocytosis ($12–15 \times 10^9$/litre). Serum bilirubin concentrations between 17 and 68 μmol/litre (1–4 mg/dl) should raise the suspicion of a stone in the bile duct. Modest rises in the serum alkaline phosphatase, transaminases, and amylase may also be seen. Ultrasound of the gallbladder is the critical investigation.

The *differential diagnosis* includes perforated peptic ulcer, acute pancreatitis, retrocaecal appendicitis, perforated carcinoma or diverticulum of the hepatic flexure of the colon, liver abscess, cardiac infarction, and pneumonia with right-sided pleurisy.

Complications

Gangrene of the gallbladder is suggested by pain, tenderness, and fever progressively increasing or persisting for longer than 24–48 h. In the elderly and obese, perforation of the gallbladder can occur without definite signs. Perforation into an adjacent viscus may produce a cholecystenteric fistula and may lead to gallstone ileus.

Cholangitis is suggested by intermittent high temperatures, often accompanied by rigors. It usually follows the passage of a stone into the bile duct.

Treatment

Acute cholecystitis usually subsides in a few days with conservative management with intravenous fluids, pethidine or nalbuphine and atropine, together with tetracycline or ampicillin or a cephalosoporin. Cholecystectomy is done either in a few days after symptoms have settled or 2–3 months later; if symptoms recur in this period, surgery is done without delay and immediate operation is mandatory if sepsis or gangrene or perforation develop.

Chronic cholecystitis

This usually develops insidiously, but can follow an acute attack. It is characterized by chronic inflammation and thickening of the gallbladder wall. In addition to stones the gallbladder may contain a brown sediment ('biliary mud').

Cholesterolosis describes the deposition of yellow specks of cholesterol in the pink gallbladder wall (strawberry gallbladder); it is usually asymptomatic but about 50 per cent of affected patients develop gallstones.

Symptoms and signs

Some patients complain of bouts of constant right hypochondrial or epigastric pain. In biliary colic, the height of the pain is separated by 15–60-min intervals, bouts lasting several hours or as little as 15–20 min. It may radiate to the right shoulder or the back. More commonly the symptoms are vague and ill-defined, and include abdominal discomfort and distension, nausea, flatulence, and intolerance of fatty foods. There may be tenderness over the gallbladder and a positive Murphy's sign. The presence of stones may be revealed by plain X-ray ultrasound or ERCP.

The differential diagnosis includes peptic ulcers, hiatus hernia, irritable bowel syndrome, chronic relapsing pancreatitis, and tumours of the stomach, pancreas, colon, or gallbladder.

Complications

These include acute exacerbations, passage of stones into the bile duct, pancreatitis, cholecystenteric fistula formation and gallstone ileus, and rarely carcinoma of the gallbladder. Occasionally, the accumulation of mucus and gallstones produces hydrops of the gallbladder, which is characterized by a tender mass without the symptoms of acute cholecystitis.

Treatment

Established cases require cholecystectomy. When the diagnosis is in doubt, a conservative approach of weight reduction and a low-fat diet is worth trying. Oral bile-acid therapy may also be considered (see above).

Prognosis

Chronic cholecystitis carries a good prognosis. Cholecystectomy should have a mortality below 1 per cent, but if it is done indiscriminately on patients with 'dyspeptic' symptoms who happen to have incidental gallstones the results will be unpredictable and often unsatisfactory.

Choledocholithiasis

About 15 per cent of patients with cholelithiasis have common duct stones. This proportion rises with age so that in the elderly nearly 50 per cent of patients with cholelithiasis may have common duct stones. Stones may develop in the bile duct in diseases causing chronic biliary obstruction, such as benign bile-duct strictures and sclerosing cholangitis.

Clinical features

The classical triad of symptoms is right upper abdominal pain, jaundice, and fever. The abdominal pain is typically colicky, severe, and persists for hours, often associated with vomiting. Fever and rigors indicate cholangitis. Jaundice is variable and is often intermittent. The urine is dark due to conjugated bilirubin and the faeces are pale. Frequently, the amount of pigment in the faeces varies. Itching may be prominent. However, common bile-duct stones may also be silent, especially in the elderly. Alternatively, only one of the triad of symptoms may be present. The liver is moderately enlarged and there may be tenderness in the right upper quadrant. Prolonged biliary obstruction lasting months or years eventually leads to biliary cirrhosis with portal venous hypertension and liver cell failure.

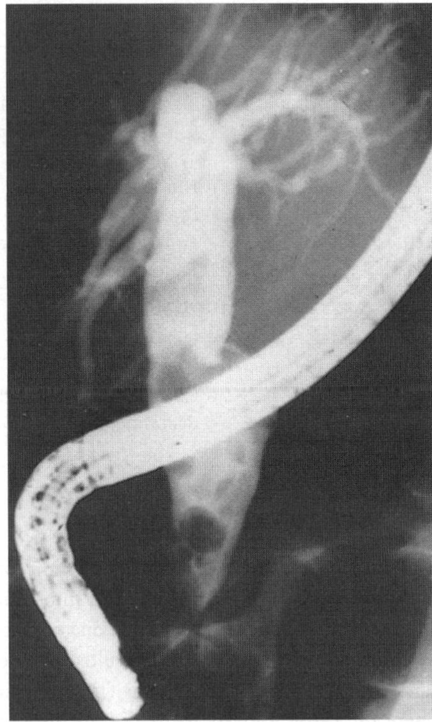

Fig. 4 Choledocholithiasis. An endoscopic retrograde cholangiogram shows multiple faceted radiolucent stones in a dilated bile duct. The gallbladder has not been opacified.

Investigations

Liver function tests show a cholestatic pattern. The prothrombin time may be prolonged due to inadequate absorption of vitamin K. Blood cultures should be made repeatedly during the fevers to isolate the organism and determine sensitivities.

Ultrasonography demonstrates biliary dilatation, and may show the stones but often fails to do so when they obstruct the lower end of the bile duct. Cholangiography by ERCP is required in these patients (Fig. 4). Common bile-duct stones should be removed by endoscopic sphincterotomy before cholecystectomy.

Differential diagnosis includes carcinomas of the head of the pancreas, bile duct, and ampulla of Vater (Table 1). Intrahepatic diseases may also cause a cholestatic jaundice; these include viral and alcoholic hepatitis, drugs, and pregnancy.

Treatment

The optimal treatment is endoscopic sphincterotomy to remove bile-duct stones, followed by laparoscopic cholecystectomy. Endoscopic removal of common duct gallstones without cholecystectomy is appropriate in patients unfit for surgery. Open exploration of the common bile duct is required if gallstones are too large to be removed endoscopically (>2 cm).

Table 1 Causes of bile-duct obstruction

Intrinsic causes	*Extrinsic causes*
• Common bile-duct gallstones	• Carcinoma of the pancreas
• Cholangitis	• Carcinoma of the ampulla of Vater
• Carcinoma of the bile duct	• Metastatic carcinoma
• Carcinoma of the gallbladder	• Lymphoma
• Benign post-traumatic stricture	• Pancreatitis (acute and chronic)
• Sclerosing cholangitis (primary and secondary)	• Pancreatic cysts
• Haemobilia	*Congenital causes*
	• Biliary atresia
	• Choledochal cyst
	• Congenital intrahepatic biliary dilatation (Caroli's disease)

Postcholecystectomy syndromes

A proportion of patients continue to complain of symptoms such as pain in the right upper quadrant, flatulence, and intolerance of fatty foods, probably as a consequence of the wrong diagnosis being made before surgery, In others, surgery may have resulted in a benign post-traumatic biliary stricture or residual calculi. There remains a group of patients where the cause appears to be due to disorders such as long, dilated cystic-duct remnants, amputation neuromas of the cystic duct, and spasm or stenosis of the sphincter of Oddi. Manometry of the biliary tract may be of value when the latter diagnoses are suspected.

Bacterial cholangitis (suppurative cholangitis)

This is usually associated with common bile-duct calculi and benign biliary strictures. Malignant strictures produce complete obstruction and the bile remains sterile. Other conditions associated with cholangitis are biliary enteric fistulas, sclerosing cholangitis, and congenital intrahepatic biliary dilation (Caroli's disease). Organisms usually cultured in these infections include *E. coli, Streptococcus faecalis, Proteus vulgaris* staphylococci, bacteroides, aerobacter, and anaerobic streptococci.

Clinical features and treatment

Malaise, fever, and rigors are followed by pain, vomiting, jaundice, and itching. The urine turns dark and the faeces pale. Recurrent attacks are common. Hepatic abscesses may result. Repeated blood cultures are made during the fever to isolate the organisms. Culture of a liver biopsy fragment may also yield the organism. The main element of treatment is drainage of the biliary tract. Additionally, appropriate antibiotics such as cefuroxime and metronidazole are given. For recurrent attacks of cholangitis, tetracycline, amoxycillin, or cephalexin are usually effective.

Infestations

Infestations with *Ascaris lumbricoides* and *Clonorchis sinensis* are particular problems of the Far East. Both lead to cholangitis. Infestation with *C. sinensis* predisposes to bile-duct carcinoma and primary liver cancer. *Fasciola hepatica* may be encountered as a cause of cholangitis in Europe during wet summers.

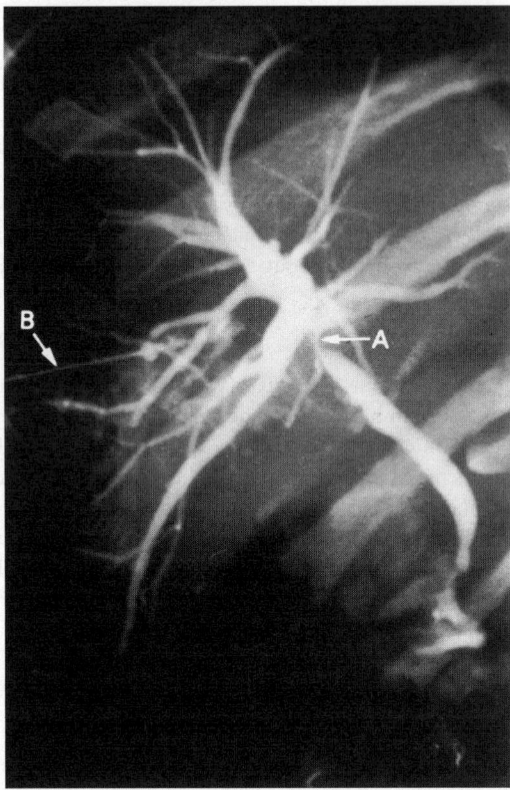

Fig. 5 Carcinoma of the bile duct. PTC shows a stricture (A) high in the bile duct at the porta hepatis. The intrahepatic bile ducts are moderately dilated. The transhepatic track of the 'skinny' needle used for the PTC is also visible (B).

Benign biliary strictures

In about 95 per cent of patients these are a consequence of biliary-tract surgery. The remainder are caused by gallstones eroding the bile duct and, rarely, blunt injury to the abdomen. The precise delineation of the stricture requires ERCP or PTC. Treatment is by skilled surgery.

Malignant biliary stricture

This is most commonly due to adenocarcinoma of the head of the pancreas but may also be caused by adenocarcinomas of the bile ducts, of the ampulla of Vater, and rarely of the gallbladder. Occasionally, the cause is lymph node enlargement at the porta hepatis due to malignant metastases or lymphoma.

Symptoms and signs

Cancers of the pancreas and biliary tree (Fig. 5) usually affect the middle aged and elderly. The onset is insidious with deepening jaundice, itching, and weight loss. A dull, nagging upper abdominal pain that radiates to the back is common. Cholangitis is unusual. Examination reveals a deeply jaundiced patient, often excoriated from scratching. The liver is enlarged but not tender. If the malignant obstruction is below the level of the cystic duct, the gallbladder is distended and may be palpable (Courvoisier's law). The urine is dark and the stools pale. In cancer of the ampulla of Vater a film of blood on the pale stool may give it a silvery colour ('silver stools').

Investigation

Liver function tests reveal a cholestatic pattern. The serum bilirubin may be very high (600 μmol/litre; 35 mg/dl). A microcytic hypochromic anaemia indicates blood loss from the tumour. An ultrasound or CT scan examination will reveal dilatation of the biliary tree and may demonstrate the level of the obstruction, but bile-duct carcinoma frequently causes obstruction at the porta hepatis and the extrahepatic biliary tract appears non-dilated. It is then important to establish the diagnosis precisely, by ERCP or PTC. Most of these patients are best treated by endoscopic or percutaneous biliary stents rather than surgery (see below).

Treatment

Small tumours confined to the head of the pancreas and ampulla of Vater may be treated curatively by a Whipple's operation, but the great majority can only be treated palliatively with a bypass procedure such as a cholecystojejunostomy. The prognosis for these patients is poor. An alternative is endoscopic or percutaneous transhepatic introduction of stents through the biliary stricture. The prostheses may block after about 3 months and need to be replaced.

Other causes of bile duct obstruction

Pancreatitis may obstruct the common bile duct where it passes through the head of the pancreas. Transient jaundice is common in acute pancreatitis, owing to compression by oedema. In chronic pancreatitis, especially alcoholic, persistent jaundice can develop, probably as a consequence of pancreatic fibrosis. Pancreatic cysts may rarely cause extrinsic compression of the bile duct. Haemorrhage into the biliary tract is uncommon but may follow trauma, liver biopsy, biliary tumours, and gallstones. The diagnosis of these conditions relies on accurate cholangiography (usually ERCP).

Sclerosing cholangitis

Sclerosing cholangitis is the description applied to multiple strictures and bead-like dilatations of the intrahepatic and extrahepatic biliary tree. It is discussed in detail in Chapter 5.34.

Further reading

Chapman, R.W. (1991). Aetiology and natural history of primary sclerosing cholangitis—a decade of progress? *Gut*, **32**, 1433–5.

Johnston, D.E. and Kaplan, M.M. (1993). Medical progress; prognosis and treatment of gall stones. *New England Journal of Medicine*, **328**, 412.

Sherlock, S. and Dooley, J. (1997). *Diseases of the liver and biliary system.* Blackwell Science, Oxford.

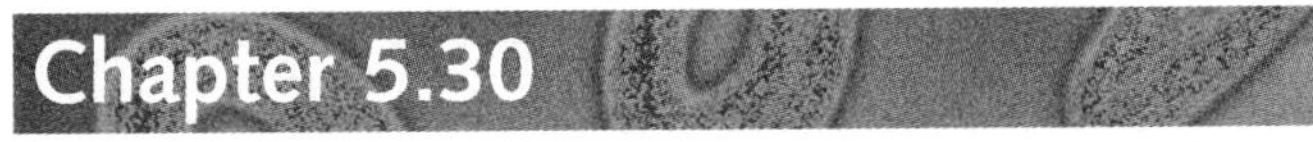

Chapter 5.30

Jaundice

E. Elias

The physiology and biochemistry of bilirubin metabolism is described in OTM3, pp. 2054–6.

Causes and pathophysiology of jaundice

Jaundice may result from excessive production or reduced hepatic uptake of unconjugated bilirubin, reduced hepatic conjugation of bilirubin or reduced excretion of conjugated bilirubin (Fig. 1).

Excessive production of bilirubin occurs in the haemolytic anaemias. It also may occur in patients with a marked degree of ineffective erythropoiesis and intramedullary destruction of red-cell precursors, as for example, in thalassaemia and pernicious anaemia.

Reduced uptake of bilirubin: A defect in the transfer of bilirubin to the hepatocyte may explain the unconjugated hyperbilirubinaemia associated with severe congestive heart failure, portocaval shunts, and the action of certain drugs including rifampicin.

Reduced hepatic conjugation of bilirubin is the cause of jaundice in premature infants and occurs in Gilbert's syndrome and the Crigler–Najjar syndrome, where it results from a specific deficiency of glucuronosyl transferase.

Reduced excretion of conjugated bilirubin occurs rarely because of congenital defects of hepatic excretion in the Dubin–Johnson and Rotor syndromes. Commonly, it is a consequence of hepatocellular injury as in viral hepatitis or drug jaundice; inflammatory, granulomatous, or neoplastic infiltration of the liver, or extrahepatic bile duct obstruction by gallstones, pancreatic carcinoma, and other disorders.

Clinical approach to the jaundiced patient

Urine testing differentiates between unconjugated and conjugated hyperbilirubinaemia. If bilirubin is absent from the urine, the detection of excess urinary urobilinogen, splenomegaly, anaemia, reticulocytosis, and a family history of anaemia suggest a haemolytic cause for jaundice. If there is no haemolysis or ineffective erythropoiesis, and other 'liver function tests' are normal, the patient may be fasted for 48 h to differentiate between benign hepatic hyperbilirubinaemia (see below) and liver disease such as inactive cirrhosis.

If bilirubin is present in the urine, the common causes are hepatitis and obstruction of the biliary system. In viral hepatitis, jaundice is usually preceded by a prodromal phase involving anorexia, nausea, and aversion to smoking, sometimes with an influenza-like illness. When the features of hepatitis are absent, jaundice may be due to cholestasis of which pruritus is the most typical symptom. Severe

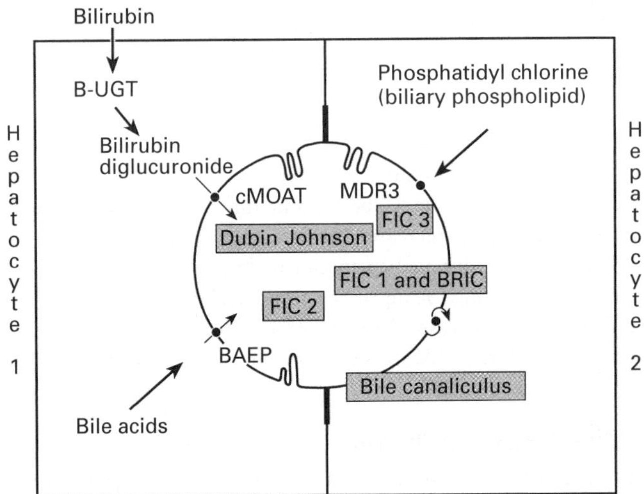

Fig. 1 Causal mutations affect cMOAT (multiorganic anion transporter) in the Dubin–Johnson syndrome; the bile acid export pump (BAEP) in FIC 2 (familial intrahepatic cholestasis); and 2 flippases which maintain asymmetry of membrane bilayer phospholipids and selective biliary phosphatidyl choline secretion, the MDR3 in FIC 3 and a chromosome 18 product in FIC 1 and benign recurrent intrahepatic cholestasis.

abdominal pain of abrupt onset preceding jaundice by a couple of days suggests gallstone obstruction. Fever in association with bilirubinuria is strong evidence of obstructive cholangitis. Painless cholestatic jaundice in the absence of urinary urobilinogen with a palpable gallbladder usually indicates a neoplastic cause (Courvoiser's law). When jaundice and bilirubinuria are accompanied by none of the features mentioned above, and 'liver function tests' are otherwise normal, one of the rare familial causes of conjugated hyperbilirubinaemia is probable.

Chronic liver disease may be suggested by its classical physical signs. Absence of such signs in a jaundiced patient with an enlarged, irregular, hard liver suggests the presence of an infiltrative disorder, usually a secondary neoplasm.

Deficiency of bilirubin UDP-glucuronosyltransferase (B-UGT)

The *ugt1* locus is 100 kb long, containing at least 10 exons and by a mechanism of alternative splicing encodes at least three functional enzymes with identical UDPGA binding sites but different substrate specificities. In Gilbert's syndrome the hepatic B-UGT activity is decreased to about 30 per cent of normal. A common inheritance has been found to be autosomal recessive with a seventh TA repeat rather than the normal six in the TATAA box of the promoter region. Heterozygotes have normal bilirubin levels. Mutations causing Crigler–Najjar may affect either the substrate or UDPGA binding domain and may thus be specific for bilirubin or affect conjugation of various phenolic substrates.

Gilbert's syndrome

Gilbert's syndrome refers to mild unconjugated hyperbilirubinaemia in the absence of liver disease or overt haemolysis. Its prevalence is some 1–2 per cent of the population. Some patients complain of non-specific symptoms such as abdominal pain, weakness, and malaise. Plasma bilirubin levels fluctuate markedly, but are usually not sufficiently high to produce jaundice. Conventional 'liver function tests' are normal. Liver histology is grossly normal. The diagnosis is based on demonstration of unconjugated hyperbilirubinaemia with otherwise normal 'liver function tests' and no overt haemolysis. Plasma bilirubin levels approximately double in both normal individuals and those with Gilbert's syndrome when dietary intake is reduced to 1680 J (400 cal) daily for 48–72 h. The percentage increase is similar in normal and Gilbert's subjects; however, the increment and final value is much higher in Gilbert's, and this may be diagnostically useful because such increases are not seen in patients with hyperbilirubinaemia due to hepatocellular disease or cirrhosis. As an alternative to fasting, 50 mg of nicotinic acid may be injected intravenously. An increase of unconjugated serum bilirubin of more than 17 μmol/litre is highly suggestive of Gilbert's syndrome. The prognosis is excellent.

Crigler–Najjar syndrome

The Crigler–Najjar syndrome results in severe unconjugated hyperbilirubinaemia in the absence of any other evidence of hepatic dysfunction or haemolysis. There are two distinct groups: types I and II.

In *type I* there is a complete absence of UDPGT (bilirubin uridine diphosphate glucuronate glycuronyl transferase) activity. Severe unconjugated hyperbilirubinaemia occurs in the neonatal period, leading to kernicterus and early death in most infants. Consanguinity is common in the parents of affected offspring, suggesting an autosomal recessive mode of inheritance. Heterozygotes are usually not jaundiced.

Type II is associated with only partial deficiency of UDPG activity, and embraces those unconjugated hyperbilirubinaemias of hepatic origin that are intermediate between Gilbert's syndrome and type I. Jaundice is usually of less acute onset and less severe than in type I, and bilirubin levels can be reduced by phenobarbital treatment. Jaundice is not always apparent in early childhood and kernicterus is rare. Familial occurrence is common. Gilbert's syndrome is frequently found in relatives.

Conjugated hyperbilirubinaemia

The Dubin–Johnson syndrome

Although many patients complain of vague symptoms of anorexia, malaise, easy fatiguability, right hypochondrial pain, and occasional diarrhoea, most are asymptomatic until jaundice is discovered. This may be brought on by pregnancy or oral contraceptives, or the diagnosis may only be made during family studies. The genetic defect affects the canalicular multi-organic anion transporter (MOAT) which is absent from the canalicular membrane in this condition.

The level of plasma bilirubin varies widely and fluctuates in individuals. Bilirubin and excess urobilinogen are found in the urine in the absence of any haemolysis or abnormalities of 'liver function tests'. The pattern of bromsulphthalein clearance is also helpful diagnostically. Early disappearance of plasma bromsulphthalein appears normal and retention at 45 min may not be markedly deranged. However, levels subsequently rise so that at 90 min they exceed those at 45 min, due to reflux of glutathione-conjugated bromsulphthalein. The diagnosis may be confirmed by measurement of urinary coproporphyrin excretion. In homozygous patients the ratio of urinary coproporphyrin I to coproporphyrin III is at least 4:1, compared with a ratio of approximately 1:3 in normal subjects. Intermediate ratios are found in heterozygous carriers.

The liver is deeply pigmented. Histologically, liver cells contain much granular pigment that is not bilirubin and has been variously ascribed to lipofuscin and melanin. There is no recognized treatment for the condition, which is benign.

Rotor's syndrome

Rotor described the familial occurrence of conjugated hyperbilirubinaemia in natives of the Philippines due to uptake and storage defects of bilirubin. Other liver function tests are normal.

Intrahepatic cholestasis

Intrahepatic cholestasis may result from primary biliary cirrhosis, sclerosing cholangitis or parasitic infestations, but may also reflect secretory failure at the level of the hepatocellular canaliculus without obstruction. This latter form is seen in drug-induced cholestasis and occasionally in alcoholic or viral liver disease. The biochemical features include marked elevation of plasma alkaline phosphatase (and 5′-nucleotidase) with elevation of serum bile acids, cholesterol and conjugated bilirubin. Loss of intestinal bile acids may cause steatorrhoea and, if prolonged, deficiencies of vitamins A, D, E, and K. Classical symptoms are pruritus with pale stools and dark urine. Liver histology in acute complete obstruction shows oedematous portal tracts, bilirubin in hepatocytes and plugs of inspissated bile within canaliculi. Prolonged partial obstruction is suggested by accumulation of copper-associated protein within periportal hepatocytes, bile ductular proliferation at the edge of portal tracts and portal fibrosis.

Vanishing bile-duct syndrome

Severe progressive cholestasis may ensue in conditions that destroy bile ducts of predominantly interlobular size. The process is always insidious in conditions such as primary biliary cirrhosis, primary sclerosing cholangitis, sarcoidosis, and mucoviscidosis but can also occur either insidiously or abruptly in liver allograft rejection, graft-versus-host disease and extremely rarely in Hodgkin's disease and cholestatic drug reactions.

Benign recurrent intrahepatic cholestasis (BRIC)

This rare condition is characterized by recurrent attacks of cholestasis in the absence of any mechanical biliary obstruction and with restoration of normal hepatic structure and function between attacks. The first attack usually occurs during childhood or adolescence: attacks last for several weeks or months and are separated by intervals of normality lasting many months or years. Pruritus usually precedes jaundice and may sometimes subside without it.

Cholestasis may cause steatorrhoea and hypoprothrombinaemia with bruising. Cholangiography rules out mechanical obstruction and histological examination of the liver reveals centrilobular cholestasis. The affected gene is responsible for familial intrahepatic cholestasis (FIC) 1 (see below).

Ursodeoxycholic acid is useful both for prophylaxis and in controlling attacks in some patients. There is no convincing benefit from corticosteroids or cholestyramine.

Familial intrahepatic cholestasis (FIC)

Genetic defects affecting bile canalicular transporter function are described for three syndromes. In FIC 1 and FIC 2 bile acid secretion is seriously impaired and the serum gammaglutamyl transferase (GGT) is normal. In FIC 3, the phosphatidylcholine flippase activity is lost, phospholipid is absent from bile and serum GGT is high.

The product of a locus on chromosome 18q21–22 is thought to be partially inactivated in benign recurrent intrahepatic cholestasis but more severely defective in FIC 1 in which cholestasis is typically progressive and fatal.

Cholestasis of pregnancy

Intrahepatic cholestasis occurs in some women during pregnancy, usually in the third trimester. Hypochondrial pain is uncommon and pruritus is much more common than jaundice. There may be steatorrhoea and hypoprothrombinaemia is corrected by parenteral administration of vitamin K. Cholestasis usually resolves rapidly after parturition. Incomplete resolution may indicate underlying disease, such as primary biliary cirrhosis, that has been unmasked by pregnancy.

There is a strong tendency for cholestasis to recur in subsequent pregnancies or on taking oral contraceptive steroids. There is a relatively strong familial tendency, although the mode of inheritance is unclear. Spontaneous labour occurs prematurely and, although outcome is usually benign, there is an increased risk of fetal distress and unexplained stillbirth.

Reports of benefit from treatment with *S*-adenosyl methionine lack confirmation. Ursodeoxycholic acid reverses liver dysfunction and pruritus in some patients, but its protective effect on the fetus remains to be determined. Early delivery following confirmation of fetal lung maturity is recommended, at least in those with a prior history of fetal distress or stillbirth.

Contraceptive steroid-induced cholestasis

Pruritus progressing to jaundice occurs in some women taking oral contraceptive steroids. Symptoms usually appear during the first three monthly cycles, and recede spontaneously when 'the pill' is discontinued. Oral contraceptive steroids should be avoided in women with a prior history of cholestasis of pregnancy or benign recurrent intrahepatic cholestasis. Rarely, progressive biliary disorders such as primary biliary cirrhosis or sclerosing cholangitis may first become symptomatic due to the unmasking effect of contraceptive steroids and also constitute contraindications to their use.

Further reading

Arias, I.M. (1998). New genetics of inheritable jaundice and cholestatic liver disease. *Lancet*, 352, 82–3.

Borra, P. and Elias, E. (1992). The vanishing bile duct syndrome. *British Journal of Surgery*, 79, 604–5.

Knox, T.A. and Olans, L.B. (1996). Liver disease in pregnancy. *New England Journal of Medicine*, 335, 569–76.

Sherlock, S. and Dooley, J. (1997). *Diseases of the liver and biliary system*. Blackwell Science, Oxford.

Tranne, M., Meier, P.J., and Boyer, J.L. (1998). Mechanisms of disease: molecular pathogenesis of cholestasis. *New England Journal of Medicine*, 339, 1217–27.

Chapter 5.31

Clinical features of viral hepatitis

H. C. Thomas

At least five viruses cause hepatitis (A–E) without significant damage to other organs. These agents, which are described in Section 16, may cause an acute (A–E) or chronic (B–D) hepatitis, the latter sometimes leading to cirrhosis and hepatocellular carcinoma. Other viruses causing hepatitis include Epstein–Barr, cytomegalovirus, herpes simplex, herpes zoster, coxsackie A and B, measles, Lassa fever, Marburg fever, and Ebola viruses.

Acute viral hepatitis

Clinical features

Many patients present with an influenza-like syndrome associated with malaise and arthralgia. These symptoms last a few days and are followed by clinical and biochemical evidence of hepatocellular necrosis. The first biochemical signs are increased concentrations of aspartate and alanine aminotransferases; to between three- and 50-fold the normal range. Conjugated bilirubinaemia then follows in some cases and is associated with leakage of this water-soluble

Table 1 Clinical features of viral hepatitis

	HAV	HBV	HCV	HDV	HEV
Transmission	Enteral	Parenteral	Parenteral	Parenteral	Enteral
Incubation period (days)	15–50	28–160	14–160	28–160 (coinfection of HBV + HDV)	20–40
Severity of hepatitis	Increases with age (rarely icteric in childhood)	50 per cent icteric	Rarely icteric	Usually icteric	Severe, with high mortality in pregnant women
Progression to chronic disease	Never	At birth: >90 per cent >2 years <5 per cent	80 per cent	Coinfection: <5 per cent Superinfection: >95 per cent	Never
Risk of hepatocellular carcinoma	None	High in cirrhotics	High in cirrhotics	High in cirrhotics	None

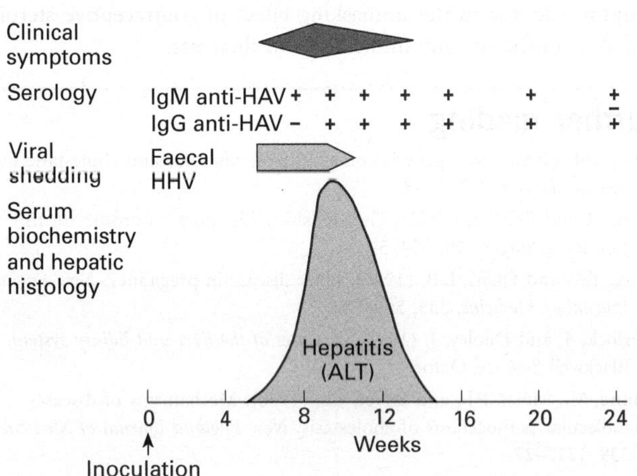

Fig. 1 Hepatitis A: clinical and virological course. HAV is shed into the faeces before clinical presentation and before appearance of IgM anti-HAV.

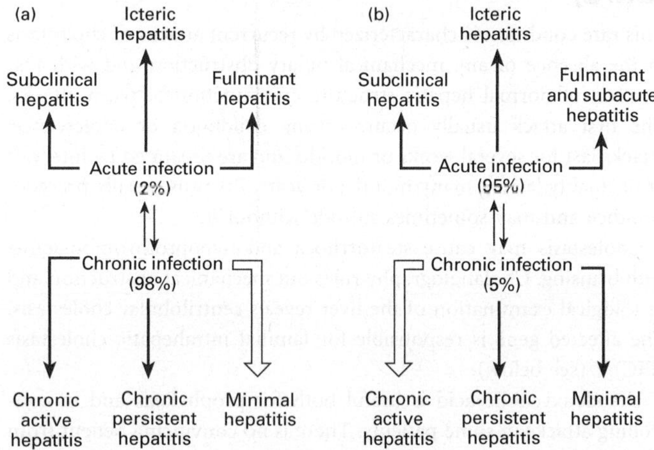

Fig. 2 Clinical syndromes occurring after HBV infection in (a) neonates, (b) children (over 2 years old) and adults. CAH, chronic active hepatitis; CPH, chronic persistent hepatitis.

pigment into the urine, causing it to darken. In patients who develop intrahepatic cholestasis, the alkaline phosphatase will rise and the patient subsequently develops pruritus and pale stools.

In many patients hepatitis is mild and they do not develop jaundice which is most common in B infection and least in patients with hepatitis C (Table 1). Once jaundice has appeared there is often rapid improvement, although in the rare syndrome of fulminant or subfulminant hepatic failure, deterioration continues and proceeds within either 1 week (fulminant) or 8 weeks (subfulminant) to liver failure and coma.

Specific features of different forms

Hepatitis A virus (HAV) infection is enterically transmitted and is most common in countries where hygiene is poor. Faecal contamination of drinking water is the usual source of infection. The incubation period is between 15 and 50 days, and a febrile onset is commonly seen. In young people the disease is usually anicteric, but from middle age onwards it may cause a severe hepatitis, often with deep icterus. Intrahepatic cholestasis is common.

The diagnosis is made by demonstration of IgM anti-HAV in the patient's blood (Fig. 1), which is present within 10 days of the onset of viraemia. This is followed by an IgG antibody response that is lifelong and confers protective immunity. Direct isolation of the virus in faeces is rarely used.

Bed-rest does not accelerate recovery. The patient should be allowed to undertake a level of exercise consistent with the symptoms. No antiviral compounds active against this agent are available.

Family contacts should be offered either an injection of pooled globulin, or active immunization with vaccine. A heat-inactivated, whole-virus vaccine is now available. The immune response to this vaccine is rapid and is sufficient to either prevent or reduce the infection. It should also be used to protect travellers and high-risk groups in developed countries.

Hepatitis B is transmitted by contact with infected body secretions (saliva, urine, and plasma). Prodromal symptoms of fever and arthralgia with malaise are common, followed by increase in serum transaminases to concentrations usually between 300 and 800 u/litre. In approximately half of the cases, jaundice will follow.

Persistent hepatitis B virus (HBV) infection occurs with differing frequency dependent on the age of exposure (Fig. 2). Exposure at birth invariably results in persistent infection. Up to half of these children will develop cirrhosis with or without liver-cell cancer and will die of the complications. Infection between birth and 2 years of age results in a persistent infection in 40 per cent of cases and these

Table 2 Diagnosis of viral hepatitis

	Acute infection	Chronic infection	Recovered infection
HAV	IgM anti-HAV	Not seen	IgG anti-HAV
HBV	HBsAg IgM anti-HBc(high titre, 19S)	HBsAg IgG anti-HBc; IgM anti-HBc in low titre usually 7S)*	IgG anti-HBs IgG anti-HBc
HCV	IgM anti-HCV IgG anti-HCV	IgG anti-HCV (polymerase chain reaction is used to detect HCV-RNA to differentiate)	IgG anti-HCV
HDV	Coinfection (HBV and HDV): IgM anti-HDV IgM anti-HBc	Superinfection (HDV on HBV): IgM anti-HDV IgG anti-HBc	IgG anti-HDV IgG anti-HBs
HEV	IgM anti-HEV	Not seen	IgG anti-HEV

*This low titre 7S IgM anti-HBc is not detectable by the standard IgM anti-HBc assay which utilizes dilute serum.

children run the same risks. From 2 years of age onwards, persistent infection is rare involving only 2–5 per cent, but approximately 25–50 per cent of these will develop cirrhosis and run the risk of hepatocellular carcinoma.

Diagnosis of acute infection involves the identification of hepatitis B surface antigen (**HBs**) in serum (Table 2), which is also present in chronic infection. The acute disease is differentiated from the chronic by the presence of high-titre IgM anti-HBc (HB core antigen). During the first month the infected liver cell secretes the viral protein HBe; its presence in serum indicates intense viraemia and infectivity. After approximately 4 weeks, there is seroconversion from HBe antigen to anti-HBe, associated with resolution of the hepatitis, clearance of the virus from serum and, usually, recovery. Some patients remain HBs positive because virus sequences have become integrated into cellular DNA, continuing to encode for the envelope proteins of the virus but without production of virus particles.

Management of the acute hepatitis is conservative. Patients must be followed until HBsAg antigen is cleared and they have developed anti-HBs. Patients who remain HBe antigen positive after 1 month or HBs positive for longer than 6 months will remain HBs antigen positive and will require further management. Monthly monitoring differentiates recovering acute from the chronic infection.

Prevention of secondary spread is important. Sexual and close family contacts should be vaccinated with the recombinant subunit envelope (HBsAg) vaccine. Over 95 per cent will develop protective immunity after three injections spaced over 6 months. A minority, more frequent among older people, will not develop antibody, and will probably remain susceptible to infection.

Hepatitis C virus (**HCV**) infection is parenterally transmitted (Table 1). The majority of patients develop hepatitis within 14–160 days of exposure. The disease is invariably anicteric and can be diagnosed by screening for elevated serum transaminases. The usual prodromal symptoms of fever and malaise may occur at the beginning of the hepatic phase.

Only 20 per cent of patients recover. The remainder develop persistent viraemia with hepatitis. One in five develops cirrhosis and runs the risk of hepatocellular carcinoma. The rate of progression of the disease is slow, over 20–40 years.

Antibodies to the virus can be detected at various times after infection. Diagnosis in the acute phase is difficult; antibodies to the nucleocapsid proteins (anti-c22) are the first to appear but may be delayed for 3–6 months (Fig. 3). Those to the non-structural proteins (NS3 and NS4) appear even later. Viraemia can be detected by polymerase chain reaction techniques as early as 2 weeks after exposure.

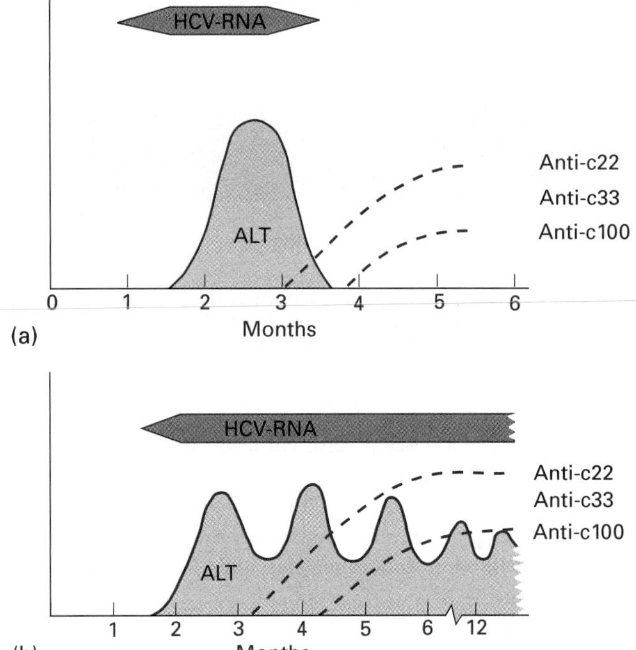

Fig. 3 (a) Acute hepatitis C. (b) Acute progressing to chronic hepatitis C (80 per cent of cases) (c22: nucleocapsid; c33: NS3; c100: NS4).

Patients with severe symptoms may require bed-rest, but the majority need only monitoring of transaminases to identify those going on to develop persistent infection. Sexual transmission may occur, but the risk is much lower than with hepatitis B. Transmission from mother to infant occurs infrequently.

Hepatitis D only replicates in patients already infected with hepatitis B, commonly among hepatitis B carriers in the Mediterranean area. In northern Europe it is only seen in intravenous drug abusers and haemophiliacs.

The delta virus requires the envelope proteins of hepatitis B to produce infectious virions. Infection may occur at the same time as HBV (Fig. 4(a)). Ninety-five per cent of patients under these circumstances clear both viruses; 5 per cent go on to persistent infection with both agents, and have a rapidly progressive disease. Hepatitis B carriers may be superinfected with delta virus (Fig. 4(b)).

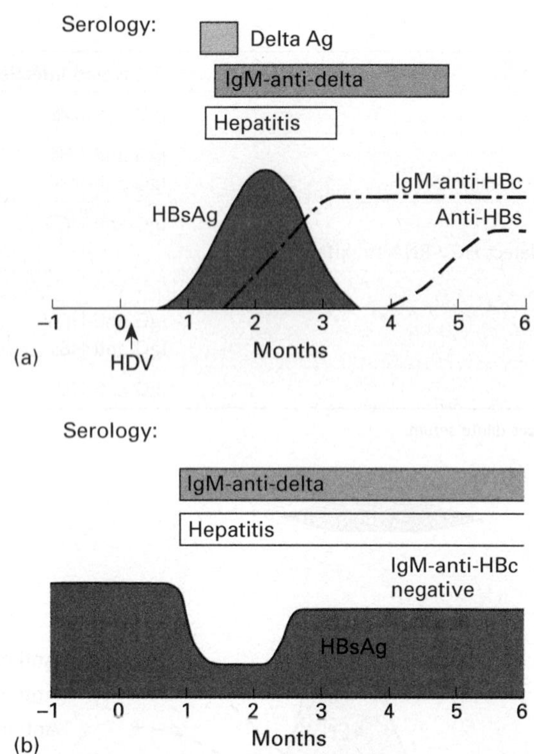

Fig. 4 Coinfection and superinfection with hepatitis D virus (**HDV**): (a) coinfection results in the development of IgM anti-HBc and IgM anti-HDV; (b) superinfection of an HBV carrier with HDV results in IgM anti-HDV in the absence of IgM anti-HBc.

The majority of them develop persistent delta virus infection, with a rapidly progressive course.

Sexual and family contacts should be immunized with the HBsAg subunit vaccine. Immunization against hepatitis B protects against both B and delta virus coinfection. Hepatitis B carriers cannot be protected against HDV superinfection.

Hepatitis E is enterically transmitted and is common in Africa and Asia. Infection usually follows faecal contamination of drinking water. The incubation period is approximately 20–40 days. A febrile illness is followed by an elevation of transaminases. Intrahepatic cholestasis is reported in approximately one-third of patients. Pregnant women suffer a particularly severe disease. Persistent infection has not been described. The diagnosis involves screening for IgM antibodies or immunoelectronmicroscopy. The management is along the lines for hepatitis A. No vaccines are currently available.

Other viruses

Cytomegalovirus and Epstein–Barr virus infections are commonly seen in immunocompromised individuals.

Chronic viral hepatitis

Chronicity is defined when hepatitis continues without improvement for longer than 6 months. Inflammation of the intrahepatic biliary tree may occur to a minor degree. The diagnosis is made by liver biopsy, which should not be undertaken earlier than 6 months after the acute episode, but may be indicated when there is no evidence of an acute hepatitis and the duration of abnormalities are consistent with a chronic disease that has already progressed to a severe stage. In some cases, fresh frozen plasma may be needed to correct coagulopathy before biopsy can be safely undertaken, or transjugular hepatic biopsy may be tried.

Several factors may initiate chronic hepatitis. These include persistent viral infection (B and C viruses). Other non-viral conditions include an autoimmune or drug-induced hepatitis (oxyphenisatin, methyldopa, isoniazid, and nitrofurantoin), alcohol, and Wilson's disease.

Chronic persistent hepatitis

The histological diagnoses of chronic persistent, chronic active, and chronic lobular hepatitis are still used to describe the lobular distribution of the inflammatory infiltrate. However, there is an increasing tendency to divide the disease into mild, moderate, and severe chronic hepatitis and then to specify the aetiology, i.e. chronic hepatitis B, chronic autoimmune hepatitis, etc.

This diagnosis can only be made by liver biopsy. The histological picture is of a mononuclear cell infiltrate of the portal tracts with no spill-over into the periportal area. There may be areas of focal liver cell necrosis in the lobule, and in these cases the histological picture should be described as chronic persistent hepatitis with a lobular component.

Patients are asymptomatic, with no physical signs of chronic liver disease. The concentrations of aminotransferases are increased by approximately two to five times. The bilirubin, alkaline phosphatase, serum albumin, globulin, and prothrombin time are always normal. Some cases present 6 or more months after an episode of acute hepatitis. Others come to clinical attention on biochemical screening. A few cases are attributable to HBV infection but most cases are due to hepatitis C.

The majority of cases do not progress, but HBs antigen-positive patients who have evidence of active viral replication (HBe antigen positivity) may progress slowly to active hepatitis and cirrhosis over many years. These patients may need antiviral therapy (see below). Twenty per cent of patients with chronic hepatitis C progress to cirrhosis and they may also require antiviral therapy.

Chronic lobular hepatitis

The histological picture is virtually identical to that of acute lobular hepatitis, chronicity being recognized by biochemical follow-up. The hepatic lobule is infiltrated from portal to central areas with chronic inflammatory cells and there are scattered areas of necrosis of hepatocytes (focal necrosis).

Patients are usually asymptomatic but some may be icteric with general malaise. The course is often fluctuating. A viral aetiology is usual (hepatitis B or C), but in some cases, high titres of smooth muscle and nuclear antibodies suggest an autoimmune aetiology. The biochemical picture is similar to that seen in acute hepatitis. A low serum albumin and prolonged prothrombin time indicate severe disease.

Hepatitis B-induced chronic lobular hepatitis has a variable prognosis from a benign to a rapid progression to cirrhosis. That due to hepatitis C may have a more benign course. Patients with autoimmune disease also have a benign prognosis.

Antiviral therapy is logical when B or C virus infection can be established, but experience is inconclusive. In patients with autoantibodies, the value of immunosuppressant therapy is difficult to assess; controlled studies have not been done.

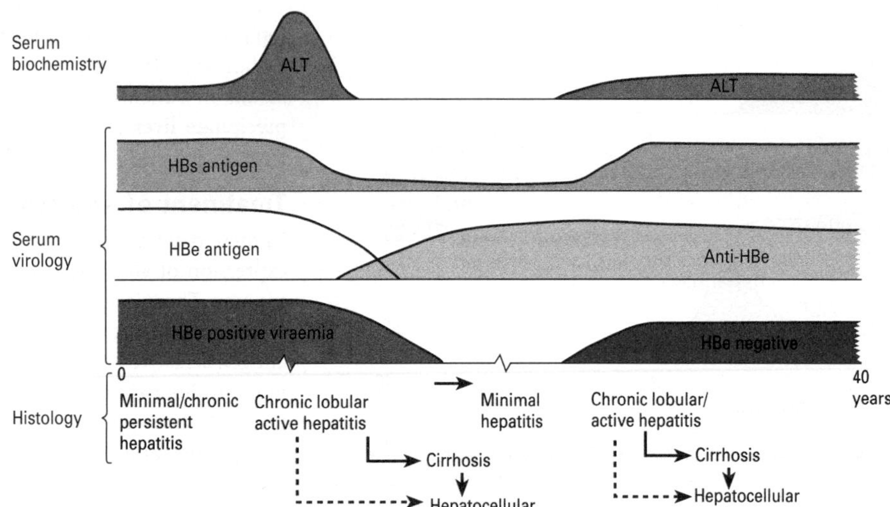

Fig. 5 Clinical course of chronic hepatitis B. Note that the natural history of this chronic infection may arrest at any stage: the patient may remain in the stage of HBe positive viraemia or never enter the stage of HBe negative viraemia. The HBe positive and negative stages of viraemia may run into each other.

Chronic active hepatitis

In this disease there is mononuclear and plasma-cell infiltration of the portal and periportal areas of the liver. The limiting plate is breached by the infiltrate and there is 'piecemeal' necrosis of the adjacent hepatocytes. Groups of hepatocytes ('rosettes') are surrounded by chronic inflammatory cells. When liver cells are destroyed, the reticulin framework may collapse. This may be followed by collagen accumulation and regeneration of hepatocytes, resulting in disorganization of the lobular architecture and the development of a coarse, macronodular cirrhosis. This picture may be accompanied by varying degrees of chronic lobular hepatitis and occasionally by cholangitic features. When the necrosis is severe, bands of necrotic tissue may extend from one portal tract to another or to the central vein (bridging necrosis), a picture usually seen in subacute hepatic necrosis, with fluid retention and encephalopathy between 1 and 2 months after the onset of acute hepatitis.

The histological entity of chronic active hepatitis may be the result of the same pathogenetic processes that cause chronic persistent hepatitis: only the viral causes will be dealt with here.

HBV-induced chronic hepatitis (chronic hepatitis B) may produce chronic persistent, lobular, or active hepatitis and up to 50 per cent of patients progress to develop cirrhosis, some developing primary hepatocellular carcinoma. In a few patients, usually those with chronic persistent hepatitis or inactive cirrhosis, extrahepatic pathology—polyarteritis nodosum or membranoproliferative glomerulonephritis—may be evident, perhaps related to the deposition of viral antigen/antibody complexes.

The factors that determine whether an individual suffers an acute or chronic infection are not known; nor is the mechanism of liver damage in chronically infected patients.

Patients with chronic hepatitis B are initially HBe antigen positive with intense viraemia and little inflammatory necrosis of infected hepatocytes (Fig. 5). Over months and years the inflammatory liver disease may become more severe, with destruction of the hepatocytes supporting viral replication. As a result, the viraemia diminishes and, eventually, HBe antigen is cleared and antibody appears. During HBe antigen/antibody seroconversion there is usually an exacerbation of the hepatitis and in some cases, cirrhosis will develop. In many patients the appearance of anti-HBe is associated with resolution of the hepatitis. The continued production of HBs antigen in such cases is dependent on the presence of viral DNA integrated into cellular DNA sequences. The HBs antigen-positive patient with anti-HBe in the serum and normal transaminases is called the 'normal carrier'.

Patients who have developed cirrhosis run an increased risk (200-fold) of developing hepatocellular carcinoma many years (7–40) after infection. In a few cases, HBV promoters are reportedly inserted into cellular DNA upstream of proto-oncogenes (*erb-*, c-*myc*) and cellular genes controlling cell division. Alternative mechanisms such as trans-activation of cellular proto-oncogenes by viral proteins probably contribute to malignant transformation. Approximately half of hepatocellular carcinomas secrete alpha-fetoprotein: screening for elevated serum concentrations, together with ultrasonographic scanning allows the early detection of such tumours, which may then be resected.

In some 'normal carriers', after months or years, viraemia reappears but HBe antigen is not secreted by the infected liver cell. This variant of the virus has undergone genetic mutation preventing synthesis of the precore/core molecule from which HBe antigen is derived. The appearances of this mutant virus, common in the Mediterranean, Asia, and the Far East, is associated with increased hepatitis and progress to cirrhosis

Clinical features

The majority of patients are asymptomatic, detected by testing for HBs antigenaemia for blood donation, or on routine screening. They usually have chronic persistent hepatitis or are carriers with a histologically normal liver, and more rarely have chronic active hepatitis or cirrhosis. They rarely give a history of acute hepatitis. Infection during the neonatal period or in early childhood is common in the Tropics and Far East, but probably of lesser importance in western Europe and North America, where infection probably occurs in the second and third decades of life as a result of sexual contact or drug abuse. Some patients present late in the course of the infection, usually with the complications of cirrhosis.

The importance of hepatitis B infection as a cause of chronic active liver disease varies considerably in different countries. In the United Kingdom, Western Europe, and North America it accounts for less than 5 per cent of the clinically overt cases. In tropical Africa, India, Japan, and China it is probably the most common cause.

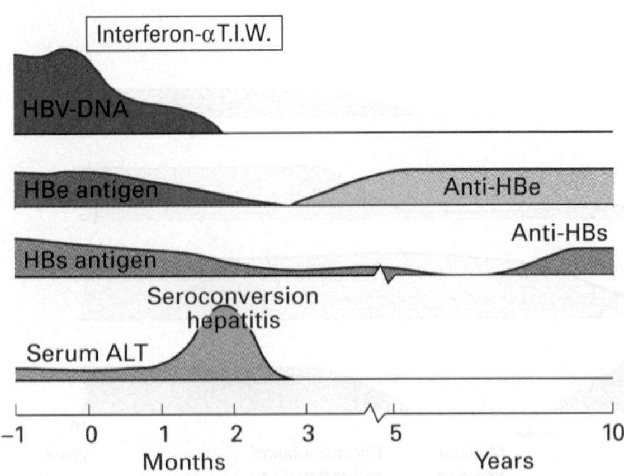

Fig. 6 Treatment of chronic HBe antigen-positive hepatitis with interferon-α. Note that HBe antigen/antibody seroconversion is preceded by exacerbation and is followed by resolution of the hepatitis. Clearance of HBs antigen is often delayed for 5 or more years.

Management

Initial assessment requires the determination of: (a) the level of viral replication; (b) the severity and type of inflammatory liver disease; and (c) the degree of fibrosis or cirrhosis.

The level of replication determines infectivity. Blood from HBe antigen-positive patients is highly infectious. These patients may then infect sexual partners by oral or genital contact. HBe antigen-positive mothers have a 95 per cent probability of infecting their infants. HBs antigen-positive patients who are HBe antibody positive are of much lower infectivity.

The level of inflammatory activity will influence prognosis. Those with severe chronic active hepatitis or active cirrhosis have progressive disease and should be offered appropriate therapy (see below). Those with chronic persistent hepatitis and inactive cirrhosis should only be treated if they have evidence of active viral replication (HBe antigen positivity) and, therefore, a high level of potential infectivity.

Assessment of the degree of fibrosis is of prognostic value only. Patients with cirrhosis should be screened every 6 months for early hepatocellular cancer.

Treatment of HBe antigen-positive patients

Alpha interferons have been shown to cause transient inhibition of viral replication and, in 40 per cent of cases, treatment for several (3–6) months has produced permanent inhibition with conversion from HBe antigen to antibody (Fig. 6), followed up to several years later by clearance of HBs antigen. Clearance of HBe antigen is followed by reduced inflammatory activity and histological resolution of the hepatitis. Patients with high concentrations of transaminases and severe chronic active hepatitis on biopsy are most likely to respond, while those with minimal hepatitis have only a 20 per cent chance of seroconversion.

Nucleoside analogues such as adenine arabinoside 5′-monophosphate have activity against HBV but are of limited value due to neurotoxicity. The reverse transcriptase inhibitor, lamivudine, reduces HBV titres substantially and if continued for one or more years is associated with improved liver histology and infrequently HBe antigen/antibody conversion (10–15 per cent cases). Drug resistant variants have emerged in some patients. Several additional drugs of this type are under evaluation (lobucavir, adejovir, famciclovir) and combination therapy may ultimately be the best approach.

Immunosuppression is contraindicated in patients with active viral replication, but prednisolone 'priming'—a 4-week course, rapidly withdrawn—followed by interferon-α for 3 months may improve results in patients with minimal hepatitis. 'Rebound hepatitis' may precipitate liver failure in cirrhotic patients who should not be so treated.

Treatment of anti-HBe-positive patients

In these patients continued HBs antigenaemia is usually the result of expression of viral sequences that are integrated into the hepatocyte genome. There is usually no replication of HBV and therefore antiviral therapy is not appropriate, but in 50 per cent of patients with HBe antigen-negative viraemia and hepatitis, interferon-α may be valuable in controlling viraemia. Lamivudine given long term may prove the most effective approach to this group.

Superinfection with the delta virus may have occurred and be responsible for continued liver damage. No effective therapy has been developed. Concurrent infection with HCV should be excluded, particularly in drug abusers.

Prognosis

The natural history of hepatitis B chronic active disease is variable. In a few cases progress to cirrhosis is rapid but in most the evolution is slow. Chronic active hepatitis may become chronic persistent hepatitis and active cirrhosis may change to inactive cirrhosis.

Hepatitis C virus-induced chronic hepatitis

Eighty per cent of patients develop chronic infection and hepatitis, 20 per cent of whom develop cirrhosis. These patients are at risk of hepatocellular carcinoma. In Britain, 0.1–0.5 per cent of the population are infected with this virus. It is a common cause of chronic liver disease hitherto called cryptogenic hepatitis. Before screening blood for HCV, most cases of post-transfusion hepatitis were caused by this virus, but in the United Kingdom, sporadic, community-acquired, non-A, non-B hepatitis is not due to this agent: these patients usually recover and do not develop chronic disease. In contrast, in the United States, sporadic hepatitis is usually due to HCV infection and chronic hepatitis is rather common. Many of these patients are abusing drugs.

Clinical features

Hepatitis C is a relatively mild, usually asymptomatic illness. The transaminases fluctuate rapidly during the early course of the illness, the peak values becoming gradually lower (Fig. 3(b)). This pattern was prominent in haemophiliac patients infected by HCV transmitted by factor VIII concentrates. About 80 per cent of them developed chronic hepatitis. Factor VIII concentrates are now rendered safe by heat inactivation.

Rare reports of hepatitis developing after blood transfusion or plasma donation are due to HCV infection transmitted by donation of blood by patients in the incubation period of the infection prior to developing anti-HCV.

Smooth muscle and nuclear antibodies may be found in patients with chronic active hepatitis or cirrhosis, but the titres are much lower than in autoimmune chronic active hepatitis and cirrhosis.

Management and prognosis

The rate of progression of the disease is variable. In 20 per cent of cases, cirrhosis develops in 20–25 years but in the majority the prognosis is good.

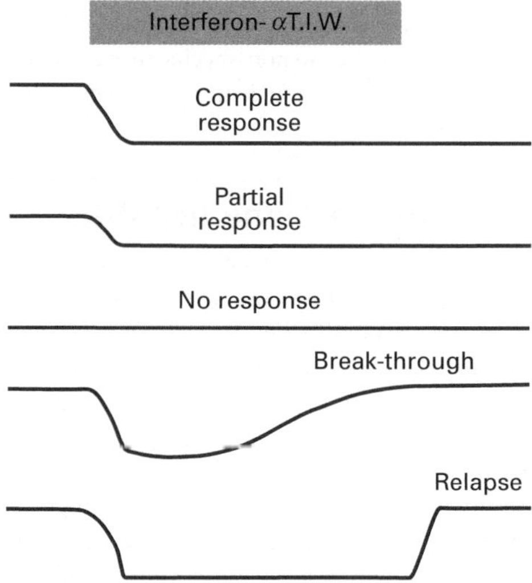

Fig. 7 Treatment of chronic HCV infection with interferon-α (usually for 6–12 months). The graphs show the pattern of transaminase change. Viraemia can be determined by polymerase chain amplification of HCV-RNA from serum. Patients with a complete response clear HCV-RNA from their serum: this response is seen in 20 per cent of patients treated. Addition of ribavirin reduces the relapse rate with interferon-α, giving sustained response rates of 40 per cent.

Interferon-α (3–5 megaunits thrice weekly for 6–12 months) has normalized transaminases in 50–85 per cent of cases but relapse is common (60 per cent) (Fig. 7). Long-term control is seen in about 10–20 per cent of treated patients. The addition of ribavirin to a 12-month course of interferon-α markedly reduces the relapse rate giving sustained response rates of 40 per cent. Protease inhibitors are in development.

Further reading

Desmet, V.J., Gerber, M., Hoofnagle, J.H., Manus, N.I., and Scheuer, P.J. (1994). *Hepatology*, **19**, 1523–19.

Eddleston, A.W.L.F. (1997). Hepatitis B and health care workers. *Lancet*, **349**, 1339–40.

Lee, W.M. (1997). Hepatitis B virus infection. *New England Journal of Medicine*, **337**, 1733–45.

Poynard, T., Bedossa, P., and Opolon, P. (1997). Natural history of liver fibrosis progression in patients with chronic hepatitis C. *Lancet*, **349**, 825–32.

Sherlock, S. and Dooley, J. (1997). *Diseases of the liver and biliary system.* Blackwell Science, Oxford.

Autoimmune liver disease

Chapter 5.32

Autoimmune hepatitis

I. G. McFarlane and A. L. W. F. Eddleston

Autoimmune hepatitis, previously called 'lupoid' or 'autoimmune chronic active' hepatitis is an unresolving, predominantly periportal hepatitis, usually with hypergammaglobulinaemia and tissue auto-antibodies, which is responsive to immunosuppressive therapy in most cases.

Presenting features and natural history

The patient conforming most closely with the early description of 'lupoid' hepatitis is typically a young woman, who presents with either an acute hepatitis or a chronic illness characterized by lethargy, epigastric pain, arthralgia and/or myalgia, oligomenorrhoea, fluctuating jaundice, and a cushingoid appearance with striae, hirsutism, and acne. Cutaneous manifestations of chronic liver disease and signs of cirrhosis may be present. Early studies described the serious nature of the disease, with up to 80 per cent mortality at 5 years when untreated.

Today, it is recognized that autoimmune hepatitis can present at any age and also affects males, although females still predominate (4:1). There are two peaks of onset: peripubertally and between the fourth and sixth decades of life (Fig. 1). In this broader spectrum of patients, signs and symptoms vary widely—from the classical presentation described above to the completely asymptomatic patient whose disease may be revealed only incidentally during routine health screening or investigation of some other condition. About 25 per cent of patients never develop jaundice. There is often a history of other autoimmune disorders, particularly thyroid disease and rheumatoid arthritis, in the patient or their first-degree relatives. Lethargy (often profound) is a prominent feature and may be the dominant symptom. Thus autoimmune hepatitis should be considered in the differential diagnosis of 'chronic fatigue' syndromes.

The disease is usually more active and more difficult to control in younger patients. Older patients tend to have a milder disease that is generally easier to manage. Approximately 30 per cent already have cirrhosis when they first present and a further 30 per cent will subsequently develop cirrhosis despite apparently satisfactory control of their disease. Occasionally, patients may present with a severe acute, uncontrollable hepatitis and require urgent referral for liver transplantation. None the less, recent long-term follow-up studies indicate that overall 10-year survival is now greater than 90 per cent and that, for the majority of patients who are carefully managed (including those with cirrhosis), life expectancy is probably not

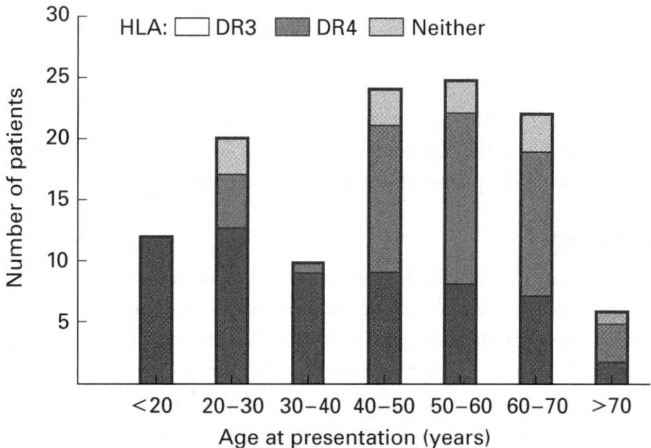

Fig. 1 Distribution according to age at presentation and HLA-DR3 and HLA-DR4 status of 118 adults with autoimmune hepatitis attending the Institute of Liver Studies, King's College Hospital, London, UK. *(Reproduced with permission from Gut 1998;* ***42****: 599–602.)*

significantly different from that of an age- and sex-matched normal population.

Diagnosis and laboratory investigations

There are no features that are pathognomonic of the condition. Diagnosis depends on the presence of a combination of suggestive abnormalities and requires that all other possible causes of liver disease have been excluded by appropriate investigations. A definitive diagnosis cannot be made without a liver biopsy. It has been recommended that patients should be classified as having *definite or probable* autoimmune hepatitis according to how closely their presenting features conform to those of classical disease.

Serum biochemistry

Serum biochemical abnormalities show a typically 'hepatitic' pattern, with elevated serum aminotransferase activities and bilirubin concentrations and usually only mild elevations in serum alkaline phosphatase. Gammaglutamyl transferase activities may also be elevated (sometimes quite markedly) but are of uncertain clinical significance. Serum aminotransferase activities vary widely, from mildly abnormal to more than 50 times the upper normal limits, even in patients presenting with histologically active disease. Importantly, a low serum aminotransferase does not necessarily equate to mild or inactive disease.

Immunoglobulins and autoantibodies

Hyperglobulinaemia with selective elevation of serum IgG is a characteristic feature. Serum IgM and IgA are usually normal but IgM may be elevated. About 80 per cent of patients present with significant titres ($\geq$1:40) of antinuclear (**ANA**) and/or smooth muscle (**SMA**) autoantibodies, as determined by indirect immunofluorescence on appropriate substrates. A further 3–4 per cent have type 1 liver–kidney microsomal (**LKM-1**) antibodies that react with the cytochrome P450 isoform IID6, usually in the absence of ANA and SMA. Up to 90 per cent also have circulating perinuclear staining antineutrophil antibodies (**pANCA**). A number of other autoantibodies reacting with components that are more specifically related to the liver also occur frequently but tests for these are currently available in only a few specialist centres. Patients with antimitochondrial antibodies should not be considered to have autoimmune hepatitis.

The ANA typically give so-called 'homogeneous' immunofluorescent staining of nuclei. Other patterns (perinuclear, nucleolar, or speckled) are frequently seen but appear to have no clinical significance. The SMA react with a variety of cytosketetal proteins, most notably F-actin. Reliance on anti-actin specificity can, however, lead to missed diagnoses of autoimmune hepatitis.

Histology

The typical morphological features are those of an interface (periportal or periseptal) hepatitis with a marked portal and periportal, predominantly lymphoplasmacytic, necroinflammatory infiltrate with piecemeal necrosis of hepatocytes. In the more severe cases there is often formation of liver cell rosettes and lobular (intra-acinar) involvement with portal–portal or portal–septal bridging necrosis. Patients with evidence of bile duct damage or well defined granulomas should not be considered to have autoimmune hepatitis. Other changes, including lymphoid aggregates, steatosis, deposits of copper or iron, or bile ductule proliferation, may sometimes be seen, especially in the later stages of the disease and in patients with cirrhosis, but are generally considered to be too non-specific to exclude autoimmune hepatitis, except when they are sufficiently prominent to be suggestive of a different aetiology.

Subtypes of autoimmune hepatitis

It has become common practice to subdivide autoimmune hepatitis into type 1 (ANA $\pm$ SMA positive) and type2 (LKM-1 positive)disease. The latter presents predominantly in children and young adults (almost always females) and tends to be more often associated with polyendocrinopathy (thyroiditis, insulin-dependent diabetes, hypoparathyroidism, and hypoadrenalism) than type 1 disease. The presentation is also more often acute, even fulminant, with severe histological features and a marked propensity to progress rapidly to cirrhosis. However, this classification is not exclusive. As noted above, type 2 cases comprise only a small proportion of all patients with autoimmune hepatitis seen in most clinical practices—even in continental Europe, where type 2 tends to be more common.

The large majority of young females who present with severe disease are in fact type 1. Several other subdivisions based on serum autoantibody profiles have been proposed but these have no proven clinical utility and have not been widely adopted.

Overlaps with other conditions

Features of autoimmune hepatitis, particularly mild to moderate hyperglobulinaemia and circulating autoantibodies, can be seen with variable frequency in acute or chronic viral hepatitis, Wilson's disease, α_1-antitrypsin deficiency, primary biliary cirrhosis, primary sclerosing cholangitis, alcoholic liver disease, non-alcoholic steatohepatitis, and in some idiosyncratic reactions to a wide range of drugs. Interface hepatitis on liver biopsy can also be quite frequently seen in these conditions, but there are usually other morphological changes that are not normally associated with autoimmune hepatitis (see above). However, primary sclerosing cholangitis in children often presents initially with features that are indistinguishable from those of florid autoimmune hepatitis.

Clinical management of overlap cases can be problematic because corticosteroids, which are the standard treatment for autoimmune hepatitis (see below), are usually of little benefit or are contraindicated in these patients and failure to introduce appropriate therapy promptly in some conditions such as Wilson's disease can have serious consequences. On the other hand, interferon therapy for chronic viral hepatitis can exacerbate underlying autoimmune disorders. None the less, recent evidence suggests that in most cases of viral hepatitis with autoantibodies it is generally safe to use interferon therapy, but patients need to be monitored carefully.

Differential diagnosis

This involves serological screening for hepatitis A, B, and C viruses and a careful drug and alcohol history. Tests for other viruses (such as cytomegalovirus and Epstein–Barr virus) that occasionally cause hepatitis are not usually essential but may also be considered. Serum copper and ceruloplasmin concentrations should be measured and, if abnormal, slit-lamp examination for ocular Keyser–Fleischer rings and urinary copper estimations after D-penicillamine challenge should be performed to exclude Wilson's disease. The serum concentration of α_1-antitrypsin should be measured and the phenotype (if available).

An elevated serum IgM together with a markedly raised serum alkaline phosphatase should raise suspicions of primary biliary cirrhosis. Cholangiography may be required to exclude primary sclerosing cholangitis.

Patients without AIVA, SMA, or LKM-1 antibodies

Up to 20 per cent of autoimmune hepatitis patients present without ANA, SMA, or LKM-1 antibodies and are sometimes included within the spectrum of 'cryptogenic chronic liver disease'. Diagnosis in these cases can be made on the combination of a 'hepatitic' pattern of serum biochemical abnormalities, elevated serum IgG, the finding of interface hepatitis on liver biopsy (without other changes suggestive of a different aetiology), and careful exclusion of other causes of liver disease. A history of other immunological disorders in the patient or family adds weight to the diagnosis. Testing for pANCA may be helpful. Such patients are indistinguishable from ANA/SMA/LKM-1 positive cases with respect to variability in severity of disease, response to treatment, or prognosis.

Pathogenesis

The aetiology of autoimmune hepatitis is unknown but is believed to relate to underlying defect(s) in immunological control of autoreactivity to liver cells. In north European caucasoids, the disease is strongly associated with inheritance of the HLA Al-B8-DR3 haplotype and particularly with the DR3 allotype. In DR3-negative patients, there is a secondary association with HLA-DR4. These markers are also associated with other autoimmune diseases. DR3-positive patients are generally younger and have more severe disease, while DR4 is associated with an older age at presentation (Fig. 1) and with milder disease. In Japan, where DR3 is very rare in the normal population, the association is almost exclusively with DR4 and almost all patients are in the older age group.

It is assumed that some triggering factor is required to initiate the disease in genetically susceptible individuals. Instances of the development of autoimmune hepatitis following infections with the hepatitis A, Epstein–Barr, measles, and other viruses are now well documented. Idiosyncratic reactions to several drugs, including oxyphenisatin, methyldopa, and the antibiotic minocycline, can mimic autoimmune hepatitis and may trigger the disease in predisposed subjects.

Mechanisms of hepatocyte damage

The final effector mechanism of liver cell damage in autoimmune hepatitis has not yet been fully elucidated. Direct T-cell cytotoxicity against liver cells appears not to be the major mechanism in patients, and existing evidence favours an antibody-dependent cellular cytotoxic reaction directed at liver-specific antigen(s) on hepatocytes. A major putative target autoantigen has been identified, namely the asialoglycoprotein receptor (**ASGPR**), which seems to be preferentially expressed on the surfaces of periportal hepatocytes *in vivo*. Most patients have CD4+ T cells that recognize this antigen and more than 90 per cent of those with active disease have high titres of circulating autoantibodies against ASGPR. However, other target autoantigens may be important and it is possible that localized cytokine production and apoptotic mechanisms initiated by antigen-specific CD4+ T cells in the liver may also be involved.

Treatment

If the patient is symptomatic, has an aminotransferase activity of greater than three times the upper normal limit, is jaundiced, or has florid activity with bridging necrosis on liver biopsy, immunosuppressive therapy is clearly indicated. On the other hand, if the patient is asymptomatic, with no histological evidence of lobular involvement and/or bridging necrosis and only a mildly elevated serum aminotransferase, the decision whether to treat is more difficult. However, because this is a naturally fluctuating condition and patients with so-called 'mild' disease can have periodic flares that can accelerate progression to (or exacerbate existing) cirrhosis, many authorities believe that some form of therapy should be offered.

The standard approach is to induce remission with prednisone or prednisolone at 0.5 mg/kg bodyweight. Higher doses may occasionally be required, especially in young patients with severe disease, but the risk of undesirable side-effects is greatly increased. When the aminotransferase has fallen to less than twice upper normal limit (usually within 2–8 weeks), the dose is decreased to 0.25 mg/kg. Azathioprine (50–75 mg/day) is usually added for its 'steroid-sparing' effect. This should be done early (within the first few weeks), partly to ascertain whether the patient will tolerate the drug (about 10 per cent do not) but mainly because it takes 3–6 months to become fully effective. When the aminotransferase becomes normal, the steroid dose can be slowly reduced (in decrements of 2.5 mg monthly) to a maintenance level of between 5 and 10 mg/day (with azathioprine at 50–75 mg/day). Patients should then be maintained on this regimen for at least 2 years before any further changes in treatment are contemplated, unless complications arise.

After 2 years, if the patient has remained asymptomatic with consistently normal aminotransferase levels, a liver biopsy should be performed to confirm histological remission. Consideration may then be given to slowly withdrawing all treatment. However, patients often relapse (even after many years in remission) and careful long-term follow-up is essential. An alternative approach is to increase the dose of azathioprine to 2 mg/kg per day before gradually withdrawing the steroids and then to maintain the patient on the higher dose of azathioprine alone. Mild to moderate arthralgia lasting a few months is frequently experienced following steroid withdrawal. Azathioprine induces myelosuppression in about 10 per cent of patients, usually within a few weeks or months of starting the drug, but it is important to distinguish between this and the leucopenia and thrombocytopenia which is often seen in autoimmune hepatitis (especially in patients with cirrhosis and splenomegaly). Accordingly, full blood counts should be done frequently, particularly during the first 6 months of treatment.

Steroid 'insensitivity'

About 10 per cent of patients never achieve remission with corticosteroids and a similar proportion become unresponsive after an initial response. Non-compliance or only partial compliance with therapy (which is difficult to monitor) may be a factor. In some cases, remission can be induced with higher doses (prednisolone, 1 mg/kg per day) but more often there is progressive liver failure and early referral for liver transplantation is indicated. In any event, review of the diagnosis is worthwhile and alternative therapy needs to be considered. There are no large-scale controlled clinical trials of the use of other immunosuppressive drug regimens for autoimmune hepatitis but there are reports that oral budesonide, D-penicillamine, cyclophosphamide, cyclosporin, or ursodeoxycholic acid are effective in some cases. Additionally, a good response to tacrolimus has been reported in patients presenting with steroid unresponsive autoimmune hepatitis who have been listed for liver transplantation.

Further reading

International Working Party Report. (1995). Terminology of chronic hepatitis. *American Journal of Gastroenterology*, **90**, 181–9.

Johnson, P.J. and McFarlane, I.G. (1993). Meeting report: International autoimmune hepatitis group. *Hepatology*, **18**, 998–1005.

Chapter 5.33

Primary biliary cirrhosis

M. F. Bassendine

Primary biliary cirrhosis is a chronic, cholestatic, inflammatory liver disease most commonly seen in middle-aged women. The cause is unknown but evidence suggests that autoimmune phenomena are involved, with a strong association with autoantibodies predominantly to mitochondria but, also in a minority of cases, to nuclear factors. The disease has an insidious onset and patients with early disease are usually only recognized following the incidental discovery of antimitochondrial antibodies or elevated levels of serum alkaline phosphatase. Progression is slow but eventually many patients develop cirrhosis and, ultimately, death may occur from liver failure or complications of cirrhosis, such as bleeding oesophageal varices. In Britain its prevalence is between 100 and 240 per million and in Europe it is one of the commonest indications for liver transplantation.

Aetiology and pathogenesis

Genetic factors are suggested by familial clustering in siblings, twins, parents, and cousins. A high familial incidence of autoantibodies, including antimitochondrial antibodies, has been noted. There is no association with major histocompatibility complex (**MHC**) class I antigens but several associations with class II have been reported, in particular HLA-DR8, with a two- to sixfold increase in patients compared with controls. Data on MHC class III associations are conflicting.

Some 90 per cent of patients have antibodies to mitochondria, the major autoantigens being components of pyruvate dehydrogenase complex (**PDC**) (Table 1). Aberrant cell surface expression of the immunodominant autoantigens (PDC-E2 and/or E3 binding protein) has been found on biliary epithelial cells of patients suggesting that antibody-mediated cytotoxicity may contribute to tissue damage.

Other autoantibodies against nuclear antigens are found in a minority of patients. Nuclear antigens reacting with these disease-specific autoantibodies include an integral glycoprotein of the nuclear-pore membrane (gp210) and nucleoporin p62 (Table 1), but as yet little is understood of the way in which the autoimmune response is induced or the effector mechanisms that cause tissue damage. Co-existing abnormalities include raised levels of IgM, depletion of C4 and aberrant expression of MHC class II antigens on biliary epithelial cells; these could be a cause of consequence of liver damage. CD8+ cytotoxic T cells play a significant part in the destructive lesion of the bile ducts, infiltrating the portal tract and appearing adjacent to biliary epithelial cells at the time of maximal damage. The role of the other effector systems is less clear.

Table 1 Disease-specific autoantigens in primary biliary cirrhosis

	Molecular weight ($\times10^3$)	Sera reacting to antigen (%)
Mitochondrial antigens		
Pyruvate dehydrogenase complex:		
E2 acetyltransferase	74	94
Protein X (E3 binding protein)	52	94
E1α decarboxylase	41	40
E1β decarboxylase	36	10
2-oxoglutarate dehydrogenase complex:		
E2 succinyl transferase	50	53
Branched-chain 2-oxo-acid dehydrogenase complex:		
E2 acyltransferase	50	89
Nuclear antigens		
Glycoprotein of the nuclear-pore membrane	210	10
Nucleoporin p62	62	32
Protein with dot-like distribution within cell nuclei	100	27

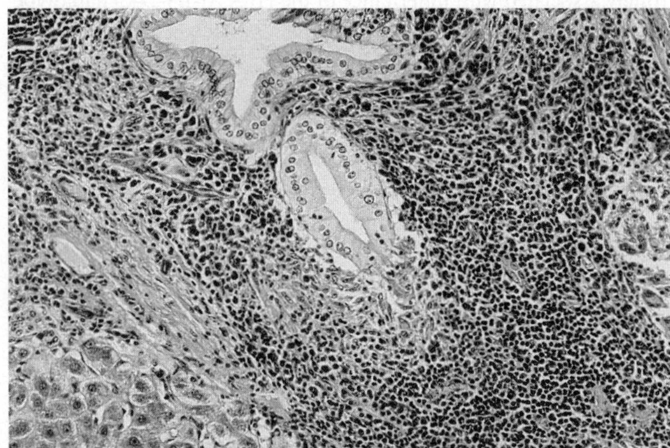

Fig. 1 Bile-duct lesion in primary biliary cirrhosis. There is granulomatous destruction of a medium-sized bile-duct radicle in which the epithelium appears hyperplastic. Epithelioid macrophages are surrounded by a chronic inflammatory cell infiltrate. Haematoxylin and eosin.
(By courtesy of A.D. Burt.)

Pathology

The characteristic early lesion is inflammatory duct destruction. Later there is fibrosis, often patchy, and eventually frank cirrhosis. The morphological classification has four stages, albeit with overlap in different parts of the liver. In stage 1, the duct lesion is florid (Fig. 1) with the epithelium irregular, hyperplastic, or ulcerated. There is a heavy infiltrate of lymphocytes, plasma cells, and neutrophils, with

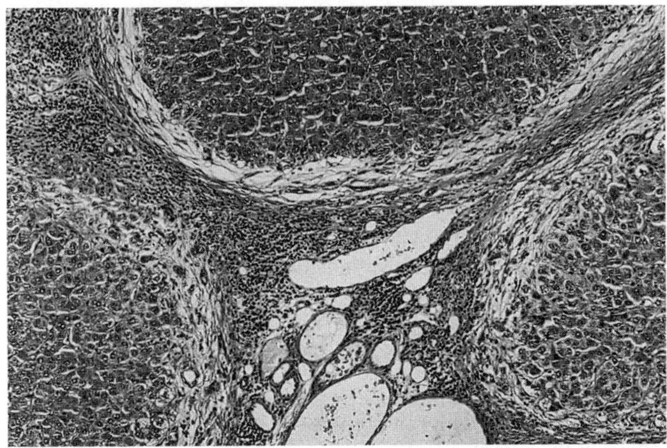

Fig. 2 Stage 4 primary biliary cirrhosis: an established micronodular cirrhosis; the halo effect seen around the nodules is a characteristic feature of biliary cirrhosis. Haematoxylin and eosin.
(By courtesy of A.D. Burt.)

occasional eosinophils. Aggregates of histocytes with granulomas ranging from foci of epithelioid cells to rounded lesions with multinucleated giant cells are present. In stage 2 there is duct destruction and replacement by lymphoid aggregates with fibrosis. In stage 3 there is relatively little inflammation, and fibrous septa extend from the portal tract. In stage 4 there is cirrhosis, paucity of bile ducts, and lymphoid infiltration (Fig. 2). Mallory bodies similar to those seen in alcoholic liver disease may be present and there is excess stainable copper-binding protein, a reflection of the cholestasis.

Clinical features

Over 90 per cent of patients are women, usually between the ages of 40 and 60 years. Patients with early disease may complain only of fatigue or symptoms of coexisting autoimmune disease. Those with more advanced disease have evidence of cholestasis with jaundice, pruritus, light stools, easy bruising, and weight loss. Occasionally, patients present with gastrointestinal bleeding from oesophageal varices. Pruritus may first be noticed during pregnancy or when the patient is on the contraceptive pill.

Findings on examination vary widely. At one extreme, there may be no abnormality, whereas at the other the patient is jaundiced, with scratch marks and signs of long-standing cholestasis. The planus form of xanthoma occurs characteristically as xanthelasmas around the eyes and in the palmar creases. Tuberous lesions develop late on the extensor surfaces around the knees, elbows, wrists, ankle, and on pressure points such as buttocks. Occasionally they affect tendon sheaths and nerves, producing xanthomatous peripheral neuropathy.

The liver is usually enlarged and firm, and splenomegaly may be present, with or without portal hypertension. Spider naevi and palmar erythema are less frequent than in alcoholic cirrhosis. Bleeding from oesophageal varices is a late complication, as are liver failure and fluid retention. Steatorrhoea occurs primarily in advanced cholestasis, leading to the malabsorption of fat-soluble vitamins, especially D, and thus to osteomalacia. Osteoporosis is also well recognized. Deficiency of vitamin K sometimes results in easy bruising or other haemorrhagic phenomena. Clubbing of the fingers and leuconychia are rare. There is an increased incidence of gallstones and peptic ulceration. Male patients with cirrhosis are at increased risk of primary hepatocellular carcinoma.

Associated diseases

These include scleroderma, Sjögren's syndrome, seropositive and seronegative arthropathy, thyroiditis, and renal tubular acidosis. The CRST syndrome, pulmonary fibrosis, and coeliac disease have also been reported.

Diagnosis

The diagnosis is based on the clinical findings, the histology, and serological and biochemical changes. A positive antimitochondrial antibody may antedate all other abnormalities. Liver function tests reflect cholestasis with increases in serum alkaline phosphatase and gammaglutamyl transferase, but only modest change in transaminases. At presentation total serum bilirubin is usually normal or only modestly increased. The serum globulins are usually raised, particularly the IgM, but the serum albumin is usually maintained until late in the disease. Other tests such as erythrocyte sedimentation rate, cholesterol, and autoantibodies other than antimitochondrial are less specific. Liver biopsy is mandatory.

The main differential diagnosis is from other causes of cholestasis. Ultrasonography and computed tomography are necessary to exclude extrahepatic biliary obstruction or gallstones. Endoscopic retrograde cholangiopancreatography (ERCP) may be necessary for patients without detectable mitochondrial antibody, many of whom have a positive antinuclear factor and may be thought to have 'autoimmune cholangitis'. There is an overlap with autoimmune chronic active hepatitis, distinguished by liver histology, while primary sclerosing cholangitis will be evident on ERCP.

Course and prognosis

The long-term prognosis is poor, but the course is variable and patients without symptoms may remain well for years. Once symptoms develop, several biochemical and histological features have prognostic significance. There is an inverse relation between serum bilirubin and survival, and most models also use age, albumin, and presence of cirrhosis or a marker of advanced liver disease such as increased prothrombin time.

Treatment

Earlier diagnosis combined with difficulty in predicting clinical course in asymptomatic patients has led to uncertainty as to which patients should be treated, when treatment should be started, and what is the best treatment to administer. The agents that have been assessed are shown in Table 2. At present ursodeoxycholic acid is generally considered to be the treatment of choice; it is not only safe but also effective in improving biochemical features of primary biliary cirrhosis and survival free of liver transplantation in patients with moderate or severe disease.

Itching can be an intolerable symptom and the first line of treatment is usually with cholestyramine. Improvement in itching has also been reported with rifampicin and opioid antagonists (nalmifene and naloxone). There is no indication for a fat-free diet unless the patient has symptoms related to steatorrhoea or xanthelasma with high serum cholesterol levels. Supplementation with medium-chain triglycerides may be necessary if adequate weight or nutrition cannot be sustained. A prolonged prothrombin time is treated with intramuscular vitamin K, 10 mg monthly. Injections of vitamin A (100 000 i.u.) and vitamin

Table 2 Therapeutic agents evaluated in primary biliary cirrhosis

Agent	Dosage	Comment
Immunosuppressive		
Cyclosporin	3–4 mg/kg/day	Improved hepatic function but renal toxicity and hypertension
Methotrexate	15 mg/week	Under evaluation Some benefit but toxicity possible
Prednisolone	30→10 mg/day	Improved hepatic function in one small study
Azathioprine	0.5–2 mg/kg/day	Minor benefits ?Improved survival
Chlorambucil	0.5–4 mg/day	Potentially toxic Benefits unclear
Antifibrotic		
Colchicine	1–1.2 mg/day	Minor benefits
Malotilate	1.5 mg/day	Minor benefits
Cupruretic		
D-penicillamine	250–1000 mg/day	No convincing benefit Excessive toxicity
Bile acid		
Ursodeoxycholic acid	10–15 mg/kg/day	Improvement in biochemistry and survival free of liver transplantation

D (100 000 i.u.) are usually given every 2 months in jaundiced patients and vitamin E supplements may also be required. Osteomalacia is rare, given such treatment but prevention of osteoporosis is more difficult; oral calcium 1 g daily may be combined with cyclical diphosphonates if there is evidence of progressive bone loss.

The complications of portal hypertension and of liver failure are treated appropriately. Liver transplantation is now the accepted treatment for end-stage primary biliary cirrhosis. Debate continues as to whether the disease recurs post-transplant. Referral to a transplant centre should be considered as the bilirubin approaches 100 μmol/l.

Further reading

Jones, D.E.J., James, O.F.W., and Bassendine, M.F. (1998). Primary biliary cirrhosis: Clinical and associated autoimmune features and natural history. *Clinics in Liver Disease*, 2, 265–82.

Poupon, R.E., Lindor, K.D., Cauch-Dudek, K., Dickson, E.R., Poupon, R., and Heathcote, E.J. (1997). Combined analysis of randomized controlled trials of ursodeoxycholic acid in primary biliary cirrhosis. *Gastroenterology*, 113, 884–90.

Chapter 5.34

Primary sclerosing cholangitis

R. W. Chapman

Primary sclerosing cholangitis is a chronic cholestatic liver disease characterized by an obliterative inflammatory fibrosis of the biliary tract. It may lead to bile-duct obstruction, biliary cirrhosis, hepatic failure and, in some patients, cholangiocarcinoma. It is now more widely recognized and is the second most common reason for liver transplantation in Britain.

The accepted criteria for diagnosis are: (a) generalized beading and stenosis of the biliary system on cholangiography (Fig. 1); (b) absence of choledocholithiasis or a history of bile-duct surgery; (c) exclusion of bile-duct cancer. Cholangitis can also be secondary to a number of predisposing factors including previous bile-duct surgery, biliary stones, intrahepatic infusion of 5-fluorodeoxyuridine, injection of formalin into hepatic hydatid cysts, and **AIDS** (probably by way of infection by cytomegalovirus or cryptosporidium).

Aetiology

The cause remains unknown, but there is a close association with inflammatory bowel disease, particularly ulcerative colitis and genetic and immunological factors are probably important. The data suggest that *HLA-DR3/DRW52a*, *HLA-DR2*, and ulcerative colitis are separate independent risk factors. Both *HLA-DRw52a* and *HLA-DR2* encode for amino acids in the HLA β-chain that may enhance antigen presentation by the HLA molecule to the T-cell receptor.

The disease is characterized by hypergammaglobulinaemia, often with a disproportionate elevation of serum IgM concentrations in

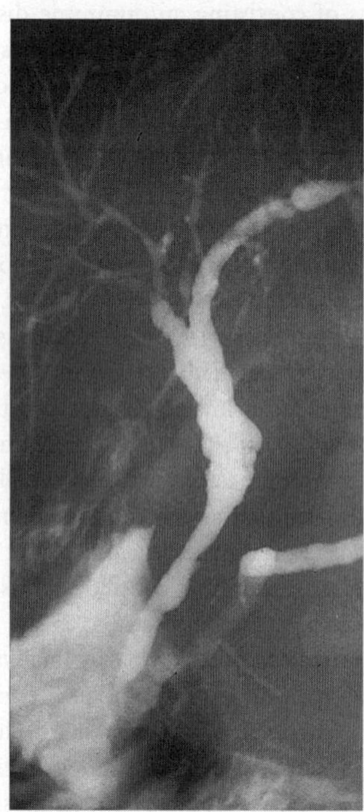

Fig. 1 Cholangiogram showing the typical features of primary sclerosing cholangitis with stricturing and dilatation of the intra- and extrahepatic biliary tree.

adult patients, and IgG in children. Smooth-muscle antibody and antinuclear factor are also found in approximately one-third of patients, usually in low titres. A cytoplasmic antineutrophil antibody has also been found in 80 per cent of patients with primary sclerosing cholangitis and in 30 per cent of those with ulcerative colitis. Unlike Wegener's granulomatosis, the antigen has yet to be identified.

Other immunological abnormalities include elevated circulating immune complexes, activation of complement via the alternate pathway, reduced levels of T-suppressor cells, and infiltration of portal tracts by mononuclear cells predominantly activated T lymphocytes.

The overall evidence suggests the disease to be immunologically mediated, and triggered in genetically susceptible subjects by unidentified toxic or infectious agents.

Clinical features

There is a male/female ratio of 2:1. The majority of patients present between the ages of 25 and 40 years, although the disease may be diagnosed at any age. Many patients are asymptomatic when the diagnosis follows detection of a raised plasma alkaline phosphatase. Others have fatigue, intermittent jaundice, weight loss, right upper quadrant abnormal pain, or pruritus. Acute cholangitis is rare unless following instrumentation of the biliary tree. Physical examination is often normal but there may be jaundice or hepatosplenomegaly.

Diagnosis

The serum alkaline phosphatase is often raised to greater than three times normal, and mild elevations in liver transaminases are seen in the majority of patients. Serum bilirubin is not usually elevated until late in the disease. Levels of bilirubin and alkaline phosphatase may fluctuate widely in an individual patient. Hypoalbuminaemia is unusual until the disease becomes advanced. Increased serum IgM concentrations are seen in about half of the symptomatic adult patients, but high concentrations of IgG are always found in children.

In addition to the serum antineutrophil antibodies, low levels of antinuclear antibody and smooth-muscle antibody may be found in approximately one-third of patients, but mitochondrial antibodies are absent.

The cholangiographic appearances on endoscopic retrograde cholangiopancreatography (**ERCP**) are usually diagnostic and consist of multiple, irregular stricturing and dilatation (beading of the intrahepatic and extrahepatic biliary ducts) (Fig. 1). Occasionally, involvement is localized to the intrahepatic system, and even more rarely, only the extrahepatic ducts may be involved. Small diverticula are found along the common bile duct in about 20 per cent of patients and are pathognomonic.

Pathological features

The histological appearances of liver are not usually diagnostic, although some form of biliary disease can usually be identified. The characteristic early features are periductal 'onion skin' fibrosis and inflammation, portal oedema, and bile ductular proliferation resulting in the expansion of the portal tracts (Fig. 2). Later, fibrosis spreads into the liver parenchyma, leading inevitably to biliary cirrhosis. Obliterative cholangitis leads to replacement of the intralobular bile ducts by connective tissue—the vanishing bile-duct syndrome. In addition, piecemeal necrosis, copper-binding protein, cholestasis, and occasional portal phlebitis may be present.

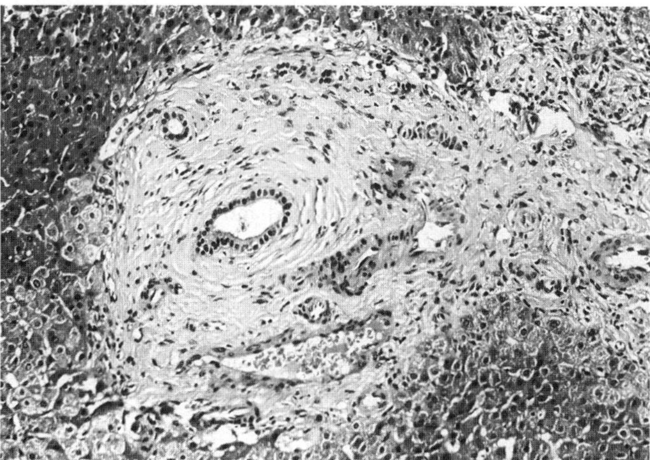

Fig. 2 The hepatic histological changes of early primary sclerosing cholangitis showing a concentric (onion skin) fibrosis around the bile ducts.

Table 1 Diseases associated with primary sclerosing cholangitis

Ulcerative colitis	Sjögren's syndrome
Crohn's colitis	Angioimmunoblastic lymphadenopathy
Chronic pancreatitis	Histiocytosis X
Retroperitoneal fibrosis	Autoimmune haemolytic anaemia
Riedel's struma	
Retro-orbital tumours	
Immunodeficiency states	

Association with other diseases

A large number of diseases have been associated with primary sclerosing cholangitis (Table 1). The most important is ulcerative colitis, symptoms of which usually precede those of cholangitis, but sometimes the liver disease is detected first. The outcome of the cholangitis is unrelated to the activity or severity of the colitis and colectomy has no effect on the course of the cholangitis. The association with Crohn's disease is much less common (less than 1 per cent) and then only with Crohn's colitis.

Natural history and prognosis

The course is highly variable. The median survival from presentation to death or liver transplantation is approximately 10–12 years. The majority die in hepatic failure following deepening cholestatic jaundice, but approximately 10–30 per cent of patients with long-standing cholangitis die from bile-duct carcinoma. Unfortunately, no factors predict which patients will develop this cancer.

Treatment

There is no curative treatment. Pruritus is best managed by cholestyramine and replacement of fat-soluble vitamins is necessary when patients become jaundiced. Broad-spectrum antibiotics should be given for acute attacks of cholangitis. If cholangiography shows obstruction to the main extrahepatic bile ducts, the best approach is to stent the obstruction, by the percutaneous transhepatic route or at ERCP. Balloon dilatation of the strictures before stenting may prove useful in a minority of patients.

Small biliary stones and biliary sludge can lead to a rapid clinical or biochemical deterioration. Endoscopic sphincterotomy with extraction of the biliary debris can then be beneficial.

Specific treatment has included trials of corticosteroids, immunosuppressive drugs, cholecystogogues, and antibiotics, either alone or in combination. The results have been universally disappointing, although assessment of treatment is difficult because the clinical course fluctuates. Metabolic bone disease may be accelerated by corticosteroids and they should not be used. Small uncontrolled trials have suggested that ursodeoxycholic acid may improve symptoms and reduce the abnormalities in markers of cholestasis and the drug is free of side-effects.

The role of hepatobiliary surgery remains controversial. Good results have been claimed for the resection of the extrahepatic biliary tree followed by biliary reconstruction with silastic transhepatic stents. Controlled trials are needed to confirm efficacy of these and other surgical techniques.

Liver transplantation is the only option available in young patients with advanced liver disease. Recent results have been encouraging, with 4-year survival rates of 80–90 per cent. There have only been a few case reports of recurrence in the transplanted liver.

Further reading

Chapman, R.W., *et al.* (1980). Primary sclerosing cholangitis—a review of its clinical features, cholangiography and hepatic histology. *Gut*, **21**, 870–7.

Chapman, R.W. (1991). Aetiology and natural history of primary sclerosing cholangitis—a decade of progress? *Gut*, **32**, 1433–5.

Farrant, J.M., *et al.* (1991). Natural history and prognostic variables in primary sclerosing cholangitis. *Gastroenterology*, **100**, 1710–17.

Sherlock, S. and Dooley, J. (1997). *Diseases of the liver and biliary system.* Blackwell Science, Oxford.

Chapter 5.35

Alcoholic liver disease and non-alcoholic steatosis hepatitis

O. F. W. James

Alcoholic liver disease

Only 10–30 per cent of heavy, persistent, alcohol drinkers develop cirrhosis, although well over 50 per cent have fatty livers. Individual susceptibility depends on many factors. The contribution of nutrition remains controversial, but is seems possible that both undernutrition and obesity act synergistically with direct alcohol toxicity to increase the likelihood of liver damage. High alcohol consumption in patients infected with hepatitis C virus also increases the possibility of severe liver disease.

In a large group of males with alcoholic cirrhosis, average alcohol consumption was 160 g/day (equivalent to over two bottles of wine, 4.5 litres of normal strength lager or two-thirds of a bottle of spirits) over 8 years. In females the corresponding figure was 110 g/day. It seems likely that almost no risk of significant alcohol-related liver damage exists below about 40 g/day equivalent to 30 units per week in men, rather less in women, assuming no other associated risk factors. Current 'sensible' limits recommended in the UK are 21 units (200 g) for men and 14 units (130 g) for women, but these figures are arbitrary.

Susceptibility to alcoholism and to alcoholic liver damage each have genetic components; probably one in three alcoholics will have at least one parent who is alcoholic. Analysis of twin studies suggests hereditability of excess drinking of alcohol in the range of 0.3–0.6 (where 0 = no hereditability, 1.0 = complete hereditability).

Pathology

Fatty liver is the first histological lesion; it occurs in most heavy drinkers at one time or another, but is completely reversible on alcohol withdrawal. More serious is alcoholic hepatitis, which may occur in up to 40 per cent chronic ethanol abusers. The most severe changes are seen in the perivenular area; including ballooning and necrosis of liver cells, in some of which Mallory bodies may be seen; pericellular fibrosis around hepatic venules ('chicken wire' fibrosis); and a patchy inflammatory-cell infiltrate, mainly polymorphs, often only seen around a few hepatocytes. Ultimately, fibrous septa link hepatic veins to portal veins and regeneration occurs, disturbing normal liver architecture with the formation of nodules and cirrhosis.

Clinical features

Symptoms and signs of alcoholic liver disease (Table 1) correlate only very broadly with underlying histology or abnormal tests of liver function.

Patients with *fatty liver* may have no symptoms or complain only of nausea and malaise. Liver function tests may be mildly deranged but in severe cases, there may be cholestasis or even, very rarely, liver failure and portal hypertension.

Mild *alcoholic hepatitis* is often indistinguishable clinically from fatty liver, with which it usually coexists, but in more severe cases anorexia, nausea, abdominal pain, and weight loss may develop. Severe alcoholic hepatitis, with or without cirrhosis, is a medical emergency; patients are at risk of ascites, bleeding, and encephalopathy. They may also become infected—urinary tract infection, pneumonia, spontaneous bacterial peritonitis, or septicaemia. Detection of such infection is complicated by the fever and leucocytosis caused by the liver disease itself. Those most severely affected may develop profound cholestasis and hypoglycaemia.

The picture in established *cirrhosis* is variable. In some who have stopped drinking there may be no symptoms and liver function tests may be near normal. More often, patients suffer malaise and will have lost weight and show classical physical signs (Table 1), may be jaundiced, and may bleed from varices. Zieve's syndrome of marked jaundice from a combination of cholestasis and haemolysis with hyperlipidaemia is rare.

History and investigation

Many patients are reluctant to admit their alcoholism, even when liver disease is gross (see Section 14). Liver function tests are often unhelpful in establishing severity, except at the late stage. Early abnormalities may include raised serum γ-glutamyl transferase and macrocytosis. Measurement of blood or urinary ethanol is helpful if high levels are found. There may be a disproportionate elevation of serum aspartate transaminase compared to alanine transaminase.

Table 1 Clinical signs of alcoholism

Undernutrition
Thin arms and legs (reduced muscle mass), frequently with swollen abdomen Red tongue Dry, scaly, cracked skin (zinc and/or essential fatty-acid deficiency)
Endocrine
Gynaecomastia Testicular atrophy Loss of body hair Signs of pseudo-Cushing's (red face, hump, striae)
Face/skin
Parotid enlargement Spider naevi Paper-money skin Easy bruising Dupuytren's contracture
Neuromuscular
Tremor Proximal myopathy Painful peripheral neuropathy Specific neurological syndromes Memory loss and cognitive impairment
Cardiovascular
Hypertension Signs of heart failure (cardiomyopathy) Hyperdynamic circulation (in advanced liver disease)
Bone
Unexplained rib fractures on chest radiographs Spinal osteoporosis (often in men)
General
Signs of personal neglect Smell of drink

Table 2 Alcoholic liver disease discriminant function

Discriminant function (number) = [4.6 × (prothrombin time – control PT) + serum bilirubin (mg%)

Over 32 = poor prognosis

Serum ferritin may be very elevated in active heavy drinkers. Alcoholism is a common cause of combined hyperlipidaemia, indeed serum may be very hyperlipaemic. Liver biopsy allows confirmation of histological severity and exclusion of other pathologies. White-out on colloid liver scan implies severe alcoholic hepatitis.

Prognosis

Prognosis is above all related to whether the patient continues to drink or stops. In patients with fatty change alone the outlook is excellent, provided patients stop or substantially cut down drinking, although some may progress to more advanced liver disease. Mild alcoholic hepatitis has a similar prognosis to fatty change. In severe, acute alcoholic hepatitis, whether or not superimposed upon cirrhosis, there is a 12–50 per cent mortality within 6 months of presentation. Particularly adverse features are raised bilirubin level and abnormal blood clotting. This had led to the use of a discriminant function to help assess prognosis and decide upon treatment (Table 2). In alcoholic cirrhosis overall survival at 5 years is about 50 per cent, among abstainers 70 per cent, and in those who continue to drink 35 per cent. A second important prognostic feature is age at presentation. In a recent UK study, 3-year survival was 77 per cent in patients under the age of 60, and 46 per cent in those presenting over that age. Nutrition (possibly reflecting socio-economic status) also influences survival. Unfortunately, hepatocellular cancer can arise in patients with long-standing, often inactive, alcoholic cirrhosis, particularly men.

Treatment

The best treatment remains total withdrawal of alcohol and subsequent long-term abstinence in all patients with liver disease worse than moderate fatty change alone, in which case, very moderate drinking after a period of abstinence may be an option. Good prognostic features include recognition of the problem by the patient, a supportive family, steady employment, and willingness to accept treatment. No other treatment is required for patients with fatty liver or mild alcoholic hepatitis.

Severe alcoholic hepatitis

Meta-analysis of more than 10 trials of high-dose corticosteroid treatment added to conventional therapy has led to the following recommendations. In patients with discriminant function over 32 (Table 2) but who have no overt sepsis or active bleeding, 40 mg prednisolone for 21 days probably provides a 20 per cent improvement in mortality. Insulin and glucagon, anabolic steroids, colchicine, enteral and parenteral nutrition, and a variety of other so-called 'hepato-protective drugs' have all been used in trials but without real evidence of benefit with respect to mortality.

Cirrhosis

Treatment is directed against its complications, particularly portal hypertension, ascites, spontaneous bacterial peritonitis, and encephalopathy.

Transplantation

The indications for transplantation in alcoholic cirrhosis are similar to those for other endstage liver diseases (see later), with the caveat that even in advanced alcoholic cirrhosis, abstention can lead to enormous clinical improvement and long-term survival. Many transplant units consider patients only after a 6-month period of abstention, both to detect patients in whom transplantation is no longer necessary and to exclude individuals who continue to drink heavily. Estimated 5-year survival following transplantation is now over 70 per cent.

Non-alcoholic steatosis hepatitis

This is increasingly recognized as an important distinct clinical entity, originally described in, usually, very, obese females and in diabetics, or patients with hyperlipidaemia, also in patients following jejunoilial bypass surgery for obesity. This condition is now recognized in individuals of both sexes who are only marginally obese but who may have changed weight recently. Patients often present because of detection of abnormal liver function tests. It is important to make this diagnosis both for prognostic reasons and to clearly state the non-alcoholic nature of this disease in an individual for purposes of employment and insurance.

Pathology

This is identical to alcoholic liver disease, most patients having simple steatosis, others develop an alcoholic hepatitis-like appearance with or without fibrosis, a small proportion (perhaps 5–10 per cent) develop cirrhosis.

Clinical features

Most are asymptomatic but are 'accused' of having alcoholic liver disease. Up to 40 per cent have persistent right upper abdominal pain and may complain of lethargy and malaise. About 5–10 per cent, usually very obese and diabetic, develop cirrhosis with its complications.

Investigations

Patients must have a history of high alcohol consumption exhaustively excluded as a cause for their liver disease. Liver function tests show raised serum transaminases, unlike alcoholic liver disease serum alanine transaminase is raised compared with aspartate transaminase. Serum γ-glutamyl transferase is also raised. Liver ultrasound shows a fatty appearance but cannot reliably distinguish the extent of fibrosis.

Prognosis

This is excellent except in the small proportion of those who develop cirrhosis where complications and clinical course are as for other causes of cirrhosis.

Treatment

No treatment has yet been proven to be effective. Probably slow weight reduction, a reduced fat diet, and a period of abstinence from any alcohol consumption are most effective.

Further reading

Day, C.P. and Bassendine M.F. (1992). Genetic predisposition to alcoholic liver disease. *Gut*, **33**, 1344–7.

Hislop, W.S., *et al.* (1983). Alcoholic liver disease in Scotland and north-eastern England; presenting features in 510 patients. *Quarterly Journal of Medicine*, **206**, 232–3.

Sherlock, S. and Dooley, J. (1997). *Diseases of the liver and biliary system.* Blackwell Science, Oxford.

Chapter 5.36

Cirrhosis, portal hypertension, and ascites

N. McIntyre and A. K. Burroughs

Cirrhosis is a diffuse 'septal' fibrosis of the liver, with regenerative parenchymal nodules and a disturbed intrahepatic circulation; fibrous sheets link portal tracts (portal–portal fibrosis), central zones (central–central), and/or portal tracts and central zones (portal–central). It results from prolonged, widespread, hepatocellular necrosis, which may have many causes, and may be absent or minimal if the causative factor is no longer operative. One classification is based on aetiology (Table 1). The most important causes are chronic infection with the hepatitis viruses B and C, and prolonged alcohol abuse.

The term 'compensated cirrhosis' implies that the patient is without serious complication, while 'decompensated' patients have more severe biochemical or clinical evidence of impaired liver function.

Pathology and pathophysiology

Cirrhotic livers are firm and may be large, of normal size, or small and shrunken. The surface is nodular, but the size of the nodules is very variable. Increased resistance to portal blood flow increases portal venous pressure. Venous collaterals may develop, allowing some blood to pass from the portal to the systemic circulation without traversing the liver. The spleen enlarges due to the high splenic vein pressure.

Histology

'Micronodular' cirrhosis, is usually obvious in a needle-biopsy specimen, as the nodules are uniformly small. In 'macronodular' cirrhosis the nodules are variable in size and may be more than 10 mm in diameter: it may be difficult to diagnose from a needle biopsy specimen (Fig. 1). Cell necrosis, evidence of active regeneration, and cellular infiltration indicate that the aetiological agent is still active. Special stains may demonstrate, for example, infection with hepatitis B and D, excessive iron stores, or the presence of α_1-antitrypsin globules.

Clinical features—symptoms

Cirrhosis can be present without symptoms or signs. Jaundice is usually absent, but indicates decompensation due to continued damage or the use of a drug affecting bilirubin metabolism, the effect of a recent blood transfusion, or another cause of jaundice, such as biliary obstruction. Malaise, easy fatiguability, and tiredness are common. Anorexia when severe is an ominous sign unless caused by a drug or another treatable condition. Weight loss is an unusual presenting feature, but is common in end-stage cirrhosis. Nausea is common but vomiting is unusual unless there is hepatocellular decompensation. Abdominal pain or discomfort is usually felt in the right upper quadrant or over the right lower ribs but may be epigastric. There is

Table 1 Causes of cirrhosis

Alcohol	***Biliary tract disease (prolonged)***
Chronic viral infection—HBV, HBV + HDV, HCV	Extrahepatic biliary obstruction
Drugs and toxins	Intrahepatic biliary obstruction:
Autoimmune chronic liver disease	Primary biliary cirrhosis Primary sclerosing cholangitis
Metabolic disorders	***Venous outflow obstruction***
Haemochromatosis	Veno-occlusive disease
Wilson's disease	Budd–Chiari syndrome
α_1-antitrypsin deficiency	Cardiac failure
Cystic fibrosis	Obesity/diabetes mellitus
Glycogen storage disease	Intestinal bypass for obesity
Galactosaemia	Sarcoidosis
Hereditary fructose intolerance	Syphilis
Hereditary tyrosinaemia	Indian childhood cirrhosis
Ornithine transcarbamylase deficiency	Hereditary haemorrhagic telangiectasia
Byler's disease	Cryptogenic
Abetalipoproteinaemia Porphyria	?Schistosomiasis, malnutrition, mycotoxins

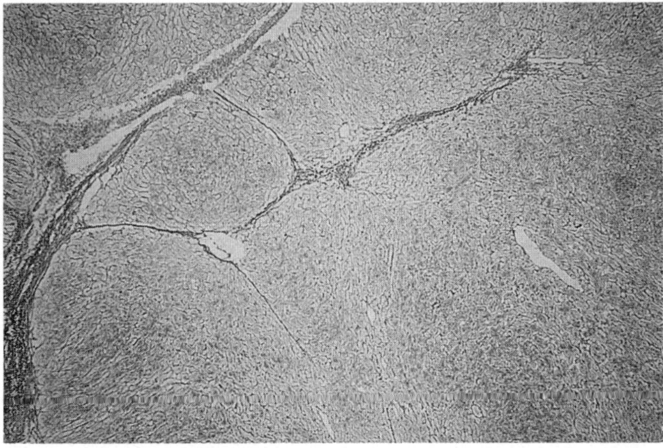

(a)

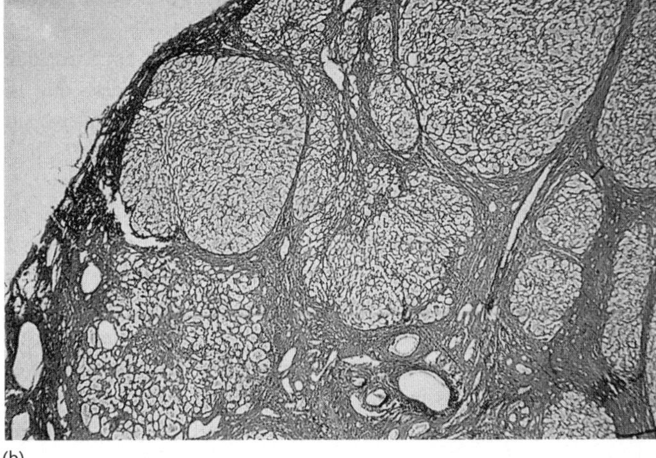

(b)

Fig. 1 (a) Clear-cut micronodular cirrhosis. (b) Fibrous septa suggestive of nodule formation compatible with macronodular cirrhosis.

rarely an obvious cause, unless a tumour has developed, when spread to the liver surface may cause 'pleuritic' pain. Pain or discomfort can also occur with gross splenomegaly or tense ascites. Increased frequency of defaecation, with soft or loose stools occurs particularly in alcoholics, but more severe diarrhoea should suggest another cause. Black stools suggest upper intestinal bleeding. Constipation is unusual but may precipitate encephalopathy in patients with decompensated cirrhosis. Fluid retention causes swelling of the ankles and legs and/or ascites (see below). Dyspnoea may be caused by gross ascites, anascitic hydrothorax, or by associated disorders such as fibrosing alveolitis, pulmonary arteriovenous shunting, and pulmonary hypertension. Pruritus, an important symptom in primary biliary cirrhosis may also occur in other types of cirrhosis, but it is rare in alcoholic liver disease. There may be spontaneous bleeding or easy bruising, related to abnormal clotting or thrombocytopenia or both. Fever is common and may reflect infection but may have no obvious cause. Rigors suggest bacteraemia. Impotence, more common and more severe in alcoholic cirrhosis, is often accompanied by loss of libido. Women often complain of amenorrhoea or oligomenorrhoea and may be sterile. Painful muscle cramps are common and seem unrelated to diuretic therapy or to electrolyte disturbances. They may respond to quinine sulphate. Depression is common. Hepatic encephalopathy is described below.

Physical signs

Most patients with cirrhosis look well until late in the disease, when muscle wasting and loss of adipose tissue may be prominent. A sudden worsening of the patient's condition should suggest an infection (especially bacteraemia or spontaneous bacterial peritonitis) or gastrointestinal bleeding; a more gradual deterioration results from hepatic decompensation or the development of hepatocellular carcinoma.

Overt jaundice suggests hepatic decompensation. Conjunctival pallor may result from recent gastrointestinal bleeding, or from iron-deficiency anaemia due either to chronic blood loss or to inadequate iron supplementation after an earlier variceal haemorrhage. Evidence of 'dehydration' with reduced skin turgor over the sternal manubrium, even when there is ascites and/or dependent oedema is usually a consequence of diuretic therapy. Postural hypotension may result from hypovolaemia.

Cyanosis may result from intrapulmonary shunting. Mild clubbing is common, particularly in primary biliary cirrhosis and when there is associated hypoxia and pulmonary hypertension. Hypertrophic osteoarthropathy may also be present.

Large and numerous spider naevi suggest alcoholic liver disease. Other signs of chronic liver damage include white spots, 'paper money' skin, and erythema of the thenar and hypothenar eminences ('liver palms'). Excessive bruising may be noted when hepatocellular function is poor. Petechial haemorrhages may be found over the lower legs and on the arms or abdomen, suggesting thrombocytopenia due to hypersplenism.

Many cirrhotics, particularly those with primary biliary cirrhosis or haemochromatosis, show widespread melanin pigmentation with local areas of hyperpigmentation, particularly at sites of minor trauma or irritation. Vitiligo occurs with autoimmune chronic liver diseases. Lichen planus, commonly associated with primary biliary cirrhosis, also appears to have a higher prevalence in other types of liver disease.

Gynaecomastia is found in some males. It may result from sex hormone imbalance, or as a side-effect of spironolactone. Testicular atrophy is common, particularly in alcoholic liver disease or haemochromatosis, and is usually accompanied by thinning of body hair and other signs of feminization.

Dupuytren's contracture is more common in alcoholic cirrhotics than in the general population. It is related to alcoholism, not to cirrhosis.

Two signs of particular importance are the flapping tremor of hepatic encephalopathy, and the Kayser–Fleischer ring of Wilson's disease.

Ascites is often associated with peripheral oedema which, when gross, may involve the abdominal wall and genitalia. Abdominal wall venous collaterals are a particularly important sign of cirrhosis and of other types of portal hypertension. Their significance is discussed below.

A firm, cirrhotic liver is usually easy to feel when it is enlarged, but it may be palpable in the epigastrium alone, or below the right lower ribs. Its shape may be markedly deformed and this occasionally causes diagnostic confusion. The spleen is often palpable, and may be very large, but it is not usually palpable in alcoholic cirrhotics. With tense ascites it is sometimes possible to feel an enlarged liver or spleen by 'dipping'.

Auscultation may reveal an arterial bruit over the liver (suggesting a hepatocellular carcinoma or alcoholic hepatitis), a 'venous hum' (in patients with portal hypertension and rapid, turbulent flow in collateral veins), or a 'friction rub' over the liver or spleen the former suggesting tumour invasion of the visceral peritoneum, the latter splenic infarction.

Investigations

Liver function tests

Aspartate aminotransferase (**AST**) and alanine aminotransferase (**ALT**) levels may be normal if the causative agent is no longer active or after effective therapy. In alcoholic cirrhosis (and hepatitis) the AST/ALT ratio is often 2 or greater, due in part to a relative reduction of ALT. Indeed, ALT levels may be normal when there is an obvious elevation of AST. A ratio in excess of 2 is also seen with other types of cirrhosis, as the AST/ALT ratio tends to rise with the transition from chronic hepatitis to cirrhosis.

The serum total bilirubin is often normal, but an increase in bilirubin load, with blood transfusion or an episode of haemolysis, or the use of drugs that impair bilirubin transport, such as oestrogens or androgenic steroids, may cause an increase and result in jaundice. An increase in bilirubin with no obvious cause suggests hepatic decompensation; it is an important prognostic feature in assessment for transplantation.

In most patients the serum alkaline phosphatase is either normal or only modestly elevated, except in biliary cirrhosis when it is usually markedly increased.

A low serum albumin is usually attributed to reduced hepatic albumin synthesis, but the albumin pool may be increased and synthesis normal or even high. Other factors also affect plasma albumin—gastrointestinal or renal loss, increased catabolism, altered vascular permeability or overhydration.

Other tests

Hyponatraemia usually results from excessive administration of water (and a reduced ability to excrete a water load), or with diuretic therapy. Hypernatraemia is rare but can occur with gastrointestinal bleeding (due to an urea diuresis), use of lactulose, or with severe fluid restriction and increased insensible water loss.

Serum potassium concentrations are usually normal. Low levels result from diuretic therapy, a poor diet, vomiting, or diarrhoea. Hyperkalaemia occurs with renal failure, and with the use of potassium-retaining diuretics.

Hypomagnesaemia occurs, particularly in alcoholics and decompensated patients, but is not usually accompanied by clinical evidence of magnesium deficiency. Increased urinary loss of magnesium may result from secondary hyperaldosteronism, or the use of loop diuretics.

In well-compensated cirrhosis the serum urea is usually normal. In decompensated cirrhosis, urea production falls and the serum urea is then low. Mild renal failure can occur without the serum urea rising above the normal range; this can be identified by an increased serum creatinine. Renal failure is common, due to diuretic therapy, hypotension (with bleeding or infection), or the development of the hepatorenal syndrome.

Fasting blood glucose is usually normal, but most cirrhotics are insulin resistant, and have postprandial hyperglycaemia. Overt diabetes mellitus is more common than in the general population.

Lecithin cholesterol acyltransferase (**LCAT**), an enzyme secreted by the liver, catalyses formation of cholesteryl ester in plasma. With end-stage disease, plasma LCAT activity falls; there is a decrease in cholesteryl ester and total cholesterol, while free cholesterol is normal or increased. In primary biliary cirrhosis the total cholesterol may reach very high levels.

Mild anaemia is common, due in part to hypersplenism. More severe anaemia results from overt bleeding or from iron deficiency. Target cells are usually visible on blood films, and in rare cases acanthocytes are found in association with features of haemolytic anaemia.

The mean corpuscular volume (**MCV**) may be high with liver disease, and very high in alcoholics, but may be normal if there is a concomitant iron deficiency. Measurement of serum iron and total iron-binding capacity may identify haemochromatosis. Serum ferritin is of less value for identifying iron deficiency as it may be normal or high due to hepatocellular damage.

The white-cell count tends to fall in patients with cirrhosis, due to hypersplenism. The platelet count is usually low, also due to hypersplenism. Changes in coagulation factors are considered in Chapter 3.33.

Diagnosis and differential diagnosis

When a patient presents with clinical signs of liver disease the first step is to establish whether it is acute or chronic. Some physical signs are strongly suggestive of cirrhosis (e.g. spider naevi, liver palms, gynaecomastia, ascites and oedema, and abdominal venous collaterals). Diseases other than cirrhosis presenting with a palpable liver and/or spleen are listed in Table 2. Disorders associated with portal hypertension and/or ascites are considered in the relevant sections below.

A definitive diagnosis requires a liver biopsy. When the prothrombin time is prolonged or the platelet count low liver biopsy is rarely justified in high-risk patients simply to establish the presence of cirrhosis. A diagnosis may still be made on clinical grounds, with strong confirmatory evidence from ultrasonography, computed tomography (CT) scanning, or peritoneoscopy. Oesophageal varices on endoscopy suggest cirrhosis, but there may be another cause of portal hypertension (see below).

It may be important to distinguish between chronic hepatitis and cirrhosis, particularly if the underlying cause is treatable.

Identifying the cause of cirrhosis

Wilson's disease, haemochromatosis, and autoimmune disease must always be considered. The cause is sometimes obvious on clinical grounds or it may be identified from biochemical and serological investigations (see Table 3). Liver biopsy can establish some causes of cirrhosis with a high degree of probability if specific stains are used, or if chemical measurements are made on the tissues (Table 4).

Searching for complications

Portal hypertension and ascites are considered below.

Hepatic encephalopathy is considered in Chapter 5.37. It is not the only cause of cerebral disturbance in cirrhotics; others include drugs, alcohol, hypotension, and renal failure. Alcoholics may develop Wernicke–Korsakoff syndrome due to thiamine deficiency, alcohol withdrawal problems, or hypoglycaemia. It is particularly important to detect a subdural haematoma, which may result from unrecognized trauma.

Table 2 Other conditions often presenting with a palpable liver and/or spleen

Some other forms of congestive splenomegaly
Primary biliary cirrhosis
Sclerosing cholangitis
Biliary atresia
Chronic active hepatitis
Graft-versus-host disease
Granulomatous hepatitis
Storage disorders
Cystic fibrosis?
Schistosomiasis
Nodular regenerative hyperplasia
Gaucher's disease
Niemann–Pick disease
Hurler's syndrome
Lymphomas and leukaemias
Extramedullary haemopoiesis
Histiocytosis X
Leishmaniasis
Amyloid
*Other conditions with a palpable spleen alone**
Congestive splenomegaly
Portal venous obstruction/thrombosis
Splenic tumours and cysts
Infections (infectious mononucleosis, septicaemias, bacterial endocarditis, tuberculosis, malaria, trypanosomiasis, AIDS, congenital syphilis, splenic abscess)
Rheumatoid arthritis (Felty's syndrome)
Systemic lupus erythematosus
Immune haemolytic anaemias, thrombocytopenias, and neutropenias

*See also Section 3.

Table 3 'Routine' investigations for identifying the cause of cirrhosis

Investigation	Cause
HBV, HDV and HCV markers	Chronic viral infection
ANA (to ds-DNA); SMA (anti-actin); LKM-1 Ab; Ab to SLA	Autoimmune chronic hepatitis (see Chapter 5.32)
Antimitochondrial antibodies (M2, M4, M8, M9) (ELISA techniques for purified AMA)	Primary biliary cirrhosis (see Chapter 5.33)
Serum copper and caeruloplasmin, urinary copper, Kayser-Fleischer rings	Wilson's disease
Serum iron and iron-binding capacity, serum ferritin	Haemochromatosis
Serum α_1-antitrypsin,	α_1-chymotrypsin
α_1-Antichymotrypsin and	α_1-chymotrypsin deficiency
Detailed drug history	Drug-induced cirrhosis (see Chapter 5.41)

AMA, antimitochondrial antibody; ANA, antinuclear antibody; ELISA, enzyme-linked immunosolvent assay; SLA, soluble liver antigen; SMA, smooth muscle antibody.

Table 4 Special tests that may be made on liver tissue in investigation of cirrhosis

Special stains
Perl's stain for iron
DPAS (periodic acid–Schiff stain after diastase digestion) for α_1-antitrypsin globules
PAS (without diastase digestion) for glycogen
Biochemical measurements
Copper (Wilson's disease, Indian childhood cirrhosis)
Iron (haemochromatosis)
Glycogen
Fructose 1-phosphate aldolase (hereditary fructose intolerance)

Hepatocellular carcinoma is one of the most serious complications of long-standing cirrhosis. The best treatment is resection if the tumour can be detected early. For this reason, patients with cirrhosis should be screened at regular intervals (4–6-monthly) with measurement of serum α-fetoprotein and the use of ultrasound. CT scanning is useful in some cases. Up to 15 per cent of cirrhotics without a carcinoma have an increased concentration of serum α-fetoprotein, but the elevation is generally minor compared with that seen with hepatocellular carcinoma.

Infections or *gastrointestinal bleeding* are important causes of acute deterioration. Both conditions may cause tachycardia, hypotension, tachypnoea, mild fever and/or confusion, and impaired renal function with oliguria. With bacterial infections the white cell count may be lower than expected, due to hypersplenism. Fresh petechiae suggest bacteraemia; there may be evidence of intravascular coagulation. Volume expansion may be necessary to maintain the blood pressure. Cultures should be taken of blood, urine, ascites, intravenous drip lines and insertion sites. As soon as bacterial infection is suspected a third-generation cephalosporin should be started. Deterioration may also result from infections such as spontaneous bacterial peritonitis, or urinary or chest infections.

Management

Some causes of cirrhosis have specific treatments, e.g. immunosuppression for autoimmune chronic hepatitis, penicillamine for Wilson's disease, venesection for haemochromatosis, and abstention from alcohol for alcoholic cirrhosis.

Patient education Patients, or their relatives, should be advised to seek help quickly for deepening jaundice, fever/rigors, haematemesis and/or melaena, ankle or abdominal swelling, or signs of confusion.

Diet Most cirrhotics should eat a normal mixed diet. Fat restriction is necessary only for troublesome steatorrhoea. The dietary management of ascites and oedema is considered below, and the management of hepatic encephalopathy in Chapter 5.37. Although short-term protein restriction may be needed for acute attacks of encephalopathy, long-term restriction should be avoided in order to avoid protein depletion.

Patients with alcoholic hepatitis and/or cirrhosis should abstain from alcohol, but there is no evidence that abstention significantly affects outcome in non-alcoholic cirrhotics who drink in moderation.

Foreign travel Cirrhotics can take standard prophylaxis for malaria, and can be actively immunized against bacterial and viral diseases, but may have a reduced immune response. Non-immune cirrhotics should probably be vaccinated against hepatitis A and B, particularly if visiting endemic areas.

Drugs and liver disease Patients with cirrhosis often need to take drugs many of which are metabolized, and/or excreted by the liver. Drugs that are removed in relatively large amounts during their first passage through the liver (e.g. propranolol, labetalol, pentazocine, morphine, lidocaine, verapamil, nifedipine, and ergotamine tartrate), when given to cirrhotics with portal-systemic shunting may cause toxicity unless given in reduced dosage. Ergot derivatives are particularly dangerous and may cause peripheral gangrene. Drugs that are metabolized by the liver tend to accumulate when liver function is impaired, unless repeated doses are given at less frequent intervals. Many patients are unduly sensitive to pethidine and benzodiazepines as well as morphine.

For simple analgesia, paracetamol is the drug of choice but no more than 3 g/day (six tablets) should be given long-term. Codeine is also useful, as it has a smaller first-pass uptake than most other opiates, but it can accumulate and cause cerebral depression. Aspirin and other non-steroidal anti-inflammatory drugs should be avoided. D-propoxyphene is of doubtful efficacy and may be hepatotoxic.

For hypertension, β-blockers are the drugs of choice, having an additional, beneficial effect on portal hypertension. Calcium antagonists tend to show a marked first-pass effect, and small doses should be used initially. Thiazide diuretics should be avoided: they enhance kaliuresis, may precipitate encephalopathy, and impair glucose tolerance.

Subclinical vitamin deficiencies are relatively common. Routine prescription of water-soluble vitamins is sensible in normal doses, but large doses of nicotinamide or nicotinic acid should be avoided.

Oral contraceptive pills are relatively contraindicated. Oestrogens reduce the excretory capacity for bilirubin. Long-term use of the pill is associated with an increased (although small) risk of hepatic-vein thrombosis, gallstones, hepatic adenoma, and hepatocellular carcinoma. A low-dose oestrogen or a progestogen-only preparation can be tried after the risks are explained. Serum bilirubin and aminotransferases should be monitored regularly (weekly for 1 month, monthly for the next 3 months, and every 3 months thereafter): if the test results deteriorate the drug should be stopped. Similarly, hormone replacement therapy can be given, with careful monitoring.

Transplantation The good results now being achieved with liver transplantation have changed the approach to the management of end-stage liver disease (see Chapter 5.39).

Portal hypertension

Anatomy and physiology of the portal circulation

The portal circulation is represented in Fig. 2, which shows the main sites of obstruction. In health portal vein flow is about 900–1200 ml/min, and portal venous pressure about 5–10 mmHg, only a little higher than that in the inferior vena cava. Vascular resistance to portal flow is thus very low.

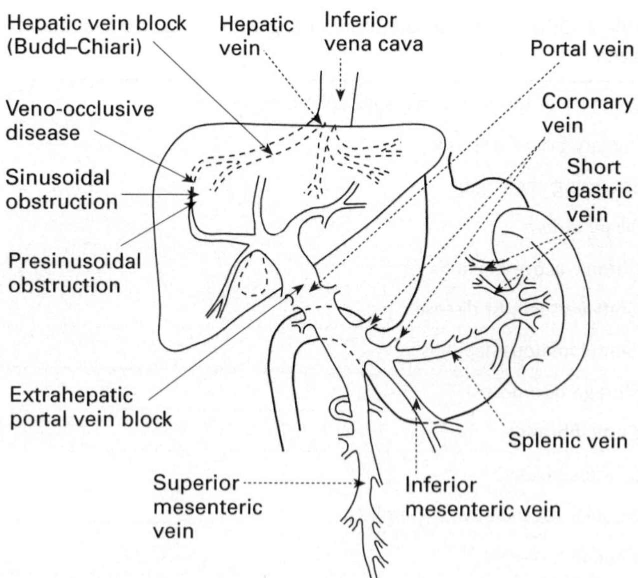

Fig. 2 A diagrammatic representation of the main tributaries of the portal vein, and the sites of obstruction to portal flow causing portal hypertension.

Definition and causes of portal hypertension

Portal hypertension may be defined as an increase in resting portal venous pressure above 12 mmHg, but it may rise as high as 50 mmHg. There are many causes (Table 5). It can be classified as 'presinusoidal', 'sinusoidal', or 'postsinusoidal'. Measurements of hepatic venous pressure are useful for determining the site of resistance; the hepatic venous-pressure gradient (**HPVG**) is the difference between the wedged hepatic venous pressure (**WHVP**) and the free hepatic venous pressure. With presinusoidal portal hypertension, due to a blocked portal vein or narrowing of the smaller intrahepatic portal vein branches, the WHVP is normal. Portal hypertension in cirrhosis is considered to be 'sinusoidal' (with a high WHVP and HPVG), but the exact site of the increased resistance is not clear.

Consequences

An elevated portal venous pressure distends the veins proximal to the block and the spleen enlarges. Capillary pressure rises in organs drained by the obstructed vein; fluid exudation and lymph flow both increase. Small anastomoses connecting the portal and systemic circulations may enlarge and allow portal blood to pass directly into the systemic circulation. The extent of collateral flow is variable, as are the routes taken by the diverted blood.

There are three main types of anastomosis:

1. Veins at the oesophagogastric junction shunt blood from the left gastric and short gastric veins into the inferior oesophageal plexus and on to the superior vena cava via the azygous system. 'Varices' are dilated submucosal veins projecting into the lumen of the oesophagus and stomach. They tend to develop in cirrhosis when the HPVG rises above 12 mmHg, and often cause gastrointestinal bleeding. Anastomoses at the anorectal junction rarely cause bleeding.
2. Venous channels from retroperitoneal viscera may communicate directly with systemic veins on the posterior abdominal wall.

Table 5 Causes of portal hypertension

Extrahepatic obstruction of portal vein and its tributaries
Portal-vein thrombosis (idiopathic, umbilical and portal sepsis, malignancy, hypercoagulable states, pancreatitis)
Splenic-vein thrombosis
Hepatic venous outflow 'obstruction'
Suprahepatic
Budd–Chiari syndrome (see Table 8)
Constrictive pericarditis
Right heart failure
Smaller hepatic veins and venules
Veno-occlusive disease (due to ingestion of pyrrolizidine alkaloids; antileukaemic drugs, radiation)
Sclerosing hyaline necrosis
Hepatic causes (in some cases there may be presinusoidal and sinusoidal resistance to flow)
Presinusoidal
Schistosomiasis
Idiopathic portal hypertension
Primary biliary cirrhosis (early stage)
Sarcoid
Myeloproliferative diseases
Arsenic, vinyl chloride
Fibropolycystic disease (including congenital hepatic fibrosis)
Sinusoidal
Cirrhosis
Chronic active hepatitis
Alcoholic hepatitis and fatty liver
Nodular regenerative hyperplasia
Partial nodular transformation
Increased hepatic blood flow (rare causes)
Tropical splenomegaly syndrome
Haematological and other conditions with massive splenomegaly
Hepatoportal arteriovenous fistula

3. The obliterated umbilical vein and paraumbilical veins may open up, allowing blood to pass from the left branch of the portal vein to the umbilicus and thence into abdominal-wall veins. Anterior abdominal-wall collaterals also occur where adhesions exist between abdominal viscera and the parietal peritoneum, or at ileostomy or colostomy sites. Localized varices may be related to previous surgical operations.

Thrombosis of individual tributaries of the portal vein causes local venous hypertension; with splenic-vein block, oesophageal and gastric varices may result. When hepatic veins are occluded (Budd–Chiari syndrome), collaterals open up within the liver; blood tends to be diverted through the caudate lobe whose short hepatic veins drain directly into the inferior vena cava.

Clinical signs

The spleen is usually palpable, and may be very large in young patients, in patients with extrahepatic portal block, and in those with small, shrunken livers. In alcoholic cirrhosis the spleen is less often palpable.

Prominent abdominal-wall veins are often found, and are easier to see if the skin of the abdominal wall is stretched. Veins radiating away from the umbilicus indicate that the block is distal to the main portal vein branches (usually due to cirrhosis).

With extrahepatic portal-vein block there are no abdominal-wall collaterals (as the pressure in the left branch of the portal vein is not elevated). However, if abdominal surgery has been performed, adhesions between viscera and the abdominal wall may result in the development of surface collaterals, radiating from the scar. These can result from intrahepatic portal hypertension or from portal-vein block.

When hepatomegaly and ascites are present with signs of inferior vena caval obstruction they suggest coexisting obstruction of hepatic veins (the Budd–Chiari syndrome), which may also cause narrowing of the cava due to pressure from an enlarged caudate lobe. The sudden development of 'umbilical' collaterals in a patient with cirrhosis suggests an acute hepatic-vein block.

A venous hum, loudest during inspiration, is sometimes heard over large upper abdominal collaterals ('Cruveilhier–Baumgarten syndrome') and there may be an accompanying thrill.

Investigation

The finding of oesophageal and gastric varices on endoscopy confirms the diagnosis of portal hypertension. In a patient without varices, portal hypertension can be confirmed by wedged hepatic venous pressure (see above). Direct measurement of portal pressure, by splenic puncture or transhepatic cannulation of a portal vein branch is rarely needed. Intravariceal pressure, which is slightly lower than portal, can be measured endoscopically.

Liver biopsy may reveal cirrhosis (and sometimes its cause), hepatic outflow obstruction, schistosomiasis, or congenital hepatic fibrosis. 'Normal' histology may be found with idiopathic portal hypertension, nodular regenerative hyperplasia, partial nodular transformation, or with macronodular cirrhosis, but the most likely cause of portal hypertension with a normal biopsy is extrahepatic portal venous obstruction.

The site of the block can be demonstrated by examining the venous phase of a coeliac or superior mesenteric arteriogram, by splenic portography following injection of dye into the splenic pulp, or by retrograde portography via a hepatic vein.

Ultrasound and CT may show changes of portal hypertension and give clues to its cause. Doppler ultrasound can show the direction of flow in individual vessels, and allows quantitation in major vessels. Magnetic resonance imaging is also valuable for investigating the hepatic vasculature.

Hepatic venography is helpful when hepatic-vein block or idopathic portal hypertension are suspected.

Management

Gastrointestinal bleeding

The most common source is from oesophageal varices. Other sources are gastric varices, portal hypertensive gastropathy, sclerotherapy ulcers, peptic ulcers, and oesophageal or gastric erosions which are common in alcoholics. Bleeding from rectal varices is rare.

Table 6 Pugh-Child's grading of the severity of liver disease

Clinical and biochemical measurements	Points scored for increasing abnormality		
	1	2	3
Encephalopathy*	None	1 and 2	3 and 4
Ascites	Absent	Slight	Moderate
Bilirubin (μmol/l)	34	34–51	>51
Albumin (g/l)	>35	28–35	<28
Prothrombin (s prolonged)	1–4	4–6	>6
For primary biliary cirrhosis bilirubin (μmol/l)	<68	68–170	>170

*According to grading of Trey *et al.* (1966). *New England Journal of Medicine*, **274**, 473.

Treatment of acute variceal haemorrhage

Acute variceal haemorrhage is often severe and there may be repeated bleeding over days or weeks. Initially, the severity of the bleeding, and the degree of hepatic dysfunction (Table 6), should be assessed. The average mortality with variceal bleeding is less than 10 per cent in grade A patients, about 25 per cent in grade B, and 50 per cent or more in grade C.

At least one large-bore venous cannula must be inserted, together with a central venous line. Colloid may be needed while waiting for cross-matched whole blood. After restoring the systolic pressure to 80–90 mmHg, packed cells should be given to maintain the haemoglobin at 10 g/dl and the urine output at 40 ml/h or more. Fresh frozen plasma is only needed to correct the effect of a large transfusion of stored blood. Platelet transfusions have only a transient effect, but are indicated when there is massive transfusion or a profound basal thrombocytopenia. Vitamin K (10 mg, IV) should be given.

The major complications of variceal bleeding are: pneumonia due to aspiration, hepatic encephalopathy, infection (septicaemia or peritonitis), water and electrolyte imbalance, and malnutrition. Prophylaxis with third-generation cephalosporins given intravenously reduces the risk of infection. There may be need for enteral or parenteral feeding.

Specific therapy

Vasoactive drugs to promote splanchnic arteriolar constriction The following regimens are effective: (a) *vasopressin* (0.20–0.40 units/min for 24–48 h) with nitroglycerin (by infusion or patch); the systolic pressure should be maintained at 100 mmHg or more; (b) *glypressin* (2 mg every 6 h for 24–48 h); (c) *somatostatin* (250 μg/h for 2–5 days); *octreotide* (50 μg/h for 2–5 days). Somatostatin or octreotide have fewer side-effects, can be given for longer; and may reduce early rebleeding.

Balloon tamponade The most frequently used tube has two balloons: the oesophageal balloon compresses the oesophageal varices; the gastric one prevents laryngeal obstruction due to upward movement of the oesophageal balloon, and may occlude some gastric varices and control bleeding from oesophageal varices. Before insertion the patient should be head down in the left lateral decubitus position. There should be suction facilities to cope with a massive haematemesis. If the patient is uncooperative or comatose, tracheal intubation is necessary. External traction is not necessary. Bleeding is controlled in at least 90 per cent of cases. Tamponade should not be maintained for more than 12 h.

Endoscopic therapy Endoscopic sclerotherapy is the mainstay of acute management. The sclerosant can be injected into the varix, or alongside it. Tissue adhesive (bucrylate) or fibrin may be useful for gastric varices. For oesophageal variceal bleeding a single session of sclerotherapy is effective in over 65 per cent of cases; the success rate is at least 85 per cent with two sessions. No more than two sclerotherapy sessions should be used in a 5-day period; this minimizes oesophageal complications, and allows endoscopic banding ligation or a later surgical transection to be done. Complications such as mediastinitis, deep oesophageal ulceration and stenosis, occur in less than 2 per cent of cases in experienced hands. Endoscopic banding ligation of oesophageal varices has fewer complications than sclerotherapy in the long term but has no advantage in the emergency situation.

Portal-systemic shunting Emergency portal-systemic shunting has a high mortality and is now rarely done. Transjugular intrahepatic stenting (**TIPS**) achieves shunting without surgery. Preliminary data suggest that it is very effective for control of bleeding, but may cause encephalopathy if the liver disease is decompensated. It has a high rate of thrombosis within 12 months.

Oesophageal staple transection This is as effective as emergency sclerotherapy with no difference in mortality, but is now rarely used as bleeding can be controlled with TIPS.

Prevention of variceal rebleeding

Cirrhotic patients who survive their first variceal bleed have a 70 per cent or more chance of rebleeding. Rebleeding is most frequent in the first 6 weeks. Surgery, TIPS, endoscopic therapy, and β-blockers all reduce the frequency of rebleeding but have variable effects on mortality. Portal-systemic shunts reduce risk of rebleeding to 10 per cent or less but do not prolong survival. They all increase the risk of encephalopathy least with distal spleno-renal shunts. TIPS has an average rebleed rate of 30 per cent over time, but this depends on how frequently the TIPS is monitored for blockage, as this is the cause of the rebleeding. Repeated sclerotherapy drops the rebleeding rate to about 50 per cent and reduces mortality. Banding ligation of varices results in less rebleeding and causes fewer complications than sclerotherapy. Meta-analysis shows a reduction in rebleeding with β-blockers, to about 50 per cent, and suggests a lower mortality compared with no treatment. The portal hypotensive effect of β-blockers may be enhanced by adding isosorbide mononitrate, which lowers intrahepatic resistance. No advantage accrues by combining β-blockers with sclerotherapy.

Primary prevention of gastrointestinal bleeding

Surgical shunts or sclerotherapy have shown no overall benefit, and mortality was increased in several studies. However, primary prevention studies of β-blocker therapy have shown a reduction in bleeding from varices and portal hypertensive gastropathy, and have suggested a decrease in mortality.

Ascites

Depending on the cause, ascites may appear gradually or accumulate rapidly. When it is a presenting feature in cirrhosis, particularly in young patients, Wilson's disease should be suspected. Moderate ascites may cause no symptoms. Larger amounts may cause abdominal discomfort. Hernias may appear or enlarge. Gross ascites may cause

Table 7 Causes of ascites

Venous hypertension	*Infections*

• Cirrhosis
• Congestive heart failure
• Constrictive pericarditis
• Hepatic venous outflow'obstruction'
(a) Hepatic-vein block (Budd–Chiari syndrome)
(b) Veno-occlusive disease
• Portal-vein block (acute thrombosis)
	• Tuberculous peritonitis
	• Fungal (candida, cryptococcus)
	• Parasitic (strongyloides, entamoeba)
	Miscellaneous
	• Chylous ascites
	• Bile ascites
	• Pancreatic ascites
	• Urinary ascites
	• Ovarian disease
	  • Meig's syndrome
	  • Struma ovarii

Hypoalbuminaemia (may be contributory in above causes, especially cirrhosis) • Nephrotic syndrome • Malnutrition and protein-losing enteropathy *Malignant disease* • Secondary carcinomatosis • Lymphomas and leukaemias • Primary mesothelioma	• Ovarian overstimulation syndrome • Myxoedema • Pseudomyxoma peritonei • Eosinophilic gastroenteritis • Whipple's disease • Sarcoidosis • Starch peritonitis • Systemic lupus erythematosus

diaphragmatic elevation and breathlessness, particularly when there is an associated pleural effusion.

Physical signs

The important physical signs are: bulging of the flanks; dullness to percussion in the flanks (while the umbilical region may be hyper-resonant); shifting dullness; and a fluid thrill. None of these signs is reliable in doubtful cases, when paracentesis, ultrasound, or CT scanning may confirm the diagnosis.

Dependent scrotal or abdominal-wall oedema may be present even when excessive diuretic therapy has reduced intravascular volume (with loss of skin turgor over the upper sternum and evidence of pre-renal failure from an inappropriate rise in blood urea in relation to creatinine concentration).

Ascites is not the only cause of marked abdominal swelling. Massive ovarian or hydatid cysts, and occasionally pregnancy with hydramnios can be confusing as they may be associated with a fluid thrill.

Causes of ascites

The causes are presented in Table 7. Constrictive pericarditis (with ascites, hepatosplenomegaly, and little or no peripheral oedema) is often mistaken for cirrhosis, as is the Budd–Chiari syndrome. Most of the other diseases can be diagnosed if their presence is suspected, often by examination of the peritoneal fluid (see below) or by percutaneous peritoneal biopsy.

Examination of the ascitic fluid

Diagnostic paracentesis is done by aspirating through a small needle inserted in the flank. In ascites due to portal hypertension or hypoalbuminaemia the fluid is clear and straw coloured. Turbid ascites may indicate infection; chylous or pseudochylous ascites is a milky colour. Blood-stained ascites is usually due to malignancy but may occur with tuberculosis, pancreatitis, hepatic-vein thrombosis, recent abdominal punctures, or with a 'bloody tap'.

Low-protein ascites (<25 g/l) is usual in portal hypertension or hypoalbuminaemia. A higher-protein ascites is usually found with malignancy, tuberculosis, pancreatitis, or myxoedema. A high ascitic-fluid amylase suggests pancreatic ascites; a low glucose (relative to blood) is found in malignant ascites. Cytological examination may reveal malignant cells, and a high concentration of carcinoembryonic antigen is of diagnostic value even in the absence of malignant cells. The triglyceride content should be measured when the ascites is milky. It is low in pseudochylous ascites, but a high level indicates true chylous ascites, usually due to malignant or inflammatory lymphatic obstruction, or to trauma, but also common in the ascites of nephrotic syndrome. Chylous ascites in cirrhosis may be due to rupture of overloaded lymphatics.

Complications of ascites

Spontaneous leakage from a large umbilical hernia requires surgical repair. Some patients develop a pleural effusion; usually right-sided. It results from passage of fluid through small holes in the diaphragm.

Spontaneous bacterial infection of ascitic fluid is usually due to a single enteric organism, occurs in 10–15 per cent of patients with ascites, and is sometimes associated with bacteraemia. Abdominal pain and tenderness may occur but cases often present with general malaise or fever, hypotension, or hepatic encephalopathy. Certain diagnosis requires bacterial culture of ascitic fluid. Culture-negative ascites is common, but a white-cell count of ascitic fluid in excess of 500/mm^3, or a neutrophil count over 250 mm^3 strongly suggests infection which should be treated immediately by a third-generation cephalosporin given over 5 days. Prophylaxis with a daily quinolone antibiotic should be used to prevent recurrence

Pathogenesis of ascites in liver disease

Renal salt and water retention, hypoalbuminaemia, portal hypertension, and increased hepatic lymph production must all contribute, but the precise reasons for renal sodium retention, secondary hyperaldosteronism, increased plasma vasopressin and sympathetic activation are not clear. The concept of lack of 'effective' plasma volume with peripheral arteriolar vasodilatation is now widely favoured.

Management

Most patients with ascites have avid urinary sodium retention (<10 mmol/day). Some have a diuresis with bed-rest and/or moderate dietary sodium restriction. If renal function is good, there is usually a good response to diuretics. Patients are then comfortable on a sodium intake of about 60 mmol/day. A strict low-salt diet is unpalatable. Medicines rich in sodium and potassium should be avoided. In renal impairment the response to sodium restriction and diuretics is poor; hyponatraemia may develop, which requires water restriction to about 1 litre/day. The prognosis is then poor.

Diuretic therapy

Spironolactone is the drug of choice, at an initial dose of 100 mg daily; increased if necessary by 100–200 mg every third day, up to a dose of 800 mg/day. Hyperkalaemia can occur and potassium supplements should be avoided, unless obvious potassium depletion is present. Some men develop reversible gynaecomastia, when triamterene (100–500 mg/day) or amiloride (10–60 mg/day) can be tried. If no diuresis results with spironolactone, frusemide should be added, starting with 40 mg on alternate days. Hypokalaemia may occur despite concurrent use of a potassium-sparing drug, and supplements may then be necessary. Hyponatraemia may develop or worsen and metabolic alkalosis may occur.

The diuretic response should be limited to salt loss of 50–100 mmol/day more than intake; or to a weight loss of about 0.5–1.00 kg/day. Rapid fluid loss may result in deterioration in renal function. Hepatic encephalopathy is often precipitated by diuretics.

If diuresis does not result from combined diuretic therapy, paracentesis is standard therapy for tense or refractory ascites, and when electrolyte changes or hypovolaemia limit the use of diuretics. Total paracentesis can be carried out; 6–8 g of albumin or colloid equivalent should be infused for every litre of ascitic fluid removed to prevent renal failure.

Ascitic fluid can be concentrated and reinfused, in order to conserve plasma proteins and intravascular volume. Longer-term, a shunt can be inserted between the peritoneum and a jugular vein. Both methods have good effects in some patients, but there is a high morbidity and mortality due to infection, consumption coagulopathy, pulmonary oedema, and variceal bleeding. In some patients TIPS results in control of ascites, but patient selection is difficult. It is very effective for cirrhotic hyavothorax.

Treatment of other forms of ascites

Surgery is required for constrictive pericarditis, ovarian tumours, and biliary and urinary ascites. Antimicrobials are needed for infective causes and thyroxine for myxoedema. Medium chain triglyceride substituted for long chain reduce the triglyceride concentration in chylous ascites but does little for fluid accumulation and surgery for obstructed lymphatics is rarely possible. Malignant ascites may be improved by intraperitoneal injection of cytotoxic drugs, colloidal radioactive gold, or phosphate. Immunotherapy with intraperitoneal 0K-432 (derived from *Streptococcus pyogenes*) is helpful in the short term in 60 per cent of patients. Otherwise, treatment is by paracentesis or creation of a peritoneo-venous shunt. Ascites of any cause may respond, at least partially to diuretics.

Budd–Chiari syndrome (hepatic vein obstruction) and veno-occlusive disease

Budd–Chiari syndrome results from obstruction of the major hepatic veins, usually from thrombosis. A thrombogenic disorder, including paroxysmal nocturnal haemoglobinuria, is responsible in about 75 per cent of cases. These and other causes are listed in Table 8.

There is an associated thrombosis in the inferior vena cava in up to 20 per cent of cases, and in the portal vein in about 10 per cent.

Hepatic congestion is worst around the hepatic vein radicles and causes necrosis. Acute portal hypertension may develop if the process is widespread. If congestion is unrelieved fibrosis results, leading to chronic portal hypertension and eventually cirrhosis. The thrombosis is often asynchronous, with late changes in some areas, and recent changes in others. In many cases the caudate lobe enlarges and obstructs the inferior vena cava, making it difficult to perform a side-to-side portacaval shunt.

Table 8 Causes and associations of Budd–Chiari syndrome and veno-occlusive disease

Budd–Chiari syndrome
Haematological disorders—polycythaemia rubra vera, other myeloproliferative disorders, paroxysmal nocturnal haemoglobinuria, sickle cell anaemia, prothrombotic disorders, antithrombin III deficiency, protein C, protein S, activated protein C deficiency (Factor V Leiden) antiphospholipid antibody
Tumours—hepatocellular carcinoma, renal-cell carcinoma, adrenal carcinoma, leiomysarcoma of inferior vena cava or right atrium, carcinoma of stomach or pancreas
Drugs—oral contraceptives, antitumour drugs (doxorubicin, vincristine, vinblastine, etc.)
Pregnancy and post-partum period
Infections—amoebic abscess, aspergillosis, other fungal infections, hydatid cysts, schistosomiasis, syphilis
Membranous webs (common in the Far East)
Trauma
Miscellaneous—inflammatory bowel disease, protein-losing enteropathy, nephrotic syndrome, sarcoidosis, mixed connective tissue disease, nodular regenerative hyperplasia, Behçet's syndrome
Veno-occlusive disease
Pyrrolizidine alkaloids (plants of Crotalaria, Senecio, and Heliotropium families)
Irradiation
Antitumour and immunosuppressive drugs (cytarabine, carmustine, mitomycin, azathioprine).
Graft-versus-host disease following bone marrow transplantation, following liver transplantation

The speed and extent of hepatic-vein thrombosis determine the presentation and prognosis. A few patients present with fulminant liver failure, and high aminotransferase levels; without intervention death usually occurs within 2 weeks. About 25 per cent of cases evolve over a month or so, with rapid onset of ascites, abdominal pain (and jaundice in about half). The most common presentation is with progressive ascites over weeks or months, and tender hepatomegaly in the later stages. Dependent oedema is due to caval compression or thrombosis. Jaundice is unusual, and there may be little disturbance of liver function tests. Variceal bleeding can occur across the spectrum of the outflow block syndrome, and the emergency treatment is similar to that for cirrhotics.

Ultrasound usually confirms hepatic vein thrombosis. The hepatic veins and inferior vena cava should be examined by venography, and the portal vein by superior mesenteric angiography. These investigations help to plan surgery. A liver biopsy, if necessary by the transjugular route, evaluates fibrosis and necrosis, and to help to estimate reversibility of liver injury.

If there are no contraindications anticoagulants should be given. Ascites is treated in standard fashion, but is often refractory. Balloon dilatation may relieve obstruction if a venous web has been detected.

Patients with a patent portal vein, and without significant fibrosis or marked obstruction of the cava, should have a portacaval shunt. In patients operated on within 16 weeks of onset of symptoms the results are good, with a long-term survival of about 85 per cent. After a shunt procedure anticoagulation should be continued.

When the inferior vena cava is blocked a mesoatrial shunt or TIPS can be used; if it is patent, but severely compressed, a stent can be placed across its intrahepatic portion.

Liver transplantation should be considered for all patients with fulminant presentation or with severe forms of the Budd–Chiari syndrome, particularly if there is fibrosis and/or marked necrosis on biopsy, and if hepatocellular failure persists because a shunt has thrombosed.

Veno-occlusive disease

This term describes non-thrombotic luminal narrowing of small intrahepatic tributaries of the hepatic veins. The clinical picture mimics the Budd–Chiari syndrome, with acute, subacute, and chronic presentations. Causes are ingestion (in 'bush teas') of pyrrolidizine alkaloids found in plants of the Crotalaria, Senecio, and Heliotropium families, but there are other causes (Table 8). Some acute cases improve spontaneously, but many are progressive and fatal. Some improve with antifibrinolytic therapy. Liver transplantation has been used successfully.

Further reading

Martin, P-Y., Gines, P., and Schrier, R.W. (1998). Mechanisms of disease. Nitric oxide as a mediator of hemodynamic abnormalities and sodium retention in cirrhosis. *New England Journal of Medicine*, **339**, 533–41.

Mitchell, M.C., *et al.* (1982). Budd-Chiari syndrome: etiology, diagnosis and management. *Medicine*, **61**, 199–218.

Pagliaro, L., *et al.* (1992) Prevention of first bleeding in cirrhosis: a meta-analysis of non-surgical randomised clinical trials. *Annals of Internal Medicine*, **117**, 59–70.

Tito, L., *et al.* (1990). Total paracentesis associated with intravenous albumin management of patients with cirrhosis and ascites. *Gastroenterology*, **98**, 146–51.

Sherlock, S. and Dooley, J. (1997). *Diseases of the liver and biliary system*. Blackwell Science, Oxford.

Stanley, A.J., *et al.* (1998). Haemodynamic parameters predicting haemorrhage and survival in alcoholic cirrhosis. *Quarterly Journal of Medicine*, **91**, 19–25.

Chapter 5.37

Hepatocellular failure

E. A. Jones

Hepatocellular failure is the syndrome resulting from severe impairment of the function of hepatocytes. Its main manifestations are hepatic encephalopathy (**HE**), an haemorrhagic diathesis, fluid retention (ascites) and hepatocellular jaundice. The duration of hepatocellular dysfunction before the onset of overt failure is variable, ranging from a few days to many years.

Definitions

Acute liver failure. The syndrome of hepatocellular jaundice, elevated serum levels of aminotransferases and prolongation of the prothrombin time associated with an acute liver disease.

Table 1 Clinical stages of hepatic encephalopathy

Stage	Mental status	Asterixis	EEG changes
I (prodrome)	Slow mentation and affect; decreased attention; untidiness; irritability, inverted sleep rhythm	Usually absent	Often lacking
II impending coma)	Drowsiness; agitation; lethargy, inappropriate behaviour; inability to perform mental tasks, loss of sphincter control; confusion; slurred speech; disorientation	Present	Generalized slowing
III	Stupor; somnolent but rousable; incoherent speech; fits of rage; restlessness	Usually present	Always present
IV	Coma; with (IVA) or without (IVB) response to painful stimuli	Usually absent	Always present

Fulminant hepatic failure (FHF). The syndrome of acute liver failure complicated by encephalopathy occurring within 8 weeks of the onset of liver disease, or encephalopathy and a plasma factor V level of less that 50 per cent of normal occurring less than 2 weeks after the onset of jaundice.

Subfulminant hepatic failure. The syndrome of acute liver failure with encephalopathy and a plasma factor V level of less than 50 per cent of normal occurring 2 weeks to 3 months after the onset of jaundice.

Late-onset liver failure. The syndrome of acute liver failure complicated by encephalopathy occurring 8–24 weeks after the onset of liver disease.

Chronic hepatocellular failure. Chronic hepatocellular disease (e.g. cirrhosis) complicated by at least one of the four main manifestations of hepatocellular failure.

Aetiology

The most common causes of acute liver failure or FHF are viral hepatitis and drugs that induce hepatocellular necrosis (e.g. paracetamol, halothane). Chronic hepatocellular failure may complicate any progressive chronic hepatocellular disease or any lesion causing chronic hepatic central venous congestion.

Cardinal manifestations

Hepatic encephalopathy (HE)

HE is a complex reversible neuropsychiatric syndrome associated with hepatocellular failure and increased portal-systemic shunting of blood. The spectrum of psychiatric and neurological abnormalities is protean and can range from subtle mental changes to deep coma (Table 1). Subclinical HE is the term used when routine neurological examination in a patient with chronic liver disease is normal, but psychometric and/or neuro-electrophysiological tests reveal abnormalities that are potentially reversed by effective treatment for HE. During overt encephalopathy there is often increased muscle tone with cogwheel and neck rigidity. Asterixis (liver flap) can usually be elicited in precoma stages. The mouth may be difficult to open. Myoclonic twitchings may occur and plantar responses may be

Table 2 Factors that may precipitate hepatic encephalopathy

Factor	Comments
Oral protein load Upper gastrointestinal haemorrhage Constipation	Gut factors contribute to hepatic encephalopathy
Diuretic therapy Paracentesis Diarrhoea and vomiting	Dehydration, electrolyte and acid-base imbalance
Hypoglycaemia Hypotension Hypoxia Anaemia	Factors with adverse effects on both liver and brain function
Sedative/hypnotic drugs	Benzodiazepines and barbiturates enhance the action of GABA
Azotaemia	Increased synthesis of ammonia in gut
Infection	May induce dehydration and increased protein catabolism
General surgery	—

GABA, gamma-aminobutyric acid

extensor. With progression there is increased slowing of the electroencephalogram waveform and an increase followed by a decrease in its amplitude, and tendon reflexes tend to increase and subsequently decrease.

Encephalopathy complicating chronic liver disease may be acute or chronic. Acute encephalopathy in a cirrhotic patient is usually associated with one or more clearly definable precipitating factors (Table 2). The term chronic portal-systemic encephalopathy (**PSE**) is often applied when HE is persistent or episodic in a patient with chronic liver disease. It may be precipitated by a surgically created portal-systemic shunt or by a transjugular intrahepatic portal-systemic stent.

The encephalopathy of liver failure is considered to be metabolic in origin with a multifactorial pathogenesis. There is increased delivery of gut-derived nitrogenous substances to the systemic circulation as a consequence of impaired extraction by the failing liver and increased intrahepatic and/or extrahepatic portal-systemic shunting of blood. Some of these substances are neuroactive and can traverse the blood–brain barrier. Of perhaps many pathogenic factors, two that appear to be important are increased levels of ammonia and increased GABAergic neurotransmission. The latter is known to be associated with impaired motor function and decreased consciousness, two of the cardinal features of HE. Factors that may be responsible for potentiating GABAergic tone in liver failure include an accumulation of natural benzodiazepine agonist ligands in the brain, and increased availability of GABA at $GABA_A$ receptors due to increased plasma-to-brain transfer of GABA and impaired reuptake of GABA from the synaptic cleft. In addition, ammonia, at the modestly increased concentrations that occur in most patients with liver failure, has been shown recently to have the ability to enhance GABAergic neurotransmission by directly interacting with the $GABA_A$ receptor complex and synergistically potentiating the action of agonist ligands of the complex. In contrast, higher concentrations of ammonia, similar to those that occur in the congenital hyperammonaemias, suppress inhibitory neurotransmission and hence induce neuro-excitatory effects. Such concentrations may occur in FHF and may account for the psychomotor agitation and seizures that occasionally complicate this syndrome.

Haemorrhagic diathesis

The pathogenesis is again multifactorial. The predominant factor is impaired hepatocellular synthesis of blood clotting factors, which is reflected in prolongation of the prothrombin time and bruises around venepuncture sites. Thrombocytopenia may reflect the hypersplenism of portal hypertension (see Chapter 5.36), but in the fulminant syndrome abnormalities of platelet structure and function may occur and may accentuate prolongation of the capillary bleeding time. Spontaneous bleeding occurs most commonly from the upper gastro-intestinal tract and not necessarily from gastro-oesophageal varices.

Ascites

Ascites due to hepatocellular failure is invariably associated with portal hypertension (see Chapter 5.36). Hepatocellular failure due to a primary hepatocellular disease (e.g. cirrhosis, subfulminant hepatic failure) is associated with sinusoidal portal hypertension. Ascites associated with lesions causing impaired hepatic venous drainage may or may not be associated with hepatocellular failure.

Hepatocellular jaundice

The jaundice of the hepatocellular failure has an orange tint. It is a conjugated hyperbilirubinaemia due to impaired secretion of conjugated bilirubin into the bile canaliculi. In acute hepatitis a deep conjugated hyperbilirubinaemia may occur in the absence of prolongation of the prothrombin time and other manifestations of hepatocellular failure, but in chronic (non-cholestatic) liver disease conjugated hyperbilirubinaemia usually reflects the degree of hepatocellular failure and is associated with prolongation of the prothrombin time.

Other features

Increased susceptibility to infections

Bacterial and/or fungal infections commonly complicated acute or chronic hepatocellular failure, e.g. spontaneous bacterial peritonitis in a cirrhotic patient with ascites (see Chapter 5.36). Bacteraemia may occur in the absence of fever, rigors, or a substantial leucocytosis.

Foetor hepaticus

Foetor hepaticus is the term applied to a particular odour of the breath that may be detected in patients with appreciable portal-systemic shunting and/or hepatocellular failure. It has been attributed to gut-derived, sulphur-containing compounds and has been described as a sweetish, slightly pungent or faecal smell, similar to that of a rotten apple, mice, or a freshly opened corpse.

Acid–base and electrolyte changes

A wide range of acid–base and electrolyte changes occur in hepatocellular failure. Hyponatraemia is usually attributable to impaired renal free-water clearance and failure of the sodium pump; hypernatraemia is likely to be iatrogenic. A respiratory alkalosis due to hyperventilation is common in FHF. Loop diuretics commonly precipitate a hypokalaemic metabolic alkalosis.

Cerebral oedema and raised intracranial pressure (ICP)

Cerebral oedema and raised ICP often occur *pari passu* with encephalopathy in FHF. These complications are present in about 80 per cent of patients with FHF and stage IV encephalopathy. Possible pathogenic factors include increased blood-to-brain transfer of fluid (vasogenic), a failure of cellular osmoregulation (cytotoxic), and expansion of the extravascular space (interstitial or hydrocephalic). Herniation of the brain due to raised ICP is a major cause of death in FHF. Clinical signs that may be associated with raised ICP include psychomotor agitation, hypertension, hyperventilation, vomiting, fever, and increased muscle tone.

Hypoglycaemia

Severe hypoglycaemia occurs in about 40 per cent of patients with FHF and may exacerbate encephalopathy. It is due primarily to impaired hepatic glucose release secondary to glycogen depletion.

Cardiovascular changes

Hepatocellular failure is associated with systemic vasodilatation and an hyperdynamic circulation. Cardiac output is increased, peripheral vascular resistance decreased, blood pressure reduced, and splanchnic and capillary flow increased, but perfusion of the renal cortex is decreased. Features of an hyperdynamic circulation include abounding pulse, capillary pulsation, vasodilated extremities, a praecordial heave, and an ejection systolic murmur. The increased cardiac output and hypotension have been attributed to an increased vascular capacitance and hence relative hypovolaemia with low jugular venous pressure. Cardiac arrhythmias are common in patients with FHF in stage IV encephalopathy.

Hepatorenal syndrome

Renal failure of uncertain pathogenesis, but not attributable to hypovolaemia, is a common complication of hepatocellular failure. It is typically functional (haemodynamic) and associated with intense renal arterial vasoconstriction, reduced glomerular filtration, and oliguria. Impaired renal function in this syndrome is reversed following liver transplantation or transplantation of a kidney into a recipient without liver disease. The degree of renal failure is a reflection of the degree of hepatocellular failure. Acute tubular necrosis may supervene. Plasma urea and creatinine may not be reliable indices of renal function in FHF; hepatic synthesis of urea is decreased and tubular secretion of creatinine increased.

Hepatopulmonary syndrome

Hepatocellular failure may be associated with intrapulmonary peripheral vascular dilatation, decreased pulmonary vascular resistance, hypoxaemia, and cyanosis. The hypoxaemia is attributable to abnormal ventilation–perfusion ratios and diffusion capacity. Oxygen does not diffuse readily into the centre of dilated vessels and increased cardiac output limits the time for gas exchange. Hypoxaemia is some patients with cirrhosis is attributable to pulmonary arteriovenous shunts and is not reversible by 100 per cent oxygen. FHF may be complicated by pulmonary oedema.

Skin changes

Certain skin changes in a patient with chronic liver disease raise the possibility of incipient or overt hepatocellular failure. These include spider naevi, palmar erythema, 'paper money' skin, and white nails.

Endocrine changes

Some male patients with cirrhosis develop signs of feminization, but gynaecomastia may be induced by spironolactone rather than liver disease *per se*.

Hypoalbuminaemia

In chronic liver disease the degree of hypoalbuminaemia reflects both decreased hepatic synthesis and an increase in plasma volume.

Diagnosis

The syndrome of hepatocellular failure consists of a clinical spectrum from acute liver failure at the one extreme to decompensated chronic hepatocellular disease at the other. A patient dying of hepatocellular failure may exhibit any combination of the four cardinal manifestations with or without complicating sepsis.

Hepatic encephalopathy

This clinical diagnosis is made by excluding other causes of encephalopathy in a patient with severe hepatocellular disease. No individual abnormal clinical or laboratory finding is specific for HE. Serum biochemical tests reflect the underlying liver disease; they are helpful in the differential diagnosis of encephalopathies and in the detection of factors that may precipitate HE. Plasma ammonia levels correlate poorly with the clinical stage of encephalopathy and are not useful in the management, but an elevated level may confirm an hepatic origin of an undiagnosed encephalopathy.

Haemorrhagic diathesis

The most important laboratory marker is a prolonged prothrombin time, uncorrected by parenteral vitamin K.

Ascites

Ultrasonography of the abdomen, which can detect as little as 100–200 ml of intraperitoneal fluid, is indicated if the presence of ascites is in doubt on physical examination. For ascites to be attributed to hepatocellular failure, it is necessary to exclude non-hepatic causes.

Hepatocellular jaundice

The conjugated hyperbilirubinaemia of hepatocellular failure has to be distinguished from that of congenital and acquired intrahepatic cholestatic disease (e.g. drug-induced cholestasis, primary biliary cirrhosis, primary sclerosing cholangitis), acquired large-duct biliary obstruction (e.g. due to stones, strictures, pancreatitis, neoplasms), and the rare congenital conjugated hyperbilirubinaemias, in which other routine biochemical liver tests, including the prothrombin time, are normal. An ultrasound of the liver is useful for the detection of dilated bile ducts due to large-duct biliary obstruction. Unconjugated hyperbilirubinaemia is not a feature of hepatocellular failure.

Pathology

Hepatic histology in acute liver failure or FHF usually reveals massive or confluent hepatocellular necrosis, and, much less commonly, when the mechanism is impaired hepatocellular mitochondrial function (due to, for example, acute fatty liver of pregnancy, tetracycline, valproic acid) microvesicular hepatocellular steatosis without displacement of nuclei. Hepatic histology in chronic hepatocellular failure usually reveals either a cirrhosis (common) or the consequences of chronic coral venous congestion. Alzheimer type 2 astrocytosis may be found in the brain of patients who died from chronic liver failure. The hepatorenal syndrome is not associated with gross pathological changes in the kidney.

Course and prognosis

Acute hepatocellular failure

In patients with acute liver failure, who do not develop encephalopathy, complete recovery is the rule. FHF is associated with a high mortality, but, with improvements in intensive care, the proportion of patients that survive with medical care alone has increased substantially. Factors that tend to be associated with a particularly poor prognosis include encephalopathy that is severe and prolonged, severe coagulopathy, age less than 5 or more than 40 years, certain causes (hepatitis C, drugs other than paracetamol), development of a major complication, diminishing liver size, convulsions, cardiac arrhythmias, and marked foetor hepaticus. The course of FHF has been divided into five phases.

(i) *Pre-encephalopathy.* Encephalopathy is preceded by a progressively increasing prothrombin time.

(ii) *Encephalopathy.* Death is most likely to occur during this phase and may be attributable to acute liver failure with progressive encephalopathy, or a major complication such as an upper gastrointestinal haemorrhage, cerebral oedema, sepsis, or renal failure.

(iii) *Hepatic regeneration.* In the absence of liver transplantation, the ability of the liver to regenerate is the key factor determining the outcome. Evidence of hepatic regeneration, e.g. rising serum level of α-fetoprotein, is not usually apparent until at least 10 days after the onset of FHF, and death due to a complication may occur at a time when hepatocellular function is improving. Recovery is usually heralded by a decreasing prothrombin time followed by an improvement in encephalopathy.

(iv) *Cholestasis.* Profound cholestasis may develop 2–3 weeks after a patient has regained consciousness and is associated with large hepatic regeneration nodules.

(v) *Long-term sequelae.* In survivors complete restoration of normal hepatic function and structure is the rule. Long-term sequelae, including neurological sequelae, are rare.

Chronic hepatocellular failure

In chronic liver disease encephalopathy is likely to be reversible if overall hepatocellular function tends to be well maintained and/or if a correctable precipitating factor can be identified. Conjugated hyperbilirubinaemia in cirrhosis due to non-cholestatic disease or alcoholic hepatitis is associated with a poor prognosis. A rising serum conjugated bilirubin in a patient with chronic cholestatic disease may reflect progress of the disease and/or development of hepatocellular failure, When ascites first develops in a patient with cirrhosis 1-year survival is about 50 per cent and 5-year survival about 20 per cent. Survival after the onset of hepatorenal syndrome is usually only a few weeks or months.

Management

A treatment of proven efficacy for the cause of the hepatocellular failure should be instituted if available, e.g. *N*-acetylcysteine following an overdose of paracetamol, antiviral therapy if viral infections other than viral hepatitis are implicated and termination of pregnancy in acute fatty liver of pregnancy. Any drugs that might have contributed to hepatocellular failure are stopped, and liver-disease-associated abnormal pharmacokinetics and pharmadynamics of drugs must be taken into account. The possibility of liver transplantation must always be considered.

Table 3 Treatment of hepatic encephalopathy

Treatment	Comments
1. Correction or removal of precipitating factors	Mandatory
2. Institution of manoeuvres to minimize absorption of nitrogenous substances: Dietary protein restriction; Evacuation of the bowel; non-hydrolysed disaccharide (lactulose or lactitol) and/or oral broad-spectrum antibiotic (e.g. neomycin)	Routine
3. Reduction of portal-systemic shunting	Rarely practical
4. Direct reversal of neuropathophysiology (e.g. flumazenil)	Experimental

Chronic hepatocellular failure

The underlying liver disease is irreversible. Management consists of trying to reduce the manifestations of hepatocellular failure, especially encephalopathy and ascites, treating complicating infections, and assessing suitability for liver transplantation.

Hepatic encephalopathy

The four principles of management are summarized in Table 3. The first of these is mandatory, the second routine, the third rarely practical and the fourth experimental. Consideration of pathogenic mechanisms provides rationales for treatments that reduce ammonia levels (e.g. arginine, ornithine, sodium benzoate) and/or decrease GABAergic neurotransmission (e.g. flumazenil). In acute encephalopathy enteric protein intake is completely withheld until the mental state improves. In chronic encephalopathy with protein intolerance, dietary protein intake is reduced (but not <40 g/day to avoid negative nitrogen balance), a non-hydrolysed disaccharide may be given in doses that induce two or three semi-formed bowel actions daily, and precipitating factors are carefully avoided. If there is intolerance of non-hydrolysed disaccharides, a broad-spectrum antibiotic may be given with careful assessment of side-effects. A new therapeutic approach is to give a drug which reverses contributory neuropathophysiological events in the brain. The benzodiazepine antagonist, flumazenil, is an example of such a drug. Intravenous bolus injections of flumazenil are associated with transient ameliorations of encephalopathy in about 60 per cent of patients with cirrhosis.

Ascites

See Chapter 5.36.

Acute hepatocellular failure

Prevention

Examples of prevention include vaccination against hepatitis B to reduce the incidence of fulminant hepatitis B, avoiding re-exposure to an agent that induced an idiosyncratic hepatic reaction (e.g. halothane) and administering *N*-acetylcysteine after a paracetamol overdose.

Acute liver failure

Frequent monitoring is required when the prothrombin time is prolonged. As soon as encephalopathy develops or levels of blood clotting factors fall below 50 per cent of normal, it is prudent to refer the patient promptly to a specialized liver unit with facilities for liver transplantation.

Fulminant and subfulminant hepatic failure

The patient is considered to have potentially reversible disease and to be potentially infectious. Treatment is designed to buy time for hepatic regeneration to take place and avoid iatrogenic deterioration. Conventional intensive monitoring and care for the unconscious patient together with barrier nursing are instituted. Caloric intake is maintained by infusing hypertonic dextrose into a central vein. Major complications are treated promptly. Psychomotor agitation should be managed by restraint in a quiet room with avoidance of sedatives.

Specific problems

Susceptibility to infections

In FHF, intensive microbiological monitoring is necessary. Antibiotics, other than nephrotoxic aminoglycosides, are given promptly when infections are diagnosed and to cover invasive procedures.

Haemorrhagic diathesis

No prophylactic treatment is routinely advocated other than parenteral vitamin K given empirically. Infusion of platelets and fresh frozen plasma may be indicated to cover invasive procedures. Maintaining gastric pH above 5.0 by administering an H_2-antagonist may decrease transfusion requirements for upper gastrointestinal haemorrhage in FHF.

Acid–base and electrolyte disturbances

Acidosis requires treatment of the cause. Potassium chloride supplementation is required for hypokalaemia. Salt replacement is not required for hyponatraemia unless there is clear evidence of excessive losses of sodium (dilutional hyponatraemia with a relative or absolute excess of water is much more common).

Cerebral oedema and raised ICP

Encephalopathy in FHF may be compounded by other factors, including the effects of cerebral oedema and raised ICP. To minimize the risk of precipitation of an increase in ICP patients are nursed in a quiet room with the trunk and head elevated to 30°. Clinical signs of raised ICP are unreliable and there is increasing application of direct monitoring of ICP, usually when stage III encephalopathy has developed or the patient has become a candidate for liver transplantation. Such monitoring requires the invasive procedure of creating a burr hole through the skull and the placement of an epidural or subdural pressure transducer. The cerebral perfusion pressure should be maintained at a minimum of 60 mmHg and the ICP less than 25 mmHg. Raised ICP (up to 60 mmHg) may be reduced by intravenous mannitol (in the absence of hyperosmolality and azotaemia) and/or a barbiturate (pentobarbital or thiopentone).

Hypoglycaemia

It is necessary to measure blood glucose frequently in FHF to detect hypoglycaemia early and correct it promptly. Large amounts of dextrose are occasionally required.

Cardiovascular changes

Blood pressure should be maintained, if possible without the use of ionotropes. Hypotensive or vasodilator drugs may adversely affect ICP. Arrhythmias are minimized by correcting acid–base and electrolyte disturbances.

Hepatorenal syndrome

Blood volume should be optimized by cautiously infusing 20 per cent albumin without overloading the circulation. Any therapeutic agent that may have contributed to the syndrome is discontinued. For severe acid–base/electrolyte disturbances, fluid overload or azotaemia ultrafiltration or dialysis may be undertaken, but with care because of concomitant cardiovascular instability and coagulopathy.

Hepatopulmonary syndrome

No attempt should be made to correct hyperventilation. Oxygen is given for hypoxaemia. Endotracheal intubation is recommended in FHF with the onset of stage III encephalopathy. Assisted mechanical ventilation may be indicated and positive end-expiratory pressure should be avoided.

Temporary hepatic support

The rationale for providing temporary hepatic support for a patient with FHF is based on the assumption that the hepatic lesion is potentially reversible and that survival may occur provided the patient can be kept alive long enough for hepatic regeneration to take place. An effective method of providing temporary hepatic support should not only maintain the general condition of the patient but also prevent life-threatening complications. Criteria for selecting patients with FHF that would benefit from treatment with artificial liver support have not been agreed and the biochemical disturbances arising from impaired metabolic, synthetic, and biliary secretory function of the liver in FHF, that need to be corrected, have not been clarified. The provision of temporary hepatic support has no place in the management of chronic irreversible liver disease, except in the context of preparing a patient for liver transplantation. Prior to liver transplantation such treatment may reduce operative mortality and increase waiting time for a donor liver. None of the temporary hepatic supports systems that have been devised so far has been shown to have a favourable risk/benefit ratio in the management of patients with hepatocellular failure.

Further reading

Basile, A.S., Jones, E.A., and Skolnick, P. (1991). The pathogenesis and treatment of hepatic encephalopathy: Evidence for the involvement of benzodiazepine receptor ligands. *Pharmacological Reviews*, **43**, 27–71.

Blei, A.T. and Butterworth, R.F. (ed.) (1996). Hepatic encephalopathy. *Seminars in Liver Disease*, **16**, 233–338.

Williams, R. (ed.) (1996). Fulminant hepatic failure. *Seminars in Liver Disease*, **16**, 341–449.

Chapter 5.38

Primary liver tumours

I. M. Murray-Lyon

Hepatocellular carcinoma

This occurs as a single mass or as scattered nodules. In some 80 per cent of patients there is pre-existing cirrhosis but some cases arise in young adults without cirrhosis.

Epidemiology

In western Europe and North America the annual incidence is about 1–2 per 100 000 population, but it is becoming more common. In Africa and South-east Asia the incidence is 20–30 times higher. In areas of high incidence the peak age is in the third and fourth decades but in Europe and North America most cases occur in the fifth and sixth decades.

Aetiology

Some 10–15 per cent of patients with cirrhosis will develop hepatocellular carcinoma in western Europe and the USA, and perhaps more in Africa and Asia where the underlying cause is more commonly hepatitis B or C. Rare cases may follow prolonged use of the oral contraceptive pill or the radioactive contrast agent Thorotrast. In parts of Africa and the Far East there is evidence implicating aflatoxin contamination of food.

Hepatitis B is now recognized to have an important part in the development of hepatocellular carcinoma, especially in areas of high incidence (see also Chapter 5.31). The virus can be identified in tumour as well as the surrounding liver and integration of viral DNA in the genome of hepatocellular carcinoma has been shown. In areas of high endemicity of hepatitis B virus (**HBV**) as well as exposure to aflatoxins, mutation of the *p53* gene on chromosome 17 is a frequent finding.

Hepatitis C is also closely linked with the development of hepatocellular carcinoma, especially in Japan, Italy, and Spain. Almost all cases are associated with cirrhosis. Prospective studies indicate the latent period before tumour development may be as long as 25–30 years.

Clinical features

In high-incidence areas, patients usually present with a short history of right upper abdominal pain, often associated with fever and weight loss. There may be considerable abdominal swelling due to liver enlargement, with or without ascites. Sometimes catastrophic intraperitoneal bleeding occurs, owing to tumour rupture. In low-incidence areas the disease often presents as a general deterioration in the health of a patient already known to have cirrhosis. There is usually hepatomegaly and a bruit may be heard over the liver. Rare non-metastatic systemic manifestations include hypoglycaemia, hypercalcaemia, and porphyria cutanea tarda.

Investigations

Raised levels of α-fetoproteins are found in about 80 per cent of patients and tend to be higher in Africa and the Far East. Concentrations of above 500 ng/ml (normal 1–10 ng/ml) in a patient with liver disease are highly suggestive of hepatocellular carcinoma but

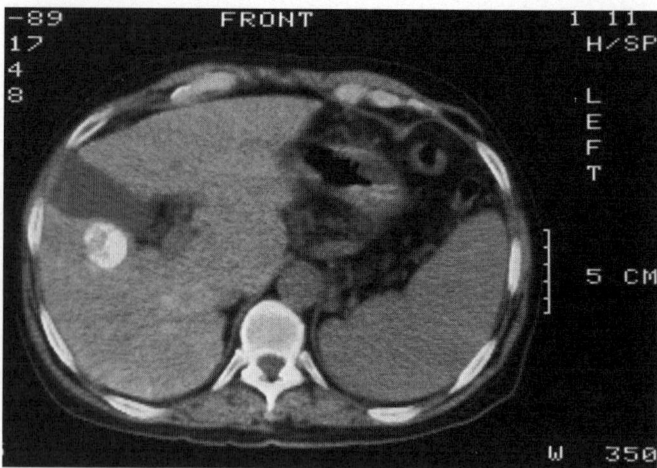

Fig. 1 CT scan of upper abdomen 10 days after Lipiodol angiography showing a cirrhotic liver with Lipiodol retained in a hepatoma *(by courtesy of Dr John Karani).*

high plasma levels are found in some patients with germinal-cell tumours of the testis and ovary as well as occasional patients with carcinoma of the stomach or pancreas, usually with hepatic metastases. Below 500 ng/ml there is a diagnostic 'grey zone', for such levels may be found in patients with severe viral hepatitis and active cirrhosis. Sequential readings are then helpful.

Other tumour markers have been described, including an abnormal vitamin B_{12}-binding protein (which is usually present with the fibrolamellar histological variant), and tumour-specific alkaline phosphatase and ferritin.

Liver imaging

Real-time ultrasound picks up hepatocellular carcinoma in 85–90 per cent of cases. False-negative results usually occur in patients with tumours of less than 2 cm diameter. Computed tomography (**CT**) scanning is probably no more accurate than ultrasound but sensitivity can be increased by combining it with a variety of arteriographic techniques (see below). Hepatic arteriography gives information on the anatomical distribution of the tumour and the vascular anatomy which are essential if surgical resection is contemplated, and provides opportunity for intra-arterial chemotherapy and hepatic artery embolization. The sensitivity of arteriography can be increased by combining it with simultaneous CT scanning with late films to show the portal venous system. The technique of Lipiodol angiography followed by CT scanning 10–14 days later can visualize tumours as small as 2–3 mm in diameter (Fig. 1). Magnetic resonance imaging has recently gained considerable specificity and sensitivity by the use of liver-specific contrast agents.

Liver biopsy

For definitive diagnosis, this is essential, although not always possible because of prolongation of the prothrombin time. The diagnosis can be considered highly likely without biopsy if the α-fetoprotein level is greater than 500 ng/ml and the hepatic arteriogram shows a tumour circulation.

Screening

Screening by α-fetoprotein assay and abdominal ultrasound should be considered for those at risk (cirrhosis or chronic infection with HBV or hepatitis C virus (**HCV**). Early tumours can be detected and survival may be prolonged in Far East patients, but benefits from screening in Europe are less certain.

Prognosis

Mean survival in most series is about 4 months, and patients with cirrhosis have a poorer prognosis. Encapsulated tumours and the fibrolamellar histological variant have a better prognosis.

Treatment

Curative

Only complete resection or orthotopic transplantation hold out any chance of cure. Resection is possible in only about 10 per cent of cases. In the presence of cirrhosis the extent of resection it is limited as liver regeneration is defective. Most units restrict transplantation to patients with tumours less than 4 cm in diameter.

Palliation

External-beam irradiation alone has not produced consistent improvement and results are no better when used in combination with cytotoxic drugs.

Cytotoxic drugs such as doxorubicin (Adriamycin) have produced worthwhile regression, but only 20–30 per cent of cases respond. Plasma α-fetoprotein concentrations fall in patients with responsive tumours and there is no point in continuing treatment if the levels are unchanged or rise. Mitozantrone (Novantrone) gives a similar response rate and has the advantage of fewer toxic side-effects.

Percutaneous ethanol injection into the tumour under ultrasound guidance causes tumour necrosis. Repeated injections may be given. The best results are obtained with tumours less than 3 cm diameter and the survival figures are comparable with those of limited surgical resection.

Cryotherapy and laser ablation techniques are currently under evaluation.

Lipiodol-targeted chemotherapy and radiotherapy is a process where cytotoxic drugs are emulsified with Lipiodol and delivered directly into the liver at selective hepatic arteriography. The duration of action of the drugs may be prolonged because of the retention of Lipiodol in the tumour. Lipiodol has been used in the same way to deliver ^{131}I to the tumour. Early clinical experience is encouraging.

Transcatheter arterial embolization with material such as gel foam can be achieved at the time of hepatic arteriography and may result in substantial tumour necrosis, particularly in highly vascular tumours, which derive the bulk of their blood supply from the hepatic artery. In patients with decompensated cirrhosis and those with portal vein occlusion the procedure is contraindicated. While such treatment may result in tumour necrosis, shrinkage, and symptomatic improvement, controlled trials have not shown that survival is prolonged.

Cholangiocarcinoma

Carcinoma may arise in any part of the biliary tree. Two varieties occur in the liver—a peripheral form, with multiple nodules often scattered throughout both lobes, and a hilar form usually situated at the confluence of the right and left hepatic ducts. This invades locally and causes obstruction of the biliary tree. This tumour is much less common than hepatocellular carcinoma and accounts for about 7–10 per cent of primary malignant tumours, except in the Far East where it makes up about 20 per cent. The peak age is in the sixth and seventh decades.

Aetiology

Thorium dioxide (Thorotrast) is a well-recognized but rare cause of the intrahepatic variety of tumour. In the Far East, infestation with one of a variety of distomes (*Clonorchis sinensis, Opisthorchis viverrini*) is commonly related.

Patients with long-standing ulcerative colitis occasionally develop carcinoma in the biliary tract and the risk is about 10 times greater than for the general population. Patients with total involvement of the colon of more than 10 years duration are the ones usually affected and the tumour may develop some years after panproctocolectomy. Various types of cystic disease of the biliary tree such as congenital hepatic fibrosis, polycystic disease of the liver, and Caroli's disease may all be complicated by the development of malignant change. The role of gallstones in extrahepatic cholangiocarcinoma is debated.

Symptoms and signs

In the peripheral intrahepatic type, patients present with upper abdominal pain, anorexia, malaise, and weight loss. With hilar tumours, jaundice is an early feature. Hepatomegaly is usual and splenomegaly may be found.

Diagnosis

The liver function tests show cholestatic features. α-Fetoprotein concentrations are usually normal or only slightly raised and tests for HBV and HCV infection are negative. Ultrasonography and CT scanning may demonstrate the tumour and with hilar lesions show dilatation of the intrahepatic biliary tree. Biliary-tree obstruction in the hilum may be demonstrated by percutaneous transhepatic cholangiography or by endoscopic retrograde cholangiopancreatography (ERCP).

Prognosis

Average survival from diagnosis is about 4–6 months, but if biliary drainage can be achieved in patients with hilar tumours, the prognosis is considerably better.

Treatment

For the peripheral tumours the principles of treatment are the same as for hepatocellular carcinoma (see above) but the response to chemotherapy is disappointing.

Hilar tumours may sometimes be resectable with re-anastomosis of the biliary tree or anastomosis of jejunum to the biliary tree in the hilum. A stent can be placed through the growth at laparotomy, at ERCP, or via the percutaneous transhepatic route. Radiotherapy may also produce useful symptomatic relief, and high-dose local irradiation has been given within the biliary tree by means of iridium-192 wire. Excellent palliation can be achieved by these procedures and survival for 1–2 years is not unusual. Liver transplantation is seldom performed because of a high risk of recurrence.

Angiosarcoma (Kupffer-cell sarcoma; malignant haemangioendothelioma)

This is a rare tumour consisting of malignant endothelial cells supported on a reticulin framework. It is often multifocal and may arise in a cirrhotic liver. It occurs in patients who were exposed to Thorotrast 15–25 years earlier, and chronic exposure to arsenic has also been implicated. The tumour has also been found in workers in the vinyl chloride industry. A few cases have occurred in long-term androgen takers but in the majority of patients no aetiological factor has yet been identified. Patients present with abdominal pain and hepatic enlargement and blood-stained ascites is common. This is a highly malignant tumour and curative resection is rarely possible. No form of palliative treatment has so far proved effective.

Other primary malignant tumours

These are extremely rare and include fibrosarcoma, leiomyosarcoma, and lymphoma.

Hepatic metastases

The liver is a favoured site for metastatic spread. Ultrasound should pick up tumours greater than 1 cm in diameter but in one large autopsy study, metastatic deposits were all less than 2 cm in diameter in one-third of the cases. 'Blind' liver biopsy is positive in only about 50 per cent of cases but accuracy can be increased by target biopsy at the time of ultrasonography. Liver function tests may be normal, but as the tumour mass enlarges, the alkaline phosphatase usually rises.

The prognosis is worst when there is extensive liver replacement by tumour. The site of primary growth is also relevant and deposits from colorectal cancer have a better prognosis (untreated mean survival, 9–12 months) than most other tumours.

Treatment

The range of possible treatments is the same as has been discussed for hepatocellular carcinoma. Partial hepatectomy to remove a solitary deposit may occasionally lead to prolonged survival or cure and the results are best in patients with colorectal cancer. A special situation exists with respect to hepatic metastases from the carcinoid tumour. This is often slowly growing and the main problem is the distress caused by flushing and diarrhoea. Resection of tumour bulk without any attempt at total removal often gives symptomatic relief, as does embolization. Transplantation should be considered.

Chemotherapy

The choice of drugs will be determined by the origin of the primary tumour. The most common drug used for deposits from gastrointestinal cancer is 5-fluorouracil but responses are infrequent (10–15 per cent) and short lasting. Better results are achieved when 5-fluorouracil is combined with folinic acid and with continuous infusion by portable pump.

Ligation of the hepatic artery at laparotomy or embolization at the time of hepatic arteriography are occasionally used for patients with severe pain.

Benign tumours

Haemangioma

This is the most common benign tumour and is usually asymptomatic, being found incidentally either during ultrasonography or CT scanning. Occasionally, it may cause abdominal pain or shock due to rupture. Rarely it may be associated with thrombocytopenia, hypofibrinogenaemia, or microangiopathic haemolytic anaemia.

Hepatic adenoma

The incidence of this tumour seems to have increased markedly since the introduction of the oral contraceptive pill and most reported cases have occurred in females who have been on the pill for 5 years or more. Even so the risk for the individual is infinitesimal. Patients are often asymptomatic and a mass is discovered on physical examination but some complain of upper abdominal pain and others present acutely with shock due to intraperitoneal bleeding. The tumour is usually solitary but may be multiple. There is little or no disturbance in liver function and α-fetoprotein concentrations are normal. A filling defect is seen on the isotope scan and hepatic arteriography demonstrates a highly vascular mass. In some cases the tumour has regressed after withdrawal of the pill but surgical resection is usually recommended because of the risk of intraperitoneal bleeding and the occasional development of malignant change.

Focal nodular hyperplasia

This is a benign condition that is frequently confused with the hepatic adenoma. It is much more frequent in women but no relation to the contraceptive pill has been established. The liver mass is usually solitary and is divided into nodules by bile duct- containing fibrous tissue septa that radiate out from a central focus. It is usually asymptomatic but rupture with intraperitoneal bleeding occasionally occurs. The prognosis is excellent and malignant change is not recorded. Distinction from hepatic adenoma may be possible with careful imaging and needle biopsy but surgical excision may be recommended for diagnostic certainty.

Other benign tumours

These are very much rarer and include fibroma, lipoma, leiomyoma, and cystadenoma.

Further reading

Bruix, J. (1997). Treatment of hepatocellular carcinoma. *Hepatology*, **25**, 259–62.

Mathurin, P., Rixe, O., Carbonell, N., *et al.* (1998). Review article: overview of medical treatment in unresectable hepatocellular carcinoma—an impossible meta-analysis? *Alimentary Pharmacology and Therapeutics*, **12**, 111–26.

Chapter 5.39

Liver transplantation

R. Williams

Transplantation of the liver is now a remarkably successful procedure (Fig. 1) and the number of operations performed annually has increased markedly since the early 1980s (Fig. 2), but a decreasing number of donors is limiting any further increase.

Selection of patients and pretransplant evaluation

Transplantation should be considered whenever a patient with a progressive or otherwise fatal liver disorder is no longer able to enjoy a reasonable existence, although still well enough to withstand the trauma of the surgery involved. Almost every type of end-stage liver disease has been treated by transplantation.

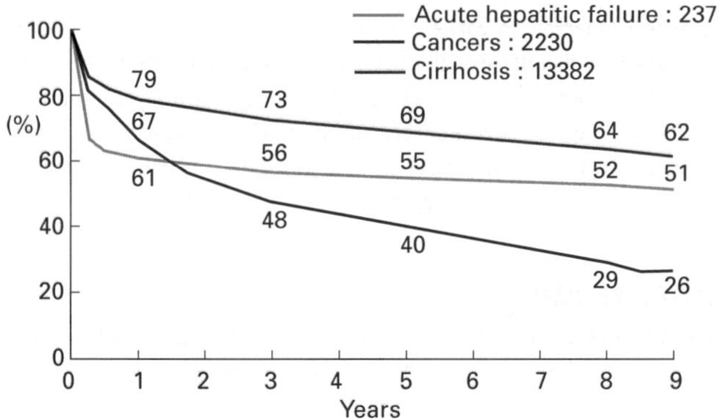

Fig. 1 Nine-year survival curves for 17 982 adult patients transplanted during the period January 1988 to December 1997
(reproduced by courtesy of Professor R. Adam, Director, European Liver Transplant Registry).

Specific diseases

Malignant tumours of the liver

A high rate of tumour recurrence has led to a decrease in the frequency of liver grafting for malignancy. None the less, the younger patient with a relatively slow-growing primary hepatocellular carcinoma may be a suitable candidate. The fibrolamellar variant, which tends to metastasize late, is one of the more favourable histological types. Hepatoma development in the long-standing cirrhotic, recognized at an early presymptomatic stage is another favourable indication. The risk of tumour recurrence is related to the size of the tumour at the time of transplantation and is low with tumours less than 3 cm in diameter (often found incidentally). Even with moderately sized tumours (4–8 cm diameter) over 40 per cent are cured and in some of the others long periods of palliation are obtained. Extrahepatic spread must be excluded, as far as is possible, before transplantation. Needle biopsy should be avoided when liver transplantation is being considered, as the subsequent appearance of tumour in the needle tract is well described.

Cirrhosis

In primary biliary cirrhosis transplantation should be considered once the serum bilirubin is greater than 150 μmol/l, or if patients are disabled by osteodystrophy, severe pruritus, or uncontrollable variceal haemorrhage. Cases of chronic encephalopathy from cirrhosis (usually of cryptogenic variety) with a large spontaneous or shunt-induced collateral circulation can also respond well to transplantation. Another indication in all types of cirrhosis is recurrent variceal haemorrhage when other measures have failed.

In cryptogenic cirrhosis and active chronic hepatitis the proper timing of the operation is difficult. Low, intermediate, and high-risk cases (depending on encephalopathy, ascites, nutritional status, serum bilirubin, prothrombin time, and age) have different survival rates over 1 year ranging from 90 per cent in low risk to 50 per cent in high-risk subjects.

Poorer early survival in cirrhotic cases due to hepatitis B is due to recurrence of infection sometimes causing acute liver failure (fibrosing cholestatic hepatitis). This risk is reduced by the use of long-term prophylactic specific immunoglobulin for time of transplantation. Recurrence of infection is virtually universal after transplantation for hepatitis C virus cirrhosis but in only about 25 per cent is associated clinical disease of significance. In alcoholic cirrhosis, excellent results can be achieved but only in carefully selected patients.

Budd–Chiari syndrome

In severe cases where cirrhosis has developed, transplantation gives more benefit long term than a side-to-side shunt and offers the chance of greater long-term benefit. Long-term anticoagulation after the transplant is mandatory.

Inborn errors of metabolism

Grafting may be curative in several congenital disorders in which the primary defect arises in the host liver and leads to its irreversible damage. These include α_1-antitrypsin deficiency, some glycogen storage disorders, galactosaemia, and Wilson's disease. Combined liver and heart transplantation can be successful when there is severe heart failure in familial hypercholesterolaemia; LDL receptors in the donor liver are sufficient to correct the hyperlipidaemia. In patients with renal failure from primary hyperoxaluria, a combined liver/kidney transplant corrects abnormal oxalate pools by providing the defective hepatic enzyme.

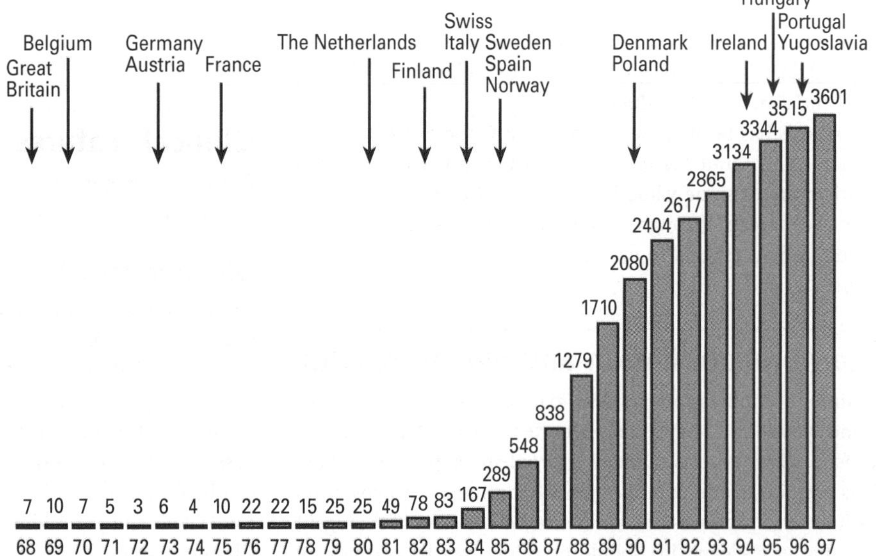

Fig. 2 The evolution of liver transplantation over the period May 1968 to December 1997
(reproduced by courtesy of Professor R. Adam, Director, European Liver Transplant Registry).

Acute liver failure

Selection of cases is based on criteria derived from a multivariate analysis of prognostic indicators (survival rates with intensive care can reach 39–67 per cent for hepatitis A and B and paracetamol overdoses). Patients with non-A, non-B fulminant hepatitis or idiosyncratic drug hepatotoxicity have the highest mortality. Reported 1-year survival figures for those transplanted vary depending on state at time of operation for 60–75 per cent.

Donor-recipient matching, organ preservation, and surgical techniques

These problems are addressed in OTM3, pp. 2113–4.

Rejection and immunosuppression

The liver is rejected less aggressively than are skin, kidneys, or heart. However, occasional instances of hyperacute liver rejection occur and the liver can be damaged by acute and chronic rejection. Most centres use prednisolone in combination with cyclosporin or FK506 (Tacrolimus) for initial immunosuppression. Oral dosage with these agents (mioral-microemulsified preparation) is 10 mg/kg per day, the dose being adjusted subsequently so as to maintain a trough blood concentration of 100–150 ng/ml (cyclosporin) and 10–15 (FK506). Long-term maintenance regimens vary, either cyclosporin or FK506 being used in combination with both prednisone and azathioprine or one or other of these agents, or with cyclosporin or FK506 alone in cases where the drug is well tolerated. A new immunosuppressive drug, mycophenolate mofelit is being used in place of azathioprine to reduce doses of cyclosporin or FK506 in cases where nephrotoxicity from those agents develops.

Acute rejection is common between the seventh and fourteenth postoperative day. The diagnosis may be confirmed by liver biopsy. Liver biopsy is also essential in the diagnosis of later rejection. Acquired hepatitis virus infection of the graft, particularly cytomegalovirus, will require histological as well as serological confirmation; it responds in most instances to ganciclovir, which in some centres is also used prophylactically in recipients receiving cytomegalovirus-positive grafts. An oral and effective preparation of ganciclovir is now available. Ultrasonographic examination is useful in distinguishing obstructive jaundice from rejection or hepatitis infection of the graft. The treatment of acute rejection is with a course of intravenous Solu-Medrone, 1 g daily for 3 days. Repeated episodes may be followed by chronic rejection of the vanishing bile-duct type.

When cirrhosis has been caused by hepatitis C there is a high rate of reinfection of the graft (as in the case of hepatitis B). Interferon and ribaviricin are of some value in such cases. Cases of hepatitis B recurrence that break through prophylactic treatment with immunoglobulin often respond to use of antiviral agents lamivudine or famiciclovir.

Long-term rehabilitation and overall results

Chronic immunosuppression renders patients susceptible to infections, and cyclosporin can produce hypertension, renal impairment, and headache. Osteoporosis, already a problem in primary biliary cirrhosis is a troublesome complication of continued corticosteroid therapy. FK506 also produces renal impairment and dose of this agent (as well as that of cyclosporin) should be minimized by addition of other agents referred to earlier. In those who survive beyond 1 year, rehabilitation is usually excellent. One-year survival figures are running at 75–80 per cent for elective operations, with 5-year survival of 65–70 per cent. Recurrence of the underlying disease is common in hepatitis B and C but rare in primary biliary cirrhosis and in autoimmune chronic active hepatitis.

Further reading

Cosimi, A.B. and Bailin, M.T. (1994). Liver transplantation. *Oxford textbook of surgery*, (ed. Morris, P.J. and Malt, R.A.), pp. 680–96. Oxford University Press.

Sherlock, S. and Dooley, J. (1997). *Disease of the liver and biliary system.* Blackwell Science, Oxford.

Wright, T.L. *et al.* (1992). Recurrent and acquired hepatitis C viral infection in liver transplant recipients. *Gastroenterology*, **103**, 317–000.

Chapter 5.40

Hepatic granulomas

G. M. Dusheiko

Hepatic granulomas are not uncommon findings in patients who have liver biopsies; they are found in 3–10 per cent of 'blind' liver biopsies at general hospitals. They may be accompanied by other signs of inflammation, including bile-duct damage, vasculitis, cholestasis, and fibrosis. Granulomas are usually found throughout the liver, but are generally clustered near portal tracts; there may be associated necrosis within the granuloma. Caseous necrosis is associated with tuberculosis, but similar necrosis may be found in sarcoidosis. Other forms of necrosis, including purulent or eosinophilic, occur, depending upon the cause.

There are many different causes; frequently the disorder is part of a generalized disease process, and the differential diagnosis can be difficult (Table 1). The most common specific causes are infective. Drugs and toxins, and specific liver diseases (particularly primary biliary cirrhosis), are also important. Sarcoidosis and tuberculosis are apparently the most common causes of granulomatous hepatitis, but in some series, idiopathic granulomatous hepatitis confined to the liver is relatively common.

Clinical features

Fever is the major presenting manifestation, irrespective of the cause. Other features vary according to the underlying disease.

Diseases associated with hepatic granulomas

Among *infective causes*, granulomatous hepatitis due to atypical mycobacteria is recognized with increasing frequency in immunosuppressed patients and those with AIDS. In the case of AIDS other causes of hepatitic granulomas are lymphomas, cytomegalovirus, histoplasmosis, toxoplasmosis, or cryptococcal infection. Further discussion of the many other infective, chemical, and drug-related causes can be found in OTM3, pp. 2121–2. A list of drugs which have been associated with granulomatous hepatitis is shown in Table 2 (see also Chapter 5.41).

Table 1 Causes of hepatic granulomas

Infections	Chemicals
Mycobacteria:	Beryllium
Tuberculosis (typical and atypical)	Copper
Leprosy	***Drugs***
Bacteria:	(see Table 2)
Brucellosis	***Immunological disorders***
Tularaemia	Sarcoidosis
Yersiniosis	AIDS
Proprioni/listeriosis	Bowel and liver disease
Melidiosis	Crohn's disease
Whipple's disease	Ulcerative colitis
Spirochaetes:	Primary biliary cirrhosis
Syphilis	Hypogammaglobulinaemia
Fungi:	Systemic lupus erythematosus
Blastomycosis	Polymyalgia rheumatica
Histoplasmosis	***Idiopathic***
Cryptococcosis	Granulomatous hepatitis
Protozoa:	***Enzyme defects***
Leishmaniasis	Chronic granulomatous disease of children
Toxoplasmosis	***Neoplasia***
Metazoa:	Lymphoma
Schistosomiasis	Carcinoma
Visceral larva migrans	***Miscellaneous***
Rickettsia:	BCG vaccine
Q fever	
Boutonneuse fever	
Viruses:	
Epstein–Barr virus	
Cytomegalovirus	
Hepatitis A	
Helminths	

Table 2 Drugs causing hepatic granulomas (see Chapter 5.41)

Allopurinol	Oxyphenbutazine
Beryllium	*p*-Aminosalicylic acid
Carbamazepine	Perhexiline maleate
Chlorpromazine	Phenylbutazone
Chlorpropamide	Phenytoin
Clofibrate	Procainamide
Contraceptive steroids	Quinidine
Diazepam	Silicon
Diphenylhydantoin	Starch
Halothane	Sulphonamides
Hydralazine	Sulphonylureas
Hydrochlorothiazide	Talc
Methyldopa	Tolbutamide
Nitrofurantoin	

For source see OTM3, p. 2123.

Sarcoidosis is the most common non-infectious cause of hepatic granulomas. Twenty per cent of patients with sarcoidosis have hepatomegaly, and hepatic granulomas are found in two-thirds of cases submitted to liver biopsy. Patients often have splenomegaly. The granulomas, which are all at the same stage of development, cluster in the portal tracts, embedded in dense fibrous tissue. Central necrosis is less obvious than in tuberculosis. The lesions are often up to 2 mm in diameter.

Systemic disease including erythema nodosum may be present. Fever and malaise are common and in symptomatic patients corticosteroid therapy may be necessary; the response is usually, but not always, good. Rare complications of hepatic sarcoidosis include cholestasis, portal hypertension, and progressive liver disease. These complications are most often seen in black males, who present with jaundice, pruritus, and hepatosplenomegaly. The serum alkaline phosphatase is elevated and the serum aminotransferases increased two- to fivefold. Ductopenia is seen on liver biopsy. The disease associated with portal hypertension has a poor prognosis, and is not responsive to steroids.

In chronic granulomatous disease of childhood (see Section 3) in which phagocytic leucocytes cannot produce hydrogen peroxide, granulomas in the liver are common apart from the characteristic liability to chronic infection.

Neoplasia Epithelioid granulomas occur in Hodgkin's and non-Hodgkin's lymphoma, even in the absence of malignant deposits in the liver. Granulomas are also found in specific carcinomas.

Miscellaneous Bacille Calmette–Guérin (BCG) vaccination may produce intrahepatic granulomas; probably an immunological response to antigens of the vaccine. They have been reported in patients who have had intravesical instillation of BCG for bladder cancer, and may respond to corticosteroids. Granulomas have also been reported in polymyalgia rheumatica, Still's disease, and regional enteritis. A type of granuloma may be formed in fatty liver when fat-laden cells rupture.

Investigation of the cause of hepatic granulomas

Laboratory abnormalities are often not specific or diagnostic. The erythrocyte sedimentation rate (ESR) is frequently elevated, as is the serum alkaline phosphatase. Patients may have mildly elevated concentrations of alanine transaminase. Hyperglobulinaemia may be present. Elevated serum bilirubin concentrations are unusual, and the prothrombin time is usually normal. A liver biopsy confirms the pathological diagnosis, and may even indicate the cause of the disease. Other morphological features may be helpful, for example damage to bile ducts in primary biliary cirrhosis. In some patients, the lesions are found unexpectedly, but the cause may be found histologically (for example, schistosomiasis). Associated hepatic changes, or special stains, such as Ziehl–Neelsen for mycobacteria, silver staining for fungi or immunostaining for specific organisms, may be diagnostic. There may be other useful morphological features including eosinophils, purulent lesions, or an associated vasculitis. Alternatively, the diagnosis may be obvious from other features.

In cases in which the cause is obscure, investigations should search for sarcoidosis, tuberculosis, brucellosis, histoplasmosis, syphilis, leprosy, cytomegalovirus, Epstein–Barr virus, schistosomiasis, berylliosis, lymphoma, Crohn's disease, primary biliary cirrhosis, AIDS, or drug reactions. After all that, some 10 per cent of cases remain undiagnosed.

Treatment

Identified underlying disease cause should be treated. Any drugs incriminated should be stopped. In idiopathic granulomatous hepatitis, the response to corticosteroids is often prompt. Treatment is started with 40–60 mg of prednisone daily. This improves symptoms, subdues the fever, and reduces the hepatic granulomas. The alkaline phosphatase and ESR improve. Alternate-day corticosteroids can be used after initiating treatment. The dose is gradually lowered over a period of months.

If there is concern over unproven tuberculosis, a trial of antituberculous therapy may be necessary. Corticosteroids can be added if there is no response in 2 months. Isoniazid prophylaxis can be added. Fever may recur every time steroids are stopped. Indomethacin may also alleviate fever, and cyclophosphamide therapy for idiopathic hepatic granulomatosis may be indicated in patients in whom prednisone is contraindicated.

Further reading

Cunningham, D., Mills, P.R., Quigley, E.M.M., *et al.* (1982). Hepatic granulomas: Experience over a ten year period in the west of Scotland. *Quarterly Journal of Medicine*, **51**, 162.

Guckian, J.C. and Perry, J.E. (1969). Granulomatous hepatitis: an analysis of 63 cases and a review of the literature. *Annals of Internal Medicine*, **65**, 1081–100.

Salti, M.B., *et al.* (1990). Hepatic granuloma in Saudi Arabia: a clinicopathological study of 59 cases. *American Journal of Gastroenterology*, **85**, 665–74.

Sartin, J.S. and Walker, R.C. (1991). Granulomatous hepatitis: a retrospective review of 88 cases at the Mayo Clinic. *Mayo Clinic Proceedings*, **66**, 914–18.

Chapter 5.41

Drugs and liver damage

J. Neuberger

Drug-induced liver injury is relatively uncommon but unless recognized early may cause death. Of 1600 adverse reactions to drugs in England over 1 year, 3.5 per cent involved the liver and 7 per cent of these were fatal. Most reactions are of jaundice and hepatitis; the more common are due to halothane, antibiotics such as penicillins, anti-inflammatory drugs, and oral contraceptives. In most instances, withdrawal of the drug will lead to resolution of the liver damage. Almost all patterns of liver disease can be induced by drugs (Table 1) and some drugs may be associated with more than one type of reaction.

The diagnosis of drug-induced liver damage is largely circumstantial and by exclusion of other causes of liver disease. The temporal association between the onset of damage and timing of drug exposure, and the response to drug withdrawal (Table 2), and the known patterns of drug reaction all help in establishing the drug as the cause. Rarely, the presence of specific serological markers may help. For example, an antibody to trifluoroacetylated proteins is found in halothane-associated hepatitis. Use of a clinical challenge is rarely justified, may be misleading, and may prove fatal.

Acute hepatitis

The range varies from a mild subclinical elevation of serum transaminases to fulminant hepatic failure. Many drugs have been associated with acute liver failure (Table 3). Clinically, the picture may be indistinguishable from that of viral hepatitis. Occasionally, pain may be so severe as to lead to the mistaken diagnosis of acute cholecystitis. Serum aminotransferases are raised and prolongation of the prothrombin time and jaundice may occur in more severe cases. Histologically, the appearances vary from a mild focal necrosis to massive liver cell damage. In some cases, paracetamol for example, the damage is predominantly centrilobular, whereas in others, such as α-methyldopa, the whole lobule is affected. Steatosis, granulomas, and eosinophilia are variable features. The most common causes of drug-associated fulminant hepatic failure are paracetamol overdose and halothane hepatitis. There is a current increase in liver failure due to drugs such as 'Ecstasy'.

The development of abnormalities of liver function during prolonged drug use poses particular problems, as for example, with antituberculous therapy. Derangement of serum aminotransferases occurs in approximately 10 per cent of patients and, if the drug is continued, up to 10 per cent of these develop severe hepatic necrosis. Identification of those patients who will develop severe hepatic failure is difficult and the clinician has to decide whether the risks of continuing therapy outweigh the potential benefits. Drugs such as

Table 1 Patterns of hepatic drug reactions

Hepatitis	
Fulminant	Halothane
Acute	
Subacute	
Chronic	Methyldopa, nitrofurantoin
Cholestatic	Phenothiazine, erythromycin
Granulomatous	
Cirrhosis	
Cholestasis	
Bland	Anabolic steroids, oestrogens
Vanishing bile-duct syndrome	Chlorpromazine
Sclerosing cholangitis	Floxuridine
Granulomas	Sulphonamides, phenylbutazone, allopurinol
Steatosis	
Microvesicular	Valproic acid, tetracycline
Macrovesicular	Methotrexate, amiodarone
Tumours	
Adenoma	Oral contraceptive, anabolic steroids
Carcinoma	Oral contraceptive
Angiosarcoma	Thorium dioxide, arsenicals
Cholangiocarcinoma	Thorium dioxide
Vascular	
Peliosis	Oestrogens
Budd–Chiari syndrome	Oestrogens
Veno-occlusive disease	Azathioprine, urethrane
Fibrosis	Vitamin A, arsenicals

Table 2 Establishing the diagnosis of drug-associated liver damage by the pattern of symptoms, their timing, and the effect of withdrawal

	Suggestive	Compatible	Incompatible		
	From onset	From onset	From cessation	From onset	From cessation
Hepatitis					
Initial treatment	5–90 days	<5 or >90 days	<15 days	Drug taken after onset	>15 days
Subsequent	1–15 days	>15 days	<15 days	Drug taken after onset	>15 days
Acute cholestasis					
Initial treatment	5–90 days	>5 or >90 days	<1 month	Drug taken after onset	>1 month
Subsequent	1–90 days	>90 days	<1 month	Drug taken after onset	

After Danan (1990).

heparin are commonly associated with abnormal liver enzymes but very rarely with liver disease.

Hepatic drug reactions are classified into predictable and idiosyncratic (Table 4). Predictable reactions are dose dependent;. The classic example is paracetamol toxicity.

Variations in susceptibility may be a consequence of genetic variations in drug metabolism. Well-recognized genetic polymorphisms include variations in the cytochrome P450 isoenzymes, drug oxidation, acetylation, and hydroxylation. Age, too, is associated with differences in susceptibility to toxicity. Children may metabolize drugs differently from adults. Those taking enzyme inducers such as alcohol, rifampicin, or phenobarbitone are at a greater risk of increased metabolism of the drug and hence of forming toxic metabolites. Those with reduced glutathione stores, due to fasting, malnutrition or associated disease, may be at greater risk of developing toxicity as detoxification mechanisms are impaired. Finally, liver disease itself may alter susceptibilities to drug toxicity.

Idiosyncratic drug reactions are dose independent and may be due either to metabolic idiosyncrasy or the involvement of immune mechanisms. Immune involvement is suggested by a rapid onset after subsequent exposure and the appearance of markers such as peripheral or intrahepatic eosinophilia, granulomas, circulating immune complexes, autoantibodies, and other autoimmune phenomena. Two drugs have been well studied with respect to immune-mediated hepatitis—halothane and tienilic acid. Halothane hepatitis occurs rarely and after multiple exposures. Risk factors include female sex, obesity, and repeated or subsequent exposure within 3 months. Immune involvement is suggested by an increased incidence of organ non-specific autoantibodies, peripheral eosinophilia and circulating immune complexes, and the presence of antibodies reacting with a variety of halothane-associated liver cell macromolecules. Tienilic acid-associated hepatitis is associated with a circulating liver/kidney microsomal antibody that reacts with the cytochrome P450 and cytochrome $2c_3$; antibodies to cytochrome $1a_w$ are associated with hydralazine hepatitis. Cross-reaction between two drugs may occur. Thus, halothane sensitization may predispose to toxicity from other halogenated hydrocarbon anaesthetic agents such as isoflurane.

Acute cholestatic hepatitis

Histologically, the liver shows dilated sinusoids with cholestasis often predominating in the centrilobular region. There may be an associated portal inflammation and liver cell necrosis. In the majority of cases there is rapid resolution following withdrawal of the drug, although with chlorpromazine and other phenothiazines the cholestasis may

Table 3 Main drugs causing hepatocellular necrosis

Anaesthesia
Chloroform
Cyclopropane
Enflurane
Ethyl ether
Fluroxene
Halothane
Isoflurane
Methoxyflurane
Trichloroethylene
Vinyl ether

Antineoplastic
Carmustine
Chlorozotocin
Cyclophosphamide
Cytarabine
Hydroxycarbamide
Mithramycin
Procarbazine
Streptozotocin
Vincristine

Cardiovascular disease
Captopril
Enalapril
Frusemide
Hydralazine
Methyldopa
Nicotinic acid
Papaverine
Quinidine
Tienilic acid

Gastroenterological
Chenodeoxycholic acid
Disulfiram
Omeprazole
Salazosulphapyridine

Endocrine disease
Acetohexamide
Carbutamide
Flutamide
Metahexamide
Propylthiouracil

Neuropsychiatric diseases
Amitriptyline
Bromocriptine
Carbamazepine
Dantrolene
Desipramine
Ferpexide
Imipramine
Iproniazid
Isaxonine
Lergotrile
Levodopa
Loxapine
Methylphenidate
Nomifensine
Pemoline
Peogamide
Phenacetamide
Phenelzine
Pheniprazine
Phenoxypropperazine
Phenytoin
Phethenylate
Tetrahydroaminoacridine
Valproate
Viloxazine

Nutritional and metabolic diseases
Clofibrate
Fenofibrate
Gemfibrozil
Nicotinamide

Radiological examinations
Iodipamide
Iopanoic acid

Rheumatic and musculoskeletal diseases
Allopurinol
Aspirin
Baclofen
Benorilate
Benoxaprofen
Clometacin
Dantrolene

continued

Table 3 *continued*

Infectious and parasitic disease	Glafenine
p-Aminosalicylic acid	Paracetamol
Amodiaquine	Piroxicates
Carbenicillin	Salicylates
Ciprofloxacin	***Skin diseases***
Clindamycin	Etretinate
Co-trimoxazole	Methoxsalen
Dapsone	Povidone–iodine
Dideoxyinosine	Tannic acid
Fluconazole	***Others***
Fusidic acid	Cocaine
Hycanthone	Ecstasy
Isoniazid	
Ketoconazole	
Levamisole	
Mebendazole	
Mepacrine	
Minocycline	
Oxacillin	
Piperazine	
Sulphonamides	
Zidovudine	

take up to 1–2 years to resolve. Many drugs cause a mixed hepatitis, where there are features both of cholestasis and liver cell damage (Table 5).

Bland cholestasis

Bland cholestasis is characterized by cholestasis in the absence of hepatitis and is due to specific interference with bile secretion. The two main groups of drugs associated with this condition are oral contraceptives, oestrogens, and anabolic steroids. Other drugs are listed in Table 6.

Steatosis

Steatosis may be micro- or macrovesicular. Differentiation is important because the clinical features and outcomes are different (Table 7).

Microvesicular steatosis

The fat is distributed in small lipid droplets; the hepatocellular nucleus is not displaced. There may be an associated hepatitis. Extensive microvesicular steatosis may lead to a serious clinical syndrome with haemorrhage, syncope, hypotension, lethargy, coma, or hypoglycaemia. In some cases, renal failure and pancreatic inflammation may occur. Serum aminotransferases and bilirubin are not greatly increased, although the prothrombin time may be greatly prolonged.

Table 4 Cholestasis of acute hepatitis associated with drugs

Type	Onset	Reaction to re-exposure	Dose effect	Reproducible in animals	Hypersensitivity features
Predictable	Rapid	Rapid	++	+	–
Idiosyncratic	Variable	Delayed	+/–	–	–
	Variable	Rapid	–	–	+

Table 5 Main drugs causing mixed or cholestatic hepatitis

Cancer	
Aminoglutethimide	Cisplatin
Arabinoside	Cyclosporin
Azathioprine	Cytosine
Chlorambucil	Mitomycin
Chlorozotocin	Streptozotocin
Cardiovascular disease	
Ajmaline	Phenindione
Captopril	Prajmaline
Diltiazem	Procainamide
Disopyramide	Propafenone
Flecainide	Quinine
Hydralazine	Spironolactone
Methyldopa	Verapamil
Mexiletine	Warfarin
Nifedipine	
Gastroenterological diseases	
Cimetidine	Ranitidine
Penicillamine	
Endocrine diseases	
Acetohexamide	Methimazole
Carbimazole	Propylthiouracil
Chlorpropamide	Tamoxifen
Glibenclamide	Thiouracil
Metahexamide	Tolbutamide
Infectious and parasitic diseases	
p-Aminosalicylic acid	Nitrofurantoin
Arsphenamine	Phenazopyride
Cefalexin	Quinine
Chloramphenicol	Rifampicin
Cloxacillin	Sulphadiazine
Co-trimoxazole	Sulphonamides
Erythromycin	Tiabendazole
Griseofulvin	Troleandomycin
Nalidixic acid	Tryparsamide
Neuropsychiatric diseases	
Amitriptyline	Iprindole
Bromocriptine	Isocarboxazid
Carbamazepine	Mianserin
Chlordiazepoxide	Phenobarbital
Chlorpromazine	Phenytoin
Desipramine	Prochloperazine
Diazepam	Promazine
Fluphenazine	Thioridazine
Flurazepam	Triazolam
Haloperidol	Trifluoperazine
Imipramine	Zimelidine

continued

Table 5 *continued*

Rheumatic and musculoskeletal diseases	
Allopurinol	Kebuzone
Baclofen	Naproxen
Colchicine	Oxyphenbutazone
Diclofenac	Penicillamine
Diflunisal	Phenopyrazone
Fenbufen	Phenylbutazone
Feprazon	Piroxicam
Flurbiprofen	Probenecid
Gold salts	Propoxyphene
Ibufenac	Proquazone
Ibuprofen	Sulcindac
Indomethacin	Zoxazolamine
Skin diseases	
Isotretinoin	

Table 6 Drugs causing acute cholestasis

Antimicrobials	***Anti-inflammatory/ analgesic drugs***
Amoxycillin/clavulanic acid	Benoxaprofen
Cephalosporins	Dextropropoxyphene
Co-trimoxazole	Diflunisal
Erythromycin	Gold
Flucloxacillin	Naproxen
Griseofulvin	Phenylbutazone
Ketoconazole	Piroxicam
Nitrofurantoin	D-Penicillamine
Novobiocin	***Anticonvulsants***
Rifampicin	Carbamazepine
Sulphones	Phenobarbitone
Thiobendazole	Phenytoin
Triacetyloleandromycin	***Psychiatric drugs***
Trimethoprim	Amitryptyline
Antithyroid drugs	Chlordiazepoxide
Carbimazole	Chlorpromazine
Methimazole	Flurazepam
Thiouracil	Imipramine
Hypoglycaemics	Haloperidol
Chlorpropamide	Nomifensine
Glibenclamide	Prochlorperazine
Tolbutamide	Thioridazine
Anticancer drugs	Zemeldene
Azathioprine	***Cardiovascular***
Busulphan	Ajmaline
Chlorambucil	Captopril
Cytarabine	Chlorthalidone
Steroids	Disopyramide
Aminoglutethimide	Hydralazine
C17 anabolic sex steroids	Nifedipine
Danazol	Thiazides
Stanozolol	Verapamil
Tamoxifen	***Others***
Cytokines	Allopurinol
Interleukin 2	Cimetidine
Tumour necrosis factor	Cyclosporin A
	Phenindione
	Ranitidine
	Warfarin

Table 7 Drugs inducing steatosis

Microvesicular	*Macrovesicular*
Amineptine	Asparaginase
Aureomycin	Glucocorticoids
Pirprofen	Methotrexate
Tetracycline	
Valproate	

Table 8 Drug-related vascular diseases of the liver

Veno-occlusive disease	*Perisinusoidal fibrosis*
Azathioprine	Arsenicals
Mercaptopurine	Azathioprine
Pyrrolizidine alkaloid	Mercaptopurine
Thioguanine	Methotrexate
	Vitamin A
Budd–Chiari syndrome	
Actinomycin	
Dacarbazine	
Oral contraceptive	

Macrovesicular steatosis

This is less serious. The hepatocyte contains a large droplet of fat, which displaces the nucleus to the periphery. Liver function tests are usually only minimally deranged.

Granulomatous hepatitis

This is described in Chapter 5.40.

Phospholipidosis

Phospholipids accumulates in liver cell lysosomes. The major associated drugs, perhexiline and amiodarone, are cationic, amphiphilic compounds that accumulate within the liver cell lysosomes, where they form complexes with phospholipids. Accumulation can be detected by immunohistochemistry or electron microscopy. The extent to which these complexes accumulate in patients without toxicity remains uncertain.

Non-alcohol steatohepatitis syndrome (see also Chapter 5.35)

Long-term treatment with perhexiline, amiodarone, diltiazem and nifedipine may be associated with a syndrome clinically and histologically identical to alcoholic hepatitis. There may be hepatomegaly, jaundice, ascites, and encephalopathy.

Fibrotic and vascular disease (Table 8)

Perisinusoidal fibrosis

Collagen accumulates within the space of Disse. This may be asymptomatic or lead to hepatomegaly and portal hypertension. The most

Table 9 Malignant hepatic tumours associated with drugs

Hepatocellular carcinoma	*Angiosarcoma*
Anabolic/androgenic steroids	Anabolic/androgenic steroids
Oral contraceptive	Arsenicals
Thorium dioxide	Thorium dioxide
Cholangiocarcinoma	
Thorium dioxide	

common drug causes are large doses of vitamin A given for prolonged periods, or methotrexate. In the former, the liver shows hyperplasia of the Ito cell as a consequence of vitamin A accumulation. Serum concentrations of vitamin A may be normal, even in the presence of marked liver damage.

Peliosis hepatitis

This is a histological diagnosis characterized by blood-filled cavities, bordered by hepatocytes, which may be distributed throughout the liver. The major drugs involved are the anabolic steroids, androgenic steroids, azathioprine, vinyl chloride, and pyrazolide derivatives. The condition is often asymptomatic.

Hepatic venous damage

The Budd–Chiari syndrome may be associated with the use of oral contraceptives and some antineoplastic drugs such as dacarbazine, doxorubicin, and cyclophosphamide. Obstruction of the small veins leads to hepatic veno-occlusive disease, initially described in association with ingestion of the pyrrolizidine alkaloids present in Senecio plants but also seen in patients treated with immunosuppression, especially with organ transplantation.

Hepatic tumours (see also Chapter 5.38)

Hepatocellular adenoma has been associated with the use of oral contraceptives and anabolic steroids. Hepatocellular carcinoma is also associated with the anabolic and androgenic steroids, oral contraceptives, and thorium dioxide. Although the risk of malignancy increases with the prolonged use of oral contraceptives, up to eightfold after 8 years, the overall risk is extremely small. Angiosarcomas and cholangiosarcomas may also be related to drugs, although the association is less clear-cut (Table 9)

Chronic disease

Cirrhosis and chronic hepatitis

Some of the drugs associated with the development of cirrhosis and chronic hepatitis are listed in Table 10.

Intrahepatic chronic cholestasis

In some instances of drug-related cholestasis such as that associated with Augmentin or flucloxacillin, jaundice or cholestatic liver function tests persist for 6 months or more (Table 11), and some drugs may be associated with a chronic vanishing bile-duct syndrome, which may be indistinguishable from primary biliary cirrhosis. A syndrome virtually identical to primary sclerosing cholangitis can be induced by infusion into the hepatic artery of floxuridine for the treatment of intrahepatic malignancy. A vanishing bile-duct syndrome has been associated with carbamazepine, thiobendazole, flucloxacillin, haloperidol, ajmaline, cyproheptidine, and chlorpromazine. There has been a suggestion that primary biliary cirrhosis is associated with the use of benoxaprofen.

Table 10 Main drugs causing subacute hepatitis, chronic hepatitis, or cirrhosis

Acetohexamide	Methotrexate
Amiodarone	Methyldopa
Amodiaquine	Nicotinic acid
Aspirin	Nitrofurantoin
Benzarone	Oxyphenisatin
Busulphan	Perhexiline
Chlorambucil	Propylthiouracil
Cimetidine	Tienilic acid
Clometacin	Urethrane
Dantrolene	Valproate
Diclofenac	Isoniazid
Iproniazid	Vitamin A

Table 11 Causes of chronic cholestasis

Phenothiazines	*Sulphonylureas*
Especially chlorpromazine	Carbutamide, tolbutamide
Tricyclic antidepressants	*Antimicrobials*
Amitriptyline, imipramine	Cloxacillin, dicloxacillin, flucloxacillin
Sex steroids	*Others*
Methyl testosterone, norandrosterone	Arsenicals, cyproheptidine, haloperidol, thiobendazole, troleandomycin, piroxicam

Further reading

Danan, G. (1990). Consensus meeting. Criteria of drug induced liver disorders. *Journal of Hepatology*, **11**, 272–6.

Lewis, J. and Zimmerman, H. (1989). Drug induced liver disease. *Medical Clinics of North America*, 73, 775–96.

Sherlock, S. and Dooley, J. (1997). *Diseases of the liver and biliary system*. Blackwell Science, Oxford.

Chapter 5.42

Miscellaneous disorders of the gastrointestinal tract and liver

D. P. Jewell

Cystic disorders of the bowel

There are a variety of disorders of the small and large bowel associated with cyst formation. All of them are rare and present major diagnostic and therapeutic problems.

Colitis cystica

Colitis cystica superficialis occurs in patients with pellagra and has also been reported in adult coeliac disease. The presenting feature is usually diarrhoea and the condition is characterized by the presence of small mucus-filled cysts that lie superficially to the muscular layer of the colon. The disease seems to respond to therapy for pellagra. In colitis cystica profunda the cysts occur below the muscular layer of the colon. It is usually characterized by cramping lower abdominal pain, tenesmus, and diarrhoea associated with blood and mucus in the stools. The diagnosis is made by sigmoidoscopy, rectal biopsy, and barium enema examinations. Treatment consists of local surgical excision.

Pneumatosis cystoides intestinalis

This disorder is characterized by the presence of multiple, gas-filled cysts in the wall of the colon and, less frequently, the small intestine. The stomach and mesentery may also rarely be affected. The condition is usually seen in middle-aged patients and may be associated with obstructive airways disease or pyloric obstruction. It has also been found in association with mesenteric vascular disease, small bowel tumours, and Whipple's disease, following small bowel surgery, and after sigmoidoscopy or colonoscopy.

Pneumatosis cystoides can be an incidental finding during radiological examination of the abdomen. However, it can present with lower abdominal pain, recurrent diarrhoea, rectal bleeding, tenesmus, and obstructive symptoms. The cysts can frequently be detected at sigmoidoscopy and rectal biopsy specimens may show the characteristic giant cells that frequently line the cyst walls. Double-contrast radiology is the best method to establish the diagnosis but computed tomography scans may detect serosal or mesenteric cysts.

If the patient has no abdominal symptoms, no treatment is necessary. For symptomatic patients, The most effective therapy is oxygen, 60–70 per cent given by a face mask or a nasal catheter. Hyperbaric oxygen may rarely be indicated. The aim is to wash out the nitrogen from the cysts and replace it with oxygen, which can be resorbed, with collapse of the cysts. Other treatments include metronidazole, a low-carbohydrate diet, and an elemental diet. Surgical resection may be necessary for patients who do not respond and for those with severe obstructive symptoms, especially if there is a suspicion of volvulus.

Microscopic and collagenous colitis

Collagenous colitis usually present in the fifth and sixth decade, mostly in women, but can occur in young adults as well as in the elderly. A watery diarrhoea accompanied by abdominal cramps, wind, distension, and nausea are the usual symptoms. The diarrhoea can be severe and is often secretory in nature. There may be mucus but bleeding is not a feature. Despite severe symptoms, these patients are usually well, with a good appetite, and they do not lose weight. There are no abnormal physical signs and, on sigmoidoscopy, the rectal mucosa is hyperaemic with some oedema and granularity. These changes occur throughout the colon but are usually patchy and never severe. The diagnosis is made on a colonic biopsy. There is a thickened band of subepithelial collagen exceeding 12 μm compared with the normal thickness of 2–6 μm. It is of maximal thickness in the right colon and tends to become thinner more distally—there may rectal sparing, which may lead to misdiagnosis if only the rectum is biopsied. There is a patchy and variable inflammatory infiltrate in the lamina propria. The disease is confined to the colon and does not extend into the ileum. It is therefore a separate entity to collagenous sprue.

Microscopic colitis shares the same clinical features but the mucosa always looks normal at colonoscopy. Nevertheless, histological examination shows a diffuse inflammatory infiltrate throughout the lamina propria with no architectural changes of the glands. A characteristic feature is the marked increase in intraepithelial lymphocytes, which clearly separates this disease from ulcerative colitis. This feature has led some clinicians to use the term 'lymphocytic colitis'. A microscopic colitis can be seen in some patients with untreated coeliac disease and others receiving non-steroidal anti-inflammatory drugs. These possibilities need to be excluded before the diagnosis of microscopic colitis can be made.

Both disorders have a variable clinical course and the symptoms can spontaneously remit and relapse. Treatment is difficult. Antidiarrhoeal agents, such as loperamide, should be used initially but, if no response is seen, then 5-aminosalicylic acid compounds or oral corticosteroids can be tried. If symptoms persist, dietary exclusion and an elemental diet are sometimes helpful. Other treatments tried include metronidazole, cholestyramine, and mepacrine.

Many of these patients are labelled as having an irritable bowel syndrome. Neither disease progresses to a frank ulcerative colitis.

Intramural bleeding

The most common cause is anticoagulant therapy. Occasionally, intramural haematomas form in patients with coagulation defects such as haemophilia or in conditions such as vasculitis. The usual presentation is with abdominal pain and symptoms of intestinal obstruction and bleeding. The diagnosis is made by barium examination and the condition can usually be treated conservatively with blood replacement and, if necessary, nasogastric suction.

Endometriosis

Intestinal involvement is most common in those parts of the bowel adjacent to the uterus and fallopian tubes, particularly the rectosigmoid colon. The mucosa of the bowel is seldom penetrated and therefore gastrointestinal bleeding is unusual. If the rectosigmoid region is involved, there may be cyclic pains in the rectum and, occasionally, mild diarrhoea and tenesmus. Implants in the small intestine may produce symptoms of obstruction or volvulus. However, endometriosis affecting the intestine is frequently asymptomatic and many of the symptoms attributed to this condition are more often caused by an irritable bowel syndrome.

The diagnosis requires a thorough pelvic examination to demonstrate tender nodules in the rectosigmoid region or in the rectovaginal area, but ultimately depends on biopsy. Laparoscopy is often helpful. The differentiation from carcinoma may be difficult and when in doubt surgical exploration should be carried out.

The management of this condition requires expert gynaecological help, but mild symptoms are probably best managed by analgesics and sedation. More severe cases may require hormonal therapy (danazole, gestrinone, or gonadorelin analogues).

Malakoplakia

This is a rare granulomatous disease involving the urinary tract and occasionally the colon or stomach. Histologically the condition is characterized by the presence of histiocytes containing dark inclusions that are periodic acid-Schiff positive and seem to contain both calcium and iron. Colonic malakoplakia is usually found as an incidental finding in elderly debilitated individuals, quite often in association with a malignant disease of the colon. Occasionally it presents as a systemic illness with fever, diarrhoea, and other gastrointestinal symptoms. It can only be diagnosed by histological examination of the bowel. There is no effective treatment.

Isolated ulcers of the large intestine

Caecal ulcers can present with abdominal pain, either acute or chronic, and may be a cause of an acute abdomen. Laparotomy may show perforation or local abscess formation. More commonly, they present with bleeding. Similar ulcers may occur elsewhere in the colon, especially at the flexures.

Solitary rectal ulcer syndrome is usually found in young adults, mostly in women, but can arise at any age. The ulcers are most commonly on the anterior wall, can be multiple and can be sufficiently extensive to encircle most of the rectum. There may be an associated anterior-mucosal prolapse. Symptoms include rectal bleeding, tenesmus, and abdominal and rectal pain. Many of these patients have a history of constipation and straining. The ulcer usually has a greyish base, but, there may be just an area of inflamed mucosa or the ulcer can be a polypoid lesion simulating a carcinoma. In either case, a biopsy should allow the correct diagnosis. Histologically, there is often evidence of ischaemia but the characteristic feature is hypertrophy of the muscularis mucosae with smooth-muscle fibres extending between the crypts towards the epithelium. There may be considerable fibrosis.

Treatment is often difficult. Correction of constipation is important and patients should be warned not to strain. Topical treatment with 5-aminosalicylic acid or corticosteroids may be helpful but there are no controlled data to confirm their efficacy. For patients with continuing and disabling symptoms, anorectal physiological measurements should be made because there may be evidence of denervation of the pelvic-floor muscles. A defecating proctogram should also be obtained to demonstrate whether the anorectal angle changes when the patient attempts to empty the rectum and to record the degree of mucosal prolapse. Surgical therapy such as an anterior and posterior rectopexy may be helpful.

Stercoral ulcers occur in association with faecal impaction and are most commonly found in the sigmoid–rectal area. Most patients are elderly but they can occur in any patient who is severely constipated. The common symptoms are nausea, abdominal distension and pain, anorexia—and there may be overflow incontinence. The ulcers are frequently asymptomatic but may be a cause of anaemia from chronic blood loss. They are normally revealed because of an acute bleed or a perforation. Treatment of these acute complications requires surgery but, otherwise, the ulcers are treated by relieving the faecal impaction.

Acute colonic pseudo-obstruction (Ogilvie's syndrome)

This syndrome describes a massive and acute dilatation of the caecum and right colon in the absence of organic obstruction or inflammatory disease of the colon. It may occur following intra-abdominal surgery, but can also happen in any sick patient. Most patients have a constant, rather dull pain with marked abdominal distension and they frequently vomit. There is constipation but usually patients continue to pass wind and some may actually have diarrhoea. On examination, there is a distended and tympanitic abdomen that is tender to the point of mild rebound tenderness. Bowel sounds are variable but are rarely absent. The diagnosis is made on a plain radiograph of the abdomen.

The danger is that of a colonic perforation if treatment is not instituted immediately. Intravenous fluids and electrolytes are given together with nasogastric suction. Any drugs that might be implicated (e.g. tricyclic antidepressants, anticholinergics) are stopped. Rectal tubes and enemas are often used but their value is dubious. If the dilatation does not resolve, decompression can sometimes be achieved by colonoscopy but as it is dangerous to prepare the colon the procedure is difficult. Surgical decompression with a caecostomy may be needed, which may be accompanied by resection if there is an obviously ischaemic segment of colon.

Melanosis coli and related disorders

Melanosis coli results from the presence of dark pigment in large mononuclear cells or macrophages in the lamina propria of the mucosa. The condition is thought to result from faecal stasis and the use of anthraquinone cathartics such as cascara or senna. Chronic cathartic abuse may also cause radiological changes of the colon characterized by loss of haustral markings and appearances resembling multiple strictures. These changes have to be distinguished from those of ulcerative colitis, Crohn's disease, and other inflammatory bowel diseases.

Miscellaneous vascular disorders of the liver

Acute cardiac failure and shock

Reduced hepatic blood flow causes ischaemia primarily in the centrilobular area, and may cause necrosis there. Deranged liver function tests may result and in severe causes, jaundice.

Chronic venous congestion

A persistently elevated central venous pressure results in hepatic venous congestion and hepatomegaly. The associated histological changes are of centrilobular congestion with surrounding fatty change ('nutmeg liver'). If the disorder is long standing, there may be progressive fibrosis extending peripherally from centrilobular to portal areas. The serum bilirubin level is usually increased and there may be a slight elevation in the serum alkaline phosphatase and in the transaminases. True cirrhosis of the liver with regenerative nodules is very rare, as is portal hypertension; it is very unusual to find oesophageal varices in patients with cardiac cirrhosis.

Hepatic arterial occlusion

This rare condition usually follows surgical trauma but has been found in association with arteritis and bacterial endocarditis. There is an acute onset of pain in the upper abdomen, tenderness over the liver, and progressive shock and liver failure. Most cases have a fatal outcome.

Septic venous thrombosis of the portal system

This results from infection anywhere in the abdominal cavity leading to pylephlebitis of the portal venous system. It may occasionally result from a systemic septicaemia or from inflammatory disorders of the bowel. The acute phase has features related to the underlying abdominal sepsis. This is followed by high fever, worsening abdominal pain, and rigors. There may be obvious evidence of septic embolization to the liver, with abdominal pain and hepatic tenderness with mild jaundice. Occasionally, multiple large intrahepatic abscesses may develop. The condition should be suspected in any patient with abdominal sepsis who develops an acute systemic illness with abdominal pain and deranged liver tests. Management consists of intensive antibiotic treatment directed particularly towards Gram-negative organisms and micro-aerophilic streptococci. In some patients portal venous thrombosis may develop.

Protein-losing enteropathy

Rarely, hypoproteinaemia may result from excessive loss of plasma proteins into the gastrointestinal tract. All plasma proteins are affected; those showing the greatest reduction in concentration are the ones with the longest half-lives, including albumin. The resulting oedema is largely due to the low albumin. This is an important condition to recognize because the oedema or ascites may overshadow the intestinal symptoms and hence the underlying conditions are easily missed. These include a wide variety of inflammatory or neoplastic disorders of the small bowel and abdominal lymphatic system, and allergic disorders involving the small bowel. Severe protein loss occurs mainly in lymphatic disorders and in Ménètriér's disease, a curious condition characterized by the presence of giant gastric rugae.

The diagnosis is made by determining the rate of loss of protein into the intestine using a radioactive label, usually, ^{51}Cr albumin, or ^{67}Cu-labelled caeruloplasmin. The proportion of radioactivity in the stool is measured during the succeeding 4 days; 0.7 per cent is taken as the upper limit of normal. Alternatively, measurements of α_1-antitrypsin in the stool has been shown to be a useful marker of protein-losing enteropathy, without necessitating radioactive labelling. Treatment is directed towards raising the plasma albumin and correction of the underlying disorder.

Jejunoileal bypass

The majority of patients with massive obesity have fatty infiltration of the liver. Following jejunoileal bypass, 55 per cent of them show further fatty change due entirely to an accumulation of triglyceride. There is frequently a mild elevation of liver enzymes in serum. Acute liver failure may develop in a few patients and is associated with considerable mortality. It is thought to be due to bacterial colonization of the included and excluded small intestine with the production of 'hepatotoxins', which are then absorbed. Treatment consists of intravenous amino acids and broad-spectrum antibiotics. If the condition recurs, the ileal bypass must be reversed.

A micronodular cirrhosis may develop 1–6 years after a bypass. The liver often shows appearances similar to those induced by alcohol. If liver function deteriorates, small bowel continuity should be restored. Patients may still progress to liver failure and death, but there are reports of the cirrhosis arresting or even reversing.

Parenteral nutrition and the liver

Abnormalities of serum liver enzymes and bilirubin are commonly seen in patients receiving total parenteral nutrition (see Chapter 8.4).

Further reading

Adibi, B.A. and Stanko, RT. (1984). Perspective on gastro-intestinal surgery for the treatment of morbid obesity: The lesson learned. *Gastroenterology*, **87**, 1381.

Dockerty, M.B. (1972). Primary malakoplakia of the colon. *Mayo Clinic Proceedings*, **47**, 114.

Sherlock, S. and Dooley, J. (1997). *Diseases of the liver and biliary system.* Blackwell Science, Oxford.

Section 6
Metabolic disorders

Contents

Chapter 6.1

The inborn errors of metabolism: general aspects

R. W. E. Watts

There are between three and four thousand known unifactorially inherited diseases, the inheritance of which is largely Medelian and results from mutations in the DNA. A small number of mitochondrial proteins have their structures encoded in the mitochondrial DNA so that genetic information for them is passed on from generation to generation in a non-Mendelian manner, being transmitted only through the female line. This arises because the spermatozoal cytoplasm, including its mitochondria, is entirely lost at fertilization. Both the Mendelian and the mitochondrially inherited diseases stem from single mutations within a cistron (the functional unit of DNA) which directs the synthesis of a single specific polypeptide. Among them are the inborn errors of metabolism in which the mutation affects a protein with a metabolic function such that a characteristic clinical and biochemical phenotype results, and in which the metabolic lesion can be identified.

Heterogeneity in the inborn errors of metabolism

The individual inborn errors of metabolism are defined on the basis of the phenotype, including the specific enzyme lesion, and by their pattern of inheritance. Close study of any particular inborn error of metabolism reveals unexpected heterogeneity. This is due to: (1) multiple allelism; (2) mutations at different gene loci affecting the structure of different polypeptide chains in a single enzyme protein; (3) mutations at different gene loci affecting different proteins with similar catalytic functions; (4) differences in the overall genetic background against which the single mutation acts; and (5) environmental factors. Early diagnosis and management lies in the field of paediatrics, but only those disorders which reach the care of the adult physician are discussed in detail here. Further information can be found in OTM3 and other standard texts.

Carrier state diagnosis

In relation to the inherited diseases, a carrier is defined as: 'An individual, who possesses, in the heterozygous state, the gene determining an inherited disorder, and who is essentially healthy at the time of study'. This includes individuals carrying the gene for a recessive disorder (e.g. phenylketonuria) and those carrying the gene for a dominant disorder, but in which symptoms occur in later life (e.g. Huntington's chorea).

The general approaches to carrier state diagnosis are: (1) the detection of minor clinical, radiological, and clinicopathological abnormalities; (2) the demonstration of levels of enzyme activity in tissue which are intermediate between those observed in individuals homozygous for the abnormal and the normal forms of the enzyme respectively; (3) the demonstration of intermediate levels of a characteristic metabolite in an accessible body fluid; (4) the demonstration of mosaicism with respect to the product of the mutant x-linked gene in the case of sex-linked recessive disorders; and (5) direct gene analysis using either a specific gene probe or a linked restriction fragment length polymorphism (RFLP).

The rapidly expanding use of gene sequencing in medicine has demonstrated the breadth of molecular heterogeneity at the DNA level in what are regarded as homogeneous single gene defects. Although this may help to explain phenotypic heterogeneity, it adversely affects the value of the method for carrier detection unless the number of mutations that produce the disease is small, ideally unity, or unless the number of mutations that produce the disease is small, ideally unity, or unless the specific mutation that causes the disease in a particular family is known from genomic DNA analysis of the index case.

Chapter 6.2

Glycogen storage diseases

T. M. Cox

Defects in the enzymatic steps for the synthesis, utilization, degradation or glycogen lead to its pathological storage. Accumulation of glycogen may be generalized or involve certain tissues selectively; the glycogen may then have a normal or aberrant structure.

Glycogen metabolism

The individual enzymatic steps for the formation and breakdown of glycogen are summarized in Fig. 1 and discussed in OTM3 (pp. 1339–41). Table 1 indicates the enzymes involved in specific diseases.

Glycogen synthesis

Inherited deficiency of glycogen synthase activity is associated with reduced storage of liver glycogen and fasting hypoglycaemia. Branching enzyme activity is essential for the formation of the compact spherical molecules of glycogen especially in liver. It transfers a minimum of six α-1,4-linked glucose units from the distal ends of glycogen chains to a 1,6 position on the same or a neighbouring chain. Deficiency of branching enzyme leads to the accumulation of abnormal molecules that are partially resistant to degradation.

Glycogen breakdown

Debranching enzyme cleaves the unique glucosyl-tyrosine linkage that anchors the terminal reducing glucose unit to glycogenin. Deficiency of debranching enzyme leads to the storage of glycogen that possesses short outer chains, 'limit dextrin'.

Glucose 6-phosphatase exists as a multicomponent complex in the endoplasmic reticulum of hepatocytes and, to a lesser extent, renal tubular cells—it is not found in muscle. The system contains glucose 6-phosphatase, several proteins that facilitate transport of glucose, glucose 6-phosphate, and phosphate, as well as other stabilizing and regulatory moieties. Several genetic defects in this compartmentalized system affect overall glucose 6-phosphatase activity: they are associated with severe hypoglycaemia, metabolic acidosis, and hepatic disease.

Glucose 6-phosphate obtained from the breakdown of glycogen in skeletal muscle is used directly in glycolysis. Defects of muscle phosphorylase lead to a defective supply of adenosine triphosphate (ATP), especially during ischaemic exercise. There is a failure of conversion of glycogen to lactate, and exercise-induced muscle cramps

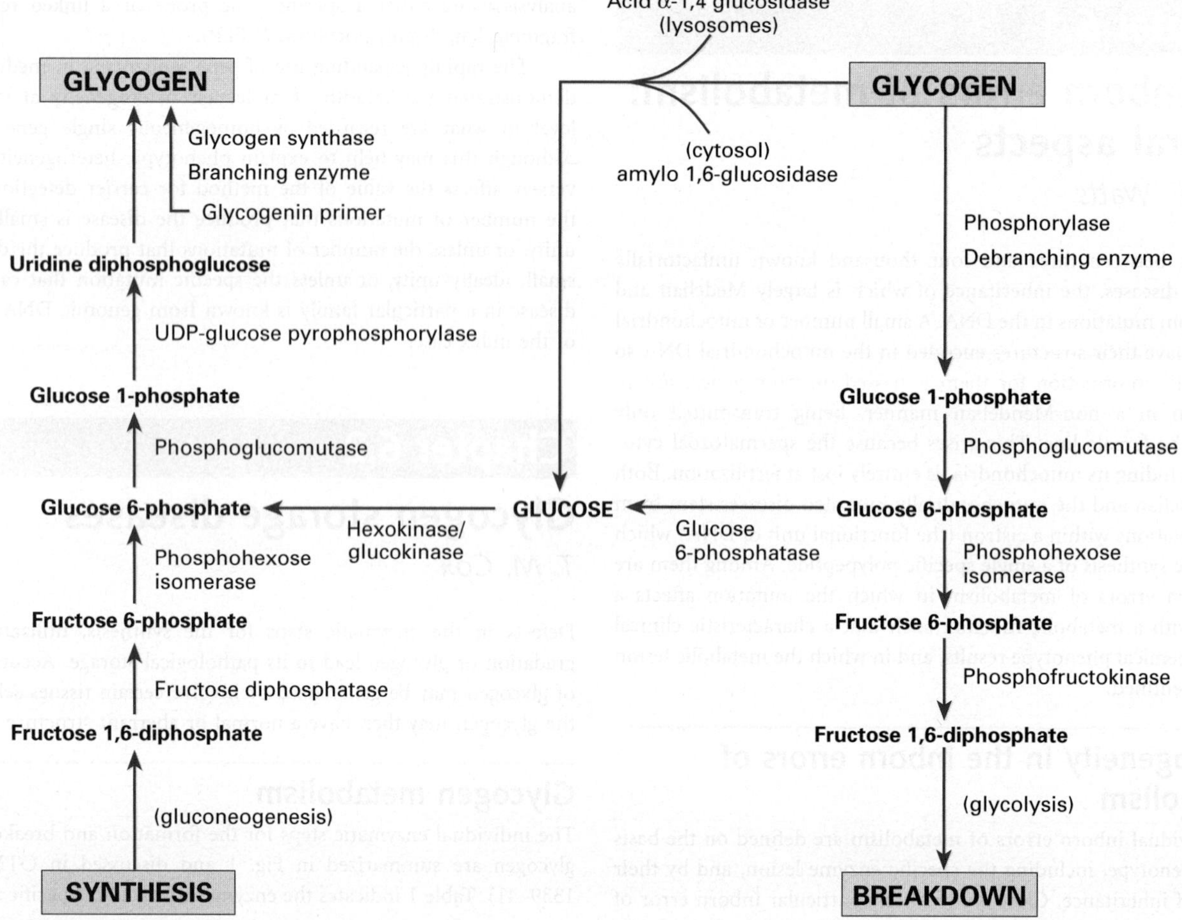

Fig. 1 The synthesis and degradation of glycogen.

reflect mild muscle necrosis with increased accumulation of glycogen. Phosphofructokinase-1 catalyses an irreversible step in the glycolytic pathway and is a key regulatory enzyme. Inherited defects that render it inactive or affect its positive allosteric regulation by the effectors AMP and fructose 2,6-diphosphate resemble muscle phosphorylase deficiency. Because deficiency of phosphofructokinase affects the metabolism of endogenous glycogen as well as carbon units derived from extracellular glucose, the symptoms of phosphofructokinase-1 deficiency are more severe and of earlier onset than muscle phosphorylase deficiency. As expected, glucose 6-phosphate, fructose 6-phosphate, and glycogen, accumulate in the muscle cells.

Breakdown of glycogen in liver and skeletal muscle is brought about by the concerted activities of phosphorylase and debranching enzyme in the cytoplasm. Phosphorylase is activated by phosphorylation in response to hormonal or neural stimulation—a complex process that is mediated by phosphorylase kinases. Phosphorylase kinase is a multisubunit protein with regulatory, catalytic, and calcium-binding subunits that are encoded on separate genes. Separate isoforms are found in liver and muscle. The final common pathways for the regulation of phosphorylase kinase involve protein kinase A (cAMP-dependent protein kinase), calcium and kinase activation of calmodulin, and protein phosphatases 1 and 2A. Another enzyme, acid α-1,4-glucosidase, has an important role in the metabolism of glycogen. This lysosomal hydrolase is present in all cells except erythrocytes and, although it has no relation to glycolysis, its deficiency causes a generalized disorder in which muscle disease, especially of the heart, is usually severe. Deficiency of acid α-glucosidase is associated with rapidly progressive cardiac hypertrophy with hepatic enlargement and generalized muscle weakness. Skeletal muscle symptoms may be prominent in patients with the infantile or late-onset forms of this condition, but disease progression is usually rapid except in older adults. Acid α-1,4 glucosidase deficiency was the first inborn lysosomal disease to be clearly recognized and represents a prototype for the other storage diseases: intracellular vesicles containing glycogen represent lysosomes distended by an undegradable substrate that accumulates as a result of autophagy. The accumulation of glycogen in lysosomes indicates that glycogen fragments are constantly being synthesized and taken up for degradation.

Diagnosis of glycogen storage disease

In the liver

The diagnosis may be suspected in infants and children with hepatomegaly, growth retardation, and hypoglycaemia, which is not invariable. In many cases a glucagon stimulation test (20 μg/kg intramuscularly) fails to induce the normal (> 2 mmol/l) rise in blood glucose, but, for prognosis, future antenatal diagnosis and to direct treatment, definitive diagnosis by biopsy is warranted. Direct assay of liver tissue for glycogen and fat content as well as enzymatic analysis is desirable. Histochemical and electron microscopic study of glycogen structure provides useful additional information. Where

Table 1 Diseases of glycogen storage

Designation number	Enzymatic defect	Affected tissues	Principal manifestations	Diagnostic tissue
von Gierke's disease (Cori Type I)	Glucose 6-phosphatase[a]	Liver, kidney	Usually severe: liver and kidney enlargement	Liver Intestinal mucosa
			Hypoglycaemia, acidosis, bleeding tendency, growth failure, hyperlipidaemia, hyperuricaemia	
Pompe's disease (Type II)	Acid α-1,4-glucosidase (lysosomal)	Generalized especially heart, muscles and liver.	Usually severe: adult cases (mild) generalized hypotonia, cardiomegaly, weakness, and arrhythmias	Liver, muscle, myocardium, fibroblasts leucocytes, amniotic fluid cells
			Mild cases respond to high-protein diet	
Forbes–Cori disease or limit dextrinosis (Type III)	Debranching enzyme	Liver and usually muscle[b]	Often mild: hepatomegaly, hypoglycaemia, progressive muscle weakness in adults. Ketosis – lactic acidosis and hyperuricaemia absent	Liver, (muscle), fibroblasts, amniotic fluid cells
Andersen's disease or amylopectinosis (Type IV)	Branching enzyme	Liver.[b] Rare variant, polyglucosan disease, affects peripheral nerves[b]	Severe: hepatosplenomegaly in infancy; death from cirrhosis and portal hypertension. Polyglucosan variant affects adults	Liver, leucocytes, (peripheral nerves)
McArdle's disease (Type V)	Muscle phosphorylase	Skeletal muscle	Exercise-induced muscle cramps	Muscle (lactate production absent)
Hers' disease (Type VI)	Liver phosphorylase	Liver	Moderate to severe hepatomegaly with hypoglycaemia in childhood	Liver, leucocytes
Tarui's disease (Type VII)	Muscle phosphofructokinase	Muscle, red cells	Marked weakness and stiffness after exertion, haemolytic anaemia	Erythrocyte, muscle
			(Glucose 6-phosphate and fructose 6-phosphate also accumulate)	(Lactate production absent)
Type VIII	Unknown	Liver, brain	Very rare. Hepatomegaly. Progressive neural degeneration and death in childhood	Liver/brain
Type IX	Phosphorylase b kinase	Liver	Mild hepatomegaly. Variable hypoglycaemia. Sex-linked and autosomal recessive forms.	Liver, leucocytes
Type O	Glycogen synthase	Liver	Very rare. Severe fasting hypoglycaemia: seizures before feeds. Failure of glucagon response. Reduced or absent glycogen	Liver
	Phosphoglucoisomerase	Red cells	Very rare. Haemolytic anaemia. Excess glycogen in liver and erythrocytes	Red cells
	Lactate dehydrogenase	Muscle	Resembles McArdle's disease. Very rare.	Muscle
	Phosphoglycerate kinase	Muscle	Resembles McArdle's disease. Very rare.	Muscle
	Lactate dehydrogenase	Muscle	Resembles McArdle's disease. Very rare.	Muscle

[a]Designations beyond Type V are extensions of Cori's classification; beyond Type VII they are controversial.

[b]Several defects described in components of the glucose 6-phosphatase system (see text). NB. Enzyme activity may be normal in tissue after freeze-thawing.

[c]Abnormal glycogen structure – total glycogen concentration may be normal.

possible, open wedge-biopsy of the liver should be carried out to obtain sufficient material for diagnosis and ensure haemostasis.

The histological diagnosis of certain variants of Type I glycogen storage disease requires fresh tissue since analysis of freeze-thawed material disrupts the integrity of the microsomal enzyme system and, by rendering it permeable to glucose 6-phosphate, overcomes the biochemical lesion (see OTM3, p.1341.) Thus, where defects of glycogen storage are suspected, it is essential to seek the prior advice of a laboratory that is competent to carry out the appropriate investigations using fresh and deep-frozen biopsy material.

In muscle

Forearm exercise tests are useful for detecting defects in skeletal muscles that interfere with the metabolic pathway from glucose and glycogen to lactate. In the absence of oxygen, glycolysis is the sole means by which ATP may be generated and glucosyl units derived from glycogen, rather than glucose obtained from the plasma, is the preferred energy source. Defects in glycolysis (glycogenosis type VII and other enzyme deficiencies) cause similar symptoms. Exercise-induced cramps may occur in the purine pathway disorder, myoadenylate deaminase deficiency, which may be also diagnosed safely by exercise testing. Unlike the earlier test devised by McArdle these provocative tests do not induce rhabdomyolysis.

After 30 min rest, blood is taken from the antecubital vein of the non-exercising arm and a small sphygmomanometer cuff placed around the other wrist is inflated to 200 mmHg. A second standard cuff around the upper arm to be tested is inflated to mean arterial pressure and the patient squeezes as powerfully as possible 120 times over 2 min. Immediately afterwards, the second cuff is inflated to 200 mmHg. Blood is drawn through a needle placed in the antecubital vein of the exercising arm 2 min after completing the exercise and the upper cuff is released. To complete the test, five further samples are drawn at 1-min intervals. The samples are transported rapidly to the laboratory for analysis of lactate and ammonia. Reduced or absent generation of lactate is characteristic of glycogenolytic and glycolytic defects that affect muscle; in contrast, plasma levels of ammonia (as well as inosine and hypoxanthine) increase greatly in patients with glycogenosis types III, V, and VIII. These abnormalities reflect excessive degradation of purines that occurs in the exercising muscles of patients in whom there is a disturbance of ATP generation. Measurement of ammonia release as well as lactate production also adds discriminatory value to the exercise test, as it controls for low levels of lactate release that result merely from inadequate exercise during performance of the test. The test also may identify myoadenylate kinase deficiency: in such patients lactate production is normal but failure to utilize the purine cycle to conserve intracellular nucleotides and provide alternative substrates for energy production, is shown by the failure of venous ammonia concentrations to rise.

Pompe's disease is a generalized disorder that predominantly affects skeletal and cardiac muscle. Carbohydrate metabolism is otherwise normal and phosphorylysis of cytosolic glycogen in the liver is sufficient to maintain euglycaemia. The diagnosis may be suspected on the basis of cardiac and liver enlargement in an infant with respiratory distress and hypotonia. Macroglossia is frequent and the electrocardiogram shows left axis deviation, a short P-R interval and broad QRS complexes. In adults proximal weakness occurs in the limb girdles—associated with wasting and later, swelling and breathing difficulties. Muscle enzyme activities e.g. LDH and creatine kinase are usually elevated in the serum. Myopathic changes—occasionally with pseudomyotonic discharges—are observed on electromyography and the diagnosis is revealed by biopsy, which shows vacuolar myopathy and massive deposits of glycogen in and between myofibrils. Under the electron microscope, free and lysosomal α-glycogen particles are observed. Enzymatic deficiency of acid α-1,4-glucosidase is readily confirmed in cultured amniocytes and all tissues except erythrocytes.

Definitive diagnosis of muscle glycogenoses depends on biopsy with histochemical, ultrastructural, and biochemical analyses. Biopsy should be carried out after liaison with the laboratory so that, if necessary, tissue can be stored frozen for further study and enzymatic analysis. Biopsy and electromyography may be needed to differentiate suspected glycogen storage diseases from other myopathies including Duchenne's dystrophy, Kugelberg-Welander disease, dystrophia myotonica, and mitochondrial and secondary disorders of muscle such as polymyositis.

Individual glycogen storage diseases

The main features of these disorders are surveyed and summarized in Table 1. Brief accounts of selected conditions are set out below.

von Gierke's disease

Glucose formation from glycogen and gluconeogenesis is defective and affected infants develop hypoglycaemia on fasting or as a result of intercurrent infection or other stress. The liver is enlarged at birth. It contains excess glycogen and shows gross infiltration with fat but cirrhosis and portal hypertension are rare. In contrast, growth retardation often combined with obesity, is common. The kidneys are enlarged by glycogen deposition. Progressive focal glomerulosclerosis and proximal tubular failure with a secondary Fanconi syndrome may also occur. Stress and starvation provoke acidotic attacks with marked lactic acidaemia. Poor metabolic control causes growth arrest; hyperuricaemia and gout; marked hypertriglyceridaemia and hypercholesterolaemia with raised VLDL and normal LDL cholesterol concentrations in the plasma and prolonged bleeding time related to an acquired von Willebrand-like defect affecting the platelets. Patients with defects of the glucose 6-phosphate translocase system (type 1B) are prone to bacterial infection: there is neutropenia and neutrophil migration and chemotaxis are impaired. These patients may develop episodes of severe diarrhoea in association with granulomatous infiltration of the colonic mucosa. Partial deficiencies of the glucose 6-phosphatase system lead to variable clinical expression and subtypes of Type I glycogen storage disease have been demonstrated in patients presenting with glucagon-unresponsive hypoglycaemia with or without liver enlargement in adult life. Adult patients or children with uncontrolled disease develop hepatic adenomas; frank hepatocellular carcinomata occur.

Metabolic disturbance

Hypoglycaemia in von Gierke's disease is often asymptomatic and tolerance of it improves with increasing age. Residual production of glucose probably occurs by lysosomal hydrolysis of glycogen and recycling through the glycogen synthase-debranching enzyme pathway, but metabolic adaptation of the brain, which can use lactate as an alternative substrate, is very important. Hypertriglyceridaemia is induced by increased provision of reduced nictotinamide adenine dinucleotide (NADH) and reduced nicotinamide adenine dinucleotide phosphate (NADPH), glycerol and acetyl-coenzyme A (CoA) because of enhanced flux through glycolysis and underutilization of gluconeogenic precursors. Malonyl-coenzyme A, derived from acetyl-coenzyme A, inhibits the carnitine acyltransferase system and blocks the oxidation of fatty acids; thus ketosis does not occur. Lactic acidaemia results from stimulation of glycolysis at the level of phosphofructokinase by high concentrations of glucose 6-phosphate (and hence fructose 6-phosphate). Lactate cannot be recycled in the liver to form new glucose and lactic acidosis results. Lactate competes with urate for excretory pathways in the kidney and thus contributes to the hyperuricaemia. Uric acid is also overproduced in the liver: it arises from degradation of purine nucleotides by adenosine monophosphate (AMP) deaminase. The deaminase is activated when the concentration of free phosphate falls as a result of sequestration in sugar phosphate esters.

Treatment

The main objective is to maintain euglycaemia: most of the other metabolic abnormalities are thereby corrected and the prognosis improves.

In later childhood and in adult patients, metabolic control can be maintained by the use of raw corn starch that serves as a source of glucose slowly released by hydrolysis. 1 to 2 g/kg is given orally every 4 to 6 h as a suspension in water.

In type Ib glycogen storage disease it is vital to avoid intercurrent infection, and prophylactic antimicrobial drugs may therefore be necessary. Patients with type Ia disease may require treatment for their bleeding tendency. The bleeding diathesis is associated with a qualitative defect of platelet function, prolonged bleeding time and reduced factor VIIIc and vW factor activities. These abnormalities and the haemorrhagic tendency respond to administration of 1-deamino-8-D-arginine vasopressin (DDAVP) at 0.3 μg/kg infused in 50 ml of saline over 30 min intravenously. Correction of the bleeding disorder lasts for several h and is useful for the treatment of bleeding after trauma or surgery.

Failure of metabolic control in type I glycogen storage disease appears to be associated with tissue complications: hepatic adenomata or malignant transformation, renal disease due to hyperfiltration, focal glomerulosclerosis, and postinfective scarring. Lately, an inflammatory disorder of the colon, resembling granulomatous colitis, has been recognized in type Ib disease. Long-term follow-up care with monitoring of biochemical parameters of kidney function and periodic ultrasonic examination of the liver is necessary. Continuing failure of growth, enlarging hepatic adenomata or progressive renal failure raise the question of organ transplantation. Several successful renal, as well as hepatic, allografts have been carried out in this condition using DDAVP infusions to control haemorrhage. However, as regression of most complications, including hepatic adenomata, can be achieved by strict dietary measures, transplantation should be reserved for patients in whom nutritional treatment has failed. Survival into adult life (and parenthood) can be now expected.

Type II glycogen storage disease

Pompe's disease is usually a rapidly-progressive disorder with effects on the heart, skeletal muscle, and nervous system. Affected children usually die within the first year or two of life and no measures (including bone marrow transplantation) other than supportive therapy are beneficial. In the mildly affected adult, progression may be very slow. Trials of enzyme-replacement therapy using recombinant acid α-glucosidase mannose-phosphate lysosomal recognition signal are under way and have been predicated on promising trials conducted in animal models of this disorder.

Type III glycogen storage disease

The clinical manifestations of Forbes-Cori's disease resemble Type I glycogenosis, especially in infants, who present with hypoglycaemia, short stature, and hepatomegaly. Mild progressive myopathy, occasionally with signs of hypertrophic cardiomyopathy, may occur. Generally the signs of liver disease regress during maturation and myopathy improves also with nutritional therapy as outlined for von Gierke's disease. Protein supplements, which may provide additional sources of energy, appear to benefit the muscle disorder.

Type IV glycogen storage disease

Deficiency of branching enzyme in Anderson's disease gives rise to the deposition of an abnormal glycogen in many tissues. Severe inflammation occurs in the liver, resulting in cirrhosis, with splenomegaly due to portal hypertension. This fatal disorder is characterized by failure to thrive, hepatosplenomegaly, jaundice, and hypotonia. Diagnosis is based on the appearances of the liver biopsy and abnormal glycogen structure shown by histochemical and biochemical analysis. Deficiency of branching enzyme is demonstrable in leucocytes. No definitive therapy is available but a few patients have survived hepatic transplantation without the development of neuromuscular or cardiac complications in up to 7 years after the procedure. Generally the prognosis is poor; most patients die before the age of 4 years with liver failure, variceal bleeding, and intercurrent infection.

Type V glycogen storage disease

This disorder is characterized by the late onset of muscle fatigue and cramps during adolescence or early adult life. Hepatomegaly is absent. Strenuous exercise may induce episodic myoglobinuria and biochemical evidence of rhabdomyolysis. Occasionally acute myoglobinuric renal failure may result. Muscle biopsy may show abnormal muscle fibres with necrosis, atrophy, and hypertrophied fibres alongside. The course of this disease is benign; ingestion of glucose or pre-exercise administration of glucagon may partially ameliorate the symptoms but avoidance of strenuous exercise is advisable.

Type VI glycogen storage disease and phosphorylase b kinase deficiency

These disorders cause hepatomegaly, intermittent hypoglycaemia, and markedly increased liver glycogen content. Although many polypeptides constitute the intact phosphorylase b kinase complex (encoded on autosomes and the X-chromosome), glycogen mobilization is usually only partially defective. X-linked phosphorylase b kinase deficiency is the most frequent variant and is associated with growth retardation, mild ketosis, and hyperlipidaemia in childhood. The symptoms improve with age and the disorder is compatible with a normal life expectancy. Cirrhosis of the liver is very rare and the incompleteness of the defect is shown by almost normal hyperglycaemic responses to glucagon administration. Rare autosomal variants of phosphorylase kinase deficiency affecting liver and muscle or restricted to skeletal or cardiac muscle have been documented. These subtypes are associated with hypotonia or cardiac failure, respectively. Treatment of liver phosphorylase or kinase deficiency with frequent feeding to avoid hypoglycaemia may be needed but the general prognosis is good so that intensive nutritional therapy is rarely indicated. No specific treatment for the isolated cardiac form of kinase deficiency is known but if the diagnosis can be established, cardiac transplantation could be considered.

Type VII glycogen storage disease

This disorder, which is most frequent in patients of Japanese or Russian Ashkenazi ancestry, closely resembles Type V muscle glycogenosis but severe symptoms usually come to light in childhood. There may be hyperuricaemia which is aggravated by exercise. Deficiency of red cell phosphofructokinase leads to chronic haemolysis. Decreased 2,3-diphosphoglycerate synthesis resulting from the metabolic block has been noted and probably contributes to exercise-induced symptoms by reducing oxygen delivery. No specific therapy for this disorder is known—in contrast to McArdle's disease, glucagon or glucose infusions do not improve exercise tolerance. Indeed, carbohydrate-rich meals aggravate the symptoms, presumably by diminishing the concentration of non-esterified fatty acids in plasma, which serve as the alternative source of muscle energy production. Several very rare variants of phosphofructokinase deficiency are known including a late-onset form which causes fixed muscle weakness in middle-aged subjects.

Glycogen synthase deficiency

Deficiency of glycogen synthase is very rare and causes deficiency of glycogen formation in the liver. It is, therefore, a disorder of storage rather than a true glycogenosis. The condition causes severe interprandial hypoglycaemia. Biopsy examination of the liver shows fatty infiltration and depletion of glycogen: uridine diphosphate-pyrophosphorylase, phosphorylase, glucose 6-phosphatase activities are normal but glycogen synthase is absent. Glucose polymers and uncooked cornstarch are effective therapy.

Further reading

Chen, Y-T, Cornblath, M., and Sidbury, J.B. (1984). Cornstarch therapy in Type I glycogen storage disease. *New England Journal of Medicine*, 310, 171–5.

Chen, Y-T. and Burchell, A. (1995). Glycogen storage diseases. In : *The Metabolic and Molecular Bases of Inherited Disease*, 7th edn, (ed. C.R. Scriver, A.L. Beaudet, W.S, Sly, and D. Valle). New York, McGraw-Hill, pp. 905–34.

de Barsy, T. and Hers, H.-G. (1990). Normal metabolism and disorders of carbohydrate metabolism. *Ballière's Clinical Endocrinology and Metabolism*, 4, 499–522.

Chapter 6.3

Inborn errors of fructose metabolism

T. M. Cox

Three inborn errors of fructose metabolism are recognized: (1) essential or benign fructosuria due to fructokinase deficiency; (2) fructose 1,6-diphosphatase deficiency; and (3) hereditary fructose intolerance (fructosaemia). The normal metabolism of fructose is shown in Fig. 1 and discussed in OTM3, p.1345.

Essential (benign) fructosuria

This is a rare disorder (estimated frequency 1 in 130~000) of little clinical consequence. It is an autosomal recessive condition and manifests itself by the presence of a reducing sugar in the blood and urine, especially after meals rich in fructose. It results from deficiency of fructokinase activity in the liver and intestine. Fructose metabolism occurs slowly as a result of conversion to fructose 6-phosphate by hexokinase in adipose tissue and muscle, so that when plasma concentrations remain high postprandially, large amounts of fructose appear in the urine. Essential fructosuria may be confused with diabetes mellitus if the nature of the mellituria is not defined but with the use of glucose oxidase strips this is now unlikely. No treatment beyond recognition and explanation is necessary.

Fructose 1,6-diphosphatase deficiency

This very rare, recessively-inherited disorder presents with hypoglycaemia, ketosis, and lactic acidosis in early infancy. Severe, sometimes fatal, acidosis is associated with infection and starvation and most cases have presented within the first few days of life or in the neonatal period (see OTM3, p.1346). The deficiency of fructose 1,6-diphosphatase causes failure of gluconeogenesis in the liver. The muscle isozyme of fructose 1,6-diphosphatase is not affected. The first infant that is affected by fructose diphosphatase deficiency in a given pedigree may succumb before the diagnosis is established, and in any case fares worse than siblings for whom the appropriate diet and prompt control of the condition are instituted. The response to treatment is favourable, however, and fructose diphosphatase deficiency is ultimately compatible with a benign course and with normal growth and development.

Dietary control and avoidance of starvation is the mainstay of treatment. Minor infections and injuries require prompt attention. The diet should exclude excess fat; sorbitol, sucrose and fructose must be strictly avoided. Medications and syrups containing fructose, sucrose or sorbitol present a special danger. A diet excluding these sugars but containing 56 per cent calories as carbohydrate with 32 per

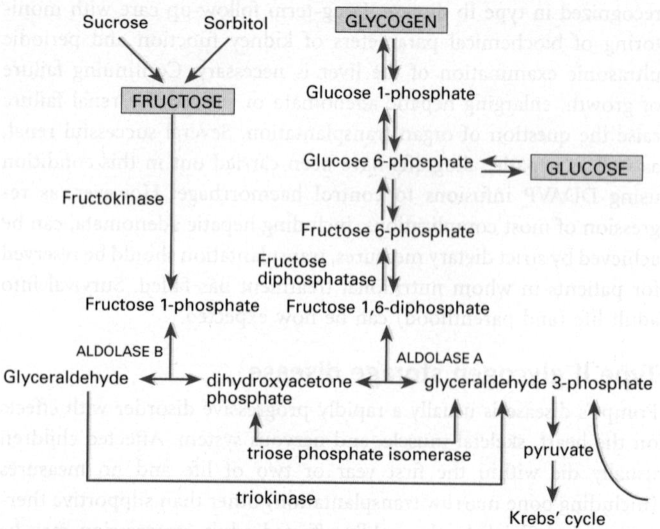

Fig. 1 Fructose metabolism.

cent calories as fat and 12 per cent as protein has produced normal growth and development. Acute episodes of acidosis or hypoglycaemia are controlled rapidly by intravenous administration of glucose with or without bicarbonate as required.

Hereditary fructose intolerance (fructosaemia)

This disorder has an estimated frequency of 1 in 18000 births in the UK. An autosomal recessive abnormality, it manifests itself first in early infancy but the effects of clinical disease may not be recognized until late childhood or adult life. Provided the diagnosis is made before visceral damage occurs, it responds completely to an exclusion diet.

The cardinal features in infancy are vomiting, diarrhoea, abdominal pain, and hypoglycaemia, which are induced by consumption of foods, drinks, or medicines that contain fructose or the related sugars, sucrose or sorbitol. Hypoglcaemia is accompanied by lactic acidosis, hyperuricaemia, and hyperphosphataemia. Episodes usually occur within 30 min of feeds that contain large quantities of fructose or sucrose. Continued ingestion of noxious sugars is associated with renal tubular disease, liver damage with jaundice, defective blood coagulation, and coma leading to death. Survival is dependent on recognition of the effects of fruit and sugar by the mother or, especially in older infants, by vomiting or forcible rejection of food.

Infants that survive weaning develop a strong aversion to sweet-tasting foods, vegetables and fruits. This usually affords protection against the worst effects of fructose and sucrose but abdominal symptoms with bouts of tremulousness, irritability, and altered consciousness due to hypoglycaemia usually continue. Many cases escape diagnosis in infancy and childhood but the risk of illness, related to dietary indiscretion, remains throughout life. These patients show a striking reduction in or absence of dental caries.

A syndrome of chronic sugar intoxication has also been recognized in older children and adolescents with hereditary fructose intolerance. General lack of vigour and developmental retardation are prominent features. Hypoglycaemia, though obvious after heavy fructose loading, may be insignificant after chronic low-level exposure in older children. Similarly, tests of hepatic and renal function may be only mildly abnormal. Persistent ingestion of fructose and sucrose is toxic to the kidney and liver, so that renal tubular acidosis (occasionally with calculi) as well as hepatosplenomegaly are frequently detectable in the younger patients. Severe growth retardation may be accompanied by rachitic bone disease that complicates the proximal renal tubular disturbance. Growth retardation responds to dietary treatment and is usually accompanied by regression of the other manifestations.

Provided that organ failure and serious tissue injury do not supervene, patients with hereditary fructose intolerance recover rapidly when the offending sugars are completely withdrawn. Normal growth and development can be secured in children if less than 40 mg/kg fructose equivalents are ingested daily.

Metabolic defect

Hereditary fructose intolerance is caused by a deficiency of aldolase B in the liver, small intestine, and proximal renal tubule. These tissues suffer injury as a result of persistent exposure to fructose. In the absence of fructose 1-phosphate splitting activity of aldolase B, the intracellular pool of inorganic phosphate is depleted. Fructose 1-phosphate then accumulates in a milieu where free inorganic phosphate is reduced: there is competitive inhibition of aldolase A and inhibition of phosphorylase activity so that glycogenolysis and gluconeogenesis are impaired. Thus challenge with fructose leads to hypophosphataemia and hypoglycaemia that is refractory to glucagon or infusion of gluconeogenic metabolites such as glycerol or dihydroxyacetone. High concentrations of fructose 1-phosphate cause feedback inhibition of fructokinase, thereby limiting the incorporation of fructose in the liver. When fructosaemia exceeds about 2 mmol/l in peripheral blood, fructosuria results. Although assimilation of fructose by the specialized pathway is blocked, only a small fraction of the fructose load is recovered in the urine. 80 to 90 per cent is taken up by adipose tissue and muscle, where it can be alternatively metabolized by phosphorylation to fructose 6-phosphate.

Electrolytic disturbances occur during challenge with fructose. Hypokalaemia, sometimes causing muscle weakness, results from acute renal impairment with defective urinary acidification. There is a defect of proximal tubule function with bicarbonate wasting and acidosis. Increases in serum magnesium concentrations probably result from breakdown of magnesium-ATP complexes, as a result of degradation by adenosine deaminase. Significant ingestion of fructose is thus also accompanied by marked hyperuricaemia.

Pathology and molecular genetics

Chronic ingestion of fructose causes fatty change and increased glycogen deposition in the liver together with hepatocyte necrosis and intralobular and periportal fibrosis. Fully developed cirrhosis results from continued exposure, probably caused by a lysosomal reaction to intracellular deposits of fructose 1-phosphate. Fatal administration of fructose or sorbitol parenterally is associated with the abrupt onset of hepatorenal failure associated with bleeding. Histological examination shows hepatic necrosis in these cases. Loss of cellular functions, for example in the proximal renal tubule, is probably caused by depletion of ATP resulting from the arrested metabolism of fructose by the specialized pathway. The source of the severe abdominal pain that follows ingestion of fructose is unknown, but stimulation of visceral afferent nerves by local release of purine nucleotides or lactate may be responsible.

Studies of the genetic basis of aldolase B deficiency show point mutations affecting the function of the enzyme. One particular mutation, $Ala^{149} \rightarrow Pro$, which disrupts residues in a substrate-binding domain of aldolase B, is prevalent in Europe and accounts for most alleles responsible for intolerance of fructose.

Diagnosis

If fructose intolerance is considered, sucrose, sorbitol, and fructose should be excluded completely before definitive tests can be carried out. Remarkable improvement may be seen within a few days but the differential diagnosis includes pyloric stenosis, galactosaemia, hepatitis, renal tubular disease, Wilson's disease, and tyrosinosis.

The intravenous fructose tolerance test is the bench mark for diagnosis: 0.25 g/kg (0.2 g/kg in infants) of D+ fructose is infused as a 20 per cent solution over a few min and blood samples for potassium, magnesium, phosphate, and glucose are taken at regular intervals over 2 h. Epigastric and loin pain accompany the infusion and hypoglycaemic coma may occur. Since the hypoglycaemia does not respond to glucagon, glucose for parenteral injection should be available. The test must be carried out with medical personnel at

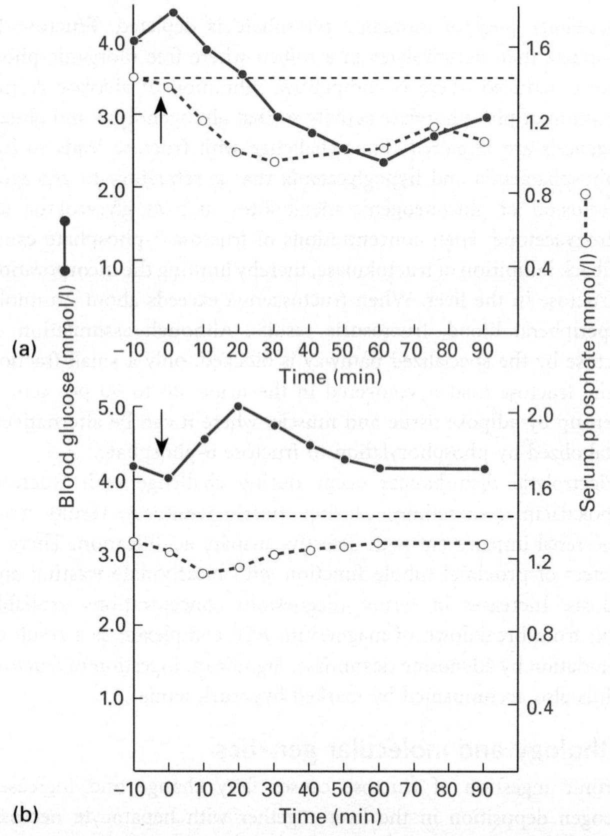

Fig. 2 (a) Intravenous fructose tolerance tests in a woman aged 39 with hereditary fructose intolerance proven by fructaldolase essay and DNA analysis and (b) an age- and sex-matched control subject with alcohol-related episodic hypoglycaemia.

hand: oral challenge with fructose or sucrose may produce severe pain and shock. It is best avoided. Responses differ between individuals and hypoglycaemia is usually milder in adults. Thus typical responses in hereditary fructose intolerance and a control subject are depicted in Fig. 2.

Aldolase B deficiency may be demonstrated by enzymatic analysis of biopsy samples obtained from the liver or small intestinal mucosa. Biochemical assay of fructaldolases characteristically demonstrates reduced or absent fructose 1-phosphate cleavage activity with a partial deficiency of fructose 1,6-diphosphate aldolase. Fructaldolase deficiency may accompany other parenchymal disease of the liver and these assays may be of limited value in the acutely ill or jaundiced patient.

Direct diagnosis is now possible in European patients by examination of aldolase B genes for the presence of common mutations responsible for the disease in this population.

Treatment

Dietary treatment of fructose intolerance alleviates the disorder but requires almost complete exclusion of sucrose, fructose and sorbitol. Daily consumption of sugar should be reduced to less than 40 mg of fructose equivalents per kilogram body weight (i.e. 2–3 g for an adult). The ubiquity of fructose and its cogeners in the Western diet presents serious difficulties. Adult patients have usually restricted their consumption of fructose to less than 20 g daily and the source of the residual sugar may be difficult to establish. For this reason, the advice of an experienced dietitian should be sought (Table 1). Particular care needs to be taken with sugar-coated pills and, especially, liquid medications for paediatric use, as large amounts of fructose, sucrose, and sorbitol are frequently present. Patients with hereditary fructose intolerance may lack folic acid and vitamin C. Vitamin supplements are recommended, especially during pregnancy but, as with other medicines, care has to be taken to avoid harmful sugars contained in the preparation: Ketovite®; (Paines and Byrne, Ltd., Surrey, England) is a satisfactory source of these vitamins.

Table 1 Food items not allowed for patients with hereditary fructose intolerance and fructose diphosphatase deficiency

Table sugar
Fruit sugar, all fruit and fruit products, including tomatoes
Sorbitol
Honey, syrup, treacle, molasses
Diabetic foods
Chocolate, sherbet
Preserves, jams, and marmalade
Frankfurters, honey-roast, and sweet-cured ham
Processed cheese spreads
Cream and cottage cheese with chives, pineapple, etc.
Flavoured milks and yoghurts
Wheatgerm, brown rice, bran
Breakfast cereals
Coffee essence, powdered milk
Carbonated sweet drinks
Allspice, nuts, coconut, carob, peanut butter
Mayonnaise, pickles, salad dressings, sauces
Some potatoes (especially stored, new potatoes)
Most legumes

Further reading

Ali, M., Rellos, P., and Cox, T.M. (1998). Hereditary fructose intolerance. *Journal of Medical Genetics*, 35, 353–65.

Bell, L. and Sherwood, W.G. (1987). Current practices and improved recommendations for teaching hereditary fructose intolerance. *Journal of the American Dietitic Association*, 87, 721–8.

Chapter 6.4

Disorders of galactose and pyruvate metabolism and pentosuria

T. M. Cox

Galactose disorders

Galactose is principally derived from lactose in the diet by the action of mucosal lactase in the small intestine. After absorption, it serves as a source of glucose and is a component of many membrane glycoproteins and glycolipids.

The conversion of galactose to glucose involves reactions that lead to the formation of glucose 1-phosphate, which can enter the main pathways of carbohydrate metabolism, directly (Fig. 1). Three inborn errors of galactose metabolism are recognized: (1) galactokinase deficiency; (2) galactose 1-phosphate uridyl transferase deficiency; and (3) uridine diphosphate-4-epimerase deficiency.

Galactokinase deficiency: 'galactose diabetes'

Failure to phosphorylate galactose at the 1-carbon position in the liver and other tissues impairs its clearance from the blood so that the free sugar and its metabolites, galactonic acid and galactitol appear in the urine. Homozygous deficiency of galactokinase occurs with an approximate frequency of 1 in 100 000 live births.

Clinical features

Precocious formation of cataracts in infants and children is characteristic and some heterozygotes develop cataracts before the age of 40 years. When blood concentrations are high, galactose is taken up by the lens and converted to galactitol by aldose reductase: subsequent toxic or osmotic effects lead to swelling and irreversible damage to lens fibres. Patients with galactokinase deficiency persistently excrete reducing sugar in their urine but apart from possible confusion with diabetes mellitus, this has no apparent significance.

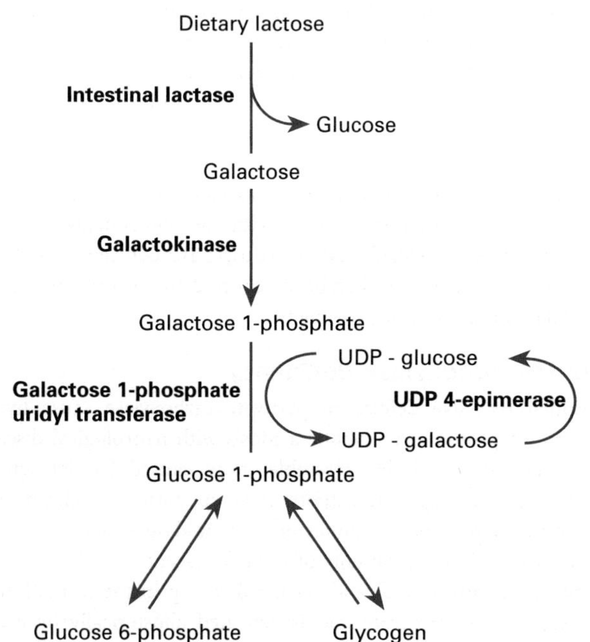

Fig. 1 Galactose metabolism.

Diagnosis and treatment

Galactokinase deficiency should be suspected in infants or children with cataracts and reducing sugar unreactive with glucose oxidase strips should be sought in the urine. Definitive diagnosis by enzymatic assay of galactokinase in erythrocytes or cultured fibroblasts differentiates the disorder from classic galactosaemia. Treatment with a strict lactose-galactose exclusion diet prevents cataract formation.

Galactose 1-phosphate uridyl transferase deficiency: galactosaemia

When patients who lack uridyl transferase ingest lactose, there is a significant rise in intracellular galactose 1-phosphate, as well as blood galactose concentration. The severe consequences of classical galactosaemia result from the toxic effects of galactose 1-phosphate principally in cells of the liver, proximal renal tubule, and brain. The exact mechanism of toxicity is unknown.

Clinical and pathological features

Vomiting or diarrhoea, jaundice, and hepatomegaly usually occur in the first few weeks of life. There is failure to gain weight, subcutaneous bruising, and cataracts may be apparent at 1 month of age, by which time abdominal distension with ascites has developed. Mental retardation does not become manifest until later in the first year of life and varies in severity. Many patients develop severe infections with *Escherichia coli* during the neonatal period.

Some patients may come to light in childhood, or even adult life, because of varying degrees of mental retardation and cataracts. Hepatomegaly and intermittent galactosuria are usually present and often there is a history of feeding difficulties during the neonatal period.

Tests of liver function are non-specifically deranged: histological examination shows lobular fibrosis, fatty change, bile ductular proliferation, and progression to frank cirrhosis. Involvement of the proximal renal tubule is shown by generalized aminoaciduria and occasionally a full-blown Fanconi syndrome. The brain shows non-specific signs of injury with gliosis and Purkinje cell loss in the cerebellum. Female patients with galactosaemia have a high incidence of gonadal failure with ovarian atrophy. No evidence of gonadal failure has been found in male patients.

Genetic studies

Galactosaemia is transmitted as an autosomal recessive trait with an overall estimated frequency of 1 in 62000. In black patients from the United States a relatively mild disorder has been reported that is probably due to an unstable enzyme variant; uridyl transferase activity is absent from their red cells but amounts to some 10 per cent of normal in samples of liver and small intestinal tissue. Individuals with the Duarte variant possess about half-normal enzyme activity in erythrocytes but remain asymptomatic.

The human galactosyl-1-phosphate uridyl transferase gene maps to human chromosome 9p13 and encodes a protein of molecular weight 43 000 Da. Molecular analysis of the transferase gene indicates that most patients with classical galactosaemia harbour mis-sense type mutations. Several other variant transferase enzymes have been described.

Diagnosis

Galactosaemia may be suspected in an infant with growth failure, cataracts, liver disease, aminoaciduria, mental retardation, and especially where reducing sugar is present in the urine. The occurrence of unexplained bacterial sepsis, especially if due to *E. coli* infection in a newborn infant is another feature.

Definitive diagnosis relies on the determination of galactose 1-phosphate uridyl transferase activity in red cells or leucocytes by means of a specific enzymatic assay. Reliable testing for heterozygotes can be carried out in the parents of a child that has died before the diagnosis has been confirmed and, in some parts of the world, neonatal screening for elevated blood galactose and galactose 1-phosphate concentrations is carried out routinely.

Treatment

Without strict dietary treatment most patients with galactosaemia die in early infancy, although some may survive with liver disease and mental retardation beyond childhood. The course of galactosaemia is altered strikingly upon withdrawal of lactose (and galactose). However, lactose is present in many non-dairy foods and advice from an experienced dietician as well as meticulous attention to detail, is required to eliminate it completely. Despite reports that galactose may be reintroduced as the patient develops, lifelong strict adherence to the exclusion diet should be advocated. In subsequent pregnancies of heterozygous mothers who have had affected children there is evidence that premature cataracts can be avoided in the fetus if the intake of lactose is restricted.

Prognosis

The acute manifestations respond quickly to dietary therapy and cataract formation is prevented. A proportion of patients have significant neurological deficits despite prompt and conscientious treatment. Ovarian failure and elevated galactose 1-phosphate concentrations in patients apparently ingesting no lactose or galactose raises the possibility that an endogenous pathway of galactose 1-phosphate formation from pyrophosphorlysis of uridine diphosphate-galactose may occur. This may also explain the late emergence of neurological disease in treated patients.

Uridine diphosphate 4-epimerase deficiency

Autosomal recessive epimerase deficiency is very rare but may be identified during screening for classic galactosaemia. In most cases no symptoms are apparent and follow-up studies have confirmed the usually benign nature of this anomaly. However, a few cases of marked deficiency of uridine diphosphate-4-epimerase have been discovered in patients otherwise manifesting the classic features of galactosaemia. As a complete deficiency of the epimerase would lead to an absolute lack of uridine diphosphate-galactose for glycosphingolipid synthesis, the ingestion of very small quantities of galactose has been recommended in this unusual disorder so that brain development and biosynthesis of essential galactosides can proceed.

Pentosuria

Pentosuria is a rare autosomal recessive trait but its frequency in Ashkenazi Jews may be as high as 0.05 per cent. It is caused by enzymatic deficiency of L-xylulose reductase in the oxidative pathway of glucuronate metabolism and 1 to 4 g of xylulose and L-arabitol appear continuously in the urine: this has no clinical significance except that it may lead to the incorrect diagnosis of diabetes mellitus should tests for reducing sugar be carried out on the urine. Xylulose does not react with urinary test strips based on the glucose oxidase method.

Inborn errors of pyruvate metabolism

Pyruvate dehydrogenase deficiency

This is the most common cause of lactic acidosis in newborn infants and children, but it is also associated with neurodegenerative syndromes in later life. Pyruvate dehydrogenase exists as a multi-enzyme complex representing the products of ten distinct genes. Defects in one subunit of pyruvate dehydrogenase itself (E1α) account for most patients so far investigated, although defects in dihydrolipoyl dehydrogenase (E3) are also described. The pyruvate dehydrogenase complex catalyses the conversion of pyruvate to acetyl coenzyme A within mitochondria. The accumulated pyruvate may either be reduced to lactate or transaminated to alanine so that hyperalaninaemia and varying degrees of lactic acidaemia occur. Very rare defects in dihydrolipoyl dehydrogenase are associated with deficiency of branched-chain keto acid dehydrogenase. Failure to carry out oxidative reactions in regions of the cortex and midbrain causes neuronal death and deficiency of 4-carbon intermediates may critically impair neurotransmitter synthesis. Definitive diagnosis depends on enzymatic assay in skin fibroblasts.

Severe deficiency of pyruvate dehydrogenase affects intrauterine development and causes marked acidosis (blood lactate > 10 mmol/l) at birth with early death. Survivors develop a variety of neurological disorders including microcephaly, quadriplegia, fits, blindness, cerebellar ataxia, choreoathetosis, and in some reaching adult life spinocerebellar degeneration (see OTM3, p.1351).

A high fat, low carbohydrate, ketogenic diet may ameliorate the biochemical abnormalities but little clinical improvement can be expected. Responses to high-dose thiamine have been reported in patients with partial enzymatic deficiency, notably where ataxia and abnormal eye movements reminiscent of Wernicke's encephalopathy were conspicuous. In rare patients with the autosomally recessive condition due to dihydrolipoyl dehydrogenase deficiency, oral administration of lipoic acid has been reported to correct the organic acidaemia with clinical improvement.

Pyruvate carboxylase deficiency

Autosomal recessive defects in pyruvate carboxylase cause hypoglycaemia or profound metabolic acidosis with neurological disease. The manifestations closely resemble those caused by deficiencies of pyruvate dehydrogenase activity. A severe form, associated with hyperammonaemia and citrullinaemia and rapid onset of liver damage is found particularly in patients of French descent.

Pyruvate decarboxylase catalyses the first step in the formation of oxaloacetate from pyruvate and is activated allosterically by acetyl coenzyme A. Thus, hypoglycaemia would be expected only after glycogen stores had been depleted. Krebs' cycle intermediates may become depleted so that there is insufficient synthesis of neurotransmitters. There may also be a reduced supply of aspartate for the arginosuccinate synthase reaction of the urea cycle. Patients with severe deficiency may present with the Leigh syndrome (necrotizing encephalomyopathy with lactate/pyruvate acidosis) or hypotonia and neurological retardation. Ataxia and abnormal ocular movements suggest midbrain disease resembling Wernicke's encephalopathy. Hypoglycaemia and acidosis occur during intercurrent infection or during starvation.

The condition is suspected when acidosis and neurological disease occur in infants, especially in the presence of hypoglycaemia. Specific diagnosis requires enzymatic assay in fibroblasts and this can be used for carrier detection. Disorders of pyruvate metabolism may be mimicked biochemically by mitochondrial diseases and acquired deficiencies of thiamine or biotin. Biotin therapy has been disappointing in pyruvate carboxylase deficiency but occasional responses to high-dose lipoic acid and thiamine treatment, which may stimulate the pyruvate metabolism by the dehydrogenase complex, have been recorded.

Episodes of acidosis are treated with intravenous sodium bicarbonate and glucose may be required for hypoglycaemia. Ketogenic diets containing 50 per cent fat and 20 per cent carbohydrate ameliorate the biochemical disturbance and delay the onset of neurological disease: in some patients administration of glutamate and aspartate, that may act as a source of oxaloacetate, appear to have been beneficial.

Further reading

Cornblath, M. and Schwartz, R. (1991). Disorders of galactose metabolism. In : *Disorders of Carbohydrate Metabolism in Infancy and Childhood* (3rd edn), pp. 295–324. Blackwell Scientific, Boston.

Robinson, B.H. (1995). Lactic acidemia (disorders of pyrovate carboxylase, pyruvate dehydrogenase). In: *The Metabolic and Molecular Bases of Inherited Disease* (7th edn) (ed. R. Scriver, A.L. Beaudet, W.S. Sly, and D. Valle). pp. 1479–500. McGraw-Hill, New York.

Chapter 6.5

Inborn errors of amino acid and organic acid metabolism

D. P. Brenton and P. J. Lee

Amino acid metabolism and genetic defects (see also OTM3 (pp. 1352–54)

Amino acids are derived from dietary protein, but eight of them cannot be synthesized. These 'essential' amino acids and their minimal requirements are shown in Table 1. Stool nitrogen losses are only about 1 g/day and bacterial protein accounts for much of this. Renal conservation of amino acids is extremely effective. Amino acids taken in excess of requirement are not stored but used for energy. After the removal of the amino group for conversion to ammonia and urea, the carbon skeletons degrade to major metabolic intermediates such as acetyl coenzyme A, acetoacetyl coenzyme A, pyruvate, or to citric acid cycle intermediates (Fig. 1) via individual amino acid pathways. Amino acids are referred to as glucogenic when their carbon skeletons degrade to intermediates used in gluconeogenesis, and ketogenic when their degradation products can form ketone bodies. Degradative enzymes frequently have important coenzymes and inherited defects of catabolism may be due to defects of the apoenzymes or their vitamin coenzymes. Table 2 offers a biochemical classification of the genetic defects of amino acid metabolism.

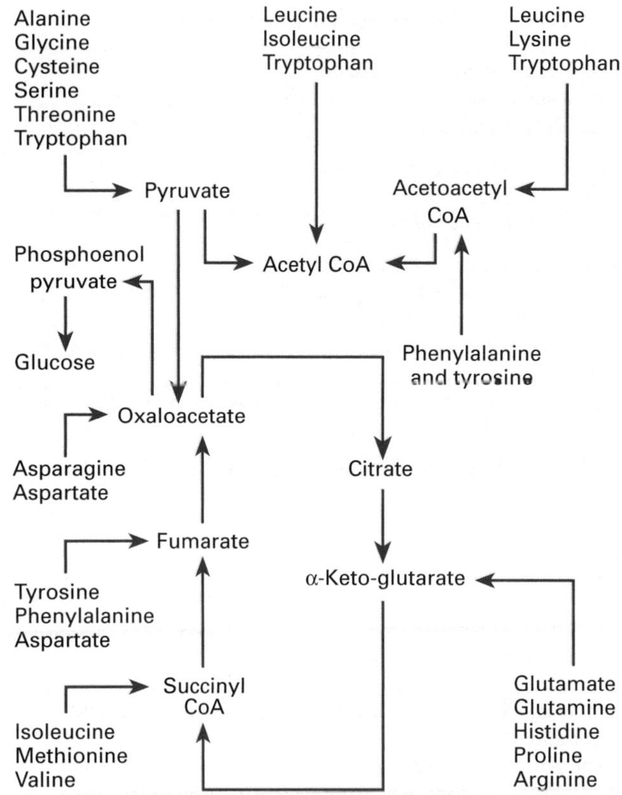

Fig. 1 Amino acids as a source of energy. The multiple entry points to the citric acid cycle for the metabolites of carbon chain catabolism.

Table 1 The essential amino acids in man with recommended dietary intakes

	Infants (mg/kg/day)	Adults (mg/kg/day)
Leucine	161	14.0
Isoleucine	70	10.0
Valine	93	10.0
Methionine*	58	13.0
Phenylalanine*	125	14.0
Threonine	87	7.0
Lysine	103	12.0
Tryptophan	17	3.5
Histidine	28	Not essential

*Requirements are lowered by the inclusion in the diet of cystine or tyrosine, respectively.

Table 2 A biochemical classification of amino acid disorders

The defects of amino acid transport intestinal and renal across cellular membranes
Defects of the amino group metabolism primary urea cycle defects secondary interference of urea cycle function
Defects of carbon chain metabolism those close to the parent amino acid with raised amino acid concentrations but mild or no acidosis those further down the pathway with organic acid accumulation and acidosis those at the end of the degradative pathways which may also involve catabolism of carbohydrates or fats
Defects primarily of major vitamin coenzymes pyridoxine vitamin B_{12} biotin biopterins

Table 3 A classification of aminoaciduria

Overflow aminoaciduria (secondary to high plasma amino acid concentrations)	
generalized	increased plasma concentrations of many amino acids, e.g. acute liver necrosis or amino acid infusions
specific	increased plasma concentration of one or a few amino acids
Renal aminoaciduria (with normal plasma amino acid concentrations)	
generalized	the Fanconi syndrome; early premature infants
specific	(i) basic aminoaciduria with or without cystine; lysinuric protein intolerance; cystinuria (ii) neutral aminoaciduria; the Hartnup syndrome (iii) glycine iminoaciduria; the normal neonatal pattern; genetic iminoglycinuria

Aminoacidurias (Table 3)

The generalized aminoacidurias

The Fanconi syndrome

There are four components to the Fanconi syndrome: (1) characteristic low molecular weight proteinuria; (2) tubular transport defects; (3) metabolic bone disease, rickets, or osteomalacia; (4) slow loss of glomerular function. Glycosuria, generalized aminoaciduria, and phosphaturia are a classic triad. The conservation of sodium, potassium, bicarbonate, and urate is impaired and the plasma concentrations of the last three decreased. Many examples of the Fanconi syndrome are not primarily disorders of amino acid metabolism but are the effects of exogenous or endogenous toxins (Table 4).

The dominantly inherited Fanconi syndrome

This disorder, of unknown cause, characteristically presents in the second to fourth decade and slowly evolves in late adult life when renal failure may be advanced. The clinical presentation is commonly with rickets or osteomalacia, which require treatment with calcitriol. Potassium, sodium bicarbonate, and phosphate supplements may also be needed (see Chapter 12.31).

Table 4 The inherited causes of the Fanconi syndrome. Acquired causes are due to heavy metals, drugs, dysproteinaemias, and some immunological disorders of the kidney

Idiopathic
Cystinosis
Hereditary fructose intolerance
Tyrosinaemia type I
Fanconi Bickel syndrome
Galactosaemia
Glycogen storage disease type I
Oculocerebrorenal syndrome of Lowe
Wilson's disease
Cytochrome *c* oxidoreductase deficiency

The oculocerebrorenal syndrome of Lowe

This is an X-linked disease characterized by dwarfism, profound mental retardation, and blindness secondary to cataracts, microphthalmos, and glaucoma. The tubular defect includes proteinuria, but not usually glycosuria, aminoaciduria with relative sparing of the branched chain amino acids, and may result in renal rickets. The OCRL1 gene is on the long arm of the X chromosome and codes for inositol polyphosphate 5-phosphatase.

Cystinosis

Cystinosis results from defective carrier-mediated transport of cystine through the lysosomal membrane, which may rupture due to cystine crystallization. In the proximal renal tubule this leads to the Fanconi syndrome. The severe infantile form presents after a few months of life with polyuria, thirst, salt and water depletion, hypokalaemia, and proximal renal tubular acidosis. Hypophosphataemia and impaired 1-hydroxylation of 25-hydroxycholecalciferol contribute to florid rickets.

Photophobia develops with the accumulation of cystine crystals in the cornea and retinopathy. Hypothyroidism is common and renal failure leads to death by 10 years of age unless treated by renal transplantation. Growth is impaired and sexual development is late. Intelligence is normal. In transplanted patients retinopathy and visual loss may progress. Cerebral cortical atrophy occurs in some and memory defects have been described. The spectrum of defects is likely to widen in long-term transplant survivors.

Diagnosis is based on the clinical features and the Fanconi syndrome. Cystine crystals in the cornea can be seen with a hand lens or a slit lamp in an older child and can also be found in bone marrow aspirates. Analysis of peripheral leucocytes or fibroblasts for their cystine content is possible in a few laboratories.

Variant forms

A benign adult form presents with photophobia due to corneal crystals. There may also be crystals in the bone marrow and leucocytes but the kidney is spared and life expectation is normal. An intermediate form is like the classic infantile form but presents in late childhood or early adult life.

Biochemistry

It is probable that all tissues accumulate cystine, but not equally, and some (e.g. muscle and brain) never seem to develop crystals. Cultured fibroblasts and leucocytes have values 50 to 100 times normal and concentrations in leucocytes are higher in the intermediate than the benign form, and highest in the severe form. The intralysosomal cystine originates from proteins catabolized within the lysosome and extracellular cystine transported into the cell. Cystine egress from the lysosome is defective.

Genetics

The disease is an autosomal recessive. The incidence is about 1 in 200 000 live births. Heterozygotes are clinically normal but have raised leucocyte cystine concentrations. Patients have been found to have novel mutations in a gene coding for a lysosomal membrane protein on the short arm of chromosome 17.

Prenatal diagnosis

This has been achieved using cultured amniocytes and measuring ^{35}S cystine uptake, or by direct analysis of chorionic villus samples for cystine content. Mutation analysis may be used in the future.

Treatment

Renal losses of salt, bicarbonate, and potassium may require initial intravenous replacement, but oral supplements, including phosphate suffice later although the need for them may be substantial. Phosphate alone may not heal the rickets without the addition of calcitriol. Oral cysteamine, or phosphocysteamine, given in divided doses, depletes leucocyte cystine and gives improved growth and preservation of renal function. Cysteamine eye drops have been used in very young children to clear corneal crystals. The role of cysteamine in preventing the consequences of cystine accumulation in non-renal tissues after transplantation is under study. Dialysis and/or renal transplantation are required for renal failure. Transplanted kidneys do not accumulate cystine. Thyroxine is needed for hypothyroidism. Growth hormone treatment increases height but has been reported to hasten the need for renal replacement. Plasma carnitine concentrations are often low and can be increased to normal by the use of supplements, but this may not help any muscular weakness.

Specific aminoacidurias

Cystinuria

Failure of renal tubular reabsorption of the dibasic amino acids cystine, lysine, arginine, and ornithine leads to the formation of cystine stones in the urinary tract, which may be silent or present with pain, haematuria, obstructive nephropathy, and infection. The condition is described more fully in Chapter 12.31.

Lysinuric protein intolerance

Defective ornithine, lysine, and arginine transport affects the renal tubule and intestine with only minor defects of cystine transport. Stones do not form. There is evidence of amino acid deficiency. At weaning, vomiting and diarrhoea begin. Failure to thrive and poor appetite are common with poor growth. Occasional intermittent hyperammonaemic encephalopathy occurs. Osteoporosis may cause vertebral collapse. Interstitial lung disease causes breathlessness, cough, fever and reduced arterial PO_2. Intellect is normal or mildly impaired. Pregnancy is associated with haemorrhage during labour.

Biochemistry

Plasma concentrations of arginine, ornithine, and lysine are low but citrulline, alanine, and glutamine are increased. Renal clearance values for lysine are 20 to 30 times normal and renal losses may be up to 1 g/day. Less marked increases of orthinine and arginine excretion are found but cystine increases are minor. Intracellular peptide hydrolysis liberates lysine, which cannot be transported across the basolateral membrane, the site of the transport defect. A deficiency of intramitochondrial ornithine due to a transport defect across the mitochondrial membrane may impair the urea cycle, causing hyperammonaemia and orotic aciduria (see below).

Genetics

The disease is an autosomal recessive with a high incidence in Finland (1 in 60 000). The gene has been localized to chromosome 14q coding for a permease-related protein. Prenatal diagnosis has not been described.

Treatment

Hyperammonaemia can be largely prevented by a low protein diet but this does not correct lysine deficiency and oral lysine supplementation causes diarrhoea. ε-*N*-acetyl lysine has been tried; plasma lysine concentrations rise but there is no agreement on its use, and cost and availability are a problem. Oral citrulline (2.5 to 8.5 day) corrects ornithine and arginine deficiency and lowers plasma ammonia by priming the urea cycle. Acute hyperammonaemic crises are managed with intravenous glucose and intravenous or oral sodium benzoate or phenylbutyrate. The cause of the serious interstitial pneumonia is not clear.

Neutral aminoaciduria: the Hartnup syndrome

This is an autosomal recessive disorder of neutral amino acid transport across the luminal brush border membrane of kidney and intestine. Clinical effects include a light-sensitive pellagra-like rash on exposed skin, cerebellar ataxia, and mental disturbance. Most patients with this disorder remain normal, however. Affected individuals may respond to nicotinamide whose relative deficiency is attributed to losses of the precursor amino acid tryptophan and its impaired intestinal absorption. Bacterial action on unabsorbed tryptophan generates indoles, which appear in the stools and urine and are characteristic of the disorder.

Defects of the urea cycle

Amino acids taken in excess of need are catabolized and the amino group effectively converted to urea. Hyperammonaemia is one of the major metabolic abnormalities in urea cycle defects but is not unique to them (Table 5).

The formation of urea

Nearly all waste nitrogen disposal—10 to 12 g/day—is in the form of urea synthesized in the liver from ammonium ions (NH_4^+) and the α-amino nitrogen of aspartic acid. The ammonium nitrogen is incorporated into the first committed synthetic step to urea formation—the production of carbamyl phosphate for which *N*-acetyl glutamine is believed to be regulatory. The α-amino nitrogen of aspartic acid comes from many amino acids during their transamination reactions with oxaloacetic acid. It is incorporated during the formation of argininosuccinic acid. Ornithine nitrogen is not incorporated into urea. Bicarbonate provides the carbon moiety of urea but this is probably not important in acid:base balance.

The generation of ammonium ions within the liver, once attributed to the deamination of glutamate by glutamate dehydrogenase, probably depends on transamination reactions linking glutamate to the

Table 5 Causes of hyperammonaemia

Urea cycle defects
Transport defects of intermediates of the urea cycle
lysinuric protein intolerance
hyperornithinaemia-hyperammonaemia-homocitrillinuria syndrome
Organic acidurias
branched chain organic acid defects
propionic acidaemia and methylmalonic acidaemia
pyruvate carboxylase or dehyrogenase deficiencies
multiple carboxylase deficiencies
glutaric aciduria type II
acyl coenzyme A dehydrogenase deficiencies
Drugs
valproate encephalopathy
Reye's syndrome
Liver disorders
cirrhosis of variable aetiology
portal systemic shunts
Transient neonatal hyperammonaemia

urea cycle. Within the liver a number of other amino acids are deaminated and may be a source of ammonium for urea synthesis. Ammonium ions are released into the renal vein by the action of renal glutaminase on glutamine.

The extrahepatic urea cycle enzymes

The urea cycle synthesizes arginine but hepatic transplantation for urea cycle defects does not correct low plasma concentrations of citrulline and arginine. The intestine also can synthesize citrulline with the mitochondrial parts of the cycle. Other tissues contain only some of the urea cycle enzymes. Citrulline transported to a variety of tissues with the cytosolic components of the cycle can be used to synthesize arginine via argininosuccinic acid. This extrahepatic synthesis of arginine may be crucial to the body's needs.

The inherited defects of the urea cycle and ornithine

Four of the five inherited defects of the urea cycle have common clinical features but arginase deficiency is different. The abbreviations CPSD, OTCD, ASD, ALD, and AD stand for deficiencies of carbamyl phosphate synthetase, ornithine transcarbamylase, argininosuccinic acid synthetase, argininosuccinic acid lyase, and arginase, respectively. Leaving aside AD, any may present with hyperammonaemic encephalopathy in the neonatal period. Less often this may occur in previously fit adolescents or adults. Some children just present with epilepsy and mental retardation. AD most often presents with the latter features and spastic quadriparesis. The biochemical features are in Table 6. Ornithine transcarbamylase deficiency (OTCD) is by far the most commonly encountered urea cycle disorder and is described in detail below. Some information on others is in Table 6. Clinically they have much in common but coma with raised ammonia is less common in AD, which presents with mental retardation, epilepsy and progressive spastic quadriparesis.

Clinical and biochemical features of OTCD

Most patients present in the neonatal period; a minority present later with occasional late childhood and early adult presentation. In the neonatal form, after a period between 24 and 72 hours of normality, poor feeding, lethargy and vomiting develop. If unrecognized, this proceeds to unresponsiveness and coma. In males, the situation is mostly fatal but survivors suffer intellectual and neurological impairment. Females who present neonatally can do better than the males, but may end up quite handicapped. A plasma ammonia concentration greater than 800 μmol/l invariably results in severe brain damage.

Older patients may present with mental retardation and epilepsy, but more commonly as intermittent episodes of encephalopathy. Female heterozygotes have even presented with hyperammonaemic encephalopathy and occasionally death, after childbirth following symptomless pregnancy. Hemizygous males may also present later in childhood or adolescence with encephalopathy and first attacks can still be fatal.

Biochemically, it is important to recognize that hyperammonaemia is often preceded by raised plasma glutamine and alanine with a reduction in arginine concentration. Acutely there may be raised transaminases and prolonged prothrombin time reflecting hepatic dysfunction.

Genetics and diagnosis

The differential diagnosis of hyperammonaemia is shown in Table 5. OTCD may be diagnosed from the clinical features and abnormal plasma amino acids, but can be confirmed by enzymatic assays on liver biopsy material When a DNA diagnosis is not possible, protein loading with serial measurement of urinary orotic acid, and plasma ammonia and amino acids can be helpful, but must be carried out in a centre with experience to ensure safety. Similarly, the allopurinol load test, with subsequent measurement of urinary orotic acid and orotidine, has been used to assess female carrier status. It is certainly more acceptable and safer than a protein load, but may fail to identify some carriers.

The gene is on the short arm of the X chromosome. A variety of gene mutations, both deletions and point mutations, have been described. Mutational analysis is useful as it allows for asymptomatic carrier detection and antenatal diagnosis. It has also highlighted the phenotypic variation of affected members within the same pedigree. These can range from neonatal death, through intermittent encephalopathy in childhood to asymptomatic adult males. Linkage studies have also been used in antenatal diagnosis and even fetal liver biopsy and enzyme assay when no useful genetic information has been available.

Treatment

The management of acute encephalopathy involves the suppression of catabolism by stopping dietary protein intake and increasing carbohydrate intake, mostly as an intravenous infusion of 10–20 per cent dextrose. Insulin can be useful in this situation as an anabolic agent and to control blood glucose. In the neonatal period, venovenous haemofiltration is often necessary to control hyperammonaemia, but nitrogen excretion can also be increased by the administration of intravenous or oral sodium benzoate and sodium phenylbutyrate. Sodium benzoate conjugates to glycine to form hippurate which is readily excreted in the urine, sodium phenylbutyrate is metabolized to phenyl acetate which conjugates to glutamine before being excreted. Arginine should also be given as this becomes an essential amino acid in OTCD because of the enzyme defect.

Maintenance treatment involves restriction of natural protein intake to the minimum necessary for growth and development, together

Table 6 A general approach to the biochemical disturbances in the urea cycle defects

	Normal	CPSD	OTCD	ASD	ALD	AD
Plasma ammonia	15–40 μmol/l	Up to 25×	Up to 25×	Up to 10–15×	Up to 10×	Up to 2–3×
glutamine	350–650 μmol/l	2–3×	2–3×	2–3×	2–3×	2×
alanine	200–400 μmol/l	2–3×	2–3×	2–3×	2–3×	2×
citrulline	10–30 μmol/l	Low	Low	up to 200×	Increased	Normal
arginine	30–90 μmol/l	Low	Low	Low	Low	Up to 15×
argininosuccinate	Not detectable	None	None	None	400–600	None
Urine orotic acid	2–6 mg/day	Not increased	Increased	Increased	Increased	Increased
Urine amino acids	—	—	—	Citrulline	ASA	Arginine/cystine lysine

AD, arginase deficiency; ALD, argininosuccinic acid lyase deficiency; ASD, argininosuccinic acid synthetase deficiency; CPSD, carbamyl phosphate synthetase deficiency; OTCD, ornithine transcarbamylase deficiency.

with supplementation of vitamins, minerals, and trace elements. Oral arginine, sodium benzoate, and sodium phenylbutyrate often need to be taken on a regular basis. During intercurrent illness, an emergency regimen of oral glucose polymer (15–20 per cent solution) and the regular medications should be taken every 2 hours. If this is not tolerated, readmission to hospital for parenteral treatment is necessary sooner rather than later. Parents learn to recognize decompensation very quickly.

The definitive treatment for OTCD is hepatic transplantation which has been performed in a few cases. The difficulty in deciding whether this is indicated is that hyperammonaemia may already have resulted in brain damage, or if not, affected individuals may be quite well. In the future, hepatocyte transplantation may be a viable alternative. It should be noted that valproate therapy is contraindicated in OTCD as it may precipitate hyperammonaemic coma even in previously asymptomatic individuals.

Defects of ornithine metabolism

These are not defects of the urea cycle but are included here for convenience. Ornithine is a non-protein amino acid upon which the synthesis of urea takes place and which is regenerated once the urea moiety is split off. It is also produced when arginine reacts with glycine to produce guanidinoacetate, the precursor of creatine. Ornithine δ-amino transferase produces glutamic semialdehyde, which cyclizes to pyrroline 5-carboxylic acid, which is also produced from proline. The decarboxylation of ornithine produces the diamine putrescine. Ornithine δ-amino transferase deficiency (gyrate atrophy) and hyperornithinaemia with hyperammonaemia and homocitrullinuria are summarized in Table 7.

Table 7 Disorders of ornithine metabolism

Ornithine-δ-amino transferase deficiency (gyrate atrophy)	
Clinical	Choroidal and retinal atrophy (atypical retinitis pigmentosa); cataracts; mild proximal myopathy in some.
Biochemistry	Raised concentration of ornithine in plasma, CSF and aqueous humour; high urinary arginine and lysine. Decreased enzyme activity in liver/muscle biopsy tissues.
Genetics	Autosomal recessive; gene locus on chromosome 10: two pseudogenes on the x chromosome
Treatment	Pyridoxine 500 mg per day or less may retard deterioration. So may the technically difficult approach of using a low arginine diet.
Hyperornithinaemia plus hyperammonaemia and homocitrullinuria (HHH)	
Clinical	Intermittent hyperammonaemic encephalopathy. Impairment of intellect of variable degree; epilepsy.
Biochemistry	Raised plasma ornithine concentration; intermittent hyper-ammonaemia; increased urinary orotic acid and citrulline.
Genetics	Probably autosomal recessive; gene locus unknown.
Treatment	Dietary protein restriction to 1 g/kg body weight per day; ornithine supplements. Extra citrulline and sodium phenyl butyrate may help in adults.

The disorders of carbon chain metabolism

Defects of phenylalanine metabolism

The hyperphenylalaninaemias are a group of disorders characterized by defective hydroxylation of phenylalanine to tyrosine and plasma phenylalanine values above the normal fasting range of 40–80 μmol/l. An adult phenylalanine intake is about 3–4 g/day, one-quarter of which is incorporated into protein and three-quarters hydroxylated to tyrosine (Fig. 2). Adults need about 1 g/day, but in classic severe phenylketonuria (PKU) health is maintained on half this. Transamination to phenylpyruvic acid and decarboxylation to phenylethylamine assume much greater importance in phenylketonuria because they occur only at elevated phenylalanine concentrations.

Classic phenylketonuria

Clinical

Untreated, phenylketonuria almost invariably causes severe mental retardation, with IQ values only occasionally above 60, and most often well below, and plasma levels of phenylalanine greater than 1000 μmol/l. Inexplicably, a few patients have normal IQ values and some female patients have been discovered only because of abnormalities in their offspring (see below). Both microcephaly and epilepsy are common. About one in 20 untreated patients develop neurological problems in adult life, usually spastic paraparesis but sometimes extrapyramidal features. Pigmentary deficiency in the iris and hair are other features of the untreated disease and so is eczema.

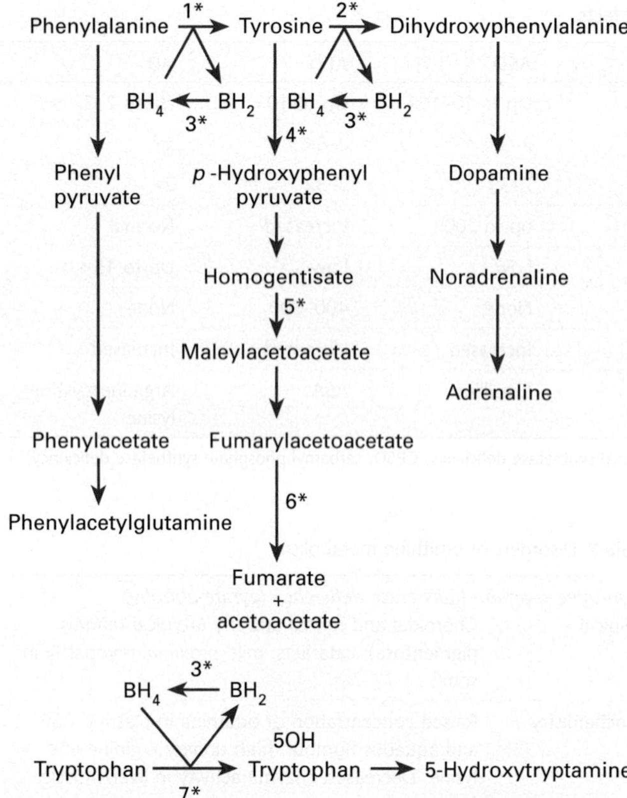

Fig. 2 The metabolism of phenylalanine and tyrosine and the role of tetrahydrobiopterin. The asterisked enzymes are: 1, phenylalanine hydroxylase; 2, tyrosine hydroxylase; 3, dihydrobiopterin reductase; 4, tyrosine amino transferase; 5, homogentisic acid oxidase; 6, fumaryl acetoacetate hydrolyase; and 7, tryptophan hydroxylase.

Milder variants

Mutations with greater residual enzyme activity produce phenylalanine values of 300 to 1000 μmol/l. Those over 400 μmol/l should be treated.

Biochemistry

Plasma phenylalanine concentrations are elevated 20–60 times normal. Phenylpyruvic acid in the urine gives the disease its name and a green colour in the ferric chloride test. The defective enzyme phenylalanine hydroxylase, which requires tetrahydrobiopterin as a cofactor, has been found only in the liver in man. It has never been found in brain of any species.

Pathophysiology

Phenylalanine itself is probably the damaging agent but there is controversy over the mechanism. High phenylalanine concentrations are associated with impaired brain growth and probably fewer nerve cells. Phenylalanine inhibits an enzyme important in sulphation of myelin intermediates and myelin formation is abnormal. Transport of other amino acids is reduced at the blood–brain barrier and at the placenta by high phenylalanine concentrations. In addition, many *in vitro* biochemical processes (e.g. protein synthesis) are impaired by high phenylalanine concentrations. Patients with classic phenylketonuria also have low cerebrospinal fluid concentrations of homovanillic acid and 5-hydroxyindoleacetic acid, indicative of possible deficiency of dopamine, noradrenaline, and 5-hydroxytryptamine. Dietary treatment restores normal concentrations in the cerebrospinal fluid.

Diagnosis

All newborns in the United Kingdom are screened for raised phenylalanine values on about the seventh day of life. Raised values are seen in the important variants due to defects in tetrahydrobiopterin synthesis and these must be excluded as they require specific treatment. Transient neonatal hyperphenylalaninaemia must also be distinguished from permanent forms.

Genetics

The disease is an autosomal recessive whose incidence in Western countries is 1 in 8000–12 000 live births. It is rare in Finland and Japan. One in 50 people carry a mutant gene on chromosome 12. These include splicing mutations, deletions, and mis-sense mutations. The majority of patients are compound heterozygotes. There is growing information on which genotypes cause the most severe functional defects in the enzyme. Over 400 mutations have been described.

Treatment

Protein intake is reduced to provide just what is necessary for growth and development while keeping the plasma phenylalanine between 120 and 360 μmol/l with regular monitoring. These are lower phenylalanine values than were once recommended because outcome in terms of IQ is closely related to the control of abnormally high values. Persistently low values may also adversely affect outcome. Despite normal or near normal IQ results, subtler neuropsychological defects have been described in well treated patients.

In infancy, milk restriction with supplements is relatively easy. Later it is necessary to introduce other foods on an exchange basis using tables that define the weight of the food containing 1 g of protein (roughly 50 mg phenylalanine). Fruits and some vegetables very low in protein are allowed freely. Adults with classic phenylketonuria tolerate only three to four exchanges, which provide about the same amount of phenylalanine as the free foods. These diets are supplemented with phenylalanine-free amino acid mixtures, minerals, and vitamins.

Patients generally have not suffered when diets have stopped at 15 or 16 years of age. However, there is no follow-up of a substantial number with respect to IQ change who have been off diet for 10 years or more, and there is concern about possible neurological deterioration. A small number of patients in adult life have developed spastic paraparesis, epilepsy, or extrapyramidal features. All these have cerebral MRI changes, as do an appreciable proportion of those without such manifestations.

Maternal phenylketonuria

The adverse effects of maternal hyperphenylalaninaemia on the fetus are shown in Table 8. Microcephaly and congenital heart disease in the offspring of mothers returning to diet at the seventh or eighth week emphasizes the need for preconception diet. Even if starting diet very early in the first trimester (5 to 6 weeks) lowers the incidence of impaired brain development, an increased risk certainly remains to brain and heart.

The ratio of fetal to maternal phenylalanine plasma levels is around 1.5–1.7 because of active placental transport. Maternal values should be controlled at between 100 and 300 μmol/l, which requires very careful monitoring twice weekly. Some values will rise above this in

Table 8 The incidence of abnormalities in the offspring of phenylketonuric mothers

	Maternal phenylalanine concentration (mg/100 ml (× 60 = μmol/l))			
	20	16–19	11–15	3–10
Mental retardation	92 (172)	73 (37)	22 (23)	21 (29)
Microcephaly	73 (138)	68 (44)	35 (23)	24 (21)
Congenital heart disease	12 (225)	15 (46)	6 (33)	0 (44)
Birth weight < 2500 g	40 (89)	52 (33)	56 (9)	13 (16)

Percentage figures with sample size in parentheses (from Lenke, R.L. and Levy, H.L. (1980), with permission from *New England Journal of Medicine*). **303**, 1202–8.

the critical first trimester when tolerance is very low and nausea restricts calorie intake. Dietary tolerance in the mother increases from about week 18 due to increased requirement for growth by the fetus and uterus, but also probably because phenylalanine hydroxylase in the fetal liver can be detected early in the second trimester. Lower maternal phenylalanine values result in neonates of higher birth weight and larger head circumference.

Defects of biopterin metabolism

In the hydroxylation of phenylalanine the cofactor tetrahydrobiopterin (BH_4) is consumed and must be regenerated. A deficiency of tetrahydrobiopterin adversely affects the function not only of phenylalanine hydroxylase, but also of tyrosine hydroxylase and tryptophan hydroxylase. Tyrosine hydroxylation is needed for the synthesis of noradrenaline and dopamine, and tryptophan hydroxylation for the production of 5-hydroxytryptamine. The supply of this coenzyme is impaired in several enzyme defects. All produce hyperphenylalaninaemia, which may not be marked, and all produce progressive neurological disability despite a low phenylalanine diet. About 1 to 2 per cent of newborns with abnormally raised phenylalanine values have a deficiency of tetrahydrobiopterin.

Dihydropteridine reductase (DHPR) deficiency

DHPR is a tetramer of four units, each of 25000 Da. It has a wide distribution in tissues. Deficiency results from an autosomal recessive genetic defect. The clinical features are those of progressive neurological deterioration and psychomotor retardation, epilepsy, pyramidal and extra pyramidal dysfunction, especially the latter. Calcification occurs in the cerebral hemispheres. Diagnosis is best confirmed by assay for the enzyme on red cells. Prenatal diagnosis can be performed on cultured amniocytes. The gene is on chromosome 4p with various mutations described.

Treatment comprises a low phenylalanine diet and use of l-dopa, 5-hydroxytryptophan and in some cases folinic acid. Early treatment gives good results.

Guanosine triphosphate cyclohydrolase deficiency and 6-pyruvoyltetrahydrobiopterin synthase deficiency

The clinical features are similar to those of dihydropteridine reductase deficiency. Tetrahydrobiopterin is used in treatment because, in the presence of dihydropteridine reductase, it can be regenerated from dihydrobiopterin. However, the clinical outcome is not assured and there is concern that tetrahydrobiopterin does not easily enter the central nervous system. Treatment, therefore, is also being attempted with low phenylalanine diet, l-dopa, and 5-hydroxytryptamine.

Disorders of tyrosine metabolism

The steps in tyrosine metabolism are outlined in Fig. 2. They are the means of production of the catecholamines, dopamine, and the principal pigments of hair and skin.

Tyrosinaemia type I

Deficiency of fumarylacetoacetate hydrolase is the cause of this autosomal recessive disorder resulting in a raised plasma levels of tyrosine and often also of methionine. The defective gene has been located to chromosome 15. The disease presents acutely in the early weeks of life with failure to thrive, vomiting, hepatomegaly, fever, oedema, and epistaxis. Death from hepatic failure occurs within the first year of life but some survive several years with chronic liver disease, renal tubular Fanconi syndrome, hypophosphataemic rickets, and sometimes abdominal pain and neuropathy suggesting acute intermittent porphyria. One-third of these milder cases develop hepatocellular carcinoma. Diagnosis is confirmed by the raised plasma levels of tyrosine and succinyl acetone together with raised urinary δ-aminolaevulinic acid. Treatment trials in specialized centres with the agent NTBC are changing the prognosis although hepatic transplantation may still be required in some patients.

Tyrosinaemia type II

This is due to deficiency of tyrosine aminotransferase which catalyses the formation of *p*-hydroxyphenylpyruvic acid. Deficiency results in plasma tyrosine levels 10–20 times normal. Corneal erosions and dendritic ulcers may form in infancy with later scarring, nystagmus, and glaucoma. Skin lesions include blistering, hyperkeratosis, and pain in palms and soles. Mental retardation is inconstant but language defects, impaired co-ordination, and self-mutilation may be more common. Skin and eye problems improve with a low tyrosine and phenylalanine diet, but there is little information on the effects of such treatment on neurological manifestations.

Alkaptonuria

This autosomal recessive disorder due to a deficiency of homogentisic acid oxidase has an incidence of some 1 in 200 000 although it is more common in some areas, notably Czechoslovakia. The responsible gene is on chromosome 3q with various mutations in the gene. The enzyme deficiency leads to an accumulation of homogentisic acid with affected individuals excreting 4 to 8 g/day in the urine. The acid produces a false positive for glucose in the 'Clinitest' reaction but the mixture then darkens rapidly because of the alkaline pH. There is no reaction with the standard dipstick tests for glucose.

Urine is usually normal when passed, but darkens on standing to deep brown or almost black. The pigment is thought to be a polymer derived from homogentisic acid. Abnormal pigmentation is seen in cartilage, tendons, ligaments, heart valves, and the sclera and pigmented stones are common in the prostate. Joint cartilage becomes thin and fragmented and intervertebral discs calcify. Back pain begins in the second or third decade and involvement of the hips, knees, and shoulders follows. By the fifth decade the lumbar spine is usually rigid and other joints seriously affected.

Table 9 A classification of albinism according to whether the hair bulbs have tyrosinase activity (positive) or not (negative)

	Oculocutaneous (tyrosinase negative)	Oculocutaneous (tyrosinase positive)	Ocular
Hair colour	White	White	Normal
Skin colour	Pink	Yellow tan White	Normal
Pigmented naevi	0	No tan +	+
Risk of skin cancer	+++	+++	Normal
Eye colour	Grey to blue	Blue to yellow brown	Normal range
Fundal pigment	0	0	0
		+	+
Photophobia	+++	++	+++
Nystagmus	+++	++	+++
Visual acuity	Severely impaired	Impaired	Impaired
Genetics	AR	AR	X-linked or AR

AR, autosomal recessive.

The diagnosis depends on clinical features and simple urine tests. Homogentisic acid can be detected by chromatography and quantitated by gas–liquid chromatography or high pressure liquid chromatography.

Although a low protein diet will reduce the production of homogentisic acid and low phenylalanine, tyrosine diets would reduce it still further, there is no good case for such an approach. Ascorbic acid may slow the rate of oxidation of homogentisic acid to pigment but there are no data on its clinical effects.

Albinism

Tyrosinase deficiency in melanocytes prevents the conversion of *p*-hydroxyphenylalanine to dihydroxyphenylalanine and thence to dopaquinone, the precursor for pigment formation in the skin, the iris, the fundus, and the inner ear. The absence of pigment is the characteristic of the group of disorders referred to together as albinism. It is a complex group of 10 or more types. The manifestations are primarily in the skin and eye. The gene is on chromosome 11q; multiple mutations have been described. Pigment abnormalities are also due to other genes in some patients.

The three main types are compared in Table 9. However, two points worth noting are: (1) oculocutaneous albinism may also occur in association with a bleeding tendency—the Hermansky Pudlak syndrome; and (2) in association with the leucocyte killing defect—the Chédiak-Higashi syndrome. Ocular albinism, too, in some genetic forms, occurs in association with nerve deafness.

Oculocutaneous albinism is characterized by structural optic tract defects. Most of the fibres at the optic chiasma cross over so there are few ipsilateral fibres and poor binocular vision. The geniculate bodies and the radiation onwards to the cortex are also structurally abnormal. The inner ear lacks pigment that is normally said to be protective against noise trauma. The predisposition to squamous carcinoma of the skin is important. Further details are in Table 9.

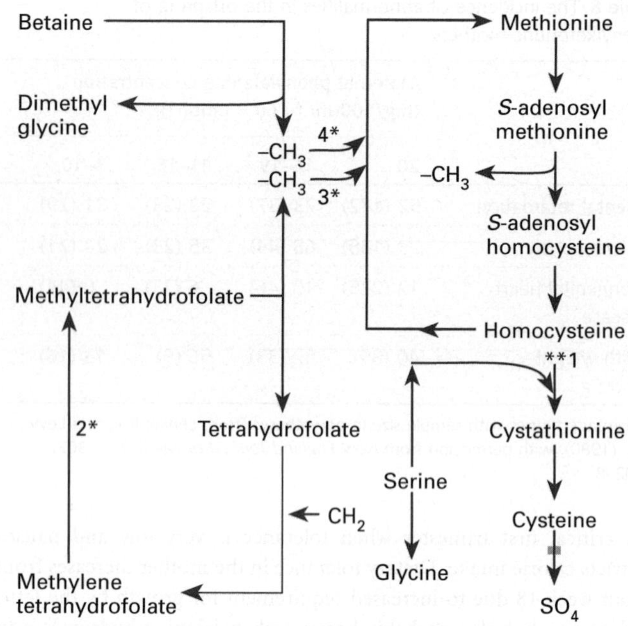

Fig. 3 The trans-sulphuration pathway from methionine to cysteine is shown on the right and the remethylation of homocysteine on the left. Asterisked enzymes are: 1, cystathionine synthase; 2, methylene tetrahydrofolate reductase, 3, methionine synthase; and 4, betaine methyl transferase.

Disorders of sulphur amino acid metabolism

The trans-sulphuration pathway transfers the sulphur of methionine to serine to produce cysteine (Fig. 3). Methionine adenosyltransferase produces *S*-adenosylmethionine, the donor in a variety of methylation reactions. In creatine formation alone adult males may utilize more methyl groups than provided by dietary methionine. *S*-Adenosyl homocysteine is cleaved to homocysteine, the sulphhydryl compound in reversible equilibrium with its disulphide homocystine. Half of the homocysteine formed goes through the trans-sulphuration pathway and the other half takes a methyl group from betaine (betaine methyltransferase) or 5-methyltetrahydrofolic acid (methionine synthase). The latter is a cobalamin-dependent enzyme which is functionally impaired in defects of vitamin B_{12} metabolism. The remethylation of homocysteine is also impaired if the activity of the reductase that generates 5-methyltetrahydrofolate (5-MTF) is inadequate.

When accumulation of homocystine results from defects of homocysteine remethylation plasma methionine concentrations are low. They are high when homocysteine accumulates from impaired activity of cystathionine synthase, which forms the thioether cystathionine, an intermediate subsequently cleaved to produce the sulphydryl compound cysteine. Further metabolism of cysteine produces inorganic sulphate for excretion.

Cystathionine synthase (CS) deficiency (homocystinuria)

This disease is due to lack of cystathionine synthase, an enzyme located on chromosome 21 with 15 mutations already described. The disease is an autosomal recessive with a birth incidence of about 1 in 40 000. Enzyme concentrations in affected individuals range from 0–10 per cent in homozygotes and in obligatory heterozygotes is less than 50 per cent of normal. The enzyme contains firmly bound pyridoxal phosphate, and some patients are helped by treatment with pyridoxine (see later). In homocystinuria there is an accumulation of homocysteine (difficult to measure), homocystine (to 50–200 μmol/l) and methionine (100–500 μmol/l). The urinary excretion of homocystine is usually some 200–1000 μmol per day.

Clinical

The classic clinical features in the older child and adult are mental retardation, lens dislocation, a thrombotic tendency, and skeletal abnormalities. Mental retardation, affecting two-thirds is sometimes gross but more commonly IQ values are around 65. Others are in the normal range with a few high values. Pyridoxine (B_6) responsive patients have generally higher IQ values than non-responsive patients. Seizures affect about one-fifth and a few patients show extrapyramidal features, sometimes with severe involuntary movements. Psychiatric disturbances have been described but an increased frequency of schizophrenia is unproven.

Lens dislocation is acquired, usually in the preschool years, but later dislocation is well recognized especially in pyridoxine-responsive patients, and a few have not developed it even in adult life. Monocular and binocular blindness have been relatively frequent due to secondary glaucoma, staphyloma formation, buphthalmos, and retinal detachment.

The skeletal abnormalities include osteoporosis and spontaneous crush vertebral fractures. The common abnormalities seen in Marfan's syndrome—high arched palate, pectus excavatum or carinatum, genu valgum, pes cavus or planus, scoliosis—are all well recognized in homocystinuria (see OTM, p. 3084). Arachnodactyly is less common and the fingers not infrequently (and elbows occasionally) show mild flexion contractures. Skeletal disproportion with a crown pubis length less than the pubis heel length is usual (Fig. 4).

Pathology

Thromboembolism is a major cause of morbidity and the main cause of the relatively high premature mortality. Thromboses have been described in a wide variety of arteries and veins (cerebral, coronary, mesenteric, renal, and peripheral). About 50 per cent are in peripheral veins with associated pulmonary emboli in many. Postoperative and postpartum thrombotic risks are high. Premature atheromatous vascular degeneration and arterial aneurysm formation have been described.

Homocysteine may interfere with cross-linking in collagen. Degeneration of zonular fibres around the lens causes the lens dislocation but these fibres are not collagen. Defects in fibrillin may be important in cystathionine synthase deficiency. There is still no accepted explanation for the relationship of homocystine/homocysteine to endothelial damage, platelet abnormalities, thromboses, and vascular change. Heterozygotes for the enzyme defect may be disposed to premature vascular disease and thrombosis. Finally, although the cerebral hemispheres normally have a high concentration of cystathionine, which is reduced in cystathionine synthase deficiency, this is not considered a cause of the mental deficiency, and neither does diffuse vascular disease seem relevant to this problem.

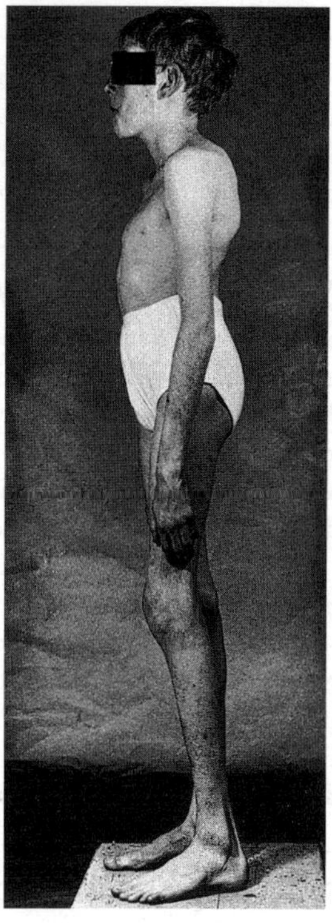

Fig. 4 Child with cystathionine synthase deficiency. Note the kyphosis and short trunk.

Treatment

Oral pyridoxine may rapidly reduce methionine and homocystine to near normal values. It is the first treatment to try, using 150–300 mg/day in the older child or adult and reducing the dose if a response is achieved. Very large sustained doses (1000 mg/day or more) in adults may cause peripheral neuropathy. A very low protein diet with a system of exchanges is appropriate for those not responding to pyridoxine and requires a methionine-free amino acid supplement, minerals, and vitamins. Biochemical control may only be achieved in older children and adults on natural protein intakes of 5–10 g/day. Cystine supplementation of diets should be considered in patients partially responsive to pyridoxine. Both folic acid (5–10 mg/day) and betaine (up to 6 g/day) can further reduce plasma homocystine levels but may produce large elevations of plasma methionine. Low red cell folate values and even megaloblastic anaemia occur. Low serum vitamin B_{12} values have also been found.

Genetics and antenatal diagnosis

The gene is on chromosome 21q with multiple defects described. This has so far rested on enzyme assays on cultured amniotic cells. It is likely that genotype analysis will supersede this.

Methylene tetrahydrofolate reductase deficiency

Neurological features predominate with psychomotor retardation, seizures, abnormalities of gait, and psychiatric disturbance in this autosomal recessive disease. Presentation occurs from early to late childhood. The risk of vascular disease is high. At autopsy dilated ventricles and low brain weight have been seen; thromboses may be present in arteries and veins. Demyelination occurs and the changes may resemble the classic findings of subacute combined degeneration seen in vitamin B_{12} deficiency. Calcification of the basal ganglia occurs. Plasma methionine concentrations are below normal and plasma homocystine concentrations in the range 20–200 µmol/l with an excretion of 15–600 µmol/day. In diagnosis homocystine is easily missed at low concentrations but this is the important clue.

Methionine synthase deficiency

This enzyme transfers a methyl group from methyltetrahydrofolate to homocysteine. Methyl cobalamin is the required coenzyme. This metabolic step may be impaired by an apoenzyme defect or defects in cobalamin metabolism, some of which limit only the formation of methyl cobalamin. Other cobalamin defects are considered under methyl malonic acidaemia. The characteristic clinical findings are developmental delay and megaloblastic anaemia, but the onset may be in later in childhood with dementia and spasticity. Retinal degeneration, cardiac defects, and haemolysis have been described. Biochemical findings include low plasma methionine and raised homocystine in plasma and urine.

Polymorphisms of the gene on chromosome 1q are common and may predispose to vascular risk in otherwise normal subjects.

Other defects of sulphur amino acid metabolism

Sulphite oxidase deficiency, cystathionase deficiency, and methionine adenosyl transferase deficiency are described in OTM3, p. 1367, where there is additional information on the defects described above.

Defects of glycine metabolism

Folate and activated 1-carbon units

Tetrahydrofolate carries 1-carbon units—methyl, methylene, methenyl, formyl, or forminino—bonded to the N-5 or N-10 nitrogen atoms and the units are interconvertible. 1-Carbon units are donated from the tetrahydrofolate derivatives in a variety of syntheses. New 1-carbon units are accepted by tetrahydrofolate in degradative reactions, of which the most important is the conversion of serine to glycine. As serine can be formed from 3-phosphoglycerate, carbohydrates are the ultimate source of 1-carbon units. Glycine in turn can be cleaved by a complex enzyme system of four mitochrondrial proteins.

Non-ketotic hyperglycinaemia

The various forms of this disorder are all autosomal recessively inherited, and are due to defects in the glycine clearage system. The defects result in raised plasma glycine levels (600–1200 µmol/l) and concentrations in CSF reach some 20 times normal. Large amounts of glycine are found in urine.

Neonatal presentation is with lethargy, fits, and vomiting proceeding to coma. Mortality is high at this stage and survivors do not develop intellectually. Fits persist and spastic cerebral palsy results. A form presenting later in childhood causes spastic paraparesis with modestly raised CSF glycine levels; optic atrophy and cerebellar signs have been described. Diagnosis rests on the analysis of plasma and CSF glycine. Enzyme assays on chorionic villi and amniotic fluid glycine:serine ratios are used in antenatal diagnosis.

Treatment is very unsatisfactory. Some central nervous system damage may be prenatal. Plasma glycine levels can be lowered

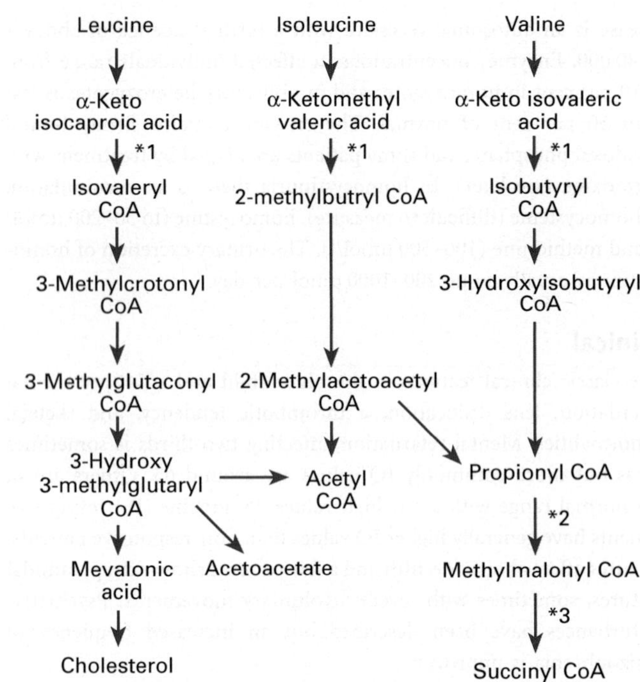

Fig. 5 Branched chain amino acid metabolism. Transamination produces the keto acids (top), all of which are metabolized by the branched chain α-keto dehydrogenase complex (asterisked) 1. 2, Propionyl coenzyme A carboxylase; and 3, methylmalonyl coenzyme A mutase.

by exchange transfusion or peritoneal dialysis but without clinical improvement. Low protein diets have only a limited effect. '1-Carbon units' in the form of methionine or *N*-formyltetrahydrofolate have not helped. The combination of sodium benzoate and diazepines, which compete for glycine receptors in the central nervous system has lowered plasma and cerebrospinal fluid levels of glycine and reduced seizures without clearly improving prognosis. A favourable clinical response to tryptophan therapy has been reported and another NMDA receptor blocker, dextromethorphan, has had variable success.

Defects in branched chain amino acid metabolism

Leucine, isoleucine, and valine collectively make up 10–15 per cent of animal protein and are catabolized by transamination to the corresponding keto acids, 2-keto-isocaproic, 2-keto-3-methylvaleric and 2-keto-isovaleric acids (Fig. 5). In all tissues except the liver aminotransferase activity exceeds α-ketodehydrogenase activity. The resulting keto acids are largely transported back to the liver for subsequent metabolism. The oxidative decarboxylation of these branched chain keto acids is analogous to the oxidative decarboxylation of pyruvate and α-ketoglutarate to acetyl coenzyme A and succinyl coenzyme A, respectively.

Branched chain ketoaciduria (BCKA) maple syrup urine disease

This autosomal recessive disease results from genetic defects in the α-ketodehydrogenase system, resulting in very high concentrations of leucine, isoleucine, and valine in plasma and urine with metabolic acidosis and the characteristic smell of maple syrup in urine. The incidence is about 1 in 120 000 in Europe but a figure as high as 1 in 1000 has been recorded in a Mennonite community. A number of genes are involved (see OTM3, pp. 1369).

In the classic disease poor feeding and sleepiness progress to coma and apnoea in the neonatal period. Hypoglycaemia and hyperammonaemia may occur. Mortality is high. Survivors show dystonia, other neurological abnormalities, and psychomotor retardation. Milder cases may present later, sometimes with intermittent symptoms provoked by infection or excessive protein intake. Between attacks biochemical findings are normal in such cases. Diagnosis is dependent on assay of plasma amino acids.

Treatment

A high calorie intake, given parenterally as 10–20 per cent dextrose suppresses nitrogen catabolism in the acutely ill. An amino acid mixture excluding leucine, isoleucine, and valine can be introduced by nasogastric tube to provide 2 g protein/kg/day. Normal protein sources are omitted until acid concentrations fall towards normal. Exchange transfusion and peritoneal dialysis have been used. Dietary treatment is lifelong but needs frequent adjustments. The aim is to reduce plasma leucine, isoleucine, and valine concentrations to about twice their normal values. Coma carries a poor prognosis for subsequent central nervous system development. The incidence of impaired intellect and neurological handicap is high and special schooling will be necessary. Responsiveness to thiamine (10–20 mg/day) has also been described in a few patients. It is claimed that large doses (up to 500 mg/day) improve some cases.

Genetics and prenatal diagnosis

Prenatal diagnosis has been based on enzyme assays in cultured amniocytes or chorionic villus samples. The β-ketoacid dehydrogenase complex is determined by three genes on different chromosomes with over 50 different mutations described. Other genetic defects have been described causing isolated hypervalinaemia or hyperleucinaemia–isoleucinaemia, indicating either separate amino transferases in man or different mutations affecting different substrate binding sites in a common enzyme.

The organic acidaemias in branched chain amino acid metabolism

The catabolic steps outlined in Fig. 5 illustrate the formation of isovaleric acid, propionic acid, and methylmalonic acid, each of which accumulates in one of the three more common organic acidaemias. In the further metabolism of two of these acids there are important vitamin coenzymes—biotin for priopionyl coenzyme A carboxylase and cobalamin for methylmalonyl coenzyme A mutase. Vitamin B_{12} has a complex metabolism but is required in only two metabolic steps—the remethylation of homocysteine to methionine and the conversion of methylmalonyl coenzyme A to succinyl coenzyme A. An outline of cobalamin metabolism in the body is shown in Fig. 6.

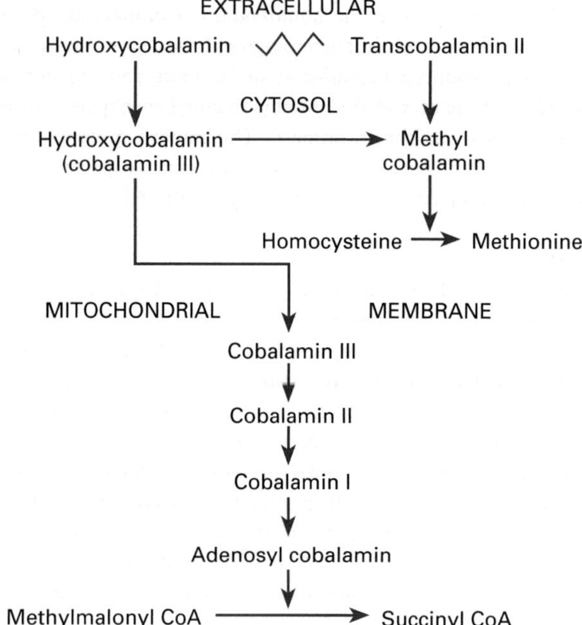

Fig. 6 Naturally occurring cobalamin is converted in the cytosol to methyl cobalamin, or by successive valency reductions of the cobalt moiety within the mitchondria adenosyl cobalamin is eventually formed.

Isovaleric, propionic, and methylmalonic acidaemias

Biochemistry

Isovaleric acidaemia is due to a deficiency of isovaleryl coenzyme A dehydrogenase and is characterized by the excretion in the urine of isovaleric acid, isovalerylglycine, 3-hydroxy isovaleric acid, and isovalerylcarnitine.

Isolated propionic acidaemia is due to a deficiency of the apoenzyme for propionyl CoA coenzyme A carboxylase, a biotin-requiring enzyme, which converts proprionyl coenzyme A to methylmalonyl coenzyme A. Characteristically, plasma and urine propionate values are raised with the formation of methylcitrate from the condensation of propionyl coenzyme A with oxaloacetate. Propionylcarnitine excretion is increased.

Methylmalonic acidaemia is due to deficient activity of methylmalonyl coenzyme A mutase, the enzyme converting methylmalonyl coenzyme A to succinyl coenzyme A, which requires adenosyl cobalamin. Two apoenzyme defects are described, one with virtually zero activity and one with residual activity of 2–75 per cent of normal. Two genetic defects in the formation of adenosyl cobalamin have been described. One affects the formation of both adenosyl and methyl cobalamin, resulting in methylmalonic aciduria and homocystinuria. The other affects only adenosyl cobalamin, and only methylmalonic aciduria occurs. Patients with severe apoenzyme defects excrete up to 5–6 g/day of methylmalonic acid with high blood concentrations up to 6 mmol/l. Propionate also accumulates in the blood and is excreted together with methylcitrate. Survivors may develop chronic renal failure in later childhood.

Genetics

All three diseases are autosomal recessive. Isovaleryl coenzyme A dehydrogenase has a single locus on the long arm of chromosome 15. Different enzyme variants cause phenotypic variation but severe neonatal and intermittent forms have been described in the same family. Propionyl coenzyme A carboxylase has the subunit structure α_6/β_6. The α-subunit gene is on chromosome 13 and the β subunit gene is on chromosome 3. Defects in the α-chain (which binds the biotin) are associated with 50 per cent enzyme activity in heterozygotes and 1–5 per cent activity in homozygotes. Homozygous β-chain defects are similarly severe but heterozygotes have near normal activity. β-Chains are produced in half-normal amounts and are normally produced in excess of α-chains. Methyl malonyl coenzyme A mutase has a gene locus on chromosome 6. The mutant mutase with no residual enzyme activity has no detectable enzyme protein, either because none is made or because it is highly unstable.

Clinical

The neonatal syndrome in which there may be acidosis, hyperammonaemia, hyperglycinaemia, and hypoglycaemia is commonly fatal. Poor feeding, respiratory distress, tonal changes, apnoea, and coma are characteristic. A more chronic form is recognized, with anorexia, failure to thrive, psychomotor retardation, hypotonia, and weakness. Cardiomyopathy has been reported.

The intermittent clinical forms present as recurrent attacks of encephalopathy and ataxia with normality between attacks. Changes in blood glucose may again be confusing. Acute attacks may be followed by neurological abnormalities of pyramidal or extrapyramidal nature. Leucopenia and thrombocytopenia sometimes occur.

Diagnosis

Diagnosis rests upon the detection of the relevant organic acids in blood and urine, their conjugates or their carnitine esters. For prenatal diagnosis isovaleric acid in amniotic fluid is measured by stable isotope dilution analysis, and isovaleryl coenzyme A dehydrogenase can be measured in cultured amniocytes. For propionic acidaemia the measurement of methylcitrate in amniotic fluid and enzyme assay in cultured amniocytes has been used. Similar approaches to prenatal diagnosis in isolated methylmalonic acidurias have used the measurement of methylmalonate acid in amniotic fluid and enzyme assays or studies of adenosyl vitamin B_{12} metabolism in cultured amniocytes.

Treatment

Initial treatment of severe neonatal syndromes involves exchange transfusion, peritoneal dialysis, feeding with intravenous glucose, and later enteral tube feeding with low protein mixtures omitting the critical amino acid. Supplements of glycine and carnitine are helpful and the catabolic state may respond to the use of insulin and growth hormone. Hydroxycobalamin is useful in methylmalonic acidaemia. Low protein diets are needed in long-term survivors and sodium bicarbonate helps in countering residual metabolic acidosis. Combined liver and renal transplantation has been used in methylmalonic acidaemia when renal failure has occurred. Further details are given in OTM3, pp. 1731–32.

Defects of lysine metabolism

The main pathway of lysine catabolism is via saccharopine to acetyl coenzyme A and others less important. Glutaryl coenzyme A dehydrogenase catalyses the conversion of glutaryl coenzyme A to crotonyl coenzyme A and its defects are serious disorders. Other lysine degradation defects are of uncertain clinical consequence.

Glutaric aciduria type I

Glutaryl coenzyme A dehydrogenase deficiency is an autosomal recessive disorder with varying residual enzyme activity and several mutations have been described. This results in an accumulation of glutaryl coenzyme A (also derived from tryptophan degradation), increasing glutaric acid concentrations in plasma and urine, and increasing concentrations of 3-hydroxyglutarate and glutaconic acid. These are all inhibitors of glutamic acid decarboxylase, which may explain the low γ-aminobutyric acid concentrations in the central nervous system. Glutaryl carnitine is excreted in the urine even when free glutaric acid is absent. Systemic acidosis occurs in acute attacks with ketosis and hypoglycaemia.

Retarded motor development in the first year of life with hypotonia is followed by ataxia, athetosis, and other involuntary movements. Acquired motor skills such as walking and writing are slowly lost in the childhood years. Severe dystonia and pyramidal defects with extensor or flexor spasms occur. Dysarthria renders speech unintelligible. Intercurrent infection precipitates acidosis, seizures, coma, and paralysis, from which recovery is incomplete. The overall picture might be regarded as dystonic cerebral palsy. Computed tomography scans have revealed progressive cerebral atrophy and hyperlucency of the caudate nucleus. Subdural effusions may occur and have wrongly been attributed to non-accidental injury.

This cause of progressive dystonic cerebral palsy is usually indicated by the organic acids in plasma and urine. Sometimes the organic acids have not been detected, particularly between acute attacks. Enzyme assays on leucocytes or fibroblasts are then indicated.

Genetics and treatment

Prenatal diagnosis has been carried out by finding glutaric acid in the amniotic fluid and enzyme assay on cultured amniocytes. Many mutations have been described in the glutaryldehydrogenase gene on chromosome 14.

Treatment with low protein diets reduce glutaric acid excretion. Carnitine supplementation corrects low plasma levels which are

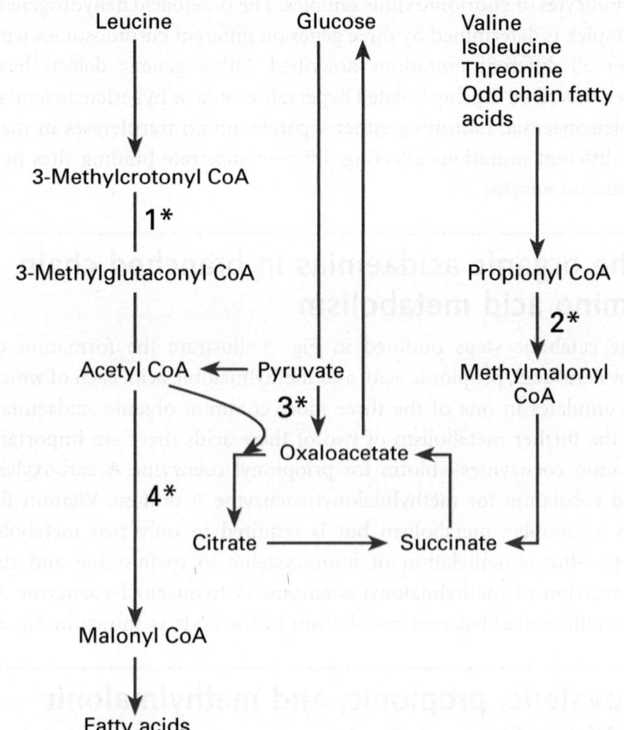

Fig. 7 Important carboxylases in amino acid metabolism. Asterisked enzymes are: 1, 3-methylcrotonyl coenzyme A carboxylase; 2, propionyl coenzyme A carboxylase; 3, pyruvate carboxylase; and 4, acetyl coenzyme A carboxylase.

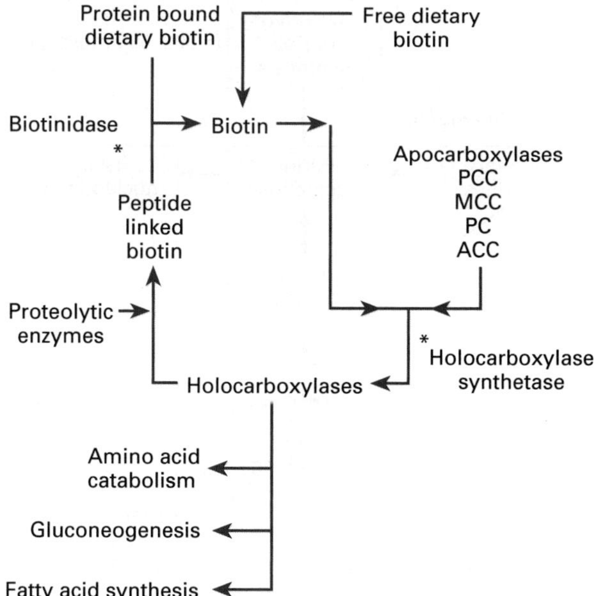

Fig. 8 The metabolism of biotin. MCC (3-methylcrotonyl coenzyme A) and PCC (propionyl coenzyme A carboxylase) are important in amino acid catabolism, and PC (pyruvate carboxylase) is important in gluconeogenesis, and ACC (acetyl carboxylase) in fatty acid synthesis. Important enzymes are asterisked.

secondary to losses from glutaryl carnitine excretion. Riboflavin has been reported to diminish glutaric acid excretion in some patients, the rationale being that increased flavine adenine dinucleotide might stabilize the enzyme. Baclofen has also been studied because it activates γ-aminobutyric acid receptors but no treatment has proved of any clinical benefit.

Defects in the final stages of carbon chain metabolism

These are characterized by complex organic acidurias.

Biotin dependent carboxylation: multiple carboxylase deficiency

Biotin is important in transferring a 1-carbon unit (carbon dioxide) to acceptor molecules. Defects in biotin metabolism disturb the function of four enzymes—pyruvate carboxylase, acetyl-coenzyme A carboxylase, proprionyl coenzyme A carboxylase, and 3-methylcrotonyl coenzyme A carboxylase (Fig. 7). These apoenzymes are converted to holoenzymes by the attachment of biotin, which needs the catalytic activity of holocarboxylase synthetase (Fig. 8). When the holoenzymes are degraded biotinidase frees and conserves the biotin. It also liberates dietary biotin from proteins in the gastrointestinal tract. In its absence biotin deficiency occurs.

Biotin dependent carboxylation fails if either the holocarboxylase synthetase or biotinidase are deficient leading to a variable and complex organic aciduria. Both respond biochemically to biotin treatment although existing clinical damage may not be reversible. Neonatal presentations include acidosis, seizures, skin rash, alopecia, coma and death. Less severe presentations are known in older patients with developmental delay, ataxia, seizures and hypotonia.

Glutaric aciduria type II

Biochemical defects at the very end of the catabolic chain have been described where electrons are transferred from the flavin containing acyl CoA dehydrogenases to the electron transporting chain. At this level the catabolic defects involve fatty acid degradation also. The organic aciduria is complex but includes glutaric acid. Presentations may be neonatal, severe, and fatal or delayed and milder with encephalopathy (like Reye's syndrome) or lipid myopathy (see OTM3, pp. 1373–4).

Further reading

Blau, N., Duran, M., and Blaskovics, M.E. (1996). *Physician's guide to the laboratory diagnosis of metabolic diseases.* Chapman and Hall, London.

Brusilow, S.W. and Maestri, N.E. (1996). Urea cycle disorders: diagnosis, pathophysiology, and therapy. *Advances in Pediatrics*, **43**, 127–70.

Fernandes, J., Saudubray, J.-M., and van den Berghe, G. (1995). *Inborn metabolic diseases. Diagnosis and treatment*, 2nd edn. Springer-Verlag, Berlin.

Fowler, B. (1997). Disorders of homocysteine metabolism. *Journal of Inherited Metabolic Diseases*, **20**, 270.

Scriver, C.R., Beaudet, A.L., Sly, W.S., and Valle, D. (1995). *The metabolic and molecular bases of inherited disease*, 7th edn. McGraw-Hill, New York.

Chapter 6.6

Disorders of purine and pyrimidine metabolism

G. Nuki

Ribonucleotides and deoxyribonucleotides are the monomeric building blocks from which nucleic acids (RNA and DNA) are constructed. Each nucleotide consists of a heterocyclic ring derived from a purine or pyrimidine base to which a pentose sugar and phosphate group have been added. Purine and pyrimidine nucleotides, nucleosides, and bases are key substrates, cofactors, and regulatory molecules in almost every branch of human metabolism, and ATP and other purine nucleotides provide the energy needed for many metabolic processes. Purines and pyrimidines are required for transcription, translation, and protein synthesis. Purine compounds play an essential physiological role in membrane signal transduction and as neurotransmitters, vasodilators, and mediators of platelet aggregation and hormone action.

Gout (see also Chapter 10.6)

Gout is the term used to describe a group of disorders in which clinical problems result from tissue deposition of crystals of monosodium urate monohydrate from hyperuricaemic body fluids. Major clinical manifestations include:

1. acute inflammatory arthritis, tenosynovitis, bursitis, or cellulitis;
2. chronic, erosive, deforming arthritis associated with periarticular and subcutaneous urate deposits (tophi);
3. nephrolithiasis and urolithiasis;
4. chronic renal disease and hypertension.

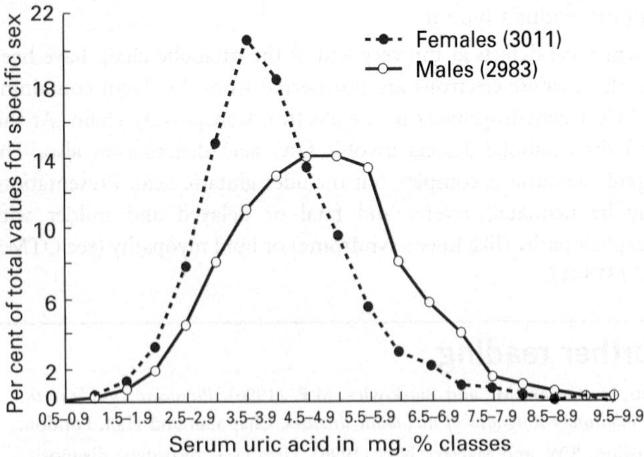

Fig. 1 Distribution of serum urate values in male and female populations of Tecumseh, Michigan, 1959–60.
(For source see OTM3, p. 1377.)

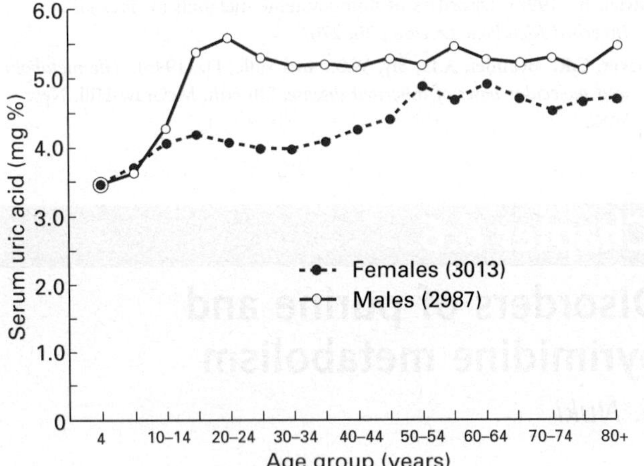

Fig. 2 Sex- and age-specific mean serum urate values in the population of Tecumseh, Michigan, 1959–60.
(For source see OTM3, p. 1377.)

Hyperuricaemia alone is not sufficient for the development of clinical disease. Tissue deposition of crystals of monosodium urate and resulting clinical symptoms and signs of gout usually only follow prolonged elevation of serum urate. Hyperuricaemia can result from increased purine intake, turnover, or production, from decreased urate elimination by the kidneys, or from a combination of these. The rheumatological features of gout are described in Chapter 10.6.

Serum urate levels

Serum urate concentrations are distributed in the community as a continuous variable (Fig. 1). Mean values are higher in men than in women and the sex-specific distribution curve is broader for males than females, with skewing to the higher end of the scale in both sexes. Serum levels rise in boys at puberty and then remain virtually unchanged throughout adult life. In girls the pubertal rise is smaller and the serum level only approaches that of males after the menopause (Fig. 2).

There are significant variations of serum urate levels in different ethnic groups. The Maoris of New Zealand and the Polynesians of the Western Pacific, for example, have high levels. Although polygenic control of serum urate levels is well established, environmental factors are also important. Members of the Chinese community in Taiwan have lower serum urate levels than those in Malaysia or British Columbia; Filipinos resident in the United States have higher levels than those in the Philippine Islands; and urban South African Negroes have significantly higher levels than those in rural communities. These differences result from a less than average capacity to increase the renal excretion of urate when the purine load is increased. The association of high serum urate levels with high purine and protein intake, alcohol consumption, weight, body bulk, and social class suggest that in most communities environmental factors are the major determinants of the serum urate. Hyperuricaemia is discussed further in Chapter 10.6.

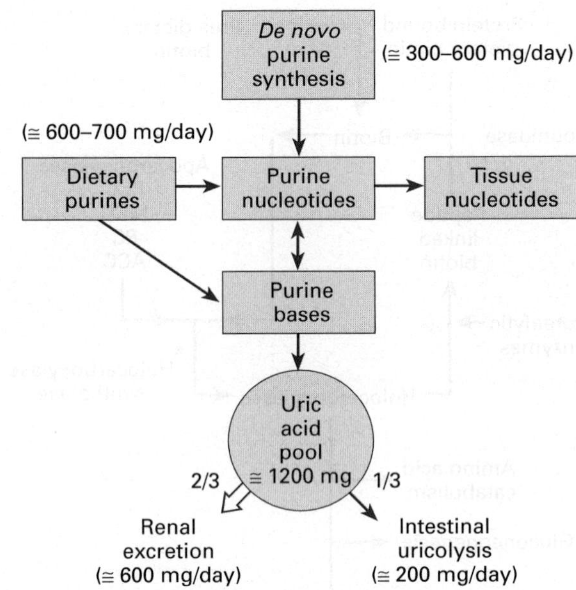

Fig. 3 The uric acid pool; origins and disposal in normal man.

Uric acid metabolism

Plasma and tissue urates are derived from the catabolism of purine nucleotides synthesized *de novo* and from dietary purines. The miscible pool of urate in normal individuals ranges from 0.9 to 1.6 g, of which about 60 per cent is replenished daily from the catabolism of newly synthesized purines. Two-thirds of the urate formed each day is eliminated by the kidney and one-third via the gastrointestinal tract (Fig. 3).

Purine nucleotide synthesis

Purine synthesis is regulated by a balanced interaction of a number of biochemical pathways (Fig. 4) (see OTM3, pp. 1377–8).

Uric acid excretion (see also Chapter 10.21)

On an unrestricted diet, excretion in the urine can exceed 1000 mg/day. Although 100 to 200 mg are secreted daily into the gastrointestinal tract, where it is degraded by bacterial uricolysis, an approximate estimate of synthesis can be made by measuring uric acid excreted in the urine on an isocaloric purine-free diet. Twenty-four h urine excretion of more than 600 mg (3.6 mmol) on a 2600 calcium, 70 g protein, purine-free diet or 10 mg/kg body weight/day on a low-purine diet strongly suggests an increase in *de novo* purine synthesis or increased turnover of cellular purine nucleotides. Accurate assessment of the rate of *de novo* purine synthesis requires measurement

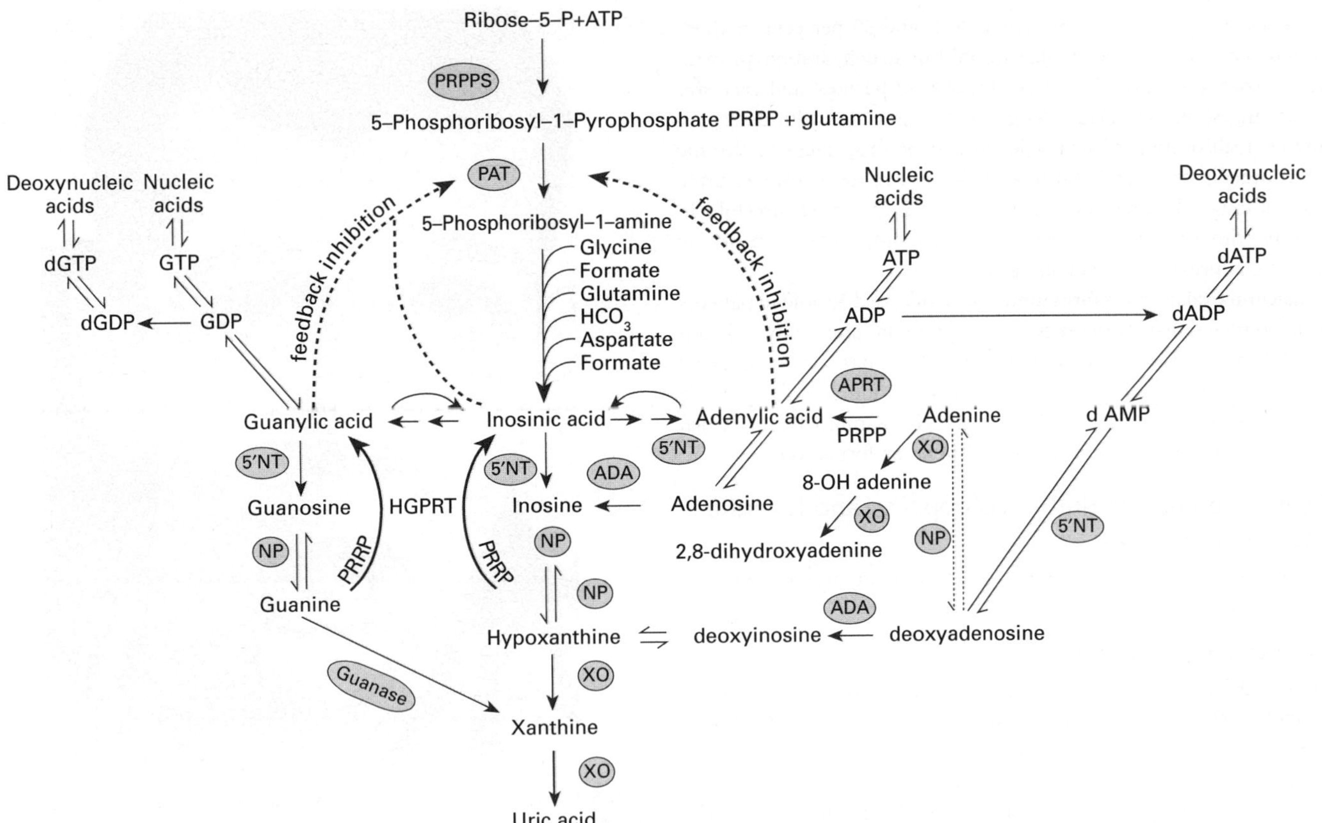

Fig. 4 Pathways of purine metabolism in humans. ADA, adenosine deaminase; APRT, adenine phosphoribosyl transferase; HGPRT, hypoxanthine-guanine phosphoribosyl transferase; NP, nucleoside phosphorylase; 5'-NP, 5'-nucleotidase; PAT, phosphoribosyl pyrophosphate amidotransferase; PPRPS, phosphoribosyl pyrophosphate synthetase; XO, xanthine oxidase.
(For source see OTM3, p. 1378.)

of ^{14}C-glycine incorporation into urine uric acid with simultaneous administration of ^{15}N- uric acid to correct for extrarenal disposal.

Renal handling of uric acid has four components; glomerular filtration, proximal tubular reabsorption, tubular secretion, and post-secretory reabsorption (Fig. 5). Glomerular ultrafiltration is complete as there is no significant protein binding of urate *in vivo*. Proximal tubular reabsorption occurs by an active transport mechanism closely linked to, or identical with, the tubular reabsorption of sodium.

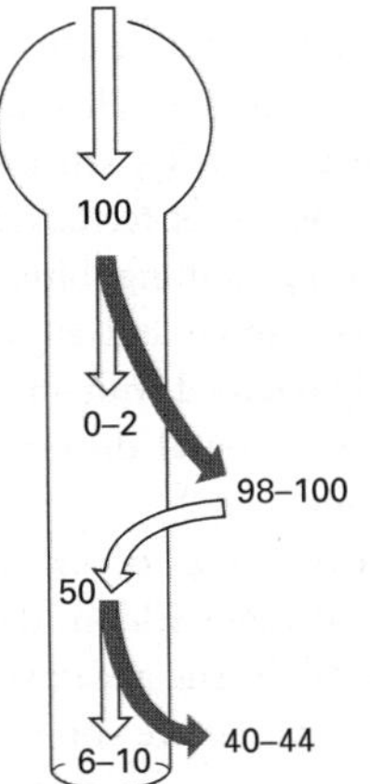

Fig. 5 Four-component model for the renal handling of urate in the human kidney. Numerical values indicate hypothetical orders of magnitude of the transport processes. (*For source see OTM3, p. 1379.*)

Evidence for active secretion comes from inherited and pharmacologically induced tubular defects in which urate clearance can exceed inulin clearance. The paradoxical effect of high- and low-dose aspirin on uric acid excretion can be explained by differential effects on active secretion and reabsorption. Low-dose aspirin blocks urate secretion with consequent hyperuricaemia while high-dose therapy also blocks reabsorption and results in a net increase in uric acid excretion. Postsecretory reabsorption of urate is suggested by the fact that pre-treatment with probenecid, which inhibits tubular reabsorption of urate, prevents the decrease in uric acid excretion that normally follows administration of low-dosage aspirin or pyrazinamide. Renal clearance of urate in normal subjects ranges from 6 to 9 ml/min.

Hyperuricaemia may be the result of increased urate production, decreased renal excretion, or a combination of both mechanisms (see Chapter 10.6).

Urolithiasis (see also Chapter 12.23)

In the UK uric acid stones account for 5 per cent of all renal calculi and 10 per cent of patients with gout have a history of renal colic. In Israel, uric acid calculi are responsible for 40 per cent of cases of nephrolithiasis and 75 per cent of patients with primary gout develop renal calculus disease. Urine uric acid concentration is the most important aetiological factor and in temperate climates this is mainly determined by urate production and purine ingestion. The prevalence of renal stones in patients with primary gout is 20 per cent in patients excreting up to 200 mg of uric acid/24 h and 50 per cent in those excreting more than 1100 mg/day. In addition to dehydration, primary purine overproduction, increased turnover of purines, and excessive purine ingestion, uric acid calculi may be associated with defects in tubular reabsorption of uric acid, uricosuric drug therapy, chronic diarrhoeal diseases, and ileostomy, the last as a result of lowered urine pH. Although the incidence of urolithiasis is increased threefold in persons with asymptomatic hyperuricaemia, only 20 per cent of uric acid stone formers are hyperuricaemic.

Calcium oxalate stone formation is also increased 30-fold in patients with gout and hyperuricosuria is common in non-gouty calcium stone formers. Uric acid crystals themselves may act as epitaxial nucleation sites for calcium oxalate stone formation. It is also possible that colloidal uric acid adsorbs urinary glycosaminoglycans which normally act as endogenous inhibitors of stone formation.

Acute and chronic urate nephropathy and juvenile gouty nephropathy

These are discussed in Chapter 10.21 and an account of lead nephropathy can be found in OTM3, p. 3261.

Other clinical associations

Gout and hyperuricaemia are often associated with obesity, heavy alcohol intake, hyperlipoproteinaemia, impaired glucose tolerance, and ischaemic heart disease in men but not in women. Obesity may be the major linking factor. Men with gout are on average 15 to 20 per cent overweight, and the prevalence of hyperuricaemia in the community rises from 3 per cent in those whose weight is on the 20th percentile to 11 per cent in those above the 80th percentile.

Hypertriglyceridaemia occurs in more than 75 per cent of patients with gout, and hyperuricaemia in a similar proportion of individuals with hypertriglyceridaemia. Non-gouty family members are not affected and heavy alcohol intake and obesity are both predisposing factors.

Hypertension occurs in 25 to 50 per cent of patients with gout, while hyperuricaemia is a feature in one-third of untreated hypertensive patients and two-thirds of those receiving thiazide therapy. Impaired glucose tolerance and ischaemic heart disease are associated with gout and obesity rather than with asymptomatic hyperuricaemia and there is no good evidence to suggest that hyperuricaemia alone is a risk factor for diabetes mellitus or myocardial infarction.

In women the clinical stereotype is often one of a lean and abstemious postmenopausal woman with mild renal insufficiency, who has received diuretic drugs for many years. Polyarticular involvement is more common and hypertriglyceridaemia is not a feature.

Hyperuricaemia and gouty arthritis may preceed the development of renal failure in patients with polycystic kidney disease, and about one-third of patients with this disease develop gouty arthritis. The basis for this association may be abnormal tubular reabsorption of urate, and similar mechanisms may account for the increase in gout and hyperuricaemia seen in patients with medullary sponge kidney and cystinuria.

Inborn errors of purine metabolism

Lesch-Nyhan syndrome

Severe cellular deficiency of hypoxanthine-guanine phosphoribosyl transferase (HPRT) is associated with primary purine overproduction, hyperuricaemia, and gout, together with a neurological syndrome comprising choreoathetosis, spasticity, a variable degree of mental deficiency, and a striking behavioural disturbance characterized by self-mutilation (Fig. 6).

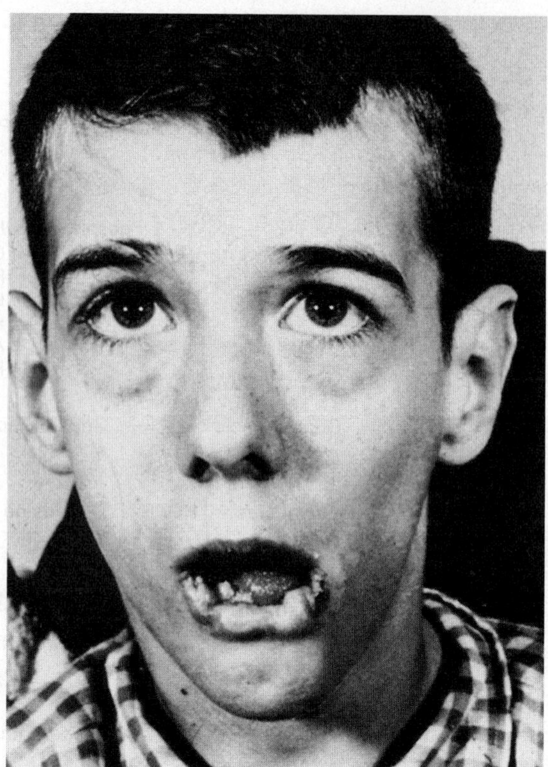

Fig. 6 Boy with Lesch-Nyhan syndrome showing evidence of self-mutilation of lips
(by courtesy of Dr J.E. Seegmiller).

Clinical expression of disease is virtually limited to males. Babies appear normal at birth but mothers may observe the presence of orange crystals in the diapers. Occasional vomiting and hypotonia is followed by a delay in motor development at the age of 3 to 4 months. The characteristic pyramidal and extrapyramidal signs which eventually progress to severe spasticity and choreoathetosis are seldom apparent before 1 year and the compulsive behavioural disturbance can commence at any time between the ages of 2 and 16 years. Episodes of involuntary and occasionally unilateral self-mutilation come and go without any clear relationship to endogenous or environmental factors. These episodes are often associated with agitation and anxiety which can be partially relieved by physical restraint to prevent finger biting. In some cases self-mutilation of the lips can only be prevented by extraction of teeth. Aggression towards others may take the form of hitting, spitting, biting, and abusive language, typically accompanied by a smile and an apology. The majority of boys affected are mentally retarded with an IQ in the range 40 to 65, but the severity of the behavioural disturbance is unrelated to the degree of mental deficiency.

Haematuria and renal colic may occur during the first decade of life but gouty arthritis and tophi seldom develop before puberty. A macrocytic or frankly megaloblastic anaemia is an occasional feature. Death from infection or renal failure commonly occurs between the ages of 20 and 30 years.

Biochemical findings

HPRT catalyses the reactions:

$$\text{Hypoxanthine} + \text{PP-ribose-P} \xrightarrow{Mg^{2+}} \text{inosine 5}'\text{-phosphate} + \text{PPi}$$

$$\text{Guanine} + \text{PP-ribose-P} \xrightarrow{Mg^{2+}} \text{inosine 5}'\text{-phosphate} + \text{PPi}$$

Deficiency results in accelerated production of uric acid with greatly increased urine uric acid excretion (0.15–0.75 mmol/kg/24 h) and a characteristically high urine uric acid:creatinine ratio. The serum urate is usually, but not invariably, raised, in the range 0.42 to 0.9 mmol/l.

Concentrations of phosphoribosyl pyrophosphate (PP-ribose-P) are raised and there is severe deficiency of HPRT in red cell lysates, in leucocytes, cultured fibroblasts, amniotic fluid cells, and other tissues such as liver and brain. Associated abnormalities include increased activity of adenine phosphoribosyl transferase, inosine monophosphate dehydrogenase, and the pyrimidine enzymes orotate phosphoribosyl transferase and orotidine 5′-phosphate decarboxylase. It seems probable that accelerated *de novo* purine biosynthesis *in vivo* is primarily due to the effect of increased availability of PP-ribose-P on the rate-limiting amido transferase enzyme rather than decreased feedback inhibition by purine nucleotides.

The biochemical basis for neurological dysfunction remains uncertain. Morphological abnormalities have not been detected in post-mortem studies of the brain but it seems reasonable to assume that accumulation of purine metabolites, rather than deficiency of purine nucleotides, interferes in some way with neurotransmitter function in the brain-stem. The demonstration of decreases in dopamine, homovanillic acid, dopa decarboxylase, and tyrosine hydroxylase activity in the dopamine-terminal-rich regions of the putamen and the caudate nucleus suggest that there may be secondary abnormalities of terminal arborization of dopaminergic neurones.

The biochemical basis for the megaloblastic anaemia also remains unclear. In isolated cases the anaemia has been shown to respond to adenine rather than to folic acid.

Genetics—prenatal detection and prevention

Lesch-Nyhan syndrome is an X-linked disorder which is only fully expressed in males. Asymptomatic carrier females can be detected by hair root analysis or by finding HPRT-positive and HPRT-negative populations of cells in fibroblast cultures from skin biopsies. Using these techniques, only four out of 47 mothers were homozygous normal, suggesting a lower than expected ratio of new to established mutations. Culture of amniotic fluid cells following amniocentesis allows the detection of affected males *in utero*.

Biochemical studies of normal human HPRT have revealed a variety of HPRT variants. Although much of the heterogeneity appears to be the result of post-translational modification, there is evidence of true genetic heterogeneity in patients. In the majority of cases complete absence of enzyme activity is associated with absence of protein cross-reacting with antibody to normal enzyme (CRM-negative mutants) but CRM-positive mutants with absent catalytic activity have also been detected, providing evidence of structural gene mutations. Amino acid sequencing shows a whole spectrum of mutations at the HPRT locus, resulting in cells with varying amounts of residual enzyme activity and HPRT with altered substrate affinities. Indeed, the level of HPRT activity in red cells from some patients overlaps the range of activities seen in some families with gout and overproduction of purines alone. Heterozygote carriers can show modest increases in the rates of *de novo* purine biosynthesis, increases in uric acid excretion, and occasionally asymptomatic hyperuricaemia.

More than 50 HPRT mutants have been characterized at the DNA and mRNA level. Four independent mutational events representing three unique base substitutions have been described within the codon for Arg 51 and a single base substitution has been found within the codon for Ala 50. Approximately 40 per cent of HPRT point mutations are estimated to occur in exon-3 within two regions. This work has contributed to the development of earlier and more reliable methods for antenatal diagnosis using DNA analysis.

Treatment

Allopurinol is mandatory in all affected subjects. Serum and urine uric acid levels are thus lowered, but total purine excretion is not reduced in Lesch-Nyhan syndrome as it is in patients with gout and purine overproduction. Nevertheless gouty arthritis, urate stone formation, and urate nephropathy can be effectively prevented and the possibility of xanthine stone formation is minimized by ensuring adequate hydration and urine flow. Hypouricaemic drug therapy does not, however, influence the neurological manifestations or the behavioural disturbance. Diazepam, haloperidol, and other sedatives can be helpful in managing the extrapyramidal movements, but tooth extraction and physical restraint with splints and bandages are often required to control the compulsive self-mutilation.

Partial HPRT deficiency

Severe familial X-linked gout with minor or absent neurological features may be associated with partial deficiency of HPRT. These patients usually present with uric acid calculi or gouty arthritis in adolescence or adult life. In about 25 per cent there is a mild neurological disturbance. In some families this resembles a *forme fruste* of Lesch-Nyhan syndrome with disorders of movement and compulsive behaviour. In others there has been a history of convulsions, mental retardation, and a spinocerebellar syndrome. As in the Lesch-Nyhan syndrome, macrocytosis and megaloblastic marrow changes may be observed.

Biochemical findings and genetics

Serum uric acid levels are high and there is evidence of primary purine overproduction with urine uric acid excretion usually in excess of 5 mmol/24 h and a uric acid:creatinine ratio greater than 0.75 unless renal insufficiency has already supervened. HPRT activity in erythrocyte lysates is usually in the range 0.01 to 30 per cent of normal, with similar levels of residual enzyme activity in individuals from the same family. Identical phenotypes have, however, been reported where red blood cell HPRT was undetectable or apparently normal. In the latter instances structural gene mutations led to subtle abnormalities of HPRT protein with an altered K_M for PP-ribose-P in one case and abnormal sensitivity to feedback inhibition by purine nucleotides in the other. These cases illustrate how the clinical features of disease associated with HPRT deficiency cannot be reliably predicted from simple assays of erythrocyte HPRT alone. Phenotypic expression is, however, always similar within each family; typical Lesch-Nyhan syndrome and X-linked gout without neurological features never occur in related patients.

Intracellular concentrations of PP-ribose-P and pyrimidine nucleotides are increased and there is increased activity of adenine phosphoribosyl transferase, inosine monophosphate dehydrogenase, orotate phosphoribosyl transferase, and orotidine 5′-phosphate decarboxylase in erythrocyte lysates.

As in Lesch-Nyhan syndrome, there is genetic heterogeneity. Most of the mutations are associated with normal mRNA and immunologically detectable defective HPRT. Point mutations in genomic DNA have been identified.

Carrier detection of heterozygotes is as for Lesch-Nyhan syndrome but amniocentesis, prenatal detection, and preventive abortion are not justified. Treatment is with allopurinol.

Adenine phosphoribosyl transferase (APRT) deficiency

$$\text{Adenine} + \text{PP-ribose-P} \xrightarrow{Mg^{2+}} \text{Adenosine 5}'\text{-phosphate} + \text{PPi}$$

Severe homozygous deficiency of APRT is associated with the formation of renal calculi of 2,8-dihydroxyadenine. While most cases present in early childhood with or without acute renal failure, some remain free from symptoms of renal lithiasis until middle age. This rare autosomal recessive disorder is not associated with primary purine overproduction, hyperuricaemia, or gout, although the renal calculi are invariably mistaken for uric acid stones if only standard laboratory methods of stone analysis are used. Homozygous APRT deficiency is characterized by increased urinary excretion of polyamine-derived adenine and its metabolites 8-hydroxyadenine and 2,8-dihydroxyadenine. Renal stone formation can be successfully prevented by administration of allopurinol, but care must be taken to reduce the dose in patients with renal failure.

As many as 1 per cent of the normal population may be heterozygotes with partial APRT deficiency which is not usually associated with clinical disease, but 2,8-dihydroxyadenine urine lithiasis has recently been described in Japanese patients.

Phosphoribosyl pyrophosphate synthetase (PPRPS) overactivity

$$\text{Ribose 5-phosphate} + \text{ATP} \xrightarrow{Mg^{2+} + Pi} \text{PP-ribose-P} + \text{AMP}$$

A number of families have been described in which X-linked gout and severe primary purine overproduction are associated with structural enzyme mutations resulting in superactive PP-ribose-P synthetase (PPRPS). In some, increased enzyme activity is associated with abnormal resistance to feedback inhibitors while in others superactive PPRPS appears to be associated with an increased *Vmax* or affinity for ribose-5-phosphate.

Affected males develop uric acid lithiasis or gouty arthritis in childhood or early adult life. Hyperuricaemia is often severe and in the range 0.5 to 1 mmol/l, with urine uric acid excretion of 5 to 15 mmol/24 h. Heterozygotes remain asymptomatic, although purine synthesis *de novo* is increased.

In some families the disorder presents in childhood with associated neurological features such as motor and mental retardation, ataxia, hypotonia, and disturbed development of speech. Polyneuropathy, intracerebral calcifications, and dysmorphic facial features have also been described, and in one family deafness was an associated clinical feature both in affected males and their heterozygous mothers.

Heterozygotes can be identified by studies in cultured skin fibroblasts but amniocentesis, prenatal diagnosis, and preventive abortion are not justified in this condition.

The hyperuricaemia, primary purine overproduction, and uricosuria can be controlled well with allopurinol.

Glucose 6-phosphatase deficiency

$$\text{Glucose 6-phosphate} + H_2O \rightarrow \text{Glucose} + \text{Pi}$$

Severe deficiency of glucose 6-phosphatase (glycogen storage disease type I, von Gierke's disease) is associated with marked hyperuricaemia from infancy (see Chapter 6.2 and OTM3, p.1342). Gouty arthritis may become a problem before the age of 10 years, and chronic tophaceous gout with renal involvement can be a major cause of morbidity in those lucky enough to survive to adult life, unless preventive measures are taken. Xanthomata frequently develop over the buttocks and extensor surfaces of the extremities and need to be distinguished from tophi.

Renal clearance of uric acid is decreased but the urine uric acid: creatinine ratio is frequently greater than 0.75 and glycine incorporation into urine uric acid is increased. Thus hyperuricaemia is a consequence of both decreased urate excretion secondary to competitive inhibition of renal tubular urate secretion by lactate and excessive purine synthesis *de novo*. It has been suggested that the accelerated purine synthesis which occurs in these patients may result from increased availability of phosphoribosyl pyrophosphate following shunting of metabolites through the pentose phosphate pathway, but more recent evidence points to accelerated purine degradation following recurrent glycogenolysis and depletion of ATP.

Myogenic hyperuricaemia

Hyperuricaemia, particularly following exercise, is also a feature of glycogen storage disease with primary muscle involvement (debranching enzyme deficiency (GSD type III), myophosphorylase deficiency (GSD type V), and phosphofructokinase deficiency (GSD type VII)). In each of these hyperuricaemia results from excessive degradation of muscle ATP following exercise because of lack of carbohydrate substrates necessary for the synthesis of muscle ATP.

Fructose intolerance (see also Chapter 6.3)

Fructose ingestion and infusion are associated with hyperuricaemia, accelerated purine synthesis, and catabolism in normal subjects, and hyperuricaemia is a feature in patients with hereditary fructose intolerance. The finding of clinical gout in three out of nine subjects with heterozygous deficiency of aldolase B has led to the suggestion that this relatively common genetic trait (1/250 in Great Britain) could be responsible for a significant proportion of cases of familial gout.

Adenylosuccinase deficiency

SAICA – ribotide → AICA – ribiotide + fumarate
Adenylosuccinic acid → AMP + fumaric acid

Adenylosuccinase deficiency has recently been associated with an infantile autistic syndrome characterized by the presence of succinyl purines in the plasma, urine, and cerebrospinal fluid. Psychomotor retardation occurs before the age of 2 years and autism, axial hypotonia, and normal tendon reflexes are characteristic. Self-mutilation can also be a feature and there is evidence of cerebellar hypoplasia on CT scanning. The diagnosis is suggested by the finding of aspartic acid and glycine in body fluids and confirmed by the identification of succinyl adenosine and SAICA riboside by HPLC. Tissue studies show partial enzyme deficiency in the liver, kidney, and muscle, as well as lymphocytes and fibroblasts but not red cells. Adenylosuccinase deficiency is associated with a secondary increase in purine nucleotide synthesis and/or a decrease in degradation. It is inherited as an autosomal recessive. Patients with growth retardation have been shown to benefit from the administration of adenine (10 mg/kg/day) together with allopurinol.

Adenylate deaminase deficiency

$$AMP \rightarrow IMP + NH_3$$

AMP deaminase deficiency leads to reduced entry of adenine nucleotides into the purine nucleotide cycle during exercise, with resultant muscular weakness and muscle cramps following exercise. Symptoms begin in early childhood. Physical and neurological abnormalities are limited to some decrease in muscle mass, hypotonia, and a little muscle weakness. Laboratory abnormalities include a modest rise in creatine phosphokinase in some but not all patients, non-specific abnormalities of the electromyogram, absence of ammonia in venous blood following exercise, and a complete absence of the enzyme on histochemical analysis of the muscle biopsy. The condition is inherited as an autosomal recessive.

Patients are advised to avoid vigorous exercise to prevent rhabdomyolysis, and administration of oral ribose (2–60 g/day) has been found to be beneficial in some cases.

Xanthine oxidase deficiency

$$Hypoxanthine + H_20 + 0_2 \rightarrow xanthine + H_20$$
$$Xanthine + H_20 + 0_2 \rightarrow uric\ acid + H_20$$

Hereditary xanthinuria is a rare autosomal recessive disorder in which severe deficiency of xanthine oxidase is associated with hypouricaemia and excessive urinary excretion of xanthine and hypoxanthine. Some affected patients remain free from symptoms throughout their lives, the condition only being detected by finding a low serum urate on routine biochemical testing. In others the formation of xanthine calculi has been associated with renal colic, a mild myopathy, and crystal synovitis.

Plasma uric acid levels are usually less than 1 mg/100 ml and urinary uric acid excretion is less than 50 mg/24 h. Plasma oxypurines are correspondingly raised in the range 0.1 to 1.0 mg/100 ml and urine oxypurine excretion may be as high as 500 mg/24 h. Assays of hepatic or intestinal xanthine oxidase usually show no detectable activity but cases with as much as 10 per cent (liver) and 25 per cent (intestine) residual activity have been recorded.

Not all patients with xanthine stones have xanthine oxidase deficiency or even increased oxypurine excretion. Treatment is usually restricted to maintaining a high fluid intake. Since xanthine solubility increases at higher pH, oral administration of alkali can be considered in recurrent stone formers. Allopurinol should be considered in those patients with residual enzyme activity, as hypoxanthine is significantly more soluble than xanthine.

Other causes of hypouricaemia

Hypouricaemia due to reduced uric acid formation occurs in patients with deficiencies of PP-ribose-P synthetase and purine nucleoside phosphorylase as well in hereditary xanthinuria, allopurinol therapy, and severe hepatic disease. More commonly, however, hypouricaemia results from increased excretion, which may be associated with isolated or more generalized defects of renal tubular transport, and particularly with drug therapy of various kinds (Table 1).

Table 1 Causes of hypouricaemia

Decreased production of uric acid	Increased excretion of uric acid
Purine enzyme defects	Isolated defects in renal tubular handling
Xanthine oxidase	Idiopathic (dalmatian dog mutation)
PP-ribose-P synthetase	Malignant diseases
Purine nucleoside phosphorylase	Hepatic diseases
Severe hepatic disease	Generalized defects in renal tubular transport (Fanconi syndrome)
Acute intermittent porphyria	Idiopathic
Drugs	Wilson's disease
Allopurinol	Carcinoma of bronchus
	Multiple myeloma
	Lymphomas
	Hepatic disease and alcoholism
	Hyperparathyroidism
	Heavy metal poisoning
	Cystinosis
	Galactosaemia
	Hereditary fructose intolerance
	Drugs
	Uricosuric agents (e.g. probenecid, sulphinpyrazone, benzbromarone)
	Radiographic contrast agents
	NSAID with uricosuric properties (e.g. phenylbutazone, azapropazone, high-dose aspirin)
	Oestrogens
	Glyceryl guaiacholate
	Coumarin anticoagulants
	Outdated tetracycline

Inborn errors of purine metabolism in immunodeficiency

Deficiency of purine nucleoside phosphorylase, of 5'-nucleotidase, and of adenosine deaminase are each associated with immunodeficiency.

Inborn errors of pyrimidine metabolism

There are three major pathways of pyrimidine metabolism in man, *de novo* synthesis, salvage, and degradation (Fig. 7).

Pyrimidine biosynthesis

The *de novo* pathway of pyrimidine biosynthesis consists of a series of six enzymatic reactions coded for by three structural genes which lead to the formation of orotic acid, orotidine monophosphate (OMP) and uridine monophosphate (UMP). Cytidine monophosphate (CMP) and thymidine monophosphate (TMP) are derived from UMP by a series of enzymatic steps before phosphorylation to their respective di- and triphosphates and synthesis of RNA and DNA. UMP and TMP are also synthesized by uridine kinase, thymidine kinase, and uracil phosphoribosyl transferase.

The pyrimidine nucleotide monophosphates are degraded to the nucleosides cytidine, uridine, and thymidine by 5'-nucleotidase.

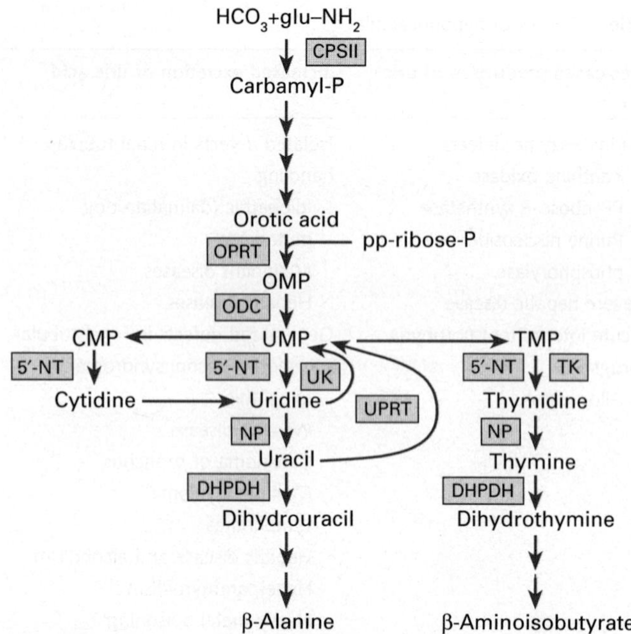

Fig. 7 Pathways of pyrimidine metabolism in humans. CPS, carbamyl phosphate synthetase II; OPRT, orotate phosphoribosyl transferase; ODC, orotidine monophosphate decarboxylase (OPRT+ODC form UMP synthase); 5′-NT, pyrimidine 5′-nucleotidase; NP, pyrimidine nucleoside phosphorylase; DHPD, dihydropyrimidine dehydrogenase; UK, uridine kinase; UPRT, uracil phosphoribosyl transferase; TK, thymidine kinase.

Cytidine is deaminated to uridine, and uridine and thymidine are further degraded to the pyrimidine bases uracil and thymine by pyrimidine nucleoside phosphorylase. Further catabolism leads to the formation of β-alanine and β-aminoisobutyrate and metabolic incorporation in the citric acid cycle.

UMP synthase deficiency

Orotate phosphoribosyl transferase (OPRT) and orotidine monophosphate decarboxylase (ODC) constitute the single bifunctional enzyme UMP synthase.

$$\text{Orotic acid} + \text{PP-ribose-P} \rightarrow \text{OMP} + \text{PPi}$$
$$\text{OMP} \rightarrow \text{UMP} + CO_2$$

Hereditary orotic aciduria is an autosomal recessive disorder associated with homozygous deficiency of UMP synthase. Massive overproduction of orotic acid results from loss of feedback inhibition of rate-limiting carbamyl phosphate synthetase II, by pyrimidine nucleotides, and deficiency of pyrimidine nucleotides is associated with inhibition of cell division, megaloblastic anaemia, and retardation of growth and development.

The disease presents soon after birth with a hypochromic, megaloblastic anaemia which is resistant to haematinics. If the diagnosis is delayed, the disorder is associated with retardation of growth and psychomotor development. Urinary orotic acid excretion is increased 200–1000-fold (1–1.5 mg/24 h) and orotic acid crystalluria may follow dehydration. Other clinical features have included strabismus, cardiac malformations, and increased susceptibility to infections.

The diagnosis can be confirmed by red blood cell enzyme assays which show low but detectable levels of OPRT and ODC (hereditary orotic aciduria type I) or ODC alone (hereditary orotic aciduria type II). Kinetic studies of the fibroblast enzyme have suggested structural gene mutations. Treatment is with uridine (100–150 mg/kg/day) which is converted to UMP by uridine kinase (Fig. 7). The haematological response to treatment is prompt and consistent but some patients have been left with neurological impairment, possibly because of delay in commencing therapy.

Orotic aciduria is also found in patients with urea cycle defects, lysinuric protein intolerance, PP-ribose-P synthetase deficiency, and deficiency of purine nucleoside phosphorylase. Mild increases in urine orotic acid also occur in normal pregnancy and in patients receiving treatment with allopurinol.

Dihydropyrimidine dehydrogenase (DHPDH) deficiency

$$\text{Uracil} \rightarrow \text{dihydrouracil}$$
$$\text{NADPC} \circlearrowleft \text{NADPH}$$
$$\text{Thymine} \rightarrow \text{dihydrothymine}$$

Homozygous deficiency leads to the accummulation of uracil and thymine in body fluids. Affected children may present with hypertonia, hyperreflexia, and mental deficiency, or with epilepsy and autistic features. Others have remained asymptomatic until adult life and then presented with severe toxic side-effects (pancytopenia, stomatitis, diarrhoea, and neurological symptoms) following cancer chemotherapy with 5-fluorouracil, which is normally metabolized by the same enzyme.

Uracil and thymine are elevated in plasma and cerebrospinal fluid, and urinary excretion of the pyrimidine bases is greatly increased (uracil, 2–10 mmol/g creatinine; thymine, 2–7 mmol/g creatinine). There is complete absence of enzyme activity in white blood cells, liver, and fibroblasts. There is no effective treatment for this condition and the prognosis is very variable.

Further reading

Simmonds, H.A., Duley, J.A., Fairbanks, L.D, and McBride, M.B. (1997). When to investigate for purine and pyrimidine disorders. Introduction and review of clinical and laboratory indications. *Journal of Inherited Metabolic Diseases*, 20, 214–26.

Hershfield, M.S., Arredondo-Vega, F.X., and Santisteban, I. (1997). Clinical expression, genetics and therapy of adenosine deaminase (ADA) deficiency. *Journal of Inherited Metabolic Diseases*, 20, 179–85.

Chapter 6.7

Porphyrin metabolism and the porphyrias

K. E. L. McColl, S. Dover, E. Fitzsimons, and M. R. Moore

The porphyrias are inherited disorders involving the biochemical pathway of porphyrin haem biosynthesis. Although comparatively rare, they may mimic many other common conditions. Porphyrin metabolism may also be disturbed in a variety of other disorders including iron deficiency, alcohol excess, lead poisoning, and hereditary tyrosinaemia.

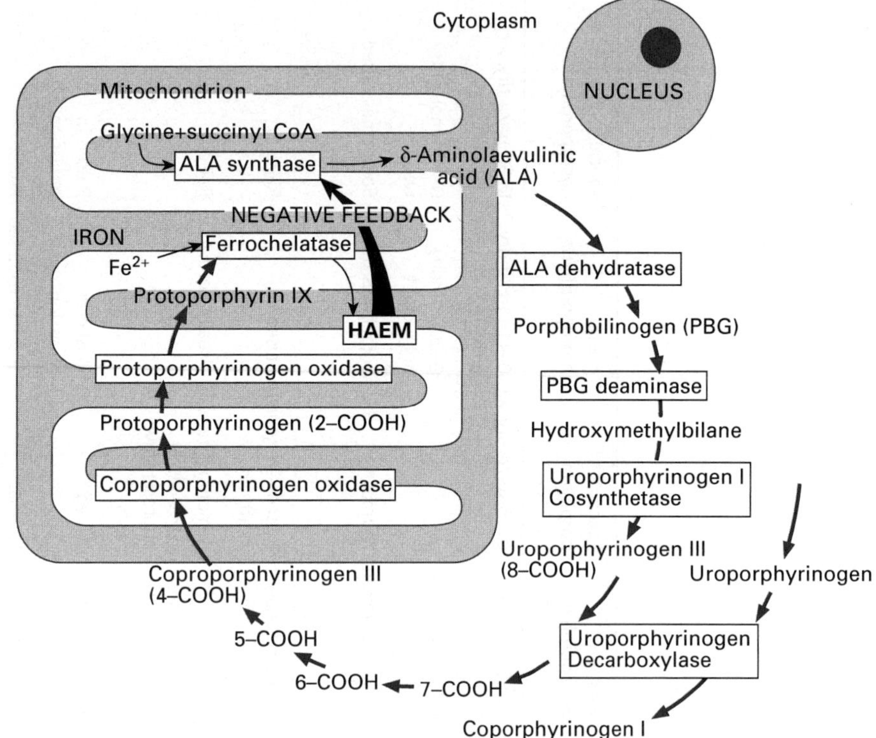

Fig. 1 Haem biosynthesis within the cell. This figure shows how haem is synthesized from the precursors glycine and succinyl CoA and the different compartmentation of the stages of the pathway in the mitochondrion and in the cytoplasm. Control of the pathway is maintained by haem acting by negative feedback on ALA synthase. Any of the series I isomer porphyrins synthesized will be excreted. The biosynthetic intermediate is the porphyrinogen and not the porphyrin.

Classification

Clinically, the porphyrias can be divided into acute (acute intermittent porphyria, variegate porphyria, hereditary coproporphyria) and non-acute (porphyria cutanea tarda, erythropoietic protoporphyria, and congenital porphyria). The acute porphyrias present with severe attacks of neurovisceral dysfunction associated with the overproduction and increased urinary excretion of the porphyrin precursors δ-aminolaevulinic acid (ALA) and porphobilinogen. Patients with variegate porphyria and hereditary coproporphyria may, in addition, experience cutaneous photosensitivity associated with the overproduction of porphyrins. In the non-acute porphyrias there is only overproduction of porphyrins and not of porphyrin precursors and, therefore, patients present only with cutaneous photosensitivity.

Biochemistry

Haem biosynthesis occurs in all metabolically active cells. It's control has been most fully documented in hepatic tissue (Fig. 1). The process starts with the condensation of glycine and succinyl coenzyme A to form δ-ALA under the control of δ-ALA synthase. A series of enzymes then controls the conversion of δ-ALA to porphobilinogen and then to the various porphyrins. Finally, iron is inserted into protoporphyrin by ferrochelatase to form haem. The rate of the pathway is regulated by the activity of the initial enzyme δ-ALA synthase, which is under negative feedback control by haem.

The various porphyrias are due to deficiencies of individual enzymes in the pathway of haem biosynthesis, which impair the production of haem with a compensatory increase in activity of δ-ALA synthase. As a consequence, there is overproduction and increased excretion of the haem precursors formed prior to the enzyme defect. Excess δ-ALA and porphobilinogen are excreted in the urine, whereas the porphyrins are mainly excreted in the faeces via the bile. In the acute porphyrias there is overproduction of all the porphyrins and porphyrin precursors formed proximal to the enzyme defect, but in the non-acute diseases there is overproduction of all porphyrins formed prior to the enzyme defect, but no overproduction of porphyrin precursors. The reason for this lack of overproduction of precursors is unclear, but may be due to a compensatory increase in the activity of porphobilinogen deaminase in addition to increased activity of δ-ALA synthase. The pattern of overproduction and excretion in the various porphyrias is shown in Table 1. In the acute porphyrias and in porphyria cutanea tarda, the liver is the main source of overproduction, in congenital porphyria the marrow is the main source, and in erythropoietic protoporphyria porphyrins are overproduced by both the liver and marrow.

Molecular biology

Complementary DNA clones have been obtained for eight of the nine enzymes of haem biosynthesis and the structures of the corresponding genes have been determined. The enzymes of the biosynthetic pathway have all now been mapped to specific chromosomes (Table 2).

The genetic basis of reduced activity of porphobilinogen deaminase in acute intermittent porphyria is related to a marked heterogeneity of mutations; most are single base changes on exons 10 and 12, and include substitutions and deletions. These have resulted in amino acid substitution, splicing defects, and premature insertion of stop codons. The marked genetic heterogeneity characterizing each of the porphyrias makes it difficult as yet to use molecular biological approaches in screening programmes.

Prevalence

The prevalence of the various forms of porphyria varies widely from country to country. In Scotland, 1 in 50 000 has some form of

Table 1 Normal values and abnormal porphyrin and precursor patterns in the porphyrias

	Erythrocyte protoporphyrin	Erythrocyte coproporphyrin	Urinary aminolaevulinic acid	Urinary porphobilinogen	Urinary uroporphyrin	Urinary coproporphyrin	Faecal X porphyrin	Faecal protoporphyrin	Faecal coproporphyrin
Normal levels	0–50 μg/dl cells	0–4.2 μg/dl cells	0–5.3 mg/day	0–3.6 mg/day	0–41 μg/day	0–280 μg/day	0–15 μg/g dry wt	0–113 μg/g dry wt	0–50 μg/g dry wt
SI units	0–900 nmol/l	0–64 nmol/l	0–40 μmol/day	0–16 μmol/day	0–49 nmol/day	0–432 nmol/day	—	0–200 nmol/g dry weight	0–76 nmol/g dry weight
Acute intermittent porphyria	Normal	Normal	Raised—very high in attack	Raised—very high in attack	Usually raised	Sometimes raised	Normal	Sometimes raised	Sometimes raised
Variegate porphyria	Normal	Normal	Raised in attack	Raised in attack	Sometimes raised	Sometimes raised	Raised—very high in attack	Raised	Raised
Hereditary coproporphyria	Normal	Sometimes raised in attack	Raised only in attack	Raised only in attack	Sometimes raised in attack	Usually raised—always raised in attack	Sometimes raised especially in photosensitive cases	Usually normal	Raised
Cutaneous hepatic porphyria	Normal	Normal	Normal	Normal	Raised—very high in attack	Slightly raised	Raised	Raised in remission	Raised in remission
Congenital porphyria	Usually raised	Usually raised	Usually normal	Usually normal	Raised	Sometimes raised	Normal	Sometimes raised	Raised
Erythropoietic protoporphyria	Raised—usually very high	Sometimes slightly raised	Normal	Normal	Normal	Normal	Normal	Usually raised	Normal

Table 2 Details of the enzymes which are defective in the different forms of porphyrias and related disorders and their chromosomal location

Names (abbreviation) (synonyms)	Chromosomal location	Related porphyria or other disease
5-Aminolaevulinate synthase (ALA.S)	3p21	
Erythroid ALA-synthase (eALA.S)	Xp11.2	X-linked sideroblastic anaemia
ALA dehydratase (ALAD) [porphobilinogen (PBG) synthase]	9q34	Plumboporphyria
PBG deaminase (PBGD and ePBGD) (hydroxymethylbilane synthase) (uroporphyrinogen I synthase)	11q23	Acute intermittent porphyria
Uroporphyrinogen cosynthase (URO COS)	10q26	Congenital porphyria
Uroporphyrinogen decarboxylase (UROD)	1p34	Porphyria cutanea tarda
Hepatoerythropoietic porphyria		
Coproporphyrinogen oxidase (COPRO O) (coproporphyrinogenase)	9	Hereditary coproporphyria
Protoporphyrinogen oxidase (PROTO O)	14	Variegate porphyria
Ferrochelatase (FERRO C) (haem synthase)	18q21.3	Erythropoietic protoporphyria

porphyria, with a predominance of acute intermittent porphyria and porphyria cutanea tarda. In South Africa the prevalent form of the disease is variegate porphyria, with a possible incidence of 1 in 1000 in the white population, while the Bantu suffer mainly from porphyria cutanea tarda.

The acute porphyrias

Acute intermittent porphyria

This is the most common and most severe form of the acute porphyrias. Although the genetic trait is inherited in an autosomal dominant fashion, manifest disease is more common in females, with a female/male ratio of about 5:1. This is probably due to hormonal fluctuations precipitating clinical attacks. The highest incidence of onset of symptoms is between puberty and 30 years of age and attacks are most common in the third decade. In one-third of reported cases there is no family history; the condition probably having remained latent or unidentified for several generations. The frequency and severity of attacks vary considerably from patient to patient. In a proportion, the disease remains latent throughout life, even in the presence of precipitating factors. Others experience frequent and sometimes life-endangering attacks even in the absence of extrinsic precipitating factors.

Underlying biochemical disorder

Partial deficiency of porphobilinogen deaminase results in excess formation and urinary excretion of δ-ALA and porphobilinogen. There is also increased excretion of uroporphyrin in the urine. Excretion of these haem precursors is always increased during clinical attacks but may be either normal or increased in remission (see Table 2).

Features of the porphyric attack

The prevalence of symptoms and physical signs in patients presenting with an acute porphyric attack is shown in Fig. 2.

Abdominal pain is the most frequent of the *gastrointestinal manifestations*, occurring in 95 per cent of attacks. It is often severe, requiring parenteral narcotic analgesics. The pain is usually felt diffusely over the abdomen and often radiates round the back. Abdominal examination may be normal or reveal mild generalized tenderness, sometimes associated with a degree of muscle guarding. Bowel sounds are normal. Anorexia usually occurs and there is often associated nausea and vomiting. Some patients develop delayed gastric emptying and a succussion splash may be elicited. Constipation is usually present. Abdominal radiographs are usually normal, although in some patients dilatation of the colon may be seen. Patients presenting with their first attack may be misdiagnosed as suffering from an acute abdomen. Unnecessary anaesthesia and laparotomy may result in a fatal outcome.

Neuropathy may be the presenting feature and complicates more than 50 per cent of attacks. Motor involvement is most common but paraesthesiae may also occur. The paralysis usually starts peripherally and then spreads proximally; however, in some patients shoulder girdle involvement may be the first manifestation. The neuropathy may progress rapidly, resulting in respiratory embarrassment.

Psychiatric manifestations are common and include agitation, mania, depression, hallucinations, and schizophrenic-like behaviour. Psychiatric manifestations may persist between attacks.

Tachycardia and hypertension disproportionate to the pain are usual manifestations of *autonomic dysfunction*. Other manifestations of autonomic dysfunction, such as profuse sweating, pallor, and pyrexia, may occur. Hyponatraemia due to inappropriate secretion of antidiuretic hormone complicates a proportion of attacks and sometimes presents with convulsions or deterioration in conscious level following intravenous fluid therapy.

Diagnosis of acute porphyric attack

The disorder should be considered in any patient presenting with unexplained abdominal pain. A helpful clue is the passage of dark urine due to the excessive excretion of haem precursors. If the urine is left standing in the light, the discoloration becomes more pronounced. The diagnosis is confirmed by demonstrating excess porphobilinogen in the urine. A useful side room test for excess porphobilinogen is to add an equal volume of Ehrlich's aldehyde reagent to the patient's urine. This causes a red discoloration that remains in the upper aqueous layer following the further addition of chloroform.

Factors which may precipitate acute porphyria

Various factors may precipitate attacks of acute porphyria in subjects with the genetic trait. These include drugs, alcohol, fasting, hormones, and infection. Drugs are the most common precipitating agents. A list of those believed to be unsafe in patients with acute porphyria is given in Appendix 1 and of drugs thought to be safe in Appendix 2. Pregnancy and oral contraceptives may precipitate attacks and some women experience regular attacks commencing in the week prior to the onset of menstruation.

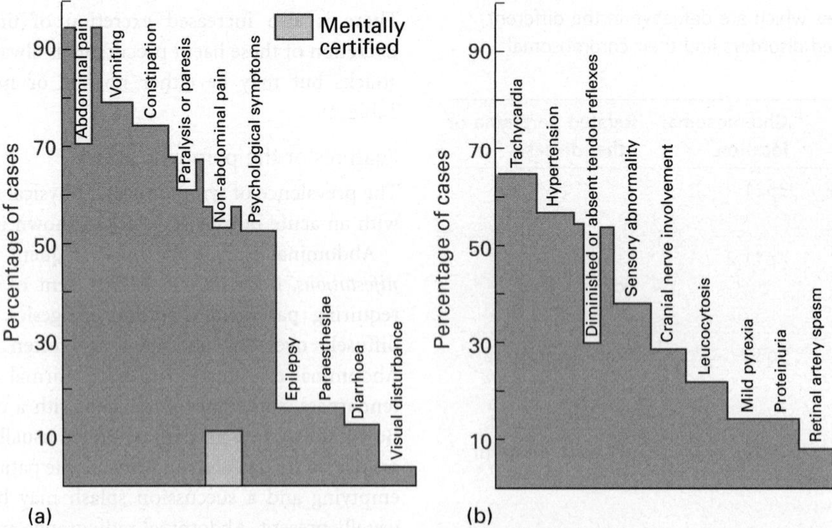

Fig. 2 (a) Prevalence of symptoms, and (b) incidence of physical signs, blood, and urine findings in 50 cases of acute intermittent porphyria.

Management of the acute attack

An attack of acute porphyria still carries a significant mortality. A successful outcome largely depends on early diagnosis, removal of precipitating factors, and provision of intensive support. In addition the administration of haem may speed recovery.

Nutrition

The patient must have a high carbohydrate intake. In mild attacks, glucose polymer drinks, such as Caloreen (Roussel) or Hycal (Beecham Products) may suffice. In more severe cases, 2 litres of 20 per cent dextrose should be infused every 24 h into a large peripheral vein or via a central line.

Control of pain

For severe pain, pethidine, or opiates may be required. The pain can be refractory to even very large doses of intravenous narcotic analgesics, and signs of respiratory and cardiovascular system depression then appear before pain relief is obtained. Some report that the only time the pain goes away is when they are asleep. This observation may be used to advantage by encouraging sleep for several h by combining chloropromazine or promazine with the analgesics. Some continue to complain of chronic abdominal pain unaccompanied by any other symptom between attacks. This can be very difficult to manage and the risk of narcotic addiction is high. Although a psychological element may be a factor in some, the pain is clearly genuine in others.

Tachycardia and hypertension

These features thought to be the result of sympathetic overactivity, should be controlled with propranolol. The dose should be titrated against its effect and frequently a very large one is required.

Convulsions

Their onset may be a sign of hyponatraemia which can be corrected by strict fluid restriction. Convulsions usually settle as the attack resolves but some patients continue to suffer them outside the acute attack. As all the commonly employed anticonvulsants may precipitate attacks, management of such cases is extremely difficult.

Neuropathy

All patients should be examined regularly for evidence of developing peripheral neuropathy. This may progress rapidly leading to quadriplegia and bulbar and ventilatory paralysis. When signs of peripheral neuropathy are present the expiratory peak flow rate should be monitored regularly. If there is any reduction, blood gases should be checked and the patient nursed in an intensive care unit. Even in patients in whom there is widespread paralysis requiring assisted ventilation for many months, good functional recovery can still be expected.

Haematin therapy

Haem preparations will bind to haemopexin and albumin in the plasma and are taken up by the liver. There they suppress activity of δ-ALA synthase and thereby reduce the overproduction of porphyrins and the precursors formed prior to the enzyme block. The most suitable preparation is haem arginate (Normosang, Leiras) administered intravenously in a dose of 3 mg/kg/day for 3 or 4 days. In some patients this results in phlebitis around the injection site. It also causes slight prolongation of the prothrombin time and should be avoided in any patient with a coagulopathy.

The clinical response to haem therapy is difficult to assess. There has only been one placebo-controlled trial and it did not show a statistically significant benefit. Numbers in the trial were small and severity of attacks variable. The biochemical changes induced by haematin therapy can be prolonged by the co-administration of tin-protoporphyrin, which inhibits the breakdown of haem by haem oxygenase. A significant side-effect of tin-protoporphyrin is cutaneous photosensitivity, which may persist for several weeks. For this reason it may not be suitable for use in the porphyrias in which cutaneous photosensitivity is a feature.

Prevention of attacks

Patients must be counselled concerning the avoidance of precipitating factors. They should be given a booklet indicating which drugs are safe and which are unsafe. Their family doctor must be fully informed and given advice about prescribing drugs. Patients should wear a bracelet or necklace indicating that they have porphyria.

Some women experience regular attacks in the week prior to the onset of menstruation and all forms of contraceptive pill may trigger attacks. There is some benefit from treating these patients with the long-acting analogue of luteinizing hormone releasing hormone, Buserilin, which can be administered nasally. This therapy may cause osteoporosis and bone density should be monitored. Attacks in pregnancy occur early and during the puerperium. They should be treated in the usual manner. No information is available concerning the effects of haem arginate on the fetus. The vast majority tolerate pregnancy well with a successful outcome for mother and child.

Surgery and anaesthetics

Provided appropriate precautions are taken, most patients with acute porphyria can tolerate surgery and general anaesthesia. Atropine and morphine may be used as premedication. Intravenous ketamine has been found to be a safe alternative to thiopentone. Cyclopropane and ether are safe inhalation agents in respect of the porphyria. Nitrous oxide used in conjunction with intravenous narcotics may be a more acceptable alternative. Suxamethonium and D-tubocurarine can be used and diamorphine, morphine, pethidine, or fentanyl are suitable for controlling postoperative pain. Epidural may be preferable to general anaesthesia, in which case bupivincaine is the local anaesthetic of choice. To prevent an attack being induced by fasting, an intravenous infusion of dextrose should be begun prior to surgery and continued until the patient is able to take an adequate diet.

Long-term complications

A small proportion of patients develop chronic hypertension. In addition, a small minority develop chronic renal failure. The cause is not clear.

Screening of relatives

Blood relatives should be screened for latent disease in order that they can be advised about necessary precautions if positive. Urinalysis will only pick up 50 per cent of latent cases and analysis of the activity of porphobilinogen deaminase in erythrocytes is more definitive.

Variegate porphyria and hereditary coproporphyria

These may present with attacks identical to those of acute intermittent porphyria, provoked by the same precipitating factors and managed in the same way. They are also inherited in an autosomal dominant fashion. The underlying defect in variegate porphyria is deficiency of protoporphyrinogen oxidase activity and in hereditary coproporphyria of coproporphyrinogen oxidase activity. There is marked overproduction of porphyrins as well as of porphyrin precursors (Table 1), with resultant susceptibility to cutaneous photosensitivity, which is most marked in sunny climates (Fig. 3). There is no specific treatment for the skin photosensitivity, although β-carotene treatment has been suggested. Barrier creams may be useful. The dermatological features often subside as the amount of circulating porphyrin is reduced.

Chester porphyria

There is deficiency of both porphobilinogen deaminase and protoporphyrinogen oxidase. In some of the patients the excretion pattern and clinical manifestation is identical to acute intermittent porphyria whereas in others it resembles variegate porphyria.

Plumboporphyria or δ-aminolaevulinic acid dehydratase deficiency porphyria

The biochemical presentation is of excess urinary excretion of δ-ALA analogous to that found in lead poisoning, although blood lead levels are normal. The activity of δ-ALA dehydratase is depressed. This genetic trait is inherited as an autosomal dominant. In the few cases described to date acute features are similar to those of acute intermittent porphyria. All clinically manifest cases have been homozygotes.

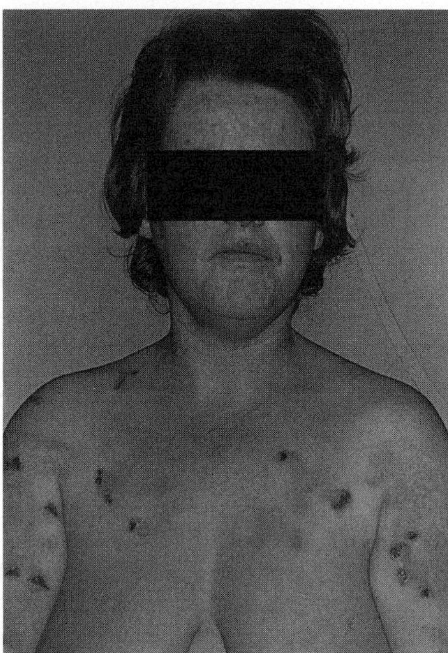

Fig. 3 Bullous eruption which developed over the exposed skin of a woman with hereditary coproporphyria after sunbathing.

The non-acute porphyrias

Porphyria cutanea tarda

Otherwise called cutaneous hepatic porphyria or symptomatic porphyria, this is predominantly an acquired disease, but there may be some genetic predisposition. A familial pattern is evident in a few patients, with the disorder being inherited as an autosomal dominant. The biochemical abnormality lies in hepatic uroporphyrinogen decarboxylase. Diagnosis is by the analysis of the porphyrin excretion pattern in which the dominant finding is an increased urinary uroporphyrin excretion (Table 1). The urinary porphyrin precursors δ-ALA and porphobilinogen are never elevated.

Cutaneous manifestations

The most striking and consistent clinical feature is bullous dermatosis on exposure to sunlight. The lesions are encountered on exposed areas such as the scalp, face, neck, and backs of the forearms and hands. They usually start with erythema, and progress to vesicles that become confluent to form bullae. Haemorrhage may occur into the bullae, which heal, leaving scars. Pruritus is often troublesome. There may be local pitting oedema at the site of the skin lesion. Increased fragility of the skin is an important feature and in less severe cases may be the only clinical sign. Hyperpigmentation is common and women often complain of hirsutism. Histological examination of the skin shows gross hyaline swelling in the walls of the capillaries in the upper curium of the bullae. Monochromator studies demonstrate that light of about the same wavelength as that absorbed by the porphyrin molecule (400 nm) will cause skin lesions in the porphyric patient.

Underlying hepatic disease

There may be evidence of hepatic disease both clinically and biochemically. Liver function tests in nearly all cases are abnormal. Serum iron and transferrin saturation are usually increased, and there may be an accelerated plasma iron turnover with early uptake of radioactive iron by the liver. Histological examination of the liver reveals features of the whole spectrum of alcoholic liver disease, although occasionally liver damage is minimal and non-specific. Siderosis is almost invariable and an underlying active chronic hepatitis may rarely be present. There is a 25 per cent incidence of diabetes mellitus, and some association with systemic lupus erythematosus and chronic active hepatitis. More than 90 per cent of patients admit to excessive alcohol consumption. Oestrogenic steroids are also implicated in some cases. An outbreak that occurred in Turkey in 1956 was traced to seed wheat dressed with hexachlorobenzene. Other polychlorinated hydrocarbons have also been implicated in the production of this toxic form of porphyria cutanea tarda. A neoplastic subgroup is secondary to benign or malignant primary liver tumours.

Management

The clinical features are reduced and even reversed by withdrawal of alcohol. Correction of iron overload by venesection brings about clinical remission. Weekly venesection of 500 ml is carried out until clinical remission occurs or until the haemoglobin level falls below 12 g/dl. A rising urinary uroporphyrin level is a useful index of the requirement for further venesection. A small dose of chloroquine 125 mg twice weekly results in increased urinary excretion of uroporphyrin with an associated fall in plasma and tissue levels and symptomatic improvement. The mechanism of its action is not clear.

Congenital porphyria

Congenital porphyria, also known as erythropoietic porphyria or Gunther's disease is extremely rare. It is inherited in an autosomal recessive manner, with evidence that the defect lies at the level of uroporphyrinogen cosynthetase. Symptoms usually begin during the first few years of life, although the disease can occasionally present in middle age. The skin reaction to sunlight is more severe than that of porphyria cutanea tarda. Pruritus and erythema are the initial features, followed by vesicle and bullous formation. The bullae rupture, leaving ulcers that frequently harbour secondary infection. Eventually the ulcers heal leaving scars. The severity of the lesions varies considerably but the result in most cases is devastating. Dystrophic changes in the nails may cause them to curl and drop off. Scarring of the skin on the hand may produce a claw-shaped deformity; lenticular scarring may lead to blindness. Hypertrichosis may be seen on the face, arms, and legs. Eyebrows and eyelashes may become thick and long. Pigmentation may be marked. The teeth become brownish-pink (erythrodontia) due to their high porphyrin content. A number of patients also develop anaemia and splenomegaly. The bone marrow reveals normoblastic hyperplasia; a proportion of erythrocyte precursors fluoresce red in ultraviolet light due to high porphyrin content. The peripheral blood film shows a normocytic normochromic anaemia with polychromasia. There is usually a moderate reticulocytosis with Howell–Jolly bodies; leucopenia and thrombocytopenia may occur when the spleen is large. Splenectomy may improve the anaemia and can reduce the degree of photosensitization. Treatment with chloroquine reduces erythrocyte fragility and diminishes the photosensitization. Bone marrow transplantation should be considered in severe cases as it theoretically offers the chance of a cure.

Erythropoietic protoporphyria

This form of erythropoietic porphyria, also known as erythrohepatic protoporphyria, is much more common than congenital porphyria. It is inherited as an autosomal dominant and symptoms may occur at any age. Diagnosis can be made by demonstrating fluorescence in a proportion of red cells (fluorocytes) in the peripheral blood and confirmed by measurement of greatly increased erythrocyte and faecal protoporphyrin (Table 1). The clinical features are mainly cutaneous with pruritic urticarial swelling and redness of the skin on exposure to sunlight. The most distressing symptom is a burning sensation of the affected parts, which may be unbearable. There may also be an eczematous skin reaction with scarring. Systemic manifestations are not usually severe, but hepatic involvement can occur. Liver function tests should be monitored in all patients and liver biopsy performed on the first sign of disturbance. There is also a tendency to the formation of protoporphyrin-containing gallstones. β-Carotene taken orally is an effective protective measure against the solar sensitivity. This may produce some yellowing of the skin after prolonged treatment, which may be made cosmetically acceptable by concurrent ingestion of canthaxanthin. The mode of action of β-carotene involves quenching of activated porphyrin triplet states, but it does not affect the biochemical pattern of the disease. Retardation of the progress of the liver lesions may be attempted by interruption of the enterohepatic circulation of protoporphyrin by bile salt sequestering agents such as cholestyramine. Liver failure occasionally develops and can be treated with liver transplantation.

Other diseases associated with abnormal porphyrin metabolism

Lead poisoning (see Chapter 12.25)

Lead poisoning leads to accumulation of protoporphyrin in erythrocytes and increased urinary excretion of δ-ALA and coproporphyrin. The elevated protoporphyrin chelated by zinc is retained in the erythrocyte, which may explain the absence of photosensitivity. The disorder is due to the inhibition by lead of δ-ALA dehydratase, coproporphyrinogen oxidase, and ferrochelatase. An increase in the activity of the rate-controlling enzyme δ-ALA synthase results.

Anaemia is due in part to the depressant effect of the lead on haem biosynthesis, though haemolysis and depression of globin synthesis are also important. Abdominal pain, constipation, and peripheral neuropathy occur in lead poisoning and are also seen in acute attacks of hepatic porphyria. Diminution in activity of erythrocyte δ-ALA dehydratase and elevated erythrocyte protoporphyrin levels are the most sensitive measures of lead poisoning, although others, such as raised urinary δ-ALA and coproporphyrin, are more frequently used.

Alcohol

Chronic alcoholics have an increased urinary excretion of coproporphyrin, mainly isomer 3, but normal urinary excretion of uroporphyrin, δ-ALA, and porphobilinogen. Ethanol has been shown to alter the activities of a number of the enzymes of haem biosynthesis. The alterations in haem biosynthesis may also be relevant to ethanol-induced sideroblastic anaemia in which there is increased activity of δ-ALA synthase in bone marrow.

Other conditions

In hereditary tyrosinaemia excess urinary δ-ALA is excreted because δ-ALA dehydratase is inhibited by succinyl acetone and, like the acute porphyria and lead poisoning, this disease is associated with neurobehavioural disturbance. In liver disease there may be increased urinary excretion of coproporphyrin predominantly the I isomer. In

Table A1 Drugs that are unsafe for use in acute porphyria

- Alcuronium
- **∗Alphaxolone:A**
- **Alphadolone**
- Alprazolam
- Aluminium preparations
- Amidopyrine
- Aminoglutethimide
- Aminophylline
- Amiodarone
- (Amitriptyline)
- (Amphetamines)
- **∗Amylobarbitone**
- Antipyrine
- Auranofin
- Aurothiomalate
- Azapropazone

- Baclofen
- **∗Barbiturates**
- **∗Bemegride**
- Bendrofluazide
- Benoxaprofen
- Benzbromarone
- (Benzylthiouracil)
- Bromocriptine
- Busulphan

- Captopril
- **∗Carbamazepine**
- **∗Carbromal**
- **∗Carisoprodol**
- (Cefuroxime)
- (Cephalexin)
- (Cephalosporins)
- (Cephradine)
- (Chlorambucil)
- **∗Chloramphenicol**
- **∗Chlordiazepoxide**
- Chlormezanone
- Chloroform
- **∗Chlorpropamide**
- (Cimetidine)
- Cinnarizine
- Clemastine
- **∗Chlorpropamide**
- (Clobazam)
- (Clomipramine HCl)
- (Clonazepam)
- Clonidine HCL
- Clorazepate
- Cocaine
- (Colistin)
- (Co-Trimoxazole)
- Cyclophosphamide
- Cycloserine
- Cyclosporin

- Danazol
- Dapsone
- Dexfenfluramine
- Dextropropoxyphene
- Diazepam
- Diazepam
- **∗Dichloralphenazone**
- Diclofenac Na
- Diethylpropion
- Dihydralazine
- **∗Dihydroergotamine**
- Diltiazem
- **∗Dimenhydrinate**
- **∗Diphenhydramine**
- (Dothiepin HCl)
- Doxycycline
- (Dydrogesterone)

- Econazole nitrate
- **∗Enalapril**
- Enflurane
- **∗Ergot compounds**
- Ergometrine maleate
- Ergotamine tartrate
- **∗Erythromycin**
- Ethamsylate
- **∗Ethanol**
- Ethionamide
- Ethosuximide
- Etidocaine
- Etomidate

- Fenfluramine
- **∗Flucloxacillin**
- **∗Flufenamic acid**
- Flunitrazepam
- Flupenthixol
- Flurazepam
- **∗Frusemide**

- **∗Glutethimide**
- Glipizide
- Gramicidin
- **∗Griseofulvin**

- (Haloperidol)
- **∗Halothane**
- **∗Hydantoins**
- Hydralazine
- (Haloperidol)
- **∗Hydrochlorothiazide**
- **∗Hydroxyzine**
- Hyoscine

- **∗Imipramine**
- Iproniazid
- Isometheptene mucate
- (Isoniazid)

- Ketoconazole

- Lignocaine
- **∗Lisinopril**
- Lofepramine
- Loprazolam
- Loxapine
- Lysuride maleate
- Lysuride maleate

- Maprotiline HCl
- Mebeverine HCl
- (Mefenamic acid)
- Megestrol acetate
- Mepivacaine
- **∗Meprobamate**
- Mercaptopurine
- Mercury compounds
- Mestranol
- (Metapramine HCl)
- Methamphetamine
- Methohexitone
- Methotrexate
- Methoxyflurane
- Methsuximide
- **∗Methyl dopa**
- **∗Methyl sulphonal**
- **∗Methyprylone**
- Methysergide
- **∗Metoclopramide**
- Metyrapone
- Mianserin HCl
- Miconazole
- (Mifepristone)
- Minoxidil

- Nalidixic acid
- Natamycin
- (Nandrolone)
- (Nicergoline)
- **∗Nifedipine**
- **∗Nikethamide**
- Nitrazepam
- (Nitrofurantoin)
- Nordazepam
- Norethynodrel
- (Nortriptyline)
- Novobiocin

- **∗Oral contraceptives**
- **∗Orphenadrine**
- (Oxazepam)

- Oxybutynin HCl
- Oxycodone
- **∗Oxymetazoline**
- Oxyphenbutazone
- Oxytetracycline

- Paramethadione
- **∗Pentazocine**
- Perhexiline
- Phenacetin
- Phenelzine
- **∗Phenobarbitone**
- Phenoxybenzamine
- Phensuximide
- (Phenylbutazone)
- Phenylhydrazine
- **∗Phenytoin**
- **∗Phenytoin**
- **∗Piroxicam**
- **∗Pivampicillin**
- Prenylamine
- **∗Prilocaine**
- **∗Primidone**
- (Probenecid)
- **∗Progesterone**
- Promethazine
- (Propanidid)
- **∗Pyrazinamide**
- Pyrrocaine

- Quinalbarbitone

- Rifampicin

- Simvastatin
- Sodium aurothiomalate
- Sodium oxybate
- (Sodium valproate)
- Spironolactone
- Stanozolol
- Succinimides
- Sulphacetamide
- **∗Sulphadimidine**
- Sulphadoxine
- Sulphamethoxazole
- **∗Sulphasalazine**
- Sulphonylureas
- Sulphinpyrazone
- Sulpiride
- Sulthiame
- Sultopride

- Tamoxifen
- **∗Terfenadine**
- Tetrazepam
- **∗Theophylline**
- **∗Thiopentone**
- Thioridazine
- Tilidate
- Tinidazole
- Tolazamide
- Thioridazine
- Tolbutamide
- Tranylcypromine
- Trazodone HCl
- Trimethoprim
- (Trimipramine)
- Troxidone

- Valpromide
- Veralipride
- **∗Verapamil**
- Viloxazine HCl

- Zuclopenthixol

These drugs have been classified as 'unsafe' because all have been shown to be porphyrinogenic in animals or *in vitro* systems, or to have been associated with acute attacks in humans.

() Drugs in parentheses are those in which there is conflicting experimental evidence of porphyrinogenicity—some positive, some negative.

∗Those marked in **bold** with an asterisk have been associated with acute attacks of porphyria.

Table A2 Drugs thought to be safe for use in acute porphyria

α-Tocopheryl-acetate
Acetazolamide
Acetylcholine
Actinomycin D
Acyclovir
Adrenaline
Alclofenac
Allopurinol
Amethocaine
Amiloride
Aminocaproic acid
Aminoglycosides
Amoxycillin
Amphotericin
Ampicillin
Ascorbic acid
Aspirin
Atenolol
Atropine
Azathioprine

β-Carotene
Beclomethasone
Benzhexol HCl
Biguanides
(Bromazepam)
Bromides
Bumetanide
Bupivacaine
Buprenorphine
Buserelin
Butacaine SO_4

Canthaxanthen
Carbimazole
(Carpipramine HCl)
Chloral hydrate
(Chlormethiazole)
(Chloroquine)
(Chlorothiazide)
Chlorpheniramine
Chlorpromazine
Ciprofloxacin
Cisplatin
Clavulanic acid
Clofibrate
Clomiphene citrate
Cloxacillin
Co-codamol
Codeine phosphate
Colchicine
(Corticosteroids)
Corticotrophin (ACTH)
Coumarins
Cyclizine
Cyclopenthiazide
Cyclopropane
(Cyproterone acetate)

(Cyproterone acetate)
Danthron
Desferrioxamine
Dexamethasone
(Dextromoramide)
Dextrose
Diamorphine
Diazoxide
Dicyclomine HCl
Diflunisal
Digoxin
Dihydrocodeine
Dimercaprol
Dimethicone
Dinoprost
Diphenoxylate HCl
Dipyridamole
(Disopyramide)
Domperidone
Doxorubicin HCl
Droperidol

Ethacrynic acid
Ethambutol
(Ethinyl oestradiol)
Ethoheptazine citrate
Etoposide

Famotidine
Fenbrufen
(Fenofibrate)
Fenoprofen
Fentanyl
Flucytosine
Flumazenil
Flurbiprofen
(Fluvoxamine maleate)
Folic acid
Fructose
Fusidic acid

Gentamicin
Glucagon
Glucose
Glyceryl trinitrate
Guanethidine

(Haloperidol)
Heparin
Hexamine
(Hydrocortisone)

Ibuprofen
Indomethacin
Insulin
Iron

(Ketamine)

(Ketamine)
Ketoprofen
Ketotifen

Labetalol
Lithium salts
Loperamide
(Lorazepam)

(Mebendazole)
Mecamylamine
Meclofenoxate HCl
Mefloquine HCl
(Melphalan)
Mequitazine
Metformin
Methadone
(Methotrimeprazine)
Methylphenidate
Methyluracil
Metoprolol
(Metronidazole)
Mianserin
(Midazolam)
Minaprine HCl
Minaxolone
Morphine

Nadolol
(Naproxen sodium)
Nefopam HCl
Neostigmine
Nitrous oxide
Norfloxacin

Ofloxacin
Oxybuprocaine
(Oxyphenbutazone)
Oxytocin

(Pancuronium bromide)
Paracetamol
Paraldehyde
Penicillamine
Penicillin
Pentolinium
Pethidine
Phenformin
Phenoperidine
Phentolamine mesylate
Piracetam
Pirbuterol
Pirenzepine
Pizotifen
(Prazosin)
(Prednisolone)
Primaquine
Procainamide HCl

Procainamide HCl
Procaine
Prochlorperazine
Proguanil HCl
Promazine
Propantheline Br
Propofol
Propranolol
Propylthiouracil
(Proxymetacaine)
Pseudoephedrine HCl
Pyridoxine
(Pyrimethamine)

Quinidine
Quinine

(Ranitidine)
Reserpine
Resorcinol

Salbutamol
Senna
Sodium bromide
Sodium Ca EDTA
Sodium fusidate
Sorbitol
Streptomycin
Sulindac
Sulfadoxine
Suxamethonium

Temazepam
Tetracaine
(Tetracyclines)
Thiouracils
Thyroxine
Ticarcillin
Tienilic acid
Timolol maleate
Tranexamic acid
Triacetyloleandomycin
Triamterene
Triazolam
(Trichlormethiazide)
Trifluoperazine
Trimetazidine HCl
Tubocurarine

Vancomycin
(Vincristine)
Vitamins

Warfarin sodium

Zidovudine
Zinc preparations (topical)

Each drug in parentheses () has had conflicting evidence of experimental porphyrinogenicity. Occasionally positive, but mainly negative—none of the drugs in this list has been associated with human porphyric attacks.

Note

While very great care has been taken in the compilation of this list and the drug information is given in the belief that it is correct at the time of publication, all information contained herein and opinions expressed must be taken as information and opinions given for general guidance only. The authors hereby disclaim for themselves, the Porphyrias Service, the University of Glasgow, and the Greater Glasgow Health Board, all responsibility for any misstatement or for the consequences to any person of any person acting in reliance on any statement or opinion contained herein. Medical practitioners and patients must make their own decisions in the circumstances of the particular case about therapy appropriate in any case of acute porphyria.

DRUG NAMES GIVEN HEREIN ARE APPROVED NAMES, NOT TRADE OR COMMON NAMES the Dubin–Johnson syndrome the ratio of coproporphyrin isomer I to isomer 3 is markedly increased in the urine (>80 per cent) possibly as a result of deficiency of hepatic uroporphyrinogen III cosynthase and increased activity of porphobilinogen deaminase. In Rotor syndrome total urinary excretion of coproporphyrin is markedly increased and consists predominantly of coproporphyrin isomer I. In the unconjugated hyperbilirubinaemia of Gilbert's syndrome depressed activity of protoporphyrinogen oxidase and increased activity of δ-ALA synthase has been noted in peripheral leucocytes. Increased urinary excretion of porphyrin-like substances has been found in a varying proportion of psychiatric patients not having porphyria. The association between this biochemical finding and the psychiatric disorder is not known.

Appendix 1: Drugs that are unsafe for use in acute porphyria

The drugs in Appendix 1 (Table A1) have been classified as 'unsafe' because all have been shown to be porphyrinogenic in animals or *in vitro* systems, or to have been associated with acute attacks in humans.

Appendix 2: Drugs thought to be safe for use in acute porphyria

The drugs in Appendix 2 (Table A2) are thought to be safe for use in acute porphyria.

Further reading

Elder, G.H., Hift, R.J., and Meissner, P.N. (1997). The acute porphyrias. *Lancet*, **349**, 1613-17.

Scarlett, Y.V. and Brenner, D.A. (1998). Porphyrias. *Journal of Clinical Gastroenterology*, **27**, 192-6.

Chapter 6.8

Lysosomal storage diseases

R. W. E. Watts

Lysosomes are subcellular organelles containing hydrolases with low optimum pH values ('acid hydrolases'), which catalyse the degradation of macromolecules which are either derived from the metabolic turnover of structural cellular components or have entered the cell by endocytosis. The products of this process leave the lysosomes by specific efflux processes. In most of the lysosomal storage diseases an inborn error of metabolism affects a specific lysosomal enzyme so that either undegraded or partial degraded macromolecules accumulate in the lysosomes. The engorged lysosomes distort the internal architecture of the cell, disturb its function, and inhibit the activities of other lysosomal enzymes, so that macromolecules other than those related to the primary enzyme deficiency also accumulate.

Cystinosis (cystine storage disease) and Salla disease, *N*-acetylneuraminic (sialic) acid storage disease are due to metabolic lesions involving the relevant specific efflux processes.

Lysosomal enzymes are glycoproteins that are subject to exocytosis and reuptake by endocytosis. The protein moieties are synthesized on the rough endoplasmic reticulum and the oligosaccharide side chains are added in the Golgi apparatus. The addition of a terminal mannose 6-phosphate residue is necessary if the enzyme molecule is to be correctly routed into the lysosomes, and if it is to be available for receptor-mediated reuptake from the interstitial fluid. This mannose 6-phosphate residue is referred to as the enzyme's recognition marker.

Sphingolipidoses

The sphingolipid molecule contains a hydrophobic portion ceramide (*N*-acylsphingosine) and either a hydrophilic mono- or oligosaccharide chain in the case of the gangliosides, or phosphorylcholine in the case of sphingomyelin. The galactose residues are sulphated in the sulphatides. The sphingolipids are degraded by a series of lysosomal hydrolases and deficiencies of the individual enzymes cause the degradation products, which are characteristic of each disease (Fig. 1, Table 1), to accumulate intralysosomally. The different diseases and different variants of the same disease have characteristic organ distribution patterns of the abnormal storage products. The diseases in which there is an abnormal sphingolipid accumulation in the neuronal cells of the central nervous system, and therefore in the ganglion cells of the retina also, show retinal degeneration, which is particularly apparent at the macula, causing pallor of this part of the retina with a central red area (the cherry-red spot); pigmentary retinal changes are also found in some cases. The cherry-red spot is a useful clinical pointer to the sphingolipidoses with neuronal involvement.

The main features of these disorders are shown in Table 2. Further details may be found in OTM3, pp. 1427–30, although Gaucher disease is described here.

Gaucher disease (glucocerebrosidosis, glucocerebrosidase deficiency)

There are three clinical types of Gaucher disease: type 1, chronic non-neuronopathic (adult); type 2, acute neuronopathic (infantile) and; type 3, subacute neuronopathic (juvenile). All have hepatosplenomegaly and large (20–100 μm in diameter) glucocerebroside-containing reticuloendothelial histiocytes (Gaucher cells) in the bone marrow. These cells have a crumpled-silk appearance in stained preparations. Increased amounts of glucocerebroside occur in the plasma and erythrocytes.

Type I is the most common and has an especially high incidence in Ashkenazi Jews (1:2500 births). It may present with hepatosplenomegaly in childhood, although the main disabilities occur later. The spleen and liver become very large and the spleen may undergo torsion and infarction. Grey–brown pigmentation of the forehead, hands, and pretibial region is characteristic. Wedge-shaped yellow–brown discoloration of subconjunctival areas (pingueculae) develop in the region of the corneoscleral junction. Bone growth and mineralization are deficient and the skeletal manifestations such as pain, pathological fractures, bone infarcts, and avascular necrosis of the femoral heads may dominate the clinical picture. It is sometimes relatively mild and confined to the Ehrlenmeyer flask-like expansion of the lower ends of the femura. Anaemia is due to a combination of bone marrow replacement, hypersplenism, and haemorrhage associated with thrombocytopenia. The serum level of non-prostatic acid phosphatases is increased.

Thrombocytopenia, hypersplenism, recurrent painful splenic infarction, and abdominal discomfort due to a greatly enlarged spleen are indications for splenectomy. Enzyme replacement therapy with

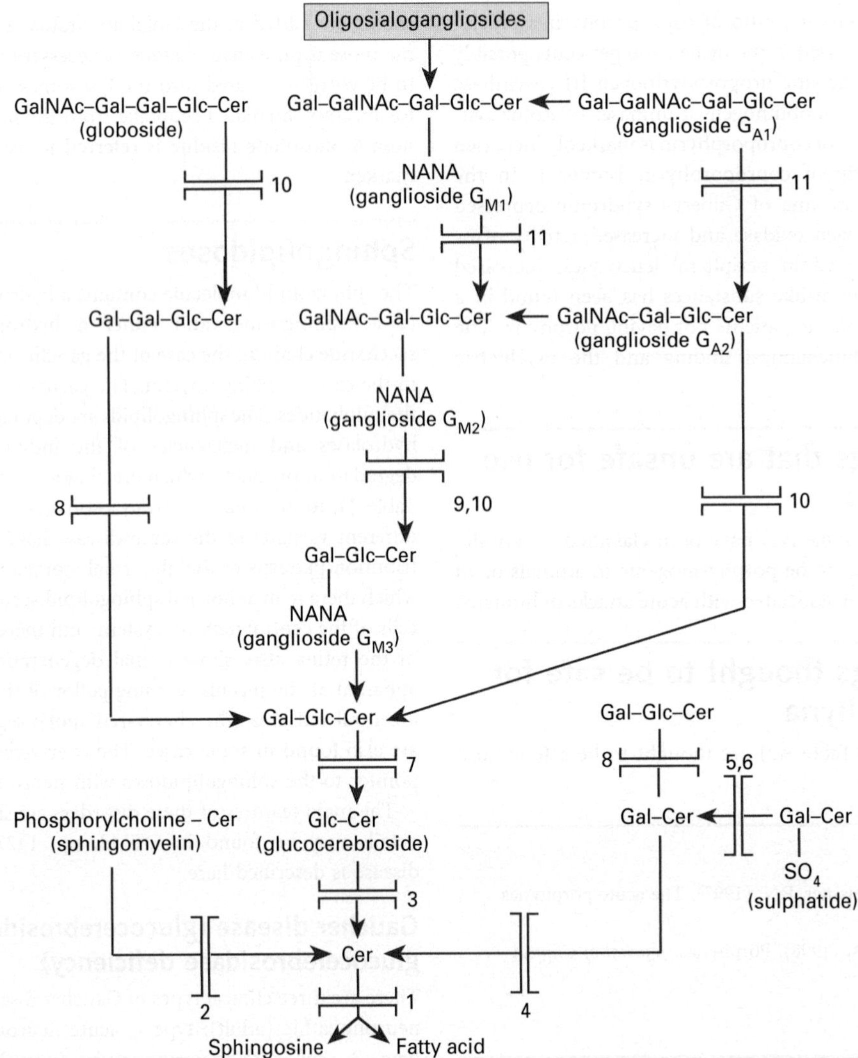

Fig. 1 Sphingolipid catabolism and the abbreviated structures of the sphingolipids which accumulate in the sphingolipidoses. The numerals indicate the metabolic blocks in the individual sphingolipidoses and correspond to those used in Table 1. Oligosialogangliosides are gangliosides with either 2, or 3, *N*-acetylneuraminic acid residues per molecule as opposed to the monosialogangliosides (G_M series) and asialogangliosides (G_A series). Cer, ceramide; Glc, glucose; Gal, galactose; GalNAc, *N*-acetylgalactosamine; NANA, *N*-acetylneuraminic acid (sialic acid). G_{M3} gangliosidosis is due to reduced activity of the transferase which converts the G_M series gangliosides to the more highly sialylated G_D and G_T series (oligosialogangliosides).
[Redrawn from Watts, R.W.E and Gibbs, D.A. (1986). Lysosomal storage diseases: Biochemical and clinical aspects. Taylor and Francis, London.]

macrophage-targeted glucocerebrosidase (alglucerase) is now a recognized treatment. Haematological improvement, reduction in the hepatosplenomegaly, and improvement in the skeletal lesions have been documented. Treatment with the biphosphonate disodium pamidronate reduces bone resorption, improves calcium balance, and maintains or improves bone density in both the axial and peripheral skeleton. Bone marrow transplantation is indicated in patients in whom infiltration of the bone marrow presents the main threat to life.

Patients with acute neuronopathic (type II) Gaucher disease have hepatosplenomegaly, and show developmental delay and retrogression by age 6 months. There are fits, focal neurological signs, and pulmonary infections due to infiltration of the lung parenchyma by Gaucher cells. These patients die in the first year of life. The subacute neuropathic (type III) cases present in later childhood and may survive into adult life with a variable degree of intellectual impairment, focal neurological manifestations, and seizures, as well as the systemic manifestations of the disease.

Mucopolysaccharidoses

The mucopolysaccharidoses are a group of seven inborn errors of metabolism in which the activity of one of the exoglycosidases which catalyse the sequential removal of individual carbohydrate groups from the mucopolysaccharides (glycosaminoglycans) is deficient. They have a combined incidence of about 1:10 000 births and their nomenclature, biochemistry, genetics, and main clinical features are summarized in Tables 3 and 4. All are inherited as autosomal recessives, except Hunter disease, which is sex-linked recessive. The term dysostosis multiplex is now used for the skeletal changes demonstrated radiologically in this group of disorders. The term lipochondodystrophy, which was formerly used because it was thought

Table 1 The sphingolipidoses

No. in Fig. 1	Systematic name	Eponymous and/or other generally used name	Main storage compound	Enzyme deficiency	Biochemical diagnosis	Chromosome assignment
1	Ceramidosis	Farber disease	Ceramide	Ceramidase (EC 3.5.1.23)	Ceramide in skin nodules. Enzyme in leucocytes, fibroblasts	Not assigned
2	Sphingomyelinosis	Niemann–Pick disease	Sphingomyelin	Sphingomyelinase (EC 3.1.4.12)	Enzyme in leucocytes, fibroblasts	17
3	Glucocerebrosidosis	Gaucher disease	Glucocerebroside	β-Glucocerebrosidase (EC 3.2.1.45)	Glucocerebroside in liver, erythrocytes. Enzyme in leucocytes, fibroblasts	1q21
4	Galactocerebrosidosis	Krabbe disease	Galactocerebroside	Galactocerebroside β-galactosidase (EC 3.2.1.46)	Enzyme in serum, leucocytes, fibroblasts	17
5	Sulphatidosis	Globoid cell leucodystrophy Metachromatic leucodystrophy	Cerebroside sulphates	Arylsulphatases A (cerebroside sulphatase) (EC 3.1.6.1)	Enzyme in leucocytes, fibroblasts, hair bulbs, plasma	22q13.31→q ter
6	Mucosulphatidosis	Multiple sulphatase deficiency syndrome	Cerebroside sulphates	Arylsulphatases A, B, C and steroid sulphatase (? sulphate receptor protein)	Enzymes in leucocytes, fibroblasts, urine. Dermatan and heparan sulphates in urine	22q13.31→q ter
			Steroid sulphates			Not assigned
7	Lactosylceramidosis	–	Lactosylceramide	Ceramide-lactoside β-galactosidase	Enzyme in fibroblasts. Lactosyl-ceramide in erythrocytes, plasma, bone marrow, urine sediment	Not assigned
8	α-Galactosyl-lactosylceramidosis	Fabry disease, Anderson–Fabry disease Angiokeratoma corporis diffusum	α-Galactosyl-lactosylceramide	α-Galactosidase A (EC 3.2.1.22)	Enzyme in leucocytes, hair bulbs, fibroblasts, tissue biopsy. Trihexoside in urine deposit	Xq22
9	G_{M2}-gangliosidosis type A_OB_H	Tay–Sachs disease	Ganglioside G_{M2}	β-d-Hexosaminidase A (α-subunit) (EC 3.2.1.30)	Enzymes in leucocytes, fibroblasts, plasma	15q25→q25.1
10	G_{M2}-gangliosidosis type A_OB_O	Sandhoff disease	Ganglioside G_{M2} Globoside	β-d-Hexosaminidases A and B (β-subunit) (EC 3.2.1.30)	Enzymes in leucocytes, fibroblasts, plasma	5q13
11	G_{M1}-gangliosidosis	–	Ganglioside G_{M1}	G_{M1} ganglioside β-galactosidase (EC 3.2.1.23)	Enzymes in leucocytes, fibroblasts, urine	3p14→cen

The materials listed under biochemical diagnosis are those which have been most frequently used for this purpose.

The enzyme defect is usually more generally demonstrable. Enzymological prenatal diagnosis is usually possible using either amniocytes or chorionic villus samples.

Table 2 Lysosomal storage diseases (see also Table 1 for enzyme deficiencies, characteristic storage products and biochemical diagnosis

Systematic name	Trivial name	Variant	Clinical features
Ceramidase deficiency	Farber's disease	Severe	Present at age 2–3 months. Hoarse cry. Arthropathy. Pulmonary infiltration. Severe mental handicap. Seizures. Thickened heart valves. Hepatosplenomegaly and lymphadenopathy inconstant. Grey retinal area with cherry red spot at the macula (±). Die in early childhood
		Mild	Slower evolution. A few survive to teenage without mental handicap.
Sphingo-myelinosis	Niemann–Pick disease	Type A (acute neuronopathic)	Present at 6–12 months. Hepatosplenomegaly. Lymphadenopathy. Psychomotor regression. Seizures. Opalescent corneae and retinae. Brown yellow skin discoloration. Cherry red spot at macula in 50 per cent. Foamy macrophages. Die by age 2 years.
		Type B (chronic non-neuronopathic)	Present in childhood. Hepatosplenomegaly. Lymphadenopathy (±). *No* neuropsychiatric disabilities. Osteopathy (±). Prolonged nerve conduction times (±). Macula reddish brown. Impaired liver function (±) and hepatosplenomegaly in adult life. Foamy macrophages. Variable survival into adult life.
		Type C (chronic neuronopathic)	Psychomotor delay and retrogression in early childhood. Inco-ordination. Myoclonus seizures. Cholestasis (±). Die in late childhood or adolescence.
		Type D (Nova Scotia variant)	Resemble type C. Common ancestry in western Nova Scotia.
		Type E (adult non-neuronopathic)	Present in adult life. Hepatosplenomegaly. Foamy macrophages in marrow. No neurological involvement. Mild osteopathy (+). Cherry red spot at macula (±).
Galactosyl ceramide lipidosis	Krabbe's disease. Globoid cell leukodystrophy	Infantile	Usual type, present at age 2–9 months. Die before age 3 years. Developmental delay and retrogression. Optic atrophy. Deafness. Long tract signs.
		Juvenile	Present in late childhood. Unusual type. Die within a few years.
Sulphatidosis	Metachromatic leucodystrophy	Late infantile	Present age 1–4 years. Progressive flaccid, and/or spastic paresis, incoordination, hyporeflexia. Severe psychomotor retrogression to vegetative state. Optic atrophy. Cherry red spot at macula.
		Juvenile	Present late childhood or adolescent. Intellectual deterioration. Emotional disorders. Pareses. Dystonia.
		Adult	Present as adults with psychosis, dementia, seizures and paresis. Slow peripheral nerve conduction. Metachromatic deposits in sural nerve biopsy.
Multiple sulphatase deficiency	Mucosulphatidosis	–	Resemble late infantile metachromatic leucodystrophy, plus dysmorphic features (resemble Hurler phenotype). Hepatosplenomegaly. Dysostosis multiplex. Ichthyosis (as in steroid sulphatase deficiency). Dermatan and heparan sulphaturia.
Lactosyl ceramidosis	–	–	Age 2 years. Psychomotor delay and retrogression. Optic atrophy. Progressive destruction of neuraxis. Hepatosplenomegaly. Generalized lymphadenopathy. Death within 1 year.
Fabry disease. Anderson–Fabry disease	Glycosphingolipid lipidosis. Ceramide trihexosidosis.		X-linked inheritance. Full expression in male hemizygotes. Female heterozygous carriers express mild manifestations or are asymptomatic. Crystalline trihexoside is birefringent (Maltese cross appearance) in corneal epithelium, urine and renal glomeruli and tubules 'foamy renal cells' (renal biopsy), myocardium, autonomic ganglia, Schwann cells. Usually present in childhood or early adulthood. Burning pain and paraesthesia in extremities aggravated by heat, cold, physical exertion and fever. Acute gastrointestinal symptoms. Raynaud phenomenon. Musculoarticular pain. Angiokeratoma corporis diffusum especially on lower trunk and thighs. Corneal and lenticular opacities. 'Cart-wheel' corneal dystrophy. Ischaemic heart disease, cardiac valvular lesions, pulmonary infiltrations, avascular bone necrosis. Males die in 4th or 5th decades of renal failure, cardiovascular or ischaemic heart disease. Females show milder renal lesions on renal biopsy, and corneal lesions.
G_{M2} gangliosidosis	Tay–Sachs disease	Infantile G_{M2} gangliosidosis (hexosaminidase isoenzyme A deficiency)	Incidence 1:2000 in Ashkenazi Jews. Onset at 6 months. Progressive psychomotor regression, with seizures, blindness and deafness. Die in a vegetative state by age 3 years. Cherry red spot at macula. Rapid abnormal head enlargement. Doll-like facies, startle reaction. Rectal biopsy shows G_{M2} ganglioside in autonomic ganglia.

Table 2 *continued*

Systematic name	Trivial name	Variant	Clinical features
–	–	Juvenile G_{M2} gangliosidosis (hexosaminidase isoenzyme A deficiency)	Present age 2–6 years. Ataxia, dysarthria, spasticity, dystonia, seizures, blindness, cherry red spot at macula. Die late childhood or teens.
–	–	Adult G_{M2} gangliosidosis (hexosaminidase A deficiency)	Slowly progressive. Difficulty in walking with muscular atrophy, inco-ordination, dystonia and dysarthria. In adult life, intellect and vision unaffected.
–	Sandhoff's disease	G_{M2} gangliosidosis with deficiency of isoenzymes A and B	Indistinguishable from rapidly evolving Tay–Sachs disease.
G_{M1} gangliosidosis	Generalized ganglio-sidosis	Infantile	Onset first weeks of life. Death before 2 years. Psychomotor retardation, with hypotonia, seizures, blindness and deafness. Spastic quadriplegia. Dysmorphic features (coarse physiognomy, frontal bossing, depressed nasal bridge). Hepatosplenomegaly. Dysostosis multiplex.
–	–	Adult	Dysarthria, ataxia and spasticity. Mild intellectual impairment.

that the stored material was a lipid, has been abandoned. The primary abnormal storage products are carbohydrate polymers. These produce secondary changes in lysosomal function, including some impairment of ganglioside turnover. The tissue deposits of highly sulphated mucopolysaccharides stain metachromatically. Mucopolysaccharide deposits in relation to the meninges can cause hydrocephalus, spinal cord compression, arachnoid cysts, and radiculopathies in all of the mucopolysaccharidoses. Leucocytes contain mucopolysaccharide inclusion bodies (Alder–Reilly bodies) in all of the mucopolysaccharidoses. The precise enzymological diagnosis is made on either leucocytes or cultured fibroblasts and prenatal diagnosis on either cultured amniotic cells or chorionic villus samples.

Mucolipidoses

The term mucolipidosis describes a group of patients with clinical features that are a mixture of those encountered in the sphingolipidoses and the mucopolysaccharidoses and who do not have abnormal mucopolysacchariduria. It includes patients with: (a) neuraminidase (sialidase) deficiency, termed mucolipidoses I and IV; (b) two groups of patients with deficiency of uridine diphosphate-*N*-acetylglucosamine:lysosomal enzyme precursor *N*-acetylglucosamine phosphate transferase who are termed mucolipidoses II (I-cell disease) and III (pseudo-Hurler polydystrophy), respectively (Tables 5 and 6). All of the mucolipidoses are inherited in an autosomal recessive manner.

Mucolipidoses I and IV are classic lysosomal storage diseases due to deficiency of an enzyme which normally degrades a macromolecule. The metabolic lesion in mucolipidoses II and III blocks the phosphorylation of the terminal mannose residue of the oligosaccharide side chain of the lysosomal hydrolases. This deprives them of the recognition marker, mannose 6-phosphate, which enables them to be guided from their site of synthesis on the rough endoplasmic reticulum to the lysosomes, and to be taken up from an extracellular location by receptor mediated pinocytosis.

Mucolipidosis II (I-cell disease)

A severe Hurler disease-like phenotype is present in infancy except that corneal clouding and hepatosplenomegaly are mild and gum hypertrophy is particularly prominent. The dysostosis multiplex is severe and the patients usually die during the first 5 years of life. Prenatal but not carrier state diagnosis is possible.

Mucolipidosis III (pseudo-Hurler polydystrophy)

These patients usually present at 4–5 years of age because of progressive arthropathy. Their intelligence is usually in the low–normal or mildly handicapped range and they develop dysostosis multiplex, spinal deformities, atlantoaxial subluxation, nerve entrapment syndromes, cardiac valvular lesions, and corneal clouding in later childhood. Visceromegaly is not a prominent feature. Cultured fibroblasts show I-cell type inclusions. Prenatal but not carrier state diagnosis is possible.

The neuraminidase (sialidase) deficiencies

Mucolipidosis I is referred to with the other glycoproteinoses. Mucolipidosis IV, in which the catalytic activity of the enzyme with respect to cleavage of neuraminyl residues from gangliosides G_{M3} and G_{D3} is deficient, presents with progressive psychomotor retardation during the first 2 years of life. The patients usually die in later childhood. The neurological picture includes muscle hypotonia, truncal ataxia, and the signs of an upper motor neurone lesion. Corneal clouding is marked and appears early. There is neither visceromegaly nor dysostosis multiplex.

Glycoproteinoses

The glycoproteinoses are a group of four autosomal recessively inherited inborn errors of metabolism in which the metabolic lesion causes faulty degradation of the oligosaccharide side chains of glycoproteins.

Sialidosis (mucolipidosis I): the cherry-red spot/myoclonus syndrome, is due to the deficiency of *N*-acetylneuraminic hydrolase, which cleaves

Table 3 The mucopolysaccharidoses

McKusick's classification	Eponymous name	Enzyme deficiency	Excreted glycosaminoglycans	Organs mainly affected	Facial appearance	Chromosome assignment
IH	Hurler	α-l-iduronidase (EC 3.2.1.76)	Dermatan sulphate	Central nervous system	Classical Hurler appearance	22pter→q11
			Heparan sulphate	Skeleton Viscera		
IS	Scheie	α-l-iduronidase (EC 3.2.1.76)	Dermatan sulphate	Skeleton (mild relative to Hurler)	Coarse features ± (Not specifically Hurler-like)	22pter→q11
			Heparan sulphate	Viscera (mild relative to Hurler)		
IH/S	Hurler/Scheie	α-l-iduronidase (EC 3.2.1.76)	Dermatan sulphate	Phenotype intermediate between Hurler and Scheie diseases	Coarse features ± (Not specifically Hurler-like)	22pter→q11
II	Hunter	Iduronate sulphate sulphatase	Heparan sulphate Dermatan sulphate	Central nervous system	Micrognathism Hurler-like	Xq28
			Heparan sulphate	Skeleton Viscera Mild and severe phenotypes reported		
III A	Sanfilippo A	Heparan *N*-sulphatase	Heparan sulphate	Central nervous system	Not characteristic	Not assigned
III B	Sanfilippo B	*N*-acetyl-α-d-glucosaminidase (EC 3.2.1.50)	Heparan sulphate	Central nervous system	Not characteristic	Not assigned
III C	Sanfilippo C	Acetyl-CoA:α-glucosaminide *N*-acetyltransferase	Heparan sulphate	Central nervous system	Not characteristic	?14 ?21
III D	Sanfilippo D	*N*-acetylglucosamine 6-sulphate sulphatase	Heparan sulphate	Central nervous system	Not characteristic	12q14
IV A	Morquio A	*N*-acetylgalactosamine 6-sulphate sulphatase	Keratan sulphate	Skeleton	Not characteristic	Not assigned
IV B	Morquio B	β-galactosidase	Keratan sulphate	Skeleton	Not characteristic	3pter→p21
V*	–	–	–	–	–	–
VI	Maroteaux–Lamy	*N*-acetylgalactosamine 4-sulphatase (Aryl sulphatase B) (EC 3.1.6.1)	Dermatan sulphate	Skeleton Mild and severe phenotypes reported	Hurler-like	5q12→q13
VII	–	β-glucuronidase (EC 3.2.1.31)	Dermatan sulphate	Central nervous system	Hurler-like	7q11→q21
	Viscera		Heparan sulphate	Skeleton		

*Originally Scheie disease which was reclassified as mucopolysaccharidosis IS when the enzyme defect was shown to be the same as that in Hurler disease. The possibility that Hurler and Scheie diseases are due to allelic mutations and that the intermediate Hurler/Scheie phenotype (mucopolysaccharidosis IH/S) is due to double heterozygosity for the allelic mutations concerned has been widely proposed. The Hurler/Scheie phenotype could also be due to homozygosity for a third allelic mutation at the same gene locus.

Table 4 The mucopolysaccharidoses (see also Table 3 for the characteristic enzyme deficiencies, storage products and biochemical diagnosis

Systematic name	Trivial name	Clinical features
Mucopolysaccharidosis I	Hurler disease	Diagnosis at 6–12 months suggested by psychomotor delay and early dysmorphic features (facies, corneal clouding, loss of lumbar lordosis). Dwarfism apparent by 2–3 years. Die by aged 10 years. Fully developed phenotype comprises coarse physiognomy, thick, stiff skin and cartilages, depressed nasal bridge, anteroposterior bony ridge on the forehead, macrocephaly, chronic upper respiratory tract infections, hyperplastic gums, macroglossia, poor dentition, stiff, straight hair, deafness, impaired vision (corneal clouding, glaucoma, retinal degeneration), hydrocephalus, hepatosplenomegaly, and psychomotor regression.
Mucopolysaccharidosis II	Hunter disease	Resemble Hurler disease except for the almost universal absence of corneal clouding. Most die in the teenage years. Mild variants may survive into the 4th decade with low or near-normal intelligence.
Mucopolysaccharidosis III	Sanfilippo disease	Four biochemically distinct types (see Table 2) which are indistinguishable clinically. Severe mental deterioration with hyperkinesia. Accelerated physical growth and coarse scalp hair.
Mucopolysaccharidosis IV	Morquio disease	Severe dysostosis multiplex, lumbodorsal gibbus, hypoplastic odontoid, spinal chord compression, broad mouth, widely spaced teeth, pectus carinatum, fine corneal opacities, cardiac valvular lesions, hepatosplenomegaly, hypermobile joints. *Normal intellect*, facies characteristic but *not* Hurler-like.
Mucopolysaccharidosis VI	Maroteaux–Lamy disease	Resemble Hurler disease, mild intermediate and severe variants are recognized. Variable degree of intellectual impairment.
Mucopolysaccharidosis I-S	Scheie disease	Arthropathy, cardiac valvular lesions, hydrocephalus (±). Cervical myelopathy, radiculopathy, arachnoid cysts and nerve entrapment are characteristic features. Mental handicap is not feature. Cases commonly present in adult life.
Mucopolysaccharidosis I H/S	Hurler–Scheie disease	Phenotype intermediate between Hurler and Scheie disease. Present in late childhood with survival into adult life.
Mucopolysaccharidosis VII	–	Resemble Hurler disease.

Table 5 The mucolipidoses

Mucolipidosis number	Alternative name	Metabolic lesion	Clinical features
I	Sialidosis	Deficient neuraminidase (sialidase EC 3.2.1.18) activity with respect to glycoprotein substrates	Two clinical types: 1. Normosomatic, myoclonus and cherry red spot appearance of the macula lutea 2. Dysmorphic, resembles Hurler disease Resembles very early onset Hurler disease
II	I-cell disease	Failure to phosphorylate terminal mannosyl residues of the glycoprotein lysosomal hydrolases due to deficiency of uridine-*N*-acetylglucosamine: lysosomal enzyme precursor *N*-acetyl-glucosamine phosphate transferase. This deprives these enzymes of their recognition markers for transfer from the rough endoplasmic reticulum into the lysosomes and for receptor-mediated pinocytic uptake into cells	
III	Pseudo-Hurler polydystrophy	As for mucolipidosis II	Resembles either intermediate severity Maroteaux–Lamy disease, or some cases of Scheie disease
IV	Berman's disease	Deficient neuraminidase activity with respect to ganglioside substrates (GM_3 and GD_{1a})	Progressive neurological deterioration beginning in infancy. Hypotonia, pyramidal and extrapyramidal signs. Corneal clouding. No visceromegaly. Not dysmorphic

Table 6 The mucolipidoses, glycoproteinoses, acid lipase deficiencies, and glycogenosis Type II: nomenclature, enzyme deficiencies, and chromosome assignments

Systemic or more commonly used name	Eponymous or other alternative name	Enzyme deficiency	Chromosome assignment
Mucolipidosis I	Sialidosis	Neuraminidase (EC 3.2.1.18) with respect to glycoprotein substrates	Not assigned
Mucolipidosis II	I-cell disease	UDP-GlcNAC:glycoprotein GlcNAc-1-phosphotransferase	4q21→q23
Mucolipidosis III	Pseudo-Hurler polydystrophy	UDP-GlcNAc:glycoprotein GlcNAc-1-phosphotransferase	4q21→q23
Mucolipidosis IV	–	Neuraminidase (EC 3.2.1.18) with respect to ganglioside substrates	Not assigned
Fucosidosis	–	α-Fucosidase (EC 3.2.1.51)	1p34
Mannosidosis	–	α-Mannosidase (EC 3.2.1.24)	19p13.2→q12
Aspartylglycosaminuria	–	1-Aspartamido-β-*N*-acetyl-glucos-amine amidohydrolase (EC .2.2.11)	4q21→4qter
–	Wolman's disease	Acid lipase (EC 3.1.1.3)	10q25
Cholesteryl ester storage disease	–	Acid lipase (EC 3.1.1.3)	10q25
Glycogenosis II	Pompé disease	α-1,4-glucosidase (EC 3.2.1.20)	17q23

sialic acid from oligosaccharides, glycoproteins, and glycolipids. The urine contains large amounts of sialic-acid-rich oligosaccharides. The patients are divided into type 1 and type 2 according to the absence or presence of dysmorphic features and mental deterioration. Infantile (onset at or below 1 year of age) and juvenile (onset at 8–15 years) variants of type 2 are recognized. The type 1 patients present at between 8 and 15 years with visual failure and action myoclonus, and have the cherry-red spot at the macula. They appear normal, and have normal or near normal intelligence. In type 2 patients, the features and skeletal abnormalities resemble those of Hurler disease. These patients also have spasticity and ataxia, as well as the cherry-red spot at the macula and myoclonus. Seizures may occur in both types. Visceromegaly is rare except in the infantile variant of type 2. Vacuolated mononuclear cells ('foam cells') are seen in the blood and/or bone marrow in most cases. Sialidosis can be diagnosed prenatally and in the carrier state.

Aspartylglycosaminuria is due to deficiency of aspartyl-glucosaminidase, which catalyses the hydrolysis of the linkage between asparagine and *N*-acetylglucosamine splitting the carbohydrate from the polypeptide chain of glycoproteins. The patients excrete large amounts of aspartylglucosamine in their urine. Most patients have been Finnish. They present with psychomotor delay at about 1–5 years and become severely retarded with some degree of motor incoordination. Coarse facial features, optic lens opacities, mild dysostosis multiplex, hypermobile joints, short stature, and cardiac systolic murmurs are other features. Hepatosplenomegaly is not a characteristic finding. Aspartylglucosaminuria can be diagnosed prenatally and in the carrier state.

Mannosidosis is due to deficiency of α-mannosidase, which cleaves terminal mannosyl residues from the carbohydrate moieties of glycoproteins. Mannose-rich oligosaccharides are excreted in the urine and accumulate in the cells of the brain, viscera, and connective tissues. The more severely affected patients, who present at 3–12 months, die in childhood. Less severely affected patients present at 1–4 years and die as young adults. The main clinical features are psychomotor delay, the development of severe mental handicap, coarsened facial features, hepatosplenomegaly, posterior 'spoke-like' cataracts, deafness, and dysostosis multiplex. Clinically, the patients resemble Hurler disease more or less closely. Prenatal and carrier state diagnoses are possible.

Fucosidosis is due to deficiency of α-fucosidase, which cleaves terminal fucosyl residues from the oligosaccharide side chains of the glycoproteins. The external appearances, visceromegaly and skeletal changes resemble those seen in Hurler disease. Severe and mild variants are recognized. Psychomotor delay and regression evolve rapidly in the former group, who also show increased sweat sodium and chloride and die in early or mid-childhood. The mild cases have angiokeratomas resembling those seen in Fabry disease, there is less neurological damage, normal sweat salinity, and they survive longer. The erythrocyte and saliva Lewis blood group antigen (Le^a and Le^b) titres are raised and the abnormal tissue glycoconjugates have Lewis blood group activity. These findings reflect the failure to cleave fucosyl residues from glycoproteins. Heterozygotes for the abnormal gene causing fucosidosis can be identified and prenatal diagnosis is possible.

Salla disease and infantile sialic acid storage disease

Salla disease is characterized by the excretion of large amounts of free sialic acid in the urine. Few cases have been reported in non-Finnish people. Psychomotor delay becomes apparent towards the end of the first year and most cases become severely handicapped mentally. Dysarthria, dyspraxia, abnormal tendon reflexes, ataxia, and athetosis are common features. Life expectancy seems not to be greatly reduced. The biochemical defect is failure to transport sialic acid (*N*-acetylneuraminic acid) derived from the breakdown of sialic-acid-containing glycoconjugates out of the lysosomes. The inheritance is autosomal recessive.

Infantile free sialic acid storage disease is a severe variant of Salla disease in which the patients are more severely affected present earlier and die in the first years of life.

Prenatal diagnosis has been achieved in both diseases; there is no specific treatment for either.

Acid cholesteryl ester hydrolase (lysosomal acid lipase) deficiency (Wolman's disease and cholesteryl ester storage disease)

Wolman's disease and cholesteryl ester storage disease are due to allelic mutations. There are two isoenzymes of lysosomal acid lipase; only one of these, the 'A' isoenzyme is lacking in Wolman's disease and cholesteryl ester storage disease. Lysosomal acid lipase catalyses the hydrolysis of low density lipoprotein-bound cholesteryl esters and triacyl glycerides but not phospholipids. The liberated cholesterol is transferred to cellular membranes where it: (a) suppresses the activity of 3-hydroxyl-3-methylglutaryl-coenzyme A reductase, which regulates the rate of cholesterol synthesis; (b) reduces low-density lipoprotein receptor synthesis and hence suppresses further transport of low density lipoprotein-cholesteryl esters into the cell; (c) stimulates fatty acyl coenzyme A:cholesterol acyltransferase, which catalyses cholesterol re-esterification with oleic (9:10) and other C_{14}–C_{18} saturated and monounsaturated fatty acids as opposed to the linoleic acid (9:10, 12:13) with which cholesterol is esterified when it enters the cell. Therefore, failure to liberate cholesterol from low density lipoprotein-bound cholesteryl esters in lysosomal acid lipase deficiency will secondarily augment cholesterol synthesis, the uptake of more low-density lipoprotein-bound cholesteryl esters, and the esterification of newly synthesized cholesterol. Lysosomal acid lipase deficiency can be demonstrated in leucocytes, fibroblasts, and amniotic cells.

Wolman's disease is the clinically more severe phenotype presenting in the first weeks of life with vomiting, diarrhoea, failure to thrive, hepatosplenomegaly, and intestinal malabsorption with marked adrenal gland enlargement and calcification. The infants usually die before the age of 6 months.

Cholesteryl ester storage disease follows a more benign course and may not be detected until adult life. There are widespread intralysosomal cholesteryl ester and triglyceride deposits, although hepatomegaly may be the only clinical abnormality. Hypercholesterolaemia is common and there may be severe premature atherosclerosis. No specific treatment is available.

The main differential diagnoses of cholesteryl ester storage diseases are: (a) Tangier disease (familial high-density lipoprotein deficiency); (b) familial lecithin cholesterol acyl transferase deficiency; (c) neutral lipid storage disease and; (d) type I glycogen storage disease.

Other lysosomal storage diseases

Cystinosis and Pompe's disease are reviewed with inborn errors of amino acid metabolism (see Chapter 6.5) and the glycogen storage diseases, respectively (see Chapter 6.3).

Inborn errors of metabolism with non-lysosomal storage of phytanic acid, β-sitosterol, and cholestanol

Phytanic acid storage disease (Refsum's disease)

Refsum's disease is an autosomal recessively inherited disease in which the long chain aliphatic alcohol phytol cannot be degraded beyond the stage of the corresponding acid because the peroxisomal enzyme, phytanic acid 2-hydroxylase, is deficient. Phytanic acid accumulates in the plasma, blood cells, and tissues. The peripheral nerves show segmental demyelination with hypertrophy due to concentric Schwann cell proliferation. Symptoms begin in the second decade and the course may be either relapsing or steadily progressive. The main abnormalities are: mixed motor and sensory polyneuropathy, cerebellar ataxia, pigmentary degeneration of the retina with failing night vision (retinitis pigmentosa), pupillary abnormalities, nerve deafness, anosmia, ichthyosis, cardiomyopathy, and epiphyseal dysplasia (short fourth metatarsal, syndactyly, hammer toe, pes cavus, osteochondritis dessicans).

The cerebrospinal fluid protein level is raised without a pleocytosis. A chlorophyll-free diet may produce clinical improvement and it should be begun as early in life as possible because established demyelinating lesions are irreversible. Plasmapheresis is useful in the initial stages in order to reduce the body burden of phytanic acid as quickly as possible, the low levels then being maintained by dietary restriction.

Although the heterozygous carriers for Refsum's disease can be identified by their 50 per cent oxidation rate for phytanic acid in cultured fibroblasts, they are asymptomatic and do not accumulate phytanic acid. Some degree of phytanic acid accumulation also occurs in some of the other peroxisomal enzyme deficiency diseases (see Chapter 6.9).

Phytosterolaemia (sitosterolaemia; sitosterol storage disease)

These patients present in childhood or early adult life with tendon and subcutaneous xanthomas. There is hypercholesterolaemia in about half the cases. Other inconsistent manifestations include xanthelasma, corneal arcus, premature atherosclerosis, haemolysis associated with abnormally shaped spherostomatocytic erythrocytes, hypersplenism, abnormal platelets, and arthropathy. There is hyperabsorption of a wide range of plant and shell-fish sterols which are all closely related to cholesterol and, like cholesterol, their esterification is catalysed by lecithin:cholesterol acyltransferase. Some of the absorbed sterols are normally converted to bile acids and this process may also be defective in β-sitosterolaemia. The plant sterols become widely distributed in the body, although unesterified cholesterol is the main constituent of the xanthomas. Histologically, the xanthomas resemble those seen in familial hypercholesterolaemia and cererbrotendinous xanthomatosis. The available data are compatible with autosomal recessive transmission. Plant sterols should be excluded from the diet and cholestyramine administered in order to bind bile acids in the gastrointestinal tract. This accelerates the synthesis of bile acids and accelerates the metabolism of the absorbed plant sterols.

Cholesterol storage disease (cerebrotendinous xanthomatosis)

Cerebrotendinous xanthomatosis is an autosomal recessively inherited disorder due to deficiency of the enzyme which catalyses the hydroxylation of cholestanol (5,6-dihydrocholesterol). This reaction is on the pathway of bile acid synthesis. The metabolic lesion reduces the feedback inhibition of cholesterol 7α-hydroxylase and thereby accelerates the synthetic pathway via cholesterol and cholestanol. Patients present in childhood or early adult life with tendon xanthomas, progressive mental handicap, and disseminated neurological lesions due to xanthomas in the brain with associated demyelination, premature atherosclerosis, and cataracts. There are granulomas (xanthomas) in most organs, and these contain cholesterol and cholestanol. The plasma concentration of cholestanol is elevated but cholesterol and other lipid concentrations are usually normal. Treatment with chenodeoxycholic acid which inhibits bile acid synthesis reduces the plasma cholestanol concentration. This approach offers the prospect of arresting or preventing xanthoma formation and cerebral damage.

Further reading

Neufeld, E.F. (1991). Lysosomal storage diseases. *Annual Review of Biochemistry*, 60, 257–80.

See also References included in Chapter 11.8, OTM3, pp. 1437–8.

Chapter 6.9

Peroxisomal disorders

R. B. H. Schutgens and R. J. A. Wanders

Peroxisomal disorders comprise a number of genetic diseases that result from an impairment of one or more metabolic functions catalysed by peroxisomes (microbodies). Peroxisomes are cellular organelles present in every human cell except for the mature erythrocyte. Like mitochondria and chloroplasts, they arise by growth and division of pre-existing peroxisomes, rather than by budding from the endoplasmic reticulum. Peroxisomes contain no DNA, so that all peroxisomal proteins must be coded for by nuclear genes, a number of which have been cloned and characterized. All peroxisomal proteins investigated so far are synthesized on free ribosomes and are imported post-translationally into peroxisomes.

Functions of peroxisomes, including peroxisomal oxidation and respiration, are summarized in Table 1; further discussion can be found in OTM3, pp. 1438–9. Table 2 provides a tentative classification of peroxisomal disorders; among them are a number which do not allow survival into adult life. These include childhood and neonatal adrenoleucodystrophy, acylcoenzyme A oxidase deficiency, dihydroxyacetone phosphate acyl transferase deficiency and Zellweger syndromes. Those allowing longer survival are described below.

Table 1 Functions of peroxisomes mammalian cells

Catabolic functions
Hydrogen peroxide-based cellular respiration
β-Oxidation of:
long chain fatty acids (C_{16}–C_{22}; saturated/unsaturated)
very long chain fatty acids (C_{22}–C_{26}; saturated/unsaturated)
branched chain fatty acids
prostaglandins
xenobiotics with an acyl side chain
Phytanic acid catabolism*
l-Pipecolic acid oxidation
Purine catabolism
Polyamine catabolism
Anabolic functions
Ether–lipid biosynthesis*
Cholesterol biosynthesis
Bile acid biosynthesis*
Dolichol biosynthesis
Glyoxylate transamination

*Only part of this pathway is localized in peroxisomes.

Adrenomyeloneuropathy

This is one phenotype of a relatively common X-linked recessive disorder affecting nervous system white matter and the adrenal cortex. The disease is characterized by slowly progressive spastic paraparesis, impaired vibration sense in the legs, sphincter disturbance, peripheral neuropathy and varying degrees of sexual dysfunction. Some 15 per cent of female heterozygotes develop moderately severe spastic paraparesis, but of late onset and milder than in affected males. A diagnosis of multiple sclerosis is often offered in error in symptomatic carriers of this X-linked disorder. Some early cases have abnormalities only detected by magnetic resonance imaging techniques, but are at risk of later overt neurological disease.

The responsible gene encodes a peroxisomal integral membrane protein of an as yet unknown function which is a member of the adenosine triphosphate-binding cassette transporter protein superfamily. The patient gene mutations are heterogeneously distributed over the functional protein domains.

The mean age of onset is about 28 years with a range from 14 to 60 years. Some 70 per cent of these patients have primary adrenal insufficiency and 20 per cent low testosterone levels also. An 'Addisons only' form has been recognized recently. Hormone replacement cures the adrenal problem. Dietary restriction of very long chain fatty acids with addition of oleic and erucic acid can ameliorate the biochemical abnormalities in plasma, but does not improve the neurological manifestations. Bone marrow transplantation has been performed in a few childhood cases with relative success especially when given to

Table 2 Classification of peroxisomal disorders

A. Disorders with a deficiency of a single peroxisomal enzyme activity; peroxisomes present
1. Disorders of peroxisomal β-oxidation
X-linked adrenoleucodystrophy and variants
trihydroxycholestanoyl-coenzyme A oxidase deficiency
acyl-coenzyme A oxidase deficiency (pseudoneonatal adrenoleucodystrophy)
bi (tri) functional protein deficiency
peroxisomal thiolase deficiency (pseudo-Zellweger)
Adult Refsum disease
2. Other disorders
acatalasaemia
hyperoxaluria type I
glutaryl-coenzyme A oxidase deficiency
dihydroxyacetone phosphate acyltransferase deficiency
B. Disorders with a deficiency of multiple peroxisomal enzyme activities; peroxisomes present in fibroblasts
rhizomelic chondrodysplasia punctata
Zellweger-like syndrome
C. Disorders with a general deficiency of peroxisomal functions (disorders of peroxisome biogenesis)
No functional peroxisomes
Zellweger (cerebrohepatorenal) syndrome
neonatal adrenoleucodystrophy
Infantile Refsum disease

boys still free of neurological manifestations, but follow up has been short and long-term results are unknown.

Reliable biochemical procedures are available for the early prenatal detection of the disease in male fetuses.

Acatalasaemia/hypocatalasaemia

Catalase is part of a cluster of antioxidant enzymes which normally act to protect cells against oxygen free radicals (O_2^-).

Acatalasaemia is a rare autosomal recessive inborn error of metabolism in which the homozygotes have extremely low or even undetectable levels of catalase activity in erythrocytes. Other tissues may display variable levels of enzyme deficiency. In liver, catalase is present within peroxisomes in which it plays an essential part in oxidation reactions.

Acatalasaemia has a world-wide distribution but it has been particularly studied in Japan, Switzerland, and Israel. It is genetically heterogeneous. In general, it is a relatively benign disease without neurological involvement. In some younger Japanese patients it is associated with ulcerating, often gangrenous, oral lesions (Takahara disease) but has no other serious manifestations. None of the Swiss acatalaemics had oral gangrene or any other health problem related to the deficiency. Heterogeneity in severity at the tissue level, dietary factors, and differences in oral flora are important factors. Surgical treatment with excursion of any necrotic areas and antimicrobial therapy is followed by satisfactory healing in severely affected cases.

Primary hyperoxaluria type I

Patients usually present during the second decade of life with recurrent calcium oxalate nephrolithiasis and nephrocalcinosis due to the deficiency of the peroxisomal enzyme alanine:glyoxylate aminotransferase in liver. The disorder is described in detail in Chapter 6.12.

Adult Refsum disease (see also Chapter 6.8)

Patients usually present beyond the first decade of life with retinitis pigmentosa, peripheral polyneuropathy, cerebellar ataxia, and elevated cerebrospinal fluid protein, although this classical triad of abnormalities is not seen in every patient. The deficiency of phytanoyl-coenzyme A hydroxylase explains the severe accumulation of phytanic acid in plasma of virtually every patient. Elimination of phytanate and its precursors from the diet can be beneficial; weight loss can be associated with a paradoxical rise in plasma phytanate levels and an accompanying clinical relapse.

Rhizomelic chondrodysplasia punctata

This is an heterogeneous group of bone dysplasias in which non-specific punctate epiphyseal and extra-epiphyseal calcifications can be found in radiological studies. Two major types are the rhizomelic type with an autosomal recessive mode of inheritance and the autosomal dominant Conradi–Hünermann type. Abnormal peroxisomal functions have only been found in the rhizomelic form.

The gene (PEX 7) for the classical rhizomelic type has been cloned and characterized. The gene product is the PTS (peroxisome targeting signal) 2 receptor protein; a mutation resulting in C-terminal truncation of PEX 7 protein and a non-functional receptor is found in all patients.

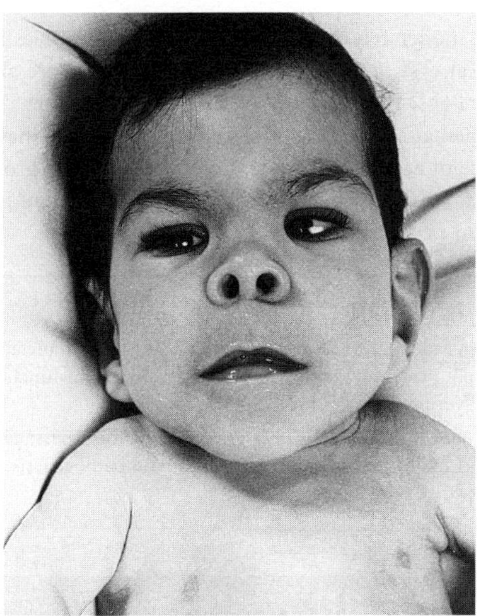

Fig. 1 The craniofacial characteristics of a rhizomelic chondrodysplasia punctata patient
(by courtesy of Dr B. Jaume, Palma de Mallorca, Spain).

Two other types are recognized that present with the same phenotype but do have a different biochemical basis. Type 2 is caused by a deficiency of dihydroxyacetonephosphate acyltransferase and type 3 by a deficiency of alkyldihydroxyacetonephosphate synthase.

Clinical characteristics

Patients have a typical facial appearance (Fig. 1), a striking symmetrical shortening of the proximal limbs, severely disturbed endochondrial bone formation and coronal clefts of vertebral bodies of the spine, and severe psychomotor retardation. Most patients have ichthyosis and cataracts. They can survive until the second decade of life. The biochemical abnormalities include deficiency of the two peroxisomal enzymes essential for the *de novo* plasmalogen biosynthesis, dihydroxyacetone phosphate acyltransferase and especially alkyl-dihydroxyacetone phosphate synthase, a deficiency of phytanic acid oxidase and a defect in the maturation of the peroxisomal 3-oxoacyl-coenzyme A thiolase enzyme protein. Biochemical diagnosis is based on the finding of decreased plasmalogen levels in erythrocyte membranes, elevated plasma phytanic acid levels, the finding of precursor (44 kDa) peroxisomal rhiolase in fibroblasts, and normal profiles of the plasma very long chain fatty acids and bile acids, respectively. The multiple biochemical abnormalities are presumably due to one underlying biochemical defect probably at the level of an impairment of the post-translational import of several newly synthesized proteins into peroxisomes. Prenatal diagnosis has been performed by measuring one or more of the specific parameters in cultured chorionic villous fibroblasts or in cultured amniocytes. No effective treatment for is available.

Infantile Refsum disease

Infantile Refsum disease includes the most mildly involved patients with disordered peroxisomal biogenesis. Distinct abnormalities are absent in the neonatal period. Most patients survive the first decade of life and show some psychomotor development. All have sensorineural hearing loss and pigmentary degeneration of the retina. Patients usually have moderately dysmorphic features and hypoplastic adrenals. Renal cortical cysts and chondrodysplasia punctata are absent. Peroxisomes are absent or seriously diminished in number.

Complementation analyses with cultured fibroblasts have revealed the existence of at least 10 different complementation groups within this category, indicating that mutations in many different genes result in a defect in peroxisome biogenesis.

Further reading

Motley, A.M. *et al.* (1997). Rhizomelic chondrodysplasia punctata is a peroxisomal protein targeting disease caused by a non-functional PTS2 receptor. *Nature Genetics*, **15**, 337–80.

Powers, J.M. and Moser, H.W. (1998). Peroxisomal disorders: genotype, phenotype, major neuropathologic lesions, and pathogenesis. *Brain Pathology*, **8**, 101–20.

Chapter 6.10

Trace metal disorders

C. A. Seymour

Trace elements in the body

By convention, trace elements are present in amounts less than 0.005 per cent of body weight (Table 1). About 15 are known to be essential for health and have various roles in cells and tissues of the body. Deficiency and toxicity states are often insidious, with the former being particularly important in the developing fetus or neonate. Gastrointestinal absorption, on the one hand, and excretion in urine and bile, on the other, are the mechanisms by which concentrations of trace elements are normally regulated.

The process of absorption of iron from the intestine, which regulates body iron content, is a good model for a number of other trace metals. Absorbed iron is bound to different proteins, for example transferrin, and is then in a rapidly exchangeable pool in equilibrium with ferritin, in which iron is stored and from which it is more slowly exchanged. Transfer of iron to plasma transferrin is rapid, whereas its passage in the reverse direction is slow. Iron absorption also affects intestinal transport of other chemically related metals (zinc, copper, cobalt, and manganese) by competition depending on their affinity for mucosal transferrin. Absorption of cobalt and manganese is increased in states of iron deficiency and a high dietary intake of these metals may inhibit iron absorption.

Table 1 Trace elements: elements present in amounts less than 0.005 per cent of body weight

Essential	Less essential	Toxic	No functional/ toxic effects
Copper	Arsenic	Cadmium	Barium
Iodine	Cobalt	Lead	Bromine
Iron	Chromium	Mercury	Gold
(Magnesium)	Fluoride	Plutonium	Rubidium
Manganese	Molybdenum		Silver
Selenium	Nickel		
Zinc	Silicon		
	Tin		
	Vanadium		

The other regulatory site in trace metal homeostasis is via excretion in the bile (cf. copper and zinc). Genetic defects in transport systems (cf. iron in haemochromatosis and copper in Wilson's and Menkes diseases) as well as hepatobiliary disease can be expected to cause deficiency or toxicity of trace metals.

Various roles for trace metals are outlined in Table 2. Both deficiency and toxicity of certain trace elements (iron, copper, selenium, and cadmium) may interact with hormonal and cell-mediated immune responses, as well as being cofactors for bacterial growth. This may result in the spread of bacterial and viral infections.

Trace elements and cell damage

Cell and tissue injury and death are often mediated by the presence or incomplete removal of free radicals produced by the cellular reduction of oxygen to water. Incomplete removal of these molecules may lead to lysosomal, microsomal, and peroxisomal membrane damage, as well as interaction with polyunsaturated fatty acids which may also trigger a further series of damaging reactions. Trace elements such as copper, zinc, manganese, selenium, and cobalt are essential to the function of free-radical scavenging enzymes, as well as to mitochondrial and adenosine triphosphate (ATP)-generating systems.

Trace metal disorders

Copper

Copper is in relative excess in most diets. It is a prosthetic element of many metalloenzymes playing a vital part in mitochondrial energy generation, melanin formation, and cross-linking of collagen and elastin. Acquired copper deficiency is rare because of the efficiency of the liver in maintaining copper homeostasis. Excretion into bile is dependent on incorporation into caeruloplasmin (copper-binding protein); toxic accumulation is infrequent and arises only with genetic defects in these homeostatic mechanisms (cf. Wilson's disease and Menkes disease).

Copper homeostasis

Total body copper is in the range of 50–150 mg, of which some 8 per cent is found in the liver. Copper is probably stored in this major site within lysosomes in association with metallothionein. High concentrations are also found in the brain, kidney, heart, and bone.

About 2–5 mg of copper is absorbed from the diet each day, and is transported loosely bound to albumin, this moiety accounting for about 10 per cent of circulating copper. Net uptake of copper (about 40–60 per cent) reflects its differential binding to low molecular weight ligands present in saliva, gastric, and duodenal juice, and high molecular weight ligands present in bile. The regulatory mechanisms involved in intestinal copper transport are still unknown, although binding occurs to two cytosolic proteins, one similar to superoxide dismutase, and the other metallothionein. Although metallothionein and active transport of copper–amino acid complexes are involved in absorption, there is no evidence that overall copper homeostasis is controlled at the intestinal site.

Table 2 Clinical features and treatment of some trace metal disorders

(a) Trace metal toxicity

Element	Metabolic role	Organ/tissue affected	Disorder	Clinical features	Specific treatment
Copper	Free radical scavenging enzymes	Red cells Liver CNS-basal ganglia	**Primary** Wilson's disease	Haemolysis, anaemia Hepatitis, cirrhosis	Chelation: Penicillamine Trientine
	Mitochondria Collagen synthesis			CNS: Kayser-Fleischer rings Dysarthria, tremor Parkinsonian-like Osteoarthritis Renal tubular acidosis	Ammonium thiomolybdate Zinc acetate (normally adjunct to other chelators) Liver transplantation
			Indian childhood cirrhosis	Jaundice Hepatitis and cirrhosis	Liver transplantation
			Biliary atresia	Jaundice Hepatitis and cirrhosis	Liver transplantation
			Secondary Primary biliary cirrhosis Sclerosing cholangitis Chronic acute hepatitis	Jaundice Hepatitis and cirrhosis	Ursodeoxycholic acid Liver transplantation
Iron	Haemoglobin Iron stores Red cell formation	Red cells Liver Spleen Bone marrow	**Primary** Genetic haemochromatosis	Cirrhosis Hypersplenism Diabetes Osteoarthritis	Phlebotomy Chelation: desferrioxamine
		Endocrine organs	**Secondary** Thalassaemias Alcoholic cirrhosis Porphyria cutanea tarda Sideroblastic anaemia	Cirrhosis Hypersplenism	Chelation: desferrioxamine + phlebotomy

Maintenance of homeostasis depends uniquely on excretion in bile, with about 1.5–1.7 mg excreted daily; some (*c.* 0.7 μg/day) is excreted in urine. Gastrointestinal secretions contain small amounts but, because of their volume, probably account for a significant amount of luminal copper. Any interruption in the secretion of bile, such as in primary biliary cirrhosis or biliary atresia, leads to copper accumulation in the liver, and subsequently in other tissues as the liver becomes cirrhotic. In bile, copper is bound to low and high molecular weight complexes, and intestinal reabsorption of biliary copper is negligible.

Copper deficiency

Copper deficiency may occur in genetic and acquired forms, although both are rare. *The acquired form* may occur in malnourished children, adults with severe malabsorption syndromes, in patients on regular total parenteral nutrition, or in patients regularly taking chelating agents (penicillamine) as treatment for rheumatoid arthritis. The diagnosis rests on low serum copper measurements associated with reduced serum caeruloplasmin, hypochromic microcytic anaemia, and evidence of bone demineralization.

The genetic form (Menkes disease) is an X-linked recessive disorder resulting in abnormalities in copper metabolism associated with malfunction of a number of key enzymes (for example lysyl oxidase, superoxide dismutase, cytochrome oxidase, and dopamine β-hydroxylase). Most tissues, except the liver, have a normal or increased copper content. Major features of the disease which results in death by the age of 3–5 years are shown in Table 2. A fuller account is provided in OTM3, pp. 1417–19.

Copper overload or toxicity

Chronic copper toxicity in man occurs in two major forms: (a) the primary inherited form, in which it accumulates in and damages the liver, later the nervous system and other tissues, giving rise to hepatolenticular degeneration, or Wilson's disease; (b) the secondary form, in which it accumulates as a consequence of chronic cholestasis, either congenital (biliary atresia or Indian childhood cirrhosis) or acquired (primary biliary cirrhosis). Amounts of hepatic copper may then be similar to those found in Wilson's disease, but some damage has always preceded the excessive deposition. In chronic active hepatitis, smaller amounts of accumulated copper exacerbate preceding hepatocyte injury.

Wilson's disease (hepatolenticular degeneration)

This is an autosomal recessively inherited disorder due to an abnormal gene located on chromosome 13. Pathognomonic features include hepatic copper accumulation (>25 μg/g dry weight) in association with reduced or absent circulating caeruloplasmin (<200 mg/dl), and reduction in biliary excretion of copper (<1.5 mg/day). These defects result in copper accumulation in the body, initially within hepatocytes and then, as damage leads to cirrhosis and portal hypertension in the

Table 2 *continued*

(b) Trace metal deficiency					
Element	**Metabolic role**	**Organ/tissue affected**	**Disorder**	**Clinical features**	**Specific treatment**
Copper	As (a)	Hair Skin CNS development	**Primary** Menkes disease	Neonatal death Kinky, steely hair Cutis laxis, dermatitis CNS degeneration Anaemia, neutropenia Bone changes secondary to reduced cross-linking elastin/collagen Skin/skeletal abnormalities Aortic aneurysm Abnormal lung development	Copper replacement (copper histidine)
			Secondary Total parenteral nutrition Nutritional deficiency		
Iron	As (a)	Bone marrow Red cells Skin, hair, nails	**Primary** Iron deficiency	Anaemia (microcytic) Ischaemic effects on organs/tissues	Iron supplement Ascorbic acid (low dose)
			Secondary Iron deficiency		
Manganese	Mitochondrial function Mucopoly-saccharide synthesis	CNS Skeletal	**Primary** Manganese deficiency *in utero*	Early noenatal death	Manganese replacement
			Secondary Total parenteral nutrition	CNS: irreversible ataxia Inner ear otolith abnormality	
			Nutritional deficiency	Skeletal: anomalous inner ear calcification	
Selenium	Free radical scavenging enzymes (glutathione peroxidase)	Muscle Skeletal	Keshan disease Kashin-Beck disease	Congestive cardiomyopathy Osteoarthropathy Muscle weakness/pain	Sodium selenite replacement
Zinc	?	Skin CNS Gastrointestinal system Reproductive system	**Primary** Acrodermatitis enteropathica Sickle-cell disease	Growth retardation Congenital malformation Chromosome aberration Alopecia CNS Mental lethargy Emotional disorder Convulsions	Zinc sulphate Zinc replacement Zinc acetate
			Secondary Gastrointestinal tract Crohn's disease Malabsorption syndromes Liver disease	Gastrointestinal tract Weight loss/anorexia Diarrhoea Skin Bullous/pustular dermatitis Increased infections Impaired wound healing Oligospermia	

central nervous system, eye, kidneys, and other organs. If untreated, the disorder results in cirrhosis and extensive central nervous system damage, with a fatal outcome within a few years of onset of the symptoms. Chelating therapy prevents progression of the disease and may also reverse some neurological and eye abnormalities.

Incidence Wilson's disease has a prevalence of 1 in 30 000 with a carrier frequency of 1 in 90. The abnormal gene is present in all racial groups studied so far and a higher incidence has been noted in Arabs, natives of southern Italy, Jews of eastern Europe, Japanese, Chinese, and Indians, as well as in communes with a high rate of consanguineous marriages. There is no known human leucocyte antigen association.

Genetics The demonstration of a linkage between the locus for Wilson's disease and the esterase D enzyme localized the gene mutation to chromosome 13. DNA restriction length polymorphism studies have further localized the position to 13q14–q21. Expression studies of this gene reveal a 7.5 kb transcript which is expressed strongly in the liver, kidney, and placenta and weakly in heart, brain, lung, muscle, and pancreas. Mutation analysis has also revealed four disease-specific mutations (two transversions and two frameshift mutations) affecting different domains of the putative protein. These correlate with distinct Wilson disease haplotypes. Identification of the Menkes disease gene mutation, coding for a transporter protein, has raised the possibility that the abnormal gene of Wilson's disease may code for a defective liver-specific copper transporter protein. A 1411 amino acid protein has been predicted from the cDNA sequence which, as a cation-transporting P-type ATPase, has close homology with the predicted protein product of the Menkes disease gene. These proteins additionally share similarity with caeruloplasmin in having six potential copper-binding motifs.

The link with reduced or absent plasma caeruloplasmin is still uncertain, as the caeruloplasmin gene has been mapped to chromosome 3q25. However, mRNA for caeruloplasmin is reduced in Wilson's disease, but not sufficiently to account for the variable reduction in plasma caeruloplasmin. In addition, the presence of intracellular caeruloplasmin, even when plasma caeruloplasmin levels are reduced or absent, suggests that the critical defect is likely to be post-translational.

Detection of gene carriers in families is now possible by development of several highly polymorphic microsatellite markers tightly linked and in linkage disequilibrium with the Wilson's disease locus, if one affected sibling and parents are available for genotyping. Using polymerase chain reaction for detection of these markers, haplotypes associated with the defective gene can be detected even if only traces of DNA are available, and the carrier status of siblings can be determined. In contrast, carrier data by mutation analysis would be difficult because of allelic heterogeneity.

Clinical features Wilson's disease may be clinically undetectable until 5 years of age. However, during this period copper accumulates in the liver without clinical signs, and excess copper in red cells may present as chronic haemolytic anaemia or an episode of acute haemolysis. In 90 per cent of patients, the disease presents with juvenile hepatic disease or with neurological/psychiatric manifestations. About 40 per cent present with a spectrum of liver disease, from acute to chronic hepatitis, or with abnormal liver function tests without clinical findings. Copper initially accumulates in the hepatic cytosol, then, as saturation occurs, in mitochondria and eventually in lysosomes prior to biliary excretion, while some copper is released to the circulation bound to caeruloplasmin. If this redistribution occurs rapidly, patients may develop fulminant hepatic failure or intravascular haemolysis. Copper accumulation in, and damage to, mitochondria precedes the accumulation in hepatic lysosomes and leads to cirrhosis. Continued extrahepatic redistribution increases as portal hypertension and shunting of blood from liver occurs. At this stage neurological, psychiatric, ophthalmological, and renal damage occurs due to increasing copper deposition.

Clinical presentations (1) *Haematological.* Presentation with non-spherocytic, Coombs-negative intravascular haemolysis may occur in 10–15 per cent of patients with Wilson's disease. Severe haemolysis may also accompany fulminant hepatitis.

(2) *Hepatic.* Before puberty, symptoms and signs of mild hepatic dysfunction are common, and if they coincide with abdominal pain and haemolysis, Wilson's disease should be suspected. Some 10 per cent of patients have pigment gallstones, suggesting previous episodes of haemolysis. The more usual presentation, however, is with chronic liver damage progressing to cirrhosis. In the early stages, patients are vaguely unwell, but later develop more specific features of liver dysfunction such as nausea, easy bleeding, fluid retention, and jaundice. Portal hypertension develops, with progressive hepatic insufficiency with splenomegaly, gastro-oesophageal varices, and ascites. Patients are often investigated incorrectly for other causes of splenomegaly, such as idiopathic thrombocytopenic purpura. About 1–30 per cent of patients present with a picture of chronic active hepatitis, when the diagnosis of Wilson's disease may be missed as plasma caeruloplasmin levels may increase to within the normal range, along with the secretion of acute phase reacting proteins. A minority of patients present with fulminant hepatitis and encephalopathy, sometimes just after starting chelating therapy. In these the prognosis is poor unless the liver is transplanted. It is notable that hepatocellular carcinoma is rare in the cirrhosis of Wilson's disease, unlike the situation in haemochromatosis.

(3) *Neurological and psychiatric.* Onset is usually in childhood or adolescence but may be delayed as late as the fifth decade. The first symptoms frequently lead to psychiatric referral with conduct disorder, personality change, or frank psychosis. Common initial neurological symptoms include tremor of any type, dysarthria and drooling (Fig. 1) chorea, dystonic spasms and posturing or akinesia and rigidity. Without treatment progression is inevitable with dementia, increasingly severe dysarthria and dysphasia and increasing rigidity, akinesia and dystonia leading to contractions and immotility. Vision, hearing, and sensation are not affected and tendon reflexes and plantar responses are usually normal. Fits may occur in a minority of cases. A Kayser–Fleischer ring may be seen in the cornea with the naked eye and is always present in those with neurological symptoms on slit-lamp examination. It consists of a ring of greenish-brown copper pigment deposited around the margin of the cornea in Descemet's membrane (Plate 1). A sunflower cataract due to copper in the lens may also be seen. In those with neurological deficits there need be no clinical evidence of liver disease but a history of hepatitis or jaundice may be found and liver function tests are often abnormal.

(4) *Renal.* Renal tubular acidosis due to damage by copper in proximal and/or distal tubules is not uncommon. Osteomalacia and rickets may occur as a result of tubular loss of phosphate. Aminoaciduria and nephrocalcinosis may also occur.

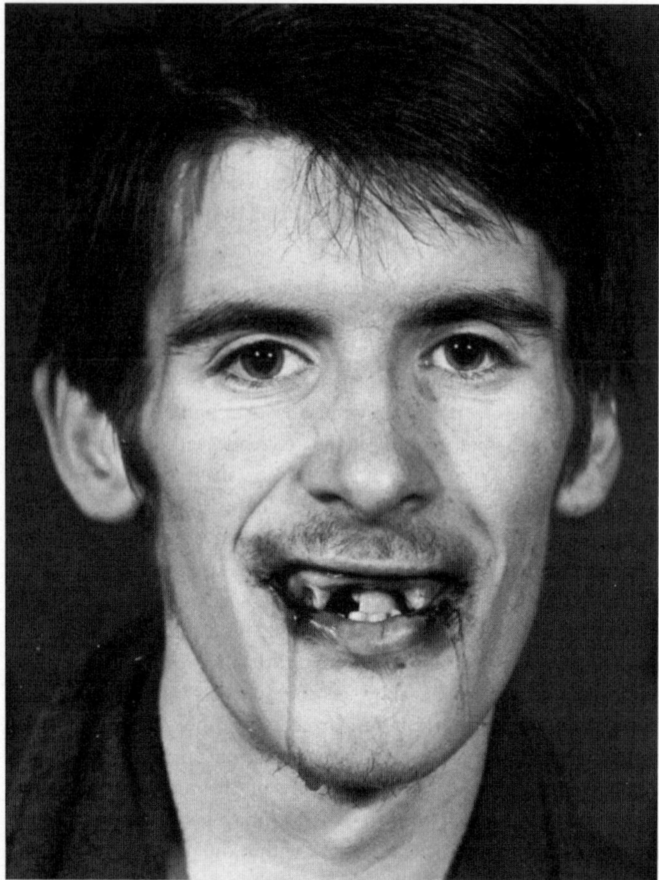

Fig. 1 The facies of a 20-year-old man with severe Wilson's disease, causing a severe pseudobulbar palsy with marked dysarthria and dysphagia, as well as a generalized akinetic–rigid syndrome.

(5) *Joints.* Early osteoarthritis of the spine (Scheuermann's disease), is not uncommon, but polyarthritis as well as hypermobile joints and chondromalacia patellae are also recognized.

(6) *Skin.* The skin may be hyperpigmented appearing slightly grey with a bluish appearance of the lanulae of the nails.

(7) *Cardiac.* Cardiac abnormalities have been noted rarely, with hypertrophy (but not cardiomyopathy) associated with interstitial fibrosis, small-vessel sclerosis, and perivascular myocarditis, which may lead to congestive cardiac failure.

(8) *Endocrine disturbances.* Endocrine disturbances are mainly due to liver dysfunction, with gynaecomastia in men and menstrual disturbance in women, with some infertility. Most women conceive easily once they have been treated and excess copper removed.

Pathology Histological changes vary with the amount of copper accumulated. The liver is most affected. The precise sequence of hepatocyte change is not certain and there may be few changes in liver lobular structure in the asymptomatic patient. Early changes comprise pericellular fatty droplet infiltration of cytoplasm and 'glycogen' degeneration of the nuclei, with copper distributed diffusely in the cytoplasm. Concurrently, or preceding these changes, mitochondrial, microsomal, and peroxisomal abnormalities are seen. Some of the lipid is contained within lysosomes. Progression from fatty infiltration to cirrhosis occurs at variable rates; either patients develop inflammatory changes indistinguishable from chronic active hepatitis, or cirrhosis may develop with little inflammatory infiltrate. Once

Table 3 Normal and Wilson's disease parameters

	Normal	Wilson's disease
Serum		
Caeruloplasmin (mg/dl)	25–40	< 25
Copper (μmol/l)	11–24	3–10
Urine		
Copper (μg/24 h)		
untreated	< 40	100–1000
treated (penicillamine)	100–600	1500–3000
Hepatic copper		
(μg/g dry weight)	15–55	250–3000

cirrhosis has occurred, the ultrastructural changes are not specific for Wilson's disease except that more copper is found within pericanulicular lysosomes (about 25 per cent) than in any other intracellular compartment. Despite increased hepatic copper content, histochemical stains for copper (rubeanic acid) or copper-associated protein (orcein) are of little value in diagnosis and do not correlate well with the degree of copper overload.

In the brain pathological effects of copper are widespread and striking in the globus pallidus and putamen but are non-specific except for cystic changes in the region of the internal capsule, which can be detected by computed tomography or nuclear magnetic resonance scans. Copper also accumulates in the renal cortex accounting for generalized proximal tubular dysfunction. In bone a wide variety of lesions have been described, due to the toxic effect of copper on chondroblasts and on collagen formation.

Diagnosis The majority of patients with Wilson's disease have Kayser–Fleischer rings and low plasma caeruloplasmin concentrations. Detection of anaemia, haemolysis, and disturbed hepatocellular function are all important diagnostic clues. Specific investigations are necessary to confirm the diagnosis and in monitoring the effects of treatment (Table 3). The activity and concentration of serum caeruloplasmin is reduced or absent (<25 mg/dl) in 95 per cent of patients. There is overlap of caeruloplasmin levels in Wilson's disease, in obligate heterozygotes, and in normal subjects in the lower range of normal distribution. Non-caeruloplasmin copper is loosely bound to albumin or amino acids (5–12 μg/dl) and is increased in untreated Wilson's disease. Twenty-four-hour urinary excretion of copper is always increased in untreated disease (>70–100 μg/day), although this may also occur in other liver diseases, such as chronic active hepatitis and primary biliary cirrhosis. Special care is needed when collecting the urine samples to avoid contamination. Measurement of urinary copper excretion is also important in monitoring the effects of chelating therapy, where, early in treatment, urine levels may rise to 2000 μg/day and fall to less than 100 μg/day as the copper overload is reduced. In normal individuals, the copper concentration in liver varies between 15 and 55 μg/g dry weight of liver. In untreated patients, the concentration is greater than 250 μg/g dry weight, and in heterozygotes the range is between 55 and 250 μg/g dry weight. Increased hepatic copper occurs also in secondary copper overload, such as Indian childhood cirrhosis, primary biliary cirrhosis, sclerosing cholangitis, and chronic active hepatitis. Measurement of the incorporation of radiocopper into caeruloplasmin is helpful in distinguishing patients with suspected Wilson's disease when diagnosis is uncertain, for example when caeruloplasmin levels are normal, or when liver biopsy

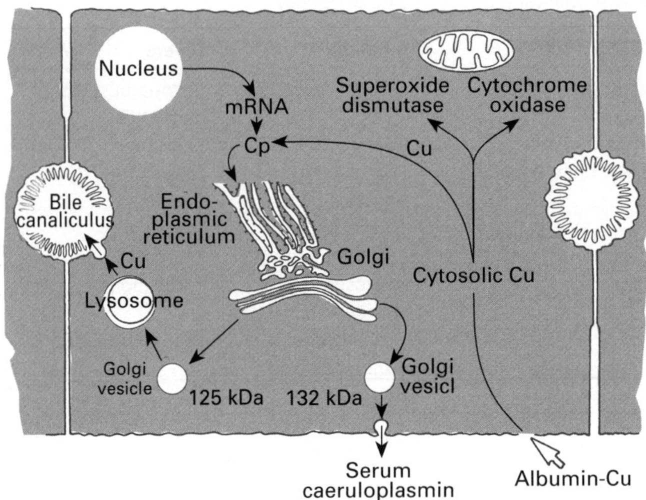

Fig. 2 Caeruloplasmin secretion and excretion in a normal hepatocyte indicating different molecular forms. White arrow shows site of defect in Wilson's disease.

is contraindicated. Measurement of incorporation of orally administered radiocopper into caeruloplasmin at 1, 2, 3, and 48 h distinguishes clearly between normal patients and those with Wilson's disease, in whom little or no radiocopper is incorporated into newly synthesized caeruloplasmin.

Basic defect Several hypotheses have been advanced to explain the primary defect of failure of biliary excretion of copper. Reabsorption of biliary copper from the intestine in Wilson's disease is not increased. Only recently has the link been made between defective biliary excretion and reduced plasma caeruloplasmin (Fig. 2).

It is now clear that the liver produces caeruloplasmin and that the defect in this glycoprotein in Wilson's disease must be post-translational. Evidence of reduced amounts of hepatic mRNA for caeruloplasmin has not yet been linked to the underlying metabolic defect. The demonstration that there are different molecular forms of caeruloplasmin, a 132 kDa form found in plasma and a 125 kDa form in bile which is reduced or absent in Wilson's disease, lends support for a post-translational abnormality. It also suggests that caeruloplasmin may play more than a secondary part in the underlying metabolic defect. The localization of the defect to the biliary tract may be the result of the liver synthesizing a high-affinity copper-binding protein or of a deficiency in synthesis of a biliary copper-binding protein. The latter possibility is supported by the reduced amounts of the 125 kDa caeruloplasmin in bile and liver in Wilson's disease. An abnormality of hepatic lysosomes, known to participate in intracellular processing and excretion of copper to bile has also been suggested.

As the metabolism of copper in the liver of neonates is similar to that of patients with untreated Wilson's disease, it has been suggested that a mutation in a 'controller' gene is responsible for repression of normal adult copper metabolism in the fetus and that Wilson's disease results from a failure to switch from the positive balance in the fetus and neonate to the normal balance of the adult. It is also possible that the Wilson's disease gene codes for an altered specific membrane copper transporter.

Pathogenesis of the liver lesion Copper, in free ionic form, is toxic to hepatocytes. Although the retained copper accumulates in lysosomes, there is no evidence that copper-filled lysosomes are fragile. In contrast, copper-containing mitochondria are more fragile, and it is likely that the mechanism of copper-induced hepatocyte damage is due to mitochondrial damage, reducing oxidative phosphorylation.

Management d-Penicillamine (dimethylcysteine) is effective in removing copper from patients with Wilson's disease. The optimum time for treatment is in the early stages, and all patients with the disease should be treated even if asymptomatic. Treatment must be lifelong, unless patients have had a liver transplant. A majority of symptomatic patients improve or have an almost complete resolution of their symptoms. Patients who discontinue treatment may relapse rapidly and die. Management also involves general care of any liver disease and anaemia, and investigation of the family and siblings of the propositus.

A low-copper diet and copper chelating agents are essential to induce a state of negative copper balance. d-Penicillamine is still the drug of first choice, although triethylene tetramine and ammonium thiomolybdate can be alternatives. Divided daily doses of penicillamine range from 500 mg to 2 g, depending on the response. Larger doses are required initially and should be reduced as urinary copper excretion falls. Progress can be monitored by clinical improvement, 24-h urine copper and serum copper measurements, blood and platelet counts, and urinalysis for protein and aminoaciduria, in addition to clinical examination and slit-lamp examination of the cornea. Triethylene tetramine dihydrochloride (trientine), given orally in divided daily doses of 750 mg–2 g, can be used when penicillamine is not tolerated or causes side-effects. As copper is mobilized from different body pools, trientine causes a rise in the serum-free copper concentration.

Oral zinc is a third agent used in treatment. It may act by promoting gastrointestinal excretion of copper by inhibiting copper absorption in a competitive way, or by inducing synthesis of metallothioneins within the enterocyte and hepatocyte which would bind copper to form mercaptides. Copper would then remain as a complex within the enterocyte, to be excreted in faeces as cells turn over or to be transferred to the portal circulation. Zinc (150 mg) is given orally either as the sulphate or the acetate form in divided doses 1 h before meals. There is still some doubt as to whether zinc can be used alone as therapy for Wilson's disease or only as an adjunct to chelating agents. There is evidence that using zinc concurrently with penicillamine may reduce treatment-induced fulminant hepatic failure.

Liver transplantation is an attractive option as it corrects the metabolic defect in the liver. With limited resources it is reserved for young patients with severe hepatic and neurological damage. Patients who have had liver transplants no longer need chelating therapy, and at least two case reports have claimed complete reversal of extensive neurological impairment after transplantation. In fulminant hepatic failure, a prognostic index based on prothrombin time, bilirubin, and transaminase determines whether the patient is suitable for transplantation.

Women with cirrhosis due to copper toxicity have an increased risk of infertility, abortion, stillbirth, and premature delivery. Conversely, once chelation therapy has reduced the copper overload, successful pregnancies occur and chelating agents do not appear to harm the fetus or cause fetal copper deficiency.

Screening of family members Screening of children should be after 3 years of age. It should include slit-lamp examination of the eyes, liver function tests, and assay of serum caeruloplasmin. If the results are suggestive of Wilson's disease, liver biopsy and quantitative measurement of hepatic copper should follow.

Side-effects of therapy Adverse effects of penicillamine are not uncommon. In the first few weeks of therapy, 20 per cent of patients may develop hypersensitivity with a maculopapular rash, lymphadenopathy, granulocytopenia, and thrombocytopenia. In these situations, the drug should be discontinued immediately, and when reintroduced it should be at much lower dose (0.25 g/day) and with steroid cover. A nephrotic syndrome may occur in as many as 3–7 per cent. Much rarer are reports of a Goodpasture-like syndrome or drug-related systemic lupus erythematosus.

Skin lesions are not uncommon with long-term chelation therapy, and patients may develop lax skin due to inhibition of elastin and collagen cross-linking in the subcutaneous tissues. The rarest form is elastosis perforans serpiginosa. Trientine has been used much less, but has also been associated with rashes and systemic lupus erythematosus nephritis. The major problem with zinc therapy is gastrointestinal intolerance, which may inhibit iron absorption, causing a microcytic anaemia; it may also alter phagocytic activity against bacteria and affect lipoprotein metabolism.

Prognosis Prognosis is best in the asymptomatic individuals who are detected early, often by the meticulous screening of families of index cases. Poor progress is more likely in patients with severe liver damage, including acute fulminant hepatic failure, and acute neurological disease and dystonia. In addition, in the presence of cirrhosis, even when copper-depleted, risks of variceal bleeding and intercurrent infections remain.

Chronic cholestatic syndromes

Intra- and extrahepatic obstruction to bile excretion affects copper excretion and causes its accumulation in the liver. Liver damage due to congenital or acquired abnormalities precedes the copper retention, which increases with the duration of cholestasis and exacerbates hepatocyte damage.

Iron

Abnormalities of iron metabolism and associated clinical features are described elsewhere (see Chapter 3.16).

Zinc

Zinc is an essential trace element required for RNA and DNA synthesis and for the function of some metalloenzymes. Deficiency is associated with malnutrition especially in those eating cereal proteins high in phosphate and phytate. It becomes manifest quickly in individuals with increased requirements, such as growing infants, children, and pregnant women (see Chapter 8.2). About 20–30 per cent (12–15 mg/day) is absorbed in the duodenum, where it competes with iron for binding to mucosal sites. Absorption is also reduced by calcium, phytate, and fibre. Daily losses occur through the gastrointestinal tract (1.2 mg/day) with less in urine and insensible losses. The clinical spectrum of zinc deficiency varies from severe to mild, as shown in Table 4. Prenatal zinc deficiency has a particularly rapid effect on the fetus, causing intrauterine death or low birth weight. Congenital malfunction and hyperplasia of the oesophageal mucosa are also common. Persistent zinc deficiency causes postnatal behavioural problems and the low zinc content of tissues may cause chromosomal aberrations and decreased synthesis of DNA and proteins, such as pulmonary surfactant and pancreatic proteins.

Table 4 Clinical features of zinc deficiency

Mild	Moderate	Severe
Oligospermia	Growth retardation	Bullous/pustular dermatitis
Weight loss	Hypogonadism	Keratitis
↑ Hyperammonaemia	Skin changes	Alopecia
	Anorexia	Diarrhoea
	Mental lethargy	Weight loss
	↓ Wound healing	Emotional disorder
	Neurosensory disorders	↑ Infections
	Taste abnormalities	Fatal if untreated
	Abnormal dark adaptation	

Zinc is found in a number of organs (liver, kidney, bone, retina, prostate, and muscle). It is carried in plasma mainly bound to albumin, but other proteins such as caeruloplasmin and α_2-macroglobulin also have a strong affinity for it. About 70 metalloenzymes require zinc but not all are sensitive to deficiency. Alkaline phosphatase in bone, carboxypeptidase in pancreas, and deoxythymidine kinase in connective tissue are among the sensitive forms. Zinc also interacts with iron, copper, calcium, lead, and cadmium, competing with these trace elements for binding sites.

Certain hormones, thymosin, somatomedin, and testosterone, are zinc dependent. It has a part in inhibiting histamine release from mast cells, and has other anti-inflammatory actions on phagocytic cells and platelets as well as interfering in cell-mediated immunity. Zinc ions are protective against free-radical injury, although the mechanism is uncertain.

Zinc has a specific part in the nucleus of cells, where it stabilizes native RNA, promotes catalytic activity of RNA polymerases, and is essential for the function of at least two of the chromatin proteins involved in transcription. Deficiency appears to alter chromatin to a more compact form which is far more accessible to hydrolytic enzymes. An essential part of gene expression is binding of a regulatory protein to the recognition sequence of an appropriate gene and it now seems that a commonly used structural motif for DNA recognition is the 'zinc finger'. Putative 'zinc fingers' are present in the structures of many regulatory proteins.

Diagnosis

Body zinc status can be assessed by measurement of zinc in plasma and urine, although in severe deficiency white cell or platelet zinc concentrations probably give a more accurate assessment. A zinc tolerance test (using oral challenge of 200 mg zinc sulphate) is useful in detecting abnormalities of absorption, but will not distinguish between a malabsorption state causing zinc deficiency or one where malabsorption is caused by the zinc deficiency (cf. acrodermatitis enteropathica). Measurement of the activity of zinc-dependent enzymes may also be helpful, as may measurements of serum thymulin and plasma metallothionein concentrations.

Treatment

Zinc replacement can be given as the sulphate or acetate, the former causing less gastrointestinal upset. The nutritional requirement is in the order of 10–15 mg/day. Zinc is absorbed more efficiently as a salt than from the normal diet. Replacement is normally with the sulphate

30–150 mg/day taken orally. More rarely, zinc deficiency in association with hepatic cirrhosis, and particularly hepatic encephalopathy, can respond to zinc acetate, 600 mg/day in divided doses.

Selenium

Selenium is an essential element for key free-radical scavenging enzymes such as glutathione peroxidase, which reduce hydrogen peroxide and a range of lipid peroxides which could potentially damage cell membranes. It is absorbed from the gastrointestinal tract as a water-soluble complex in a process which is not regulated. Selenium is normally excreted in urine via direct methylation. In toxic situations, a differently methylated metabolite is excreted. Selenium concentrations are highest in the liver and kidneys, perhaps reflecting their part as organs of storage and excretion. The standard replacement dose of selenium is difficult to assess, as daily recommended intake is between 50 and 200 μg for an adult, and for the pre-term infant, a minimum requirement of 1 μg/kg per day has been suggested. Supplementation of total parenteral nutrition fluids to supply selenium at a level of 1 μg/kg per day is recommended. Thus a normal daily intake of 100 μg in total parenteral nutrition fluids is needed to maintain levels at about 100 ng/ml. Selenium is usually replaced in the form of selenious acid, and a dosage of 100 μg/day is administered intravenously for 21–31 days. Selenium toxicity is rare but occurs in parts of America where there is a high content in the soil. The major clinical features are alopecia and nail deformities. Deficiency is associated with two human diseases which occur in the East, particularly in China.

Keshan disease

This is a cardiomyopathy where multifocal necrosis and fibrosis of the myocardium is combined with muscle weakness and myalgia. It is improved by administration of sodium selenite. It is unknown whether this condition is due entirely to selenium deficiency and whether this interacts with a genetic deficiency of selenium-dependent glutathione peroxidase; or whether interaction with a virus component occurs. Some protection has been claimed for prophylactic dosing with 150 mg/day of selenium, given as selenomethionine.

Kashimbeck disease

This endemic osteoarthropathy occurring in East Asia and China, is characterized by chronic osteoarthrosis affecting fingers, toes, and long bones and is found in children aged between 5 and 12 years. It is a progressive disorder which results in deformity and growth retardation. Some improvement has been noted with sodium selenite treatment.

Chromium

This is an essential element in carbohydrate and lipid metabolism, where deficiency due to insufficient intake results in clinical features indistinguishable from those of non-insulin-dependent diabetes and associated vascular disease. It is absorbed from the diet, by a mechanism similar to that of iron uptake, in very small amounts (1 p.p.m.) and is excreted through the kidneys at a rate that is increased by exercise, physical trauma, and diets high in refined sugars. Its precise part in glucose metabolism is unclear, but chromium may increase the expression of insulin receptors.

Manganese

It is absorbed in constant amounts from the duodenum, which are increased in cirrhotic or iron-deficient patients. This may be due, in part, to an increase in transport binding proteins which participate in a transport of iron and manganese. Manganese absorption is reduced by the presence of phytates, calcium, and phosphates in the diet. Once absorbed, it is transported bound to α_2-macroglobulin in the portal circulation and is taken up by the liver and excreted in bile. It also interacts with iron metabolism in that a proportion is bound to transferrin and released in circulation for uptake by other tissues.

Manganese is an essential component of several proteins/enzymes involved in intermediary metabolism (arginase and pyruvate carboxylase), in free-radical scavenging (Mn-superoxide dismutase), and in transport proteins (calmodulin-dependent protein phosphatases). It may also be involved in glucose homeostasis, and perhaps participates in second-messenger interactions (phosphorylation, dephosphorylation cascades), and signal transduction systems coupled to specific receptors. It also affects calcium fluxes across cell membranes in excitable and other tissues (liver and pancreas), playing a part in intracellular calcium fluxes in mitochondria.

Manganese deficiency may be associated with joint disease (congenital dislocation of the hips) and osteoarthritis, but the mechanisms are not certain.

Other trace metal toxicity syndromes

Aluminium toxicity deserves a brief mention but is covered more fully elsewhere (see Chapter 12.30 and Section 9). Aluminium absorption is similar to that of iron, and it comes from water, additives, and contamination by utensils and containers. Foods such as herbs and leaves contain small quantities, but processed foods contain very little (<5 μg/g). Most adults absorb about 1–10 mg/day and can cope with this by excretion in urine. It is present in serum is in very small amounts, with levels less than 10 μg/ml. Toxicity may arise from contamination of food, the use of aluminium containing antacids and phosphate binders, or in dialysis solutions used in treatment of renal failure.

A good example of acute aluminium poisoning occurred when 20 tons of concentrated aluminium sulphate were discharged into a water reservoir. The initial toxic symptoms were gastrointestinal disturbances, skin rashes, and mouth ulcers. Long-term effects on brain, bones, and joints, such as have been reported with aluminium toxicity in dialysis, were thought to be unlikely. There has been no evidence of any of the long-term effects. Aluminium salts can cause hypersensitivity reactions, but only when given by injection or in relation to the work-place, not by oral ingestion. They may deposit in bone, and about 30–80 mg may accumulate during a lifetime, half of which will be found in bone as this is a protective mechanism, removing aluminium from circulation when the levels become elevated.

Postmortem reports on the brains exposed to chronically increased levels of aluminium in dialysis fluid have shown the effects of chronic aluminium poisoning. Aluminium enters the brain at a slow rate by an iron-uptake system (transferrin-related transport), accumulating in the cortex and hippocampus, which are selectively vulnerable to Alzheimer's disease. In some patients with prolonged exposure to high blood aluminium, β-amyloid protein is deposited in the brain as lesions which may be precursors of senile plaques, one of the major neuropathological features of Alzheimer's disease; but no neurofibrillary tangles, the other hallmark of this disease, have been found. In addition, miners exposed over years to inhalation of aluminium particles to reduce silicotic lung disease, showed a dose-related declining cognitive function, and treatment with desferroxamine, removing the aluminium, slowed the progress of this disorder.

Further reading

Yarze, F., Martin, P., Munoz, S.J., and Friedman, LS. (1992). Wilson's disease: current status. *American Journal of Medicine*, 92, 643–54.

See also references within Chapter 11.7, OTM3.

Chapter 6.11

Lipid and lipoprotein disorders

P. N. Durrington

Lipid physiology

Triglycerides (triacylglycerols)

These are formed by the esterification of glycerol with fatty acids which have a hydrocarbon group attached to a carboxyl group. Generally, the hydrocarbon part is present in a long chain. Naturally occurring fatty acids usually have even numbers of carbon atoms, most of them linked by single bonds. Those with double bonds are termed unsaturated, whereas those with only single bonds are the saturated fatty acids. Fatty acids with one double bond are termed mono-unsaturated and those with more, polyunsaturated. Each double bond creates the possibility of two stereoisomers according to whether the hydrogen atoms of the –CH=CH–; are both on the same side of the double bond (*cis-*) or on the opposite sides (*trans-*). Naturally occurring fatty acids are mostly *cis*-isomers.

Triglycerides in adipose tissue provide our principal energy store. The body of a 70 kg man of ideal body weight contains some 15 kg of stored triglycerides, representing 135 000 cal (560 000 J) of energy which would permit survival during total starvation for up to 3 months [compare this with 225 mg of glycogen, present in the same man representing only 900 cal (3800 J)]. Each gram of adipose tissue yields almost 8 cal (33 J) of energy, whereas tissues containing cells packed to capacity with glycogen would not even approach a yield of 1 cal (4.2 J) for each gram.

For other organs to utilize the energy in adipose tissue the stored triglyceride must first be hydrolysed to give its constituent glycerol and non-esterified fatty acids, a process known as lipolysis. This is accomplished by adipose tissue lipase, an intracellular enzyme, which is inhibited by insulin (see OTM3, p. 1400).

The products of lipolysis are released into the circulation. The non-esterified fatty acids become bound to albumin. Normally their circulating concentration is 300–800 mmol/l (8–23 mg/dl), but this falls when insulin is secreted following a meal and rises in starvation when insulin secretion is low. Their importance in transporting lipid energy should not be underestimated, even at low concentrations, since their half-life in the circulation is only 2–3 min and their turnover is thus 100–200 g/day, even more in starvation and in diabetes.

Non-esterified fatty acids can be oxidized to acetyl-coenzyme A (CoA) by some tissues, such as muscle and liver, and then entered into the Krebs (carboxylic acid) cycle. Other tissues, which in the fed state rely on glucose as an oxidative substrate, cannot directly utilize non-esterified fatty acids. During starvation these tissues are supplied with water-soluble ketone bodies (acetone, acetoacetate, β-hydroxybutyrate), which the liver produces by partial oxidization (β-oxidation) of non-esterified fatty acids transported to it from adipose tissue. These ketone bodies, which can readily be entered into the Krebs cycle by tissues lacking the ability to oxidize fatty acids, constitute the second system for the transport of lipid energy. They are vital for survival when dietary energy is at a premium, but are also the cause of diabetic ketoacidosis when the insulin production is insufficient to suppress the flux of non-esterified fatty acids from adipose tissue, so that the production of ketone bodies takes place at a faster rate than they can be respired. The amount of insulin required to decrease blood glucose increases in the presence of high levels of circulating non-esterified fatty acids.

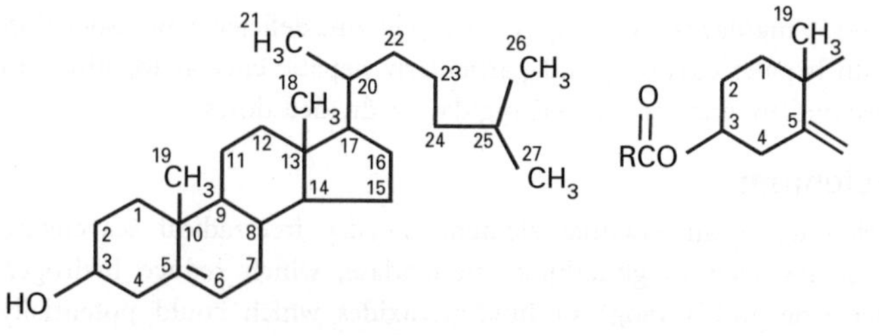

(a) Cholesterol (b) Cholesteryl ester

Fig. 1 The structure of free cholesterol and cholesteryl ester.

Phospholipids

These also have at least one fatty acyl group esterified to an alcohol and one phosphate group linked both to the alcohol and to another organic compound. The glycerolipids have glycerol as the alcohol. Examples of these are phosphatidylcholine (lecithin) and lysophosphatidylcholine (lysolecithin). Another abundant class of phospholipids are the sphingolipids, such as sphingyomyelin. Phospholipids are essential components of cell membranes.

Cholesterol

Cholesterol is also an essential component of cell membranes, where it allows the phospholipid molecules to pack more closely, increasing membrane rigidity. It is also a precursor for the synthesis of steroid hormones, vitamin D, and bile acids. It is present in arterial fatty streaks and in atheromatous plaques (see below). Cholesterol is an alcohol and may be unesterified as free cholesterol or esterified with a fatty acyl group (Fig. 1).

Lipoprotein physiology

Lipoprotein structure

The general structure of lipoprotein molecules is globular (Fig. 2). The physicochemical considerations, which govern the arrangement of their constituents, are similar to those involved in the formation of mixed micelles in the lumen of the intestine. Thus, within the outer part of the lipoprotein are found the more polar lipids, the phospholipids and free cholesterol, with their charged groups pointing out towards the water molecules. The physical role of bile salts, which are also in the outer layer in the mixed micelle, is assumed by proteins, so that the surface of a lipoprotein structurally resembles the outer

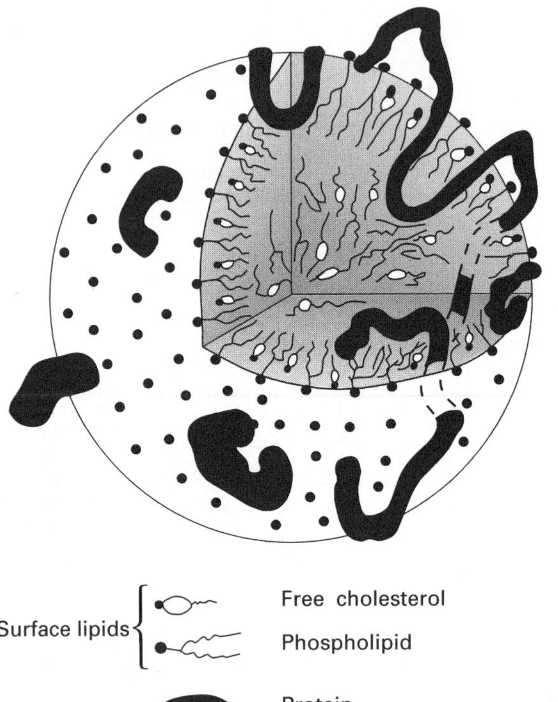

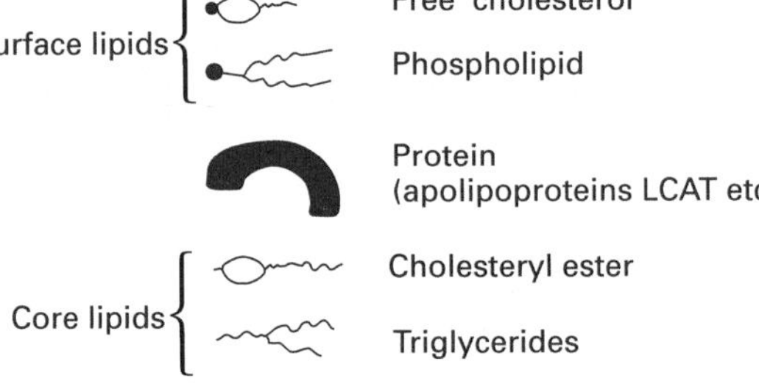

Fig. 2 Lipoprotein structure. The most hydrophobic lipids (triglycerides, cholesteryl esters) form a central droplet-like core, which is surrounded by more polar lipids (phospholipids, free cholesterol) at the water interface. Apolipoproteins are anchored by their more hydrophobic regions, with their more polar regions often exposed to the surface.
(Reproduced from Durrington 1995, with permission.)

half of a cell membrane. Within the core of the lipoprotein particle are the more hydrophobic lipids, the esterified cholesterol and triglycerides. These form a central droplet, to which are anchored, by their hydrophobic regions, the surface-coating molecules, phospholipids, free cholesterol, and proteins. The exception to this general structure is newly formed high-density lipoprotein (**HDL**), which lacks the central lipid droplet and appears to exist as a disc-like bilayer, consisting largely of phospholipids and proteins.

The protein components of lipoproteins are the apolipoproteins some of which have a largely structural role and others are major metabolic regulators. Enzymes are also found as components of lipoproteins. The leading example is lecithin:cholesterol acyltransferase located on the HDLs, which are also its site of action.

Lipid transport from liver and gut to peripheral tissues

The products of fat digestion (fatty acids, monoglycerides, lysolecithin, and free cholesterol) enter the enterocytes from the mixed micelles. They are re-esterified in the smooth endoplasmic reticulum. There, long-chain fatty acids (>14C) are esterified with monoglycerides to form triglycerides and with lysolecithin to form lecithin. Free cholesterol is esterified by acyl-CoA:cholesterol *O*-acyltransferase.

The triglycerides, phospholipids, and cholesteryl esters are then combined with an apolipoprotein, known as apo B_{48}, in the enterocyte. The lipoproteins thus formed are secreted into the lymph (chyle) and are termed chylomicrons. They are large (diameter >75 nm; density <950 g/l) and are rich in triglycerides, but contain only relatively small amounts of protein. They travel through the lacteals to join lymph from other parts of the body and enter the circulation via the thoracic duct. In addition to cholesterol absorbed from the diet, the chylomicrons may also receive cholesterol that has been newly synthesized in the gut or transferred from other lipoproteins present in the lymph and plasma. The newly secreted, or nascent, chylomicrons receive C apolipoproteins from HDL, which in that respect appears to act as a circulating reservoir, since later in the course of the metabolism of the chylomicron, the C apolipoproteins are transferred back to the HDL pool. The chylomicrons also receive apolipoprotein E (apo E), although the manner in which they do so is unclear. Unlike other apolipoproteins, which are synthesized either in the liver or the gut, or both, apo E is synthesized (and perhaps secreted) by a large number of tissues: liver, brain, spleen, kidney, lungs, and adrenal gland.

Once the chylomicron has acquired apo CII, it is capable of activating lipoprotein lipase (Fig. 3(a)). This enzyme is located on the vascular endothelium of tissues with a high requirement for triglycerides, such as skeletal and cardiac muscle (for energy), adipose tissue (for storage), and lactating mammary gland (for milk). Lipoprotein lipase releases triglycerides from the core of the chylomicron by hydrolysing them to fatty acids and glycerol, which are taken up by the tissues locally. In this way the circulating chylomicron becomes progressively smaller. Its triglyceride content decreases and it becomes relatively richer in cholesterol and protein. As the core shrinks, its surface materials (phospholipids, free cholesterol, C apolipoproteins) become too crowded and they are transferred to HDL. The cholesteryl ester-enriched, triglyceride-depleted product of chylomicron metabolism is known as the chylomicron remnant. The apo B_{48}, present from the time of assembly, remains tightly anchored to the core throughout. The apo E also remains and regions of its structure are exposed, permitting chylomicron remnant catabolism via the 'remnant receptor' of the liver and the low-density lipoprotein (**LDL**) receptors (also called apo B_{100}/E receptors), which can be expressed by virtually every cell in the body, including the liver. It is possible that apo E is inhibited from binding to its receptors earlier in the metabolism of chylomicrons, because its receptor-binding domain is blocked by apo CIII. Remnants are largely removed from the circulation by the liver. Although the clearance of these particles via the LDL receptor is theoretically possible, this route is not likely to contribute greatly to remnant uptake in the adult.

The liver itself secretes triglyceride-rich very low-density lipoprotein (**VLDL**). Teleologically, this allows the supply of triglycerides to tissues in the fasting state as well as postprandially. VLDL particles are somewhat smaller than the chylomicrons (diameter 30–45 nm; density <1006 g/l). Once secreted they undergo exactly the same sequence of changes as chylomicrons with the exception that in humans the liver, unlike the gut, does not esterify cholesterol before its secretion, most of which is secreted in the VLDL as free cholesterol. It undergoes esterification in the circulation. Free cholesterol is transferred to HDL along a concentration gradient. There it is esterified by the action of lecithin:cholesterol acyl transferase, changing the hydroxyl group in the 3-position of cholesterol to a fatty acyl group. This it selectively removes from the 2-position of lecithin to give lysolecithin. The fatty acyl group in this position is generally unsaturated and the cholesteryl

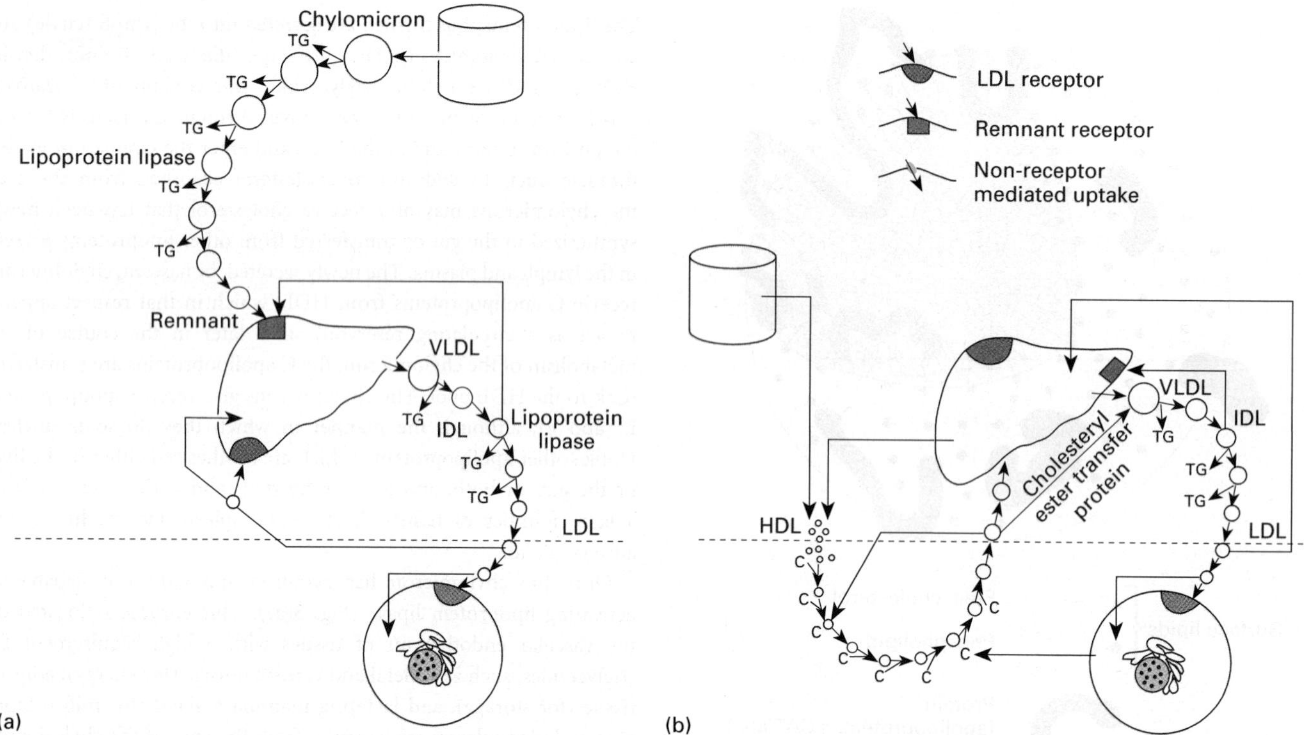

Fig. 3 Metabolism of (a) triglyceride-rich lipoproteins secreted by the gut and liver; and (b) hepatic triglyceride-rich lipoproteins and lipoproteins transporting cholesterol to and from the tissues.

esters thus formed are frequently cholesteryl oleate or cholesteryl linoleate. Familial deficiency of lecithin:cholesterol acyltransferase is a rare disorder, in which HDL fails to mature, and circulating free cholesterol levels increase. It leads to anaemia, corneal opacities, proteinuria, and renal failure.

Esterified cholesterol on HDL is transferred back to VLDL. Cholesteryl ester transfer protein in plasma transports cholesteryl ester from HDL to VLDL, in exchange for triglycerides in VLDL. This contributes to the removal of core triglycerides from VLDL, although the major mechanism for the removal of triglycerides from VLDL is lipolysis catalysed by lipoprotein lipase.

Another major difference between VLDL and chylomicrons is that the apolipoprotein B produced by the liver in humans is not apo B_{48}, but almost entirely apo B_{100}. As in the case of chylomicrons, the quantum of apo B packaged in the VLDL remains tightly associated with the particle until its final catabolism and its amount does not vary after secretion. It is probable that each molecule of VLDL contains one molecule of apo B_{100}. The apo B_{100} produced in the liver contains the protein sequence necessary to bind to the LDL receptors, whereas that produced by the gut, although derived from the same gene, does not.

The circulating VLDL particles become progressively smaller as their core is removed by lipolysis and surface materials are transferred to HDL. In normal humans most of the VLDL is converted to smaller LDL particles through the intermediary of intermediate density lipoprotein (IDL). This has a density of 1006–1019 g/l and possesses apo E. In this latter respect it is similar to chylomicron remnants. Hepatic lipase may be important in the conversion of IDL to LDL.

LDL particles, which are relatively enriched in cholesterol, but are small enough (diameter 18–25 nm; density 1019–1063 g/l) to cross the vascular endothelium, serve to deliver cholesterol to the tissues. Their concentration in the extracellular fluid is probably about 10 per cent of that in the plasma. Cells require cholesterol for membrane repair and growth and as a precursor for steroid hormone and vitamin D synthesis.

LDL is able to enter cells by two routes making a major contribution to its catabolism: one which is regulated according to the cholesterol requirement of each individual cell, and one which appears to depend almost entirely on the extracellular concentrations of LDL. The first of these two routes is by the cell-surface LDL receptor, which specifically binds lipoproteins that contain apolipoprotein B_{100} or E. This receptor, although capable of binding apo E-containing lipoproteins, in practice usually binds largely to the apo B_{100}-containing lipoproteins of which LDL is the most widely distributed. After binding, the LDL-receptor complex is internalized within the cell, where it undergoes lysosomal degradation. Its apo B is hydrolysed to its constituent amino acids, and its cholesteryl ester is hydrolysed to free cholesterol. The release of this free cholesterol is the signal by which the cellular cholesterol content is regulated precisely by three co-ordinated reactions. First the enzyme, which is rate-limiting for cholesterol biosysthesis (3-hydroxy, 3- methyl-glutaryl CoA reductase), is repressed, thus effectively centralizing cholesteryl biosynthesis to organs such as the liver and gut. Secondly, the synthesis of the LDL receptor itself is suppressed. Thirdly, acyl-CoA:cholesterol *O*-acyltransferase is activated so that any cholesterol that is surplus to immediate requirements can be converted to cholesteryl ester, which, because of its hydrophobic nature, forms into droplets within the cytoplasm and is thus conveniently stored. The effect of the lysosomal release of free cholesterol on the expression of the LDL receptor contrasts with its effect on the hepatic remnant receptor, which is not subject to any similar down-regulatory process. Free cholesterol released by lysosomal digestion of cholesteryl ester-rich, apo E-containing lipoproteins entering the hepatocyte via the remnant receptor does not influence its own expression; it will, nevertheless, down-regulate the hepatic LDL receptors. Defective LDL uptake by the LDL receptor is the basis of familial hypercholesterolaemia (see below).

The other important mechanism by which LDL cholesterol may enter cells is by a non-receptor-mediated pathway: LDL binds to cell membranes at sites other than those where the LDL receptors are located and some of it passes through the membrane by pinocytosis. HDL is able to compete with LDL for this type of cell membrane association. The absence of a receptor means that the 'binding' is of low affinity and thus, at low concentrations, LDL entry by this route may have little significance. However, unlike receptor-mediated entry, non-receptor-mediated LDL uptake, is not saturable, but continues to increase with increasing extracellular LDL concentrations. When LDL levels are relatively high, entry of cholesterol into the cells by this route may thus assume greater quantitative importance than that via the LDL receptor, which will be both saturated and down-regulated. This appears to be the situation in the typical adult consuming a high fat diet, whose LDL cholesterol is high. Only about one-third of LDL is then catabolized by receptors and two-thirds by non-receptor-mediated pathways. In hypercholesterolaemia, even more is catabolized via the non-receptor pathway (four-fifths in patients heterozygous for familial hypercholesterolaemia, virtually all in homozygotes, see below).

LDL may also be removed from the circulation by a number of receptors other than the classical LDL receptor. Probably these are responsible for the catabolism of only relatively minor amounts of LDL, but two such receptors present on the macrophage have excited considerable interest, because they may lie at the heart of atherogenesis. They are the beta-VLDL receptor, a modified LDL receptor, which allows the uptake of the beta-VLDL from patients with type III hyperlipoproteinaemia (see below), and the acetyl-LDL receptor, which permits the uptake of modified LDL by macrophages. Uptake at both these receptors is so rapid *in vitro* that foam cells resembling those in arterial fatty streaks are formed. On the other hand, uptake of unmodified LDL by the macrophage via the LDL receptor is too slow for foam cell formation. Modifications, which permit LDL uptake at the acetyl-LDL receptor include acetylation (hence its name) but also oxidation, which may occur *in vivo* and is of potential relevance to atherogenesis (see below). A third class of receptors present on the macrophage, the oxidized LDL receptors, have also recently been described.

Lipoprotein (a)

The precise location of lipoprotein (a) [Lp(a)] in LDL and HDL_2 varies from individual to individual, as does its serum concentration. It may be undetectable in some people or present at concentrations equalling those of LDL in others. The protein moiety of Lp(a) like that of LDL contains apo B_{100}, but, in addition, apolipoprotein (a) [apo(a)]. This is a huge homologue of plasminogen, in which part of the plasminogen protein sequence (the kringle 4 domain) is repeated many times. The number of these repeats, which is determined at a genetic locus adjacent to the plasminogen gene, determines the molecular mass of apo(a), and individuals expressing polymorphisms with fewer kringle 4 repeats have the highest serum concentrations of Lp(a). Lp(a) is associated with the risk of coronary heart disease (**CHD**) in people of European origin, particularly when serum cholesterol levels are also raised and when there is a family history of premature CHD if concentration is also greatly increased in renal disease. It does not possess fibrinolytic activity, but it has been suggested that it may interfere with thrombolysis. Because Lp(a) binds to a wide variety of cells and connective tissue matrices, it is retained in the arterial wall longer than LDL and is thus more likely to undergo oxidative modification and macrophage uptake, leading to atheroma (see below).

Transport of cholesterol from tissues back to liver

Cholesterol is transported out of the gut and liver in quantities which greatly exceed its peripheral catabolism. Therefore, except when the requirement for membrane synthesis is high, for example during growth or active tissue repair, the greater part of the cholesterol transported to the tissues must be returned to the liver for elimination in the bile, or for reassembly into lipoproteins. The return of cholesterol from the tissues to the liver is termed 'reverse cholesterol transport'. It is less well understood than the pathways by which cholesterol reaches the tissues, but it may well be critical to the development of atheroma. HDL is very likely to be intimately involved in this.

The precursors of plasma HDL (nascent HDL) are probably disc-shaped bilayers composed largely of protein and phospholipid secreted mainly by the gut and liver (Fig. 3(b)). These are converted to the spherical, mature form of HDL by the action of lecithin:cholesterol acyltransferase. HDL components are also derived from surplus material (phospholipids, free cholesterol, and apoproteins) of triglyceride-rich lipoproteins released during lipolysis. Apolipoproteins AI and AII, which are the major apolipoproteins of HDL, and apolipoprotein E have been identified in nascent HDL. Other apolipoproteins and the bulk of its lipid are acquired as it circulates through the vascular and other extracellular fluids.

HDL is a small particle compared with the other lipoproteins (diameter 5–12 nm; density 1063–1210 g/l) and easily crosses the vascular endothelium, so that its concentration in the tissue fluids is much closer to its intravascular concentration than is the case for LDL. Because the serum HDL cholesterol concentration is only about one-quarter that of the LDL, it is often wrongly assumed that its particle concentration is lower. In fact, the particle concentrations of HDL and LDL in human plasma are often similar, and in the tissue fluids there are several times as many HDL molecules as those of other lipoproteins unless the capillary endothelium is fenestrated. Generally, therefore, cells are in contact with higher concentrations of HDL molecules than of any other lipoprotein.

Cells may express receptors for HDL, particularly HDL_3, which might permit the transfer of cholesterol out of the cell. Passage across the cell membrane may not simply depend on such receptors, however, as free cholesterol can cross by diffusion. Factors regulating the balance between intracellular cholesterol esterification and free cholesterol (activities of acyl-CoA:cholesterol *O* acyltransferase and cholesterol esterase) may also be important. Apo E synthesized within certain cells may be instrumental in transporting cholesterol out on to HDL.

Once outside the cell, free cholesterol must be re-esterified to be transported in any quantity in the core of lipoproteins. Therefore, cholesterol must at some stage on its return journey to the liver reside on HDL, the site of lecithin:cholesterol acyltransferase activity. However, once cholesterol has been esterified and packed into the core of HDL, simple clearance of the whole lipoprotein particle by the liver is not the route by which most cholesterol is returned to it. This is because LDL equivalent to 1500 mg of cholesterol is produced each day, whereas the rate of catabolism of the HDL apolipoproteins AI and AII would permit less than 200 mg of HDL cholesterol to be returned each day. Therefore: (a) the liver must be capable of selectively removing cholesterol from HDL and then returning the particle to the circulation with most of its apolipoproteins intact, or (b) the cholesterol in HDL must be transferred to another lipoprotein class which is capable of being cleared in quantity by the liver, or (c) a class of HDL, which contains little apo AI or AII, must be cleared by the liver at a much greater rate than the bulk of HDL (see OTM3, p. 1404).

HDL is not a single homogeneous species; it is known to be a mixture of particles differing in size, in lipid and apolipoprotein composition, and in function. Two peaks are seen in the analytical ultracentrifuge, the less dense HDL_2 and the more dense, HDL_3. HDL_3 may be converted to HDL_2 by the acquisition of cholesterol, HDL_3 thus being a precursor of HDL_2. Whereas antisera to apo AI precipitate virtually all of HDL, antisera to AII do not, suggesting that some molecules of HDL contain AI and AII, whereas others contain AI only. The AI-only HDL molecules, which predominate in HDL_2, may arise from different metabolic channels than do the AI/AII particles. Apo E-containing HDL may also have a different metabolic fate. Furthermore, HDL may contain other molecular species with overlapping density ranges, such as Lp(a).

Disorders produced by raised levels of lipoproteins

Within populations there is an exponential relationship between serum cholesterol and the incidence of CHD. This depends on the LDL cholesterol which comprises some 70–80 per cent total cholesterol in men and a little less in women. The greater part of the rest of the cholesterol in serum is on HDL, and the concentration of this HDL cholesterol is inversely related to the likelihood of developing CHD. The pathogenesis of atherosclerosis is discussed in Chapter 2.7.

Normal serum lipid concentrations

In Britain the median serum cholesterol for a middle-aged man is 6.1 mmol/l and deaths from CHD comprise about 40 per cent of total mortality at this age. In China the average for men of middle age is 2 mmol/l less, and CHD accounts for less than 5 per cent of their deaths.

Conventionally, the normal range for a variable in a particular population is chosen to include values between the 2.5 and 97.5 percentiles, or sometimes the 1 and 99 percentile, on the assumption that 19 of 20 of the population, or 49 of 50, respectively, are normal. The implication in a medical context must also be that those people in the normal range are healthy. In the case of cholesterol, the healthy range must therefore be that of a society in which CHD is uncommon. Thus an optimal serum cholesterol is 5.0 mmol/l (approximately 200 mg/dl) or less. A level of 6.3 mmol/l (250 mg/dl) (at the 75th percentile in the United States) is considered to indicate 'moderate risk' and 6.7 mmol/l (270 mg/dl), which is the 90th percentile in the United States, 'high risk'. Some caution is required in using this concept. The risk of fatal CHD in an American middle-aged male population whose serum cholesterol is 5 mmol/l (200 mg/dl) over the next 6 years is about 6 in 1000. At 6 mmol/l (250 mg/dl) it is about doubled, but that is only 10 in 1000, and at 7 mmol/l (270 mg/dl) it is still less than 15 in 1000. Thus, although these levels may be of great importance for public health initiatives aimed at reducing the cholesterol level in societies in which the risk of CHD is high, the clinician must be wary about overtreating men with cholesterol at these levels, if it is their only risk factor for CHD, but the risk conferred by a particular level of cholesterol increases considerably when it is combined with another risk factor.

An upper limit of normality for fasting serum triglycerides is often regarded as 2.2 mmol/l (200 mg/dl). This is close to the 90th percentile for men and the 95th percentile for women. For serum HDL cholesterol a lower limit of normality of 0.9 mmol/l (35 mg/dl) is frequently quoted, which is close to the 10th percentile for men and between the 5th and the 10th percentile for women.

Table 1 The Fredrickson/WHO classification of hyperlipoproteinaemia

Type	Lipoprotein increased	Lipids increased
I	Chylomicrons	Triglycerides
IIa	LDL	Cholesterol
IIb	LDL and VLDL	Cholesterol and triglycerides
III	beta-VLDL (=IDL + chylomicron remnants)	Cholesterol and triglycerides
IV	VLDL	Triglycerides
V	Chylomicrons and VLDL	Cholesterol and triglycerides

The Fredrickson/WHO classification

The hyperlipoproteinaemias can be classified according to which of chylomicrons, VLDL, LDL, or beta-VLDL are in excess (Table 1). The Fredrickson/WHO classification causes great confusion, largely because it is difficult to remember and is frequently wrongly regarded as a diagnostic classification when it is simply a way of reporting which of the serum lipoproteins are elevated. It is usually sufficient to remember that when cholesterol alone is elevated there is a type IIa hyperlipoproteinaemia. When both cholesterol and triglycerides are elevated the hyperlipoproteinaemia is generally type IIb, but occasionally it is type V (the serum will look milky if it is) and rarely type III. Type I is extraordinarily rare. An isolated increase in fasting serum triglycerides almost invariably signifies type IV hyperlipoproteinaemia.

All hospital laboratories, in addition to measuring cholesterol and triglyceride levels, should also measure HDL cholesterol in patients in whom treatment of hyperlipoproteinaemia with drugs is under consideration. Particularly in women, an elevated level of cholesterol may result from a relative excess of high HDL cholesterol and thus not signify any increased risk of CHD. High serum HDL cholesterol is associated with longevity, so it cannot be regarded as hyperlipoproteinaemia in the pathological sense. Low HDL cholesterol is associated with an increased cardiovascular risk, particularly if total serum cholesterol and triglycerides are also elevated.

Primary hyperlipoproteinaemias

Primary hyperlipoproteinaemias in which there is hypercholesterolaemia (type IIa)

Serum cholesterol levels exceeding 6.5 mmol/l are common in adults in Britain and much of Europe, the United States, Australia, and New Zealand. In Britain, for example, 25–30 per cent of middle-aged people have levels exceeding this, and the proportion in the United States is at least 10 per cent. Most of this hypercholesterolaemia does not represent the effect of any single cause, but is due to some combination of diet, obesity, and individual susceptibility. The latter is partly genetic, probably involving more than one gene (polygenic hypercholesterolaemia). At the very top end of the cholesterol distribution are to be found individuals who have the less common monogenic condition, familial hypercholesterolaemia.

Familial hypercholesterolaemia

Heterozygous familial hypercholesterolaemia

Familial hypercholesterolaemia is dominantly inherited. The heterozygous form of the condition affects about 1 in 500 people in Britain and the United States. In some populations, such as the Lebanese Christians, the Afrikaner and Cape-coloured peoples of South Africa, and French Canadians, it is considerably more common. In yet other populations, such as Africans who have not intermingled with Europeans it is rare.

Typically, the serum cholesterol in adult heterozygotes is 9–11 mmol/l (350–450 mg/dl). The lipoprotein phenotype is usually IIa, but occasionally there is a moderate increase in fasting serum triglycerides to produce a IIb pattern. There is a tendency for HDL cholesterol to be at the lower end of the range, particularly if triglycerides are elevated.

The clinical hallmark of familial hypercholesterolaemia is the presence of tendon xanthomas (Plate 1). These appear in heterozygotes from the age of 20 onwards. The most common sites are in the tendons overlying the knuckles and in the Achilles tendons. They may also be found in the extensor hallucis longus and triceps tendons, and occasionally others. It is also common to find subperiosteal xanthomas on the upper tibia where the patellar tendon inserts. The skin overlying tendon xanthomas is of normal colour and they do not appear yellow. The cholesteryl ester deposits are deep within the tendons, but feel hard because they are fibrotic. It is not uncommon for those in the Achilles tendons to become inflamed from time to time. More generalized tendinitis may follow rapid therapeutic reduction in serum cholesterol levels. Tendon xanthomas occur in only two disorders apart from familial hypercholesterolaemia and these are so rare as not to pose any diagnostic difficulty. They are cerebrotendinous xanthomatosis, in which plasma cholestanol is elevated and deposited in tendons, and phytosterolaemia (beta sitosterolaemia), in which there is abnormal intestinal absorption of plant sterols, which are then deposited in tendons (see Chapter 6.8).

Corneal arcus is also frequent in familial hypercholesterolaemia but it is not uncommon to encounter patients with familial hypercholesterolaemia who have florid tendon xanthomas, but no arcus. Xanthelasmata palpebrarum, although occurring with greater frequency and at a younger age in familial hypercholesterolaemia, affect only a minority of heterozygotes. Xanthelasmata are not specific for any particular type of hypercholesterolaemia and occur in polygenic hypercholesterolaemia, pregnancy, primary bilary cirrhosis, and hypothyroidism. They are also common in middle-aged women, often overweight, with no very marked increase in serum cholesterol, if any. They may run in families apparently independently of hypercholesterolaemia.

Identifying familial hypercholesterolaemic heterozygotes as early as possible is important, because of their risk of CHD. Untreated, over half of affected men die before the age of 60. It is not uncommon for men to have their first myocardial infarction or develop angina in their thirties and occasionally even earlier. Some 15 per cent of women with familial hypercholesterolaemia die of CHD before the age of 60 years and the majority have symptomatic coronary disease by that age. Perhaps as many as 10 per cent of women have some evidence of cardiac ischaemia before their menopause. However, whereas it is exceptional for a man with familial hypercholesterolaemia to live to 70 without symptomatic CHD, almost a quarter of women do so. This accounts in large part for the reason why a family history of premature CHD is absent in as many as one-quarter of patients discovered to have familial hypercholesterolaemia on screening, or in men who are discovered to have familial hypercholesterolaemia when they present with a heart attack in early life: the condition has been inherited from their mother, who has herself not yet developed coronary symptoms.

Those families which develop CHD particularly early tend to have low serum HDL cholesterol and increased fasting triglycerides. Serum Lp(a) is increased in familial hypercholesterolaemia and any familial tendency to run a high level of Lp(a) is exacerbated in those members who also have familial hypercholesterolaemia. The apo E_4 genotype (see below) is also associated with more aggressive atheroma in familial hypercholesterolaemia.

There is an increased risk of atheroma in other parts of the arterial tree in heterozygous familial hypercholesterolaemia, but this is strikingly less than in the coronary arteries. Some heterozygotes have aortic systolic cardiac murmurs due to deposits of atheroma in the aortic root, sometimes involving the aortic cusps.

Homozygous familial hypercholesterolaemia

Most cases of homozygous familial hypercholesterolaemia occur in societies in which consanguineous marriages and heterozygous familial hypercholesterolaemia are frequent. The chance of marriage between unrelated heterozygotes in countries such as the United Kingdom or United States is 1 in 500^2, and each of their children would stand a 1 in 4 chance of being homozygotes. Assuming no adverse effect on the survival of the conceptus, an incidence of homozygous familial hypercholesterolaemia of 1 in 10^6 births would be predicted. It is thus a rare condition in these countries.

Clinically the homozygous disease is characterized by the development of cutaneous xanthomas in childhood. These may be present in the first year of life or may not develop until late childhood. They are typically orange–yellow, subcutaneous, planar xanthomas, occurring on the buttocks, antecubital fossae, and the hands, frequently in the webs between the fingers. Tuberose subcutaneous xanthomas on the knees, elbows, and knuckles are also a feature. Serum cholesterol is typically greater than 15 mmol/l (600 mg/dl). Myocardial infarction and angina frequently occur in childhood, sometimes even in infancy. Atheromatous deposits at the aortic root, invariably present by puberty, are so marked as to produce significant aortic stenosis, which contributes to the risk of sudden death. Death before the age of 30, and often considerably younger, was the rule before the advent of plasmapheresis and similar techniques for the extracorporeal removal of LDL (see below).

Polyarthritis, predominantly affecting the ankles, knees, wrists, and proximal interphalangeal joints, is common.

The metabolic defect in familial hypercholesterolaemia

Normally the plasma half-life of LDL is 2.5–3 days, whereas in familial hypercholesterolaemia heterozygotes it is 4.5–5 days, and even longer in homozygotes. Heterozygotes express only about half the LDL receptors of a normal person. Homozygotes have between none and 25 per cent of normal receptor activity. The mutations in the LDL receptor gene (chromosome 19) produce either receptors with no binding activity (receptor negative; the receptor is not synthesized, is not transported to the cell surface, or cannot be internalized after binding to LDL) or because, although the mutation allows some LDL to be bound and to enter the cell, this occurs only slowly because the binding site is abnormal (receptor defective). Some 200 mutations have been described and undoubtedly more exist. Three mutations account for 90 per cent of familial hypercholesterolaemia in Afrikaners. In Britain and the United States, however, the most frequent of these mutations is likely to occur in no more than 3–4 per cent of patients. This means that the prospect of developing a DNA test for this condition in most countries is unrealistic. It also means that only in populations with a small number of mutations, or where intermarriage is common, are clinical homozygotes truly homozygous in the sense that both their LDL gene mutations are identical. Most will be mixed heterozygotes. Some of the heterogeneity of the severity of the syndrome relates to the nature of the two LDL mutations present. The worst prognosis is associated with inheritance of two receptor-negative mutations, and the best is with two receptor-defective mutations. The type of receptor mutation in heterozygotes is also probably of some importance, but here it is blurred against a background of other acquired or genetic factors, which can find expression over a much longer time than in homozygotes.

A small proportion (3 per cent) of patients, who clinically have the same features as heterozygotes, do not have an LDL receptor defect, but a mutation of apolipoprotein B in which glutamine is substituted for arginine at amino acid residue 3500, which is part of the LDL receptor binding domain. This disorder has been termed familial defective apo B_{100}. It probably has a frequency of 1 in 500 to 600 in Britain and the United States, but only the minority of affected individuals have tendon xanthomas and typically the serum cholesterol associated with it is about 8.0 mmol/l (310 mg/dl), which is less than in most heterozygotes for familial hypercholesterolaemia.

Common or polygenic hypercholesterolaemia

There is overlap between the range of LDL cholesterol levels encountered in familial hypercholesterolaemia and those due to the commoner, polygenic hypercholesterolaemia, but it is probable that the risk at a given level in familial hypercholesterolaemia is greater than in the polygenic form. This may be because in the familial condition the hypercholesterolaemia has been present since birth, whereas the polygenic form is frequently not fully developed until the third or fourth decade. Furthermore the familial type is associated with increased serum concentrations of Lp(a).

Estimates of how much different levels of cholesterol contribute to the overall cumulative male mortality from CHD by the age of 60 years are given in Table 2. The majority of such premature deaths come from the middle part of the cholesterol distribution, and therefore it has been argued that if a significant reduction in the incidence of CHD is to be achieved efforts to lower cholesterol cannot simply be confined to those individuals whose plasma cholesterols lie at the upper end of the distribution. Nevertheless because the number of people in the middle range is so huge (the vast majority of whom are not at increased risk of premature CHD), a different strategy must be applied to reducing their cholesterol from that applied to those in the upper part of the cholesterol distribution. This is the 'low-risk' or 'population' strategy, which aims to lower serum cholesterol by public health measures. Some patients from the middle range of cholesterol are, however, at much greater individual risk because they have other risk factors for CHD. The most potent of these is that the individual already has CHD. In middle-aged myocardial infarction survivors, serum cholesterol is an important indicator of cardiac prognosis (Fig. 4(a)). Lipoproteins are also the most important risk factors for occlusion of coronary artery bypass grafts after the initial postoperative period. Factors such as cigarette smoking, hypertension, and diabetes also increase the risk any level of cholesterol. A family history of CHD at an early age in a first-degree relative also increases the likelihood of CHD, and part of this effect is independent of other risk factors. The combination of all these factors with a relatively modestly increased serum cholesterol level can increase individual risk to a level where clinical intervention is as justified as it is with more marked elevations in serum cholesterol.

Table 2 Estimates of the proportion of men in the United Kingdom dying before the age of 60 years from coronary heart disease (CHD) according to their serum cholesterol and whether they have the familial hypercholesterolaemia (FH) clinical syndrome

Serum cholesterol (mmol/l)	Risk of death before the age of 60 (per 1000)	Percentage of UK male population with these cholesterol levels	Percentage of UK male population dying before the age of 60 from CHD with these cholesterol levels
<5	25	10	0.25
5–6	30	35	1.05
6–7	43	40	1.72
7–8	55	10	0.55
8–9	74	4	0.30
>9	130	1	0.13
Heterozygous FH	500	0.2	0.1
Total			4.1

Death up to 60 in men is chosen because of limited data about cholesterol in older age groups and in women and about morbidity. The combined CHD death and non-fatal symptomatic CHD rate is probably two to three times that of CHD death.

Metabolic defect in polygenic hypercholesterolaemia

There is generally overproduction of VLDL by the liver. If this is rapidly converted to LDL there is no increase in serum triglyceride levels. The LDL receptor mechanism is probably overloaded in many individuals and in any case appears to catabolize only about one-third of LDL, so that the build-up of cholesterol in most patients is not due to any defect in the LDL receptor, but the inability of non-receptor-mediated catabolism to cope. Obesity and a high fat diet (particularly saturated fat) are probably the major reasons for the enormous differences in the prevalence of polygenic hypercholesterolaemia in different parts of the world. Undoubtedly, however, individual responses to diet vary tremendously and there is probably a complex interplay between dietetic and genetic factors. The rise in cholesterol with age, which occurs in both men and women until the climacteric, seems less evident in societies where the cholesterol level is, for dietetic reasons, lower. There is an impression that dietary modification aimed at lowering cholesterol in middle age in societies where serum cholesterol is high does not

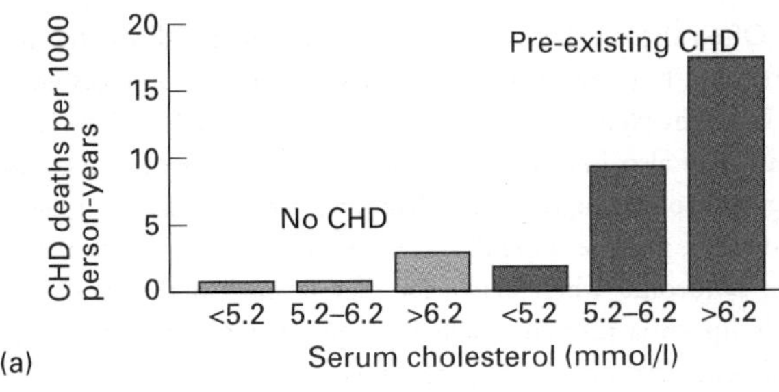

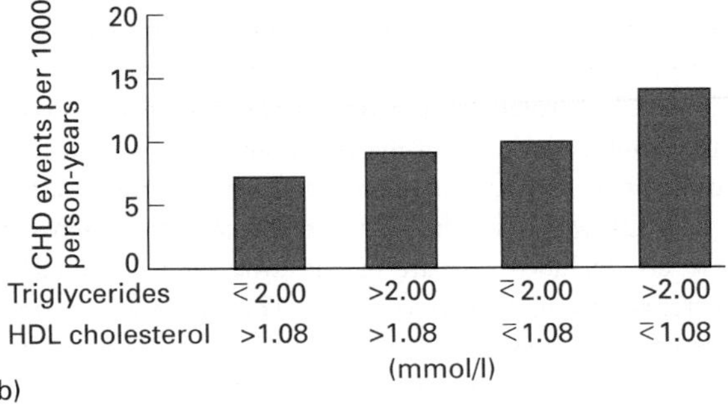

Fig. 4 (a) The risk of subsequent fatal myocardial infarction in survivors of myocardial infarction according to their serum cholesterol concentration (data from Pekkanan *et al.* 1990, see OTM3, p. 1415). (b) The likelihood of developing CHD in patients with moderately raised serum cholesterol concentrations (on average 6.9 mmol/l) is increased when serum triglyceride levels are also raised and HDL cholesterol concentrations decreased *(data from Manninen et al. 1989, see OTM3, p.1415).*

reduce it to the extent that might be anticipated from populations habitually consuming such a diet. Whether this is simply a matter of non-compliance or represents some permanent change in metabolism caused by a high fat diet in early life is at present uncertain.

Primary hyperlipoproteinaemias in which there is hypercholesterolaemia combined with hypertriglyceridaemia

Type III hyperlipoproteinaemia

Type III hyperlipoproteinaemia has several synonyms: broad beta disease, floating beta disease, dysbetalipoproteinaemia, and remnant removal disease. It is rare, probably occurring in fewer than 1 in 5000 people. It is due to the presence in the circulation of increased amounts of chylomicron remnants and IDL, often collectively termed beta-VLDL. This is the result of decreased clearance of these lipoproteins at the hepatic remnant (or apo E) receptor. There is an increase in both the serum cholesterol and fasting triglyceride concentrations. Typical levels are 7–12 mmol/l (270–470 mg/dl) for cholesterol and 5–20 mmol/l (450–1800 mg/dl) for triglycerides. Often the molar concentrations of cholesterol and triglycerides are similar, and this may be a clue that a patient has type III. Occasionally the condition is associated with marked hypertriglyceridaemia due to overwhelming chylomicronaemia.

Xanthomas are present in more than half of the patients. Characteristic are striate palmar xanthomas and tuberoeruptive xanthomas (Plate 2). Striate palmar xanthomas may simply be an orange–yellow discoloration within the creases of the skin of the palms of the hands. They may be more florid and appear as raised, seed-like lesions (sometimes even larger) in the skin creases of the palms, fingers, and flexor surfaces of the wrists. Tuberoeruptive xanthomas are raised yellow lesions, usually on the elbows and knees. They may be nodular or cauliflower-like, often surrounded by smaller satellites. Sometimes they may be found over other tuberosities, such as the heels and dorsum of the interphalangeal joints of the fingers. They resolve entirely with successful treatment.

Type III hyperlipoproteinaemia is rare in women before the menopause, perhaps because hepatic remnant particle uptake is enhanced by oestrogen, but may occur in men by early adulthood. It is generally an autosomal recessive condition with variable penetrance. In all cases there appears to be a mutation or polymorphism of the apo E gene, which impairs the receptor binding of apo E. The commonest is a polymorphism, called apo E_2, in which cysteine is substituted for arginine at position 158 of the amino acid sequence. At least 90 per cent of patients are homozygous for E_2. More often than not, however, apolipoprotein E_2 homozygosity, which is present in around 1 per cent of the population, does not itself impose such a severe strain on lipoprotein metabolism that hyperlipoproteinaemia develops: its combination with some other disorder, leading to overproduction of VLDL or some additional catabolic defect, is required. This explains the association with diabetes and hypothyroidism. More often the additional stimulus to hyperlipoproteinaemia is obesity or the co-inheritance of a polygenic tendency to hypertriglyceridaemia. Rarer mutations of apo E have been described; more severe is a mutation leading to apo E deficiency, which in homozygotes does not require other factors for the expression of the phenotype. Heterozygous apo E deficiency finds little clinical expression, but, interestingly, mutations directly involving the receptor-binding domain of apo E (amino acids 124–150) produce the phenotype even in heterozygotes (dominant expression), implying that such mutations are a greater handicap to receptor clearance than mutations in which one gene is not producing apo E.

Type III undoubtedly causes accelerated atherosclerosis in the coronary, femoral, and tibial arteries. Intermittent claudication occurs at least as frequently as CHD and the incidence of the latter is about the same as that in familial hypercholesterolaemia.

In the presence of typical xanthomas, the diagnosis is not difficult. When these are absent the diagnosis must be made in the laboratory. Type IIb or V hyperlipoproteinaemia can give similar serum lipid levels. Polyacrylamide isoelectric focusing can identify apo E_2 homozygosity and this, in the presence of hyperlipidaemia, makes type III virtually certain. Rarely, the apo E mutation does not affect the electrical charge of apo E, or affects only one gene so that apo E_2 homozygosity is not found. The only way then to confirm the diagnosis is to send plasma to a centre that can provide ultracentrifugation to identify the cholesterol-rich VLDL (beta-VLDL) typical of type III. It is also important in these circumstances to exclude paraproteinaemia, which can produce both hyper- and hypolipoproteinaemia and can mimic type III.

Type IIb hyperlipoproteinaemia

The common lipoprotein phenotype associated with a combined increase in serum cholesterol and triglycerides is IIb. In the majority of people with this, in whom it is primary, the cause is probably a polygenic tendency exacerbated by acquired nutritional factors, such as obesity. A few patients will have tendon xanthomas, indicating familial hypercholesterolaemia (see above). The great majority will not. Cardiovascular risk is greater for any given level of cholesterol when the serum triglyceride concentration is also elevated (Fig. 4(b)). Often the HDL is low, which further compounds the risk. Some authorities believe that there is a specific syndrome, in which there is a combined increase in serum cholesterol and triglycerides and greatly increased coronary risk. They term this familial combined hyperlipidaemia. In this, multiple lipoprotein phenotypes occur in different family members: some IIa, some IIb, some IV, or occasionally even V. It is likely that what is being observed is the genetic tendency for hypercholesterolaemia and hypertriglyceridaemia running in the same family to combine in some members and not in others, and that when this occurs in a family susceptible to coronary disease a particularly high premature mortality ensues. However, until the arguments about whether familial combined hyperlipidaemia is a distinct genetic entity are resolved the message is that hypertriglyceridaemia (especially when HDL cholesterol is low) is an additional factor increasing the risk of hypercholesterolaemia, and that when these are combined with a family history of premature CHD the outlook is bleak unless the condition is detected and treated.

Primary hyperlipidaemias in which hypertriglyceridaemia predominates

Severe hypertriglyceridaemia (types I and V)

Diagnosis and underlying mechanism

In any circumstance in which the serum triglycerides exceed 11 mmol/l (1000 mg/dl), chylomicrons in addition to VLDL will be major contributors to the hyperlipidaemia, even when the patient is fasting. This is because chylomicrons and VLDL compete for the same clearance mechanism (lipoprotein lipase). The lipoprotein phenotype is usually type V. This severe hypertriglyceridaemia generally ensues when an increase in hepatic VLDL production either familial or secondary to, for example, obesity, diabetes, alcohol, or oestrogen administration is associated with decreased triglyceride clearance, which again may be genetic or acquired, for example hypothyroidism, β-blockade, or diabetes (which can cause both an overproduction of VLDL and decreased lipoprotein lipase activity). With the clearance mechanism already overloaded with VLDL, the rise in serum triglyceride levels when chylomicrons enter the circulation following a fatty meal may be tumultuous and they may spend days rather than hours in the circulation. The serum takes on the appearance of milk and triglyceride levels may exceed 100 mmol/l (9000 mg/dl). Thus a patient, who might otherwise have a fasting serum triglyceride level of 5 mmol/l, can, with the injudicious use of alcohol or the development of diabetes, achieve extraordinarily high serum triglyceride levels. Overall the frequency of severe hypertriglyceridaemia [>11 mmol/l (1000 mg/dl)] is probably no more than 1 in 1000 in adults and less in children.

Rarely, severe hypertriglyceridaemia is caused by a genetic deficiency in lipoprotein lipase activity. This is inherited as an autosomal recessive trait. Usually it is due to mutations in both lipoprotein lipase genes (homozygous) but occasionally to a genetic deficiency of apolipoprotein CII, the activator of lipoprotein lipase. In familial lipoprotein lipase deficiency severe hypertriglyceridaemia may be encountered in childhood. Occasionally, in children and young adults presenting for the first time, it produces type I hyperlipoproteinaemia, in which only serum chylomicron levels are elevated. It is not known why the VLDL is not also raised, but with advancing age the increase in both VLDL and chylomicrons, which might be expected if lipoprotein lipase is ineffective, becomes the rule.

Physical signs in severe hypertriglyceridaemia

Tuberoeruptive xanthomas are characteristic. These appear as yellow papules on the extensor surfaces of the arms and legs, buttocks, and back. Often there is hepatosplenomegaly. Imaging shows the liver to be fatty, and bone marrow biopsy may reveal macrophages engorged with lipid droplets (foam cells). Because the triglyceride-rich lipoprotein may also interfere with the determination of transaminases, giving spuriously high values, liver disease, in particular alcoholic liver disease, may be difficult to exclude other than by the resolution of the syndrome when a low-fat diet is instituted. Other features include lipaemia retinalis (pallor of the optic fundus, with both the retinal veins and arteries appearing white).

Complications of severe hypertriglyceridaemia

Atheroma is not a complication of familial lipoprotein lipase deficiency, but it does complicate severe hypertriglyceridaemia in which there is some lipoprotein lipase activity, albeit diminished. It is difficult to make a precise estimate of the risk from the hyperlipidaemia *per se* because it is so frequently associated with insulin resistance or frank diabetes, which are themselves risk factors for atherosclerosis. If these are included as part of the syndrome, both CHD and peripheral arterial disease are common. The reason for the complete absence of lipoprotein lipase removing the risk of atheroma is not known, but it may be because the incidence of diabetes is not increased in familial lipoprotein lipase deficiency, because fibrinogen and factor VII activity are not increased, or because the conversion of VLDL and chylomicrons to the atherogenic IDL and remnant lipoproteins, respectively, is impaired in the absence of lipoprotein lipase.

Although atheroma is not directly due to the high levels of triglyceride-rich lipoproteins, other complications are. Acute pancreatitis may occur when serum triglyceride levels exceed 20–30 mmol/l (2000–3000 mg/dl) (see above). The diagnosis may not be confirmed by detecting increased serum amylase activity, because falsely low values may be encountered due to interference by triglyceride-rich lipoproteins in the laboratory method. All laboratories should inspect serum for milkiness before reporting normal or only moderately raised serum amylase activity in patients with severe abdominal pain. Some patients do not develop acute pancreatitis, even when serum triglyceride levels exceed 100 mmol/l (9000 mg/dl). Others, who are more susceptible, experience recurring acute episodes. Chronic pancreatitis is not a feature.

Recurrent abdominal pain, not typical of pancreatitis, sometimes occurs in patients prone to marked hypertriglyceridaemia. It may mimic irritable bowel syndrome. Severe abdominal pain may also sometimes be the result of splenic infarction.

Pseudohyponatraemia is another problem. Spuriously low serum sodium values are reported, because much of the volume of the serum aliquot on which the measurement is made is occupied by lipoproteins as opposed to water. When the serum triglycerides exceed 40–50 mmol/l (3500–4500 mg/dl) spurious serum sodium levels of 120–130 mmol/ are reported and can be misinterpreted; and a patient already seriously ill with pancreatitis, or occasionally uncontrolled diabetes, will then be made more so by infusion of isotonic saline or, worse, hypertonic saline.

Focal neurological syndromes such as hemiparesis, memory loss, and loss of mental concentration may complicate extreme hypertriglyceridaemia, perhaps because of a sluggish cerebral microcirculation caused by the high concentrations of chylomicrons in the blood. Paraesthesiae, especially in the feet, may also be an occasional feature, even in the absence of diabetes. Sicca syndrome and polyarthritis have also been described, but undoubtedly the commonest articular association is gout (see below).

Table 3 The more common causes of secondary hyperlipoproteinaemia

Endocrine	Diabetes mellitus Thyroid disease Pregnancy
Nutritional	Obesity Alcohol excess Anorexia nervosa
Renal disease	Nephrotic syndrome Chronic renal failure
Drugs	β-Adrenoreceptor blockers Thiazide diuretics Steroid hormones Microsomal enzyme-inducing agents Retinoic acid derivatives
Hepatic disease	Cholestasis Hepatocellular dysfunction Cholelithiasis
Immunoglobulin excess Hyperuricaemia	Paraproteinaemia

Moderate hypertriglyceridaemia (type IV)

Fasting serum triglyceride levels in the range 2.2–5.0 mmol/l (200–450 mg/dl) in the absence of an elevated cholesterol level are commonly encountered, principally the result of obesity. Diabetes and an excess of alcohol are other important causes. Sometimes hypertriglyceridaemia is present in a fit, non-obese person with none of these factors. Family studies may then reveal similar increases in relatives, when the condition is called familial as opposed to sporadic hypertriglyceridaemia.

Raised levels are associated with the risk of CHD, but there is little evidence that the triglyceride itself is causal and much of the association might be because of associated low levels of HDL, raised cholesterol, or glucose intolerance. Hypertriglyceridaemia increases the coronary disease risk of any associated increase in serum cholesterol [Fig. 4(b)], but present evidence would not favour its treatment in the absence of hypercholesterolaemia. Occasionally, levels of 5 mmol/l (450 mg/dl) or less must be treated, if they occur in patients prone to periodic exacerbations associated with acute pancreatitis. Generally, levels exceeding 10 mmol/l justify therapy, but for levels between 5 and 10 mmol/l clinical judgement must apply. In diabetes, evidence that serum triglycerides are an independent risk factor for CHD justifies therapy at lower levels than in non-diabetics after improvements in diet and glycaemic control have been exhausted as a means of decreasing triglyceride levels.

Secondary hyperlipoproteinaemias

Secondary hyperlipoproteinaemias are listed in Table 3. When a disease causing hyperlipidaemia is combined with primary hyperliproteinaemia, the two frequently synergize to produce marked hyperliproteinaemia. The best-known example of this is diabetes mellitus; in the United Kingdom and the United States, CHD is the most common cause of premature death in diabetics.

Diabetes mellitus

The dominant hyperlipidaemia in diabetes is hypertriglyceridaemia. This is more likely to be associated with hypercholesterolaemia and with decreased HDL cholesterol in type 2 diabetes, but the risks of CHD and peripheral arterial disease are increased in both types 1 and 2 diabetes. This may be because in both disorders the hypertriglyceridaemia results not simply from an increase in VLDL, but also from an increase in IDL and a small triglyceride-rich, cholesterol-depleted LDL particle. As neither of these may contribute greatly to an increase in lipids, the term dyslipoproteinaemia is particularly aptly applied in diabetes. Also, plasma fibrinogen levels, which are increased in both types of diabetes relate to serum triglyceride levels. Although lipoprotein abnormalities in type 1 diabetes may be less frequent than in type 2, the risk of CHD in type 1 is more often compounded by the presence of proteinuria. In diabetes uncomplicated by proteinuria, the risk of CHD is about two to three times that of non-diabetic people of a similar age. Proteinuria increases the risk by as much as 40 times.

Insulin resistance may be present in non-diabetic, usually obese, people who are still able to secrete sufficient insulin to maintain control of blood sugar, but in such people there is often hypertriglyceridaemia with low HDL cholesterol and hypercholesterolaemia, hypertension, and increased risk of CHD. This syndrome is often referred to as the insulin resistance syndrome (syndrome X) or chronic cardiovascular risk syndrome. A proportion of people with this condition ultimately develop diabetes, sometimes not until after they have already developed CHD.

Diabetic women, particularly those with type 2 disease, tend to have a distribution of adipose tissue resembling that of obese men, being mostly around the abdomen and waist, rather than the more female pattern which involves the buttocks and thighs, but leaves the waist relatively small. Relative protection from CHD is largely lost by diabetic women, and this may result from this androgenization. Many women with a similar body habitus, but who have not yet developed diabetes, are insulin resistant, hypertensive, have hyperlipidaemia, and have an associated increased risk of CHD.

Other secondary hyperlipoproteinaemias

Obesity alone causes hypertriglyceridaemia (usually type IV) and usually exacerbates any primary hyperlipidaemia. There is often hypercholesterolaemia as well as hypertriglyceridaemia. The exception appears to be familial hypercholesterolaemia, which is not associated with obesity. Alcohol excess also causes hypertriglyceridaemia. Weight loss is generally associated with decreases in serum cholesterol and triglyceride levels. Anorexia nervosa is paradoxical in that it may be associated with quite marked elevations of serum cholesterol.

In hypothyroidism, serum LDL cholesterol and, less frequently, serum triglycerides are raised. HDL levels tend to be increased. There is decreased receptor-mediated LDL catabolism and lipoprotein lipase activity may be decreased. Hypothyroidism should always be considered in the diagnosis of hyperlipidaemia, and it is particularly important to exclude it when marked hyperlipidaemia occurs in women and in diabetic patients.

Renal disease is an important cause of secondary hyperlipidaemia. In nephrotic syndrome the major lipoprotein disorder is a rise in serum LDL cholesterol. In chronic renal failure hypertriglyceridaemia is produced by an increase in both VLDL and in LDL triglycerides. Haemodialysis, chronic ambulatory peritoneal dialysis, and high-energy diets exacerbate the hyperlipidaemia. Following renal transplantation, many of the lipoprotein abnormalities resolve if good renal function is established, but corticosteroid therapy, weight gain, antihypertensive therapy, and perhaps cyclosporin treatment allow hyperlipidaemia to persist in about one-quarter of patients. Lp(a) is markedly elevated in renal disease, even after transplantation.

Drugs are a common cause of hyperlipidaemia. β-Blockers without intrinsic sympathomimetic activity raise triglycerides and lower HDL cholesterol. Thiazide diuretics tend to increase both cholesterol and triglycerides. These effects may be relatively small in people whose serum lipids are not elevated at the outset, but in patients with hypertriglyceridaemia or with diabetes they may be substantial. Oestrogens tend to raise serum triglycerides, but will often lower LDL cholesterol after the menopause. They also raise serum HDL. Androgens have the opposite effect, decreasing triglycerides, raising LDL cholesterol, and lowering HDL. They may contribute to premature cardiac death in athletes unwise enough to use them in training. Glucocorticoids increase serum LDL cholesterol and triglycerides and often HDL cholesterol. Retinoic acid derivatives used in the management of skin disorders cause hypertriglyceridaemia. Phenytoin and phenobarbitone raise serum HDL cholesterol.

Cholestatic liver diseases produce hypercholesterolaemia. This is not due to an increase in apo B-containing LDL, but to an abnormal lipoprotein, designated lipoprotein X (LpX), produced largely as the result of reflux of biliary phospholipids into the circulation. Xanthelasmata are common in biliary obstruction and other xanthomas occasionally develop. In the later phase of chronic biliary obstruction, when secondary biliary cirrhosis and hepatocellular disease sets in, hepatic lipid biosynthesis plummets and the hyperlipidaemia of biliary obstruction resolves. Hepatocellular diseases may be associated with moderate hypertriglyceridaemia, probably because of impaired hepatic lipoprotein clearance. HDL concentrations are markedly decreased and lecithin:cholesterol acyltransferase activity is low. This defect in cholesterol esterification may contribute to the complications of liver failure.

Hyperuricaemia is present in as many as half the men with hypertriglyceridaemia. It may lead to gout, particularly if such patients are receiving diuretic therapy.

Management of hyperlipoproteinaemia

Clinical trials have established beyond all question that reduction in serum cholesterol decreases both coronary morbidity and mortality. Until recently, though, there was doubt as to whether dietary or drug therapy might reduce total mortality or cardiovascular mortality by as much as would be anticipated; and there were concerns about increased death from non-cardiovascular causes. Five major clinical trials of statin drugs have altered this perspective. Three of these (4S, CARE, and LIPID) were secondary and two (WOSCOPS and AFCPS/TexCAPS) were primary prevention trials. They lasted from 5 to 6 years and all showed a decrease in new coronary events of about one-third. A decrease in the risk of cerebral infarction was also evident in LIPID. There was no increase in non-CHD mortality associated with treatment. This means that all the patients with established coronary disease or other major atherosclerotic disease whose serum cholesterol exceeds 5.0 mmol/l (200 mg/dl) should generally receive statin drugs. Their value in primary prevention is also clearly established, but the level of risk at which they should be used in this context is more controversial.

The absolute risk of coronary events in these trials spanned a range from 4.5 per cent per year to 1 per cent per year. The number of patients requiring treatment to prevent one event was substantially lower in the trials with the higher rates of new events. This has fuelled much discussion about the level of CHD risk at which statin therapy can be considered cost-effective, particularly in countries such as Britain in which high CHD risk is so prevalent. A consensus is emerging that this occurs when the annual CHD risk is 2 per cent or greater. The cost of statins will become less and this figure may be revised downwards in future, but this will also depend on the associated costs of the clinical services required to institute and monitor treatment which are not likely to become cheaper. The essential point to grasp is that the decision to treat hyperlipidaemia is not based simply on any particular cholesterol value, but on an assessment of individual risk of coronary disease. For instance, a 35-year-old man with a cholesterol level of 9.00 mmol/l (350 mg/dl) and no other risk factors, has a risk of CHD similar to a man of the same age, who has a serum cholesterol concentration of only 6.5 mmol/l (250 mg/dl), but who is a smoker with moderate hypertension. The identification of patients with gross hypercholesterolaemia and of those with more modest increases in serum cholesterol combined with multiple risk factors (smoking history, hypertension, diabetes or impaired glucose tolerance, low HDL cholesterol, bad family history or premature menopause) or established coronary disease or other major atherosclerotic disease (myocardial infarction is the leading cause of death in patients with cerebrovascular disease or peripheral arterial disease) allows the targeting of cholesterol-lowering management to high-risk individuals. Calculations of coronary risk using the various charts, tables, or computer programs which are becoming available can be helpful in management decisions, but a single level of absolute risk of coronary disease (be it 2 per cent per year or some other level) cannot be the only indicator of the need for therapy, partly because in some patients, for example with diabetes complicated by proteinuria or with familial hypercholesterolaemia, the risk is underestimated, but also because many younger patients with a high lifetime expectancy of coronary disease would be neglected while at the other end of the age range the majority of the elderly population would qualify for cholesterol-lowering medication, because age is such a potent risk factor.

Dietary management

Dietary advice should be given to people whose serum cholesterol exceeds the optimal level of 5.2 mmol/l (200 mg/dl). Again the rigour with which this is possible in the United Kingdom, where 85 per cent of middle-aged people have cholesterol levels exceeding this level must to some extent be determined by individual risk.

The principal aims are to reduce obesity and to decrease saturated fat consumption. In the non-obese, advice should focus on decreasing saturated fat to below 10 per cent of energy intake and substituting it with a mixture of unrefined carbohydrate and monounsaturated and polyunsaturated fats (Table 4). Polyunsaturates should not alone replace saturated fat, because it is not certain that in large amounts they do not have harmful long-term effects. Increasingly, oils rich in the monounsaturated oleic acid are being encouraged. Mucilaginous fibre in fruit, vegetables, and oats may have a small hypocholesterolaemic effect. Dietary cholesterol itself, usually has little influence on serum cholesterol levels. Foods rich in plant sterols may help to lower serum cholesterol. Avoiding coffee is probably pointless. The epidemiological evidence indicating that alcohol is protective against CHD is strong enough to justify encouraging moderate indulgence. Evidence that wines are preferable to spirits and red to white wine is now in doubt. Alcohol can also lead to obesity and to exacerbation of hypertriglyceridaemia and a trial of abstinence should

Table 4 Dietary fatty acids and their sources

Saturated	
Myristic	Pork, beef,
Palmitic	sheep fat, and
Stearic	dairy products
Monounsaturated	
Oleic	Olive oil, rapeseed oil
Polyunsaturated	
Linoleic	Sunflower, safflower,
Eicosapentaenoic	corn, soyabean oil
Docosahexaenoic	Fish oil

All can contribute to obesity. Saturated fats lead to raised cholesterol and triglyceride levels. Oleic acid and linoleic acid decrease LDL cholesterol and often triglycerides. Oleic acid is widely distributed in foods rich in saturated fats, but these sources are not helpful in a diet designed to decrease saturated fat intake. Fish oil decreases triglycerides, but does not decrease LDL cholesterol.

be considered in the patient with hyperlipidaemia suspected of over-indulgence.

This diet is suitable also for treatment of moderate hypertriglyceridaemia as well as for the management of diabetes. The patient with severe hypertriglyceridaemia, however, must limit the production of chylomicrons and so any fat in the diet must be avoided. Often a 25–30 g low-fat diet can be employed, but occasionally even lower fat intakes must be achieved. Lipid-lowering drugs are frequently ineffective in patients with severe hypertriglyceridaemia, whereas diet is particularly effective.

Drug therapy of hyperlipidaemia

Patients with established CHD or other significant atherosclerotic disease

Secondary prevention trials provide evidence of overall benefit for lipid-lowering treatment. Drugs are indicated therefore in patients with CHD should their cholesterol level persist above 5.2 mmol/l (200 mg/dl) [LDL cholesterol >3.4 mmol/l (130 mg/dl)] despite diet. Similar evidence also applies to at least some patients following cerebral infarction. It is probably also reasonable to extend this policy to patients with peripheral arterial, aortic, or significant carotid atherosclerosis, because angiographic studies demonstrate favourable effects and because this type of disease is closely associated with risk of CHD.

Familial hypercholesterolaemia and type III hyperlipoproteinaemia

The high risk of CHD justifies the use of lipid-lowering drug therapy. Few patients with familial hypercholesterolaemia will achieve adequate reduction of serum cholesterol with diet alone. Many with type III hyperlipoproteinaemia can, however. Often when their cholesterol is 6.5 mmol/l, their triglyceride levels are still elevated, indicating that significant beta-VLDL is still present in the circulation. The indication for drug therapy should therefore probably be at about 6.00 mmol/l in this group.

Diabetes mellitus

The low rate of CHD in diabetic patients in countries where cholesterol levels are generally low justifies the use of lipid-lowering therapy. Men and women should have equal consideration. Diet (particularly the avoidance of obesity) and improvements in glycaemic control can improve serum lipid levels dramatically. Lipid-lowering drugs are indicated if a cholesterol level above 5.2 mmol/l persists.

Multiple risk factors

The risk of CHD in patients with additional adverse factors, whose serum cholesterol remains elevated despite diet, justifies the use of lipid-lowering drugs. Just how high the risk needs to be, and how it can be determined, is a persisting problem as was previously discussed. The decision should be made depending on individual circumstances. The case is stronger in men whose cholesterol persists above 5.2 mmol/l than in women. This, combined with hypertension or a bad family history, or a long smoking history, may justify the use of lipid-lowering treatment in men. Two of these factors would be required in most women. The finding of raised triglycerides and a low HDL cholesterol in combination with raised cholesterol also militates in favour of drug therapy when other risk factors for CHD are present. It is always important to seek evidence of existing CHD.

Markedly elevated cholesterol with no other risk factors and no clearly identifiable genetic syndrome

Many people fall into this category, but they are not at sufficiently high risk of CHD to justify lipid-lowering drug therapy unless serum cholesterol is at least 8.0 mmol/l despite diet. Even then, many women do not require such therapy because they have relatively high HDL cholesterol, and it is reasonable not to introduce it in the absence of risk factors in women unless the total cholesterol/HDL cholesterol ratio exceeds 7 and total cholesterol exceeds 8 mmol/l. If women in this category are peri- or postmenopausal, the possibility of prescribing hormone replacement therapy should be considered. It often decreases LDL and may increase HDL cholesterol and it may have a beneficial effect in preventing CHD, although randomized clinical trial evidence to support this view is required. In men, in whom high levels of HDL are less commonly encountered, it is reasonable to advocate lipid-lowering therapy if the total cholesterol exceeds 8 (or the LDL cholesterol is >6 mmol/l) and probably at somewhat lower levels if serum triglyceride levels are also raised.

Lipid-modifying drugs

A single measurement of cholesterol concentration should never be the reason for advising either dietary or drug therapy. Laboratory results are usually ± 10 per cent of the true mean value, but can be less accurate, particularly in the case of portable 'on-site' analyses.

Non-fasting cholesterol measurements are satisfactory for the management of patients responding to diet, but when drug therapy is under consideration, at least two, and preferably three, fasting determinations of cholesterol, triglycerides, and HDL cholesterol are necessary (serum cholesterol and HDL cholesterol levels are not affected by meals, but serum triglyceride levels are). Abnormal values of HDL and triglycerides would favour drug therapy, and their concentrations may influence the choice of drug. Serum thyroxine should be measured if there is any suspicion of hypothyroidism and some advocate its measurement in all patients whose serum cholesterol exceeds 8 mmol/l (310 mg/dl).

3-Hydroxy-3-methylglutaryl-CoA reductase inhibitor drugs now generally known as statins (atorvastatin, cerivastatin, fluvastatin, lovastatin, pravastatin, simvastatin) have become the most widely used cholesterol-lowering drugs because of their effectiveness and the clinical trial evidence in their favour. As well as their potent LDL cholesterol-lowering properties statins have a triglyceride-lowering effect which, although generally less than their effect on LDL cholesterol, is of clinical value in combined hyperlipidaemia. There is a small incidence of myositis associated with their use. This is most likely when they are combined with fibrates, cyclosporin, or antibiotics such as erythromycin. The latter should be avoided in patients receiving statin therapy, but with adequate supervision the risk of myositis is not so great as to preclude the use of statins in combination with fibrates or cyclosporin when clinically indicated in high-risk patients with combined hyperlipidaemia or in cardiac and renal transplant patients, respectively. Serum creatine kinase should then be regularly monitored. In patients receiving statin monotherapy creatine kinase should be measured about 6 weeks after its introduction and after any increase in dose. Thereafter, it is probably reasonable to measure creatine kinase only if patients report muscle aching, which they should be warned to do. Minor excursions of creatine kinase activity into the abnormal range are fairly frequent in ambulant people and so those occurring on statin therapy are not necessarily drug related. Statins may be used in patients with renal disease, but are contraindicated in liver disease.

Bile-acid sequestrating agents (cholestyramine, colestipol) lower cholesterol, but may exacerbate hypertriglyceridaemia. Their principal use is now as an adjunct to statin therapy in patients with marked hypercholesterolaemia responding inadequately to statin monotherapy. A dose (two sachets) is best taken well soaked in fruit juice before breakfast. In larger, more frequent doses these agents often cause nausea, heartburn, and constipation. In children and women of child-bearing potential, who have heterozygous familial hypercholesterolaemia and in whom drug treatment is considered essential, they are preferred to statins because of their long safety record (certainly if combined with folic acid supplements). On the other hand, because of their gastrointestinal side-effects, compliance is often poor and alienation from the clinic may occur so that increasingly children and younger women are left off drug treatment in order that the boys may promptly receive statin therapy in early adulthood and the women when they have completed their families.

The fibrate drugs (bezafibrate, ciprofibrate, clofibrate, fenofibrate, gemfibrozil) primarily lower serum triglycerides. Their cholesterol-lowering action is largely due to reductions in VLDL cholesterol. Clofibrate is no longer used because it encourages cholelithiasis. They are often highly effective in type III hyperlipoproteinaemia and useful in type V hyperlipoproteinaemia. They may also be used in the management of combined hypercholesterolaemia and hypertriglyceridaemia. Generally, in such patients advantage should be taken of the stronger evidence for benefit from statins and one of these should be the initial agent of choice unless the triglyceride levels are particularly high or type III hyperlipoproteinaemia is present. There is, however, clinical trial evidence that fibrates can reduce CHD risk when triglycerides as well as cholesterol are raised. Thus in particularly high-risk patients such as those with diabetes and CHD the addition of fibrate to statin therapy is justified when triglyceride values persist above 4 mmol/l (350 mg/dl). Fibrates must be avoided in patients with disturbed hepatic or renal function.

Nicotinic acid (niacin) can be used to lower serum cholesterol and triglyceride levels. Unpleasant flushing can be minimized if aspirin is taken before the nicotinic acid. There are many other side-effects and liver function must be monitored. Nicotinic acid has not found great favour outside the United States, but it is enjoying renewed interest because, unlike other lipid-lowering drugs, it is effective in lowering serum Lp(a). Acipimox, an analogue, has a similar spectrum of action to the fibrate drugs and causes less flushing. Probucol lowers HDL cholesterol more markedly than LDL. Despite its undoubted antioxidant properties, it requires further clinical evaluation before it can be regarded as beneficial in its overall action. Fish oil, despite its triglyceride-lowering properties, does not lower LDL cholesterol. Preparations which concentrate its long chain fatty acid components (eicosapentaenoic and docosapentaenoic acid) are more potent in lowering triglycerides, but clinical trial evidence that they reduce coronary risk is required.

Non-pharmacological lipid-lowering treatment

Extracorporeal removal of LDL is available in many centres for severe hypercholesterolaemia, usually homozygous familial hypercholesterolaemia in which it improves survival. Plasmapheresis or LDL apheresis, using systems that absorb LDL, are the two methods employed. Plasmapheresis and most LDL apheresis methods also lower serum Lp(a). They must be repeated every 2–4 weeks. Occasionally, patients with homozygous familial hypercholesterolaemia have also been treated with liver transplantation to provide an organ with normally functioning LDL receptors. Partial ileal bypass surgery has been used to treat heterozygous familial hypercholesterolaemia (it is ineffective in homozygotes), but with the advent of more effective lipid-lowering drugs this is now only exceptionally necessary.

Hypolipoproteinaemia

Hypolipoproteinaemia is an increasing clinical problem, because more cases are being discovered as a result of population screening for high cholesterol. People who have had a low serum cholesterol level all their lives do not seem to be at any disadvantage unless the decrease is profound, as in abetalipoproteinaemia; but when the condition is discovered for the first time it is often difficult to be sure that the low cholesterol is not due to an acquired disease, such as malignancy or malabsorption.

Some with serum cholesterol levels about 1.0–3.5 mmol/l (40–140 mg/dl) will have heterozygous familial hypobetalipoproteinaemia, which is an autosomal dominant condition in which a truncated apo B mutation occurs. The condition is benign. However, homozygous hypoapobetalipoproteinaemia and abetalipoproteinaemia (inherited as an autosomal recessive; site of mutation unknown, but not the apo B gene itself), which produce more profound hypocholesterolaemia, are associated with retinitis pigmentosa, unusually shaped erythrocytes (acanthocytes), a syndrome resembling Friedreich's ataxia (preventable with fat-soluble vitamin administration), steatorrhoea (which can create diagnostic confusion with other causes of malabsorption leading to secondary hypocholesterolaemia), and fatty liver.

Analphalipoproteinaemia (Tangier disease) is a very rare disorder associated with virtually absent HDL, reduced LDL cholesteryl ester, and cholesteryl ester deposition throughout the body, leading to enlarged orange–yellow tonsils and adenoids, lymph node enlargement, hepatosphenomegaly, bone marrow infiltration (thrombocytopenia), orange-brown spots on the rectal mucosa, neuropathy, and corneal cloudiness. A less severe form of this disorder (fish-eye disease) has been described. In another disorder, combined deficiency of the apolipoproteins AI and CIII due to a DNA rearrangement affecting the transcription of both their genes, which are clustered together on chromosome 11, leads to markedly decreased serum HDL levels, accelerated atherosclerosis, and corneal opacities. Some believe that a much more common genetic HDL deficiency is the cause of HDL cholesterol levels in the lower 10 per cent of the frequency distribution. Evidence for this contention is incomplete.

Further reading

Brunzell, J.D. (1995). Familial lipoprotein lipase deficiency and other causes of the chylomicronaemia syndrome. In *The metabolic and molecular bases of inherited disease* (7th edn) (ed. C.R. Scriver, A.L. Beaudet, W.S. Sly, and D. Valle), pp. 1913–32. McGraw-Hill, New York.

Durrington, P.N. (1995). *Hyperlipidaemia. Diagnosis and management* (2nd edn). Butterworth Heinemann, Oxford.

Goldstein, J.L., Hobbs, H.H., and Brown, M.S. (1995). Familial hypercholesterolaemia. In *The metabolic and molecular bases of inherited disease* (7th edn) (ed. C.R. Scriver, A.L. Beaudet, W.S. Sly, and D. Valle), pp. 1981–2030. McGraw-Hill, New York.

Mahley, R.W. and Rall, S.C. (1995). Type III hyperlipoproteinaemia (dysbetalipoproteinaemia): the role of apolipoprotein E in normal and abnormal lipoprotein metabolism. In *The metabolic and molecular bases of inherited disease* (7th edn) (ed. C.R. Scriver, A.L. Beaudet, W.S. Sly, and D. Valle), pp. 1953–80. McGraw-Hill, New York.

Wood, D., Durrington, P.N., Poulter, N., McInnes, G., Rees, A., and Wray, R. (1998). Joint British recommendations on prevention of CHD in clinical practice. *Heart*, **80** (Suppl 2), S1–29.

Chapter 6.12

Disorders of oxalate metabolism

R. W. E. Watts

The oxalate anion is metabolically inert in humans and its overall metabolism can be represented by a single compartment model (Fig. 1) in which the oxalate metabolic pool is somewhat larger than the extracellular fluid volume. The normal plasma oxalate concentration is 1–3 μmol/l and shows a circadian rhythm, being lowest in the morning and highest in the evening with superimposed postprandial rises. Urinary excretion does not normally exceed 450 μmol/24 h in adults. The results in children are similar if they are adjusted to a standard body surface area (1.73 m^2). Adult levels of excretion are reached when the child is about 14 years old. Urinary excretion also rises during the waking hours and shows seasonal variations related to dietary oxalate and calcium intake and the effects of vitamin D. Oxalate in the plasma and tissues is of both dietary and biosynthetic origin. Beans, beetroot, celery, chocolate, cocoa, nuts, rhubarb, strawberries and tea have a particularly high oxalate content.

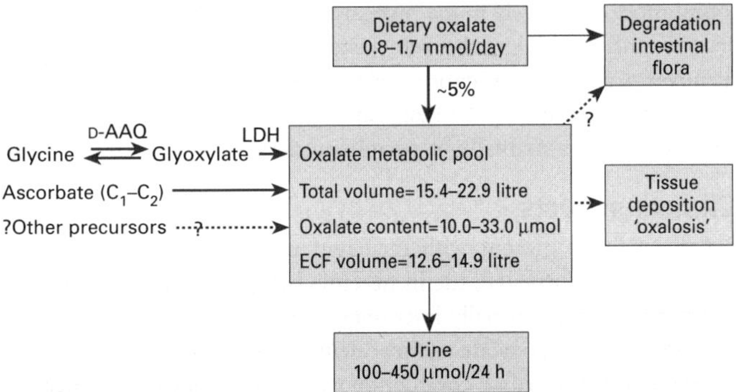

Fig. 1 The one-compartment model of oxalate metabolism in humans. The numerical values relate to adults and the data for the oxalate metabolic pool have been normalized to a body surface area of 1.73 m^2. The proportion of the dietary oxalate, which is absorbed, depends on whether it is ingested in an ionizable form and on the calcium content of the intestinal tract. AGT, alanine : glyoxylate aminotransferase (EC 2.6.1.44); D-AAO, d-amino acid oxidase (glycine oxidase, EC 1.4.3.3); LDH, Lactate dehydrogenase (EC 1.1.1.27). The metabolic pathway from glycine to oxalate is a minor component (not more than 1 per cent) of the total metabolic turnover of glycine. The system is normally in equilibrium and there is no tendency for oxalate to be deposited in the tissues. Perturbation of the system with expansion of the oxalate metabolic pool occurs in renal failure and when there is either overproduction or overabsorption. Overt oxalosis only occurs when renal failure is combined with one of these other pathophysiological factors.

The only important biosynthetic sources of oxalate in humans are glycine via the glyoxylate anion, and the C_1–C_2 fragment of ascorbate. The claim that the artificial sweetening agent, diethylene glycol, is converted to oxalate in humans has not been confirmed.

The absorption of oxalate from the small intestine involves both an active carrier mediated transport system with oxalate-chloride exchange and passive diffusion. It is greatly influenced by the calcium ion concentration in the gut lumen, being reduced when this is high and vice versa. The kidney handles oxalate by 100 per cent filtration at the glomerulus, tubular secretion involving active transport into the lumen, and passive back-diffusion into the peritubular capillaries. The ratio of oxalate clearance to glomerular filtration rate is normally about 1.2, indicating net tubular secretion.

Apart from acute oxalic acid poisoning, diseases attributable to oxalate occur when calcium oxalate stones form in the urinary tract and when this salt crystallizes in either the renal parenchyma (calcium oxalate nephrocalcinosis) or in other tissues (oxalosis).

The disorders of oxalate metabolism are due to either overproduction or excessive absorption of oxalate. Reduced renal excretion does not cause oxalosis unless one of these other pathophysiological processes is also operating. Conversely, increased oxalate biosynthesis and hyperabsorption do not cause oxalosis unless recurrent oxalate urolithiasis and nephrocalcinosis have impaired renal function to the point where there is superadded oxalate retention. The risk of oxalosis developing is greatly increased when the glomerular filtration rate decreases to about 25 ml/min per 1.73 ms^2. Hyperoxaluria is the hallmark of the disorders of oxalate metabolism; Table 1 lists its causes.

Primary hyperoxaluria type I

Biochemistry

Primary hyperoxaluria type I is due to autosomal recessively inherited deficient activity of hepatic peroxisomal alanine:glyoxylate aminotransferase. This enzyme appears to be confined to the liver and Fig. 2 shows the location of the metabolic lesion with some related metabolic reactions. There are four genetic variants (Table 2). The group of patients in whom the enzyme is mislocated, being mitochondrial and not peroxisomal, is of particular interest. This defect is attributed to a mutation that alters the peptide leader sequence that guides the enzyme from its site of synthesis on the rough endoplasmic reticulum to the correct organelle. It is present in about one-third of the patients with residual enzyme catalytic activity and appears to be unique among the inborn errors of metabolism.

The chromosomal assignment of the alanine:glyoxylate aminotransferase gene is 2q37.3. The coding region of about 10 kb pairs is organized into 11 exons and 10 introns. The gene has been sequenced and several different mutations identified. Most attention has been paid to explaining the misrouting phenomenon. It appears that a critical mutation, which produces a Pro_{11}Leu amino acid substitution,

Table 1 The hyperoxalurias

Primary
Type I Hyperoxaluria due to hepatic peroxisomal alanine:glyoxylate aminotransferase (AGT;EC 2.6.1.44) deficiency. Associated with hyperglycollic aciduria in about 75 per cent of cases
Type II Hyperoxaluria due to glyoxylate reductase (D-glycerate dehydrogenase, EC 1.1.1.29) deficiency. Always associated with l-glyceric aciduria
Type III Hyperoxaluria due to intestinal hyperabsorption (primary absorptive hyperoxaluria). Not associated with any other abnormal organic aciduria
Secondary
Enteric
jejunoileal ileal bypass small intestine resection blind loops diffuse disease of the small intestine (e.g. Crohn's disease) chronic pancreatic and biliary tract disease Oxalate ingestion (acute poisoning)
Excessive intake of ascorbic acid
Ethylene glycol poisoning
Adverse reaction of methoxyfluorane inhalation
Adverse reaction to xylitol infusion
Glycine irrigation (after transurethral prostatectomy)
Aspergillus infection
Pyridoxine (vitamin B_6) deficiency

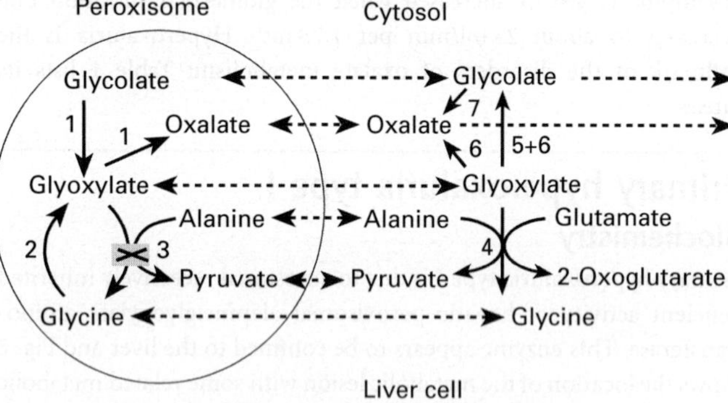

Fig. 2 The site of the metabolic lesion in primary hyperoxaluria type I (reaction 3 in this diagram). The outer rectangle represents the plasma membrane of the hepatocyte and the circle represents the membrane of a peroxisome. The solid arrows show enzyme-catalysed metabolic pathways and the broken arrows indicate diffusion pathways. The enzymes catalysing the reactions are: 1, glycollate oxidase (L-2 hydroxyacid oxidase; EC 1.1.3.1); 2, glycine oxidase (d-amino acid oxidase; EC 1.4.3.3); 3, alanine : glyoxylate aminotransferase (serine : pyruvate aminotransferase, EC 2.6.1.44); 4, (glutamate : glyoxylate aminotransferase EC 2.6.1.4); 5, glyoxylate reductase (d-glycerate dehydrogenase, EC 1.1.1.26); 6, lactate dehydrogenase (EC 1.1.1.27); 7, glycollate dehydrogenase (EC 1.1.1.79). Glyoxylate reductase is the site of the metabolic lesion in type II primary hyperoxaluria.
(Reproduced with permission from the Journal of Inherited Metabolic Disease, ***12****, 214. Copyright ©; Society for the Study of Inborn Errors of Metabolism and Kluwer Academic Publishers 1989.)*

Table 2 Genetic heterogeneity in primary hyperoxaluria type I

Pyridoxine responsive and non-responsive variants
Residual catalytic activity present or absent
Immunologically demonstrable enzyme present (CRM^+) or absent (CRM^-)
Alanine:glyoxylate aminotransferase mislocated into mitochondria as opposed to its normal location in peroxisomes

affects the conformation of the amino terminus peptide sequence of the protein molecule in such a way that it becomes more alpha-helical, therefore more like the recognition sequence of a true mitochondrial protein and is recognized as such by specific receptor sites on the mitochondrial membrane. However, a second mutation producing a $Gly_{170}Arg$ substitution is necessary for this to occur. Normal alanine: glyoxalate aminotransferase is a dimeric protein and it must dimerize for peroxisomal uptake. The $Gly_{170}Arg$ substitution impairs dimerization and thus allows mitochondrial uptake.

Pathology

In the early stages, the pathological findings are confined to the kidney and comprise a variable degree of hydrocalycosis and hydronephrosis with multiple calculi. Interstitial deposits of calcium oxalate, which mainly form later, cause severe renal fibrosis and shrinkage. Renal hypertension and chronic interstitial nephritis are often present, and the tubules may be blocked by aggregates of calcium oxalate crystals, particularly if the terminal illness has been associated with a hypotensive-oliguric episode. The characteristic rosette-like calcium oxalate monohydrate crystals are highly birefringent and easily recognized under a polarizing microscope. Their full extent will only be observed if unfixed tissues are examined or if non-aqueous fixatives are used, but they are usually sufficiently insoluble for some to remain and be apparent after routine fixation in formol-saline. They are found most extensively in the myocardium, tunica media of muscular arteries and arterioles, the rete testes, and at sites of rapid bone turnover. Careful examination reveals a few crystals associated with the arterial supply of all organs and tissues. Similar deposits have been found intra-axonally in peripheral nerves.

Clinical aspects

Patients usually present with recurrent urolithiasis during the first decade and, if untreated, die in uraemia before they are 20 years old. The terminal phase usually lasts only a few months and is associated with dense calcium oxalate nephrocalcinosis and with the development of oxalosis. Intracardiac conduction defects may develop. Ischaemic lesions occur on the extremities, particularly in the pulps of the fingers and toes, and are attributable to the extensive crystallization of calcium oxalate in the walls of small arteries and arterioles. Progressive peripheral neuropathy and mononeuritis multiplex are associated with calcium oxalate deposition within axons as well as in the walls of the vasa nervorum. These manifestations, as well as a wider range of oxalotic features, occur particularly in patients in whom the terminal renal failure has been treated by haemodialysis, peritoneal dialysis, or by an unsuccessful renal transplantation. The additional manifestations include livedo reticularis, subcutaneous calcinosis which may ulcerate, retinal changes (white flecks, exudates, infarcts, yellow crystalline deposits especially along the courses of the renal arteries, black 'geographic' lesions at the macula), dilated

Table 3 The clinical grading of patients with primary hyperoxaluria

	Grade					
	1	2	3	4	5	6
Passage of stones	–	+	±*	±*	±*	±*
Stones/nephrocalcinosis on imaging	–	–	+	±*	±*	±*
Stone removal procedure	–	–	–	+	±*	±*
Impaired overall renal function	–	–	–	–	+	+
Renal support or replacement	–	–	–	–	–	+

*Usually present.

cardiomyopathy, synovitis and a painful osteodystrophy with dense osteosclerosis, deformation, and stress fractures (especially in the vertebrae).

A few cases present during the first months of life with seizures, advanced renal failure, and dense nephrocalcinosis, but few if any calculi (the infantile type). Another small group (the adult type) follow a benign course, presenting in adult life and surviving into the fourth and fifth decade with only occasional stone formation. The amount of oxalate excreted and the age at which renal failure develops are not very closely correlated.

A few patients present with severe uraemia and may give no history of urolithiasis. Others present with symptoms arising from oxalosis rather than renal disease, involving principally the heart, arteries, bones, and nerves. The severity of the overall clinical picture for a particular patient can be expressed in terms of a six-point scale (Table 3). Considering this in relation to the patient's age, pyridoxine responsiveness and the plasma and urine oxalate concentrations gives a guide to prognosis.

Diagnosis

This should be considered in any child with urinary stones or nephrocalcinosis and in adults with recurrent calcium oxalate stones for which no alternative explanation has been found, especially if the clinical history extends back into childhood. The presence of calcium oxalate crystals in the urinary centrifuged deposit is not a specific diagnostic sign; 24-h urinary oxalate excretion is more helpful. About 75 per cent of patients have an associated hyperglycollic aciduria. The definitive diagnosis is made by assaying alanine:glyoxylate aminotransferase activity on a liver biopsy which can also be examined by immunoelectron microscopy to establish whether the enzyme protein is present and its intracellular location. Liver biopsies have been used for prenatal diagnosis as early as the seventeenth week of pregnancy. The plasma oxalate concentration should be determined when the patient is first evaluated and subsequently as a guide to prognosis. A progressive rise indicates an increasing risk of oxalosis developing. In renal failure not due to hyperoxaluria there is a linear regression relationship between plasma oxalate and creatinine, and a plasma oxalate value that is high for the corresponding creatinine level is a valuable pointer to oxalate overproduction (or overabsorption). Early oxalosis is usually clinically silent. The possibility of identifying potentially useful diagnostic mutations in the gene is being actively explored.

Treatment

Patients should drink sufficient fluid to maintain a measured urine volume of at least 3 litres every 24 h. The diet should be low in oxalate and calcium and have minimum intakes of vitamins C and D.

The effect of pharmacological doses (150–1000 mg/day) of pyridoxine on the urinary oxalate excretion should be assessed over three 1-week periods—pretreatment, on-treatment, and post-treatment—with assays of urinary oxalate and creatinine on each 24-h urine collection. If the urinary oxalate decreases appreciably, pyridoxine should be continued indefinitely. A favourable response can probably be anticipated in between about 10 per cent and 30 per cent of cases.

Orthophosphates (e.g. Phosphate-Sandoz®) equivalent to 2 g of elemental phosphorus per day and magnesium oxide or hydroxide (e.g. 200 mg magnesium oxide) are recommended as non-specific inhibitors of crystal growth. The doses used should be sufficient to produce a material increase in the urinary excretion of either phosphate or magnesium.

Patients who are pyridoxine resistant ultimately require liver transplantation to correct the metabolic lesion, and renal transplantation if they are approaching end-stage renal disease. Planning for liver transplantation should begin when the glomerular filtration rate falls to below 20 per cent of the mean predicted normal value to minimize oxalosis and reduce the risk of oxalate deposition in the grafted kidney. After a successful liver transplant, the hyperglycollic aciduria returns to normal immediately, the plasma oxalate value normalizes over the course of a few weeks or months, and the urinary oxalate excretion returns to normal over the course of 1 or more years, depending on the size of the oxalate deposits that are gradually mobilized from the tissues. Should endstage renal failure occur before liver transplantation, neither haemodialysis nor peritoneal dialysis can keep up with the rate of oxalate production, but either treatment may limit further deposition of oxalate pending transplantation. These palliative measures should be instituted early and carried out more vigorously than in other forms of renal failure. A renal transplant performed while the glomerular filtration rate is in the 15–20 ml/min per ms^2 range can 'buy time', during which liver transplantation can be organized, but the long-term prognosis for such a grafted kidney is usually very poor. Residual catalytic activity and/or partial pyridoxine responsiveness would be expected to improve the prognosis for an isolated renal graft.

Treatment of the urinary stones

Surgical intervention should be the minimum necessary to relieve obstruction and every effort should be made to avoid removing functioning renal tissue. Unsuspected collections of stones may be found in the lower ureter on abdominal radiographs. Nephroscopic lithotomy, endoscopic lithotripsy with ultrasonic, electrohydraulic, and laser techniques, as well as extracorporeal shock-wave lithotripsy can be used to deal with asymptomatic stones and with obstructive uropathy as soon as it is diagnosed. If these techniques are available then early stone removal or disruption is recommended in order to avoid obstructive uropathy later but it is possible that nephrocalcinotic kidneys may be more easily damaged by shock-waves than normal or purely fibrotic kidneys. Open surgery should be avoided as far as possible.

Table 4 The relevance of different treatment modalities to the different types of primary hyperoxaluria

	Type I	Type II	Type III
Diet			
low oxalate	+	+	+
low calcium	+	+	–
low vitamin C	+	+	+
low vitamin D	+	+	+
Hydration	+	+	+
Inhibition of crystal growth (administration of MgO, $Mg(OH)_2$ or orthophosphate)	+	+	+
Oxalate binding agents	–	–	+
Thiazides	–	–	+
Pyridoxine	+	–	–
Dialysis	+	+	+
Renal transplantation	+	+	+
Hepatic transplantation	+	–	–

See OTM3, p. 1448 for source

Primary hyperoxaluria type II

Primary hyperoxaluria type II is due to autosomal recessive deficiency of glyoxylate reductase (d-glycerate dehydrogenase). This enzyme is cytosolic, widely distributed and the enzymological diagnosis can be made on peripheral blood leucocytes. The hyperoxaluria is accompanied by l-glyceric aciduria. The clinical features, complications, and pathological findings are the same as those of primary hyperoxaluria type I. There have been no reports of biochemical and genetic heterogeneity. Table 4 summarizes and contrasts the treatments that are available for the three types of primary hyperoxaluria. Enzyme replacement by organ transplantation has not been attempted in type II, although if the liver proved to contain the major part of the total body's glyoxylate reductase activity liver transplantation might be beneficial. The expression of the enzyme in leucocytes suggests that bone marrow transplantation from a fully histocompatible sibling might also be an option.

Primary hyperoxaluria type III

Patients with primary hyperoxaluria type III do not have an associated hyperglycollic or l-glyceric aciduria and have, therefore, to be distinguished from the approximately 25 per cent of type I patients with isolated hyperoxaluria. The diagnosis rests on: firm evidence of normal intestinal anatomy and absorptive function; the demonstration of excessive oxalate absorption; normal hepatic alanine : glyoxylate aminotransferase levels. The urinary oxalate excretion (usually 1–2 mmol/24 h) is similar to that in some patients with type I and type II, and type III patients are at risk of urinary stones, renal failure, and oxalosis. The metabolic lesion has not been identified precisely, but it might involve an oxalate-chloride exchanger in the small intestine. Thiazides reduce the urinary oxalate excretion in type III. Treatment is by a low oxalate diet with oxalate binding agents such as cholestyramine, and calcium ions (given as calcium carbonate). A marine hydrocolloid preparation (Ox-absorb®) has recently been developed as an intestinal oxalate binding therapeutic agent.

Enteric hyperoxaluria

Enteric hyperoxaluria is an uncommon but potentially serious complication of the diseases listed in Table 1. It can cause extensive urolithiasis with nephrocalcinosis and renal failure. Expansion of the oxalate pool has been demonstrated and there is the same potential for oxalosis developing as in the primary hyperoxalurias. Treatment depends upon reducing dietary oxalate intake, the use of oxalate binding agents, and correcting the steatorrhoea.

Further reading

Allan, A.R., Thompson, E.M., Williams, G., Watts, R.W.E., and Pusey, C.D. (1996). Selective renal transplantation in primary hyperoxaluria type I. *American Journal of Kidney Diseases*, 27, 891–5.

Watts, R.W.E. (1997). Primary oxaluria. *Hyperoxaluria Internationalis*, **59**, 203–13.

Chapter 6.13

Diabetes mellitus

J. I. Bell and T. D. R. Hockaday

Definition

Diabetes mellitus is a state of chronic hyperglycaemia, classically associated with excessive thirst, increased urine volume, and weight loss. Over time, particular types of tissue damage may develop. It can be produced by different disease processes, for as well as types I and II, the two forms commonly found in the UK, diabetes may also be secondary to other diseases such as pancreatitis (acute or chronic), haemochromatosis, and a number of endocrine disorders producing excessive levels of cortisol (Cushing's syndrome), growth hormone (acromegaly), glucagon (glucagonoma), or adrenaline (phaeochromocytoma).

Diagnostic emphasis has been based on blood glucose levels, and in addition to 'diabetes' a milder level of hyperglycaemia, denoted 'impaired glucose tolerance', has been defined by the World Health Organization (WHO) (Table 1). However, it is difficult to produce a single definition because of the different aetiologies and varying severity and manifestations of diabetes. The fundamental defect is in insulin secretion and/or action. In the classical young onset form of the disorder (type I), there is often near-total insulin deficiency, with inevitable widespread metabolic changes. In the older age onset form (type II), there is diminished and/or delayed insulin secretion in response to glucose combined with varying degrees of diminished effectiveness of circulating insulin. When there is associated obesity, insulin resistance predominates. Therefore diabetes can be seen as a state of diminished insulin action due to its decreased availability or effectiveness in varying combinations.

Arguments can be advanced in favour of the term impaired glucose tolerance rather than 'chemical diabetes', to distinguish hyperglycaemia without clinical symptoms or signs from more severe

Table 1 Degrees of hyperglycaemia

Mild	Moderate	Severe
Impaired glucose and insulin control (sophisticated tests necessary)	Impaired glucose tolerance (WHO) (temporary or permanent)	Diabetes mellitus (WHO) (temporary or permanent)
	Chemical diabetes	Clinical diabetes
		Liability to retinopathy and nephropathy
	Increased risk of ischaemic heart disease	More pronounced risk of ischaemic heart disease

hyperglycaemia with symptoms and/or signs. The former is a mild version of the diabetic defect, whether progressive or not; 2 to 5 per cent of those so classified do advance to 'diabetic' (WHO) glucose levels annually. Hence, although few subjects with impaired glucose tolerance initially show typical forms of diabetic tissue damage, many do so later as they progress to higher glucose levels.

Diagnosis

Diagnosis depends on measurement of glucose levels in the blood. Glucose tolerance testing was introduced when the measurement of blood glucose was much less accurate than it is today. It involves measuring the rise and subsequent fall of blood glucose values after drinking 75 g of glucose dissolved in water within 10 min. Venous or capillary blood glucose is measured every 30 min from the start of the drink for 2 to 2.5 h (the defining glucose values vary according to which type of sample is used). The 2 h value is generally the most informative, and the test is often performed with just initial overnight fasting and the 2 h values. Indeed, with precise blood glucose measurement, the fasting value alone is very indicative of glucose tolerance.

When the symptoms are clear cut, random or fasting glucose levels will be notably raised and diagnostic. The exact defining levels are a matter of opinion and vary from time to time. It is most useful to give the recommendations from the current World Health Organization paper (1988) (Table 2); although this differs from the 'in place' WHO 1985 statement, it has important similarities (but some differences) from the American Diabetes Association's 1997 suggestions. Basically, the threshold for diagnosis has been lowered, and the abnormal zone between normality and the threshold for impaired glucose tolerance recognized as at least potentially pathological.

The differences between plasma and whole-blood glucose concentrations, and between capillary and venous levels, are too often ignored. Whole-blood values are about 10 to 15 per cent lower than those of plasma, and capillary values are 7 per cent higher than venous values in the fasting state and 8 per cent higher after a glucose load. These differences are important because clinical laboratories may use venous plasma whereas bedside monitoring techniques use capillary whole blood or plasma.

Glucose levels vary with nutritional state and are raised by infection, sterile inflammation, psychological upset, and medicaments such as glucocorticoids or thiazide-type diuretics and adrenergic β-blockers impair glucose tolerance.

The hyperglycaemic exposure associated with diabetic microangiopathy seems higher than that associated with macroangiopathy. Table 3 lists the important types of diabetic tissue damage. Different types may interact, for instance in the aetiology of diabetic foot ulcers to which poor arterial supply (macroangiopathy), diseased small blood vessels (microangiopathy), loss of feeling from sensory neuropathy, and disordered regulation of blood flow in small vessels owing to autonomic neuropathy all contribute, together with abnormality of the connective tissue collagen. Similarly, in the ischaemic heart disease of diabetes, abnormal cardiac collagen, autonomic neuropathy, and microangiopathy of the vasa vasorum may all add to the effects of the dominant lesion of coronary arteriosclerosis.

The disease processes of diabetes

Type I diabetes (once termed juvenile onset) is the result of an autoimmune destruction of the islets of Langerhans. It typically presents before 30 years, but can occur at any age. Islet-cell antibodies are usually found in the plasma for a period of 1–2 years after diagnosis, but in a minority (perhaps 20 per cent) these may persist. The latter (type Ib) are particularly liable to suffer other autoimmune diseases. Most type I patients are 'insulin dependent' because of the severe degree of β-cell destruction. Without insulin injection they will become ketoacidotic within days or a few weeks, lapse into coma, and die.

A variety of disease processes may give rise to the type II syndrome. Some patients with maturity-type onset diabetes of the young have a variety of abnormalities of the glucokinase gene, which is important in the metabolism of glucose in both hepatic and pancreatic β-cells. A few others with mild type II features secrete an abnormal insulin of reduced potency through an inherited error. There is also evidence that the pathogenesis of the majority of type II patients is influenced by deficient fetal nutrition, probably more often resulting from placental deficiencies than from maternal malnutrition affecting the development of β-cell function. This hypothesis is based on the demonstration of increased risk of ischaemic heart disease, hypertension, hyperlipidaemia, and impaired glucose tolerance or diabetes around the age of 60 years in those with a small birth weight. These data call into question the extent of the genetic contribution to the very strong concordance of type II diabetes among identical twins.

Perhaps because of an abnormality in insulin production or chronic elevated glucose levels, a very insoluble polymer derived from amylin forms between the β-cells. This amyloid deposit may well contribute to the islet destruction but is probably not the only mechanism of β-cell glucotoxicity.

Those born in the tropics, particularly India and East Africa, may show destruction of the islets of Langerhans resulting from an initially exocrine pancreatic lesion caused by multiple small calculi in the finer branches of the pancreatic duct; the whole process is known as tropical fibrocalculous disease and can cause great weight loss or stunted development. Thus, although clearly distinct in the exact lesion, it has similarities with diabetes secondary to acute or chronic pancreatitis in developed countries.

Malnutrition may influence the expression of several types of diabetes, but is not thought a fundamental causative factor (except perhaps to the fetus or perinate). Hence, WHO suggests that 'malnutrition' and 'protein-deficient' diabetes be no longer recognized as special entities.

Classification

Two classifications have appeared in recent years. The first separates type I primary diabetes from type II and secondary diabetes, while

Table 2 Values for diagnosis of diabetes mellitus and other categories of hyperglycaemia

	Glucose concentration (mmol/l (mg dl))		
	Whole blood		Plasma[a]
	Venous	Capillary	Venous
Diabetes mellitus			
Fasting	≥6.1 (≥110)	≥6.1 (≥110)	≥7.0 (≥126)
Or			
2-h post glucose load	≥10.0 (≥180)	≥11.1 (≥200)	≥11.1 (≥200)
or both			
Impaired glucose tolerance (IGT)			
Fasting concentration (if measured)	<6.1 (<110)	<6.1 (<110)	<7.0 (<126)
And			
2-h post glucose load	≥6.7 (≥120) and <10.0 (<180)	≥7.8 (≥140) and <11.1 (<200)	≥7.8 (≥140) and <11.1 (<200)
Impaired fasting glycaemia (IFG)			
Fasting	≥5.6 (≥100) and <6.1 (<110)	≥5.6 (≥100) and <6.1 (<110)	≥6.1 (≥110) and <7.0 (<126)
2-h (if measured)	<6.7 (<120)	<7.8 (<140)	<7.8 (<140)

[a] Corresponding values for capillary plasma are: for diabetes mellitus, fasting ≥7.0 (≥1226), 2-h ≥12.2 (≥220); for impaired glucose tolerance fasting <7.0 (<126) and 2-h ≥8.9 (≥160) and <12.2 (<220); and for impaired fasting glycaemica ≥6.1 (≥110) and <7.0 (<126) and if measured 2-h <8.9 (<160).

For epidemiological or population screening purposes, the fasting or 2-h value after 75 g oral glucose may be used alone. For clinical purposes the diagnosis of diabetes should always be confirmed by repeating the test on another day unless there is unequivocal hyperglycaemia with a metabolic decompensation or obvious symptoms. Glucose concentrations should not be determined on serum unless red cells are immediately removed, otherwise glycolysis will result in unpredictable under-estimation of the true concentrations. It should be stressed that glucose preservatives do not totally prevent glycolysis. If warm blood is used, the sample shuld be kept at 0–4°C or centrifuged immediately, or assayed immediately.

Table 3 Types of diabetic tissue damage

Microangiopathy (particularly retina, kidneys)
Macroangiopathy (accelerated arteriosclerosis (distally), e.g. ischaemic heart disease, cerebrovascular disease, intermittent claudication or gangrene of feet)
Neuropathy (autonomic, sensory, motor)
Ocular cataracts
Inelastic collagen (e.g. Dupuytren's contractures)

the second separates insulin-dependent diabetes (IDDM) from non-insulin-dependent diabetes (NIDDM) (see Table 4).

These classifications have different aims. It is insidiously easy to equate, for instance, type I diabetes with IDDM. Although many patients fall into both categories, others belong to one only. The type I-type II classification attempts to assign a pathogenetic mechanism although the two mechanisms may not be mutually exclusive. People can be afflicted very severely or very mildly by either. Different degrees of severity of type I diabetes range from a classic ketoacidosis-prone patient dependent upon daily injections of insulin to, much less commonly, a type I subject (also afflicted by autoimmune damage to islet cells) with mildly raised fasting plasma glucose but no glycosuria. This second subject at this stage is not liable to ketoacidosis and so would be classified as having NIDDM.

The IDDM-NIDDM classification applies to the metabolic state of a subject at one instant, and can change with time. Thus the second subject described above could well progress from NIDDM to IDDM. During this progression there could be a phase without risk of ketoacidosis although treated by insulin. He would then be in the not uncommon state of a subject with NIDDM who is treated with insulin. This conjunction is much more common among type II patients, where the proportion given insulin varies considerably from country to country (and from clinic to clinic).

The clinical characteristics and markers for types I and II diabetes are given in Table 4. None is absolute, and there is much debate as to whether pathogenesis is the same in most type II patients. The natural history of the Type II clinical condition in the young often does not resemble that of 'classical' type II diabetes; hyperglycaemia does not increase as rapidly as might be expected, and probably as a consequence patients are relatively immune from microangiopathic and neuropathic tissue damage. Some of these patients have an abnormality of the glucokinase gene, and are now best considered separately, with other recognized genetic defects (Tables 5 and 6). Other rare subsets depend on genetically dependent flaws in insulin synthesis, which result in the production of weakly active insulin, or inherited abnormalities of the insulin receptor.

In Tables, 5, 6, and 7 we present the new WHO proposals for classification of the diabetic (hyperglycaemic) states, many previously regarded as secondary diabetes, including a number of inherited syndromes, ranging from DIDMOAD (diabetes insipidus, diabetes mellitus, optic atrophy, and deafness) via the progeria of Werner's syndrome to the obesity usual in both the Laurence-Moon-Biedl and Prader-Willi syndromes. It is suspected that in conditions with abnormal connective tissue (for example Werner's syndrome and ataxia telangiectasia) there may be abnormalities involving interaction between insulin and insulin-like growth factors and/or their receptors. Diabetes (usually IDDM) may also accompany the various mitochondrial myopathy syndromes, as may a variety of other endocrine defects.

Diabetes, or often just impaired glucose tolerance, has been associated with a variety of neurological or muscular diseases (for example motor neurone disease and dystrophia myotonica), at least when they are severe. This may be a consequence of the associated marked muscular wasting.

Table 4 Simplified classification of diabetes mellitus and kindred states

Type	Alternative name	Clinical characteristics	Aetiological features
Ia	Insulin-dependent diabetes (IDDM) Juvenile onset diabetes Ketosis-prone diabetes	In early phase retain some endogenous insulin secretion and may have honeymoon phase Later have no endogenous insulin Develop ketoacidosis when insulin withdrawn or with stress states Mostly young, often markedly thin at diagnosis	(i) Association with HLA types (e.g. DR3, DR4) (ii) Generally cytoplasmic and complement-fixing islet cell antibody positive at diagnosis but later becomes negative
Ib	As for type Ia	Higher percentage of females and older age of onset than type Ia	Also: (i) Close association with other autoimmune endocrinopathies (ii) Persistent islet cell antibodies (iii) Presumed autoimmune aetiology
II (non-obese)	Non-insulin-dependent diabetes (NIDDM) Maturity onset diabetes of the young, now non-insulin-dependent known as diabetes of the young	Always measurable insulin present Tendency to insulin resistance Ketosis not provoked by insulin withdrawal but may become ketoacidotic with severe illness Onset usual above age of 40	(i) Heterogeneous aetiologies (ii) Familial aggregation (iii) Environmental factors
II (obese)	As for type II (non-obese)	Hyperinsulinaemic and insulin resistant Rarely if ever ketotic	(i) Related to obesity (ii) Glucose tolerance often normal after weight lost (iii) Probably different aetiology from type II (non-obese)
III	Malnutrition-related diabetes Tropical diabetes J-type K-type Z-type	Often underweight with history of malnutrition Mostly restricted to tropical countries and non-caucasians May have severe insulin resistance Often associated with exocrine malfunction and pancreatic fibrocalculous disease Endogenous insulin secretion intermediate between types I and II	Alcohol may be important Malnutrition and cassava consumption also implicated (Z-type)
Other types- Secondary diabetes Pancreatic disease		Pancreatectomized subjects are insulin dependent	Chronic pancreatitis Pancreatic calcification Pancreatomy
Hormonal		Obvious signs of steroid excess Associated with skin rash Diabetes mild Obvious signs and symptoms of particular hormone excess	(i) Corticosteroid excess (exogenous or endogenous) (ii) Glucagonomas (iii) Acromegaly (iv) Thyrotoxicosis (v) Phaeochromocytoma (vi) ?Hypothalamic lesions
Drug-induced			(i) Diuretics (ii) Catecholaminergic agents, e.g. salbutamol
Insulin-receptor abnormalities			(i) Congenital lipodystrophy (ii) Associated with acanthosis nigrans (iii) Autoimmune insulin receptor antibodies

Table 4 *continued*

Type	Alternative name	Clinical characteristics	Aetiological features
Genetic syndromes			Glycogen storage disease Ataxia telangiectasia DIDMOAD syndrome Huntingdon's chorea Laurence-Moon-Biedl syndrome Werner's syndrome Prader-Willi syndrome
Impaired glucose tolerance	Asymptomatic diabetes Borderline diabetes Chemical diabetes Latent diabetes Subclinical diabetes	Increased risk of macrovascular disease and of later diabetes Likely to be obese	Mild glucose intolerance from any cause
Gestational diabetes		Diagnosis as for IGT or more severe forms of glucose intolerance	Pregnancy: normal glucose tolerance test beforehand but may have been abnormal in previous pregnancy
Potential abnormality of glucose tolerance	Prediabetes	Strong family history Mother of big baby	

Table 5 Aetiological classification of disorders of glycaemia[a]

Type 1 (beta-cell destruction, usually leading to absolute insulin deficiency) Autoimmune Idiopathic
Type 2 (may range from predominantly insulin resistance with relative insulin deficiency to a predominantly secretory defect with or without insulin resistance)
Other specific types (see Table 3) Genetic defects of beta-cell function Genetic defects in insulin action or structure Diseases of the exocrine pancreas Endocrinopathies Drug- or chemical-induced Infections Uncommon forms of immune-mediated diabetes Other genetic syndromes sometimes associated with diabetes
Gestational diabetes[b]

[a] As additional subtypes are discovered it is anticipated that they will be reclassified within their own specific category.

[b] Includes the former categories of gestational impaired glucose tolerance and gestational diabetes.

Presenting features

The classic symptoms of hyperglycaemia are polyuria, thirst, weight loss, and lassitude. Weight loss may be severe in patients with IDDM, and in type II diabetes it is often substantial even though the patient is still obese. Pruritus vulvae is a frequent symptom in women. Balanitis, sometimes causing paraphimosis, is much less common but can be severe. Other non-specific symptoms are the appearance or exacerbation of cramp in the calves or feet, and tingling in the fingers. Some complain of a loss of appetite, but others develop a craving, particularly for sweet foods. Occasionally, crystallized glucose can be seen as white spots on the shoes of elderly males. Patients are often constipated, and develop a change in lens refraction which causes visual blurring.

Pathognomic types of tissue damage, such as background diabetic retinopathy (see Plate 2, The eye and disease), or associated clinical findings, such as cardiac infarction or cataract, may lead to detection of hyperglycaemia in neglected or imperceptive subjects.

Pathogenesis

Type I diabetes mellitus

Immune mechanisms

Type I diabetes results from immunologically mediated damage to the β-cells in the pancreas. This process may occur over many years and probably results from environmental influences in genetically susceptible individuals.

Lymphocyte infiltration of islets has been seen in postmortem material obtained early in the disease. Most type I patients have circulating autoantibodies to β-cell antigens, including insulin and glutamic acid decarboxylase, as well as anti-islet-cell antibodies. Lymphocyte subsets in peripheral blood are altered in patients with type I diabetes. At a genetic level, HLA alleles are also implicated, providing further evidence that they are responsible for activating the immune response to specific peptides (and hence are labelled immune response genes).

There has been much speculation about the possible role of a viral pathogen in the immune response. Seasonal variation in frequency and young age of onset are consistent. Coxsackie and mumps viruses are two candidates, but many others, including retroviruses, have been implicated. Because of the potentially long natural history of β-cell damage (up to 10 years), observations at the time of endstage β-cell failure are unlikely to reveal useful information about an initiating role of such infectious pathogens.

Genetic susceptibility

Susceptibility to type I diabetes has a substantial genetic component. The disease runs in families, with sibling risk of developing the disease

Table 6 Other specific types of diabetes

Genetic defects of beta-cell function	Endocrinopathies
• Chromosome 20, HNF4α (MODY1) • Chromosome 7, glucokinase (MODY2) • Chromosome 12, HNF1α (MODY3) • Chromosome 13, IPF-1 (MODY4) • Mitochondrial DNA 3243 mutation • Others	• Cushing's syndrome • Acromegaly • Phaeochromocytoma • Glucagonoma • Hyperthyroidism • Somatostatinoma • Others
Genetic defects in insulin action	***Drug- or chemical-induced***
• Type A insulin resistance • Leprechaunism • Rabson-Mendenhall syndrome • Lipoatrophic diabetes • Others	(see Table 4)
	Infections
	• Congenital rubella • Cytomegalovirus • Others
Diseases of the exocrine pancreas	***Uncommon forms of immune-medicated diabetes***
• Fibrocalculous pancreatopathy • Pancreatis • Trauma/pancreatectomy • Neoplasia • Cystic fibrosis • Haemochromatosis • Others	• Insulin autoimmune syndrome • (antibodies to insulin) • Anti-insulin receptor antibodies • 'Stiff man' syndrome • Others
	Other genetic syndromes
	(see Table 5)

Table 7 Other genetic syndromes sometimes associated with diabetes

Down's syndrome
Friedreich's ataxia
Huntington's chorea
Klinefelter's syndrome
Lawrence-Moon-Biedl syndrome
Myotonic dystrophy
Porphyria
Prader-Willi syndrome
Turner's syndrome
Wolfram's syndrome
Others

substantially greater than in the normal population (6 per cent versus 0.4 per cent), but the pattern of inheritance is complex. Twin studies suggest that approximately one-third of susceptibility is genetic, but do not consider contributions from somatic genetic events that may differ in twins, including T-cell receptor and immunoglobulin genes, nor do they account for shared environment, perhaps particularly intrauterine or immediately postnatal.

The complex pattern of inheritance, the relatively high frequency of non-familial disease, and the increasingly rapid reduction in risk for first-, second-, and third-degree relatives all suggest that multiple loci are involved. Two loci encoding susceptibility have been defined, HLA and insulin (INS), although together these account for no more than 30 per cent of total genetic susceptibility. HLA has by far the largest effect defined to date, with the risk to siblings rising to 12 per cent if they are HLA identical. Of the 15-fold increase in relative risk in siblings, approximately 25 per cent is accounted for by HLA alone. INS contributes less to the genetic susceptibility; in some populations this effect is predominant in individuals with HLA DR4.

HLA was originally implicated with the locus alleles B8 and B15. These were subsequently shown to be in strong linkage disequilibrium with alleles in the class II region that mediated disease susceptibility. Approximately 90 per cent of caucasian type I diabetics carry either HLA DR3 or DR4 specificities compared with 45 per cent of the general population. There is a pronounced heterozygous effect, whereby DR3 and DR4 heterozygotes have an increased susceptibility compared with DR3,3 or DR4,4 homozygotes. Other HLA haplotypes (DR1, DR8, and DR5) give a more modest susceptibility. Protection is provided by the HLA-DR2 haplotype.

Identification of the precise molecular basis of HLA-mediated susceptibility has been hampered by strong linkage disequilibrium across the region. Evidence of a role for HLA-DQ molecules was provided by the correlation between the disease and HLA-DQ sequences at position 57 of the β-chain. This correlation, as well as similar correlations with α-chain sequences, provides evidence that the structural context of the DQ binding site usually dictates the HLA-mediated disease susceptibility. However, this correlation is not valid in all ethnic populations. Other evidence demonstrates an important role for HLA DR alleles in determining susceptibility. HLA-DR and HLA-DQ effects together account for the majority of HLA-mediated disease susceptibility.

The INS locus on chromosome 11p is flanked on the upstream side by a multiple repeat of 14 base pairs. Variations in the length of this repeat correlate with disease susceptibility. The shorter repeats are associated with the disease, and this region has been shown to be linked to familial disease. The short and long repeat classes are in tight linkage disequilibrium with a set with 10 single-base-pair polymorphisms within and adjacent to the INS locus. The mechanism of this disease susceptibility has not been clearly defined, but is likely to depend on variations in INS gene regulation.

Epidemiology

The worldwide incidence of type I diabetes varies greatly. In some Scandinavian countries it is as high as 35 per 100 000 per year, while in Japan it is only 2 per 100 000 per year. The disease is predominantly one of white Caucasian populations and is relatively rare in both oriental and black populations. Accurate data for Africa are unavailable, but the risk is possibly less than 3 per 100 000 per year. The high incidences in Scandinavia and the UK contrast with much lower ones in France and Italy. An environmental factor which varies with latitude has been suggested, but several exceptions argue strongly against it. Figures in Sardinia are similar to those in Scandinavia, while the incidence in Iceland is closer to the usual Mediterranean figures. The incidence in Estonia which is ethnically extremely similar to the Finns, is approximately one-third of that seen in Finland. These figures argue against a gradient of disease from north to south in Europe, but they are not easily explained by either genetic or environmental factors alone.

Migration studies suggest that environmental factors play a substantial role in the geographical variation of disease incidence.

Environmental factors

Twin data support environmental factors as the main influences on susceptibility, although no individual contributor has yet been identified. The possible role of viruses is mentioned above, but perhaps the only viral infection with a definite link is congenital rubella. Type I diabetes is commoner in individuals who have suffered from congenital rubella, as are other autoimmune disorders such as thyroid and Addison's disease. Rubella-associated diabetes is found predominantly in populations with the same HLA susceptibility alleles as non-rubella-associated diabetes and is associated with the same immunological abnormalities.

Toxins have been suggested but the evidence is unconvincing. *N*-nitroso derivatives are known to destroy β-cells, and some have been directly implicated in both neurotoxicity and diabetes after fatal poisoning. Nitrates and nitroso compounds in the diet have also been suggested.

Exposure to cow's milk in early life is a third factor which has been much debated. It has been suggested that the rising incidence of the disease may correlate with the declining prevalence of breast-feeding, but there are local anomalies. The most impressive data show that patients with type I diabetes have antibodies to cow's milk albumin that react to a β-cell surface protein.

Type II diabetes mellitus

The apparent prevalence varies with the thoroughness of testing, particularly in the proportion of the elderly that are tested. When the WHO definition is used, it may be as high as 40–50 per cent in some populations of Polynesian–Micronesian stock. The prevalence in the UK was once believed to be 2 per cent of the population, but recent studies suggest values of 8 to 12 per cent, depending on ethnic mix. Patients typically present between 50 and 65 years of age, but may be as young as 15 to 20 years or of any age above 65.

There are four major hypotheses (not mutually exclusive) for pathogenesis.

Genetic

Evidence for genetic influence is based on familial incidence, supported by identical twin studies, with concordance varying from below 60 to above 85 per cent, although the interpretation of these results is questionable (see below). A substantial number of genetic abnormalities have been linked with type II diabetes, involving genes with products of metabolic importance (for example glucokinase variants, glycogen synthetase variants) or hormonal importance (for example, abnormal insulin, gross increase in the proinsulin to insulin ratio), or genes with an unknown product, (for example mitochondrial DNA deletions and duplications). The last category often show maternal inheritance. The mitochondrial defects may be more common than yet realized because there is more mutant mitochondrial DNA in muscle, which is a relatively non-dividing tissue, than in peripheral blood cells, but the latter have been studied much more. Clinically, the diabetes associated with mitochondrial DNA abnormalities may be linked with myopathy or deafness and is associated with an A to G mutation in position 3243 of leucine tRNA. This appears to interfere with the synthesis of leucine tRNA and also with its ability to bind a transcription termination factor. This mutation appears quite common in a large set of families, particularly those with some evidence of sensory hearing disturbance.

These genetic defects are not be a good model for the majority of Type II patients because their hyperglycaemia often presents at a relatively young age and is relatively non-progressive. Again, many of these patients are not obese, unlike the majority of type II patients.

If there is a genetic cause for the overweight majority, it would seem to be multifactorial. Candidate genes might contribute to either insulin resistance or insulin deficiency. In both cases functional mutations have been identified that account for the disease phenotype in a small number of patients. The major genes, accounting for larger subsets of the population, remain to be identified. The disease displays substantial genetic heterogeneity, and hence characterization of some of the genetic factors responsible is likely to be extremely difficult.

The existence of ethnic populations with an extremely high prevalence of the disease (Pima Indians or Nauruans) suggests that genetic polymorphisms may have been selected in these populations to allow them to have adapted to survive more effectively during earlier periods of prolonged food scarcity. Subsequent exposure of such populations to Western diets might leave them at a substantial metabolic disadvantage in coping with the high-carbohydrate high-fat diets of the developed world.

The first mutations to be associated with type II diabetes were those of the insulin receptor gene. Several specific syndromes exist where extreme insulin resistance is evident. Leprechaunism is a congenital disorder associated with glucose intolerance and extremely high insulin levels. The Rabson–Mendenhall syndrome is associated with insulin resistance, acanthosis nigricans, ectodermal abnormalities (teeth and nails), and pineal hyperplasia. Type A insulin resistance, which is a syndrome consisting of insulin resistance, acanthosis nigricans, and hyperandrogenism, is commoner in females. These patients all have impaired glucose tolerance associated with hyperinsulinaemia. All these syndromes are associated with mutations in the insulin receptor gene including non-sense mutations, deletions, splicing defects, and single-base-pair substitutions. They may result in defects in receptor synthesis, receptor transport, insulin binding, transmembrane signalling, or receptor recycling. In some cases these mutations correlate specifically with the type and severity of insulin resistance seen.

Severe forms of insulin resistance are associated with homozygocity for insulin receptor mutations, but heterozygous patients occasionally have more modest degrees of insulin resistance consistent with a diagnosis of type II diabetes. The frequency of insulin receptor mutations in the population is unknown. Based on the incidence of leprechaunism, at least 0.1 per cent of the population are heterozygous for insulin receptor mutations, and this figure may be as much as 10 times higher. However, even this higher figure suggests that insulin receptor mutations are more important in the rare syndromes of severe insulin resistance than in the commoner forms of type II diabetes.

Patterns of type II diabetes that are consistent with a dominant mode of inheritance have been known since the description of maturity onset diabetes of the young (MODY). This disorder is characterized by early onset of mild hyperglycaemia in families associated with three different single gene defects for MODY 1, 2, and 3. Large family pedigrees have been useful in identifying other genetic factors. The first such localization revealed a linkage to the regions surrounding the adenine deaminase locus on chromosome 20, a locus important in only a small subset of pedigrees with Type II diabetes of the young. The glucokinase locus has been shown to be an important factor in approximately half such pedigrees. The mutations in glucokinase cluster round the active side of the molecule where glucose is bound. They are found predominantly in pedigrees with maturity-type onset diabetes of the young, but occasionally families with more conventional type II diabetes have such mutations, and association studies have suggested that mutations may be associated with the disease in black and Creole populations. The overall contribution of glucokinase mutations to type II diabetes is unlikely to account for more than 1 per cent of the disease.

Adaptation to early environment

If the genetic structure is important, so is the expression of those genes. The great majority of cell divisions occur in early life, and habitual patterns of gene expression or physiological function may be established according to the environment at that time. These considerations accord with observations by Barker and colleagues that hyperglycaemia at the age of about 60 years is commoner in those with lower birthweights, and that low birthweight (or low weight at the age of 1 year) is associated with both lower insulin and 32–33 split proinsulin levels, particularly during an oral glucose tolerance test, and decreased insulin sensitivity. It is possible that those who have been exposed to prenatal and perinatal metabolic deprivation grow and function differently and so are more liable to the ill effects of excess food in adult life.

Pancreatic amyloid

Deposits of amylin or islet amyloid polypeptide are found outside the surviving β-cells of the morbid islet in Type II diabetes and may be concentrated near the islet's small blood vessels. Amylin is also present within lysosomes of β-cells and damages β-cells where its spiky projections abut them. Amylin is secreted from β-cells together with insulin. It has been detected in plasma, but at levels about two orders of magnitude below those at which disturbed muscle metabolism with insulin insensitivity has been reported in animals following its injection. There is stronger evidence that it has a paracrine influence within the islets, inhibiting insulin secretion. One hypothesis is that if amylin is secreted to excess (or differs in fine structure), it may polymerize in the intercellular spaces of the islets. Amylin is a vasodilator with similarities to calcitonin-gene-related polypeptide, and therefore could influence islet blood flow. It remains to be demonstrated whether islet amyloid deposits are primary or secondary influences in β-cell failure in type II diabetes.

β-Cell overstimulation

When β-cells are strongly stimulated for any length of time they secrete more proinsulin per unit insulin secreted. It has been suggested that this disturbance, possibly allied to a constitutional abnormality in the cellular processing of proinsulin, damages β-cells. The overstimulation is ascribed to the excess food intake that must have occurred during the development of obesity in typical type II patients. The crucial question is whether obesity precedes glucose/insulin disturbance or whether the basic abnormality itself generates obesity.

Metabolic basis of diabetes mellitus

The intermediary metabolism of carbohydrate, fat, and protein substrates is disturbed in diabetes. The osmotic diuresis of glycosuria carries sodium, potassium, calcium, and magnesium out of the body, so that mineral balance is also disturbed. However, the cationic loss is much greater if ketonuria is present because acetoacetate and 3-hydroxybutyrate are relatively strong acids for organic compounds, with $pK = 5.5$.

Carbohydrate metabolism

The organs most closely involved in blood glucose control are the liver, the pancreas, and muscle. Disease of any of these may impair glucose tolerance, but sustained hyperglycaemia always implies some failure of insulin secretion whose main action in this respect is the inhibition of hepatic glucose release and of gluconeogenesis.

The liver takes up excess glucose from the gut and stores it as glycogen or uses the acetyl-CoA resulting from oxidation cellular for fatty acid synthesis. This increases hepatic triacylglycerides and other lipids, and these will later be released as low density lipoproteins and cholesterol esters. When blood glucose drops the liver releases glucose, in the short term by glycogenolysis to glucose 6-phosphate and hence glucose, but in the longer term from gluconeogenesis and the sparing of hepatic carbohydrate by using triacylglycerides as the principal source of hepatic acetyl-CoA for energy. The substrates for gluconeogenesis are lactate, glycerol, and amino acids. Lactate comes principally from skeletal and cardiac muscle and from the gut. It is released during any muscular exercise in which the work rate exceeds the available oxygen and so anaerobic metabolism supports activity. It may also be released, perhaps initally as pyruvate, whenever the rate of glucose uptake is very high. Glycerol is released from adipose tissue during lipolysis, while amino acids leave muscle during fasting. Alanine can be considered as 'aminated lactate', taken up by muscle in the digestive phase in excess of its needs and released later to be deaminated in the liver. The amino acids fall into two main groups, glucogenic (for example alanine, glutamate, aspartate) and ketogenic (for example valine, leucine), depending upon whether the carbon skeleton remaining after deamination is converted into 3-C pyruvate or a 4-C ketoacid. When there is gross insulin deficiency, net protein degradation in muscle increases markedly and the plasma concentration of all the amino acids rises.

Hepatic gluconeogenesis occurs from phosphoenol pyruvate, generated via malate but not directly from acetyl-CoA. Hence non-esterified fatty acids are not net substrates for gluconeogenesis, while the 3C compounds are.

Glycaemia is also affected by the rate of glucose removal in the periphery. This may or may not be insulin dependent. Insulin-independent uptake comprises uptake into insulin-insensitive tissue, and that component of increased uptake into insulin-sensitive tissue that results from hyperglycaemia rather than hyperinsulinaemia. This last division is artificial in health because a high glucose concentration should be accompanied by a high insulin level. However, in a typical inadequately controlled but not acutely ill diabetic patient, the rate of peripheral glucose disposal is approximately normal because the increased uptake due to hyperglycaemia balances the effects of reduced insulin action. The potential of insulin for effective action is much less when blood glucose is either very high or very low than it is around the usual levels of 3.5–6 mmol/l because of the steep rise of insulin levels over that range of the dose-response curve (Fig. 1).

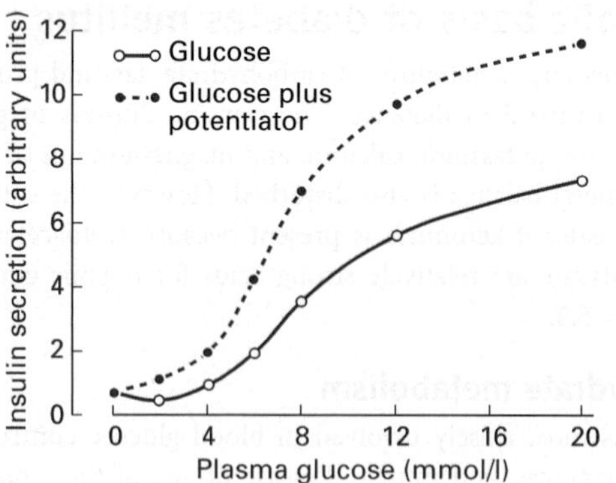

Fig. 1 Dose-response curve of plasma glucose and insulin secretion.

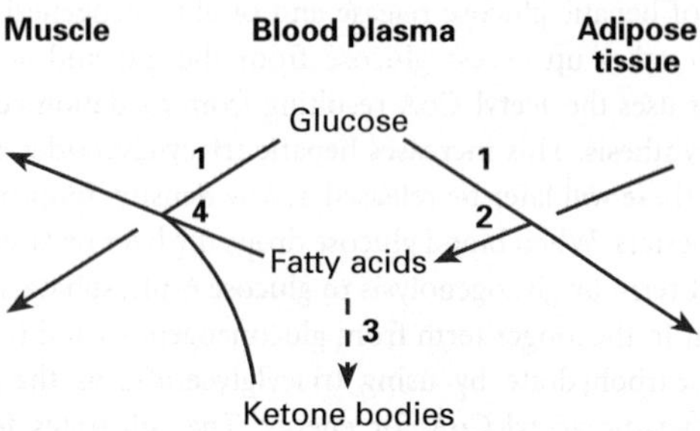

Fig. 2 Glucose fatty-acid cycle, blood phase. 1. Uptake of glucose by muscle and adipose tissue. 2. Release of fatty acids from adipose tissue to plasma albumin. 3. Formation of ketone bodies from fatty acids by liver. 4. Uptake of fatty acids and ketone bodies by muscle.

The rate of glucose disposal is also affected by the plasma levels of non-esterified fatty acids in that their cellular uptake depends on their plasma concentration. High concentrations inhibit the uptake of glucose. These properties are the basis of the glucose–fatty acids cycle (Fig. 2), which somehow reflects the competition for the hydrogen from these substrates to combine with oxygen.

The low insulin levels of the fasting state allow a steady release of glucose to sustain normoglycaemia. They also allow steady release of non-esterified fatty acids from adipose tissue via hormone-sensitive lipase activity, and in the fasting resting state these acids are the main body fuel with the respiratory quotient RQ around 0.7. Any sudden increased activity will be supported by muscle glycogen. Increased gluconeogenesis, and hepatic glucose release, are then necessary to sustain exercise, particularly the capacity to sprint. Intramuscular lipolysis of triacylglycerides may also be useful. A plasma insulin concentration of only 10–20 mU/l is adequate for the effective restraint of lipolysis and hepatic glucose release, in contrast with the 100–200 mU/l required for the maximum uptake of glucose by skeletal muscle.

Lipid metabolism

Normal lipid metabolism is discussed in Chapter 6.11.

Insulin is important in lipid metabolism because it activates adipose tissue lipoprotein lipase and inhibits adipocyte-hormone-sensitive lipase. Deficient insulin action has two effects on the adipose tissue: first, impaired degradation of both chylomicra and VLDL particles with an increase in the remnant chylomicra and large VLDL particles: second, through decreased inhibition of hormone-sensitive lipase, there is an increased flux of non-esterified fatty acids to the liver as a potential source of hepatic cell triacylglyceride, and of both VLDL and ketone bodies leaving the liver. Hence diabetics show high VLDL levels, and less abnormality in cholesterol than in triglyceride concentrations. HDL cholesterol levels are reduced but, like the raised VLDL levels, return towards normal with improved glycaemic control. LDL levels are usually normal, although they tend to increase with gross hyperglycaemia.

Insulin biosynthesis

Insulin is synthesized in the β-cells of the islets of Langerhans, initially on the rough endoplasmic reticulum as a large precursor, preproinsulin, of molecular weight 11 500 Da. This has a very short half-life, for it is split almost immediately to yield a long polypeptide chain, proinsulin, of molecular weight 9000 Da, which is held in an overlapping circle by two disulphide bridges. At the Golgi apparatus the proinsulin is packed into granules surrounded by a single membrane layer. The connecting or C-peptide part of the molecule is then split off, but not always cleanly; indeed, an appreciable amount of 32–33 split proinsulin is found in plasma. The characteristic double chain of insulin, C-peptide, and such split products remain in the granule, where a small amount of proinsulin is also found. The β-cell granules migrate via the microtubular-microfilamentary system from the Golgi apparatus to the cell surface where the vesicular membrane fuses with the outer cell membrane to discharge C-peptide in a 1:1 ratio with insulin together with small amounts of proinsulin and its split products. Perhaps 10–15 per cent of insulin leaves the cell via another constitutive pathway which does not involve a secretory granule and in which the ratio of proinsulin (intact or split) to insulin may not be the same as in the secretory pathway.

When a β-cell has not been strongly stimulated for some time, there are many secretory vesicles close to the cell membrane at its secretory pole. Discharge of these can permit a large first-phase secretion in response to a strong stimulus. When the cell is continuously stimulated it takes 90 to 120 min for newly synthesized preproinsulin to yield secreted insulin; meanwhile secretion is sustained by degradation of preproinsulin which has already been formed and movement of the products to the secretory surface. Such new synthesis presumably underlies the observations that, with time, β-cells respond more strongly to a given raised level of glucose than early in this prolonged second phase of secretion. Such persistent hyperglycaemia also increases the β-cell insulin response to other secretagogues, for example isoprenaline or gastrointestinal peptide.

The insulins of different species show remarkable similarities, with much cross-reaction of antibodies, although fish insulins are not neutralized by antibodies to bovine or porcine insulin.

Insulin secretion

Glucose is the prime stimulus and acts via generation of ATP, certainly through oxidative metabolism of the hexose, but possibly also via an active receptor on the cell surface. Other metabolites active in evoking secretion are glyceraldehyde phosphate, fructose 2,6-biphosphate, and branch chain amino acids and corresponding ketoacids. Stimulation leads to an increased outward flux of potassium through the voltage-sensitive potassium channel. This activates an inward movement of calcium to increase its cytosolic concentration which may also be raised by purely intracellular mechanisms. A variety of substances, for example gastrointestinal peptide and some prostaglandins, although not themselves strong stimuli to insulin secretion, potentiate the action of glucose or other direct stimuli (Table 8).

Table 8 Stimulators and inhibitors of insulin secretion

	Mechanism	Glucose required
Stimulators		
Glucose	?Glucoreceptor ?Metabolite ±Calcium shifts	
Glucagon	↑Cyclic AMP	+
Gut hormones (GIP)	↑Cyclic AMP	+
β-Adrenergic agents	↑Cyclic AMP	+
Prostaglandins	↑Cyclic AMP	+
Leucine	?Membrane effect ?Metabolite	–
Other amino acids (arginine)	?	+
Fatty acids	?	–
Ketone bodies	?	–
Acetylcholine	?Ca^{2-} shifts	–
Vagal stimulation		
Inhibitors		
α-Adrenergic agents	↓Cyclic AMP	–
Sympathetic nerve stimulation		
Dopamine	?Ca^{2-} shifts	–
Serotonin	?Ca^{2-} shifts	–
Somatostatin	?	

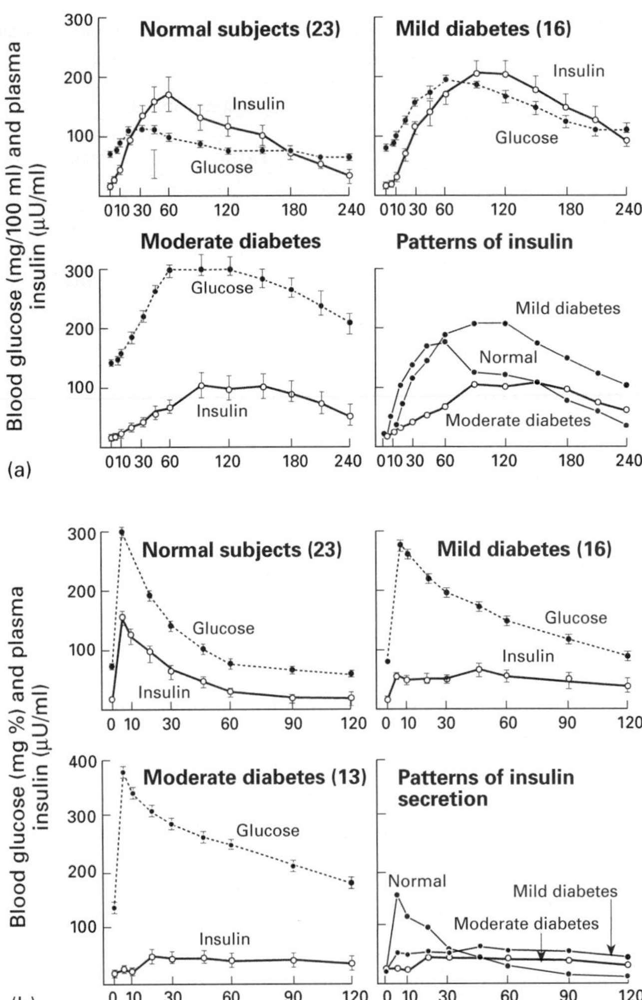

Fig. 3 (a) Oral glucose tolerance test (1.75 g/kg body weight), showing blood glucose and plasma insulin values for 4 h in non-diabetic healthy subjects and 'mild' and 'moderate' diabetics (fasting blood glucose below 11 mM). (b) Intravenous glucose tolerance tests (0.5 g/kg body weight injected over 5 min) for 2 h in the same people as in Fig. 4(a).
(Reproduced from Seltzer et al. (1967). Journal of Clinical Investigation, ***46****, 323, with permission.)*

The stimulatory action of sulphonylurea drugs depends on their binding to the voltage-sensitive potassium channel at a point distinct from ATP, with consequent activation of the channel. β-Adrenergic agents probably also act through the cyclic AMP mechanism, but both stimulatory acetylcholine and inhibitory dopamine and serotonin probably act more directly on the cytoplasmic calcium level. Another inhibitory agent is somatostatin which is secreted by the islet D-cells. There are probably other important paracrine influences within the islets, as yet little understood, because glucagon promotes insulin secretion, insulin may promote glucagon secretion, and somatostatin inhibits both.

Neural regulation of insulin secretion is active *in vivo*, with vagal action stimulatory, and adrenergic activity on balance inhibitory. Vagal discharge is probably responsible for the cephalic pre-first phase of insulin secretion which occurs when a meal is seen or smelt before any food has been ingested.

Secretion occurs in two phases. The first is fast, probably resulting from the release of granules already formed near the cell surface. If the stimulus is sustained, there is a subsequent slower second phase in which much of the insulin is newly synthesized. In humans the two phases are not seen clearly unless a constant stimulus is applied, as with a constant glucose infusion. Early in type II diabetes there is usually some diminution in the first phase and a slight delay in a sustained second phase, but a normal response to non-glucose stimulus such as arginine. In type I and more severe type II diabetes, the first phase is generally entirely absent, and in type I the second phase is greatly diminished and eventually disappears. Some of these features are illustrated in Fig. 3.

The earliest insulin secretion precedes ingestion which is followed by release of gut hormones and absorption of glucose. Together these cause a steady rise to peak after 45–60 min. Absorbed amino acids have a synergistic effect with that of glucose. As food absorption is completed, the stimulus to secretion falls and plasma levels return to baseline after 2–3 h.

In the fasting state basal insulin secretion is controlled in part by the plasma glucose concentration and in part by neuroregulation. In addition, as levels of non-esterified fatty acids and ketone bodies rise, there will be a slight increase in secretion which damps down lipolysis. Basal insulin secretion is crucial to the restraint of catabolism. It is normally phasic with a cycle length of about 13 min and a variability of 20 per cent of the mean value from trough to peak. A given amount of insulin has a greater effect if infused phasically rather than at a steady rate. Phasic secretion allows a higher concentration of insulin to reach the far end of each hepatic sinusoid intermittently.

Table 9 Plasma concentration of insulin and its precursors in normal subjects and those with glucose intolerance, all non-obese (approximate values for both fasting levels and those from an oral glucose tolerance test)

	Normal subjects			IGT subjects		
	Fasting	Peak	Peak time (min)	Fasting	Peak	Peak time (min)
Insulin						
Immuno-reactive						
mU/l	6	50	30	7	52	90
pmol/l	40	340	30	50	365	120
'True' 2 site immunoradio-metric (pm/l)	35	300	30	40	310	90–120
C-peptide (pmol/l)	500	1800	60	550	2000	120
Proinsulin (pmol/l)	4	14	120	6	23	120
32–33 split proinsulin (pmol/l)	3	7	120	3	18	120
Glucose (mmol/l)	4.5	8.5	60	6	10	90

It would require perhaps twice the secretory rate to achieve this concentration constantly because about half the insulin reaching the liver is cleared in one passage.

Insulin reaches the liver via the portal vein at a concentration three to ten times that in the systemic circulation. About 40 per cent is extracted in a single passage through the kidney, while smaller amounts are removed in the lung and by muscle. The half-life of insulin in the circulation is 4–5 min with a metabolic clearance rate of 1.2–1.4 l/min and an apparent distribution space of approximately 10–13 litres in people of average build.

C-peptide is secreted in equimolar amounts with insulin. It is not metabolized by the liver so that measurement in peripheral blood gives a better index of pancreatic β-cell function than does peripheral insulin measurement, with the reservation that, since C-peptide has a half-life of 20–35 min, it cannot be used to follow short-term changes. It is degraded and excreted by the kidney, and its use to assess insulin secretion requires precise analysis of its renal handling.

Table 9 gives typical values of the circulating concentrations of insulin and its related molecules in systemic venous blood, both after overnight fasting and in response to an oral glucose tolerance test.

The insulin receptor

Insulin binds to specific cell-surface receptors in fat, muscle, liver, and brain. The receptors are postulated to comprise a symmetric tetrameric complex of glycoproteins with a molecular weight of approximately 350–400 kDa. There are two subunits, each of 125 kDa, and two smaller subunits, each of 90 kDa, with disulphide linkages between them.

The receptors display 'negative co-operativity', a form of feedback control in which the affinity of unoccupied receptors for insulin decreases with increasing number of occupied receptors. They also down-regulate in number in the presence of hyperinsulinaemia, with the converse in hypoinsulinaemic states. The classical example of down-regulation is obesity. If such patients diet, there is an immediate increase in affinity followed by a slower increase in receptor number. Regulation of receptor number may be protective in obesity due to hyperphagia, when the resultant reduced response to insulin would limit triglyceride synthesis and deposition. However, a vicious circle can result, with more and more insulin secreted to overcome the fall in receptor number and activity. This imposes an unusually high work-load on the secretion of insulin by β-cells which can lead to cellular failure and damage.

After binding, the insulin receptor complex is internalized as a vesicle which fuses with lysosomes in which both insulin and the receptor are degraded.

The receptor acts as a protein kinase which is inactive when unoccupied but activated by the binding of insulin. This results in autophosphorylation of a tyrosine residue, which may be linked to the further phosphorylation of neighbouring proteins. Further steps in intracellular action are less certain, but some involve diacylglycerol and some various phosphatidylinositols.

Assay of insulin

Insulin antibodies used in immunoassay detect all compounds containing the epitope with which the antibody reacts. Several such substances may be present in plasma including some of the insulin precursor molecules. This may result in overestimation of the amount of true insulin present depending on the antibody used (Table 9).

Importance of metabolic control

The main aims of therapy for diabetics are to relieve symptoms of hyperglycaemia or hypoglycaemia and to prevent the long-term complications from tissue damage (Table 10).

There is now conclusive evidence that tight control of blood glucose, together with meticulous control of blood presure, can prevent or delay diabetic complications (UK Prospective Diabetes Study (UKPDS)).

Both the duration and degree of hyperglycaemia are important to the risk of developing tissue damage, but some patients—perhaps some 10 per cent of those with IDDMs—maintain markedly raised glucose levels for decades but none the less are free from clinically evident tissue damage. Others come within the usual targets for good glycaemic control but nevertheless develop severe complications. The former may go 40 years from diagnosis without clinical tissue damage. They are characterized by three features: they are not obese, they

Table 10 The chronic complications of diabetes

Complication	Possible causes
Macroangiopathy (arteriosclerosis, myocardial disease)	Hyperglycaemia Hyperlipidaemia Hyperinsulinaemia Smoking ?Increased growth hormone levels ?Platelet and other vascular factors
Microangiopathy (retinopathy, nephropathy, capillary basement membrane thickening)	Hyperglycaemia Protein (basement membrane) glycosylation Insulin deficiency
Neuropathy	Hyperglycaemia Sorbitol accumulation Deficient myoinositol Myelin glycosylation
Diabetic cataract	Hyperglycaemia Sorbitol accumulation Protein glycosylation
Collagen change	Glycosylation

have blood pressure on the low side of normal, and they have long-lived non-diabetic relatives.

Clearly other factors, probably genetic, in addition to hyperglycaemia are important in determining diabetic tissue damage. Relationships between blood pressure and liability to nephropathy or retinopathy, and to survival, have been found in many studies.

Subjects with impaired glucose tolerance show markedly increased liability to ischaemic heart disease, but not so much as known diabetics. This may reflect duration as well as severity of hyperglycaemia. Overall, studies have not shown such a clear relationship between glycaemia and liability to cardiac damage as has been found for retinopathy and nephropathy, perhaps because of greater interactions with other risk factors, such as hyperlipidaemia or hypertension.

Diabetics with proteinuria have a 10 times greater rate of death from cardiac disease than those without proteinuria, and there is also evidence of an increased risk for those with microalbuminuria compared with those with normal urinary albumin excretion.

In diabetic lesions in retina and kidney there appears to be an earlier phase depending on the degree of hyperglycaemic exposure and individual susceptibility, and a later phase in which tight glycaemic control does not significantly reduce the rate of deterioration. It may be that initial exposure to hyperglycaemia results in thickening of the basement membrane and increased permeability. In the later phase what is filtered through the damaged capillary walls may become critical. Diabetics have higher mean capillary pressures in extremities than non-diabetics; this could be another important determinant of progression of retinal and glomerular damage.

Practical consequences

Glycaemic control which is as near normal as possible should be instituted immediately after diagnosis and then maintained except under the following conditions.

1. Concomitant hypoglycaemic attacks seem more dangerous than the risk of future tissue damage.

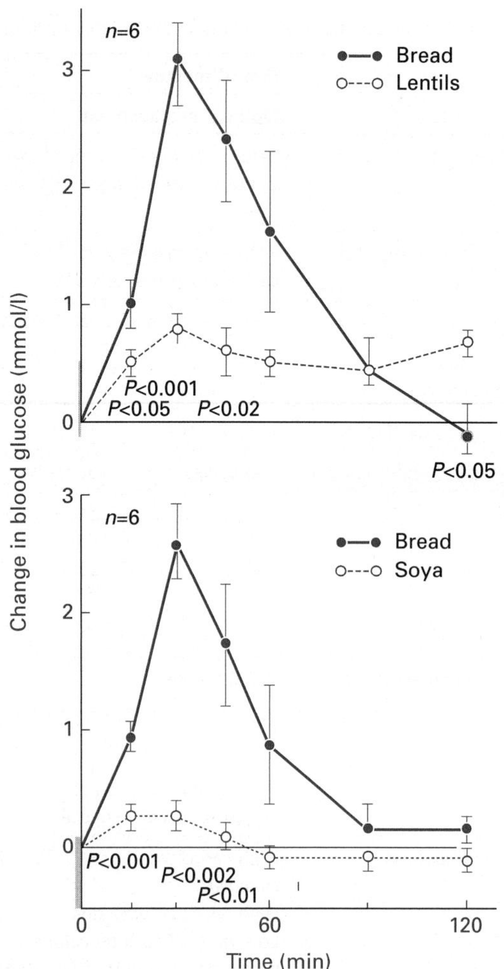

Fig. 4 Rise in blood glucose concentrations in six healthy volunteers after meals containing 50 g carbohydrate as wholemeal bread or lentils (top) or wholemeal bread and/or soya beans (bottom).
*(Reproduced from Jenkins. (1980). British Medical Journal, **281**, 16, with permission.)*

2. A severe degree of microangiopathic tissue damage has already occurred, in which case other approaches, such as control of hypertension, may become relatively more important.
3. If, after 20 or 30 years of relatively high glycaemic levels, there is virtually no clinically evident diabetic tissue damage, the risks of hypoglycaemia should be balanced against the small advantage that might accrue from meticulous control.

Treatment of diabetes mellitus

Aims of therapy

Management is not aimed solely at glycaemic control (Tables 11 and 12). Its scope ranges from those in whom symptomatic relief alone seems the most appropriate goal to those in whom maximal prophylaxis against future tissue damage is the aim.

Diet

In type II diabetes, obesity is a common contribution to relative pancreatic failure, through associated increase in insulin resistance. Successful management depends on weight loss by way of a low

Table 11 Aims of management of patients with diabetes mellitus

Factor	Aim of therapy: Optimal management		Compromised prophylaxis		Symptomatic management
Blood glucose	Fasting: below 6.0 mmol/l usually 2 h postprandial: below 8.0 mmol/l usually		Fasting: <8 mmol/l usually 2 h postprandial: <11 mmol/l usually		Under 12 mmol/l
Glycosylated haemoglobin	Within normal range of local laboratory (mean ±2 SD)		Mean ±4 SD		Neglect
Glycosuria	Absent (if normal renal threshold)		Fasting: absent postprandial ≤0.25%		<1%
Plasma cholesterol	<5.2 mmol/l		<6.2 mmol/l		Neglect
Plasma triglyceride (fasting)	<2.0 mmol/l		<3.5 mmol/l		Neglect
Blood pressure, upper limits (mmHg)	<50 years*	>50 years*	<50 years*	>50 years*	As for general population, or neglect unless renal or cardiovascular disease
Systolic	135	145	145	150	
Diastolic	80	85	85	90	
Tobacco	None		<5 cigarettes/daily No limit pipe		<20 cigarettes/daily No limit pipe
Obesity (body mass index)	<27.0 kg/m²		<30.0 kg/m²		<33.0 kg/m²
Exercise	Walk for at least 30 min 4 days weekly (or alternatives)		Active job *or* walk for at least 30 min once weekly (or alternative)		As wished
Alcohol	Not >2 units/day usual Not >4 units/day special		Not >4 units/day usual Not >6 units/day special		As wished, up to social limits
Dietary modifications	High carbohydrate (>45–50% total calories) High 'viscous' fibre diet Low fat (<35% total calories) Increased unsaturated fats (P:M:S = 2:2:3) Limited 'quick' carbohydrate, only at meal end 6 intakes daily Limit calories according to BMI and exertion		Ample carbohydrate (>45% total calories) High fibre diet, some 'viscous' Limit fat (<35% total calories) Increased unsaturated fats (P:M:S = 1:1:2) Limited 'quick' carbohydrate 6 intakes daily Limit calories according to BMI and exertion		Limit calories according to BMI
Expectation of hypoglycaemia	Mild symptoms if meal delayed or unusual exercise without extra food		Only if exceptional exertion or starvation		Avoid

*Values require more precise adjustment acording to actual age.

calorie diet (see Table 13), but much encouragement will be necessary to maintain this over any length of time.

In type I diabetes emphasis on the need for a low carbohydrate intake became widespread following the discovery of insulin. There were two good reasons to doubt the validity of the approach: first, diabetics in Africa or India often showed sustained good control of glucose levels despite following their local high carbohydrate diets; second, since a low carbohydrate diet was likely to be high in fat, it might contribute to hyperlipidaemia and so substantially to the development of macroangiopathy.Low carbohydrate diets were seriously questioned only with the renewed interest in natural or high fibre diets which showed that a high carbohydrate diet, avoiding excess of quickly absorbed forms, achieved at least as good glycaemic control in diabetics as did the traditional low carbohydrate regimen.

The second fallacy came from the emphasis on chemical analysis of food 'on the shelf' without any thought as to how it was dealt with in the body. Diets were based on building blocks of 10 g portions of carbohydrate regardless of their composition. Eventually it was realized that what mattered was the effect of the food on the blood glucose of the recipient, and that this would be greatly influenced by the speed of its passage through and digestion within the gut. How a particular food is cooked can affect its rate of absorption, which is clearly illustrated by the greater rise in blood glucose when the juice from a particular weight of apples is drunk than when the apples are taken as a purée, which is greater again than if the apples are eaten raw.

Studies in which dietary fibre was added to meals showed lower blood glucose rises and lower insulin concentrations in both normal and diabetic subjects owing to a delay but not an overall decrease in absorption. This effect may be useful in preventing both hypoglycaemia in insulin-treated diabetics and reactive hypoglycaemia in non-diabetics (Fig. 4). The viscous fibres (for example pectins from fruits or galactomannans from legumes) are much more effective

Table 12 Glycaemic treatment and its monitoring for diabetic patients according to use of insulin and therapeutic aim

Type of patient	Aim of therapy: Optimal management	Compromised prophylaxis	Symptomatic management
Insulin-dependent			
Mode of insulin treatment	At least two, often three, perhaps four subcutaneous injections daily *or* continuous subcutaneous pump with preprandial boosts.	One or two subcutaneous injections daily	One subcutaneous injection daily if adequate
Mode of monitoring	2 × 5/day BG profile weekly 2 BG tests daily on other days 2 Urine tests 4 days a week	2 BG tests on 4 days weekly *or* 2 BG tests on 2 days and 2 urine tests on 5 days	4 BG tests weekly *or* 2 urine tests 4 days a week
Non-insulin dependent (even if insulin treated)			
Hypoglycaemic treatment	Insulin (1 or 2 subcutaneous injections daily) if oral hypoglycaemics inadequate. Oral hypoglycaemics if diet alone inadequate	As for 'optimal'	Insulin only if acceptable, and probably once daily Oral hypoglycaemics as required
Mode of monitoring	1 × 5/day BG profile weekly 2 BG tests daily or other days 2 Urine tests on 4 days/week	2 BG tests thrice weekly *or* 2 BG tests on 1 day and 2 urine tests on 5 days weekly	4 BG tests weekly *or* 2 urine tests on 4 days a week

than the fibrous fibres (for example bran). Viscous fibres are also effective in lowering cholesterol levels.

The delayed absorption is accompanied by earlier satiety, increased feelings of epigastric fullness, and abdominal distension with borborygmi together with increased rectal flatus and looser bulkier stools, but such symptoms lessen greatly within 3 months. Concentrations of some viscous fibres are available (for example, Guar gum from the cluster bean of India, already used as a thickener for gravy), but some people find much viscous fibre repugnant because of its 'slimy' or 'gummy' feel, and this revulsion is not easily lost with time. 'Mouth feel' is also associated with viscosity, so that the most effective fibre concentrates are likely to be unpalatable to many people.

An increase in the viscous fibre content of the diet can be achieved by two methods. First, natural foods rich in these substances can be made predominant constituents of the diet, so a high legume content is useful because galactomannans are their main storage carbohydrate. The pectins of cell walls (particularly fruits) form another major group, and to some extent galactomannans and pectins have additive qualities. The other approach is to take concentrates of viscous fibre as capsules or, more usually, by adding them to meals or incorporating them into particular foods.

To obtain the best results from these dietary changes, quickly absorbed simple sugars should be limited in amount and taken late in a meal.

Another consideration is that the diet of a diabetic must contain a proper intake of vitamins and minerals. Fruits and vegetables contain compounds that may act as antioxidants and help to remove free radicals. Their presence in the diet is associated with a reduction in both coronary arteriosclerosis and cancer. Thus the amount of fruit currently recommended is greater than might be expected from a consideration of its content of simple sugars alone.

Specific considerations

The most important nutritional approach to a typical type II diabetic is to restrict caloric intake (Table 13), although energy expenditure is also important. The possibility of weight loss depends principally on the strength of motivation (see Chapter 8.3). There should be a substantial emphasis in the timing as well as the content of meals in patients treated with insulin. The action of oral sulphonylureas seems to be much less dependent on the exact time at which they are taken.

Restriction of sodium intake may reduce the risk of hypertension and measures to regulate the blood lipids are also important. Diabetics are probably no more liable to hypercholesterolaemia than non-diabetics, but a deficiency of effective insulin action increases liability to hypertriglyceridaemia.

Dietary advice may need to be amended in the presence of renal failure. Any reduction in protein should not be compensated mainly by fat; many nephropaths die from ischaemic heart disease. It has also been argued that at early stages of renal damage, evidenced by microalbuminuria, progression of the renal lesion may be reduced by a decrease in dietary protein to about 0.6 g/kg body weight.

Ethanol

There is no reason why diabetics should not enjoy alcohol in moderation. The weekly intake should probably not much exceed 21 equivalents for men or 14 for women. The carbohydrate in sweet wines or liqueurs is quickly absorbed, which means that these should be avoided, as should sugar-containing mixers such as tonic water, other than in low calorie form. Ethanol is a potent inhibitor of gluconeogenesis and may be responsible for hypoglycaemia after 2–3 h if it is taken without food or 4–8 h after a small meal if it is taken in excess. Alcoholic flushing is greatly increased by chlorpropamide, and to a lesser extent by some other sulphonylureas.

Practical advice

1. Each insulin-taking diabetic must work out the right balance between extra food and extra exercise. Walking for an hour would be expected to increase carbohydrate requirements by about 20 g, while more active exercise such as playing tennis or football may require at least 40 g of carbohydrate per hour. This is best taken

Table 13 Menus for three specimen diets

Meal	1000 kcal	CHO (g)	1500 kcal	CHO (g)	2500 kcal	CHO (g)
Breakfast	Fresh orange segments	40	Fresh grapefruit, half	38	Large bowl Puffed Wheat® with milk (150 ml) (or medium helping Puffed Wheat®+one banana)	73
	One Weetabix® with skimmed milk (130 ml) Wholemeal toast: one slice with margarine Tea with skimmed milk (20 ml)		Small bowl All-Bran® with skimmed milk (150 ml) Wholemeal toast: one slice with margarine Tea with skimmed milk (20 ml)		Wholemeal toast: one slice with baked beans One glass of milk (150 ml)	
Mid-morning	Tea with skimmed milk (20 ml)	1	Tea with skimmed milk (20 ml) One apple	12	Tuna and cucumber sandwiches from two slices wholemeal bread Tea with milk (20 ml)	30
Lunch	Butter beans, sweetcorn, and ham salad Lemon juice dressing One apple Tea with skimmed milk (20 ml)	37	Tuna and cucumber sandwiches from two slices wholemeal bread One small banana and a small carton of natural yoghurt Tea with skimmed milk (20 ml)	53	Beef and bean hot pot Rice and pineapple condé Low calorie squash	81
Mid-afternoon	Coffee with skimmed milk (40 ml)	2	Coffee with skimmed milk (40 ml) One wholewheat cracker biscuit	10	One wholewheat fruit scone Coffee with milk (40 ml) One apple	29
Evening meal	Lean roast lamb: two slices Sugar-free mint sauce Garden peas and carrots One large jacket potato Stewed pear with cinnamon Low-calorie squash	42	Red bean and lamb casserole One large jacket potato Runner beans Fresh fruit jelly Diabetic squash	86	Vegetable and pasta soup Red bean and cheese flan Red cabbage salad with yoghurt dressing Orange fruit jelly Coffee with milk (40 ml)	90
Bedtime	Skimmed milk as tea/hot milk/ coffee (40 ml) Two rye crispbreads (Ryvita®)	15	Skimmed milk as coffee/hot milk (50 ml) One digestive biscuit	13	One tall glass unsweetened fruit juice (or one glass milk) Two digestive biscuits	39
Total		137		212		342
Total calories from carbohydrate		55%		57%		55%

as extra food at a preceding meal, but small amounts may be taken as quickly absorbed carbohydrate just before the exercise or halfway through it.

2. Food should be spread out throughout the day, and those taking conventional insulin therapy should have three main meals and three snacks. Older patients who wake regularly during the night may have a small intake then.
3. Meals should consist of foods that are slowly digested and absorbed. Simple sugars (glucose, sucrose) should be confined to small amounts taken with meals (for example 5–10 g). Exceptions are treatment of hypoglycaemia and illness, particularly gastro-intestinal.
4. The carbohydrate content of the diet should provide 50–55 per cent of the total calories, although in individual meals this can vary as widely as from 30–60 per cent.
5. Patients should aim at a ratio of polyunsaturated to mono-unsaturated to saturated fatty acids of around 2:2:3, and be advised to restrict intake of eggs to a maximum of eight a week, to limit the consumption of hard cheese, and to keep the intake of other high cholesterol foods such as shellfish at a modest level. Fat should not contribute more than 35 per cent to total calorie intake.
6. The need for a regular pattern of eating should be stressed in insulin-dependent diabetics on fixed insulin regimens.

Three specimen diets, with calorie contents of 1000, 1500, and 2500 kcal, are given in Table 13. Approximately 1000–1200 kcal/day should be advised when the body mass index exceeds 30.0 kg/m^2, 1500 kcal/day for a body mass index of 27.5–29.9 kcal/day, and 2000 or more for a body mass index of less than 27.5 kcal/day, but the optimum amount will depend on exercise, muscularity, and height.

Sulphonylureas

Sulphonylureas act in two different ways. They sensitize the β-cell to the stimulatory effect of glucose on insulin secretion, causing a leftward shift in the dose-response curve of secretion against glucose concentration. The metabolism of glucose within pancreatic β-cells generates ATP which binds with a receptor on cell-membrane voltage-dependent potassium channels to favour a potassium efflux which stimulates an influx of calcium leading to insulin secretion. The sulphonylureas bind at a different site from ATP to this same potassium channel with an avidity proportional to their potency as hypoglycaemic agents. Sulphonylureas may also upregulate insulin receptors and increase their number. This receptor action may be relatively short lasting and the effective β-cell mass is also likely to decrease with time, so that the effectiveness of these drugs also tends to fall *pari passu*.

The main argument about the use of the sulphonylureas is the extent to which they can be replaced by proper dieting, or indeed interfere with this. Long-term weight loss alone always improves glucose tolerance, often to a degree that makes sulphonylureas superfluous and improved control of glycaemia achieved by the use of suphonylureas may result in weight gain and associated increased insulin resistance.

The American University Group Diabetes Program implied an excessive risk of cardiovascular deaths in diabetics if they had been treated with a fixed dose of tolbutamide (500 mg three times daily) together with their diet. This concern has been largely dissipated with greater understanding of the imperfections of this trial and how the data may be more clearly interpreted. Such risk from tolbutamide or other sulphonylureas has not been seen in a number of other studies, particularly the UKPDS.

Toxic effects

The sulphonylureas can cause a wide range of allergic reactions, particularly on the skin. Some are particularly associated with rare but severe bone marrow depression. This has most often been reported with more than 500 mg of chlorpropamide daily, a dose that would rarely be exceeded today. All can produce hypoglycaemia, rarely severe enough to cause unconsciousness. But this can happen, under special circumstances, for example in synergy with β-adrenergic blocking agents or monoamine oxidase inhibitors; when displaced from binding plasma proteins by another drug (for instance dicoumarins or salicylates); or in the neonate if the agent was unwisely administered to the pregnant mother within a few days of delivery. The risk is generally greater for longer-acting agents, and is enhanced by hepatic or renal disease. This may be one mechanism underlying the risk of severe and prolonged nocturnal hypoglycaemia in some elderly persons given long-acting preparations.

Administration

The commonly used sulphonylureas are listed in Table 14. Although there is no advantage in adding a second sulphonylurea when a maximum dose of one has already been prescribed, it is reasonable to supplement a small dose of a long-acting agent with a quick-acting drug, for instance before a large evening meal or regularly before breakfast in those with a marked morning hyperglycaemic surge.

Chlorpropamide and tolbutamide are usually as effective as any of the more expensive second-generation agents. Gliquidone may be more suitable in the presence of renal impairment, as it is mostly metabolized in the liver with excretion of its metabolites in the bile. Glymidine is a sulphapyrimidine rather than a sulphonylurea and so may be acceptable when sensitivity to a sulphonylurea proves to be a group phenomenon.

Indications for sulphonylurea prescription will depend mostly on the ability of a type II diabetic to initiate and sustain dietary effort, and in the physician's aim of glucose control. Continuing β-cell deterioration in type II diabetes will be a major cause of secondary failure as is increased insulin resistance with time. About 30 per cent of those on sulphonylureas will be transferred to insulin treatment within 4 years. Sulphonylureas are contraindicated in young thin type I patients, particularly if they are ketotic, but some slow-onset type I diabetics can achieve adequate glucose control on sulphonylureas without insulin for many years.

Biguanides

Biguanides are believed to act by reducing ion exchange across membranes, decreasing the efficiency of cellular metabolism. Both hepatic gluconeogenesis and the yield of chemical energy from peripheral utilization of glucose are decreased, with a resulting fall in blood glucose. The same properties may underlie the toxic effects of these agents which range from generalized lassitude and vague muscular discomfort to the serious complication of lactic acidosis. Lactic acidosis, although rare, is particularly liable to occur with phenformin therapy; hence this agent is no longer available in many countries. It is also more likely when there has been an acute reduction in hepatic blood flow, for example after myocardial infarction, pulmonary embolus, or Gram-negative septicaemia, but is also predisposed to by excess alcohol intake or leukaemia. Since the biguanides are largely eliminated by the kidney, renal impairment is another contraindication to their use. The risk of lactic acidosis is least with metformin but the dose should probably not exceed 500 mg three times daily or 850 mg twice daily.

The principal roles of biguanides are first, as an initial oral agent, especially in the obese, and secondly together with a sulphonylurea when either agent alone, together with dietary advice, has failed to produce satisfactory glucose control. Such a state is often an indication for transfer to insulin, but combined sulphonylurea–biguanide therapy is a useful method of attempting continued oral treatment, particularly if symptomatic relief rather than strict glycaemic control is the aim. The biguanides remain active after months or years of therapy, and their efficacy shows little dependence on the residual effective β-cell mass.

Other oral hypoglycaemic agents

Certain herbal preparations, for example kerala, are widely used in India and are weakly hypoglycaemic, and onion extract is also weakly active. A number of pharmaceutical agents are under construction, but either have only a weak action (eg hypolipidaemic agents such as acipimox) or may have unwelcome side-effects.

Reduction of tissue damage

Apart from the need for tight control of blood glucose and arterial pressure and attention to other risk factors for arteriosclerotic disease, various drug therapies have been suggested.

Aldose reductase inhibitors

There is as yet no convincing evidence that any of these agents are beneficial in humans.

Aminoguanidine

Aminoguanidine interferes with the development of advanced glycosylation end-products and the consequent cross-linking of protein

Table 14 Major oral hypoglycaemic agents available in the United Kingdom

	Daily dose range (mg)	t_{max} (h)	*ti* (h)	No. of daily doses	Site of metabolism
Sulphonylurea					
Acetohexamide	250–1500	1–2	1.3–4.5	1–3	Liver
Chlorpropamide	100–500	1–7	33–43	1	Most excreted unchanged in urine
Glibenclamide	2.5–20	1–2	6–10	1–3	Liver
Glibornuride	12.5–75	2–4	8–9	1–2	Liver
Gliclazide	80–240	4–8	10–12	1–3	95% liver
Glipizide	2.5–30	0.5–2	3–7	2–3	90–95% excreted unchanged
Gliquidone	30–180	2–3	–	1–3	95% liver meta-bolites excreted in bile
Glymidine	500–2000	1–2	5–8	1–2	?
Tolazamide	100–1000		7	1–3	Liver
Tolbutamide	1000–3000	3–4	7	2–3	Liver
Biguanide					
Metformin	500–1700	2–4	12–20	1–3	Excreted unchanged in urine

chains. Its use has not progressed beyond the treatment of experimental diabetes in small laboratory animals.

Polyunsaturated fatty acids (ω-6)

The N6 series of polyunsaturated fatty acids are important nutrients and potential therapeutic agents. Steps in the conversion of linolenate to arachidonate may be deficient in diabetic patients, and so D-linolenate has been tried (as evening primrose oil), particularly against diabetic neuropathy. There is uncertain evidence of prevention of slowing of nerve conduction but no clear evidence of clinical efficacy. More general polyunsaturated fatty acid supplements have decreased the development of diabetic retinopathy, particularly of the advanced type, but the benefit could be limited to those with hyperglycaemia of a level unacceptable by present standards.

Insulin therapy

Types of insulin available

The various insulin preparations have three main characteristics—species of origin, purity, and duration of action—and to these may be added concentration, now fixed in the UK at 100 IU/ml.

Species

Bovine and porcine insulins have long been the mainstays of therapy, but now synthetic human insulin has become available. It differs from porcine only at the amino acid in position 30 of the β-chain. Bovine insulin differs at two other sites—amino acids 8 and 10 of the α-chain. The potency of the three insulins is very similar. A small difference in solubility leads to slightly quicker absorption of the human preparations. Bovine is now used much less frequently because of its greater antigenicity, and porcine is also used less.

Purity

Insulin prepared by acid–ethanol extraction of porcine or bovine pancreas also contained small amounts of other pancreatic hormones, such as glucagon, pancreatic, polypeptide, and vasoactive intestinal polypeptides, as well as insulin dimers and degradation products, and significant amounts of proinsulin (1–4 per cent). In the last 30 years, purer preparations have become available; the less pure the preparation the greater is the antigenicity. Highly purified bovine insulin is slightly more antigenic than is porcine; human preparations are slightly less antigenic still. Antibodies to insulin have been recognized for nearly 30 years in the plasma of insulin-treated diabetics. The antigenicity resides mainly in insulin-like molecules, either natural or degraded, particularly proinsulin. Substances that prolong the action of insulin (for example protamine and zinc), also appear to increase antigenicity, perhaps acting as adjuvants.

Are insulin antibodies clinically significant? One effect could be to retard the action of quick-acting insulins, with a later sustained release which may be unwanted. Insulin doses are on average less in patients with low antibody titres. Insulin antibodies may also shorten the honeymoon phase of low insulin requirement early in the course of type I diabetes. They cross the placenta and may increase hypoglycaemia in the neonates of diabetic mothers. The suggestion that insulin antibodies are implicated in the development of diabetic tissue damage, particularly retinopathy and nephropathy, has not been substantiated.

Duration of action and pharmacokinetics

Insulins given subcutaneously can be divided into short-acting, intermediate, and long-acting preparations. The duration of action depends on the site of injection. Intravenous insulin has a half-life in the plasma of 4–5 min and an effective half-life of 20 min, and so must be infused continuously to produce a sustained effect. Only short-acting insulins should be used intravenously, as longer-acting preparations are particulate and carry a theoretical risk of embolism. The half-life of crystalline (short-acting) insulin given intramuscularly is approximately 2 h. In day-to-day use insulin is given subcutaneously, with a plasma half-life for the quick-acting preparations of 2 to 4 h in diabetics already treated with insulin but less in normal subjects. The onset of action varies from 15 to 60 min, with peak effects at 2 to 6 h and some effect for up to 8 h, although this may exceed 12 h in patients with high antibody levels.

Absorption from subcutaneous sites is variable both within and between subjects and the same dose may have quite different effects on different days in the same patient. Human insulin preparations seem to be absorbed slightly more rapidly than porcine, which in turn is absorbed more rapidly than bovine.

An important influence on the rate of absorption is the tissue blood flow, and this varies with ambient temperature and site of injection. Absorption is quicker from the abdomen than from the arm, which in turn is quicker than from the thigh. A consistent approach is important. Depth of injection is also important—shallow injections are absorbed more rapidly than deeper ones, provided that the former are not intradermal and the latter are not intramuscular. Exercise, particularly of the injected part, as well as massage or hot baths, can also speed absorption.

Variations in absorption rate also apply to the intermediate and long-acting insulins. Indeed, the variability between and within patients is then greater. There are several intermediate preparations. The duration of action varies from 16 to 30 h with peak effect at 5 to 12 h. The tard and lente insulins depend on zinc, whilst protamine is used for the isophane insulins. Both these agents may increase antigenicity.

The long-acting insulins have a broad peak of maximum effect and a duration of action of up to 3 days. They can be used to give a constant background of insulin. Because of the long half-life several days may be required to achieve stability. The human ultralente preparation is considerably shorter-acting than the more antigenic bovine ultralente insulin, and in some patients may not last adequately even for 24 h.

Mixed insulin preparations are also available. These are useful when less than optimal control is sought or when mixing insulins proves difficult.

Routine use of insulins

If the patient is simply to be kept asymptomatic, a once-daily regimen is acceptable. A single dose of an intermediate insulin of the lente or isophane type, particularly the latter, carries little risk of nocturnal hypoglycaemia. It may be necessary to add a short-acting insulin if there is severe post-breakfast hyperglycaemia. Once-daily therapy may also be successful in type II diabetics who are not controlled satisfactorily by oral agents by using, for example, a mixture of short-acting and intermediate insulins. If there is persistent fasting hyperglycaemia, an additional evening injection may be required.

Most type I diabetics require two or three injections daily to try to reproduce the natural peak levels during and after meals with basal concentrations preprandially. Some patients can be dealt with satisfactorily using a twice-daily mixture of short-acting and intermediate insulins. Guidelines for modifying twice-daily insulin therapy are shown in Table 15. The absorption of even short-acting insulin is slower than the physiological pancreatic responses to a meal. More important, circulating levels do not return to baseline sufficiently quickly. However, some of these disadvantages can be countered by appropriate dietary adjustments. Thus a small breakfast, with the carbohydrate mostly slowly absorbed, followed by an equivalent carbohydrate load 2 h later as a snack can match the profile from a short-acting insulin injection given in the morning. Similar dietary adjustments can be made at other times of the day.

The day is usually divided into unequal portions with respect to insulin injections; the morning injection may be at 7 a.m. and that before the evening meal between 5.30 and 6.30 p.m, with the latter covering the larger nocturnal fraction of the 24-h period. Many patients on twice-daily therapy have morning hyperglycaemia, but if additional intermediate insulin is given in the early evening, there may be nocturnal hypoglycaemia. Hence a longer-acting insulin is required in the evening, or the evening meal should be later, or a different insulin regimen is required. One successful manoeuvre is to give short-acting insulin alone before the evening meal and an intermediate insulin at bedtime. Another pattern is the twice-daily or thrice-daily injection of short-acting insulin against a background of long-acting insulin. Frequent, even four times daily, injections of short-acting insulin may be particularly helpful for labile diabetics, those with early rapidly advancing tissue damage, the pregnant diabetic, or the diabetic requiring maximum flexibility in lifestyle. More frequent injections are well accepted.

Multidose pen injectors have been a help to many patients, increasing flexibility when they are away from home. They carry the insulin for many injections in cartridges, thus obviating the necessity to draw up each dose.

When a change is made from less pure to more pure preparations, the new preparation may be more potent so it is prudent to reduce the dose by 20 per cent if the daily total is more than 0.9 units/kg body weight and by 10 per cent if it is less.

Practical aspects of insulin therapy

Emphasis should be placed on the correct injection technique. Neutral short-acting and isophane-type insulins can be mixed in the same syringe. The smaller dose should be drawn up first. The rotation of injection sites should be taught. Rapidly absorbing sites, such as the abdomen or arm, are used in the morning and more slowly absorbing sites, such as the thigh or buttocks, in the evening when more prolonged action is required. If given 30 min before eating, the upstroke of the resulting plasma insulin profile begins to match the physiological rise, but in some patients the interval between injection and eating may need to be 40–45 min. When patients are first started they should inject 20 min before eating, with the interval increased if necessary as indicated by blood glucose tests 90–150 min after the meal. A different injection site should be used for each of at least 20 consecutive injections, because repeated injections in one place predispose to lipohypertrophy.

Initial dosage of insulin

The two main indices of the required total daily dose are the prevailing blood glucose and height and weight. An inital small dose can help in deciding on the succeeding one. Another approach is to calculate the first dose from formulae based on body mass index and prevailing glucose concentration. The disadvantage here is that the recommended doses are the means of a range of effective doses, and in a small proportion of patients a dose that is only 80 per cent of that given by the formula may be correct. Therefore some patients are liable to suffer hypoglycaemia if the formulae are adhered to rigidly. A compromise between the two approaches is probably best. If a formula is used, it is wise to start with doses that are about 80 per cent of those calculated. If no formula is available, the patient should start on a total daily dose of 0.5 units/kg body weight, initially using a relatively rapidly acting insulin in several dividing doses. The requirement a few days after the start of therapy is usually less than that needed to control the initial hyperglycaemia.

Complications of insulin therapy

The complications of insulin therapy are listed in Table 16. Hypoglycaemia is by far the commonest. The probable time for an attack

Table 15 Guide to modification of twice-daily (short-acting and intermediate) insulin regimen

	Prebreakfast	Prelunch	Pre-evening meal	Bedtime
Persistent hyperglycaemia (>10 mmol/l) or glycosuria (>0.5%)	↑Evening* intermediate 2–4 units	↑Morning short-acting 2–4 units or decrease† breakfast or mid-morning snack	↑Morning intermediate 2–4 units or decrease† afternoon snack	↑Evening short-acting 2–4 units or decrease† evening snack
Persistent hypoglycaemia	↓Evening intermediate 2–4 units	↓Morning short-acting 2–4 units or †increase mid–morning carbohydrate	↓Morning intermediate 2–4 units or †increase afternoon carbohydrate	↓Evening short-acting 2–4 units or †increase evening meal carbohydrate
Symptomatic or BG <4 mmol/l				

BG, blood glucose

*This may result in nocturnal hypoglycaemia in which case the evening intermediate insulin should be moved to bedtime

†Carbohydrate should be increased or decreased in approximately 10 g amounts.

Table 16 Complications of insulin therapy

Hypoglycaemia	Local allergy
Antibody formation—?	Generalized allergy
impaired control,	Insulin resistance
transplacental transfer	Insulin oedema
Lipoatrophy	Sepsis
Lipohypertrophy	

of hypoglycaemia is often predictable, for instance late morning or late afternoon in patients taking mixed insulins twice daily. Hypoglycaemia is generally correctly recognized by patients, but long-standing and/or older diabetics may lose their typical warning symptoms. The family and workmates of a diabetic should be instructed in both the symptoms and signs of hypoglycaemia and in the action to be taken.

Lipodystrophy is much less common than it was. It is commonest when less pure insulins are used. It may be due to immunogenic components which lead to the formation of either immune complexes or IgE antibodies which bind locally and so stimulate lipolysis. It is treated by injecting a purer insulin into the centre or edge of the atrophic area until this fills.

Lipohypertrophy is commoner than lipoatrophy when patients are treated with highly purified insulins. It is due to repeated injection at the same site and presumably results from continued lipid synthesis in response to a high local concentration of insulin. It is prevented by proper rotation of injection sites, and disappears with time if the patient stops injecting into the affected area.

Insulin allergy, either local or general, is rare. The local form comprises pruritic, erythematous, indurated, and occasionally painful lesions subsequent to insulin injection. There are three distinct types. The commonest is a biphasic IgE-dependent reaction called the late-phase reaction. Arthus-type or delayed reactions also occur. Insulin impurities and the retarding agents zinc and protamine have all been implicated as causative agents. The incidence is much decreased by the use of highly purified insulins. The first step in treatment is to ensure that the lesions are not due to faulty technique, for example intradermal injection. Skin testing with different insulins, including zinc-free preparations, can then be used to find a non-reactive preparation. Oral antihistamines may also be useful. Local steroid therapy may be necessary, and the appropriate steroid can be mixed with the insulin before injection, for example 1 mg of prednisolone per millilitre of insulin preparation. Generalized allergy is extremely rare and presents classically. The antigen is usually insulin itself, and the β-chain of all commonly used insulins induces the response. It responds to conventional desensitization regimens.

Insulin resistance can be defined as a daily intake of more than 1.5 units/kg body weight. It is now relatively uncommon in type I diabetics in the UK but before insulins of high purity were available, it was much commoner and most cases were due to high levels of antibodies. Obesity is the most common non-immunological cause. In the case of immunologically based resistance, the preparation should be changed to highly purified human insulin. Failing this, systemic prednisolone may be useful, but only when the resistance is severe, because of its diabetogenic properties and other side-effects. Other forms of insulin resistance include antireceptor antibodies or elevated levels of counter-regulatory hormones.

Pseudo-insulin resistance has been recognized among patients who are overtreated with insulin, hence becoming hypoglycaemic and thus eating excessively in response, only to become hyperglycaemic and so have their insulin dose increased. Hepatomegaly is a rare clinical feature. A dramatic improvement in glycaemic level and stability can be obtained by drastic reduction of the insulin dose and appropriate dietary advice.

Insulin oedema is rare but is extremely troublesome when it does occur. It is seen when strict glycaemic control is achieved in markedly hyperglycaemic and underweight diabetics. Marked pitting oedema may develop within 3 to 4 days of the start of insulin therapy but resolves spontaneously usually 5 to 10 days later. Occasionally the condition is so severe that pulmonary oedema occurs. The cause is unknown.

Alternative methods of insulin delivery

The main aim has been a system that will respond to ambient blood glucose by automatic provision of an appropriate insulin dose, for example via an insulin infusion pump. This delivers soluble insulin subcutaneously using a fine cannula with a needle inserted under the skin which is resited every 24–48 h. A background infusion is given at a predetermined rate (0.5–1.2 units/h on average). Extra boluses are delivered as desired at mealtimes, using an override switch or a manual drive. Much more sophisticated programmable pumps with long-lasting insulin reservoirs are also available. Pumps or open-loop devices should only be used in conjunction with appropriate education and self-monitoring (see below). Their untutored use has resulted in disaster due to hypoglycaemia or ketoacidosis.

Pumps can also be used to deliver insulin intravenously. This route has been used occasionally in patients with brittle diabetes, but the risks of septicaemia and thrombosis are considerable. It is logical to implant the pump to reduce the possibility of infection. This has been done but alterations in the infusion rate remain a problem. A potentially more useful route is via the peritoneal cavity, mimicking secretion from the pancreas into the portal venous system. Peritoneal insulin is used routinely in diabetics undergoing chronic ambulatory peritoneal dialysis. Intraperitoneal infusion from either external or implanted pumps also results in good glycaemic control with less peripheral hyperinsulinaemia.

Two major new developments are under way. The first aims at the production of an artificial endocrine pancreas comprising a glucose sensor, a small computer programmed to respond to both absolute levels of, and changes in, glucose concentration, and an insulin infusion pump directed by the computer. Effective systems are available, but they are large, expensive, and extracorporeal. The outstanding problem is the lack of a glucose sensor which is reliable and can function for a lengthy period *in vivo*.

Pancreatic transplantation has been successfully achieved, particularly with segmental grafts, but with poor long-term endocrine function. Autologous islet transplants have been used more successfully in patients made diabetic by total pancreatectomy for chronic pancreatitis. Several have been independent of insulin for up to 3 years.

Exercise

Exercise affects glycaemic levels and so is a major factor influencing day-to-day food and insulin requirements. It can be harnessed as a tool for glycaemic control, particularly in non-insulin-treated patients in whom replacement of adipose tissue by muscle will increase the sensitivity to insulin. In non-diabetics, the consumption of glucose increases rapidly on exercise. Muscle utilization increases independently of variations in insulin levels. There is a parallel increase in hepatic glucose production, resulting from associated increases in glucagon and catecholamine secretion, and often a slight drop in insulin levels. Consequently, plasma glucose levels alter little. Several of these responses are absent in type I diabetics, so that in the well-controlled diabetic glucose levels fall and hypoglycaemia may result unless treatment is modified. Paradoxically, in the poorly controlled diabetic blood glucose rises with exercise because of insulinopenia. Muscle glucose uptake does not increase normally, but hepatic production increases supranormally. There may also be a profound increase in ketone body levels—exercise ketosis. There is also increased insulin absorption from subcutaneous injection sites during exercise, particularly if the injection has been made into the exercising limb.

In the mildly overweight subject it is probably wisest to decrease insulin before exercise. The lean diabetic should take extra carbohydrate before starting and more may be necessary during prolonged exercise. The extra carbohydrate required varies considerably from person to person, but may be surprisingly large. If exercise is to last only 1–2 h, a rough and ready rule is to take 20 g of fairly quickly absorbed carbohydrate before exercise and hourly during it. If it is prolonged and strenuous 40 g of carbohydrate per hour may well be needed, at least half of which should be in a quick-acting form. Hypoglycaemia may occur several hours after exercise, and patients with autonomic neuropathy may have both diminished exercise capacity and a highly abnormal metabolic response.

A fall in blood glucose with exercise also occurs in type II diabetics.

Education

Self-management should be the watchword for both type I and type II patients. A well-taught patient will know when to seek professional help. In the elderly or long-standing diabetic, education in care of the feet is mandatory. Simple booklets, films, and audiovisual aids are helpful, but frequent reinforcement is necessary. A team of teaching nurses and dietitians may well make the greatest impact; a phone-in service is often useful.

Monitoring of therapy

Urinary glucose

Passing a test strip through the urine stream is the quickest and easiest of all urinary glucose tests. Glucose-specific methods such as Diastix and Diabur are preferable.The renal threshold for glucose varies between 7 and 12 mmol/l. In general, if results are positive, blood glucose values are at least twice normal; if negative, there is no indication whether blood glucose is at the low or high end of the normal range. However, urinary glucose does reflect glycaemia over several hours. When control is erratic, a method (Diabur test strips) which measures up to 5 g of glucose per 100 ml urine is useful in indicating the degree of glycosuria. More crudely, urine diluted 1:1 with water can be tested approximately. There is also some benefit from periodic 24-h quantitative measurement of urinary glucose.

Urinary ketones

The routine measurement of urinary ketones is not necessary in the majority of type I diabetics or in any type II diabetic. The test is useful for home monitoring of labile ketosis-prone diabetics. The available methods measure only acetone and acetoacetate and not the quantitatively important 3-hydroxybutyrate. Because of this and limited sensitivity, blood ketones may be elevated by a factor of 10–20 before the urinary test is positive. A high urinary concentration interferes to a practically important extent with the interaction of glucose with Diastix, which should therefore never be relied on in a sick patient suspected of ketoacidosis (Ketodiastix or Ketodiabur should be used instead).

Urinary protein

The threshold sensitivity of Albustix is some 200mg/dl. Persistent albuminuria at this level, in the absence of sustained infection, is crucial evidence of nephropathy and a poor prognosis. More sensitive methods have been developed to measure smaller amounts (microalbuminuria). The concentration of albumin varies substantially with urinary dilution, so that either a timed urine collection is made or the urinary creatinine concentration is measured simultaneously and the albumin-to-creatinine ratio calculated. Exercise can increase urinary albumin in the absence of nephropathy, so that analysis is best performed on a timed overnight urine collection or a spot urine passed on rising from sleep. The thresholds for abnormality may still be too high, but are currently taken as about 20–30 μg/min for the mean of three timed specimens, or 2–3 mg/mmol for the albumin-to-creatinine ratio from three early morning specimens.

Blood glucose

It is of little value to measure random blood glucose routinely at a diabetic clinic. Fasting and timed postprandial measurements are more useful. Fasting blood glucose in type II diabetics reflects overall glycaemic control accurately but is limited in usefulness if performed only two or three times per year.

The only useful way to assess control in Type I patients is to obtain a blood glucose profile with measurements before and after each main meal. This can be done in a day clinic, but home blood glucose monitoring has revolutionized assessment. There are two main forms; in one, blood from a finger-prick added to test strips, then washed off and the resulting colour read visually, so that there is no need to issue all patients with meters. However, meters are useful if greater accuracy is required, during initial education, to reduce observer bias, or for colour-blind patients. Secondly, non-colorimetric measurement by an electric current generated on the test strip is now possible. Patients use small lances (Monolets) with or without an additional spring-loaded device (Autolets or Autoclix) to draw blood, and many are prepared to do this 10 to 12 times each week. One common protocol is for the patient to measure blood glucose before and after each main meal and at bedtime on one weekday and one weekend day each week, with fasting and bedtime samples on the other days. Alternatively, tests are performed four times daily on 2 or 3 days per week with intermittent urine testing. Such frequent testing is unnecessary in type II diabetics, for whom periodic fasting and postprandial sampling is adequate.

Glycated haemoglobin

Measurement of glycated protein can provide useful evidence of overall glycaemic control. Haemoglobin A is glycated post-translationally and non-enzymatically at the terminal valine of the β- chain. This produces haemoglobin A1c. There are two further minor glycation fractions, haemoglobin A1a and haemoglobin A1b. It is important to be accurate in describing the analytical method used, for glycated haemoglobin A1 (all three types) is present in rather larger quantities than the more relevant haemoglobin A1c. Values should never be used without knowing the mean and standard deviation of the particular laboratory for a population found to be normal by simultaneous blood glucose measurement. Many then take the mean plus two standard deviations as indicating the rough limit between overall normoglycaemia and hyperglycaemia.

The percentage of haemoglobin A that is glycated is directly proportional to the time that the red cells have been exposed to glucose, and to the glucose concentrations. Measurement of the glycated haemoglobin fraction gives an integrated picture of the mean blood glucose level during half the average lifespan of the red blood cells, i.e. 60 days. The result will be unduly low if the lifespan of the red blood cell is appreciably shortened, and this must be taken into account.

Colorimetric methods can be automated and so may be much cheaper than other tests for HβA1c, but they are less reliable and more likely to be affected by interfering substances such as uric acid or large amounts of vitamin C. The costs of more accurate measurements have resulted in attention to other techniques, such as colorimetric measurements of serum fructosamine. If this method is used, the result is best expressed per unit of plasma albumin, but the albumin half-life may change substantially with a variety of physiological and pathophysiological events.

It is possible for a normal or minimally raised value of glycated haemoglobin to be obtained from patients suffering frequent and dangerous episodes of hypoglycaemia if these are balanced by other episodes of excessive hyperglycaemia. The assay is of particular value in assessing those patients who give over-optimistic reports of the results of their home assessment of glucose levels and explain away high glucose levels on the day of the clinic visit by intercurrent infection or some other transient upset.

Diabetic tissue damage

The development of microangiopathic lesions requires higher sustained glucose levels than those associated with an increased risk of macroangiopathy. The proper target now appears to be to achieve blood glucose values below 6.0 mmol/l fasting and a maximum of 8–9 mmol/l throughout the day. Reduction in the mean value for haemoglobin Alc from 9 to 7 per cent decreased the development of significant retinopathy in a primary prevention cohort by 75 per cent (from 36 to 9 per cent of subjects after 7 years) while in a secondary prevention cohort (recruited a mean of 9 years after diagnosis and with at least minimal retinopathy already present) significant deterioration in retinopathic appearance was reduced by 55 per cent (from 40 to 18 per cent of subjects after 7 years). Approximately similar reductions were seen in nephropathy as judged by microalbuminuria or clinical grade albuminuria, and in neuropathy. Such experience in type I patients in America has now been mirrored among type II patients in the UK prospective diabetes study (UKPDS) in which an 11 per cent reduction in HβA1c reduced microvascular endpoints by 25 per cent. There was no difference in outcome whether the initial therapy was with insulin or sulphonylureas.

Diabetic nephropathy causing renal failure in type I patients occurs mainly in those under the age of 50 who have had diabetes diagnosed less than 30 years previously. However, foot ulceration, particularly if mainly ischaemic in origin, is rare under the age of 45 but is increasingly common thereafter, up to at least age 70. This is predominantly a lesion of type II diabetics. Visual disturbance in this group is more likely to be due to cataract or exudative retinopathy than to proliferative retinopathy, which is found mainly in type I diabetics, often accompanying nephropathy. Such differences may explain the trough in age-corrected diabetic mortality seen between the ages of 45 and 55 years, at which stage the more vulnerable type I diabetics will have died whereas little damage will yet have developed in type II diabetics.

There has been an improvement in the prognosis of diabetic patients in the last 20 years. This cannot be explained purely by improved care of such problems as myocardial infarction, peripheral vascular disease, renal failure, or developing retinopathy. It probably reflects improved glycaemic control, as well as better and more active antihypertensive and hypolipidaemic treatment. Older data indicate the average expectation of life of a type I diabetic diagnosed younger than 30 years to be 29 years, with only half of them reaching the age of 50. A third of such patients had severe renal failure, although several of these died from coronary artery disease which altogether accounted for at least half the group. Expectation is now at least 35 years, with over 60 per cent reaching the age of 50.

The mortality rate of type I diabetics is about five times greater than that of the general population, with the relative risk being greater the younger the patient. It is difficult to state an exact rate for type II diabetics as this depends on accurate detection, which is a particular problem in studies undertaken before the definition of impaired glucose tolerance came into use. Recent estimates range around an increased mortality of around 40 per cent. Older insurance company figures were near to 300 per cent, but were not unbiased. Whatever the precise figures, the risk is larger the younger the patient.

Table 17 Principal causes of death in diabetics (mainly Type I)

	Joslin Clinic 1966–1968	UK survey of deaths in diabetics under 50 years old (via death certificate)
Cardiovascular		
Cardiac causes (%)	54.6	35
Cerebral (%)	10.0	7
Other (%)	1.6	+—
Renal (%)	8.0	17
(Diabetic nephropathy (%))	(6.0)	
Infections (%)	5.9	2
Cancer (%)	12.8	7
Hepatic cirrhosis (%)	1.5	2
Hyperglycaemic coma (%)	1.0	16
Hypoglycaemia (%)	0.7	4
Suicide (%)	0.3	+—
Others (%)	3.6	10
Respiratory (%)		5
Chronic neurological (%)		3

NB A greater proportion of Type II patients will die of cancer.

One study of deaths of diabetics aged under 50 showed that the great majority occurred above age 40, mostly from cardiac infarction but also from renal failure in the long-term type I diabetic. Some 15 per cent were the result of acute metabolic derangement, either hyperglycaemic or hypoglycaemic (Table 17).

Diabetic nephropathy

The risk of nephropathy in type I diabetics appears to be 30–40 per cent and similar figures are probably applicable to type II patients. The mechanism remains uncertain, although data suggest that there is a significant inherited component to susceptibility. This subject is discussed further in Chapter 12.9.

Diabetic eye disease

Some 30 years ago diabetic eye disease was the main cause of blindness in the UK between the ages of 20 and 65 years, largely due to retinopathy or cataract. Other less frequent causes are glaucoma associated with rubeosis iridis and thrombotic occlusion of the retinal vein or artery. The prevalence of open-angle glaucoma is probably increased in diabetics.

Retinopathy (see Plates 2, 4, 5 and 6, The eye and disease)

Diabetic retinopathy almost certainly has a multifactorial pathogenesis. There are changes in the endothelial cells, thickening of the capillary basement membranes, and a decreased number of intramural pericytes, together with tissue hypoxia and increased retinal blood flow. All these, together with increased permeability of the blood–retina barrier, are the most likely factors underlying the occurrence of haemorrhages, exudates, and oedema.

Somehow the retinal changes lead to blockage of capillaries and arterioles with reduced blood flow and non-perfusion of certain areas. The veins draining these may become uneven in diameter and show increased tortuosity, while vessels close to the non-perfused area show abnormal permeability with a risk of development of surrounding oedema and fatty deposits (the basis of retinal exudates). New blood vessels develop at the margins of such areas. There is little risk of serious visual loss from peripheral neovascularization or from small degrees of neovascularization which are not associated with previous haemorrhage, but marked neovascularization (particularly on or very close to the optic disc) is associated with rapidly advancing disability. The stimulus for such neovascularization is believed to arise from ischaemic retina and presumably reaches the affected vessels by diffusion.

Retinopathy can be divided into three types:

(1) 'background' retinopathy which is harmless in itself and is often present without substantial alteration for many years, but is nearly always observed before either of the other two;

(2) proliferative retinopathy which is associated with neovascularization, vitreous haemorrhage, fibrous overgrowth, retinitis proliferans, and retinal detachment;

(3) exudative retinopathy which only threatens vision severely when the macula lutea is involved by either oedema or exudates.

Background retinopathy

This has a number of ophthalmoscopic features ranging from small red dots (microaneurysms or dot haemorrhages) to much larger, although still usually regular, red 'blot haemorrhages'. There may also be small areas of exudate, either cottonwool spots (areas of retinal ischaemia) or small 'fatty' exudates, either circular or crescent-shaped and usually slightly yellow in colour. There may be an increase in the size and tortuosity of the veins.

The momentum of deterioration may be established early and then be relatively resistant to close glycaemic control. This accords with the increase in retinopathy, particularly cottonwool exudates, seen in patients with established background retinopathy brought rapidly to normoglycaemia by continuous subcutaneous infusion. This degeneration is transient, and tight glycaemic control carries no ill effects after 2 or 3 years (and indeed may have some benefit). However, the aim is to prevent substantial amounts of retinopathy from ever developing by ensuring that there is adequate glycaemic control throughout. Various studies indicate an almost continuous relationship between glycaemic control and the prevalence of background retinopathy such that a fasting plasma glucose level of 6 mmol/l, a mean glucose level of 8.5 mmol/l, or a glycated haemoglobin A1c value of 7.5 per cent should markedly restrain the development of background retinopathy, while a haemoglobin A1c value below 8 per cent should markedly restrict the development of proliferative retinopathy (Fig. 5).

Proliferative retinopathy

This is dominated by neovascularization and evidence of preretinal, usually vitreous, haemorrhage. Neovascularization is recognized by an increased density of fine arteriolar elements arranged in a disorganized fashion, as in a crazy lattice. Such areas are often smaller than a quarter of the optic disc, but may be larger and are often widespread throughout the retina. They are particularly likely to be seen close to the disc or even on it. Vitreous haemorrhages vary widely in size, but are rarely as small as a typical subhyaloid haemorrhage. They usually resolve over 2 to 4 months, with complete remission even if the initial loss of vision was complete. However, any single haemorrhage, and particularly repeated haemorrhages, may become 'organized', with forward spread of fibrous elements, often as a sheet running at right angles to the retina. This is liable both to cause a retinal detachment

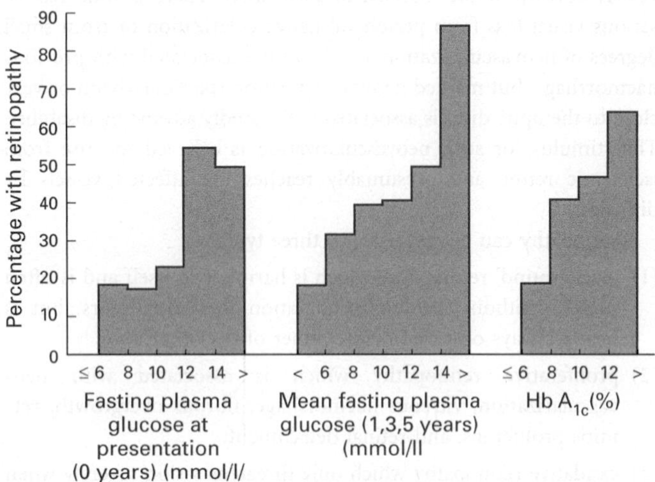

Fig. 5 Effects of control of blood glucose on diabetic retinopathy 7 to 9 years after diagnosis of NIDDM patients.

and to be a source of further vitreous haemorrhage, as the vessels growing forward over these fibrous sheets are particularly fragile.

No single feature of diabetic proliferative retinopathy is unique, but the evolution of retinal change is characteristic. Similar features are seen in hypertensive retinopathy and in the reaction to ischaemic areas of retina as are present after fat embolus, in sickle-cell disease, after venous occlusion, and in the hyperviscosity syndrome.

Hypertension exacerbates background and proliferative retinopathy, but smoking is believed to exacerbate only the latter. There have been claims that increased ocular tension may retard the development of retinopathy, but this is unproven.

Exudative retinopathy

This may present as either macular oedema or macular exudates or, much less seriously for vision, with exudates away from the macula. Macular oedema is the most difficult to recognize ophthalmoscopically. The retina shows a glazed appearance, with some diminution of vascular calibre and number, which is not necessarily accompanied by any obvious focal feature such as haemorrhage or exudate. Exudates are particularly liable to occur as crescents just lateral to the macula, but they may be sited anywhere. They should be distinguished from the usually smaller and highly refractile cholesterol deposits in the walls of vessels, particularly where they bifurcate. These indicate vascular change but are usually less directly related to visual disturbance. Fluorescein angiography may be particularly helpful in assessing the probable course of oedema or exudates by indicating the nature of the vascular pattern close to them and whether there is markedly increased permeability. This can be particularly helpful in deciding whether to coagulate vessels believed to be responsible for the formation of perimacular exudates. While exudative retinopathy is usually accompanied by background haemorrhagic lesions, when exudates occur alone the patient often has clinical features more typically linked with macro- rather than microangiopathy.

Management

The corrected visual acuity should be assessed in each eye separately in every diabetic 1 to 3 months from diagnosis to allow any temporary, refractile disturbance (due to rapid onset of hyperglycaemia) to settle. The fundi should be examined after pupillary dilation because about a third of abnormalities are missed in examination through undilated pupils. In patients aged under 40, checks should be carried out at intervals of 2 years until 10 years after diagnosis when annual checks should start. Annual review is wise in all those diagnosed over the age of 40 years. Some 4 per cent of diabetics have clinical retinopathy at diagnosis, and some 15 per cent on retinal photography, and nearly all these are type II patients aged at least 50 years. Younger patients are more prone to develop proliferative retinopathy, and older patients to show exudative changes with insidious visual disturbance from macular exudate or oedema. A minority (perhaps 10–15 per cent of type I patients) can be diabetic for 40 or 50 years without any ophthalmoscopic sign of retinopathy. Background retinopathy commonly develops 10 to 20 years after the disease is recognized, but may never progress to threaten vision. Minor ophthalmoscopic features (such as microaneurysms) may disappear, but this does not always indicate improvement for fluorescein angiography may show reduced perfusion. However, even fluorescein examination often shows that the deterioration ceases spontaneously. Proliferative retinopathy may become much worse during pregnancy, but such deterioration usually regresses substantially after delivery unless an irreversible lesion has occurred.

Treatment given early is more effective than at a late stage. It is not known whether photocoagulation can be beneficial at the stage of mild background retinopathy, but probably the main demand is for improved glycaemic control.

Treatment

Blood glucose must be controlled as closely as possible.

1. The fasting blood glucose needs to be consistently 6.0–6.5 mmol/l.
2. Hypertension and hyperlipidaemia need meticulous control (Table 11).
3. The retina can be photocoagulated by either xenon or argon arcs. The treatment is paradoxical in that it mimics the disease by reducing blood flow. The aim is to preserve the function of the crucial central retinal areas, even if this involves destruction of less important peripheral regions. Photocoagulation has been shown to be effective in randomized controlled trials and has been associated with a decrease of some 60 per cent over the following 5 years in the incidence of blindness both in patients with severe proliferative retinopathy and when perimacular lesions threatened function. Once retinitis proliferans has become established, or retinal detachment has occurred, or large exudates have developed close to the macula, photocoagulation has no effect. Similarly it is probable that improved glycaemic control will no longer retard deterioration once substantial retinopathy is established.
4. Vitrectomy has been developed as a treatment for blindness due to unresolved vitreous haemorrhage and as a treatment of retinal detachment subsequent to vitreous haemorrhage. Specialist opinion will be required before diabetics who have been blind in one eye for as long as 5 years are considered to have irreversible loss of sight.
5. Pituitary ablation was used before photocoagulation was available, to prevent the production of growth hormone and perhaps prolactin, although the exact role of diminished gonadotrophin secretion was never fully elucidated. In two small studies hypophysectomy was beneficial against severe proliferative retinopathy, but it is unsuitable for patients aged over 40 years

and is only feasible when there is unusually well-preserved renal function despite severe retinopathy.

Ocular cataract

The metabolic or 'snowflake' cataract of poorly controlled juvenile diabetics may be seen at first diagnosis of type I diabetes, but more often after a few years of poor glycaemic control. It may be very severe, causing blindness within a few days, but it can be reversed by early successful blood glucose control. Such a cataract can be extracted if it progresses, but this is rarely necessary.

The overall prevalence of common senile cataract seems no higher among diabetics than non-diabetics, but the former develop it earlier. It extends more rapidly and interferes more with vision among diabetics. Around 50 per cent of diabetics diagnosed more than 20 years previously have some lens opacity visible on examination, while the frequency of cataract extraction among diabetics is perhaps six times that in the general population. Operative results are almost as good in diabetics as in non-diabetics, although particular care must be taken to guard against infection. Lens opacities are more common in diabetic women than in men, and women show a faster progression.

A dense cataract makes it difficult to know whether diabetic retinopathy may have developed during its maturation, but blindness after extraction is less commonly caused by retinopathy than by operatic complication or failure in those known retinopaths from whom a lens is removed.

Other abnormalities

Severe hypertriglyceridaemia usually related to ketoacidosis may produce lipaemia retinalis, but this resolves within a few days with metabolic control and is not dangerous.

Rubeosis iridis is caused by proliferative microangiopathy of the iris and is usually seen only in patients with severe retinopathy. The lesion may interfere with normal drainage of aqueous humour from the anterior chamber and can lead to acute glaucoma and blindness if untreated.

Retinal artery or venous thrombosis may be commoner among diabetics than in the general population.

Neuropathy

Diabetic peripheral neuropathy affects the axonal processes of somatic and autonomic neurones (Table 18). It is debatable whether there is also primary neuropathy within the central nervous system. An increased liability to cerebral and presumably spinal arterial disease is widely accepted, as is the possibility of damage due to hypoglycaemia, particularly to certain layers of the cerebral cortex.

Peripheral neuropathy is both common and symptomatic, but it is more often annoying than life-threatening. It contributes to much of the foot ulceration of diabetics and is the cause of the uncommon Charcot's neuroarthropathy. Autonomic neuropathy is also essentially a nuisance initially, but later causes major morbidity and may even result in fatal complications. Thus, although severe postural hypotension is uncommon, disorders in the motility of stomach, large bowel, or urinary bladder can all be distressing, and predispose to infection or malnutrition, as well as carrying a poor prognosis. Impotence is particularly distressing. Cardiac autonomic neuropathy may lead to fatal dysrhythmia.

The most important factor in the development of neuropathy is probably the duration of diabetes. In diabetics aged 40 years or more, who have been diagnosed for at least 20 years, it is uncommon for there to be no evidence of peripheral neuropathy even though it may have little ill effect. The frequency of excruciating dysaesthesiae has been estimated at 3 per cent, that of incapacitating proximal neuropathy in at least one leg at 7 per cent, that of feet so numb that they are at real risk of traumatic ulceration at 24 per cent, that of diabetic bowel disturbance at 28 per cent, and that of impotence (males only) at 40 per cent. In contrast, each clinic of 1–2000 patients will usually contain only two or three patients with severe postural hypotension at a time and urinary retention severe enough for operation is rare.

Table 18 Diabetic neuropathies

Type	Structure involved	Main parts affected
Radiculopathy	Nerve root	
Mononeuropathy	Mixed spinal or cranial nerve	Single dermatome
	Nerve terminal	Arm, leg, cranial nerves III, IV, VI, X, XII
Polyneuropathy	Sensory and motor fibres	Feet
Proximal motor	Motor fibres	Quadriceps, gluteal muscles, hamstrings
	?Ventral horn cells	
Autonomic neuropathy	Sympathetic ganglia and fibres	Cardiovascular Gastrointestinal Bladder Impotence

Treatment, at least of newly diagnosed type I diabetics, can produce substantial improvement within 3 to 4 weeks although normality is not restored. Recent studies of large-fibre peripheral neuropathy in the legs have shown a positive correlation between glycaemic control over 5 years and the average degree of deterioration in vibration sense. This applied across a range of mean fasting glucose of 5–12 mmol/l. However, glucose levels are not the only factor contributing to the neuropathy. The pathogenesis is multiple. In addition to vascular lesions and segmental demyelination, there are abnormalities of both axoplasmic transport and the mechanism generating the action current, and perhaps also of the nodal membranes. Table 18 summarizes a classification of diabetic neuropathy.

Clinical features and management

Peripheral sensory neuropathy

Large-fibre disease may be detected clinically by loss of ankle jerks and decreased vibration sense. Likely symptoms are numb feet, with the feeling of walking on a bed of feathers or on a thick pile carpet. Loss of joint position sense is rarely severe enough to affect walking but can progress to produce a pseudotabetic picture. Gross loss of position sense contributes to Charcot's neuroarthropathy but in this loss of pain appreciation is more important.

Damage to small fibres alters pain sensation and probably underlies the unpleasant dysaesthesiae which range from feelings of numbness or compression via bizarre sensations of warmth or cold to tingling, pricking, and irritability. In a few patients the discomfort is excruciating. Small fibre damage also reduces or abolishes temperature sensation.

Most patients show a combination of large and small fibre involvement, but occasionally one or the other predominates sometimes almost to the exclusion of the other.

Most dysaesthesiae become more obtrusive as the patient settles for sleep or later in the night. Management consists in a combination of simple sedation or analgesia with identification of exacerbating physical factors. Many find relief by sleeping with their feet exposed, but others are helped more by bedsocks. Again, several are helped by raising the foot of the bed, while in others raising the head is more successful. There is no relationship between which manoeuvre will be successful and the presence or absence of foot pulses, except that an erythromelalgic picture with retained and even bounding peripheral pulses, and a reddish-blue but often cool foot is more likely to be helped by cool surroundings and foot elevation.

One comforting aspect of prognosis is that, as the neuropathy worsens the dysaesthesiae lessen, but then the need to take good care of the feet becomes critically important. Patients should inspect otherwise invisible parts of the foot each evening to ensure absence of any break in the skin or consequent infection. If their vision is impaired, they must ask relatives or friends to do this for them.

The hands are only rarely seriously involved clinically, although paraesthesiae of recent onset are more common at diagnosis in the hands than the feet, and diabetics are possibly more liable than others to nocturnal or early morning tingling of the fingers. Uncommonly a painful swollen hand with discoloured clammy skin, altogether suggestive of rheumatoid arthritis, may develop (diabetic cheiroarthropathy). The typical joint deformities of rheumatoid arthritis are absent, while muscle wasting is more localized. Such hands may suggest the causalgic syndrome and are presumably due to neuropathy involving vasomotor nerves. Sympathectomy is not a successful treatment of this or other forms of diabetic dysaesthesiae.

Femoral neuropathy (proximal motor neuropathy: diabetic amyotrophy)

This is typically of rapid onset and is very rare in young type I diabetics. In those over 50 years it usually causes weakness at the hip and knee, but seldom affects those on insulin treatment. It develops within a few days or sometimes more suddenly. Within weeks or months the other leg is often affected, but one is usually substantially worse. The thighs may be uncomfortable or even intensely painful. There may or may not be accompanying peripheral sensorimotor neuropathy. The lesion can be severe enough to prevent walking, even with a supporting frame. Rising from a chair or climbing stairs is often very difficult. However, there is excellent long-term prognosis, for within 12 to 24 months the patient is usually walking again, albeit with one or two sticks, because a substantial but mostly incomplete recovery is the rule.

The affected muscles waste and uncommonly fasiculate. The tendon jerk is lost or reduced to a flicker. There is no reason to believe that forced or excessive exercise speeds recovery, but passive movement is essential to preserve the neighbouring joints, and some practice in voluntary effort is almost certainly a help. It is very rare for the proximal shoulder muscles to be affected.

More widespread and even entirely distal motor lesions may be seen along with marked weight loss. This is sometimes termed 'diabetic cachexia' and may be severe enough to provoke an over-zealous search for malignancy. These lesions may represent pressure palsies of vulnerable nerves. This condition is usually seen in insulin-dependent type I patients, sometimes quite soon after diagnosis.

Diabetic mononeuropathy

Typical pressure mononeuropathies are common in diabetics, and are typically seen in the median nerve in the carpal tunnel, the lateral popliteal nerve just below the knee, the cervical spinal roots as they pass through the spinal foramina, and the first thoracic root if a cervical rib (or corresponding fibrous structure) is present. Sometimes it is probable that the lesion results from a vascular accident to a peripheral or cranial nerve. Its onset is then sudden and occasionally, when the nerve has a substantial somatic sensory component, is accompanied by a severe lancinating pain of very short duration. The cranial nerves most often affected are the oculomotor nerves, particularly III or VI. Substantial recovery from the resulting ophthalmoplegia can be expected in some 3–6 months. Mononeuritides of the hypoglossal, recurrent laryngeal, or intercostal nerves have also been described.

Autonomic neuropathy

Postural hypotension

This is rare but can be dramatic, with syncope and collapse on standing at its worst. After a spell of heavy glycosuria with loss of sodium and water, the circulating blood volume may have dropped and postural hypotension be more likely. A similar exacerbation may occur 30 min to 2 h after subcutaneous injection of insulin owing to increased transcapillary passage of albumin, again with a reduction in circulating blood volume although by no more than 5 per cent. The vasodilatation that occurs during hot weather or a febrile illness may exacerbate symptoms similarly, as may a temporary disturbance caused by spinal herpes zoster.

Treatment is by simple measures. Changing from a lying to a sitting position should be done cautiously, by sitting on the edge of the bed and exercising the legs for a min before standing. This is particularly necessary if patients wake at night to pass urine. Sitting on the lavatory during and after micturition may prevent associated syncope. Glycosuric natriuresis should be avoided. Otherwise treatment is as described under chronic autonomic failure (see Chapter 13.7). Elastic bandages or antigravity suits must be applied with caution if there is impairment of the arterial supply to the feet.

Impotence (see also Chapter 7.11)

Diabetics may become impotent insidiously or suddenly through failure of the autonomic functions controlling erection. Libido is normal, and there is often other evidence of autonomic neuropathy. Again, there is often accompanying somatic sensory neuropathy, but autonomic neuropathy may be present without clinical evidence of this. The cremasteric or bulbocavernous reflexes may be tested; their absence certainly supports the diagnosis of organic neuropathic impotence but their presence by no means excludes it. Diabetic autonomic neuropathy is sometimes the cause of retrograde ejaculation.

The differential diagnosis is from behavioural, psychic, or functional impotence and other organic causes, of which the most important are pelvic arteriosclerosis and endocrine disease of either the testes or the pituitary.

Functional impotence is common, and may stem from emotional disturbance from the diagnosis of diabetes itself, especially if the patient has heard that the disease may produce impotence. Onset of type I diabetes of any severity may cause a temporary organic impotence because of general weakness and the catabolic state, and this may be confused with long-term disability. Balanitis at the time of diagnosis or later may also lead to undue anxiety over erection and intercourse, which may also occur in the husbands of diabetics with pruritus vulvae. Later in the disease a temporary period of impotence, from intercurrent disease, exacerbation of hyperglycaemia, or functional causes, may be made permanent by overwhelming anxiety. Impotence occasionally arises from a horror that any children may develop diabetes.

A careful history is important in management, regarding both erections and possible causes of emotional upset in either the marriage or the patient. Normal nocturnal penile plethysmography gives good evidence of an adequate neurovascular mechanism and allows substantial reassurance, particularly by showing the tracing to the patient. Much depends upon the attitude of the partner, and it is important that she should not confuse a temporary or even long-lasting period of impotence with loss of affection. Marriage guidance counselling should be freely recommended. However, the plasma prolactin concentration should first be determined to exclude hyperprolactinaemia as a rare cause, and other endocrine tests should be performed if there are suggestive features.

Effective treatment of organic impotence is now often possible, but all methods depend upon a reasonable arterial supply to the penis. Pelvic angiography may show feasibility of arterial surgery or angioplasty, but the affected vessels may be too small for this to be possible.

Older treatments of the impotence of autonomic neuropathy involved application of a partial vacuum, using a plastic cylinder surrounding the penis and a hand-operated extractor pump, or self-injection of a smooth-muscle relaxant (papaverine) or, less usually, an α-adrenergic blocker (for example phentolamine) into the corpora cavernosa. The second method requires careful education of the patient and trial as to the correct dose and carries the risks of priapism, thrombosis, or a corpora cavernosal infection. Newer methods offer further benefit and convenience , but have yet to be fully evaluated. Oral sildenafil has helped diabetic men, but the relative contributions of psychic and neuropathic factors to their impotence was not clear. It is important to remember the increased incidence of cardiac disease among diabetics. Both oral and local dermal application of other vasodilators is also under study. There are now strong indications that sexual arousal and vaginal lubrication are impaired in diabetic women through neuropathy.

Diabetic diarrhoea

This is usually intermittent, occurring for a few days and then disappearing for weeks or months, but gradually increasing in frequency as the condition worsens. The motions are typically watery with mucus and only small amounts of faecal material, but the first one or two motions of a cluster may be fairly normal. Typically, diarrhoea begins in the early morning with up to 10 further motions during the day, and often settles by evening. However, a burst of diarrhoea may begin at any time, and in some there is undue frequency of defaecation soon after meals. There is rarely pain, but there may be abdominal distension. It is rare for particular foods to precipitate attacks.

Differential diagnosis includes the irritable bowel syndrome or other more serious causes of diarrhoea, but particularly pancreatic steatorrhoea. Also, many patients with type I diabetes eventually show deficient pancreatic exocrine function, and although it is rare for this to progress severely enough to produce clinical steatorrhoea, it may cause some malabsorption. Malabsorption usually causes weight loss, which autonomic diarrhoea does not. There is an increased prevalence of gluten enteropathy among type I diabetics.

The pathogenesis may depend upon incomplete digestion in an abnormal upper alimentary tract, altered bowel flora, or motor disturbance of the colon. The exact roles of the parasympathetic, sympathetic, and peptidergic nervous systems are uncertain, as is the possibility of disturbance in gastrointestinal hormonal production and response.

Codeine is usually an effective treatment, but this should become the main prop only if there is not a good response to a 5-day course of a broad-spectrum antibiotic such as metronidazole, neomycin, a cephalosporin, or tetracyline. Another course should be equally successful on recurrence, which often follows a few months later. Increased dietary bulk is usually helpful.

Diabetic gastroparesis can produce a gastric stagnation that is almost as severe as pyloric stenosis, and can cause intermittent vomiting or a succussion splash on examination. However, it is usually asymptomatic except for feelings of upper abdominal distension after meals. It probably leads to diabetic diarrhoea as a result of the production of irritant compounds in the sluggishly moving contents of the dilated viscera. It causes erratic glucose control in that the rate of absorption of meals becomes unpredictable. Breath hydrogen studies may indicate abnormal flora of colonic origin in the small bowel, and culture of duodenal aspirates may also reveal abnormal flora. Direct gastric motility studies are also useful.

Treatment of gastroparesis is by cisapride (10 mg twice or three times daily) or by metoclopramide in the same dose, or by cholinergic or anticholinesterase drugs. The last-mentioned may relieve many of the visceral effects of diabetic autonomic neuropathy but usually only partially or when it is mild; they also have side-effects, particularly on visual focusing and salivation.

Severe gastroparesis has a grave prognosis (50 per cent mortality within 2 years in one early study). The danger is mostly through an association with other severe manifestations of diabetic tissue damage but perhaps also through cardiac autonomic disturbance.

Sluggish motility of the gallbladder in long-standing diabetes may contribute to either gallstone formation or impaired digestion.

Urinary retention

This may result from impaired urinary bladder motility. Treatment is by education in abdominal straining and by trial of anticholinesterase or cholinergic agents, with only secondary consideration of self-catheterization. Surgery to the bladder neck can relieve retention, but often only at the risk of dribbling incontinence. Electrical devices to stimulate bladder contractility are disappointing.

Gustatory sweating

Rarely, on starting a meal, a diabetic has diffuse sweating and reddening of the face and blush area. Particular foods, such as cheese, may precipitate attacks in some.

Pupillary reflexes

These may be sluggish or absent.

Cardiac autonomic disturbance

It is difficult to know how serious this is. Electrocardiographic studies show frequent failure of the normal cardiac acceleration with deep breathing, standing, or mental arithmetic, and a plethora of manoeuvres has been used to illustrate this. Simple clinical tests include measurement of the R-R interval on the ECG during sleep or on slow deep breathing, or determining the ratio of the R-R interval on standing to that when lying down. Thus the ratio of the R-R interval at the 30th beat after standing compared with that at the 15th beat should be 1.0 or more. The more severe the abnormality, the more likely is the presence of other forms of autonomic neuropathy. Patients often have a moderate resting tachycardia, presumably due to vagal neuropathy, but such a finding is not rare in elderly non-diabetics, particularly if there is cardiomyopathy. Indeed, the usual response for age-matched non-diabetics should always be clearly established for any of these tests. This condition may contribute to postural hypotension.

It is not known whether autonomic neuropathy contributes to sudden death from cardiac dysrhythmia, but there is strong circumstantial evidence that patients with marked cardioneuropathy are at risk of sudden death from cardiorespiratory arrest following anaesthesia.

Collagen disturbance and skin problems

Tissue damage may result from increased glycation of collagen, with consequent change in its physical properties. Few clinical consequences are obvious, but Dupuytren's contracture is more frequently found in diabetics than others. A tendency to slight flexion of the hand is often seen, even in quite young diabetics of several years' standing. This is due to a change in collagen, perhaps particularly in periarticular membranes and ligaments, and may be associated with a waxy appearance of the skin. Thickening of the knuckle-pads of the first interphalageal joint is also common. The foot may also be affected, as shown particularly in the hammer toe deformity.

It is unknown how much collagen disturbance contributes to diabetic dermopathy, which presents mainly as trivial pigmented macules found particularly on the shins and usually regarded as the result of past trauma. These areas neither ulcerate nor cause discomfort. Secondly, a curious blistering can occur in diabetics through accumulation of serous fluid in a horizontal split in the epidermis, similar to that which may occur in non-diabetics after deep coma from intoxication. In diabetics the blisters may be precipitated by exposure to cold or wet, but sometimes occur without obvious cause. The sterile fluid within them may be mildly bloodstained. The lesions are best treated conservatively, but if the blister is large the fluid should be aspirated with a thin needle. Even then the pierced overlying skin is best left in place, at least until some repair of the base of the blister has occurred, when the overlying and then dead skin should be removed. The only indication to remove the overlying skin straight away is an infection of the contained fluid, but this is rare.

Necrobiosis lipoidica diabeticorum presents as painless areas, usually on the anterior aspects of the lower leg and typically 2 to 8 cm long. Although red at first, established lesions are yellowish in colour, often with slightly raised edges. Rarely, they become infected and then they are slow to heal, with difficulty in removing all infection. They persist for many years, typically in type I diabetics between 15 and 40 years old. Curiously, similar lesions are seen in non-diabetics, where their genesis is unknown. On biopsy in diabetics, microangiopathy is nearly always found in the underlying dermis.

Granuloma annulare is commoner among diabetics than in the general population, although the reason is unknown. Diabetics are also unduly liable to certain skin infections, particularly by fungi. Candida causes vulvovaginitis, but is seen also in the webs of the fingers and toes. These infections are all much more likely if there is poor glycaemic control; otherwise, treatment is with topical antifungal agents or sometimes, when there is a reservoir of colonic Candida, oral nystatin may be required for recurrent vulvar infection. Nail-plate infections by dermatophytes, giving onychomycosis, are more common. Fungal infections may cause fissuring, providing an entry for bacterial infection which can precipitate gangrene in a foot with compromised circulation. Tinea pedis should be aggressively managed by oral griseofulvin or ketoconazole in patients with poor circulation. Phycomycetes should always be suspected if a diabetic ulcer is unduly slow to heal. Occasionally, diabetics with gross hyperglycaemia may develop a rare but serious deep mycotic infection with mucormycosis. This typically involves the linings of the nasopharynx where black crusting or pus is seen on the turbinates, nasal septum, or pallet. Infection may spread to the nasal sinuses or the orbit. Treatment is by aggressive debridement of necrotic tissue and intravenous amphotericin.

The frequent yellowing of the nails of diabetics is not usually the result of dermatophytosis. It probably results from glycation.

Diabetic foot disease

Different types of diabetic tissue damage interact and combine in the feet, giving a wide variety of lesions ranging from relatively harmless dysaesthesiae to fulminating infections and widespread ulceration. Ulcers or ischaemic or dead tissue can develop in the absence of appreciable neuropathy, but never without some circulatory disturbance. However, this may be slight, with neuropathy the main cause of the lesion. Reduction in blood flow may be the consequence of macro- or microangiopathy. There may also be a contribution from autonomic neuropathy.

Infections of painless traumatic abrasions of neuropathic feet have the best prognosis. They occur particularly after trauma to the sole, which becomes progressively infected. The poor eyesight of elderly diabetics exacerbates this problem. The spreading infection may cause acute local vascular damage as a result of endarteritis obliterans, which leads to cell death and faster spread of the infection, resulting in wet gangrene. This contrasts with the dry gangrene that occurs with ischaemia of uninfected tissue, although such dead tissue may be secondarily infected to produce a wet state. Infarction of the toes may be due to thrombosis, for instance of the deep plantar arch or its prime branches. Less commonly it is due to an embolus, either from a fibrillating heart or of grumous material discharged from an arteriosclerotic ulcer of the abdominal aorta or more distal large vessel. Another serious lesion is the Charcot neuroarthropathic foot, which is grossly distorted, usually at the tarsal level, but remarkably painless.

Preventive management is as important as correct treatment of established lesions; chiropodists are key agents. The main aim is to prevent excessive pressure on particular areas of skin. Corns and callosities, or even areas of excessive keratinization on the soles or heels, may warn of this. Static footprints can be of help in identifying individual risk sites, while pressure measurements during walking can be made using specialized equipment.

Treatment of diabetic foot disease

Debridement

This must be thorough, extensive, and readily repeated. Drainage of infection must be ensured by opening out narrow sinuses into deep-lying pus, as well as saucerizing more superficial lesions. Radiographic evidence of bony infection is an immediate indication for amputation of such tissue, for however successful conservative management of osteomyelitis may be in the young and healthy, antibiotics alone rarely succeed in diabetic feet.

Antibiotics

Local antibiotic application is generally avoided, as it is liable to cause local skin sensitivity. Culture of pathogens from the surface of otherwise well-healing lesions is not an indication for systemic antibiotics, but they should be used if the infection invades surrounding tissue, and particularly if there is generalized disorder such as fever or deterioration in glucose control. The most difficult organisms to treat are Pseudomonas and Proteus, and their elimination usually depends on local therapy, which may include antiseptics such as iodine soaks or acriflavin. If there is excessive granulation tissue lotions such as acerbin may help.

Pain relief

This should be effective and repeated, as pain is vasoconstrictive.

Improved vascular supply

Before any substantial amputation of tissue, vascular repair to improve the blood supply should be considered. Vascular surgery has advanced to tackle some blocks distal to the arterial trifurcation just below the knee. Hence a palpable popliteal artery no longer excludes successful vascular repair, although it still lowers the chances. In perhaps 10 to 15 per cent of patients likely to undergo a mid-tarsal or more severe amputation, there may be a vascular lesion worth treating by surgery. Lumbar sympathectomy may relieve the pain from a diabetic foot, and occasionally aid healing, but the improved blood flow is probably only temporary.

Anaemia should be treated, and oedema from coincident heart failure should be appropriately managed. Elevation of an oedematous foot can reduce swelling, but may also reduce arterial perfusion if this is severely compromised.

Glycaemic control

Blood glucose levels above 10 mmol/l must be avoided, as they are associated with impaired function of the leucocytes, both polymorphonuclear and mononuclear. Insulin will often be required in those not previously receiving it, if only temporarily.

Amputation

The indications are as follows.

Life-threatening infection is a rare indicator for amputation but is particularly so if there is surgical crepitus or air within the tissues, revealed by radiography, indicating a gas-forming organism.

Removal of dead tissue is essential unless the patient is not thought able to withstand amputation, or if one or two toes have undergone dry gangrene when it may be best to leave them to wither and slowly separate spontaneously, when the bare area exposed to possible infection will be much smaller than after surgery. Osteomyelitic bone is usually best removed but there are reports of healing on long-term antibiotic treatment. This will require a healthy blood supply, good general condition of the patient, and close co-operation with bacteriologists to know what the infecting organisms are, including those in the bone, so that antibiotics may be changed accordingly.

Intractable pain is rarely a problem with infections, but sometimes results from dry gangrene or severe ischaemia.

Lifestyle needs range from the inability of a wage-earner to have the long period of rest necessary for conservative management, to undue boredom and deterioration of personality in an old person excessively confined.

Successive anaesthetics over a short period in an elderly and infected patient may be lethal, so it is important to be as accurate as possible in predicting the final outcome. Hence, one may be radical where the small bones of the forefoot are concerned, and cosmetic considerations for the elderly to conserve the phalanges of a toe whose metatarsal has mostly been removed are misplaced. The difficulty arises with the decision between a mid-tarsal amputation and an amputation a little below the knee. The amount of background diabetic tissue damage in these patients nearly always prevents success of Syme's amputation at the ankle.

Diabetic macroangiopathy

Diabetic heart disease

Several different processes contribute to diabetic heart disease. Accelerated coronary artery disease is the commonest. Although abnormalities in plasma lipids and hypertension account for much of this, the diabetic state itself, and indeed that of impaired glucose tolerance, also contribute perhaps through microangiopathy of the vasa vasorum and perhaps through changes in vessel wall collagen and others produced by protein glycation. Structural narrowing of the lumen may then be worsened by thrombus formation on the endothelial lining. Diabetics have increased plasma concentrations of some coagulative factors, for example fibrinogen and von Willebrand's factor, and their platelets have an increased sensitivity to aggregatory stimuli. The endothelium is also abnormal in its functional metabolism with regard to nitric oxide, plasminogen activator and its inhibition, and platelet-derived factors.

The increase in fibrosis and the change in the nature of the connective tissue act outside the coronary circulation to reduce the contractile power of the myocardium which becomes increasingly rigid, so producing diastolic heart failure. The first evidence of diabetic heart disease often comes from flattening or inversion of the T waves over the left ventricular leads on the ECG. This may develop in the absence of angina pectoris or any episode suggestive of infarction, and it may not worsen greatly in an exercise tolerance test.

A greater proportion of cardiac infarcts are painless in patients with diabetes than in non-diabetics and angina may also be less in diabetics. Therefore an exercise test is as important as are symptoms. The T-wave relationship with the 'sudden death' syndrome among diabetics is also uncertain but a long Q-T interval in the ECG is associated with such deaths.

The management of ischaemic heart disease among diabetics differs little from that generally employed. The minor disadvantages of β-blockers for diabetics do not prevent the use of selective agents such as atenolol. The hypoglycaemic action of aspirin when combined with sulphonylureas is so slight that this should never prevent its use. Coronary angiography is more likely to show multiple lesions with a tendency to be relatively distal in the arterial tree, but many patients are suitable for arterial bypass or angioplasty.

The 1-month mortality after cardiac infarction is increased some two- to threefold among diabetics. Patients treated by sulphonylureas seem to be more vulnerable than those given insulin or managed by diet alone. The infarct precipitates a phase of hyperglycaemia for 1–5 days, and short-acting insulins should be used as supplements to usual therapy, aiming at control of the blood sugar to between 7 and 10 mmol/l.

Diabetics can also develop a cardiomyopathy not evidently of ischaemic origin.

Hypertension in diabetics

Much thought has been given to whether hypertension or renal disease comes first among diabetics. For type I patients, the evidence from microalbuminuria suggests mild renal involvement first; for many type II patients the two appear to develop in parallel, or hypertension is present first.

Poorly controlled hypertension is likely to accelerate the rate of progress of both diabetic nephropathy and retinopathy. Therefore antihypertensive treatment must be particularly meticulous. The preferred antihypertensive agents are the ACE inhibitors, the α-adrenergic antagonists, and selective β-blockers. The thiazide diuretics tend to impair glucose tolerance as well as elevate blood lipids. Effective treatment of hypertension improves mortality, total and cardiac, and reduces renal impairment and accelerated retinopathy. Usually a combination of several antihypertensive agents is necessary to lower the blood pressure to the target values of 140/80 mmHg.

Special problems

Infection

Diabetics with poor glycaemic control are particularly prone to develop severe bacterial or fungal infections. Approximately half the cases of ketoacidosis in known diabetics are due to infection. There are three aspects of the problem: first, the effect of infection on metabolism; second, the increased liability to serious infections in hyperglycaemic diabetics; third, those infections which occur specifically with much increased frequency in diabetics.

Metabolic effects of infection

Infections lead to a stress response, with increased secretion of cortisol, glucagon, and catecholamines. These increase insulin resistance and blood glucose concentration and, in the absence of a normal insulin response, also increase ketogenesis. In the type II diabetic there may be a temporary need for exogenous insulin, and in the type I patient insulin requirements may rise dramatically. Infected patients often stop eating and may mistakenly decrease their insulin. Even when no food is taken the daily dose of insulin should be as much as or more than usual. Every effort should be made to maintain a reasonable calorie intake, if necessary purely in liquid form, for example lemon squash with 20 g of sucrose, glucose, or honey every 2 h, or Ribena or Lucozade, or milk with added sucrose. If food intake is likely to be erratic, it may be easier to rely on several injections per day of quick-acting soluble insulins, but this does not take into account the increase in the basal insulin requirement. Hence those on Ultratard and Actrapid should increase the Ultratard dose by some 20 per cent and decrease the Actrapid by about the same number of units initially, but the latter should be divided between three injections instead of the usual one or two. Blood tests will then indicate whether adjustments, up or down, are necessary in the total daily dose.

Host defences against infection in diabetes

Chemotaxis and phagocytosis are defective in both hyperglycaemic and ketoacidotic diabetics, and the microbicidal activity of polymorphonuclear leucocytes may also be impaired. Abnormalities are consistently found when fasting blood glucose levels exceed 10 mmol/l making the case for rigorous glycaemic control in any patient with an infection.

Table 19 Infections associated with diabetes mellitus

Urinary tract infections* (females):	cystitis, pyelonephritis, perinephric abscess*, acute papillary necrosis*, fungal urinary tract infection
Mucocutaneous candidiasis	
Furunculosis (staphylococcus)	
Gram-negative pneumonia, staphylococcal pneumonia*	
Tuberculosis*	
Foot-ulcer-related infections*	
Cryptococcosis, histoplasmosis, blastomycosis, coccidioidomycosis	
Rhinocerebral mucormycosis*	
Malignant otitis external*	
Cholecystitis*	
Influenza*	

*Proven associations; the remainder are possible or suggested associations.

Specific infections in diabetes

Some of the infections proved or suggested to be particularly associated with diabetes are shown in Table 19. The prevalence of bacteriuria is three times higher in diabetic than non-diabetic women. Poor glycaemic control is not the only factor; abnormal bladder function from autonomic neuropathy can also be important. Pyelonephritis, perinephric abscesses, and papillary necrosis are also associated with diabetes, particularly when there has been poor glycaemic control.

Impaired motor function, secondary to autonomic neuropathy, is one reason for the increased liability to cholecystitis, together with altered cholesterol and bile salt metabolism.

An association between tuberculosis and diabetes mellitus has long been suspected, with a greater incidence in poorly controlled diabetics.

Fungal infections are also frequently associated with poorly controlled diabetes. *Candida albicans* is the most common agent, particularly in females who present with vaginal or vulval candidiasis. Candidial infections of the bladder and skin are also found. Other fungal infections are rarer but can be catastrophic, such as rhinocerebral mucormycosis.

Cutaneous infections are more common in poorly controlled diabetics. The rare but severe malignant otitis externa due to *Pseudomonas aeruginosa* should probably be included in this group. In most cases infections in diabetics respond to standard therapy, provided that the glucose levels are simultaneously brought under good control.

Anaesthesia and surgery

Surgical procedures probably carry both increased morbidity and mortality. Coincident cardiovascular disease and obesity contribute, as does autonomic neuropathy.

Even with modern anaesthetics there is generally an increase in secretion of cortisol and catecholamines, although halothane does not increase the latter. There is an initial decrease in insulin secretion, in those still capable of producing it, and an increase in insulin resistance, although the effects of anaesthesia are small when compared with the metabolic upset of surgery itself. These effects are avoided by spinal anaesthesia, provided that it is not accompanied by excessive hypotension.

Table 20 The management of insulin-treated diabetics during surgery

Preoperative
1 Admit to hospital 2–3 days before operation
2 Stop long-acting insulins and stabilize on either twice-daily short-acting and intermediate insulins or thrice-daily short-acting insulin with intermediate insulin in the evening
3 Monitor blood glucose (bedside methods) before and after each main meal and at bedtime
4 Aim to maintain fasting blood glucose <8 mmol/l, and other values between 4 and 10 mmol/l
5 Check urea, electrolytes, and renal, cardiovascular, and neurological systems
Perioperative
1 Schedule operation for early in the day
2 Check fasting glucose. If ^{3}13 mmol/l, delay operation
3 Omit morning insulin and breakfast
4 Start infusion of glucose–insulin–potassium (see Table 29) as early as possible and at least 1 h preoperatively
5 If operation delayed more than 2 h from onset of infusion, recheck blood glucose and adjust infusion if necessary
6 Recheck blood glucose at end of operation (and during lengthy operations) and modify regimen if necessary
7 Check K^+ as in point 6
Postoperative
1 Check glucose every 2–4 h and K^+ every 6 h, then twice daily
2 Continue infusion until first meal taken; restart subcutaneous insulin at preoperative dose 1 h before infusion stopped
3 Consider total parenteral or gastrointestinal nutrition if oral refeeding not recommenced within 48 h

SC, subcutaneous.

Surgery causes an immediate neuroendocrine response with release of ACTH, cortisol, catecholamines, growth hormone and glucagon. Insulin levels may fall owing to inhibition by catecholamines and other factors, with a loss of responsiveness to glucose. The end result is hyperglycaemia proportional to the severity of surgery. During and after surgery the mobilization of lipids is less than would be expected, particularly in fasting patients. Thus there is a dependence on glucose for oxidative metabolism, and so an increased utilization of amino acid for gluconeogenesis. The increase in cortisol also increases protein catabolism.

These changes will be exaggerated in the non-insulin-treated diabetic, where insulin secretion is already compromised and insulin resistance is present. In the untreated insulin-dependent diabetic the endocrine changes will lead to severe hyperglycaemia, ketoacidosis, and major loss of protein.

Management of insulin-treated diabetics undergoing surgery

A guideline to pre-, per-, and postoperative management is shown in Tables 20 and 21. The defined aim is to maintain blood glucose between 5 and 10 mmol/l. The infusion (Table 21) should be continued until the first meal has been taken, when subcutaneous insulin may be reinstituted but begun at least 1 h before the infusion is discontinued because of its relatively slow absorption and the rapid decay in plasma insulin level once the infusion has stopped.

There are several ways in which the insulin can be given. The safest method is to put it directly into the bag or bottle of intravenous dextrose. In this case variations in infusion rate will affect all components equally, and wide glycaemic swings are less likely.

Insulin resistance is common, and is most severe during and following cardiopulmonary bypass surgery. In this case the standard glucose–insulin–potassium infusion should be used preoperatively, but insulin alone should be infused during surgery when as much as 20 units/h may be needed, with the amount being determined by frequent glucose monitoring. A combined glucose–insulin infusion should be restarted at the end of the operation, but insulin requirements will continue to be high for the next 24 hours.

Other infusions should be given through separate lines. If requirements result in potential fluid overload, half the volume of 20 per cent dextrose can be used instead of the 10 per cent preparation.

Day admissions for minor procedures present a separate problem. They should not be encouraged for insulin-treated patients, but may be dictated by lack of beds. Patients should come to the hospital early in the day, omitting their usual insulin and breakfast. Blood glucose should then be checked. If it is less than 13 mmol/l, and above 6 mmol/l, the patient can go immediately to theatre and return to the day ward to be given insulin and breakfast as usual. Blood glucose can be checked once more, and the patient can return home in the late afternoon. The alternative is to start an infusion on admission, and this will apply to all patients with fasting blood glucose above 13 mmol/l. The infusion is then continued until the first postoperative meal when short-acting insulin is given. Usual therapy is reinstituted with the evening meal, after which the patient may return home.

Table 21 Insulin infusion regimen for pre-, per- and postoperative management of diabetes during surgery

1 Add 15 units short-acting insulin (soluble)+10 mmol KCl to 500 ml 10% glucose (dextrose)
2 Run 25–50 ml through infusion tubing before attaching to patient
3 Infuse at 100 ml/h
(If there is need to limit fluids, use double amounts of insulin and KCl in 20% glucose and infuse at 50 ml/h)
If blood glucose >10 mmol/l increase insulin by 4 units/500 ml; check blood glucose 2 h later; increase by further 4 unit increments as necessary
If blood glucose <5 >3 mmol/l decrease insulin by 4 units/500 ml; check blood glucose 2 h later; decrease by further 4 unit decrements as necessary (if glucose <3 mmol/l, stop insulin for 1 h)

Management of non-insulin-treated diabetics undergoing surgery (Table 22)

Blood glucose both pre- and postoperatively should be checked every 2 to 4 h. After major surgery it is probably safest to use thrice-daily insulin for 1 or 2 days when refeeding begins before attempting reconversion to sulphonylureas or therapy with diet alone. These patients are particularly at risk of cardiovascular illness and meticulous attention should be paid to potassium, fluid balance, and myocardial function.

Table 22 The management of non-insulin-treated diabetics during surgery

Minor operations	
Diet-treated	If BG ≤10 mmol/l treat as non-diabetic If BG >10 mmol/l treat with insulin infusion regimen during operation
Oral agent treated	1. Stop biguanides and long-acting sulphonylureas 2–3 days preoperatively Stabilize on diet alone or short-acting sulphonylureas
	2. If BG ≤10 mmol/l on day of operation treat as non-diabetic If BG >10 mmol/l treat with insulin infusion regimen during operation
Major operations	
Diet-treated	Admit to hospital 2 days before operation
	1. If BG ≤7 mmol/l, treat as type I diabetic on day of surgery
	2. If BG >7 mmol/l treat with short-acting insulin three times daily preoperatively; treat as type I diabetic on day of surgery
Oral agent treated	1. Stop all oral agents 2 days preoperatively
	2. Treat with short-acting insulin three times daily>
	3. Treat as type I diabetic on day of surgery
Postoperative management	
	1. Minor surgery: recommence usual therapy with first meal
	2. Major surgery: Convert to subcutaneous insulin two times daily with first oral feeding; recommence oral agent or diet-alone therapy 24–48 h later

BG, blood glucose; SC, subcutaneous.

Emergency surgery in diabetes

In nearly all cases there is some metabolic disturbance and sometimes frank ketoacidosis. The trap of abdominal pain consequent to the ketoacidosis in younger patients, which disappears with rehydration and insulin therapy, must be emphasized. One important guide is that if vomiting precedes abdominal pain, the latter is more likely to be due to ketoacidosis.

The first priority is to assess glycaemic and acid–base status. While results are awaited a saline infusion should be started and nasogastric suction applied where appropriate. If moderate or severe ketoacidosis is confirmed, the operation should be delayed for 4–5 h if possible whilst rehydration and standard therapy for ketoacidosis is applied (see below). In all such cases hourly blood glucose monitoring is desirable. Insulin resistance is likely and a higher insulin infusion rate will be required (0.5–0.8 units/g glucose compared with the usual 0.3 units/g).

Brittle diabetes

Only about 1–2 per cent of diabetics truly fall into this category. The causes fall into five main groups: therapeutic errors, intercurrent illness, accessible emotional causes, self-induced (or carer-induced), and unknown aetiology.

Commonest is therapeutic error by either the physician or the patient. For example attempts to achieve morning normoglycaemia in a totally insulin-deficient patient by once-daily therapy can cause repeated severe hypoglycaemia in the late afternoon or evening. Similarly, nocturnal hypoglycaemia can be produced by over-enthusiastic increases in intermediate insulin in the late afternoon. This may lead to extra food intake, and early morning hyperglycaemia. Imperfect dietary advice can also result in wide glycaemic fluctuations. Equally, the patient can generate the brittle state by erratic exercise and lack of dietary compliance. Somogyi described the phenomenon of reduction in overall glycosuria by lowering the dose of insulin. This could result from clinically silent hypoglycaemia provoking a increased food intake. Suggestions that an undetected period of hypoglycaemia could trigger a counter-regulatory response, with subsequent hyperglycaemia, have been much debated.

The second most likely cause is intercurrent illness, infection, endocrine disorder, or pancreatic disease. The commonest occult infective cause worldwide is probably tuberculosis. The brittle state always resolves with cure of the infection. Endocrine causes include hyperthyroidism, Addison's disease, and hypopituitarism. Amongst pancreatic causes are pancreatectomy, which is predictable from the lack of pancreatic glucagon, chronic pancreatitis, and, more obviously, pancreatic steatorrhoea.

The third and fourth causes may well be linked. Home disturbances and family conflict may cause glycaemic instability. It is not certain how much of this is due to a neuroendocrine disturbance and how much to manipulative behaviour. This type of brittle diabetes is not uncommon in adolescence, may disappear spontaneously when the psychosocial problems resolve, or may occasionally respond to psychotherapy or family group therapy. The liability to premenstrual hyperglycaemia, most marked in adolescence and sometimes episodic monthly before menarche, certainly has an endocrine basis.

The fourth group is the most difficult to deal with and is estimated to have a prevalence of one per 1000–2000 type I diabetics in the UK. The majority of such patients are female aged between 14 and 26 years, and the onset is soon after menarche. They are all mildly overweight, which may be secondary to overeating in response to intermittent hypoglycaemia. The majority require large subcutaneous doses of insulin with considerable day-to-day variation in requirement. Many have intermittent sluggish insulin absorption from subcutaneous injection possibly due to varied subcutaneous blood flow and shallow injection. Some respond well to intravenous insulin.

Measurement of plasma insulin concentrations has shown that a notable proportion produce the situation deliberately. There may also be evidence of manipulation by the carer, whether a parent or nurse (Munchausen's syndrome by proxy). Although sophisticated manipulative patients may produce alarming metabolic swings, they usually ensure that help is available in time to provide proper therapy. One frequent feature is that introduction of new techniques of insulin administration are followed by a period of relative stability until a manipulative patient has worked out what is happening. Sometimes such improved glycaemic control breaks a vicious circle and the restored physical well-being is so welcome that a return to conventional treatment may then be successful.

By definition one cannot describe the last group. Some may be due to fluctuating concentrations of antibodies against insulin receptors. Measurement of plasma insulin in relation to effect can be useful.

Adolescence

Features of diabetes particular to adolescence include unusually large daily variations in energy output, variability in the nature and timing of meals, and generally increased emotional and hormonal turmoil. The anabolism of growth may disturb metabolism more than is realized.

Adolescent patients are often highly motivated, but equally are readily discouraged. Some girls experience particular problems around menarche. Either during the first few menstrual cycles, or at approximately monthly intervals before onset of menstruation, rapid deterioration in glycaemic control may occur. So far no convincing hormonal explanation has been advanced. This remains an important but usually relatively short-lived conundrum. Prescription of oral contraceptives (low oestrogen) for a few months sometimes helps. Rapid response with extra insulin to incipient loss of control is important.

Another special problem arises at the time of cessation of upward growth. If the energy intake necessary for growth continues after it has ceased, larger doses of insulin may become customary which sustain the food intake at a time when it would have fallen in the healthy adolescent. Obesity then develops. The growth spurt early in puberty poses the opposite problems; failure to increase caloric intake as necessary to fuel the initial spurt can result in well-controlled glycaemia but failure in growth.

Coma in diabetics

Hypoglycaemic coma (see Chapter 6.14)

At least one-third of insulin-treated patients suffer an episode severe enough to cause loss of consciousness at some time, 10 per cent have such coma annually, and, at some stage, 3 per cent suffer recurrent attacks so frequently as to be incapacitating. Hypoglycaemia also occurs in those taking sulphonylureas but true coma is uncommon in these patients.

Diagnosis

Usually there are important clues in the history: the patient is a known diabetic, on insulin, and has probably been completely normal as little as 15 or 30 min before the onset of stupor. There may have been a phase of typical symptomatic hypoglycaemia or of abnormal behaviour, usually mild confusion and sluggish speech, but occasionally wild and aggressive. On examination the patient is not dehydrated, hyperventilating, nor ketotic. The most important evidence is of insulin injection sites. There may be non-specific helpful physical signs, such as symmetrically dilated pupils (which react normally to light) and tachycardia, but a drenching sweat is often the most useful. The condition has to be distinguished from non-metabolic comas; the neck is not stiff, but the plantar reflexes may be upgoing. A rapid measurement of the blood glucose is essential in any undiagnosed comatose patient.

Hypoglycaemic episodes are more likely to occur several hours after the last meal or after unusual physical exertion but attacks do not always occur classically.

Self-administered insulin overdosage is always a possibility, as are errors in the preparation of the insulin dose. There has been unjustified concern that human insulin has unique properties favouring hypoglycaemia.

Different people have different thresholds for neuroglycopenia, and that threshold alters in the same patient under different circumstances. It is affected by the rate of glycaemic fall (the faster, the higher), by the size of the fall (the bigger, the higher), and by the habitual glycaemic levels for 36 to 60 h (the higher, the higher the threshold). There is a tendency for 'hypoglycaemic unawareness' to develop in patients with increasing duration of diabetes. The cause is uncertain, although developing autonomic neuropathy with failure of normal catecholamine release may be implicated, as may increasing α-cell damage with failure of glucagon release.

Symptoms

These are discussed more fully in Chapter 6.14. As symptoms develop diabetics may resist advice to take sugar from onlookers and great firmness may be needed to achieve intake of quickly absorbed carbohydrate.

The frequency of undetected nocturnal hypoglycaemia is difficult to assess, but a value below 2.0 mmol/l probably occurs at least annually in a third of insulin-treated patients. Patients sometimes wake in the morning with grossly disturbed bedclothes, or even lying on the floor, without any memory of upset during the night. Alternatively, a throbbing headache may be the only residue. Hypoglycaemia may precipitate epilepsy, either by day or by night, but this is rare and not always realized during sleep. Anticonvulsants do not seem to protect against epilepsy which occurs as a complication of diabetic hypoglycaemia.

The amount of cumulative brain damage that results from recurrent hypoglycaemia is difficult to assess, but most studies indicate mild impairment of higher mental function in any insulin-treated patients suffering over 5 to 10 years two or three attacks annually, which are severe enough to require help from others.

Treatment

It is vital that no fluid be put into the mouth of a patient who is so comatose that he or she cannot swallow properly. A patient in such a state requires an intravenous injection of concentrated glucose, usually 20 ml of 50 per cent initially. The alternative is intramuscular injection of 1 mg glucagon by a relative or other carer. This may increase the blood glucose sufficiently to allow oral glucose to be given, but it does not help some comatose patients and is often less effective than intravenous glucose. While it has a real place in the management of the stuporose, it should never be allowed to delay the call for help that will lead to the administration of intravenous glucose. It has the great advantage of providing some independence to the family unit, and whenever possible a family member should be trained in glucagon injection. A paste containing glucose may be rubbed into the buccal mucosa to give some help.

After the administration of intravenous glucose, the patient usually comes round within a minute or two, but then may lapse back into stupor or sleep. If there has been no substantial response to the first injection within 5 min, a further intravenous injection of 20 ml of 50 per cent glucose should be given. There is no point in increasing the dose further, but if the patient still does not respond a continuous intravenous infusion of 5 per cent glucose in water (or 4 per cent glucose in N/5 saline) should be started. The blood glucose should be checked by glucose oxidase strips and confirmed in the laboratory.

If consciousness is still abnormal after an hour, further treatment should be considered. There is no objective evidence that high dose glucocorticoid treatment or any other measure against cerebral oedema is beneficial, but equally none that they do harm, although the steroids will increase the insulin dose required in management over the next 24 to 48 h. Many physicians use such agents.

After recovery from a severe attack a patient may be best managed either by continuous intravenous insulin or by frequent injections of small doses of short-acting insulin. The routine daily dose of insulin should be decreased by at least 4 units when it is resumed unless there is some obvious explanation for the hypoglycaemic episode.

Hyperglycaemic comas

The majority of patients with major hyperglycaemia are not comatose, but confused or stuporose. Type I diabetics generally suffer ketoacidotic hyperglycaemia, while type II diabetics may present with or without ketosis. In the UK as many as 70 deaths occur annually from hyperglycaemic coma in those under 50 years old, and the mortality in this condition increases with age to approximately 50 per cent in those over 70. These emergencies occur perhaps once in 200 patients each year, but as particular patients may contribute several events, rather fewer individuals are affected annually. Ketoacidosis is relatively common in girls around menarche who may suffer repeated attacks at intervals of 1 or 2 months.

The mortality from ketoacidosis remains as high as 3 to 10 per cent in hospitals that admit all emergencies. If individual factors are examined for their correlation with mortality, age is the most important. Associated illnesses (such as overwhelming infection, cardiac infarction, and pulmonary embolism) are also dominant; the elderly are more likely to present with coma accompanied (and very likely precipitated) by such associated conditions. The depth and duration of coma are also prognostic factors. The clinical state of the patient is of greater prognostic influence than their disturbed biochemistry. The blood urea concentration is a more important guide than the blood glucose, the blood ketones, the plasma bicarbonate, or the arterial pH.

The biochemical feature most related to the depth of unconsciousness is plasma osmolality; the blood glucose concentration and the degree of acidosis or ketosis correlate poorly with disturbed unconsciousness.

The onset of severe ketoacidosis is linked indirectly to depletion of total body water, sodium, and potassium, and no doubt major changes in the intracellular electrolytes. The levels of the catabolic and hyperglycaemic hormones increase markedly to magnify the crisis.

Non-ketotic coma occurs in older patients in whom there tends to be less severe insulin deficiency, and defective renal function leads to greater losses of water and electrolytes when there is persistent heavy glycosuria.

Ketoacidotic hyperglycaemic coma

The three cardinal clinical features of ketoacidotic hyperglycaemic coma are signs of extracellular volume and intracellular water depletion, air hunger with an increased depth and rate of breathing, and ketosis. Some can identify the last of these by the typical sickly sweet smell on the breath, but 20 per cent cannot detect this usefully and the sensitivity of the remaining 80 per cent varies greatly. The degree of ketosis can also be readily assessed either by testing the urine or by centrifuging heparinized blood and testing the clear supernatant with Ketostix or Ketodiabur. The acid-base disturbance is discussed in Chapter 6.17.

When a history is available this varies from several weeks to a few days, and is often shorter in those already on insulin treatment. Occasionally excessive physical activity precipitates ketoacidosis in someone already severely hyperglycaemic from marked insulin deficiency. There may have been weight loss, fatigue, excessive thirst, and polydipsia with polyuria. Other cardinal features are anorexia or vomiting, with or without diarrhoea. The onset of vomiting is always a threatening symptom and is particularly useful as a warning in those already known to be diabetic. An uncommon but well-recognized symptom is abdominal pain, which is likely to occur in younger patients as a dull persistent severe discomfort often affecting the whole abdomen but usually centred on the umbilicus. It may cause unjustified suspicions of an abdominal emergency.

The patient is likely to have a rapid pulse of low volume and low systolic pressure. There may be postural hypotension, certainly because of volume depletion, and perhaps because of temporary autonomic neuropathy which may also contribute to vomiting and diarrhoea. Significant postural hypotension in a markedly hyperglycaemic and ketonuric young patient, however alert and physically active, should always indicate the need for immediate parenteral fluid treatment. Infection of the urinary tract or other sites, for example ischiorectal, dental, or perinephric abscess, should be sought.

Certain physical signs may be unexpectedly absent during ketoacidosis. Thus, even if there is a pyogenic infection, there is usually no fever until insulin treatment has been given for 6 to 12 h. Indeed, some patients may be hypothermic initially. Again, classical signs of consolidation in patients with lobar pneumonia may not be elicited even though the radiograph shows lung shadows. The blood leucocyte count is of no help in assessing the likelihood of an infection, for the metabolic disturbance itself can cause a severe (95 per cent) polymorphonuclear leucocytosis of up to 30×10^9/l.

Differential diagnosis

Table 23 shows guidelines for diagnosis. The main differentials are:

Any other illness with overventilation

Uraemic or lactic acidosis is the commonest. Hyperventilation from salicylate overdosage is another possibility, but the most confusing picture is *Claude Bernard's 'piqure' diabetes* which is a short-lived hyperglycaemia from a lesion in the region of the fourth ventricle. It probably results from massive discharge of the sympathetic division of the autonomic nervous system. The accompanying hyperventilation is due to irritation of pathways involved in respiration, and such overbreathing produces a respiratory alkalosis rather than the usual metabolic acidosis. Determination of the arterial pH is decisive, as the bicarbonate concentration will be low in both instances. Patients with such fourth-ventricle lesions may have mild ketonaemia because of reduced food intake and a degree of hypermetabolism (possibly with fever), and their conscious state will also be disturbed. The hyperglycaemia of piqure diabetes settles spontaneously in 6 to 12 h, and unless the glucose concentration is watched carefully unnecessary insulin treatment can cause a rapid swing to hypoglycaemia. The fall in glucose is unaccompanied by any improvement in consciousness, unlike the situation in diabetes. Hypoglycaemia may then further worsen central nervous function. Fourth-ventricle lesions are often accompanied by neck stiffness, but a degree of meningism may also occur in ketoacidosis. If there is doubt, a lumbar puncture will differentiate.

Table 23 Differential diagnosis of coma in diabetics

	Blood glucose* (mmol/l)	Plasma ketones†	Dehydration	Hyperventilation	Blood pressure
Hypoglycaemic coma	≤2	0	0	0	Normal
Severe diabetic ketoacidosis	>13	+ to +++	+++	+++	Normal or low
Hyperglycaemic hyperosmolar non-ketotic coma	>13	0 to +	++++	0	Normal or low
Lactic acidosis	Variable	0 to +	0 to +	+++	Low
Non-metabolic comas	Normal to high	0 to +	0 to +	0 to +	Variable

*Assessed with Visidex or BM-Glycemie 20–800 R.

†Assessed with Ketostix.

Non-ketotic hyperglycaemic states

Of the features discussed above, only dehydration is present. Glucose levels should be checked in any stuporose or even confused patient, particularly if old. Unilateral signs of central nervous system abnormality do not exclude the diagnosis, for if a metabolic disturbance coincides with asymmetry of cerebral blood flow focal neurological signs may be present.

Many ketoacidotic patients are markedly hyperosmolar. The differences in management depend upon arterial blood pH and plasma sodium.

Investigation

Initially, blood urea, plasma sodium and potassium, and arterial pH should all be measured in addition to glucose and ketones. Arterial pO_2 is surprisingly low initially, in perhaps 20 per cent of patients even below 8 Torr. Heart rate, blood pressure, respiratory rate, and level of consciousness must be recorded. The discrepancy between the warmth of the abdominal wall and the tip of the nose is a guide to impaired peripheral circulation.

Blood glucose and potassium levels should be reassessed 1 h after the start of insulin treatment and, unless the clinical course is convincingly satisfactory, arterial pH and blood urea should be remeasured after 3 h together with glucose and potassium. The last two should also be measured after 5 h. Crucial targets are normality of the plasma potassium concentration, and the level of blood glucose (about 12 mmol/l) at which glucose should be added to the intravenous infusion.

Treatment

Treatment is summarized in Tables 24 and 25.

Fluid

The basis of treatment is the replacement of water, sodium, insulin, and potassium. Normal saline (0.9 per cent) should be given rapidly, for example 0.5 litres in the first 20 min and 2.5 litres in the next 3 h, with infusion of 500 ml hourly thereafter to a total of about 5 litres (or until a normal circulation is present and obvious clinical features of dehydration have disappeared). The use of hypotonic sodium chloride is indicated only when there is marked hypernatraemia, for example an initial plasma sodium concentration of 150 mmol/l or higher, and even then not initially (see below).

A report of a plasma sodium concentration under 110 mmol/l should raise suspicion of pseudohyponatraemia due to gross lipaemia which may be missed if the plasma is not looked at after centrifugation. A clinical clue to this may be lipaemia retinalis, in which the small retinal vessels are yellow.

The central nervous system in ketoacidosis is unduly liable to oedema. Hence the osmolality of the extracellular fluid should be kept relatively high but if plasma sodium concentration exceeds 149 mmol/l, half-normal physiological saline should be infused after 2 litres of normal saline to prevent further hypernatraemia. Hypernatraemia is particularly liable to occur in non-ketotic patients. If the blood pressure is unduly low (below 90 mmHg systolic) and/or the peripheral circulation is little improved 2 h after start of treatment, a plasma expander should be infused.

Insulin

The necessary actions of insulin in diabetic ketoacidosis are to inhibit inappropriate gluconeogenesis and excessive adipose tissue lipolysis. Concentrations of 60–80 mU/l are the aim during treatment because, with the high glucose concentrations, a maximum uptake of glucose by peripheral tissues can then be achieved, with a decrease in blood glucose of 3–5 mmol/l/h. Insulin can be administered either by hourly intramuscular injection or by continuous intravenous infusion.

Intramuscular regimen

An initial injection of 20 IU of short-acting insulin should be followed by a further 6 IU hourly. It is important that the injections are intramuscular and not subcutaneous. If blood glucose has not dropped by 5 mmol/l after 2 h, a change to the intravenous route is indicated together with reassessment of fluid status.

Intravenous

After an initial bolus of 6 IU of crystalline insulin the same amount (6 IU) is infused hourly in adults. This is best given by a pump. Absorption of insulin to the walls of syringes or tubing occurs but is not a clinical problem. The recommended rate of insulin administration should be doubled if glucose falls by less than 5 mmol/l in the first 2 h. The rate of fall is remarkably constant in individual patients, and allows a rough and ready prediction of when intravenous glucose should be infused, which is at a blood glucose between 10 and 15 mmol/l. This serves both to provide necessary fuel to a starving patient and further to reduce the chances of cerebral oedema. The intravenous glucose is best given as 500 ml of 4 per cent dextrose in 0.18 per cent saline (one-fifth normal) every 4 h.

Insulin can then be continued by intravenous infusion at 2–4 IU/h. If the intramuscular route has been used, the injections may be changed to 6 IU every 2 h; alternatively subcutaneous injections of 12 IU insulin can be given every 4 h. The intravenous route should be used only as long as it is necessary to give intravenous fluids on

Table 24 Management of diabetic hyperglycaemic comas

Initial assessment	
Clinical examination	Hydration, respiration, pulse, blood pressure, consciousness, signs of infection
Biochemical	Bedside: glucose, ketone body test strips, ECG Laboratory: glucose, Na^+, K^+, urea arterial pH, PO_2
Treatment	
Fluid	1 litre of 150 mmol/l saline in 30 min; 1 l/h for next 2 h, then 0.51/h until 5–7 l given in total, when give 500 ml 2–4 hly, but change to 4% glucose in 30 mmol/l saline, 500 ml every 4 h, when blood glucose 10–15 mmol/l. If plasma Na^+ >150 mmol/l use hypotonic saline after early isotonic saline. Consider use of central venous catheterization
Insulin	IV regimen. 6 unit IV bolus, then 6 units/hour continuously IV; change to 2–4 units/h continuous IV when dextrose infusion commenced; change to subcutaneous with first meal IM regimen; 20 units intramuscular (or 10 ml IM/10 units IV) initially, then 6 units every h; change to 6 units every 2 h or 12 units subcutaneous every 4 h when dextrose infusion commenced
Potassium	Start at 13–20 mmol/l/hour in saline just after first insulin; adjust rate according to plasma values (26 mmol/h if plasma K^+ 3–4 mmol/l, 39 mmol/h if K^+ < 3 mmol/l, 10 mmol/h if K^+ 5–6 mmol/l, stop IV potassium if plasma K^+ >6 mmol/l)
Bicarbonate	Give 100 mmol+20 mmol KCl in 20–40 min if pH <7.0; repeat after 60–90 min if pH still <7.0 Give 50 mmol+10 mmol KCl if pH <7.1 but >7.0 or if patient distressed by hyperventilation

IV, intravenous; SC, subcutaneous; IM, intramuscular.

Table 25 General measures in the treatment of diabetic hyperglycaemic coma

1. Nasogastric tube in unconscious patients
2. Continuous venous pressure line in patients with cardiovascular disease
3. Plasma or plasma expanders in persistent hypotension
4. Low dose subcutaneous heparin in comatose, obese, or severely hyperosmolar patients, provided that there is no contraindication
5. Antibiotics if infection detected or suspected
6. ECG; cardiac monitor as guide to K^+ therapy
7. Bladder catheterization if prolonged failure to pass urine
8. Frequent monitoring of pulse, blood pressure, respiration, conscious state

other grounds. Feeding should be encouraged as soon as possible, beginning with small quantities of simple fluids.

Potassium

Patients in diabetic ketoacidosis have a total body deficit of potassium averaging 500 mmol and sometimes more than twice this. A major action of insulin is to increase tissue potassium uptake. Therefore once insulin treatment has been started, it is safe to infuse potassium provided that both the potassium and the insulin will reach the tissues. The only contraindication to early potassium supplementation is a grossly inadequate circulation, such that potassium added to a small circulating blood volume does not reach enough cells for its uptake to be increased effectively by insulin. It is also only in patients with such an inadequate circulation that there is a real risk of acute tubular necrosis, with the possibility of prolonged anuria or oliguria. Obviously this makes ill-judged potassium administration potentially dangerous, but this is much less so now that peritoneal dialysis and haemodialysis are more widely available.

Even though a quarter of the patients admitted with diabetic ketoacidosis are hyperkalaemic initially potassium should be given a few minutes after intravenous insulin and about 10 min after intramuscular insulin, with the exceptions noted above. In the first hour 10–13 mmol/l potassium chloride can be given safely, by which time the initial potassium concentration should be available. At this stage another sample should be sent for assay, as the change over the first hour helps greatly in the prediction of future doses, which can be altered accordingly. With resalination and insulin treatment plasma potassium may fall fast, particularly from high values. Thus a drop from 6.4 to 5.2 mmol/l may occur in the first hour, even though 13 mmol/l potassium was given. If concentration is between 3 and 4 mmol/l the rate of intravenous infusion can be increased to 26 mmol/l/h, while if it is below 3 mmol/l at least 40 mmol/l/h should be given.

Low initial plasma potassium concentrations are most common in the newly diagnosed, when the period of kaliuresis is likely to have been considerably longer than in those already on insulin, and in patients treated with a thiazide or similar diuretics. Such patients may require 400–600 mmol of potassium in the first 12 h of treatment.

Potassium should be started orally as soon as fluids can be taken, initially as potassium-rich fluids such as meat soups, fruit juice, or milk. Particular attention must be paid to potassium replacement when intravenous bicarbonate is given (see below).

Bicarbonate (see Chapter 6.17)

This is a contentious aspect of treatment. The advantages of bicarbonate infusion are reduction in metabolic acidosis and consequent relief of distressing hyperventilation. If acidaemia is severe (pH < 7.0), tissue function may be impaired with a negative inotropic effect on the heart, peripheral vasodilatation, and depression of the central nervous system. However, bicarbonate infusion also has the disadvantages of favouring hypokalaemia and a leftward shift in the dissociation curve of oxyhaemoglobin so that oxygen less readily reaches the tissues. The dissociation curve is approximately normal on admission of ketoacidotic patients, despite the marked acidosis which, by the Bohr effect, would be expected to have moved the curve to the right. However, the right shift is approximately balanced by decreased red-cell 2,3-diphosphoglycerate. If the metabolic acidosis is rapidly corrected, the curve will shift to the left as the 2,3-diphosphoglycerate deficit persists for 24 to 72 h after treatment starts. In addition, after bicarbonate infusion a metabolic alkalosis often appears as ketonaemia disappears. This is rarely severe enough to disturb health, but it shows that the amount of bicarbonate needed is often less than that given.

Ketosis disappears through oxidation of the ketone bodies in the periphery, coincident with inhibition of their further formation in the liver once insulin has checked the typical excessive lipolysis. The drop in concentration of these organic acids is faster than the rise in bicarbonate concentration of the plasma, and usually a mild hyperchloraemic acidosis occurs for a short while during replacement therapy.

Therefore bicarbonate should not be given as long as the peripheral circulation is grossly restricted, for it will almost certainly reduce oxygen delivery to the periphery. However, once sufficient saline has been given to restore a reasonable circulation, 100 mmol sodium bicarbonate should be given over 20 min if pH is below 7.0, and 50 mmol in the same time if it is between 7.1 and 7.0. Such bicarbonate should be accompanied by an extra 20 mmol of potassium chloride per 100 mmol of bicarbonate. Arterial pH should be measured 60–90 min later to decide whether more bicarbonate is needed (with the amount judged similarly).

Hyperosmolar hyperglycaemic non-ketotic coma

The patient should be treated in similar fashion to the classical ketoacidotic case, but the following special points should be noted:

1. Approximately half such patients are hypernatraemic, so that hypotonic fluid replacement may be necessary although not initially. In general, total fluid requirements are likely to be greater (but so is the risk of cardiac failure).
2. There is an increased likelihood of thrombotic events, so that prophylactic anticoagulation should be seriously considered.
3. Smaller amounts of potassium are required than in ketoacidotic patients. A replacement rate of 10–13 mmol/h is probably adequate.
4. Blood glucose levels are likely to be extremely high, so that restoration of normoglycaemia will take many hours, but, as with ketoacidotic patients, too great a rate of fall of glucose levels could be harmful because of the effects of osmotic disequilibrium on the central nervous system.

General management

An unconscious patient should be nursed semiprone until a thin nasogastric tube has been passed and any gastric content aspirated. Frequently this is of large volume. If aspiration into the lungs has occurred, anti-inflammatory doses of glucocorticoid should be given. The intubation should be done as soon as possible, for such aspiration is often fatal, and gastric stasis not uncommon in these patients.

An ECG should always be recorded early in case an acute (and possibly painless) cardiac infarction has precipitated the metabolic emergency; serial records can help assess electrolyte recovery via the T-waves.

Urethral catheterization has no place early in management as it readily introduces infection, unless a distended bladder makes the patient restless.

Central venous catherization is best confined to patients in whom there is real suspicion of cardiac embarrassment, as when intravenous fluid is rapidly administered to those with known cardiac disease, or to the aged. If there is any suspicion of deterioration from fluid infusion, a central line should be inserted but should be removed as soon as possible in order to reduce the risk of infection. Failure of the heart rate to decrease during treatment can indicate cardiac insufficiency, but another cause may be the uncommon deterioration in pulmonary function that can occur 4 to 8 h after treatment starts. This is associated with a radiographic appearance like that of pulmonary oedema and a marked drop in arterial pO_2. Medium or coarse crepitations are heard over the lung fields, quite unlike the fine moist crepitations of left-sided heart failure. If the condition is severe enough to warrant artificial ventilation, pulmonary compliance is very low. The cause of such stiff lungs is uncertain, but may result from interstitial pulmonary oedema or, alternatively, from a disseminated intravascular coagulation particularly affecting the lungs. The possibility of interstitial oedema has led to arguments about whether it is the the oncotic pressure of the plasma that matters in this state, and some would advocate the use of colloids in this situation.

It is probably wiser to confine the use of anticoagulants to high risk patients, such as those in deep coma, those with a known history of venous thrombosis, the very obese, and the very hyperosmolar. Subcutaneous heparin injections should not be started until 4 to 6 h after admission, which will allow some time for clinical assessment.

While routine use of antibiotics has been suggested, prescription on more positive grounds is probably preferable. When diabetes newly presents as a metabolic emergency, infection is rarely a precipitating cause. Also, bacterial infection is rare in known diabetics who present after 2 or 3 days of vomiting, particularly if admission has been precipitated by marked reduction in their usual insulin dose. However, infection, for example an ischiorectal abscess or a relatively small foot ulcer at the mouth of a sinus leading to a deeper collection of pus, should be sought avidly. Whether or not there is intraperitoneal infection when there is abdominal pain, conservative treatment by intravenous fluids, antiobiotics and insulin, together with gastric aspiration, is best for at least the first 4 to 6 h. If the abdominal features are purely metabolic, there should then be substantial improvement; if peritonitis is present, a fever is then likely to have appeared and the patient's condition will probably have worsened rather than improved. Surgery, for however good a cause, is dangerous in the presence of severe ketoacidosis, which should be dealt with first. With current antibiotics, intravenous fluids, and gastric aspiration, little will be lost on the surgical side by such delay but a great deal will be gained medically. If antibiotics are to be given, blood, urine, and throat swabs should first be taken for culture.

Further reading

Cooper, M.E. (1998). Pathogenesis, prevention, and treatment of diabetic nephropathy. *Lancet*, **352**, 213–19.

Edelman, S.V. (1998). Importance of glucose control. *Medical Clinics of North America*, **82**, 665–87.

Mogensen, C. E. (1998). Combined high blood pressure and glucose in type 2 diabetes. *British Medical Journal*, **317**, 693–4.

Nathan, T. (1998). Some answers, more controversy from UKPDS. *Lancet*, 352, 832–3.

Kahu, C. R. and Weir, G. C. (1994). *Joslin's Diabetes Mellitus* (13th edn). Lea and Febiger, Philadelphia.

Turner, R.C. (1998). The UK Prospective Diabetes Study. A review. *Diabetes Care*, 21(suppl. 33), C35–8.

Chapter 6.14

Hypoglycaemia

*R. C. Turner**

Hypoglycaemia is an uncommon cause of symptoms in adults, apart from diabetic patients on insulin or sulphonylurea therapy; but any curious attack, in which a low plasma glucose concentration is found, should be investigated as some of the causes of hypoglycaemia can be life-threatening, yet are readily treatable.

Pathological hypoglycaemia

Spontaneous hypoglycaemia can be divided into two main categories:

1. Fasting hypoglycaemia which only occurs after several hours without food. It always indicates an identifiable underlying disease.
2. Reactive or postprandial hypoglycaemia occurs 2–5 h after meals. These patients never have hypoglycaemia during a fast, although occasionally patients with fasting hypoglycaemia may have a reactive component. Reactive hypoglycaemia usually occurs in the absence of organic disease.

Clinical features

Hypoglycaemic symptoms are unusual unless the plasma glucose falls to less than 2.5 mmol/l. However, the threshold varies from person to person. Patients with prolonged hypoglycaemia (from an insulinoma, for example, or a diabetic patient chronically overtreated with insulin), have a lower threshold, and can have a plasma glucose of 1 mmol/l for several hours without symptoms. At the other extreme, a diabetic who has had prolonged hyperglycaemia may get adrenergic symptoms if the plasma glucose concentration is rapidly lowered towards normal.

Adrenergic symptoms usually predominate, particularly when the plasma glucose falls rapidly. Adrenaline is secreted (together with the other counter-regulatory hormones including glucagon, growth hormone, and cortisol) and induces pallor, sweating, tremor, and palpitation.

Neuroglycopenic symptoms occur when the brain has insufficient glucose resulting in poor concentration, slow movements, dysarthria, double vision, tingling around the mouth, transient strokes, fits, and coma in a variety of combinations. Each patient may have a characteristic group of symptoms. The features may resemble ethanol intoxication. Poor judgement and inco-ordination can be especially dangerous if the patient is driving, swimming, or near to dangerous machinery. Neuroglycopenic symptoms predominate when chronic hypoglycaemia occurs, because the threshold to adrenergic symptoms is then lowered.

Treatment

The treatment of acute hypoglycaemia is discussed in Chapter 6.13. Glucagon is not effective when there is hepatic dysfunction, as in ethanol-induced hypoglycaemia when hepatic glycogen is depleted. Glucagon should not be given to a patient with an insulinoma, as it may stimulate more insulin secretion and induce greater hypoglycaemia.

Sequelae of hypoglycaemia

Short-duration hypoglycaemia does not produce obvious, permanent neurological sequelae, which are rarely apparent after hypoglycaemic coma of less than 4 h duration. Occasionally, normal recovery occurs in patients who have been unconscious for more than 24 h, although they may be drowsy and confused for several days. Nevertheless, prognosis for recovery of cerebral function deteriorates with increasing duration of coma. Brain damage is more likely if hypoglycaemia is accompanied by hypoxaemia or hypotension. Cerebral oedema may be a secondary factor and mannitol or high-dose dexamethasone therapy sometimes appears to expedite recovery. Prolonged severe hypoglycaemia can lead to cortical atrophy and prolonged coma or dementia, but seldom causes death unless complicated by fits or inhalation of vomit. The degree to which multiple, short-duration hypoglycaemic comas can cause insidious brain damage is uncertain, but clinically apparent neurological deterioration is only recognized in those patients who, for some reason, have experienced in the order of hundreds of events.

Fasting hypoglycaemia

Diagnosis

Anybody with an unexplained 'funny turn' or transient stroke should promptly have blood glucose measurement with a glucose-oxidase strip. The results are semiquantitative, and if 'low' (<4.0 mmol/l), blood samples should be taken for laboratory assay of glucose and insulin. A fasting plasma glucose of less than 3.5 mmol/l is likely to be pathological. If a patient is recovering from a hypoglycaemic episode by the time a blood sample is taken a level of 4–5 mmol/l may be found, in part due to secretion of adrenergic and other stress hormones. Thus a normal value after an attack may not exclude an episode of hypoglycaemia. Different laboratories have different normal ranges, and this makes definition difficult.

Table 1 lists the differential diagnosis, and details of specific diseases are given below. In adults most of the causes of fasting hypoglycaemia, other than insulinoma can be recognized clinically by history and examination. Liver disease, Addison's disease, or hypopituitarism are usually clinically obvious. An extrapancreatic tumour is usually large, and either palpable or easily seen on radiography. Ethanol-induced hypoglycaemia only occurs in patients who have had a prolonged fast, and can usually be excluded by the history. Thus, an adult with proven fasting hypoglycaemia, who is otherwise well, will usually have an insulinoma, or be self-administering insulin or a sulphonylurea. Other possibilities are primary adrenocorticotrophic hormone (ACTH) or growth hormone deficiency, an occult sarcoma, or autoimmune anti-insulin or anti-insulin receptor antibodies.

Any disease or drug that inhibits glycogenolysis or gluconeogenesis may lead to fasting hypoglycaemia. They can be divided conveniently into categories: (a) excess insulin-like activity, and (b) non-insulin-induced hepatic dysfunction. The plasma insulin during spontaneous hypoglycaemia is the key investigation, and measurement of plasma 3-hydroxybutyrate is also helpful.

Excess insulin or insulin-like activity [for example insulin-like growth factor (IGF) -II, or insulin receptor antibodies] inhibit both hepatic glucose and ketone-body production, so patients do not have

* It is with regret that we must report the death of Dr R. C. Turner.

Table 1 The differential diagnosis and investigation appropriate to either fasting hypoglycaemia or postprandial hypoglycaemia in adults

Fasting attacks
Exclude clinically
Hypopituitarism
Addison's disease
Ethanol ingestion after a fast
Cirrhosis of the liver and acute hepatic failure
Sarcoma (including chest radiography, plain abdomen radiography)
Availability of insulin/sulphonylurea for self-administration
Severe heart failure or renal failure
Septicaemia, e.g. shigellosis or malaria
Aspirin, β-blocker, pentamidine, or other drugs
Any autoimmune disease, including thyrotoxicosis treated by methimazole
Surgical removal of phaeochromocytoma
Investigations
No ketonaemia during hypoglycaemia
Insulinoma
Inordinately raised plasma insulin and C-peptide during hypoglycaemia:
during spontaneous episode after an overnight fast insulin suppression test with C-peptide assay during prolonged fast
Fasting plasma proinsulin
Self-administration of sulphonylurea
Investigation results as for insulinoma
Tablets in patient's possession
Plasma sulphonylurea assay
Self-administration of insulin
Available insulin supply
Insulin antibodies
During 'spontaneous' hypoglycaemia, low plasma C-peptide with high plasma insulin
Autoimmune insulin antibodies
Detected with immunoassay
During 'spontaneous' hypoglycaemia, low plasma C-peptide with high plasma insulin
Autoimmune insulin receptor antibodies
Hypoglycaemia with low plasma insulin and C-peptide
Send plasma for insulin receptor-binding studies
Sarcoma hepatoma, or other solid tumour
Hypoglycaemia with low plasma insulin and C-peptide
Send plasma for IGF-II assay
Often ketonaemia during hypoglycaemia
Pituitary/adrenal failure
Plasma cortisol and growth hormone during hypoglycaemia
Pituitary stimulation tests
ACTH response to corticotrophin-releasing factor
Synacthen test (6 days' administration for isolated ACTH deficiency)
Ethanol
Plasma ethanol during hypoglycaemia
Postprandial attacks
Exclude clinically
Gastric surgery
Mild diabetes
Think of possibility of fasting hypoglycaemia
Investigations
Extended oral glucose tolerance test with either capillary blood or 'arterialized' venous samples from the back of a warm hand.
Home blood glucose sampling with memory meter or filter paper blots and a diary

ACTH, adrenocorticotrophic hormone.

ketonuria, ketosis, or raised 3-hydroxybutyrate levels. Ketonaemia is a feature of starvation or ethanol-induced hypoglycaemia, because the low plasma insulin levels secondary to the hypoglycaemia allow free fatty acid release and ketone-body production. Insulinomas might be expected to give a high insulin and low 3-hydroxybutyrate level after an overnight fast, but a normal 3-hydroxybutyrate level is usually found. The insulin immunoassay can be used to detect the presence of insulin antibodies, from self-administration of bovine or porcine insulin or autoimmunity.

Insulinomas

There is a low incidence of insulinoma (approximately 4/million/year) but it is the most common cause of fasting hypoglycaemia in non-diabetic subjects admitted to hospital. The tumours are semi-autonomous and maintain insulin secretion in the presence of hypoglycaemia, which suppresses normal β-cell function. The persistent basal insulin secretion by insulinomas inhibits hepatic glucose efflux and thus causes hypoglycaemia. Insulinomas can occur at any age, the median being in the sixth decade. The aetiology is usually unknown, although when associated with multiple endocrine neoplasia (see below) the inherited tendency is mediated by a deletion of part of chromosome 11q. In sporadic insulinomas, deletions of both alleles of the retinoblastoma gene have been reported.

Patients characteristically present with drowsiness on waking, which is relieved by a sweet drink or breakfast. They may present to a neurologist, because of confusional states or 'funny turns' (including paraesthesiae, diplopia, faintness, light headedness, fits, or an apparent stroke that is secondary to hypoglycaemia). Symptoms can occur several hours after a meal, particularly associated with exercise, for example prior to lunch after a busy morning's shopping. The tumours grow very slowly, and patients have often had symptoms for several years. Nevertheless, cognitive impairment is very unusual. Most patients have no change in weight, but a few find symptoms can be prevented by frequent meals and become obese. There are no abnormal physical signs when the patient is normoglycaemic.

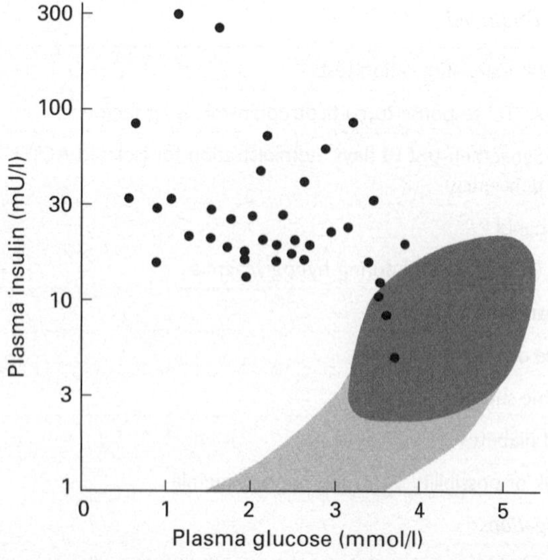

Fig. 1 Inordinately raised fasting plasma insulin concentrations after an overnight fast in 31 patients with insulinomas (each shown as a black square). The dark shaded area is the normal fasting plasma glucose and insulin range, and the lighter area the normal suppression of plasma human insulin in response to hypoglycaemia. The majority of patients with insulinomas have a diagnostic high plasma insulin during their spontaneous hypoglycaemia. Those with normal fasting plasma glucose fail to suppress their plasma insulin to below 1.5 mU/l during a hypoglycaemic suppression test.

(Adapted from Turner, R.C. (1976). Hypoglycaemia: Proceedings of the European Symposium, Rome. Hormone and Metabolic Research **6**, *40.)*

The tumours are usually small, 0.5–5 cm diameter, and occur in any part of the pancreas. Ectopic insulinomas rarely, if ever, occur. The tumours can be well or poorly differentiated histologically, often secreting more proinsulin than insulin. They respond subnormally to meals, and blood glucose after a meal or an oral glucose tolerance test may paradoxically be moderately high (for example 10 mmol/l). Although immunostaining may show a few other islet cells containing glucagon, somatostatin, gastrin, ACTH, or other hormones, it is rare for these to be secreted or to cause symptoms, even in the 5–10 per cent of insulinomas which are malignant.

The diagnosis of or exclusion of an insulinoma is needed in any patient with suspected fasting hypoglycaemia. Insulinomas are primarily diagnosed by a suppression test. Normally, hypoglycaemia inhibits insulin secretion, the plasma insulin level being less than 1.5 mU/l for a fasting plasma glucose of less than 2 mmol/l (normal range 3–13 mU/l at normal fasting plasma glucose concentrations). The possible investigations are:

(1) *Overnight fasting plasma glucose and insulin measurements.* Patients with insulinomas in effect do their own suppression tests, as 90 per cent have marked hypoglycaemia after just an overnight fast. Their plasma insulin concentration, which induced the hypoglycaemia, is inordinately high in relation to the normal plasma glucose/insulin relationship (Fig. 1). If the fasting plasma glucose is below 2.5 mmol/l, a plasma insulin concentration greater than 5 mU/l is diagnostic. Values greater than 3 mU/l are suggestive and indicate an additional suppression test.

(2) *Overnight plasma pro-insulin measurement.* A high proportion of pro-insulin is secreted by insulinomas. Its diminished biological effect, compared with insulin, means that patients with normal fasting plasma glucose concentrations still have inordinately high pro-insulin concentrations. Thus, the ideal screening test is measurement of one or two fasting samples for pro-insulin. However, pro-insulin assays are not widely available.

(3) *Admission for 2-day fast.* This is time-consuming and uncomfortable for patients, and is rarely needed now that dynamic tests are available. During the fast, it is important to maintain exercise to try to induce hypoglycaemia. Blood samples are taken every 6 h for insulin, C-peptide and laboratory glucose assay, and are monitored promptly. If hypoglycaemia, below 2.5 mmol/l, occurs at any time during the fast, an additional blood sample should be taken for glucose, insulin, C-peptide, cortisol, growth hormone, and 3-hydroxybutyrate assay. A plasma or urine sample for sulphonylurea assay may be indicated. After a 72-h fast, normal subjects have a plasma C-peptide concentration below 0.1 nmol/l, whereas in those with insulinomas it exceeds 0.2 nmol/l when the fasting glucose levels are less than 2.8 mmol/l. The plasma for C-peptide assay has to be kept at 4°C, and frozen at −20°C as soon as possible, because it is susceptible to degradation if blood or plasma is kept at room temperature, whereas insulin and pro-insulin are remarkably stable, even at room temperature. Once hypoglycaemia has been induced, a blood sample should be taken 30 min later for cortisol and growth hormone assay, as a test of pituitary/adrenal function. If a dynamic test (see below) suggests an insulinoma, but spontaneous hypoglycaemia has not been documented, a fast is required. A fast is also needed if a dynamic suppression test is normal, but the clinical suspicion of hypoglycaemia is sufficiently high that one needs to exclude rare causes such as autoimmune hypoglycaemia or isolated ACTH or growth hormone deficiency.

(4) *Dynamic suppression test.* Insulin is administered over a 2-h period to induce hypoglycaemia (for example, 0.05 U/kg per h intravenously) and plasma C-peptide, which is secreted on an equimolar basis with each insulin molecule, is measured to monitor endogenous β-cell secretion. An intravenous cannula should be used to ensure venous access in the unlikely event of a fit. When the plasma glucose is below 2.5 mmol/l, the test can be terminated. At that glucose level, the plasma C-peptide should suppress to below 50 per cent of the basal level and to less than 150 pmol/l.

(5) *Stimulation tests are no longer used.*

Localization and excision of insulinomas

Abdominal ultrasound and computed tomography (CT) scans only detect large tumours and are usually not helpful. Magnetic resonance imaging (MRI) is more sensitive but might not detect small tumours. Insulinomas have somatostatin receptors and tumours of diameter 3 mm can be detected with a gamma camera following intravenous labelled octreotide. Specificity and sensitivity have not yet been assessed. The need for accurate pre-operative localization has been reduced by the efficiency of intra-operative ultrasound and it is reasonable to proceed directly to surgery if this technique is available.

Endoscopic ultrasonography can detect small tumours, particularly in the head of the pancreas. Coeliac axis angiography can localize an adenoma in 60–70 per cent of patients, with additional superior mesenteric artery angiography required for adenomas in the uncinate lobe of the head of the pancreas. When the tumour is visible on angiography, it is usually large enough to be found easily at operation. It is doubtful whether angiography is now ever warranted.

Percutaneous transhepatic cannulation of the portal vein for multiple blood sampling of effluent from the pancreas in the portal, splenic, and superior mesenteric veins is only needed if there has been a failed operation and other investigations have been inconclusive. High localized plasma insulin concentrations indicate the position of the tumour, but many venous samples are needed. In a normal subject, the pulsatility of basal insulin secretion provides variable levels that may imply a tumour. The test should only be done in patients in whom a suppression test has confirmed the diagnosis, as the insulin secretion from the rest of the pancreas is suppressed by chronic hypoglycaemia, and this aids localization. In addition, it is advantageous if the blood glucose is low–normal (about 3–5 mmol/l) during the investigation to assist inhibition of secretion of insulin from the normal pancreas.

Surgical therapy and intraoperative ultrasound

Surgical excision of the tumour is the main therapy for fit patients. The majority of insulinomas can be palpated at operation, even if they were not detected preoperatively, although mobilization of the pancreas may be required. Direct operative ultrasonography is of great assistance, the tumour, appearing as a dense area with a surrounding non-reflective halo. The insulinoma can then be enucleated, with care being taken not to damage the exocrine pancreatic duct in the posterior part of the pancreas.

Repeated measurement of the plasma glucose concentration, with a rise following excision of the tumour, has been suggested to be helpful in confirming excision. A lack of rise indicate that other tumours are still present. This technique is not completely reliable, particularly if the anaesthetist has to give blood or other glucose-containing fluid. It can take 30–60 min for the plasma glucose to rise after excision, and the technique is probably only indicated if multiple tumours have been found.

If an insulinoma cannot be found, distal pancreatectomy should not be undertaken, as the tumour is most likely to be hidden in the head of the pancreas. Biopsy of the tip of the pancreas to exclude β-cell hyperplasia or nesidioblastosis should be performed. Then the patient should be referred to a centre that undertakes endoscopic ultrasonography or labelled octreotide scanning.

Medical treatment

Hypoglycaemic attacks can usually be prevented by frequent fibre-containing meals, including during the night if necessary. Somatostatin infusion (up to 300 μg/day), with physiological glucagon replacement, can be used in the short term if attacks are very severe. Octreotide injections are often unsuccessful, as suppression of glucagon and growth hormone secretion can aggravate the hypoglycaemia. Diazoxide therapy, 150–800 mg/day, will relieve symptoms in about 50 per cent of patients. However, it may induce nausea, rashes, and, in women, hirsutism. Sodium retention can be counteracted with a thiazide diuretic. Despite its limitations, medical treatment may be preferable to an operation in the elderly, or in other patients in whom surgery is undesirable.

Multiple endocrine neuroplasia (see also Chapter 7.14)

It is unusual for insulinomas to be part of a multiple endocrine neoplasia (**MEN**) type 1 syndrome, but measurement of plasma calcium to detect hyperparathyroidism is indicated, particularly if there is a family or personal history of other endocrine neoplasia. If MEN 1 is present, there is a greater chance of multiple adenomas or malignancy.

β-Cell hyperplasia

There have been a few reports of β-cell hyperplasia or β-cell adenomatosis as a cause of hypoglycaemia in adults. Most are poorly documented and depend on a non-quantitative, subjective interpretation of islet size. Many of these patients have probably had an occult insulinoma, but diffuse islet abnormality can occur rarely in adults.

Malignant insulinomas

These account for 5–10 per cent of insulinomas, and often such patients already have hepatic metastases at presentation. The undifferentiated tumour usually is inefficient at secreting insulin, and large hepatic or lymph node metastases are present before the tumour bulk is sufficient to induce enough insulin secretion to produce symptoms. It is rare for the tumours to secrete other peptides giving symptoms, although 75 per cent secrete β-choriogonadotrophin. Symptoms from the secretion of ACTH, gastrin, vasoactive intestinal polypeptide, or the mediators of the carcinoid syndrome can occur.

Diazoxide and somatostatin, given by intravenous infusion, or subcutaneous injections of octreotide are usually of little benefit. 'Debulking' by surgical excision of large hepatic metastases, or by infarcting them by selective arterial catheterization can give relief of symptoms for several months.

Streptozotocin, particularly combined with 5-fluorouracil, can dramatically decrease the size of the tumour and its deposits, and temporarily relieve persistent hypoglycaemia. Relapse usually occurs within a year, but some patients are free of symptoms for 2 or 3 years. Streptozotocin can cause renal failure, and the dose has to be titrated carefully, for example 500 mg/m^2 streptozotocin and 400 mg/m^2 5-fluorouracil intravenously given on alternate days for 10 days, stopping the course if albuminuria or hepatic or bone marrow dysfunction occur. The course can be repeated every 2–3 months for three to four courses, with a 6-month wait to assess the effect or side-effects. Mithramycin, carboplatin, cyclophosphamide, and α-interferon have also been used.

Death eventually ensues from uncontrollable hypoglycaemia or from metastases, but the tumours sometimes grow slowly. When other therapy fails, patients can become dependent on a continuous glucose infusion through a central intravenous catheter.

Factitious hypoglycaemia

Some patients surreptitiously take either insulin or a sulphonylurea drug. A secondary gain to the patient is usually not obvious, and other hysterical or psychiatric symptoms may not be apparent. The patients usually deny self-administration and are remarkably plausible.

Until recently, insulin self-administration was easily detected because impure insulin preparations induce insulin antibodies, which can be shown with a suitable modification of the insulin immunoassay. The availability of pure pork and human insulins, which are seldom immunogenic, make detection more difficult, but if a blood sample is taken when the patient has a hypoglycaemic episode, the presence of immunoreactive insulin in the absence of immunoreactive C-peptide, confirms the exogenous origin.

Self-medication with sulphonylureas presents exactly like an insulinoma with similar lack of suppression of insulin or C-peptide in response to hypoglycaemia. These patients are usually detected only because of clinical suspicion leading to the finding of the sulphonylurea tablets. The wide variety of sulphonylureas available makes the detection in plasma or urine difficult, although immunoassays for individual agents are provided by several manufacturers. If an overdose of sulphonylurea has been taken, therapy with diazoxide or somatostatin is feasible.

Sarcoma, hepatoma, and other tumours

Fasting hypoglycaemia can occur with low-grade malignant tumours of many cell types, the most common being retroperitoneal fibrosarcoma and mesothelioma. The tumours are large, usually weighing 2–4 kg, the smallest recorded being 310 g. The syndrome can also arise from some epithelial cell tumours, such as malignant hepatoma, cholangioma, and adrenocortical tumours. The tumours are usually obvious either on palpation of the abdomen or on chest or abdomen radiography, CT scan, or MRI.

Patients with mesotheliomas or sarcomas do not have ketosis, as hypoglycaemia is caused by excess secretion of an insulin-like growth factor, IGF-II. The patients have low–normal concentrations of IGF-I. Increased expression of the mRNA for IGF-II in the tumour may be an oncogenic factor that induced the tumour to develop. The tumour can secrete a large precursor, a proinsulin-like peptide, pro-IGF-II, and a specific immunoassay for the first 21 amino acids of the E-domain can be diagnostic. The peptide circulates predominantly with IGF binding proteins as a small, 50-kDa complex rather than as the usual 150-kDa complex, and this increases its bioavailability through the capillaries. The hypoglycaemia is resistant to treatment other than by taking regular, fibre-containing meals; eventually intravenous glucose infusion may be necessary. Operative removal stops the hypoglycaemia, but recurrence is common even if the lesion was reported histologically to be benign.

Autoimmune hypoglycaemia

Insulin receptor antibodies

Patients with insulin receptor antibodies usually present with a rare variant of insulin-resistant diabetes, because these antibodies bind with insulin receptors and displace the binding of insulin. However, sometimes the antibodies activate the receptor and cause an insulin-like effect and fasting hypoglycaemia. Autoimmune hypoglycaemia is rare and tends to occur in middle-aged women, but can occur in either sex at any age. Such antibodies can be detected by assaying the patient's plasma or serum for antibody binding to insulin receptors. The insulin receptors on the patient's red cells may be occupied by antibody and unable to bind labelled insulin *in vitro*. The hypoglycaemia is resistant to treatment except by plasmapheresis and immune suppression, including prednisolone therapy. The condition often remits spontaneously and can transmute to the production of predominantly blocking antibodies, giving rise to insulin-resistant diabetes.

Insulin antibodies

Antibodies to insulin can lead to the accumulation of antibody-bound insulin, which dissociates to maintain higher-than-normal free insulin levels. Hypoglycaemia occurs either 5–7 h after a meal, or many hours later as fasting hypoglycaemia. The C-peptide concentrations can then be low, even though insulin levels are high. The condition may be more common in Japanese patients, particularly in those treated for thyrotoxicosis with antithyroid drugs containing an –SH group. Patients often, but not invariably, have other autoimmune disease and have the HLA-DR4 antigen. The antibodies are usually polyclonal but can be monoclonal. If symptoms are not controlled by frequent meals and α-glucosidase inhibitors, immunosuppression with prednisolone, or even plasmapheresis, may be needed.

Acute infections

Septicaemia

Hypoglycaemia occasionally occurs with severe infections in children or the elderly. Gram-negative septicaemia is the most common cause; in particular, *Shigella* dysentery. Infections with streptococci or *Haemophilus influenzae* can also cause hypoglycaemia. The pathophysiology is unclear, but may be due to a combination of acute calorie deprivation, high metabolic demands from fever, and hepatic dysfunction. Accompanying medication, such as β-blockers or calcium antagonists, can reduce hepatic glucose efflux. Preceding cirrhosis or renal failure may make a patient susceptible. Ketonuria is not found. Hypoglycaemia may also accompany hypotension in severe meningococcal disease as part of adrenal failure from Waterhouse–Friderichsen syndrome.

Malaria

Hypoglycaemia can occur with fulminant *Plasmodium falciparum* infection and is usually caused by hyperinsulinaemia stimulated by quinine therapy. Hypoglycaemia can be found in milder infections in pregnancy, partly because of the greater glucose demand of the fetus and partly because the β-cells may be more responsive to quinine. Large amounts of glucose may be needed to prevent hypoglycaemia. Suppression of insulin secretion by somatostatin is an alternative therapy. Hypoglycaemia can also occur without quinine therapy and is then probably due to the mechanisms described above.

Ethanol-induced hypoglycaemia

The oxidation of ethanol in the liver reduces the NAD^+ to NADH (nicotinamide adenine dinucleotide), and the altered redox potential means that gluconeogenesis from lactate is no longer possible. Glycogenolysis is not affected, so ethanol has little effect on plasma glucose concentration in those who are eating meals and have glycogen stores. However, after a 24-h fast, when the glycogen is depleted, ethanol consumption causes marked hypoglycaemia. As hypoglycaemia is due to decreased hepatic glucose efflux accompanied by low plasma insulin concentrations, these patients characteristically have ketonuria and raised plasma ketone-body levels. Ethanol-induced hypoglycaemia is usually only seen in alcoholics who drink and do not eat.

Children, with their greater proportional turnover of fuel supply, can have ethanol-induced hypoglycaemia after a few hours without food, sometimes with fatal consequences. In the wider world, except for preterminal starvation, ethanol is probably the most common cause of fasting hypoglycaemia.

Severe liver disease

Only gross liver disease is severe enough to deplete hepatic glucose efflux and induce hypoglycaemia. Hypoglycaemia is more a feature of acute hepatic coma than of uncomplicated cirrhosis or other liver disease. When hypoglycaemia does occur in cirrhosis, interaction with ethanol or drug therapy is usually a feature (see below). Hypoglycaemia associated with a hepatoma is discussed above.

Endstage renal failure

Hypoglycaemia can occur following intraperitoneal dialysis, when it may follow termination of the high glucose concentration-containing peritoneal infusion, which has stimulated insulin secretion and decreased glucagon secretion. Hypoglycaemia can also occur in end-stage renal failure *per se* and should be suspected if there is a change of mental or neurological status. It is often a marker of multisystem failure, including hepatic failure. Acute calorie deprivation and drugs, such as ethanol, β-blockers, salicylates, or disopyramide are often implicated; hypoglycaemia rarely occurs in uncomplicated renal failure.

Heart failure

Hypoglycaemia in elderly patients with severe heart failure is well recognized. It is usually due to a combination of fasting, ethanol, certain drugs (see below), and possibly hepatic congestion.

Cortisol deficiency

Patients with deficiency of cortisol production from Addison's disease, pan-hypopituitarism, or isolated ACTH deficiency, have slightly low fasting plasma glucose concentrations. Frank hypoglycaemia may be precipitated by exercise but usually only develops after missing meals. Patients presenting with persistent vomiting are particularly at risk. Hypoglycaemia may be provoked by ethanol in the absence of the usual 24-h fast needed to deplete liver glycogen. Half the patients with this condition present with fasting hypoglycaemia that clinically mimics an insulinoma. It is important to treat the hypoglycaemia with hydrocortisone as well as with glucose.

Patients with Addison's or pituitary disease can usually be diagnosed because of associated symptoms and signs. The characteristic findings are of a low plasma glucose accompanied by a low insulin, but without gross ketonuria. Plasma cortisol measurements are of considerable value. The diagnosis is made by lack of an ACTH or cortisol response to hypoglycaemia or corticotrophin-releasing factor.

Growth hormone deficiency

Isolated growth hormone deficiency occasionally induces hypoglycaemia, but it is even less common than isolated ACTH deficiency. Hypoglycaemia also occurs in Laron dwarfism, in which a defect of IGF-I production is associated with high plasma growth hormone levels.

Pregnancy

The metabolic demands of the fetus mean that even with short periods of fuel deprivation there is accelerated starvation, with the plasma glucose reducing to 3 mmol/l and resultant moderate ketonaemia. It is rare to develop symptomatic hypoglycaemia. Placental lactogen may have developed evolutionarily as a protective mechanism. Nevertheless, illness in pregnancy causing acute calorie deprivation sometimes induces hypoglycaemia, which may be aggravated by the use of β_2-adrenoreceptor agonists given to retard premature labour.

Drugs

Salicylates and non-selective β-blockers sometimes induce hypoglycaemia even when given in normal pharmacological doses, particularly in children and in the elderly when illness prevents feeding. The cause is uncertain, but they may both directly prevent hepatic glucose efflux. Salicylate may also enhance insulin secretion. This effect of salicylate is distinct from Reye's syndrome, which is an idiosyncratic response to aspirin in children, leading to acute liver failure and encephalopathy. Drugs for treating arrhythmia, particularly disopyramide, have also been implicated. Pentamidine induces β-cell death and subsequent release of stored insulin. Hypoglycaemia is common following intravenous pentamidine and can also occur after inhalation of a pentamidine aerosol. Hypoglycaemia due to quinine has been mentioned above.

Reactive postprandial hypoglycaemia

Alimentary hypoglycaemia

Several operations (such as partial gastrectomy and pyloroplasty) can give rise to rapid gastric emptying, with brisk absorption of glucose and prompt release of enteric insulin-stimulating hormones. These induce greater than normal insulin release, which can induce hypoglycaemia 1.5–3 h after a meal. This needs to be distinguished from the 'dumping' syndrome 30 min after a meal, which is probably induced by increased secretion of gastroenteric peptides such as neurotensin, vasoactive intestinal polypeptide, and motilin, and is not related to hypoglycaemia.

All forms of reactive hypoglycaemia are likely to benefit from therapy with an α-glucosidase inhibitor, such as acarbose or miglitol. These drugs delay absorption of disaccharides and starch from the jejunum. When they are used, subsequent hypoglycaemia has to be treated with glucose and not sucrose. The dose needs to be kept below that which hinders the ileal as well as the jejunal enzyme, to prevent carbohydrate transfer to the colon where bacteria can digest the carbohydrate and cause flatulence.

Incipient diabetes

Patients with diabetes, usually of maturity-onset type with near-normal fasting plasma glucose levels, occasionally present with postprandial hypoglycaemia 3–5 h after a meal. An initial subnormal insulin response to a meal leads to hyperglycaemia which may eventually stimulate sufficient insulin release to produce reactive hypoglycaemia. The symptoms disappear as β-cell function decreases and fasting hyperglycaemia ensues.

Idiopathic reactive hypoglycaemia

This is the most frequently diagnosed form of postprandial hypoglycaemia in the USA, whereas it is not commonly accepted in the UK. Patients are often of an anxious disposition, and the possibility that non-specific symptoms may be due to hypoglycaemia seems in some patients to aggravate their symptoms. The 'diagnosis' is often made on a suggestive history and is 'confirmed' by a 5 h oral glucose tolerance test. The condition is markedly overdiagnosed because use of venous blood samples taken from the cubital fossa during an oral glucose test can spuriously indicate hypoglycaemia. Glucose uptake by forearm muscle can give a venous plasma glucose concentration of 2 mmol/l when the arterial glucose concentration is normal at 4 mmol/l. It is not unusual for the venous plasma glucose level to fall to 2.5–3.0 mmol/l (44–52 mg/100 ml), between 90 and 150 min after a glucose tolerance test, and such levels are often overinterpreted. Thus, postprandial hypoglycaemia should only be confirmed by taking plasma glucose levels after a normal meal or an oral glucose tolerance test by arterialized blood from a vein on the back of a warmed hand or from finger-tip or ear-lobe capillary blood samples. The diagnosis should only be made when proven low arterialized glucose levels are accompanied by symptoms that improve as the plasma glucose rises.

Patients in whom this condition is suspected, with a low plasma glucose level during a glucose tolerance test, do not usually show abnormal low glucose concentrations after taking mixed meals. Confirmation of low blood glucose levels at the time of symptoms may be achieved by the patient putting blood on a special filter paper for laboratory testing, or by use of home blood-glucose monitoring with a memory meter. A parallel diary of symptoms is helpful.

The few patients who show true reactive hypoglycaemia are usually underweight or of normal weight. Some have been reported to have a greater than normal initial insulin response to meals. One patient has been reported to have abnormal hepatic glucose 6-phosphatase activity.

The plasma insulin or proinsulin concentration measured during a reactive hypoglycaemic episode may still be raised from secretion induced by a previous meal, and the diagnostic criteria for insulinomas that apply to fasting hypoglycaemia should not be applied to postprandial hypoglycaemia.

Hypoglycaemia in childhood

A brief account of the causes and management is given in OTM3, pp. 1511–12.

Further reading

Service, F.J. (1997). Hypoglycaemia. *Endocrinology and Metabolism Clinics of North America*, **26**, 937–55.

Veneman, T.F. and Erkelens, D.W. (1997). Clinical review 88: hypglycaemia unawareness in non-insulin-dependent diabetes mellitus. *Journal of Clinical Endocrinology and Metabolism*, **82**, 1682–4.

Chapter 6.15

Amyloidosis

M. B. Pepys and P. N. Hawkins

Amyloidosis is a disorder of protein metabolism, which may be either acquired or hereditary, characterized by extracellular deposition of abnormal protein fibrils. Many different proteins can form amyloid fibrils (Tables 1 and 2). In addition, the deposits contain glycosaminoglycans, some of which are tightly associated with the fibrils, and also a non-fibrillar plasma glycoprotein, amyloid P component (AP). Small focal, clinically silent, amyloid deposits in the brain, heart, seminal vesicles, and joints are a universal accompaniment of ageing. However, systemic or significant local amyloid deposits usually accumulate progressively, disrupting the structure and function of affected tissues and leading inexorably to organ failure and death. No treatment yet exists which specifically causes resolution, but intervention which reduces availability of the protein precursors of amyloid fibrils may lead to regression.

Amyloid deposits in the brain and cerebral vessels are a central part of the pathology of Alzheimer's disease, while amyloid is present in the islets of Langerhans of the pancreas in all patients with type 2 diabetes mellitus. Amyloid deposition in the bones, joints, and periarticular structures eventually affects most patients who are on long-term haemodialysis for end-stage renal failure. Systemic amyloidosis complicating myeloma and other B-cell dyscrasias, or chronic infections and inflammatory diseases, is very important because the diagnosis is often difficult and the prognosis is poor, but effective treatments are increasingly available. Hereditary amyloidosis is very rare, except in a few geographic foci, but its diversity is remarkable. Its importance derives both from its poor clinical prognosis and from its value as a model for understanding the pathogenesis of amyloid deposition.

Although there are some correlations between fibril protein type and clinical manifestations, there are also many forms in which there is little or no concordance between the fibril protein, or the genotype of its precursor, and the clinical phenotype. There are genetic and/or environmental factors, which are distinct from the amyloid fibril protein itself, which determine whether, when, and where clinically significant amyloid deposits form. The nature of these important determinants of amyloidogenesis is obscure.

Reactive systemic, AA, amyloidosis

Associated conditions

Amyloid A protein (AA) amyloidosis occurs in association with chronic inflammatory disorders, chronic local or systemic microbial infections, and malignant neoplasms. In western Europe and the United States the most frequent predisposing conditions are rheumatic and connective tissue diseases (Table 3). Amyloidosis complicates up to 10 per cent of cases of rheumatoid arthritis and juvenile rheumatoid arthritis (JRA). It is exceptionally rare in systemic lupus erythematosus, and in ulcerative colitis in contrast to Crohn's disease. Tuberculosis and leprosy are important causes, particularly in the major endemic areas. Chronic osteomyelitis, bronchiectasis, chronically infected burns and decubitus ulcers as well as the chronic pyelonephritis of paraplegic patients are other well recognized associations. Hodgkin's disease and renal carcinoma are the malignancies most commonly associated.

Clinical features

AA amyloid involves the viscera but may be widely distributed without causing clinical symptoms. It most commonly presents with non-selective proteinuria due to glomerular deposition, and may cause nephrotic syndrome before terminating in end-stage renal failure. Haematuria, isolated tubular defects, nephrogenic diabetes insipidus, and diffuse renal calcification occur rarely. Acute renal failure may be precipitated by hypotension and/or salt and water depletion, and may be associated with renal vein thrombosis. The second most common presentation is with organomegaly, e.g. hepatosplenomegaly or thyroid enlargement. Deposits are almost invariably widespread at the time of presentation. Involvement of the heart and gastrointestinal tract is frequent, but rarely causes functional impairment.

The mean duration of chronic rheumatic diseases such as rheumatoid arthritis, ankylosing spondylitis, or JRA before amyloid is diagnosed is 12–14 years, although it can present much sooner. For most patients the prognosis is closely related to the presence of renal involvement, found in 70 per cent or more, and is poor. Fifty per cent of patients with AA amyloid die within 5 years of diagnosis. By 15 years a further 25 per cent are dead, but the remainder have a better prognosis. Availability of chronic haemodialysis and transplantation prevents early death from uraemia *per se*, but the extensive amyloid deposition in extrarenal tissues causes the prognosis in these patients to be less favourable than in those with end-stage renal failure of other aetiology.

Table 1 Acquired amyloidosis syndromes

Clinical syndrome	Fibril protein
Systemic AL amyloidosis, associated with immunocyte dyscrasia, myeloma, monoclonal gammopathy, occult dyscrasia	AL fibrils derived from monoclonal immunoglobulin light chains
Local nodular AL amyloidosis (skin, respiratory tract, urogenital tract, etc.) associated with focal immunocyte dyscrasia	AL fibrils derived from monoclonal immunoglobulin light chains
Reactive systemic AA amyloidosis, associated with chronic active diseases	AA fibrils derived from serum amyloid A protein (SAA)
Senile systemic amyloidosis	Transthyretin derived from plasma transthyretin
Focal senile amyloidosis: atria of the heart	Atrial natriuretic peptide
brain	β-protein
joints	Not known
seminal vesicles	Seminal vesicle exocrine protein
prostate	β_2-microglobulin
Non-familial Alzheimer's disease, Down syndrome	β-protein derived from β-amyloid protein precursor (APP)
Sporadic cerebral amyloid angiography	β-protein derived from β-amyloid precursor protein (APP)
Inclusion body myositis	β-protein derived from β-amyloid precursor protein (APP)
Sporadic Creutzfeldt–Jakob disease, kuru (transmissible spongiform encephalopathies, prion diseases)	Prion protein derived from prion protein precursor
Type II diabetes mellitus	Islet amyloid polypeptide (IAPP), amylin, derived from its precursor protein
Endocrine amyloidosis, associated with APUDomas	Peptide hormones or fragments thereof (e.g. precalcitonin in medullary carcinoma of thyroid)
Haemodialysis-associated amyloidosis; localized to osteoarticular tissues or systemic	β_2-microglobulin derived from high plasma levels
Primary localized cutaneous amyloid (macular, papular)	?Keratin-derived
Ocular amyloid (cornea, conjunctiva)	Not known
Orbital amyloid	Not known

Amyloidosis associated with immunocyte dyscrasia, AL amyloidosis

Almost any dyscrasia of cells of the B-lymphocyte lineage, including multiple myeloma, malignant lymphomas and macroglobulinaemia, and 'benign' monoclonal gammopathy, may be complicated by immunoglobulin light chain (AL) amyloidosis. In some cases amyloid may be the only evidence of the dyscrasia. Amyloid occurs in up to 15 per cent of cases of myeloma and in a lower proportion of other malignant B-cell and plasma cell disorders. The incidence in 'benign' monoclonal gammopathy is probably about 5–10 per cent. Most patients with AL amyloid have a monoclonal paraprotein or free light chains in serum or urine. However, some patients present in the absence of detectable abnormal protein in serum or urine. The finding of immunoglobulin gene rearrangement in bone marrow, or even peripheral blood, sometimes confirms a monoclonal gammopathy in the absence of protein abnormality apart from the amyloid. If there is no previous predisposing inflammatory condition or family history of amyloidosis, it is likely that such apparently 'primary' cases of amyloidosis are related to an immunocyte dyscrasia and that analysis of the fibrils will show them to be AL in type. Sometimes the paraprotein manifests after diagnosis of amyloid, and subnormal levels of some or all serum immunoglobulins or increased numbers of marrow plasma cells may provide less direct clues.

Clinical features

AL amyloid usually occurs over the age of 50, but may be seen in young adults. It is more common in men than in women, and in Caucasians than in non-Caucasians. Uraemia, heart failure, or other effects usually cause death within a year of diagnosis. Patients with myeloma complicated by amyloid have a significantly worse prognosis than those with myeloma alone.

The heart is affected in 90 per cent of AL patients, in 30 per cent of whom cardiac dysfunction is the presenting feature and in up to 50 per cent of whom it is fatal. Restrictive cardiomyopathy with right ventricular failure and arrhythmias due to involvement of the conducting system are common. Sensitivity to digoxin may cause fatal arrhythmias. Renal AL amyloid has the same manifestations as renal AA amyloid, but the prognosis is even worse. Gut involvement may cause motility disturbances (often secondary to autonomic neuropathy), malabsorption, perforation, haemorrhage, or obstruction. Macroglossia is quite frequent and is almost pathognomonic. Hyposplenism sometimes occurs in both AA and AL amyloidosis. Painful sensory polyneuropathy with early loss of pain

Table 2 Hereditary amyloidosis syndromes

Clinical syndrome	Fibril protein
Predominant peripheral nerve involvement, familial amyloid polyneuropathy. Autosomal dominant	Transthyretin genetic variants (most commonly Met30, but over 30 others described)
Predominant peripheral nerve involvement, familial amyloid polyneuropathy. Autosomal dominant	Apolipoprotein AI *N*-terminal fragment of genetic variant Arg26
Predominant cranial nerve involvement with lattice corneal dystrophy. Autosomal dominant	Gelsolin, fragment of genetic variant Asn187 or Tyr187
Non-neuropathic, prominent visceral involvement (Ostertag-type) Autosomal dominant	Apolipoprotein, *N*-terminal fragment of genetic variant Arg26 or Arg60
Non-neuropathic, prominent visceral involvement (Ostertag-type) Autosomal dominant	Lysozyme genetic variant Thr56 or His67
Non-neuropathic, prominent visceral involvement (Ostertag-type) Autosomal dominant	Fibrinogen α-chain genetic variant Val526 or Leu554
Predominant cardiac involvement, no clinical neuropathy. Autosomal dominant	Transthyretin genetic variants Thr45, Ala60, Ser84, Met111, Ile122
Hereditary cerebral haemorrhage with amyloidosis (cerebral amyloid angiopathy). Autosomal dominant	
Icelandic type (major asymptomatic systemic amyloid also present)	Cystatin C, fragment of genetic variant Glu68
Dutch type	β-protein derived from genetic variant β-amyloid precursor protein Gln693
Familial Alzheimer's disease	β-protein derived from genetic variant β-amyloid precursor protein Ile717, Phe717 or Gly717
Familial dementia – probable Alzheimer's disease	β-protein derived from genetic variant β-amyloid precursor protein Asn670, Leu671
Familial Creutzfeldt–Jakob disease, Gerstmann–Sträussler–Scheinker syndrome (hereditary spongiform encephalopathies, prion diseases)	Prion protein derived from genetic variants of prion protein precursor protein 51–91 insert, Leu102, Val117, Asn178, Lys200
Familial Mediterranean fever, prominent renal involvement. Autosomal recessive	AA derived from SAA
Muckle–Well's syndrome, nephropathy, deafness, urticaria, limb pain	AA derived from SAA
Cardiomyopathy with persistent atrial standstill	Not known
Cutaneous deposits (bullous, papular, pustulodermal)	Not known

Table 3 Conditions associated with reactive systemic (AA) amyloidosis

Chronic inflammatory disorders	bronchiectasis
rheumatoid arthritis	decubitus ulcers
juvenile chronic arthritis	chronic pyelonephritis in
ankylosing spondylitis	paraplegics
psoriasis and psoriatic	osteomyelitis
arthropathy	Whipple's disease
Reiter's syndrome	
adult Still's disease	*Malignant neoplasms*
Behçet's syndrome	Hodgkin's disease
Crohn's disease	renal carcinoma
	carcinomas of gut, lung,
Chronic microbial infections	urogenital tract
leprosy	basal cell carcinoma
tuberculosis	hairy cell leukaemia

and temperature sensation followed later by motor deficits is seen in 10–20 per cent of cases and carpal tunnel syndrome in 20 per cent. Autonomic neuropathy may occur alone or together with the peripheral neuropathy. Skin involvement takes the form of papules, nodules, and plaques usually on the face and upper trunk, and involvement of dermal blood vessels results in purpura spontaneous or after minimal trauma. Articular amyloid affecting large joints usually occurs in association with myeloma or presents as asymmetrical arthritis affecting the hip or shoulder. Infiltration of the glenohumeral articulation occasionally produces the characteristic 'shoulder pad' sign. A rare but serious manifestation is an acquired bleeding diathesis that may be associated with deficiency of factor X and sometimes also factor IX, or with increased fibrinolysis. It does not occur in AA amyloidosis, although in both AL and AA disease there may be serious bleeding in the absence of any identifiable factor deficiency.

Senile amyloidosis

Senile systemic amyloidosis

Up to 25 per cent of old people have microscopic, clinically silent systemic deposits of transthyretin (TTR) amyloid involving the heart and blood vessel walls, smooth and striated muscle, fat tissue, renal papillae, and alveolar walls. The spleen and renal glomeruli are rarely affected and the brain is not involved. Occasionally, more extensive

Table 4 Cerebral amyloidosis

Age-related amyloid angiopathy with or without intracerebral deposits
Hereditary amyloid angiopathy of meningeal and cortical vessels associated with cerebral haemorrhage: (a) Icelandic type; (b) Dutch type
Hereditary amyloid angiopathy affecting the entire central nervous system
Alzheimer's disease: sporadic, familial or associated with Down's syndrome
Cerebral amyloid associated with prion disease:
sporadic spongiform encephalopathy: Creutzfeldt–Jakob disease
familial prion disease: familial Creutzfeldt–Jakob disease. Gerstmann–Sträussler–Scheinker disease and atypical familial prion disease
prion disease in animals
Familial oculoleptomeningeal amyloidosis

deposits in the heart cause significant impairment of cardiac function and may be fatal.

Senile focal amyloidosis

Microscopic and clinically silent amyloid deposits of different fibril types, localized to particular tissues, are very commonly present in old people. Deposits of β-protein (see below) amyloid in cerebral blood vessels and intracerebral plaques seen in 'normal' elderly brains may or may not be the harbinger of Alzheimer's disease. Amyloid deposits are present in most osteoarthritic joints at surgery or autopsy, but neither their clinical significance nor biochemical nature are known. The corpora amylacea of the prostate are composed of β_2-microglobulin (**β^2M**) amyloid fibrils. Amyloid in the seminal vesicles is derived from an as yet unidentified exocrine secretory product of the vesicle cells. Isolated deposits of cardiac atrial amyloid contain atrial natriuretic peptide.

Cerebral amyloidosis

The brain is a very common site of amyloid deposition (Table 4), although it is never affected in any form of acquired systemic visceral amyloidosis. In familial amyloid polyneuropathy due to the TTR Met30 variant, cerebrovascular amyloid has been reported, but intracerebral deposits and clinical brain involvement have not. However, familial oculoleptomeningual amyloid is caused by other variant TTRs. The major forms of brain amyloid are confined to the brain and cerebral blood vessels with the single exception of cystatin C amyloid in hereditary cerebral haemorrhage with amyloidosis, Icelandic type, in which there are major though clinically silent systemic deposits.

Alzheimer's disease

Intracerebral and cerebrovascular amyloid deposits are hallmarks of the neuropathological diagnosis. The amyloid fibrils are composed of β-protein, a small cleavage product derived from the large β-amyloid precursor protein (**APP**). A further hallmark is the neurofibrillary tangles located within neuronal cell bodies and processes. These have a characteristic ultrastructural morphology of paired helical filaments and, although they bind Congo Red and then give pathognomonic green birefringence when viewed in polarized light, they differ structurally from all other known amyloid fibrils. Their main constituent is an abnormally phosphorylated form of the normal neurofilament protein, *tau*. Most causes of Alzheimer's disease are sporadic and of late onset, after age 65, but some come from families with an autosomal dominant pattern of inheritance and early onset. In about 20 families with such early-onset disease there are mutations in the APP gene on chromosome 21, and most other kindreds have mutations in the presenilin 1 (chromosome 14) and presenilin 2 genes (chromosome 1). All these mutations are associated with increased production from APP of the amyloidogenic form of β-protein (Aβ 1–43) and, together with the fact that all individuals with Down syndrome (trisomy 21) develop Alzheimer's disease if they survive into their forties, this provides a strong link between β-protein, amyloid deposition, and pathogenesis of Alzheimer's disease, although the mechanisms responsible for neuronal loss remain unclear. Another gene, *ApoE4* (chromosome 19), encoding one of the three isoforms of apolipoprotein E, is strongly associated with predisposition to develop Alzheimer's disease and with increased amounts of amyloid and neuronal damage in the brain. In addition to the amyloid deposits composed of β-protein, there are much more extensive 'amorphous' deposits of β-protein throughout the brain. These do not contain amyloid fibrils and therefore do not stain with Congo Red, and are detectable only by immunohistochemical staining. Their significance is unknown.

Senile cerebral amyloidosis and amyloid angiopathy

The cerebral blood vessels contain amyloid, consisting of β-protein, in up to 60 per cent of aged brains of non-demented individuals and there may also be focal intracerebral amyloid plaques of the same fibril type. These deposits are usually clinically silent and may or may not be harbingers of Alzheimer's disease, had the patients survived long enough. Sometimes the amyloid angiopathy is more extensive and it is a rare but important cause of cerebral haemorrhage and stroke, to be distinguished from atherosclerotic cerebrovascular disease.

Hereditary cerebral haemorrhage with amyloidosis; hereditary cerebral amyloid angiopathy

Icelandic type

Cerebrovascular amyloid deposits composed of a fragment of a genetic variant of cystatin C are responsible for recurrent major cerebral haemorrhages starting in early adult life in members of families originating in western Iceland. There is autosomal dominant inheritance and appreciable but clinically silent amyloid deposits are present in the spleen, lymph nodes, and skin. There is no extravascular amyloid in the brain and the neurological deficits of patients who survive are compatible with their cerebrovascular pathology. Multi-infarct dementia is common.

Dutch type

In families originating in a small region on the Dutch coast the autosomal dominant inheritance of recurrent normotensive cerebral haemorrhages starting in middle age, is due to deposition of a genetic variant of β-protein as cerebrovascular amyloid. There are also 'amorphous' β-protein deposits in the brain and early senile plaques, without congophilic amyloid cores. Multi-infarct dementia occurs in survivors but some patients become demented in the absence of stroke. Amyloid outside the brain has not been reported.

Cerebral amyloid associated with prion disease

Sporadic and familial Creutzfeldt–Jakob disease, the familial Gerstmann–Sträussler–Scheinker syndrome, and Kuru are caused by the prion protein, and are closely related to the animal diseases, scrapie, transmissible encephalopathy of mink, elk, and male deer, and bovine spongiform encephalopathy. The neuropathology in this group of disorders sometimes includes cerebral prion amyloid, but its significance is not clear. Prion abnormality is clearly related to the cause of the encephalopathy, but amyloid *per se* is evidently not necessary for expression of the neurological disease.

Hereditary systemic amyloidosis

Familial amyloid polyneuropathy

Familial amyloid polyneuropathy is an autosomal dominant syndrome with onset at any time from the second to the seventh decade, characterized by progressive peripheral and autonomic neuropathy and varying degrees of visceral involvement affecting especially the vitreous of the eye, the heart, kidneys, thyroid, and adrenals. There are usually amyloid deposits throughout the body involving blood vessel walls as well as the connective tissue matrix and the pathology is due to these deposits. Apart from major foci in Portugal, Japan, and Sweden, familial amyloid polyneuropathy has been reported in most ethnic groups throughout the world. There is considerable variation in the age of onset, rate of progression, and involvement of different systems, although within families the pattern is usually quite consistent. There is remorseless progression and the disorder is invariably fatal. Death results from the effects and complications of peripheral and/or autonomic neuropathy, or from cardiac or renal failure.

Familial amyloid polyneuropathy is caused by mutations in the gene for TTR, formerly known as prealbumin, the most frequent of which causes Met for Val substitution at position 30 in the mature protein, but over 60 other amyloidogenic mutations have been described. There is no correlation between the underlying mutation and the clinical phenotype. Furthermore, the TTR mutations are not always penetrant, asymptomatic Met30 homozygotes over the age of 60 having been reported. Familial amyloid polyneuropathy may also rarely be due to a mutation in the apolipoprotein AI (apoAI) gene.

Familial amyloid polyneuropathy with predominant cranial neuropathy

Originally described in Finland but now reported in other ethnic groups, this autosomal dominant hereditary amyloidosis presents in adult life with cranial neuropathy, lattice corneal dystrophy, and distal peripheral neuropathy. There may be skin, renal, and cardiac manifestations and microscopic amyloid deposits are widely distributed in connective tissue and blood vessel walls, although life expectancy approaches normal. The mutant gene responsible encodes a variant of the actin-modulating protein, gelsolin. Individuals homozygous for the mutation have severe renal amyloidosis in addition to the usual neuropathy.

Non-neuropathic systemic amyloidosis, Ostertag type

In this rare autosomal dominant syndrome of major systemic amyloidosis without clinical evidence of neuropathy, the patterns of organ involvement and overall clinical phenotype vary between families. The kidneys are often most severely affected, but the heart, spleen, liver, bowel, connective tissue, and exocrine glands, may all be involved. There is inexorable progression to death or organ failure requiring transplantation. Clinical presentation is usually in early adulthood, although in a few kindreds it may be as late as the sixth decade. The amyloid proteins identified so far are genetic variants of apolipoprotein AI, lysozyme, and the α-chain of fibrinogen.

Cardiac amyloidosis

Cardiac amyloidosis, without other systemic involvement or neuropathy, progressing inexorably to death, is associated with TTR gene mutations (see Table 2). In a large Danish family with autosomal dominant TTR Met111 cardiac amyloid, deposition starts only in adult life a few years before the clinical presentation, despite presence of the variant TTR from birth.

Recurrent polyserositis (familial Mediterranean fever—Chapter 6.16)

Untreated familial Mediterranean fever is eventually complicated in a high proportion of cases by typical systemic AA amyloidosis. Furthermore, a subset may present with AA amyloidosis before they have experienced any clinical attacks of the inflammatory disease. It is not clear why this should occur but it is possible that they may have been mounting an acute phase response to subclinical manifestations. The absence of amyloid in Armenians and the lower incidence in Ashkenazis is another illustration of the unknown genetic factors, other than the fibril protein itself, which determine clinical amyloidosis.

Haemodialysis-associated amyloidosis

Almost all patients with end-stage renal failure who are maintained on haemodialysis for more than 5 years develop amyloid deposits composed of β_2M. These deposits are predominantly osteoarticular and are associated with carpal tunnel syndrome, large joint pain and stiffness, soft tissue masses, bone cysts, and pathological fractures. Renal tubular amyloid concretions may also form. Furthermore, in some patients more extensive deposition occurs, most commonly in the spleen but also in other organs, and a few cases of death associated with systemic β_2M amyloid have been reported. The β_2M is derived from the high plasma concentrations, which develop in renal insufficiency and are not cleared by dialysis. This type of amyloid also occurs in patients on continuous ambulatory peritoneal dialysis and has been reported in one patient with chronic renal failure who had never been dialysed.

Endocrine amyloidosis

Many tumours of APUD cells which produce peptide hormones have amyloid deposits in their stroma. These are probably composed of the hormone peptides and in the case of medullary carcinoma of the thyroid the fibril subunits are derived from procalcitonin. In insulinomas the amyloid fibril protein is the same as the fibril protein in the amyloid of the islets of Langerhans in type II, maturity onset, diabetes. This peptide (islet amyloid polypeptide, or amylin), shows appreciable homology with calcitonin gene-related peptide.

Rare localized amyloidosis syndromes

Amyloid deposits localized to the skin occur in both acquired and hereditary forms. Primary localized cutaneous amyloidosis presents in adult life as macular or papular lesions, the fibrils of which may be derived from keratin. Hereditary cutaneous amyloid lesions are rare, of unknown fibril type and sometimes associated with other, non-amyloid, multisystem disorders. Amyloid deposits in the eye cause local problems in the cornea (corneal lattice dystrophy) or conjunctiva, while orbital amyloid presents as mass lesions which can disrupt eye movement and the structure of the orbit. In one such case the fibril protein has been identified as a fragment of IgG heavy chain but otherwise the proteins involved in these non-hereditary conditions have not been characterized.

Localized foci of AL amyloid can occur anywhere in the body, in the absence of systemic AL amyloidosis, the most common sites being the skin, upper airways and respiratory tract, and the urogenital tract. They may be associated with a local plasmacytoma or B-cell lymphoma producing a monoclonal immunoglobulin, but often the cells, which must be present to produce the amyloidogenic protein, are inconspicuous. The clinical problems caused by these space-occupying amyloidomas are usually cured by surgical resection, but this is not always possible.

Amyloid fibril proteins and their precursors

The physical chemistry and structure of amyloid fibric proteins and their many precursors (AL, AA, TTR, β-protein, cystatin C, Gelsolin, ApoAI, lysozyme, amylin, β_2 microglobulin, glycosaminoglycans and amyloid P component) in relation to the deposition of amyloid material are discussed on pp. 1518–1522 of OTM3.

Diagnosis and monitoring of amyloidosis

Until recently amyloidosis was an exclusively histological diagnosis, and green birefringence of deposits stained with Congo Red and viewed in polarized light the gold standard, with immunohistochemical staining the simplest method for identifying the fibril type. However, biopsies provide extremely small samples and therefore can never provide information on the extent, localization, progression or regression of deposits. A major advance has been the development of radiolabelled serum amyloid P (SAP) as a specific tracer for amyloid.

Histological diagnosis of amyloid

When amyloidosis is suspected, biopsy of rectum or subcutaneous fat is the least invasive. Amyloid is present in these sites in more than 90 per cent of cases of systemic AA or AL. Alternatively, a clinically affected tissue may be biopsied directly. Congo Red staining, and the resultant green birefringence when viewed with high intensity polarized light, is the pathognomonic test for amyloid. The amyloid fibril protein may then be identified by immunohistochemical staining.

Antibodies to serum amyloid A protein always stain AA deposits, similarly with anti-β_2M antisera and haemodialysis-associated amyloid. In AL amyloid the deposits are stainable with standard antisera to κ or λ in only about half of all cases. Staining of TTR, β-protein, and prion protein amyloids may require pretreatment of sections with formic acid or alkaline guanidine or deglycosylation. However, demonstration of amyloidogenic proteins in tissues does not, on its own, establish the presence of amyloid. Congo Red staining and green birefringence are always required and immunostaining may then enable the amyloid to be classified.

Electron microscopy alone is not sufficient to confirm the diagnosis, as amyloid fibrils cannot always be convincingly identified ultrastructurally. Failure to find amyloid in a biopsy does not exclude the diagnosis because of sampling error.

Non-histological investigations

Two-dimensional echocardiography showing small, concentrically hypertrophied ventricles, generally impaired contraction, dilated atria, homogeneously echogenic valves, and 'sparkling' echodensity of ventricular walls can be diagnostic of cardiac amyloidosis, but some of these signs may be absent despite histologically confirmed involvement.

In cases of known or suspected hereditary amyloidosis it is important to identify the gene defect (see OTM3, Chapter 11.13.1).

Serum amyloid P component as a specific tracer in amyloidosis

The universal presence in amyloid deposits of AP, derived from circulating SAP component, is the basis for use of radioisotope-labelled SAP as a diagnostic tracer in amyloidosis. No localization or retention of labelled SAP occurs in healthy subjects or in patients with diseases other than amyloidosis. However, in patients with amyloidosis, the tracer rapidly and specifically localizes to the deposits, in proportion to the quantity of amyloid present, and persists there without breakdown or modification. The dose of radioactivity administered (<4 mSv) is well within accepted safety limits. In addition to high resolution scintigraphs, the uptake of tracer into various organs can be precisely quantified and, together with highly reproducible metabolic data on the plasma clearance and whole body retention of activity, the progression or regression of amyloid can be monitored serially and quantitatively.

Management of amyloidosis

Although no treatments yet exist that specifically promote the mobilization of amyloid, there have been substantial recent advances in the management of systemic amyloidosis, in particular active measures to support failing organ function while attempts are made to reduce the supply of the amyloid fibril precursor protein. Serial SAP scintigraphy, in more than 1000 patients with various forms of amyloid, has confirmed that control of the primary disease process, or removal of the source of the amyloidogenic precursor, usually results in regression of existing deposits and recovery or preservation of organ function. This strongly supports aggressive intervention, and relatively toxic drug regimens or other radical approaches can be justified by the poor prognosis. Such an approach, leading to reduced morbidity and improved survival, is the basis for the establishment of the NHS National Amyloid Centre. However, clinical improvement in amyloidosis is often delayed long after the underlying disorder has remitted, reflecting the very gradual regression of the deposits that is now recognized to occur in most patients. Continuing production of the APP should be monitored as closely as possible long term, to determine the requirement for and intensity of treatment for the underlying primary condition. In AA amyloidosis this involves frequent estimation of the plasma serum AA level, and in AL amyloidosis requires monitoring of monoclonal plasma cell proliferation and immunoglobulin light chain production.

The treatment of AA amyloidosis ranges from potent anti-inflammatory and immunosuppressive drugs in patients with rheumatoid arthritis, to life-long prophylactic colchicine in familial

Mediterranean fever, and surgery in conditions such as refractory osteomyelitis and Castleman's disease tumours. The alkylating agent chlorambucil can induce rapid and complete remission of inflammatory activity in many patients with rheumatoid and juvenile chronic arthritis, but its use must be considered very carefully as it is not licensed for this indication, it is potentially carcinogenic, and it causes infertility.

Treatment of AL amyloidosis is based on that for myeloma, although the plasma cell dyscrasias in AL, are often very subtle. Prolonged low-intensity cytotoxic regimens such as oral melphalan and prednisolone are beneficial in about 20 per cent of patients. Dose-intensive infusional chemotherapy regimens such as vincristine, doxorubicin (Adriamycin), and dexamethasone ('VAD'), and autologous peripheral blood stem-cell transplantation are presently being evaluated with far more promising early results.

The disabling arthralgia of β_2M amyloidosis may respond partially to non-steroidal anti-inflammatory drugs or corticosteroids, but even the most severe symptoms usually vanish rapidly following renal transplantation. The basis for this remarkable clinical response is unclear because, although transplantation rapidly restores normal β_2M metabolism, regression of β_2M amyloid may not be evident for many years.

Hepatic transplantation is effective in familial amyloid polyneuropathy associated with TTR gene mutations as the variant amyloidogenic protein is produced mainly in the liver. Successful liver transplantation has now been reported in hundreds of patients with this condition and, although the peripheral neuropathy usually only stabilizes, autonomic function can improve substantially and the associated visceral amyloid deposits have been shown to regress in most cases. Important questions remain about the timing of the procedure but, so far, early intervention seems advisable.

Supportive therapy remains critical in systemic amyloidosis, with the potential for delaying target organ failure, maintaining quality of life and prolonging survival while the underlying process can be treated. Rigorous control of hypertension is vital in renal amyloidosis. Surgical resection of amyloidotic tissue is occasionally beneficial but, in general, a conservative approach to surgery, anaesthesia and other invasive procedures is advisable. Should any such procedure be undertaken, meticulous attention to blood pressure and fluid balance is essential. Amyloidotic tissues may heal poorly and are liable to bleed. Diuretics and vasoactive drugs should be used cautiously in cardiac amyloidosis because they can reduce cardiac output substantially. Dysrhythmias may respond to conventional pharmacological therapy or to pacing. Replacement of vital organ function, notably dialysis, may be necessary and cardiac, renal, and liver transplant procedures have a role in selected cases.

Further reading

See OTM3, p. 1524

Chapter 6.16

Recurrent polyserositis (familial Mediterranean fever, periodic disease)

M. Eliakim

Recurrent polyserositis is a genetic disorder characterized by bouts of abdominal pain and fever. Pleurisy and arthritis, affecting one or more joints, occur in more than half the cases. The disease exhibits a preference for Jews, Arabs, Armenians, and Turks but may affect subjects of any ethnic group. It is frequently familial and is inherited by autosomal recessive transmission. Prognosis is generally good, but some subjects still develop amyloidosis with nephropathy.

The nomenclature of recurrent polyserositis is subject to controversy. The term 'familial Mediterranean fever' has been used widely, although it fails to convey the recurrent character of the disorder and the symptoms due to serosal inflammation. The disease is not limited to the Mediterranean region any more than are thalassaemia and brucellosis; the latter also known as Mediterranean fever. The term 'familial' is inadequate, as many other hereditary disorders with familial clustering are not referred to as 'familial'. Periodic disease implies recurrence at regular intervals and a close relationship to other periodic disorders. In fact, the paroxysms of recurrent polyserositis occur usually at irregular intervals. The term 'recurrent polyserositis' is preferable because it seems to convey most closely the main characteristics of the disease.

Racial and ethnic distribution

Apart from Jews, Armenians, Arabs, and Turks it has been reported in subjects of many other nationalities and races. More than 90 per cent of the Jewish patients are of either Sephardic or Iraqi origin. Sephardic Jews are those whose ancestors left Spain in the fifteenth century and were dispersed over various North African, Middle Eastern, and South American countries, while Iraqi Jews are descendants of the Babylonian Jews exiled to Mesopotamia about 2600 years ago. Most of the Sephardic patients originate from North African countries.

Mode of inheritance

Inheritance is by autosomal recessive transmission. The incidence of multiple familial occurrence varies between 20 and 40 per cent in families reported in different series. The disease usually occurs in several members of one generation. The incidence in families with healthy parents has been reported to be 18 per cent, and that in families with one affected parent, 36 per cent. With full penetrance, the expected figures would be 25 and 50 per cent respectively. The lower figures observed can be explained by incomplete penetrance of the gene, or alternatively, by later appearance of the disease in some of the children. The disease is slightly more prevalent in males (1.7–1.0). The male predominance has not been explained adequately, but may be accounted for by the milder form of disease leading to undiagnosed cases in females. Partial penetrance in females is an alternative explanation. The frequency of the gene in Sephardic and

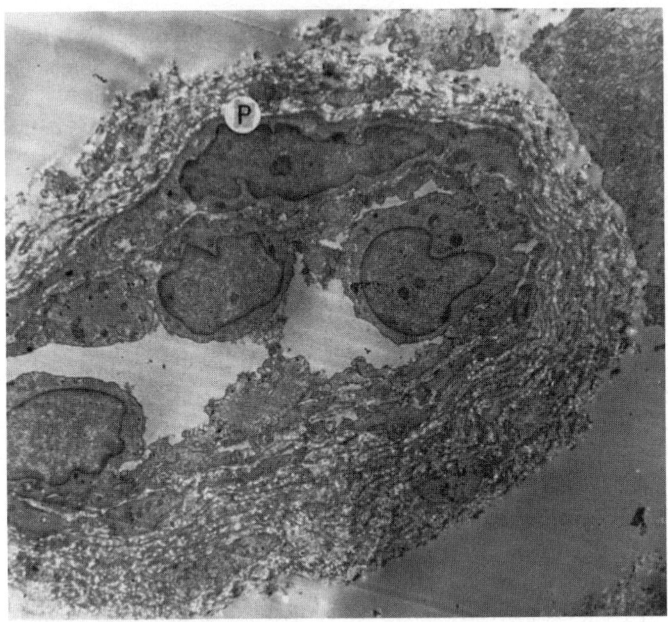

Fig. 1 Electron microscopic picture of a synovial blood vessel with a pericyte (P) and cell processes in between the many basement membrane layers. *(Reproduced from Eliakim, M. et al. (1981). Recurrent polyserositis (familial Mediterranean fever, periodic disease). Elsevier/North Holland Biomedical Press., Amsterdam, by permission.)*

Iraqi Jews has been calculated to be 1 in 45 and the homozygous incidence 1 in 2000. The respective figures for the Armenian population in Lebanon are 1 in 32 and 1 in 1000. The human leucocyte antigen system has been studied in a smaller number of subjects but no associations have been found. Recently, the gene that causes recurrent polyserositis in non-Ashkenazi Jews has been located in the short arm of chromosome 16.

Pathology

The underlying pathological lesion is hyperaemia and an acute non-bacterial inflammatory reaction, affecting mainly the serous membranes. Adhesions, when present, are thin and mechanical ileus is extremely rare. Microscopically, the most striking finding is marked hyperaemia and a cellular infiltrate consisting of varying proportions of neutrophils, lymphocytes, monocytes, and, sometimes, plasma cells and eosinophils. The picture is different from infective inflammation in that it is not as purulent. The reaction seems to originate in the serosa and may not reach the mucosa. The inflammatory exudate concentrates around the venules and arterioles, some of which have thickened walls. In the synovia, pannus formation and extensive intra-articular damage may occur. Ultrastructural studies of synovial biopsies have shown that the most prominent vascular change is thickening of the basement membrane, which is organized in many concentric, closely arranged layers, separated by a less dense ground substance (Fig. 1). It has been suggested that reduplication of the basement membrane is due to repeated episodes of cell death and regeneration, each lamina representing the residue of one cell generation.

Aetiology and pathogenesis

The aetiology is unknown. The blood vessels seem to be the primary target. The pathogenesis of the vascular lesion is, however, obscure. Most authors tend to relate recurrent polyserositis to the 'collagen' disorders. The similarity between the former and systemic lupus erythematosus is sometimes striking. The incidence of atopic allergy, rheumatic fever, glomerulonephritis. Schönlein–Henoch purpura, and periarteritis nodosa is higher in recurrent polyserositis than in the general population. High serum immunoglobulin levels, circulating immune complexes, and lymphocytotoxins have been demonstrated in patients suffering from the disease. Results of additional immunological studies are still controversial. It has been suggested that C5a-inhibitor deficiency in joint and peritoneal may have a role in pathogenesis.

Clinical manifestations

Symptoms start in the first decade of life in about 50 per cent of cases and before the age of 20 years in at least 80 per cent. Only 1 per cent may manifest the first symptoms after the age of 40. Almost all have attacks of abdominal pain, often originating in one area, but spreading over the whole abdomen within a few hours. The temperature rises to 38–40°C with tachycardia, and about one-quarter of the patients report a chill. The attack usually reaches its peak in 12 h. The clinical picture is that of acute peritonitis, manifested by exquisite abdominal tenderness, involuntary rigidity, rebound tenderness, and diminished peristalsis. Constipation is the rule and vomiting is frequent. Patients frequently flex their thighs and lie motionless to relieve the pain. The crisis resolves spontaneously and is usually over within 24–48 h. The temperature returns to normal after a variable period of 12 h–3 days and the pain subsides gradually. The attacks recur, usually at irregular periods of several days to several months. Spontaneous remissions may last years. The severity of the pain varies from mild discomfort to that in severe generalized peritonitis. Mild attacks may be afebrile. In pregnant women, the attacks usually abate spontaneously after the second trimester. After the first attacks, many patients avoid visits to the emergency wards because they fear aggressive treatment. They learn to caution their physicians against performing unnecessary surgery and request symptomatic relief of pain.

Pleurisy

More than 50 per cent have pleuritic chest pain, localized in the lower part, more frequently on the right than on the left, and radiating to the abdomen and the shoulders. Suppression of breath sounds over the affected side is usual but pleural friction is exceptional. A small effusion is occasionally detected in the costophrenic angle.

Arthritis

Arthritis is common, its incidence varying between 24 and 84 per cent in various reported series. Sephardic Jews seem to be affected more frequently than patients of other ethnic origins. Several clinical forms have been identified. Rheumatic fever is more common in patients with recurrent polyserositis and has to be differentiated from the forms typical of the disease. Most patients manifest an asymmetric, non-destructive mono- or oligoarthritis affecting the large joints. The knees and ankles are affected about three times more often than the hips, shoulders, feet, and wrists. Involvement of small joints is very rare. The affected joint becomes painful and swollen but local redness and heat are not pronounced and may be absent. The synovial fluid is usually turbid but it forms a good mucin clot. The white cell content ranges between 15 000 and 30 000 polymorphonuclear cells per mm^3 and the fluid is always sterile. The symptoms intensify during the first 24–48 h but may last as long as a week. Usually, one, or mostly two, large joints are affected at a time. However, when the attacks are frequent, involvement of one joint may start before the symptoms from the previous joint have subsided, and the impression of migratory arthritis is created. The clue to the differential diagnosis may lie in the temperature curve, which shows high peaks lasting 1–3 days. In about 5 per cent of the cases, the acute attack fails to resolve and the symptoms may persist several weeks or even months before they abate with no residual damage. About 2 per cent of the patients develop a chronic destructive mono- or oligoarthritis affecting most frequently the hip or the knee. Permanent organic damage results from one protracted attack or from repeated short attacks. Marked abnormalities may result and surgical treatment may be necessary. Sacroiliitis, frequently asymptomatic, has been described in a considerable number of patients. The radiographic changes include loss of cortical definition, sclerosis with or without bone erosion, and fusion of the joints.

Skin rash

Skin rash occurs in 10–20 per cent of the cases. The typical lesion resembles erysipelas, which appears invariably over the extensor surfaces of the legs below the knees, over the ankle joints, or the dorsum of the foot. The skin becomes bright-red, hot, swollen, and painful. The rash is usually unilateral and its border may or may not be sharply defined. It resembles cellulitis and frequently prompts initiation of antibiotic therapy. Fever and arthralgia or arthritis are frequently present. The symptoms intensify rapidly and then fade within 2–3 days without any therapy. On biopsy the epidermis shows mild acanthosis and hyperkeratosis, while the dermis contains an inflammatory exudate consisting of polymorphonuclear cells, lymphocytes, and some histiocytes concentrated mainly around the blood vessels. Nodular rashes, Schönlein–Henoch purpura, and urticaria are also encountered.

Other manifestations

Attacks of pericarditis appear occasionally and there may be severe headache. Transient electrocardiographic signs of myopericarditis and non-specific electroencephalographic abnormalities have been observed during paroxysms. Severe myalgia has been reported and muscle atrophy adjacent to affected joints is not infrequent. Numerous attacks in children may lead to growth retardation. Colloid bodies are often found in the eye grounds and the spleen is palpable in more than one-third of patients.

Laboratory investigations

There are no specific laboratory criteria for the diagnosis of recurrent polyserositis. There may be transient microscopic haematuria during attacks. Persistent albuminuria is due to renal amyloidosis or, more rarely, glomerulonephritis. The white blood count usually rises to 12 000–18 000/mm^3 during attacks and the differential count remains normal or shows mild neutrophilia. Persistent leucocytosis is frequent in the presence of amyloidosis. Mild anaemia may occur. The erythrocyte sedimentation rate, rises during attacks, usually to between 40 and 60 mm after 1 h and the plasma fibrinogen level to more than 5 g/l. Other serum protein changes include inversion of the albumin-globulin ratio, a rise in α_2 and, less consistently, gammaglobulin and a rise in IgG, IgA, and IgM. Liver function tests are normal, although a mild and transient hyperbilirubinaemia has been reported. Bacteriological and serological examinations of blood, throat, urine, stool, peritoneal and joint exudates reveal no abnormal findings. The Rose–Waaler and latex globulin fixation tests are negative as are the laboratory markers of systemic lupus erythematosus.

Amyloidosis (see also Chapter 6.15)

Amyloidosis occurs more frequently in Sephardic Jews and Turks and is rare in non-Sephardic Jews and Armenians. Patients who develop it have a higher familial incidence, more frequent joint involvement, and skin rashes. The first sign of amyloidosis is massive albuminuria. Within several years, nephrotic syndrome and advancing renal failure develop. Renal vein thrombosis is a frequent complication, signalled by a rapid decline of renal function. Patients die within 3–13 years unless treated by haemodialysis and renal transplantation. Rectal biopsy will confirm the diagnosis in 70 per cent of the cases. On autopsy, amyloid deposits are found in the kidneys, intestines, adrenals, heart, ovaries, pancreas, and muscles. In most organs the deposition is perivascular. A marked decrease in new cases of amyloidosis has occurred since the advent of colchicine therapy. Genetic factors probably explain the greater incidence in Sephardic Jews. Indeed a form of familial amyloidosis occurs in this ethnic group in the absence of symptoms of recurrent polyserositis.

Differential diagnosis

During the initial attacks, most patients are wrongly diagnosed as suffering from appendicitis or cholecystitis. Erroneously explorative laparotomy is performed frequently but cholecystitis, diverticulitis, pancreatitis, and perforation of peptic ulcer are unlikely to occur before the age of 30. Helpful hints in the differential diagnosis are the early fall of the temperature, the history of previous attacks, a positive family history, and the ethnic origin of the patient. A high plasma fibrinogen and a normal amylase are of additional help. Recurrent pleurisy may occasionally simulate pulmonary embolism. Joint attacks are frequently misdiagnosed as septic arthritis. The main feature of the arthritic attacks is their episodic occurrence, starting during childhood or adolescence. The temperature curve is typical, the leucocyte count in the synovial fluid rarely exceeds 30 000/mm^3, and the fluid is always sterile. The destructive form of arthritis may be mistaken for juvenile rheumatoid arthritis or tuberculous arthritis but the diagnosis should present no difficulties. The association of fever, arthritis, splenomegaly, and skin rashes may suggest the diagnosis of systemic lupus erythematosus. However, accepted criteria for this disease will not be met, in particular, antinuclear factor and other laboratory data tests are always negative and the leucocyte count is usually high. In cases of doubt, a therapeutic trial with colchicine is indicated. Indeed, suppression of attacks is the only reliable diagnostic test.

Treatment

Colchicine has been established as the only effective treatment both for recurrent attacks and for prevention of amyloidosis. A daily dose of 1.0–1.5 mg will prevent the attacks in 95 per cent of the cases. Short courses of colchicine taken at the onset of attacks have been reported to suppress the symptoms but continuous therapy is more reliable. The mechanism of the action of colchicine is not established.

Pregnancy is no longer considered a contraindication for continuing colchicine therapy.

Prognosis

Recurrent polyserositis is a relatively benign disease which does not affect life expectancy, unless amyloidosis appears. Children are frequently physically underdeveloped because of the recurrent fever, nausea, and vomiting. Colchicine therapy seems to provide, for the first time, relief of much suffering for many patients, and opens a new horizon as a potential drug for the prevention of amyloidosis. The prognosis of patients with amyloidosis on chronic dialysis seems to be similar to that of patients with renal failure due to other causes.

Further reading

Ben-Chetrit, E. and Levy, M. (1998). Familial Mediterranean fever. *Lancet*, **351**, 659–64

Livnch, A., Langevitz, P., Zemer, D., *et al.* (1996). The changing face of familial Mediterranean fever. *Seminars in Arthritis and Rheumatism*, **26**, 612–27.

Prias, E., Aksentijevich, I., Gruberg, L., *et al.* (1992). Mapping of a gene causing familial Mediterranean fever to the short arm of chromosome 16. *New England Journal Medicine*, **326**, 1509–13.

Samuels, J., Aksentijevich, I., Torosyan, Y, *et al.* (1998). Familial Mediterranean fever at the millenium. Clinical spectrum, ancient mutations, and a survery of 100 American referrals to the National Institutes of Health. *Medicine*, 77, 268–97.

Chapter 6.17

Disturbances of acid–base homeostasis

R. D. Cohen and H. F. Woods

The normal acid burden

In resting humans arterial blood pH (pH_a) is normally tightly maintained between 7.36 and 7.42, as a result of control of arterial partial pressure of CO_2 ($PaCO_2$) and plasma bicarbonate between the limits 4.7–5.7 kPa and 24–30 mmol/l, respectively. Intracellular pH is also controlled and varies between tissues within the range 6.3–7.4, depending on prevailing physiological circumstances, although lysosomes are very acid (pH 5). Most physiological and clinical disturbances shift, or tend to shift, pH in the acid direction, and are due to the accumulation of hydrogen ions (H^+) derived from metabolism. Table 1 shows the approximate order of magnitude of the various sources of endogenous acid in moles of hydrogen ions per day in a resting normal human.

The many extracellular and intracellular buffers, notably haemoglobin, other proteins, bicarbonate, and phosphate, play a transient part in counteracting pH changes but normally the acid burdens are quantitatively eliminated in the middle or long term. They have been grouped into three classes according to the mode of elimination (Table 1). Carbon dioxide derived from cellular respiration is much the largest potential generator of hydrogen ions, the burden from lactic and other organic acid production and urea synthesis being approximately 10 times less and that derived from the metabolism of sulphur- and phosphorus-containing compounds is a further order of magnitude lower. Disposal of CO_2 is dependent on adequate respiratory function. The metabolism of sulphur-containing amino acids in the diet eventually results in the production of sulphuric acid, and phosphoric acid may be derived from many sources. Both of these acids are non-volatile and excretion of hydrogen ions from them may occur in the urine, virtually entirely in combination with urinary buffer.

The organic acids (Table 1) have pK values much less than blood pH and are, therefore, present in blood as the organic acid anions rather than as the undissociated acid, the equivalent amount of hydrogen ions, which was formed at the site of production of these acids, having titrated blood bicarbonate and other buffers. The organic acid anions (lactate, 3-hydroxybutyrate, acetoacetate, and fatty acids) are non-volatile but may be eliminated by metabolism. Figure 1 shows an example of the general principle that when these organic acid anions are metabolized to electroneutral products (e.g. glucose, or CO_2 and water), hydrogen ions are consumed and bicarbonate is regenerated. Hydrogen ions from organic acids can also be eliminated by the urinary route, but this is under normal circumstances a much slower process than the metabolic route. In the case of the ketone bodies, for which the renal threshold is quite low, substantial amounts can be lost in the urine when their plasma concentration is elevated. Although maximally acid urine (pH 4.5) results in about half of the urinary ketone body excretion being as the undissociated acid, the remaining free anion moiety represents loss of potential alkali from the body, because by escaping into the urine it eludes eventual metabolism to bicarbonate.

Comment on the unconventional appearance in Table 1 of urea synthesis as a source of acid burden is made in OTM3, pp. 1534–5. But, despite the large quantitative differences in the burden due to the three classes of acid in Table 1, their correct elimination is in a sense equally important, for no class is able substantially to use a disposal route normally associated with another class. The distinction lies in the potential rate at which the clinical state may become critical when a disposal route is deranged. Thus it has been calculated that total failure of elimination of CO_2 would result in critically severe acidosis in 30 min. Observations in clinical lactic acidosis suggest that elimination of the lactate removal mechanisms would take several hours to produce a lethal acidosis; in acute renal failure several days may elapse before acidosis becomes a major problem.

Normally the production and elimination of each class of acid are balanced. The homeostasis of arterial blood pH that this balance provides is given quantitative expression in the Henderson–Hasselbalch equation:

$$pH = 6.1 + \log_{10} [(HCO_3^-]/0.225 \times PaCO_2]$$

where $PaCO_2$ is the partial pressure of arterial CO2 expressed in kiloPascals (kPa). The constancy of arterial bicarbonate ions (HCO_3^-) is maintained by the removal of class II and III acids and by ureogenesis (see OTM3, pp. 1534–5) and that of the partial pressure of arterial CO_2 by the lungs, thereby fixing arterial blood pH within a narrow normal range.

Definitions

The terminology of acid–base disturbances has always been confused. Here we use the terms acidaemia and alkalaemia to indicate that the

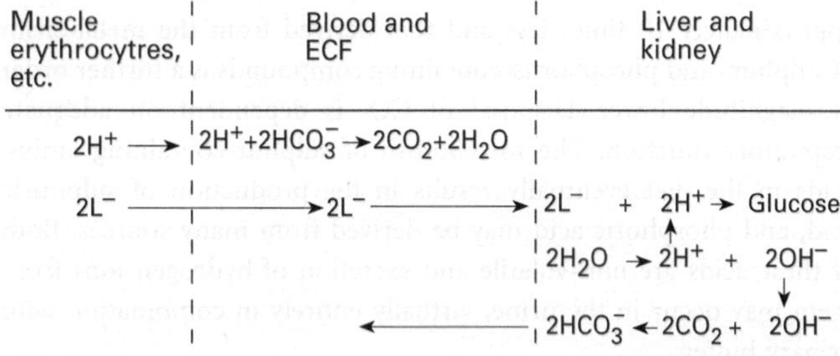

Fig. 1 A scheme, using lactate conversion to glucose as an example, showing how the conversion of an organic acid of low pK to an electroneutral substance consumes H^+ and regenerates HCO_3^-. The lactate ion is shown as L^-.

arterial blood pH is lower or higher than the normal range, respectively. The term acidosis is used to encompass both the situation where the arterial blood pH is low, and also that in which, although arterial blood pH is normal, the nature of the responsible disturbance is such that if compensatory mechanisms had not operated, arterial blood pH would be low. An equivalent definition applies to alkalosis. Most acid–base disturbances are due to imbalance of production and removal of hydrogen ions derived from the endogenous sources classified in Table 1. However, some are due to ingestion or infusion of excessive amounts of acids or bases (particularly bicarbonate). When the primary disturbance is related to abnormal CO_2 elimination, the acidosis or alkalosis is termed 'respiratory'. All other primary disturbances (i.e. those due to disturbances of class II and III acid production or removal, including those of ureogenesis), are termed 'metabolic' or 'non-respiratory'. The term 'primary' is used to contrast with 'secondary' disturbances, which are compensatory in nature. Thus metabolic acidosis is compensated for by hyperventilation due to stimulation of the respiratory centre, and consequently the arterial partial pressure of CO_2 is lowered; respiratory acidosis is compensated for by metabolic events which result in elevation of plasma bicarbonate.

The diagnosis of acid–base disturbances

The clinical manifestations of acid–base disturbances are described later. They are rather non-specific and may not be evident until the disturbance is quite severe. Thus, although clinical features may provide the first indication of a disturbance of acid–base homeostasis, accurate characterization, both qualitatively and quantitatively, requires laboratory investigation. Measurement of pH and $P\text{aCO}_2$ on arterial, or arterialized venous blood is the most definitive procedure. Additional useful information may be obtained from measurement of plasma sodium, potassium, chloride, and bicarbonate, and subsequent calculation of the anion gap.

Measurement of pH_a and $P\text{aCO}_2$

Blood gas analysers measure pH and $P\text{aco}_2$ and calculate bicarbonate from the Henderson–Hasselbalch equation. Interpretation of the results is best achieved by the use of an acid–base diagram, which has arterial blood pH on one axis and $P\text{aco}_2$ in the other. Diagrams which use the concentration of arterial bicarbonate ions $[HCO_3^-]_a$ instead of either arterial blood pH and $P\text{aco}_2$ are less suitable, as arterial bicarbonate ion concentration is calculated from arterial blood pH and $P\text{aco}_2$ and is not only affected by the errors in both the latter measurements, but also by the fact that pK_a in the Henderson–Hasselbalch equation is subject to some poorly understood variations in blood from severely ill patients.

The acid–base diagram shown in Fig. 2 has bands drawn in to show the range of expected response to uncomplicated acid–base disorders. The shaded square represents the approximate limits of arterial blood pH and $P\text{aco}_2$ in normal individuals. Thus a patient with uncomplicated metabolic acidosis will have values lying in the band marked metabolic in the region to the left and above the shaded area; the metabolic band is the envelope of measurements of arterial blood pH and $P\text{aco}_2$ from patients recorded in the literature with uncomplicated metabolic acidosis or alkalosis. The band marked acute respiratory is the 95 per cent confidence range of values obtained in normal individuals voluntarily hyperventilating or breathing air/

Table 1 Production and elimination of hydrogen ions

Class		Daily production (mol)	Source	Excreted in breath	Metabolic removal possible	Normal organ of elimination
I	CO_2	15	Tissue respiration	+	–	Lungs
II	*Organic acids and urea synthesis*					
	Lactic	1.2	Muscle, brain erythrocytes, skin, etc.	–	+	Liver (50 per cent), kidneys, heart
	Hydroxybutyric and acetoacetic	0.6*	Liver	–	+	Many tissues (not liver)
	Free fatty acids (FFA)	0.7	Adipose tissue	–	+	Most tissues
	H^+ generated during urea synthesis	1.1†	Liver	–	+	Most tissues (see text) small fraction in urine
III	*'Fixed acids'*					
	Sulphuric	0.1	Dietary sulphur-containing amino acids	–	–	Urinary excretion (partly)
	Phosphoric	0.1	Organic phosphate metabolism			

The daily production rates for the organic acids are calculated from results obtained in resting 70 kg man after an overnight fast, and are proportioned up to 24 h values.

*Because of ingestion of food during daytime and consequent suppression of FFA and ketone body production, the values for these acids may be considerable overestimates.

†On 100 g protein diet.

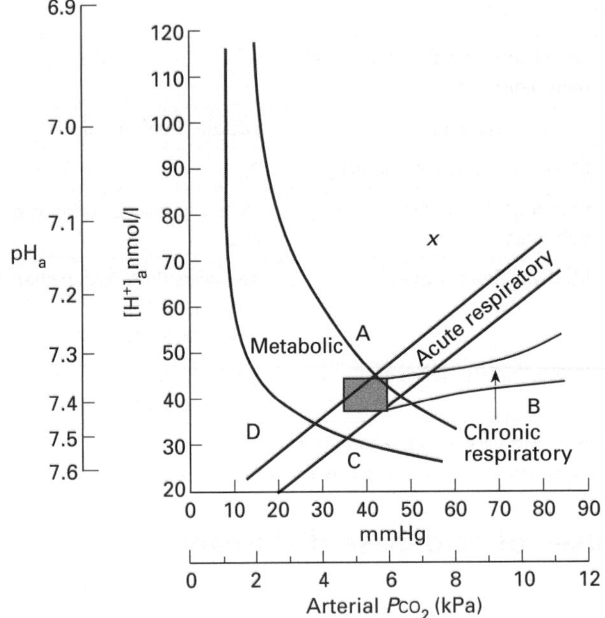

Fig. 2 For explanation see text. Pco$_2$ = partial pressure of CO_2.

CO_2 mixtures for short periods of time. As, after a few days of CO_2 retention in respiratory acidosis, an increase in plasma bicarbonate produces substantial or complete compensation, the response expected in chronic respiratory acidosis is different from the acute response, the presence of the extra bicarbonate reducing the fall in pH for a given rise in Paco$_2$.

Figure 2 therefore also includes the uncomplicated response to chronic respiratory acidosis. The band for metabolic alkalosis (to the right of and below the shaded region) is restricted, extending only a short distance along the Paco$_2$ axis, because compensation by hypoventilation for metabolic alkalosis is often poor, perhaps because hypoxia sets a limit to compensating hypoventilation and also because a number of conditions causing metabolic alkalosis may be associated with intracellular acidosis, which could stimulate the respiratory centre. Marked hypercapnia is, however, occasionally seen in metabolic alkalosis.

The arterial blood pH and Paco$_2$ measurements in some patients will not fall within any of the defined bands shown in Fig. 2. Such patients have a mixture of acid–base disorders. Thus a patient whose arterial blood pH and Paco$_2$ is represented by the point '*x*' has mixed respiratory and metabolic acidosis (e.g. a patient with an exacerbation of chronic bronchitis and coexistent diabetic ketoacidosis). It may be noted that a disturbance lying in sectors A or C results from the combination of two primary acid–base conditions; in sectors B and D one of the two disturbances could be compensatory for the other. The diagram not only permits the diagnosis of acid–base disorders, but by serially plotting results the course of an individual patient's disturbance and its response to treatment may be closely followed.

Contemporary acid–base analytical equipment usually also provides at least two further acid–base variables if the haemoglobin concentration is also known. These are the 'standard bicarbonate' and the 'base excess' or 'base deficit' variables. The standard bicarbonate represents what the plasma bicarbonate would be if the blood had a normal Paco$_2$ (5.33 kPa, 40 mmHg) rather than its actual value. Standard bicarbonate was introduced in an attempt to provide a measurement which was independent of respiratory disturbance and thus to provide an estimate of underlying pure metabolic disturbance. 'Base deficit' represents the amount of alkali in mmol required to restore the pH of 1 litre of the patient's blood *in vitro* to normal at Paco$_2$ 5.33 kPa and might at first sight be considered a quantitative measure of metabolic acidosis. Unfortunately, the titration curve of blood *in vitro* is different from when it is circulating *in vivo*, as in the latter situation the interstitial and intracellular fluids are in equilibrium with blood and may gain or lose bicarbonate from it; in addition their buffering capacity differs from that of blood. These considerations detract from the usefulness of base excess or deficit as a guide either to diagnosis or therapy. Further difficulties arise from ambiguities in the interpretation of base excess or deficit. Thus a patient with chronic respiratory acidosis will have a high standard bicarbonate and a base excess due to compensatory renal retention of bicarbonate. It could be said, therefore, that this patient has simultaneously a respiratory acidosis and a metabolic alkalosis, as a base excess indicates the latter. This way of regarding the situation, which is quite widely adopted, is confusing, and is not compatible with the definitions of acidosis and alkalosis given here, which are intended to indicate the direction of the primary disturbance. For these reasons the acid–base diagram shown in Fig. 2, which is based entirely on directly measured variables is preferable.

Use of the anion gap

The main electrolytes routinely measured in plasma are sodium (Na^+), chloride (Cl^-), potassium (K^+), and bicarbonate (HCO_3^-). The sum of the measured cations ($Na^+ + K^+$) normally exceeds that of the measured anions by about 14 mmol/l (reference range 10–18 mmol/l). This difference is known as the 'anion gap' and is attributable largely to negatively charged proteins but also to phosphate, sulphate, and some organic acids. Calculation of the anion gap is principally of value in the differential diagnosis of metabolic acidosis and in following the progress of therapy. Metabolic acidoses may be divided broadly into those with normal and those with high anion gap.

Metabolic acidoses with normal anion gap

These are due to the direct loss of bicarbonate, either through the gut (e.g. diarrhoea, pancreatic fistulae, ureterosigmoidostomy) or through the kidney (e.g. renal tubular acidosis, acetazolamide therapy) or, rarely to the ingestion or infusion of hydrochloric acid or substances effectively giving rise to it (e.g. ammonium chloride, arginine hydrochloride). When bicarbonate is lost more chloride is retained by the renal tubules; thus low plasma bicarbonate is accompanied by hyperchloraemia and the anion gap remains unaltered. In the case of hydrochloric acid intake bicarbonate is titrated and replaced by chloride.

Metabolic acidoses with high anion gap

These are due to the ingestion or endogenous generation of acids, usually organic, whose anions are not routinely measured. Plasma bicarbonate is titrated and the anion gap is now widened by the presence of these unmeasured anions. The principal causes are ketoacidosis, lactic acidosis, uraemic acidosis, and poisoning by salicylates. In uraemic acidosis the anion gap seldom exceeds 28 mmol/l, but considerably higher values may be found in severe lactic acidosis and ketoacidosis. There are also causes of raised anion gap other than metabolic acidosis, for example therapy with sodium salts of relatively strong acids (e.g. lactate, acetate) and high-dose sodium carbenicillin therapy, and respiratory or metabolic alkalosis.

Table 2 High anion gap metabolic acidoses

	Associated serum acid anions*
(i) *Predominant ketoacidosis*	
Diabetic ketoacidosis	*3-hydroxybutyrate*, acetoacetate, lactate
Starvation ketoacidosis	*3-hydroxybutyrate*, acetoacetate, lactate
Alcoholic ketoacidosis	*3-hydroxybutyrate*, acetoacetate, lactate
Ketotic hypoglycaemia of childhood	*3-hydroxybutyrate*, acetoacetate, lactate
(ii) *Predominant lactic acidosis*	
Type A lactic acidosis	
Exercise	*Lactate*
Postepileptic	*Lactate*
Shock (traumatic, haemorrhagic, cardiogenic, septic)	*Lactate*
Severe hypoxia.	*Lactate*
Type B lactic acidosis	
Biguanide-associated (phenformin, buformin, metformin)	*Lactate*, 3-hydroxybutyrate
Ethanol-associated	*Lactate*, 3-hydroxybutyrate
Following recovery from diabetic ketoacidosis	*Lactate*
Fructose, sorbitol, or xylitol infusion	*Lactate*
Other poorly characterized acquired lactic acidoses	*Lactate*
Severe liver disease	*Lactate*
Leukaemia and reticulosis	*Lactate*
Paracetamol poisoning	*Lactate*
Thiamine deficiency	*Lactate*
Type I glycogenosis	*Lactate*
Hepatic fructose 1,6-diphosphatase deficiency	*Lactate*
Lactic acidosis associated with metabolic myopathies	*Lactate*
Pyruvate carboxylase deficiency	*Lactate*
Other poorly characterized hereditary lactic acidoses	*Lactate*
d(–) lactic acidosis due to lactobacillus ingestion	*Lactate*
(iii) *Conditions with imperfectly defined source of acidoses*	
Uraemic acidosis	Phosphate, sulphate, etc.
Salicylate poisoning (acidotic phase)	Salicylate lactate, ketoacids
Methanol poisoning	*Formate, lactate*
Ethylene glycol poisoning	Lactate, glycolate, oxalate
Paraldehyde poisoning	?
Reye's syndrome	Lactate
Jamaican vomiting sickness (ackee poisoning)	?
Glutaric aciduria type II	Lactate, free fatty acids
Ethylmalonic-adipic aciduria	?
Propionyl CoA carboxylase deficiency	Higher ketoacids, propionic acid
Methylmalonic aciduria	Ketoacids (including higher ones), lactate, methylmalonate
β-Ketothiolase deficiency	Methylhydroxybutyrate, methylacetoacetate

*The predominant acid anion is shown in italics.

Except when otherwise stated, lactate refers to the l(+)isomer.

Causes of acid–base disturbance

The most diverse problems of aetiology and classification arise in metabolic acidosis. Table 2 classifies those conditions associated with high anion gap metabolic acidosis and divides them into those in which the predominant unmeasured anion is lactate, ketoacids, or other less well-defined acid anions. The term 'ketoacid' is loosely used to refer both to a ketoacid itself (e.g. acetoacetic acid) and its reduced derivative (e.g. 3-hydroxybutyrate). High anion gap acidosis is often due to a mixture of acids, but where possible the predominant acid has been indicated in *italic type*. The acid anions actually identified in plasma can often only account for part of the acidosis. The common form of uraemic acidosis is the best example of this. Table 3 lists metabolic acidoses with normal anion gap classified according to whether they are due to gut or renal bicarbonate loss, or to ingestion or infusion of acidifying agents.

Metabolic alkalosis (Table 4) is due either to ingestion or infusion of excessive alkali in circumstances (e.g. poor renal function) when it cannot be excreted, or to loss of acid, either from the stomach as in pyloric stenosis, or in the secretion of an inappropriately acid urine. Most of the causes of the latter are related to the complex disturbances occurring in potassium and chloride deficiency. The metabolic alkalosis seen in fulminant hepatic failure has not been explained but may be due to failure of urea synthesis, and consequent failure to neutralize bicarbonate derived from metabolism of the carbon skeletons of amino acids. *Respiratory acidoses* (Table 5) are due to problems at one or more of three levels, namely, the lungs and airways, the neuromuscular and mechanical aspects of respiration, and the central nervous system. *Respiratory alkalosis* (Table 6) is nearly always due to some form of stimulus to the respiratory centre, whether it be psychogenic, reflex, chemically induced, or due to a local lesion; the exception is deliberate or inadvertent hyperventilation during anaesthesia or other occasions when assisted ventilation is used.

The consequences of acid–base disturbances

Respiratory effects

Both metabolic acidosis and acute respiratory acidosis induced by breathing high partial pressure of CO_2 gas mixtures result in hyperventilation. Deep sighing respiration (Kussmaul breathing) is a familiar sign of metabolic acidosis. The degree of hyperventilation

Table 3 Normal anion gap metabolic acidoses

(i) *Gastrointestinal bicarbonate loss* Diarrhoea Pancreatic fistula
(ii) *Ureteroenterostomy*
(iii) *Renal causes* Renal tubular acidosis (**RTA**) (a) *Gradient distal type, type I RTA)* Primary transient, in infancy permanent (childhood or adult) Secondary In hypergammaglobulinaemia and some autoimmune states Amphotericin B therapy Vitamin D intoxication Hyperthyroidism Carnitine palmitoyl transferase (type I) deficiency (b) *Bicarbonate wastage (proximal type, type II RTA)* Primary isolated as part of idiopathic Fanconi syndrome Secondary Hyperthyroidism Vitamin D deficiency Uraemia (occasionally) Dysproteinaemic states (myeloma, Sjögren's syndrome) Heavy metal poisoning (cadmium, mercury) Outdated tetracycline Renal transplant rejection Hereditary disorders (e.g. cystinosis, Wilson's disease, hereditary fructose intolerance, galactosaemia, Lowe's syndrome) Acetazolamide treatment (c) *Type IV RTA (hyperkalaemic)* Hypoaldosteronism, aldosterone insensitivity Types I and II pseudohypoaldosteronism Hyporeninaemia Diabetes Pyelonephritis Potassium sparing diuretics Angiotensin converting enzyme inhibitors Non-steroidal anti-inflammatory drugs. As part of moderate renal insufficiency
(iv) *Ingestion or infusion of acidifying agents* Ammonium chloride Arginine hydrochloride, hydrochloric acid Intravenous feeding with solutions containing excess cationic amino acids
(v) *Rapid intravenous hydration* (dilutional acidosis)

achieved is dependent on factors which are related both to the magnitude and the rate of development of the acid–base disturbance. pH control of ventilation is determined both by the pH perceived by the carotid and aortic body chemoreceptors and by chemoreceptors in the medulla which appear to monitor the pH of brain extracellular fluid (**ECF**). In the steady state, brain ECF pH is closely similar to that of cerebrospinal fluid (**CSF**). Sudden development of metabolic acidosis, resulting in low arterial blood pH and plasma bicarbonate, induces hyperventilation by stimulating the carotid and aortic body chemoreceptors and $Paco_2$ is thus lowered. However, the first effect on brain ECF pH is to raise it, as brain ECF $Paco_2$ is lowered, because CO_2 is rapidly equilibrated across the blood–brain barrier. In contrast, it takes many hours for the brain ECF bicarbonate concentration to fall in response to the lowering of plasma bicarbonate because movement of bicarbonate across the barrier is very much slower than that of CO_2. The temporary alkalinization of brain ECF pH in the presence of systemic metabolic acidosis somewhat offsets the ventilatory drive provided by the peripheral chemoreceptors. In the longer term, brain ECF and CSF pH are tightly controlled and their initial high pH in acute metabolic acidosis is eventually restored to normal or slightly below normal. This removes the partial inhibition of ventilatory response and the degree of hyperventilation increases. Though clinical circumstances usually prevent the observation of this sequence of events, the opposite effect, namely the persistence of hyperventilation after restoration of normal arterial pH during the therapy of metabolic acidosis is commonly seen. In this situation systemic alkalinization has suppressed the peripheral chemoreceptors, raising $Paco_2$ and thus causing paradoxical acidification of brain ECF and CSF. Over 24 h may elapse before the resulting persisting

Table 4 Causes of metabolic alkalosis

Ingestion or infusion of alkali in excess of excretory ability	
Milk-alkali syndrome	
'Alkaline overshoot' during therapy of high anion gap acidoses	
Forced alkaline diuresis therapy of salicylate and barbiturate poisoning	
Loss of acid inappropriately (gastric or renal routes)	
Pyloric stenosis, self-induced persistent vomiting	
Potassium depletion (other than in tubular acidosis)	Frequently associated
Chloride depletion	Frequently associated
Hyperaldosteronism	Frequently associated
'Contraction alkalosis'	
Rapid diuresis	
?Failure of ureogenesis	
Fulminant hepatic failure	

Table 5 Causes of respiratory acidosis

1.	*Structural and mechanical pulmonary disease* Chronic obstructive airways disease Severe asthma (uncommonly) Large airway obstruction
2.	*Neuromuscular and mechanical problems* Acute ascending polyneuritis (Guillain–Barré) Poliomyelitis Acute porphyria Myasthenia gravis Motor neurone disease Muscular dystrophies Traumatic 'flail chest' Ankylosing spondylitis Severe kyphoscoliosis Gross obesity, often in association with sleep apnoea Muscle relaxant drugs
3.	*Respiratory centre disorders* Organic disease affecting respiratory centre Numerous respiratory centre depressant drugs e.g. opiates, barbiturates, benzodiazepines, anaesthetic agents Respiratory arrest

Table 6 Causes of respiratory alkalosis

Spontaneous or psychogenic hyperventilation
Reflex hyperventilation (e.g. in pulmonary disease and pulmonary embolism)
Other stimuli to respiratory centre
(*a*) Via chemoreceptors
Low inspired oxygen concentration (e.g. high altitude)
Alveolo-capillary diffusion block
Right to left shunt
Carbon monoxide poisoning
(*b*) Via drugs or metabolites
Salicylate poisoning
Acute liver failure
(*c*) After recovery from metabolic acidosis
(*d*) Local lesion affecting centre
Overventilation during anaesthesia or other assisted ventilation

hyperventilation ceases. In acute and chronic respiratory acidosis the ventilatory manifestations of phased events equivalent to those seen in metabolic acid–base disorders are seldom given full expression, because the respiratory disease usually prevents this. In chronic CO_2 retention direct depression of the respiratory centre occurs, and the respiratory response to increments of $Paco_2$ becomes progressively lost, ventilation becoming increasingly dependent upon hypoxic drive.

Cardiovascular effects

On the heart

Acidosis has adverse effects on cardiac contractility and alkalosis smaller but opposite effects. The negative inotropic effects are particularly related to changes in cardiac intracellular pH and are experimentally found to be rather greater in acute respiratory than in acute metabolic acidosis. These effects are due to a combination of mechanisms connected with excitation–contraction coupling and energy supply; among other mechanisms, acidosis inhibits the inward slow calcium current during the action potential and the release of calcium from sarcoplasmic reticulum, and depresses glycolysis. The consequence is that circulatory collapse is often seen after some hours of severe metabolic acidosis not primarily due to shock. Mild to moderate acidosis may not be associated with negative inotropic effects due to the protective effect of catecholamine release, which is increased in acidosis. Patients receiving blocking drugs are thus potentially more susceptible to the effects of acidosis on cardiac function.

On the peripheral vasculature

Cerebral arterioles are very sensitive to the pH of brain ECF, being dilated when it falls and constricted by increases. The cerebrovascular resistance is therefore subject to similar phased responses to different types of acute acid–base disturbances as is ventilation, due to the differential time response of brain ECF, Pco_2, and bicarbonate to acute systemic changes. Dilatation is also the response of most systemic arterioles to acidosis, although this response may be modified or offset completely by catecholamine effects. The peripheral veins, however, constrict in acidosis, resulting in a shift of blood from the peripheral capacitance vessels to the central circulation.

Effects on intermediary carbohydrate metabolism and nitrogen balance

Glycolysis is inhibited by acidosis and stimulated by alkalosis, due to the effects of intracellular pH on phosphofructokinase, a rate-limiting enzyme of glycolysis. Respiratory alkalosis might, therefore, be expected to raise blood lactate, but in normal individuals the effect is very small, no doubt due to removal of lactate by the liver. However, in the presence of severe liver disease gross elevation of blood lactate may be seen in association with respiratory alkalosis and the increased production of lactic acid may partially compensate for the alkalosis.

Hepatic gluconeogenesis from lactate is inhibited by severe acidosis due to an effect on the step between pyruvate and oxaloacetate. This phenomenon could be responsible for perpetuating and worsening lactic acidosis.

Acidosis shifts nitrogen balance towards a more negative stance; it has been shown that the negative nitrogen balance of chronic acidotic renal failure may be alleviated by treatment with bicarbonate.

Effects on blood oxygen uptake and delivery

One of the factors determining pulmonary oxygen uptake and tissue oxygen delivery is the position of the blood oxygen dissociation curve with respect to the ordinate (the oxygen saturation) and abscissa (the partial pressure of oxygen; PO_2). Right shifts of this curve improve unloading of oxygen in the tissues, but, in the presence of low inspired oxygen concentration or pulmonary disease, impair oxygen uptake in the lungs; left shifts have the opposite effect. The position of the curve is determined by three ligands capable of interacting with haemoglobin, namely, hydrogen ions, CO_2, and 2,3-bisphosphoglycerate (2,3-BPG). Increases in the concentration of any of these result in a shift to the right. The effects of changes in extracellular hydrogen ions (Bohr effect) and CO_2 are immediate and operate through changes in intraerythrocytic hydrogen ions and CO_2. In addition, an increase in intraerythrocytic hydrogen ions (i.e. fall in pH) inhibits the synthesis of 2,3-BPG and encourages its breakdown. In diabetic ketoacidosis erythrocyte 2,3-BPG may be decreased by as much as 90 per cent. Opposite effects occur in alkalosis. These reactions are, however, very slow in comparison with the immediate Bohr effect.

The effect of these timing differences on oxygen delivery during the course of acid–base disturbances may be exemplified by the changes occurring during the development and treatment of acute metabolic acidosis. Initially, the acute acidosis causes a right shift and hence improved oxygen delivery. After several hours the 2,3-BPG level falls, thus restoring the position of the curve approximately to normal. If the patient is now rapidly treated with alkali, the Bohr effect results in an immediate shift to the left; it may be many hours, even up to 2–3 days, before 2,3-BPG concentrations are restored. The sudden deterioration in oxygen delivery caused by alkalinization could have adverse clinical effects unless the effect of shift in the curve is counteracted by other factors—such as increase in tissue blood flow.

Effects on the nervous system

These are a result of many factors, including changes in cerebral blood flow and oxygen dissociation (see above) and other mechanisms less well characterized. Severe acidosis is frequently associated with a variety of degrees of impairment of consciousness, varying from mild drowsiness to coma. The degree of disturbance is not closely related to systemic pH, and the mechanism is not understood. Attempts to relate this effect of acidosis to CSF pH have proved unsuccessful. The excitability of neuromuscular tissues is in general increased by alkalosis and decreased by acidosis. Tetany is a common feature of respiratory alkalosis, and may also be seen when a chronic metabolic acidosis is corrected in a patient with low plasma calcium, a combination of events which may occur in renal failure. Epileptic attacks in those prone to them are precipitated by alkalosis and suppressed by acidosis.

Effects on potassium homeostasis (see also Chapter 12.4)

Effects on the kidney

The kidney is a major organ of acid–base control and many of its responses to acid–base disturbances are therefore geared to their correction. Acidosis causes a marked increase in renal gluconeogenesis, primarily due to increased activity of phosphoenolpyruvate carboxykinase. The increased gluconeogenesis is thought to be causally linked with the increase of renal ammoniagenesis which is a crucial part of the renal response to acidosis. The ammoniagenic response to acidosis also depends on an adequate supply of ammonium precursors to the kidney, and an intact ammonium production mechanism within the tubular cells. The main precursor of renal ammonium is glutamine and substantial changes take place in glutamine metabolism in acidosis. Glutamine release from liver and skeletal muscle is increased and disposal of glutamine nitrogen is shifted away from urea production in the liver to ammonium excretion in the kidney. This is due not only to the stimulatory effects of acidosis on renal ammoniagenesis, but also to direct inhibition of urea production, thus tending to counteract the acidosis. In addition, chronic acidosis also results in the increased activity of renal glutaminase, the critical enzyme of ammoniagenesis.

Most textbooks of physiology state that the kidneys are capable during acidosis of increasing their effective acid secretion from a typical normal value of 100 mmol/day to about 500 mmol/day. This assertion, however, is based on calculating the daily urinary acid excretion as: (titratable acid + ammonium − bicarbonate) in urine. Here 'titratable acid' refers mainly to hydrogen ions carried in phosphate buffer and is typically, in millimolar terms, about 25–30–per cent of the ammonium excretion. Bicarbonate excretion is normally small except in alkaline urine. During acidosis, further titration of the phosphate buffer produces a modest increment in effective hydrogen ion excretion, but ammonium excretion may increase five-fold or more, and it is this latter effect which has largely given rise to the quoted values for total hydrogen ion excretion during acidosis. But, if it is incorrect to regard the ammonia/ammonium system as a urinary buffer (see OTM3, pp. 1534–5), then the classic explanation of the renal response to acidosis must be incorrect. The alternative view, is that the increased ammonium excretion in acidosis results in diversion of nitrogenous substrate from urea synthesis, and consequent counteraction of acidosis. The ability of the kidney to excrete ammonium and thereby activate this mechanism depends on its ability to lower the urinary pH to the normal minimum of 4.5–5.3, as well as upon the adaptive mechanisms described in the previous paragraph.

In alkalosis other than that due to potassium chloride, and extracellular volume depletion, large quantities of bicarbonate are excreted in the urine, the maximum pH of which is about 8.

Effects on bone

Bone acts as a buffer in chronic metabolic acidosis, in that leaching out of a calcium carbonate phase in bone and exchange of extracellular phosphate for carbonate within the apatite crystal result in the neutralization of hydrogen ions. The first of these mechanisms gives rise to a negative calcium balance in chronic metabolic acidosis and in chronic uraemic acidotic subjects calcium balance can be restored by treatment with sodium bicarbonate. Renal tubular acidosis and the acidosis of ureterosigmoidostomy lead to osteomalacia, which can be corrected by alkali therapy alone.

Effects on leucocytes

Severe acidosis is often associated with marked leucocytosis, unrelated to the presence of infection. Counts of up to 60 000/mm^3 have been recorded in lactic acidosis and high values are also common in diabetic ketoacidosis.

Effects on the distribution of metabolites and drugs

When weak acids and bases are distributed between body compartments by non-ionic diffusion, pH differences between the two compartments will determine their relative concentrations. Weak bases are concentrated in the more acid ones, and weak acids in the more alkaline compartments. Examples of physiological metabolites thus affected are ammonia (weak base) and urobilinogen (weak acid). The urinary excretion of ammonium is thus markedly increased in acid urine and that of urobilinogen decreased. Examples of drugs exhibiting this behaviour are salicylates and phenobarbitone, which are both weak acids; so that their fractional renal excretion in the case of poisoning, is much increased by alkalinizing the urine.

Major syndromes of metabolic acidosis

For renal tubular acidosis see Chapter 12.31.

Uraemic acidosis

Metabolic acidosis of varying degree is a classical feature of both acute and chronic renal failure and has traditionally been attributed to failure to excrete hydrogen ions derived from 'fixed acids'—class III acids of Table 1. The remaining nephrons are usually able to lower the urinary pH to the normal minimum value, but occasionally failure of proximal bicarbonate reabsorption prevents achievement of the minimum urinary pH until the plasma bicarbonate has been substantially lowered, and, if the primary condition giving rise to the overall glomerulotubular failure has principally affected the renal papilla, some intrinsic acidification defect may exist. However, the fact that acidification is usually normal means that the phosphate buffers in the urine can be fully titrated; titratable acid excretion is therefore commonly normal in the steady state, even though phosphate excretion often has to be maintained by a high plasma phosphate and secondary hyperparathyroidism. The excretion of ammonium is, however, low, presumably both because of loss of glutaminase containing proximal tubules and because the supply of glutamine is curtailed by impairment of renal blood flow. The classic explanation of the acidosis of renal failure has therefore been that the diminished supply of ammonia lowers the ability of the tubular contents to buffer secreted hydrogen ions and that the minimum pH of the urine is therefore attained before the normal content of buffered hydrogen ion is achieved. However, as the ammonium cannot act as a urinary buffer (see **OTM3, pp. 1534–5**), an alternative explanation is that the nitrogen which, in renal insufficiency fails to be excreted as ammonium, is diverted to the liver where it is converted into urea, with hydrogen ion production as a result. The acidosis of acute or chronic renal failure is therefore due to overproduction of urea, not to failure of excretion of hydrogen ions in the urine as ammonium. The elevation of anion gap in uraemic acidosis is usually relatively modest, and the unmeasured anions have not been well characterized, but include minor contributions from phosphate and sulphate. When there is proximal bicarbonate wastage, the anion gap may not be grossly raised, and chloride may be reabsorbed instead of bicarbonate, giving rise to moderate hyperchloraemia.

Diabetic ketoacidosis

The pathogenesis of hyperglycaemic ketotic diabetic coma is described elsewhere (see Chapter 6.13). Only the acid–base disturbance will be discussed here. Though the acidosis has been conventionally regarded as being due mainly to overproduction of ketoacids by the liver, recent evidence has suggested that, although the anions of ketoacids are indeed generated in the liver, the hydrogen ions are wholly or partly derived from other tissues.

Diabetic ketoacidosis has usually been regarded as an high anion gap metabolic acidosis in which extracellular bicarbonate has been simply titrated by the ketoacids. If this were the case, the fall in plasma bicarbonate should roughly equal the rise in anion gap and the plasma concentration of ketoacids, but the situation is frequently more complex. Patients in ketoacidosis with well-preserved renal function tend to have an elevation of anion gap which is much less than the fall in bicarbonate. This appears to be due to the loss of large quantities of ketoacid anions in the urine and concomitant retention of chloride and hyperchloraemia which, together with the urinary loss of ketones, results in a relatively low elevation of anion gap compared with the bicarbonate deficit. Patients who have relatively poor renal function, because of dehydration, lose much smaller quantities of ketoacid anions in the urine and present with a more classical high anion gap metabolic acidosis. Some of the severest cases of diabetic ketoacidosis produce an arterial pH value as low as 6.8. The minimum possible urinary pH is achieved (4.5–5.3). About half the urinary ketoacids are undissociated and some hydrogen ions are lost in this way. Those patients who have presented with an high anion gap tend to recover their plasma bicarbonate concentration more rapidly on treatment, as they have lost less ketoacid anions in the urine and therefore less potential alkali than those presenting with relatively normal anion gaps.

Metabolic alkalosis can follow ketoacidosis when vomiting has been severe and when excessive amounts of bicarbonate have been infused to treat the acidaemia. In such circumstances, although arterial blood pH may initially be returned to normal, the quantity of ketoacid anions remains high as does the anion gap. When the ketoacid anions are metabolized metabolic alkalosis ensues.

Lactic acidosis, may either develop during therapy, or play a major part in the original pathogenesis. During the therapy, if the blood sugar is falling satisfactorily and the blood ketone concentration is also decreasing, the persistence of a severe metabolic acidosis points to the possibility of supervening lactic acidosis. This is relatively rare, but much more common (in 5–10 per cent of cases) is a significant contribution to the initial metabolic acidosis by the accumulation of lactic acid to concentrations of 5 mmol/l or above, particularly when there is shock, hypoxia, or infection. In most cases these concentrations fall with successful treatment but may, on occasions, rise further later.

The question of the use, or not, of bicarbonate in ketoacidosis is discussed above and in Chapter 6.13.

Lactic acidosis

Nature and classification

In health, the concentration of lactate in venous blood at rest varies within the narrow limits of 0.6–1.2 mmol/l. It is lower after fasting and rises after meals. In severe physical exercise the concentration may rise to 10–20 mmol/l or above, rapidly returning to normal after it. Lactic acid has a pK of 3.86 and thus over the physiological range of pH is virtually completely dissociated, so that the generation of the lactate ion in body tissues is accompanied by a similar amount of hydrogen ion.

Lactate excess can be divided into two groups: (a) hyperlactataemia, in which there is raised lactate without change in blood pH, and (b) lactic acidosis, when the lactate accumulation is sufficient to lower the blood pH. The acidosis is seldom significant unless blood lactate exceeds 5 mmol/l. Cases of lactic acidosis fall into two groups. In type A, which is much the most common, there are signs of poor tissue perfusion with or without hypoxia. Patients with haemorrhagic or cardiogenic shock provide good examples. Type B patients do not have signs of tissue hypoxia or underperfusion except as a secondary and late event. These cases can be further subclassified into those occurring as a result of the administration of certain drugs, chemicals, and toxic compounds, and those in which the patient has an inherited metabolic defect which results in lactate accumulation (Table 2). Many of the causes listed in this table are rare, being the subject of single case reports. Most information has been collected from patients with shock (type A) or those associated with biguanide therapy—usually phenformin (type B). The condition has been almost exclusively confined to the accumulation of the natural l(+) isomer of lactic acid. Although humans have the capacity to metabolize the *d*-isomer, it is not a product of normal metabolism, but a small amount is ingested in food and produced by bacterial metabolism in the gut. A few cases of *d*-lactic acidosis in humans have been described due to excessive *d*-lactic acid production in the gut, related to the presence of an unusual distribution of bacterial flora commonly associated with short gut syndromes.

The presentation in type B lactic acidosis is fairly uniform. Symptoms in order of frequency include: hyperventilation or dyspnoea, stupor or coma, vomiting, drowsiness, and abdominal pain. The onset is usually rapid over a few hours with a deterioration in consciousness which varies from mild confusion to coma and may, in the early stages, be accompanied by profound lethargy. Although by definition there is no initial poor tissue perfusion or hypoxia, patients with severe type B lactic acidosis commonly become shocked after a few hours.

Lactic acidosis has been described in association most frequently with diabetes mellitus (especially in association with biguanide therapy), liver disease, renal impairment, acute pancreatitis, bacterial infections, septicaemia, leukaemia, and lymphoma. These associations may alert the clinician to lactic acid as the cause of a metabolic acidosis. There will be a high anion gap but the definitive diagnosis depends on the identification of lactate as the cause. Measurement of lactate in blood is simple, rapid, and specific through the use of enzymic spectrophotometric micromethods.

Pathogenesis

Lactic acidosis must be due to: increased lactate production; impaired lactate utilization; or a combination of these two.

Up to 70 per cent of the total daily lactate production of about 1.2 mol/24 h per 70 kg body weight in resting humans is taken up by the liver. Many patients with liver disease have an elevated resting blood lactate concentration and their ability to dispose of an exogenous lactate load is impaired. Some 30–40 per cent of patients with lactate acidosis have evidence of liver disease and thus many explanations of the pathogenesis of lactic acidosis have centred upon the liver. Before lactic acidosis can develop in liver disease the extent of the impairment must be severe or increased production must be present. Phenformin caused an unacceptably high incidence of type B lactic acidosis increasing lactate production in the splanchnic bed and decrease hepatic lactate uptake. Increased peripheral production of lactic acid may also be involved. Phenformin has now been withdrawn, but metformin is still widely used. The incidence of lactic acidosis during metformin therapy is an order of magnitude less than for phenformin, but occasional severe and fatal cases are still seen, nearly always in patients with renal insufficiency. Metformin should not be administered to such patients, or to those at particular risk of suffering a decrease in renal function during intercurrent illness.

Increased lactate production is probably the main factor in type A lactic acidosis but impaired utilization is also involved. The latter may be a result of impaired blood flow and energy supply in those tissues usually removing lactate and organs which usually remove lactate may produce it in the presence of shock. Infusion of fructose, sorbitol, or xylitol have all been associated with lactic acidosis and during fructose infusion the liver becomes a site of net lactate production because a major portion of the infused substrate is metabolized to lactate at a rate which is greater than the removal capacity of the extrahepatic tissues. In the cases described in association with malignant disease, the increased lactate production consequent upon the high glycolytic capacity of malignant tissue is probably important.

Overall the prognosis of lactic acidosis is poor, the mortality being very high in type A cases where their survival is clearly related to the blood lactate concentration on presentation. A blood lactate concentration of 9 mmol/l or greater is accompanied by a mortality of 80 per cent or greater. In the type B cases, the mortality is substantial, depending on the aetiology, but lower than in type A cases.

Acidosis associated with alcohol (ethanol) ingestion

In normal subjects, relatively modest ethanol ingestion after a 12–24-h period without adequate food intake may result in quite severe hypoglycaemia. Because of the poor or absent calorie intake, liver glycogen reserves have fallen to a low level and maintenance of blood glucose depends solely on gluconeogenesis from lactate and other substrate. Ethanol inhibits gluconeogenesis by diversion of NAD^+ for its own metabolism; lactate therefore accumulates and a significant, although usually mild, lactic acidosis may be seen. Administration of glucose and refeeding is all that is needed, but the hypoglycaemic element of this syndrome may be dangerously severe.

In chronic alcoholics, many of whom have significant hepatic damage, a range of acid–base disorders may be seen. In alcoholic ketosis, there is a history of a longer period of heavy alcohol ingestion, culminating in a few days of severe vomiting, and (usually) cessation of alcohol intake for that reason. A few of these patients have significant acidosis due to ketoacid accumulation, but in others, metabolic alkalosis results from vomiting. Administration of glucose and rehydration is usually adequate to deal with the metabolic disturbance in both situations. Occasionally, particularly when alcohol intake has not stopped, moderate or severe lactic acidosis occurs, related to liver damage, the direct effect of ethanol on gluconeogenesis, and other intercurrent factors such as gastrointestinal haemorrhage. Alcohol may precipitate hepatic encephalopathy in those prone; respiratory alkalosis is commonly seen in these patients, due, it is suggested, to direct stimulation of the respiratory centre by ammonium and amines responsible for encephalopathy.

Methanol and salicylates

The acidosis of methanol ingestion and of salicylate poisoning are described in Chapter 18.1.

Principles of treatment of acid–base disorders

Acute metabolic acidosis

The main difficulty is in assessing the relative risks of bicarbonate treatment against the advantages. The main potential advantages are improvement in cardiac performance, redistribution of blood volume away from the central circulation, correction of hyperkalaemia, restoration of hepatic lactate removal, and alleviation of distressing hyperventilation. Disadvantages lie in short-term adverse effects on the oxygen dissociation curve, and, in the case of lactic and ketoacidosis, the production of 'alkaline overshoot' due to metabolism of the organic acids after the arterial blood pH has been normalized.

Major controversies have arisen concerning the use of sodium bicarbonate as an alkalinizing agent in acute metabolic acidosis. The value of such therapy depends very much on the cause of the metabolic acidosis and also on the particular circumstances of individual patients. There are a few situations in which sodium bicarbonate is clearly beneficial, and these are summarized below.

1. *Metabolic acidosis in severe renal failure.* Sodium bicarbonate here may correct hyperkalaemia by inducing the shift of potassium into the cellular compartment. It may also relieve distressing hyperventilation and may make time for definitive renal support therapy to be introduced. If the patient is already fluid-overloaded, bicarbonate may cause pulmonary oedema and should be used only with caution. If the patient is dehydrated the isotonic solution (1.4 per cent) is the solution of choice.
2. *In severe diarrhoea (cholera).* When metabolic acidosis is due to dehydration and alkali loss sodium bicarbonate is superior to sodium chloride. Severe peripheral venoconstriction will have displaced blood volume towards the lungs. The administration of sodium chloride may thus induce pulmonary oedema before the volume depletion has been corrected. Sodium bicarbonate appears to relieve the peripheral venoconstriction and full replacement is thus made less hazardous.
3. *In exacerbations of renal tubular acidosis.* Sodium bicarbonate is of clear value in this situation, but it is of the utmost importance to correct hypokalaemia before alkali therapy, or at least in conjunction with it, and with frequent monitoring of plasma potassium.

It is in the treatment of lactic acidosis, particularly type A, and in diabetic ketoacidosis that the uncertainty of the value of bicarbonate therapy principally lies. In a number of animal models, treatment with bicarbonate has been shown to produce less favourable haemodynamic and metabolic results than equivalent amounts of sodium chloride. In the only available randomized cross-over trial of sodium bicarbonate versus sodium chloride in critically ill patients with lactic acidosis due to shock, there was no advantage of one therapy over the other and increases in cardiac output were transient.

In circulatory insufficiency the partial pressure of CO_2 of mixed venous blood may be much greater than in arterial blood, which is often normal. On occasion, intravenous bicarbonate therapy exaggerates this difference by titrating protons in the venous blood, thereby generating CO_2. It has been argued on the basis of *in vitro* experiments that this will result in dangerous cellular acidosis by rapid diffusion of CO_2 into cells, despite extracellular alkalinization by the slower diffusing bicarbonate (so-called 'paradoxical intracellular acidification'). There is, however, little evidence of such an effect *in vivo*, and it could in any case be obviated by administering bicarbonate slowly. A more plausible concern, born out in experimental studies, is related to acute left shift of the oxygen dissociation curve of haemoglobin in patients whose erythrocyte 2,3-BPG has been depleted by more than a few hours of acidosis.

The following practical guidance to therapy is empirical and largely based on current practice rather than proper trials:

1. *Diabetic ketoacidosis.* Provided arterial blood pH is not below 7.0, bicarbonate treatment is not indicated. Rehydration and insulin therapy result in improved renal function, a fall in ketone body production and increase in ketone body metabolism, all of which contribute to the correction of the acidosis. When arterial blood pH is less than 7.0, many give just sufficient bicarbonate to bring arterial blood pH above 7.0, with careful attention to changes in plasma potassium, but there is no evidence which indicates this is better than rehydration and insulin alone. If bicarbonate is given, it is essential that it should be isotonic (1.4 per cent). To give hypertonic bicarbonate would merely exacerbate the already present hyperosmolality. The amount required only seldom exceeds 0.5–1 litre, given intravenously over 60–90 min. More bicarbonate creates an 'alkaline' overshoot.
2. *Lactic acidosis.* The most common dilemma is in type A lactic acidosis, due to shock. Of paramount importance is the correction of hypovolaemia and cardiogenic and other factors which are the primary causes of the condition. Such correction will relieve tissue anaerobism and promote intracellular metabolism of lactate, with consequent alkalinization and regeneration of bicarbonate. Whether bicarbonate can trigger or hasten this process is uncertain, and the only trial which addresses this question usefully offers no support for this idea. Nevertheless, the possibility of bicarbonate helping in some circumstances cannot be ruled out. If it is given, it should be given relatively slowly, as the isotonic solution (unless there is fluid overload), and probably only sufficient to raise arterial blood pH to a 'safe' level (e.g. 7.1–7.2). It is particularly in the situation of circulatory insufficiency that the effect of rapid blood alkalinization on the haemoglobin oxygen dissociation curve might be deleterious, since the impaired oxygen release to the tissues cannot be compensated for by an increase in blood flow.

In the special case of the acidosis of cardiac arrest the previous priority given to infusion of sodium bicarbonate has disappeared, because of lack of evidence of efficacy and the risk of alkaline overshoot when lactate is metabolized on restoration of circulation. Hypertonic sodium bicarbonate is now only recommended as a secondary treatment after prolonged arrest.

The amount of bicarbonate, if given, should be determined by an iterative process of administration of a relatively small quantity (e.g. 80 mmol), followed by reassessment of the clinical condition and arterial blood pH, and partial pressure of CO_2 with the aid of serial plots on Fig. 2 before repeating the cycle. Attempts to calculate the amount of alkali needed from the 'base excess' have little validity both for reasons outlined earlier and, because the primary cause of proton accumulation may still be operative, such estimates can in no way replace the need for repeated clinical and biochemical monitoring.

There has been interest in the use of alkalinizing agents other than sodium bicarbonate. Of these alternatives, sodium lactate has the disadvantage that lactate has to be metabolized before the alkalinizing effect occurs and in some patients lactate metabolism is impaired. Trishydroxyaminomethane has the theoretical advantages of dealing with intracellular as well as extracellular acidosis, and does not involve the administration of a sodium load, but, hypoglycaemia and adverse effects on the renal tubules are possible complications of its use and its place is uncertain. Another agent for treating lactic acidosis is sodium dichloroacetate, which increases the metabolism of lactate and results in cell alkalinization. However, a recent multicentre trial of sodium dichloroacetate in patients with lactic acidosis, most of whom were receiving pressor or inotropic therapy, showed no haemodynamic or survival advantage of the drug over a sodium chloride-treated control group, despite reducing blood lactate levels and slightly increasing arterial pH.

Metabolic alkalosis

It is seldom necessary to treat metabolic alkalosis by direct attempts at acidification. However, occasions arise when a severe metabolic alkalosis unrelated to potassium and chloride deficiency may need treating because of tetany or suspected effects in the cerebral circulation. In such rare instances oral ammonium chloride or intravenous infusion of arginine hydrochloride may be indicated.

Further reading

Gluck, S.L. (1998). Acid–base. *Lancet*, **352**, 474–9.

Hood, V.L. and Tannen, R.L. (1998). Protection of acid-base balance by pH regulation of production. *New England Journal of Medicine*, **339**, 819–26.

Williams, A.J. (1998). ABC of oxygen: assessing and interpreting arterial blood gases and acid-base balance. *British Medical Journal*, **317**, 1213–16.

Chapter 6.18

Metabolic effects of accidental injury and surgery

R. Smith

The metabolic response to injury is the result of many sequential processes. The first, and the most important, is the effect of the injury itself, producing pain, blood loss, volume depletion, and tissue damage. Second is the neuroendocrine response, leading to the production of readily utilizable metabolic fuels, such as glucose, fatty acids, and ketone bodies. Third is variable food deprivation; and fourth is immobility, which leads to loss of muscle and skeletal mass. To these can be added the metabolic effects of sepsis and burns.

Severe injury and complicated surgery lead to complex nutritional deficiencies which require prevention and correction and, although the biochemical effects of injury are not simply those of starvation, they have similarities (Table 1). Severe injury is characterized by an increase in circulating catecholamines and cortisol, by initial

Table 1 Similarities and differences between the effects of injury and starvation

	Total starvation	Injury	Starvation and injury
Weight loss	++	+	+++
Nitrogen loss	+	++	+++
Blood glucose	↓	↑	↑
Blood alanine	↓	↓	↓
Blood BCAA[a]	↑	↑	↑
Endocrine response Catecholamine	↓	↑	↑
Cortisol	↓	↑	↑
Insulin	↓	↓ (early)	↓
Metabolic rate	↓	↑	↑
Ketonaemia	++	Variable	Variable
Water and sodium	Early loss	Retention	Retention
Potassium loss	+	++	+++

[a] BCAA; branched chain amino acids—leucine, isoleucine, and valine.

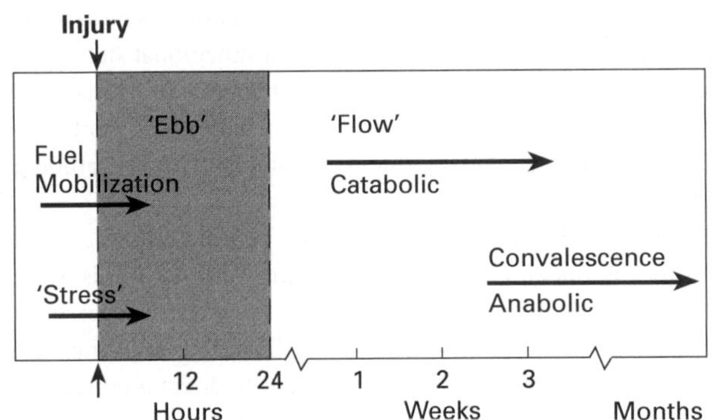

Fig. 1 A diagram of the phases of response to injury in humans. The time-scale is variable and the phases merge into each other. Fuel mobilization and the neuroendocrine response may begin in anticipation of injury.

hyperglycaemia, and by a greater eventual loss of muscle-derived protein and nitrogen than in starvation alone. In total starvation, weight loss will be more rapid than in uncomplicated injury, but it will be most severe where injury and starvation are combined.

The biochemical effects of injury are related both to its severity and nature; and increase in the following order: elective surgery, multiple injuries, sepsis, and burns. In humans the phases originally proposed by Cuthbertson (Fig. 1) are less easy to define than in animals. In the immediate 'ebb' phase the organism is reacting to the injury; rapid neuroendocrine changes occur, and there is an equally rapid mobilization of body fuels. The thermoregulatory response varies and is influenced by the ambient temperature. In survivors this early phase is followed by a 'flow' phase in which biochemical processes accelerate and energy production, metabolic rate, and temperature increase, leading to eventual recovery with catabolism giving way to anabolism and tissue repair.

The length of these phases varies according to many factors, particularly the severity of injury, and some attempt has been made to relate the early biochemical changes to the subsequent outcome. These biochemical changes are begun and orchestrated by the complex neuroendocrine response to injury.

Neuroendocrine response to injury

The neuroendocrine response has been more fully studied in experimental animals than in injured humans. Those components mobilizing metabolic fuels include increased activity of the sympathetic nervous system, increased secretion of hypothalamic hormones which stimulate adrenocorticotrophic hormone (ACTH) production, and the release of vasopressin. The sympathetic system increases adrenaline (epinephrine) and glucagon secretion and suppresses that of insulin; vasopressin has its main influence on water balance, but may have other effects; and increased secretion of ACTH produces a wide range of metabolic effects.

ACTH is released in response to all noxious stimuli. Acute injury may also stimulate the production of endorphins, prolactin, and intermediate lobe peptides. Vasopressin release is increased by only some forms of injury. The production of other pituitary hormones (growth hormone, thyrotrophins, and gonadotrophins), may also be variably affected. In prolonged stress with continuing production of ACTH, gonadotrophin production is inhibited.

The ways in which the production of vasopressin and ACTH are controlled and stimulated by injury differ. Vasopressin secretion is stimulated by an increase in osmolality or by a reduction in blood volume. Emotional trauma, anaesthetics, and visceral manipulation during operation are also recognized causes. The control of ACTH secretion is influenced by corticotrophin-releasing factors, but also by vasopressin, which may act synergistically. There are probably also other unidentified components. Together they stimulate the production of pro-opiomelanocortin, and other peptides. The main metabolic effect of ACTH is through the production of glucocorticoids.

Thermoregulation after injury

Heat production and loss after injury, is most marked after extensive burns. Their cause is debated. In addition to the changes in fuel utilization, there are important alterations in hypothalamic thermoregulation. Insight into these processes in humans has come from the use of mobile calorimeters. Contrary to the data from animal work, there is no clear evidence of a reduction of basal metabolic rate. Indeed, in patients undergoing elective surgery the metabolic rate tends to increase in the first 24 h postoperatively. There is, however, an inhibition of thermoregulation and failure of shivering, despite a fall in whole-body temperature. In the later response to injury there is an increase in core temperature and in basal metabolic rate. This increase, only moderate after multiple fractures, is more marked after head injury, and is greatest after extensive burns. The large increase in evaporative water loss from the burned surface is compensated for by an increase in heat production, but the two events are not closely related. Even in the absence of burns the increase in heat production after injury may be prolonged and may lead to marked weight loss.

Water and electrolytes

The secretion of aldosterone, cortisol, and vasopressin are all increased after injury. There is usually a retention of water in excess of sodium, and a dilutional hyponatraemia which may be associated with potassium deficiency. This relatively simple picture is often complicated by fluid and blood loss and their intravenous replacement. If the effects of injury are prolonged and recovery is delayed, body composition may alter considerably, with an increase in water relative to both lean body mass and body weight, and a continuing loss of intracellular electrolytes such as magnesium, potassium, and zinc. The causes of these changes are not fully understood. It is important to remember that after surgery or injury hyponatraemia rarely means sodium deficiency.

Glycogen and fat

The earliest metabolic result of the neuroendocrine responses of the hypothalamic pituitary axis and of the sympathetic nervous system to noxious stimuli is the mobilization of body fuels by the breakdown of glycogen (from liver and muscle) and fats (triacylglycerols). Because of its immediacy, this occurs in the 'ebb' phase. The production of glucose from the amino acids of muscle protein, associated with negative nitrogen balance, is a later event (in the 'flow' phase).

Mobilization of glycogen results mainly from the marked increase in catecholamines, an increase in glucagon, and a deficiency of insulin relative to the hyperglycaemia produced by injury. The main contribution to glucose comes from hepatic glycogen.

After injury there is an increase in the concentration of free fatty acids and glycerol. Lipolysis is stimulated mainly by the increase in catecholamines, although many other hormones (glucagon, ACTH, growth hormone) may also stimulate lipolysis at a sufficiently high concentration. The rate of lipolysis is high in all severities of injury, but the ketone body levels are variable. The hepatic conversion of free fatty acids to ketone bodies depends particularly on the ratio between glucagon and insulin, and is increased when this ratio is also increased. In those who do not develop hyperketonaemia subsequent protein breakdown and gluconeogenesis may be increased compared with hyperketonaemic subjects.

Substrate turnover

The immediate neuroendocrine response to injury produces an excess of readily available energy from glycogen and fat. Teleologically this is wasteful unless the energy can be utilized. However, despite hyperglycaemia there is evidence of a reduced uptake of glucose early after injury, whereas the uptake of free fatty acids is probably increased. The response to sepsis appears similar in some respects to that of injury, although most studies have been done in experimental endotoxaemia in animals.

In the flow phase the carbohydrate fuels have been utilized, and energy is derived from fat and protein (see below). There is hypermetabolism and increased nitrogen excretion. The relative contribution of fuels to this is related to the available nutritional source. Protein contributes less than 20 per cent to the metabolic rate even under the most catabolic conditions. Where large amounts of glucose are given (as in parenteral nutrition) the effects are complex and unexpected.

In normal people the administration of large amounts of glucose leads to net lipogenesis, but this does not occur after injury when the infusion of glucose does not completely suppress hepatic glucose production, and the respiratory quotient does not rise above 1.0, which implies continuing oxidation of fat. There is a large increase in oxygen consumption and in metabolic rate. These changes may be due to persistent sympathetic overactivity. A major problem is the fate of the infused glucose, especially as storage as glycogen is impaired in both injured and septic patients.

Protein metabolism

A major deleterious effect of injury is loss of protein, mainly from skeletal muscle, which begins soon after injury and leads to a negative nitrogen balance which is maximal on the second or third post-traumatic day. The negative nitrogen balance is proportional to the severity of the injury and is accentuated and prolonged by sepsis, burns, and immobility. Nitrogen loss is most marked after severe injury in a previously fit young adult. It is reduced in the elderly and also by an increase in the external temperature to the thermoneutral zone (28–32°C). Its extent is not always appreciated; the loss of 15 g of nitrogen/day (which is not unusual) is equivalent to nearly 100 g of protein or 400 g of lean tissue. Nitrogen loss depends on the balance between synthesis of protein and its catabolism. Much work has been done to identify the relative contributions of changes in synthesis and breakdown. In some conditions both may alter in the same direction (both reduced in starvation, both increased in exercise-induced hypertrophy); but after injury the changes are diverse and depend on its severity and nutritional state. After mild injury, synthesis and breakdown both appear to be depressed and both increase with severity of injury, although the increase in breakdown is more marked. At some stage, which depends on the initial nutritional status, breakdown exceeds synthesis. Skeletal muscle synthesis is primarily controlled, whereas in liver and other gastrointestinal proteins the processes of breakdown are under physiological and pathological control.

Synthesis and breakdown of muscle are both decreased in patients after surgical operations. In severe injury and in sepsis there is evidence of both increased synthesis and breakdown (measured by 3-methylhistidine). After burns, 3-methylhistidine excretion is also considerably increased; this is likely to be due to direct muscle damage.

Parenteral nutrition can lessen the fall in synthetic rate after injury, and claims have been made that the branched-chain amino acids (leucine, isoleucine, and valine) also have specific effects on protein synthesis.

Important changes occur in the circulating concentrations of amino acids after injury. For instance that of alanine, a major precursor for gluconeogenesis tends to fall after the first day; in contrast, the concentration of the branched-chain amino acids may remain considerably increased, and is highest after severe injuries where hyperketonaemia does not develop. The reason for these changes is not clear. There are also changes in the intramuscular glutamine concentrations which always fall in sepsis and after injury. This observation has led to its use, as a possible specific stimulator of protein synthesis.

Injury also has effects on plasma protein concentrations. Many, such as albumin, transferrin, and prealbumin fall, whereas others, the 'acute phase' plasma proteins (C-reactive protein, fibrinogen, for example) increase. Recent work points to the likely importance of cytokines, such as interleukin-6 and tumour necrosis factor in the acute phase response.

There is little doubt about the deleterious effects of prolonged protein loss. Apart from loss of weight, of muscle tissue, and of muscle strength, there is delayed healing of wounds, susceptibility to infection, and hypoproteinaemic oedema. Continuing loss of nitrogen appears to increase the mortality rate.

Immobility

The mass of both the skeleton and of voluntary muscle depends on the mechanical forces to which they are subjected. Most patients are immobilized after injury. After a minor operation, such as a hernia repair, this may be of no significance, but after multiple fractures immobility produces widespread effects. In the skeleton there is a fall in the rate of new bone formation and an apparent increase in bone resorption. It is not known how bone cells perceive mechanical stimuli; *in vivo* these cells are likely to be the osteocytes. The muscles of immobilized limbs rapidly waste, but it is not clear whether this is due to a failure of synthesis or an increase in myofibrillar breakdown, or both. Neither skeletal nor muscular wasting can be satisfactorily prevented or reversed until mobility is restored.

Sepsis and burns

The metabolic effects of sepsis are poorly understood. They are known to increase nitrogen loss and 3-methylhistidine excretion and to worsen prognosis. Myofibrillar breakdown rate is increased. The most extreme post-traumatic biochemical and endocrine changes occur in the burned patient. In addition to the injury itself there is excessive fluid loss from the damaged surfaces and an increase in metabolic rate. The energy requirements are high and may be difficult to satisfy.

Tissue repair and recovery

Repair begins at the time of injury with the control of haemorrhage and the production of local hormones leading to cell migration, with eventual fibroblast proliferation, scar formation, and fracture repair. The factors that initiate, control, and terminate repair processes are largely unknown. There is similar ignorance about the detailed control of whole-body recovery, although an increase in mobility, return of appetite, and sufficient sleep appear to be basic requirements.

Further reading

Furst, P., Pogan, K., and Stehle, P. (1997). Glutamine dipeptides in clinical nutrition. *Nutrition*, **13**, 731–7.

Plank, L.D., Connolly, A.B., and Hill, G.L. (1998). Sequential changes in the metabolic response in severely septic patients during the first 23 days after the onset of peritonitis. *Annals of Surgery*, **228**, 146–58.

Section 7
Endocrine disease

Contents

The pituitary

Chapter 7.1

Anterior pituitary disorders

M. O. Thorner

Pituitary anatomy

The pituitary is located in the sella turcica (Fig. 1) within a dense lining layer of connective tissue, the dura. Superiorly it is covered by the diaphragma sellae which has a 5 mm wide central opening which is penetrated by the hypophyseal stalk. In some subjects this opening is much wider, and is thought to allow transmission of pulsations of the cerebrospinal fluid pressure, leading to the development of the 'empty sella syndrome', or cisternal herniation.

The pituitary measures 13 mm transversely, 9 mm anteroposteriorly, and 6 mm vertically. Its weight is approximately 100 mg, somewhat more in women than in men; it enlarges during pregnancy and may then weigh 0.9–1.0 g.

Several structures may be affected by an enlarged pituitary gland. The lateral walls of the sella are close to the cavernous sinuses containing the internal carotid arteries, the oculomotor (III), trochlear (IV), and abducens (VI) nerves, and first and second divisions of the trigeminal (V) nerve. The sphenoid sinus lies anteriorly and inferiorly to the pituitary and is separated from it by the thin inferior portion of the sella, which may be eroded, allowing extension into the sinus when a pituitary tumour enlarges. The optic chiasm lies directly above the diaphragma sellae, in front of the hypophyseal stalk and is vulnerable to suprasellar growth of a pituitary tumour. The tuber cinereum of the hypothalamus and the third ventricle of the brain lie above the roof of the sella. Space-occupying lesions arising in or above the pituitary may compress and compromise the tuber cinereum, causing hypothalamic/hypophyseal dysfunction which is usually manifest as hypopituitarism associated with mild hyperprolactinaemia.

The blood supply to the pituitary is complex and plays an important role in delivering hypothalamic hormones to the gland. The superior and two inferior hypophyseal vessels originate from the internal carotid arteries. The hypothalamic hormones are produced in neurones which originate in various parts of the hypothalamus and terminate at the infundibulum. There they permeate through fenestrations in capillaries to enter the portal circulation which transports them to the capillaries in the anterior pituitary. The portal circulation provides approximately 80–90 per cent of the blood supply to the anterior lobe, the remainder being provided by arterial blood from superior hypophyseal arteries. The neurohypophysis receives its blood supply from the inferior hypophyseal arteries. Venous blood leaves the pituitary through adjacent venous sinuses to enter the internal jugular veins bilaterally. Under certain circumstances, unidirectional blood flow, from the hypothalamus to the anterior pituitary may be reversed to produce ultrashort loop feedback by pituitary hormones on several hypothalamic centres. The anterior lobe has no direct innervation except for a few sympathetic nerve fibres which reach it along blood vessels.

Hypothalamic–pituitary regulation

Each pituitary hormone is regulated by substances which are synthesized in the hypothalamus and transported from the median eminence to the anterior pituitary via the hypothalamic–pituitary portal circulation to bind to specific high-affinity cell membrane receptors of the relevant pituitary cells. With the possible exception of prolactin, all anterior pituitary hormones are also regulated by the hormones secreted by their target glands. Normal pituitary function is therefore tightly regulated by interaction and integration of signals from both the brain and the periphery. When a target gland fails, negative feedback is reduced, augmenting secretion of the trophic hypothalamic hormone, as well as reducing secretion of any tonic hypothalamic inhibiting hormone, negative feedback occurring at both pituitary and hypothalamic levels. Additionally, 'short loop' feedback, in which pituitary hormones are probably transported back to the hypothalamus, reduces further secretion by reducing hypothalamic stimulation (Fig. 2).

All anterior pituitary hormones are secreted in a pulsatile fashion, so that accurate assessment of function often requires more than one measurement.

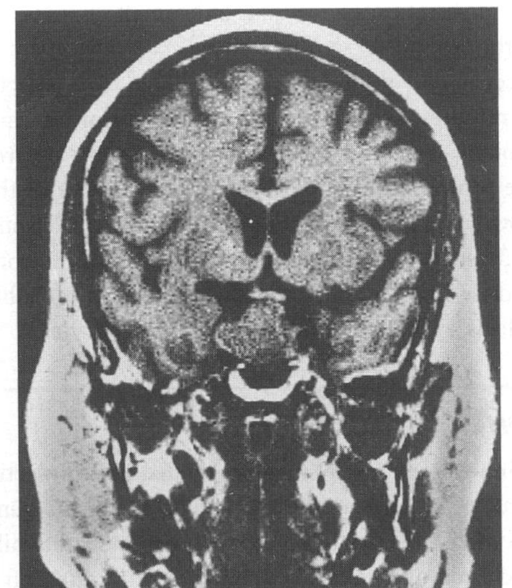
(a)

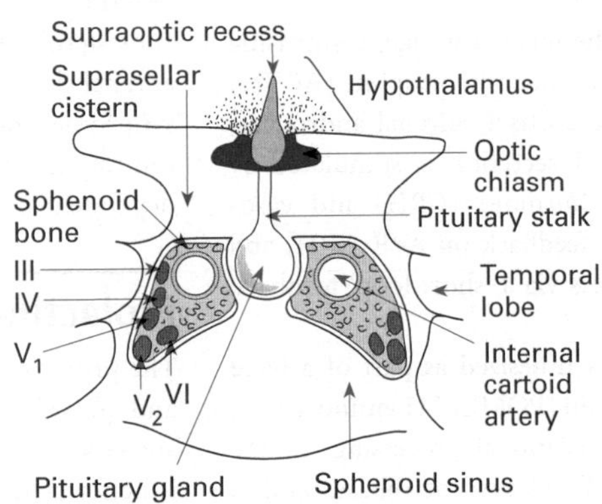

(b)

Fig. 1 (a) MRI scan of the normal pituitary fossa. See also diagram in Fig. 1(b). (b) Diagram of the normal pituitary fossa. The pituitary gland is bordered laterally by the cavernous sinus which contains the internal carotid artery and cranial nerves III, IV, V_1, V_2, and VI. The optic chiasm lies immediately above the pituitary gland and is separated from it by a cerebrospinal fluid-filled cistern. Note the location of the sphenoid sinus and temporal lobes.
(Modified and reproduced with permission from Lechan, R.M. (1987). Neuroendocrinology of pituitary hormone regulation. Endocrinology and Metabolism Clinics of North America, **16**, *475–502.)*

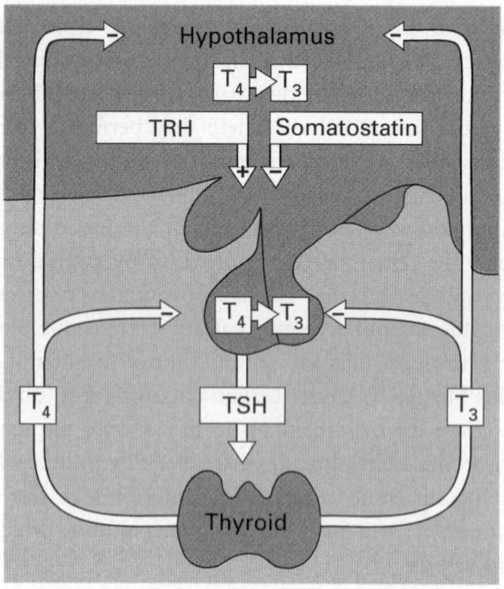

Fig. 2 Schematic representation of the hypothalamic–pituitary–target gland axis. Hypothalamic hormones regulate pituitary hormone secretion which in turn stimulates target gland hormone production. Peripheral hormones feed back on the hypothalamus and pituitary to modulate secretion in a classical negative fashion. For example, hypothalamic thyroid releasing hormone (TRH) stimulates pituitary release of thyroid stimulating hormone (TSH) which stimulates thyroidal hormone release. Thyroid hormones inhibit TRH and TSH in the hypothalamus and pituitary, respectively.
(Modified and reproduced with permission from Reichlin, S. (1987). Neuroendocrine control of pituitary function. In Clinical endocrinology: an illustrated text (ed. G.M. Besser and A.G. Cudworth), pp. 1.1–1.14. J.B. Lippincott, Philadelphia.)

Anterior pituitary ontogeny

Immunohistochemical studies indicate that five phenotypically distinct cell types appear sequentially during anterior pituitary ontogeny. The order of appearance is: corticotrophs, producing pro-opiomelanocortin (POMC); thyrotrophs, producing thyroid stimulating hormone (TSH); gonadotrophs, producing luteinizing hormone (LH) and follicle stimulating hormone (FSH); somatotrophs, producing growth hormone (GH); and lactotrophs, producing prolactin. The coexpression of GH and prolactin in precursor cells prior to the appearance of the mature lactotroph cell and in a subpopulation of mature anterior pituitary cells suggest that prolactin and GH genes are regulated by related factors.

Hormones

Corticotrophin

Corticotroph cells reside primarily in the median wedge, comprising some 10 per cent of the cells there. Adrenocorticotrophin (ACTH) stimulates the adrenal cortex to secrete cortisol, adrenal androgens, and mineralocorticoids. Pituitary ACTH secretion is stimulated by hypothalamic corticotrophin-releasing hormone (CRH) and vasopressin (AVP). Cortisol exerts negative feedback on AVP, CRH, and ACTH secretion; additionally, ACTH acts via a 'short loop' feedback to suppress CRH secretion.

ACTH, a 39 amino acid peptide, is synthesized as part of a large precursor molecule, pro-opiomelanocortin (POMC; 241 amino acids), which undergoes considerable post-translational processing. In the human pituitary POMC is enzymatically cleaved at dibasic amino acids, predominantly into β-lipotrophin, ACTH, joining peptide, and an amino-terminal peptide. In the intermediate lobe, ACTH is cleaved into melanocyte stimulating hormone (α-MSH), ($ACTH_{1-13}$) and corticotrophin-like peptide ($ACTH_{8-39}$), and β-lipotrophin into lipotrophin (LPH) and β-endorphin. Because these peptides are derived from the same precursor molecule, they are secreted in equimolar amounts, but circulating concentrations do not vary in tandem because their half-lives are different.

Regulation of secretion

To stimulate ACTH secretion, CRH binds to high-affinity receptors on corticotrophs, stimulates the accumulation of cAMP, and activates protein kinase A, resulting in rapid release of ACTH and related peptides and in increased POMC gene transcription and synthesis. The magnitude of the response to exogenous CRH depends on the time of day and the prevailing level of circulating glucocorticoids; for instance, the cortisol response is greater in the afternoon than in the morning. Exogenous glucocorticoids inhibit both the ACTH and cortisol responses to CRH, whereas metyrapone, by reducing cortisol secretion, enhances them. AVP alone is a weak secretagogue for ACTH, but acts synergistically with CRH.

ACTH is secreted in bursts increasing in frequency after 3–5 h of sleep and maximal in the last hours before awakening and the hour thereafter. The circadian rhythm of ACTH secretion is regulated by a number of factors, one of the most important being light. In normal subjects, ACTH concentrations decline through the morning, reaching a nadir in the evening. This rhythm is disrupted by a major time shift, as occurs with transmeridian jet travel and physical stress; for example, trauma, major surgery, fever, hypoglycaemia, and burn injury, increase both ACTH and cortisol secretion. Increased cortisol secretion also occurs during psychological stress, for instance in anticipation of physical activity, during mental activity, and in patients with anorexia nervosa and depression, but not in schizophrenia or chronic anxiety. Glucocorticoids reduce the ACTH response to CRH by inhibiting POMC gene transcription and synthesis, as well as CRH and AVP synthesis and release in the hypothalamus.

ACTH actions

The actions of ACTH at the adrenal are mediated through specific high-affinity cell membrane receptors. Activation of adenylate cyclase leads to accumulation of intracellular cAMP, increases in protein kinase A activity, phosphorylation of a number of proteins, and to increased synthesis and secretion of cortisol, only small amounts of which are stored in the adrenal.

ACTH has both acute and prolonged actions. The acute effects, which occur within minutes, are stimulation of conversion of cholesterol to pregnenolone and an increase in the supply of free cholesterol ester. The prolonged effects promote maintenance of the adrenal size (and growth) by increasing protein synthesis. In Nelson's syndrome and in Addison's disease, when circulating ACTH concentrations are extremely high, pigmentation of the skin is probably dependent on the effects of ACTH and β-LPH on melanocytes.

Prolactin–growth hormone family

The prolactin–growth hormone family may be divided into prolactin and growth hormone (GH) subfamilies. A single prolactin gene appears on chromosome 6. The human growth hormone subfamily is better characterized and consists of five members, all located on a 78 kilobase section of chromosome 17. They include the normal

GH gene, a GH variant gene, two expressed chorionic somatomammotrophin genes, and an incompletely characterized chorionic somatomammotrophin-like gene, which is thought not to be expressed. The GH-variant gene codes for a protein different from GH by 13 amino acids.

Prolactin

Human prolactin consists of 199 amino acids, only 16 per cent of which are homologous with those of GH. The lactotroph cell has a wide distribution throughout the pars distalis and constitutes from 10 per cent of the cells in men, to 30 per cent in multiparous women.

Regulation of prolactin secretion

Prolactin secretion varies under different physiological conditions. It is secreted in an episodic manner, regulated by hypothalamic dopamine, and by various prolactin releasing factors (PRF). Dopamine acts by stimulating the lactotroph D2 receptor which inhibits adenylate cyclase, and thereby inhibits both prolactin release and synthesis. The putative prolactin releasing factors include TRH, vasoactive intestinal peptide (VIP), and PHM-27, a peptide with structural homology to VIP. VIP is produced in the anterior pituitary cells and has been proposed to act as an autocrine or paracrine regulator of prolactin secretion.

Normal base-line serum prolactin concentrations are less than 20 μg/l in adults; in men they are usually less than 10 μg/l. Circulating levels are lowest at midday, with a modest increase during the afternoon. Marked increases in concentration occur shortly after the onset of sleep, whenever that takes place, but peak levels are seen during the middle to end of the night.

Prolactin synthesis is also affected by direct effects of oestrogen on prolactin gene expression. Concentrations are higher in normal premenopausal women than in men, and they rise during menarche in girls, and during pregnancy. Following delivery, maternal prolactin concentrations decline into the normal range over the course of the first 3 months if breast feeding does not occur. With suckling, maternal prolactin rises, with the greatest response just after delivery. If breast feeding is intermittently supplemented with bottle feeding the increase wanes, although normal levels are sufficient to sustain established lactation. Prolactin levels increase in women during sexual stimulation and in both men and women in response to stress.

Hyperprolactinaemia occurs with any disruption of the hypothalamus, the hypothalamo/hypophyseal stalk, or administration of drugs which interfere with dopamine synthesis or action. In some patients with primary hypothyroidism there may be mild hyperprolactinaemia due to increased hypothalamic TRH secretion. Thyroid hormone replacement may then require months for prolactin to decline to normal.

Actions of prolactin

Specific receptors for prolactin are present in many tissues, including the liver, ovary, testis, and prostate, but the main site of action is the mammary gland, where it initiates and maintains lactation. Lactation is inhibited during pregnancy by high concentrations of oestrogen and progesterone. The rapid fall in concentrations of these after delivery enables prolactin to act unopposed, and to initiate lactation. Dopamine agonists can be used to inhibit prolactin secretion, and thereby lactation, after delivery.

The physiological functions of prolactin at other sites is poorly characterized, but both the hyperprolactinaemia of pregnancy and lactation and pathological hyperprolactinaemia are associated with suppression of the hypothalamic–pituitary–gonadal axis. This is likely to be due to prolactin-mediated inhibition of pulsatile gonadotrophin releasing hormone (GnRH) secretion.

Growth hormone

Human GH is a non-glycosylated, single-chain, 191 amino acid, 22-kDa protein with two intramolecular disulphide bonds. Approximately 75 per cent of pituitary GH is in this form and some 5–10 per cent in a 20 kDa form, the latter produced by alternate splicing of the mRNA that deletes the codons for amino acids 32 to 46 from the RNA. Growth hormone is present in several different forms in the anterior pituitary.

The somatotroph cells, which secrete GH, make up about 50 per cent of the hormone-producing adenohypophyseal cells and occupy the lateral wings. They are remarkably stable and their number, morphology, and immunoreactivity are unchanged by age or by various diseases. GH is synthesized and stored in somatotrophs and accounts for as much as 30 per cent of the protein in these cells.

The hormone circulates in several forms, including a 22 kDa, a 20-kDa form, and at least one acidic form. Additionally, a mixture of GH oligomers (up to pentamer) can also be detected in peripheral blood. The proportions of GH variants in the circulation are broadly similar to those in the pituitary, except that the 20 kDa form and oligomeric forms are more predominant in the circulation, due to slower metabolic clearance rates. During pregnancy GH-V (from the placenta) is produced and peripheral blood levels rise to peak levels in the second and third trimesters when pituitary GH secretion is suppressed.

Growth hormone receptor

The cDNA of the human GH receptor encodes 638 amino acids and has homology with the prolactin receptor. In the middle of the protein there is a sequence of 24 hydrophobic amino acids representing the transmembrane domain, dividing the molecule into extracellular and intracytoplasmic domains of approximately equal size. Abnormalities in the cDNA encoding this GH-receptor is found in many children with Laron dwarfism.

Growth hormone binding protein

The binding protein in plasma which is identical to the extracellular domain of the human GH receptor is also absent from the plasma of Laron dwarfs.

Forty-five per cent of 22 kDa GH and 25 per cent of 20 kDa GH are complexed with binding proteins. When circulating GH concentrations are consistently above 10–20 μg/l, a progressively smaller proportion is linked to the binding protein. Protein-bound GH persists 10 times longer in plasma than monomeric GH and its volume of distribution is also larger. The plasma concentrations of the binding proteins appear to remain fairly constant with wide variability among individuals.

Regulation of growth hormone secretion

Growth hormone is secreted in a pulsatile fashion, regulated by two hypothalamic hormones, growth hormone releasing hormone (GHRH) and somatostatin (SRIF). GHRH is necessary for GH synthesis, increasing transcription of GH messenger RNA within minutes by increasing cyclic AMP. SRIF appears to be particularly important

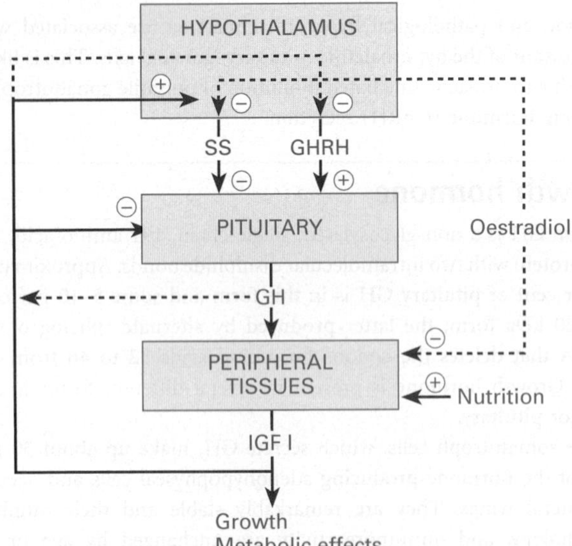

Fig. 3 Schematic illustration of regulation of serum GH secretion. *(Reproduced with permission from Thorner, M.O., Vance, M.L., Horvath, E., and Kovacs, K. (1992). The anterior pituitary. In Williams textbook of endocrinology, 8th edn (ed. J.D. Wilson and D.W. Foster), p. 231. W.B. Saunders, Philadelphia.)*

in the timing and amplitude of GH pulses but has no effect on synthesis.

Figure 3 illustrates this regulation of GH secretion. The somatotroph is also regulated by negative feedback at the pituitary itself by circulating insulin-like growth factor (IGF-I) and by 'short loop' feedback on the hypothalamus by GH. The amount of GH secreted is greatest during adolescence and decreases with age. Premenopausal women have higher rates of production than do young men.

The pattern of GH secretion is dependent upon a number of factors. Increased secretion during puberty suggests that gonadal steroids, particularly oestradiol, are important regulators. Secretion is enhanced by sleep, with levels highest during slow-wave sleep and lowest during rapid eye movement (REM) sleep. Hyperglycaemia in normal subjects acutely suppresses GH secretion, while in poorly controlled type 1 diabetics levels are increased. Similarly, although acute increases in free fatty acid concentrations inhibit GH release, fatty acid levels are increased during starvation or fasting when GH secretion is augmented. Growth hormone secretion is also augmented in insulin-dependent diabetes mellitus, and hepatic cirrhosis. Certain amino acids, particularly arginine and leucine, also stimulate secretion. In contrast, secretion is suppressed in obesity.

While exercise, stress, and some neurogenic factors stimulate GH secretion, emotional deprivation can inhibit its release in children and lead to diminished linear growth. Central α-adrenergic agonists (for instance clonidine) stimulate GH secretion, and β-antagonists augment the efficacy of various GH stimuli. Dopamine agonists stimulate secretion in normal subjects. Acetylcholine agonists also stimulate, while agents which lower acetylcholine tone suppress release. Stimulation of GH by sleep, dopamine agonists, α-adrenergic agonists, glucagon, and by amino acids is inhibited by cholinergic muscarinic blocking drugs, which are considered to act at the level of hypothalamus or the median eminence. GH secretory responses to a number of stimuli are augmented after pretreatment with oestrogens. The role of serotonin in human GH secretion is unclear. Endogenous or exogenous opiates probably do not directly influence GH secretion, but nalorphine and an enkephalin analogue (DAMME, FK33824) stimulate secretion through naloxone-sensitive mechanisms. The pharmacological agent, growth hormone-releasing peptide (GHRP), developed from an enkephalin series of peptides, is a potent GH releasing agent, whose mechanism of action is unknown. A unique receptor for the GHRPs has been cloned. GHRP acts through this GH–secretagogue receptor.

Growth hormone actions

Although many of the effects of GH are mediated by somatomedins there are probably direct actions of GH, as well those mediated through IGF-I (somatomedin C) and IGF-II. Each of these is a single-chain peptide with a high degree of homology with human proinsulin. Serum concentrations of IGF-I are markedly elevated in acromegaly and reduced in GH deficiency; IGF-II levels are unaffected in acromegaly and only modestly reduced in GH deficiency, suggesting that IGF-I is the important mediator of GH action; that IGF-I feeds back to inhibit GH secretion lends support to this hypothesis. The site of IGF-I production and the significance of circulating levels are the subject of controversy.

Growth hormone is described as 'anabolic', 'lipolytic', and 'diabetogenic'. When administered to GH-deficient children and adults it produces positive nitrogen balance, decreased urea production, redistributed body fat, and reduced carbohydrate utilization without development of diabetes. These effects may also occur in normal subjects and have led to the experimental use of GH in attempting to reverse some of the metabolic changes associated with ageing and catabolic illness.

Glycoprotein hormone family

The three anterior pituitary glycoprotein hormones are thyroid stimulating hormone (thyrotrophin; TSH), luteinizing hormone (lutrophin; LH), and follicle stimulating hormone (follitrophin; FSH). Each consists of two non-covalently bound subunits: the α-subunit is common to all three hormones, while the β-subunit is unique for each hormone and confers biological specificity. There is considerable microheterogeneity of the carbohydrate constituents of the individual hormones, which leads to heterogeneity in receptor affinity, biological potency, and metabolic clearance.

The α-subunits are approximately 20–22 kDa in molecular weight, have 92 amino acid residues, and contain two N-linked carbohydrate groups. The TSH β-subunit is approximately 18 kDa, consists of 110 amino acids, and contains one N-linked complex carbohydrate. Both TSH α- and β-subunits are negatively regulated by thyroid hormone. Thyroid hormone receptors bind to the 5' flanking regions of α- and TSH β-subunit genes; which thyroid hormone receptor, and whether it acts directly or by interacting with transacting factors, remains to be elucidated. Free serum α-subunits are secreted and are present in concentrations equivalent to those of combined TSH, LH, and FSH. Free serum β-subunit concentrations are much lower and are usually close to the level of detectability in conventional assays.

Thyrotroph cells and TSH

Thyrotroph cells are the least common anterior pituitary cell type (about 5 per cent) and are located in the anteromedial portion of the gland.

Secretion of TSH is regulated both by hypothalamic and circulating thyroid hormones. Hypothalamic TRH stimulates TSH release. If the

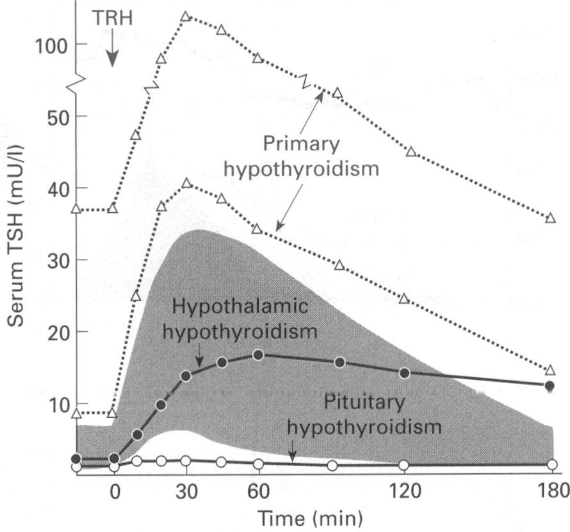

Fig. 4 Serum TSH changes after TRH administration in normal subjects (shaded area) and in patients with primary hypothyroidism, hypothalamic disease, and pituitary hypothyroidism. Patients with hypothalamic disease may have a delayed TSH response to TRH.
(Modified and reproduced with permission from Utiger, R.D. (1986). Tests of the thyroregulatory mechanisms. In The thyroid, 5th edn (ed. S.H. Ingbar and L.E. Braverman), p. 516. J.B. Lippincott, Philadelphia.)

hypothalamic pituitary stalk is interrupted, secondary hypothyroidism develops and TSH secretion is reduced, but not absent. Somatostatin and dopamine can inhibit TSH secretion and it is likely that they regulate the circadian rhythm of TSH.

Thyrotrophin secretion is regulated principally by feedback by thyroid hormones, which act at the hypothalamic level to inhibit TRH synthesis as well as at the pituitary to inhibit TSH secretion. Intracellular tri-iodothyronine in thyrotroph cells regulates TSH secretion. Thyrotrophin is secreted in a pulsatile fashion, with low-amplitude peaks, and in a circadian fashion. Levels may rise before the levels of T_4 and T_3 decline below the normal range; in hypothalamic/pituitary disease the TSH level may be in the 'normal' range but be inappropriately low for the circulating concentration of thyroid hormone.

TRH administration has been used as a diagnostic test for TSH reserve; to amplify the TSH signal, to distinguish between low, normal, and high TSH levels, and to assess feedback inhibition by peripheral thyroid hormone levels. Figure 4 illustrates the TSH responses to TRH in normal subjects, patients with primary hypothyroidism, and pituitary and hypothalamic hypothyroidism. In the patient with elevated thyroid hormone levels and detectable 'normal' TSH levels, the absence of a TSH response is compatible with either hyperthyroidism or a thyrotrope adenoma (see below), while a positive response may suggest pituitary resistance to thyroid hormone. The actions of TSH are discussed in Chapter 7.3.

Gonadotrophins

LH β-, FSH β-, and hCG β-subunits

Both LH β- and FSH β-subunits are composed of 115 amino acids and have two carbohydrate side-chains. The structure of the β-subunit of LH is similar to that of human chorionic gonadotrophin (hCG) except for an additional 32 amino acids and additional carbohydrate residues on the carboxyl end of the β-subunit of hCG. A terminal sialic acid is frequently present on the carbohydrate side-chains of hCG-β and FSH β. Sialic acid is not necessary for receptor binding but decreases the metabolic clearance of these hormones in contrast to TSH and LH (which do not have sialic acid side-chains).

In men and in menstruating women, the pituitary contains approximately 700 IU of LH and 200 IU of FSH. After menopause, the content of pituitary LH rises approximately two- to threefold, but there is no change in FSH content, although both LH and FSH are synthesized in the gonadotroph cell. hCG is present in small amounts in the pituitary.

Regulation of LH and FSH secretion

Secretion from gonadotroph cells is regulated by the integration of the GnRH signal from the hypothalamus and feedback effects of gonadal steroids and peptides (e.g. inhibin). GnRH interacts with a membrane receptor to regulate both LH and FSH release and synthesis. The frequency and the amplitude of GnRH pulses are important in differentially regulating LH and FSH secretion. Both LH and FSH pulse secretion are maintained with one GnRH pulse per hour, while higher GnRH pulse frequencies initially increase the frequency of LH pulses and the basal LH concentrations. In contrast, when the GnRH pulse frequency is decreased to once every 3 h, FSH secretion is preferentially stimulated. Gonadal steroids and peptides alone are ineffective alone in stimulating release, their actions being dependent on the presence of GnRH.

Gonadal steroids

Oestradiol can inhibit GnRH secretion from the hypothalamus and thereby reduce pituitary gonadotrophin secretion but it can also act in a positive manner, which may be a result of both direct effects at the pituitary level and at the hypothalamus to enhance GnRH secretion.

Progesterone regulates gonadotrophin secretion by slowing the GnRH pulse generator.

Androgens suppress GnRH secretion by the hypothalamus, an effect best exemplified in patients with testicular feminization syndrome with an androgen receptor defect.

Gonadal peptides

Peptides produced in the gonad have important feedback effects on gonadotrophin secretion, and possibly other pituitary hormones. *Inhibin* is a member of a large family of glycoprotein hormones and growth factors. It is synthesized by Sertoli cells of the testis, granulosa cells of the ovary, the placenta, pituitary gonadotrophs, and the brain. Gonadal secretion of inhibin is regulated by gonadotrophins, growth factors, and by gonadal steroids, and inhibin exerts a negative feedback control of FSH secretion.

Activin is a hetero- or homodimer of the inhibin β-subunit. It stimulates FSH synthesis and secretion. *Follistatin* is a single-chain glycosylated polypeptide produced in the ovary. It selectively decreases levels of FSH β mRNA, and inhibits FSH secretion *in vitro*, and may act by binding to activin.

The physiology of LH and FSH

The regulation of LH and FSH secretion is unique in that the pulsatile pattern of gonadotrophin and GnRH secretion are necessary for normal gonadal stimulation. Gonadal development is regulated by gonadotrophin secretion. Prior to puberty, the release of FSH is greater than that of LH; this is reversed at puberty. The reason for the preferential release of LH to FSH or vice versa is uncertain, but may reflect inhibin secretion. It is likely that the major restraint on GnRH secretion originates in the central nervous system.

The development of the human hypothalamo-pituitary gonadotrophin–gonadal axis may be divided into five stages: fetal, early infancy, late infancy, late prepubertal period, and puberty.

Fetal, infantile, and childhood patterns are described in OTM3, p. 1580.

Late prepubertal period

Both the intrinsic CNS inhibitory influences and the sensitivity of the hypothalamus and pituitary to gonadal steroids decrease, resulting in an increased set point and a resultant increased amplitude and frequency of GnRH pulses. Initially these pulses are most prominent during sleep. There is an increase in gonadotroph sensitivity to GnRH, increased secretion of FSH and LH, and increased gonadal responsiveness to FSH and LH, with resultant increase in gonadal hormone secretions.

Puberty

A further decrease occurs in both the CNS restraint of the hypothalamic 'GnRH pulse generator' and the sensitivity of negative feedback by gonadal steroids. The prominent sleep-associated increase in episodic secretion of GnRH gradually changes to the adult pattern of one pulse approximately every 90 min; the pulsatile pattern of LH follows this GnRH pattern. Progressive development of secondary sex characteristics occurs and spermatogenesis is initiated in boys. In girls, at mid- to late puberty, the capacity for oestrogen positive feedback develops and this culminates in a midcycle LH surge and ovulation.

Menstrual cycle

The minimum requirements for the changes in gonadotrophin secretion during the menstrual cycle can be generated by the pituitary under invariant pulsatile GnRH stimulation (e.g. GnRH pump therapy at one fixed dose administered hourly for the full cycle of 28 days). This suggests that the feedback effects of gonadal steroids and peptides can occur at the pituitary level. Although this minimum requirement is definite, it is likely that under physiological conditions there are other regulators, including the hypothalamus. During the menstrual cycle changes occur in the frequency, amplitude, and mass of GnRH bursts secreted into the portal circulation.

Figure 5 shows FSH, LH, 17-OH progesterone, progesterone, and basal body temperature changes during the human menstrual cycle synchronized around the day of the midcycle preovulatory peak. LH levels rise slightly during the follicular phase, peak at the time of the midcycle surge, and then decline during the luteal phase of the cycle. FSH concentration begins to rise during the late luteal phase, increases during early follicular phase of the next cycle, and declines just before the midcycle FSH surge. This midcycle FSH surge is more modest than that of LH. FSH levels then decline during the luteal phase to increase again prior to the next menses. The frequency of LH peaks varies with different phases of the menstrual cycle. The greatest number of LH peaks occurs during the late follicular phase, and the fewest during the luteal phase of the cycle, with an intermediate number during the early follicular phase.

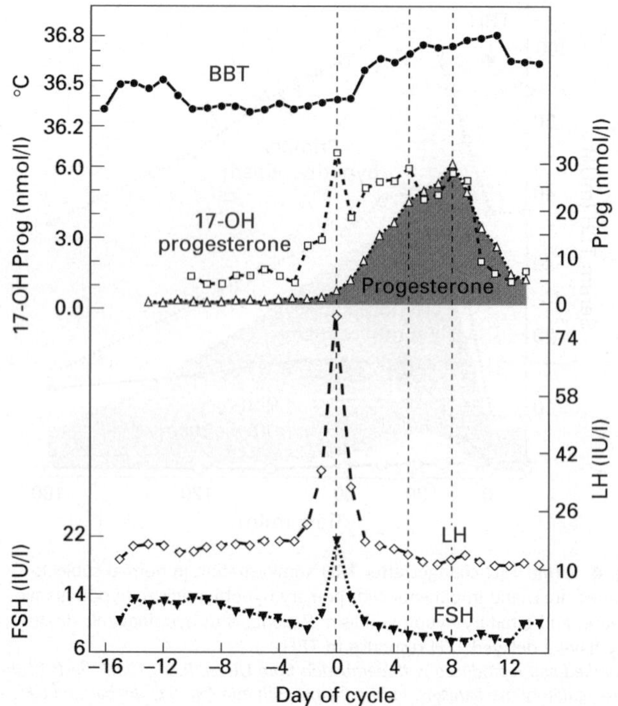

Fig. 5 Mean daily plasma FSH, LH, progesterone, and 17-OH progesterone concentrations and basal body temperature during 16 presumptively ovulatory cycles from 15 young women.
(Modified and reproduced with permission from Ross, G.T., Cargiu, C.M., Lipsett, et al. (1970). Pituitary and gonadal hormones in women during spontaneous and induced ovulatory cycles. Recent Progress in Hormone Research, **26***, 1–62.)*

LH and FSH actions

LH is primarily responsible for the regulation of sex steroid production by Leydig cells of the testis and the ovarian follicles. The preovulatory LH surge observed in women produces rupture of the follicle and luteinization. FSH stimulates gametogenesis; in the male it also stimulates Sertoli cells which have an important role in spermatogenesis. In the female FSH is important for follicular development. FSH also stimulates the production of LH receptors.

Pituitary diseases

Pituitary tumours account for 10–20 per cent of intracranial tumours, and are classified as microadenomas (diameter < 10 mm) or macroadenomas (diameter > 10 mm). The patient with a pituitary tumour presents with symptoms of a mass lesion, or with endocrine dysfunction, or both. Endocrine dysfunction may comprise hyperfunction or hypofunction, or a combination of the two.

Clinical manifestations

Pituitary mass

The symptoms of a sellar mass (Fig. 6) include headache or symptoms secondary to compression of intracranial nerves: visual field disturbances, ophthalmoplegia, and, occasionally, compression of the first or second branch of the trigeminal nerve, giving rise to facial pain. The extent of the abnormality depends upon the size of the tumour and its position. Thus, microadenomas may be asymptomatic except for producing endocrine dysfunction. A macroadenoma which extends inferiorly may also be asymptomatic other than headache, while a superior extension with abutment on the optic chiasm may produce visual field defects. Visual disturbance occurs during the course of illness in about 60 per cent of patients with macroadenomas. Bitemporal hemianopia is the classic finding, but any visual disturbance can occur, depending on the extent of suprasellar extension

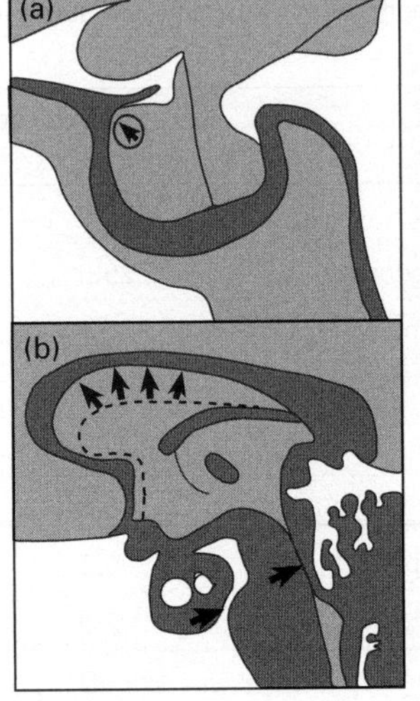

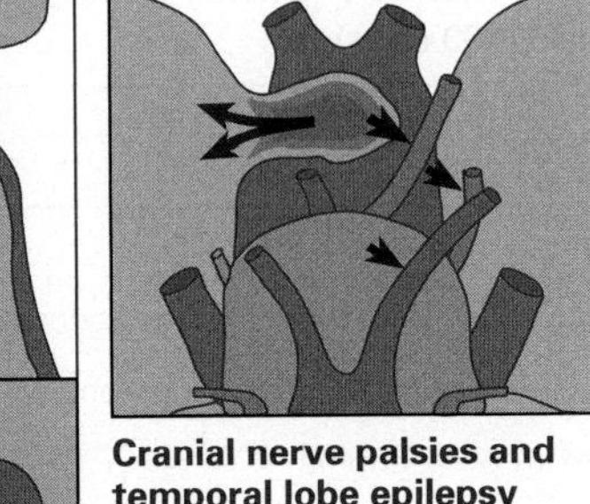

Cranial nerve palsies and temporal lobe epilepsy
Lateral extinction of tumour

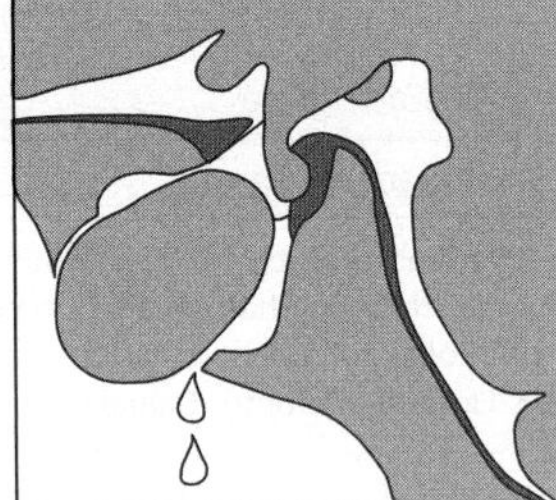

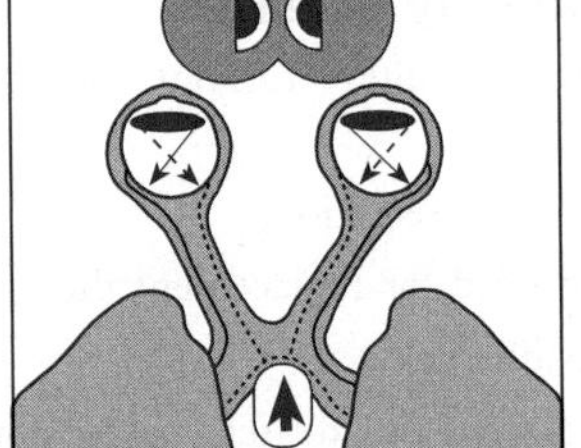

Fig. 6 Various symptoms of a pituitary tumour in addition to hypopituitarism. Headaches are only rarely caused by hydrocephalus. Visual field defects caused by extension of the tumour are readily plotted using the Goldmann perimeter.
(Modified and reproduced with permission from Wass, J.A.H. (1987). Hypopituitarism. In Clinical endocrinology: an illustrated text (ed. G.M. Besser and A.G. Cudworth) pp. 2.1–2.14 J.B. Lippincott, Philadelphia.)

and the location of the optic chiasm, whether prefixed or postfixed. A pituitary tumour can produce diminished visual acuity, scotoma, quadrantic defects, and total blindness of one or both eyes. The fibres of the optic nerve course along a precise path, depending on their site of origin in the retina. Those from the temporal halves of the retina (for nasal vision) do not cross, but course posteriorly along the ipsilateral optic tract. Those from the nasal half (for temporal vision) cross in the chiasm and course posteriorly along the contralateral optic tract. Even when bitemporal hemianopia is present it is often asymmetrical.

Headache from pituitary tumour can be variable and is often nonspecific. While it may be occipital, retrorbital pain or bitemporal headaches are more typical, which are sometimes worse on awakening and generally improve over the course of the day, and are often ameliorated by analgesics. Very large pituitary tumours or a suprasellar hypothalamic tumour (for example, craniopharyngioma) may extend sufficiently superiorly or posteriorly to compress either the foramen of Munro or the aqueduct of Sylvius. The former leads to obstruction of the lateral ventricles and the latter to obstruction of the cerebrospinal fluid flow from the third ventricle to the fourth. This leads to hydrocephalus, involving the lateral ventricles or the lateral and third ventricles, respectively. Extensive lateral extension may produce dysfunction of the third, fourth, the first and second divisions of the fifth, and the sixth cranial nerves.

If the tumour extends inferiorly, the patient may have no symptoms or may develop sphenoid sinusitis, producing pain. Rare complications include CSF rhinorrhoea or recurrent meningitis from erosion of the sella turcica and loss of the barrier between CSF and the exterior. Giant tumours may extend into the temporal lobes, causing temporal lobe epilepsy, and occasionally can extend to the cerebral peduncles and give rise to motor and/or sensory disturbances.

Table 1 Clinical features of adult GH deficiency syndrome

Clinical features
Mixed truncal and generalized adiposity
Increased waist:hip ratio
Reduced strength and exercise capacity
Thin, dry skin; cool peripheries; poor venous access
Cold intolerance
Impaired psychological well being: poor general health impaired emotional reaction depressed mood impaired self-control anxiety reduced vitality and energy increased social isolation

Modified and reproduced with permission from Cuneo *et al.* (1992).

Manifestations of anterior pituitary hormone deficiencies

Total or selective hypopituitarism may occur in patients with pituitary adenomas, with parasellar diseases (see below), in those who have had pituitary surgery or radiation, or following head injury. The most common symptom in both men and women is cessation of gonadal function. Secondary hypogonadism may result from LH and FSH deficiency, but may also occur with hyperprolactinaemia. The classic finding is progressive loss of pituitary hormone secretion in the following order: gonadotrophin (LH, FSH), GH, TSH, ACTH, but variations occur and some patients may have ACTH and/or TSH deficiency as the initial presenting feature. Prolactin deficiency is uncommon and is usually caused by pituitary infarction.

Growth hormone deficiency in the adult

GH has a number of important modulatory physiological actions in the adult, including partitioning of nutrients and energy and maintenance of muscle mass. The clinical features of adult GH deficiency syndrome are shown in Table 1. Short-term GH administration to GH-deficient adults appears beneficial for restoration of muscle mass, skin-fold thickness, and nutrient utilization.

Causes of adult GH deficiency include tumours of the hypothalamus or pituitary, other intracranial tumours (optic nerve glioma, for example), hypopituitarism secondary to cranial irradiation, head injury, or infection/inflammation. Growth hormone deficiency may also occur in the setting of severe psychosocial deprivation.

Gonadotrophin deficiency

This results from either a pituitary defect or the lack of hypothalamic GnRH stimulation of the gonadotrophe. It may be due to hypothalamic disease, disease of the pituitary stalk, or a functional abnormality as occurs with hyperprolactinaemia, anorexia nervosa, secondary adrenal insufficiency, or secondary hypothyroidism.

Gonadotrophin deficiency often occurs early in the course of development of hypopituitarism. In adolescents, it presents with delayed or arrested puberty. In women it is manifest by infertility, menstrual disorder, or amenorrhoea. The low gonadotrophin levels result in low serum oestradiol levels in the range of the follicular phase of the menstrual cycle. Hypo-oestrogenaemia is often associated with lack of libido and dyspareunia; long-standing oestrogen deficiency produces breast atrophy, unless the cause is hyperprolactinaemia. Long-standing oestrogen deficiency of any aetiology causes osteopenia.

In men, hypogonadism is often undiagnosed since the syndrome develops slowly and the patient often discounts the diminished libido and impotence as a function of 'age'. As in women, gonadotrophin deficiency may result from hyperprolactinaemia (see below). Low gonadotrophin concentrations result in serum testosterone levels in the prepubertal range. Testicular size may decrease and consistency may be soft. Acquired gonadotrophin deficiency is a rare cause of male infertility. Spermatogenesis is often well preserved and the significant abnormality in semen analysis is a reduced ejaculate volume, which is a function of the testosterone concentration. Beard growth and muscle bulk may also be reduced, and with long-standing hypogonadism osteopenia also develops. Hypogonadal men and women often develop fine wrinkling of the skin of the face, particularly around the mouth and eyes, a sign now considered to reflect GH deficiency.

Thyrotrophin deficiency (see also Chapter 7.3)

Secondary hypothyroidism usually occurs relatively late in the development of hypopituitarism and is usually characterized by malaise, weight gain, lack of energy, cold intolerance, and constipation. The degree of hypothyroidism depends upon the duration of thyrotrophin deficiency, but is rarely as profound as that of primary hypothyroidism.

Corticotrophin deficiency

Secondary adrenal failure may occur as an isolated deficiency, or may occur late in the course of the development of panhypopituitarism. The symptoms are essentially the same as those of Addison's disease, but differ in two important respects. Because of preserved mineralocorticoid secretion, these patients may not experience an adrenal crisis. In contrast to patients with Addison's disease, these patients have a pale and sometimes slightly sallow complexion; corticotrophin levels are low. Common symptoms are malaise, loss of energy, anorexia, and weight loss. Postural hypotension and orthostatic dizziness may be present. These patients are often misdiagnosed as malingerers. Women tend to lose secondary sexual hair and libido, while men have preserved secondary sexual hair unless there is coexistent gonadotrophin deficiency. Severe cortisol deficiency may result in hypoglycaemia and hyponatraemia. These patients, particularly those with panhypopituitarism, may deteriorate gradually and a relatively trivial illness may then precipitate circulatory collapse, coma, or a hypoglycaemia-induced seizure.

Morphological classification of pituitary adenomas

Pituitary tumours are now classified by immunocytochemical staining and electron microscopic appearances. Table 2 shows the functional morphological classification of pituitary adenomas and their prevalence in unselected surgical specimens.

Table 2 Prevalence of pituitary adenoma types in unselected surgical material (1960 cases)

	Prevalence (%)
Prolactin producing adenoma	26.2
Null cell adenoma, including oncocytoma	25.5
Growth hormone producing adenoma	14.1
Corticotroph adenoma	10.0
Gonadotroph adenoma	9.3
Growth hormone and prolactin producing adenoma	6.6
Silent corticotroph adenoma, subtypes I, II, III	5.3
Unclassified adenoma	2.0
Thyrotroph adenoma	1.0

Frequency is based on careful electron microscopic analysis. Many adenomas contain more than one hormone by immunocytochemistry. To date, the frequency of plurihormonal adenomas is not clarified. (Data kindly provided by K. Kovacs, St Michael's Hospital, Toronto, Canada.)

Evaluation of suspected pituitary disease

The evaluation of the patient with a pituitary tumour should determine:

(1) Presence and type of hormone hypersecretion;

(2) Any hormonal deficiencies and need for replacement therapy;

(3) Presence of any visual abnormalities;

(4) Pituitary anatomy including presence of extrasellar extension.

Assessment of hypothalamic pituitary function

A number of aspects need to be considered. These include interpretation of the level of the pituitary hormone in relation to that of the target hormone, the pulsatile secretion of anterior pituitary hormones, and specific factors that affect the concentration of each (for example, time of day, stress, fed or fasting, asleep or awake, stage of development). In general, screening for hyperfunction and hypofunction can usually be achieved by clinical assessment and drawing a single basal blood sample to measure pituitary and target organ hormone levels. More subtle abnormalities require more sophisticated studies.

Plasma ACTH

Because of the short half-life of plasma ACTH, the sample must be collected into a cold syringe, placed in an EDTA tube, immediately centrifuged at 4°C, and the plasma frozen immediately. ACTH secretion is pulsatile, with a circadian rhythm, and it increases during stress. Results must therefore be interpreted with knowledge of time of sample collection, whether it was drawn from an indwelling cannula (in place for at least 2 h), whether the patient was stressed, and whether exogenous synthetic glucocorticoids were administered. A simultaneously obtained plasma cortisol sample is necessary to interpret the plasma ACTH concentration. Practically, much information is obtained from a plasma cortisol measurement alone. The plasma cortisol is a good index of hypothalamic–pituitary–adrenal function. An 8 a.m. cortisol between 10 and 20 μg/dl effectively excludes adrenal insufficiency, although it does not assess ACTH reserve.

Table 3 Provocative tests of GH secretion

1. Insulin, 0.15 U/kg body weight, causes a peak GH response in 45–60 min. A physician should be in attendance. Severe hypoglycaemic symptoms should be reversed with intravenous glucose
2. Arginine hydrochloride, 0.5 g/kg body weight in normal saline, is administered intravenously over 30 min. GH peak occurs at 45–60 min
3. Levodopa (> 30 kg body weight; 500 mg; 15–30 kg; 250 mg; < 15 kg; 125 mg) is given orally. Transient nausea is common and vomiting may occur. Side-effects are minimized if patient is kept supine in a quiet room. Peak GH response usually occurs between 45 and 90 min
4. Glucagon, 1 mg, is given intramuscularly. Peak GH usually occurs 2–3 h later. Nausea and vomiting may result

See OTM3, p. 1584 for source.

Serum thyrotrophin

Ultrasensitive assays of TSH now distinguish between low, normal, and high levels and have decreased the need for dynamic function tests (see Chapter 7.3) .

Serum growth hormone

A random serum GH measurement is usually not helpful. To evaluate deficiency a stimulation test is required (Table 3) and a suppression test, for example the oral glucose tolerance test, if hypersecretion is suspected. Since the bursts of spontaneous GH secretion may occur at any time of day, timing of the sample is not helpful. GH is a stress hormone and secretion increases in response to psychogenic or physical stress or to pain. The serum IGF-I provides an overall index of GH secretion and is particularly useful as a screening test for acromegaly. Growth hormone secretion is increased after fasting for 24 h, in type 1 diabetes mellitus, in anorexia nervosa, and in hepatic failure, and is reduced in obesity. Secretion increases during puberty and is then greater in girls than in boys; this increase is accompanied by an increase in the serum IGF-I concentration. During pregnancy, GH secretion is progressively suppressed by the GH variant secreted by the placenta, but serum IGF-I concentrations are increased, indicating a biological effect of the placental hormone.

Serum LH and FSH

In men the levels of these hormones, despite their pulsatile secretion, are within a fairly narrow range; marked abnormalities are therefore easily diagnosed from a single blood sample, particularly when interpreted with the clinical findings, simultaneous testosterone levels, and possibly semen analysis.

In women the situation is more complex because of the marked changes in gonadotrophin secretion during different phases of the menstrual cycle. Clinically, measurement of serum LH and FSH in a woman who is not taking an oral contraceptive and who has regular menstrual cycles almost begs the question; a normal menstrual cycle with documentation of a normal luteal phase serum progesterone concentration effectively excludes significant gonadotrophin dysfunction. In amenorrhoeic women it is important to measure the serum LH and FSH concentrations, and simultaneous serum 17β-oestradiol, prolactin, and hCG concentrations. In this manner, the following diagnoses can be made:

(1) Primary ovarian failure with the resultant increase in LH and FSH (FSH > LH) with usually prolactin normal or low;

(2) Hyperprolactinaemia, with an elevated prolactin, normal or follicular phase LH, FSH, and 17β-oestradiol levels;

(3) Pregnancy with a positive hCG test, normal or high prolactin; high LH (if hCG cross-reacts in the assay), and high 17β-oestradiol.

Serum prolactin

Concentrations increase in the early hours of the morning, particularly just before awakening, and rise in response to psychological and physical stress, including pain. They also rise in response to nipple stimulation and may increase during sexual intercourse. Prolactin secretion is increased in response to oestrogens, and during pregnancy levels may increase to 3600–9000 mIU/l (200–500 μg/l).

A random prolactin, drawn by venepuncture, is useful if the level is normal, or markedly elevated. A concentration greater than 4500 mIU/l (250 μg/l) is almost certainly diagnostic of a prolactinoma, and further measurements are unnecessary. A more mildly elevated level (for example, 450 mIU/l (25 μg/l)) is likely to reflect the stress of venepuncture or of the physical examination, including examination of the breasts. In this situation, it is necessary to repeat the measurement once or twice. Alternatively, samples can be obtained from an indwelling venous cannula after a rest period of 2 h; samples should be obtained at 20 min intervals over the ensuing 2 h. If the prior elevation was a result of stress, results are usually normal. Although prolactin concentrations vary during the day, with lower levels observed in the afternoon, the time of day is not critical.

Dynamic tests of pituitary function

The combined anterior pituitary test

Simultaneous administration of four hypothalamic releasing hormones with measurement of target pituitary hormone concentrations permits assessment of pituitary reserve without need for admission to hospital. The four hypothalamic hormones are administered intravenously (sequentially) over 20 s. The doses are: GnRH, 100 μg; TRH, 200 μg; CRH, 1 μg/kg; and GHRH, 1 μg/kg. The normal pituitary hormone response ranges have been established. Useful information is obtained from samples drawn at −30, 0, 15, 30, 60, 90, and 120 min for measurement of ACTH, TSH, LH, FSH, GH, and prolactin. Results can be interpreted only in light of the circulating levels of the target gland hormones. Baseline samples are obtained at 08.00 h for cortisol, thyroxine, T_3-resin uptake, oestradiol (amenorrhoeic women), testosterone (men), and IGF-I.

If the pituitary hormone response is normal, in the setting of an appropriate peripheral target hormone level, then pituitary reserve is likely to be normal. An absent response to an hypothalamic hormone may be a result of absent or dysfunctional pituitary cells or because of increased negative feedback by the peripheral hormone. An example of the latter situation is an absent TSH response to TRH in thyrotoxicosis. An absent or diminished pituitary response may also result from a lack of priming because of insufficient exposure to the hypothalamic hormone (for example isolated gonadotrophin deficiency, which in most instances results from GnRH deficiency). The administration of CRH may also be useful in distinguishing between ectopic ACTH production and Cushing's disease. However, there are exceptions, and differentiating between these two conditions still remains difficult. Over 70 per cent of presumed GH-deficient children (usually due to GHRH deficiency) have an increase of serum GH to greater than 7 μg/l when GHRH is administered. In those who do not, an adequate GH response may occur after repeated GHRH injections.

Insulin tolerance test

The insulin tolerance test is the most widely used test to determine ACTH and GH reserve. The contraindications are: 08.00 hour basal plasma cortisol less than 5 μg/dl, history of a seizure disorder, altered mental status, or ischaemic heart disease. If the 08.00 h plasma cortisol is less than 5 μg/dl the patient has adrenal failure and requires a test to distinguish primary from secondary adrenal failure. Hypoglycaemia may precipitate fits in a patient with a seizure disorder or myocardial infarction in a patient with ischaemic heart disease. An alternative test such as metyrapone administration should be performed in such patients.

The test must be performed only when a physician is present. Before insulin administration, clinical assessment and ECG must be performed and interpreted and the 08.00 h plasma cortisol of greater than 5 μg/dl documented. The test and symptoms of hypoglycaemia must be explained in detail to the patient, who should have fasted from midnight, but may have taken water *ad libitum.* A venous cannula is placed about 1 h prior to commencement of the test, which should take place in the morning. Blood is drawn for blood glucose, plasma cortisol (and, if indicated, for corticotrophin), prolactin, and GH at −30, 0, 30, 45, 60, and 90 min. At 0 min, 0.15 units/kg of soluble or Actrapid® insulin is injected intravenously. Pulse rate, blood pressure, and clinical observations are made at the times of blood sampling. During the initial 30 min after the injection there are often no symptoms, but between 30 and 45 min sweating, tachycardia, drowsiness, and hunger usually occur. If there are no signs of hypoglycaemia and the blood glucose has not fallen to less than 2.2 mmol/l (40 mg/dl), a second dose of insulin, 0.3 units/kg, is administered. In the event of adverse effects (e.g. a fit) the hypoglycaemia is reversed with intravenous glucose, and 1 mg dexamethasone administered intravenously. Sampling should continue until the end of the test. In patients known to have insulin resistance (e.g. acromegaly) a dose of 0.3 U/kg may be used initially. However, if doubt exists, it is safer to start with the standard dose and then double it.

Interpretation

Clinical signs of hypoglycaemia and a blood glucose of less than 2.2 mmol/l (40 mg/dl) are required for the ACTH and GH levels to be interpretable. If these two criteria are fulfilled, the plasma cortisol should rise to greater than 580 nmol/l (21 μg/dl) and GH should increase to above 10 (in children) and 3 (in adults) μg/l.

Oral glucose tolerance test

The test is performed to diagnose or exclude acromegaly since growth hormone secretion is inhibited by acute hyperglycaemia. The patient fasts from midnight and is allowed to take water *ad libitum.* A cannula is placed in a forearm vein 1 h before the test. Blood samples for blood glucose and serum GH are obtained at −30, 0, 30, 60, 90, and 120 min after 75 g glucose has been given by mouth. Serum GH by immunoradiometricassay should then decrease to less than 2 μg/l.

The development of ultrasensitive chemiluminescence assays which measure GH concentrations as low as 0.002 μg/l will probably lead to re-evaluation of the normal GH response to oral glucose. The new criteria using this assay are: suppression of GH to less than 0.06 μg/l in men and to less than 0.71 μg/l in women.

Pituitary imaging

Computerized tomography (CT) and MRI techniques image the pituitary gland directly and, with respect to MRI, the structures surrounding it. Since pituitary enlargement may occur without enlargement of the sella, a normal skull radiograph or sellar tomograms do not exclude a pituitary mass. Cerebral angiography may occasionally be required prior to surgical intervention, but has no place in the initial evaluation unless there are no facilities for MRI or CT. MRI is superior to CT because the optic chiasm is easily visualized and can be distinguished from the diaphragma sellae, vascular structures (including aneurysms) can be seen, and any lateral tumour extension can be delineated (Fig. 7).

A comparison of patients with a surgically proven microadenoma demonstrated that the MRI scan detected the microadenoma and its correct location in 100 per cent of cases; but only 50 per cent of cases were detected on CT. A pituitary microadenoma on MRI scan may range from 1.5–10 mm in diameter. Deviation of the infundibulum away from the side of the tumour may be observed. Macroadenomas (> 10 mm) tend to have signal characteristics that are similar to those of the normal gland, but may contain cystic or haemorrhagic areas. Intravenous administration of gadolinium-diethylenetriamine penta-acetic acid (Gd-DTPA) produces prompt enhancement of the normal pituitary which is maximal after approximately 30 min; adenomas enhance more slowly and persistently than the normal gland. The use of Gd-DTPA and coronal images increases the probability of identifying a small lesion and should be used in all studies in which a pituitary tumour is suspected. MRI may also successfully identify a non-pituitary intrasellar mass such as a meningioma or internal carotid artery aneurysm. Very small tumours may not be detectable. This is particularly true for patients with Cushing's disease where only 83 per cent of the tumours are detectable by MRI.

Neuro-ophthalmological evaluation

Visual acuity and visual fields should be assessed at the initial examination, most commonly by use of a Snellen chart and estimation of visual fields by confrontation. Confrontation testing with a red coloured object (e.g. tip of a pen) may reveal subtle visual field loss. A normal clinical examination does not exclude abnormalities which are only detectable using perimetry. In patients with visual symptoms or evidence of optic chiasm compression on MRI or CT scan, the extent of visual field compromise must be documented using automated perimetry.

Permanent loss of vision or visual field defect(s) usually results from long-standing nerve compression, but the relationship between duration of compression and permanency of damage is not known. If vision from one eye is normal, the patient may fail to notice any abnormality or describe the vision as dim or foggy. Vision is usually lost gradually, except in the case of haemorrhage into the tumour (pituitary apoplexy), when it may be sudden with loss of central vision and development of bitemporal field defects, ophthalmoplegia, and changes in mental function.

Visual acuity may range from 20/20 to near or complete blindness. Loss of perception of colour, particularly red, and a decreased pupillary light reaction may accompany decreased visual acuity. If the optic nerve has been compromised for 6 weeks or more optic disc pallor may be present and occurs in 30–70 per cent of patients with large tumours.

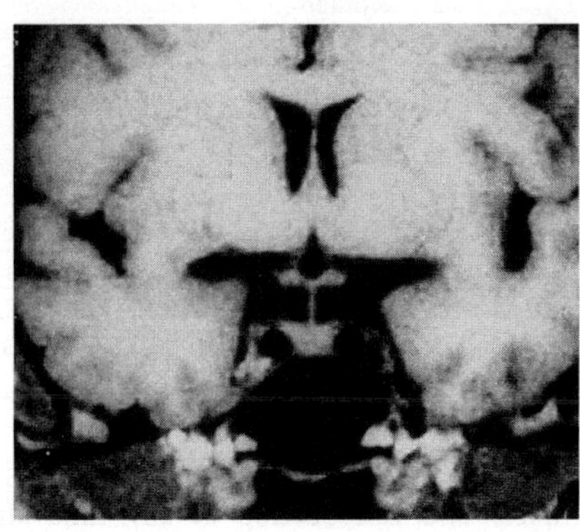

(a)

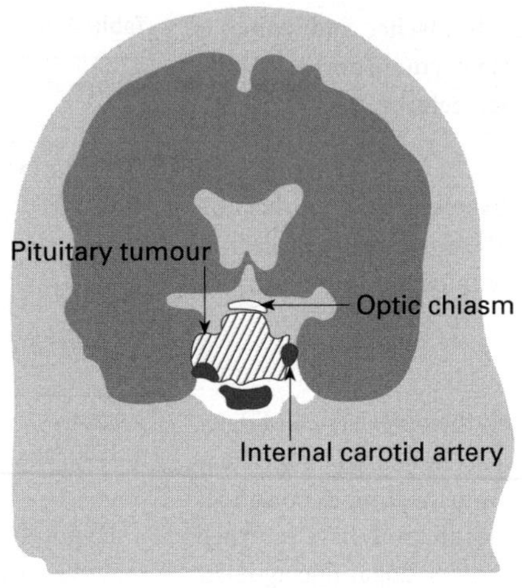

(b)

Fig. 7 (a) Coronal MRI scan demonstrating a large pituitary tumour extending laterally into both cavernous sinuses and superiorly abutting the optic chiasm. (b) Schematic drawing demonstrating a large pituitary tumour extending laterally into both cavernous sinuses and superiorly abutting the optic chiasm.
(For source see OTM3, p.1586.)

Ophthalmoplegia, the result of lateral extension of the tumour, is less common. Involvement of the cavernous sinus occurs in up to 15 per cent of patients, but is clinically apparent in only a minority of these. Symptoms include diplopia and/or ptosis or altered facial sensation. Depending on the degree of cavernous sinus invasion, cranial nerves III, IV, VI, and the first and second divisions of V may be damaged, most commonly III.

Successful decompression of the optic nerves and chiasm, either by surgical resection or shrinkage of the tumour by medical therapies, is often accompanied by marked improvement in visual function, usually occurring within hours or days of surgery, continuing thereafter for some months. Visual abnormalities may worsen in some 4–10 per cent after surgical decompression. The trans-sphenoidal approach carries the least risk of such deterioration. The prognosis is best in those with a short history and absence of clinical evidence of optic atrophy.

Hormone replacement therapy

Cortisol deficiency

Cortisol deficiency is usually treated by oral administration of 20 mg hydrocortisone on awakening and 10 mg at 6 p.m. Some patients require an additional 10 mg at lunch time, while others, particularly very small patients, may require a lower dose of 10 mg on awakening and 5 mg at 6 p.m. Alternatively, synthetic glucocorticoids may be used; prednisone, 5 mg on awakening and 2.5 mg at 6 p.m., or dexamethasone, 0.5 mg on awakening. During stress, whether psychological or physical, fever, and during illness, the dose should be increased to an equivalent of hydrocortisone 20 mg every 6–8 h. More severe illness may require intravenous administration of hydrocortisone in a dose of 100 mg intravenously every 4 h.

Thyroid hormone deficiency

Thyroid hormone replacement should not be given until the hypothalamic–pituitary–adrenal axis has been assessed since in a cortisol deficient subject it may precipitate an adrenal crisis. Deficiency is treated with L-thyroxine; 0.075–0.15 mg once daily. The dose is adjusted according to the clinical response but measurement of the serum tri-iodothyronine level aiming at the middle or upper part of the normal range can also be helpful.

Gonadal steroids

Gonadal steroids are required for hypogonadal patients in whom hyperprolactinaemia is not the cause, and for patients who do not desire fertility.

Testosterone enanthate for hypogonadal men is usually given intramuscularly, 200 mg every 2 weeks or 300 mg every 3 weeks. It is advisable to begin with a low dose (50 mg every 2 weeks, for example) to avoid breast tenderness, gynaecomastia, or excessive and painful erections. This can then be doubled every 2 weeks until the patient is receiving a full dose. Alternative preparations of testosterone replacement therapy are available including oral testosterone undecanoate and skin patches.

There are numerous regimens for oestrogen replacement in hypogonadal women. If the uterus has not been removed, oestrogens are administered cyclically with appropriate progestogens; a convenient choice is a low dose (containing 30 μg ethinyl oestradiol) oral contraceptive preparation. Alternatively, oestrogen can be given for 3 weeks out of four and a small dose of progestogen administered for the third week; for instance conjugated oestrogen 0.625 mg daily for 3 weeks together with medroxyprogesterone acetate 5 mg or 10 mg daily for the last 7 or 10 days.

Growth hormone

Recombinant DNA-produced preparations of natural sequence GH are now available for GH deficient children. GH is now approved for replacement in GH-deficient adults, although trials of its efficacy are currently under way.

Pituitary surgery

Trans-sphenoidal surgery is the technique of choice and much increases the chances of selective removal to leave the normal tissue intact and functional. Decompression of the pituitary fossa from below, also allows a recurrence to extend inferiorly instead of laterally or superiorly.

Indications for pituitary surgery

Pituitary apoplexy

Minor haemorrhage into a pituitary tumour probably occurs quite frequently and may be clinically insignificant; many such cases are probably not diagnosed. However, a severe haemorrhage leading to prostration, visual disturbance, profound headache, and coma is a neurosurgical emergency. If sudden visual compromise occurs, neurosurgical intervention is mandatory (see below).

Pituitary tumour

Therapy is indicated if pituitary tumours hypersecrete or if they are large enough to produce mass effects. With the exception of prolactin-secreting adenomas, most authorities recommend trans-sphenoidal surgery as the first intervention.

Failure of other therapies

Patients who have undergone previous failed therapies are candidates for surgery, for example, those with acromegaly not cured by pituitary radiation. Patients with a prolactinoma in whom the tumour continues to grow also may require surgery even if prolactin levels have returned to normal. Intolerance to bromocriptine or other dopamine agonists is another indication for surgery. Additionally, prolactinomas are not always fully responsive to treatment with dopamine agonists. Surgery is then often helpful in reducing the bulk of the tumour allowing potentially a better response to medical therapy.

Results of pituitary surgery

These are usually good, particularly in patients with suprasellar extension and visual abnormalities. Improvement in visual field abnormalities occurs in over 80 per cent of such patients, progression of visual disturbance is arrested in 16 per cent, but there is deterioration in 4 per cent. The endocrine results of pituitary surgery are discussed below.

There are few complications, but every operation carries a risk, which is lowest in patients with microadenomas and highest in patients who have had previous therapy. The incidence of postoperative hypopituitarism is 3 per cent in patients with microadenomas but increases with invasiveness of the tumour. The experience of the surgeon is a key factor in determining the outcome of surgery.

Pituitary radiation

Currently, pituitary radiation is administered only to patients with residual disease following surgery or in patients unable to undergo surgical resection. The techniques used include conventional supervoltage therapy, yttrium implantation, stereotactic radiosurgery with alpha particles or proton beam therapy, or a single high dose of focused radiation from the gamma knife unit. The choice is made according to the size and location of the tumour (proximity to the optic chiasm and cavernous sinus) and the available resources. Conventional supervoltage therapy is the approach most commonly used, administered in daily fractions 5 days per week over 4 or 5 weeks. Yttrium implantation involves surgical placement of radioactive yttrium-90 seeds into the pituitary and is now used in very few centres. Alpha particle and proton beam radiotherapy can only be used to treat small tumours and require a cyclotron for the energy source. Focused radiation using the gamma knife unit is also limited to treatment of small tumours and is not widely available.

The results of these treatments are broadly similar, with the exception of gamma knife unit therapy in which there is inadequate information for comparison with other techniques. Most studies have demonstrated that very few patients have progression of disease after radiotherapy. Partial reduction in hormone hypersecretion may occur within 3–6 months of therapy, but a complete response requires at least 5 years, and more often is delayed until 10 years after treatment.

Table 4 Symptoms associated with hyperprolactinaemia

Women	Men	Men and postmenopausal women
Galactorrhoea (30–80%)	Galactorrhoea (< 30%)	Visual field abnormalities
Menstrual irregularity	Impotence	Headache
Infertility		Extraocular muscle weakness Anterior pituitary malfunction

A variable incidence of galactorrhoea is reported in different studies. See OTM3, p. 1589 for source.

Hypopituitarism is an expected consequence of radiotherapy; it may be partial or complete and can develop at any time after treatment. In one study, 50 per cent of patients treated with conventional supervoltage radiation developed hypopituitarism within 26 months of therapy. Other series indicate that at least one-third of patients develop pituitary deficiencies within 2–3 years, the incidence increasing with length of follow-up.

Other complications of radiotherapy include damage to the hypothalamus, optic chiasm, and/or optic nerve(s) or other cranial nerves, vascular damage, resulting cerebral ischemia, seizures, and development of a pituitary or brain malignancy.

Pituitary tumours

Prolactinoma

Hyperprolactinaemia, the result of excessive prolactin production by the lactotropes, is the most common anterior pituitary disorder. The natural history of a prolactinoma is not precisely known, but the majority grow slowly, usually over years. Autopsy studies have suggested that 23–27 per cent of the general population may have an asymptomatic microadenoma. Serial observations of untreated patients with a microadenoma indicate that a minority have a significant increase in serum prolactin and/or in tumour size, while in the majority there is either no change or a decrease in serum prolactin concentrations over time. The aetiology is unknown but analyses of tumour DNA indicate a monoclonal origin.

Clinical features

The presentation varies according to the patient's age and sex, the duration of hyperprolactinaemia and, if present, the size of the tumour. Men and postmenopausal women usually come to medical attention because of symptoms of a pituitary mass, such as headache and disturbances of vision. Table 4 illustrates the common clinical features, among which hypogonadism is almost invariable. Women of reproductive age commonly seek medical attention because of delayed menarche, disturbance of menstrual function, or infertility. Galactorrhoea is present in 30–80 per cent of these women, a symptom which is less common in those with long-standing amenorrhoea, probably reflecting prolonged oestrogen deficiency. Other features of oestrogen deficiency include decreased libido, vaginal dryness, and dyspareunia. In the majority of premenopausal women the cause of hyperprolactinaemia is a microadenoma.

In men, hypogonadism may be complete or partial, producing decreased libido, complete or partial impotence and/or infertility. Many hyperprolactinaemic men report 'normal' sexual function and realize there was dysfunction only after successful treatment. When hypogonadism has been long-standing, beard and body hair may be decreased and the testes are usually soft but of normal size (> 12 ml volume). Galactorrhoea occurs in 14–33 per cent of affected men, but its presence may require vigorous breast manipulation; gynaecomastia is uncommon. In those with arrested puberty a female body habitus may be evident and the testes are usually small (< 12 ml volume) and soft. Symptoms other than decreased libido (which affects 83 per cent) include adiposity (69 per cent), apathy (63 per cent) and headache (63 per cent). Although in the majority of men seeking treatment for sexual dysfunction the cause is psychogenic, some 8 per cent have hyperprolactinaemia, emphasizing the importance of measuring the serum prolactin concentration in such patients.

A pituitary tumour may be found coincidentally when a CT or MRI scan is obtained because of head trauma or for evaluation of headaches. A less common presentation is that of severe headache and/or prostration secondary to haemorrhage into a previously undiagnosed pituitary tumour (see above).

Complications

A tumour which extends beyond the confines of the sella turcica most commonly produces headache and visual abnormalities. The classic presentation is with a bitemporal hemianopia from compression of the optic chiasm by a tumour which has extended superiorly. Lateral extension into the cavernous sinus causes impaired oculomotor function involving the cranial nerves III, IV, VI, and the first and second divisions of V, either singly or in combination. Occasionally, very large tumours may extend into the temporal lobe of the brain, increasing the risk of fits.

Compression of normal pituitary tissue by a large tumour may result in disturbance of secretion of other pituitary hormones, resulting in GH, ACTH, LH, FSH, or TSH deficiency, singly or in combination. The most common deficiency in patients with large prolactinomas is most probably that of GH, but this has not been systematically studied. Hyperprolactinaemia is associated with impaired pulsatile gonadotrophin release, probably by alteration of hypothalamic GnRH secretion and resulting in gonadal insufficiency which is reversible with reduction of prolactin secretion. Both men and women with chronic hyperprolactinaemia have decreased bone density, when compared with age-matched normal subjects.

Diagnosis and endocrine evaluation

A full drug history is important since a number of medications may produce hyperprolactinaemia (see Table 5). A single prolactin measurement may be sufficient to diagnose a prolactinoma if the value is high enough, for example greater than 3600 mIU/l (200 μg/l). A mildly increased concentration of 400–1200 mIU/l (20–60 μg/l) may reflect pulsatile secretions or the effects of breast examination; it is prudent therefore to obtain several measurements before making the diagnosis of true hyperprolactinaemia. A morning cortisol concentration may be used to screen for adrenal function, but a normal value does not assess hypothalamic–pituitary reserve and a stimulatory test such as insulin-induced hypoglycaemia or metyrapone administration is necessary to determine if the hypothalamic–pituitary–adrenal axis is intact. Induction of hypoglycaemia can also be used to determine GH reserve. Additional helpful studies include measurement of plasma testosterone (in men) and oestradiol (in women).

Table 5 Causes of hyperprolactinaemia

Causes
Hypothalamic disease
Tumour, e.g. metastases, craniopharyngioma, germinoma, cyst, glioma, hamartoma
Infiltrative disease, e.g. sarcoidosis, tuberculosis, histiocytosis X, granuloma
Pseudotumor cerebri
Cranial radiation
Pituitary disease
Prolactinoma
Acromegaly
Cushing's disease
Pituitary stalk section
Empty sella syndrome
Other tumours, e.g. metastases, non-secretory, gonadotroph adenoma, meningioma
Intrasellar germinoma
Infiltrative disease, e.g. sarcoidosis, giant cell granuloma, tuberculosis
Drugs
Dopamine receptor antagonists, e.g. chlorpromazine, fluphenazine, fluorperazine, haloperidol, perphenazine, promazine, domperidone, metoclopramide, sulpiride
Other drugs
Antihypertensives, e.g. alpha methyldopa, reserpine, verapamil
Oestrogens
Opiates
Cimetidine
Primary hypothyroidism
Chronic renal failure
Cirrhosis
Neurogenic, e.g. breast manipulation, chest wall lesions, spinal cord lesions
Stress, e.g. physical, psychological
Idiopathic

See OTM3, p. 1590 for source.

A raised serum prolactin must be interpreted in conjunction with MRI or CT scanning of the pituitary to determine whether the hyperprolactinaemia is a result of a prolactinoma or is a secondary phenomenon. A prolactin concentration of 3600 mIU/l (200 μg/l) or greater, in the presence of a macroadenoma (> 10 mm), is most likely caused by a prolactinoma. Conversely, a prolactin concentration of less than 3600 mIU/l (200 μg/l) in the setting of a large pituitary tumour is most likely to be caused by compression of the pituitary stalk, resulting in interference with dopamine transport from the hypothalamus to the gland. This distinction is particularly important in selecting appropriate therapy, since dopamine agonists will reduce serum prolactin in both instances, but will not shrink the tumour which has caused secondary hyperprolactinaemia. Prolactin-secreting microadenomas do not usually increase prolactin concentrations beyond 3600 mIU/l (200 μg/l). Hyperprolactinaemia can also be caused by non-pituitary intracranial lesions. Craniopharyngiomas, meningiomas, ectopic pinealomas, metastatic tumours, or third ventricle tumours do not usually increase prolactin concentrations above 2000 mIU/l (100 μg/l).

Treatment

Medical therapy

Successful treatment of a prolactinoma is most often and easily accomplished with administration of a dopamine agonist, but there may be an additional need for surgery and/or radiotherapy in some cases.

Bromocriptine has been shown to lower serum prolactin to normal in 64–100 per cent, to improve galactorrhoea in 57–100 per cent, and to return menses and ovulation to normal in 57–100 per cent of patients. The results of treatment in patients with macroadenomas are similar to those with microadenomas, except that in some with large tumours, a longer time is required to lower the serum prolactin to normal.

Reduction in tumour size with improvement in visual abnormalities usually occurs before the serum prolactin returns fully to normal. Some 76–100 per cent of patients can expect a reduction in tumour size, and visual field defects improve in 90 per cent, often before any demonstrable decrease in tumour size assessed by CT or MRI.

The usual dose of bromocriptine is 2.5 mg three times daily. When prolactin concentrations have been reduced to normal, the dose may be reduced to 2.5 mg twice daily and continued suppression may be expected with this reduced dose. Some patients have been given larger doses (e.g. 20–30 mg/day) in resistant cases but there is no conclusive evidence that these larger doses are any more effective than the standard regimen.

Other currently available dopamine agonists include lisuride, pergolide, metergoline, cabergoline, and a non-ergot preparation, mesulergine. These drugs act by direct stimulation of pituitary cell membrane dopamine receptors (DA 2) to inhibit prolactin secretion. The most common side-effects of dopamine agonists are nausea and orthostatic hypotension, which occur commonly on initiation of treatment and can be minimized by beginning with a small dose, given with food, increasing gradually over 1–2 weeks. Less common side-effects include headache, fatigue, nasal stuffiness, abdominal cramping, and constipation. Hallucinations and psychosis have also been observed; the incidence of psychosis was 1.3 per cent in one study of 600 patients, the symptoms including auditory hallucinations, delusions, and mood changes that abated when the dopamine agonist was discontinued. Concomitant alcohol ingestion may exacerbate the symptoms of nausea and abdominal discomfort.

Most patients require long-term treatment, and withdrawal usually results in recurrent hyperprolactinaemia and re-expansion of the tumour but it is occasionally possible to stop treatment in a patient with a microadenoma or no demonstrable tumour.

Pregnancy in women with hyperprolactinaemia

Fertility in treated patients is identical to that of other women of the same age. A recommendation for women attempting to become pregnant is that barrier contraception should be used until the patient has had two or three regular cycles, so that cycle length can be determined. After discontinuation of mechanical contraception, a serum β-human chorionic gonadotrophin (β-hCG) measurement is obtained to confirm pregnancy as soon as there is a delay in expected menses. This regimen allows for early diagnosis of pregnancy so that dopamine agonist therapy can be discontinued, although bromocriptine is not associated with an increased risk of multiple pregnancies, spontaneous abortion, ectopic pregnancy, trophoblastic disease, or congenital malformation. Tumour expansion during pregnancy may occur, particularly in women with macroadenomas. Clinically significant enlargement has been estimated to occur in 1.4 per cent of women with microadenomas and approximately 16 per cent of those with macroadenomas, but these are almost certainly overestimates. When significant tumour enlargement has occurred bromocriptine is effective but alternatives include surgical resection or high dose corticosteroid therapy. Patients with macroadenomas treated with bromocriptine continuously during pregnancy do not have tumour-related complications.

Men with prolactinomas

Men treated with a dopamine agonist have improvement in libido and potency. Some note marked improvement in function early in treatment, before the testosterone concentration becomes normal. The semen analysis can be expected to improve with lowering of prolactin to normal and restoration of normal pulsatile gonadotropin (LH, FSH) secretion.

Resistance to dopamine agonist therapy

A few patients have a partial response or no response to this therapy, probably dependent on the number and affinity of dopamine receptors in the tumour. Failure to respond leads to consideration of surgical resection.

Surgical therapy

Trans-sphenoidal resection of the adenoma is the most frequently employed approach and is associated with better results and less morbidity than is craniotomy. Although surgical resection offers the potential cure, this is only accomplished in a minority of patients with large tumours and is associated with a definite risk of recurrence in all patients. Patients with microadenomas (< 10 mm) treated surgically at centres where the procedure is frequently performed have a normal postoperative serum prolactin concentration in 60–80 per cent of cases, while in patients with macroadenomas (> 10 mm) this is achieved in 0–40 per cent of patients. The most important factors predictive of successful surgery are the preoperative serum prolactin concentration and the tumour size. Recurrence rates in patients with a microadenoma range from 10–50 per cent for up to 5 years of follow-up and from 0–91 per cent of those with a macroadenoma followed for up to 5 years.

Radiation therapy

Pituitary radiation is rarely used as primary treatment of a prolactinoma. Although it is effective in preventing further growth or expansion of the tumour, it is much less effective in promoting a prompt reduction of the serum prolactin concentration.

Acromegaly

The estimated prevalence of acromegaly is 38–69 per million, with an annual incidence of 3–3.3 per million. The percentage of acromegalics in pituitary surgical series is about 15 per cent. It is seen with equal frequency in men and women, and may occur at any age, but is diagnosed most frequently in the fourth and fifth decades of life. When it occurs prior to puberty, gigantism develops; this is an extremely rare syndrome and it accounts for less than 5 per cent of acromegalics. In about 6 per cent of patients, acromegaly may occur as a part of multiple endocrine neoplasia type 1 syndrome.

In over 99 per cent of cases, acromegaly results from a primary pituitary adenoma, but in a very few, less than 1 per cent, it results from excessive production of GHRH which causes somatotroph hyperplasia and possibly tumour formation. GHRH secretion occurs in gangliocytomata (eutopic; either hypothalamic or pituitary) or peripheral tumours (ectopic). One case of ectopic GH secretion by a pancreatic islet cell tumour has been described.

Most evidence suggests that acromegaly due to somatotroph adenoma is a primary pituitary disease. The tumour is circumscribed and the remaining pituitary is normal without evidence of somatotroph hyperplasia. Additionally, after successful removal of the tumour recurrence is rare.

Point mutations in α_s, the GTP-binding subunit of the stimulatory regulator of adenyl cyclase (G_s), have been found in about half of somatotroph tumours, demonstrating that adenylate cyclase is constitutively activated. Somatotroph tumours are monoclonal in origin.

Clinical features

Symptoms usually begin insidiously and anatomical changes develop gradually and go unnoticed until complications develop so that diagnosis is often delayed for up to 15–20 years.

The tumour mass may produce headaches and/or visual disturbances, including a visual field defect or diplopia from ophthalmoplegia. Hypopituitarism may occur if the tumour is very large when gonadal dysfunction is more common than hypothyroidism and secondary adrenal insufficiency. The symptoms and signs of excessive secretion of GH are the most common presentation, gigantism before puberty and acromegaly after it. Acromegaly is characterized by thickening and oiliness of the skin, particularly of the face. Facial changes include thick lips, exaggerated nasolabial folds, thickening of the scalp, giving rise to the development of deep folds, which are visible on skull radiograph or CT scan—cutis verticis gyrata. Acanthosis nigricans may also occur. The vocal cords thicken which, in conjunction with sinus enlargement, results in a deep and resonant voice. The overall appearance and a deep voice give acromegalic women a rather masculinized appearance often associated with mild hirsutism. The hands and feet enlarge; rings become tighter, cannot be removed and may have to be cut off. Increased foot size is manifested particularly by an increase in the shoe width. An increase in both soft tissue and skull mass leads to increased head, and therefore, hat size. The calvarium of the skull thickens; hyperostosis frontalis is common and frontal sinuses expand resulting in protrusion of the brows ('frontal bossing'). The zygomatic arch enlarges to produce prominence of the cheek bones and relative hollowness of the temporal fossae, particularly evident after successful treatment when the soft tissues regress. The mandible grows in length and breadth, which leads to protrusion of the lower jaw, malocclusion, and development of temporomandibular arthritis. The changes in the lower jaw and the temporomandibular arthritis are sometimes the particular feature leading to the diagnosis of acromegaly.

Arthralgia is present in 62–75 per cent of acromegalic patients and arthropathy in 16–62 per cent. Between 10 and 40 per cent of patients have joint disease severe enough to limit daily activities. The knees, hips, and shoulders are most frequently affected, while elbows and ankles are relatively spared. The spine may also be affected, with the lumbosacral region most commonly involved. The initial symptoms are of joint stiffness, particularly of the hands; this may reflect the increase of subcutaneous tissue which is reversible with reduction of circulating GH concentration. In addition to changes in the soft tissues, there may be thickening of the shafts of the metacarpals, metatarsals, and phalanges. Tufting of the ends of the terminal phalanges develops with exostoses of the bones of the hands and feet.

Early in the course of the disease, joint spaces are increased secondary to cartilage proliferation. The synovial and periarticular swelling produces joint swelling without effusion. Cartilage degeneration is often sufficiently disabling as to require joint replacement.

Backache is common, especially when associated with dorsal kyphosis. Disc spaces are increased and anterior osteophytes are common. Spinal mobility is normal or increased since the discs are resilient and paraspinal ligaments become hypertrophied and lax. The characteristic barrel chest is caused by a combination of the changes in the vertebrae and the ribs.

High levels of GH are associated with excessive sweating, particularly of the face, head, hands, and feet; hyperhidrosis may be the presenting symptom. The increase in soft tissue mass may produce a carpal tunnel syndrome, which is a very common presentation of acromegaly.

Galactorrhoea is common in acromegalic women, but rare in men. Hyperprolactinaemia occurs in up to 40 per cent of acromegalics but in its absence galactorrhoea is idiopathic or the result of the lactogenic effects of GH. Between 32 and 87 per cent of acromegalic women under the age of 45 years have menstrual abnormalities and decreased libido, and 27–46 per cent of acromegalic men are impotent; these features probably relate to the high frequency of hyperprolactinaemia and the lactogenic effects of GH.

Other features of acromegaly include enlargement of the thyroid, sometimes with palpable nodules. Other organs increase in size. The skin, particularly of the palms of the hands and soles of the feet, is often moist. Multiple skin tags are frequently present and correlate with the occurrence of colonic polyps.

Complications

Metabolic and endocrine

Hypersecretion of growth hormone induces insulin resistance and glucose intolerance, which occurs in 29–45 per cent of cases; clinical diabetes mellitus is present in 10–20 per cent. The higher the GH levels the more likely is diabetes, but the HLA phenotype, a family history of diabetes, and duration of acromegaly do not appear particularly to influence its development.

Hypertriglyceridaemia occurs in 19–44 per cent of acromegalic patients and hepatic triglyceride lipase and lipoprotein lipase activities are decreased but return towards normal after successful treatment.

Respiratory

A threefold increase in respiratory deaths occurred in one study of morbidity and mortality, probably dependent on associated narrowing of the airway. Exacerbation of upper airway narrowing during an upper respiratory tract infection may result in acute dyspnoea and stridor. Difficult intubation during induction of anaesthesia and airway obstruction from an enlarged tongue following extubation are not uncommon. Many acromegalic patients suffer from the obstructive sleep apnoea syndrome, not always corrected by cure of acromegaly.

Cardiovascular

Acromegaly is associated with an increased rate of death from hypertension and cardiomyopathy. Indeed, cardiovascular disease is the most common cause of death in acromegalics. Since these patients often have hypertension and/or diabetes it is difficult to determine whether the cardiac disease is secondary to these disorders or due to a specific acromegalic cardiomyopathy. An autopsy series of 27 cases revealed myocardial hypertrophy in 93 per cent, interstitial fibrosis of the myocardium in 85 per cent, and lymphomononuclear myocarditis in 59 per cent. Echocardiography has shown cardiac enlargement, usually with an increase of left ventricular mass, in 80 per cent of patients, apparently independent of hypertension or known ischaemic heart disease. The severity of these abnormalities does not consistently correlate with GH levels, but the duration of the disease may be important. After restoration of normal GH levels the cardiac abnormalities may improve in some patients.

Hypertension occurs in 18–41 per cent of acromegalics and has been associated with higher mean GH concentrations and prolonged duration of acromegaly; it is usually mild and its pathophysiology is poorly understood. Rarely, the hypertension may result from an associated phaeochromocytoma or aldosterone-secreting adenoma.

Calcium and bone metabolism

Serum 1,25-dihydroxyvitamin D concentrations are increased, while 25-hydroxyvitamin D levels are low and those of parathyroid hormone and calcitonin are normal. The increase in 1,25-dihydroxyvitamin D concentrations occurs as a result of GH stimulation of renal 1α-hydroxylase activity. The net effect is an increase in intestinal calcium absorption and hypercalciuria; serum calcium levels are normal unless coincidental hyperparathyroidism is present. Growth hormone increases tubular phosphate reabsorption with resultant hyperphosphataemia in approximately 50 per cent of acromegalics. Urolithiasis occurs in 6–12.5 per cent. Acromegaly is associated with increased bone turnover. Bone density in acromegalics is increased; osteoporosis does not occur unless hypogonadism is also present.

Neuromuscular

Although acromegalics have a muscular appearance they are often weak. The precise cause of this weakness is unknown; a myopathic process has been suggested. The bony changes of the vertebral column may cause nerve root compression at the vertebral foramina, giving rise to lumbar radiculopathy. Spinal stenosis and an amyotrophic-like syndrome may occur. Carpal tunnel syndrome occurs in 35–45 per cent of patients.

Colonic polyps and malignancies

A recent prospective study identified an increased incidence of colonic polyps in acromegalic patients. Although several retrospective studies have suggested an increased incidence of gastrointestinal malignancies, a survey of mortality in 194 acromegalic patients did not reveal an increased mortality from malignant neoplasms, a finding confirmed by other studies on prevalence of malignant disease in acromegaly.

Biochemical evaluation

Serum IGF-I concentration

The serum IGF-I concentration is the best screening test for acromegaly; an elevated value suggests excessive GH secretion, except during pregnancy or puberty when IGF-I levels are normally increased. Serum IGF-I levels are increased in acromegaly compared with age- and sex-matched normal subjects and vary minimally, thus providing a reliable index of GH secretion during the previous 24-h period. Reliability of IGF-I assays is variable, so that proper interpretation of results requires knowledge of the assay used. The predominant IGF-I binding protein, IGF-BP3, is positively regulated by GH and may well be a further useful marker of GH secretion. Serum IGF-I should be used as an initial screen, as an index of disease activity, and to assess efficacy of therapy.

Oral glucose and insulin tolerance test

The definitive test to diagnose acromegaly is failure of serum GH to decrease to less than 2 μg/l after ingestion of glucose. Other tests that have been proposed include administration of TRH, GnRH, L-DOPA, and other dopamine agonists which produce different (paradoxical) effects in acromegalic patients compared with normal subjects. These responses are not as uniform as is the abnormal response to oral glucose, and therefore are not routinely used.

Insulin-induced hypoglycaemia is used in acromegalic patients to evaluate the hypothalamic–pituitary–adrenal axis. Patients with acromegaly have insulin resistance and frequently require higher doses of insulin to decrease the blood glucose to interpretable levels.

Differential diagnosis

This includes a primary pituitary micro- or macroadenoma (99 per cent of cases), and GH hypersecretion stimulated by eutopic (hypothalamic tumour) or ectopic (peripheral tumour) GHRH. However, radiological studies cannot distinguish between an enlarged pituitary with an adenoma and an enlarged hyperplastic gland and no patient with hypothalamic acromegaly from a GHRH-secreting hypothalamic tumour has yet been diagnosed antemortem. Ectopic GHRH secretion, although very rare, is more common than eutopic and should be suspected in a patient with acromegaly and elevated circulating GHRH levels (normal less than 100ng/l; but in the μg/l range in ectopic GHRH cases). The most likely peripheral sites are the pancreas, lung, thymus, adrenal (in association with phaeochromocytoma), or gastrointestinal tract, but occasionally no ectopic source can be found. If an ectopic tumour is identified, surgical resection is curative provided there are no metastases. Patients with metastatic disease are responsive to octreotide therapy (see below).

Surgical therapy of pituitary macro- or microadenomata

The outcome is dependent on the size of the tumour and the expertise of the neurosurgical team. The presence of an intrasellar microadenoma (< 10 mm diameter) offers the greatest possibility for a cure. Results are less good for macroadenomas (> 10 mm diameter), particularly when there is suprasellar extension or extension into the cavernous sinus, although a substantial reduction in tumour mass and immediate improvement in visual abnormalities, headaches, and symptoms of excessive GH are to be expected.

Trans-sphenoidal surgery achieves a basal postoperative GH concentration of less than 5 μg/l in approximately 60 per cent of patients in the best centres. While a basal serum GH of less than 5 μg/l may be indicative of successful surgery, the oral glucose tolerance test is a more accurate method to evaluate postoperative GH secretion.

The serum IGF-I concentration should be measured before and after surgery. Although GH concentrations decline rapidly after tumour removal, clearance of IGF-I, complexed with a binding protein, may require several months. Even if all tests of GH secretion are normal postoperatively, some patients relapse, emphasizing the need for careful follow-up. The precise incidence of recurrence is not known, but probably ranges from 0–13 per cent over 2–3.5 years.

Surgical mortality is rare. Permanent diabetes insipidus follows surgery in 1–9 per cent of patients.

Radiation therapy

Pituitary radiation is most frequently administered in patients with persistent disease following surgery, but it has a limited ability to effect a prompt reduction in tumour size or in hormone hypersecretion.

Medical therapy

Bromocriptine improves clinical symptoms (70–90 per cent) and reduces GH concentrations during chronic treatment (approximately 70 per cent), but reduction of serum GH to less than 5 μg/l occurs in only a minority. Other effects include improvement in diabetic control or glucose intolerance, resolution of hyperprolactinaemia (if present), and improvement in visual field abnormalities. A larger dose is required to treat acromegaly than to treat hyperprolactinaemia; usually 10–20 mg per day (or higher) in divided doses, 4 times per day. A small dose should be used initially, with a gradual increase to minimize side-effects. Bromocriptine is particularly useful for treatment of patients with residual postoperative disease.

Somatostatin analogue

Somatostatin is a 14 amino acid cyclic peptide present in the brain, hypothalamus, pancreas, and in the gastrointestinal tract. In the hypothalamus it inhibits GH release, and intravenous administration of somatostatin produces a prompt reduction in serum GH concentrations in normal subjects and in patients with acromegaly. After cessation of the infusion, there is a rapid rise in serum GH, and a rebound hypersecretion in some acromegalics. Somatostatin must be administered by continuous intravenous infusion because its half-life is less than 3 min, thus making it impractical for clinical use. Octreotide, an 8 amino acid cyclic peptide analogue of somatostatin, has a serum half-life of approximately 90 min and suppresses GH release for up to 8 h in normal subjects and in acromegalic patients. Given subcutaneously it is 20-fold more suppressive of GH release than is the native peptide, and 22 times more suppressive of GH release than of insulin release. Despite its greater selectivity for GH, insulin release is decreased for approximately 3 h after administration, and postprandial hyperglycaemia may occur.

Octreotide has been used to treat acromegaly and other hypersecretory endocrine tumours since 1984. Several studies in a limited number of acromegalic patients, usually treated briefly, indicate that most patients have improvement in symptoms and signs and a reduction in serum GH and IGF-I concentrations, and a small number have had a reduction in pituitary tumour size. While some patients have suppression of GH and IGF-I concentrations to normal, others have only a partial suppression, a heterogeneity of response which is most likely dependent upon the density of somatostatin receptors on the adenoma and the binding affinity for octreotide.

The recommended octreotide dose is 100 μg every 8 h, but, some patients have adequate GH suppression with 100 μg/day, and others require as much as 1500 μg/day in divided doses. Some patients have a better response to continuous subcutaneous infusion than with intermittent injections. A good clinical response occurs in 70–88 per cent of patients; however, a mean 24-h GH concentration less than 5 μg/l is achieved in only about 50 per cent of patients. IGF-I concentrations are normalized in 45–68 per cent of patients. Additionally, a small number have greater GH suppression with the combination of octreotide and bromocriptine. The precise dose and frequency of administration should be adjusted according to the patient's response.

Octreotide inhibits gallbladder contractility and this may facilitate formation of gallstones. The incidence of gallstone formation or sludge during octreotide therapy is about 20 per cent. Since postprandial gallbladder motility is decreased by octreotide, a potential method of decreasing the risk of gallstone formation is administration of the drug 2–3 h after meals.

Prognosis

There are no studies which demonstrate that treatment of acromegaly leads to a reduction in the increased morbidity and premature mortality associated with this condition despite reversal of adverse metabolic effects. Earlier diagnosis and modern treatment are likely to improve outcome.

Cushing's disease

Cushing's syndrome, referred to as Cushing's disease when it is caused by an adenoma of the corticotroph cells of the anterior pituitary, or more rarely by corticotroph hyperplasia, is discussed in Chapter 7.6.

Nelson's syndrome

Nelson's syndrome is the result of accelerated growth of an underlying ACTH-secreting pituitary adenoma in patients who have undergone bilateral adrenalectomy for Cushing's disease. These patients develop symptoms of a mass, including headaches, visual field defects, and external ophthalmoplegia. The very high ACTH levels cause hyperpigmentation in the distribution of that seen in Addison's disease. The syndrome presumably results from the removal of the negative feedback of excessive cortisol from the adrenal glands. Its estimated incidence varies from 10–50 per cent. Some studies, but not all, suggest that the syndrome is preventable by external pituitary irradiation prior to or at the time of adrenalectomy.

The condition is suspected from the characteristic history and physical findings. Plasma ACTH levels are extremely high, often ranging from 220 pmol/l (1000 pg/ml) to 2202 pmol/l (10 000 pg/ml) or higher. However, the level of ACTH does not accurately reflect the size or aggressiveness of the tumour, the presence of which is confirmed by CT or MRI scan.

These tumours are locally invasive and grow rapidly, and urgent pituitary surgery by the trans-sphenoidal route is the preferred treatment. Pituitary irradiation is useful in those with residual tumour after surgery. ACTH secretion by the tumour is responsive to endogenous CRH and AVP. Thus, by optimizing negative feedback to the hypothalamus by both using a long-acting glucocorticoid and by judicious timing of its administration to reverse the normal glucocorticoid rhythm, hypothalamic stimulation of the tumour can be minimized; a suggested regimen is dexamethasone 0.5 mg on retiring. This approach has not been fully evaluated but it seems logical.

Glycoprotein-producing adenomata

Thyrotroph adenoma

The TSH adenoma is the least common type of pituitary tumour, representing less than 1 per cent of cases, and the only glycoprotein tumour producing a characteristic clinical syndrome. Common clinical features include symptoms referable to the pituitary mass lesion and/or hyperthyroidism with goitre. The tumour also frequently secretes free α-subunit, so that a molar ratio of α-subunit to TSH of greater than 1 is helpful in distinguishing a TSH-secreting adenoma from other forms of hyperthyroidism. Other secretory products of thyrotroph adenomas may include GH or prolactin. The diagnosis of acromegaly or hyperprolactinaemia may then only be evident when the patient seeks care for symptoms of hyperthyroidism. Increased concentrations of T_3 and T_4 are then associated with inappropriately normal or elevated serum TSH concentration measured by sensitive assays. Concentrations may be markedly increased; but values of less than 10 mU/l occur in 30 per cent of patients. It is in these cases that measurement of the serum α-subunit is particularly helpful. This assay also helps to exclude the syndrome of pituitary resistance to thyroid hormone in which serum concentrations of TSH (but not those of the α-subunit) are inappropriately increased in the setting of hyperthyroxinaemia. Administration of TRH may also help distinguish between these rare conditions. TRH given to patients with TSH-secreting tumours does not increase TSH, whereas the response in pituitary resistance to thyroid hormone is often exaggerated.

The ideal treatment of a TSH-secreting adenoma is surgical resection, but complete resection may not be possible and there may be a need for postoperative irradiation. Preliminary reports indicate that treatment with octreotide may lower serum TSH concentrations, but antithyroid drugs have to be used in some cases.

Gonadotroph adenoma

Gonadotroph adenomata are identified by either increased serum LH, FSH, and/or α-subunit concentrations or by *in vitro* studies of surgical specimens. The precise prevalence of gonadotroph adenomata is unknown. In a series of 139 men with macroadenomas, 24 per cent were gonadotroph tumours; 17 per cent had hypersecretion of FSH, either alone or in combination with LH α-, LH β-, and FSH β-subunits, and 7 per cent had hypersecretion of only the α-subunit. The majority of these men, 87 per cent, presented with visual impairment indicative of a large tumour. Other series report a lower prevalence of gonadotroph adenomata (<5 per cent).

The glycoprotein hormone most commonly secreted is FSH, accompanied or not by an increase in circulating α-subunit concentrations, which also occurs in association with tumours producing the LH β-subunit. Hypersecretion of intact LH occurs less commonly and an apparent increase in serum LH may also be the result of assay cross-reactivity with free α-subunit or LH β. In the majority of men with this kind of adenoma the serum testosterone concentration is either normal or below normal, since intact LH is not being produced. Hormone measurements then show inappropriately normal serum LH concentrations in the setting of reduced testosterone production; but when intact LH is produced, the serum testosterone concentration is above normal.

Administration of TRH may be helpful in diagnosis, since approximately 50 per cent of patients with a gonadotroph adenoma have an increase in LH or FSH after TRH stimulation. The FSH and LH responses to exogenous GnRH are variable; approximately 50 per cent of patients with an FSH-secreting tumour have an increase in serum FSH concentrations; an increase in serum LH occurs less frequently.

Gonadotroph adenomata are most commonly diagnosed in middle-aged men. It is not known if these tumours truly occur more frequently in men or whether they are more difficult to diagnose in women, for instance in the case of a postmenopausal woman with a pituitary tumour in whom increased LH and FSH levels are attributed to the menopause. The distinction between a non-secretory adenoma and a gonadotroph adenoma may then not be possible clinically or biochemically and may only be decided by electron microscopic or immunocytochemical studies of the excised tumour.

Diagnostic difficulty arises in men when the serum testosterone is below normal and the serum immunoreactive LH is increased from increased free α-subunit or LH β secretion with assay cross-reactivity; this pattern may then erroneously suggest the diagnosis of primary gonadal failure. The possibility of a gonadotroph tumour should always be considered in such a case if there is a history of headache or change in vision, when MRI or CT of the pituitary is indicated.

The initial treatment of a gonadotroph tumour is surgical resection, particularly if visual function is abnormal. Trans-sphenoidal surgery improves vision in the majority and may correct hormonal hypersecretion, hypogonadism, and the abnormal gonadotrophin response to TRH. Persistent hormonal hypersecretion and the presence of residual tumour may require postoperative pituitary radiation treatment. Medical treatment of gonadotroph adenomata has involved the use of bromocriptine, octreotide, and more recently, long-acting GnRH agonist and antagonist analogues.

Non-secretory adenoma

Apparently non-functioning pituitary tumours (chromophobe adenomas) have been reported in 25–30 per cent of cases. However, on morphological examination, these tumours often contain secretory granules, suggesting hormone synthesis and storage. Immunocytochemical and electron microscopic studies have identified many of them as gonadotroph, α-subunit, or corticotroph tumours, and immunocytochemistry and molecular biological techniques have revealed combinations including hCG-α, LH-β, FSH-α, TSH-β, and ACTH. The absence of increased serum hormone concentrations in such cases has been attributed to abnormal post-translational processing or the lack of specific glycoprotein subunit assays.

The majority of patients are diagnosed with symptoms and signs of a macroadenoma (headache, visual disturbance) or of hypopituitarism. These tumours occur most commonly in men and in postmenopausal women. A mild or moderate elevation of serum prolactin less than 1800 mIU/l (< 100 μg/l) often occurs and is thought to reflect stalk compression.

Pretreatment evaluation to determine hormone hypersecretion should include measurement of serum prolactin, IGF-I, LH, FSH, TSH, and α-subunit, and when assays are available, LH β-, FSH β-, and TSH β-subunit concentrations. The need for hormone replacement, particularly of cortisol and thyroxine, should be assessed by measuring basal thyroxine, cortisol and testosterone (men) concentrations. A normal morning cortisol concentration does not exclude secondary adrenal insufficiency and an insulin-induced hypoglycaemia or metyrapone test is required for accurate assessment. The precise anatomy of the tumour is best assessed by a gadolinium-enhanced MRI scan or coronal CT scan with contrast.

The treatment for a non-secretory tumour is surgical excision, usually via the trans-sphenoidal approach. Residual tumour is usually treated with postoperative supervoltage radiation. If the patient is unable to undergo surgery or the tumour is asymptomatic and intrasellar (uncommon) and vision is normal, pituitary radiation with careful monitoring of pituitary function, tumour size, and vision is an alternative. The response to pituitary radiation is similar to that of other pituitary tumours; prompt reduction in tumour size is rare but additional growth may be inhibited.

Medical treatment with the dopamine agonist drugs has been used in a small number of patients. Non-secretory tumours do possess high-affinity membrane-bound dopamine receptors, but they are fewer in number than in prolactin-secreting tumours, so that this approach is mostly unsuccessful.

Non-pituitary sellar masses

A number of lesions occur in the region of the hypothalamus and pituitary that are not pituitary tumours. These include craniopharyngioma, hypophysitis, apoplexy, aneurysm, Rathke's pouch cyst, arachnoid cyst, germinoma, chordoma, optic nerve glioma, reticulosis, meningioma, and secondary deposits. Only the first four will be discussed, as the management of the others follows standard medical lines. It is important to make the correct diagnosis since therapy is often quite different. Specifically, the trans-sphenoidal approach can be disastrous for some lesions, such as an internal carotid artery aneurysm. The advent of modern imaging techniques has greatly facilitated accurate diagnosis prior to therapeutic intervention.

Craniopharyngioma

A craniopharyngioma, or Rathke's pouch tumour, arises from embryonic squamous cell rests which persist after the upward migration of stomodeal epithelium to the anterior pituitary. Since a tumour may arise from any position along the craniopharyngioma canal, it may be intrasellar or extrasellar. The tumour is usually well encapsulated and composed of cystic and solid components. The cysts may be multiloculated and contain dark brown, oily fluid. These tumours may occur at any age, but are most common in children, accounting for 5–10 per cent of primary brain tumours in children. Approximately one-quarter are diagnosed after the age of 40 years.

Clinical presentation

Children are usually diagnosed because of growth failure, visual disturbance or with symptoms of increased intracranial pressure (headache, vomiting, somnolence). In adults most have visual symptoms or have visual abnormalities on examination. About 30 per cent also have disturbance of intellectual function which may cause dementia. Most also have some degree of hypopituitarism. Growth hormone and gonadotrophin deficiency are most common, but secondary hypothyroidism and corticotrophin deficiency are seen in more than 50 per cent. Diabetes insipidus may occur after surgical resection of the tumour.

Craniopharyngiomas are characteristically suprasellar. They may extend inferiorly into the sella turcica causing destruction of bony margins of the sella and dorsum sellae. They may also extend superiorly into the third ventricle, producing hydrocephalus from block at the foramen of Monro. Calcification of the tumour occurs in 70–90 per cent of children and 40–60 per cent of adults and is detectable on a CT scan, but not on an MRI scan. The solid portion of the tumour may enhance on CT scan after administration of intravenous contrast. The high cholesterol content of cyst fluid produces a characteristic MRI signal which may also aid diagnosis.

The primary treatment is surgical resection, which may be associated with considerable morbidity and mortality, usually from the standard surgical approach (craniotomy) and from diabetes insipidus and other hypothalamic–pituitary dysfunction. Recurrence is a definite risk. Since these tumours are relatively radioresistant and grow slowly, it is difficult to assess the efficacy of radiotherapy.

With increasing use of CT and MRI scans more relatively asymptomatic patients with a craniopharyngioma are being diagnosed. These patients present a therapeutic dilemma since a craniotomy is associated with substantial risks. If the patient is asymptomatic, an argument can be made for an anticipatory approach with careful follow-up, including a repeat imaging study at 6 months or 1 year. The interval between scans may be doubled if there has been no increase in tumour size.

Lymphocytic hypophysitis

This is a rare disorder of lymphocytic infiltration of the pituitary, associated with complete or partial hypopituitarism, a pituitary mass, and occurrence almost exclusively in women, often during pregnancy or in the postpartum period. A maternal death rate of approximately 50 per cent, most likely due to unrecognized secondary adrenal failure, emphasizes the need for consideration of this diagnosis in a pregnant or postpartum woman with symptoms of headache, visual disturbance, weakness, and fatigue.

Lymphocytic hypophysitis was first described in an autopsy specimen in 1962; fewer than 30 cases have been reported subsequently. Most of them were in the second or third trimester of pregnancy or up to 7 months postpartum. The clinical presentation was of symptoms and signs of pituitary dysfunction, frequently hypocortisolism, and of a pituitary mass. Pituitary deficiencies have included ACTH, TSH, LH, FSH, and vasopressin, either alone or in combination; an increased serum prolactin occurred in 50 per cent. The most common symptoms and signs of the mass were headache in the majority and visual field loss in 32 per cent. In those patients who underwent imaging studies, suprasellar extension of the mass was present in 64 per cent. Although the majority of women had permanent destruction of all or part of the pituitary and required chronic hormone replacement therapy, a report of one patient who had transient hypopituitarism of 12 months' duration suggests that total pituitary destruction may not always occur. These patients should therefore be evaluated at regular intervals to determine the necessity for continued hormone replacement.

The aetiology of lymphocytic hypophysitis is unknown, but several studies have suggested an autoimmune cause. Antipituitary antibodies were present in the sera of some women and others had other autoimmune endocrine disorders, including thyroiditis and adrenalitis. Another proposed aetiology is virus-induced autoimmune destruction of the gland as suggested by studies in animals. The common association with pregnancy has been attributed to increased exposure to pituitary antigens or changes in maternal immunological status.

Diagnosis requires surgical biopsy and histological examination of the tissue. Diffuse infiltration with lymphocytes and plasma cells, some areas of follicles with germinal centres, and destruction of normal pituitary cells are the characteristic morphological changes. The differential diagnosis of light microscopic findings includes sarcoidosis, syphilis, tuberculosis, granulomatous hypophysitis, and postpartum haemorrhagic infarction. Electron microscopy demonstrates the characteristic interdigitation of lymphocytes and pituitary cells, fusion of lysosomes and secretory granules, and swollen mitochondria indicative of oncocytic transformation. Treatment comprises the replacement of identified hormonal deficiencies.

Suprasellar germinoma (ectopic pinealoma)

This highly malignant tumour has no sex preponderance and appears to have an increased prevalence in Japan. It has been diagnosed in patients aged between 6 and 41 years, but is very rare over the age of 30 years. This tumour is of hypothalamic origin and is curable by radiotherapy. It is vital that the correct diagnosis is made, thus avoiding an unnecessary and likely destructive operation.

The tumour may originate in the ventral region of the hypothalamus, in association with a pineal tumour (either metastatic or multifocal origin), in the anterior third ventricle or, more rarely, in the pituitary fossa to mimic a pituitary tumour. Because of rapid growth and large size it often compresses the optic nerves and chiasm and extends inferiorly into the pituitary and sella. Extension into the third ventricle produces hydrocephalus.

Clinical presentation and diagnosis

At the time of diagnosis, diabetes insipidus is present in 83 per cent, visual disturbance in 78 per cent, headache in 50 per cent, and endocrine abnormalities, including growth retardation in 39 per cent and hypogonadism in 17 per cent of cases. Other symptoms include anorexia in 28 per cent and nausea and vomiting in 11 per cent of cases, which likely reflect hydrocephalus, electrolyte disturbances, and/or secondary adrenal or thyroid failure. This tumour is malignant, often multifocal, and may metastasize not only within the CNS, but extracranially, and also outside the CNS. For these reasons, staging is very important.

The radiological appearances are not distinctive. Usually a large mass is observed in the third ventricle, which extends superiorly and inferiorly. It may enhance with intravenous contrast on CT scan.

In addition to performing the same tests as in a patient with a pituitary tumour, serum β-hCG should be measured and if elevated is suggestive of a germinoma. If the level is undetectable, germinoma is not excluded and a cerebrospinal fluid sample should be obtained for cytological examination and measurement of glucose, protein, β-hCG and alpha-fetoprotein. Expected results are malignant cells, elevated serum protein, and increased concentrations of hCG and alpha-fetoprotein. This is sufficient to make the diagnosis, which is confirmed by the rapid reduction in the size of the lesion with as little as 5 Gy of radiation.

Therapy

The first step is to correct any hormonal deficiencies. If there is likely to be a delay in obtaining the results, glucocorticoid and thyroid hormone replacement should be given; these can always be discontinued if the results are normal. Diabetes insipidus should be promptly treated with desmopressin. If the thirst centre is intact and if the patient is alert, he/she will usually be able to drink an adequate amount of fluid, but loss of thirst does occur and leads to great difficulty in maintaining water balance.

Because of the location of this tumour and its propensity to metastasize in the CNS, surgery is not likely to effect a cure. It may be required to relieve hydrocephalus, but the risk of seeding tumour cells must be considered and it should be only performed if high-dose steroids and radiation therapy have failed. Any surgery of the hypothalamus can potentially damage remaining hypothalamic centres. If the diagnosis is uncertain, a therapeutic trial of 5 Gy radiation may be administered. If within 14 days the tumour decreases in size, the diagnosis is confirmed since other types of masses are not that sensitive to radiation therapy. A full course of radiation therapy to the whole brain and spinal cord is then recommended. If there is evidence of peripheral metastases, chemotherapy may also be indicated. Cis-platin based chemotherapy appears to hold promise; in children and adolescents this may be followed, in good responders, with a lower dose of radiotherapy to avoid adverse effects of radiation therapy.

Pituitary apoplexy

Pituitary apoplexy is classically defined as an acute, life-threatening infarction of the pituitary gland. Haemorrhagic infarction most commonly occurs in the presence of a pituitary tumour but may also occur spontaneously in a normal gland, after obstetric haemorrhage (Sheehan's syndrome), in the setting of increased intracranial pressure or systemic anticoagulation therapy. Other predisposing factors include diabetes mellitus, bleeding disorders, following pituitary radiation, pneumoencephalography, carotid angiography, mechanical ventilation, trauma, and upper respiratory infection. Sheehan's syndrome may result from occlusive arterial spasm of the arteries supplying the anterior lobe and infundibulum. After a period of complete ischaemia, revascularization and vascular congestion with thrombosis of the anterior lobe is observed.

Pituitary infarction usually produces anterior pituitary dysfunction, which may be permanent or transient, with the degree of impairment being dependent upon the amount of tissue destruction. Hormone deficiencies include GH (88 per cent), gonadotrophins (58–76 per cent), and corticotrophin (66 per cent). Secondary hypothyroidism occurs in 42–53 per cent and abnormal prolactin secretion is present in 67–100 per cent. Diabetes insipidus is uncommon, occurring in only 2–3 per cent of patients.

The precise incidence of pituitary infarction and haemorrhage is unknown. In unselected autopsy studies, infarction of more than 25 per cent of the gland was present in 1–3 per cent of specimens. The frequency of apoplexy in patients with a known pituitary tumour was 17 per cent in one series of 560 patients undergoing pituitary surgery; 8 per cent had no clinical symptoms of haemorrhage. Imaging studies of patients with a known pituitary tumour using CT and MRI scans indicate that intratumoural haemorrhage can occur without clinical evidence of apoplexy. The pattern of tumour growth, the size of the tumour, and the amount of haemorrhage and oedema within the gland determine the clinical symptomatology.

Infarction with haemorrhage and oedema may cause rapid expansion of the lesion with compression of surrounding structures and abnormal neurological function. In a conscious patient, the initial symptom is usually a severe retro-orbital headache which is frequently accompanied by nausea and vomiting. Extravasation of blood or necrotic tissue into the subarachnoid space may cause meningeal irritation, fever, alteration of consciousness, or coma. Superior expansion produces compression of the optic chiasm and/or optic nerve(s) with development of visual field loss and/or decreased visual acuity. Lateral expansion into the cavernous sinus may produce dysfunction of cranial nerves III, IV, VI, and the first division of cranial nerve V, most commonly the third nerve. If expansion causes mechanical compression of the carotid siphon against the anterior clinoid process, hemispheric dysfunction, including seizures and hemiplegia, may result. Hemispheric dysfunction may also occur with vasospasm secondary to irritation from subarachnoid haemorrhage.

Evaluation of a patient with a sudden change in sensorium, headache, ophthalmoplegic or visual loss, or prostration should include an immediate imaging study of the pituitary area and orbits, either a non-contrast enhanced CT scan or an MRI scan. A CT scan may be superior to visualize intratumoural haemorrhage within the first few days of the event, but an MRI scan is more sensitive in detecting and following the haemorrhage in the subacute stage.

If pituitary apoplexy is suspected, the patient should be presumed to have anterior pituitary insufficiency and treated accordingly. Blood should be obtained for measurement of serum cortisol and thyroxine, and glucocorticoid treatment should be instituted immediately. The dose must be adequate for the stress of the illness and presumptive cerebral oedema (for example dexamethasone 2 mg every 6 h). If there are significant visual deficits or altered sensorium, neurosurgical intervention may be required. Immediate surgical decompression of the haemorrhage and tumour affords the opportunity for recovery of visual deficits and alleviation of increased intracranial pressure. After recovery from surgery the patient should undergo a complete endocrinological evaluation to determine the nature and degree of residual hormone deficits. Since these may be transient, re-evaluation is sensible several months after the event.

Surgical decompression may not be necessary in the setting of normal sensorium and visual function. The patient should be treated with glucocorticoid replacement, and needs serial ophthalmological and imaging examinations.

Further reading

Cuneo, R.C., Salomon, F., McGauley, G.A., and Sonksen, P.H. (1992). The growth hormone deficiency syndrome in adults. *Clinical Endocrinology* (Oxford), **37**, 387–97.

Melmed, S., Braunstein, G.D., Horvath, E., *et al.* (1983). Pathophysiology of acromegaly. (Review.) *Endocrinology Reviews*, **4**, 271–90.

Orth, D.N. and Kovacs, W.J. (1998). The adrenal cortex. In *Williams textbook of endocrinology*, 9th edn (ed. J.D. Wilson, D.W. Foster, H.M. Kronenberg, and P.R. Larsen), pp. 517–664. W.B. Saunders, Philadelphia.

Thapar, K. and Laws, E.R., Jnr (1995). Pituitary tumors. In *Brain tumors* (ed. A.H. Kaye and E.R. Laws, Jnr). Churchill Livingstone, London.

Thorner, M.O., Vance, M.L., Laws, E.R., Jnr, *et al.* (1998). The anterior pituitary. In *Williams textbook of endocrinology*, 9th edn (ed. J.D. Wilson, D.W. Foster, H.M. Kronenberg, and P.R. Larsen), pp. 249–340. W.B. Saunders, Philadelphia.

Vance, M.L. (1994). Hypopituitarism. *New England Journal of Medicine*, **330**, 1651–62.

Chapter 7.2

The posterior pituitary (see also Chapter 12.2)

P. H. Baylis

Neuroanatomy of the posterior pituitary

The two major peptides secreted by the posterior pituitary are arginine vasopressin (AVP), the antidiuretic hormone of most mammals including man, and oxytocin. Both are synthesized principally in magnocellular neurones of the supraoptic and paraventricular nuclei of the hypothalamus (Fig. 1). Neuronal pathways from these nuclei pass to the posterior pituitary; the median eminence of the hypothalamus; the brainstem and spinal cord; the floor of the third ventricle; and throughout the brain substance.

Afferent sensory tracts to the nuclei control peptide synthesis and secretion. Osmotically sensitive cells in the organum vasculosum of the lamina terminalis (OVLT), the putative osmoreceptor, situated in the anterior hypothalamus, transmit information mainly to the supraoptic nucleus. AVP secretion is also influenced by baroregulatory afferents from the great vessels in the chest and heart, and oxytocin by sensory input from the nipples and female genital tract.

Chemistry of arginine vasopressin and oxytocin

Both AVP and oxytocin are nonapeptides. Their genes are located on chromosome 20, only a few kilobases apart, and, interestingly, are transcribed in opposing directions. Three exons encode the large precursor molecule which contains signal peptide, nonapeptide with its specific neurophysin (the carrier protein within the neuronal tracts), and, for AVP, a glycoprotein moiety. Following synthesis in the cell bodies of the hypothalamic nuclei, the precursors are processed as they migrate along the tracts to secrete AVP or oxytocin separate from their specific neurophysins into the systemic circulation from the posterior pituitary, or into the portal blood from the median eminence to influence anterior pituitary function.

The molecular weights of AVP and oxytocin are 1084 and 1007 Da, respectively. Both circulate unbound to proteins and have short half-lives of the order of 5–15 min. AVP is metabolized principally in the liver and kidneys, and oxytocin in the uterus, liver, and kidneys.

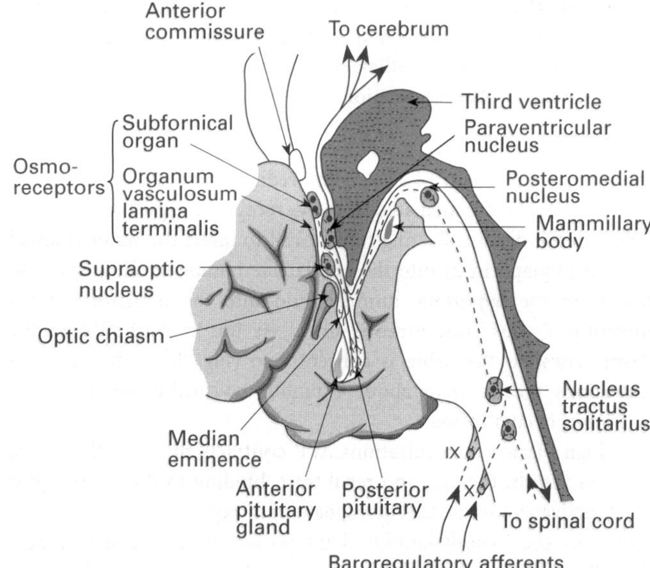

Fig. 1 Schematic representation of the posterior pituitary, supraoptic, and paraventricular nuclei, and surrounding neuroanatomical structures. Major efferent pathways (—) pass to the posterior pituitary, the median eminence, floor of the third ventricle, brainstem, spinal cord, and brain substance. Afferent sensory pathways (- - -) arise from the osmoreceptors and brainstem nuclei. IX and X, glossopharyngeal and vagus nerves).

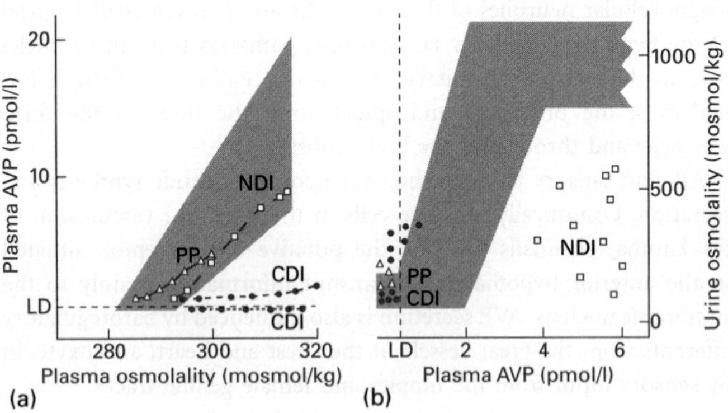

Fig. 2 (a) Relationship between plasma AVP and osmolality after infusion with hypertonic saline. Shaded area represents the normal response, patients with cranial diabetes insipidus (CDI (●)), nephrogenic diabetes insipidus (NDI (□)), and primary polydipsia (PP (△)). (b) Relationship between urine osmolality and plasma arginine vasopressin after dehydration. Shaded area represents the normal response, CDI, NDI, PP. LD, limit of detection of the AVP assay.

Arginine vasopressin

Physiology

Control of arginine vasopressin secretion

The principal determinant of AVP secretion is blood osmolality, which is sensed in the region of the OVLT. There is an exquisitely sensitive linear relationship between increasing plasma osmolality and AVP release (Fig. 2(a)). As the concentration of AVP in the plasma rises, renal water excretion is reduced, thus lowering plasma osmolality, a mechanism which maintains plasma osmolality within the narrow range of 284–295 mosmol/kg.

Reductions in blood pressure and/or volume stimulate AVP release in an exponential manner, which can result in a massive release of this hormone following severe acute hypotension. Baroreceptors in the carotid arteries, aorta, heart, and great veins mediate the pressure/volume changes via the vagus and glossopharyngeal nerves, the brainstem nuclei, and hypothalamus. Nausea and/or emesis are also potent stimuli of AVP secretation.

Actions of AVP

The main renal action of AVP is the reduction of solute-free water excretion. Its effect is mediated by the V_2 receptor coupled to adenylate cyclase in the distal collecting tubular cell to insert the water channel proteins (aquaporin 2) into the cellular membrane to allow water to flow from the hypotonic luminal fluid into the hypertonic renal interstitium, thus concentrating urine. As the level of AVP in the plasma rises, so the urine is concentrated (Fig. 2(b)), but at concentrations greater than about 4 pmol/l no further urinary concentration occurs in man.

At high plasma concentrations AVP contracts the smooth muscle of blood vessels, the gut, and renal tract, binding to the V_{1a} receptor which activates the inositol phosphate pathways.

AVP in the hypothalamopituitary portal circulation acts synergistically with corticotrophin releasing factor to stimulate adrenocorticophin release from the anterior pituitary gland (V_{1b} receptor).

Thirst

In addition to a normal AVP osmoregulatory system and a healthy kidney responsive to this hormone, normal water homeostasis is dependent on a thirst mechanism. This is particularly evident when the body continues to lose water despite maximal urine concentration when a mechanism to increase fluid intake is essential. The osmoregulatory control of thirst appreciation is similar to that of AVP. Thirst osmoreceptors, probably distinct from AVP osmoreceptors, are sited in the anterior hypothalamus.

Table 1 Causes of cranial diabetes insipidus

Causes
Familial
Dominant (rarely recessive) inheritance
DIDMOAD syndrome[a]
Acquired
Idiopathic
Trauma (neurosurgery, head injury)
Tumour (craniopharyngioma, large pituitary tumour, germinoma, metastasis to hypothalamus, pinealoma)
Granuloma (sarcoidosis, histiocytosis X, eosinophilic granuloma)
Lymphocytic infiltration of neurohypophysis
Infection (meningitis, encephalitis)
Vascular (aneurysm, infarction, sickle-cell anaemia, Sheehan's syndrome)

[a] DIDMOAD; diabetes insipidus, diabetes mellitus, optic atrophy, deafness.

Disorders of AVP secretion

Deficiency of AVP

Cranial diabetes insipidus results from decreased secretion of osmoregulated AVP. Patients develop polyuria (urine volumes 3–20 l/24 h) and polydipsia. They rely upon an intact thirst mechanism and adequate fluid to maintain water homeostasis. Destruction of at least 80 per cent of the hypothalamic neurones is necessary before symptoms appear. The causes of cranial diabetes insipidus are given in Table 1. The familial causes are very rare, some of which are due to point mutations in the AVP. At least 30 per cent of all cases are idiopathic.

Diagnosis of cranial diabetes insipidus

Abnormal thirst and polyuria may be caused by vasopressin deficiency, renal resistance to the antidiuretic effect of vasopressin, or primary increased drinking (primary polydipsia; compulsive polydipsia). The fluid deprivation test is the most commonly used investigation to distinguish these three disorders, although confusing results from the test occur frequently.

Confirmation of polyuria (urine output greater than 3 l/24 h) is wise prior to performing the fluid deprivation test (Table 2). Patients who fail to concentrate urine to above 750 mosmol/kg after dehydration, but do so following desmopressin, have cranial diabetes insipidus. Unfortunately, many patients with this disorder have equivocal results. A definitive diagnosis of cranial diabetes insipidus can be made by infusing 5 per cent hypertonic saline to increase plasma osmolality. Subnormal plasma AVP values confirm the diagnosis (Fig. 2(a)). The other causes of polyuria can be differentiated by AVP measurements (Fig. 2(a,b)).

Alternatively, a carefully supervised therapeutic trial of low dose desmopressin may suggest a diagnosis of cranial diabetes insipidus, with such a patient improving symptomatically and remaining normonatraemic, in contrast to those with nephrogenic diabetes insipidus whose symptoms and biochemistry fail to improve, and those with primary polydipsia who become progressively hyponatraemic.

Table 2 Fluid deprivation test

Preparation of patient Fluid intake encouraged during the night before the test Light breakfast—no tea, coffee, alcohol, smoking for 12 h before or during the test Constant supervision of the patient throughout the test
Response to dehydration No fluid for up to 8 h—dry snacks allowed Patient weighed hourly—stop test if there is a 5 per cent loss of initial body weight Urine samples hourly—measure volume and osmolality Blood drawn hourly—measure plasma osmolality (and plasma AVP if possible)
Response to exogenous vasopressin After dehydration, administer desmopressin (DDAVP®) 2 µg intramuscularly Urine samples at 3, 5, and 16 h after desmopressin—measure volume and osmolality Blood drawn at 5 and 16 h—measure plasma osmolality Patient allowed to eat and drink up to twice the urine volume passed during dehydration

Treatment of cranial diabetes insipidus

Desmopressin (DDAVP®) is the treatment of choice. It is administered orally (100–1000 µg daily in divided doses), intranasally at a dose of 5–40 µg once to three times daily, or parenterally up to 4 µg daily. Desmopressin is a long-acting synthetic analogue of AVP with no pressor activity and twice the antidiuretic action of the natural hormone. Hyponatraemia is the only significant adverse effect due to overdosage. Lysine vasopressin is rarely given as it has a short period of action (4 h) and possesses pressor activity that can lead to renal or intestinal colic. There is no place for the chlorpropamide, thiazides, clofibrate, or carbamazepine in the treatment of cranial diabetes insipidus.

Syndrome of inappropriate antidiuresis

The commonest cause of normovolaemic hyponatraemia (see also Chapter 12.2) is the syndrome of inappropriate antidiuresis (SIAD), due most often to posterior pituitary or ectopic secretion of AVP which is persistent and inappropriate in relation to the normal physiological mechanisms that regulate its release.

SIAD presents with hyponatraemia (serum sodium less than 130 mmol/l). Moderate chronic hyponatraemia (serum sodium 120–130 mmol/l) is usually asymptomatic, but clinical features became increasingly severe as the serum sodium approaches 100 mmol/l. They range from mild anorexia and nausea, through symptoms of drowsiness, cramps, and confusion, to convulsions, coma, and death. Rapid falls in serum sodium lead to clinical features at higher absolute sodium values.

Diagnosis of SIAD

The diagnosis should only be made if the criteria established by Bartter and Schwartz are fulfilled (Table 3). Although detectable plasma AVP is consistent with the diagnosis of SIAD it is not in itself diagnostic. A large number of conditions and drugs have been purported to cause this syndrome, some of which are given in Table 4.

Osmoregulatory studies on patients with SIAD have indicated two common patterns of AVP secretion. The first shows erratic release of AVP with dissociation between plasma osmolality and the hormone; the second indicates AVP secretion with increasing plasma osmolality but occurring around a lower absolute plasma osmolality, i.e. a shift to the left of the normal relationship.

Table 3 Cardinal features of the syndrome of inappropriate antidiuresis

Hyponatraemia with appropriately low plasma osmolality
Urine osmolality greater than plasma osmolality
Persistent excessive renal sodium excretion
Absence of hypotension, hypovolaemia, and oedema-forming states
Normal renal and adrenal function

Table 4 Some causes of the syndrome of inappropriate antidiuresis

Malignant disease	*Central nervous system disorders*
Carcinoma	Meningitis, encephalitis
Lymphoma	Head injury
Leukaemia	Brain tumour, abscess
Thymoma	Subarachnoid haemorrhage
Sarcoma	Cerebral thrombosis
Mesothelioma	Guillain–Barré syndrome
Chest disorders	*Miscellaneous*
Pneumonia	Drugs: AVP, chlorpropamide, carbamazepine, cytotoxics, oxytocin
Tuberculosis	Miscellaneous
Empyema	Porphyria
Asthma	ACTH deficiency
Pneumothorax	Acute psychosis
Positive-pressure ventilation	Idiopathic

Treatment of SIAD

The underlying cause should be treated whenever possible (Table 4). Mild chronic asymptomatic hyponatraemia (serum sodium greater than 120 mmol/l) does not necessarily require specific therapy. If hyponatraemia is life-threatening or associated with significant clinical features, therapy is necessary. Fluid restriction to about 500 ml/24 h may be all that is required in mild cases. Drugs (for example, phenytoin) to suppress neurohypophyseal AVP secretion have met with limited success. The antidiuretic action of AVP may be blunted by democlocycline (600–1200 mg daily) or the more toxic and less reliable lithium; both induce nephrogenic diabetes insipidus. The linear nonpeptide V_2 antagonist, OPC-31260, appears to be a specific aquaretic drug of great therapeutic promise. Infusion of hypertonic saline to increase serum sodium in *chronic* hyponatraemia is dangerous, and may cause demyelination.

Whatever method is used to raise serum sodium in chronic hyponatraemia, it is essential that the rate of increase is no greater than 0.5 mmol/l/h or 10 mmol/l/24 h. Rapid correction can lead to osmotic demyelination in central pontine and/or extrapontine structures. Neurological sequelae or death may occur up to 4 days after correction of hyponatraemia (see Chapter 12.2).

Thirst deficiency

Hypodipsia or adipsia is an uncommon condition due to damage to the anterior hypothalamic thirst osmoreceptors, which leads to chronic hypernatraemia (serum sodium greater than 150 mmol/l). Causes include vascular lesions (such as haemorrhage from an anterior communicating artery aneurysm), hypothalamic metastatic or granulomatous disease, or trauma. Defective osmoregulation of AVP may also occur, greatly complicating management.

A complete osmoreceptor defect leads to intra- and extracellular dehydration causing life-threatening hypernatraemia (serum sodium up to 190 mmol/l). Slow rehydration is vital to avoid cerebral oedema, convulsions, and death. Long-term therapy is difficult but requires controlled fluid intake of 2–3 l/24 h to maintain constant body weight.

In 'essential' hypernatraemia, osmoregulation of thirst and AVP secretion is maintained around plasma osmolalities higher than normal, i.e. a shift to the right (Fig. 2(a)). Hypernatraemia is discussed in greater detail in Chapter 12.2.

Oxytocin

Control of oxytocin secretion

The precise physiological control of oxytocin release is poorly defined. Stimulation of the nipple leads to oxytocin secretion and milk ejection of the lactating breast (the suckling reflex), which is probably mediated by spinothalamic afferent fibres. The Ferguson reflex, release of oxytocin following cervical distension of the pregnant uterus, may initiate parturition.

Actions of oxytocin

The effects of oxytocin are confined mainly to pregnancy and the postpartum period. In addition to contraction of myoepithelial cells surrounding breast ducts, oxytocin stimulates contraction of the uterine myometrium, binding to specific receptors. During pregnancy, the numbers of these receptors increase, and the placenta secretes an enzyme, oxytocinase, which degrades avidly circulating oxytocin and AVP. It is unlikely that oxytocin is the sole initiator of labour, but plasma oxytocin concentrations increase substantially during its final stages, to expel the placenta and maintain uterine contraction.

There are no significant physiological actions of oxytocin in men or non-pregnant, non-lactating women. Even in pregnancy the role of oxytocin does not appear to be essential, as patients with posterior pituitary hormone deficiency have normal pregnancy, labour, and lactation. No disorders of oxytocin deficiency or excess have been described, despite the occurrence of some tumours synthesizing and releasing oxytocin ectopically.

Clinical use of oxytocin

Infusion of oxytocin in increasing doses is used routinely to initiate and maintain labour. A significant adverse effect can occur when high doses are administered with large volumes of intravenous fluid, which causes rapid profound acute hyponatraemia, leading to convulsions. This is due to low-affinity binding of oxytocin to the arginine vasopressin V_2 renal receptor, resulting in antidiuresis.

Further reading

Baylis, P.H. (1998). Disorders of water balance. In *Clinical endocrinology*, 2nd edn (ed. A. Grossman), pp. 265–78.

Fried, L.F. and Palevsky, P.M. (1997). Hyponatremia and hypernatremia. *Medical Clinics of North America* **81**, 585–609.

Robertson, G.L. (1995). Diabetes Insipidus. Clinical disorders of fluid and electrolyte metabolism. *Endocrinology and Metabolism Clinics of North America* **24**, 549–72.

Verbalis, J.G. (1992). Hyponatraemia: endocrinologic causes and consequences of therapy. *Trends in Endocrinology and Metabolism* **3**, 1–7.

The thyroid

Chapter 7.3

The thyroid gland and disorders of thyroid function

A. M. McGregor

Structure of the thyroid

The thyroid gland consists of two lobes connected by an isthmus, with the normal adult gland in an iodine replete population weighing 15–20 g. The gland is attached to the anterior and lateral aspects of the trachea by loose connective tissue such that the isthmus lies just below the cricoid cartilage. The recurrent laryngeal nerves lie in the grooves between the lateral lobes and the trachea and the lateral extent of the thyroid lobes are marked by the carotid sheaths and sternocleidomastoid muscles. The gland is supplied by the superior and inferior thyroid arteries on each side, and has both adrenergic and cholinergic innervation.

The basic functional unit of the thyroid gland is the follicle (Fig. 1). These hollow, spherical structures ranging in size from 15–500 μm

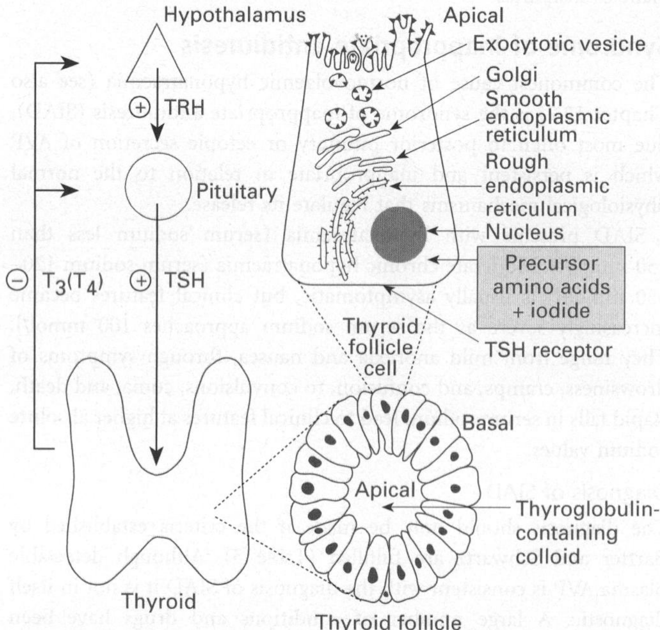

Fig. 1 The basic functional unit of the thyroid gland is the thyroid follicle which is involved in the synthesis and storage of thyroglobulin and its iodination to form thyroid hormones. These processes are closely regulated by interaction between the thyroid and the hypothalamic–pituitary axis.

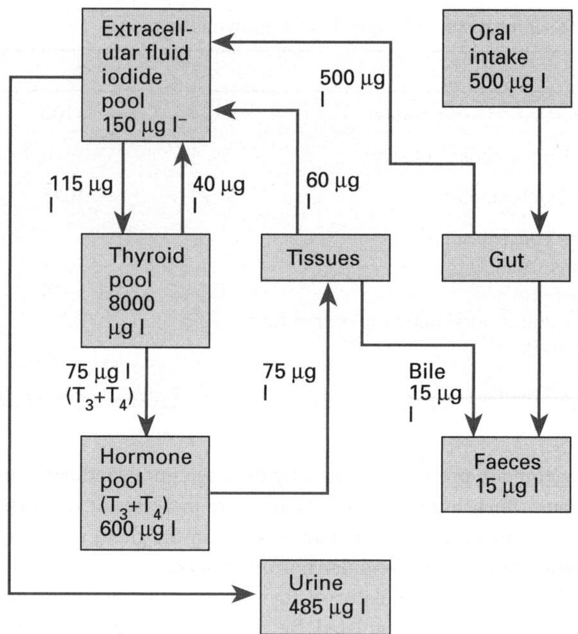

Fig. 2 Iodine metabolism in a healthy subject ingesting 500 μg of iodine daily.

in diameter are surrounded by a basement membrane. The wall of the unit is made up of a single layer of thyroid follicular cells, which are cuboidal when quiescent. The lumen of the follicle contains the proteinaceous colloid which is normally the major constituent of the thyroid mass and serves as the primary site of storage of thyroglobulin. The rich capillary network surrounding the follicles and the high blood flow through the gland ensure easy access of thyroid hormone to the circulation. Interspersed between the thyroid follicles are the parafollicular C cells which secrete calcitonin.

Function

Iodine metabolism (Fig. 2)

The thyroid requires iodide for hormone synthesis. Adequate dietary intake of iodide is therefore essential. Although mechanisms for conserving iodine exist, in iodine deficiency they are not always capable of preventing depletion. When natural levels of iodide are insufficient the iodination of water or food products, such as bread and salt, ensure adequate intake. Medications, diagnostic agents, and dietary supplements are also potential sources of iodine.

Iodine intake varies widely across the world. In western Europe a level of 200 μg/day is considered optimal, although the range of intake in adults across areas of the world in which iodine deficiency is not severe enough to impair thyroid hormonogenesis is from 50–1000 μg/day. Iodine is almost completely absorbed in the gastrointestinal tract where it enters the inorganic iodide pool in the extracellular fluid. Provided renal function is normal, inorganic iodide is rapidly cleared from the extracellular fluid with a half-life of about 2 h. Besides dietary iodide, a small contribution to the extracellular fluid iodide pool is made by iodide released following the deiodination of thyroid hormones in peripheral tissues and the leak of inorganic iodide from the thyroid gland. Iodide clearance from the extracellular pool is via the thyroid and the kidney. The thyroid is able to regulate the amount of iodide it clears, taking up only as much as is required for hormone synthesis. In so doing it is able to buffer itself against marked changes in dietary iodide intake, taking up relatively less from the extracellular pool when iodide is ingested in excess and relatively more when intake declines.

The major iodine pool in the body is the organic component synthesized by the thyroid follicular cell and stored as iodinated thyroglobulin in the colloid within the follicular lumen. When dietary iodine intake is in the range of 500 μg daily an equivalent amount will be cleared into the urine over the same period in its inorganic form. On this intake the removal of iodide from the extracellular pool by the thyroid ensures the maintenance of a thyroid pool of iodine of about 8000 μg which turns over slowly at about 1 per cent/day. From this pool the thyroid secretes about 75 μg of organic iodine per day in the form of the thyroid hormones, predominantly thyroxine (T_4) with a small amount of triiodothyronine (T_3), and this intravascular pool of thyroid hormones contains about 600 μg of iodine. Cellular uptake of thyroid hormones is of the order of 75 μg of iodine per day, of which about 60 μg re-enters the extracellular fluid iodide pool following intracellular deiodination of the thyroid hormones, and the remainder of the iodine is excreted in the faeces.

Thyroid hormone synthesis and secretion

A poorly characterized (trapping) mechanism ensures that sufficient iodide is available for hormone formation. This process is enhanced by thyroid stimulating hormone, thyrotropin (TSH) and is responsive to the glandular content of organic iodine. The mechanism for concentrating iodide is shared by perchlorate and pertechnetate.

Once iodide is trapped within the thyroid follicular cell, it is rapidly oxidized in the presence of hydrogen peroxide by thyroid peroxidase. Oxidation is followed by the incorporation of the resulting reactive intermediate into the tyrosine residues of thyroglobulin (iodide organification). Thyroid peroxidase is predominantly localized on the apical border of the thyroid cell where organification probably occurs.

Oxidation and organification of iodide result in the formation of hormonally inactive iodotyrosines (monoiodotyrosine and diiodotyrosine). The coupling of these leads to the formation of the hormonally active iodothyronines T_4 and T_3. The synthesis of T_4 results from the fusion of two molecules of diiodotyrosine, whereas that of T_3 results from the coupling of one molecule of monoiodotyrosine with one of diiodotyrosine. Thyroid peroxidase plays a key role, not only in the catalysis of the iodination of tyrosyl residues in thyroglobulin but also in the coupling of iodotyrosyl residues to form T_4 and T_3.

Thyroglobulin, the main precursor of thyroid hormones, is a large glycoprotein molecule present in the follicular luminal colloid in multiple forms, with the major source of thyroid hormone being the 19S molecule with a molecular size of 660 kDa. There are approximately three to four T_4 molecules per mole of human thyroglobulin under conditions of normal iodination, but only one in five molecules of human thyroglobulin contains a T_3 residue. Following transcription and processing of thyroglobulin mRNA and its ribosomal translation, the resulting polypeptide chain is extruded into the endoplasmic reticulum and glycosylated during transport to the Golgi apparatus. Packaging of the thyroglobulin into exocytotic vesicles in the Golgi apparatus then allows the transport of the protein in these vesicles (which also contain membrane-bound thyroid peroxidase) to the apical surface of the follicular cell, where the contents are released into the colloid-containing follicular lumen. The process of thyroglobulin biosynthesis and exocytosis is regulated by TSH.

Table 1 Situations that impair T_4 to T_3 conversion

Physiological	Pharmacological
Fetal/early neonate	Propylthiouracil
Pathological	Glucocorticoids
Fasting/malnutrition	Propranolol
Severe systemic illness	Amiodarone
Hepatic or renal impairment	Iodinated radiographic contrast media
Trauma	
Postoperative hypercatabolic state	

For thyroid hormone to be secreted into the circulation, thyroglobulin from the large colloid reservoir needs to re-enter the thyroid follicular cell where it undergoes proteolytic cleavage with the release of T_4 and T_3, which leave the thyroid follicular cell at its basal surface to enter the capillary circulation. This process is activated by TSH with the formation of pseudopodia induced on the apical surface of the follicular cells which engulf colloid to produce colloid-containing endocytotic vesicles within the follicular cell. The subsequent fusion of enzyme-containing lysosomes with these droplets leads to the hydrolysis of thyroglobulin and the liberation of the iodotyrosines from the thyroglobulin.

Thyroid hormone transport and metabolism

Of the iodothyronines circulating in the plasma, T_4 is the most abundant and is the only one that arises solely by direct secretion from the thyroid gland. Very little T_3 is secreted, most of it in plasma being derived from the peripheral conversion of T_4 by enzymatic monodeiodination. Of the remaining iodothyronines and their derivatives, of importance is reverse T_3, which is generated almost entirely in the peripheral tissues from T_4. Within the circulation, T_4 and T_3 are reversibly bound to a variety of proteins synthesized by the liver including thyroxine-binding globulin, thyroxine-binding prealbumin, transthyretin, and, to a smaller extent, albumin. Of the thyroid hormones present in the plasma, only about 0.04 per cent of T_4 and 0.4 per cent of T_3 circulate in the unbound state (free). Of the binding proteins, thyroxine-binding globulin is responsible for the transport of about 75 per cent of T_4. Changes in binding protein concentration, or in the ability of these proteins to bind thyroid hormones, are important considerations in the context of the interpretation of measurements of thyroid hormones in plasma.

The most important pathway for the metabolism of T_4 is its conversion to the biologically active hormone T_3. Up to 90 per cent of T_3 production results from deiodination of T_4, which utilizes up to 40 per cent of the secreted T_4. Virtually all the reverse T_3 is produced by the mono-deiodination of T_4, accounting for a further 40 per cent of the secreted T_4, the remaining 20 per cent being excreted in the urine or faeces. Other deiodination reactions of T_4 and T_3 lead to the generation of inactive products. A number of factors impair the peripheral conversion of T_4 to T_3 (Table 1).

The fractional rate of turnover of T_4 is normally about 10 per cent per day (half-life 6.7 days). This relatively slow rate is a reflection of the extent to which T_4 is bound. In contrast, T_3 is cleared rapidly from plasma (Table 2) with a turnover rate of about 60 per cent per day (half-life 0.75 days).

Regulation of thyroid function

The thyroid participates with the hypothalamus and pituitary in a classical feedback control system (Fig. 1 and Chapter 7.1). Fluctuations in secretion are prevented in part by the large intraglandular store of hormone which buffers the effects of acute increases or decreases in synthesis. Autoregulatory mechanisms within the gland maintain the constancy of the intraglandular hormone pool.

Table 2 Comparison of T_3 and T_4 in a euthyroid human

	T_3	T_4
Production rate (nmol/day)	34	100
Relative metabolic potency	1	0.3
Body pool (nmol)	71	1023
Serum concentration		
Total (nmol/l)	1.2–2.8	70–150
Free (pmol/l)	3–9	9–25
Fraction of total hormone in free form ($\times 10^{-2}$)	0.3	0.02
Half-life (days)	0.75	7.0

TSH is the major regulator of thyroid structure and function. Its secretion, in turn, is regulated by thyrotropin releasing hormone (TRH) from the hypothalamus which stimulates the pituitary thyrotroph to release and later synthesize TSH.

TSH is composed of a 14 kDa α-subunit in common with LH, follicle stimulating hormone (FSH) and human chorionic gonadotropin (hCG), and a specific β-subunit. It is secreted in both 1–2-hourly pulses and with a circadian rhythm which is characterized by a nocturnal surge which precedes the onset of sleep. By binding to the TSH receptor on the thyroid follicular cells, TSH activates thyroid function, predominantly through adenylate cyclase. A number of key elements of thyroid cell function have been demonstrated to be responsive to TSH stimulation; these include iodide transport and organification, the release of thyroglobulin into the follicular lumen, increased pseudopod formation on the apical cell border allowing endocytosis of colloid, lysosome maturation, thyroid hormone secretion, and, with chronic stimulation, hyperplasia and thyroid growth. Autoregulatory control mechanisms are assumed to be at work when the level of TSH remains constant.

The influence of iodine on the rate of thyroid hormone synthesis is determined by the amount and duration of administration of iodine. With increasing doses given acutely, the initial increase in the organification of iodine is followed by a decrease (the acute Wolff–Chaikoff effect). As a result, overproduction of thyroid hormone is prevented. Chronic repeated lower dose iodide administration allows 'escape' from this process, thus preventing the development of goitrous hypothyroidism. Pharmacological doses of iodine will, in addition, rapidly inhibit thyroid hormone release. This acute effect occurs much more rapidly than is seen with the Wolff–Chaikoff effect and the mechanism remains uncertain.

Thyroid hormone action

The cellular site of action for thyroid hormones is within cell nuclei (Fig. 3). The discovery of multiple thyroid hormone receptor isoforms and the characterization at the molecular level of their structure and function have greatly clarified the mode of action of thyroid hormones and allowed the elucidation of mechanisms that result in syndromes of thyroid hormone resistance. The thyroid hormone receptors, which have been named α and β, map to human chromosomes 17 and 3, respectively. They belong to a family of similar cell-protein receptors,

Fig. 3 Thyroid hormone action.

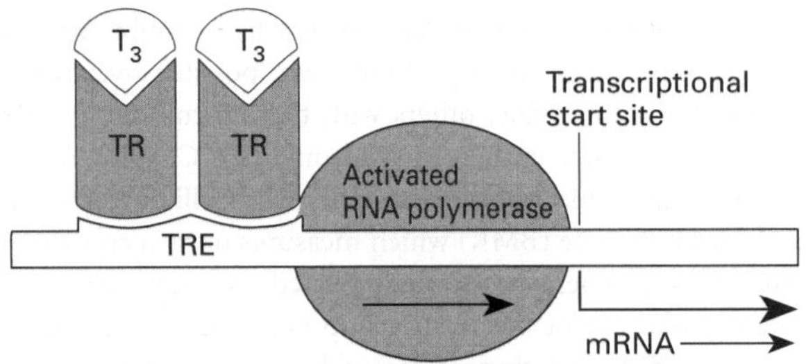

Fig. 4 Diagrammatic representation of gene activation through interaction of the thyroid hormone receptor (TR)–thyroid hormone (T_3) complex with the DNA sequence of the thyroid hormone response element (TRE). Depending on the target gene, thyroid hormone receptor auxillary proteins (TRAP) interact with the T_3–TR complex to augment their binding to the TRE and either enhance or inhibit gene activation.

which include the glucocorticoid, mineralocorticoid, oestrogen, androgen, progesterone, vitamin D, and retinoic acid receptors. All possess a well-conserved DNA-binding domain and a hormone-binding domain. Two peptide loops (zinc fingers) which project from the surface of the protein in the DNA-binding domain interact with specific DNA response elements, and it is through this interaction that thyroid hormones coupled to their receptor regulate gene function. Several thyroid hormone receptor (TR) isoforms are produced by alternative splicing, with the principal TRβ isoforms being β-1 and β-2 and those for the TRα gene being α-1 and α-2. TRα-2 does not function as a true thyroid hormone receptor. The most highly regulated TR isoform is the TRβ-2 which is expressed only in the pituitary gland and in selective areas of the central nervous system. TRα-1 is particularly abundant in skeletal muscle and brown fat, TRα-2 in the brain, and TRβ-1 is more homogeneously distributed with high levels in the brain, liver, and kidney.

It is likely that all thyroid hormone-dependent processes are initiated by the interaction of the hormone with the nuclear receptor and the subsequent interaction of the thyroid hormone–thyroid hormone receptor complex with the DNA sequence of the thyroid hormone response element (Fig. 4). In this context thyroid hormones influence a number of metabolic processes by their action on a variety of enzymes; the metabolism of substrates, vitamins, and minerals; the secretion and degradation rates of virtually all other hormones and the response of their target tissues to them. They stimulate calorigenesis, protein synthesis, all aspects of carbohydrate and lipid metabolism, increasing the demands for coenzymes and the vitamins from which

Table 3 Situations in which the binding of T_4 by thyroxine-binding globulin is impaired

Increased binding	Decreased binding
Genetic	Genetic
Pregnancy	Androgens
Neonate	Anabolic steroids
Oestrogens	Glucocorticoids
Tamoxifen	Acromegaly
Hepatitis, cirrhosis	Nephrotic syndrome
Perphenazine	Severe systemic illness
Opiates	Protein malnutrition
Acute intermittent porphyria	

they are derived, and in so doing have an impact on every tissue and organ system in the body.

Investigation of structure and function

Thyroid hormones

The normal ranges for circulating thyroid hormones are 70–150 nmol/l for total T_4 and 1.2–2.8 nmol/l for total T_3. Total T_4 discriminates well between hyperthyroidism, hypothyroidism, and the euthyroid state, but total T_3 measurements are of little value in suspected hypothyroidism because in this condition the levels of total T_3 are often within the normal range. They may, however, be of value in patients suspected of being hyperthyroid, when they may rise before changes in total T_4 levels are detectable. Total hormone measurements of T_4 and T_3 will vary with alterations in thyroid hormone binding protein concentrations (Table 3). Methods are now available for the assay of free thyroid hormones. Normal ranges are 9–25 pmol/l for free T_4 and 3–9 pmol/l for free T_3. Although radioimmunoassays are available for the measurement of reverse T_3, its measurement is rarely required.

Thyroglobulin

Thyroglobulin is present at low levels (up to 30 pmol/l) in the circulation of normal individuals. The major clinical value of its measurement is in the management of patients with differentiated thyroid carcinoma (see Chapter 7.4).

Thyroid gland iodine metabolism

The only means of assessing thyroid function directly is by the use of a tracer dose of a radioactive isotope of iodine and measurement of its fractional uptake by the gland. Following the administration of an oral preparation of radiolabelled iodine, a γ-scintillation counter is used to measure radioactivity over the area of the thyroid 24 h later, when the tracer uptake is near maximum. In patients with hyperthyroidism, uptake is likely to be higher much earlier and an additional measurement is therefore performed at 6 h. Variations in dietary iodine intake will determine the normal range of the radioactive iodine uptake so that high values do not always indicate thyroid hormone overproduction.

The efficiency of thyroid organification is examined using the discharge of radioactive iodine from the thyroid in response to the administration of potassium perchlorate. Two to three hours after an oral dose of radio-iodine, 0.5 g of potassium perchlorate is given orally in solution and its effect on radioactive iodine uptake is assessed. In normal subjects no further uptake of radio-iodine by the thyroid occurs and less than 5 per cent of the accumulated iodide is discharged during the succeeding hour. Where an iodide organification defect exists, diffusion of iodine out of the thyroid continues, reflected by an increased discharge of radioactivity.

Thyroid imaging

Radionuclide scanning allows the localization of functioning and non-functioning thyroid tissue. A number of isotopes of iodine and $^{99}Tc^{m}$ pertechnetate have been used. Because pertechnetate is not organified following concentration by the thyroid, it diffuses rapidly out of the gland and this, together with its short physical half-life (6 h), makes the radiation delivered to the thyroid by a standard dose very low and allows imaging 20–30 min after the dose has been given. An important consideration when using pertechnetate is that some tumours of the thyroid appear to be functioning when examined by pertechnetate but are cold with radio-iodine.

Ultrasonography can demonstrate diffuse or localized enlargement of the gland and provide assessments of change in size. The sensitivity of the technique allows detection of nodules which are not clinically palpable. When these nodules are solitary the significance of their detection in this way is as yet unresolved. The major role of ultrasonography is in the differentiation of cystic from solid lesions in the thyroid and when a solitary nodule can be shown to be purely cystic this considerably reduces the likelihood of it being malignant.

The demonstration by radio-isotope scanning of a solitary cold nodule, which is then shown by ultrasonography to be solid, demands further investigation. Fine-needle aspiration biopsy coupled with cytological examination then provides a simple, safe, and rapid means for diagnosis.

Hypothalamic–pituitary–thyroid axis

Third-generation immunometric assays now detect TSH levels of 0.01 mU/l, improving the accuracy of diagnosis of both primary and secondary thyroid disorders. Patients with TSH levels above 5.0 mU/l are likely to have primary hypothyroidism and symptomatic hyperthyroidism is almost always present when levels below 0.01 mU/l are recorded. Since immunometric assays commonly use mouse-derived monoclonal antibodies for the assay of TSH, it is important to be aware of the uncommon presence in the patients' sera of endogenous antibodies to mouse immunoglobulin, which may produce a spuriously high TSH result in normal individuals and an apparently normal result in patients who are hyperthyroid. Difficulties also arise in the group of patients in whom TSH levels lie between 0.01 mU/l and 0.1 mU/l, in whom there is no clinical evidence of hyperthyroidism. These patients may have conditions such as euthyroid multinodular goitre, ophthalmic Graves' disease, or a solitary autonomous nodule. In rare patients in whom mild clinical evidence of hyperthyroidism is accompanied by a modest elevation in TSH confirmed by a different assay technique, the failure of the TSH to respond to TRH administration suggests a TSH-producing tumour. A disproportionate increase in the concentration of the TSH α-subunit as compared with the β-subunit provides further evidence of a likely pituitary tumour.

There is now little need for the TRH infusion test, but in patients with clinical evidence of hypothyroidism with low plasma concentrations of T_4, but without increase in TSH, damage to the hypothalamic–pituitary axis may be confirmed by an absent, delayed, or subnormal response of TSH to TRH. When hyperthyroidism is suspected clinically and free thyroid hormone levels are equivocal, a sensitive TSH measurement may lie between 0.01 and 0.1 mU/l. The TSH response to TRH may then be subnormal or absent, and this is seen particularly in patients with solitary autonomous nodules, euthyroid Graves' disease with ophthalmopathy, patients with treated hyperthyroid Graves' disease and some of their relatives, a significant number of patients with multinodular goitre, and many patients receiving replacement or suppressive therapy with exogenous thyroid hormone. In this grey area, clinical judgement ultimately determines the appropriate management.

Peripheral effects of thyroid hormones

A reliable method of assessing the effects of thyroid hormones in peripheral tissues would be of value in situations in which clinical features and biochemical results leave diagnosis in doubt. Such cases include possible subclinical hypothyroidism, possible overtreatment of patients taking thyroxine, others with thyroid tumour resistance, and those with the sick euthyroid syndrome (see Chapter 7.16). No good test is yet available, but the best approach is still measurement of the basal metabolic rate (BMR) which measures oxygen consumption converted into an energy equivalent related to body surface areas. Other tests make use of the relationship between muscle relaxation after a contraction and thyroid status by measuring the speed of relaxation of the Achilles tendon reflex, which is prolonged in hypothyroidism and shortened in hyperthyroidism. Tests of myocardial contractility have also been developed and the best validated is the measurement of the interval between the initiation of the QRS complex on the ECG and the arrival of the pulse wave in the brachial artery at diastolic pressure (QKd). This is shortened in hyperthyroidism and prolonged in hypothyroidism. All three of these measures are altered by a number of non-thyroidal states, so that they can only be interpreted with circumspection. The serum cholesterol is usually elevated in hypothyroidism and decreased in hyperthyroidism and the serum creatinine phosphokinase may be increased in the hypothyroid state. It is suggested that absent serum sex hormone binding globulin and absent serum ferritin responses to administered thyroxine are likely to be associated with generalized resistance to thyroid hormone.

Thyroid autoantibodies

The autoimmune thyroid diseases span a spectrum which ranges from clinically and biochemically overt hyperthyroidism to clinically and biochemically overt hypothyroidism. Within the spectrum are included euthyroid Graves' disease with ophthalmopathy, transient postpartum thyroid dysfunction, and transient syndromes of altered thyroid function in neonates. The commonest cause of hyperthyroidism is Graves' disease which is due to TSH receptor antibodies. Goitrous (Hashimoto's thyroiditis) and atrophic (primary myxoedema) thyroiditis are the commonest causes of hypothyroidism in areas of adequate iodine intake. Thyroid destruction in these diseases is predominantly the result of cell-mediated mechanisms, but antibodies to thyroid peroxidase, and those that bind the TSH receptor without stimulating it (TSH receptor blocking antibodies), may well have a role in contributing to their pathogenesis (Table 4). It seems highly unlikely that antibodies to thyroglobulin, although present in 80 per cent of patients with autoimmune thyroiditis, and in some 35 per cent of patients with newly diagnosed hyperthyroid

Table 4 Autoantigens in autoimmune thyroid disease

	Thyroglobulin	Thyroid peroxidase	Thyroid stimulating hormone receptor
Protein	Iodinated glycoprotein	Haemoprotein enzyme	G-binding protein-linked receptor
Glycosylated	+	+	+
Function	Biosynthetic precursor of T_3 and T_4	Catalyses iodination and coupling of tyrosine to yield T_3 and T_4	Receptor for TSH
Thyroid location	Follicular lumen	Membrane-bound cell surface (apical)	Membrane-bound cell surface (basal)
Molecular weight	Circulation 660 000	Exo/endocytotic vesicles 105 000; 110 000	86 000
Amino acids	2748	TPO-1 933; TPO-2 876 Alternatively spliced products	764 (excludes 20aa signal sequence)
Regions	–		
extracellular	–	842 (TPO-1)	418
transmembrane	–	29	265 (seven transmembrane domains)
intracellular	–	62	81
Chromosome location	8	2	14
Homologies	Acetylcholinesterase	Myeloperoxidase	LH/hCG, FSH receptors

For abbreviations, see text.

Graves' disease, have any role in the pathogenesis of autoimmune thyroid disease. Thyroid peroxidase antibodies are present in almost all those with autoimmune thyroid disease at some stage in the disease process.

Thyroid stimulating hormone receptor antibodies

There are two approaches to the assay of these antibodies. In the radioreceptor technique, antibody activity is measured by the degree of inhibition of the binding of radiolabelled TSH to preparations of thyroid membrane or of purified TSH receptors. This method gives no indication of the functional nature of the antibody. The other techniques involve an assessment of the biological activity of TSH antibodies measured by their ability to stimulate thyroid cells in a variety of preparations; the measurement of cell activation is then most easily assessed by the generation of cAMP. Other systems allow the detection of antibodies that block function. These can be shown by their preincubation with thyroid cells, blocking the subsequent effects of TSH and the resultant stimulation of cAMP production.

Assessment TSH receptor antibody activity provides information on the pathogenesis of atrophic thyroiditis in patients with primary myxoedema, among whom this antibody activity may contribute to the development of thyroid failure in up to 30 per cent of patients. Of greater importance is the recognition that since TSH receptor antibodies can cross the placenta, babies born to mothers with high enough levels of this antibody activity are at risk of either developing transient neonatal hyper- or hypothyroidism.

Disorders of the thyroid

Clinical assessment

In the history, evidence of possible exposure to ionizing radiation, of iodide ingestion in the form of food preparations, such as those derived from seaweed, or of iodine-containing medications, such as amiodarone, is of considerable importance. Other agents (e.g. lithium carbonate) may affect thyroid function other than by way of iodine content. In large areas of the world low dietary iodide intake is common and leads to iodine deficiency goitre (endemic goitre). A family history of goitre, altered thyroid function, and a personal and family history of other organ-specific autoimmune diseases may be helpful, particularly of insulin-dependent diabetes, pernicious anaemia, vitiligo, and myasthenia gravis.

Examination of the thyroid should be performed while standing behind the patient and palpating with the fingertips of both hands. Having identified the cricoid cartilage, the isthmus of the thyroid should be identifiable just below it. The extent of the gland is then assessed by determining the lower borders of the lateral lobes and the rest of the outline of the gland. This process can be enhanced by asking the patient to swallow sips of water at regular intervals during the procedure with the physician palpating the gland as it moves up and down in the neck in response to swallowing. It is important not only to assess the size and consistency of the gland but also the presence or absence of nodules within it. The thyroid may be tender or, rarely, exceedingly painful to touch. A search should be made of the neck for enlarged local lymph nodes. Auscultation over the thyroid in patients with hyperthyroidism may reveal a bruit. A thyroglossal cyst moves upwardly on protrusion of the tongue. Transillumination of large nodules may allow the discrimination between a solid and cystic mass. If palpation of the neck fails to reveal a gland in the expected position there may be a retrosternal goitre; elevation of the arms above the head may then cause venous obstruction by further compromising the thoracic inlet so causing facial congestion and in addition respiratory distress (Pemberton's sign). Displacement of the trachea and inspiratory stridor may also be signs indicating compression of the trachea by retrosternal goitre or of a goitre extending retrosternally. Hoarseness of the voice requires consideration of possible involvement of the recurrent laryngeal nerve, most usually by a malignant thyroid lesion.

Thyroid hormone excess

A number of conditions lead to the development of hyperthyroidism (Table 5). The prevalence of this disorder is approximately 20 per

Table 5 Causes of hyperthyroidism

Common	Uncommon
Graves' disease (diffuse toxic goitre)	Hyperthyroid phase of Hashimoto's thyroiditis
Toxic multinodular goitre	Neonatal hyperthyroidism
Toxic solitary adenoma	Iodine-induced
Thyroiditis subacute, viral, de Quervain's silent, painless postpartum	Thyrotoxicosis factitia Hydatidiform mole, choriocarcinoma TSH-secreting pituitary adenoma Metastatic thyroid carcinoma (follicular) Struma ovarii (thyroid-tissue-containing teratoma)

Table 6 Clinical features associated with hyperthyroidism

General Heat intolerance Sweating Fatigue Apathy Tremor Diffuse goitre* Nodular goitre	*Neuromuscular* Fatiguability Restlessness Muscle weakness—proximal Choreoathetosis Hypokalaemic periodic paralysis Myasthenia gravis*
Cardiovascular Palpitation Dyspnoea Angina Tachycardia Atrial fibrillation Heart failure	*Psychiatric* Irritability Nervousness Agitation Emotional lability Psychosis
Gastrointestinal Weight loss despite ↑ appetite Diarrhoea, steatorrhoea Vomiting	*Dermatological* Pruritus Palmar erythema Pretibial myxoedema* Hair thinning Onycholysis Vitiligo* Acropachy*
Genitourinary Polyuria and polydipsia Amenorrhoea Infertility	*Ocular* Lid lag/lid retraction Ophthalmopathy*

*Symptoms and signs which may occur in patients with Graves' disease.

1000 in females and 2 per 1000 in males. The presentation of the disease with a variety of symptoms and signs (Table 6) depends on its severity, duration, aetiology, age of the patient, and the presence or absence of disease in other organs. Confirmation of the diagnosis requires laboratory assessment. Hyperthyroidism is indicated by elevated concentrations of free or total T_4 and T_3 in the presence of an undetectable level of TSH. Uncommonly, T_3 values are elevated despite normal T_4 values (T_3 toxicosis). The presence of thyroid autoantibodies in conjunction with a diffuse goitre, and evidence of increased uptake in an isotope scan, makes the cause of the hyperthyroidism almost certainly due to Graves' disease. A radioisotope scan also allows the demonstration of a solitary toxic nodule or of a toxic multinodular goitre.

Table 7 American Thyroid Association abridged classification of the eye changes (ophthalmopathy) associated with Graves' disease

Class	Definition*
0	No physical symptoms or signs
1	Only signs (upper lid retraction, stare, lid lag, proptosis to 22 mm)
2	Soft tissue involvement (symptoms and signs)
3	Proptosis > 22 mm
4	Extraocular muscle involvement
5	Corneal involvement
6	Sight loss (optic nerve involvement)

*Initial letters of the definitions provide a useful mnemonic: 'NO SPECS'.

Graves' disease

Graves' disease is the most common cause of hyperthyroidism (75 per cent of all cases in the UK). It is characterized by a diffusely enlarged thyroid gland, hyperthyroidism, ophthalmopathy (Table 7), and, uncommonly, dermopathy (pretibial myxoedema). The exact aetiology of the condition remains unknown, but it is an organ-specific autoimmune disease with a strong familial predisposition, occurring much more commonly in females and with a peak incidence between the ages of 20 and 40 years. It is associated with other organ-specific autoimmune diseases and is characterized by associations with particular major histocompatibility complex (HLA) antigens, with different associations being reported for different racial groups. Lymphocytic infiltration of the thyroid gland is a hallmark of the autoimmune process. The process leading to hyperthyroidism depends on the presence of antibodies against the thyroid follicular cell surface membrane TSH receptor, usually of the IgG1 subclass. Binding to the TSH receptor activates the adenylate cyclase system, and thus stimulates thyroid function. The levels of antibody correlate with thyroid function and, in the offspring of mothers with high levels of antibodies, passage of them across the placenta leads to transient neonatal hyperthyroidism.

Toxic multinodular goitre

This usually occurs in an older age group with a long-standing multinodular goitre. Hyperthyroidism may be precipitated by the administration of iodides. The gland is characterized by structural and functional heterogeneity and functional autonomy. Thyroid hormone overproduction is usually much less marked than in Graves' disease, so that the clinical presentation is less dramatic. Thyroid function tests may confirm hyperthyroidism but a subgroup of patients with TSH levels between 0.01 and 0.1 mU/l are defined as having thyroid autonomy without hyperthyroidism.

Toxic solitary adenoma

Less than 2 per cent of patients presenting with hyperthyroidism are found to have a solitary toxic adenoma. These solitary nodules usually occur in patients in their 30s and 40s. Laboratory investigation depends on the stage of the disease. At first the only evidence of abnormality may be borderline suppression of the serum TSH level. Later a thyroid scan will demonstrate localization of radio-isotope to the nodule, with suppression of uptake by the surrounding normal thyroid; plasma concentrations of T_3 and T_4 will be increased. Histologically these lesions are almost always benign follicular adenomas.

Thyroiditis

Subacute thyroiditis, also known as granulomatous giant cell or de Quervain's thyroiditis, is due to a viral infection of the thyroid gland, often following an upper respiratory infection. The disease is uncommon and may be mistakenly diagnosed as pharyngitis. Mononuclear cell infiltration of follicles with follicular disruption and loss of colloid are characteristic and may be confused with autoimmune thyroiditis. In contrast to the classical autoimmune histology is the presence of multinucleate giant cells. Colloid may be present within these or leak into the interstitium. The follicular changes progress to granuloma formation. Follicular destruction leads to the release of preformed hormone, often with clinical and biochemical evidence of hyperthyroidism. The radioactive iodine uptake is low and new thyroid hormone synthesis is impaired.

Once stores of preformed hormone are depleted, clinical and biochemical evidence of hypothyroidism may follow. Ultimately thyroid function returns to normal. Apart from transient changes in thyroid function the characteristic presentation is with pain in the thyroid which may be accompanied by fever. The pain may be excruciating and some enlargement of the gland occurs. The erythrocyte sedimentation rate (ESR) is markedly elevated during the active phase of the disease.

Hyperthyroidism may also occur in painless (silent) thyroiditis, when biopsy reveals lymphocytic rather than subacute thyroiditis; but subacute thyroiditis can also be painless. Silent thyroiditis is also associated with a markedly decreased radioactive iodine uptake in the absence of excess iodide intake and with a transient hyperthyroid phase followed by one of transient hypothyroidism. The thyroid may be enlarged during the disease but is not tender to touch. The disease is almost certainly autoimmune in origin, with the characteristic lymphocytic infiltration of the gland, the presence of antithyroid antibodies, and HLA associations (at least in the postpartum variant of this syndrome) similar to those observed in autoimmune thyroid disease.

Other causes of thyroid hormone excess

A hydatidiform mole or a choriocarcinoma can stimulate thyroid function as a result of the high levels of human chorionic gonadotropin (hCG) secreted by the tumour. Thyroid overactivity in conjunction with a normal or elevated level of TSH suggests the possibility of a TSH-secreting pituitary adenoma, confirmed by the absence of any features of autoimmune thyroid disease, the presence of a mass in the pituitary fossa, the elevated concentration of free TSH α-subunits, and the failure of TSH to respond to TRH. In a rarer group of patients, biochemical evidence of hyperthyroidism is due to resistance to thyroid hormone and is associated, if anything, with tissue deficiency rather than excess of thyroid hormone; this problem is addressed later. The ingestion of iodine can lead to iodine-induced hyperthyroidism, particularly in patients with autonomously functioning thyroid nodules. Assessment of radioactive iodine uptake will demonstrate this to be low and urinary iodine excretion is greatly increased. Less commonly, even normal individuals given large doses of iodine may develop iodine-induced hyperthyroidism.

Epidemics of exogenous thyrotoxicosis can occur when large quantities of animal thyroid tissue, for example from beef, are used in the preparation of hamburgers. The surreptitious ingestion of excessive quantities of thyroid hormone (thyrotoxicosis factitia) characteristically occurs in individuals with an underlying psychiatric background and usually with some medical knowledge and access to such preparations. In both of the latter situations, a radioactive iodine uptake assessment of the thyroid shows absence or reduced uptake of the isotope.

Table 8 Causes of euthyroid hyperthyroxinaemia

Causes
Increased thyroxine-binding globulin concentration
Familial dysalbuminaemic hyperthyroxinaemia
Increased T_4 binding to thyroxine-binding prealbumin or anti-T_4 antibodies
Thyroid hormone resistance
Non-thyroidal illness (sick euthyroid)
Acute psychiatric illness
Hyperemesis gravidarum
Medication, e.g. amiodarone
Exogenous T_4 administration

The situations in which T_4 levels are elevated in the absence of clinical evidence of hyperthyroidism are shown in Table 8.

Treatment

Antithyroid drugs

The major group of drugs used for the treatment of hyperthyroidism are the thionamides. Carbimazole is the most widely used in the UK whereas in the US propylthiouracil or methimazole are the agents of choice. They all inhibit both oxidation and organification, thus leading to a state of intrathyroidal iodine deficiency and inhibition of thyroid hormone synthesis. In addition, propylthiouracil inhibits the conversion of T_4 to T_3 in the periphery. All these compounds are weakly immunosuppressive and this effect may contribute to the control of Graves' disease by reducing the levels of TSH receptor antibodies.

Carbimazole is usually begun at a dose of 40 mg daily and this can be given as two 20 mg tablets once daily. Since these agents inhibit the synthesis but not the release of thyroid hormone, a reduction in secretion does not occur immediately but only after glandular stores have been depleted. Patients only improve some 4–8 weeks after commencing therapy. Subsequent management is either by 'titration' of the dose against the clinical and biochemical response, which requires fairly frequent reassessment of the patient; alternatively, a blocking and replacement regimen can be used, in which carbimazole is maintained at a dose of 40 mg once daily with thyroxine (50–150 μg/day) being added once thyroid function is under control. There is evidence to suggest that maintaining a high dose of carbimazole in this way may contribute to controlling the disease by having the greatest effect on the autoimmune process, in addition to its effects on thyroid hormone synthesis, and once a patient is stabilized on such a regimen the need for regular follow-up is considerably decreased.

In Europe, patients presenting with the first episode of hyperthyroid Graves' disease under the age of 40 years have been treated with a course of antithyroid drugs. Following the blocking and replacement regimen for 6–12 months, between a third and half the patients achieve lasting remission. Factors that predict the likelihood of long-term remission at the end of a course of drug therapy are a small goitre, a decrease in goitre size during treatment, a normal serum TSH level, and disappearance of TSH receptor antibody activity from the serum. Patterns of subsequent management of those who relapse are changing; in Europe in particular, and in the UK to a lesser extent, partial thyroidectomy was once the treatment of choice for those under the age of 40. There is now more widespread use of radio-iodine, irrespective of the patient's age, as has been long-standing common practice in the US.

All the thionamides produce similar side-effects. The most common is an itchy maculopapular skin rash, occurring in up to 5 per cent of patients. Although it may settle spontaneously, should this fail to occur it is worth trying to switch from carbimazole to propylthiouracil or vice versa. Other less common adverse reactions include arthralgia, myalgia, neuritis, hepatitis, thrombocytopenia, nausea and vomiting, lymphadenopathy, and fever. All of these may resolve spontaneously or after changing treatment to another thionamide, but it is often better to proceed to surgery or radio-iodine treatment. The most important ill-effect of these agents is agranulocytosis, which is seen in less than 1 per cent of patients. It tends to occur early in the course of treatment and is accompanied by fever, sore throat, mouth ulcers, and other evidence of infection. Patients should be advised of this rare but serious complication and should, if these symptoms develop, discontinue the drug immediately and seek medical advice urgently. Agranulocytosis occurs rapidly but recovers provided that the drug is stopped quickly. Any patient who has developed this complication should not be treated with a thionamide again.

Partial thyroidectomy

Surgery is very effective in relieving hyperthyroidism, and mortality and morbidity are exceedingly low. Patients should be made euthyroid prior to surgery by the use of carbimazole for at least 2–3 months before the operation and by the addition of Lugol's solution (0.1–0.3 ml three times a day) for 10 days immediately prior to the operation. One-year follow-up figures suggest that 80 per cent of patients are euthyroid, about 15 per cent have developed hypothyroidism, and 5 per cent have relapsed. Less than 1 per cent develop hypoparathyroidism or damage to the recurrent laryngeal nerve. With longer follow-up, up to half the patients may go on to develop hypothyroidism, particularly those who had high levels of antithyroid peroxidase antibody prior to treatment. Transient hypothyroidism following surgery is not uncommon and thyroxine replacement should be withheld until the physician is confident that the patient is indeed permanently hypothyroid. The only other important complication of surgery is bleeding into the operative site and, although this is exceedingly rare, it can be rapidly fatal if not recognized and treated urgently.

Radio-iodine

Radio-iodine is simple and cheap and is as effective as surgery acting via the radiation-induced destruction of thyroid follicular cells. An acute inflammatory response in the thyroid with follicular cell death is followed by fibrosis, vascular narrowing, and lymphocytic infiltration. The principal long-term consequence of radio-iodine therapy is hypothyroidism, which occurs in most patients despite all efforts to titrate the dose against various parameters of thyroid function, size, or iodine uptake. It was once thought that this therapy might lead to thyroid malignancy, leukaemia, or teratogenic effects. Long-term follow-up over a number of years has failed to provide any evidence that there is an increased risk of any of these possibilities. There is a move, therefore, particularly in the US, to reduce the age limit for giving it from 40, so that in some centres radio-iodine is now used for children and adolescents. Side-effects from the administration of radio-iodine are minimal and uncommon. Transient soreness over the thyroid may occur. Ill effects of radiation to the parathyroids, particularly at higher dosage, has rarely been reported to lead to clinically overt hypoparathyroidism. In patients with severe hyperthyroidism, thyrotoxic crisis has been reported to occur following radio-iodine, so glandular hormone stores of such patients should be depleted by administration of antithyroid drugs for several weeks before radio-iodine. Carbimazole should be withdrawn 5 days before the dose of radio-iodine, and can be given again a few days after it, if indicated. Pregnancy is an absolute contraindication to radio-iodine, and should be avoided until 6 months after the last dose, because of the effects on the fetal thyroid. Doses are now given on a arbitrary basis in a range between about 185 and 555 MBq orally. Good control of thyroid function is unlikely for some 2–3 months after the dose, so it is often necessary to prescribe carbimazole or a β-blocker for this short time. Failure to control the disease with a first dose of radio-iodine may require the administration of a second one 6 months later. Long-term follow-up is essential because of the ultimate development of hypothyroidism in almost all patients. An alternative approach, which has the advantage of making such follow-up unnecessary, is to seek to achieve thyroid ablation initially with a large enough dose of radio-iodine to ensure that hypothyroidism is induced early. Patients can then be treated with thyroxine replacement and need not be followed thereafter.

β-Blockers

These agents are effective in resolving some of the manifestations of hyperthyroidism such as tremor, palpitation, sweating, and tachycardia. They work rapidly if an adequate dose is given. They serve as a useful adjunct at the start of treatment with thionamides or following radio-iodine when they help to control peripheral manifestations of hyperthyroidism before antithyroid treatment becomes effective. Propranolol can be used in a dose of 40–80 mg by mouth every 8 h, but is contraindicated in patients with asthma or with congestive cardiac failure.

The management of hyperthyroidism without the features of Graves' disease varies with the cause. In toxic multinodular goitre the only indication for antithyroid drugs is the presence of severe hyperthyroidism, when the disease is best controlled with antithyroid drugs before treatment by radio-iodine. Larger doses of radio-iodine may need to be given than those used in Graves' disease (555–1100 MBq). Surgery is indicated in patients with large goitres, particularly in those in whom there is concern about obstructive features or where it is feared that these might develop following radio-iodine treatment. In patients with solitary toxic adenomas the treatment of choice is again radio-iodine, with the same alternative available as for a toxic multinodular goitre if the disease is severe or the nodule particularly large. Doses of radio-iodine similar to those used in Graves' disease are often adequate. The ultimate risk of hypothyroidism in patients with nodular goitres following radio-iodine is much lower than that in Graves' disease.

In patients with subacute thyroiditis, aspirin may be all that is required although in more severe cases glucocorticoids may be of benefit. Uncommonly, antithyroid drugs may be indicated if the hyperthyroid phase induces marked disease. In patients with molar pregnancies, the treatment is to remove the lesion, and the same applies to pituitary tumours secreting TSH. Iodine-induced hyperthyroidism is often difficult to manage. Even after discontinuation of the exogenous source of iodide, if this is possible (and it may not be, for example in patients taking amiodarone), the uptake of radio-iodine by the thyroid gland remains low. Control may be achieved with large doses of antithyroid drugs given for 6–9 months, perhaps best combined with 750 mg of sodium perchlorate to inhibit the thyroid iodide trap.

Thyrotoxic crisis

Thyrotoxic crisis or thyroid storm is a rare but serious complication most commonly occurring in patients with Graves' disease, when it is a manifestation of the severity of the hyperthyroidism. Its onset is often abrupt and it occurs in patients whose hyperthyroidism has either been treated inadequately or not at all. Often it is precipitated by factors such as infection, trauma, following radio-iodine treatment, and childbirth. The patient is markedly hypermetabolic, with fever, profuse sweating, and marked tachycardia, which may progress to congestive cardiac failure and pulmonary oedema. The patient is restless with a marked tremor and may develop delirium or frank psychosis; further progression to coma may result. Nausea, vomiting, and abdominal pain are often present, as is hypotension. Unrecognized, the condition is fatal. In controlling the severe hyperthyroidism there is a need both to inhibit hormone synthesis and release and to block adrenergically mediated effects of thyroid hormones. Large doses of carbimazole (up to 60 mg a day, if necessary by nasogastric tube) should be used, but propylthiouracil at doses of 300–400 mg every 4 h may be preferable because of its additional effects in inhibiting the peripheral conversion of T_4 to T_3. In the absence of evidence of cardiac insufficiency, propranolol at doses up to 80 mg every 6 h can be given orally. The most urgent requirement is to administer iodine in order to block acutely the release of thyroid hormones from the thyroid. This is best given after the administration of the antithyroid drug, so that the latter is present to inhibit the synthesis of new thyroid hormone from the iodine load. Lugol's solution is given at a dose of 5 drops every 6 h. Additionally, large doses of dexamethasone (2 mg orally every 6 h) are given, both to provide glucocorticoids in a time of crisis and because dexamethasone inhibits hormone release from the thyroid and the peripheral conversion of T_4 to T_3. Coupled with these medications, correction of hydration and of any other metabolic anomalies is essential. Separate manoeuvres may need to be directed at lowering the body temperature, although salicylates should be avoided because, by competing with thyroid hormones for sites on binding proteins, they increase the free hormone concentration.

Graves' ophthalmopathy

Patients with Graves' disease frequently develop ophthalmopathy, which usually occurs within 12 months of the onset of hyperthyroidism but less commonly may precede or accompany the onset of the disease. On rarer occasions, it is seen in patients who have never been clinically hyperthyroid and even in some who present with hypothyroidism. The pathogenesis remains uncertain. Some observations suggest that it is mediated by an autoimmune process directed primarily at the orbital extraocular muscles. The presence and severity of the eye disease both appear to be associated with cigarette smoking. Patients present with a number of symptoms, including pain, watering of the eyes, photophobia, and blurred or double vision. A variety of physical signs are associated with the disease, including proptosis, lid retraction and lid lag, periorbital oedema, extraocular muscle functional impairment, conjuctival oedema and injection, and exposure keratitis, which may lead to corneal ulceration, visual field defects, impaired visual acuity, and papillo-edema. When there is doubt about the diagnosis, ultrasound or a CT of the orbits reveals the characteristic enlargement of the extraocular muscles, with the medial and inferior rectus most usually involved. Since hypothyroidism has an adverse effect on ophthalmopathy, management of hyperthyroid Graves' disease should be designed to ensure that hypothyroidism does not develop and, if it does, is recognized early and treated promptly. In most patients symptoms of ophthalmopathy are mild and require no treatment, beyond advice about wearing protective glasses against bright lights, wind, or cold air. Elevation of the head of the bed at night and the use of conjunctival lubricants such as 1 per cent methylcellulose may be of benefit if there is incomplete closure of the eyelids when sleeping. When the disease progresses, the major therapies are designed either to reduce the volume of the orbital soft tissues medically or to expand the space within which the soft tissues and the globes sit, by surgically decompressing the orbit. High-dose steroids, with or without cyclosporin, have been effective in controlling the disease but both these medications carry with them significant side-effects. Dexamethasone, 4 mg 6 hourly initially, reducing by 4 mg every 48 h until the total daily dose is 4 mg is a reasonable regimen during the first week. Thereafter transfer on to prednisolone and its very gradual reduction is necessary. The addition of cyclosporin may improve results; the standard starting dose is 10 mg/kg body weight continued for some 3–10 months. External radiation to the orbits in conjunction with corticosteroids is more effective than radiotherapy alone, and is particularly effective in treating relatively acute disease. Where glucocorticoids alone or in conjunction with external radiation fail to halt the progression of the disease, and particularly if loss of vision is threatened, orbital decompression is the only alternative. A number of different surgical approaches are used. Although this procedure will relieve the acute situation and allow considerable regression of proptosis, once the disease process settles there is often a need for surgical correction of the resulting extraocular muscle dysfunction.

Thyroid hormone deficiency

The causes of hypothyroidism are shown in Table 9. The onset may be insidious and the symptoms and signs reflect the fact that thyroid hormone deficiency affects every tissue in the body (Table 10).

Presentation

In the adolescent precocious puberty may occur and there may be enlargement of the sella turcica in addition to short stature. In adults common features include tiredness, lethargy, weight gain, constipation, cold intolerance, muscle cramps, menstrual irregularities, cold dry skin, husky voice, and slow relaxing reflexes (Table 10). In patients with primary hypothyroidism a reduction in the total and free thyroxine level is accompanied by an increase in the serum TSH. Measurement of serum total or free T_3 levels are usually of little help in making the diagnosis since these are often within the normal range at a time when the serum T_4 concentration is decreased. In this context it is important to remember that there may be low levels of T_3 in euthyroid patients when they are seriously ill with non-thyroidal systemic illness (see below). In patients with secondary hypothyroidism with low levels of total or free T_4, the TSH level may be decreased or normal or only slightly elevated.

Table 9 Causes of hypothyroidism

Causes
Primary
Lymphocytic (autoimmune) thyroiditis
Hashimoto's (goitrous) thyroiditis
Atrophic thyroiditis; primary myxoedema
Postpartum thyroid dysfunction
Silent, painless thyroiditis
Iatrogenic (for hyperthyroidism)
Post-radio-iodine
Following partial thyroidectomy
Antithyroid drugs
Non-thyroidal medication
Lithium
Amiodarone
Iodine excess
Iodine deficiency (endemic goitre)
Congenital (sporadic)
Thyroid agenesis
Thyroid maldescent
Dyshormonogenesis
Riedel's thyroiditis
Secondary
Hypothalamic–pituitary disease/damage
Peripheral resistance to thyroid hormone

Table 10 Clinical features associated with hypothyroidism in the adult

General	*Mental state*
Lethargy	Mental slowing
Easy fatiguability	Inability to concentrate
Weight gain	Poor memory
Cold intolerance	Hypersomnolence
Pallor or yellow skin	Depression
Goitre	Psychosis (myxoedema madness)
Hyperlipidaemia	
Puffy face and hands	
	Neuromuscular
Cardiovascular	Weakness
Angina	Muscle cramps
Bradycardia	Paraesthesiae
Cardiac failure	Hoarseness
Pleural effusion	Deafness
Pericardial effusion	Cerebellar ataxia
Low voltage complexes (ECG)	Delayed reflexes
	Entrapment neuropathies
Gastrointestinal	
Constipation	*Haematological*
Ascites	Anaemia-iron or folate deficiency
Ileus	Pernicious anaemia
Genitourinary	
Water retention	*Dermatological*
Menorrhagia	Dry skin
Infertility	Vitiligo
Hyperprolactinaemia	Alopecia
	Erythema ab igne

Primary hypothyroidism

Previous treatment for hyperthyroidism with either radio-iodine or by partial thyroidectomy cannot be overemphasized as a common cause of primary hypothyroidism.

Hypothyroidism with or without development of a goitre may follow the chronic ingestion of iodine in either organic or inorganic form. Similarly, a number of non-iodine-containing compounds may lead to hypothyroidism, with or without a goitre, including lithium, which decreases thyroid hormone synthesis.

Lymphocytic thyroiditis

In areas of the world where iodine intake is adequate, autoimmune lymphocytic thyroiditis is the commonest cause of hypothyroidism. It is more common in women than men, and occurs particularly in the age group between 30 and 50 years. There is often a family history of autoimmune thyroid disease, or of other organ-specific autoimmune diseases in the patient or in his or her relatives. The two major variants of lymphocytic thyroiditis are distinguished most easily by the presence or absence of a goitre. Patients with Hashimoto's thyroiditis have enlargement of the thyroid, whereas those with idiopathic or primary myxoedema (atrophic thyroiditis) have no goitre. In the presence of biochemical evidence of hypothyroidism, the demonstration of circulating autoantibodies to thyroglobulin and thyroid peroxidase make autoimmune lymphocytic thyroiditis the likely cause. There is also a small subpopulation of patients with primary myxoedema in whom antibodies which bind to the TSH receptor block its activation (TSH receptor blocking antibodies), thereby probably playing an important role in the development of impaired thyroid function.

Lymphocytic thyroiditis is uncommonly associated with pain and tenderness of the gland; differentiation from subacute thyroiditis is helped by the demonstration of high levels of thyroid autoantibodies in the former and an elevated ESR in the latter. Riedel's thyroiditis, predominantly seen in middle-aged women, may uncommonly be associated with low levels of thyroid autoantibodies. The aetiology is unknown. Biopsy of the thyroid reveals extensive fibrosis which often extends into adjacent structures. Fibrosis elsewhere, particularly retroperitoneally, may also be seen. The enlarged thyroid is rock-hard and symptoms result from the local fibrotic invasion of surrounding structures.

Endemic goitre and cretinism

Endemic goitre occurs in areas of environmental iodine deficiency and may afflict as many as 200 million people throughout the world. It is particularly prevalent in mountainous areas. Most individuals with endemic goitre are not hypothyroid and this may be because of the increased synthesis of T_3 at the expense of T_4. The incidence and severity of endemic goitre and the biochemical state of the individual depend primarily on the degree of iodine deficiency. Iodine supplementation, either in the form of iodine-enriched table salt, injections of iodized oil, or the introduction of iodine to communal drinking water, reduces the incidence of endemic goitre. Endemic cretinism develops in the offspring of mothers living in severe endemic goitre areas of the world. The mother usually has a goitre.

Thyroid hormone biosynthetic defects

A number of rare inherited disorders of thyroid hormone biosynthesis may lead to goitrous hypothyroidism. Most of the defects appear to be inherited as autosomal recessive conditions (see OTM3, pp. 1615–16).

Hypothalamic–pituitary disease

The commonest causes of secondary hypothyroidism are postpartum pituitary necrosis (Sheehan's syndrome) or tumours of the pituitary or adjacent structures. In the latter group craniopharyngiomas are particuarly common (see Chapter 7.1).

Treatment

Patients with symptomatic hypothyroidism require treatment with thyroxine. A dose of 100–150 µg/day is effective in most patients; this can be taken as a single daily dose since the half-life of the drug is long (7 days). Symptomatic improvement occurs within 2–3 weeks of beginning treatment, although it may take several weeks longer before the serum TSH returns into the normal range. Replacement doses of thyroxine should aim ultimately to achieve TSH values within the normal range, and serum T_4 values towards the upper end of the normal range. There has been concern in the past few years about the possibility that overreplacement with thyroxine, particularly in women, may be associated with reducing bone density, but occasional patients require more thyroxine than might be expected and this may reflect normal variations in absorption. Rarely the diagnosis of coeliac disease is made in patients requiring suprapharmacological doses of thyroxine because of their malabsorption. The dose of thyroxine may need to be increased in some patients during pregnancy.

Particular care is needed in beginning treatment in the elderly and in those with a history of heart disease. In patients with coronary artery disease low levels of circulating thyroid hormone may protect the heart against increased demands that would otherwise result in increasing angina. In such patients appropriate therapy for their coronary artery disease should be considered before beginning thyroxine. When thyroxine is given it should be begun at a low dose (25 µg daily or on alternate days) and be increased cautiously every 4 weeks until euthyroidism is achieved.

Myxoedema coma

Myxoedema coma is an uncommon complication of long-standing hypothyroidism and is typically seen in the elderly, often precipitated by severe infection, therapy with sedative agents, or by inadequate heating during cold weather. It is has a high mortality. It is characteristically associated with depression of the level of consciousness, and hypothermia. Alveolar hypoventilation leading to carbon dioxide retention and a dilutional hyponatraemia are often seen. Early recognition of the condition and its management are essential. The latter is complicated by the sluggish circulation and hypometabolism. General supportive measures include intravenous fluids, antibiotics, ventilation, and slow rewarming. Thyroid hormone replacement is best given as an intravenous bolus of 100 µg of T_3, because of its rapid action. Thereafter a reasonable dose is 20 µg three times a day. It is worth covering the initial treatment period with hydrocortisone (100 mg daily) to protect against the possibility of associated adrenocortical insufficiency.

Simple, non-toxic goitre

Simple or non-toxic goitre is diagnosed when thyroid enlargement is not associated with altered function and is not due to an inflammatory or neoplastic process. It is not usually seen in an area of endemic goitre. The pathogenesis of this condition remains uncertain. In the majority of patients, TSH levels are not elevated, and claims that there may be thyroid growth stimulating immunoglobulins have not been substantiated. These goitres occur much more commonly in women and particularly at puberty and during pregnancy. Patients present usually because of thyroid enlargement. Thyroid function tests are normal, although the serum thyroglobulin concentration is often raised. Thyroid autoantibodies are negative. In managing the condition, thyroxine has been advocated in patients in whom there is biochemical evidence of a detectable or mildly raised TSH; the dose should not induce hyperthyroidism. Usually this fails to reduce the size of the goitre and if there are associated symptoms, particularly obstructive ones, surgery may be required. Postoperative replacement therapy should be given to reduce the likelihood of recurrence.

Non-thyroidal illness

In patients who are severely ill, alterations, primarily in the transport and peripheral metabolism of thyroid hormones, induce biochemical changes, the physiological significance of which remain uncertain but which make the interpretation of tests of thyroid function difficult. In this situation, the serum T_3 concentration is reduced, often markedly so, and this is accompanied (if measured) by an increase in the concentration of reverse T_3. These changes result from a reduction in 5-monodeiodination of T_4 and reverse T_3. Although alterations in the binding of thyroid hormones in plasma occur in this situation, there is not, as might be expected, a normal or increased level of free T_3 because of the marked reduction in total T_3. The more severe the illness, the lower will be the serum T_3 concentration. In early illness there may be no change in the total or free T_4 concentration, but both decline with progression of the non-thyroidal illness. The TSH level in this group of patients is characteristically within the normal range. The interpretation of thyroid function tests in this group of patients may be further complicated by medication given during their severe illness. Of particular importance are glucocorticoids, which reduce TSH secretion from the pituitary and, therefore, reduce thyroid hormone secretion.

Management has been shown not to be improved by the administration of thyroid hormone. As and when the patient recovers, there is a recovery in thyroid function, usually preceded by a small rebound in TSH secretion, so that serum TSH levels may be mildly elevated until thyroid hormone levels have returned to the normal range.

In patients with acute psychiatric illness, particularly schizophrenics, serum total and free T_4 concentrations are frequently noted to be elevated. These changes, if present, precede the introduction of medication and there is often an absent TSH response to TRH, although usually with a sensitive assay the basal TSH remains detectable. If the TSH is suppressed, there may be concern that the patient is hyperthyroid, but again these changes in thyroid function return to normal once the patient's psychiatric illness is brought under control.

Resistance to thyroid hormones

In adult patients with goitre, or children and adolescents with short stature, hyperactivity, or learning disabilities, thyroid function tests

Table 11 Thyroid hormone resistance; possible mechanisms to explain the phenomenon

Structurally abnormal hormone
Reduced accessibility of hormone to tissue due to binding/interaction with another substance
Cell membrane defect
Impaired metabolism of a hormone precursor
Defective receptor for hormone
Postreceptor abnormalities

Hormone resistance represents a situation in which inappropriately elevated levels of hormone occur in a setting in which the accompanying biological/clinical manifestations are inappropriate.

may demonstrate elevations of total and free T_4 and T_3 in the presence of a non-suppressed serum TSH. Having excluded the possibilities of alterations of thyroid hormone binding proteins, drugs, or intercurrent illness, the possibility of resistance to thyroid hormone needs to be considered. In such cases patients are not clinically hyperthyroid. A number of mechanisms may underlie such cases (Table 11). The lack of accurate measures of the peripheral effects of thyroid hormones on target tissues makes it exceedingly difficult to determine whether there is true evidence of deficiency of thyroid hormone action. To date, two major subgroups of patients with evidence of thyroid hormone resistance have been defined by defects at the level of the thyroid hormone receptor. Most such patients have generalized tissue resistance to thyroid hormone, but there is a smaller group in whom resistance is confined to the pituitary. This last condition is characterized by evidence of hypermetabolism and, in addition, is more commonly sporadic. In the generalized syndrome, the pattern of inheritance is autosomal dominant in the majority of families described. Variability in the clinical manifestations among affected members suggests that the syndrome encompasses a wide variety of defects at various stages of thyroid hormone action. Once it is suspected, diagnosis is aided by tests that measure the effects of doses of T_3 on concentrations of serum sex hormone binding globulin, ferritin, cholesterol, triglycerides, and creatinine phosphokinase. In addition, assessment of the sleeping pulse rate, the basal metabolic rate, echocardiography, and deep tendon relaxation time may all help to demonstrate evidence of peripheral tissue hypothyroidism.

With the cloning of the nuclear T_3 receptor, a number of different point mutations in the thyroid hormone receptor β-gene have been identified in various families with the generalized syndrome, resulting in substitutions of a single amino acid in the T_3-binding domain. The ability to identify these mutations provides a means for potential prenatal diagnosis which is of particular importance in families where there is evidence of growth and mental retardation. In the majority, however, an increase in the endogenous supply of thyroid hormone adequately compensates for the degree of tissue resistance. Therefore, in these patients, only identification of the cause of the abnormal thyroid function is necessary so they are not treated erroneously for hyperthyroidism, and there is no requirement for treatment with thyroid hormone.

Further reading

Bartalena, L., Marcocci, C., Bogazzi, F., *et al.* (1998). Relation between therapy for hyperthyroidism and the course of Graves' ophthalmopathy. *New England Journal of Medicine* 338, 73–8.

Glinoer, D. (1993). Maternal thyroid function in pregnancy. *Journal of Endocrinological Investigations* 16, 374–8.

Wartofsky, L., Sherman, S.I., Gopal, J., *et al.* (1998). The use of radioactive iodine in patients with papillary and follicular thyroid cancer. *Journal of Clinical Endocrinology and Metabolism* 83, 4195–203.

Chapter 7.4

Thyroid cancer

M. C. Sheppard

Prevalence

In the UK, thyroid cancer accounts for less than 0.5 per cent of new malignancies and less than 0.5 per cent of cancer deaths; in contrast, the prevalence of thyroid nodules is considerable. The Whickham survey, from the north-east of England, reported that thyroid enlargement was present in up to 10 per cent of the population, being four times more common in females than males. Similarly, the Framingham study in the US found that 4.2 per cent of the surveyed population had a thyroid nodule. The presence of nodular thyroid disease may be even more common than suggested by such surveys, since in postmortem studies up to 50 per cent of the population are found to have either single or multiple nodules, many of which are very small. Furthermore, ultrasound studies have revealed discrete nodules in up to 50 per cent of the population beyond the fifth decade of life. Thyroid cancer is reported to occur in approximately 10 per cent of thyroid nodules which have been selected for surgery on clinical grounds, although the risk of malignancy is lower in multinodular goitre than in solitary nodules. Cancer rates are much lower in small nodules such as those noted incidentally at ultrasound scanning or autopsy.

Aetiological factors

While ^{131}I given as treatment for hyperthyroidism or as a scanning agent is not associated with an increased risk of thyroid cancer, epidemiological studies have confirmed a relationship between radiation and thyroid nodules and neoplasms. These data are derived from the previous practice of treating a wide range of benign conditions during childhood with external irradiation of the head and neck as well as from studies of exposed individuals in the Marshall Islands and at Hiroshima. The risk of developing thyroid nodules and thyroid cancer is greater for women and is inversely related to the age at which radiation exposure occurs. Almost all cancers are well differentiated, nearly all being papillary in type. A high proportion (30–40 per cent) of patients with nodules after radiation are found to have thyroid cancer at the time of surgery and thus surgery should be performed for most palpable thyroid nodules.

Another environmental risk is iodine deficiency, probably operating through the action of thyroid stimulating hormone (TSH), but Graves' disease does not increase the risk.

Normal and neoplastic thyroid tissues express a variety of proto-oncogenes, growth factors, and growth factor receptors. Mutated forms of the H-*ras*, K-*ras*, and N-*ras* oncogenes are found in thyroid neoplasms; benign and malignant tumours have the same mutations, but the abnormalities are more frequent in the cancers. Therefore, these mutations are not of diagnostic use but may have a role as prognostic factors. Activated forms of the rearranged *ret* proto-oncogene (*ret/ptc*) are found in papillery carcinomas.

Clinical presentation

Most patients present with an otherwise asymptomatic nodule noticed incidentally, or the nodule is detected on routine physical examination. A family history of goitre or thyroid dysfunction usually suggests a benign disorder; if, however, this includes medullary thyroid carcinoma, phaeochromocytoma, or the multiple endocrine neoplasia syndrome, thyroid cancer is more probable. Age is important because nodular thyroid disease is uncommon in childhood and its presence should be viewed with suspicion. Similarly, there appears to be a greater risk of malignancy in nodules developing over the age of 60. A particularly relevant feature is whether the nodule developed or increased in size while the patient was on suppressive doses of thyroid hormones. Local symptoms such as dysphagia, dysphonia, dyspnoea, and haemoptysis may suggest oesophageal or tracheal involvement by a thyroid cancer, although such symptoms may occur in association with a benign goitre, especially if multinodular. Local pain in the neck or pain radiating to the jaw or ear may occur. The physical characteristics are, on the whole, poor predictors of malignancy, although some features, such as the presence of lymph nodes or obvious fixation to local structures, may be of diagnostic value. Patients may present with advanced disease with evidence or metastases to lungs, bone, or liver, and in some cases without clinically obvious thyroid pathology. Well-differentiated follicular carcinoma causing thyrotoxicosis is a very rare entity.

Laboratory tests

There is no laboratory test of value in distinguishing benign from malignant lesions of the thyroid. It is, none the less, important to assess thyroid function in patients presenting with nodular thyroid disease because the presence of hyperthyroidism is rarely associated with malignancy. Equally, it is important to exclude hypothyroidism, when, as in Hashimoto's thyroiditis, the firm goitre may raise suspicion of malignancy. The presence of thyroid autoantibodies may also be helpful, although there appears to be an increased risk of lymphoma in Hashimoto's thyroiditis. Serum thyroglobulin concentrations are often elevated in patients with differentiated thyroid cancers, but are also elevated in endemic goitre, multinodular goitre, benign adenoma, Graves' disease, and Hashimoto's thyroiditis. Measurement of serum thyroglobulin is of value in the follow-up of treated differentiated thyroid cancer.

Imaging tests

Neither isotope nor ultrasound scanning techniques have sufficient diagnostic accuracy to be used as single investigations on which to base management.

Technetium scanning

A solitary thyroid nodule can usefully be characterized by either reduced or enhanced uptake compared with that of the surrounding normal tissue. Whilst the great majority of thyroid cancers are hypofunctioning, only 20 per cent of cold nodules are cancers, the remaining 80 per cent being benign lesions, including cysts, colloid nodules, adenomas, degenerative nodules, and thyroiditis. Hypofunctioning lesions warrant further investigation, usually biopsy. The incidence of cancer in a cold nodule within a multinodular goitre is lower than in a solitary nodule, but the risk in such lesions is still sufficiently high that needle biopsy is warranted for such lesions that are dominant, hard, or rapidly growing. Autonomously functioning (hot) thyroid nodules are so rarely malignant that neither biopsy nor surgical removal is indicated.

Table 1 Thyroid malignancy

Papillary carcinoma	Lymphoma
Follicular carcinoma	Medullary carcinoma
Hürthle cell carcinoma	Metastasis
Anaplastic carcinoma	

Iodine scanning

Radio-iodine is given by mouth as sodium iodide. Imaging is usually performed 18–24 h after administration, at which time the majority of radioactivity within the thyroid is present as radio-iodotyrosine residues on thyroglobulin, reflecting hormonogenesis. The imaging patterns for radio-iodine scanning of the thyroid are similar to those of Tc^{m}, in that nodules demonstrating radio-iodine uptake greater than that of surrounding issue are almost invariably benign. Hypofunctioning nodules carry a higher risk of malignancy, although most are benign. The disadvantages of iodine scanning are the expense of the isotope and inconvenience to the patient because of the necessity of two visits. There are no advantages over the use of technetium.

Ultrasound

High-resolution imaging of thyroid nodules is most often used to determine whether the lesion is cystic or solid and whether it is solitary. True cysts of the thyroid are benign. However, they are uncommon and most large nodules contain areas of cystic or haemorrhagic degeneration. Although solitary nodules pose a greater risk of malignancy than multiple nodules, the finding of additional nodules does not eliminate the potential for malignancy or the need for further evaluation.

Needle biopsy

Given an experienced cytopathologist, fine-needle aspiration has largely replaced radioisotope and ultrasound imaging in the initial preoperative evaluation of most patients with thyroid nodules. Preoperative diagnosis expedites definitive treatment and facilitates counselling of patients. Risks associated with fine-needle aspiration are few, but false negative results can result from sampling error.

Another problem is that fine-needle aspiration cannot reliably distinguish between a follicular adenoma and a follicular carcinoma. New techniques such as DNA amplification combined with gene analysis, flow cytometry with chromosome ploidy analysis, or cell cycle analysis, may, when combined with traditional cytology, improve diagnostic accuracy. The histopathological patterns of thyroid cancers are shown in Table 1.

Papillary thyroid carcinoma

Papillary thyroid carcinoma is the most frequently diagnosed malignant thyroid tumour; in 25 retrospective analyses of 12 855 treated cases of differentiated thyroid cancer from North and South America, Japan, and Europe, papillary thyroid carcinoma comprised 50–89 per cent of these cases (average, 74 per cent). Papillary thyroid carcinoma and follicular cancer are more common in women (3:1) and although occurring at all ages, are rarest in childhood. Papillary cancers are most frequent in the third and fourth decades, whereas follicular cancers tend to occur in older individuals.

Papillary cancers are locally invasive, rarely encapsulated, and may have areas of cystic degeneration. They often appear multifocal, small foci being scattered elsewhere in the gland. Some papillary cancers are small (< 1 cm in diameter) and are often referred to as occult. At the other extreme is the diffuse papillary type, often sclerosing, which infiltrates the whole thyroid; it usually occurs in children and young adults. The presence of small papillary cancers has been demonstrated in 6–13 per cent of autopsied American patients. These occult papillary tumours rarely undergo transition to clinically evident carcinomas.

The two most controversial topics in the management of papillary thyroid carcinoma are the extent of thyroid surgery that is optimal and the indications for postoperative radio-iodine therapy. Surgery is the primary mode of treatment and unless there is clear evidence of contralateral disease or of metastasis, simple lobectomy is the preferred option. Those advocating near-total thyroidectomy do so because papillary cancers are often multifocal and follow-up is rendered easier. Patients in whom lymph nodes are involved often require removal of these but block dissection is usually unwarranted. There is no consensus with regard to the use of ^{131}I in patients with small, solitary lesions, but radio-iodine has a clear role in the management of residual disease or established metastases. Some authorities recommend ^{131}I ablation for nearly all patients with papillary cancer, others reserving this treatment for only a few very high-risk patients. In those most commonly affected, that is aged between 20 and 40 years, papillary cancer is a relatively benign condition, with 10- to 20-year recurrence rates of 5–10 per cent, and death rates of 2–5 per cent. Cervical lymph node involvement is relatively common at presentation but because local treatment (surgery or ^{131}I administration) is effective, the prognosis is not adversely affected. Unfortunately, in individuals aged over 40 years, papillary cancers often progress by slowly invading local structures.

Follicular thyroid carcinoma

Follicular thyroid carcinoma is uncommon, accounting for about 15 per cent of all thyroid cancers. In approximately 15 per cent of patients, distant metastases are already present at diagnosis, whereas follicular thyroid carcinoma only occasionally involves regional nodes. Distant metastases ultimately develop in approximately 20 per cent of patients, the most common sites being lung and bone.

Appearances of follicular cancers range from almost normal-looking follicles to sheets of cells with only an occasional follicle; the tumours are not multifocal. One of the most difficult distinctions in thyroid cytology is the differentiation between benign follicular adenomas and encapsulated low-grade or minimally invasive follicular carcinomas. In view of this cytological examination cannot replace surgery in this situation. Most cytopathologists will report follicular neoplasms to be suspicious, although a relatively small minority prove to be truly malignant when examined histologically. Preponderant opinion favours total thyroidectomy as the procedure of choice in follicular thyroid carcinoma, although prospective data are not available and studies showing that total thyroidectomy improves survival are retrospective and conflicting.

Routine remnant ablation is accepted practice in follicular thyroid carcinoma because of its aggressive behaviour. Most endocrinologists recommend total body scanning using 5–10 mCi of ^{131}I 6 to 8 weeks after total thyroidectomy. If significant uptake is noted in the thyroid bed, ablation of these remnants may destroy microscopic tumour left behind at surgery and by removing all functioning tissue will allow more efficient later visualization and treatment of any metastases with radio-iodine.

The prognosis is poor in metastatic follicular thyroid carcinoma, with 5- and 10-year mortality rates of about 60 and 80 per cent, respectively. Studies of metastatic differentiated thyroid cancer have shown that survival is improved in patients treated with radio-iodine, compared with those in whom treatment cannot be given because the tumour fails to concentrate the radio-isotope. Poor prognostic features include older age, greater degrees of invasiveness, distant metastases, and possibly an abnormal chromosomal number (aneuploidy) within tumour tissue.

Hürthle cell carcinoma

Hürthle cell carcinoma comprises only about 3–6 per cent of all differentiated thyroid cancers. Hürthle cells (also known as oxyphil or Askanazy cells) are large polygonal cells with pleomorphic hyperchromatic nuclei and eosinophilic granular cytoplasm. Most malignant Hürthle cell tumours are considered to be variants of follicular carcinoma and are primarily a disease of adults, most patients being diagnosed in the fourth to seventh decade with a predominance in women. This condition is associated with previous head and neck irradiation. As in the case of follicular carcinomas, cervical lymphadenopathy is infrequent but distant metastatic disease is present in 10–15 per cent of patients at the time of the initial diagnosis. The most common metastatic sites are lung and bone. Pathological distinction between benign and malignant Hürthle cell tumours may be extremely difficult and requires demonstration of vascular, or full-thickness, capsular invasion in a surgical specimen. Hürthle cells are commonly found in benign thyroid disorders. Because these cytological features are difficult to interpret, surgical resection of lesions when cytology reveals the presence of Hürthle cells is commonly recommended, total thyroidectomy being the treatment of choice for patients with histologically malignant lesions. Radioactive iodine is generally ineffective in treatment of metastatic disease because of a lack of uptake of ^{131}I by the metastases. Hürthle cell carcinoma is a relatively aggressive thyroid tumour and is associated with a 5-year mortality rate of about 80 per cent.

Anaplastic carcinoma

Anaplastic carcinoma accounts for only 5–14 per cent of primary malignant thyroid neoplasms but is very aggressive, with a 5-year survival rate of 7 per cent and a mean survival period of 6 months from diagnosis. The peak incidence of the disease is in the seventh decade of life. Anaplastic carcinoma is characterized by rapid growth of a mass in the neck that was not present before, or by a rapid growth in a pre-existing thyroid tumour. The mass is usually firm or hard and fixed to the underlying structures. The skin overlying the tumour may also undergo necrosis. Large anaplastic carcinomas almost always encroach on the trachea, but to varying degrees. Severe respiratory obstruction may occur. Frequently the tumour is fixed to the larynx and nearby major vessels. Because of infiltration into these structures, the mass does not move with swallowing. Vocal cord paralysis can occur, as well as obstruction of the superior vena cava. Enlargement of the neck lymph nodes occurs early. Anaplastic thyroid carcinoma is very resistant to any form of therapy and is rarely cured. The best survival results have been obtained with a combination of total thyroidectomy, resection of lymph nodes, external irradiation, and chemotherapy. Neither radioactive iodine nor thyroid hormone treatment significantly alters the course of the disease. There is no consensus on the selection of chemotherapeutic regimens.

Lymphomas

Lymphoma may affect the thyroid primarily, or may involve the gland as part of a systemic disease. Thyroid lymphoma is uncommon, accounting for only 1–2 per cent of all thyroid malignancies. It rarely occurs under the age of 40 years and has a female predominance of approximately 4:1. Patients usually present with a short history of enlargement of the thyroid. The gland is often firm and may appear to be fixed to adjacent tissues. Regional lymph nodes may be enlarged because of lymphoma involvement. The majority of patients are euthyroid although some are hypothyroid secondary to autoimmune thyroiditis. Follow-up studies have estimated that the relative risk of thyroid lymphoma in patients with autoimmune thyroiditis is 60–80 times greater than in controls. The nature of this relationship is unknown.

Fine- and large-needle biopsies are the initial diagnostic procedures. The vast majority of thyroid lymphomas are non-Hodgkin's in type. Non-involved areas of thyroid tissue may be normal or altered by a concomitant autoimmune thyroiditis. Radiotherapy alone appears to be an excellent treatment for disease limited to the thyroid, with or without cervical lymphadenopathy. Results for patients with mediastinal extension treated by radiotherapy alone are unsatisfactory, when the addition of combination chemotherapy is indicated.

Follow-up evaluation

All patients require suppressive thyroxine therapy following definitive treatment for thyroid cancer (usually 200 μg/day). The degree of suppression of serum TSH concentration needed to minimize tumour recurrence rates is as yet unclear but most clinicians would aim for a level below the normal range of the assay. Following radio-ablation of the thyroid, patients should have a total body radio-iodine scan at 6–12 months to document successful ablation, but the optimal frequency of subsequent scans is uncertain. It is essential to withdraw thyroid hormone therapy prior to such investigation.

Serum thyroglobulin measurement is a valuable tumour marker. Patients with known differentiated papillary or follicular thyroid cancers who have undergone definitive treatment have normal or undetectable serum thyroglobulin concentrations in the absence of residual tumour, but elevated levels in the presence of metastases or recurrence. Measurement at regular intervals, often while thyroxine treatment is continued, allows radio-iodine scans to be confined to patients in whom the thyroglobulin result or clinical evidence suggests recurrence.

Medullary thyroid carcinoma (see also Chapters 7.5 and 7.15)

This arises from the parafollicular or C cells of the thyroid and constitutes about 3–5 per cent of all thyroid cancers. These tumours secrete calcitonin which provides a useful diagnostic criterion and a marker to monitor response or relapse after treatment. In cases of doubt, calcitonin secretion may be enhanced by infusion of calcium, pentagastrin, or ingestion of alcohol. Medullary carcinoma forms part of the multiple endocrine neoplasia type 2 syndrome, the genetic basis of which has now been characterized. Genetic and biochemical tests are likely to be complementary.

Further reading

Burman, K.D. (ed.) (1995). Thyroid Cancer I. *Endocrinology and Metabolism Clinics of North America* **24**, 4.

Burman, K.D. (ed.) (1995). Thyroid Cancer II. *Endocrinology and Metabolism Clinics of North America* **25**, 1.

Suarez, H.G. (1998). Genetic alterations in human epithelial thyroid tumours. *Clinical Endocrinology* **24**, 531–46.

Chapter 7.5

Disorders of calcium metabolism

J. A. Kanis

Distribution and function of calcium

Plasma calcium

The concentration of plasma calcium in health is maintained within a very narrow range, varying by less than 5–10 per cent, despite the large movements of calcium across gut, bone, kidney, and other tissues. Several hormones, including parathyroid hormone and calcitriol (1,25-dihydroxyvitamin D_3; 1,25$(OH)_2D_3$), regulate the ionized fraction of plasma calcium (approximately 50 per cent of total plasma calcium; Table 1) by modulating calcium fluxes to and from the extracellular fluid. In turn, the secretion rates for these hormones are regulated in part by the calcium concentration of the extracellular fluid, thereby completing a negative feedback loop.

Changes in plasma calcium are usually due to changes in the total amount of calcium in the extracellular fluid, since there is a free distribution of ionized calcium throughout the compartment. Within the plasma compartment, however, approximately half of the calcium

Table 1 Distribution of plasma calcium

Ultrafilterable calcium (53%)	
Ionized calcium	47%
Complexed calcium	
Phosphate	1.5%
Citrate	1.5%
HCO_3, etc.	3%
Protein-bound calcium (47%)	
Albumin	37%
Globulin	10%
Total plasma calcium (2.12–2.6 mmol/l)	100%

is bound to proteins, mainly albumin, and the binding is pH dependent. Major changes in plasma protein concentrations, the presence of abnormal proteins, and large shifts in extracellular hydrogen ion concentration can therefore affect the amount of calcium that is bound to protein, so that the estimation of total plasma calcium may not accurately reflect the ionized concentration. These changes have important clinical consequences. Thus, the paraesthesiae seen in patients with hyperventilation syndrome are associated with a decreased ionized calcium concentration due to alkalosis, but total plasma calcium is normal. Also, the infusion of alkali into patients with long-standing metabolic acidosis (for example, those with chronic renal failure) may precipitate hypocalcaemic convulsions due to a decrease in ionized calcium, without changing the total plasma calcium.

In the absence of severe acidosis or alkalosis, the major factor influencing plasma calcium concentrations is the quantity of albumin present. Failure to account for protein binding may result in the erroneous diagnosis of hypercalcaemia in conditions where increased concentrations or abnormal plasma proteins are found, for example, dehydration, prolonged venostasis, and myeloma. Also, in hypoproteinaemic states total plasma calcium may be low, though ionized calcium is normal. Similarly, in such disorders total plasma calcium may be normal and mask true hypercalcaemia.

Since the ionized plasma calcium is the physiologically relevant fraction, ideally this should be measured, but the present methods are often unreliable and not widely available. Many formulae have been proposed for predicting the ionized calcium from the total plasma calcium, by 'correcting' the total plasma calcium for a given protein value. These methods depend on the concurrent measurement of total proteins, albumin, or specific gravity of plasma. None is entirely satisfactory but a widely used adjustment factor for ionized calcium is to subtract from the measured plasma calcium 0.02 mmol/l for every 1 g/l that the plasma albumin exceeds 40 g/l, provided the sample is withdrawn without venostasis. A similar addition is made when the plasma albumin is less than 40 g/l. Many laboratories now report 'corrected' plasma calcium or 'ionized' plasma calcium, but these are at best a guide to the true ionized calcium concentration.

A small proportion of total plasma calcium is complexed with cations such as phosphate, citrate, and bicarbonate (see Table 1). The calcium that is normally filtered by the kidney includes this portion as well as ionized calcium. In several disorders this proportion of complexed, ultrafilterable calcium is increased (e.g. in disorders of acid–base, phosphate, and citrate metabolism).

Principles of regulation of plasma calcium

The total amount of calcium in the extracellular fluid is dependent upon movements of calcium to and from the extracellular fluid. The major fluxes occur across the gut, bone, and kidneys. (Fig. 1). There is a significant exchange of calcium between extracellular fluid and bone; in normal human adults between 1 and 2 per cent of total body calcium is exchanged over a few days. This represents 1000 or 2000 mmol, which is a substantial amount considering that the extracellular fluid contains somewhat less than 20 mmol as ionized calcium. This exchangeable pool may therefore be very important in plasma calcium homeostasis, although how these large movements are subject to metabolic regulation is controversial.

These large and rapid fluxes should be distinguished from the movements of calcium that occur in bone as a result of mineralization

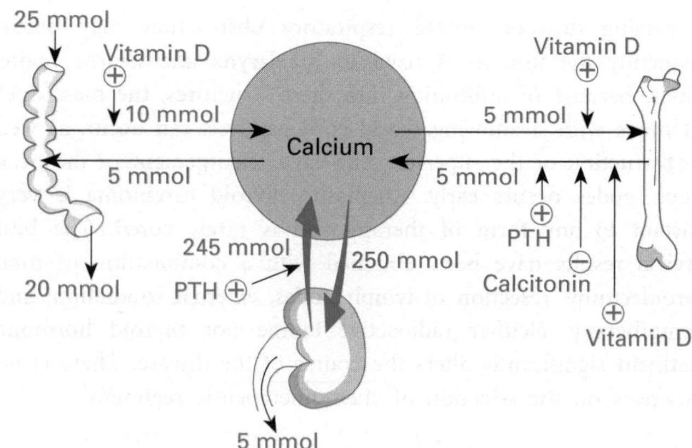

Fig. 1 Major fluxes of calcium (mmol/day) in a healthy adult. Exchange of calcium in the extracellular fluid occurs across bone, gut, and the kidneys. The net balance for calcium equals the net absorption minus the losses of calcium in faeces and urine, which in a healthy adult is zero. The major fluxes of calcium are regulated by the regulating hormones. Parathyroid hormone (PTH) increases renal tubular reabsorption of calcium and bone resorption, calcitonin inhibits bone resorption, and vitamin D augments intestinal absorption of calcium. The precise role of vitamin D in augmenting bone resorption and mineralization *in vivo* is unclear (1 mmol = 40 mg calcium).

and bone resorption. These account for only a fraction of the total calcium exchange between extracellular fluid and bone, the remainder occurring across the large surface area of osteocytes and their canaliculi without synthesis or destruction of bone matrix. Approximately 10 per cent of the adult skeleton is thought to be renewed each year by remodelling, although this is not uniformly distributed throughout the skeleton; for example, cancellous bone has a faster turnover than cortical bone, so that disturbances of bone turnover commonly have greater and earlier effects at cancellous than at cortical sites.

Calcium is lost from the body by urinary and intestinal excretion, and to a lesser extent in sweat, and enters by intestinal absorption and renal tubular reabsorption of glomerular filtrate. The true intestinal absorption of calcium is greater than the net absorption because some calcium is returned to the gut in biliary, pancreatic, and intestinal secretions. Thus, from an average daily dietary intake of 25 mmol, approximately 10 mmol is absorbed. This is offset by intestinal secretion amounting to approximately 5 mmol daily, leaving a net transport into the extracellular fluid pool of 5 mmol. Apparent and real fluxes across the gut can be measured by tracer and balance studies.

The kidney is a major site for calcium excretion. A large amount of calcium is filtered (see Fig. 1), but most of this is reabsorbed, leaving only some 5 mmol for urinary excretion. Several hormones, particularly parathyroid hormone, alter renal tubular reabsorption of calcium, small changes in which have profound effects on the extracellular fluid concentration. Losses in sweat can be as high as 8 mmol daily under extreme conditions but are usually insignificant.

In mature adults who are neither gaining nor losing calcium, bone and soft tissues contribute neither a net gain nor loss of calcium to the extracellular fluid; the amount of bone resorbed exactly matches the amount formed. Also, the net amount of calcium absorbed by the gut matches the urinary excretion. Because plasma and intracellular calcium levels are controlled within a narrow range, changes in bone mass are reflected as changes in the external balance for calcium. For example, during growth, when there is a net daily gain of calcium to be incorporated into the skeleton, plasma and intracellular concentrations of calcium are normal. In the long term, therefore, the total body balance of calcium reflects exactly the skeletal balance for calcium (in this case positive calcium balance). Negative balance begins at middle age. Between the age of 25 and 45 the body should be neither gaining nor losing calcium, so that inflow and outflow of calcium are matched.

The transport of calcium between the extracellular fluid and bone, gut, and kidneys is regulated by a variety of factors, including several hormones (see Fig. 1). These hormones can be subdivided into 'controlling hormones' and 'influencing hormones'. The controlling group comprise PTH, calcitonin, and vitamin D metabolites, and the production of each is altered in response to changes in ionized calcium concentrations. The influencing hormones are thyroxine, growth hormone, and adrenal and gonadal steroids, the secretion of which is determined primarily by factors other than changes in plasma calcium.

Major regulating hormones

Parathyroid hormone

The actions of PTH serve to increase plasma calcium in an efficient negative feedback hormonal loop, and the major stimulus to secretion is a fall in the ionized fraction of plasma calcium.

In humans there are usually four parathyroid glands, two embedded in the superior poles of the thyroid and two in the inferior poles. There is considerable individual variation, both in site and number. Parathyroid tissue is occasionally found in the mediastinum. Each gland, approximately the size of a match head, comprises chief cells, with clear cytoplasm and larger oxyphil cells.

PTH is released as a single peptide chain containing 84 amino acids (molecular weight 5500). It is synthesized as a prohormone which contains an additional six amino acids at its amino-terminal end. A further precursor form, pre-pro-PTH, containing a total of 150 amino acids, has been identified in studies *in vitro*. The site of synthesis of the precursor hormone is the rough endoplasmic reticulum of the chief cells. The function of the oxyphil cells is unknown. The precursor forms of PTH are probably converted to the 84 amino acid polypeptide before secretion from the gland in secretory granules.

Only the first 32 to 34 amino acids, reading from the amino-terminal end, are necessary for biological activity. There is evidence that cleavage occurs naturally, partly in the liver, to produce a short amino-terminal fragment with biological activity and a larger inactive carboxy-terminal fragment. This cleavage may be necessary for PTH to act on bone. There are also many less well-characterized circulating fragments of PTH. The liver and kidney are important sites for degradation. For example, the C-terminal fragment normally cleared by the kidney may be increased in chronic renal failure, although the circulating levels of biologically active PTH may be normal. This may cause problems in interpretation of results since the C-terminal fragment is the major component measured in some assay systems. Sensitive assays for the intact PTH molecule have been developed but are not yet universally used.

Secretion of PTH

The major physiological stimulus to the secretion of PTH is a fall in the plasma ionized calcium concentration whilst a rise suppresses secretion. Many other factors are known to influence secretion, including β-adrenergic agonists, vitamin D metabolites, growth hormone and somatostatin, vitamin A, prostaglandins, prolactin, aluminium, and divalent cations such as magnesium and strontium. With the exception of magnesium and aluminium, the physiological or clinical relevance of these factors is uncertain. In the presence of chronic hypomagnesaemia, the release of PTH from parathyroid tissue is impaired, and this, together with an impaired target organ response to PTH, accounts for the hypocalcaemia occasionally observed in magnesium deficiency.

Actions of PTH

The target organ actions of PTH include effects on bone, kidney, and indirectly on gut. PTH acts on the proximal and distal tubules of the kidney to increase the renal tubular reabsorption of calcium and to depress the tubular reabsorption of phosphate. This leads to a rise in plasma calcium and fall in plasma phosphate. Inhibition of proximal tubular reabsorption of phosphate appears to be mediated by cyclic AMP as a result of activation of adenylate cyclase in the renal cortex. PTH also decreases the proximal renal tubular reabsorption of bicarbonate which leads to increased excretion of bicarbonate ions and to an hyperchloraemic acidosis. A mild metabolic acidosis is commonly seen in primary and secondary hyperparathyroidism, whereas in hypoparathyroidism there may be a metabolic alkalosis. Alkalosis may also be observed when the secretion of PTH is suppressed, for example by hypercalcaemia due to malignant disease affecting the skeleton. In this example the alkalosis is also partly due to the release of buffer from bone. It is possible that the acidosis induced by PTH augments calcium release from bone.

PTH has a further important effect on the kidney, to stimulate the 1α-hydroxylase enzyme responsible for the production of 1,25-dihydroxyvitamin D_3 (calcitriol) from calcidiol. This potent metabolite of vitamin D increases calcium absorption from the gut and possibly releases calcium from the bone. Thus, the various effects of PTH on the kidney and gut appear, either directly or indirectly, to increase the extracellular fluid concentration of calcium. Other effects of PTH on the kidney include decreased proximal tubular reabsorption of sodium and increased amino acid excretion.

The major effect of PTH on bone is to increase its resorption, by increasing the activity and numbers of osteoclasts. There is evidence, however, that PTH also increases bone formation, suggesting that its major effect on the skeleton is to increase bone turnover.

Calcitonin

Calcitonin is a peptide hormone containing 32 amino acid residues with a disulphide bond between cystine residues in positions 1 and 7. A major stimulus to its secretion is an increase in the serum concentration of calcium. Many of its actions serve to lower serum calcium, principally by inhibiting osteoclast numbers and activity.

Calcitonin is produced from the parafollicular (C-cells) of the thyroid. There are several differences in amino acid composition of the calcitonins from different species and the salmon hormone resembles the human more than other mammalian calcitonins and is more potent in man than the human hormone itself. Extrathyroidal sites for calcitonin production have been demonstrated in the thymus, adrenal, and the pars intermedia of the pituitary gland.

Many agents are known to affect the secretion of calcitonin in addition to calcium. These include gastrointestinal hormones, such as glucagon and gastrin, β-adrenergic agents, and whisky. It is widely believed that calcitonin is a calcium-regulating hormone with a

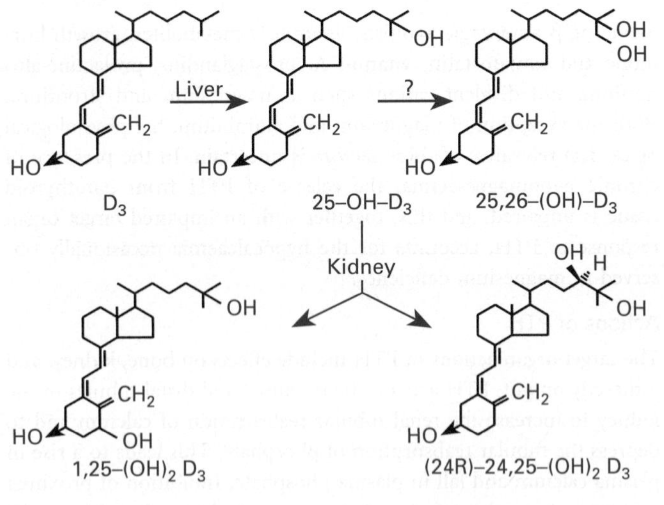

Fig. 2 Steps in the metabolism of vitamin D. The site of synthesis of 25-hydroxyvitamin D_3 (calcidiol) is in the liver. The active form of vitamin D (1, $25(OH)_2D_3$; calcitriol) is made in the kidney and placenta. Secalciferol (24, $25(OH)_2D_3$) is synthesized in several tissues, but the kidney is probably the major site. The site of synthesis and function of $25,26(OH)_2D_3$ is unknown.

negative feedback loop controlled by plasma calcium and acting in the opposite way to that of PTH, but its physiological role is unclear. One difficulty of ascribing any such role is that calcitonin deficiency (total thyroidectomy) or excess (medullary carcinoma of the thyroid) are associated with only minor disturbances in skeletal or calcium homeostasis.

The major clinical interest in calcitonin is its pharmacological use as an inhibitor of bone resorption and turnover for the treatment of osteoporosis, Paget's disease, and of hypercalcaemia associated with increased bone resorption. Assay of calcitonin is useful in the diagnosis of medullary carcinoma of the thyroid and for the screening of members of families with this disease.

Vitamin D

Vitamin D_3 (cholecalciferol) is derived from the diet and from the skin by ultraviolet irradiation of 7-dehydrocholesterol. Vitamin D_2 (calciferol) is a product originally derived from the ultraviolet irradiation of plant sterols and is used to supplement the diet, particularly in margarine. In most respects the two are comparable in their metabolism and their actions.

Following photochemical conversion from 7-dehydrocholesterol, vitamin D is transported in plasma bound to a specific α-globulin (vitamin D binding protein). It is fat soluble and dietary sources are absorbed primarily from the duodenum and jejunum into the lymphatic circulation. A large amount of the vitamin may be stored in adipose and muscle tissues.

Before exerting biological effects, vitamin D undergoes a series of further metabolic conversions (Fig. 2). The first step involves its conversion in liver to 25-hydroxyvitamin D ($25OHD_3$; calcidiol) which is the major circulating vitamin D metabolite. Its measurement provides an index of vitamin D nutrition, when serum values of less than 5 ng/ml (12.5 nmol/l) indicate deficiency. There is a marked seasonal variation in its serum concentration, with a peak in late summer and a trough in late winter, reflecting exposure to ultraviolet irradiation. In northern Europe, serum values in winter commonly approach those associated with deficiency states. A proportion of the calcidiol formed is secreted into the intestinal lumen, some of which may be available for reabsorption.

The next step is further hydroxylation to calcitriol (1,25-dihydroxyvitamin D_3), secalciferol ($24,25(OH)D_3$), or $25,26(OH)D_3$. The kidney is the major, if not sole, site for 1α-hydroxylation, a point of considerable importance in the pathogenesis of vitamin D resistance in renal failure. The production of calcitriol is enhanced by deficiency of vitamin D, calcium, or phosphate as well as by a variety of hormones, including PTH, oestradiol, prolactin, and growth hormone. The rise in calcitriol concentrations during pregnancy is partly due to increased synthesis of vitamin D binding protein.

The production of secalciferol (also largely by the kidney) is favoured under conditions which inhibit synthesis of calcitriol, such that a reciprocal relationship is commonly observed between their respective production rates. Secalciferol may have a physiological role in cartilage, bone, or parathyroid homeostasis. Many other vitamin D metabolites have been identified in serum but their metabolic function, if any, is unclear.

Calcitriol has a serum half-life measured in hours and a normal plasma concentration of approximately 30 pg/ml in adults. Higher concentrations are observed in growing children and during late pregnancy and lactation. Serum values of calcidiol and secalciferol are 1000-fold and 100-fold greater than those of calcitriol, and both of these have a long biological half-life in the circulation.

Actions of vitamin D

The principal effects of calcitriol are to increase intestinal absorption of calcium and phosphate and to increase resorption of bone mineral and matrix. Although lack of vitamin D in humans is associated with defective mineralization of cartilage and bone, the question of whether or not vitamin D and its metabolites directly increase mineralization of bone is unsettled. From a teleological viewpoint, the action of calcitriol can be thought of as increasing the availability of calcium and phosphate for mineralization. Alternatively, its function may be to maintain extracellular concentrations of calcium and phosphate in concert with PTH.

Receptors for calcitriol have been found in many other tissues apart from bone and gut. These include skin, breast, salivary, and parathyroid tissue. In the case of the parathyroid glands tissue there is evidence that calcitriol decreases the synthesis of PTH.

A striking weakness of skeletal muscles, particularly of the pelvic and shoulder girdles, is a well-described feature of vitamin D deficiency, reversible following treatment with vitamin D or one of its metabolites. The mechanisms of the effects of vitamin D on muscle function are unknown but may involve calcium transfer across the sarcoplasmic reticulum, modifications in the metabolism of troponin C, or be mediated by way of hypophosphataemia or changes in intracellular phosphate. There are several other poorly understood trophic effects of vitamin D, particularly on cellular differentiation, endocrine secretion, growth, the maintenance of intestinal mucosa, and on the maturation of collagen and cartilage.

Other hormones

Growth hormone (see also Chapter 7.1)

Changes in growth hormone secretion have very little effect on plasma calcium and the occasional finding of hypercalcaemia in acromegalic patients should alert one to the possibility of coexisting primary hyperparathyroidism (pluriglandular syndrome). Hypercalciuria is more common and may be related to increased synthesis of calcitriol.

Thyroid hormones

In the adult, thyrotoxicosis is associated with hypercalciuria, hypophosphataemia, augmented bone turnover, osteoporosis, and occasionally hypercalcaemia, probably due to direct effects of thyroid hormones on bone.

Adrenal steroids

Adrenal insufficiency is occasionally accompanied by hypercalcaemia, probably due to haemoconcentration and to increased renal tubular reabsorption of calcium because of extracellular volume depletion. The ability of corticosteroids to decrease plasma calcium in some forms of hypercalcaemia has been used for many years as a diagnostic aid (see below), but the mechanism of action is uncertain.

Sex steroids

Male or female sex hormones may influence the amount of calcium present in the skeleton at the time of maturity, and administration of oestrogen reduces the rate of bone loss in postmenopausal osteoporosis. Oestrogens also lower plasma calcium, an effect more marked in postmenopausal women with hyperparathyroidism or hypercalcaemia from carcinoma of the breast. Hypercalcaemia is also occasionally seen with the use of tamoxifen, an oestrogen inhibitor, when used in the treatment of carcinoma of the breast.

Gastrointestinal hormones

Gastrin secretion is increased in hyperparathyroidism, due to its stimulation by hypercalcaemia. Large doses of glucagon may induce hypocalcaemia by inhibiting bone resorption, either directly or by stimulating the secretion of calcitonin.

Osteoclast activating factors

Several factors derived from leucocytes are potent bone-resorbing agents. These include lymphotoxin, tumour necrosis factors, and interleukin-1α and -1β. Their physiological importance is unknown, but the production of leucocyte-derived factors is increased in haematological neoplasias and may be responsible for the hypercalcaemia and bone loss seen in myeloma, which is characteristically sensitive to treatment with corticosteroids. Prostaglandins and procathapsin D may be important in the activation of osteoclasts in solid tumours. In addition, transforming growth factors and the PTH-related protein are causes of generalized bone resorption (see below).

Sites of calcium regulation

Intestine

Intestinal absorption of calcium is episodic and is dependent on an adequate supply delivered in an available form to the intestinal mucosa. The availability of calcium for absorption depends on many dietary factors. For example, excess phosphorus, lipids, and phytates bind calcium and render it unavailable for absorption, which depends both on active transport and diffusion processes occurring throughout the length of the small intestine and to a lesser extent in the colon. The major site for active transport is the duodenum and upper part of the jejunum. However, because the duodenum is relatively short compared to the entire length of the gastrointestinal tract, more calcium is probably absorbed at sites distal to the duodenum at normal dietary intakes than within the duodenum itself.

At very low intakes of calcium, net absorption may be negative since endogenous faecal calcium secretion may exceed the amount absorbed. In malabsorption syndromes loss of endogenous faecal calcium is probably due to poor absorption of digestive-juice calcium.

Adaption to variations in dietary intake of calcium allow net absorption to remain relatively constant over a fairly wide range of intake, probably regulated by calcitriol which stimulates the synthesis of a calcium-binding protein (calbindin) in addition to an intestinal alkaline phosphatase. The mechanism involves the translocation of calcitriol plus its receptor protein to the nucleus to stimulate the synthesis of messenger RNA and new protein synthesis.

There is good evidence that calcium and phosphate can be absorbed separately from each other, and calcitriol has independent effects to enhance the absorption of each. Unlike the absorption of calcium, which is closely regulated, the proportion of the dietary phosphate absorbed remains relatively constant at approximately 80 per cent of the intake over a wide range. This explains in part the fluctuations in plasma phosphate seen after a meal and underlines the need to study phosphate metabolism under controlled conditions.

A variety of tests are available to study calcium and phosphate absorption, including metabolic balance and the use of tracer techniques. A 24-h urine collection for calcium provides an indirect index of absorption, provided it is assumed or known that the net flux of calcium across bone is zero. The expression of excretion as a ratio of creatinine excretion standardizes somewhat for variations in body weight and for incomplete urine collections.

Increased intestinal absorption of calcium is found in pregnancy, during lactation, and in hyperparathyroidism, sarcoidosis, and idiopathic hypercalciuria due to increased production of calcitriol. Conversely, malabsorption of calcium is often caused by low levels of calcitriol, for example in hypoparathyroidism, vitamin D deficiency states, and in chronic renal failure. Calcium malabsorption is also seen in untreated coeliac disease where a target tissue for calcitriol has been destroyed.

Kidneys

Renal tubular reabsorption of calcium in the kidneys is a complex process. The total amount reabsorbed is the result of several mechanisms in various parts of the nephron and can be estimated by subtracting the amount of calcium excreted by the kidneys from the filtered load. The filterable calcium is approximately 60 per cent of total plasma calcium, and the filtered load represents the product of the glomerular filtration rate and the filterable calcium (approximately 200–250 mmol/day).

In health there is a curvilinear relationship between plasma calcium and renal excretion. The renal excretion may be expressed per unit of glomerular filtration to take account of variations in this rate (Fig. 3). Any value below the line depicting the normal relationship would indicate an increase in the net tubular reabsorption of calcium, and values above the lines denote decreased tubular reabsorption. When calcium excretion is measured in the fasting state, this will reflect more closely calcium derived from skeletal sources. An important corollary is that the estimation of urinary calcium excretion does not give information concerning renal tubular reabsorption unless the filtered load is also known. Some normal ranges for these values are shown in Table 2.

The assessment of renal tubular reabsorption in this way has several limitations since ultrafilterable calcium is rarely measured, and its derivation from total plasma calcium may be difficult in disorders of acid–base metabolism, dysproteinaemia, and renal damage. In health, approximately 97 per cent of the calcium filtered by the kidney is reabsorbed. Many hormones influence renal tubular reabsorption,

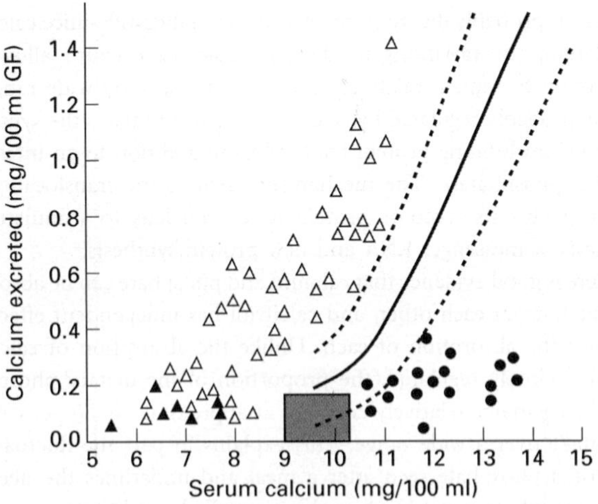

Fig. 3 Relationship between urinary calcium excretion (expressed as mg/100 ml of glomerular filtrate) and serum calcium in health and disorders of parathyroid function. The solid and dashed lines denote the mean values (+ 2 SD) obtained in normal subjects during calcium infusions. The shaded area represents the normal basal range. Patients with primary hyperparathyroidism (•) lie to the right of the line describing normal subjects, indicating increased renal tubular reabsorption for calcium. In contrast, patients with hypoparathyroidism (▲, untreated; △ during calcium infusion) lie to the left of the normal line, indicating decreased renal tubular reabsorption for calcium. Note that the determination of calcium excretion alone (without concurrent measurement of serum calcium) does not give information concerning renal tubular reabsorption for calcium. Note also that hypoparathyroid patients, not infused with calcium, and many hyperparathyroid patients, have normal values of calcium excretion. *(For source see OTM3, p.1628.).*

Table 2 Typical normal adult ranges for some simple biochemical measurements used in the investigation of patients with disorders of calcium homeostasis

Measurement	Units	Reference range
Plasma		
Total calcium	mmol/l	2.12–2.60
Ionized calcium	mmol/l	1.10–1.35
Fasting inorganic phosphate	mmol/l	0.6–1.5
Urine		
Calcium	mmol/24 h	M 2.5–10
	mmol/24 h	F 2.5–9.0
Phosphate	mmol/24 h	16–32
Total hydroxyproline	µmol/24 h	M 55–250
	µmol/24 h	F 75–430
Fasting urine		
Calcium/creatinine ratio	mmol/mmol	0.10–0.32
Calcium excretion	mmol/l GF	0.04
TmP/GFR	mmol/l	0.8–1.35
Total hydroxyproline/creatinine	µmol/mmol	< 40

M or F denotes sex; TmP/GFR, tubular maximum for phosphate reabsorption; GF, glomerular filtrate.

of which PTH is probably the most important. In mild primary hyperparathyroidism, the hypercalcaemia is due mainly to increased renal tubular reabsorption. Conversely, in hypoparathyroidism the low

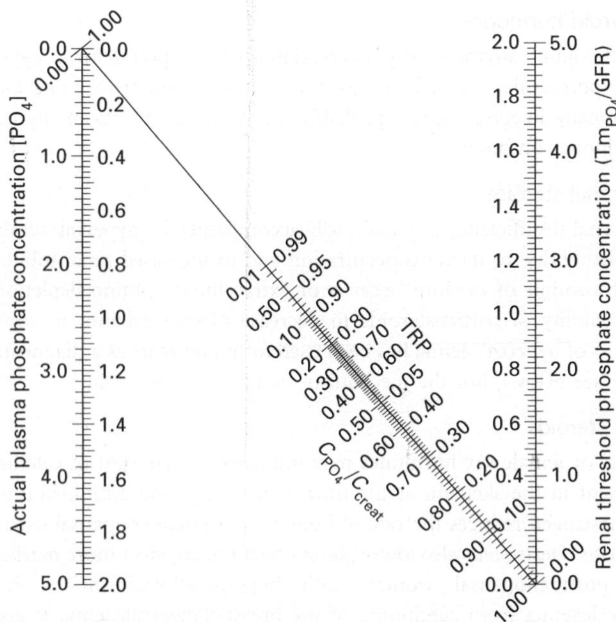

Fig. 4 Nomogram for the derivation of TmP/GFR (estimate of phosphate reabsorption) from simultaneous measurements of tubular reabsorption (TRP) or the ratio of the clearance of phosphate to the clearance of creatinine (CPO_4/ Creat) and plasma phosphate (PO_4). TRP can be calculated from the concentrations of phosphate and creatinine in plasma; the urine volume is not required:

$$\frac{\text{Phosphate clearance}}{\text{Creatinine clearance}} = \frac{\text{urine phosphate} \times \text{plasma creatinine}}{\text{plasma phosphate} \times \text{urine creatinine}}$$

A straight line through the appropriate values of plasma phosphate and TRP or phosphate/creatinine clearance passes through the corresponding value of TmP/GFR. TmP/GFR and phosphate are expressed in the same units. The scale in units of the figure is arbitrary. *(For source see OTM3, p. 1628).*

plasma calcium is in part due to decreased renal tubular reabsorption.

Plasma phosphate varies more than plasma calcium and its concentration is set mainly by the kidney. Unlike serum calcium, the vast majority of inorganic phosphate is ultrafilterable (90 per cent). The measurement of renal tubular reabsorption of phosphate may be used in clinical investigation, for example in the diagnosis of hyperparathyroidism. There are several methods available to calculate phosphate reabsorption; the best is probably an estimation of TmP/GFR (tubular maximum for phosphate reabsorption). This examines the relationship between filtered load and renal excretion which, like that for calcium reabsorption, is curvilinear at physiological concentrations. A nomogram has been produced for deriving this measurement (Fig. 4). Phosphate reabsorption is increased by growth hormone, in hypoparathyroidism, and in phosphate deprivation. It is low in several inherited or acquired renal tubular disorders, and may also be influenced by drugs such as corticosteroids.

Both calcium and phosphate excretion are influenced by other factors, notably sodium excretion, extracellular fluid volume expansion, and by the administration of diuretics. Infusion of sodium chloride increases the excretion of both calcium and phosphate, an effect which contributes to its value in the treatment of hypercalcaemia.

Bone

The processes of bone formation, its mineralization, and resorption and their disorders are described in Section 9.

Integrated responses

In considering plasma calcium homeostasis, it is useful to separate acute from chronic changes. When the system is disturbed a steady response occurs which adjusts the system to produce a new steady state. Deviations of plasma calcium away from its normal value are rapidly corrected by alterations in the secretion and synthesis of the regulating hormones. PTH can be considered the fast-acting component of the regulatory system, whereas vitamin D is responsible for adaptation over a longer time. The rapid control of plasma calcium by PTH is mainly due to its ability to regulate renal tubular reabsorption and possibly by effects on the rapid exchange of calcium in bone. After parathyroidectomy, the fall in plasma calcium can be largely accounted for by the continued loss of calcium into urine until a new steady state is achieved in which calcium excretion is the same as its starting value but takes place at a much reduced filtered load of calcium. During the transient state when plasma calcium is falling, urinary excretion of calcium will increase. In contrast, when a new steady state is established, urinary calcium excretion will fall to normal despite a lower level of plasma calcium.

A further example of the difference between the steady and transient state is seen during the infusion of calcium. During a calcium infusion (or, for example, increased absorption of calcium from the gut or increases in bone resorption not mediated by PTH) plasma calcium rises. If the rate of calcium entry into the extracellular fluid is constant, concentrations of plasma calcium will not rise indefinitely but only until the rate of efflux of calcium from the extracellular fluid pool (into bone, gut, and other tissues, but mainly from the kidney) matches the rate of influx. At this point, extracellular calcium levels a new steady state will prevail. The infusion of calcium would result in the suppression of secretion of PTH and a decrease in the renal tubular reabsorption of calcium. This increases the rate at which a new steady state is achieved, and also decreases the final concentration of plasma calcium obtained.

Hyperparathyroidism

Definitions

Hyperparathyroidism can be classified into primary, secondary, tertiary, and ectopic (pseudo-) hyperparathyroidism.

Primary hyperparathyroidism implies hyperfunction of one or more parathyroid glands which results in a change in the set point for the control of plasma calcium such that plasma calcium values are higher than normal.

Secondary hyperparathyroidism is due to prolonged hypocalcaemia, such as is seen in vitamin D deficiency or chronic renal failure, which results in increased secretion of PTH and hyperplasia of the parathyroid glands. The biochemical and skeletal lesions which result are a reflection of the underlying disorder, hypocalcaemia, as well as high circulating levels of PTH. The skeletal abnormalities seen, for example, in vitamin D deficiency, represent a combination of hyperparathyroidism, phosphate deficiency, and varying degrees of osteomalacia. Secondary hyperparathyroidism can be cured by treatment which restores the plasma calcium to normal. Concentrations of PTH fall rapidly but the involution of parathyroid hyperplasia may take many months. More detailed considerations of secondary hyperparathyroidism are found in the sections on disorders of vitamin D metabolism (see below), on renal bone disease (see Chapter 12.30), and on osteomalacia (see Section 9).

Table 3 Causes of primary hyperparathyroidism; chief-cell hyperplasia is associated with multiple endocrine abnormalities

Single adenoma	83.0%
Multiple adenoma	4.3%
Carcinoma	1.7%
Hyperplasia clear cell	7.6%
chief cell	3.6%

Tertiary hyperparathyroidism is a term used to denote those patients with long-standing secondary hyperparathyroidism who develop autonomous gland function and hypercalcaemia. This is most commonly seen after renal transplantation, but may also be observed in patients with long-standing malabsorption or chronic renal failure. The term 'autonomous secretion' is a misnomer since PTH can be suppressed by calcium infusion, or further augmented by lowering plasma calcium. Tertiary hyperparathyroidism therefore implies a change in the set point with respect to the calcium control of PTH secretion. In this disorder, plasma calcium and PTH are both raised and treatment includes parathyroidectomy and the management of the cause.

Pseudohyperparathyroidism describes the elaboration of PTH-like material in association with certain malignancies, particularly of the lung, giving rise to biochemical abnormalities not unlike those of primary hyperparathyroidism.

Primary hyperparathyroidism

Primary hyperparathyroidism is usually due to a single parathyroid adenoma of the chief cells of the parathyroid gland. More rarely it is due to diffuse hyperplasia or multiple adenomata (Table 3). Hyperplasia and adenoma may be difficult to differentiate histologically. Carcinoma is very rare. The most common presentation (50–70 per cent of cases) is asymptomatic hypercalcaemia. Prevalence is estimated as between 2 and 10 per 10 000 of the population, occurring with greatest frequency between the fourth and sixth decades of life, when it is twice as common in females as in males. At other age groups the sex incidence is roughly equal. The cause of primary hyperparathyroidism is unknown, but in women it appears to be unmasked by the menopause. An increased risk occurs some years following irradiation of the head and neck.

The usual biochemical abnormality is an increase in the circulating concentration of both PTH and calcium. There are, however, instances where patients with proven adenoma have normal total serum calcium levels or intermittent hypercalcaemia. Conversely, patients may have values of PTH within the laboratory reference range which in the presence of hypercalcaemia are inappropriately high. Thus, primary hyperparathyroidism can be defined as a circulating level of PTH that is inappropriately high for the prevailing level of plasma calcium (Fig. 5). In some instances, the patient with primary hyperparathyroidism may be normocalcaemic because of coexistent vitamin D deficiency.

The renal tubular reabsorption for calcium is enhanced at any given filtered load in primary hyperparathyroidism (see Fig. 3). There is often also increased bone resorption and increased intestinal absorption of calcium due to the stimulation of calcitriol production. These factors will tend to increase the 24-h urinary excretion calcium. Although resorption of bone is commonly enhanced in primary

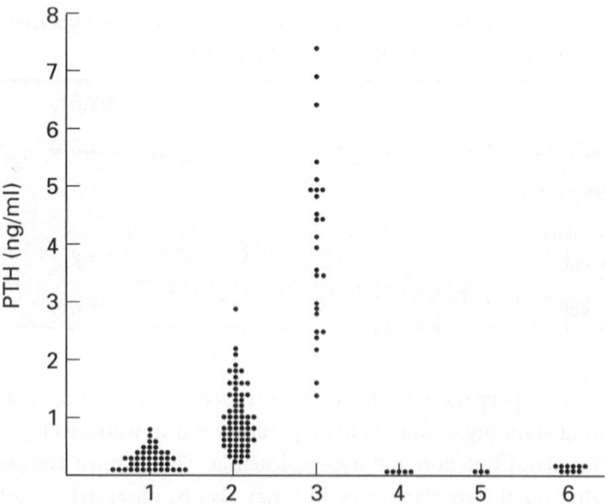

Fig. 5 Plasma values of parathyroid hormone in normal subjects (group 1) and patients with hypercalcaemia (2–6). Patients with surgically proven hyperparathyroidism (groups 2 and 3) have higher levels of PTH, but there is an overlap with the normal range. However, these patients were hypercalcaemic, indicating that values of PTH were inappropriately high for the plasma calcium. Thus, patients with vitamin D intoxication (group 4), idiopathic hypercalcaemia of infancy (group 5), and patients with skeletal metastases and hypercalcaemia (group 6) have very low or undetectable levels of PTH.
(For source see OTM3, p.1631).

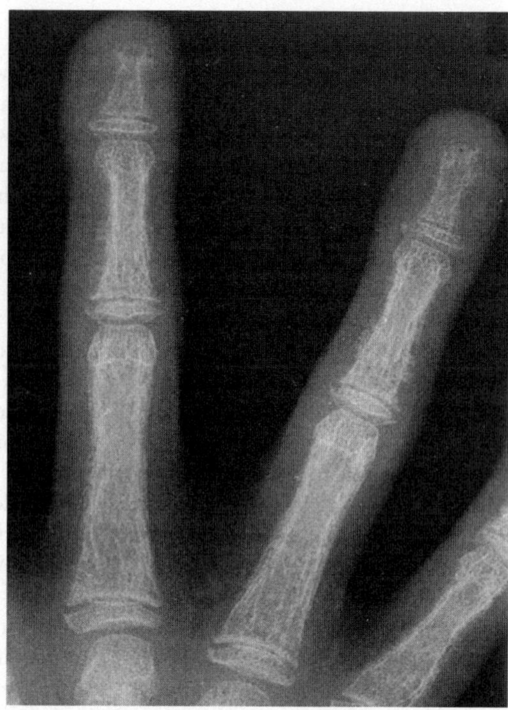

Fig. 6 Radiographic features of hyperparathyroid bone disease. Note the marked subperiosteal bone resorption involving the terminal phalanges. Note also the cortical porosity.

hyperparathyroidism, so too is bone formation, reflected as an increase in alkaline phosphatase. Thus the skeletal balance of calcium is usually normal, but at the expense of an increased bone turnover. Bone loss may occur, however, particularly in patients with severe disease and in female patients with coexisting postmenopausal osteoporosis. Calcium-containing renal stones are also a feature of primary hyperparathyroidism.

Clinical features

Up to 50 per cent of patients present with renal stone disease, and primary hyperparathyroidism accounts for approximately 5 per cent of patients with renal stones.

Bone disease is usually apparent on histology of bone but it is rarely overt. Biochemical indices of increased bone turnover (raised alkaline phosphatase and increased urinary hydroxyproline excretion) are found in up to 50 per cent of patients. Radiographic manifestations of primary hyperparathyroidism occur in less than 2 per cent of patients; in these hyperparathyroidism is severe, and sometimes due to parathyroid carcinoma; renal calculi are uncommon in this group. The characteristic radiographic feature of hyperparathyroidism is subperiosteal erosion of bone (Fig. 6). The skeleton may also be diffusely osteoporotic or osteosclerotic, although the latter findings are usually confined to patients with severe and long-standing secondary hyperparathyroidism.

Cystic lesions in bone may also be found in primary hyperparathyroidism, 'brown tumours' which may result in pathological fracture. In the skull, extensive bone resorption may give a mottled 'salt and pepper' appearance on radiographs. Subperiosteal erosion is most frequently noted in the hands, with resorption of the phalangeal tufts, and on the radial borders of the middle phalanges. The distal ends of the clavicles are also commonly involved by resorption but are more difficult sites to examine radiographically. The loss of the lamina dura and the appearance of brown tumours in the mandible are late complications. Bone pain and tenderness are seen in primary hyperparathyroidism but are more common in secondary disease.

Although in one-third of patients hypercalcaemia will have been an incidental finding, many present with symptoms of hypercalcaemia including nausea, vomiting, thirst, fatigue, and constipation; muscles and ligaments may become hypotonic. Hypercalcaemia induces polyuria, and this may lead to dehydration or polydipsia. The raised plasma calcium and dehydration may also lead to nephrocalcinosis and progressive chronic renal failure (see Chapter 12.23). Calcification may also occur in other sites, such as cartilage (pseudogout) and blood vessels. Periarticular soft tissue calcification is more commonly seen in hyperparathyroidism due to renal failure. Calcification in the cornea is reflected as band keratopathy and conjunctival deposits cause a 'red eye' with local inflammation.

Peptic ulceration is seen in 5–10 per cent of patients, possibly related to hypercalcaemia-induced secretion of gastrin. Acute or chronic pancreatitis is also associated with hyperparathyroidism and calcification of the pancreas may be evident on radiography or on radionuclide scanning.

Neurological disturbances attributable to hypercalcaemia range from behavioural disorders and mood variation to organic psychosis, dementia, and focal neurological lesions. Proximal myopathy is an unusual feature and may be due to concurrent phosphate depletion.

Hypercalcaemia is occasionally seen in Paget's disease, particularly during immobilization, and may be associated with primary hyperparathyroidism.

There is a familial form of hyperparathyroidism and suspicion should be alerted when hyperparathyroidism is found in young adults or children. It has an autosomal dominant mode of transmission. It may occur without other abnormalities but is frequently part of the pluriglandular syndrome. It may be associated with pituitary or pancreatic tumours, with peptic ulceration and gastric hypersecretion, or with tumours of the adrenal cortex (multiple endocrine neoplasia type 1). Combinations of hyperparathyroidism, medullary carcinoma of the thyroid, phaeochromocytoma, carcinoid tumours, and mucosal and cutaneous neurofibromata also occur (multiple endocrine neoplasia type 2).

Familial benign hypercalcaemia is also an autosomal dominantly inherited form of hypercalcaemia. The aetiology is unknown, but is associated with increased renal tubular reabsorption of calcium and normal, rather than low, circulating PTH. It is important to recognize the disorder since parathyroidectomy is rarely of benefit or required.

Diagnosis

The characteristic feature of primary hyperparathyroidism is a raised plasma calcium in the presence of high or normal circulating values of PTH. The majority of patients also have low values of serum phosphate due to decreased renal tubular reabsorption of phosphate. The estimation of TmP/GFR (see Fig. 4), however, does not always discriminate various groups of patients with hypercalcaemia. Less common laboratory findings in hyperparathyroidism include aminoaciduria, hypomagnesaemia, elevated erythrocyte sedimentation rate (ESR), and a shortening of the QT interval on the electrocardiogram. A monoclonal increase in immunoglobulins has also been described and does not, therefore, necessarily indicate myelomatosis.

In the majority of patients, the diagnosis is straightforward and rests on the finding of an increase in plasma calcium, increase (or lack of suppression) in plasma PTH, reduction in tubular reabsorption of phosphate, and an increase in renal tubular reabsorption of calcium. The finding of augmented intestinal calcium absorption and high values of calcitriol, hyperphosphatasia, or increased urinary excretion of hydroxyproline support the diagnosis. Renal failure may make the interpretation of these tests difficult.

A diagnostic difficulty among patients with renal calculi is encountered in distinguishing between hyperparathyroidism and idiopathic hypercalciuria. In the case of idiopathic hypercalciuria, plasma calcium is always normal but there are also well-documented cases of patients with parathyroid adenoma in whom plasma calcium lies within the normal range. The administration of a thiazide diuretic such as bendrofluazide, which increases renal tubular reabsorption of calcium, will induce persistent hypercalcaemia in patients with primary hyperparathyroidism and may aid in the identification of such patients.

Hypercalcaemia in malignant disease may occasionally be due to the production of a PTH-related protein and other factors by the tumour itself. This syndrome may occur in the absence of skeletal metastases. Other causes of hypercalcaemia are discussed later in this chapter. A variety of tests have been advocated to distinguish these disorders, including the hydrocortisone suppression test, but are now obsolete with the development of better immunoassays for PTH.

In hyperparathyroidism, a metabolic acidosis is commonly found which is reflected by a low plasma bicarbonate and a high plasma chloride.

Treatment

A moderate increase in plasma calcium may lead to progressive renal impairment and severe hypercalcaemia may cause an immediate threat to life when parathyroidectomy is urgently indicated. At the other extreme, many patients with primary hyperparathyroidism have mild hypercalcaemia (plasma calcium < 3.0 mmol/l) without symptoms. Opinion varies on whether such patients should undergo parathyroidectomy, but it is probably wise to err in the favour of surgery since many of the symptoms of hypercalcaemia are subtle and not always appreciated until after removal of excess parathyroid tissue. The aims of surgery are to remove the adenoma or to resect sufficient hyperplastic parathyroid tissue to render the patient euparathyroid.

The surgical management of patients with primary and tertiary hyperparathyroidism can be difficult because of the variable anatomy of the parathyroids and problems with the differentiation between multiple gland hyperplasia and single gland adenoma. A common approach is to identify all cervical parathyroid tissue, since more than one parathyroid gland is affected in an appreciable minority of patients (Table 3). On the other hand, the majority of patients with primary hyperparathyroidism have a single adenoma and some surgeons, on finding an adenoma, undertake no further exploration. In cases of diffuse hyperplasia the tendency is to remove three and a half glands. This has become a standard treatment for the secondary hyperparathyroidism of renal disease requiring resection. Alternatively, total parathyroidectomy may be undertaken, followed by transplantation of parathyroid tissue into the forearm muscles. Whatever the strategy employed, the operative implantation of radiopaque markers at sites of remaining parathyroid tissue is helpful in case re-exploration is required.

Venous sampling for assay of PTH can be used as a preoperative localizing procedure for abnormal parathyroid tissue, but is most useful after failed surgery, although there may be difficulties with the interpretation of PTH data due to variations in venous drainage from the parathyroids, particularly after previous surgery. This approach is particularly useful for detecting mediastinal tumours. Other techniques of variable value include thallium pertechnetate scanning, CT, ultrasonography, and the use of methylene blue at operation to discolour the glands.

After surgery, plasma calcium should be measured at least daily for the first few days. Post-operative tetany is common in patients who have significant bone disease; they should be treated peroperatively with intravenous calcium (10 per cent calcium gluconate, 10–30 ml in 1 litre of saline), and, at the same time vitamin D should be begun, as calcitriol, alfacalcidol, or dihydrotachysterol since these agents work quickly and with precision. Hypocalcaemia usually lasts for only a few days, but may persist on occasion for weeks of even months. Permanent hypoparathyroidism is rare.

Medical treatment can be considered in some asymptomatic patients with only borderline or mild hypercalcaemia. Oestrogens and progesterone can lower plasma calcium in postmenopausal women with modest hypercalcaemia. Clodronate can be given by mouth for long periods, but the long-term effects are disappointing. Oral cellulose phosphate with calcium restriction may transiently lower plasma calcium. Neutral phosphate has been used in doses between 1 and 2.5 g daily, but may cause diarrhoea and extraskeletal calcification. Overall, there is little place for these approaches. The situation is different when the problem is very severe hypercalcaemia, which needs correction before surgery. In that situation saline-induced calciuresis and intravenous biphosphonates should be used.

Hypoparathyroidism

Definitions

Hypoparathyroidism results in hypocalcaemia and hyperphosphataemia arising from the defective secretion or action of PTH

Table 4 Major causes of hypoparathyroidism

Cause
Inadequate secretion of PTH
Surgical—thyroid, parathyroid, and radical neck surgery
Familial
Sporadic
DiGeorge's syndrome
Suppression of PTH secretion from normal parathyroid glands
Neonatal—from maternal hypercalcaemia
Severe magnesium depletion
Defective end-organ response to PTH
Pseudohypoparathyroidism types I and II

(the latter is termed pseudohypoparathyroidism). Serum phosphate is raised due to an increase in TmP/GFR. Hypocalcaemia is due to a decrease in tubular reabsorption of calcium (Fig. 3), to inhibition of osteolytic transfer of calcium from bone, and to a decrease in intestinal absorption of calcium since PTH deficiency reduces synthesis of calcitriol.

General clinical features

Hypocalcaemia may cause carpopedal spasm, paraesthesiae of the face, fingers, and toes, and occasionally abdominal cramps. Latent tetany may be detectable by tapping of the fifth facial nerve, resulting in contraction of the facial muscles (Chvostek's sign) or by inducing carpal spasm following occlusion of the arterial circulation of the forearm (Trousseau's sign). Chvostek's sign has limited clinical usefulness since approximately 5 per cent of the normal population have a positive response. The neurological changes which accompany profound hypocalcaemia include irritability, emotional lability, impairment of memory, generalized lethargy, and convulsions which are usually of the grand mal type. Occasionally petit mal is a presenting feature. Papilloedema occasionally associated with increased intracranial pressure is another rare manifestation of hypocalcaemia. A prolonged QT interval on the ECG may be associated with partial insensitivity to digoxin.

Cataracts are common consequences of chronic hypocalcaemia. Soft tissue calcification is not infrequent and has a curious predilection for the basal ganglia or subcutaneous tissue. If hypocalcaemia occurs in early life and is sustained, dental abnormalities such as blunting of the roots of the teeth and enamel dysplasia occur. Nails may be malformed, brittle, and have transverse grooves. Other ectodermal changes which may be found include a dry rough skin. Certain clinical features are associated with particular forms of hypoparathyroidism; these are discussed below since they aid with the differential diagnosis.

Causes (Table 4)

Hypoparathyroidism most commonly results from thyroid, parathyroid, or laryngeal surgery. The incidence after thyroidectomy varies enormously, depending on the surgeon, the length of the follow-up, and the criteria used for diagnosis. Surgical hypoparathyroidism may be latent for many years, sometimes becoming manifest in association with increased calcium demands such as pregnancy and lactation.

Idiopathic hypoparathyroidism is a relatively rare condition associated with absence, fatty replacement, or atrophy of parathyroid glands. In the familial form it may be inherited as a sex-linked recessive, autosomal recessive, or autosomal dominant with variable penetrance. The sporadic form, occurring at any age, may be associated with pernicious anaemia, Addison's disease, or candidiasis. Addison's disease and candidiasis may also occur, but less commonly, in the familial form. These observations, together with the presence of antibodies to parathyroid tissue, suggest that these are autoimmune disorders. Children with idiopathic hypoparathyroidism have impaired growth and malformations of the nails and teeth. Idiopathic hypoparathyroidism is also associated with intestinal malabsorption, steatorrhoea, and osteomalacia.

Rarely hypoparathyroidism may result from infiltration of the parathyroid glands by iron in haemochromatosis, copper in Wilson's disease, or from the invasion of parathyroid tissue by malignant metastases. In DiGeorge's syndrome there is a congenital absence of parathyroid glands. It is associated with immunological deficiencies (thymic aplasia) and is a consequence of failure of development of the third and fourth branchial pouches from which the parathyroids and thymus arise. Patients with this syndrome usually die in early childhood from hypocalcaemia, severe infections, or both.

The presence of neonatal tetany should alert one to investigate the mother for primary hyperparathyroidism, when maternal hypercalcaemia may have suppressed the fetal parathyroids. Hypoparathyroidism has also been reported following ^{131}I treatment for hyperthyroidism.

Pseudohypoparathyroidism

Pseudohypoparathyroidism results from the resistance of one or more target tissues to the actions of PTH. The physiological control of PTH secretion is intact, in the sense that PTH levels are appropriate for the degree of hypocalcaemia. There is an association between pseudohypoparathyroidism and somatic abnormalities. These include short stature, round face, short neck, and shortening of the metacarpals and metatarsals. Characteristic radiographic findings include shortening of the fourth, fifth, or all metacarpals and metatarsal bones (Fig. 7). These features are not invariably found in pseudohypoparathyroidism and may rarely be present in idiopathic hypoparathyroidism. An X-linked dominant inheritance has been postulated but reports of male to male transmission suggest that a recessive inheritance pattern may also occur. Pseudohypoparathyroidism is also associated with hypothyroidism due to a selective deficiency of thyroid stimulating hormone. Other associated disorders include diabetes mellitus and gonadal dysgenesis.

The resistance to PTH may be partial or complete. In type I disease neither phosphaturia nor increased urinary cyclic AMP production is stimulated during the infusion of PTH. This type is further subdivided into those with somatic and other endocrine disorders (type Ia) and those without (type Ib). In type II, infusion of PTH causes a marked rise in urinary cyclic AMP without a phosphaturic response. In yet other patients, the responsiveness to PTH may be restored by calcium infusion. Not all target tissues need be affected, and occasionally pseudohypoparathyroidism may be associated with radiographically obvious osteitis fibrosa, indicating skeletal sensitivity to PTH.

Pseudopseudohypoparathyroidism

Rarely the somatic features of pseudohypoparathyroidism may be found in patients with normal plasma concentrations of calcium and phosphate. This condition is termed pseudopseudohypoparathyroidism. PTH values are usually normal but may be raised. There are patients with pseudopseudohypoparathyroidism who are relatives of patients with pseudohypoparathyroidism and who indeed may undergo transitions from hypocalcaemia to normocalcaemia or vice

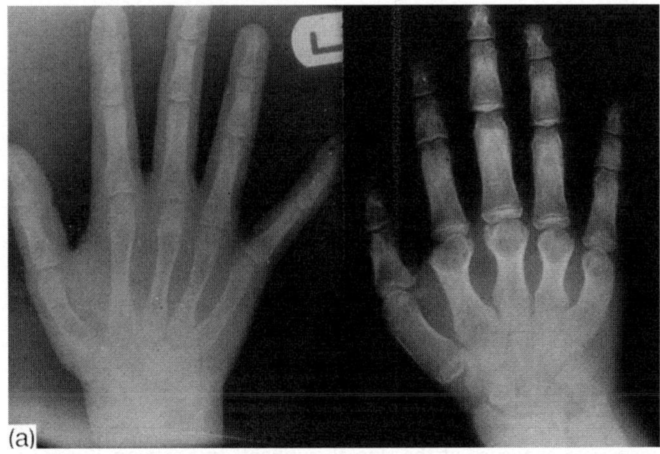

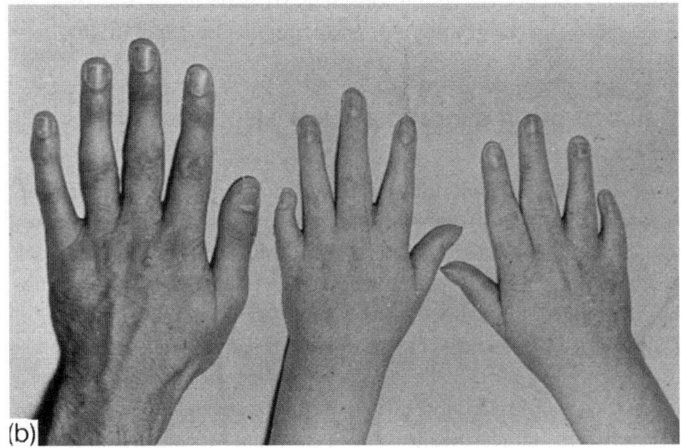

Fig. 7 Brachydactyly in a patient with pseudopseudohypoparathyroidism. The radiograph on the left-hand side shows a normal hand for comparison.

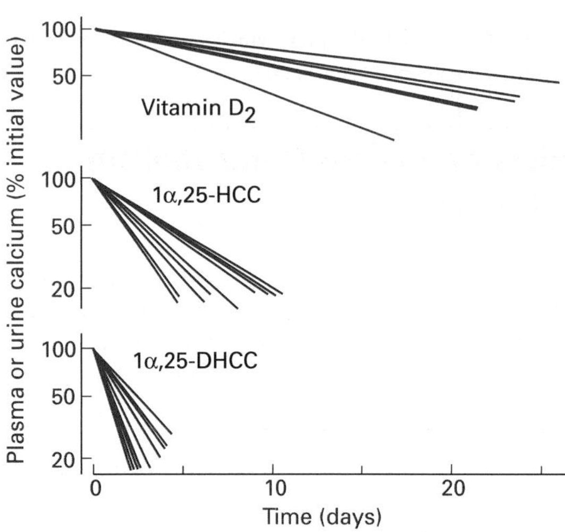

Fig. 8 The rate of reversal of biological effects after stopping treatment with vitamin D compounds. The fall in plasma or urine calcium is shown on a logarithmic scale. Note that the reversal of vitamin D toxicity is more rapid in the case of 1,25-dihydroxyvitamin D (1,25-DHC; calcitriol) and its synthetic analogue 1-hydroxyvitamin D (1-HCC; alfacalcidol) than seen with vitamin D_2.
(For source see OTM3, p. 1635).

versa. It is notable that cataracts may develop in patients with pseudopseudohypoparathyroidism who have a consistently normal plasma calcium, suggesting that mechanisms other than hypocalcaemia are responsible for this feature.

Diagnosis

The diagnosis of hypoparathyroidism is based on the finding of hypocalcaemia and hyperphosphataemia in the absence of renal failure, osteomalacia, or malabsorption. The clinician should be aware of the association of hypocalcaemia secondary to magnesium deficiency. A history of previous neck surgery or physical examination usually indicates the underlying cause. The finding of Addison's disease, pernicious anaemia, candidiasis, atypical epilepsy, or bizarre mental symptoms should alert one to the possibility of hypoparathyroidism. Apart from rare forms of vitamin D deficiency, the only other disorder commonly associated with hyperphosphataemia and hypocalcaemia is chronic renal failure. Measurement of plasma creatinine easily resolves this possibility. The differential diagnosis and investigation of hypocalcaemia is discussed below. The 24-h excretion secretion of urinary calcium is commonly low but the fasting urinary calcium excretion is usually normal. In order to distinguish the various forms of idiopathic and pseudohypoparathyroidism, more detailed investigation, including the measurement of PTH and the responses to exogenous PTH, are required. The principles of treatment, however, are similar for all forms of hypoparathyroidism although the doses required of the vitamin D-like agents used may vary.

Treatment

The priorities of treatment are to restore normal circulating values of calcium and phosphate. This is not often attainable with the use of calcium supplements alone but they are commonly used (1–1.5 g daily) in conjunction with vitamin D or its metabolites. The use of intravenous calcium (10–30 ml of 10 per cent calcium gluconate in 500 ml or 1 litre of saline) may be required in patients with tetany. In the past, the most commonly prescribed vitamin D preparation has been calciferol (vitamin D_2) in doses from 0.25–20 mg daily (10 000–800 000 units). One of the disadvantages of vitamin D_2 is that the onset and reversal of its action are very slow (Fig. 8). Thus it is very difficult to titrate the dose according to requirements, and inadvertent hypercalcaemia may take weeks or months to resolve. The 1α-hydroxylated derivatives of vitamin D (calcitriol, alfacalcidol, and dihydrotachysterol) all have a more rapid onset and offset of action. The daily maintenance dose required of these agents is 1–2 μg in the case of alfacalcidol and calcitriol, and 0.25–2 mg of dihydrotachysterol. Occasionally higher doses are required. High doses may also be used at the start of treatment. It is mandatory to follow plasma calcium closely to avoid toxicity in the first 2–3 weeks of treatment and at least once every 6 months in patients on stable doses. The requirements for vitamin D and its derivatives may vary, particularly when the defect in PTH secretion is incomplete. Treatment may be required for concurrent hypomagnesaemia and other endocrinopathies when present. Intercurrent illness, pregnancy, and the use of antacids, thiazide diuretics, ammonium chloride, anticonvulsants, and acetazolamide may alter the requirements for vitamin D.

The prognosis of adequately treated hypoparathyroidism is excellent. It is, however, unclear whether or not cataracts can be prevented. Major difficulties with long-term vitamin D treatment include prolonged hypercalcaemia, which may lead to renal stone formation and progressive renal failure.

Disorders of vitamin D metabolism

Hypervitaminosis D

Vitamin D toxicity

Vitamin D toxicity is not uncommon and is usually iatrogenic. Hypercalcaemia is the result of increased intestinal absorption of calcium and increased bone resorption. Plasma phosphate is commonly also elevated due to similar effects on phosphate transport. If overdosage is prolonged, there may be progressive loss of bone. The effects of prolonged hypercalcaemia are discussed in the sections on hypercalcaemia (see below) and hyperparathyroidism (see above), but the effects on the kidney are the most important. Vitamin D preparations should be stopped when hypercalcaemia is confirmed or suspected. The rate of fall of plasma calcium depends upon the agent used. The biological half-life of vitamins D_2 and D_3 may be months or even years, particularly when pharmacological amounts have been used over prolonged periods, resulting in high body stores (Fig. 8). A long half-life of several weeks is also seen with calcidiol.

The principles of treatment include the general management of hypercalcaemia (see below) but corticosteroids are particularly efficacious when the cause is vitamin D toxicity. In life-threatening situations, particularly in the face of renal impairment, patients may require haemodialysis or peritoneal dialysis.

Increased production of calcitriol

Factors augmenting the synthesis of calcitriol include hypophosphataemia, hypocalcaemia, and excessive secretion of PTH. Abnormally high values of calcitriol have been reported in patients with primary hyperparathyroidism and account for the increased calcium absorption in this disorder. Increased calcium absorption in acromegaly may also be due to increased production of calcitriol. Approximately one-third of patients with idiopathic hypercalciuria have increased serum values of calcitriol. The hypercalcaemia of sarcoidosis is associated with high circulating values of calcitriol and also has a seasonal incidence, being more common in the summer months. Plasma levels of calcidiol are normal, reflecting increased 1α-hydroxylation of 25-hydoxycholecalciferol by the granuloma. A similar syndrome of excess calcitriol production occurs in other granulomatous disorders (such as berylliosis, candidiasis, tuberculosis, leprosy, cat-scratch disease, and silicon-induced disease) and occasionally in human T-cell leukaemia virus (HTLV)-associated adult T-cell lymphoma.

Defective production of vitamin D metabolites

The hallmarks of vitamin D deficiency include defective mineralization of bone and retardation of growth. Simple vitamin D deficiency is associated with hypocalcaemia, hypophosphataemia, and high plasma activity of bone-derived alkaline phosphatase; but in the early stages of vitamin D deficiency, plasma calcium may be normal. The hypocalcaemia is caused by malabsorption of calcium from the gut and a decrease in the calcium efflux from bone. Hypocalcaemia stimulates PTH secretion and the hypophosphataemia is due to secondary hyperparathyroidism (decreased TmP/GFR) as well as malabsorption of phosphate. Indeed, it is possible that defective mineralization of bone is due, in part, to phosphate depletion.

Not all cases of osteomalacia or rickets result from deficiency of vitamin D or its metabolites. For instance, in X-linked or sporadic hypophosphataemia (vitamin D-resistant rickets) defective mineralization of bone is probably due to abnormalities in phosphate transport rather than to impaired metabolism of vitamin D. Conversely, deficiency of calcitriol does not invariably lead to osteomalacia. Thus, osteomalacia is an unusual finding in hypoparathyroidism and is not invariably seen in end-stage chronic renal failure, even though plasma values of calcitriol are reduced in both these disorders. The clinical manifestations of osteomalacia, its investigation and differential diagnosis are discussed in Section 9.

Privational vitamin D deficiency

Simple vitamin D deficiency may be due to dietary deficiency or inadequate exposure of the skin to sunlight. In northern Europe it commonly occurs in young children, particularly at the time of adolescence, in the immigrant Asian population, and in the very old.

Malabsorption syndromes (see also Chapters 5.6–5.13)

Patients with long-standing malabsorption are likely to develop osteomalacia. Not all such patients have symptomatic steatorrhoea and further investigation, such as intestinal biopsy or the determination of faecal fat excretion, may be necessary. The pathophysiology of the disorder is related in part to malabsorption of vitamin D, which is fat soluble, but in patients with active disease the intestinal cells themselves have been destroyed and hence the vitamin D deficiency is partly related to the destruction of one of its target organs. The absorption of calcifidiol is also decreased in patients with intestinal disease, including those with small bowel resection, and it has been suggested that there is a defect in the enterohepatic circulation of calcifidiol. An increased prevalence of osteomalacia is also seen in patients with liver disease and those with partial gastrectomy. Malabsorption of vitamin D may contribute to the former but the cause of osteomalacia after partial gastrectomy remains somewhat of a mystery and may be more related to malabsorption of calcium.

Reduced availability of calcifidiol

Vitamin D is hydroxylated in the liver to form 25-hydroxyvitamin D. It might be expected that severe liver disease could impair this hydroxylation, and there is some evidence that the prevalence of osteomalacia is higher in patients with liver disease than in normal subjects. However, osteoporosis is more common though osteomalacia may be erroneously suspected because of hyperphosphatasia and reduced serum phosphate due to the liver disease. There is little direct evidence for defective 25-hydroxylation in liver disease. Low values of calcidiol, when found, may be due to malabsorption or a poor dietary intake of vitamin D.

Osteomalacia has been associated with the administration of anticonvulsant drugs such as phenobarbitone and phenytoin, which are potent inducers of hepatic microsomal enzymes. Increased metabolic degradation of vitamin D to inactive metabolites is unlikely to be the sole mechanism and drug-induced target organ resistance is a major feature.

A convincing role for abnormal metabolism of calcifidiol is seen in the nephrotic syndrome. Certain features of vitamin D deficiency are common, such as reduced plasma calcium, hypocalciuria, and decreased intestinal absorption of calcium, even when the glomerular filtration rate is normal or increased. The hypocalcaemia is partly related to the low plasma concentrations of albumin which occur as a consequence of protein losses in the urine, but ionized calcium is also low, as are values of calcifidiol due to losses of the vitamin D-binding protein in the urine.

Reduced availability of calcitriol

Chronic renal failure, pseudohypoparathyroidism, and hypoparathyroidism are disorders in which the conversion of calcidiol to calcitriol is impaired. Serum values of calcitriol are low, and physiological quantities of calcitriol reverse some of the biochemical abnormalities, whereas pharmacological amounts of vitamin D_3 are required to achieve the same response. Not all these disorders are associated with osteomalacia. In the case of parathyroid disorders, the low values of calcitriol are probably due to hyperphosphataemia as well as reduced secretion of PTH, or, in the case of pseudohypoparathyroidism, a resistance of renal tissue to respond to PTH. In chronic renal failure, low values of calcitriol reflect the destruction of the renal tissue which converts calcidiol to calcitriol.

Patients with vitamin D-dependency rickets have all the features of vitamin D deficiency except that vitamin D must be given in very large doses to correct the biochemical and skeletal abnormalities (10 000–50 000 units daily). Pharmacological doses of calcidiol are also needed, whereas physiological doses of calcitriol (1 μg daily) cure the disorder. It is thought that some of these patients have a defective 1α-hydroxylase enzyme system. However, there are patients with similar biochemical characteristics who have normal or even high levels of circulating calcitriol—the vitamin D equivalent of pseudohypoparathyroidism. This rare condition, sometimes associated with alopecia and other somatic abnormalities, has been described as vitamin D-dependent rickets type II. It reflects an inherited defect of the vitamin D receptor associated with target tissue resistance to calcitriol. An even rarer form of calcitriol deficiency is seen in patients with benign mesenchymal tumours. This is commonly associated with hypophosphataemia. It is important to identify such patients since resection of the tumour, if feasible, reverses the osteomalacia.

Other disorders

It is probable that target tissue resistance to the action of vitamin D metabolites is an important component of the osteomalacia associated with anticonvulsant treatment and with intestinal disorders.

Osteomalacia associated with phosphate deficiency is unrelated to defects in the metabolism of vitamin D, but some renal tubular disorders are associated with a profound metabolic acidosis which might impair the activity of the renal 1α-hydroxylase. In some such cases, correction of the acidosis alone without phosphate supplements may lead to healing.

Low serum values of calcitriol have also been described in postmenopausal and corticosteroid-induced osteoporosis. In the elderly, bone loss associated with ageing or menopausal loss of oestrogens is commonly aggravated by vitamin D deficiency giving rise to secondary hyperparathyroidism. It is treated with vitamin D (800 units daily) and calcium supplementation of the diet. It is possible that a component of age-related bone loss is due also to impaired renal 1α- hydroxylation or target tissue resistance to calcitriol.

Disorders of calcitonin secretion

Medullary carcinoma of the thyroid (see also Chapter 7.15)

Increased secretion of calcitonin occurs in medullary carcinoma of the thyroid, a malignant disorder of the C-cells. The majority of patients present with a thyroid mass, often with palpable cervical lymph nodes. The tumour may spread to the mediastinum, but spread beyond the neck and mediastinum usually occurs late, with the lungs, liver, adrenal glands, and bones being the most common sites. Metastases to bones are sometimes osteoblastic. The tumour may be associated with other endocrine abnormalities such as phaeochromocytoma and hyperparathyroidism—multiple endocrine adenoma syndrome (MEA Type II). Severe diarrhoea may occur which is probably related to the synthesis of prostaglandins or serotonin. Hypocalcaemia is very rare.

Calcitonin is consistently produced by medullary carcinomata of the thyroid, and the measurement of serum calcitonin or its flanking peptide katacalcin is of value in establishing the diagnosis, the presence of metastases, and in following the effects of treatment. These assays are also of value in family studies for tracing asymptomatic cases. A number of other humoral agents may be synthesized by the tumour, including prostaglandins, 5-hydroxytryptamine, and adrenocorticotrophic hormone (ACTH). The last may give rise to Cushing's syndrome. Other genetically related disorders include multiple mucosal neuromata, ganglion neuromatosis of the gastrointestinal tract, marfanoid features, muscular weakness, and a high arched palate.

Treatment is surgical, but it is advisable to screen for phaeochromocytoma preoperatively and, if present, this should be dealt with first. Because of the high proportion of adrenaline produced by these tumours, β-adrenergic blockade should be used in addition to α-adrenergic blockade during surgery. In the presence of distant spread it may still be worth resecting a large tumour mass to control severe diarrhoea or Cushing's syndrome.

Partial or total thyroidectomy is indicated in family members if raised basal plasma levels of calcitonin or katacalcin are demonstrated, or if exaggerated responses to provocative tests of calcitonin secretion (with whisky, pentagastrin, or calcium infusion) are shown.

Other disorders

High values of calcitonin have also been demonstrated in patients with hypercalcaemia and a variety of non-thyroidal tumours such as oat-cell carcinoma of the lung, carcinoma of the breast, and in chronic renal failure.

Hypercalcaemia

Differential diagnosis

The causes of hypercalcaemia are summarized in Table 5. The most common cause in hospitalized patients is malignant disease. Bone lesions and hypercalcaemia are most frequently seen in patients with tumours of the breast, lung, thyroid, and kidney. Carcinoma of the prostate commonly involves bone but induces osteoblastic lesions in 90 per cent of patients, and hypercalcaemia is rare. Hypercalcaemia can develop rapidly in patients with malignancy and initiate a vicious cycle of increasing nausea, vomiting, dehydration, and impaired renal function, all of which accelerate the rise in serum calcium. These patients often have an hypochloraemic metabolic alkalosis, whereas

Table 5 Causes of hypercalcaemia

Common
Artefactual: hyperproteinaemia due to venous stasis, hyperalbuminaemia (dehydration, intravenous nutrition), hypergammaglobulinaemia (myeloma, sarcoidosis)
Neoplasia: carcinoma with skeletal metastases (e.g. breast, lung), carcinoma without skeletal metastases (humoral hypercalcaemia of malignancy), haematological disorders (myeloma, HTLV-associated lymphoma)
Primary hyperparathyroidism
Rare
'Tertiary' hyperparathyroidism—transplantation, chronic renal failure, malabsorption
Vitamin D toxicity
Vitamin D 'sensitivity'—sarcoidosis, other granulomatous disorders, ?hypercalcaemia of infancy
Immobility—Paget's disease, adolescence
Milk-alkali syndrome
Thyrotoxicosis
Thiazide diuretics
Adrenal failure
Phaeochromocytoma
Familial hypocalciuric hypercalcaemia
Haemodialysis: high dialysate calcium, aluminium toxicity
Some other drugs, e.g. vitamin A
Acute renal failure
VIPoma
Familial hypocalciuric hypercalcaemia

hyperchloraemic acidosis is more common in primary hyperparathyroidism. Serum phosphate concentrations are variable, depending on the presence or absence of malnutrition, disturbed renal function, and increased bone resorption.

The causes of hypercalcaemia in malignancy arise by several mechanisms. Most commonly the cause is widespread destruction of bone by metastases. In such cases the secretion of PTH is suppressed. Tumours can also secrete peptides such as PTH-related protein and tumour growth factors which cause a generalized increase in bone resorption or increase renal tubular reabsorption of calcium. PTH-related protein is a 141 amino acid hormone (molecular weight 16 000), sharing sequence homology with PTH at its amino terminus. Like PTH, it increases bone resorption and renal tubular reabsorption of calcium. It is secreted by many solid tumours, including squamous carcinomas of the lung, oesophagus, head and neck, and breast. It may cause hypercalcaemia in the absence of skeletal metastases (humoral hypercalcaemia of malignancy) but may also contribute to hypercalcaemia in patients with focal lytic lesions.

The investigation and diagnosis of primary hyperparathyroidism has been discussed previously (see above). The majority of other causes may be accurately detected by a good history (including a full drug history) and the measurement of plasma calcium, phosphate, proteins, ESR, and creatinine, and an estimate of tubular reabsorption for phosphate. Radiography and bone scans are helpful in detecting malignant disease not otherwise clinically apparent.

Renal manifestations

Acute hypercalcaemia causes a high flux of calcium through the renal tissues with epithelial cell degeneration, necrosis and calcification, and the tubules become obstructed. Calcium deposits may also be found in glomeruli and blood vessels. There is impairment of urine-concentrating ability with resistance to ADH. High levels of calcium ions either impair the ability of the ADH receptor to bind to ADH, or the ability of the hormone-receptor complex to activate adenylate cyclase. In addition, impaired sodium chloride reabsorption in the ascending limb of Henle's loop may contribute by reducing medullary accumulation of solutes, so interfering with water reabsorption.

Acutely this state of nephrogenic diabetes insipidus causes dehydration which is aggravated by nausea and vomiting resulting in additional salt depletion. Chronic hypercalcaemia leads to interstitial calcification and fibrosis, most marked in the renal medulla. It is sometimes associated with renal tubular losses of potassium and bicarbonate.

The severity of hypercalcaemic nephropathy roughly parallels the degree of hypercalcaemia, and serum concentrations above 3.5 mmol/l indicate a risk of serious renal dysfunction.

Treatment

Apart from dealing with the cause urgently, there are a number of ways in which severe hypercalcaemia can be ameliorated. Plasma levels of calcium at 3.0 mmol/l in the presence of renal impairment, or at 3.5 mmol/l regardless of symptoms require urgent treatment.

Parenteral rehydration and saline calciuresis

The first step is to correct the deficit of salt and water by rapid infusion of normal saline and to continue at a rate dependent on the degree of hypercalcaemia, and renal and cardiac function. Most patients will tolerate 3–6 litres of normal saline per 24 h, and the resulting calciuresis may be greatly enhanced and the risk of pulmonary oedema reduced by the coincident use of a loop diuretic. Usual doses range from 40 mg of frusemide twice daily by mouth to 40 mg intravenously 2 hourly in the most severe cases. This combined approach can increase urinary calcium to some 25 mmol and reduce plasma calcium by some 1.0–1.5 mmol/l per day.

Biphosphonates

If the above approach does not reduce plasma calcium below 3.5 mmol/l biphosphonates are indicated. The agents of choice in the UK are sodium clodronate or disodium pamidronate; in the US, where clodronate is not available, editronate and pamidronate are most commonly used.

These agents are given by intravenous infusion, clodronate 300 mg in 500 ml of normal saline over 2 h for periods not exceeding 10 days, or 1500 mg as a single infusion. The dose of pamidronate should be adjusted to the prevailing plasma calcium concentration as shown in Table 6. The total dose of pamidronate may be given as a single infusion, or in individual doses, but should not exceed 90 mg in a single course of treatment. Editronate is also given intravenously in saline in a dose of 7.5 mg/kg body weight over a 4-h period daily for 3–7 days. A reasonable target in using these agents is to reduce plasma calcium to below 3.0 mmol/l.

Oral doses of these drugs can be used in chronic cases and although editronate can cause osteomalacia, this ill effect seems less likely with clodronate or pamidronate.

Table 6 Recommended doses of pamidronate according to plasma calcium concentrations

Plasma calcium (mmol)	Dose
Less than 3.0	15–30 mg in 125–250 ml saline in 2 h
3.0–3.5	30–60 mg in 25–500 ml saline in 4 h
3.5–4.0	60–90 mg in 500–1000 ml saline in 8–24 h
More than 4.0	90 mg in 1000 ml saline in 24 h

Table 7 Causes of hypocalcaemia

Low plasma albumin: malnutrition, liver disease, etc.
Vitamin D deficiency or resistance
Chronic renal disease
Hypoparathyroidism, pseudohypoparathyroidism
Magnesium deficiency
Acute pancreatitis
Drugs, e.g. calcitonin, phosphate, diphosphonates, some chemotherapeutic agents, and chelators of calcium
Carcinoma, particularly of the prostate

Corticosteroids

Prednisolone 20 mg 8-hourly by mouth or hydrocortisone 150 mg 8-hourly intravenously can be effective in treating the hypercalcaemia of vitamin D intoxication, sarcoidosis, and in some cases of lymphoma or myeloma, but are ineffective in other cases.

Phosphate

Oral phosphate preparations (for example phosphate-Sandoz; dose equivalent 500 to 1500 mg—16 to 48 mmol—of elemental phosphorus) and oral fluids can be given if nausea and vomiting are not prominent, but the effects on plasma calcium are small and larger doses cause diarrhoea.

Mithramycin

At doses of 25 mg/kg body weight intravenously, this drug inhibits bone resorption and lowers plasma calcium in 2–3 days, but carries the risk of myelotoxicity, hepatotoxicity, and nephrotoxicity.

Calcitonin

The effects of this agent are rapid but relatively weak and short-lasting. Salmon calcitonin is less immunogenic than other forms and is given by slow intravenous infusion (5–10 units/kg body weight over at least 6 hr).

Newer agents

Octreotide 50 mg per day subcutaneously has been shown to reduce malignancy-associated hypercalcaemia, possibly by inhibiting PTH-related peptide release.

Hypocalcaemia and tetany

The more common causes of hypocalcaemia are shown in Table 7, most of which have been discussed earlier. Tetany may develop in the presence of alkalosis, and potassium and magnesium deficiency, as well as in hypocalcaemia. Hyperventilation alters the protein binding of calcium such that the ionized fraction is decreased, and may therefore cause hypocalcaemic tetany in the face of normal plasma calcium. Hypocalcaemic tetany may also occur during the administration of alkalis. This is particularly prone to occur during the treatment of acidotic patients with bicarbonate, particularly those with chronic renal failure in whom total plasma calcium may be low. Alkalosis may also occur in intestinal disorders where excess alkalis are ingested or there is excessive loss of gastric acid. Alkalotic tetany is diagnosed by an increase in plasma bicarbonate and an alkaline urine. The principles of treatment are those of the underlying disorder.

Further reading

Kebebew, E. and Clark, O.H. (1998). Parathyroid adenoma, hyperplasia, and carcinoma: localization, technical details of primary neck exploration, and treatment of hypercalcemic crisis. *Surgery and Oncology Clinics of North America* 7, 721–48.

Marx, S., Spiegel, A.M., Skarulis, M.C., *et al.* (1998). Multiple endocrine neoplasia type 1: clinical and genetic topics. *Annals of Internal Medicine* 129, 484–94.

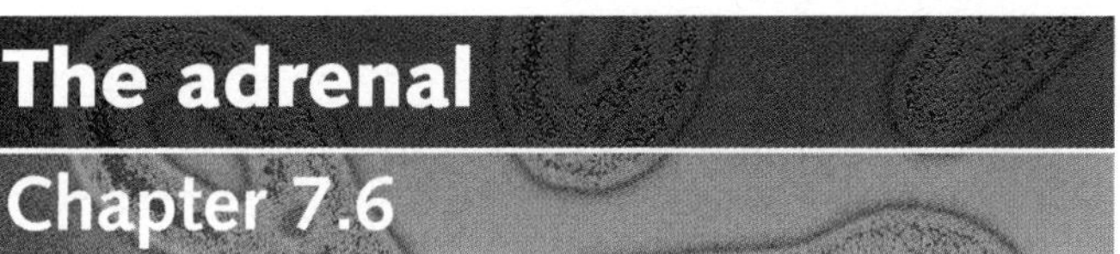

The adrenal

Chapter 7.6

Adrenocortical diseases

C. R. W. Edwards

Three main types of hormone are produced by the adrenal cortex—glucocorticoids (cortisol, corticosterone), mineralocorticoids (aldosterone, deoxycorticosterone), and sex steroids (mainly androgens). The biochemical pathways involved in their synthesis are shown in Fig. 1.

Adrenocortical diseases are relatively rare but their importance lies in their morbidity and mortality if untreated, coupled with the relative ease of diagnosis and the availability of effective therapy. The diseases are most readily classified on the basis of whether there is hormone excess or deficiency (Table 1) usually the result of disturbed secretion of hormones. More uncommonly the defect may relate to a change in corticosteroid metabolism (for example effects of liquorice or carbenoxolone) or to defective receptors (for example glucocorticoid resistance syndromes, pseudohypoaldosteronism).

Glucocorticoid excess

Cushing's syndrome comprises the symptoms and signs associated with prolonged exposure to inappropriately elevated free plasma glucocorticoid levels. This definition takes into account the elevated corticosteroid levels which may be found in severely depressed patients but which appear to be appropriate to the condition (there is some evidence for glucocorticoid resistance in depression) and the increased total (but normal free) glucocorticoid levels found when there is an increase in circulating cortisol binding globulin.

Classification of Cushing's syndrome

The condition is most readily classified into those causes that are ACTH-dependent and those that are not (Table 2). The term Cushing's *syndrome* is used to describe all causes; that of Cushing's *disease* is reserved for pituitary-dependent cases in recognition of the original

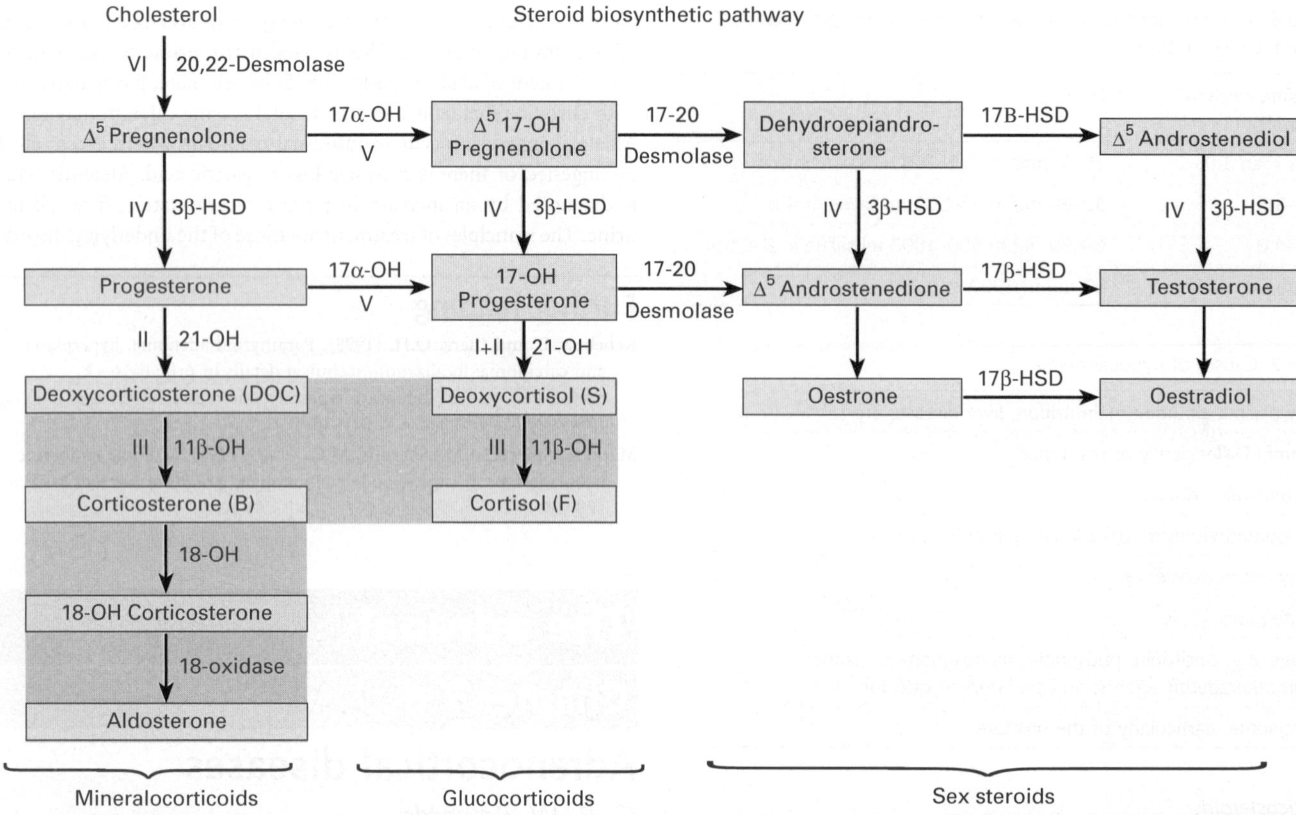

Fig. 1 Pathways of adrenocortical steroid biosynthesis. The shaded area shows the affected steroids in a patient with salt-wasting 21-hydroxylase deficiency.

Table 1 Adrenocortical diseases

Glucocorticoid excess	**Mineralocorticoid deficiency**
Cushing's syndrome	Congenital adrenal hyperplasia
Glucocorticoid deficiency	Cholesterol desmolase
Primary	3β-ol dehydrogenase
Congenital adrenal hyperplasia	21-OHase
21-OHase	Congenital adrenal hypoplasia
Classical 3β-ol dehydrogenase	Disorders of terminal part of aldosterone biosynthetic pathway
17α-OHase	Pseudohypoaldosteronism
Cholesterol desmolase	Isolated renin deficiency
11β-OHase	Addison's disease
Addison's disease	**Adrenal androgen/oestrogen**
Hereditary adrenocortical unresponsiveness to ACTH	Excess
	Non-classical 3β-ol
Secondary	Non-classical 21-OHase
Hypothalamic/pituitary disease	PCO, tumours
Mineralocorticoid excess	Deficiency
Aldosteronism	17α-OHase
Other mineralocorticoids	17,20 lyase
Glucocorticoid resistance	Adrenopause
	Testicular feminization

Ohase = hydroxylase.

Table 2 Classification of causes of Cushing's syndrome

ACTH-dependent
Iatrogenic (treatment with $ACTH_{1-39}$ or Synacthen®, $ACTH_{1-24}$)
Cushing's disease (pituitary)
Ectopic ACTH syndrome
Ectopic CRF syndrome
?Macroscopic nodular adrenal hyperplasia
ACTH-independent
Iatrogenic (e.g. pharmacological doses of prednisolone, dexamethasone, etc.)
Adrenal adenoma
Adrenal carcinoma
Carney's syndrome
McCune–Albright syndrome
Gastric inhibitory polypeptide (GIP) adrenal hypersensitivity
Alcohol

CRF, corticotrophin releasing factor.

description (Plate 1). There is an additional, rather poorly defined, group of patients with ACTH-independent Cushing's syndrome but in whom there is bilateral adrenal disease, when the adrenals are usually enlarged and frequently contain multiple nodules. It is likely that there are several different pathologies in this subgroup. In some there may be local adrenal production of a factor which enhances the response to ACTH. Alternatively, abnormal processing of the ACTH precursor molecule, pro-opiomelanocortin, may be important as the N-terminal part of this molecule appears to play a role in adrenal growth. In some patients there may be stimulating immunoglobulins, whereas in others a somatic mutation in the stimulatory G-protein may result in continuous activation of adenyl cyclase, thus stimulating constant stimulation by ACTH.

There is also a small group of patients in which food stimulates cortisol secretion. These patients' adrenal glands have enhanced sensitivity to the normal postprandial increase in gastric inhibitory polypeptide (GIP) (see below).

Another poorly understood condition is alcohol-induced pseudo-Cushing's syndrome, in which the glucocorticoid excess associated with high alcohol intake resolves when the patients stop drinking (see below).

ACTH-dependent causes

Cushing's disease

Bilateral adrenocortical hyperplasia with widening of the zona fasciculata and reticularis in this disease is ACTH dependent. The release of ACTH from the pituitary is normally controlled by CRF acting synergistically with AVP. Despite some data suggesting that these two hypothalamic agents might be involved in the excessive production of ACTH, there is abundant evidence that at presentation the condition is pituitary- rather than hypothalamus-dependent. Thus, rare cases that have been treated by stalk section have not been cured, whereas selective removal of a microadenoma usually results in cure, gradual recovery of suppressed adjacent corticotrophs, and a very low recurrence rate.

There may be different subgroups of patients with pituitary-dependent Cushing's disease. Analyses of cortisol secretion over 24 h have shown two patterns, hypo- or hyperpulsatile, the latter perhaps hypothalamic in origin and the former pituitary-dependent.

The histopathology of pituitary adenomas from patients with Cushing's disease has been correlated with the outcome of operation and hormonal characteristics prior to surgery. In one group the adenomas contained argyrophilic nerve fibres and in nearly all of them cortisol secretion rates reverted to normal after surgery, a rare finding in the other groups. Conversely, bromocriptine did not affect preoperative ACTH and cortisol levels in this group, but suppressed them in the majority of patients whose tumours were free of the argyrophilic fibres, suggesting that the former may arise from the anterior pituitary and the latter from the intermediate lobe.

Of particular clinical interest has been the small group of patients with cyclical Cushing's syndrome. In this condition periods of excess cortisol production (for example 40 days) are followed by intervals of normal production (for example 60–70 days). Some of these patients have a paradoxical rise in plasma ACTH and cortisol when treated with dexamethasone, and occasional patients show benefit with dopamine agonist (bromocriptine) or serotonin antagonist (cyproheptadine) therapy. In many of these patients basophil adenomas have been removed, some with long-term cure, but in others subsequent bilateral adrenalectomy has been required.

One other piece of evidence militates against Cushing's disease being a primary hypothalamic disease. Basophil hyperplasia is very uncommon and in up to 90 per cent of cases properly examined there is a corticotroph microadenoma of monoclonal origin.

Ectopic CRF production

This is a very rare cause of pituitary-dependent Cushing's. However, a number of cases have now been described in which a tumour (for example medullary thyroid, prostate carcinoma) has been shown to contain CRF but not ACTH, contrasting with the much more common situation in which a tumour contains both ACTH and CRF. Ectopic CRF production may explain the metyrapone responsiveness and suppression with high-dose dexamethasone found in some patients with the ectopic ACTH syndrome.

Table 3 Tumours associated with the ectopic ACTH syndrome

Tumour type	Approximate incidence (%)
Small cell lung carcinoma	50
Non-small cell lung carcinoma	5
Pancreatic tumours (including carcinoids)	10
Thymic tumours (including carcinoids)	5
Lung carcinoids	10
Other carcinoids	2
Medullary carcinoma of thyroid	5
Phaeochromocytoma and related tumours	3
Rare carcinomata of prostate, breast, ovary, gallbladder, colon	10

Ectopic ACTH syndrome

Cushing's syndrome may be associated with non-pituitary tumours producing ACTH, most commonly a small cell carcinoma of bronchus (Table 3). These conditions are described further in Chapter 7.16.

Macroscopic nodular adrenal hyperplasia

In about 20–40 per cent of patients with Cushing's disease there is bilateral adrenocortical hyperplasia associated with one or more nodules. Such nodules are a trap for the unwary (see below) as they may be mistaken for primary adrenal tumours. It has been suggested that this condition may be a transitional stage between a pituitary-dependent condition and an autonomous adrenal tumour. An alternative explanation is that the nodules result from an autocrine or paracrine mechanism with either excess local production of growth factors or altered processing of N-terminal pro-opiomelanocortin (N-POC); this has been shown to be involved in adrenal growth. N-POC has also been found to enhance markedly the corticosteroid response to ACTH.

ACTH-independent causes

Adrenal adenoma and carcinoma

With the exclusion of iatrogenic Cushing's syndrome, adrenal adenomas are responsible for about 10 per cent of cases and carcinomas for about the same. Carcinomas are the commonest cause of Cushing's syndrome in children.

Carney's syndrome

This is an autosomal dominant condition comprising mesenchymal tumours (especially atrial myxomas), spotty skin pigmentation, peripheral nerve tumours, and various endocrine tumours, one of which may be Cushing's syndrome. The adrenals then contain multiple, small, pigmented nodules. The condition has been described as pigmented multinodular adrenocortical dysplasia. There is evidence to suggest that it results from stimulation by ACTH receptor antibodies.

McCune–Albright syndrome

In this condition fibrous dysplasia of bone and cutaneous pigmentation may be associated with pituitary, thyroid, adrenal, and gonadal hyperfunction. The adrenal hypersecretion may produce

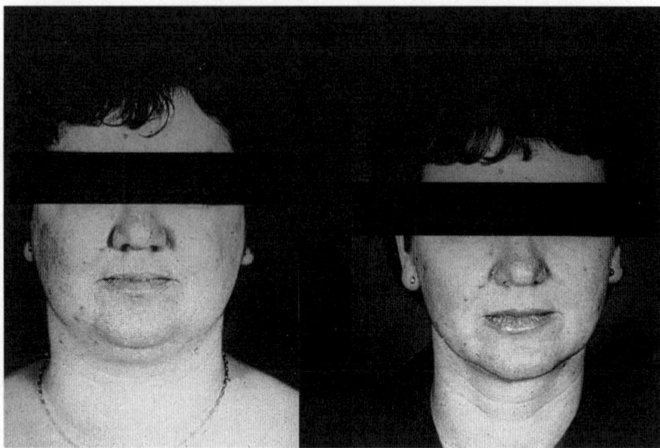

Fig. 2 Typical facies of a Cushing's patient before and after treatment.

Cushing's syndrome. The underlying abnormality is a somatic mutation in the α-subunit of the stimulatory G protein which is linked to adenyl cyclase. The mutation results in the G protein being constitutively activated (that is, in the adrenal mimics constant ACTH stimulation). As the mutation occurs in fetal life, there is a mosaicism of cells with some containing, and others not, the mutation. In the adrenal such a mutation leads to associated local nodule formation.

GIP hypersensitivity

Two patients have been described with nodular hyperplasia, ACTH-independent Cushing's syndrome, and enhanced adrenal responsiveness to GIP. This food-dependent form of Cushing's syndrome results from the normal increase in GIP after eating. The adrenocortical tissue of these patients responded *in vitro* to low doses of GIP suggesting that in them adrenal GIP receptors are linked to steroidogenesis. The clinical syndrome is related to food intake and fasting can produce adrenal insufficiency.

Alcohol-associated pseudo-Cushing's syndrome

The frequency and pathogenesis of this condition in which ACTH is normal or suppressed remain unknown. With abstinence from alcohol the abnormalities rapidly revert to normal.

11β-hydroxysteroid dehydrogenase (11β-OHSD), the enzyme responsible for converting cortisol to inactive cortisone, is inhibited by alcohol *in vitro*. The effects of alcohol could therefore be due to a direct effect on the enzyme in the liver and possibly also in the CNS where the enzyme appears to be involved in negative feedback control of ACTH.

Clinical features of Cushing's syndrome

The classical features of Cushing's syndrome with centripetal obesity, moon face, hirsutism, and plethora are well known (Fig. 2), but this gross clinical picture is not always present. The commonest symptoms and signs are listed in Table 4 together with the incidence of other commonly associated conditions. Weight gain and obesity are the commonest symptoms, but the distribution of fat is not invariably centripetal; a 'buffalo hump' is present in about half the patients.

Gonadal dysfunction is very common, with menstrual irregularity in females and loss of libido in males. Hirsutism is frequently found in female patients, as is acne. All these features tend to be present more in patients with adenoma than in those with bilateral adrenal hyperplasia.

Table 4 Prevalence of symptoms and signs in Cushing's syndrome

Symptoms	**Signs**
Weight gain (91%)	Obesity (97%)
Menstrual irregularity (84%)	truncal (46%)
Hirsutism (81%)	generalized (55%)
Psychiatric (62%)	Plethora (94%)
Backache (43%)	Moon face (88%)
Muscle weakness (29%)	Hypertension (74%)
Fractures (19%)	Bruising (62%)
Loss of scalp hair (13%)	Striae (56%)
Other findings	Muscle weakness (56%)
Hypertension (74%)	Ankle oedema (50%)
Diabetes (50%)	Pigmentation (4%)
overt (13%)	
abnormal GTT (37%)	
Osteoporosis (50%)	
Renal calculi (15%)	

For source of data see OTM3, p. 1644.

Table 5 Discriminant index in diagnosis of Cushing's syndrome

	Discriminant index
Bruising	10.3
Myopathy	8.0
Hypertension	4.4
Plethora	3.0
Hirsutism	2.8
Red striae	2.5
Menstrual irregularity	1.6
Truncal obesity	1.6
Generalized obesity	0.8

For source of data see OTM3, p. 1644.

Depression and lethargy are among the commonest psychiatric problems, but poor concentration, paranoia, and overt psychosis are also well recognized.

Most patients with long-standing Cushing's syndrome have lost height because of osteoporotic vertebral collapse. Pathological fractures, either spontaneous or after minor trauma, are not uncommon. Rib fractures, in contrast to those of the vertebrae, are often painless.

The plethoric appearance of the patient with Cushing's syndrome is secondary to the thinning of the skin and is not due to true polycythaemia. Such thinning is also the cause of typical red-purple livid striae which are found most frequently on the abdomen but may also be present on the upper thighs and arms.

The myopathy of Cushing's involves the proximal muscles of lower limb and shoulder girdle and the two features best discriminating Cushing's syndrome from simple obesity have been shown to be bruising and myopathy (Table 5). Hypertension is common.

Pigmentation is rare in Cushing's disease but common in the ectopic ACTH syndrome. However, in some pituitary tumours there is abnormal processing of the pro-opiomelanocortin ACTH precursor molecule, with resulting pigmentation.

Infections are more common in Cushing's patients. Glucose intolerance may be a predisposing factor, with overt diabetes being

Table 6 Tests used in the diagnosis and differential diagnosis of Cushing's syndrome

Diagnosis
Does the patient have Cushing's syndrome?
Circadian rhythm of plasma cortisol
Urinary free cortisol excretion*
Low-dose dexamethasone suppression test*
Insulin tolerance test
Differential diagnosis
What is the cause of the Cushing's syndrome?
Plasma ACTH
Plasma potassium
High-dose dexamethasone suppression test
Metyrapone test
Corticotrophin releasing factor
Inferior petrosal sinus ± selective venous sampling for ACTH
CT/MRI scanning of pituitary/adrenals
Scintigraphy
Tumour markers

*Valuable outpatient screening tests (see text).

present in up to one-third of patients in some series. Cataracts, a well-recognized complication of corticosteroid therapy, seem to be uncommon, except as a complication of diabetes.

Special features of Cushing's syndrome

Children

In children, in addition to the above features, growth arrest is almost invariable. In addition, androgen excess may result in precocious puberty.

Adrenal carcinomas

In addition to the usual features patients may present with abdominal pain or with secondary deposits. Excess secretions of androgens in females may cause virilization with clitoromegaly, breast atrophy, deepening of the voice, temporal recession, and severe acne. Excess mineralocorticoid may cause hypertension with hypokalaemic alkalosis.

Ectopic ACTH syndrome

If this is due to a small cell lung carcinoma, patients are commonly pigmented and have lost weight, features suggesting Addison's disease, but the associated hypokalaemic alkalosis and glucose intolerance should distinguish. Patients with benign tumours present with the typical features of Cushing's syndrome.

Investigation of patients with suspected Cushing's syndrome

There are two stages in the investigation of a patient with suspected Cushing's syndrome. (1) Does the patient have Cushing's syndrome? (2) If so, what is the cause?

Diagnostic tests (Table 6)

Circadian rhythm of plasma cortisol

In normal subjects plasma cortisol levels are at their highest first thing in the morning and reach a nadir at around midnight. This circadian rhythm is lost in patients with Cushing's syndrome. In the majority of patients the 09.00 h plasma cortisol is normal with raised nocturnal levels. Random morning plasma cortisol levels are therefore of little value in diagnosis. Also, various factors such as stress of venepuncture, intercurrent illness, and admission to hospital may result in normal subjects losing their circadian rhythm. It is therefore good practice to not measure plasma cortisol until the patient has been in hospital for 48 h. A morning sample is then taken at 09.00 h together with plasma for the subsequent measurement of ACTH if other tests suggest Cushing's syndrome (see below for the importance of 08.00 h versus 09.00 h sampling). The midnight sample should be taken with the patient having been asleep; prior warning is not sensible as an apprehensive patient without disease who has not been asleep will often have an elevated plasma cortisol.

The ideal is to measure free cortisol, but few laboratories can do this. As more than 90 per cent of plasma cortisol is protein bound, conventional assays can be affected by drugs or conditions which alter cortisol binding globulin (CBG) levels. In normal subjects, not on oestrogens, midnight plasma cortisol is usually less than 180 nmol/l.

It is important to recognize two pitfalls in the interpretation of circadian data. The first is the pulsatile nature of cortisol secretion in some patients and the second relates to the difficulty of investigating patients with cyclical Cushing's syndrome, who may have long intervals of normal cortisol secretion.

Urinary free cortisol excretion

Urinary free cortisol is an integrated measure of plasma free cortisol. It is a useful outpatient screening test for Cushing's syndrome, but has the disadvantage of requiring timed urinary collections. This can be obviated by measuring the cortisol–creatinine ratio, and can be further refined by measuring this ratio on the first urine specimen passed on waking. This should reflect the time during the 24-h cycle when there is the greatest difference between patients with Cushing's syndrome and normal subjects. Using radio-immunoassay, the upper limit of normal for cortisol–creatinine ratio in an early morning specimen of urine is about 50 with a false negative rate of 5–6 per cent and false positive 1 per cent. Obese subjects have an increased cortisol production rate and but their urinary free cortisol is usually normal (false positive rate 5 per cent) as there is an increase in metabolism of cortisol to cortisone.

Measurement of urinary 6β-hydroxycortisol may be useful in diagnosis, especially in mild cases. This enzyme is induced by glucocorticoid excess, resulting in a disproportionate rise in its urinary excretion in comparison to cortisol.

Dexamethasone suppression tests

In normal subjects administration of a supraphysiological dose of glucocorticoid results in suppression of ACTH and hence of cortisol secretion. In Cushing's syndrome of whatever cause there is a failure of this suppression when low doses of dexamethasone are given. Dexamethasone is used as it does not cross-react in the assays commonly used for the measurement of plasma cortisol.

Dexamethasone suppression tests are thought to have 97–100 per cent sensitivity in the diagnosis of Cushing's syndrome. In normal subjects the postdexamethasone immunoreactive plasma cortisol is usually less than 50 nmol/l. Drugs such as phenytoin or rifampicin are a cause of false positive tests by way of their capacity to induce liver enzymes which increase the metabolic clearance rate of dexamethasone.

The overnight test is used to screen outpatients. Dexamethasone is given at midnight. The plasma cortisol is then measured at 08.00 h or 09.00 h. A dose of 1.5 or 2 mg gives a 30 per cent false positive rate, whereas after 1 mg this is reduced to 12.5 per cent with a false negative rate of less than 2 per cent. This test therefore has high sensitivity but low specificity, and further investigation is often required.

The next step is to carry out the more reliable 48-h test, in which plasma cortisol is measured at 09.00 h on day 0 and 48 h later. Dexamethasone is given in a dose of 0.5 mg 6 hourly for 48 h, with the last dose given 6 h before final blood sample. It is useful to collect 2 × 24-h urines for free cortisol prior to dexamethasone and then continue collection for the 2 × 24 h on the drug. This test is reported as having a 97–100 per cent true positive rate and a false positive of less than 1 per cent.

Insulin tolerance test

Patients with severe depression may show many of the biochemical features of Cushing's syndrome (loss of circadian rhythm of plasma cortisol, increased urinary free cortisol, failure of cortisol suppression with low-dose dexamethasone). Conversely, patients with Cushing's syndrome are frequently depressed. It is thus important in a depressed patient to take particular care in distinguishing the two conditions. In normal subjects and patients with severe endogenous depression insulin-induced hypoglycaemia results in a rise in ACTH and cortisol levels, a response usually not seen in Cushing's syndrome. It is important to make sure that there is adequate hypoglycaemia (i.e. blood glucose less than 2.2 mmol/l). In patients with Cushing's it may be necessary to give as much as 0.3 U soluble insulin/kg body weight, in comparison to 0.15 U/kg in normal subjects. The value of this test is limited by the observation that there is a rise in ACTH and cortisol in some 20 per cent of Cushing's patients.

Differential diagnostic tests

Plasma ACTH

Having determined that the patient has Cushing's syndrome, the first step in the differential diagnosis is to decide whether the condition is or is not dependent on ACTH. In normal subjects random morning samples contain a range of plasma ACTH concentrations from 9–77 ng/l; the range is much narrower (9–24 ng/l) if samples are taken only between 09.00 and 09.30. In comparison, in patients with Cushing's *disease* the ACTH concentrations at this time ranged from 39–109 ng/l. In patients with the ectopic ACTH syndrome, plasma ACTH levels are almost invariably elevated (Fig. 3). In benign causes such as a bronchial carcinoid the levels may overlap with the levels found in Cushing's disease, but with small cell lung tumours and other malignant causes much higher levels of ACTH may be found. Levels are usually undetectable in adrenal tumours.

The problem patients are those in whom plasma ACTH levels are low normal or intermittently detectable. This may occur in macronodular hyperplasia, when assymmetry of the adrenals on imaging may lead to a wrong diagnosis of adrenal adenoma and unilateral adrenalectomy performed inappropriately (Fig. 4).

Plasma potassium

Hypokalaemic alkalosis is nearly always found in patients with the ectopic ACTH syndrome, but is present in fewer than 10 per cent of patients with Cushing's disease. Patients with the ectopic syndrome not only usually have higher plasma cortisol levels but also have impaired conversion of cortisol to cortisone. This results in a failure of the normal renal mechanism which prevents cortisol gaining access

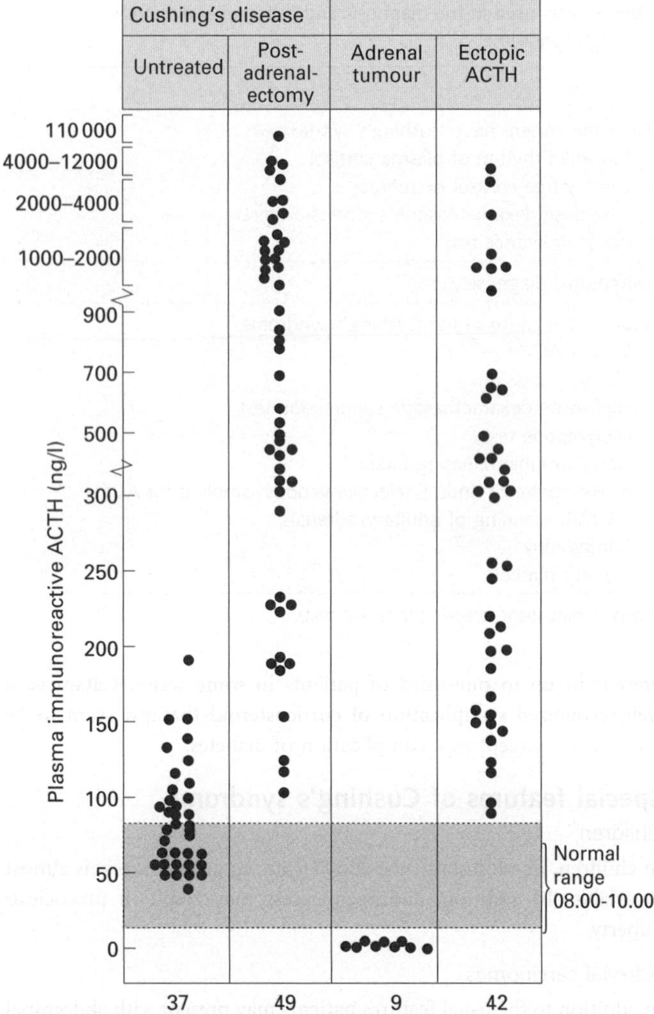

Fig. 3 Immunoreactive N-terminal ACTH levels in plasma samples taken between 08.00 and 10.00 h in normal subjects (hatched area), and patients with Cushing's disease either untreated or postadrenalectomy, patients with adrenal tumours, and in the ectopic ACTH syndrome.
(By courtesy of Professor Lesley Rees.)

to non-specific mineralocorticoid receptors (see apparent mineralocorticoid excess syndrome, below). In addition, these patients have higher levels of ACTH-dependent deoxycorticosterone.

High-dose dexamethasone suppression test

In Cushing's disease cortisol levels do not suppress with low-dose, but do with high-dose dexamethasone (2 mg 6 hourly for 48 h). Plasma cortisol is measured at 0 and + 48 h. Alternatively, 8 mg dexamethasone is given orally at 23.00 h and plasma cortisol taken at 08.00 h on the same day (basal sample) and at 08.00 h on the following morning. In both these tests greater than 50 per cent suppression of plasma cortisol in comparison to the basal sample defines a positive response which is found in 90 per cent of those with Cushing's disease but only in 10 per cent with the ectopic ACTH syndrome.

The variable absorption of dexamethasone has prompted the introduction of a 5-h dexamethasone infusion test (1 mg/h). With this, plasma cortisol at 5-h shows a fall of greater than 190 nmol/l (in comparison to a mean of three basal values) in all patients with

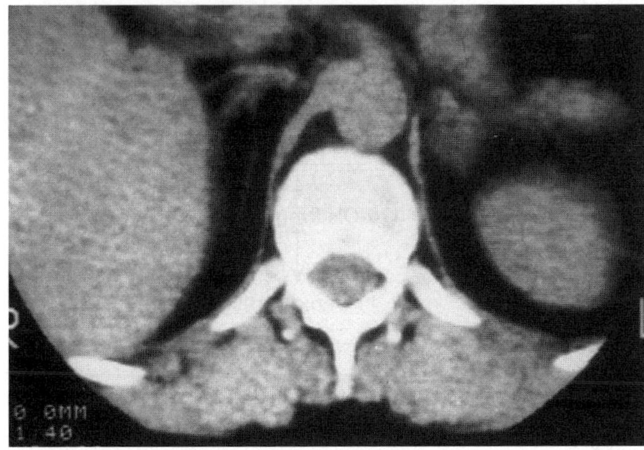

Fig. 4 CT scan of adrenals in patient with asymmetrical nodular hyperplasia. The macronodule on the left was initially thought to be an adrenal tumour. The biochemistry indicating ACTH-dependent Cushing's was ignored and a unilateral adrenalectomy performed without cure of the hypercortisolism. Further investigation confirmed Cushing's disease and a selective pituitary microadenomectomy resulted in cure.

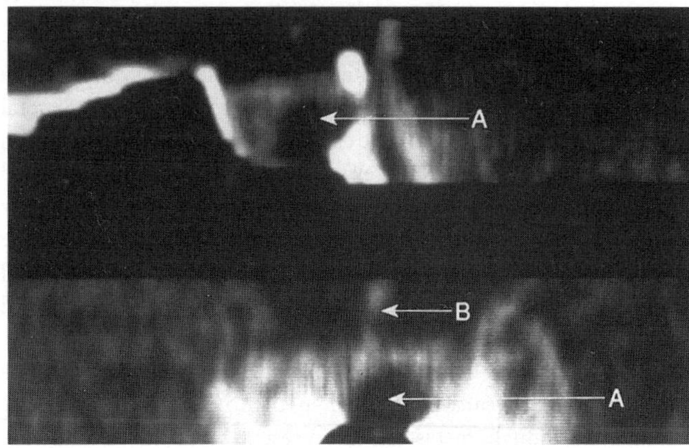

Fig. 5 Typical CT scan of pituitary in patient with Cushing's disease, showing hypodense microadenoma (A) in lateral view (top) and anteroposterior view (AP) (bottom). The pituitary stalk can be identified (B) in the AP view.

Cushing's disease but in only occasional patients with the ectopic ACTH syndrome.

Metyrapone test

Metyrapone blocks the conversion of 11-deoxycortisol to cortisol and deoxycorticosterone to corticosterone (Fig. 1). This lowers plasma cortisol and, via negative feedback control, increases plasma ACTH. This in turn stimulates an increase in the secretion of adrenal steroids proximal to the block. Metyrapone is usually given orally in a dose of 750 mg 4 hourly for six doses, starting at 08.00 h. The value of this test is in doubt. It does not reliably distinguish between Cushing's disease and the ectopic ACTH syndrome, but when the results of ACTH assay and CT scanning are equivocal, many clinicians still perform it. Details of the test and its interpretations are given in OTM3, p. 1647.

In patients with adrenal adenomas or carcinomas, ACTH is suppressed and metyrapone has little effect. Problems of interpretation arise in macronodular hyperplasia (see OTM3, p. 1647).

CRF test

After taking a basal blood sample for ACTH and cortisol at 08.00 h, further samples for ACTH and cortisol are then taken every 15 min for 2–3 h after administering CRF in a dose of 100μ or 1μ/kg body weight given intravenously.

In normal subjects, CRF produces a rise in ACTH and cortisol, and this response is exaggerated in Cushing's disease. It is typically absent in the ectopic ACTH syndrome and in patients with adrenal tumours. In distinguishing pituitary-dependent Cushing's from the ectopic ACTH syndrome the response of ACTH to CRF has a specificity of 90 per cent, and with cortisol as the endpoint, 95 per cent. An ACTH increase of 100 per cent over basal or a cortisol rise of 50 per cent eliminates a possible diagnosis of the ectopic ACTH syndrome.

As with the other tests, patients with macronodular hyperplasia may present a problem in diagnosis and show no response to CRF. In the obese and depressed the CRF response is either normal or reduced.

Inferior petrosal sinus sampling/selective venous catheterization

As blood from each half of the pituitary drains into the ipsilateral inferior petrosal sinus (IPS), catheterization of both sinuses with simultaneous sampling of IPS venous blood can distinguish a pituitary from an ectopic source of ACTH and aid in the lateralization of a pituitary microadenoma (see OTM3, p. 1648).

CT/MRI scanning of pituitary and adrenals

CT or MRI techniques have revolutionized the investigation of Cushing's syndrome. However, the results of the imaging must always be interpreted in the light of the biochemical results if mistakes are to be avoided.

The classic CT features of a pituitary microadenoma are a hypodense lesion after contrast, associated with deviation of the pituitary stalk and a convex upper surface of the pituitary gland (Fig. 5). About 90 per cent of ACTH-secreting pituitary tumours are microadenomas (i.e. less than 10 mm in diameter), and CT is inaccurate for the detection of lesions less than 6 mm in diameter. The sensitivity of CT scanning of the pituitary is therefore relatively low (20–60 per cent) with a similar specificity. MRI is better, with sensitivity of about 70 per cent and specificity of 87 per cent.

The results of CT scanning of the adrenals are much better than those for the pituitary. Adrenal tumours causing Cushing's syndrome are usually greater than 1.5 cm in diameter. With tumours of this size MRI has no diagnostic advantage over CT. Asymmetrical nodular hyperplasia may lead to a false diagnosis of adrenal adenoma (Fig. 4). 'Incidentalomas' are present in up to 8 per cent of normal subjects, and thus adrenal imaging should not be performed unless biochemical investigation suggests a primary adrenal cause.

Adrenal scintigraphy

The most commonly used agent is ^{131}I-6β-iodomethyl-19-norcholesterol. In patients with adrenal adenomas the isotope is taken up by the adenoma but not by the contralateral suppressed adrenal. With adrenal carcinomas the tumour uptake is very low, and as the opposite adrenal is suppressed the usual result is lack of image in either adrenal area. Adrenal scintigraphy is useful in patients with suspected adrenocortical macronodular hyperplasia, in which CT scanning may be misleading by suggesting unilateral pathology, whereas with isotope scanning the bilateral adrenal involvement is identified.

Treatment of Cushing's syndrome

Untreated, some 50 per cent of patients with Cushing's syndrome die within 5 years. *Adrenal adenomas* should be removed by unilateral adrenalectomy, with 100 per cent cure rate, but following operation it may take many months or even 1–2 years for the suppressed contralateral adrenal to recover. It is wise, therefore, to give slightly suboptimal replacement therapy with dexamethasone 0.5 mg in the morning, with intermittent measurement of 08.00 h plasma cortisol prior to taking dexamethasone. When the morning plasma cortisol is above 180 nmol/l, dexamethasone can be stopped.

Adrenal carcinomas have a very poor prognosis and most patients are dead within 2 years. It is usual to try to remove the primary tumour even though metastases are present so as to enhance the response to the adrenolytic agent *o,p'*-DDD (see below). Radiotherapy to the tumour bed and to some metastases, such as those in the spine, may be of limited value.

The treatment of *Cushing's disease* has been transformed by the improvements in trans-sphenoidal surgery. Bilateral adrenalectomy had an appreciable mortality even in the best centres (about 4 per cent) and morbidity. The major risk was the subsequent development of Nelson's syndrome. These patients also required life-long replacement therapy with hydrocortisone and fludrocortisone. Nowadays bilateral adrenalectomy is reserved for the occasional patient with Cushing's disease in whom no pituitary tumour can be found, or when pituitary surgery has failed, or where the condition has recurred.

Following selective removal of a pituitary microadenoma by trans-sphenoidal surgery, the surrounding corticotrophs are normally suppressed. In these cases plasma cortisol levels are also suppressed postoperatively and glucocorticoid replacement therapy is required. Using the dexamethasone regime after removal of an adrenal adenoma described above, there is usually (but not invariably) gradual recovery of the hypothalamic–pituitary–adrenal axis. The incidence of post-operative hypopituitarism in the best centres is low (about 10 per cent). Transient diabetes insipidus occurs in about 20 per cent of patients, but the permanent condition is rare.

Fewer patients are now treated by irradiation. In children pituitary irradiation appears to be effective but in adults the long-term results have been very poor, with remission rates usually lower than with trans-sphenoidal surgery, a variable time to onset of effect, and a higher incidence of hypopituitarism. Radiotherapy is now therefore reserved for patients not responding to pituitary microsurgery or when pituitary surgery is contraindicated and bilateral adrenalectomy has been performed, or with established Nelson's syndrome.

Treatment of the *ectopic ACTH syndrome* depends on the cause. If the tumour can be found and has not spread, then its removal can lead to cure. However, the prognosis for small cell lung cancer associated with the ectopic ACTH syndrome is poor. The cortisol excess and associated hypokalaemic alkalosis and diabetes mellitus can be ameliorated by medical therapy (see below). The treatment of the small cell tumour itself will also, at least initially, produce improvement. Sometimes, if the ectopic source of ACTH cannot be found, it may be necessary to perform bilateral adrenalectomy.

Medical treatment of Cushing's syndrome

Several drugs have been used in the treatment of Cushing's syndrome. Their site of action is shown in Fig. 6. *Metyrapone* has been most commonly used, often to control the condition prior to definitive therapy. The effective dose has to be determined by measuring either plasma or urinary free cortisol. The aim should be to achieve a mean plasma cortisol of about 300 nmol/l during the day or a normal urinary free cortisol. Usual doses range from 250 mg twice daily to 1.5 g every 6 h. Nausea can be helped by giving the drug with milk.

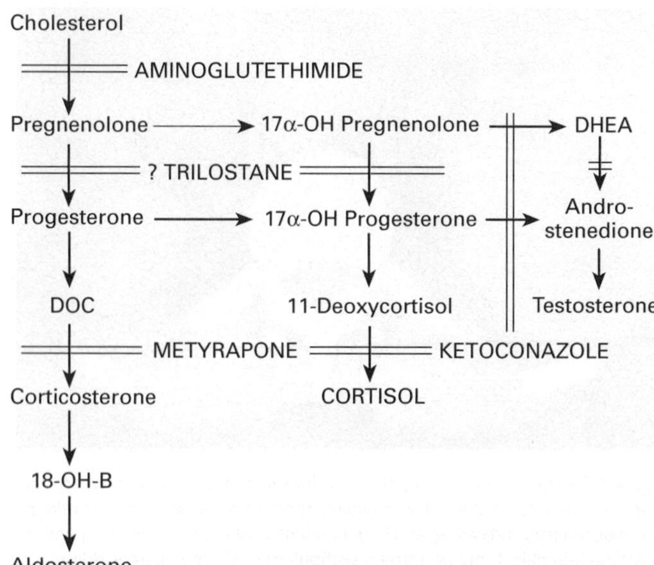

Fig. 6 Medical treatment of Cushing's syndrome: site of action of various drugs.

Aminoglutethimide is a more toxic drug which in high dose blocks earlier in the steroidegenic pathway and thus affects the secretion of steroids other than cortisol. In doses of 1.5–3 g daily (start with 250 mg 8 hourly) it commonly produces nausea, marked lethargy, and a high incidence of skin rash.

Trilostane, a 3β-hydroxysteroid dehydrogenase inhibitor, is ineffective in Cushing's disease, as the block in steroidogenesis is overcome by the rise in ACTH. However, it can be effective in patients with adrenal adenomas.

Ketoconazole blocks a variety of cytochrome P450-dependent enzymes and thus lowers plasma cortisol levels. High doses (400–800 mg daily) are required in Cushing's syndrome. Abnormal liver function tests occur in some 14 per cent and a small number of deaths have been reported.

o,p'-DDD is an adrenolytic drug which is taken up by both normal and malignant adrenal tissue, thus causing adrenal atrophy and necrosis. Because of its toxicity it has been used mainly in the management of adrenal carcinoma and only rarely in Cushing's disease. In daily doses of up to 8 g it is sometimes possible to control glucocorticoid excess and may have some beneficial effect on tumour growth. The drug will also produce mineralocorticoid deficiency. Patients may therefore require both glucocorticoid and mineralocorticoid replacement therapy. Problems such as fatigue, skin rashes, and gastrointestinal side-effects are common.

Glucocorticoid deficiency

Primary and secondary hypoadrenalism

Glucocorticoid deficiency can can occur as a result of a deficiency of ACTH (secondary hypoadrenalism) or to a defect in the adrenals (primary hypoadrenalism; Addison's disease). Congenital adrenal hyperplasia is considered separately (see Chapter 7.7).

Table 7 Aetiology of Addison's disease

Tuberculosis
Autoimmune Sporadic Polyglandular deficiency type I (Addison's disease, chronic mucocutaneous candidiasis, hypoparathyroidism, dental enamel hypoplasia, alopecia, primary gonadal failure) Polyglandular deficiency type II (Schmidt's syndrome) (Addison's disease, primary hypothyroidism, primary hypogonadism, insulin-dependent diabetes, pernicious anaemia, vitiligo) Metastatic tumour
Lymphoma
Amyloid
Intra-adrenal haemorrhage (Waterhouse–Friederichsen syndrome) following meningococcal septicaemia
Haemochromatosis
Adrenal infarction or infection other than tuberculosis (especially AIDS)
Adrenoleucodystrophy
Adrenomyeloneuropathy
Hereditary adrenocortical unresponsiveness to ACTH
Bilateral adrenalectomy

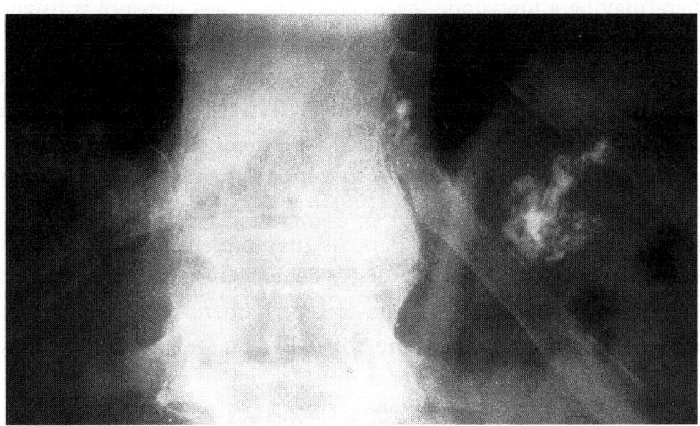

Fig. 7 Plain radiograph of the abdomen showing adrenal calcification in a patient with tuberculous Addison's disease.

Primary hypoadrenalism

Addison's disease

This is a rare condition with an estimated incidence in the developed world of 0.8 cases per 100 000 population. The causes are listed in Table 7. The incidence of tuberculous Addison's disease has gradually fallen, and autoimmune adrenalitis now accounts for more than 70 per cent of cases.

In tuberculous disease the adrenals are initially enlarged with extensive epithelioid granulomas and caseation. Calcification eventually ensues in most cases (Fig. 7). Both the cortex and the medulla are affected.

In autoimmune adrenalitis the glands are atrophic with loss of most of the cortical cells. Some hypertrophied eosinophilic compact cells remain. The medulla is usually intact. The adrenal antibodies react with the 21-hydroxylase enzyme and are found in virtually all newly diagnosed cases of autoimmune Addison's disease, and in 70–80 per cent of patients the antibodies can still be found 10 years later; they are not found in other causes of the condition, but may be present in 1–2 per cent of patients without Addison's disease but who have other organ-specific autoimmune conditions. Follow-up of these patients shows that about one-third will develop adrenal insufficiency in the next 10 years.

Patients with Addison's disease may also have antibodies which cross-react with steroid-producing cells in the ovary, testis, and placenta, and are distinct from the antibodies specific for the 21-hydroxylase enzyme. These are found in nearly all patients with both Addison's disease and primary ovarian failure, in one-third of type II polyglandular deficiency, and three-quarters of type I. Type I is an autosomal recessive condition in which adneurocortical insufficiency is associated with chronic cutanerns candidiasis, hypoparathyroidism and a variety of other conditions. Type II (Schmidt's syndrome) comprises Addison's disease, hypoparathyroism, primary hypogruadism, insulin dependent diabetes and vitiligo. The antigen recognized is a common cytoplasmic antigen (either 17α-hydroxylase or side-chain cleavage enzyme) found in the adrenals and gonads. In patients with associated pernicious anaemia the autoantigen is the gastric parietal cell Na^+/K^+ATPase.

Recent evidence suggests that many Addisonian patients also produce immunoglobulins which block the effect of ACTH. Their binding site could be the ACTH receptor. The role that they play in producing adrenal insufficiency is unknown.

With the exception of tuberculosis and autoimmune adrenal failure, other causes of Addison's disease are rare. Adrenal metastases are often found at postmortem examinations but adrenal insufficiency from these is uncommon. Necrosis of the adrenals with intra-adrenal haemorrhage may result from bilateral adrenal vein thrombosis. This may be due to infection, trauma, or hypercoagulability. Intra-adrenal bleeding may be found in any cause of severe septicaemia. When this is due to meningococcus the association with adrenal insufficiency is known as the Waterhouse–Friederichsen syndrome.

X-linked adrenoleucodystrophy, due to a deficiency of the preoxisomal enzyme lignoceroyl-COA lipase is described in OTM3, pp. 1439–40. Adrenocortical deficiency is common in this condition which usually results in death by 12–15 years of age. The adult form of the disease, adrenomyeloneuropathy is discussed in Chapter 6.9.

Another rare disease is hereditary adrenocortical unresponsiveness to ACTH. In this condition the renin–angiotensin–aldosterone axis is intact and children may present either with neonatal hypoglycaemia or later with increasing pigmentation, often with enhanced growth velocity. This condition has recently been shown to be due to a point mutation in the ACTH receptor and is inherited as an autosomal recessive.

Secondary hypoadrenalism (ACTH deficiency)

This is most often due to a sudden cessation of exogenous glucocorticoid therapy or a failure to give glucocorticoid cover for intercurrent stress in a patient who has been on long-term glucocorticoid therapy. Such therapy suppresses the hypothalamic–pituitary–adrenal axis, with consequent adrenal atrophy. Whereas the adrenal may recover with exogenous ACTH therapy, the suppression of the hypothalamus and pituitary may last for months after stopping glucocorticoid treatment. In addition to the magnitude of the dose of glucocorticoid, the circadian timing of the doses may affect the degree

Table 8 Aetiology of secondary hypoadrenalism (ACTH deficiency)

Exogenous glucocorticoid therapy
Pituitary pathology
Selective removal of ACTH-secreting pituitary adenoma
Radical hypophysectomy for Cushing's disease
Pituitary surgery for other pituitary tumours
Pituitary apoplexy
Large pituitary adenoma
Granulomatous disease (tuberculosis, sarcoid, eosinophilic granuloma)
Secondary tumour deposits (breast, bronchus)
Postpartum pituitary infarction (Sheehan's syndrome)
Pituitary irradiation (effect usually delayed for several years)
Idiopathic isolated ACTH deficiency
Hypothalamic pathology
Surgery for hypothalamic lesions (e.g. craniopharyngioma) or for pituitary tumours with large suprasellar extension
Craniopharyngioma
Head injury
Cranial irradiation
Third ventricular tumours or cysts
Granulomatous disease
Secondary tumour deposits

of adrenal suppression. Thus prednisolone in a dose of 5 mg given last thing at night and 2.5 mg in the morning may produce marked suppression of the hypothalamic–pituitary–adrenal axis, whereas 2.5 mg at night and 5 mg in the morning may produce a minimal effect. This is because the larger evening dose blocks the early morning surge of ACTH.

Some of the causes of secondary hypoadrenalism are given in Table 8. With the exception of glucocorticoid therapy, the other conditions are rare. In many of these, other pituitary hormones are deficient in addition to ACTH, so that the patient presents with partial or complete hypopituitarism. The clinical features of hypopituitarism usually make this a relatively easy diagnosis to make, but isolated ACTH deficiency is readily missed.

Clinical features of adrenal insufficiency

The most obvious feature differentiating primary from secondary hypoadrenalism is skin pigmentation, which is nearly always present in primary adrenal insufficiency (unless of short duration) and absent in secondary. The pigmentation is seen in sun-exposed areas, recent rather than old scars, axillae, nipples, palmar creases, pressure points, and in mucous membranes (buccal, vaginal, vulval, anal). In autoimmune Addison's disease there may be associated vitiligo (Fig. 8).

The cause of the pigmentation has long been debated. Three molecules derived from pro-opiomelanocortin contain melanocyte stimulating hormone (MSH) sequences, N-terminal pro-opiomelanocortin (γ-MSH), ACTH, (α-MSH), and β-lipotrophin (β-MSH). All three are elevated in Addison's disease, but the relative contribution made by each to the pigmentation is unclear.

Patients with primary adrenal failure usually have both glucocorticoid and mineralocorticoid deficiency. In contrast, those with secondary adrenal insufficiency have an intact renin–angiotensin–aldosterone system. This accounts for differences in salt balance in the two groups of patients, which in turn result in different clinical presentations.

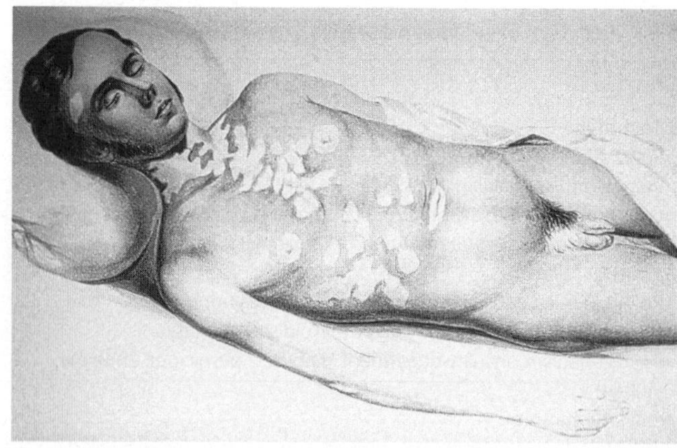

Fig. 8 Vitiligo in one of Thomas Addison's original patients. This was the only one in which he failed to get permission for a postmortem examination *(see OTM3, p.1654 for source).*

Primary adrenal failure may present with hypotension and acute circulatory failure (Addisonian crisis). Anorexia may be an early feature, which progresses to nausea, vomiting, diarrhoea, and, sometimes, abdominal pain. These crises may be precipitated by intercurrent infection or by stress, such as a surgical operation. Alternatively, the patient may present with the rather vague symptoms of weakness, easy fatiguability, weight loss, nausea, intermittent vomiting, abdominal pain, diarrhoea or constipation, general malaise, muscle cramps, and symptoms suggestive of postural hypotension. There may be a low-grade fever. The lying blood pressure is usually normal but almost invariably the pressure falls on standing.

In secondary adrenal insufficiency the presentation may relate to deficiency of hormones other than ACTH. In particular, gonadal failure is common, either because of hyperprolactinaemia or gonadotrophin deficiency. In Sheehan's syndrome there may be prolactin deficiency, with failure of lactation. If there is both ACTH and growth hormone deficiency, patients may present with episodes of hypoglycaemia. Secondary hypothyroidism is usually a late feature in the development of hypopituitarism. If there is isolated ACTH deficiency, the patient may present with malaise, weight loss, and other features of chronic adrenal insufficiency.

Laboratory investigation of hypoadrenalism

Measurement of plasma electrolytes may give the first clue to the diagnosis. In established primary adrenal insufficiency hyponatraemia is present in about 90 per cent of cases and hyperkalaemia in 65 per cent. The blood urea concentration is usually elevated. In secondary adrenal failure there may be a dilutional hyponatraemia with normal or low blood urea. Eosinophilia and an elevated erythrocyte sedimentation rate (ESR) may be pointers to the diagnosis. Hypoglycaemia has been found in up to 50 per cent of patients with chronic adrenal insufficiency.

Basal plasma cortisol and urinary free cortisol levels are often in the low normal range and cannot be used to exclude the diagnosis. For primary adrenal insufficiency the definitive tests are either the simultaneous measurement of plasma cortisol and plasma ACTH (when the ACTH level is disproportionately elevated in comparison to the plasma cortisol) or the measurement of the plasma cortisol response to exogenous ACTH. The typical ACTH levels found in primary and secondary adrenal insufficiency are shown in Fig. 9.

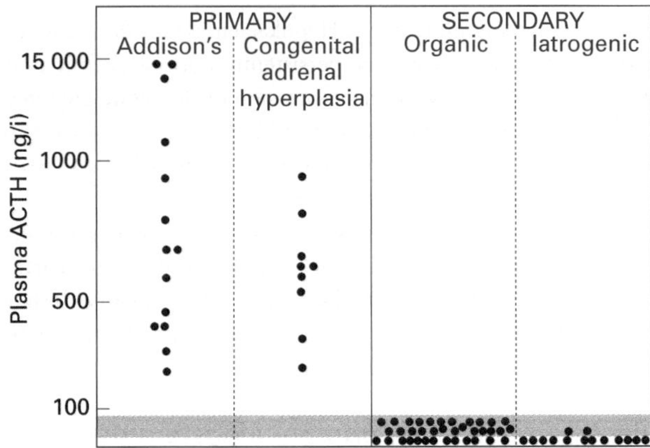

Fig. 9 Morning N-terminal immunoreactive ACTH values in patients with hypoadrenalism. The reference range is indicated by the horizontal lines *(by courtesy of Professor L. H. Rees).*

The commonest ACTH stimulation test involves the intramuscular or intravenous administration of 250 μg of tetracosactrin (Synacthen®). Plasma cortisol levels are measured at 0, 30, and 60 min. In normal subjects the plasma cortisol at 30 min is at least 550 nmol/l. The peak level rather than the increment is the most sensitive in detecting adrenal insufficiency. Levels less than 550 nmol/l in response to the acute administration of Synacthen® are found in both primary and secondary adrenal insufficiency. These two conditions can be distinguished either by measuring ACTH or by performing a prolonged stimulation test, usually involving administration of depot tetracosactrin in a dose of 1 mg by intramuscular injection, with measurement of plasma cortisol at 0, 4, and 24 h. In normal subjects the plasma cortisol at 4 h is greater than 1000 nmol/l and the 24-h value shows little further increase. Patients with secondary hypoadrenalism show a delayed response with usually a much higher value at 24 than at 4 h. In primary hypoadrenalism there is no response at either time. With further injections of depot tetracosactrin the difference between primary and secondary becomes even more obvious, with a progressive increase in plasma cortisol in secondary and no response in primary.

Another difference between these two conditions is in the renin–angiotensin–aldosterone axis. In primary hypoadrenalism there is normally mineralocorticoid deficiency with elevated plasma renin activity and either low or low normal plasma aldosterone.

The insulin hypoglycaemia test remains one of the most useful in assessing ACTH and growth hormone reserve (see Chapter 7.1).

If the tests confirm primary hypoadrenalism, it is important to determine its cause. Antibodies against the 21-hydroxylase antigen can now be demonstrated. Others, such as those blocking either ACTH-induced adrenal DNA synthesis and/or cortisol secretion, are more difficult to detect. In autoimmune Addison's disease it is also important to look for other organ-specific autoimmune disease.

In long-standing tuberculous adrenal disease there may be adrenal atrophy with calcification (Fig. 7). This is most readily detected by CT scanning. At an earlier stage the adrenals may be enlarged and tuberculosis will then need to be distinguished from haemorrhage or neoplasm. CT and MRI appear to be equally good in diagnosing adrenal haemorrhage, but CT may be better for differentiating acute inflammatory from metastatic disease.

Treatment of acute adrenal insufficiency

This is an emergency, and treatment should not be delayed while waiting for proof of diagnosis. However, in addition to measurement of plasma electrolytes and blood glucose, samples for ACTH and cortisol should be taken before giving corticosteroid therapy.

Hydrocortisone, 100 mg should be given intravenously 6 hourly. If this is not possible, the intramuscular route should be used. In the shocked patient 1 litre of normal saline should be given intravenously over the first hour. Because of possible hypoglycaemia, it is normal to give 5 per cent dextrose saline. The subsequent saline and dextrose therapy will depend on biochemical monitoring and the patient's condition. Clinical improvement, especially in the blood pressure, should be seen within 4–6 h. It is important to recognize and treat any associated condition, such as an infection, which may have precipitated the acute adrenal crisis.

After the first 24 h the dose of hydrocortisone can be reduced, usually to 50 mg intramuscularly 6 hourly for the second 24 h and then, if the patient can take by mouth, to oral hydrocortisone, 40 mg in the morning and 20 mg at 18.00 h. This can then be rapidly reduced to the normal replacement dose of 20 mg on waking and 10 mg at 18.00 h.

With high-dose hydrocortisone therapy it is not necessary to give additional mineralocorticoid replacement. However, when the hydrocortisone dose is reduced it may be necessary in primary adrenal failure to add this in the form of fludrocortisone acetate, the mineralocorticoid activity of which is about 125 times that of hydrocortisone. The usual replacement dose is 0.05–0.1 mg daily (see below).

If the patient is not critically ill, an acute ACTH stimulation test can be performed but this can be delayed and carried out with the patient on dexamethasone which does not interfere with the plasma cortisol assay.

Chronic replacement therapy

Patients with primary adrenal failure may require both glucocorticoid and mineralocorticoid replacement, but those with secondary disease require glucocorticoid alone. The usual daily dose of glucocorticoid is hydrocortisone 30 mg per day, given as 20 mg on waking and 10 mg at 18.00 h. Some patients require more than this and others less. Inadequate treatment may lead to persistent pigmentation and elevation of ACTH levels.

Patients should be advised to double the dose of glucocorticoid in the event of intercurrent febrile illness, accident, or severe mental stress. If the patient is vomiting and cannot take by mouth, parenteral hydrocortisone must be given urgently. For minor surgery, 100 mg hydrocortisone hemisuccinate is given with the premedication. For major operations this is then followed by the same regimen as for acute adrenal insufficiency but without the saline replacement. If a patient on replacement therapy is given enzyme inducing drugs such as rifampicin or phenytoin, the replacement dose of hydrocortisone will need to be increased. The same is also true in pregnancy as the oestrogen-induced rise in cortisol-binding globulin will decrease the free cortisol.

The patient on glucocorticoid therapy should be advised to register for a MedicAlert bracelet or necklace and should carry a 'Steroid card'.

Mineralocorticoid replacement is not always necessary in Addison's disease but postural hypotension and/or hyperkalaemia, should be

Table 9 Mineralocorticoid excess syndromes

Aldosterone
Primary hyperaldosteronism
Conn's syndrome—aldosterone-producing adrenal adenoma (APA)
Angiotensin II-responsive APA
Primary adrenal hyperplasia
Aldosterone-producing adrenal carcinoma
Glucocorticoid-suppressible hyperaldosteronism
Secondary hyperaldosteronism
Mineralocorticoids other than aldosterone
17α-hydroxylase deficiency
11β-hydroxylase deficiency
Deoxycorticosterone
Corticosterone
Congenital apparent mineralocorticoid excess syndromes
Acquired apparent mineralocorticoid excess syndromes
Ectopic ACTH syndrome
Glucocorticoid resistance
Exogenous mineralocorticoids
Abnormal renal tubular ionic transport (pseudoaldosteronism)
Liddle's syndrome

treated by fludrocortisone 0.1–0.2 mg/day. The adequacy of this replacement can be monitored by measuring blood pressure and plasma electrolytes.

Mineralocorticoid excess

The syndromes of mineralocorticoid excess can be due to excess of aldosterone (primary or secondary aldosteronism), of other mineralocorticoids, or abnormal renal tubular function (Table 9).

Primary aldosteronism

Since Conn's original description of a patient with hypertension, neuromuscular symptoms, and hypokalaemia associated with an aldosterone-producing adrenal adenoma, it has been recognized that the same clinical and biochemical picture may be produced by other conditions in which there is aldosterone excess without adenoma. Measurement of plasma renin activity is the key to distinguishing primary aldosteronism (in which plasma renin activity is low or undetectable) from secondary, in which it is usually elevated. The exception to this is in patients with idiopathic hyperplasia of the zona glomerulosa, in which there is marked enhancement of the adrenal responsiveness to angiotensin II. Thus although this appears to be a form of primary aldosteronism with elevated aldosterone and low plasma renin activity, it is actually a type of secondary aldosteronism (see OTM3, p. 1656).

In about 60 per cent of patients with apparent primary aldosteronism an adenoma is found. Most of the remainder will have bilateral adrenal hyperplasia. Aldosterone-producing adrenal carcinomas are rare (3–5 per cent of aldosterone-producing adrenal tumours).

Glucocorticoid-suppressible hyperaldosteronism (familial hyperaldosteronism type I)

This syndrome has an autosomal dominant mode of inheritance and most commonly presents with the discovery of hypertension in asymptomatic young individuals. Hypokalaemia may be a clue to the diagnosis, but some patients are persistently normokalaemic despite marked aldosterone excess with suppression of the renin–angiotensin system. Another form of familial hyperaldosteronism (familial hyperaldosteronism type II) is not glucocorticoid suppressible and may, in some patients, be due to an adenoma.

In the glucocorticoid-suppressible disorder (type I) aldosterone secretion is under ACTH control and can be reduced by glucocorticoid therapy. This disease results from the ectopic expression of aldosterone synthase in the zona fasciculata, an enzyme normally only found in the zona glomerulosa (see OTM3, pp. 1656–7).

Presenting features of primary aldosteronism

The majority of patients are asymptomatic and present with hypertension and hypokalaemia. A minority of patients will have symptoms related to hypokalaemia such as muscle weakness, polyuria, and polydipsia secondary to nephrogenic diabetes insipidus, paraesthesiae, and occasionally tetany due to the decrease in ionized calcium associated with the hypokalaemic alkalosis. Whilst susceptibility to hypokalaemia is a consequence of the hyperaldosteronism, it is now recognized that many patients with this disease may be normokalaemic, perhaps particularly among those who have a low salt intake. Hypokalaemia may be exacerbated or precipitated by diuretic therapy, and in one series 62 per cent of patients with primary aldosteronism became normokalaemic when their thiazide diuretic was stopped.

Diagnosis

Hypokalaemic alkalosis in an hypertensive patient suggests the diagnosis. Confirmation then comes from the demonstration of increased aldosterone secretion together with low or suppressed plasma renin activity. Hypokalaemia retards aldosterone secretion, and if potassium is less than 3 mmol/l supplementation should be given before measuring aldosterone. Some antihypertensive drugs have long-term effects on the renin–angiotensin axis and thus should be stopped several weeks before testing (Table 10).

Plasma aldosterone is measured at 08.00 h with the patient having been lying down for 30 min. Alternatively, 24-h urinary aldosterone excretion can be measured. Both plasma renin activity and aldosterone are affected by posture and sodium intake, so plasma renin activity samples should be taken under the same controlled conditions as aldosterone, with sodium intake estimated by measurement of 24-h urinary sodium excretion.

Measurement of the aldosterone-renin ratio helps to overcome problems in controlling posture, sodium intake, and drug therapy. In patients with aldosterone-producing adenomas the ratio (plasma aldosterone pg/ml and plasma renin activity ng/ml/h) is above 400, whereas in essential hypertensive patients it is less than 200. Secondary hyperaldosteronism is characterized by elevated plasma aldosterone with a normal ratio.

Various dynamic tests have been used to further investigate aldosterone secretion in suspected primary aldosteronism. These have usually involved some form of salt loading and/or exogenous mineralocorticoid administration. The rationale is that plasma volume expansion in normal subjects will suppress plasma aldosterone concentrations, but not in primary aldosteronism. This is true in aldosterone-producing adenoma, but patients with idiopathic hyperplasia may show suppression.

Table 10 Drugs and the renin–angiotensin–aldosterone axis

Drug	Effect	Action
Spironolactone	↑ PRA especially in idiopathic hyperplasia	Stop 6 weeks before tests
Oestrogens	↑ Plasma renin substrate	Stop 6 weeks before tests
ACE inhibitors	↑ PRA ↓ aldosterone in idiopathic hyperplasia and secondary aldosteronism	Stop 2 weeks before tests
Diuretics other than spironolactone	↑ PRA	Stop 2 weeks before tests
Non-steroidal anti-inflammatory drugs	Retain sodium ↓ PRA	Stop 2 weeks before tests
β-Adrenoceptor-blocking drugs	↓ PRA	Stop 2 weeks before tests
Calcium-channel-blocking agents	↓ Aldosterone	Stop 2 weeks before tests

ACE, angiotensin-converting enzyme; PRA, plasma renin activity.

Differential diagnosis

A number of tests can be used to distinguish between the various causes of primary aldosteronism and these are described in OTM3, pp. 1657–9. The most useful include assessment of the effects of posture on renin and aldosterone, of dexamethasone on plasma aldosterone, and measurement of urinary 18-hydroxy cortisol. The gold standard for confirming a unilateral functioning adenoma is bilateral adrenal vein catheterization. High levels of aldosterone are then found on the side or the tumours with contralateral suppression. This is a very difficult technique; easier but less definitive is adrenal scintigraphy using ^{131}I- or ^{75}Se-labelled metabolic precursors of aldosterone when unilateral uptake is expected in the case of adenomas. Drugs such as spironolactone must be stopped for 6 weeks before scanning. It is important to look at sequential isotope uptake rather than at one single time point. In one series nearly half the patients with an adenoma had bilateral uptake and a quarter of those with hyperplasia markedly asymmetrical uptake. When dexamethasone has been given to suppress ACTH, early unilateral uptake (less than 5 days) suggests adenoma and early bilateral uptake, hyperplasia. It has been calculated that the accuracy of scintigraphy is about 72 per cent.

CT and MRI imaging of the adrenals can detect tumours but do not assess their function. Modern CT can accurately diagnose tumours down to 7 mm in diameter. There have been few comparisons of CT with MRI but the latter is probably more sensitive.

Aldosterone-producing adrenal carcinoma

This may be suspected clinically as the tumours may produce cortisol or androgens in addition to aldosterone. Further clues would be a CT scan which shows either a tumour greater than 4 cm in diameter or with calcification.

Treatment

Glucocorticoid-suppressible hyperaldosteronism

Initial therapy is with dexamethasone in the lowest dose necessary to suppress ACTH (start with 0.5 or 0.75 mg on going to bed and 0.25 mg on waking). The plasma aldosterone, cortisol, plasma renin activity, electrolytes, and blood pressure can be used to assess the efficacy of therapy. It is not unusual to find that the initial effective control of blood pressure diminishes, so that additional therapy with spironolactone or amiloride is required.

Aldosterone-producing adenoma

Before surgery treatment with spironolactone 400 mg/day lowers blood pressure, returns plasma potassium levels to normal, and increases renin secretion to stimulate the atrophic zona glomerulosa in the contralateral gland and thus avoids aldosterone deficiency after removal of the adenoma. Overall, about 60 per cent of patients with adenomatous disease become normotensive within a month of surgery, and 75 per cent within a year.

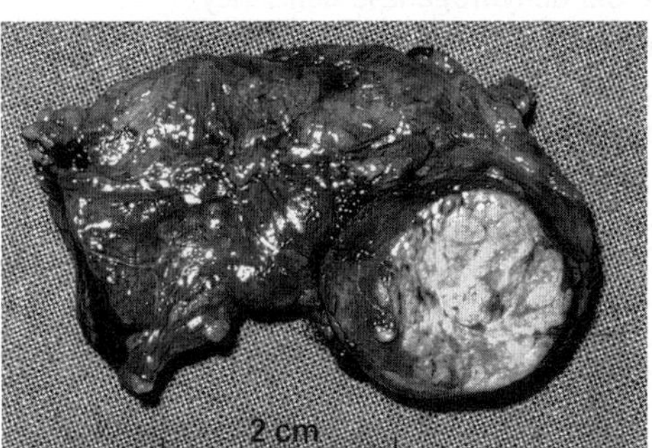

Fig. 10 Typical Conn's adenoma.

The typical Conn's adenoma is canary yellow (Fig. 10). Comparison of surgery with long-term spironolactone suggests that surgery is more effective in lowering blood pressure to normal. If medical treatment is required long term, spironolactone remains the drug of choice. After initial high-dose therapy it is often possible to reduce this to a maintenance dose of 25–50 mg/day. However, even with this dose patients may get unacceptable side-effects. These include impotence, gynaecomastia, and menorrhagia. Such patients should be given amiloride in a dose of up to 40 mg daily.

Idiopathic hyperaldosteronism and primary adrenal hyperplasia

Surgery is contraindicated in patients with idiopathic hyperaldosteronism as even bilateral adrenalectomy is not curative. It would seem likely that the small minority who have responded to surgery have had primary adrenal hyperplasia. The usual therapy for idiopathic hyperaldosteronism is to start with spironolactone or amiloride. These drugs will correct the hypokalaemia but not usually the hypertension. The latter will often respond to the addition of an angiotensin-converting-enzyme inhibitor or a calcium-channel-blocking drug. Spironolactone is more often effective in lowering blood pressure in primary adrenal hyperplasia than in idiopathic hyperaldosteronism.

Aldosterone-producing adrenal carcinoma

This has a poor outlook regardless of therapy (5-year survival 25 per cent). Treatment is with unilateral adrenalectomy usually together with *o,p′*-DDD (see above).

Mineralocorticoids other than aldosterone

Deoxycorticosterone and corticosterone

With the exception of congenital adrenal hyperplasia (see Chapter 7.7), only a few patients have been described who have isolated production of deoxycorticosterone or corticosterone. Rarely, adenomas may produce deoxycorticosterone alone and aldosterone secretion is suppressed. More commonly, an aldosterone-producing adrenal adenoma will also produce deoxycorticosterone in excess. Occasional patients will have elevated levels of deoxycorticosterone with normal levels of aldosterone. Some of these have adenomas with intermittent aldosterone secretion. Most pure corticosterone-producing adrenal tumours have been carcinomas.

Congenital apparent mineralocorticoid excess syndrome (11β-hydroxysteroid dehydrogenase deficiency)

This is a rare condition in which there is hypertension, hypokalaemia, and suppression of the renin–angiotensin–aldosterone axis. 11β-hydroxysteroid dehydrogenase is the enzyme that interconverts active cortisol to inactive cortisone. The liver isoform of the enzyme converts cortisone to cortisol and the renal isoform cortisol to cortisone. The kidney enzyme protects the mineralocorticoid receptors in the distal nephron from local effects of cortisol. This receptor has an equal affinity for cortisol and aldosterone, and given the 100-fold excess of circulating cortisol over aldosterone it would be expected that the receptor would be largely occupied by cortisol. Under normal circumstances this does not happen as 11β-hydroxysteroid dehydrogenase in the distal nephron cells prevents cortisol from reaching the receptor. If, however, the enzyme is either congenitally deficient or inhibited, cortisol reaches the receptor and produces gross mineralocorticoid excess. Congenital deficiency presents in childhood with severe hypertension and has a high morbidity and mortality. The condition is diagnosed by the clinical and biochemical picture, with suppression of both plasma renin activity and plasma aldosterone, together with an elevated ratio of urinary cortisol to cortisone metabolites. Spironolactone may improve the plasma electrolyte changes, but rarely controls the hypertension. Dexamethasone has a much higher affinity for the glucocorticoid than for the mineralocorticoid receptor and by lowering plasma cortisol may be a useful treatment given in low doses. It is usually necessary to add further drugs, such as an ACE inhibitor with a diuretic to achieve full control of blood pressure.

Acquired apparent mineralocorticoid excess—liquorice

Hypertension, hypokalaemia, and suppression of both plasma renin activity and aldosterone can be found in patients who take excess liquorice or carbenoxolone. These agents are potent inhibitors of 11β-hydroxysteroid dehydrogenase and thus block the renal conversion of cortisol to cortisone. Treatment is to stop the excessive ingestion of liquorice or carbenoxolone.

Ectopic ACTH syndrome

Patients with ectopic ACTH syndrome are almost always hypokalaemic probably because of impaired conversion of cortisol to cortisone in the kidney. The inhibitor of 11β-hydroxysteroid dehydrogenase is probably an ACTH responsive steroid other than cortisol. A small number of patients lack the stigmata of Cushing's syndrome. They are resistant to suppression of cortisol with low-dose dexamethasone but respond to high doses. The increased ACTH levels lead to increased adrenal production of androgens and deoxycorticosterone with features of androgen and/or mineralocorticoid excess. Treatment with a dose of dexamethasone adequate to suppress ACTH (usually 3 mg/day) results in a fall in adrenal androgens and often return of plasma potassium and blood pressure to normal. Some have been found to have point mutations in the steroid-binding domain of the glucocorticoid receptor.

Table 11 Causes of mineralocorticoid deficiency

Adrenal hypoplasia
Congenital adrenal hyperplasia
Pseudohypoaldosteronism types I and II
Hyporeninaemic hypoaldosteronism
Aldosterone biosynthetic defects (corticosterone methyl oxidase deficiency types I and II)
Addison's disease
Drug induced

Exogenous mineralocorticoids

The administration of large doses of hydrocortisone, fludrocortisone, deoxycorticosterone (often as the acetate), or 9α-fluoroprednisolone will produce hypertension and hypokalaemia with suppression of the renin–angiotensin–aldosterone axis. With the exception of prolonged high-dose hydrocortisone or inappropriately high mineralocorticoid replacement therapy, it is unusual to see this in clinical practice. However, severe mineralocorticoid excess can result from 9α-fluoroprednisolone, prescribed as a spray for chronic rhinitis or as topical therapy for eczema.

Abnormal renal tubular ionic transport (Liddle's syndrome)

Liddle described a familial syndrome which simulated primary aldosteronism but in which aldosterone was suppressed. Spironolactone therapy was ineffective but an inhibitor of renal tubular ionic transport (triamterene) resulted in a natriuresis with potassium retention and return of the blood pressure to normal. An alternative drug is amiloride. Patients with this syndrome have a mutation of the β-subunit of the highly selective type I epithelial sodium channel. 11β-Hydroxysteroid dehydrogenase deficiency can be readily distinguished by the urinary cortisol : cortisone metabolite ratio and by its electrolyte response to high-dose spironolactone.

Mineralocorticoid deficiency

These syndromes (other than Addison's disease) are listed in Table 11.

Disorders of the terminal part of the aldosterone biosynthetic pathway—isolated aldosterone deficiency

Failure of conversion of corticosterone to 18-hydroxycorticosterone or of 18-hydroxycorticosterone to aldosterone results in salt-wasting (Fig. 1). A number of genetic defects in the critical enzymes have been described (see OTM3, p. 1662). Patients present at birth with salt-wasting (hyponatraemia, hyperkalaemia, and fluid depletion).

Pseudohypoaldosteronism

In this condition there is a failure of the normal tissue responsiveness to mineralocorticoids. The usual presentation is with severe salt-wasting and failure to thrive in infancy. The condition is heterogeneous and may be transmitted as an autosomal dominant. The salt-wasting nearly always improves with age.

Another group of patients with so-called pseudohypoaldosteronism type II has been described. These have mineralocorticoid-resistant hyperkalaemia but do not have the salt-wasting of the type I condition (Gordon's syndrome). There appears to be excessive reabsorption of chloride by the distal nephron, which then affects mineralocorticoid-dependent potassium and hydrogen ion secretion, resulting in hyperkalaemia and acidosis. The increased sodium chloride reabsorption results in hyperchloraemia, hypertension, and suppression of plasma renin activity. A similar condition has been described in obstructive uropathy.

Hyporeninaemic hypoaldosteronism

Various renal diseases have been associated with damage to the juxtaglomerular apparatus and hence renin deficiency. Of these the most common is diabetic nephropathy. The usual picture is of an elderly patient who presents with hyperkalaemia (often severe) or resultant symptoms of recurrent arrhythmias. The hyperkalaemia is associated with acidosis, and mild to moderate impairment of renal function. Plasma renin activity and aldosterone are low and fail to respond to sodium depletion, the erect posture, or frusemide administration.

Treatment of the renin deficiency is with fludrocortisone in the first instance, to replace aldosterone, together with dietary potassium restriction. However, these patients are not salt depleted and may become hypertensive with fludrocortisone. In this case the addition of a loop-acting diuretic such as frusemide is appropriate.

Further reading

Barzon, L., Scaroni, C., Sonino, N., *et al.* (1999). Risk factors and long-term follow-up of adrenal incidentalomas. *Journal of Clinical Endocrinology and Metabolism* **84**, 520–6.

Newell-Price, J., Trainer P., Besser, M., and Grossman, A. (1998). The diagnosis and differential diagnosis of Cushing's syndrome and pseudo-Cushing's states. *Endocrine Reviews* **19**, 647–72.

Pang, S. (1997). Congenital adrenal hyperplasia. *Endocrinology and Metabolism Clinics of North America* **26**, 853–91.

Chapter 7.7

Congenital adrenal hyperplasia

I. A. Hughes

Congenital adrenal hyperplasia comprises a family of inherited disorders of adrenal steroidogenesis. They have in common the net effect of an insufficient production of cortisol and/or aldosterone which leads to increased trophic stimulation by ACTH and hyperplastic adrenals. Genital abnormalities are not a feature of all the adrenal enzyme deficiencies so that the term, adrenogenital syndrome, has now largely been abandoned.

The pathways of adrenal steroidogenesis and the required enzymes are illustrated in Fig. 1, Chapter 7.6. Deficiency of 21-hydroxylase activity is the cause of congenital adrenal hyperplasia in more than 90 per cent of cases. Here, the accounts of this and other forms of congenital adrenal hyperplasia deal largely with presentation and management in older children and adults; other texts should be consulted for description of these disorders in infancy.

21-Hydroxylase deficiency

The classical presentation is with ambiguous genitalia in infancy; the female fetus becomes virilized *in utero* as a result of excess adrenal androgen production. Aldosterone biosynthesis is deficient in up to 75 per cent of cases, but clinical signs of salt depletion are seen in only some 50 per cent. Late-onset forms are also recognized. Precocious puberty and tall stature result from the growth-promoting effects of adrenal androgens. In males, testes remain pre-pubertal in size (less than 4 ml in volume)—a useful feature to distinguish from other causes of precocious puberty associated with excess gonadotrophin secretion. In females, pubic hair growth may appear early; hirsutism and menstrual dysfunction occur after puberty, and infertility can be a presenting feature. Male infertility is also recognized, usually related to uncontrolled salt-wasting, as well as to suppression of testicular testosterone production resulting from suppression of LH by excessive adrenal androgens.

Diagnosis

The diagnosis of 21-hydroxylase deficiency in the later-onset forms usually requires an ACTH stimulation test to amplify marginally elevated basal values for adrenal steroid concentrations. Following a 250 µg bolus injection of tetracosactin, plasma 17OH-progesterone concentrations are inappropriately elevated. In females the conditions

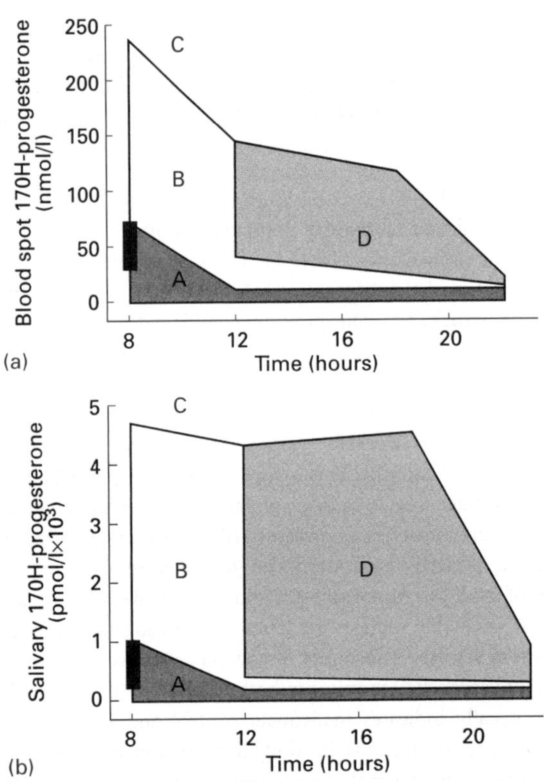

Fig. 1 Nomograms to monitor control in congenital adrenal hyperplasia using (a) blood spot and (b) saliva 17OH-progesterone profiles. Areas A, B, and C represent good, poor, and extremely poor control, respectively; area D indicates overlap of B and C areas. The shaded bars denote a range of 17OH-progesterone values at 0800 h which avoids overtreatment. *(Reproduced with permission of Archives of Disease in Childhood.)*

Table 1 Parameters to monitor treatment in congenital adrenal hyperplasia

Clinical	Linear growth velocity Weight gain Striae formation Blood pressure Skeletal age
Biochemical	Profiles of 17OH-progesterone, androstenedione Plasma testosterone Plasma renin activity Urinary steroid metabolites

should be standardized so that the test is performed during the early follicular phase of the menstrual cycle and preferably following a small dose of dexamethasone given the night before. The differential diagnosis in females includes other adrenal enzyme deficiencies, particularly 3β-hydroxysteroid dehydrogenase deficiency and polycystic ovarian syndrome.

Treatment

Surgical reconstruction of the external genitalia is required in the virilized female infant with congenital adrenal hyperplasia. Medical treatment requires replacement doses of hydrocortisone and 9α-fludrocortisone (for salt-losers) adjusted according to body size. The hydrocortisone dose should be doubled or trebled in times of stress, such as an infection or for a surgical procedure. Prednisolone and dexamethasone are both longer-acting glucocorticoids which appear to be useful for treatment in the postpubertal age group. Dexamethasone is often used as a single daily dose (0.5 mg) and appears to regulate menses more efficiently in the young adult female patient. Some girls, however, develop side-effects, such as excessive weight gain and striae formation on quite small doses of dexamethasone.

Monitoring treatment

Several clinical and laboratory parameters can be used to monitor treatment at various ages (Table 1). The rate of linear growth is the main clinical yardstick of control before puberty. A delicate balance has to be struck between providing sufficient glucocorticoid replacement to reduce excess androgen secretion (which causes rapid growth) and to avoid the effect of excessive glucocorticoid treatment (which causes growth suppression). Linear growth in the older infant and child provides a useful yardstick of control when height is measured every 6 months. This is supplemented by periodic measurement of bone age from a radiograph taken of the left hand and wrist. Androgens are powerful stimulators of epiphyseal maturation and changes in skeletal maturation can be detected over quite short periods of time. It is important to avoid an excessive bone age advance since this inevitably reduces the length of growing time and leads to adult short stature. The onset of the pubertal growth spurt is an important yardstick to monitor in both sexes, while delayed menarche in girls usually indicates inadequate control and increased plasma testosterone concentrations. In adult life, regular menses and ovulation in the female and normal spermatogenesis in the male are reliable clinical indicators of adequate control.

Some of the laboratory investigations listed in Table 1 are used to refine the degree of control by clinical indices. A profile of plasma 17OH-progesterone based on measurements performed on three to four samples collected throughout the day is a useful measure of control, now that assays are available in capillary blood samples spotted on to filter paper and in saliva samples. It has been possible to derive nomograms which indicate the degree of control based on profiles of 17OH-progesterone (Fig. 1). Similar analyses can be performed for androstenedione used as a marker of control. Testosterone has less of a pronounced diurnal rhythm than adrenal steroids and random plasma measurements are useful to monitor control in infants, children, and adult females but are of no value as an index of control in pubertal boys and adult males. It should be possible to monitor control with ACTH measurements, but this is seldom used in practice. Serum electrolytes are an insensitive index of the adequacy of mineralocorticoid replacement, but the periodic measurement of plasma renin activity can be useful. Elevated levels may indicate the need for 9α-fludrocortisone treatment even if the patient has had no overt evidence of salt loss. In such cases, the patient may have compensated by adjusting to a high salt intake when they would be at risk as a result of severe gastrointestinal losses or severe diarrhoea, or in excessive heat when losses of salt in sweat may be considerable.

Outcome in treated 21-hydroxylase deficiency

The survival rate for the salt-wasting form has improved in recent years, but male infants in particular still die in infancy from salt-losing crisis because the diagnosis has been missed. Achieving normal growth has long been a problem in management. There has been an increased recognition of the importance of the type and dose of glucocorticoid to use, the need to provide adequate mineralocorticoid replacement, and the use of newer assays to monitor control in more detail. A generation of patients treated in this way has yet to reach adulthood, but even so, final height is invariably lower than expected based on parental target height. Fertility is reduced in adult females. Evidence that sexual intercourse is unsatisfactory in some females because of an inadequate vaginoplasty is a contributory factor, as well as the presence of anovulatory cycles when medical treatment is insufficient. These problems are potentially remediable so that adequately treated females with this condition should expect to be fertile. Adult males who stop taking glucocorticoid replacement may develop oligospermia; this is usually reversed when treatment is restarted. Testicular tumours may also occur when treatment is stopped because of hyperstimulation of adrenal-rest cells by ACTH.

Genetics of 21-hydroxylase deficiency

Congenital adrenal hyperplasia is an autosomal recessive condition. In the case of 21-hydroxylase deficiency, linkage studies have shown the gene encoding the enzyme to be closely linked with the genes encoding the major histocompatibility complex on the short arm of chromosome 6. Further details are provided in OTM3, p. 1666.

Prenatal diagnosis and treatment

Prenatal diagnosis of 21-hydroxylase deficiency is now more reliable, even when the index case within an affected family is not available for study. Chorionic villus sampling at around 10 weeks' gestation is used to provide a DNA sample for mutational analysis as well as determining the sex of the fetus. Amniocentesis is now performed earlier in gestation so that the concentration of 17OH-progesterone in amniotic fluid can also be measured as an indication of 21-hydroxylase deficiency.

There is an option to offer prenatal treatment with dexamethasone, given to the mother in order to prevent virilization of an affected female fetus. Treatment needs to start as early as 6 weeks' gestation because fetal adrenal steroidogenesis is established early. The usual daily dose of dexamethasone is 20 μg/kg maternal body weight, divided in three equally spaced doses. The diagnosis is confirmed or excluded at the time of chorionic villus sampling and treatment is continued to term only if an affected fetus is female. Male infants with congenital adrenal hyperplasia are not virilized at birth. The success of treatment has been variable with the limited number of cases reported. Partial virilization is still liable to occur when treatment is started too late, interrupted for any reason, or the dexamethasone dose is inadequate. Maternal oestriol levels should be suppressed (fetal adrenal steroids provide the substrate for formation of this oestrogen) as should the concentration of 17OH-progesterone and testosterone determined in amniotic fluid collected in mid-trimester. In ideal circumstances, one can anticipate normal external genitalia in treated females or, at least, a marked reduction in virilization compared with the previously affected female infant within the family. Treatment is not without side-effects to the mother. These can include excessive weight gain, formation of striae, hypertension, and glucose intolerance which are all reversible when treatment is stopped. No fetal malformations have been reported and early growth and development in those infants who were treated before birth has been normal. It is essential that the offspring of all treated pregnancies are monitored into adult life in order to determine whether glucocorticoid effects on the fetus increase the later risk of glucose intolerance and hypertension.

Incidence

The world-wide incidence of 21-hydroxylase deficiency is estimated to be 1 in 14 000 live births, and is unusually high in the Yupik Eskimos of south-western Alaska. Newborn screening programmes for congenital adrenal hyperplasia have not been universally adopted. Affected females should be recognized at birth by careful physical examination, while there is debate whether it is justifiable to screen for affected males, not all of whom would be at risk of life-threatening adrenal insufficiency. It has been decided not to add this to the list of conditions currently screened for after birth in the UK.

Other forms of congenital adrenal hyperplasia

P_{450}scc deficiency

This extremely rare form of the condition has also been variously called cholesterol desmolase deficiency and lipoid adrenal hyperplasia. The latter term illustrates a feature of lipid accumulation which can lead to massive enlargement of the adrenals. Since cholesterol cannot be converted to pregnenolone, the production of all classes of steroid hormones is deficient in gonadal as well as in adrenal tissue. Glucocorticoid and mineralocorticoid insufficiency is particularly severe and leads to infant death unless recognized and treated early. Affected males have female external genitalia or perhaps minimal virilization because of failure to synthesize testosterone. Milder cases which have survived infancy untreated are recorded. Plasma steroid and urinary steroid metabolite levels are uniformly low and show no response to exogenous ACTH stimulation. The gene encoding P_{450}scc is designated CYP11A and, in all cases studied with P_{450}scc deficiency, no mutations have been found. The defect in this form of congenital adrenal hyperplasia has now been identified as resulting from mutations in StAR, *St*eroid *A*cute *R*egulatory protein. This is a transport protein which is involved in the mobilization of cholesterol across the mitochondrial membrane.

3β-Hydroxysteroid dehydrogenase deficiency

3β-hydroxysteroid dehydrogenase/isomerase (3βHSD) is a non-P_{450} enzyme which is required for the conversion of Δ^5 to Δ^4 steroids in both adrenal and gonadal tissue. Two closely linked and highly homologous genes control the expression of two isoenzymes. The type I enzyme is expressed predominantly in the placenta and peripheral tissues, whereas the type II enzyme is expressed in the adrenals, testis, and ovary. Deficiency of 3βHSD activity results in severe glucocorticoid and mineralocorticoid deficiency. Genital abnormalities occur in affected males and females. The production of weak androgens by the testis (dehydroepiandrosterone, androstenediol) is insufficient to produce adequate virilization in the male, but their production by the adrenal does virilize the external genitalia in an affected female. The diagnosis is confirmed by demonstrating elevated concentrations of steroid precursors (particularly 17OH-pregnenolone) in plasma and their metabolites in urine.

The molecular basis of 3βHSD deficiency has been characterized in a number of affected families. Mutations such as nonsense and frame shifts have only been found in the type II 3βHSD gene while the type I gene was normal. This probably explains why some patients with 3βHSD deficiency may show normal or elevated levels of Δ^4 steroids such as 17OH-progesterone and androstenedione, particularly following ACTH stimulation. Significant amounts of type I 3βHSD enzyme activity in peripheral tissues produce sufficient amounts of active androgens to virilize some males at puberty. It has been suggested that a late-onset or non-classical form of 3βHSD deficiency is a common cause of hirsutism in adult females. This is based on an increase in the ratio of Δ^5 to Δ^4 steroids following ACTH stimulation. However, no mutations have been identified in either type I or type II 3βHSD genes.

17α-Hydroxylase deficiency

A single $P_{450}17\alpha$ enzyme catalyses 17α-hydroxylase and 17,20-lyase reactions. Both are required for the synthesis of sex hormones, whereas only 17α-hydroxylase activity is required to synthesize cortisol. Mineralocorticoid biosynthesis is not dependent on the presence of the $P_{450}17\alpha$ enzyme, so that ACTH-stimulated, low renin hypertension is a typical feature of $P_{450}17\alpha$-hydroxylase deficiency. This occurs in both males and females and is accompanied by a hypokalaemic metabolic alkalosis. Lack of adequate sex hormone production leads to a variable phenotype in affected males, ranging from female genitalia to an ambiguous appearance or features of a hypospadic male. Females have lack of development of secondary sexual characteristics and primary amenorrhoea.

The biochemical pattern in this enzyme deficiency shows increased concentrations of corticosterone, deoxycorticosterone, and progesterone, with decreased levels of testosterone, oestradiol, and plasma renin. More detailed measurements of steroid can delineate patterns indicative of deficiencies of either 17α-hydroxylase or 17,20-lyase activities alone, or as a combination of both. Many examples of this enzyme deficiency have now been described, with the majority involving a deficiency of both activities. The human CYP17 gene is made up of eight exons, and a range of mutation types has been discovered in affected patients. One of the more frequent mutations observed is a 4 bp duplication in exon 8 which, as a result of altering the reading frame, leads to a shortened carboxy-terminal sequence. Expression studies of the mutant protein show absence of both 17α-hydroxylase and 17,20-lyase activities. This is consistent with biochemical findings and a female phenotype in affected males and females.

11β-Hydroxylase deficiency

This is a second form of congenital adrenal hyperplasia that leads to hypertension. The enzyme is required for the terminal conversion of 11-deoxycortisol to cortisol, and for the conversion of deoxycorticosterone to corticosterone. The consequences of increased ACTH stimulation are salt and water retention, low-renin hypertension, and virilization, because of the increased production of deoxycorticosterone and adrenal androgens. Virilization seems to be more profound compared with that observed in 21-hydroxylase deficiency. Prepubertal breast development is another unexplained feature. Hypertension usually develops in older childhood and does not necessarily correlate with the levels of deoxycorticosterone. Hypokalaemia is not a constant finding.

The diagnosis is confirmed by elevated concentrations of 11-deoxycortisol and deoxycorticosterone in plasma and their tetrahydro metabolites in urine. Plasma concentrations of androstenedione, testosterone and 17OH-progesterone are increased, although the levels of the last steroid are not as high as in 21-hydroxylase deficiency. Treatment requires glucocorticoid replacement only, although a salt-wasting state may develop transiently when plasma deoxycorticosterone levels initially fall. Hypertension should be glucocorticoid-reversible but specific antihypertensive treatment may be necessary. Milder or late-onset forms of 11β-hydroxylase deficiency are also described. As with 21-hydroxylase deficiency, virilization in affected females can be prevented with prenatal glucocorticoid treatment.

The P_{450}c11 isoenzymes are encoded by two genes, labelled CYP11B1 and CYP11B2, respectively. They are 93 per cent identical in predicted amino acid sequences. Both genes are functional but only the CYP11B1 gene is expressed at high levels in normal adrenals. Transcripts are controlled mainly by ACTH and, to a lesser extent, by angiotensin II. The expression of CYP11B2 in the adrenal is much less and is controlled only by the presence of angiotensin II. It was originally thought that a single 11β-hydroxylase enzyme was involved in both cortisol synthesis and the production of aldosterone via 18-hydroxylase and 18-methyloxidase (or corticosterone methyloxidase II) activities. Now it is realized that the product of CYP11B2 first hydroxylates corticosterone and then oxidizes 18OH-corticosterone in order to produce aldosterone. The isoenzyme is variously termed corticosterone methyloxidase II, 18-methyloxidase, or aldosterone synthase (P_{450}aldo). Deficiency of 11β-hydroxylase activity accounts for about 5 per cent of congenital adrenal hyperplasia cases in general, but the incidence is higher (about 1 in 6000 births) in Moroccan Jews. A single base change mutation in exon 8 of the CYP11B1 gene has been reported. This alters the haem-binding sequence which is a unique and conserved feature of all cytochrome P_{450} enzymes.

Further reading

Bose, H.S., Sugawara, T., Strauss, J.F., and Miller, W.L. (1996). The pathophysiology and genetics of congenital lipoid adrenal hyperplasia. *New England Journal of Medicine* 335, 1870–8.

Hughes, I.A. (1998). The masculinized female and investigations of abnormal sexual development. *Clinical Endocrinology and Metabolism* 12, 157–71.

Lajic, S., Wedell, A., Bui, T.-H., *et al.* (1998). Long-term somatic follow-up of prenatally treated children with congenital adrenal hyperplasia. *Journal of Clinical Endocrinology and Metabolism* 83, 3872–80.

Speiser, P.W. and White, P.C. (1998). Congenital adrenal hyperplasia due to steroid 21-hydroxylase deficiency. *Clinical Endocrinology* 49, 411–17.

White, P.C., Curnow, K. M., and Pascoe, L. (1994). Disorders of steroid 11β-hydroxylase isozymes. *Endocrine Reviews* 15, 421–38.

The reproductive system

Chapter 7.8

Ovarian disorders

H. S. Jacobs

Approach to the patient with ovarian disorders

Synchronization of the changes in the ovary and uterus and the hypothalamic–pituitary unit is complex, and the ovulation cycle is vulnerable to disturbances at any level of endocrine organization. Ovarian cyclicity may also be disrupted by a deterioration in general health, a protective mechanism that prevents reproduction occurring in circumstances adverse to fetal development.

Information about the regularity of the menstrual cycle is relevant in women concerned about fertility because the chance of conception is directly related to the rate of ovulation. Oligomenorrhoea (interval between menstrual periods of more than 6 weeks but less than 6 months) is usually a consequence of the polycystic ovary syndrome (see below); amenorrhoea (no periods for more than 6 months) has a broader spectrum of causes (see Tables 1 and 2). The duration of a menstrual disturbance is relevant both to its cause and its consequences. For example, a history of delayed menarche implies the disturbance was present from the age of 12, a common finding in women with polycystic ovary syndrome. A history of weight fluctuation is important because weight loss, often in the context of mild (and denied) anorexia nervosa, is a common cause of amenorrhoea and weight increase a common precipitant of the clinical expression

Table 1 Causes of primary amenorrhoea in 90 consecutive cases seen in the author's clinics

Cause	Percentage
Premature (primary) ovarian failure	36
Hypogonadotrophic hypogonadism	34
Polycystic ovary syndrome	17
Hypopituitarism	4
Congenital anomalies	4
Hyperprolactinaemia	3
Weight-related amenorrhoea	2

Table 2 Causes of secondary amenorrhoea in 570 consecutive cases seen in the author's clinics

Cause	Percentage
Polycystic ovary syndrome	36
Premature (primary) ovarian failure	24
Hyperprolactinaemia	17
Weight-related amenorrhoea	10
Hypogonadotrophic hypogonadism	6
Hypopituitarism	4
Exercise-related amenorrhoea	3

of polycystic ovary syndrome. Bulimia may also cause either of the above conditions.

The association of amenorrhoea with galactorrhoea implies hyperprolactinaemia. Symptoms of oestrogen deficiency (flushing and sweating attacks and/or vaginal dryness and discomfort during intercourse) imply an increased risk of osteoporosis. Symptoms of hyperandrogenism (seborrhoea, acne, and excessive hair growth) are, in most cases, caused by polycystic ovary syndrome. It is preferable to use the term 'unwanted hair' rather than 'hirsutism' to avoid debate about what is and what is not truly excessive. Whether or not treatment of unwanted hair is justified is a matter for judgement. There is often concern that the development of unwanted hair presages a sex change. Patients with such anxieties need a clear explanation of the underlying disorder and reassurance that treatment is available.

If there has been previous use of an oral contraceptive, it is relevant to determine whether it was used for contraception or to correct a menstrual disturbance. An oral contraceptive does not cure such a disturbance, which is therefore likely to recur when it is stopped; nor does oral contraception cause amenorrhoea after it has been discontinued, i.e. there is no such thing as 'post-pill amenorrhoea'. Amenorrhoea occurring after discontinuation of the pill therefore needs the same investigation as in any other case of amenorrhoea.

Most women with menstrual disturbances want reassurance about their present or future fertility. The failure to ovulate as an explanation for infertility is clearly dependent on age. Many older women need advice about the long-term effects of oestrogen deficiency and the wisdom of hormone replacement therapy.

Amenorrhoea

While the classification is usually into primary (the patient has never menstruated) or secondary amenorrhoea (interval between periods more than 6 months), most of the common causes can present as either (Tables 1 and 2). With the exception of structural abnormalities, such as an absent uterus, differences between primary and secondary amenorrhoea are outweighed by similarities, so here they are considered primarily in terms of aetiology.

In young women with primary amenorrhoea there may have been congenital abnormalities in the development of the ovaries, genital tract, or external genitalia, or a perturbation of the normal process of puberty. Investigations should be considered when menstruation has not occurred by the age of 16 in the presence of normal secondary sexual development, or by the age of 14 in its absence.

Developmental abnormalities

Developmental abnormalities of the müllerian duct, the external genitalia, and the problems of intersexual abnormalities are dealt with elsewhere (see Chapter 7.12).

Gonadal dysgenesis

The commonest cause of gonadal dysgenesis is Turner's syndrome in the severest form of which a 45XO karyotype is associated with a characteristic phenotypic appearance. Typically, patients are short with cubitus valgus, webbed neck, low hairline, shield chest, and widely separated nipples. The palate is often arched and the 4th metacarpal may be short. Lymphoedema and multiple naevi are common. External genitalia are immature and axillary and pubic hair absent or scanty. Coarctation of the aorta occurs in some 10–20 per cent and hypertension independent of that abnormality appears more common than in the general population. The condition is found in some 1 in 2500 female births. Although spontaneous and, indeed, ovulatory cycles occasionally occur, particularly if there is chromosomal mosaicism, in the long term premature ovarian failure is inevitable. The karyotype should be determined, as the presence of a Y chromosome in an individual with gonadal dysgenesis necessitates the removal of residual gonadal tissue because of an increased risk of malignancy.

Serum gonadotrophin concentrations are elevated compared with those of normal girls of the same age, and may approach the menopausal range. Oestrogen levels are low, the uterus is small, and bone densitometry shows significant skeletal decalcification; a history of spontaneous fracture is common. In addition to a search for associated cardiovascular and renal abnormalities, autoimmune thyroiditis should be excluded.

Management includes initiation of low-dose oestrogen therapy at the time puberty would normally have occurred, starting with no more than 5 μg of ethinyl oestradiol per day to promote breast development without prejudicing linear growth. The dose is gradually raised over 12–18 months. Maintenance therapy is with a cyclical oestrogen–progestogen preparation (such as an oral contraceptive), as regular withdrawal bleeding is necessary to prevent endometrial hyperplasia and the risk of malignancy. It is now possible to provide women with Turner's syndrome with fertility through ovum donation, although the shortage of oocytes remains an important and usually critically limiting factor.

Hypothalamic causes of amenorrhoea

Hypothalamic hypogonadotrophic hypogonadism may be functional or organic, and occur in an isolated form or in association with more widespread endocrine defects, as in patients with infiltrating (sarcoidosis, tuberculosis), expanding (craniopharyngioma), or traumatic (head injury) lesions of the hypothalamus. Lesions of the pituitary stalk are increasingly recognized.

Kallmann's syndrome

Isolated deficiency of secretion of gonadotrophin releasing hormone (GnRH) occurs in Kallmann's syndrome of hypogonadotrophic hypogonadism associated with hyposmia and sometimes colour blindness. Other defects, such as unilateral renal agenesis and a disorder of movement (hereditary bimanual synkinesis), may be associated.

Kallmann's syndrome occurs sporadically and as an inherited condition, of which the X-linked recessive form is the commonest.

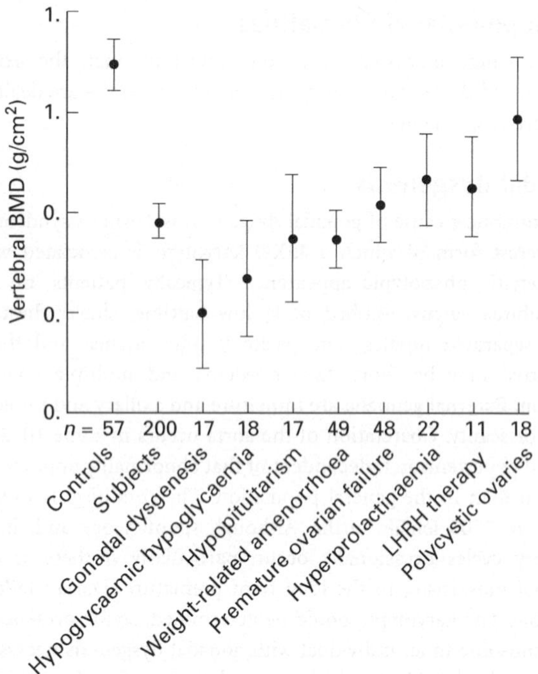

Fig. 1 Vertebral bone mineral density measurements in 200 young women with amenorrhoea, arranged by diagnosis. With the exception of the bone mineral density measurements in the women with polycystic ovary syndrome, the bone mineral density measurements of all other groups were significantly below those of the controls.

The X-linked syndrome is thought to arise from a genetically determined defect of the embryonic migration of olfactory and GnRH-producing neurones from the anlage of the olfactory lobes into the hypothalamus. The cause in non-X-linked Kallmann's syndrome is not yet known.

The condition presents with delayed puberty and primary amenorrhoea. Characteristically the patient cannot smell curry or the difference between tea and coffee. There are signs of marked oestrogen deficiency, usually amounting to sexual infantilism. Overall, the stature of adults with Kallmann's syndrome is normal, although the patient will not have experienced a pubertal growth spurt so skeletal proportions are abnormal.

Investigations reveal subnormal serum gonadotrophin and oestradiol concentrations. Ultrasound of the pelvis shows the small uterus and ovaries, and bone densitometry reveals marked skeletal demineralization (Fig. 1).

Management involves induction of pubertal maturation, initially with small doses of oestrogen (not more than 5 μg/day of ethinyl oestradiol) to optimize breast development. Delay in recognition and treatment impairs full development. Surgical referral for breast augmentation is appropriate if development is inadequate after a year's treatment with gradually increasing doses of oestrogen. Maintenance hormone treatment is with an oral contraceptive preparation. Bone densitometry should be repeated after a year to ensure that the dose of oestrogen is adequate (an increase of 5–6 per cent/year for 2–3 years should be obtained). Treatment with pulsatile GnRH or gonadotrophin injections allows an excellent prognosis for fertility.

Functional hypogonadotrophic hypogonadism

Weight-related amenorrhoea

When, for any reason, body fat content falls below 17 per cent, or body mass index below 19, amenorrhoea is usual. This latter figure assumes an average amount of exercise; for competitive athletes, particularly in track events, the figure would be higher.

The neuroendocrine mechanisms underlying the necessity for this degree of nutritional reserve are uncertain, but result in impaired secretion of gonadotrophins, particularly luteinizing hormone (LH), together with reduced insulin and insulin-like growth factor I levels and therefore lowered insulin drive to the ovaries and pituitary. The consequent anovulation is protective because it avoids the occurrence of reproduction in adverse circumstances.

Investigation and management of weight-related amenorrhoea

Women with weight-related amenorrhoea have subnormal serum gonadotrophin (particularly LH) and oestradiol concentrations, with small ovaries and a small uterus on ultrasound scanning. Skeletal demineralization is the rule, except in those with coexisting polycystic ovaries (see below).

Management involves explanation, identification of psychiatric conditions for which specialist advice is needed, and correction of oestrogen deficiency. Optimally the latter is achieved through weight gain alone. Oestrogen deficiency may, however, be so severe that if the patient is unable to put on weight, it may be advisable for her to take oestrogen in the form of an oral contraceptive. When the question of fertility is concerned, however, induction of ovulation using drugs should be eschewed until the patient's weight has returned to normal to avoid nutritional risks to the unborn child (and adult). In the event, when a normal body mass index is regained, induction of ovulation is rarely required.

Pituitary causes of amenorrhoea

Hyperprolactinaemia

While a non-functioning pituitary tumour sometimes causes amenorrhoea, the commonest pituitary cause is hypersecretion of prolactin. Hyperprolactinaemia may be caused by a prolactinoma, by a non-functioning pituitary tumour that compresses the pituitary stalk or hypothalamus, by dopaminergic antagonist drugs (phenothiazines, metoclopramide, and domperidone are the most frequent), by primary hypothyroidism, or it may be idiopathic. Prolactinomas account for about 60 per cent of cases of hyperprolactinaemia, the exact proportion depending on the sensitivity of the method of investigation. The subject is discussed further in Chapter 7.1.

Ovarian causes of amenorrhoea

Primary ovarian failure

Primary ovarian failure occurs normally at the menopause because of the process of atresia (Fig. 2) that results in almost complete depletion of oocytes and follicles by about the age of 50. If the rate of atresia is faster than normal, the causes of which are discussed below, depletion of oocytes and follicles occurs prematurely and 'age-inappropriate' or 'premature' ovarian failure develops.

Oocytes do not divide once they have been laid down in the ovary. Thus, unlike the testis, the ovary has a finite complement of germ cells. Oocytes 'used' in the process of ovulation account for a minute proportion of those that are lost, and it can be seen from Fig. 2 that most atresia occurs during intrauterine life when endocrine influences are least important. The process of atresia is controlled genetically.

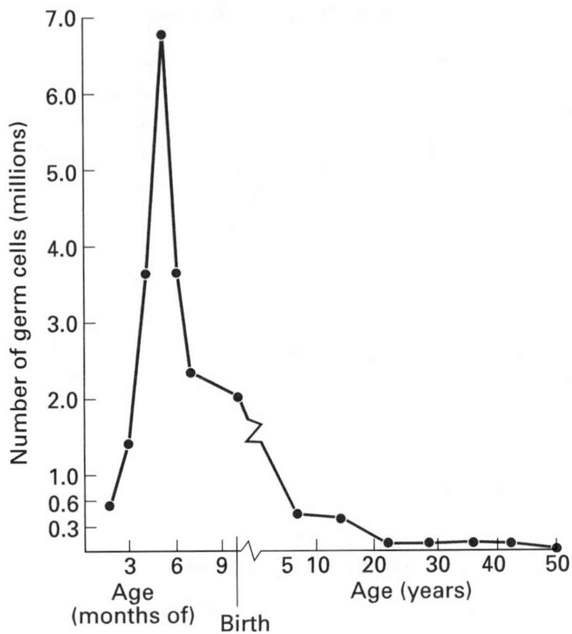

Fig. 2 The number of oocytes in the gonads in relation to age. Note that the maximum rate of atresia occurs before birth.
(After Baker, T.G. (1963). Proceedings of the Royal Society (Biology), **158**, *417.)*

Table 3 Causes of primary ovarian failure in 320 cases seen in the author's clinics

Cause	Number	Percentage
Idiopathic	169	52.6
Turner's syndrome	73	22.7
Autoimmune disease*	22	6.9
Anticancer chemotherapy	21	6.5
'Resistant ovaries'	10	3.1
Surgery	7	2.2
Radiotherapy	6	1.9
Galactosaemia	6	1.9
Familial	3	0.9
Miscellaneous	4	1.2

*Sixteen had primary hypothyroidism and six had Addison's disease. Three of these patients had diabetes mellitus.

Loss of the second X chromosome, as in 45 XO Turner's syndrome, and destruction of genetic material by ionizing irradiation or anticancer chemotherapy are therefore predicted causes of premature ovarian failure (Table 3). Viral infections, such as mumps oophoritis, and the accumulation of compounds such as galactose and its metabolites (as in galactosaemia) can damage the ovary directly. The association of premature ovarian failure with autoimmune disorders such as thyroiditis, adrenalitis, and diabetes mellitus, has led to the hypothesis that many cases are autoimmune in origin. While reliable tests are not widely available, autoantibodies to ovarian cells, oocytes, or gonadotrophin receptors have been reported in up to 80 per cent of cases of premature ovarian failure, a result consistent with the author's finding of thyroid and adrenal autoantibodies in almost half of the patients remaining after those with chromosomal causes had been excluded. Finally, the presence in the follicular fluid of toxic pollutants from tobacco smoke, such as cotinine, a cogener of nicotine, may account for the earlier menopause that occurs in women who smoke cigarettes.

The symptoms of primary ovarian failure are those of oestrogen deficiency, together with infertility. Investigation reveals raised serum gonadotrophin and subnormal oestradiol concentrations. While the serum LH is often elevated in patients with polycystic ovary syndrome, a rise in the follicle stimulating hormone (FSH) concentration always suggests primary ovarian failure. Autoantibodies should be sought as their presence alerts the clinician to the possible development of pluriglandular endocrine failure. Pelvic ultrasound shows undetectable or small ovaries and a small uterus. Bone densitometry usually reveals significant demineralization.

Patients with premature ovarian failure usually require hormone replacement therapy, the indications and precautions being the same as for those of an age for a normal menopause. In some women there may be a spontaneous return of ovulatory menstrual cycles, albeit usually temporary, and therefore pregnancies do sometimes occur. Treatment with glucocorticoids or immunosuppressive drugs for women with autoimmune ovarian failure has occasionally proven successful, but formal controlled trials are lacking and this treatment cannot be recommended. The ovaries do not respond to further stimulation with gonadotrophins and so the only chance of child-bearing for most of these women is through ovum donation. The problems of supplies of donor oocytes are formidable.

Resistant ovary syndrome

This ill-defined syndrome refers to women with amenorrhoea and elevated serum gonadotrophin concentrations in whom, paradoxically, oestrogen levels are well maintained. The persistent secretion of oestradiol suggests persistence of ovarian follicular activity, an implication confirmed by ultrasound assessment of the ovaries or occasionally by histology and by the occasional and unpredictable occurrence of pregnancy. The ovaries do not respond to further stimulation with exogenous gonadotrophins. While both cause and prognosis remain obscure, the condition is most easily understood as a transitional phase on the way to primary ovarian failure.

Polycystic ovary syndrome

A full description of polycystic ovary syndrome is given later. Its clinical expression, typically dating from the time of puberty, involves a menstrual disorder (usually oligomenorrhoea but amenorrhoea in 26 per cent of cases), hyperandrogenization, and weight increase.

The indications for treatment of amenorrhoea in women with polycystic ovary syndrome depend upon the patient's needs. For women who wish to conceive, induction of ovulation is required, combined with attempts to reduce insulin drive to the ovaries by diet and exercise. For women needing contraception, an oestrogen–progestogen pill is appropriate, the choice of preparation depending on the degree of associated unwanted hair. The oral contraceptive is also appropriate for women troubled by the lack or unpredictability of menstruation. For the remainder, it is acceptable to remain amenorrhoeic, provided annual ultrasound scans of the endometrium show that overstimulation has not occurred.

Investigation of amenorrhoea

The patient's stature, her nutritional status, the presence of unwanted hair (male pattern or the lanugo of anorexia nervosa) or acanthosis nigricans, and the physical stigmata of oestrogen deficiency are important parts of the physical examination. Pelvic ultrasound reveals the ovarian dimensions and whether they have the characteristic internal echoes of polycystic ovaries and the size and degree of endometrial thickening of the uterus. Hormone assays reveal subnormal serum oestradiol levels associated with elevated (primary ovarian failure) or subnormal (hypogonadotrophic hypogonadism) gonadotrophin concentrations. Assessment of white blood cell karyotype and measurement of autoantibodies is undertaken in patients with primary ovarian failure. Bone densitometry may reveal significant demineralization of spine and hips. Radiological assessment of the pituitary is undertaken in patients with hyperprolactinaemia.

Treatment of amenorrhoea

In addition to correcting the cause whenever possible, management is directed at minimizing the consequences of long-term oestrogen deficiency. When the cause cannot be corrected, oestrogen replacement therapy, usually in the form of an oral contraceptive, is appropriate. Outcome should be monitored by ensuring that sufficient oestrogen is administered to cause withdrawal bleeds and that there is an improvement in bone density if skeletal demineralization has been demonstrated.

Hyperandrogenization

Normal hair growth and androgen production in women

At birth the fetus is covered in lanugo hair which rapidly disappears and is not seen again unless anorexia nervosa develops, although very rarely such hair appears as a non-metastatic complication of malignancy. Prepubertal children grow soft, short and fair vellus hair, which, together with scalp, eyebrow, and eyelash hair, is known as non-sexual hair. In response to the secretion of adrenal androgens at puberty, both boys and girls develop terminal hair in the axillae and lower pubic triangle (ambosexual hair). Terminal hair is long, pigmented, and coarse. In boys the further increase of (testicular) androgen secretion leads to the development of terminal hair in the upper pubic triangle and on the face, chest, abdomen, and arms and legs.

Perception of hairiness depends in part on its distribution and in part on its character and pigmentation. While there is racial variation in the density of hair follicles (native Americans and Orientals having few and women from the Mediterranean littoral having many follicles per unit area of skin), it is the development of male-pattern hair in women which constitutes hirsutism.

The sources of androgens in normal women are shown in Fig. 3, from which it can be seen that 50 per cent of directly secreted and 75 per cent of peripherally derived testosterone normally originate from the adrenal cortex. Testosterone circulates specifically bound to sex hormone binding globulin (SHBG), from which it disassociates and diffuses into target tissues, where it is either 5α reduced to a more powerful androgen, dihydrotestosterone, or aromatized to oestradiol. The dihydrotestosterone-nuclear protein receptor complex associates with its specific DNA receptor to cause androgen-specific protein synthesis and the expression of androgen action.

Synthesis of SHBG, whose concentration largely determines the total serum testosterone concentration, takes place in the liver, stimulated by thyroxine and inhibited by insulin and to a lesser extent by androgens. The rate of clearance of SHBG is reduced by oestrogen.

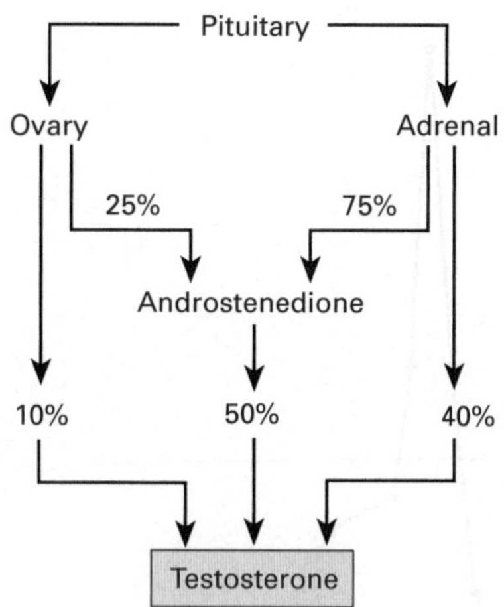

Fig. 3 Sources of androgens in normal women.

Clinical hyperandrogenization

Hyperandrogenization in women is manifest as seborrhoea, persistent acne, and the development of a male pattern of distribution and quality of hair. Male-pattern scalp hair loss may also occur, particularly in women with male family members who are bald. Clitoromegaly and increased muscle bulk are signs of severe and usually long-standing overexposure to androgens.

Although defects in adrenal steroid biosynthesis (congenital and late-onset adrenal hyperplasia), Cushing's syndrome, and adrenal androgen-secreting tumours may all cause oversecretion of androgens, and therefore present with hirsutism, the commonest cause by far is polycystic ovary syndrome, in which condition there is an increase in the direct ovarian secretion of androgens.

Polycystic ovary syndrome

Polycystic ovaries are readily identified by pelvic ultrasound, because they are larger than normal (average volume three times that of normal ovaries) and have a highly echo-dense central stroma in which cysts of 6–8 mm diameter are arranged around the circumference (Fig. 4).

Patients commonly present in their late teens or early twenties, complaining of the consequences of hyperandrogenization or of a menstrual disturbance (Table 4). Infertility is caused by failure of ovulation, although hypersecretion of LH is also important. Obesity, often associated with an increase in the ratio of waist to hip circumference, is the third classical feature.

Endocrine features

The classical profile is of hypersecretion of LH and androgens, with normal circulating FSH, prolactin, and thyroxine concentrations although there is heterogeneity of the hormonal changes. In more than 1500 cases, 44 per cent had an elevated serum LH and 22 per cent an elevated serum total testosterone concentration. Levels of LH were raised most commonly in the women complaining of infertility, and of testosterone in those complaining of hirsutism.

The nature of the primary disturbance underlying these findings is uncertain. A central problem is a failure of the polycystic ovary to convert androgens, made in excessive amounts by the abundant theca and interstitial cells of the hyperplastic ovarian stroma, into oestrogens. The androgens (predominantly androstenedione and testosterone) are then released into the circulation and converted in the skin to

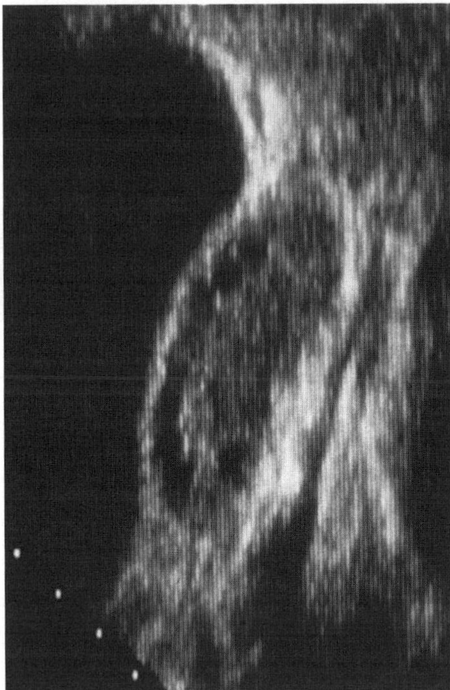

Fig. 4 Transabdominal ultrasound image of polycystic ovary. Note the enlarged ovary with the echo-dense central stroma and the necklace of cysts around the circumference.

Table 4 Clinical features in 1500 patients with ultrasound-diagnosed polycystic ovaries seen in the author's clinics

Skin and appendages	*Fertility status*
Hirsutism (61%)	Untested (67%)
Acne (24%)	Primary infertility (20%)
Alopecia (8%)	Secondary infertility (9%)
Acanthosis nigricans (5%)	Proven fertility (4%)
Menstrual cycle	*Body weight*
Normal cycle (25%)	Body mass index less than 20 (13%)
Oligomenorrhoea (45%)	Body mass index 20–25 (normal) (52%)
Amenorrhoea (26%)	Body mass index over 25 (35%)
Frequent cycles (3%)	
Menorrhagia (1%)	

Note: Some patients had more than one symptom, so the figures do not add up to 100 per cent.

dihydrotestosterone. In liver and fat tissue they are converted into oestrogens at a rate which increases with the degree of obesity. The high levels of oestrogen (predominantly oestrone) inhibit secretion of FSH and may stimulate secretion of LH. The former effect contributes to persistent anovulation and the consequent lack of progesterone (which in the normal luteal phase limits the proliferative action of oestradiol) means that the action on the uterus of the normally weak oestrogen oestrone is unopposed. These patients are consequently at risk from endometrial hyperplasia and neoplasia. The raised levels of LH stimulate the excessive numbers of theca and interstitial cells to oversecrete androgens. In addition, it is thought that exposure of the ovaries to high levels of LH at inappropriate times of the cycle impairs fertility through an action on the developing oocyte. The above model does not, however, explain its variable clinical presentation. It is likely that environmental factors lead to differing expression of the underlying, probably inherited, abnormality.

Many patients with the polycystic ovary syndrome, particularly those who are anovulatory, hypersecrete insulin in association with variable degrees of insulin resistance. Three types of insulin resistance in patients with polycystic ovary syndrome are presently recognized. Type A results from one of a number of mutations in the gene that encodes the insulin receptor. The consequence is a defect in transmission of the insulin signal anywhere along the pathway from the extracellular binding of insulin to its target tissue, to phosphorylation of the intracellular receptor-associated tyrosine kinase. Type B results from circulating autoantibodies to the extracellular domain of the insulin receptor. Type C insulin resistance, probably mediated by postreceptor defects, is by far the commonest and is the form associated with obesity. The clinical clue to the presence of severe hyperinsulinism is the presence of acanthosis nigricans.

Excessive insulin secretion occupies a central role in expression of the polycystic ovary syndrome. Thus receptors for insulin and insulin-like growth factor I have been identified in the ovary, and their stimulation sensitizes the ovary to stimulation by gonadotrophins, observations that may provide insight into the deleterious effects of obesity because, as body weight rises, secretion of insulin increases further. Although insulin receptors are down-regulated by exposure to persistently high levels of insulin, there is evidence that receptors for the insulin-like growth factors are maintained.

Hypersecretion of insulin inhibits hepatic synthesis of sex hormone binding globulin which results in an apparent disparity between circulating testosterone concentrations and the degree of hirsutism. The concentration of unbound testosterone, and by implication the testosterone production rate, is then very high despite serum total testosterone concentrations which may be within the normal range. Hypersecretion of insulin also has adverse effects on serum lipids (tendency to lower HDL2 concentrations) and high rates of coronary artery disease, hypertension, and diabetes have been reported.

Other ovarian causes of hirsutism

Hyperthecosis

This condition is probably best regarded as a severe form of polycystic ovary syndrome and is characterized by the presence of islands of luteinized theca cells within the ovarian stroma at a distance from follicles. The clinical features include very marked hypersecretion of androgens and of insulin.

Ovarian tumours

Androgen-secreting tumours of the ovary are derived from sex cord or stromal cells and include Sertoli–Leydig cell tumours (arrhenoblastomas), hilar cell tumours, lipoid cell tumours, and adrenal rest tumours. Other non-hormone-secreting tumours (Brenner, cystadenoma, and cystadenocarcinoma) have been reported to stimulate androgen secretion by the surrounding ovarian stroma. These conditions are all very rare causes of hirsutism.

Diagnosis of hyperandrogenism

Adrenal causes of hyperandrogenization are discussed in Chapters 7.6 and 7.7 but much more common is hypersecretion of androgens by polycystic ovaries. While an ovarian tumour is suggested by a short history of rapidly advancing hirsutism, amenorrhoea, and a

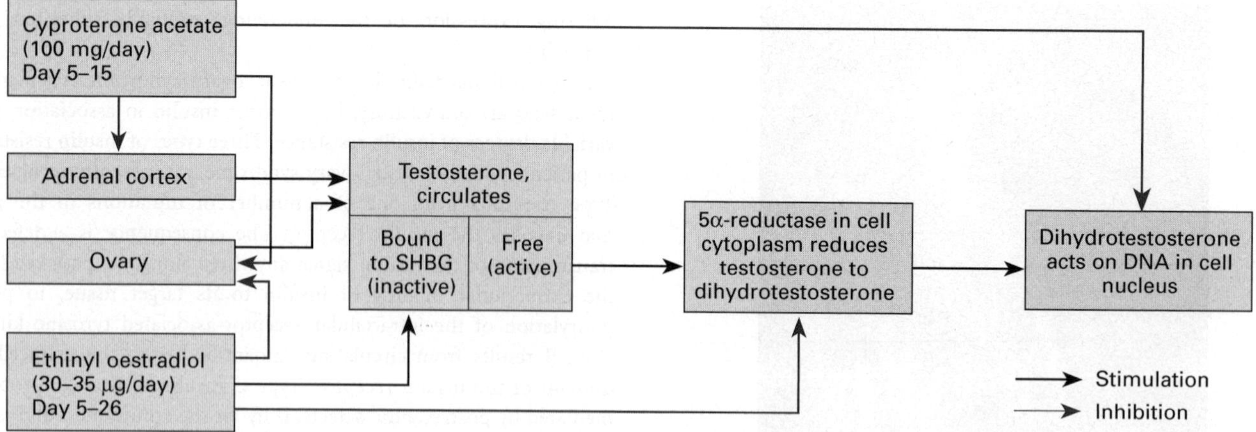

Fig. 5 The use of cyproterone acetate and ethinyloestradiol in the treatment of hirsutism. In the author's practice, ethinyloestradiol is usually replaced with Dianette®, a conveniently packaged formulation of ethinyloestradiol (35 μg) and cyproterone (2 mg).
(After Medicine International 1989.)

serum testosterone concentration in the male range, such lesions are rare; indeed, a serum testosterone concentration exceeding 10 nmol/l is more commonly associated with polycystic ovary syndrome and severe insulin resistance than with the development of an ovarian tumour.

Pelvic ultrasound will detect polycystic ovaries or ovarian tumours. In those with polycystic ovaries the serum total testosterone concentration reflects in part the testosterone production rate, and in part the serum sex hormone binding globulin concentration; it should be interpreted in light of the patient's body weight, and a concentration within the normal range should not therefore be dismissed in women who are overweight. Serum LH concentrations are often raised, but the FSH level is normal. Serum prolactin concentrations are modestly elevated (up to 2500 mU/l) in 15 per cent of patients with polycystic ovary syndrome.

A small number of patients with hirsutism have no diagnosable cause of cutaneous virilism. Labelled 'idiopathic hirsutism', these patients may have enhanced sensitivity of androgen-dependent tissues, perhaps caused by increased dermal activity of the 5α-reductase enzyme.

Management of hirsutism

The preferred drug treatment of hyperandrogenization is by administration of cyproterone acetate. This steroid is a peripheral antiandrogen, a progestogen, and a mild glucocorticoid. In combination with oestrogen, it suppresses gonadotrophin secretion and so reduces the secretion of ovarian androgens; the combination is also contraceptive. The glucocorticoid activity may reduce secretion of adrenal androgens. Finally, the drug blocks uptake of the dihydrotestosterone-protein complex by the DNA acceptor protein in the nucleus of androgen-sensitive cells, and so acts as a peripheral antiandrogen.

Cyproterone is administered cyclically, together with oestrogen, given most conveniently in the form of Dianette® (Fig. 5). Seborrhoea and acne usually clear up in about 6 weeks but it takes 12–18 months to realize the maximum improvement of unwanted hair. Cosmetic treatment is continued while on the medication, the impact of therapy being assessed by a reduction in the number of episodes of electrolysis required.

High doses of cyproterone, such as those used in treatment of carcinoma of the prostate (200–300 mg per day continuously) can have adverse effects on the liver and liver function tests should be checked twice yearly when such doses are used. As symptoms remit, the dose of cyproterone is reduced until the patient is taking the lowest dose compatible with symptomatic relief. Eventually, treatment with Dianette® alone is usually sufficient.

In patients not responding to this regimen, newer antiandrogens, such as flutamide, may be tried. Since pure antiandrogens are not contraceptive the patient must be warned of possible feminizing effects on a male fetus if they are taken inadvertently during pregnancy. They are therefore optimally prescribed with an oral contraceptive.

Infertility

Infertility can be defined as absence of conception after a year of unprotected intercourse but it is most logically evaluated in relation to normal fertility. The maximum conception rate per ovulation is 25–30 per cent, so that cumulative conception rates are usually about 60 per cent after 6 months and 85 per cent after a year. Other than mechanical bars to conception (for example gynaecological problems such as occluded Fallopian tubes), the important factors that reduce a woman's fertility are her age and any condition that reduces the number of ovulations per unit time. The central strategy of medical management of female infertility is therefore the diagnosis and treatment of anovulation. An additional strategy is to ensure that ovulation, and thus conception, occurs in as favourable an environment as possible.

Ovulation is usually inferred retrospectively by detection of a corpus luteum, indexed endocrinologically either by measurement of serum progesterone concentrations or indirectly by the effects of progesterone on basal body temperature or endometrial histology. Ovulation can be predicted ultrasonically by detecting the development of a preovulatory follicle of average diameter 20–22 mm, followed by its collapse and replacement by a solid structure, i.e. corpus luteum. The preovulatory surge of LH can be detected by the patient herself using one of a number of commercially available immunological urine tests. These methods are used to determine whether anovulation can account for a couple's infertility and whether treatment has actually resulted in ovulation; prediction of ovulation is helpful for

Table 5 Induction of ovulation

Hypothalamic level
Enchance secretion of GnRH
Weight increase
Suppression of hyperprolactinaemia: bromocriptine, pituitary surgery
Antioestrogens: clomiphene citrate, tamoxifen
Replace secretion of GnRH
Pulsatile GnRH therapy
Pituitary level
Enhance secretion of gonadotrophins
Pulsatile GnRH therapy
Replace gonadotrophins*
Human menopausal gonadotrophin: 75 IU FSH and 75 IU LH per ampoule
Follitropin: 75 IU FSH, less than 0.4 IU LH per ampoule
Human chorionic gonadotrophin: ampoule size varies

*More purified urinary extracts and recombinant versions of FSH and LH are now available.

timing investigations and maximizing the chance of conception by ensuring that intercourse occurs around the time of ovulation.

Conception rates after the age of 35 are only half of those before the age of 25. Demographic changes in northern Europe (median maternal age at first birth in the United Kingdom is now 27 years) have resulted in a steady increase in the number of couples requesting consultations for infertility.

The causes of amenorrhoea are discussed above. All except primary ovarian failure are correctable (and that condition is treatable by oocyte donation) so the fertility prognosis for this group of patients is excellent. The commonest cause of oligomenorrhoea is polycystic ovary syndrome, and while patients with this condition usually ovulate readily in response to treatment, in about 40 per cent hypersecretion of LH impairs fertility, despite the occurrence (spontaneously or as a result of treatment) of otherwise normal ovulation. The mechanism is uncertain but may involve an adverse effect of the high levels of LH on completion of the final stages of oocyte maturation.

Failure to ovulate despite (more or less) regular menstrual cycles is an unusual but recognized cause of infertility.

Induction of ovulation

Table 5 shows the agents commonly used and the endocrine level at which they exert their actions. Antioestrogens enhance hypothalamic secretion of GnRH by competing with oestrogen receptors, thus simulating oestrogen deficiency. The drug is taken for 5 days and provokes gonadotrophin secretion and thence follicular development. The most commonly used preparation is clomiphene, which is a racemic mixture, one isomer having oestrogenic and the other antioestrogenic activity. Most patients with polycystic ovary syndrome ovulate in response to clomiphene.

In patients not responding to antioestrogens, pituitary secretion of gonadotrophins can be enhanced by injection of synthetic GnRH. It is administered in a pulsatile fashion, usually by the subcutaneous route, the injections being given at 90-min intervals by a portable miniaturized pump.

For patients with destructive lesions of the pituitary, gonadotrophin secretion can be replaced by injections of LH and FSH. At present, the preparations available are extracted from human urine and are either mixtures of equal amounts of FSH and LH bioactivity (human menopausal gonadotrophin) or compounds with varying ratios of bioactivity. Because of the substantial amounts of non-hormonal protein contained in the extracts, the injections are given intramuscularly. More purified preparations and those synthesized by recombinant technology can be given subcutaneously. Follicular development is induced by the injections of FSH and LH; ovulation is triggered and the corpus luteum is maintained by a single injection of human chorionic gonadotrophin (HCG) which has LH-like bioactivity and a very long half-life.

The objective of treatment is unifollicular ovulation with full-term delivery of a single infant. The response is monitored by ultrasound assessment of the ovaries and uterus and by measurement of plasma oestradiol concentrations. HCG is administered according to strict criteria (for example, by ultrasound not more than three follicles of diameter equal to or greater than 16 mm, or six follicles equal to or greater than 14 mm diameter). Complications include multiple birth and the ovarian hyperstimulation syndrome. The latter condition occurs almost entirely in women with polycystic ovary syndrome who have received high-dose and inadequately monitored gonadotrophin therapy. It results from massive follicular luteinization and so only occurs after ovulation has been triggered by HCG or, very rarely, by a spontaneous LH surge. Symptoms usually appear 5–10 days after administration of HCG. In its mildest form it consists of ovarian enlargement and discomfort but in the more severe forms abdominal distension, nausea, vomiting, and diarrhoea develop. As a result of increased vascular permeability, protein-rich fluid accumulates in the peritoneal and sometimes the thoracic cavity; hypovolaemia develops, associated with haemoconcentration, decreased central venous pressure, low blood pressure, and tachycardia. The patient develops tense ascites, respiration is embarrassed, and urine formation is suppressed. A hypercoagulable state may develop with the risk of cerebral and peripheral venous thrombosis and embolism.

In managing this syndrome, its self-limiting nature should be borne in mind. Treatment is designed, first, to maintain blood volume while correcting fluid and electrolyte balance; second, to avoid thromboembolic phenomena (by full heparinization if severe hypercoagulability is detected); and, third, to relieve abdominal and pulmonary symptoms (by paracentesis under ultrasound control).

Further reading

Berchuck, A., Cirisano, F., Lancaster, J.M., *et al.* (1996). Role of BRCA1 mutation screening in the management of familial ovarian cancer. *American Journal of Obstetrics and Gynecology* **175**, 738–46.

Dunaif, A. (1997). Insulin resistance and the polycystic ovary syndrome: mechanism and implications for pathogenesis. *Endocrine Reviews* **18**, 774–800.

Kalantaridou, S.N., Davis, S.R., and Nelson, L.M. (1998). Premature ovarian failure. *Endocrinology and Metabolism Clinics of North America* 27, 989–1006.

Sourander, L., Rajala, T., Raiha, I., *et al.* (1998). Cardiovascular and cancer morbidity and mortality and sudden cardiac death in postmenopausal women on oestrogen replacement therapy (ERT). *Lancet,* **352**, 1965–9.

Chapter 7.9

The breast

H. S. Jacobs

Gynaecomastia

Gynaecomastia is defined as benign enlargement of the male breast caused by proliferation of the glandular components. The distinction is made from enlargement by fat tissue by examining the patient in the supine position: the breast is held between thumb and forefinger and the fingers gently moved towards the nipple. A firm or rubbery, mobile disc-like mound of tissue arising concentrically from beneath the nipple and areola indicates the presence of gynaecomastia. The most important condition that needs to be excluded is carcinoma of the male breast. Cancer usually presents as a unilateral eccentric mass that is hard and fixed to underlying tissue; it may be associated with skin tethering, nipple discharge, or axillary lymphadenopathy. Mammography and fine-needle aspiration are helpful in the differential diagnosis but if doubt remains biopsy is appropriate. While cancer of the male breast is rare, it has to be recognized that it is 16 times more common in those with Klinefelter's syndrome than in other men. Other causes of gynaecomastia are not, however, associated with an increased risk of breast cancer.

Pathogenesis

Microscopically, breast tissue in each sex appears identical at birth. It remains quiescent until puberty when, in boys, the ducts and surrounding mesenchymal tissue transiently proliferate, only to involute and ultimately to atrophy. Gynaecomastia is characterized by initial proliferation of the fibroblastic stroma and ductal system. Progressive fibrosis and hyalinization then occur in association with regression of the epithelial components. These regressive changes occur even if the stimulus (for example, oestrogen treatment) continues. When gynaecomastia has been present for more than a year, clinical regression is rarely complete, because the fibrosis persists even when the cause has been removed.

Since oestrogens stimulate and androgens inhibit development of breast tissue, gynaecomastia arises whenever there is an imbalance between these hormones. An alteration in the ratio of free androgen to free oestrogen, rather than a specific concentration of either, is thought to underlie almost all cases.

In men 98 per cent of testosterone is directly secreted by the testes, whereas the origin of oestrogen is more complex (Fig. 1): thus only about 15 per cent of oestradiol and less than 5 per cent of oestrone are directly secreted. The remainder of both is produced by extraglandular conversion of androgenic precursors in peripheral tissues. There is also substantial interconversion of oestrone and oestradiol. Directly secreted oestradiol in normal men rarely amounts to more than 6 μg/day, but when luteinizing hormone (LH) levels are persistently high, substantial amounts may be directly secreted by the testis.

Causes

Physiological gynaecomastia occurs at three times of life: the first is neonatally in response to transplacental passage of oestrogens. The second is during puberty for reasons that are not clear, and the third is in elderly men, probably because of the decline in Leydig cell function that occurs normally with age.

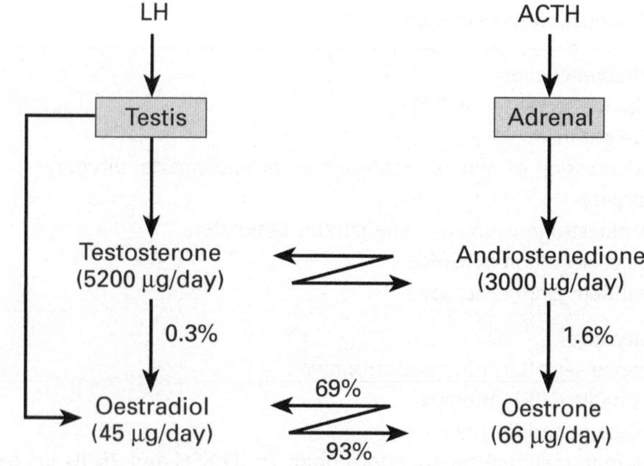

Fig. 1 Sources of oestrogen in men.

Pathological gynaecomastia is caused by a deficiency of testosterone formation or action, enhanced production of oestrogen, drugs, and unknown causes.

Testosterone deficiency

The commonest cause is Klinefelter's syndrome, about half the cases of which develop gynaecomastia at the time of puberty. The serum testosterone concentration is usually about 50 per cent of normal. Other congenital causes of testosterone deficiency include defects in testosterone biosynthesis and congenital anorchia. Acquired causes include viral orchitis (usually mumps), trauma, neurological disease (myotonia dystrophica and spinal cord lesions), and renal failure. Androgen resistance syndromes (for example, testicular feminization) are associated with high rates of secretion of testosterone and oestradiol; because of the large amounts of precursor (testosterone) there is also excessive extragonadal conversion of androgens to oestrogens.

Increased secretion

Testicular tumours, such as Leydig and Sertoli cell tumours, may secrete androgens and oestrogens autonomously; gonadotrophin secretion is therefore suppressed and azoospermia is common. These tumours may be too small to be detected clinically but ultrasound can be very helpful. Some testicular tumours, for example choriocarcinomas, secrete human chorionic gonadotrophin (hCG) which then stimulates oestrogen secretion by the contralateral testis. hCG may also be secreted by non-testicular tumours such as a bronchogenic carcinoma.

True hermaphroditism may be associated with gynaecomastia because of oestrogen secretion by the ovotestis.

Increased extragonadal production of oestrogens

Adrenal disease

Congenital adrenal hyperplasia caused by 21 hydroxylase, 3β or 17β steroid dehydrogenase deficiencies results in increased availability of adrenal androgen for peripheral aromatization. Adrenal carcinoma may be associated with massive oestrogen production, usually caused by extraglandular aromatization of the enormous amounts of androgen secreted by the tumour, but occasionally the oestrogen is directly secreted.

Liver disease

Cirrhosis, particularly alcoholic cirrhosis, is typically associated with gynaecomastia, testicular atrophy, and impotence. Plasma and urinary excretion of oestrogen is increased. The mechanism is in part decreased hepatic extraction of androstenedione, and consequently an increase in its extrasplanchnic aromatization, and partly reduced testosterone secretion by the testes. The gynaecomastia of starvation and refeeding may also be related to disturbed liver function.

Drugs

Oestrogens and oestrogen-like drugs

The most familiar is the use of oestrogen in the treatment of advanced carcinoma of the prostate. Pollution of food (via injected animals) and cosmetic products by oestrogen has been reported. Treatment with digitalis glycosides may cause gynaecomastia, the drug acting either as an oestrogen or as an oestrogen precursor.

Drugs that enhance oestrogen secretion

Treatment with hCG and clomiphene can increase oestrogen secretion. The development of gynaecomastia in men treated with hCG usually indicates that the dose has been too high.

Drugs that inhibit testosterone secretion

Ketoconazole, an antifungal agent that is also used in the management of certain forms of Cushing's syndrome, blocks steroid synthesis in Leydig cells and, if a high dose is maintained, gynaecomastia may result.

Spironolactone causes gynaecomastia in as many as 50 per cent of men treated with 150 mg/day. The drug suppresses testosterone synthesis (by inhibiting 17,20 desmolase) but it also acts as a peripheral antiandrogen.

Drugs that block testosterone action

Cyproterone acetate and flutamide are two antiandrogens used in the management of advanced prostatic disease, which usually produce gynaecomastia. Cimetidine, but not ranitidine, is antiandrogenic and is associated with a significant risk of gynaecomastia.

Although, in most series, between 50 and 75 per cent of cases of gynaecomastia are labelled idiopathic because no endocrinopathy can be identified, there are increasing reasons to suspect that environmental pollution, either with oestrogens or antiandrogens, is responsible for many of the cases.

Diagnosis

The history should include enquiry about drugs as well as possible environmental exposure to oestrogens and antiandrogens. Examination should include the testes. While small, firm testes are characteristic of Klinefelter's syndrome, asymmetrical enlargement suggests a Leydig cell tumour (most readily diagnosed by ultrasound). Evaluation of alcohol intake and liver function is appropriate. Endocrine assessment should include measurement of testosterone, oestradiol, gonadotrophins, and dehydroepiandrosterone sulphate (a high level suggests adrenal disease) concentrations.

Treatment

Once gynaecomastia has been present for about a year, treatment is unlikely to lead to a reduction in breast size because of the fibrosis that usually develops by this time. Surgery is then the mainstay of treatment. The psychological effects of persistent breast development in adolescent boys may be severe and surgery should be considered at an early stage. Medical therapy with androgens or antioestrogens produces uncertain effects and can only be expected to have much benefit if administered early in the course of the disorder. Gynaecomastia caused by oestrogen treatment, as in the management of prostatic disease, can be prevented by pretreatment with low-dose irradiation of the breasts.

Galactorrhoea

Galactorrhoea is defined as a persistent discharge of milk or milk-like secretion in the absence of parturition, or beyond 6 months postpartum in a non-nursing mother. There are essentially two types of galactorrhoea—spontaneous or present on expression only. In the latter case the menstrual cycle is usually intact and an endocrine cause is rarely found. It is spontaneous galactorrhoea that is associated with hyperprolactinaemia and amenorrhoea.

In the puerperium there is a clear correlation between the amount of prolactin released in response to suckling and the volume of milk secreted. In contrast, in galactorrhoea, no such relation exists, presumably because the breasts have not been prepared for lactation by the oestrogen- and progesterone-rich environment of pregnancy. In women with amenorrhoea caused by hyperprolactinaemia, for example, only about 20 per cent have galactorrhoea. Thus the evaluation of galactorrhoea nowadays is essentially the evaluation of hyperprolactinaemia.

Management

The essential investigation is the measurement of serum prolactin. The management of hyperprolactinaemia is outlined in Chapter 7.1. A number of drugs can cause hyperprolactinaemia, including many psychotropic agents (e.g. phenothiazines, tricyclics), verapamil, methyldopa, and reserpine. For women with non-hyperprolactinaemic galactorrhoea the important advice is first to stop expressing the milk, the second is the reassurance that it is not a sign of cancer, or a risk factor for it, and the third is a trial of drug therapy with bromocriptine. In the author's experience, after they have received appropriate reassurance, patients with non-hyperprolactinaemic galactorrhoea rarely need drug therapy. Such patients are, however, very sensitive to the adverse affects of the drug, and side-effects are common, even with low doses.

Further reading

Berchuck, A., Carney, M., Lancaster, J.M., *et al.* (1998). Familial breast-ovarian cancer syndromes: BRCA1 and BRCA2. *Clinical Obstetrics and Gynecology,* 41, 157–66.

Haney, A.F. (1997). Galactorrhea. *Current Therapy in Endocrinology and Metabolism,* 6, 393–6.

Chapter 7.10

Disorders of male reproduction

F. C. W. Wu

Physiology

The adult testis subserves two functions—the production of androgens and of spermatozoa (Fig. 1). These functions are dependent on trophic hormones from the hypothalamus and anterior pituitary which are sensitive to the negative feedback of testicular hormones (see Chapter 7.1). Androgens are essential for the differentiation, growth, and

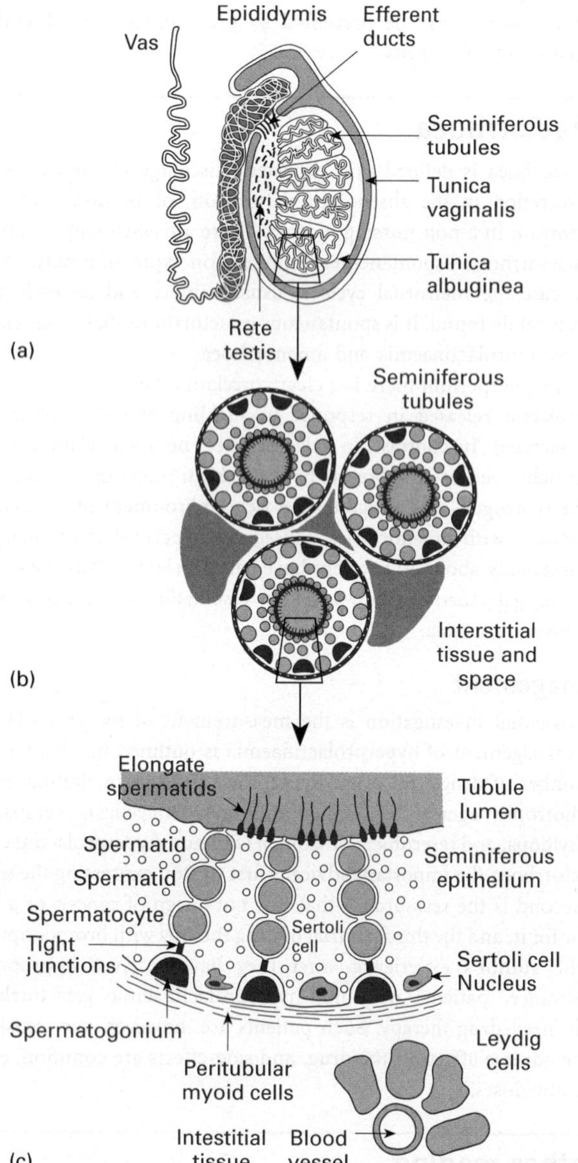

Fig. 1 (a) Human testis, epididymis, and vas deferens showing efferent ducts leading from the rete testis to the caput epididymis and the cauda epididymis continuing to become the vas deferens. (b) Cross-section through a seminiferous tubule showing central lumen, seminiferous epithelium, and interstitial space containing Leydig cells. (c) Anatomical relationships in the seminiferous epithelium between germ cells (spermatogonia, spermatocytes, and spermatids), Sertoli cells, peritubular myoid cells, and Leydig cells.

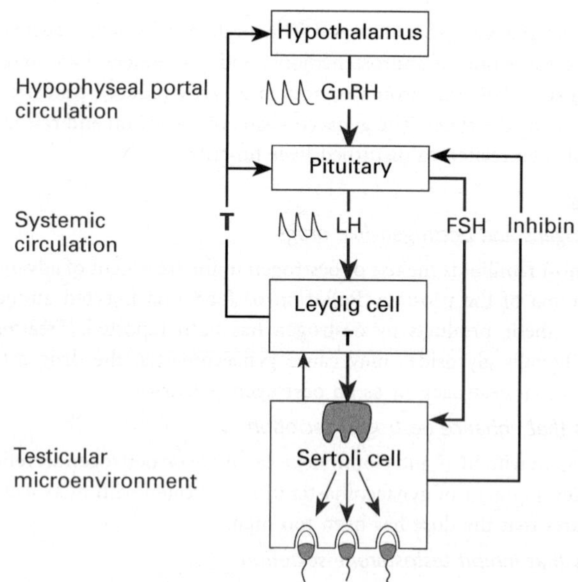

Fig. 2 Functional relationships in the hypothalamic–pituitary–testicular axis and testicular microenvironment. GnRH is secreted into the hypophyseal circulation in an episodic manner, which is reflected by an LH pulse in the systemic circulation. Blue arrows represent positive stimulation and black arrows negative feedback.

function of the epididymis, seminal vesicles, prostate, male secondary sexual characteristics, and sexual potency.

The pulsatile pattern of LH concentrations in the circulation reflects intermittent hypothalamic gonadotrophin releasing hormone (GnRH) secretion. LH stimulates biosynthesis of androgenic steroids by binding to specific surface membrane receptors on the Leydig cells. This activates the cyclic-AMP/protein kinase mechanism which mobilizes cholesterol substrate and promotes the conversion of cholesterol to pregnenolone so beginning the process which results in the formation of testosterone. Testosterone exerts the major negative feedback action on gonadotrophin secretion by restricting the frequency of GnRH release from the hypothalamus and by reducing the amplitude of LH response to GnRH.

Sixty per cent of circulating testosterone is bound to sex hormone binding globulin (SHBG), 38 per cent to albumin, and 2 per cent is free. Free and albumin-bound fractions constitute the major bioavailable portion of the circulating hormone. Androgen action is mediated through specific binding to intranuclear receptors, which increase transcription of androgen-responsive genes in target cells. In the fetal external genitalia, prostate, and facial hair follicles, full activation requires the local metabolism of testosterone by 5α-reductase to 5α-dihydrotestosterone, an androgen which is at least tenfold more potent than testosterone.

The androgen synthetic and spermatogenetic functions in the testis are closely interlinked. The paracrine action of testosterone within the testis is crucial, together with follicle stimulating hormone (FSH), for the initiation and maintenance of spermatogenesis and hence fertility. In response to these trophic signals, the Sertoli cells of the seminiferous tubules provide the physical framework and chemical milieu for the developing germ cells which are embedded in their cytoplasm. The Sertoli cells secrete inhibin, a group of related glycoprotein hormones, which inhibits FSH secretion by the pituitary (Fig. 2).

Spermatogenesis comprises repetitive cytodifferentiation in the seminiferous epithelium whereby cohorts of undifferentiated diploid germ cells (spermatogonia) multiply and transform into haploid spermatozoa (Fig. 1). Mitotic divisions of stem cells form populations of spermatogonia which, at regular intervals of 16 days, differentiate into primary preleptotene spermatocytes to initiate meiosis. Meiotic reduction divisions of spermatocytes generate round spermatids which then transform into compact, elongated spermatids with condensed DNA in the head and a tail capable of propelling beating movements. Mature spermatozoa are finally released from Sertoli cell cytoplasm into the tubular lumen around 74 days after their initial development from spermatogonia.

Male reproductive disorders

Male hypogonadism results from androgen deficiency usually, but not invariably, due to the failure of Leydig cell function. Concomitant impairment of spermatogenesis is also likely since the seminiferous tubules will also be androgen deficient or directly involved by the same pathological process. Infertility, on the other hand, is usually an isolated abnormality of spermatogenesis where patients seldom show any clinical evidence of androgen deficiency. The causes of hypogonadism, infertility, or the two together are shown in Table 1.

Hypogonadism

Clinical features

Prepubertal testosterone deficiency will present with delayed puberty. Eunuchoid body proportions (arm span greater than height and heel-pubis exceeding crown-pubis lengths by at least 5 cm) develop due to the continued growth of long bones allowed by the delayed closure of their epiphyses and failure of the testosterone-induced spinal growth in late puberty.

A postpubertal onset leads to regression of spermatogenesis, diminished sex drive and erection, loss of ejaculation, muscle atrophy and low stamina, decreased secondary sexual hair and frequency of shaving. No change is, however, observed in body and penile proportions or voice. The clinical diagnosis of male hypogonadism in the adult is generally not difficult since the clinical features of androgen deficiency are characteristic. However, because the symptoms and signs develop very insidiously, it is common for patients to present only after many years following the onset of hypogonadism. Furthermore, a patient who has never been adequately androgenized may not be aware that his secondary sexual function is subnormal. In contrast, young adults will often be troubled by severe and intractable hot flushes from acute withdrawal of androgens after surgical or traumatic/inflammatory castration.

Additional clinical findings

These are specific to the underlying cause and may thus be useful in identifying the aetiology of hypogonadism. The clinical symptoms and signs of hypothalamic–pituitary tumours and of hyperprolactinaemia are discussed in Chapter 7.1. Primary testicular failure is suggested by a history of orchitis, testicular trauma, surgery, torsion, or irradiation and chemotherapy.

Drugs which may interfere with pituitary–testicular function include cyproterone acetate, flutamide, ketoconozole, cimetidine, and spironolactone. Abuse of alcohol may lower testosterone concentrations through a direct effect on Leydig cells. Testicular atrophy and gynaecomastia, found in 50 per cent of men with hepatic cirrhosis, are due to altered androgen steroid metabolism, increased concentrations of sex hormone binding globulin, and increased oestrogen production.

Neurological diseases can be associated with hypogonadism. Postpubertal atrophy of the seminiferous tubules occurs in 80 per cent of patients with dystrophia myotonica; variable degrees of androgen deficiency also exist. Hypogonadotrophic hypogonadism is associated with familial cerebellar ataxia, Laurence–Moon–Biedl and Prader–Willi syndromes. Defective spermatogenesis is common in paraplegia or quadraplegia following spinal injury, presumably because of the inability to maintain a low scrotal temperature.

Specific conditions

Klinefelter's syndrome is the commonest cause of male hypogonadism, with an incidence of 2 per 1000 live births. It is a developmental disorder of the testis resulting from the presence of an extra X chromosome. The most common karyotype is 47 XXY but rarer variants include 46 XY/47 XXY mosaic, multiple X + Y, and the so-called XX male syndrome. Accelerated atrophy of germ cells before puberty gives rise to sterility and small, firm testes. The degree of Leydig cell defect is very variable, ranging from the fully virilized male presenting with infertility to the eunuchoidal youth who fails to complete sexual maturation. Other features include gynaecomastia, tall stature (longer lower body segment), learning difficulties, and autoimmune endocrinopathies.

Kallmann's syndrome—with an incidence of 1 in 7500 males is described in Chapter 7.8.

Investigations

Confirmation of hypogonadism

Measurement of basal testosterone, LH and FSH, and prolactin, by repeated frequent sampling over 1–2 h if necessary, is all that is required for the diagnosis of male hypogonadism. Patients with androgen insensitivity syndromes have elevated testosterone with high LH.

Assessment of the hypothalamic–pituitary–testicular axis

Pathologies in the hypothalamus and pituitary will give rise to low or low-normal gonadotrophins and low testosterone. In these conditions the potential for stimulating testicular function by exogenous gonadotrophin or GnRH replacement is maintained. Conditions affecting the testes result in elevated gonadotrophin levels with low plasma testosterone. Failure of spermatogenesis with reduced testicular size is commonly associated with a rise in FSH alone. Inhibin cannot be measured easily for diagnostic purposes at present.

Human chorionic gonadotrophin (hCG) stimulates Leydig cell steroidogenesis, and plasma testosterone increases in response. Its use can be helpful in detecting the presence of functional testicular tissue in patients with impalpable testes, assessing functional reserve of the testes prior to treatment with exogenous gonadotrophin or GnRH, and in differentiating hypergonadotrophic hypogonadism from rare patients who produce immunologically detectable but biologically inactive LH in excess.

Assessment of the pituitary

Patients with hypogonadotrophic hypogonadism without the stigmata of Kallmann's syndrome must undergo full pituitary functional and anatomical assessment to exclude an underlying pituitary tumour.

Other investigations

Suspected Klinefelter's syndrome should be confirmed by chromosome karyotyping on peripheral blood lymphocytes. Ultrasound is useful in locating ectopic or intra-abdominal testes. Androgen-receptor studies on biopsied genital skin fibroblasts or DNA analyses of the androgen receptor gene are required to confirm the diagnosis of androgen resistance in the testicular feminization syndrome (see Chapter 7.12).

Treatment

Androgen replacement

The mainstay of treatment of the hypogonadal male is androgen replacement. Although hypogonadotropic patients have the potential

Table 1 Aetiologies of male reproductive disorders

(a) Hypogonadism and infertility	
Hypothalamic	*Target tissues*
Isolated GnRH deficiency	Androgen insensitivity syndromes (testicular feminization)
Kallmann's syndrome	5α-reductase deficiency
Male anorexia nervosa	Steroidogenic enzyme deficiencies
	Systemic diseases
Pituitary	Chronic debilitating illnesses (cardiac failure, uncontrolled diabetes, neoplasia)
Craniopharyngioma	Liver cirrhosis
Pituitary adenoma	Chronic renal failure
Hyperprolactinaemia	Thyrotoxicosis
Cranial irradiation	
Haemochromatosis	*CNS diseases*
Transfusion siderosis	Prader–Willi syndrome
Sarcoidosis/tuberculosis/histiocytosis X	Laurence–Moon–Biedl syndrome
Biologically inactive LH	Familial cerebellar degeneration
Testicular	*Drugs/chemicals*
Congenital steroidogenic enzyme deficiencies	Digitalis, spironolactone,
Klinefelter's syndrome and variants	Cyproterone acetate, flutamide
Testicular agenesis (congenital anorchia)	Ketoconazole, cimetidine
Testicular torsion	
Surgical orchidectomy	
Testicular trauma	
Testicular tumour	
Male Turner's syndrome	
(b) Infertility	
Testicular	*CNS diseases*
Idiopathic hypospermatogenesis	Dystrophia myotonica
Varicocele	Spinal cord injury
Cryptorchidism	
Orchitis	*Drugs/chemicals*
Irradiation	Cytotoxic chemotherapy
	Sulphasalazine, nitrofurantoin
Post-testicular	Anticonvulsants
Sperm antibodies	Anabolic steroids, oestrogens
Immotile cilia (Kartårgener's) syndrome	Ethanol, opiates, cannabis
Young's syndrome	Pesticides, fungicides, amoebicides
Agenesis of epididymides and vasa	Heavy metals
Postinfection obstruction	
Accessory gland infection	
Retrograde ejaculation	
Coital insufficiency	

for fertility, gonadotrophin or pulsatile GnRH therapy should only be employed when there is a requirement for fertility, because of the expense and complexity of these regimens. Previous testosterone treatment does not jeopardize a subsequent response to gonadotrophin so that younger hypogonadotrophic subjects should be treated by testosterone to initiate and maintain virilization and sexual function.

Parenteral testosterone administration

Testosterone esters are the most widely used but at dose regimens generally recommended, unphysiologically high levels are invariably observed 24–48 h after each injection, followed by an exponential fall to subnormal levels before the next injection. Most commercially available injectable preparations contain combinations of short- and longer-acting esters, but these inevitably produce exaggerated peak concentrations which are best avoided. Single-agent preparations containing long-acting esters (e.g. testosterone enanthate, 200 mg every 2 weeks) are therefore recommended.

Testosterone implants containing 100 or 200 mg of crystalline testosterone are inserted under local anaesthesia into the subcutaneous space of the lower anterior abdominal wall by means of a trocar and obturator. Peak testosterone levels are usually achieved at 2–4 weeks. A 600–800 mg dose will provide relatively stable levels of plasma testosterone within the physiological range, which gradually decline towards the base-line over 4–6 months.

Oral testosterone administration

The absorption of testosterone undecanoate is variable, but can be improved by administration with food. After a single 40-mg oral dose, peak concentrations are usually observed 4–6 h later and return to baseline after 10 h. To maintain testosterone within the adult physiological range, 40 mg of testosterone undecanoate three to four times daily is required.

Mesterolone is a weak androgen which is metabolized by the liver slowly; its use in hypogonadal patients as physiological replacement cannot be recommended.

Transdermal testosterone application

Testosterone is incorporated in a patch applied either to the shaved scrotal skin or on the back, and changed daily. With daily application, plasma levels can be maintained within the adult physiological range throughout the 24 h. The scrotal application gives elevated levels of 5α-dihydrotestosterone as a result of the abundant 5α-reductase activity in genital skin, a disadvantage not seen with non-scrotally applied systems. Early indications regarding clinical efficacy are favourable but long-term safety and acceptability are as yet unproven.

Choice of androgen preparations

The choice depends on patient preference, available facilities, and requirement for dosage adjustments. The invasive nature of the implantation procedure, the long duration of action, and the difficulties in removal make this less than ideal for the induction of puberty in adolescents and the initiation of treatment in androgen-naive young adults, where a more gradual and flexible increase in dose is desirable. For these reasons, testosterone implant is usually reserved as maintenance treatment in young adults, replacement having been initiated with intramuscular or oral preparations. Almost all patients respond well to testosterone enanthate 200 mg every 2 weeks, 300 mg every 3 weeks, or Sustanon 250® every 2–3 weeks. Monitoring of treatment is best gauged by clinical response and documenting plasma testosterone in the mid-normal range 7 days after a dose of testosterone enanthate or 6–8 weeks after testosterone implant.

Safety and side-effects

Side-effects seem very rare but may include acne, transient priapism, gynaecomastia, fluid retention, and a clinically insignificant increase in haematocrit. The potential risk for cardiovascular disease through alteration of lipid metabolism, and exacerbation of underlying prostatic disease in hypogonadal men on androgen replacement is currently not known. Periodic digital or ultrasound examination of the prostate and measurement of circulating prostate specific antigen should be performed in patients over the age of 50 maintained on androgens. Obstructive sleep apnoea may rarely complicate androgen therapy; those particularly at risk are older, obese men with thick necks and high upper airways resistance, identified by a raised haematocrit and a propensity to snore.

Infertility

Some 8–15 per cent of couples experience involuntary infertility. Of these, male factors alone are estimated to be responsible in 30 per cent and contributory in a further 20 per cent. Thus, male infertility may affect 5 per cent of men of reproductive age.

Idiopathic hypospermatogenesis

Male infertility implies a failure to fertilize the normal ovum arising from the deficiency of functionally competent sperm at the site of fertilization. In most instances, this is associated with defective spermatogenesis, giving rise to absent or low sperm output, and abnormal spermiogenesis, giving rise to spermatozoa with poor motility (asthenozoospermia) and/or abnormal morphology (teratozoospermia). The pathophysiology of hypospermatogenesis remains very poorly understood. Over three-quarters of patients with male infertility due to poor semen quality do not have any clearly identifiable cause. Reduced velocity or vigour of sperm motility may be due to metabolic/functional defects or structural malformations in the axonemal complex of the sperm tail. Rarely, absent or extremely low sperm motility (with normal sperm density) may result from the absence of dynein arms (Na/K ATPase) of the sperm tail. This is associated with similar defects in respiratory cilia and a history of chronic respiratory infection, bronchiectasis, and sinusitis (immotile cilia syndrome). In addition, some of these patients have situs inversus (Kartagener's syndrome). Abnormal sperm morphology may indicate defective spermiogenesis. An extreme example is the failure of acrosome development leading to the formation of round-headed spermatozoa (globozoospermia).

Chromosome disorders

Abnormal chromosome karyotypes are found in 15 per cent of azoospermic patients, 90 per cent of whom have Klinefelter's syndrome (47 XXY). Other chromosomal abnormalities encountered include reciprocal X or Y autosomal translocations, XYY and XX males, reciprocal and Robertsonian autosomal translocations, supernumerary autosomes, and inversion of autosomes. Microdeletions of the azoospermic factor locus in chromosome Yq11.22–23 have been reported in some azoospermic patients.

Cryptorchidism

The lower temperature in the scrotum is a prerequisite for normal spermatogenesis. Undescended testes are exposed to the harmful effects of the higher temperature in the abdomen and inguinal region. Spontaneous descent of the testis rarely occurs after 1 year. A testis which is not permanently in a low scrotal position by the age of 2 will have sustained damage to the seminiferous epithelium. Orchidopexy after 2 years of age for undescended testes does not improve fertility. For these reasons, treatment should ideally be undertaken between 1 and 2 years of age. Human chorionic gonadotrophin or intranasal GnRH are currently being used increasingly for early treatment of cryptorchidism. If hormonal treatment is unsuccessful, orchidopexy can be carried out. Undescended testes can be a feature of hypogonadotrophic hypogonadism and intersexual states. The risk of testicular tumour in a patient with a history of undescended testis, whether successfully treated by orchidopexy or not, is four- to tenfold higher than in the general population.

Varicocele

The significance of varicocele in male infertility remains controversial. Reflux of blood in the internal spermatic vein, usually involving the left side from the renal vein, gives rise to distension of the pampiniform venous plexus and reduction in ipsilateral testicular volume, associated with varying degrees of non-specific histological abnormalities in both testes. Increased scrotal temperature, hypoxia, and exposure of the testes to adrenal metabolites have been postulated as possible mechanisms by which spermatic vein reflux can induce seminiferous tubular damage. Since varicoceles can be detected clinically in 15 per cent of young fertile men, it must not be assumed that this condition is invariably or solely responsible for infertility without carefully excluding other possible aetiologies.

Sperm autoimmunity

Immunological infertility is caused by sperm-membrane-bound IgA antibodies found in around 5 per cent of men presenting with infertility. Predisposing conditions include vasectomy, testicular injury/inflammation, genital tract infection/obstruction, and family history of autoimmune disease. Male patients with significant sperm antibody usually have severely suppressed fertility potential due to sperm agglutination, poor sperm transit through cervical mucus, and blocked sperm-oocyte fusion.

Genital tract infection

Infection in the lower genital tract is a major cause of male infertility. Chlamydia, gonococci, Gram-negative enterococci, and the tubercle bacillus are the usual pathogens. If not treated promptly, inflammation of the accessory glands and excurrent ducts may give rise to disturbed function, formation of sperm antibody, and permanent structural damage with obstruction in the outflow tract. Asymptomatic prostatitis due to occult and usually focal infection is best diagnosed by transrectal ultrasound examination of the prostate.

Excurrent duct obstruction

Vasectomy and previous genitourinary infections are the most common causes of obstructive azoospermia. Rare congenital abnormalities include bilateral agenesis of the Wolffian duct-derived structures, corpus/cauda epididymis, vas deferens, and seminal vesicles, characterized by impalpable scrotal vasa and low volumes (< 1 ml) of acidic non-coagulating ejaculate (prostatic fluid) devoid of fructose and sperm. These patients have mutations in the cystic fibrosis (CFTR) gene and are considered to have a genital form of cystic fibrosis, while all males with typical cystic fibrosis also have the same congenital maldevelopment of Wolffian ducts. In Young's syndrome, epididymal obstruction is due to progressive inspissation of amorphous secretion in the lumen. In these patients, the high incidence of chronic sinopulmonary infection and bronchiectasis is presumably the consequence of the same abnormality in the respiratory tract.

Coital disorders

Inadequate coital technique (including the use of vaginal lubricants with spermicidal properties, e.g. vaseline), low frequency, and faulty timing of intercourse may contribute to continuing infertility but are rarely the only aetiological factor in the infertile couple. Erectile and ejaculatory failure may be caused by many different conditions (see below).

Diagnosis

History

Previous surgery such as herniorrhaphy in childhood, trauma, or torsion suggests possible damage to the vas or testis. A history of cryptorchidism or genitourinary infections is important. Painful ejaculation, haematospermia, and pain in the perineum suggest chronic infection in the prostate and seminal vesicles. Delayed puberty suggests possible gonadotrophin deficiency. A history of recurrent chest infection, sinusitis, or bronchiectasis may be obtained in patients with epididymal obstruction (Young's syndrome), immotile cilia syndrome, and agenesis of the vasa (cystic fibrosis). Chronic disorders such as renal failure, liver disease, malignancy, diabetes, and multiple sclerosis are associated with a variety of testicular and sexual dysfunctions. Patients should be asked about episodes of pyrexia within the past 12 weeks because of transient suppression of spermatogenesis. Enquiry should also be made about occupational or environmental exposure to testicular toxins and radiation, current medications, previous treatment, or the use of recreational drugs. It is important to establish that vaginal intercourse takes place with appropriate frequency and timing without the use of vaginal lubricants.

Examination

Height, weight, body habitus, and secondary sexual development must be assessed. Measurement of testicular volumes by comparison with Prader's orchidometer provides a convenient clinical index of seminiferous tubular mass. Normal adult testicular volume is between 15 and 35 ml. Testicular volume is a key finding in differentiating between azoospermia due to seminiferous tubular failure (reduced volumes) and that arising from excurrent duct obstruction (normal volume). Testicular size is also a useful indicator of the degree of testicular development in hypogonadotrophic patients. If not in the scrotum, the lowest position of the testes should be defined. Irregular contour, induration, or abnormal consistency of the testis suggest previous orchitis, surgery, or malignancy. Special attention should also be paid to the palpation of the epididymis and scrotal vas. An enlarged and tense caput epididymis may be palpable in cases of obstructive azoospermia. Irregularity and induration of the epididymis and vas suggest previous infection. In congenital agenesis of Wolffian duct-derived structures, the scrotal vasa are either impalpable or extremely thin. The patient should also be examined standing so that varicoceles can become visible (grade 3) or palpable (grade 2), or be detected as a venous impulse in the spermatic cord during Valsalva manoeuvre (grade 1). Rectal examination may reveal an irregular contour or abnormal consistency and tenderness in the prostate in the presence of chronic prostatitis and enlarged seminal vesicles.

Investigations

Semen analysis of sperm density, percentage of motile sperm, quality of sperm movements, and sperm morphology, provide a semiquantitative index of fertility potential. Although a variety of tests of sperm function, such as sperm movement analyses, mucus penetration, acrosome reaction, sperm-zona binding, and hamster oocyte penetration have been devised, none is sufficiently reliable and accurate to be used routinely in clinical practice. The continuing lack of a reliable quantitative and objective measure of sperm-function is a major obstacle in patient management.

Plasma FSH is useful in distinguishing primary from secondary testicular failure and in identifying patients with obstructive azoospermia. In the presence of azoospermia or oligozoospermia, an elevated FSH, particularly with reduced testicular volume, is presumptive evidence of severe and usually irreversible seminiferous tubular damage. Low or undetectable FSH (usually associated with low LH and testosterone, with clinical evidence of androgen deficiency) is suggestive of hypogonadotrophism. Conversely, azoospermia with normal FSH and normal testicular volume usually indicates the presence of bilateral genital tract obstruction. Testosterone and LH measurements are only indicated in the assessment of the infertile male when there is clinical suspicion of androgen deficiency, Klinefelter's syndrome, or sex steroid abuse. High concentrations of LH and testosterone should raise the possibility of abnormalities in androgen receptors, while the opposite suggests hypogonadotrophism. Hyperprolactinaemia is not a recognized cause of male infertility but prolactin measurement should be undertaken if there is clinical evidence of sexual dysfunction (particularly diminished libido) or pituitary disease leading to secondary testicular failure. Measurement of oestradiol is rarely indicated except in the presence of gynaecomastia.

Chromosome karyotyping should be carried out in patients with azoospermia, testicular atrophy, and elevated FSH, primarily to confirm the diagnosis of Klinefelter's syndrome. The need for testicular biopsy has largely been superseded by the use of plasma FSH in recent years to differentiate between primary testicular failure and obstructive lesions. Undetectable or very low levels of seminal fructose provide evidence to corroborate the clinical diagnosis of vasal and seminal vesicle agenesis or blocked ejaculatory ducts in the presence of obstructive azoospermia. An increase in the number of peroxidase-positive white cells in the semen is indicative of genital tract infection. Semen culture and detection of micro-organisms to identify infective pathogens are difficult because of the bactericidal properties of seminal plasma and urethral and skin commensals. Transrectal ultrasound has been advocated to diagnose asymptomatic chronic prostatitis. Sperm antibodies are detected by a mixed agglutination reaction. These will attach to motile sperm carrying specific IgA on the surface of the sperm head or tail.

Treatment

Potentially treatable infertility

In patients with inflammatory bowel diseases changing treatment from sulphasalazine to 5-aminosalicylic acid removes sulphapyridine which is toxic to the testis.

Patients with hypogonadotrophic hypogonadism can discontinue androgens and start hCG (2000 IU intramuscularly twice weekly) given alone for 6–12 months. If there is no sperm in the ejaculate at the end of 12 months, human menopausal gonadotrophin, which contains both FSH and LH, should be added at 75 IU intramuscularly thrice weekly. The outcome of treatment is variable but, in general, around 70 per cent should show some degree of spermatogenesis and 50 per cent can be expected to achieve pregnancies. In patients with hypothalamic GnRH deficiency, pulsatile GnRH replacement is accomplished by battery-driven portable infusion minipumps which can automatically deliver a subcutaneous dose of GnRH at a set time interval of 120 min; the patient has to wear this device continuously. The outcome of this treatment is very similar to that obtained with exogenous gonadotrophin therapy.

Active infection in the genital tract should be treated by appropriate antibiotics (erythromycin, doxycycline, or norfloxacin) given for 4 weeks to both the patient and his partner. Bypass of epididymal obstruction with microsurgical techniques of epididymovasostomy have been reported to produce high pregnancy rates. It is now possible for sperm to be aspirated directly from the caput epididymis or efferent ducts proximal to the site of obstruction for use in assisted fertilization procedures in patients with obstructive azoospermia and agenesis of the vasa. The latter group should have genetic counselling beforehand because of the risk of cystic fibrosis in any offspring.

Infertility due to the presence of antibody to sperm can be treated by immunosuppression with high-dose prednisolone 0.75 mg/kg/day or prednisolone 20 mg twice a day on days 1–10 and 5 mg on days 11–12 of the partner's cycle for 3–6 cycles. Side-effects are common and controlled trials have not been able to confirm the efficacy of such treatment. Intrauterine insemination of 'washed' sperm and *in vitro* fertilization have been increasingly applied to immunological male infertility.

Varicocele can be treated either by surgical ligation of the internal spermatic vein(s) above the internal inguinal ring or by transfemoral embolization of the internal spermatic vein(s). The results are inconsistent. Until an adequate prospective controlled trial is carried out, the significance of varicocele and its treatment in male infertility must remain an open question.

If semen of good quality can be obtained with masturbation, vibrators, or electroejaculation from patients with various coital dysfunctions, and functional spermatozoa recovered from alkalinized bladder urine of appropriate osmolality from the patient with retrograde ejaculation, artificial insemination can be reasonably successful.

Subfertility due to idiopathic hypospermatogenesis

Pregnancies can occur in some cases without treatment, albeit with a much reduced probability, depending on the duration of infertility, age, and coexisting subtle abnormalities in the female partner in addition to the defects in sperm quality. Although a wide variety of empirical treatments have been tried, none has been shown to be effective when assessed in controlled therapeutic trials. *In vitro* fertilization is increasingly applied to treat male infertility and, in patients with moderate oligozoospermia, fertilization rates of 30 per cent can be effected, with live birth rates of 8–10 per cent per treatment cycle. Those with severe and multiple defects in semen fluid have significantly poorer results. Microinjection of a single spermatozoon directly into the oocyte cytoplasm can achieve remarkably high fertilization and live birth rates (55 and 26 per cent, respectively) even with the most severely abnormal samples. This promises to be a useful technique for overcoming extreme oligozoospermia and obstructive azoospermia when sperm can be aspirated.

Untreatable sterility

Patients with azoospermia, atrophic testes, and elevated FSH have irreversible primary seminiferous tubular failure and are, to all intents and purposes, sterile. They should be informed of their prognosis and counselled regarding the options of continuing childlessness, adoption, and donor insemination.

Erectile impotence

Erectile failure may be caused by androgen deficiency, hyperprolactinaemia, neurological disorders such as autonomic neuropathy (usually complicating diabetes), multiple sclerosis and spinal injuries, vascular disease involving pelvic vessels, retroperitoneal and bladder-neck surgery, medications (commonly α- and β-adrenergic antagonists, psychotropic agents), alcohol abuse, severe systemic disease, psychological dysfunctions (including depression), and problems in personal relationships. Loss of libido characterizes androgen deficiency and hyperprolactinaemia while preservation of normal spontaneous morning erections are suggestive of psychogenic impotence. Ejaculatory abnormalities may be associated with erectile failure in neurological and drug-induced cases. Management should aim to correct any reversible underlying disease (e.g. prolactinoma) or substitute offending medications. Androgen treatment is only indicated in patients with plasma testosterone in the hypogonadal range. Vacuum devices and intracavernosal injection of vasodilator agents such as papaverine or prostaglandin E_1 have been used in the management of neurogenic and vasculogenic impotence but are now likely to be replaced by Viagra. Psychosexual therapy can benefit those with psychogenic impotence.

Further reading

Goldenberg, M. M. (1998). Safety and efficacy of sildenafil citrate in the treatment of male erectile dysfunction. *Clinical Therapeutics*, 20, 1033–48.

Hargreave, T. and Ghosh, C. (1998). Male fertility disorders. *Endocrinology and Metabolism Clinics of North America* 27, 765–82, vii–viii.

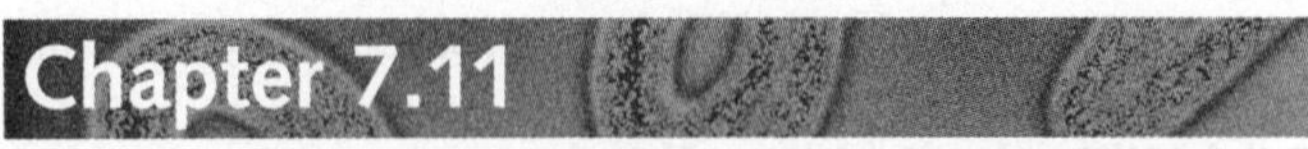

Chapter 7.11

Disorders of sexual function

K. E. Hawton

In physical illness

Disorders of sexual function may be associated with a wide range of physical illnesses because of direct interference with the anatomical or physiological mechanisms associated with sexual desire or response, by pathological processes or medication, or because of psychological reactions to physical disorders or treatment. Problems very often result from a combination of physical and psychological factors. Almost every physical illness is likely to have some effect on sexual function, whether this be due to reduction in sexual interest because of general debility, or to more direct effects of pathological processes on sexual arousal and performance. Sexual function often returns to normal after resolution of the physical condition, but several medical conditions may result in permanent impairment of sexual function; some of the most important of these are considered below.

Medical conditions causing sexual problems

Endocrine disorders

Diabetes mellitus

Erectile dysfunction occurs in 35–40 per cent of male diabetics. It is not closely related to the duration of diabetes and is sometimes the presenting symptom. This problem is usually permanent, although transient erectile difficulty may occur during episodes of poor diabetic control. Explanation that the problem is due to diabetes and not to some other factor (e.g. loss of attraction) can be of some reassurance. The problem is discussed further in Chapter 6.13.

There is some uncertainty about the effects of diabetes on female sexuality. Most studies report reduced vaginal lubrication in a substantial proportion of diabetic women. A synthetic lubricant is then often helpful. Overall it appears that diabetes is less likely to cause major sexual problems in women than in men.

Hypogonadism

Testicular production of androgens may be greatly reduced by disorders such as Kleinfelter's syndrome, undescended testes, mumps in adulthood, hepatic cirrhosis, and neoplastic disease, which can directly or indirectly impair testicular activity. Although hypogonadism occurring in adulthood will lead to sexual problems in some men, others surprisingly suffer little or no reduction in sexual drive or erectile performance. Investigation of men who are hypogonadal as a result of testicular malfunction will reveal elevated serum gonadotrophins (follicle stimulating hormone and luteinizing hormone (LH)) and low testosterone (hypergonadotrophic hypogonadism). Hormone replacement therapy is usually effective in restoring sexual function.

Pituitary disease

Hypopituitarism may impair sexual function because of reduced gonadotrophin production. In such cases both serum gonadotrophins and testosterone will be below normal levels (hypogonadotrophic hypogonadism). Hyperprolactinaemia may be accompanied by erectile dysfunction particularly where serum prolactin levels are very high and testosterone levels are reduced.

Cardiovascular disorders

Sexual problems are particularly common in patients with cardiac disease, especially those with angina or who have suffered myocardial infarction. Sexual activity usually ceases for several weeks after myocardial infarction. Many patients never resume sexual relations in spite of a return to other normal activities. In others the frequency of activity may be reduced compared with the preinfarct level. In some men both erectile and ejaculatory difficulties occur; less is known about the consequences for women who have had infarcts.

The physiological effects of sexual activity in patients who have suffered myocardial infarction are similar to those found with regular activities such as climbing a flight of stairs so that most patients with ischaemic heart disease should be able to enjoy normal sexual relations without risk. In many cases sexual problems in people with cardiac disease are the result of psychological factors such as fear of relapse, loss of desire, and depression. In addition the spouse may fear relapse, or feel guilty about expressing his or her sexual needs. Failure to discuss these problems may contribute to these difficulties.

Individuals who suffer from cardiovascular disorders are at increased risk of sexual dysfunction resulting from abnormalities of the pelvic vasculature.

Neurological disorders

Involvement of any of the neurological mechanisms responsible for sexual arousal and response are likely to cause sexual problems. Erection is primarily mediated by parasympathetic activity in S2–4 under the control of a sacral erection centre. Another centre in the thoracolumbar portion of the cord influences erectile response via sympathetic fibres. Both centres are moderated by facilitatory and inhibitory influences from the brain and act in unison to produce erections. The localization of higher centres that control sexual arousal and response is obscure but thalamic, hypothalamic, and limbic systems appear to be involved.

Ejaculation occurs in two phases, emission of semen to the posterior urethra and expulsion by muscular contraction. Emission results from sympathetic activity mediated by a lumbar ejaculation centre. The process of emission stimulates another ejaculation centre in the sacral cord, and expulsion then occurs because of the resulting activation of motor nerves. Both centres are moderated by cerebral influences. Although the neurological pathways controlling female sexual response are less well understood, they are assumed to correspond to those in the male.

Spinal cord damage

Disturbed spinal cord function likely to affect sexual response may occur with injury, tumours, multiple sclerosis, inflammatory processes, and congenital defects such as spina bifida. The results of such damage depend on whether the lesion is complete or incomplete, and whether it affects upper or lower motor neurones. Broadly speaking, erection is more likely to return the higher the cord lesion, and ejaculation more likely the lower the lesion. If disturbed sexual function continues for more than 6 months after injury, it is unlikely to resolve. Although orgasm usually returns with ejaculation the sensation is often altered. Interference with spinal autonomic pathways may cause sterility due to elevation of testicular temperature. Electrically induced ejaculation shortly after injury can be used to produce semen, which can be deep frozen and stored for possible use later in artificial insemination.

Little is known concerning the effects of spinal cord damage on female sexual function, except that total transection of the cord causes absence of orgasm.

The psychological sequelae of physical disablement and the attitudes of staff towards spinal injury patients are important determinants of subsequent sexual adjustment.

Damage to higher neurological centres

Focal cerebral lesions may cause sexual problems when there is paralysis, or when the frontal regions are damaged. Hypothalamic, limbic, and temporal lobe lesions may cause erectile dysfunction. Hyposexuality is often found in patients with epilepsy, particularly complex partial seizures. This may be attributable more to anticonvulsant medication than to the neurological disorder.

Other conditions

Sexual function may be disrupted by many other conditions, including gastrointestinal disorders, particularly where an ileostomy or colostomy is necessary, diseases of the genital organs (e.g. hypospadias and Peyronie's disease), painful arthritides, respiratory conditions that limit exercise tolerance, and chronic renal failure. Chronic alcohol abuse may cause erectile dysfunction due to peripheral neuropathy or hypogonadism.

The effects of medication

Many drugs can affect sexual interest and function. The effects of some of the more important of these are summarized in Table 1. In men, broadly speaking, drugs that have sympathetic inhibitory activity are likely to impair ejaculation, and those with parasympathetic inhibitory activity are likely to disrupt erectile function. Some drugs, especially anticonvulsants such as phenytoin and carbamazepine, induce increased plasma hormone binding globulin, thus causing a reduction in free testosterone. Less is known about the effects of most medication on female sexuality.

Sexual problems due to psychological reactions to physical illness

Reactions of the individual

Some patients may develop a sexual problem following an illness because of anticipation, albeit unjustifiable, that the illness has impaired sexual capacity. Others fear that sexual activity may cause relapse, harm, or pain. Severe illness, particularly where disfiguring surgery has been necessary, may cause an individual to doubt his or her attractiveness and to fear rejection. Sexual desire is usually reduced in depression, which is a common sequel to serious illness.

The partner's reaction

A patient's partner may also fear the potential consequences of sexual activity. There may be guilt about sexual desires that appear to conflict with concern for the patient's physical health. Consequent restrictions on sexual activity may cause resentment and friction.

The nature of the relationship

How couples adjust to the effects of illness depends particularly on their previous sexual relationship. Poor adjustment is likely when there are inhibitory attitudes and difficulty discussing sex. Physical illness brings some partners closer together. For others it results in alienation because of resentment about changes in roles necessitated by disability or because the afflicted partner is found unattractive due to physical change or depression.

Attitudes of the medical profession

The ways in which the implications of physical illness are dealt with by medical personnel may be important determinants of subsequent sexual adjustment. Advice concerning sexual activity should be part of general rehabilitation counselling.

Management and prevention of sexual problems related to illness

These are often a matter of common sense and do not necessarily require special training.

Assessment

Advice should be based on individual assessment in relation to the likely effects of the illness. If sexual dysfunction is already established, the relative contributions of organic, pharmacological, and psychological factors must be considered.

The nature of the dysfunction should be clarified first, particularly what aspect of sexuality (desire, arousal, or orgasm) is primarily affected. In cases of erectile dysfunction it should be established whether or not erections occur under any circumstances (e.g. on wakening, with masturbation). Careful enquiry concerning medication and possible alcohol abuse is always necessary.

During physical examination of a man, the physician should be alert to signs of hypogonadism. Blood pressure, peripheral pulses, deep reflexes, and sensation in the lower limbs must be tested. In some centres nocturnal penile tumescence recording is available, diminution or absence of erection during rapid eye movement sleep suggesting, but not confirming, organic aetiology for erectile dysfunction. Possible vascular disorder of the genitals can be investigated by penile blood pressure measurement, corpus cavernosography, and other radiological studies of the pelvic vasculature. Local neurological causes of erectile dysfunction may be confirmed by testing of the sacral nerve provoked potentials. When an abnormality of sex hormone production is suspected, serum testosterone, LH, and prolactin should be measured. The possibility of diabetes mellitus must always be considered.

In assessing psychological factors, enquiry should be made about the patient's previous sexual adjustment, current anxieties (especially about his or her illness), and the partner's sexual adjustment, attitude to the problem, and willingness to help in overcoming it. It is usually essential to interview the partner.

Treatment

Explanation and advice

The physician must explain the nature of the problem in simple terms both to the patient and, whenever possible, the partner. The relative contributions of both physical and psychological factors must be made clear. Advice should then be given as clearly as possible and might usefully be supplemented by written information. If irreversible

Table 1 Drugs which can affect sexuality

Drug group	Examples	Reported effects on sexual function: Desire	Arousal	Orgasm
Anticholinergic	Probanthine		Erectile dysfunction	
Antidepressants				
Tricyclics	Imipramine		Erectile dysfunction	Delayed ejaculation or orgasm
Serotonin reuptake inhibitors	Fluoxetine			Delayed/absent ejaculation or orgasm
Monoamine oxidase inhibitors	Phenelzine		Erectile dysfunction	Delayed ejaculation or orgasm
Antihypertensives				
Central acting ganglion blockers	Methyldopa	Reduced	Erectile dysfunction	Delayed ejaculation
	Hexamethonium		Erectile dysfunction	Failure of ejaculation or retrograde ejaculation
α-Blockers	Indoramin			Inhibited emission
β-blockers	Propranolol	Reduced	Erectile dysfunction	
Adrenergic blockers	Guanethidine		Erectile dysfunction	Failure of ejaculation or retrograde ejaculation
Anti-inflammatory	Indomethacin	Reduced		
Antiparkinsonian	L-Dopa	Increased		
Diuretics				
Thiazides	Bendrofluazide		Erectile dysfunction	
Hormones				
Androgens	Testosterone	Increased in females		
Corticosteroids	Prednisolone	Reduced	Erectile dysfunction	Delayed ejaculation
Oestrogens	Oestradiol	Reduced in males	Erectile dysfunction	Delayed ejaculation
Major tranquillizers				
Phenothiazines	Thioridazine	Reduced	Erectile dysfunction	
	Chlorpromazine	Reduced	Erectile dysfunction	
	Flupenthixol	Reduced	Erectile dysfunction	
Butyrophenones	Haloperidol	Reduced	Erectile dysfunction	

physical damage to sexual anatomy has occurred, then alternative forms of sexual behaviour may be suggested. A useful general principle is to encourage a couple to re-establish their sexual relationship gradually, perhaps starting with general caressing, in order to establish a relaxed atmosphere before fully resuming their sexual relationship. This is particularly helpful for couples faced by the problem of adjusting to the effects of an acute debilitating illness. When doctors feel unable to provide such advice themselves then responsibility might be delegated to a suitably trained non-medical member of the team.

Hormone replacement

Hormone replacement therapy will be required for patients with hypogonadism. Testosterone can be given intramuscularly, orally (testosterone undecanoate), or by skin patches. The transdermal route probably provides a more physiologically normal hormone profile. LH releasing hormone can be provided for patients with hypopituitarism, and bromocriptine sometimes restores erectile dysfunction resulting from hyperprolactinaemia.

Special treatments for erectile dysfunction

During recent years several advances have occurred in the treatment of erectile dysfunction of organic aetiology. The most important has been the introduction of sildenafil (Viagra). This is an oral drug that enhances relaxation of smooth muscle in the corpus cavernosum through inhibition of the cyclic guanosine monophosphate phosphodiesterase (cGMP) enzyme, thus enhancing cGMP activity and thereby nitric oxide function in smooth-muscle relaxation. Unlike most other physical treatments, sildenafil results in erections mainly in response to physical and psychogenic stimulation. Clinical trials have shown that it is highly effective in patients with erectile dysfunction resulting from psychogenic and neurological disorders and moderately so in patients with certain other chronic disorders such as diabetes.

Another physical treatment involves intracavernosal injections of vasoactive drugs (e.g. papaverine, prostaglandin E_1). These usually elicit erections even when there is severe organic impairment. Men are taught to inject themselves. The vacuum constriction device is a further approach. Erection is elicited through creation of a vacuum in a plastic cylinder which is placed over the penis. A rubber constriction ring is then slipped off the device around the base of the penis in order to restrict outflow from the penile venous system, following which the cylinder is removed. The constriction ring may obstruct ejaculation (but not orgasm) and should not be left in place for more than half an hour in case of anoxic damage to the penis. Penile implants (semirigid or inflatable) offer another alternative for men with permanent organic erectile dysfunction. They should be reserved for young men with erectile dysfunction due to disorders such as Peyronie's disease or priapism.

Whenever one of these physical methods of treatment is considered it is important to counsel both partners in attitudes and expectations. Without this there is a significant risk that the treatment will not be used effectively and even that it may have a detrimental effect on a relationship.

Referral to a specialist in sexual problems

This may be necessary for patients whose problems result from complex psychological factors, and have failed to respond to simple counselling. Such sexual problems resulting from either psychological causes, or psychological complications of physical disorders, are often helped by sex therapy. In this approach both partners are seen together and a graduated series of activities suggested including, first, non-genital caressing, later, genital caressing and, finally, resumption of sexual intercourse. Psychological barriers interfering with the relationship are identified, information about sexuality is provided when ignorance is an important factor, and particular emphasis is placed on helping partners communicate freely with each other about their sexual anxieties and needs. The results of sex therapy are reasonable, with as many as two-thirds of patients deriving considerable benefit. The Relate organization in the UK has a large number of counsellors training in treating sexual problems.

There are far fewer specialists in sexual medicine in the UK than in the US, where multidisciplinary clinics for people with sexual problems exist. Some psychiatrists and psychologists specialize in this area of work, particularly for people with sexual problems that are primarily psychological in aetiology. Some urologists take a broad interest in male sexual dysfunctions, not just in the use of intracavernosal injections. Sexual problems resulting from endocrine disorders are best managed by endocrinologists or other medical practitioners specializing in sexual medicine.

While general practitioners are increasingly treating patients with erectile dysfunction of primarily organic aetiology, specialist referral is often advisable, especially where sophisticated physical assessment procedures may be required and the most appropriate treatment is unclear. Some urologists specialize in this area of work.

Further reading

Bancroft, J. (1989). *Human sexuality and its problems* (2nd edn). Churchill Livingstone, Edinburgh.

Gregoire, A. and Pryor, J.P. (1993). Impotence: an integrated approach to clinical practice. Churchill Livingstone, Edinburgh.

Hawton, K. (1985). *Sex therapy: a practical guide.* Oxford University Press, Oxford.

Schover, L.R. and Jensen, S.B. (1988). *Sexuality and chronic illness: a comprehensive approach.* Guilford Press, New York.

Disorders of development

Chapter 7.12

Normal and abnormal sexual differentiation

M. O. Savage

Most disorders of sexual differentiation are genetically determined and are associated with an ambiguous appearance of the external genitalia. Description of clinical syndromes can now be supplemented by analysis of the biochemical and molecular nature of the defects that cause them.

Table 1 Classification of intersex states

Female pseudohermaphrodite: virilization of genetic female with ovaries
Male pseudohermaphrodite: incomplete virilization of genetic male with testes
True hermaphrodite: individual with ovarian and testicular tissue

Physiology of fetal sexual differentiation

The fetal testis is essential for male development. Specific genes on the short arm of the Y chromosome code for testis determination, and hence contribute to testicular differentiation. Testicular Leydig cells synthesize and secrete testosterone from 8 weeks of gestation, aided by stimulation with placental human chorionic gonadotrophin (hCG). Testosterone diffuses locally to maintain and virilize the Wolffian ducts which become the vas deferens, seminal vesicles, and epididymis. Antimüllerian hormone, or müllerian-inhibitory factor is secreted at the same time by testicular Sertoli cells to inhibit the formation of the uterus, fallopian tubes, and upper vagina.

In androgen-dependent tissues, testosterone is converted to dihydrotestosterone which virilizes the external genitalia. Peripheral androgen action depends on the binding of the androgen in the target tissues to a receptor controlled by an X chromosome.

In the female, ovarian development and external gonadal development occurs spontaneously. Genital development in both sexes is completed by 20 weeks of fetal life.

Classification of intersex states

The classification that forms the basis of clinical assessment and management depends on gonadal morphology (Table 1).

Female pseudohermaphroditism

Female pseudohermaphrodites have 46 XX karyotypes with normal ovaries and müllerian structures, but the external genitalia are virilized. The aetiology is given in Table 2. The degree of genital ambiguity can range from enlargement of the clitoris or fusion of the posterior labia to a completely male appearance, depending on the timing of androgen production and the concentration of androgens in the fetal circulation.

Virilization by fetal androgens

Congenital adrenal hyperplasia

The commonest cause of ambiguous genitalia in the newborn female is a recessively inherited enzyme defect of cortisol synthesis, with diversion of intermediates to androgen production. 21-Hydroxylase deficiency, 11β-hydroxylase deficiency and 3β-hydroxylase deficiency are described in Chapter 7.7.

Other causes of fetal virilization

Virilization of the external genitalia by a maternal ovarian or adrenal androgen-secreting tumour is a rare cause of female pseudohermaphroditism which can also result from maternal intake of progestogen preparations. A number of dysmorphic childhood syndromes may also be associated with virilized female genitalia.

Table 2 Aetiology of female pseudohermaphroditism

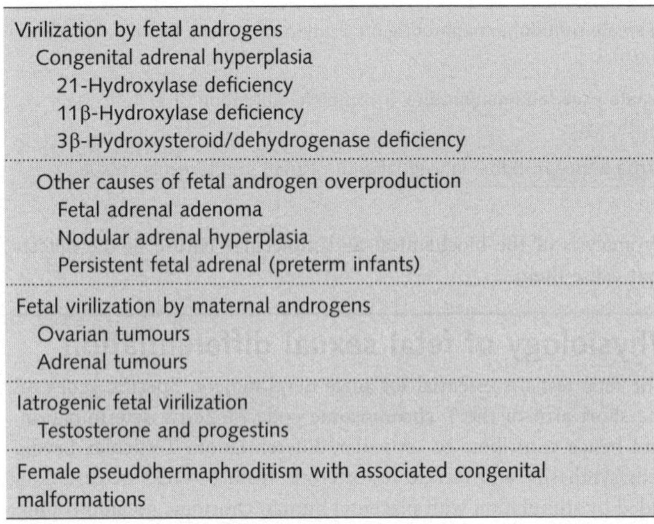

Aetiology
Virilization by fetal androgens
Congenital adrenal hyperplasia
21-Hydroxylase deficiency
11β-Hydroxylase deficiency
3β-Hydroxysteroid/dehydrogenase deficiency
Other causes of fetal androgen overproduction
Fetal adrenal adenoma
Nodular adrenal hyperplasia
Persistent fetal adrenal (preterm infants)
Fetal virilization by maternal androgens
Ovarian tumours
Adrenal tumours
Iatrogenic fetal virilization
Testosterone and progestins
Female pseudohermaphroditism with associated congenital malformations

Table 3 Aetiology of male pseudohermaphroditism

Aetiology
Impaired Leydig cell activity
Inborn errors of testosterone biosynthesis
Deficient formation of pregnenolone
3β-Hydroxysteroid dehydrogenase deficiency
17α-Hydroxylase deficiency
17,20-Desmolase deficiency
17β-Hydroxysteroid dehydrogenase deficiency
Leydig cell hypoplasia
Androgen insensitivity syndromes
Androgen receptor defects
Complete testicular feminization
Incomplete testicular feminization
Reifenstein syndrome
Infertile male syndrome
Post-receptor resistance
5α-Reductase deficiency
Incomplete differentiation of testes with deficient testosterone and antimüllerian hormone production
Mixed gonadal dysgenesis
Dysgenetic male pseudohermaphroditism
XY pure gonadal dysgenesis
Drash syndrome
Other forms
Iatrogenic male pseudohermaphroditism
Associated with other congenital anomalies
Persistent müllerian structures

Male pseudohermaphroditism

Male pseudohermaphroditism arises as a result of a disturbance of male genital development in patients with testes and a 46 XY karyotype. The genital anomaly can vary from apparently female to male external genitalia with a small penis or perineal hypospadias. The three main aetiological groups (Table 3) are impaired Leydig cell activity, peripheral androgen insensitivity, and deficient testosterone and antimüllerian hormone production by incompletely differentiated testes.

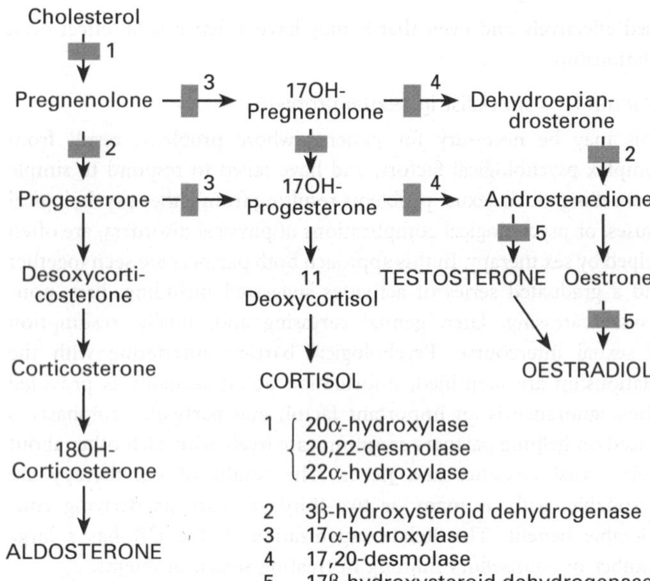

Fig. 1 Enzyme defects in testosterone biosynthesis.

Impaired testicular secretion of testosterone

Inborn errors of testosterone biosynthesis

These rare disorders (Fig. 1) lead to defective testosterone synthesis during the critical period of fetal sexual differentiation. The result is inadequate testosterone secretion, either locally to virilize the Wolffian ducts to form the vas deferens, seminal vesicles, or epididymis, or peripherally to virilize the external genitalia. Synthesis of antimüllerian hormone, being a glycoprotein rather than a steroid, is unaffected. When the enzyme deficiency, inherited as an autosomal recessive trait, is situated early in the biosynthetic pathway, adrenal steroid synthesis may also be affected.

Deficient formation of pregnenolone

Three closely related microsomal enzymes (20α-hydroxylase, 20,22-desmolase, and 22α-hydroxylase) are necessary for the conversion of cholesterol to pregnenolone. Deficiency of one of these enzymes leads to impaired synthesis of cortisol, aldosterone, and testosterone.

Deficiency of 3β-hydroxysteroid dehydrogenase or 17α-hydroxylase

These conditions are described in Chapter 7.7.

Deficiency of 17,20-desmolase

This rare defect is related to 17-hydroxylase deficiency as both enzyme activities are coded by the same gene. Impaired virilization may be variable in degree. Biochemically, identification of the defect relies on elevation of plasma 17-hydroxyprogesterone, 17-hydroxypregnenolone, and urinary pregnanetriolone.

Deficiency of 17-ketosteroid reductase (17β-hydroxysteroid dehydrogenase)

Patients with this defect are born with female-looking external genitalia and a phallus closely resembling a normal clitoris. There is a high prevalence within the Arab population of the Gaza Strip. The enzyme defect interferes with conversion of androstenedione to testosterone, adrenal steroid synthesis being unaffected. There is elevation of the androstenedione to testosterone ratio, particularly after hCG stimulation. Subjects are usually raised as girls; however, gender

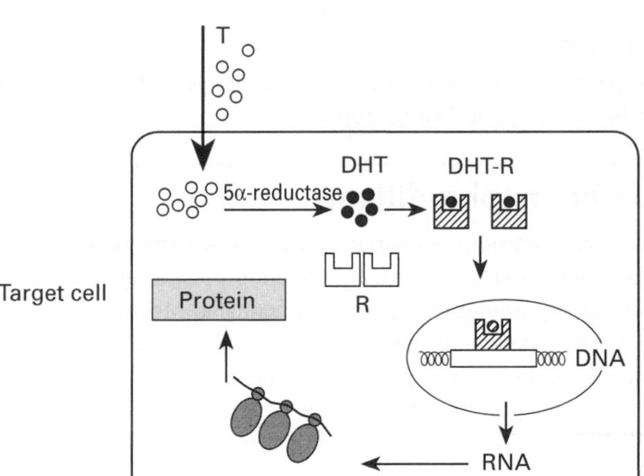

Fig. 2 Scheme of intracellular androgen action (for source see OTM3, p. 1692). T, testosterone; DHT, dihydrotestosterone; R, receptor.

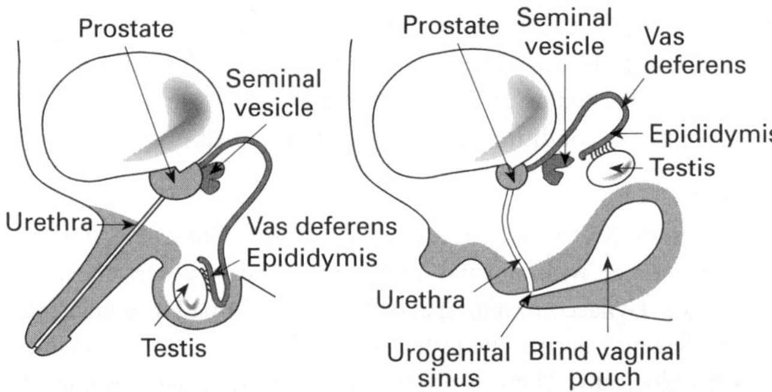

Fig. 3 Roles of testosterone and dihydrotestosterone in male sexual differentiation in the normal male (left) and the patient with 5α-reductase deficiency (right). Testosterone, heavy shading; dihydrotestosterone, light shading.

conversion to male has been described, coinciding with the marked virilization which occurs at puberty.

Androgen insensitivity syndromes

Mechanisms of androgen action

Free testosterone enters the target cell by a passive mechanism (Fig. 2). Inside the cell, some is reduced to dihydrotestosterone by 5α-reductase. Testosterone or dihydrotestosterone bind to specific receptor proteins to form an androgen-receptor complex which enters the cell nucleus and, after transformation into a DNA binding state, binds to specific nucleotide sequences which promote transcription of messenger RNA, resulting in virilization.

Although testosterone and dihydrotestosterone bind to the same receptor, each performs a different role in androgen physiology (Fig. 3). Testosterone regulates secretion of luteinizing hormone (LH), virilizes the Wolffian ducts during fetal life, and may be essential for spermatogenesis. Dihydrotestosterone is responsible for formation of the external genitalia and prostate, and for most secondary sexual effects, such as hair growth and enlargement of the genitalia.

Mechanisms of androgen insensitivity

The syndromes of androgen insensitivity probably account for the majority of cases of male pseudohermaphroditism. There are three main forms. The most common is an X-linked cystolic androgen receptor defect. This may be manifested by a broad clinical spectrum from complete androgen insensitivity to a virtually normally formed male with infertility. The second form is known as receptor-positive resistance, where a similar spectrum of clinical defects is associated with apparently normal receptor function. Thirdly, 5α-reductase deficiency is an autosomally inherited enzyme defect resulting in impaired conversion of testosterone to dihydrotestosterone in the target cell.

Androgen receptor defects

These defects may be expressed clinically as four main phenotypes, two predominantly female and two male. The female forms are complete and incomplete testicular feminization and the male are the Reifenstein syndrome and the 'infertile male' syndrome.

Complete testicular feminization

The typical patient with complete androgen insensitivity presents after puberty with primary amenorrhoea, or before puberty with inguinal hernias and palpable testes. The phenotype and psychosexual orientation is female. Breasts develop as in a normal woman, but pubic and axillary hair is scanty and the vagina is blind-ending due to regression of müllerian structures, which are virtually always absent. Wolffian structures are usually absent and the gonads show Leydig cell hyperplasia with no spermatogenesis. There is a significant risk of gonadal malignancy occurring after puberty, when gonadectomy is recommended.

Incomplete testicular feminization

This and the two subsequent syndromes come into the category of incomplete androgen insensitivity. Here there is more virilization than in the complete form, usually seen as clitoral enlargement and labial fusion. At puberty, feminization is dominant, with some further virilization apparent.

Reifenstein syndrome

The phenotype is predominantly male with severe perineal hypospadias. Virilization at puberty is more marked than in the two previous conditions, but is nevertheless incomplete and associated with gynaecomastia. Several pedigrees with family members affected according to an X-linked pattern have now been described. The degree of clinical abnormality within families may be very variable.

The infertile male syndrome

This condition represents the male end of the spectrum of androgen insensitivity. There is a normal male phenotype except for a rather small penis and small testes and possibly gynaecomastia. The main expression of the androgen receptor defect is oligospermia and infertility.

Hormonal features

The hormonal features of androgen receptor defects are essentially common to the four variants. Plasma testosterone may be elevated in infancy but is normal during the remainder of the prepubertal period. At puberty, plasma testosterone, oestradiol, and sex hormone binding globulin levels are elevated. Plasma gonadotrophins are normal in childhood but both LH and follicle stimulating hormone levels are consistently elevated during and after puberty, due to insensitivity of the hypothalamic androgen receptor.

5α-Reductase deficiency

This autosomal recessive disorder is characterized by impaired conversion of testosterone to dihydrotestosterone in androgen-dependent

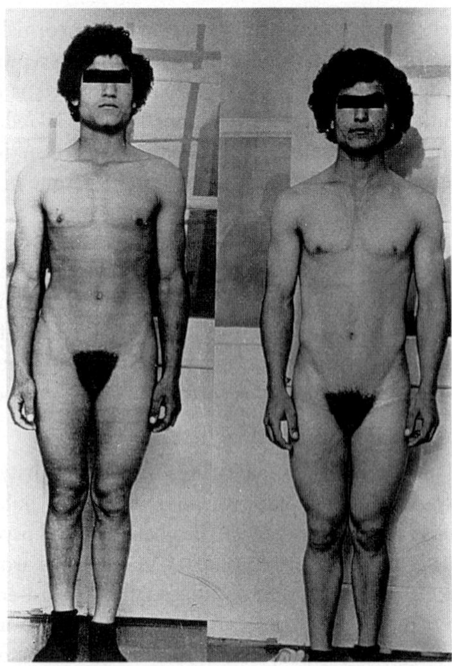

Fig. 4 Two Greek Cypriot brothers with 5α-reductase deficiency.

target cells. It occurs principally in areas of high consanguinity. The clinical features comprise male internal genital structures and female external genitalia. Fetal dihydrotestosterone-dependent development is abnormal, resulting in a rudimentary phallus and absent prostate. The Wolffian structures develop normally, and the testes differentiate with spermatogenesis capable of progressing to the spermatozoa stage. Most subjects are raised as females but gender conversion to male occurs at puberty, coinciding with striking virilization of body habitus (Fig. 4) and male psychosexual orientation. Virilization during and after puberty, however, is incomplete, as the penis remains small and body and facial hair is sparse.

The hormonal features comprise low plasma dihydrotestosterone with normal testosterone. There is also elevation of the ratio of 5β:5α androgen metabolites (i.e. aetiocholanolone to androsterone) in urine.

Male pseudohermaphroditism related to abnormal testicular differentiation

Incomplete differentiation of the fetal testes due to a defect of the Y-chromosomal genes responsible for testicular determination may cause genital ambiguity. Incompletely formed or dysgenetic testes secrete insufficient testosterone and antimüllerian hormone for normal male development. A number of clinical syndromes exist in this category.

Dysgenetic male pseudohermaphroditism

In this syndrome there are bilateral dysgenetic testes, persistent müllerian structures, cryptorchidism, and poorly virilized external genitalia.

Mixed gonadal dysgenesis

Here there is asymmetrical gonadal differentiation with a testis present on one side and a streak gonad on the other. The internal structures are also asymmetrical, reflecting the endocrine function of the ipsilateral gonad. Many patients have a mosaic XO/XY karyotype and features of Turner's syndrome.

Drash syndrome

This syndrome combines dysgenetic testes, genital ambiguity, glomerulonephritis, and Wilms' tumour.

True hermaphroditism

In true hermaphroditism ovarian and testicular tissue are both present in the same individual. The most common presenting symptoms are abnormal appearance of the external genitalia. Most patients have a 46 XX karyotype: about half are pure 46 XX and about a third are mosaics or chimeras with 46 XX cell lines, i.e. 46 XX/46 XY. A few patients with a pure 46 XY karyotype have been reported. Occasional familial cases of true hermaphroditism have been described in the literature.

Other 46 XX intersex states

Pure gonadal dysgenesis

This disorder, which may be familial, is usually associated with female external genitalia. Clitoromegaly is sometimes present. The gonads are streaks and the karyotype may be 46 XX or XY. 46 XY gonadal dysgenesis, inherited as an X-linked recessive or male-limited autosomal dominant condition, has also been described.

XX male

A number of XX males have been described. These are normal-appearing males with normal intelligence and male psychosexual orientation. Gynaecomastia, sparse facial hair, small genitalia, and hypospadias may occur. The testes are small and resemble Klinefelter testes histologically. There is absence of spermatogenesis, leading to sterility. Families have been reported containing both an XX male and a 46 XX true hermaphrodite.

Gonadal neoplasia and intersex states

A number of intersex disorders carry an increased risk of gonadal tumours. Two important risk factors are the presence of dysgenetic gonadal tissue and a Y chromosome. Intra-abdominal gonads are more susceptible than scrotal glands. The commonest tumour is a gonadoblastoma which is a premalignant lesion but can progress to an invasive tumour.

Clinical and laboratory assessment of patients with intersex states

Clinical assessment

The general appearance of the external genitalia, while important in deciding the appropriate gender, is of very little help in defining the aetiology of the disorder. The principles of clinical assessment are shown in Table 4. A history of a similar disorder in other family members may shed light on the likely diagnosis. The most important aspect of the examination is careful palpation of the gonads.

If no gonads are palpable, the most likely diagnosis is female pseudohermaphroditism due to congenital adrenal hyperplasia, and this is virtually certain if symptoms of salt loss develop. Other possible disorders are true hermaphroditism or male pseudohermaphroditism with intra-abdominal gonads. When both gonads are palpable in the scrotum or labial folds, the patient is likely to be a male pseudohermaphrodite, and measurement of plasma androgens will indicate whether the aetiology is a testicular or peripheral defect. A true hermaphrodite with bilateral ovotestes may also present in this way.

Table 4 Patient with intersex state: clinical assessment

Family history, general examination for dysmorphic features
Examination of external genitalia
No gonads palpable
Female pseudohermaphrodite: congenital adrenal hyperplasia (21-hydroxylase deficiency)
Male pseudohermaphrodite
One gonad palpable
Abnormal gonadal differentiation
Mixed gonadal dysgenesis (XO/XY)
True hermaphroditism
Two gonads palpable
Male pseudohermaphrodite
Impaired testosterone biosynthesis
Androgen receptor defect
5α-Reductase deficiency
True hermaphroditism

Table 5 Patient with intersex state: laboratory assessment

No gonads palpable Karyotype, plasma 17-hydroxyprogesterone, 11-deoxycortisol
One gonad palpable Karyotype, hCG test, gonadal biopsy, pelvic ultrasonography, laparotomy
Two gonads palpable Karyotype, hCG test (hCG 1000 units daily × 3), plasma testosterone, dihydrotestosterone, dihydroepiandrosterone, androstenedione on days 0 and 4
Molecular analysis of the androgen receptor gene
Sinogram

The presence of only one palpable gonad or asymmetry of the perineum is suggestive of mixed gonadal dysgenesis; true hermaphroditism with asymmetrical gonads is the other differential diagnosis.

Laboratory assessment (Table 5)

The karyotype must be determined in all intersex patients. If no gonads are palpable, determination of plasma 17-hydroxyprogesterone will confirm or exclude 21-hydroxylase deficiency. In 11β-hydroxylase deficiency the plasma 11-deoxycortisol concentration is elevated. The infant with two palpable gonads needs an hCG stimulation test to assess testicular androgen secretion. Basal and poststimulatory concentrations of testosterone, dihydrotestosterone, and androstenedione should distinguish a disorder of testosterone biosynthesis from a syndrome of androgen insensitivity.

If one gonad is palpable, gonadal biopsy may be helpful, particularly if ovarian tissue is suspected. Pelvic ultrasonography or exploratory laparotomy for identification of internal genital structures may also be indicated. In any patient with incomplete virilization, urethrography should be performed to identify a vaginal cavity communicating posteriorly with the urethra.

Medical management

Choice of gender

Parents are usually shocked to learn that there is doubt as to the sex of their child. The decision as to the appropriate sex-of-rearing is based mainly on the appearance of the external genitalia and on the likely pattern of secondary sexual development at puberty and should be taken jointly with the parents. The gender should be assigned as soon as possible; however, in some cases of severe ambiguity, there is a case for waiting to assess the effect of early treatment with depot testosterone (25–50 mg at monthly intervals) on phallic growth as a guide to androgen responsiveness.

The concept that, once established, gender identity and role are more or less fixed has now been questioned. Although change of gender may be extremely difficult, the possibility of gender conversion should be viewed with an open mind in the individual subject who, because of spontaneous virilization or feminization at puberty, finds existence in their original gender intolerable.

Sex hormone therapy

Long-term treatment with androgens to promote phallic growth in early childhood has fallen into disrepute because of the acceleration of bone maturation, which leads to loss of ultimate growth potential. While standard testosterone treatment is effective for inducing pubertal development in males with androgen-responsive syndromes, it is of limited value in patients with androgen insensitivity. Induction of full masculization in these patients is still very unsatisfactory. It has, however, been demonstrated that some further virilization in adult patients may be effectively induced using supraphysiological doses of depot testosterone (500 mg weekly). Effects, albeit slow to appear, were seen specifically in penile length and facial and body hair growth.

Further reading

Hines, M. (1998). Abnormal sexual development and psychosexual issues. *Baillière's Clinical Endocrinology and Metabolism* **12**, 173–89.

Saenger, P. (1996). Turner's syndrome. *New England Journal of Medicine* 335, 1749–54.

Chapter 7.13

Disorders of growth

M. A. Preece

The normal curve of growth

The upper panel of Fig. 1 shows the height distance curve for a typical male from birth to 18 years of age. In the lower panel the growth data are converted to provide a record of height velocity in cm/year. This representation of growth is particularly useful as it shows more detail and is more immediate. The growth velocity in any one year is a more sensitive measure of events that have occurred in that year than is the coincident height distance datum.

Disorders of growth

Growth disorders are predominantly problems of childhood, but patients seen by the adult physician are inevitably left with a legacy of events which have occurred before maturity. In many cases where the condition was successfully treated during childhood there may be no residual problem with stature in adult life. In contrast, there are many situations where this outcome is not achieved and there is

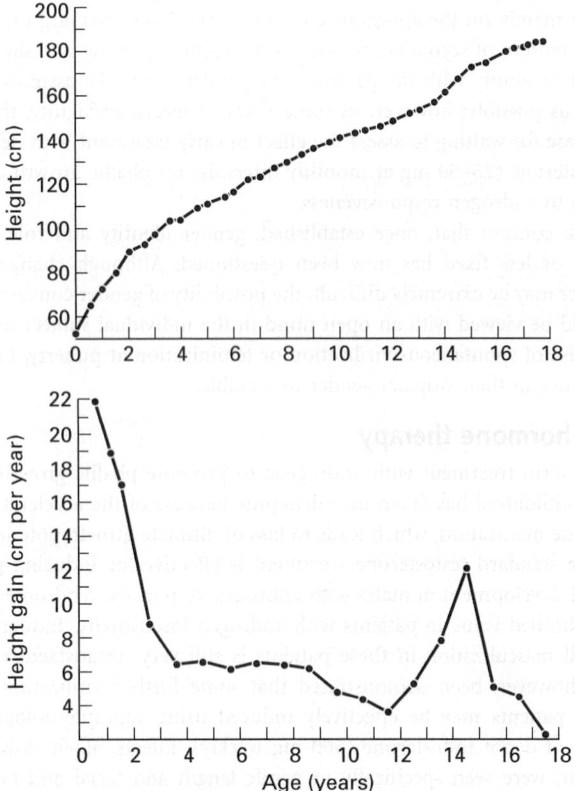

Fig. 1 The growth in height of an individual boy from birth to 18 years of age. The top panel shows the height attained or distance curve and the lower panel shows the data replotted as height gain or growth velocity. *(See OTM3, p. 1695 for details of source.)*

Table 1 Critical heights (cm) for male and female adults in the United Kingdom

	3rd Centile	50th Centile	97th Centile
Females	152.7	163.9	175.2
Males	165.2	177.8	190.4

a persistent problem requiring attention in the adult clinic. The importance of the various underlying disorders is different and what follows reflects this.

Short stature

Definition

What is considered as short stature is essentially arbitrary. It is usually considered as a height that falls below the third centile for the relevant population; values for adults are given in Table 1. Difficulties arise in patients whose height lies close to these limits. In this situation the perceptions of the patient may greatly colour the situation and its management. The important decision then is whether or not the apparent short stature is a symptom of a disorder that requires attention.

Classification of short stature (Table 2)

Familial short stature

This relatively common condition is among the most difficult to manage. The parents are usually of comparable size and the child's stature simply reflects genetic inheritance. This apparently straightforward situation may be made difficult because current social pressures. Many parents and their children find it hard to accept the situation and want a different diagnosis or some treatment to increase growth.

Table 2 Major groups of disease processes leading to short stature

Familial short stature
Constitutional delay of growth and/or puberty
Intrauterine growth retardation
Environmental short stature
Chronic paediatric disease
Endocrine disease
Genetic/chromosomal disorders
Dysmorphic syndromes
Bone dysplasias

Diagnosis

The child will be at or below the third centile for height with a normal growth velocity measured over 1 year. The predicted adult height is calculated by a method that takes into account skeletal maturity, and should lie within a range of 10 cm above or below the mid-parental height centile, which represents the 3rd to 97th centiles for that family.

The general medical picture is of good health and no abnormalities are found on general examination. In this situation no investigations are necessary other than the assessment of skeletal maturity for the prediction of adult height.

Management

It is often difficult to persuade the patient and the family that there is no medical problem. Even when this is achieved, there is often a wish to change the prognosis for height. In recent years there have been many clinical trials of recombinant human growth hormone in this situation. While definitive data are still scarce, there is increasing evidence that although a short-term acceleration of height velocity is almost always achieved, this is not maintained, and adult height is unchanged. When such treatment is started after the age of 11 years this is moderately certain, but there remains some uncertainty if the recombinant human growth hormone is started at younger ages (6–8 years). Even if this is more successful, there remains a considerable debate about the ethics and cost-effectiveness of such treatment of normal healthy children.

Intrauterine growth retardation

Many of those born small for gestational age reach normal centiles for height and weight, but a significant number do not, although they will have grown at a normal velocity. Puberty in such cases tends to be prompt and the adolescent growth spurt attenuated, so that less growth is achieved in the teenage years than expected. Recombinant human growth hormone has been used in some cases, but is still under trial. Early results suggest short-term benefit, but in many skeletal maturation is accelerated and predicted mature height is probably unchanged.

Environmental short stature

Children's growth may be adversely affected by their environment other than by malnutrition or infection. Emotional or physical abuse or neglect may sometimes present in the most bizarre of ways, often imitating other organic disorders such as growth hormone insufficiency. It is most common in young children but may rarely present in young teenagers and, strikingly, may present in a single child in a family where the other children thrive.

This is a diagnosis which is easy to miss. In its most classical form it presents as an apparently straightforward diagnosis of growth hormone insufficiency although there will often be additional features of bizarre eating habits, behavioural abnormalities, or other evidence of abnormal family dynamics. In many where an initial diagnosis of growth hormone insufficiency is made, treatment with recombinant human growth hormone is started, often with early success. However, the accelerated growth soon falters and during the subsequent reappraisal the real diagnosis is uncovered.

Endocrine investigations are often misleading. Once the suspicion is raised the only way to confirm the diagnosis is a period of time away from the family environment, either by a hospital admission or by short-term fostering. A period of accelerated growth (initially weight gain followed by height growth) makes the diagnosis. There is then the need for a detailed social and psychiatric appraisal of the family.

With proper management in childhood those who have suffered from environmental short stature should not present medical problems in adult life. However, it is highly likely that there may be continuing psychological problems and particularly the possibility of subsequent abuse of one or more of their own children.

Chronic paediatric disease

Any child with a long-standing chronic disease will show some degree of growth disorder if the primary disease is less than optimally managed. This may be due to the disease itself or to its treatment; the use of high doses of systemic corticosteroids is a particularly important example of the latter. However, it is very unusual for such a child to present with short stature as the primary symptom. Notable exceptions to this rule are some gastrointestinal diseases, for example, coeliac and inflammatory bowel disease.

In some situations adjunct therapies, such as recombinant human growth hormone in chronic renal failure, are being studied within clinical trials. The long-term benefits of such treatments are far from clear at present.

Hypothyroidism

In any undiagnosed short child there should always be a high degree of suspicion of the possibility of juvenile hypothyroidism. The classical features of adult disease are usually absent and poor growth may be the only abnormality. Typically the child grows with a very low velocity, rapidly crossing centiles and falling progressively further away from the third centile. General medical examination may be normal unless the disease is long established and severe when such symptoms and signs are no different to those in adults.

Striking delay in skeletal maturation is often seen; to the unwary this may lead to an incorrect diagnosis of constitutional delay of growth and/or puberty, as the degree of maturational delay will usually be sufficient to apparently explain the height deficit. For this reason there should be a low threshold for performing thyroid function tests.

Thyroid replacement with L-thyroxine is straightforward, with an initial dose of 100 μg/m^2/day. The prognosis for height is generally very good, except in those diagnosed and treated well into puberty, when the outcome is less satisfactory.

Growth hormone insufficiency

Congenital and acquired forms present differently. In the first case failure of normal growth can usually be detected within the first year of life, but acquired insufficiency can lead to abnormally slow growth at any age before maturity. In the latter situation the assessment of height velocity assumes far greater importance as height may remain within the normal centiles for several years before the child becomes overtly short and below the third centile.

Particularly noteworthy is the pattern of growth in children receiving cranial or craniospinal irradiation as this may be rather different from other causes of growth hormone insufficiency. In both cases there may be associated early puberty, particularly with radiation doses below 2400 cGy, leading to a rather confusing picture as the early but rather attenuated adolescent growth spurt may mask the onset of growth hormone insufficiency. When the spine is involved in the radiation field there may be a combination of growth hormone insufficiency and direct damage to the spinal epiphyses, with subsequent failure of spinal growth which is not due to the endocrine abnormalities and not responsive to endocrine replacement.

The degree of short stature can range from relatively mild to very severe, depending on the degree of insufficiency, the age of onset, and parental heights. As in many short stature disorders, the parents' heights still modify the expression of the disorder such that children with growth hormone insufficiency born to tall parents will tend to be more normal in height than those with equivalent disease born to shorter parents.

The diagnosis is confirmed by a variety of endocrine measurements (discussed in Chapter 7.1). Growth hormone insufficiency may be isolated or part of a wider constellation of pituitary hormone deficiencies, and it is important to check thyroid and adrenal function at an early stage. Gonadotrophin deficiency is difficult to confirm prior to the age of puberty, and it may not be until puberty fails to occur spontaneously that suspicion is raised.

The treatment of growth hormone insufficiency with recombinant human growth hormone, 15–30 IU/m^2/week (0.6–1.2 IU/kg/week; 1 IU = 0.37 mg pure protein), by daily subcutaneous injection. The growth velocity is the best indicator of response and it should show a clear acceleration, usually to 10 cm/year or more. A poor response indicates the need to review the diagnosis. Treatment is continued until growth is complete.

Growth hormone receptor deficiency

This very rare disorder closely mimics severe growth hormone insufficiency but in the case of receptor deficiency there is excessive secretion of GH by the pituitary. The GH receptor, which is either absent or non-functioning due to one of several mutations in the receptor gene, is inherited according to an autosomal recessive pattern. Until now it has been untreatable but clinical trials of recombinant IGF-I look promising.

Adrenocortical excess

An excess of circulating corticosteroids is a potent cause of growth failure, whether due to endogenous overproduction or exogenous medication. Iatrogenic glucocorticoid excess can be related to overuse of topical steroids for atopic disease, inhaled locally active steroids for asthma, and powerful dermatological preparations for eczema as well as to oral treatment. The management of the growth failure is entirely dependent on reducing the dose of corticosteroid or, in the case of oral therapy, using alternate day dosage.

Table 3 Principal causes of tall stature

Familial tall stature
Pituitary gigantism
Sotos syndrome
Marfan syndrome
Homocystinuria

Turner's syndrome (see also Chapter 7.8)

Turner's syndrome is relatively common (about 1 in 2500–3500 female births). The classical features, including coarctation of the aorta, lead to early diagnosis but a large number of affected girls only have subtle clinical signs, and in them short stature may be the presenting feature. Diagnosis is confirmed by chromosomal analysis, which may reveal a 45 X karyotype with complete absence of one X chromosome; a more subtle structural abnormality of one X, such as an isochromosome; or a mosaic combination of cells with different chromosomal complements.

Untreated girls with Turner's syndrome reach adult heights of between 134 and 156 cm but this is dependent on their parents' heights; girls from tall families will be relatively tall for the diagnosis, even reaching into the lower part of the normal range. Puberty is usually, but not always, absent.

Treatment for both the short stature and the lack of puberty is possible. A typical regimen would be the slow introduction of ethinyl oestradiol at about 12–13 years of age in a dose of 1 μg/day increasing to doses of 20–30 μg/day over 2 years (see Chapter 7.8). Significant growth benefit can also be achieved by the combined use of recombinant human growth hormone (20–30 IU/m^2) and the mild anabolic steroid, oxandrolone (1.25–2.5 mg/day).

Tall stature

Excessive tallness can be defined in a complementary way to short stature and is equally arbitrary. In practical terms, boys find difficulty in accepting heights above 200 cm, whereas most girls find 185 cm the limit. Pathological causes of tall stature are very rare. The major causes are listed in Table 3.

Familial tall stature is more or less the mirror image of familial short stature. There is often an element of advanced maturation with a skeletal age that exceeds chronological age by several years and early pubertal development. The diagnosis is made by clinical appraisal, including knowledge of parental heights and the demonstration that predicted adult height is appropriate for the family. Exclusion of other potential causes is often possible on clinical grounds, but the exclusion of excessive GH secretion may be necessary.

The calculation of a predicted adult height, which because of the advanced skeletal maturation is often less than the family fears, may be all that is necessary as the expected height is then acceptable. If this is not the case, then other pharmacological treatments may need discussion. At present these are unsatisfactory, although high-dose ethinyl oestradiol (100–300 μg/day) has been advocated in girls, in an attempt to accelerate skeletal maturation. However, the benefits are far from certain and there may be quite unpleasant side-effects, such as water retention. The long-term safety of this treatment is also unproven.

The use of testosterone in boys, in an analogous manner to oestrogen use in girls, is of even less value and is probably contraindicated.

Pituitary gigantism with excessive GH secretion is extremely rare but does occasionally require specific exclusion, usually by demonstration of normal suppression of GH secretion to undetectable levels by oral glucose (1.75 g/kg). Serum IGF-I concentrations will usually be high, but may overlap the normal range.

The Marfan syndrome is characterized by the disproportionately long limbs and digits (arachnodactyly), and is usually associated with a high-arched palate and pectus excavatum. It is an important diagnosis to make because of the risk of eye problems and dissection of the aortic root and arch (see Section 9).

Sotos syndrome and the other dysmorphic causes of tall stature are even rarer, and can usually be diagnosed on other criteria. They are not considered further here.

Further reading

Hintz, R.L., Attie, K.M., Baptista, J., and Roche, A. (1999). Effect of growth hormone treatment on adult height of children with idiopathic short stature. Genentech Collaborative Group. *New England Journal of Medicine* 340, 502–7.

Tolis, G. (1996). The role of somatostatin agonistic analogs in the treatment of acromegaly. *Metabolism* 45(8 Suppl. 1), 109–10.

Chapter 7.14

Puberty

R. J. M. Ross and M. O. Savage

Normal puberty

The hypothalamic gonadotrophin releasing hormone (GnRH) pulse generator is essential for normal puberty, and the cues that switch it to pubertal mode include, most importantly, age and maturation of the central nervous system, environmental factors such as stress, social factors (probably the reason for an earlier onset of puberty in Western countries), and metabolic factors such as nutrition.

The onset of puberty is characterized by an increase in basal luteinizing hormone (LH) levels and in the amplitude and frequency of LH pulses independent of gonadal changes. Gonadal activation stimulated by the rise in gonadotrophin (LH and follicle stimulating hormone (FSH)) secretion results in rising levels of sex steroids. Apart from their action on sexual maturation, gonadal steroids have a direct effect in stimulating skeletal growth and also a central action in stimulating increased growth hormone (GH) production. A consistent pattern of hormonal changes results in a relatively constant pattern of growth and pubertal development, characterized in girls by the development of breasts, pubic hair, and the onset of menstruation, and in boys by an increase in testicular volume, genitalia size, and the appearance of pubic hair.

Timing of puberty

Disorders of puberty can be classified by the timing of onset of sexual characteristics into either precocious or delayed puberty. Precocious puberty is characterized by signs of sexual maturation appearing less

Table 1 Causes of precocious puberty

Isolated thelarche and isolated pubarche
True precocious puberty (pituitary gonadotrophin dependent)
Idiopathic
sporadic
familial
CNS abnormalities
congenital (e.g. hydrocephalus)
acquired (e.g. irradiation, surgery, and infection)
tumours, including hypothalamic hamartomas, gliomas, and pineal tumours
Hypothyroidism
Pseudoprecocious puberty (pituitary gonadotrophin independent)
McCune–Albright syndrome (polyostotic fibrous dysplasia)
Adrenal disorders
adenomas and carcinomas
congenital adrenal hyperplasia
Gonadal disorders
ovarian cyst
ovarian tumours
testotoxicosis
Leydig cell tumour
Ectopic gonadotrophin producing tumours
dysgerminoma, hepatoblastoma, teratoma, chorionepithelioma
Exogenous sex steroids

than 2.5 standard deviations (SD) from the mean; before 8 years in a girl and before 9 years in a boy. In Western society puberty is considered delayed when there are no signs of pubertal maturation in a girl aged 13.2 years (2SD) or boy aged 14.2 years. As a simple working rule, if there are no signs of puberty at 14 years of age investigation should be considered.

Precocious puberty

Precocious puberty can be classified into true (pituitary gonadotrophin dependent) or pseudo- (pituitary gonadotrophin independent) precocious puberty (Table 1). In true precocious puberty there is activation of the hypothalamic–pituitary axis and thus the normal pattern of puberty is preserved. In pseudoprecocious puberty, for example that caused by an adrenal adenoma, the normal pattern of puberty is lost. Pseudoprecocious puberty may be isosexual, with appropriate male or female puberty, or heterosexual, when there is virilization of a girl, as in congenital adrenal hyperplasia, or feminization of a boy, as in an oestrogen-producing Leydig cell tumour.

Precocious puberty presents much more commonly in girls than boys, and in the majority of girls no organic cause is found and it is idiopathic and sporadic. In contrast, in boys idiopathic precocious puberty is rare and, although there are families with familial true precocious puberty, most commonly it is due to CNS tumours, either hypothalamic hamartomas or gliomas, or dysgerminomas (Table 1).

The investigation of precocious puberty is first directed towards distinguishing between a true, pseudo, isosexual, or heterosexual condition. History and examination will help establish whether there is a normal pattern of pubertal development, as in true precocious puberty, or an abnormal pattern as seen in pseudoprecocious puberty. In girls, ultrasound of the pelvis will demonstrate the effect of oestrogens on uterine size and define the appearance of the ovaries. Measurement of the gonadotrophin response to GnRH should be made, as should basal measurements of β-human chorionic gonadotrophin, adrenocorticotrophic hormone, adrenal steroids (including cortisol, 17-hydroxyprogesterone, DHEA-S, and androstenedione), testosterone, oestrogen, and thyroid hormones. Steroid profiles may also be made on urine collections. Skeletal maturation should be determined by measuring the bone age.

True precocious puberty

In true precocious puberty the gonadotrophins will reflect a pubertal response to GnRH with a greater rise of LH than FSH. In the normal prepubertal child there is only a small rise in the gonadotrophins and the response of FSH is greater than that of LH. In pseudoprecocious puberty the gonadotrophins are usually suppressed unless true puberty has also been initiated, which may occur due to excessive sex steroid secretion from any cause. Acquired hypothyroidism is associated with increased levels of FSH and may result in breast development and menstruation in girls and testicular enlargement in boys. These patients usually have stunted growth and the diagnosis is easily made by the measurement of thyroid stimulating hormone (TSH). Once a diagnosis of true precocious puberty is made, appropriate scanning of the hypothalamic–pituitary axis should be performed using MRI.

Pseudoprecocious puberty

The further investigation of pseudoprecocious puberty depends on the findings of the original screening tests. Adrenal tumours will be associated with increased production of adrenal steroids which is not suppressed by a low-dose dexamethasone suppression test. CT or MRI scanning will pick up adrenal carcinomas (usually greater than 6 cm in diameter) and most adenomas, although on occasion venous catheter sampling is required. Congenital adrenal hyperplasia in girls usually presents early with virilization and ambiguous genitalia, but may present later in boys with virilization and tall stature, but prepubertal testes. Ovarian tumours are best detected by ultrasound scanning, as are testicular tumours. The McCune–Albright syndrome (polyostotic fibrous dysplasia) is an unusual cause of precocious puberty in girls which may manifest initially as autonomous ovarian activity, but this may be succeeded by true precocious puberty. It is due to a mutant G protein α-subunit resulting in a constitutively active cAMP second-messenger system. Patients have patches of *café au lait* pigmentation with a ragged border and fibrous dysplasia of the bones.

Testotoxicosis is an unusual inherited disorder (activating mutation of the LH receptor), characterized by pubertal levels of testosterone, pubertal-sized testes, and a suppressed hypothalamic–gonadal axis. Tumours producing human chorionic gonadotrophin (hCG) can be detected by the measurement of hCG and scanning of appropriate sites, including the gonads, liver, and pineal gland.

Treatment

The aims of treatment are to remove the primary cause; to treat the psychosocial consequences; to allow normal puberty; and to promote normal growth.

Children with precocious puberty appear much older than they are and this can result in considerable psychological difficulties and behavioural problems. Growth is stimulated both by a direct action of sex steroids on skeletal maturation and by the induction of GH secretion. This early maturation of the skeleton results in early fusion of the epiphyses, and although the child is initially tall his or her ultimate height may be very short.

Girls with only slightly advanced pubertal development often require no treatment because puberty only advances slowly, and they do not have a significant loss in height potential. GnRH analogues are now the treatment of choice in true precocious puberty. They act by down-regulating the GnRH receptor and switching off the secretion of LH and FSH. GnRH analogues have been produced as nasal sprays, and monthly intramuscular and subcutaneous depot injections. Depot injections have proved the most effective. GnRH may produce an initial period of stimulation, which can be prevented by giving concomitant treatment with cyproterone acetate (100 mg/m^2/24 h for the first 6 weeks). Occasionally the acute suppression of oestrogen production at the start of treatment will precipitate an oestrogen-withdrawal bleed.

Cyproterone acetate, a peripherally acting antiandrogen, is the drug of choice for the treatment of pseudoprecocious puberty. A dose of 50–100 mg daily is effective in halting the progress of the physical features of puberty, and is useful in suppressing menstruation. It is a weak glucocorticoid and may suppress ACTH and the adrenal glands. An alternative treatment is ketoconazole which blocks several steps in adrenal steroid synthesis, including testosterone. However, it occasionally causes severe hepatic dysfunction.

Any effective treatment of precocious puberty will slow the growth rate by the consequent reduced secretion of sex steroids and GH. Patients treated to arrest puberty have longer to grow, but their reduced growth rate and already reduced growth potential mean that, despite the use of GnRH analogues, they will not achieve the height of which they were originally capable. Studies to see if GH treatment can promote better growth during the treatment of precocious puberty have been disappointing.

Delayed puberty

The causes are summarized in Table 2. The individual conditions which may cause it are discussed in other parts of this book. Here, discussion is limited to the management of constitutional delay of growth and adolescence.

Constitutional delay of growth and adolescence (CDGA)

CDGA occurs in otherwise normal adolescents who have relatively short stature, delayed puberty and bone age, and a height prognosis appropriate in relation to their parents. It presents far more frequently in boys than girls and is the commonest cause of delayed puberty in boys, with Turner's syndrome being the commonest in girls. CDGA needs to be distinguished from isolated gonadotrophin deficiency, but this is rarely easy as gonadotrophins are low with a low or prepubertal response to GnRH in both conditions. A positive family history may indicate CDGA, and associated anosmia suggests Kallmann's syndrome. If in doubt and treatment is indicated, then the patient should be reassessed after therapy (see below) to see if puberty then progresses without treatment.

Psychological problems are common in children with delayed puberty and short stature. Delayed puberty may be associated with a reduced spinal bone density, putting adults at risk of bone fracture later in life. Thus, there are good reasons for treating this condition, which may be considered as a variant of normal growth.

Table 2 Causes of pubertal delay

Causes
Hypogonadotrophic hypogonadism (low LH and FSH)
Constitutional delay in growth and adolescence (CDGA)
sporadic
familial
Chronic diseases
Crohn's, renal failure, thalassaemia
Malnutrition
Coeliac disease, cystic fibrosis, anorexia nervosa
Hypothalamic–pituitary
Hypopituitarism (idiopathic, tumours, craniopharyngiomas)
Isolated LH and FSH deficiency (Kallmann's, Prader–Willi, and fertile eunuch syndromes)
Isolated GH deficiency
Leptin deficiency or mutations
Hyperprolactinaemia
Polycystic ovarian disease
Exercise (gymnasts)
Hormonal
Hypothyroidism, Cushing's syndrome
Hypergonadotrophic hypogonadism (high LH and FSH)
Congenital
Chromosome abnormalities (Turner's and Klinefelter's syndromes)
Gonadal dysgenesis/agenesis
Steroid hormone or receptor deficiency (5α-reductase deficiency and testicular feminization)
Acquired
Radiotherapy, surgery, chemotherapy, trauma, torsion, autoimmunity

Intervention with sex steroids or anabolic steroids is safe and brings forward the timing of the growth spurt without reducing height potential. The object of treatment is to stimulate normal puberty and maximize linear growth. In boys a reasonable starting dose of testosterone esters is 25–50 mg monthly, increasing gradually to 250 mg every 4 weeks, although puberty may be induced more rapidly over a 6-month period and the course of treatment may be as short as 3 months. Oral Oxandralone (unlicensed but available on a name patient basis from Searle, UK), 2.5 mg daily, will similarly increase growth velocity.

In girls, ethinyloestradiol at an initial dose of 2–10 μg daily can later be increased to 10–20 μg daily, with the addition of progesterone when the oestrogen dose has reached 20 μg (for example, medroxy-progesterone acetate 5 mg on days 1–14 of the calender month).

Further reading

Kulin, H.E. (1996). Delayed puberty. *Journal of Clinical Endocrinology and Metabolism* 81, 3460–4.

Merke, D.P. and Cutler, G.B., Jr. (1996). Evaluation and management of precocious puberty. *Archives of Disease in Childhood* 75, 269–71.

Chapter 7.15

Non-diabetic pancreatic endocrine disorders and multiple endocrine neoplasia

P. J. Hammond and S. R. Bloom

Pancreatic endocrine tumours

Pancreatic endocrine tumours (islet cell tumours, gastroenteropancreatic tumours) are rare. The commonest, insulinomata and gastrinomata, occur with an annual incidence of one per million, with others having an incidence of less than 1 per 10 million. Functioning tumours usually present with the symptoms of hormone excess. They may secrete the pancreatic hormones insulin, glucagon, and somatostatin, or ectopic hormones such as gastrin, vasoactive intestinal polypeptide (VIP), or parathyroid hormone related peptide (PTHrP). Non-functioning tumours can reach a large size in an apparently well patient. They were once often mistakenly identified as adenocarcinomata, but are now increasingly diagnosed as a result of detection of their secretion of functionally inactive peptides, such as pancreatic polypeptide and neurotensin, or immunohistochemical staining for neuroendocrine markers, such as chromogranin and neurone-specific enolase. They probably account for 50 per cent of all pancreatic endocrine tumours.

Natural history

These tumours were originally described as APUDomata because it was thought that they had a common origin from neural crest cells with the ability to perform amine precursor uptake and decarboxylation (APUD). This theory has since been disproved, and it has been proposed that the neuroendocrine and mucosal endocrine cells of the gastroenteropancreatic axis are derived from a common bipotential endoplacal stem cell.

The genetic basis for the development of sporadic pancreatic endocrine tumours is largely unknown. However, about 25 per cent of them, particularly gastrinomata and insulinomata, occur as part of the familial autosomal dominant multiple endocrine neoplasia type 1 (MEN 1) syndrome (see below), in which allelic deletion in the q13 region of chromosome 11 is found, and loss of heterozygosity for this region has been demonstrated in some patients with sporadic gastrinoma and insulinoma.

Islet cells are pluripotential with respect to peptide production. Thus 70 per cent of tumours are associated with elevated pancreatic polypeptide levels, and in a small proportion of cases other hormones, particularly gastrin, may become elevated and cause secondary syndromes during the course of the disease. Altered processing of peptide precursor molecules may result in a variety of molecular weight forms of the same peptide being secreted, and not all the immunoreactive peptide is bioactive. This can have clinical implications: for example large molecular forms of glucagon (enteroglucagon) can cause villous hypertrophy and slowed intestinal transit, and large forms of somatostatin have been reported to cause hypoglycaemia, rather than the hyperglycaemia usually associated with the somatostatinoma syndrome.

Table 1 Causes of elevated gut hormones other than pancreatic endocrine tumours

All hormones	Glucagon
Non-fasting sample	Hepatic failure
Chronic renal failure	Oral contraceptives and danazol
Gastrin	Stress
Hypercalcaemia	Prolonged fast
Achlorhydria	Familial hyperglucagonaemia
G-cell hyperplasia	Pancreatic polypeptide
Vasoactive intestinal polypeptide	Elderly
Hepatic cirrhosis	Pernicious anaemia
Bowel ischaemia	Hypercalcaemia
	Neurotensin
	Fibrolamellar hepatoma

The majority of pancreatic endocrine tumours are slow-growing and prolonged survival is often possible, even in the presence of metastatic spread, the median survival being about 5 years. However, some patients have rapidly spreading disease, particularly those with non-functioning tumours, whose median survival is little over 2 years. Early in the disease, morbidity and mortality result from the effects of peptide hypersecretion rather than tumour bulk. The unpredictable nature of these tumours makes it difficult to give an accurate prognosis, occasional patients surviving for decades, and, combined with their rarity, this has made it difficult to assess the efficacy of different therapeutic strategies.

Diagnosis

Pancreatic endocrine tumours can usually be diagnosed by hormonal radio-immunoassay of a single fasting plasma sample, but certain syndromes require confirmatory tests. Several conditions other than tumour are associated with increased circulating gut hormone levels (Table 1), particularly renal failure, but the elevations are usually more modest than those associated with tumour syndromes.

Most glucagonomata, non-functioning tumours, and pancreatic VIPomata and somatostatinomata are large (greater than 2 cm), may be calcified, and have metastasized to the liver in the majority of cases. Such tumours are easily localized by abdominal CT scanning and ultrasonography. However, localization of tumours producing more active hormones, which are therefore detected earlier in their development, may be difficult: for example, 40 per cent of gastrinomata and insulinomata are microadenomata, less than 1 cm in diameter. Insulinomata often occur in the distal two-thirds of the pancreas, and over 90 per cent of gastrinomata are found in the gastrinoma triangle, bounded by the third part of the duodenum, the neck of the pancreas, and the porta hepatis, about 20 per cent of these being in the duodenum. CT scanning and meticulous highly selective angiography (Fig. 1) will localize 70 per cent of these microadenomata; MRI may be more sensitive. Transhepatic percutaneous portal venous sampling is a good method of detecting hormone gradients, but cannot give accurate enough resolution to assist the surgeon in most cases, and is an expensive procedure not without risk. Endoscopic ultrasonography may be more sensitive than conventional imaging, with a resolution of 2 mm and a detection rate of over 75 per cent for tumours in the pancreatic head, but detection is poorer for lesions of the pancreatic tail and duodenum. Intraoperative ultrasonography has a sensitivity of over 90 per cent for pancreatic tumours, and endoscopic transillumination of the duodenum may allow the surgeon to detect an occult

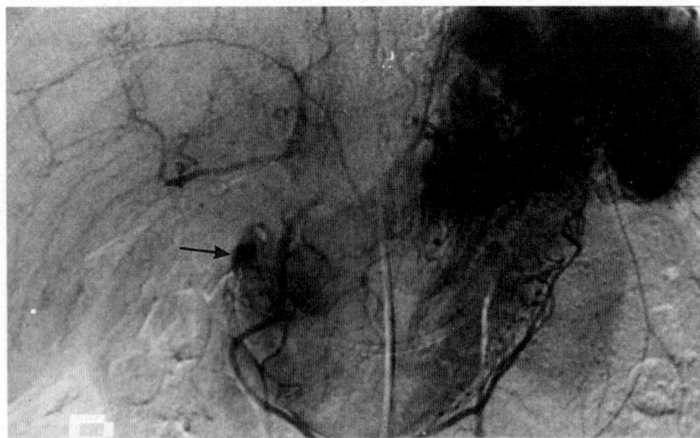

Fig. 1 Venous phase of coeliac axis angiogram demonstrating gastrinoma blush in duodenal wall (arrowed).

gastrinoma. Functional radiological localization has been described for both insulinomata and gastrinomata. Injection of calcium or secretin into the artery supplying the tumour causes a marked rise in insulin or gastrin levels, respectively, in the hepatic vein, and allows equivocal lesions to be verified, or the site of unlocalized lesions to be more accurately predicted. Radiolabelled somatostatin analogues have proved useful in demonstrating the extent of metastatic disease, and may assist in the localization of extrapancreatic VIPomas, but are ineffective in detecting microadenomata.

Confirmation of the diagnosis can be made by immunocytochemical analysis of resection specimens or liver biopsies, in addition to conventional histology.

Treatment

Sporadic tumours without evidence of metastatic spread should be resected if possible. Surgical cures have been reported for a few patients with hepatic metastases amenable to enucleation, and liver transplantation has been successful in some patients with metastatic disease confined to the liver.

In the majority of patients, surgical cure is not possible. Until the terminal stages of the disease palliation is directed at reducing the symptoms of hormone excess in those with functional tumours. This can be achieved by reducing tumour bulk and/or inhibiting hormone secretion or action. Reduction of tumour bulk surgically is usually precluded by the operative morbidity. A variety of chemotherapy regimens have been reported as effective. The standard one consists of streptozotocin and 5-fluorouracil, with response rates of 80 per cent for functioning tumours, VIPomata responding particularly well, and about 50 per cent for non-functioning tumours. The combination of doxorubicin and streptozotocin has recently been reported to be more effective. Other agents advocated are dacarbazine for glucagonomata, and cisplatin and etoposide for anaplastic tumours. Response rates after embolization of the hepatic arterial supply liver metastases are between 60 and 80 per cent.

Inhibition of hormone release and action is achieved by using subcutaneous octreotide given in three doses daily. The clinical sequelae of peptide hypersecretion are often greatly diminished 24 h after the first injection, but patients become progressively resistant over many months or years.

Tumour syndromes

Gastrinoma

Sixty per cent of gastrinomata are malignant, 50 per cent of patients having metastases at the time of diagnosis, and up to 30 per cent have the MEN 1 syndrome. The majority of tumours are pancreatic, but between 20 and 40 per cent are duodenal, and these are usually microadenomata, as little as 1 mm in diameter. Sporadic duodenal microgastrinomata are solitary, but in those patients with MEN 1 they are usually multiple and associated with pancreatic microadenomata. Apparent primary lymph node gastrinomata may represent metastases from duodenal microgastrinomata.

The syndrome is the result of excess gastrin-stimulated gastric acid secretion. This causes severe, multiple peptic ulcers, which are usually duodenal, but may occur in the oesophagus and jejunum, and are often associated with haemorrhage, perforation, and stricture formation. Diarrhoea and steatorrhoea, due to acid inactivation of small bowel enzymes and mucosal damage, may be prominent, frequently preceding ulcer disease by 12 months or more.

Diagnosis requires the demonstration of a raised fasting gastrin concentration, while off H_2-blockers or omeprazole, associated with increased basal gastric acid secretion. Hypergastrinaemia and raised acid output may also arise from retained antrum following partial gastrectomy or the rare condition of G-cell hyperplasia. The intravenous secretin test distinguishes these conditions from gastrinoma. In the presence of a gastrinoma, gastrin levels are elevated by at least 50 per cent following secretin, while there is no such increase in association with G-cell hyperplasia or retained antrum. Furthermore, gastrin levels are increased in response to a test meal in the latter conditions but not in association with a gastrinoma.

Localization of microgastrinomata may be aided preoperatively by endoscopic ultrasound or selective arterial secretin injection, or intraoperatively by ultrasonography or duodenotomy with transillumination and palpation.

Localized non-metastatic tumours should be resected, and regular attempts at localization should be made for occult tumours. Omeprazole, which almost completely inhibits gastric acid production in all cases, has transformed the management of these patients, and offers the best palliation for those with metastatic disease. It is acid-labile and so initially should be administered with an H_2-blocker.

VIPoma

VIPomata arise in the pancreas in 90 per cent of cases. The remaining tumours are mainly gangliomata or ganglioneuroblastomata originating in the sympathetic chain or adrenal medulla, and these tumours are especially common in children. Most extrapancreatic tumours are benign, but 50 per cent of pancreatic VIPomata have metastasized at the time of diagnosis, usually to local lymph nodes and the liver.

The features of the VIPoma (Verner–Morrison, pancreatic cholera) syndrome are shown in Table 2. Large-volume diarrhoea without steatorrhoea is the cardinal symptom, most patients excreting more than 3 litres daily, with volumes of over 20 litres described. It is often intermittent at first, but in severe crises the volume loss coupled with the vasodilatory effects of VIP and the associated hypokalaemia may precipitate cardiovascular collapse.

Hypokalaemia results from stool loss and activation of the renin–angiotensin system, and may be profound. The loss of bicarbonate in the stool leads to acidosis which may mask the true potassium

Table 2 Features of the VIPoma syndrome

Clinical features	Biochemical features
Secretory diarrhoea	Raised plasma VIP
Severe dehydration and weakness	Hypokalaemic acidosis
Hypotension and cardiac standstill	Hypochlorhydria
Abdominal colic	Hypercalcaemia—probably due to PTHrP
Flushing	Hypomagnesaemia
Weight loss	Glucose intolerance

deficit. Achlorhydria or hypochlorhydria occurs in over 50 per cent of patients and distinguishes this diarrhoeal syndrome from that associated with gastrinoma. In up to 50 per cent of cases there is glucose intolerance as a result of the glucagon-like actions of VIP. Other features include hypercalcaemia, probably due to PTHrP secretion and exacerbated by dehydration; hypomagnesaemia due to stool loss; and flushing of the head and neck, which can occur on tumour palpation and may be associated with a marked fall in systemic blood pressure. In advanced cases extreme weight loss may occur.

VIPomata are usually associated with markedly raised plasma VIP concentrations, but because the half-life of VIP in circulation is only 2 min, the diagnosis is best confirmed by the finding of elevated circulating histidine methionine, which is produced from the prepro-VIP molecule, is more stable in plasma, and is co-secreted by VIPomata. Pancreatic polypeptide levels are elevated in 75 per cent of cases and neurotensin in 10 per cent. Ganglioneuroblastomata may secrete noradrenaline and adrenaline and so be associated with elevated urinary catecholamines and their metabolites. VIPomata are usually large and so localization is rarely a problem.

Patients with non-metastatic disease should have surgical resections, and this is feasible in the majority of ganglioneuroblastomata. Chemotherapy provides very effective palliation for those with metastatic disease, and the excellent response to streptozotocin and 5-fluorouracil makes the use of other agents, particularly α-interferon, unnecessary. Similarly, hepatic embolization is not usually indicated for metastatic VIPomas. Acute VIPoma crises should be managed with fluid and electrolyte support, and central venous pressure monitoring. A number of drugs, including prednisolone, indomethacin, metoclopramide, lithium carbonate, and opiates, have been used to treat the diarrhoea, but have been superseded by octreotide. Ninety per cent of patients respond to octreotide with reduction of diarrhoea almost to normal and resolution of the electrolyte imbalance within 48 h. Unfortunately, the median duration of response to octreotide alone is less than 1 year, and so its use is probably best combined with chemotherapy.

Glucagonoma

Glucagonomata are α-cell tumours of the pancreas which secrete various forms of glucagon and other peptides derived from the preproglucagon molecule. They have an estimated annual incidence of 1 in 20 million, with a marginal female preponderance, and invariably present in adulthood. Over 70 per cent of patients have metastases at the time of diagnosis.

The characteristic feature is the rash of *necrolytic migratory erythema*, which occurs in almost all patients, although it often remains undiagnosed for many years. It usually starts in the groins and perineum, migrating to the distal extremities. The initial lesions are erythematous patches, which become raised and may be associated with bullae. These lesions break down and gradually heal, often leaving an area of hyperpigmentation, only to recur in another site. All mucous membranes may be involved, commonly leading to angular stomatitis, cheilitis, and glossitis. The cause of the rash is unknown; it has been reported in a few patients without glucagonomata, who either had coeliac disease or cirrhosis, both of which may have led to elevation in glucagon and glucagon-like peptides. Other common features of glucagonomata include impaired glucose tolerance, progressive weight loss, venous thrombosis, normochromic normocytic anaemia, bowel disturbance and nail dystrophy. Mental slowness, depression, and paraneoplastic neurological syndromes have also been described.

The diagnosis is confirmed by demonstrating raised fasting plasma glucagon concentrations, usually by ten- to twentyfold. Localization is almost never a problem, since tumours are invariably large and pancreatic, with metastases in the majority of cases. Barium studies often show a thickened jejunal and ileal mucosa due to the trophic effects of large forms of glucagon on the small bowel. Fifty per cent of tumours produce pancreatic polypeptide and co-production of gastrin and insulin has been described. Skin biopsies show necrolysis of the stratum Malpighi of the epidermis in early lesions, but only a non-specific dermatitis at later stages.

Surgical cure of glucagonomata is rarely possible although liver metastases may be resectable or treated by liver transplantation. Surgery is complicated by the tendency to venous thrombosis, the catabolic effects of glucagon, and anaemia. A significant proportion of glucagonomata fail to respond to the combination of streptozotocin and 5-fluorouracil, and in these cases dacarbazine or hepatic embolization may be necessary. Octreotide is particularly effective in treating the rash, with resolution usually occurring within the first month of treatment and persisting for at least 6 months, but it has little impact on the other features of the syndrome. Other simple treatments for the rash are topical or oral zinc and a high-protein diet. The thrombotic tendency, which can result in fatal pulmonary emboli, is refractory to conventional anticoagulation, but aspirin or dipyridamole may be of benefit.

Somatostatinoma

Somatostatinomata are extremely rare, with an estimated annual incidence of about 1 in 40 million. Fifty per cent of these tumours are pancreatic, the remainder arising in the duodenum. Approximately 50 per cent of duodenal somatostatinomata occur in association with neurofibromatosis type I (von Recklinghausen's disease) and these tumours are usually periampullary. Pancreatic tumours usually present late with hepatic metastases, but duodenal tumours are frequently identified earlier as a result of local effects such as obstruction of the ampulla of Vater, intestinal obstruction, or haemorrhage.

The somatostatinoma syndrome is characterized by the triad of cholelithiasis, diabetes mellitus, and steatorrhoea, the latter occurring in almost all patients with pancreatic tumours. These features result from the inhibitory actions of somatostatin on gallbladder contraction and secretion, insulin secretion, and pancreatic exocrine secretions. Hypoglycaemia has also been described, possibly due to larger molecular forms of somatostatin having a greater inhibitory effect on counterregulatory hormones than on insulin. Other features of the syndrome include hypochlorhydria, anaemia, postprandial fullness, and weight loss. The full syndrome is rarely seen in association with duodenal somatostatinomata, gallbladder disease being the only common manifestation.

Circulating levels of somatostatin are usually elevated greater than tenfold in association with pancreatic tumours, but the smaller duodenal tumours are associated with much lower levels. Multiple molecular weight forms of somatostatin may explain unusual clinical features. Localization is rarely a problem, barium examinations or endoscopy identifying duodenal lesions.

Surgical resection of duodenal tumours is usually curative. Pancreatic tumours have almost always metastasized by the time of diagnosis and so palliation with chemotherapy or hepatic embolization are the only therapeutic options.

Pancreatic polypeptide, neurotensin, and other hormones

Pancreatic polypeptide (PP) can be extracted from almost all pancreatic endocrine tumours and is secreted by up to 75 per cent of them. The finding of elevated circulating PP in association with other tumour syndromes indicates a pancreatic source, but PP has no recognized physiological role so that pure PPomas can be regarded effectively as non-functioning tumours. Similarly neurotensin, which is elevated in 10 per cent of VIPomata, does not cause a characteristic syndrome.

Hypercalcaemia is a feature of the VIPoma syndrome and may also occur in association with pancreatic endocrine tumours without other hormone syndromes. Secretion of PTHrP by pancreatic endocrine tumours has now been reported in a number of cases. It is probable, therefore, that almost all cases of hypercalcaemia in association with pancreatic endocrine tumours are mediated by PTHrP. In these patients the hypercalcaemia responds to both octreotide and bisphosphonates.

There have also been reports of acromegaly and gigantism caused by growth hormone releasing hormone (GHRH) secretion by pancreatic endocrine tumours. Treatment for these patients has included surgical resection, octreotide therapy, and liver transplantation.

Corticotrophin releasing hormone may be produced by pancreatic endocrine tumours, but only causes Cushing's syndrome when the tumour also secretes corticotrophin (ACTH). Other peptides produced by islet-cell tumours include neuropeptide Y, neuromedin B, calcitonin gene-related peptide, bombesin, and motilin, but these are not associated with recognized clinical syndromes.

Non-functioning tumours

These may account for half of all pancreatic endocrine tumours. They usually present late with symptoms attributable to tumour bulk, such as anorexia and weight loss, or to effects on local structures, such as obstructive jaundice or intestinal obstruction or haemorrhage. They are often mistakenly diagnosed as adenocarcinomata, but the presence of elevated circulating gut hormones, such as pancreatic polypeptide or neurotensin, and the use of immunocytochemical analysis can point to the correct diagnosis. Non-functioning tumours usually respond poorly to chemotherapy, but hepatic embolization may be beneficial. They have a poor prognosis as a result of their late presentation and lack of response to therapy.

Multiple endocrine neoplasia

The MEN syndromes (MEN 1 and MEN 2) are familial conditions with an autosomal dominant pattern of inheritance and a high degree of penetrance. The genetic defect in MEN 2, previously localized to chromosome region 10q11.2, has been identified, but that underlying MEN 1 has been mapped only to a specific chromosomal region. Identification of specific gene defects in these syndromes may provide novel therapeutic options for tumour prevention in affected individuals.

Multiple endocrine neoplasia type 1 (MEN 1)

MEN 1 is characterized by the association of parathyroid hyperplasia, pancreatic endocrine tumours, and pituitary adenomas. The prevalence of the condition has been estimated at about 1 in 10 000. The genetic abnormality fits the 'two-hit' model, whereby there is a germline mutation of the MEN 1 gene on one chromosome, followed by a somatic deletion of the same region on the other, leading to loss of heterozygosity for that allele and subsequent tumour formation. Loss of heterozygosity for the long arm of chromosome 11 has also been found in some sporadic parathyroid adenomas and pancreatic endocrine tumours, implying that the MEN 1 gene is a proto-oncogene. A substantial proportion of MEN 1 cases arise through sporadic mutations, and these patients present between the third and fifth decades, while familial cases can be identified earlier through screening.

Parathyroid hyperplasia and adenomata

Hyperparathyroidism is the presenting feature of MEN 1 in the majority of patients, and occurs in almost all cases. All four glands are diffusely hyperplastic and there may be nodule formation. Whether true adenomata develop remains controversial. Subtotal parathyroidectomy is almost always followed by recurrence, so total parathyroidectomy is preferred, either with autotransplantation of one gland to the forearm, which can later be removed if hyperparathyroidism recurs, or with immediate replacement therapy with 1α-hydroxycholecalciferol.

Pancreatic endocrine tumours

Pancreatic endocrine tumours occur in about 70 per cent of patients with MEN 1, and usually present between the ages of 15 and 50 if not identified by screening. They account for most of the morbidity and mortality of the syndrome. Over 60 per cent of tumours are gastrinomata and about 30 per cent are insulinomata, the two co-existing in about 10 per cent of cases. VIPomata have rarely been described and there are only isolated reports of glucagonomata, but non-functioning tumours may occur frequently. Diffuse hyperplasia of the pancreas is usually seen, similar to the parathyroid, and in the majority of cases there are multiple adenomata, most of which are less than 1 cm in diameter. Duodenal microgastrinomata are very common, probably accounting for almost half of all MEN 1 associated gastrinomata, and are usually multiple, with up to 15 separate tumours described.

The surgical approach to pancreatic endocrine tumours in MEN 1 is controversial. Surgical cure is best achieved by removing the pancreas and duodenum with adjacent lymph nodes, but such an aggressive approach is only justified in families in which the pancreatic disease has been extremely malignant, and in these kindreds should be performed only when pancreatic disease is biochemically apparent. An alternative, potentially curative, approach is to perform a subtotal pancreatectomy with enucleation of palpable tumours in the head and careful exploration for duodenal lesions, which should also be resected. A more conservative strategy is to enucleate gross lesions to reduce the risk of developing metastatic disease and then control hormonal syndromes with appropriate medical therapy. The latter approach is probably appropriate for gastrinomata because omeprazole is such an effective treatment, but for insulinomata, where medical therapy is often unsuccessful and symptoms usually recur after enucleation alone, more aggressive surgical management may be the best option. The treatment of metastatic disease is the same as in sporadic cases.

Pancreatic endocrine tumours associated with MEN 1 are less malignant than sporadic tumours and carry a better prognosis, with a median survival of 15 years compared to 5 years for patients with sporadic tumours.

Pituitary adenomata

The true incidence of pituitary adenomata in MEN 1 is disputed. They are detected by screening in 30 per cent of patients, but are found at autopsy in 50 per cent of patients. Unlike the pancreas and parathyroid, there does not appear to be diffuse pituitary hyperplasia, and loss of heterozygosity for the MEN 1 locus is much less common in pituitary tumours than in parathyroid and pancreatic lesions.

Prolactinomata are the commonest tumours, occurring in about two-thirds of cases, with acromegaly accounting for about 30 per cent, and other functioning tumours being rare. Treatment is the same as for sporadic pituitary tumours.

Other lesions

Lesions in other tissues have been reported in association with MEN 1, but their relationship to the syndrome remains controversial. Carcinoid tumours occur in about 10 per cent of cases, and are often found in the pancreas, but are rarely symptomatic. Lipomata occur in a significant proportion of patients and act as a marker for affected individuals. Adrenal nodular hyperplasia occurs more commonly than in normals and as in them there is no associated excess hormone secretion.

Screening

The screening of first- and second-degree relatives lowers the age of detection of the syndrome by about 20 years and may allow curative surgery which would be expected to prolong survival.

The most useful screening investigations are a serum calcium, fasting gastrin, and prolactin, although a full gut hormone screen is usually performed. The most sensitive markers of pancreatic disease appear to be basal and test-meal stimulated pancreatic polypeptide and gastrin, and basal insulin and proinsulin, identifying lesions at least 3 years before there are any radiological abnormalities. The syndrome rarely develops before the age of 5 or after the age of 70, and so screening should be performed annually from 5–65, and at longer intervals thereafter. Eighty per cent of affected individuals will have been identified by the fifth decade. Screening of patients with apparently sporadic pancreatic endocrine tumours for evidence of MEN 1 is also probably justified, especially in those with gastrinomata or insulinomata. There is little evidence to support screening in those with sporadic pituitary tumours. MEN 1 is present in 15 per cent of all patients with hyperparathyroidism, but screening for MEN 1 is not currently warranted.

Genetic linkage analysis has greater than 95 per cent predictive accuracy, and in most families a haplotype associated with the mutant allele can be found. If three markers can be identified, the accuracy improves to greater than 99 per cent. However, at present the use of this technique alone for detection of gene carriers cannot be advocated.

Multiple endocrine neoplasia type 2 (MEN 2)

MEN 2 is the association of medullary cell carcinoma of the thyroid (MTC) and phaeochromocytoma. In type 2A or Sipple's syndrome, parathyroid hyperplasia may occur; type 2B is associated with mucosal neuromata and marfanoid habitus. In addition, there is a familial form of MTC without other features. Germline mutations of the *ret* proto-oncogene have been identified in all three syndromes. In MEN 2A and familial MTC mutations occur in the extracellular domain, and in MEN 2B a single mutation in the tyrosine kinase domain has been demonstrated. The MEN 2 phenotypes reflect the tissue expression of *ret*. Tumours in affected individuals are heterozygous for the *ret* mutation, the only known dominantly inherited proto-oncogene. It is likely that activation of *ret* leads to hyperplasia in affected tissues and that a somatic mutation in another oncogene is required for carcinogenesis. Thus loss of heterozygosity for the short arm of chromosome 1 has been described in phaeochromocytomas and MTC associated with MEN 2. New mutations are uncommon in MEN 2A, but account for about 50 per cent of cases with MEN 2B. Patients with MEN 2A not identified by screening usually present in the fourth and fifth decades, while those with 2B present much earlier due to their characteristic phenotype.

Medullary cell carcinoma of the thyroid (MTC) (see also Chapter 7.5)

MTC is a tumour of the C cells of the thyroid, which secrete calcitonin, and this acts as a tumour marker. Twenty-five per cent of cases are familial. The incidence of MTC in MEN 2 is probably 100 per cent. Familial MTC alone is the most benign form of MTC; in association with MEN 2B, MTC is the most malignant form of the disease. In MEN 2 the initial thyroid lesion is C-cell hyperplasia. All forms of hereditary MTC are bilateral, with multifocal tumours, usually occurring at the junction of the upper third and lower two-thirds of the thyroid. Metastases are invariably present when tumours are already palpable.

In MEN 2A, screening, measuring pentagastrin-stimulated calcitonin, probably identifies all cases before MTC has developed. This allows total thyroidectomy to be performed at the stage of hyperplasia or microscopic tumour, which is curative in all patients. In MEN 2B, thyroidectomy with lymph node clearance should be performed at the earliest possible age in individuals with the phenotypic features. In those patients not identified by screening, thyroidectomy should still be performed, unless distant metastases, usually to lung or liver, are present. Spread to local lymph nodes is near inevitable in this group for whom the prognosis is poor, with recurrent disease in about 20 per cent of patients with clinically occult MTC and in over 60 per cent of those with palpable tumours. It is particularly poor in MEN 2B presenting with clinically apparent MTC. Their 10-year survival is about 50 per cent, and death from metastatic disease in the mid-twenties is common.

Phaeochromocytoma

Phaeochromocytoma is familial in 5 per cent of cases, 20 per cent of whom have MEN 2. Fifty per cent of individuals with MEN 2 develop phaeochromocytoma. About 70 per cent are bilateral, almost all are benign, and they are rarely extra-adrenal. The initial lesion is adrenal medullary hyperplasia, followed by nodule formation and then multiple, multifocal phaeochromocytomata.

MEN 2-associated phaeochromocytomata are characterized by excessive adrenaline secretion, so that palpitation and other β-adrenergic

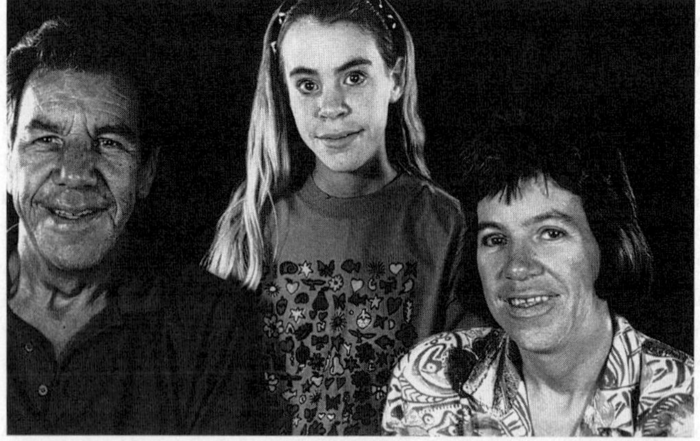

(a)

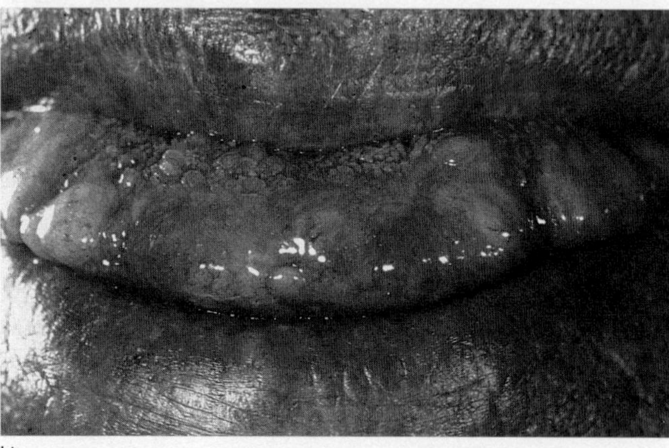

(b)

Fig. 2 (a) Characteristic phenotype of MEN 2B showing facial appearance. (b) Characteristic phenotype of MEN 2B showing mucosal neuromas on tongue.

symptoms predominate initially, with hypertension a late feature. Treatment is bilateral adrenalectomy, since the incidence of bilateral disease is high, and the mortality from phaeochromocytoma in MEN 2 about 15 per cent, usually due to sudden death. If an adrenal lesion is identified at the same time as MTC, the adrenalectomy should be performed first.

Other features of MEN 2A

Parathyroid hyperplasia occurs in up to 80 per cent of patients with MEN 2A, but less than 20 per cent have hypercalcaemia. Parathyroidectomy should be performed in those with hypercalcaemia and in those without it grossly enlarged glands should be removed at the time of thyroidectomy. Cutaneous lichen amyloidosis, often preceded by intense pruritus, has been described in two kindreds.

Other features of MEN 2B

The characteristic phenotype of marfanoid habitus and mucosal neuromata (Fig. 2) identifies affected individuals and allows early intervention. Neuromata are commonly ocular and oral, causing whitish-yellow or pink nodules on the anterior aspect of the tongue, lips, and eyelids, with thickening of the mucosa and often eversion of the lower lids. The nasal bridge may be broadened, pedunculated neuromata are found on cheek mucosa, and the corneal nerves are thickened and medullated. Involvement of peripheral motor and sensory nerves can cause a peroneal muscular atrophy type picture. Intestinal ganglioneuromatosis affects about 75 per cent of cases. Neuromata involve the autonomic nerves of both the myenteric and submucosal plexi and can cause poor suckling with failure to thrive, altered bowel habit, recurrent pseudo-obstruction, toxic megacolon, and occasionally dysphagia and vomiting, possibly due to achalasia. Almost all patients have a marfanoid habitus, usually associated with skeletal abnormalities, particularly slipped femoral epiphyses. Delayed puberty is the other common feature of the syndrome.

Screening

The screening investigations are a pentagastrin stimulation test, measurement of 24-h urinary metanephrines and catecholamines, and of plasma calcium. Screening should commence at the age of 3 years and continue annually until the age of 35 after which it can be performed less frequently. Urinary metanephrines and catecholamines identify at least 95 per cent of phaeochromocytomas. Genetic linkage analysis has 98–99 per cent predictive accuracy, and in individuals identified as at low risk less frequent screening is reasonable. In families in whom a mutation has been characterized affected individuals can be identified by mutation screening.

Other syndromes associated with endocrine neoplasia

There are other syndromes which overlap with the MEN syndromes. Phaeochromocytomata may be associated with pancreatic islet-cell tumours alone, or in combination with other syndromes: von Hippel–Lindau syndrome is associated with a high incidence of phaeochromocytomata, islet-cell tumours, cerebellar haemangioblastomata, retinal angiomata, and renal cell carcinoma; neurofibromatosis type I (von Recklinghausen's syndrome) is often associated with phaeochromocytoma and, rarely, with duodenal somatostatinoma and medullary thyroid carcinoma; and phaeochromocytoma may be associated with prolactinoma as a mixed MEN syndrome.

Further reading

Trump, D., Farren, B., Woodrug, C., *et al.* (1996). Clinical studies of multiple endocrine neoplasia type I (MEN 1). *Quarterly Journal of Medicine*, 89, 653–69.

Chapter 7.16

Endocrine manifestations of non-endocrine disease

J. A. H. Wass

A number of different endocrine syndromes may develop in association with diseases that are not primarily disorders of an endocrine gland. In most instances the cause is a tumour, usually but not invariably malignant, that develops in tissue not normally the site of the particular hormone synthesized.

Many different hormones can be secreted ectopically by neoplasms arising in a variety of organs, notably the bronchus, breast, pancreas, kidney, thyroid, thymus, ovary, as well as in mesenchymal tissue. Although a particular endocrinopathy may be associated with a specific type of tumour in a particular organ, such a relationship is not invariable. Indeed, many neoplasms elaborate more than one hormonal substance at the same or at different times, and thus may produce a mixed endocrine picture. Furthermore, the amount of ectopic hormone(s) produced may fluctuate from time to time (for example, cyclical Cushing's syndrome in ectopic ACTH secretion). Sometimes the changes induced by the ectopic hormone mimic very closely those found in the true endocrinopathy. In others the picture is less characteristic, for instance in ectopic ACTH production by small cell lung cancer when the course of the illness may be too rapid for the classical features of Cushing's syndrome to develop, and hypokalaemic alkalosis with diabetes mellitus predominates.

The amino acid sequences of hormones of ectopic origin generally resemble closely those of their normally occurring counterparts (except parathyroid hormone (PTH) and parathyroid hormone related protein PTHrP), but there is a tendency for a greater proportion of higher molecular weight precursors, or subunits and fragments, to be associated with an ectopic origin.

Prevalence

Clinical syndromes are less common than biochemical or hormonal abnormalities. The prevalence of ectopic production of ACTH, corticotrophin-releasing hormone (CRH), (PTHrP), calcitonin, human chorionic gonadotrophin (HCG), prolactin, or growth hormone, without clinical manifestations, is high when extensive assays are applied to patients with cancer.

Hypercalcaemia in the absence of detectable bony metastases due to PTHrP is the most common abnormality. It occurs in about 15 per cent of patients with squamous cell carcinoma, usually of the bronchus, and carcinoma of the kidney, breast, or ovary. The syndrome of inappropriate antidiuresis (SIAD), associated with a small cell lung cancer is reported in 40 per cent of such cases. Cushing's syndrome due to ectopic ACTH or CRH secretion occurs in about 5 per cent of patients with small cell lung cancer, and in association with other neoplasms. Biochemical accompaniments of Cushing's syndrome in the absence of the clinical features are much more common, occurring in 50 per cent of patients with small cell lung cancer.

Pathogenesis

A variety of hypotheses for ectopic hormone synthesis and secretion have been made. None explains all of the observed facts. All cells inherit an identical complement of DNA, and have all the coded information required for the synthesis of all proteins and peptides. The normal inability of non-endocrine tissue to synthesize hormones is ascribed to 'repressors' that mask specific segments of the DNA molecule. It is possible that when a cell becomes malignant this repression becomes ineffective, allowing the unmasked DNA to synthesize proteins or peptides 'foreign' to the cell concerned. Such a 'de-repression' hypothesis does not explain why certain tumours are more prone to secrete particular ectopic hormones. Another hypothesis suggests that there are a small number of special proliferative cells in normal mature tissues that have fetal characteristics with the ability to produce peptide hormones—a process of 'dysdifferentiation' rather than 'de-repression'. The role of oncogenes in modulating this expression remains to be clarified.

Hypercalcaemia without osseous metastases

PTHrP is the cause of tumour-associated hypercalcaemia in a large number of patients. It shares homology between positions 2 and 13 of the 84 residues of PTH, and acts on PTH receptors to increase bone resorption and decrease renal excretion of calcium. The gene is located on the short arm of chromosome 12; that of PTH is on chromosome 11. PTHrP is made by squamous carcinomata as well as renal, bladder, ovary, breast, pancreas, and skin carcinomata and lymphomata. Two-site immunoradiometric assays of PTH which detect the whole molecule show high levels in primary hyperparathyroidism and low ones in patients with excessive PTHrP secretion.

Other factors can be involved in hypercalcaemia unassociated with osseous metastases. 1,25-Dihydroxy vitamin D_3 is not uncommonly made by lymphoproliferative tumours, which are either high grade or widely disseminated. Transforming growth factor α (TGFα), which stimulates osteoclastic bone resorption, is also made by squamous carcinoma, renal and breast carcinomata. Some tumours co-secrete both TGFα and PTHrP. Interleukin-1, which is a very powerful stimulator of osteoclastic bone resorption, is also made by squamous carcinomata as well as some haematological malignancies. Tumour necrosis factor (TNF) and lymphotoxin also stimulate osteoclastic bone resorption. These related cytokines cause hypercalcaemia *in vivo*, and lymphotoxin is produced by cultured myeloma cells *in vitro* and accounts for the hypercalcaemia seen in this condition. Prostaglandins of the E series have also been implicated in the process of hypercalcaemia, particularly in breast cancer, but they are an uncommon cause of it.

Syndrome of inappropriate antidiuresis (SIAD)

This syndrome, is usually, but not invariably, associated with high levels of circulating arginine vasopressin. Other, as yet unidentified, antidiuretic substances are sometimes involved. Diagnostic criteria and management are described in Chapter 7.2.

Ectopic ACTH secretion

Pro-opiomelanocortin (POMC) is a 31 kDa precursor for both ACTH and β-lipotrophin as well as of other polypeptides derived from it, including γ-lipotrophin and β-endorphin. A variety of non-pituitary tumours are capable of secreting POMC-derived peptides accounting for between 15 and 20 per cent of patients with Cushing's syndrome. Approximately 50 per cent of these ectopic ACTH-producing tumours are in the lung and the rest are present in a variety of other tissues (Table 1). Some tumours, particularly pancreatic islet cell tumours which are seldom (< 5 per cent) associated with Cushing's syndrome, can, in addition to ACTH, also secrete a number of other hormones, including insulin, gastrin, and glucagon (see Chapter 7.15). This accounts for the usefulness, when screening for ectopic ACTH, of measuring tumour markers, other hormones, or compounds which may be co-secreted, the presence of which raises the suspicion of an ectopic hormone-secreting tumour. Very rarely, CRH is secreted ectopically in association with ACTH.

Table 1 Types of neoplasm causing ectopic POMC (ACTH) secretion

Small cell carcinoma of the bronchus
Bronchial carcinoid
Thymic carcinoid
Islet cell pancreatic tumour
Phaeochromocytoma
Medullary carcinoma of the thyroid

Table 2 Response to tests used to differentiate ectopic ACTH secretion from Cushing's disease

	Ectopic ACTH (% of cases)	Cushing's disease (% of cases)
Hypokalaemia < 3.2 mmol/l	100	10
Diabetes mellitus	78	38
Dexamethasone 8 mg/day (no suppression)	89	22
No response to metyrapone	50	36
CRH test excessive		
response	0	> 90

For source see OTM3, p. 1713.

Presentation

In patients with small cell lung cancer who have a rapidly progressive tumour, the physical features of Cushing's syndrome may not have time to develop. The major features are weight loss, proximal muscular weakness, polyuria, thirst, oedema, carbohydrate intolerance, and sometimes pigmentation. Hypokalaemic alkalosis is characteristic and in part due to the very high cortisol levels. Corticosterone and 11-deoxycorticosterone may also be produced in excess. The 11β-hydroxysteroid dehydrogenase enzyme may also function abnormally, causing decreased renal inactivation of cortisol and corticosterone. The serum cortisol level is usually greatly elevated (> 1000 nmol/l). The plasma ACTH level is also raised (> 200 μg/l) beyond the levels seen in pituitary-dependent Cushing's disease.

When the ectopic sources are other than a small cell lung cancer, the clinical picture may be quite indistinguishable from Cushing's disease, the features of which may antedate by months or years any evidence of a tumour. The degree of elevation of ACTH is less marked than with small cell lung cancer and is proportional to tumour size. Some carcinoid tumours may be small and difficult to locate. The real problem is to differentiate ectopic ACTH secretion from pituitary-dependent disease (Table 2). Hypokalaemic alkalosis (< 3.2 mmol/l) remains the most useful test in the differential diagnosis. High-dose dexamethasone (8 mg/day, 2 mg 6 hourly for 2 days) is useful, but the metyrapone test is not. CRH may be used as a stimulation test; the response is flat in ectopic ACTH secretion and exaggerated in most patients with pituitary-dependent disease. CT of the chest or abdomen will often reveal the source of ectopic secretion. If not, selective venous catheterization and sampling may help. The presence of other tumour markers, for example hCG, calcitonin, and alpha-fetoprotein, may also suggest an ectopic source of ACTH.

Treatment

Removal of the primary growth or its control with radiotherapy or chemotherapy will relieve the endocrine manifestations. A relapse may occur if metastases develop. When it proves impossible to control a primary tumour, adrenocortical hypersecretion may be reduced by metyrapone (500–4000 mg daily). Aminoglutethimide (1000–1500 mg/day) may also be used, but frequently causes a skin rash. Ketoconazole (400–800 mg/day), which can cause fatal liver damage, and op-DDD are also useful. RU-486, a glucocorticoid antagonist at the receptor level, has been used as palliative therapy for some patients (10–30 mg/kg/day). Octreotide (0.3 mg subcutaneously/day), has also been used in the treatment of ectopic ACTH syndrome associated with metastatic gastrin-secreting pancreatic islet cell carcinoma.

Bilateral adrenalectomy, optimally done laparoscopically, is an alternative approach, but frequently it is not practical for patients with rapidly progressive metastatic disease. It may be possible to embolize the arterial supply of the adrenal gland if patients are not suitable surgical candidates for adrenalectomy.

Hypoglycaemia

Malignant tumours not derived from pancreatic islet cells may be associated with hypoglycaemia. Usually the tumour is large and of mesenchymal origin, arising in the abdomen or thorax. Histology shows a mesothelioma, a fibrosarcoma, or other sarcoma such as a leiomyosarcoma. Other neoplasms associated with hypoglycaemia are haemangiopericytoma, hepatoma, adrenal carcinoma, lung carcinoma, Wilms' tumour, and colonic carcinoma. The cause of hypoglycaemia is insulin-like growth factor II (IGF-II). Circulating IGF-II levels are usually normal, but there is an increase in the large molecular weight (10–15 kDa) molecules. The matter is discussed further in Chapter 6.14.

Ectopic chorionic gonadotrophin secretion (Table 3)

In normal circumstances hCG circulates only during pregnancy, arising from the syncytiotrophoblast. The excess is usually clinically silent. In the first decade of life, ectopic hCG production may cause isosexual precocious puberty in boys with hepatoblastoma. Intracranial teratoma, choriocarcinoma, and pinealoma are also associated with ectopic hCG secretion. In men this may be associated with gynaecomastia. In some this is due to co-secretion of oestrogen which may, in women, be associated with dysfunctional uterine bleeding.

hCG is a useful tumour marker in gestational trophoblastic disease (choriocarcinoma) and in some men with testicular tumours, giving an early warning of recurrent disease. In some patients, most commonly with choriocarcinoma and massive elevation of hCG, the latter, through its weak thyroid stimulating hormone (TSH) activity may cause goitre and mild hyperthyroidsim. This most frequently occurs in women and is not associated with eye signs.

Ectopic human placental lactogen

Human placental lactogen (hPL), also called human chorionic somatomammotropin (hCS), is a trophoblastic hormone not normally produced. It may be secreted ectopically, often together with oestradiol

Table 3 hCG in sera of patients with malignant tumours

Tissue	Percentage of cases with ectopic secretion of hCG
Breast	21
Lung	10
Gastrointestinal tract	18
Pancreas (more commonly hCG-α)	33
Stomach	22
Liver	21
Small intestine	13
Large intestine	12
Biliary tract	11
Ovary (adenocarcinoma)	40
Testis	62
Seminoma	38
Embryonal cell carcinoma	58
Choriocarcinoma	100
Mixed	73

For source see OTM3, p. 1715.

and hCG, most commonly in association with lung tumours. It is associated with gynaecomastia in men.

Extrapituitary acromegaly and diseases associated with abnormal growth hormone secretion

Less than 2 per cent of patients with acromegaly have ectopic growth hormone releasing hormone (GHRH) production. Besides the pancreas, lung carcinoid tumours, small cell lung cancer, and phaeochromocytoma may produce GHRH ectopically and cause acromegaly by stimulation of the pituitary somatotrophs to produce hyperplasia. These tumours are usually clinically apparent and GHRH levels in the circulation are elevated. GHRH can also be secreted by hypothalamic hamartomas, and cause pituitary somatotroph hyperplasia.

In McCune–Albright syndrome, polyostotic fibrous dysplasia of bone occurs in association with gonadotrophin-independent sexual precocity and growth hormone and prolactin secreting pituitary adenomas, autonomous adrenal hypercortisolism, and primary hyperthyroidism (see Chapter 7.6).

Ectopic growth hormone secretion has been reported in patients with bronchial, pancreatic, and gastrointestinal carcinoma. Breast carcinoma and ovarian tumours may also occasionally secrete growth hormone, but without clinical manifestations.

Ectopic prolactin secretion

Prolactin may be secreted by bronchial carcinoma and renal cell carcinoma; the usual endocrine manifestation is galactorrhoea. Difficulties in diagnosis may arise unless the underlying tumour is obvious. In most instances the hyperprolactinaemia will be attributed to a prolactin-secreting adenoma, but suspicion of an ectopic source should arise when the prolactin level is not lowered by bromocriptine treatment.

Ectopic calcitonin secretion

Increased serum calcitonin levels are encountered in a variety of cancers apart from medullary carcinoma of the thyroid. The most common of these are small cell lung cancer, leukaemia, and neoplasms of the breast and pancreas. Ectopic calcitonin may differ from the normal hormone in having more high molecular weight components; it does not cause symptoms and does not produce hypocalcaemia.

Ectopic renin secretion

Ectopic secretion of renin has been described in association with cancer of the lung, pancreas, and ovary. The clinical picture is usually dominated by the underlying neoplasm, but the patient has hypertension and hypokalaemia. When the underlying cause cannot be eradicated, the use of an ACE inhibitor will control the hypertension.

Ectopic aldosterone secretion

Hypertension and hypokalaemia related to ectopic secretion of aldosterone from a non-adrenal neoplasm have been described in patients with ovarian tumours. The aberrant production of a steroid rather than a peptide is presumably due to biochemical change in the ovarian steroidogenic cells. Attention is likely to be focused on a suspected lesion of the adrenal zona glomerulosa because the hyperaldosteronism is associated with low plasma renin activity. The ovarian lesion may initially be clinically silent and only revealed by pelvic ultrasonography.

Further reading

Bishop, A.E. and Polak, J.M. (1996). Gastrointestinal endocrine tumours. Pathology. *Baillière's Clinical Endocrinology and Metabolism* **10**(4), 555–69.

Guise, T.A. (1997). Parathyroid hormone-related protein and bone metastases. *Cancer* **80**(8 Suppl.), 1572–80.

Miller, M. (1997). Inappropriate antidiuretic hormone secretion. *Current Therapy in Endocrinology and Metabolism* **6**, 206–9.

Sharma, O.P. (1996). Vitamin D, calcium, and sarcoidosis. *Chest* **109**, 535–9.

Section 8
Nutrition

Contents

Chapter 8.1

Nutrition requirements

R. Smith and W. P. T James

It is not easy to calculate the amounts of all nutrients needed to maintain optimum function. Committees have produced reports that estimate the average nutrient requirement of healthy children of different ages and for adults. These estimates tend to be somewhat conservative and their derivation is often quite complex.

The reasons why some people have a greater need for nutrients than others are unclear, but presumably include genetic factors. The range of needs in a healthy population can be estimated by a variety of techniques. These assess the intake needed to keep the body's stores, biochemical function, or cellular saturation with a nutrient (such as a vitamin) at a maximum. The criteria of adequacy therefore vary and there can be much debate as to the most appropriate index for specifying a 'healthy' level for the intake of a vitamin or mineral. Requirements will also vary for dietary reasons, for instance intake of inhibitors of absorption, for physiological reasons, e.g. growth or pregnancy, and for others such as illness. It may be necessary to specify all these before one can obtain a reasonable estimate of a patient's true need.

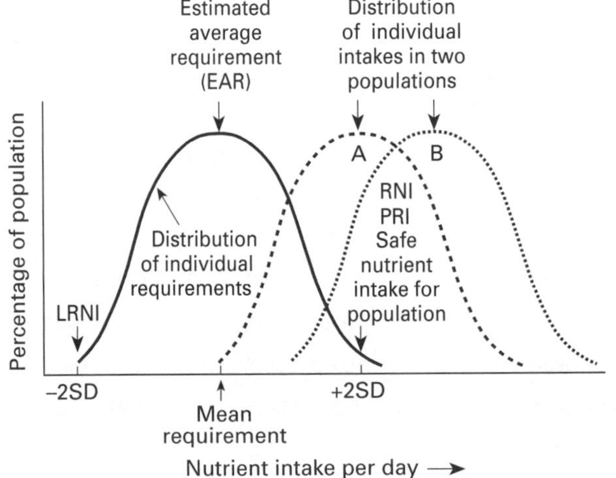

Fig. 1 Assessing the probability of nutrient deficiency. Note that the average requirement of energy is the value taken to estimate a group's energy needs. This differs from all other nutrients, where an allowance for the 2 SD range of individual need is estimated before specifying the 'safe intake' or 'reference nutrient intake' (RNI). LNRI, lower reference nutrient intake (UK); RNI, reference nutrient intake (UK); PRI, population reference intake (EU).

Examples of increased needs include: an increase for vitamin A in measles; of vitamin D in people on high cereal diets; of vitamin C in smokers; of folate supplements before conception and in early pregnancy to avoid neural tube defects; of zinc supplementation in severe diarrhoea and additional iron in many situations to prevent anaemia, and for optimal development of the infant brain.

The United Kingdom Department of Health published revised dietary reference values (**DRVs**) in 1991. The range of intakes were based on an assessment of the distribution of requirements for each nutrient. Figure 1 provides an illustration of the relationship between these estimated requirements of healthy individuals and the observed nutrient intakes in two populations. The upper limit of a population's needs is calculated as the mean + 2 SD, as this covers the estimated needs of 97 per cent of the population. This reference nutrient intake (**RNI**) is also considered the 'safe intake'; below this an increasing proportion of the population is at risk of deficiency. The European Union estimates have a different nomenclature. The average adult male requirement rather than the population reference intake (**PRI**; Fig. 1) is proposed for labelling foods. Thus when a portion of cereal is described as providing 30 per cent of the recommended dietary allowances, this meant 30 per cent of the *estimated upper limit* of the adult male's needs, but will now become 30 per cent of the *average* healthy males' requirement.

Tables 1 and 2 specify the reference nutrient intakes of vitamins and minerals for healthy people. In Fig. 1, population A is not particularly well fed, as about half are eating less than the RNI. Those individuals with low constitutional needs for a particular nutrient will remain healthy, but those with a high requirement will be inadequately fed. In the absence of known individual requirements, everybody with an intake below the RNI is considered to be at risk. Population B, on the other hand, is rather better off, with about

Table 1 Reference nutrient intakes for vitamins in adolescents and adults

Age	Thiamine	Riboflavine	Niacin[d]	Vitamin B_6[e]	Vitamin B_{12}	Folate	Vitamin C	Vitamin A	Vitamin D
Males									
11–50 years	0.9–1.0	1.2–1.3	15–17	1.2–1.4	1.2–1.5	200	35–40	600–700	[b]
Females									
11–50+ years	0.7–0.8	1.1	12–14	1.0–1.2	200	35–40	600	[b]	
Pregnancy	+0.1[c]	+0.3	[a]	[a]	[a]	+100	+10	+100	10
Lactation									
0–4 months	+0.2	+0.5	+2	[a]	+0.5	+60	+30	+350	10
4+ months	+0.2	+0.5	+2	[a]	+0.5	+60	+30	+350	10

[a] No increment.

[b] After age 65 the RNI is 10 mg/day for men and women.

[c] For last trimester only.

[dc]Nicotinic acid equivalent.

[e] Based on protein providing 14.7 per cent of estimated average requirement (**EAR**) for energy.

Table 2 Reference nutrient intakes for minerals in adolescents and adults (mg/day)

Age	Ca	P[b]	Mg	Na[c]	K[d]	Cl[e]	Fe	Zn	Cu	Se	I
Males											
11–50 years	1000–700	775–550	280–300	1600	3100–3500	2500	11.3–8.7	9.0–9.5	0.8–1.2	45–75	130–140
Females											
11–50 years	800–700	625–550	280–270	1600	3100–3500	2500	14.8[f]–8.7	9.0–7.0	0.8–1.2	45–60	130–140
Pregnancy	a	a	a	a	a	a	a	a	a	a	a
Lactation											
0–4 months	+550	+440	+50	a	a	a	a	+6.0	+0.3	+15	a
4+ months	+550	+440	+50	a	a	a	a	+2.5	+0.3	+15	a

[a] No increment.

[b] Phosphorus RNI is set equal to calcium in molar terms.

[c] 1 mmol sodium = 23 mg.

[d] 1 mmol potassium = 39 mg.

[e] Corresponds to sodium 1 mmol = 35.5 mg.

[f] Insufficient for women with high menstrual losses where the most practical way of meeting iron requirements is to take iron supplements.

Table 3 Reference nutrient intakes for protein in adolescents and adults

Age	Reference nutrient intake[a] (g/day)
Males	
11–14 years	42.1
15–18 years	55.2
19–50 years	55.5
50+ years	53.3
Females:	
11–14 years	41.2
15–18 years	45.0
19–50 years	45.0
50+ years	46.5
Pregnancy[c]	+6
Lactation[c]	
0–4 months	+11
4+ months	+8

[a]These figures, based on egg and milk protein, assume complete digestibility.

[b]No values for infants 0–3 months are given by WHO. The RNI is calculated from the recommendations of COMA.

[c]To be added to adult requirement through all stages of pregnancy and lactation.

15 per cent of the population at risk. Many of the intakes proposed in Tables 1 and 2 are based on the concepts depicted in Fig. 1, but often the information on the range of individual need is scanty.

Table 3 gives the RNI for protein. In pregnancy and lactation additions are specified to compensate for the growth of the fetus and allow adequate breast-milk production. Energy requirements are different from other nutritional requirements because no allowance can be made for the 2 SD range shown in Fig. 1. If all people were fed to intakes at the highest level (i.e. 2 SD of the full range) almost all would gain weight, whereas if all were fed the *average* some would gain weight, some lose, and some remain stable. Recommendations are therefore set as the average of energy requirements for any population and these are given in Table 4. An estimate of adult energy needs may be made by calculating the likely basal metabolic rate (BMR) for age, weight, and sex as in Table 5. This rate can then be multiplied by a simple factor to allow for varying levels of physical activity as shown in Table 6. For example, the BMR of a 25-year-old male weighing 65 kg would be: $(65 \times 0.063) + 2.896 = 6.99$ MJ/day (from Table 5). If this young man works in an office with only light activity, but is moderately active in his non-working h, then his average energy requirement would be: $6.99 \times 1.5 = 10.485$ MJ/day (from Table 6). Energy needs decline with age and inactivity.

Table 4 Estimated average requirements (**EARs**) for energy in adolescents and adults

Age	EARs (MJ/day (kcal/day))	
	Males	Females
11–14 years	9.27 (2220)	7.92 (1845)
15–18 years	11.51 (2755)	8.83 (2110)
19–50 years	10.60 (2550)	8.10 (1940)
51–59 years	10.60 (2550)	8.00 (1900)
60–64 years	9.93 (2380)	7.99 (1900)
65–74 years	9.71 (2330)	7.96 (1900)
75+ years	8.77 (2100)	7.61 (1810)
Pregnancy		+0.80 (200)[a]
Lactation		
1 month		+1.90 (450)
2 months		+2.20 (530)
3 months		+2.40 (570)
4–6 months (group 1)[b]		+2.00 (480)
4–6 months (group 2)[c]		+2.40 (570)
>6 months (group 1)		+1.00 (240)
>6 months (group 2)		+2.30 (550)

[a]Last trimester only.

[b]Exclusive breast-feeding for 3–4 months followed by active weaning.

[c]Breast-feeding primary source of nourishment for 6 months or more. Limited complementary feeds after 3–4 months.

Table 5 Equations for the prediction of basal metabolic rate (Department of Health 1991)

	Age range (years)	Prediction equation BMR (MJ/day) per kg body weight	95% confidence limits (MJ/day)
Males	10–17	0.074 (wt) + 2.754	±0.88
	18–29	0.063 (wt) + 2.896	±1.28
	30–59	0.048 (wt) + 3.653	±1.40
	60–74	0.0499 (wt) + 2.930	(N/A)
	75+	0.0350 (wt) + 3.434	(N/A)
Females	10–17	0.056 (wt) + 2.898	±0.94
	18–29	0.062 (wt) + 2.036	±1.00
	30–59	0.034 (wt) + 3.538	±0.94
	60–74	0.0386 (wt) + 2.875	(N/A)
	75+	0.0410 (wt) + 2.610	(N/A)

N/A, not available.

Table 6 Basal metabolic rate multiples for light, moderate, and heavy activity

Non-occupational [[col1]]activity level	Occupational activity level					
	Light		Moderate		Heavy	
	M	F	M	F	M	F
Non-active	1.4	1.4	1.6	1.5	1.7	1.5
Moderatively active	1.5	1.5	1.7	1.6	1.8	1.6
Very active	1.6	1.6	1.8	1.7	1.9	1.7

Excess of nutrients

The concepts and tables set out above deal with the need to avoid a deficiency state. Excessive intakes other than of vitamins A or D are rarely considered a problem. For many nutrients adaptive mechanisms in the intestine tend to limit the effects of any dietary excess, e.g. of calcium or iron; water-soluble vitamins are readily excreted in the urine and excess protein can be metabolized readily. However, an excess intake of some other nutrients may be harmful if ingested for many months or years. What is needed to avoid problems that develop from high intakes of saturated fatty acids, *trans* fatty acids, sugar, or salt, is even more difficult to quantify than the reference values for vitamins or minerals. Table 7 shows the recommendations given by the UK Department of Health's *Dietary Reference Values* in 1991 for fats and carbohydrates.

Further reading

Department of Health (1991). *Dietary reference values for food energy and nutrients for the United Kingdom.* Report of the panel on Dietary Reference Values of the Committee on Medical Aspects of Food Policy; Report on Health and Social Subjects, 41. HMSO London.

Garrow, J. and James, W.P.T. *Human nutrition and dietetics,* (9th edn). Churchill Livingstone, Edinburgh.

World Health Organisation (1990). *Diet, nutrition and the prevention of chronic diseases.* Report of the WHO Study Group, Technical Report Series 797. World Health Organisation, Geneva.

Table 7 Dietary reference values for fat and carbohydrate for adults as a percentage of daily total energy intake (percentage of food energy)

	Individual minimum	Population average	Individual maximum
Saturated fatty acids		10 (11)	
cis-Polyunsaturated fatty acids	6 (6.5)	10	
n-3	0.2		
n-6	1.0		
cis-Monosaturated fatty acids		12 (13)	
trans Fatty acids		2 (2)	
Total fatty acids		30 (32.5)	
Total fat		33 (35)	
Non-milk extrinsic sugars	0	10 (11)	
Intrinsic and milk sugars and starch		37 (39)	
Total carbohydrate		47 (50)	
Non-starch polysaccharide	12	18	24

The average percentage contribution to total energy does not total 100 per cent because figures for protein and alcohol are excluded. Protein intakes average 15 per cent of total energy. Many individuals will derive some energy from alcohol, and this has been assumed to average 5 per cent. Average figures are given as percentages both of total energy and, in parentheses, of food energy.

Chapter 8.2

Severe malnutrition

M. H. N. Golden

Introduction

Nutritional state often critically alters the expression and course of disease as well as its response to treatment. Indeed, malnutrition often accompanies disease, which is the major reason for morbidity and mortality. Up to half of all patients admitted to hospital suffer from some degree of malnutrition.

Primary malnutrition is seen most frequently in the young child, the elderly, and particular groups such as prisoners and the mentally subnormal. Secondary malnutrition accompanies any disease which disturbs appetite, digestion, absorption, or utilization of nutrients. In poor countries malnutrition-associated disease is the major cause of death; it stunts the physical and mental development of the majority of the population. In more advanced societies it accompanies a wide variety of social, psychiatric, medical, and surgical conditions. Slight dementia, grief, physical frailty, deterioration of eyesight, hearing, or teeth, social isolation, and the degenerative diseases combine to make malnutrition common in the elderly.

The term protein energy malnutrition has been used to cover a number of clinical conditions in both adults and children. These include failure to thrive, marasmus, cachexia, phthisis, nutritional dwarfism, kwashiorkor, and nutritional or famine oedema. The large number of terms used reflects emphasis on particular clinical features. Notwithstanding the clinical differences, most of the physiological, biochemical, and body compositional features are common to all varieties of malnutrition. The term protein energy malnutrition is best avoided; it carries the false implication that protein and/or energy deficiencies are the direct cause of all the conditions grouped under this rubric. Aetiologically neutral terms such as undernutrition or malnutrition, qualified as necessary, are more appropriate.

Nature of nutritional deficiency

If a growing animal is given a diet devoid of iron, there is an initial consumption of stores followed by clinical signs characteristic of iron deficiency: the concentration of iron in the tissues is markedly reduced, but there is no effect on growth or body weight. If such an animal is given a diet devoid of zinc there is an immediate cessation of growth and then loss of weight. After death from zinc deficiency, the concentration of zinc in the major tissues is normal; the animal has died from a nutrient deficiency without any direct evidence of depletion of the nutrient. This may appear confusing. However, in both iron and zinc deficiency the total amount of each within the body is less than normal, but in the case of iron the reduced amount is contained within a normally sized body whereas in the case of zinc the body size has contracted and hence the concentration is maintained. There is clearly a fundamental difference between these two responses to deprivation of a single nutrient. Most nutrients can be classified into those that give an iron-like (type I) or a zinc-like (type II) response (Table 1). The characteristics of the two types of deficiency are summarized in Table 2.

Table 1 Classification of nutrients according to whether the response to a deficiency is a reduced concentration in the tissues (type I) or a reduced growth rate (type II)

Type I	Type II
Selenium	Nitrogen
Iodine	Sulphur
Iron	Essential amino acids
Copper	Potassium
Calcium	Sodium
Manganese	Magnesium
Thiamine	Zinc
Riboflavin	Phosphorus
Ascorbic acid	Water
Retinol	
Tocopherol	
Calciferol	
Folic acid	
Cobalamin	
Pyridoxine	

Table 2 Characteristics of the two types of nutritional deficiency

Type I	Type II
Tissue level variable	Tissue level fixed
Used in specific pathways	Ubiquitously used
Characteristic physical signs	No characteristic signs
Late or no growth response	Immediate growth response
Stored in body	No body store
Buffered response	Responds to daily input
Not interdependent	Control each other's balance
Little excretory control	Sensitive physiological control

Type I deficiency

Most physicians consider deficiency of an essential nutrient in terms of a type I deficiency. The diet is deficient; with the low intake there is a reduction in the tissue concentration; the dependent metabolic pathways are compromised, giving rise to characteristic clinical signs and symptoms. The diagnosis is straightforward and can be achieved by measuring the concentration of the nutrient in a suitable tissue, testing the appropriate metabolic pathway, and demonstrating the effect of replacing the nutrient.

Type II deficiency

The position with respect to the type II nutrients is quite different giving rise to both conceptual and practical difficulties in the understanding, definition, diagnosis, and treatment of these deficiencies.

Type II nutrients are the building blocks of tissues which cannot be sustained without their necessary complement. A deficiency of any one of them results in catabolism of the tissue and loss of all its components. Resynthesis can only take place in the presence of adequate amounts of all components. Such nutrients are interdependent. They have characteristic ratios that vary over quite a narrow range and are required in the diet in approximately the same ratios as they occur in the body.

An understanding of these particular nutrients is integral to the problem of malnutrition.

1. The response to a deficiency (growth failure with a mild deficiency and weight loss with more profound deficiency) is the same for each type II nutrient. Therefore, nutritional growth failure or weight loss *per se* cannot identify which particular nutrient is lacking. The response to a prolonged mild deficiency of any of the type II nutrients is stunting. Acute deficiency leads to tissue loss and wasting. Mild chronic deficiencies are more common than severe acute deficiencies, so that stunting is more common than wasting. About half the world population of children are stunted whereas only 5–10 per cent are wasted.
2. Because whole tissues are being broken down, all other nutrients which are in excess relative to the deficient nutrient must be metabolized and excreted; they are not stored. Thus the balance between the various type II nutrients in the diet is important, as a deficiency in any one of them results in a negative balance for all of them. For example, if potassium is omitted from a parenteral feeding regimen, the patient will lose nitrogen, zinc, phosphorus, and magnesium; but type I nutrients, such as calcium, will not necessarily be in negative balance.
3. If the diet is deficient in any type II nutrient, mechanisms to conserve that nutrient are activated avidly. Thus it is difficult to demonstrate signs of such a deficiency in the non-growing animal

by dietary means alone; usually there must be a coincident pathological loss of the nutrient (for example, diarrhoea or renal disease). For this reason the rate of weight gain is the major determinant of the dietary requirement of a type II nutrient. For example, children given a diet providing just enough energy for them to maintain body weight, without growing, are able to remain in zinc balance and maintain plasma zinc concentration with an intake of only 1.3 mmol Zn/kg per day. When the same children are gaining weight rapidly, their plasma zinc concentration falls precipitously despite a 10-fold increase in the amount of zinc consumed (14 mmol Zn/kg per day); at this level, the zinc supply limits lean tissue synthesis. No other sign, apart from growth failure and weight loss, is expected from a deficiency of one of these nutrients, unless the deficiency is very profound. There is an apparent paradox in that a diet which has a sufficiently low concentration of a type II nutrient to give clinical signs other than growth failure will affect the elderly first, then adults, and finally children. This is a consequence of the higher energy requirement of the child. The protein requirement of a child for the maintenance of body weight is about the same as that for an adult (0.6 g/kg per day); however, the maintenance energy requirement for the child is about 400 kJ/kg per day while that for the adult is about 160 kJ/kg per day. Hence an adult must have a diet which supplies 6 per cent of the energy as protein to maintain body weight, whereas a child only requires about 2.4 per cent of the energy as protein if he or she is not gaining weight. Therefore, type II deficiency in children is expected to cause growth failure only, unless the child has a disease which causes a pathological loss of the nutrient.

4. As growth rate is the major determinant of the requirement for type II nutrients, a 'catch-up' effect might be expected as a result of restoration of an adequate intake which could be used as a diagnostic test. This does not necessarily happen. The initial deficiency will result in loss of all the type II nutrients, irrespective of which caused the original problem. Therefore, a catch-up response to the supply of only the deficient nutrient will be transient.
5. Common to a deficiency of each type II nutrient is anorexia, which is related to the relative surfeit of other nutrients, particularly amino acids which need to be metabolized and excreted to prevent toxicity. Data on specific dietary intake cannot be interpreted without intervention because a large or small intake may be caused by a deficiency of a nutrient which is not being considered. Conceptually, refusal to eat a diet which leads to disordered metabolism makes sense; there is then a metabolic preference for consumption of one's own tissues to satisfy nutritional demands. This strategy may in the short term restore metabolic balance, but in the longer term leads to severe malnutrition. As growth will be limited by intake of the most deficient nutrient, it is only possible to have an effective 'deficiency' with one type II nutrient at a time—the limiting nutrient. The other nutrients develop a deficit, but this is silent and there is no positive response to any of them. When a dietary supplement is given, which does not contain all the nutrients required for new tissue synthesis, the rate of growth will be determined by the most limiting nutrient in the new diet, not in the original diet or in a supplement alone. Indeed, an incomplete supplement can make a deficiency worse by diluting the original diet.

Table 3 Classification of malnutrition in adults by body mass index (BMI)

BMI	
>20	Normal
18.5–20	Marginal
17–18.5	Mild malnutrition
16–17	Moderate malnutrition
<16	Severe malnutrition

6. Conventional techniques to try to make a diagnosis of deficiency of a specific type II nutrient, are likely to mislead. There is little point in performing a muscle biopsy and measuring concentrations because of the effects of the associated loss of whole tissue. If a change in the nutrient concentration is detected in the biopsy, that change is just as likely to be due to deficiency of another type II nutrient or a metabolic alteration unrelated to nutrition as to deficiency of the nutrient of concern.

The type II nutrients have always posed problems to clinicians and nutritionists because of difficulty in diagnosis. The non-specificity of weight loss and the lack of confirmatory tests of an inadequate intake have led these nutrients to be largely ignored and their importance to be grossly underestimated. As a group, their deficiency is responsible for malnutrition in half the world's children and to unrecognized problems of ill health in many others.

Classification of malnutrition

Any classification should have the practical use of either identifying those individuals who require intervention or examining the prevalence of malnutrition in a community. The system should identify those most at risk, should be simple, and should be accepted internationally.

Children

The various classifications (for example, Gomez, Wellcome and Waterlow) are discussed in OTM3, pp. 1280–1.

Adults

Body mass index

Stunting in adults usually represents chronic undernutrition in childhood. It is more useful to define an index of 'thinness'. The most useful measure is the body mass index, defined as weight (in kilograms) divided by the square of height (in metres). Table 3 gives values for defining adult grades of malnutrition. The same index is used to define grades of obesity.

Some sick adults cannot stand to have their height measured, and the measurement is not useful in those with kyphosis or scoliosis. Several proxy measures for height can be used. Although arm span is claimed to be equal to height, this is only valid in those about 1.6 m tall. Clinically, the most useful measurement is the demispan. This is measured as the distance from the middle of the sternal notch to the tip of the middle finger in the coronal plane. Both sides should be measured; if there is a discrepancy the measurements should be repeated before taking the longest demispan. Height (in metres) in both males and females can then be calculated from the formula Height $= 0.73\ (2 \times \text{demispan}) + 0.43$.

Table 4 Classification of adult malnutrition by mid upper arm circumference

Circumference (cm)	
Male	
≥23	Normal
<23	Malnourished
Female	
≥22	Normal
<22	Malnourished

Mid upper arm circumference

The mid upper arm circumference can be used to grade the degree of body wasting. Appropriate cut-off points are given in Table 4.

Clinical features

Severe malnutrition can broadly be divided into three clinical syndromes: marasmus, kwashiorkor, and nutritional dwarfism. They often coexist in the same individual and the clinical features frequently reflect a mixed picture.

Marasmus

The patient with classical marasmus has obviously lost weight, with prominent ribs, zygoma, and limb joints, gross loss of muscle mass, particularly from the limb girdles, and almost no subcutaneous fat. The skin, which is thin and atrophic, lies in redundant folds. The pinched look of the face gives the patient an 'old man' look.

Kwashiorkor

Typically, a child aged 1–2 years with fine friable discoloured hair develops a typical skin rash, oedema, and hepatomegaly. He is apathetic when undisturbed and irritable when picked up. Kwashiorkor develops abruptly. The history of swelling, loss of appetite, and mood change is of a few days only; sometimes there is a history of repeated bouts of swelling but this is uncommon.

Nutritional dwarfism

On casual observation the nutritional dwarf may appear perfectly normal. It is only when the age of the patient is known that the short stature becomes apparent. Dental development is less retarded than height, so that facial shape can be inappropriate for size.

Oedema

Pitting oedema is the *sine qua non* for making the diagnosis of kwashiorkor. The extent of sodium and water retention is variable. It is commonly 10–30 per cent of body weight but may reach 50 per cent in severe cases. The oedema is usually dependent and periorbital. Small accumulations may be found post mortem in the pericardium, pleura, and peritoneum, but large effusions are uncommon; if a serous effusion is present, the possibility of an associated condition such as tuberculosis should always be considered. Adults with kwashiorkor are more likely to have serous effusions. In severe cases the entire body and internal organs are oedematous.

Circulation

The retained sodium and water are not distributed evenly through the extracellular compartments. Depletion of the intravascular volume usually accompanies the enormous expansion of the interstitial space. This maldistribution give rise to the anomalous statement that an oedematous patient can be 'dehydrated'. This is incorrect, and the term 'hypovolaemic' should be used. The use of the word 'dehydration' has led physicians to treat these patients incorrectly with rehydration solutions. The hypovolaemia is a form of toxic shock and should be treated as such.

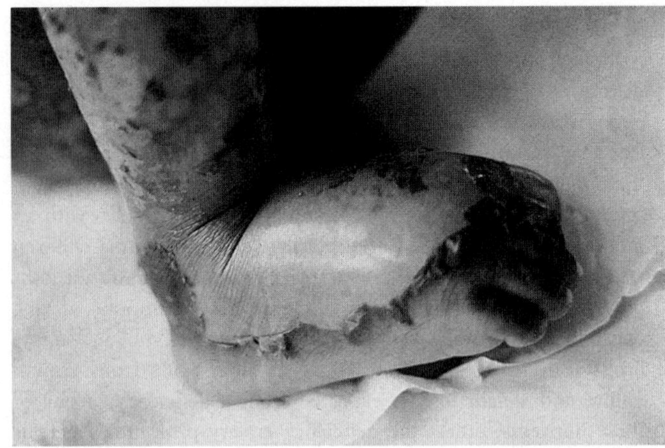

Fig. 1 Oedema and superficial skin stripping in a child with kwashiorkor.

Hepatomegaly

The liver may extend to the iliac brim; it is smooth, firm, and not usually tender. The enlargement is due to fat accumulation, mainly as triglyceride. Indications of liver dysfunction such as petechiae or very slight hyperbilirubinaemia are serious prognostic signs. Splenomegaly is very unusual in uncomplicated malnutrition: where it occurs it is likely to be associated with particular infections such as malaria, kala azar, or human immunodeficiency virus (HIV).

Anorexia

Loss of appetite is a common feature of all forms of severe malnutrition. The most probable underlying causes are infection, type II nutrient deficiency, and liver dysfunction, usually all three.

Mood and behaviour

Children have an altered affect. Classically they are apathetic when left alone and cry when they are picked up. When they cry, they emit a characteristic monotonous 'bleat' or loud groan rather than a normal 'bawl'.

A series of stereotyped self-stimulating repetitive movements are frequently displayed, typical of psychosocial deprivation and absent stimulation. One of the most damaging types of self-stimulating behaviour is rumination. When alone, the child regurgitates the last meal and then re-swallows it; inevitably some is lost. Ruminating children tend to be more alert.

Skin

In kwashiorkor there are a series of sequential changes, the appearance and progression of which are not unlike sunburn. These usually occur over the course of a few days. Often the different stages are present simultaneously in different parts of the body. The skin first becomes darker in colour, particularly over pressure areas and places exposed to minor trauma. The superficial dermal layers then dry like thin parchment and split when stretched to reveal pale areas between the cracks—crazy pavement dermatosis (Fig. 1). The dry cracked layer then peals off, leaving extremely thin hypopigmented skin. If it is gently pinched between the fingers numerous small wrinkles appear showing how thin and atrophic the epidermis is. The skin is very friable and ulcerates or macerates, particularly in the flexures, the perineum, and behind the ears. In severe cases it may appear as if the child has been burnt.

Atrophy of the skin in the perineum leads to severe napkin dermatitis, particularly in children or the elderly with diarrhoea or incontinence. The perineum should be left exposed to dry without napkins. Application of a barrier such as zinc and castor oil ointment, petroleum jelly, or paraffin gauze dressing (tulle gras) to raw areas helps to relieve pain and prevent infection. Management should be the same as that used for burns. In countries with limited resources the affected areas can be bathed in a dilute solution of 1 per cent potassium permanganate for 10–15 min daily; this dries the lesions and inhibits colonizing organisms. The zinc supplement contained in the diet may be insufficient in these patients, as zinc deficiency almost always accompanies severe skin lesions. These patients should always be given systemic antibiotics.

Hair

There is atrophy of the hair roots of the scalp, and the hair which is thin, straight, and lifeless can be plucked out easily and painlessly. Some patients go completely bald. In patients with naturally curly hair the curls may be lifted up by the new straight hair to give the appearance of trees with straight trunks and a canopy—the 'forest sign'. The hair may change colour to red, brown, grey, or blond. It may become banded (the flag sign) if there are successive bouts of malnutrition interspersed with periods of normal growth. Unlike the hair on the scalp, the eyelashes become long and luxuriant. There may also be excessive growth of lanugo hair. In adults pubic and axillary hair is lost and male patients need to shave less frequently.

Cheeks

Fullness of the cheeks, so-called jowls, is commonly associated with oedematous malnutrition. The cause is unknown; it is not usually due to parotid enlargement, although painless enlargement can occur, particularly in malnourished adults.

Gynaecomastia

Breast enlargement is particularly likely to occur in patients with gross hepatomegaly.

Bone

There is almost always an enlargement of the costochondral junctions giving a 'rickety rosary'. The cause may be related to abnormalities of vitamin D metabolism, or to vitamin C or copper deficiency. Harrison's sulci and other chest deformities from lung infections are quite common. Radiography always reveals marked osteopenia.

Abdominal swelling

The abdomen is usually protuberant. This is due to gas in the intestine rather than the enlarged liver. Frequently, the abdominal wall is sufficiently thin for peristalsis to be easily visible. Bowel sounds are high pitched and infrequent. In newly admitted patients there is often a succussion splash from the atonic bowel.

Other features

The tympanic membranes are white and thickened (tympanosclerosis). The tonsils are atrophic, and there is frequently oral

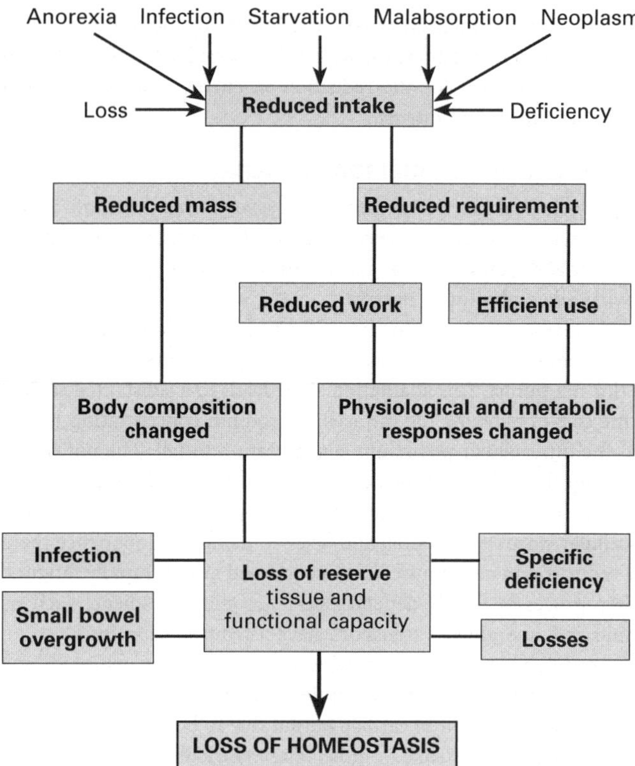

Fig. 2 Schema showing the changes that occur in severe malnutrition.

candidiasis. Angular stomatitis, lingual atrophy, follicular hyperkeratosis, eye signs characteristic of vitamin A deficiency, and other signs of specific type I nutrient deficiencies occur frequently.

Pathophysiology

The sequence of events that occur in any malnourished individual is illustrated in Fig. 2. The defects reinforce each other in a cyclical way. The initial reduction in dietary intake may be due to psychiatric illness, anorexia of any cause, infection, neoplasia, drug intoxication, type II nutrient deficiency, famine or starvation, upper intestinal disease, malabsorption, or other losses of nutrients from the body.

Reduced mass

The first effect of such a reduced intake is a reduction in body mass which forms the basis for the various anthropometric classifications of malnutrition.

Reduced requirement

As weight is lost, nutritional requirements are reduced; this can continue until a new equilibrium is established at a level where the lower intake becomes sufficient to sustain the reduced mass. There is also a relative reduction in requirement so that each gram of body tissue requires less energy. This component of the reduced requirement is substantial, and is achieved over weeks or months by metabolic adaptation. Ingested food is used more efficiently; for example a much higher proportion of the amino acids released from protein during tissue breakdown are reused to synthesize tissue instead of being oxidized. The mechanisms that conserve nutrients in the body are activated and biochemical pathways involving futile cycles are curtailed. The most important adaptation is in work performed by the tissues and in their enzymatic machinery. In the well-nourished there is an excess metabolic capacity; this is sacrificed in malnutrition and this is the basis for the reduction in energy requirements and functional capacity of organs.

Physiological and metabolic changes

No physiological function is 'normal' in severe undernutrition. Spontaneous physical activity is severely curtailed. No discretionary activity is performed; adults sit in a state of suspended animation, only moving when absolutely necessary.

A fundamental adaptation is slowing of the sodium pump. Normally, about one-third of basal energy requirements are consumed by this ion pump. This adaptation alone leads to a substantial saving, at the cost of allowing the intracellular sodium concentration to rise and the intracellular potassium concentration to fall. The potassium lost from the cell cannot be accommodated in the extracellular fluid and is excreted. Slowing of the sodium pump also leads to a reduction in cellular electrical potential and delay in its restoration; hence there is a reduction in neuromuscular function and muscle rapidly fatigues. Other processes which depend upon a sodium gradient, such as amino acid and glucose transport, have a reduced capacity.

A considerable saving in energy expenditure is also achieved by a reduction of about 40 per cent in the intensity of protein turnover.

There is a reduction in cardiac output due to both a lowered heart rate and a lowered stroke volume. The ventricular function curves (stroke work versus pressure) are altered so that the point of maximum performance occurs at a lower mean pressure; these patients are easily precipitated into heart failure.

The maximum concentrating and diluting ability of the kidney is severely restricted. There is a very limited capacity to excrete free hydrogen ions, titratable acid, and ammonia in response to an acid load. There is also a severe limitation of the ability to excrete sodium, particularly in response to an expanded extracellular fluid volume. During the early phase of treatment, when the sodium pump is recovering and the excess intracellular sodium is being exported to the extracellular compartment, acute circulatory overload and sudden death can easily occur if renal function recovers more slowly than the sodium pump.

The motility of the whole intestine is reduced so that transit time in the small intestine is increased. There is a reduction in gastric acid, bile, and pancreatic enzyme production. The cellular enzymes and transport systems for nutrient absorption are compromised and the mucosa becomes flattened; mitotic figures in the crypts become rare. That the defect is one of capacity and not a specific abnormality is demonstrated by the observation that absorption at low rates of presentation is relatively normal, whereas at high rates the digestive and absorptive capacity is overwhelmed.

The malnourished patient becomes poikilothermic. Even a modest reduction to 21 °C or elevation to 33 °C in environmental temperature may lead to hypothermia or pyrexia respectively. Normal individuals increase their oxygen consumption in response to a cool environment in order to maintain body heat by either non-shivering or shivering thermogenesis. Malnourished patients reduce their oxygen consumption in response to a cool environment (Fig. 3); they never shiver.

Marked changes in hormonal balance occur in malnutrition. Growth hormone levels are usually elevated in association with a low insulin concentration and a reduced insulin response to a test meal. Levels of insulin-like growth factors 1 and 2, catecholamine, and

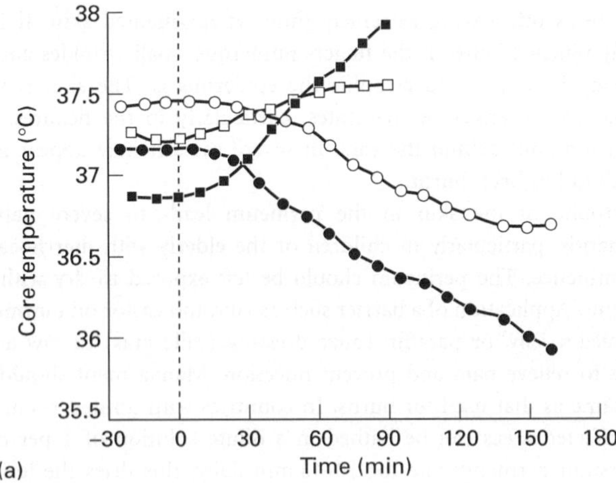

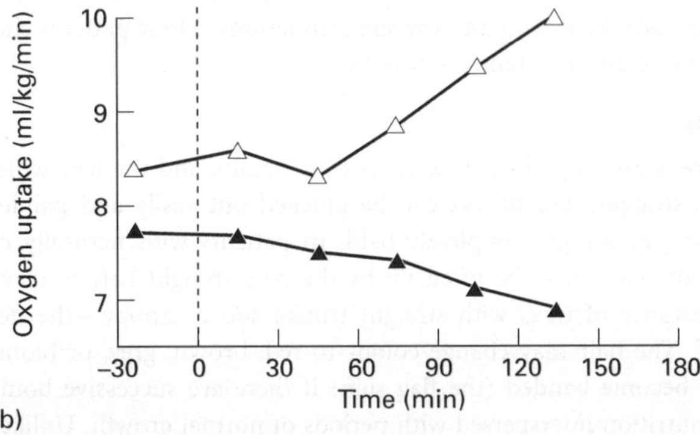

Fig. 3 (a) Response of the body temperature of malnourished children (closed symbols) and recovered children (open symbols) to changes in environmental temperature (squares 33 °C; circles 21 °C); (b) the oxygen consumption upon exposure to a cool environment in malnourished and recovered children. It should be noted that normal children have a higher body temperature and oxygen consumption in a thermoneutral environment.

glucagon are low. Cortisol levels tend to be high. Levels of both free and bound thyroxine and tri-iodothyronine are low. There are also diminished responses to injected hormones, with downregulation of most receptors. Although there is glucose intolerance, glucose levels are generally lower than normal, due partly to liver dysfunction and partly to a marked reduction in gluconeogenesis.

The febrile, acute phase, and inflammatory responses, and the immune system also partake in the reductive adaptation; they are either absent or severely blunted in seriously malnourished patients.

Body composition

Most tissues contribute to the loss of weight, but not equally. Subcutaneous fat may virtually disappear and muscle mass is often reduced by more than half. Skin and intestine are also disproportionately affected, whereas the viscera and the central nervous system are relatively well preserved.

The chemical composition of the body is altered because of the absolute and relative changes in the size of its organs and as a consequence of the reductive adaptations themselves. Thus the change in activity of the sodium pump invariably leads to increased total body sodium and reduced total body potassium, irrespective of the patient's state of hydration or the serum electrolyte concentrations.

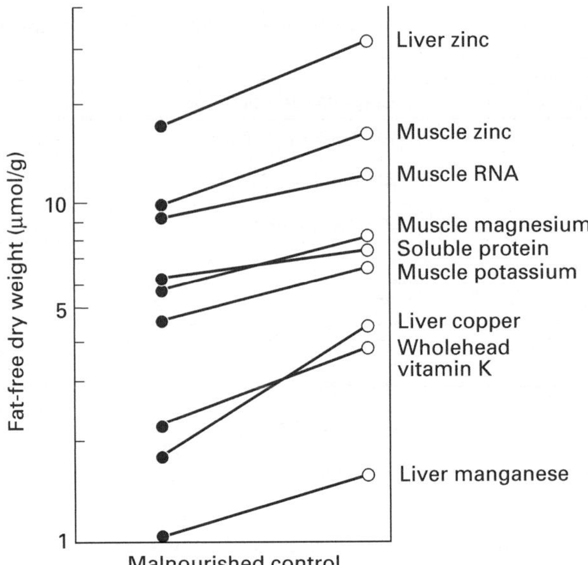

Fig. 4 Cellular constituents in malnourished and recovered children. The values are expressed per unit fat free dry weight multiplied by various factors of 10.

When oedema is also present, the malnourished patient has increased extracellular as well as intracellular sodium levels; like the Biblical Lot's wife, these patients become 'pillars of salt'.

The reduction in the metabolic activity of cells leads to a reduction in the levels of enzymes, soluble protein, and RNA that are synthesized and maintained by the cell. Most of the trace elements are used to form integral parts of these cellular components. They cannot be retained in the tissues in isolation when the parent proteins are not required. Thus there is a proportionate reduction in the tissue concentration of zinc, copper, manganese, and magnesium (Fig. 4). It would, therefore, be a mistake to measure one component of the tissue and conclude that there was a specific deficiency of that element. Nevertheless, during reversal of the adaptation, the deficits in all these components have to be made good before any weight gain can occur. Iron is an exception. There is an increased concentration of tissue iron in most forms of severe malnutrition, although not in patients with chronic blood loss.

Vicious cycles

The curtailment of inflammatory and immune responses results in repeated or, more usually, chronic infections. An atonic gut, achlorhydria, and poor secretion of IgA and bile salts combine to allow normal intestinal flora, both bacteria and fungi, to overgrow the small intestine and stomach. These organisms directly damage the intestine, deconjugate bile salts, and exacerbate any malabsorption. Unless they are suppressed, diarrhoea may worsen when additional food is given. The gas produced and the intestinal stasis is the reason for abdominal swelling in malnutrition.

The diarrhoea and repeated infections give rise, in turn, to specific nutrient deficiencies, particularly of mineral elements. When the integrity of the skin is breached, bedsores, fistulae, and indolent traumatic or surgical lesions develop.

The consequences of infections, small bowel overgrowth, malabsorption, nutrient losses, and thermal stress in a patient adapted to malnutrition is to exacerbate anorexia and further reduce intake. The adaptations are reinforced and physiological function is increasingly compromised. The patient then reaches a self-perpetuating stage where increasing anorexia and organ dysfunction leads to rapid deterioration and death.

Treatment regimens must always work within the patient's limited metabolic capacity while the reductive adaptations are reversed dietetically. Disequilibrium syndromes can lead to sudden unexpected death during early refeeding, even in previously obese patients who have been undergoing a prolonged period of energy restriction. Such illness and death are related to the disordered physiology rather than the precise degree of wasting. For this reason, clinical signs and features such as anorexia as well as anthropometric criteria, should be used in decisions to admit and treat these patients.

Oedematous malnutrition

Oedematous malnutrition is an acute illness. Patients that appear quite well may, over the course of a few days, become extremely irritable, progress through the various stages of skin lesions to give an appearance indistinguishable from burns, develop an enlarging liver, and then suddenly blow up with oedema. They have then overall retention of sodium but hypovolaemia and a low blood pressure. In its severe form, the clinical picture is not dissimilar from that of toxic shock syndrome. There is also evidence of profound incompetence of the immune system.

Patients with nutritional oedema, without the wasting or stunting of marasmus may not show the reductive adaptations characteristic of other forms of severe malnutrition. Other features point to roles for infection, cytokines, and free radicals. There is increased excretion of urinary nitrate, a measure of whole-body nitric oxide production rate. The circulating levels and urinary excretion of the leukotrienes are also increased. There is a reduction in cellular glutathione concentration, a key intermediate in protection from the effects of free radicals. Measurement of the ratio of NADPH to NADP show a marked cellular deficit in reducing equivalents. Furthermore, an unusually large proportion the sulphydryl groups on proteins are oxidized.

The high intracellular sodium and low potassium concentrations are produced by a different mechanism from the slowing of the sodium pump of marasmic patients. The sodium pump is more active than normal in oedematous malnutrition but the cell membranes are much more leaky to sodium and potassium.

Protein synthesis is disrupted. Electron microscopy shows a marked reduction of the protein synthetic machinery. Hepatic export proteins are not made at a sufficient rate to maintain their circulating concentrations. The reduction in lipoprotein synthesis accounts for the large accumulation of triglyceride in the liver.

Most textbooks ascribe kwashiorkor to protein deficiency, but this concept is now untenable. Protein deficiency does not account for the abnormalities; further, experimental protein deficiency does not reproduce the clinical features of kwashiorkor, although it does result in stunting and wasting. The oedema can resolve completely on a very low protein diet with no change in plasma albumin level, and no differences have been found in the protein contents of the diets of those who develop kwashiorkor and those who develop marasmus.

Investigations

The history and examination usually provide most of the necessary information. The laboratory has a relatively minor part to play, and is used for the identification of infection and confirmation of type I nutrient deficiencies.

Urine should always be cultured and obtained by suprapubic aspiration if there are perineal lesions.

Tuberculosis is common; its diagnosis presents special difficulties as the Mantoux test is usually negative despite the presence of active disease. Acid-fast bacilli can sometimes be recovered from laryngeal aspirate or from gastric washings. The optic fundi should be carefully examined for characteristic retinal tubercles. The chest radiograph should be scrutinized carefully for small tuberculous lesions, although infection causes much less shadowing than in the well-nourished and may even be absent in the presence of bronchopneumonia. It is important to recognize interstitial lymphocytic pneumonia (HIV associated) because it is specifically treated with steroids which are otherwise contraindicated.

The blood should be examined for malarial parasites, and faeces for ova and parasites. Testing for sickle-cell disease is important in many communities. Changes in haematocrit often give clues to the distribution of fluid between the intravascular and interstitial compartments. Plasma concentrations of sodium and potassium are not necessarily related to whole-body content; hyponatraemia is common and is a bad prognostic sign.

Therapy should be based on clinical criteria, guided by frequent reappraisal.

Management

There are two main criteria for admission to residential care:

(1) the presence of anorexia of more than a few days duration.

(2) failure to respond immediately to a trial of outpatient management in the presence of (a) oedema, regardless of weight, or (b) less than 75 per cent weight for height and less than 60 per cent weight for age, or less than 70 per cent weight for height.

Treatment is divided into several phases: an initial 1 or 2 days when the immediate threats to life are managed and treatment is initiated; an intermediate phase of about a week during which reversal of the metabolic abnormalities is expected, a rehabilitation phase of 4–6 weeks of intense feeding to return to a normal body composition, and finally a follow-up phase.

The acute phase

The immediate need is to treat infections, restore electrolyte balance, and start to reverse the physiological changes without overloading the limited capacity of the heart, kidney, intestine, or liver.

If the patient has true dehydration, this must be treated with extra fluid, but the diagnosis and treatment of dehydration one of the most difficult aspects of management. First, signs of dehydration such as sunken eyes, poor skin elasticity, dry mouth, and lack of tears are all unreliable as they are themselves features of malnutrition. The only signs that can be used are those of a compromised circulating volume and an observed loss of fluid. Second, there is more sodium inside the cells than normal and, if there is oedema, there is also excess extracellular sodium. Third, the patients are very vulnerable to the ill effects of overhydration; fatal heart failure is common during the early stages of treatment. Fourth, there is nearly always some element of 'toxic shock' arising from infections. For these reasons, oral rehydration fluids are only given for a short time in limited amounts to restore the circulating volume before feeds are given.

Table 5 Composition of an oral rehydration solution suitable for use in malnourished children (OFUM)

Component	Concentration per litre
Sodium	45 mmol (45 mEq)
Potassium	40 mmol (40 mEq)
Magnesium	3 mmol (6 mEq)
Glucose	10 g
Sucrose	25 g
Osmolality	291 mOsm
Zinc	300 mmol (19.5 mg)
Copper	45 mmol (2.9 mg)
Selenium	0.6 mmol (47 mg)

The rehydrating solution should have a lower sodium content (45 mmol/l) and higher potassium content (40 mmol/l) than is used for normally nourished patients. The oral solution recommended by the WHO should not be used. Because magnesium, zinc, and phosphorus are also depleted, solutions which contain these ions as well as the major electrolytes are particularly useful. A suitable formula is given in Table 5. Intravenous treatment is dangerous and, if given, needs close monitoring.

One of the critical differential diagnoses in malnourished patients with low tissue perfusion is between dehydration and toxic shock. Toxic shock is the most difficult complication to treat successfully; it accounts for a large proportion of deaths. The veins and capillaries dilate, cardiac muscle is weakened, and blood pressure falls. Renal perfusion is reduced to a level at which the kidney cannot excrete the end-products of metabolism. The intestine fails to absorb and then secretes fluid; bowel movement diminishes and petechial bleeding occurs throughout the intestine. Liver perfusion is reduced so that gluconeogenesis becomes ineffective and the blood sugar falls. The metabolic stress of processing dietary protein can provoke liver failure and high protein diets are dangerous. There is a clouding of consciousness with a progressive decrease of awareness, which results from poor cerebral perfusion, hypoxia, electrolyte disturbance, and hypoglycaemia. The low perfusion of the tissues reduces the metabolic rate to a stage where there is insufficient heat to maintain body temperature.

Management depends on the maintenance of cardiac output, the removal of the source of the toxin by treating infection, the prevention of hypoglycaemia and hypothermia, the strict avoidance excess fluid or protein, the provision of nutrition, and the correction of deficiencies.

The principle of dietary management in the acute stage is to give enough to prevent hypoglycaemia and hypothermia, to prevent any further tissue catabolism, and to allow the patient to begin to reassemble cellular enzymes; this must be done within the capacity of the intestine, liver, and other organs. At this stage, not only may the functional capacity be easily exceeded, but deficiencies and nutrient imbalances may be aggravated if too much food is given. Children are given not less than 80 kcal/kg per day and not more than 100 kcal/kg per day; in adults the intake should be 30–40 kcal/kg per day.

The diet must be divided into many small portions fed at hourly, 2-hourly, or 3-hourly intervals. It should not be given less frequently than 4-hourly during a complete 24 h period. At this

Table 6 The desirable nutrient intake (per kg body weight) from the diet during the acute and intermediate phases of treatment

Nutrient		
Water	120–140 ml	120–140 ml
Energy	420 kJ	100 kcal
Protein	1–2 g	1–2 g
Electrolytes Sodium	<1.0 mmol	<23 mg
Potassium	>4.0 mmol	>160 mg
Magnesium	>0.6 mmol	>10 mg
Phosphorus	2.0 mmol	60 mg
Calcium	2.0 mmol	80 mg
Trace minerals Zinc	30 mmol	2.0 mg
Copper	4.5 mmol	0.3 mg
Selenium	60 nmol	4.7 mg
Iodine	100 nmol	12 mg
Water-soluble vitamins Thiamine	70 mg	70 mg
Riboflavin	200 mg	200 mg
Niacin	1000 mg	1000 mg
Pyridoxine	70 mg	70 mg
Cobalamin	100 ng	100 ng
Folic acid	100 mg	100 mg
Ascorbic acid	10 mg	10 mg
Pantothenic acid	300 mg	300 mg
Biotin	10 mg	10 mg
Fat-soluble vitamins Retinol	150 mg	150 mg
Calciferol	3 mg	3 mg
Tocopherol	2.2 mg	2.2 mg
Vitamin K	4 mg	4 mg
Lipids Total lipid	25–55% energy	
n-6 fatty acids	4.5% energy	
n-3 fatty acids	0.5% energy	

stage the number of feeds that have to be given and the risks of hypoglycaemia and hypothermia necessitates feeding throughout the night and residential care. In the extremely ill patient, the diet is given continuously via a nasogastric drip; intravenous feeding can be used in specialized centres in rich countries but the principles of management are the same.

The diet should contain every essential nutrient (all the minerals, particularly potassium and magnesium, vitamins, protein, and energy) (Table 6); if any one of these is not given in adequate amounts the patient will not recover. However, no nutrient should be present in great excess as this will cause metabolic stress. For patients with liver

Table 7 Formula F75 for use in the acute phase and F100 for use in the intermediate and rehabilitation phases of treatment of severely malnourished children

Ingredient	F75	F100
Dried skim milk	25 g	80 g
Sugar	60g	50 g
Dextrimaltose/rice starch	60 g	–
Vegetable oil	20 g	60 g
Mineral mix	To give the concentrations in Table 6	
Vitamin mix	To give the concentrations in Table 6	
Water	To 1000 ml	To 1000 ml
Energy (kcal/100 ml)	75	100
Protein (% energy)	4.8	11.4
Carbohydrate (% energy)	71	36
Fat (% energy)	25	53
Sodium (mmol/100 ml)	0.6	1.9

dysfunction, toxic shock, severe anorexia, or oedema a formula (Table 7) with limited amounts of protein and sodium is used at a rate of 132 ml/kg per day (5.5 ml/kg per h). For other children the F100 diet can be given during the acute phase. This is most easily formulated to provide 1 kcal/ml with additional water in the acute and intermediate phases.

Infections

The usual signs of infection in the malnourished are unobtrusive or absent; infection expresses itself as apathy, drowsiness, hypothermia, hypoglycaemia, and death. Almost all malnourished children have infections, and many have multiple ones such as urinary tract infection, otitis media, tuberculosis, cytomegaloviral infection, **AIDS**, dengue, giardiasis, and cryptosporidiosis. There is overgrowth of the small intestine with organisms normally present in the colon, and commensals, such as *Staphylococcus epidermidis*, become invasive. Infection of the lower respiratory tract is particularly common.

Early effective treatment is important in preventing toxic shock, and improving the response to feeding. Blind broad-spectrum antimicrobial treatment is recommended for all patients with severe malnutrition. Some believe that antibiotics should only be prescribed for clearly identified infection. This approach is only justifiable for senior experienced staff who carefully and personally closely monitor their patients. Microbiologists often advocate specific treatment of the particular pathogenic organisms that they have isolated; this can be dangerous in malnourished patients because of the probable presence of multiple organisms, the need to suppress commensals, and failure to sample most of the potential sites of infection.

Candidiasis

Most malnourished children have candidiasis. Even when the mouth is free of lesions, it may occur in the oesophagus, stomach, and rectum, as well as on any damp moist skin. Oral nystatin suspension is effective and nystatin cream should be applied to cutaneous lesions. Systemic candidiasis should be treated with ketoconazole.

Measles (herpes and other systemic viral infections)

The mortality rate of severely malnourished patients with measles is very high. Measles vaccine should be given to all malnourished children on admission to reduce the risk of cross-infection. Severe cases are often deficient in vitamin A (particularly associated with death from measles).

Vitamin deficiency

In regions where measles or vitamin A deficiency is known to occur, vitamin A should be given routinely to all malnourished children on admission in a single dose. The patients are usually also deficient in folic acid and should receive 5 mg orally on admission. Many are deficient in riboflavin, ascorbic acid, pyridoxine, thiamine, and vitamins D, E, and K. Where specific deficiencies are known to be common, the amounts in the diet can be increased, but therapeutic doses should be given to those with clinical signs.

Hypoglycaemia

All malnourished patients are prone to develop hypoglycaemia which can occur when a patient has not been fed for as short a time as 4–6 h. A low body temperature, lethargy, limpness, and clouding of consciousness are usually the only features, although rigidity, twitching, or convulsions may occur; sweating and pallor, are unusual. Often the only sign before death is drowsiness. There should be a high index of suspicion of this diagnosis. If the patient can drink, glucose in water, sugar in water, or a formula feed should be given and the response observed. Otherwise a rapid bolus injection of about 1 ml/kg body weight of sterile 50 per cent glucose should be given intravenously followed by a nasogastric infusion of 10 per cent glucose or sucrose. If the intravenous dose cannot be given, about 50 ml of 10 per cent glucose or sucrose in water should be given nasogastrically. When the patient regains consciousness, an oral feed of a milk preparation or glucose in water should be given immediately, followed by frequent oral feeds to prevent recurrence.

Hypothermia

Hypothermia is a consequence of a low metabolic rate, and frequent feeding is crucial in the management of susceptible patients. The ideal temperature for the care of malnourished patients is 25–30 °C (77–86 °F). Newly admitted patients should not be nursed near windows or in draughts; windows should always be closed at night. Malnourished patients should always be properly covered with clothes and blankets. Washing should be kept to a minimum and done during the day, followed by immediate drying.

When the rectal temperature is below 35.5 °C (94.9 °F) or the under-arm temperature below 35 °C (95 °F), the patient should be warmed. This is best done by placing a lamp near (but not in contact with) the patient's body or placing warm (not hot) water bottles on the groins and underarms outside the clothes and blankets. Body temperature must be measured every 30 min during rewarming, as these patients may rapidly become hyperthermic. All hypothermic patients must also be treated for coincidental hypoglycaemia.

Severe anaemia

Blood transfusion is rarely indicated unless the haemoglobin concentration less than 5 g per 100 ml or haematocrit below 15 per cent. Patients with severe anaemia need a slow blood transfusion of about 10 ml/kg body weight of whole blood or packed cells over a period of about 3 h. If the patient has heart failure, or it is feared as a complication, blood should be given by exchange transfusion.

Congestive heart failure

This is a common complication of overhydration, severe anaemia, blood transfusion, plasma transfusion, or of formulae that have a high sodium content. It can also occur during early recovery when the extra food that is given causes sodium to come out of the cells to be resorbed into the circulation at a faster rate than can be excreted by the kidney. Heart failure may be more common in areas where the diet is low in selenium.

The first important symptom is an increasing respiratory rate but heart failure has then to be differentiated from respiratory infection and toxic shock. This may be difficult and the patient must be re-examined at very frequent intervals after any treatment is started, so that the diagnosis can be revised if improvement is not rapid. Later signs are respiratory distress, rapid pulse, venous engorgement, cold hands and feet, and a purple discoloration under the fingernails and tongue.

When heart failure is diagnosed, treatment for it should take precedence over feeding; all oral intake and intravenous fluids should be stopped. A loop diuretic given intravenously may be effective, but the renal response may be substantially reduced in very malnourished patients. In such cases venesection (5 ml/kg) is a reasonable emergency approach. The withdrawn blood should be kept sterile in a syringe for retransfusion if the patient's condition deteriorates as a result of this treatment. More often there is an improvement, in which case further venesection is justified, always provided that the total volume of blood removed does not exceed 10 ml/kg. Although this is a very effective treatment in the appropriate circumstances, it should only be used by those with considerable experience. As malnourished patients have a low level of total body potassium and are frequently hypokalaemic, digitalis is rarely used. Trials of agents such as angiotensin-converting enzyme inhibitors have not been conducted in heart failure associated with malnutrition.

When heart failure is due to severe anaemia the treatment is the same, except that 10 ml/kg of red cell concentrate (or whole blood) is transfused in combination with venesection.

Intermediate phase

The beginning of a return of appetite is the signal to begin the intermediate phase of treatment. Appetite is used as a barometer of progress. Great care must be taken not to overload the patient at this stage. A source of energy must be provided which is marginally above the patient's requirement for maintenance, allowing a small excess for tissue repair. This is achieved by giving not less than 80 and not more than 100 kcal/kg per day. When the patient is taking the diet well the formula can be changed from F75 to F100 (Table 7). The end of the intermediate phase is marked by the full return of appetite and hunger, usually after 2–7 days.

There are two ways of reducing the load that is given to the intestine and liver at any one feed. One is to reduce the concentration of the feed while keeping the volume constant (e.g. half-strength feeds). This method is not recommended: it either results in the patient receiving insufficient total energy or such large volumes of dilute feed that vomiting occurs. The preferred method is to keep the composition of the diet constant, to reduce the size of each feed, and to give feeds more frequently.

Because these patients may not able to express thirst, their requirement for water may not be met from the formula alone. Extra water can then be provided by nasogastric feeding.

Milk intolerance

Milk intolerance is uncommon but can be diagnosed if there is copious watery diarrhoea which improves when milk intake is reduced and recurs with its reintroduction. In such cases, milk formulae can be partially or totally substituted by other liquid foods.

Rehabilitation phase

The patient's physiological responses are still abnormal and capacity to eat is still limited. If that capacity is exceeded, there will be a corresponding reduction of appetite. At this stage more food than is necessary for mere maintenance is required. There are still deficits of potassium, magnesium, zinc, and other essential nutrients, and so it is necessary to take in greatly increased amounts of all these (as well as protein and total calories) to allow anabolism.

The transition between the intermediate and the rehabilitation phase is achieved by increasing intake by, say, 10 ml per feed until the patient starts to refuse to finish the feed. Time must be spent to encourage the patient to try to finish each feed; the attitude of the attendants is crucial; the patient should never be left alone to 'take what he wants'. As weight is gained appetite and requirements steadily increase.

During rehabilitation children should take a minimum of 130 kcal/kg per day and adults a minimum of 70 kcal/kg per day. Fat malabsorption is then a frequent cause of failure to gain weight at the expected rate, but the fat content of the diet should only be decreased if diarrhoea is clearly shown to be dependent on dietary fat. It is appropriate to maintain patients on the formula until they have achieved a normal weight for height (children) or a body mass index of at least 18 (adults). They then enter the discharge phase of treatment.

Assessing progress

Patients should be weighed daily. It is useful to set out the target weight for height (children) or body mass index (adults). Weight gain should be about 5–20 g/kg per day (usually about 10–15 g/kg per day).

Emotional and psychological stimulation

It is a major psychological trauma for a child to be separated from its mother and normal surroundings. The best person to be with the child is the mother. When children have reached the rehabilitation phase, they can be allowed out of their cots to play with others for prolonged periods. The risk of cross-infection is not increased substantially.

Affection and tenderness are insufficient in themselves. Psychological stimulation through play programmes which start in hospital and continue after discharge can substantially reduce mental retardation.

The hospital should provide a large fenced area, with mats on the floor, where the children can play. Brightly coloured mobiles should be hung over every cot. Hospital rooms should be brightly coloured with cheerful decorations. Care must be taken to avoid sensory deprivation; the children's faces must not be covered, they must be able to see and hear what is going on around them, and they should not be wrapped or tied to prevent them moving around. Toys must always be available.

Preparation for discharge

The family and community should be equipped to prevent recurrence. A home visit should guide the decision to discharge. When the patient has been abandoned or the social and economic conditions at the home are hopeless, appeals should be made for foster homes or other forms of community support.

Education cannot be left to the last few days before discharge. Parents or those responsible should be taught about the causes of the patient's malnutrition and how to prevent it in the future.

Children must be vaccinated in accordance with the local health regimen and provision made for booster doses to be given at the appropriate time. There should also be a strategy for tracing those children that fail to attend follow-up appointments.

If severely malnourished patients are tested for HIV, this should be at discharge. A positive HIV test may lead the staff to treat the patient differently (or not at all) and to fail to follow up after discharge. HIV testing is needed for epidemiological and prognostic purposes but not for the management of individual cases (except interstitial lymphocytic pneumonia); the result should only be available to the doctor in charge and procedures to maintain confidentiality are essential.

Further reading

Golden, M.H. (1991). The nature of nutritional deficiency in relation to growth failure and poverty. *Acta Paediatrica Scandinavica*, **374**, 95-110.

Waterlow, J.C. (1992). *Protein-energy malnutrition.* Edward Arnold, London.

Chapter 8.3

Obesity

J. S. Garrow

Relationship between overweight and mortality and morbidity

As early as 1913 the Society of Actuaries showed that overweight was an important predictor of decreased longevity. At intervals since, the Metropolitan Life Insurance Agency has published tables of 'desirable weight' for men and women of a given height, the most recent of which was the Build Study 1979. In some publications the range was subdivided according to large, medium, and small frame size, but there is no agreement about how frame size should be measured, nor is there evidence that this refinement improves the accuracy with which mortality, or total body fat, can be predicted for a person of given age, sex, and height.

There is international consensus that tables showing weight for height can conveniently be replaced by a single index: weight (kg) divided by the square of height (m^2). This is called Quetelet's index (QI). QI and body mass index (BMI) are terms that can be used interchangeably. Here the QI notation will be used. Figure 1 shows the general relationship of QI to mortality ratio: the curve is J-shaped, with a minimum mortality ratio in the QI range 20–25 kg/m^2 for both men and women.

The effect of age and cigarette smoking on desirable weight for longevity

The nadir of the curve in Fig. 1 changes with age: between 20 and 50 years it increases linearly from 20 to 25 kg/m^2 which, in a person 1.73 m tall, implies an increase from 60 to 75 kg. This does not mean that there is a health benefit from a gain of 15 kg during adult life. Several confounding factors operate. First, some people who are very overweight at age 20 will already have died by the age of 50. Secondly, the degenerative diseases which are the main cause of excess mortality in obese people take many years to develop, and are therefore more likely to limit life expectancy in a young person than an old one. Thirdly, malignant disease, bowel diseases, and chronic infections tend to cause weight loss and thus increase the mortality ratio in the lower weight ranges. Finally, with increasing age the distribution of fat in the body alters towards a greater proportion intraperitoneally, compared with subcutaneous sites, and this has adverse metabolic consequences, discussed below.

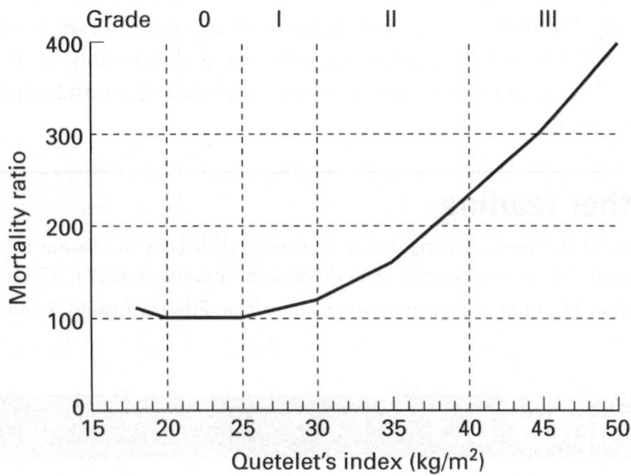

Fig. 1 Mortality ratio in young adults: minimum value is in the range 20–25 kg/m^2. Values of 30 and 40 kg/m^2 mark the boundaries between obesity grades I, II, and III.

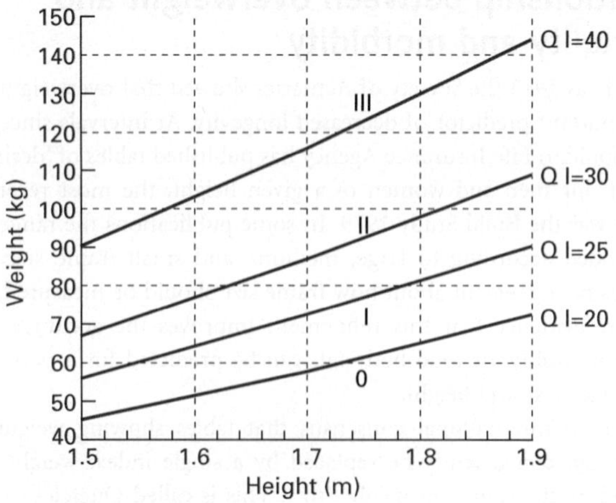

Fig. 2 Weight to height relationship which defines the grades of obesity shown in Fig. 1
(from Garrow 1993, see OTM3, p. 1314).

Table 1 Comparison of the cost, difficulty, and accuracy of methods for measuring total fat (TF), or intra-abdominal fat (IAF) in human subjects

Method	Cost	Difficulty	Accuracy TF	Accuracy IAF
Whole-body density	B	A	A	?
Total body water	B	B	B	?
Total body potassium	A	B	B	?
Neutron activation analysis	A	A	B	?
Quetelet's index	E	E	C	?
Skinfolds	E	D	C	D
Electrical impedance	D	D	C[a]	?
Near-infrared reactance	D	E	E	?
Waist/hip circumference	E	E	D	C
CT or NMR imaging	A	A	B	A

A, highest; E, lowest; ?, not specifically measured.

[a] Tetrapolar bioelectrical impedance combined with anthropometry gives a better estimate than either method used alone.

Cigarette smoking is also associated with decreased weight and increased mortality, but a large survey has shown that whereas the relation of QI to mortality risk among men or women who smoke 20 cigarettes a day is increased to about 150 per cent of that of non-smokers of the same age, the shape of the curve is little changed. It is salutary to advise smokers who dare not stop for fear of weight gain that the health risk of smoking 20 cigarettes a day is similar to that of gaining 20 kg in weight. As weight gain on stopping smoking is usually far less than 20 kg it is preferable to stop smoking.

Operational definition of obesity in adults

It is evident from Fig. 1 that obesity can be arbitrarily divided into three grades. Figure 2 shows bands of weight and height which define these grades: it is a form of presentation which obese patients find easy to understand, and on which it is possible to indicate both their present situation, and also a reasonable target weight which they might try to achieve.

Relationship between overweight and fatness

Overweight is not necessarily synonymous with excess fatness. In 1940 in the United States there was widespread concern because some nationally famous footballers were refused for service as aircrew because they exceeded weight limits. National composure was restored by showing that their excess comprised muscle and not fat.

Methods for measuring total body fat

The three classical methods for measuring body fat in living subjects depend on the assumption that body weight is the sum of the weight of fat and the weight of a mixture of non-fat

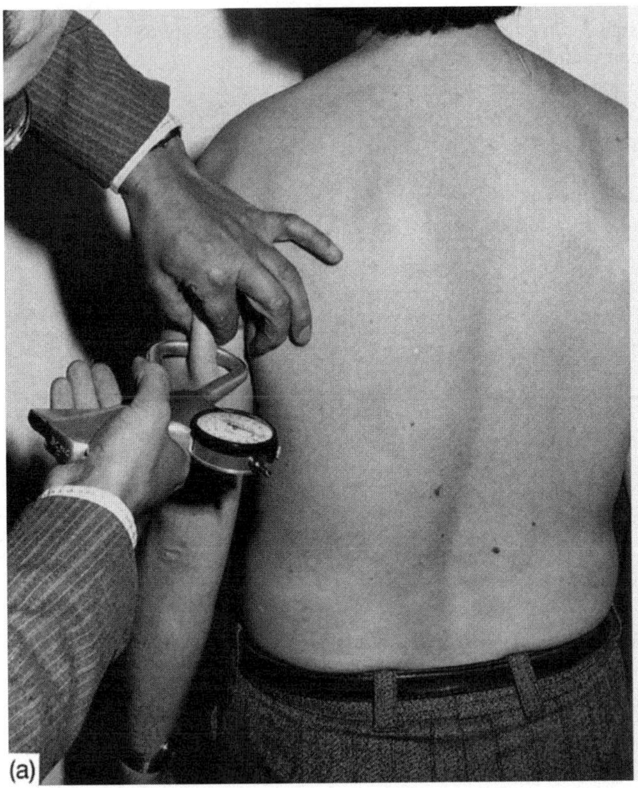

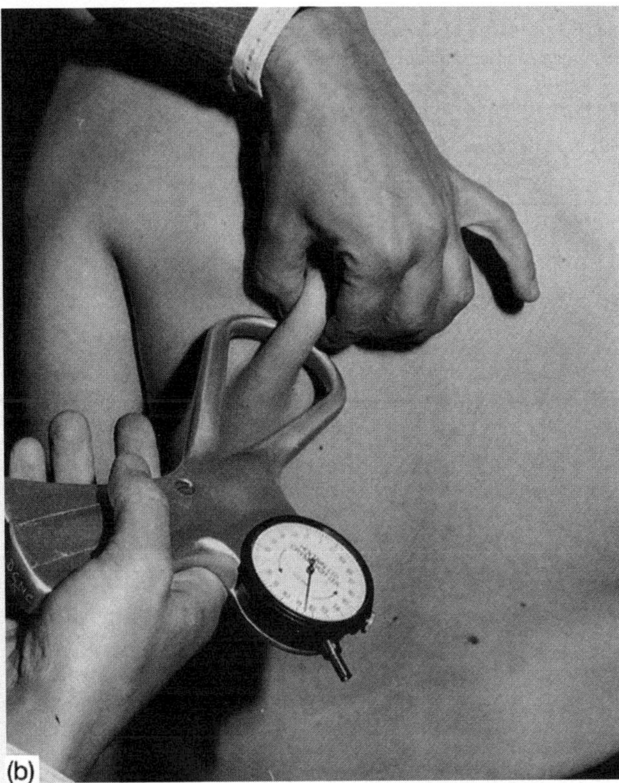

Fig. 3 The measurement of skinfold thicknesses (a) The point at which the skinfold is taken on the arm is measured as half the distance between the acromial and the olecranon processes. A fold of skin and subcutaneous tissue is taken by pinching the tissue between thumb and forefinger as shown and initially placed 2 cm apart. It is essential to maintain the grip with the left hand as shown while the right hand relaxes pressure completely on the handle of the callipers. Above a reading of 20 mm the measurement may decrease despite a firm hold with the left hand. In this case the reading should be taken 2 s after the calliper is applied. The biceps reading is taken in the same plane but at the front of the arm with the hand supinated. The suprailiac measurement is also taken on the left side in the mid-axillary line just above the iliac crest.
(Callipers are obtainable from Holtain Ltd, Crosswell, Crymych, Dyfed, UK.) (b) Technique for subscapular measurement.

components (called fat-free mass) which has some constant characteristic. This assumption, although necessary, is not quite true. For research purposes, when an accurate estimate of body fat is required, it is preferable to use two or more methods which involve different assumptions about the measurable characteristics of fat-free mass. The advantages and disadvantages of available methods are summarized in Table 1, and further details can be found in OTM3, pp. 1303–6. In ordinary clinical practice, the simplest methods are by the use of QI, skinfold thickness, or computed tomography or nuclear magnetic resonance imaging.

Quetelet's index

QI provides a satisfactory measure of obesity in people who are not hypertrophied athletes, in which case it overestimates, or old, in which case it underestimates fatness.

Skinfolds

Normally most adipose tissue is in a subcutaneous layer, the thickness of which can be estimated by measuring a skinfold, as illustrated in Fig. 3. Individuals differ in the proportion of fat at different subcutaneous sites, but the sum of skinfolds at biceps, triceps, subscaplar and suprailiac sites yields an estimate of body fat as shown in Table 2 : the error is about 2 kg. The method is inexpensive, but requires a skilled observer, and is not applicable to very obese people whose skinfolds do not fit between the jaws of the measuring calliper.

Methods for measuring the distribution of body fat

The health risks associated with obesity relate mainly to that portion of body fat which is within the peritoneal cavity. The following methods yield information about this.

Waist/hip circumference ratio

Waist circumference is the minimum circumference between the costal margin and iliac crest, measured in the horizontal plane, with the subject standing. Hip circumference is the maximum circumference in the horizontal plane, measured over the buttocks. The ratio of the former to the latter provides an index of the proportion of intra-abdominal fat. The average value for men is about 0.93 with a range of 0.75–1.10, and for women 0.83 with a range from 0.70 to 1.00. The risk of metabolic complications of obesity (diabetes, hypertension, heart disease) is increased with increasing intra-abdominal fat. The threshold waist circumference at which this risk is increased in Caucasian men is 94 cm, and it is substantially increased above 102 cm. Among women the corresponding threshold circumferences are 80 cm and 88 cm.

Table 2 Percentage body fat predicted by the sum of biceps, triceps, subscapular, and suprailiac skinfolds

Skin-folds (mm)	Percentage fat: Males (age in years) 17–29	30–39	40–49	50+	Females (age in years) 16–29	30–39	40–49	50+
15	4.8				10.5			
20	8.1	12.2	12.2	12.6	14.1	17.0	19.8	21.4
25	10.5	14.2	15.0	15.6	16.8	19.4	22.2	24.0
30	12.9	16.2	17.7	18.6	19.5	21.8	24.5	26.6
35	14.7	17.7	19.6	20.8	21.5	23.7	26.4	28.5
40	16.4	19.2	21.4	22.9	23.4	25.5	28.2	30.3
45	17.7	20.4	23.0	24.7	25.0	26.9	29.6	31.9
50	19.0	21.5	24.6	26.5	26.5	28.2	31.0	33.4
55	20.1	22.5	25.9	27.9	27.8	29.4	32.1	34.6
60	21.2	23.5	27.1	29.2	29.1	30.6	33.2	35.7
65	22.2	24.3	28.2	30.4	30.2	31.6	34.1	36.7
70	23.1	25.1	29.3	31.6	31.2	32.5	35.0	37.7
75	24.0	25.9	30.3	32.7	32.2	33.4	35.9	38.7
80	24.8	26.6	31.2	33.8	33.1	34.3	36.7	39.6
85	25.5	27.2	32.1	34.8	34.0	35.1	37.5	40.4
90	26.2	27.8	33.0	35.8	34.8	35.8	38.3	41.2
95	26.9	28.4	33.7	36.6	35.6	36.5	39.0	41.9
100	27.6	29.0	34.4	37.4	36.4	37.2	39.7	42.6
105	28.2	29.6	35.1	38.2	37.1	37.9	40.4	43.3
110	28.8	30.1	35.8	39.0	37.8	38.6	41.0	43.9
115	29.4	30.6	36.4	39.7	38.4	39.1	41.5	44.5
120	30.0	31.1	37.0	40.4	39.0	39.6	42.0	45.1
125	30.5	31.5	37.6	41.1	39.6	40.1	42.5	45.7
130	31.0	31.9	38.2	41.8	40.2	40.6	43.0	46.2
135	31.5	32.3	38.7	42.4	40.8	41.1	43.5	46.7
140	32.0	32.7	39.2	43.0	41.3	41.6	44.0	47.2
145	32.5	33.1	39.7	43.6	41.8	42.1	44.5	47.7
150	32.9	33.5	40.2	44.1	42.3	42.6	45.0	48.2
155	33.3	33.9	40.7	44.6	42.8	43.1	45.4	48.7
160	33.7	34.3	41.2	45.1	43.3	43.6	45.8	49.2
165	34.1	34.6	41.6	45.6	43.7	44.0	46.2	49.6
170	34.5	34.8	42.0	46.1	44.1	44.4	46.6	50.0
175	34.9					44.8	47.0	50.4
180	35.3					45.2	47.4	50.8
185	35.6					45.6	47.8	51.2
190	35.9					45.9	48.2	51.6
195						46.2	48.5	52.0
200						46.5	48.8	52.4
205							49.1	52.7
210							49.4	53.0

Data of Durnin and Womersley 1974.

Table 3 Time trends in the prevalence (%) of obesity (QI > 30) in representative samples of men and women

Country	Year	Age range	Men	Women
England	1980	16–64	6.0	8.0
	1987		8.0	12
	1991		12.7	15.0
	1994		13.2	16.0
	1995		15.0	16.5
The Netherlands	1987	20–59	6.0	8.5
	1995		8.4	8.5
Sweden	1980	16–84	4.9	8.7
	1988		5.3	9.1
USA	1960	20–74	10.0	15.0
	1978		12.0	14.8
	1991		19.7	24.7
Australia	1980	25–64	9.3	8.0
	1989		11.5	13.2
Japan	1976	20+	0.7	2.8
	1993		1.8	2.6
Brazil	1975	25–64	3.1	8.2
	1989		5.9	13.3
Samoa (urban)	1978	25–69	38.8	59.1
	1991		54.8	76.8
Samoa (rural)	1978		17.7	37.0
	1991		41.5	59.2

Data for UK 1995 from Prestcott-Clarke and Primatests (1997) and for other countries from WHO (1998).

Imaging techniques by computed tomography or magnetic resonance

A series of 20 transverse scans provides a very good estimate of the amount and distribution of body fat. This is the gold standard.

Prevalence of obesity in the United Kingdom and other countries

Surveys of height and weight in a nationally representative sample of adults in the UK were performed in 1980, 1987, 1991, 1994, and 1995. The data are summarized in Table 3 and show an alarming, progressive, increase in the prevalence of obesity over these 15 years. Similar trends are evident in each of the other countries studied and in each case the prevalence is higher in women than in men.

The broad risk of morbidity associated with degrees of overweight (or underweight), according to BMI is shown in Table 4.

Aetiology of obesity

Considerations of energy balance

Typically, a person who is 15 kg overweight has 100 000 kcal (25 MJ) more energy stored than a person of normal weight. This situation cannot have arisen unless the overweight person had an energy intake

Table 4 Classification of overweight in adults according to BMI

Classification	BMI (kg/m^2)	Risk of comorbidities
Underweight	< 18.5	Low (but risk of other clinical problems increased)
Normal range	18.5–24.9	Average
Overweight	> 25	
Pre-obese	25–29.9	Increased
Obese class I	30.0–34.9	Moderate
Obese class II	35.0–39.9	Severe
Obese class III	> 40.0	Very severe

Data from WHO 1998.

which was greater by this amount, or an energy output which was less by this amount, or some combination of these two factors.

Energy intake in obese versus lean persons

Obese people who seek medical help have invariably at some time tried to diet, and have been dissatisfied with the result. They believe that the problem must be one of reduced requirements, rather than excessive intake. A diet history tends to confirm this view, as the best a dietitian can do is to calculate from the food which the patient recalls (or records) having eaten. Over a week or two this record may be quite accurate, but it is rarely both accurate and typical of habitual intake. Many studies have shown that when the energy output of obese patients is measured by calorimetry, or by the doubly labelled water technique, the recorded energy intake would have been incapable of maintaining the obese state, and so was inaccurate.

Energy output in obese versus lean people

Studies of energy expenditure on groups of lean and obese subjects have shown consistent results. In both groups, resting metabolic rate accounts for about 70 per cent of total daily energy output (range 62–76 per cent); and there is no difference between obese and lean subjects in this respect. However, the total energy expenditure of the obese group is 124 per cent (range 121–128 per cent) of the lean group. The magnitude of the difference between the groups depends on the weight difference: on average, weight differences in women are associated with a difference in daily energy expenditure of about 12 kcal (50 kJ)/kg, and among men of about 15 kcal (63 kJ)/kg. The main determinant of resting metabolic rate is fat-free mass. Formulae by which resting metabolic rate can be predicted from weight, age, and fat-free mass are given in Table 5.

Mechanisms that maintain energy balance: set-point theory

Maintenance of energy stores is essential for survival in times of famine. Several physiological mechanisms tend to maintain energy balance. Energy intake is to some extent controlled by the sensations of hunger and satiety, but these are readily overridden if there is unlimited supply of varied palatable food. Changes in energy intake also directly affect output: the increase in metabolic rate which occurs during 4 h after a meal is equivalent to about 10 per cent of the ingested energy: this is the metabolic work of assimilating the meal. Energy output increases by about 6 per cent during overfeeding and decreases similarly during underfeeding: the mechanism for this adaptive thermogenesis is not fully understood, but probably involves thyroid and catecholamine metabolism. Finally, weight change causes changes in energy output as described above. These factors combine to buffer large changes in energy balance when the food supply alters.

Table 5 Prediction of resting metabolic rate (RMR, kcal/24 h) in adults

1. From age and weight (W, kg) (data of Schofield 1985)		
Age (years)	Men	Women
18–30	RMR = 15.1W + 693	RMR = 14.8W + 488
31–60	RMR = 11.5W + 872	RMR = 8.13W + 846
> 60	RMR = 11.7W + 588	RMR = 9.08W + 660
2. From fat-free mass (FFM, kg), fat mass (FM, kg), and age (A, years) (data of Ravussin *et al.* 1991)		
RMR = 13.9FFM + 6.3FM − 4.4A + 941 (men)		
RMR = 13.9FFM + 6.3FM − 4.4A + 794 (women)		

Table 6 Percentage of biological (or, in parentheses, adoptive) parents who were overweight or obese, according to the weight class of the adoptee

Weight class of adoptee	Thin	Medium	Overweight/ obese
Mean QI of adoptee	17.8	23.0	31.4
Percentage of overweight parents			
Mother			
biological	18	35	41
(adoptive)	(34)	(37)	(35)
Father			
biological	35	38	49
(adoptive)	(57)	(53)	(45)

Data of Stunkard *et al.* (1986).

There is persuasive evidence in laboratory rodents that particular strains have a set point of weight, to which they tend to return after over- or underfeeding. The evidence for a similar effect in man is very weak.

Genetic predisposition to obesity

Obesity tends to run in families, but that might imply either genetic or environmental influences. Table 6 shows the results of a study of the weight status of 540 adult Danish adoptees for whom information was available about the build of both biological and adoptive parents. In general, adoption studies indicate that about 10–30 per cent of variation in obesity is heritable, but the mechanisms are not well understood. Adult offspring of obese parents do not have a significantly reduced metabolic rate compared with the offspring of lean parents.

Social factors associated with obesity or rapid weight gain

In developed countries there is an inverse relationship between obesity and socio-economic status, especially among women. The view that obesity in disadvantaged sections of society is caused by a diet of cheap food lacks experimental support: it is true that fruit and fresh vegetables are relatively expensive, and lacking in the diet of poorer people, but food of high-energy density, such as meat and cream, are also expensive. The cheapest diet that will provide the daily requirements of nutrients is based mainly on cereals, and is monotonous: both of these characteristics normally lead to undereating, not overeating.

Recent research has indicated the factors associated with rapid weight gain (defined as an increase of > 5 kg in 5 years). In a survey of 12 000 Finnish men and non-pregnant women aged 25–64 years, 15.1 per cent of men and 17.5 per cent of women were in this category. The characteristics in which they differed significantly from the weight-stable members of the population were: a lower level of education, chronic disease, little physical activity at leisure, and heavy alcohol consumption. Weight gain was also observed among those who got married or stopped smoking.

Mechanisms by which obesity causes disease

Obesity is not only a marker of raised plasma cholesterol, hypertension, and non-insulin-dependent diabetes mellitus, but is a cause of these risk factors.

Insulin insensitivity and its consequences

Obese people are insulin resistant and, if their capacity to secrete insulin is limited, very liable to develop non-insulin-dependent diabetes mellitus. Intra-abdominal fat is especially important in causing insulin insensitivity, as its high lipolytic activity releases high concentrations of free fatty acids into the portal circulation. A high alcohol intake is associated with increased intra-abdominal fat. Insulin insensitivity is the key abnormality in 'syndrome X' in which it is associated with hypertension, high low-density lipoprotein cholesterol, low high-density lipoprotein cholesterol, and an increased risk of atheroma formation.

Metabolic effects of a large adipose mass

A large adipose mass has three other important effects which predispose to diseases:

Aromatase converts androgens to oestrogens, and in an obese person there is more aromatase in adipose tissue than in the gonads. This probably accounts for the menstrual problems, polycystic ovaries, and infertility which are often seen in obese women; infertility in obese men; and the excess risk of sex-hormone-sensitive cancers: of the colon, rectum, and prostate in men, and of the endometrium, cervix, ovary, and breast in women.

Cholesterol stores in adipose tissue greatly increase the rate of cholesterol excretion in the bile, leading to its supersaturation in obese people, predisposing to gallstones, cholecystitis, and to gall-bladder cancer.

The mechanical load of excess weight decreases exercise tolerance and predisposes to inactivity, itself a contributor to insulin insensitivity. The increased load also contributes to osteoarthritis of weight-bearing joints, with a further decrease in exercise tolerance.

Effects of weight loss in obese people on mortality and morbidity

Life insurance companies have consistently found that obese people who lose weight into the normal range, thereafter have an improved life expectancy. This is not totally satisfactory evidence that weight loss reduces the mortality risk in obese people, because those who lose weight in order to enjoy a reduced life insurance premium are self-selected, and probably not typical of all obese people. They may also have altered other habits, such as cigarette smoking and physical activity.

Weight loss in the general population is associated with a decrease (and weight gain an increase) in blood pressure, in plasma lipoprotein cholesterol fractions, triglycerides, fasting glucose, post-prandial glucose, and uric acid. However, data on the effect of weight loss on mortality have been equivocal, probably because they did not differentiate between voluntary and involuntary weight loss, the latter perhaps caused by disease.

Clinical significance of weight cycling

Individuals who maintain a constant weight over many years have a lower risk of death (particularly from cardiovascular disease) than individuals of the same age, sex, and weight who show large fluctuations in weight. It may be that the weight cycling is itself injurious to health, as it may imply alternating periods of starvation and overeating, both of which are known to impair insulin sensitivity. It may also be that people who undergo periods of weight loss and regain are manifesting a personality trait which is associated with an increased risk of cardiovascular disease. Whatever the explanation it is reasonable to conclude that treatment for obesity which causes weight to be lost and then regained is not helpful, and possibly does more harm than not losing weight in the first place.

Social issues: the anti-diet movement

Particularly in the United States, but increasingly in other countries, there is a movement which opposes any attempt to get obese people to lose weight. The argument is based on the belief that dieting causes so much anguish, to so little good effect, that it is unjustified, but the balance of evidence does not support this view.

Treatment of obesity

Expectations by patient and therapist

The obese patient usually comes to the doctor wanting to know why previous treatments failed, and to be given a different treatment which works better.

Too many doctors assume that all that is required is to send the patient off with a diet sheet. Others assume that past dietary failure is evidence of some metabolic disorder resulting in an extensive trawl through all known hormone assays. Others offer a sympathetic acknowledgement that the condition is untreatable. The truth lies somewhere between these extremes. Successful treatment of obesity requires patience and motivation on the part of both patient and therapist.

Clinical history relevant to obesity

Table 7 sets out 10 essential questions to which answers are required before starting to advise an obese patient.

1. *Target weight* Beware the patient who hopes to reduce from a QI of greater than 30 to one of less than 20 kg/m^2: such a target is very difficult to achieve, and carries no health benefit if it is achieved. It is reasonable to try to help such a patient to achieve QI 25 kg/m^2, but no less.

Table 7 Ten essential questions to ask an obese patient

Concerning the patient's target weight
1. What weight do you think you should be?
2. In what way would you benefit if you were (weight given as answer to question 1)?
3. Is your present weight the most you have ever been?
Concerning the patient's perception of dieting
4. Are you on a diet at present?
5. What is the longest time you have kept strictly to a reducing diet?
6. What rate of weight loss do you expect to achieve if you keep to a diet?
7. Do you expect to lose weight without dieting?
Factors which may make dieting more difficult
8. Who does the shopping/cooking at home?
9. What work do you do?
10. Are you on any medication at present?

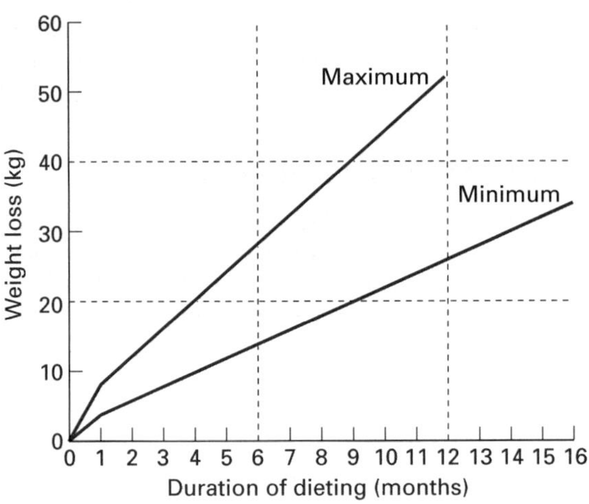

Fig. 4 Range of desirable weight loss in obese people. Younger, taller, male, and severely obese patients should aim at the upper line, and older, shorter, female, and less overweight patients the lower line.
(From Garrow 1993, see OTM3, p.1314.)

2. *Expected benefit* Some, such as relief from shortness of breath or painful knees, are realistic expectations following weight loss.
3. *Maximum weight* A patient who now weighs 100 kg, but who weighed 130 kg 6 months ago, is far more sophisticated about methods of weight loss than a patient who has never weighed more than 100 kg.
4. *Is the patient on a diet now?* If so it is necessary to find out what it is, and why the results are unsatisfactory. If not it is necessary to find out why not. (Question 7 may throw further light on this.)
5. *Length of time on diet* If the patient has never kept to a diet for more than a few days it is not surprising that little weight has been lost.
6. *Expected rate of weight loss* The appropriate range of rates of weight loss is shown in Fig. 4: those who are younger, taller, and more overweight may aim for the higher limit, while those who are older, shorter, and less overweight should be satisfied with something near the lower limit. For the first month of dieting the rate of weight loss is more rapid due to the loss of glycogen and the water bound to it. Subsequently the optimum rate of weight loss is 0.5–1.0 kg (1–2 lb)/week, which represents an average energy deficit of 500–1000 kcal (2–4 MJ)/day. The disadvantages of energy deficits greater than 1000 kcal/day are that there may be excessive loss of lean tissue, it becomes difficult to provide the essential nutrients, it is unnecessarily unpleasant, and there will have to be further large adjustments when the target weight is achieved to find a suitable diet to maintain the new weight. The disadvantages of deficits less than 500 kcal/day are that it takes too long for the subject to reach target weight.
7. *Weight loss without dieting* Occasionally, patients believe that modern medicine has developed techniques which escape the thermodynamic imperatives. Unless they are disillusioned on this point no progress will be made.
8. *Who cooks/shops?* Many patients have to eat food prepared by other people, or have to cook for other people.
9. *The patient's job* Working differing shifts, or working in a catering environment, may add considerably to the difficulty of dieting.
10. *Medication* It is important to consider modifying hypoglycaemic medication in a diabetic who wishes to lose weight. Psychotropic drugs affect the ability of the patient to achieve successful dieting, and some have acquired inappropriate prescriptions for thyroid hormone.

It is necessary to agree a plan concerning the target weight, the length of time which it is likely to take to achieve it (Fig. 4), and how the target weight, once achieved, can be maintained. Expectations must be realistic. One of the tasks of the therapist is to restore the patient's self-esteem.

Dieting relationship trap

Initially, the patient is pleased to find a doctor who is willing to help. All goes well so long as satisfactory weight loss is achieved, but the time then comes when the patient returns having not lost weight, or even having regained it. This may precipitate feelings of unworthiness, leading to the invitation to the doctor to discharge the patient. The correct response at this point is to agree with disappointment, to assure the patient that steady weight loss uninterrupted by set-backs is virtually unknown, and to try to identify the factors that precipitated the problem; above all to provide encouragement, not criticism. On the other hand, it is possible to carry sympathy too far. There is little to be gained from regular monthly meetings at which the lack of any weight loss is noted, the difficulty of dieting is agreed, but nothing is done to increase the chance of success next time.

Matching treatment strategy to degree of obesity

Table 8 shows the treatment strategies which should be considered for different grades of obesity. The first choice is usually a conventional reducing diet.

Dietary advice

The diet should provide 500–1000 kcal/day less than the maintenance energy requirements in order to achieve weight loss at the rate shown in Fig. 4. It must also provide the essential nutrients, so it is logical to seek to restrict those food items which provide energy but little else of nutritional importance, such as sucrose and alcohol. It is also

Table 8 Matching treatment strategy of the degree of obesity

Treatment	Grade of obesity			
	III	II	I	0
Diet				
Starvation	No	No	No	No
Very-low-calorie	Poss	No	No	No
Conventional	Yes (1)	Yes (1)	Yes (1)	No
Milk only	Yes (2)	Yes (2)	Poss	No
Jaw wiring + waist cord	Yes (3)	Poss	No	No
Gastric exclusion surgery	Poss	No	No	No
Drugs				
Anorectic	Poss	Poss	No	No
Thermogenic	No	No	No	No
Physical training	No	Poss	Yes (2)	Yes
Reassurance	No	No	Poss	Yes

Yes, appropriate treatment, and figure in parentheses indicates order of preference; No, inappropriate; Poss, possible in some circumstances.

desirable to restrict intake of fat, partly because fat is a concentrated energy source, and partly because there is evidence that fat has a lower satiating capacity than isoenergetic quantities of carbohydrate or protein. The foods that are not restricted are fruit, vegetables, and whole-grain cereals. Protein intake should be adequate to avoid unnecessary loss of lean tissue. Some patients prefer exactly specified diets, whereas others prefer flexibility.

Frequency and timing of meals

Traditionally, patients are advised to have small, frequent meals, and this policy seems to decrease hunger compared with a regimen of less frequent larger meals. It is probably useful for patients to establish a formal pattern of eating meals at specified times, as continuous snacking makes it difficult to establish control over total energy intake.

Behaviour therapy

The mere recording of a food diary is associated with some weight loss in most people. Such a food diary is also useful for the dietitian.

Weight-loss groups

The initial assessment should be one-to-one with a dietitian, but later there are advantages in working with groups of about 10–15 who benefit from being associated with others in a similar situation, and from hearing answers to problems raised by other members of the group.

Very-low-calorie diets

Commercial diets that provide the recommended daily amounts of micronutrients with minimal energy are attractive to patients wishing to lose weight rapidly. The disadvantage is that rapid weight loss is associated with excessive loss of lean tissue.

Exercise

Physical activity increases energy expenditure, fitness, and sensitivity to the action of insulin. Although élite athletes can maintain very high levels of energy expenditure for sustained periods, the maximum rate of work of the average non-athlete is about 6 kcal (25 kJ)/min over 1 h. The average resting metabolism is about 1 kcal (4 kJ)/min, so after 1 h the jogger will have used about 360 kcal, while his twin who remained at rest used 60 kcal, so the net cost of an hour's jogging is about 300 kcal. This is probably the upper limit of the increase in energy expenditure which it is realistic to expect overweight people to achieve by exercise. However, exercise alone is not an effective method for achieving weight loss, nor of significantly altering the proportions of fat and lean issue in the body.

Anorectic drugs

Three types of medication are intended to reduce hunger. Bulk fillers, such as guar gum, reduce food intake if taken in sufficient quantity, but the discomfort involved in taking effective quantities make them generally unacceptable. Drugs related to amphetamine have a significant anorectic effect, but the risks of abuse and psychosis require that their prescription is closely controlled. D-fenfluramine, which in any event was poorly effective has now been withdrawn because of toxic effects especially on heart valves.

Drugs to inhibit digestion and absorption of food from the gut

The amylase inhibitor xenecal (Orlistat) decreases the absorption of dietary fat by about 30 per cent, and causes increased weight loss during the first 6 months of administration in placebo-controlled trials. Its place in the treatment of obesity is not yet established.

Surgical treatment of obesity

This is not an alternative to dieting, but a method for trying to enforce it. The exception is apronectomy, but this is really only appropriate as a cosmetic operation in severely obese patients who have already lost a considerable amount of their excess fat. Cutting, or sucking, fat from subcutaneous sites is advertised as a cosmetic procedure, but the amount of fat that can be removed is trivial in comparison with the total excess in a patient who has important obesity. In many cases the cosmetic result from an attempt to remove significant quantities of subcutaneous fat is very unsatisfactory.

Bypass operations and gastric stapling

In the bypass operation the gut is cut and rejoined so that the majority of the bowel is short-circuited. The objective is to produce some degree of malabsorption, so that some of the food is not absorbed, and also so that a large intake provokes severe diarrhoea.

Gastric stapling closes off all but a small pouch at the fundus, which empties through a small stoma into the main body of the stomach, so only about 50 ml of food can be taken at a time. Typically, patients lose about one-third of their excess weight in the year after operation, but there is then a tendency for weight regain.

Weight loss is somewhat greater after the bypass than after the stapling operation, but at the cost of greater metabolic complications, and a greater risk of nutrient deficiencies. Both operations are reversible, but weight gain after reversal is rapid and almost universal.

The relative advantages and disadvantages of bypass operations and gastric stapling have been reviewed in a Consensus Statement (1991), the main points of which were:

1. Patients seeking therapy for severe obesity for the first time should be considered for treatment in a non-surgical programme, with integrated components of a dietary regimen, appropriate exercise, and behavioural modification and support.

2. Gastric restrictive or bypass procedures could be considered for the well-informed and motivated patient with acceptable operative risks.
3. Patients who are candidates for surgical procedures should be selected carefully after evaluation by a multidisciplinary team with medical, surgical, psychiatric, and nutritional expertise.
4. The operation should be performed by a surgeon experienced with the appropriate procedures and working in a setting with adequate support for all aspects of management and assessment.
5. Lifetime medical surveillance after surgical therapy is a necessity.

Gastric balloon

Balloons have been inserted into the stomach to reduce gastric capacity without the hazards associated with abdominal operations in obese people. The results have been disappointing; weight loss is small and not sustained, and the risk of ulcerating the gastric mucosa is significant.

Jaw wiring

With this procedure the patient can drink, but not chew, and as liquid diets tend to have a low-energy density patients often lose weight. Weight loss of about 36 kg in 9 months can be achieved, but is not sustained when the wires are removed. The procedure is not justified unless it is combined with some method for helping the patient to maintain the weight loss (see below).

Maintenance of weight loss

It is likely that a patient who reduces from, say, 100 kg to 70 kg and then goes back to eating 'normally' will return to their original weight. Previously, obese people who have lost weight benefit from a device that warns them of weight gain, which may be a spouse, or flatmate, or a favourite pair of jeans. Alternatively, this monitoring function can be performed by a nylon cord fixed round the waist which becomes tight if excessive weight is gained.

Prevention of obesity

As about one-third of the adult population in the UK is already overweight, the opportunities for primary prevention of obesity lie mainly with primary school children. The idea that fatness is determined in infancy by the number of fat cells is no longer tenable: fat babies often do not become fat children, and many fat children were not fat babies. However, fatness at age 13 years is a strong predictor of adult fatness, so the optimum time to prevent obesity is in the interval between 5 and 12 years.

Further reading

See OTM3, pp. 1313–4.

Chapter 8.4

The use of enteral and parenteral nutrition

M. Elia

Preventing and treating malnutrition and the indications for artificial nutritional support

There are many simple things that the clinician can do to help those at risk of malnutrition. Nausea may be helped by an antiemetic. Dysphagia due to an oesophageal stricture may be helped by the provision of sloppy or liquid meals rather than solid foods. Pain relief may improve appetite. Dedicating time to feeding weak and elderly patients may do much to prevent the development of malnutrition.

In some patients it is obvious that artificial nutritional support is necessary from the time of the first consultation; for instance, those who are unconscious (and likely to remain so for a long period), or are unable to swallow or have intestinal failure. Others will have been subjected to major surgery, and thus prevented from eating for a week or more until the anastomosis has adequately healed. Some patients receiving aggressive chemotherapy develop severe inflammation of the mucous membranes of the mouth and other parts of the gastrointestinal tract, so that artificial nutritional support (enteral or parenteral) may be required shortly after the start of treatment.

Whenever the gut is available, oral or enteral nutrition should be used because it is simpler, cheaper, and more physiological than parenteral nutrition. The enteral route also has the advantage of maintaining the integrity of the 'gut barrier', which prevents bacteria and associated endotoxins from entering the systemic circulation. Some general and specific recommendations about the use of enteral tube feeding are given in Table 1. Some of these also apply to parenteral nutrition, but only when the gut is not available for feeding, as in prolonged gastrointestinal failure in the form of ileus, peritonitis, severe and recurrent pancreatitis, high intestinal fistulae, short bowel syndrome, or severe inflammatory disease of the intestine. The use of parenteral nutrition in the postoperative period is discussed below.

Peripheral venous infusions of nutrients have often been associated with the rapid development of phlebitis and venous occlusion, complications reduced by infusing solutions of lower osmolarity, through suitable fine-bore catheters. Small doses of heparin and/or corticosteroids and vasodilatory glycerine trinitrate skin patches may help. However, peripheral parenteral venous feeding has obvious limitations for patients with poor peripheral venous access, and for patients requiring prolonged infusions of hypertonic solutions.

Nutritional requirements

Protein and energy

Recommendations about nutrient intake depend on the disease activity and nutritional state. Figure 1 shows the effects of increasing nitrogen intake on nitrogen balance in subjects who are close to energy equilibrium. Normal individuals in energy balance achieve nitrogen balance at a mean intake of 0.1 g N/kg. The World Health Organization

Table 1 Guidelines for the use of enteral nutrition in the adult patient[a]

1. Clinical settings where artificial enteral nutrition should be a part of routine care
(a) Greater than 10% weight loss with little or no oral intake for the previous 5 days
(b) Less than 50% of the required oral nutrient intake for the previous 7–10 days
(c) Severe dysphagia or swallowing-related difficulties, e.g. head injury, strokes, motor neurone disease
(d) Major, full-thickness burns
(e) Massive small bowel resection in combination with parenteral nutrition (in patients with 50–90% small bowel resection, enteral nutrition is given to hasten gut regeneration and return to oral intake)
(f) Low-output enterocutaneous fistulae (& 60;500 ml/day)[b] (elemental diets may hasten closure of fistula)
2. Clinical conditions where enteral nutrition would normally be helpful
(a) Major trauma (see 1(a) and 1(b))
(b) Radiation therapy (see 1(a) and 1(b))
(c) Mild chemotherapy (see 1(a) and 1(b))
3. Clinical settings where enteral nutrition is of limited or undetermined value
(a) Intensive chemotherapy (parenteral nutrition is often indicated)
(b) Immediate postoperative period or poststress period (especially if an adequate oral intake will be resumed within 5–7 days)
(c) Acute enteritis
(d) Less than 10% remaining small intestine (parenteral nutrition is usually indicated)
4. Clinical settings in which enteral nutrition should not be used
(a) Complete mechanical intestinal obstruction
(b) Ileus or intestinal hypomotility
(c) Severe uncontrollable diarrhoea
(d) High-output fistulae
(e) Severe acute pancreatitis
(f) Shock
(g) Aggressive nutritional support not desired by the patient or legal guardian, and such action being in accordance with hospital policy and existing law
(h) Prognosis not warranting aggressive nutritional support

[a] Based on the American Society of Parenteral and Enteral Nutrition Board of Directors (ASPEN) (1987).

[b] If the fistula is proximal, the feeding should be distal. If the fistula is distal, sufficient proximal length must be present to allow sufficient absorption. Fistulae due to malignancy, radiation, and distal obstruction are unlikely to close spontaneously.

recommends a minimum of 0.12 g N/kg. A greater intake produces little improvement in nitrogen balance in normal subjects. In contrast, depleted individuals, particularly those without associated inflammatory or infective disease, continue to achieve a progressively greater positive balance as the nitrogen intake is increased.

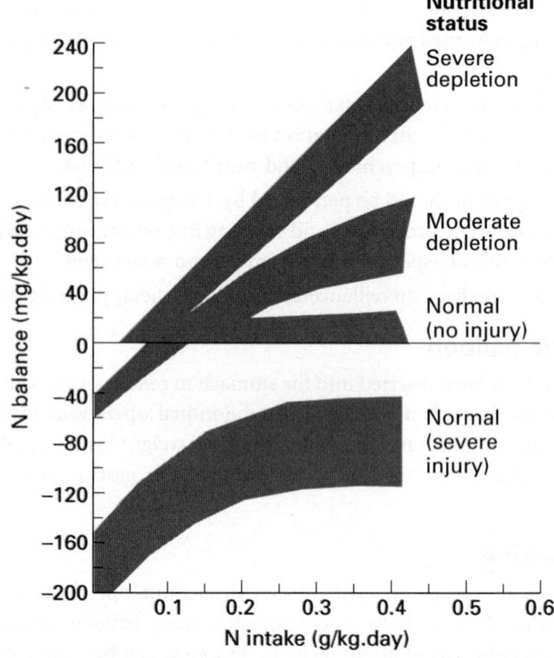

Fig. 1 Relationship between N intake (1 g N = 6.25 g protein) and N balance in subjects who are receiving sufficient energy to be close to energy balance (see text) (based on Elia 1982; Elwyn 1993).

Negative nitrogen balance in catabolic states is due to a combination of the disease itself, of immobility, and the effect of some drugs such as steroids. The catabolic response is usually greatest within the first few days of injury, but in burned patients it may continue for weeks. In normally nourished catabolic patients who are close to energy balance, an increase in nutritional intake results in improved nutritional balance. However, as Fig. 1 indicates, the curve of nitrogen intake versus nitrogen balance is shifted downwards and to the right. Many patients become malnourished following a severe catabolic injury, so that the response to nutrient intake is intermediate between malnutrition uncomplicated by disease, and severe injury uncomplicated by malnutrition.

From these different responses emerge some approximate recommendations for nitrogen intake in patients (Fig. 2). The recommended energy intake varies with the clinical state. In well-nourished individuals who are likely to receive nutritional support for considerable periods of time, it is sensible to aim for energy balance. In the depleted patient, it is desirable to achieve a positive energy balance (as well as a positive nitrogen balance); whereas in obese individuals, loss of adiposity (while limiting the loss of lean tissue) is desirable.

Concepts about the energy requirement of hospitalized patients have changed over the past 10–20 years, so that much less energy-providing food is now generally prescribed than previously. This change is due to a combination of factors. One is past over-reaction to the frequent and severe malnutrition which was present before artificial nutritional support became widely practised. Another concerns errors in the interpretation of measurements of metabolic rate. For example, measurements made while patients are receiving large quantities of nutrients will include the thermic effects of the nutrients; therefore, it is incorrect to ascribe any hypermetabolism detected to the disease itself. It is also incorrect to estimate energy requirements for long periods of time based on measurements made over short

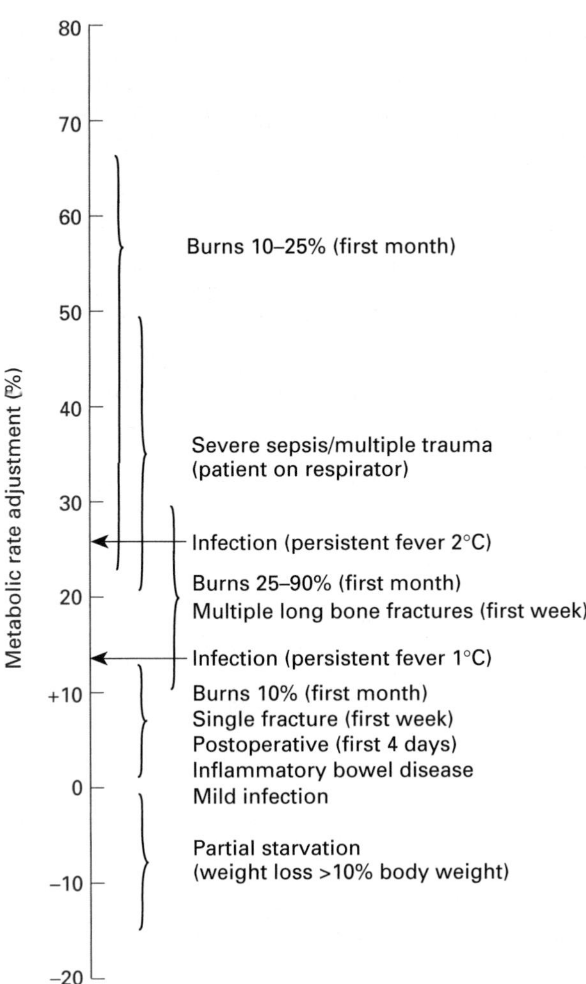

Fig. 2 Guidelines for estimating the approximate energy and nitrogen (N) requirements (1 g N = 6.25 g protein) for an adult patient receiving artificial nutritional support (based on Elia 1990).

intervals, especially those obtained during peak hypermetabolism. Furthermore, the effect of pyrexia on energy requirements should not be doubly accounted, as has been done by some, as it is already included in the measurement of basal metabolic rate. Another reason stems from change in the clinical management of certain groups of patients. The practice of nursing burned patients in a thermoneutral temperature (26–30 °C) and surgically removing necrotic skin tissue, instead of leaving it until it scabs, has contributed to a reduction in energy expenditure.

In addition, disease is associated with a reduction in physical activity which is often more than sufficient to offset any increase in basal metabolic rate due to disease. Even in ambulatory patients receiving parenteral nutrition in hospital and at home, measurement of total 24-h energy expenditure using tracer techniques has often been found to be only 1700–2300 kcal/day.

Finally, administration of excess nutrients can increase the likelihood of metabolic complications (e.g. hyperglycaemia, hypermetabolism, increased CO_2 production, and abnormal liver function tests). This, together with animal studies suggesting that overfeeding produces a greater mortality in sepsis, has alerted clinicians to the possible dangers of overprescribing nutrients.

Table 2 Approximate electrolyte content of intestinal effluents (mmol/l)

	Sodium	Potassium	Bicarbonate	Chloride
Gastric	60	15	–	90
Pancreatic	140	5	90	75
Biliary	140	5	35	100
Small intestinal	100	10	25	100
Diarrhoea	60	30	45	45

Energy requirement varies substantially with body size, nutritional status, and disease activity. Approximate estimates are given in Fig. 2. Most hospitalized adult patients require between 1500 and 2500 kcal and between 10 and 15 g N/day. In prescribing artificial feeding it is often possible to approximate the requirements to the contents of three or four standard regimens, to monitor the patient's progress, and to adjust accordingly. In some conditions it may be sensible to reduce the intake below normal, for example, in the obese, and the intake of protein may be reduced or even temporarily stopped in hepatic encephalopathy. In renal failure it may also be restricted to reduce uraemia or to avoid dialysis or to increase the interval between dialyses. Fluid restriction in some patients may limit the quantity of nutrients that can be administered. In this case, a compromise between the general clinical needs and nutrient needs is necessary.

Fluid

Usually 1.5–3.0 litres of fluid are given to adults receiving enteral or parenteral nutrition, but the intake may vary both above and below this. Particularly high fluid and electrolyte provision is necessary in patients with large-output intestinal fistulae and those with burns. In other situations fluid is restricted, partly because the patient may already be receiving some for other purposes, and/or because of the presence of oedema, renal, hepatic, or cardiac failure, or a recent head injury. In the intensive care unit, fluid intake is often guided in part by central venous pressure measurements. Changes in body weight from one day to the next are particularly helpful in the assessment of fluid requirement as these predominantly reflect changes in fluid balance.

Minerals and trace elements

For most adults receiving artificial nutrition, the intake of sodium and potassium is 50–100 mmol/day. Chloride intake is similar to that of sodium, and phosphate is usually prescribed at a dose of 20–40 mmol/day, but mineral requirements vary considerably. Sodium restriction is necessary in renal, hepatic, and cardiac failure. Extra is required in patients with increased loss of gastrointestinal fluid. The additional requirements can be predicted (Table 2). Loss of 1 litre of gastrointestinal fluid may more than double the sodium requirements while affecting potassium requirements much less. The latter may be increased by excessive renal losses and may double in patients receiving amphotericin B. Adequate amounts of potassium and phosphate, which are predominantly intracellular ions, are also necessary during repletion of lean tissue, when deficiencies can make the nitrogen balance substantially more negative.

The recommended intakes of calcium, magnesium, and many trace elements are quite different for oral/enteral nutrition compared with intravenous nutrition (Table 3), because the gut only absorbs a proportion of these nutrients, sometimes less than 10 per cent.

Prolonged intravenous administration of trace elements at the dose recommended orally may result in toxicity.

The requirements of trace elements in various diseases are not clearly established, although patients with intestinal fluid losses may have greater requirements for zinc (Table 3, footnote) and to a lesser extent, chromium. Patients on intravenous nutrition may require a fivefold increase in the amount of zinc for every litre of gastrointestinal fluid lost, and a twofold increase in the case of chromium.

Vitamins

In contrast to the lower requirements of trace elements given intravenously than those given orally, the reverse is true for vitamins (Table 4). Vitamins are generally absorbed to a much greater extent than most trace elements, and their requirement probably increases in many diseases; some patients are also deficient in vitamins prior to the start of treatment. In addition, some vitamins may degrade during the preparation and storage of parenteral nutrition solutions. For example vitamin A, riboflavin, and vitamin K are photosensitive, and vitamin C may degrade in the presence of trace elements, oxygen, and copper. Thiamine can degrade in the presence of sulphate, which is used as a preservative, and vitamin A palminate may be adsorbed on some plastic storage bags or administration sets.

Manufactured enteral feeds have a long shelf-life and contain trace elements and vitamins. Parenteral feeds have a shorter shelf-life and vitamins and trace elements are often added shortly before use because of concern about stability. Vitamin K need not be added routinely and particular care must be taken in patients who are on anticoagulants.

Table 3 Recommended daily oral and parenteral intakes of calcium, magnesium, and trace elements in adults

Mineral or trace element	Oral (mg)[a] Men	Women	Intravenous (mg)[b]
Calcium	800	800	240–400
Magnesium	350	280	140–290
Iron	10	15	1–2
Zinc	15	12	2.5–4.0[c]
Copper	1.5–3.0	1.5–3.0	0.5–1.5
Iodine	0.15	0.15	0.1–0.2
Manganese	2–5	2–5	0.15–0.8[e]
Fluorine	1.5–4.0	1.5–4.0	1–3
Chromium	0.05–0.20	0.05–0.20	0.007–0.013[e]
Selenium	0.070	0.055	0.03–0.06
Molybdenum	0.075–0.25	0.075–0.25	0.015–0.030

[a] Recommended dietary allowances (National Research Council 1989). The values are for adult males (79 kg) and non-pregnant, non-lactating women (63 kg) aged 25–50 years. Values for those aged >50 years are generally identical. Some values are indicated as ranges because there is less information on which to base precise recommendations.

[b] Based on American Medical Association (1989), Shenkin and Wretlind (1977), Elia (1990).

[c] Add 2 mg in acute catabolic state and 12–17 mg/litre of intestinal effluent lost.

[d] Add 20 mg/l of intestinal fluid lost.

[e] These doses, especially those at the upper end of the range, are probably overestimates as they have been reported to result consistently in supraphysiological concentrations.

Table 4 Recommended oral and parenteral intake of vitamins in adults

Vitamin	Oral (mg)[a] Men	Women	Parenteral (mg)[b]
Water soluble			
Thiamine (B_1)	1.5	1.1	3.0
Riboflavin (B_2)	1.7	1.3	3.6
Niacin (B_5)	19	15	40
Pyridoxine (B_6)	2.0	1.6	4.0
Folate (B_9)	0.2	0.18	0.4
B_{12}	0.002	0.002	0.005
Pantothenic acid (B_3)	(4–7)	4–7	15
Biotin (B_7)	(0.03–0.1)	(0.03–0.1)	0.1
Ascorbic acid (C)	60	60	100
Fat soluble			
Vitamin A[c]	1	0.8	1.0
Vitamin D[d]	0.005	0.005	0.005
Vitamin E[e]	10	8	10
Vitamin K	0.08	0.65	–

[a] Recommended dietary allowances (National Research Council 1989). The values relate to adult males (79 kg) and non-pregnant, non-lactating females (63 kg) aged 25–50 years. Values for those aged >50 years are similar to those indicated. Some values are indicated as ranges because there is less information on which to base allowances.

[b] Based on American Medical Association (1979).

[c] Retinol equivalents: 1 retinol equivalent = 6 mg β-carotene.

[d] As cholecalciferol: 10 mg cholecalciferol=400 IU vitamin D.

[e] α-Tocopherol equivalents (TE): 1 mg D-α-tocopherol = 1 αTE.

Sufficient quantities of this vitamin are normally synthesized in the gut, but a weekly intramuscular dose is often recommended, especially in those receiving antibiotics that affect the metabolism of intestinal bacteria. More frequent doses may be given to patients with liver disease who have a coagulation problem and are at risk of gastrointestinal bleeding. Vitamin B_{12} is not generally given, but in patients requiring long-term nutritional support, monthly injections should be administered.

Although the stores of some trace elements and vitamins are large, and deficiencies are not likely to develop for months or possibly years (vitamin A, vitamin D, vitamin B_{12}), reserves of mainly water soluble vitamins (e.g. thiamine, riboflavine) are very small. It is therefore usual to give a mixture of trace elements and vitamins from the outset of nutritional support even if this is likely to be required for only 1–3 weeks.

Complications of artificial nutritional support: prevention, treatment, and monitoring

Parenteral

Mechanical

The insertion of a central venous catheter, usually into the subclavian vein, causes pneumothorax in 2–3 per cent of cases. Lying the patient head down while changing feeds and checking the position of locks prevents air embolism.

Occlusion of the catheter may result from reflux of blood into the catheter, but also from coagulation of the feed, especially when all-in-one solutions, which include lipid, are infused. The incidence of catheter blockage depends on the period of use, the diameter, and type of catheter (soft polyurethane and Teflon catheters are said to have a lower risk of thrombosis than rigid polyethylene catheters). In patients that have cyclic nocturnal feeding, flushing the catheter with heparin (e.g. 50 U/ml) at the end of feeding reduces the risk of thrombosis. Some recommend routine inclusion of heparin (2–3 U/ml) in the parenteral nutrition solution to prevent both catheter and local venous thrombosis.

Several methods may be tried to unblock an occluded catheter. Gentle suction may remove the clot. It may be lysed by inserting a solution of urokinase (5000 U/ml) for about 1 h. Alcohol (50 per cent) may be used in a similar way to dissolve lipid-associated occlusions. Insertion of hydrochloric acid (1 M) into the catheter is another potentially effective method.

Infections

Catheter-related infection remains an important complication. Typically the organisms are derived from the skin (e.g. *Staphylococcus aureus*; *S. epidermidis*), although a variety of other organisms from the systemic circulation, including Gram-negative organisms and fungi, may seed on to the catheter tip, in the presence of a fibrin clot. Catheter-related sepsis can largely be avoided by the use of aseptic techniques during insertion of the catheter and during the change of feeds, and by avoiding the use of the central venous catheter for purposes other than feeding, such as blood sampling, or administration of drugs and blood.

When catheter-related sepsis is strongly suspected, the catheter should be removed. Blood cultures taken both from the central venous line and a peripheral vein, and a swab from the catheter entral site, may help to identify the causative organism, and the likelihood that it is related to the catheter. The procedure of tunnelling the line under the skin, from its site of insertion to the anterior chest wall, makes dressing and care of the catheter easier, and the location is often more comfortable to the patient. However, there is little evidence that the use of a tunnelling procedure reduces the incidence of sepsis.

Multilumen catheters are used in some patients because of the need for multiple uses (sampling and administration of blood, and the infusion of drugs). They have advantages in patients with limited peripheral venous access, but probably become infected more frequently than single-lumen catheters which are used solely for parenteral nutrition.

Metabolic complications

Fluid and electrolyte abnormalities are common during parenteral nutrition. Zinc deficiency may impair wound healing and produce dermatitis. Magnesium deficiency may lead to neuromuscular excitability and tetany, and can produce hypocalcaemia which is not corrected by calcium administration.

Hyperglycaemia is common but can be managed by reducing the intake of glucose ($\pm$ increase in lipid intake) or by administering insulin, either as a constant infusion or by intermittent subcutaneous or intramuscular injections, at a dose determined by blood glucose concentrations. Particularly high glucose concentrations may occur if the rate of infusion of nutrients is not adequately regulated. Without the use of an infusion pump the rate of infusion may increase severalfold to cause severe hyperglycaemia, hyperosmolarity, headaches, vomiting, and impaired consciousness.

Increased glutamate oxaloacetate transaminase, glutamic pyruvic transaminase, and alkaline phosphatase are commonly observed. These are frequently due to the underlying disease but other factors may be involved: infusion of lipid or excess glucose (leading to hepatic steatosis); bacterial overgrowth in the intestine; and biliary sludge and gallstones. The prolonged absence of oral intake during parenteral nutrition fails to stimulate normal gallbladder contraction and this is probably the major factor responsible for the development of biliary sludge. Investigation may be necessary on occasion to discover the underlying pathology.

Phosphate and essential fatty acid deficiencies may arise from inadequate provision in parenteral nutrition solutions. Phosphate deficiency can cause muscle weakness and impair utilization of protein. It also causes hypercalcaemia and, in the long term, can produce bone disease. Essential fatty acid deficiency produces alopecia, thrombocytopenia, anaemia, and a skin rash as early as 6 weeks after starting intravenous nutritional support without fat. It is diagnosed by an increase in the triene to tetraene ratio (> 0.4) as, in the absence of linoleic acid, oleic acid is metabolized to eicosatrienoic acid. The condition is more likely to develop in patients receiving continuous rather than intermittent parenteral nutrition, because essential fatty acids from the endogenous lipid stores are continually prevented from being released by hyperinsulinaemia. The deficiency syndrome is rapidly reversed by administering an intravenous lipid. Regular application to the skin of oils containing essential fatty acids allows sufficient absorption to treat or prevent this syndrome.

In patients intolerant of lipid (e.g. patients with hyperlipidaemia and some with renal or hepatic disease or diabetes) hypertriglyceridaemia results. This may affect the assays of a number of standard biochemical tests, and dilute other plasma constituents (e.g. pseudohyponatraemia). Visual inspection of plasma for lipid several hours after cessation of the lipid infusion can alert the clinician to this problem. Measurement of plasma triglycerides provides a more accurate assessment.

Lipid infusion has been implicated in affecting the function of some organs. For example, hepatic steatosis may cause abnormal liver function tests, and lung deposition in patients with respiratory distress can impair pulmonary function by reducing the permeability of the lung to gases.

Excessive administration of glucose may also have adverse respiratory effects. This is because glucose produces 30 per cent more CO_2/MJ than fat, and an even greater amount of CO_2/MJ when there is net lipogenesis from carbohydrate. Furthermore, excessive administration of glucose increases energy expenditure (dietary induced thermogenesis) to a greater extent than fat. In patients with impaired pulmonary function this may precipitate respiratory failure, or impair weaning of a patient with respiratory failure from a respirator. However, with the typical amount of glucose infused in most patients this is probably not an important problem, and the use of high-fat regimens generally have little or no advantage.

Metabolic bone disease is an occasional problem associated with long-term home parenteral nutrition. Several factors may contribute, including corticosteroid therapy, chronic use of heparin, the underlying disease, immobility, and possibly intoxication with aluminium. Excess amino acid intake has also been implicated. Some studies have reported that the bone histology is not dissimilar to that of osteomalacia, although paradoxically it has been reported that administration of vitamin D can make the condition worse.

Trace element and vitamin deficiencies may occur in patients on long-term parenteral nutrition; for example, copper, zinc, iron, selenium, chromium, and molybdenum. Several vitamin deficiencies have been described, including biotin deficiency (eczematous dermatitis, hair loss, depression, anorexia), and night blindness due to lack of vitamin A. Usually this is due to the prescription of insufficient amounts, but excessive losses of intestinal effluents may also be responsible.

Enteral nutrition

The commonest complications of enteral feeding include nausea or vomiting (10–20 per cent), abnormal bloating and cramps, diarrhoea (5–30 per cent), and constipation (but mainly in long-term feeders at home). Delayed gastric emptying, a feature of postoperative abdominal surgery, head injury, or severe sepsis may lead to accumulation of feed in the stomach, resulting in nausea and vomiting. This problem can be prevented by administering the feed directly into the small intestine. In those at risk, gastric pooling can be checked by intermittent aspiration through tubes with a sufficiently wide bore.

Continuous infusion of feed into the stomach can prevent the sudden disturbance associated with bolus feeding. The use of an infusion pump to control delivery prevents gastric flooding. Pharmacological agents that stimulate gastric emptying, such as metoclopramide or erythromycin, may help in susceptible individuals. Erythromycin acts by stimulating the motilin receptor on the smooth muscle of the stomach and small intestine. In unconscious patients and those with an impaired swallowing reflex, vomiting may lead to aspiration pneumonia, as can gastro-oesophageal regurgitation.

Despite the high incidence of diarrhoea, the mechanism is not entirely understood. It is often associated with antibiotic therapy. Lactose intolerance is uncommon as most enteral feeds are free of lactose. Over-rapid delivery of nutrients may lead to diarrhoea, especially if the delivery is postpyloric. A number of other factors have been implicated, including bacterial contamination of enteral diets, an underlying gastrointestinal disease, the use of laxatives, lack of dietary fibre, and neuroendocrine reflexes whereby the administration of feed in the stomach or upper small intestine cause secretion of fluid in the small and large bowel. Drugs such as codeine phosphate or loperamide may help.

Constipation may be a problem, particularly in elderly, inactive subjects. Lack of fibre may contribute.

Several metabolic disturbances have been described; hyperglycaemia in glucose-intolerant subjects; rebound hypoglycaemia after sudden withdrawal of feed; disturbances in plasma potassium, depending on the patient's renal and gastrointestinal function and the potassium content of the feed; hypophosphataemia during refeeding; and abnormalities of liver function which are generally of little clinical significance, but may be due to the underlying disease, drug therapy, or fatty infiltration associated with malnutrition. Refeeding malnourished subjects may produce hypophosphataemia and hypokalaemia as lean tissues containing these electrolytes are accreted.

Trace element deficiencies do not normally occur in patients on long-term enteral feeding but discrepancies have been found between the manufacturers' stated content of some trace elements (copper, zinc, iron, manganese) and the measured content, which was sometimes less than the recommended dietary allowance.

The complications of enteral nutrition at home are similar to those in hospital, but there are a number of frequent but minor problems. Flushing of the tubes with water at the end of each feed helps to prevent blockage and a blocked tube may be unblocked by flushing it with water in the first instance, followed by a warm solution of sodium bicarbonate or by digesting the coagulated feed with pancreatic enzymes. Coca-Cola® may also be effective in unblocking tubes. If a gastrostomy or enterostomy tube has been dislodged, it must be replaced quickly because the stoma may rapidly close up and make further access difficult.

Regurgitation of feed in patients with impaired gastro-oesophageal function, can lead to aspiration pneumonia. This can be avoided by administering the feed with the upper part of the body elevated to an angle of about 30°, or in those with a particularly high risk it is best to administer the feed directly into the small intestine.

Nutritional aspects of some specific conditions and situations

Acquired immune deficiency syndrome (AIDS)

Acute weight loss is usually a consequence of acute infection, whereas more chronic loss is usually associated with an enteropathy. Food intake is usually decreased during acute infections. In advanced disease, decreased intake is often associated with opportunistic infections in the mouth, pharynx, and oesophagus, which may cause pain and dysphagia. Antifungal and antiviral drugs can cause nausea, vomiting, and anorexia. Dementia in advanced AIDS, may make dietary assessment and management particularly difficult. Anxiety, apathy, and depression are common and may lead to self-neglect.

Support should begin with general advice about diet, but it may need to progress to the use of supplements and, occasionally, enteral tube feeding or parenteral nutrition. The enteral route is preferable when the gastrointestinal tract is functional. Lactose-free feeds and low-fat feeds (with medium-chain triglycerides) are often used in an attempt to improve dietary tolerance, especially in those with an enteropathy. A large proportion of patients with AIDS take supplements of vitamins and trace elements. In some cases, this may lead to toxicity.

Severe burns

Severe burns provide one of the most catabolic stimuli to humans and the injury response may persist for weeks or months. The nutritional requirements of such patients are greater than for most other catabolic states (Fig. 2) and artificial nutritional support is usually necessary.

Feeding through a nasogastric tube is often well tolerated, but may be restricted because of early gastric stasis and occasionally ileus. In most patients gastrointestinal motility improves within 2–4 days, but it is important to aspirate the gastric contents intermittently, especially in the early phase, to ensure that there is no gastric pooling. Extra fluid is often necessary to match the increased fluid losses from the skin surface. The extent to which vitamin and trace element requirements are increased after burns is poorly defined.

Enteral feeds are not always tolerated because of persistent ileus or associated problems such as intra-abdominal injury, sepsis, smoke inhalation, and multiorgan failure. Some patients then need both enteral and parenteral nutrition.

Head injury

Delayed gastric emptying frequently lasts for more than 10 days after severe head injury. This may be due to the head lesion alone, but it may also be due to associated abdominal trauma. Traditional nasogastric feeding may not provide the full nutritional requirements within 1–2 weeks. The impaired level of consciousness and poor or absent swallowing reflex also means that gastric pooling and aspiration are not uncommon. Parenteral nutrition has been used routinely in some centres, which have reported improved nutritional and clinical outcome in comparison with intermittent bolus feeding through a nasogastric tube, but emphasis should still be placed on enteral feeding, because of its protective effect in preventing mucosal atrophy and bacterial translocation from the gut. Improved methods of delivering nutrients enterally include pump-assisted delivery and the use of metoclopramide and erythromycin, to stimulate gastric emptying. Feeds can also be made directly into the small intestine.

Cytotoxic therapy, bone marrow, and intestinal transplantation

Aggressive cytotoxic therapy or radiotherapy may result in inflammation of the mucous membranes of the gastrointestinal tract from mouth to rectum. Swallowing then becomes painful and diarrhoea a problem. A nasogastric tube is often uncomfortable to such patients, and bleeding may occur from friction with the inflamed mucosa, especially in those with thrombocytopenia. Parenteral nutrition is therefore often necessary.

There is interest in the use of specific nutrients or bioactive substances to protect the mucosa of the gut from damage by cytotoxic drugs or radiotherapy. Large doses of intravenous glutamine (30–40 g/day) may be beneficial to patients undergoing transplantation, but other work with glutamine supplementation has not been so conclusive. Graft-versus-host reactions may also be accompanied by gastrointestinal symptoms. Severe, prolonged, watery diarrhoea, amounting to several litres a day, presents a serious problem.

Parenteral nutrition is usually necessary after intestinal transplantation, partly because the pre-existing bowel disease produces malnutrition, and partly because it is necessary to ensure that sufficient time has been allowed after surgery to ensure that anastomoses have adequately healed, and that mucosal integrity has recovered. Fluid electrolyte and trace elements may need to be given in increased amounts to balance the increased loss associated with gastrointestinal effluents.

Perioperative nutrition

Many studies have been undertaken to assess whether perioperative nutritional support reduces the complication rate after surgery. They have produced conflicting results partly because of the multiple other factors that affect outcome (age, sex, severity of disease, skill of the surgeon, nursing care, and presence or absence of a nutrition team, and preoperative nutritional status).

The largest trial of perioperative parenteral nutrition (The Veterans Affairs Total Parenteral Nutrition Co-operative Study Group 1991) involved several hundred patients undergoing elective abdominal and thoracic surgery. The routine administration of parenteral nutrition (from up to 2 weeks before surgery and at least 3 days after surgery) provided no overall benefit. However, in the subgroup of patients who were severely malnourished, perioperative nutritional support decreased the non-infective complications from 42 per cent to between 5 and 23 per cent (depending on the method used to define malnutrition). This and other studies emphasize the importance of patient selection for nutritional support.

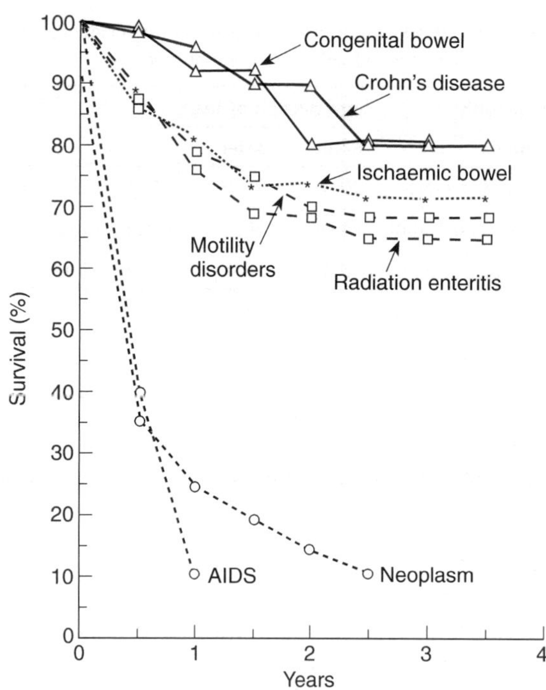

Fig. 3 Survival of different groups of patients receiving home parenteral nutrition
(For source, see OTM3, p. 1325).

Home nutritional support

In 1993 more than 30 per cent of the total artificial nutritional support in Britain (mainly enteral tube feeding) took place in the community, and it is likely that the trend towards more home care will continue to increase. In the United States there are probably more patients receiving enteral tube feeding outside than in hospital. In other countries the trend towards home care has been limited by the lack of an adequate infrastructure and organization. Artificial nutritional support at home has a number of advantages over treatment in hospital. Patients frequently feel more comfortable at home. Affected adults frequently go to work and children attend school. Treatment at home is cheaper and frees beds for the use of others.

Indications for home artificial nutrition

Patients or carers must be able to perform the necessary tasks to a sufficiently high standard. Whether enteral or parenteral nutrition is used depends on whether the gastrointestinal tract is available for the digestion and absorption of nutrients.

Home parenteral nutrition

Crohn's disease (with or without fistulae), short bowel syndrome, motility disorders (such as systemic sclerosis, and pseudo-obstruction), congenital bowel disease, and radiation enteritis provide important indications. Others include patients with malignancy (usually those with intestinal obstruction) and some with AIDS who are unable to tolerate enteral nutrition.

Table 5 Effect of introducing a nutrition team on the incidence of complications (%) associated with parenteral nutrition

Percentage with complication	Introduction of team: Before	After	
Catheter-related sepsis	25.0	3.6	Mean of nine studies
Mechanical complications	24.0	6.5	Mean of four studies
Metabolic complications	29.1	12.4	Mean of three studies

Home enteral tube feeding

The major indications are those associated with swallowing difficulties. These may be obstructive or due to neurological disorders (for example, multiple strokes, Parkinson's disease, motor neurone disease, multiple sclerosis, and primary muscle diseases that affect swallowing).

Management

Psychological evaluation

Many patients find the concept of a need for artificial nutritional support for months or years daunting, but given appropriate support their fears and anxieties frequently subside. It is always essential to involve family members (or carer) and contact with patients who are already on home treatment may do much to reassure. School-age children also have particular difficulties, but careful counselling and the use of nocturnal feeding alone, frequently allows them to adjust, attend school, and lead a reasonably normal life.

Training

Patients and their carers must learn the basic principles of nutritional support and of asepsis. They should know how to programme the infusion pump, how to add solutions to the feed, how to connect and disconnect the feeds to the catheter/tube, how to change dressings, how to recognize problems, such as a blocked catheter and infection, and how to recognize hyper/hypoglycaemia, measure blood glucose, and screen for glycosuria. A trial of home nutritional support over a weekend may be a useful way of assessing the patient's ability to cope. An assessment of the home environment is essential before discharge. Patients and their carers must have a telephone number to contact in an emergency, with advice available day or night.

Outcome

Home parenteral nutrition

The most extensive analysis of outcome of patients on home parenteral nutrition is illustrated in Fig. 3. For a variety of conditions (congenital bowel disease, Crohn's disease, motility disorders of the gut, and radiation enteritis), there is a substantial mortality in the first 2 years (10–30 per cent), but few deaths occur after this period. The mortality is usually due to the underlying condition, although a few deaths arise from the complications of parenteral nutrition. Mortality in patients receiving home parenteral nutrition for AIDS and malignancy is inevitably high, so that treatment should only be offered to those in whom there is good reason to expect a substantial consequent improvement in the quality of life.

A survey in Britain has revealed that 40 per cent of patients on home parenteral nutrition were independent, able to be fully employed and to look after their families. Fewer than 10 per cent were severely disabled and heavily dependent on others.

Home enteral tube feeding

There is much less information about the outcome of patients receiving home enteral tube feeding. In one survey an overall mortality of 45 per cent was reported over a period of 2 years. Rates were particularly high for adults who had a malignancy or cerebrovascular disease, as well as for children with major congenital defects. In another study of elderly patients (median age, 76 years) who had suffered from strokes and neurological conditions affecting swallowing, mortality was as high as 50 per cent within the first year.

Despite this high mortality, the quality of the remaining life of affected individuals frequently improves.

Monitoring

Nutritional assessment is based on changes in growth, or oedema-free body weight, but changes in skinfold thickness and arm muscle circumference (see Chapter 8.3) and a variety of biochemical parameters may also be used. The need for blood counts, urea and electrolytes, and liver function tests varies. They are more often required for those given parenteral nutrition. Measurements of trace elements and vitamins are sensible for patients receiving long-term parenteral nutrition, but this may not be necessary for those receiving well-formulated enteral feeds.

The role of nutrition teams in the management of patients in hospital and at home

A nutrition team, consisting of a clinician, a specialist nurse, dietitian, pharmacist, and possibly others, such as a chemical pathologist and bacteriologist minimizes the incidence of complications associated with nutritional support, avoids unnecessary nutritional support, and reduces wastage of feeds. The reduction in the incidence of catheter-related sepsis alone, from a rate of 25 per cent to 3 per cent (Table 5), has substantial implications. It is regrettable that currently only some 25–30 per cent of British hospitals have set up such a team.

Further reading

Mataresse, L.E. and Gottschich, M.M. (ed.). (1998). *Contemporary nutrition support practice. A clinical guide.* W.B. Saunders, London.

Payne-James, J., Grimble, G., and Silk, D. (ed.) (1995). *Clinical practice.* Edward Arnold, London.

Rombeau, J.L. and Rolandelli, R.H. (ed.) (1997). *Enteral and tube feeding,* 3rd edn. W.B. Saunders, London.

and see OTM3, p. 1326.

Section 9

Disorders of the skeleton

Contents

Section 9

Disorders of the skeleton

R. Smith

The physiological, biochemical, and histological background of skeletal tissues, important in the understanding of bony disorders, is discussed in OTM3, pp. 3055–64 and also in the *Oxford Textbook of Rheumatology*, (2nd edn), pp.421–40. Here accounts are confined to specific disorders.

Osteoporosis

In osteoporosis there is a reduction in the amount of bone per unit volume without a change in its composition; and this disorder can be further defined as a reduction in bone mass by more than 2.5 standard deviations (SD) below the mean for a young adult population, or as a reduction in the amount of bone sufficient to predispose to fracture. Osteopenia defines a reduction between 1 and 2.5 SD. The microarchitectural changes in bone are seen particularly in trabecular bone, and mediated by bone cell activity. The trabeculae become thinner and non-weight-bearing bone is selectively removed by mechanisms which vary according to the cause of the osteoporosis, leading to increased fragility.

Bone mass and fracture

Bone mass reaches a peak at about 30 years of age, and is higher in men than in women and in negroids than in caucasians. From young adult life bone is lost progressively in men at a steady rate, and in women rapidly after the menopause for some 10 years and then at the same rate as men. Endosteal resorption of bone dominates over new periosteal bone formation and the increase in external diameter is less than the internal expansion. Peak bone mass depends on the interaction between genetic and mechanical factors, modified by nutritional and endocrine influences (Fig. 1).

Bones that are used are denser than those that are not, and bone loss in later life is delayed, to a variable extent, by exercise. Additional calcium intake increases peak bone mass and reduces subsequent loss. The most important hormones determining peak bone mass are the sex hormones; and varying degrees of oestrogen lack in the growing skeleton cause bone loss. The effects of the interaction of these nutritional, mechanical, and endocrine factors on bone mass is particularly seen in anorexia nervosa (nutrition and oestrogen lack) often associated with excessive exercise. The vertebral bone density of some competitive female athletes can be low rather than high compared with age-matched normal women, demonstrating that the beneficial effects of mechanical stress on the skeleton are at least blunted by hormone lack.

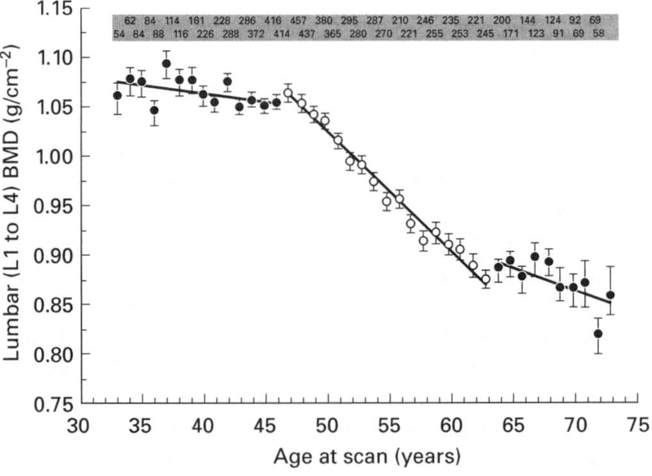

Fig. 1 The relationship of bone mineral density of the spine to age in 8789 caucasian women who have never taken HRT. The data are expressed as mean ± 1 SEM at each year (from Shipman *et al.* 1999, with permission).

Fractures are more frequent in women than men because they reach the fracture threshold earlier and live longer.

Below a certain bone density fractures become more likely (theoretical fracture threshold).

The likelihood of fracture is directly and linearly related to bone density, but there is an overlap in the bone densities of those who fracture and those who do not. Thus in groups of subjects, the mean bone density in those who sustain a femoral neck fracture is not more than 1 SD lower than in those who do not. This means that the measurement of bone density in a population of postmenopausal women will not detect a significant proportion who are liable to fracture. Measurement of bone density ('osteoporosis screening') of populations is not medically or economically worthwhile. This does not mean that in the individual patient measurement of bone density is useless, since low bone density is the most important risk factor for fracture.

The reason why bone density and fracture are not more closely related is that fracture depends on more than bone mass. An important cause, especially in the elderly, is falling. This may be increased by the physical and mental frailty of later years, by hypothermia, drugs and alcoholism, and by environmental factors. Some investigations suggest that falling is more important than osteoporosis in causing fracture in the elderly.

Fractures at three main sites—vertebrae, femoral neck, and forearm—are those most often related to osteoporosis. The composition of the bone differs at these sites, with vertebral bone being predominantly trabecular and hip predominantly cortical. Vertebral fractures occur in younger adults more than hip fracture, probably because bone loss occurs more rapidly from the vertebral site. The frequency of both fractures increases with age, but in the immediate perimenopausal years bone loss is largely due to excess bone resorption and vertebral fractures predominate; later, reduced osteoblast activity reduces new bone formation and femoral neck fractures become important. The difference between the two groups (type I and II) and the proposed causes are outlined in Table 1.

Fractures of the forearm in mixed trabecular and cortical bone do not show an increase in incidence with ageing. This may be because this type of fracture often results from putting out the arm to prevent a fall, and in the elderly, the reflex to do so is diminished.

The medical and economic effects of femoral neck fracture are considerable; for instance it has been estimated that 20 per cent of all orthopaedic beds in the UK are occupied by elderly women with hip fractures, and that after a femoral neck fracture up to 25 per cent of patients are dead 6 months later and the majority are disabled. The annual cost of such fractures in the US approaches \$16 billion.

Table 1 The different causes of bone loss and fracture after the menopause

	Type I	Type II
Age (years)	51–75	70
Sex ratio (F:M)	6:1	2:1
Type of bone loss	Mainly trabecular	Trabecular and cortical
Rate of bone loss	Accelerated	Not accelerated
Fracture sites	Vertebrae (crush) and distal radius	Vertebrae (multiple wedge) and hip
Parathyroid function	Decreased	Increased
Calcium absorption	Decreased	Decreased
Metabolism of 25-OH-D to 1,25-$(OH)_2D_3$	Secondary decrease	Primary decrease
Main causes	Factors related to menopause	Factors relating to ageing

Table 2 The main causes and types of osteoporosis

Age-related	***Nutritional***
• Postmenopausal	• Anorexia nervosa
• Elderly	• Starvation
Not age-related	• Coeliac disease
Immobility	***Genetic***
• General	• Osteogenesis imperfecta
• prolonged bed rest, neurological injury, space flight	• Familial and racial (Oriental, Caucasian)
Local	***Lifestyle (risk factors)***
• rheumatoid arthritis	• Smoking
	• Alcohol
Endocrine	***Idiopathic***
• Oestrogen lack	• Pregnancy-related osteoporosis
• Oophorectomy	• Juvenile osteoporosis
• Hysterectomy	• Osteoporosis in young adults
• Obsessional athletes	***Other***
• Early menopause	• Mastocytosis
• Testosterone lack in young men	• Heparin administration
• Cushing's syndrome, spontaneous or iatrogenic	• Cytotoxic agents
• Thyrotoxicosis	
• Hypopituitarism	

Measurement of bone mass

All methods depend on the assumption that the bone is normally mineralized, since they measure the amount of calcium and do not detect changes in the organic bone matrix. Apart from radiological assessments of cortical thickness and density compared with standards such as aluminium wedges, current methods are single and dual photon densitometry, quantitative CT scanning, and dual X-ray absorptiometry (DxA), and of these DxA is the most widely used.

The single photon forearm technique is relatively inexpensive and reproducible; dual photon methods are more expensive. CT methods result in a high dosage of radiation, while dual X-ray absorptiometry methods are rapid and do not require a replaceable isotope source. Bone mineral density (BMD) is expressed as the amount of mineral within a given area and the result is expressed as an area density.

Although various differences have been recorded in accuracy and reproducibility, other factors influence the choice of method. If one is concerned with density at a particular site, it is important to measure the density at that site. However, spinal bone density (measured by DxA) will, in general, be a more sensitive indicator of bone loss (and gain) than other sites, and most useful in sequential studies in individuals. Hip DxA has less artefactual errors than spine DxA.

Causes of osteoporosis

The main causes are shown in Table 2, but many patients have more than one. Osteoporosis occurs most commonly in postmenopausal and elderly women, (age-related bone loss). When it is not clearly related to age it is often associated with accelerated bone loss. Rarely, this occurs in childhood, in adolescence, and also in young adults, sometimes associated with pregnancy in women. Accelerated bone loss may also occur as the result of immobility, endocrine disease, chromosomal disturbances, and a number of other conditions. In some of these there is also a reduction in peak bone mass. Bone loss is increased by excessive smoking and alcohol consumption, lack of exercise, early menopause, and excessive thinness.

Symptoms and signs

The features differ according to the site. The most common is deformity and loss of height due to vertebral collapse. This may be noticed more by others than by the patient. Original height may be determined by measurement of the span. In the young vertebral collapse is accompanied by deformity of the chest and protrusion of the manubrium sterni. Sudden vertebral collapse is usually related to a recognized event, for instance moving heavy furniture; it produces severe and localized pain, and tenderness to percussion. However, collapse frequently occurs without symptoms. Examination will then confirm loss of trunk height, thoracic kyphosis, proximity of the ribs to the iliac crest, and a transverse abdominal crease.

Radiology

Plain films do not detect osteoporosis until there is a considerable loss of bone, and they are mainly useful in detecting structural collapse. In the vertebrae, fractures due to osteoporosis appear as irregular anterior wedging affecting some vertebrae and not others. The end plates may be biconcave but this change does not have the uniformity of distribution seen in osteomalacia, except where it occurs in the young skeleton as in juvenile osteoporosis or in osteogenesis imperfecta. Different grades of vertebral fracture are defined, from a moderate loss of anterior height through conspicuous anterior wedging to complete flattening of the whole vertebra. Various changes are also described in osteoporotic bones before fracture. These include loss of the horizontal trabeculae in the vertebrae with apparent accentuation of those in the vertical direction and reduction of cortical thickness in the long bones with progressive loss of trabeculae, particularly at the upper end of the femur. In the vertebrae, herniation of the disc through the end plate causes a 'Schmorl's node'; it is said by some that this is unrelated to osteoporosis. In severe or acute

Table 3 The main differential diagnosis of osteoporosis

Multiple myeloma: especially in men; high erythrocyte sedimentation rate, monoclonal gammopathy, light chains in the urine, plasma cells in the marrow, sometimes hypercalcaemia
Metastatic carcinoma: breast, bronchus, prostate, kidney, thyroid
Osteomalacia: may coexist with osteoporosis, especially in the elderly; identify by biochemistry and bone biopsy
Hyperparathyroidism: occasionally associated with generalized osteoporosis; biochemistry diagnostic
Osteogenesis imperfecta: distinguish by family history, blue sclerae, wormian bones

osteoporosis (as with immobilization), the endosteal surface of peripheral bones may appear scalloped, and the mineral loss has a 'spotty' or 'rain-drop' appearance. Osteoporosis is said not to affect the skull except where it is due to an excess of adrenal cortical steroids.

Biochemistry

Biochemical measurements are usually normal, but recent immobility in a young person considerably increases the urine calcium excretion, and after the menopause the ratios of calcium and of hydroxyproline to creatinine in the urine after an overnight fast may both be increased, reflecting increased bone resorption. Recent long-bone fracture may slightly increase plasma alkaline phosphatase.

When the osteoporosis is due to an underlying disorder, the biochemical changes reflect this; for example in thyrotoxic bone disease the plasma calcium, phosphate, alkaline phosphatase, and the urinary hydroxyproline excretion may all be increased. Patients with active osteoporosis may be in negative calcium balance.

Measurement of plasma procollagen peptides and cross-linked collagen-derived peptides in the urine is widely used in research to assess the rate of bone formation and resorption respectively.

Other investigations

Bone biopsy is not necessary to confirm osteoporosis, but is useful to exclude coexisting or alternative bone disease. It should then be combined with bone marrow aspiration to exclude haematological disorders, especially in the young.

Isotope scanning may show fresh fractures, and helps to exclude such problems as multiple secondary deposits.

The role of bone density measurements (see above) is not yet established. Recommended indications are to confirm a radiological suggestion of osteoporosis, to provide a baseline measurement for treatment, to aid with decisions about hormone replacement therapy, and in research.

Diagnosis

There are two steps; first to establish that osteoporosis is present and that other significant bone diseases are absent (Table 3), and secondly to try to establish its cause—since there are some which can be improved by treatment. Osteoporosis itself should be readily distinguished from other forms of bone disease because of its usually normal biochemistry, and from other causes of loss of trunk height and vertebral collapse by examination of the patient, the peripheral blood, the bone marrow, and if necessary the bone itself.

Table 4 Usual daily doses of oestrogens and progestogens used in hormone replacement therapy

Oral preparations	
Oestrogens	
micronized oestradiol-17β	1–2 mg
oestradiol valerate	1–2 mg
oestrone sulphate	1.5 mg
conjugated equine oestrogens	0.625–1.25 mg
Progestogens	
DL-norgestrel	0.15 mg
norethisterone acetate	0.7–1.0 mg
dydrogesterone	10–20 mg
medroxyprogesterone acetate	5–10 mg
Non-oral preparations	
Oestrogens	
transdermal oestradiol-17β	0.05–0.1 mg
oestradiol-17β implant	25–50 mg (6-monthly)
Progestogens	
transdermal norethisterone acetate	0.25 mg

Types of osteoporosis

Age-related bone loss

Bone loss occurring in the first decade after the menopause should be distinguished from 'senile' or 'elderly' osteoporosis, since the causes are probably different. In the early postmenopausal years the main cellular abnormality is excess bone resorption due to oestrogen deficiency whereas later defective new bone formation becomes relatively more important.

Management of age-related osteoporosis

Patients often have unnecessary worries about osteoporosis, because of the widespread publicity about it, when reassurance and explanation may be necessary. In prevention it is important to build up an optimum bone mass in early years by exercise, adequate nutrition (especially calcium), and the avoidance of risk factors. In practice the opportunities to do this have usually disappeared, so that the main steps are to prevent any further bone loss and, where possible, to stimulate effective new bone formation. Moderate weight-bearing exercise (and the avoidance of immobility) encourages new bone formation and reduces osteoclastic bone resorption.

There is increasing evidence of the usefulness of additional calcium in the prevention of bone loss. A total intake of 1–1.5 g daily is now recommended. This does not provide an alternative to hormone replacement therapy in the early postmenopausal years, but may reduce bone loss (and fracture rate) in later years in women, and also in men.

There seems little doubt that hormone replacement therapy prevents further bone loss at whatever postmenopausal age it is given. It also appears to reduce femoral neck fracture rate. However, because bone loss is most rapid in the first 10 postmenopausal years, it is most effective if given during that time. Usual doses are shown in Table 4. Oestrogen given on its own increases the risk of endometrial cancer, and this risk is abolished by giving cyclical progestogen. Long-term oestrogen appears to increase the incidence of breast carcinoma, but the relative risk is small and debated (values of 1.3–1.7 have been given). There is also a very small increase in thromboembolic events. A number of epidemiological observations have shown that oestrogen alone significantly reduces cardiovascular deaths. A study of 59 000 nurses also suggests no loss of benefit from adding progestogen. At present, therefore, hormone replacement therapy is widely recommended to prevent bone loss, both before and after fracture.

Within the past few years the bisphosphonate, disodium etidronate, has been given in a cyclical manner (together with oral calcium) to prevent bone loss by suppression of osteoclastic bone resorption. This treatment is licensed for treatment of established vertebral osteoporosis with vertebral collapse. A more potent aminobiphosphonate, alendronate, is now widely used to prevent bone loss and reduce fracture rate. Calcitonin also reduces bone resorption when given by injection (which has side-effects) and also by nasal inhalation, but any increase in bone mass will only be temporary. This does not seem to be so for hormone replacement therapy or cyclical etidronate treatment.

Sodium fluoride stimulates the osteoblasts to form new bone and increases bone density. However, the newly formed bone is woven and mechanically unsound. In osteoporotic patients given sodium fluoride, vertebral bone density increases, but fractures do not decrease. There is, however, a controversy about the effects of different doses of fluoride.

Other agents have also been used in the treatment of osteoporosis; thiazides reduce urine calcium excretion and femoral neck fracture rate; and vitamin D or its metabolites may also reduce the fracture rate (particularly in those with malabsorption of calcium). The usefulness of the 1–34 amino acid fragment of parathyroid hormone has yet to be established.

Osteoporosis not related to age

Immobility contributes to many forms of osteoporosis. This immobility may be local, around inflamed joints or fractured limbs, or it may be general. Rapidly progressive osteoporosis follows severe injury in the young associated with enforced immobilization. This is due to a sudden 'uncoupling' of bone resorption and formation, which may produce hypercalcaemia or hypercalciuria; radiographically there is a spotty 'rain-drop' form of rarefaction. Similar events probably occur in space travel. Treatment is difficult, but the osteoporosis will improve when mobility is resumed.

Osteoporosis and pregnancy

Women occasionally develop vertebral fractures during pregnancy. Pain in the back and kyphosis are noticed near term or shortly after delivery. The pain generally improves after 2 or 3 months and the loss of height may cease; follow-up bone density measurements show a slow improvement towards normal. Further vertebral collapse in subsequent pregnancies is unusual. This very rare form of osteoporosis may be associated with failure of the normal changes in calciotrophic hormones which appear to protect the maternal skeleton during pregnancy. The relationship to transient regional osteoporosis, which particularly affects the femoral necks in pregnancy, is obscure.

Osteoporosis in the young

Osteoporosis with structural collapse can occur during growth. The particular form that occurs around puberty (idiopathic juvenile osteoporosis) is usually self-limiting. Growth rate is reduced and shortness of the trunk with kyphosis due to vertebral fracture may develop. There is pain in the back which may follow injury. There may be metaphyseal fractures at the ends of the long bones which can be confused with Looser's zones. Such fractures are associated with pain in the ankles and difficulty in walking. Excessive bone resorption has been reported but decreased bone formation also occurs. The cause of the condition is unknown. Although it is generally associated with the rapid growth of adolescence, similar conditions occur in childhood. Except in rare cases, it is not progressive and the bones may return to a nearly normal structure within a few years, especially in the spine, although spinal deformity often persists (Fig. 2). The real incidence of this condition may be underestimated; it could account for a number of cases of idiopathic kyphosis. The condition most difficult to distinguish from it is mild osteogenesis imperfecta (see below), especially where the characteristic family history and blue sclerae are absent, and the rare osteoporosis–glioma syndrome.

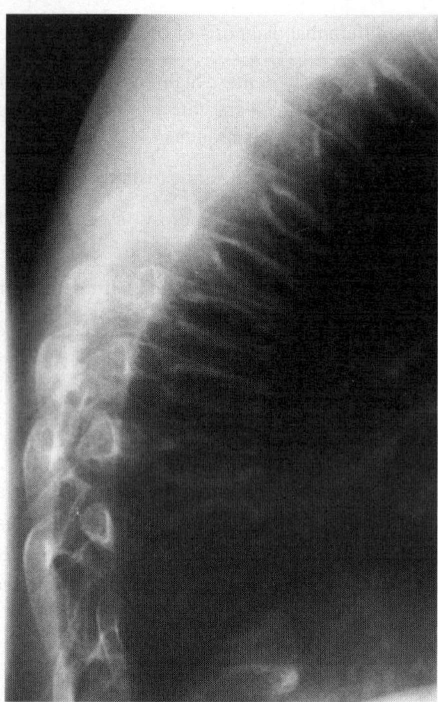

Fig. 2 Widespread vertebral collapse in an 11-year-old boy with idiopathic juvenile osteoporosis.

Osteoporosis and endocrine disease

Thyroid bone disease

In thyrotoxicosis bone turnover is excessive, bone resorption is more increased than bone formation, and after many years of thyroid overactivity significant osteoporosis may occur. There may be hypercalcaemia, hyperphosphataemia, and an increase in plasma alkaline phosphatase; hypercalciuria and increased urinary hydroxyproline also occur. Since thyrotoxicosis is often recognized early, significant bone disease is uncommon.

Corticosteroids and osteoporosis

Osteoporosis is a common complication of Cushing's syndrome or of prolonged administration of corticosteroids. In patients treated with corticosteroids there is not a close association between corticosteroid dose and osteoporosis, although the duration of treatment and reduction in bone mass are significantly related. However, there is wide individual variation, and in some subjects vertebral collapse may occur within a month or so of starting corticosteroid therapy.

The main effect on the skeleton is to reduce osteoblast activity and bone formation. This appears to be direct; indirect suppression of bone formation also results from the inhibitory action of corticosteroids on the pituitary, affecting the production of oestrogen and testosterone. Early in corticosteroid treatment there is also an increase in osteoclast resorption secondary to intestinal malabsorption of calcium and hypercalciuria.

In children excess glucorticoids particularly affect the vertebrae and, in contrast to other forms, the skull. There is also excessive callus formation around fractures. Such fractures may occur in the same regions as Looser's zones (pubic rami, ribs), and be relatively painless.

The pituitary and osteoporosis

Hypopituitarism in childhood produces infantilism. The epiphyses fuse very late and the rarefied bones tend to collapse in adult life. Acromegaly is often said to be a cause of osteoporosis because of the radiographic appearance of the skeleton, but there is little other evidence of this.

Hypogonadism

Bilateral oophorectomy in young women is a well-recognized cause of severe osteoporosis. There is also some evidence that in a significant proportion of women oestrogen deficiency follows a year or so after hysterectomy, despite leaving the ovaries *in situ*.

Bone mass is similarly reduced in young women with anorexia nervosa, and in others in whom illness results in temporary amenorrhoea.

In men, hypogonadism is a potentially reversible cause of osteoporosis and should always be considered in a young patient. Treatment with testosterone derivatives is important. Interestingly osteoporosis has been described in a man with a mutation in the oestrogen receptor.

Osteoporosis and chromosomal abnormalities

The most common chromosomal cause of osteoporosis is probably Turner's syndrome. In those with chromosomal mosaics there may be no symptoms apart from growth failure and delayed puberty. In Down's syndrome osteopenia is described in childhood which does not persist after adolescence.

Other possible causes of osteoporosis

Osteoporosis may occur in association with alcoholism, liver disease, chronic heparin administration, and rheumatoid arthritis. It is said to occur more frequently in cigarette smokers and in thin people. Recent studies demonstrate that diabetics do not have clinically significant osteoporosis. Osteoporosis in osteogenesis imperfecta, homocystinuria, and scurvy are dealt with separately.

Osteomalacia and rickets

Osteomalacia results from a lack of vitamin D or a disturbance of its metabolism; in the growing skeleton it is referred to as rickets, and the terms are often used interchangeably. Very rarely, severe calcium deficiency can lead to rickets. Inherited hypophosphataemia and a number of other renal tubular disorders may also cause rickets without clear evidence of abnormal vitamin D metabolism.

The main histological feature of osteomalacia is defective mineralization of bone matrix. Understanding of osteomalacia relies on knowledge of vitamin D metabolism (Fig. 3). Two aspects require emphasis. The first is the quantitative importance of vitamin D synthesis in the skin in comparison with that in the diet, and the second concerns the relative role of different vitamin D metabolites.

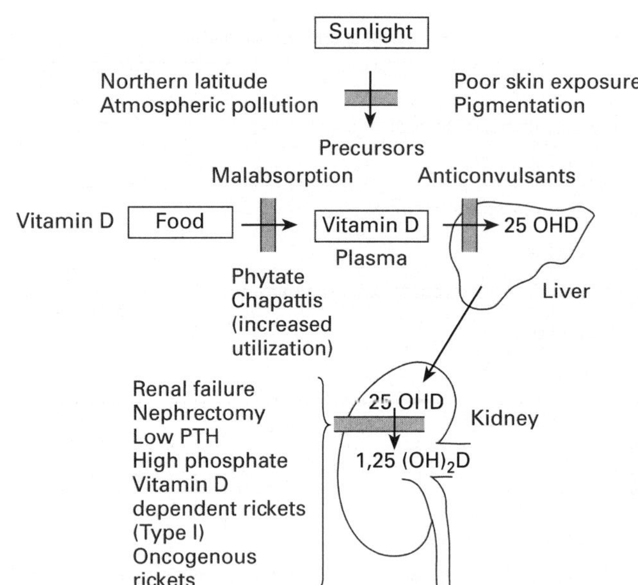

Fig. 3 The causes of rickets and osteomalacia related to the sources and metabolism of vitamin D.

The measurement of circulating concentrations of 25-hydroxy-vitamin D (25(OH)D) as an index of vitamin D status has identified those groups (Asian immigrants and the elderly) most at risk from vitamin D deficiency. Secondly the causes of osteomalacia can now be partly understood in terms of its metabolites, and the major importance of 1,25$(OH)_2$D (1,25-dihydroxy-vitamin D) is established. However, the effects of giving vitamin D cannot be ascribed to the actions of 1,25$(OH)_2$D alone, and probably include other biologically active derivatives, such as 25-hydroxy-vitamin D (25(OH)D) and possibly 24,25-dihydroxy-vitamin D (24,25$(OH)_2$D).

Pathology

The features of osteomalacia can be predicted largely from the known calciotropic effects of vitamin D. Examination of undecalcified bone shows wide osteoid seams with many birefringent lamellae of collagen covering more of the bone surface than normal, and absence of the 'calcification front'. The absence of this front is important since excessive osteoid may also be found in conditions other than osteomalacia, such as hypophosphatasia, Paget's disease of bone, and thyrotoxicosis, where the calcification front is normal; in these disorders the increase tends to be in the amount of bone surface covered rather than in the thickness of osteoid. Excess osteoid also occurs when certain bisphosphonates, such as etidronate, or aluminium accumulate in the skeleton. In rickets the main change is disorganization of the growth plate.

There appears to be no difficulty in laying down bone matrix collagen, but it cannot be properly mineralized.

Causes

There are many causes of osteomalacia (and rickets), some of which are very rare. They may conveniently be divided into three main groups: nutritional, malabsorptive, and renal (Table 5). Most can be understood in terms of vitamin D metabolism (Fig. 3). In the elderly and in some immigrant communities the intake of vitamin D in the food is often deficient and requirements may be increased; the absorption of vitamin D is poor in coeliac disease, after partial

Table 5 The main causes of rickets and osteomalacia

Lack of vitamin D
Deficient synthesis in the skin
Low intake in the diet
Probably increased requirement
Malabsorption
Gluten-sensitive enteropathy (coeliac disease)
Gastric surgery
Bowel resection
Intestinal bypass surgery
Biliary cirrhosis
Renal disease
Renal-tubular disorders
inherited hypophosphataemia (vitamin D-resistant rickets)
others[a]
Renal glomerular failure
renal osteodystrophy
dialysis bone disease
Others
Anticonvulsant osteomalacia
Tumour rickets
Vitamin D-dependent rickets
Phosphate-deficiency rickets

[a] Table 6.

gastrectomy, intestinal resection or bypass, and in biliary disease. The intestinal absorption of calcium is reduced by phytate and chapattis which may also increase vitamin D requirements (see below). Endogenous synthesis of vitamin D in the skin is poor in towns and northern cities in the UK, and is reduced by pigmentation of the skin. The 25-hydroxylation of calciferol may be impaired in some chronic liver diseases, and anticonvulsants may induce hepatic enzymes which degrade vitamin D. The 1α-hydroxylation of 25(OH)D is reduced or absent in renal failure (see Chapter 12.30), after nephrectomy, in hyperphosphataemia, parathyroid insufficiency, in type I vitamin D-dependent rickets and probably in some bone tumours. Many patients have more than one cause for osteomalacia; in the elderly person vitamin D intake is poor, exposure to sunlight is limited, and renal glomerular failure progressive. Reduced exposure to sunlight is a frequent consequence of physical immobility.

Clinical features

The main symptoms of osteomalacia are bone pain and tenderness, skeletal deformity, and proximal muscle weakness, often accompanied by the features of the underlying disorder and by those of hypocalcaemia. In severe osteomalacia all the bones are painful and tender, often sufficiently so to disturb sleep. The tenderness can be particularly marked in the lower ribs and may also be accentuated over Looser's zones. Deformity is most often seen in rickets when the effects of vitamin D deficiency are superimposed on a growing skeleton. The linear growth rate is reduced, there is bowing of the long bones, enlargement of the costochondral junctions (rickety rosary), and bossing of the frontal and parietal bones. Later osteomalacia may produce a triradiate pelvis, a gross kyphosis, and corresponding deformities of the chest.

Proximal muscle weakness is an important symptom. Its cause is unknown and it is more marked in some forms of osteomalacia than in others. Most commonly there is a waddling gait, a difficulty in getting up and down stairs, out of low chairs, and in and out of small cars. In the elderly, weakness may make walking impossible and suggest paraplegia. In younger subjects muscular dystrophy may be simulated.

Features of the underlying disorder include anaemia, tiredness, and steatorrhoea in coeliac disease; pigmentation, thirst, and nocturia in renal failure. Occasionally hypocalcaemia may cause spontaneous tetany; in children the manifestations of carpopedal spasm, stridor, and fits are more dramatic than in the adult.

Measurement of the body proportions is useful. Thus patients with inherited hypophosphataemia and rickets have relatively short limbs, whereas those with late-onset osteomalacia will have a relatively short trunk.

Biochemistry

The detailed biochemical changes differ according to cause. In vitamin D deficiency or malabsorption there is a low plasma calcium and phosphate, a low urine calcium, and an increase in the plasma alkaline phosphatase level. Initially hypocalcaemia may be the only abnormality. Later, with secondary hyperparathyroidism, the plasma calcium returns towards normal, the plasma phosphate falls, and the alkaline phosphatase increases. In inherited hypophosphataemia (vitamin D-resistant rickets) plasma phosphate is low, but the plasma calcium is normal and the alkaline phosphatase may also be normal. Renal glomerular failure causes an increase in the plasma phosphate, urea, and creatinine, and hypocalcaemia, and in the rare renal tubular syndromes there may be a marked systemic acidosis. In patients with osteomalacia the urine should always be examined for the presence of glucose and protein. If these are present, it is important to check for the aminoaciduria characteristic of renal tubular disorders.

Radiology

In rickets the main abnormalities are at the ends of the long bones, where the width of the growth plate is increased, and the metaphysis is widened, cupped, and ragged (Fig. 4); periostitis of the distal ends of the long bones, such as the radius and ulna is common. The radiological hallmark of active osteomalacia is the Looser's zone (Fig. 5). This is a ribbon-like area of defective mineralization, which may be found in almost any bone but is seen particularly in the long bones, the pelvis, and the ribs, and also around the scapulae. Looser's zones may be bilateral and symmetrical; in bones such as the femur they occur on the medial border of the shaft or neck and are usually single, in contrast to the multiple fissure fractures on the lateral convexity of the bone in Paget's disease. In osteomalacia the vertebral bodies are often uniformly biconcave, to produce an appearance likened to a fish spine. Additionally, in renal glomerular osteodystrophy, the end plates may become relatively more dense than the rest of the vertebral body, to produce the so-called 'rugger jersey' spine. In the adult with inherited hypophosphataemia the bones may also become deformed, buttressed, and dense; in this disorder calcification of the tendons and ligaments at their insertions (enthesiopathy) and of the vertebral ligaments can produce an appearance

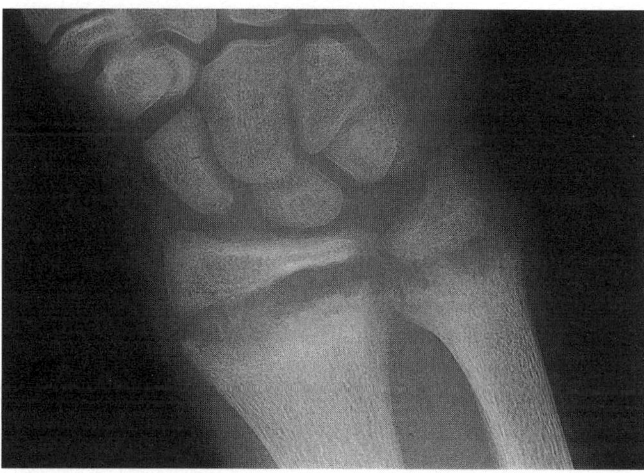

Fig. 4 The radiological appearance of rickets. The growth plates are widened and the metaphyses cupped and ragged.

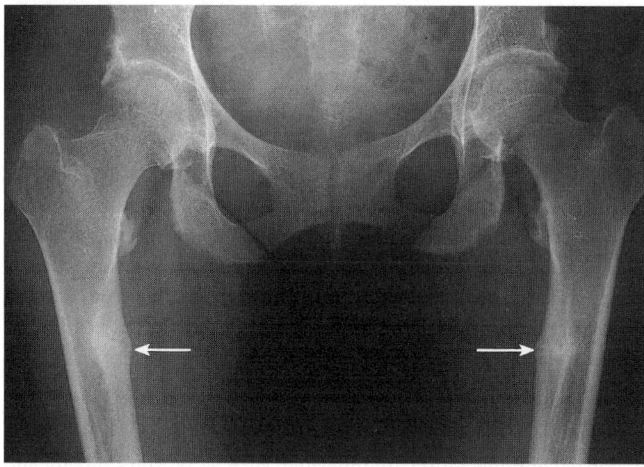

Fig. 5 To demonstrate the bilateral Looser's zones on the medial border of the femora in a woman with osteomalacia due to adult Fanconi's syndrome.

similar to that of ankylosing spondylitis. Ossification of the ligamenta flava narrows the spinal canal and compresses the spinal cord and its roots. This is well shown on CT scans. In patients with osteomalacia and hypocalcaemia the radiological features of secondary hyperparathyroidism appear with subperiosteal bone resorption which affects the phalanges, the pubic symphysis, and the outer ends of the clavicles.

An isotope scan may be very useful in osteomalacia, demonstrating multiple pathological fractures often not seen on the plain films.

Bone biopsy

The diagnosis of osteomalacia is often clear without examining the bone. Where doubt exists, a transiliac biopsy examined before and after decalcification will demonstrate the failure of mineralization and the wide osteoid seams.

Other investigations

Further investigation may be necessary to identify the cause of osteomalacia. Thus patients with vitamin D-deficient rickets or osteomalacia will have a low plasma 25(OH)D. In vitamin D-dependent rickets, measurement of circulating $1,25(OH)_2D$ will be necessary to sort out absence of the 1α-hydroxylase (type 1) from resistance to $1,25(OH)_2D$ (type 2). Further, CT scanning may help to identify the presence of a mesenchymal tumour causing hypophosphataemic osteomalacia.

Diagnosis

Osteomalacia must be distinguished from other forms of metabolic bone disease, from other causes of proximal muscle weakness, and from other disorders causing bone pain. In patients with proximal muscle weakness, Cushing's syndrome, thyrotoxic myopathy, muscular dystrophy, neoplastic neuropathy, dermatomyositis, and polymyositis all need to be considered.

Treatment

Rickets and osteomalacia should respond rapidly to vitamin D (or to its metabolites) in an appropriate dose, which is a useful way of confirming the diagnosis. Increased mobility with increase in muscle strength may be the first clinical response, despite a temporary increase in bone pain. Biochemically, plasma phosphate and urine hydroxyproline are the first to increase. The alkaline phosphatase level may show a temporary rise and then falls slowly to normal.

The effective dose and choice of preparation depends on the cause of the osteomalacia. That due to vitamin D deficiency will respond to microgram doses, but it is often useful to give considerably more than this, such as calciferol 1.25 mg daily for 1–2 weeks only. Where there is doubt about compliance, vitamin D may be injected intramuscularly in one large dose (up to 15 mg = 600 000 units). Lack of response to microgram doses suggest that the osteomalacia is not due to simple vitamin D deficiency but, for instance, to malabsorption or renal failure. It is particularly in the last group that the 1α-hydroxylated metabolites of vitamin D are effective.

Particular forms of osteomalacia and rickets

Nutritional osteomalacia

In the UK nutritional osteomalacia occurs particularly amongst the elderly and in Asian immigrants of all ages. In the elderly the high incidence is mainly due to poor exposure to sunlight and to a low intake of vitamin D, and may be contributed to by the effects of drugs such as anticonvulsants and by increasing renal glomerular failure. The frequency of osteomalacia in patients with fractures of the femoral neck is higher than previously suspected, but figures of up to 30 per cent are probably overestimates. Osteomalacia should always be excluded in elderly people with bone disease, and particularly in those with femoral neck fractures. When in doubt, a therapeutic trial with vitamin D is often useful, since it can be difficult to diagnose osteomalacia in elderly people.

Asian immigrants to the UK develop osteomalacia and rickets more often than the indigenous population. They tend to live in northern cities away from sunlight and women especially do not expose their skin to the limited ultraviolet light. Where dermal synthesis of vitamin D is limited, dietary factors become more important, and it is particularly those on a meat-free diet containing chapattis who develop osteomalacia.

25(OH)D levels can be very low in Asian immigrants. They increase in the summertime, when there may be spontaneous healing of rickets.

Osteomalacia and malabsorption

Coeliac disease is a relatively common cause of malabsorbtive osteomalacia. Osteomalacia can also follow classic partial gastrectomy, but the incidence is debated and its cause is probably multifactorial: post-gastrectomy subjects tend to take little vitamin D in their diet and

Table 6 Renal tubular disorders, rickets, and osteomalacia

Inherited hypophosphataemia
Adult-onset hypophosphataemic osteomalacia
Renal tubular acidosis
Inherited
Proximal (bicarbonate wastage)
Distal (H^+ gradient defect)
Acquired
Ureterocolic anastomosis
Multiple renal tubular defects (Fanconi's syndrome)
Inherited
Cystinosis
Oculocerebrorenal syndrome (Lowe's syndrome)
Wilson's disease
Galactosaemia
Acquired
Cadmium poisoning
Multiple myeloma
Ifosfamide toxicity

there is defective calcium absorption. Osteomalacia is rare after vagotomy and pyloroplasty, but it can follow removal of long segments of small intestine for conditions such as Crohn's disease, and complicates some intestinal bypass operations used for extreme obesity.

Osteomalacia and liver disease

In liver disease osteomalacia is uncommon, except in biliary cirrhosis; prolonged cholestasis may also contribute: there may be also malabsorption of vitamin D or defective 25-hydroxylation.

Anticonvulsant osteomalacia

This has been attributed to the induction by the anticonvulsants of hepatic enzymes which metabolize vitamin D to biologically inactive derivatives. However, epileptic patients in institutions are often deficient of vitamin D because they are deprived of sunlight, and osteomalacia in such patients probably has several causes.

Osteomalacia and renal tubular disease

It is important to distinguish the osteomalacia and rickets of renal glomerular failure from that attributable to renal tubular disorders. Bone disease in renal glomerular failure (renal osteodystrophy) is dealt with elsewhere (see OTM3, p. 3334).

Many renal tubular disorders lead to osteomalacia (Table 6) (see also Chapter 12.31).

Vitamin D-resistant rickets (inherited hypophosphataemia)

This is normally inherited as an X-linked dominant characteristic, in which the main abnormality is hypophosphataemia due to a reduction in the maximum renal tubular reabsorption of phosphate. The mutant gene (the PEX gene) has now been identified. The way in which this leads to the renal phosphate abnormality is unknown. $1,25(OH)_2D$ concentrations are within the normal range; since hypophosphataemia would normally increase 1α-hydroxylation this suggests a reduced sensitivity of the 1α-hydroxylase. Children with hypophosphataemic rickets are unlike patients with other forms of rickets. They present with deformity but are otherwise well, without muscle weakness; however, growth is defective and eventual height is usually less than 150 cm. Apart from hypophosphataemia there may be no other abnormality in biochemical values routinely available, and the plasma alkaline phosphatase can be normal for age. Radiographs show severe rickets, and later the bones are often dense with buttressing and exostoses. Enthesiopathy with ossification of the ligamenta flava can lead to paraplegia. Ligamentous calcification may also contribute to deafness. Abnormal teeth in this disorder cause periapical translucencies and may lead to abscesses.

For many years the mainstay of treatment was large doses of vitamin D; this posed a continuous danger of vitamin D poisoning and did not correct the eventual short stature. When oral phosphate is given in addition to vitamin D, there is an improvement in growth rate, but the condition does not appear to respond to phosphate alone. More recently it has been shown that combined oral phosphate and $1,25(OH)_2D$ produces healing of both epiphyseal and trabecular bone, and this is now the recommended treatment. This combination produces bone healing and may increase eventual stature. However, it is still unusual for affected patients to have a final height of more than 1.5 m (5 ft).

Genetics

Because the defect is inherited as a dominant on the X chromosome, an affected mother transmits the condition to 50 per cent of her children regardless of their gender. All the daughters of an affected father will have the disease, but none of his sons. In general, affected sons have a more severe disease and some affected daughters may be asymptomatic.

Other forms of renal tubular rickets and osteomalacia

Other rare causes of renal tubular rickets and osteomalacia with generalized aminoaciduria are inherited, such as Wilson's disease and the X-linked oculocerebral renal syndrome, or acquired, such as multiple myeloma, cadmium poisoning, and the toxic effects of ifosfamide, used in the treatment of childhood malignant disease. A persistent acidosis with resultant osteomalacia may be inherited or acquired from ureterosigmoid anastomosis.

Tumour rickets

A rare form of hypophosphataemic rickets or osteomalacia occurs in patients who have mesenchymal tumours, often of a particular pathological type, namely sclerosing haemangioperiocytomas or non-ossifying fibromas. In any adult who develops hypophosphataemic osteomalacia, particularly with prominent myopathy, a tumour should be considered. The disorder is improved by oral phosphate and cured by removal of the tumour. The way in which the tumour induces hypophosphataemia and subsequent osteomalacia is unknown, but current evidence suggests that it interferes with renal 1α-hydroxylation of 25(OH)D, since the circulating levels of $1,25(OH)_2D$ are abnormally low and rapidly return to normal when the tumour is removed. Rarely, hypophosphataemic osteomalacia may occur in adults with neurofibromatosis and polyostotic fibrous dysplasia. Oncogenous osteomalacia has also been described in prostatic and oat-cell carcinoma.

Vitamin D-dependent rickets

Patients with these rare, recessively inherited forms of rickets show the features of severe rickets without vitamin D deficiency. There are at least two types of vitamin D-dependent rickets. In type I the activity of the renal 1α-hydroxylase is reduced so that the concentration of $1,25(OH)_2D$ is abnormally low. However, it can be increased by large doses of the native vitamin, which shows that the enzyme block is not complete. In type II there is an end-organ resistance to $1,25(OH)_2D$, which is present in high concentrations. In both forms there is severe rickets and myopathy from infancy; in type II, lifelong total alopecia is a striking feature. Vitamin D-dependent rickets type I responds to very large doses of vitamin D or physiological doses of $1,25(OH)_2D$; type II may also respond to large doses of vitamin D or its metabolites, or to prolonged intravenous calcium, but some recorded cases suggest that recovery occurs spontaneously with age.

The $1,25(OH)_2D$ receptor defects responsible for the end-organ resistance in type II are due to a variety of point mutations in the gene for the 1,25 receptor, either at its steroid- or DNA-binding domains. Type II vitamin D dependent rickets is also known as hereditary $1,25(OH)_2$ vitamin D resistant rickets (HVDRR).

Phosphate deficiency rickets

If patients take a large amount of phosphate-binding drugs, such as aluminium hydroxide, a form of hypophosphataemic osteomalacia may develop. This differs clinically from inherited hypophosphataemic osteomalacia by the presence of severe muscle weakness. Other biochemical features include increased calcium absorption with hypercalcuria, associated with an increase above the normal concentration of $1,25(OH)_2D$.

Paget's disease of bone

Paget's disease of bone (osteitis deformans) is the most common of the metabolic bone diseases next to osteoporosis. Its hallmark is excessive and disorganized resorption and formation of bone. Its cause is unknown.

Pathophysiology

The natural history of Paget's disease is similar to that of a multicentric neoplasm or a slow virus disease which begins in young adult life. Electron microscopy shows virus-like inclusion bodies in the osteoclasts of patients with Paget's disease. Immunofluorescence studies suggest that these could represent the measles or respiratory syncytial virus. Another candidate is the canine distemper virus. The results of polymerase chain reaction amplification of reverse transcribed DNA from Paget's tissue to identify the putative virus are controversial.

Genetic studies demonstrate linkage to chromosome 18 (as in familial expansile osteolysis) in some families but exclude it in others.

Histology shows multinucleate osteoclasts which appear to be resorbing bone, and busy osteoblasts which appear to be replacing it; these activities are closely linked. There is also excess fibrosis in the marrow. The bone matrix is laid down in all directions and partially loses its birefringence and strength. Mineralization may be defective, probably because of the excessive rate at which the organic bone matrix is laid down. The cement lines and the mosaic appearances of the bone result from the tidemarks of resorption followed by formation. Osteosarcoma which occurs in Paget's disease is presumably the result of the excessive and prolonged activity of the bone cells. Pagetic bone is large, vascular, and deformed. Its physical characteristics depend on the stage of the disorder, and it may be hard or soft. In any case, it fractures more readily than normal.

Table 7 The radiological prevalence of Paget's disease

	Prevalence (%) of Paget's disease	
	Men	Women
Preston	8.6	6.3
Bolton	7.7	6.4
Blackburn	8.8	3.8
Bradford	7.9	3.6
Hull	7.6	3.1
Southampton	6.6	3.6
Bath	5.3	4.7
Stoke	4.7	4.2
York	5.8	2.5

These data are based on more than 500 patients in each town. The age-standardized incidence is always higher in men than in women. The high incidence in Lancashire towns is not explained. For source see OTM3, p. 3075.

Incidence

Paget's disease occurs in about 3–4 per cent of subjects over 40, is more common in men than in women and its frequency increases with age. It is not unknown in younger people. In Britain about 750 000 people may have Paget's disease, of whom fewer than 5 per cent have symptoms. It seems to be an Anglo-Saxon affliction, being very rare in countries such as Scandinavia and Japan. Within England early radiological surveys showed that it occurs most often in Lancashire towns and in northern industrial regions (Table 7). It is also more frequent in recent British immigrants to Western Australia than in the Western Australian population, but less frequent than in those relatives who remained in Britain. Such studies do not distinguish between the effect of environment and heredity. In a disorder as common as Paget's disease many striking examples of 'familial' Paget's disease occur by chance. Recent studies suggest a decline in its prevalence.

Clinical features

Pain, deformity, fracture

The bone itself may be painful, or pain may be due to arthritis of a nearby joint, to an associated fracture, or to the development of sarcoma. It has been suggested that there is a specific type of hip joint disorder associated with Paget's disease. Bone pain could be due to stretching of the periosteum, since this part of the bone (and the vessels within bone) contain nerves sensitive to pain. Clinically, the affected bones are enlarged, deformed, and warm. The enlargement is well seen in bones such as the tibia and the skull; in the former the bone is typically bowed forwards; the latter shows a characteristic enlargement of the vault which is said to look like a soft beret, or 'tam-o'-shanter', which appears to descend over the ears. Other long bones may become bent and a kyphosis may develop. Although any bones can be affected, including the maxilla and the phalanges, the most common sites for Paget's disease are the pelvis and the spine. Fracture may be the first symptom of undiagnosed Paget's disease, for instance at the junction of a resorbing front with normal bone, or across a fissure fracture (see Fig. 6).

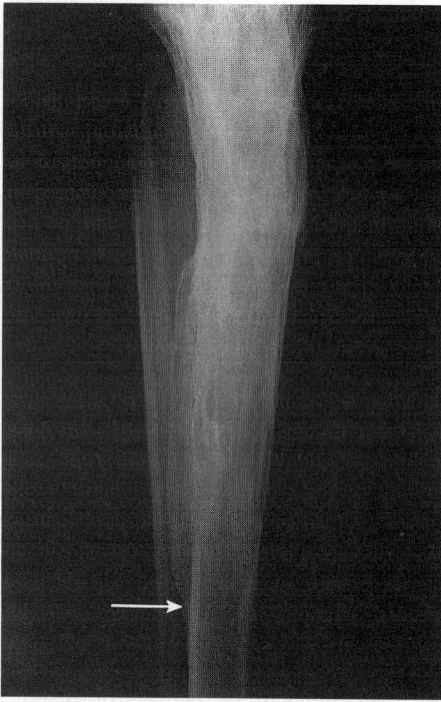

Fig. 6 A healed fracture proximal to a resorbing front (arrowed) in a pagetic bone: proximal to the area of resorption the cortex is thickened and the bone widened by disorganized formation of new bone.

Deafness and nerve compression

Deafness in Paget's disease is one of its most disabling symptoms and responds little to treatment. It has many causes, of which nerve compression is only one.

Most nerves can be compressed by enlarging pagetic bone. The spinal cord is particularly at risk, due to the combined effects of increased bone mass, vertebral collapse, and excessive vascularity. Paraplegia or cauda equina lesions may occur. Alterations in the shape of the skull may produce multiple cranial nerve palsies and brainstem lesions, with dysphagia, dysarthria, and ataxia. Basilar invagination with obstruction of cerebrospinal fluid drainage can lead to internal hydrocephalus, raised intracranial pressure, and confusion.

Heart failure

In severe Paget's disease cardiac output is considerably increased, due to the excessive vascularity of the affected bones, but there is no convincing evidence of large arteriovenous shunts within the skeleton. The heart failure which results may be of the high-output variety, but this is rare. Since heart failure and Paget's disease of bone are common in the elderly, their occurrence together is usually coincidental.

Sarcoma

In the past the incidence of sarcoma in Paget's disease has sometimes been overestimated; it probably occurs in 1 per cent or less of those with symptoms. Paget's sarcoma often occurs in the humerus, although Paget's disease itself is most common in the pelvis and spine. Sarcoma should be considered in a patient known to have Paget's disease if pain has developed for the first time, or worsened, or if deformity has altered. Radiologically, the appearance of the pagetic bone alters, with evidence of bone destruction (Fig. 7); the tumours occur most often in the medulla. Lytic lesions are more common than sclerotic; periosteal reaction is uncommon; and radionuclide diphosphonate scans often show areas of decreased uptake (contrasting with the increased uptake of the underlying pagetic bone).

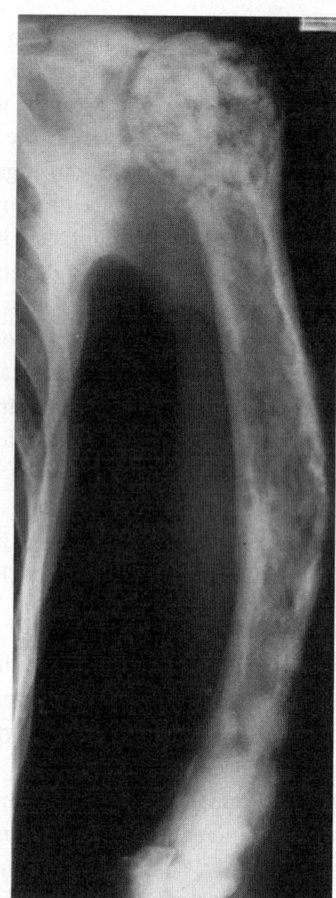

Fig. 7 A sarcoma in the upper end of the left humerus in a man of 70 with Paget's disease. The destructive lesion in the proximal humerus has been treated with radiotherapy; there are secondary deposits around the distal end of the bone.

Biochemistry

There is a marked increase in the level of plasma alkaline phosphatase, derived from the overactive osteoblasts, which is roughly related to the extent of clinical and radiological involvement. In contrast, the acid phosphatase (derived partly from osteoclasts) is only slightly increased. The rapid turnover of bone matrix collagen increases the urinary hydroxyproline in proportion to the increase in alkaline phosphatase. The plasma calcium and phosphate are normal; hypercalcaemia suggests coexistent hyperparathyroidism, malignant disease, or immobility.

Radiology

The radiological appearances of Paget's disease are legion. The most characteristic is an increase in size of the affected bone. Resorption predominates early in the disease and in the young patient. A resorbing front may be seen in a long bone (as a flame-shaped area) or in the skull (as 'osteoporosis circumscripta'). Excessive resorption is inevitably followed by disordered formation, and at this stage the bone becomes thick and deformed. In elderly subjects multiple partial fractures (microfractures, fissure fractures) are common on the deformed convex surface of long bones (Fig. 6), particularly the femur and tibia.

The use of bone-scanning agents (such as $^{99}Tc^{m}$-labelled disodium etidronate (EHDP)) has been particularly informative in Paget's disease. Affected bones take up the isotope avidly, which demonstrates both the extent of the bone lesions and the effects of treatment.

Diagnosis

The diagnosis of Paget's disease is usually obvious. It may initially be confused with osteomalacia because of the high plasma alkaline phosphatase; bone biopsy is then useful. An elevated plasma calcium should suggest additional hyperparathyroidism or malignant disease. In prostatic carcinoma with osteoblastic bone secondaries the dense bones are not enlarged (as they are in Paget's disease) and the acid phosphatase is considerably and disproportionately increased in relation to the alkaline phosphatase. Of many other conditions with similar radiological appearance, fibrous dysplasia (see below), in which the alkaline phosphatase may also be slightly increased, may be difficult to distinguish; in the generalized form the unilateral bone lesions, pigmentation, and sexual precocity (in the female) are characteristic. Another rare disorder usually mistaken for Paget's disease is fibrogenesis imperfecta ossium (see below), where the bone trabeculae are thickened without bony enlargement and there are multiple abnormal fractures.

Treatment

Medical treatment

Patients with pain associated with Paget's disease should first be treated with a simple analgesic. Where possible it should be determined whether the pain is directly due to the bone disease or to associated arthritis. In those who have pain due to bone disease despite analgesia, or have the complications of deformity, nerve compression, deafness, or heart failure, specific treatment aimed at the pagetic bone should be considered. This should also be considered in the young person with Paget's disease to prevent further progress. There is no evidence that the rapid course of pagetic sarcoma is altered by any treatment. Of the many agents previously tried in Paget's disease, such as aspirin, fluoride, and corticosteroids, only three are currently in use, mithramycin, bisphosphonates, and calcitonin. Mithramycin is now rarely used. It may rapidly abolish pain, but the effect is usually temporary. It has been used on its own or in combination with bisphosphonates or calcitonin.

The bisphosphonates are a series of compounds with a P-C-P structure resistant to the naturally occurring phosphatases and pyrophosphatases. They are effective orally or parenterally and reduce excessive bone turnover in Paget's disease. The first bisphosphonate used, ethane-l-hydroxy-l,l-bisphosphonate (disodium etidronate, EHDP, Didronel®), also interferes with mineralization if given in high doses (20 mg/kg body weight); subsequent derivatives, dichloromethylene bisphosphonate (Cl_2MDP) and 3-amino-hydroxy-propylidine-l,l-bisphosphonate (APD, pamidronate) do not appear to do this. According to their dose, the bisphosphonates may take up to 6 months to produce their effect on symptoms, histology, and biochemistry. The recommended dose for EHDP is 5 mg/kg/day for up to 6 months. It also has been used in combination with calcitonin, and together these agents suppress Paget's disease more effectively than when given alone. The biochemical effects of EHDP may last for a long time (possibly several years) after the drug is stopped. Both Cl_2MDP and APD effectively suppress resorption in Paget's disease without disturbing mineralization.

The calcitonins have been used for the treatment of Paget's disease, and salmon calcitonin is the most effective form. Various dose regimens are used, among which 100 IU three times a week is average. Injected calcitonin may produce nausea and vomiting; if side-effects are troublesome, it is best given in the evening with an antiemetic. Its main effects are in the first 3 months of treatment, and continued treatment is ineffective, especially when the alkaline phosphatase level has ceased to decline. Antibodies to calcitonin do develop but are not necessarily related to calcitonin 'resistance'.

Indications for the bisphosphonates and calcitonins are different. Calcitonin is preferred to treat bone pain, for osteolytic Paget's disease, and for preoperative treatment (below). Some evidence suggests that calcitonin may halt the progression of deafness. Spinal cord compression is also alleviated. Calcitonin can also be given preoperatively to reduce excessive bleeding when operations such as total hip replacement have to be done on pagetic bone.

The majority of pagetic patients who require treatment are now given a bisphosphonate. Many new bisphosphonates of increasing potency have been developed. These include alendronate (amino-butane bisphosphonate) and tiludronate (chloro-4-phenyl thio-methylene bisphosphonate).

Surgical treatment

Fractures through pagetic bone require the usual surgical treatment, although union may be delayed. Where fracture occurs through a deformed bone, this deformity should be corrected. In addition, elective osteotomy and intramedullary nailing may be considered for severe long bone deformity. Spinal cord compression not responding to medical treatment requires surgery. Rarely, hydrocephalus may require a ventriculojugular shunt.

Parathyroids and bone disease

This subject is addressed in Chapter 7.5.

Osteogenesis imperfecta: the brittle bone syndrome

Osteogenesis imperfecta is said to occur in about 1 in 20 000 births; since the milder forms may never be diagnosed, this could be an underestimate. It is a leading cause of lethal short-limbed dwarfism and crippling skeletal dysplasia. There is no convincing evidence of different racial frequency. Many patients do not fit easily into the Sillence classification (Table 8), and in some hypermobility and features of the Ehlers-Danlos syndrome (see below) are dominant.

Pathophysiology

Osteogenesis imperfecta involves those tissues that contain the major fibrillar collagen, type I. These include particularly bone and dentine, but also the sclerae, joints, tendons, heart valves, and skin. The pathology in bone varies with the type and severity of the disease, with age, previous fracture, and surgery. The skeletal effects of osteogenesis imperfecta are most severe in the lethal forms (type II) and at the region of the growth plate. There is faulty conversion of apparently normal mineralized cartilage to defective bone matrix. The collagen fibres are thin but show the normal striated pattern. The endoplastic reticulum of the osteoblasts is dilated by retained mutant collagen. In type III, which is less severe, there are variable amounts of woven immature bone, with disorganized trabeculae and an apparent excess of osteocytes—as in other forms of the disorder. At the growth plate there are multiple islands of cartilage in the epiphyses and metaphyses. Accounts of the bone pathology in type IV are sparse.

Table 8 Current clinical classification of osteogenesis imperfecta

Type	Clinical features	Inheritance
I	Few fractures Normal stature Prominent extraskeletal features Little or no deformity	Autosomal dominant
II	Multiple fractures Perinatal lethal, short limbs	New dominant mutations
III	Bones deform with age Extreme short stature Dentinogenesis imperfecta common Sclerae less blue with age	Some new mutations Some recessive
IV	Moderate bone deformity and short stature Sclerae normal colour	Autosomal dominant

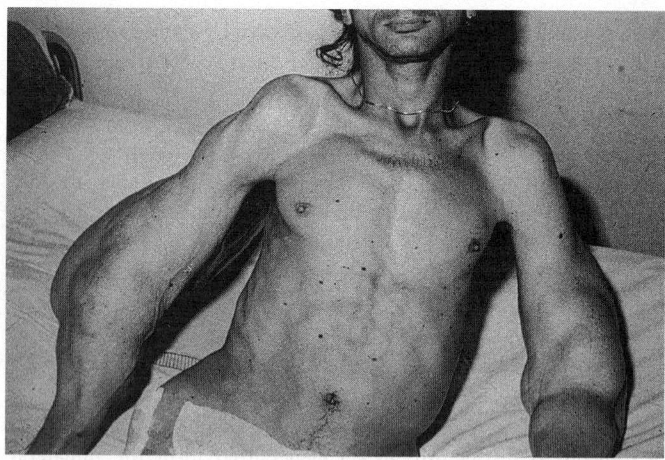

Fig. 8 The appearance of hyperplastic callus in a patient with osteogenesis imperfecta.

In mild, type I osteogenesis imperfecta there is a reduction in the amount of bone (and hence in measured bone mineral density) and defective bone formation at the cellular level, such that the osteoblasts each make approximately half as much bone collagen as normal. The result is an osteoporotic bone with an apparent excess of osteoblasts and osteocytes. This appearance of 'hyperosteocytosis' suggests an increase in bone turnover rate. The overall bone structure is otherwise normal, apart from occasional woven bone. In affected dentine, the odontoblasts produce short, branched dentinal tubules and fill in the dental pulp. In the ear, the auditory ossicles may be imperfect or fractured.

The reduction in collagen is repeated in non-skeletal tissues. Thus, the sclerae are thin (leading to their blueness since the pigmented coat of the choroid becomes visible), the tendons are gracile and weak, the thin heart valves may become incompetent, and the aortic root dilated.

Clinical features

Type I is the most frequent and least serious form, and accounts for 60 per cent of all patients with the disorder. Fractures can occur in the perinatal period or even be delayed until the early perimenopause. After the menopause the overall fracture rate has been recorded at seven times more than in the normal population, and the vertebral bone mineral content in adults with type I osteogenesis imperfecta has been found to be 70 per cent of normal.

Childhood fractures in type I osteogenesis imperfecta may be numerous, but rarely lead to deformity unless treated inappropriately. Any type of fracture can occur; they become less frequent with age. Overall, fractures are more frequent in the lower limbs. Significant scoliosis is rare. The skull shows interesting changes; in addition to multiple wormian bones, the vault may overhang the base, leading to basilar impression requiring surgical correction.

Clinical dentinogenesis imperfecta occurs in only some patients; the appearance varies widely and affects some teeth more than others; the teeth are discoloured and the normal enamel fractures easily from the dentine, leading to rapid erosion of both the first and second dentition. Blueness of the sclerae is a particularly important physical sign. The cause of the frequently early arcus is unknown. The cardiac manifestations are also important, not only because of their effects but because tissue fragility makes surgery dangerous. Aortic incompetence, aortic root widening, and mitral valve prolapse all occur. Patients with osteogenesis imperfecta often show hypermobile joints.

Type II is nearly always lethal but the severity does differ: some children may be born dismembered whereas others may (rarely) survive the perinatal period to later merge into the type III form. Not all infants with multiple fractures at birth succumb immediately. Perinatal death results from the mechanical uselessness of the skeleton, which leads to respiratory failure or intracranial haemorrhage.

Type III causes most clinical difficulty, since its cause and forms of inheritance are obscure and its disability is severe and progressive. During the early years of life, progressive deformity affects the skull, the long bones, the spine, chest, and pelvis; the deformity is associated with fractures but can probably occur without them. The radiological appearance of the bones changes rapidly with age. The face appears triangular, with a large vault, prominent eyes, and small jaw. The sclerae may be blue in infancy but take on a normal colour in childhood. Eventual disability and deformity is considerable. Such patients rarely walk, even after multiple operations, and have a very short stature (-4 to -6 standard deviations (SD) below the mean). The changes in the long bones are often bizarre, with long, thin diaphyses and comparatively wide metaphyses. Cartilaginous islands often develop at the end of the long bones in the epiphyses and the metaphyses, spreading into the diaphysis, giving the appearance of 'popcorn' bone. Early death may occur from respiratory infections superimposed on the restrictive reduction in vital capacity associated with severe kyphoscoliosis. Progressive deformity requires specialized orthopaedic care.

Type IV is clinically intermediate between type I and type III and is inherited as a dominant trait. The sclerae are of normal colour after infancy. Overall stature is reduced and disability is variable. The rare complication of hyperplastic callus occurs most often in this form (Fig. 8). This begins with a swollen, painful, and vascular swelling, most often over the long bones, an increase in plasma alkaline phosphatase, and sometimes a systemic illness.

Diagnosis

In the perinatal period, the concern is with alternative causes of lethal short-limbed dwarfism. In the first few years of life, 'the battered baby syndrome' is the main differential diagnosis. The distinction between osteogenesis imperfecta and non-accidental injury is legally important and can be difficult.

In late childhood and adolescence idiopathic juvenile osteoporosis needs to be distinguished. This begins during growth with fractures of the long bones, reduction in growth rate (due to vertebral collapse), and metaphyseal compression fractures. In adult life, mild osteogenesis imperfecta may go unrecognized.

Collagen biochemistry

In type I osteogenesis imperfecta there appears to be a null allele for collagen I, so that only 50 per cent of collagen is produced but this is of normal composition. Lethal osteogenesis imperfecta (type II) may result from large gene deletions, but more commonly from single base changes in COL1A1 or COL1A2. The effect on the triple helix appears to be most marked when the substitution occurs near the carboxy-terminal end of the chain, when the substituting amino acid is large, and when it occurs in the α1- rather than the α2-chain. Such mutations delay helix formation and render collagen structurally unsound. Such abnormalities are common in type II osteogenesis imperfecta and less well defined in type III, which may rarely result from failure to synthesize α2-chains. Type IV is most often due to changes in the α2-chain.

The mutant locus for osteogenesis imperfecta can now be followed through large, dominantly inherited families providing the basis for accurate prenatal diagnosis from a chorionic villus biopsy.

Genetic advice

Parents who have had an infant with osteogenesis imperfecta need advice about further pregnancies. Where the mutant gene is dominant (type I and IV) and where one parent is clearly affected, the likelihood of affected children is 50 per cent. Difficulties arise where neither parent is clinically affected and in the lethal and progressive deforming varieties of the brittle bone syndrome. It is impossible then to give an accurate prediction of the likelihood of another affected child. However, there are some guidelines. Where one offspring of clinically unaffected parents has a form of osteogenesis imperfecta which fits into type I or type IV, this is likely to be a new dominant mutation and risk of a further affected child is probably no more than normal. In the case of type II disease, the evidence is that the great majority (if not all) result from a new dominant mutation. To allow for the possibility of germ-line mosaicism the likelihood of phenotypically normal parents having a second baby with type II disease is put at approximately 7 per cent.

The recurrence risk in type III is unknown. If recessive inheritance, which is very rare, is included in the definition, it is 25 per cent; if not, it is considerably less.

Germ-line and somatic cell mosaicism are important factors in the inheritance and expression of osteogenesis imperfecta. This accounts for those pedigrees where a phenotypically normal man has two babies with lethal osteogenesis imperfecta by separate partners. Somatic mosaicism likewise provides one (but not the only) explanation for phenotypic variability and differing tissue expression.

Prenatal diagnosis

This may be done from the second trimester by ultrasound and appropriate radiographs, and in the first trimester by analysis of fetal DNA from a chorionic villus biopsy (see OTM3, p.3082). The choice depends on clinical circumstances.

Confident diagnosis by ultrasound is possible only in the more severe forms of osteogenesis imperfecta (types II and III).

Prognosis and management

It is in those severely affected survivors classified as type III that management will be a lifelong and specialized problem. Such individuals are of normal intelligence and prolonged admission to hospital, either for repeated surgery or for investigation, should not necessarily take precedence over education. Intramedullary rodding to correct deformity and improve mobility should be very selective since the bones are often so abnormal as to take little advantage from such procedures. An organized programme of rehabilitation is important. There is no convincing evidence that medical treatments such as fluoride (to increase bone formation) or calcitonin (to decrease bone resorption) have any beneficial effect. Intermittent intravenous bisphosphonate (in the form of 3-amino-hydroxypropylidine-l,l-bis-phosphonate (APD)) may produce corresponding increases in bone density. Improvement in symptoms, bone mineral density, and bone histology are also described. The non-skeletal features of osteogenesis imperfecta, such as dentinogenesis imperfecta, aortic incompetence, and deafness also require management.

The Marfan syndrome

This disorder is dominantly inherited. Its major effects are on the skeleton, cardiovascular, and ocular systems. There is considerable phenotypic variation. In the typical patient, the overall height is increased (relative to unaffected siblings or a matched population) and the limbs are long relative to the trunk (so that the crown to pubis measurement is less than pubis to heel). Long, thin fingers (arachnodactyly) are common. Together with hypermobility, this disproportion forms the basis of clinical signs of variable utility. However, not all patients with Marfan's syndrome are long and thin. The skeletal phenotype differs from one family to another and within families. Asymmetric anterior chest deformity is associated with either depression or prominence of the sternum. Scoliosis is common, may be severe, and worsens during preadolescent growth as in the idiopathic form. The hard palate is often narrow and high-arched (gothic).

Dislocation of the lens is the main ocular feature of Marfan's syndrome (see Plate 16, The eye and disease). Typically, this occurs upwards or sideways (in contrast to the downward dislocation in homocystinuria), and this may be present at birth or occur later. Dislocation causes the unsupported iris to wobble on movement (iridodinesis). Less important ocular features are squint, myopia, and retinal detachment. The axial length of the globe is increased and the cornea tends to be flattened.

The most severe complication of the Marfan syndrome is dilatation of the ascending aorta leading to aortic incompetence and dissection. Progressive widening of the aorta can be readily measured by serial echocardiography. Less well known manifestations include cutaneous striae, herniae, spontaneous pneumothorax, and dural ectasia. The mean life expectancy in Marfan's syndrome is reduced by nearly 50 per cent, predominantly due to cardiovascular catastrophe.

Pathophysiology

Marfan's syndrome is caused by mutations in the epidermal growth factor-like regions of the fibrillin gene on chromosome 15. Fibrillin is the major constituent of the microfibrillar system and of the suspensory ligament of the lens; and it is also associated with elastin-containing tissues such as the aorta. This explains the association between dislocation of the lens and dissection of the aorta. The aorta dilates at its proximal part at the sinuses of Valsalva, and returns to normal diameter below the innominate artery, unless a dissection is present. The cusps of the aortic valve do not close efficiently. Dissection is most often above the aortic valves in the area of greatest dilatation. The dissection may progress forwards or backwards. Retrograde dissection may tear the attachment of the coronary arteries and rupture into the pericardial sac. Histopathology shows a reduction in elastic fibres which are swollen and fragmented. The valve cusps are usually diaphanous and redundant. In the eye the suspensory ligament of the lens is disorganized.

Diagnosis

At present, there is no certain biochemical way of excluding or confirming Marfan's syndrome and in those with few clinical features and no family history, the diagnosis can be difficult. The diagnostic criteria are often revised.

In the absence of an unequivocally affected first-degree relative, evidence of involvement of the skeleton, together with at least two other systems, and one major manifestation is necessary; when one first-degree relative is affected, involvement of at least two systems, with one major manifestation preferred, confirms the diagnosis. Homocystinuria (see below), which has a recessive mode of inheritance, should be excluded. Other important alternative diagnoses include congenital contractural arachnodactyly, familial tall stature, isolated mitral valve prolapse, familial or isolated annulo-aortic ectasia, and Stickler's syndrome. The latter is a dominantly inherited connective tissue disorder that affects the eyes, ears, and skeleton with severe myopia in childhood, sensorineural hearing loss from adolescence, and degenerative arthritis from early adult life. The diagnosis can be made at birth if cleft palate and micrognathia are present. There is considerable phenotypic variation. In some families the disorder is linked to mutations in the type II collagen gene.

Contractures can occur in Marfan's syndrome but are of a late onset. In congenital contractural arachnodactyly, which is inherited as an autosomal dominant trait, contractures involving the hands, feet, and larger joints are present from birth and tend to improve. Abnormal ears are described. Limited studies suggest that this disorder involves mutations of an additional fibrillin gene on chromosome 5.

Treatment

Major clinical manifestations require attention. Scoliosis may be progressive and severe, particularly in adolescence. Bracing is largely ineffective and operative stabilization may be necessary. Excessive height in girls may be prevented by giving oestrogen together with progestogen in the prepubertal years. Marked sternal deformity may need correction for cosmetic or cardiopulmonary reasons, but opinions on the value of surgery vary widely. It is rarely necessary to remove dislocated lenses unless they prolapse into the anterior chamber, but myopia should be corrected. The main decisions concern the management of the cardiovascular problems; when and if to operate on the dilated ascending aorta or to replace incompetent valves, and whether aortic dilatation can be prevented by reducing the intermittent force on its walls due to left ventricular systole. Current evidence suggests that giving a β-blocker has a significant beneficial effect on aortic dilatation. Progressive aortic widening (measured regularly by echocardiography), together with progressive aortic incompetence and left ventricular strain provide strong indications for replacement of the proximal aorta by a prosthesis. Mitral valve replacement may also be necessary.

Since both aortic and mitral valves are susceptible to endocarditis, prophylactic antimicrobials must be given at the time of dentistry.

Genetic advice

Genetic advice is at present based on clinical observations and the knowledge that inheritance is of the autosomal dominant pattern. There is no close association between the type and position of the mutation and clinical severity.

Ehlers-Danlos syndrome

This syndrome initially included only those conditions with the common clinical features of abnormal velvety hyperelastic skin which healed poorly, hyperextensible joints, and lax ligaments. However, the disorders included in this syndrome have now been increased and have brought with them additional specific features, amongst which is vascular rupture, especially in type IV Ehlers-Danlos syndrome, associated with various mutations in type III collagen. In the currently expanded Ehlers-Danlos syndrome the skeleton is particularly affected in types VI and VII (Table 9).

Homocystinuria

Homocystinuria is phenotypically similar to Marfan's syndrome but with a different cause and additional important complications. It is due to a deficiency of cystathionine β-synthase, an enzyme whose gene is located on chromosome 21, and which contains firmly bound pyridoxal phosphate (vitamin B_6). Homocystinuria is inherited as an autosomal recessive condition and is described more fully in Chapter 6.5.

Alkaptonuria (see also Chapter 6.5)

In this rare autosomal recessive disorder, decreased activity of homogentisate oxidase leads to accumulation of homogentisic acid in the urine and increased pigmentation (ochronosis) in cartilage and connective tissues. Mutations in the gene for the defective enzyme have now been described. Darkening of the urine, alkaptonuria, is due to the presence of 2,5-dehydroxyphenylacetic acid derived from the oxidation and polymerization of homogentisic acid. Polymerization increases in alkaline urine and is slowed down by antioxidants such as vitamin C. The structure of the pigment which causes ochronosis is not known. It is granular or homogeneous and may occur within or outside the cell. It is said to be associated with a reduction in lysyl hydroxylase in the tissue concerned, and impairment of the cross-links of collagen.

The most important effects of this disease are on the spine (Fig. 9) and later on the larger joints. The intervertebral discs lose height and subsequently calcify; they may also herniate acutely. The spine becomes rigid and short and the lumbar lordosis is lost. In the large joints, such as the knees, shoulders, and hips, there are effusions and loose bodies. The symphysis pubis may be affected but not the sacroiliac joints. Ochronotic 'arthritis' is described with episodes of acute inflammation which resemble those of rheumatoid arthritis. Calcification of the aorta is an additional feature.

The diagnosis of alkaptonuria—often made late—should be suspected where there is a premature disc degeneration, even if there is no excessive darkening of the urine. Early degenerative arthritis

Table 9 Classification and clinical features of the Ehlers-Danlos syndrome

	Type	Inheritance	Skin extensibility and fragility	Bruising	Joint mobility	Other significant features	Biochemical defects
I	Gravis	Dominant	Gross	Severe	Generalized gross	Prematurity Molluscoid pseudotumours Musculoskeletal deformity	?Abnormal collagen fibrils and fibre packing
II	Mitis	Dominant	Mild	Mild	Moderate, often limited to hands and feet	None	Not known
III	Benign hypermobile	Dominant	Variable, usually minimal	Mild	Generalized gross	Recurrent joint dislocations Osteoarthritis Skilled contortionists	Not known
IV	Ecchymotic (arterial or Sack-Barabas type; includes acrogeria)	Dominant or recessive	Thin pale skin with prominent veins	Gross	Minimal limited to digits	Rupture of great vessels and bowel Elastosis perforans serpiginosa	In synthesis, secretion, and structure of type III collagen
V	X-linked	X-linked	Moderate with variable fragility	Variable	Mild	Floppy value syndrome	Lysyl oxidase deficiency (unconfirmed in other patients)
VI	Ocularscoliotic (hydroxylysine deficient disease)	Recessive	Moderate	Moderate	Generalized gross	Scoliosis Microcornea Ocular fragility	Procollagen lysyl hydroxylase deficiency
VII	Arthrochalasis multiplex congenita	Recessive	Moderate	Moderate	Severe	Short stature Congenital dislocations	N-terminal cleavage sites for procollagen peptidase mutated
VIII	Periodontitis	Dominant	Minimal with marked fragility	Mild	Moderate limited to digits	Advanced generalized periodontitis	Not known
IX	X-linked skeletal Bowed long bones	X-linked recessive	Moderate	Moderate	Moderate	Occipital exostoses Deformed clavicles	Abnormal copper metabolism

suggests the disease, confirmed by finding deeply pigmented articular cartilage at the time of operation. In those patients with lifelong discoloration of the urine, the differential diagnosis is from other rare causes of urinary pigmentation. The urine of a patient with alkaptonuria contains reducing substances and will therefore give a positive result suggesting glycosuria except where glucose oxidase is used. An increase in homogentisic acid in the urine and plasma confirms the diagnosis.

Hypophosphatasia

This rare disorder which occurs in all races has similarities to rickets and osteomalacia. It is due to a reduction in the tissue non-specific alkaline phosphatase (TNSAP) which leads to defective mineralization and a triad of biochemical disturbances; increased urinary phosphoethanolamine, plasma pyrophosphate, and plasma pyridoxal phosphate. Hypophosphatasia has been estimated to occur in 1 in 100 000 live births in Toronto.

Pathophysiology

The biochemical changes result directly from the alkaline phosphatase deficiency. Various mutations have been described in the alkaline phosphatase gene on chromosome I. There is often also hypercalcaemia and hypercalciuria in childhood, and up to half affected children and adults have an increase in plasma phosphate levels. Hyperphosphataemia is also described in carriers in whom increased urinary pyrophosphate excretion is more reliable than urinary phosphoethanolamine as a marker.

Histological examination of bone shows an excess of osteoid with abnormal tetracycline labelling without evidence of secondary hyperparathyroidism. Matrix vesicles do not contain alkaline phosphatase or hydroxyapatite crystals. The primary dental defect is in

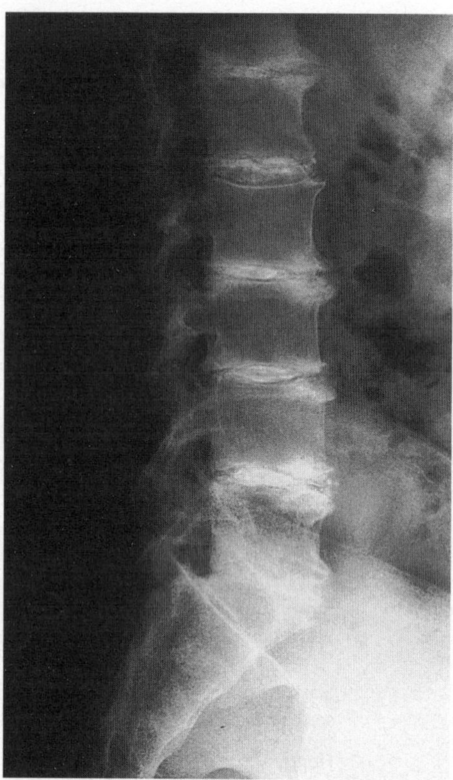

Fig. 9 The appearance of the spine in a man with alkaptonuria. There is universal calcification of the intervertebral discs.

the cementum; additionally, the predentine is widened and the dentinal tubules are enlarged and few.

Clinical features

Four clinical types provide a continuous spectrum from a lethal perinatal disorder to an asymptomatic disease in adults. The first is an important cause of lethal short-limbed dwarfism.

The infantile form (within the first 6 months) results in hypotonia, failure to thrive, hypercalcaemia, and hypercalciuria. Clinical rickets appears and the fontanelle looks wide but there is a functional synostosis. Craniostenosis can produce optic atrophy, exophthalmos, and raised intracranial pressure requiring surgery.

The most variable expression occurs in childhood. Early loss of deciduous teeth, due to defective cementum, may be the only feature (ondontohypophosphatasia). The pulp chambers are enlarged, the root canals short (shell teeth). If bone disease is present, walking is delayed and deformities occur, for instance bow legs, knock knees, short stature, and enlargement of the epiphyses at the wrist, knees, and ankles.

In the adult progressive stiffness, pain in the bones, and apparent 'stress' fractures can occur. Approximately 50 per cent of such patients have a history of bone disease resembling rickets, or premature loss of deciduous teeth, or both in childhood. There may also be premature shedding of adult teeth, short stature, and abnormal skull shape. Recurrent poorly healing metatarsal fractures occur. Partial fractures of the long bones characteristically occur on the convex outer surface (in contrast to the concave inner position of the Looser's zones in osteomalacia), most often in the upper one-third of the femoral shaft, and are often bilateral; other sites include ribs, tibia, and ulna. They may be unaltered for years or increase in size and eventually fracture. Secondary hyperparathyroidism is not seen. Chondrocalcinosis is common and in a proportion is associated with clinical pyrophosphate gout (pseudogout).

Management

Premature synostosis leading to raised intracranial pressure requires surgical relief. Hypercalcaemia may be dealt with by reducing dietary calcium and by giving prednisone. Replacing the defective enzyme by the transfusion of alkaline phosphatase-rich plasma does not produce consistent results. Another theoretically possible approach is the transfusion of bone marrow stromal cells. Intramedullary rods may prevent and treat fractures of the long bones. Dental abnormalities, which can occur in biochemically normal members of hypophosphatasia families, require treatment.

Prenatal diagnosis of a severely affected child can be made by ultrasound. There is also reduced alkaline phosphatase activity in the amniotic fluid cells.

Lysosomal storage diseases (see also Chapter 6.8)

This large group of diseases is due to various inborn errors which affect the function of specific lysosomal enzymes normally responsible for the breakdown of a variety of complex molecules. The skeleton is significantly involved in only a proportion of them. They include some mucopolysaccharidoses and Gaucher's disease.

The Hurler syndrome (MPS IH)

This is the most severe type of mucopolysaccharidosis. The enzyme defect is recessively inherited and all patients have the same appearance, to which the term gargoylism was previously applied. Death often occurs in late childhood, commonly due to pneumonia or to coronary artery disease associated with mucopolysaccharide deposits.

The physical features include proportionate short stature, a typical facial appearance, a short neck with a lumbar gibbus and chest deformity, and a protuberant abdomen. The facial features are coarse and ugly, with flattening of the nasal bridge, large open mouth and tongue, and often with hypertrophied gums over enlarged alveolar ridges. The eyes are prominent with corneal clouding. There is noisy breathing and variable deafness. The vault of the skull may show scaphocephaly or acrocephaly. Other striking features include the stiff, broad trident hands and the large abdomen with hepatosplenomegaly. Radiographs show the abnormal shape of the skull, the slipper-shaped sella turcica, the beaking of the vertebrae with the thoracolumbar kyphosis, and the bullet-shaped phalanges. Similar but less severe features are seen in the Hunter syndrome, inherited as an X-linked recessive.

The Morquio syndrome (MPS IV)

In this disorder the orthopaedic manifestations are striking, and intelligence is normal. Although the disorder is probably heterogeneous and only a proportion of cases excrete an excess of keratan sulphate in the urine, the skeletal changes are uniform. In the first years of life the child becomes progressively more deformed and dwarfed. Characteristically the neck is short, the sternum is protuberant, and there may be a flexed stance with knock knees. There is a striking loss of muscle tone in comparison to the stiffness of MPS IH; hypermobility and a loose skin are features. Radiographs in infancy show a spine similar to that of Hurler syndrome, but later flattening of the vertebrae with anterior beaking lead to relative shortening of the trunk. The small bones of the hands are very different from those of MPS IH and the metacarpals show diaphyseal constriction.

Importantly the odontoid may be hypoplastic, leading to atlantoaxial instability, compression of the long spinal tracts, and paraplegia.

Gaucher's disease (see also Chapter 6.8)

This is a very rare lysosomal storage disorder in which glucocerebroside-containing reticuloendothelial histiocytes accumulate within the bone marrow. It is recessively inherited and largely restricted to Ashkenazi Jews, where the incidence of the adult form (type I) is about 1 in 2500 births. The skeletal manifestations are often severe and disabling. They vary from a characteristic symmetrical failure of remodelling in the lower femora (Erlenmeyer-flask appearance) to diffuse and localized bone loss and osteosclerotic and osteonecrotic lesions, which cause pain and pathological fracture.

Skeletal dysplasias

The term skeletal dysplasia has been used to cover a wide range of generalized disorders of the skeleton affecting both cartilage and bone. It is now correct to distinguish the chondrodysplasias, which primarily affect cartilage from such disorders as diaphyseal hyperostosis and assorted dense bone diseases, where the cause is unknown. Osteopetrosis is a well-defined and separate disorder of osteoclast function.

Most chondrodysplasias are familial, and many are rare. They are more fully described in atlases and orthopaedic texts. Defects in some of the chondrodysplasias mirror those in osteogenesis imperfecta, with the mutant collagen being type II (cartilage collagen) rather than type I. Others involve different collagens and non-collagen connective tissue components.

Clinical features

Precise diagnosis other than in achondroplasia can be difficult. One convenient classification is a clinical one (Table 10). Most patients with skeletal dysplasias have restricted growth, and most are short limbed. The bodily proportions of skeletal dysplasias will provide a clue about whether the limbs are mainly affected, or the spine, or both. In the short-limbed group, achondroplasia and achondroplasia-like dwarfs are the most typical. Those without conspicuous dwarfing include various inherited epiphyseal dysplasias, diaphyseal dysplasias, and some metaphyseal dysplasias. An alternative classification, not based on height, groups the dysplasias according to whether they are predominantly epiphyseal or metaphyseal, whether the spine is predominantly involved, and whether single limbs or segments are involved. Since the biochemical courses of many chondrodysplasias are now known, a classification into dysplasia families according to mutations is possible. Radiographs, taken as soon as possible and, where possible, consecutively, are essential to determine whether the metaphyses of the long bones or the epiphyses are primarily affected.

Osteopetrosis (marble bones disease, see below) is here dealt with separately as a disorder of bone cell biology. Other sclerosing disorders of bone, in some of which biochemical abnormalities have been described (Engelmann's disease, van Buchem's disease), receive brief mention.

Table 10 Clinical classification of the main chondrodysplasias with short stature

Disproportionate	*Proportionate*
Short limbs	Mucopolysaccharidoses
Lethal	*Without obvious short stature*
Type II osteogenesis imperfecta	Multiple epiphyseal dysplasia
Hypophosphatasia	Diaphyseal dysplasias
Achondrogenesis	Some metaphyseal dysostoses
Thanatophoric dwarfism	*With increased limb length*
Not lethal	Marfan syndrome
Achondroplasia	Homocystinuria
Short limbs and trunk	Some diaphyseal dysplasias
Pseudoachondroplasia	*Sclerosing bone dysplasias*
Diastrophic dwarfism	*Others*[a]
Kneist disease	Fibrodysplasia ossificans progressiva
Short trunk	Polyostotic fibrous dysplasia
Spondyloepiphyseal dysplasia	

[a]Many obscure disorders can be added to this list.

Achondroplasia

This is the prototype of short-limbed short stature. It is inherited as an autosomal dominant, with a high mutation rate and the incidence increases with paternal age. It is due to an activating mutation in the transmembrane region of fibroblast growth factor receptor 3. How this mutation leads to the skeletal problems is not yet clear. Until recently any undiagnosed patient with excessively short limbs had the label of achondroplasia. This explains the previous apparent high frequency of achondroplasia and its apparently excessive mortality, since different forms of lethal short-limbed dwarfism were included. The true incidence and natural history are therefore not well defined.

There is a failure of the epiphyseal growth cartilage, and bulbous masses of cartilage appear at the ends of the long bones. In contrast, periosteal and membrane bone formation and bone repair are normal. This selective effect on growth cartilage accounts for the skeletal deformity.

Achondroplasia can be diagnosed at birth or within the first year of life, when the disparity between the large skull and short limbs becomes obvious. There is a striking disproportion between the trunk of normal length and the short arms and legs. Thus the finger tips may only come down to the iliac crest. The shortness of the limbs particularly affects the proximal segment. The limbs themselves look very broad, with abnormally deep creases, and the hands are trident-like. In contrast to the short limbs is the enlarged bulging vault of the skull, the small face, and flat nasal bridge or 'scooped out' glabella. There is a marked lumbar lordosis and also sometimes some wedging of the upper lumbar vertebrae, which may later lead to a thoracolumbar kyphosis. Radiological features include metaphyseal irregularity and flaring in the long bones, irregular and late-appearing epiphyses, a pelvis which is narrow in its anteroposterior diameter, with short iliac wings and deep sacroiliac notches, and a spine which shows progressive narrowing of the interpeduncular distance from above downwards, which is the reverse of normal.

Children with achondroplasia are of normal intelligence, and the complications of this disease arise particularly from the skeletal disproportion. This may lead to early osteoarthritis, to obstetric difficulties and the need for caesarian section, to hydrocephalus, and to paraplegia. Eventual height can vary between about 80 to 150 cm. Narrowing of the spinal canal producing symptoms of spinal stenosis is common. Bilateral leg lengthening partially to correct the symmetrical short stature is possible but is tedious with significant complications.

Homozygous achondroplasia (the offspring of two affected parents) is severe and lethal. In the condition of hypochondroplasia the skeletal disproportion and the spinal abnormalities are less and the skull is unaffected.

Achondroplasia-like dwarfs

For the details of these and other causes of short-limbed dwarfism the reader should consult more specialized texts (see also Table 10). Those which most closely resemble achondroplasia at birth are thanatophoric dwarfism, achondrogenesis, severe hypophosphatasia and type II osteogenesis imperfecta. All can be distinguished radiologically.

Spondyloepiphyseal dysplasias

This is a heterogeneous group of disorders in which the spine is predominantly affected and the short stature is largely due to shortness of the trunk. The most severe type is spondyloepiphyseal dysplasia (SED) congenita; milder forms are referred to as SED tarda. At least some are due to mutations in Type II collagen.

There are various forms of inheritance. **SED tarda** is often X-linked. In affected males the disproportionately short trunk becomes obvious at adolescence. Failure of ossification in the anterior part of the ring epiphyses leads to central and posterior humps on the upper and lower parts of the flattened bodies. The condition needs to be distinguished from multiple epiphyseal dysplasia, which predominantly involves the epiphyses of the long bones.

SED congenita can be diagnosed at birth because of the short stature associated with a short trunk. There may be a close resemblance to Morquio's disease (MPS IV). The severe form may be distinguished from the age of about 4 years. The appearance of the capital femoral epiphyses is delayed (in some patients it may never be seen, except by arthrography). Marked lumbar lordosis, waddling gait, back pain, and progressive disproportion may occur. The odontoid is hypoplastic, kyphoscoliosis may develop, and the interpeduncular distances of the vertebrae do not increase in the lumbar region. Because of all these changes paraplegia may occur. Myopia and retinal detachment are other features.

There is a form of SED, **pseudoachondroplasia**, which resembles achondroplasia because of the short limbs but the facial appearances are normal. The short stature becomes obvious from about 2 years of age. Lumbar lordosis and scoliosis may develop. The tubular bones are short with irregular metaphyses and small, deformed epiphyses. Hypermobility is marked and early osteoarthritis occurs. The mutation affects the cartilage oligomeric protein.

Proportionate dwarfism

Although it is important clinically to classify short stature into proportionate and disproportionate (Table 10), there are many skeletal conditions in which this distinction is difficult to make. Hypophosphataemic rickets, mucopolysaccharidoses, vitamin D-dependent rickets, and osteogenesis imperfecta may come into both categories.

Bone dysplasias without conspicuous short stature

The height of patients with multiple epiphyseal dysplasia may only be slightly reduced. Although many epiphyses are affected, the spine is virtually normal. There are also variable forms of inheritance.

In patients with multiple hereditary exostoses (often referred to as diaphyseal aclasis) there is a juxtaepiphyseal disorder of bone growth, limited to bones developed in cartilage, which gives rise to cartilage-capped exostoses that point away from the joint. The disorder is due to mutations in the tumour suppressor genes. Inheritance is autosomal dominant and stature is normal.

The metaphyseal disorders are rare; some, such as the Jansen type of metaphyseal dysostosis do cause severe dwarfing. In others with less severe growth disturbance, such as Type Schmid, rickets is simulated, and confusion with inherited hypophosphataemia is possible. In progressive diaphyseal dysplasia (see below) the limbs are disproportionately long.

Sclerosing disorders of bone

Apart from marble bones disease (see below) the experience of most physicians of the osteoscleroses is limited by their extreme rarity.

Engelmann's disease (progressive diaphyseal dysplasia: Camurati-Engelmann disease)

This rare condition is inherited as an autosomal dominant. It affects endocrine and muscular systems in addition to the skeleton, where the main feature is a variable but progressive endosteal and periosteal thickening of the diaphyses of the long bones. In severely affected subjects the spine, skull, and axial skeleton are all affected. The cause is unknown.

There is a waddling broad-based gait, muscle wasting and weakness, loss of subcutaneous tissues, and pain in the legs during childhood. The appearance is characteristic; the head is large with a prominent forehead and proptosis, the muscle mass is reduced, and the bones are palpably thickened. Cranial nerve palsies, deafness, and blindness with raised intracranial pressure can occur. Puberty is delayed. Bone pain resistant to analgesia is often a presenting and troublesome feature.

Radiographic appearances vary, from limited thickening of the diaphyses (often in the lower extremities) to widespread new bone formation, affecting all bones, including the skull.

The increased bone turnover causes a moderate increase in plasma alkaline phosphatase and urinary hydroxyproline levels. There may be a markedly positive calcium balance, associated with hypocalcaemia and hypocalciuria. Hyperphosphataemia has been recorded.

Pathological examination confirms gross thickening of the bone with disorganization of internal structure and external shape. The peripheral subperiosteal new bone is woven. The muscles show non-specific type II fibre atrophy.

In the differential diagnosis the proximal myopathy and abnormal gait simulate muscular dystrophy. The radiographic appearances are diagnostic, although idiopathic hyperphosphatasia may present some difficulties.

The course of this disorder is unpredictable and remission of symptoms may occur during adolescence or adult life, so it is difficult to assess treatment. Bone pain may respond to corticosteroids in small, alternate-day doses. Etidronate (20 mg/kg daily) has produced hypocalcaemic tetany but intermittent administration is reported to reduce pain. It is recorded that limb pain may be relieved by surgical removal of a cortical window in the diaphysis.

Pyknodystosis

Pyknodystosis has an autosomal recessive inheritance, with parental consanguinity in some 30 per cent of subjects. It has some similarities to osteopetrosis. It is due to mutations in the gene for cathepsin K, an enzyme used by the osteoclast to resorb bone. Marked reduction in stature with short limbs is a particular feature.

The vault of the skull is large, the face and chin small, the palate high-arched, and the teeth crowded, with retained deciduous teeth. The anterior fontanelle (and other cranial sutures) are typically open. The fingers may appear to be clubbed because of associated acro-osteolysis. The chest is deformed with kyphoscoliosis and pectus excavatum. Recurrent fractures of long bones occur, and occasionally rickets. Radiologically, there are similarities to osteopetrosis with generalized osteosclerosis and fractures. However, the osteosclerosis is uniform; there are no defects of modelling and no endobones. In addition to delayed closure of the cranial sutures there are also wormian bones; the bony fragility, wormian bones, and blue sclerae simulate osteogenesis imperfecta.

Idiopathic hyperphosphatasia

This very rare condition is also labelled juvenile Paget's disease. It has autosomal recessive inheritance. The long bones are abnormal, thickened, and bowed from the first year of life, and the skull may be enlarged. Muscular weakness is common and the plasma alkaline phosphatase level is continuously very high.

Sclerosteosis

This condition is due to an autosomal recessive trait. There is progressive overgrowth and sclerosis of the skeleton, including the skull and the mandible. There are similarities to van Buchem's disease (endosteal hyperostosis), but the skeletal problems are more severe and there is often syndactyly. Prophylactic craniectomy may be necessary to reduce the increased intracranial pressure.

Van Buchem's disease

In this rare hyperostosis, endosteal thickening of the shafts of the long bones is associated with generalized hyperostosis, including the base of the skull and the mandible. Bilateral facial nerve weakness, deafness, and optic atrophy may ensue. Severe recessive and mild dominant forms are described.

Osteopetrosis (marble bones disease)

Marble bones disease or osteopetrosis (Albers-Schönberg disease) is a heterogeneous disorder with a widespread increase in bone density. The basic defect lies in the osteoclasts which, for various reasons, are unable to resorb mineralized bone. Two main forms have been distinguished; recessively inherited severe osteopetrosis causing death in childhood; and the dominantly inherited mild form, in which the diagnosis can be made on radiological grounds alone. This distinction is not absolute and two distinct dominantly inherited forms exist, as well as intermediate forms. Deficiency of carbonic anhydrase II can also cause osteopetrosis associated with cerebral calcification, growth failure, and mental simplicity.

Severe osteopetrosis

In severe recessively inherited osteopetrosis there is widespread increased density of the bones without modelling or remodelling. This produces the Erlenmeyer-flask deformity of the metaphyses. The increase in bone density is often intermittent, producing alternating bands of sclerosis. The increase in bone mass leads to a reduction in bone marrow space with a leucoerythroblastic anaemia and hepatosplenomegaly. It also produces nerve compression, with blindness, deafness, hydrocephalus, delayed tooth eruption, and osteomyelitis. Fracture of the dense bones is common. The affected infant is short with an apparently large head with frontal bossing, hepatosplenomegaly, and knock knees. The plasma calcium appears to alter with the dietary intake and may be sufficiently low to contribute to rickets. The acid phosphatase concentration is increased. Secondary hyperparathyroidism leads to an increase in calcitriol levels. Apart from transplantation of bone marrow, as a source of normal osteoclasts, from an appropriate donor, other forms of medical treatment deal only with complications; these include surgery for fractures, blood transfusions for anaemia, and antibiotics for frequent infections.

Mild osteopetrosis

The mild forms vary from subjects with an increased number of fractures affecting both the long bones and the small bones of the hands and feet, to those in which the disorder is so mild that the diagnosis is made by radiology alone. There are more severe forms of dominantly inherited osteopetrosis with nerve compression, deafness and blindness, and anaemia at times of increased physiological requirement, such as pregnancy. Other established features include osteomyelitis and facial nerve palsy.

Two dominantly inherited forms have been described; one with uniformly dense bones with sclerosis of the cranial vault and the spine and no increase in plasma acid phosphatase, and another with variable bone density (giving rise to an endobone appearance, Fig. 10) and lack of modelling, with a significant increase in plasma acid phosphatase.

Carbonic anhydrase II deficiency

Carbonic anhydrase II deficiency is associated with osteopetrosis, renal tubular acidosis, cerebral calcification, some degree of mental retardation, growth failure, and dental malocclusion. Carbonic anhydrase II is found in the kidney, brain, red cells, and elsewhere, and its gene is on chromosome 22. Deficiency is autosomal recessively inherited, and apparently normal parents of affected offspring have 50 per cent of normal carbonic anhydrase II levels within their red cells. The bone disease is not distinguishable from other forms of osteopetrosis, and fractures occur until adulthood. There is always growth retardation, and height may be more than four standard deviations below the mean. The bone age is also delayed. Radiographic appearances improve in adult life.

The renal tubular acidosis is mixed, both proximal and distal. Cerebral calcification affects the basal ganglia within the first decade. It increases during childhood to include the cortical grey matter and is similar to that occurring in idiopathic or pseudohypoparathyroidism. Histology of bone shows unresorbed calcified cartilage and osteoclasts without a ruffled border.

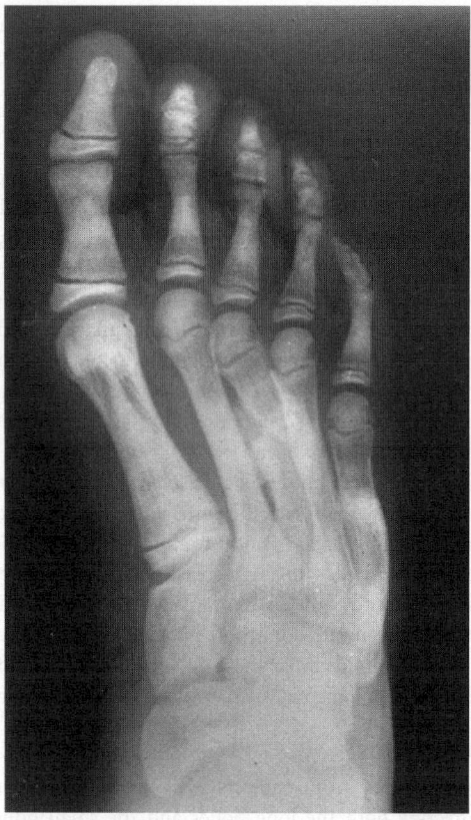

Fig. 10 The appearance of the bones in a boy with dominantly inherited osteopetrosis and raised acid phosphatase. There are variations in bone density ('endobones') with recent and old pathological fractures.

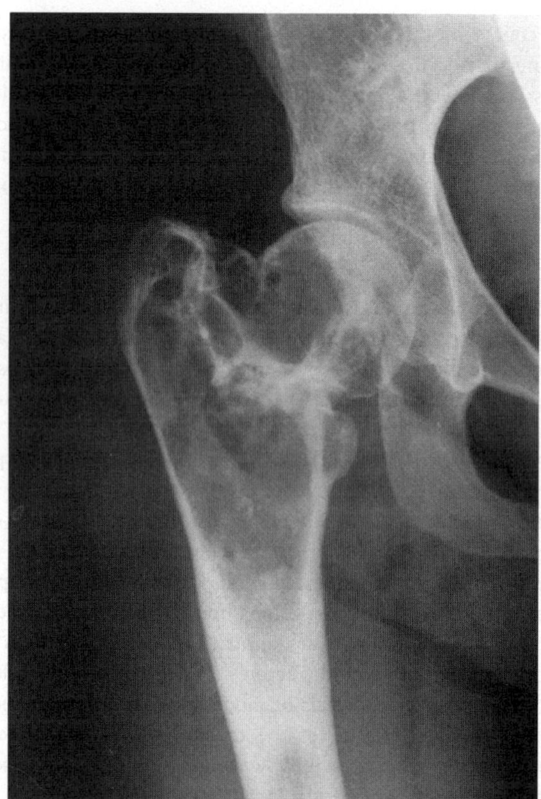

Fig. 11 Polyostotic fibrous dysplasia in a woman of 23 years. A large cyst in the upper femur led to a spontaneous fracture which subsequently united with conservative treatment. Two ribs on the same side of the body show similar abnormalities. Puberty was precocious but pigmentation absent.

The diagnosis should be considered in any neonate with renal tubular acidosis. Genetic counselling is possible since adult heterozygotes have reduced levels of the enzyme in their red cells.

Treatment is symptomatic; it is possible that correction of the renal tubular acidosis temporarily increases the rate of growth.

In the differential diagnosis of osteopetrosis there are many disorders with an excessive amount of bone in various parts of the skeleton; these include other skeletal dysplasias, Caffey's disease (infantile cortical hyperostosis) which causes a temporary increase in bone density from birth, myelofibrosis, renal glomerular osteodystrophy, inherited hypophosphataemia, and fluorosis in adult life.

Fibrous dysplasia

Fibrous dysplasia of bone is a condition in which areas of fibrous tissue, either single or multiple, are found within the skeleton. This results from a widely distributed postzygotic activating mutation in the gene for the alpha subunit of the G-protein signalling system. All forms of fibrous dysplasia appear to have the same cause, the effect of which is determined by the distribution of the cells carrying the mutation (ie the mosaicism).

Monostotic fibrous dysplasia

This disorder is relatively common in orthopaedic practice. Although the lesions may occur in any bones, and particularly in the facial bones and ribs, the most frequent presenting symptom at any age is a fracture, often of the upper end of the femur (Fig. 11). The biochemistry is usually normal, and the diagnosis is made from the radiographic and pathological appearances. There is a smooth-walled translucent area within the bone, often with thinning of the cortex and sometimes with associated deformity. Pathologically, areas of abnormal fibrous tissue area are found, with the appearance of fibromata, associated with woven bone and wide osteoid seams. The differential diagnosis is from other causes of bone cysts, from Paget's disease, and from hyperparathyroidism with osteitis fibrosa cystica. Treatment is largely surgical with stabilization of fractures and correction of deformity.

Polyostotic fibrous dysplasia

Interest in this condition, in which the bone lesions are multiple, arises from its frequent association with pigmentation and sexual precocity, especially in females (McCune–Albright syndrome). The bone lesions and the brown pigmentation are typically associated in position (but not in extent), and may be restricted to one side of the body. Sexual precocity is said to be present in up to 50 per cent of females with polyostotic disease, and is then the presenting complaint. Where sexual precocity is not a feature, deformity and fracture are often the first symptoms. Gross deformity of the upper femur and femoral neck produces the 'shepherd's crook' appearance. Asymmetry of the long bones and of the skull are also seen; and in about half of the cases the base of the skull may be thickened. The macular pigmentation tends to have smooth borders (in contrast to those of neurofibromatosis) and often does not cross the midline. The bone lesions tend to increase in size and number, but less rapidly after growth has ceased. The endocrine hyperfunction—sexual precocity, thyrotoxicosis, acromegaly, and Cushing's syndrome—is attributable to the activating mutation, which also causes pigmentation because of its effect on the melanophores. The skeletal lesions may cause complications such as optic nerve spinal cord compression, and may be associated with hypophosphataemic osteomalacia. Sarcoma formation has been reported, but only after irradiation.

Both the plasma alkaline phosphatase and the urinary hydroxyproline may be slightly increased and the plasma phosphate slightly reduced. The bone pathology is similar to the monostotic form, but it is said that cartilage- and fluid-filled cysts are more common. Microscopically there is an abundance of woven bone and an increase in osteoblasts and osteoclasts. The cortex and marrow may be virtually replaced by fibrous tissue, so that the bones are very fragile. Healing is rapid with abundant callus formation. Radiologically the bones are deformed, the cortex may be difficult to detect, and the medullary bone takes on a 'ground-glass' or 'smoky' appearance.

The main differential diagnosis is from osseous neurofibromatosis; in this condition there is also pigmentation, bone deformity, and sometimes hypophosphataemic osteomalacia. The borders of the pigmentation are less smooth than in fibrous dysplasia, and there are other cutaneous features of neurofibromatosis; the bone deformity in neurofibromatosis can be quite bizarre, with overgrowth or undergrowth of isolated bones. In neurofibromatosis the characteristic spinal change is a very sharp upper thoracic kyphoscoliosis. Finally, neurofibromatosis often shows clear evidence of dominant inheritance whereas fibrous dysplasia is not inherited (presumably because an activating G protein mutation in the germline would be lethal).

Medical treatment of the bone disease is unsatisfactory. Calcitonin has been used in an attempt to prevent progression, without significant result.

Recent work suggests that intravenous pamidronate (APD) may improve symptoms and ameliorate the bone disease.

Ectopic mineralization

Deposition of calcium in the soft tissues (ectopic calcification) and on ectopic bone matrix (ossification) has many causes (Table 11). There are some in which calcification and/or ossification are associated with biochemical abnormalities, but often the cause is unknown.

Ectopic calcification without bone formation

Calcification can result from previous damage in soft tissues (dystrophic calcification) or from an increase in the circulating calcium phosphate product (metastatic calcification as, for instance, in advanced renal osteodystrophy). The distribution of the calcification varies inexplicably with its cause; for example, in hypoparathyroidism there is subcutaneous and basal ganglia calcification and in hyperparathyroidism vascular calcification, suggesting that metastatic calcification is not only related to the Ca:P product. Calcification and ossification may also coexist.

Dystrophic calcification

This occurs in disorders involving connective tissue, such as alkaptonuria (intervertebral discs), pseudoxanthoma elasticum (blood vessels), systemic sclerosis, and dermatomyositis, and also after infection, tumours, and trauma. In systemic sclerosis, subcutaneous calcification, often around the phalanges (calcinosis circumscripta) may be part of the CRST syndrome. In dermatomyositis, sheets of subcutaneous calcification can be deposited some time after the initial inflammatory episode characterized by a systemic illness and painful weak muscles; the calcification can be very extensive (calcinosis universalis), but can also disappear rapidly, sometimes in adolescence. Rarely this is associated with hypercalcaemia.

Table 11 The main causes of ectopic mineralization

Calcification without bone formation
Dystrophic; secondary to tissue damage
Metastatic; secondary to biochemical abnormalities
Hypocalcaemia
Hypercalcaemia
Hyperphosphataemia
Hypophosphataemia
Calcification with bone formation (ectopic ossification)
Acquired
After injury
After neurological damage
In tumours
Other disorders
Inherited
Fibrodysplasia (myositis) ossificans progressiva
Familial osteoma cutis

Metastatic calcification

Calcification and hypocalcaemia

This occurs in idiopathic and postsurgical hypoparathyroidism, as well as in pseudohypoparathyroidism, and also in pseudopseudohypoparathyroidism, where the skeletal abnormalities of pseudohypoparathyroidism coexist with normal biochemistry. There may be extensive subcutaneous calcification, calcification within the basal ganglia (and outside it), and cataract formation.

Calcification and hypercalcaemia

There are many causes of hypercalcaemia; ectopic calcification occurs frequently in hyperparathyroidism (especially associated with renal glomerualar failure and hyperphosphataemia), prolonged vitamin D intoxication, and hypercalcaemic sarcoidosis. The ectopic mineral is deposited in the conjunctivae, sclerae, medium-sized blood vessels, and subcutaneous tissue.

Calcification in hyperphosphataemia

Idiopathic hyperphosphataemia is a rare autosomal recessive disorder with an increase in the maximal tubular reabsorption of phosphate and an inappropriate increase in plasma $1,25(OH)_2D$ concentration. Masses of ectopic mineral which form around the joints from childhood (tumoural calcinosis) may discharge through the skin. Treatment with large oral doses of aluminium hydroxide or other phosphate-binding agents can reduce the plasma phosphate and the size of the deposits.

Calcification in inherited hypophosphataemia

A particular feature of X-linked inherited hypophosphataemia is widespread calcification and ossification of ligaments and tendons at their insertions into the periosteum (so-called Sharpey fibres). This is termed an enthesiopathy. Calcification and new bone formation in the ligamenta flava may produce spinal cord compression.

Idiopathic soft tissue calcification

This includes calcific tendinitis and calcinosis circumscripta of unknown cause.

Ectopic ossification

Acquired ectopic ossification

Post-traumatic ossification

Local ossification can occur after total hip replacement. The quoted incidence varies widely, depending on the method used to detect it. It is said to occur more often in men than in women and in certain individuals; for instance, where ossification follows hip replacement on one side, it is likely to occur if the contralateral hip is also replaced. The reason for this is unknown and there is no confirmed association with HLA-B27. The bone mainly forms in the hip abductors and ossification is classified according to its severity. Disodium etidronate may delay mineralization, but only while it is being given, and non-steroidal anti-inflammatory drugs are also useful. A small dose of radiotherapy may also delay ectopic ossification after total hip replacement.

Ossification after neurological injury

Extensive myositis ossificans can occur 1–4 months after injuries to the head or spinal cord, but in muscles distant from the injury such as the major muscles of the thigh. Affected muscles become swollen, red, and warm, and, unless the cord lesion is complete, pain and tenderness also occur. At this time the differential diagnosis may include cellulitis, arthritis, and thrombophlebitis. Radiological calcification is initially absent (appearing at about 6 weeks or more after the injury) but an isotope bone scan will show increased uptake before that. Later there is progressive mineralization with the eventual appearance of organized bone. Because the bone affects the major periarticular muscles, it leads to joint fixation, particularly of the hips. The plasma alkaline phosphatase may be increased in the early stages.

Attempted surgical removal of ectopic bone is often difficult and produces little increase in movement. The ectopic bone recurs, especially if it is removed too early. Oral disodium etidronate at full dose (20 mg/kg/body weight daily) may delay the onset of mineralization, but only while it is being given. Likewise, the prevention of further ectopic bone formation after its removal may be delayed by non-steroidal anti-inflammatory drugs or radiotherapy, which should be commenced as soon as possible.

Myositis ossificans can also occur after other neurological diseases, such as poliomyelitis and meningitis, and also after prolonged coma. The reason why ectopic ossification occurs after head injury is unknown; interestingly head injury is associated with an increased rate of fracture healing and excessive callus formation. In such patients the serum contains increased mitogenic activity for osteoblast-like cells; the source of this activity is unknown, but there could be an increase in bone morphogenic proteins.

Other causes of ossification

Ossification can coexist with calcification of the spinal ligaments in hypoparathyroidism. The enthesiopathy in inherited hypophosphataemia (vitamin D-resistant rickets) is a form of ectopic ossification. Ossification of the posterior longitudinal ligament and sternoclavicular hyperostosis is particularly described in Japan. Ligamentous ossification has been noted in patients treated with vitamin A analogues, such as etretinate, for dermatological disorders. The term osteoma cutis covers a number of rare conditions of uncertain cause. Finally, ectopic bone may complicate varicose veins, chronic venous insufficiency, and surgical incisions.

Inherited ectopic ossification (fibrodysplasia ossificans progressiva)

The main inherited cause of ectopic ossification is myositis ossificans progressiva, a disorder which appears to arise from a defect in bone cell biology. Histology suggests that the connective tissue within muscles is primarily involved and therefore the alternative term, fibrodysplasia ossificans progressiva, is widely used.

The condition is exceedingly rare, with an incidence of about 1 per million which increases with paternal age. Since patients rarely reproduce, most represent new mutations. The few family histories demonstrate that the unidentified mutant gene is inherited as a dominant with full penetrance but variable expression. Diagnosis depends on the combination of progressive myositis, leading to ossification in the major skeletal muscles, and characteristic bony abnormalities.

Pathophysiology

Initially there is oedema and cellular infiltration throughout the muscle, with myofibrillar breakdown. Later endochondral ossification leads to mature bone, within which is haemopoietic marrow. Information on the earliest histological appearances is scanty because biopsies are often taken after the acute phase of myositis; for this reason there is still doubt about the primary lesion. Ectopic ossification occurs when mesenchymal or stromal cells take on the behaviour of osteoblasts. The cause of this is unknown. There is some evidence of overactivity of components of the bone morphyogenetic protein system.

Clinical features

Episodes of myositis are the non-skeletal hallmark of this disease. Typically the affected muscle becomes swollen and hard, sometimes following injury; after a week or two these features subside, but the apparent improvement is followed in a month or so by ossification within the muscle and progressive joint fixation. Myositis usually begins in the upper paraspinal muscles. By late childhood or adolescence ossification will have occurred within the muscles around the shoulders, hips, and knees, to fix these joints and to complete the disability. The large, striated muscles are affected; ossification does not involve the small muscles of the hands and feet, the diaphragm, the cardiac, or the smooth muscles. Ossification in the muscles around the jaw may fix it almost completely. Although the overall sequence of ossification is characteristic from large upper paraspinal to lower limb muscles, it varies considerably in its rate. For instance, neonates may have sufficient ossification to produce torticollis while, in contrast, late and slow ossification producing stiffness may delay the correct diagnosis until adolescence. Likewise, there may be long symptom-free periods.

The diagnostic skeletal abnormalities affect the big toes (Fig. 12) (and to a lesser extent the thumbs), the cervical spine (Fig. 13), and the metaphyses. The big toes are always abnormal; in the infant, bony changes produce bilateral hallux valgus and, in the adult, fusion produces a short fixed monophalangic big toe. In the cervical spine the vertebral bodies are small and the laminae large. Both are variably fused; and this fusion is independent of nearby ossification of the cervical muscles. The femoral necks are short and wide and there are exostoses from the metaphyses.

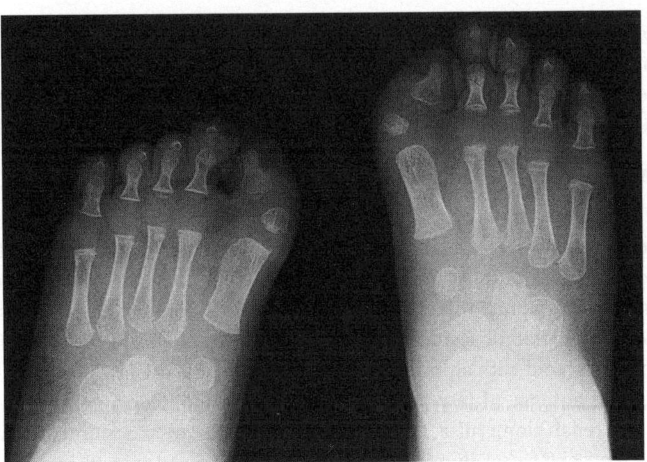

Fig. 12 The abnormal short big toes in an infant with fibrodysplasia ossificans progressiva.

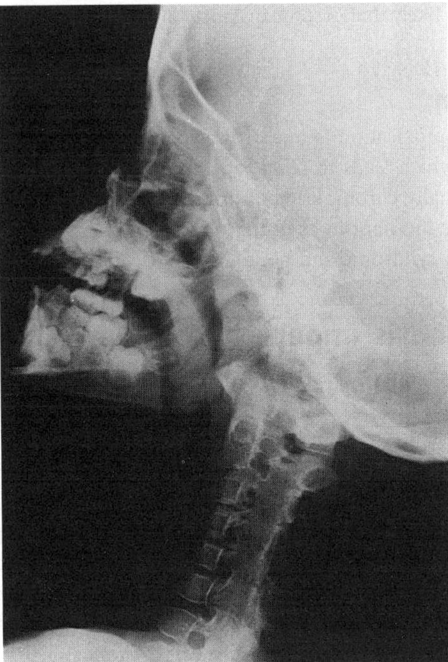

Fig. 13 Fusion of the cervical spine in a young woman with fibrodysplasia ossificans progressiva.

Rare clinical features include early onset baldness, difficulty in hearing, and mental retardation.

Differential diagnosis

In childhood, myositis may be mistaken for soft-tissue sarcoma; and a biopsy showing oedema and increased cellularity may support this or suggest an aggressive fibromatosis. Painful swelling of the masticatory muscles simulates mumps, and progressive stiffness with a fixed abnormal neck suggests the Klippel–Feil syndrome or childhood rheumatoid arthritis.

Management

Since the onset of myositis is quite unpredictable, it is almost impossible to assess the effect of any form of therapy. Corticosteroids have been used, sometimes associated with symptom-free periods. Sometimes myositis follows injury, which should be avoided where possible. It seems likely, but difficult to prove, that myositis is inevitably followed by ossification. It is to prevent or slow down this ossification that the bisphosphonate EHDP (disodium etidronate) can be given in full doses (20 mg/kg/body weight daily by mouth) but there is little evidence that this is effective. In children continued high-dose etidronate interferes with mineralization, disorganizes the growth plates, and delays fracture healing so that it is not an acceptable long-term treatment. Surgical removal of ectopic bone is technically difficult. It rarely produces the expected increase in mobility and recurrence cannot be prevented.

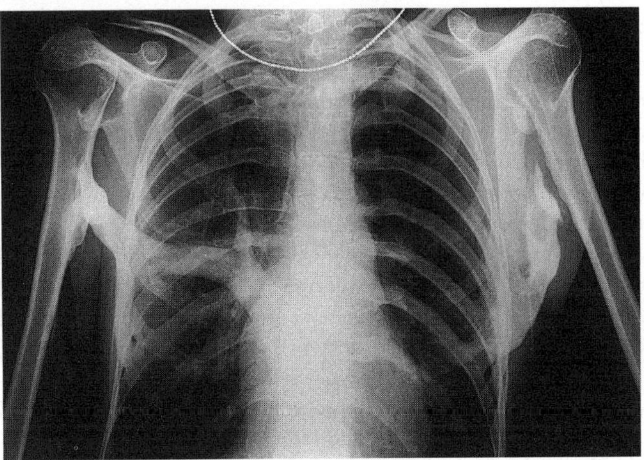

Fig. 14 Extensive ectopic ossification in the paraspinal muscles fixing the shoulders in a patient with fibrodysplasia ossificans progressiva.

The eventual disability produced by fibrodysplasia ossificans progressiva is severe (Fig. 14). The body moves as in one piece with the legs usually fixed in partial extension. All major joints become completely fixed. The help of a specialized rehabilitation centre is essential.

Progressive osseous heteroplasia

In this very rare disorder, intramembranous bone forms in the subcutaneous fat and connective tissues. This typically begins in a lower limb in childhood and progresses. Extensive surgery may be necessary. The cause is unknown.

Assorted bone disorders

The haemoglobinopathies

Skeletal abnormalities result from a hyperplastic bone marrow and overactivity of the osteoblasts, so that the skull, facial bones, and long bones are thickened. Additional features include collapse of the weight-bearing bones and disorganization of the joints following bone infarction. In β-thalassaemia an increase in osteoid thickness has been described which resembles that of osteomalacia.

Parenteral nutrition

Prolonged parenteral nutrition can produce a form of bone disease with similarities to osteomalacia. The main symptom is periarticular bone pain, particularly in the ankles. Histology shows impaired mineralization of bone, and biochemistry an increase in plasma alkaline phosphatase, in urinary calcium, and sometimes in plasma calcium. The radiographic appearances suggest osteoporosis. There are several probable causes for this disorder; aluminium intoxication may contribute.

Fluorosis

Deposition of excess fluoride in the skeleton can result from an excess in the diet (endemic fluorosis), from industrial exposure (during the manufacture of aluminium, steel, and glass, and from exposure to the dust of fluoride-containing rock), and from the administration of sodium fluoride in treatment. The most severe effects are seen in endemic fluorosis, well described from the Punjab.

There is considerable disability, with spinal rigidity, restricted movements of the joints, and flexion deformities of the hips and knees. There is a generalized increase in bone density (with loss of the normal corticomedullary junction), and the tendons, ligaments, and sometimes muscles may be mineralized. This can produce compression of the spinal cord and its roots, with progressive neurological disability. Increased levels of fluoride can affect the enamel of developing teeth, producing chalky-white patches, yellow-brown discoloration, and other defects.

The diagnosis of fluorosis depends on the radiographic changes and an increased urinary excretion of fluoride. Bone biopsy shows an increase in new bone formation with an increase in the width of osteoid borders. There is also an increase in fibrous tissue and bone resorption. When the biopsy includes an area of tendinous insertion, this may be mineralized.

Sodium fluoride has been given to treat osteoporosis and produces increased vertebral density. This does not increase vertebral bone strength and may lead to an increase in appendicular bone fracture. The new bone induced by fluoride appears to be mainly woven in character and imperfectly mineralized. Clinical usefulness of this treatment depends, in part, on the dose used.

Vitamin A

Retinoic acid and its derivatives have profound effects on osteoblast function. Vitamin A poisoning produces characteristic periostitis in the young skeleton, and the prolonged use of retinoids for the treatment of skin disease, such as psoriasis and ichthyosis, leads particularly to calcification of the spinal ligaments, causing stiffness and reduced mobility. There is a resemblance to Forestier's disease (diffuse idiopathic skeletal hyperostosis).

Vitamin D

Vitamin D poisoning can result from inappropriate therapy or accidental over-consumption. This leads to hypercalcaemia without detectable effects on the skeleton. The main opportunities for overdose exist when potent preparations of vitamin D are used inappropriately. Chronic vitamin D overdosage leads to soft-tissue calcification, especially in the arteries and kidneys. After several years progressive stiffness in the spine, major joints, and feet lead to difficulty in walking. Radiographs show ligamentous calcification.

Lead (see also Chapters 12.21 and 18.1)

Lead deposition in the growing skeleton produces a radiologically dense line near the growth plate. When exposure has been intermittent, or the condition has been treated, this may be a single, relatively narrow line, which is superseded by apparently normal bone. If exposure to lead recurs, a further line will appear.

Such lines lead lines are an important clue to lead poisoning in infants and children up to about the age of 6 years. They occur most commonly around the knees, wrists, and ankles, and appear after about a month of chronic poisoning. The diagnosis of lead poisoning is confirmed by an increase in plasma and urinary lead. There are other causes of radiologically dense metaphyses. These include other heavy metals—bismuth, mercury, or phosphorus; vitamin D intoxication and idiopathic hypercalcaemia of infancy; cretinism; and healing rickets.

Aluminium (see also Chapter 12.30)

The accumulation of aluminium in the skeleton in patients in some renal units where the aluminium content of tap water was high led to the occurrence of 'dialysis bone disease'. The clinical features included proximal myopathy, multiple painful spontaneous fractures with radiographic evidence of bone loss, histological evidence of excess osteoid with aluminium deposition near the calcification front, and an absence of response to vitamin D metabolites.

In renal glomerular failure, aluminium may also accumulate in patients given oral aluminium hydroxide to reduce plasma phosphate. Aluminium bone disease can also occur in patients on prolonged parenteral nutrition.

The pathology of aluminium bone disease is not fully understood, but it seems likely that in some instances aluminium reduces osteoblast activity.

Cadmium

Cadmium intoxication is one of the acquired causes of the Fanconi syndrome which leads to renal tubular rickets or osteomalacia.

Exceptionally, chronic lead poisoning can also produce osteomalacia by the same mechanism as cadmium, and copper 'poisoning' causes the Fanconi syndrome and bone disease of Wilson's disease.

Fibrogenesis imperfecta ossium

This is a very rare, apparently acquired disorder, characterized by excessive bony fragility due to the replacement of normal bone with a fibre-deficient, poorly mineralized matrix. The cause is unknown. The main clinical feature has been pathological fractures first presenting in adult life. In most patients, progressive disability has followed, with more fractures which fail to unite. Radiologically, the trabeculae throughout the skeleton appear to be thickened. There is also ectopic mineralization around large joints and tendon insertions. Plasma calcium and phosphate are normal, but the alkaline phosphatase is moderately raised. In the urine, monoclonal light chains may be present. The diagnosis is confirmed by the examination of undecalcified bone. This shows defective mineralization and wide osteoid seams suggesting severe osteomalacia, but the osteoid is not birefringent under polarized light and the normal structure of bone collagen under electron microscopy is absent. The differential diagnosis is from those disorders which produce widespread coarse trabeculation throughout the skeleton, and those which produce the histological changes of osteomalacia. In the first category, Paget's disease of bone, renal glomerular osteodystrophy, and fluorosis should be excluded, and in the second, axial osteomalacia has some similarities; in this very rare osteosclerotic disorder, both histology and radiographs suggest that the osteomalacia is limited to the spine, pelvis, and ribs.

Treatment to date has been largely empirical. The occasional finding of an excess of plasma cells in the bone marrow, or a monoclonal gammopathy, or light-chain proteinuria, has led to apparently successful treatment with melphalan and prednisolone. Where surgery is indicated for fractures, particularly of the femoral neck, this is difficult because of the extreme fragility of the bones.

Although it seems likely that the defect may be related to an acquired disorder of bone collagen, no consistent abnormality has been detected.

Sudeck's atrophy (algodystrophy or sympathetic reflex dystrophy)

This is a syndrome, usually involving hands or feet, comprising local pain, tenderness, and swelling with accompanying vasomotor instability. It usually follows minor trauma, but some patients remember no precipitating event. Those suffering severely from the syndrome often show a particular personality type, being very dependent, anxious, and depressed. It may also follow medical conditions such as myocardial infarction, stroke, or herpes zoster. When looked for carefully it may complicate as many as 25 per cent of cases of Colles' fracture. The early oedema and erythema can be followed by subcutaneous atrophy, worsening of the pain, and local flexion contractures and osteoporosis. The pathophysiology is obscure, but there appears to be an abnormal reflex arc mediated by the sympathetic nervous system, with a consequent disturbance of the microcirculation.

The most common sites of involvement are the limb extremities, although it is also recognized in the knee and even hip or spine. When the shoulder and hand is involved, especially after myocardial infarction, it is called the shoulder–hand syndrome. The vasomotor instability classically begins with warm red skin with local swelling and sweating. Later comes a cold phase with the affected area cold, clammy, and cyanosed. From an early phase local joint movements are limited and painful.

Radiological changes (Fig. 14) appear late with patchy osteoporosis with a subchondral lucent line initially, progressing to severe local osteoporosis.

Algodystrophy is nearly always a transient condition resolving after a few months, but it can be progressive and chronically disabling. Early recognition and treatment is important. It is essential to maintain mobility despite pain and here good physiotherapy is the key. Pain may be helped by non-steroidal anti-inflammatory agents. Regional sympathetic blockade by medical or surgical techniques can be effective, but only if given early before the trophic changes. Other measures have been proposed including courses of corticosteroids, calcitonin and β-blockers, but good evidence that these are useful is lacking.

Further reading

Bilezikian, J.P., Raisz, L.G., and Rodan, G.A. (1996). *Principles of bone biology.* Academic Press, San Diego.

Chapurlat, R.D., Delmas, P.D., Liens, D., and Meunier, P.J. (1997). Long term effects of intravenous panudronate in fibrous dysplasia of bone. *Journal of Bone and Mineral Research* ,**12**, 1746–52.

Delmas, P.D. and Meunier, P.J. (1997). The management of Paget's disease of bone. *New England Journal of Medicine,* **336**, 558–66.

De Paepe, A., Devereux, R.B., Dietz, H.C., Hennekam, R.C.M., and Pyeritz, R.E. (1996). Revised diagnostic criteria for the Marfan syndrome. *American Journal of Medical Genetics,* **62**, 417–26.

Favus, M.J. (1996). *Primer on the metabolic bone disease and disorders of mineral metabolism,* (3rd edn). Lippincott-Raven, Philadelphia.

Francke, U. and Furthmayr, H. (1994). Marfan's syndrome and the other disorders of fibrillin. *New England Journal of Medicine,* **330**, 1284–385 (editorial).

Horton, W.A. (1996). Molecular genetic basis of human chondrodysplasias. *Endocrinology and Metabolism Clinics of North America,* **25**, 683–97.

Hosking, D., Meunier, P.J., Ringe, J.D, Reginster, J-Y., and Gennari, C. (1996). Paget's disease of bone: diagnosis and management. *British Medical Journal,* **312**, 491–4.

Marcus, R., Feldman, D., and Kelsey, J. (1996). *Osteoporosis.* Academic Press, San Diego.

Olsen, B.J. (1998). 'A rare disorder, yes; an important one, never'. *Journal of Clinical Investigation,* **101**, 1545–6 (editorial).

Pope, F.M. and Smith, R. (1995). *Color atlas of inherited connective tissue disorders.* Mosby-Wolfe, London.

Rowe, P.S.N. (1997). The PEX gene: its role in X-linked rickets, osteomalacia, and the bone mineral metabolism. *Experimental Nephrology,* **5**, 355–63.

Shafritz, A.B., Shore, E.M., and Gannon, F.H. (1996). Overexpression of an osteogenic morphogen in fibordysplasia ossificans progessiva. *New England Journal of Medicine,* **355**, 555–61.

Shipman, A. J., Guy, G.W.G., Smith, I., Ostlere, S., Greer, R., and Smith, R. (1999). Vertebral bone mineral density, content and area in 8,789 women aged 33–73 years who have never had hormone replacement therapy. *Osteoporosis International,* **9**, 420–6.

Smith, R. (1998). Fibrodysplasia (myositis) ossificans progressiva. *Clinical Orthopaedics and Related Research,* **346**, 7–14.

Smith, R. (1998). Bone in health and disease. In: *Oxford textbook of rheumatology* (2nd edn) (ed. P.J. Maddison, D.A. Isenberg, P. Woo, and D.N. Glass), pp. 421–40. Oxford University Press, Oxford.

Smith, R., Athanason, N.A., Ostlere, S.J., and Vipond, S.E. (1995). Pregnancy associated osteoporosis. *Quarterly Journal of Medicine,* **85**, 865–78.

Whyte, M.P. (1992). Hereditary metabolic and dysplastic skeletal disorders. In: *Disorders of bone and mineral metabolism* (ed. F.L. Coe and M.J.Favus), pp. 977–1026. Raven Press, New York.

Section 10
Rheumatology

Contents

Chapter 10.1

Introduction

P. Dieppe and P. T. Dawes

Rheumatic disorders are extremely common. Back pain occurs in a large proportion of the population, and severe attacks, sufficient to interrupt work or leisure activities, are frequent in developed countries, particularly in young adults. Furthermore, a large percentage of the population will suffer from some form of transient periarticular disorder (such as 'tennis elbow' or a 'frozen shoulder') at some stage in their life. Osteoarthritis causes problems in up to 10 per cent of the adult population, and inflammatory arthropathies are present in about 2–3 per cent.

These diseases cause major problems in the provision of health care; about 1 in 5 of all consultations with a general practitioner are caused by disorders of the locomotor system, and rheumatic diseases are responsible for 30 per cent of all physical disability, and about 60 per cent of the burden of severe disability in older people.

An holistic approach is needed to help patients with chronic, painful, disabling disorders.

Family and others involved may need to participate in therapy, and rheumatologists often as the co-ordinators of a team, normally including physiotherapists, occupational therapists, specialist nurses, and community-based health-care workers.

Clinical presentation and diagnosis

Patients may present with swollen, painful, stiff joints, or in more subtle ways with non-specific pains, arthralgias, or myalgias. There may be systemic involvement with fever, sweating, malaise, fatigue, weight loss, and anorexia. Alternatively some rheumatic diseases may present when an associated organ becomes involved, for instance when acute uveitis unmasks a case of previously undiagnosed ankylosing spondylitis. All patients with an acute rheumatic disease must be asked about any prodromal event such as an upper respiratory tract infection, diarrhoeal illness, genitourinary infection, insect bite, or recent vaccination, as well as drug usage, family history and ethnic origin, and dietary, social, and occupational factors. Some forms of rheumatic disease, systemic lupus erythematosus for example, can be precipitated by drugs (such as hydralazine), and many forms of arthritis have a genetic predisposition and racial preferences. It is essential to assess the effect of the disease on daily activities; Can the patient climb the stairs, get outside his or her home, or go shopping? Have they become socially isolated? How many different people have they been able to see in the last week? Can they independently transfer from bed, chairs, toilet, and cope with self-hygiene? Are they able independently to cook, feed, and dress themselves? Who is at home and what support do they provide? Is their job at risk, and are they financially embarrassed?

The ill effects of chronic rheumatic diseases may be compounded by associated anxiety or depression. An assessment of the mental attitude and motivation in patients with conditions like fibrositis and other chronic pain syndromes is always important. There may also be problems with sexual activity consequent on the disease or the patients perception of it. Correcting (when possible) these emotional and social problems can be just as important as pharmacological treatment of the patient with complex chronic disabling disease.

Key articular symptoms

It is important to establish how a symptom started, whether the onset was sudden or gradual, and if episodic, self-limiting, or persistent and progressive. Precipitating or relieving factors such as overuse and exercise, rest, emotional stress, temperature, sunlight, and treatment should be identified as well as the pattern and extent of musculoskeletal involvement. Other important issues concern the first joint to be affected, how many are now affected, whether or not joint pains have migrated, and whether the joint involvement has been symmetrical or asymmetrical. It is also important to determine whether the major disability is due to pain, stiffness, or weakness.

Pain

In osteoarthritis pain is often worse at the end of the day and after activity, and is relieved by rest; whereas in active inflammatory diseases it tends to be worse after rest, particularly in the morning, and may improve with exercise. Joint abnormalities often cause referred pain; for example, disease of the cervical spine can present with shoulder pain, shoulder disease with upper arm pain, lumbar spine lesions with hip or thigh pain, and hip disease with knee pain.

Stiffness

A joint may be stiff either because of mechanical deformity or because of a local inflammatory process. In chronic arthritis stiffness is often due to a combination or both of these factors. Early morning stiffness is a feature of all inflammatory synovial diseases and its duration is often recorded (usefully) as a measurement of disease activity. Acute or subacute onset of severe bilateral shoulder and pelvic girdle stiffness in the early morning in an elderly patient should always arouse suspicion of polymyalgia rheumatica. Transient joint stiffness after rest occurs in osteoarthritis. With increasing age, joints often become stiffer and complaints of stiffness may be a particular feature of Parkinson's disease, not always clinically obvious.

Swelling

Swelling of joints may be due to bony hypertrophy, synovitis, intra-articular fluid, or a swollen periarticular structure. Unlike tenderness, objective evidence of swelling indicates organic disease. Occasionally, patients complain of swelling which is not confirmed by examination and the clinician must then question closely to establish or refute its presence. In general, synovial swelling is most pronounced on the extensor surface of joints where the capsule is more distensible.

Loss of function

Impaired function is often due to a combination of pain, stiffness, tendon and joint damage, neurological impairment, and muscle weakness. Patients with such chronic disability often under-report their problems and loss of function from a joint does not always relate to deformity. Some patients, for instance, complain of their joint 'giving way'. This occurs commonly with the knee and may indicate intra-articular pathology or muscle weakness. If the primary complaint is of weakness, observations of gait and ability or otherwise to sit up from a supine position with arms folded across the chest will help assessment of any primary muscle disease. Patients who describe a loss of function out of proportion to the physical findings often are found to have compounding psychological problems.

Key extra-articular symptoms

Raynaud's phenomenon

Symptoms are usually bilateral, affect fingers more often than toes, and are provoked by cold, albeit sometimes by a very small change in temperature. They comprise numbness, tingling, and burning, with three sequential colour phases of pallor, cyanosis, and finally, erythema on recovery. Raynaud's phenomenon is often idiopathic, especially in young women, but is associated with many of the connective tissue diseases, particularly systemic sclerosis in which it is the initial complaint in over 70 per cent of patients.

Skin and mucous membranes

Rashes that often fluctuate with symptoms occur with rheumatic fever, erythema nodosum, adult and juvenile Still's disease, and connective tissue diseases, particularly systemic lupus erythematosus, when they may be photosensitive. Psoriasis may be missed when quiescent or hidden, for example in the natal cleft or scalp. Circinate balanitis in Reiter's disease may be asymptomatic, is not always admitted, and specific examination for it is important. Oral ulceration may be a feature or Reiter's and Behçet's disease as well as the connective tissue disorders; Sjögren's syndrome will cause a dry mouth (xerostomia), when oral hygiene may be poor.

Eyes

Patients should be asked whether they have ever had red, gritty, or painful eyes. Conjunctivitis occurs in Reiter's disease, uveitis in the other spondyloarthropathies, episcleritis (painless), scleritis (painful), and keratoconjunctivitis sicca in rheumatoid and related diseases. Disturbance of vision and blindness can occur in giant cell arteritis. Rarely, tenosynovitis in rheumatoid disease can affect the occular muscles and cause diplopia.

Gastrointestinal

Transient diarrhoea precipitating a reactive arthritis may have been relatively mild. Chronic bowel symptoms including diarrhoea, blood loss, and malabsorption should arouse suspicion of an enteropathic arthritis secondary to ulcerative colitis, Crohn's, Whipple's, or coeliac disease. Oesophageal reflux and dysphagia are common symptoms of systemic sclerosis; dysphagia may also be a prominent symptom in polymyositis and also occurs in Sjögren's syndrome secondary to a dry mouth or even an oesophageal web. Acute abdominal pain from mesenteric ischaemia or, on occasion, cholecystitis due to ischaemia occur in the vasculitic syndromes, particularly polyarteritis nodosa.

Cardiorespiratory

Episodes of pericardial and/or pleuritic chest pain may indicate the presence of a connective tissue disease. Asthma may be a feature of Churg–Strauss syndrome or polyarteritis. Musculoskeletal chest pain is a common feature of the spondylarthropathies. Breathlessness may indicate associated pulmonary fibrosis or a cardiac defect such as aortic regurgitation in the spondylarthropathies. Chronic nasal, sinus, or middle-ear diseases are usual in Wegener's granulomatosis and may also complicate relapsing polychondritis.

Genitourinary

Symptomatic urethritis or an asymptomatic urethral discharge may point to a diagnosis of Reiter's disease. Testicular pain is sometimes a feature of polyarteritis. Dyspareunia occurs in Sjögren's syndrome. Miscarriages, particularly in the second trimester may be one important clue to the presence of the antiphospholipid antibody syndrome.

Neurological

Peripheral neuropathies, particularly an entrapment neuropathy (e.g. carpal tunnel syndrome) may be early features of inflammatory synovitis. A history of migraine, depression, psychoses, dementia, or stroke may point to a diagnosis of systemic lupus erythematosus, vasculitis, or the antiphospholipid antibody syndrome. Headaches, scalp tenderness, and jaw claudication are well-recognized features of giant-cell arteritis.

Examination

Comparison between the two sides of the body, looking for asymmetry in colour, deformity, swelling, function, and muscle, wasting, can be helpful. Separate and careful examination of gait, arms, legs, and finally spine is a useful routine, perhaps best performed by the examiner undertaking the movements and then asking the patient to copy them.

Gait

The patient should be observed while walking, turning, and walking back, looking for smoothness and symmetry of leg, pelvis, and arm movements, normal stride length, and the ability to turn quickly.

Arms

Inspection from the front allows assessments of shoulder girdle muscle bulk and symmetry. After placing both hands down by the side with elbows straight in full extension, the patient should attempt to place both hands behind the head and then push elbows back, to test the glenohumeral, acromioclavicular, and sternoclavicular joints. Hands should be examined palms down and fingers straight to detect swelling or deformity. It is important to assess movements of pronation/supination and grip, and placement of the tip of each finer on to the tip of the thumb in turn allows evaluation of normal dexterity. Discomfort in response to squeezing across the second to fifth metacarpals suggests synovitis.

Legs

Observation of the standing patient reveals any gross knee, hindfoot, midfoot, or forefoot deformity. Later examination on the couch should include flexion of each hip and knee while holding the knee to test normal movement and help detect knee crepitus. Each hip should be passively internally rotated in flexion, and the knee carefully examined for the presence of fluid in the joint. Synovitis in the feet is best detected by squeezing across the metatarsals. The soles of the feet may show callosities; keratoderma blennorrhagicum may be present in patients with Reiter's syndrome.

Spine

This is best examined with the patient standing. A view from behind detects lateral spinal curvature, differences in the levels of iliac crests, and any asymmetry in paraspinal and girdle muscle bulk. Lateral flexion of the cervical spine can be assessed by asking the patient to place his or her ear on the tip of the shoulder on either side. Tenderness over the midpoint of the supraspinatus muscle suggests the presence of fibrositis.

Table 1 Common causes of acute monoarticular arthritis

Crystal arthritis—gout, pseudogout, calcific periarthritis
Septic arthritis
Haemarthrosis
Traumatic synovitis
Foreign-body synovitis—plant thorn

Table 2 Common causes of acute polyarticular arthritis

Rheumatoid arthritis
Palindromic arthritis
Reactive arthritis—Reiter's disease, rheumatic fever
Gonococcal arthritis
Post-viral arthropathies—rubella, parvovirus, hepatitis B
Adult and childhood Still's disease
Psoriatic arthritis and association spondylarthropathies
Systemic lupus erythematosus
Paraneoplastic syndromes
Polymyalgia rheumatica

Anteroposterior curvature of the spine is best observed from the side. Lumbar spine and hip flexion are easily assessed when patients bend to touch their toes with knees straight.

Clinical presentations

Peripheral joints

Peripheral arthritis may present as a monoarthritis or polyarthritis, which may either be acute (Tables 1 and 2) or chronic. Often there is overlap; monoarthritis may have an acute exacerbation and may, with time, become polyarticular. Many types of chronic polyarthritis may start with an acute onset.

Monoarthritis

Certain causes of acute monoarthritis show a preference for particular joints; for instance gout in the first metatarsophalangeal joint, pseudogout in the knee, calcific periarthritis in the shoulder, haemarthroses in the knees, foreign body synovitis in the feet (plant-thorn synovitis). Distribution is often in a lower limb in Reiter's disease and the spondylarthropathies, and in an upper limb in gonococcal arthritis. Palindromic rheumatism (self-limiting attacks lasting 1–2 days) often starts in the knees, shoulders, or small joints of the hand. Swelling and pain in a single joint arising on it own or as part of a generalized arthritic state should always raise the possibility of septic arthritis. The most critical test is the examination of the synovial fluid for the presence of infectious agents or crystals.

Polyarthritis

Detection of early synovitis (Table 3) is paramount in the management of certain disease, such as early rheumatoid disease, where there is mounting evidence that treatment is most efficacious if instituted early.

Table 3 Detection of early synovitis in the absence of major joint deformity

1. Evidence of vasospasm in the fingers can be detected by stroking the dorsum of the examiner's hand across the patient's palm and fingers to detect swelling and a distal temperature drop
2. Proximal interphalangeal joint skin discoloration and local joint tenderness suggests synovitis.
3. The knuckles of a clenched fist should be white and stand out clearly with no infilling between them.
4. Squeezing across all four metacarpophalangeal joints together may elicit tenderness.
5. Pain elicited by forcibly stressing the inferior radio-ulnar joint at the extremes of pronation/supination often indicates early wrist movement.
6. When the elbow is held in full extension a bulge of synovium may be detected just above the radial head
7. Small effusions in the knee can be detected by pressure on the lateral side of the joint, when any fluid present is moved to produce a contralateral bulge.
8. Pressure across the heads of the metatarsals may detect local tenderness, reflecting synovitis.

Spine

Spinal disease can be broadly categorized into inflammatory and non-inflammatory types, although the differentiation is not always clear-cut.

Inflammatory spinal pain

Sleep disturbance due to back pain should arouse suspicion of ankylosing spondylitis, infection, Paget's disease, or malignancy. Vertebral collapse gives rise to acute unremitting, progressive, and severe pain associated with localized tenderness. Spinal stiffness, worse in the morning and relieved by exercise, suggests ankylosing spondylitis; tenderness of the sacroiliac joints when pressure is applied downward and outward on the iliac crests of the supine patient, or discomfort elicited or by placing the flexed knee on to the opposite shoulder suggests an associated sacroiliitis. Schobers test of flexibility of the spine, is performed on the erect patient; a mark is made on the middle of the back at the level of the posterior iliac crest (approximately L5) and a point 10 cm above. If the increase in the distance between these two points on maximum forward flexion is less than 3 cm, spondylarthritis is the likely cause of symptoms.

Non-inflammatory spinal pain

Pain due to degenerative spinal disease is worse with overuse and weight bearing, and improved by rest. The symptoms are often episodic with periods of acute exacerbation followed by improvement. Spinal movements are impaired, and during the acute episodes there may be scoliosis and associated paraspinal muscle spasm. Degenerative spinal disease is often associated with neurogenic symptoms. Pain, weakness, paraesthesiae, or numbness radiating into the arm or leg are caused by nerve compression, have a dermatome distribution, and are aggravated by movements which irritate the nerve root, such as straight-leg raising and sciatic and femoral nerve stretch tests.

Wasting of muscles, loss of power, and impaired reflexes and sensation may be present. Spinal cord claudication from a localized or diffuse spinal stenosis classically presents with weakness in the legs on walking with the patients having to sit down for relief of symptoms; this contrasts with the patient with peripheral vascular claudication, who gets relief at rest by standing. Patients with spinal claudication often walk with a flexed spine and adopt a 'simian' posture as this increases the spinal canal diameter.

Soft tissue

Soft tissue symptoms may be due to a localized anatomical problem, with or without an associated systemic disease, or be the result of a condition such as fibrositis. Localized periarticular tenderness from epicondylitis, such as tennis elbow (lateral epicondyle) or golfer's elbow (medial epicondyle), can be confirmed by appropriate movements, such as forced extension of the wrist which exacerbates tennis elbow pain. Enthesitis describes an area of pain arising from inflammation at a bony interface with a joint capsule, ligament, or tendon, and can be a feature of the spondylarthropathies, for example plantar fasciitis. Localized ligamentous problems around a joint can also be aggravated by an appropriate stress test; for example, tenderness around the medial aspect of the knee due to ligamentous strain will be aggravated by stressing the joint into a valgus position. A more diffuse tenderness around the joint line is more likely to occur with intra-articular disease. Tendons may become diffusely painful and swollen from repetitive trauma, chronic infection, or from synovial diseases such as rheumatoid disease and pigmented villonodular synovitis. Pain from inflamed tendons may be elicited by specific stress tests such as Finkelstein's test for De Quervain's tenosynovitis (extensor tendon of the thumb). Tendons should be palpated during movement to detect crepitus, nodules, and triggering. Tenderness around joints may be due to a superficial bursitis with obvious swelling, as in prepatellar bursitis, or be in the deeper tissues when less obvious, for example subtrochanteric bursitis of the hip. Diffuse swelling around a joint may be due to local oedema or be part of an inflammatory process such as leakage of synovial fluid from a ruptured popliteal cyst, causing symptoms and signs suggestive of venous thrombosis. Periarticular soft tissue hypertrophy may be due to a lipoma or a more diffuse fatty swelling, as seen in the tender medial fat pad syndrome of obese middle-aged ladies' knees, or the benign fibrofatty pads seen over the proximal interphalangeal joints of the fingers (Garrod's pads). Periarticular swellings also occur with arthritis and may be due to gouty tophi, or the nodules of rheumatoid disease and rheumatic fever, xanthomas, calcific deposits associated with systemic sclerosis, or rarities such as multicentric reticulohistiocytosis. If fibrositis is suspected, trigger points and specific sites of tenderness should be sought, particularly in the lateral neck strap muscles, the belly of the trapezius, the epicondylar area, the medial aspect of the knee, and over the greater trochanter of the femur. Hypermobility can cause arthralgia and is detected by the ability to appose the thumb to the forearm, to hyperextend fingers, elbows, knees, by subluxation of patella, and the ability of affected patients to place palms of hands on the floor with knees fully extended.

Further reading

Dawes, P.T. (1995). History and examination techniques. In: *Collected reports on the rheumatic diseases* (ed. RT.C. Butler and M.I.V. Jayson), pp. 3–10. Arthritis and Rheumatism Council for Research, Chesterfield, UK.

Grahame, R. and Sargent, J.S. (1998). Evaluation, signs, and symptoms. In: *Rheumatology* (ed. J.H. Klippel and P.A. Dieppe), pp. 1.1–14.8. Mosby International, London.

Chapter 10.2

Rheumatoid arthritis

B. P. Wordsworth

Rheumatoid arthritis is generally regarded as an autoimmune disease but details of its pathogenesis remain unclear. Its prevalence is remarkably consistent world-wide (approximately 1 per cent) with a few important exceptions that have helped to highlight environmental influences and the role of the immune response genes. Inflammation of the synovial joints leading to the destruction of joints and periarticular tissues is the most obvious clinical and pathological characteristic of the disease, but a wide variety of extra-articular features can also develop. A remarkable characteristic of the condition is that it is confined to humans, being virtually unknown in any other species.

Aetiology

Rheumatoid arthritis has a complex multifactorial aetiology. There is considerable evidence for an important genetic component. Twin studies indicate a concordance rate of 20 per cent in monozygotic twins, although this figure is probably influenced by the severity of the disease in the proband. Thus, concordance rates may be lower when the index twin has mild, non-erosive disease but as high as 40 per cent if only index twins with erosive, rheumatoid factor-positive disease are considered. Confirmation of an important genetic contribution comes from comparing monozygotic and dizygotic twins, as disease concordance is approximately five times higher in the former despite their presumably similar exposure to environmental influences. However, susceptibility to rheumatoid arthritis must be determined predominantly by non-genetic factors as concordance rates are substantially lower than 50 per cent.

The pan-global distribution of rheumatoid arthritis could be explained by the involvement of an ubiquitous organism. However, strong supporting evidence for this concept is lacking. Although rheumatoid arthritis has many similarities to reactive arthritis, in which a wide range of different Gram-negative organisms are known to trigger the disease, infection at sites distant from the joints has not been identified, in spite of claims that infections of the urinary tract (*Proteus* sp.) may be more common in patients with rheumatoid arthritis than in healthy controls.

Likewise, no particular organism has ever been found reproducibly in the joints of patients with rheumatoid arthritis, although there have been sporadic reports of the isolation of viruses (rubella, parvovirus), atypical mycobacteria, and mycoplasma.

Some populations appear to be at unusually high or low risk of developing rheumatoid arthritis. Such observations could be explained by genetic or environmental differences. For example, the prevalence of the disease is very low in much of Africa. In the case of the South African black population there is strong support for an environmental influence: in the rural areas this ethnic group has the same low prevalence of the disease as elsewhere in rural sub-Saharan Africa, but this is greatly increased in those who have migrated to the townships where the prevalence is similar to that in the population of European descent. In contrast, the high prevalence (5 per cent more) in the Yakima and Chippewa Amerindians is more likely to be, at least in part, genetically determined. Both these tribes have a high frequency (c. 70 per cent) of HLA class II alleles associated with susceptibility to rheumatoid arthritis (DR4 in the Chippewa and DR6dW16 in the Yakima).

The genetic component of rheumatoid arthritis has been clarified by studying families, and from the definition of specific genetic markers associated with the disease. The risk to the first-degree relatives of probands with mild, non-erosive, seronegative disease (2–3 per cent) is little greater than in the risk in the general population. In contrast, the prevalence of rheumatoid arthritis among the first-degree relatives of probands with erosive, seropositive disease may be as high as 15 per cent, underlining the importance of genetic factors in determining disease severity. Estimates of the risk to the siblings of affected individuals range between 4 and 10 per cent, but there may be a delay, of decades even, before the development of the disease in the second sibling. Increasingly, interest in the genetic component of rheumatoid arthritis has focused on immunogenetic factors, particularly the immune response genes in the major histocompatibility complex on chromosome 6.

Immunopathology

In the early stages of rheumatoid arthritis the most obvious histological changes are confined to the synovial microvasculature, which shows evidence of endothelial damage, infiltration by polymorphonuclear leucocytes, and obliteration by thrombus. In the chronic phase, polymorphonuclear leucocytes are less obvious but the synovium is infiltrated by large numbers of inflammatory cells (macrophages, T and B lymphocytes, dendritic cells, and plasma cells). Among the lymphocyte population, B cells appear to be somewhat under-represented while T cells with the CD4+ (helper/inducer) phenotype are increased, particularly in the perivascular areas. The plasma cells in the subsynovium synthesize large quantities of immunoglobulin, much of which is IgM and IgG rheumatoid factor (i.e. immunoglobulin with reactivity to self-IgG). The precise role of these autoantibodies in the pathogenesis of the disease is not clear, but their ability to form immune complexes that can activate complement could be important in either initiating or prolonging local inflammation within the joint. Evidence for complement activation in the inflamed joints and serositis associated with rheumatoid arthritis is demonstrated by the presence of complement breakdown products such as C3a and C5a, both highly potent chemotactic agents for polymorphonuclear leucocytes and powerful mediators of inflammation. Rheumatoid factors are not specific for rheumatoid arthritis, being found in some 5 per cent of the normal population (usually in low titre) and in other diseases, particularly chronic infections such as tuberculosis, leprosy, and osteomyelitis. Their presence may precede the development of rheumatoid arthritis by months or even years, while in a minority of cases classical IgM rheumatoid factor may be persistently absent or only detectable long after the development of the disease.

Several observations suggest that the inflammatory reaction in rheumatoid arthritis is a T-cell-mediated phenomenon. First, there is a clear physical association between CD4-positive T cells and dedicated antigen-presenting cells (dendritic cells and cells of the macrophage/monocyte lineage) in the perivascular areas of the synovium. Second, certain therapeutic measures, including thoracic duct drainage, total body lymphoid irradiation, and, perhaps, the use of anti-CD4 monoclonal antibodies are associated with a decline in circulating T-cell numbers as well as clinical improvement. Third, cyclosporin, which is primarily directed against CD4-positive T cells is effective in rheumatoid arthritis. Finally, a role for a selected population of T cells might be inferred from the limited array of HLA class II antigens (e.g. DR4, DR1) that are strongly associated with rheumatoid arthritis. Most of these cells are activated and have a mature (CD45Ro) phenotype but, somewhat surprisingly, it has been difficult to demonstrate increases in the levels of cytokines (interleukin-2, interleukin-4, and γ-interferon) that might have been expected in the synovium and synovial fluid. One explanation for these findings might be that there is an accumulation of an unusual lymphocyte subset in the synovium. In contrast, large quantities of macrophage-derived cytokines (interleukin-1, tumour necrosis factor-α) are present, perhaps indicating an important part for the macrophage in the synovial inflammation. Preliminary trials of the efficacy of chimeric antitumour necrosis factor antibodies have proved promising.

Unusual glycosylation patterns of immunoglobulins have been observed in patients with rheumatoid arthritis, similar to those which may be seen in mycobacterial infections and sarcoidosis. Curiously, these changes in glycosylation have also been noted in the unaffected spouses of those with the disease. It has been suggested that this may render self-immunoglobulins potentially immunogenic, leading to the development of rheumatoid factors, but this is speculative. A reduced capacity to oxidize certain sulphur-containing compounds has also been described in patients with rheumatoid arthritis. Whether either of these phenomena is of primary importance is not known, but both have been used successfully as predictors of progression to chronic rheumatoid arthritis in patients with signs of early inflammatory joint disease.

Immunogenetics

Susceptibility to rheumatoid arthritis is associated with the immune response (**HLA**) genes in the major histocompatibility complex. The products of these genes are cell-surface glycoproteins that play a fundamental part in the binding of peptide antigens and their presentation for recognition by T cells.

The class I antigens (HLA-A, -B, and -C) are present on all nucleated cells and are particularly important in the immune surveillance of viral infections. The class II antigens (HLA-DR, -DQ, and -DP), in contrast, are found only on certain cells specialized in antigen presentation, such as dendritic cells, macrophages, and also B lymphocytes.

The observation that affected sibling pairs tend to inherit HLA haplotypes in common from their parents more frequently than would be expected by chance incriminates a gene (or genes) linked to HLA in susceptibility to rheumatoid arthritis. Furthermore, in most populations there are strong associations with specific alleles at the HLA-DRB1 locus which encodes the DRβ chain. Thus, the relative risk associated with alleles at this locus, defined serologically, ranges from nearly twofold for DR1 to over sixfold for DR4. The most likely explanation for this lies in the structure of the HLA molecule, in which polymorphic amino acid residues are concentrated around the antigen-binding site (Fig. 1). Those molecules which are associated with the disease share considerable homology in this region which is likely to have considerable influence on the range of peptide antigens that can be bound by particular HLA molecules. This is most clearly exemplified by the differential association of the various allelic

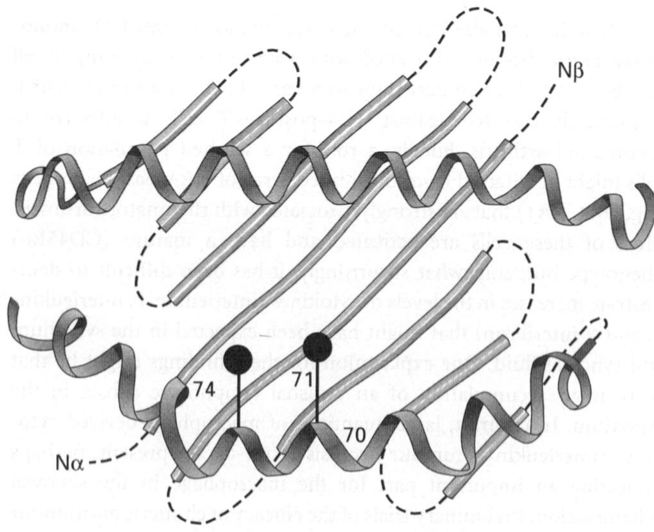

				67			70	71			74	
		Dw14	Asp	Leu	Leu	Glu	Gln	Arg	Arg	Ala	Ala	Val
Susceptible	DR4	Dw15	–	–	–	–	–	–	–	–	–	–
		Dw4	–	–	–	–	–	Lys	–	–	–	–
	DR1		–	–	–	–	–	–	–	–	–	–
	DRw10		–	–	–	–	Arg	–	–	–	–	–
	DR6	Dw16	–	–	–	–	–	–	–	–	–	–
Not susceptible	DR4	Dw10	–	Ile	–	–	<u>Asp</u>	<u>Glu</u>	–	–	–	–
		Dw13	–	–	–	–	–	–	–	–	<u>Glu</u>	–
	DR2		–	Phe	–	–	<u>Asp</u>	–	–	–	–	–

Fig. 1 Schematic representation of some HLA-DR molecules positively or negatively associated with rheumatoid arthritis. Charged amino acid substitutions (underlined) at positions 71 and 74 in the antigen binding-site are crucial in influencing susceptibility among the DR4 subtypes.

Table 1 Differential association of rheumatoid arthritis with the various subtypes of HLA-DR4 in the UK. HLA-Dw4 and -Dw14 are positively associated while Dw10 and Dw13 are negatively associated

	n	Dw4	Dw14	Dw10	Dw13
DR4-positive controls	185	119 (64%)	53 (29%)	7 (4%)	15 (8%)
DR4-positive rheumatoid arthritis	178	133 (74%)	66 (37%)	0	2 (1%)
Probability	0.02	0.05	<0.01	0.01	

subtypes of DR4 with rheumatoid arthritis where even one amino acid substitution in this region is sufficient to abrogate susceptibility to the disease (Table 1).

The association between DR4 and rheumatoid arthritis is strongest in the more severe variants of the disease. In community-based studies, which tend to include many milder cases, the association may be weak or even absent; in patients with erosive, seropositive disease 70 per cent of patients are likely to be DR4 positive, compared with about 25 per cent of the normal Caucasian population; in the Felty syndrome the frequency of DR4 is over 90 per cent. Furthermore, in the more severe forms of rheumatoid arthritis there is an increased frequency of the Dw4 subtype of DR4 (up to 90 per cent in the Felty syndrome) and also of DR4 homozygotes, the majority of whom have the Dw4/Dw14 genotype. It is likely that HLA accounts for no more than 30 per cent of the total genetic effect in rheumatoid arthritis, although no other genes contributing to susceptibility have yet been defined.

Table 2 American College of Rheumatology criteria for rheumatoid arthritis

1. Morning stiffness of at least 1 h
2. Arthritis of three or more joint areas
3. Arthritis of hand joints
4. Symmetric arthritis
5. Rheumatoid nodules
6. Serum rheumatoid factor positive
7. Typical radiographic changes in the hand and wrist

Criteria 1–4 must have been for at least 6 weeks.

Clinical features

Rheumatoid arthritis is a systemic disorder characterized by a chronic inflammatory synovitis which typically affects the peripheral joints but may affect any synovial joint in the body. In addition to the articular features that are the hallmark of the disease, many other tissues may also be affected, although this, like the severity of the articular disease, is highly variable. It is a disease of exacerbations and remissions, the clinical variability of which suggests that it might represent the end result of a number of different disease pathways. Diagnosis is based on the aggregation of a series of common clinical features rather than any specific pathognomonic abnormality: until there is a fuller understanding of the aetiology of the disease the possibility that the single diagnosis 'rheumatoid arthritis' masks considerable heterogeneity cannot be excluded.

The development of various classifications, based predominantly on clinical criteria, has been of benefit in the study of the epidemiology and aetiology of the disease. The diagnostic criteria developed by the American Rheumatism Association in 1958 have been used widely. They allow the recognition of three grades of rheumatoid arthritis according to the number of diagnostic criteria present ('classical', seven or more criteria of 11; 'definite', five criteria; 'probable', three criteria). However, the specificity of these criteria for rheumatoid arthritis is considerably increased if the milder variants are excluded. For this reason the 1987 American College of Rheumatology criteria, corresponding approximately to the 1958 'classical' and 'definite' groups, are now generally employed (Table 2). In individuals presenting with early inflammation of the joints, these criteria have proved good predictors of those likely to progress to chronic destructive rheumatoid arthritis.

Disease prevalence and onset

Rheumatoid arthritis may occur at any age but has a peak incidence in the fifth decade. The lifetime incidence of the disease in women (1.8 per cent) is three times that in males (0.5 per cent) and the prevalence of the disease in women over 65 years old is more than 5 per cent. The sex difference is most pronounced (as high as 6:1) in those with early-onset disease but is almost equal by the age of 65. The disease starts twice as commonly in winter, but whether this represents a non-specific effect, such as the increased sensitivity to joint symptoms, or a more specific process, such as the precipitation of vasculitis, is not clear. Several distinct patterns of onset are recognized which can be of some use in predicting the prognosis.

Palindromic onset

In about one-fifth of patients with rheumatoid arthritis, persistent joint disease may be antedated by repeated attacks of acute self-limiting synovitis, affecting a variable number of joints. Typically, the inflammation develops over a few hours and is accompanied by erythema and swelling of the affected joints but resolves completely within 48–72 h, leaving no residual features. About 50 per cent of individuals who suffer from attacks of palindromic rheumatism ultimately develop chronic rheumatoid arthritis, and they can usually be identified by the presence of rheumatoid factor in the blood, although this may not be present at the outset. The number of joints involved is usually small but increases with time and with the onset of persistent joint disease. If joint symptoms are sufficiently frequent to be troublesome during the palindromic phase, they can often be controlled by intramuscular gold injections or D-penicillamine (often in low doses) as in the case of established rheumatoid arthritis.

Explosive onset

In about 10 per cent of cases the onset of the disease is very rapid, even overnight, with severe symmetrical polyarticular involvement. Many patients with this type of onset do surprisingly well in the long term.

Systemic onset

This is particularly common in middle-aged men in whom non-articular features may dominate the clinical picture. Fever, myalgia, weight loss, anaemia, pleural effusions, and vasculitic lesions may be severe, sometimes in the absence of marked joint pathology. Although rheumatoid factor is usually present in high titres, it is often necessary to exclude other causes such as other connective tissue disorder, malignancy, or infection.

Insidious onset

The majority of cases of rheumatoid arthritis develop insidiously over weeks or months, with gradually increasing joint involvement. This pattern of onset, which is seen in up to 70 per cent of cases, is associated with a relatively poor prognosis. Progression from predominantly peripheral small-joint disease to the involvement of the more proximal joints, including the knees and hips, is the most common pattern. However, the subset of patients with the earliest joint involvement is in the knees and wrists are particularly likely to be positive for IgA rheumatoid factor.

Polymyalgic onset

Limb girdle muscle symptoms may precede the onset of an overt arthropathy, particularly in the elderly. Not all patients with this pattern are rheumatoid-factor positive and it may be difficult to distinguish with certainty from polymyalgia rheumatica. It is therefore of considerable interest that both these conditions are associated with the HLA-DR4 antigen. The initial response to corticosteroid therapy in these cases is impressive but is less well maintained as progressive synovitis supervenes.

Mono- and pauci-articular onset

In young women there may initially be very limited joint involvement, particularly involving the knees. While there is no doubt that a proportion of these cases go on to develop full-blown rheumatoid arthritis, many do not. It is therefore important to exclude other potential causes of monoarthritis, such as low-grade infection or pigmented villonodular synovitis. Intermittent hydrarthrosis causes effusions which recur with remarkably consistent periodicity in the absence of pronounced systemic or joint inflammation. The erythrocyte sedimentation rate and C-reactive protein are normal and joint fluid white cell counts are typically less than 200/mm^3. Patients with such limited joint disease who are persistently seronegative for rheumatoid factor usually pursue a benign course and probably represent an entirely different type of joint disease from classical rheumatoid arthritis.

Joint features

Rheumatoid arthritis is typically a distal, symmetrical, small-joint polyarthritis involving the proximal interphalangeal and metacarpophalangeal joints of the hands, the wrists, metatarsophalangeal joints, ankles, knees, and cervical spine. The shoulders, elbows, and hips are less frequently involved, but can be a major source of morbidity. Any synovial joint in the body may be affected, including the cricoarytenoid and the temporomandibular joints. In addition, periarticular synovial structures, such as bursae and tendon sheaths, are commonly inflamed.

It may be difficult to distinguish between symptoms and signs of joint disease due to inflammation and those that result from secondary mechanical problems arising from joint destruction. This is an important distinction as it will often dictate the most appropriate form of treatment. Anti-inflammatory and disease-modifying drugs may be appropriate in the early inflammatory phase, but the use of analgesics and physical approaches, such as splints or corrective surgery, would be more likely to aid patients with severe joint damage.

The most common symptoms described by patients are pain and pronounced stiffness. The latter frequently exhibits a diurnal rhythm, worse on rising in the morning and then recurring towards the evening. Gentle activity may alleviate the symptoms but is followed by stiffening or 'gelling' with subsequent inactivity. The affected joints are frequently tender, swollen, and warm and there may be limitation of both active and passive movement. Muscle wasting serves to accentuate the local swelling of the joint, which is in part due to proliferation of the synovial tissue and in part to synovial effusion within the joint. Progressive destruction of the articular cartilage, subchondral bone, and periarticular soft tissues eventually combine to produce the characteristic deformities seen in long-standing rheumatoid arthritis.

In parallel with these clinical changes there are characteristic radiological appearances which may be helpful in the diagnosis of early rheumatoid arthritis and in monitoring its progress (Fig. 2). In the early stages of the disease it is common for the first evidence of erosions to be in the feet, and these should always be included in diagnostic views. Radiological changes include:

1. soft-tissue swelling;
2. juxta-articular osteoporosis;
3. loss of joint space due to erosion of the articular cartilage;
4. bone erosions at the points of attachment of the synovium; and
5. joint deformities.

Upper limbs

Hands and wrists

The appearance of the hands in classical rheumatoid arthritis is highly characteristic. However, there are numerous potential patterns of

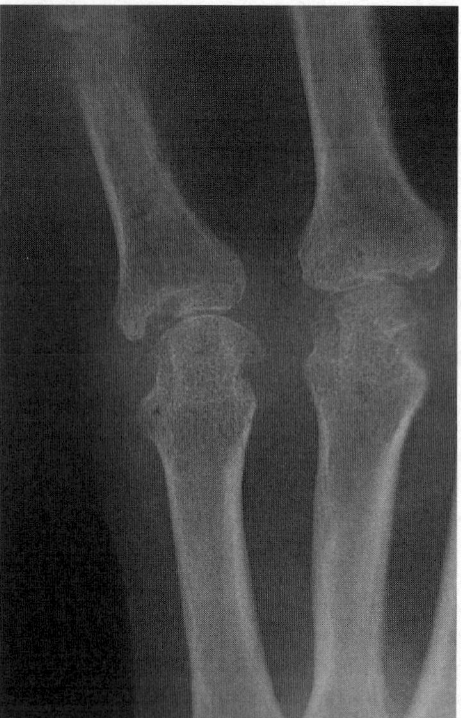

Fig. 2 Typical radiological features of rheumatoid arthritis in the metacarpophalangeal joints, showing osteoporosis, joint space narrowing, periarticular erosions, and angular deformity.

deformity, and distinction from other arthropathies is occasionally difficult. Early in the disease there may be soft-tissue swelling around the affected joints. Involvement of the proximal interphalangeal joints give a spindle-shaped appearance to the fingers, and soft-tissue swelling can be observed over the ulnar styloid, and in the second and third metacarpophalangeal joints. Distal interphalangeal joint involvement is less common (about 15 per cent of cases) but rheumatoid arthritis may sometimes be superimposed on pre-existing osteoarthritis of these joints.

Tenosynovitis of the long flexor tendons in the palm of the hand may exacerbate stiffness of the fingers and cause 'trigger finger'. This may be associated with palpable crepitus over the tendon on active or passive movement of the corresponding finger. Similar synovitis at the wrist within the flexor retinaculum may cause compression of the median nerve with the typical features of carpal tunnel syndrome. Tinel's sign is sometimes positive but relatively insensitive. Phalen's sign (pressure over the carpal tunnel with the wrist in flexion) may be more useful, not only because it is more frequently positive but also because it reproduces the symptoms accurately. The diagnosis can be confirmed by nerve conduction studies.

On the dorsal surface of the wrist, synovitis of the extensor tendons is common and may lead to rupture (Fig. 3). A 'dropped finger' affecting the little finger is an important indication for surgical exploration and synovectomy, as it may presage the progressive rupture of the rest of the extensor communis tendon. Similar rupture of the extensor pollicis longus and extensor indicis proprius may occur.

Persistent synovitis with erosion of the articular surfaces, weakening of the joint capsules, and muscle weakness, with or without tendon rupture, will inevitably lead to deformities. There are several commonly occurring variants:

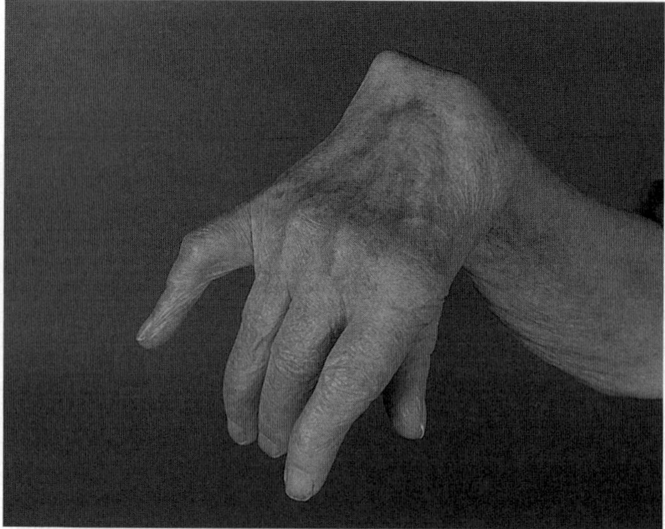

Fig. 3 'Bull's horn' deformity due to rupture of the extensor communis tendon from synovitis near the ulnar styloid. Selective sparing of the extensor indicis proprius and extensor digiti minimi tendons has in this instance preserved the ability to point the index and little fingers independently.

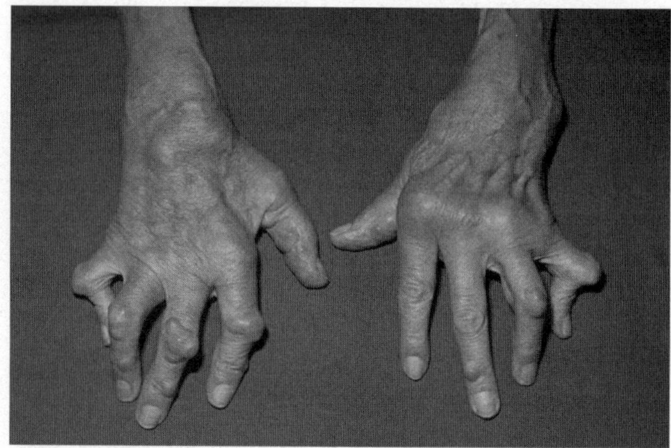

Fig. 4 Volar and ulnar subluxation of the fingers at metacarpophalangeal joints which results, respectively, from the relative strength of the long flexors and the ulnar direction of pull arising from both the long flexors and extensors. Cutaneous nodules are present on the fingers.

Volar subluxation of the fingers at the metacarpophalangeal joints occurs as a result of destruction of the articular cartilage, and subsequent instability of these joints. As the flexor tendons provide the strongest force acting across these joints progressive subluxation towards the palm may develop, leaving the metacarpal heads relatively prominent.

Ulnar deviation and subluxation of the fingers is the result of instability of the metacarpophalangeal joints. The fingers may tend to drift in an ulnar direction because of the ulnar vector of the action of both the flexor and extensor finger tendons. The process may be exacerbated by radial deviation of the carpus and also by ulnar subluxation of the extensor tendons if the supports which usually hold them in place over the centre of the metacarpophalangeal joints are weakened by synovitis (Fig. 4).

Swan neck deformities occur following volar subluxation of the proximal phalanges at the metacarpophalangeal joints, with subsequent contracture of the intrinsic muscles which become extensors rather than flexors of the proximal interphalangeal joints. Compensatory flexion of the distal interphalangeal joint occurs as a result of a tenodesis effect as the flexor digitorum profundus tendon is stretched over the hyperextended proximal interphalangeal joint.

Boutonnière (button-hole) deformity occurs when a chronic effusion within the proximal interphalangeal joint stretches or even ruptures the dorsal slip of the extensor hood, allowing dorsal migration of the joint through the discontinuity. A similar process at the carpometacarpal joint of the thumb may give rise to the Z-thumb deformity.

The piano-key sign can be detected when weakening of the distal radio-ulnar ligament by synovitis allows the distal ulna to migrate dorsally so that it overrides the radius (caput ulnae syndrome). The ulna can be depressed by pressure like a piano key (while the patient emits a note!). Progressive destruction of the carpal joints may be followed by volar subluxation and ultimately ankylosis.

Carpal collapse and fusion may occur late in the disease, particularly in those with an early-onset rheumatoid arthritis, when instability of the wrist may lead to collapse of the carpal bones, causing foreshortening of the carpus and, ultimately, spontaneous fusion of the wrist.

Elbows and shoulders

Involvement of the elbows is less common than of the wrist but severe destruction may occur, leading to pronounced deformity and disability. The radiohumeral joint is more commonly symptomatic than the humeroulnar joint and presents problems particularly with pronation/supination. Periarticular structures (olecranon bursa, ulnar nerve) may also be affected by synovitis and subcutaneous nodules are commonly found on the extensor surface of the forearm close to the elbow.

Pain around the shoulder may arise from the glenohumeral joint itself, periarticular structures (particularly the subacromial bursa), the acromioclavicular joint, or the cervical spine. Frequently more than one cause may coexist, necessitating careful evaluation of the anatomical cause of the pain if appropriate treatment is to be applied. There may be inflammation of the subacromial bursa or supraspinatus tendon in addition to glenohumeral joint synovitis, producing a typical painful arc syndrome. Involvement of the acromioclavicular joint can give rise to pain particularly with overhead activities, and is associated with localized tenderness. Referred pain from the neck or cervical radiculopathy may closely mimic shoulder pathology but tends to persist at rest. In late disease of older people, severe destruction of the shoulders can occur, with loss of the whole of the head of the humerus.

Lower limbs

Feet and ankles

Involvement of the feet is common from an early stage of the disease. It frequently gives rise to problems which go unrecognized despite the fact that they can often be overcome relatively simply by the provision of the appropriate footwear. Active synovitis of the metatarsophalangeal joints, with or without effusions, leads to spreading of the forefoot and a marked increase in width, necessitating a larger shoe fitting. Collapse of the transverse arch of the forefoot causes the weight to be taken predominantly on the second and third metatarsal heads rather than the first and fifth which is customary (Fig. 5). Patients frequently complain of pain arising in the ball of the foot (metatarsalgia) which can vary in intensity from 'walking on pebbles' to 'like walking on broken glass'. Dorsal subluxation of the toes leads to their progressive defunctioning for weight bearing and commonly causes pressure problems as they rub against the shoe uppers. In addition, the specialized weight-bearing skin and subcutaneous tissue lying under the metatarsal heads is drawn forward to be replaced by unprotected skin, which becomes hyperkeratotic in response to repeated loading. The resulting plantar callosities exacerbate the pain of the metatarsalgia and may require regular chiropody. Hallux valgus almost invariably develops as a consequence of the spreading of the forefoot and the bowstring effect from the extensor hallucis longus.

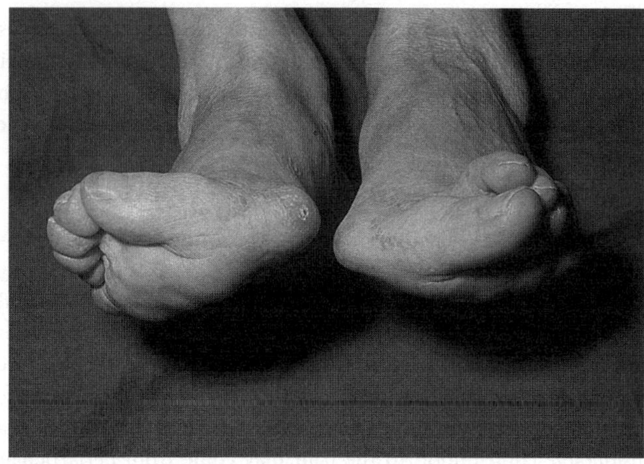

Fig. 5 Forefoot deformity is common from an early stage of rheumatoid arthritis as a result of destruction of the normal transverse arch by synovitis of the metatarsophalangeal joints.

Involvement of the ankle joint in isolation is rare but may occur in association with disease of the subtalar and midtarsal joints, which occurs in two-thirds of patients. Valgus deformity of the hindfoot is usual and may be exacerbated by rupture of the tibialis posterior tendon which buttresses the medial aspect of the ankle. Associated collapse of the medial longitudinal arch of the foot may add to the resulting mechanical problems, which include severe pain around the lateral aspect of the ankle from joint compression. Extensive synovitis, particularly of the long flexor tendons, may lead to compressions of the medial plantar nerve in the tarsal tunnel.

Knees

Involvement of the knee is an important and relatively common cause of disability from an early stage in the disease because of its role in load bearing. Synovial proliferation is usually most obvious in the suprapatella pouch and there may be pronounced wasting of the quadriceps as a result of reflex muscle inhibition. Synovial effusion typically produces posterior knee pain in the early stages by stretching the posterior capsule of the joint. This may lead to the development of a popliteal cyst communicating with the joint via a valve-like opening which does not easily allow fluid back into the joint. Rupture of the joint or a popliteal cyst may cause extravasation of highly irritant synovial fluid into the calf where the inflammation and swelling may mimic a deep vein thrombosis. These two pathologies can sometimes coexist because there may be partial obstruction to the venous return by the presence of an extensive popliteal cyst.

Tricompartmental damage to the articular surfaces of the knees is the usual outcome of late disease and may cause severe instability of the joint as the collateral and cruciate ligaments become lax. Valgus deformities of the knees are the usual consequence of loading such unstable joints, and are often combined with a degree of fixed flexion deformity. Pain may also arise from periarticular structures, such as the insertion of the collateral ligaments which are chronically under strain in the unstable knee joint. Even in the end stages of destruction of the knee joint it may be possible to afford the patient considerable relief by attention to specific anatomical sites of injury.

Hips

Involvement of the hips in rheumatoid arthritis is relatively uncommon overall (c. 25 per cent) but is a major source of morbidity in those patients with more severe disease. Pain is usually experienced in the groin and the buttock but may radiate to the knee, sometimes mimicking knee arthritis. Rotation and abduction of the hip are reduced before flexion, but ultimately fixed flexion deformity of the joint may occur. Even in patients with advanced hip arthritis a considerable contribution to the pain may come from periarticular tissues, in particular trochanteric bursitis. Typically, this is associated with tenderness over the grater trochanter (which may stop the patient lying on that side), and pain on adduction of the hip which may be referred to the lateral aspect of the knee. In late disease these may be relatively sudden collapse of the femoral head, with a severe increase in pain and disability, necessitating joint replacement.

Axial skeleton

Involvement of the sacroiliac joints is rare in rheumatoid arthritis. However, spinal arthritis is common, up to 80 per cent of patients demonstrating radiological evidence of the disease in the cervical spine. This may be asymptomatic but the most frequent result is painful limitation of movement, often in several planes. The most common radiological abnormalities consist of osteoporosis, erosion of the sygapophyseal joints, erosion of the vertebral end plates, and loss of disc space in the absence of florid osteophytosis.

There may be evidence of atlantoaxial subluxation in up to 25 per cent of patients attending hospital, but less than one in four of these will be symptomatic. In the normal joint the odontoid peg is closely opposed to the posterior aspect of the anterior arch of the atlas by a network of ligaments, including the cruciate, posterior longitudinal, and alar ligaments. Instability of the atlantoaxial joints results from erosion of the odontoid peg or rupture of the supporting ligaments and will be apparent on lateral radiographs of the cervical spine taken in flexion and extension. Lateral or vertical subluxation of the atlantoaxial joint may also occur. Separation of the odontoid peg from the arch of the atlas by 4 mm or more is abnormal. The risk of cord compression is greatest in males, in those with a subluxation exceeding 8 mm, and where there is also vertical subluxation of the atlantoaxial joint. Minor degrees of atlantoaxial subluxation can be relatively well tolerated because the cervical canal is relatively wide at this level. Subaxial subluxation presents a serious risk of cord compression because the cervical canal there is narrower.

Serious erosive change in the cervical spine is more likely in patients who have pronounced peripheral joint disease and in those on corticosteroids. Erosion, when present, usually develop within 2 years of the onset. Symptoms suggestive of atlantoaxial disease include high cervical pain radiating to the occiput and temporal regions, exacerbated by neck movements. There may be audible or palpable clunking on flexion, and inability to place the chin on the sternum is a useful screening test. At its worst, compression of the cervical cord or vertebral blood vessels may lead to quadriplegia or sudden death. More commonly it causes shooting pains in the arms or legs, weakness, and unsteadiness of gait or sphincter disturbance. A mild spastic weakness in the arms or legs may be difficult to detect in a patient whose limbs have already been rendered weak and stiff by arthritis, but pathologically brisk tendon jerks, a positive Hoffman sign, or upgoing plantar response are important signs. Loss of proprioception, vibration sense, and balance may indicate significant damage to the posterior columns, but can be difficult to distinguish from the peripheral neuropathy that is common in rheumatoid arthritis.

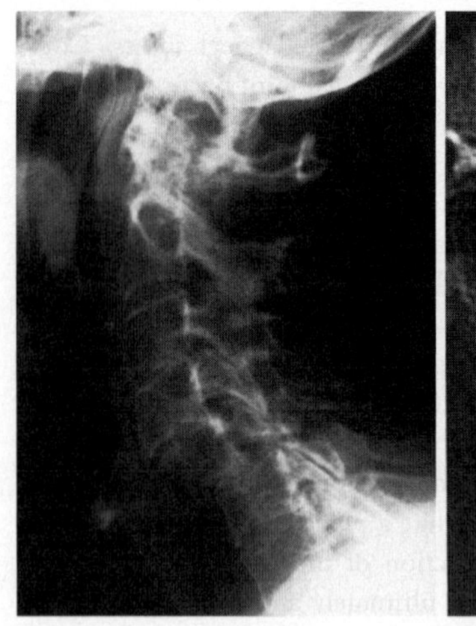
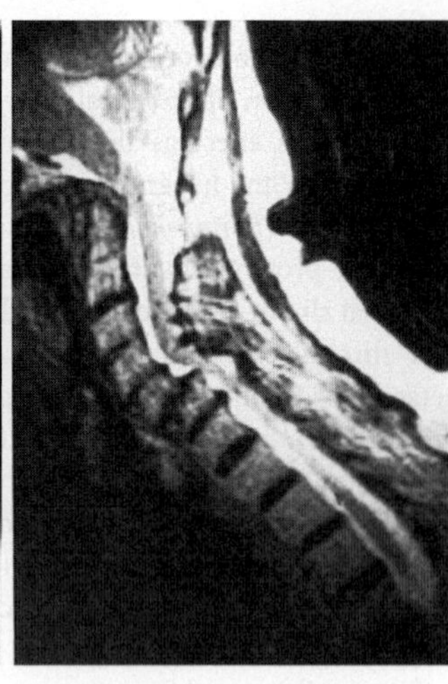

Fig. 6 Subaxial subluxation of the cervical spine (C5/6) with compression of the spinal cord. The loss of disc height and subluxation in the absence of marked osteophytosis on the standard radiographs (left) is typical of rheumatoid arthritis. Magnetic resonance imaging (right) reveals the extent of the spinal cord compression.

Acute subluxation of the cervical spine with neurological signs will initially require immobilization with skeletal traction. A proportion of cases will improve with such conservative measures but most will be left with marked residual neurological impairment and handicap. It has been estimated that atlantoaxial subluxation is responsible for as many as 5 per cent of all deaths in rheumatoid arthritis. However, although there may be pre-existing radiological evidence of atlantoaxial subluxation in a small proportion of these, it is rare for overt cervical myelopathy to have developed. The most common indication for fusion is intractable pain, and it is notoriously difficult to predict individuals at risk of catastrophic neurological damage on the basis of symptoms and physical examination alone. Patients with atlantoaxial slip of 8 mm or more should certainly be considered for posterior fusion, particularly if there is also evidence of vertical migration of the joint or if neurological signs suggestive of myelopathy are present. Magnetic resonance imaging provides an accurate, non-invasive method of assessing the degree of compromise to the spinal cord that can be particularly useful in patients with subaxial subluxation (Fig. 6).

Other joints

Hoarseness of the voice may occasionally be caused by effusion within the cricoarytenoid joints. Temporomandibular joint disease causes pain on chewing and may particularly restrict opening of the mouth. Discitis can occur in the lumbar as well as the cervical spine.

Extra-articular features

The majority of patients with rheumatoid arthritis exhibit at least some extra-articular features and these tend to be more numerous and more severe in those with high titres of rheumatoid factor in the blood. These systemic features are highly variable, ranging from the fairly trivial (e.g. episcleritis, subcutaneous nodules) to the potentially life-threatening (e.g. systemic vasculitis, pleuropericarditis). Actuarial studies indicate that rheumatoid arthritis significantly reduces life expectancy. This is not explained by the effects of progressive immobility alone but by the systemic nature of the illness. Long-term studies suggests that rheumatoid arthritis itself is either responsible directly or contributes to death in about one-third of patients. This effect appears to be particularly pronounced in seropositve middle-aged men with pronounced extra-articular features.

The extra-articular disease may pursue a course quite dissociated from the joint disease. For example, systemic vasculitis may appear for the first time when joint synovitis has been suppressed by disease-modifying drugs.

The precise cause of many of the extra-articular features of rheumatoid arthritis remains to be elucidated. However, three major pathological phenomena dominate the disease: inflammation of membranes (pleura, pericardium and others as well as the synovium), nodule formation, and vasculitis. Nodules correlate with titres of IgM rheumatoid factor, and vasculitis appears to depend more on the formation of IgG-containing immune complexes. Combinations of these phenomena explain most extra-articular events.

Rheumatoid nodules

Subcutaneous and intracutaneous nodules are a hallmark of the disease, occurring in about one-quarter of patients. They are discrete, firm, non-tender swellings varying from a few millimetres to several centimetres in size, and in rare instances, usually in seropositive males, they may occur in the absence of typical articular disease (rheumatoid nodulosis). They occur most frequently on the extensor surface of the forearm and olecranon, site where repeated minor trauma from leaning could initiate their formation. They also commonly occur around tendons, including the Achilles, the flexor and extensor tendons of the fingers, and over the sacrum. Sometimes superficial nodules may break down with ulceration of the surrounding skin.

Histological examination of these nodules reveals central fibrinoid necrosis surrounded by palisades of fibroblasts and chronic inflammatory cells, suggesting a combination of proliferative and destructive tissue responses.

Rheumatoid nodules may also develop in many other tissues including the eye (scleromalacia), pleura, pericardium, and parenchyma of the lungs and heart (where they may be found at autopsy in as many as 10 per cent of patients). They sometimes occur on the vocal cords and very occasionally they may cause dysfunction of the heart valves or conducting tissue. The Caplan syndrome, describing the combination of massive pulmonary fibrosis and pulmonary nodules, was first described in a miner with rheumatoid arthritis but it may also develop, following occupational exposure to inorganic dusts (e.g. silica, asbestos), in seropositive individuals without arthritis. Such intrapulmonary nodules may be mistaken for other pathology, including tumours or abscesses, particularly if they break down and cavitate.

Anaemia

A moderate normochromic normocytic anaemia is an almost invariable finding in active rheumatoid arthritis. A number of factors related to the inflammatory process probably contribute. Iron may be sequestered in an unusable form (haemosiderin) by the reticuloendothelial system; there may be ineffective erythropoiesis and red blood cell survival is reduced; haemodilution may occur as a result of increased blood volume. The potential influence of increased levels of cytokines (interleukin-1 and interleukin-6) and blunted erythropoietin responses are the foci of research interest. The potential therapeutic role of recombinant erythropoietin has not yet been established.

The most important practical consideration is the differentiation of iron-deficiency anaemia secondary to gastrointestinal haemorrhage from the anaemia of chronic disease. This may be particularly difficult when the two coexist. As a general rule, a microcytic hypochromic blood picture indicates iron deficiency and should be investigated and treated as such. In the chronic anaemia of rheumatoid disease the blood picture is usually normocytic and normochromic or hypochromic (but rarely microcytic). Assessment of the bone marrow iron stores is the most reliable indicator of iron deficiency but is rarely necessary if the mean corpuscular volume, serum iron-binding capacity, and ferritin are used in combination. Iron-binding capacity is typically reduced in active rheumatoid arthritis: normal or slightly raised levels in the presence of a low serum iron are therefore highly indicative of iron deficiency. In contrast, as part of the acute phase response, ferritin levels are typically elevated in active rheumatoid arthritis unless there is iron deficiency. The typical anaemia of chronic disease correlates closely with the sedimentation rate as a marker of disease activity and does not respond to iron, folic acid, or vitamin B12. In contrast, suppression of the disease by corticosteroids appears to mobilize iron stores rapidly, resulting in increased haemopoiesis and a subsequent rise in haemoglobin concentration.

Platelets

The platelet count is commonly increased to levels greater than 5×10^5 in active disease and this may also occur when there is active bleeding from the intestine. In contrast, the platelet count may be low in the Felty syndrome or as a result of marrow toxicity from antirheumatic drugs.

Vasculitis

Vascular lesions are evident at autopsy in as many as 25 per cent of individuals with rheumatoid arthritis, with an equal sex incidence. Many different sizes of blood vessels may be affected. The resulting clinical spectrum of disease is therefore highly variable. Intimal hyperplasia of the small terminal digital vessels causes very limited cutaneous lesions (nailfold infarcts, rashes, and splinter haemorrhages) and has a generally good prognosis in the absence of other signs suggestive of more severe systemic involvement. In contrast, severe life-threatening systemic tissue infarction (widespread cutaneous ulceration, infarction of the bowel, mononeuritis multiplex) may develop if there is involvement of the larger blood vessels by leucocytoclastic or necrotizing vasculitis. This may be indistinguishable from polyarteritis nodosa with fibrinoid necrosis of the intima and infiltration of the outer layers by lymphocytes and occasional polymorphonuclear leucocytes.

Vasculitis is more common in patients with high levels of IgM rheumatoid factor and severe joint disease, although the activity of the synovitis and extra-articular disease is often temporally dissociated. Its incidence increases with the duration of the disease, but occasionally it may be present from the outset, even, rarely, in the absence of joint disease. It is possible that the vasculitis may be initiated by IgG rheumatoid factor containing immune complexes deposited in the vessel walls, as these can activate complement.

Vasculitis is increased somewhat in patients in whom antinuclear antibody can be detected and correlates more closely with raised circulating levels of IgG than IgM rheumatoid factor. In some patients with vasculitic features there may be detectable circulating cryoglobulins and low concentrations of complement in plasma.

Rheumatoid vasculitis is associated with significant mortality but this can be significantly reduced with appropriate therapy. Oral or intravenous pulses of corticosteroids alone are probably ineffective but, regimens based on intermittent boluses of cyclophosphamide coupled with corticosteroids appear to induce effective and sustained suppression similar to that obtained in other forms of necrotizing vasculitis.

Lung involvement

Several patterns of lung disease may occur.

Pleurisy has an incidence of about 1 per cent overall, but pleural effusions due to rheumatoid arthritis may go undetected. Pleural involvement is five times more common in men than in women and often needs differentiation from other causes, particularly when other systemic features, such as weight loss and fever, are present. The fluid has raised protein, low glucose, and low complement levels and is typically positive for rheumatoid factor. The cell count is high due to the presence of lymphocytes, macrophages, and, to a lesser extent, multinucleate giant cells, including comet cells. Pleural biopsy may reveal rheumatoid granulomas, like an 'opened-out rheumatoid nodule', but typically there is the appearance of non-specific inflammation which does not allow differentiation from other causes of pleurisy.

Nodules are more common in the upper than the lower zones and may be single or multiple. Cavitation may occasionally lead to haemoptysis, and tissue diagnosis can usually be obtained by percutaneous or trans-bronchial needle biopsy without recourse to thoracotomy.

Pulmonary fibrosis is common in rheumatoid arthritis but is often subclinical. Ten per cent of patients have radiological evidence of fibrosis and many more have evidence of impaired vital capacity and gas transfer. Classical fibrosing alveolitis occurs in 2 per cent of patients with rheumatoid arthritis and causes progressive dyspnoea, clubbing of the fingers, fine late-inspiratory crepitations, and lower-zone reticulonodular shadowing on the chest radiograph. It carries a 5-year mortality of 50 per cent and responds poorly to treatment with corticosteroid, D-penicillamine, or cytotoxic agents.

Obliterative bronchiolitis is a rare but rapidly progressive and fatal process manifesting with an acute onset of breathlessness. Widespread small airways obstruction is present in the absence of alveolar fibrosis and there is little evidence of inflammation. Many patients with rheumatoid arthritis have evidence of airways obstruction irrespective of their smoking habits. Bronchiectasis also appears to be more common in those with the disease and to pre-date its onset.

Cardiac involvement

This is more common in men and is frequently subclinical. Small pericardial effusions can be found by ultrasonography in up to half those patients with seropositive nodular disease admitted to hospital but this represents the severe end of the disease spectrum. The true overall prevalence is probably between 5 and 10 per cent. Clinically symptomatic pericarditis has an annual incidence of about 0.4 per cent and may occur at any stage of the disease. However, potentially life-threatening complications such as tamponade or constrictive pericarditis are very rare.

Valvulitis may be apparent at autopsy in 20 per cent of cases but is rarely symptomatic during life. Granulomatous thickening of the cusps of the aortic valve occurs more frequently than in the mitral valve but only rarely produces incompetence of the valve. Acute aortic regurgitation following perforation of one of the cusps is described and may need emergency valve replacement.

Autopsy studies reveal a patchy myocardial fibrosis in about one-sixth of patients and myocardial nodules can be found in some patients. Although evidence of a small-vessel vasculitis may be apparent at post mortem in 20 per cent of patients, the incidence of myocardial infarction resulting from necrotizing vasculitis during life seem to be very low. However, there is an excess cardiac mortality among patients with rheumatoid arthritis that appears to be caused through ischaemic heart disease, although the precise mechanisms involved are not clear.

Eye involvement (see Plate 23, The eye and disease)

This is common in rheumatoid arthritis and may be due to localized tissue involvement or as part of a more generalized disorder involving the exocrine glands—*Sjögren's* syndrome. *Episcleritis* usually appears as a raised lesion in the anterior sclera with hyperaemia of the deeper layers. The lesions are often transient but may be associated with vasculitis elsewhere. Low-grade discomfort is not uncommon and may require the use of topical corticosteroids. *Scleritis* is less common but potentially more serious as it may lead to progressive thinning of the sclera (scleromalacia) and even perforation. Treatment with systemic corticosteroids is usually required. *Keratolysis* (corneal melting) and *limbal guttering* are rare complications of vasculitis of the circumcorneal vessels, which can also cause perforation. Exceptionally there may be diplopia resulting from stenosing tenosynovitis of the superior oblique tendon (Brown's syndrome).

Sjögren's syndrome is characterized by diffuse infiltration of the exocrine glands and other tissues by lymphocytes, resulting in destruction and glandular insufficiency. The syndrome occurs in one-fifth of patients with rheumatoid arthritis (secondary Sjögren's syndrome). Typical syndromes consist of pain, erythema, grittiness in the eyes, photosensitivity, and stickiness associated with adherent strands of mucus. Secondary bacterial infection is relatively common due to the loss of lysozymes, bacteriostatic agents normally present in tears. Corneal damage may occur. Extraglandular involvement is less common in secondary Sjögren's syndrome that in the primary disease, but half of those with rheumatoid arthritis exhibit at least some degree of parotid gland enlargement. General malaise is common and cutaneous vasculitis, peripheral neuropathy, renal tubular acidosis, interstitial pulmonary fibrosis, and myositis may all coincide. Lymphoproliferation occurs in one-quarter of all patients (particularly those with primary disease), and there is a measurable excess of individuals who subsequently develop lymphoma.

In difficult cases the diagnosis may be aided by the following: lymphocytic infiltration of labial salivary glands on biopsy; the presence of anti-salivary gland antibodies; reduced secretion of saliva measured by cannulation of the parotid or submandibular ducts; abnormalities of the parotid ductular architecture at sialography. Rheumatoid factor is almost invariably positive and 70 per cent of patients are also positive for antinuclear factor.

Peripheral nerve involvement

This is common in rheumatoid arthritis but is quite frequently masked by the severity of the joint disease. Entrapment neuropathies have already been considered and are amendable to treatment by corticosteroid injection and other measures to relieve local pressure. A mild glove and stocking sensory neuropathy is relatively common in rheumatoid arthritis but is usually benign. In contrast, the presence of a mixed sensorimotor neuropathy or mononeuritis multiplex is indicative of underlying vasculitis of the vasa nervorum and dictates the use of high-dose corticosteroid therapy with cyclophosphamide as outlined above.

Muscle involvement

In rheumatoid arthritis muscle involvement is usually attributed to the reflex inhibition and wasting resulting from severe joint pain. Focal lymphocytic infiltration may be present on muscle biopsy, but its relevance to symptoms is in doubt and there is no increase in muscle enzyme concentrations in the serum to suggest active myositis in all but a tiny minority of patients. It is important to remember that some drugs used in the treatment of the disease may cause a myopathy (e.g. corticosteroids, antimalarials) and that D-penicillamine is well documented to cause myasthenia gravis in some patients.

Liver involvement

This is evident in about 10 per cent of patients with active disease. There may be mild hepatosplenomegaly and asymptomatic elevation of the serum alkaline phosphatase but liver biopsy rarely shows specific changes. Minor degrees of fatty change, Kupffer cell hyperplasia, and lymphocytic infiltration of the portal tracts may be seen. The potential hepatotoxicity of many drugs used in the treatment of rheumatoid arthritis should be recalled, particularly high-dose salicylates, sulphasalazine, good salts, and antimalarials.

Renal involvement

This is less of a problem in rheumatoid arthritis than might be expected from analogy with other disorders associated with vasculitis, such as systemic lupus erythematosus and polyarteritis nodosa. Renal biopsy studies have consistently failed to reveal evidence of renal vasculitis. Renal papillary necrosis and interstitial nephritis occasionally occur and are probably related, at least in part, to the use of non-steroidal analgesics. IgA nephropathy associated with elevated serum levels IgM and IgA is described in rheumatoid arthritis but is probably no more common than in age-matched controls.

Gold salts and D-penicillamine can cause proteinuria due to membranous glomerulonephritis in about 10 per cent of patients. This may persist for up to 2 years after the drug has been stopped but rarely progresses to frank nephrotic syndrome.

Bone involvement

This occurs in the vicinity of the joints, where juxta-articular osteoporosis is an early feature. It also occurs as a more generalized phenomenon, partly as a result of the relative immobility of patients with severe arthritis but particularly in those receiving corticosteroids. Osteoporotic fractures are common and may occur at sites such as the pubic rami or ankle where they mimic exacerbations of the joint disease. Fractures of the long bones may develop with minimal trauma and are particularly common where there is a pre-existing angular deformity of the limb. A small proportion of patients may develop osteomalacia. However, its prevalence in patients with rheumatoid arthritis is probably no greater than in similarly handicapped, age-matched populations who also receive little exposure to direct sunlight and have diets poor in vitamin D.

The Felty syndrome

Lymphadenopathy is common in patients with rheumatoid arthritis, biopsies showing nodular hyperplasia. It is most obvious in patients with the Felty syndrome (rheumatoid arthritis, splenomegaly, and leucopenia). Other extra-articular features include anaemia, thrombocytopenia, persistent vasculitic leg ulceration, cutaneous pigmentation, weight loss, and recurrent infection. It is uncommon (less than 1 per cent of all cases) and rarely develops in patients who have had the disease for less than 10 years. It also seems to be particularly uncommon in certain ethnic groups, including Greeks and Chinese. This may reflect the weaker association of rheumatoid arthritis with the Dw4 antigen in these populations, as this marker is present in about 85 per cent of individuals with the Felty syndrome in the UK.

Susceptibility to recurrent infection is closely related to the absolute neutrophil count, which may be less than 100/mm^3. Antineutrophil antibodies may be detected in a proportion of cases, but the pathogenesis of the Felty syndrome is uncertain. Inadequate granulopoiesis, sequestration in the bone marrow, excessive margination of the circulating polymorphonuclear leucocytes, and destruction in the spleen have all been invoked. Splenectomy usually results in a temporary increase in the neutrophil count but does not provide reliable protection against recurrent infection. It is probably best reserved for those cases in which severe anaemia is due to hypersplenism. The potential role of recombinant granulocyte colony-stimulating factors remains to be evaluated.

Clinical course of the disease

The outcome of rheumatoid arthritis is unpredictable and observations in hospital populations are an unreliable guide to the clinical picture in the disease overall. Many patients with mild disease are never referred to hospital and may run a relatively benign, self-limiting course. Ten-year follow-up of patients admitted to hospital suggests that 25 per cent will remain fit for most activities, 40 per cent will exhibit moderate functional impairment, 25 per cent will be severely disabled, and 10 per cent will be wheelchair bound.

An adverse outcome is suggested by an insidious, progressive onset of the symptoms, pronounced extra-articular disease (including nodules), the early development of erosions and failure to respond adequately to anti-inflammatory analgesics. Relatively severe disease also correlates with the presence of high titres of circulating rheumatoid factor and the presence of the HLA-DR4 antigen (particularly DR4 homozygosity). Although it is standard practice to begin treatment at an early stage in patients with more aggressive joint disease, evidence that this approach really does have a major influence and modifying effect on the long-term degree of disability and handicap is equivocal.

Complications

Septic arthritis (see Chapter10.7) is a serious complication of rheumatoid arthritis, with a mortality rate of 25 per cent in some series. It is typically monoarticular but may be polyarticular in a quarter of cases. The expected clinical features (fever, rigors, neutrophil leucocytosis, and local inflammation of the joint) are frequently blunted or absent. Staphylococci account for three-quarters of all infections and may cause very rapid destruction of the articular surface if left untreated. In addition to systemic antibiotics, daily aspiration of the purulent synovial fluid at least is required. Open surgical drainage is sometimes necessary, particularly if the diagnosis has been delayed.

Rheumatoid arthritis is the commonest cause of AA amyloidosis in the UK. Its prevalence on rectal biopsy may be as high as 5 per cent, but rapidly progressive disease is very unusual. Suppression of disease activity with disease-modifying agents is probably as effective as the use of cytoxic agents, although chlorambucil may be helpful, particularly in juvenile rheumatoid arthritis and Still's disease.

Differential diagnosis

When present in its classical form the diagnosis of rheumatoid arthritis presents few problems. However, particularly during the early stages, it may be difficult to distinguish from other, sometimes self-limiting, inflammatory arthropathies. For this reason it is probably best to be guarded about the diagnosis if there is any significant doubt. This is particularly true when rheumatoid factor is absent.

Viral infections are commonly associated with transient arthralgias and sometimes more prolonged attacks of synovitis. Numerous types of bacterial infection may also be followed by reactive arthropathies, and serological tests may confirm recent infection. These syndromes can usually, but not invariably, be distinguished from rheumatoid arthritis by the history, but a strongly positive test for rheumatoid factor is undoubtedly the most useful discriminatory laboratory test. In practice it is rare for there to be much difficulty distinguishing the seronegative spondylarthropathies from rheumatoid arthritis, with the exception of psoriasis. This may be associated with an identical arthritis to seronegative rheumatoid arthritis and may sometimes develop before skin lesions (psoriatic arthritis without psoriasis), although there is usually a family history in such cases. Peripheral joint involvement in ankylosing spondylitis may be confusing, particularly in children, in whom it frequently antedates overt spinal disease. However, the asymmetrical pauciarticular lower limb distribution contrasts starkly with the polyarticular distribution typical of juvenile-onset rheumatoid arthritis.

Widespread synovitis commonly occurs in systemic lupus erythematosus but, although joint deformities may develop, bony erosion is very unusual. Rheumatoid factor is often present in low titre in addition to antinuclear antibodies, but evidence of renal disease, photosensitivity, mouth ulcer, pleuropericarditis, and the presence of anti-DNA antibodies should clarify the diagnosis.

About 10 per cent of patients with gout have polyarticular disease from the outset but this tends to have an asymmetrical distribution and predilection for the lower limbs, in particular the great toe. Negative tests for rheumatoid factor plus the demonstration of an elevated plasma urate level are suggestive, but the demonstration of urate crystals within the affected joints provides the definitive test. Gout may also preferentially affect joints involved by osteoarthritis itself, can usually be distinguished without too much difficulty. However, rheumatoid arthritis superimposed on osteoarthritis can be difficult unless there are raised titres of rheumatoid factor.

The several forms of juvenile chronic arthritis can usually be distinguished from juvenile-onset rheumatoid arthritis by the absence of rheumatoid factor and the distinctive pattern of joint involvement. Still's disease has a systemic onset with fever, neutrophilia, rash, lymphadenopathy, and hepatosplenomegaly. Rheumatoid factor is absent and the systemic features of the disease may pre-date the onset of joint symptoms by weeks or even months. It is uncommon in adults but may cause severe systemic upset requiring extensive investigation to exclude other connective tissue disorders, sepsis, or malignancy.

Management

Effective management of the patient with any but the mildest form of rheumatoid arthritis requires a multidisciplinary approach. Accurate diagnosis is essential for the early application of appropriate forms of therapy, the education of the patient in joint protection, and for counselling in adapting to disability and planning adequate social support.

In addition to standard pharmaceutical preparations, there are many other options for amelioration of symptoms, some orthodox and others not. Most patients seek relief from proprietary medicines and heterodox treatments such as copper bracelets, acupuncture, and various dietary regimens at some time in their illness. The value of many of these has undergone little rigorous testing but should not be discounted entirely.

The value of physical measures is well established. Acutely inflamed joints benefit from rest which may be accomplished either with bed-rest or splintage of the affected joints, depending on the clinical context. Local application of heat or cold to affected joints and gentle massage are also frequently effective, and can be combined with stretching exercises to prevent the development of deformities, consequent upon tendon and joint contractures. Regular exercise to strengthen muscles can help to stabilize damaged joints and should be initiated as early in the disease as practicable to prevent excessive muscle wasting. Many varieties of supporting splints are available to allow patients to continue to use joints that have been rendered painful or unstable by arthritis, and access to good orthoses may revolutionize the life of a patient, even with severe disease. In particular, careful attention to footwear with the provision of 'depth' shoes with soft uppers and adequately supporting insoles is important, both for immediate comfort and the prevention of future deformities.

Patients with more severe disabilities often benefit greatly from a careful assessment of the home environment, with advice on how to save labour and the provision of aids to give a mechanical advantage for specific tasks. Wheelchairs are often viewed negatively by patients and doctors alike but may greatly increase the range of activities and mobility open to the patient, thereby reducing the potential for social isolation.

Drug treatment

First-line drugs

These should include simple analgesics, such as paracetamol, codeine, and dextropropoxyphene. If these are effective, they should be used in preference to other non-steroidal anti-inflammatory drugs (NSAIDs) because of their relative safety. Many patients with mild or quiescent disease may require only intermittent analgesia.

A large number of NSAIDs are available with a broadly similar pattern of efficacy and side-effects, but there may be differences in response between individual patients. Many of the newer variants have prolonged half-lives which give a more sustained action, even allowing a single daily dosage regimen. Others may rely on sustained slow-delivery systems to achieve the same effect, despite the relatively short half-life of the drug being administered. It is logical to develop familiarity with a small selection of these drugs, including representatives from different chemical groups (Table 3). It is most appropriate to prescribe only one drug at a time and to use an adequate dose before abandoning it as ineffective. The use of nocturnal suppositories (indomethacin, diclofenac, naproxen) for the relief of morning stiffness is one particular exception to this general rule.

Table 3 Chemical groupings of the non-steroidal anti-inflammatory analgesics

Phenylacetic acids (propionic acids)	Ibuprofen, fenoprofen, ketoprofen, flurbiprofen
Indoleacetic acids	Indomethacin, sulindac
Heterocarboxylic acids	Aspirin, salicylsalicylic acid, diflunisal
Naphthalenenacetic acids	Naproxen
Oxicams	Piroxicam, tenoxicam
Pyrazolidinediones	Phenylbutazone, oxyphenbutaxone

Before embarking on long-term administration of these drugs it should be clear that there is a definite benefit to the patient, and the requirements for these drugs in the light of varying disease activity and symptoms should be critically reviewed periodically. The potential for serious adverse side-effects should not be underestimated. Gastrointestinal problems alone are very common, particularly as a result of superficial mucosal erosion, which may cause dyspepsia and haemorrhage. The relationship with chronic gastroduodenal ulceration is less clear-cut but it is important to remember that almost half of all patients admitted to hospital with acute gastrointestinal bleeding are taking NSAIDs.

Second-line drugs

These are believed to exert an influence on the underlying pathological processes involved in rheumatoid arthritis. In contrast to the first-line drugs, they may retard the progression of erosive joint damage, but their effects are not usually apparent until they have been taken for at least 2–3 months. Commonly used second-line drugs include gold salts, D-penicillamine, antimalarials (hydroxychloroquine), and sulphasalazine. They are most appropriately used in patients who have evidence of widespread synovitis with inadequate control of symptoms by first-line drugs. Patients with advanced secondary degenerative changes and mechanical deformity are unlikely to respond to this form of therapy. Highly active disease limited to one or two joints may be best managed in the first instance by local measures, such as intra-articular corticosteroid injection, splintage, or synovectomy (surgical or radiochemical).

The effectiveness of these second-line agents can be monitored not only by the demonstration of improvement in such clinical parameters as pain, morning stiffness, and grip strength, but also by a fall in the erythrocyte sedimentation rate, platelet count, level of rheumatoid factor, and acute-phase reactants. They should only be continued where a clear beneficial effect can be demonstrated after an adequately prolonged trial, because of the wide range of potential ill-effects. These include skin rashes, bone-marrow toxicity, and mouth ulcers (with gold, D-penicillamine, and sulphasalazine), nephrotic syndrome (gold and D-penicillamine), hepatitis (gold and sulphasalazine), and retinopathy (antimalarials). Accordingly, careful monitoring (e.g. urinalysis, full blood count, and liver function) for side-effects is essential when these drugs are prescribed. After 1 year, about two-thirds of patients started on second-line drugs will be doing well, while the remainder will have stopped the drugs because of side-effects or lack of efficacy.

Third-line drugs

These include azathioprine, cyclophosphamide, chlorambucil, and methotrexate, all of which can modify the course of rheumatoid arthritis. Low-dose methotrexate (7.5–15 mg weekly), in particular, has found a firm place in treatment, and in many centres is used frequently as a second-line agent. In low dose it does not have the hepatotoxicity otherwise associated with its use; bone-marrow suppression is uncommon, but occasionally severe episodes of pneumonitis occur.

Corticosteroids are highly potent inhibitors of the inflammatory response that can have dramatic effects on the synovitis of rheumatoid arthritis. Unfortunately, the plethora of unwanted side-effects strictly limits their usefulness. Nevertheless, about a quarter of hospital outpatients ultimately receive corticosteroids, usually in doses less than 10 mg daily, and such an approach may be highly effective in keeping patients mobile and independent when other drugs have failed.

A number of forms of experimental therapy have proved of some benefit in the treatment of rheumatoid arthritis, although their use is restricted to a few centres. These include total lymphoid irradiation, thoracic duct drainage, anti-CD4 monoclonal antibodies, and antibodies directed against the lymphocyte cell-surface determinant, Cdw52.

Surgery

Many aspects of the disease are amenable to surgical correction, and access to good orthopaedic services is critical to its management. The main indications for surgical intervention are to relieve pain, to correct deformity, to reduce instability, and to increase the effective range of movement and function.

Soft-tissue procedures

These include the repair of ruptured tendons, tendon transfers, decompression (carpal tunnel), or transfer of nerves (ulnar nerve at the elbow).

Synovectomy

This can be a useful procedure in joints with persistent active synovitis, particularly when the damage to the articular surface is relatively mild. It is also frequently performed in conjunction with excision arthroplasties (proximal radial head, lower end of ulna, forefoot arthroplasty).

Arthrodesis

This still plays a useful part in the surgical management of arthritis despite the loss of movement that it necessarily produces. It is particularly useful for the painful wrist or finger, and can correct pain and instability in the ankle and thumb. Fusion of the cervical spine may be essential to prevent catastrophic neurological damage to the cervical spinal cord.

Joint replacement arthroplasty

This has revolutionized the treatment of patients with severe arthritis of the large, weight-bearing lower limb joints. Total hip replacement is successful in 95 per cent of individuals, although ultimately revision due to loosening of the prosthesis and pain may be necessary. For this reason it is wise to consider using an uncemented prosthesis in individuals under the age of 60. Thromboembolism in the post-operative phase is rare in patients with rheumatoid arthritis compared with those with osteoarthritis. Sepsis occurs occasionally and can be a disastrous complication which may require removal of the prosthesis. The introduction of partially constrained total condylar prostheses for the knee has increased the success from replacement of this joint to rates similar to those of the hip, although postoperative mobilization and recovery tends to be a little slower.

Replacement of other joints such as the elbow and shoulder may be highly successful in many patients but is less predictable. It should therefore be reserved for individuals with severe pain and limitation of movement. Prosthetic replacement of the wrist and ankle is not yet satisfactory and pain relief is better achieved in most cases by arthrodesis.

Further reading

Li, E., Brooks, P., and Conaghan, P.G. (1998). Disease-modifying anti-rheumatic drugs. *Current Opinion in Rheumatology*, 10, 159–68.

Scott, D.L., Shipley, M., Dawson, A., *et al.* (1998). The clinical management of rheumatoid arthritis and osteoarthritis: strategies for improving clinical effectiveness. *British Journal of Rheumatology*, 37, 543–4.

Sewell, KL. (1998). Rheumatoid arthritis in older adults. *Clinics in Geriatric Medicine*, 14, 475–94.

Verhoeven, A.C., Boers, M., and Tugwell, P. (1998). Combination therapy in rheumatoid arthritis: updated systematic review. *British Journal of Rheumatology*, 37, 612–19.

Chapter 10.3

Seronegative spondylarthropathies

C. J. Eastmond

Introduction

The concept of seronegative spondylarthritis as an inclusive group of diseases is based upon:

- inflammatory arthritis with a negative IgM rheumatoid factor
- common clinical features
- increased prevalence of radiological sacroiliitis
- familial aggregation
- association with HLA–B27

The diseases included and their HLA-B27 frequencies are shown in Table 1.

Ankylosing spondylitis

Definition and diagnostic criteria

Criteria for the diagnosis of ankylosing spondylitis have been established, but they are more applicable to epidemiological studies than to the clinical diagnosis of an individual case. Diagnosis is usually made on the basis of inflammatory back pain with radiological evidence of sacroiliitis in the absence of evidence of microbial infection. Inflammatory back pain is commonly of insidious onset, with persistent low back or buttock pain for more than 3 months, together with early morning stiffness and improvement with exercise. In most cases symptoms arise before the age of 40 years.

Table 1 Diseases included in seronegative spondylarthropathies and their respective HLA-B27 frequencies

	HLA-B27 +ve(%)
Ankylosing spondylitis	80–96
Psoriatic arthritis	4.5–27
with sacroiliitis	9–77
Reactive arthritis	80–90
Reiter's syndrome	65–96
Enteropathic synovitis	
Ulcerative colitis	C
Crohn's disease	C
Intestinal bypass	C
Chronic inflammatory bowel disease with ankylosing spondylitis	28–72
Uveitis	56
Whipple's disease	30
Behçet's syndrome	C
Undifferentiated	?

C, Control population frequency.

Prevalence

Racial variation in the prevalence of ankylosing spondylitis closely matches that of HLA-B27. In white European and North American populations the prevalence lies between 1 in 250 and 1 in 100 males, but is less frequent in females, male/female ratio about 5:1.

Aetiology and pathogenesis

Approximately 90 per cent of Caucasians with ankylosing spondylitis are HLA-B27 positive, contrasting with a general population frequency of about 8 per cent. It is possible that HLA-B27 is not itself important in the pathogenesis of the disease, but no evidence has been produced to support the alternative proposition that a linked gene is responsible. The association with HLA-B27 has given rise to a number of ideas regarding pathogenesis, although all at present remain hypotheses. The main suggestions are centred around molecular mimicry, receptor theories, and abnormal host defence mechanisms.

Molecular mimicry theories emphasize shared amino acid residues between HLA-B27 and *Klebsiella* species or other organisms, perhaps resulting in:

1. this shared molecular structure leading to an impaired immune response and hence to disease;
2. the shared structure leading to the production of antibodies directed against self, resulting in disease; or
3. proteins encoded by the pathogen resulting in antibody formation against self structures in joints and entheses.

In the third model, HLA-B27 is required to bind peptide from the pathogen or self and present this to the immunocompetent cell with resultant disease.

In the original receptor theory, HLA-B27 was proposed as a receptor for *Klebsiella* and other bacterial cell products. An alternative possibility is that bacterial plasmids may transfect HLA-B27 positive cells to express new determinants specific for ankylosing spondylitis, resulting in HLA-B27 being a specific receptor rather than non-specific as in the original theory. Finally, there may be abnormal host

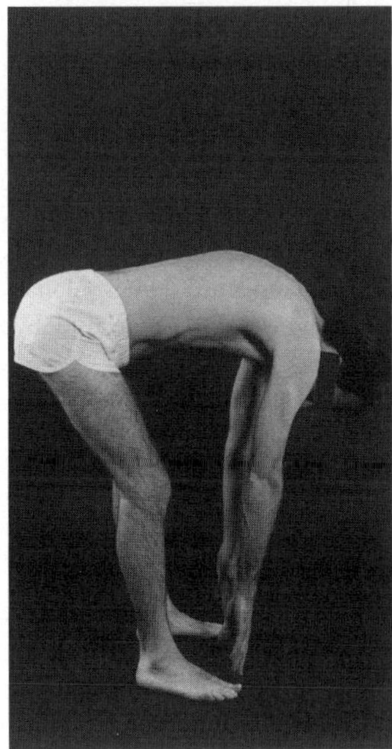

Fig. 1 Limitation of spinal forward flexion. Note the flat lumbar spine.

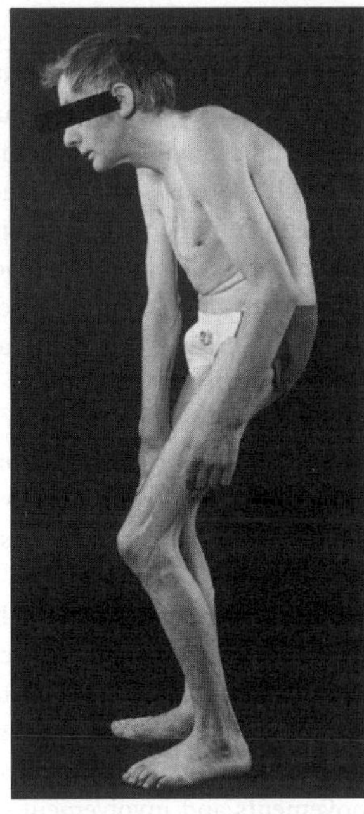

Fig. 2 Advanced ankylosing spondylitis with marked thoracic kyphosis and flexion deformity of the hip.

defence mechanisms related to the presence of HLA-B27 (or products of closely linked genes) which in a more generalized way lead to a defective immune response.

Clinical features

The initial symptoms predominantly affect people under the age of 40 with a strong male predominance, and classically comprise pain and stiffness in the low back, buttocks, and the back of the upper thighs, more marked in the mornings, eased by moderate exercise and activity, tending to recur with rest or inactivity. Some patients experience disturbance of sleep because of these symptoms and many find lying in bed after waking uncomfortable. Radiation of the pain into the thighs is classically bilateral but may be unilateral and can mimic sciatica; it rarely goes much below the knee and virtually never into the foot. There are no associated paraesthesiae. Cough impulse pain may be present. Initially limitation of spinal movement may not be evident, particularly in mild cases; but once it begins it involves movements in all planes, to include lateral flexion as well as forward flexion and extension. There is frequently a flattening of the lumbar lordosis or an inability to reverse this on forward flexion (Fig. 1). Scoliosis may or may not be present but is not usually a marked feature. With more advanced disease a thoracic kyphosis develops, with concomitant restriction or thoracic rotation and chest expansion due to involvement of the costovertebral and costotransverse joints. In advanced and severe cases movements of the cervical spine are also restricted in all planes, usually with dramatic limitation of lateral flexion. The combination of a thoracic kyphosis and cervical stiffness may lead to difficulties with forward vision or marked hyperextension of the cervical spine (Fig. 2).

There is peripheral joint involvement in some 30–40 per cent of patients during the course of disease and this is a presenting feature in 10–20 per cent of patients. This type of onset is more common in younger patients, particularly teenagers. Initial diagnosis is difficult if back symptoms are absent. The joints most commonly involved are those of the lower limb, particularly the knees and ankles. There may be dactylitis of the toes and involvement of the hip. In the upper limb the shoulders and wrists are most commonly involved with comparative sparing of the small joints of the hands. The temporomandibular joints may be affected, as may the sternoclavicular and manubriosternal joints. Joint involvement is usually oligoarticular and asymmetrical. The junctional areas between ligament or tendon and bone (entheses) are characteristically involved, particularly at the heel at the insertions of the plantar fascia and the Achilles tendon to the calcaneum. This enthesopathy is associated with pain, tenderness, and sometimes swelling. Other sites include the iliac crests, ischial tuberosities, and greater trochanters. It tends to be an early feature of the disease but may occur at any time and is often associated with other peripheral joint involvement.

Acute anterior uveitis occurs at any time in the course of the disease and is seen in up to 20 per cent of patients. Recurrent attacks are common, occurring in 60 per cent of affected patients. Either eye may be affected in separate episodes but simultaneous bilateral involvement is uncommon.

Limitation of chest expansion results in a restrictive pulmonary defect, partially compensated for by diaphragmatic movement. It is often associated with a rather flat-looking chest and a pot-belly. Approximately 1 per cent of patients with advanced disease will develop apical pulmonary fibrosis and cavitation radiologically similar to the appearance of tuberculosis. Superinfection with *Aspergillus* may occur.

Aortic regurgitation secondary to aortitis has been found in approximately 1 per cent of patients, usually in those with advanced severe disease. Atrioventricular block is also a recognized association. There is a definite but weak association with IgA nephropathy.

A cauda equina syndrome may complicate advanced disease with resultant disturbance or bladder and bowel function. In most cases myelographic examination reveals lumbar diverticulae.

Some patients have associated psoriasis or chronic inflammatory bowel disease. Ileocolonoscopy studies have recently revealed ileal ulceration in a high proportion of patients with ankylosing spondylitis and other seronegative spondylarthritides. The significance of this finding has yet to be fully determined.

Laboratory and radiological features

The radiological hallmark of ankylosing spondylitis is sclerosis and erosion of both sides of both sacroiliac joints over an extensive segment, most marked in the lower half (Fig. 3). When these changes are combined with classical clinical features the diagnosis is straightforward. Lesser degrees of radiological abnormality of the sacroiliac joints are more difficult to interpret, and in early and mild disease there may be no radiological abnormality for several years, making early diagnosis difficult.

In established disease, bony bridging (syndesmophytes) occurs between the vertebrae (Fig. 4), usually first observed in the upper lumbar spine and increasing with progression of the disease. Preceding or coinciding with syndesmophyte formation, squaring of the lumbar vertebrae is often observed in lateral radiographs, with loss of the normal anterior concavity. This may be preceded by an eroded sclerotic (Romanus) lesion at the upper or lower border of the vertebrae best seen on lateral films. In advanced cases syndesmophyte formation will extend throughout the spine. Ligamentous calcification may occur, resulting in linear calcification joining the posterior spinus

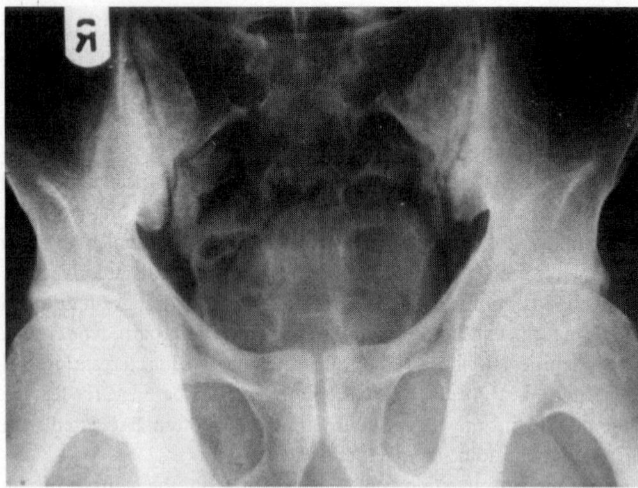

Fig. 3 Radiological sacroiliitis. Note the sclerosis and erosions on both the ilial and sacral sides of the joint.

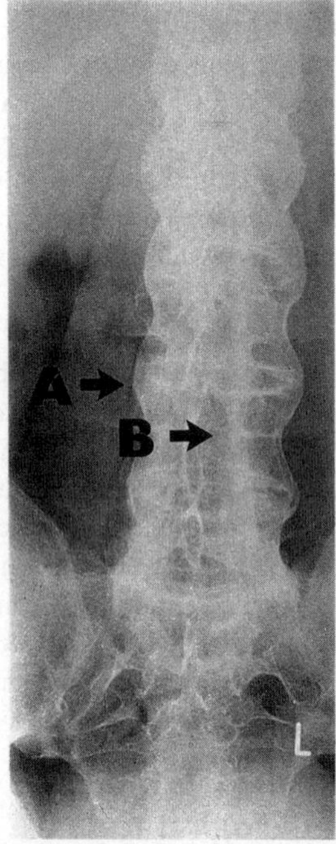

Fig. 4 (a) Lumbar spinal syndesmophytes and (b) linear posterior ligamentous calcification, in ankylosing spondylitis.

processes and laminae, best seen in the anteroposterior radiograph (Fig. 4).

The erythrocyte sedimentation rate (ESR) and C-reactive protein are raised in only 25–30 per cent of patients. Less commonly there may be raised plasma concentrations of immunoglobulins, particularly IgA. Mild degrees of normochromic normocytic anaemia are common but are not usually as profound as in rheumatoid arthritis. Abnormalities of the liver function tests, particularly the alkaline phosphatase and γ-glutamyl transferase, are also well recognized but are not usually severe.

Treatment

There is no cure for ankylosing spondylitis. Control of symptoms can usually be achieved by the use of one of the non-steroidal anti-inflammatory drugs combined with a daily programme of mobilizing, postural, and chest expansion exercises. These may help to limit the degree of subsequent spinal stiffness and deformity. Intra-articular depot corticosteroids can be useful for short-term improvement of peripheral synovitis. Slow-acting antirheumatic drugs are ineffective, although there is some evidence to suggest that sulphasalazine may be useful in patients responding inadequately to non-steroidal anti-inflammatory drugs. The response is probably better for peripheral arthropathy than for spinal disease. The recommended dose is sulphasalazine 1–1.5 g twice daily, and the response will be delayed by 2–4 months from initiation of therapy.

Regular daily exercises may need to be supplemented by specific physiotherapy for exacerbations or when there is increased spinal stiffness. Regular swimming is recommended as additional exercise. Contact sports are usually best avoided, particularly for those with more advanced disease.

Braces and corsets should be avoided. They do not limit spinal deformity nor reverse it. For severe kyphosis, lumbar osteotomy may be valuable in some cases. Osteotomy at higher levels is particularly hazardous and requires assessment by a surgeon fully familiar with the procedure and its complications. Combined restriction of spinal movements and involvement of hips is particularly disabling. When hip involvement is painful, a good out-come can be anticipated from hip joint replacement. Persistent peripheral arthropathy involving single joints, such as a knee joint, may require synovectomy if painful and disabling.

Prognosis

The few long-term follow-up studies performed have indicated that the majority of patients do well, with about 90 per cent either fully independent or minimally disabled. This is despite some 40 per cent of patients having severe spinal restriction. Early onset of peripheral arthritis or the presence of iritis is associated with more severe spinal restriction.

The longer-term prognosis can probably be determined after about 10 years of disease. Seventy-four per cent of those with mild restriction at 10 years do not progress further, and 80 per cent of those found to have severe spinal restriction after prolonged follow-up had marked spinal restriction after 10 years' duration. Those who do not develop hip involvement within the first 10 years appear to retain normal hips thereafter.

Long-term follow-up of manual workers with ankylosing spondylitis indicates that one-third are unable to continue working after 25 years. Of those still in employment, at least half are doing the same job, whereas a slightly smaller proportion have had to change to lighter work. For those with less physically demanding jobs a higher proportion are able to remain in work.

A third to a half of deaths are due to cardiovascular causes. There is a 2.5–4 to threefold excess mortality due to respiratory causes. Radiotherapy is not currently used as a form of treatment, but studies of those who have previously received it demonstrate an overall two-thirds excess mortality, with a fivefold increase in death due to leukaemia and a 60 per cent excess of death due to carcinoma in the irradiated sites. The mortality is highest among those who have received radiotherapy late in the course of the disease.

The effect of pregnancy is less predictable than in rheumatoid arthritis, with the disease being unaffected in over one-half of patients, a quarter being worse, and a fifth improving during pregnancy. Slightly less than a half of patients suffer a mild postpartum flare. There is no evidence that pregnancy affects the overall course of the

Table 2 Categories and characteristic features of psoriatic arthritis

Categories	Characteristic features
Distal interphalangeal (predominantly but not exclusively)	Asymmetry
Asymmetrical	Dactylitis
Symmetrical	Distal interphalangeal joints
Mutilans	Oligoarticular
Spinal	Radiological/clinical sacroiliitis

disease, or that the disease itself affects the course of pregnancy or the fetus.

Psoriatic arthritis

Psoriatic arthritis is characterized by a peripheral inflammatory polyarthritis associated with the presence of psoriasis and the absence of IgM rheumatoid factor. Psoriatic nail dystrophy is strongly associated and radiological sacroiliitis may be present.

Prevalence

Psoriasis affects about 1.6 per cent of the general population and seronegative arthritis occurs in some 6.8 per cent of these patients. These figures form part of the case for psoriatic arthritis being a distinct entity. No formal epidemiological studies have been conducted but its prevalence is estimated to be 0.1 per cent.

Clinical features

Psoriatic arthritis has been divided into five subgroups (Table 2). Their relative frequency tends to vary between series and may reflect different methods of ascertainment.

In addition, patients may develop overlap between these subgroups during follow-up. It is probably more useful to identify those characteristics which distinguish psoriatic arthritis as a separate clinical entity from rheumatoid arthritis (Table 2 and Fig. 5). Additionally, many patients have relatively self-limiting episodes rather than persistent destructive synovitis, although the latter does occur.

There is a poor correlation between the presence or severity of arthritis and the severity and extent of psoriasis; or between the activity and time of onset of arthritis and psoriasis. There is a closer relationship between the onset of the nail dystrophy and the arthritis. In addition, nail dystrophy occurs in 85 per cent of patients with psoriatic arthritis, contrasting with only 20 per cent of patients with uncomplicated psoriasis. Nail dystrophy occurs more commonly in those patients with distal interphalangeal joint involvement than other patterns of joint disease. Several patients demonstrate a close association between involvement of individual finger distal interphalangeal joints and the corresponding nail. Features of nail dystrophy which are particularly helpful in diagnosis are onycholysis in the absence of infection or trauma and large numbers of nail pits. Horizontal ridging may also be helpful diagnostically, but usually only when associated with one of the other two features. Longitudinal ridging of the nail is not a specific associated feature.

Occular inflammation has been documented in 30 per cent of patients with psoriatic arthritis. Acute anterior uveitis is particularly prevalent in patients with radiological sacroiliitis (15 per cent) and those with ankylosing spondylitis (18 per cent). It does, however, occur in 6 per cent of patients with only peripheral arthritis. Non-suppurative conjunctivitis has been documented in 10–20 per cent of patients. Episcleritis and keratoconjunctivitis sicca are seen occasionally.

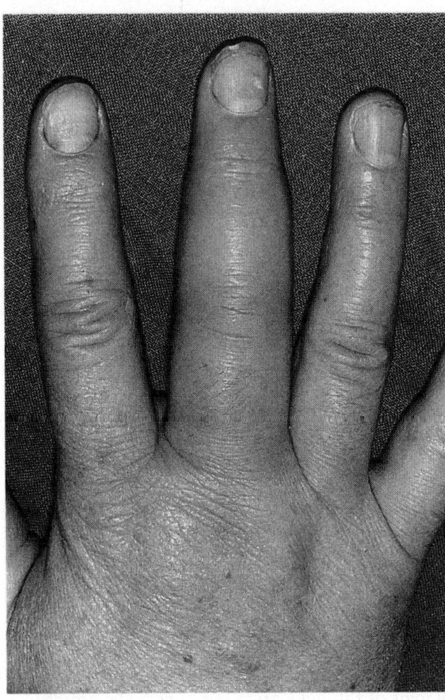

Fig. 5 Dactylitis of the finer in psoriatic arthritis. Note the uniform swelling of the whole digit.

The differential diagnoses can include any other form of arthritis. Some patients have an acute onset involving only one joint, in which case, sepsis and crystal arthritis must be excluded by appropriate synovial fluid examination. The symmetrical form of psoriatic arthritis needs to be distinguished from rheumatoid arthritis on the basis of the presence or absence of other extra-articular features more characteristic of rheumatoid arthritis, in addition to the presence or absence of IgM rheumatoid factor.

Laboratory and radiological features

In common with other inflammatory arthropathies, the acute-phase reactants (such as ESR and C-reactive protein) are often raised. This may not occur if only one or two small joints are involved. Anaemia is not as common or marked as in rheumatoid arthritis. By definition, IgM rheumatoid factor is absent. There may be mild elevations of the alkaline phosphatase and γ-glutamyl transferase, particularly in patients with widespread and active disease.

The distribution of radiological changes on the whole reflects the clinical distribution, characteristically involving the distal interphalangeal joint of the fingers with asymmetrical involvement of these and other joints. The small joints of the hands and feet will generally show radiological changes before the larger joints. Periarticular osteoporosis is less severe than in rheumatoid arthritis. Erosion, joint-space narrowing, and, later, sclerosis occur. There may be periosteal elevation along the shafts of the phalanges. A characteristic pencil-in-cup deformity may occur with resorption of the distal end of the next distal phalanx (Fig. 6). When widespread, these changes conform to the classical arthritis mutilans. Rarely, the severity of bone resorption may be such that individual finger or toe

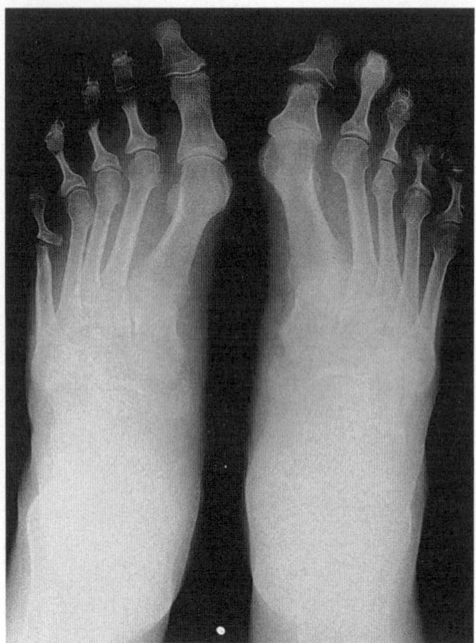

Fig. 6 Radiological appearances of the pencil-in-cup changes at the interphalangeal joint of the right great toe in psoriatic arthritis.

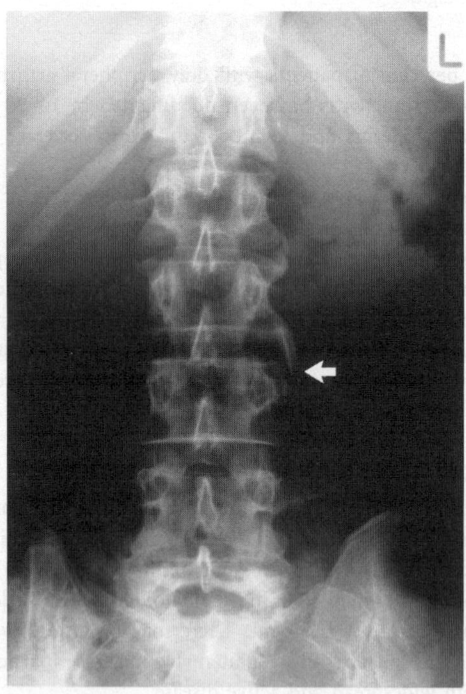

Fig. 7 Coarse syndesmophyte in psoriatic spondylitis.

phalanges seem to disappear. This would be clinically evident as a telescoping digit.

Sacroiliitis demonstrable by radiology occurs in 20–30 per cent of patients. Spinal changes with bony bridging (syndesmophytes) occurs in a lesser proportion of patients and also in those who have predominant spinal disease. Characteristically, the syndesmophytes are more coarse than in classical ankylosing spondylitis and they may be asymmetrical. Coarse syndesmophyte formation has been described in the absence of sacroiliitis (Fig. 7).

Treatment

The majority of patients improve with the use of non-steroidal anti-inflammatory drugs given together with judicious use of intra-articular depot corticosteroid. The latter is most useful when only one or two larger joints are involved or there is localized flexor tenosynovitis in the hand.

In patients with more persistent or active disease not adequately responding to these measures, the use of selected slow-acting drugs is appropriate. The antimalarials should be avoided as they may exacerbate psoriasis. There is little or no evidence to suggest that penicillamine has any useful effects, but intramuscular gold can be helpful without any increased risk of mucocutaneous toxicity. Sulphasalazine is efficacious in some patients. In addition, cytotoxic agents such as methotrexate and azathioprine can be used with benefit, and may additionally improve psoriasis itself. Cyclosporin has recently been reported to be beneficial.

Systemic corticosteroids are not used routinely as psoriasis may flare when they are withdrawn; they may, however, need to be used occasionally for persistently active disease which has not responded to other treatment.

Local treatment of the skin has no effect on the arthropathy. There is no conclusive evidence that PUVA therapy (psoralen with ultraviolet light) or etretinate have any predictable benefit on the arthropathy, although occasional patients have been found to improve coincident with these treatments.

Bedrest for short periods during episodes of active synovitis is appropriate, but joints should be mobilized early to reduce the risk of fibrous ankylosis and improve muscle tone and power. If there is spinal involvement, it is essential for patients to also carry out a similar programme of exercises to that used in ankylosing spondylitis.

Prognosis

There have been few long-term follow-up studies of this disease. In general, the prognosis is better than in rheumatoid arthritis. One 8-year follow-up found 60 per cent of those with psoriatic arthritis in work, compared with only 36 per cent of those with rheumatoid arthritis; 23 per cent of the psoriatic arthritics were disabled, compared with 43 per cent of rheumatoid arthritics. In a further study, 11 per cent of psoriatic arthritics were severely or very severely disabled. Psoriatic arthritis improves during pregnancy in the majority of patients. There is no adverse effect on the course of the pregnancy or on the fetus.

Reactive arthritis

Definition

The arthropathy of reactive arthritis is of a similar pattern to that seen in Reiter's syndrome, and it is sensible to consider these two disorders together. They both represent a sterile synovitis associated with recent infection at a distant site. There may or may not be extra-articular features. The features defining Reiter's syndrome are the presence of synovitis, urethritis, and conjunctivitis, occurring within a short time of each other.

Prevalence

Epidemiological studies of gastroenterological causes of reactive arthritis and Reiter's syndrome have shown that 1–2 per cent of a population exposed to a specific trigger infection may develop articular

Table 3 Reactive arthritis and Reiter's syndrome

Common precipitating features	Characteristic features of the arthropathy	Characteristic extra-articular features
Chlamydia *Salmonella* spp. (not *S. typhi* or *S. paratyphi*) *Campylobacter jejuni* *Shigella flexneri* *Yersinia* spp.	Oligoarticular Asymmetrical Dactylitis Enthesitis (especially heels) Low back/buttock pain (inflammatory sacroiliitis)	Conjunctivitis[a] Urethritis[a] Circinate balanitis Oral ulceration Acute anterior uveitis Keratoderma blennorrhagicum Dystrophic nails Fever

[a] Features defining Reiter's syndrome.

disease. Similar studies of patients with non-specific urethritis suggest a similar frequency for articular disease in this group.

Aetiology and pathogenesis

The infective causes of reactive arthritis and Reiter's syndrome can be divided into those of gastrointestinal or of urogenital origin (Table 3). The delay between symptoms of the initial gastrointestinal infection and arthropathy may vary from 3 to 30 days. The serum IgA levels are increased during active disease and antigen-specific IgA levels are increased for longer in those who develop arthropathy compared with those who do not. Bacterial cell wall fragments have been demonstrated within synovial fluid and membrane in the arthropathy associated with *Chlamydia*, *Salmonella*, and *Yersinia*. Whether these fragments are present in a free form or as immune complexes is not currently determined, although the latter seems likely.

There is enhanced synovial fluid T-cell responsiveness to causative bacterial antigens, suggesting a specific intra-articular immune response. However, synovial fluid lymphocytes are predominantly CD4 rather than CD8 cells. The latter would normally be expected to be the responding T-cell subset in relation to class I antigens such as HLA-B27, which is strongly associated with reactive arthritis and Reiter's syndrome. As with ankylosing spondylitis, the precise role of HLA-B27 remains undetermined, nor is it clear whether or not the mechanism in these two diseases is similar.

Clinical features

Certain characteristics (Table 3) are common to both reactive arthritis and Reiter's syndrome. In the latter, urethritis normally pre-dates other features. Conjunctivitis is either simultaneous with urethritis or follows very quickly thereafter, with arthropathy the third feature to develop, although this is not always the sequence. In sexually acquired Reiter's syndrome the urethritis is due to *Chlamydia* in 60 per cent of patients. Urethritis following gastrointestinal infection is sterile. Conjunctivitis is usually sterile, although secondary infection may occur. Some patients with so-called 'incomplete Reiter's' do not demonstrate all features of this classical triad. It may therefore be preferable to use the term reactive arthritis to encompass all patients and qualify this according to the presence of individual extra-articular features. Other extra-articular features are shown in Table 3. Oral ulceration may be due to multiple aphthae or a superficial erosive ulceration (Fig. 8) somewhat similar in appearance to balanitis (Fig. 9).

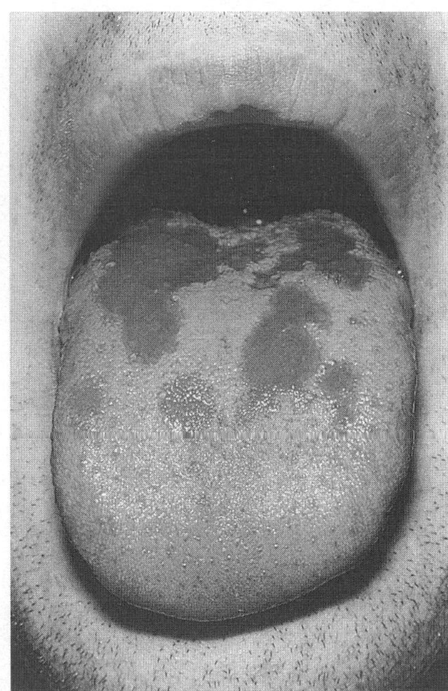

Fig. 8 Ulceration of the tongue in Reiter's syndrome.

This form of oral ulceration is usually symptomless as is balanitis. Symptoms alone may not differentiate between severe conjunctivitis and mild acute anterior uveitis. The latter occurs during the acute episode in some 10 per cent of patients and requires expert ophthalmic assessment and treatment. Acute anterior uveitis may also pre-date or succeed by several years an episode of Reiter's syndrome. Keratoderma blennorrhagicum (Fig. 10) affects less than 10 per cent of patients. It is usually seen in patients who are systemically unwell and is rare in patients without the full triad of Reiter's syndrome; it is most common in the soles of the feet, but may also affect the palms. In severe cases it may extend to other areas of the skin. Nail dystrophy is usually more florid, often with onycholysis and hyperkeratosis, than that occurring in psoriasis. Fever may be present on its own or in association with other extra-articular features. Its presence requires the exclusion of coincidental infection, both systemic and articular.

Investigations

During the active phase the ESR and acute phase reactants are raised. There may be anaemia broadly reflecting the overall severity and degree of systemic illness. Abnormalities of liver function tests, particularly alkaline phosphatase and γ-glutamyl transferase, are not uncommon in active disease.

By the time arthropathy has developed there is often no continuing bacteriological evidence of active infection. This should, however, be sought by appropriate urethral and stool cultures. If sexually acquired disease is suspected, it is important to seek evidence for coincidental gonorrhoea and syphilis. In some circumstances it will be necessary to test for human immunodeficiency virus (HIV) infection.

Serum agglutinin tests are available for the currently known causes. They are not entirely reliable but may be an adjunct to diagnosis when titres are high, rise over the first 2 weeks, or fall over the succeeding months.

During the acute phase it is uncommon to find any radiological abnormality of the joints. In the small number of patients who have persisting disease, radiological erosions may occur, particularly in the

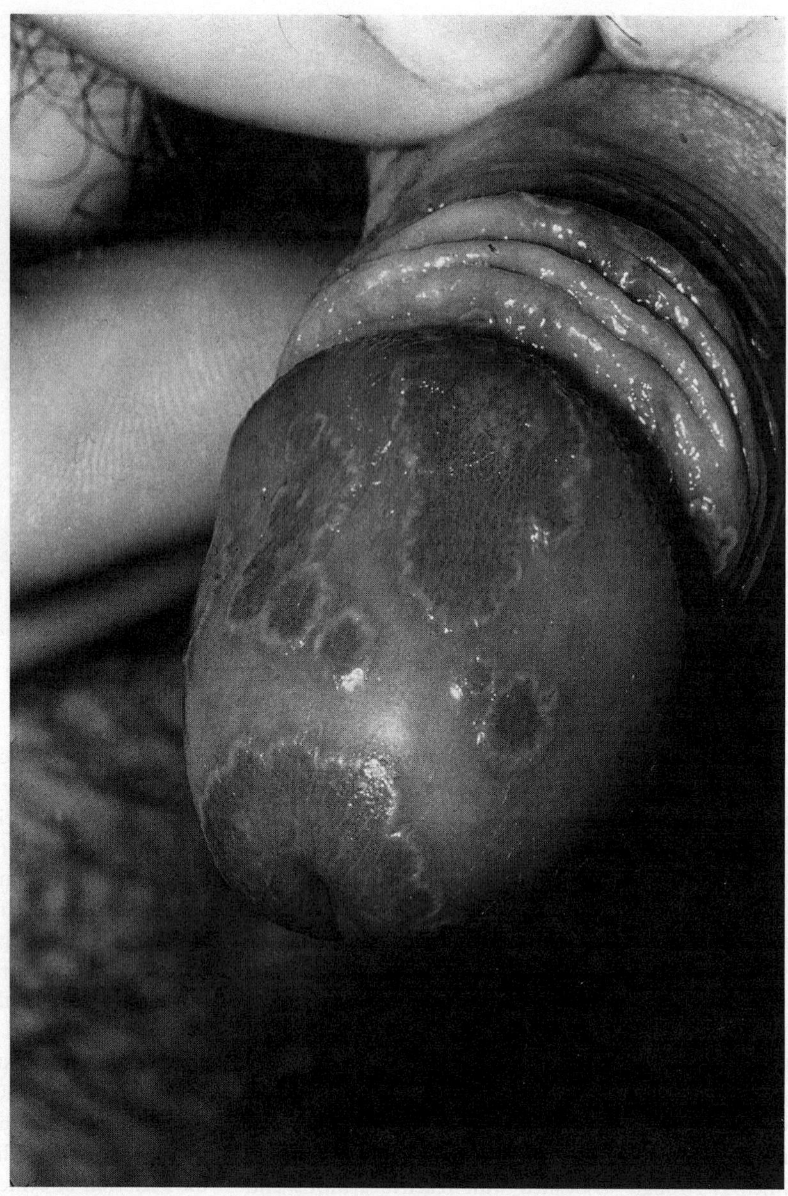

Fig. 9 Circinate balanitis in Reiter's syndrome.

metatarsophalangeal joints and around the heel entheses (Fig. 11). Some patients develop radiological sacroiliitis, and a small proportion of these may acquire spinal disease. The syndesmophytes are then often coarse and asymmetrical, resembling those of psoriatic spondylitis rather than those of classical ankylosing spondylitis.

Treatment

The joints should be rested during the acute phase. Effusions in the larger joints should be aspirated. Non-steroidal anti-inflammatory drugs help to reduce pain and stiffness. If effusions are recurrent, intra-articular depot corticosteroids can be useful if intra-articular infection has been excluded.

Secondarily infected conjunctivitis requires local antibiotic treatment; otherwise hypromellose may be used to reduce symptoms. The help of an ophthalmologist is required if acute anterior uveitis is present or suspected.

There is no current evidence that treatment of gastrointestinal infection or infective urethritis alters the course of the arthropathy, although active urethritis, gonorrhoea, or syphilis require treatment in their own right. Local hygiene is required for balanitis, and, if it is, severe, 1 per cent hydrocortisone ointment can be applied with benefit.

Oral ulceration usually responds to antiseptic and local anaesthetic mouth washes; local corticosteroid preparations may be needed if pain is persistent. Any coincidental fungal infection should be treated.

It is important during the acute phase to maintain muscle tone and power with isometric exercises and, as soon as the active inflammatory joint disease improves, to mobilize the joints. Spinal exercises similar to those used in ankylosing spondylitis can be useful in patients with symptomatic sacroiliitis.

A small proportion of patients develop chronic inflammatory joint disease; for them sulphasalazine 2–3 g daily may be helpful, but benefit may be delayed for 2–4 months. Azathioprine and methotrexate have also been used with benefit, but it is important to ensure that there is no coincident HIV infection before considering these, in view of their adverse effects on the course and prognosis of HIV-associated disease.

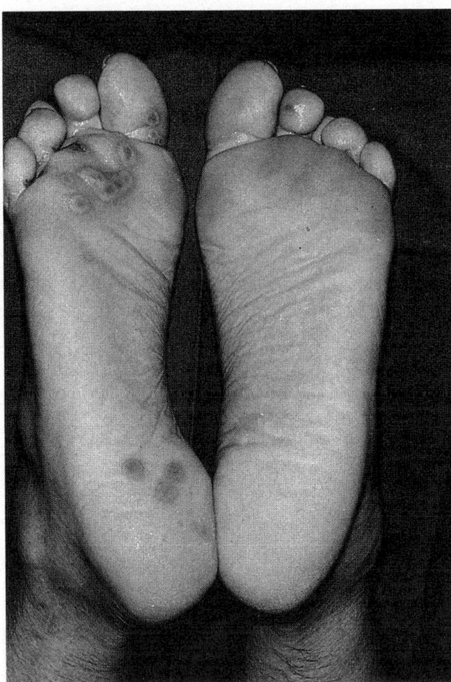

Fig. 10 Keratoderma blennorrhagicum in Reiter's syndrome

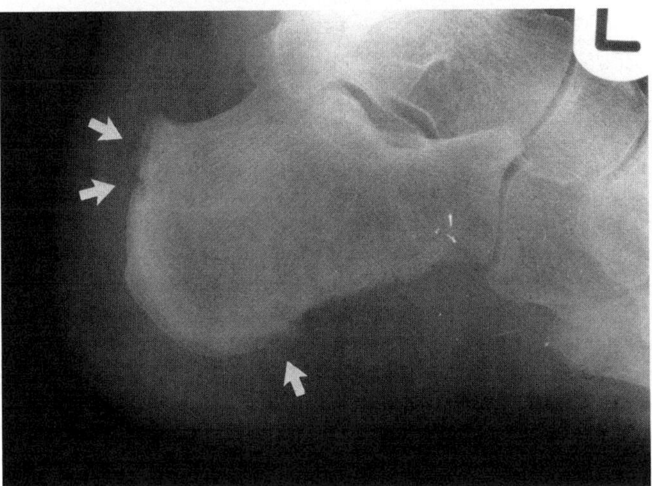

Fig. 11 Erosion at the insertions (entheses) of the Achilles tendon and plantar fascia in Reiter's syndrome.

Prognosis

Some patients have a short, acute illness lasting only a few weeks, rarely leading to any residual disability. More commonly, the active phase of inflammatory joint disease lasts between 3 and 6 months. With resolution of the clinical features, the laboratory features also return to normal. Some such patients may continue to have arthralgia, rarely sufficient to warrant the use of anti-inflammatory agents. Active arthritis can extend to beyond 6 months in a few patients, who are then at risk of developing erosive disease. Classical psoriatic arthritis may also develop in some patients whose initial manifestations include severe systemic Reiter's syndrome and keratoderma blennorrhagicum. The prognosis in this situation is usually poor, and slow-acting or immunosuppressive drugs are commonly required. Recurrences after full recovery do occur, and as it is not always possible to identify an infecting organism at the time, it is difficult to determine whether there has been reactivation of previous disease or reinfection with an unidentified organism. There is evidence that Reiter's syndrome may be especially severe and associated with more severe extra-articular features in those who have coincident HIV infection and acquired immune deficiency syndrome.

Enteropathic synovitis

Aetiology and pathogenesis

Enteropathic synovitis, a sterile synovitis, occurs in 10 per cent of patients with ulcerative colitis and in 10–20 per cent of patients with Crohn's disease. It has also been found in 8–30 per cent of those treated by intestinal bypass surgery for morbid obesity. The mechanism is unknown, but may be related to increased permeability of the inflamed intestinal mucosa to intraluminal antigens. Experimental models of intestinal bypass arthropathy have demonstrated IgA immune complexes associated with blind loops, and complexes of IgA and secretory IgA have been found in individuals with bypass arthropathy.

Clinical features

Chronic inflammatory bowel disease

The arthropathy has a predeliction for lower limb joints, particularly knees and ankles but upper limb joints can also be involved. Dactylitis of the toes is characteristic. Classically, the arthropathy relapses and remits in association with exacerbations and remissions of bowel disease. Joint destruction does not occur. Exceptionally, Crohn's granulomas have been observed in synovial membranes leading to a persistent arthropathy and joint destruction.

The arthropathy is frequently associated with other complications, in particular uveitis, episcleritis, and conjunctivitis, erythema nodosum, pyoderma grangrenosum, and oral ulceration (especially in Crohn's disease), and clubbing of the fingers.

Sacroiliitis and ankylosing spondylitis

This also occur with an increased frequency in patients with inflammatory bowel disease and in their relatives. These cases are also associated with HLA-B27 but in lower frequency (28–72 per cent) than in classical ankylosing spondylitis. There is no association between the severity of chronic inflammatory bowel disease and the presence, absence, or severity of sacroiliitis and ankylosing spondylitis. The course of the spinal disease is independent of that of the bowel disease.

Bypass surgery

This also tends to affect lower limb joints, particularly the knees and ankles, although fingers and shoulders may be involved. It usually occurs within 1 year of the bypass procedure. Males are more commonly affected than females. The pain is usually intense, with only slight swelling. Joint destruction does not occur, and there is no association with sacroiliitis. Eighty per cent of patients with arthropathy have associated cutaneous features which may be macular, papular, pustular, urticarial, or erythema nodosum.

Treatment

Enteropathic synovitis associated with chronic inflammatory bowel disease

Control of synovitis is associated with successful medical treatment of the bowel disease. In ulcerative colitis removal of the affected colon leads to complete remission of the arthropathy. Complete surgical exclusion of disease is not possible in Crohn's disease and the arthropathy may therefore continue despite surgical treatment if medical treatment cannot fully control the disease. The additional use of non-steroidal anti-inflammatory drugs may be useful, but some of these may aggravate the bowel disease. In large joints, aspiration of synovial fluid and local injection of depot corticosteroid may be helpful while other measures are undertaken to control the bowel disease.

Ankylosing spondylitis and sacroiliitis should be treated in the same way as ankylosing spondylitis occurring independently of bowel disease (see above).

Intestinal bypass arthropathy

Antibiotics and non-steroidal anti-inflammatory drugs, respectively, may be useful in eliminating bacterial overgrowth and reducing synovitis. The syndrome can be fully reversed with corrective bowel surgery.

Prognosis

The prognosis of enteropathic synovitis is largely dependent on that of the bowel disease. It is not usually destructive, with the rare exception of intra-articular granuloma formation in Crohn's disease, when systemic treatment with immunosuppressives and steroids may be helpful. The prognosis for ankylosing spondylitis and sacroiliitis is similar to that for the spinal disease in the absence of bowel disease (see above).

Whipple's disease (see also Chapter 5.11)

This disease predominantly affects middle-aged male Caucasians. HLA-B27 was present in 30 per cent of one reported series. Arthropathy is a presenting feature in 60 per cent of patients and occurs in 90 per cent during the course of the disease, being either oligoarticular or polyarticular. Occasionally, it may precede other manifestations by more than 10 years. It is rarely erosive and is frequently migratory. It tends to fluctuate independently of the gastrointestinal symptoms. Sacroiliitis has been found in 7 per cent of patients and ankylosing spondylitis in 4 per cent.

Diagnosis is confirmed by periodic acid-Schiff (PAS)-positive staining material in joint fluid and macrophages in the lamina propria of the intestine. Many other tissues may also have PAS-positive staining material. The finding of bacterial cell fragments on electron microscopy adds further confirmation. Treatment is with prolonged courses of penicillin, 500 mg four times per day; tetracycline, 500 mg four times per day; or erythromycin, 500 mg four times per day. Relapse may occur if treatment is stopped prematurely.

Behçet's syndrome

This chronic relapsing syndrome or oral ulceration, genital ulceration, and uveitis is more fully discussed in Chapter 10.16.

Synovitis occurs in some 40 per cent of patients (Table 4). The synovitis is subacute or chronic, involving large and small joints. It particularly affects the knees and ankles, and is usually oligoarticular or monoarticular. Erosive change is rare. Symptomatically it responds to corticosteroids. Sacroiliitis is a rare association.

Undifferentiated spondylarthritides

Clinical observation has led to the necessity of defining a group of undifferentiated seronegative spondylarthritides. Ankylosing spondylitis may have a peripheral joint onset in 10 per cent of patients, especially in teenagers in whom radiology of the sacroiliac joints is unreliable; arthropathy may precede the onset of the dermal manifestations of psoriasis; Crohn's disease may be initially silent and present with arthropathy; and 50 per cent of patients with gastrointestinal infection may have no intestinal symptoms, but a proportion still develop reactive arthritis.

The clinical features suggestive of a seronegative spondylarthritis are shown in Table 5 and 6. The evolution of the disease may allow more precise diagnosis with time; but long-term follow-up studies of such patients have not been undertaken. Treatment and prognosis are largely dependent upon the most likely cause. Non-steroidal anti-inflammatory drugs, joint aspiration, and injection with depot corticosteroid, periods of immobilization, and physiotherapy will be effective for most. Appropriate slow-acting or cytotoxic drugs may be required.

Table 4 The clinical features of Behçet's syndrome and their frequency

	Percentage
Oral ulceration	100
Genital ulceration	74
Uveitis	52
Synovitis	40
Cutaneous vasculitis (similar to erythema nodosum)	54
Meningoencephalitis	30
Large artery aneurysms	
Phlebitis	
Discrete intestinal ulcers	

Table 5 Characteristic features of seronegative spondylarthritis

Oligoarthritis
Lower limb predominance
Asymmetry
Enthesitis
Dactylitis
Back/buttock pain and stiffness
Family history of a seronegative spondylarthritis or associated disease

Adult Still's disease

This is a rare disease of unknown prevalence, which is unlikely to be more than 1 per 100 000 population. It principally affects young adults aged between 16 and 35 years. It has the same characteristics as systemic juvenile chronic arthritis. Its cause is unknown, although in a small number of cases there has been evidence to suggest a preceding viral infection, principally of echovirus or rubella. There is no association with HLA-B27. Studies suggest association with HLA-B14 and DR7, BW35 and CW4 and DR4. The principal criteria for diagnosis are given in Table 7. It is essential to exclude infection and primary haematological disease such as lymphoma and leukaemia.

Table 6 European Seronegative Spondarthritis Group criteria for undifferentiated spondylarthritis

1.	Inflammatory-type back pain: ≤40 years age at onset insidious onset improvement with exercise early morning stiffness ≥3 months' duration Or
2.	Asymmetrical lower-limb synovitis Plus two of:
(a)	Positive family history: ankylosing spondylitis psoriasis acute anterior uveitis reactive arthritis chronic inflammatory bowel disease
(b)	Psoriasis
(c)	Chronic inflammatory bowel disease
(d)	Urethritis preceding by ≤1 month
(e)	Acute diarrhoea preceding by ≤1 month
(f)	Alternating buttock pain
(g)	Definite radiological sacroiliitis

Table 7 Diagnostic criteria for adult Still's disease

Each of:	
1.	Quotidian fever >39°C
2.	Arthralgia/arthritis
3.	Negative rheumatoid factor
4.	Negative antinuclear factor
Plus two of:	
(a)	Leucocytosis $>15\times10^9$/l
(b)	Evanescent macular/maculopapular rash
(c)	Serositis (pleuritic/pericarditic)
(d)	Hepatomegaly
(e)	Splenomegaly
(f)	Generalized lymphadenopathy

In some patients it is necessary to consider the differential diagnoses of sarcoidosis and endocarditis.

Initial treatment should be with high-dose non-steroidal anti-inflammatory drugs, such as aspirin, indomethacin, or naproxen. If unsuccessful, or if there are severe systemic features, anaemia, pericarditis, or myocarditis, corticosteroids are usually required. High doses may be needed initially, but the aim should be to achieve a maintenance dose of less than 15 mg of prednisolone per day and finally to discontinue corticosteroid treatment within 6 months of its commencement. For patients failing to respond adequately to corticosteroids, or requiring more prolonged treatment, it may be necessary to consider slow-acting antirheumatic drugs or cytotoxic agents. No adequate trials of these have been performed in adult Still's disease but there are anecdotal reports of success with intramuscular sodium aurothiomalate, penicillamine, antimalarials and sulphasalazine. Cytotoxic agents have rarely been used, but there are anecdotal reports of improvement with azathioprine, chlorambucil, cyclophosphamide, or methotrexate.

Although initially considered to be a relatively benign disease, it is now recognized that 50 per cent of patients have progressive joint disease, particularly involving the wrists and hind feet leading to carpal and tarsal fusion, respectively. In addition, systemic complications including disseminated intravascular coagulation, acute hepatic failure, sometimes in combination with associated renal failure, cardiac tamponade, constrictive pericarditis, myocarditis, endocarditis, severe lung disease, peritonitis, and amyloidosis, have all been reported. There have been single case reports of panophthalmitis, status epilepticus, and polymyositis and rhabdomylosis.

Further reading

Maddison, P.J., Isenberg, D.A., Woo, P., and Glass, D.N. (ed.) (1998). *Oxford Textbook of Rheumatology*, (2nd edn), Section 5, pp. 1037–99. Oxford University Press, Oxford.

Chapter 10.4

Osteoarthritis

C. W. Hutton

Osteoarthritis is an enigmatic condition. Fatalism about the process being simply due to 'wear and tear' and old age has delayed systematic study. However, present knowledge of osteoarthritis allows a more rational approach to its management, underlines its importance as a public health problem, and delineates the directions for future research.

The concept of osteoarthritis

As osteoarthritis is poorly understood, it is difficult to define. Some features are recognized as important in diagnosis but whether they are necessary or sufficient remains controversial. Historically, it was recognized from morbid anatomy and later radiographic changes. Some forms were characterized by loss of articular cartilage associated with bone increase ('hypertrophic'), in contrast to that associated with bone loss ('atrophic'). With the recognition of the role of chronic infection and the evolution of the diagnosis of inflammatory arthritis the 'atrophic' group became well defined. A rump of disease remained associated with bone proliferation that can loosely be described as osteoarthritis. The age association and premature development of osteoarthritis after trauma meant that it was seen as a degenerative process.

Osteoarthritis is a chronic condition, and although it may develop acutely, current knowledge is primarily based on observations made at a single time in the evolution of the disorder. Short-term follow-up studies are few and long-term studies exceptional.

A current pathological definition of osteoarthritis is 'a disease process of synovial joints characterized by focal areas of loss of hyaline articular cartilage, associated with increased activity in marginal and subchondral bone'. These features, when severe, result in the characteristic radiographic changes of reduced interbone distance

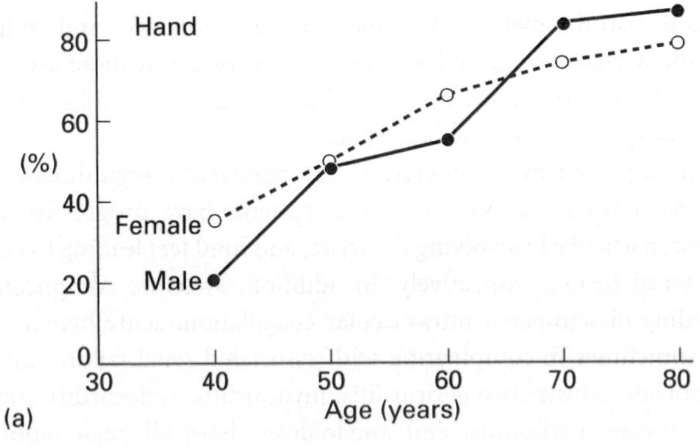

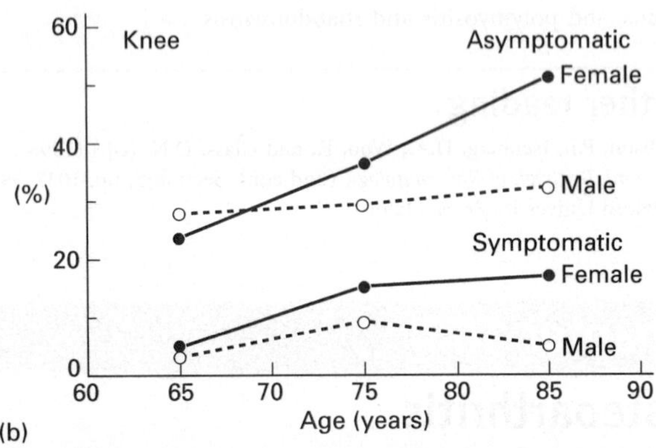

Fig. 1 The relationship of age to increasing prevalence of radiographic osteoarthritis at different joints groups. Radiographic prevalence of osteoarthritis in (a) the hand and (b) the knee.

(joint space narrowing), osteophyte formation, and subchondral sclerosis and cysts. A proportion of people with these changes develop symptoms, including use-related pain in the affected joints, with stiffness after inactivity.

The sites most frequently affected are knees, hips, certain joints of the hands, and the spinal apophyseal joints. Various clinical subgroups have been proposed, both on the basis of joint site, and on presumed aetiology. Osteoarthritis is often described as 'secondary' if a clear abnormality is associated with it, and 'primary' if there is no obvious association.

Epidemiology

Prevalence: age, sex, and pattern of joint involvement

Population-based studies show a low prevalence in all joint sites in young adults. In the commonly affected joints (hands, knees, hips, spine) prevalence rates rise steeply with age so that radiographic changes are almost universal in the elderly. Some joints, such as the ankle, are rarely affected. Radiographic osteoarthritis also depends on race and gender. In Caucasians, osteoarthritis of the hip has a roughly equal sex incidence, contrasting with the 2:1 excess in females of knee and hand osteoarthritis. Some of the less commonly affected sites, such as the elbow, are affected more commonly in males (Fig. 1).

Symptomatic osteoarthritis is less common than radiographic change, many damaged joints remaining asymptomatic. It has been estimated that the overall adult prevalence of symptomatic osteoarthritis is 1 per cent, with some 10 per cent of the over-sixties affected. Common clinical patterns include lone hip osteoarthritis in younger males, knee and hand disease in middle-aged, obese females, and involvement of several joints in the elderly.

Table 1 Factors associated with osteoarthritis: severity, symptoms and incidence

Strong:	Age, sex, familial, geographical, major joint trauma
Weak:	Chondrocalcinosis, occupation, obesity
Uncertain:	Hypermobility, osteoporosis

Risk factors

If 'wear and tear' were to be the cause of osteoarthritis there should be a close correlation with joint trauma. Untreated fractures through a joint do result in a high frequency of subsequent osteoarthritis, but population studies have failed to show a clear relationship of osteoarthritis to previous trauma.

Studies of occupational groups such as footballers, parachutists, and ballet dancers give confusing results but development of disease at unusual sites, for example at the ankle in footballers and ballet dancers, and 'miners elbow', suggest repetitive trauma is important. This is supported by studies of mill-workers, showing that the pattern of hand osteoarthritis reflects their repetitive occupation. Knee disease is increased by previous major knee injury and occupations involving frequent bending; and hip osteoarthritis is increased in farmers.

Systemic factors

Osteoarthritis is now thought to be due to a combination of systemic influences leading to a predisposition to joint damage, and local biochemical influences, which dictate the distribution and severity of the condition (Table 1).

Obesity is an important risk factor for osteoarthritis of the knees and has weak associations with hip and hand disease. It is unclear how much of its effect is systemic, and how much is biomechanical.

Hypermobility is another predisposing factor that may involve general as well as local factors. In contrast, osteoporosis has a negative association with hip osteoarthritis. Other evidence of systemic predisposition comes from the geographical and genetic data outlined below.

Geography

Osteoarthritis is present in all populations, but patterns vary in different populations (Fig. 2). Sadly there are no population migration studies to help define whether this variation is from environmental rather than genetic factors, although anthropological studies suggest that the pattern of disease has been different in different cultures and at different times. In addition, endemic forms of osteoarthritis are seen in certain parts of the world:

Kashin–Beck disease

In Manchuria and along the Amur River there is a high prevalence of a severe disease developing in adolescence with interphalangeal joint, wrist, and metacarpophalangeal stiffness, swelling, and pain. There is irregular epiphyseal growth and premature focal ossification. By early adult life a severe premature osteoarthritis develops with involvement of elbows, knees, and ankles. Hip involvement is uncommon. Histologically there is zonal necrosis of the growth plate. Environmental toxicity by trace metals or mycotoxins has been suggested as a cause.

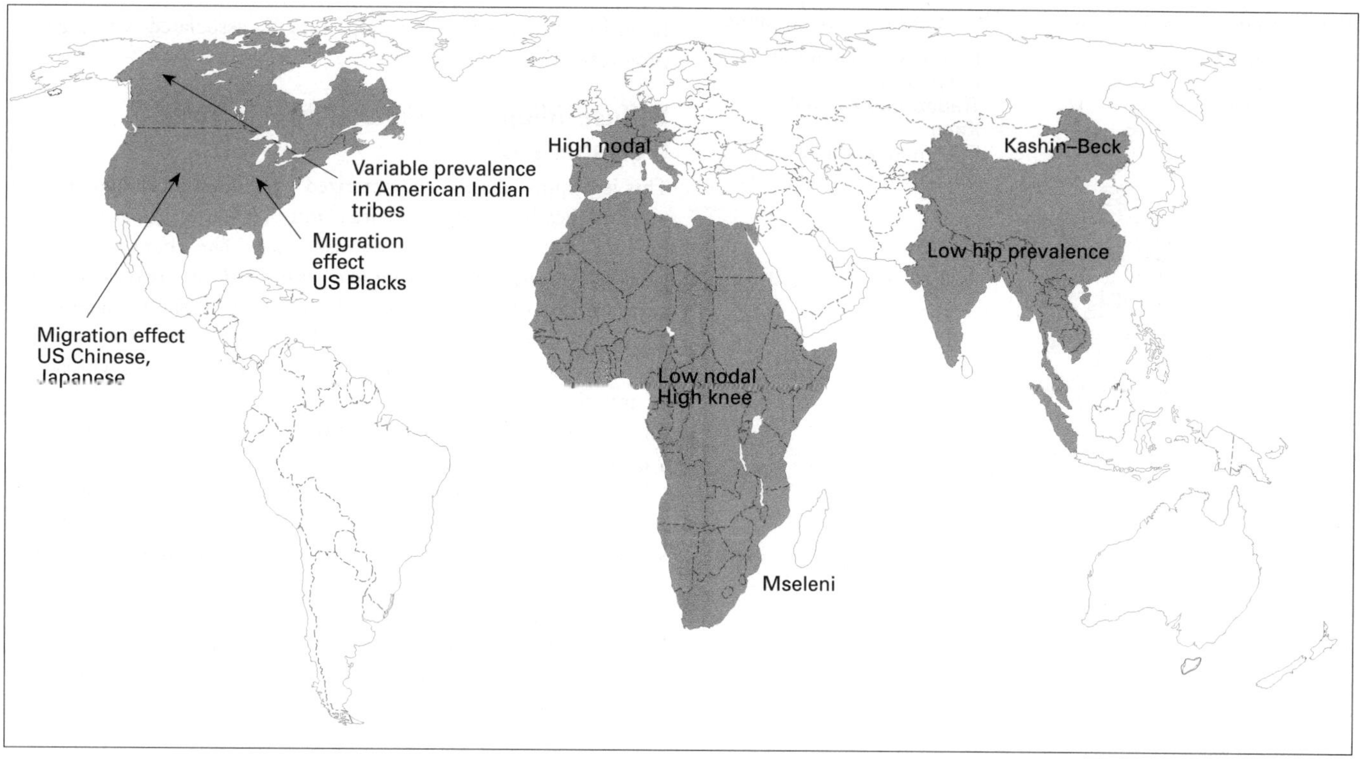

Fig. 2 The geography of osteoarthritis.

Table 2 Heredity disorders associated with premature osteoarthritis

Mucopolysaccharidosis type I, aa; II, X; IV, aa
Familial chondrocalcinosis, Aa
Multiple epiphyseal dysplasia, Aa, aa
Spondyloepiphyseal dysplasia tarda, X
Ehlers–Danlos syndrome types I and III, osteo-onychodystrophy (nail-patella syndrome), Aa
Progressive hereditary arthro-ophthalmopathy (Sticker's syndrome), Aa

aa = Autosomal recessive.

AA = Autosomal dominant.

X = Sex-linked.

Mseleni disease

In Natal there is a high prevalence of hip disease with protrusio acetabuli, associated with ankle, knee, shoulder, and elbow involvement; it appears to have a genetic basis.

Genetics

Genetic factors are important in the development of osteoarthritis (Table 2). This is apparent in that 'secondary' osteoarthritis can result from developmental and metabolic disorders like the chondrodysplasias, congenital dislocation of the hip, and ochronosis. Indications of the genetic basis of 'primary' osteoarthritis come from twin studies, family studies, and molecular genetics.

Specific and possible polygenetic effects are shown by a familial tendency, particularly for generalized nodal osteoarthritis, concordance in identical twins, and the identification of an abnormality in the type II collagen gene in a few families with premature osteoarthritis.

Subgroups

Osteoarthritis is not a single entity. The risk factors outlined above vary with joint site (Fig. 3); thus knee disease has strong associations with obesity and the female sex, whereas hip osteoarthritis has an equal sex incidence, little or no link to obesity, and a strong association with farming. This indicates that osteoarthritis of each of the major joint sites should be regarded as a different disorder. In addition, the implication of having developed osteoarthritis in different sites varies—in general, hip and knee osteoarthritis produce much more pain and disability than does upper limb disease. Subgroups of osteoarthritis can also be distinguished, independent of risk factors and site of joint involved: examples are illustrated in Fig. 4.

Generalized osteoarthritis

There is controversy as to whether or not there is a 'generalized' form of osteoarthritis. This has been suggested from clinical and epidemiological studies, and it has been defined as involvement of three or more joint groups. If this is a true entity, a common predisposing factor should result in osteoarthritis developing in all joints; such a pattern should, therefore, be a feature of known generalized problems like collagen gene defects. However, there are marked differences in the frequency of individual joint involvement which remain unexplained. The alternative hypothesis is that joints in which it is common for osteoarthritis to develop will be involved, so as to give a generalized pattern purely by chance.

Generalized osteoarthritis is often diagnosed when it involves the distal interphalangeal joints, knees, apophyseal joints of the

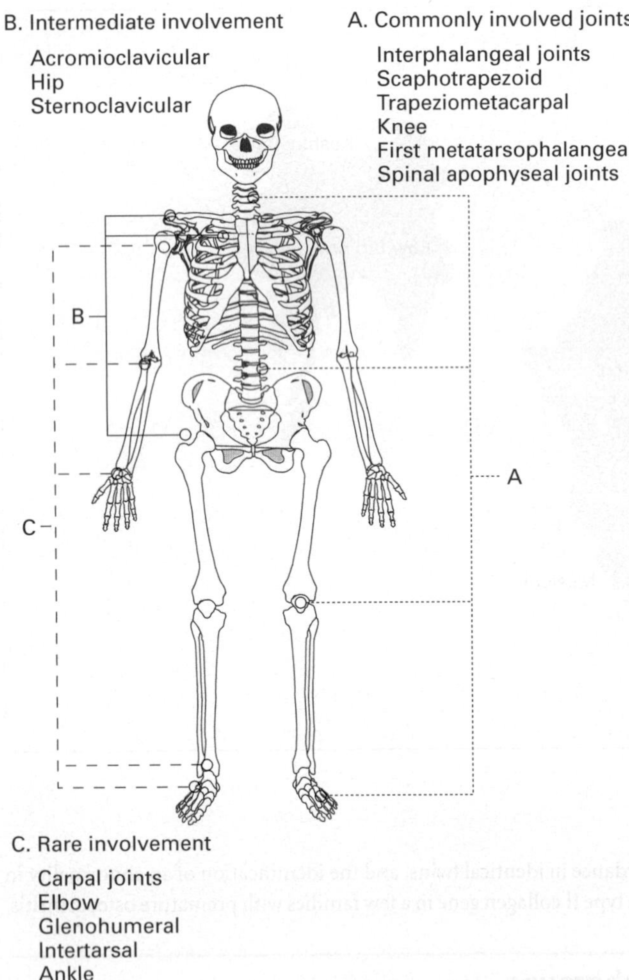

Fig. 3 The pattern of involvement at different joints.

spine, and first metatarsophalangeal joints. Bony swellings in the distal interphalangeal joints (Heberden's nodes) may form insidiously or from a hyaluronate-filled cyst that may be painful and warm. Nodal disease appears more common in women, with a strong familial pattern. The joint involvement is strikingly asymmetrical, with individual finger joints going through different phases of evolution of the disease; some becoming quiescent and non-painful while others become inflamed and active. This type of nodal hand osteoarthritis is common in women around the menopause and has been termed 'menopausal' osteoarthritis. Polyarticular hand osteoarthritis may be associated with marked inflammation of the joints and the pattern of destruction may include erosive damage. This has led to some cases being classified as 'inflammatory' or 'erosive' osteoarthritis of the hand. Ankylosis of the interphalangeal joints can also occur.

Atrophic/hypertrophic osteoarthritis

Classification of osteoarthritis according to the bone changes seen on radiographs suggests two polar groups: atrophic and hypertrophic disease—atrophic being rapidly progressive, associated with apatite crystal deposition, and more common with increasing age, while more subchondral sclerosis and osteophytosis (seen in the hypertrophic group) may be associated with a better prognosis.

Diffuse idiopathic skeletal hyperostosis (Forestier's disease)

This is a spinal disease characterized by exuberant 'flowing candle wax' ossification bridging at least four vertebral disc spaces, with no loss of vertebral height or disc space. The changes are most marked in the lower thoracic spine. It is associated with calcification of anterior spinal ligament without sacroiliitis, although there may be para-articular osteophytes. There may be ligamentous calcification around peripheral joints, with whiskering of muscle insertions. It is a common, age-related disorder with an estimated adult prevalence rate of 3.8 per cent in men and 2.6 per cent in women.

Although diffuse idiopathic skeletal hyperostosis is most often asymptomatic, backache, stiffness, and pain or tenderness at osseous spurs has been described. It is associated with obesity and diabetes. Spinal encroachment can cause myelopathy, and large cervical osteophytes may cause dysphagia. There may be an association between diffuse idiopathic skeletal hyperostosis and the hypertrophic type of peripheral joint osteoarthritis, but this remains controversial.

Charcot's joints

Destructive osteoarthritis associated with a proliferative bone response is sometimes seen in patients with diabetes mellitus, syringomyelia, meningomyelocele, and neurogenic syphilis. It is non-inflammatory, often with a haemorrhagic effusion. It is probably due to neurovascular, not neurotraumatic change.

'Secondary' osteoarthritis

Osteoarthritis may develop following any process damaging a joint (Table 3). In Paget's disease and osteopetrosis the most common site of osteoarthritis is in the hip. Ochronosis, due to an abnormality of homogentisic acid oxidase results in the deposition of homogentisic acid in connective tissues such as cartilage, and degenerative changes are seen in the spine (with disc calcification), in the knee, shoulder, and hip. Haemochromatosis results in degenerative disease in the metacarpophalangeal, interphalangeal, and shoulder joints, often with pyrophosphate deposition. In Wilson's disease 50 per cent of adults show osteoarthritis changes in metacarpophalangeal joints, wrists, elbows, hips, and knees, and these are associated with periarticular osteopenia.

The localization of osteoarthritis—within and between joints

The commonly affected sites are the spine, hips, knees, hands, and feet. In the spine the atlantoaxial joint, apophyseal joints in the mid-cervical and low lumbar regions, and oncovertebral joints are most vulnerable, probably because these are the sites of greatest stress. Three different radiographic patterns have been identified in the hip joint: concentric, superior pole, and medial pole disease (Fig. 5; see also Fig. 4), illustrating the fact that osteoarthritis localizes to specific sites within a joint, as well as to different joint sites. Similarly, at the knee, osteoarthritis may affect the medial tibiofemoral or patellofemoral com-

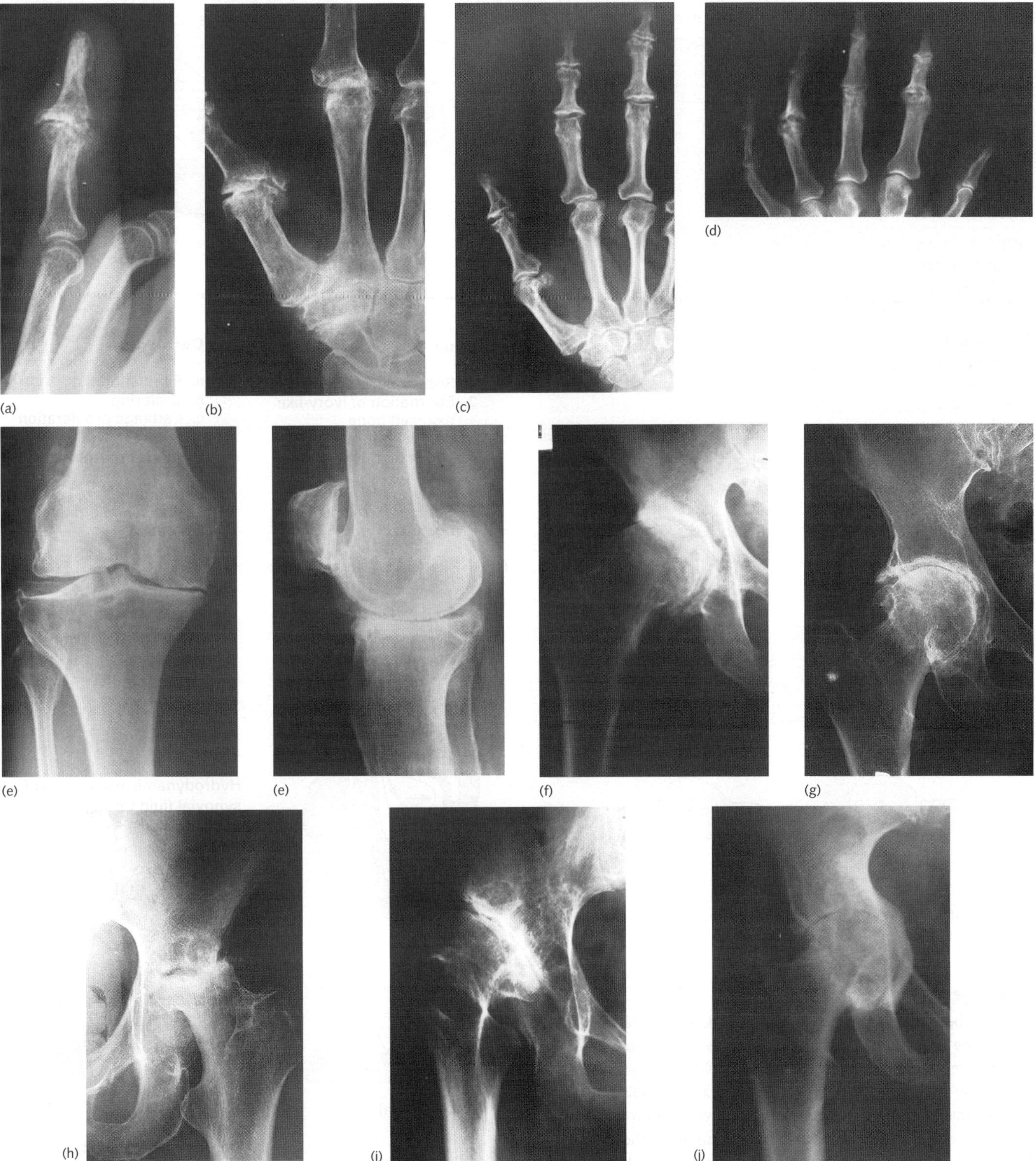

Fig. 4 Examples of subgroups of osteoarthritis. (a) The Heberden's node. (b) Scaphotrapezoid, trapeziometacarpal, and metacarpal osteoarthritis in haemochromatosis. (c) Acromegalic hand osteoarthritis. Note joint space widening. (d) Interphalangeal erosive osteoarthritis. (e) Knee osteoarthritis. Anterior and lateral views. (f) Superior pole hip osteoarthritis. (g) Medial pole hip osteoarthritis. (h) Atrophic hip osteoarthritis. (i) Osteoarthritis in congenital dislocation of the hip. (h) Concentric osteoarthritis of the hip with protrusio acetabulae.

partments, and in the hand the only sites to be affected commonly are the thumb base (trapezometacarpal and scaphotrapezial joints) and the distal interphalangeal joint. The base of the big toe (first metatarsophalangeal) is the major site involved in the foot.

Pathology

Changes occur throughout an affected joint and can be identified at macroscopic, microscopic, and biochemical levels (Fig. 6).

Table 3 Conditions favouring later development of osteoarthritis

Infection, inflammation
Trauma
Frostbite
With abnormal development Congenital dislocation of the hip Slipped upper femoral epiphysis Perthe's disease
With bone disease Paget's disease Osteopetrosis Avascular necrosis of bone
In metabolic and endocrine disease Acromegaly Ochronosis Haemochromatosis Wilson's disease

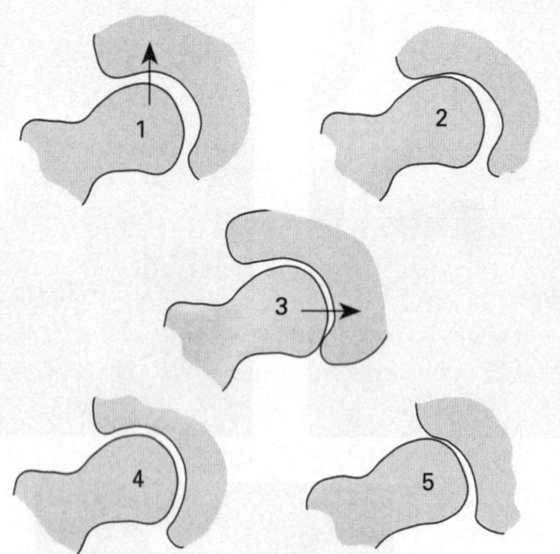

Fig. 5 Classification of osteoarthritic hip. (1) Normal. (2) Superior pole. (3) Medial pole. (4) Concentric. (5) Dysplastic.

Cartilage

Cartilage becomes fibrillated, thins, and develops craters. These changes are usually focal within the joint, becoming more extensive with progression. Areas of new cartilage proliferation may be seen, particularly in association with osteophytes and fibroblast invasion from the marrow. There is invasion by blood vessels into the cartilage across the subchondral plate, and reduplication to the tide mark delineating change in the calcified cartilage layer. Chondrocytes may appear grouped in nests, and other areas have empty lacunae. Fibrocartilage menisci disintegrate.

The hallmark of osteoarthritis is the change in bone; osteophyte formation, sclerosis, and cyst formation. The subchondral plate and trabecular network thicken. Cortical bone thickens, particularly in the hip to 'buttress' the femoral neck. The cartilage surface may be lost and the exposed bone becomes eburnated—thick and ivory-like. Bony outgrowths, osteophytes develop; there may be formation of subchondral cysts (Fig. 7). The marrow becomes hyperaemic and big

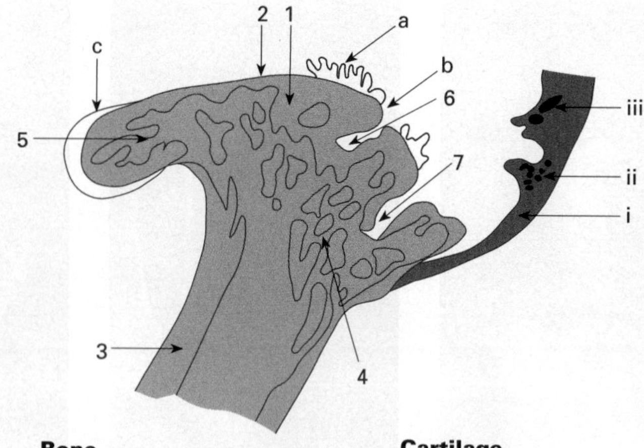

Bone

1. Subchondral sclerosis
2. Eburnation of ivory-like exposed bone
3. Cortical buttressing
4. Trabecular hypertrophy
5. Osteophyte
6. Cysts
7. Structural collapse and fracture

Cartilage

a. Fibrillation
b. Cratering
c. Cartilage proliferation

Synovial membrane

i. Fibrosis
ii. Patchy inflammation
iii. Debris

Fig. 6 Pathological features of osteoarthritis.

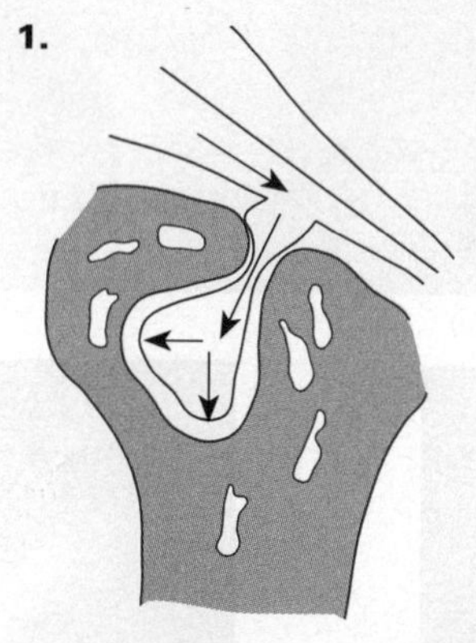

Hydrodynamic excavation of synovial fluid through a cartilage cleft

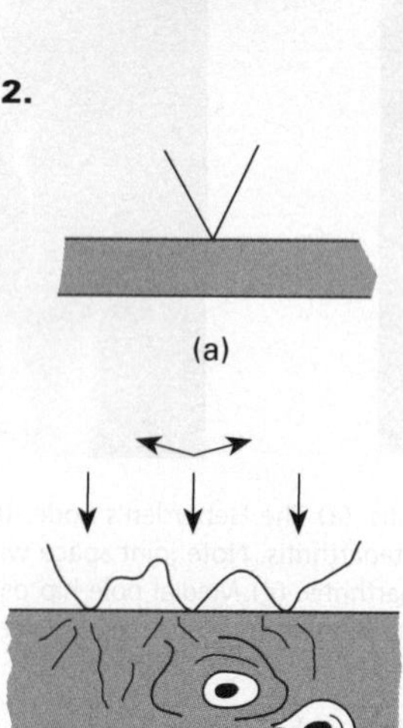

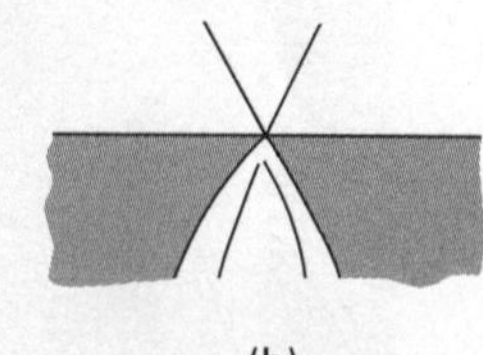

2. Focal peak forces kill bone
   (a) Normal cartilage dissipates load as an incompressible 'fluid'
   (b) No cartilage gives focal peak loading
   (c) Complex point loading and dynamic loading maps vulnerable areas of intense stress that form cysts

Fig. 7 The formation of bone cysts.

sinusoids develop. Late stages of the disease are associated with collapse of the subchondral bone.

Synovium and periarticular structures

The synovium is usually bland. It may contain bone debris, foci of mild, chronic inflammation, and proliferation of fibrous tissue. Tendons hypertrophy and there is wasting of muscle. The synovial fluid may increase in volume and become less viscous. It may contain cartilage and bone debris in addition to crystals, including pyrophosphate and apatite.

Aetiology

Mechanical considerations

How joints malfunction and how to modify such malfunction must be considered in a mechanical context. Essentially, joints allow stable, controlled movement of a system of levers under load. The power for movement from muscle is transmitted through tendons to bone. Systems must be designed to reduce wear of moving surfaces and control fatigue of components during life. Movement with excessive load induces wear. The coefficient of friction in the joint surface is below 0.02, but once damage has started this may change. In gel and fluid phases there is also a possibility of cavitation damage. Considerable uncertainty exists whether wear is a problem in normal joints. One possibility is that cartilage continues to grow *pari passu* with wear.

If loading on a bone increases, the bone will hypertrophy, and the highest loads will produce a fracture: either a fatigue (stress) fracture or a catastrophic disintegration. The transmission of force across non-congruent surfaces results in non-uniform distribution of stress. This distribution will change with movement but results in localized intense foci of force that may prevent viable cell function with resultant development of focal cysts. Cartilage acts like a fluid and disperses load to counteract these forces. However, photoelastic models demonstrate that a change in the character of the cartilage may prevent this dispersion of stress. Cyst formation may result from hydrodynamic stress transmitted through cartilage fissures into bone.

The distribution of cartilage fibrillation in the hip, knee, and elbow in pathological studies shows a focal development in areas of relative disuse; the less loaded areas. For example, the hip areas covered by the acetabulum are less affected than a zone in the periphery and around the fovea. This runs counter to the concept that stressed areas should develop change first, and suggests the reverse; that inadequate loading may be a cause of damage. The lack of data on stress distribution *in vivo* underlies the difficulty of identifying whether or not loading keeps the surface intact and inadequate loading induces damage.

The vulnerability of the system to develop these changes and capacity to tolerate damage is a function of the design of joints. These include factors determining the configuration of the joint and its material composition. Degenerative change will therefore be provoked by factors such as failure of remodelling, design limitation, defects in materials, and control of development.

A unifying hypothesis of osteoarthritis therefore emerges as a common pathway that can be triggered by any damage to a joint, and accelerated by a wide range of factors, although it is difficult to identify independent variables in each case.

Repair

Osteoarthritis may be considered as an ill result of the process of joint repair. The cartilage may not regenerate perfectly as the joint adapts to damage and maintain function. The anabolic processes in bone, particularly osteophyte growth, are part of this response. In progressive osteoarthritis the repair process is inadequate.

Biochemistry

In experimental osteoarthritis there is an initial increase in cartilage hydration and resultant swelling. There must be a change in the collagen network that restrains the proteoglycan matrix for this to occur. It is unclear how the network of collagen type II is damaged, but changes occur in proteoglycan turnover, altering the size and charge density of cartilage macromolecules, and thus the behaviour of matrix. The increase in chondroitin sulphate resembles the proteoglycan composition of developmental cartilage. Antibodies recognizing epitopes on these 'juvenile' molecules may offer a method of monitoring the progress of osteoarthritis. Proteoglycans may also be important in determining the development of a joint. The limb bud is rich in dermatan sulphate, but with cartilage formation chondroitin sulphate synthesis is turned on. With maturation there is a decrease in chain length. In ageing, at least in bovine cartilage, this is associated with an increase in dermatan sulphate formation and increased synthesis of type II cartilage. These changes may be mediated by cytokines and hormones. The chondrocyte also has oestrogen, growth hormone, and somatomedin receptors. For the anabolic response, a switch on of genes controlling cell proliferation and synthesis, changes in the stability of mRNA, or decreased catabolic degradation must occur. Growth factors such as insulin-like growth factor, platelet-derived growth factor, and transforming growth factor β, may be involved in this control.

Clinical features

Osteoarthritis causes pain and joint malfunction.

Pain

Pain must result from changes in the bone or periarticular structures, as hyaline cartilage contains no nerves. Ligamentous strain and inflamed bursae and synovial tissue may also contribute. Pain is characteristically worse on loading, and may be due to secondary effects on loaded tissue such as the bone marrow. In severe disease, night pain is a particular feature.

Malfunction

In joints involved with locomotion, malfunction limits mobility and causes instability, stiffness, secondary muscle weakness, and pain. Lower limb disease, particularly of the hip and knee, results in major difficulties with steps, stairs, and walking. Upper limb involvement is uncommon, except around the thumb and interphalangeal joints, resulting in restricted manipulation. In the spine osteoarthritis contributes to postural deformity and causes pain.

Management (Fig. 8)

There is a dearth of data from controlled trials but prevention is attempted by early detection of congenital deformity of the hip and improving the management of fractures. Exercise and avoidance of

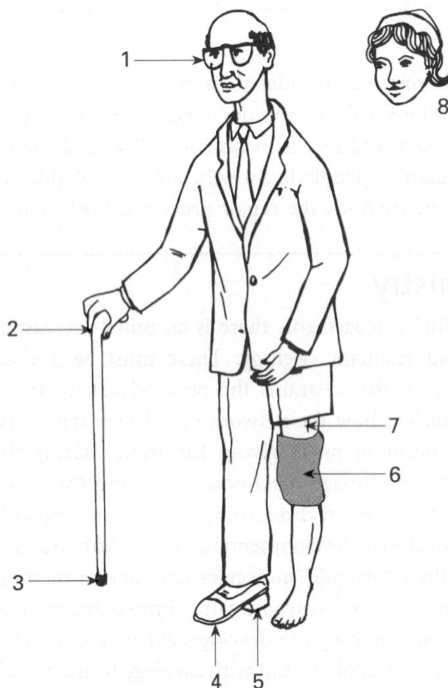

1. Correction of any problem likely to affect handicap: eyesight, inappropriate medication.
2. Correct stick length in contralateral hand to painful leg.
3. Ferrule with rubber grip.
4. Rocker sole for hallux rigidus, wide deep fitting shoe for hallux valgus.
5. Heel raise to correct leg length inequality.
6. Knee support splint.
7. Good quadriceps and corrected knee flexion deformity.
8. Happy, informed, and supported carer.

Fig. 8 Management of the patient with osteoarthritis.

obesity are other measures despite lack of data on their effectiveness.

Of particular importance is the need to assess the degree of handicap in relation to other problems. For example, if the patient has poor sight, is on inappropriate medication, is under stress, or is isolated, the osteoarthritis may result in much greater handicap than would otherwise be the case. The psychological response to the disease, possible difficulties in sexual relationships, and the impact on work and leisure activities are important issues, not always properly addressed.

A joint that is unstable and painful may be made less painful and more stable by physiotherapy and appropriate aids. Wheelchairs and adaptations, such as bath rails and stair lifts, may make it possible to maintain independence. Walking sticks can be remarkably helpful, but only if used properly. For a painful hip or knee, holding the stick in the contralateral hand transfers the weight off the painful joint; for instability, use in the most reassuring hand is appropriate. Splinting to correct instability, correction of varus or valgus at knee and ankle, use of a rocker sole to ease hallux rigidus pain, or a heel raise for leg inequality, all allow reduction of symptoms at low risk. Many people with osteoarthritis find great relief from use of shoes with good shock absorbing insoles, which can reduce pain related to joint loading.

Also important is the correction of the secondary effects of a flexion deformity or muscle wasting. In the knee, quadriceps wasting produces a weak leg with a perception of instability and loss of confidence in movement. Getting up from a chair and using stairs become difficult. If there is knee flexion, the gait is abnormal and the inequality of leg length tends to weight the painful knee. Exercise, including hydrotherapy, continuous passive motion, and splinting, may correct any deformity, as well as strengthening muscles. Quadriceps exercises have been shown to be an effective way of reducing pain and increasing mobility in people of all ages with osteoarthritis of the knee.

Modifying pain

In osteoarthritis, drug-related pain control is rarely good, either with simple analgesics, or with non-steroidal anti-inflammatory agents, which carry a risk of gastropathy. Pain is multifactorial, with exacerbation from mood, fear, and uncertainty which may be helped by education and support. Improved sleep, combined with physical treatment, may reduce the need for analgesics. Soft-tissue pain may be underdiagnosed, and may follow postural change induced by deformity. Joint pain and swelling may respond to local steroid injection. However, the limited number of controlled studies only show a transient effect. Injection of proteoglycans may also have a pain modifying effect. Postural pain may alter with changes in work environment, or advice on posture, sitting, and lifting. Uncontrolled pain remains the major indication for surgery.

Surgery

Arthroplasty has transformed the outlook for people with severe osteoarthritis of the hip and knee, but for other joints is still experimental, partly because of the technical problem of surgery and partly from the lack of understanding of the natural history of the disease in most joint sites.

Other procedures to ease symptoms may be appropriate, particularly in high-risk patients. In the hip, a Girdlestone's operation may control pain and allow some mobility. Osteotomy of the knee, and adductor muscle release at the hip, may allow treatment in younger people as well as correcting contributing deformity. Arthroscopy with lavage of debris and meniscal cartilage debridement may ease knee locking and reduce symptoms for a period. Joint fusion will give a pain-free joint albeit at the cost of immobility.

Investigation

The diagnosis is usually clear from history and examination, confirmed if necessary by imaging. Serology and crystallography of synovial fluid may be important in excluding other inflammatory disease, and investigation is occasionally necessary to exclude underlying metabolic causes. Radiographs remain the major way to assess the bone response and definition of osteoarthritis. Their limitation is poor definition of soft tissues and lack of information about cartilage unless contrast agents are used. Isotope bone scans show increased activity in osteoarthritic joints and can have some prognostic value, but do not contribute to diagnosis or management. Cartilage can be imaged by magnetic resonance, and major advances in this technique, such as magnetization transfer, are likely to make this more valuable. Methods of following the osteoarthritic process by tracking biochemical markers of the different processes are also being developed.

Further reading

Bellamy, N. (ed.) (1997). Osteoarthritis. *Baillière's Clinical Rheumatology*, Vol. 11, No. 4.

Buckwalter, J.A. and Lohmander, S. (1994). *Journal of Bone and Joint Surgery (USA)*, 76(9), 1405–18.

Creamer, P. and Hockberg, M.C. (1997). *Lancet*, **350**, 503–8.

Chapter 10.5

Crystal-related arthropathies

M. Doherty

Diversity and terminology

A large number of crystals have been associated with acute synovitis, chronic arthropathy, or periarticular syndromes (Table 1). In practice only urate pyrophosphate and basic calcium phosphates (mainly hydroxyapatite) crystals are commonly encountered.

The taxonomy of these conditions is not universally agreed. Difficulties arise from poor understanding of pathogenesis, historical extrapolation from gout to other crystal-related conditions, and multiple terms for the same clinical syndrome. Possible relationships between crystals and disease are outlined in Fig. 1. A 'crystal-deposition disease' is defined as a pathological condition associated with mineral deposits which contribute directly to the pathology. This is probably the situation for all manifestations of gout, for acute syndromes associated with pyrophosphate crystals, and for acute apatite periarthritis. The role of non-urate crystals in chronic arthropathy, however, is unclear and confounded by the following observations.

Table 1 Crystalline particles associated with joint disease

Intrinsic
Monosodium urate monohydrate
Calcium pyrophosphate dihydrate (monoclinic, triclinic)
Calcium phosphates basic: hydroxyapatite, octacalcium phosphate, tricalcium phosphate acidic: brushite, monetite
Calcium oxalate
Lipids cholesterol lipid liquid crystals Charcot–Leyden (phospholipase) crystals
Cystine
Xanthine, hypoxanthine
Protein precipitates (e.g. cryoglobulins)
Extrinsic
Synthetic corticosteroids
Plant thorns (semicrystalloid cellulose), especially blackthorn, rose, dried palm fronds
Sea-urchin spines (crystalline calcium carbonate)
Methylmethacrylate

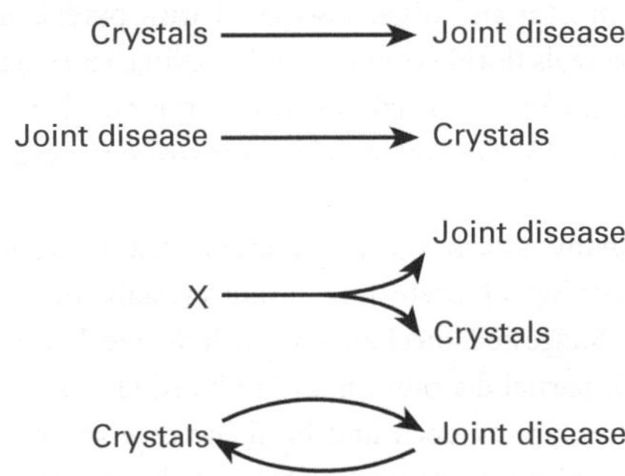

Fig. 1 Possible relationships between crystals and joint disease.

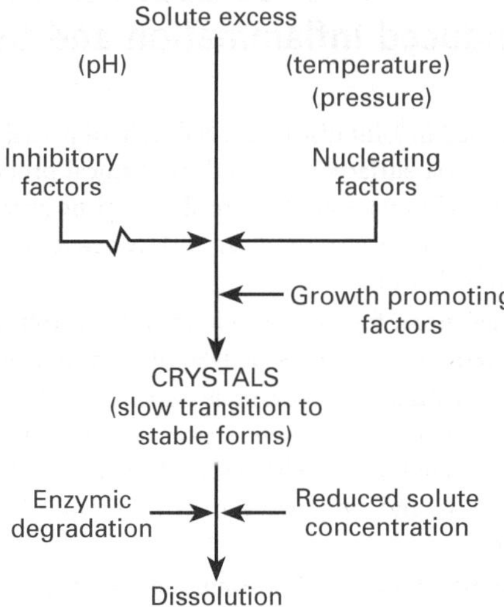

Fig. 2 Factors affecting crystal formation.

1. Most crystals lack disease specificity and occur in a variety of clinical settings, often unaccompanied by symptoms or other abnormality.
2. Crystal deposition may coexist with other rheumatic disease, most commonly osteoarthritis, and often follows rather than precedes articular damage.
3. Combined deposition of several crystal species is common ('mixed crystal deposition').

For descriptive purposes, confusion may be avoided by itemizing the crystal, the site of involvement, and the clinical syndrome (for example, chronic urate olecranon bursitis, acute pyrophosphate arthritis of the knee).

Crystal deposition and clearance

Many factors determine crystal formation and dissolution (Fig. 2). High solute concentrations alone are often insufficient to initiate crystal formation, and the presence of nucleating factors that aid initial particle formation and the balance of growth-promoting and inhibitory factors are equally important. Little is known of such tissue factors, although they may in part explain:

1. the characteristic limited distribution of different crystals within the body;
2. the frequency of mixed crystal deposition (via epitaxial nucleation and growth of one crystal on another); and
3. non-specific predisposition to crystal formation in osteoarthritic tissues (via accompanying alterations in proteoglycan, collagen, and lipid).

Formation of crystals *in vivo* is a dynamic, although usually slow process. At any time the crystal load will depend on the rate of formation, the rate of dissolution, and trafficking of crystals away from their site of formation (via 'shedding' from preformed deposits with secondary uptake by synovial and other cells).

Crystal-induced inflammation and tissue damage

Crystals implicated in joint disease are stable, hard particles that exert biological effects via surface-active and mechanical properties. With respect to acute inflammation, they are all phlogistic agents in a wide range of *in vitro* and *in vivo* systems. Surface-active interaction has been demonstrated with:

1. humoral mediators, for example complement activation via classical and alternative pathways; activation of Hageman factor;
2. cell-derived mediators, for example superoxide production and release of lysozymes, chemotactic factor, and lipoxygenase-derived products of arachidonic acid by neutrophils; release of interleukin-1, interleukin-6, and tumour necrosis factor by monocytes and synoviocytes;
3. cell membranes, for example membranolysis of lyosomes, erythrocytes, and neutrophils; non-lytic platelet and neutrophil secretory responses.

In general, urate is the most inflammatory, followed by pyrophosphate, then apatite, and the less common crystals. In general, marked surface irregularity and high negative surface charge correlate with inflammatory potential. Some surface effects result from direct crystal contact but others are mediated via absorbed protein, particularly immunoglobulin. Although absorbed IgG may enhance inflammation, most other protein binding is inhibitory.

Less is known of chronic crystal-induced tissue damage. Postulated effects include persistent synovial inflammation, altered cell metabolism, and deleterious mechanical effects from large deposits. Evidence for activation of inflammatory mediators in chronic 'granulomatous' reaction often occurs around large accretions. The physiochemical effects of hard, highly charged crystals embedded within cartilage, or occurring as wear particles at the surface, are largely unknown.

Gout

The biochemical and metabolic disturbances which underlie gout are also discussed in Chapter 6.6. Here the account concerns the rheumatological manifestations of disturbed uric acid metabolism and their management. Nephrolithiasis, urolithiasis, chronic renal disease, and hypertension are discussed elsewhere.

Monosodium urate crystals are undoubtedly the causal agents in gout, usually depositing in previously normal tissues and eliciting acute inflammation and eventual tissue damage. Their effective removal halts progression and results in 'cure'.

Epidemiology

Gouty arthritis occurs predominantly in post-pubertal males and is seldom seen in women before the menopause. The known incidence varies with populations from 0.2 to 0.35 per 1000. The self-reported prevalence increases with age from 2.4 per 1000 in men aged 18–44 to 34.4 per 1000 for men and 0.05 per 1000 for women. In addition to male sex, risk factors include obesity, excess alcohol consumption, lead exposure, hypertension, renal insufficiency, the use of diuretic drugs, and a family history of gout.

Clinical aspects

The natural history of untreated gout evolves through four clinical phases: asymptomatic hyperuricaemia, acute gout, intercritical gout, and chronic tophaceous gout.

Table 2 Incidence of gout by uric acid level in men

Serum uric acid (mg/dl)	5-year cumulative incidence	Incidence (per 1000 person years)
<6	0.5	0.8
6–6.9	0.6	0.9
7–7.9	2.0	4.1
9–9.9	9.8	43.2
>10	30.5	70.2

Asymptomatic hyperuricaemia

Serum is saturated with monosodium urate at a concentration of 7 mg per 100 ml (0.42 mmol/l), but much higher concentrations may remain in stable supersaturated solution for long periods. Hyperuricaemia is arbitrarily defined as a concentration greater than two standard deviations from the mean of 7 mg per cent (0.42 mmol/l) for adult males in the UK and USA. The majority of hyperuricaemic subjects are without symptoms throughout their lives. The incidence of gout by serum urate levels in men is shown in Table 2.

Urate crystals preferentially deposit in connective tissues in and around synovial joints, favouring the lower rather than the upper limbs. Deposits occur first in articular cartilage, most commonly of the first metatarsophalangeal and small joints of the feet and hands (Plate 1). Later they develop in synovial capsules and periarticular soft tissues, with progressive involvement of more proximal sites. Urate crystals probably take months or even years to grow *in vivo* to a detectable size, implying a long asymptomatic phase in gouty subjects.

The first presentation of gout is usually acute synovitis, although an insidious onset of chronic arthropathy or nodular deposits ('tophi') occasionally occurs without preceding attacks.

Acute attacks—the classical syndrome

In almost all initial episodes a single peripheral joint is involved. This is the first metatarsophalangeal joint ('podagra') in 50 per cent of first attacks and 70 per cent of all attacks. Other common sites are the ankle, mid-tarsal joints, knees, small hand joints, wrist, and elbow. The axial skeleton and large central joints are rarely involved and never as the first site.

Attacks often wake the patients in the early morning with localized irritation and aching. Within just a few hours the joint and surrounding tissues are swollen, hot, red, shiny, and extremely painful. The patient cannot bear even bedclothes to touch the joint and often describe it as 'the worst pain ever experienced'. Inflammation is maximal within 24 h and often associated with pyrexia and malaise. Examination reveals florid synovitis, and swelling, extreme tenderness, and overlying erythema. If left untreated, the attack resolves spontaneously over 5–15 days, often with pruritus and desquamation of overlying skin.

Although many attacks occur spontaneously, certain situations encourage shedding of preformed urate crystals and triggering of acute attacks. Suggested mechanisms include mechanical loosening (local trauma); partial dissolution and reduced crystal size (initiation of hypouricaemic treatment); and local increase in cytokines which encourage inflammatory responses to crystals and facilitate crystal escape via alterations in cartilage matrix (intercurrent illness, surgery).

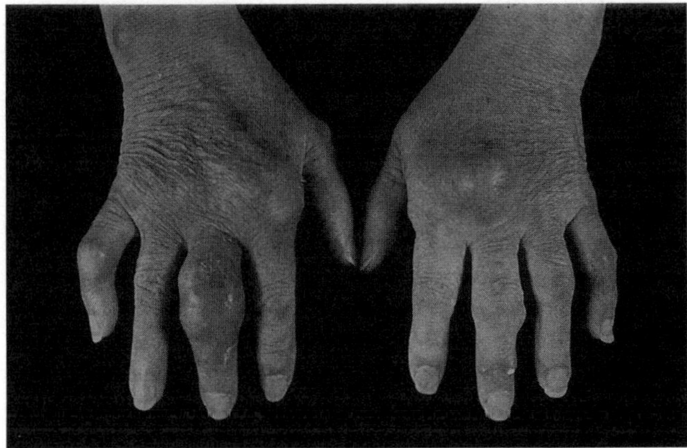

Fig. 3 Chronic tophaceous gout affecting the hands. Note the eccentric nature of the tophi and the asymmetry between sides.

Atypical attacks

These may manifest as tenosynovitis, bursitis, or cellulitis. Many patients describe mild episodes of discomfort without swelling lasting a day or so ('petite attacks'). Ten per cent of all attacks involve more than one joint; sometimes acute gout, by triggering the acute phase response, provokes migratory attacks in other joints over subsequent days ('cluster attacks'). Polyarticular attacks are rare, usually occurring after a long history of recurrent attacks; marked systemic upset, fever, and confusion may dominate the clinical picture.

Intercritical periods

These are asymptomatic intervals between attacks. Some patients never have a second attack, in others the next episode occurs after may years; in most, however, a second attack occurs within 1 year. Subsequently, the frequency of attacks and number of sites involved gradually increase with time. Later attacks are more often pauci- or polyarticular and more severe. Eventually, recurrent attacks and continuing urate crystal deposition cause joint damage and chronic pain; the interval between the first attack and development of chronic symptoms is variable, but averages about 10 years. The principal determinant is the serum uric acid—the higher it is, the earlier and more extensive the development of joint damage and tophaceous deposits.

Chronic tophaceous gout

Large crystal deposits ('tophi') produce irregular firm nodules, principally around extensor surfaces of fingers, hands, ulnar surface of forearms, olecranon bursae, Achilles tendons, and first metatarsophalangeal joints; the cartilaginous helix of the ear is classically, but rarely, affected. Marked asymmetry, both locally and between sides, is particularly characteristic (Fig. 3); urate crystals beneath the skin may give a 'chalky' appearance. If untreated, tophi can enlarge into gross knobbly swellings that may ulcerate; discharging material is white and gritty and associated with local inflammation (erythema, pus) even in the absence of secondary infection. If extensive, tophi may rarely involve the eye, eyelids, tongue, larynx, or heart (causing conduction defects and valvular dysfunction).

Joints most commonly involved with signs of damage (restricted movement, crepitus, deformity) and varying degrees of synovitis are the first metatarsophalangeal joints, mid-foot, small finger joints, and wrists. As with tophi, joint involvement is usually asymmetrical. Occasionally, gross destruction may occur in the feet and hands, and less commonly other sites. Acute attacks may become less of a feature as chronic symptoms become established. If untreated, the combination of extensive joint destruction and large tophi may cause grotesque deformities, particularly of the hands and feet. Ankylosis is a rare late event. Although axial involvement is rare even in later stages, gouty involvement of hips, shoulders, spine, and sacroiliac joints, and spinal cord compression by tophi are all reported.

Classification and pathogenesis

Traditional classification into primary or secondary gout depends on defined predisposing factors for hyperuricaemia. Most gout is primary. In 75–80 per cent of those with primary disease, hyperuricaemia is associated with impairment of excretion of uric acid; urate clearance is significantly reduced (mean 3.6 ml/min), while creatinine clearance is normal. This could be the result of a decreased filtered load, increased reabsorption or decreased secretion. As urate is not bound significantly to plasma proteins, one or both of the latter mechanisms must be operative.

Increased uric acid production and excretion are found in 10–15 per cent of patients with gout. In the majority the basis for increased synthesis of purines is unknown, but in a few there is evidence of a specific inherited purine enzyme defect (see Chapter 6.6). In some 10 per cent of gouty patients seen in hospital hyperuricaemia results from an increased turnover of performed purines and in a few, accelerated *de novo* purine synthesis may be a subordinate manifestation of an inherited enzyme defect.

Secondary gout usually results from chronic diuretic therapy and presents in older subjects (>65 years). This form often associates with osteoarthritis, acute attacks are less prominent and presentation is often with painful, sometimes discharging deposits in Heberden's and Bouchard's nodes.

Investigations and diagnosis

The history and signs of classical acute or chronic tophaceous gout are highly characteristic, and with a raised serum uric acid a strong presumptive diagnosis is readily made. However, definitive confirmation requires demonstration of urate crystals by compensated polarized light microscopy of fluid from a gouty joint, bursa, or tophus. Synovial fluid in acute attacks is typically turbid with diminished viscosity and greatly elevated cell count (>90 per cent neutrophils); chronic gouty fluid is more variable, but occasionally appears white due to the high crystal load. Only a few drops collected directly on to a slide are required for crystal identification. Monosodium urate crystals are seen readily as strongly birefringent (negative sign) needle-shaped crystals, 5–20 μm in length, within cells or occurring freely in fluid; in tophaceous material they occur as dense, tightly packed sheets. During intercritical periods, aspiration of an symptomatic first metatarsophalangeal joint or knee still often permits urate crystal identification.

Hyperuricaemia is confirmed if two or more fasting serum uric acid levels exceed the normal range for the patient's age and sex. In primary gout of young onset, determination of undersecretion or overproduction of uric acid is best undertaken by measuring total urinary excretion on a low purine diet, but a quick guide is given by the creatinine/uric acid ratio estimated on a single urine sample (normally <0.5). In young overproducers, a purine enzyme defect becomes more likely and should be sought (see Chapter 6.6). Assessment of renal function (creatinine, urea, electrolytes, urine testing) should always be undertaken. Measurement of fasting lipoprotein

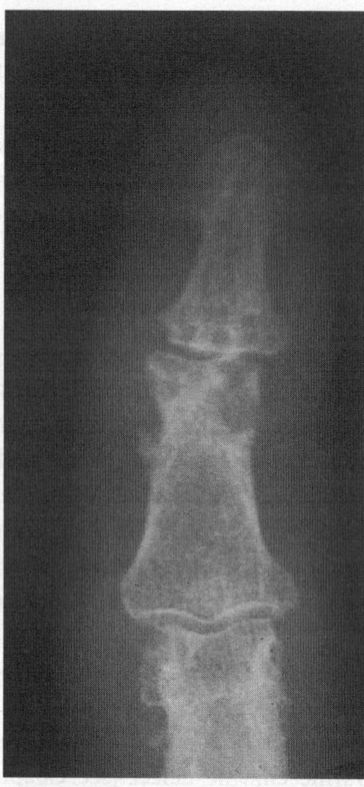

Fig. 4 Characteristic radiographic changes of established gout in a finger; joint space loss and cystic change at the distal interphalangeal joint, 'pressure erosions' with overhanging bony 'hooks' at both interphalangeal joints, and eccentric soft-tissue swelling at the proximal joint.

concentrations should be made in all patients with primary gout. An intercritical full blood count and measurement of erythrocyte sedimentation rate (ESR)/viscosity should detect any underlying myeloproliferative disease. During acute attacks a marked acute phase response (high ESR, neutrophil leucocytosis, thrombocytosis, elevated C-reactive protein) is usual; modest elevations of ESR also accompany chronic gout.

Radiographs supplement the clinical assessment of structural damage but may also aid diagnosis; in early disease they are usually normal. During acute gout, non-specific soft-tissue swelling (rarely juxta-articular osteopenia) may be evident. After repeated attacks, and in chronic disease, joint space narrowing, sclerosis, cysts, and osteophytes (that is the changes of osteoarthritis) become more frequent in feet and hands. Gouty 'erosions' are a less common but more specific abnormality, occurring as para-articular 'punched-out' bone defects with well-demarcated sclerotic margins, overhanging hooks of bone, and retained bone density (Fig. 4). They are typically asymmetric, eccentric lesions positioned away from the 'bare area' of the joint, contrasting with more symmetrical, ill-defined marginal erosions (with osteopenia) of rheumatoid. Tophi appears as eccentric soft-tissue swellings, occasionally with patchy calcification due to epitaxial growth of apatite. In late disease, severe destructive change with osteopenia may occur and distinction from rheumatoid or other conditions becomes more difficult.

Differential diagnosis

Acute attacks

Sepsis and other crystal-associated synovitis are the main considerations. Furthermore, gout and sepsis may coexist, as may urate and calcium pyrophosphate deposition (particularly in elderly subjects). Examination of aspirated fluid for both crystals and sepsis (Gram stain, culture) is the only sure way of obtaining the correct diagnosis. In ill patients particularly, a wider search for sepsis may be indicated (for example blood and urine cultures). With less classic attacks, other conditions that may be considered include psoriatic and acute Reiter's arthropathy, acute sarcoid arthropathy, traumatic arthritis, palindromic rheumatism, and exacerbation of osteoarthritis.

Chronic tophaceous gout

Other causes of arthritis and perarticular swellings/nodules that may require differentiation are rheumatoid arthritis, general nodal osteoarthritis, xanthomatosis with arthropathy, and multicentric reticulohistiocytosis. Gout is usually less symmetrical in distribution than these conditions and, except for hyperlipidaemia, acute attacks are not a feature. Nodal osteoarthritis, of course, may coexist with gout. Aspiration (joint fluid, nodules) and plain radiographs readily facilitate correct diagnosis.

Treatment

Acute gout

The treatment aim is pain relief by reducing inflammation and intra-articular hypertension. Alteration of uric acid levels is postponed until the attack has resolved. Rapid relief of pain may be obtained with a quick-acting, non-steroidal anti-inflammatory drug (NSAID), given in full dosage. Although indomethacin has a long tradition in this context, it is preferably avoided in the elderly due to its frequent renal, gut, and nervous system side-effects.

Oral colchicine is effective within a few hours (1 mg immediately, followed by 0.5 mg every 6 h until symptoms abate). Unfortunately, at these doses diarrhoea, nausea, and abdominal cramps are common, causing the patient 'to run before he can walk'. Colchicine, however, is a useful alternative if NSAIDs are contraindicated. Intravenous colchicine is particularly toxic and should never be used.

Joint aspiration often provides dramatic immediate relief by reducing intra-articular hypertension. Intra-articular steroid is useful for large joints such as the knee, or when NSAIDs or colchine are contraindicated or unsuccessful. In difficult cases, joint lavage may terminate an attack, and for troublesome polyarticular attacks there is anecdotal support for the use of intramuscular steroid.

Long-term management

Modification of provoking factors

In early primary gout, gradual weight loss, reduction in alcohol consumption, and avoidance of toxins (low-dose aspirin, lead) alone may be sufficient. Similarly, in diuretic-induced gout stopping the diuretic may prove possible and be all that is required.

Hypouricaemic drug therapy

Indications for drug therapy are:

1. recurrent, troublesome acute attacks;
2. presence of tophi;
3. bone or cartilage damage;
4. coexistent renal disease, uric acid urolithiasis;
5. very high uric acid levels (particularly with overproduction or hypoexcretion).

The aim is to maintain the serum uric acid well within the normal range (preferably the lower half). The logical drugs would be allopurinol for overproducers and uricosurics for underexcretors. In practice, however, allopurinol is the drug of choice, permitting flexible tailoring of doses to reduce urate levels below the solubility limit. Allopurinol inhibits xanthine oxidase and often also depresses *de novo* purine synthesis. The starting dose is 100–300 mg daily, which is then adjusted within the range 100–900 mg daily according to the serum uric acid level (initially checked monthly). In patients with renal insufficiency, particularly the elderly, excretion of the active metabolite oxypurinol is delayed; the starting dose should therefore be 100 mg daily and adjustments made more cautiously. The uricosurics probenecid (0.5–1.0 g twice a day) and sulphinpyrazone (100 mg, three to four times daily), which prevent proximal tubular reabsorption of urate, are rarely used, and have partly been replaced by uricosuric NSAIDs (for example, azapropazone 600 mg, twice a day). Because of their symptomatic benefit, compliance with NSAID uricosurics is good; a drawback is the usual spectrum of NSAID side-effects. Uricosurics are alternatives to allopurinol in patients with normal renal function but are contraindicated in those with renal impairment, urolithiasis, or gross overproduction of uric acid.

Acute attacks may be provoked during the first few months of hypouricaemic treatment. Prophylactic colchicine (0.5 mg, twice a day) or a standard dose of NSAID given for the first 2–3 months of treatment largely avoids such attacks. Uricosuric NSAIDs do not require such cover. With any uricosuric, high fluid intake and urine alkalinization in the early week of treatment are recommended to avoid uric acid deposition within the kidney. Serious side-effects are unusual with any hypouricaemic drug. Rare problems include toxic epidermal necrolysis, vasculitis and acute interstitial nephritis (allopurinol), nephrotic syndrome (probenecid), and hepatitis and marrow suppression (both drugs). Important interactions with allopurinol occur with coumarin anticoagulants (due to hepatic microsomal enzyme inhibition) and purine analogues (such as azathioprine), which are inactivated by xanthine oxidase. Associated hypertension should be treated, but preferably not with diuretics.

Pyrophosphate arthropathy

Deposition of calcium pyrophosphate dihydrate crystals (Ca_2, P_2O_7, $2H_2O$) is common age-related phenomenon. These crystals preferentially deposit within fibrocartilage and are the most common cause of cartilage calcification (chondrocalcinosis). This may occur in otherwise normal cartilage or in association with structural change and clinical arthropathy—'pyrophosphate arthropathy'. A causal role for pyrophosphate crystals in acute inflammation is accepted but their role in chronic arthropathy is unclear. The strong association/overlap with osteoarthritis has led some to consider the arthropathy not as a crystal deposition disease but as a 'subset' of osteoarthritis, with calcium pyrophosphate a 'process' marker associating with a hypertrophic articular response.

The prevalence of *radiographic* chondrocalcinosis is rare under 50 years of age, but rises from 10 to 15 per cent in those aged 65–75, to 30 to 60 per cent in those over 85, showing female preponderance (relative risk 1.33) and association with osteoarthritis (relative risk 1.52 at the knee). No epidemiological data exist for pyrophosphate *arthropathy*, but the mean age of presentation is about 65–75 with female preponderance (about 2–3:1), particularly in older patients.

Clinical features

Common presentations are acute synovitis, chronic arthritis, or incidental finding. Other presentations are rare.

Acute synovitis ('pseudogout')

This is the most common cause of acute monoarthritis in the elderly. Attacks may occur as isolated events or superimposed on a background of chronic symptomatic arthropathy. Most occur spontaneously but provoking factors include intercurrent illness, surgery, and local trauma. Although any joint may be involved, the knee is by are the most common site, followed by the wrist, shoulder, and ankle. Concurrent attacks in several joints are uncommon (<10 per cent of cases).

The typical attack develops rapidly with severe pain, stiffness, and swelling, becoming maximal within 6–24 h of onset. Examination reveals a very tender joint with signs of florid synovitis (increased warmth, tense effusion, restricted movement with stress pain) and often overlying erythema. Fever is common and elderly patients may appear unwell or mildly confused. Attacks are self-limiting, usually resolving within 1–3 weeks.

Chronic pyrophosphate arthropathy

This common condition affects mainly elderly women and targets the same large and medium-sized joints as pseudogout. Knees are the usual and most severely affected joint. Presentation is with chronic pain, stiffness, and functional impairment ($\pm$superimposed acute attacks). Symptoms usually relate to just a few joints, although examination often reveals more widespread abnormalities. Affected joints show signs of osteoarthritis (crepitus, bony swelling, restricted movement) with varying degrees of synovitis (often most marked at the knee, radiocarpal, or glenohumeral joint). Knees typically show abnormality of two or three compartments; valgus or varus deformity may occur. Although symptoms and signs are those of osteoarthritis, chronic pyrophosphate arthropathy may often be distinguished from uncomplicated osteoarthritis by:

1. the joint distribution: in osteoarthritis wrist, glenohumeral, ankle, elbow, and mid-tarsal involvement are uncommon;
2. the often marked inflammatory component; and
3. superimposition of acute attacks.

The outcome for chronic pyrophosphate arthropathy is generally good particularly when small and medium-sized joints are involved. Most progression that occurs is slow and occurs in the knees, hips, or shoulders. Occasionally severe, rapidly progressive destructive arthropathy develops at these sites; this is virtually confined to very elderly women and associates with severe pain, recurrent haemarthrosis (shoulder, knee), and occasional joint capsular rupture.

Incidental finding

Clinical or radiographic evidence of pyrophosphate arthropathy and chondrocalcinosis are not uncommon incidental findings in the elderly, and may confound the cause of regional pain if a thorough history and examination are not undertaken.

Uncommon presentations

Acute tendinitis (triceps, Achilles), tenosynovitis (hand flexors, extensors), and bursitis (olecranon, infrapatellar, retrocalcaneal) occur uncommonly, usually in patients with widespread chondrocalcinosis. Median and ulnar nerve compression at the wrist may accompany flexor tenosynovitis. Rare tophaceous deposits of pyrophosphate usually present as solitary lesions in areas of chondroid metaplasia.

Classification and associations

Calcium pyrophosphate deposition can be hereditary, associated with metabolic disease or, most commonly, associated with osteoarthritis.

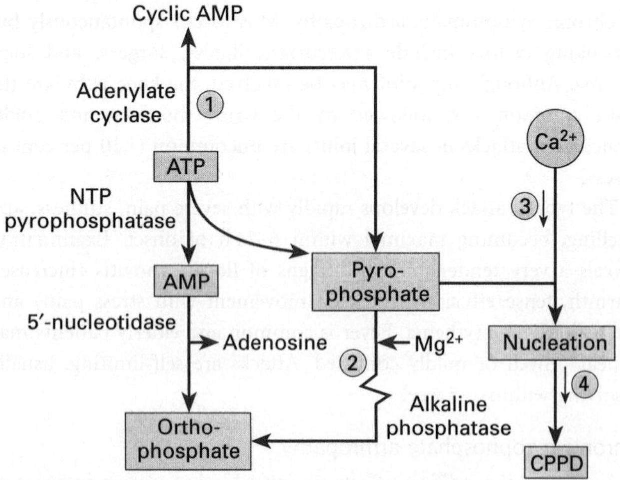

Fig. 5 Simplified scheme of extracellular pyrophosphate metabolism, showing putative sites of interaction by metabolic diseases. Hyperparathyroidism 1, 2, 3; haemochromatosis, 2, 4; hypophosphatasia, 2; Wilson's disease, 2, 4; and hypomagnesaemia, 2.

Familial predisposition

This is reported from many countries and different ethnic groups. Two clinical phenotypes occur: early-onset (third to fourth decade) florid polyarticular chondrocalcinosis with variable severity of accompanying arthropathy; and late-onset (sixth to seventh decade) oligoarticular chondrocalcinosis (mainly knee) with arthritis resembling sporadic disease. The pattern of inheritance varies, although autosomal dominance is usual. The mechanism of familial predisposition remains unclear and may differ between families; a primary cartilage abnormality that promotes pyrophosphate crystal nucleation and growth (Swedish and Japanese families), and a generalized abnormality of pyrophosphate metabolism resulting in local increase in cartilage levels (French and American kindreds) have both been reported. Gene localization to two sites (on chromosomes 5p and 8q) are reported in UK and North and South American families, and may shortly lead to elucidation of the mechanism of crystal deposition.

Metabolic disease associations

Inorganic pyrophosphate (PPi) is a by-product of many biosynthetic reactions, with a turnover of several kilograms per day. Much extracellular PPi derives from adenosine triphosphate via the action of nucleoside triphosphate pyrophosphatase, and is rapidly converted to orthophosphate by pyrophosphatases (particularly alkaline phosphatase). (Fig. 5). A number of metabolic diseases associate with calcium pyrophosphate dihydrate deposition (Table 3). Suggested mechanisms include:

1. reduced PPi breakdown by alkaline phosphatase, due to (a) reduced levels; (b) inhibitory ions (calcium, iron, copper), or; (c) impaired complexing with magnesium;
2. enhanced nucleation by iron or copper;
3. increased calcium concentration; and
4. increased production of pyrophosphate through stimulation of adenylate cyclase by parathyroid hormone.

Osteoarthritis and joint insult

Several observations support a relationship between osteoarthritis and pyrophosphate crystal deposition, the latter often following rather than preceding joint damage. However, a negative association exists

Table 3 Metabolic diseases associated with calcium pyrophosphate dihydrate (**CPPD**) crystal deposition

	Chondro-calcinosis	Pseudo-gout	Chronic CPPD arthropathy
Definite associations			
Hyperparathyroidism	+	+	−
Haemochromatosis	+	+	+
Hypophosphatasia	+	+	−
Hypomagnesaemia	+	+	−
Possible associations			
Hypothyroidism	+	−	−
Gout	+	+	−
X-linked hypo-phosphataemic rickets	+	+	+
Familial hypocalciuric hypercalcaemia	+	−	−
Wilson's disease	+	−	−
Ochronosis	+	−	−
Acromegaly	+	−	−

in the case of rheumatoid arthritis, with atypical radiographic features in coexistent disease (retained bone density, marked osteophyte, cyst, and bone remodelling) suggesting that the primary association of crystal deposition is with hypertrophic tissue response/osteoarthritis and not joint damage *per se*. The explanation for this association is unknown. Synovial fluid PPi levels are increased when pyrophosphate has been deposited. Crystals form in pericellular sites and associate with lipid, proteoglycan depletion, and adjacent hypertrophic chondrocytes containing lipid granules; it is therefore possible that reduction of inhibitors (such as proteoglycan) and increase in promotors (such as lipid) may combine to co-promote pyrophosphate crystal formation in active osteoarthritic tissue.

Investigations and diagnosis

Critical investigations are synovial fluid analysis and plain radiographs. In pseudogout aspirated fluid is often turbid or blood-stained with an elevated cell count (>90 per cent neutrophils); fluid from chronic pyrophosphate arthropathy shows variable characteristics. Compensated polarized microscopy reveals calcium pyrophosphate crystals as weakly birefringent (positive sign) rhomboids or rods, about 2–10 μm long, but they are less readily identified and often less numerous than those of monosodium urate; examination of a spun deposit may increase detection.

Radiographic changes relate both to calcification and arthropathy. Chondrocalcinosis signifies extensive deposition and is not always evident; it mainly affects fibrocartilage (particularly knee menisci, wrist triangular cartilage, symphysis pubis), less commonly hyaline cartilage (Fig. 6). Although occasionally monoarticular, it usually affects several sites. Calcification of capsule, synovium, and tendons is less common. Chondrocalcinosis and calcification may increase or decrease with time, diminishing chrondrocalcinosis often accompanying crystal 'shedding' or cartilage loss.

Changes of arthropathy are those of osteoarthritis: cartilage loss, sclerosis, cysts, and osteophytes but certain characteristics suggest pyrophosphate:

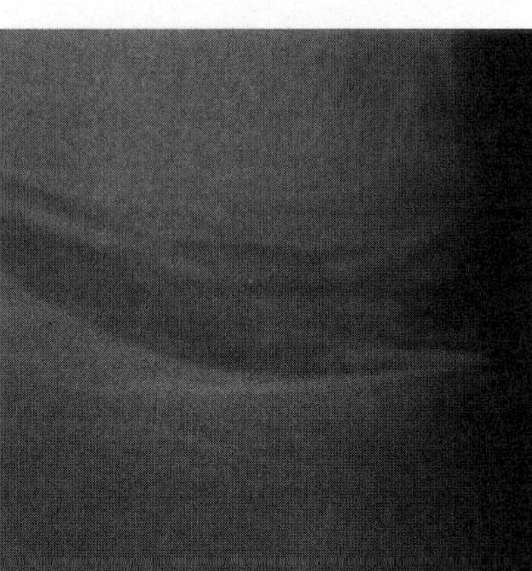

Fig. 6 Radiographic chondrocalcinosis of the knee, affecting meniscal fibrocartilage (central, triangular) and hyaline cartilage (linear, parallel to bone).

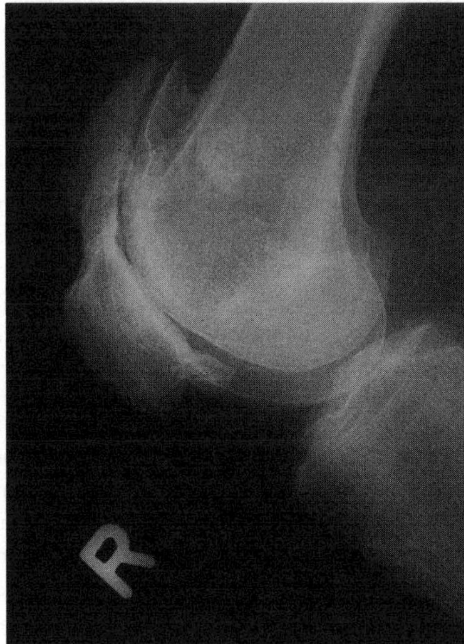

Fig. 7 Lateral knee radiograph showing predominant patellofemoral involvement by 'hypertrophic' osteoarthritis characteristic of pyrophosphate arthropathy.

1. distribution between and within joints that is atypical of osteoarthritis (for example, glenohumeral disease; isolated or predominant patellofemoral or radiocarpal involvement);
2. prominence of osteophytes and cysts; and
3. prominent osteochondral bodies

Such combined features may present a distinctive 'hypertrophic' appearance even in the absence of chondrocalcinosis (Fig. 7). In destructive arthropathy, marked cartilage and bone attrition with fragmentation and loose osseous bodies may resemble a Charcot joint.

Metabolic predisposition is rare and routine screening of all patients is unrewarding but and a search is warranted in the following circumstances:

1. early-onset arthritis (<55 years);
2. florid polyarticular chondrocalcinosis; or
3. presence of additional clinical or radiographic clues.

A reasonable screen would include serum calcium, alkaline phosphatase, magnesium, ferritin, and liver function tests.

Differential diagnosis (Table 3)

The principal differential diagnosis for pseudogout is sepsis or gout (both of which may coexist with pyrophosphate crystal deposition). Gram stain and culture of joint fluid should be undertaken even when pyrophosphate ($\pm$urate) crystals are identified. Marked blood-staining may lead to consideration of other causes of haemarthrosis (especially a bleeding disorder or subchondral fracture).

Chronic pyrophosphate arthropathy is usually readily distinguished from rheumatoid by the synovial fluid and radiographic findings, the infrequency of severe systemic upset, absence of extra articular features, and only modest acute-phase response. Proximal stiffness due to glenohumeral involvement may suggest polymyalgia rheumatica, although clinical examination and near normal ESR should exclude the diagnosis. Destructive pyrophosphate arthropathy may simulate a neuropathic joint, although such joints are severely symptomatic and neurological abnormality is absent.

Treatment

Pseudogout

As pseudogout usually affects only one or a few joints in elderly patients, local therapy is preferred. Aspiration alone often relieves symptoms, but may be combined with intra-articular steroid in florid cases. Simple analgesics and NSAIDs give additional benefit but should be used cautiously in the elderly. Joint lavage is reserved for troublesome steroid-resistant cases. Colchicine is effective but rarely warranted. Triggering illnesses (for example, chest infection) will require appropriate treatment. Rapid mobilization should be instituted once the synovitis is settling.

Chronic pyrophosphate arthropathy

There is no specific therapy, and treatment of underlying metabolic disease does not influence outcome. Aims are to reduce symptoms and maintain or improve function. This may include education of the patient in appropriate use of the affected joints, reduction in obesity, improvement of muscle strength, use of stick or other walking aid, and surgery for severe disease. Chronic synovitis may be improved by intermittent steroid injection or intra-articular radiocolloid (yttrium-90). Simple analgesics are generally preferable to NSAIDs, but both should be used with caution in older patients.

Other crystal-related disorders

Apatite-associated syndromes

Hydroxyapatite is the principal bone mineral. Apatites or basic calcium phosphates (partially carbonate-substituted hydroxyapatite, octacalcium phosphate, rarely tricalcium phosphate) are also the usual mineral to deposit in extraskeletal tissues (for example, tuberculous lesions, arteries). Abnormal calcification generally results from an elevation of the calcium phosphate product, causing widespread 'metastatic' calcification, or alteration in the balance between inhibitory and promoting tissue factors, resulting in local 'dystrophic' calcification. In rheumatic diseases abnormal deposition of calcium phosphates may occur in periarticular tissues (particularly tendon); hyaline cartilage, in association with osteoarthritis; or subcutaneous tissues and muscle, principally in connective tissue diseases. Apatite crystals are too small (5–500 nm) to be seen by light microscopy.

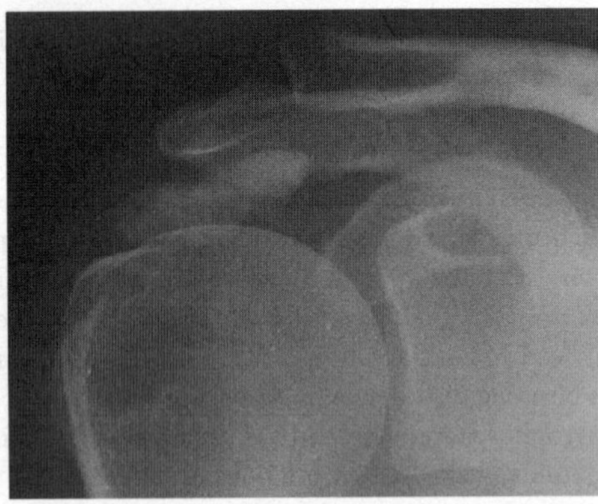

Fig. 8 Shoulder radiograph showing florid supraspinatus tendon clarification (calcific periarthritis).

Particles may aggregate, however, to form spherulites visible by light microscopy. Confirmation of basic calcium phosphates requires sophisticated analytical techniques and most diagnoses are based on radiographic calcification or non-specific staining of joint fluid or histological material.

Acute calcific periarthritis

Apatite disposition in the supraspinatus tendon (Fig. 8) is a relatively common incidental finding (about 7 per cent of adults). It occasionally results in severe acute inflammation of the subacromial bursa, periarticular tissues, or joint itself. Periarticular sites around the greater trochanter, the foot, or the hand are less commonly affected.

Acute episodes may follow local trauma or occur spontaneously. Within a few hours pain and tenderness are often extreme and the area appears swollen, hot, and red. Modest systemic upset and fever are common. Sepsis is usually considered first but the diagnosis is made following radiographic demonstration of calcification. If the lesion is aspirated, thick white fluid containing many apatite aggregates may be obtained. The condition usually resolves spontaneously over 1–3 weeks, often accompanied by radiographic dispersal of modest-sized calcifications (crystal 'shedding'). NSAIDs ameliorate symptoms and attacks can be abbreviated by aspiration and injection of steroid. Large deposits may require surgical removal. Calcific periarthritis can result from metabolic abnormality (renal failure, hyperparathyroidism, hypophosphatasia), but measurements of serum calcium, alkaline phosphatase, and creatinine are usually normal. Rare families are predisposed to calcific periarthritis at multiple sites with no evidence of altered calcium phosphate product.

Osteoarthritis and apatite-associated destructive arthritis

Modest amounts of basic calcium phosphates are commonly found in synovial fluid from osteoarthritic joints, in isolation or with calcium pyrophosphate crystals ('mixed crystal deposition'). Whether apatite plays any part in inflammatory exacerbations, or associates with severity or progression of osteoarthritis remains uncertain.

The uncommon condition 'apatite-associated destructive arthritis' is often considered a subset of osteoarthritis. It is virtually confined to elderly women and affects the hip, shoulder ('Milwaukee shoulder'), or knee. It has the general appearance of severe large joint osteoarthritis but is particularly characterized by:

1. rapid progression, often leading to severe pain and disability within a few months of onset;
2. development of marked instability;
3. large, cool, effusions;
4. an atrophic radiographic appearance with marked cartilage and bone attrition and little osteophyte or bone remodelling.

Aspirated fluid has normal viscosity and a low cell count but contains large amounts of apatite aggregates, seen readily on light microscopy following non-specific calcium staining (alizarin red, acidic pH). The differential diagnosis may include sepsis (excluded by synovial fluid culture), late avascular necrosis, or neuropathic joint. The pathogenesis of this condition remains unclear. Although apatite particles could contribute to tissue damage by stimulating release of collagenase and other proteolytic enzymes from synovial cells, it is most likely that the apatite is non-contributory and principally reflects the severity of subchondral bone attrition. The outcome is poor and inevitably requires surgical intervention.

Other apatite syndromes

Tophaceous periarticular apatite deposition may occur in patients with chronic renal failure. Apatite has also been incriminated in the occasional erosive interphalangeal arthropathy seen in such patients.

Other crystals

Cholesterol

Cholesterol crystals may induce acute synovitis, acute tenosynovitis, and chronic xanthomatous tendinitis in hypercholesterolaemic subjects. Cholesterol and other lipid crystals may also occur as a non-specific finding in chronic synovitis, most commonly due to rheumatoid arthritis: in this situation the lipid probably derives from cellular debris and its pathogenic significance is uncertain.

Oxalate

Oxalate crystals may cause acute and chronic articular and periarticular syndromes occurring in association with either primary familial oxalosis (types I and II) or secondary oxalosis (see Chapter 6.12). Chronic renal failure managed with dialysis is the commonest cause of secondary oxalosis, particularly if ascorbic acid supplementation has been given. Acute symmetrical interphalangeal and metacarpophalangeal arthritis, with or without tenosynovitis, and digital calcific deposits are the usual manifestation; large joint involvement, chondrocalcinosis, and tophaceous periarticular masses are less common. Calcium oxalate crystals may also induce life-threatening organ involvement, with peripheral vascular insufficiency and digital necrosis, myocardiopathy, peripheral neuropathy, and aplastic anaemia.

Extrinsic crystals

These are a rare cause of locomotor problems. Acute flares following intra-articular injection of corticosteroids are uncommon but may represent iatrogenic crystal-induced inflammation. Penetrating injuries involving plant thorns and sea-urchin spines may cause acute and chronic inflammatory synovitis, periostitis, or periarticular lesions which only resolve following surgical removal of the crystalline material.

Further reading

Smyth, C.J. and Holers, V.M. (ed.) (1999). *Gout, hyperuricaemia and other crystal associated arthropathies.* Marcel Decker, New York.

Schumacher, H.R. (1998). Crystals and osteoarthritis. In *Osteoarthritis* (ed. K.D. Brandt, M. Doherty, L.S. Lohmander), pp. 137–43. Oxford University Press, London.

Chapter 10.6

Back pain and periarticular disease

I. Haslock

Aches and pains in the musculoskeletal system are common features of everyday life. Each year about 40 per cent of the population develop such symptoms. Sixty per cent of these symptoms do not lead to medical consultation, but about 8 million people consult their general practitioner each year. The commonest locomotor symptom is pain in the back, with 15 per cent of the adult population reporting at least 3 days' back pain annually.

Approach to the patient with back pain

Traditional medical diagnosis aims to attribute a pathological cause to the patient's symptoms through a process based on the history, physical examination, and appropriate investigations. These three diagnostic processes are equally important in elucidating the cause of back pain, but several complicating features interfere with the simplicity of the deductive process. For example, comparisons of patients with acute back pain who consult a doctor with those who manage their own symptoms reveals no significant difference in clinical findings between the two groups. There is no agreed pathological cause for the symptoms in 85 per cent of cases, but there are large numbers of medical and non-medical specialists in the care of back pain who offer precise and superficially convincing detailed explanation and consequential therapies, which have rarely been exposed to scientific evaluation. Outcome appears to relate more to factors such as educational level and perception of illness than to diagnostic categories or treatment methods. Further complexity is added when, as is often the case, ideas about the pain being caused by an incident, accident, or occupation are present, with attendant interference from legal or compensatory processes. Attempts to dissociate these 'non-medical' factors has led to the development of an examination system which encompasses the distinction of a series of inappropriate clinical signs as well as those that might relate to an organic cause. In particular, dramatic and non-anatomical descriptions of unvarying pain accompanied by widespread superficial tenderness, lumbar pain on axial loading or simulated rotation, and jerky giving-way on motion assessment all alert the examiner to the contribution of 'illness behaviour' to the patient's symptoms.

Pathology

The behaviour of the spine is that of a flexible rod, whose function is to absorb loads and permit movement while protecting the spinal cord and emerging nerve roots. The intervertebral discs are designed to allow absorption of loads. The synovial apophyseal joints are angled so that the appropriate movement is facilitated—flexion/extension, side flexion, and rotation in the cervical spine; predominantly rotation in the dorsal spine, and predominantly flexion/extension and side flexion in the lumbar region. The normal spine posture is vertical, with cervical and lumbar lordoses and mild thoracic kyphosis; this alignment facilitating absorption of impact loads during walking and running.

The intervertebral disc comprises an outer annulus fibrosus comprising tough, obliquely arranged collagenous fibres surrounding a thick gelatinous nucleus pulposus. This provides a good shock-absorbing mechanism, which becomes less efficient with age as the nucleus becomes more fibrotic.

The apophyseal joints may be involved as part of any inflammatory polyarthritis, and are particularly important in ankylosing spondylitis. They are also prone to osteoarthritis, especially when loading is abnormal as a result of degeneration and narrowing of the adjacent disc, or in a more widespread fashion from alignment abnormalities such as scoliosis.

Spondylosis describes the association of degeneration and narrowing of the disc space with the development of osteophytic lipping at the adjacent vertebral margin. There is often secondary osteoarthritis in the associated apophyseal joints.

Prolapse of the intervertebral disc occurs when the nucleus pulposus is no longer contained within the annulus but bulges through it. Because of the increased curvature of the posterolateral border of the vertebra, prolapse takes place preferentially at this site, which is adjacent to the emerging spinal nerve roots. The force distribution throughout the spine is such that the L5–S1, then the L4–L5, discs are by far the most commonly affected, although prolapse can occur at any level. Root pressure at these sites gives rise to pain and neurological signs in the ipsilateral leg (sciatica). The second commonest site of prolapse is at the posterior margin of the disc where the extruded nucleus presses on the tightly bound posterior spinal ligament. This causes pain without lateralizing signs, and, if large, may result in cord or, more usually, cauda equina compression, leading to interference with bladder function and sphincter competence. More chronic disc protrusion associated with degeneration can lead to spinal stenosis. This causes symptoms of 'cord claudication' with pain in the legs on exertion. The canal diameter is increased by flexion, which explains the characteristic symptom that cycling is easier than walking, or that the patient bends forward in order to hurry.

The integrity of the bony spinal canal may be interrupted at the pars interarticularis, either because of a congenital defect or trauma. The resultant forward slippage of the vertebra is called spondylolisthesis.

The bony spine and its attendant articulation is surrounded by powerful muscles and ligaments, with a particularly complex ligamentous array at the junction with the pelvis. Both local and referred pain may arise from irritation of these structures, illustrated by the range of responses produced by irritation of these structures after local injection of hypertonic saline. It is assumed that a great deal of back pain arises from these structures, but the nature of the nociceptive insult, the precise attribution of symptoms to sites, and the appropriate treatment for these putative insults are all obscure.

In addition to the mechanical causes of back pain described above, the spine may be the site of infection or tumour. The classical spinal infection was tuberculosis; haematogenous spread to a disc expanded through the vertebral end plates into the two adjacent vertebrae. This led to vertebral body collapse with preservation of the posterior spinal elements resulting in severe angulation—the gibbus. Infection is now most commonly with staphylococci, with streptococci becoming increasingly important, and more exotic infections occur in the immunocompromised and in those with acquired immune deficiency syndrome. Primary malignancy may occur, but is less common than secondary, particularly from breast, bowel, and prostate. Myeloma

Table 1 Neurological signs in the legs

Nerve root	Pain and distribution	Weakness	Sensory loss	Reflexes
S1	Buttock	Eversion and plantar flexion of foot	Lateral foot	Ankle jerk diminished
	Back of thigh			
	Back of calf			
L5	Buttock	Dorsiflexion of hallux	Dorsum of foot	
	Back and side of thigh			
	Lateral calf	Eversion of foot		
L4	Lateral thigh	Inversion of foot	Medial calf	Knee jerk diminished
	Medial calf			

may present with back pain. Pain from infection and malignancy is often both severe and unvarying. Pain which lacks periodicity and association with activity, especially unremitting night pain, raises the suspicion of a sinister cause.

Acute low back pain

The majority of the estimated 23 million episodes of back pain occurring in Britain annually are acute. The sudden onset may be associated with an incident such as bending, lifting, or turning. Pain is usually in the lumbar area and often radiates to one or both legs.

In evaluating treatment, it is important to know the natural history of acute back pain. Only a minority of sufferers come to medical attention, and of those who do consult a general practitioner, 40 per cent recover each week. Thus by 3 weeks 80 per cent of acute episodes have settled, irrespective of the intervention used. A short period of rest—2 or 3 days is as effective as 2 weeks—followed by progressive resumption of activity is the treatment of choice. Paracetamol or co-dydramol provide adequate analgesia for most patients. Severe pain may require an intramuscular analgesic. Non-steroidal anti-inflammatory drugs given intramuscularly are as effective as narcotics, and avoid the risk of constipation. Where muscle spasm is severe, intramuscular diazepam is valuable.

Extensive evaluation is only needed when there is disturbance of bladder or bowel function which might indicate a massive central disc protrusion. Examination under these circumstances should include reflexes, power, and sensation in the lower limbs, including the saddle area particularly. The relevant motor and sensory signs shown in Table 1.

Persistence of acute back pain

If the pain fails to settle with simple measures, or the symptoms become more severe, a full physical evaluation is needed. The pain may present in the back, in the affected leg alone, or in both. Persistence of sciatica with resolution of the back pain deserves just as much attention as when back pain persists. The presence of a cough impulse—dysaesthesiae in the leg produced by raising the intrathecal pressure by coughing or sneezing—demands further investigation.

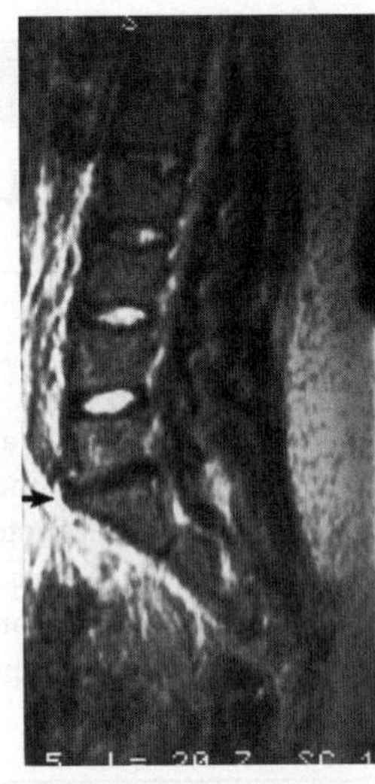

Fig. 1 MRI scan showing a degenerate L5/S1 disc.

Clinical examination

The patient must stand undressed and the spinal posture is noted. Flexion, extension, and side flexion are observed for range and symmetry. Finger–floor distance, often suggested as a measure of spinal flexion, is an inconsistent blend of spinal and hip movement, and should never be used. The patient then lies down to allow neurological examination of the legs. The most important sign to seek is restriction of straight leg raising (Lasague's sign). Although straight leg raising to 90 degrees is usually quoted as normal, not everyone can achieve this. Comparison with the contralateral side is valuable, but restriction to less than 75 degrees is almost always significant, and below 45 degrees strongly suggestive of disc prolapse. Increasing the pressure on the irritated sciatic nerve by sharply dorsiflexing the foot at the limit of straight leg raising (the sciatic stretch test) produces extra pain. Finally, there should be a general examination to look for signs that suggest infection or malignancy. This should include examination of the breasts in women and the prostate in men. Non-mechanical disease may be accompanied by severe, local spine tenderness.

Investigation

Investigation will be guided by the physical signs. Plain radiographs are rarely of value in mechanical back pain, as some degree of disc degeneration is almost universal with increasing age, and the severity of the radiological signs bears almost no relationship to the symptoms. They can, however, show major anatomical abnormalities, spondylolisthesis, vertebral collapse, or malignancies producing isolated or multiple lesions, usually destructive but occasionally sclerotic. If the history and neurological signs indicate the possibility of nerve root compression or central disc protrusion a computed tomography (CT) scan is the most generally available next investigation. Disc protrusion or other anatomical abnormalities are well shown, but nervous tissue is better shown by magnetic resonance imaging (MRI) (Fig. 1). The role of myelography is now very restricted. Some surgeons feel it gives greater pre-operative information, although good quality MRI is as valuable. Myelography may be needed where MRI is unsuitable because of extensive local metal implants or severe claustrophobia preventing its use. A raised erythrocyte sedimentation rate (ESR) or plasma viscosity, a raised white cell count, raised alkaline or acid phosphatase, and a monoclonal band on electrophoresis of plasma are all indications of serious disease. Isotope bone scanning is the most useful way of identifying infective or malignant lesions, with CT and MRI scanning providing complementary methods of delineating them, and CT-guided percutaneous biopsy providing histological material.

Chronic back pain

The proportion of patients developing chronic back pain is small, but their symptoms may last for many years, producing significant disability. They are often referred to specialists in many disciplines, undergoing many fruitless investigations. Chronicity is as much caused by social and psychological factors as by underlying pathology. Re-referral to hospital is often precipitated by events such as refusal or downgrading of benefits. The major obligation is to take a careful history to ensure no new features suggesting a new cause of pain are present, and to undertake and document a careful clinical examination. Without new guiding symptoms, reinvestigation of patients with chronic back pain is almost invariably unrewarding.

Treatment

Patients found to have non-mechanical causes for back pain, such as infection or malignancy, require treatment guided by underlying diagnosis.

Persistent acute pain

Patients with persistent mechanical back pain first require an explanation of their symptoms. Phrases such as 'spinal arthritis' should be avoided, as they imply chronicity and inevitable incapacity, and inhibit recovery. A progressive re-educative exercise regimen should be accompanied by postural correction and advice regarding lifting and work. 'Back schools' designed to convey this advice are found in a lot of physiotherapy departments, but many people fail to respond to group activities such as these. Patients should be encouraged to lose weight if obese, and take regular exercise; swimming would be ideal. Although corsets may be helpful in the short term, their long-term use should be discouraged as it tends to cause paraspinous muscle weakness.

Analgesia should be simple, non-costive, and given for the shortest possible duration. Non-steroidal anti-inflammatory drugs are often prescribed. Their use is illogical in the absence of demonstrated inflammation, but they are sometimes helpful. Manipulation often helps mobilize the patient in the early stages of treatment. Various 'schools' of manipulation appear to offer no differential advantage. Many patients have some intermittent residual back pain. Whether this is considered tolerable will depend on personality and occupation.

Patients with neurological symptoms and signs often show spontaneous recovery. Manipulation, epidural injection, and out- or in-patient traction may all be useful in settling symptoms. Surgery should only be considered where conservative treatment has failed. Discectomy can now be undertaken as a day patient or overnight stay procedure. It is particularly effective in relieving sciatica, less so in relieving back pain. Spinal stenosis may require more radical discectomy and laminectomy and spondylolisthesis may require surgical fixation especially in the young and athletic.

Chronic pain

The treatment of chronic back pain follows the same principles, but is unsatisfactory. Approaches such as the 'school of bravery' attempt to persuade the patients to 'push through' their pain and increase their physical capability. Skilled psychological input helps this approach. Very rarely surgery, usually in the form of spinal fusion, may be helpful, especially when degenerative disease has led to spinal instability. Many patients continue to be regular attendees to their family doctor, chronic consumers of analgesics, and frequent visitors to physiotherapy departments and pain clinics.

Pain in the dorsal spine

Mechanical dorsal spine pain is less common than lumbar pain, but does occur and may radiate around the chest wall. Examination of the dorsal spine is best done with the patient seated. A dorsal kyphosis is common, especially in those who bend forward at work. Fixed kyphosis accompanies osteoporosis. The 'gibbus' caused by spinal tuberculosis may be seen in some older patients, and in some patients who have had osteoporotic crush fractures. Severe local tenderness may be caused by fracture, sepsis, or malignancy. Referred pain from penetrating peptic ulcer, carcinoma of the pancreas, pancreatitis, and occasionally gallbladder disease may be felt in the dorsal region, so the history and examination must be appropriate for these conditions.

Investigations

The radiological appearances of spondylosis and of diffuse idiopathic skeletal hyperostosis are too ubiquitous to be discriminating in dorsal pain. Osteoporotic wedging or crush fractures, sepsis, or malignancy may be seen on radiography and confirmed by scintigraphy, CT, or MRI. Measurement of ESR, white cell count, and plasma alkaline phosphatase concentration also aids these diagnoses. Myeloma may produce single or multiple lesions, and plasma protein electrophoresis and urinary Bence Jones proteins should be included in the diagnostic work-up of the ill patient with dorsal pain.

Treatment

Mechanical dorsal pain is treated by posture correction, which is difficult, and active exercises. These may be enabled by mild simple analgesia. Osteoporosis with or without fracture requires appropriate treatment (see Section 12), as do malignancy and sepsis. Acute dorsal disc protrusion requiring surgery is extremely rare.

Pain in the cervical spine

Radiological changes of spondylosis are almost universal in those over 35 years, but correlate as poorly with symptoms as do similar changes in the lumbar region. Cervical pain is often associated with spasm in the trapezius, paraspinous muscles, and the muscles of the scalp. These in turn are frequently caused by poor posture, especially at work, and emotional trauma. Osteophytic lipping may occasionally impinge on surrounding structures such as the oesophagus or the vertebral vessels. Symptoms radiating to the arms are common in patients with neck pain, the dysaesthesiae often following a non-anatomical pattern. Distinct radiculopathy raises the suspicion of nerve compression by disc protrusion or impinging osteophytes. MRI is then the investigation of choice.

Treatment

This involves reassurance, especially when head pain occurs, and an exploration of physical and emotional lifestyle causes for muscle spasm. Local and general methods to induce relaxation are valuable, and the use of a soft collar at night is helpful in diminishing pain. A daytime collar is often used as a badge of disability and encourages perpetuation of symptoms. Simple analgesics or short courses of non-steroidal anti-inflammatory drugs may be helpful. Physiotherapy may help alleviate pain, but should be supplemented by a long-term home exercise and postural correction regimen.

Periarticular disorders

The shoulder

The complex interrelationships of the muscles, tendons, and bursae related to the shoulder joint, together with its wide range of movement, appear to make it particularly vulnerable to the development of pain and restriction. Unfortunately, there is considerable confusion in the nomenclature of shoulder disease, with different authorities referring to the painful restricted shoulder syndrome as capsulitis of the shoulder, periarthritis, adhesive capsulitis, frozen shoulder, rotator cuff lesion, and subacromial or subdeltoid bursitis. Subtle differences among these 'different' entities are often described but appear to be of little practical importance. However, increasing use of ultrasound examination of the shoulder is providing greater insights into local pathology and a more structured approach to treatment.

Examination of the painful shoulder usually reveals diminished abduction and rotation, both active and passive, with reversal of the normal scapulohumeral rhythm of movement. Tenderness may be related to the anterior part of the shoulder joint, the subacromial region or the posterior aspect of the shoulder. There is often muscle spasm, particularly of the upper fibres of the trapezius, leading to pain in the neck, and pain may also be referred to the deltoid muscle and the medial condyle of the elbow as well as being felt diffusely around the whole of the shoulder girdle.

Pathologically, the primary lesion appears to be tearing fibres at the insertion of the rotator cuff with secondary inflammation, both in relation to the healing fibres and in the subacromial bursa. As movement may exacerbate the pain, the limb tends to be held to the patient's side with consequent adhesion formation both within the joint and between the surrounding soft tissues structures.

Treatment is by reduction of pain, muscle spasm, and inflammation using non-steroidal anti-inflammatory agents and physical methods such as infrared radiation or ice. Thereafter the shoulder is re-mobilized, the accent being on teaching an active home exercise regimen which gradually but progressively increases the range of pain-free movement. Full relief of symptoms takes up to 2 years to accomplish and the range of movement is rarely normal after an episode of capsulitis, although an adequate functional range is usually achieved. Resolution of symptoms may be accelerated by local corticosteroid injection in the rotator cuff, the joint itself, or into the subacromial bursa. Occasionally, manipulation, either under the influence of diazepam or general anaesthesia, is used to regain movement in a recalcitrant joint.

More localized lesions occasionally form part or all of the painful stiff shoulder syndrome. A painful arc of abduction between about 45 degrees and 90 degrees can be associated with calcification in the supraspinatus tendon, the pain being related to the position in which the calcified portion is squeezed between the humeral head and the acromion. Patients with this condition can hold their arm fully elevated if it is passively moved to that position, but are inhibited from achieving elevation by the painful arc, and tend to drop the arm suddenly as the pain strikes rather than achieving smooth depression from an elevated position. Treatment is by local corticosteroid injection, ultrasound application to disrupt the calcium deposit, or, occasionally, surgical removal of the deposit.

Bicipital tendinitis is differentiated by the finding of local tenderness over the insertion of the long head of the biceps and pain on resisted flexion of the pronated forearm. Local corticosteroid infiltration into the paratendon is usually effective, but care must be exercised not to inject into the body of the tendon as this may lead to its rupture.

The elbow

Pain related to the common extensor origin on the lateral epicondyle is called tennis elbow, and the less common syndrome of pain related to the common flexor origin on the medial epicondyle is called golfer's elbow. Both of these are overuse phenomena, usually relating to easily identifiable, often sporting, activities, as their names imply. Tearing of muscle fibres near bony insertions, or pulling up of the periosteum in that area, sets off a low-grade inflammatory reaction. There is local tenderness and pain occurs when the muscles are brought into action. Ideally, the precipitating movement should be avoided and the elbow rested, but this is usually advice the patient will not, or cannot, follow. It is important in relation to all overuse injuries in sportsmen to examine the player's technique in conjunction with an experienced coach. Many such overuse injuries are the result of bad technique, and coaching to correct the technique is as important as medical treatment, for if faulty style is not eliminated recurrence is inevitable. Local corticosteroid injection is often helpful in reducing the pain, although several injections may be necessary. Both manual frictions, applied by a physiotherapist, and ultrasound have also been used effectively in these conditions. Rarely, surgery is required to achieve full symptom relief, especially where lifting of the periosteum has led to formation of a spicule of new bone which is often both palpable and visible on radiographs.

The wrist and hand

Tenosynovitis of the wrist and hand occurs as part of inflammatory disease such as rheumatoid arthritis, but may occur as a discrete entity as the result of overuse. The extreme example of this is cane-cutter's disease, a severe form of tenosynovitis of the wrist extensors suffered by sugar-cane cutters in the harvesting season. Lesser degrees of the same condition are associated with racquet sports and unaccustomed house-painting. As the thumb is, functionally, half the hand, the extensors of the thumb are particularly prone to develop overuse inflammation. Clinically the affected tendon sheath becomes painful, especially on use, tender and swollen, and exhibits soft crepitus on movement. The overlying skin is often red and warm. The thickening induced by swelling of the tendon sheath may become sufficient, especially as it becomes more chronic, to prevent smooth running of the tendon. This condition is known as stenosing tenovaginitis, or, in relation to the thumb extensors and abductors, de Quervain's disease. Treatment of simple tenosynovitis is by rest, either in a splint or a plaster cast. Resolution may be aided by injection of corticosteroid into the tendon sheath, but significant obstruction requires surgical release of the stenotic sheath.

Tenosynovitis is recognized as an occupational disease, and patients with non-specific pain in their forearms, felt during their work, often described it as 'teno' in the knowledge that this diagnosis implies compensation. Non-specific use-related pain and fatigue in the fore-arms associated with non-specific physical signs such as diffuse tenderness has been called 'repetitive strain syndrome' or sometimes 'repetitive strain injury', this latter term confirming the patients' feelings about the causation. These symptoms are common in workers making repetitive movements, especially keyboard operators. The complexity of the disease was demonstrated by the epidemic that occurred in Australia when it became recognized as an industrial disease. Many repetitive workers suffer similar symptoms, which the majority simply tolerate, and which can be relieved by minor changes in working posture or practice, including short periods of rest, in well-motivated people.

The thigh and knee

Subtrochanteric bursitis produces symptoms that are often diagnosed as hip pain. The pain is felt in the lateral side of the thigh and is exacerbated by hip movement. Examination reveals local tenderness just distal to the great trochanter, and the symptoms are relieved by local corticosteroid injection, which may need to be repeated two or three times to achieve complete resolution. This syndrome is often related to abnormalities of the gait, and these need to be eliminated to ensure persistent resolution of the symptoms.

The prepatellar bursa becomes inflamed when subjected to repeated trauma—beat knee of miners, housemaids' knee, or clergyman's knee—painful swelling distal to the lower pole of the patella. This area becomes red and oedematous and secondary infection may occur. Local injection is less effective in this site and excision is frequently required.

Ligamentous injuries to the knee are common accompaniments of sport and recreation. Pain may be accurately located at the medial or lateral side, but more diffuse pain and swelling may make differentiation from an internal derangement difficult. Local tenderness and swelling occurs, usually related to the tibial attachments of the medial or lateral ligaments, and pain may be produced on stressing the appropriate ligament by flexing the knee to about 20 degrees and then forcibly abducting or adducting the leg with the thigh fixed. Local corticosteroid injection, frictions, ultrasound, and muscle strengthening may all be effective, but sever strains require a period of immobilization in a Robert-Jones bandage, or plaster of Paris. Muscle wasting, in the quadriceps especially, takes place with extreme rapidity when the knee is immobilized. To some extent this can be prevented by isometric exercises in the plaster, but it is of great importance not to allow vigorous use of the leg, either in sport or at work, until muscle strength and bulk have been progressively restored by graded exercise, or further sprains around the knee will inevitably occur.

Fat pads related to the knee, especially the medial side, may be painful either in isolation or as part of Durcum's disease. Local treatment with pain-relieving physiotherapy methods or infiltration with local anaesthetics such as bupivacaine, sometimes mixed with Hyalase® is often effective. Intravenous infusions of lignocaine may help intractable or widespread symptoms.

The leg and ankle

The calf can be the site of sudden rupture of tendons, usually the plantaris, or of parts of gastrocnemius muscle belly. The patient feels sudden pain in the calf, with local tenderness and swelling. Plantaris rupture is of no significance and requires only an antalgesic heel raise until the pain subsides. Achilles tendon or gastrocnemius rupture requires surgical repair. The ankle is prone to sporting ligamentous injuries and also those arising from accidents such as stepping awkwardly off kerbs. The stability of the ankle joint is almost entirely dependent on the integrity of the surrounding ligaments, and minor tears in them may produce serious problems, resulting in a chronically 'weak' or unstable ankle. The ankle is also particularly prone to swelling after injury, as the hydrostatic pressure here is very high, and ligaments may be stretched or disrupted as a result of this. Strains or partial tears of the ankle ligaments should, therefore, be treated by immobilization in a tight bandage or plaster of Paris for a short period (2 or 3 days) followed by assessment of the severity of the damage and subsequent therapy aimed to reduce oedema and improve muscle tone. Post-traumatic rehabilitation with special attention to fine balancing movements, most easily stimulated by use of a wobble-board, is essential if recurrent strains are to be avoided.

The foot

Bursal lesions in the foot are common. The great toe is subject to valgus deviation, especially when ill-fitting shoes are worn which force the great toe into valgus and cause rubbing on the lateral surface of the metatarsophalangeal joint. Inflammation of the bursa at this position produces a bunion. Treatment is by prophylaxis—avoiding ill-fitting shoes—local pressure relief by padding, or surgical correction of the hallux valgus. The calcaneal bursa, between the Achilles tendon and the calcaneum, may become inflamed, often in conjunction with Achilles tendinitis. This latter condition produces heel pain and the swollen Achilles tendon sheath is easily visible and palpable and is often red. This condition usually arises as a result of overuse, and may be exacerbated or caused by local pressure. Unfortunately, the heel-tabs on running shoes which are often claimed to protect against this problem appear to be the prime cause of it. Rest and infiltration of corticosteroid into the paratendon are effective forms of treatment, but especially in sportsmen, it is important to modify the footwear to prevent recurrence. A rarer overuse condition is central core degeneration of the Achilles tendon. Here the tendon itself is swollen, and at operation is found to contain a degenerate central core which requires excision.

The longitudinal arch of the foot is maintained by the long plantar (spring) ligament. Laxity of this ligament produces a flat foot. Pain felt at the insertion of the ligament into the calcaneum occurs as part of the enthesopathy of seronegative spondylarthritis but also as an isolated, idiopathic condition. Plantar spurs may be seen on radiographs of these patients, but well-defined spurs are of no pathological significance, occurring as often in normal subjects as in patients with heel pain; in contrast, fluffy spurs are indicative of the presence of an inflammatory process. Initially, treatment is by removing impact trauma by use of sorbo heel pads. If this fails, local corticosteroid injection may be effective, although this procedure is painful. Surgery may be necessary.

Metatarsalgia, or pain felt under the metatarsal heads, is a common accompaniment of rheumatoid arthritis, but also occurs as an isolated idiopathic complaint. Overuse and inappropriate footwear are the usual precipitating causes. Treatment is by use of a metatarsal bar attached to the sole of the shoe or appropriately padded insoles. Morton's metatarsalgia is a variant of this condition caused by neuroma formation in the digital nerve at the level of the metatarsal heads. Careful examination reveals the tenderness to be located in the web space between the toes rather than under the metatarsal heads. Treatment is by local anaesthetic and corticosteroid injection or, more usually, surgical excision of the neuroma.

Generalized musculoskeletal pain

Increasing numbers of patients present with 'pain all over'. A careful history and detailed clinical examination is required to sort such patients into different categories.

Sorting out generalized musculoskeletal pain

Inflammatory joint disease may present as diffuse pain rather than localized articular symptoms. Examination reveals signs of rheumatoid arthritis, ankylosing spondylitis, or other arthritides. The symptoms of the diffuse connective tissue diseases are often rather non-specific, reflecting the generalized nature of these disorders. A careful history must be coupled with examination for features such as Raynaud's phenomenon, rashes, or vasculitis. Polymyalgia rheumatica is particularly prone to present as a rather non-specific illness with diffuse pain in older people.

Rheumatic complaints associated with general medical disorders are often characterized by diffuse aching or pain. Thyroid disorder, both hyper- and hypothyroidism, and diabetes are particularly prone to present in this way. Metabolic bone disease may cause diffuse pain, although it should be noted that osteoporosis, even when severe, is not intrinsically painful, and should not be blamed for pain in the absence of fractures.

Although many patients assume all their musculoskeletal symptoms have a simple common cause, this is often not the case. Soft-tissue rheumatic disorders are very common, and they coincide commonly. They also coincide with common articular disease such as osteoarthritis or spondylosis. A careful history and examination might, for example, reveal that a patient with pain 'from head to toe' has got cervical spondylosis to explain his neck and shoulder pain, tennis elbow causing symptoms in one arm and carpal tunnel syndrome in the other, trochanteric bursitis causing thigh pain, and flat feet producing chronic aching in the feet and ankles. Such combinations are not rare, and the individual components should be treated individually rather than by the blanket diagnosis 'rheumatism'—or even worse—'arthritis'—being followed by the unthinking prescription of a non-steroidal anti-inflammatory drug.

Increasingly, 'pain all over' is attributed to the group of syndromes variously called postviral fatigue syndrome, fibromyalgia, or myofascial pain syndrome, which in some aspects blends into myalgic encephalomyelitis. This group of syndromes is characterized by severe diffuse pain, morning stiffness, subjective swelling, especially in the hands, incapacitating fatigue, and often severe resultant disability. They are occasionally preceded by a viral infection. The only significant physical finding is of multiple tender spots in muscles and ligaments. There is an association with irritable bowel syndrome and tension headaches, and many patients have psychological disturbance, particularly depression. Despite many theories of causation, the aetiology of these conditions remains obscure. Treatment is unsatisfactory, the only helpful therapies appearing to be antidepressants coupled with a progressive exercise programme aimed at improving aerobic fitness and improving function. This group of diseases is unique in that membership of the relevant patient's association appears to produce a worse prognosis.

Further reading

Bennett, R. (1998). Fibromyalgia, chronic fatigue syndrome, and myofascial pain. *Current Opinion in Rheumatology*, **10**, 95–103.

Burton, A.K. and Waddell, G. (1998). Clinical guidelines in the management of low back pain. *Baillière's Clinical Rheumatology*, **12.1**, 17–35.

Doherty, M., Hazleman, B.L., Hutton, C.W., Maddison, P.J., and Perry, J.D. (1992). *Rheumatology examination and injection techniques.* W.B. Saunders, London.

Palmer, K., Coggon, D., Cooper, C., and Doherty, M. (1998). Work related upper limb disorders: getting down to specifics. *Annals of the Rheumatic Diseases*, 57, 445–6.

Peterfy, C.G. (1998). Imaging techniques. In *Rheumatology* (2nd edn), (ed. J.H. Klippel and P.A. Dieppe), pp. 14.1–14.18. Mosby, London.

Chapter 10.7

Septic arthritis

M. H. Seifert

Many different organisms can cause septic arthritis, including bacteria, fungi, viruses, and spirochaetes.

Bacterial arthritis

Pathogenesis

Joints become infected most often by haematogenous spread of microorganisms from a remote site or less commonly, as a result of direct penetration by instrumentation or trauma. Once in the joint the organism multiplies in the synovium and can usually be recovered from the synovial fluid or synovium itself. The resultant pathophysiological sequence is the same for all bacterial infections in joints. The synovial membrane is extremely vascular and the microorganisms soon migrate from the vascular compartment into the interstitial space where the reaction to the infection varies markedly, depending on the amount and type of organism present, its virulence, and the host's defence mechanisms. The bacteria multiply and set off a cascade of inflammation in the synovium and synovial fluid. Proteolytic enzymes are released by activated polymorphonuclear leucocytes and these destroy the articular cartilage first by altering the proteolycan matrix and then destroying the collagen superstructure, with resultant deformation of cartilage. With the increase in synovial fluid the intra-articular pressure rises. Other synovial tissues, such as bursae and tendon sheaths, also suffer from this inflammatory damage, but it is the destruction of articular cartilage that causes the most serious sequelae to septic arthritis, and dictates the urgency of treatment (Table 1). The septic stage must be halted urgently prior to collagen loss and chondroycte death to prevent cartilage destruction and joint damage.

Predisposing causes

Although previously more common in young children, joint sepsis is now found increasingly in the elderly and in those with chronic illness such as malignancy, diabetes, alcoholism, or anaemia. Intravenous drug abusers and immunosuppressed patients are also predisposed to septic arthritis. Chronic joint disease due to rheumatoid arthritis, crystal synovitis, trauma, or surgery also increases the risk of infection (Table 2).

Infecting organisms

A wide variety of bacteria can cause septic arthritis, but some particular organisms have varying predilection for different age groups and

Table 1 Sequence of joint destruction in bacterial arthritis

1. Synovial membrane hypertrophy (a) Infiltration by polymorphonuclear cells (PMNs) (b) Release from PMNs of proteolytic enzymes (c) Activation of lining cells (d) Cartilage erosions by membrane proliferation
2. Synovial fluid accumulates Pressure necrosis of cartilage
3. Articular cartilage destruction (enzymatic and bacterial) (a) Proteoglycan depletion (b) Collagen degradation
4. Bone involvement

Table 2 Predisposing causes of non-gonococcal bacterial arthritis

Systemic disease
Chronic liver disease
Diabetes mellitus
Cancer
Chronic renal disease
Sickle-cell anaemia
Systemic lupus erythematosus
Chronic arthritis, joint trauma
Rheumatoid arthritis
Trauma, arthroscopy, joint replacement
Gout
Systemic immunosuppressive medications
Intravenous drug abuse
Infection with the human immunodeficiency virus

predisposing causes. For example, *Staphylococcus aureus* is more likely to be found in the septic joints of children aged between 2 and 15 years and the elderly, than *Haemophilus influenzae*, which is more likely to be encountered in children under 2 years of age. In rheumatoid arthritis *Staphylococcus aureus* is the likely cause of secondary infection, while in acute leukaemia a Gram-negative bacillus is most common. In the years of sexual activity *Neisseria gonorrhoeae* is the likely cause, and infections of joints due to streptococci and Gram-negative organisms, such as enterobacteria and *Pseudomonas aeruginosa*, can occur at any age. Specific clinical pictures are recognized to be associated with particular organisms, including brucella, gonococci, and meningococci (see Section 16).

Clinical features

The onset is generally abrupt with the development of severe pain and inflammation over a few days. Weight-bearing joints, particularly the knee, are most commonly involved in adults. Less common are the small joints of the hands and feet. Although usually monoarticular, polyarticular involvement is well recognized, particularly with streptococcal infections. Most patients have a fever, although it can be low grade or absent; rigors are not common unless there is bacteraemia. Movement of the involved joint is painful and restricted and examination reveals swelling, heat, and joint tenderness, sometimes, but not always, with erythema of the overlying skin.

Differential diagnosis

Acute arthritic disorders such as gout, pseudogout, palindromic rheumatism, rheumatic fever, or trauma with haemarthrosis may be confused with infectious arthritis. Systemic symptoms such as fever or chills and marked leucocytosis are, however, uncommon or less marked in these conditions. Pre-existing joint disease such as rheumatoid arthritis may cause difficulty in recognizing the development of a septic joint. Any patient with rheumatoid arthritis who has a joint that is inappropriately swollen and hot should be suspected of having developed sepsis in that joint, and whenever there is this possibility the joint must be aspirated promptly.

Bacterial and joint fluid examination

After a complete medical and physical examination, paying particular attention to potential portals of entry of infection, such as the skin, nasal passages, middle ear, lungs, rectum, urethra, and pelvis, it is essential for the joint to be aspirated. This is of vital diagnostic value but also removes debris and destructive enzymes and relieves pain by reducing the joint pressure. The laboratory should be warned that the aspiration is to be performed in order that the fluid may be inoculated into appropriate culture media while still warm. Samples of fluid should be placed in sterile tubes for culture and into heparinized containers for cell counting. The fluid should also be examined under polarized light microscopy for crystals of gout or pseudogout. Infected synovial fluid usually appears purulent and thick with a high white cell count of predominantly polymorphonuclear leucocytes, but occasionally the fluid is not obviously purulent and there may be only modest increases in the cell count. The fluid should be Gram stained and inoculated into appropriate media.

Other potential sites of infection should be sought, and culture from skin, nasopharynx, sputum, urine, and stool obtained routinely. At least two blood cultures for aerobic and anaerobic organisms should be obtained. These may yield positive results when culture of synovial fluid is negative. Cerebrospinal fluid should be cultured when clinically indicated. Occasionally, all these cultures are negative despite joint sepsis, especially if antimicrobial treatment has been initiated prior to joint aspiration.

Radiological examination

Early in the course of infection radiographs of the affected joint are normal or show only the changes of soft tissue swelling and the presence of effusions. Films at this stage are useful, however, to compare with later ones which characteristically reveal juxta-articular osteoporosis, followed by joint space narrowing resulting from destruction of articular cartilage. Vertebral bone and disc destruction can occur within weeks of infection. Sacroiliac joint infection is predominantly unilateral. Radioisotope scanning using either gallium or technetium is particularly useful in detecting sepsis in deep joints such as the hip, shoulder, and spine, as are computed tomography or magnetic resonance imaging (MRI), especially where there is suspicion of osteomyelitis. MRI has been shown to detect the early changes in infected joints, especially in cartilage.

Treatment

General

A septic joint is extremely painful and the natural reluctance of the patient to move it should be respected. A splint helps to reduce pain and, by immobilization, to control inflammation. This should be only a temporary measure and physiotherapy must be started early to prevent stiffness, contractures, and muscle wasting. Pain is relieved by aspirating as much synovial fluid as possible, daily or more frequently if the fluid reaccumulates rapidly. When this is a persistent problem, it is helpful to wash out the joint with physiological saline. It is sometimes difficult in shoulder and hip joints to eliminate sepsis, particularly when there are loculated pockets of fluid; then it may be necessary to establish open surgical drainage, a procedure which should always be considered in the absence of clinical or laboratory signs of improvement despite 4–7 days of adequate antimicrobial therapy. Consultation from the outset with an infectious disease specialist and an orthopaedic surgeon is invaluable in planning treatment.

Antimicrobial treatment

This should be initiated as soon as the diagnosis of septic arthritis is made, and even before the infecting organism has been identified. A preliminary estimate of the type of micro-organism can be made on the result of the initial Gram stain smear of the synovial fluid. Parenteral antimicrobials should be continued for at least 7–14 days, and because some Gram negative and staphylococcal infections are slow to respond, it is often necessary to continue for 4–6 weeks. Parenteral administration of antimicrobials provides maximal serum and synovial fluid concentrations, and there is no indication for intra-articular injections, which can cause a chemical synovitis and may even introduce further infection. Improvement is indicated by a decrease in the frequency of the need for joint aspiration and the return to normal of the joint fluid. A progress chart recording temperature, the volume and content of aspirated fluid, the results of repeated Gram stains, and the antimicrobial prescribed is helpful in assessing the response to therapy.

Suppurative arthritis, sometimes monoarticular, is a rare feature of brucellosis and of infection with *N. gonorrhoeae* or *N. meningitidis.*

Arthritis due to mycobacteria and fungi

Mycobacterial and fungal arthritis are characterized by a slowly progressive evolution of symptoms and signs. Constitutional symptoms may be few, and extra-articular involvement absent. It is therefore not surprising to find a long delay between the onset of symptoms such as pain and the final diagnosis. Patients with unexplained chronic monoarthritis or with spondylitis and chronic tendinitis with erythema nodosum should be considered as potentially infected.

Tuberculous arthritis

Although there has been a steady decline until recently in the prevalence of tuberculosis in advanced countries, there is a huge morbidity and mortality in the developing world, and the disease is being seen more frequently in accultured societies. The disease has changed from being one of children and young adults to one that affects all ages. In the UK, tuberculosis is particularly common among Asian immigrants, often with atypical presentation. Rheumatological presentations include tendon sheath involvement and dactylitis, but half the cases of skeletal tuberculosis occur in the spine, while the rest involve the hip, knee, ankle, and wrist. There is often an absence of active pulmonary disease, although in 40 per cent there is radiological evidence of previous infection. The most frequent symptom is pain on movement, and gross synovial proliferation with effusion is a common sign. Predisposing trauma may have been noticed, and there is an association with debilitating diseases, alcoholism, drug addiction, and acquired immune deficiency syndrome. The tuberculin skin test is usually positive and this should be included in the investigation of any unexplained monoarthropathy. Radiological features of skeletal tuberculosis are not pathognomonic. Soft-tissue swelling and diffuse osteoporosis of the bone appear early. Later cystic lesions develop initially adjacent to joints with little periosteal reaction. The joint space tends to be preserved until gross adjacent cortical bone destruction has developed. There is no osteophyte formation.

Spinal tuberculosis (Pott's disease)

Fifty per cent of skeletal tuberculosis occurs in the spine, often in the absence of pulmonary or extrapulmonary disease. The lower thoracolumbar area is most often involved. Infection typically starts at the margin of adjacent vertebral bodies and invades the disc spaces early. These spaces narrow with vertebral collapse and consequential kyphosis or gibbus formation. Cold paraspinous abscesses may develop and dissect along the spine, causing multiple sites of destruction with skip areas in the vertebral column and ribs, and pointing in the neck, groin, or chest wall. There is overlying muscle spasm, nerve root irritation, and spinal cord involvement in 10–25 per cent of patients.

Peripheral tuberculous arthritis

This is usually monoarticular, and the hip is a common site. In children the initial complaints are of pain in the groin with a limp and the hip held in flexion and abduction when at rest. Later, destruction of the femoral neck and acetabulum occurs with the appearance of a cold abscess pointing to the outer thigh. In the knee and other peripheral joints pain is the prominent symptom, with synovial swelling and warmth. The majority of patients have both bone and synovial infection. Non-specific symptoms of low-grade fever and weight loss frequently occur, but florid reactions such as high fever, night sweats, malaise, and anorexia are limited to patients with concomitant pulmonary or miliary tuberculosis.

Synovial fluid findings include elevated protein and, in 50 per cent, a low sugar content. There is a polymorphonuclear leucocytosis in the blood and the white cell count varies widely. In 80 per cent of cases synovial fluid cultures are positive but a higher yield is obtained by culturing synovial biopsy tissue. In 90 per cent of cases caseating granulomas and acid-fast bacilli are found on microscopic examination.

Treatment

There is debate about the number and choice of drugs to use and the duration of treatment, although all would agree the need for at least two drugs. One favoured regimen is the combination of isoniazid, ethambutol, and rifampicin, at least for the first 6–8 weeks. Overall, treatment should continue for 18–24 months and should be adjusted in the light of the sensitivity of the organism. Surgical intervention has been recommended to clean infected synovium and to deal with a spinal abscess, to secure an unstable spine, or to provide material for culture and sensitivity testing.

Atypical mycobacterial arthritis

A heterogeneous group of organisms usually having a low pathogenicity for humans, shares some of the characteristics of infection with *Mycobacterium tuberculosis.* Pulmonary and joint disease is indistinguishable from that produced by the tubercle bacillus. The pathological lesions are also similar and diagnosis depends on the isolation of the organism and analysis of growth characteristics and biochemical and serological properties. Previous joint disease and compromise of immune defences predispose to these infections. Treatment may prove difficult and resistance to antituberculous drugs results in more recourse to surgical intervention than with *M. tuberculosis* infection. The problem of drug resistance by these organisms dictates that a number of drugs must be used in combination before sensitivity data are available.

Fungal arthritis

Fungi invade bone locally to cause septic arthritis and only rarely is fungal arthritis the result of haematogenous spread. Diagnosis usually requires synovial biopsy, because culture from synovial fluid is difficult and serological tests are disappointing. Synovial fluid changes are non-specific. A chronic joint destruction occurs. Radiologically, the lesions resemble other forms of granulomatous infection, such as tuberculosis.

Coccidioidomycosis

Coccidioides immitis infection is endemic in the south-western United States and Mexico. Following inhalation, in one-third of previously fit patients there is a transient arthralgia with erythema nodosum, fever, and malaise. Within a month all symptoms resolve without residual arthritis. Dissemination occurs in a small percentage of patients, and of these, 20 per cent have bone and joint involvement. The affected joints are ankles, knees, and, less commonly, the feet and wrists. The chronically infected joint has a thick, grey synovial membrane with serous or purulent fluid and often a discharging sinus. Diagnosis, often delayed, is made by identification of the organisms in the synovium or by culture from these tissues. Treatment is by surgical synovectomy and intravenous amphotericin B. Intra-articular amphotericin B has also been used.

Blastomycosis

Blastomyces dermatitidis is endemic in the Mississippi and Ohio River basins. The fungus gains entry through the lungs, causing a mild flu-like illness, but in some cases more florid pulmonary and cutaneous lesions develop. Up to 50 per cent of patients systemically infected also develop bone and joint lesions. Most of the joint infection is from osteomyelitic spread, although primary arthritis without bone disease also occurs. Joints commonly involved are the ribs, vertebrae, long bones, and skull. Because the organisms are so numerous, synovial fluid examination frequently reveals the yeast-like organisms. Treatment is with amphotericin B.

Sporotrichosis ('rose grower's arthritis)

Penetration of the skin by a thorn or other plant material carrying *Sporothrix schenckii* may result in the development of cutaneous sporotrichosis. Rarely, there is a systemic infection secondary to the cutaneous lesions, and in 8 per cent of these an arthritis develops. Large joints are most frequently involved, although other joints and tendon sheaths can also be infected. Delay in diagnosis averages 2 years and can result in irreversible joint damage. Cultures of synovial fluid and tissue yield *Sporothrix*. Serological tests may be suggestive but not diagnostic. Treatment is with intravenous or intra-articular amphotericin B.

Candidiasis

This is now perhaps the most common fungal arthritis in the UK, due to an increased incidence of systemic candidiasis in the compromised host. Nevertheless, bone and joint infection is rare. The knee is the most frequently involved joint and usually the adjacent bone is infected. Treatment is with amphotericin B, accompanied by appropriate measures to improve immunological defences whenever possible.

Viral arthritis

A number of viral infections can be associated with later development of arthritis; these include hepatitis B, rubella, parvovirus, group A arboviruses, mumps, varicella zoster, and vaccinia.

Hepatitis B

Arthritis occurs in approximately 50 per cent of people infected with hepatitis B, often together with a skin rash and the prodromal features of the infection. There is a sudden onset of arthritis which is usually polyarticular and symmetrical with involvement characteristically of the small joints of the hands. These joint symptoms last for a few weeks and are often associated with tendinitis. Fifty per cent of patients with arthritis also develop a pruritic urticarial rash on the legs. These features have disappeared by the time jaundice develops. During the prodrome, surface antigen (**HBsAg**) is present in the blood in excess over antibody (**anti-HB**) and immune complexes containing both these are present, together with depressed C4 and CH50 serum complement levels. With resolution of the arthritis there is disappearance of HBsAg, normalization of complement, and increase of anti-HB. Tests for HBsAg are positive in both blood and synovial fluid during the arthritic phase, but become negative as the arthritis resolves and the tests for anti-HB become positive. There are few other significant haematological abnormalities and synovial fluid analysis is also unrewarding. The arthritis is helped by salicylates and varies in duration from a few days to several weeks.

Rubella

In naturally acquired rubella infection, arthritis is extremely common. Ninety per cent of women infected with the virus develop a symmetrical polyarthritis affecting the small joints of the hands, wrists, and knees in a distribution similar to that of rheumatoid arthritis. The arthritis is self-limiting and rarely lasts more than 3 weeks. As well as the characteristic morbilliform rash and lymphadenopathy, a carpal tunnel syndrome may develop. Tests for rheumatoid factor may be positive and the virus has been isolated from synovial fluid. Rubella virus has also been isolated from the synovial fluid of some patients with an inflammatory polyarthritis in the absence of clinical evidence of rubella and it has been suggested that some form of rubella infection may be the primary pathogenic event in the aetiology of the chronic arthritis in these patients.

Parvovirus

The parvovirus (PV) demonstrated to cause disease in humans is PV B-19 and at least 30 per cent of adults in Great Britain have antibodies to it by the age of 16. PV B-19 is associated with an acute and chronic arthropathy in adults with either clinical or inapparent infections. Common features of this complication in adults include a symmetrical polyarthropathy involving small joints of hands, wrists, and knees. Prodromal symptoms are reported in under half the cases, when an

IgM and IgG response to B-19 can be measured. Adult females are more frequently affected in a ratio of 4:1. Within 2–8 weeks joint symptoms resolve, but occasionally persistent disease develops.

Arboviruses

The most common manifestations of arboviral diseases are fever, arthritis, or arthralgia, and rash. The three main arbovirus infections causing arthritis are epidemic polyarthritis of Australia, Chikungunya, and O'nyong-nyong.

Epidemic polyarthritis of Australia

This is caused by the Ross River virus and transmission to humans is via the mosquito. Outbreaks have been reported in New South Wales, and the north and south of eastern Australia. An incubation period of 10 days is followed by fever, malaise, myalgia, and 2 days later an urticarial rash which is associated with lymphadenopathy and arthritis. Young adult women are more frequently affected and the small joints of the hands, ankles, and wrists are involved. A maculopapular rash often develops on the trunk, fading after a week. There are no specific investigations and the Ross River virus has only been isolated once from the blood of a patient. The arthritis clears after 2 or 3 weeks, sometimes longer, and aspirin gives partial relief of symptoms.

Chikungunya (Swahili for 'he who walks doubled up')

This epidemic infectious arthritis occurs in wide areas of Africa, southern India, and southern Asia. There is acute onset of fever, chills, and arthritis involving the knees, wrists, fingers, and lumbar spine. The arthritis lasts from 5 to 7 days and sometimes recurs for months. A maculopapular rash develops on the trunk or extremities and follows the arthritis by 4 or 5 days. The chikungunya virus can be recovered from blood within 3 days of the onset of symptoms, but its recovery from synovial fluid has never been reported. Aspirin and non-steroidal anti-inflammatory drugs help the symptoms.

O'nyong-nyong ('joint breaker')

This virus is transmitted by mosquitoes and results in a disease characterized by the acute onset of fever with severe joint pains, headaches, rash, and lymphadenopathy. Epidemics occur in East Africa and have the added complication of conjunctivitis and eye pain. The virus is similar to that of chikungunya and has been isolated from the blood of only a few patients.

Arthritis associated with miscellaneous viruses

Mumps

Arthritis in young adult males is well recognized and occurs 10 days after the onset of parotitis. The arthritis is migratory and lasts for 2 weeks, leaving no residual joint damage.

Chicken-pox

Characteristic swelling and heat in the knees occurs very rarely a few days after the typical vesicular rash. The arthritis resolves after a few weeks. The virus has never been recovered from the synovial fluid.

Infectious mononucleosis

Arthritis rarely occurs in patients with infectious mononucleosis. Large joints are involved and the arthritis settles within a week.

Retroviruses

Some patients infected with human immunodeficiency virus, have been shown to have a polyarthritis. Although this is likely to be a reactive arthritis, the virus has been isolated from synovial fluid in infected patients.

Arthritis due to spirochaetal infections

Syphilitic arthritis

Bone and adjacent joints can be affected in both congenital and acquired treponemal infection, but this is rare. Congenital syphilis can present in the first weeks of life as osteochondritis or epiphysitis with pseudo-paralysis of a limb and para-articular swelling. Eventual complete fracture of the epiphysis may occur. From the age of 8 to 16 painless effusions of the knees can develop (Clutton's joints). These may be confused with an inflammatory polyarthritis, although there is little pain or loss of function. Mild stigmata of congenital syphilis, such as interstitial keratitis, Hutchinson's teeth, or nerve deafness may be present, and synovial biopsy shows lesions suggestive of microgummata. Acquired syphilis presents in its secondary stage with arthralgia and arthritis. As well as back pain, large joints are involved and painful effusions occur in the knees. Tenosynovitis and periostitis are common, and the latter can be identified on bone scan. Other stigmata of secondary syphilis such as rash, mucous plaques, alopecia, and lymphadenopathy should also be sought. In tertiary syphilis it is common to find periostitis of the tibia and the clavicle. The ossification that follows produces a characteristic lacy pattern of the bone. Joint disease results from the spread of gummatous infiltration from the bone. Charcot (neuropathic) joints associated with tabetic lesions usually present as a monoarthropathy. There is progressive enlargement, effusion, and instability of the painless joint with marked crepitus. The knee is the most frequent site, followed by the hip and the ankle. Serological tests for syphilis are strongly positive in all patients in these latter two stages of the disease.

Lyme disease

Lyme disease is a tick-borne, immune-mediated inflammatory disease caused by the spirochaete *Borrelia burgdorferi*. A characteristic rash of erythema chronicum migrans has been reported in 25 per cent of patients prior to the development of the arthritis. Joint manifestations occur in approximately half the patients, mostly affecting the knees. This initially lasts for 1 week but recurrent attacks may follow. In a small minority chronic arthritis develops years after the initial manifestations of Lyme disease. Immune complexes and cryoglobulins have been detected in both serum and synovial fluid. The erythrocyte sedimentation rate is frequently elevated.

Penicillin clears the skin disease and shortens the duration of arthritis. Non-steroidal anti-inflammatory drugs and intra-articular steroids also help. Other manifestations of the disease and their management are discussed in Chapter 16.67.

Further reading

Kaandorp, C.J., Krijnen, P., Moens, H.J., *et al.* (1997). The outcome of bacterial arthritis: a prospective community based study. *Arthritis and Rheumatism*, 40, 884–92.

Ryan, M.J., Kavanagh, R., Wall, P.G., and Hazelman, B.L. (1997). Bacterial joint infections in England and Wales: analysis of bacterial isolates over a four year period. *British Journal of Rheumatology*, 36, 370–3.

Sack, K. (1997). Monoarthritis: differential diagnosis. *American Journal of Medicine*, 102 (1A), 30S–4S.

Chapter 10.8

Miscellaneous conditions

B. Hazleman

Joint symptoms may be either the presenting feature, or major component of many conditions. Some of the less well recognized associations are described below.

Dermatological disorders

Acne arthralgia and arthritis

Severe acne may be associated with myalgias, arthralgia, and non-septic joint effusions. Large joints are usually involved. Most reported cases have been in young males. There is a tendency for improvement with resolution of the acne. The arthritis associated with acne resembles psoriatic arthritis or rheumatoid arthritis. These patients have severe acne, palmar and plantar pustules, hyperostotic reactions (particularly in the clavicles and sternum), sacroiliitis, and peripheral inflammatory arthritis.

Erythema nodosum

Joint manifestations occur in about 75 per cent of patients with erythema nodosum. Arthralgia is more common than synovitis and can precede the appearance of skin lesions. A symmetrical synovitis occurs in one-third of patients, usually involving the knees and ankles, but can involve wrists, elbows, small joints of the hands, and shoulders. The affected joints are painful, tender, and stiff, with synovial thickening and effusion. The presence of erythema nodosum around the ankles may be confused with involvement of these joints, because of the redness and swelling with pain and stiffness on movement which arise from the skin and subcutaneous lesions. The synovitis is self-limiting and non-erosive. Anti-inflammatory drugs usually provide effective relief, but corticosteroid therapy may be necessary.

Haemangioma of synovium

True haemangiomas of the synovium or joint capsule are rare and most are associated with soft-tissue vascular abnormalities, particularly arteriovenous malformations or skin vascular lesions. The most common symptoms include unilateral intermittent joint pain and enlargement with subsequent limitation of movement. Therapy for a localized haemangioma of the joint is excision of the tumour. However, those lesions associated with soft-tissue vascular malformations may recur due to the extensive vascular abnormalities. Radiation therapy has been advocated in such cases, with mixed results.

Pyoderma gangrenosum

This painful, non-infective, ulcerating skin lesion may be associated with ulcerative colitis, rheumatoid arthritis, a para-proteinaemia, or occur without an identifiable underlying disorder. A seronegative, progressive, symmetrical erosive polyarthritis has been described, and about 30 per cent of patients have arthralgia or arthritis. The arthritis may develop before and is unrelated to the activity of the skin lesion. It is unlike rheumatoid arthritis in that joints involved include the first carpometacarpal and terminal interphalangeal joints, in addition to the elbows, temporomandibular joints, and cervical spine. Depressed complement levels in synovial fluid suggest immune complex deposition, but skin histology does not reveal arteritis or immune complex deposition.

Sweet's syndrome

The characteristic tender, red or purple, discrete skin plaques are associated with myalgias, arthralgias, or non-inflammatory joint effusions, manifestations which usually resolve over 2–3 months. Sjögren's syndrome and a facial rash have been reported to coincide in some cases, causing confusion with systemic lupus erythematosus.

Endocrine and metabolic disorders

Amyloid arthropathy (see also Chapter 6.15)

Articular involvement has been described most frequently in cases of myeloma associated amyloidosis, and is also present in primary generalized amyloidosis. In most instances, the associated monoclonal protein is either a κ Bence Jones protein or an intact immunoglobulin with a κ light chain. Arthropathy is not a significant feature of secondary (AA) amyloidosis nor of familial amyloidosis.

Amyloid arthritis can mimic a number of rheumatic diseases, presenting as it does with a symmetrical peripheral arthritis associated with nodules, morning stiffness, and fatigue. Small and large joint involvement can occur. The initial symptoms of pain and stiffness are associated later with soft-tissue flexion contractures of the hands. The joints are often swollen, firm, and occasionally mildly tender, but without redness or severe tenderness. The shoulder may be prominently involved, giving the appearance of a 'padded shoulder'. Subcutaneous nodules are present in 70 per cent of patients. An associated carpal tunnel syndrome is often present; amyloidosis should always be excluded in cases of apparently idiopathic carpal tunnel syndrome occurring in middle-aged and elderly men, by histopathological examination of tissue removed at operation.

Synovial fluid analysis usually reveals a non-inflammatory fluid but staining of sediment by Congo red and examination under polarized light may reveal amyloid deposits in fragments of synovial villi. Radiographs show osteoporosis or lytic lesions, but erosions are rare. Large deposits in bone simulate neoplasms.

Hyperlipoproteinaemia and joint symptoms

Type II hyperlipoproteinaemia may cause a migratory polyarthritis affecting small and large peripheral joints which resembles rheumatic fever. Xanthomas may produce tendon nodules and involve bone with the formation of peri-articular bone cysts. In type IV hyperlipoproteinaemia the onset of musculoskeletal symptoms occurs later than those in type II, most usually in the early forties. The most frequent joint complaints are of morning stiffness, pain on movement, or joint tenderness. There is little evidence of joint inflammation, despite the intensity of joint pain.

Hyperparathyroidism

This may present with musculoskeletal complaints. Arthralgia then usually affects hands, wrists, and, when persistent, is an indication for parathyroidectomy. Muscle weakness and pain may also be a prominent feature, affecting over 50 per cent of patients; improvement can follow parathyroidectomy. Arthropathy may be due to subchondral bone lesions due to bone disease with loss of the integrity of the subchondral plate. Other causes include associated gout and pseudogout with chondrocalcinosis. The mechanism by which chondrocalcinosis occurs in primary hyperparathyroidism is not understood. Osteitis fibrosa cystica usually manifests as bone pain, but is declining in frequency with earlier diagnosis.

Ochronosis (see Section 6)

In ochronosis or alkaptonuria, homogentisic acid accumulates in cartilage, causing it to become leathery and rigid, and thus prone to rapid degeneration. This affects the spinal joints in particular, the disc spaces becoming thin and ragged. Any peripheral joint may also be affected and severe disability may result. The diagnosis is usually obvious, homogentisic acid appearing in the urine causing it to go black on exposure to the light or on alkanization. The deposits in the cartilage of the ear or in the sclera also become blackened when exposed to light. The treatment is that of osteoarthrosis, but in the absence of the capacity to correct the underlying metabolic abnormality it is largely ineffective.

Wilson's disease (see Chapter 6.10)

Chondrocalcinosis occurs, as does bone fragmentation at the joint margins, with irregularity and sclerosis of the underlying bone. Osteochondritis and chondromalacia patellae have also been described.

The pathogenesis of the arthropathy is not understood, although copper inhibits pyrophosphatase. Joint manifestations do not correlate with other features of the disease. A lupus-like syndrome with an inflammatory polyarthritis is a known but rare accompaniment of penicillamine therapy.

Gastroenterological disorders

Coeliac disease

Well-recognized musculoskeletal manifestations of coeliac disease include metabolic bone disease, muscle weakness, and a seronegative arthritis which improves on a gluten-free diet. The variant pattern of arthritis affecting the hip, knee, and shoulder most frequently makes identification difficult, particularly as 50 per cent of patients have no bowel symptoms. Malaise, weight loss, and a low serum folate are useful clinical pointers.

Hepatic disorders and arthritis

Polyarthritis or arthralgia occurs in 25 per cent of patients with chronic active hepatitis. An acute self-limiting arthritis affecting large joints is described with viral hepatitis, and about 4 per cent of patients with alcoholic cirrhosis suffer from arthropathy during their illness. An erosive inflammatory arthritis commonly accompanies primary biliary cirrhosis. The arthritis is non-deforming and usually asymptomatic. The erosions are symmetrical and involve the distal small joints of the hands. Bone lesions similar to those seen in hyperlipoproteinaemia have been described and tend to be periarticular rather than true joint lesions.

Haematological disorders

Anaphylactoid (Henoch–Schönlein) purpura

This syndrome can present predominantly with arthritis, particularly in children. In general the joint involvement is mild, consisting of transient, non-migratory synovitis with synovial swelling, pain, and stiffness, usually affecting more than one joint. The ankles, knees, hips, wrists, and elbows are usually affected, with a tendency to lower limb involvement. The synovial fluid is inflammatory in character. Joint destruction does not occur. The disease usually settles in 4–6 weeks without sequelae, but may recur.

Coagulation defects

Acute haemarthrosis is the most constant feature of severe haemophilia and, in the majority, preceding trauma does not occur. The incidence an severity of haemarthrosis are closely related to the severity of the coagulation defect in this disease and in Christmas disease. Joint bleeding usually begins before the age of 5 years and tends to recur repeatedly during childhood, after which it becomes less frequent. The preponderance of knee, elbow, and ankle bleeds over those into other joints is pronounced, and is presumably because these are hinge articulations, subject to angulatory and rotatory strain. Haemarthroses tend to occur in cycles, perhaps because of associated hypertrophy and vascularity of the synovial membrane. If haemarthrosis is not treated early or adequately, it will progress with synovial proliferation and atrophy of surrounding muscles.

In acute haemarthrosis the joint becomes hot, painful, swollen, and very tender, often with preceding sensations of prickling, increased warmth, and stiffness in the joint. Pain is the most disabling complaint and is due to a local irritant effect of blood and also to joint distension. The joint is usually held in flexion to a degree in which the volume of the joint is maximal and the intrascapular pressure minimal.

Immediate treatment is indicated comprising clotting factor replacement and immobilization. Prompt replacement therapy alone is sufficient in the majority. Pain is relieved by splinting and analgesics when necessary. Joint aspiration may be required if the haemarthrosis is under tension.

Permanent joint damage depends upon the frequency of bleeding into a joint and the length of time that blood remains there. The end-stages of haemophilic arthropathy have features in common with both degenerative joint disease and long-standing rheumatoid arthritis. Joint function is lost and motion is severely restricted. There is often an associated flexion deformity, and subluxation, joint laxity, and alignment abnormalities are not uncommon. Hyperaemia of epiphyseal plates with resultant irregular overgrowth and periarticular fibrosis, both contribute to the deformity and loss of function. Once chronic joint changes have developed, treatment depends of physiotherapy, orthotic appliances, corrective plasters/traction, and reconstructive surgery.

Haemochromatosis

The patient with haemochromatosis who develops arthritis is nearly always a man over the age of 50. Although other features of the disease usually antedate arthritis, it can occasionally be the presenting complaint, when the first symptoms are usually in the second and third metacarpophalangeal joints, becoming more severe in the dominant hand. Early, there is minor pain on flexion of the fingers, with bony swelling of the involved joints, as in degenerative arthritis. Later, other small joints in both hands may be involved, with bony swelling and deformity, but ulnar deviation does not occur. In a few patients more severe progressive changes take place, especially in the hip joints. Superimposed on this slowly progressive degenerative joint disease there may be attacks of acute synovitis due to pyrophosphate arthropathy. This usually involves the knees, but can involve several joints at the same time, leading to a mistaken diagnosis of rheumatoid arthritis.

The earliest radiological change is the appearance of small cysts in the metacarpal heads; prominent cystic changes can be seen in the carpal bones. In the shoulder, subchondral sclerosis occurs, and in the hips cystic changes with loss of cartilage. The most striking change is that of chondrocalcinosis affecting the knee most commonly; extra-articular sites of calcification include the tendo Achilles, the ligamentum flavum, and intervertebral discs.

Calcification in articular cartilage in the intervertebral disc is due to deposition of calcium pyrophosphate dihydrate. Iron and haemosiderin can be found in the chondrocytes and synovium of untreated cases. The mechanism by which the arthritis occurs is unknown. A direct relationship with iron overload is supported by reports of identical joint lesions in secondary haemochromatosis. Pyrophosphatase inhibition by the metal ions has been cited as a possible mechanism, but does not explain the distribution of the joint changes, with a predilection for the metacarpophalangeal joints, which differs from that seen in other types of chondrocalcinosis. Venesection is disappointingly ineffective in influencing the arthritis.

Haemoglobinopathies

Sickle-cell disease is by far the most common haemoglobinopathy to produce rheumatic symptoms, but they are seen also in patients with sickle-C haemoglobin, sickle-thalassaemia, and sickle-F haemoglobin. Expansion of the bone marrow occurs in all haemoglobinopathies associated with haemolysis but, except when secondary mechanical problems have developed, these changes are asymptomatic. Gout and hyperuricaemia occur in about 40 per cent of adults with sickle-cell disease. Patients with sickle-cell disease are susceptible to bacterial infections or osteomyelitis or, less frequently, septic arthritis. The bone pains in sickle-cell crises are due largely to infarction. Aseptic necrosis of the head of the femur is the most disabling complication. Similar aseptic necrosis occurs at the humeral head, tibial condyles, and occasionally other sites, these lesions may also complicate thalassaemia. Joint effusions involving the knee and resulting from infarction of the synovium usually occur during crises and are far more common that either gout or septic arthritis.

Hypogammaglobulinaemia

Primary hypogammaglobulinaemia is associated with a non-erosive inflammatory synovitis in 10–30 per cent of patients. It resembles rheumatoid arthritis with symmetrical pain, stiffness, tenderness, and synovial swelling occurring in the small and medium-sized peripheral joints. The synovitis can be transient or persist for many years with continuing tenderness and effusion. Little evidence of permanent joint damage is seen. Subcutaneous nodules are occasionally found. The histology of synovium and subcutaneous nodules differs from that of rheumatoid arthritis, in that plasma cells are absent. Tests for rheumatoid factor are negative. Patients with hypogammaglobulinaemia are also prone to develop septic arthritis.

Leukaemia

Joint symptoms include symmetrical or occasionally migratory polyarthritis, arthralgias, and bone pain and tenderness. Sixty per cent of patients with lymphocytic leukaemia have joint symptoms, usually involving large peripheral joints. Acute lymphoblastic leukaemia in young children can mimic Still's disease with fever, lymphadenopathy, and splenomegaly. An acute suppurative arthritis or haemarthrosis can occur; but aching in the limbs is more common due to subperiosteal infiltration. Joint symptoms with a leukaemoid reaction in young children with infections, lymphoma, or neuroblastoma, may cause diagnostic confusion.

Lymphoma

Bone pain is a common symptom. Synovial reaction is rarely caused by direct invasion; but is most often associated with adjacent bone disease.

Serum sickness

A generalized polyarthritis may occur some 2–16 days after the therapeutic injection of foreign serum accompanied by fever, rash, and headache. There may be transient proteinuria. These patients should be treated with antihistamines or corticosteroids.

Neoplastic disorders

The polyarthritis of carcinoma

A polyarthritis resembling rheumatoid arthritis may be presenting manifestation of malignancy, particularly in elderly men. Although most often confused with rheumatoid disease, it has been mistaken for adult Still's disease when associated with unexplained fever. Improvement of the joint symptoms parallels the successful treatment of the underlying tumour, and recurrence of the joint symptoms is associated with re-appearance of the tumour. Arthritis is most common in patients with carcinoma of the bronchus, prostate, or breast. Other rheumatic disorders that may be complications of malignancy include polymyositis, secondary gout, necrotizing vasculitis, systemic sclerosis, and a syndrome resembling polymyalgia rheumatica.

Hypertrophic osteoarthropathy

This syndrome consists of chronic proliferative periostitis of the long bones, clubbing of the fingers or toes, or both, and oligo- or polyarticular synovitis. It can be primary or secondary. Diseases associated with it are usually neoplastic, inflammatory, or infectious, involving the pulmonary, cardiovascular, gastrointestinal, or hepatobiliary systems. Most cases relate to intrathoracic disease, particularly lung neoplasia. The reported incidence in primary lung tumours varies from less than 1 per cent to 10 per cent, and is seen less in small-cell carcinomas. The cause is uncertain. A circulating vasodilator normally inactivated by the lungs may be involved. Relief of symptoms as well as signs may be achieved by vagotomy.

Neurological disorders

Algodystrophy (reflex sympathetic dystrophy)—Sudeck's atrophy

Algodystrophy describes a condition characterized by pain, vasomotor disturbance, and tophic changes usually affecting part, or the whole, of a limb. There are many synonyms, including some that refer to the autonomic features, such as reflex neurovascular atrophy. In other synonyms, for instance Sudeck's atrophy and regional migratory osteolysis, the radiological changes are highlighted. The common association with trauma is emphasized by the term post-traumatic dystrophy. Involvement in particular locations has led to the use of terms such as shoulder–hand syndrome and transient osteoporosis of the hip. This confusing army of terminologies represents an attempt to describe a disorder that is poorly understood and that represents a spectrum of acute, subacute, and chronic clinical manifestations, some of which may be atypical and of varying severity.

Typical features include burning pain, hyperaesthesiae, vasomotor changes, hyperihidrosis, and trophic changes. It can occur at all ages, in females more than males, and its incidence probably increases with age until late middle-age. The condition frequently follows an injury, but in up to 50 per cent of cases there may be no identifiable precipitating cause. Metabolic changes, such as occur in pregnancy, diabetes, and hyperlipidaemia, may contribute to the disorder. Essentially, the diagnosis is a clinical one. Severity of pain out of proportion to the preceding injury and its persistence is characteristic.

Physiotherapy aimed at restoring movement and function, and hence desensitizing abnormal reflex changes, remains the main treatment. When identifiable, the underlying disorder should be treated. Physical therapy alone may be effective, but pain can make patient co-operation difficult. Analgesics may help but further measures are frequently required. Sympathetic blockade is the best way of suppressing the sympathetic hyperactivity, but multiple blocks are often required and the effect may be short-lived. Stellate ganglion or lumbar sympathetic chain blockade is achieved by infiltration with a long-acting anaesthetic such as bupivacaine hydrochloride. Guanethidine can be incorporated into an intravenous regional Bier block. These techniques are likely to be most effective given early and combined with an active intensive rehabilitation programme. Early treatment is most successful, before reflex patterns, tissue changes, and any (common) psychological response to chronic pain become relatively fixed. Algodystrophy was originally described as a self-limiting condition but in many cases it persists for years, sometimes with major disability.

Neuropathic joints: synonym, Charcot's joints

Loss of joint sensation renders that joint liable to develop a gross osteoarthrosis with prolific new bone formation and marked instability (Charcot's joints). The condition is seen in association with tabes dorsalis, syringomyelia, and diabetes mellitus, but may also occur in association with paraplegia. Charcot–Marie–Tooth disease, myelomeningocele, and leprosy. An associated pyrophosphate arthropathy leads to inflammation. The joints are usually painless, although the diabetic tarsal neuropathic joint may be painful and present a clinical and radiological appearance suggestive of sepsis.

Renal disorders

Renal transplantation and haemodialysis

Joint disorders occurring in patients given renal replacement therapy include septic arthritis, acute episodic synovitis, and acute calcific periarthritis. In those receiving renal transplants, a transient synovitis may develop in the early postoperative period. Avascular necrosis affecting the head of the femur or lower femoral condyle is a later complication.

Disorders of uncertain aetiology

Recurrent polyserositis (familial Mediterranean fever) (see Chapter 6.16)

The joint symptoms consist of episodic, recurrent attacks of synovitis marked by pain and swelling of the joint. Although less frequent than the attacks of serositis, they are experienced by 75 per cent of the patients, and, in one-third, they are the presenting feature. In some patients they may be the only feature for years, in other they dominate the clinical picture because of their severity and resulting incapacity. Protracted attacks persisting for months sometimes occur. The joints most commonly affected are the knees, ankles, and hips; occasionally more than one joint is involved and recurrent attacks usually involve the site affected originally. Fluid from the affected joint shows a high polymorphonuclear cell count and is sterile.

One of the typical features of the disease is the propensity for recovery of the joints after what appears to have been a potentially damaging arthritis. There is no treatment available to abort an attack once it has started and complete bed rest and anti-inflammatory drugs, including corticosteroids, provide no demonstrable effect. Colchicine therapy prevents attacks.

Multicentric reticulohistiocytosis

This is a rare systemic disease of unknown aetiology, with a large number of synonyms. It is characterized by an infiltration of lipid-laden histiocytes and multinucleated giant cells into various tissues. The onset of the disease is usually insidious, with almost two-thirds presenting with a polyarthritis. Skin nodules may precede the arthritis or appear concurrently. Middle-aged females are most commonly affected. Rapid development of a severe incapacitating, deforming arthritis is well recognized. The interphalangeal joints are most frequently involved but other joints, including the spine, may be affected. In contrast to rheumatoid arthritis, the distal interphalangeal joints are commonly involved. Radiographs show 'punched out' bone lesions in the early stages, followed later by severe destructive changes.

Nodules appear most frequently on the face and hands, but can occur in any part of the body. They can range in number from a few to hundreds, and are light copper to reddish-brown in colour. Mucosal surfaces are also frequently involved. Associated malignant disease has been reported in 20–30 per cent of patients. There is no satisfactory treatment.

Pigmented villonodular synovitis

This is a hyperplastic overproduction of the synovial tissue of the joints, tendon sheaths, bursae, or the fibrous tissue adjacent to the tendons. It may present in the diffuse villous or villonodular form or in the localized nodular form. The localized nodular form is found almost exclusively in the tendon sheaths and peritendinous tissue. The diffuse villous and the localized nodular form are found with equal frequency in the joints. Paratendinous localized nodular synovitis (usually in the hand) is frequent, whereas diffuse villonodular synovitis is rare. It is usually found in adults with a maximum incidence between 20 and 40 years of age.

In localized nodular tenosynovitis the patient complains of a nodule in relation to a tendon sheath. It is generally not painful and is never greater than 3 cm in diameter. It causes pain only when it becomes enlarged and compresses surrounding structures, or after trauma. Impairment of tendon function is usually mild and late in the course. The histological findings of crowded and confluent nodules of yellow to brown colour are unmistakable.

The symptoms of diffuse villonodular synovitis are initially mild but long in duration. Often the diagnosis is made years after the onset of symptoms. The principal symptoms are diffuse synovial thickening, mostly confined to the knee, with recurrent effusions. The synovial fluid is often brown in colour, and the synovium itself is also brown, a feature which distinguishes it from all other conditions. The synovial membrane is greatly thickened, with long villi and numerous nodules. Macrophages from affected joints contain haemosiderin pigment.

Surgical excision of the localized nodular form is not associated with recurrence, but in the diffuse villonodular forms complete surgical excision is difficult or impossible. An yttrium synovectomy is often the first line of therapy, and radiotherapy is sometimes used to complement surgery. It is not clear whether these treatments reduce the incidence of relapse.

Sarcoidosis

Arthritis is the most frequent rheumatological manifestation of sarcoidosis, occurring in up to 37 per cent of patients. It is three times more common in females. An acute onset is most common. Frequently associated with erythema nodosum and hilar lymphadenopathy, the synovitis is symmetrical, migratory, and most frequently affects the knees and ankles, proximal interphalangeal joints, wrists, and elbows; monoarthritis is unusual. The arthritis reaches maximal intensity with 3 days and may last from 2 weeks to 4 months. Joint deformity and destruction does not occur.

Chronic sarcoid arthritis may occur at any time in the course of the disease and may occur with acute exacerbations over a period of years. This is more common in those of African ancestry and is usually accompanied by other signs of sarcoidosis. Biopsy of synovial membrane may reveal granulomas. Radiological changes appear late, and therefore are of limited diagnostic value. The joint space may become narrowed, and mottled rarefactions and multiple 'punched out' cystic lesions can be seen in the metacarpals and phalanges.

Acute synovitis responds to salicylates or, if necessary, corticosteroids. The response to corticosteroid therapy in the chronic group is poor.

Tietze's syndrome and costochondritis

Both these disorders are characterized by inflammation of one or more costal cartilages at the costochondral junction, but the less common Tietze's syndrome is associated with local swelling while costochondritis is not. The cause is unknown; violent coughing and direct trauma are suspected of playing a part; although there is often no history of trauma. Patients of all ages can be affected. In Tietze's syndrome one or more tender lumps of the upper costal cartilages gradually develop. A single costal cartilage is involved in 80 per cent of patients, the second and third being most affected. Deep breathing and coughing may produce local pain. The lumps are firm and somewhat tender, but not warm. The onset of pain may be acute or insidious. Investigations show no evidence of a generalized disorder, and only non-specific minor inflammatory changes are found on biopsy. The course is variable; there may be spontaneous remission, or painless lumps may persist for years. If the pain is troublesome, local injections of lignocaine and/or corticosteroid preparations may give relief.

The diffuse nature of costochondritis and its occurrence in an older age group make it more likely that it will be confused with visceral pain. Costochondritis is too diffuse to inject but anti-inflammatory drugs are often effective. These syndromes should not be confused with sepsis or rheumatoid arthritis involving the manubriosternal joint.

Chapter 10.9

Connective tissue disorders and vasculitis: an introduction

C. M. Black and D. G. I. Scott

The spectrum of diseases

The connective tissue diseases comprise a group of syndromes of unknown aetiology affecting as many as 1 person in 40, often with a predilection for the female sex. Included are systemic lupus erythematosus, polymyositis and dermatomyositis, Sjögren's syndrome, scleroderma, overlap syndromes, and the vasculitides.

These disorders have in common evidence for an autoimmune pathogenesis, which in most instances is linked to the major histocompatibility locus HLA-DR. Several can be precipitated or mimicked by exposure to drugs or chemicals in the environment, as in drug-induced lupus or scleroderma-like illnesses. A high level of suspicion may be necessary in order to recognize these diseases, particularly in their evolutionary stages. The symptoms and signs are often diffuse and involve several systems, for example arthralgias, myalgias, breathlessness, chest pains, headaches, malaise, weight loss, dry eyes and mouth, nasal discharge, fever, skin rashes, and hair loss.

The autoantibody profile may add considerable weight to the clinical features, but it must be remembered that a low titre of antinuclear antibody is found in a small percentage of the normal population (1–2 per cent) and is found more frequently in older people; that some antibodies, such as U1–RNP, are found in more than one connective tissue disease and p-ANCA (antineutrophil cytoplasmic antibody) is found in more than one form of vasculitis.

Many patients (perhaps some 20 per cent of cases) do not fit easily into one disease entity: these may have true overlap syndromes, most common are scleroderma/systemic lupus erythematosus, scleroderma/polymyositis, and systemic lupus erythematosus/rheumatoid overlaps; or they have insufficient features for an established diagnosis, in which case the term undifferentiated connective tissue syndrome is a more accurate description of the clinical state. Attempts to classify these diseases are also complicated by the fact that many of them are heterogeneous and contain several subsets.

Immunopathogenesis

Recent findings in immunogenetics and the identification of disease-specific antibodies show promise for identifying specific biochemical and biological markers which are strongly linked to disease, part of a disease or a process within the disease. The products of several major histocompatibility complex (MHC) genes appear to play an important part and some are associated with multiple HLA antigens. Systemic lupus erythematosus is associated with a null allele at C4A (poor prevention of amino-rich immune complex formation and dissolution) and with MHC class II antigens (often on the same A1, B8, C4Q0, DR3, DR52, DQ2 haplotype). Mixed connective tissue disease, in contrast, has a strong single antibody type association (to the message and/or protein for RNP) and a strong single MHC class II association with an HLA-DR4 subgroup epitope (also shared with HLA-DR2).

All these diseases have associations with genetic polymorphisms in the MHC region. In general, there are MHC class II associations with the production of IgG autoantibodies. It is not known how these antibodies relate to pathogenesis but they do help in subset definition. The presence of IgG antibodies and the known role of MHC class II in peptide presentation to CD4 T cells support an important role for helper T cells in these diseases. Several of the strategies for immune intervention in connective tissue disorders utilize agents that affect the proportion of CD4 cells.

The triggers that initiate the connective tissue diseases are still poorly understood but may represent a genetically determined host response to external factors. Scleroderma, for instance, is associated with the use of solvents and other chemicals, whereas drugs of various kinds can induce both systemic lupus erythematosus and scleroderma.

The mechanisms by which autoimmune processes cause damage are numerous, ranging from antibody and immune-complex-mediated injury, to damage orchestrated by activated T cells, monocytes, macrophages, or mast cells, either directly or through their products, such as cytokines.

General clinical considerations

Connective tissue diseases present to a variety of clinicians, most commonly rheumatologists, nephrologists, or dermatologists, but not uncommonly to neurologists, infectious disease physicians, haematologists, chest physicians, or cardiologists; sometimes the major clinical features determine a surgical referral. Increasing specialization in medicine may hinder early diagnosis, sometimes with serious or fatal consequences.

Urgent problems

When faced with a patient with possible connective tissue disease, it may be more important to assess the severity of the disorder and the specific organ dysfunction involved than to try to find a diagnostic label. This is particularly so when delay in treatment leads to serious and irreversible morbidity or death. Some presentations constitute a medical emergency. Chief among those for the nephrologist is rapidly progressive glomerulonephritis (systemic lupus erythematosus, polyarteritis, Wegener's granulomatosis) associated or not with lung haemorrhage; or the scleroderma renal crisis. For the neurologist, urgent presentations include fits, disturbed consciousness level, focal neurological signs, and occasionally acute transverse myelitis. Myocardial infarction can be the result of vasculitic illnesses; pericarditis can produce tamponade; and acute myocarditis may induce complex arrhythmias or severe heart failure. Pneumonitis due to systemic lupus erythematosus can be life-threatening if unrecognized and treated only with antimicrobials. Acute venous or arterial thrombosis complicating the antiphospholipid antibody syndrome can affect any organ, whereas polyarteritis affecting gut vasculature can result in an 'acute abdomen'. In all these conditions prompt treatment is essential; too often physicians hesitate to treat because of a lack of certainty in diagnosis.

Diagnosis

In 'classical' cases there is no difficulty, but clinical features are not always characteristic, and many change with time. Laboratory investigations sometimes conflict with clinical features, and vice versa. When a connective tissue disorder is suspected, it is common to use the presence or absence of an antinuclear antibody or extractable nuclear antigen as a screening test. Although this is a satisfactory approach in many cases, the result must not be assessed without close consideration of all the other clinical and laboratory findings. The type of staining of antinuclear antibodies, although not specific, often gives a clue to the diagnosis (Table 1). Extractable nuclear antibodies also have some common associations with specific diseases (Table 2). Anti-Scl-70 is one of the most specific of these in its association with diffuse cutaneous scleroderma, and anticentromere antibodies correlate best with benign limited scleroderma and the **CREST** (Calcinosis, Raynaud's phenomenon, oEsophageal involvement, Sclerodactyly, and Telangiectasia) syndrome.

One variety of the antineutrophil cytoplasmic antibody (c-ANCA) is relatively closely associated with Wegener's granuloma, but the p-ANCA is much less specific and has been found in microscopic polyarteritis, idiopathic crescentic glomerulonephritis, and a variety of other vasculitic syndromes, including Churg–Strauss syndrome, adult Henoch–Schönlein purpura, and the vasculitis of rheumatoid arthritis.

Table 1 Antinuclear antibodies

Staining pattern	Clinical association
Homogeneous	SLE
Rim	SLE
Speckled	Overlap syndromes, Sjögren's
Nucleolar	Scleroderma

SLE, systemic lupus erythematosus.

Table 2 Common antibodies seen in connective tissue diseases

Antibody	Disease
Anti-dsDNA	SLE
Anti-Sm	SLE
Anti-U_1RNP	SLE, overlap syndrome (MCTD)
Anti-Ro	SLE, Sjögren's
Anti-La	SLE, Sjögren's
Anticentromere	Limited cutaneous scleroderma (CREST)
Anti-Scl-70	Diffuse cutaneous scleroderma
Anti-Jo-1	Polymyositis, lung involvement
c-ANCA	Wegener's granulomatosis
p-ANCA	Microscopic PAN, other vasculitides
Anticardiolipin	SLE with thrombosis, miscarriages, etc.

ANCA, antineutrophil cytoplasmic antibody; MCTD, mixed connective tissue disease; PAN, polyarteritis nodosa; SLE, systemic lupus erythematosus.

Chapter 10.10

Vasculitis

C. M. Lockwood*

The primary systemic vasculitides are characterized by the presence of inflammation and necrosis of the blood vessels themselves, with disease outside the vasculature being subordinate to this. As such they are distinct from the secondary forms of vasculitis, which arise in the context of other pathology, for example close to a necrotic tumour or downstream from an abscess cavity. According to the site and size of vessel involved, a number of eponymously defined primary vasculitic syndromes have been recognized. Difficulties with classification have arisen, leading to different terminologies being used for the same vasculitides in Europe and the United States (see OTM3, pp. 3010–11). The simple classification used here is largely a morphological one, based on the size of vessel involved and the presence or absence of granulomas near the vasculitic lesions (Table 1).

Consensus has now been reached that the term 'microscopic polyangiitis' should be used to indicate that a venulitis and capillaritis may be present, as well as inflammation of small arteries, in those conditions previously described as microscopic polyarteritis or hypersensitivity angiitis. Polyarteritis nodosa and microscopic polyangiitis are now identified as separate syndromes and other small vessel vasculitides have emerged as entities, based largely on the pattern of organ involvement and, to a varying extent, distinctive associated pathology. Thus Henoch–Schönlein purpura is characterized by its gastrointestinal, kidney, joint, and skin symptomatology, with distinctive IgA deposition in kidney, gut, and skin; Wegener's granulomatosis by the granulomatous involvement of the upper respiratory tract, lungs, and kidneys; and Churg–Strauss syndrome by its asthma and peripheral eosinophilia. Most recently, Kawasaki disease has been recognized as a childhood vasculitis in which aneurysmal dilation of affected medium-sized arteries, particularly the coronary vessels, can have substantial clinical and pathological consequences.

The vasculitides can be divided into those involving the small vessels and the large-vessel vasculitides. The reasons for this segregation are twofold: first, there is growing evidence that autoimmune mechanisms may play an important part in the pathogenesis of small-vessel vasculitis, and, second, that similar therapeutic strategies may be useful in their management.

Table 1 Classification of the systemic vasculitides

	With granulomas	Without granulomas
Large vessel	Takayasu's disease Giant cell arteritis	
Medium vessel		Polyarteritis nodosa Kawasaki disease
Small vessel	Wegener's granulomatosis	Microscopic polyangiitis
	Churg–Strauss syndrome	Henoch–Schönlein purpura

*It is with regret that we report the death of Dr. C. M. Lockwood in 1999.

With the availability of new diagnostic tests, the prevalence of small vessel vasculitis can now be appreciated. Based on clinical criteria, together with the serological identification of their associated specific circulating autoantibodies, an overall incidence rate of small vessel vasculitis of 40 per million has been derived from general population studies. This is almost certainly an underestimate, firstly, because patients with biopsy proven vasculitis do not necessarily completely fulfil all the clinical criteria, and secondly, because patients with their wide ranging manifestations of vasculitis, may present to any medical discipline, not just that performing the study. An annual incidence of 100 per million seems more likely, of which Wegener's granulomatosis forms the largest diagnostic category.

Aetiology and pathogenesis

The aetiology of the small-vessel vasculitides is poorly understood. A genetic predisposition, viral or bacterial infectious agents, as well as abnormal responses to drugs, have been suggested as important factors. A weak genetic linkage of systemic vasculitis with DQQw7 has been reported but not yet confirmed by other studies. Hepatitis B infection has been associated with polyarteritis nodosa and the virus identified in both circulating immune complexes and vasculitic lesions, although whether, because of the infectious load, the virus is deposited ubiquitously in any immune complex has yet to be determined. That environmental factors, such as microbial pathogens, may be important is suggested by the seasonal incidence of vasculitis, with a peak in winter in the North American population. However, whether these environmental factors are initiators or amplifiers of injury is uncertain as, for example, there is a well-documented association of vasculitis relapse after episodes of intercurrent infection. Better evidence supports the role of drugs in producing vasculitis. Both hydralazine and propylthiouracil have been reported to cause a clinical vasculitis characterized by the associated development of autoantibodies to neutrophil cytoplasmic antigens. Withdrawal of the drugs was accompanied by disappearance of the vasculitic lesions. Experimental models indicate a predisposing role for genetic factors and an exacerbating one for accompanying infection.

Antineutrophil cytoplasmic antibodies in systemic vasculitis

A major advance in understanding of the small-vessel vasculitides has come with the identification of antineutrophil cytoplasmic antibodies (ANCAs) in a variety of vasculitic syndromes. They can be found in the majority of untreated patients with Wegener's granulomatosis, microscopic polyangiitis, and Kawasaki disease, as well as to a variable extent in Churg–Strauss syndrome and polyarteritis nodosa. Their immunochemical properties and pathophysiological effects have led to the belief that they are important in pathogenesis.

Initially these autoantibodies were characterized by the pattern of indirect immunofluorescence which was produced when sera from patients were overlaid on to immobilized normal human polymorphonuclear leucocytes. Two binding specificities were recognized: the first a cytoplasmic granule immunofluorescence with an interlobular accentuation (c-ANCA) and the second a perinuclear (p-ANCA) pattern. Subsequently, the molecular nature of the ligands was identified, the target of c-ANCA being proteinase 3, those giving p-ANCA comprising a number of different molecules, including myeloperoxidase (the most frequent) as well as elastase, lysozyme, lactoferrin, and cathepsin G. Clinical correlation has shown that antiproteinase 3 antibodies are closely associated with the development of Wegener's granulomatosis. However, although antimyeloperoxidase antibodies are associated with the development of microscopic polyangiitis, the association is not as close as that for antiproteinase 3 antibodies and Wegener's granulomatosis: antimyeloperoxidase antibodies have been described in a number of conditions, particularly chronic inflammatory gastrointestinal lesions, such as sclerosing cholangitis, chronic active hepatitis, ulcerative colitis, and Crohn's disease. In none of these is a primary vasculitis a dominant component. Furthermore, conditions indistinguishable from microscopic polyangiitis have been described in association with ANCA with specificity for elastase, cathepsin G, and lactoferrin. When indirect immunofluorescence was the only diagnostic test available, false-positive ANCA tests were occasionally recorded in acquired immunodeficiency syndrome and other chronic infections, such as infective endocarditis, but such false-positives have not been substantiated using molecularly defined antigens.

Levels of ANCA have been shown to correlate with disease activity, and have been used by some as a guide to management. Nevertheless, there are certain patients in whom high ANCA levels persist, despite little evidence of disease activity and there are others in whom vasculitis activity continues in the absence of detectable ANCA. Thus rising titres of ANCA should be viewed with caution and only to alert the physician to extra vigilance and readiness to treat early.

Antineutrophil cytoplasmic antibodies in pathogenesis

ANCA can stimulate polymorphonuclear leucocytes directly, by binding to membrane-expressed proteinase 3 and myeloperoxidase. Neutrophil adhesion is increased through upregulation of the expression of the adhesion molecule CD18 and eventual activation brings about the release of injurious oxygen free radicals. Thus the neutrophil may mediate endothelial cell injury and so initiate vasculitis. Other work has focused on the ability of cytokines, particularly tumour necrosis factor, to orchestrate the expression of proteinase 3 on the surface of the endothelial cell. This ligand is then the target for ANCA-mediated cytolysis. Another school of thought has suggested that ANCA may inhibit the complexing of neutrophil enzymes with their physiological inactivators, such as α_1-antitrypsin.

Wegener's granulomatosis

Wegener's granulomatosis is a necrotizing granulomatous vasculitis which involves both the upper and lower respiratory tracts. Typically this is accompanied by a small-vessel vasculitis affecting the kidney, and to a variable extent by a vasculitis in other organs. Circulating autoantibodies to neutrophil cytoplasmic antigens, usually to proteinase 3, can be found in most untreated patients at presentation.

Clinical presentation

Most patients have a background of non-specific symptoms such as malaise, weight loss, fever, and night sweats together into a rise in erythrocyte sedimentation rate (ESR) and C-reactive protein. The disease has an equal sex incidence and no ethnic group is exempt. The course is variable; some patients have indolent disease which takes months or years to declare itself, during which long periods occur when the patient is relatively symptom-free; others develop fulminating life-threatening organ failure within weeks. Because any organ may be involved, the patient may be seen first by a wide range of specialists, so that a varying spectrum of clinical involvement may be reported. However, with the predilection of the vasculitis to affect the airways, usually respiratory-tract symptoms and signs predominate.

Upper respiratory tract

Bloody, foul-smelling nasal discharge, paranasal sinus pain, nasal ulceration, and septal perforation as well as eventually a saddle nose deformity, may be present. Involvement includes the development of chronic suppurative otitis media, due to Eustachian tube blockage and occasionally painless deafness, due to eighth nerve involvement. Hoarseness or stridor may also be a feature due to granulomas developing on the vocal chords or vasculitis in the trachea producing tracheal stenosis, respectively. Granulomatous space-occupying lesions in the sinuses may erode locally, leading to fistula formation, and bacterial superinfection may be a significant clinical problem wherever the mucosal epithelium is breached.

Lower respiratory tract and lungs

Chronic non-productive cough, dyspnoea, pleurisy, and haemoptysis may all reflect vasculitic injury and or development of granulomas in the airways or lung parenchyma. Occasionally, formation of exuberant endobronchial granulomatous tissue can occlude the airway and lead to segmental collapse, or more rarely an obliterative bronchiolitis may spread, sleeve-like along the bronchi or bronchioles. The extension of this into the alveolar spaces, either as a capillaritis or as a necrotizing granulomatous pneumonic process, may bring about a rapid deterioration in pulmonary function and is an ominous development. The characteristic picture on chest radiograph is of nodules or larger masses which may cavitate and are often misdiagnosed as tuberculosis or malignancy. Transient pulmonary infiltrates or more permanent changes of pulmonary fibrosis may also be found.

Renal involvement

The disease causes a glomerulonephritis which may present quietly with proteinuria and haematuria. Renal biopsy at this stage may only show a minor focal proliferative glomerulonephritis. The tempo of the renal disease is unpredictable and sudden deterioration in renal function, in the presence of red cell casts in the urine, may indicate the development of an acute focal necrotizing glomerular capillaritis with crescent formation and the clinical cause of rapidly progressive renal failure. Capillaritis may also be found in the peritubular vessels when the histological picture is that of a granulomatous tubulo-interstitial nephritis.

The eye

Conjunctivitis, uveitis, and scleritis all occur in Wegener's disease, but the finding of proptosis, due to retro-orbital development of granulomatous vasculitis forming a pseudotumour, is a rare but important manifestation.

Other manifestations

Most patients experience generalized myalgias and arthralgias at some stage in the disease; less frequently a symmetrical polyarthritis may develop. Occasionally, the arthritis may be restricted to one or few joints. Joint deformity is not a feature. A variety of lesions can be found in the skin. These may vary from nailfold infarcts and purpuric rashes to isolated ulcers, vesicles and papules. Biopsy occasionally discloses granulomas typical of Wegener's disease. Mononeuritis multiplex is the commonest neurological lesion but occasionally, central nervous system abnormalities are found, including meningeal involvement and stroke. Involvement of the heart is rare, but pericarditis and coronary arteritis have been reported, as well as arrhythmias attributed to granulomas in the conducting tissues. Very rarely,

Wegener's granulomatosis has been described in the breast, ureter, vagina, cervix, and parotid gland.

'Limited' Wegener's granulomatosis is the term given to the condition where there is only restricted involvement evident clinically, and in most patients it describes disease limited to the upper respiratory tract. Sometimes this situation may persist for many years before progression to other organ involvement occurs; occasionally subclinical disease is only discovered at autopsy. There was an impression that limited Wegener's disease ran a more benign course and was easier to treat, but milder forms of the generalized disease also exist and so the prognostic and therapeutic distinction is no longer evident.

Diagnosis

The diagnosis may be suspected clinically from the combination of upper or lower airways disease, renal involvement and malaise, fever, night sweats, and weight loss. Histological evidence of a typical granulomatous vasculitis is often hard to obtain in life. Usually the kidney provides the most suitable tissue, although transbronchial biopsies are also useful. In the kidney the diagnostic requirement is the demonstration of focal necrosis of the glomerular capillary wall in the absence of any other primary glomerular pathology. The differential diagnosis then lies between other small-vessel vasculitides, such as microscopic polyangiitis and Henoch–Schönlein purpura, systemic lupus erythematosus, or Goodpasture's syndrome. Immunofluorescence may be helpful in this differential as mesangial deposits of IgA are characteristic of Henoch–Schönlein disease and glomerular and extraglomerular capillary immunoglobulin deposits of any isotype, as well as complement, are found in lupus nephritis. Linear deposits of IgA along the glomerular basement membrane are the hallmark of antiglomerular basement membrane nephritis. Glomerular immunoglobulin deposits, if found at all, are typically scanty in Wegener's granulomatosis or microscopic polyarteritis, (pauci-immune nephritis). Because granulomas are rarely found in the kidney, further distinction between these two disorders has to depend on the clinical context and ANCA specificity (see above).

Other abnormal laboratory findings include almost invariably, normochromic normocytic anaemia, neutrophil leucocytosis, thrombocytosis, and evidence of an acute-phase response (raised ESR and C-reactive protein), as well as, in 80 per cent of patients, a polyclonal increase in immunoglobulins and, in 50 per cent, a positive rheumatoid factor.

Differential diagnosis

Idiopathic 'lethal' midline granuloma may present with features suggestive of Wegener's disease limited to the head and neck. This condition is now thought to be a variant of a T-cell lymphoma which is locally invasive and found elsewhere other than the head and neck. Unlike Wegener's disease, it may produce destructive ulceration of facial tissues, although both can erode through upper airways. Laboratory tests reflect the absence of inflammatory vasculitis with near normal ESR or C-reactive protein and absence of neutrophilia or thrombocytosis.

Lymphomatoid granulomatosis is extremely rare but closely resembles Wegener's granulomatosis in its multisystem distribution. It differs from Wegener's disease in the nature of the blood vessel involvement, with an absence of an inflammatory infiltrate: instead the vessel destruction appears to be mediated by infiltrates of lymphocytes of either T- or B-cell lineage. In approximately half the patients lymphomatous transformation eventually occurs. A raised C-reactive protein, ESR, and neutrophilia are unusual.

Microscopic polyangiitis

Microscopic polyangiitis is a small-vessel vasculitis which may affect any organ, either individually or in multisystem fashion. Disease limited to a single organ is well described for kidney, gut, and skin, although evolution to a multisystem disease may occur up to several years after presentation. Circulating autoantibodies to a variety of neutrophil cytoplasm antigens, predominantly myeloperoxidase, can be found in many patients.

Clinical presentation

The disease has an equal sex incidence and is not restricted by age or race. Fever, night sweats, weight loss, and profound malaise are common and it may be some weeks before organ-specific symptoms arise. In one-third of patients an influenza-like prodromal illness may have occurred prior to presentation.

Renal involvement

The kidney is almost always involved in microscopic polyangiitis, and up to 100 per cent of patients in some series had proteinuria and haematuria; glomerulonephritis may be mild, moderate or run a rapidly progressive course. It is not possible to predict the outcome, based on the level of plasma creatinine at referral. Renal biopsy usually, but not always, reflects the severity of the vasculitis the presence of focal necrosis of glomerular capillary walls supporting the diagnosis. Idiopathic rapidly progressive nephritis is often a *forme fruste* of microscopic polyangiitis limited to the kidney, which should be treated in the same way as generalized polyangiitis.

Lung involvement

This may present with cough, pleurisy, dyspnoea, or haemoptysis. Radiologically there may be transient or segmental atelectasis. The most serious complication is lung haemorrhage which can be profuse and occasionally fatal.

Other manifestations

Purpuric rashes are common and splinter haemorrhages may be found. Arthralgia is frequent and usually symmetrical; arthritis is less usual and joint deformation is not a feature. Mononeuritis multiplex is a particularly debilitating complication. Gastrointestinal symptoms may include non-specific abdominal pains, diarrhoea, or gastrointestinal haemorrhage. Patients with microscopic polyangiitis do not frequently have nasopharyngeal or ocular symptoms, in contrast to patients with Wegener's granulomatosis: nor do they have asthma and flitting pulmonary infiltrates, as in Churg–Strauss syndrome; nor do they present with severe hypertension and large organ perforation infarction, as may occur in polyarteritis nodosa.

Diagnosis

This may be suspected in a patient in whom symptoms of malaise, fever, weight loss, and night sweats are not accounted for by an infective or neoplastic aetiology and in whom there is evidence of multiple organ dysfunction. Confirmation may come from biopsy of the affected organ, of which the best is usually the kidney. Segmental vascular necrosis with an inflammatory cell infiltrate at any site may provide a useful clue, although changes may also be seen near epithelial surfaces which have been breached due to a variety of causes, infective, traumatic, or neoplastic, or in association with other pathologies such as tumour, abscess cavity formation, or in other connective tissue diseases such as rheumatoid arthritis and systemic lupus erythematosus. The finding of focal segmental necrosis of glomerular capillary walls restricts the diagnosis to microscopic polyangiitis or to Wegener's granulomatosis, systemic lupus, Goodpasture's syndrome, cryoglobulinaemia, or Henoch–Schönlein purpura. The first four of these have distinctive circulating immunoglobulins, autoantibodies to proteinase 3, DNA, glomerular basement membrane, or cryoglobulins, respectively. All have characteristic deposits of immunoglobulin in the renal biopsy except microscopic polyangiitis and Wegener's granulomatosis, where such deposits are not found.

The detection of ANCAs (see above) helps to the laboratory diagnosis. Usually these have specificity for myeloperoxidase, but occasionally identical clinical syndromes present with autoantibodies to other neutrophil cytoplasmic antigens, such as lactoferrin, elastase, and cathepsin G. In the right clinical context, the detection of these antibodies is very helpful, but it must be remembered that autoantibodies with similar specificities may be found in a number of other conditions which are not primary vasculitides, for example, inflammatory gastrointestinal diseases, such as chronic active hepatitis, sclerosing cholangitis, Crohn's disease, and ulcerative colitis. Other laboratory investigations, which are almost invariably abnormal, include a normochromic normocytic anaemia, raised ESR or C-reactive protein, and a neutrophilia. Frequently there is thrombocythaemia as well as hyperglobulinaemia, and occasionally positive rheumatoid factors may be found.

The major differential diagnoses are pyrexia of unknown aetiology (**PUO**) malignancy or covert infection. It may be difficult as a vasculitic rash can occur in any of these, for example associated with sarcoid or endocarditis in those with PUO, with carcinoma or leukaemia in those with malignancy, or with tuberculosis or syphilis in those with infection. All of these disorders may also show additional multisystem involvement. These diagnostic problems underscore the importance detection of ANCA, which is not a feature of any of the above.

Polyarteritis nodosa

Polyarteritis nodosa is a vasculitis of medium-sized arteries in which aneurysm formation is frequent. The clinical manifestations reflect the size of vessel involved: infarction may affect the gut, renal, or cerebral vasculature. Moderate to severe hypertension is common, as is an overlap with microscopic polyangiitis. Circulating ANCAs are rarely found, and when present may indicate the coincident development of the smaller-vessel vasculitis. An association with hepatitis B antigenaemia is evident in certain populations.

Clinical presentation

The disease may present at any age and is more common in men (male to female ratio 2:1). Tachycardia, fever, and weight loss are frequent and may be accompanied by striking events such as an acute abdomen, myocardial infarction, juvenile stroke, or severe hypertension.

Renal involvement

Extraglomerular arteritis rarely occurs alone and often a glomerular capillaritis similar to microscopic polyarteritis results in proteinuria, haematuria, and urinary casts. Malignant hypertension or frank haematuria may reflect the contribution of arterial ischaemia or infarction due to larger-vessel vasculitis. Progressive renal failure is common.

Cardiac involvement

Coronary arteritis is an important cause of intractable heart failure or of myocardial infarction and other cardiac complications include the development of an acute vasculitic pericarditis. Renovascular hypertension is also a well recognized complication.

Gastrointestinal tract

Typically, the presentation is with severe abdominal pain or gastrointestinal haemorrhage due to mucosal ulceration or perforation. Polyarteritis may also affect single organs, producing acute cholecystitis, pancreatitis, or appendicitis. Liver involvement may produce a hepatitic presentation or even hepatic necrosis. There is no distinctive clinical entity associated with hepatitis B polyarteritis.

Skin

Cutaneous involvement may vary from vasculitic purpura or urticaria to subcutaneous haemorrhage with gangrene. Palpable nodules, which may occur near to the course of superficial arteries are a distinctive feature. These may reach the size of a large pea, and can persist from days to months. Rarely these small 'nodosed' aneurysms may cause the surrounding skin to ulcerate.

Other manifestations

Arthralgias and myalgias are frequent. Neurological manifestations are rare, but stroke due to cerebral vasculitis or visual disturbance due to retinal aneurysms and haemorrhage (visible fundoscopically) are striking. Mononeuritis multiplex is secondary to arteritis of the vasa nervorum. Rarely, the vasculitis affects ovaries, testes, epididymis, and bladder.

Diagnosis

It is unusual for the disease to present without clinical features to suggest a microscopic polyangiitis but a superimposition of substantial dysfunction of any of the major organs, together with hypertension, are useful pointers to the diagnosis which may be confirmed by angiography or by histology of affected tissue.

There are no specific laboratory tests, but most patients have a normochromic normocytic anaemia, raised ESR or C-reactive protein, and neutrophilia. Microscopic polyangiitis is in the differential diagnosis, but the size of vessel involved in polyarteritis nodosa is shared by two other diseases. Thrombotic thrombocytopenic purpura is readily identified by the presence of thrombocytopenia and intravascular haemolysis; and Degos disease, an occlusive arterial disease affecting skin, gastrointestinal tract, and brain, is distinguished by its skin lesions, which are distributed centrifugally towards the extremities and undergo a typical course starting as pink–grey papules which then develop a depressed scaly centre surrounded by an elevated red margin.

Henoch–Schönlein purpura

This condition is described in Chapter 12.10. Its characteristic features generally allow confident diagnosis, but on occasion its features may overlap with, or more closely mimic, the conditions described here.

Churg–Strauss syndrome

This is probably a variant of polyarteritis in which there is a granulomatous necrotizing vasculitis predominantly affecting the lungs and to a lesser extent other organs. Typically, patients present with asthma and eosinophilia with clinical evidence of multisystem vasculitis.

Clinical presentation

Marked constitutional disturbance is frequent at presentation. Asthma is the feature which distinguishes Churg–Strauss syndrome from the other vasculitides; it is often severe and usually pre-dates the development of systemic vasculitis. Transient pulmonary infiltrates may be seen radiologically. There may be disturbance of bowel habit and abdominal pain due to gut vasculitis. Biopsy usually shows an eosinophilic infiltrate which may be present extensively throughout the gastrointestinal tract. There is occasionally involvement of other organs similar to that seen with microscopic polyangiitis. Mononeuritis multiplex and coronary vasculitis may prove particularly refractory to treatment.

Diagnosis

This may be suspected in a patient with asthma and evidence of multisystem vasculitis. Confirmation comes from demonstration of vasculitis on biopsy in which the affected tissues frequently show eosinophilic infiltrates. Moderate ($<20 \times 10^9$/l) peripheral eosinophilia is common. In occasional patients ANCAs, with specificity for myeloperoxidase, are to be found. The main disorder to consider in the differential diagnosis is the hypereosinophilic syndrome that accompanies endomyocardial fibrosis (Löffler's endocarditis). In this condition hypereosinophilia may be intense (usually $>20 \times 10^9$/l) and the eosinophils are morphologically abnormal, displaying loss of granules and vacuole formation. Asthma is rare in the hypereosinophilic syndrome, and although involvement of other organs with eosinophilic infiltrates may occur, rarely is there evidence of overt vasculitis.

Relapsing polychondritis

This is a rare condition in which a small vessel vasculitis predominantly affects cartilaginous structures such as the pinna of the ear, nasal cartilage, larynx, and trachea.

Clinical presentation

Males and females are equally affected and the onset is most frequent in the seventh decade; untreated it carries a poor prognosis. Fever, weight loss, and malaise are common at the onset. Tenderness, inflammatory swelling, and eventual destruction of the cartilage, often in cyclical fashion, are the main features. There may be gross deformation of the pinna of the ear, a saddle nose, and stridor due to collapse of the larynx or trachea. Involvement of the heart valves or aorta may produce heart failure or aneurysm, respectively. Other manifestations include episcleritis and monoarticular arthropathy as well as, infrequently, evidence of small-vessel vasculitis in other organs.

Diagnosis

The diagnosis is usually made on clinical grounds, with biopsy showing necrotizing vasculitis and cartilage destruction in affected tissue. There is no specific laboratory test, but normochromic anaemia, a marked acute-phase response, and leucocytosis are frequent.

Table 2 Direct complications of conventional immunosuppression in Wegener's granulomatosis ($n = 158$)

Cyclophosphamide		Prednisolone	
Female infertility	57%	Cushingoid features	100%
Cyclophosphamide cystitis	43%	Cataracts	21%
Hair loss	17%	Fractures	11%
Bladder cancer	3%	(aseptic necrosis 3%)	
Myelodysplasia	2%	Diabetes mellitus (requiring insulin 3%)	8%
Development of malignancy*	↑×2.4		
Development of bladder cancer*	↑×33		

*Related to age- and sex-matched population (after Hoffman *et al.* 1992).

Kawasaki disease

This childhood form of systemic vasculitis is described in Chapter 10.17.

Treatment of the systemic vasculitides

Cytotoxic drugs and steroids are the mainstays of treatment. Cyclophosphamide and prednisolone are combined, at high dose, in an induction regimen which is followed after 2 months by a lower dose, maintenance regimen in which other immunosuppressive agents may substitute for cyclophosphamide. The latter regimen should be continued long term, as particularly in Wegener's granulomatosis remissions are slow to achieve and relapses are frequent. There is thus substantial morbidity due not only to the vasculitis but also to the cumulative toxicity of therapy (Table 2).

Cyclophosphamide at 3 mg/kg body weight (rounded down to the nearest 50 mg) is suitable for the induction regimen. This dosage should be lowered or discontinued temporarily if the total white cell count falls to less than 4.0×10^9/l, or the neutrophil leucocyte count falls to less than 2.0×10^9/l. Cytotoxic therapy should also be modified if severe infection occurs. In patients aged 55 years or over, a lower induction dose of 2 mg/kg is often given because of the greater susceptibility of the elderly to bone marrow immunosuppression and infection. Steroids are given at high dose, initially prednisolone 60 mg/day, tapering at weekly intervals until at 2 months (when possible) the patient is receiving 10 mg/day. Cyclophosphamide can usually be substituted by the same dose of azathioprine at 2 months when steroid treatment may be converted to an alternate-day regimen. Both drugs may then be withdrawn gradually at 12 months at least in some patients.

Monitoring disease activity

Standard tests of organ function should be used to monitor the effect of treatment on disease activity. Serial measurements of the C-reactive protein and the ESR (less useful), are guides as to whether the vasculitis has been brought under control. Both are non-specific, being elevated during intercurrent infection or by other causes of inflammation as well as by vasculitis. ANCA measurements may help to monitor treatment but some patients have persistently raised ANCA levels despite no evident disease activity, and vice versa. A small number of patients have undetectable ANCA but continuing vasculitis.

Other therapeutic strategies

Use of pulsed dose cyclophosphamide (0.75-1.00 g intravenously) or prednisolone (500 mg–1 g, i.v.) has been advocated but recent evidence suggests that pulsed cyclophosphamide is less effective at maintaining remission than oral cyclophosphamide. Furthermore, the active metabolites of cyclophosphamide are in part renally excreted, so that in patients with nephritis, lower-dose oral therapy should allow more accurate titration of dose.

For patients who are intolerant of cyclophosphamide, the most useful drug is azathioprine. Where disease activity is not controllable by either, methotrexate or cyclosporin A, have been tried. Some patients benefit, but there is no substantial evidence to warrant their use as first-line agents.

Trimethoprim–sulphamethoxazole has enjoyed a vogue for the management of systemic vasculitis, particularly Wegener's granulomatosis, but with the advent of better diagnostic criteria, careful exclusion of intercurrent infections (particularly a problem in Wegener's affecting the upper respiratory tract), and study of controls given trimethoprim–sulphamethoxazole alone, doubts have been cast over the efficacy of this agent.

In patients who have fulminating vasculitis intensive plasma exchange may be beneficial. There is now evidence that such an approach may benefit patients with severe renal vasculitis (requiring dialysis support), lung haemorrhage due to pulmonary vasculitis, or in coma due to cerebral vasculitis.

For patients with intractable vasculitis, resistant to conventional immunosuppression, a few reports now point to the value of more specific forms of immunotherapy, such as pooled high-dose intravenous immunoglobulin, 0.4 g/kg per day for 5 days (believed to exert one of its immunomodulatory effects through anti-idiotypic control of B-cell function) or humanized monoclonal antibody therapy which targets T cells.

Response to treatment

Wegener's granulomatosis and microscopic polyangiitis

Approximately 75 per cent of patients with Wegener's granulomatosis and microscopic polyangiitis treated with cytotoxic drugs and steroids will ultimately achieve complete remission. Sixty per cent of patients with microscopic polyangiitis may achieve this within 2 months but only 50 per cent of those with Wegener's do so in 12 months. The rate of relapse does not appear to differ between the two disorders, affecting approximately 50 per cent of patients. Periods of remission may last several years.

Henoch–Schönlein purpura

Most cases of childhood Henoch–Schönlein purpura resolve spontaneously within 2–3 weeks. Relapses do occur within the first 2 years, but are usually self-limiting and permanent sequelae are rare. For those with progressive disease, some physicians prescribe short courses of steroids alone, or, for resistant cases, similar regimens to those used for the other small-vessel vasculitides, but results are usually disappointing.

Polyarteritis nodosa and Churg–Strauss syndrome

Treatment for both conditions generally follows a similar pattern to that for small-vessel vasculitis, (with the minor variation that high-dose steroids may be effective when given alone initially). Results of therapy and often less good that is the case in other vasculitides.

Further reading

de Groot, K. and Gross, W.L. (1998). Wegener's granulomatosis: disease course, assessment and extent and treatment. *Lupus*, 7, 285–91.

Hoffman, G.S. and Specks, U. (1998). Antineutrophil cytoplasmic antibodies. *Arthritis and Rheumatism*, **41**, 1521–37.

Schmidt, W.H. and Gross, W.L. (1998). Vasculitis in the seriously ill patient: diagnostic approaches and therapeutic options in ANCA-associated vasculitis. *Kidney International*, **64** (Suppl.), 539–44.

Trentham, D.E. and Le, C.H. (1998). Relapsing polychondritis. *Annals of Internal Medicine*, 129, 114–22.

Tse, W.Y., Cockwell, P., and Savage, C.O. (1998). Assessment of disease severity in systemic vasculitis. *Postgraduate Medical Journal*, 74, 1–6.

Chapter 10.11

Systemic lupus erythematosus and related disorders

M. L. Snaith and D. A. Isenberg

This disease has a broad spectrum of clinical features (Table 1). Patients with minor forms may continue with near normal health for many years, but eventually most present to a dermatologist, rheumatologist, or nephrologist. Treatment with corticosteroids and immunosuppressives has improved life expectancy in recent years, but systemic lupus erythematosus (SLE) is still a serious and potentially fatal disorder.

Epidemiology

The disease is encountered world-wide and can affect any race but is most commonly found among women of child-bearing years. The

Table 1 The common clinical features in systemic lupus erythematosus, by system

System	Clinical features
Musculoskeletal	Arthralgia, arthritis, myositis, tendinitis
Cardiorespiratory	Pleurisy, pericarditis, endocarditis, myocarditis, atelectasis, 'shrinking lungs'
Nervous system	Polyneuritis, cranial nerve lesions, migraine, spinal cord lesions, cerebritis, epilepsy, stroke, chorea
Urogenital	Cystitis, primary ovarian failure, miscarriages
Renal	Glomerulonephritis, tubular syndromes
Vascular	Raynaud's, vasculitis, arterial and venous thromboses
Constitutional	Fever, fatigue, anorexia, nausea
Haemopoietic	Anaemia (haemolytic or normochromic–normocytic), thrombocytopenia, lymphopenia, leucopenia, splenomegaly, lymphadenopathy
Mucocutaneous	Mucositis/ulcers, rashes, photosensitivity, alopecia
Ocular	Uveitis, retinal lesions

Table 2 A summary of the 1982 American Rheumatism Association revised criteria for the classification of systemic lupus erythematosus

Criterion	Definition
Malar rash	Fixed erythema, flat or raised
Discoid rash	Erythematous raised patches with adherent keratotic scaling and follicular plugging
Photosensitivity	By history or observation
Oral ulcers	Observed by a physician, usually painless
Arthritis	Non-erosive; two or more joints
Serositis	Pleuritis or pericarditis
Renal disorder	Proteinuria >0.5 g/24 h or casts
Neurological disorder	Seizures (not otherwise explained) *or* psychosis
Haematological disorder	Haemolytic anaemia *or* leucopenia *or* lymphopenia *or* thrombocytopenia
Immunological disorder	Lupus erythematosus cells *or* anti-native DNA *or* anti-Sm *or* biological false positive test for syphilis
Antinuclear antibody (ANA)	ANA positive, in the absence of possible drug induction

highest frequencies and severity are in women of Afro-Caribbean, Chinese, Asian, and South American Indian ancestry. Reported incidences of new cases range from 4.8 cases per 100 000 population in Sweden to 7.6 per 100 000 in San Francisco. Prevalence ranges from 36 in Europeans, to 90 in Asians, and up to 200 per 100 000 in Afro-Caribbeans. The frequency seems highest among young black females in the United States and the Caribbean. Indigenous West Africans appear to be less affected than descendants of West Africans in North America or the Caribbean.

In the absence of a single screening test with a high specificity and sensitivity for SLE, classification criteria have aided the study of its epidemiology. The American College of Rheumatology (**ARA/ACR**) criteria are shown in Table 2. The convention of using four ARA criteria, whether present simultaneously or sequentially, to classify patients as having definite SLE has been helpful, but patients with fewer than four criteria may still have lupus. Presentation differs between different races, for example with regard to the expected frequency of skin disease or fever.

Influence of hormones and age

The majority of patients with SLE are female (overall ratio 9:1 female/male), but this ratio is less in older patients and possibly in certain racial groups. In male and probably also female patients, there is an abnormal degree of 16-hydroxylation of oestriol. There is a relatively high frequency of SLE in Klinefelter syndrome and in lupus-prone mice the disease can be manipulated by alteration in the androgen/oestrogen status of the animals. The pattern of disease at onset in patients over the age of 50 differs from that in younger patients. Apart from the lower ratio of females to males, the disease seems to be less aggressive. The age of onset is, on average, higher in Caucasians than in those of African descent. There are few data on patients followed through the menopause to ascertain whether the disease changes its characteristics with this change in hormonal environment.

Lupus in children, which is unusual, is broadly similar to the disease in adults, except that major haematological manifestations, positive antibodies to DNA, Sm, and RNP are commoner and higher doses of steroids tend to be required for control. Neonatal lupus or congenital heart block may result from transplacental passage of maternal antibody (anti-Ro or anti-La).

Clinical course

The disease is usually episodic. Flares may be superimposed on an increasing burden of disability. Examples are: increasing hand deformity, cutaneous scarring, intellectual blunting or renal failure. If the patient survives the more active phases of the disease, amelioration may come with advancing years, but as overall survival improves, other problems are burgeoning, such as osteonecrosis or coronary vascular disease. Both are related to high dose or long duration of steroid treatment but also to continuing active disease. Spontaneous remission is more likely to occur in younger patients presenting acutely. In those with advanced renal disease, the non-renal features may regress, perhaps because of uraemic immune suppression. The same is true after successful renal transplantation, in this case perhaps because of the associated immunosuppressive therapy.

Clinical features

Constitutional

Undue fatiguability can often be marked, as with other autoimmune disorders; it may be due to coincident hypothyroidism or fibromyalgia. Unstable disease may also be characterized by weight change (gain or loss) and low-grade fever. Lymphadenopathy, which can be gross enough to mimic lymphoma, may precede disease flare.

Cutaneous and mucosal

The skin is affected in over 70 per cent of cases: rashes range from erythematous lesions resembling a drug reaction to severe ulceration and scarring. Unusually rapid hair loss often heralds a flare, can proceed to alopecia and, ultimately, scarring. The characteristic 'butterfly rash' is seen in up to 40 per cent of patients (Plate 1). It involves the blush area, perhaps because of the particular vascular reactivity in this part of the face, because of local susceptibility to vasculitis, or as a consequence of particular exposure to the sun in the area. Additional cutaneous features include non-specific rashes, apparently allergic or hypersensitive drug-induced rashes (particularly to sulphur-containing compounds and antibiotics), urticaria, and bullous lesions. About 50 per cent of patients with SLE are photosensitive, especially marked in the subgroup of subacute cutaneous lupus erythematosus (Plate 2), which is associated with anti-Ro antibodies. Oral ulceration is a common feature of active disease but may be relatively painless. A painful throat may accompany a flare.

Vascular involvement

Twenty to 30 per cent of patients have Raynaud's phenomenon (compared with up to 15 per cent of the general population). Nail-fold capillaritis, dermal infarcts, and other minor forms of vasculitis can extend to ulceration and major vessel thrombosis, especially in the context of a coagulopathy (see below).

Musculoskeletal system

Over 90 per cent of patients experience arthralgia, arthritis, or tendinitis. Joint erosions are not characteristic of SLE but deformity

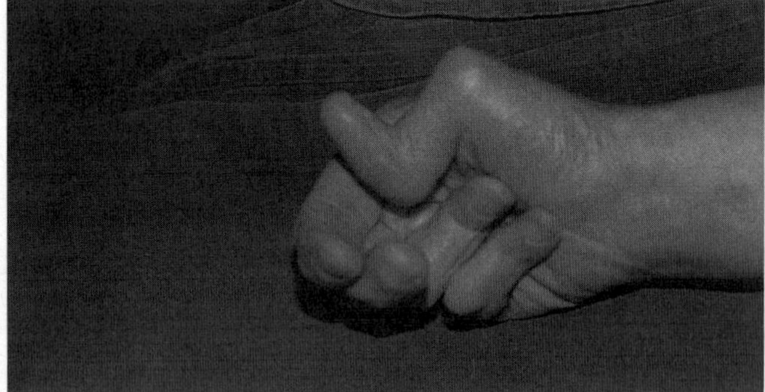

Fig. 1 Tendon contractures of the hand, including the Z-deformity of the thumb.

resulting from joint capsule or tendon contracture may mimic rheumatoid arthritis. The Z-deformity is characteristic (Fig. 1). Tendinitis may be acute and painful and joint effusion may be painfully tense. Avascular (aseptic) osteonecrosis most frequently affects the subchondral cancellous bone of the femoral head, but other sites include the shoulder, knee, or other joints, especially now that minor degrees can be detected with isotope bone scans or magnetic resonance imaging. It is associated with prolonged high-dose steroid treatment.

Renal involvement (see also Chapter 12.15)

The presentation may be with rapid onset of an acute nephritic and/or nephrotic syndrome, or with asymptomatic haematuria or proteinuria. Urinalysis is crucial in patients with lupus: simple stick testing for protein and blood should be accompanied, in positive cases, by direct microscopy of a fresh uncentrifuged specimen of urine. A small group of patients experiences insidious loss of glomerular function as part of the antiphospholipid syndrome (see below) without haematuria or proteinuria. The major histopathological finding is then of multiple small glomerular thrombi rather than glomerulonephritis. Such patients may be better treated by anticoagulants than by immunosuppressive agents.

Neurological involvement

The central nervous system is obviously involved in about 20 per cent of patients in most series, but a much larger proportion is affected in a more subtle way; patients will say that they feel 'distant', a form of depersonalization. There is difficulty in deciding whether a patient with, for example, severe headache, can be said to have cerebral involvement. Patients may have classical or atypical migraine; visual phenomena (teichopsia or scotomata) may feature without headache. Less doubt arises in patients with strokes, cranial nerve palsies, fits, chorea, long-tract signs, or organic confusional states, all of which may occur as single manifestations or as part of a multifaceted clinical syndrome. There is evidence for increasing loss of intellectual function with cerebral atrophy in some patients with long-term cerebral lupus. The peripheral nervous system is less commonly involved, but spinal infarction can give rise to paraplegia.

Cardiorespiratory system

The most common manifestation is serositis. A history of an unexplained episode of pleurisy some years prior to multisystem disease is common. Acute chest pain with shortness of breath may be due to basal atelectasis, with apparent lung shrinkage. The pain can be confused with infective pleurisy, pulmonary infarction, or, in patients with steroid-induced osteoporosis, dorsal vertebral collapse. Primary pulmonary hypertension is a rare manifestation. Pericarditis may be acute and symptomatic, or identified only on cardiac ultrasound. Valvular involvement and Libman–Sachs endocarditis are less common clinical features, but Doppler ultrasound studies suggest a greater prevalence than previously recognized, particularly among patients with severe disease.

Gastrointestinal involvement

Sterile peritonitis is a rare example of serositis. Vasculitis may cause mesenteric infarction, usually in the presence of skin vasculitis. Pancreatitis is uncommon but can be severe. Elevated concentrations of transaminases are common, but may be drug induced, as inflammatory hepatitis is unusual. An episode of diarrhoea may precede a flare of disease, but it is unclear if this represents a disease manifestation or an incidental infection triggering a flare.

Anaemia and cytopenias

Normocytic, normochromic, or hypochromic anaemia are frequent. Lymphopenia and neutropenia are disease manifestations, the former being particularly an indicator of propensity to disease and leucopenia more often associated with active disease, although it may also be drug-induced. Leucocytosis is not necessarily observed in an infected lupus patient. Pancytopenia is well recognized, as is immune thrombocytopenia, which may be the mode of presentation. There are broadly four types of immune thrombocytopenia in lupus.

1. Rapid onset, with counts falling to below $10 \times 10^9/l$, usually responsive to steroid treatment.
2. Progressive severe, resistant to steroids alone and requiring considerable support with pooled immunoglobulin infusions, danazol, cytotoxic treatment, and possibly splenectomy (see below).
3. Chronic low grade, with counts ranging from about 30 000 to 100 000 without need for aggressive management.
4. Immune thrombocytopenia, presenting as a prodrome of systemic disease.

The lupus anticoagulant and the antiphospholipid syndrome

False positive Wasserman reactions or VDRL tests have long been recognized in SLE, as have an increased rate of early miscarriage with retention of normal fertility, and the Sneddon syndrome comprises livedo reticularis with cerebral thrombosis. A connection between these and other features, including thrombocytopenia, depends on the presence of antibodies to negatively charged phospholipids (e.g. cardiolipin or phosphatidyl serine). These may coincide with other antibodies and clinical SLE, or with features of the primary antiphospholipid syndrome, or may be found in isolation. The antibodies may be detected by functional tests for the lupus anticoagulant, such as the dilute Russell viper venom test, or serologically by anticardiolipin (ACL) antibodies. Clinical manifestations of the syndrome include thrombosis, recurrent miscarriage, thrombocytopenia, and haemolytic anaemia. Deep vein thrombosis without an obvious precipitating cause may be complicated by thromboembolism; Budd–Chiari syndromes and renal vein thrombosis are described elswhere. Less common is arterial thrombosis, but this may affect any artery. An association with stroke in young people is particularly well-recognized, but events in the retinal, coronary, renal, brachial, femoral, and more distal arteries can also occur and are not always diagnosed promptly, particularly if other features (laboratory or clinical) of SLE are absent. These antibodies may be considered directly pathogenic or as markers of the causative antibody. In the appropriate clinical context, with persisting IgG ACL antibodies, treatment by long-term anticoagulation is warranted. A caveat is that such antibodies have also been described in such chronic disorders as syphilis or leprosy and antiphospholipid antibodies (usually IgM) may appear transiently after acute infections (e.g. viral pneumonia, Epstein–Barr virus, viral hepatitis, measles, chicken-pox, Lyme disease, and many others). These infection-associated antibodies are not associated with clinical manifestations and do not require treatment.

The erythrocyte sedimentation rate may not correlate well with disease activity, and may be normal with, for example, marked cerebral involvement. Other patients may appear quite well with a raised rate, which then probably reflects involvement of the coagulation cascade or hyperglobulinaemia. The C-reactive protein (**CRP**) level, commonly raised in other inflammatory rheumatic disorders, tends to be normal in patients with active SLE unless they have active synovitis, heart, or lung involvement. A raised level in SLE implies concurrent infection. CRP estimation is, therefore, useful in the evaluation of the lupus patient with fever.

Complement deficiency may be inherited or acquired. Inherited deficiency (e.g. C2 or C4) carries an increased risk of developing SLE, but not necessarily of severe disease. A low level of complement components (CH50, C4, C3) is found in most patients with active renal disease, but is less predictably helpful in other presentations. It is evidence of increased complement consumption, but there may also be reduced synthesis. Levels of breakdown products (e.g. C3d) fluctuate with disease flare.

About 2.5 per cent of patients have a negative antinuclear antibody (ANA). They are characterized by prominent cutaneous disease and variable joint, kidney, and neurological involvement. Despite the absence of conventional ANA, antibodies to Ro or La antigens may be found.

Antibodies to DNA are commonly raised in patients with active lupus nephritis, less frequently when other systems are the major site of disease. Disease flare may be predicted by a rise (and in some cases, subsequent falls) in the level of anti-DNA antibodies. Enzymatic assays (enzyme-linked immunosorbent assays) are now readily available, but users should be aware of the rather different affinity and avidity of antibodies detected with these methods compared with those using radioactively labelled DNA in immunoprecipitation (Farr) assays. The micro-organism *Crithidia lucilliae* has contributed usefully to diagnosis: it is used as the substrate in a highly specific immunofluorescent assay for double-stranded DNA. Antibodies to single-stranded DNA are not specific for SLE but do correlate with disease activity.

Clinical subgroups

Various subgroups can be discerned within the heterogeneous spectrum of lupus. These patients tend to run to type and there are reasonably clearly defined autoantibody associations with the clinical syndromes, summarized in Table 3.

Specific organ involvement

Renal complications of SLE are picked up by conventional tests of renal function. Renal biopsy may help in planning treatment and assessing prognosis (see Chapter 12.15). In chronic disease renal biopsy can help to detect evidence of potentially reversible pathology, whereas if there is much scarring and little acute inflammation it may not be useful to persist with potentially toxic immunosuppression.

Table 3 Autoantibody associations with clinical syndromes in systemic lupus erythematosus

Clinical syndrome	Typical autoantibody profile
Nephritis, photosensitivity, serositis	Anti-dsDNA
Photosensitivity (subacute cutaneous lupus erythematosus)	Anti-Ro/La
Neonatal lupus syndromes	Anti-Ro/La
Coagulopathy, thrombocytopenia, miscarriages, CNS syndromes	Lupus anticoagulant, antiphospholipid
Overlap features such as Raynaud's, myositis, and cardiopulmonary lesions	Anti-RNP (certain epitopes)
Drug-induced lupus (serositis, rashes, fever)	Antihistone

This table is presented in order to indicate that, contrary to the sometimes apparently random profusion of autoantibodies and clinical features, there is some consistency. These clinical syndromes are not necessarily found in their entirety in any individual patient, nor are the antibodies always found with the syndromes. Therefore, it is still appropriate to recognize the overall complex as SLE, within which are several recognizable subgroups.

Chest radiograph and respiratory function tests aid assessment in those with lung involvement. Magnetic resonance imaging scanning is superior to computed tomography in detecting focal lesions in cerebral white matter in those with neurological features. Serial psychological tests are useful in detecting and monitoring cognitive dysfunction.

Skin biopsy is helpful not only in the assessment of a rash in a patient with lupus, but also in diagnosing a patient with suspected lupus, with or without a rash. Clinically normal skin should be biopsied in such a patient: the presence of immune complexes (C3 and immunoglobulin) in a linear band at the dermo-epidermal junction is very suggestive of SLE (Plate 3). Lymph node biopsy may reveal the unusual but characteristic pattern of lymphorrhexis.

Management concerns

Patients with lupus tend to be female and relatively young. The social implications in relation to family and work are important. The patient may wish to become pregnant; or if she has already completed her family, her children are still likely to be young and dependent upon her. Questions of family planning, contraception, primary or secondary infertility, and social support are all considerations in the overall management.

Contraception, family planning, and pregnancy

Possible oestrogen effects on SLE in some patients raise doubt over oestrogen contraception. It should certainly be avoided in the context of a thrombotic tendency. Barrier methods should be used where possible. Intrauterine contraceptive devices maybe contraindicated in those with a bleeding tendency. Progesterone contraception is an alternative, but slightly less certain, strategy.

Pregnancy in systemic lupus erythematosus

Pregnancy in patients with SLE was once thought to be accompanied by a greater risk of flare in the puerperium, but this is now considered to have been due to selection bias. Whether or not pregnancy affects the disease depends largely on the disease activity at the time of conception. Flares are less frequent in those in remission at the start of pregnancy. Maternal deaths are rare but especially vulnerable are those with active renal disease at the onset of pregnancy. The outcome is worse in patients with a pre-pregnancy plasma creatinine above 150–200 mmol/l. Timing, therefore, requires careful consideration. Those in the early stages of disease cannot be assured of long-term remission. On the other hand, delay into the late thirties adds the age-related problems of pregnancy. This aspect of care requires full discussion with the patient, her partner, her physician, obstetrician, and often haematologist.

Although prednisolone and azathioprine appear safe in pregnancy, antimalarials can cause fetal ototoxicity and warfarin teratogenesis. The ideal is to have the patient in remission, on low doses of prednisolone and perhaps azathioprine.

Aspirin has been shown to be of value to those undertaking pregnancy with the antiphospholipid syndrome, but suppression of ACL antibody by immunosuppression is rarely successful. Attempts to reduce, with plasmapheresis, levels of antibody in patients with recurrent Ro-associated fetal problems have been unsuccessful.

It may be difficult to distinguish active lupus from pre-eclampsia, particularly during the third trimester, in patients with hypertension and proteinuria. Pre-eclampsia does not cause joint, skin, or pleuritic problems; nor is it associated with signs of active glomerular disease such as the presence of red cell casts in the urinary sediment, lowered C3, or rising anti-DNA antibody levels: so serological monitoring is helpful in this situation.

Despite all these potential problems, many women with SLE undergo successful pregnancy without ill effect either to themselves or their offspring. There is no evidence of reduced fertility in SLE (aside from cyclophosphamide-induced gonadal atrophy), but abortion, fetal retardation, premature labour, and perinatal death are all more common in those with impaired renal function, hypertension and the antiphospholipid syndrome

Neonatal SLE is a rare complication of maternal SLE, arising from the transfer of maternal antibodies. Features may include congenital heart block, classical discoid skin lesions, and more rarely haemolytic anaemia or thrombocytopenia. The skin and haematological problems are transient and do not usually present a major difficulty. Heart block, however, may lead to heart failure *in utero* and fetal hydrops; a pacemaker may be required early after delivery. Up to 80 per cent of mothers who deliver a child with congenital heart block have antibodies to the cytoplasmic antigens designated Ro or La (SSA or SSB). Neonatal heart block is found in babies of about 1 in 20 mothers with anti-Ro/La antibodies, who may have no clinical symptoms or perhaps features more suggestive of Sjögren's syndrome than of SLE. Anti-Ro persists in affected babies for several months. Occasionally, neonatal disorders of this kind are the first indication of a previously unsuspected disorder in the mother.

Treatment

Immunosuppression and corticosteroids are not always necessary. The range of treatments which may be appropriate for patients with SLE is indicated in Table 4. It is not prescriptive. In one individual, for example, tendinitis may be treated effectively with an injection of corticosteroid and an accompanying skin rash may respond to hyroxychloroquine. In another patient, active nephritis may necessitate systemic steroids and immunosuppression. Antimalarial drugs (hydroxychloroquine 200–400 mg/day or chloroquine 250–250 mg/day) are often effective for skin rash, arthralgia, fever, fatigue, or serositis. The dose may be increased to 600 mg/day in the case of hydroxychloroquine for short periods, as the risk of retinopathy is much less than in the case of chloroquine. Smaller doses are required for those weighing less than 50 kg. Regular ophthalmic monitoring is mandatory for patients taking chloroquine long term, but is probably unnecessary for hydroxychloroquine.

High protection factor ultraviolet barrier cream is essential for those with known photosensitivity and is advisable for any patient with a fair skin exposed to the sun.

Anti-inflammatory agents, aspirin, and non-steroidal anti-inflammatory drugs may on their own control minor arthralgia or may usefully supplement immunosuppression in more severe joint symptoms. Aspirin or full anticoagulation is necessary and preferable to immunosuppression in those with recurrent thrombosis in the antiphospholipid syndrome; some patients combining the latter with SLE may require both approaches.

Minor degrees of thrombocytopenia do not require treatment, but life-threatening thrombocytopenia resistant to immunosuppression may respond to danazol or to intravenous stabilized gammaglobulin; the role of splenectomy is controversial but seems most successful when combined with immunosuppression.

Raynaud's syndrome may respond symptomatically to calcium channel blockers or other vasodilator. Warming the hands prior to going out into cold weather and using gloves (which can be electrically heated) is helpful. Occasional patients develop severe digital ischaemia and even gangrene. Some of these respond, if only partially, to infusions of prostacycline or calcitonin gene-related peptide.

Treatment of an acute crisis

Acute or rapidly deteriorating renal function, evidence of cerebral lupus, major haemolysis, or thrombocytopenia are indications for aggressive treatment, combining high doses of prednisolone with cyclophosphamide or azathioprine and in the case of severe thrombocytopenia, i.v. immunoglobulin. There are trial data showing the efficacy of pulsed methyl prednisolone 500 mg–1 g given intravenously daily for 3 days, combined with cyclophosphamide (i.v. pulses or orally 2.5 mg/kg per day). The regimen (at least initially) is quite well tolerated. Smaller doses given intravenously or intramuscularly may be as effective; indeed, pulses of oral prednisolone can be effective and are cheaper than intravenous boluses. Plasma exchange has been used in severe unremitting disease, but evidence for its benefit is lacking. Azathioprine (1.0–2.5 mg/kg) is a useful steroid-sparing maintenance immunosuppressive therapy. Methotrexate is less well tested in lupus, but its value in treating inflammatory myositis or severe synovitis in rheumatoid arthritis has led to its use in SLE, particularly in those intolerant of cyclophosphamide or azathioprine.

Precautions

A single intravenous dose of 0.75–1.0 g of methyl prednisolone preceding 0.5–1.0 g of cyclophosphamide reduces but does not eliminate the need for antiemetics such as metoclopramide or ondansetron. A high fluid intake during infusion of cyclophosphamide combined with Mesna (sodium mercaptoethane sulphonate) reduces the risk of bladder toxicity. The nadir of the white cell count following cyclophosphamide is at about 10 days; hence it is usually advisable leave a gap of 2 weeks between infusions.

Table 4 Problem-directed treatment in systemic lupus erythematosus

	Analgesics	NSAID	Local steroid	Physical therapy	Vascular modifiers	Antimalarials	Corticosteroids	Immuno-suppression	Adjunctives[a]
Arthralgia	(+)	+				+	(+)		
Synovitis	(+)	+	+	+		+	(+)	(+)	(+)
Tendinitis		+	+	(+)					
Vasospasm					+				
Photosensitivity			(+)			+			+
Vasculitis					(+)	(+)	+	(+)	
Thrombosis					(+)		(+)		+
Serositis	(+)	(+)				+	(+)	(+)	
Pneumonitis							(+)	(+)	
Myositis				+			+	(+)	
Neuropathies				(+)			+	(+)	(+)
Cerebritis							(+)	(+)	(+)
Convulsions							(+)	(+)	+
Nephritis							+	+	(+)
Cytopenias							(+)	(+)	(+)
Sicca syndrome						(+)	(+)	(+)	(+)

[a] Adjunctives include (for example) local treatments for rashes or sicca symptoms, transfusions, intravenous globulin for cytopenias, etc.

+, Of clear therapeutic value; (+), of less certain effectiveness, or under specific circumstances.

This table illustrates the range of treatments which may be appropriate for patients with SLE. It is *not* prescriptive. In one individual, for example, tendinitis may be treated effectively with just a local intralesional injection of corticosteroid, and an accompanying skin rash may respond to hydroxychloroquine. In another patient active nephritis may necessitate systemic steroids and immunosuppression, rendering an antimalarial superfluous. The importance of physical therapy as part of a programme of rehabilitation in patients with locomotor or neurological disability must not be overlooked.

Table 5 Drugs which can induce systemic lupus erythematosus

Hydralazine	Phenytoin
Procainamide	Sulphonamides
Bleomycin	Cephalosporins
Minocycline	Quinidine
Isoniazid	Thiouracil
Methyl dopa	Asparaginase

Drug-induced lupus syndromes

A number of drugs may induce lupus syndromes (Table 5). Susceptibility is associated with HLA-DR3, slow acetylation and complement deficiencies. The drug-induced syndrome includes rashes, fever, and serositis, but rarely nephritis or cerebritis. Once the causative drug is removed the clinical features remit but the ANA remains for many months. The ANA specificity may be to histones. There seems to be no risk of exacerbating established disease by the addition of a drug know to be capable of inducing a drug-related SLE syndrome.

Table 6 Prevalence of autoantibodies in systemic lupus erythematosus

Autoantigen	Prevalence (%)	Autoantigen	Prevalence (%)
dsDNA	40–90	Cardiolipin	20–50
ssDNA	50–70	Lupus anticoagulant	15–20
Histones	50–70	IgG Fc	20–30
Sm	5–30	Thyroglobulin	10–30
RNP	25–35	Thyroid microsomes	10–30
Ro/SSA	25–35	Red cell membrane	5–10
La/SSB	10–15	(Coombs' test)	
poly(ADP-ribose)	50–70		

The wide ranges may be accounted for by differences in laboratory technology and also in the populations of patients studied in the various reported series. For example, anti-Sm antibodies are found predominantly in black populations and only rarely in white Europeans.

Autoantibodies and cellular immunology in systemic lupus erythematosus

The serological hallmark of lupus is the presence of circulating autoantibodies which directed against a range of nuclear, cytoplasmic, and plasma membrane antigens (Table 6). Many cellular abnormalities have also been identified (for the more important, see Table 6, OTM3, p. 3025). Increase B lymphocyte activation contributes to hyperglobulinaemia. CD4 and CD45 Ro T cells are reduced, which may contribute to the failure of T cells to suppress hyperactive B cells.

Additional T-cell defects may underlie their impaired responsiveness in SLE. Dysregulation of apoptosis is a candidate in the aetiopathogenesis of autoimmune disease, including SLE. Fas and Fas ligand function appear normal, but aberrations in Bcl-2 have been reported, also in clearance of apoptotic material. In view of the relationship with photosensitivity, it is of relevance that ultraviolet light can induce expression of normally conserved nuclear antigens on the surface of keratinocytes. Other abnormalities, such as in cytokine production (e.g. raised interleukins-6 and -10, but reduced interleukin-2) are described in OTM3, pp. 3025–6.

Genetic factors

The lower prevalence of lupus in West Africans than in Americans of African descent, indicates an environmental contribution to the inherited risk. Among monozygotic twins a concordance rate for lupus is about 30 per cent, compared with 5 per cent for dizygotic twins.

Lupus is strongly associated with deficiencies of the early components of the classical pathway of complement, notably C1, C4, and C2. Two alleles are inherited for each complement component, so deficiencies may be partial or complete (homozygous). Congenital deficiencies of C2 and C4 are often in linkage disequilibrium with HLA-DR3 and -DR2, known to be associated with lupus. C4 is composed of two distinct but homologous proteins, C4A and C4B. A single null C4A allele increases the relative risk for lupus by a factor of 3, and two null alleles by a factor of 17.

The complement receptor CR1 is present on peripheral B lymphocytes, erythrocytes, monocytes, and tissue macrophages. The expression of CR1 on these cells is reduced in patients and their healthy relatives. This is thought to be an acquired phenomenon. The extent of the CRI deficiency appears to correlate with disease activity.

Among Caucasians those expressing the HLA-A1, B8, DR3 haplotype are approximately 10 times more likely to develop lupus. The haplotype also appears to be in linkage disequilibrium with a null allele of C4A. In Japanese people, however, the disease is more strongly associated with DR2. Other weaker associations with tumour necrosis factor (and certain T-cell receptor polymorphisms) are also evident.

Over 20 different DNA antibody idiotypes have been identified. Some of these, including the 16/6 Id and Id GN2, are found frequently (in more than 40 per cent of patients) on the immunoglobulins in the serum of lupus patients or deposited in their kidneys, suggesting that such idiotypes may be involved in the immunopathology of lupus. The identification of these and other idiotypes in the healthy relatives of lupus patients, albeit at much lower frequencies, also suggests that their expression is inherited. However, it is also clear that idiotypes first identified on antibodies binding to DNA are not confined to antibodies with this antigen-binding specificity. Indeed, the expression of, for example, the 16/6 idiotype on anti-*Klebsiella* antibodies and the 3I idiotype on anti-pneumococcal antibodies points strongly to a link between autoimmunity and infectious disease.

Further reading

Denbury, S.D., Carbotte, R.M., and Denburg, J.A. (1997). Psychological aspects of systemic lupus erythematosus: cognitive function, mood and self-report. *Journal of Rheumatology*, **24**, 998–1003.

Godfrey, T., Khamashta, M.A., and Hughes, G.R. (1998). Therapeutic advances in systemic lupus erythematosus. *Current Opinion in Rheumatology*, **10**, 435–41.

Hahn, B.H. (1998). Antibodies to DNA. *New England Journal of Medicine*, **338**, 1359–68.

Pisetsky, D.S., Gilkeson, G., and St Clair, E.W. (1997). Systemic lupus erythematosus: diagnosis and treatment. *Medical Clinics of North America*, **81**, 113–28.

Stratta, P., Canavese, C., Ferrero, *et al.* (1997). Guidelines to looking at antiphospholipid antibodies in systemic lupus erythematosus. *Nephron*, **76**, 400–5.

Chapter 10.12

Systemic sclerosis

C. M. Black

Systemic sclerosis is a disease which results in widespread damage to small blood vessels and fibrosis in both the cutaneous tissue and the internal organs. Consequent disability may be minimal or life-threatening. Skin thickening is the hallmark of the disease. Historically, the term 'scleroderma' (Plate 1) has encompassed both the skin lesions of systemic sclerosis (Table 1) and the heterogeneous group of dermal fibrotic conditions known as localized scleroderma in which vascular and internal organ involvement are absent (Table 2). A transition from localized scleroderma to systemic sclerosis is excessively rare, as is the coexistence of the two diseases. Environmental and chemical agents have been implicated in the development of systemic sclerosis (Table 3) and many conditions have scleroderma-like features, e.g. amyloid, carcinoid, and scleromyxoedema (Table 4).

Table 1 Spectrum of systemic sclerosis

1. **'Pre-scleroderma'**
Raynaud's phenomenon plus nailfold capillary changes and circulating antinuclear antibodies (topoisomerase I, anticentromere, nucleolar).
2. **Diffuse cutaneous systemic sclerosis**
Onset of skin changes (puffy or hidebound) within 1 year of onset of Raynaud's phenomenon
Truncal and acral skin involvement
Presence of tendon friction rubs
Early and significant incidence of interstitial lung disease, oliguric renal failure, diffuse gastrointestinal disease, and myocardial involvement
Nailfold capillary dilatation and capillary drop out
Antitopoisomerase I (Scl-70) antibodies (30% of patients)
3. **Limited cutaneous systemic sclerosis**
Raynaud's phenomenon for years (occasionally decades)
Skin involvement limited to hands, face, feet, and forearms (acral) or absent
A significant (10–15 years) late incidence of pulmonary hypertension, with or without interstitial lung disease, skin calcifications, telangiectasia, and gastrointestinal involvement
A high incidence of anticentromere antibody (ACA) (70–80%)
Dilated nailfold capillary loops, usually without capillary dropout
4. **Scleroderma sine scleroderma**
Raynaud's phenomenon +/–
No skin involvement
Presentation with pulmonary fibrosis, scleroderma renal crisis, cardiac disease, gastrointestinal disease
Antinuclear antibodies may be present (Scl-70, ACA, nucleolar)

Table 2 Localized scleroderma

Morphoea types:	plaque guttate bullous morphea profunda (subcutaneous) nodular (keloid) generalized
Linear types:	*en coup de sabre* facial hemiatrophy
Morphea ←→	eosinophilic fasciitis

Table 3 Chemical agents implicated in the development of scleroderma

Organic chemicals aliphatic hydrocarbons, e.g. vinyl chloride, trichlorethylene aromatic hydrocarbons, e.g. benzene, toluene
Epoxy resins
Toxic oil (aniline-treated rape-seed oil)
Silica, in stone masons, coal miners, gold miners
Foam insulation (urea-formaldehyde)
Drugs, e.g. L-tryptophan, bleomycin, cocaine, pentazocine, and appetite suppressants
Augmentation mammoplasty, silicone, paraffin

Table 4 Scleroderma-like syndromes

Immunological/ inflammatory	Chronic graft-versus-host disease, eosinophilic fasciitis, overlap syndromes (with rheumatoid arthritis, systemic lupus erythematosus syndrome, for example) undifferentiated connective tissue disease
Metabolic	Sclerodema of Buschke } with or without Scleromyxoedema } paraproteinaemia Insulin-dependent diabetes mellitus (digital sclerosis) Carcinoid syndrome Acromegaly Lichen sclerosis et atrophicus Acrodermatitis chronica atrophicans Amyloidosis
Inherited	Phenylketonuria Porphyrias Premature ageing syndromes—progeria, Werner's syndrome
Localized systemic sclerosis and visceral diseases	Idiopathic pulmonary fibrosis Amyloidosis Sarcoidosis Infiltrating carcinomas Infiltrating cardiomyopathy Oesophageal and intestinal hypomotility syndromes

In some patients the disease is not clearly defined, there being in addition features of other connective tissue disorders.

The disease is global in distribution and appears to affect all races. It strikes 18 people per million in the UK every year, and 20 per million in the United States. Age, sex, race, and genetic factors all influence development. Systemic sclerosis is the only connective tissue disease in which several environmental factors have been implicated as initiating factors, and the finding of antinuclear antibodies in the serum of spouses of patients with the disease adds weight to the supposition of environmental influences.

Systemic sclerosis usually begins between the ages of 30 and 60, although it is also found in children and may strike the elderly. It affects women approximately four times as often as men, and this ratio increases during the child-bearing years. It is slightly more common in the Afro-American than the Caucasian, and more severe in the non-Caucasian patient. Scleroderma usually occurs in a sporadic fashion, and familial occurrence is unusual but it, or other connective tissue disorders, has been reported in the families of patients with systemic sclerosis; this, and the increased incidence of antinuclear antibodies in blood relatives (particularly females) suggests a genetic susceptibility related to the human leucocyte antigen (**HLA**) system.

The typical patients presents with Raynaud's phenomenon, often with other complaints such as swollen hands, tight skin, and painful joints and muscles. Swallowing difficulties may be an early symptom, and the challenge is then to detect those patients destined to have a progressive and complicated course as opposed to those whose disease will remain mild. The duration, both of Raynaud's phenomenon and of other symptoms and signs, helps place the patient in one of the two major subsets (Table 1): the relatively benign and at worst slowly progressive limited cutaneous systemic sclerosis or the aggressive diffuse cutaneous form. Patients with the rarer scleroderma *sine* scleroderma often have Raynaud's phenomenon and express the appropriate antibodies; they lack changes in the skin but not in other tissues susceptible to the change of sclerosis. Within the spectrum overall should be included patients who appear to have primary Raynaud's phenomenon, but with positive autoantibodies and abnormal nailfold capillaries; these patients may be developing more classical systemic sclerosis.

Raynaud's phenomenon

Raynaud's phenomenon is an episodic event characterized by pallor, cyanosis, suffusion, and/or pain in the fingers, toes, ears, nose, or jaw in response to cold or stress. It affects 3–10 per cent of the adult population world-wide and has a predilection for females. About 1 per cent of those showing the phenomenon develop a connective tissue disease, the most common of which is scleroderma. Other conditions associated with Raynaud's include cervical rib, vibration white finger, hypothyroidism, and uraemia. It is important to make an accurate diagnosis; Raynaud's is intermittent and is not usually the cause of cold extremities, chilblains, or digital ulceration. Associated symptoms such as rash, ulcers, changes in skin texture, calcium deposits in skin, painful swollen joints, myalgia, muscle weakness, difficulty in swallowing, or breathlessness would indicate that the primary condition has developed into one of the connective tissue disorders, if not systemic sclerosis itself.

Limited cutaneous scleroderma

This was formerly described as the CREST syndrome (Calcinosis circumscripta, Raynaud's, Esophagus, Sclerodactyly, and Telangiectasia) and is the most common form of the disease, accounting for some 60 per cent of cases overall. The patient is usually female,

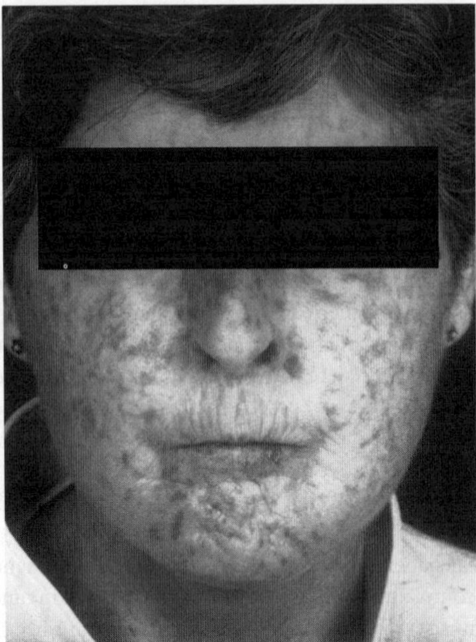

Fig. 1 This patient shows the typical facial features of scleroderma—microstamina, thickened shiny skin, and beaking of the nose, with telangiectasia on lips and forehead, and alopecia.

between 30 and 50 years old. Raynaud's phenomenon will already be long-standing in such a patient, often of up to 20 years' duration. Skin changes are noticed, but at first disturbing only from a cosmetic point of view. She will often complain of swelling of her hands with some thickening of the skin or the fingers, with local pain which may extend to the wrist with some of the features of a carpal tunnel syndrome. The bilateral nature of the problem, with furrowing and puckering around the mouth as well as telangiectases on the face and anterior chest and painful crusting lesions on the fingertips, should lead to the correct diagnosis (Fig. 1). The patient may also complain of dyspepsia from reflex oesophagitis.

Diffuse cutaneous scleroderma

Patients with this form, often only have a very short history of Raynaud's phenomenon, which may indeed have arisen concurrently with other symptoms and signs and sometimes will have followed the skin changes. These patients (less than 40 per cent of the total) are often in their fourth decade, although the range extends from the first to the eighth; they are more likely to be male. The onset of the disease is often abrupt with diffuse, bilateral, and sometimes itchy and painful swelling of the fingers, arms, feet, legs, and face. Rapid weight loss and fatigue are common and the muscles may be weak. Oesophageal symptoms are frequent as is exertional dyspnoea. If the patient presents at a later stage, i.e. 2–3 years after onset, widespread skin thickening with painful joint contractures, muscle wasting, and digital ulcers are usually the major complaints, along with those related to disease of the internal organs. Headaches, blurring of vision, and significant hypertension may portend a hypersensitive renal crisis, and requires immediate action (see OTM3, pp. 3198 and 3290–1 and Chapters 12.10 and 12.28).

Scleroderma *sine* scleroderma

These patients are the most difficult group to recognize. They may or may not have Raynaud's phenomenon, but never have the skin changes of scleroderma: common presenting problems include oesophagitis, malabsorption, pseudo-obstruction, renal failure, cardiac arrhythmias, and interstitial drug disease.

Physical examination

Raynaud's phenomenon

Most patients with Raynaud's destined to develop systemic sclerosis will have done so within the first 2 years of the onset of the phenomenon. After this time, fewer than 5 per cent will develop it. The clinical examination must include the nailfold capillaries, looking for typical changes that are highly predictive of the subsequent development of sclerosis. There are several ways to do this:

1. with the naked eye—only occasionally rewarding;
2. with an ophthalmoscope or other form of magnification (some workers regard this method as having a sensitivity equal to that of microscopy); and
3. capillary microscopy, which is highly sensitive and also allows for a permanent photographic recording of a row of horizontal capillary loops at the nailfold, just proximal to the cuticle.

On microscopy two morphological patterns may be seen, either dilatation of many loops, or 'giant' loops associated with avascular areas without visible capillaries. The latter pattern is associated with diffuse disease. The capillary patterns appear early and are remarkably constant over time. Taken together with the presence of specific autoantibodies, they can detect more than 95 per cent of patients in a stage transitional to the full-blown disease.

Limited cutaneous systemic sclerosis

Early in the disease there is non-pitting oedema of the fingers (sausage-shaped fingers) which after several weeks or months is gradually replaced by skin thickening. The thickening occurs in the dermis and is accompanied by epidermal thinning, leading to a loss of skin creases, hair, and secretions but the skin involvement in this subset is minimal. It may thicken and become shiny but it is not usually so closely adherent to the underlying structures that mobility of tendons, joints, and muscle is severely impaired—in sharp contrast to findings in the diffuse disease. Involvement does not spread proximally on to the trunk, but the face should be examined for thin, tightly pursed lips and microstomia. The most striking cutaneous finding is digital and facial telangiectasis. Other evidence of structural vascular change is to be seen in the fingertips, where small areas of ischaemic necrosis or ulceration are common, often leaving pitting scars and pulp atrophy. The reabsorption of the tufts of the terminal phalanges, suspected clinically and confirmed on radiography, is also presumed to be due to ischaemia. These patients also often develop intracutaneous and subcutaneous calcification in the fingers, particularly on the digital pads, and periarticular tissues such as the pre-patella area and olecranon bursa. Such calcinotic masses vary in size from tiny lumps to large masses in the forearms and legs. They are often complicated by ulceration of overlying skin, extrusion of calcium, and secondary bacterial infection.

In an early case the patient may be otherwise healthy, but if the disease has been present for more than 10–15 years, two major complications may arise: small bowel involvement and pulmonary hypertension. The former may result in malabsorption, anaemia, marked weight loss, oily, bulky, offensive stools, and abdominal distension. This complication, except for those few patients who have a functional ileus (pseudo-obstruction) has a slower clinical evolution than that of pulmonary hypertension. Severe pulmonary arterial hypertension is found in up to 10 per cent of patients in the limited cutaneous subset, and is not secondary to pulmonary interstitial fibrosis, which in such patients is either absent or mild. In addition to marked dyspnoea, these patients develop right ventricular hypertrophy, an accentuated pulmonary component of the second heart sound, and eventually signs of right heart failure. The prognosis is extremely poor and mean duration of survival from detection is only 2 years.

Diffuse cutaneous scleroderma

The clinical findings in diffuse scleroderma depend on the stage of the disease. At the onset, which is often abrupt, examination will usually reveal cold, painful, swollen hands, with the swelling and stiffness already extending into the arms, the feet, and the lower legs, the face, and the trunk. The oedematous phase is usually replaced within a few months by the indurative phase, when the skin becomes tight and shiny, and bound to underlying structures. Hyperpigmentation or hypopigmentation accompanies the skin thickening in many patients.

The natural history of skin involvement is quite different from that in the limited form of the disease, and can be mapped semi-quantitatively, by the measurement of the degree and extent of cutaneous thickening in multiple sites, from which is derived a skin score. In diffuse scleroderma, the skin score increases rapidly at first and often peaks after 1–3 years. This rapid progression is accompanied by impaired mobility in tendons, joints, and muscles. The contractures and stretching of the skin over the bony points often lead to painful ulcers which are slow to heal. The most frequent site for the ulcers are the proximal interphalangeal joints; the elbows and malleoli of the ankles are other favoured sites.

In its earliest stages diffuse scleroderma may be confused with an acute inflammatory arthropathy, particularly if Raynaud's phenomenon is absent. The oedematous puffy skin is often accompanied by symmetrically stiff, painful joints (hands, feet, ankles, knees, and wrists) but the classic synovitis of rheumatoid arthritis is usually absent. A sign which must be carefully sought in this group is a tendon friction rub which has a distinctive leathery crepitus: it may be elicited over elbows, knees, fingers, wrists, and ankles, during joint movement. These are ominous signs, frequently antedating a rapid increase in cutaneous involvement, or the onset of visceral disease. A carpal tunnel syndrome may be present due to a flexor tenosynovitis at the wrist. Mild muscle disease is common; not usually accompanied by an increase in plasma creatine phosphokinase or inflammatory changes on muscle biopsy. It is also non-progressive. A few patients have florid changes of polymyositis, and are usually classified to have an overlap syndrome. As with limited disease, evidence of structural vascular damage may be found in the nailfold capillaries and the digital pads, and can be extensive.

It is the timing of the onset of visceral disease that distinguishes the patient with diffuse from the one with limited scleroderma; the signs of, for example, gastrointestinal involvement are similar in both subsets (Table 5), but occur earlier in the diffuse form of the disease. Lung involvement (Table 6) occurs in 70 per cent of patients, and is the most common cause of death directly related to scleroderma. It has two components: interstitial lung disease and pulmonary hypertension. The hypertension is either secondary to lung fibrosis and then mild; or severe and associated with limited cutaneous scleroderma. Unfortunately, patients with interstitial lung disease often have few clinical signs, although careful auscultation may reveal fine bilateral basal crepitations. Primary heart disease in scleroderma consists of pericarditis with or without effusion, heart failure (left or bi-ventricular), or arrhythmias. (Table 7). Again, clinical signs are not common. Symptomatic pericarditis is unusual and heart failure occurs in less than 5 per cent of patients. Arrhythmias are often symptomless.

The regular recording of the blood pressure is particularly important in early diffuse disease (less than 5 years' duration). Between 15 and 20 per cent of these patients develop a scleroderma renal crisis, with the abrupt onset of malignant hypertension. Clinical features include visual difficulties with retinopathy, severe headaches, seizures, or left heart failure. Normotensive renal failure has been reported and is often accompanied by severe microangiopathic haemolytic anaemia. Renal crisis may also be precipitated by sudden severe volume depletion in a susceptible patient who has had clinically undetected reduced renal blood flow (see Chapter 12.28).

Disease course

Patients with *limited disease* have an 'early phase' that lasts about 10 years, when the picture is usually dominated by Raynaud's phenomenon, pitting scars, digital ulcers, and telangiectiasiae. Later there may be worsening of the vascular disease, both cutaneously and in the pulmonary circulation. Pulmonary interstitial disease, usually more indolent than that seen in the diffuse form, can also occur as a late complication. Gut involvement may worsen with time, and oesophageal strictures, malabsorption, pseudo-obstruction, and anal incontinence are all potential late and troublesome events in this subset.

During the early phase of *diffuse disease* (the first 5 years), the patient is fatigued and loses weight. Hypertensive renal crisis is a real risk and rapid progression of pulmonary and cardiac disease may occur. Arthritis, myositis, and tendon involvement can be most marked at this time. After 5 years, considered to be the late stage of diffuse disease, the constitutional symptoms settle down, the skin and musculoskeletal problems have usually reached a plateau, and there is progression of existing visceral disease but reduced risk of new organ involvement. These differences in pattern and natural history influence evaluation and therapy.

Pathogenesis

The pathophysiology of systemic sclerosis includes immunological, vascular, and connective tissue abnormalities. The concept of an initial immune attack on the endothelial cell and fibroblast or other component of the extracellular matrix is an attractive one. Currently, the precise relationship between these components is unknown. They may represent separate processes, different target responses to a common process, or a sequential event with the initial target being the endothelial cell and the resultant factors acting on the fibroblast to cause fibrosis (Fig. 2).

The use of the laboratory

Any patient with Raynaud's phenomenon may develop scleroderma; the identification of one of the scleroderma-specific autoantibodies has been shown to be a useful predictor. The anticentromere antibody has a predictive value for the development of the limited cutaneous

Table 5 Gut involvement in scleroderma

Region	Disorder	Symptom	Investigation	Treatment
Mouth	Sicca syndrome	Dry mouth	Salivary gland biopsy	Artificial saliva
Oesophagus	↓ Motility	Dysphagia	Oesophageal scintiscan	Domperidone Metoclopramide Cisapride
	↓ Lower oesophageal sphincter pressure → Reflux	Retrosternal discomfort/pain	Endoscopy Barium swallow	Omeprozole
	Stricture	Dysphagia	Endoscopy	Dilatation and omeprazole
Stomach	Ulceration secondary to NSAIDs	Dyspepsia	Endoscopy	H_2 blockers then misoprostol
	Gastric paresis	Anorexia, nausea/vomiting, early satiety	Scintigram	Metoclopramide
Small bowel	Hypomotility, stasis/bacterial, overgrowth, adynamic ileus pseudo-obstruction	Weight loss, abdominal, distension, steatorrhoea episodes of abdominal pain and distension	Ba follow-through, hydrogen breath test or ^{14}[C] glycocholate breath test jejunal aspiration, 3-day faecal fat, plain abdominal radiograph	Antibiotics (anti-anaerobes) Metoclopramide/cisapride Pancreatic supplements Total parenteral nutrition
	Small bowel ulcers secondary to NSAIDs	Chronic anaemia, abdominal pain	Small bowel enema	Misoprostol
	Pneumatosis intestinalis	Diarrhoea and blood, benign pneumoperitoneum	Plain abdominal radiograph	Oxygen
Large bowel	Sigmoid/rectal hypomotility	Alternating constipation/ diarrhoea	Barium enema	Dietary manipulation+stool expanders (e.g. ispaghula)
	Colonic wide-mouthed pseudodiverticulae	Rare perforation	Barium enema	(Resection)
	Anal sphincter involvement	Anal incontinence	Rectal manometry	??Stimulation

Table 6 Pulmonary disease in scleroderma

Disorder	Symptoms	Signs	Investigations	Therapeutic possibilities
Pulmonary fibrosis	Dry cough	↓ Chest expansion	Chest radiography	Steroids +/−
	Dyspnoea	Basal crepitations	Lung function tests High-resolution CT scan DTPA scan Bronchoalveolar lavage Lung biopsy	cyclophosphamide, azathioprine, D-penicillamine, cyclosporin, α-interferon Intravenous or intra-arterial prostacyclin
Pulmonary hypertension	Dyspnoea Ankle oedema	Loud P_2 right ventricular heave	Chest radiography Doppler-echo cardiography cardiac catheter	Nifedipine ?ACE inhibitor
Rare complications				
Bronchiectasis				Antibiotic treatment if necessary
Spontaneous pneumothorax				Try to avoid a tube
Lung carcinoma (squamous, adeno-carcinoma, small cell)				Use drugs and radiotherapy; most cases unsuitable for surgery

disease (sensitivity 60 per cent, specificity 98 per cent) and Scl-70 for the diffuse subset (sensitivity 38 per cent, specificity 100 per cent). Other autoantibodies, notably those to nucleolar antigens, are also relatively specific for scleroderma, and the proportion of patients having one or more antibody is over 80 per cent of the total. Some of these antibodies have been shown to have correlations with class II major histocompatibility complex polymorphisms. A summary of the clinical and laboratory characteristics of patients according to serum autoantibody type is shown in Table 8. Although these antibodies are good markers of individual subsets, a pathogenic role for

Table 7 Cardiac involvement in scleroderma

Disorder	Effect	Frequency	Symptom	Investigation	Treatment
Pericardial involvement	Pericardial effusion	10–15% clinically 35% at autopsy More common in localized than diffuse scleroderma	Chest pain Dyspnoea	Chest radiography Electrocardiography Echocardiography	NSAIDS Steroids Rarely drainage
Myocardial fibrosis	Congestive cardiac failure Arrhythmias	30–50% More common in diffuse than localized	Dyspnoea Oedema Atypical chest pain Palpitation	Thallium scan MUGA scan Holter monitor	Diuretics Calcium channel blockers Antiarrhythmics
Myocarditis failure	Congestive cardiac Ankle oedema	Rare Echocardiography	Dyspnoea	Electrocardiography	Corticosteroids

MUGA = multiple uptake gated acquisition scan.

Again, clinical signs are not common. Acute symptomatic pericarditis is unusual, congestive cardiac failure occurs in less than 5 per cent of patients, and arrhythmias are often asymptomatic.

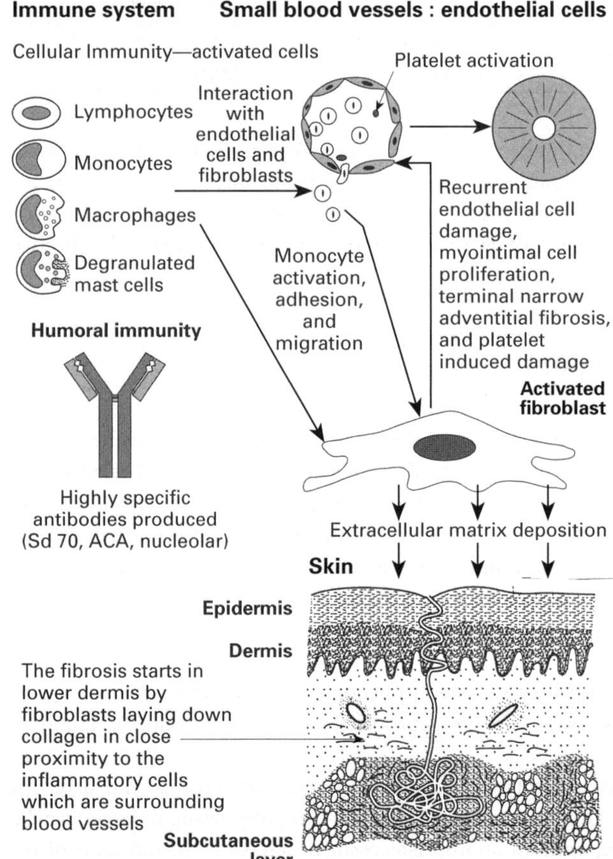

Fig. 2 Pathophysiology of systemic sclerosis.

them has yet to be assigned: there is evidence for either molecular mimicry or an antigen-driven process.

Other less specific serological abnormalities include hypergammaglobulinaemia, the presence of immune complexes, low concentrations of complement components, and a weakly positive rheumatoid factor. Antibodies to SSA/Ro and SSB/La are found in 50 per cent of scleroderma patients who also have Sjögren's syndrome, and are nearly always found in patients with glandular lymphocyte infiltration rather than fibrosis. Once the patient has developed full-blown disease other investigations will be needed to assess function of small bowel, lung, heart, and kidneys. In a patient with limited cutaneous disease, only a few of these tests need to be repeated regularly; the longer the disease has been present, the greater the need for monitoring for pulmonary hypertension and for small bowel disease.

The monitoring of the diffuse syndrome is quite different. In the first 3 to 4 critical years of the disease, patients need monthly serum creatinine and urinary microscopy and measurements every 3 months creatinine clearance and monitoring of cardiac and lung function every 6 months.

Lung disease is a current major challenge. Chest radiography is not sufficiently sensitive to identify early involvement. Pulmonary function tests, particularly exercise ones, are more sensitive, but neither they nor chest radiography provide a guide to the course of the disease in the lung. The combined use of thin section (3 mm) high-resolution computed tomography (CT) (Fig. 3), bronchoalveolar lavage, and **DTPA** scans is beginning to provide much earlier diagnosis and indices of progression (see OTM3, pp. 3033). Bronchoalveolar lavage identifies patients with an alveolitis often before the onset of symptoms or abnormalities on chest radiography or in pulmonary function tests. DTPA scans, particularly serial ones, may become useful predictors of progression or improvement.

Other organ involvement

Neurological involvement is uncommon, but in the late stages of limited cutaneous disease a small proportion of patients develops unilateral or bilateral trigeminal neuralgia. Impotence is also a major problem for males with the diffuse syndrome. It usually occurs 1–2 years after the onset and is thought to have an neurovascular cause which is refractory to treatment.

Dryness of the mucus membranes is common and dyspareunia frequent. Hypothyroidism occurs in as many as 50 per cent of patients with systemic sclerosis and is frequently missed. Some patients have antithyroid antibodies but lymphocytic infiltration in the gland is uncommon, fibrosis being the more typical finding.

Table 8 Serum autoantibodies with clinical and laboratory correlates

Antigen	Antinuclear antibody staining pattern	HLA associations	Frequency in all patients (%)	Clinical associations	Organ involvement
Scl-70 Topoisomerase 1	Speckled	DR5 (DR11) DR3/DR52a DQ7 DQB1	15–20	Diffuse	Lung fibrosis
ACA centromere	Centromere (kinetochore)	DR1 (DQ5) DQB1 DR4 (D13 subtypes)	25–30	Limited	Pulmonary hypertension
RNA I and III	Speckled/nucleolar	?	20	Diffuse	Renal Skin
U_3RNP	Nucleolar	?	5	Overlap Mixed	Pulmonary hypertension Muscle
U_1RNP	Speckled	?	10	Limited overlap Afro-Caribbeans	Muscle
Th (To)	Nucleolar	?	5	Limited	Pulmonary hypertension Small bowel
PM-Scl	Nucleolar	DR3 DR52	3–5	Overlap Mixed	Muscle

Survival

The 5-year cumulative survival rate ranges from 34 to 73 per cent. Even prolonged survival does not protect against an increased mortality risk, which continues over time for at least 15 years. Factors which adversely affect outcome are increasing age, being male, extent of skin involvement, and heart, lung, and renal disease. Survival has altered little in the past 50 years, reflecting the lack of any truly effective therapy.

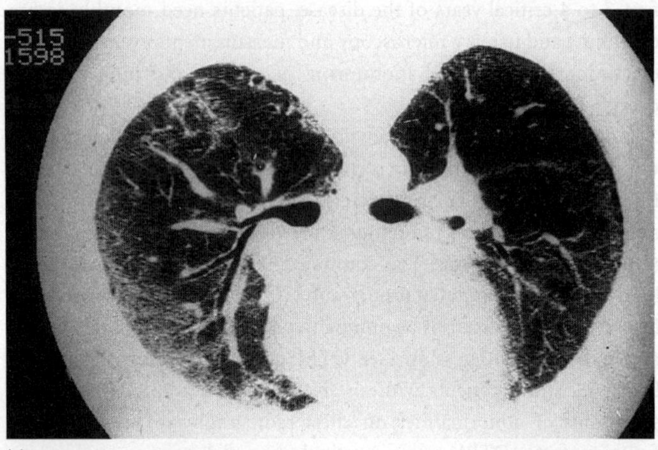

(a)

(b)

Fig. 3(a)(b) Thin section CT scan images illustrating: (a) the ground glass appearance of early pulmonary involvement posteriorly, associated with a normal chest radiograph. (b) Extensive honeycomb shadowing and cystic air spaces involving both lower lobes, with corresponding chest radiographic appearances of advanced interstitial lung disease (bibasilar reticulonodular shadowing).
((With grateful acknowledgement to Drs A. Wells, R. du Bois, and B. Strickland, Departments of Respiratory Medicine and Radiology, Royal Brompton National Heart and Lung Hospitals (Chelsea).)

Treatment

Scleroderma is a chronic disease, difficult to manage, and patients are often pessimistic at the onset. The first responsibility of the physician is therefore to discuss with the patient and relatives the particular form of his or her disease. An adjunct to such discussion is provided by the excellent publications available through patient support groups, and these should be recommended. Current treatments include management of Raynaud's phenomenon, some aimed to modify the immune system and encroaching fibrosis and the approach to specific organ problems. A graded scheme for the management of Raynaud's phenomenon with some of the drugs in current usage and the appropriate surgical procedures is found in Table 9.

Many patients find lanolin and other oils, creams, and bath oils helpful for moisturizing the skin. Unsightly telangiectiasiae can be covered with an appropriate cosmetic preparation. Infection of ulcerated fingers must be treated promptly, and troublesome calcinotic

Table 9 Treatment of Raynaud's phenomenon

Stages of Raynaud's phenomenon	Recommended treatment
Simple short attacks	Warmth, heating appliances No smoking or β-blockers Fish oil and evening primrose oil
Frequent prolonged attacks interfering with daily living often accompanied by digital infarcts	Calcium-channel blockers, e.g. nifedipine, diltiazem, felodipine, isradipine, norcardipine Transdermal glyceryl trinitrate AcE inhibitor, e.g. captopril Ketanserin—selective $5HT_2$ receptor antagonist reducing 5-hydroxytryptomine (5HT)-induced vasospasm and platelet aggregation
Severe prolonged attacks with ulceration and incipient gangrene	Prostacyclin infusion
Secondary infection	Antibiotics, surgery (e.g. debridement, nail removal, nail bed removal)
Gangrene	Amputation—auto, surgical
Surgical measures	Cervical sympathectomy—should be avoided Lumbar sympathectomy—still has a place for Raynaud's phenomenon of the lower limb Digital sympathectomy for severe pain and ulceration of fingers or toes: may be used in conjunction with intravenous prostacyclin

Table 10 Drugs currently used in treatment of scleroderma

Drug	Mechanism of action	Efficacy in trials	
		Uncontrolled	Controlled (double blind)
D-Penicillamine	Forms a complex with hydroxylysine aldehyde and lysine groups needed for formation of stable collagen cross-links, so reducing collagen production	Yes: lung, skin, renal	?
Interferon α and γ	Specific inhibitory effect on collagen production by fibroblasts, possibly by elimination of a subpopulation of high-collagen-producing fibroblasts, or by inhibiting procollagen mRNA synthesis	Yes	?
Cyclosporin	Alters early immune response by reducing IL-2 production ? via reduced m-RNA transcription; also reduction in IL-1 from monocytes	Yes	?
Methotrexate	Folic acid antagonist	Yes	?
Azathioprine	Purine antagonist—thus reducing DNA synthesis	?	?
Cyclophosphamide + prednisolone	Alkylating agent Immunosuppressant	+ Yes for arthralgia, myositis	?
Plasmapheresis + prednisolone and cyclosporin	Removes immune complexes and vasoactive substances	Alone no good ? in combination	
Pentoxifylline	Reduces fibroblast proliferation and synthesis of collagen glycosamino-glycans and fibronectin	Yes	?
Antithymocyte globulin	Disruption of T-cell activity early in disease, may reduce cytokine production and hence fibroblast activation	Yes	?
Photopheresis	Extracorporeal exposure of blood to photoactivated 8-methoxypsoralen to reduce activity of aberrant T cells	Yes	?
Factor XIII	Inhibits collagen synthesis	Yes	?

deposits may be removed surgically. The role of physiotherapy, exercises, and splinting is controversial—if these therapies are to be of any use they must be started at the onset and performed regularly.

Prevention or attenuation of renal failure by the use of angiotensin-converting enzyme inhibitors has been reported in a few patients, but there is no effective treatment for vascular insufficiency and fibrosis in the lung, heart, and gastrointestinal tract.

A number of drugs have been tried and largely found wanting (Table 10).

Overlap syndromes

Some patients have features overlapping with those of other connective tissue diseases. A variety of terms such as mixed connective tissue disease, undifferentiated connective tissue syndrome, and overlap syndromes have emerged to describe such patients. Whether or not mixed connective tissue disease is a true entity as first suggested in the 1970s is controversial. Sharp described patients with some of the features of polymyositis, lupus, and scleroderma who ran a benign course with no pulmonary, cerebral, or renal involvement, and no vasculitis. They supposedly responded well to low-dose steroids, and could be identified by the presence of antibody with a specificity for nuclear U1 ribonucleoprotein (**RNP**) antigen. However, neither the clinical features, the laboratory tests, nor the response to therapy have proven to be specific, and these patients do not fulfil the definition of and diagnostic criteria for a single disease. Neither do they fall within the 'overlap syndromes' assuming the definition for this subset to be the coexistence of two separate diseases. These patients do not 'conform'. Many with long-term follow-up develop major internal organ involvement and evolve into a defined connective tissue disease. RNP antibodies can be found in patients with scleroderma or systemic lupus erythematosus.

The typical patient with this syndrome presents with Raynaud's phenomenon, puffy hands, arthralgia, myositis, abnormal oesophageal motility, and lymphadenopathy. Over a period of a few years, the skin may become thickened, telangiectiasiae and calcinosis may appear, and signs and symptoms of interstitial lung disease emerge; such a patient has developed scleroderma. Another patient with similar initial findings may develop alopecia, photosensitivity, mouth ulcers, renal disease, antibodies to dsDNA and has developed systemic lupus erythematosus. Patients who remain undifferentiated (about 50 per cent at 5 years) are almost invariably a subset carrying HLA-DR4, the exceptions carrying HLA-DR2. Whether these observations imply the presence of a single disease entity remains unclear.

Further reading

Jacobson, S., Halberg, P., Ullman, S., *et al.* (1998). Clinical features and serum antinuclear antibodies in 230 Danish patients with systemic sclerosis. *British Journal of Rheumatology*, 37, 39–45.

Mitchell, H., Bolsten, M.B., and LeRoy, E.C. (1997). Scleroderma and related conditions. *Medical Clinics of North America*, **81**, 129–49.

Spencer-Green, G., Alter, D., and Welch, H.G. (1997). Test performance in systemic sclerosis, anti-centromere and anti-Scl-70 antibodies. *American Journal of Medicine*, **103**, 242–8.

Chapter 10.13

Sjögren's syndrome

P. J. W. Venables

Sjögren's syndrome comprising the triad of dry eyes, dry mouth, and rheumatoid arthritis is characterized by inflammation and destruction of exocrine glands, principally the lachrymal and salivary glands. The syndrome is now classified as primary when it exists on its own, or secondary when associated with other disease, such as rheumatoid arthritis, systemic lupus erythematosus, systemic sclerosis, polymyositis, and primary biliary cirrhosis. The syndrome has also been described in chronic graft-versus-host disease, after bone marrow transplantation and in infection with human T-lymphotropic virus (**HTLV**)-1 and human immunodeficiency virus (**HIV**)-1.

Aetiology and pathology

The aetiology and Sjögren's syndrome is not known, but is often considered to be related to an interaction between genetic and environmental factors, leading to autoimmunity. Primary Sjögren's syndrome is strongly associated with HLA-DR3 and the linked genes B8 and DQ2 and the C4A null gene. The syndrome occurring with HIV infection, which has been termed diffuse infiltrative lymphocytosis syndrome is associated with alleles of HLA-DR5 and -DR6, with a decreased frequency of HLA-B35.

Obvious candidates for triggering autoimmunity are viruses which infect the salivary glands; Epstein–Barr virus and cytomegalovirus have been the main subjects of investigation, with conflicting results. Epstein–Barr virus has been detected in biopsies of parotid and labial glands, but it remains controversial whether or not the virus has truly triggered the lymphocytic infiltration and inflammation. Because Sjögren's syndrome can be caused by HIV and HTLV-1 there has been much recent speculation that an unknown retrovirus could cause idiopathic disease.

The cardinal pathological features are inflammation and destruction of salivary tissue. In the primary and connective-tissue-associated syndrome the infiltrating cells are mainly CD4-positive T cells, found largely around ducts and acini. In cases associated with HIV-1 infection, the infiltrating lymphocytes are CD8-positive T cells, but the simple microscopic appearances are very similar. Scattered interstitial plasma cells are common, but are also seen in the glands of normal people. The destructive changes are predominantly of duct dilatation, acinal atrophy, and interstitial fibrosis. These latter findings can also be seen in biopsies of glands in patients without Sjögren's syndrome, particularly in the elderly, and cannot be regarded as specific.

Clinical features

Sjögren's syndrome is nine times more common in women than men and its onset is at any age from 15 to 65. Patients rarely complain of dry eyes, but rather a gritty sensation, soreness, photosensitivity, or intolerance of contact lenses. In early disease excessive watering or deposits of dried mucus in the corner of the eye and recurrent attacks of conjunctivitis may occur. The dry mouth is often manifest as the 'cream cracker' sign, inability to swallow dry food without fluid, or the need to wake up in the night to take sips of water. About half of patients complain of intermittent parotid swelling, sometimes

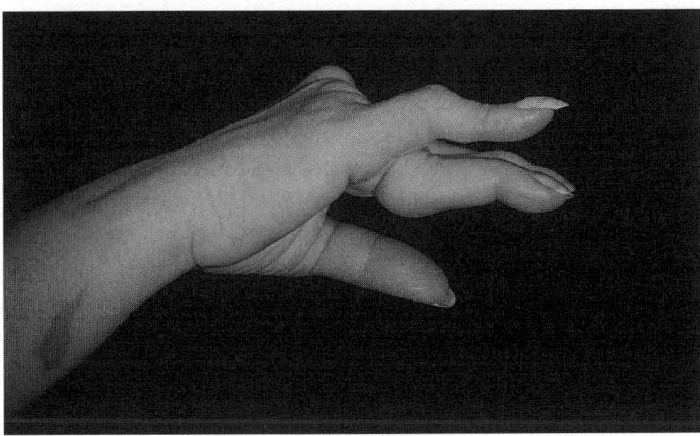

Fig. 1 Hands of a patient with long-standing primary Sjögren's syndrome, showing correctable swan-necking deformities similar to the Jaccoud-like arthritis seen in systemic lupus erythematosus.

misdiagnosed as recurrent mumps. When the swelling is excessively painful it is often due to secondary bacterial infection. Xerostomia can be detected as a diminished salivary pool, a dried fissured tongue, often complicated by angular stomatitis and chronic oral candidiasis. The eyes may be reddened and roughened due to shallow erosions in the conjunctiva. Occasionally, the front of the eye is eroded to reveal stands of underlying collagen leading to the appearance of filamentary keratitis.

Other exocrine glands may be affected. Dry nasal passages and upper airways may lead to recurrent bouts of sinusitis, a dry cough, and possibly, a higher than expected frequency of chest infections. Dry skin and dry hair are symptoms frequently elicited by questioning. About 30 per cent of patients have diminished vaginal secretions and may present with dyspareunia. Involvement of the gastrointestinal tract leads to reflux oesophagitis or gastritis due to lack of protective mucus secretion, and some patients complain of constipation which may be attributed to defective mucus in the colon and rectum. Pancreatic failure, leading to malabsorption syndromes, occurs rarely. Endocrine disease in the form of a higher than expected frequency of thyroid autoimmunity also occurs. Whether this is part of the same pathological process is debatable. Nevertheless, it underlines the importance of checking thyroid function from time to time in patients with Sjögren's syndrome. The possibility of underlying infection with HIV or HTLV-1 should always be borne in mind and appropriate serological tests ordered where indicated.

Systemic manifestations

Two-thirds of patients with primary disease, complain of fatigue and depression. Occasionally, weight loss and fever mimicking an occult malignancy may be the presenting symptoms, particularly in the elderly. Other features include an arthritis which resembles the Jaccoud-like arthritis of systemic lupus erythematosus (Fig. 1). Raynaud's phenomenon occurs in about 50 per cent of patients, although a true vasculitis is less common. Waldenström's benign hypergammaglobulinaemic purpura affecting the lower legs is found in patients with very high IgG levels. Patients may present with polymyalgia rheumatica or, much less frequently, polymyositis. Pleurisy occurs in about 40 per cent , and a high prevalence of pulmonary function abnormalities has been described, although these are rarely clinically significant. A wide range of neurological diseases, including findings resembling multiple sclerosis, have been described, although these appear to be rare in unselected populations. Peripheral neuropathies are relatively common, particularly mononeuritis multiplex mediated by vasculitis. Interstitial nephritis leading to renal tubular acidosis or nephrogenic diabetes insipidus occurs in about 30 per cent of patients; the manifestations are usually subclinical but may lead to hypokalaemia causing muscular weakness or, occasionally, nephrocalcinosis. Lymphomas, almost always of B-cell lineage, are a characteristic but unusual feature. They occur in about 5 per cent of patients in referral units and are particularly found in patients with high levels of immunoglobulins, autoantibodies and cryoglobulins. As the lymphoma develops, the immunoglobulin levels often fall and the autoantibodies become undetectable. Women of child-bearing age are at increased risk of giving birth to babies with congenital heart block, by way of transplacental transfer of anti-Ro and -La antibodies, which are thought to have a pathogenic effect on the developing conduction system.

In secondary Sjögren's syndrome the sicca symptoms are less severe than in primary disease. In rheumatoid arthritis with Sjögren's syndrome, extra-articular manifestations, such as digital infarcts and subcutaneous ulcers are more frequent. In systemic lupus erythematosus, those with Sjögren's syndrome have a lower frequency of renal disease and a relatively good prognosis.

Diagnostic tests

Keratoconjunctivitis sicca can be detected by Schirmer's test, tear break-up time, and Rose Bengal staining, and xerostomia by a reduced parotid salivary flow rate and by reduced uptake and clearance on isotope scans. It is important to remember that both salivary and lachrymal function decline with age and may be impaired in conditions other than Sjögren's syndrome. One cause of diagnostic confusion arises from treatment with drugs with anticholinergic side-effects, the most frequent being the tricyclic antidepressants.

Biopsy of the labial glands from behind the lower lip provides the most definitive diagnostic test. The area is anaesthetized with lignocaine containing adrenaline and an incision 1.5 cm long allows access to five to 10 glands, 2–4 mm in diameter, which are removed by simple blunt dissection. A diagnosis of Sjögren's syndrome depends on finding foci of periductular infiltrates of at least 50 lymphocytes and/or plasma cells at a density of more than one focus/4 mm^2.

The majority of patients have a raised erythrocyte sedimentation rate (**ESR**), and a mild normocytic anaemia with leucopenia in about 50 per cent. A remarkable feature of primary Sjögren's syndrome is the high level of IgG, which can be up to 50 g/1. Complement levels are usually normal, although C4 can sometimes be reduced, because of the link between Sjögren's syndrome and the C4A null gene. Anti-Ro and/or anti-La antibodies occur in about 50 per cent of patients with the primary syndrome; although of relatively low sensitivity, they are of great diagnostic help when present. Rheumatoid factors occur in all forms of Sjögren's syndrome and their detection in primary disease is a common reason for misdiagnosing rheumatoid arthritis. Similarly, antinuclear antibodies can occur. Both rheumatoid factors and antinuclear antibodies, although not diagnostically specific, can help in distinguishing true Sjögren's syndrome from non-autoimmune causes of sicca symptoms. Anti-salivary gland antibodies have been described in patients with Sjögren's syndrome and rheumatoid arthritis, but this assay is not widely available and has not established itself as a useful diagnostic test.

Table 1 Questionnaire for eliciting the main ocular and oral symptoms of Sjögren's syndrome (see OTM3, p. 3038 for source)

Ocular symptoms: a positive response to at least one of the three selected questions:
1. Have you had daily, persistent, troublesome dry eyes for more than 3 months?
2. Do you have a recurrent sensation of sand or gravel in the eyes?
3. Do you use tear substitutes more than three times a day?
Oral symptoms: a positive response to at least one of the three selected questions:
1. Have you had a daily feeling of dry mouth for more than 3 months?
2. Have you had recurrently or persistently swollen salivary glands as an adult?
3. Do you frequently drink liquids to aid in swallowing dry food?

Diagnostic criteria

Current criteria depend on the demonstration of keratoconjunctivitis sicca, xerostomia, and a positive labial gland biopsy. Criteria, resulting from a European study, are probably the most thoroughly evaluated and simplest to apply. They are based on a short questionnaire (Table 1) of ocular and oral symptoms. Other essential criteria are ocular signs (by Schirmer's test or Rose Bengal staining), lymphocytic infiltrates on lip biopsy, salivary gland involvement (scintigraphy, sialography, or decreased salivary flow rate); and demonstration of serum autoantibodies (rheumatoid factors, antinuclear antibodies, and/or Ro or La antibodies).

Treatment

Simple measures can help preserve the integrity of the cornea as well as the gums and teeth. Tear substitutes, such as hypromellose eye drops, are the mainstay of treatment of the dry eye and it is worth trying several different types before settling on the most suitable preparation. Where thick mucus strands are a particular problem, topical acetylcysteine may help. Eye ointments, particularly at night, can help lubricate sticky eyes. Bacterial infection should be treated immediately with chloramphenicol ointment or drops. Some benefit can be achieved by preventing evaporation of tears by fitting side panels to spectacles. Temporary or permanent occlusion of the canaliculi or, rarely, tarsorraphy may help to retain tears within the conjunctival sac.

Dry mouth may be treated by saliva substitutes, now available as convenient sprays. Candidal infections are extremely common in Sjögren's syndrome and are often missed. They are best treated with prolonged courses of anticandidal drugs, such as fluconazole, 50 mg daily for 10 days. Attention to dental hygiene may help to prevent the premature caries which is a common problem.

Attempts to treat the underlying disease with steroids or cytotoxic drugs is ill-advised unless there are systemic complications. Fever and weight loss often respond well to a low dose of steroids. Serious systemic complications such as polymyositis, mononeuritis multiplex, or fibrosing alveolitis are treated with steroids and cytotoxic drugs as in other connective tissue diseases. Other second-line agents for rheumatoid arthritis, such as gold or sulphasalazine, are associated with a high frequency of side-effects. The arthritis of primary Sjögren's syndrome may be treated with anti-inflammatory drugs, or hydroxy-choloroquine. Recently, hydroxycholoroquine has attracted interest as a possible treatment for the fatigue of Sjögren's syndrome, although controlled clinical trials are still awaited to address this issue. Small-scale studies have shown that treatment with hydroxycholoroquine (400 mg daily) lowers the ESR and immunoglobulins suggesting a disease-modifying effect.

Further reading

Fox, R.I. (1997). Sjögren's syndrome. Controversies and progress. *Clinics in Laboratory Medicine*, 17, 431–44.

Fox, R.I., Tornwall, J., Marruyama, T., and Stern, M. (1998). Evolving concepts of diagnosis, pathogenesis and therapy of Sjögren's syndrome. *Current Opinion in Rheumatology*, **10**, 446–56.

Manthorpe, R., Asmuseen, K., and Oxholm, P. (1997). Primary Sjögren's syndrome: diagnostic criteria, clinical features and disease activity. *Journal of Rheumatology*, **24** (Suppl. 50), 8–11.

Price, E.J. and Venables, P.J.W. Aetiopathogenesis of Sjögren's syndrome. *Seminars in Arthritis and Rheumatism*, 25, 117–33.

Chapter 10.14

Polymyositis and dermatomyositis

J. Walton

These names have been given to clinical syndromes produced by combined degenerative and inflammatory changes in skeletal muscle. In some instances skin and mucous membranes are also involved, when the condition is called dermatomyositis, but often the main brunt of the disease falls upon the skeletal muscles (see also OTM3, pp. 4156–58 and Section 13).

Aetiology

Although the syndrome may embrace several diseases of varying aetiology, in most cases the pathological process is clearly autoimmune. It was once customary to group together polymyositis and dermato-myositis, but in several respects the two conditions are different. Thus polymyositis is due to a lymphocyte-mediated autoimmune process in which sensitized T4 and T8 cells invade and destroy skeletal muscle; the typical histological picture is one of muscle fibre necrosis and regeneration with interstitial and perivascular infiltration with such cells, identified by monoclonal antibodies. In dermatomyositis, the intramuscular blood vessels may be damaged by circulating immune complexes and the autoimmune process is humoral rather than cell-mediated. Vasculitis is common as is perifascicular atrophy of muscle fibres.

Clinical features

These syndromes are seen in patients of all ages and in both sexes. The peak incidence is in middle life. Acute polymyositis in adults is uncommon but dermatomyositis is much more so; it sometimes occurs in childhood. The latter is characterized by generalized muscular pains and weakness of comparatively rapid progression, associated often with a widespread erythematous rash on the face, limbs, and trunk. the proximal limb muscles are more severely affected than the distal. The affected muscles are tender and patients are often ill and febrile; the respiratory muscles may be involved and the illness may end fatally within a few weeks or months. Subacute polymyositis is much more common. In such cases muscular pain and tenderness and symptoms of constitutional upset are often absent, and the presenting features are those of progressive weakness, and moderate atrophy of the muscles of the shoulder and pelvic girdles. This clinical picture can resemble closely that of muscular dystrophy, save for the fact that in polymyositis all the proximal limb muscles are usually weakened, and the deltoid, for instance, is not spared; furthermore, the neck muscles are often weak, dysphagia and a Raynaud phenomenon in the hands are common (although these two features occur more often in dermatomyositis), and the muscular weakness is often greater than the degree of atrophy would suggest. This form of subacute polymyositis is particularly common in middle and late life.

When dermatomyositis occurs in childhood or adolescence there are often minor skin changes on the face and the hands and fingers, resembling those of early systemic sclerosis or acrosclerosis. In some cases, the skin lesions resemble those of lupus erythematosus, while in others there may be associated evidence of another connective tissue disease such as rheumatoid arthritis. Subcutaneous and intramuscular calcification (calcinosis universalis) is common in childhood dermatomyositis. Many cases of dermatomyositis in middle and late life develop in association with malignant disease in the lung or in some other organ. The relationship between adult polymyositis and malignant disease is much less striking and may indeed not be significant.

Diagnosis

A raised erythrocyte sedimentation rate may be helpful but this test is normal in more than a third of cases. The serum creatine kinase activity and immunoglobulins are also often raised, but in most cases final diagnosis depends upon a combination of the clinical findings, electromyography, and muscle biopsy.

Prognosis and treatment

The prognosis of polymyositis and dermatomyositis is variable. Some acute cases are eventually fatal, despite modern treatment. A few subacute cases in childhood have been known to remit spontaneously and even to recover incompletely; others enter a chronic stage with the development of fibrous contractures in the muscles and severe deformity (chronic myositis fibrosa). Most subacute cases occurring in adult life are progressive. Many remit completely or partially when treated with prednisone and immunosuppressive drugs, but maintenance therapy may have to be continued for many years. Plasma exchange can be useful as a temporary measure in acute dermatomyositis; and in some intractable cases of polymyositis whole-body irradiation has been successful. Treatment is considered further in OTM3, pp. 4156–58 and Section 13).

Related conditions

Eosinophilic myositis is clinically similar and is steroid responsive, as are granulomatous myositis (resembling sarcoidosis of muscle) and localized nodular myositis, a focal form of polymyositis which causes painful swellings in one or more muscles. An eosinophilic fasciitis giving a scleroderma-like syndrome has been described in patients receiving L-tryptophan for treatment of depression. Inclusion-body myositis, which is more common in older age groups, often affects distal limb muscles predominantly and is insidiously progressive in most cases, usually uninfluenced by steroids and immunosuppressive agents. Histologically, ringed vacuoles and intranuclear filamentous inclusions are characteristic of the latter condition (also see Ch. 25.5 in OTM3, pp.4154-9 and Section 13).

Chapter 10.15

Polymyalgia rheumatica and giant-cell arteritis

A. G. Mowat

Polymyalgia rheumatica and giant-cell arteritis (GCA) are common debilitating conditions that may represent opposite ends of a disease spectrum, but as they appear to present with different clinical symptoms and signs and demand different treatment, it is best to describe them separately.

Polymyalgia rheumatica

Polymyalgia rheumatica occurs predominantly in patients over the age of 60 years. There is marked pain and stiffness in the shoulder and pelvic girdles associated with variable systemic symptoms and elevated C-reactive protein (CRP) and erythrocyte sedimentation rate (ESR). While an incidence of some 50 per 100 000 of the population aged 50 years and over has been accepted for hospital referrals on both sides of the Atlantic, careful study of a defined elderly population has shown an incidence of 1.5 per cent which exceeds that of any other inflammatory rheumatic disease in the elderly.

Although the most common age group involved is that between 60 and 70 years, a third of patients are under 60 years old. Initial symptoms are seldom seen before 45 years or after 80 years, The male to female ratio is 1:2. The onset is often dramatic, with some patients giving the precise date of their first symptoms, and in most cases it is fully developed within a month. Pain and stiffness is usually localized to muscles, although tenderness is not as severe as in myositis. There may be additional tenderness involving periarticular structures. The onset is most common in the shoulder girdle, spreading to involve both shoulders, the pelvic girdle, and proximal muscles with striking symmetry. Involvement of distal muscles is unusual. Immobility is most severe on waking; a characteristic complaint is a need to roll out of bed, often with the aid of a spouse. Such morning stiffness may persist for hours. Most patients look unwell and complain of general malaise, fatigue, and depression. Anorexia and weight loss can be striking, often suggesting neoplasia while night sweats and fever are frequent and occasionally are the presenting feature,

The extent of joint involvement is disputed: an incidence of mild inflammatory polyarthritis varying from 0 to 100 per cent being recorded. Almost any joint may be affected. particularly knee and finger joints, but because the arthritis is mild and non-deforming some argue that central joint involvement, which may be the basis for

Table 1 Validation of diagnostic criteria for polymyalgia rheumatica

Discriminatory feature	Sensitivity* (%)	Relative value †
Shoulder pain and/or stiffness bilaterally	86	155
Onset duration 2 weeks or less	88	151
Initial ESR >40 mm/h	74	149
Stiffness duration >1 h	80	141
Age 65+ years	70	139
Depression and/or weight loss	58	130
Upper-arm tenderness bilaterally	36	132

*Sensitivity (%) = individuals with disease with positive test/all individuals with disease

Specificity (%) = individuals without disease with positive test/all individuals without disease

†Relative value = sensitivity + specificity (range 0–200)

After H.A.Bird *et al.* (1979). *Annals of the Rheumatic Diseases*, **38**, 434–9

Table 2 Differential diagnosis of polymyalgia rheumatica

Infection	Joint disease
Viral	Osteoarthritis
Brucellosis	Rheumatoid arthritis
Tuberculosis	Connective tissue diseases
Endocarditis	
	Others
Bone disease	Neoplasia
Osteoporosis	Muscle disease
Osteomalacia	Fibromyalgia syndrome
Paget's disease	Chronic fatigue syndrome
Senile hyperostotic spinal ankylosis	Parkinsonism
	Hypothyroidisin

the referred pain patterns, is underdiagnosed. Distinctive radiographic erosion is claimed in some central joints (e.g. sternoclavicular), while isotopic and arthroscopic studies of the shoulder support this contention. Carpal tunnel syndrome is an occasional accompaniment.

Laboratory findings

An acute phase response (raised ESR, CRP) is typical. The elevation in ESR, often to more than 100 mm/h should not be overinterpreted as polymyalgia rheumatica accounts for only 2 per cent of such high values. Although untreated patients with a normal ESR do exist, 40 mm/h has good diagnostic value. A mild hypochromic normocytic anaemia is common. Rheumatoid factor shows a low incidence of positivity consistent with the patient's age. Serum values of liver enzymes, alkaline phosphatase, and γ-glutamyl transferase are elevated in most patients, and can be correlated with the ESR and disease severity. Liver biopsy shows only a mild cellular infiltrate and minor changes in the bile canaliculi.

Despite the prominent muscle symptoms, electromyographic (EMG) studies and serum muscle enzyme values are normal while changes on sequential muscle biopsy are non-specific largely due to disuse. While several studies have shown changes in the absolute number and percentage of activated CD8 T cells and interleukin receptors, these have not provided diagnostic or therapeutic correlation.

Differential diagnosis

Polymyalgia rheumatica remains a clinical diagnosis. Several diagnostic criteria have been validated over the years but the first remains practical: the seven best discriminatory features are shown in Table 1: three or more criteria are required. Differential diagnosis includes a wide range of conditions (Table 2). Infection may be viral or bacterial, with miliary tuberculosis and infective endocarditis causing confusion. Bone diseases may be difficult to separate as they are common in this elderly group and the alkaline phosphatase is raised in polymyalgia rheumatica. This is also the case with neoplastic disease, which may be associated with myalgia even in the absence of secondary spread to bone. Primary muscle disease can be distinguished by EMG, biopsy, and enzyme values, but joint disease, particularly osteoarthritis, rheumatoid arthritis, and other connective tissue diseases, all of which may start with a polymyalgic pattern lasting for some months in older patients, cause confusion.

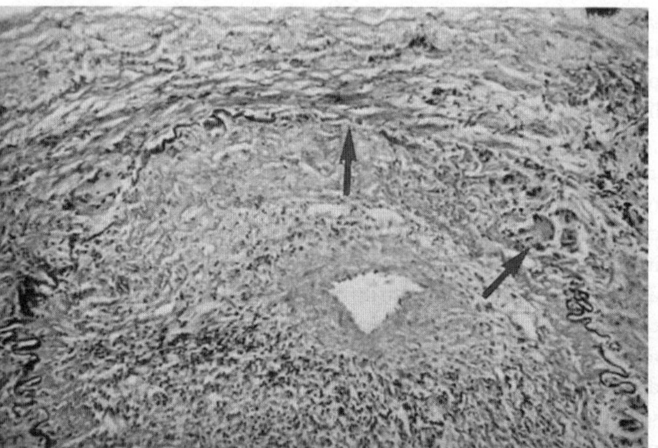

Fig. 1 Photomicrograph of a temporal artery biopsy showing giant cells, mononuclear infiltrate, and disruption of the internal elastic lamina.

Aetiology and pathogenesis

No distinctive pathophysiological mechanisms have been found. Polymyalgia rheumatica may include several different conditions, which are only due to arteritis in 15 per cent of cases. A prodromal malaise and a possible summer/winter peak incidence has promoted an unrewarding search for infective causes. The evidence for a central arthritis affecting clavicular, shoulder, and sacroiliac joints comes from a study which reproduced the usual pain patterns by injecting hypertonic saline into these joints. In those with proven arteritis, which need not be confined to the temporal and other central vessels, but can be found in larger arteries all over the body, a similar pattern of referred pain can be implicated. An immune destruction of the internal elastic lamina is supported by finding circulating immune complexes, together with immunoglobulins, complement deposition, and mononuclear cell infiltrate adjacent to the lamina (Fig. 1).

Although polymyalgia rheumatica is found world-wide, it is more common in Caucasians, particularly those of Scandinavian extraction, The infrequency of the disease in spouses argues against environmental factors, while familial aggregation and an association with HLA DR4

Table 3 Suggested treatment of polymyalgia rheumatica (PMR) and giant cell arteritis (GCA)

	Prednisolone (mg/day)		
	Weeks 1–4 (4 weeks)	Weeks 5–6 (2 weeks)	Weeks 7–8 (2 weeks)
PMR	20	15	10
GCA	40	30	20

suggests both genetic and immunological mechanisms, possibly similar to seronegative rheumatoid arthritis.

Treatment

A decade ago, the average delay to diagnosis and treatment was 6 months. Now, greater awareness and the fear of the GCA link and possible blindness has led to overdiagnosis and over-treatment, and the commonness of middle-age muscle ache has been forgotten. It is a myth that a prompt or dramatic response to corticosteroid confirms a diagnosis; many of the listed differential diagnoses show a similar response. Nevertheless corticosteroids are the drugs of choice.

As the average duration of symptoms is 2–3 years, with some persisting for 7 or more years, corticosteroid side-effects are commonly recorded. Thirty-five to 75 per cent of patients with polymyalgia rheumatica show fluid retention, weight gain, diabetes or osteoporosis. Many clinicians now advocate starting therapy appropriate to the patient's age and wishes, to prevent osteoporosis at the outset of corticosteroid therapy. Higher initial ESRs tend to be associated with longer duration of disease and a greater risk of osteoporosis. Suggested corticosteroid regimens for the first 2 months are shown (Table 3).

The gradual reduction of corticosteroid treatment over 2 years minimizes the risk of relapse; most clinical problems and associated diagnostic doubts appear to be caused by fluctuating corticosteroid dose. ESR and CRP do not respond reliably to help in adjusting dosage or in predicting relapse. A few patients can be managed on non-steroidal anti-inflammatory drugs, but the value of poorer and slower symptom control and the risk from different side-effects is debatable. Azathioprine 50 mg twice daily or methotrexate 10 mg/ week may be helpful in steroid sparing, although the clinical trial evidence is not striking.

Relationship of polymyalgia rheumatica to giant cell arteritis

For more than 20 years a common cause has been suggested, emphasized by the term polymyalgia arteritica, and based upon the similar clinical and laboratory features. This has led some to search hard for arterial biopsy evidence lest the patient suffer visual features of GCA. Because the arteritis may be patchy and hence missed, attempts have been made to increase the sensitivity of biopsy site selection—angiography, sonography, isotope studies, magnetic resonance imaging—without success, However, prospective studies emphasize the difference between the conditions, even if part of a spectrum, and the lack of need for biopsy studies in clear polymyalgia rheumatica. In GCA biopsy proof underpins the need for higher and sustained steroid therapy.

Table 4 Clinical presentation and features of giant-cell arteritis (percentage of cases affected)

Chief presentation		Clinical features	
Symptoms of temporal arteritis	30%	Signs of temporal arteritis	90%
Polymyalgia rheumatica	27%	Polymyalgia rheumatica	55%
Weight loss, malaise	14%	Weight loss, malaise	50%
Fever	13%	Visual disturbance	40%
Visual disturbance	6%	Fever	32%
Headache	4%	Cranial features	24%
Anaemia	4%	Peripheral neuropathy	12%
Claudication (leg)	2%	Claudication (leg)	7%

Giant-cell arteritis

Giant-cell (cranial, senile, or temporal) arteritis, which is rare before the age of 50 years, chiefly affects those between 65 and 75 years with a male/female ratio of 1:2. An annual incidence of biopsy-proven disease among those aged 50 years or more of 18 per 100 000 (25 per 100 000 for women and 10 per 100 000 for men) has been recorded in the United States and Scandinavia, with the rate for women appearing to rise. The features of GCA are protean, but typical ones are shown in Table 4. The diagnosis depends upon clinical suspicion in less typical cases. As with polymyalgia rheumatica, the onset may be dramatic and the condition always becomes fully developed over a few weeks, although the delay in diagnosis may be months. The malaise, fever, and anaemia are similar to those in polymyalgia rheumatica; the differences are in the vascular symptoms. The majority have temporal features with headache, scalp sensitivity, and tender thickened arteries; the classical nodular red streaks are unusual. Overwhelming generalized headache and the feared complication of irreversible loss of vision are more readily recognized. The clinical features listed emphasize temporal arteritis. A wide range of cranial manifestations reflects the involvement of larger arteries with an internal elastic lamina in the face, neck, and brain base but not in the cerebral vessels. They include headache, scalp tenderness, skin necrosis, jaw claudication while talking or chewing, tongue pain and claudication, and face and neck pain with nerve damage. The visual manifestations, which include blurred vision, amaurosis fugax, transient and permanent blindness, diplopia, and visual hallucinations, are due to ischaemic changes in the ciliary arteries causing optic neuritis or infarction, with a smaller number of cases being due to central retinal artery thrombosis. Fifteen per cent have evidence of arteritis elsewhere, with intermittent claudication, peripheral neuropathy, widespread vessel tenderness with bruits, myocardial ischaemia and damage, and occasionally an aortic syndrome with valve disease. Stroke due to brain-stem vascular disease is uncommon, accounting for only l–2 per cent of such cases. In contradistinction to other vasculitides, renal involvement is rare.

Laboratory features

These are the same as in polymyalgia rheumatica. Temporal artery biopsy is the definitive diagnostic test. A 2-cm segment of a tender artery will provide positive histology in 70 per cent of cases. The rate may been enhanced by taking longer segments or by the biopsy of other tender scalp vessels. While biopsy confirmation of the diagnosis is important, it should not be a reason for withholding steroids, as characteristic pathological features persist for at least 2 weeks after treatment has begun, and some argue scar change never clears.

Differential diagnosis

As the diagnosis of GCA depends upon a positive biopsy, the differential diagnosis does not include other causes of headache, neck pain, anaemia, and weight loss. The vasculitis of rheumatoid arthritis or systemic lupus erythematosus affects arterioles and is associated with other disease features, particularly arthritis and characteristic immunological tests. Polyarteritis affects small arteries with cutaneous, abdominal, and renal rather than cranial features and the histology is distinctive. Although cranial and central nervous system features occur in Wegener's granulomatosis, involvement usually includes characteristic lesions of the respiratory tract. Takayasu's arteritis, in which the pathological lesions mimic those of GCA, is confined to the aortic arch and its major branches and occurs chiefly in young oriental women (see Chapter 2.35).

Treatment

Corticosteroids are mandatory; immunosuppressive therapy has no direct effect and the modest steroid sparing rarely warrants the additional hazard. While doses of prednisolone up to 100 mg/day are often advocated, careful sequential studies indicate that lower doses are quite satisfactory (Table 3). Ophthalmologists, who are likely to see patients with established visual effects or threatening features in the second eye, may use higher doses or methylprednisolone infusions. Dosage reduction must be gradual and be judged solely on clinical features as acute phase responses are no guide. Most should have achieved a maintenance dose of 10 mg/day after 1 year. Subsequently, the known persistence of disease in a significant proportion for 4 years or more and the possible recurrence of symptoms, including blindness, even a year after corticosteroid withdrawal argues for very gradual dosage reduction. Unfortunately, there are no predictors of these risks. Accordingly, the hazards of therapy are even greater than in polymyalgia rheumatica and require preventive treatment for osteoporosis. Despite all the problems, GCA does not reduce life expectancy.

Further reading

Achkar, A.A., Lie, J.T., Hunder, G.G., O'Fallon, M., and Gabriez, S.E. (1994) How does previous corticosteroid therapy affect the biopsy findings in giant-cell arteritis? *Annals of Internal Medicine*, 120, 987–92.

Bird, H.A., Esselinckx, W., Dixon, A.St.J., Mowat, A.G., and Wood, P.H.H. (1979) An evaluation of criteria for polymyalgia rheumatica. *Annals of the Rheumatic Diseases*, 38, 434–9.

Gonzaley-Gay, M.A., Garcia-Porrua, C., and Vazquez-Caruncho, M. (1998) Polymyalgia rheumatica in biopsy proven giant-cell arteritis does not constitute a different subset but differs from isolated polymyalgia rheumatica. *Journal of Rheumatology*, 25, 1750–5.

Myklebust, G. and Gran, J.T. (1996) A prospective study of 287 patients with polymyalgia rheumatica and temporal arteritis: clinical and laboratory manifestations at onset of disease and at time of diagnosis. *British Journal of Rheumatology*, 35, 1161–8.

Chapter 10.16

Behçet's disease

T. Lehner

Behçet's disease is a recurrent, multifocal disorder which usually persists over many years. Initial descriptions of the disease comprised oral and genital ulcers and uveitis, but a number of other clinical features are now added, notably skin, joint, neurological, and vascular manifestations. This creates considerable difficulty in diagnosis.

Diagnostic criteria, based on data from 914 patients with the disease, require the presence of oral ulcers plus any two of the following: genital ulcers, defined eye lesions, defined skin lesions, or a positive skin pathergy test. These criteria (Table 1) show better discrimination in sensitivity, specificity, and relative value than did their predecessors. A large number of important clinical manifestations of Behçet's disease have not been included (Table 2) because their lower frequency does not contribute to the accuracy of diagnosis.

Epidemiology

A striking feature of the disease is the high prevalence in Japan (up to 1 in 10 000). It is also high in countries bordering the Mediterranean: Italy, Greece, Turkey, Israel, Egypt, Lebanon, Syria, Jordan, Saudi Arabia, as well as Algeria and Tunisia. In the UK a possible prevalence of 1 in 170 000 compares with 1 in 800 000 in the US.

Although the disease may develop at any age, the most common onset is in the third decade. It can start in childhood with orogenital ulcers, followed by other manifestations years or decades later. Male predominance is found in most series, but this may vary from 2:1 in Japan to 9:1 in the Middle East. Increased familial prevalence has been recorded frequently, and there is evidence for an immunogenetic basis for the disease.

Aetiology

The cause is unknown but an immunogenetic basis has now been established. HLA-B51 is significantly associated with Behçet's disease and as with other HLA disease associations, there are at least two interpretations of these findings: (1) the HLA antigen might function as a specific receptor for viruses (or pathogens), or (2) the antigenic

Table 1 Criteria for diagnosis of Behçet's disease: recurrent oral ulcers plus any two of the four other manifestations

Recurrent oral ulcers	Minor aphthous, major aphthous, or herpetiform ulcers which recurred at least three times a year
Recurrent genital ulcers	Ulcers or scarring
Eye lesions	Anterior uveitis, posterior uveitis, or cells in the vitreous on slit-lamp examination; or retinal vasculitis
Skin lesions	Erythema nodosum, pseudofolliculitis, papulopustular lesions, or acneiform nodules in postadolescent patients not on corticosteroid treatment
Positive pathergy test	Read by physician at 24–48 h

Table 2 Clinical manifestations of Behçet's syndrome

Mucocutaneous
Recurrent oral ulcers: aphthous or herpetiform
Recurrent genital ulcers: vulval, vaginal, penile, or scrotal
Skin lesions: pustules, erythema nodosum, perianal ulceration, erythema multiforme
Arthritic
Polyarthritis of predominantly large joints
Polyarthralgia of large joints
Neurological
Brainstem syndrome, resembling minor strokes
Meningomyelitis or meningoencephalitis
Organic confusional syndromes
Multiple sclerosis-like disorder
Ocular
Uveitis with or without hypopyon
Iridocyclitis
Retinal vascular lesions
Optic atrophy
Vascular
Venous thrombosis
Aneurysms
Gastrointestinal
Abdominal pain, diarrhoea, distension, nausea, anorexia
Others
Pulmonary: haemoptysis
Renal: asymptomatic proteinuria and haematuria

determinants of some pathogens might mimic the HLA antigens. A viral aetiology, particularly herpes simplex, has been suggested, and there is evidence that a variety of streptococci might be implicated by way of heat shock proteins (see OTM3, pp. 3043–4).

Lymphocytic infiltration in and around small blood vessels, T-cell proliferative responses to four specific peptides derived from the sequence of the 65 kDa heat shock protein, and the presence of circulating immune complexes in 40–60 per cent of Behçet patients point to immune mechanisms in this disease which are discussed further in OTM3, p. 3044.

Unlike most autoimmune diseases, nuclear, thyroid, and gastric autoantibodies are not found in greater proportion in Behçet's disease than in the normal population. Rheumatoid factor is also negative, even in patients with joint involvement.

Clinical features (Fig. 1)

The patients are often generally well and only complain of the localized lesions, but they may present with acute exacerbation of malaise, fever, dysphagia, and loss of weight. Other manifestations are listed in Table 2.

Recurrent oral ulcers are the presenting feature in most but not all patients. They can be of the minor or major aphthous or herpetiform type (Fig. 1). Such ulcers are common in the general population and usually give rise only to local discomfort so may be missed in the history. The least severe minor aphthous ulcers are found in 67 per cent of the neurological and 76 per cent of the ocular types of Behçet's disease, whereas the most severe type of major aphthous ulcers are found in 40 and 64 per cent, respectively, of the mucocutaneous and arthritic types. Herpetiform ulcers are found mostly in the mucocutaneous type (45 per cent). An essential feature is that the ulcers recur frequently, at intervals of weeks or months, but this varies from one patient to another. The long-cherished view that oral ulcers in Behçet's disease are rather severe and associated with scarring is no longer tenable. The clinical manifestations can be readily recognized and differentiated from those of similar disorders. The pharynx can also be the site of aphthous ulcers which tend to be rather large, shallow, and covered with a fibrinopurulent exudate.

Genital ulcers are found in most patients and can be of the three types described for oral ulcers (Fig. 1). They affect females more commonly than males, and scars may follow healing in either sex. Females develop recurrent ulcers on their labia or vagina and they suffer from disabling dysuria and dyspareunia. Males develop recurrent ulcers on the penis or scrotum, again with dysuria and pain on sexual intercourse (Fig. 1); some develop epididymo-orchitis.

Skin lesions vary, but diffuse pustular lesions on the face and particularly the back are most common. Erythema nodosum may affect the limbs or other parts of the body (Fig. 1). Occasionally, erythema multiforme is found. Both females and males may develop perianal ulcers and, curiously, these may present in the young, well before genital ulcers have appeared.

Ocular lesions are the most serious manifestations. Relapsing uveitis, with or without hypopyon (Fig. 1), iridocyclitis, retinal vascular lesions, and optic atrophy are common. Relapsing conjunctivitis, keratitis, and choroiditis are also features. Gross retinal vascular changes affect both arteries and veins, and fluorescein angiography is particularly helpful in such cases. Both eyes tend to be involved in 90 per cent of patients, within a period of 2 years of onset of symptoms in one eye. Visual prognosis is then poor, as useful vision (less than 6/60) is lost in about half the patients within 4 years of onset of the ocular symptoms.

Neurological features are found in 10–25 per cent of patients. Transient or persistent brainstem syndromes resemble minor strokes. Transient focal cerebral syndromes and spinal cord involvement are also found, as are meningomyelitis or meningoencephalitis and organic confusional syndromes. Multiple sclerosis-like features have been described. The cerebrospinal fluid sometimes shows pleocytosis and raised protein concentrations but more often is normal. Computed tomography scanning does not often reveal abnormalities but the electroencephalogram can show slowing of basic rhythm. Magnetic resonance imaging (**MRI**) is the most sensitive and reliable examination. It may show atrophy of the cerebral cortex, cerebellum or brainstem and enlarged sinuses; high-intensity signals may be recorded in the pons, brainstem, or the midbrain; and demyelinating processes may be found in the pons and medulla. MRI can help to differentiate Behçet's disease from multiple sclerosis and other neurological diseases, as well as in assessing the response to treatment.

The prognosis of Behçet's disease with neurological features used to be poor, with mortality of about 40 per cent before 1970. The

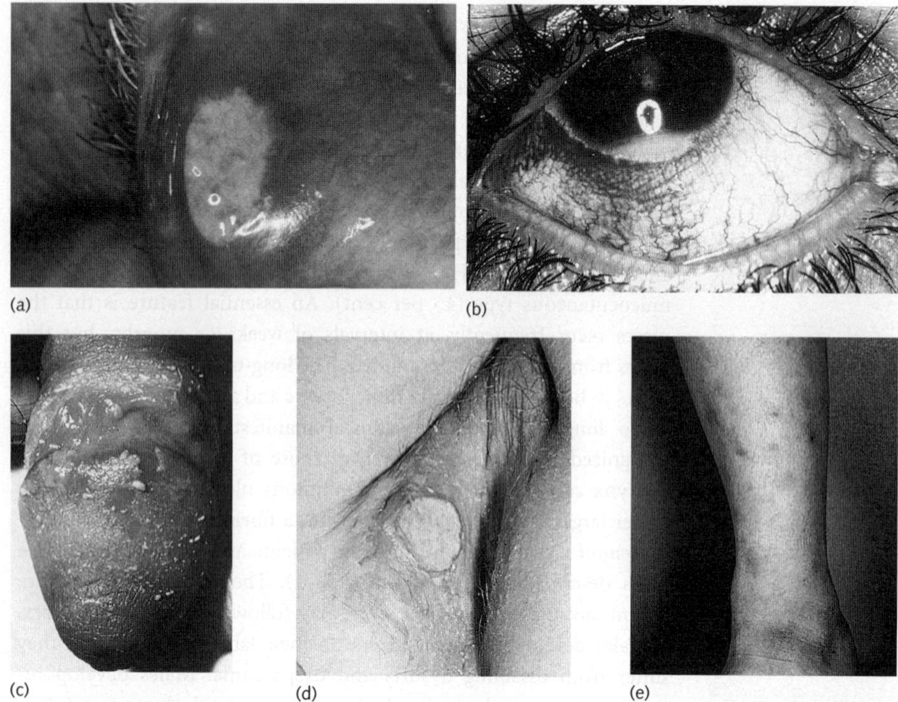

Fig. 1(a)–(e) Behçet's disease: (a) oral ulcer, (b) hypopyon in the eye, (c) ulceration of the head of the penis, (d) vulval ulcers, (e) multiple erythema nodosum lesions of the leg.

prognosis has recently been improved, although whether this can be attributed to steroid and/or cytotoxic agents remains uncertain.

Arthritis or arthralgia occurs in about half the patients with Behçet's disease, at irregular intervals and usually in more than one joint. The knees, ankles, and elbows are most commonly involved, and less frequently the joints of the hands, feet, shoulders, and hips. Effusions, especially in the knees, cause considerable disability. Erosive changes visible on radiography are some changes, but can occur in the hips, wrists, and elbows.

Vascular lesions Recurrent thrombophlebitis of leg veins is a significant feature of Behçet's disease, ascribed to decreased plasma fibrinolytic activity. Less frequently, superior or inferior vena cava and sagittal sinus thrombosis may develop. Arterial aneurysms have also been reported.

Gastrointestinal manifestations are ill-defined. The Japanese literature records diarrhoea, distension, nausea, and anorexia in more than half the patients. Radiological examination has revealed abnormalities affecting predominantly the small intestine: dilatation, gas and fluid retention, segmentation and thickening of intestinal folds. However, a British series failed to identify consistent gastrointestinal manifestations, although various transient symptoms were noted in 13 of 70 patients. Patients with inflammatory bowel disease are excluded from the diagnosis of Behçet's disease by the Mayo Clinic, although they may fulfil current criteria for that diagnosis.

Renal involvement has not been established. A small number of patients have been reported with Behçet's disease and amyloidosis affecting the kidneys, and few also with glomerulonephritis. It is doubtful if these renal changes can be considered as primary manifestations. Asymptomatic proteinuria and haematuria without evidence either of amyloidosis or nephritis have also been reported in a small number of patients.

Pulmonary manifestations have been reported occasionally, usually with haemoptysis. In some of these patients, pulmonary tuberculosis has been suspected.

Diagnosis

There are no definitive criteria for the diagnosis and the various schemes suggested rely on the association between two, three, or four clinical features (Table 1). The spectrum of the disorder can be divided into four types.

1. Mucocutaneous disease which involves oral and genital ulcers with or without skin manifestations.
2. Arthritic type, in which joint involvement is combined with some or all of the mucocutaneous manifestations.
3. Neurological type, with some or all of the features in (1) and (2).
4. Ocular type, with some or all of the features described in (1), (2), and (3).

Thrombosis can be found in any one of the four types as can some of the other inconsistent features.

The pathergy test, whereby a sterile subcutaneous puncture (without injection of any material) elicits a pustular reaction within 24–48 h, has been used as a diagnostic test in the Middle Eastern countries and in Japan. Raised levels of acute-phase reacting proteins are non-specific but the C9 level is particularly useful in monitoring the course of the disorder. The T-cell proliferative response stimulated by four specific peptides derived from the mycobacterial 65 kDa heat shock proteins has been used as a diagnostic test. However, at present it is performed only in specialized laboratories.

Stevens–Johnson syndrome may mimic Behçet's disease but the recurrences are less frequent and tend to be seasonal, the ulcers are large and shallow, the lips are often covered with haemorrhagic crusts, and the skin may show typical lesions of erythema multiforme.

Treatment

The management of patients with Behçet's disease can be difficult. Oral and genital ulcers often respond to topical application of steroids or tetracycline or both. Uveitis is also initially treated with local steroids. However, at some stage, systemic prednisolone is usually administered, with a starting dose of 30–60 mg/day which is rapidly brought down to a minimum effective maintenance dose of about 10 mg/day. There is usually a prompt response, although a small core of patients are resistant. Azathioprine is often used with prednisolone (2–3 mg/kg body weight daily) and apart from its steroid-sparing function, may have additional beneficial effects. Colchicine has been particularly advocated by Japanese and Turkish physicians in a dose of 0.5 mg twice a day. Cyclosporin (2.5–5 mg/kg body weight) should be used in patients with unresponsive uveitis in spite of possible serious side-effects. Chlorambucil has also been successful in the treatment of uveitis, but side-effects have limited its application. Thalidomide has recently been found to be effective in the treatment of orogenital ulcers, but the teratogenic effect of this drug may severely restrict its use.

Further reading

Lehner, T. Behçet's disease. (1996). In *Oxford Textbook of Medicine*, (ed. D. J. Weatherall, J.G.G. Ledingham and D.A. Warrell), pp. 3043–4. Oxford University Press, Oxford.

Chapter 10.17

Kawasaki disease

T. Kawasaki

Kawasaki disease is an acute febrile eruptive disease commonly occurring in infants and children under 5 years of age first described in 1967. Its synonym is: infantile acute febrile mucocutaneous lymph-node syndrome. Originally, the prognosis was believed favourable, but there is a fatality rate of 0.3–0.5 per cent, and autopsy findings reveal unique pathological features, such as coronary artery aneurysms with thrombosis in many cases. As this disease cannot be differentiated histopathologically from infantile periarteritis nodosa, which has rarely been reported in American and European literature, it is still unclear whether it is a new entity or had previously been overlooked.

The disease has attracted attention because asymptomatic coronary artery lesions (mainly aneurysms) have remained as sequelae in 5–10 per cent of patients, causing sudden death, myocardial infarction, or mitral insufficiency, probably due to papillary muscle dysfunction.

Clinical manifestations

The clinical features can be classified into principal and subsidiary. At least five of the six principal features should be present for the diagnosis, although four features are enough, provided coronary aneurysms are identified by echocardiography or coronary angiography.

Principal features

These comprise:

1. Fever for 5 days or more.
2. Bilateral congestion of conjunctiva without conjunctivitis.
3. Dryness, redness, and fissuring of the lips and inflammation of the oral cavity.
4. Acute non-purulent swelling of cervical lymph nodes.

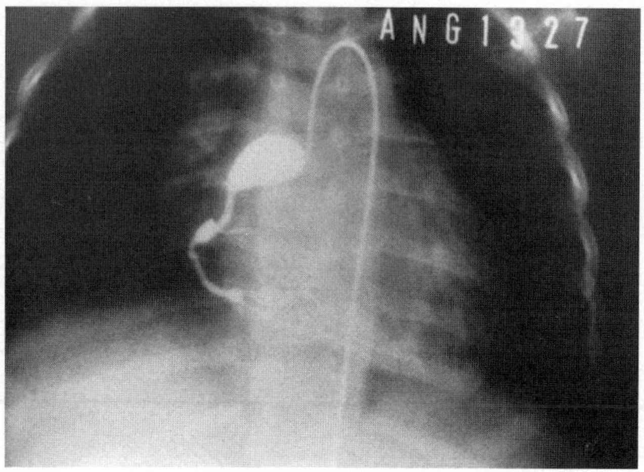

Fig. 1 Multiple aneurysms of a coronary artery in Kawasaki disease.

5. Skin rash comprising morbilliform, scarlatiniform, urticarious, or erythema multiforme-like lesions.
6. Reddening of the skin of palms and soles with oedema fading to produce desquamation.

Subsidiary features

Cardiac manifestations include pericarditis, coronary artery disease and arrhythmias. Coronary aneurysms occur in 40 per cent of cases in the first 10–20 days and decline thereafter to some 10 per cent by 60 days (Fig. 1). Aneurysms less than 4 mm across tend to regress and heal; those 8 mm or more often stenose and occlude. Between these diameters, regression is possible. In general, stenosis and occlusion are commonest in large saccular and cylindrical lesions. In all patients angiography is advisable from 1 to 3 months from the onset.

Gastrointestinal problems include diarrhoea, cholecystitis, and jaundice with disturbed liver function. A leucocytosis, high erythrocyte sedimentation rate, and C-reactive protein are usual. Other problems include transient proteinuria, cough, arthralgia, arthritis, and aseptic meningitis. Facial palsy, hemiplegia, and encephalopathy have also been reported.

Pathological findings

This is an acute inflammatory disease with systemic angiitis which is distinguishable from classic periarteritis nodosa. Coronary aneurysms are usually present at autopsy (Fig. 2). The angiitis is characterized by acute inflammation with no or mild fibrinoid necrosis. Its course can be classified into four stages according to the duration of the illness:

Stage 1 (1–2 weeks from onset) shows perivasculitis and vasculitis of microvessels, small arteries, and veins. There is inflammation of the intima, externa, and perivascular areas in the medium- and large-sized arteries. Oedema and infiltration with leucocytes and lymphocytes is also present.

Stage 2 (2–4 weeks from onset) shows less inflammation in the vessels. Aneurysms are present with thrombus and stenosis in the middle-sized arteries, especially in the coronary arteries.

Stage 3 (4–7 weeks from onset) shows further subsidence of inflammation in the vessels. Granulation may occur in the medium-sized arteries.

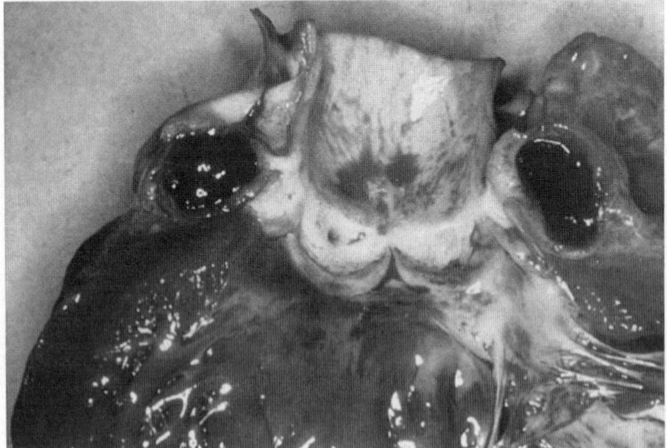

Fig. 2 Postmortem findings in Kawasaki disease. This 9-month-old boy died suddenly at 49 days after the onset of the illness. A large aneurysm of the coronary vessels is shown.

Stage 4 (more than 7 weeks from onset) reveals scar formation and intimal thickening with aneurysms, thrombus, and stenosis in the medium-sized arteries.

Other lesions include myocarditis involving conduction systems, pericarditis, endocarditis, and inflammation of almost all organs. All these lesions are frequently seen in stages 1 and 2, but rarely in stage 4.

Ischaemic heart disease usually occurs in stages 2–4. The major cause of death in stage 1 is myocarditis, including inflammation of conduction systems. In stages 2 and 3, the causes are ischaemic heart disease, rupture of an aneurysm (rare), and myocarditis. In Stage 4, there may be ischaemic heart disease and, in rare cases, heart failure due to mitral insufficiency.

Epidemiology

Between 1970 and 1992 a total of 116 848 cases (67 815 males and 49 033 females, M/F = 1.4) have been reported, including 392 (0.03 per cent) deaths. The number of cases reported has been steadily increasing since 1971. Since 1974 a number of cases have been reported from Korea, China, the US, Canada, Germany, France, the UK, and other countries. However, reports from the developing countries are still few.

Aetiology

Human leucocyte antigen typing specific to Kawasaki disease or other genetic factors has not been confirmed. The disease may be a unique clinical reaction pattern to several agents, just as a variety of agents may trigger such disorders as Reye's, Guillain–Barré, or Stevens–Johnson syndromes.

Treatment

High-dose gammaglobulin treatment for the acute phase is now accepted as the best way to prevent coronary artery abnormalities. The recommended regimen is 200 mg/kg per day plus 50 mg/kg aspirin per day for 5 days. A regimen of a single dose of 1 g/kg of intravenous gammaglobulin has also been reported, repeated if there has been relapse. After the acute phase, aspirin in a dose of 3–5 mg/kg per day for 2 months is recommended. If coronary artery complications remain, aspirin should be continued until two-dimensional echography or angiography show normal vessels. When gammaglobulin is not available during the acute phase, a good regimen is with aspirin, 30–50 mg/kg per day, plus prednisolone 2 mg/kg per day for 1–2 weeks.

Further reading

Dhillon, R. *et al.* (1993). Management of Kawasaki disease in the British Isles. *Archives of Disease in Childhood*, **69**, 631–6.

Chapter 10.18

Cryoblobulinaemia

S. A. Misbah

The term cryoglobulinaemia refers to the presence in blood of immunoglobulins that reversibly precipitate in the cold (4°C; Fig. 1(a)), redissolving at higher temperatures (37°C). Three distinct types of cryoglobulins have been recognized on the basis of their immunoglobulin composition and associated diseases (Table 1). Type I cryoglobulins are composed entirely of monoclonal immunoglobulin (usually IgM or IgG) and account for approximately 25 per cent of all cryoglobulins. Type II, which are made up of a mixture of monoclonal IgM exhibiting rheumatoid factor activity and polyclonal IgG, constitute up to 25 per cent of all cryoglobulins, whereas the remaining 50 per cent are made up from type III cryoglobulins, which are composed entirely of polyclonal immunoglobulins (IgM rheumatoid factor and polyclonal IgG).

Usually cryoprecipitation only occurs below a temperature of 10°C, although a thermolabile type I cryoglobulin may sometimes precipitate in the syringe soon after venepuncture if the syringe has not been prewarmed to 37°C. The precise reason(s) for the cryoprecipitation of immunoglobulins is not known. It is plausible to suggest that temperature-dependent conformational changes in paraproteins might account for the cryoprecipitation of type I cryoglobulins, but the evidence for this is conflicting. Analysis of immunoglobulin light chains of mixed (types II and III) cryoglobulins suggests a correlation between the presence of certain subgroups of κ variable region chains and cryoprecipitability. Biochemical abnormalities noted include instability of disulphide bonds linking heavy chains and siliac acid deficient side chains, but no single structural abnormality has provided a unifying explanation for cryoprecipitability.

Aetiology

In the majority of patients with cryoglobulinaemia an underlying malignant paraproteinaemia, lymphoma, autoimmune disease, or infection is evident. Type I cryoglobulinaemia is typically associated with plasma cell dyscrasias, with only a small minority of patients failing to show evidence of underlying lymphoproliferative disease. In mixed cryoglobulinaemia (types II and III) detailed clinical investigation fails to uncover associated disease in up to one-third of patients, originally classified as having idiopathic or mixed essential cryoglobulinaemia.

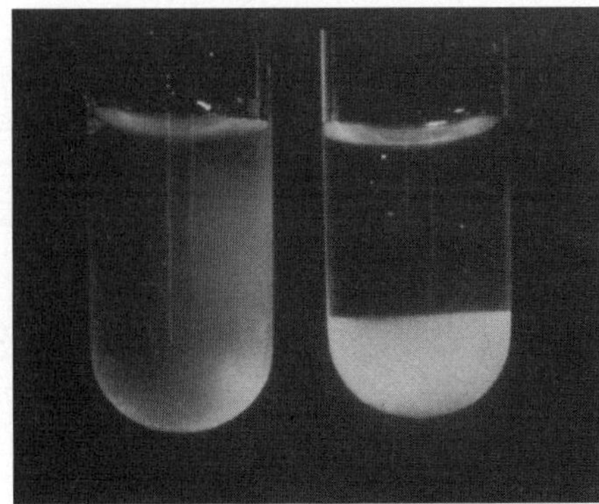

(a)

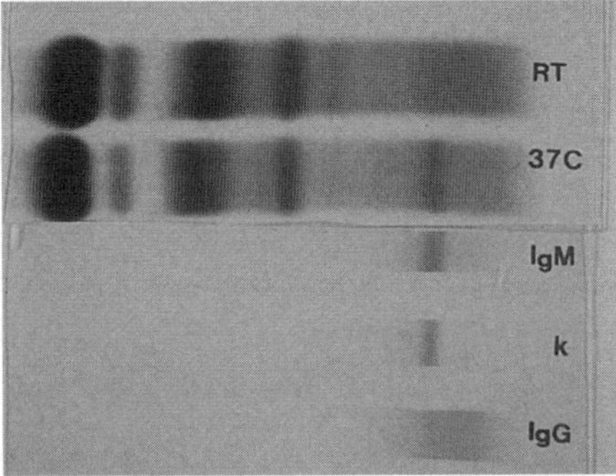

(b)

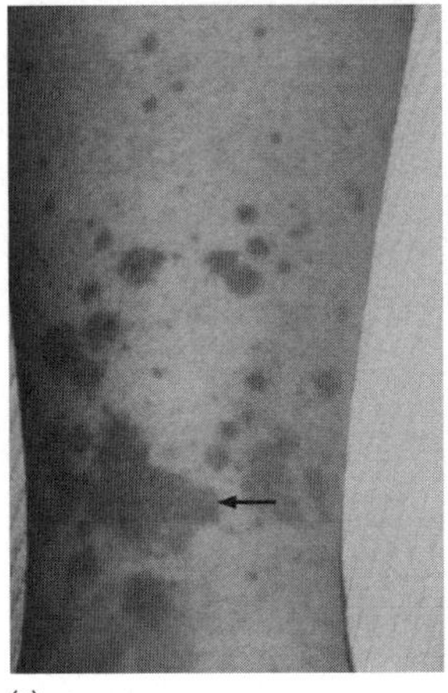

(c)

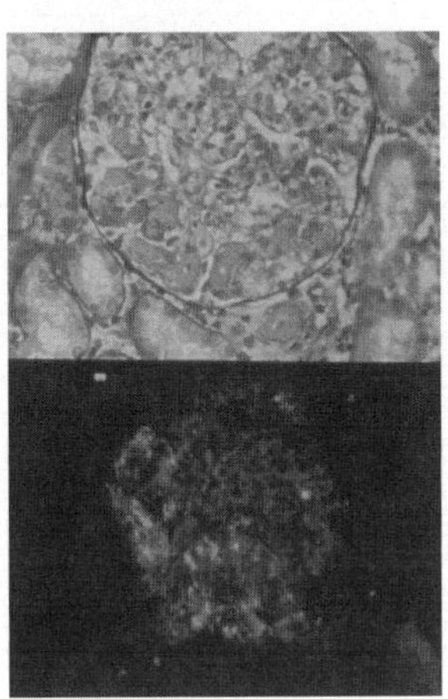

(d)

Fig. 1(a) (d) Clinical and laboratory manifestations of mixed cryoglobulinaemia in a patient with hepatitis C (reproduced with kind permission from Misbah, S.S. (1998). In *The science of laboratory diagnosis* (ed. J. Crocker and D. Burnett) (Fig. 48:8), Isis Medical Media). (a) Stored serum showing cryoprecipitate after 24 h incubation at 4°C (right of panel), redissolving on heating to 37°C (left of panel). (b) Zone electrophoresis of serum collected at 37°C shows the redissolved cryoprecipitate as a discrete band in the gamma region which on immunofixation is shown to be composed of monoclonal IgM κ and polyclonal IgG. Note absence of γ band on zone electrophoresis of sample collected at room temperature (RT) from the same patient. (c) Characteristic purpuric rash on lower limbs; arrow indicates an area of palpable purpura (reproduced with kind permission from Shakil, A.O, Bisceglie, A.M. (1994). *New England Journal of Medicine*, **331**, 1624). (d) Renal biopsy showing eosinophilic glomerular deposits of cryoglobulin ('pseudothrombi') on routine haematoxylin and eosin examination (left of panel) corresponding to coarse deposits (right of panel) of IgG on immunofluorescence.
(Reproduced with kind permission from Graham A. (1992). Arthritis and Rheumatism, ***35****, 1107, Fig. 5)*

The immunopathogenesis of cryoglobulinaemia is poorly understood. A wide range of primary antigen–antibody complexes has been detected in the cryoprecipitates of type II and III cryoglobulins, in addition to the complex of rheumatoid factor and IgG. This has led to the view that the formation of mixed cryoglobulins is the end result of a sequence of events driven by an antibody response to either infective agents or endogenous antigens, as in systemic lupus erythematosus.

Features of lymphoproliferative disease such as monoclonal B-cell populations in bone marrow, clonal immunoglobulin gene rearrangement in peripheral blood lymphocytes, and idiotypic cross-reactivity between monoclonal IgM rheumatoid factors characteristic of the disease, may also occur in type II cryoglobulinaemia. However, overt lymphoma only develops in a minority of such patients. Recent studies suggest that 60–80 per cent patients with type II cryoglobulinaemia have underlying hepatitis C virus infection.

Clinical features

The clinical signs of cryoglobulinaemia are due to a combination of vascular obstruction and inflammation induced by immune complexes. Type I cryoglobulins may occur in either sex and are characterized by Raynaud's phenomenon, arterial thrombosis, gangrene, and retinal haemorrhage. Mixed cryoglobulins affect females in particular and present with diverse clinical features due to deposition of precipitable immune complexes in blood vessels, causing systemic vasculitis (Table 2). The triad of skin, renal, and joint disease is of particular importance. Cutaneous vasculitis is seen in virtually all patients, with prominent lower limb purpura, often progressing to ulceration (Fig. 1(c)). Biopsies of affected areas show leucocytoclastic vasculitis with deposition of immunoglobulins and complement. Membranoproliferative glomerulonephritis with immunoglobulin and complement deposition occurs in about 50 per cent of all patients with mixed cryoglobulinaemia (Fig. 1(d)). Distinctive features include marked glomerular monocytic infiltration, amorphous Congo-red-negative eosinophilic deposits in capillaries and a double contoured basement membrane due to interposition of monocytes. These features in a renal biopsy of a patient with apparent 'idiopathic glomerulonephritis' should prompt a search for cryoglobulins. Nephrotic syndrome and hypertension are common sequelae.

Although arthralgia is seen in three-quarters of all patients with mixed cryoglobulinaemia, frank arthritis with deformity is uncommon. Impaired liver function with a wide variety of histological changes, ranging from chronic persistent hepatitis to cirrhosis, occurs in up to 70 per cent of patients, a finding of interest in view of the strong association with hepatitis C infection in type II cryoglobulinaemia.

Investigation of suspected cryoglobulinaemia

Meticulous attention to the collection of blood samples is vital. Blood should be collected into a plain tube without anticoagulant and immersed into a flask containing water at 37°C, followed by immediate transfer to the laboratory. Failure to collect samples at 37°C enables the cryoglobulin to precipitate out with the blood clot and hence escape detection. Blood samples are centrifuged at 37°C and serum stored at 4°C for 5–7 days, with daily inspection for the presence of

Table 1 Classification of cryoglobulins

	Levels of cryoglobulin	Composition	Disease associations
Type I	>5 mg/ml Cryocrit >1–30 per cent	Monoclonal immunoglobulin, usually IgM or IgG	• Waldenström's macroglobulinaemia • Myeloma, lymphoproliferative disease
Type II	1–5 mg/ml Cryocrit <1–10 per cent	Monoclonal IgM rheumatoid factor plus polyclonal IgG *	Infections • Bacterial: endocarditis • Viral: hepatitis C, hepatitis B, Epstein–Barr, cytomegalovirus
Type III	<1 mg/ml Cryocrit <1 per cent	Polyclonal IgM rheumatoid factor plus polyclonal IgG	• Spirochaetal: Lyme disease, syphilis • Fungal: coccidioidomycosis • Parasitic: malaria • Autoimmune disease: systemic lupus erythematosus, rheumatoid arthritis, Sjögren's, scleroderma • Idiopathic: mixed essential cryoglobulinaemia

*There is considerable overlap in the disease associations for types II and III cryoglobulins.

a cryoprecipitate. Most significant cryoglobulins are evident within 24–72 h.

A quantification of the cryoprecipitate (cryocrit) and typing by immunoelectrophoresis at 37°C follows (Fig. 1(b)). In patients with type I cryoglobulin, appropriate investigations for plasma cell dyscrasias and lymphoproliferative disorders should be carried out. The presence of type II and III cryoglobulin should instigate a search for underlying autoimmune disease or infective agents stimulating an immune response, in particular hepatitis C. The presence of IgM rheumatoid factor with marked depletion of early serum complement components (C4, Clq) due to activation of the classical pathway by immune complexes is highly suggestive of mixed cryoglobulinaemia and occurs in over 90 per cent of patients. Patients with an unexplained low serum C4 and renal or skin disease should be investigated for cryoglobulinaemia. Cryoglobulins interfere with the routine measurements of serum immunoglobulins, leading to artefactually low levels; they may also interfere with routine full blood count analysis by automated Coulter counters leading to spurious apparent leucocytosis and thrombocytosis. Collection and analysis of samples at 37°C prevents such errors.

Management

The aims of treatment are to treat the underlying disease and to reduce the concentration of cryoglobulin. In type I cryoglobulinaemia treatment of the associated plasma cell dyscrasia or lymphoma is often combined with regular plasmapheresis to remove cryoglobulins. The presence of type II or III cryoglobulin should instigate a search for underlying autoimmune disease or infective agents stimulating an immune response, in particular, hepatitis C.

Until recently, patients with unexplained types II and III cryoglobulinaemia and progressive renal or hepatic disease were treated with immunosuppressive treatment in the form of steroids and cytotoxic agents. With the recognition of high prevalence of hepatitis C virus in type II cryoglobulinaemia, antiviral therapy with α-interferon has replaced blanket immunosuppression as the treatment of choice. Plasmapheresis remains a useful adjunct, particularly as a short-term measure in the management of acute exacerbations. The long-term outcome of patients with mixed cryoglobulinaemia is largely determined by the extent of renal disease.

Table 2 Frequency of clinical features in 50 patients with mixed cryoglobulinaemia

	Number	(%)
Female	33	(66)
Purpura	50	(100)
Arthralgia	35	(70)
Leg ulcers	15	(30)
Raynaud's phenomenon	11	(22)
Abdominal pain	9	(18)
Sjögren's syndrome	7	(14)
Sensorimotor peripheral neuropathy	10	(20)
Liver disease	35	(70)
Renal disease	26	(54)
Hypertension	17	
Oedema	20	
Azotaemia	13	
Nephrotic syndrome	6	
Haematuria	24	
Proteinuria		
>4 g/day	5	
1–4 g/day	17	
>0.5–<1 g/day	3	

See OTM3, p. 3051, for source.

Further reading

Trendelenburg, M. and Schifferli, J.A. (1998). Cryoglobulins are not essential. *Annals of Rheumatic Disease*, 57, 3–5. A recent editorial review summarizing conceptual changes in our understanding of cryoglobulinaemia in the light of hepatitis C.

Section 11
Diseases of the skin

Contents

Section 11

Diseases of the skin

T. J. Ryan

The structure of the skin

The skin consists of the epidermis from which grow hair, nails, and sweat glands and its supporting dermis lying on a layer of fat. The epidermis is a stratified squamous epithelium consisting of a germinative basal layer adherent to the basement membrane and giving rise to successive layers of differentiating cells which synthesize the insoluble protein keratin. Keratins are the intermediate filaments of the cytoskeleton found in epithelial cells which serve as a scaffold in these cells and contribute to cell integrity. The epidermis is infiltrated by a number of dendritic cells including the melanocytes and Langerhans cells that internalize HLA-DR molecules from the cell membrane and are involved in antigen processing.

The rich vasculature has a generous reserve to meet the requirements of wounding and repair, so common at the surface. Dilatation can increase blood flow 100-fold, assisting thermoregulation. Macromolecules and cells leave the dermis through the lymphatic system, which arise in an elastic network at the junction of the upper and middle dermis. The lymphatic system is responsive to hydrostatic forces and to movement of the solid components of the dermis by massage or compression. The dermis also supports the extremely complex innervation, essential for sensations of touch and pain. All the main constituents of the dermis, collagen, and elastic fibrous proteins embedded in the mucopolysaccharide ground substance, are secreted by the fibroblast.

Functions of the skin and 'skin failure'

'Skin failure' can be disastrous. The skin is the largest organ of the body and being on the surface, it is continually exposed to injury. It is not only displayed, but also fondled, and together with the hair and nails, is an organ of sexual attraction. It has to be both supple and strong because it is bent, stretched, trodden upon and compressed, as well as scratched and prodded. It must have a capacity to repair itself fully to form a physical barrier impervious to excess water loss or to damage from the environment. It must resist wear and tear. These functions are impaired in skin diseases, making those affected more vulnerable and less able to reconstitute themselves after damage, as well as causing them social embarrassment.

The skin is capable of presystemic metabolism of drugs and other substances applied topically and can generate toxic metabolites. It can synthesize vitamin D from calciferol in the presence of sunlight. Cytokines, important to the skin, include interleukins, interferons, and transforming growth factors. A range of peptides, complement factors, eicosanoids, and platelet activating factors are present in the epidermis, involved in intracellular communication. The epidermis readily forms vascular endothelial growth factor (vascular permeability factor) which has a major effect on the upper dermis.

Colouring or decolouring, tattooing, distorting and stretching and, of course, adorning with jewellery and clothing, are all part of the skin's appeal. It is well known that blushing or cold sweats and pallor are skin reflections of the mind. Practitioners of indigenous or fringe medicine, the witch doctor, as well as almost every lay person recognizes the link between anxiety and skin disease. The principal anxieties resulting from skin disease are fear of being infectious, unclean, and ultimately, unwelcome. If one considers what may happen to a patient with leprosy, such fears are well founded. Common diseases such as dermatitis and psoriasis, affect personal autonomy—(1) to move around and manipulate the environment, (2) to service oneself, (3) to resist normal stresses and traumas, (4) to groom oneself, and (5) to organize oneself emotionally or to care for one's home, work, or family and experience education and employment.

It is often said that people do not die of skin disease, but only accidents are a more common cause of death in males aged between 20 and 30 than, for instance, melanoma. Squamous epithelioma of the lip and angioedema of the upper respiratory tract are other causes. Burns are one of the commonest causes of death, as well as one of the commonest accidents, particularly for children in the developing world. Blistering disorders such as pemphigus vulgaris, widespread impetigo, or epidermolysis bullosa are life-threatening diseases. Erythroderma, due to eczema or psoriasis, commonly results in failure of body temperature control, and more rarely, in uncontrollable protein losing enteropathy. In the tropics, many die from uncontrolled skin infections.

Patients with skin disease are unemployable in any job in which they are in the public eye, or involved in food preparation. For the many whose skin is vulnerable to the minor wear and tear of quite ordinary living, there is a long list of jobs which should be discussed. Sufferers from atopic eczema avoid occupations such as hairdressing, food handling, and mechanical engineering. For the less skilled, unemployment may be the consequence. Wear and tear of the skin is the most common consequence of work, and those who have lowered resistance are unable to work. Communities with many such people, have a higher mortality from other life-threatening events, like childbirth, neonatal survival, or protection from the climate.

Because our skin is on the surface, it is on display. Through it, we make contact with others. It is observed and touched. If there are defects in it observers may not like what they see and will not touch. Isolation causes earlier death.

The greatest handicap of all is to be unwelcome. Whether this is real or imagined, it is the commonest social effect of skin disease. Skin disease is extremely common. In one study of 20 000 Americans, 60 per cent had an important skin condition, and in about 10 per cent, the condition limited activity and there was a physical handicap. Diseases of the skin account for almost half of all reported cases of industrial illness, and are the commonest reasons for consultation in rural health centres. Often skin complaints exist for more than 5 years. Diseases of the hands are the greatest handicap.

History taking

The following is a suitable basis for taking a history from a patient with skin problems:

1. How long have you had it; exactly when did it start; have you had it before?
2. Which part of your skin was first affected; where were you when it started; what were you doing?
3. How did it progress, to what sites, and what was there before?
4. Does it come and go; how long does each individual lesion last?
5. Does it itch; is it painful, tender, numb?

6. Does it develop blisters or clear fluid?
7. Does anything make it better?
8. Does anything make it worse?
9. What ointments, creams, lotions, or bath oils have you used? Have you had any medicine or injections?
10. Has anyone else you know got it; does it run in your family; do any other diseases like asthma, eczema, or hay fever run in your family?
11. Have you had any previous illnesses?

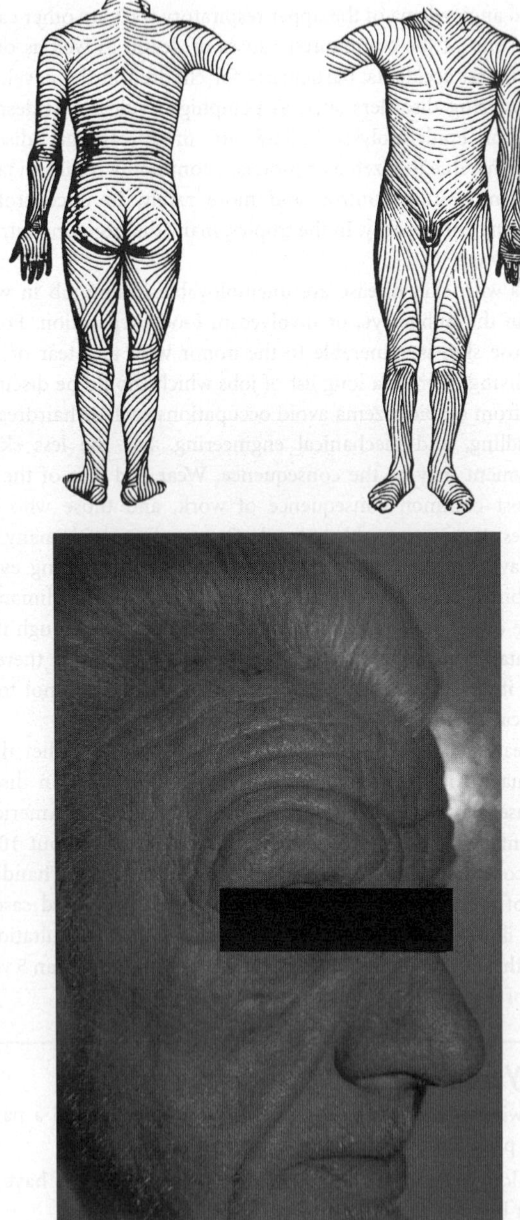

Fig. 1 When excising lesions of the skin, it is helpful to follow lines of tension and to be aware of the elasticity of the skin. (a) On the trunk and limbs Langer's lines may be helpful. (b) On the face it is most important to follow the lines of facial expression. The patient should be encouraged to smile and frown in order to ascertain where the wrinkles are and to provide a guide for lines of tension along which biopsies could extend.

Physical examination

The patient must be undressed. A full examination may include a look at the genitalia and the mouth, but even if the rash is diagnosable at a glance and a history is not obtainable, it is important to speak to patients. Remember that they have a handicap and respond to a sympathetic hearing as well as to a careful examination.

One should keep looking until something is recognized. Often much of a rash is atypical but somewhere there should be a classical physical sign. Good lighting is essential, sunlight is the best.

Touch assures the patient there is no abhorrence and that contagiousness and uncleanliness are insignificant. Papules are palpable, macules are not. Compression distinguishes between purpura and telangiectasia. It reveals much about the depth of the lesion and its consistency.

Investigations

Biopsy

The lesion chosen for biopsy should not be modified by excoriation, therapy, or secondary infection. Small lesions should be totally excised, removing skin in the shape of an ellipse along lines of stretch known as Langer's lines (Fig. 1). In subjects prone to keloids it is best to avoid the sides of the face, neck, sternal region, and shoulders. It is often useful to biopsy the edge of the lesion so that it can be compared with adjacent normal-looking skin. An appropriate fixative is 10 per cent formalin for at least 12 hours.

The histological report may include the following terms:

Hyperkeratosis: thickening of the horny layer usually resulting from retention and increased adhesion of epidermal cells.

Parakeratosis: cell nuclei in the horny layer usually resulting from a high rate of cell turnover as in psoriasis.

Spongiosis: separation of prickle cells by oedema fluid, i.e. the epidermis looks like a sponge—a feature of eczema.

Acantholysis: loss of cohesion between prickle cells and isolation, and balloon-like appearance of individual epidermal cells, a feature of pemphigus.

Liquefaction: degeneration and rupture of basal cells—characteristic of lupus erythematosus, lichen planus, and erythema multiforme.

Pigmentary incontinence: the shedding of melanin from the epidermis into the dermis following injury to the basal layer.

Elastotic degeneration: changes in dermal collagen which occur in light-exposed and ageing skin. Whorled masses of disorganized elastin-staining fibres replace normal collagen.

Fibrinoid degeneration: deposition of eosinophilic material which resembles fibrin.

Necrobiosis: a type of focal necrosis of collagen which leads to the formation of a palisading granuloma, i.e. macrophages lining up like a fence around the necrotic material.

Lichenoid: a heavy infiltrate of white cells hugs the epidermal interface with the dermis and fills the upper dermis.

Immunofluorescence examination: IgG is found intercellularly in the epidermis in pemphigus. Linear deposits of Ig and complement are found at the dermoepidermal junction in pemphigoid, while IgA occurs in the same distribution in linear IgA dematosis. Granular IgA and often complement are found in dermal papillae in dermatits herpetiformis.

The basis of rashes

Some rashes are distributed with a constituent of the skin, e.g. hair follicles in folliculitis (Fig. 2), sweat glands in prickly heat, sebaceous glands in acne vulgaris, dermatomes in herpes zoster, or annular and reticulate patterns as in some rashes determined by vascular anatomy.

Inflammation near the surface of the skin usually damages the epidermis so that vesiculation and scaling become features of the response, whereas deep dermal or subcutaneous inflammation merely produces 'lumps' known as nodules.

Some classical distributions are shown in Fig. 3; Table 1 illustrates some well-known morphological terms and Figs 4 and 5 show some other shapes.

External contact infections such as cattle ringworm or the primary chancre are frequently asymmetrical whereas psoriasis or secondary syphilis is usually exactly symmetrical.

Injury to the skin from contact dermatitis usually has the distribution of contact; in cases due, for example, to mascara, gloves, or shoes, there will be symmetry, but casually brushing against a noxious plant will produce bizarre asymmetrical patterns.

External irradiation from the sun spares skin beneath the lobes of the ear and under the chin, whereas an airborne pollen dermatitis will not spare such areas but may have a similar cut-off point below the collar.

Factors determining or modifying skin disease

Changes of skin with age, sex, and race

Newborn

Birth marks are usually first noticed in the newborn but some, like cavernous haemangiomas, may not be present on the first day. Certain epidermal or pigmented naevi and some neurofibromas do not appear until puberty.

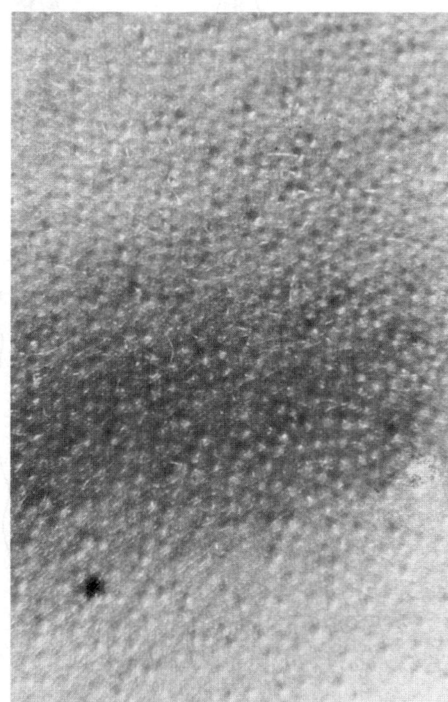

Fig. 2 Perifollicular hyperkeratosis having the distribution of the hair follicle.

Old age

Most elderly people have multiple skin problems, including seborrhoeic eczema, intertrigo, and dermatophytosis. Probably the principal characteristic of elderly skin is its inhomogeneity or the increased diversity that develops with age. Some changes are endocrine related, such as hirsutism and baldness. Others are more specifically age-related, like dryness, decreased sweating, or poor healing of superficial wounds. Dry, scaly, rough skin occurs in about 80 per cent of people over the age of 75 and there are disparities in the size and thickness of the epidermis and in its pigmentation. Seborrhoeic warts, actinic injury, Campbell de Morgan spots, and dilatation and derangement of superficial venules are common features.

Genetic or age related loss of control of malignant change and the cumulative exposure to solar radiation explains neoplasia of the skin. Degenerative disease of the vascular system explains venous ulcers and arterial ischaemic diseases. In one study, after controlling for age, sex, and sun exposure, premature wrinkling increased with years of smoking. Heavy smokers were 4.7 times more likely to be wrinkled than non-smokers.

Is it due to malnutrition?

The skin is 8 per cent of body weight and uses up about one-eighth of the body's protein; hence it is affected early in malnutrition. Dryness of the skin and hyperpigmentation are early signs. At birth, malnutrition is seen as loss of vernix and maceration. The skin is wrinkled and peeling with deficient subcutaneous fat.

Older people develop a mild ichthyosis with hyperkeratosis. The stratum corneum is unsupple and cracks appear in the horny surface, particularly on the front of the legs (eczema craquelée) (Fig. 6).

Malnutrition usually results from mixed deficiencies including protein loss. There is weight loss, weakness, and emaciation. Anaemia, oedema, sore tongue, and dry, thin hair are often featured.

Vitamin A deficiency should be thought of when there are dry eyes and perifollicular hyperkeratosis. Vitamin B deficiency causes a dermatitis of seborrheoic distribution particularly of the nasolabial folds, scrotum, and vulva. The lips are dry, cracked, crusted, or ulcerated; the tongue is sore and smooth. Nicotinic acid deficiency or pellagra causes the triad of dementia, diarrhoea, and dermatitis. Early signs are prominent sebaceous follicles of the nose. The erythema is a characteristic dusky brown in light-exposed areas and the dermatitis is well marginated. In the dark skin the lesions are relatively depigmented but equally well marginated. Vitamin C deficiency causes perifollicular haemorrhages, painful bruising, woody oedema of legs, and failure of wound healing. In the dark skin it may appear that the skin is stretched and shiny. Coiled hairs are an early sign but they are common in the normal population especially in the elderly. Swollen and bleeding gums are an important sign but occur only in those with teeth.

Protein deficiency is common in all forms of malnutrition, but where it is supplemented by carbohydrate and there is no active starvation, a characteristic disease is recognizable. In children this is typified by kwashiorkor. Features of protein deficiency include:

(1) erythema as in a second-degree burn;

(2) dry hyperkeratotic hyperpigmented scales;

(3) peeling like enamel paint, cracking like crazy pavement;

(4) it is maximal over pressure areas; and

(5) there is straightening and reddening of the hair.

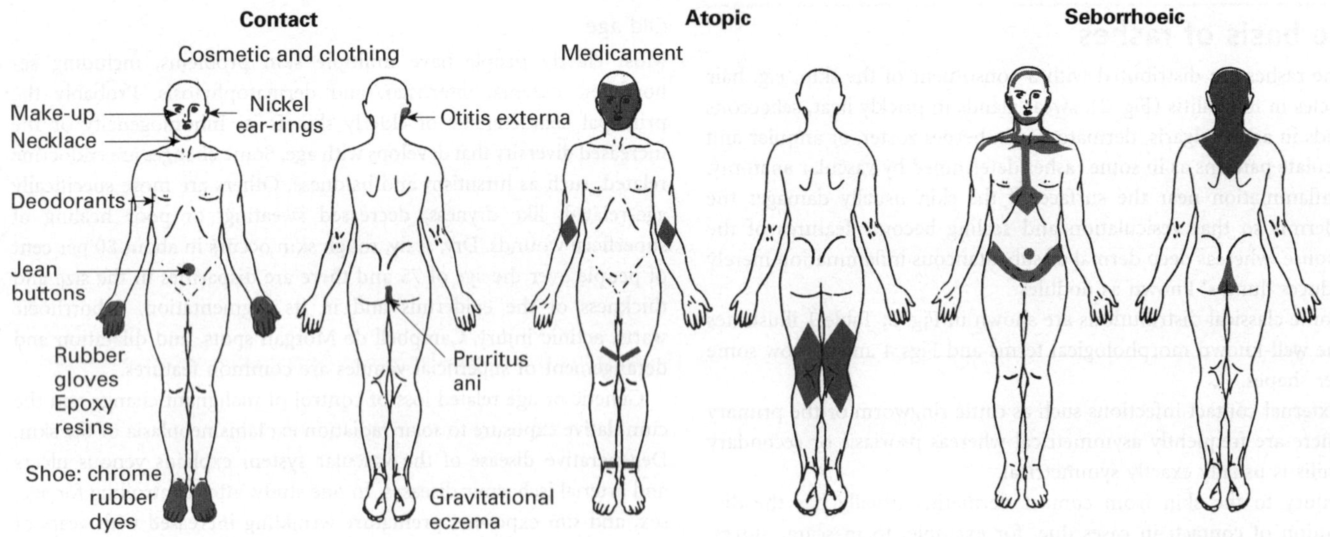
Contact
Cosmetic and clothing
Make-up
Necklace
Nickel
ear-rings
Deodorants
Jean
buttons
Rubber
gloves
Epoxy
resins
Shoe: chrome
rubber
dyes
Atopic
Medicament
Otitis externa
Pruritus
ani
Gravitational
eczema
Seborrhoeic

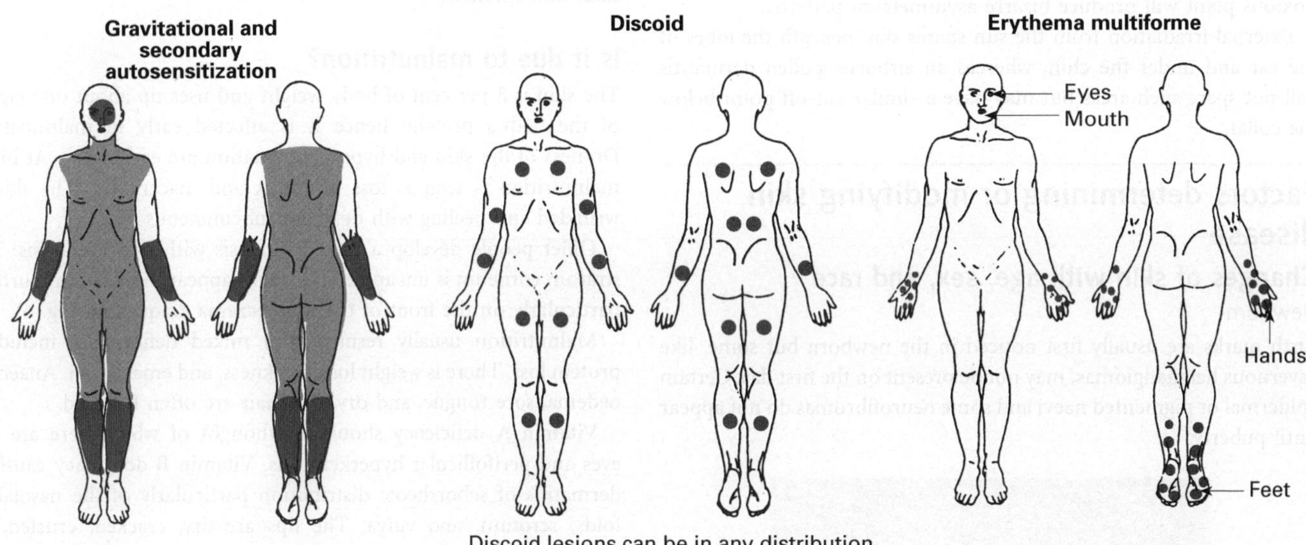
Gravitational and
secondary
autosensitization
Discoid
Discoid lesions can be in any distribution
but they tend to be symmetrical and coin-sized
Erythema multiforme
Eyes
Mouth
Hands
Feet

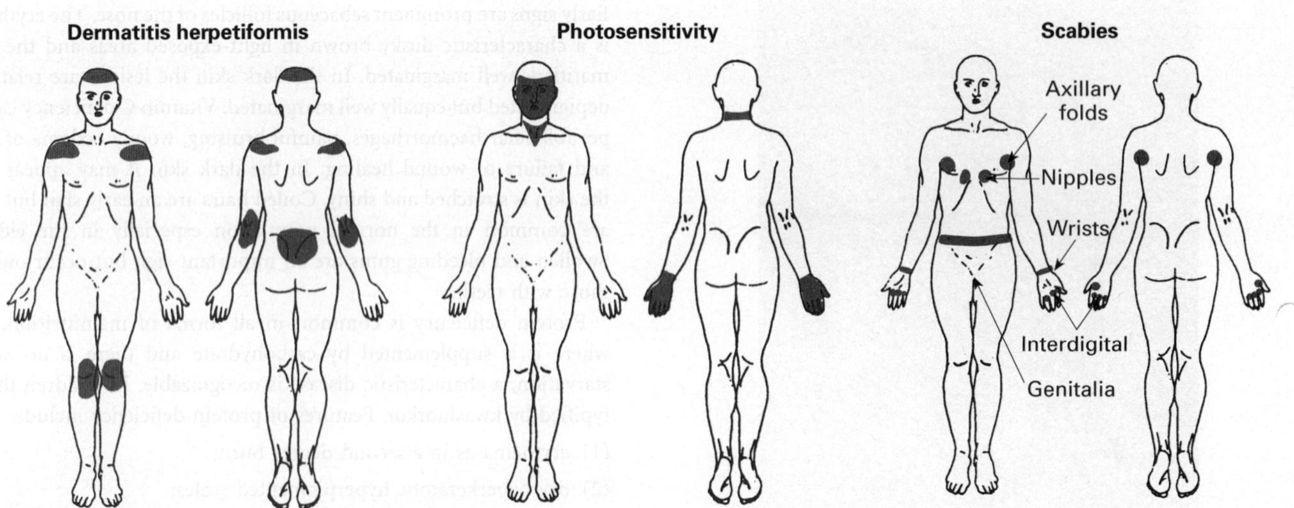
Dermatitis herpetiformis
Photosensitivity
Scabies
Axillary
folds
Nipples
Wrists
Interdigital
Genitalia

Fig. 3 Distribution of rashes.

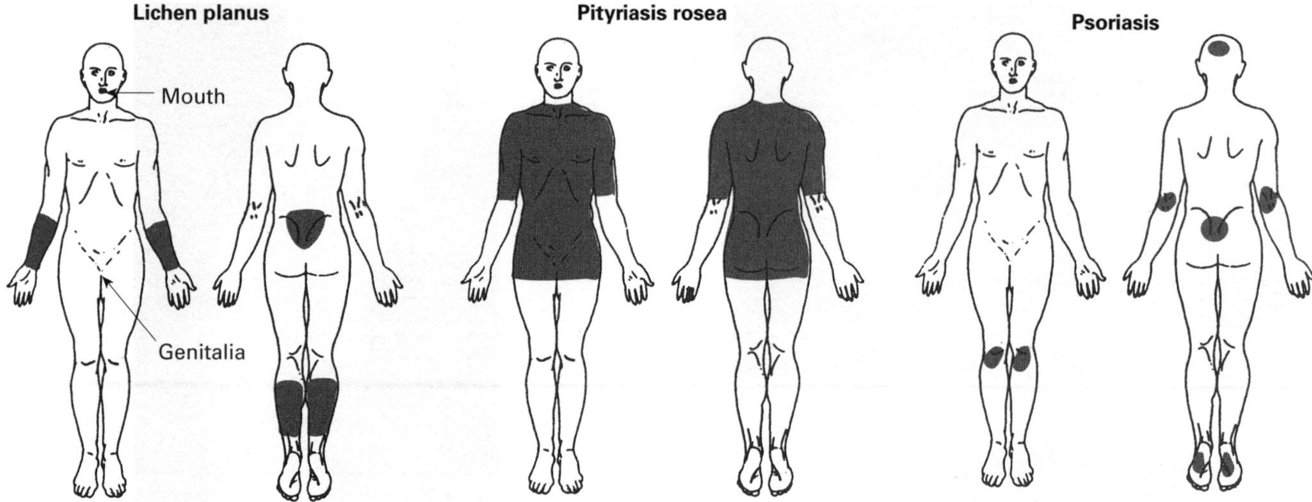

Fig. 3

Table 1 Some morphological terms

A *macule* is flat without change in surface marking or texture—it may be merely redness, purpura, or melanin
A *papule* is a circumscribed, palpable elevation or a thickening of the epidermis or of the upper dermis by infiltration or oedema
A *plaque* is a disc-shaped lesion often as a result of the coalescence of papules
A *nodule* is a circumscribed palpable mass larger than 1 cm in diameter and usually consisting of oedema, malignant or inflammatory cells filling the dermis or subcutaneous tissue. Some are small and painful, others are juxta-articular
Vesicles and bullae are visible accumulations of fluid (often the lay person uses the term blister to include wealing in which there are no visible accumulations other than swelling). Vesicles are small, while bullae are larger than 1 cm
Annular lesions result from spreading infiltrations or healing centre often with refractoriness due to such factors as raised tissue pressure or scarring preventing vasodilatation or leakiness in the centre of the lesions. Vascular patterns in the skin have a reticular or annular anatomical distribution
Linear lesions are due to external scratches, developmental or anatomical distribution of lymphatics, blood vessels, or nerves

Ultraviolet radiation and the sun

Ultraviolet rays are classified into three ranges. UVB (290 to 320 nm) penetrates and is of high energy and hence damages and produces sunburn. UVA (black light 320–400 nm) is of lower energy but it is penetrating and usually it is only damaging in the presence of sensitizers such as drugs, porphyrins, or plant juices. The shortest is UVC (200 to 290 nm), which is non-penetrating and accounts for the damage to the skin in mountain climbers or from some ultraviolet lamps, especially those used for sterilization.

On the head, nose, and cheeks, there is often sparing below the eyebrows, under a forelock, beneath and behind the ears, and below the chin. The sides and back of the neck are picked out but there is a sharp border to the sun damage where the collar shields the skin from sunlight. The backs of the hands and dorsum of the feet are often caught by the sun but there may be some tolerance of such skin previously exposed and tanned so that skin not so tolerant is clearly more damaged. Heat from the sun lowers the itch threshold at sites of vasodilatation. The condition phytophotodermatitis is a rash in the distribution of actual contact with plant juices on which the sun then acts and produces a burn. The pattern of such casual contact from plants or perfumes is often streaky and bizarre.

White skin and the sun

Exposure to sunlight is a major cause of ageing of the skin and of degenerative diseases of the epidermis and dermis that accompany age (Fig. 7). In Australia, South Africa, and the south-western USA, solar keratosis, basal cell epitheliomata, chronic solar cheilitis, and squamous carcinoma (Fig. 8) are the commonest cause of referral to the dermatologist (Table 2). Even children are not completely immune and those who burn easily and still persist in exposing themselves regularly to the sun will inevitably suffer gross changes in their skin, even at an early age.

Malignant melanoma

The incidence of this tumour is increasing. In Scotland it rose between 1979 and 1989 by 3.4 to 7.1 per 100 000 in men, and 6.6–10.4 per 100 000 in women. Most lesions were on the female leg or on the male trunk. High melanocytic naevi counts are associated with a greater incidence of melanoma, as is prominent freckling. Naevi increase during childhood, peaking in early adulthood. The counts have been shown to increase at an earlier age in caucasians who live closer to the equator where sun exposure is greater. Early recognition is important since it allows the tumour to be detected before it has developed depth. At depth greater than 0.76 mm, the prognosis worsens, from a 95 per cent 5-year survival to 80 per cent, and with a tumour thickness greater than 3.5 mm, the prognosis sharply worsens to 40 per cent 5-year survival. Survival from malignant melanoma is determined by early detection and early adequate surgery. The recommended width of the margin at excision should be 0.5 cm for *in-situ* lesions, 1 cm for invasive melanoma, and up to 2 cm for more than 1 mm in depth. Less than half of melanomas emerge in a previously

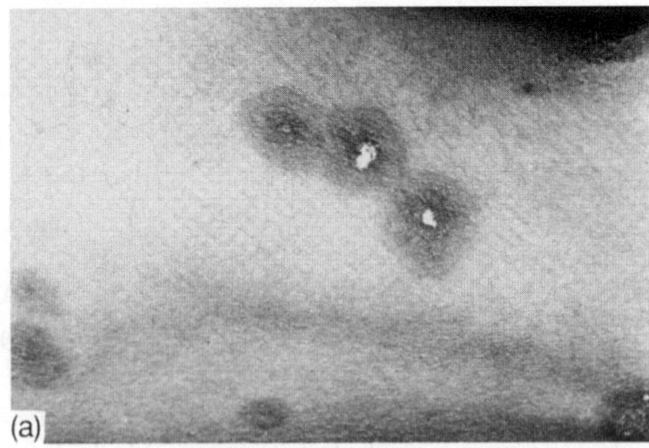

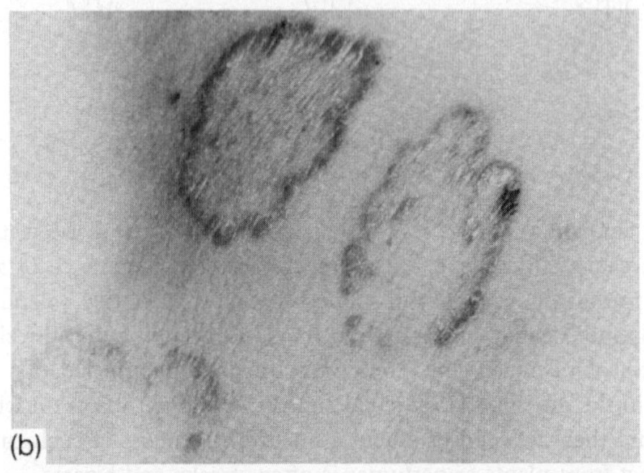

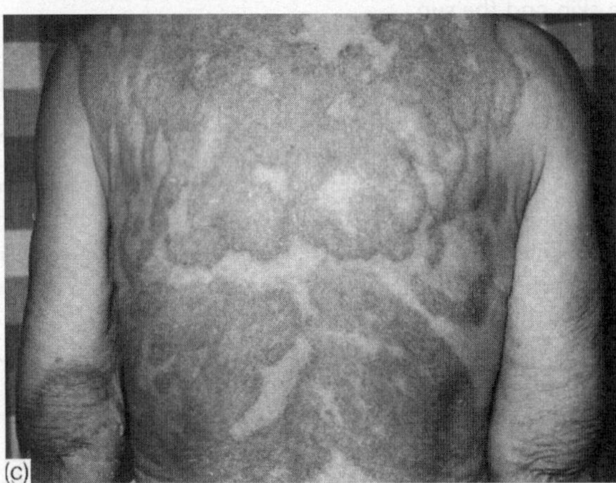

Fig. 4 (a) An example of the 'target' lesion of erythema multiforme. (b) Healing of the centre of the lesion is a feature of many skin diseases, including fungus infections and, in this case, psoriasis. (c) Annular erythema in lupus erythematosus with Ro antibody. This pattern of widespread erythema is also observed in association with underlying malignancy.

recognized mole or lentigo (Fig. 9) or in a giant hairy naevus. About 10 per cent of giant congenital pigmented naevi become malignant. However, opinion is divided as to whether all congenital pigmented naevi should be removed prophylactically. Those with a family history of multiple pigmented naevi and malignant melanoma, should avoid the sun and use sun-screening agents. The most important diagnostic factors are rapid and recent change in growth rate, irregularity of margin, colour, or depth. In addition, the development of a new pigmented lesion after puberty is an important clue (Plates 1–9).

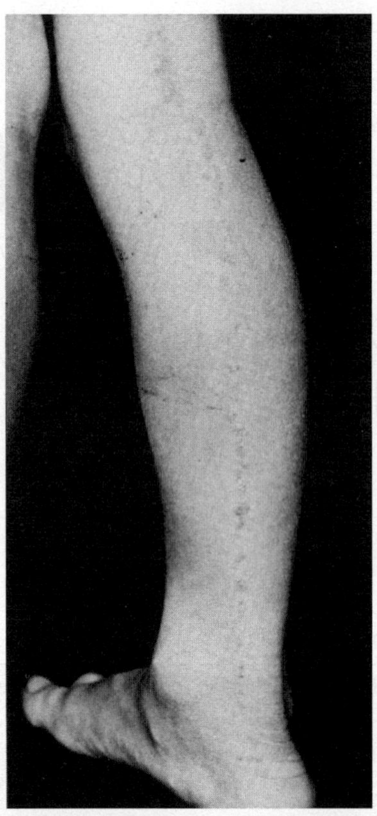

Fig. 5 Example of a linear distribution, in this case lichen planus. The distribution does not conform to a dermatome and the exact cause of the linear lesions remains largely unexplained.

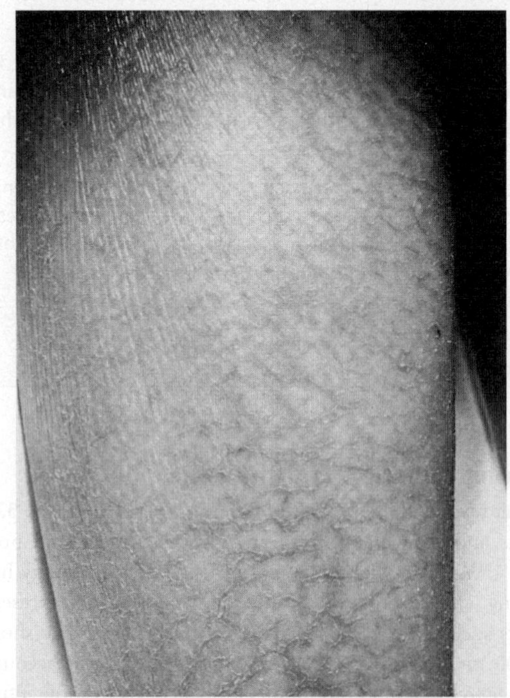

Fig. 6 An early and common sign of malnutrition of the skin, especially in the elderly, is cracking of a well-made stratum corneum giving a pattern of eczema craquelée.

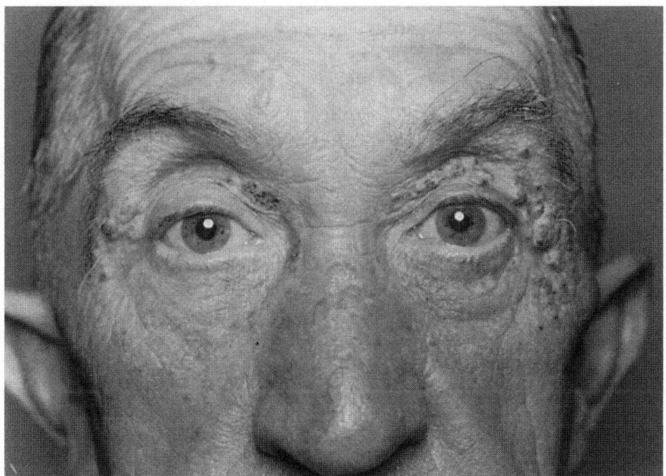

Fig. 7 Prominent sebaceous glands and comedo formation in solar elastosis.

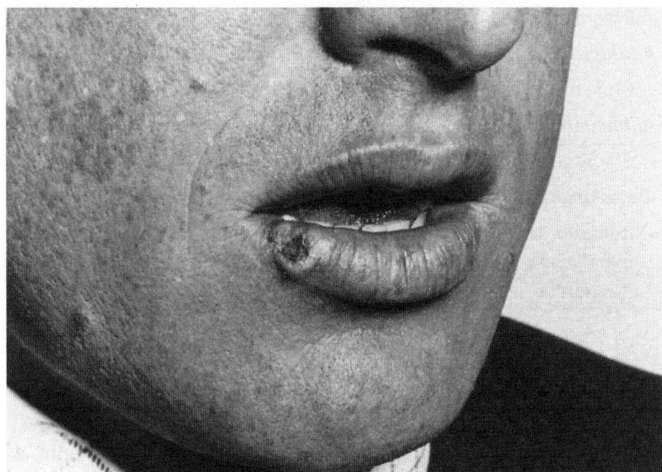

Fig. 8 Squamous epithelioma of lower lip as a consequence of sun exposure.

Rashes due to sun or artificial light and associated ultraviolet rays

Sunburn is initially an erythema at about 6–8 hours after exposure and may progress to blistering and later peeling; if the exposure is excessive, redness may begin as early as 2 hours.

Solar urticaria is an erythema and wealing immediately on exposure to sun, often of sites not habitually exposed to the sun.

Polymorphic light eruption is a variant of sunburn. Instead of erythema there is itchy papular or eczematous responses about 6 to 8 hours after exposure, which may persist for several days (Fig. 10). There are several variants including a lymphoma-like pattern with heavy lymphocytic infiltrates.

Actinic prurigo Sun-induced prurigo shares features with atopic eczema, polymorphic light eruption, and persistent light eruption due to photosensitivity agents in the environment. It is common, and probably genetically determined, in American Indians. It is chronic and initially seasonal. Urticarial plaques develop a few hours after ultraviolet exposure and are followed by a persistent eczematous rash, not always confined to exposed skin.

Exacerbation or localization of other dermatoses is characteristic of pellagra, Hartnup's disease, lupus erythematosus, Darier's disease,

Table 2 Clinical features of chronic sun exposure

Elastosis	Less elastic, more fragile, yellowish, furrowed; Telangiectasia, venous lakes, spider angiomas; Prominent sebaceous glands (Fig. 7); Linear and stellate scars; Idiopathic guttate melanosis
Keratosis	10 per cent precancerous; Yellow-brown hyperkeratosis on a red telangiectatic background—the scale is not laminated as in psoriasis but firmly adherent and removal is painful; unlike lupus erythematosus, it bleeds when the scale is removed; Cutaneous horn common; Annular lesions frequent; Bleed easily when scratched
Solar cheilitis	Lower lip; yellow-white thickenings; Scaling and crusting; Fissuring
Basal cell epithelioma	Central erosion; Telangiectasia runs over the edge; Pearl-like border; Cystic, pigmented, or sclerotic forms
Squamous epithelioma	Indurated beyond the visible margin (Fig. 8); Ulcerated, hyperkeratotic, or granulomatous; Crusted and horny; Hard, elevated, or undermined edge
Keratoacanthoma	Rapid growth: 4–6 weeks; Sharply defined hemispherical; Central horny core which may leave a crater; 2–12 months disappears spontaneously; Scarring may be considerable
Bowen's disease	Often single with a well-defined edge; Usually red scaly or crusted plaques; Often slightly pigmented
Malignant melanoma	Change in depth of pigmentation (either darkening or loss) irregular notched border; Growth changes, satellites; Bleeding, itching, or ulceration; Family history of atypical multiple pigmented naevi

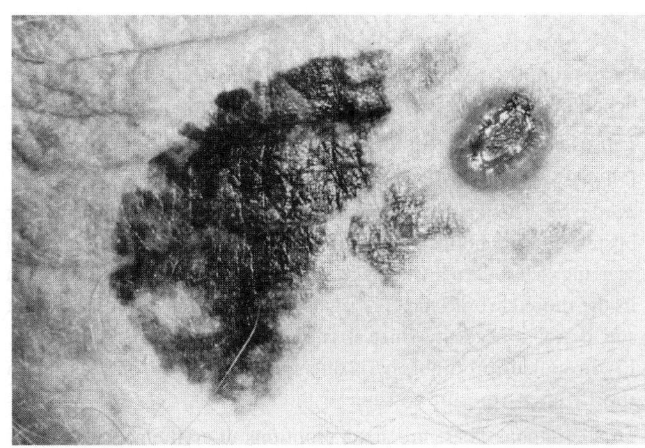

Fig. 9 The features of malignancy in this melanoma are an irregular notched border, variation in colour from red to black, variation in depth, or a history of recent change.

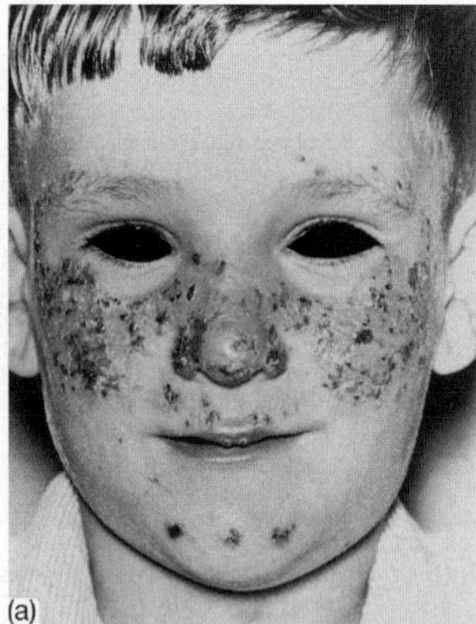

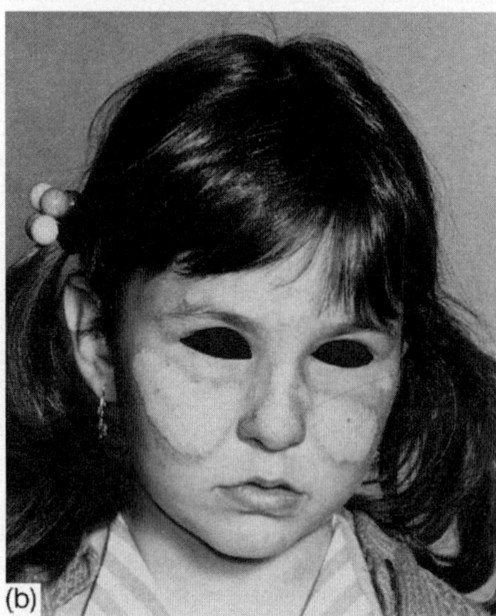

Fig. 10 Two patterns of altered response to sunburn wavelengths: (a) an eczematous prurigo with excoriations; (b) a plaque-like form not unlike lupus erythematosus.

herpes simplex, rosacea, scleroderma, erythema multiforme, actinic lichen planus (psoriasis) (sometimes), and lymphocytoma.

Ultraviolet rays may diminish antigen surveillance by reducing the population of Langerhans cells.

Porphyria The rash of exposed areas is a swelling, bruising, or blistering often noticed immediately after exposure. There is pitted scarring, scleroderma-like thickening, pigmentation, and hirsutism in the more chronic stages. Fragility of the skin is a feature. Bright sun is not a necessity since it is due to the UVA and blue light. Erythropoietic protoporphyria often presents as a burning sensation shortly after exposure to sun.

Drug eruptions These are acute eruptions of erythema, swelling or blistering like severe sunburn but not dependent on bright sun since UVA is often responsible. They are often dose dependent as with psoralens in PUVA therapy. Ingestion of a spinach (Atriplex) also causes photosensitivity (see Table 3). Some present only as deep pigmentation.

Table 3 Photosensitivity to drugs

Sulphonamides and related chemicals

- Antibacterial group: sulphathiazole, long-acting sulphonamides
- Diuretics: chlorothiazide, hydrochlorothiazide, quinethazone
- Antidiabetic: sulphonylureas, carbamides
- Rarely: paraphenylenediamine, procaine group of anaesthetics

Antibiotics

- Tetracyclines; tetracycline, dimethylchlortetracycline (Ledermycin®)
- Declomycin chlortetracycline (Aureomycin®)
- Griseofulvin

Antiarrhythmic

- Amiodarone

Phenothiazines

- Chloropromazine, promazine, trimeprazine, meprazine, promezathine hydrochloride

Other psychotrophic drugs

- Chlordiazepoxide

Antihistamines not of phenothiazine structure

- Diphenhydramine

Antimalarials

- Chloroquine

Occasional, rare, or of historical interest

- Isoniazid, psoralens, stilbamidine 9-aminoacridine, eosin, trypaflavine, methylene blue, rose bengal, frusemide, nalidixic acid (Negram®)

Xeroderma pigmentosum is the term given to several genetic diseases in which repair of DNA is defective. Children develop severe redness and swelling up to 72 hours after exposure. Chronic injury results in keratosis, telangiectasia, irregularities of pigmentation, and even, in childhood, the early development of cancers and melanomas. Severe sunburn in infancy must be investigated by fibroblast DNA repair studies because future protection from sun can much reduce the incidence of subsequent malignancy. There are at least 10 variants with three known different chromosome locations. The mechanisms include a failure of DNA excision repair of ultraviolet-induced thymidine dimers. Variants with postreplication repair defects are described. The incidence of different tumour types is determined by the gene defect.

Persistent light eruption is the term given to sensitivity to light induced by agents previously applied to the skin, often years before. Drugs eliciting light sensitivity are listed in Table 3.

Investigations

Patients should be asked about family history, drug or food ingestion, exposure to perfumes, occupation, and how and when exposure took place. It is important to know whether glass or cloud is protective. Although testing to light may be done with a variety of light sources, especially in photobiology units, sunlight is a natural source that can be used by blacking out the skin of the back of the trunk and exposing it by opening 'windows' at 5 min intervals.

Prophylaxis

Health education in schools should emphasize that burning in the sun is not related to heat. It is maximal at midday and protection is essential mainly through avoidance by using clothing. Sunscreens are effective if properly used, i.e. they must be applied evenly, thoroughly, and well before exposure, but they are not a substitute for avoidance.

Management

Protection from light for those with sensitivity to UVB includes advice on the time of day and season likely to be harmful. Most patients can safely take an early morning or late afternoon bathe. Those with severe sensitivities such as xeroderma pigmentosum can be saved from all ill-effects by diligent protection, including appropriate clothing. Indeed, clothing and household shade are the best protections for children sensitive to the sun, but a wet T-shirt can transmit ultraviolet rays; tightly woven silks and cottons are more effective than loose weave yarns or wool. Glass windows and certain plastics are protective against shorter wavelengths. Natural pigment and thickening of the epidermis accounts for normal tolerance.

Sunscreening agents include thick pastes or creams such as titanium dioxide; these are popular with skiers but prevent tanning. They are most useful for lip protection. Some have a number indicating the protection factor. Sunscreening agents may reflect light and invisible lotions or creams containing *p*-aminobenzoic acid in 70 per cent alcohol absorb ultraviolet rays and allow gradual tanning.

β-Carotene and mepacrine are pigments that can be taken by mouth. Aspirin, by inhibiting prostaglandin synthetase, reduces the erythema from sunburn.

Drug eruptions

Adverse reactions account for 3 per cent of hospital admissions and 14 per cent of medical resources. Thirty per cent of hospital patients develop adverse reactions. In developing countries cheap drugs such as sulphonamides are the commonest cause of adverse reactions.

Drug rashes are essentially blood borne and therefore often have a symmetrical urticarial, erythematous, or purpuric and ischaemic pattern determined by vascular anatomy. Less likely is a 'primary epithelial' reaction in the initial stages and so scaling or even the vesiculation of eczema as a first manifestation of a drug rash would be unusual. The exceptions are well known and include the intraepidermal immunologically induced 'pemphigus' rash of penicillamine, rifampicin, and captopril, especially when the first of these is used to treat rheumatoid arthritis, and the cell-mediated hypersensitivity to epidermal protein and drug haptens in a person previously having a contact dermatitis to a local antihistamine or sulphonamide. The psoriasis-like rash of various β-blockers, or the scaly eruption particularly of the scalp from methyldopa, are exceptions.

Nevertheless if a rash looks like eczema, it is probably not caused by a drug. If it is an erythema and urticaria, it may well be. Later stages of the rash are frequently complicated by a secondary epidermal reaction so that diagnosis should be made on the initial manifestation. An increased frequency of adverse reactions to drugs has been reported in HIV-positive patients.

Unlikely or likely drugs

It may be helpful to rule out unlikely offenders such as digoxin, paracetamol, steroids, other hormones, and vitamin and electrolyte supplements. In any drug group there are likely and less likely offenders. Thus of antibiotics, oxytetracycline, nystatin, and erythromycin are not under suspicion but dichlortetracycline is a common cause of a photosensitivity rash, and in infectious mononucleosis ampicillin is almost invariably responsible for a characteristic bright pink maculopapular rash.

Timing

Timing is useful when trying to establish mechanisms such as anaphylaxis or the Arthus phenomenon. The patient should be asked about previous reactions to drugs. In the absence of such history, and especially if the drugs were new to the patient, it would be unlikely to cause a rash within the first few days of administration. An exception is the way drug eruptions develop in combination with infections. A cough mixture or co-trimoxazole may produce an extremely severe erythema within 2 or 3 days of the intake. Erythema multiforme or Stevens-Johnson syndrome occasionally occurs surprisingly early after a drug's administration and one suspects that the disease for which the drug was given may have prepared the host in some way. Where there is a known hypersensitivity to the drug, the immunological response can be very rapid.

Slow excretion, genetically determined or due to depot injections, can explain slow recovery from an eruption. When examining a list of drugs taken by a patient, those added within the previous month are the most likely to have caused the rash. However, interference with metabolic pathways by drugs may take many months to produce a rash, as for example, isoniazid and the production of pellagra.

Many patients do not admit to taking a drug, perhaps because it was never prescribed but was borrowed from a neighbour or bought over the counter and therefore considered to be harmless. Drug rashes usually fade after withdrawal of the drug—exceptions include pemphigus from penicillamine.

Transient susceptibility

The best example is urticaria. Many people with chronic urticaria are susceptible for many months, and during that time, the rash may be triggered by prostaglandin synthetase inhibitors, such as aspirin or indomethacin. It is possible that certain acute erythemas require both a drug and an infection to provoke the rash, so the underlying disease of the patient should always be taken into account. Diseases such as psoriasis or dermatitis herpetiformis may go into spontaneous remission and at such time they are less likely to be provoked by drugs. Psoriasis is expected to be made worse by β-blockers, lithium, or chloroquine, but this is unpredictable and not a reason for withholding them. Dermatitis herpetiformis is provoked by iodine so readily that it should be avoided if possible.

Specific drug eruptions

The most common diagnostic problem is a toxic urticating erythema which begins like measles without the upper respiratory and conjunctival prodromal signs. Over a number of hours, red indurated papules erupt (Fig. 11) and, unlike urticaria, persist for days, ultimately involving the epidermis and producing scales. After the first 2 to 3 days the rash tends to become fixed but there may be mild bleeding of the skin with overlying slight peeling. This rash appears 8 to 10 days after the ingestion of the drug. Fever and arthropathy may be associated. Causes include ampicillin, phenylbutazone, phenothiazine, co-trimoxazole, diazides and sulphonylureas, gold, phenylbutazone,

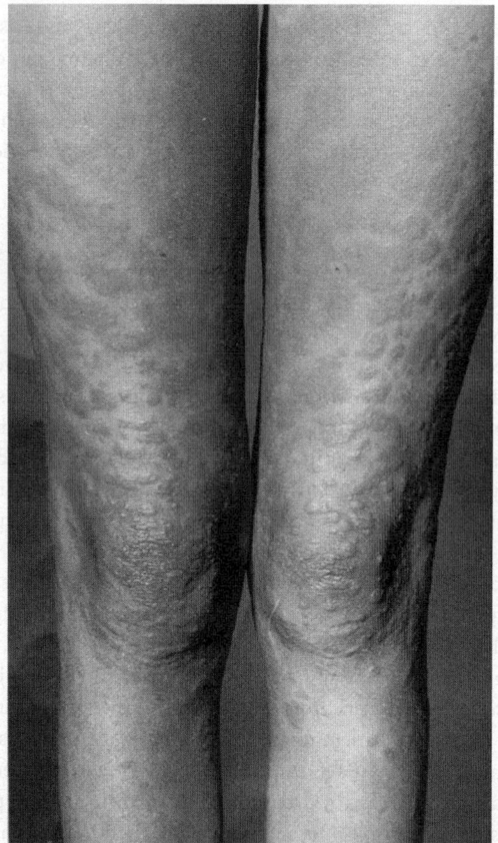

Fig. 11 One of the most common drug eruptions, initially a bright pink papular eruption, symmetrical and becoming confluent. This case is due to ampicillin.

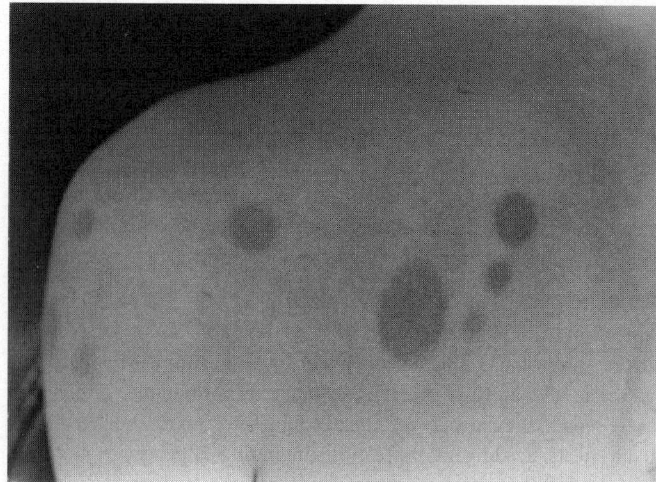

Fig. 12 Fixed drug eruption due to phenolphthalein present in a laxative. Such an eruption characteristically appears within half a day of taking the causative drug and the site affected is the same on every occasion. Violaceous annular lesions are common and may persist for several weeks.

Table 4 Drugs causing fixed drug eruptions

• Phenazone (synonym: antipyrine), dipyrine	• Quinine and derivatives
• Phenolphthalein	• Tetracyclines
• Barbiturates: phenytoin	• Oxyphenbutazone, pyrazolones
• Sulphonamides	• Chlordiazepoxide
• Dapsone, iodides	

indomethacin, allopurinol, hydantoins, sulphonylureas, and *p*-aminosalicyclic acid. Exfoliative dermatitis is the end result.

Ampicillin and amoxycillin

Ampicillin rash appears 5–14 days after treatment of an infection. Thus the rash is often seen after the course of the drug has been completed. It begins on the extensor aspects of the limbs and has a morbilliform or maculopapular pattern which becomes confluent. It is a bright pink-reddish colour and may become purpuric and desquamate. In the pigmented skin such features are usually recognizable. The rash occurs in 5–7 per cent of all recipients and is the usual consequence of prescribing the drug in infectious mononucleosis, cytomegalovirus, or lymphatic leukaemia.

β-Blockers

These cause a psoriasiform scaly eruption that may be modified by basal cell necrosis. A hyperkeratotic scale is more adherent than in psoriasis and often slightly yellowish. The palms and soles, elbows, and knees are particularly favoured.

Lupus erythematosus

Lupus erythematosus, like erythemas or necrotizing vasculitis, are most commonly caused by hydralazine, phenytoin, practolol, penicillamine, and isoniazid. Many other drugs have been incriminated. Drug-induced lupus erythematosus is reversed by withdrawal of the drug, but it recurs when it is readministered.

Photosensitivity

This occurs in light-exposed areas such as the face, neck, forearms, or the dorsum of the feet. It is usually due to long-wave UVA and so glass and cloud are not necessarily protective. However, photosensitivity does occur more often on a bright spring or summer midday. The resulting phototoxic eruption begins as an erythema and, as with severe sunburn, can become bullous or, as in the case of amiodarone, result in blue-grey pigmentation. The problem drugs are listed in Table 3.

Fixed drug eruption

This eruption is easy to recognize as it is usually annular and erythematous (Fig. 12), it frequently blisters, and after resolution of the acute phase, may be a dull purple-brown colour caused by macrophage transport of melanin to the dermis. It is fixed in site and whenever the subject takes the causative drug the eruption begins within a few hours and in exactly the same site as was affected on a previous occasion. The tongue and the glans penis are common sites. In pigmented races very dark pigmentation remains between attacks. Purgatives, blood cleansers and tonics, and many other homely remedies may contain phenolphthalein, which in most countries is the commonest cause. Causative drugs are listed in Table 4.

The investigation of fixed drug eruption is a little easier than for most other drugs since it is safe to test. Many patients are not aware of the significance of many of the drugs they take as analgesics, laxatives, and tonics, and therefore a very searching history is necessary.

Management of drug eruptions

Stop all drugs likely to have caused the eruptions. Readministration of the drug is possible for most drug eruptions other than those that cause anaphylactic shock, but it is usually at a risk of considerable

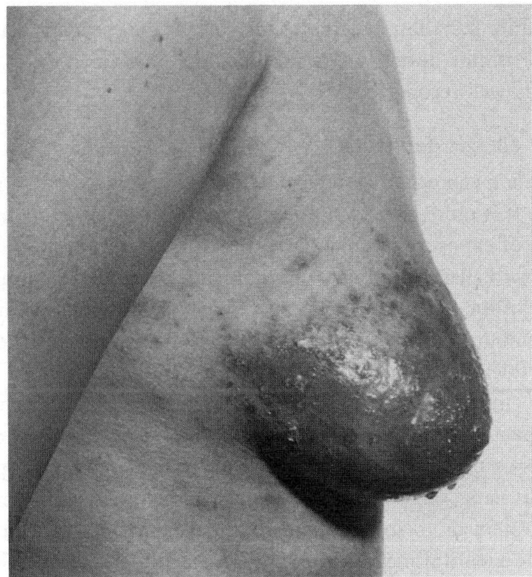

Fig. 13 Acute dermatitis is characterized by an oedematous epidermis in which vesiculation, oozing, and crusting are the principal features. The borders are often ill-defined, while the centre of the lesion is confluent.

morbidity and it should be considered only if essential to the patient. Skin tests are not helpful, as a risk of dangerous anaphylaxis, false negatives, and lack of knowledge of the antigen, makes skin testing useless. Where there is a medicament dermatitis due to contact, then patch testing is helpful. Blood tests are of no help.

Dermatitis

Definition

Dermatitis is the commonest of reaction patterns in the skin. The term is used especially for a reaction of the skin to external injury as in 'industrial' or in 'contact' dermatitis. Eczema has a similar meaning but is used more often for endogenous or constitutional dermatitis.

Clinical features

Dermatitis has both dermal and epidermal components. There are signs confined to the dermis such as swelling, heat, itchiness, tenderness, and redness, but at the same time the epidermis proliferates and therefore thickens and produces scale. The oedema in the dermis extends to the epidermis, swells the cells, and separates them giving the histological appearance of a sponge, known as spongiosis, and frequently this results in vesicles which distinguish dermatitis from other proliferative states of the epidermis such as psoriasis. Acute weeping exudation occurs when the vesicles burst (Fig. 13). In dermatitis itching is usually severe.

The reaction pattern of dermatitis is not homogeneous. It is made up of papular elements of different ages and size sometimes confluent in the centre (Fig. 14) with widely scattered satellite papules or vesicles. The scales are of varied size and broken by excoriation, exudate, and even pinpoint haemorrhages.

A secondary factor prominent in the pigmented skin is loss of melanin so that the skin is depigmented. In later or more chronic stages the dermis is darkened by 'incontinence' of pigment so that thickened chronic epidermal plaques may contain increased pigment in the underlying dermis. Chronic scratched skin has a brownish violaceous colour due to the combination of pigment, vasodilatation, and epidermal thickening.

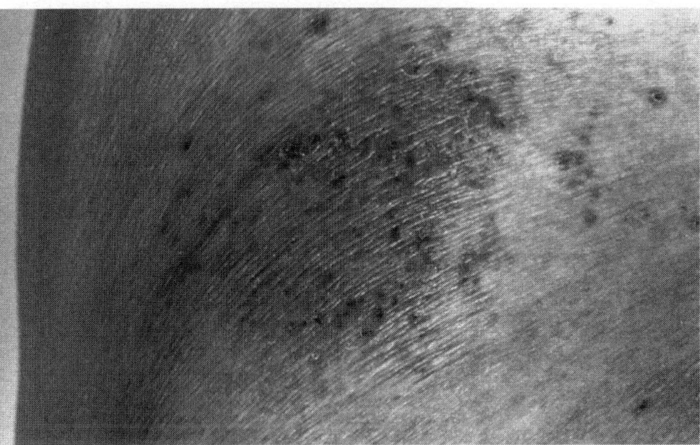

Fig. 14 Dermatitis is comprised of papules which are confluent in the centre and become vesicular or evidently excoriated. Oedema makes the line markings in the skin more prominent. There are satellite lesions beyond an ill-defined border.

For reasons unknown, dermatitis of the foot frequently provokes a response in the hand. Thus, vesicular eczema of the hands often follows a fungus infection of the feet, and varicose eczema of the lower legs often spreads to the forearms and face.

Contact dermatitis

Wear and tear or primary irritant

Contact dermatitis is one of the greatest public health problems. It particularly affects the hands. Wear and tear, known as irritant dermatitis, is the commonest cause of hand dermatitis. In other words, simple irritation from external agents accounts for by far the greatest proportion of skin disease (and less than one-fifth of such involvement is due to allergy). Indeed in industry, most outbreaks of dermatitis are not due to allergy but to the introduction of irritants into the work process or changes in the environment such as humidity or excessive drying. Industrial or occupational dermatitis are terms that indicate what may happen to the skin through its everyday exposure.

It is important to distinguish between wear and tear, taking into account different degrees of toughness or vulnerability, and allergic contact dermatitis, since their aetiology and management are different. A skin that is worn is dry and unsupple. Deep cracks occur through the normally resilient and elastic stratum corneum. Underlying epidermal cells and the dermis are no longer protected and the cracks become secondarily infected (Fig. 15).

An irritant can be defined as a chemical that in most people is capable of producing cell damage if applied for a sufficient time and in a sufficient concentration. Many persons at home or in industry are in daily contact with various chemicals over long periods. They work in wet or extremely dry conditions with skin cleaners, alkalis, acids, cutting fluids, solvents and oxidants, reducing agents, enzymes, and medicaments. The skin is also worn and irritated by cold and heat, sun, pressure, scratching, or friction of various kinds from tools or clothing. There are many variables which influence its toughness or vulnerability. It can be immature in the newborn or worn out in the aged. The most important cause of lowered resistance is constitutional disease such as the ichthyotic skin of old age (Fig. 16), atopic eczema, or psoriasis. Heredity of mainly polygenic type influences dermatitis by an effect on the constitution of the skin. There is as yet only little evidence in man of a hereditary factor in contact allergic dermatitis, neither HLA studies not twin studies

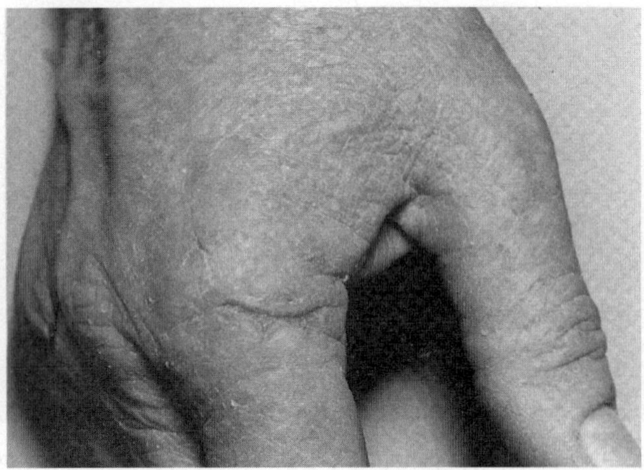

Fig. 15 Chronic dermatitis causes irregular thickening of an inhomogeneous epidermis. The texture of the stratum corneum varies so that it is firmly attached at some points but exfoliates with small scales at others. Loss of moisture causes decreased suppleness, cracking over joints, and exposure of deeper epidermal cells. This causes irritation of the dermis at the bottom of the deep crevasses.

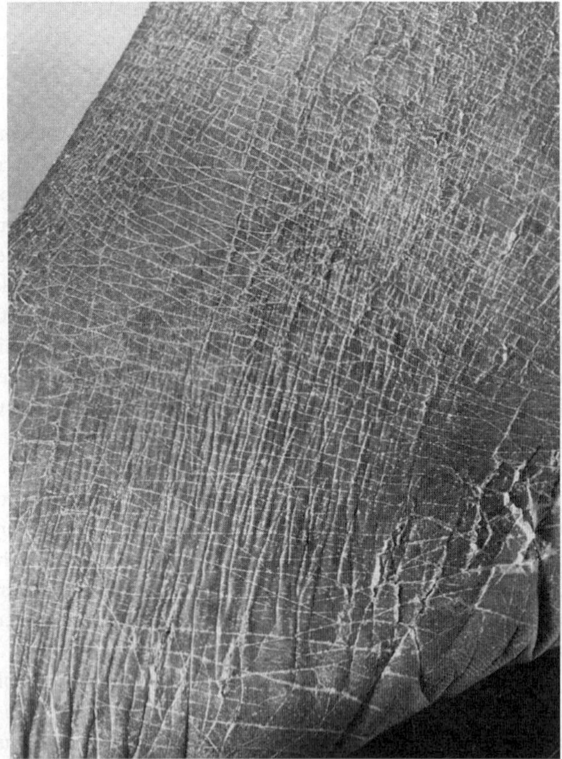

Fig. 16 Chronically thin and slowly turning-over epidermis results in a closely knit stratum corneum which is firmly adherent but cracks excessively. It is characteristic of elderly, malnourished, or ichthyotic skin. Such skin is less resistant to primary irritants.

having confirmed such a role in man as compared to animal studies.

Contact urticaria

This is an acute swelling developing within a few minutes to half an hour of contact with certain agents. In atopic eczema there is an especial susceptibility to this phenomenon but it is also well recognized in non-atopic subjects and is particularly common as a result of the application of cosmetics. Many agents commonly applied to the skin will produce irritation in certain sites, such as the eyelids or scrotum, and this is not always an immunological phenomenon. It is increasingly well recognized.

Contact allergic dermatitis

Sensitization can occur 7–10 days after the first contact with a potent allergen. It is more usually, however, a consequence of many months or years of exposure to small amounts of allergen. Once sensitized, contact with allergen can produce dermatitis within 24–48 hours and all areas of the body are equally susceptible. Sensitivity can vary due to the amount of exposure, the degree of penetration of the skin, and the tolerance of the immune system.

It is believed that certain allergens, such as nickel and chrome, have a greater affinity for the skin than others. This is in part due to the easier recognition and assimilation by the epidermal macrophages known as Langerhans cells. The allergen binds to epidermal microsomal protein or to some cell surface marker or to serum proteins which are plentiful in the epidermis. It is a complex of the allergen with such protein that is recognized as foreign. The T lymphocyte ultimately recognizes the complex but the macrophage is a necessary intermediary. Suppression of Langerhans cells by ultraviolet rays diminishes cell-mediated immunity. Genetic factors play a part in the recognition process. Once recognized, T-cell proliferation occurs in the paracortical area of the lymph node. On re-exposure sensitized lymphocytes release lymphokines. The mechanisms of lymphocyte stimulation include some role for suppressor and effector cells. The role of antibodies, some of which are clearly specific for the same antigen, is also unknown. The inflammatory reaction resulting from recognition is variable and dependent on other pharmacological agents including secretions from the mast cell and on prostaglandins. Some of the variability of response, such that persons are consequently labelled as more or less allergic, depends on these secondary factors and can be modified by various conditional factors, including anxiety and the hormonal status of the monthly menstrual cycle.

Contact dermatitis sensitizers

Causes of contact uricaria Dander, saliva, or serum of internal organs of many laboratory animals; egg white or yolk; fish and shellfish; various insects giving rise to cotton seed itch, copra itch, grocers' itch, millers' itch, etc.; caterpillars, pteropods, schistosomes; jellyfish; a glycoprotein in human seminal fluid; root vegetables, citrus fruits; nuts; spices; pollens; exotic woods; numerous common weeds; α-amylase; flour; amniotic fluid and other proteins; latex gloves.

Cosmetics Perfumes and preparations containing tars, formaldehyde, and Dowicil, vaseline dermatitis in the Bantu, deodorants, and in the hair industry, glyceryl monothioglycollate (acid perms), bleaches, ammonia persulphate.

Clothing and textile dermatitis Clips containing metal (Fig. 17), e.g. jeans buttons, rubber in elastic, dyes, azodyes or *p*-phenylenediamine, chrome, and formaldehyde. Shoe dermatitis: rubber additives (mercaptobenzothiazole or butyl phenol formaldehyde); adhesives and dyes.

Foods Animal feeds including antibiotics, plants and fruits, garlic, cinnamon, onion, and lemon or orange, shellfish, species of fish contaminated by algae.

Plastics Acrylic and epoxy polymers or resins, adhesive tape, spectacle frames, bonding agents, dentures, hearing aids, bone cement, artificial fingernails, sealants, printing plates, and inks. Epoxy resins for steel

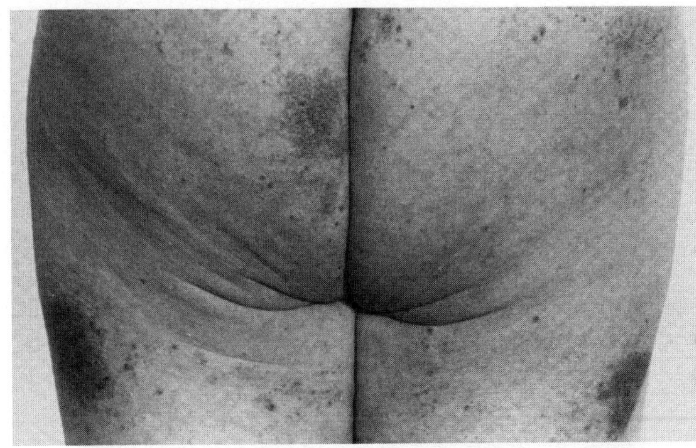

Fig. 17 Contact dermatitis due to garments containing nickel. The diagnosis is made by observing how the distribution of the rash corresponds to the distribution of the contact with the causative agent.

pipes and ships, powder paints, electrical insulation adhesives, construction of concrete and steel buildings, and for the surface of roads and bridges.

Rubber Accelerators: thiuram, mercaptobenzothiazole, and guanides; antioxidants including monobenzyl ether of hydroquinone; rubber gloves, tyres, or rubber linings; the contraceptive sheath, shoes, fingerstalls, masks, particularly in motorbike or scuba-diving pursuits, elastic bands, bicycle or golf-club handles, and rubber sheets or cushions. Anaphylaxis is recorded from type I sensitivity to rubber latex surgical gloves.

Colophony Rosin for paper size adhesives, inks, underseal cables, Elastoplast®, violin rosin, and cosmetics; medicaments (Zambuk®, Secaderm® salve, or ilonium).

Plants and wood Primula obconica, the chrysanthemum or ragweed plants, known as the Compositae or daisy family, the cashew family, such as poison ivy, poison oak, poison dogweed, elder or sumac, mango, wax, or lacquer trees; wood dermatitis; resins or lichens, liverworts, and moss, or insect parasites.

Medicaments Local anaesthetics, lanolin and cetylsteacyl alcohols, antibiotics and antiseptics, antifungal compounds, and antihistamines. Topical corticosteroids (hydrocortisone, hydrocortisone 17-butyrate, budesonide).

Metal Nickel in electroplating, enamels, and glass, ear-rings, buttons and clips, money or pots and pans.

Patch testing

The principle of patch testing is to apply to the skin the agent to which the patient may be sensitive, but avoiding irritants, and observe its effect on cell-mediated immunity. It involves:

(1) applying the agent on a carrier material such as aluminium foil over filter paper covered by adhesive tape;
(2) using a concentration in white soft paraffin in water or ethyl alcohol which is non-irritant; for most chemicals 0.1–1 per cent (in the case of cosmetics or medicaments the concentration used in the whole product is suitable);
(3) applying to the back, which is more consistent in its response than arms or legs, and removing the covering adhesive tape and filter paper 2 hours before reading; and
(4) reading at 2 and 4 days.

Treatment of contact dermatitis

Elimination of known irritants or allergens must be attempted but, as in the case of poison ivy in the US or some of the Compositae in Asia, complete avoidance may be impossible. For less severe allergens, such as chrome or nickel, the skin can settle to a tolerable degree merely by removing obvious sources in clothing or jewellery. In industry cleanliness and ventilation in working environments should be encouraged and less allergenic materials substituted. Anti-inflammatory agents, such as steroid creams, are always of help and can help the affected stay at work, particularly for short periods, such as during the training of hairdressers or nurses.

Severe chronic allergy can be relieved by immunosuppressive drugs such as azathioprine. For nickel dermatitis where life has become intolerable, chelating agents such as Antabuse®, or nickel-free diets have been used.

Atopic eczema

This is a constitutional disorder of the skin affecting 1–3 per cent of the population. It is one of the most common diseases of childhood and one of the main reasons for loss of work in industry. It accounts for about 50 per cent of hand eczema. It is inherited through several genes affecting the capacity to produce reagenic antibody reactions to the environment as well as the itch and consequent response to scratching.

Allergic respiratory disease affects about 50 per cent of eczema sufferers, and 70 per cent of patients are aware of other family members with the disease; for 90 per cent the disorder starts within the first 9 years of life. In the majority, the eczema gradually improves but the skin remains vulnerable to physical and chemical irritants throughout life.

Pathogenesis

Atopic disease is essentially imbalance in immunology with depressed Thy 1 T-cell function. Atopic dermatitis and the associated elevated IgE is associated with an *in vivo* up-regulation of the interleukin-4 (IL-4), IL-4 receptor pathway. As bacterial infections become less overwhelming, epidemiological studies incriminate urbanization, pollution, central heating, and middle class culture to explain a very much higher incidence in some European cities.

Immunology

Skin tests by pricking various antigens into the skin result in weal and flare responses that are often multiple and strongly positive. However, there is a poor correlation between the skin test response and the activity of the eczema which may be even in remission in, for example, the hayfever season in spite of strong reactivity to skin testing with grasses.

The role of food allergy is difficult to test accurately in such a fluctuating and multifactorial disease. Neither prick tests nor allergen-specific IgE tests can be used to predict those most likely to benefit from dietary elimination. Exclusive breast feeding is of benefit but not necessarily due to avoidance of factors in the diet.

Humoral immunity

IgE reagenic antibody is elevated in over 80 per cent of patients with atopic dermatitis, often to over 2000 units/ml. There is an increased frequency of the presence of specific reagin (RAST) to numerous allergens in the sera of atopics.

Reactivity of immune system

About 80 per cent of atopics have an excessive reactivity of the immune system. They react to certain foods and to house dust with immediate itching and swelling of the tissues. The agents to which

90 per cent of atopic patients react differ from those usually encountered in allergic disease. They include a number of animal and vegetable proteins from milk, meat, and corn. Eczema itself is most typically a consequence of delayed or cell-mediated immunity but in the case of the atopic skin there seems to be depression of T-cell function leading to a greater susceptibility to viral, bacterial, and fungal infections. Herpes simplex, vaccinia, warts, *Staphylococcus aureus*, and *Trichophyton rubrum* infections are most favoured; 90 per cent of atopic subjects carry *Staphylococcus aureus* in their skin, compared to 10 per cent of normal subjects.

Characteristics

The principal characteristics of atopic eczema are described below.

A low itch threshold

Indeed a diagnosis should not be made if there is no history of itching. Besides the usual causes of itching, many minor irritants, such as wool of clothing or changes in climate, cause scratching. Scratching causes excoriations and ulceration as well as thickening of the epidermis and swelling and redness of the underlying dermis. The broken surface is sore and further irritated by soaps, some ointment bases such as sorbic acid, sea-water, or citric fruit juices.

Dry and lined skin

In non-excoriated areas the skin is often dry and lined. This is more obvious in hard water areas with temperate climates. About 70 per cent of adult patients have a hand dermatitis and such hand dermatitis usually spares the palms. In adults also, nipple eczema may be a problem during breast feeding. It seems that there is a deficiency in sweating and sebum excretion which leads to chapping, wear, and tear, particularly from solvents or water. In industry, occupational dermatitis from primary irritants is commonly due to an underlying atopic eczema. Other features of atopic dryness are keratosis pilaris which is a perifollicular hyperkeratosis.

Vasodilatation

In the popliteal and cubital fossae the vasculature too readily vasodilates, heating the skin and hence inappropriately lowering the itch threshold. When scratched, rubbed, or stretched, the skin blanches for a few minutes, beginning 12–15 seconds after injury. This is in part due to upper dermal precapillary shutdown and also to persistent inflammatory oedema. Deeper vessels often dilate so that the skin is warm. This combination of hot but pale skin accounts for the itching as well as the atopic pallor.

Clinical features

Itching is the chief feature and becomes apparent during the first 2–6 months of life. The face is usually first affected and scratching begins between the second and third month. Sore lips from licking and chapping as well as conjunctivitis with ectropion are common; 70 per cent of patients have a skin fold or wrinkle just beneath the margin of the lower lid of both eyes (Fig. 18). When the child begins to crawl, the exposed surfaces such as the knees and hands become most involved. The papules are scratched and become exudative and secondary infection associated with lymphadenopathy is a common finding. Lymphadenopathy can sometimes be so gross as to lead to suspicion of some dire malignant disease. From 18 months onwards the sites most characteristically involved are the flexures of the elbows, knees, sides of neck, wrists, and ankles (Fig. 19). Local areas of lichenified skin may persist at such sites, and the face, too, may be heavily lichenified. Rubbing of the eyes is not the whole explanation of why keratoconus and anterior subcapsular cataracts are featured in severe cases. Seasonal influences on the disease are in part climatic, due to sunlight and humidity, but probably even more related are seasonal allergies. Pollen is a feature of spring and early summer, while house dust seems to be a feature of late summer.

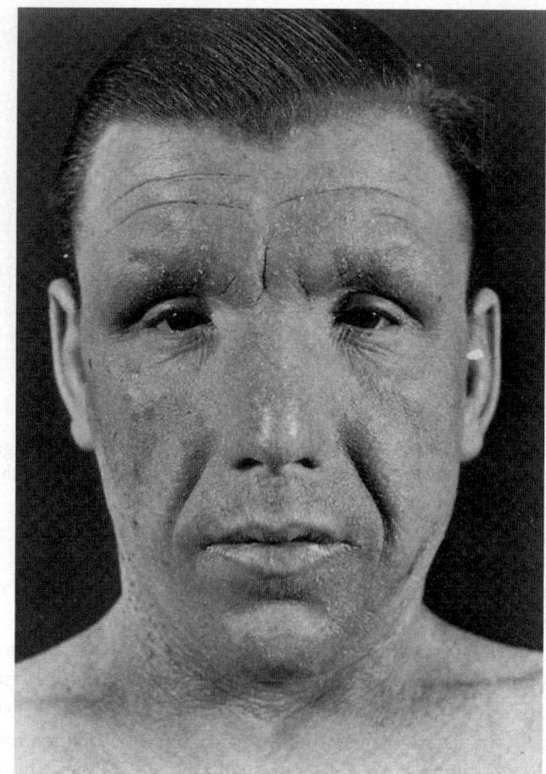

Fig. 18 Atopic eczema in an adult, showing the characteristic skin fold of the lower eyelid and the loss of eyebrow hair, as well as the thickening of the skin due to rubbing.

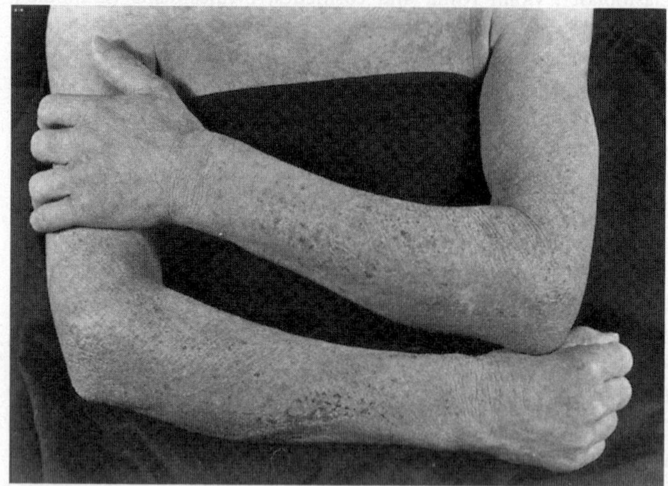

Fig. 19 Typically thickened and excoriated skin of the chronic prurigo of atopic eczema.

Associated disorders

Hayfever and asthma occur in 30–50 per cent of patients. Drug reactions of the anaphylactic type are more common and abdominal symptoms due to food allergy are frequently described. Contact urticaria is common. Alopecia areata is associated.

Prognosis

Most children develop their eczema within the first 6 months of life but about one-fifth of patients may have a delayed onset, even into adult life. There is, in general, a tendency for gradual improvement. Complete clearance without breakdown when in contact with skin irritants is unusual but most people are clear by the time they are teenagers.

Management

This is a multifactorial disease and all factors have to be managed. It is useful for parents to have access both to the doctor and nurse as well as to the literature provided by patient groups. All factors which cause irritation of the skin should be even more avoided in the atopic, and these include various primary irritants such as soap, wool, and extremes of climate. Moisturization of the skin is good but evaporation is bad. Wet wrapping is the application of wet dressings over moisturizing creams. These are then covered by dry dressings. Washing with liberal soap substitutes based on emulsifying ointments is mostly helpful and these are most effective if applied at least four times a day. The common-sense avoidance of jobs in which there is a large amount of primary irritants should be advised. Fortunately smallpox vaccination is no longer compulsory, but it is difficult to avoid the occasional contact with herpes simplex, molluscum contagiosum, and other viruses affecting the skin. If there is an immunological defect, then it remains difficult to know how to remedy this. The role of food allergy is difficult to determine in such a fluctuating and multifactorial disease. While breast feeding is to be recommended for all infants, it may be especially important for babies with a strong family history of eczema. Breast milk has a lower antigen load than cow's milk and is rich in IgA which may modify the absorption of food antigens. Breast feeding should continue for an extra 3–4 months, since any supplement exposes the immature gut to foreign protein. The mother should avoid eggs and cows' milk, since foreign protein can be transmitted through her milk. Where breast feeding is not possible, milk substitutes are second-best since they are expensive and require care to prevent bacterial contamination. Some paediatricians believe cows' milk should be avoided for 1 year and eggs for 18 months.

Some patients appear to benefit from a regime of antigen avoidance. Neither RAST tests nor skin-patch tests are reliable in selecting patients who are helped by dietary modification, since even those known to benefit from antigen avoidance may not show specifically raised IgE nor positive skin tests.

Elimination diets must be assessed carefully to obtain complete avoidance with, at the same time, adequate nutrition, and since they are not without risk in this respect, they should be reserved for the most severely affected children. Some authors recommend avoidance of egg, chicken, milk, and artificial colouring agents or preservatives. Goat's milk is not now in favour on nutritional grounds. Careful studies of the use of Chinese herbal teas have shown significant improvement in generalized dry eczema in children, but users should be aware of the potential hepatotoxicity of these drinks.

Other allergens in the environment that can be shown to be important for some children include the house-dust mite. Avoidance includes eliminating clothing and furniture that are dust collecting and the use of vacuum cleaning rather than brushing. A cold and dry environment discourages the mite.

Topical therapy

Apart from the liberal use of emollients, steroid creams are effective antipruritics (see Tables 6 and 7 later666). There has been some fluctuation in the amount they have been prescribed over the past few years. Certainly there was a period in which overprescription resulted in systemic side-effects as well as local atrophy of the skin. Withholding of steroids, on the other hand, deprives the child of the one effective therapy. Short, sharp bursts of effective therapy with strong steroids may be entirely justified, but prolonged daily usage is bound to lead to complications. Secondary infection is so common and bacterial allergy is so important that vigorous treatment of infection is justified and systemic antibiotics should be given according to the sensitivities of the bacteria from time to time. Erythromycin is especially valuable; mupirocin, topically, is as effective. The matter of climatic therapy remains unpredictable; undoubtedly a change of climate does effect great improvements in some children. It may be exposure to sunlight or to the sea or to a mountain top.

Severe cases of eczema, as with asthma, may have to be controlled by systemic steroids, either in the form of prednisolone or corticosteroid injections. This may be simply to help the patient over an acute period but a few patients may require treatment for several years. Cyclosporin controls severe eczema but there is little long-term benefit. Traditional herbal remedies are popular and carefully controlled studies have shown some benefits from Chinese medicinal plants.

Other patterns of dermatitis

Infected dermatitis

The staphylococcus is particularly responsible. This is most frequently seen as a rather well-demarcated patch of eczema with crusting and scaling on an exposed area. There may be small pustules on an advancing edge; it is seen around discharging wounds, around ulcers, and occasionally around a paronychia or in a flexure, subject to sweating and maceration; it is particularly common around the ear or at sites of occlusion such as under a hat band or between the toes. An underlying pediculosis may be one trigger. Black skin seems commonly to develop a similar condition principally affecting the shins. Management includes the use of local antiseptics and wet soaks, or dyes, such as gentian violet, combined with an appropriate systemic antibiotic.

Seborrhoeic dermatitis

This is an unsatisfactory term but it is a recognizable disease affecting mainly the flexures in the distribution of the head, neck, upper chest, axillae, and groin. The aetiology is unknown but the distribution does appear to be in the areas of sebaceous activity. Breakdown of the skin occurs spontaneously but is activated by bacterial infection and by other primary irritants. There is a strong association with neuroleptic-induced parkinsonism as well as with AIDS. *Pityrosporum orbicularis* may be the responsible pathogen. In AIDS the oval blastosphere is predominant, whereas in pityriasis versicolor, the hyphal form is increased. The most characteristic lesion is a dull or yellowish-red and greasy plaque with a marginated scale. It is most likely to involve hair-bearing areas and particularly the scalp that has considerable dandruff; it spreads on to the face and involves the nasolabial folds and eyebrows. It affects the axillae and groins with well-defined brownish-red scaly areas deep into the folds, on the front of the chest, and in the middle of the back there may be small brown follicular papules covered by greasy scales or multiple discrete patches, or rarely a widespread eruption resembling pityriasis rosea with oval lesions with peripheral scale. Severe cases of seborrhoeic dermatitis develop marked crusting and scaling, particularly of hair-bearing areas and the genitalia. Otitis externa is one manifestation. The disorder tends to recur and may be chronic.

Management includes an attack on local infection and removal of crusts with wet soaks. Preparations, such as vioform hydrocortisone, sulphur, and ichthammol in a variety of water-miscible bases, usually in 1–2 per cent concentrations, have been traditionally prescribed. Lithium succinate ointment is recently favoured. Imidazoles control Pityrosporum overproduction which is thought to play some part in the diathesis.

Nummular eczema

The main feature of this eczema is that it is discoid or composed of coin-shaped lesions scattered, often symmetrically, over the body. They are intensely vesicular and intensely itchy. They are undoubtedly endogenous, sometimes as a reaction pattern to a localized primary irritant such as an insect bite, although occasionally sensitivity to metals, such as nickel or chrome, may produce a similar picture. Secondary infection is common.

Asteatotic eczema

This is usually associated with drying out of the skin. It is particularly found in the elderly or those suffering from a minor degree of malnutrition (see Figs. 6 and 16). It is seen particularly when there is a change of habitat, as in admission to a centrally heated hospital and enforced nudity. The essential feature is the drying out and cracking of the skin over certain exposed areas, such as the backs of the hands and the fronts of the legs. It gives an appearance of crazy paving with deep fissures. It is aggravated by soaps and other irritants and by scratching. It responds very well to humidifiers and emollients as well as to a weak steroid.

Pityriasis alba

This is a pattern of eczema quite common in children, often with darker skins, in which a very low-grade dry eczema with shedding of pigment gives rise to a white patch of skin. It may be associated with drying out—reduced sebum—around the hair follicles, known as keratosis pilaris.

Pruritus

Pruritus implies that itching is the primary complaint without visible evidence of lesions predisposing to itch. Of course, itching is the most prominent symptom in skin disease and tends always to evoke scratching or rubbing (insect bites are the most common cause of pruritic skin lesions). It is subjective and for any one skin disease varies from individual to individual. It is induced by a number of agents including histamine, bradykinin, bile salts, and proteases, and is potentiated by prostaglandin E. It can be disassociated from pain in hypoalgesia. Central neurological and emotional psychiatric factors control the threshold to itch or pain. Awareness is a complex attribute modifying or intensifying the response to the itch. The itch itself may cause irritability, depression, or the attitude of the masochist who wears a 'hair shirt'. Thinly myelinated nerves in lateral spinothalamic tracts and secondary neurones to the thalamus relay both pain and itch and the cerebral cortex can modify these responses.

Itching is usually worse when the skin is heated to normal body temperature and when there is little else to distract one—a combination common at night.

The itch of different dermatoses evokes different types of scratching. Urticaria is rarely scratched but usually rubbed or pinched perhaps because the exact site of the itch is difficult to pinpoint. Where intense itching is located exactly it is often persistent and deeply excoriated.

Parasites are an important cause of pruritus but those experienced at examining the skin will usually observe primary urticarial or papular lesions in among the scratches. Onchocerciasis, trichinellosis, and schistosomiasis cause severe pruritus, usually with marked eosinophilia as well as urticaria, prurigo, and depigmentation. In onchocerciasis, loss of elasticity and the development of a leather-like skin hanging in folds is one consequence.

Causes of pruritus (without skin lesions)

A common factor is dryness and desiccation of the stratum corneum, common in the elderly and worse in winter. The threshold of itching is lowered by isolation, including the common accompaniments of ageing such as blindness, deafness, and loneliness. Paroxysmal itching may originate in the central nervous system and provoke deep scratching which is pleasurable but injurious. It is a feature of cocaine addiction.

Sweat retention also causes intense pruritus such as prickly heat. The intense pruritus of scabies with much excoriation requires a very careful search for burrows especially in well-groomed persons in the early stages of the disease. Head lice may similarly be elusive and the hair rather than the scalp is the principal hiding place; in the early stages the insect lies very close to the scalp. The classical nit is a relatively late stage. People insulating their roof with fibreglass may suffer from pruritus due to almost invisible spicules of fibreglass.

Aquagenic pruritus

This occurs after contact with water—fresh, salt, or sweat. In some it is from the moment of contact and lasts 15 minutes. In others, it is less immediate and longer lasting. Some have been helped by acetylcholine or histamine antagonists or by ultraviolet rays. In the elderly, a common similar reaction due to rapid drying out after prolonged hydration is helped by shortening the period of hydration.

Generalized pruritus and systemic disease

Hepatic disease

Obstructive jaundice causes severe pruritus especially in biliary cirrhosis. Because bile salts rather than bilirubin are responsible for the itch, the degree of jaundice need not to be great, as in the oestrogen-induced pruritus of pregnancy or from the contraceptive pill, and with chlorpromazine and testosterone.

Blood disease

Iron deficiency causes itching even when the patient is not anaemic. There is often some thinning of hair. Polycythaemia is frequently associated with itching, particularly after a hot bath. Lymphatic leukaemia and Hodgkin's disease can cause persisting pruritus before they become clinically overt.

Carcinoma of the internal organs

Carcinoma of the bronchus in particular may present with generalized pruritus.

Chronic renal failure

Itching is not a feature of acute renal failure or even of malignant hypertension, however uraemic. In chronic pyelonephritis and chronic glomerulonephritis, the patients usually suffer greatly from pruritus. Haemodialysis does not necessarily relieve it. Parathyroidectomy, for reasons that remain obscure, relieves itching in those in whom removal is necessitated by secondary hyperparathyroidism. The cause of pruritus in renal failure is unknown but dryness of the skin is one factor, and there are also increased numbers of mast cells in the skin.

Endocrine disease

Pruritus is sometimes a presenting symptom of diabetes mellitus but mostly this is localized principally to the vulva. About 1 in 10 patients with hyperthyroidism complain of itching. Dry skin in hypothyroidism often itches.

Management of pruritus

Overheating should be avoided as should vasodilators such as alcohol and hot drinks. Calamine lotion is used as a cooling agent. Evaporation is increased by the enhanced surface area provided by the powder. Dryness of the skin should be discouraged by emollients. In hospital a moist microenvironment can be enhanced by the wearing of clothes. Too frequent bathing should be discouraged unless emulsifying ointments are added to the bath as soap substitutes. Proprietary bath oils are more cosmetically acceptable but tend to be expensive for regular daily use. The treatment of the cause of the pruritus is obviously indicated where possible. Antihistamines act principally through their sedative effect and they reduce the awareness. Plasma exchange has been used to control sweats and pruritus. The anion exchange resin cholestyramine, 6–8 g daily, or oral activated charcoal helps the pruritus of liver disease and sometimes also its use in chronic renal disease or polycythaemia has been helpful. Suberythema doses of UVB irradiation twice weekly, and even natural sunlight, help pruritus somewhat unpredictably. They have been used to treat the itching of uraemia and of certain acute exanthems such as pityriasis rosea. Hydroxyethyl rutosides (Paroven®) have been advocated in renal failure. The H_2-receptor antagonist cimetidine is sometimes helpful in Hodgkin's disease; 1 per cent menthol and 1 per cent phenol have a mild anaesthetic effect and promote a sensation of cooling. Nails should be kept short and occlusive bandaging may reduce the vicious circle of itch and skin damage.

Are insects biting?

Insects cause many cases of prurigo or papular urticaria, especially in the rainy season in hot countries. Flea bites and such like are grouped and since no insect knows how to bite symmetrically, the pattern of scratched lesions can be identified as exogenous. The human flea is found on the skin only transiently and it is the patient's environment that may need to be treated often by agents which are best not applied to the skin.

Cheyletiella mites from dogs, cats, and other pets are picked up by a strip of transparent sticky tape applied to the pet's skin several times, especially where there is any mange from canine scabies. Birds' nests in the eaves may be one source. Stored cereals, fruits, and other vegetable matter sometimes contain mites as does house dust.

In scabies, most of the rash is a hypersensitive response taking about 3 weeks to develop. The characteristic burrows (Fig. 20) at the front of the wrist and between the fingers or on the areolae of the breasts are not necessarily themselves a cause of pruritus. Widespread scabies has been reported in renal transplant patients receiving azathioprine and prednisolone. Persistent cutaneous granulomas following treatment for scabies or other parasitic infections are not a sign of persistence of the live insects but may be an immune reaction to the dead parts—mouth parts and other insect antigens may cause persistent lesions for more than 3 months in about 20 per cent of patients.

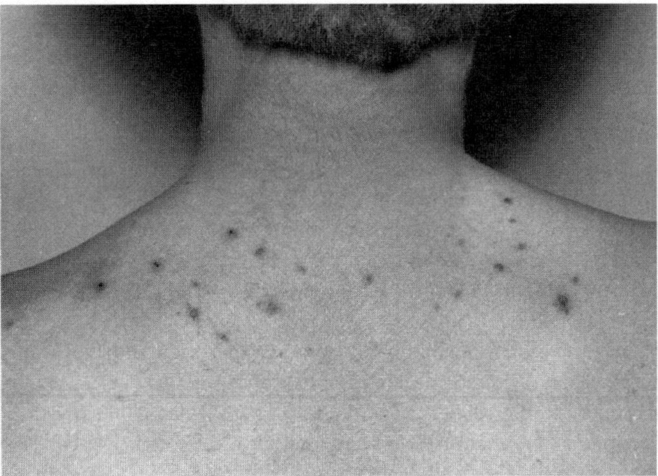

Fig. 20 The diagnostic feature of scabies. The burrow of the mite in the horny layer of the epidermis. The dark spots are the haemoglobin in the belly of the mite.

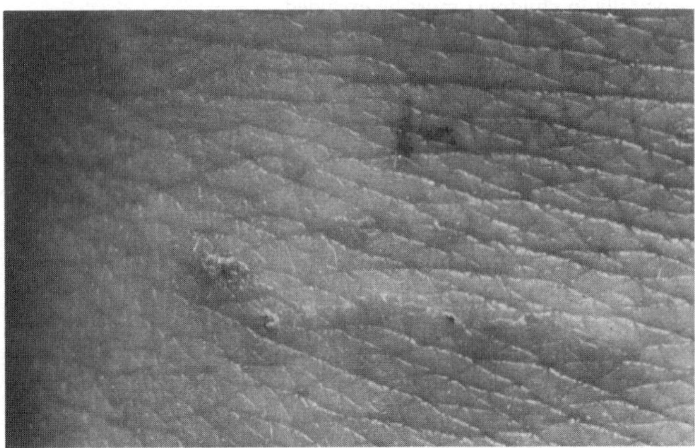

Fig. 21 Prurigo nodularis is a form of scratched lesion which is very exactly localized. The upper back is a common site for such persistent excoriation.

Irritable papules at sites of contact with insects, such as the face, lap, or arms, are a feature of infestation from lapdogs and other pets. These may simulate eczema or dermatitis herpetiformis and, being a hypersensitivity reaction rather than a bite, there are no puncta but necrotic centres may develop.

Delusions of parasitosis are best treated with antipsychotics.

Localized pruritus

Localized intensely itchy areas of skin having no obvious causation are a common problem . The nape of the neck, upper back (Fig. 21), genitalia, lower leg, elbow, and outer thigh are easily accessible sites liable to persistent rubbing and scratching. The injury to the skin results in thickening, purple-brown violaceous coloration due to dilated vessels and postinflammatory pigmentation. The normal line marks of the skin are exaggerated and excoriations are usually numerous. This is termed lichen simplex or neurodermatitis.

Nodular prurigo is an unexplained reaction to scratching, evoking severe very localized pruritus. The nodules are 1–2 cm in diameter and scattered over accessible areas. It is sometimes a consequence of atopic eczema or parasite infestation. Freezing with liquid nitrogen is helpful but in pigmented races depigmentation may result.

Local steroids are helpful and anything which protects the skin from scratching may eventually allow healing. Occlusive tape or bandaging is occasionally helpful but secondary infection is a problem, especially in hot countries. Intralesional injection with triamcinolone causes rapid resolution in some cases but this may be only temporary.

Pruritus ani and pruritus vulvae

Pruritus ani is common, from soiling of the perianal skin. Haemorrhoids, fissures, and fistulae contribute to this. Diabetes mellitus, trichomoniasis, or candidiasis are among the commonest causes of pruritus vulvae. Pruritus ani and vulvae can be part of an orogenital syndrome due to vitamin B deficiency; eczema and angular cheilitis are associated.

Sufferers use a large number of agents to relieve the pruritus, some of which cause contact dermatitis. Pruritus vulvae may be caused by sensitivity to the rubber of condoms or spermicidal jelly or even to deodorants. Local anaesthetics and local steroids are much used. The latter encourage secondary infections with fungus or yeasts; these usually spread on to the buttocks and down the thighs.

Skin diseases, such as psoriasis, seborrhoeic dermatitis, lichen planus, lichen sclerosis and atrophicus, and threadworm infection (especially in children) must be excluded.

Perianal soiling requires cleaning of the area immediately and an hour or two later. Weak local steroids often mixed with anticandida or antiseptic agents (e.g. timodine) are the mainstay of treatment.

Psoriasis

In temperate zones psoriasis affects 2 per cent of the caucasian population. It is less common in sunny climates and in pigmented skins. The mode of inheritance is debated, but there is evidence of dominant and polygenic patterns.

Pathogenesis

There is a tenfold increase in epidermal cell proliferation. The cells pass upwards through the epidermis at a faster rate and seem not to have time to produce a horny layer. The cells remain nucleated even when exfoliated. The increased turnover is triggered by neutrophils, which are attracted in large numbers into the epidermis. Streptococcal antigens are cross-reactive with skin antigens and stimulate an autoimmune response. A role for lymphocytes is supported by the exacerbation of psoriasis in AIDS, its control by cyclosporin, and the possible immunosuppressive effects of other effective therapies, such as corticosteroids or PUVA. Psoriasis in AIDS is most pronounced at intermediate levels of immunodeficiency, and is diminished or lost in terminal profound immunodeficiency.

Koebner phenomenon

The Koebner phenomenon is a term given to psoriasis developing in traumatized skin.

Clinical appearance

Psoriasis can affect all age groups but has a peak age of onset in the young adult. The commonest lesion is a sharply marginated plaque with silvery scales (Fig. 22). These mask the underlying redness from tortuous convoluted capillaries which lie close to the surface of the skin. The edges of the lesion are usually the most active and there is commonly clearing in the centre (Fig. 23).

Sites most commonly affected are the elbows, knees, and scalp which normally have a higher rate of epidermal turnover. The face is less often affected. Spontaneous fluctuations are common and remissions occur in about one-third of cases per annum. There are several well-recognized patterns and it is important to examine the patient thoroughly until a completely recognizable lesion of psoriasis can be detected.

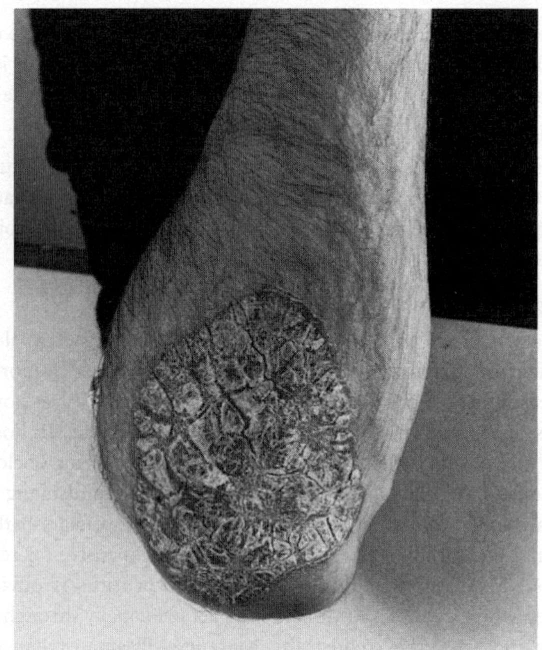

Fig. 22 A plaque of psoriasis, showing the silvery scales, well-defined border, and predilection for the elbow.

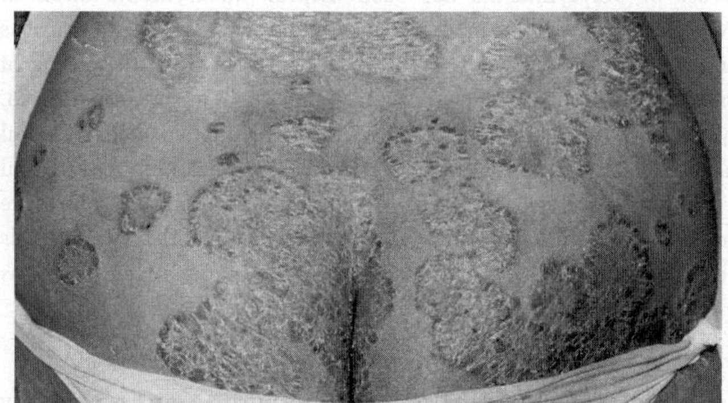

Fig. 23 Psoriasis that is less stable than in Fig. 22. The lesions are erupting and more active at the periphery while healing in the centre.

Guttate psoriasis

This term is derived from gutta meaning a drop. The skin looks as though it has been splashed by the psoriasis. It often follows a streptococcal sore throat or vaccination and is especially common in children. The lesions are scattered over the entire body and tend to be no more than a few millimetres in diameter. They may include the face and are often red slightly scaly spots. They appear less well defined and less obviously covered by silvery scales than in classic types of psoriasis. In the absence of a family history the prognosis tends to be good.

Nummular discoid

This is probably the commonest form of psoriasis and coin-shaped lesions of various sizes (Fig. 24) are scattered over the body in a completely symmetrical distribution. Such lesions are usually well defined and chronic.

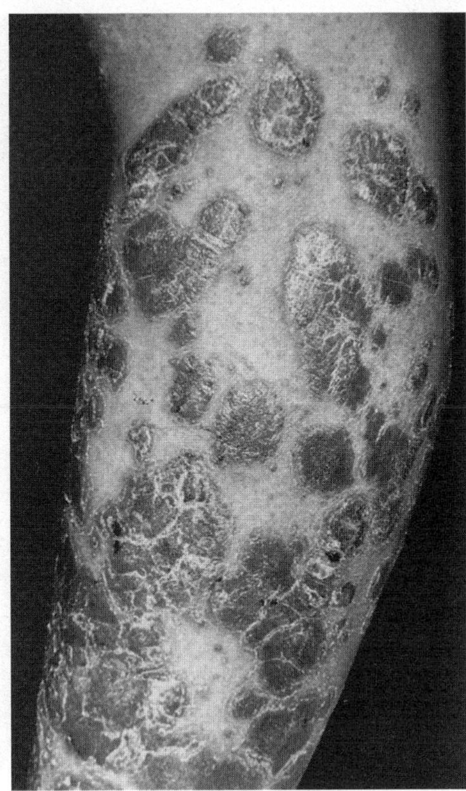

Fig. 24 Discoid lesions still well defined but almost becoming confluent.

Palmar and plantar psoriasis

This may be typical of lesions elsewhere but there is often a modification of the psoriasis due to the nature of the palmar and plantar skin. The scales tend to be more adherent and less silvery and they are more likely to develop deep cracks because of the thickness of the epidermis at these sites. Neutrophils tend to collect into larger abscesses trapped by the thicker surface layers of the stratum corneum. The sterile pustules so formed are often the most obvious feature. This pattern may be seen as part of a more generalized disease but in many cases it affects only the hands and feet. There is some evidence that it is a different disease without the above mentioned HLA associations and without obvious increase in the rate of epidermal turnover. It is an occasional and acute response to infection and is then known as pustular bacterid.

Psoriasis of the nails

Pinpoint pitting is usual but can be seen in other disorders affecting nail growth. Onycholysis with a salmon-pink discoloration of the base of the uplift of the nail is probably even more characteristic. Sometimes the nail growth is distorted, thickened and friable, and difficult to distinguish from a fungus disorder affecting the nail.

Flexural psoriasis

When psoriasis affects the groins, natal cleft, or axillae, it is usually less scaly. The bright red plaques are shiny and liable to cracking and maceration. They may be very well defined.

Erythroderma (Plate 10)

This may present as a medical emergency due to fluid loss, septicaemia, or loss of body temperature. The elderly may develop high-output cardiac failure. Oedema is a consequence of capillary leak, low albumin, and heart failure. When psoriasis affects the entire skin there is generalized redness, the well-defined margins are lost and the scales are exfoliated profusely. The erythroderma may be indistinguishable from that found in eczema or lymphoma. When the normal protective function of the skin is lost, bacteraemia is common. The loss of water is difficult to estimate and prerenal failure can develop very rapidly. The vasodilatation and the obstruction to the sweat ducts by the proliferating epidermis results in impaired thermoregulation. Hyperthermia is very common in hot climates; hypothermia can occur in cold climates. Internal organs such as the gut and liver may be impaired and loss of protein both from the skin and the gut is an important complication.

Generalized pustular psoriasis

In this condition, which is relatively rare, waves of bright erythema develop within a few hours with a fever, arthropathy, and leucocytosis. Myriads of pustules quickly develop and equally quickly disappear. This disorder may occur in the absence of a previous history of psoriasis and even occasionally as a viral exanthem. However, most commonly it is only a complication of psoriasis that has been treated by systemic or local steroids. It is an acute rebound phenomenon of steroid withdrawal. A rare cause is hypoparathyroidism.

Arthropathic psoriasis

See Section 10.

Management

The aim is to depress epidermal cell turnover without irreversibly damaging the skin or other organs.

Local steroids

Steroid creams and ointments are the first line of treatment because they are so easy to use. A few plaques of psoriasis on the elbows, knees, or scalp may be treated by daily application, and in about one-third of patients the lesions are controlled within 1–2 weeks and remain under control even when the application ceases. The stronger fluorinated steroids or betamethasone valerate are the most effective. One-third of patients need to continue once or twice weekly application and another third show no improvement even with twice daily application. In all those in whom these stronger steroids have to be continued, complications gradually develop including skin atrophy and gradual extension of the psoriasis.

Tar

Tar is effective and safe but its smell, colour, and stain make it cosmetically unsatisfactory.

Dithranol

Dithranol is more effective than coal tar especially if the plaques are large, well-defined, and few in number. It is more irritant, but can be diluted and then the concentration gradually increased. The dithranol is mixed in zinc oxide and salicylic acid paste (Lassar's paste) in concentrations of 0.1, 0.25, 0.5, 1, or 2 per cent.

Other agents

Calcipotriol, a vitamin D analogue, is a safe and cosmetically acceptable, effective topical treatment, inhibiting proliferation and enhancing epidermal differentiation. It is applied twice daily at a rate of not more than 100 g/week. It is irritant for about 10 per cent of users. Fish-oil supplements (eicosapentanoic acid capsules for 10 weeks) are helpful for itching.

Phototherapy

Natural sunlight is helpful in about 75 per cent of patients and probably accounts for a decreased incidence of psoriasis in sunny climates. UVB is a useful substitute. Its effectiveness can be increased by prior bathing in, or an application of, tar which sensitizes the skin to the UVB.

PUVA therapy was introduced for psoriasis 10 years ago. The combination of long-wave ultraviolet rays (UVA or black light) with eight methoxypsoralen tablets 0.5 mg/kg taken 2 hours before exposure produces effective clearance and a bronze skin in most patients. Recurrences are no less frequent than with other forms of therapy. Dryness, atrophy, and other expected changes of irradiation are a consequence. The risk of skin cancer is as yet difficult to estimate but it is not insignificant.

Systemic therapy

ACTH or prednisolone provide short-term control but are best avoided because psoriasis may rebound when they are withdrawn, and side-effects, including irreversible vertebral osteoporosis, are common. It may be life-saving in generalized erythroderma or pustular psoriasis in the elderly. Methotrexate is the most favoured antimitotic or immunosuppressive agent. Carefully monitored and given intermittently, the serious side-effects of liver fibrosis are slow to develop and may be justified in the older patient. Marrow suppression is rarely a problem.

Retinoic acid is helpful in some more difficult cases and is the treatment of choice in generalized and pustular psoriasis. It is relatively free of serious side-effects but the effective dose is often a cause of annoying dry mouth, sore lips, and conjunctivitis, as well as skin irritation and erosions, and the high levels of blood lipids induced by the drug are potentially a long-term hazard. It is teratogenic; contraception must be guaranteed for at least 2 years after discontinuing the drug. Hyperostosis is another long-term side-effect.

Cyclosporin is a highly effective treatment of severe psoriasis. The principal side-effects are hypertension and nephrotoxicity. The dose should not exceed 5 mg/kg if these side-effects are to be controlled.

Other keratodermas

Pityriasis rubra pilaris, ichthyosis hystrix, and erythrokeratoderma are probably inherited, occasionally as a dominant gene but more often as a recessive. Involvement of the face is more characteristic than is the case in psoriasis (Fig. 25). The palms and soles often have a thickened yellow appearance. Nails are less often pitted and quite often show subungual keratosis. A follicular prominence is characterisitc of pityriasis rubra pilaris (Fig. 26); the extensor surfaces are favoured and so the knees and elbows are often involved, as in psoriasis. The management of these conditions is difficult and, in the case of the erythrokeratodermas, retinoic acid has become the treatment of choice. This is taken by mouth but side-effects of dry mouth and eyes and some soreness of the skin may be sufficiently annoying for the patient to opt for living with his or her disease.

Pityriasis rosea

The natural history and clustering of cases suggests that it is an infectious disease. It tends to occur in spring and autumn and in any one individual does not recur. Recurrent or prolonged eruptions of similar nature may be a variant of seborrhoeic eczema. The initial lesion or herald patch is usually on the trunk or proximally on the limbs. It is well-defined, oval, erythematous, and scaly. It precedes the generalized eruption by 3–10 days. The rash of pityrisasis rosea is characterized by oval lesions orientated in the line markings of the skin of the trunk. The lesions develop a collarette of scales after 1 week. The rash may spread upwards to the neck and down the arms and legs, usually fading as it reaches below the elbows and knees. It lasts 3–6 weeks. Pruritus may be intense. Slight lymphadenopathy and fever rarely accompany the developing rash.

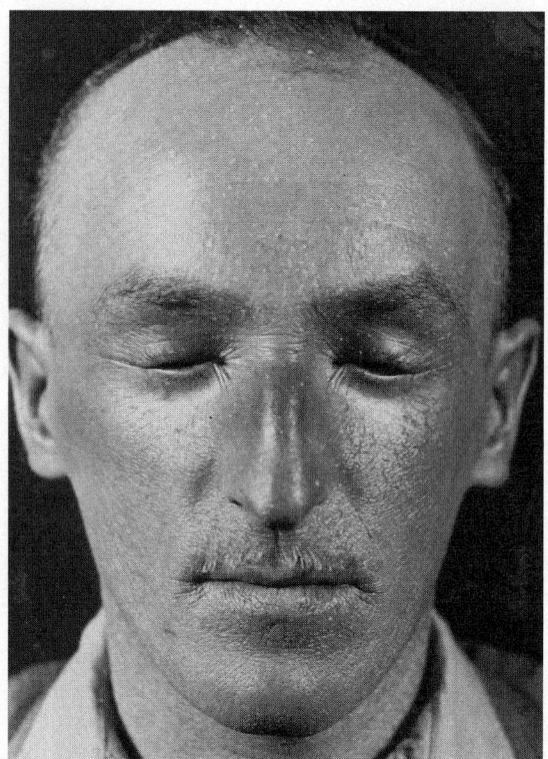

Fig. 25 Pityriasis rubra pilaris, a disorder showing some similarities to psoriasis but differing in its predilection for the face. There is some shrinkage of tissues around the eyes so that ectropion and incomplete closure of the eyelids has developed. This is also a characteristic of the disorder.

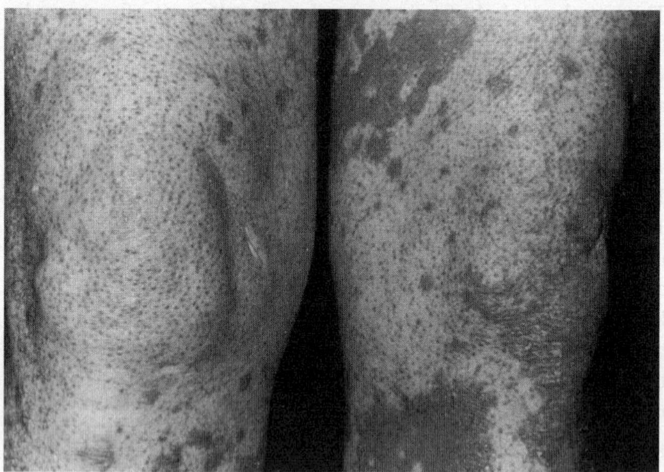

Fig. 26 Pityriasis rubra pilaris is primarily a disorder of the follicular epithelium.

Lichen planus and lichenoid eruptions

Lichen planus and lichenoid eruptions are characterized by violaceous papules which are usually flat-topped and shiny and heal leaving pigmentation. The histology includes damage to the basal layer of the epidermis and an intense infiltration of lymphocytes and a few histiocytes situates immediately below the epidermis (Fig. 27). A T-cell-mediated LD4+ attack on the epidermis may be triggered by

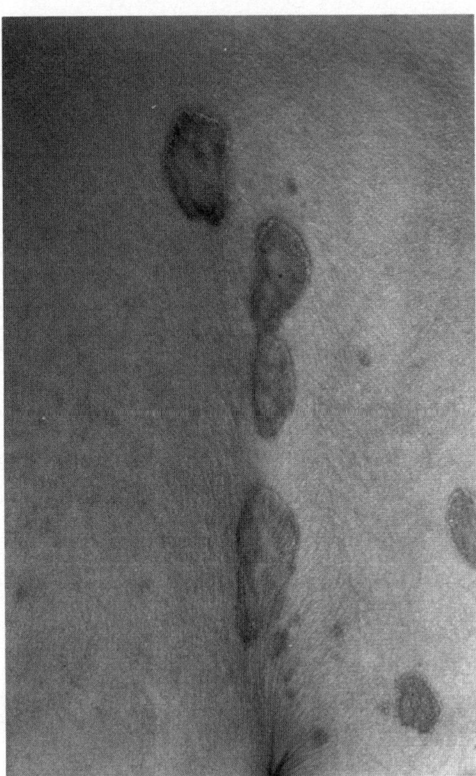

Fig. 27 Lichen planus may heal in the centre, leaving atrophy and pigmentation. The edge is slightly raised; this gives rise to the annular form of the condition.

viral, drug, or neoplastic processes. Lichen planus thus presents a model for the elimination of damaged and normal keratinocytes. Cytokines, γ-interferon, and tumour necrosis factor-β play a critical role. Lymphocytes and keratinocyte molecules subserving adhesion are activated and, in the mouse, lichen planus can be blocked by monoclonal antibodies. The disturbances in the growth of the epidermis that result from this damage range from extreme atrophy with ulceration and almost no epidermal cell turnover to considerable hypertrophy and hyperkeratinization, giving rise to thick nodules meriting the name hypertrophic lichen planus. Most cases are seen between the ages of 30 and 60 and it is extremely rare in children. More erosive forms are seen in the elderly, and pigmented skin tends to develop more hypertrophic varieties.

Clinical features

The classical lesion is a shiny, violaceous flat-topped papule (Plate 11). Small white dots or lines in such papules are termed Wickham's striae. The papules may become confluent and heal in the centre, giving rise to annular (Fig. 27) lesions or plaques. This may result in either atrophic skin or extreme hypertrophy. In lesions of mouth or of the glans penis a lacy-white appearance (Fig. 28) is common. Lichen planus is one cause of scarring alopecia. Healing of the lesion is often followed by pigmentation. Warty hyperkeratotic lesions may be very persistent, as may ulceration, particularly of the peripheries or of the mucosa of the mouth. The initial lesions are commonly on the front of the wrists, in the lumbar region, or around the ankles. Involvement of the nails produces longitudinal linear depressions.

Prognosis

The mean age of onset is the fifth decade. It may be very explosive or insidious. Most cases clear slowly but two-thirds take up to a year so to do; 85 per cent of clearance is in 18 months. Mucuous membrane lesions or extremely hypertrophic lesions on the legs often persist for years, and there is risk of squamous epitheliomatous changes, particularly in ulcerated mucosal lesions.

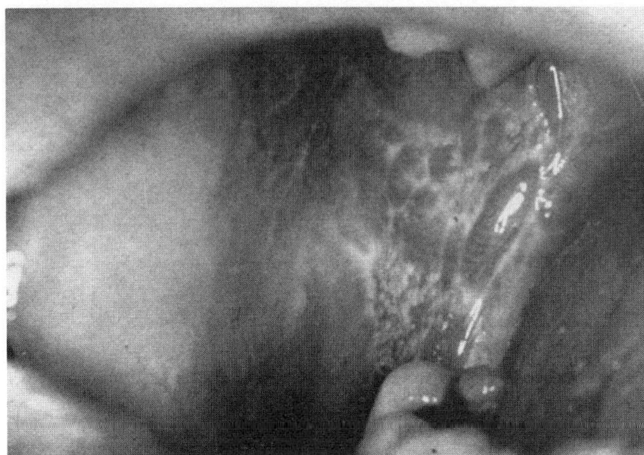

Fig. 28 Lichen planus of the mouth is one cause of mucosal whiteness. Unlike candidiasis the lesions cannot be removed by scraping. They are characteristically 'lacy' in appearance.

Treatment

Treatment is mainly aimed at the relief of the itching, and local steroid creams are perhaps the most effective. Occasionally, for a very severe widespread lichen planus, a course of prednisolone is justified. Probably it does not influence the course of the disease but merely its intensity. As with all itching conditions of the skin, cooling evaporating lotions such as calamine lotion may be helpful. In the mouth local steroid creams, particularly those manufactured for the mouth containing orabase, can be prescribed. A spray such as that used in asthma may be a more convenient way of administering steroid to the mucosa of the mouth, emphasizing that its use is without inhalation.

Acne vulgaris

Acne vulgaris is the most common disease of the skin affecting teenagers and consequently affecting those who are most conscious of their body image. It is a disorder of the pilosebaceous follicles which are most numerous on the face and upper trunk.

Aetiology

There are three main processes contributing to acne:

(1) increased sebum excretion;

(2) pilosebaceous duct obstruction; and

(3) inflammation.

Under the influence of local metabolism of sex hormones, androgens stimulate an increase in the size of the sebaceous glands and hence, more sebum. These large glands themselves produce more androgen metabolites through the activity of 5-α-reductase. One effect of these metabolites is a partnership with resistant bacteria to produce keratinization and hence blockage of the pilosebaceous duct. The organisms responsible are *Propionibacterium acnes*, *Staphylococcus epidermidis*, and *Pityrosporum ovale*. Acne may also be drug-induced, particularly secondary to steroids, iodides, lithium, phenytoin, streptomycin, and isoniazid.

Sebaceous gland activity is regulated by hormones and, in particular, by androgens from the testes and adrenals, which stimulate, and

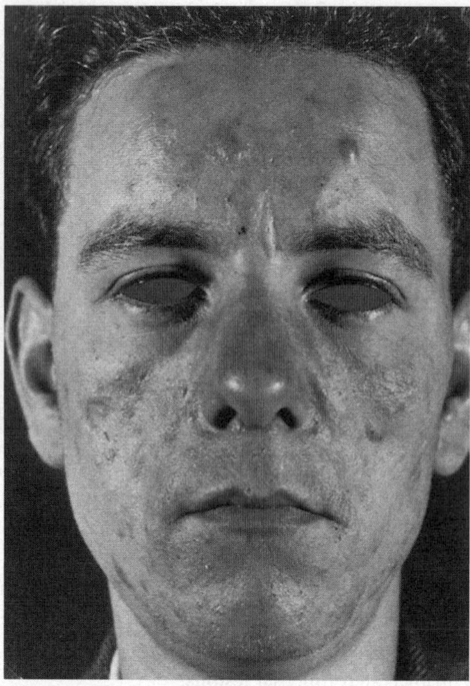

Fig. 29 Greasiness of the skin is a common accompaniment of acne, as is comedo formation, or 'blackheads', as seen on the forehead of this young man. Whether either are wholly responsible for the consequent inflammation and scarring also seen in this photograph is debatable.

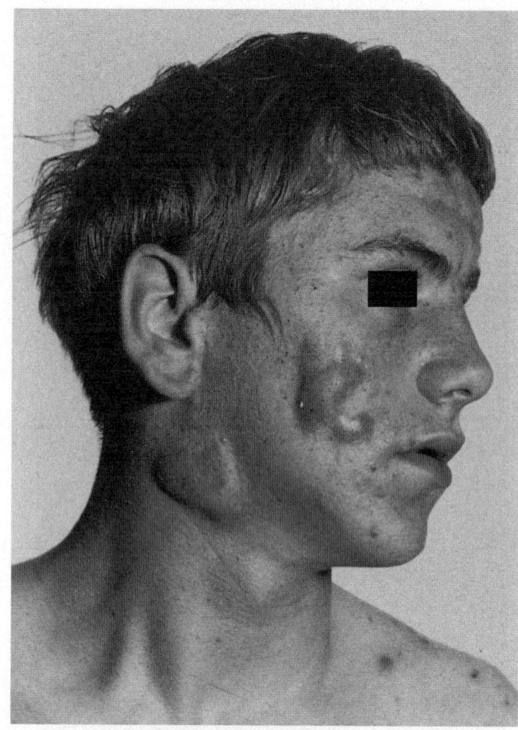

Fig. 30 Large cystic lesions are the most disfiguring aspect of acne vulgaris.

oestrogens, which seem to suppress activity. In the adult male the glands are normally maximally stimulated and acne is more severe in boys than in girls. The skin itself is a major site for androgenic conversion similar to that observed in the prostate gland and in the male genitalia. Dihydrotestosterone rather than testosterone may be the end-organ effector and it is formed within the target cells where it stimulates lipogenesis as well as mitosis. Eunuchs do not develop acne. Oestrogens reduce the size of sebaceous glands and sebum production is diminished.

Clinical features

The closed comedo is the first stage of acne and appears as tiny white nodules below the surface seen especially when the skin is stretched. These may rupture giving rise to irritation of the dermis, i.e. inflamed papules, or form the open comedo or blackhead by pushing open the mouth of the follicle (Fig. 29). The black material is melanin; blackheads are blacker in dark skins and white in the albino; the melanin is transferred to the keratinocytes before they are shed into the sebaceous follicle. Acne cysts (Fig. 30) occur as the result of ballooning of the distended follicle, and often the walls of the cyst and hair and sebaceous apparatus are destroyed. Adjacent cysts often form fistulae and sinuses, which rupture, displacing epithelium in the dermis, forming irregular channels or foreign-body reactions.

Atrophic or hypertrophic scars of all types may be seen, and often excoriations, picking, and squeezing contribute to the irregularities of pigment and to the epidermal or dermal thickening. Rarely, young males develop suppurative and highly inflamed lesions in the skin over the chest with pain, fever, and accompanying polyarthralgia, probably mediated by immune mechanisms and the activation of complement.

Acne usually presents before the menarche and clears after a few years. A more persistent form—particularly affecting the chin—may be seen in persons up to middle age, especially in women who have premenstrual exacerbations. Most women with adult acne also have the polycystic ovary syndrome.

Acne is induced by iodides and bromides, steroids, androgens, barbiturates, phenytoin, and phenothiazines.

Cosmetics

In many parts of the world cosmetics contribute to acne and the lesions may be confined to the site of application. Vaseline-type preparations or medicated oil in shampoos in young women with long hair, are a well-known cause.

Management

Local preparations All local preparations produce some erythema and occasional pustulation before the acne comes under control. Sulphur is a time-honoured agent, producing local irritation and causing peeling. It is helpful for pustules and may not be so good for comedones which precede pustulation, often by several months. Comedones are reduced by retinoic acid and by 10 per cent salicylic acid in ethanol. Sunlight is a popular therapy and it is undoubtedly helpful for some patients. The tanning effect may be a purely cosmetic form of camouflage. However, there is clinical and experimental evidence that in some patients comedones are increased in number after exposure to sunlight.

Long-acting oxidizing antiseptics such as benzoyl peroxide reduce sebum excretion, reduce comedo production, and inhibit *P. acnes in vitro*. They are the topical treatment of choice, are a mild irritant, and produce peeling after several days' application. It is best to start sparingly with 5 per cent and later to increase the amount applied or the concentration to 10 per cent.

Retinoic acid helps the lining cells of the follicle to slough off without plugging the follicle. It is applied in a cream or a lotion or gel, and is indicated for comedones rather than for pustules or cysts. It is irritant and causes redness and peeling. Its effect is not unlike sunburn and should not be used when there is undue sun exposure, either in the summer bather or the winter skier.

Oral therapy

Oral tetracycline is the mainstay of treatment of acne if simple measures have not resulted in clearance. Erythromycin and clindamycin (now usually prescribed as a lotion) are also effective but tetracycline is exceptionally safe. The only side-effect is the discoloration of teeth in the fetus and in children. Anorexia nausea, colic, or vaginal candidiasis are rare. Provided they are taken on an empty stomach, one or two tetracycline tablets taken daily control acne. Rarely Gram-negative folliculitis occurs, particularly around the nose or in persistent cysts. This results in sudden worsening with considerable inflammation and may warrant a course of ampicillin. Severe inflammatory and cystic acne respond to a zinc sulphate citrate complex taken with meals. Acute severe inflammatory disease also responds to prednisolone.

Oestrogen

Oestrogens have to be given in excessive amounts (50 mg or more of ethinyl oestradiol per day in women or 50 mg/day in the male) to have an effect in acne.

Acne is made worse by 19-nor-testosterone derivatives in the contraceptive pill. Cyproterone 17 acetate up to 100 mg for the first 10 days of the cycle plus ethinyl oestradiol 50 mg for 21 days, is used to block the receptor sites for dihydrotestosterone. This antiandrogen effect works only if the drug is given systemically and no topical preparation has proved effective. Small doses of prednisolone suppress androgen activity.

13-*cis*-Retinoic acid up to 1 mg/kg is the most effective treatment of acne. However, vitamin A-type toxicity is usual, including dryness and peeling of the lips and conjunctivae; raised blood lipids, muscle aches, and pains may also occur. The most serious problem is teratogenicity. The drug is incompletely metabolized and can be damaging to the fetus for many months after discontinuing its intake and so contraception is essential for female patients. The Diane® contraceptive pill, which contains 50 mg ethinyl oestradiol with only 2 mg cyproterone acetate, is partially effective if taken for many months. In resistant cases additional cyproterone acetate taken on days 5–14 of the menstrual cycle will improve the effectiveness. Combinations with oxytetracycline show advantages but contraception is less secure. In pregnancy acne can occasionally be severe. The treatment of choice is erythromycin.

Pigmentation

The principal pigments in the skin include melanin, which is black, phaeomelanin, which is reddish-yellow, haemoglobin and its by-products bilirubin, biliverdin, and haemosiderin which produce colours of yellow, green, red, and brown. Longer wavelengths such as red penetrate deeper and are absorbed by melanin. Since blue does not penetrate so deeply it is not absorbed and is reflected back and therefore dermal pigment appears blue—hence blue naevus. Immediate darkening may occur within minutes of the skin being exposed to sunlight. Over a number of days increased pigment production is associated with epidermal thickening and retention of pigment.

Some pigmented lesions are naevi, others result from 'incontinence' of pigment which increases the amount of pigment in the dermal macrophages and is commonly post-inflammatory.

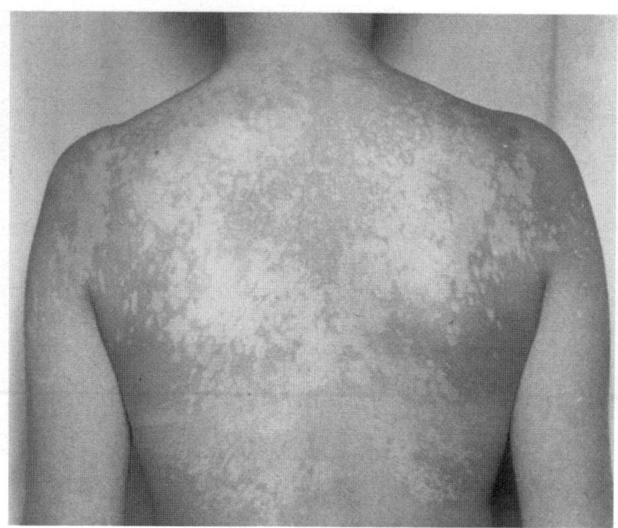

Fig. 31 Pityriasis versicolor due to the organism *Malassezia furfur* causes redness and slight brownish coloration of very pale, white skin. In dark or sallow skin it causes depigmentation. It favours the upper trunk.

Pigmentation as a feature of systemic illness especially endocrine dysfunction affecting the melanocyte stimulating hormone. Where malnutrition and infections are common, protein and vitamin deficiency, as well as cachexia from a variety of causes, account for disturbances in the colour of the skin.

'Tinea' or pityriasis versicolor is due to a superficial fungus known as *Malassezia furfur*. It usually affects the upper trunk and may spread on to the neck or on to the arms. The lesions are slightly scaly, off-white, pink, and brown. Pityriasis is the term for a bran-like powdery scale and versicolor implies the variation in the colouring (Fig. 31).

In leprosy, hypomelanosis is a feature of tuberculoid and borderline tuberculoid types (see Section 16). Light touch and later pinprick sensation are impaired. There is often lack of sweating and there may be loss of hair. An adjacent enlarged peripheral nerve may be palpable, and this may be mistaken for an enlarged lymph node.

Depigmentation

Leucoderma is a term used for any whiteness of skin, and ranges from a mild hypopigmentation to complete loss of pigment as in vitiligo. Pityriasis versicolor (Fig. 31), leprosy (see Plate 13), and syphilis are important infectious causes of depigmentation. Pinta should be suspected in people from central or southern America. The late stage resembles vitiligo. Naevus anaemicus is a hypovascularity of the skin observed in white skins. It is not a disorder of melaninization.

Vitiligo

The melanocytes are destroyed and the affected skin is totally depigmented. In many parts of the world where skins are deeply pigmented, it is a principal cause of attendances at a dermatology department. It affects up to 1 per cent of the UK population but 8.8 per cent in India. It presents during the first decade in 25 per cent of those affected. Except in those people unable to protect themselves from bright sunlight, the disability is purely cosmetic, but causes more concern and social handicap than almost any other common disease. However, an association with other autoimmune diseases and a family history is found in one-third of cases. The cause is unknown and the melanocyte seems to be damaged by some as yet unidentified antibody or toxin. There is a 20–30 per cent incidence of vitiligo in those who develop melanoma.

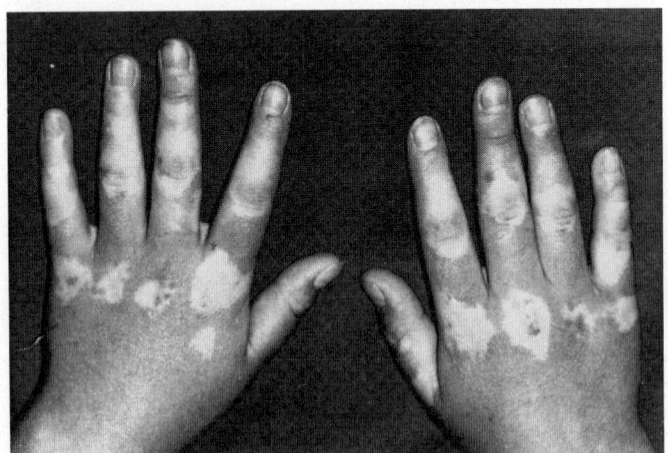

Fig. 32 Vitiligo is complete depigmentation and not merely hypopigmentation; it often begins at sites of minor trauma such as the knuckles. As with all essentially endogenous disorders it is symmetrical.

Clinical features The initial depigmentation is often at sites of trauma, particularly of the knuckles of the hands and sometimes around a naevus (Fig. 32). The face and neck are usually affected early. In white-skinned people the first complaint is often in the summer when the unaffected skin is at its darkest from sun exposure. There is usually marked symmetry; the axillary folds and genitalia are commonly affected; the eye is not involved. The depigmentation of the lesion is ultimately total and should cause no confusion with the hypopigmentation of diseases such as leprosy. Only in the earlier stages of vitiligo is there hypopigmentation but such areas are never anaesthetic as in leprosy. Pigment may accumulate and be well defined at the borders of the lesion, giving a hyperpigmented edge. Melanocytes of hair follicles are usually unaffected and repigmentation, when it occurs, is often from such sites.

The clinician should be aware of the associations with diabetes mellitus, pernicious anaemia, Addison's disease, myxoedema, or thyrotoxicosis. Less than one-third of patients show spontaneous repigmentation. In most, the loss of pigment gradually extends. Depigmentation of the vulva, penis, and neck is sometimes persistent and of a localized variety, and need not necessarily progress to generalized vitiligo and should be distinguished from the more atrophic lichen sclerosis of those sites.

Management Offering advice on camouflage with matching of the skin using appropriate mixtures gives the patients an opportunity to help themselves, especially on important social occasions. Dihydroxyacetone is the basis of many suntan lotions, but again it is difficult to apply satisfactorily without overpigmenting the adjacent unaffected skin.

Patients should be told to avoid occupations which injure the skin. For those whose skin is almost completely depigmented the cosmetic effect of removing the remaining pigment is sometimes preferred.

Psoralens, methoxy- or tripsoralen, are taken by mouth 2 hours before exposure to light or may be applied topically 30 minutes before exposure. The simplest regimen is a combination of meladinin paint and sunlight. It is necessary to test reactivity with short-time exposure and always to expose the skin at the same time of the day in order not to burn the skin by unexpectedly high intensity of UVA. The chances of remission are not much greater than those from natural responses and treatment successes may take 2–3 years to accomplish.

As might be expected from an autoimmune disorder, local steroid preparations are sometimes helpful. They have been advocated in combination with psoralens but therapeutic triumphs are difficult to assess, and the requirement to use these agents for years rather than days makes side-effects very likely. Local steroids are sometimes used to stabilize a rapidly progressive early stage of the disease.

Other forms of depigmentation (postinflammatory)

Albinism

This is a group of at least six genetically distinct syndromes determined not by absence of melanocytes but by their inability to synthesize melanin. There are a number of associated defects affecting vision, hearing, and the delivery of lysosomes.

Halo naevi

These are characterized by loss of pigment around benign or very rarely malignant melanocytic naevi. They are a common first sign of vitiligo. Antibodies against the cytoplasm of malignant melanoma cells are found in the serum of patients with halo naevi. The naevus need only be removed if there is a progressive enlargement, bleeding, and irregularities of the pigment within the centre of the naevus.

Post-inflammatory depigmentation

This is probably the commonest cause of leucoderma. The lesions are not as white as in vitiligo and they are sometimes known as pityriasis alba. It is in fact a variant of a dry eczema and causes mild hypopigmentation. It may be sharply circumscribed and have a halo of surrounding inflammation. It is usually slightly scaly and there is follicular prominence due to hyperkeratosis. The cheeks and upper arms are most commonly affected and atopic children are the most frequent sufferers.

In some parts of the world discoid lupus erythematosus is a common cause of depigmentation. It is preceded by the itching, deep violet erythema of light-exposed skin. Hair loss of the scalp is common. This is usually of scarring type.

Nails

Nails grow continuously throughout life. Normal fingernails grow at the rate of approximately 1 cm in 3 months but toenails take anything from 9–24 months to grow as much. The nails grow more rapidly in psoriasis and more slowly in cold, ischaemia, or severe systemic illness.

Koilonychia is a term for a spoon-shaped depression of the nail plate, sometimes brittle, found in iron deficiency or in overusage of solvents such as nail varnish remover or detergents. It is also a consequence of repetitive trauma such as vibration, or in the case of toenails, from kicking or walking up a hill pushing a trolley, known as rickshaw boy's nail.

Onycholysis is due to premature separation of the nail plate as seen in psoriasis, infection, thyroid disease, and UVA exposure. Trauma from excessive handwashing or keratolytics are other causes.

Clubbing is an increased angle between the nail fold and nail plate and a spongy matrix which is easily depressed. There is increased curvature of the nail and swelling of the terminal phalanx.

Onychogryphosis is great horny thickening and curving often due to trauma. Sometimes it is a consequence of ischaemia or neglect.

Pits are most frequently found in any quantity as a result of psoriasis. Lesser degrees are found in eczema. Fine stippling is seen

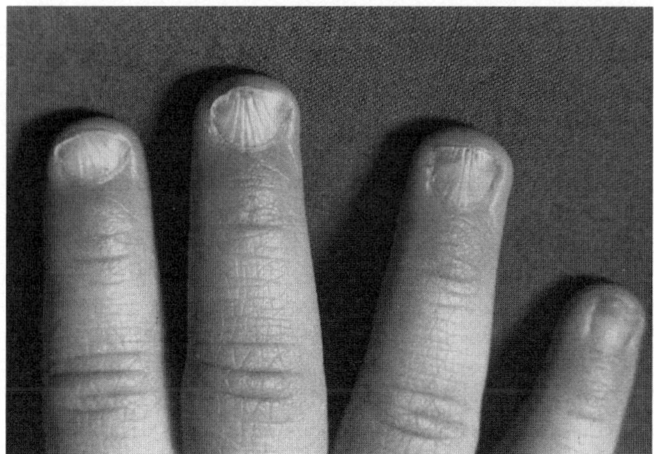

Fig. 33 Longitudinal ridging is usually due to decreased growth, and the nails are often thin and poorly made (idiopathic dystrophy).

in alopecia areata and longitudinal pits and thinning are seen in lichen planus.

Ridges or grooves are seen in psoriasis, eczema, and fungus infection. Longitudinal central grooves may be due to habit of picking at the base of the thumb, but occasionally it is idiopathic (Fig. 33). Longitudinal white lines are a feature of the genetic dyskeratoses (Darier's and Hailey Hailey diseases). Transverse ridges result from injury to the nail fold from infection, as in paronychia or dermatitis. Systemic illness interferes with growth and such furrows are known as Beau's lines. A common cause of nail deformity producing a longitudinal depression is a mucous cyst at the base of the nail. This can be destroyed by cryotherapy or by repeated needling and extrusion of contents over a number of weeks.

Paronychia

This is most commonly due to bacterial infection or repeated irritation by water, detergents and other agents by nurses, bar tenders, and bakers. The loss of the natural seal between the nail fold and the nail plate is an important consequence. It is often due to injudicious manicuring. The use of ointments as a seal applied many times a day before using the hand is an effective therapy. Antiseptic paints are especially useful for discoloration of the nail from *Pseudomonas aeraginora* which causes black or green nails. Keeping the hands dry is advisable but difficult.

Tinea unguium

This is commonly asymmetrical, the toenails being more involved than the fingernails. Differential diagnosis from psoriasis is often difficult, but psoriasis usually involves the fingernails and usually it affects them symmetrically and is associated with terminal phalangeal arthritis. Fungal infection usually begins distally, unlike the secondary distortion of a paronychia which affects the nail in the nail bed. Softening, fragility, or thickening are further consequences of fungus infection. Microscopic examination of nail clippings after prolonged soaking in 5–10 per cent potassium hydroxide should reveal mycelia.

Toenails should only be treated only if the patient complains of the disorder and is prepared to take antifungals daily for very many months. Local fungal preparations are only rarely effective, but amorolfine nail lacquer is a recent improved formulation. Itraconazole, fluconazole, and perhaps most promising terbinafine have greatly improved management but they are given orally and may cause hepatoxicity.

Hair

The hair cycle

The life of a hair is up to about 3 years. Each hair grows about 1 cm per month (anagen phase) after which they involute, form club bed ends and shed (catagen phase). This is followed by the telogen or resting stage. Some 50–300 hairs are shed from the scalp each day. The proportion of hairs in anagen in the scalp and beard is greater in spring than in autumn. Lengthening of the eyelashes has been described in AIDS, malnutrition, and chronic liver disease. There are some 300 000 hairs on the scalp, 1 per cent of which are in catagen at any one time while the rest are completing their 3-year cycle. In systemic illness, 'shock' or a physiological state such as pregnancy, many of the older hairs may pass into catagen earlier so that a partial moult of longer hairs may occur, often a few weeks later (telogen effluvium). The hair recovers completely within a few months. Cytotoxic drugs especially cyclophosphamide, inhibit hair growth so that hair loss is a common side-effect. The effect of these drugs can be prevented by cooling the scalp with a tightly fitting ice bag for about 20 minutes while such drugs are given intravenously.

Androgen dependent baldness

Baldness (alopecia) is a consequence of androgen dependent sexual maturation, due to a shortening of the anagen phase and resulting increase of the proportion of hairs in telogen. Bitemporal recession occurs in 90 per cent of men and about 80 per cent of women. Frontotemporal loss and thinning of the vertex occurs in 25 per cent of white women by the age of 50 and 60 per cent of men at an earlier age. A family history of baldness is so common as to make it very likely that there are genetic factors involved. Most important is the influence of testosterone; it is the relative lack of testosterone in young women that accounts for their lessened tendency to develop baldness. Benign baldness of the forehead is associated with normal or slightly raised serum testosterone and a lowering of sex hormone binding globulin. Males castrated before puberty are similarly protected. Hirsuties and baldness go together.

Examination for other causes of hair loss

The scalp should be examined for evidence of disease such as scaliness, redness, injury, or scarring with its associated loss of follicles. Severe seborrhoeic eczema, which produces diffuse and excessive dandruff, is often associated with thinning. Psoriasis, on the other hand, tends to leave some scalp unaffected and mostly the hair grows well. In very thick plaques, hair may get broken off or its growth is occasionally inhibited. Lichen planus and discoid lupus erythematosus both destroy the hair follicles and produce respectively a violaceous or red colour as well as scarring. *Tinea capitis* is a common cause of hair loss in many parts of the world. The acute, painful, boggy, inflammatory swelling of cattle ringworm (kerion) is sometimes mistaken for a bacterial abscess, but closer examination shows satellite lesions which are clearly not abscesses. Kerions of the head often heal with scarring and some permanent loss of hair. Children may present with discoid patches of slightly scaly red areas of broken hairs due to other forms of animal ringworm. Fortunately most adult scalps are resistant to these. In many parts of the world *T. violaceum* is responsible in black-skinned children, and *M. canis* in white. White scales and scarring in dark heads is often due to favus. In Africa and the Middle East, favus is due to *T. schoenleinii*. Infection of the scalp with streptococcus or staphylococcus is common in parts of the world where generalized impetigo is common. The scalp may carry a persistent staphylococcus in persons who scratch or pick at their scalp, sometimes known as 'tycoon scalp'. The rash of secondary syphilis often causes a patchy pattern of hair loss scattered over the scalp like numerous 'glades in a wood'. Loss of eyebrows is a feature of lepromatous leprosy.

Common causes of diffuse hair thinning are iron deficiency, hyperthyroidism, hypopituitarism, severe illness, and drugs such as cyclophosphamide, anticoagulants, and antithyroid drugs, or poisons such as thallium. Temporary thinning is common in those on oral contraceptives.

Alopecia areata

The cause is probably multifactorial, involving heredity, autoimmunity, stress, infection, and emotional factors in the pathogenesis. The hair bulb is infiltrated by CD4 lymphocytes. There are autoimmune associations and response to immunomodulating therapy. It is not known whether a primary hair-follicle defect invokes this response. It is characterized by localized patches of complete hair loss. At the edges of the lesion there is often a short stubby hair, similar to an exclamation mark, which is due to abortive hair growth. The scalp may be slightly red but scaling is not a feature. The prognosis of a hair growth within 9 months is good for small patches on the vertex in children, but hair loss at the temples or occiput is less likely to grow well. New growth is often initially white. A strong family history and an association of atopic eczema or recurrent attacks suggest a bad prognosis. There is an association with vitiligo, thyrotoxicosis myxoedema, pernicious anaemia, and it is common in Down's syndrome. An identical picture is a consequence of secondary syphilis. Spontaneous remission is common. Intralesional steroids encourage local regrowth but atrophy of the scalp is an unpredictable side-effect and the hair often falls out again after a few months.

Coalescent hair loss results in total scalp alopecia or universal body alopecia.

Dandruff

It is normal to lose small dry scales from the surface of the skin. These tend to be slightly larger in the scalp and show up as white flecks in dark hair or dark clothing. Irritation of the scalp and mild infection with a variety of organisms, as in seborrhoeic dermatitis or high rates of turnover in psoriasis, results in excessive dandruff or pityriasis capitis. Most cases respond to regular shampooing twice weekly with preparations containing mild antiseptics, tar, sulphur, or mercury. Salicylic acid reduces scaling; a common scalp preparation is lotio acid salicyl et hydrag perchlor. The imidazoles are also prescribed.

The scalp tolerates strong steroids such as Betnovate® or Dermovate®, which are very effective for severe dandruff.

Hirsutism

Hirsutism implies a male pattern of hair growth with associated baldness. In contrast, hypertrichosis is the growth of terminal hair from vellus hair at sites not normally hairy, such as the forehead in porphyria.

Women who are menstruating normally, are pregnant, or have a family history of hairiness are unlikely to have endocrine disease. After the menopause most women develop coarse hair on the face. Some normal women may suffer from an enhanced responsiveness of the hair follicles to normal androgen levels in the blood. This is probably due to conversion by the follicle of testosterone into a more active form.

A common cause of hirsutism results from the secretion of upper limits of normal amounts of testosterone by the ovary. Such women may suffer from seborrhoea, acne, hidradenitis suppurativa, decreased fertility, and male-pattern baldness.

The adrenal gland produces 75 per cent of plasma testosterone. Hyperplasia or tumours are responsible for Cushing's syndrome and the adrenogenital syndrome. In children pseudohermaphroditism due to male-pattern development of the genitalia in a gonadal female will be a feature. In older women marked hirsutism is usually associated with virilism, failure to menstruate, and poor breast development.

Anabolic steroids, anti-oestrogenic drugs, progesterone, anticonvulsants, and the polycystic ovary syndrome (Stein-Leventhal) cause hirsutism. It is associated with obesity and infertility as well as menstrual disorders. Rarer causes include virilizing tumours of the ovary, gonadal dysgenesis, and Turner's syndrome.

The onset of amenorrhoea, acne, and hirsutism or baldness should merit examination for an enlarged clitoris. This should be followed by plasma testosterone, plasma cortisol, 24-h urinary steroid excretion, and an estimate of pituitary size by skull radiography or scan.

Hypertrichosis or lanugo hair on the face is almost always due to porphyria cutanea tarda or underlying neoplasia.

Treatment

Bleaching with 20 volume hydrogen peroxide makes dark hair on white skin less noticeable. Commercial depilatories are destroyers of hair but not of the hair root. They are highly irritant and many persons find them impossible to use. Various waxes are now available for the legs and arms, some impregnated in gauze which are easy to apply, against the grain, and to pull off with the grain. The abnormally hirsute often require professional electrolysis, which is more effective for hairs that have not been repeatedly plucked.

Cyproterone acetate (2 mg daily) is a potent antiandrogen and produces gradual improvement over a period of 6 months to 1 year, if prescribed in the early stages of hair loss of scalp or hair gain on face. Its long-term effects are not known. It is given with ethinyloestradiol (50 mg daily). Cimetidine and spirolactone may be substituted.

A combination of prednisone, ethinyloestradiol, and progesterone is helpful. The diameter of the hair is a useful measurement of response to therapy. Plucked hairs 1 cm above the root should show thickening within the range 40–120 µm at the end of 3 months and subsequently at 3-monthly intervals.

Sweating

Apocrine

Apocrine glands occur throughout the skin surface in the embryo but subsequently disappear so that they are found in the adults only in the axillae, areolae, and anogenital region. The secretions are formed by the dissolution of apocrine gland cells which are discharged in the hair follicles close to the surface of the skin. They are not active until puberty. Bacterial decomposition accounts for body odour. Washing with soap and water is the first phase of management. Deodorants reduce the bacterial flora.

Hydradenitis suppurativa

Chronic hyperactivity of the apocrine glands, disturbance of apocrine flow, and secondary infection gives rise to abscesses, sinuses, and scarring, especially in the axillae and groin. The early phase of blind boils may be responsive to antiandrogens as for hirsuties (see above). Cryosurgery is helpful; courses of antibiotics such as tetracycline three times daily for several weeks are worth trying, but wide surgical excision and grafting is often necessary.

Eccrine sweating

Humans have about 3–4 million sweat glands, equivalent in weight to one kidney. They can secrete at a maximum rate of 2 –3 l/h. The secretory coil produces a plasma-like fluid. Sodium is reabsorbed in the sweat duct.

The hands, feet, axillae, and face may sweat profusely in the absence of general sweating. Generalized sweating is a feature of fever as well as thermoregulation in a warm climate, or when the metabolic rate is increased, as in exercise or thyrotoxicosis and in acromegaly.

Eccrine sweat glands are largely innervated by unique postganglionic sympathetic fibres that release acetylcholine at the neuroglandular junction. The control centre is in the hypothalamus. It is important to consider whether the sweating is appropriate for the degree of stimulus.

Many teenagers complain of sweating of the hands and feet and a resulting odour of skin and clothing. The fear of being unwelcome increases the anxiety and subsequent sweating. It may summate with thermoregulatory sweating and therefore be worse in hot weather or at a dance. Winter clothing is often more troublesome than the loose garments of summer. Sweating of the hands and feet occurs with acrocyanosis and with some forms of keratoderma.

Segmental, unilateral sweating is often due to irritative lesions of the spine and requires a neurological opinion.

Excessive sweating contributes to tinea pedis and to eczema from footwear.

Treatment of hyperhidrosis

The total daily water loss at rest is about 500 ml but the hyperhidrosis may increase this to 12 l/day or even 3 litres in the first hour. This is faster than it is possible to drink. For this reason it is important to be aware of fluid loss and to restore water and salt in those who are sweating excessively.

Reassurance, simple advice on hygiene, washing, keeping cool, and appropriate clothing is helpful. The avoidance of obesity, and relaxation if self-conscious are basic points of management. Cotton clothing is more appropriate than non-absorbent fibres. Many shoes are now made with linings which prevent absorption and keep the foot and sock wet. Frequent changes of socks prevents bacterial overgrowth, and readjustment of footwear and the wearing of leather shoes or sandals reduces discomfort. Tranquillizers are sometimes helpful.

Local therapy

Sweating can be inhibited by applying a saturated 20 per cent solution of aluminium chloride hexahydrate to the skin. The skin should be as dry as possible and the patient as tranquil as possible since dilution of the saturated solution by sweat causes it to become irritant. It is probably most effective for the axillae when applied at night and maintenance therapy need be only once or twice weekly.

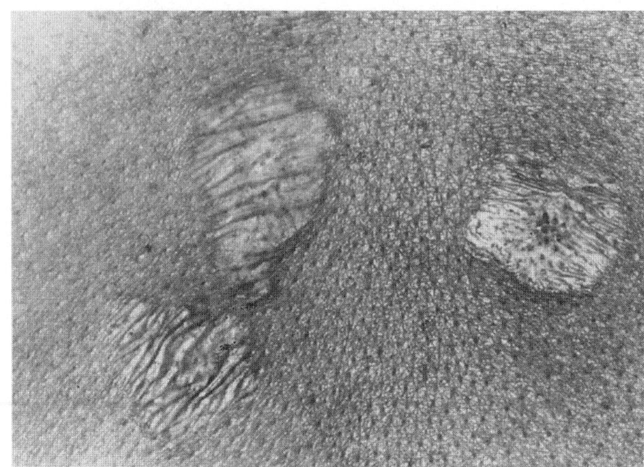

Fig. 34 Lichen sclerosis causes tissue-paper-like crinkling or atrophy of the skin. The border is often violaceous but the centre of the lesion is white.

Application of 3 per cent formalin soaks to the soles of the feet for 10 min or topical glutaraldehyde 10 per cent solution buffered to pH 7.5 are sometimes helpful. Poldine methylsulphate 3–4 per cent in alcohol is another topical agent used on the feet.

Systemic anticholinergic drugs such as propantheline, 15 mg three times daily controls sweating but may cause a dry mouth, blurred vision and even hyperthermia.

Adult intertrigo

Obesity and sweating predispose to mixed irritation and infection in the occluded skin under the breast, axillae, and groins. The affected area is moist, red, fissured, and malodorous. Attempts at keeping the site dry and free of excessive infection have been improved by preparations such as miconazole and hydrocortisone, and ZeaSORB® powder acting as a drying agent without too much caking. Washing and gentle drying is the most important therapy. Blind boils and comedones are likely to be due to hidradenitis suppurativa.

Psoriasis in the flexures is usually well defined, bright red, and, unlike at other sites, is non-scaly. It is worth treating initially for 3 days with a strong steroid because this sometimes clears the psoriasis. More often the lesions persist and strong steroids are then harmful since they cause so much atrophy. Hydrocortisone can be used but it is only mildly effective. It is important to protect the skin from excessive infection by regular washing.

Dermatitis of the genitalia is commonly due to contact with agents such as antiseptics or perfumes. Some of these are added to the bath and inadequately mixed with the water. There may be a considerable immediate contact swelling from certain deodorant sprays. Infection of mixed type may contribute to the problem. Persistent pruritus and scratching is a very common disorder and produces thickening of the skin and a range of colours from white fissured areas to pigmented and violaceous plaques.

Leucoplakia and the atrophy of lichen sclerosus et atrophicus

This is often confusing and it is possible for the skin of the genitalia to be thinned but nevertheless to be covered by a thickened scale. The lesion of lichen sclerosus is well defined (Fig. 34), white, may have a violaceous border, and small haemorrhagic blisters are common, especially in children, and should not be mistaken for sexual abuse.

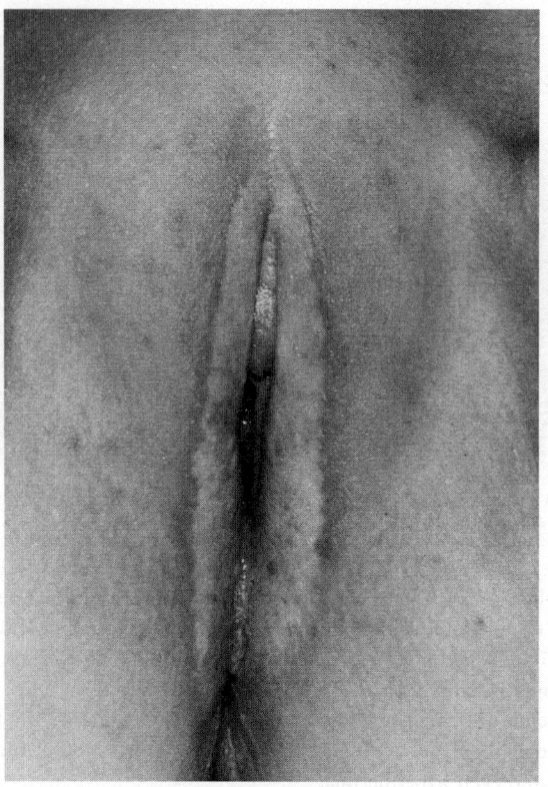

Fig. 35 Lichen sclerosis of the vulva in a child tends to clear at puberty. In the elderly it is a persistent cause of irritation.

The perianal areas are always involved, especially in children (Fig. 35). Intractable itching, burning, or soreness of perineum or genitalia is common. In young women it usually slowly improves; in older persons it persists. It responds well to high-potency local steroids.

When in doubt, a biopsy should be performed, but leucoplakia and lichen sclerosus may coexist in as many as 24 per cent of patients. In the case of leucoplakia, vulvectomy is usually advocated as there is much greater chance of the development of a squamous epithelioma.

Well-defined asymmetric plaques of red pigmented skin should be biopsied to exclude intraepidermal carcinoma to which this site is predisposed.

Urticaria

Urticaria is a transient swelling and/or flushing of the skin. The underlying vasodilatation and accumulation of tissue fluid in the dermis is due to a succession of mediators of inflammation acting mainly on the small blood vessels. The time taken to bring their effects under control varies and thus the inflammatory response varies from the very transient to more persistent inflammation overlapping with vasculitis.

Immunology

Allergens of the type commonly incriminated in sufferers from atopic disease are bound to IgE antibodies attached to the surface of the mast cells or basophils. Allergens causing this include egg white, cows' milk, house dust, dandruff, feathers, and tomatoes. It is commonly of contact type affecting the lips during eating or some other parts of the skin when in contact with animals or house dust.

The urticaria of serum sickness, penicillin reactions, the acute illness of systemic lupus erythematosus, and many infectious diseases are in part due to immune complexes.

Complement activation

While complement is activated by immunological reactions, it is also activated enzymatically by proteases such as plasmin when there are insufficient natural inhibitors of this mediator in the serum and tissues. Congenital or acquired deficiencies in inhibitor levels account for some forms of angioedema and for hereditary angioedema in particular. The activation of complement by the alternative pathway may explain some non-familial cases.

Histamine liberators

Some drugs and foods release histamine from mast cells, or at least make such release more likely by inhibiting prostaglandin activity. Mast cell stimulators include morphine, codeine, thiamine, polymyxin, and D-tubocurarine. Bee venom, strawberries, and shellfish as well as aspirin, salicylates, benzoates, and tartrazine are enhancers of an urticarial tendency, bringing it to the fore in susceptible subjects as well as occasionally initiating the eruption.

Types of urticaria

Genetic factors

Familial urticaria is a well-recognized phenomenon. Many large families of hereditary angioedema are recorded. The autosomal dominant inheritance is mediated through an absence of C1 esterase inhibitor. Familial cold urticaria is another autosomal dominant disease described in several families in the US and others have been described in France and Holland.

Contact urticaria

This is a weal and flare reaction occurring for 20–40 min after application to the skin of a number of agents. Some may be IgE mediated, such as animal dander, saliva, or seminal fluid, but most are probably non-immunological, as with the nettle or jellyfish sting, or the solar or aquagenic varieties of urticaria. Often there is a consequent or associated dermatitis, as in atopic eczema. Many of the ointments used for dermatitis contain bases such as sorbic acid or polyethylene glycol which cause an immediate stinging and slight swelling.

Cholinergic urticaria

This is characterized by numerous, superficial, small swellings which sting, smart, or itch and are surrounded by a blush lasting a few min only (Fig. 36). Probably it is mediated by an increase of receptors for acetylcholine from dorsal root nerve endings. The commonest pattern is found in adolescents and young adults and, like blushing, it is brought on by emotion, exercise, or hot baths.

Heat urticaria

This is a rare local response to heat in which histamine is released or complement is activated.

Angio-oedema

This is characterized by a few, deep, large swellings which may be tender and often itch, sometimes preceded by redness, lasting several hours or even days. Proteases such as complement, plasmin, and kinins are incriminated.

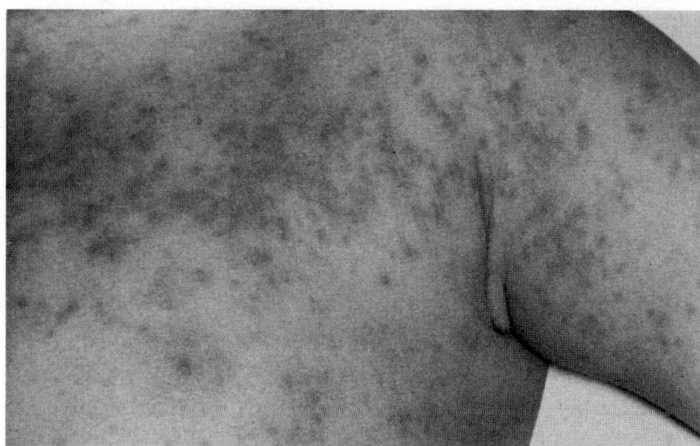

Fig. 36 Cholinergic urticaria. It is transient, lasting no more than about 15 min, and may be associated with small, superficial weals with a prominent flush. These tend to sting rather than itch.

Ordinary urticaria or hives

This is characterized by numerous weals of all sizes, and varying degrees of pallor or redness, which itch and last for 1 or more hour, but not usually more than a day. Successive lesions may account for long illness. Chronic urticaria is arbitrarily defined as continuous or recurrent lesions of more than 3 months' duration. Histamine is the principal mediator. Current evidence supports the view that skin blood vessels have both H_1 and H_2 receptors.

Time of onset

Cholinergic urticaria is like a blush and develops abruptly and instantaneously within minutes of the triggering event. Ordinary urticaria also develops within minutes of the release of the mediator but not all mediators are released instantaneously. Thus foods and certain allergens, or drugs such as aspirin, have to be digested and absorbed. Ordinary urticaria is often difficult to relate to events in the life of the patient for this reason. Delayed onset is a well-recognized phenomenon of some of the physical urticarias. Thus delayed dermographism is the development of redness and slight wealing several hours after scratching the skin. Delayed pressure urticaria is a tender swelling 2–12 hours after localized pressure injury to the skin. It is possible that the insult localizes noxious agents such as soluble immune complexes, or that mechanisms such as transient ischaemia and release of proteases bring to light homeostatic defects such as deficiency of inhibitors of complement or other proteases.

Physical urticaria

Solar urticaria develops within 30 seconds to 3 minutes of exposure to the sun. Tolerance may develop in sites habitually exposed such as the hands and feet. The differential diagnosis includes porphyria, lupus erythematosus, and photosensitivity following drug ingestion. Because the longer, more penetrating ultraviolet rays are responsible, it can occur even on a cloudy day or when the skin is protected by glass, clothing, or sunscreens.

Familial cold urticaria is an autosomal dominant disease in which the rash develops up to several hours after cold exposure from, for example, cold winds, and it usually presents in infancy. Fever and joint pains accompany the rash and there is a leucocytosis. Low levels of a chymotrypsin inhibitor have been demonstrated. It may not be induced by the application of ice to the skin.

Acquired cold urticaria occurs within a few minutes of plunging into cold water or after applying ice to the skin. Mast cells are degranulated and it is one cause of sudden death in young people.

Papular urticaria

This is the only form of urticaria to have a persistent epidermal component. Most often this is due to insect bites, and the epidermis is either damaged directly or by mediators in the upper dermis which evoke an eczematous response so that oedema of the epidermis and a proliferative repair effect results in a typical itchy and persistent papule. Such lesions are usually excoriated, whereas most urticarias are not deeply scratched but merely rubbed. They often blister.

Scaling is not a feature of urticaria, and while acute dermatitis and some erythema initially appear to be urticarial the development of scaling immediately excludes such diagnoses.

Distribution of urticaria

Cholinergic urticaria favours the head and upper trunk. Angio-oedema most commonly involves mucocutaneous junctions such as the lips, eyes, and penis. The physical urticarias clearly relate to sites of exposure. Thus solar urticaria affects the face and the dorsum of the hands, or, if tolerance is developed, it occurs at such sites that are exposed for the first time during the summer. Pressure urticaria favours the soles of the feet when walking or digging, or the backs of the thighs or lumbar region when sitting.

Investigations

A history is the most effective investigation of urticaria. An eosinophilia should alert one to parasites such as microfilaria or trichiniasis, and a raised blood sedimentation is due to a systemic illness such as sepsis, malignancy, or 'collagen' disease. Rubbing or scratching of the skin with the fingernail produces a weal and flare in the dermographic subject within 2 minutes.

Absence of C1 esterase inhibitor in the serum should be looked for in patients with angio-oedema, especially if initiated by minor surgery, associated with abdominal pains or if other members of the family affected.

About 25 per cent of cases of acute hepatitis B present with urticaria.

Foci of infection as a cause of urticaria are statistically difficult to support but dental and sinus infections continue to be described as aetiological factors based on impressive case histories.

Bee and wasp stings

See Chapter 18.2.

When should urticaria be taken more seriously?

Urticaria is life-threatening when it is part of anaphylaxis, when angio-oedema involves the upper respiratory tract, or when it is part of the systemic immune complex disease and is associated with more dire pathology such as meningococcal septicaemia or lupus erythematosus. The latter type of urticaria is recognized by its more persistent lesion, lasting at least 1–2 days and often tender and ultimately purpuric. All acute urticaria may be very widespread and accompanied by joint pains, stomach aches, and fever. If the individual lesion lasts for only a few hours it is less likely to be due to a noxious circulating trigger such as immune complex or infective organisms.

Management

Removal of the known physical factor and the known trigger is helpful, but in the majority of cases of chronic urticaria in the adult no cause is found. Food, medicines, and infectious or parasitic diseases are the commonest suspected factors, but in Europe and the US physical urticaria accounts for more than half of the patients in some series. Cold, heat, and solar urticaria often respond to the induction of tolerance by subthreshold desensitization. It is useful to try antihistamines because of much individual variation in response and in the side-effects. Antihistamines are often prescribed in too low a dosage to be effective, and patients should be encouraged to rest at home taking a rather higher dosage. The evidence that skin blood vessels have both H_1 and H_2 receptors has encouraged trials with their antagonists. At present the financial cost and large number of pills that have to be taken every day is a disadvantage. Most H_1 antihistamines are cheap and free of serious side-effects. Drowsiness is often troublesome but the variations in the response are considerable and they are otherwise effective in the majority if taken regularly to prevent the urticaria rather than to treat the existing weals. Long-acting antihistamines are worth trying when short-acting ones fail. The value of combined H_1 and H_2 blockers (4 mg cyproheptadine and 300 mg cimetidine four times daily) remains unproven but like all regimens has some individual successes. Hydroxazine (10–25 mg three times a day) is often effective in dermographism or cholinergic urticaria. Nifedipine in conjunction with antihistamines has its advocates. When the urticaria is painful and long-lasting, prednisolone is often effective and need only be given for 2 or 3 days. Avoidance of known triggers of urticaria such as aspirin, tartrazine, benzoate, and other salicylates often requires a rather complex diet.

Management of autosomal dominant hereditary angio-oedema

This should be suspected if there is a family history of angio-oedema or a few long-lasting swellings precipitated by trauma. The signs include a transient erythema followed by the oedema. There is often recurring colicky abdominal pain. The diagnosis should be confirmed by looking for low levels in the serum of α-neuroaminoglycoprotein, C1 esterase inhibitor (normal 18 ± 5 mg/100 ml).

Prophylaxis includes care to protect against trauma especially in the region of the mouth and neck after dental manoeuvres. Methyltestosterone 10 mg as linguets after breakfast and another when there is a suspicion of developing oedema often aborts attacks. Fresh plasma, containing C1 esterase, therefore, may be given before surgery or at the initiation of an attack. Unlike other forms of chronic urticaria, adrenaline, antihistamines and corticosteroids are of only a little benefit. Trasylol intravenously is an inhibitor of proteases and is sometimes helpful, as is ε-aminocaproic acid 12–18 g daily in divided dosage. The most effective treatment is danazol. This may be supplemented by fresh plasma during an attack or, if available, C1 esterase inhibitor concentrate.

Cutaneous vasculitis

Vasculitis is the response of small blood vessels to injury, ranging from a transient increase in permeability or wealing, to coagulation and necrosis of the vessel wall. It is due to agents such as immune complexes, toxins, or to physical stimuli such as cold and heat, as well as impaired perfusion.

Vasculitis is a feature of many diseases described elsewhere in this book, such as Henoch-Schönlein purpura, polyarteritis nodosa, nodular vasculitis, Wegener's granulomatosis, hypersensitivity angiitis, and allergic granulomatosis, Behçet's syndrome, pyoderma gangrenosum, purpura fulminans, thromboangiitis obliterans, erythema nodosum, chilblains, atrophie blanche, and livedo reticularis. Vasculitis overlaps with urticaria and with infarction or gangrene.

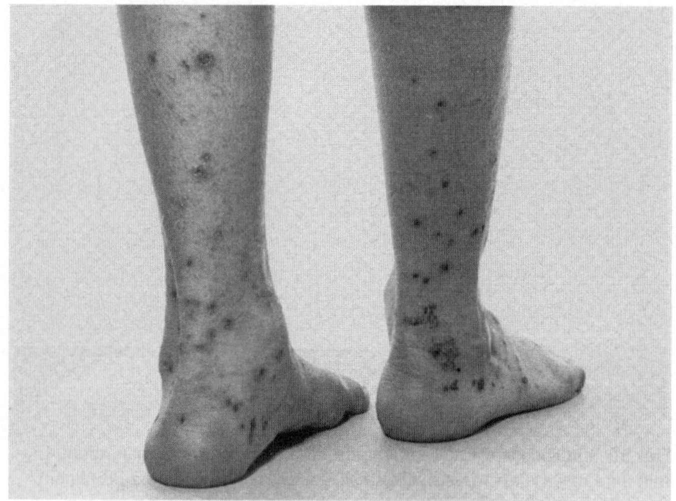

Fig. 37 Typical purpura of the lower leg of adult Henoch-Schönlein purpura. The lesions are palpable and inflammatory.

Harmful agents responsible for vasculitis

Immune complexes, infective agents, drugs, food additives, and circulating particulate matter all injure blood vessels. It is probable that these are present in small amounts in all of us some of the time, but it is likely that the injuries are often so mild as to be imperceptible and quickly repaired.

Immune complexes

The 'defensive' system which clears antigens includes complexing them with antibody and complement to make phagocytosis by macrophages more inevitable. It is a system which is used to remove damaged tissue and it is often difficult to distinguish whether damage preceded or is a consequence of the immune complex. It is the process of complexing that activates complement not the complex itself. Trapping of antigen in a tissue and its exposure to immunoglobulin and complement is determined by local events having little to do with what circulates in the bloodstream.

Diagnosis

Almost essential to the diagnosis is purpura (Fig. 37), but an urticarial lesion that is tender, lasts for more than 12 hours, and leaves a slight bruise on resolution falls within the term vasculitis. The histology of such a lesion often shows more perivascular neutrophils than the common short-lasting urticarial weal. At the other end of the spectrum is obliterative or sclerosing thromboangiitis in which total occlusion of a small vessel often prevents exudation, and because there is no neutrophilic infiltrate, there may not be such acute destruction of the vessel wall. A similar appearance may be observed in DIC and in platelet embolic diseases.

Vasculitis affecting deep dermis or fat and subcutaneous tissues most commonly produces a nodule, sometimes with redness or violaceous skin overlying it. Blistering and pustulation, when they occur as manifestations of vasculitis, are usually part of a superficial polymorphic eruption in which at least some of the lesions are palpable purpura (Fig. 38), distinguishing the eruption from other more monomorphic blistering diseases. Very heavy infiltration with

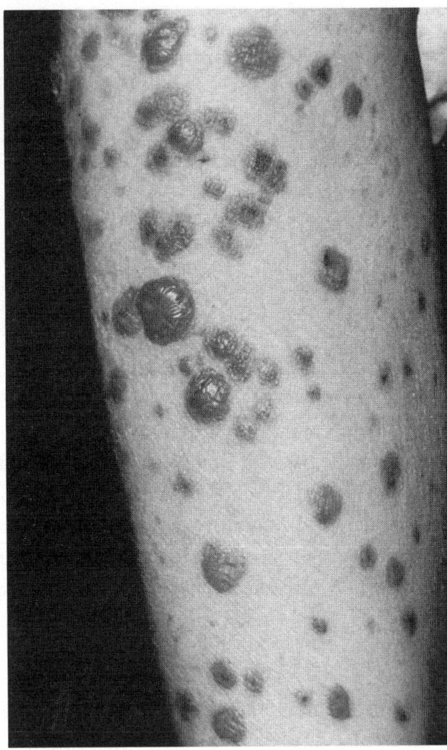

Fig. 38 The presence of blisters in vasculitis is due to the intensity of the oedema in the upper dermis; sometimes it is due to necrosis.

eosinophils is a feature of eosinophilic cellulitis which is sometimes a reaction to arthropod bites.

Vasculitis in which immune complexes have played a causative role is more likely to be leucocytoclastic—a term used to describe numerous disrupted neutrophils at the site of the damaged vessel. It is now well recognized that a mononuclear variety of vasculitis also occurs which is sometimes termed lymphocytic vasculitis and in which complement activation seems less significant but upgrading of cell wall adhesion factors is a response to cytokines and other pharmacological agents, such as histamine. It is a feature of drug eruptions and also of damage to vessels sometimes prior to the deposition of immune complexes, i.e. within 2 hours of a cutaneous capillary fragility test. In fact macrophages rather than lymphocytes could be the more injurious infiltrate, depending on the stage of maturation and their secretion. Much of the pathology of vasculitis is that of ischaemia. Whatever the cause of the damage to the vessel, there is usually some impairment of blood flow. Hypoxia and infarction are quite capable of causing equally extensive pathology.

The significance of eosinophils in some forms of vasculitis is not known and they are no guide to prognosis or therapy.

Detection of cause

Streptococcal sore throat is still the commonest precursor of vasculitis in children and otitis media, dental caries, cystitis, and sinusitis occasionally play a role; in many countries tuberculosis or leprosy is the commonest cause; bacterial endocarditis and meningococcal septicaemia are often missed. Other treatable infections occasionally causing vasculitis are syphilis, *Neisseria rickettsiae*, and mycoplasma. Although viruses usually cannot be eliminated, any history of a recent flu-like illness or vaccination may be relevant. Hepatitis B virus is a well-recognized cause.

Lupus erythematosus and rheumatoid arthritis are common causes of immune complex vasculitis, but, as mentioned above, it is the exposure of antigen so that its complexing can activate complement that is important, not the complex itself.

Drugs such as penicillin and sulphonamides have often been incriminated. Some foods may act as allergens and others have a more obscure enhancing action. Enquiries should be directed towards headache pills, throat lozenges, purgatives, health foods, any medicine given for a specific illness, and any recent intake of food or drugs to which the patient is known to be sensitive.

It is now clear that many patients have cold-precipitated immune complexes and perhaps even more have soluble immune complexes that are localized by blood stasis due to cold, pressure, vasoconstriction, or prior inflammation. The number of patients in whom an antigen has been isolated is small and in still fewer has it been possible to eliminate the antigen, except in the case of bacteria sensitive to antibiotics.

Detection of antineutrophil cytoplasmic antibodies (ANCA) is a useful for prognosis and management. They occur in those forms of systemic vasculitis such as Wegener's granulomatosis which respond to cyclophosphamide in addition to prednisolone. They may play a part in the pathogenesis of neutrophil induced vascular damage. Subtyping and serum levels provide a guide to disease severity and response to therapy.

Factors that modify the inflammatory response

These are very numerous and include any known chronic illness, such as malnutrition, diabetes mellitus, blood disorders, rheumatoid arthritis or other forms of collagen disease, chronic respiratory disease, disorders of the bowels or liver, and hypertension. Malignancy, whether carcinoma or lymphoma, is a not unusual factor and recent surgery, pregnancy, and unusual anxiety are also included.

Management

Avoid all further injury

This allows healing to take place and prevents further damage to already inflamed tissue. Rest is essential for all acute inflammation but blood stasis should be counteracted by adequate elevation and movement of the limbs. Cold and direct sunlight should also be avoided since both injure the skin and affect blood flow. Female legs are particularly at risk, depending on the fashion for long or short skirts or trousers.

Scratching, pinching, pressure, and constriction of the skin by ill-fitting clothing or bandages should not be allowed. Patients lying in bed will develop vasculitis on the buttocks, elbows, and over the greater trochanter unless they shift their position every few minutes. Venepuncture sites become inflamed in some forms of vasculitis, particularly in Behçet's disease and pyoderma gangrenosum but also in severe generalized leucocytoclastic angiitis.

Eliminate circulating noxious agents especially if antigens

Bacterial infection should be treated appropriately. Immune complex disease is sometimes treated with plasmapheresis.

Provide specific treatment

Acute short-lasting itchy weals often respond to antihistamines. Acute tender swelling due to progressive tissue oedema may need steroids. Painful swollen joints, acute optic neuritis, temporal (giant cell) arteritis, erythema nodosum, tender persistent weals, and tense painful

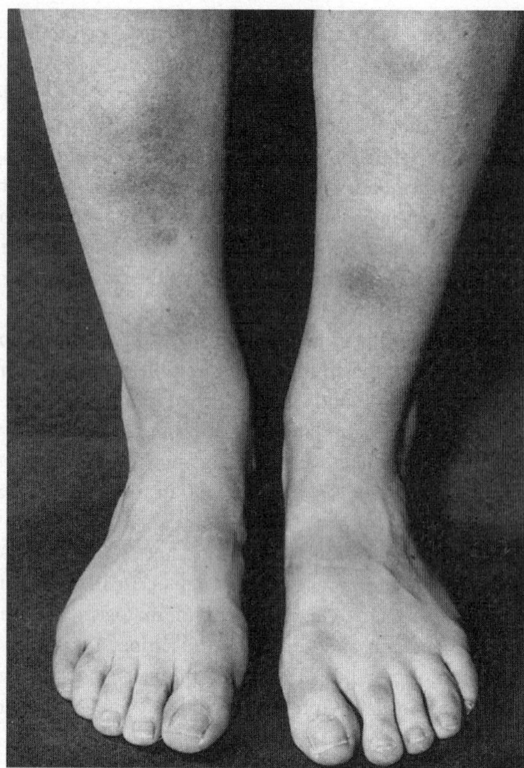

Fig. 39 Tender erythematous swelling on the front of the legs with ill-defined borders is characteristic of erythema nodosum.

swellings at the edge of pyoderma gangrenosum all usually respond to corticosteroids.

Fulminant vasculitis affecting more than one organ and brought about by a known trigger (allergens, drugs), should be treated with steroids once the cause has been eliminated. Immunosuppressive drugs such as azathioprine, cyclophosphamide, and methotrexate are used as a last resort but are of doubtful value except in granulomatous forms affecting the lung, in which they are the treatment of choice.

Erythema nodosum

There is injury to small blood vessels in the deep dermis and subcutaneous tissue but primary injury to the blood vessels from a noxious agent, such as soluble immune complexes, is difficult to prove: it is characterized by tender red swellings on the front of the shins (Fig. 39) and often also on the thighs and forearms. Bruising is common but necrosis, scarring, and atrophy of the tissues is not a feature.

Erythema nodosum is a reaction pattern to infection (viral, bacterial, and mycotic) and sometimes to drugs. Neoplasia, pregnancy, and sarcoidosis are other causes. The causes are listed in Table 5. By far the commonest is a streptococcal sore throat. Sarcoidosis, tuberculosis, ulcerative colitis and Crohn's disease are common associations. Worldwide, erythema nodosum is commonly due to lepromatous leprosy. Erythema nodosum is often preceded by or accompanied by fever, malaise, fatigue, loss of weight, and arthralgia. Although it sometimes resolves in 2–3 weeks, persistent and recurrent forms over several months may suggest an alternative diagnosis. It is important not to label the disease as polyarteritis nodosa or rheumatic fever, for instance, merely because it is persistent and the patient is ill for several months, or the blood sedimentation rate is unusually high. The number, size, and chronicity of the lesions is variable. They can be few and as large as the hand or multiple and the size of the thumb nail. They can be acute, tender, and last only a few days, or they can be chronic, less tender, and migratory, tending to heal in the centre and spread peripherally as a swollen ring. The more chronic lesions are less red and may be violaceous or any of the colours of a resolving bruise.

Table 5 Some causes of erythema nodosum

• Streptococcus	• Blastomycosis
• Tuberculosis	• Coccidioidomycosis
• Sarcoidosis	• Trichophyton verrucosum
• Lymphogranuloma venereum	• Ulcerative colitis
• Cat scratch disease	• Crohn's disease
• Ornithosis	• Leukaemia
• Epstein–Barr virus	• Hodgkin's disease
• Tularaemia	• Sulphonamides
• Histoplasmosis	• Bromides
• Yersinia	• Pregnancy and contraceptive pill
• Leprosy	

Investigations

Chest radiography is essential and the most useful for the diagnosis of sarcoid or tuberculosis.

Treatment

Recovery is to be expected. While for the first 2–3 weeks it is possible to keep the patient at rest and to prescribe acetylsalicylic acid, the difficult period is often several weeks after the initial illness when the patients have to be mobilized. Firm support bandages or stockings give some relief for persistent aching and swelling of the legs. Steroids reduce swelling and fever but do not affect the length of the illness.

Pyoderma gangrenosum

This is a necrosis of the tissues often with a heavy neutrophilic infiltrate. It is not primarily an infection, but a reaction pattern in which venous and capillary engorgement, haemorrhage, and coagulation feature prominently. The exact pathogenesis is uncertain. In many cases there is an associated depression of the immune system demonstrable by *in vitro* and clinical tests. Failure of macrophages to respond to tissue injury or to clear noxious agents is another feature. Its associations include ulcerative colitis, Crohn's disease, particularly of the colon, rheumatoid arthritis, seronegative arthritis with paraproteinaemia, Wegener's granulomatosis, and plasma cell dyscrasias including myeloma. A bullous variety is associated with leukaemia, primary thrombocythaemia, and with myelofibrosis. Up to half of the cases seen in dermatology clinics have no obvious association. Presentation is with a tender red or blue nodule suggestive of erythema nodosum, vesico pustules, or an acneiform folliculitis. The swollen red or blue edge is often acutely tender; blistering may be considerable, especially in the leukaemic variety. The necrosis follows no particular pattern and, like a carbuncle, may have multiple centres. It is usually undermined, and exuberant granulation tissue sprouts from the base of the ulcer. The calves, thighs, buttocks, abdomen, and face are favoured but no site is immune.

Dermatitis artefacta is often suspected and the personality of the patient disabled for many months may be consequently affected and encourage the suspicion. Unlike pyoderma gangrenosum which is often multiple, synergistic gangrene is more clearly associated with a recent wound, such as an operation on the gastrointestinal tract; the area of gangrene is solitary and an extension of the wound. In any form of pyoderma gangrenosum, aerobic and anaerobic bacterial culture, amoebiasis, tuberculosis, buruli ulcer, and deep fungus infections such as nocardiosis or blastomycosis should be considered.

The treatment of choice is high-dose corticosteroids by mouth. The management of underlying diseases such as ulcerative colitis or leukaemia is essential. Any suspicion of an infective causation such as amoebiasis requires the appropriate investigations and treatment. For cases responding poorly to steroids, dapsone 100 mg daily or clofazimine is worth a try. Colchicine, cyclophosphamide, and cyclosporin have their advocates. There are subacute presentations that respond to locally applied steroids by inoculation or under an occlusive dressing.

Behçet's disease

See Chapter 10.16.

Vesico-blistering diseases

A vesicle is an elevated circumscribed lesion filled with serum and sometimes blood and pus. It is usually no larger than 0.5 cm in diameter. Above this size a vesicle is called a bulla or blister.

Predisposing factors

These include congenital diseases such as epidermolysis bullosa or metabolic disorders such as porphyria.

Causes

Friction or minor knocks can produce blisters in the predisposed or at sites unaccustomed to wear and tear. The hands and feet are most often affected. Friction is increased by damp, sweating skin.

Ischaemia

Prolonged pressure obliterating blood supply for more than 2 hours causes damage to the smooth muscle of small arterioles and underlying fat. The epidermis can survive more than 6 hours of ischaemia and in cool skin with a decreased metabolism much longer periods may be survived. The unconscious or those with sensory loss, especially from barbiturate poisoning, are particularly vulnerable but most cases occur from peripheral vascular disease with acute interference of blood supply.

Acute sweat pore occlusion

This occurs especially with fever or in hot climates. Numerous small transparent vesicles are seen especially in the flexures or in parts of the body in which the stratum corneum is unduly thick. In the fingers or feet this is called pompholyx.

Burns

Burns can occur from cold as in frostbite or from cryotherapy, heat, or ultraviolet irradiation (photosensitivity from plants, porphyria, or pellagra). Dermatitis artefacta is often induced by burning the skin; it is clearly self-induced but usually denied and is often a bizarre pattern. Cigarette burns are amongst the commonest induced lesions.

Chemicals

These may be toxic, as from mustard gas or cantharidin. Sometimes an allergic dermatitis from contact also produces vesicles due to separation of the epidermal cells by inflammatory oedema. Plant dermatitis is amongst the most common cause, due to, for example, the primula in Europe and poison ivy in the US.

Fixed drug eruptions

These can cause erythema and blistering and appear and reappear at the same site whenever the causative drug is ingested; usually there is itching within 6 hours of ingestion.

Infections (see Section 16)

Viral disorders including herpes simplex, zoster, chickenpox, and smallpox, or bacterial diseases most commonly cause blisters, particularly the staphyloccus and streptococcus.

Fungus infections commonly present as blistering on the soles of the feet, and insect bites give rise to papular urticaria which often blisters on the lower legs. Arthropods, like the brown recluse spider, give rise to necrotic blisters and others, like the hairy caterpillar, will secrete a toxin in its hairs, which can produce blistering (see Chapter 18.2).

Specific skin disorders

Erythema multiforme

This, as the name implies, can present with a variety of patterns. The classical pattern affects the hands and feet more than the trunk and the lesions have an erythematous and coin-shaped presentation which is more intense and blistering in the centre—a target-shaped lesion. Several toxic erythematous eruptions overlap with the classic pattern and sometimes the classic distribution and even the target lesions are missing. Involvement of the mucosa is common so that mouth, eyes, and genitalia may be affected in varying degrees. Where the blistering and mucosal lesions are severe, the disease is termed Stevens-Johnson syndrome. This is usually associated with high fever and sometimes also anterior uveitis, pneumonia, renal failure, polyarthritis, or diarrhoea.

Aetiology

In 50 per cent of these cases the cause is not known. For the rest the commonest causes are herpes simplex, or other viruses such as orf. Infections such as mycoplasma, streptococcus, typhoid, and diphtheria may be incriminated. Drugs also cause this disorder and sulphonamides are amongst the most common. In fact, any infection and any drug can probably give rise to erythema multiforme, usually after a latent period of 1–3 weeks. Other causes include neoplasm and its treatment with drugs or radiotherapy, as well as certain other systemic diseases such as rheumatoid arthritis, lupus erythematosus, or ulcerative colitis. One of the difficulties is the overlap with the other patterns of toxic erythema and their causation. The erythema of pregnancy may sometimes be called erythema multiforme.

Pathology

There is vacuolar degeneration of the basal cells of the epidermis; vesicles develop between the cells and the underlying basement membrane. There is vasodilation and a lymphocytic infiltrate around the upper dermal vessels.

Treatment

The cause should be removed if known and systemic steroids should be prescribed if the patient is very uncomfortable and toxic. Recurrent attacks should also be treated by eliminating the cause if known, for instance, treating the earliest stage of the herpes simplex with idoxuridine and avoiding triggers like bright sunlight. Continuous acyclovir therapy is also increasingly recommended. Viral resistance and long-term side-effects of frequent or long-term usage have not so far been demonstrated.

Toxic epidermal necrolysis (Lyle's syndrome)

This is a rare variety of erythema with acute epithelial necrosis affecting all areas of the skin and is sometimes called 'scalded skin syndrome' because of its clinical appearance. It is usually acute in onset and may be preceded by various patterns of toxic erythema or blistering. Pressure and shearing stresses on the skin tend to encourage the extension of the blisters. There are two varieties of the disease: the first, originally described by Ritter, is due to a staphylococcus, often phage type 71, and particularly affecting children—the blistering and the resulting erosions are very superficial and are due to a split at the level of the stratum granulosum; the second is a drug reaction or a toxic consequence of malignant disease or its therapy. The entire epidermis is necrotic. The drugs responsible are sometimes sulphonamides, barbiturates, phenytoin, pyrazolone derivatives, or phenolphthalein, but there are also a number of other drugs more rarely blamed.

Pemphigus vulgaris

This is a blistering condition favouring the mucosa as much as the skin. It is a separation of epidermal cells above the basal layers of the epidermis always in association with an antibody having an affinity with intercellular material in the epidermis. The separated epidermal cell is large, basophilic, and rounded and is termed an acantholytic cell.

Aetiology

The pemphigus antibody will cross the placental barrier and promote neonatal blistering. It is also pathogenic *in vitro*. The antibody reacts with a specific 85 kDa protein, plakoglobin, and a 130 kDa protein in pemphigus vulgaris, but in pemphigus foliaceous it reacts with a 160 kDa protein, desmoglein. The 130 kDa polypeptide is an epidermal cadherin. Autoantibodies in pemphigus foliaceous bind to an extracellular epitope of desmoglein. The reason why this should cause loss of adhesion in the granular layer remains obscure.

It is assumed to be an autoimmune disease, possibly associated with HLA-A10 and DR4, and is found more commonly in the Jewish race. It is one of the commonest causes of admission to a skin hospital in India. The more superficial variety that affects Brazilians may or may not be a separate, genetically determined reaction pattern. The antibody that binds with complement both *in vivo* and *in vitro* is specific for an, as yet unidentified, intercellular material which activates proteases that lyse intercellular adhesive materials. Several investigators have found that the antibody frequently causes intraepithelial clefting *in vitro* in human, rabbit, and monkey epithelium. There is an association with thymoma as well as with lymphoma and carcinoma. Not surprisingly, therefore, it occurs with lupus erythematosus and myasthenia gravis.

Penicillamine has been responsible for the development of pemphigus in about 9 per cent of patients treated for rheumatoid arthritis. Captopril and rifampicin as well as meprobamate have also been incriminated.

Clinical features

Erosions of the mucosa of the mouth are the initial problem in more than half the cases. The erosions are often misdiagnosed as mouth ulcers but close examination reveals a friable mucosa with no well-defined aphthous ulcers. Actual blisters may be missed because they are so quickly eroded. On the skin the superficial nature of the blisters also determines that the principal lesion is a more painful erosion and the flaccid blisters quickly burst. The base is red and bleeds easily. The epidermis at the edge of the blister is easily dislodged by sliding pressure (Nikolsky sign). There are many reports of clinical and histological overlap with pemphigus foliaceous or pemphigoid. In all such cases pemiphigus vulgaris proves to be the final diagnosis.

Treatment

Corticosteroids are life-saving; without them the disease is one of the most dangerous in dermatology. Very high dosage is required. Prednisolone 120 mg daily is a common starting dose and failure to control the eruption within a week merits doubling of even this high dose. As soon as there are no new blisters the steroids are reduced by large increments about every 3 days. Withdrawal is more gradual below 30 mg daily. Most practitioners now add azathioprine, methotrexate, or cyclophosphamide as a steroid sparing immunosuppressant.

Pemphigoid

The bullae are subepidermal and acantholysis is not a feature. About 80 per cent of patients are over the age of 60. It is about twice as common as pemphigus. There is a specific antibody (usually IgG) for the basement membrane zone of the epidermis and this is present in about 70 per cent of patients. Complement is bound *in vivo*. The basement membrane remains in the floor of the bullae in most cases. Two large epidermal polypeptides are the major antigenic target of BP antibodies. The BP230 gene is localized to the short arm of chromosome 6 and BP180 gene to the long arm of chromosome 10. Both proteins are components of the hemidesmosome. BP180 is a transmembrane glycoprotein with an external terminal ectodomain consisting of collagen triple helical domains. It binds keratin to the hemidesmosome.

Clinical features

The initial features of pemphigoid are often non-specific and confusing. It can be eczematous or urticarial. The lesions often begin around a site of damage such as a leg ulcer or burn. After 2 or 3 weeks blisters may erupt abruptly. They favour the flexures and are tense and dome-shaped. They often contain blood. Small blisters in the mouth are rare and tend not to erode as in pemphigus. The patients are distressed by itching, and oedema of the skin may be troublesome, but their general health is usually unaffected.

Treatment

The treatment of choice is prednisolone 60–80 mg daily until there are no new blisters. Azathioprine, methotrexate, dapsone, or cylophosphamide may be used to allow a lower maintenance dose of the steroid, since morbidity in the elderly is great. Osteoporosis, gastric ulceration, and diabetes mellitus are particularly common complications of steroid therapy. However, complete remission after 1 year is common.

Dermatitis herpetiformis

This is a vesicobullous disorder associated with the granular deposition of IgA in the dermis and a usually symptomless subtotal villus atrophy of the small intestine. The IgA is believed to be derived from plasma cells in the intestine. As in coeliac disease HLA-A8/DRW 3 is associated and may be responsible for a defective Fc receptor status. It is probable that gluten hypersensitivity results in circulating immune complexes that have an affinity for material in the upper dermis; this is possibly reticulin and the Fc receptor dysfunction impairs the removal by macrophages of the immune material. Histology of the skin shows fibrin, neutrophils, and eosinophils in the dermal papillae.

Clinical features

The eruption is characterized by intensely itchy grouped papular or vesicular lesions that lie on an urticarial or erythematous base. The elbows, knees, sacrum, and shoulders are favoured (see Fig. 3) and the face and scalp are more commonly affected than in the case of pemphigus or pemphigoid. The itchy vesicles are quickly excoriated since this relieves the pruritus. The eruption waxes and wanes, sometimes being in remission for many months, but for most it remains a lifelong disorder.

Treatment

Dapsone (100–200 mg daily) or sulphapyridine (0.5 g three times daily) are remarkably effective and can be used as a diagnostic test since itchiness is relieved within 48 hours. The maintenance dose should be titrated to suit each patient. It may be as low as 50 mg dapsone weekly. Haemolytic anaemia is common on higher dosage and especially when, in some cases, 400 mg of dapsone is needed daily to control the eruption. A strict gluten-free diet controls some but not all patients; 70 per cent can omit dapsone after 2 years of such dieting.

Steroid therapy is strangely ineffective and heparin oddly effective. Inorganic arsenicals (Fowler's solution) are effective and were once very popular, and it is probably justified in elderly patients much troubled by the disease and unable to tolerate dapsone or sulphapyridine.

Abnormal vascularity of the skin, angioma, and telangiectasia

Strawberry naevi

These are almost never present at birth but may be preceded by a small area of blanching observed at that time. From a few days after birth nests of granulation tissue proliferate rapidly. After a few weeks the rate of growth becomes less rapid and some vessels become dilated and cavernous. A stable period of no growth often occurs from about 9 months to about 1 year, after which gradual absorption by fibrosis is to be expected. Management consists of reassurance of the parents and emphasis on satisfactory natural resolution.

Exceptions to this policy include involvement of the eyelid interfering with sight, in which case plastic surgery may be advised. Some large haemangiomata sequester platelets giving rise to a bleeding tendency (the Kassabach-Merrick syndrome). High-dose steroids (3 mg/kg) are life-saving. On withdrawal, rebound overgrowth may be observed, justifying a second or third course. Ulceration of the haemangioma is common, especially in the nappy area. Bleeding is easily controlled by light pressure.

Sometimes haemangiomata have a deep element in which arteriovenous shunts are a complication.

Treatment of haemangiomata has included radiotherapy; more recently, systemic steroids, pressure pads, excision, and, currently, embolization and α-interferon.

Port wine naevi

This is a pattern of vascular birth mark present at birth and usually segmental. It is unwise to make a prognosis at birth because pale naevi and segmental patterns of erythema may look similar and often fade. The majority of port wine naevi persist for life. Arteriovenous shunts and gravitational stasis often cause some increase in the vasculature in adult life. The nape of the neck is a site in which a pale plaque of macular telangiectasia is present in the majority of normal babies and persists in more than one-half of those affected.

Telangiectasia

Telangiectases are enduring dilatations of blood vessels. They are usually less than 1 mm in length and may be point-like or punctate, linear, star-like, spider, or stellate, forming flat, square, oblong, or oval plaques, or mat-like with an eccentric punctum. They blanch completely when they are compressed. Telangiectasia is not new-vessel formation—indeed new vessels in wounds are not unduly dilated.

Telangiectases are probably always secondary to mesenchymal connective tissue dysplasia but can be congenital and naevoid, acquired and genetic, i.e. familial or hereditary, as well as secondary to 'collagen' disease such as lupus erythematosus, scleroderma, or dermatomyositis, or from radiation damage.

All dilatations of small vessels are made worse by blushing, as is seen in rosacea, carcinoid, or due to oestrogen and related hormonal imbalances as in pregnancy or liver disease. They are also made worse by loss of supporting tissue as in steroid atrophy, solar elastosis, ageing, or Cushing's syndrome.

Treatment

Telangiectases are easy to camouflage with 'covermark' type of preparations but advice may need to be given on application with respect to the use of cream and powder, blends, and matching of skin colour.

Telangiectases when small and localized can be destroyed by cryotherapy, cautery, electrolysis, or laser therapy. The latter can be endoscopic. The laser specifically burns haemoglobin and it is therefore more successful in the treatment of the larger blood containing dilatations. Sclerotherapy is also possible.

Bleeding should first be treated by the simple first-aid measure of elevation and local pressure. Cautery is most effective only on a dry blanched area controlled by compression. Patients can be taught to inflate a lubricated finger cot tied over the end of a small catheter for the immediate control of severe epistaxis.

Oestrogen therapy

Oestrogen therapy is sometimes advocated, e.g. ethinyloestradiol 0.25 mg daily, and increased to 0.5 mg per day at the end of 4 weeks if epistaxis continues. However, its effectiveness is unproven by controlled trials.

Percutaneous embolization

This is increasingly used to close unwanted vasculature but it requires careful angiographic control and skilled surgeons, and has not overcome the problem of rapid recanalization and opening up of collaterals. It is nevertheless the treatment of choice for severe uncontrolled bleeding from arteriovenous shunts.

Disorders of collagen and elastic tissue

The metabolism and diseases of collagen are described in Section 9. The fundamental defects are in its chemical structure, its cross-linkage between fibres, and its distribution and quantity.

Striae

These are common; stretch is always a factor. The epidermis is thin and elastic fibres are scanty. Striae are seen on the back and thighs of adolescents during growth, especially when there has been a spurt and the child is athletic. It occurs more in girls than in boys. Striae are a feature of pregnancy and affect especially the abdomen and breasts. This is usually due to excessive adrenocortical activity. Incomplete inhibition of fibroblasts causes atrophy of collagen in response to glucocorticoids. When the collagen is ageing or degenerate as follows irradiation or in diseases such as cutis laxa or Ehlers-Danlos syndrome, striae are uncommon and may not appear even in the pregnant or those with Cushing's syndrome. Striae have also been described in chronic infections such as tuberculosis. They are a diagnostic problem only when they are newly formed in which case they may appear to be weal-like and raised. Later they flatten and become bluish-red and still later, white and depressed.

Localized fibrosis, keloids, and hypertrophic scars

The connective tissue response to cutaneous injury exceeds the limits of the needs for repair appropriate to the degree of injury at that site. This is commonly so a few weeks after injury and gives rise to hypertrophic scars. If the scar continues to hypertrophy and extends beyond the limits of the site of the injured skin, especially after a period of 3 months since the injury, then it is often termed a keloid. Such scars tend to be more tender than hypertrophic scars. Keloids tend to be familial and are commoner in negroes. They are rare in infancy and old age and tend to be less severe after the age of 30. Significant factors are the presence of foreign material in the wound and tension. Preferred areas are the ear lobes, chin, neck shoulders, upper trunk, and lower legs. Keloids in their early stages may respond to strong local steroids applied locally or intralesionally. Compression therapy is sometimes helpful, as is cryotherapy in the early stages. Most would now prefer re-excision and radiotherapy to the edges of the wounds.

Atrophy

Atrophy is characterized by thinning, loss of elasticity, loss of hair follicles, and a smooth surface to the skin. When pinched gently the skin produces fine wrinkles and may be compared to tissue paper. The upper dermal atrophy causes poor support to an atrophic vasculature and telangiectasia is often observed. At the same time there tends to be increased pigmentation within the dermis. Atrophy may be a consequence of inflammation following acute bacterial (particularly elastase-producing organisms) infection vasculitis or pancreatitis. It may be widespread as in the chronic scarring of leprosy or onchocerciasis. Some circumscribed atrophies follow an urticarial vasculitic process which is probably due to an infection which destroys elastic tissue. Perifollicular atrophy or postacne atrophy is similarly due to strains of staphylococcus which produce elastase. Syphilis is another cause of destruction of elastic tissue. Non-infectious causes include lupus erythematosus and localized scleroderma with its variants.

Deep dermal and subcutaneous atrophy

The skin loses its subcutaneous or deep dermal tissue in a number of conditions. Such skin is waxy in colour and may be yellow, pigmented, or bluish with a loss of connective tissue. Deeper vessels may become more obvious so that there is either telangiectasia or obvious cutaneous atrophy and linear stretch marks which are initially red and sometimes protrude above the surface of the skin, but later there is always marked atrophy. The skin that is atrophic may be tethered to underlying tissue or more obviously scarred. Such skin may feel hard or sclerosed.

Morphea is a localized form of scleroderma with a good prognosis for complete recovery. It is not associated with any systemic disease.

Malignant disease

Signs of underlying malignancy

Pallor, pigmentation, and pruritus are common terminal events in malignant disease but any one can also be a presenting sign. Defective immunosurveillance predisposes to infections such as candidiasis or herpes simplex and herpes zoster. Disseminated intravascular coagulation is a common terminal event of malignancy but may be a presenting sign of lymphoma, leukaemia, or carcinoma of the pancreas. Rarer diseases associated with malignancy include:

1. Acquired ichthyosis in which the skin becomes progressively drier and more scaly.
2. Dermatomyositis is commonly caused by malignancy in the white-skinned adult. In children or in black-skinned Africans it is more often a manifestation of autoimmune (collagen) disease. The muscle weakness is proximal. The skin signs include erythema, lichenoid, or psoriaform eruptions, and itching or tenderness may be considerable. Periorbital swelling and redness, as well as a streaky erythema on the backs of the fingers and ragged telangiectatic nailfolds, are other features.
3. Acanthosis nigricans is pigmentation and wartiness of the axilla and groins. There is a velvety brown thickness of the skin of the hands and at mucocutaneous junctions such as the lips.
4. Acquired hypertrichosis lanuginosa is a generalized increase in terminal hair and should be distinguished from hirsuties which is an increase in hair in sites normally associated with hair growth, such as the chin.
5. Acute onset of multiple irritable seborrhoeic warts is known as the sign of Leser-Trélat.
6. Superficial thrombophlebitis or migrating thrombophlebitis is especially associated with carcinoma of the pancreas.
7. Bullous pyoderma gangrenosum is a feature of leukaemia and myeloma.
8. Bullous disease of erythema multiforme type, or occasionally more suggestive of pemphigoid, is more likely to be associated with malignancy if the oral mucosa is involved or if immunofluorescence studies are negative.

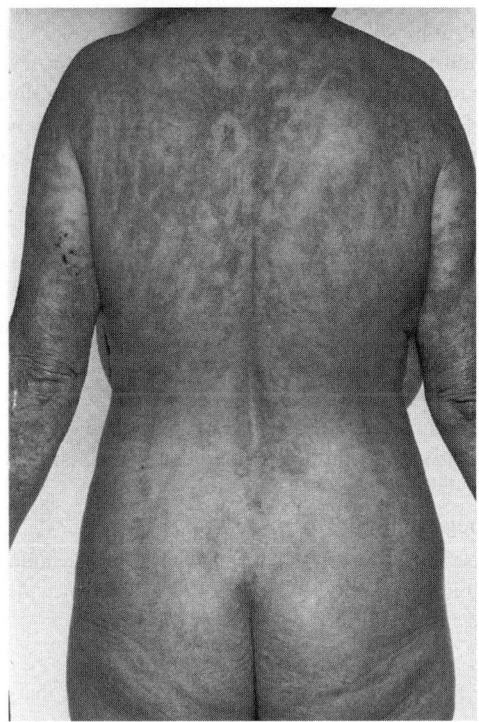

Fig. 40 Erythema gyratum repens in a patient with adenocarcinoma of the colon.

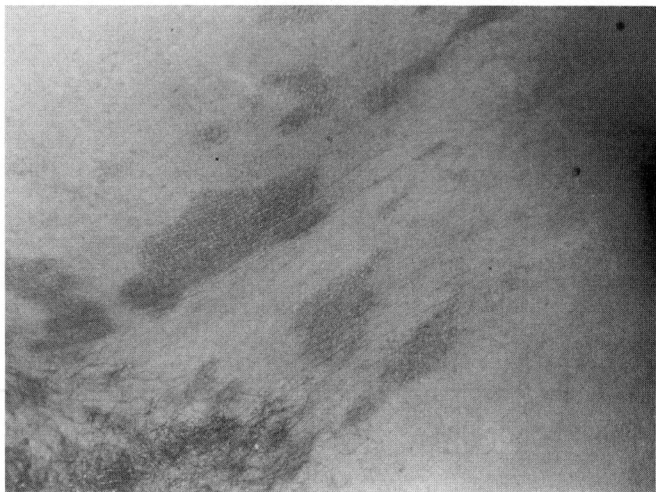

Fig. 41 Lower abdominal, persistent superficial dermatitis (parapsoriasis). These are fixed and persistent digitate (finger-like) patterns, erythematous, and slightly scaly.

9. Erythema gyratum repens (Fig. 40) is one of many patterns of erythema forming repeated concentric rings. The more bizarre and rapidly evolving the process, the more likely is it to be associated with malignancy. This is particularly so when it is generalized, oedematous, or scaling.
10. Palmar keratoses are found in association with cancer of the bladder or lung.

Cutaneous lymphoma

Skin manifestations of lymphoma have features of chronic dermatitis and psoriasis (parapsoriasis) because there is a chronic reaction in the dermis and epidermis which is often indistinguishable from other causes of such a reaction. The feature that causes suspicion is lack of symmetry in an atypical distribution. There is also inhomogeneity within the lesion. Infiltration with white cells suggesting tumour formation is one feature. Another is atrophy or thinning of the dermis, telangiectasia, and pigmentation known as poikiloderma. Persistent superficial dermatitis, previously known as parapsoriasis in plaque (benign type), consists of flat, symmetrical slightly scaly, red patches on the trunk or limbs which persist for years. They are round, oval, or finger-like and are sometimes yellowish (Fig. 41). This is now thought to be benign.

Poikiloderma atrophicans vasculare, previously known as parapsoriasis (large plaque or lichenoides), resembles radiodermatitis in that there is atrophy, telangiectasis, and reticulate pigmentation (Fig. 42). It favours areas spared exposure to natural sunlight such as the breasts or buttocks. It may be composed of small papules or large plaques of any shape. The expected outcome, often many years later, is the cutaneous T-cell lymphoma known as mycosis fungoides but Hodgkin's disease is also a possibility.

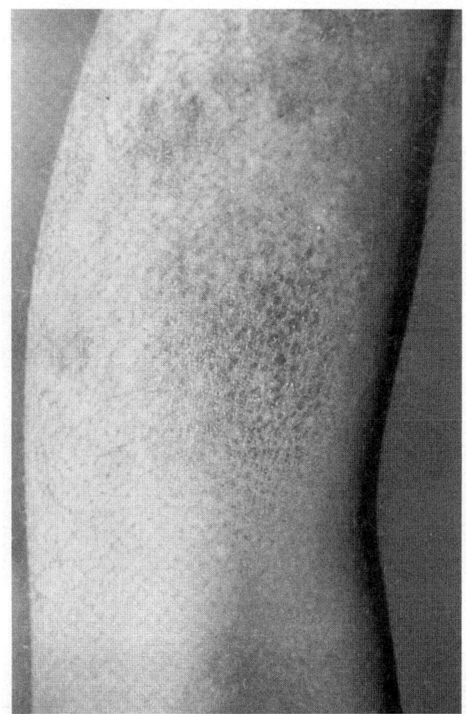

Fig. 42 Poikiloderma; atrophy, pigmentation, and telangiectasia, commonly preceding the development of lymphoma in the skin. The clinical appearance is like radiodermatitis.

B-cell lymphoma, when present in the skin, forms firm pink-red or skin-coloured tumours, often in groups coalescing to produce annular or other patterns (Fig. 43).

Lipomelanic reticulosis is a non-specific enlargement of lymph nodes associated with widespread dermatitis or erythroderma.

Mycosis fungoides is initially often no more than a non-specific dermatitis or more commonly poikiloderma atrophicans vasculare. Occasionally it is a tumour from the beginning. The lesions may be symptomless but severe pruritus is common. The affected areas become more infiltrated, scaly, and reddened (Fig. 44). Often they are annular, serpiginous, or have other bizarre shapes. Erythroderma

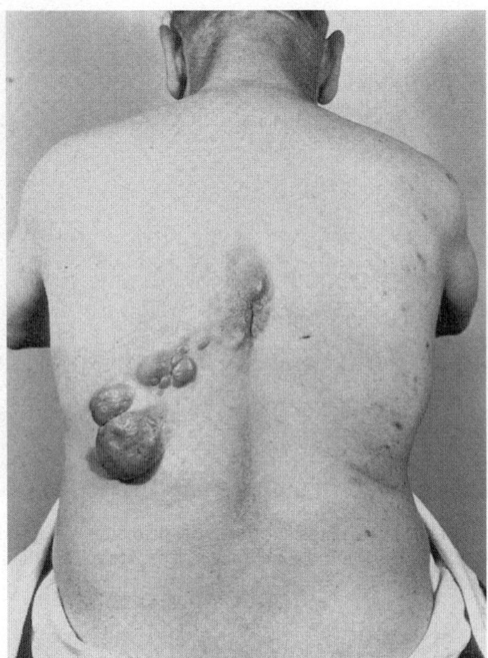

Fig. 43 Fleshy tumours grouped and arising in the dermis without epidermal hyperplasia. This is characteristic of B-cell lymphomas.

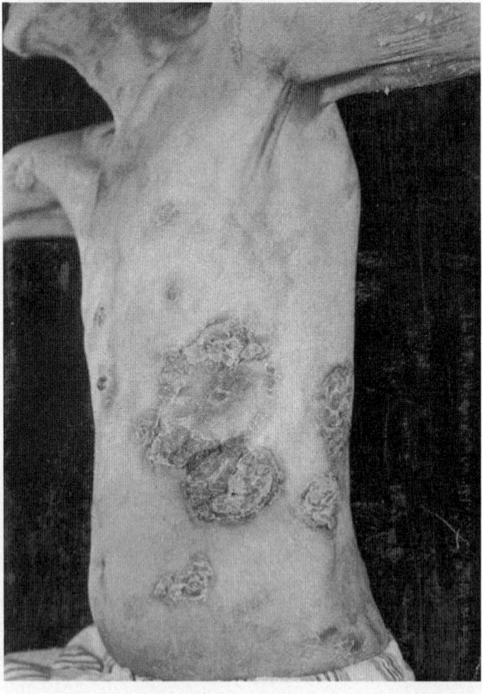

Fig. 44 Marked irregular epidermal reactivity is a characteristic response to T-cell lymphoma of the mycosis fungoides type.

and widespread ulceration is the final stage of the disease. The diagnostic histological feature is invasion of the epidermis by atypical lymphocytes, often in clusters—Pautrier abscesses—and a heavy pleomorphic infiltration of the upper dermis hugging the epidermis but causing less necrosis of individual epidermal cells than in lichen planus.

Skin manifestations of Hodgkin's disease include infiltration of the skin with nodules of the disease. Pigmentation and pruritus are common. Prurigo with deep excoriations and secondary infection is one of its most distressing manifestations. Ichthyosiform atrophy as part of the terminal wasting disease is common. The scaling is often as severe as an exfoliative dermatitis but shedding of the scale is less than that of psoriasis. Hair loss, herpes zoster, and rarely erythema nodosum are other complications.

Management of mycosis fungoides

The rate of progression is highly variable. Among patients who, at time of presentation, lack tumours, skin ulcers, or palpable lymph nodes, the prognosis tends to be very good and it is important not to overtreat.

Radiation therapy

Small-field orthovoltage radiation has been standard therapy for many years and it is very useful to control plaques and tumours resistant to other modalities.

Topical nitrogen mustard (mechlorethamine, HN_2)

This is a useful treatment for patients who have less infiltrated skin lesions. Clinical response may be slow and maintenance therapy may be required for at least 2 years.

PUVA

This is the first line of therapy for superficial lesions that are widespread. Penetration of PUVA is limited so that deep tumours are unlikely to be cleared.

Systemic chemotherapy

This is reserved for palliation in those with systemic disease and deep tumours. There is usually some initial response. Clearance for more than 1 year is unusual.

Viral warts

Warts are caused by the papovavirus (see Section 16), which enters the skin through small abrasions, particularly if the skin is moist and warm. The incubation period is probably several months. There are a number of strains of wart virus giving rise to different types of warts—common, plantar, mosaic, plane, and anogenital.

The incidence of warts is increased in immunosuppressed patients either from drugs or associated with lymphoma. Cell-mediated immunity is more certainly a factor than humoral immunity. The peak incidence is in children aged 12–16 and in recent years in Europe and the US there seems to be an increase in infection rate compared to Asia, Australia, or Africa. Twenty per cent of warts disappear within 6 months and 65 per cent in 2 years. Plane warts and mosaic warts are slow to clear.

Treatment

Warts should be treated if they are unaesthetic and uncomfortable. Spontaneous resolution is to be expected. Overall, 12 weeks is the usual time required to cure warts irrespective of the treatment used and most standard treatments do no better or worse than this. Podophyllin and formalin or salicylic acid are standard therapies.

Podophyllin 10–20 per cent in liquid paraffin or in tincture benzoic compound is painted on to anogenital warts and the area is then powdered. The podophyllin is irritant and some persons need to wash it off in 2 hours. Others have no such discomfort. It should not be used in the pregnant since absorption sufficient to damage the fetus is a possibility. The treatment is repeated at intervals of 1–3 weeks.

Formalin 10 per cent solution can be applied as a soak to multiple warts of the soles of the feet, but dryness and fissuring may be troublesome.

Salicylic acid is the most reliable chemical for treating warts. Paints or plasters containing 20–40 per cent salicylic acid are best applied after a 5-minute soak with warm soapy water and preferably after removal of excess surface keratin.

Freezing is with liquid nitrogen either in a special spray or by application from a cotton wool bud on the end of an orange-stick. The wart should be whitened for at least 20–30 seconds and blistering is a common consequence.

Local anaesthetic injected into the base of a wart to lift it up from the dermis can be followed by curettage. Compression with the thumb on immediate adjacent tissue prevents bleeding while silver nitrate is applied. The rim of horny tissues around the wart side should be cut away using scissors.

Granulomata and other infiltrations of the skin

A granuloma is a compact accumulation of cells, comprised mainly of monocytes or their variants, macrophages, epithelioid cells, and giant cells. Often there is subsequent fibrosis. Lymphocytes are more numerous in granulomata due to allergens to which the host is sensitive. Degeneration or foreign bodies encourage neutrophil and eosinophil participation.

The clinical features of granulomata are either space-occupying nodules lying in the dermis or, if close to the surface of the skin, they may be seen as yellow or brownish-red and sometimes translucent areas. The chronic changes in blood supply associated with the lesion cause a bluish colour and sometimes telangiectasia. If they are in the upper dermis, then there may be overlying epithelial hyperplasia or ulceration with extrusion of some of the granulomatous material. On the other hand, thinning of the epidermis may be considerable. In dark skins, pigmentary changes may include hypo- or hyperpigmentation.

A common cause of granulomata is persistent irritation of the skin by external trauma causing ulceration and pseudoepitheliomatous hyperplasia. Examples include granuloma fissuratum of the ear or nose due to ill-fitting spectacles. The ingrowing toenail, the pilonidal sinus, or the presence of extrafollicular but intradermal hair as is seen in the interdigital clefts of barbers, and cattle or horse dealers are other examples.

Granuloma gluteal infantum is seen in the nappy area due to incomplete resolution of an irritant rash in which steroid creams have been too extravagantly applied. Numerous agents acting as a foreign body incompletely degraded and removed are causes of chronic granulomas in the skin. They include sea urchin spines, silicates, cactus allergen, grit, and various chronic infections such as *Candida albicans*, *Trichophyton verrucosum*, coccidioidomycosis, atypical mycobacteria from fish tanks or swimming baths (Plate 12), leprosy (Plate 13), tuberculosis (Plates 14, 15), leishmaniasis, and halogen granulomas.

Sarcoidosis

See Chapter 4.28.

Urticaria pigmentosa or mastocytosis

Mast cells are normally present in the skin but the numbers vary greatly, with up to $80/mm^3$ in the upper dermis. In mastocytosis they are greatly increased in number and may be found as a single isolated mastocytoma or numerous nests scattered over the entire body, i.e. the classic urticaria pigmentosa, or diffusely throughout the entire skin. Occasionally there is systemic infiltration of all tissues including liver, spleen, and bone marrow. The mast cell releases histamine, leucotrienes, and heparin and these may have systemic effects, but it is increasingly realized that the local contribution is through its secretion of proteases.

In the infant, mastocytosis may present as blisters, but more commonly the lightly pigmented swellings in the skin are noted and observed to swell when scratched or after a hot bath or exercise. Rarely there is a generalized flushing and itching. The condition is most common in the first year of life or at birth and an onset at this age is a good prognosis for eventual complete resolution by adolescence.

In the adult a late onset is associated with diffuse plaques and telangiectasia.

Treatment

Treatment is unsatisfactory but the increasing use of H_1 and H_2 antagonists in various combinations is proving beneficial in some cases. The prognosis for eventual resolution is good in children but a solitary or troublesome single lesion in an adult can be excised. The cosmetic appearance of pigmented lesions is helped by sun exposure or by use of UVA and psoralens, but the number of mast cells is not reduced. Disodium cromoglycate helps some patients with systemic mastocytosis. The number of mast cells can be suppressed by high-potency steroids under occlusive dressings.

Granuloma annulare and necrobiosis lipoidica

A partial necrosis of the collagen and the connective tissue cells associated with immunoglobulin and complement deposition results in a lymphocytic and histiocytic response that is known as a palisading granuloma. This is entirely reversible over many months and years in granuloma annulare, but in necrobiosis lipoidica it tends to result in fibrosis and scarring. The association with insulin-dependent diabetes mellitus and AIDS is unpredictable and is to be expected in more widespread forms or in older age groups of granuloma annulare and in about 75 per cent of necrobiosis lipoidica.

In children, granuloma annulare are commonly on the knuckles (Fig. 45), fingers, and dorsum of the feet. Ears and elbows are quite frequently affected. The tendency to heal in the centre and spread centrifugally over many weeks gives rise to an annular appearance.

Necrobiosis lipoidica is commonly to be found on both shins (Plate 16). Widespread forms of granuloma annulare may be often of giant type, forming large violaceous plaques or rings. No treatment is necessary since eventual resolution of granuloma annulare is expected in 75 per cent in 2 years, but intralesional steroids probably speed resolution, particularly sometimes aborting necrobiosis lipoidica.

Management of skin disease

General principles

Acute skin lesions require rest. Limbs should be elevated because this reduces swelling. Dressings should be applied lightly and evenly to the surface and should support the inflamed area without drag or compression. All agents applied to the skin should be no stronger than necessary.

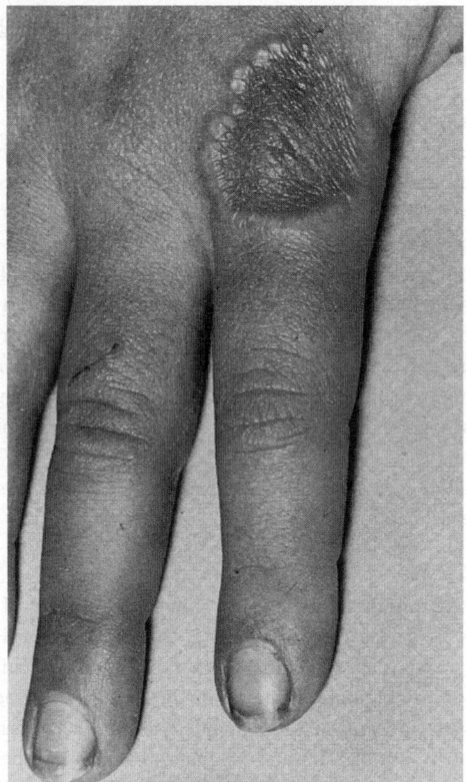

Fig. 45 Papules of granuloma annulare forming a ring around a now healed but previously affected area on the knuckle.

Elimination of the cause of the skin lesion is essential. This applies particularly to dermatitis from primary irritants or allergens, but it is also important to know and eliminate infection if possible, although this does not mean attempting to make a chronic ulcer sterile.

Damaged skin is vulnerable; it should be protected from further injury, such as scratching, rubbing, wrongly applied dressings, and unsuitable local medicaments.

Chronic skin conditions are obviously more difficult to cure, and correct diagnosis is even more important than in acute skin conditions which are likely to heal spontaneously if the cause is eliminated. A biopsy for histological analysis is often helpful and where chronic infection is a possibility, bacterial or mycological analysis is clearly indicated.

The handicap of the chronic lesion includes a feeling of being unwelcome, often leading to the accusation of 'unclean' and leading to being 'outcast'. Sympathetic questioning along the lines indicated earlier will help to relieve the patient's suspicion that the doctor is not interested in the problem. Touching the skin during examination often does more to make the patient feel that the physician cares than any other manoeuvre.

Local topical treatment

The fingertip unit

The fingertip unit is the amount of ointment expressed from a tube with a 5 mm diameter nozzle, applied from the distal crease to the tip of the index finger. One unit weighs 0.49 g and covers 286 cm^2 in males and 0.43 g which covers 257 cm^2 in females. One unit will cover an area equivalent to twice the area of the hand. Four hands is thus equivalent to two finger units, which is equivalent to 1 g.

Drugs are dissolved or suspended in bases which have properties of their own quite independent of the active ingredient. As in Table 6, bases were originally either powder, water, or grease. However, modern processes have prepared bases which are essentially much more complex than this, although still retaining the objectives of the primary agents. Powder may repel water or absorb it and allow further evaporation. Modern powders tend not to cake and abrade the skin as much as the original talc or starch. Watery lotions evaporate and cool as well as wet and dissolve. Various agents, such as alcohol or glycerine, may be added to increase any one of these properties. Creams and emulsions of oil and water (aqueous or milky) or water in oil (butter or oily) are cooling, moisturizing, and emollient. Penetration of active agents through the skin is aided by the aqueous (vanishing) oil and water creams. Ointments based on vaseline or paraffin are more occlusive and less quickly absorbed. They are better at softening dry surface scales.

There are various other preparations which are also water soluble, such as macrogels or emulsifying ointment in which a wax or animal fat is mixed with mineral oil. Pastes are powder and oil mixtures, such as talc and vaseline. They are more occlusive and protective. They are useful for slow surface release of agents such as dithranol. The addition of an active ingredient to a base often makes it unstable and hence various other agents are added as a preservative or to control pH. Further dilution usually makes the preparation still more unstable and shortens its shelf life. Much of the skill in preparing an ointment or cream or paste is in the use of the homogenizer by the pharmacist.

The actions and side-effects of topical steroids are illustrated in Table 7. Tar and dithranol preparations are discussed in the section on psoriasis.

Skin cleaning

Washing is important for reducing smell and for removing debris, but this is best done by soaking rather than scrubbing. Soaking is one of the most effective of skin treatments for oozing exudative conditions.

Emulsifying ointment is a useful soap substitute; it can be made into 'cakes' of soap or spooned out of a pot and mixed with hot water to soften it. Liberally applied it is a useful softener of crusts.

Bathing in water, often for prolonged periods several times a day, is an effective remedy for generalized soreness of the skin. The skin tends to dry excessively when all grease is removed and this can enhance pruritus. For this reason emulsifying ointments and proprietary (oilatum) oils are usually added to the bath.

The use of antiseptics in the bath is of dubious value but weak solutions of potassium permanganate 1/8000–1/16 000 can be used. The patient often uses these agents too extravagantly. High concentrations of antiseptics poured into a bath may lie on the bottom and burn the skin, especially in sensitive areas such as the scrotum.

Bacteria are best dealt with by removing crusts and other debris; soaking achieves this even without the addition of antiseptics. In intertriginous areas soaking should be followed by drying. Organisms thrive in moist crevasses such as under the breasts and in the groins or between the toes,. At such sites powders which do not cake are helpful. Many proprietary brands of powders such as ZeaSORB® can be recommended.

Smell

Malodorous necrotic skin is always very difficult to deal with. Removal of debris and dead tissues is essential. Antibiotics and local antiseptics

Table 6 Bases and their properties

Base	Site for application	Effect	Disadvantage	Examples
Watery and shake lotions (powder in water)	Acutely inflamed, wet and oozing	Drying, soothing, and cooling	Tedious to apply; frequent changes (lessened by polyethylene occlusion); powder in shake lotions may clump	Fuller's earth solution Lotio Terra silica Saline solution BPC Potassium permanganate 1/ 8000–1/18000 0.5 acetic acid in water Eusol in chlorinated lime and boric acid solution
Creams	Both moist and dry	Cooling, emollient, and moisturizing	Short bench life; fungal and bacterial growth in base; sensitivities to preservatives and emulsifying agents	Oily cream BP Aqueous cream BP, i.e. variants on water oil, and water mixes
Fatty acid, prophlene, glycol	Both moist and dry	Emollient and moisturizing	May sting when applied; occasional sensitivity to propylene glycol	FAPG base
Ointments	Dry and scaly	Occlusive and emollient	Messy to apply and soils clothing; removed with an oil	Soft white paraffin Vaseline Hydrous wool fat (lanolin) Emulsifying ointment BP
Pastes; powder/ointment mixture	Dry, lichenified, and scaly	Protective and emollient; delays absorption of grease	Messy and tedious to apply (linen or calico needed)	Zinc compound paste BP Lassar's paste BP
Dusting powders	Flexures; may be slightly moist	Lessens friction	If too wet, clumps and irritates	Talc, dusting powder BPC Zinc, starch, and talc dusting powder BPC

cut down bacterial degradation which is a cause of smell. Metronidazole 400 mg three times daily is sometimes used to reduce the smell of tumours as it is effective against various anaerobic bacteria. Charcoal dressings are also helpful.

Itching

Itching is described in the section on pruritus. Elimination of the causes are discussed therein and are always an important beginning to management. Management includes cooling, or at least, not overheating. Excessive cooling is drying and this can cause pruritus. Water-miscible creams are cooling whereas vaseline-based ointments are heating. Antipruritic agents include ichthammol, tar, menthol, camphor, phenol, local anaesthetics, and steroids (Table 7). Most of these are used in a 1 per cent concentration.

Protection of the skin from obsessional rubbing is helped by occlusive dressings in those who will tolerate them. In young children or in the adult who prefers to scratch, it is difficult to impose an occlusive regime. Cutting nails and encouraging gentle rubbing rather than scratching reduces the damage done to the skin.

Retinoids

The greatest advance in dermatological therapeutics of the last decade has been the introduction of systemic retinoids. The main retinoids available are Roaccutane® (*cis*-retinoic acid) and etretinate (retinoic acid). These modulate cell differentiation and growth, inhibit polymorphonuclear cell chemotaxis, inhibit polyamine formation, and inhibit eicosanoid formation. They are effective in acne, psoriasis, and genetic dyskeratoses. Their side-effects include teratogenesis, hyperostosis, lipidaemia, hepatitis, and various minor skin, bowel, and neurological problems previously recorded with vitamin A administration. They are prescribed in combination with other topical therapies or psoralen UVA therapy in an attempt to reduce their dosage and consequent side-effects.

Mood-controlling drugs

Apart from the value of psychotherapeutic drugs to control the secondary emotional reactions to skin disease (many such drugs are used to control skin symptoms), antipruritics are often sedative but hydroxyzine and trimeprazine are favoured. Delusions of parasitosis and obsessive concern with pruritus is relieved by pimozide.

Intertrigo

The treatment of intertrigo is essentially to protect the area from chafing and secondary infection and to encourage dryness. Underlying disorders such as diabetes mellitus or obesity must be managed along traditional lines. Infection from bacteria, Candida, or fungus requires monitoring by appropriate swabs and scrapings. Bed rest and nudity are helpful. In hot climates a fan encourages evaporation and drying. The folds of the skin should be kept apart by ventilated loose-weave dressings. Acute eczema requires bland wet lotions, steroid creams, and simple antibacterial agents such as gentian violet or vioform cream. When dry, powdering is to be encouraged. Frequent bathing is always helpful.

Hand dermatitis

To provide healing and prevent relapse of dermatitis of the hands, patients should use lukewarm water and emulsifying ointments when washing. If possible, running water is better than a prolonged soak in a bowl of detergent soap. Soap should be used sparingly and the hands thoroughly rinsed and dried carefully with a clean towel. As far as possible there should be no direct contact with detergents and

Table 7 Topical steroids

Active constituents Include hydrocortisone and synthetic halogenated derivatives of prednisolone such as beta-methasone 17-valerate, triamcinolone acetonide, and fluocinolone acetonide. Halogenation increases topical activity
Bases Available in lotions, creams, fatty acid propylene glycol base, and ointments. Over 100 preparations listed in MIMS
Penetration Readily penetrate skin via the horny layer and appendages. Form a reservoir in the horny layer. Polyethylene occlusion and the use of higher concentrations increase penetration
Metabolism Some, though probably minor,metabolism in epidermis and dermis (for example, hydrocortisone conversion and other metabolites). Leave skin via dermal vascular plexus and enter general metabolic pool of steroids. Further metabolism in liver
Excretion As sulphate esters and glucuronides
Action
Anti-inflammatory
Vasoconstrict
Decrease permeability of dermal vessels
Decrease fibrin deposition
Decrease kinin formation
Decrease prostaglandin synthesis
Depress fibroblastic activity
Stabilize lysosomal membranes
Immunosuppressive: antigen–antibody interaction unaffected but inflammatory consequences lessened (above mechanisms)
Decrease rate of epidermal turnover
Side-effects
Thinning of epidermis
Thinning of dermis
Telangiectasia and striae (due to thinning of epidermis and dermis)
Bruising (due to thinning of dermis and vascular wall fragility)
Hirsutism
Folliculitis and acneiform eruptions
May worsen or disguise infection (bacterial, viral, and fungal)
Systemic absorption (rare but, for example, occurs in infants, when applied in large quantities under polyethylene pants)
Allergy to hydrocortisone is well documented
Uses Eczema. Psoriasis in a few instances (facial, flexural, and palms/soles). Many non-infective pruritic dermatoses

Currently there are at least 60 different topical corticosteroids available in the UK which can be classified into four groups: mild, moderate, potent, and very potent. When treating skin disease, the doctor should select one from each group and test its efficacy and limitations; this should cover all contingencies. The least potent corticosteroids that gives good control should be used, starting with a mild preparation and increasing potency as required. With experience more potent corticosteroids can be used appropriately from the outset. If a very potent agent is required, it should be remembered that more than 50 g/week leads to measurable adrenal suppression. Because of the reservoir, once daily application is recommended, supplemented by frequent emollients.

Modified from Hunter, J.A.A. (1976). *Today's treatment, 7.* Blackwell Scientific, Publications, Oxford.

other strong cleansing agents, shampoos, polishes, and stain removers. Oranges, lemons, grapefruit juices, and various other irritant vegetables should be avoided. Rings should not be worn during housework or other work even when the dermatitis has healed. This is because irritants often collect under them. Rings should be cleaned on the inside frequently with a brush and left in ammonia (one tablespoon to 500 ml of water) overnight and rinsed thoroughly. If gloves are used for washing dishes and clothes, they should be plastic and not rubber since the latter often causes dermatitis. They should not be worn for more than 15–20 minutes at a time. If water happens to enter a glove, it must immediately be taken off. The gloves should be turned inside out and rinsed several times a week. Sprinkling with talc before they are used helps to dry them. Cotton gloves can be used under the plastic ones. They should only be worn a few times before they are washed.

Vulnerability

The skin in many diseases is vulnerable. This is manifested as the tendency to produce disease even from minor trauma. It is seen in the primary irritant dermatitis of the atopic eczema sufferer, the Koebner phenomenon of psoriasis, or lichen planus, the hyperreactivity of the skin to needle puncture or pressure localization in vasculitis, and in the ulceration that results from minor knocks of the skin of the legs in gravitational stasis. The skin's vulnerability is severe in epidermolysis bullosa.

The lower limbs

Management of leg ulceration

The cause of ulceration should be identified and, if possible, eliminated. (Table 8).

Elevation

Healing of leg ulceration is always helped by elevation. If there is a major degree of arterial disease so that there are absent peripheral pulses then it should not be raised more than about 23 cm above the level of the heart. In every other case emptying of the distended veins and superficial venules is helped by lying the patient in a prone position and elevating the legs to an angle of at least 45°. This is best done by placing an object such as a chair under a mattress. It is also best during the day because the patient cannot sustain such a position when asleep, but will curl up into a bundle at the top of the bed.

When stiff hips, heart failure, and obesity are factors preventing elevation of the legs, a compromise includes compression bandages (see below) and attempts to make the most of any muscle pump in the lower leg. Intermittent positive pressure inflatable bags are marketed. These are leggings that blow up and squeeze the legs at a pressure and rate that can be regulated.

Elevation is also a requirement for lymphoedema but the protein collecting in the tissues of a swollen leg usually fails to clear satisfactorily via the lymphatics. To hasten its passage out of the tissues into the lymphatics, movement such as massage, vibration, or ankle exercise are necessary. Provided the solid elements of the skin, i.e. collagen fibres, are moved, the massage or vibration need not be very sophisticated. In the absence of lymphatics the only other way protein can be removed from the tissues is by macrophages. To control venous hypertension, the pressure at the ankle should be 40 mmHg and there should be a gradient of decreasing pressure as one moves proximally. This gradient is aided by the increasing circumference of the calf. Each layer of bandage doubles the compression.

Table 8 Causes of leg ulceration

Trauma	External injuries, burns, scalds, chemical, self-inflicted, artefacts, contact dermatitis
Infections	
Viral	
Bacterial	Acute: 'desert sore', gas gangrene Chronic: buruli ulcer, tuberculosis, leprosy, swimming pool granuloma
Anaerobic	Meleney's ulcer, synergistic gangrene
Streptococcal	
Mycotic	Superficial or deep fungus
Spirochaetal	Syphilis, yaws
Leishmaniasis	
Infestations, bites	Spiders, scorpions, snakes
Metabolic	Diabetes
Vasculitis	Collagen disease, immune complex disease
Pyoderma gangrenosum	
Perniosis erythrocyanosis	
Venous	Stasis, congenital absence of veins, post-thrombotic
Atrophie blanche	
Necrobiosis lipoidica	
Neoplastic	Epithelioma, Kaposi's sarcoma, leukaemia, reticulosis, melanoma
Arteriovenous anastomoses	
Ischaemic	Scars, fibrosis, radiodermatitis
Arterial	Hypertension, temporal arteritis, atherosclerosis
Thrombosis, embolism, platelet agglutination	
Blood diseases	Coagulation, platelet disorders; impaired fibrinolysis
	Thrombocythaemia, polycythaemia
	Dysglobulinaemia, spherocytosis, sickle-cell anaemia
Neuropathic ('trophic')	Diabetes mellitus, leprosy
	Tabes dorsalis, syringomyelia, alcoholic neuropathy

Arterial disease should always be excluded by examining the arterial system, especially by taking the blood pressure in the legs and arms or by an arteriogram. Stopping smoking and keeping walking is essential therapy.

Wound dressings should encourage moist wound healing, which favours epithelial migration and the development of granulation tissue.

Movement

Inflammation is aimed at removing injurious agents and promoting healing. In acute infection or injury there is often a need for immobilization. However, such immobilization should be localized to the site of injury. Gentle passive movement of the joints and active movement of the main muscles of the leg are encouraged by wriggling the toes or ankles, or by quadriceps exercises.

Table 9 Common causes of contact dermatitis in leg ulcers

Ointment bases and preservatives	*Additives in bandages*
Wool alcohols (lanolin)	Ester gum resin
Parabens	Azo disperse yellow No. 3
Propylene glycol	Colophony
Chlorocresol	Mercaptobenzothiazole thiuram (rubber)
Ethylene diamine	
Antibacterial agents	*Self-medication*
Sodium fusidate	Caine mix (local anaesthetics)
Gentamicin sulphate	Antihistamine creams®
Neomycin	Dettol®
Soframycin®	Germolene
Quinoline mix (Vioform®)	

Dressings and bandages

The objective of bandaging is to hold the dressing in position to protect the leg from further injury and to provide a sleeve against which movement of the underlying muscles can compress and empty the superficial veins.

The control of infection—what should be put on the ulcer?

If the cause of ulceration is eliminated, then healing should take place. However, healing depends on healthy epidermis at the edge of the ulcer. Often this is damaged by proteolytic enzymes from slough and infection. Unhappily common is the damage done by irritation or sensitivity to medicaments. For this reason, simple bland therapy aimed at reducing debris should be used. Debris will float off if softened. Hard adherent crusts are usually dry. The most effective remedy is wetness, and saline is sufficient to give this, provided it is applied very frequently as a wet dressing. Surgical debridement should be performed with a scalpel or scissors if there is any non-viable tissue. This is not difficult provided one remembers that dead tissue has no sensation. In other words, trim away anything the patient is unaware of, provided the diseases causing neuropathy like leprosy and diabetes mellitus have been excluded, in which case only that which is necrotic and non-adherent should be removed. Antiseptics such as eusol, 0.5 per cent acetic acid (a teaspoon of vinegar in a pint of water), or 0.5 per cent silver nitrate in aqueous solutions are other wetting agents. While helpful to remove slough they inhibit granulation tissue and are less often recommended.

Many antibiotics are applied to ulcers and they rarely control infection. It is naive to believe that an ulcer can be made sterile. It is common for antibiotics to be inhibited rapidly by serum and debris under a bandage. It is common also for such agents to do damage to the epidermis. In this respect it is sometimes forgotten that the health of the surrounding epidermis is more important for healing than the state of the ulcer bed. Tropical phagedenic ulcers often follow trauma and relative avascularity encourages invasion by fuso-spirochetal organisms.

Contact dermatitis

Healing is often delayed and ulcers may be enlarged by damage to the surrounding epidermis from medicaments. Such dermatitis as is seen so often around the ulcer occurs either because of the medicament or due to bacterial toxins or allergy. Table 9 is a list of common causes of contact dermatitis.

Toenails

Poor sight, apathy, stiff hips, and obesity are all reasons why toenails are uncut. Clippers rather than scissors are to be recommended because they cut hard, thickened nail more effectively. The nails should be softened by soaking them in warm water for 10 minutes. Only the distal part of the nail protruding beyond the toe need be cut. Good positioning of the cutter and patient in adequate light is essential. Only very distorted nails or the foot with arteriosclerosis and the consequences of diabetes mellitus need the attention of a chiropodist where such is available.

Corns

These are due to thickening of the epidermis due to pressure from without, or from pressure from underlying bony prominences. It should be possible to avoid pressure from without by adjustment to footwear and skilful padding, so that the weight is taken on less bony areas of the foot. Surgery is sometimes necessary to remove bony prominences. The thickening of the skin is self-perpetuated and is greatly helped by careful paring away of excess keratin, avoiding damage to underlying blood capillaries which often project upwards to near the surface.

Carcinoma

Carcinoma develops in the hypopigmented margin of ulcers that have persisted for many years. Such ulcers often invade bone but rarely metastasize. Local excision and grafting is often preferable to amputation.

Surgery

Whereas in technically developed countries, amputation and a good prosthesis may convert a cripple into an active and otherwise normal person, amputation is objected to by certain races, such as the Bantu, or by certain religions, such as the Hindu. It inevitably causes them to be dejected and rejected so that they are unemployable and outcast.

Injection of superficial veins with sclerosants or their removal, is indicated only when the deep veins are patent. If the deep veins are blocked, then the superficial veins are the only venous drainage of the legs and they should be preserved. The assessment of the proportion of flow returned through the superficial veins is greatly facilitated by the Doppler flowmeter. Surgical debridement and skin grafting is often a means of quickly healing ulceration but is outside the scope of this textbook. Consideration of amputation must take into account social circumstances and the degree of subsequent aftercare.

Elephantiasis

See Chapter 2.36.

The decubitus ulcer

The decubitus ulcer is a consequence of distortion of the tissues, often due to pressure which obstructs blood flow. It occurs especially in neurological disease in which painful stimuli from tissue distortion or ischaemia is not recognized. Because the pathogenesis includes impaired perfusion by blood, anything which affects blood supply can contribute to the problem. Thus, in general, old patients who are ill or dying, and especially if they have vascular disease, are most likely to develop sores. Such sores are unusual in purely motor neurological disease with no sensory loss or in the very old who have a healthy vascular system.

Because it is distortion of the tissues rather than simply pressure that induces sores, shearing forces on the sacral area and heels are also to be taken into account. Such forces are increased by moisture from sweating or incontinence. Distortion of the tissues is enhanced by deformities such as kyphoscoliosis or contractures.

While the basis of management is relief of tissue distortion by frequent relaxation of stress and strains on the tissues, best brought about by movement, factors contributing to poor perfusion must also be attended to. These include intercurrent illness causing hypoxia, hypotension, immobility, dehydration, impairment of consciousness, or peripheral sensation. Most acute illnesses requiring admission to hospital provide the necessary criteria for the development of a decubitus ulcer within the first hours or days. The chronic sickness which determines prolonged bed rest at home rarely produces this degree of tissue ischaemia and thus the hospital nurse gets blamed for what has never occurred at home. The blame is partly misdirected because, for example, an old woman with a fractured hip may develop decubitus ulcers from immobility in the ambulance, on a hard trolley waiting for a bed, or on the operating table. Education concerning the causes of decubitus ulcer should be widely dispersed amongst all attendants.

All ill patients are best put to bed. Some of the worst pressure sores can occur while sitting in a collapsed state in a day room or during the postoperative phase of 'mobilization'. The basis of management is regular 2-hourly turning. Heavy and unco-operative patients, together with inadequate staffing, especially at night, are a constellation of factors that frequently combine so that the resources are not enough to prevent pressure sores. Good equipment to modify pressure on a bed surface is important and may include a fleece under the heels, a bed cradle to take the weight of the bed clothes, a variety of soft surfaces, and alternating pressure as in a ripple bed, preferably with large ripples.

Further reading

Braverman, I.M. (1981). *Skin signs of systemic disease*, (2nd edn). W.B. Saunders Co., Philadelphia.

Canizares, O. and Harman, R. (1992). *Clinical tropical dermatology*, (2nd edn), p. 859. Blackwell Scientific Publications, Oxford.

Champion, R.H., Burton, J.L., Burns, D.A., and Breathnach, S.M. (ed.). (1998).*Rook, Wilkinson, Ebling textbook of dermatology*, (6th edn). Blackwell Scientific Publications, Oxford.

Eisen, Z. and Wolff, K. (1999). *Dermatology in general medicine*, (5th edn). McGraw Hill, New York.

Goldsmith, L.A. (1991). *Physiology, biochemistry, and molecular biology of the skin*. Oxford University Press, New York.

McKee, P.H. (1996). *Pathology of the skin with clinical correlations*, (2nd edn). Mosby-Wolfe, London.

Ryan, T.J. (1996). Diseases of the skin. In: *Oxford textbook of medicine*,(3rd edn) (ed. D.J. Weatherall, J.G.G. Ledingham, and D.A. Warrell), pp. 3073–812.Oxford University Press, Oxford.

The year book of dermatology 1990–1998. Mosby, St Louis.

Section 12
Nephrology

Contents

Chapter 12.1

Clinical physiology of the kidney: tests of renal function and structure

K. M. Bannister and M. J. Field

Examination of the urine

Urine volume

In health there is a diurnal variation in renal function, with relative retention of both water and solute by night. Normal adults excrete between 1 and 2 litres of urine in 24 h, of which 60–80 per cent is passed by day. This rhythm may be abolished or reversed in oedematous states, in chronic renal disease, malabsorption, adrenal insufficiency, and in some cases after head injury or renal transplantation.

Polyuria, arbitrarily defined as a regular urine volume in excess of 3 litres/24 h, is most commonly caused by a high fluid intake, but is also a feature of the glycosuria of diabetes mellitus and renal failure. Less common causes include diabetes insipidus, hypokalaemia, and hypercalcaemia. It is important to distinguish true polyuria from frequency. *Nocturia*, may be defined as the passing of more than one-third of the total 24-h urine volume by night. This must be distinguished from nocturnal frequency, with which it is often confused. *Oliguria*, is defined as the production by an adult of less than 400 ml of urine/24 h.

Midstream urine samples

A reliable midstream urine sample can be collected from males after retraction of the foreskin, and from females with the labia separated by their fingers. Ideally, the genitalia should be swabbed with sterile saline but this is often impracticable. Antiseptics should be avoided if a sample is required for culture. The patient should have a full bladder and should collect the midstream specimen by moving the container in and out of a free-flowing stream.

Suprapubic bladder puncture is underutilized in the investigation of adult patients when it is difficult to obtain uncontaminated midstream specimens. The bladder should be sufficiently full to be palpable in the slim adult and dull to percussion well above the pubis in the obese. If there is doubt, a potent diuretic should be given to fill the bladder before aspiration. No local anaesthetic is needed; the urine is aspirated through a thin needle.

Diagnostic catheterization should be reserved for the infirm from whom midstream or bladder puncture specimens cannot be obtained. The risk of introducing infection is reduced by instilling 120 ml of 0.2 per cent neomycin after taking the diagnostic sample, before withdrawing the catheter.

All urine samples must be sent promptly to the laboratory or cooled in a refrigerator at 4°C if the delay is likely to be greater than 2 h.

Urinalysis

Protein

The Dipstick test is particularly sensitive to albumin, which is the main constituent of most pathological proteinurias, but is insensitive to low molecular weight proteins (for example, Bence Jones proteins). The protein content of the urine of normal individuals can rise to about 150 mg/litre when the urine is concentrated, a figure sufficient to give a trace positive result.

False positive results can occur with very alkaline urine, for example during infection with urea-splitting organisms. There is considerable observer error. Doubtful tests, and those in alkaline urine, should be checked with 25 per cent sulphosalicylic acid, which is a little less sensitive.

Any suspected abnormality should be further investigated by measuring the total protein excretion in 24-h urine collection. The upper limit of normal here is generally taken to be 150 mg.

Benign proteinuria

Postural Three to five per cent of young adults have abnormal proteinuria when up and about, but not after a period of horizontal rest. Standing in a position of exaggerated lordosis can induce significant proteinuria in a substantial proportion of people who do not otherwise show it. These findings do not reflect renal disease and do not require investigation.

Functional Abnormal proteinuria can be observed in normal people after severe exercise, in fever, or on exposure to extremes of heat or cold. Patients with cardiac failure may also have proteinuria without renal disease. After prolonged severe exercise, proteinuria, cylinduria, and microscopic haematuria may persist for as long as 24 h.

Microalbuminuria Microalbuminuria (excretion rates of 30–300 mg/day—20–200 μg/min) is a useful early marker of diabetic nephropathy—see Chapter 6.13.

Blood and myoglobin

The detector in the stick turns green in the presence of very low concentrations of either haemoglobin or myoglobin. Intact red cells produce small green spots by lysis on contact with the detector. The chemical test should always be complemented by microscopy. Absence of excess red cells when the stick test is positive should raise the possibility of myoglobinuria.

Dextrose

The test square is specific for dextrose. Although the colour depth is semiquantitative, it is not sufficiently accurate for assessment of the degree of glycosuria.

Urine pH

The pH detector square is useful in detecting infection with urea-splitting organisms, which raise urine pH to 8 or above, in alerting the observer to false positive tests for proteinuria, and in ensuring that the urine is being kept alkaline in patients with salicylate poisoning, uric acid calculi, cystinuria, and urinary infection during treatment with aminoglycosides.

Nitrate

Most Gram-negative organisms reduce nitrates to nitrites and produce a red colour in the reagent square of an appropriate 'stick'. False negative tests are common (about 30 per cent), but the test has some use in giving immediate confirmation of urinary infection and in screening large populations.

Leucocytes

Dipsticks give results in close accord with quantitative microscopy but it is important to observe the required 2-min wait before the result can be read; all other detectors can be read within 1 min.

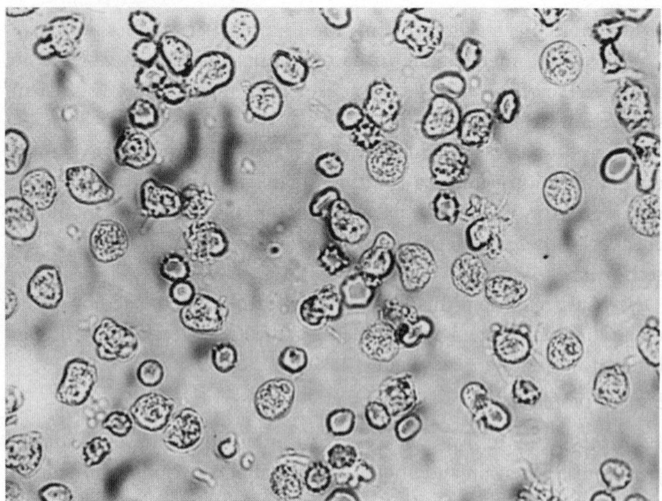

Fig. 1 Pus cells, red cells, and bacteria in an unspun urine sample from a patient with an acute urinary infection. (High power.)

Urine microscopy

The urine sample should be fresh. If this is not possible, a trace of formalin will preserve cells and casts. Boric acid (0.5 g/30 ml of urine) will also inhibit bacterial growth while maintaining viability of cellular components.

In the diagnosis of acute urinary infection a drop of urine under a coverslip can be examined under high power within about 1 min; the answer is usually obvious (Fig. 1). The heavy pyuria, often accompanied by some haematuria and visible bacilluria, is readily distinguishable from normal urine. When the answer is not clear-cut, the unspun urine may be examined in a counting chamber and the findings expressed quantitatively.

If renal disease is suspected, a centrifuged urine should be examined. The Kova® system (Boehringer, Mannheim) facilitates recognition of formed elements and gives quantitative results if the urine is a timed specimen. Twelve millilitres is spun for 2–5 min at 2000–3000 r.p.m. A pipette isolates the lowest 1 ml, and the supernatant is poured off. One drop of stain is mixed with the remaining 1 ml. A drop is placed on a slide with a counting chamber. Experienced microscopists can obtain much the same information from a qualitative examination of an unstained sediment. A thick, uncovered drop is scanned for casts, then a coverslip is added and the high power used to distinguish cells, bacilli, yeasts, and trichomonads. Illumination is kept down by lowering the condenser and closing the diaphragm. Phase contrast is necessary for the study of red cell morphology (see below).

White cells

In uncentrifuged urine, less than three leucocytes/ml is normal; three to 10, of doubtful significance; and greater than 10, abnormal. It is abnormal to find any leucocytes in a bladder-puncture sample. Not all pyuria is due to infection, nor is bacteriuria always accompanied by pyuria; the causes of a dissociation between the two are summarized in Table 1.

Red cells

Although there are a few red cells in normal urine, if there are enough to produce any count in unspun urine they are almost certainly pathological. There is considerable observer error in detecting slight haematuria; scanty red cells are often confused with small oxalate crystals, yeasts, and small air bubbles. Their presence should always be confirmed under high power, when a count of greater than 2000 red cells/ml is probably abnormal.

Phase-contrast microscopy has been used to distinguish red cells of renal origin from those coming from the lower urinary tract. Those of renal origin are said to show irregularities of size, shape, membrane spiculations, or crenation, while those from the lower tract look more normal. This technique requires skill and experience and not all are agreed of its value. Moreover, with heavy haematuria red cells tend to appear normal whatever their source.

Table 1 Dissociation between bacteriuria and pyuria

Bacteriuria without pyuria
- Asymptomatic bacteriuria (covert bacteriuria)
- Contamination

Heavy pyuria without bacteriuria
- Culture inhibited by:
  - antibacterial agent
  - specimen contaminated by antiseptic
  - wrong growth conditions for fastidious organisms
- Urinary tuberculosis
- Renal or bladder calculi
- Analgesic nephropathy
- Chemical cystitis, e.g. cyclophosphamide
- Acute glomerulonephritis
- Non-bacterial (e.g. chlamydial) infections of the urethra

Minor pyuria without bacteriuria
- Many chronic renal diseases (e.g. glomerulonephritis, polycystic disease, interstitial nephritis)
- False pyuria (not confirmed on bladder puncture)
- Vaginal discharge

Casts

These form in the lumen of the distal tubule, particularly the collecting tubule, where flow and pH are low and osmolality high. Their matrix is formed from Tamm–Horsfall mucoprotein. Cells, cell debris, and other proteins in the tubular lumen may be agglomerated and caught up in the gel to form the different varieties of cast discussed below.

Hyaline casts

These consist entirely of Tamm–Horsfall protein. These clear, colourless cylinders, are occasionally seen in the urine of normal people, particularly when it is concentrated, or after exercise. Showers of hyaline casts appear in the urine during any febrile illness and after the administration of loop diuretics.

Granular casts

These contain elements of disintegrated cells or aggregated serum proteins. Finely granulated casts (Fig. 2) occur in much the same situations as hyaline casts and have similar significance. Densely granular casts (Fig. 3) are always pathological and are particularly characteristic of chronic proliferative or membranous glomerulonephritis, diabetic nephropathy, and amyloidosis.

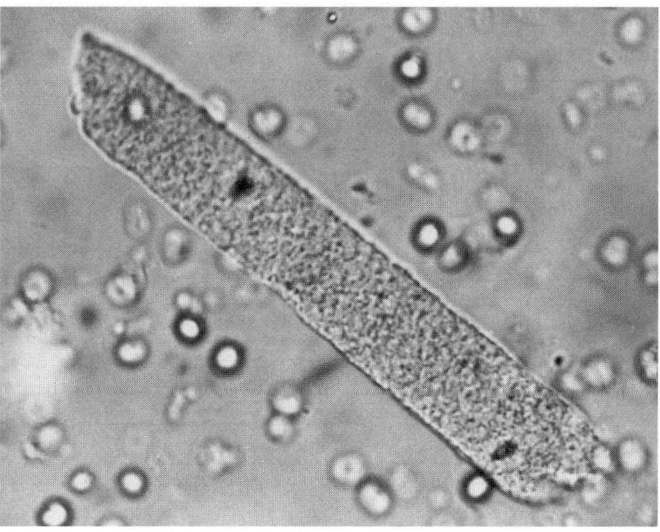

Fig. 2 A finely granular cast surrounded by red cells. (High power.)

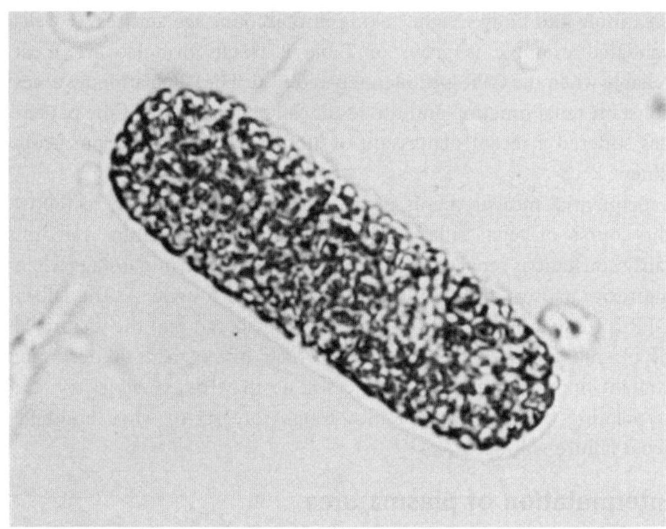

Fig. 3 A densely granular cast. (High power.)

Fatty casts

These are composed of highly refractile fat globules of varying size, often accompanied by oval fat bodies which are epithelial cells stuffed full of fat granules, and by free fat globules; they are most common when there is moderate to heavy proteinuria. Polarized light reveals the classical 'Maltese crosses' thought to be due to cholesterol esters.

Red cell casts

These are pathognomic of glomerular bleeding and can be found in large numbers in acute glomerular inflammation of any origin including malignant hypertension (Fig. 4).

Scanty red cell and granular casts are found in association with microscopic haematuria in several forms of focal proliferative glomerulonephritis. Even one red cell cast indicates a renal cause for haematuria. A thorough search of the deposit from several concentrated urine samples may be supplemented by the examination of a urine filtrate, which is stained and examined on the filter paper.

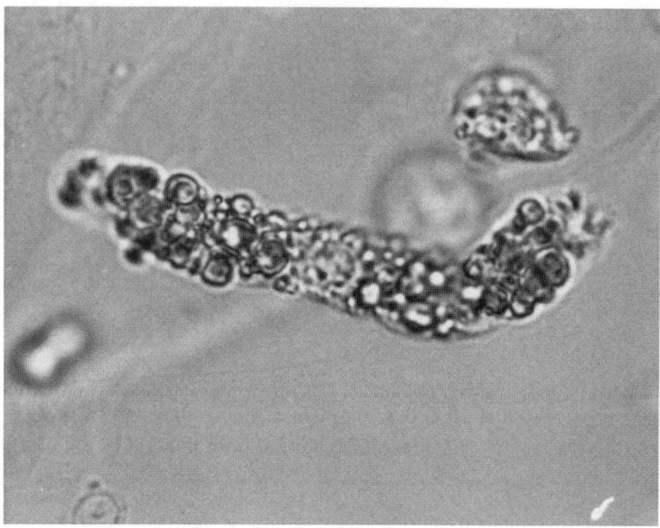

Fig. 4 A red cell cast from the urinary deposit of a patient with acute glomerulonephritis. (High power.)

White cell casts

These are relatively rare but may appear in considerable numbers during an episode of acute pyelonephritis. A few may be found in the urine in chronic pyelonephritis, and their numbers may increase in pyrexia of any cause.

Epithelial cell casts

These are found in acute tubular necrosis or acute glomerulonephritis. A commoner phenomenon is a hyaline or finely granular cast with one or two epithelial cells attached; these are seen in many forms of chronic renal disease.

Transitional epithelial cells

These are smaller than vulvar squames and of a more uniform, oval shape. They are seen in small numbers in normal urine and are sometimes plentiful in the presence of urinary infection. Clumps of transitional cells, often with bizarre nuclei, are found in bladder cancer or papilloma; they give a clue to diagnosis but their absence does not exclude it.

Estimation of glomerular filtration rate (GFR) (see also OTM3, pp. 3105–7)

GFR is estimated by measuring the clearance from plasma by the kidney of any substance completely filtered at the glomerulus and neither reabsorbed nor secreted by the tubules.

$$\text{Clearance} = \frac{\text{urinary excretion rate}}{\text{plasma concentration}} = uv/p$$

Where u and p are the concentrations in urine and plasma and v is urinary excretion rate.

Inulin clearance is the gold standard, but the chemical assay is tedious and poorly reproducible in inexpert hands. [^{51}Cr]-ethylenediamine tetraacetic acid or [^{99}Tc^{m}]diethylenetriamine-pentaacetic acid (**DTPA**) can be used instead of inulin, providing results that correlate well. DPTA also allows imaging of the kidney and is the method of choice when accurate measurement of GFR is required. The test is most accurate when renal function is normal,

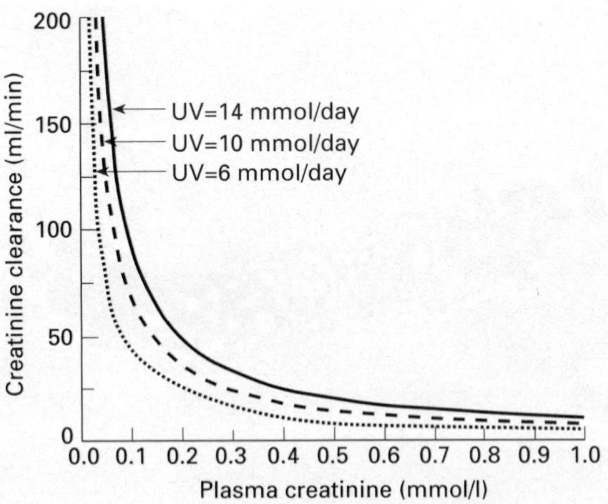

Fig. 5 Compound graph showing theoretical relationship between plasma creatinine concentration and creatinine clearance for three subjects of differing muscle mass, with creatinine excretion rates (UV) of 14, 10, and 6 mmol/day.

or near normal. In renal failure results are inaccurate and measurement of plasma creatinine is more useful (see below). DPTA clearance is most commonly used to confirm good renal function in patients, with isolated proteinuria or haematuria, when plasma creatinine concentrations are normal.

Endogenous creatinine clearance

Creatinine is a breakdown product of skeletal muscle, and maintains a nearly constant plasma concentration, proportional to the total body muscle mass, throughout 24 h. Its excretion is largely determined by glomerular filtration, and the GFR can be estimated by determining endogenous creatinine clearance. Its accuracy is limited in renal impairment, as tubular secretion of creatinine becomes then more significant, leading to overestimation.

The procedure involves collection of a precisely timed specimen of urine, with the drawing of a blood sample at some time during this period. Accuracy is best obtained using a 12- or 24-h interval. There is a high rate of error in the completeness of urine collection, leading to poor reproducibility (about ±20 per cent). For this reason, the use of creatinine clearance has declined as it gives no better an estimate of the GFR than calculation from the plasma creatinine (see below), except where this itself is prone to error (states of muscle atrophy and wasting, oedema, obesity, and pregnancy).

Interpretation of plasma creatinine

The relationship between the creatinine clearance, and the plasma creatinine concentration is a rectangular hyperbola, of the form shown in Fig. 5. Two important consequences arise from this relationship. First, very small changes in plasma creatinine concentration in the low (normal) range where the hyperbolic curve is steepest, imply, very significant changes in GFR. This makes the test a very sensitive indicator of early renal impairment, although laboratory error in this range is also proportionally greater. Secondly, individuals with differing muscle mass will fall along different hyperbolic curves. The interpretation of a given plasma creatinine must therefore be made in relation to a patient's muscle mass; for example, a value of 0.1 mmol/l might reflect a normal GFR in a well-built young man, but would indicate significant renal impairment in a frail elderly woman.

Table 2 Formulae for calculating creatinine clearance from serum or plasma creatinine

Males			
Creatinine clearance in ml/min per 70 kg	=	(145 −age in years)	−3
		serum creatinine in mg/dl)	
	=	(88(145 −age in years))	−3
		(serum creatinine in μmol/l)	
Females			
Creatinine clearance in ml/min per 70 kg		(0.85(145 −age in years))	−3
	=	(serum creatinine in mg/dl)	
		(75(145 −age in years))	−3
	=	(serum creatinine in μmol/l)	

Note: These formulae and all others studied by Hull *et al.* (1981) are inaccurate in the presence of liver disease.

(Source: Hull, J.H. *et al.* (1981).)

Formulae have been devised to relate creatinine clearance to plasma creatinine and body weight, taking into account age and sex. A well-validated example is given in Table 2. Such formulae are most reliable when the GFR is moderately reduced. The calculation assumes constant renal function and the result can be misleading if the patient has suffered a recent depression of glomerular filtration from acute illness.

Sequential measurements of plasma creatinine are used to follow the course of renal failure. The production of creatinine remains fairly constant as renal disease advances, until the terminal stage when anorexia, nausea, and vomiting lead to loss of muscle. As the fall in GFR is frequently linear over time, it is valuable to plot the reciprocal of plasma creatinine versus time, which often yields a declining straight-line relation. In some cases, it may be possible, by extrapolating this plot, to obtain a rough forecast of when endstage renal failure will occur.

Interpretation of plasma urea

Plasma urea varies reciprocally with the GFR, but there are two reasons why urea is an unsatisfactory marker of the filtration rate. First, its clearance is not a constant fraction of the filtration rate, but varies with urine flow, from less than 40 per cent of the rate at low flows to 60 per cent or more during diuresis. Secondly, a number of other (non-renal) factors, affect urea production rate within the liver. Catabolic states or therapy with corticosteroids or tetracyclines will elevate the plasma urea, as will a high dietary intake of protein, or bleeding into the gut. Conversely, urea synthesis is low during periods of low dietary protein intake, or in advanced liver disease.

Simultaneous knowledge of plasma concentrations of both urea and creatinine provide clues as to the possible contributing factors in any disturbance of GFR (Table 3).

Plasma β_2-microglobulin

β_2-Microglobulin is a low molecular weight protein of about 11 800 Da which is a surface constituent of most cells, representing the constant zone of HLA antigens. It is filtered at the glomerulus, reabsorbed almost completely in the renal tubule but catabolized in the process. It is produced at a nearly constant rate, unaffected by diet, so that its plasma concentration usually reflects the GFR. Plasma levels rise as a result of overproduction, in some malignant, immunological,

Table 3 Diagnostic significance of differential changes in plasma urea and creatinine

Plasma urea raised out of proportion to plasma creatinine
Sodium and water depletion
Heart failure
Gastrointestinal haemorrhage
High protein intake (oral or intravenous) in the presence of renal disease
Protein catabolism
corticosteroid therapy
tetracycline in overdose or in presence of renal disease
Following trauma
Pure water depletion (modest effect)
Plasma creatinine raised out of proportion to plasma urea
Some cases of rhabdomyolysis
Drugs that block creatinine secretion (aspirin, co-trimoxazole) or increase creatinine production (penacemide): (modest effect)
Plasma urea depressed out of proportion to plasma creatinine
Pregnancy
Liver failure
High fluid intake
Low protein diet
Plasma urea and creatinine raised in parallel
Chronic renal failure
Established acute renal failure

and hepatic diseases. In the absence of these it is a better guide to changes in the GFR than is plasma creatinine, but is unlikely to replace the latter as its assay is more tedious and expensive than is the automated test for creatinine.

Renal plasma flow

Renal plasma flow can be measured by clearance of paramino hippurate or radio hippurate. The measurement is largely confined to research and is seldom required in clinical practice.

Measurement of urinary concentrating ability

In chronic renal failure, the tubules of surviving nephrons are exposed to an increased osmotic load, partly because the GFR per nephron is increased and partly because the plasma concentration of solutes such as urea, sulphate, and phosphate is elevated. These osmotic effects impair urinary concentration, even if tubular function is preserved in surviving nephrons. Maximal urinary concentration can be related to GFR to deduce whether concentrating ability is disproportionately reduced, indicating tubular disease, but this approach has little practical value.

Indications for performing a concentration test are few outside suspected diabetes insipidus or perhaps analgesic nephropathy. The test is described in Chapter 12.2.

Measurement of urinary acidification

This subject is addressed in Chapter 6.17.

Urinary enzyme excretion

Enzymes present in tubular cells and easily released by injury, may be measured in urine to detect early tubular damage, for instance during exposure to nephorotoxic drugs (e.g. aminoglycoside, cisplatinum) or toxins such as cadmium or chromates. *N*-Acetyl-β-glucosaminidase is most commonly used, measured on a 'spot' urine and expressed per millimole of creatinine. β_2-Microglobulin filtered at the glomerulus and catabolized by healthy tubules may also appear in the urine in excess in tubular disease and provides an alternative.

Radiological investigations

Plain radiographs are still useful in the detection of nephrocalcinosis or radio-opaque calculi. Filling defects in the collecting system and bladder are shown well by intravenous urography, but this approach has been largely replaced by ultrasound or computed tomography (CT) scanning for the detection of abnormalities of renal anatomy and by nuclear techniques or angiography for renal arterial disease.

Contrast-associated nephropathy is a risk in patients with pre-existing renal failure, diabetes mellitus, and multiple myeloma. The risk is shared by arteriography and CT scanning but is reduced by assurance of adequate hydration and plasma volume before the procedure.

Retrograde pyelography/ureterography is useful for determining the site of complete obstruction of a ureter and for visualizing the ureter distal to the obstruction. It is particularly useful in cases of poor renal function where the kidneys and ureter are poorly seen on the intravenous urogram (IVU).

Antegrade ureteropyelography is performed by percutaneous puncture of the renal pelvis under ultrasound guidance to locate the dilated pelvis. Urine is aspirated and contrast injected. A nephrostomy tube may be left *in situ* temporarily as a drainage procedure or to allow measurement of pressure change. This procedure allows visualization of the ureter proximal to an obstruction.

Renal arteriography

The chief use is in the evaluation of renovascular disease. If renal artery stenosis is amenable to transluminal angioplasty, the dilatation (or stenting) can be performed at the same time as the arteriogram.

Other indications include suspected arterial occlusion from thrombus, embolus, dissection or trauma, screening for the aneurysms of polyarteritis nodosa, and when an intrarenal vascular lesion is suspected, as in persistent haematuria following a renal biopsy. CT and magnetic resonance imaging (MRI) scanning have now largely replaced arteriography in the evaluation of renal tumours.

Micturating cystourethrography

The usual purpose of a micturating cystourethrogram is the demonstration of vesicoureteric reflux, but it can also be used to display abnormalities of the bladder neck and urethra. The risk of subsequent urinary infection is substantial and it is sensible to administer an antibacterial for 2 or 3 days after the procedure.

Computed tomography (CT scanning)

CT scanning can reveal abnormalities of the retroperitoneal and perirenal spaces but the prime indications are to detect renal mass lesions and suspected trauma. Simple renal cysts and polycystic renal disease can be equally well diagnosed by ultrasound. CT scanning is also useful in the investigation of retroperitoneal fibrosis. The appearance of the fibrous plaque, which starts below the level of the aortic bifurcation and extends upwards, often enveloping the ureters, can usually be distinguished from lymphoma or sarcoma involving this region.

Magnetic resonance imaging

MRI offers superior soft-tissue contrast in solid renal masses. It is particularly useful in detecting tumour extension into veins. MRI angiography of the renal circulation is yet to be assessed but may have a future role in renovascular disease.

Ultrasonography

Ultrasound is independent of renal function and reveals with considerable accuracy the shape, depth from the surface, and internal architecture of the kidney and upper urinary tract. It generally detects the dilated calyces, pelvis, and ureter of the obstructed kidney, although in the presence of very recent obstruction the calyceal system may not have dilated sufficiently to make a firm diagnosis. Ultrasonography has replaced excretion urography as the screening test for polycystic disease. Perinephric lesions are readily displayed and ultrasonography is the first test for radiolucent calculi.

Nuclear renal imaging

Radionuclides (such as ^{123}I, ^{99}Tc^{m}) can be linked to compounds that depend on either glomerular filtration alone, tubular excretion, or a combination of both. These compounds can therefore provide quantitative information on these functions, in addition to dynamic images.

The main indication is in the investigation of suspected renal arterial disease, with scans best performed after treatment with an angiotensin-converting enzyme (ACE) inhibitor. In the presence of significant renal artery stenosis, glomerular filtration in the ipsilateral kidney depends on angiotensin II mediated efferent arteriolar constriction. ACE inhibition will then reduce filtration rate as glomerular transcapillary hydraulic pressure falls. A radiopharmaceutical, such as [^{99}Tc^{m}]DTPA depends for imaging on glomerular filtration and uptake will then decrease, often dramatically (Fig. 6).

Interpretation of the test depends on comparison of pre- and post-captopril studies, assessing both scintigraphic images and renal time-activity curves. The detection of bilateral renal artery stenosis is more difficult.

Assessment of individual kidney function

Nuclear renal scanning is the only non-invasive way of assessing quantitatively the contribution of each kidney to total renal function. This information is often critically important in conditions that can affect renal function unilaterally, such as reflux nephropathy, nephrolithiasis, and obstruction. Decisions about surgical intervention in such cases should depend on measurements of global GFR, individual kidney function, and sometimes function within an individual kidney (for example, upper and lower moieties of a duplex collecting system).

Renal obstruction

Diuretic renography is the best choice to answer the question of true obstruction versus a dilated but non-obstructed collecting system

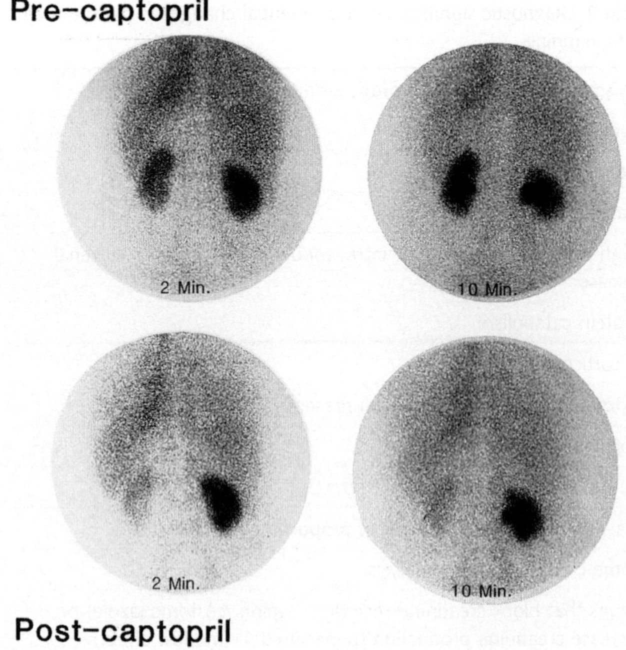

(a)

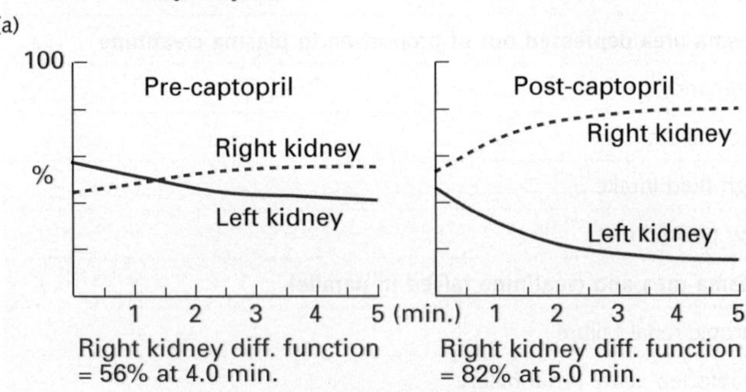

(b)

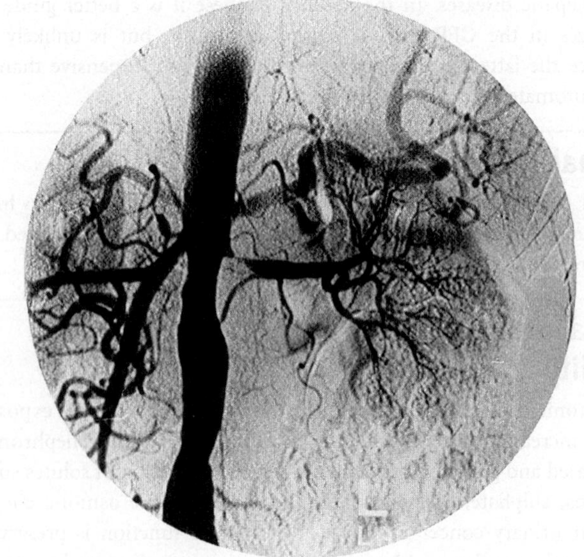

(c)

Fig. 6 (a) [^{99}Tc^{m}]DTPA renal scan, showing a dramatic fall in uptake in the left kidney following captopril administration. (b) Computed differential function of the kidneys showing a dramatic fall in uptake in the left kidney following captopril administration. (c) The renal arteriogram confirms a high-grade stenosis in the left renal artery.

revealed by ultrasound or IVU (see OTM3, pp. 3114–15 and Chapter 12.27).

Renal transplant assessment

Nuclear renal scanning can provide information on graft perfusion and function earlier than changes in blood chemistry. Infarction of the kidney is readily recognized from the scan. In uncomplicated acute tubular necrosis, renal perfusion gradually improves, but if transplant rejection or cyclosporin nephrotoxicity is superimposed, perfusion will deteriorate. Unfortunately, the nuclear renal scan is currently unable to differentiate between acute rejection and cyclosporin nephrotoxicity.

Further reading

Cameron, J.S. and Greger, R. (1998). Renal function and testing of renal function. In: *Oxford textbook of clinical nephrology*, 2nd edn. (ed. A.M. Davison, J.S. Cameron, J.-P. Grünfeld, D.Kerr, E. Ritz, and C. Winearls), pp. 38–69. Oxford University Press, Oxford.

Davison, A.M., Cameron, J.S., Grünfeld, J.-P., Kerr, D., Ritz, E., and Winearls, C. (ed.) (1998). *Oxford textbook of clinical nephrology*, 2nd edn., pp. 93–155. Oxford University Press, Oxford.

Fogazzi, G.B. and Fenili, D. (1998). Urinalysis and microscopy. In: *Oxford textbook of clinical nephrology*, 2nd edn. (ed. A.M. Davison, J.S. Cameron, J.-P. Grünfeld, D.Kerr, E. Ritz, and C. Winearls), pp. 21–38. Oxford University Press, Oxford.

See also OTM3, p. 3115.

Water and electrolyte metabolism

Chapter 12.2

Water and sodium homeostasis and their disorders

P. H. Baylis

Total body water accounts for about 60 per cent of body weight of a healthy adult, of which two-thirds is intracellular and one-third extracellular. The extracellular fluid compartment is divided into the vascular and interstitial fluid compartments, in the ratio 1:2. Thus, for a 75-kg adult, the total body water volume is approximately 45 litres, with intracellular and extracellular volumes of 30 and 15 litres, respectively; the latter comprising the blood (5 litres) and interstitial (10 litres) compartments. Sodium is the main extracellular cation, which with its anion, chloride, contributes 95 per cent of the extracellular solute. The major intracellular cation is potassium. Cell membranes are freely permeable to water but not to most electrolytes, which results in the same total solute but very different electrolyte concentrations in the extracellular and intracellular compartments (Fig. 1).

The measurement of circulating concentrations of electrolytes and glucose approximates closely to their concentrations in interstitial fluid. Total solute concentration assessed by an osmometer, is expressed as the number of osmoles of solute per kilogram (osmolality). Thus, a solution of glucose at 1 mmol/l will provide an osmolality of 1 mosmol/kg but 1 mmol/l solution of salt which dissociates completely in the solvent into its sodium and chloride ions will have an osmolality of 2 mosmol/kg. The assessment of volume, whether intravascular, interstitial, or extracellular, is more difficult and inaccurate.

The physiology of water homeostasis

Normal water balance is achieved by the inter-relationship of three major factors: vasopressin, the kidney, and thirst. Vasopressin acts on the distal renal tubules to allow the re-absorbtion of solute-free water in appropriate circumstances. The kidney is capable of wide variations of urine output, ranging from 0.5 to 20 l/24 h, but most healthy adults excrete 1–2 l/24 h. Osmotically stimulated thirst is important when the kidney is concentrating urine maximally. The extraordinary sensitivity of the function of these three factors allows plasma osmolality to be maintained within the narrow range, 285–295 mosmol/kg (equivalent to serum sodium, 137–142 mmol/l) in healthy adults.

Thirst and water intake

Primary drinking describes the situation in which as the body loses water, the increase in blood osmolality is sensed by osmotically sensitive cells in the brain, which promote thirst. Secondary drinking, which is far more common, occurs for social reasons, habit, or the need to drink with food. For the majority of adults living in temperate climates, secondary drinking ensures a state of mild water excess when water balance is maintained by regulating renal water excretion.

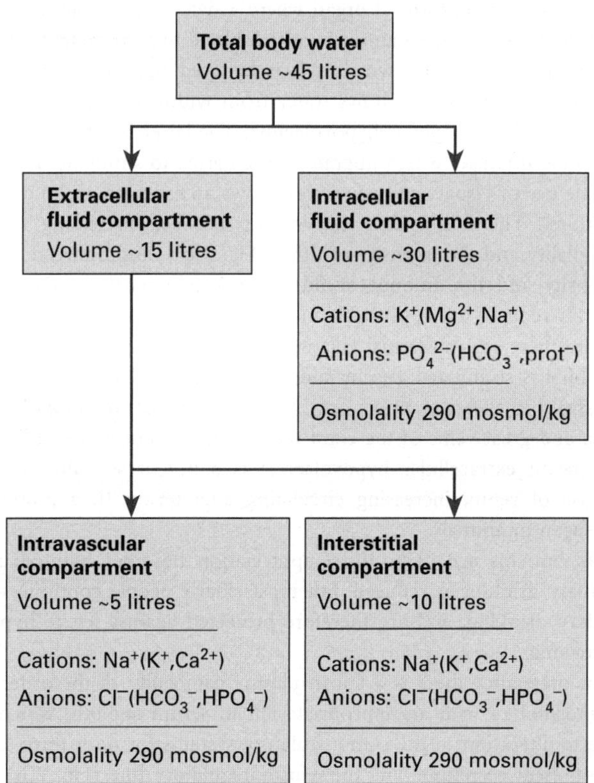

Fig. 1 Composition of body compartments. Body water is distributed uniformly throughout all compartments. Major and some minor (in parentheses) anions and cations are indicated. Osmolality remains the same inside and outside the cell.

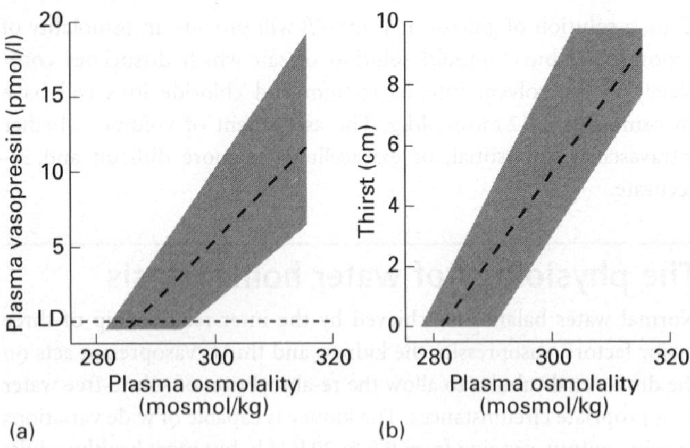

Fig. 2 (a) The relationship between plasma osmolality and plasma vasopressin during infusion of hypertonic (850 mmol/l) saline in healthy adults. There is a linear relationship between the two variables, represented by the dashed line, termed the mean osmoregulatory line for vasopressin secretion. The abscissal intercept of the line represents the threshold for vasopressin secretion, approximately 283 mosmol/kg. LD is the limit of detection of the assay, and the shaded area is the extent of the normal response. (b) The relationship between plasma osmolality and thirst intensity assessed by a visual analogue scale during the same hypertonic infusion. The dashed line is the mean osmoregulatory line for thirst, which has an abscissal intercept (thirst threshold) of 281 mosmol/kg.
*(Adapted from Thompson et al. 1986, Clinical Science, **71**, 651–6, with permission.)*

Osmoreceptors regulating thirst are situated in the anterior hypothalamus, probably in the organum vasculosum of the lamina terminalis or the subfornical organ where a defect in the blood–brain barrier exists. The mechanism by which blood hyperosmolality stimulates thirst is not known, but it is believed that the increase in extracellular osmolality draws water from within the osmoreceptor cells, resulting in cellular hypovolaemia. The latter is translated into neuronal impulses which migrate to the cortex to stimulate thirst.

The use of visual analogue scales allows an estimate of the degree of thirst. There is a clear relationship between increasing blood osmolality and the intensity of thirst (Fig. 2(b)), and between thirst intensity and the amount of fluid drunk to quench it. Drinking quickly reduces thirst, probably mediated by an oropharyngeal reflex before there are substantial falls in blood osmolality.

Thirst is stimulated also by sudden falls in blood volume (and/or pressure) in excess of 15 per cent. Low-pressure baroreceptors in the atria and great veins of the chest mediate the response. In addition, significant extracellular hypovolaemia is a potent stimulus to the release of renin, increasing circulating angiotensin II, a powerful dipsogen in animals.

As humans age, their thirst appreciation becomes blunted and primary drinking is reduced, but most elderly people continue secondary drinking, and are therefore protected against severe hypernatraemia.

In pregnancy there is a fall in plasma osmolality of the order of 10 mosmol/kg with an appropriate fall in serum sodium, which is due to alteration in the osmoregulatory systems for both thirst and vasopressin secretion. The thirst osmoregulatory line (Fig. 2(b)) is displaced to the left and runs parallel, but the abscissal intercept, the osmotic threshold for thirst, is reset to about 275 mosmol/kg. Similar changes occur with the osmoregulatory line for vasopressin secretion (see below).

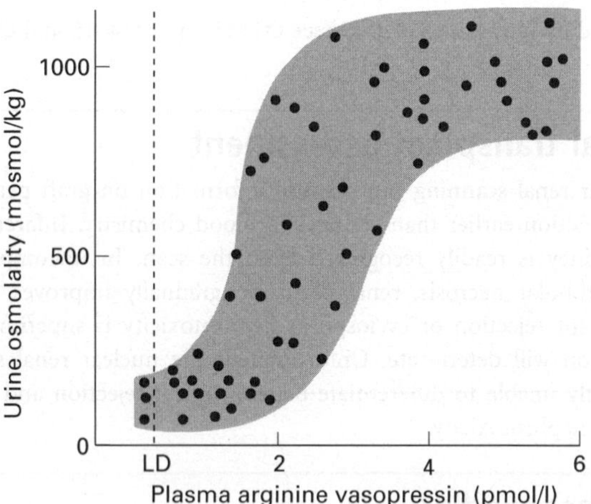

Fig. 3 The effect of vasopressin on urinary concentration during varying states of hydration in humans. Each closed circle represents a single value, and the stippled area the normal range. Values of plasma vasopressin greater than 4 pmol/l fail to increase urinary concentration further. LD is the limit of the assay.

Vasopressin and renal water excretion

Arginine vasopressin is synthesized from a large precursor molecule in the supraoptic and paraventricular nuclei of the hypothalamus, and transported in neurosecretory granules to the posterior pituitary, median eminence of the hypothalamus, and to a lesser extent to other areas of the brain and brain-stem. It is secreted into the systemic circulation from the posterior pituitary to influence renal function; and into the hypothalamopituitary portal circulation to enhance pituitary adrenocorticotrophic hormone (ACTH) secretion.

Control of vasopressin release

Secretion of vasopressin is regulated mainly by changes in blood osmolality, but can also be influenced by non-osmotic factors. The vasopressin osmoreceptors, although probably distinct from the thirst osmoreceptors, are located in the same anterior hypothalamic structures. Rising blood osmolality causes water to flow out of the osmoreceptor cells and the resulting cellular hypovolaemia is believed to initiate a neuronal signal which passes principally to the supraoptic nucleus to stimulate vasopressin secretion. There is an exquisitely sensitive linear relationship between blood osmolality and vasopressin secretion (Fig. 2(a)). The slope of the line is a measure of the sensitivity of the system and the abscissal intercept represents the threshold for vasopressin release. At plasma osmolality values less than 285 mosmol/kg (on average) vasopressin secretion is inhibited to allow a maximum water diuresis (15–20 l/24 h) with urine osmolality of 50–70 mosmol/kg (Fig. 3). Increases in blood osmolality above this threshold induce progressive vasopressin release, so that at plasma vasopressin values of 2–4 pmol/l, maximum antidiuresis occurs.

Individuals have narrowly variable thresholds and sensitivity for both thirst and vasopressin release. Circulating solutes have varying abilities to stimulate the osmoregulatory system, with sodium chloride being the most potent but glucose having little or no effect. In contrast to osmoregulated thirst, there is no blunting of the vasopressin response to osmotic stimulation with ageing. Pregnancy is associated with a lowering of the vasopressin threshold similar to the thirst threshold, which allows osmoregulation to occur about a lower set-point of 275 rather than 285 mosmol/kg.

Non-osmotic release of vasopressin may be influenced by large acute reductions in blood volume or pressure, of the order of 10–15 per cent or more, nausea and/or emesis, hypoglycaemia, and a variety of circulating substances (for example angiotensin II). Low-pressure receptors in the great veins of the chest and cardiac atria mediate the effect of hypovolaemia, while receptors in the arch of the aorta and carotid vessels sense reductions in arterial pressure. The information is carried via the vagus and glossopharyngeal nerves to the brainstem vasomotor centres and is then transmitted to the hypothalamus, principally the paraventricular nucleus. There is an exponential relationship between the fall in blood volume/pressure and vasopressin release, such that large reductions (40 per cent of normal) raise plasma vasopressin to huge values (100–500 pmol/l), which have vasoconstrictor effects. Similarly, high vasopressin concentrations can result from nausea/emesis.

Actions of vasopressin

The major action of vasopressin is to induce urinary concentration (Fig. 3). It binds to a specific V_2 renal tubular receptor on the basolateral membrane of the collecting duct. Adenyl cyclase is stimulated to produce cyclic 5′-adenosine monophosphate (**AMP**), which activates intracellular protein kinases to incorporate the water channels proteins (aquaporins) into the luminal cell membrane. Vasopressin also stimulates the transport of urea across the collecting tubule and of sodium chloride across the medullary thick ascending limb of Henle's loop, both enhancing the osmotic gradient. Renal prostaglandins reduce cyclic 5′-AMP generation, and blunt the effect of vasopressin, so that prostaglandin synthetase inhibitors augment the antidiuretic action of vasopressin. Vasopressin also binds to vascular smooth muscle receptors (V_1 receptors) that increase intracellular calcium concentrations by activation of phosphatidylinositol pathways, to cause vascular muscle contraction. High circulating concentrations are necessary to achieve pressor effects, and at physiological values vasopressin probably plays little, if any, part in maintaining blood pressure. It is, however, involved in the response to hypovolaemia/hypotension.

Vasopressin released from the hypothalamic median eminence acts as a physiological co-secretagogue of ACTH with corticotrophin-releasing factor. It binds to a modified V_1 receptor on the pituitary corticotroph to enhance ACTH release. At high concentrations, It increases circulating concentrations of factor VIII and the von Willebrand factor, by releasing them from vascular endothelium via a V_2 receptor. Specific V_2 agonists (for example, desmopressin) are used to improve haemostasis in mild haemophilia A and in von Willebrand's disease, and can be helpful in uraemic bleeding.

Physiology of sodium homeostasis

Changes in sodium balance result in alterations in blood and interstitial volumes (Fig. 1) but rarely in sodium concentration. The reason is that a rise in sodium concentration normally leads transiently to thirst, increased water intake and to vasopressin secretion to reduce renal water excretion. Extracellular osmolality is then conserved at the expense of volume.

Sodium intake

There is little regulation of sodium intake in humans, which in Western countries, is in gross excess for needs, at about 100–200 mmol/24 h. There is little sodium loss from the healthy bowel and in temperate climates sweating is minimal (sweat sodium concentration is 40–50 mmol/l). Thus, most people are in a state of potential sodium excess, which is prevented by the normal kidney but which leads commonly to salt retention in renal failure.

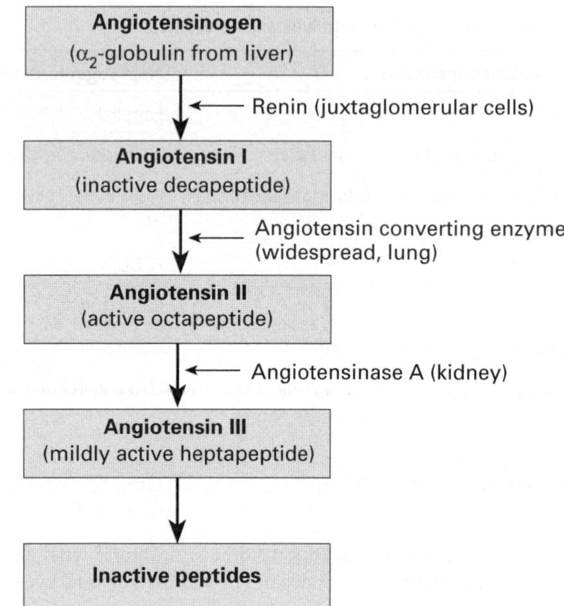

Fig. 4 The renin–angiotensin–aldosterone system. The enzyme, renin, secreted by juxtaglomerular cells of the renal afferent arterioles, acts to produce angiotensin I (inactive). The active peptides, angiotensin II and III are potent vasoconstrictors and stimulate aldosterone secretion from the adrenal cortex to expand blood volume and raise blood pressure.

Control of renal sodium excretion

Sodium balance is maintained largely by the kidneys, which are capable of excreting a very wide range of sodium, 1–500 mmol/24 h. The glomerular filtration rate of normal kidneys is 170 l/24 h, the filtrate containing some 140 mmol of sodium/l. Most of the filtered sodium is reabsorbed iso-osmotically by the proximal tubule (60–75 per cent), the remainder being reabsorbed in the medullary thick ascending limb of Henle's loop and the distal nephron, where the fine adjustment of sodium balance is largely regulated. A glomerulotubular feedback mechanism operates at the single nephron level to maintain a balance between the reabsorptive function of each nephron and the amount of sodium and fluid filtered by the glomerulus.

Renin–angiotensin–aldosterone system

Reductions of renal perfusion pressure increase renin secretion directly while baroreceptors within the great veins of the chest influence renin secretion via the sympathetic nerves. Renin catalyses the conversion of angiotensinogen to angiotensin I (Fig. 4), which, in turn, is converted into the highly active octapeptide angiotensin II. The activity of angiotensin III is about 30 per cent that of angiotensin II. These peptides influence extracellular sodium content and volume in a number of ways. Angiotensin II, which acts both locally and systemically, is a potent vasoconstrictor which readily increases systemic blood pressure, stimulates the secretion of aldosterone from the adrenal cortex to enhance sodium reabsorption in the distal nephron, stimulates thirst, and is involved in the glomerulotubular feedback mechanism.

Table 1 Causes of the polyuria–polydipsia syndromes

Cranial diabetes insipidus	Nephrogenic diabetes insipidus	Primary polydipsia
Familial	Familial	Familial
Dominant (rarely recessive) inheritance	X-linked recessive inheritance	Psychogenic (compulsive water drinking)
*DIDMOAD or Wolfram syndrome (autosomal recessive)	Autosomal recessive inheritance	Psychotic (schizophrenia, mania)
Acquired	Acquired	Idiopathic
Idiopathic	Idiopathic	Secondary
Trauma (neurosurgery, head injury)	Metabolic (hypercalcaemia, hypokalaemia)	Granuloma (sarcoid)
Neoplasia (craniopharyngioma, germinoma, pinealoma, hypothalamic metastasis, large pituitary tumour)	Vascular (sickle-cell disease)	Vasculitis
Infection (meningitis, encephalitis)	Osmotic diuresis (glycosuria, postobstructive uropathy)	Multiple sclerosis
Vascular (sickle-cell anaemia, aneurysms of anterior communicating artery, Sheehan's syndrome)	Chronic renal disease (renal failure, amyloid, sarcoidosis, pyelonephritis)	Drugs (phenothiazines, tricyclic antidepressants)
Granuloma (sarcoid)	Drugs (lithium, demeclocycline, amphotericin, glibenclamide, methoxyfluorane)	

*DIDMOAD: diabetes insipidus, diabetes mellitus, optic atrophy, deafness.

Atrial natriuretic peptide

α-Atrial natriuretic peptide, is synthesized and secreted primarily by cardiac atrial myocytes. Moderate increases in blood volume and postural changes influence its release, probably mediated by direct distension. The most important actions are on the kidney. At physiological concentrations it causes a modest natriuresis, minimal diuresis, and reduces plasma renin activity and plasma aldosterone concentration. It is also a vasodilator and reduces systolic blood pressure and cardiac contractility. Specific receptors have been identified in the kidney, on cortical glomeruli, the inner medulla, the vasa recta in the outer medulla, and the collecting duct.

It is likely that other natriuretic factors exist and there are numerous intrarenal factors that may influence sodium excretion. Local production of dopamine appears to augment natriuresis following increased dietary sodium intake. Prostaglandins, particularly prostaglandin E_2, inhibit sodium transport in the medullary thick ascending limb. The role of the renal kallikrein–kinin system is less clear.

Disorders of water and salt homeostasis

Polyuric states

Cranial diabetes insipidus

Cranial diabetes insipidus is due to decreased secretion of vasopressin. At least 80 per cent of vasopressin-synthesizing neurones must be destroyed before overt clinical features become manifest.

Aetiology

The causes are given in Table 1. Familial cases are very rare, and, in some incidences, are due to point mutations or deletions in the vasopressin gene. About 30 per cent of cases are idiopathic, of which a third have circulating antibodies to the hypothalamic neurones that produce vasopressin. Trauma to the hypothalamus or pituitary stalk is a frequent cause. After head injury, some patients follow a triple-phase response, characterized by initial polyuria for a few hours or days, followed by antidiuresis for a variable period, which progresses to permanent polyuria. Primary pituitary tumours rarely cause cranial diabetes insipidus.

Clinical features

The major clinical manifestations are polyuria, nocturia, and excessive thirst. Children may present with enuresis. In most patients the deficiency of vasopressin is partial. Urine volumes range between 3 and 20 l/24 h with random urine osmolalities less than 300 mosmol/kg. Plasma osmolality and serum sodium are usually maintained within the normal ranges because of intact osmoregulated thirst but coincident defective thirst leads to hypernatraemia and hyperosmolality. With severe polyuria the slightest urinary tract outflow obstruction can lead to hydronephrosis and hydroureter. Cranial diabetes insipidus may be masked by glucocorticoid deficiency due either to hypopituitarism or primary adrenal failure, because cortisol is necessary for the maximal diluting function of the distal nephron. Symptoms are often worsen in pregnancy due to the increase in metabolic clearance of arginine vasopressin.

Nephrogenic diabetes insipidus

In this condition the renal tubules are totally, or more often, partially, resistant to the action of vasopressin.

Aetiology

Table 1 outlines the causes. The X-linked recessive disorder is rare but very severe. Males express symptoms while females have only slightly impaired urinary concentration. Different gene mutations between families are responsible for abnormal renal V_2 receptors and loss of cyclic 5′-AMP generation. A subgroup of patients can activate adenyl cyclase but fail to stimulate intracellular events that open water channels. Congenital nephrogenic diabetes insipidus can result from genetic mutations of the aquaporins (water channel proteins) which cause an autosomal recessive form of the disorder.

Hypercalcaemia-induced nephrogenic diabetes insipidus is due in part to reduced medullary hyperosmolality and adenyl cyclase stimulation, and in part to calcium deposition with scarring of the kidney. Sustained hypokalaemia inhibits sodium–potassium co-transport in the thick ascending limb; reduces adenyl cyclase activity; increases intrarenal prostaglandin synthesis, which blunts vasopressin's antidiuretic effect; and may reduce intracellular protein kinase function.

A third of patients taking long-term lithium carbonate develop nephrogenic diabetes insipidus. Lithium blunts the generation and action of cyclic 5′-AMP in the distal nephron and may reduce osmoregulated vasopressin secretion and/or stimulate thirst. Demeclocycline also inhibits cyclic 5′-AMP generation and function.

Clinical features

Nephrogenic diabetes insipidus in adults is usually partial, with mild symptoms. Serum sodium and plasma osmolality are within the normal range, but urine osmolality is low (<300 mosmol/kg).

Primary polydipsia

Many of these patients have a psychological disturbance leading to compulsive drinking, some of whom have a lowered osmotic thirst threshold but a normal threshold for vasopressin release. Very rarely a structural hypothalamic lesion (such as sarcoidosis) is believed to be the cause of primary polydipsia (Table 1). Some drugs stimulate thirst.

Clinical features

The clinical manifestations are similar to those of cranial and nephrogenic diabetes insipidus but nocturia is less of a feature. Some may drink at a rate faster than their kidneys can excrete free water, when serum sodium tends to be lower than that of patients with cranial and nephrogenic diabetes insipidus, but many patients can drink up to 20 l/24 h and still remain normonatraemic.

Diagnostic evaluation of polyuric patients

Urine output less than 3 l/24 h with a normal serum sodium and plasma osmolality excludes significant disturbance of water balance. Plasma of glucose, calcium, and potassium concentrations should be measured. Diagnostic tests comprise: dehydration tests, measurement of plasma vasopressin after dehydration or osmotic stimulation, and a therapeutic trial of desmopressin.

Dehydration tests

These are useful in the diagnosis of severe forms of cranial and nephrogenic diabetes insipidus. The test starts in the morning. Basal samples of urine (volume and osmolality) and blood (plasma osmolality) are taken and the patient weighed. Fluid is then withheld for 8 h with regular 1–2 hourly urine and blood samples and weighing of the patient. Thereafter, 2 μg of desmopressin is injected intramuscularly. Urine samples are collected over the subsequent 16 h. This test should be stopped if there is a weight loss in excess of 5 per cent.

A guide to interpretation of the results is given in Table 2. A major difficulty arises in the differentiation of the partial diabetes insipidus disorders from each other and from primary polydipsia in which prolonged polyuria leads to a reduction in maximal renal concentrating ability by removing renal medullary interstitial solute. Direct measurement of plasma vasopressin aids diagnosis in these circumstances.

Table 2 Interpretation of results from the water deprivation–desmopressin test

Urine osmolality (mosmol/kg)		
After dehydration	**After desmopressin**	**Diagnosis**
>750	>750	Normal*
<300	>750	CDI
<300	<300	NDI
300–750	<750	Partial CDI or
		Partial NDI or PP

*Assumes that plasma osmolality remains in the normal reference range, 285–295 mosmol/kg.

CDI, cranial diabetes insipidus; NDI, nephrogenic diabetes insipidus; PP, primary polydipsia.

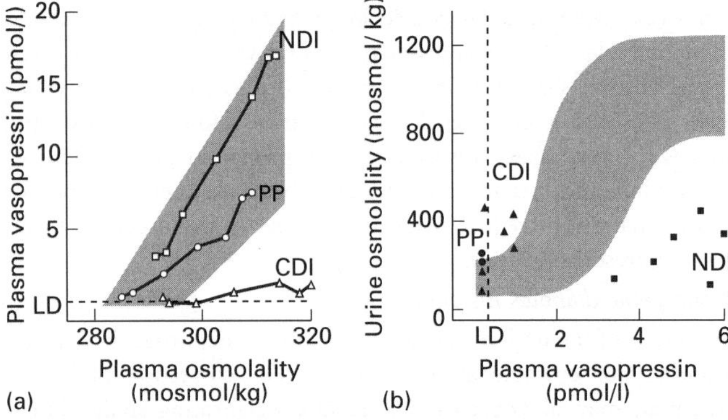

Fig. 5 (a) Relationship between plasma vasopressin and plasma osmolality during hypertonic saline infusion in typical patients with (i) cranial diabetes insipidus (CDI), (ii) nephrogenic diabetes insipidus (NDI), and (iii) primary polydipsia (PP). The shaded area represents the normal response. (b) Relationship between urine osmolality and plasma vasopressin in patients with CDI (▲;), NDI (■;), and PP (●) after a period of dehydration. The shaded area is the normal relationship under various degrees of hydration. LD represents the limit of detection of the plasma vasopressin assay.

Plasma vasopressin response to osmotic stimulation and dehydration

Measurement of plasma vasopressin and osmolality during a 2-h hypertonic (850 mmol/l) saline infusion at a rate of 0.04 ml/kg per min will diagnose precisely partial and compete cranial diabetes insipidus, as the vasopressin response to osmotic stimulation is subnormal (Fig. 5(a)). Patients with nephrogenic diabetes insipidus or primary polydipsia have results that fall within the normal range. After a period of water deprivation, the measurement of urine osmolality and plasma vasopressin will define nephrogenic diabetes insipidus (Fig. 5(b)), as vasopressin will be inappropriately elevated with respect to the low urine osmolality.

Therapeutic trial of desmopressin

If the water deprivation–desmopressin test gives equivocal results and facilities to measure vasopressin are not available, a formal therapeutic trial of desmopressin should be undertaken. Because of the potential hazard of severe water intoxication in primary polydipsia patients, the trial must be supervised in hospital. After a basal period of 3–4 days, desmopressin (1–2 μg, intramuscularly) is administered and weight urine and plasma osmolalities or serum sodium and urine volume are measured daily. Patients with cranial diabetes insipidus will be identified by a reduction of thirst, little or no weight gain, a reduction in urine flow, and normal plasma osmolality. Nephrogenic diabetes insipidus is characterized by lack of response. Those with primary polydipsia remain thirsty, continue to drink, gain weight, and become progressively hyponatraemic.

Treatment

Cranial diabetes insipidus

Mild cranial diabetes insipidus (urine volume <4 l/24 h) may only require advice to drink sufficient quantities to quench thirst. In more severe forms, the drug of choice is desmopressin, a synthetic vasopressin V_2 receptor agonist, possessing potent antidiuretic but no pressor activity, with a prolonged duration of action. It is administered intranasally by spray or tube, parenterally or orally. There are wide variations in the intranasal dose required to control symptoms, ranging between 5 and 80 μg daily. The oral dose is 100–1000 μg. Dilutional hyponatraemia can be avoided by omitting the drug 1 day each week. Desmopressin is safe in pregnancy, and is resistant to circulating placental vasopressinase. Lysine vasopressin, also given intranasally, is a shorter-acting alternative, but its pressor activity may cause intestinal and/or renal colic, increase blood pressure, and induces coronary artery vasospasm. Chlorpropamide, clofibrate, carbamazepine, and thiazide diuretics have been used, either singly or in combination, to reduce urine volume by up to 50 per cent, but are now prescribed rarely.

Nephrogenic diabetes insipidus

Correction of the underlying cause of acquired nephrogenic diabetes insipidus (for example, removal of drug or correction of hypercalcaemia) may allow recovery of renal concentrating ability, but it may take a number of weeks to resolve. Polyuria of the severe familial can be reduced by about 50 per cent using the combination of thiazide and/or amiloride diuretics with a prostaglandin synthetase inhibitor.

Primary polydipsia

There is no efficacious treatment but therapy directed towards underlying psychiatric problems may prove helpful.

Hyponatraemic states

Hyponatraemia, defined as a serum sodium less than 130 mmol/l, is a common electrolyte disturbance, affecting up to 5 per cent of hospital patients. Severe hyponatraemia (serum sodium <115 mmol/l) is rare.

Pseudohyponatraemia

Spuriously low measurements of sodium can be reported in patients with very high circulating concentrations of lipids or proteins because the volume of either contributes substantially to serum volume, but plasma osmolality is normal. The mechanism is different in severe hyperglycaemia which draws intracellular water into the extracellular space. Plasma osmolality is then elevated due to the high blood glucose.

Classification and causes of hyponatraemia

In all hyponatraemic states there is an excess of water relative to sodium, but the absolute sodium content may be high, normal, or low, resulting in excess, near normal, or reduced extracellular fluid and plasma volumes. In other than gross cases, volume status is difficult to assess clinically. Table 3 presents the pathogenesis, provides some examples of causes, and emphasizes the importance of measuring urinary sodium in the three types of hyponatraemia. In the majority of patients urine osmolalities are in excess of 300 mosmol/kg.

Large non-renal sodium losses result in the healthy kidney conserving sodium to urinary concentrations less than 10 mmol/l, and as low as 1 mmol/l. Renal losses can be due to renal diseases (analgesic nephropathy, chronic pyelonephritis, polycystic kidneys, recovery from acute tubular necrosis or after bilateral ureteric obstruction), mineralocorticoid deficiency (Addison's disease, hyporeninaemic hypoaldosteronism), or diuretic excess.

Normovolaemic hyponatraemia is usually due to the syndrome of inappropriate antidiuresis (**SIAD**; see below) or inappropriate administration of intravenous fluid in the postoperative period, and rarely to isolated glucocorticoid deficiency or severe prolonged hypothyroidism. Some individuals drink excessive volumes over short periods, for example 10 litres in 6 h, which overwhelms the kidney's capacity to excrete water.

Hypervolaemic hyponatraemia is common in severe heart failure, decompensated cirrhosis, and nephrotic syndrome when the kidney's ability to excrete free water is much reduced.

Clinical features

There may be evidence of extracellular volume depletion but some clinical manifestations are due to hyponatraemia *per se* (Table 4). The severity of these depend upon partly the actual sodium concentration and partly its rate of fall. Chronic mild hyponatraemia (serum sodium 120–130 mmol/l) is often totally asymptomatic; but a fall to only 125 mmol/l from normal values over a few hours can cause convulsions.

General principles of management

Therapy for mild hyponatraemia is often not necessary, but attention to the underlying cause frequently corrects the serum sodium concentration. In hypovolaemic hyponatraemia infusion of isotonic saline is usually sufficient, but occasionally intravascular volume expanders are required. Immediate hydrocortisone as well as intravenous saline and subsequently fludrocortisone are essential to treat Addison's disease. The treatment of normovolaemic hyponatraemia is discussed below. The approach to hyponatraemia associated with hypervolaemia is to give potent diuretics and to restrict water to less than 1 l/24 h. In cardiac failure, but not in cirrhosis, there may be benefit from angiotensin-converting enzyme inhibitors.

Acute severe hyponatraemia and myelinolysis

There is a high morbidity and mortality in patients in whom the plasma sodium concentration has fallen below 110 mmol/l, particularly when it has done so acutely. Although the underlying cause of such a change may be water intoxication from primary polydipsia in psychotic patients, or a combination of water excess and the use of amiloride-containing diuretics, the most common and always avoidable cause is iatrogenic ill-advised postoperative fluid administration. Modest hyponatraemia is common postoperatively and there are now more than 50 reports of symptomatic hyponatraemia after elective surgery in previously healthy women, all of whom died from the neurological sequelae. In the state of water intoxication, early symptoms include headache, nausea, vomiting, and later drowsiness proceeding to confusion, stupor, fits, respiratory arrest, and death.

An hyponatraemic patient with neurological features requires urgent treatment; but over-rapid correction of the sodium concentration by whatever means can result in a different, but equally severe, neurological syndrome due to local areas of demyelination, called central pontine myelinolysis or the osmotic demyelination syndrome. Features include quadriparesis, respiratory arrest, pseudobulbar palsy,

Table 3 Classification of hyponatraemia

	Hypovolaemia: deficit of *TBW; larger deficit of *ExNa		Normovolaemia; normal or slight excess of TBW	Hypervolaemia: excess of ExNa; larger excess of TBW	
	Renal loss	**Non-renal loss**		**Renal loss**	**Non-renal loss**
Aetiology (examples)	Mineralocorticoid deficiency	Vomiting	Syndrome of inappropriate antidiuresis	Acute and chronic renal failure	Cardiac failure
	Sodium-losing renal disorders	Diarrhoea	Glucocorticoid deficiency		Cirrhosis
	Diuretic excess	Burns	Hypothyroidism		Nephrotic syndrome
		Excessive sweating	Inappropriate IV therapy (5% glucose)		Inappropriate IV therapy(normal saline)
			'Sick-cell' concept		
Urinary sodium concentration (mmol/l)	>20	<10	>20	>20	<10

*TBW, total body water; ExNa, extracellular sodium; IV, intravenous.

Table 4 Clinical features of hyponatraemia

Mild	Moderate	Severe
Anorexia	Personality change	Drowsiness
Headache	Muscle cramps	Diminished reflexes
Nausea	Muscle weakness	Convulsions
Vomiting	Confusion	Coma
Lethargy	Ataxia	Death

Table 5 Criteria for the diagnosis of the syndrome of inappropriate antidiuresis

Dilutional hyponatraemia, i.e. plasma hypo-osmolality proportional to hyponatraemia
Urine osmolality greater than plasma osmolality (usually)
Persistent renal sodium excretion (>50 mmol/l)
Absence of hypotension, hypovolaemia, and oedema-forming states
Normal renal and adrenal function

mutism, and, rarely, fits. The distribution of demyelination includes most often the pons, but also, the basal ganglia, internal capsule, lateral geniculate body, and even the cerebral cortex. Death may result.

This condition usually arises 24–48 h after over-rapid correction of profound hyponatraemia, and probably results from large shifts of intracellular water consequent on rapid changes in osmotic gradient between cells and extracellular fluid. Because of adaptations to chronic hyponatraemia resulting in reduced osmolality in brain cells, myelinolysis is particularly a risk when treatment of severe hyponatraemia is delayed for more than 24 h. A number of guidelines to the management of this dangerous clinical state have been proposed. All depend on a more or less rapid rate of infusion of physiological or hypertonic saline with the following caveats.

(1) The plasma sodium concentration should not rise by more than 10–12 mmol/l per 24 h or 25 mmol/l in the first 48 h in chronic hyponatraemia, defined as hyponatraemia lasting >3 days.

(2) When the fall is known to have occurred within 12–24 h it is safe to correct more quickly than if the hyponatraemia is more chronic.

Syndrome of inappropriate antidiuresis

Inappropriate secretion of vasopressin is the most common cause of normovolaemic hyponatraemia, and accounts for about 50 per cent of all hyponatraemia. The diagnosis is established by ensuring that all the criteria of SIAD are fulfilled (Table 5). Too often only the first two criteria are met, leading to overdiagnosis. Measurement of urinary sodium is essential, which is persistently elevated (50–70 mmol/l). The final two criteria help to exclude hypo- and hypervolaemic states. Plasma vasopressin estimations are unhelpful in differentiating SIAD from other causes of hyponatraemia, because the majority of all hyponatraemic states (>90 per cent) have detectable or elevated values, due to non-osmotic release of the hormone.

Pathophysiology and causes of syndrome of inappropriate antidiuresis

A very large number of disorders has been associated with SIAD. They include a variety of neoplasic conditions, the most common being small-cell carcinoma of bronchus; non-malignant chest diseases including infections; neurological disorders (infective and vascular); drugs (cytotoxic agents, chlorpropamide, carbamazepine, antidepressants, oxytocin, and thiazide diuretics); and a miscellaneous group (porphyria, cortisol deficiency, idiopathic). The persistent natriuresis can be explained by the expanded total body-water producing a reduction in aldosterone production, an increase in circulating natriuretic factors, and a decrease in proximal sodium reabsorption.

Treatment of syndrome of inappropriate antidiuresis

Identification and successful treatment of the underlying cause will usually correct the hyponatraemia. Only in cases of chronic symptomatic or life-threatening hyponatraemia are specific measures required. Fluid restriction to 500 ml/24 h may increase serum sodium to about 130 mmol/l. If this is unsuccessful, the best approach is the induction of partial nephrogenic diabetes insipidus with demeclocycline (600–1200 mg daily in divided doses) but maximal effect may take 2 weeks to achieve. It is preferable to lithium carbonate

Table 6 Classification and causes of hypernatraemia

Hypervolaemic (excess extracellular sodium)
Accidental (salt emetics, infant feeds)
Iatrogenic (e.g. infusion of hypertonic bicarbonate or saline)
Hypovolaemic (insufficient total body water)
Decreased water intake
Hypo- or adipsia
Neoplasia of the hypothalamopituitary region
Vascular (anterior communicating artery aneurysm)
Granuloma (sarcoidosis, Langerhans cell histiocytosis)
Miscellaneous (trauma, hydrocephalus, ventricular cyst)
Reduced access to water
Travel in desert
Limitation of movement (stroke)
Coma
Acute excessive fluid loss
Gastrointestinal
Burns

which is more toxic. An alternative is the administration of frusemide (40–80 mg daily) in combination with oral sodium chloride supplementation (3 g daily). Phenytoin has occasionally proved helpful by suppressing inappropriate neurohypophysial vasopressin secretion. Infusion of isotonic or hypertonic solutions of saline are not advised because of the danger of rapid serum sodium increases causing osmotic demyelination syndrome (see above). Linear non-peptide vasopressin renal receptor antagonists are being developed.

Sick-cell concept

Hyponatraemia may develop quickly in severe trauma or overwhelming infection and in malnourished very ill patients. It is a normovolaemic state. It has been suggested that there is a shift of intracellular water into the extracellular compartment due to reduction of intracellular solute by either leakage across damaged cell membranes or enhanced intracellular catabolism, or possibly due to movement of sodium into the cell. There is no specific therapy.

Hypernatraemic states and thirst deficiency

Hypernatraemia is less common than hyponatraemia and may be defined by a serum sodium greater than 150 mmol/l (Table 6). Hypervolaemic hypernatraemia is caused by extracellular sodium excess, usually as a result of iatrogenic overdoses of sodium-containing preparations. Acute hypovolaemic hypernatraemia occurs when patients lose large quantities of hypotonic fluid. Chronic hypovolaemic hypernatraemia is the result of prolonged water deficit, usually the result of impaired or absent thirst. Diabetes insipidus may be present. The most serious cases arise from destruction of osmoreceptors both for vasopressin and for thirst. Serum sodium concentrations then may reach as high as 190 mmol/l and vary day to day considerably.

Clinical features

Hypervolaemic hypernatraemia causes severe thirst, irritability, hypotonia, and may lead to convulsions, seizures, and death. Symptoms of hypovolaemic hypernatraemia relate to extracellular and intracellular fluid loss, and the striking feature is lack of thirst. The slow development of hypernatraemia is often associated with minimal symptoms of confusion or drowsiness.

Treatment

In patients with chronic hypernatraemia, sodium concentration should be lowered only slowly with the rate of fall no faster than 10 mmol/24 h. The safest approach is with extra water by mouth, but unconscious patients require infusion of 5 per cent dextrose solutions. Patients with total loss of thirst and vasopressin osmoregulation pose major problems. They should be instructed to drink a daily volume of about 2 litres which is adjusted according to changes in daily body weight. Desmopressin may be required. Regular checks of serum sodium are essential to avoid wide fluctuations. Constant vigilance is necessary.

Further reading

Arieff, A.I. (1993). Management of hyponatraemia. *British Medical Journal*, **307**, 305–8.

Baylis, P.H. (1996). Disorders of water balance. In *Clinical endocrinology*, (2nd edn), (ed. A. Grossman), pp. 265–78. Blackwell Science, Oxford.

Ellis, S.J. (1995). Severe hyponatraemia: complications and treatment. *Quarterly Journal of Medicine*, **88**, 905–9.

Fried, L.F. and Palevsky, P.M. (1997). Hyponatraemia and hypernatraemia. *Medical Clinics of North America*, **81**, 585–609.

King, L.S. and Agre, P. Pathophysiology of the aquaporin water channels. *Annual Review of Physiology*, **58**, 619–48.

Robertson, G.L. (1995). Diabetes insipidus. Clinical disorders of fluid and electrolyte metabolism. *Endocrinology and Metabolism Clinics of North America*, **24**, 549–72.

Sterns, R.H., Spital, A., and Clark, E.C. (1996). Disorders of water balance. In *Fluids and electrolytes*, (3rd edn), (ed. J.P. Kokko and R.L. Tannen), pp 63–109. W. B. Saunders Company, Philadelphia.

Chapter 12.3

Idiopathic oedema of women

J. G. G. Ledingham

Fluid retention unrelated to cardiac, hepatic, renal, allergic, hypoproteinaemic, obstructive venous, or lymphatic disease, and occurring in the absence of sodium-retaining drugs occurs not uncommonly in women and has been labelled idiopathic oedema, cyclical oedema, or periodic oedema.

Clinical features

The cardinal features are of episodic or more constant fluid retention, aggravated by standing, with diurnal weight fluctuations exceeding 1.4 kg/day and day-to-day weight changes sometimes as much as 4–5 kg. During periods of weight gain, urine volumes may be as low as 300–500 ml/24 h, containing minimal amounts (1–20 mmol/l) of sodium. The retained fluid accumulates in the face, hands, breasts, thighs, buttocks, and tissues of the abdominal wall. Rings do not fit over the swollen fingers and the expansion in waist and breast measurements results in some sufferers keeping two sizes of brassiere. Pitting ankle oedema is uncommon but may be observed after prolonged standing. Orthopnoea and pulmonary oedema are rare complications. Constipation is common. Episodes may occur unpredictably, but emotional stress, obesity, food high in carbohydrate, as well as prolonged standing, are recognized triggers.

The condition occurs only after menarche, is seen more often in the third and fourth decade but may persist with amenorrhoea, after oophorectomy, and may continue after the menopause. Sufferers are characteristically emotionally labile and are prone to neurosis and depression. Extreme physical and mental lethargy is usual and the patient's misery during periods of retention is aggravated by the sense of bloated ugliness and distortion of appearance that she feels. Most, but not all, find access to diuretics. Hypokalaemic hypochloraemic alkalosis with hyperuricaemia may reflect diuretic abuse, and rare patients abuse purgatives as well.

Pathophysiology

There is no strong consensus of opinion about pathophysiology. There is a subset in whom overconcern with weight and appearance leads to diuretic abuse and rebound oedema when diuretics are stopped. Some of this group have features in common with anorexia nervosa. Diuretics cannot be the whole story as cases were described before potent agents became available and because withdrawal of diuretics in hospital over 2–3 weeks reverses the condition in only a few patients.

No good evidence exists of primary abnormalities in the renin–angiotensin–aldosterone system, nor in the metabolism of oestrogens or progestogens. Hyperprolactinaemia, dopamine deficiency, and high plasma adenosine monophosphate have been described in a few cases, but it is unlikely that these changes are of aetiological significance. There is evidence of an orthostatic leak of plasma volume and plasma proteins into the tissue fluids; the increase in venous blood haematocrit on standing is greater than normal, and reflects a fall in plasma volume which initiates renal salt and water retention. Diurnal weight gains amounting to 4–5 kg must reflect an abnormally high fluid intake during periods of fluid retention. The mechanism of the presumed increase in capillary permeability is unknown.

Management

Sympathetic explanation of the nature of the problem may help. Patients should be advised to avoid long periods of standing and to use supine rest to relieve oedema instead of diuretics whenever possible. Elastic stockings, put on before getting up, help to reduce the orthostatic loss of plasma volume. Obesity increases the tendency to fluid retention and some women associate exacerbation with an increase in dietary carbohydrate. Diuretics, by further decreasing an already reduced plasma volume, are an illogical treatment and should be used as sparingly as possible; but many patients' symptoms are unacceptable without some diuretic treatment. Resistance develops quickly and many patients are very difficult to wean from massive doses of loop agents, often combined with amiloride or spironolactone. Psychotherapy may help the neurotic and depressive traits but is of no proven benefit in reducing the frequency or severity of episodes of oedema. Drugs have little to offer in this condition.

Further reading

Edwards, O.M. and Bayliss, R.I.S. (1976). Idiopathic oedema of women. *Quarterly Journal of Medicine*, **45**, 125–44.

Gill, J.R. (1983). Idiopathic edema. *Seminars in Nephrology*, **3**, 205–20.

Chapter 12.4

Disorders of potassium metabolism

J. G. G. Ledingham

Physiological considerations

Potassium is present in cells in a concentration between 150 and 160 mmol/l. Total body potassium ranges between 37 and 52 mmol/kg body weight depending very largely on muscle mass, so that amounts are greater in the young than the old and in men than in women. Ninety-eight per cent of potassium is intracellular, the ratio of the intracellular to the extracellular components being a critical determinant of the membrane potential of excitable tissues. The movement of potassium into cells and the maintenance of the consequently large concentration gradient is chiefly dependent on Na-K ATPase, which extrudes sodium and takes in potassium in a ratio of 3:2. This active transport into cells is normally balanced by passive losses, largely through ion-selective potassium channels present in all cell membranes.

Dietary potassium intake in Western society normally varies between 50 and 150 mmol/day, but homeostasis can be maintained with intakes as high as 500 mmol/day. In normal circumstances, the kidney is the only important route of excretion, with only some 5–15 mmol appearing daily in the stools.

The plasma potassium concentration (normally 3.5–4.5 mmol/l) is regulated by mechanisms controlling internal as well as external balance. External balance, which determines total body potassium, is largely controlled by the kidney but with a small and sometimes important contribution by the gut. Internal balance determines the proportions of intracellular and extracellular potassium under the influence of pH, bicarbonate, aldosterone, insulin, adrenergic stimuli, glucagon, and osmolality.

Internal balance

pH and bicarbonate

The ratio of intracellular to extracellular potassium is influenced by pH and plasma bicarbonate concentrations separately, with a rise in either increasing intracellular at the expense of extracellular potassium. The hyperkalaemia of acidosis has long been attributed to an exchange of hydrogen for potassium in cells, but inhibition of the Na-K ATPase by acidosis, although countered by an associated reduction in the conductance of potassium to cell membranes, must also contribute. The degree of change in plasma potassium depends on the cause of the associated change in pH. A metabolic hyperchloraemic acidosis may increase plasma potassium by some 0.7 mmol/l for each 0.1 unit fall in pH, whereas the change associated with respiratory acidosis is considerably less, about 0.1 mmol/l per 0.1 unit change of pH. In most states of acidosis there is hyperkalaemia or at least a high plasma potassium concentration in relation to external balance; but hyperkalaemia is not a feature of post-ictal lactic acidosis.

Aldosterone

A rise in plasma potassium stimulates aldosterone secretion and a fall retards it. Although the major contribution of aldosterone in protecting against hyperkalaemia is to increase renal and, to a much lesser extent, colonic potassium excretion, it is possible that aldosterone also affects internal potassium balance; the adrenal is essential for the phenomenon whereby acute potassium loads are taken up by cells after a high potassium diet (potassium adaptation).

Insulin and glucagon

An increase in plasma potassium stimulates insulin release which might induce a net uptake of potassium into cells. High concentrations of insulin given intravenously certainly lower plasma potassium by promoting uptake into the liver and muscle but the much lower concentrations of endogenous insulin have not yet been proven to influence internal potassium balance significantly. Tolerance of potassium loads is impaired in insulin-deficient diabetics and in normal subjects infused with somatostatin, suggesting at least a permissive role for insulin in the regulation of cellular uptake of potassium.

Glucagon has been shown to increase plasma potassium concentrations independently of its effects on glucose and insulin, and, conversely, hyperkalaemia may be associated with the release of glucagon.

Adrenergic stimuli

The rise in plasma potassium concentrations resulting from an infusion of potassium chloride is increased in the presence of non-selective β-adrenergic blocking drugs, or of the α-agonist phenylephrine. Adrenaline infusions induce hypokalaemia by increasing potassium flux into skeletal muscle by β_2-activation of membrane-bound adenylate cyclase and subsequent stimulation of Na-K ATPase. Sympathetic nervous discharge also promotes a shift of potassium from extra- to intracellular fluid. β-Blocking drugs exaggerate the hyperkalaemia of exercise, while phentolamine reduces it. α-Agonists increase net loss of potassium from cells into the extracellular fluid while β-adrenergic stimuli promote hypokalaemia, particularly the β_2-selective agents such as salbutamol and terbutaline. Theophylline preparations also induce the entry of potassium into cells.

Plasma concentrations of adrenaline may rise to levels known to promote hypokalaemia after the pain and anxiety of myocardial infarction, and there are increasing reports of hypokalaemia in patients in coronary care units who have not yet been treated with potassium-losing diuretics. The hypokalaemia which may complicate delirium tremens after alcohol withdrawal is also likely to be β-adrenergically mediated.

Non-selective β-blocking drugs may increase plasma potassium significantly in some patients with chronic renal failure or with insulin-deficient diabetes mellitus.

Osmolality

Hyperosmolar states tend to increase plasma potassium by some 0.6 mmol/l per increase in osmolality of 10 mosmol/kg.

External balance

Renal control of external potassium balance

Renal tubular handling of potassium is complex, but ultimate control of urinary potassium excretion is still believed to lie in the mechanisms of potassium secretion in the distal nephron.

Proximal tubular reabsorption is in part an active process and is complete by the end of the proximal segment. Potassium then re-enters tubular fluid in the pars recta and the descending limb of Henle's loop to be reabsorbed in the thick ascending limb by sodium–potassium cotransport. Potassium in the descending limb may come from reabsorption in the collecting ducts via the medullary tissue, thereby contributing to medullary hypertonicity by a recycling process which takes place largely in the juxtamedullary nephrons. The system may contribute to the regulation of potassium excretion in several ways. Reduced potassium absorption by the thick ascending limb of Henle's loop can contribute to kaliuresis. Further, a high medullary concentration of potassium tends to decrease sodium reabsorption in the thick ascending limb; the resultant increase of delivery of sodium to the distal nephron also favours kaliuresis.

In the early distal tubule there are mechanisms of active transport of potassium into cells on both the peritubular and luminal surfaces. Movement of potassium into tubular urine at this site is dependent on electrical and chemical gradients. The luminal concentration of sodium and the nature of its accompanying anion are important factors in controlling these gradients.

In the cortical collecting ducts, potassium transport into tubular fluid is active, not strictly linked to sodium reabsorption but in some way dependent on intraluminal sodium concentration and the rate of flow of tubular fluid. Further secretion of potassium may occur in the medullary collecting ducts under conditions of metabolic alkalosis, solute diuresis, potassium loading, and facilitated by anti-diuretic hormone.

A number of factors influence distal nephron potassium secretion and determine the rate of potassium excretion in the urine.

Potassium adaptation

A chronic high potassium intake enhances distal tubular potassium secretion by a number of mechanisms, which result in a kidney able to excrete as much as 10 or 20 times more than it does in normal circumstances. In this situation, there is an increased content of Na-K ATPase and of surface area in the basolateral membranes of the cortical collecting tubules, and the colon also increases its capacity to secrete potassium, again by an increase in Na-K pumps. These changes can occur independently of an increase in plasma aldosterone concentration, but hyperaldosteronism stimulated by hyperkalaemia is required for full adaptation by the kidney to chronic, very high potassium intakes.

Sodium delivery to the distal nephron

Any condition which increases sodium delivery to the distal nephron (for example, loop diuretics, osmotic diuretics, or salt loading) enhances urinary potassium excretion. The mechanisms are not clear but relate to sodium concentrations and tubular flow rates in the distal tubules.

Aldosterone

Mineralocorticoids enhance sodium reabsorption and potassium secretion in the cortical collecting ducts by increasing Na-K ATPase

Table 1 Causes of hypokalaemia

Intracellular shifts	
• Alkalosis	• ?Aldosterone
• High-dose insulin	• Poisoning by barium salts
• β_2-Adrenergic stimulation	• Toluene intoxication (glue-sniffing)
• Theophylline overdose	
• Periodic paralysis	
Renal wasting	
• Alkalosis (metabolic and respiratory)	• Cushing's syndrome
	• Adrenogenital syndromes
• Diuretic drugs	• Bartter's syndrome
• Solute diuresis	• Liddle's disease
• Glucose	• Magnesium depletion
• Urea	• Carbenoxolone sodium
• Mannitol	• Liquorice addiction
• Saline	• Renal tubular acidosis
• Aldosteronism	• Gentamicin
• Primary	• Amikacin
• Secondary	• Carbenicillin
• Renin-secreting tumours	• Penicillin
• Acute leukaemia	
Gastrointestinal	
• Pyloric stenosis	• Chloride-diarrhoea
• Bulimia nervosa	• Villous adenoma of the rectum
• Ileostomy	• Purgative abuse
• Ureterosigmoidostomy	

activity in the basolateral membranes and by increasing the conductance of potassium in the luminal membrane of the principal cells of the collecting duct.

pH changes

Alkalosis, by increasing the uptake of potassium in the basolateral membranes and the conductance of the luminal membranes of the distal nephron, promotes kaliuresis. The reverse is the case in chronic acidosis. In addition, potassium hydrogen exchange favours renal potassium wasting in alkalosis and retention in acidosis.

ADH

The stimulation of distal tubular potassium secretion by ADH helps to prevent hyperkalaemia in oliguria secondary to dehydration. The effect is mediated by activation of sodium and potassium channels in the luminal membrane, together with an increase in Na-K ATPase activity in the basolateral membrane; the effects of ADH and aldosterone in this context are additive.

Anions

An increased delivery of poorly reabsorbable anions in the glomerular filtrate also enhances distal tubular potassium secretion by a combination of increased fluid and sodium delivery and by the enhanced transepithelial electrical potential gradient.

Hypokalaemia

Causes of hypokalaemia are listed in Table 1. Dietary deficiency alone is an uncommon cause.

Pathophysiological effects of hypokalaemia

Whether hypokalaemia is the consequence of overall potassium depletion or because of a shift of potassium into cells, there will be an increase in the ratio of intracellular to extracellular potassium, causing hyperpolarization across excitable membranes. The resultant increase in myocardial excitability can precipitate a variety of cardiac dysrhythmias ranging from unifocal extrasystoles to ventricular tachycardia or fibrillation. The toxicity of digitalis preparations is enhanced and may be associated particularly with atrial tachycardia with block and with atrioventricular dissociation. Changes in the electrocardiogram, which may be evident when plasma potassium concentrations fall below 3 mmol/l, include depression of the ST segment, flattening of the T-waves, and prominent U-waves. These changes correlate poorly with the development of serious dysrhythmias.

Marked potassium depletion impairs striated muscle function, with weakness and absent reflexes sometimes progressing to paralysis which can affect the respiratory muscles. Frank rhabdomyolysis when depletion is profound occurs particularly after exercise, but an increase in plasma creatine phosphokinase without myalgia is more common and may occur when plasma concentrations fall below 3 mmol/l. The smooth muscle of the gut is also affected, with reduced motility or frank ileus.

The effects on the kidney include nephrogenic diabetes insipidus, a fall in glomerular filtration rate, a tendency towards sodium retention, and increased renal acid excretion resulting in metabolic alkalosis. Failure to concentrate urine appears to be due to a reduction in medullary solute concentration, and resistance to ADH because of increased production of prostaglandins. The mechanism whereby very low potassium diets result in sodium retention and sometimes to oedema are not understood.

Chronic hypokalaemia is associated with the appearance of prominent vacuoles in the cytoplasm of both proximal and distal cortical tubular cells, but evidence that severe and prolonged potassium deficiency causes irreversible and progressive interstitial nephritis with consequent renal failure, is not conclusive.

The association of potassium deficiency with metabolic alkalosis, is probably a true one linked to retention of sodium and bicarbonate and most likely to be seen with coincident volume depletion. But, in most clinical states of hypokalaemic alkalosis there are other participating factors.

Specific syndromes of hypokalaemia

Vomiting

The concentration of potassium in gastric and upper intestinal secretions varies between 5 and 10 mmol/l, so that direct losses in vomitus contribute little to potassium deficiency. Major losses of chloride and acid result in hypochloraemic alkalosis, which induces a renal potassium leak. This, together with a shift of potassium from the extracellular to the intracellular fluid, is largely responsible for the hypokalaemia. Patients with pyloric stenosis may have deficits of sodium and potassium exceeding 500 mmol, of chloride rather more, and of water in excess of 5 litres. In such extreme cases, massive chloride depletion, causes 'paradoxically' acid urine despite profound metabolic alkalosis. The excretion of alkaline urine is not possible, then, until the chloride deficit has been reduced. Covert vomiting is a cardinal feature of bulimia nervosa, which in many respects resembles Bartter's syndrome (see below).

Diarrhoea

There is more potassium (50–100 mmol/l) in liquid stools than in vomitus, so that potassium deficiency from diarrhoea does not require an additional renal leak. Any condition in which stool volumes are high may cause hypokalaemia. Potassium loss is usually paralleled by loss of bicarbonate, with a resultant metabolic acidosis, so that plasma potassium concentrations do not accurately reflect the true deficit. In some cases the opposite occurs, when potassium and chloride are jointly lost with resultant metabolic alkalosis. A villous adenoma of the colon or rectum may result in profound hypokalaemia, due to disturbances of ion transport in the colonic mucosa mediated by the tumour. Similar disturbances underlie the hypokalaemia of patients with non-insulin-secreting islet-cell tumours. More common than these rarities is laxative abuse, in which hypokalaemia may be profound without a change in the acid–base balance. Ureterosigmoidostomy leads to profound hypokalaemic hyperchloraemic acidosis if urine is allowed to remain stagnant in the colon.

Diuretics

All diuretics other than those acting directly on the distal tubules tend to increase urinary potassium excretion in an amount dependent on the dose, the natriuretic response, and the degree of prevailing secondary hyperaldosteronism. Hypokalaemia may or may not occur. It is most common early in treatment but potassium concentrations rarely fall below 3 mmol/l. The loop agents are chloruretic and may cause an hypochloraemic hypokalaemic alkalosis with renal potassium wasting, correctable by supplements of potassium chloride but not of bicarbonate.

The average fall after treatment with benzothiadiazines is 0.69 mol/1litre but levels below 3.5 mmol/l have been described in some half of treated patients. Hypokalaemia can be reduced by using minimal effective doses, avoiding the longer-acting agents, reducing sodium intake, and using potassium-retaining diuretic-thiazide combinations. The need to prescribe potassium supplements routinely or not has been much debated. The risks of hypokalaemia are of cardiac arrhythmias and an enhancement of digitalis toxicity. In the longer term, impairment of carbohydrate tolerance is related to an impaired insulin secretory response to hyperglycaemia. An excellent correlation between total body potassium and impairment of insulin secretion has been described. On the other hand, most patients with modest hypokalaemia come to no particular harm and potassium supplements are variably absorbed, are a nuisance to take, and can, on rare occasions, cause jejunal ulceration and stricture formation. Most physicians would prescribe supplements of the chloride in patients who are prone to cardiac arrhythmias and in patients with severe liver disease in whom electrolyte imbalance may precipitate encephalopathy.

Bartter's syndrome

The first reported cases presented with hypokalaemic alkalosis, hyperaldosteronism without hypertension, hypertrophy and hyperplasia for the juxtaglomerular apparatus, nephrogenic diabetes insipidus, and resistance to the pressor effects of infused angiotensin II. Patients may present at any age from the neonatal period to old age. Occurrence in siblings and children of consanguineous patients suggests occasional autosomal recessive inheritance, but most cases are sporadic. The sexes are equally susceptible and evidence that the syndrome is commoner in Afro-Caribbeans is not conclusive.

Clinical findings

Heterogeneity in clinical and biochemical features reflect the heterogeneity of causative mechanisms. In some patients the condition may be asymptomatic, with biochemical abnormalities detected by chance. At the other extreme, marked hypokalaemia causes muscle weakness, polydipsia, polyuria, tetany, fits, vomiting, and, in children, stunting of growth. The cardinal features are hypokalaemic alkalosis with urinary potassium and chloride wasting and a normal, or marginally low, arterial pressure, but a proportion of cases also show hyponatraemia, hypophosphataemia (with or without rickets), hypercalciuria, hypercalcaemia, nephrocalcinosis, hypomagnesaemia, and hyperuricaemia. Urinary potassium losses may exceed the filtered load, reaching amounts as high as 400–600 mmol over 24 h in rare patients. Plasma renin activity and angiotensin II levels are high, as is aldosterone secretion, unless retarded by profound hypokalaemia. Other described abnormalities include increased urinary prostaglandin E and kallikrein, high plasma levels of bradykinin, and abnormalities of platelet aggregation.

Renal histology

A variety of abnormalities have been described, including, apart from juxtaglomerular cell hyperplasia, hypercellularity of glomeruli, periglomerular fibrosis, arteriolar sclerosis, and chronic interstitial nephritis. Primary renal damage may, in some cases, coincide with Bartter's syndrome if not be its underlying cause. Medullary interstitial hyperplasia is not now considered a feature confined to patients with true Bartter's syndrome.

Pathogenesis

Recent evidence suggests a defect in the Na-K-2Cl co-transporter in the medullary portion of the thick ascending limb of Henle's loop, resulting in impaired reabsorption of chloride and sodium at that site. Overproduction of prostaglandin E_2 is probably the non-specific result of prolonged potassium depletion.

Differential diagnosis

Primary renal tubular disorders can closely mimic Bartter's syndrome. Laxative and diuretic abuse, together with vomiting can produce all the features. Urinary chloride estimations will detect covert vomiting as in bulimia nervosa. In that condition, in purgative abuse, and in the 'rebound' chloride retaining state after diuretic abuse, urinary chloride can be as low as 1–3 mmol/24 h, whereas in Bartter's syndrome there is an *increase* in fractional chloride excretion. Diuretic abuse mimics Bartter's syndrome precisely, but can be detected by urinary assays. Villous adenoma of the rectum, renal tubular acidosis, chronic pyloric stenosis, and the effects of liquorice (see below) or carbenoxolone sodium are more easily detected.

Treatment

In some asymptomatic patients with mild biochemical disturbance, an increase in dietary potassium and supplements of potassium chloride (150–200 mmol/day) may suffice. Others can be improved by the addition of spironolactone, amiloride, or triamterene. In severe cases, particularly in children with stunted growth, prostaglandin synthetase inhibitors should be prescribed. Most experience has been gained with indomethacin, which should be given in a dose up to 2 mg/kg per day. Secondary aldosteronism is always improved, but some degree of hypokalaemia usually persists. Remarkable improvement in clinical features can be expected.

Other causes of renal potassium wasting

In primary aldosteronism, hypokalaemia is more severe in adenoma than in hyperplasia. Secondary hyperaldosteronism with hypokalaemia may complicate malignant hypertension, renal artery stenosis and the fluid retention of heart failure, cirrhosis of the liver, and nephrotic syndrome treated by diuretic agents. Cushing's syndrome may be associated with renal potassium wasting, especially if caused by carcinoma of the adrenal cortex or by a non-endocrine tumour. Adrenogenital syndromes due to 11β-hydroxylase or 17α-hydroxylase deficiency result in hypokalaemia due to overproduction of deoxycorticosterone. Renin-secreting tumours increase urinary potassium loss by stimulating hyperaldosteronism. Liquorice consumed in large amounts or chronic use of carbenoxolone produce renal potassium wasting and hypokalaemia, by inhibition of renal 11β-hydroxysteroid dehydrogenase (see Chapter 7.6). Hypokalaemia in renal tubular acidosis is described in Chapter 12.31.

Liddle's syndrome

Hypokalaemia in this rare autosomal dominant syndrome is accompanied by hypertension and suppression of the resin–aldosterone system. The condition appears to be the result of abnormalities in the genes on chromosome 16 which control the amiloride-sensitive sodium channel in the distal nephron, leading to increased sodium reabsorption at that site. Both hypertension and hypokalaemia respond to treatment with triamterene or amiloride, but not to spironolactone.

11β-Hydroxysteroid dehydrogenase deficiency

This condition is discussed in Chapter 7.6.

Acute leukaemias

Renal potassium wasting and hypokalaemia may complicate acute myeloid, monocytic, and myelomonocytic leukaemias. Increased urinary lysozyme excretion, either causing or reflecting renal tubular damage, is found in many, but not all, cases. In some patients renal tubular damage by aminoglycosides may be the cause (see below), and in others avid transmembrane transport of potassium by leukaemic cells.

Antimicrobials

Amphotericin B, gentamicin, and amikacin may cause renal tubular damage, leading on occasion to urinary potassium wasting and hypokalaemia.

Magnesium deficiency

Any cause of profound and chronic magnesium deficiency can impair renal conservation of potassium. Hypokalaemia is then difficult to correct unless supplements of potassium are combined with those of magnesium.

Hypokalaemic periodic paralysis

In this rare condition, episodes of muscle weakness or paralysis lasting up to 24 or even 72 h occur sporadically or at more regular intervals. In most cases there is a family history reflecting a Mendelian autosomal dominant inheritance. Symptoms first appear late in the first or in the second decade. Legs are affected more than arms and proximal muscles more than distal. Bulbar and respiratory musculature are rarely affected. Permanent and progressive muscle weakness may evolve in middle age. Attacks are associated with a shift of potassium from extracellular to intracellular fluid, with profound hypokalaemia, but, on occasion, the plasma potassium may be normal. Precipitating factors include rest after several exercise, large carbohydrate meals, anxiety, and an habitual high salt diet. Attacks may also occur in sleep, with the patient awaking weak or paralysed. The mechanism of the disease is unclear, but a primary defect in muscle membrane sodium conductance has been described.

Attacks can be provoked by administration of glucose and insulin or adrenaline, and prevented by diazoxide, which blocks insulin release. Long-term treatment by diazoxide is too toxic for use in this condition. A number of other treatments have been recommended, including potassium supplements, spironolactone, amiloride, and non-selective β-adrenergic blocking drugs. Acetazolamide or ammonium chloride may also prevent attacks by inducing extracellular fluid acidosis.

A very similar hypokalaemic syndrome may complicate thyrotoxicosis, especially in Oriental races (see Chapter 7.3). This variant of the condition is always corrected by reversal of the hyperthyroidism, and responds acutely to the use of β-adrenergic blocking agents.

Hypokalaemia and sudden death in Thailand

Poor socio-economic status, nutritional deficiency, and loss of electrolytes in sweat may underlie a metabolic syndrome described in young people in north-east Thailand, which includes renal stone disease, distal renal tubular acidosis, diabetes mellitus, and hypokalaemia with low dietary and urinary potassium. The importance of hypokalaemia relates to reports of sudden unexplained deaths at night, usually afflicting young, muscular men, some of whom are known to have been hypokalaemic. In some cases there has been evidence of ventricular fibrillation. Vanadium toxicity may mediate some of the metabolic changes by inhibition of Na-K ATPase and H-K ATPase.

Treatment of hypokalaemia

Potassium replacement in hypokalaemia caused by internal shifts is rarely necessary. In those cases in which there is a true deficit, the need to provide supplements or to retard urinary losses varies according to clinical circumstances. In patients with myocardial disease, there is a good case for treating all levels of hypokalaemia. In healthy subjects, most physicians will treat those in whom potassium concentrations are consistently below 3 mmol/l. The case when concentrations lie between 3.0 and 3.5 mmol/l is much less clear.

In most conditions in which oral supplements are required, there is an associated metabolic alkalosis provoking renal potassium losses which are not then corrected by the bicarbonate or citrate salts of potassium. In this situation the chloride salt is essential and can be given as an elixir but is better accepted embedded in a wax medium (Slow-K®). Bicarbonate preparations are particularly indicated when hypokalaemia is associated with acidosis, for instance in renal tubular acidosis.

Indications for rapid elevation of plasma potassium by parental infusion are few, but include hypokalaemic cardiac arrhythmias, paralysis, and hypokalaemic diabetic ketoacidosis. In every case care should be taken to assess the adequacy of renal function. No rule is absolute, but it is rarely wise to infuse potassium in a concentration exceeding 40 mmol/l, at a rate exceeding 40 mmol/h or 200 mmol/day.

Table 2 Causes of hyperkalaemia

Excessive intake
Impaired renal excretion
Renal diseases
Acute renal failure
Chronic renal failure
Renal tubular disorders (including pseudohypoaldosteronism)
Endocrine effects on the kidney
Addison's disease
Isolated hypoaldosteronism
C-21 hydroxylase deficiency
3β-hydroxydehydrogenase deficiency
Corticosterone methyloxidase deficiency
Pharmaceutical effects on the kidney
Potassium-retaining diuretics
Angiotensin-converting enzyme inhibitors
Non-steroidal anti-inflammatory agents
Cyclosporin
Changes in internal balance
Acidosis
Rhabdomyolysis
Burns
Massive death of tumour cells
Hyperkalaemic periodic paralysis
Succinyl choline
Digitalis poisoning
Malignant hyperthermia
Familial hyperkalaemic acidosis
Pseudohyperkalaemia
Haemolysed blood samples
Leukaemia with very high white cell counts
Familial pseudohyperkalaemia

Hyperkalaemia

Hyperkalaemia is less common than hypokalaemia but more dangerous. Hyperkalaemic patients may develop muscle weakness, but cardiac arrest is the major complication which most commonly occurs without premonitory symptoms. Diagnosis therefore depends on clinical suspicion, on measurement of potassium in plasma, and on the characteristic changes in the electrocardiogram (see Chapter 12.28).

Some causes of hyperkalaemia are listed in Table 2. Although renal failure, acute or chronic, underlies most cases, all too commonly there has been an iatrogenic contribution from unwise use of potassium supplements, potassium-retaining diuretics, angiotensin-converting enzyme inhibitors, and non-steroidal anti-inflammatory drugs.

Excessive intake

An individual's ability to handle an excessive intake of potassium depends mainly on renal function, but also on the phenomenon of adaptation, whereby a chronic high intake increases potassium tolerance (see above). Hyperkalaemia due solely to excessive intake of potassium by mouth in healthy people is therefore rare, but has been described after overdosage with slow-release potassium preparations. Hyperkalaemia of dietary origin is a common enough problem in the presence of renal failure, and may complicate mineralocorticoid deficiency or the inappropriate prescription of potassium-retaining diuretics. Parental infusion of potassium may cause dangerous hyperkalaemia if rates of infusion exceed 40 mmol/h or concentrations of potassium exceed 40 mmol/l or less in the presence of renal insufficiency. There is a risk of hyperkalaemia if patients with impaired renal function are transfused with stored blood, or treated with large doses of the potassium salts of penicillin.

Acute renal failure

Hyperkalaemia is to be expected in any case of acute renal failure (see Chapter 12.28), especially when the condition is associated with muscle injury, tissue necrosis, gastrointestinal bleeding acidosis, or severe infection.

Chronic renal failure

Hyperkalaemia is rarely a problem in chronic renal failure until the glomerular filtration rate falls below 15–20 ml/min. At lower levels of function, plasma potassium can usually be maintained at normal or near normal concentration by restriction of dietary intake, treatment of acidosis, and avoidance of potassium-retaining diuretics. Adaptive changes, identical to those that occur in healthy individuals on a high potassium diet, increase the capacity of surviving nephrons to excrete potassium, and similar changes in the Na-K pump numbers and potassium conductance probably also occur in colonic mucosa.

Pseudohyperkalaemia

Samples in which plasma or serum have not been promptly separated from red cells will contain excessive amounts of potassium derived from leakage out of red cells. Haemolysed samples show hyperkalaemia without long storage. Less common is the pseudohyperkalaemia associated with leukaemias when the total white cell count is so high that leakage from white and red cells together induce it within a few minutes after venesection.

Familial pseudo-hyperkalaemia may reflect an autosomal dominant inheritance of abnormal cation transport across red cell membranes. The prime feature is an abnormal net efflux of potassium from red cells stored over 2–6 h at room temperature. The leak can be prevented by storing the cells at 37°C rather than at room temperature. The blood film of these patients may show a few target cells and there is evidence of mild compensated haemolysis.

Potassium-retaining diuretics

Large doses of amiloride or triamterene (and to a lesser degree of spironolactone) may cause severe hyperkalaemia, even in healthy people with normal renal function. These drugs are particularly to be avoided in renal failure.

Adrenal insufficiency

Addison's disease is commonly associated with modest hyperkalaemia (plasma potassium 5.0–6.5 mmol/l), hyponatraemia, and a rise in blood urea. Isolated hypoaldosteronism presents the same electrolyte disturbances, but absence of glucocorticoid deficiency makes the diagnosis easy to miss (see below).

Isolated hypoaldosteronism

The commonest cause of chronic hyperkalaemia without severe renal failure is probably hyporeninaemic hypoaldosteronism. In many cases, plasma renin activity is low and unresponsive to the erect posture and sodium depletion. The associated hyperchloraemic metabolic acidosis (type 4 renal tubular acidosis) is largely the consequence of suppression of renal ammonia synthesis by hyperkalaemia. In most cases, there is also evidence of an acquired enzymatic defect in aldosterone biosynthesis with a reduced response to infusions of either angiotensin II or adrenocorticotrophic hormone (ACTH). A chronic low concentration of angiotensin II may contribute.

The plasma aldosterone concentrations may be 'normal' or low, but can be considered reduced in every case when indexed by the plasma potassium concentration. Glucocorticoid metabolism is normal.

Clinical features

Patients are usually over the age of 60 years. Vascular and ischaemic heart disease are common. Some 50 per cent of patients have been diabetic and 70 per cent have evidence of renal disease, most commonly chronic interstitial nephritis, with modest impairment of glomerular filtration rate. Symptoms may include muscle weakness, but in most cases hyperkalaemia with hyperchloraemic acidosis is detected during laboratory investigation, or the disorder declares itself with episodes of hyperkalaemic heart block, or cardiac arrest, often precipitated by vomiting or diarrhoea which tends to reduce sodium delivery and flow in the distal tubules and thus reduces renal potassium excretion. A similar course of events may follow discontinuation of potent diuretics previously overgenerously prescribed. Blood pressure is normal or even high.

The associations of this disorder with old age, diabetes, and renal disease may reflect the decreasing activity of the renin–angiotensin system with age, reduced sensitivity of the renal stretch receptors with increasing rigidity of arteriolar walls, insulin deficiency, and autonomic neuropathy.

The condition should be suspected in any patient with hyperkalaemia without obvious explanation. Investigation is complex and requires measurements of renin activity and plasma aldosterone in response to sodium deprivation, with assessment in addition of the aldosterone response to infusions of angiotensin and ACTH.

Cyclosporin treatment

In some patients treated by cyclosporin, hyperkalaemia (serum potassium 6.0–7.1 mmol/l) and acidosis may occur that are quite disproportionate to glomerular filtration rate and dietary intake. This condition is probably another variant of hyporeninaemic hypoaldosteronism and responds to treatment by fludrocortisone (see below).

Treatment

Most patients respond well to replacement therapy of 0.1–0.2 mg daily of fludrocortisone, but doses as high as 0.4 or even 1.0 mg may be needed to reduce the potassium concentration to normal, often at the cost of inducing oedema, hypertension, or cardiac failure. The failure of normal replacement doses to correct hyperkalaemia indicates a renal tubular component to the disease in some patients. In those in whom mineralocorticoids alone do not suffice, the combination of fludrocortisone with a thiazide diuretic may be successful. Supplements of sodium bicarbonate may correct acidosis and facilitate renal potassium excretion.

Congenital adrenal syndromes are discussed in Chapter 7.7

Angiotensin-converting enzyme inhibitors

The fall in angiotensin II concentrations induced by these drugs results acutely in reduced aldosterone secretion. Some elevation of plasma potassium occurs, but severe hyperkalaemia is only likely when the inhibitors are given to patients with creatinine clearances of less than 20 ml/min.

Non-steroidal anti-inflammatory substances

Inhibition of prostaglandin synthetase reduces glomerular filtration and delivery of sodium to the distal tubular exchange sites, and may interfere with renal renin secretion. These effects together are the reason for some 25 per cent of patients with chronic renal failure becoming hyperkalaemic when given indomethacin or similar agents.

Renal tubular disorders

Hyperkalaemia with impaired renal excretion of potassium may be a feature of any cause of renal tubular acidosis (see Chapter 12.31). Hyperkalaemia and acidosis disproportionate to the degree of loss of glomerular filtration rate are also occasionally seen in chronic obstructive nephropathy, in sickle-cell disease with renal involvement, in systemic lupus erythematosus, and in renal amyloidosis. More rare still are the conditions of type I and type II pseudohypoaldosteronism (discussed in OTM3, pp. 1661-2, and in Chapter 7.6).

Hyperkalaemic periodic paralysis

This disease is familial with an autosomal dominant mode of inheritance. Attacks of paralysis begin in the first decade of life, usually precipitated by rest after exercise, when pronounced hyperkalaemia is associated with a flaccid paralysis lasting from a few minutes to several hours. Bulbar muscles may be involved. Myotonia may be a striking feature and can be demonstrated by McArdle's sign. Established attacks can be reversed by salbutamol inhalation, but treatment is best given prophylactically by use of benzothiadiazine diuretics. Attacks can be aborted by ingestion of carbohydrate, but a progressive proximal myopathy can develop. A mutation in the sodium channel of adult skeletal muscle has been described.

Succinyl choline

Agents that depolarize muscle membranes increase plasma potassium by some 0.5 mmol/l in healthy subjects. In patients already at risk of hyperkalaemia, the rise after muscle relaxants may be much greater and should be considered when such patients need general anaesthesia.

Digitalis

Severe hyperkalaemia may occur after an overdose of digitalis, presumably secondary to loss of intracellular potassium, following massive inhibition of Na-K ATPase.

Malignant hyperthermia

This syndrome, is due to a genetically determined increase in calcium concentration in skeletal muscle, precipitated by inhaled anaesthetics.

Hyperthermia and rhabdomyolysis are accompanied by hyperkalaemia which may reach dangerous levels in subjects with impaired renal function.

Treatment of hyperkalaemia

The need to treat hyperkalaemia, how urgently and how aggressively, depends on its degree, whether it is stable or increasing, its cause, and most importantly on the presence or not of associated changes in the electrocardiogram. Stable concentrations under 6.0 mmol/l may not need specific therapy. Concentrations over 6.5 mmol/l with electrocardiogram (ECG) changes and levels exceeding 7.0 mmol/l constitute a medical emergency. ECG abnormalities, in order of severity, include tenting of T-waves, diminution or absence of P-waves, widening of the QRS complex, slurring of the ST segment into the T-waves, and a sine-wave pattern immediately preceding cardiac arrest (see Chapter 12.28).

If ECG changes are absent or involve only changes in P- and T-waves, intravenous glucose (50 g) and insulin (10–20) units soluble or Actrapid® will lower plasma potassium by approximately 1.0 mmol/l within 30 min, the effect persisting some 1–2 h; 50–100 ml 4.2 per cent sodium bicarbonate increases intracellular at the expense of extracellular potassium and is particularly effective when hyperkalaemia and acidosis are combined.

When the ECG changes are more advanced, intravenous 10 per cent calcium gluconate should be given over 2–5 min in whatever dose (usually 10–30 ml) is required to correct the ECG. The beneficial effects of calcium salts are evident within 2 min of infusion but are short lived.

A combination of calcium gluconate, glucose and insulin, and hypertonic bicarbonate provides control of hyperkalaemia for 2–3 h and can be supplemented, when necessary, by haemodialysis, peritoneal dialysis, or by cation exchange resins in the calcium or sodium phase. These agents in a dose of 15–20 g three or four times daily can be given by mouth or as a retention enema. Constipation, or worse, faecal impaction, may be avoided by adding 10–30 ml of a 70 per cent solution of sorbitol with each dose. Exchange resins begin to exert an effect on external potassium balance in some 1 or 2 h,

There is evidence that a variety of β_2- adrenergic agonists can be used to treat hyperkalaemia by virtue of their action in transferring potassium from the extracellular fluid into cells. There may be occasions in which this approach has advantages, but in general the established methods, which are thoroughly effective, are to be preferred.

Further reading

Botero-Velez, M. Curtis, J.J., and Warnock, D.G. (1994). Liddle's syndrome revisited - a disorder of sodium reabsorption in the distal tubule. *New England Journal of Medicine*, 330, 178–81.

Clive, D.S.M. (1995). Bartter's syndrome: The unsolved puzzle. *American Journal of Kidney Disease*, 25, 813–23.

Epstein, F.J. and Rosa, R. Adrenergic control of serum potassium. *New England Journal of Medicine*, 309, 1450–51.

Koko, J.P. (1985). Primary acquired hypoaldosteronism. *Kidney International*, 27, 690–702.

Chapter 12.5

Common clinical presentations and symptoms in renal disorders

J. S. Cameron

The patient with proteinuria

Excess protein in the urine will not be noticed unless a large amount is excreted—more than several grams per 24 h—when the urine may become frothy because protein lowers surface tension and permits foam to form.

The physiological and pathological basis of proteinuria

The glomerular filter permits a high flux of solvent (water) and does not retard the passage of molecules of up to an Einstein–Stokes radius of about 1.5 nm. Above this value, there is a gradual cut-off with increasing molecular size (Fig. 1). In health, the urinary clearance of albumin is less than 0.01 per cent, while the clearance of proteins of lower molecular weight, approaches that of the glomerular filtration rate. These findings can be modelled by the supposition of the presence of water-filled cylindrical pores of about 4.7 nm diameter occupying about 10 per cent of the glomerular filtration area; the true existence of these 'pores' is in doubt.

Figure 1 also shows that the glomerulus permits greater penetration of uncharged molecules, suggesting an effect of the high density of negative charges on the structures of the glomerular capillary wall.

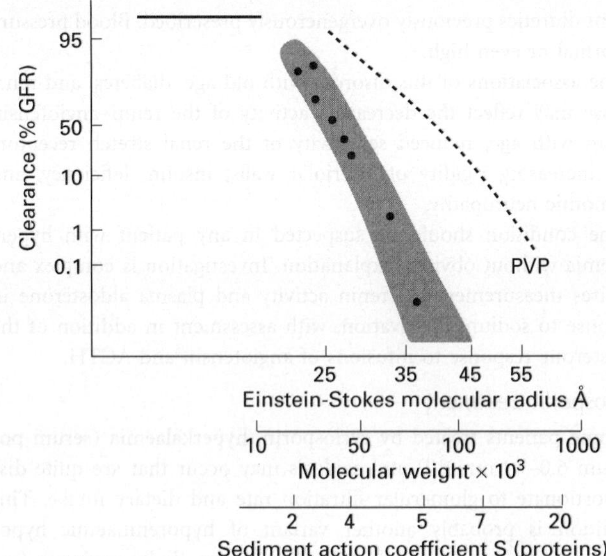

Fig. 1 The selectivity of the normal human and mammalian glomerulus to proteins, which carry a negative charge (shaded area) and polydisperse macromolecules (PVP or dextran) which are uncharged (dotted line). The glomerulus shows both size- and charge-selective properties. Urinary clearances (vertical axis) for infused proteins of various molecular weights (dots) are progressively reduced below the glomerular filtration rate as molecular weight and size (horizontal axis) increases. At any molecular size, the clearance of a neutral dextran or PVP is much greater than that of negatively charged proteins. Albumin has an Einstein–Stokes radius of 37 Å and a molecular weight of 67 kDa. (10 Å; = 1 nm).

Some degree of size discrimination ('selectivity') is preserved in all proteinurias resulting from glomerular damage, and is highest in nephrotic patients with minimal change lesions. The clearances approximate to that expected for molecular weight, so that the effects of charge seem to be subordinate for most proteinurias, despite plasma proteins (although all anionic at physiological pH) having different isoelectric points.

In diabetic nephropathy, as glomerular filtration rate falls, proteinuria reflects a gradual loss of glomerular discrimination for proteins of molecular size within the range 60–1000 kDa (Einstein–Stokes radius 3.5–20 nm). In minimal change disease, the clearance of smaller molecules of dextran (<4.8 nm) is actually decreased compared with normal clearance, while that of larger dextrans is normal or increased. A similar pattern has been found in nephrotic syndromes of varying types, including diabetes, lupus, and membranous nephropathy. These data have been interpreted in terms of a heteroporous model, which supposes the enlargement of existing pores or the appearance of larger pores in the membrane which permit the abnormal proteinuria.

A consequence of selectivity of the glomerular filter is that glomerular proteinuria consists largely of albumin, even in the most poorly selective and severely damaged glomeruli.

There is dispute about how much albumin is normally filtered but reabsorbed in the proximal tubule by endocytosis and catabolized, either in health or in disease, and thus is not reflected by the amount in the urine. There is no evidence of competition between large anionic molecules for reabsorption, but this is not true for cationic or smaller molecules.

Proteins of lower molecular weight (10–45 kDa; 1.5–3.0 nm) are filtered at rates of 1–80 per cent of the glomerular filtration rate. There is extensive reabsorption of low molecular weight protein in the proximal tubule, so that only about 100 mg/24 h are normally excreted, along with some 30–100 mg of albumin. Thus in proximal tubular damage, low molecular weight protein will predominate in the urine.

Clinical proteinuria

Normal proteinuria

The amount of protein excreted in the urine per 24 h is 80 $\pm$ 24 mg (mean $\pm$ SD), so that 128 mg/24 h represents the upper limit of normal (+2 SD). More than half of this consists of small molecular weight proteins or protein fragments, although albumin is the largest single component.

Pathological proteinuria

Proteinuria in excess can come about in three ways:

1. The glomerular filter becomes more permeable to proteins of large molecular size. This is by far the commonest cause in clinical practice (glomerular proteinuria).
2. There is a marked rise in the plasma concentration of protein, so that the amount filtered exceeds the reabsorptive capacity of the proximal tubule ('overflow' proteinuria). The only clinical circumstances in which this occurs is the excretion of immunoglobulin (Ig) G light chains and light chain fragments in myeloma, and of lysozyme in monomyelocytic leukaemia.
3. The proximal tubule is damaged so that normally reabsorbed proteins, principally of low molecular weight, pass into the urine ('tubular' proteinuria).

Glomerular proteinuria Methods for detecting excess urinary protein in 'spot' samples are discussed on p 1–2 this Section. The usual method of assessing severity of proteinuria is to measure the amount excreted in a 24-h collection. Inaccuracies in such collections are common and an alternative is to use the urine creatinine to correct protein concentration, either in the 24-h sample or in 'spot' samples. In adults, an upper limit of 0.2 mg/mg creatinine has been suggested, that is 21 mg/mmol. More than 3.5 mg protein/mg creatinine (360 mg/mmol) represents nephrotic-range proteinuria.

Tubular proteinuria All except the most specific chemical tests will miss some low molecular weight proteins, particularly immunoglobulin light chains, which are poorly precipitated in the sulphosalicylic acid test, are denatured reliably on heating and do not react with sticks. Cellulose acetate electrophoresis is particularly valuable in the diagnosis and assessment of tubular proteinuria.

Specific radioimmunoassays and enzyme-linked immunosorbent assays are available for β_2-microglobulin, but this low molecular weight protein, although a very sensitive indicator of tubular damage, is unstable in urine of normal pH. Less than 0.4 µg/l of β_2-microglobulin is present in normal urine, but many times more is found in tubular damage, or in glomerular disease with a prominent tubulointerstitial component. Lysozyme can also be used to assess proximal tubular damage: normal excretion is less than 1 mg/mmol creatinine (10 µg/mg), and α_1-microglobulin and retinol-binding protein have also been used.

Assays for κ and λ chains by immunoelectrophoresis are an essential part of the diagnosis of myeloma, and may also be found in the urine of patients with primary amyloidosis and light chain nephropathy. The problem is to remember to test for them—in the presence of good renal function their concentrations in the plasma may often be negligible, compared with their abundance in the urine.

Persistent symptomless proteinuria Isolated modest proteinuria (0.5–1.5 g/24 h), even when present in all samples tested but in the absence of haematuria, is almost always benign. The first thing to ascertain is that it is not postural and is persistent. The mild proteinuria of uncontrolled hypertension, recent exercise (which can induce several grams per litre of protein) and cardiac failure should be excluded. If renal function is normal, blood pressure is normal, and no haematuria is present, renal biopsy is not necessary, at least in the first instance. As many as 5 per cent of schoolchildren may show isolated proteinuria persisting for months or even years, which is benign in the great majority.

Proteinuria together with persistent microscopic haematuria implies the possibility of structurally damaged kidneys. In some cases this will be benign, as in resolving acute nephritis or IgA-associated nephropathy, but focal segmental glomerulosclerosis, crescentic nephritis, membranous nephropathy, or mesangiocapillary glomerulonephritis may be present. In the middle-aged or older patient amyloid or even diabetes may be found. A renal biopsy is usually necessary, especially if reduced renal function, hypertension, or both are present. In addition, some form of renal imaging will be needed, because reflux nephropathy, polycystic kidneys, and renal tuberculosis may present as haematuria with proteinuria. Serology for lupus and hepatitis B should also be performed.

An algorithm for the investigation of proteinuria is given in Fig. 2.

Selectivity of proteinuria Tests of selectivity are of limited value. They may help distinguish minimal change nephrotic syndromes from other causes but even here, they are more useful in children than in

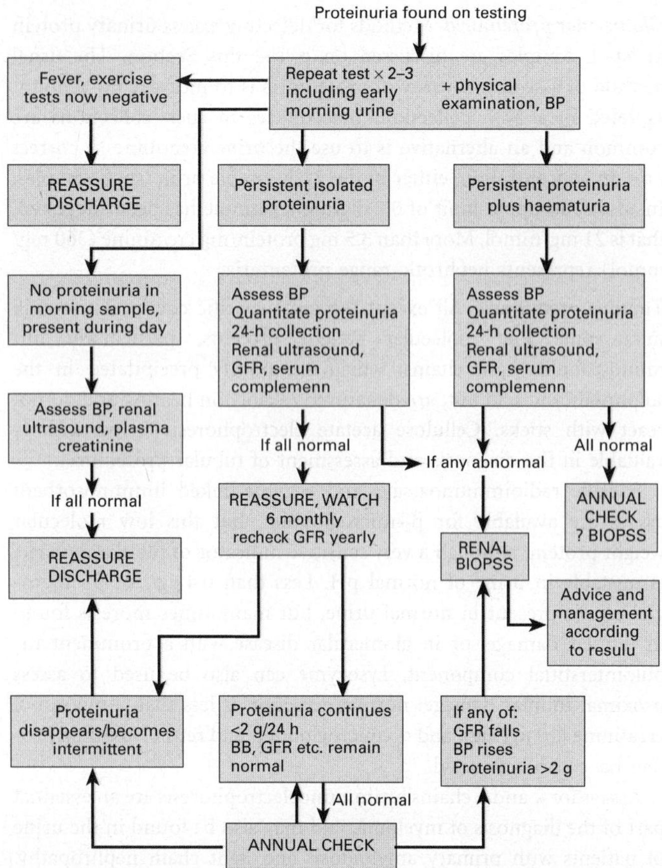

Fig. 2 An algorithm for the investigation of a patient found to have proteinuria on stick testing.

adults. A common test for selectivity is to compare the clearance of IgG with that of a protein of lower molecular weight abundant in the urine, either albumin or transferrin. This requires only a roughly simultaneous sample of plasma and a 'spot' untimed urine, as the urine volume cancels out in the relationship $C_{IgG}/C_{transferrin}$. A clearance of IgG greater than 20 per cent of transferrin or albumin represents 'non-selective' proteinuria; less than 10 per cent indicates a 'highly selective' proteinuria, suggesting a minimal change lesion, whereas the range between 10 and 20 per cent is of little discriminatory value.

The nephrotic syndrome

The nephrotic syndrome comprises a combination of profuse proteinuria, oedema, and hypoalbuminaemia. Proteinuria of more than 3–4 g/24 h for more than a few weeks is usually necessary to induce oedema with a serum albumin below 30 g/l, but there is no firm boundary between persisting heavy proteinuria without oedema and a nephrotic syndrome; many patients will cross the boundary in either direction, sometimes because of a change in salt intake or activity rather than a change in proteinuria.

In the history, attention needs to be paid to medicines ingested, prior infections, allergies, or features suggestive of a systemic disorder such as lupus. A history of macroscopic haematuria is unusual except in postinfectious or mesangiocapillary nephritis (MCGN). An associated tumour needs to be kept in mind in older patients. The family history may be revealing, as in Alport's syndrome or the Finnish form of congenital nephrotic syndrome.

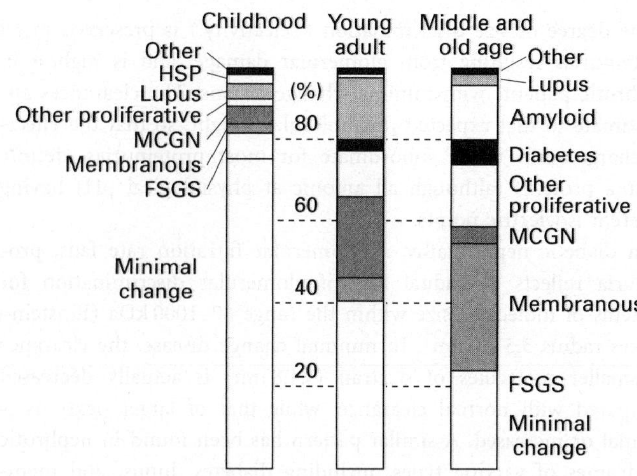

Fig. 3 The underlying histological appearances found in renal biopsies done in nephrotic patients in the developed world. During childhood, by far the most common appearance is that of minimal glomerular changes, and this appearance may be found even in the elderly. In young adults, the proportion of minimal change patients falls, and proliferative glomerulonephritis and lupus in young women form a significant proportion. In the elderly, membranous nephropathy becomes the dominant appearance together with diabetes and primary amyloidosis. The proportion of diabetics among older nephrotics is probably a considerable underestimate because many nephrotic diabetics do not have a renal biopsy. HSP, Henoch–Schönlein purpura; MCGN, mesangiocapillary glomerulonephritis; FSGS, focal segmental glomerulosclerosis.

The oedema, is soft, pitting, and dependent, often with facial swelling in the morning and ankle oedema at night. The arms may show oedema about the elbows and forearms, with wasting of the muscle in the upper arm—'Popeye' arms. Genital oedema may be massive. Xanthomas are found in patients with the most severe forms of an associated hyperlipidaemia, around the eyes or on the elbows. The oedema may extend to the pleurae, with bilateral hydrothorax, and there may be ascites. The jugular venous pressure is usually normal, and if raised gives a suspicion in older patients of amyloidosis with cardiac involvement. In the progressive disorders, hypertension and uraemia may ensue. The liver will often be enlarged, especially in younger patients.

The microscopic appearance of the urine varies from a bland sediment with no red cells and only fatty casts in the case of minimal changes, to an 'angry' sediment with abundant red cells, and red cell and granular casts in a case of mesangiocapillary or crescentic nephritis.

Investigation of nephrotic patients follows that of patients with persistent proteinuria and haematuria, discussed above. All adult nephrotics and all nephrotic children over 10 years of age should be biopsied, even if their urine shows no casts or red cells (Fig. 3). Renal imaging will be needed, and glomerular filtration rate is best assessed by an isotopic method. Proteinuria should be quantitated on several 24-h urines. Serological measurements should include a DNA antibody test, serological tests for hepatitis B and C, C3 and C4 complement concentrations, and, in older patients, a chest radiograph and protein electrophoresis searching for paraproteins.

The genesis of nephrotic oedema

The classical explanation was that renal protein loss led to a diminished plasma oncotic pressure, which in turn led to hypovolaemia and triggered salt-retaining humoral stimuli to which the kidney responded

Table 1 Complications of the nephrotic syndrome

Susceptibility to infection	Acute renal failure
Thromboses	Loss of binding proteins in urine
Hyperlipidaemia	Protein malnutrition

by avid salt retention. Observation of patients accumulating or losing oedema shows that this story can only be partially true, and the finding that most stable adult nephrotics have normal or even increased plasma volumes is further evidence against the old hypothesis. Furthermore, studies on unilateral proteinuric disease in rats and on isolated perfused kidneys have shown that the level of serum albumin is not an important determinant of salt retention, and suggest that proteinuria *per se* leads to renal salt retention.

There is an important difference between nephrotic and nephritic oedema in that, although there is retention of salt and water in both conditions, hypoalbuminaemia in the former favours peripheral oedema, whereas in the latter pulmonary oedema is more likely as intravascular volume expands as well as interstitial volume.

Management of the nephrotic syndrome

Some general measures are applicable to all nephrotics, whatever their underlying disease may be.

Salt intake should be modestly limited (to, say, 60 mmol/24 h) because stricter regimes are rarer followed. Nephrotics excrete water loads poorly, and excessive intake may precipitate hyponatraemia. Loop diuretics are often the only effective ones, although both metolazone and spironolactone may be useful as adjuncts. Sometimes very large doses will be required, as much as 500 mg twice a day of frusemide or equivalent. If this proves ineffective, patients can be admitted to hospital and a regimen of intravenous salt-poor albumin and intravenous diuretics (frusemide, 250 mg) used. Alone, the former carries the risk of pulmonary oedema and the latter the risk of hypovolaemic shock, but the two together are safe. This may need to be continued for a week or 2, and 20, 30, or even 40 litres of oedema removed.

A number of agents can reduce proteinuria, in every case at the expense of some reduction in glomerular filtration rate. ACE inhibitors have the best ratio of reduction in proteinuria to reduction in glomerular filtration rate. Non-steroidal anti-inflammatory drugs and cyclosporin present a poorer profile, the change in proteinuria and glomerular filtration rate usually being identical, and a risk of acute or irreversible renal failure being much larger than with ACE inhibitors. Both can be used together with an additive effect but increased risk of renal failure.

Dietary protein intake in nephrotics has been much debated. Protein restriction diminishes proteinuria and a high protein diet augments it. On the other hand, giving a low protein diet in a protein-wasting state runs the risk of depletion in the long term. A reasonable compromise is to advise 1 g/kg per 24 h of mainly first-class protein to nephrotic patients.

Complications and consequences of the nephrotic state (Table 1)

Infections

Primary peritonitis is particularly characteristic of nephrotic children. The onset may be insidious but is usually sudden, and should be suspected in any nephrotic child who develops abdominal pain. The diagnosis must be confirmed by microscopic examination of a Gram stain, or an immunochemical search for bacterial antigens, on ascitic fluid removed by needle. Blood cultures are usually positive, but take time to perform. Hypotension, shock, and even acute renal failure may follow rapidly, sometimes with disseminated intravascular coagulation (see below). In the past the organism was almost always *Streptococcus pneumoniae*, but other organisms, such as β-haemolytic streptococci, *Haemophilus*, and Gram-negative organisms may be found.

Cellulitis is another problem, especially in severe oedema. Organisms responsible include β-haemolytic streptococci and a variety of Gram-negative bacteria. Usually the clinical diagnosis is clear. The patient may be toxic and become shocked. Others run a more indolent course. It is difficult to stain or culture organisms from fluid aspirated from the area, but blood cultures are usually positive.

Causes of susceptibility to infection in nephrotic patients

Pneumococcal infections are also a particular problem in patients with some congenital deficiencies of the complement system, and alternative pathway activation is crucial in the phagocytosis of encapsulated organisms. Factor B, a major factor in this pathway, is lost in nephrotic urine. By 20 years of age, most adults have acquired antibodies against a variety of pneumococcal capsular antigens. Transferrin is essential for normal lymphocyte function, and acts as a carrier for a number of metals, including zinc. It too is lost in nephrotic urine.

Infections are commonest in children, reports of severe infections in adults being rare. The predominance of pneumococcal infections is striking and organisms are nearly always encapsulated. Local humoral defences may also be diluted by oedema. Immunoglobulin G provides the main defence against infection in tissues, and low concentrations are characteristic of nephrotic patients. Even so, in patients with inherited common hypogammaglobulinaemia, levels of IgG below 2 g/l are required before serious infections are seen, and such levels are rarely reached in nephrotic patients.

Treatment and prophylaxis In children there is a good case for prophylactic penicillin to avoid pneumococcal infections, at least while the child is oedematous. Antipneumococcal vaccines induce an adequate response when given in remission, but are not always protective when given during steroid therapy and are frankly defective when given shortly after cytotoxic therapy.

Successful treatment depends on anticipation and rapid diagnosis. The erythrocyte sedimentation rate is useless in nephrotic children, and the white cell count may be misleading, especially in those taking corticosteroids; C-reactive protein is more useful. Parenteral antibiotics should be begun as soon as cultures have been taken. In children, benzylpenicillin should always be a component but broad-spectrum therapy is also needed, because the pneumococcus may not be the only organism present. A cephalosporin, together with an aminoglycoside, may be used as initial 'blind' treatment in adults. Blood pressure and venous pressure need careful watching and colloid may be necessary. The risk of secondary thrombosis suggests the need for anticoagulation. Supplementary corticosteroid is essential in those taking these drugs, or who have just stopped them.

Thromboembolic complications

The prevalence of clinical *renal vein thrombosis* is about 6–8 per cent in nephrotics with membranous nephropathy and only 1–3 per cent in other forms of glomerulopathy. However, if venograms are performed, the prevalence is 10–45 per cent in membranous patients and about 10 per cent in others.

Renal venous thrombosis may present acutely, with loin pain, haematuria, renal enlargement, and deterioration in renal function; or as a slower fall-off in renal function without dramatic signs or symptoms. Otherwise, the thrombosis may be silent, being found incidentally by venography or other evaluation. Thrombosis of renal veins is frequently bilateral. About 35 per cent of patients with renal venous thrombosis will have pulmonary emboli. Nevertheless, few nephrologists undertake renal venous venography in all nephrotic patients, or even in all those with membranous nephropathy.

Overt *deep venous thrombosis* is evident in about 6 per cent of nephrotic adults and can be detected in 25 per cent if Doppler ultrasonography is used. It is much less common in childhood (0.6 per cent). Clinically diagnosed pulmonary emboli are present in 6 per cent of adult nephrotics and, if ventilation-perfusion scanning is used, as many as 12 per cent are affected. However, only a single patient in our own series comprising 2100 patient-years died of pulmonary embolism. Subclavian or axillary, jugular, iliac, portal, splenic, hepatic, sagittal sinus, and mesenteric vein thrombosis have also all been described, albeit much more rarely.

In adults arterial thrombosis is much less common than venous thrombosis. Almost every artery has been involved: aorta, femoral, coronary, pulmonary, mesenteric, cerebral, renal, ophthalmic, and carotid arteries, together with major intracardiac thrombi. Those worth investigating are those with suggestive clinical signs and those with pulmonary emboli. It has yet to be established that seeking symptomless renal venous thrombosis is useful, as its prognosis appears to be benign; and how frequently or at what intervals re-screening must be undertaken is not established. If Doppler ultrasound, computed tomography, or magnetic resonance imaging scanning can be established as reliable, much of this will change.

Abnormalities of coagulation in nephrotics Many proteins involved in clotting show altered concentrations in nephrotic patients and the possible ways in which these may promote thrombosis are complex. No certain mechanism has been identified (see OTM3, p. 3142).

Treatment and prophylaxis of thrombosis in nephrotics Patients should be mobilized and volume depletion by diuretic therapy avoided. Anticoagulation presents particular difficulties in nephrotic patients; heparin acts mainly through the activation of antithrombin III, the concentration of which is usually greatly diminished. Warfarin is albumin bound and the levels of albumin may change. Whether only some—or all—nephrotics should receive anticoagulation remains unclear. Those with symptomatic thromboses, should be anticoagulated for at least 3–6 months. At this point their serum albumin should be assessed, and if under 25 g/l, or especially if 20 g/l, anticoagulation should probably be continued until it exceeds this level. Despite the association of renal venous thrombosis with membranous nephropathy, even in these patients prophylaxis of all patients cannot be justified.

Alterations in lipid metabolism

Concentrations of cholesterol, triglycerides, and lipoproteins Total cholesterol is raised in almost all nephrotics, with a strong negative correlation with the serum albumin. Increases in fasting triglyceride levels are less common, and are found largely in the more severe cases, again correlating with depression of serum albumin.

Very low density lipoproteins and low density lipoproteins (**LDLs**) are increased in the more severe nephrotic states, and concentrations vary inversely with the serum albumin concentration. Apolipoprotein (a) concentrations are usually raised.

Data on high density lipoprotein (**HDL**) concentrations are conflicting. In most studies reduced HDL concentrations have been noted only in the most severe syndromes. HDL2 concentrations are reduced, and those of HDL3 are normal or increased, except in the most severe cases.

Causes of lipid alterations in the nephrotic syndrome The causes are still not understood in full, but both a major increase in production of all types of lipid and a minor decrease in receptor-mediated removal of lipoproteins and decrease in lipoprotein lipase occur, and abnormalities at almost every step in the production and removal of lipids have been described.

Hypoalbuminaemia was once thought to be the stimulus inducing increased liver apoprotein synthesis, but evidence that this is so in the long term is lacking.

Reduced activity of lecithin cholesterol acyltransferase has been reported, and could thereby reduce HDL production.

Treatment of lipid alterations in nephrotics Alterations in lipid metabolism in the nephrotic syndrome might induce atheromatous vascular disease. Early descriptions reported atheroma even in nephrotic children, and several small series have suggested that the incidence of myocardial infarction in nephrotics in increased. However, two case–control studies came to discordant conclusions. The question remains open, but patients with a particularly severe or prolonged course are almost certainly at extra risk.

It seems reasonable to give dietary advice to nephrotic as to any other hyperlipidaemic patient but there is no justification in treating all nephrotic patients with hypolipidaemic agents. Most remit spontaneously, are treated, or go on to develop chronic renal failure within 3–5 years. The decision to treat hyperlipidaemia or not can therefore be postponed until the decision can be made in the light of probable duration.

There are few reports of studies on dietary modification of plasma lipids, and none of the administration of omega-3 unsaturated fish oils. Neither is there any indication as to which hypolipidaemic drug may be the most useful, although the statins are effective and seem the preferable drugs at present even though their long-term benefit has yet to be shown.

Losses of binding transport proteins in the urine

A number of important plasma proteins are lost into the urine of nephrotic patients. These include transferrin, caeruloplasmin, vitamin D binding protein, thyroid-binding globulin cortisol-binding protein, and erythropoietin. Such losses appear to be of little, if any, clinical significance, although renal osteodystrophy may be increased in renal failure complicated by nephrotic syndrome and a variety of changes in calcium metabolism have been described (see OTM3, pp. 3143–4), and erythropoietin loss may be associated with anaemia.

Hypovolaemia and acute renal failure in the nephrotic syndrome

Hypovolaemia is more common in nephrotic children than in adults, even in the absence of diuretic therapy, but acute renal failure is rarely seen and is almost always associated with sepsis and/or thrombosis. In contrast the commoner acute renal failure seen in older adults is not associated with hypovalaemia, and its origins are not clear.

Renal tubular dysfunction in nephrotics

Tubular dysfunction has been described in a small number of nephrotic patients, usually with multiple proximal tubular deficiencies in reabsorption, (complete or partial Fanconi syndrome).

Proteinuria as factor in the progression of renal failure

There is a correlation between the amount of proteinuria, its persistence, and decline of renal function. There is now strong evidence that proteinuria is of itself deleterious to the kidney. Several consequences of profuse proteinuria may contribute. First, the proteinuria of intravenous protein overload causes an interstitial infiltrate, but although this describes a potential mechanism for direct toxicity of filtered albumin, it does not account for the absence of renal failure in many patients with chronic minimal change disease unresponsive to steroids. Second, hypercoagulability could promote intraglomerular thrombosis by release of platelet-derived factors. Third, hyperlipidaemia has a complex relationship with glomerulosclerosis. Mesangial cells bear LDL receptors, and there is evidence that binding of excess LDL can damage them.

The patient with haematuria

Macroscopic haematuria

The urine of macroscopic haematuria may be bright red but more often after a dwell time in the bladder it is brownish, likened to tea or Coca-Cola.

Usually, the amounts of blood lost are trivial, but the presence of clots, with or without colic, suggests bleeding from the renal pelvis, ureters or bladder, although major bleeding may also complicate polycystic kidney disease as well as renal tumours. Occasionally, heavy bleeding of glomerular origin leads to acute renal failure not related to clot obstruction; the mechanisms remains obscure.

Given the long list of causes of haematuria in Table 2, it is valuable to be able to distinguish the site of origin of the red cells. Clues include the presence of concomitant proteinuria, which almost always indicates a renal origin. The use of phase contrast microscopy to define red cell morphology in urine is described above.

Persistent symptomless isolated haematuria

The significance of this finding varies with age. In young individuals, significant disease in as few as 2 per cent of a haematuric population has been reported. Red cell casts and dysmorphic red cells imply glomerular haematuria, and in such cases renal biopsy often shows minor patterns of glomerular change, but may show thin membrane nephropathy or mesangial IgA deposition. Alport's syndrome will often present as isolated haematuria before any deafness or associated proteinuria is present.

Figure 4 gives an algorithm for the investigation of a patient with haematuria. If no red cell casts or dysmorphic cells are present and a clotting screen is normal, an intravenous urogram or ultrasound followed by a cystoscopy are usual practice, but in many young cases no abnormalities are detected.

In older patients the position is quite different. From 2 to 20 per cent of middle-aged and elderly males show microscopic symptomless haematuria, most commonly as manifestation of stones or renal tract malignancy; in them investigation is mandatory.

Persistent microscopic haematuria with associated proteinuria

Non-glomerular causes include renal tuberculosis, polycystic kidneys, papillary necrosis, interstitial nephritis, and reflux nephropathy, but glomerular disease is more likely, commonly thin membrane nephropathy or IgA or other mesangial nephropathy, as well as other

Table 2 Causes of haematuria

Disorders of coagulation	Anticoagulants Bleeding disorders (haemophilia, etc.)
Glomerular diseases	IgA nephropathy
	Endocapillary nephritis
	Alport's syndrome
	Thin membrane nephropathy
	Mesangiocapillary glomerulonephritis
	Crescentic glomerulonephritis
	Fabry's disease
	Vasculitis/lupus, etc.
Interstitial diseases	Interstitial nephritis
	Polycystic disease
Medullary diseases	Papillary necrosis from: analgesic nephropathy sickle-cell disease diabetes mellitus
	Sponge kidney
	Tuberculosis
Renal and urinary tract tumours	Wilms'
	Renal cell carcinoma
	Transitional cell lesions
	Carcinoma of prostate
	Carcinoma of urethra
Infections	Acute pyelonephritis/cystitis
	Schistosomiasis
	Urethritis
	Prostatitis
Stones	Anywhere in urinary tract
	Calcium oxalate crystalluria
	Urate crystalluria
Obstruction	NB release of obstruction
Trauma	To kidney, bladder, ureter
Miscellaneous	Hypertension
	Loin pain–haematuria syndrome
	Familial telangiectasia
	Arteriovenous malformations
	Endometriosis
	Chemical cystitis
	Meatal ulcers
	Urethral caruncle
	Foreign body
	Factitious (added blood)

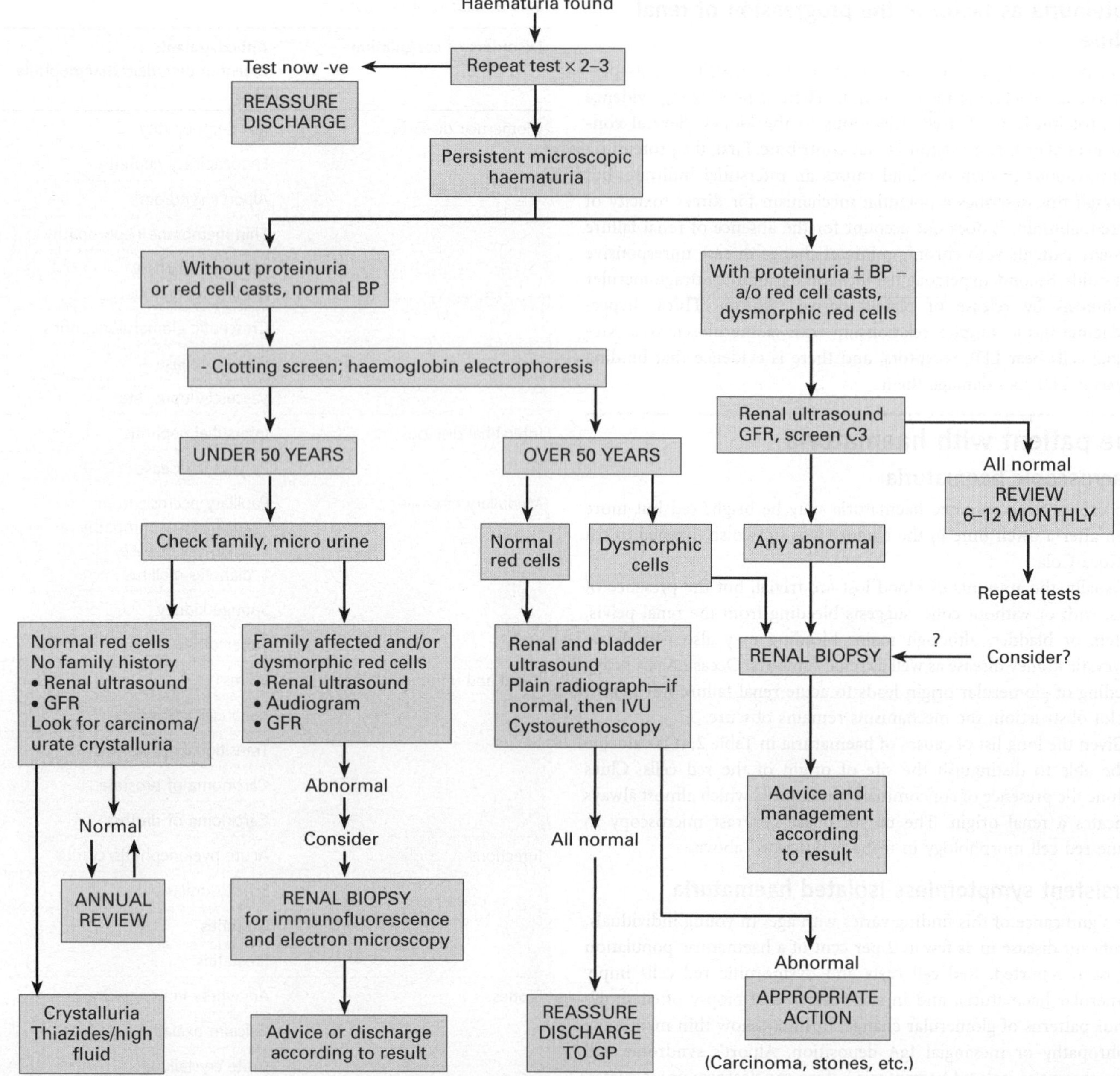

Fig. 4 An algorithm for the investigation of a patient found to have haematuria. Note the different strategies in those aged less than or more than 45 years of age.

proliferative patterns and membranous nephropathy. Patients with Alport's syndrome develop added haematuria as their glomerulopathy evolves. Renal biopsy is the critical investigation unless ultrasound or urography shows an anatomical cause.

Acute haematuria with proteinuria: the acute nephritic syndrome

Usually there is associated oliguria, circulatory overload and pulmonary oedema, hypertension (sometimes in the malignant phase); and variable, often non-pitting oedema. There is often a prodrome of an infection, either in skin or throat, arising from *Streptococcus haemolyticus;* but many other infections can precipitate this syndrome.

Most frequently some form of proliferative/infiltrative nephritis is present, particularly endocapillary nephritis or mesangiocapillary nephritis, with or without crescent formation. Sometimes a necrotizing glomerulitis with severe crescent formation is caused by a vasculitis, when purpura, arthritis, or uveitis help to make the diagnosis, but quite often the renal disease is, at least for a time, the only manifestation. Rarely, antiglomerular basement membrane disease is found. In neither vasculitic nor antiglomerular basement membrane disease is hypertension as common a problem as it is in those forms of glomerulonephritis in which glomeruli are infiltrated by monocytes.

Loin pain in parenchymal renal disease; the loin pain–haematuria syndrome

An unusual group of patients present with recurrent or persistent severe loin pain, often with intermittent or persistent microscopic haematuria but sometimes without. They are predominantly young women, and often have some connection with the practice of medicine. Many require opiates, and have disturbed personalities. It is impossible to know if this is truly the result of chronic pain. Nephrectomy is often requested and sometimes performed. Usually the pain then recurs at another site, often in the opposite kidney. In some, angiography reveals tortuous middle-sized arteries, and renal biopsy may show onion-skinning of the vessels, but this is not common.

These patients present many problems of management. Around cases of a 'typical' loin pain–haematuria syndrome cluster a more varied group with unexplained severe loin pain who behave similarly. Some have had renal colic; many seek opiates. Nephrectomy rarely solves the problem, and nor do attempts to denervate of the kidney by injection, surgical stripping of nerves, or autotransplantation. Both corticosteroids and antiplatelet drugs have been used in view of the arterial changes, but usually without effect. Management finally settles round establishing a regimen for pain relief. Transcutaneous nerve stimulation, carbamazepine, and amitriptyline are usually ineffective, and establishing a stable analgesic regimen, usually employing narcotics, is often required. Few patients have been followed long term, but the impression is that there is often remission when the patients are in their 40s and 50s, which supports hypotheses suggesting a role for oestrogens, as the vascular changes have been linked with the use of oral contraceptives.

Disorders of micturition: oliguria, polyuria

In any oliguric patient the first step in diagnosis is to establish whether the patient has had an adequate intake, has had excess extrarenal losses, is already overloaded because of failure to excrete a normal amount of intake, or has urinary tract obstruction at some level. The composition of the urine, the state of the circulation and renal perfusion, as well as the history, will help in diagnosis

The commonest cause of polyuria is a habitual high fluid intake. Diabetes mellitus, compulsive polydipsia, diabetes insipidus, hypercalcaemia, and hypokalaemia are discussed elsewhere.

Polyuria and nocturia are to be expected in any case of chronic renal failure. A major cause in this context is the increased solute load per surviving nephron. In disorders affecting the medulla more than the cortex (nephronophthisis, sickle cell disease, urinary tract obstruction, hypokalaemia) polyuria is particularly prominent.

Pain as a symptom of renal disease

Ureteric colic

Ureteric colic is acute, usually very severe, and waxes and wanes in a typical colicky pattern. Pain radiates from the loin into the abdomen, and down into the testicle, labium, or upper thigh. Vomiting is usual. Sudden relief may occur if the stone, blood clot, or sloughed papilla, moves on, only to recur when it impacts again. At the end of all this agony a surprisingly tiny, innocent looking stone may be passed. Once it has reached the bladder signs of irritation in the trigone may appear instead. The obvious differential diagnoses are appendicitis and biliary colic, if the pain is on the right side of the abdomen. Other differentials include colonic pain, especially left-sided. Ultrasound usually reveals the problem, although neither this technique nor straight radiographs of the abdomen is good at revealing small stones in the middle third of the ureter. An intravenous urogram is then the definitive investigation.

Renal pain

Renal pain is usually static, dull, constant, and felt in the loin. Sometimes there is obvious renal swelling, with or without tenderness. The commonest cause is obstruction to urinary outflow, especially at the pelviureteric junction, and may be made worse by diuretics or consumption of large amounts of fluid, or alcohol. Acute pyelonephritis will give rise to similar pain, and a rare differential diagnosis is of renal infarction by *in situ* thrombosis or embolism in the renal arterial tree. Less severe (and uncommon) renal pain may be a symptom of acute nephritic conditions and IgA nephropathy, presumably caused by distension of the renal capsule. The loin pain/haematuria syndrome is described above. Renal abscesses may be acutely tender. Renal venous thrombosis, if acute, also leads to acute renal pain. The main differential diagnosis is musculoskeletal pain, usually referred from segments D10 to D12 in the back. Renal pain, which may be intractable and require cyst puncture or nephrectomy, comes from bleeding or infection within cysts of polycystic kidneys.

Frequency and dysuria

These are among the commonest symptoms in medicine, accounting for 20/1000 patient attendances in general practice. Dysuria describes pain or scalding on the passage of urine, and a sensation of incomplete voiding which often follows the slight relief after passing urine and leads to frequent painful passage of small amounts of urine. Microscopic haematuria is usually present, and bleeding from the inflamed mucosa may be sufficient to produce macroscopic haematuria. The complaint is much more frequent in women than in men, and is frequently attributed to cystitis. Dysuria can also occur in acute pyelonephritis, but is often absent. The commonest cause is inflammation of the urethra, trigone, and bladder, most commonly with Gram-negative bacteria of gut origin.

Further reading

Cameron, J.S. (1998). The patient with proteinuria and/or haematuria. In *Oxford textbook of clinical nephrology*, (2nd edn), (ed. Davison, A.M., Cameron, J.S., Grünfeld, J.-P., Kerr, D., Ritz, E., and Winearls, C.), pp. 441–59. Oxford University Press.

Cameron, J.S. The nephrotic syndrome. In *Oxford textbook of clinical nephrology*, (2nd edn), (ed. Davison, A.M., Cameron, J.S., Grünfeld, J.-P., Kerr, D., Ritz, E., and Winearls, C.), pp. 461–92. Oxford University Press.

De Jong, P., de Zeeuw, D., and Mogensen, C.E. (ed.). (1997). Proteinuria and progressive renal disease. *Nephrology Dialysis Transplantation*, **12** (Suppl. 12) 1–85.

Niuwehof, C., Doorenbos, C., Grave, W., de Heer, F., de Leeuw, P., Zeppenfeldt, E., and van Breda Vriesman, J.C. (1996). A prospective study of the natural history of idiopathic non-proteinuric hematuria. *Kidney International*, **49**, 222–5.

Ruggenenti, P. *et al.* (1998). Urinary protein excretion rate is the best independent predictor of ESRF in non-diabetic proteinuric chronic nephropathies. *Kidney International*, **53**, 1209–16.

Primary renal glomerular disease

Chapter 12.6

Immunoglobulin A nephropathy, Henoch–Schönlein purpura, and thin membrane nephropathy

A. R. Clarkson, A. J. Woodroffe, and A. C. Thomas

Immunoglobulin A nephropathy

IgA nephropathy is now recognized as the commonest form of glomerulonephritis in the world. There are racial differences in prevalence, but where renal biopsy is widespread, IgA nephropathy is found in approximately 30 per cent of all biopsies for primary glomerular disorders. Population studies indicate an occurrence rate of 1 in 10 000, but some autopsy studies suggest an incidence between 1 in 100 and 1 in 1000.

Clinical features

IgA nephropathy is characteristically found in young males in the second or third decades of life (male to female ratio 3:1) who have recurring episodes of 'synpharyngitic' macroscopic haematuria, which usually occurs within 12–24 h of the pharyngitis and frequently is accompanied by diffuse muscle pains, loin pain, high fever, and lethargy out of proportion to the severity of the sore throat. On occasion, infections involving other mucosal surfaces may initiate the haematuria. These include bronchial, gastrointestinal, bladder, female genital tract, and breast infections. Unlike the smoky, grey-coloured urine seen 10–14 days after throat infection in post-streptococcal glomerulonephritis, urine in IgA nephropathy is frankly bloody for between 1 and 5 days. Most commonly, blood pressure is normal during these episodes, there is no periorbital or ankle oedema, and recovery is rapid. However, an acute decrease in renal function (sometimes to the extent that dialysis is needed) may accompany a haematuric episode and delay recovery. In some patients, the diagnosis is made following discovery of proteinuria or microscopic haematuria. The urinary sediment contains numerous dysmorphic erythrocytes and granular and red cell casts. Other features, such as hypertension, nephrotic syndrome, acute or chronic renal failure, and, rarely, the acute nephritic syndrome, may be the presenting problem in the remainder.

Diagnosis

Renal biopsy is the only definitive investigation; mesangial immunofluorescence for IgA and C3 is the hallmark. Variable findings include high circulating concentrations of IgA and IgA-containing immune complexes. There are no characteristic abnormalities in serum complement components.

Clinical course

In children IgA nephropathy has a good prognosis for at least a decade, and complete remission occurs in 30 per cent of them after 10 years. In the remainder, varying degrees of proteinuria, hypertension, and renal impairment may persist and only 1–3 per cent develop end-stage renal failure. In adults the outlook is worse, but development of the disease is usually slow. A small group has a rapid downhill course into renal failure over 3–5 years but more commonly renal failure develops after 15–25 years of indolent and often asymptomatic progress; 25–50 per cent of adult patients will eventually develop end-stage renal failure. Few data exist on the proportion of patients entering complete clinical remission, but estimates of 10 per cent are not unusual.

Henoch–Schönlein purpura

Henoch–Schönlein purpura is easily diagnosed by the association of arthritis, palpable purpura, gut symptoms, and glomerulonephritis; it can be viewed as a systemic manifestation of IgA nephropathy. The skin disease begins with urticarial spots on the extensor surfaces of arms and legs, especially around the ankles, buttocks, and elbows. The face and trunk are spared. Development to purpura which is often palpable occurs quickly, with some lesions coalescing to become necrotic. Resolution occurs over 2–4 weeks, but fresh crops frequently appear. Polyarthritis, often flitting, occurs in about two-thirds of patients, characteristically involving large joints (knees and ankles) and is manifest by varying degrees of pain and periarticular swelling. Resolution is usually within 10 days, but recurrence is common.

Abdominal symptoms include colicky pain, melaena, haematemesis, and obstruction due to intramural haematomas and intussusception. The most frequently observed clinical sequence is the development of one or more of the joint, gut, and skin manifestations soon after an intercurrent infection. Upper respiratory tract infections are the most frequent precipitants.

When there is renal involvement (reported frequency 20–100 per cent depending on criteria used to define it), it is usually noticed later, although examination may detect microhaematuria from the onset. Rarely, extrarenal manifestations occur a considerable time after the initial diagnosis. Recurrence may be frequent. Overt acute nephritis, nephrotic syndrome, progressive renal failure, and macroscopic haematuria are recognized more frequently in adults than in children. Prognosis in both generally depends on the severity of the initial renal disease, but progressive renal failure may develop in patients whose initial renal disease is mild.

Diagnosis

This can be confirmed by finding positive immunofluorescence for IgA and C3 within the 'vasculitic' skin lesions and the glomerular mesangia. Approximately 50 per cent of patients have elevated serum IgA concentrations, and IgA-containing immune complexes are found during the active phase of the disease.

Clinical course

Apart from intussusception, the major cause of morbidity and mortality is glomerulonephritis. Fifty per cent of children with Henoch–Schönlein purpura glomerulonephritis are in complete clinical remission after 2 years. About 30 per cent have persisting urinary abnormalities with normal renal function, while a minority (3–5 per cent) progress quickly to renal failure. Proteinuria and decreased renal function persist in the remaining 15–20 per cent, and a significant proportion of these will have developed end-stage renal failure after 10 years. Similar observations have been made in adults.

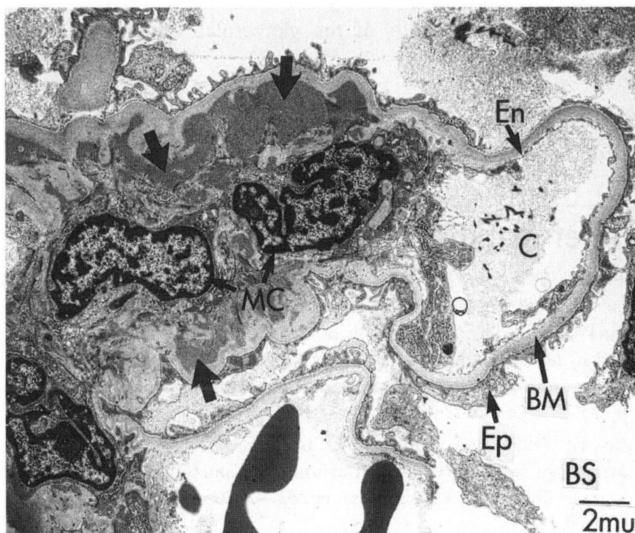

Fig. 1 Electron micrograph of glomerular capillary loop in IgA nephropathy. Numerous electron-dense deposits representing deposits of IgA can be seen within the expanded mesangium (arrows) (×5200). BM, basement membrane; C, capillary lumen; Ep, visceral epithelium; En, fenestrated endothelium; MC, mesangial cell nucleus; BS, Bowman's space.

Pathology of IgA nephropathy and Henoch–Schönlein purpura

Glomerular pathology is similar in IgA nephropathy and Henoch–Schönlein purpura, although widely variable in both. The basic lesion is a mesangial proliferative glomerulonephritis. In their mildest form the mesangial changes are focal, and much of the glomerular tuft may appear normal. More frequently there is diffuse disease, the mesangial expansion and cellular proliferation appearing like a tree trunk. Sometimes mesangiocapillary changes are apparent. Added to the mesangial lesion, three distinct types of focal segmental lesion may be seen.

The first, seen in 'active' disease consists of areas of tuft necrosis manifest by fibrin exudates and leucocyte infiltration. Small crescents are frequently associated with these lesions and, on occasion, circumferential crescents may be seen. The second consists of segmental glomerular scars with associated synechiae joining the tuft to Bowman's capsule. In long-standing disease, areas of tuft collapse and sclerosis with hyalinosis occur. These are most frequently seen in progressive disease, in which there is progressive glomerular obsolescence.

Mononuclear cells and neutrophils surround glomeruli with 'active' areas of tuft necrosis and crescents. Interstitial scarring, tubular atrophy, and hypertensive vascular changes complicate long-standing disease. Within the glomerular mesangia IgA and C3 are found by immunofluorescence or immunoperoxidase techniques. IgG and IgM are variable, as is fibrinogen. Electron microscopy reveals electron-dense deposits in paramesangial areas (Fig. 1), and occasionally in the glomerular capillary basement membranes. In the leucocytoclastic vasculitis of Henoch–Schönlein purpura deposits of IgA and C3 are found in blood vessel walls; electron-dense deposits have been demonstrated in early lesions. Deposits of IgA and C3 can also be found in dermal blood vessels of patients with IgA disease despite the absence of clinical changes.

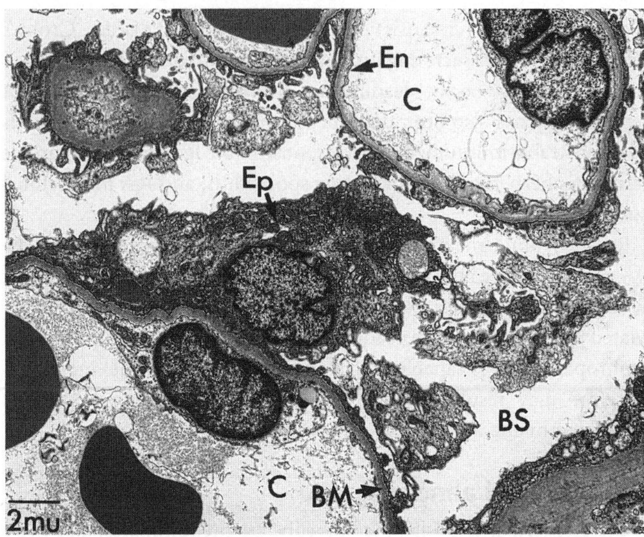

(a)

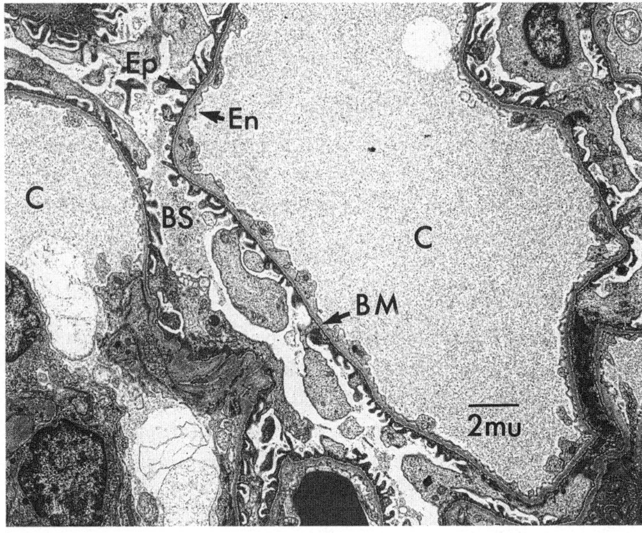

(b)

Fig. 2 (a) Electron micrographs of glomerular basement membranes, contrasting membranes of normal thickness (a) with those of patients with thin membrane nephropathy (b). The normal basement membrane thickness is in the order of 350–430 nm, whereas in the example of thin membrane nephropathy illustrated it is about 200–270 nm (×5200). BM, basement membrane; C, capillary lumen; Ep, visceral epithelium, En, fenestrated endothelium; BS, Bowman's space. (b) Electron micrographs of glomerular basement membranes, contrasting membranes of normal thickness (a) with those of patients with thin membrane nephropathy (b). The normal basement membrane thickness is in the order of 350–430 nm, whereas in the example of thin membrane nephropathy illustrated it is about 200–270 nm (×5200). BM, basement membrane; C, capillary lumen; Ep, visceral epithelium, En, fenestrated endothelium; BS, Bowman's space.

Pathogenesis of IgA nephropathy and Henoch–Schönlein purpura

A genetic susceptibility is likely. Many instances have been described of first-degree relatives with the diseases and even more relatives without disease who have similar abnormalities of IgA production *in vitro*. Associations with HLA-DR4-DQW4, and complement genes have been also described.

Increased serum IgA concentrations are found in 50 per cent of patients. IgA nephropathy and Henoch–Schönlein purpura may occur in association with (cirrhosis) of the liver and coeliac disease, Crohn's disease, and mucin-secreting carcinomas, wherein disorders of antigen processing may occur, leading to overproduction of IgA. IgA nephropathy has also been described in other diseases where there is a demonstrable immunoglobulin response of the IgA class, for example dermatitis herpetiformis, ankylosing spondylitis, and IgA monoclonal gammopathy.

Recently, abnormalities in glycosylations of the hinge region of the IgA_i molecule have been demonstrated, possibly resulting from specific deficiency of the α_i-galactosyl-transferase enzyme. Aberrantly glycosylated IgA_i adheres more readily to mesangial cells than normal IgA nephropathy and is capable of activating complement. Mesangial IgA_i therefore may result from deposition of IgA_i containing immune complexes or the abnormally glycosylated IgA_i.

Production of abnormal IgA

In the glomerular deposits, the IgA_i subclass predominates, and there is evidence that glomerular IgA is abnormally anionic. The IgA_i is derived from bone marrow cells as a result of defective mucosal immunity.

Defective immune clearance

Impaired hepatic clearance of IgA aggregates has been shown and might reflect saturation of receptors, resulting from the original load. It is still not known how the mesangial IgA deposits lead to glomerular injury (see OTM3, p. 3152).

Transplantation

IgA nephropathy recurs in kidneys transplanted into recipients whose primary disease was the same, but kidneys already with IgA nephropathy inadvertently transplanted into recipients without that disease are free of it within a few weeks of transplantation. This suggests a primary role for those factors determining mesangial IgA_i deposition rather than a primary abnormality in the kidney.

Treatment

There is no known effective treatment for these diseases. Experience with anti-inflammatory and immunosuppressive drugs is disappointing.

Thin membrane nephropathy (benign familial haematuria)

The association of haematuria with thin glomerular basement membranes is a common one, usually diagnosed in investigation of persistent, usually asymptomatic, microscopic, or 'dipstick' haematuria. Microscopy of urine reveals a significant number of dysmorphic red blood cells. Minor proteinuria may be present, but blood pressure and renal function are normal. Episodes of macroscopic haematuria occasionally occur.

Family studies support an autosomal dominant inheritance. A dilemma exists in deciding how far to investigate these otherwise well individuals. As there is no genetic marker for this condition it may be useful to make a firm diagnosis by renal biopsy in at least one member of a family, but there is no point in performing renal biopsy unless electron microscopy is available; the light microscopic features are non-specific, and immunofluorescence is not helpful. The key finding is decreased width of the glomerular capillary basement membrane (Fig. 2).

Prognosis

The condition is benign and should not compromise life insurance.

Further reading

Feehally, J. (1997). IgA nephropathy—a disorder of IgA production? *Quarterly Journal of Medicine*, **90**, 387–90.

Haycock, G.B. (1998). The nephritis of Henoch-Schonlein purpura. In: *Oxford textbook of clinical nephrology*, 2nd edn (ed. A.M. Davison, J.S. Cameron, J.-P. Grünfeld, D. Kerr, E. Ritz, and C.G. Winearls), pp.858–77. Oxford University Press, Oxford

Schena, F.P. (1998). IgA nephropathies. In: *Oxford textbook of clinical nephrology*, 2nd edn (ed. A.M. Davison, J.S. Cameron, J.-P. Grünfeld, D. Kerr, E. Ritz, and C.G. Winearls), pp. 537–70. Oxford University Press, Oxford.

Tiebosch, A.T.G.M., Frederik, P.M., van Brieda Vriesman, P.J., *et al.* (1989). Thin-basement-membrane nephropathy in adults with persistent haematuria. *New England Journal of Medicine*, **320**, 14–18.

Chapter 12.7

Idiopathic glomerulonephritis

D. Adu

Glomerulonephritis is idiopathic in most cases occurring in temperate regions. Aetiology and patterns are different in topical countries. Understanding is hampered by different systems of classification which have been based on clinical features (e.g. rapidly progressive glomerulonephritis) on aetiology (e.g. post-streptococcal) and on histology. Of these, the most helpful has been histology. Table 1, for instance, summarizes the histological features of nephrotic syndrome in both children and adults. The ways in which glomerulonephritis

Table 1 Histology of the nephrotic syndrome

Histology	Children (%)	Adults (%)
Minimal change nephrotic syndrome	76	25
Mesangiocapillary glomerulonephritis	8	14
Focal segmental glomerulosclerosis	7	9
Proliferative (including diffuse mesangial proliferation)	2	13
Membranous	2	21
Other	5	–
Systemic lupus erythematosus	–	8
Amyloid	–	7
Diabetes	–	3

For sources see OTM3, p.3161.

Children: ISKDC study (1978) (excludes secondary causes of nephrotic syndrome, such as systemic lupus erythematosus, Henoch-Schönlein purpura—about 10 per cent).

Adults. Cameron (1979).

Table 2 Clinical presentation of glomerulonephritis

Persistent microscopic haematuria
Persistent proteinuria
Nephrotic syndrome
Acute nephritic syndrome
Acute renal failure and chronic renal failure

Table 3 Idiopathic nephrotic syndrome in childhood: histology and response to steroids

Histology	Percentage of all cases	Remission with steroids (%)
Minimal change nephrotic syndrome	76	93
Mesangiocapillary glomerulonephritis	8	7
Focal segmental glomerulosclerosis	7	30
Proliferative glomerulonephritis	2	25
Diffuse mesangial proliferative glomerulonephritis	2	56
Focal and global glomerulosclerosis	1.7	75
Membranous nephropathy	1.5	0
Chronic glomerulonephritis	0.8	75
Unclassified	0.8	75

ISKDC (1978, 1981). (See OTM3, p. 3161.)

may present are limited and are summarized in Table 2. Definitive diagnosis of most forms is dependent on a renal biopsy.

Nephrotic syndrome

Children

Minimal change nephropathy is much the most likely cause of nephrotic syndrome in children aged between 1 and 6 years, particularly in the absence of microscopic haematuria, hypertension, and renal impairment and when proteinuria is highly selective (Table 3). Indeed, the probability is such that renal biopsy is not appropriate in these cases who are instead given a trial of steroid treatment. Biopsy is then reserved for those who fail to respond. Those over the age of 8 are less likely to have a steroid-responsive lesion and many of these need renal biopsy.

Adults

As only 25 per cent of adults with nephrotic syndrome have minimal change disease, renal biopsy has been considered an essential first step in management. An alternative is to give a trial of steroid treatment for 6–8 weeks, turning to biopsy only in those who have failed to respond. The latter approach will involve unnecessary treatment with a toxic drug and as renal biopsy carries little morbidity or risk in skilled hands, the former approach is still preferred.

Minimal change nephropathy, focal segmental glomerulosclerosis, and mesangial proliferative glomerulonephritis: one disorder or not?

In some children subjected to serial renal biopsy in steroid-responsive nephrotic syndrome, the histological lesion changes with time from true minimal change or mesangial proliferative disease to focal segmental glomerulonephritis (**FSGS**). This observation has raised the question of whether these entities are all variants of the same disease. In fact, those patients with minimal change evolving into FSGS who remain steroid responsive have a good prognosis, whereas those who are steroid resistant tend to progress to chronic renal failure. The prognosis is, therefore, more dependent on response to steroids than on renal histology. The arguments for and against these histological patterns reflecting different diseases are complex and unsettled.

Aetiology or minimal change nephropathy

There is an association between minimal change nephropathy and Hodgkin's disease and to a lesser degree with carcinoma. There are also reports of minimal change nephropathy in individuals exposed to bee stings, poison oak, grass pollen, and cow's milk. Some of these patients had other atopic symptoms, leading to suggestions that minimal change nephropathy might then be caused by reaginic antibodies. The evidence for this is not convincing. Non-steroidal anti-inflammatory drugs can cause an interstitial nephritis, which in some cases is accompanied by a nephrotic syndrome with renal histology showing the changes of minimal change nephropathy.

Pathogenesis of minimal change nephropathy

The responsiveness of minimal change nephropathy to steroids, cyclophosphamide, chlorambucil, and cyclosporin is evidence that this disorder is immune mediated. Impairment of lymphocyte proliferation in response to mitogens has been described, but this is also found in patients with other causes of the nephrotic syndrome. The low serum IgG and high IgM appear to be a consequence of the nephrotic syndrome *per se*. The hypothesis that proteinuria in this disorder is caused by a lymphokine produced by an abnormal clone of T lymphocytes has been studied extensively. As yet it has neither been proved nor disproved. In Europe an increased incidence of HLA-DR7 is found and in Japan the association is with HLA-DR8, suggesting a genetic predisposition to this disorder.

Pathology

On light microscopy the glomeruli appear normal and small and on electron microscopy there is effacement of epithelial-cell foot processes over the outer surface of the glomerular basement membrane. Some authors also accept a minor degree of mesangial IgM deposits and mesangial proliferation.

Clinical presentation in children

Heavy proteinuria (over 2 g/24 h) is accompanied by hypoalbuminaemia with serum albumin less than 10 g/1itre in some 38 per cent of cases. Microscopic haematuria is infrequent (22 per cent) as is hypertension (9 per cent). Oedema is variable, but ascites and hydrothorax are common. Renal impairment is unusual at presentation. These children are prone to infection and a number of other complications . In 75 per cent of patients the proteinuria is highly or moderately selective.

Treatment of minimal change nephropathy in children

Prednisolone is given at an initial dose of 60 mg/m^2 (maximum dose 80 mg) daily, reducing at 4 weeks to 40 mg/m^2 (maximum dose 60 mg) on alternate days for a further 4 weeks. More than 90 per cent respond with complete loss of proteinuria within 8 weeks.

Relapses

Sixty-six per cent of children develop at least one relapse and 40–55 per cent develop multiple relapses when steroids are discontinued, or become steroid dependent and relapse when dosage is reduced. Early frequent relapses (three or more) in the 6 months following the initial response to steroids predicts a frequently relapsing course.

Treatment of relapses

A standard regimen is prednisolone 60 mg/m^2 until the urine is free of protein for 3 days (maximum 4 weeks) and then prednisolone 40 mg/m^2 on alternate days for 4 weeks. During repeated steroid treatment of relapses, growth should be monitored. Treatment with cyclophosphamide/chlorambucil should be considered in: (a) children who are frequent relapsers; (b) children who are steroid dependent (two consecutive relapses occurring during alternate-day treatment for an earlier relapse) or who relapse within 14 days of treatment of an earlier relapse (fast relapse); (c) children in whom two of four relapses within 6 months were fast relapses; (d) children who have developed serious side-effects from steroids.

Cyclophosphamide is given in a dose of 2 mg/kg per day (ideal height for weight) for 8 weeks. Approximately 50 per cent of treated children are in remission at 2 years and 40 per cent at 5 years. Chlorambucil has also been used, but there is no evidence that it is better than cyclophosphamide. Permanent gonadal toxicity occurs with chlorambucil at a cumulative dose of 8 mg/kg. The borderline dose for permanent gonadal toxicity with cyclophosphamide is a cumulative dose of 200 mg/kg. Other acute toxic side-effects of cyclophosphamide include leucopenia, haemorrhagic cystitis, and alopecia, and an oncogenic potential is well established.

Minimal change nephropathy in adults

About 25 per cent of adults with a nephrotic syndrome have minimal change nephropathy. The mean age of onset is 40 years but the condition can occur up to the age of 60 and over.

Clinical presentation

The nephrotic syndrome is not as severe as in children. Profound hypoalbuminaemia (serum albumin <10 g/litre) is found in only 6 per cent of cases. The disease is slightly more common in men than in women with a male to female ratio of 1.3:1. More adults than children are hypertensive (30 per cent), have microscopic haematuria (28 per cent), and renal impairment at diagnosis (60 per cent).

Treatment

The response to prednisolone 60 mg/day is slightly less frequent than in children, and also slower. Eighty per cent respond but remission can take up to 16 weeks to occur. The number of relapses in adults is less frequent, at 1.7/patient, than in children, and only 20 per cent of adults develop multiple relapses or are steroid dependent. In them, cyclophosphamide is often effective in inducing a long-lasting remission. Cyclosporin is also effective in both adults and children. Patients who are steroid responsive or multiple relapsers are more likely to respond with complete or partial remissions (70–80 per cent) than patients who are resistant to steroids (40–50 per cent). This drug is effective at blood levels of 100–200 ng/ml, when nephrotoxicity and hypertension are uncommon. Relapses recur with the same frequency after cyclosporin has been discontinued as before.

Long-term outcome

In children, some 5 per cent continue to relapse into adult life. All such cases have presented before the age of 6 years. The long-term mortality rate in children ranges from 2 to 7 per cent. In adults, 6 per cent of patients are still nephrotic after a mean follow-up of 7.5 years. Reported survival in patients aged over 60 is 50 per cent at 10 years and in those aged 15–59, 90 per cent. Progression to endstage renal failure is rare in both adults and children, and occurs in 1 per cent of cases, probably due to the subsequent development of FSGS.

Table 4 Secondary focal segmental glomerulosclerosis

Alport's syndrome
Reduced renal mass
Reflux nephropathy
Remnant kidney
Healed glomerulonephritis
IgA nephropathy
Vasculitis
Diffuse proliferative glomerulonephritis
Sickle-cell disease
AIDS
Intravenous drug abuse (heroin)

Focal segmental glomerulosclerosis

Pathogenesis

In experimental models FSGS can develop from toxic injury (puromycin nephropathy), immunological injury (antiglomerular basement membrane nephritis), the nephritis of experimental lupus, and hyperfiltration injury. Some of these models have clinical counterparts and the diversity of pathogenic mechanisms may explain the variability in clinical presentation as well as responses to therapy. There are suggestions that the glomerular injury in FSGS is caused by a lymphokine. The rapid development of heavy proteinuria following renal transplantation in some patients with FSGS suggests that the glomerular injury is caused by a circulating factor.

Pathology

Focal segmental sclerosing lesions affect predominantly juxtamedullary glomeruli. These lesions are usually adherent to Bowman's capsule, with a predilection for the hilar regions. In some cases the lesions are located at the glomerulotubular junction, the so-called glomerular tip lesion. Focal areas of tubular atrophy and interstitial nephritis are prominent. On immunofluorescent microscopy deposits of IgM and C3 may be seen in the sclerotic areas. Electron microscopy shows diffuse foot process effacement in apparently unaffected glomeruli.

Primary and secondary focal segmental glomerulosclerosis

FSGS may be found early on in the course of a nephrotic syndrome, when by convention it is called primary. FSGS has also been found later in patients whose initial renal biopsy had shown minimal change (secondary). It may also be a sequel of glomerular scarring in patients with previous proliferative glomerulonephritis, and is seen in the biopsies of patients with Alport's syndrome (Table 4). It has also been found in reflux nephropathy and other conditions leading to a reduced renal mass. The sclerosing lesions in these circumstances are probably a consequence of glomerular hypertension and hyperfiltration.

Clinical presentation of focal segmental glomerulosclerosis in children

Approximately 7 per cent of children presenting with an idiopathic nephrotic syndrome have FSGS. The majority (75 per cent) present with a nephrotic syndrome, 20 per cent have persistent proteinuria, and 5 per cent haematuria as well as proteinuria. These patients differ from children with minimal change nephropathy in that two-thirds have microscopic haematuria, one-half have impaired renal function at diagnosis, and one-third are hypertensive. The proteinuria is usually poorly selective.

Clinical presentation of focal segmental glomerulosclerosis in adults

Approximately 10 per cent of adults with a nephrotic syndrome have FSGS. The clinical presentation does not differ from that in children. The mean age at onset is between 20 and 30 years, but FSGS has been found in patients aged 70.

Treatment and prognosis of classical focal segmental glomerulosclerosis

The response to steroids is poor. Only 10–30 per cent of patients respond by going into remission. This group has a good prognosis but non-responders fare badly; between 30 and 50 per cent develop endstage renal failure over 5–10 years. There is no difference in prognosis between adults and children. Patients with a nephrotic syndrome are more likely to develop endstage renal failure than those with more modest proteinuria. Cyclophosphamide has been given to some patients with FSGS resistant to steroids: useful remission was induced in 25 per cent of cases. Responsiveness to cyclosporin has been poor and has paralleled to that of steroid therapy.

Treatment of glomerular tip lesion

Patients with the glomerular tip lesion have been reported to be responsive to steroids or immunosuppression and not to progress to endstage renal failure, but these observations have not been confirmed beyond doubt.

Mesangiocapillary glomerulonephritis

Mesangiocapillary, or membranoproliferative, glomerulonephritis (**MCGN**) is a disorder that is defined by its histological appearance. It is found in approximately 8 per cent of children and 14 per cent of adults with the nephrotic syndrome.

Aetiology

In most cases the disorder is idiopathic, but a similar histological appearance may be seen in infectious endocarditis, hepatitis B and C infections, systemic lupus erythematosus, Henoch-Schönlein purpura, mixed cryoglobulinaemia, *Candida* infections, and other conditions (Table 5). Two major types of idiopathic MCGN are recognized: type I with subendothelial deposits and type II with electron dense deposits replacing the lamina densa of the glomerular basement membrane.

Table 5 Conditions associated with mesangiocapillary glomerulonephritis (MCGN)

	MCGN
Autoimmune	
• Systemic lupus erythematosus	Type I
Infection	
• Post-streptococcal	Type I
• Infective endocarditis	Type I
• Visceral abscess	Type I
• Shunt nephritis	Type I
• Schistosomiasis	Type I
• Leprosy	Type I
• Filariasis	Type I
• Hepatitis B	Type I
• Hepatitis C	Type I
• Mixed cryoglobulinaemia	Type I
• Candidiasis	Type II
Partial lipodystrophy	Type II
Miscellaneous	
• Sickle-cell disease	Type I
• Inherited complement deficiency	Types I and II
• Carcinoma	Type I
• α_1-Antitrypsin deficiency	Type I

Pathogenesis

Complement and immunoglobulin can be detected in deposits in glomeruli. In hepatitis B-associated nephritis evidence of hepatitis B virus antigen has been found in serum, in immune complexes, in cryoprecipitates, and in glomerular deposits. In cases associated with hepatitis C RNA antibodies have been found in plasma. These findings and the occurrence of complement abnormalities strongly favour a role for immune complexes, circulating or formed *in situ*. This case is strengthened by the frequent observation of subendothelial type I MCGN associated with infections.

Serum complement abnormalities

A low serum C3 is found in 60–100 per cent of patients with type II MCGN, and 36 per cent of patients with type I. Less commonly, C4 levels are low: 15 per cent in type II and 9 per cent in type I. These abnormalities indicate activation of the alternative pathway of complement. A C3 nephritic factor (**C3Nef**) is found in 60 per cent of patients with type II and 27 per cent of patients with type I MCGN. C3Nef is an IgG autoantibody directed at determinants on C3bBb, the alternative pathway convertase. Binding of C3Nef factor to C3bBb prevents its inactivation and this leads to continuous activation of the alternative pathway, with the generation of C3b and ticking over of this pathway. A small proportion of patients with both types of MCGN have been reported to have inherited deficiencies of C2, factor B, C6, C7, and C8.

Partial lipodystrophy and mesangiocapillary glomerulonephritis

A proportion of patients with partial lipodystrophy have C3Nef and develop type II MCGN and, rarely, type I MCGN. Partial lipodystrophy is a disorder in which there is asymmetrical loss of subcutaneous fat from the face, trunk, and arms, leading to a gaunt face with sunken cheeks. The disorder may follow infectious illnesses, especially measles. About 80 per cent of patients with partial lipodystrophy have a low serum C3 and 66 per cent have C3Nef. Approximately one-third of patients develop MCGN between 5 and 20 years after the onset of partial lipodystrophy, with the complement abnormalities preceding the development of nephritis.

Pathology

Type I mesangiocapillary glomerulonephritis (subendothelial) The glomeruli are increased in size and there is increased lobularity of the glomerular tuft. There is an increase in both mesangial cells and matrix, with extension of the latter between the glomerular basement membrane and the endothelium. This gives a 'double contour' appearance to the basement membrane. Crescent formation is rarely

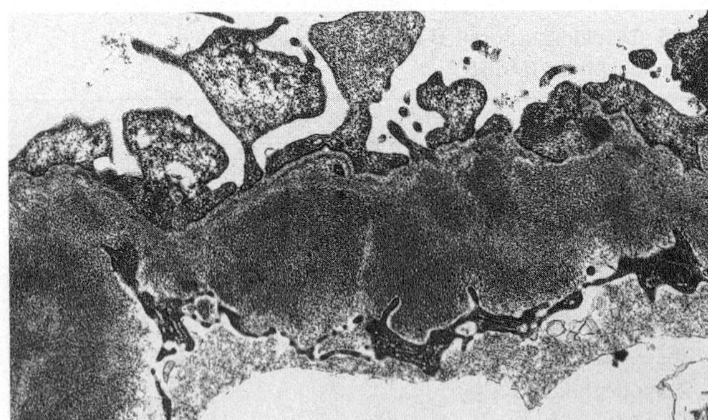

Fig. 1 Subendothelial-type mesangiocapillary glomerulonephritis. Electron-dense deposits on endothelial side of basement membrane (electron micrograph, magnification ×10 000).
(By courtesy of Dr A.J. Howie.)

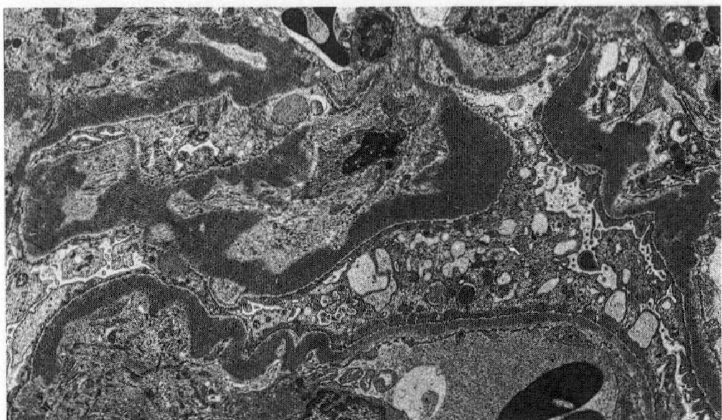

Fig. 2 Dense deposit disease. Electron-dense intramembranous material (electron micrograph, magnification ×2000).
(By courtesy of Dr A.J. Howie.)

extensive. On electron microscopy there are subendothelial and mesangial deposits (Fig. 1). Rarely, subepithelial deposits or 'humps' are seen. On immunofluorescence subendothelial deposits of IgG and C3, and less commonly Ciq, C4, IgM, and IgA, are seen.

Type II (dense deposit disease) The enlarged glomeruli are hypercellular with an increase in mesangial cells and matrix, and subendothelial extension leading to a double contour of the basement membrane. Glomerular lobularity may also be seen with crescents in about one-third of biopsies. The thickening of the glomerular capillary walls is due to replacement of the lamina densa of the glomerular basement membrane by a ribbon-like electron-dense material, that may in places be focal (Fig. 2). This material is often also present in the basement membrane of Bowman's capsule and the tubular basement membrane. In about one-third of biopsies there are subepithelial electron-dense 'humps'. On immunofluorescence deposits of C3 are seen in the mesangium. Continuous linear deposits of C3 are also seen on the basement membrane, with rare deposits of IgG, IgM, and IgA.

Clinical presentation

Type II MCGN is uncommon in infants and in old age, and has a median age of onset of 11–12 years. By contrast, the median age of onset in type I MCGN is in the twenties. Equal numbers of males and females are affected. The clinical presentations differ little between types I and II. Most frequent are a nephrotic syndrome (30–50 per cent), acute nephritis (20 per cent), or both, and less frequently the initial features are with macroscopic haematuria or asymptomatic proteinuria and/or haematuria. Approximately 30 per cent of patients are hypertensive and 40–60 per cent have renal impairment at diagnosis. Macroscopic haematuria is more common in children, whereas adults are more likely to have renal impairment and hypertension at the onset.

Treatment

There is no treatment of proven benefit in MCGN. The only controlled trial of steroids was inconclusive, and suggestions that cyclophosphamide, warfarin, and dipyridamole are beneficial have been disproved by one controlled study, but another has suggested marginal benefit from warfarin and dipyridamole, although the complication rate from bleeding was high. Antiviral agents such as alpha-interferon may ultimately prove to have a role in patients with viral-induced glomerulonephritis.

Prognosis

MCGN is slowly progressive, with the development of endstage renal failure in some 50 per cent of patients 10 years after onset. Patients with a nephrotic syndrome are more likely to develop endstage renal failure. Sclerosed glomeruli or crescents often predict more rapid development of renal failure. Serum complement levels, C3Nef, and the presence or absence of hypertension do not correlate with outcome.

Membranous nephropathy

Membranous nephropathy accounts for between 20 and 30 per cent of cases of the nephrotic syndrome in adults, and about 2–5 per cent in childhood. It is unlikely that this is a homogeneous disorder. Its aetiology (where identifiable), genetic basis, frequency as a cause of the nephrotic syndrome, and clinical evolution with or without treatment differ substantially between studies from different countries.

Aetiology

In about 20–25 per cent of adults and 35 per cent of children there is an identifiable associated condition (Table 6). Carcinoma and rarely Hodgkin's or non-Hodgkin's lymphoma, is found in between 3 and 7 per cent of patients, and this rises to 16 per cent in patients aged over 60 years. The most common carcinomas are of the bronchus, colon, kidney, breast, stomach, and prostate. Gold and penicillamine cause membranous nephropathy, more commonly in individuals who carry the HLA-DR3 gene. Approximately 3 per cent have systemic lupus erythematosus and a further 2 per cent serological features or histological changes suggestive of this disorder, which may pre-date the clinical evidence of systemic lupus erythematosus by many years. In northern Europe about 1 per cent have positive hepatitis B serology, but this association is much more common in South-east Asia and in Africa. In Europe there is a strong association with HLA-A1 B8 DR3; in Japan the association is with HLA-DR2. By contrast no such association is seen in the United States.

Pathology

There is diffuse thickening of the glomerular basement on light microscopy, usually with argyrophyllic subepithelial spikes. On immunofluorescent or immunoperoxidase microscopy this is shown to be due to the presence of immune deposits consisting of usually IgG and C3 on the subepithelial surface of the glomerular basement membrane. Mesangial proliferation, mesangial immune deposits, and IgA and C1q on immunofluorescence raises the possibility of systemic lupus erythematosus.

Table 6 Conditions associated with membranous nephropathy

Autoimmune diseases
Systemic lupus erythematosus
Rheumatoid arthritis
Drugs
Gold
Penicillamine
Captopril
Malignancy
Carcinoma (bronchus, colon, stomach, prostate, breast)
Infections
Hepatitis B
Syphilis
Filariasis
Leprosy
Miscellaneous
Autoimmune thyroid disease
Diabetes mellitus

Clinical presentation

The majority of patients are aged between 30 and 50, although some are aged up to 80 years. The male to female ratio is 2:1 to 3:1. Some 70 per cent present with a nephrotic syndrome or with asymptomatic proteinuria. Microscopic haematuria is found in 50 per cent of adults and 90 per cent of children. Macroscopic haematuria occurs in about 10–20 per cent of children but is rare in adults. About 25–40 per cent of adults and 6 per cent of children are hypertensive at diagnosis, and between 10 and 30 per cent of patients have a raised serum creatinine at diagnosis. Patients with membranous nephropathy appear to be at particular risk of developing a renal vein thrombosis.

Clinical evolution of untreated membranous nephropathy

Untreated membranous nephropathy evolves either to remission or to the development of chronic renal failure. The rate at which either outcome occurs varies in different studies. After a mean follow-up of 4.5–6 years, between 9.5 and 22 per cent of patients are in endstage renal failure, 9.5–19 per cent have significant impairment of renal function, and 23–50 per cent are in remission. Actuarial survival shows that about 75 per cent of patients are alive at 10 years and 60 per cent have functioning kidneys. Of 205 patients untreated in trials, 15 per cent were incomplete remission and only 9 per cent in renal failure after 2–5 years. Any treatment in membranous nephropathy must therefore address the wisdom of treating with toxic drugs large numbers of patients who have little risk of developing renal failure.

Steroid treatment

In the Collaborative Study in the US (1979), 72 adults with membranous nephropathy were randomized to treatment with either prednisolone (125 mg on alternate days) or placebo for 8 weeks. Deterioration of renal function, was significantly more rapid in untreated than in treated patients and a significantly lower proportion of treated patients developed renal failure. In the Medical Research Council study in the UK (1990), 107 patients with membranous nephropathy were randomized to treatment with either prednisolone (125 mg on alternate days for 8 weeks) or placebo. At 36 months there were no significant differences in plasma creatinine, creatinine clearance, and 24-h urine protein between treated and untreated patients. In a Canadian study, 158 patients were treated with either prednisolone (45 mg/m^2 per day for 6 months) or no specific treatment. No benefits were seen in renal function or proteinuria after a mean follow-up of 48 months.

Table 7 Proliferative glomerulonephritis

Focal proliferative
Systemic lupus erythematosus
Acute endocapillary proliferative
Post-streptococcal
Infective endocarditis
Leprosy
Extracapillary proliferative (crescent formation)
Idiopathic
Microscopic polyarteritis/Wegener's
Antiglomerular basement membrane antibody disease
Systemic lupus erythematosus
Henoch–Schönlein purpura
Mesangial proliferative
Idiopathic
IgA disease
Henoch–Schönlein purpura
Mesangial IgM
Systemic lupus erythematosus
Diffuse proliferative
Systemic lupus erythematosus

Steroid and chlorambucil treatment

The study of Lagrue *et al.* (1975) suggested that chlorambucil was more effective than azathioprine or placebo in the treatment of membranous nephropathy. This provided the rationale for an Italian study (Ponticelli *et al.*, 1989) in which patients were randomized to symptomatic treatment only or treatment with a regimen alternating (monthly for 6 months) high-dose methylprednisolone with chlorambucil. After a follow-up period of 31–37 months, significantly more treated than untreated patients were in remission. In addition, there had been a more than 50 per cent rise in serum creatinine in eight of 30 untreated patients, but no such change in any treated patient. A further study (1992) by the Italian group compared the effect of methylprednisolone alone to that of methylprednisolone plus chlorambucil. Those treated with the combination were more likely to have an early remission of the nephrotic state, but this advantage was no longer evident after 4 years, and there was no difference in the rates of decline of renal function between the two therapies.

Most nephrologists are hesitant to use the alternating regimen because of gonadal toxicity and the oncogenic risks of chlorambucil given to patients who might do well on no treatment. However, there may be a subgroup of patients in whom renal function deteriorates more rapidly than is the norm, when intravenous methylprednisolone or prednisolone, combined with chlorambucil or cyclophosphamide, might reverse the rate of loss of renal function. A trial of treatment is probably justifiable in this subgroup only. Identification of those patients who are most likely to do badly would be helpful in deciding whom to treat. Deterioration of renal function is more common in patients with a nephrotic syndrome, in those with tubulointerstitial fibrosis or with initial poor renal function and whose renal function has deteriorated in the first 2.5 years after diagnosis.

Proliferative glomerulonephritis

Most types of proliferative glomerulonephritis (Table 7) are described elsewhere, but the exception is mesangial IgM disease.

Mesangial IgM proliferative glomerulonephritis

There is disagreement on the significance of mesangial proliferation in patients with a nephrotic syndrome whose renal biopsies are otherwise normal. One view is that mesangial proliferation with IgM deposits defines a subset of patients with a nephrotic syndrome who respond poorly to steroids and tend to develop progressive renal failure. The opposite view is that patients with this histological appearance cannot be differentiated by their clinical behaviour or responsiveness to steroids from patients with true minimal change glomerulonephritis. Only 25–55 per cent of these patients respond to steroids and those who are resistant tend also to fail to respond to cyclophosphamide or chlorambucil. Between 3 and 20 per cent develop progressive renal failure.

Further reading

Appel, G.B. (1993). Immune complex glomerulonephritis - deposits plus interest. *New England Journal of Medicine*, 328, 505–6.

Davison, A.M., Cameron, J.S., Grünfeld, J.-P., Kerr, D., Ritz, E., and Winearls, C.G. (ed.) (1998). *Oxford textbook of clinical nephrology*, 2nd edn, vol.1, section 3. Oxford University Press, Oxford.

Nolasco, F., Cameron, J.S., Heywood, E.F., *et al.* (1986). Adult onset minimal change glomerulonephritis, a long term follow-up. *Kidney International*, 29, 1215–33.

Ponticelli, C. and Passerini, P. (1994). Treatment of the nephrotic syndrome associated with primary glomerulonephritis. *Kidney International*, 46, 595–694.

Chapter 12.8

Rapidly progressive glomerulonephritis and antiglomerular basement membrane disease

C. D. Pusey and A. J. Rees

Definition

The term rapidly progressive glomerulonephritis describes those cases which progress from onset to endstage renal failure within weeks or months. The characteristic histological appearance is of a focal necrotizing glomerulonephritis with crescent formation, and the term crescentic nephritis has been used almost synonymously. Attempts have been made to define crescentic nephritis in relation to the percentage of glomeruli involved and extent of the crescents, but there is no consensus, and a rigid definition is inappropriate because of the sampling error implicit in renal biopsy material and the fact that the biopsy represents only one stage in the evolution of the disease. The two principal causes are antiglomerular basement membrane (anti-GBM) disease and primary systemic vasculitis. Idiopathic rapidly progressive glomerulonephritis may be regarded as a renal-limited form of systemic vasculitis (see below). The syndrome may also occur in other systemic diseases, such as systemic lupus erythematosus, and may complicate most types of primary glomerulonephritis (Table 1). The diagnosis must be considered in any case of unexplained acute renal failure.

In the absence of associated systemic disease, presentation may be delayed until renal failure leads to oliguria, peripheral oedema, shortness of breath, or uraemia. Some patients complain of non-specific symptoms such as malaise, fever, myalgia, and weight loss. Macroscopic haematuria and loin pain are sometimes reported. Hypertension is uncommon in the absence of fluid overload. Microscopy of a fresh sample of urine is essential and will generally reveal many dysmorphic red cells, together with red cell and granular casts. Proteinuria is usually modest, but occasionally reaches nephrotic levels. Renal ultrasound will confirm the presence of normal-sized non-obstructed kidneys. Once rapidly progressive glomerulonephritis is suspected, renal biopsy should be performed urgently, together with appropriate serological tests (Table 2).

Management

The specific management of anti-GBM disease is considered below, and that of systemic vasculitis in Chapter 12.24. The prognosis has been greatly improved in both conditions. The major adverse effect of modern treatment is infection. The risk is particularly related to the steroid dosage, and there should be regular cultures of available material (blood, urine, sputum, peritoneal dialysis fluid, wound swabs) and a low threshold for performing relevant invasive investigations. Opportunistic infections are common, particularly with nosocomial bacteria, fungi, *Pneumocystis*, and cytomegalovirus. Treatment may need to be started on the basis of the likely diagnosis, pending microbiological results. There is no convincing evidence for the use of prophylactic antimicrobial drugs, although oral antifungal agents are widely used. It is important to ensure adequate nutrition, and to reduce the risk of upper gastrointestinal haemorrhage, by use of prophylactic H_2-antagonists. Indications for dialysis are conventional, but early treatment is preferred.

Antiglomerular basement membrane disease

Definition

'Goodpasture's syndrome', the combination of rapidly progressive glomerulonephritis and lung haemorrhage, may be due to a variety of processes, including systemic vasculitis (Table 1). Thus, the term anti-GBM disease (or Goodpasture's disease) is preferred for those cases associated with anti-GBM antibodies. An identical form of glomerulonephritis may occur without lung haemorrhage, and is included in the definition.

Table 1 Causes of rapidly progressive glomerulonephritis

Antiglomerular basement membrane disease
- Goodpasture's disease[a,b]
- Isolated antiglomerular basement membrane nephritis[a]

Primary systemic vasculitis
- Wegener's granulomatosis[a,b]
- Microscopic polyarteritis[a,b]
- Idiopathic rapidly progressive glomerulonephritis[a]
- Churg–Strauss syndrome[b]
- Polyarteritis nodosa
- Giant-cell arteritis
- Takayasu's arteritis

Systemic disorders
- Systemic lupus erythematosus[a,b]
- Essential mixed cryoglobulinaemia[b]
- Henoch–Schönlein purpura[b]
- Relapsing polychondritis
- Behçet's syndrome[b]
- Rheumatoid disease

Primary glomerulonephritis
- Mesangiocapillary glomerulonephritis[a]
- Mesangial IgA nephropathy[a]
- Membranous nephropathy

Infection-related glomerulonephritis
- Post-streptococcal (and other causes of acute proliferative) glomerulonephritis[a]
- Infective endocarditis
- Ventriculoatrial shunt infection
- Visceral abscess

Neoplastic disease
- Carcinoma
- Lymphoma (Hodgkin's and non-Hodgkin's)

Drug reactions
- Penicillamine[b]
- Hydralazine
- Rifampicin

[a] Relatively common cause of rapidly progressive glomerulonephritis in adults.

[b] Association with pulmonary haemorrhage.

Postinfectious glomerulonephritis is common worldwide but now rare in Europe.

Aetiology

Anti-GBM disease is rare, with an estimated annual incidence of 0.5–1 cases per million population. It accounts for up to 5 per cent of cases of glomerulonephritis, and 2 per cent of the endstage renal failure population. It is reported mainly in Caucasians. The disease can occur at any age, but is most frequent in the third and again in the sixth/seventh decades. Males are affected about twice as often as females.

Environmental factors

Geographical clustering of cases and peaks of incidence in spring and early summer, suggest a role for environmental factors. Viral infections and hydrocarbon exposure have been associated but the evidence for a causative role is not strong. Isolated cases have followed lithotripsy and obstructive nephropathy. There is a strong association between cigarette smoking and lung haemorrhage.

Genetic factors

There are several reports of sibling pairs, including monozygotic twins, who have developed anti-GBM disease. There are associations with particular class II HLA genes. The strongest is with HLA-DR2(DR15), with an additional association with DR4, and negative associations with DR1 and DR7. In patients with HLA-DR2, the possession of the class I gene HLA-B7 is associated with more severe glomerulonephritis. The disease is also associated with the GM1, 1, 21 (axg) immunoglobulin Gm haplotype. The disease has been described in association with systemic vasculitis, and with primary glomerulonephritis, malignancy, and drug therapy.

Pathogenesis

Autoantibodies

There is good evidence for the pathogenicity of anti-GBM autoantibodies: levels generally correlate with severity of disease; nephritis recurs in renal transplant recipients with detectable circulating antibodies; and treatment designed to lower antibody levels is often effective. Antibodies bind to GBM, distal tubular basement membrane, and Bowman's capsule, but not to other renal basement membranes. They also bind to alveolar basement membrane, and to basement membranes of the choroid plexus, lens, choroid, retina, and cochlea. This pattern of distribution explains the principal clinical features of the disease, and rarely patients with choroid plexus or retinal involvement have been described. Antibodies bind to type IV collagen, principally to the non-collagenous (NC1) domain of the α3(IV)-chain. The gene encoding this protein (COL4A3) has been cloned, sequenced, and localized to chromosome 2.

Cell-mediated immunity

The restricted specificity of the antibody response, and the strong HLA class II associations make it likely that autoantibody production is T-cell dependent. T cells from patients have been shown to proliferate *in vitro* in response to purified α3(IV)NCI. Also, infiltration of the glomeruli and interstitium by T cells and macrophages is observed on renal biopsy, suggesting a direct role for cell-mediated immunity in tissue injury.

Clinical features and diagnosis

Most presenting symptoms can be related to rapidly progressive glomerulonephritis or lung haemorrhage, although a proportion of patients complain of minor non-specific features of malaise. Tiredness and dyspnoea may be due to anaemia due to overt or covert lung haemorrhage.

The renal manifestations are similar to those of other causes of rapidly progressive glomerulonephritis (see above). Detection of circulating anti-GBM antibodies can be done rapidly by experienced laboratories and treatment may be started when antibody has been detected, but renal biopsy remains the definitive investigation. Early changes on biopsy are of a focal and segmental proliferative glomerulonephritis, progressing to a more diffuse nephritis with focal

Table 2 Selected blood tests in rapidly progressive glomerulonephritis

Specific	
Antiglomerular basement membrane antibodies	Goodpasture's disease
Antineutrophil cytoplasmic antibodies	Systemic vasculitis
Anti-dsDNA antibodies, anti-Sm antibodies	Systemic lupus erythematosus
Cryoglobulins	Essential mixed cryoglobulinaemia type II
C3 nephritic factor	Mesangiocapillary glomerulonephritis type II
Raised ASOT	Post-streptococcal glomerulonephritis
Non-specific	
Complement	
low C4, normal C3	Essential mixed cryoglobulinaemia type II
low C4 ± C3	Systemic lupus erythematosus
low C3, normal C4	Mesangiocapillary glomerulonephritis type II
low C3 ± C4	Postinfectious glomerulonephritis, mesangiocapillary glomerulonephritis type I
raised C3, C4	Systemic vasculitis
Immunoglobulins	
raised IgG, IgM	Systemic lupus erythematosus, systemic vasculitis, postinfectious glomerulonephritis
raised IgE	Churg–Strauss syndrome
raised IgA	IgA nephropathy, Henoch–Schönlein purpura
paraprotein (usually IgM)	Essential mixed cryoglobulinaemia type II
Acute phase response	
raised C-reactive protein + ESR	Systemic vasculitis
raised ESR ± C-reactive protein	Systemic lupus erythematosus
raised alkaline phosphatase, low albumin	Systemic vasculitis
Haematology	
neutrophilia, thrombocytosis	Systemic vasculitis
eosinophilia	Churg–Strauss syndrome
leucopenia, thrombocytopenia	Systemic lupus erythematosus
severe anaemia	Goodpasture's disease
moderate anaemia	Systemic vasculitis, systemic lupus erythematosus, essential mixed cryoglobulinaemia
Microbiology	
blood cultures positive	Infective endocarditis
	Ventriculoatrial shunt nephritis

Some of the non-specific tests are abnormal only in a proportion of patients.
ASOT, anti-streptolysin O titre; ESR, erythrocyte sedimentation rate.

necrosis and extensive crescent formation. There is usually accompanying interstitial inflammation. Immunofluorescence shows linear deposits of IgG along the GBM and sometimes distal tubular basement membrane. IgA and/or IgM are present in addition to IgG in up to a third of cases, and rarely IgA or IgM are deposited alone. C3 complement is detected in about two-thirds of cases. On electron microscopy there is usually irregular thickening and mottling of the GBM, with intermittent breaks in its continuity.

About two-thirds of patients have pulmonary haemorrhage. Some present with a history of intermittent haemoptysis and dyspnoea over months or years, others with massive haemoptysis or with dyspnoea alone. Almost all current smokers have lung haemorrhage whereas it is rare in non-smokers. Clinical examination can be normal or reveal tachypnoea, cyanosis, or inspiratory crackles throughout the lung fields.

The radiological appearances are non-specific, and comprise alveolar shadowing, generally in the central and lower lung fields. These changes are usually symmetrical, and often transgress the fissures. They can clear rapidly, usually within days, and no long-term sequelae are apparent radiologically. As similar appearances can result from fluid overload or infection, and as haemoptysis is not invariable, additional information may be required to detect lung haemorrhage.

Table 3 Initial treatment of antiglomerular basement membrane (anti-GBM) disease

Prednisolone 60 mg daily, reducing to 20 mg daily by 4 weeks
Cyclophosphamide 2–3 mg/kg daily (lower dose if >55 years); discontinued if white cell count <4.0 × 10^9/l or in presence of life-threatening infection
Plasma exchange 4 l daily for 5 per cent albumin; continued for 14 days or until anti-GBM antibody levels controlled; fresh, frozen plasma 400 ml given at end of exchange in presence of lung haemorrhage or within 3 days of invasive procedure

After 2–3 months, depending on response, cyclophosphamide is discontinued and prednisolone tapered.

The corrected carbon monoxide uptake, or *K*CO, is a sensitive test for it, as free haemoglobin in the alveoli leads to an increased value. A change of greater than 30 per cent from base-line usually indicates haemorrhage. Bronchoscopy confirms haemorrhage, and transbronchial biopsies may reveal intra-alveolar haemorrhage accompanied by haemosiderin-laden macrophages and alveolar cell hyperplasia. The alveolar walls may be thickened with oedema, fibrosis, and an inflammatory infiltrate. Direct immunofluorescence usually shows intermittent linear binding of IgG in areas of lung haemorrhage. Electron microscopy may show thickening and irregularity of the alveolar basement membrane.

Treatment and outcome

Untreated patients mostly die within 6 months from lung haemorrhage or renal failure. Plasma exchange is remarkably effective when combined with prednisolone and cyclophosphamide. This generally leads to resolution of pulmonary haemorrhage within a few days and recovery of renal function in all but the most severe cases. A current regimen is shown in Table 3. Plasma exchange alone has only a temporary effect, while drug therapy alone acts too slowly to be of immediate benefit. Once antibody levels have been reduced to near background they do not usually rise again, suggesting that the autoreactive lymphocytes have in some way been inactivated. Removal by plasma exchange of other potentially proinflammatory plasma components, such as complement and clotting factors, could also be important. There has only been one controlled trial. The group receiving drugs and plasma exchange had a better outcome than those receiving drugs alone, but the results were confounded by more severe renal disease in the drug-treated group. Patients treated with serum creatinine level of less than 600 µmol/litre frequently recover, whereas those treated later (especially if oliguric) have little chance of regaining renal function. Results of recent series are summarized in Table 4.

The use of bolus doses of methylprednisolone has been proposed as an alternative to plasma exchange, but this approach has not been compared with plasma exchange, and several reports suggest that it is ineffective.

Duration of treatment depends on the immunological and clinical response. In general, plasma exchange is continued until antibody levels are close to background and the patient has improved, which usually takes at least 2 weeks. Regular monitoring of serum creatinine, urine microscopy, *K*CO, radiography, and haemoglobin is required. Cyclophosphamide is continued for 2–3 months, and prednisolone tailed off by 6 months. Relapses during the initial treatment period may be provoked by the recurrence of anti-GBM antibody, or by infection, and in the case of lung haemorrhage by fluid overload or smoking. Such episodes are treated by re-introduction of plasma exchange and management of any precipitating factor. Late recurrence of the disease months or years later is rare and should be treated as for the initial episode. Some patients with significant renal impairment after treatment of the acute episode may show a progressive decline in renal function, despite absence of immunological abnormality or other obvious cause of renal damage.

Renal transplantation

Patients with anti-GBM disease can be transplanted successfully, provided they do not have circulating anti-GBM antibodies. Recurrence with graft loss occurs when circulating antibodies are present at the time of operation. Rarely, immunological recurrence has followed transplantation and antibody levels should be monitored postoperatively. It is reasonable to wait for 6 months after antibody has become undetectable before transplantation.

The development of anti-GBM disease after renal transplantation in Alport's syndrome is well recognized. Anti-GBM antibodies fail to bind to the GBM of many cases of Alport's syndrome, suggesting an absence or alteration of the Goodpasture antigen in that disorder. This is consistent with the genetic defect in Alport's which has been localized to the gene (COL4A5) encoding the α5(IV)-chain. Alport's patients may therefore develop an immune response to a 'new' antigen in the grafted kidney.

Idiopathic rapidly progressive glomerulonephritis

Crescentic nephritis without significant immune deposits or concomitant systemic disease has been termed idiopathic rapidly progressive glomerulonephritis, to differentiate it from those cases with a proposed cause or association, such as anti-GBM disease or systemic lupus erythematosus. It has also been referred to as 'pauci-immune' crescentic nephritis, because of the lack of immune deposits on immunofluorescence. Patients with this condition frequently have circulating antineutrophil cytoplasmic antibodies.

The renal lesions of systemic vasculitis have many characteristics in common with those of idiopathic rapidly progressive glomerulonephritis, and some patients with idiopathic rapidly progressive glomerulonephritis have subsequently been observed to develop features of systemic vasculitis. It is now accepted therefore that idiopathic rapidly progressive glomerulonephritis most often represents a renal-limited variant of small-vessel vasculitis. The aetiology, clinical features, and management are essentially the same as those of systemic vasculitis (see Chapter 12.24).

The response to treatment is probably similar to that in systemic vasculitis. In recent series using a combination of corticosteroids and cytotoxic drugs, the 1-year survival was generally over 70 per cent. The addition of either pulse methylprednisolone or plasma exchange appears to be of benefit in advanced cases, and dialysis-dependent patients frequently regain independent renal function. In one controlled trial, including patients with systemic vasculitis and idiopathic rapidly progressive glomerulonephritis, those receiving plasma exchange in addition to drug therapy were more likely to come off dialysis than those receiving drugs alone.

Table 4 Outcome of patients with antiglomerular basement membrane disease treated with immunosuppressive drugs and plasma exchange

Series	Percentage with independent renal function at 1 year according to initial serum creatinine level (number of cases shown in parentheses)		Notes on regimen used
	≤600 μmol/l	>600 μmol/l	
Briggs *et al.* 1979 (*n* = 15)	36 (11)	0 (4)	Only 4/15 received plasma exchange
Simpson *et al.* 1982 (*n* = 12)	70 (10)	0 (2)	8/12 received plasma exchange
Johnson *et al.* 1985 (*n* =17)	69 (13)	0 (4)	Less cyclophosphamide than in Table 3. Half received plasma exchange, but only every third day and using fresh, frozen plasma
Walker *et al.* 1985 (*n* = 22)	82 (11)	18 (11)	Slightly less cyclophosphamide and plasma exchange than in Table 3
Hammersmith 1976–88 (*n* = 56)	90 (21)	11 (35)	As Table 3, except some also received azathioprine 1 mg/kg/day

For full details of sources see OTM3, p. 3167.

Rapidly progressive glomerulonephritis in other disorders

Other causes are summarized in Table 1. Proliferative lupus nephritis generally responds well to high-dose oral steroids together with oral or intravenous pulses of cyclophosphamide. The addition of pulse doses of methylprednisolone or of plasma exchange has been proposed in severe crescentic nephritis, although neither approach has been subjected to adequate trials. In essential mixed cryoglobulinaemia with rapidly progressive glomerulonephritis, the addition of plasma exchange to immunosuppressive drugs is logical, as this will reduce the concentration of the potentially pathogenic cryoglobulin.

Further reading

Levy, J. and Pusey, C.D. (1998). Crescentic glomerulonephritis. In: *Therapy in nephrology and hypertension* (ed. Brady, H.R. and Wilcox, C.S.), pp. 145–51. W.B. Saunders, Philadelphia.

Pusey, C.D. and Rees, A.J. (ed.) (1998). *Rapidly progressive glomerulonephritis.* Oxford University Press, Oxford.

Turner, A.N. and Rees, A.J. (1998). Antiglomerular basement membrane disease. In: *Oxford textbook of clinical nephrology,* (2nd edn), (ed. A.M. Davison, J.S. Cameron, J.-P. Grünfeld, D. Kerr, E. Ritz, and C.G. Winearls), pp. 647–66. Oxford University Press, Oxford.

Renal manifestations of systemic disease

Chapter 12.9

Diabetic nephropathy

E. Ritz, D. Fliser, and M. Siebels

Definition

The hallmark of the renal lesion is a particular form of glomerulosclerosis (Fig. 1) which is associated with arteriolar hyalinosis and interstitial fibrosis. Increased urinary albumin excretion is the first clinical manifestation. Once overt albuminuria is present, diabetic nephropathy will inexorably progress to endstage renal failure. Renal involvement is more frequent in the male and is particularly frequent in patients who develop diabetes in the second decade of life.

As shown in Fig. 2, the prevalence of proteinuria for any given duration of the disease is comparable in type 1 and type 2 diabetics, and so is the prevalence of renal failure. With current improvements in management, more of the elderly type 2 diabetics survive to experience renal failure. At the time of diagnosis of type 2 diabetes up to 20 per cent of patients already have albuminuria and 30–40 per cent of patients given renal replacement therapy suffer from diabetic nephropathy.

Both renal and overall prognosis have improved so that the 10-year survival of albuminuric diabetic patients is currently approximately 80 per cent.

Albuminuria is closely linked to dyslipidaemia and elevated lipoprotein (a) (**Lp(a)**) but the excess cardiovascular risk of proteinuria is not explained by known risk factors alone. As shown in Fig. 3, the relative mortality is strikingly higher in insulin-dependent diabetics

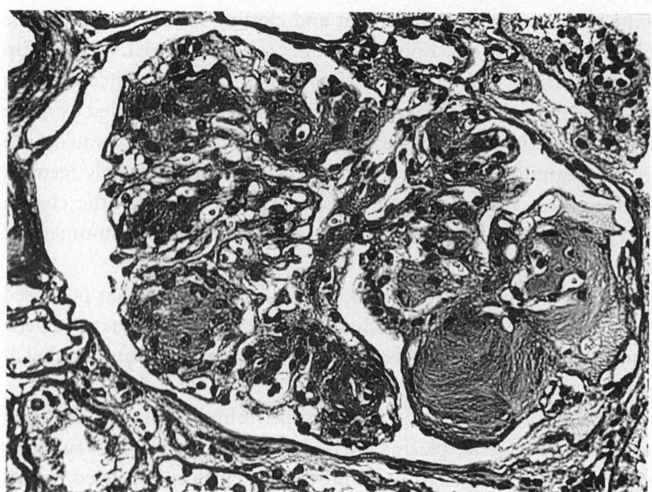

Fig. 1 Glomerulus from a patient with nodular diabetic glomerulosclerosis. Note the presence of two well developed acellular nodules in peripheral lobules (Masson trichrome stain, ×440).
(By courtesy of Professor R. Waldherr, Department of Pathology, Heidelberg.)

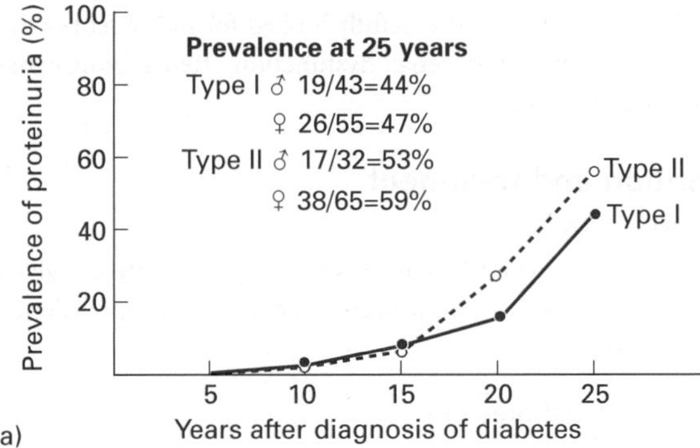

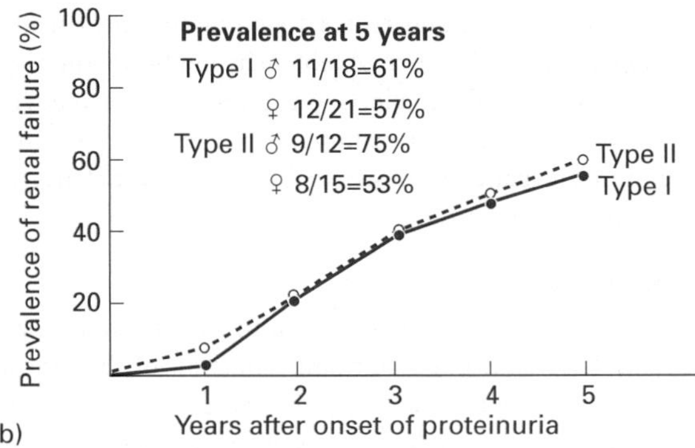

Fig. 2 Similar risk of nephropathy in type I and type II diabetes. Cumulative prevalence of persistent proteinuria in type II and type I patients (a) and cumulative prevalence of renal failure, i.e. serum creatinine 1.4 mg/dl, in proteinuric type I and type II patients (b).
(After E. Ritz et al. (1990). Hypertension pathophysiology, diagnosis and management (ed. J.H. Laragh and B.M. Brenner) pp. 1703–15. Raven Press, New York.)

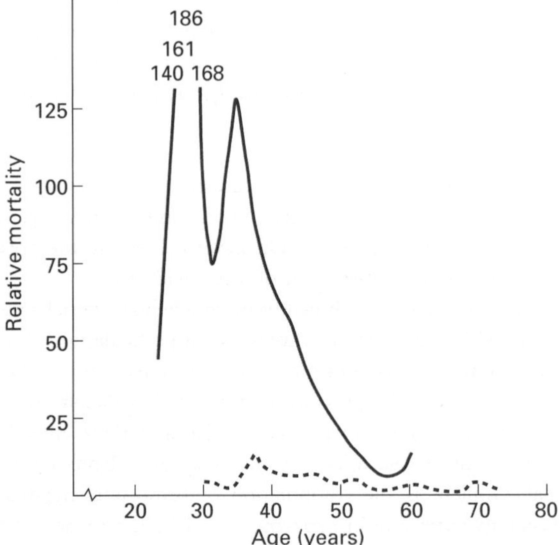

Fig. 3 Cardiovascular mortality in insulin-dependent diabetics depends on proteinuria. Relative mortality from cardiovascular disease in insulin-dependent diabetics with persistent proteinuria (—-) and without proteinuria (—-).
*(After K. Borch-Johnsen and S. Kreiner. (1987). British Medical Journal, **294**, 1651–54.)*

with proteinuria, but only marginally higher in the diabetic patient without proteinuria.

Evolution of diabetic nephropathy

Early on there is renal overperfusion, accompanied by renal and glomerular hypertrophy. These changes are only partially reversible with insulin treatment. The first evidence of nephropathy is microalbuminuria; (see below). Blood pressure then rises and renal failure ensues after a median interval of approximately 10–20 years.

Pathophysiology of diabetic nephropathy

Hyperglycaemia on its own is not a sufficient condition for the development of nephropathy. Diabetic siblings of propositi with diabetic nephropathy have an 83 per cent risk of developing nephropathy, whereas the risk is only 17 per cent for those of propositi without nephropathy. The mechanisms by which hyperglycaemia might be injurious have not been clarified. Glycation reactions may be involved. Another potential pathway is accumulation of sorbitol as a consequence of increased availability of glucose for reduction by aldose reductase in mesangial cells. Reduced glycosaminoglycan content of glomerular basement membranes is another possibility. Polyanionic substances are responsible, at least in part, for the fixed negative charges of the glomerular basement membrane and account for the charge selectivity which is responsible for restricted filtration of polyanionic macromolecules (such as albumin). Alterations of glomerular haemodynamics may also be involved.

Blood pressure in diabetic nephropathy

Patients with type 1 diabetes are usually normotensive until albuminuria has supervened. Blood pressure then starts to rise. The close relationship between elevated blood pressure and evidence of renal damage in type 1 diabetes suggests that the hypertension is the consequence of renal parenchymal changes.

The relationship between nephropathy and hypertension is more complex in type 2 diabetics. Such patients have usually been hypertensive for years and decades prior to the onset of overt diabetes. At the time of diagnosis, hypertension is found in approximately 70–80 per cent of the patients. Blood pressure rises further in those who subsequently develop nephropathy. Isolated systolic hypertension is linked to higher cardiovascular mortality even when the mean arterial pressure is normal. Lowering of blood pressure by antihypertensive agents reduces the rate of decrease of glomerular filtration.

Management of the patient with diabetic nephropathy

Clinical evaluation

Patients must be monitored regularly for the presence of albuminuria and elevated blood pressure as early indicators of nephropathy.

Albuminuria (see Chapters 12.1, 12.5)

It is best to examine early morning urine samples on at least three occasions. The diagnosis of microalbuminuria should be made only when, during a period of 6 months, three independent measurements confirm albumin excretion between 20 and 200 µg/min in morning urine specimens (approximately equivalent to 30–300 mg/24 h). The amount of albumin excreted is clearly related to blood pressure

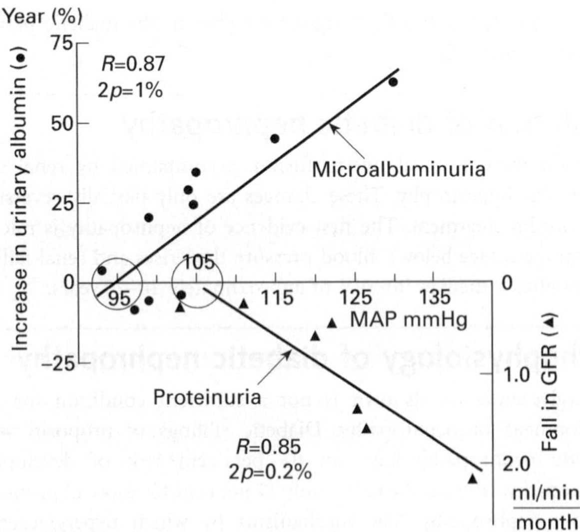

Fig. 4 Progression of microalbuminuria and loss of glomerular filtration depend on blood pressure. The graph gives the theoretical threshold of mean arterial blood pressure (MAP) for progression in microalbuminuria (95 mmHg) and the rate of decrease of glomerular filtration rate (105 mmHg) in insulin-dependent diabetic patients.
(After C.E. Mogensen. (1992). In V.E. Andreucci, and L.G. Fine (ed.) International Yearbook of Nephrology, p. 141. Springer-Verlag, London.)

(Fig. 4) and is effectively reduced by antihypertensive treatment. With progression of nephropathy, albumin excretion increases. In the later stages, proteinuria may be in the nephrotic range when a particularly adverse renal prognosis is expected.

Hypertension

It is particularly important to detect hypertension early in order to institute prompt antihypertensive intervention. If albumin excretion is elevated, an attempt to lower blood pressure by angiotensin-converting enzyme (ACE) inhibitors should be made. The target blood pressure should be lower than 140/mmHg (WHO), i.e. approximately 130/70 mmHg.

Renal function

Serum creatinine is commonly used as an index of the glomerular filtration rate, but there are particular problems with this method in diabetes; it does not adequately reflect the initial fall in glomerular filtration rate. It also seriously underestimates the magnitude of loss of glomerular filtration rate in wasted patients. On the other hand, endogenous creatinine clearance usually overestimates glomerular filtration rate. It is important to detect causes other than diabetic nephropathy when there is an unexpected increase in serum creatinine; these might include the effects of radiological contrast media, urinary tract infection with papillary necrosis, urinary tract obstruction, uncontrolled hypertension, congestive heart failure, untoward reactions to drugs (particularly non-steroidal anti-inflammatory agents and ACE inhibitors), or hypovolaemia.

Differential diagnosis

Nephropathy is rare before the tenth year of diabetes, at least in type 1 disease, and is almost always associated with retinopathy. A cause of renal dysfunction other than diabetes should be sought when the onset is unexpectedly early and when there is no evidence of retinopathy. In the elderly diabetic, atherosclerotic renal artery stenosis is common. Renal papillary necrosis, as well as intrarenal or perinephric abscess formation, must be carefully looked for in the febrile diabetic patient with pyuria and renal dysfunction. Renal biopsy may be required in some cases.

Prevention and treatment

Metabolic control

There is now good evidence that consistently good control of glycaemia will delay the onset of albuminuria and reduce its prevalence (see Chapter 6.13).

Control of arterial pressure

A number of controlled prospective trials have shown that reduction in blood pressure has attenuated or even prevented the loss of glomerular filtration rate and reduced albuminuria in patients with diabetic nephropathy. Whether or not ACE inhibitors offer specific advantage by way of their effects on glomerular haemodynamics is not yet proven, but it is common practice to give them to microalbuminuric patients in whom blood pressure starts to rise within the normotensive range.

Low-protein diet

Two studies of diabetic patients with moderately advanced nephropathy have shown a significant reduction of the rate of loss of glomerular filtration rate when dietary protein was restricted to approximately 0.6–0.8 g/kg body weight per day. Similar renal functional changes are also seen on a vegetarian diet. Malnutrition and wasting are risks of a low-protein diet in more advanced renal failure, and it is inadvisable when plasma creatinine levels exceed 500 µmol/l. Patients taking reduced dietary protein require close monitoring to detect malnutrition.

The diabetic patient with renal failure

As renal failure progresses, the requirement for insulin or oral hypoglycaemic agents tends to fall, but in a way and to a degree that is difficult to predict. Renal catabolism and excretion of insulin is reduced, prolonging its half-life, but there is a coincident trend towards insulin resistance. Consequently, frequent monitoring of blood glucose concentrations and reassessment of insulin requirements are essential. Most sulphonylurea compounds (or their active metabolites) are eliminated, at least in part, via the kidney and so there is need for particular care in the use of these agents in uraemic diabetics. Metformin should never be used in the presence of renal failure because of the risk of lactic acidosis.

There may be particular difficulty in controlling arterial pressure in diabetics with nephropathy, who are often particularly susceptible to salt and volume loads; and may require massive diuretic therapy. When control of arterial pressure is particularly difficult and renal failure advanced, it is often wise to start dialysis early to allow better correction of hypervolaemia and the associated hypertension. A particular problem is the combination of orthostatic hypotension with supine hypertension in nephropathic diabetic patients suffering from autonomic nephropathy. More than one antihypertensive agent is almost always required in advanced renal failure; a combination of diuretics (loop agents), ACE inhibitors, and calcium antagonists is often best. ACE inhibitors can cause rise in plasma potassium to dangerous levels in advanced renal failure and in the rare elderly diabetic with hyporeninaemic hypoaldosteronism.

Cardiac disease

This is extremely common in the diabetic with nephropathy and is the single most common cause of death. Ischaemic heart disease is particularly common but may remain asymptomatic because of afferent denervation. An abrupt onset of pulmonary oedema or congestive heart failure in such patients may be the first indication of severe ischaemic heart disease, particularly in the presence of renal dysfunction.

Dyslipidaemia

This is also common in the nephropathic diabetic and is more severe, at any given level of glomerular filtration, than in the non-diabetic uraemic patient. The most common feature is hypertriglyceridaemia, resulting from accumulation of very low density lipoprotein, associated with low high-density lipoprotein and inconstant elevation of cholesterol. Lp(a) is also high. Although no definite proof for the efficacy of the treatment is available, it appears sensible to advise reduced intake of saturated fat and to administer lipid-lowering agents, fibrates, or statins as indicated.

Renal replacement therapy

Diabetics, particularly elderly women, often have poor vessels with which to create vascular access. It is therefore good practice to create it early, for example when serum creatinine has exceeded 500 μmol/l. Three options are available, haemodialysis, continuous ambulatory peritoneal dialysis, or renal transplantation (isolated or combined with pancreatic or islet cell transplantation). Transplantation restores quality of life and rehabilitation best, and is the treatment of choice in the younger patient. Despite claims that continuous ambulatory peritoneal dialysis is superior to haemodialysis in the older diabetic, the two procedures give very similar results. Insulin requirements usually decrease on dialysis and volume control is more difficult in the diabetic than in the non-diabetic dialysis patient.

The major causes of death after transplantation are cardiac, specifically coronary, events. Transplantation of the pancreas from the same donor still presents a number of technical problems, and is not yet a routine procedure.

Further reading

Barnes, D.J., Pinto, J.R., and Viberti, G.C. (1998). The patient with diabetes mellitus. In: *Oxford textbook of clinical nephrology,* (2nd edn) (ed. A.M. Davison, J.S. Cameron, J.-P. Grünfeld, D. Kerr, E. Ritz, and C.G. Winearls), pp. 723–75. Oxford University Press, Oxford.

Bojestig, M., Arnquist, H.J., Hermansson, G., *et al.* (1994). Declining incidence of nephropathy in insulin dependent diabetes mellitus. *New England Journal of Medicine,* **330**, 15–28.

Diabetes Control and Complications Trial Research Group. (1995). The effect of intensive therapy on the development and progression of diabetic nephropathy in the Diabetes Control and Complications Trial. *Kidney International,* 47, 1703–20.

Zeller, K., Whittaker, E., Sullivan, L., *et al.* (1991). Effect of diatary protein restriction on the progression of renal failure in patients with insulin-dependenet diabetes mellitus. *New England Journal of Medicine,* **324**, 78–84.

Chapter 12.10

Haemolytic uraemic syndrome

G. H. Neild

Definition

The haemolytic uraemic syndrome (**HUS**) is a condition in which acute renal failure combines with thrombocytopenia, microangiopathic haemolytic anaemia, and a characteristic renovascular pathology. In the UK it is now the commonest cause of acute renal failure in children, and appears to be increasing in incidence. These features do not represent a single disease, although HUS following a diarrhoeal infection due to a verocytotoxin-producing *Escherichia coli* is the most common cause. The diarrhoeal-associated syndrome (D+ HUS) most commonly affects children under 5 years of age. In adults, HUS was once considered rare, usually associated with irreversible renal failure, but in the past decade increasing numbers of cases have been seen, associated with a diarrhoeal prodrome and recovery of renal function (Table 1). Each of the many causes of HUS (Table 2) have in common extensive endothelial injury of the renal microvasculature. Involvement of the central nervous system is increasingly recognized when the diarrhoeal prodrome has occurred.

In the closely related syndrome of thrombotic thrombocytopenic purpura (**TTP**), a similar vascular injury occurs simultaneously in many organs, and the associated haematological findings are correspondingly more severe. There is increasing recognition of overlap between HUS and TTP, especially as cases of both have now been reported following *E. coli* gut infection, in patients receiving cyclosporin, and in familial cases in HLA identical siblings. In the case of HUS there are two characteristic presentations:

1. A diarrhoeal-associated (D+) form, usually presenting acutely with bloody diarrhoea and renal failure often requiring dialysis, but usually with complete recovery of renal function.
2. A sporadic and idiopathic form (D−), which has an insidious onset, often without any prodromal illness. Severe hypertension at presentation is common and the kidneys may be irreversibly damaged. This form is usually seen in adults, may occur postpartum, and is occasionally seen in more than one member of a family.

A septicaemic illness with disseminated intravascular coagulation may present in a way suggesting HUS, but the clotting abnormalities that occur in the septicaemia syndrome (prolonged prothrombin and activated partial thromboplastin time) are absent in HUS.

Aetiology (Table 2)

E. coli producing verocytotoxin

Infection with *E. coli* 0157:H7 causes bloody diarrhoea which is commonly associated with HUS. The usual picture is of cramping abdominal pain and watery diarrhoea, followed by bloody diarrhoea without much increase in faecal leucocytes. Fever, rarely exceeding 38°C occurs in fewer than 50 per cent of the cases. The clinical features of HUS, or more rarely TTP, are most common in those under 5 years or over 65 years of age, and tend to occur some 6–10 days after the onset of diarrhoea.

Table 1 Adult haemolytic uraemic syndrome (HUS) in the United Kingdom

Prodrome	*n*	F/M	Age (year)	Hb (g/dl)	Platelets ($\times 10^9$/ml)	Recovery
Diarrhoea	19	15/4	46 (15–89)	6.8 (4.9–8.4)	40 (14–150)	17/19 (2 died)
None	19	15/4	46 (18–72)	6.6 (4.0–8.6)	55 (14–117)	12/19
Viral RTI	5	2/3	34 (28–51)	6.7 (5.6–11.3)	75 (31–106)	3/5
Other*	24					

Data on 67 adult cases of HUS reported to the UK Centre for the International HUS Registry.

Haemoglobin (Hb) and the platelets: lowest value, median, and observed range.

Recovery: dialysis independent.

RTI, respiratory-tract infection.

*Others pregnancy (4), malignancy (4), familial (2), malignant hypertension (4), cardiac transplantation (1), mycoplasma septicaemia (2), scleroderma (1), HIV (5), cyclosporin (1).

Table 2 Aetiology of haemolytic uraemic syndrome

Infections

- *E. coli* diarrhoea associated
- Shigella associated
- Neuraminidase associated
- HIV infection
- Others

Sporadic, non-infectious causes

- Idiopathic
- Familial
- Drugs
- Tumours
- Pregnancy
- Systemic lupus erythematosus
- Transplantation
- Scleroderma
- Malignant/accelerated hypertension
- Superimposed on glomerulonephritis

The bacteriology and epidemiology of enterohaemorrhagic strains of *E. coli* are described in Section 16 (and see OTM3, pp. 556–7).

Shigella

Shigella dysenteriae type I is a common cause of acute renal failure in children under 5 years of age on the Indian subcontinent. It is associated with a HUS which is characterized by a striking neutrophil leucocytosis (mean 34×10^9/l). HUS is more likely to develop if amoxycillin is given in the diarrhoeal phase.

Neuraminidase-producing organisms

HUS may occur rarely with pneumococcal infections. It is postulated that the neuraminidase produced by these organisms strips sialic acid from cell membranes and exposes the Thomsen–Friedenreich antigen ('T antigen'). There is a false positive Coombs test and erythrocytes agglutinate with anti-T sera. However, virulent strains of *Streptococcus pneumoniae* commonly produce neuraminidase and yet HUS is a very rare association.

Other infections

Gut infection with *Campylobacter* has been associated with a TTP syndrome. Sporadic cases of HUS often appear to follow mild viral infections, and several viruses have been implicated, including coxsackie, echo, and adenovirus.

Table 3 Drugs that may cause haemolytic uraemic syndrome

Contraceptive pill
Cyclosporin
Mitomycin-Candsup®
5-Fluorouracil
Deoxycoformycin (an adenosine deaminase inhibitor)
Ticlopidine

Sporadic, non-diarrhoeal causes

Idiopathic

Often, when HUS occurs in adults, no antecedent factors can be implicated.

Familial

In most cases the inheritance appears to be autosomal recessive: with childhood onset, recurrence is common and the prognosis is poor. In other families there is evidence of autosomal dominance with incomplete penetrance: there is then a male predominance, a very poor prognosis, often with malignant hypertension and severe ocular and pulmonary manifestations. In women HUS often occurs postpartum or on taking the contraceptive pill. In some families there may be a defect in the gene for complement factor H.

Drugs

The number of drugs associated with HUS has been increasing (see Table 3).

Idiopathic postpartum renal failure

This is syndrome of acute rapidly progressive renal failure occurring in the first weeks after an uncomplicated pregnancy. Blood pressure may be normal initially, but rises rapidly and may reach the malignant phase. Complete recovery of renal function is rare, some 10 per cent of patients requiring long-term renal replacement therapy. In some cases, the antiphospholipid syndrome may be the cause; rarely there is a family history of HUS.

Systemic lupus erythematosus

Rarely systemic lupus erythematosus may present as HUS with multiple organ involvement and arteriolar thrombi.

Transplantation

Sporadic forms of HUS may recur following transplantation, but not D+ HUS. A similar picture can complicate severe vascular rejection.

Systemic sclerosis

Scleroderma renal crisis may closely resemble HUS and is described in Chapter 10.12 and Chapter 12.15.

Malignant/accelerated hypertension

The association of the haematological features of HUS with malignant hypertension is well known.

HIV infection

TTP has been increasingly described in HIV-positive men, with half the patients having no symptoms of HIV-related disease. Some have a preceding history of idiopathic immune thrombocytopenia. The presenting symptoms are similar to those of classical TTP and include fever in 75 per cent of cases, central nervous system (CNS) involvement in 40 per cent, a median platelet count of 16 $\times$ 10^9/l and renal dysfunction.

Clinical manifestations: haemolytic uraemic syndrome

HUS, in children, occurs equally between the sexes, although in adults there is a female preponderance. It is rare in those of African origin and uncommon in Japan but common in Argentina. In children, there is a seasonal variation associated with hot weather. Somewhere between 75 and 100 per cent of cases follow verocytotoxin-producing *E. coli* gut infections. Sporadic cases, are usually preceded either by an upper respiratory tract infection or have an insidious onset. Although HUS was considered to involve the kidney almost exclusively, the involvement of other organs has been increasing recognized.

Renal manifestations

Microscopic haematuria is common, but gross macroscopic haematuria can occur. Typically, the urine contains 1–2 g protein/24 h, although proteinuria can be up to 10 g/day and patients have presented with a nephrotic syndrome or become nephrotic during the early recovery phase. Renal failure is variable in degree, ranging from modest to a need for dialysis.

Cardiovascular system

Patients with D+ HUS are usually normotensive but in sporadic cases (D-HUS) there may be severe hypertension and a retinopathy with haemorrhage and exudates. Significant cardiac involvement is rare but may lead to heart failure due to cardiomyopathy and myocarditis, the former particularly postpartum.

Central nervous system

Uraemia, severe hypertension, and sometimes hyponatraemia—all may contribute to a disturbance of CNS function, but it is now believed that the pathological process affects the cerebral vasculature as in TTP. Although recovery may follow severe CNS involvement, there is often residual injury with developmental retardation, focal motor deficit, and learning and behavioural problems.

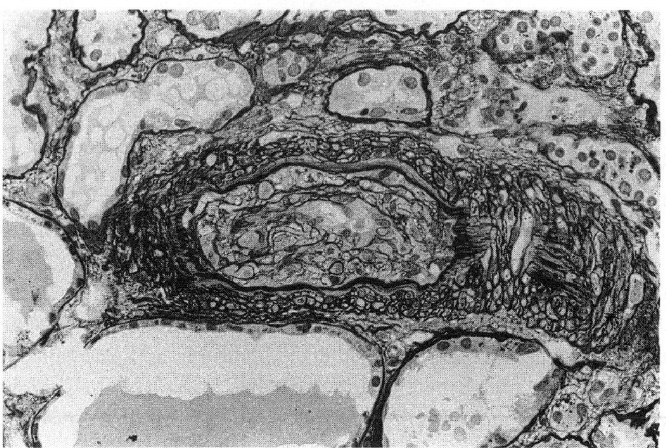

Fig. 1 An arcuate artery in which the lumen has been obliterated by intimal proliferation. The muscular wall and elastic lamina are normal (×200).

Gastrointestinal manifestations

In extreme cases there can be infarction or perforation of the bowel due to severe microvascular disease. Patients with severe colitis develop rectal prolapse. The differential diagnosis, in children, may include haemorrhagic colitis, intussusception, or Henoch–Schönlein purpura; in adults, ischaemic or inflammatory colitis. Hepatosplenomegaly may occur; pancreatic infarction leading to insulin dependence, and oesophageal involvement leading to stricture have been described.

Renal manifestations of thrombotic thrombocytopenic purpura

This condition is also discussed in Chapter 3.11. Renal manifestations range from proteinuria and microscopic haematuria to renal failure which is usually mild with plasma creatinine greater than 300 μmol/l in less than 20 per cent of cases.

Pathology

In HUS two different patterns are seen, although they may overlap. In D+ HUS there is predominantly glomerular capillary thrombosis with some arteriolar necrosis. Other forms of HUS, particularly in adults, commonly show severe intimal proliferation of arterioles and small arteries with luminal stenosis; that is, a preglomerular pathology (Fig. 1). With the former pattern, recovery is to be expected; but with the latter it is unusual. In rare cases of severe D+ HUS there may be irreversible acute cortical necrosis. Acute tubular necrosis occurs in proportion to the vascular pathology.

Pathogenesis

Endothelial cell injury is central to the pathogenesis of HUS and TTP. It is assumed that this precedes the platelet activation and consumption. Free radicals, neutrophil activation, and cytokines may all play a major part, but it is difficult at present to identify the sequence of events (see OTM3, pp. 3199–200).

Investigations

Haematological changes in haemolytic uraemic syndrome

Red cells

Although the haemoglobin concentration may fall rapidly to as low as 3 g/dl, the median values are 7–9 g/dl. The degree of anaemia is not related to acute renal failure and vice versa. The peripheral blood film shows fragmented and deformed cells (schistocytes, spherocytes). Depending on the degree of haemolysis, there will be an increase in reticulocytes, an increase in unconjugated bilirubin and plasma lactic dehydrogenase, together with a decrease in haptoglobin levels. Coombs test is negative; red cell enzymes and osmotic fragility are normal. Haemolysis may continue for 1–3 weeks.

Platelets

Platelet counts can fall to 5–20 × 10^9/l, but more usually are about 50 × 10^9/l, although at presentation 50 per cent of patients will have levels greater than 100 × 10^9/l. Red cell fragments may falsely raise 'automated' platelet counts. Thrombocytopenia usually lasts between 7 and 20 days, but the severity and duration do not correlate with the severity of the illness. In some patients it may be very brief. The thrombocytopenia in HUS is rarely severe enough to cause spontaneous bleeding.

Leucocytes

The white cell count may be over 20 × 10^9/l and can reach 30 × 10^9/l. In D+ HUS, leucocytosis greater than 20 × 10^9/l is associated with a poor outcome.

Clotting and fibrinolysis

Typically, prothrombin time and activated partial thromboplastin times are normal. Fibrin degradation products are raised and the thrombin and reptilase clotting times are therefore slightly prolonged. However, early in the disease, fibrinogen concentrations are only slightly reduced and fibrin degradation products are slightly raised. Later, fibrinogen levels may be raised. Disseminated intravascular coagulation is very rare.

Differential diagnoses

These include any cases of disseminated intravascular coagulation, Hantaviral infection, malaria due to plasmodium falciparum, some snake bites (particularly from vipers), Dengue haemorrhagic fever; but most commonly the differential will be in the spectrum between classical HUS and TTP.

Treatment

Specific treatments of TTP and, by implication of HUS is described in Chapter 3.35, but general measures, especially in relation to renal function, are of particular importance.

Hypovolaemia

Volume depletion is common and may be a consequence of diarrhoea and vomiting. In severe cases there may also be a capillary leak.

Acute tubular necrosis

Apart from hypovolaemia, there may be a nephrotoxic contribution from haemoglobinaemia or hyperbilirubinaemia. Hyperuricaemia may lead to a urate crystal nephropathy. Vigorous therapy with crystalloids and high-dose intravenous frusemide may convert patients to a polyuric phase and either avoid the need for dialysis or at least make fluid balance management easier. If the patient is still passing urine, a trial of prostacyclin infusion has some logic, although no formal study has been performed in adults. A dose of 2.5 ng/kg per min can be started and this can be gradually increased to 5 ng/kg, or higher if the drug is tolerated without troublesome hypotension or abdominal discomfort. There is no evidence, however, that prostacyclin affects the outcome.

Hypertension

Rigorous control of blood pressure is an essential feature of the management of relapsing HUS, in which such relapses are often associated with, or triggered by, increased blood pressure.

Outcome

The natural history of HUS, when preceded by a diarrhoeal illness and associated with glomerular thrombi, is one of spontaneous recovery, although there may be some residual injury. In idiopathic cases, particularly in adults, there is often major preglomerular vascular pathology and irreversible renal failure.

Further reading

Kaplan, B.S., Meyers, K.E., and Schulman, S.L. (1998). The pathogenesis and treatment of hemolytic uremic syndrome. *Journal of the American Society of Nephrology*, **9**, 1126–33.

Neild, G.H. (1994). Haemolytic uraemic syndrome: clinical practice. *Lancet*, **343**, 398–401.

Neild, G.H. and Barratt, T.M. (1997). Acute renal failure associated with microangiopathy. In *Oxford textbook of clinical nephrology*, (2nd edn), (ed. S. Cameron, A.M. Davison, J. Grünfeld, D. Kerr, and E. Ritz), pp. 1649–66. Oxford University Press.

Remuzzi, G. and Ruggenenti, P. (1995). The hemolytic uremic syndrome. *Kidney International*, **48**, 2–19.

Warwicker, P., Goodship, T.H. Donne, R.L., *et al.* (1998). Genetic studies into inherited and sporadic hemolytic uremic syndrome. *Kidney International*, **53**, 836–44.

Chapter 12.11

Infections and associated nephropathies

D. G. Williams and D. Adu

Infections of many kinds can be associated with, or be the specific cause of, all clinical syndromes of renal diseases, for example acute tubular necrosis, acute interstitial nephritis, glomerulonephritis, obstructive uropathy, and chronic renal failure. The association may be overt, as in septicaemia with acute renal failure, or covert, for example when membranous glomerulonephritis is ascribed to infection with hepatitis B. New infections affecting the kidney are appearing, either *de novo* such as AIDS-associated nephropathy, or due to geographical spread, for example Hantavirus nephropathy which is slowly progressing westward across Europe from Russia and the Far East.

Glomerulonephritis

Pathogenesis

Immune complex deposition/formation

Circulating immune complexes can be detected in many infections without a complicating nephritis but in those in which nephritis does develop, hypocomplementaemia and deposition of immunoglobulins, complement, and, in some instances, antigen in glomeruli suggest that antigen–antibody complexes have become localized in the kidney. A variant of this mechanism is the renal deposition of antigen alone, with subsequent formation of antigen–antibody complexes *in situ*. Physical characteristics of the antigens and antibody, and their complexes, such as size, antibody class and subclass, and charge, are important determinants of renal deposition.

Cross-reactive antibodies or molecular mimicry

Among the wide range of antigens presented by infectious organisms, it is likely that there will be some that are sufficiently similar to endogenous antigens to evoke an antibody response cross-reacting with renal tissues with resultant nephropathy.

Polyclonal B-cell activation

Infections usually induce an oligoclonal B-cell response, but some in addition, can stimulate a wide range of B cells whose immunoglobulins are less specific—polyclonal activation. Some of these latter antibodies may react with antigenic determinants in the host to cause renal damage by deposition of immune complexes in glomeruli.

Cell-mediated immunity

Some infection-associated nephritides are caused by lymphocytes which specifically target renal structures, particularly in infection-associated interstitial nephritis.

Post-infectious/acute endocapillary proliferative glomerulonephritis

The most common cause is an infection with group A streptococci, but other causative organisms include staphylococci, meningococci, *Streptococcus pneumoniae,* and *Shigella.* Post-streptococcal glomerulonephritis provides the typical model.

Clinical features

These develop 1–2 weeks after a streptococcal pharyngitis or 3–6 weeks after skin infection (impetigo). The disease has become uncommon in Western countries but epidemic outbreaks following secondary streptococcal infection of scabies or insect bites is a common cause in the tropics.

Presentation ranges from asymptomatic haematuria and proteinuria, through an acute nephritic syndrome at times accompanied by nephrotic features, to, rarely, a rapidly progressive glomerulonephritis. The typical patient presents with oliguria, reddish-brown urine (haematuria), proteinuria, a puffy face, and ankle oedema, often accompanied by hypertension and sometimes left ventricular failure. Headache, vomiting, and fits may complicate the rise in blood pressure. There is some degree of impairment of glomerular filtration in the majority, usually only slight to moderate, and resolving within 1–2 weeks. A nephrotic syndrome is much less common and acute renal failure is found in less than 2 per cent of affected children.

Aetiology and pathogenesis

Only certain M types (cell wall protein antigens) of Lancefield group A/β haemolytic streptococcal infections are followed by glomerulonephritis, but group C streptococci have also been associated with acute proliferative glomerulonephritis. The frequent occurrence of hypocomplementaemia supports antigen–antibody-mediated nephritis. A variety of candidate antigens have been suggested as have involvement of rheumatoid factor, antinuclear antibodies, or cross-reaction with glomerular structures by antistreptococcal antibodies.

Pathology

There is increased hypercellularity of glomeruli from mesangial proliferation and an influx of polymorphonuclear leucocytes, monocytes, and T lymphocytes with deposits of C3, IgG, and sometimes IgM in the glomerular mesangium and in large subepithelial deposits (humps) detected by immunofluorescence studies and electron microscopy. Crescents are infrequent. Rarely, there is typical mesangiocapillary glomerulonephritis which usually carries a better prognosis than does its idiopathic form.

Serology

After streptococcal pharyngitis 95 per cent of children will have an antibody response to streptolysin O, deoxyribonuclease, deoxyribonuclease B, hyaluronidase, and streptokinase. After pyoderma, antibody responses to deoxyribonuclease B are found but those to streptolysin O are infrequent. The rate of positive cultures from the site of suspected infection is low, so that failure to grow streptococci does not negate the diagnosis. Low serum concentrations of C3 occur in 80–90 per cent of cases and of C4 in a smaller proportion and, where present, last for 4–6 weeks.

Management and outcome

All patients should be given a 10-day course of penicillin or erythromycin but such treatment has no effect on the outcome of the renal illness, the management of which is based on meticulous attention to fluid balance together with diuretics and antihypertensive therapy as necessary. Very few patients will require dialysis. The acute illness usually resolves within 1 or 2 weeks, with return of normal renal function, although slight proteinuria and microscopic haematuria may persist for years in 20 per cent of patients. The long-term prognosis is good and there are few reports of resultant endstage chronic renal failure.

Nephritis associated with current infection

Infective endocarditis (see also Chapter 2.25)

Renal lesions in infective endocarditis range from focal renal infarcts, glomerulonephritis, which may be of diffuse or focal segmental proliferative types, to acute tubular damage. The most common of these is glomerulonephritis. The incidence of this complication is probably of the order of 1 per cent. Glomerulonephritis has been reported in patients with acute as well as subacute endocarditis, and has been described with all types of infecting organism. The presentation is often with an acute nephritic syndrome but some patients have only minimal urinary abnormalities. A small proportion have coincident cutaneous vasculitis and arthralgia. Low serum levels of C3 and C4 are found in approximately 50 per cent of patients and in some C3 nephritic factor can also be detected. Circulating immune complexes and cryoglobulins are found in some 50 per cent.

Pathology

Focal segmental necrotizing glomerulonephritis, mesangial proliferative glomerulonephritis, mesangiocapillary, and an endocapillary proliferative glomerulonephritis which may be accompanied by crescent formation have all been described. There is no clear association between the infecting organism and the type of glomerulonephritis. Immunohistology shows granular deposits of complement, IgG, IgA, and IgM in the glomerular basement membrane and mesangium. Electron microscopy shows subepithelial, subendothelial, and mesangial electron-dense deposits.

Treatment

Successful treatment of infective endocarditis leads to resolution of the glomerulonephritis in most cases. However, patients with extensive crescent formation may develop chronic renal failure. Deaths are usually due to the infective endocarditis and not to the renal lesion.

Shunt nephritis

Nephritis may result from infection of ventriculoatrial shunts for hydrocephalus and presents with haematuria which may be gross, and proteinuria which is often heavy enough to cause a nephrotic syndrome. Significant renal impairment is rarely present at diagnosis, but may develop in the absence of successful treatment. Fever is common, and anaemia, arthralgia, and a rash may develop. The most common infective organism is *Staphylococcus epidermidis*, but a wide variety of other organisms has also been implicated, including *Staph. aureus, Pseudomonas aeroginosa*, and diphtheroids. Glomerular deposits of IgM and C3, and in some cases of bacterial antigen with low serum complement levels and serum cryoglobulins, point to the glomerulonephritis being mediated by antigen–antibody complexes. Antibiotics alone are usually ineffective in eradicating infection. Removal of the shunt catheter usually leads to resolution of the nephritis.

Pathology

The renal lesion is usually a subendothelial mesangiocapillary glomerulonephritis with granular deposits of IgM and C3 in the mesangium and capillary walls, but other histological types, for instance focal sclerosing glomerulonephritis, occur.

Visceral abscesses

Chronic visceral abscesses, (pulmonary, subphrenic, and pelvic), may be complicated by the development of glomerulonephritis. The clinical presentation of renal disease, the types of glomerulonephritis, and the outcome with treatment resemble those seen in infective endocarditis.

Septicaemia

Staphylococcal septicaemia can cause a proliferative glomerulonephritis, particularly in intravenous drug abusers.

Typhoid fever

Salmonella typhi infection can be complicated by glomerulonephritis, which may be mesangial proliferative, diffuse proliferative, or IgA nephropathy. Glomerulonephritis increases the mortality from 5–10 per cent to 20–30 per cent.

Legionnaire's disease

Proteinuria, microscopic haematuria, and casts are found in 20–30 per cent of patients with legionnaire's disease. These features may be accompanied by mild impairment of renal function. Acute renal failure, which may be due to shock, rhabdomyolysis, endotoxaemia, and disseminated intravascular coagulation, develops in 7–14 per cent of patients. Renal biopsy typically shows an acute interstitial nephritis or acute tubular necrosis. The mortality in patients who develop acute renal failure ranges from 30 to 50 per cent.

Tuberculosis

Glomerulonephritis of different histological types, with or without detectable granulomas in the kidney, can complicate infection with *Mycobacterium tuberculosis,* most commonly in the presence of pulmonary lesions.

Hepatitis B infection

The renal complications of hepatitis B infection are found mainly in individuals with chronic disease and serological evidence of continued infection. The renal injury is probably immune mediated. The major renal lesions are membranous nephropathy and vasculitis. Membranous disease is seen particularly in children who are chronic carriers of the virus. Between 60 and 100 per cent of children with membranous nephropathy in Japan, Hong Kong, South Africa, and Zimbabwe have hepatitis B surface antigenaemia, contrasting with a rate of about 20 per cent in the US. The rates in adults are less and range from 0–4 per cent in the UK to 30–40 per cent in Hong Kong. The clinical presentation is usually with a nephrotic syndrome. Sera from almost all patients show hepatitis B surface antigenaemia, hepatitis Bc antibodies, Be antigenaemia, and Be antibodies. The histological lesion differs from idiopathic membranous disease in that, there are often subendothelial and mesangial in addition to subepithelial deposits.

Treatment and outcome

There is no treatment of proven benefit. Steroids are not helpful and, their use and withdrawal may lead to rebound hepatitis. α-Interferon and adenosine arabinoside have been used in some patients but with no conclusive evidence of benefit. The prognosis in children is good, with reported spontaneous remissions of the nephrotic syndrome in up to two-thirds of cases.

Hepatitis C-associated nephropathy

Hepatitis C infection may lead to chronic active hepatitis and cirrhosis and is the main cause of mixed essential cryoglobulinaemia. The renal presentation is with proteinuria or a nephrotic syndrome often accompanied by mild to moderate renal impairment. Diagnosis is by serology for antibodies to hepatitis C and this is confirmed by the detection of hepatitis C RNA. Cryoglobulinaemia is often found and typically serum complement levels are low and there is a positive rheumatoid factor.

Pathology

The renal lesion in mixed essential cryoglobulinaemia is a membranoproliferative glomerulonephritis type 1 but other types (e.g. focal and mesangioproliferative) have been reported and rarely there is a granulomatous renal arteritis. Immunofluorescent microscopy shows subendothelial as well as mesangial and capillary wall deposits of IgM, IgG, and C3. On electron microscopy these deposits may show the characteristics of cryoglobulins. A membranoproliferative glomerulonephritis may also develop in patients without cryoglobulinaemia.

Treatment

Treatment with α-interferon improves liver function and proteinuria and possibly renal function but relapses occur once treatment is discontinued.

HIV-associated glomerulonephritis

Glomerulonephritis may be seen early in HIV infection as well as in AIDS. The major manifestations are proteinuria, a nephrotic syndrome, and renal impairment. This complication is more common in the US than in Europe; and in intravenous drug abusers and black homosexuals than in white homosexuals. The clinical course, once a nephrotic syndrome has developed, is of evolution to endstage renal failure within a few months. It is suspected that direct viral invasion of the kidney is the basic cause; viral genome has been found in tubular and glomerular epithelia. Secondary infections, for instance with hepatitis B virus, may also play a part. There is no evidence of benefit from treatment with azidothymidine or ddI, although this has not been systematically studied. Patients have been treated with chronic haemodialysis, but survival is poor.

Pathology

The characteristic lesion is a focal segmental glomerulosclerosis often with a marked interstitial infiltrate of lymphocytes and plasma cells. Other histological types described include IgA nephropathy, mesangiocapillary, membranous, and minimal change nephropathy. Typically, on immunohistology mesangial deposits of IgM and C3 are seen.

Schistosomiasis

Just under 5 per cent of patients with *S. mansoni* infection have hepatosplenic disease, and of these about 10–15 per cent develop glomerular lesions over a period of up to 10 years. The presentation is with proteinuria or a nephrotic syndrome. In Egypt there is evidence that schistosomal glomerulonephritis is more common in individuals with concomitant chronic infections with salmonella. Treatment with antischistosomal drugs, or prednisolone and cyclophosphamide, has been of no benefit, and progression to renal failure is usual.

Pathology

A mesangial proliferative glomerulonephritis is seen in mild or early cases, and the most common histological change in advanced cases is a mesangiocapillary glomerulonephritis. The next most frequent lesion is focal segmental glomerulosclerosis. There are also infrequent reports of membranous nephropathy and proliferative glomerulonephritis. Immunohistology shows granular deposits, predominantly of IgM, but also of IgG, IgA, IgE, and C3, in the mesangium and the subepithelial and subendothelial sites. Renal amyloidosis has been described in Sudanese patients.

Leprosy

The major renal lesions are amyloidosis and glomerulonephritis, although chronic interstitial nephritis has also been described. Glomerulonephritis is found in up to 10 per cent of patients at autopsy. It tends to be more common in patients with lepromatous disease.

Pathology

The most common glomerular lesions are a mesangial proliferative glomerulonephritis, focal or diffuse proliferative glomerulonephritis, or rarely a membranous nephropathy. Immunohistology shows granular glomerular deposits of IgG, IgM, and C3 in the mesangium or on capillary walls.

Filariasis

There are several reports from India and Cameroon of an association between filariasis and glomerulonephritis. The clinical presentation is usually with a nephrotic syndrome and rarely with an acute nephritic syndrome. Treatment with diethylcarbamazine probably hastens recovery in those patients with an acute nephritic presentation but has no effect in patients with a nephrotic syndrome.

Pathology

Patients with *Wuchereria bancrofti* infection may develop a mesangial proliferative or a diffuse proliferative glomerulonephritis. In patients with loa-loa both membranous and mesangiocapillary glomerulonephritis have been reported. Onchocerciasis infections have been associated with a nephrotic syndrome due to minimal change nephropathy, mesangial proliferative glomerulonephritis, or a mesangiocapillary glomerulonephritis. On immunohistology glomerular deposits of IgG, IgM, and C3 are seen in the mesangium and capillary walls.

Malaria

An association between *Plasmodium malariae* infection and glomerulonephritis has been shown in Nigeria and Uganda, largely affecting children and young adults. Presentation is with a nephrotic syndrome, often with profound hypoalbuminaemia and ascites disproportionate to the degree of peripheral oedema. Microscopic haematuria is common and proteinuria is usually poorly selective. Immunohistology shows granular deposits of IgG and IgM. *P. malariae* antigen and antibody have been identified in the glomeruli.

Quartan malarial nephropathy is uncommon in Ghana, Senegal, and Papua New Guinea. This may be because only some strains of *P. malariae* are nephritogenic; environmental influences, genetic factors, or the effects of coincident other infections could be important. Alternatively, it is possible that whatever abnormality leads to quartan malarial nephropathy also leads to an increased susceptibility to *P. malariae* infection.

Pathology

The lesion comprises segmental glomerular capillary wall thickening with expansion of the subendothelial area. In advanced cases there is segmental and mesangial sclerosis and global glomerulosclerosis. Mesangial hypercellularity and small fibroepithelial crescents are seen infrequently. Immunohistology shows coarse granular or fine diffuse deposits of IgG, IgM, and C3 in the glomerular capillary walls. Electron microscopy shows increased basement membrane material in the subendothelial area.

Management and outcome

Antimalarial treatment does not produce remission. Only a minority with minor glomerular lesions respond to steroids. Azathioprine and cyclophosphamide are not effective, and azathioprine may worsen prognosis. Most develop progressive renal failure.

Syphilis

Secondary syphilis may rarely be complicated by a nephrotic syndrome caused by a mesangial proliferative glomerulonephritis or membranous nephropathy. Immunofluorescent microscopy shows subepithelial deposits of IgG and complement. Treatment with penicillin leads to resolution.

Table 1 Some infections rarely associated with glomerulonephritis

Bacteria	*Escherichia coli, Yersinia enterocolitica, Mycoplasma pneumoniae, Klebsiella pneumoniae*
Rickettsia	Rocky Mountain spotted fever
Viruses	Epstein–Barr virus, influenza (which has a particular association with antiglomerular basement membrane disease), cytomegalovirus, measles, varicella
Fungi	*Candida albicans, Histoplasma capsulatum*
Parasites	Toxoplasma, *Leishmania donovani*

Congenital syphilis may rarely be complicated by a membranous nephropathy with mesangial proliferation and at times crescent formation and a tubulointerstitial nephritis. The clinical presentation is with an acute nephritis or with a nephrotic syndrome. The renal lesion resolves following treatment with penicillin.

Other infections

Some of many other infections that have rarely been associated with glomerulonephritis are shown in Table 1.

Vasculitis

Hepatitis B-associated vasculitis

Hepatitis B surface antigenaemia with vasculitis has been reported in 10–40 per cent of patients in the US, 18–50 per cent of patients in France, and 4–8 per cent of patients in the UK. Renal involvement causes haematuria, proteinuria, and renal impairment. The renal lesions are indistinguishable from those of typical vasculitis and antineutrophil cytoplasmic antibody is often detectable.

Treatment and outcome

The prognosis is improved by treatment with cyclophosphamide and prednisolone. Antiviral agents such as α-interferon and adenosine arabinoside have been used in small numbers but with no compelling evidence of benefit. Unlike typical vasculitis, which tends to relapse in up to 40 per cent of cases, hepatitis B-associated vasculitis is more often a self-limiting disease.

Post-streptococcal vasculitis and other infections

A well-described but uncommon sequel of streptococcal infection is a systemic vasculitis occurring several days after the onset of skin or upper respiratory tract infection. Vasculitis can also occur in association with septicaemia caused by any organism. Heroin-associated vasculitis in intravenous drug abusers may be due to infection and septicaemia, or substances other than heroin in the mixture.

Interstitial nephritis

Interstitial nephritis associated with infections can arise by direct infection or by immune mechanisms. The usual organisms in pyelonephritis are *Escherichia coli*, *Staphylococcus aureus*, and *Proteus* species. In most cases that are treated promptly and effectively a full renal recovery is expected.

Immune-mediated interstitial nephritis

A range of infections has been associated with an acute interstitial nephritis which is characterized by a lymphocytic infiltration, without evidence of direct invasion by the micro-organisms. The clinical picture is of tubular proteinuria, microscopic haematuria, and varying degrees of renal dysfunction. Foreign antigens in the responsible organisms are thought to cause a cellular (type IV) reaction against foreign antigens in the infecting agents. Focal or diffuse infiltration of the interstitium is typical; in some patients glomerulonephritis may coexist. Most patients recover on treatment of the underlying infection.

Leptospirosis

There is renal involvement in most cases. The major histological lesions are an acute interstitial nephritis with acute tubular necrosis. Minor glomerular mesangial proliferation may be seen. Acute hypercatabolic renal failure develops in about 50 per cent. Treatment is with penicillin and erythromycin (see Chapter 16.69). Renal failure is treated by conventional methods. Most patients make a full recovery.

Haemorrhagic fever (hantavirus disease)

This disease is apparently increasing in frequency in Europe, spreading westwards. The Hantaviruses are carried by rodents and infection has occurred in laboratory workers exposed to rats. In the severe form, haemorrhage into the skin and mucous membranes is the cardinal symptom, together with myalgia, fever, and loin pain. Oliguria with microscopic haematuria and proteinuria develop 7–10 days after the onset. Acute tubular necrosis and medullary haemorrhage with mononuclear cell infiltrates are typical. There is no specific treatment but the outlook for renal function is good.

Haemolytic uraemic syndrome (see also Chapter 12.10)

This syndrome of thrombocytopenia, microangiopathic haemolytic anaemia, and acute renal failure in diarrhoea-associated epidemics is caused by verocytotoxin-producing *E. coli*. In the Indian subcontinent this syndrome may also complicate *Shigella dysenteriae* type I infection. Rare causes of the syndrome include neuraminidase-producing pneumococci and *Salmonella typhi* infection.

Acute renal failure (see also Chapter 12.28)

Severe sepsis, without nephritis, may lead to acute renal failure, typically accompanied by disseminated intravascular coagulation, most commonly from septicaemia with endotoxin-producing Gram-negative bacteria. A similar outcome may result from infections with *Staphylococcus aureus* and meningococci. Acute renal failure from gynaecological sepsis is still common in some parts of the tropics. *Plasmodium falciparum* and *Salmonella typhi* infections can lead to massive intravascular haemolysis and acute renal failure, more commonly in individuals who are glucose 6-phosphate dehydrogenase deficient. The main renal lesion in septicaemia is acute tubular necrosis but disseminated intravascular coagulation may cause thrombosis.

Further reading

Davison, A.M. (1998). Infection-related glomerulonephritis. In: *Oxford textbook of clinical nephrology*, (2nd edn) (ed. A.M. Davison, J.S. Cameron, J.-P. Grünfeld, D. Kerr, E. Ritz, and C.G. Winearls), pp. 667–87. Oxford University Press, Oxford.

Chapter 12.12

Renal amyloidosis, cryoglobulinaemia, light-chain deposition disease, and fibrillary glomerulonephritis

J. P. Grünfeld

Amyloidosis and cryoglobulinaemia are described elsewhere (Chapters 6.15 and 10.18 and OTM3, pp. 3050–2 and 3179–82).

Light-chain deposition disease

Light-chain deposition disease is characterized by the deposition of monoclonal light chains (mainly κ) in various tissues because of proliferation of an abnormal and small clone of B lymphocytes, which produces light chains, often with an abnormal structure (abnormally polymerized or glycosylated). The light-chain deposits are often widespread but the kidney is the most frequently involved organ and renal manifestations predominate. Most patients are over 50 years of age and have an underlying malignant lymphoplasmacytic disease, usually multiple myeloma. However, 20–30 per cent of them have no such overt disorder at presentation and do not develop it later in the course.

Symptoms

Proteinuria, either moderate or in the nephrotic range, often progresses rapidly or slowly to renal failure. Deposits in the heart rarely result in heart failure or arrhythmias, and liver deposits are often asymptomatic, even when associated with marked capillary dilatations with the appearance of peliosis hepatis. In patients with myeloma and light-chain deposition disease, the prognosis is determined by the severity of the myeloma. In 'idiopathic' light-chain deposition disease, some rare patients have a fulminant course with multiorgan involvement. Most patients progress more slowly to endstage renal disease and some do not develop extrarenal manifestations even after years on dialytic therapy.

Diagnosis

Monoclonal light chain antibodies are used in immunofluorescent microscopy to detect light chains, usually κ along the tubular basement membrane. By light microscopy, this membrane has a thickened and refractile appearance and appears outlined on its external aspect by ribbon-like, continuous deposits; by electron microscopy, the peritubular deposits have a granular structure. Fixation is also found in the glomerular mesangium, forming mesangial nodules in approximately 60 per cent of the patients. In the absence of an immunofluorescence study, these lesions may be misdiagnosed as nodular diabetic (Kimmelstiel–Wilson) glomerulopathy. In 'idiopathic' light-chain deposition disease, the monoclonal light chain can be detected in some patients in serum and/or in concentrated urine.

Treatment

Chemotherapy is indicated in patients with multiple myeloma. In 'idiopathic' disease, it is not established whether chemotherapy is beneficial. Recurrence of light-chain deposition disease after renal transplantation has been reported.

Fibrillary glomerulonephritis

Fibrillary glomerulonephritis is a very rare disease, characterized by the deposition of randomly arranged fibrils in the glomerular capillary wall and mesangium. These fibrils do not bind Congo red, and are wider (18–22 nm) than are amyloid fibrils. IgG4 and the C3 complement can be shown in fibrils by immunofluorescence. The presentation includes proteinuria, haematuria, and hypertension, progressing to renal failure in half the patients. No monoclonal protein is found in serum or urine. Treatment is limited to symptomatic management. The disease may recur after renal transplantation.

Immunotactoid glomerulopathy has been considered as either belonging to the same spectrum or as a separate entity. It is characterized by the crystallization of immune aggregates into tactoids resulting in the deposition of fibrils or microtubules. These structures are arranged in parallel; their diameter ranges from 30 to 40 nm. Monoclonal immunoglobulin deposition is more common in immunotactoid glomerulopathy. In addition, these patients appear to be at risk for a concomitant dysproteinaemia and/or lymphoproliferative disorder.

Further reading

Davison, A.M. Cameron, J.S., Grunfeld, J.-P., Kerr, D., Ritz, E., and Winearls, C.G. (ed). (1998). *Oxford textbook of clinical nephrology*, (2nd edn). Oxford University Press, Oxford.

Chapter 12.13

Renal manifestations of malignant disease

A. M. Davison

Renal disease can occur in patients with benign and malignant tumours and with lymphoproliferative and myeloproliferative disorders. The renal manifestations may arise as a direct effect of the tumour, or due to its systemic consequences, the secretion of tumour products, or related to tumour therapy (Table 1).

Direct renal involvement

Metastatic spread of malignant tumours to the kidney is relatively uncommon in spite of high renal blood flow. When present, metastases are usually multiple and often bilateral, presenting as either loin pain or haematuria; rarely do they cause significant impairment of renal function. In contrast, renal infiltration is present in approximately 50 per cent of patients with leukaemia and 30 per cent of those with lymphoma. The most common leukaemia to infiltrate the kidney is lymphoblastic leukaemia, which usually affects both kidneys diffusely throughout the cortex. As with metastatic disease, renal infiltration with lymphoma or leukaemia leads only uncommonly to significant renal functional impairment; and only rarely is the initial manifestation of lymphoma or leukaemia due to renal infiltration.

Tumours at the hilum of the kidney may compress the renal artery sometimes resulting in hypertension. Only very rarely is the renal vein

Table 1 Renal manifestations of malignancy

Direct effects
◆ Metastases
◆ Infiltration
◆ Obstruction
Indirect effects
◆ Electrolyte disorders
• Hypercalcaemia, hypokalaemia, hyponatraemia
◆ Acute renal failure
◆ Nephropathy
◆ Disseminated intravascular coagulation
◆ Renal vein thrombosis
◆ Hyperviscosity syndrome
◆ Fanconi syndrome
◆ Amyloidosis
Treatment associated
◆ Drug nephrotoxicity
◆ Tumour lysis syndrome
◆ Radiation

Table 2 Evidence required to demonstrate a causal relationship between malignancy and nephropathy

A close temporal relationship between the clinical presentation of the tumour and the nephropathy
Remission of nephropathy after cure or removal of tumour
Recurrence of nephropathy with recurrence of tumour
Demonstration of tumour antigen and associated antibody in glomerular deposits

involved. Ureteric obstruction may arise from external compression of the ureters by retroperitoneal or pelvic tumours or from lymphoma involving para-aortic nodes. Bladder cancer rarely causes obstruction unless it involves the trigone.

Malignant tumour nephropathy

There have been many reports suggesting an association between malignancy and nephropathy. The tumours most commonly associated with nephropathy are adenocarcinomas of the lung and gastrointestinal tract (stomach, colon, and rectum), but there are reports of many other associated tumours, frequently in single case reports. There are few reports of nephropathy in association with carcinoma of the breast. The incidence in adults is probably less than 1 per cent of patients with nephrotic syndrome. A 1976 review of 14 published series with a total of 1643 patients with nephrotic syndrome revealed six (0.4 per cent) with associated malignancy.

Demonstration of a causal relationship requires that a number of conditions should be satisfied (Table 2). A review of 93 patients with carcinoma and nephropathy showed that the nephropathy had been described within 6 months of the detection of the tumour, in 63 per cent of cases; in most diagnoses were made simultaneously, but in 23 patients the nephrotic syndrome developed more than 12 months before or 12 months after tumour diagnosis.

There are a number of reports of a prompt response between remission of the nephropathy after tumour removal but, some patients fail to improve. Recurrence of the tumour is usually associated with the recurrence of the nephropathy, but this is not invariable. The demonstration of tumour antigen and antitumour antibodies in the affected kidneys has been possible in a number of studies, and the pathogenesis of the nephropathy in the majority of patients is immunologically mediated with glomerular immune deposits formed *in situ* from antigen and antibody deposited separately. In a number of malignancies, particularly in lymphoproliferative diseases, viral antigens may be the causal agent; antibodies to Epstein–Barr virus have been demonstrated in glomeruli in Burkitt's lymphoma. Glomerular deposition of autologous non-tumour antigens has also been described.

The most common clinical presentation is with nephrotic syndrome. A wide variety of renal histological appearances have been described, although membranous nephropathy is the most common, occurring in approximately 70 per cent of patients with associated carcinoma. Mesangiocapillary glomerulonephritis has been described in association with carcinoma of the breast, bronchogenic carcinoma, and adenocarcinoma of the stomach, and lymphocytic leukaemia. The very rare association of IgA nephropathy and malignancy is most likely to be fortuitous. In patients with Hodgkin's lymphoma the most common histological finding is that of minimal change nephropathy, although membranous nephropathy and mesangiocapillary glomerulonephritis have also been described. In no instance does the glomerular appearance appear to be specific for a particular tumour nor is there any association between tumour load, or the presence of metastases and the development or severity of nephropathy.

The overall prognosis is determined more by the malignancy than the glomerular findings. In general, complete resection or remission of the malignancy is associated with remission of the nephropathy, and there may also be an improvement with a reduction in tumour mass.

Renal manifestations due to therapy

Nephrotoxicity may develop as a consequence of analgesic therapy, antibiotic therapy, or the use of cytotoxic drugs. A severe uric acid nephropathy (tumour lysis syndrome) may follow chemotherapy in patients with lymphoproliferative or myeloproliferative disorders (see Chapaters 3.28, 3.29). Radiation nephritis is now uncommon as, during such treatment, care is taken to shield the kidneys. However, in a few instances it is impossible to protect the kidney completely, and acute radiation effects may become manifest within 6–12 months of radiation, whereas chronic effects develop over the years, becoming manifest by the development of proteinuria, hypertension, and impaired renal function.

Further reading

Ponticelli, C. (1998). Oncology and the kidney. In: *Oxford textbook of clinical nephrology*, (2nd edn) (ed. A.M. Davison, J.S. Cameron, J.-P. Grünfeld, D. Kerr, E. Ritz, and C.G. Winearls), pp.2745–2753. Oxford University Press, Oxford.

Chapter 12.14

Sarcoidosis and the kidney (see also Chapter 4.27)

A. M. Davison

Sarcoidosis may involve the kidney directly or indirectly (Table 1). Most commonly, renal involvement is a consequence of hypercalcaemia (see Chapter 7.5), but acute or chronic interstitial nephritis, glomerulopathy, and a number of miscellaneous conditions may also arise. In the majority of patients, renal complications develop in those known to have sarcoidosis, and only rarely are they a presenting feature.

Granulomatous interstitial nephritis

Granulomatous interstitial nephritis most commonly presents with impaired renal function, usually chronic and slowly progressive, but some patients may present with acute renal failure. Impaired renal function is associated with mild proteinuria, which is predominately tubular. Other tubular abnormalities include glycosuria, the Fanconi syndrome, proximal and distal tubular acidosis, and nephrogenic diabetes insipidus. The pathogenesis of the tubular disorder is most likely to be related to the accompanying hypergammaglobulinaemia.

The prevalence of granulomatous interstitial nephritis is difficult to determine, as infiltration may be clinically silent and small lesions may be missed on biopsy. However, it is likely to be in the region of 15–40 per cent of patients with sarcoidosis. The lesions involve both the cortex and medulla and are similar to sarcoid granulomas found elsewhere.

At diagnosis, many patients have severely impaired renal function, but this may respond dramatically to corticosteroid therapy. The dosage most commonly employed is 1–1.5 mg/kg per day with a gradual reduction after 2 months. It is likely that prolonged therapy, up to and perhaps even exceeding a year, will be required. In some cases granulomas may progress to fibrosis with consequent tubular atrophy and renal failure may then be chronic.

Table 1 Renal consequences of sarcoidosis

Disordered calcium metabolism
• Nephrocalcinosis
• Nephrolithiasis
Interstitial nephritis
• Chronic renal failure
• Acute renal failure
Glomerulopathy
• Membranous nephropathy
• Rarely, other glomerulopathies
• Amyloidosis
Miscellaneous
• Obstructive uropathy
• Hypertension

Glomerular involvement

Sarcoidosis-associated glomerulopathy is uncommon, but when present is usually manifests as a nephrotic syndrome associated with minor haematuria and mild impairment of renal function. It occurs most commonly as a late manifestation in patients with overt sarcoidosis. In approximately 50 per cent of patients the histological appearances are those of a membranous nephropathy, although focal and segmental glomerulosclerosis, diffuse endocapillary proliferative glomerulonephritis, and crescentic nephritis have also been described. A few patients have amyloidosis. Whether or not sarcoid-associated membranous disease responds to steroids is unclear.

Miscellaneous

Another rare cause of renal involvement with sarcoidosis is obstructive uropathy due to retroperitoneal granulomas.

Further reading

Kenouch, S. and Méry, J.-P. (1998). The patient with sarcoidosis. In: *Oxford textbook of clinical nephrology*, (2nd edn) (ed. A.M. Davison, J.S Cameron, J.-P. Grünfeld, D. Kerr, E. Ritz, and C.G. Winearls), pp. 837–45. Oxford University Press, Oxford.

Chapter 12.15

Rheumatological disorders and the kidney: systemic lupus erythematosus, mixed connective tissue disease, scleroderma, Sjögren's syndrome, and rheumatoid arthritis

J. S. Cameron and D. G. Williams

Renal systemic lupus erythematosus

The pathogenesis of systemic lupus erythematosus and its general manifestations are dealt with in Chapter 10.11, and here we deal only with its effects on the kidney.

Prevalence and presentation

The proportion of patients with lupus who have renal involvement depends upon how assiduously the nephritis is sought. In most unselected series 40–60 per cent of adults and up to 80 per cent of children show clinical evidence of renal involvement. However, if renal biopsies are performed in patients with normal renal function and normal urine, the proportion approaches 100 per cent. The histological appearances in patients with clinically inapparent lupus nephritis are usually mild (see below). Clinical renal involvement is present in only about 20 per cent of adults at the time of presentation; the proportion with abnormal urine and/or renal function increases over the next 1–10 years, after which new involvement of the kidney is rare.

Table 1 Summary of World Health Organization (WHO) classification of lupus nephritis

Class	Optical microscopy	Immunohistology*
I (normal) (0–5%)	Virtually normal glomerulus	Scanty mesangial immune aggregates
II (mesangial) (15–20%)	Mesangial prominence and hypercellularity	Diffuse mesangial aggregates only
III (a) (focal) (20–30%)	Focal/segmental proliferative necrotic lesions usually on a background of diffuse mesangial hypercellularity	Diffuse mesangial aggregates
III(b)	As III(a) but much more diffuse with major disturbance of glomerular architecture focally in capillary wall	Diffuse mesangial aggregates plus segmental crescents in some glomeruli
IV (diffuse) (45–60%)	Diffuse proliferative/infiltrative glomerulonephritis plus irregular capillary wall thickening and frequent small and occasional large, crescents round glomeruli	Diffuse mesangial aggregates; diffuse capillary wall aggregates both inside and outside capillary wall
V (membranous) (10–15%)	Diffuse peripheral capillary wall thickening with little or no proliferation/infiltration	Predominant diffuse subepithelial capillary aggregates plus some mesangial aggregates in most cases

*In all forms of lupus nephritis, it is common to find IgG, IgA, IgM, C1q, C3, and C4 in the immune aggregates ('full-house' pattern), but this is by no means invariable. IgG and C3 are almost always present, and lupus is very unlikely if they are absent

An important, although unusual group of patients with lupus nephritis are those in whom the nephritis is initially the sole manifestation of the disease. This particularly applies to patients with membranous nephropathy. After a period, usually months or several years, other manifestations of lupus appear, and only then can the diagnosis be made. However, from the beginning these patients usually show positive antinuclear factor tests or the presence of anti-dsDNA antibodies, so that these should be sought in the evaluation of patients who appear to have primary nephritis, particularly young women.

Renal involvement usually becomes evident in the form of proteinuria, amounting to a full nephrotic syndrome in 50–60 per cent of patients. Although this proteinuria is usually accompanied by microscopic haematuria, visible blood in the urine is rare and lupus nephritis almost never presents with isolated haematuria. At renal presentation, 40 per cent of patients have hypertension, 50 per cent have reduced renal function, and the occasional patient presents with acute renal failure. Many patients have, in association with the interstitial component of their nephritis, modest defects of distal tubular function of which renal tubular acidosis is the most important and is often associated with hyperkalaemia.

Laboratory tests

These are described in Chapter 12.1 but there is a particular need to screen for the antiphospholipid antibody syndrome which may result in a different cause of renal dysfunction than classical lupus nephritis (see Chapter 10.11).

Renal histology in lupus nephritis

Two approaches are useful in assessing histology: the first describes the pattern of involvement of the glomerulus, and the second the activity and/or chronicity of the process. The patterns of nephritis in lupus are bewildering in their variety (Table 1). These broad categories provide only a general guide; some patients may show varying patterns in different glomeruli, and even within a single glomerulus, others are difficult or impossible to classify. The appearances on light microscopy are associated with the presence within the glomeruli of material which contains immune reactants, such as immunoglobulins and complement components. DNA and anti-DNA antibodies form only a very small proportion of this material, and their pathogenetic significance remains in doubt. The distribution of the immune material parallels the distribution of the lesions on conventional microscopy (Fig. 1).

In the interstitium there is almost always an infiltrate of monocytes and T lymphocytes, a minority of plasma cells, killer cells, and a few eosinophils. This is associated with immune aggregates in the tubular basement membranes, which are more common in severe forms. On occasion interstitial nephritis may be a dominant feature, with associated severe renal dysfunction. Varying degrees of tubular atrophy and interstitial fibrosis may be observed.

Fig. 1 (*opposite*) The appearances of the glomeruli in the nephritis of systemic lupus erythematosus as classified by the WHO. (a) Glomerulus normal to optical microscopy (class I) but with aggregates of immune reactants within the mesangium (arrows), in this case revealed by antibody directed against C1q labelled with peroxidase. The patient had fever, arthralgia, and glandular enlargement but only trivial proteinuria. (b) Obvious mesangial deposits associated with expansion of the mesangium on optical microscopy, together with a mild increase in mesangial cellularity, not visible in this preparation (WHO class II). (c) A more obvious mesangial hypercellularity, again associated with mesangial immune aggregates revealed by immunoperoxidase staining against C3. However, the peripheral capillary walls, however, show no aggregates (WHO class II). (d) WHO class III lesion with not only mesangial involvement but also a focal, predominantly necrotic, lesion containing nuclear debris (arrows). In some patients this may be associated with an overlying area of epithelial proliferation amounting to a segmental crescent. WHO class III includes a wide range of appearances, mild as here (WHO class III(a)) and also severe widespread lesions (but still predominantly focal and segmental) (class III(b)). (e) WHO class IV lesion with diffuse proliferative and infiltrative nephritis. There is a segmental crescent overlying part of the glomerulus. The capillary walls are thickened irregularly. The patient had a full nephrotic syndrome with reduced renal function and hypertension. (f) Appearance of such a glomerulus on immunohistological staining, in this case for IgG. There is mesangial deposition of the immune aggregates and also irregular deposition along the capillary walls, massively in some areas ('wire loops'). (g) A capillary loop from a class IV lesion at high power, stained with silver to show glomerular basement membranes. One of the thickened capillary loops is shown, and demonstrates the black silver-stained glomerular basement membrane, and at a subendothelial site massive clear aggregates of immune material (arrows) are present, with endothelial cells and mesangial cells completing the gross thickening of the capillary wall. (h) WHO class V membranous lesion. Although the mesangium contains immune aggregates, the most prominent lesion is a diffuse scattering of irregular-sized aggregates along the capillary walls which are on the subepithelial side of the membrane and protrude under the epithelial cells and Bowman's space. The patient was nephrotic but normotensive, with normal renal function. (See Table 1 for further identification.)

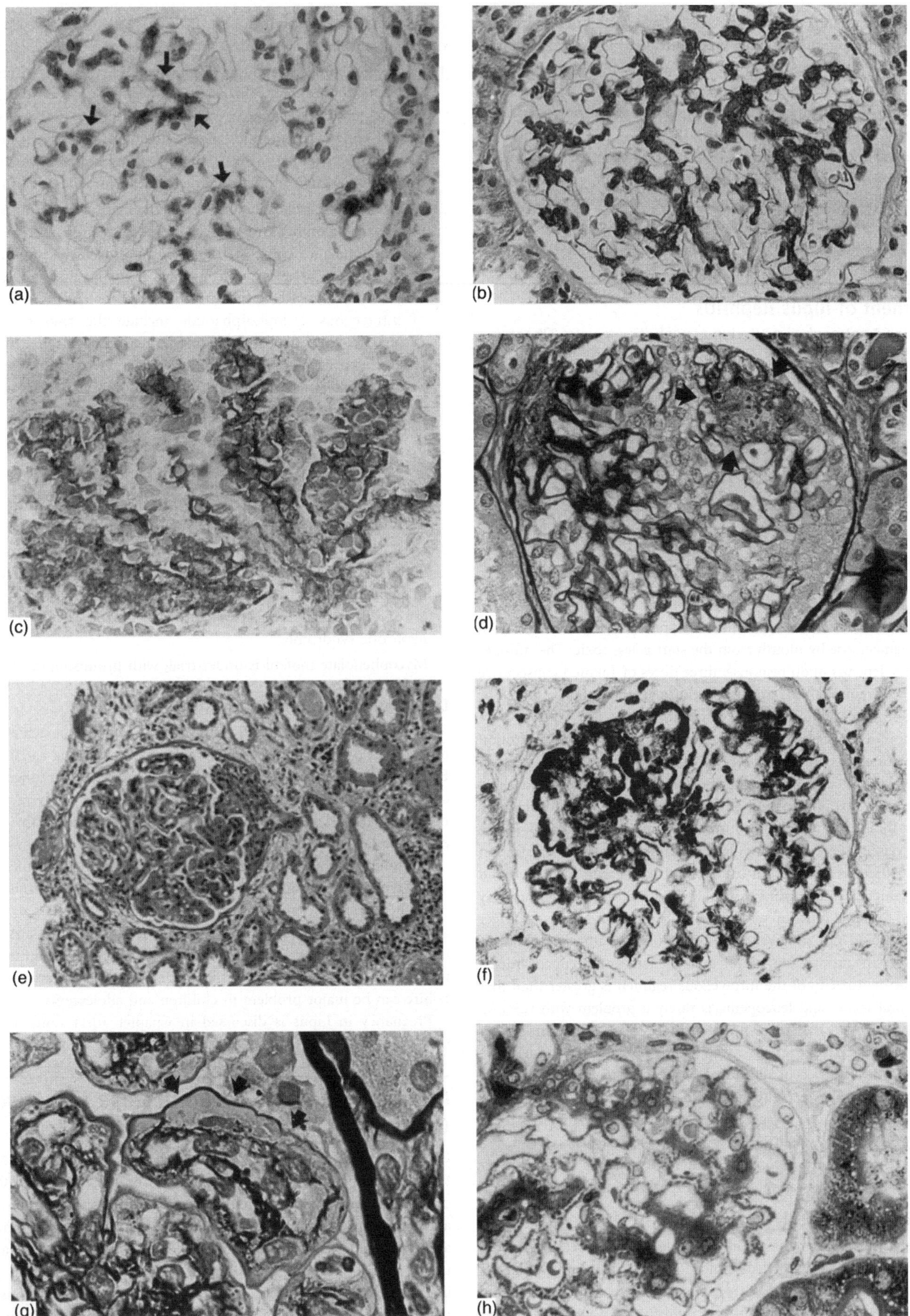

Fig. 1

Changes seen in the intrarenal vessels include immune aggregates, rarely necrotizing angiitis, and premature vascular sclerosis. Sometimes, particularly in association with antiphospholipid antibodies, thrombi may be seen in glomerular capillaries or renal arterioles, and rarely this is accompanied by a clinical picture of a haemolytic uraemic syndrome.

Assessment of activity is based on features such as necrosis, nuclear dusting from fragmented cells, glomerular thrombi, and intensity of cellular infiltrate. Chronicity is assessed by the amount of collagen (sclerosis) within the glomeruli and the interstitium. Active changes are judged to be susceptible to treatment, while sclerosis is assumed to be irreversible.

Treatment of lupus nephritis

Induction treatment of acute lupus nephritis (see also Chapter 10.11)

Induction treatment is guided by the severity of the clinical and histological picture. All patients should begin corticosteroid treatment, although some would dispute this for WHO class V patients with membranous nephropathy which tends to run an indolent course. Corticosteroids alone suffice in the initial phase for class I and II patients, and perhaps for mild class III patients. A regimen comprising a high initial oral dose (e.g. 60 mg/daily), followed by tapering doses to a maintenance treatment of 10–15 mg/daily over 8–12 weeks depending on response, has been much used, but usually results in a cushingoid patient and can cause a high incidence of infections. Large intravenous doses of methylprednisolone ('pulses') have also been used as initial therapy, and this approach coupled with a low maintenance dose by mouth from the start is less toxic. The number of pulses depends upon response; three doses of 1 g on 3 consecutive days is conventional but arbitrary, with a further similar course or courses if the condition appears resistant.

In more severe cases it is usual to use a cytotoxic agent in addition to corticosteroids. In the induction phase the choice lies between cyclophosphamide and azathioprine. No trial has compared these two drugs in this phase, and both seem effective. Cyclophosphamide quickly inhibits autoantibody formation and many prefer it in the acute phase. Despite the popularity of intravenous administration (750–1000 mg as an infusion over several hours with hydration and an antiemetic), oral dosing for 8–12 weeks at 1–3 mg/kg per day adjusted for renal function and white-cell count is as effective. Longer courses should not be given because of bladder toxicity (which is avoided by the intravenous route), gonadal damage, and oncogenicity. The marrow toxicity of the intravenous regimen is greater than that of the oral route, and leucopenia is rarely a problem with the oral regimen provided that renal function is taken into account. Newer agents such as cyclosporin and mycophenolate mofetil are under trial.

Two controlled trials of additional plasma exchange in acute disease have been performed: Neither showed definite benefit, but neither used plasma exchange as aggressively as advocates of this treatment have suggested (daily 4-litre exchanges for 7–10 days).

Intravenous pooled gammaglobulin has had some success in resistant patients, but is as yet a highly experimental approach.

Maintenance treatment

Maintenance treatment is usually feasible some 12 weeks after the acute inductive phase. Corticosteroids form the mainstay given at the lowest effective dose, aiming at prednisolone between 7.5 and 15 mg daily. This alone will often suffice in mild forms of nephritis, but in those with more resistant disease, cytotoxic agents are needed. The options available are as follows.

1. Change oral or intravenous cyclophosphamide to oral azathioprine (2–2.5 mg/kg per day). This has the advantages of low toxicity in the long term, no increase in the incidence of infections over those treated with corticosteroids alone, no gonadal toxicity, and no adverse effects on pregnancy. Complete remission, allowing withdrawal of all drugs, is rarely attained, at least for a decade or more.
2. Intravenous cyclophosphamide (750–1000 mg) every month, and then every 2months, for 1–2 years or more, again backed by low-dose maintenance corticosteroids. This approach was superior to corticosteroids alone in two controlled trials but not significantly different from corticosteroids and azathioprine. The disadvantages of intravenous cyclophosphamide include the risks of severe chronic marrow depression, considerable gonadal toxicity and teratogenicity, inability to conceive while receiving treatment and premature menopause and infertility in more than 50 per cent of patients. There is also the problem of the risk of the later development of leukaemia.
3. Methotrexate 5–15 mg orally each week. Some patients resistant to other approaches may respond to the addition of this drug. The main limitation has been hepatotoxicity, but this is not usually a major problem in the low doses appropriate here.
4. Cyclosporin at a dose of 4–5 mg/kg per day or less (monitored by blood levels) may have a role in chronic management, particularly in allowing lower doses of corticosteroids to be used. It will also reduce proteinuria in patients who have particularly severe nephrotic syndromes.
5. Mycophenolate mofetil is under trial, with promising results.

Long-term outcome and complications

Survival of renal function and of the patient can now be achieved in 80 per cent of patients with severe nephritis for as long as 10 years. Even if renal failure occurs, both dialysis and renal transplantation can be performed, and surprisingly the disease very rarely recurs in the transplanted kidney even in patients with continued active lupus elsewhere.

Complications of lupus, and of its treatment, include infections of all types, but particularly opportunistic infections, thromboses, osteonecrosis, hypertension, and neoplasia. In addition, an alarming incidence of accelerated atheroma is present in long-term survivors, the pathogenesis of which is not yet clear. Cataracts are common but usually insignificant clinically, while diabetes mellitus is rare. Growth failure can be major problem in children and adolescents.

Pregnancy in lupus is discussed in Chapter 10.11 (and see also OTM3, p. 3022).

Mixed connective tissue disease (see also Chapter 10.12 and OTM3, p. 3034)

Glomerular disease was once thought to be rare in mixed connective tissue disease, but it is now recognized to be present in 10–40 per cent of patients. The presenting features are symptomless proteinuria and haematuria in most cases; a nephrotic syndrome is uncommon and renal failure is very rare. The histological appearances are varied; the most common are membranous nephropathy, mesangial proliferative, or proliferative glomerulonephritis. A good response to corticosteroid treatment is usual, but the renal manifestations are usually mild and not progressive. Transformation into typical systemic lupus or scleroderma may be seen.

Sjögren's syndrome (see also Chapter 10.13)

Renal disease is uncommon, affecting only about 10 per cent of patients. The commonest form is a tubulointerstitial nephritis which presents particularly with renal tubular acidosis of which it is a major cause (50%) and immunosuppressive. This is more commonly distal tubular (type I) rather than proximal tubular (type II). There may be polyuria and hypokalaemia from renal potassium wasting, which may lead to muscle weakness (of which it is a major cause) and even paralysis. The kidney is infiltrated with plasma cells and CD4-positive T lymphocytes, and extensive tubular atrophy may be present. Peritubular immune aggregates of IgG and complement may be present, but severe disease can be seen in their absence. The condition is responsive to both corticosteroids and cyclophosphamide, but it is rarely justified to use these for the nephropathy alone. Otherwise, potassium supplements and sodium bicarbonate may be used. Rarely, nephrocalcinosis may appear together with renal failure.

Glomerular disease is very rare. It usually takes the form of a membranous nephropathy and occasionally a focal proliferative nephritis associated in some cases with cryoglobulinaemia and low serum complement concentrations.

Systemic sclerosis (scleroderma) (see Chapter 10.12)

Renal involvement primarily arises from the vascular changes which are central to this disease. Renal disorder is present in about one-third of patients, almost all with the diffuse form of the disease, and ranges from proteinuria, usually of modest degree, and haematuria, to slowly progressive renal failure with hypertension, to acute renal failure with accelerated hypertension ('scleroderma crisis'). The diagnosis should be suspected in all patients presenting with severe hypertension and acute renal failure, but even careful examination of the digits and face may fail to reveal any changes in the skin to begin with. Raynaud's phenomenon is a valuable clue, and immunological testing shows a positive antinuclear factor resulting from antibodies against scl 70 in a high proportion.

The most important lesion affects the blood vessels, with proliferation of endothelial cells, and deposition of glycoproteins and mucopolysaccharides within the vessel wall (Fig. 2) together with fibrinoid necrosis and reduplication of the internal elastic lamina, giving rise to the so-called 'onion skin' appearance which is particularly common in interlobular and arcuate arteries of diameter 150–500 μm. These vascular changes and renal failure can precede hypertension. The glomeruli usually only show changes due to ischaemia, but occasionally renal arteriolar thrombosis may be seen and there may be thrombocytopenia and red-cell fragmentation.

Effective control of arterial pressure, particularly by angiotensin-converting enzyme inhibitors, has reduced the mortality of scleroderma renal crisis from 100 per cent to lower levels, depending upon how early treatment is begun. There is no role for corticosteroids or anticoagulants.

If endstage renal failure supervenes, a small proportion of patients may recover some degree of renal function after several months of dialysis. Transplantation is also a possibility, but recurrence in the allograft has been reported in a few patients. The ultimate outcome depends upon involvement of other organs.

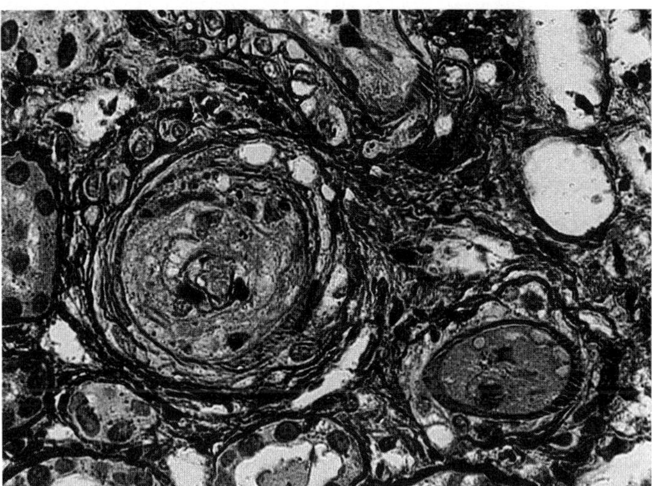

Fig. 2 Lesions in medium-sized renal arterioles in a patient with systemic sclerosis. The intima shows swelling and proliferation, so that the lumen of the vessel is completely occluded. in addition the internal elastic lamina is reduplicated, the beginnings of an 'onion skin' appearance can be seen, and the media is vacuolated and swollen. A smaller vessel to the left of the picture shows similar changes.

Rheumatoid arthritis (see Chapter 10.2)

Glomerulonephritis

Glomerulonephritis in rheumatoid arthritis is unusual. Several forms have been described. There may be mesangial proliferation with or without visible deposits of IgA and in a proportion of patients the serum IgA concentration is elevated. Whether or not this represents more than the coincidence of two relatively common conditions is unclear. Membranous nephropathy can be found in occasional patients who have never received gold or penicillamine both of which may lead to slowly reversible proteinuria or nephrotic syndrome. Again the possibility of coincidence arises, but seems unlikely. Vasculitis is common, but rarely affects the kidney. When it does, the appearances are similar to those of microscopic polyangiitis, and it also responds well to treatment with corticosteroids or cyclophosphamide.

Amyloid

See Chapter 6.15.

Further reading

Berden, J.H.M. (1997). Lupus nephritis. *Kidney International*, **52**, 538–58.

Emery, P. and Adu, D. (1998). The patient with rheumatoid arthritis, mixed connective disease, or polymyositis. In *Oxford textbook of clinical nephrology*, (2nd edn), (ed. Davison, A.M. Cameron, J.S., Grünfeld, J.-P., Kerr, D., Ritz, E., and Winearls, C.), pp. 975–86. Oxford University Press.

Lewis, E., Schwartz, M., and Korbet, S. (1999). *Lupus nephritis.* Oxford University Press, London.

Ponticelli, C., Banfi, G., and Moroni, L. (1998). Systemic lupus erythematosus (clinical). In *Oxford textbook of clinical nephrology*, (2nd edn), (ed. Davison, A.M. Cameron, J.S., Grünfeld, J.-P., Kerr, D., Ritz, E., and Winearls, C.), pp. 935–59. Oxford University Press.

Venables, P.J.W. (1998). The patient with Sjögren's syndrome and overlap syndromes. In *Oxford textbook of clinical nephrology*, (2nd edn), (ed.

Davison, A.M. Cameron, J.S., Grünfeld, J.-P., Kerr, D., Ritz, E., and Winearls, C.), pp. 987–93. Oxford University Press.

Chapter 12.16

Sickle-cell disease and the kidney

G. R. Serjeant

Homozygous sickle-cell (SS) disease results in anaemia, a hyperdynamic circulation, less deformable red blood cells, and probably widespread endothelial damage and dysfunction. These processes affect structure and function in the kidney, although medullary and glomerular involvement occur at different ages and have different implications for outcome. Other genotypes of sickle-cell disease manifest similar but less frequent and less severe changes. Even the sickle-cell trait is associated with some abnormalities of renal function.

Medullary involvement

Vascular damage

The vasa recta system of the renal medulla, with its low oxygen tension, high pH, and hypertonicity, is uniquely conducive to sickling causing disruption of the blood vessels and secondary damage to the tubules. Microradioangiographic studies have shown almost complete obliteration of the fine-vessel system of the vasa rectae, the remaining vessels being distorted into spirals, dilatations, and appearing to end blindly. These changes have been observed in SS disease in childhood and occur to a lesser extent in the sickle-cell trait in which haemoglobin S levels are only 20–45 per cent of total haemoglobin.

Tubular dysfunction

The functional effect of these changes is an inability to concentrate the urine normally, which becomes worse with age. Proximal tubular functional abnormalities include an increased secretion of urate and increased reabsorption of phosphate and of β_2-microglobulin. Distal tubular functional abnormalities include an inability to excrete an acid load, defective maximal potassium excretion, and occasionally evidence of hyporeninaemic hypoaldosteronism. The clinical significance of these changes is limited to hyposthenuria which results in larger urinary volumes, contributing to nocturia, enuresis, and possibly a tendency to dehydration.

Glomerular involvement

Large hypercellular glomeruli are characteristic of SS disease from the age of 2 years, with an increase in size with age even over the age of 40 years. The total number of glomeruli fall with age and progressive glomerular obsolescence contributes to chronic renal failure, which is common in SS disease over the age of 40 years. The large glomeruli in childhood are associated with supranormal glomerular filtration rates, effective renal blood flows, and effective renal plasma flows. All of these indices fall with age, and in many patients aged 30–40 years they are below normal, with particularly rapid declines occurring in some patients who proceed to chronic renal failure. This functional deterioration is assumed to reflect progressive glomerular loss. The mechanism of glomerular damage is unclear but contributions may come from immune complexes derived from renal tubular epithelial antigen and mechanical damage from nephron hyperfiltration. The latter concept has received support from the observation that angiotensin-converting enzyme inhibitors significantly reduced proteinuria in some affected patients.

Clinical syndromes

Nocturnal enuresis

Enuresis is common in SS disease.

Haematuria

Haematuria occurs in both sickle-cell disease and the sickle-cell trait, and is believed to result from ischaemic lesions of the renal papilla, varying from minute ulcerations to papillary necrosis. Treatment is conservative, although prolonged haematuria may require blood transfusion or, rarely, limited surgery. ε-Aminocaproic acid, which inhibits urokinase, has been effective in some cases, but it promotes clots that may obstruct the ureters and its use requires assessment in controlled trials.

Urinary tract infections

The frequency of urinary tract infections is increased in subjects with the sickle-cell trait during pregnancy, and may be increased in SS disease, although no reliable data are yet available. *Escherichia coli*, *Klebsiella*, and *Enterobacter* spp. are most commonly responsible.

Acute glomerular disease

Poststreptococcal glomerulonephritis occurs in SS disease. It is unclear whether patients are more prone to this complication, but there is evidence that it affects SS subjects at a later age than in the normal population. An association of proteinuria with leg ulceration raised the possibility that leg ulcers acted as a portal of entry for β-haemolytic streptococci, but further analysis has not supported this hypothesis.

Nephrotic syndrome

A variety of histological patterns occur with the nephrotic syndrome in SS disease, but membranoproliferative glomerulonephritis accounts for over half the adult cases. Acute glomerulonephritis frequently manifests a nephrotic picture in SS disease and the prognosis of this form is good. The prognosis of other forms of nephrotic syndrome in SS disease is generally poor, with a 50 per cent mortality within 16 months.

Chronic renal failure

This is an important contributor to illness and death among adults with SS disease, especially those over 40 years of age. It is usually insidious in onset, manifested initially only by a falling haemoglobin level, which is well tolerated until down to 3–4 g/dl. Older patients should be monitored by periodic urea and creatinine levels. Serum creatinine levels tend to be lower than normal in steady-state SS disease and renal impairment may occur with creatinine levels within the accepted normal range. It is likely that levels of 60–70 μmol/l reflect significant renal damage.

Patients may be maintained in tolerable health for years by chronic transfusion or administration of erythropoietin. Endstage renal failure may require chronic haemodialysis or renal transplantation, but there are conflicting data on outcome. Successful transplantation may be followed by striking increases in haemoglobin levels sufficient to precipitate painful crises, and recurrent sickle nephropathy may affect the transplanted kidney.

Further reading

Allon, M. (1990). Renal abnormalities in sickle cell disease. *Archives of Internal Medicine*, 150, 501–4.

Caruana, R.J. (1998). The patient with sickle cell disease. In: *Oxford textbook of clinical nephrology*, (2nd edn) (ed. A.M. Davison, J.S. Cameron, J.-P. Grünfeld, D. Kerr, E. Ritz, and C.G. Winearls), pp. 994–1015. Oxford University Press, Oxford.

Chapter 12.17

Clinical aspects of inherited renal disorders

J. P. Grünfeld

The spectrum of inherited renal disorders (and of inherited diseases with kidney involvement) is summarized in Table 1.

Autosomal dominant polycystic kidney disease

Autosomal dominant polycystic kidney disease is the most frequent inherited kidney disorder, accounts for approximately 8 per cent of cases of endstage renal failure in Western countries, and is one of the most frequent human inherited monogenic diseases (approximately 1 in 1000 individuals). The disease is characterized by the presence of multiple cysts, arising from various segments of the nephrons and involving both kidneys. The mechanisms underlying cyst formation and progression are unknown. The mutant gene responsible for 85 per cent of the cases has been identified in the short arm of chromosome 16 (PKD1 gene). *De novo* mutations are very rare. In 15 per cent of the families, the PKD2 gene located to the long arm of chromosome 4 is mutated. There is most probably a third locus, so far unidentified.

Table 1 Main groups of inherited kidney diseases

Cystic kidney diseases
Autosomal dominant polycystic kidney disease
Autosomal recessive polycystic kidney disease
Juvenile nephronophthisis–medullary cystic disease complex
Associated with multiple malformation syndrome: such as phacomatoses (autosomal dominant): tuberous sclerosis, von Hippel–Lindau's disease; or other rare syndromes
Alport's syndrome and variants
Inherited metabolic diseases with renal involvement
with glomerular involvement (such as diabetes mellitus, genetic amyloidosis, Fabry's disease) with non-glomerular involvement (such as cystinosis, primary hyperoxaluria)
Other inherited diseases
with glomerular involvement (such as congenital nephrotic syndrome, nail–patella syndrome) with non-glomerular involvement (such as nephronophthisis)
Primary immune glomerulonephritis, occasionally familial (such as IgA nephropathy)
Inherited tubular disorders
Various renal diseases with 'genetic influence' (such as reflux nephropathy, haemolytic uraemic syndrome)

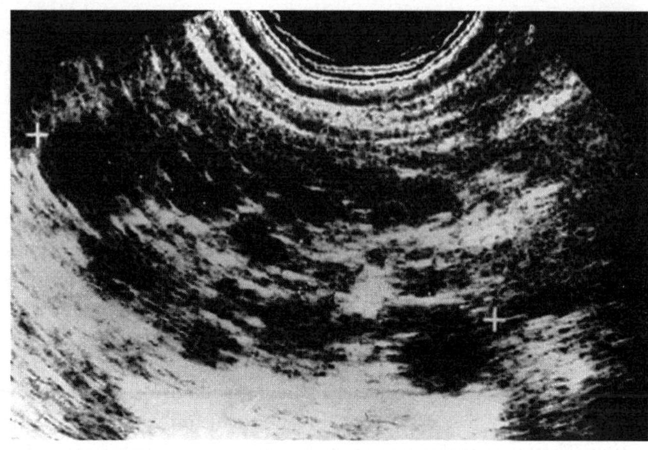

Fig. 1 Typical ultrasonographic findings in a patient with autosomal dominant polycystic kidney disease. The kidney is enlarged and contains multiple cysts of different sizes; the contralateral kidney had similar changes. The concentration of serum creatinine was 120 mmol/litre at the time of ultrasonography.
(By courtesy of Dr O. Helenon.)

The sensitivity of ultrasonography for detecting the disease is poor before 20 years of age (but the specificity is high as solitary renal cysts, *a fortiori* bilateral, are very rare at this age) (Fig. 1). In PKD1 families, false negative ultrasonographic diagnosis is very unlikely at ages above 30 years, and rare at ages 20–29 years. Thus, routine screening in asymptomatic members of affected families should not be performed before 20 years of age. In contrast, renal cysts, even bilateral, are relatively common in patients aged 50 years or more; therefore, strict criteria (multiple cysts in both enlarged kidneys and clear-cut inheritance) are required for diagnosis at this age.

Symptoms

Renal manifestations

In some patients, the disease is asymptomatic and discovered during family investigation or by chance on abdominal ultrasonography. In most cases, however, patients complain of one or more of the following symptoms at some time: renal pain due to cyst enlargement, or stone or blood clot migration; bleeding within a cyst, leading to flank pain, gross haematuria which occurs in approximately 30 per cent of the patients; fever due to upper urinary tract infection, which is more frequent in female patients or, more specifically, to cyst fluid infection. Renal stones develop in about 20 per cent of the patients; surprisingly, uric acid stones predominate.

Hypertension is a common and early finding. About 30–50 per cent of patients are hypertensive at a stage when renal function is normal. Subsequently, with the development of renal failure, up to 80 per cent become hypertensive.

Renal failure progresses to endstage between 40 and 60 years of age in most cases but, in 30 per cent of patients is reached later and in 5 per cent earlier. The disease may have a more indolent course in a substantial number of cases: 25 to 50 per cent of the affected subjects are not in endstage renal failure by 70 years of age, and some patients may reach 80 or 90 years without the need for renal replacement therapy. This information is crucial for genetic counselling.

Genetic and non-genetic factors determine renal prognosis: the renal disease progresses more slowly in PKD2 families, it progresses more slowly in women than in men, and control of hypertension may reduce the rate of progression.

Extrarenal manifestations

Liver cysts develop in 70 per cent of the patients, usually later in life than renal cysts. Liver cysts are more frequent and more diffuse in women. They are usually asymptomatic, detected by ultrasonography, but may be palpable. Cyst infection may occur particularly in dialysis or transplant patients. Massive liver involvement may cause severe discomfort in some patients, mostly females: liver function tests are usually normal.

Cardiovascular abnormalities include intracranial aneurysms and mitral valve prolapse. Subarachnoid haemorrhage or intracerebral bleeding due to rupture of intracranial aneurysm occur in approximately 1–2 per cent of the patients. Diagnosis should be suspected early in patients with recent and severe headache or with any transient focal neurological deficit. In cross-sectional studies by computed tomography (CT) or magnetic resonance angiography, intracranial aneurysms have been found in 5–8 per cent of asymptomatic middle-aged patients. The prevalence is higher in those with a family history of intracranial aneurysm. Routine screening even by non-invasive methods is not currently indicated in all patients. It seems reasonable only in certain subgroups—especially those with a family history of intracranial aneurysm or subarachnoid haemorrhage, those who have already bled from an aneurysm, and possibly, those who are to undergo major elective surgery. In high-risk groups, screening should be repeated every 5–10 years, as the cerebral vascular disease is progressive. Mitral valve prolapse is discovered in 20 per cent of patients by echocardiography, whereas it is found in only 2–3 per cent of the general population. Other cardiac valve abnormalities may also be detected. Other extrarenal defects are described. Abdominal herniae are more prevalent than in the general population. Aneurysm or dissections of large arteries may be more frequent in these patients.

Treatment

Meticulous control of hypertension is vital. Haematuria is common and should be managed conservatively, although bleeding may sometimes be prolonged over several days and even weeks. The relief of pain can be difficult. Surgical renal cyst decompression should be restricted to very selected cases. Surgery is rarely needed in the management of renal stone. Liver cyst aspirations by needle under CT guidance, fenestration, marsupialization, or resection may be needed when massive involvement gives rise to pain; and in very rare cases such patients have come to liver transplantation. Kidney infection requires prompt administration of antimicrobials. In some cases, control is not obtained, probably because agents penetrate some infected cyst fluids poorly and do not achieve adequate concentration. Lipophilic drugs, such as trimethoprim–sulphamethoxazole and ciprofloxacin, have been shown to penetrate the cyst fluid more adequately. Liver cyst infection also requires antimicrobials and drainage if infection is not controlled. Ciprofloxacin penetrates well into liver cyst fluid. The management of chronic renal failure is addressed in Chapter 12.29. The results of renal replacement therapy are similar to those obtained in other renal diseases.

Genetic counselling

The offspring of an affected subject have a 50 per cent risk of having the disease but it has a highly variable clinical course, even within a given family. Prenatal diagnosis by gene linkage studies of chorionic villi has been performed and can be considered if adequate family information is available. The demand for it has so far been very low in the light of the late onset and the variable clinical course of the disease.

Autosomal recessive polycystic kidney disease

Autosomal recessive polycystic kidney disease is a rare disorder (approximately 1:40 000), the first manifestations of which appear early in childhood. Three features characterize this disease:

1. Its recessive nature: both heterozygous parents are unaffected, with normal renal ultrasonography; parental consanguinity is found in some families; the mutant gene has been located on chromosome 6.
2. Renal cysts derive from the collecting ducts, accounting for the striations in the dilated collecting system seen on intravenous pyelography.
3. The renal disease is invariably associated with congenital hepatic fibrosis, which may be responsible for portal hypertension due to pre-sinusoidal block, or for bacterial angiocholitis due to intrahepatic bile-duct dilatation.

Diagnosis may be revealed before birth by antenatal ultrasonography. With prolonged survival, liver and renal involvement becomes prominent. Gastrointestinal bleeding due to portal hypertension may be life-threatening. Systemic hypertension is a frequent finding in the first year of life but may regress in subsequent years. Urinary tract infection is common. The rate of progression of renal failure is variable. Endstage may be reached in childhood, but slower progression to adulthood has been reported.

Alport's syndrome

This syndrome is characterized by the association of progressive haematuric hereditary nephritis and bilateral sensorineural hearing loss. Its prevalence is approximately 1 in 5000 individuals. In 85 per cent of the kindreds, the mode of transmission is compatible with X-linked dominant inheritance. In the remaining families, autosomal dominant or recessive inheritance should be considered.

Symptoms

The first manifestation is typically gross haematuria, occurring sometimes in the first year of life, recurring during childhood, and followed by permanent microscopic haematuria. Proteinuria appears later. A nephrotic syndrome, usually moderate, develops in 30–40 per cent of patients. In other cases, moderate proteinuria and microscopic haematuria are the presenting symptoms in adult patients. The disease is progressive, leading to renal failure in all affected males. The rate of progression in males is heterogeneous from one family to another, but usually homogeneous within a given family. In some families, endstage is reached at or before 30 years of age, sometimes in childhood; in the others, renal failure progresses to endstage between the ages of 30 and 60 years. As expected in an X-linked disorder, carrier females often have slight or intermittent urinary abnormalities and do not develop renal failure or develop mild renal impairment late in life but some progress to endstage as in males.

The hearing defect may be severe, but is often moderate or slight, only detected at audiometric testing. In some kindreds, familial progressive nephritis occurs, without any hearing defect.

Eye abnormalities are detected in 30–40 per and include bilateral anterior lenticonus, corneal erosions, and perimacular or macular retinal flecks which do not alter visual acuity. In some families, macrothrombocytopenia is associated with nephritis and hearing defect. In other rare kindreds the latter features are found in association with diffuse, mainly oesophageal, leiomyomatosis, and congenital cataracts.

Pathogenesis

The glomerular basement membrane is abnormally thickened with splitting of the lamina densa, thinned with focal thickening, or diffusely thin in younger children. In some patients, antigenicity of the glomerular basement membrane is abnormal in that antiglomerular basement membrane antibodies do not bind linearly along the membrane. In X-linked Alport's syndrome, the molecular defect involves the gene encoding for the α5-chain of type IV collagen which is a major component of basement membranes. Six α-chains of type IV collagen have been identified so far, differently associated in the various basement membranes (see Chapter 12.8). In Alport's syndrome, mutations have been identified in the gene encoding for the α5-chain, which has been mapped to the long arm of the X-chromosome. The Goodpasture antigen is located in the α3-chain (the gene of which has been mapped on chromosome 2). Absence or severe alteration of the α5-chain possibly prevents normal integration of the α3-chain into the glomerular basement membrane leading to the defect in antigenicity. In Alport's syndrome with leiomyomatosis, the genes encoding for α5- and α6 chains are deleted. In the autosomal recessive form, the genes encoding for α3- and/or α4-chains are defective. The cases with extrarenal abnormalities are usually not linked to the gene on chromosome 2.

Genetic counselling and treatment

This requires correct identification of the mode of inheritance. If there is X-linked dominant inheritance, affected men will not transmit the disease to their sons, whereas all their daughters will carry the mutant gene; affected women will transmit the mutant gene to 50 per cent of either sons or daughters. DNA analysis may be helpful for genetic counselling in these families.

Treatment of hypertension and supportive management of renal failure are indicated in patients with progressive disease. The results of kidney transplantation are similar to those obtained in other renal diseases. In rare cases, however, antiglomerular basement membrane crescentic glomerulonephritis develops on the graft. It is assumed that this complication is related to alloimmunization to the 'missing antigen' introduced by the transplant.

Nephronophthisis–medullary cystic disease complex

This complex represents an inherited form of chronic tubulointerstitial disorder with cysts located at the corticomedullary junction or in the medullary region, associated with tubular atrophy and interstitial fibrosis (which are non-specific lesions), and extreme thickening and multilamellation of the tubular basement membrane.

The juvenile form is a major cause of endstage renal disease in children. It is transmitted as an autosomal recessive trait; the gene has been identified and mapped to the short arm of chromosome 2. Heterozygotes are asymptomatic.

The clinical manifestations first appear at about the age of 4 years and consist of polyuria, secondary enuresis, and polydipsia, reflecting urinary concentration defect. Subsequently, renal failure, metabolic acidosis, anaemia, and growth retardation develop, and endstage renal failure is reached approximately at the age of 10–13 years. More or less severe renal salt wasting is common. The first reported cases were initially misdiagnosed as Addison's disease because of the renal salt-losing state and skin pigmentation due to renal failure. In approximately 10–15 per cent of cases, renal involvement is associated with retinal changes: tapetoretinal degeneration with or without retinitis pigmentosa, leading to blindness early or later in life (the Senior–Loken syndrome). Other extrarenal features (skeletal changes, cerebellar ataxia, and liver fibrosis) are more rarely found.

The adult form is rare and is restricted to the kidney involvement. Its mode of inheritance is usually autosomal dominant. Endstage renal failure is reached at approximately 30 years of age.

Further reading

Davison, A.M., Cameron, J.S., Grünfeld, J.P., Kerr, D.N.S., Ritz, E., and Winearls, C.G. (ed.). (1998). *Oxford textbook of clinical nephrology*, (2nd edn), Section 16.The patient with inherited disease, pp. 2375–500. Oxford University Press, Oxford.

Morgan, S.H. and Grünfeld, J.P. (ed.) (1998). *Inherited Disorders of the Kidney*, p. 632. Oxford University Press, Oxford.

Interstitial nephritides

Chapter 12.18

Urinary tract infection

*R. R. Bailey**

Introduction

Urinary tract infections are responsible for considerable morbidity, particularly in sexually active women. Except in the first year of life and after the age of 60 years, they predominantly affect females and range from asymptomatic bacteriuria to severe sepsis, often with hospital-acquired organisms, and affecting high-risk patients such as diabetics or those on immunosuppressive therapy.

Pathogenesis

The entry of bacteria into the female bladder is facilitated by the short urethra, and urinary tract infections frequently follow sexual

*It is with regret that we report the death of Dr R.R. Bailey before the preparation of this volume. His chapter in OTM3 was abbreviated by Professor J.G.G. Ledingham.

intercourse. Although the ascending route is much the commonest portal of entry, there may on occasion be haematogenous spread. The frequency of recurrence of infection is increased in women with small increases (1–10 ml) in residual urine volume which allows an inoculum of bacteria to multiply.

When diaphragms are used for contraception, the vagina is often invaded by enterobacterial organisms. This may explain an increased prevalence of *Escherichia coli* urinary tract infections in users of diaphragms. A diaphragm may also alter the angle of the bladder neck and therefore affect bladder emptying. The additional use of a spermicide may also contribute, as available preparations encourage the growth of enterobacterial organisms.

Infection due to two or more bacterial species, or to more than one serotype of *E. coli* is uncommon. A genuine mixed infection is most common in patients with multiple urinary calculi.

E. coli is the predominant urinary tract pathogen, but one-quarter of symptomatic urinary tract infections in women treated in general practice are due to *Staphylococcus saprophyticus.* The surface agglutinin of this pathogen appears to be a key determinant of virulence, permitting it to colonize the urinary tract. The third commonest pathogen in domiciliary practice is *Proteus mirabilis.* This organism invariably invades the kidney, probably because of its high motility or ability to adhere to urothelium. *Proteus* species also have the ability to split urinary urea into ammonia, which by trapping hydrogen ions leads to an alkaline urine and the risk of stone formation. Other urinary tract pathogens, and those that are more frequently seen in hospitalized patients, include *Proteus* species other than *mirabilis, Streptococcus faecalis, Klebsiella pneumoniae, Enterobacter* sp., *Acinetobacter* sp., *Pseudomonas aeruginosa,* and *Serratia marcescens.*

The bacteria responsible for urinary tract infections are invariably derived from faecal flora. In the great majority of recurrent infections the infecting organism is a different strain with each episode.

E. coli strains causing acute pyelonephritis belong to a limited number of O:K:H serotypes. They carry fimbrial adhesins, are resistant to killing by serum, and produce haemolysin. Bacterial adhesion to mucosal epithelial cells may increase persistence by reducing elimination by micturition. Infection of the upper urinary tract by these strains of *E. coli* is facilitated by attachment to receptors of the epithelial cells of the ureter and renal pelvis. Adherence may also relate to the presence of certain glycolipids in urothelial cells, which are associated with differences in P and ABO blood groups. The adhesion of pyelonephritogenic strains of *E. coli* is often mediated by P fimbriae with specificity for these glycolipids, which correspond to antigens of the P blood group system.

The aetiology of the *urethral syndrome* remains unclear. Bacterial infections with low counts of pathogens certainly occur in some women and genital (*Chlamydia trachomatis, Neisseria gonorrhoeae, Herpes simplex*) or vaginal infections (*Candida albicans, Trichomonas vaginalis*) may be contributory in others. Urethral or vulval irritation from deodorants, bubble baths, or detergents also cause dysuria as may atrophic vaginitis, resulting from oestrogen deficiency.

Clinical presentations

Symptomatic urinary tract infections

Symptoms of lower urinary tract infection include frequency, dysuria, urgency, strangury, initial or terminal haematuria, and suprapubic discomfort. Up to one-third of women suffering from frequency and dysuria, however, do not have bacteriuria (the urethral syndrome).

Acute pyelonephritis is a more serious illness. High fever (38–40°C), rigors, and loin pain are cardinal features, commonly associated with vomiting and prostration. There is usually tenderness in one or both loins. Lower urinary tract symptoms are often absent. When both kidneys are severely affected, oedema of the epithelium or the renal pelvis can result in oliguric acute renal failure. The complication of papillary necrosis is discussed below. Conditions that may simulate acute pyelonephritis include urinary tract obstruction, urinary colic, acute glomerulonephritis, renal infarction, renal vein thrombosis, and haemorrhage into a renal tumour or cyst, while the differential diagnosis should also include acute appendicitis, cholecystitis or pancreatitis, pelvic inflammatory disease, and a basal pneumonia.

Acute bacterial prostatitis presents with 'flu-like' symptoms, low backache, often few urinary tract symptoms, and a swollen, tender prostate.

More unusual presentations include pyonephrosis, or a variant of this, xanthogranulomatous pyelonephritis, which predominantly affects elderly women, and is commonly associated with calculous obstruction and infection with an organism such as *Proteus mirabilis.* In addition to loin pain and fever, these patients may have weight loss, constitutional symptoms, and a palpable renal mass. A renal carbuncle or cortical abscess is probably the result of a haematogenous infection with *Staphylococcus aureus.* The presentation is similar to that of acute pyelonephritis, or of an infected renal cyst or a perinephric abscess.

Asymptomatic (covert) urinary tract infection

Many different populations have been screened for asymptomatic bacteriuria, but with the exception of pregnancy, there is no convincing evidence to suggest that routine screening or treatment is valuable. The prevalence of this condition is between 1 and 2 per cent in schoolgirls and 3–5 per cent in adult women. It is much rarer in the male (0.05 per cent of schoolboys and 0.5 per cent of male adults). In most studies, 5–6 per cent of pregnant women have been found to have bacteriuria. If left untreated 20 per cent of these will go on to develop acute pyelonephritis, preventable in half by treatment in the asymptomatic stage. A single dose of antimicrobial suffices. Bacteriuria is recurrent in some 30 per cent, indicating the need for surveillance throughout pregnancy. Persistent recurrence can be treated safely by prophylactic trimethoprime 200 mg or nitrofurantoin 100 mg at bedtime. About 20 per cent of women with asymptomatic bacteriuria in pregnancy have a radiological abnormality of the urinary tract, particularly likely in those with recurrence. Suggestions that untreated bacteriuria is associated with an increase in premature delivery and low birth weight are now disputed. Even so, an attack of acute pyelonephritis can precipitate premature labour, can cause septicaemic shock, renal dysfunction, and perinatal death.

Diagnosis

The diagnosis of a urinary tract infection can only be proven by culturing the urine. This is the ideal, and must be done in all cases affecting infants, children, and males. It may be more cost-effective to treat women with an isolated episode with a single dose or a 3-day course, and only culture the urine if the symptoms do not resolve or recur shortly after completing treatment.

Midstream specimen

The clean-catch midstream (MSU) technique suffers from the disadvantage that some contamination of the specimen is inevitable in the female, making it necessary to quantitate the bacterial content. A single specimen with a colony count of more than 100 000/ml (>100 × 10^6/l) represents only an 80 per cent confidence level in diagnosing a urinary tract infection in a female who is asymptomatic or has only mild lower urinary tract symptoms. Multiple cultures of MSU specimens are necessary in those without symptoms. On the other hand, a count of more than 100 000 colonies/ml (>100 × 10^6/l) in an MSU from a patient with acute pyelonephritis has a confidence limit exceeding 95 per cent.

In women with marked frequency of micturition, or those infected with *Staphylococcus saprophyticus*, the bacterial count may be low. A count of greater than 1000/ml (>10^6/l) of a potential pathogen in a symptomatic female is one suggested criterion for proven infection, but many would prefer 10 000/ml (> 10 × 10^6/l). In males, a count of greater than 1000/ml (>10^6/l) may be taken to indicate true infection with a high degree of confidence.

Special problems exist in the collection of samples from the elderly, bedridden or paraplegic patients, from women who are menstruating or who have a vaginal discharge, and from patients in the postsurgical or postpartum period. For women in the puerperium, even with extremely careful urine collection, 30 per cent of MSU cultures have been demonstrated to give false positive results.

Some dipstick reagent strips now include the nitrite test and/or a test to detect leucocytes. If a patient has acute symptoms, a positive nitrite test, and pyuria it is likely that the urine is infected.

Uncentrifuged fresh urine from patients with symptomatic urinary tract infections invariably contains more than 10 leucocytes/mm^3 (>10 × 10^6/l) but of women with asymptomatic bacteriuria, only about one-half will have pyuria,

Suprapubic aspirate

Suprapubic aspiration of the distended bladder has made the diagnosis of urinary tract infection more accurate. It eliminates need for quantitative counts, as any bacteria so obtained can be regarded as significant.

Catheter specimen

In elderly women it is often difficult to obtain an uncontaminated MSU and they may not be able to hold an adequate volume of urine in their bladder for suprapubic aspiration. In such cases it may be necessary to obtain a catheter specimen.

Prostatic specimens

When prostatic infection is suspected it may be valuable to culture specimens derived from the urethra, the bladder, and the prostate separately. After cleaning the glans penis, the first few millilitres of urine are not discarded, but are collected for culture of organisms in the urethra. The midstream specimen is then deemed to reflect bladder urine. The prostate is then massaged and any secretion yielded collected with 5–10 ml or urine passed immediately after massage. Culture of the three specimens then gives some clue about localization of the infection.

Treatment

Bacterial cystitis

A single oral dose of an antimicrobial agent is as effective as a conventional short course for the treatment of uncomplicated cystitis.

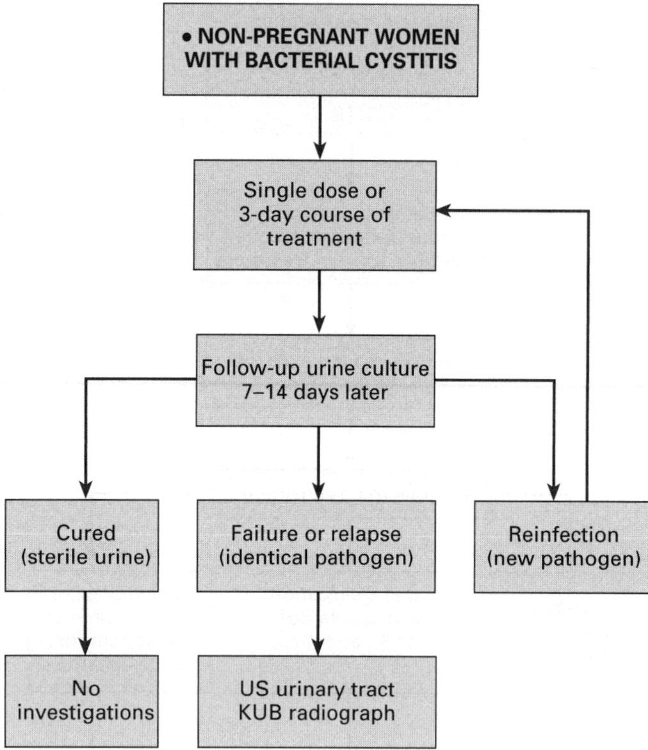

Fig. 1 A suggested algorithm for the management of non-pregnant women with bacterial cystitis (US, ultrasonography; KUB, plain abdominal radiograph, including kidney, ureter, and bladder areas).

Algorithms of management are shown in Figs 1 and 2 and the drugs best prescribed in Table 1.

An alternative is a short course of treatment (Table 2). Up to 30 per cent of *E. coli* isolated in the community and 50 per cent in hospitals are now resistant to amoxycillin, but it remains the drug of choice for treating *Streptococcus faecalis.*

Urethral syndrome

Management is unsatisfactory, but symptoms usually settle over a few days and may be improved by a high fluid intake. Alkalinization of the urine is rarely of much benefit. Antibacterial therapy appears to influence recovery in some women, but there have been no controlled studies.

Acute pyelonephritis

Patients with uncomplicated acute pyelonephritis should receive a 5-day course of treatment, preferably with at least one dose of a parenterally administered drug if vomiting is a problem (Table 3). Many need to be in hospital for rehydration, analgesia, and administration of parenteral antibiotics. Blood cultures should be taken before antimicrobial treatment is started. In particularly ill patients the choice now lies between an aminoglycosides, a 4-quinolone, or a β-lactam antibiotic.

Special problems

Chronic bacterial prostatitis

Until recently there were few antimicrobial agents that could effectively cross non-inflamed prostatic epithelium from plasma into prostatic fluid, but long-term (for example, 4–12 weeks) low-dose therapy (with, for example, nitrofurantoin, trimethoprim, norfloxacin) could

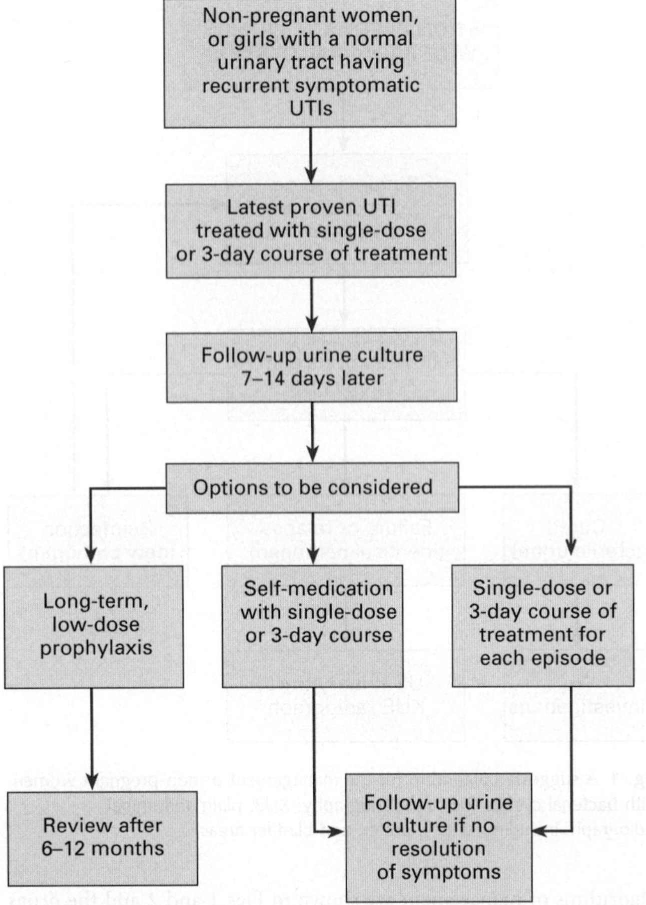

Fig. 2 A suggested algorithm for the management of either non-pregnant women or girls with a normal urinary tract who are having recurrent symptomatic urinary tract infections.

Table 1 Suggested drugs for single-dose oral treatment of bacterial cystitis or asymptomatic bacteriuria

Trimethoprim, 600 mg	Ciprofloxacin, 500 mg
Co-trimoxazole, 1.92 g	Fleroxacin, 400 mg
Norfloxacin, 800 mg	Fosfomycin trometamol, 3 g

prevent prostatic bacteria from initiating bacteriuria or even bacteraemia. However, the new quinolones penetrate prostatic tissue and are becoming established as the drugs of choice for bacterial prostatitis both acute and chronic.

Asymptomatic (covert) bacteriuria in pregnancy

Either a single 1.92 g dose of co-trimoxazole or a single 600 mg dose of trimethoprim is highly effective in treating women with covert bacteriuria between 16 and 30 weeks' gestation. If bacteriuria returns, this should be repeated and followed by prophylaxis in the form of 50 mg of nitrofurantoin each night until the puerperium (Fig. 3).

Elderly women

About one-fifth of apparently healthy elderly women have bacteriuria. In the presence of a debilitating illness and in those cared for in institutions the rate rises to between 25 and 50 per cent. Bacteriuria without symptoms is best left untreated because of the risk of inducing resistance. Symptoms may be atypical in the elderly, however, and bacteriuria in those who have become acutely confused, confined to bed, or in other ways have deteriorated should be treated. Atrophic vaginitis should be treated in elderly women with recurrent symptomatic urinary tract infections by oral or topical oestrogens.

Table 2 Drug regimens for an oral 3-day course of treatment for bacterial cystitis

Drug	Dose	Comment
Trimethoprim	300 mg q24 h	A useful agent.
Co-trimoxazole	960 mg q12 h	Should be replaced by trimethoprim alone
Nitrofurantoin	50 mg q8 h	Not effective against *Proteus* sp.
Nalidixic acid	500 mg q8 h	Not effective against *Staphylococcus saprophyticus*; superseded
Norfloxacin	400 mg q12 h	
Ciprofloxacin	250 mg q12 h	
Lomefloxacin	400 mg q24 h	
Fleroxacin	400 mg q24 h	
Cephalexin	250 mg q8 h	Useful if renal insufficiency present
Cephradine	250 mg q8 h	
Cefaclor	250 mg q8 h	
Sulphamethizole	1 g q8 h	Unfashionable
Pivmecillinam	200 mg q8 h	
Amoxycillin	250 mg q8 h	High incidence of resistance;useful for *Streptococcus faecalis*
Augmentin®	500 mg amoxycillin/ 125 mg clavulanic acid q12 h	Proving disappointing

Urinary catheters

All patients with long-term indwelling urinary catheters will have bacteriuria. The responsible pathogen(s) will be resident in the biofilm lining the catheter which is impermeable to antimicrobial agents. Catheters that are blocking up should be replaced, but the regular changing is no longer good practice provided that the patient is asymptomatic and urine is draining freely. A high fluid intake and consequent high urine flow is important. In patients managed outside hospital, clean intermittent urethral catheterization constitutes a minimal risk. Such intermittent catheterization has revolutionized the care of patients with neurogenic bladders.

Acute papillary necrosis complicating acute pyelonephritis

Some patients, usually elderly, with severe acute pyelonephritis may develop acute papillary necrosis with complicating acute renal failure. This may occur particularly in diabetics, alcoholics, and those consuming non-steroidal anti-inflammatory drugs which should always be discontinued in the presence of acute pyelonephritis.

Prophylactic or preventive treatment

Many women have troublesome recurrent or closely spaced symptomatic urinary tract infections. They may benefit from advice always

Table 3 Drug regimens for a parenteral 5-day course of treatment

Drug	Dose	
Gentamicin	Loading dose 3 mg/kg body weight; maintenance dose 1 mg/kg q8 h*	
Tobramycin	As for gentamicin*	
Netilmicin	Loading dose 2 mg/kg body weight; maintenance dose 2 mg/kg q12 h*	
Amikacin	Loading dose 15 mg/kg body weight; maintenance dose 7.5 mg/kg q12 h*	
Ciprofloxacin Lomefloxacin	100 mg q12 h 400 mg q24 h	Can be switched to oral formulation
Cefazolin	1 g q8 h	
Cephradine	1 g q8 h	
Ceftriaxone	2 g q24 h	
Aztreonam	1 g q12 h	
Ipipenem/cilastin	500 mg/500 mg q8 h	
Amoxycillin	1 g q8 h	
Clavulanic acid/amoxycillin	200 mg/l g q8 h	

*Computer-derived individualized maintenance doses can be determined—drug concentrations should be monitored; single large daily doses are now being recommended rather than divided doses.

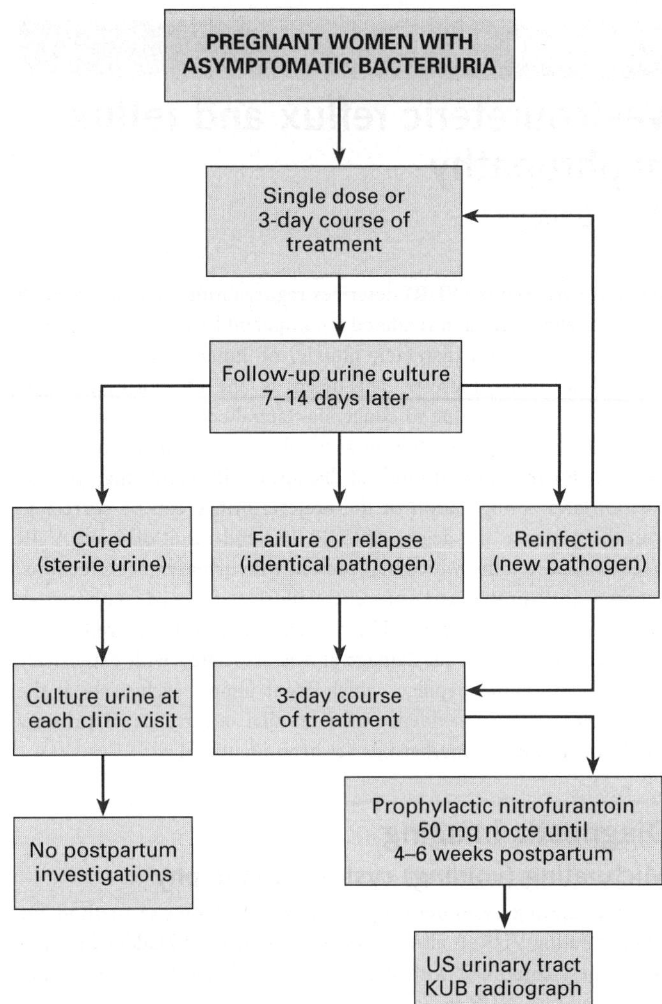

Fig. 3 A suggested algorithm for the management of pregnant women with asymptomatic bacteriuria (US, ultrasonography; KUB, radiograph—kidney, ureter and bladder areas).

to empty the bladder completely, to avoid tight clothes round the perineum and to maintain a high fluid intake, especially at night. Others are helped by applying an antiseptic cream (for example 0.5 per cent cetrimide w/w) to the periurethral area before intercourse. If these simple techniques fail, the pattern of recurrences can be interrupted by instituting prophylactic therapy after the urine has been sterilized. Nitrofurantoin (50 mg taken last thing at night after the patient has emptied her bladder) is highly effective, as are trimethoprim (100 mg), co-trimoxazole (0.24 g), and norfloxacin (200 mg). It is just as effective to give a dose on alternate nights, 3 nights a week, or in some women simply after intercourse.

Suppressive treatment

Some patients have urological abnormalities which make it impossible to sterilize the urinary tract. In some such patients, recurrent episodes of bacteraemia may occur, best managed by long-term suppressive treatment with an antimicrobial appropriate to the organism. If, however, there have been no such episodes and local symptoms are not a serious problem, suppressive treatment is best avoided because of the risk of events caused by a more resistant organism.

Investigation

Any urinary tract infection raises the question as to whether it is a marker of underlying urinary tract abnormality. Every male must have his urinary tract investigated following the first infection, but it is not cost-effective to undertake invasive investigations on sexually active women with occasional bacterial cystitis. When there is no evidence of urinary tract problems as a child, and occasional urinary tract infections respond rapidly to a single dose of an oral antimicrobial agent, and when follow-up urine specimens show no microscopic haematuria and are sterile on culture, it is unnecessary to investigate further. In contrast, after an attack of acute pyelonephritis, or if there are unusual findings, such as persistent microscopic haematuria, pyuria, or recurrence of the same organism, imaging of the urinary tract should always be undertaken.

Further reading

Johnson, C. (1991). Definitions, classification and clinical presentation of urinary tract infections. *Medical Clinics of North America*, 75, 241–52.

Chapter 12.19

Vesicoureteric reflux and reflux nephropathy

*R. R. Bailey**

Vesicoureteric reflux (VUR) describes regurgitation of urine through a vesicoureteric junction rendered incompetent by a congenital defect of either the length, diameter, muscle, or innervation of the submucosal segment of ureter. The defect is one of shortness of the submucosal segment due to congenital lateral ectopia of the ureteric orifice. As a child grows, the intravesical ureter lengthens; hence the tendency for reflux to diminish or disappear with increasing age. The position and configuration of the ureteric orifice can be correlated with the presence and degree of VUR. The end-result of severe VUR is reflux nephropathy, which may present with urinary tract infections, hypertension, proteinuria, or renal failure with small, contracted, irregularly scarred kidneys. The presence of intrarenal reflux determines the site of renal damage and is associated with extensively fused or compound papillae, which occur almost exclusively at the renal poles. There is evidence of a familial occurrence of primary VUR but no genetic marker has yet been identified.

Diagnostic imaging

Micturating (voiding) cystourethrography

The micturating cystourethrogram is the most precise method for demonstrating VUR. It also allows an assessment of bladder function and is best combined with measurements of bladder pressure and urine flow rate. VUR is classified according to the extent of ureteric filling and the degree of dilatation of the collecting system, in particular, the minor calyces. The most widely favoured classification at present is illustrated in Fig. 1.

Grade I. Ureter only.

Grade II. Ureter, pelvis, and calyces with no dilatation and normal calyceal fornices.

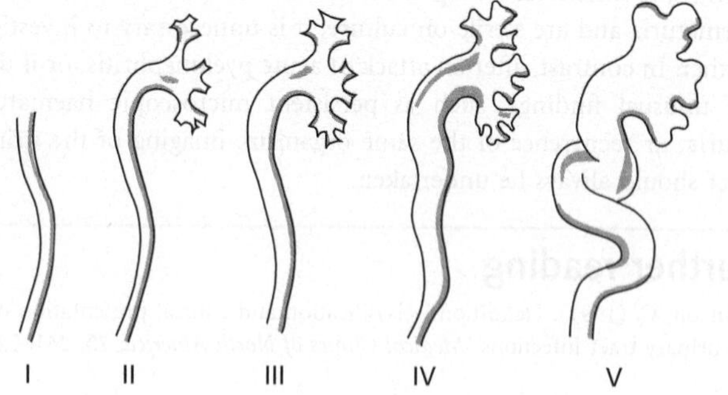

Fig. 1 Classification of grades of vesicoureteric reflux used by the International Reflux Study Committee
(reproduced from International Reflux Study Committee Report (1981) with permission).

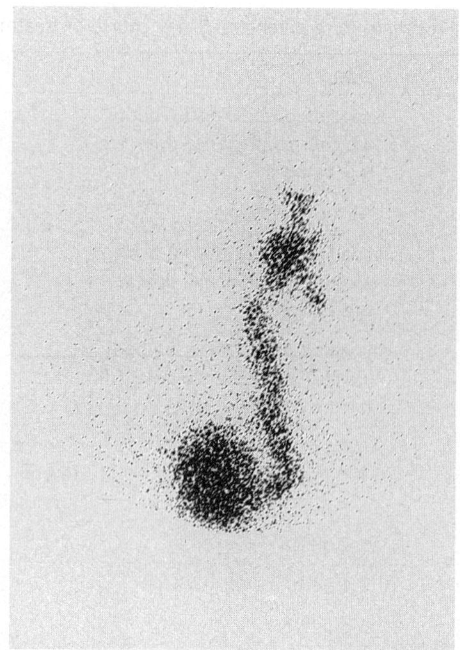

Fig. 2 Radionuclide micturating cystogram, showing vesicoureteric reflux into the left kidney. (reproduced from Bailey (1993) with permission).

Grade III. Mild or moderate dilatation and/or tortuosity of the ureter, and mild or moderate dilatation of the pelvis. No, or only slight, blunting of the fornices.

Grade IV. Moderate dilatation and/or tortuosity of the ureter, and moderate dilatation of the pelvis and calyces. Complete obliteration of the sharp angles of the fornices but maintenance of papillary impressions in the majority of calyces.

Grade V. Gross dilatation and tortuosity of the ureter, pelvis, and calyces. The papillary impressions are no longer visible in the majority of calyces.

Radionuclide micturating cystography

Radionuclide micturating cystography is ideal for the follow-up of those whose reflux has been treated surgically or managed conservatively (Fig. 2).

Dynamic ultrasonography

The findings are essentially limited to the anatomical abnormalities of dilatation of the pelvicalyceal system and ureter, and dynamic information on ureteric function. Examination of the distal ureter may reveal a widely patent ureteric orifice, while the dynamic aspects of real-time ultrasonography allow an assessment of ureteric peristalsis. A limitation is the inability to differentiate between urine passing up or down the ureter. Colour Doppler ultrasonography can localize the ureteric orifices and assess their displacement from the midline.

Intravenous urography

Intravenous urography with tomography allows renal length and cortical thickness to be measured. Papillary morphology is assessed by calyceal appearance. Full thickness scars with calyceal clubbing and retraction of the overlying cortex is seen most frequently in polar regions and is pathognomonic of reflux nephropathy (Fig. 3).

*It is with regret that we report the death of Dr R.R. Bailey before the preparation of this volume. His chapter in OTM3 was abbreviated by Professor J.G.G. Ledingham.

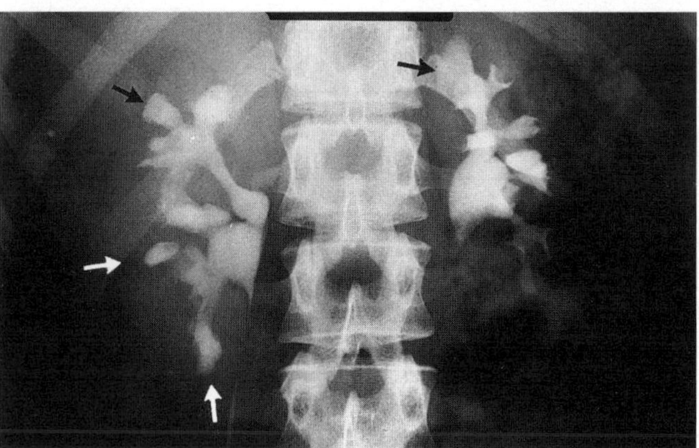

Fig. 3 Intravenous urogram in a 35-year-old woman, showing bilateral reflux nephropathy, more marked on the right side. Several focal scars (arrowed) involving the full thickness of the renal parenchyma and associated with calyceal clubbing are most obvious in the polar regions *(reproduced from Bailey (1993) with permission).*

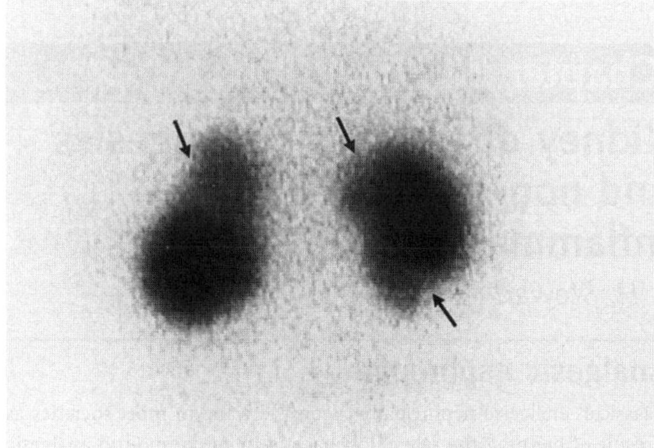

Fig. 4 Dimercaptosuccinic acid scan showing focal scars (arrowed) in both kidneys.

Occasionally, damage is more diffuse with a general reduction in cortical mass and uniform papillary change.

Radionuclide scanning

$^{99}Tc^{m}$ dimercaptosuccinic acid scans and intravenous urography are complementary investigations to detect renal scars (Fig. 4).

Natural history of vesicoureteric reflux

The severity of reflux is the most important factor determining whether renal parenchymal damage will occur. The critical period is during infancy and early childhood. Nephropathy may occur in the absence of infection.

Clinical presentations

The most frequent presentation, particularly in infants and children, is a urinary tract infection: other presentations are included in Table 1.

Urinary tract infections

Depending on age 15–60 per cent of children with urinary tract infection will be found to have some degree of reflux, and 8–13 per cent of the total will have evidence of reflux nephropathy. About 5 per cent of sexually active women with symptomatic urinary tract

Table 1 Clinical presentations

Vesicoureteric reflux
Fetal ultrasonography
Urinary tract infections
Family studies
Nocturnal enuresis or other urological complications
Associated with other congenital abnormalities
Loin pain
Reflux nephropathy
Fetal ultrasonography
Urinary-tract infections
Hypertension—benign or accelerated
During pregnancy—syndrome mimicking pre-eclampsia
Proteinuria
Renal failure
Urinary calculi
Family studies
Nocturnal enuresis or other urological complications
Associated with other congenital abnormalities

infections will have reflux nephropathy. These patients may present with either bacterial cystitis or acute pyelonephritis. The disorder may also come to attention because of the detection of asymptomatic bacteriuria in situations such as pregnancy. With increasing age, other presentations of VUR or reflux nephropathy become relatively more common

Nocturnal enuresis or other complications

Children with VUR have a high incidence of nocturnal enuresis or evidence of lower urinary tract dysfunction, such as detrusor instability or detrusor-sphincter dyssynergia. Hypospadias, undescended testicles, bifid pelvicalyceal collecting systems, ureteric duplication, pelviureteric junction obstruction, and other urological conditions may be associated with primary VUR.

Loin pain

Older patients may give a history of loin pain when their bladder is full, with worsening at the start of micturition followed by rapid relief after voiding.

Hypertension

Reflux nephropathy is the commonest cause of hypertension in childhood. Approximately 15 per cent of patients who reach adulthood will present with hypertension or its complications without a history of urinary tract infections. It may occasionally follow an accelerated course with deteriorating renal function.

Presentation during pregnancy

Apart from a urinary tract infection, the commonest presentation of reflux nephropathy in pregnancy is with a syndrome mimicking pre-eclampsia, often in the first or second trimester. Of women found to have bacteriuria during pregnancy, up to a third may have a urinary tract abnormality, the commonest of which is reflux nephropathy.

Table 2 Total number of patients entering renal replacement programmes in Australia and New Zealand and the number with end-stage reflux nephropathy, 1971 to 1991 inclusive (ANZDATA Registry, A.P.S. Disney, personal communication)

	Australia		New Zealand	
	Male	Female	Male	Female
Total number of patients	6752	5577	1283	940
Number with reflux nephropathy	405 (6.0%)	485 (8.7%)	83 (6.5%)	109 (11.6%)
Total number of patients aged <16 years	286	219	56	57
Number aged <16 years with reflux nephropathy	64 (22.4%)	55 (25.1%)	9 (16.1%)	15 (26.3%)

Urinary calculi

Patients with reflux nephropathy have an increased frequency of urinary calculi. Some of these are staghorn calculi in patients (invariably women) with uncontrolled urinary tract infections, usually with *Proteus mirabilis* or another urea-splitting organism.

Proteinuria

Persistent proteinuria is a bad prognostic feature. It indicates a complicating glomerulopathy, the histological hallmark of which is focal and segmental glomerulosclerosis with hyalinosis involving the unscarred segments of kidney, or the structurally normal contralateral kidney in patients with unilateral reflux nephropathy.

Renal failure

Reflux nephropathy is an important cause of chronic renal failure (Table 2) and all too frequently patients present with advanced uraemia but without any history of urinary tract infection.

Management

Vesicoureteric reflux

There is still controversy about the role of surgery in the treatment of VUR. It appears to have no useful effect on the incidence of infections which can be controlled satisfactorily by medical measures such as low-dose antimicrobial prophylaxis and prompt treatment of symptomatic infection.

In the context of prevention of progressive renal damage, the balance of evidence suggests that the only role for surgery is in the first few months of life and then only for those with grades III–V reflux. The only indication for antireflux surgery in the adult is the very occasional patient with severe loin pain when the bladder is full or after micturition.

Reflux nephropathy

Once nephropathy is established, surgery has no beneficial effect on subsequent renal function, but the question arises as to whether it can improve hypertension, either by antireflux surgery or by nephrectomy in cases where the lesion is unilateral. There are no data about the effects of antireflux surgery in this context, but in the occasional patient unilateral nephrectomy can improve or even cure hypertension but it is not yet possible to predict which case may benefit and which will not.

Further reading

Bailey, R.R. (1998).Vesicoureteric reflux and reflux nephropathy. In: *Oxford textbook of clinical nephrology*, (2nd edn) (ed. A.M. Davison, J.S. Cameron, J.-P. Grünfeld, D. Kerr, E. Ritz, and C.G. Winearls), pp. 2501–23. Oxford University Press, Oxford.

Birmingham Reflux Study Group (1987). Prospective trial of operative versus non-operative treatment of severe vesico-ureteric reflux in children: five years observer. *British Medical Journal*, **295**, 237–41.

Cotran, R.S. (1982). Glomerulosclerosis in reflux nephropathy. *Kidney International*, **21**, 528–34.

Chapter 12.20

Kidney disease from analgesics and non-steroidal anti-inflammatory drugs

J. H. Stewart

Analgesic nephropathy

'Classical' analgesic nephropathy is on the wane in most societies as a result of banning the sale of phenacetin or of compound analgesic preparations, but rather different syndromes caused by non-steroidal anti-inflammatory drugs (**NSAIDs**) have appeared.

The renal lesion

Papillary necrosis

The primary pathology is in the renal papilla. Initially the naked-eye appearance is virtually normal; microscopically, the lesion is confined to the central part of the inner medulla and affects only the interstitial cells, the thin ascending limb of Henle's loop, and the peritubular capillaries (cellular necrosis; basement-membrane thickening; increased ground substance). In advanced disease there is necrosis of all medullary elements, commonly with partial or total papillary separation.

Chronic interstitial nephritis

There is some atrophy of cortex overlying papillae, and hypertrophy of columns of Bertin. When papillary separation does not occur or is incomplete, there is progressive cortical atrophy with fibrosis and mononuclear infiltration, attributed to intrarenal urinary obstruction. Glomerulosclerosis and arterial intimal thickening appear later, associated with chronic renal failure.

Capillary sclerosis

This is seen immediately under the urothelium, maximally at the pelvi-ureteric junction but evident even in the bladder. It is due to repeated toxic lysis (by phenacetin metabolites) of endothelium,

Table 1 Differential diagnosis of renal papillary necrosis

Aetiology	Pathology
Toxic:	
classical analgesic nephropathy	Non-inflammatory; calcification
Ischaemic:	
diabetes	Acute inflammation; infection
urinary obstruction	Acute inflammation; infection
acute pyelonephritis	Acute inflammation; infection
sickle-cell disease	Non-inflammatory; scarring
NSAID-induced	Non-inflammatory; scarring
profound shock (especially newborn)	Acute infarction

NSAID, non-steroidal anti-inflammatory drug.

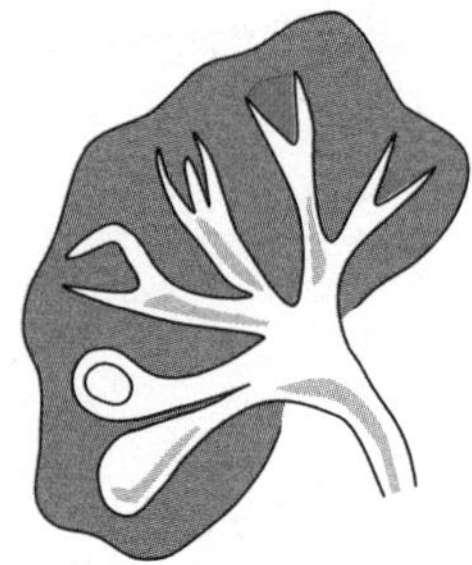

Fig. 1 A schematic drawing of the pyelographic appearances of analgesic nephropathy. From above down, the pyramids show: (i) central and (ii) total papillary calcification, (iii) central papillary cavitation, (iv) partial and (v) total papillary separation ('ring sign'), and (vi) a 'clubbed' calyx from which the papilla has been passed. Note the areas of cortical atrophy over papillae, interspersed with hypertrophied columns of Bertin.

resulting in concentric deposition of layers of basement membrane on the inside of the damaged capillary wall.

Aetiology

Preparations causing nephropathy have contained at least three ingredients, each contributing to pathogenesis: phenacetin; caffeine or codeine; and either aspirin or phenazone (or other pyrazolone). Amounts required to cause nephropathy have exceeded 1 kg (equivalent to two powders or tablets per day for 2 years) often more than that. The potential of all analgesics and NSAIDs to cause papillary necrosis is evident from testing in rodents. Some studies implicate paracetamol (acetaminophen). Aspirin alone is not a cause.

There is evidence that phenacetin, alone or with another antipyretic analgesic, is habituating, but more likely codeine or caffeine is responsible, the latter by causing withdrawal headache which then prompts taking further analgesics.

Clinical presentations

Renal papillary necrosis (Table 1)

There may be no clinical symptoms or signs. Proteinuria appears only with the onset of renal failure, when microscopy of urine usually shows casts, or red or white cells (persistent asymptomatic sterile pyuria is characteristic). Infection in or around necrotic papillae may manifest as acute pyelonephritis or indolent urinary infection. Separation of papillae may cause haematuria, colic, or obstruction, giving rise to hydronephrosis or pyonephrosis, the latter often resulting in Gram-negative septicaemia and acute renal failure.

Chronic interstitial nephritis and chronic renal failure

Impaired urinary concentration is the earliest abnormality, and distal renal tubular acidosis, salt-wasting, and hypocitraturia (possibly accounting for calcium deposition) are relatively common. Hypertension may appear late, or early and severe. Acidosis and renal osteodystrophy occur more frequently than in other chronic kidney diseases.

Urothelial cancer

Phenacetin is weakly carcinogenic in the kidney and urinary tract, and papillary necrosis is a common precursor of transitional cell carcinomas, often multiple, in the renal pelvis or bladder or both.

Diagnosis

The diagnosis is certain only if both analgesic abuse and a characteristic renal lesion can be demonstrated. The regular taking of analgesics may be denied; in such cases the detection in the urine of salicylate or *N*-acetyl-*p*-aminophenol indicates surreptitious consumption, which is almost always excessive. Papillary necrosis gives a characteristic appearance of cortical scarring and calyceal irregularity on contrast pyelography (Fig. 1). The 'wavy' renal outline and random distribution of affected calyces often will discriminate from reflux nephropathy even when papillary necrosis is not evident. Medullary sponge kidney, tuberculosis, or simple calculi must be distinguished. The pyelogram may be normal, or nearly so, in early disease or when no papillae have separated. Ultrasound or computed tomography will demonstrate calcified papillae, cortical scarring and, rarely, medullary cavitation.

Histopathology

Chronic interstitial nephritis can be diagnosed only with certainty by biopsy, but the appearances do not identify the aetiology unless papillary necrosis is seen. Voided fragments of tissue or calculi may be identified as necrotic papillae by histology.

Treatment

Complete cessation of analgesic consumption is the only specific measure. Even normal doses of NSAIDs, or of antipyretic analgesics taken regularly, may cause progression of established renal damage whatever the original aetiology.

Indolent urinary infection should be eradicated by prolonged antimicrobial therapy but its role in causing progression of renal failure is debatable. There is an increased likelihood of urothelial cancer which may develop even when analgesics are no longer taken. It is important therefore to perform regular cytological examination of the urine up to or after transplantation or maintenance dialysis.

Prognosis

Progression despite cessation of abuse occurs less in analgesic nephropathy than in chronic renal failure of other causation, but gradual deterioration is seen with focal glomerulosclerosis (indicated by proteinuria), diffuse accumulation of calcium salts in the kidneys or, more usually, continuing consumption of analgesics, overt or occult.

Prevention

Removing phenacetin from proprietary medications without its replacement by paracetamol, or prohibition from direct sale of any

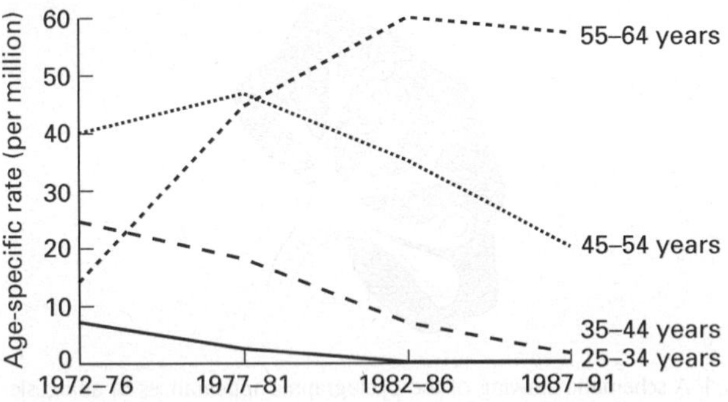

Fig. 2 The declining age-specific incidence of young and middle-aged women entering Australian endstage renal failure programmes as a result of analgesic nephropathy. Phenacetin was withdrawn in 1975, and all compound analgesic preparations in 1979. The decline occurred earlier, and was proportionately greater, in the younger age groups; much of the rise in the 55–64-year age group was due to increasing acceptance of older patients into renal failure treatment programmes.

analgesic containing more than one ingredient, has proved effective in Scandinavia, Canada, Britain, and Australia (Fig. 2).

Syndromes due to non-steroidal anti-inflammatory drugs

NSAIDs may cause functional renal failure, or acute or chronic intrinsic renal disease.

Functional renal failure

Each type of cell in the kidney elaborates one or more of the prostaglandins or thromboxane. These paracrine agents play a part in regulating blood flow. They become important when renal function is already under haemodynamic stress or chronically reduced. In such circumstances the addition of NSAIDs may precipitate an acute fall in glomerular filtration unrelated to structural damage. Mild cases are manifest only as elevation of serum creatinine or salt and water retention, but occasionally the circulatory insult is severe and prolonged enough to cause tubular, or in isolated cases, cortical necrosis.

Acute interstitial nephritis—minimal change nephrotic syndrome

The histological and clinical picture may be exclusively of either acute interstitial nephritis or minimal change nephrotic syndrome, but usually both are present.

It seems likely that this syndrome is caused by disturbance of prostaglandin-modulated production of lymphokines, or the diversion of eicosanoid metabolism towards proinflammatory leukotrienes. The resulting T-lymphocyte abnormality is manifest at two sites in the kidney. In the interstitial tissue, there is mononuclear infiltration sometimes involving tubules, with formation of granulomas occasionally. The second target is the glomerular filtration barrier—hence the minimal change nephrotic syndrome. The insidious onset of worsening renal function, together with moderate proteinuria or the nephrotic syndrome several months after starting an NSAID is characteristic. Renal biopsy will confirm the diagnosis, but often is unnecessary.

Treatment and prognosis

Not only should the offending NSAID be stopped, but all drugs of this class avoided, as the disorder appears to be a toxic rather than an allergic reaction. There is little evidence that corticosteroids help, except when granulomas are present. Nephrotic syndrome resolves spontaneously and completely within 1 month of withdrawing the drug, but recovery from acute interstitial nephritis is slow and incomplete.

Chronic interstitial nephritis

This may be a slowly evolving form of the acute disease described above, or analogous to classical analgesic nephropathy. Papillary necrosis is relatively uncommon—when present, the cause may be medullary ischaemia rather than cytotoxicity (Table 1). Only recognition that NSAIDs may be nephrotoxic even at prescribed dosage, and the performance of a biopsy to show chronic interstitial nephritis, will give the diagnosis with certainty. The majority of cases are overlooked because of the insidious nature of the chronic renal failure and the lack of urinary abnormalities.

Treatment and prognosis

Avoidance of all NSAIDs, and of antipyretic analgesics taken regularly, may protect against slow progression of chronic renal failure. The severity of renal dysfunction seems to be less than in classical analgesic nephropathy, probably because papillary necrosis occurs rarely, and endstage renal failure recognizably and primarily due to this cause is infrequent.

Toxic renal tubular necrosis

Paracetamol and glafenine (an NSAID introduced in France but not used widely elsewhere) can cause nephrotoxic tubular necrosis. In the case of paracetamol, the mechanism of toxicity probably is the same as in hepatocellular necrosis; in these cases, why the kidney rather than the liver should be the main target organ, is unknown.

Further reading

Molzahn, M., Pommer, W., De Broe, M.E., and Elseviers, M.M. (1998). Analgesic nephropathy. In: *Oxford textbook of clinical nephrology*, (2nd edn) (ed. A.M. Davison, J.S. Cameron, J.-P. Grünfeld, D. Kerr, E. Ritz, and C.G. Winearls), pp. 1129–46. Oxford University Press, Oxford.

Sandler, D.P., Burr, F.R., and Weinberg, C.R. (1991). Non-steroidal anti-inflammatory drugs and the risk of chronic renal disease. *Annals of Internal Medicine*, 115, 165–72.

Stewart, J.H. (1993). *Analgesic and NSAID induced kidney disease*. Oxford University Press, Oxford.

Wai, Y.T. and Adu, D. (1998). Non-steroidal anti-inflammatory drugs and the kidney. In: *Oxford textbook of clinical nephrology*, (2nd edn) (ed. A.M. Davison, J.S. Cameron, J.-P. Grünfeld, D. Kerr, E. Ritz, and C.G. Winearls), pp. 1147–56. Oxford University Press, Oxford.

Chapter 12.21

Gout, purines, and interstitial nephritis

J. S. Cameron and H. A. Simmonds

Chronic crystal-related interstitial nephropathy in a middle-aged male with gout was formerly common but has become rare in the past 30 years. Various factors may have contributed: a lower intake of dietary purines, a lower frequency of chronic lead intoxication, and early treatment of the majority of severely affected gouty subjects with allopurinol. Thus the relative importance of rarer forms of metabolically induced or inherited gouty nephropathy has increased, and the average age of diagnosis of gout-associated or hyperuricaemic nephropathy has decreased.

The relevant disorders of purine metabolism—glycogen storage disease type I, hypoxanthine guanine phosphoribosyl transferase deficiency, superactivity of phosphoribosyl synthetase, deficiency of adenine phosphoribosyl transferase, and hereditary xanthinuria (or xanthine oxidase deficiency) are reviewed in Chapter 6.6). Familial juvenile gout is described here.

Familial juvenile gout

Hyperuricaemia underlies juvenile gout affecting males and (unusually) females equally. The disorder, termed also familial juvenile hyperuricaemic nephropathy, is an autosomal dominant condition with high penetrance and shows two major hallmarks: hyperuricaemia disproportionate to the degree of renal dysfunction and an extremely low FE_{ur}. Clinical gout and hypertension are inconsistent features and the disease may be misdiagnosed as 'familial nephritis'. The reason for the renal damage is obscure, as there is no evidence of urate deposition in the kidney, although the absence of detectable crystals does not necessarily preclude their original presence. There is probably a defect in a gene coding for one of the anion transporters in the proximal tubule, either in the basolateral or brush border membrane. It is not yet clear whether allopurinol may protect against renal failure, but it must be given in any event in order to control the hyperuricaemia and reduce the risk of gout.

Acute and chronic renal disease associated with disorders of purine metabolism and urate handling

Acute crystal nephropathy (see Chapter 12.28)

Hyperuricosuria–hypouricaemia

Some inherited tubular disorders, either as part of the Fanconi syndrome or as one of the heterogeneous isolated tubular defects (e.g. dominantly inherited familiar renal hypouricaemia) have uricosuria as a component. FE_{ur} is usually 30–50 per cent, but in occasional cases may equal, or even exceed, the glomerular filtration rate. Almost all of these hyperuricosuric patients are symptomless, but stones have been noted in a minority, and acute renal failure has been reported after severe exercise which may be recurrent.

Chronic urate nephropathy

In classical gout, chronic urate nephropathy is more complicated and its pathogenesis more contentious than acute uric acid nephropathy. An interstitial fibrosis with vascular changes are the usual histological findings; it is rare to find urate crystals, but chronic interstitial deposits of sodium urate may occur in a few untreated subjects. They are most common in the medulla surrounded by an inflammatory infiltrate of varying age. Crystals of 2,8-dihydroxyadenine or xanthine may appear similarly in the interstitium in adenine phosphoribosyltransferase and xanthine oxidase deficiencies, respectively, and present as chronic renal insufficiency. One particular cause of gout-associated chronic renal failure is chronic lead intoxication which may be commoner than realized because a history of exposure may be absent.

Treatment

Allopurinol is the drug of choice, since uricosuric agents such as probenecid become ineffective as the glomerular filtration rate falls and FE_{ur} increases concomitantly. The dose of allopurinol must be modified from the standard 300 mg/24 h down through 200 and 100 mg/day as glomerular filtration rate falls, to the lowest dose in dialysed patients, who require only 100 mg thrice weekly.

Stones

Uric acid stones (see Chapter 12.23) are much less common today in classical middle-aged male gout than in the past. Other rare purine stones, such as those of 2,8-dihydroxyadenine in adenine phosphoribosyltransferase deficiency and xanthine in xanthine oxidase deficiency may occasionally be identified; the former are often confused with uric acid stones, but are grey and friable, unlike the yellow and hard uric acid stones. Increased urine volume, alkalinization of urine, and allopurinol are all effective in presenting recurrent uricacid lithiasis.

Further reading

Cameron, J.S., Moro, F., and Simmonds, H.A. (1998). Uric acid and the kidney. In *Oxford textbook of clinical nephrology*, (2nd edn), (ed. A.M. Davison, J.S. Cameron, J.-P. Grünfeld, D. Kerr, E. Ritz, and C. Winearls). Oxford University Press, Oxford.

Chapter 12.22

Urinary tract obstruction

L. R. I. Baker

Urinary tract obstruction at any point from the renal calyces to the exterior may result in adverse effects on renal function (obstructive nephropathy) and characteristic anatomical changes (hydronephrosis). Although dilatation of the outflow system proximal to the site of obstruction is a characteristic finding, widening of the ureter and/or pelvicalyceal system does not necessarily indicate the presence of obstruction. Causes of such anatomical abnormality in the absence of obstruction are listed in Table 1. The major causes of obstruction are listed in Table 2.

Calculi and neuromuscular dysfunction at the junction of the renal pelvis and ureter are common causes of unilateral obstruction. Prostatic obstruction, stone disease, and bladder tumours account for approximately 75 per cent of cases of bilateral obstruction in developed countries. Wide geographical variations occur in the relative incidence of some causes of obstruction, for example, schistosomiasis.

Urinary tract obstruction has been found in 3.8 per cent of a large series of routine autopsies and 25 per cent of autopsies carried out upon uraemic patients. The most important questions are whether urinary tract obstruction affects the upper or lower urinary tract, and whether it is of recent onset or is of long-standing.

Pathophysiology

Acute upper tract obstruction

During peristalsis ureteric pressure normally rises to some 10–25 mmHg, but this is not transmitted to the renal pelvis where

Table 1 Causes of non-obstructive collecting system dilatation

Anatomical variants

- Large major calyx
- Extrarenal pelvis
- Distensible system after relief of obstruction
- Pregnancy

Congenital anomalies

- Megacalyces

Vesicoureteric reflux

- Children
- Abnormality of ureteric insertion into bladder
- Adults
- Neuropathic bladder, after ileal loop diversion, following vesicoureteric surgery, after renal transplantation
- Calyceal pathology

Tuberculosis

- Caliceal cyst
- Papillary necrosis

pressures seldom rise above 4 mmHg. After obstruction pressures generated in the ureter are transmitted to the renal pelvis and parenchyma, the effect depending on the degree of obstruction and its duration.

Any change in blood flow or glomerular filtration rate resulting from ureteric obstruction has important effects on tubular pressures and flows. Time of onset of obstruction is seldom known with any precision, and methods of measurement of renal blood flow or filtration rate are indirect and depend upon tubular function, which is itself affected by urinary tract obstruction, so that concepts must depend on animal experiments. In the dog, renal blood flow falls to 50 per cent of control values 3 or 4 days after induction of complete ureteric obstruction. At 4 weeks, blood flow is about one-third that to the contralateral unobstructed kidney (see OTM3, p. 3233).

Chronic upper tract obstruction

Three months after production of experimental obstruction in dogs, base-line ureteric wall tension is increased and there is no difference between base-line and peak values of wall *tension*. By contrast, base-line and peak *pressures* within the ureteric lumen are not significantly different from control values. This is a consequence of the relationship between pressure and wall tension expressed in Laplace's law, which states that $P = K(T/R)$, where P is the transluminal pressure, K is a constant, T is wall tension, and R is the radius of the ureter. In chronic obstruction, therefore, normal intraluminal pressures are maintained as a consequence of ureteric dilatation.

These findings suggest that the major component of damage to the kidney due to obstruction occurs soon after its onset. The notion that chronic obstruction with dilatation of the ureter may be relatively benign is supported by the observation that patients with incomplete urinary tract obstruction due to congenital anomalies lose renal function only slowly.

Acute lower tract obstruction

Factors which may precipitate acute retention include a sudden diuresis, urinary infection, and drugs which have pharmacological effects upon the bladder, such as those with antimuscarinic and calcium-channel-blocking activity.

Chronic lower tract obstruction

In adult males chronic outflow obstruction to the bladder is most commonly due to benign prostatic hypertrophy. Prostatic malignancy and urethral strictures may also be responsible. In children, posterior urethral valves and urethral strictures are most often the cause. Functional obstruction may occur at the bladder neck and at the

Table 2 Some causes of urinary tract obstruction

Within the lumen	Within the wall	Pressure from outside
Calculus	Pelviureteric neuromuscular dysfunction (congenital, 10% bilateral)	Pelviureteric compression (bands, aberrant vessels)
Blood clot	Ureteric stricture (tuberculosis, especially after treatment; calculous; following surgery)	Tumours, e.g. retroperitoneal growths or glands, carcinoma of colon, diverticulitis, aortic aneurysm
Sloughed papilla (diabetes, analgesic abuse, sickle-cell disease)	Ureterovesical stricture (congenital, ureterocele, calculous, schistosomiasis)	Retroperitoneal fibrosis (peri-aortitis)
Tumour of renal pelvis or ureter	Congenital megaureter	Accidental ligation of ureter
Bladder tumour	Congenital bladder neck obstruction	Pancreatitis
	Neurogenic bladder	Retrocaval ureter (right-sided obstruction)
	Urethral stricture (calculous, gonococcal, after instrumentation)	Crohn's disease
	Congenital urethral valve	Chronic granulomatous disease
	Pin-hole meatus	Prostatic obstruction
		Tumours in pelvis, e.g. carcinoma of cervix
		Phimosis

level of the distal sphincter owing to a failure of co-ordination between bladder contraction and sphincter relaxation. The bladder wall may become increasingly compliant or the opposite may occur. The highly compliant bladder tends not to be associated with upper tract dilatation, whereas the high pressure that exists within a bladder of low compliance may be transmitted to the upper tracts and may be the cause of renal impairment.

Histopathological changes

The rise in intraluminal pressure and dilatation of the system proximal to the obstruction result in compression of the renal substance. In the early phase the kidney becomes oedematous and haemorrhagic. Tubular dilatation initially affects mainly the collecting duct and distal tubular segments. Bowman's space may be dilated.

The ducts of Bellini are first affected. Subsequently, other papillary structures are involved, and ultimately compression of cortical tissue occurs with thinning of the parenchyma. Enlargement of the kidney occurs in association with dilatation of the renal pelvis. Atrophy of the parenchyma with reduction in size of the kidney (obstructive atrophy) is believed to result from prolonged ischaemia. Slowly progressive partial obstruction tends to result in gross dilatation of the collecting system, dilated calyces, and renal pelvis surrounded by only a thin rim of parenchyma. In acute complete obstruction dilatation tends to be less marked.

In long-standing obstruction there is flattening of renal tubular epithelium, periglomerular fibrosis, interstitial fibrosis, and mononuclear cell infiltration. These changes are thought to result in part from renal ischaemia and, in part, to reflect the effects of bacterial infection (Fig. 1).

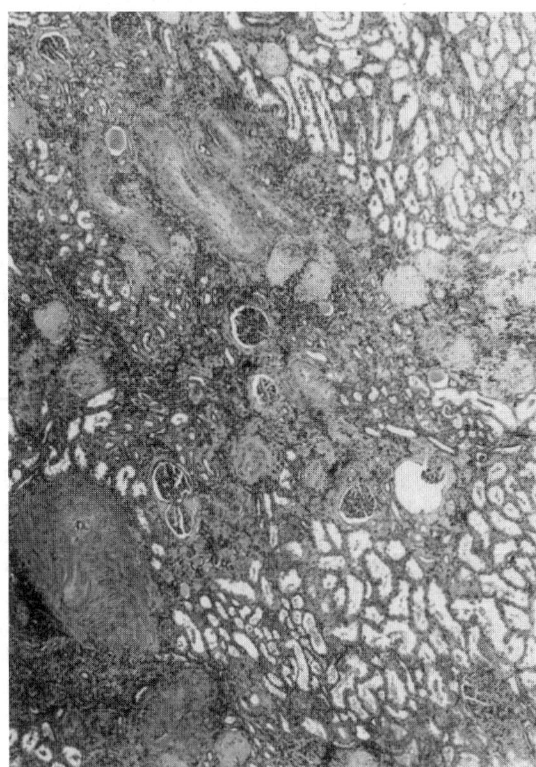

Fig. 1 Histological appearances in long-standing obstruction. Note dilated tubules, interstitial fibrosis, vessel wall thickening, and global sclerosis of some glomeruli.

Effects of obstruction upon renal function

Ureteric obstruction results in a marked fall in glomerular filtration rate, and bilateral incomplete obstruction causes progressive renal failure. Glomerular filtration must continue to some extent even after development of complete acute obstruction as a nephrogram (albeit a delayed one) can be obtained after injection of intravenous contrast medium.

In chronic partial ureteric obstruction, distal tubular function is more strikingly disturbed than is that of the proximal tubule. A characteristic feature is impaired ability to concentrate urine, resistant to the administration of antidiuretic hormone. Such patients may present with polyuria, dehydration, and hypernatraemia. There may also be a salt-losing state.

In many patients with obstructive nephropathy, urinary pH is inappropriately high for any associated degree of metabolic acidosis. This distal renal tubular acidosis is present in both unilateral and bilateral ureteric obstruction, and may be associated with hyperkalaemia.

Renal function after relief of obstruction

The relationship between duration of obstruction and the extent of recovery of renal function after its reversal is unknown. Renal blood flow increases after relief of obstruction, and glomerular filtration rate either remains the same or increases. The extent of recovery probably depends upon whether obstruction is partial or complete, the duration of it, and whether or not obstruction is complicated by bacterial infection.

A severe salt-losing state, with urinary losses as high as 300–600 mmol in 24 h, may follow relief of bilateral obstruction, leading to massive requirements for intravenous saline to prevent superadded extra-renal uraemia. Such salt loss may persist for several days, or even a week or two.

Hormonal changes induced by obstruction

Erythropoietin

Levels of erythropoietin are low in renal failure due to obstructive uropathy, but neither the degree of anaemia nor the degree of depression of erythropoietin concentration is known to differ from that occurring in chronic renal failure of similar severity and different aetiology. Erythraemia is a recognized association of chronic upper urinary tract obstruction and correction after relief of obstruction has been recorded. Erythropoietin concentrations in such patients have rarely been documented.

Vitamin D metabolism

Scant data are available in respect of vitamin D metabolism in renal failure associated with obstruction, but radiological evidence of hyperparathyroid bone disease is more common in patients with obstructive endstage renal failure, even when a correction is applied for duration and gender.

Hypertension and the renin–angiotensin system

Hypertension is more common in patients with bilateral urinary tract obstruction than in normal individuals matched for age and sex. The prevalence in unilateral obstruction is unknown.

Patients with chronic bilateral upper tract obstruction appear to have a volume-dependent form of hypertension consequent upon salt and water retention. Others with chronic unilateral obstruction and hypertension have been described in whom renal vein renin concentrations were elevated on the side of obstruction and in whom both blood pressure and renal vein renin concentration returned to normal after relief of obstruction, but there are no clinical features or preoperative investigations which will predict the outcome of such surgery.

Atrial natriuretic peptide

Atrial natriuretic peptide release is augmented in patients with bilateral ureteric obstruction and uraemia, probably owing to salt and water overload. This may contribute to postobstructive diuresis and natriuresis (see above).

Clinical features

Acute upper tract obstruction

Typically, this gives rise to pain in the flank which may radiate to the iliac fossa, inguinal region, testis, or labium. The pain may be dull or sharp, intermittent or persistent, although waxing and waning in intensity. It may be provoked by a high fluid intake, alcohol, or diuretics: this is particularly noticeable when obstruction occurs at the pelviureteric junction. Loin tenderness may be detected and an enlarged kidney felt. Signs of septicaemia may dominate the clinical picture. Complete anuria is strongly suggestive of complete bilateral obstruction or complete obstruction of a single kidney. The differential diagnosis then includes bilateral total renal cortical necrosis, acute anuric glomerulonephritis, and bilateral renal arterial occlusion.

Chronic upper tract obstruction

Patients may present with flank or abdominal pain, renal failure, or both; symptoms and signs of urinary tract infection and septicaemia may be superimposed. Rarely, presentation is with erythraemia or hypertension. A proportion of patients are asymptomatic, obstruction being found during investigation of some other condition. Polyuria often occurs in chronic partial obstruction owing to impairment of renal tubular concentrating capacity. Intermittent anuria and polyuria indicate intermittent complete and partial obstruction.

Acute lower tract obstruction

Acute urinary retention is often preceded by a history of symptoms of bladder outflow obstruction. Acute retention is typically associated with severe suprapubic pain, but this may be absent if acute retention is superimposed on chronic retention or if there is an underlying neuropathy. Patients who have had an epidural anaesthetic may develop painless acute retention. Pre-existing obstruction may have provoked changes in the bladder, such as muscle wall hypertrophy, sacculation, and diverticulum formation; these in turn predispose to persistence of lower urinary tract infection once acquired and occasionally to bladder stones. Epididymo-orchitis may occur.

Chronic lower tract obstruction

Symptoms may be minimal. Hesitancy, narrowing, and diminished force of the urinary stream, terminal dribbling, and a sense of incomplete bladder emptying are typical features. If a large volume of residual urine remains in the bladder after urination, the frequent passage of small volumes may be a prominent symptom even in the absence of infection. Incontinence of such small volumes is termed overflow incontinence. If the residual urine volume is sufficient, the bladder may be palpably distended. The apparent size and consistency of the prostate is variable. Acute complete retention of urine, usually with severe suprapubic and perineal pain, may occur.

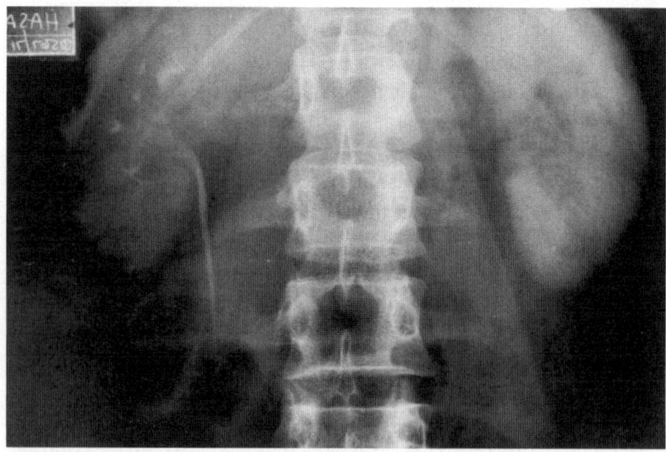

Fig. 2 Acute left ureteric obstruction. Note the increased density of the nephrogram and the absence of pyelogram on the left side 15 min after injection of contrast.

Lower urinary tract infection occurs commonly in association with bladder outflow obstruction and may precipitate acute retention. Frequency, urgency, urge incontinence, dysuria, strangury, suprapubic pain, haematuria, and cloudy, smelly urine may be present. Asymptomatic bacteriuria is common.

Investigation

Acute upper tract obstruction

Intravenous urography

Intravenous urography will confirm the diagnosis and will usually demonstrate the site, cause, and degree of obstruction. The plain film must be examined carefully for opaque calculi along the line of the ureter—calculi overlying bone are easily missed. Ureteric calculi within the bony pelvis are often impossible to distinguish from calcified phleboliths on the plain film.

A large dose of contrast, preferably of low osmolality, should be given to compensate for the lack of preparation and the probability of a low glomerular filtration rate. The recently obstructed kidney is typically enlarged and smooth in outline. The nephrogram is delayed owing to a reduction in glomerular filtration rate and the calyces and pelvis fill with contrast later than normal. The nephrogram eventually becomes more dense than normal owing to the prolonged nephron transit time. In time, the site of obstruction may become obvious owing to dilatation of the system to the level of the block (Figs 2 and 3).

Opacification may never be seen in severe acute obstruction but in most instances, filling of the pelvicalyceal system and ureter to the level of obstruction can be demonstrated on delayed films. In acute ureteric obstruction the pelvicalyceal system and ureter may be only slightly dilated. Occasionally, the only abnormality may be a ureter which remains full throughout its length to the level of the vesicoureteric junction, with this finding persisting on the full-length postmicturition film. Acute obstruction is characterized by increased excretion of contrast medium by the liver, leading to gallbladder opacification on delayed films.

If there is an obstructed nephrogram or dilatation of the pelvicalyceal system and/or ureter but no radio-dense calculus is seen, diagnosis is difficult. If the history is of recent-onset pain, the likely possibilities are: recent passage of an opaque stone; uric acid stone;

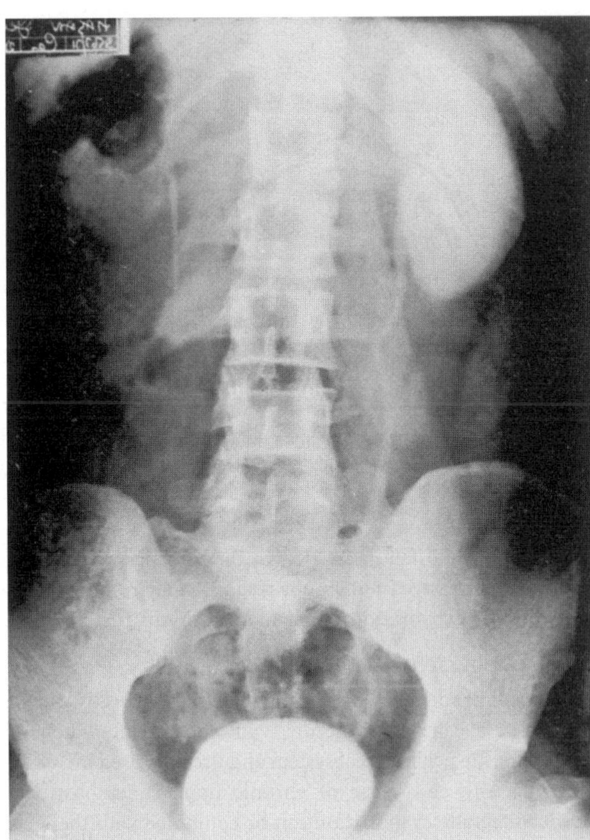

Fig. 3 Same patient as in Fig. 2. A later radiograph, showing a persistent dense nephrogram on the left. The pelivicalyceal system and ureter, which have now filled, are only slightly dilated due to the fact that obstruction is of very recent onset. The obstructing calculus at the left ureteric orifice is not visible.

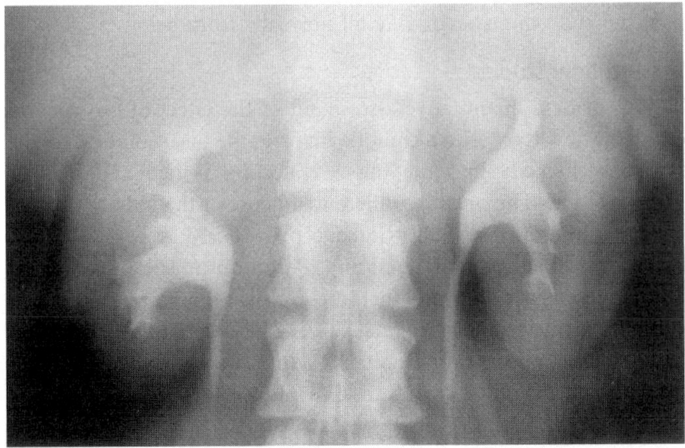

Fig. 4 Uric acid stones seen on intravenous urography as lucent filling defects in the collecting system on the left.

acute pelviureteric junction obstruction; blood clot; or sloughed papilla. Clot colic is always associated with macroscopic haematuria.

Urography shows uric acid stones as lucent filling defects (Fig. 4); similar filling defects may also occur with transitional cell tumours, sloughed papillae, or blood clots. If a persistent lucency is present, computed tomography (CT) scanning may be very helpful (Fig. 5).

When papillae are sloughed, abnormal calyces are usually seen in both kidneys, but papillary necrosis may occasionally be unilateral,

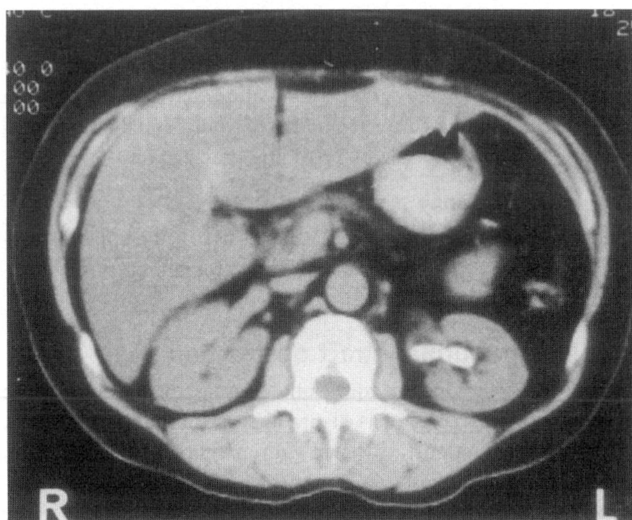

Fig. 5 CT scan clearly shows uric acid stones as opacities within the left collecting system.

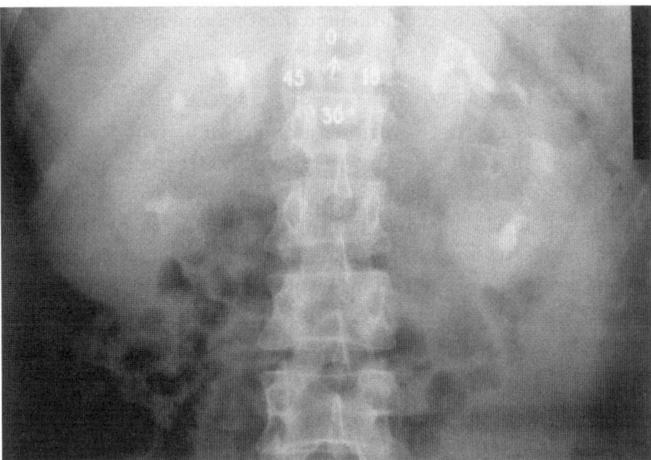

Fig. 6 Bilateral papillary necrosis with papillary calcification mimicking stones.

usually as a result of a previous episode of infection associated with unilateral obstruction, especially in diabetics. Occasionally, calcified papillae may mimic stones. (Fig. 6).

Ultrasonography

Ultrasound can define dilatation of the collecting system in the upper third of the ureter, but dilatation of the middle and lower thirds of the ureter is not easily detectable, and the dilated ureter cannot usually be followed to the level of obstruction. As dilatation is not synonymous with obstruction, and as acute obstruction can exist with only minimal dilatation, the value of ultrasonography is limited. The differentiation between collecting system dilatation due to obstruction and, for example, polycystic kidney disease, megacalycosis, and non-obstructive hydrocalycosis cannot be made ultrasonically.

Ultrasound may be used to investigate patients with suspected acute urinary obstruction if they are pregnant or have a history of contrast allergy. The risk of contrast nephrotoxicity in diabetics with moderate to severe renal impairment and in patients with myelomatosis is currently considered a relative contraindication to intravenous urography; therefore, ultrasonography has a primary role in the investigation of such patients.

Antegrade and retrograde pyelography and ureterography

If the site of obstruction is not demonstrated by intravenous urography, antegrade or retrograde examination may be helpful. Both techniques can be initiated as a method of diagnosis and then extended to provide a therapeutic role by providing drainage.

Computed tomography scanning

CT plays only a very minor part in the diagnosis of acute upper urinary tract obstruction, although the potential exists for demonstrating non-opaque stones.

Chronic upper urinary tract obstruction

The history should include questions relating to analgesic abuse (papillary necrosis, transitional cell tumours, and periureteric fibrosis), vitamin D consumption (associated with calculus formation), gout, diabetes, or renal stones. Initial investigation of unexplained impairment of renal function should include ultrasonography, together with plain abdominal radiographs and renal tomography to screen for urinary tract calculi. As ultrasound cannot distinguish between an obstructed distended system and a baggy, low-pressure dilated system, an abnormality on ultrasound must prompt further definitive investigation.

Intravenous urography

A high dose of contrast is required in renal failure and tomograms and delayed films are necessary. In chronic obstruction, films taken immediately after contrast injection will show a dilated pelvicalyceal system as a lucent 'negative pyelogram' surrounded by opacified parenchyma. Later films usually show filling of the dilated pelvicalyceal system and ureter. In very long-standing obstruction, generalized thinning of the renal parenchyma (obstructive atrophy) is typically diffuse and symmetrical, and there is associated generalized calyceal dilatation.

Computed tomography scanning

On CT the dilated collecting system appears as a multiloculate fluid collection of water density in the renal sinus. It is possible to distinguish the intrarenal collecting system from the extrarenal portion of the pelvis; this is important as obstruction can only be diagnosed on CT when there is dilatation of the intrarenal collecting system. The main value in the investigation of chronic upper tract obstruction is in defining the cause when this is unclear.

Scintigraphy

Scintigraphy provides functional evidence of obstruction. The first passage of the bolus of radioactivity reflects renal perfusion; later images provide information on renal uptake, excretion, and drainage. [^{99}Tc^{m}]diethylenetriamine penta-acetic acid which is excreted by glomerular filtration is most commonly used.

A rise in pressure in the collecting system, sufficient to result in impaired renal function, delays parenchymal clearance of tracer and emptying of the collecting system. On whole-kidney renograms, the time–activity curve fails to fall after the initial uptake peak, or continues to rise (Fig. 7). This does not enable a distinction to be made between obstructive nephropathy and retention of tracer within a large, baggy, low-pressure, unobstructed collecting system. A dynamic renal scintigram performed during frusemide-induced diuresis may be of value in this situation. Time–activity curves obtained over the renal pelvic area immediately after injection of frusemide show no significant change in the renogram. In normal subjects this is followed by a rapid fall in activity. In the presence of obstruction the half-time is prolonged but a poor response may result from poor renal function or dehydration rather than from obstruction.

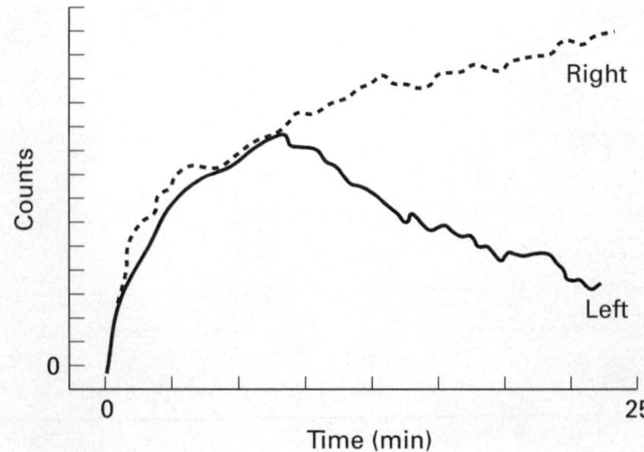

Fig. 7 Dynamic [^{99}Tc^{m}]diethylenetriamine penta-acetic acid scintigram. Note the progressive rise of the right kidney curve to a plateau, in contrast to the normal left kidney curve.

Antegrade pyelography and ureterography

Percutaneous introduction of contrast medium directly into the renal pelvis or a calyx via a needle, with subsequent radiographic examination of the pelvicalyceal system and ureter is used increasingly to define the site and cause of chronic upper tract obstruction. Diagnostic antegrade examination can be combined with therapeutic drainage of an obstructed system.

Retrograde ureterography

The technique carries the risks of infection and of septicaemia and usually requires a general anaesthetic. It should be performed only when absolutely necessary. In obstruction due to neuromuscular dysfunction at the pelviureteric junction and in retroperitoneal fibrosis, the collecting system may fill normally from below.

Pressure flow studies

These provide a quantitative assessment of the effect of obstruction on the outflow tract. The technique involves the insertion of a needle transparenchymally into the upper collecting system and bladder catheterization. The pressure differential between the kidney and the bladder is monitored while the collecting system is perfused with dilute contrast at a rate of 10 ml/min. Perfusion must be maintained for long enough to ensure that the upper urinary tract is filled. Normal systems can accommodate a flow rate of 10 ml/min without a pressure differential of more than 15 cm of water. If an obstruction is present, there will be a pressure differential of more than 22 cm of water.

Acute lower urinary tract obstruction

Most patients presenting with acute urinary retention require no investigation before treatment. Suprapubic pain coexisting with a bladder which is palpably or percussibly distended above the level of the symphysis pubis is sufficient evidence for immediate catheterization. If doubt exists, ultrasound will confirm or refute the presence of a distended bladder. Transrectal ultrasound of the prostrate can demonstrate both the size of the gland and, to some extent, the benign or malignant nature of the enlargement. An ascending urethrogram may be indicated if an attempt at urethral catheterization proves unsuccessful.

Management

Acute upper tract obstruction

The management of acute obstruction due to stones is described in Chapter 12.23. The two other most common causes are sloughed papillae and blood clots. The principles of management vary little from those for ureteric stones. In the patient with papillary necrosis, infection is a more common accompaniment of obstruction, and surgical intervention, usually with a percutaneous needle nephrostomy, is required more often. Renal parenchymal tumours and transitional cell tumours of the collecting system may both cause persistent bleeding and colic, and ablative open surgery is usually required. More difficulty is encountered when bleeding occurs from a non-malignant cause. An arteriovenous fistula may be embolized with every prospect of success. The most difficult case of recurrent bleeding to manage is that associated with papillary necrosis in sickle-cell trait or disease. (see Chapter 12.16).

Drainage of an obstructed system

If there is evidence of infection above an obstruction, drainage must be established as a matter of urgency. The patient will be pyrexial and the degree of loin tenderness will be greater than when obstruction is not associated with infection. Examination of bladder urine may be unhelpful as ureteric obstruction may prevent red and white blood cells and organisms from reaching the lower urinary tract. Leucocytosis may be present but this is not invariably the case, especially in the elderly. The choice between antegrade and retrograde intervention will depend on the facilities and expertise available. In most specialist centres there is a clear preference for the antegrade approach to provide a nephrostomy. The initial puncture may best be directed under ultrasound control using a fine needle. A retrograde ureteric catheter, in contrast, can be relied on to provide drainage at best only for a matter of days.

Chronic upper tract obstruction

Pelviureteric junction obstruction

Commonly, this appears to result from a functional disturbance in peristalsis of the collecting system in the absence of mechanical obstruction. A percutaneous procedure for managing pelviureteric junctional obstruction is a useful technique, but there is no consensus on the indications. Currently, patients with secondary pelviureteric junction stenosis, in association with stones, infection, or previous surgery, are offered this approach, whereas those with primary idiopathic obstruction are better treated by open pyeloplasty. The percutaneous operation involves a full thickness incision through the stenosed region and a stent left *in situ.*

Malignant obstruction

A wide variety of tumours may cause ureteric obstruction, either by local spread (cervix, prostate, bladder), or secondary to para-aortic nodal enlargement (lymphoma, testicular tumours). An aggressive or radical approach is almost always indicated in a patient who has received no previous treatment. Unilateral or bilateral percutaneous nephrostomies may be necessary to cover the period during which chemotherapy or radiotherapy are given. More difficulty arises when ureteric obstruction is due to recurrent tumour. Nephrostomy drainage for what is left of life significantly diminishes its quality, but may be right in certain circumstances. Open surgery can be avoided by the use of a ring nephrostomy inserted percutaneously under general anaesthesia: this provides secure long-term drainage, for years if necessary.

Urinary diversion

There are many reasons for diverting the urine into an isolated loop of ileum or colon but ureterosigmoidostomy has fallen into disfavour owing to the associated complications of infection, metabolic acidosis, and osteomalacia.

Idiopathic retroperitoneal fibrosis (peri-aortitis)

In this condition the ureters become embedded in dense fibrous tissue, with resultant unilateral or bilateral obstruction, usually at the junction between the middle and lower thirds of the ureter. The condition is progressive: initially, the fibrous tissue is fairly cellular, later becoming relatively acellular. The mechanism by which obstruction occurs is unclear, not least because of the frequent observation that contrast medium injected into the lower ureter may pass freely up to the pelvicalyceal system despite the presence of clinical, radiological, and isotopic evidence of functional urinary tract obstruction.

Pathogenesis

'Retroperitoneal fibrosis' is an unfortunate term, as there are many causes of fibrosis in the retroperitoneal area (including malignant disease of breast, colon, or prostate, for instance), and because it is anatomically misleading and says nothing about pathogenesis. Evidence now suggests that the condition is an autoimmune peri-aortitis. Histologically, atheroma, medial thinning, splits in the media, and an increase in the adventitia, which contains an inflammatory infiltrate, are seen in the abdominal aorta. The fibrous tissue itself contains macrophages and plasma cells but not polymorphs. The probable cause of the autoimmune response is leakage of material derived from atheromatous plaques in the diseased aorta.

Clinical features

The condition is three times as common in men as in women. Ages range from the third to the ninth decade, but peak incidence occurs in the sixth and seventh decades. The early clinical manifestations are not distinctive. Most commonly there is pain in a girdle-like distribution from the low back to the lower abdomen, occasionally spreading to the buttocks or thighs. Examination is usually unremarkable apart from hypertension, which is found in over 50 per cent of patients. Oedema of the legs, a palpable kidney, and hydrocele, are found in less than 10 per cent of patients. There is usually a normochromic, normocytic anaemia, and a raised erythrocyte sedimentation rate and plasma C-reactive protein, but a significant minority are normal in one or both of these respects. Proteinuria is uncommon and significant bacteriuria rare.

Diagnosis

Peri-aortic fibrosis is more common than hitherto appreciated. Diagnostic delay is the rule; in one series, 6–12 months, or even longer, elapsed from the onset of symptoms to diagnosis. In the history, enquiry should be made regarding consumption of relevant drugs, including methysergide, β-blockers, and bromocriptine, another ergot-like drug. Ultrasonography, isotopic methods, and the intravenous urogram will usually reveal findings typical of urinary tract obstruction. CT scanning will show the peri-aortic mass. The differential diagnosis includes lymphoma and various forms of cancer, including particularly those of the bladder, bowel, and cervix. A histological diagnosis should be obtained if possible, and laparotomy is often required in order to obtain a sufficiently large sample to exclude lymphoma and cancer with certainty, although a CT-guided needle biopsy may be sufficient to make a definitive diagnosis.

Management

Management of the syndrome is empirical and controversial as controlled trials of treatment are lacking. Corticosteroid therapy alone may correct obstruction, but is by no means invariably effective. Ureterolysis alone may also correct obstruction in the short term but is sometimes associated with recurrence or the development of a further obstruction in a previously unaffected kidney. Surgical relief of obstruction by ureterolysis followed by long-term corticosteroid therapy (prednisolone 20 mg daily begun when sutures are removed) has proved a reliable and successful strategy. Surgery alone should be employed in those with a particular contraindication to corticosteroid treatment. Steroid therapy alone should be reserved for patients unfit for ureterolysis. Insertion of ureteric stents to correct obstruction combined with corticosteroid therapy is gaining in popularity but there is at present no consensus as to whether this is an appropriate approach.

Prognosis

The older and the more uraemic the patient at the time of presentation, the worse is the prognosis, but if treated appropriately, most patients do well.

Follow-up

In one series of 60 patients, 10 relapsed more than 5 years after the time of diagnosis when steroid therapy had been stopped. Five patients relapsed as late as 10 years after the initial problem had apparently resolved. Lifelong follow-up is therefore mandatory. Clinical assessment, serial measurement of erythrocyte sedimentation rate or of C-reactive protein, and assessment of renal function, are appropriate. Reduction in size of the peri-aortic mass can be detected on serial CT scanning, but the usefulness of CT in monitoring disease activity is limited.

Chronic inflammatory bowel disease

Chronic inflammatory bowel disease is associated with chronic and unsuspected urinary tract obstruction in 10–15 per cent of patients. The obstruction is nearly always right-sided in patients with Crohn's disease, and a valuable clue to its existence is pain radiating down from the right iliac fossa into the right leg. The ureter is usually involved in an inflammatory mass. In contrast, in patients with ulcerative colitis the problem may occur on either side and nearly always follows colectomy. An ultrasound examination of the urinary tract to detect obstruction should be considered as part of the annual review in patients with chronic inflammatory bowel disease.

Further reading

Baker, L.R.I., Croxson, R., Khader, N., *et al.* (1992). Rate of development of ureteric obstruction in idiopathic retroperitoneal fibrosis (periaortitis). *British Journal of Urology*, **69**, 102–5.

Baker, L.R.I. and Whitfield, H.M. (1998). The patient with urinary tract obstruction. In: *Oxford textbook of clinical nephrology*, (2nd edn) (ed. A.M. Davison, J.S. Cameron, J.-P. Grunfeld, D. Kerr, E. Ritz, anad C.G. Winearls), pp. 2523–42. Oxford University Press, Oxford.

Gillenwater, J.Y. (1982). Clinical aspects of urinary tract obstruction. *Seminars in Nephrology*, **2**, 46–54.

Whittaker, R.H.L (1990). The diagnosis of upper urinary tract obstruction. *Postgraduate Medical Journal*, **66** (suppl.), 25–30.

Chapter 12.23

Urinary stone disease (urolithiasis)

R. W. E. Watts

Epidemiology

Urolithiasis is a common worldwide problem; Table 1 shows its high incidence in the UK. Many cases were previously regarded as being idiopathic when they were due to multiple small but additive risk factors. The stone recurrence rate in such cases approaches 70 per cent after 10 years.

Socio-economic development is associated with a decrease in childhood bladder stones (calcium oxalate, ammonium urate, and uric acid) and an increase in renal stone disease in adults. The composition of the diet appears to be important: high protein, high carbohydrate diets appear to increase the risk of upper urinary tract calcium oxalate stones in the relatively affluent industrial societies; and protein deprivation, increases this risk in developing regions. Stone epidemics in Europe during times of extreme deprivation after major wars have been well documented.

Urate stones predominate in some parts of the Middle East, India, and North Africa. Calcium oxalate stones are most common in some parts of South-east Asia, although ammonium urate, calcium oxalate, and calcium phosphate stones occur in all areas. Calcium oxalate or mixed calcium oxalate and calcium phosphate renal stones in adults predominate in Europe, North America, Australasia, and South Africa.

The cause of the extremely high incidence of pure calcium oxalate bladder stones in boys in northern Thailand and adjacent areas is a special case. Here the practice of partly replacing breast milk with premasticated glutinous rice (*Oryza glutinosa*) from the early neonatal period increases urinary oxalate excretion, and decreases fluid intake and urine volume and lowers urinary phosphate. Lowered urinary phosphate excretion favours calcium oxalate crystallization, and supplementing the infants' diet with orthophosphate reduces the incidence of stone formation in the young children of this region.

Industrial exposure to beryllium and cadmium are the only well-recognized industrial hazards associated with an increased incidence of urinary stone. The potassium-sparing diuretic triamterine has been reported as either the sole constituent of urinary stones or mixed with calcium oxalate. Pure triamterine stones are radiotranslucent.

Pathophysiology

Calcium-containing stones are the commonest type in the UK (Table 2). Even apparently pure calcium oxalate stones commonly contain a small central core of calcium phosphate or uric acid. Apart

Table 1 Incidence of urinary stones in the UK

Patients discharged from hospital with diagnosis of stones	1.8 per 10 000
Incidence of stones in general practice	7 per 10 000
General practice incidence of stones in males aged 45–60 years	21 per 10 000

Table 2 The composition of a series of approximately 1000 present-day renal calculi studied at the Institute of Urology, London (data kindly supplied by Dr G.A. Rose, Institute of Urology, London, England)

Type of stone	Whole sample (%)	Adult (%)	
		Males	Females
Pure calcium oxalate	39.4	47.9	22.2
Mixed calcium oxalate/phosphate	13.8	16.0	9.4
Magnesium ammonium phosphate	15.4	8.1	35.1
Stones which were virtually wholly composed of calcium and phosphate	13.2	11.3	17.8
Mixed stones containing: calcium, magnesium, ammonium, oxalate, phosphate, and uric acid	6.4	6.0	8.4
All or predominantly uric acid	8.0	8.9	1.0
Cystine	2.8	1.5	5.9
Total:	99.0	99.7	99.8

Table 3 Urinary stones: clinical presentations

Pain	Urinary tract infections
Ureteric colic	Acute (single or recurrent attack)
Lumbar ache	Chronic
On micturition	Pyonephrosis
Haematuria	Calculus anuria
Sterile pyuria	Strangury and interruption of urine stream
Asymptomatic proteinuria	
Dysuria and increased urinary frequency	

from stasis due to chronic urinary tract obstruction and infection, the main factors that predispose to stone formation are the urine volume, composition, and pH. The role of physiological inhibitors of crystallization is difficult to evaluate (see OTM3, p. 3252).

The urine of those not forming stones is in such a physicochemical state that, although crystallization of stone-forming salts will not begin spontaneously, it is likely to progress once it has been initiated. This arises because the concentrations of the ions that contribute to calcium-containing stones are such that the activity products for octacalcium phosphate, hydroxyapatite, calcium oxalate, and magnesium ammonium phosphate are between their solubility products and their formation products, or at the most only a little below their formation products. Calcium oxalate is the salt which is most likely to precipitate from normal urine on the basis of physicochemical criteria, and this agrees with the observation that calcium oxalate is the commonest constituent of urinary stones. Brushite ($CaHPO_42H_2O$) is the most likely salt to crystallize from persistently acidic urine.

Small postprandial and diurnal variations in the urinary calcium and oxalate excretions, as well as longer-term cyclic and seasonal variations occur. These can be quite small in absolute terms, but exert a marked effect on the degree of urine saturation.

Increased calcium and oxalate excretion in the summer months, with low values in the winter, are thought to reflect increased vitamin D synthesis in the skin during the summer. The diurnal variations in the degree of urine saturation due to changes in urine flow-rate, pH, and calcium and oxalate excretion, summate with seasonal factors to increase the liability to crystallization at certain times in a 24-h cycle.

Decreasing the calcium intake only may actually increase the degree of urine saturation with respect to calcium oxalate by allowing more oxalate to be absorbed and therefore excreted. This increase in the degree of urine saturation arises because the oxalate ion has a greater effect than the calcium ion on the activity product that determines the degree of urine saturation (see below).

Most calcium-containing stones are of multifactorial origin. The epidemiological risk factors include age, sex, occupation, overall nutritional status, diet, fluid intake, climate, and the presence of specific metabolic disorders. The urinary risk factors are high concentrations of calcium, oxalate, and uric acid in urine, lack of the normal diurnal rhythm of urinary pH, deficiency of crystallization-inhibiting glycosaminoglycans, and a low urine volume. Of these, the urine volume and the urinary oxalate excretion are the most important.

Genetic factors clearly play a part in the aetiology of idiopathic hypercalciuria, which is well-known to be more common in men than in women suggesting a sex-linked inherited component in its aetiology. The results of studying some unusual families in which the pattern of inheritance is very clear-cut have been rewarding from this point of view. Thus three sex-linked recessive phenotypes are associated with different mutations in the gene *GLCN-5* which maps to Xp11.22. The gene encodes a renal chloride-channel protein GLC-5. These phenotypes are: (a) Dent's disease in which hypercalciuria is associated with low-molecular weight proteinuria, other renal tubular reabsorption defects, metabolic bone disease, and progressive renal failure; (b) X-linked recessive nephrolithiasis; (c) X-linked recessive hypophosphataemic rickets. It is possible that as yet unidentified mutations in this gene may contribute to the well-known higher incidence of idiopathic hypercalciuria in men than in women.

Other genes, for example the autosomal gene (mapping to 3q21–24) which directs the calcium-sensing receptor in the parathyroid, two other autosomal recessive genes, and ROMK-1 and NKCC-2 genes which control ion transport in the thick ascending limb of Henle's loop may also contribute to the overall genetic background against which environmental factors act to produce idiopathic hypercalciuria.

Clinical diagnosis of urinary stones

Urinary stones may be either clinically silent or they may present as summarized in Table 3. Pain due to urinary stones is either a dull ache in the renal angle due to pelvicalyceal distension, or colicky and very severe, classically radiating from the loin to the groin, perineum, scrotum, or penis. An attack of ureteric colic is often associated with retching and vomiting. Stones sometimes migrate down the ureter without pain and are occasionally passed *per urethram* with little or no discomfort. A history of recurrent urinary infections, which relapse after treatment, suggests the presence of a predisposing anatomical abnormality of the urinary tract, and this is commonly a stone. Occasional patients present with fever and rigors due to infection

Table 4 Causes of generalized nephrocalcinosis

Mainly medullary (usual location)	Mainly cortical (very rare)
Primary hyperparathyroidism Idiopathic hypercalciuria Primary renal tubular acidosis Hypervitaminosis D Milk alkali syndrome Primary hyperoxaluria Sarcoidosis Chronic berylliosis Thyrotoxicosis Sulphonamide injury	Chronic glomerulo-nephritis Renal cortical necrosis ('tram-line' calcification)

proximal to an obstructing calculus. Those with impacted bilateral ureteric stones present with acute anuric renal failure.

Small stones that are voided spontaneously are generally composed of calcium oxalate. The larger calcium-containing stones usually contain appreciable amounts of phosphate. Predominantly phosphatic stones indicate past or present urinary tract infection.

Calcium oxalate stones are characteristically spiky and discoloured by altered blood, whereas phosphatic stones are generally larger, smoother, and more friable. Cystine stones are pale yellow and look crystalline. Xanthine stones are smooth, brownish yellow, and rather soft. The composition of urinary stones is markedly altered by complicating urinary infections. For example, a cystinuric patient may pass magnesium ammonium phosphate stones as well as cystine stones if there has been much infection. Similarly, the stone matrix which remains after a cystine stone has been dissolved medically may provide the basis on which a calcium oxalate stone develops subsequently.

Imaging investigations

Patients presenting with acute abdominal pain suggesting renal colic require immediate plain abdominal radiography with tomography and ultrasound examination. If these leave the diagnosis in doubt, early intravenous urography may demonstrate lesser function on the side of the lesion and/or show evidence of a filling defect or spasm of the ureter around a very small calculus. If renal function is too poor to produce a pyelogram, and ultrasound shows evidence of hydronephrosis, the obstructive lesion is well shown by percutaneous antegrade pyelography.

Uric acid, xanthine, dihydroxyadenine, and triamterine stones are characteristically radiolucent. The chemical nature of radio-opaque stones (calcium-, cystine-, and silica-containing stones) cannot be established by their radiographic appearance. The presence of multiple stones detected simultaneously, especially if they are bilateral, is generally held to indicate that they are likely to arise from a metabolic cause. Nephrocalcinosis has many causes (Table 4).

Biochemical investigations

The minimum biochemical evaluation for a patient with urolithiasis is: (a) analysis, preferably quantitative, of the stone; (b) microbiological and microscopic examination of the urine; (c) measurement of serum calcium, phosphorus, creatinine, total protein, and albumin; (d) a qualitative test for urinary cystine; (e) measurement of the pH of the first morning urine, which should be in the pH range 5.3–6.8, as a screen for possible renal tubular acidosis; and (f) measurement of the 24-h excretion of oxalate, calcium, creatinine, and uric acid with the patient ambulant and taking a usual diet and fluid intake. A dietary history may detect any gross excess of vitamin D and calcium intake.

Table 5 Final diagnosis in 708 patients with urolithiasis attending the Stone Clinic at the Institute of Urology. London (see OTM3, pp. 3254 and 3257 for source)

Cause	No. of patients	%
Idiopathic hypercalciuria	230	32.5
Chronic dehydration	132	18.6
Medullary sponge kidney	95	13.4
Urinary tract infection	52	7.3
Primary hyperparathyroidism	41	5.8
Cystinuria	28	4.0
Uric acid stones	26	3.7
High dietary oxalate	26	3.7
Renal tubular acidosis	21	3.0
Secondary hyperoxaluria	13	1.8
Primary hyperoxaluria[a]	15	2.1
Miscellaneous (immobilization, gout, Paget's disease)	29	4.1
Total	708	100

[a] This figure includes the group of patients which Embon *et al.* (1990) refer to as having mild metabolic hyperoxaluria but which may be mild variants of primary hyperoxaluria type I (alanine-glyoxylate aminotransferase (AGT: EC 2.6.1.44) deficiency). Assay of AGT on liver tissue obtained by a percutaneous needle biopsy would be needed to establish this.

Table 5 summarizes the diagnostic experience of a large stone clinic. The importance of chronic underhydration, even in a temperate climate, is apparent.

The many causes of sustained hypercalcaemia include primary hyperparathyroidism, sarcoidosis, multiple myelomatosis and other malignancies, hypervitaminosis D, and more rarely, thiazide diuretic therapy, familial hypocalciuric hypercalcaemia, thyrotoxicosis, lithium therapy, the milk alkali syndrome, Addison's disease, Cushing's syndrome, and chronic granulomatous diseases other than sarcoidosis.

Primary hyperparathyroidism and urinary stones

Primary hyperparathyroidism is responsible for 5–10 per cent of cases of calcium-containing urinary stones and about 50 per cent of patients with primary hyperparathyroidism have urolithiasis (see Chapter 7.5).

Idiopathic hypercalciuria and urinary stones

When renal stones are accompanied by high urinary calcium excretion rates and plasma calcium concentrations are normal, idiopathic hypercalciuria may be diagnosed. This is an important possible cause of urinary calculi, but there are difficulties with this diagnosis as excretion rates vary across countries; healthy young men may excrete apparently excessive amounts of calcium without forming stones; and excessive excretion of oxalate may be more commonly associated with recurrent urolithiasis than calcium. A commonly accepted upper limit of the normal level of calcium excretion is 7.5 mmol/day.

Urinary calcium excretion much over 7.5 mmol in 24 h accompanied by urinary stones is commonly treated by thiazide diuretics, which increase renal tubular reabsorption of calcium and thus reduces hypercalciuria. Amiloride also reduces urinary calcium and can be used with thiazides to reduce the likelihood of hypokalaemia. There may then be a rise in plasma calcium, but this is rarely a problem. There is also a disputed case for the use of sodium cellulose phosphate, which, by binding calcium in the gut, reduces calcium absorption; but this manoeuvre may increase urinary oxalate and may cause diarrhoea (see below). It is more important than either of these approaches to be sure of a sufficiently high fluid intake.

Medullary sponge kidney

Ectasia of the collecting tubules with enlarged renal pyramids allows small calculi to form in a characteristic pattern in this congenital disorder which may, on occasion, run in families. The condition may be unilateral, partial within a kidney and in some cases is associated with hypercalciuria and type I (distal) renal tubular acidosis. Haematuria can be macroscopic and perhaps as many as 25 per cent of cases are associated with hemihypertrophy of the limbs.

Other causes of hypercalciuria

The renal tubular dysfunction in chronic cadmium poisoning, berylliosis, and Wilson's disease may also cause normocalcaemic hypercalciuria. Although it classically causes hypercalcaemia, sarcoidosis can also be associated with normocalcaemic hypercalciuria. Hyperuricaemia, occasional aminoaciduria, and mild hypophosphataemia associated with idiopathic hypercalciuria may be attributable to renal tubular dysfunction caused by the hypercalciuria.

Intestinal disease and urinary stones

Two groups of patients with intestinal disease are predisposed to urolithiasis. Continuous loss of alkaline intestinal secretions from an ileostomy and in chronic diarrhoea makes the urine concentrated and persistently acid. This predisposes to uric acid stone formation. Malabsorption due to diffuse small intestine disease or resection leaves increased concentrations of long-chain fatty acids in the bowel lumen. These bind calcium, leaving oxalate ions available for absorption and excretion in the urine. This predisposes to hyperoxaluria and to calcium oxalate urolithiasis.

Treatment

The treatment of urinary stones has been revolutionized by the development of extracorporeal shock-wave lithotripsy and minimally invasive nephroscopic procedures. Only about 10 per cent of stone patients now require open surgery for such problems as large infected and obstructing staghorn calculi.

Ureteric stones

A ureteric stone that is causing renal colic need only be removed immediately if infection is trapped above it. Otherwise, and provided it does not cause obstruction it can be treated conservatively. Stones less than 5 mm in diameter usually pass down the ureter and can be removed or fragmented endoscopically from below. Stones that are causing obstruction should be removed without delay. If it is proposed to fragment a ureteric stone by extracorporeal lithotripsy, the stone is usually manipulated back into the renal pelvis for this procedure. Cases of ureteric stones that are being treated conservatively need regular supervision with serial abdominal radiographs, to assess migration. In the absence of obstruction it is reasonable to wait 6 weeks after stone migration ceases before intervening. A single kidney, impaired, and especially deteriorating, renal function, and bilateral ureteric stones indicate early surgical intervention. The spontaneous passage of stones is aided by maintaining a high fluid intake, sometimes augmented by short bursts of intravenous frusemide.

Pelvicalyceal stones

Single pelvicalyceal stones of diameter less than 0.5 cm do not need treatment, unless they are obstructing a calyx or are associated with infection. Those less than 2 cm in diameter not obstructing the pelvicalyceal system are suitable for extracorporeal lithotripsy alone. Those between 2 and 4 cm in diameter in a normal collecting system are also suitable for treatment by lithotripsy, provided that measures are taken to avoid obstructive complications. In these cases, a double-J ureteric stent is usually inserted preoperatively and the stone fragments then pass down the ureter around the stent. Larger calculi and those with multiple branching segments require preliminary percutaneous procedures to reduce their size ('debulking' operation). The contraindications to extracorporeal lithotripsy are: doubt about the location of the stone, calyceal stenosis, large, peripherally located stones, distal obstruction, patient morphology (weight more than 135 kg, or height less than 100 cm, skeletal deformities), uncorrectable clotting disorders, and pregnancy. Very radio-dense stones, cystine, uric acid, and rapidly growing soft stones associated with infection may all be difficult to break up with extracorporeal lithotripsy, but calcium oxalate stones and those of mixed composition usually fragment well.

The dissolution of pelvicalyceal stones by continuous irrigation, either from below or through a percutaneous nephrostomy, as a sole treatment has not gained wide acceptance, although it is used as an adjunct to extracorporeal lithotripsy and nephroscopic procedures.

Stone prevention

Biochemical causes of the stone, urinary infection, and anatomical abnormalities that obstruct the free flow of urine should be treated. All patients should drink enough to maintain a urine volume of at least 3 litres/24 h, and should check this themselves. Some of the extra fluid should be taken late at night and larger volumes are needed in tropical climates and by those who work in hot environments. It is unnecessary to specify softened water, the final urine calcium concentrations achieved with hard tap water being only slightly higher than those with calcium-free water.

Those who form uric acid stones should assess their diurnal change in urine pH by use of wide-range pH indicator papers. If they excrete persistently acid urine and do not have hyperuricaciduria, it is sufficient, in the first instance, to give enough alkali to keep the urine pH above 6. Allopurinol (100–300 mg/day) is recommended if there is proven hyperuricaciduria, or if an alkalinizing regimen fails or is inappropriate for other reasons. The degree of dietary restriction of animal protein and other purine-containing foods necessary to lower uric acid excretion greatly is unacceptable to most European patients.

Patients who have had only one calcium-containing stone, for which no cause was found, need only be advised to maintain a high rate of urine flow, to avoid self-medication with vitamins D and C and calcium-containing antacids, and to avoid more than average

Table 6 Dietary management of patients with recurrent calcium-containing stones

Fluid intake	Sufficient to produce 3 litres of urine divided approximately uniformly over the 24-h period. Tap water is satisfactory. Increase fluid intake in hot environments. Check 24-h urine volume
Calcium	Reduce milk intake to 300 ml or less per day. This also reduces lactose intake. Omit cheese and yoghurt. Aim at an approximate 17.5 mmol (700 mg)/day calcium intake
Oxalate	Restrict intake because a low calcium diet increases oxalate absorption and excretion; urinary oxalate is a major risk factor for urolithiasis. Omit rhubarb, spinach, beans, beetroot, strawberries, nuts, chocolate, cocoa, and tea (or limit to 2 cups/day)
Fruits and fruit juices	Omit those that are rich in vitamin C (an oxalate precursor). These are oranges, lemons, grapefruit, limes, and blackcurrant syrup
Protein	Limit lean meat to 225 g (approximately 0.5 lb)/day.
Carbohydrate	Sufficient for estimated calorie needs
Fibre	Include high-fibre foods
Salt	Reduce dietary sodium chloride if urinary sodium >250 mmol/24 h
Vitamin preparations	Omit vitamin D (promotes calcium absorption); omit vitamin C (oxalate precursor)
Pharmaceuticals	Omit any that are calcium salts, or which contain calcium salts, unless they are essential for the treatment of another disease. Examples are: calcium aspirin and many antacid preparations, including aluminium hydroxide preparations

intakes of dairy products and oxalate-rich beverages and fruits. The principles of the dietary management of patients with recurrent stones containing calcium salts are summarized in Table 6.

Orthophosphates and magnesium oxide (or hydroxide) have been used as non-specific inhibitors of crystallization when stones recur in spite of apparently adequate treatment, or when no more specific treatment is available. A dose equivalent to between about 1 and 2 g of elemental phosphorus per day is given in effervescent tablets (Phosphate-Sandoz®). The dose of magnesium ions should be sufficient (for example, 200 mg magnesium oxide daily) materially to increase the urinary magnesium excretion. Hypocitraturia has been identified as an aetiological factor in some cases of urolithiasis. The administration of potassium citrate or mixed citrate preparations in large doses (for example, potassium citrate equivalent to 60 mmol potassium/day) is sometimes helpful especially where alkalinization as well as the calcium complexing power of the citrate ion is desired.

Further reading

Bolino, A., Devoto, N., Enia, G., Zoccali, C., Weissenbach, J., and Romeo, G. (1993). Genetic mapping in the XP11.2 region of a new form of X-linked recessive hypophosphataemic rickets. *European Journal of Human Genetics*, 1, 269–79.

Fromyer, P.A., Sheinman, S.J., Dunham, P.B., Jones, D.B., Hueber, P., and Schröder, S. T. (1991). X-linked recessive nephrolosiasis with renal failure. *New England Journal of Medicine*, **325**, 681–6.

Hebert, S.C. (1996). Critical-clear chloride channels. *Nature*, **379**, 398–9.

Lloyd, S.E., Pearce, S.H.S., Fisher, S.E., *et al.* (1996). A common metabolic basis for three inherited kidney stone diseases. *Nature*, **379**, 445–449.

Lloyd, S.E., Pearce, S.H.S., Günther, W., Kawaguchi, H., Jentsch, T.J., and Thacker, R.V. (1997). Idiopathic low molecular proteinuria associated with hypercalciuric, nephrocalcinosis in Japanese children is due to mutations of the renal chloride channel (GLCN-5), *Journal of Clinical Investigation*, **99**, 967–74.

Pearce, S.M.S. (1998). Straightening out the renal tubule. *Quarterly Journal of Medicine*, **91**, 5–12.

Pearce, S.M.S., Trump, D., Wording, C., *et al.* (1995). Calcium-sensing receptor mutations in familial benign hypercalciuria and neonatal hyperparathyroidism. *Journal of Clinical Investigation*, **96**, 2681–92.

Watts, R.W.E. (1998). Aetiological factors in stone formation. In *Oxford textbook of clinical nephrology*, (ed. A.M. Davison, J.S. Cameron, J.-P. Grünfeld, D.N.S. Carr, E. Ritz, and C.G. Winearls), (2nd edn), pp. 1317–41. Oxford University Press, Oxford.

Wrong, O.M., Noorden, A.G.H., and Feest, T.G. (1994). Dent's disease: a familial proximal renal tubular syndrome with low molecular weight proteinuria, hypercalciuria, nephrocalcinosis, metabolic bone disease, progressive renal failure and a marked male predominance. *Quarterly Journal of Medicine*, **87**, 473–93.

Chapter 12.24

Hypertension: its effects on the kidney

*A. E. G. Raine**

Hypertension is common in patients with renal failure, and the reasons for this are discussed in Chapter 2.32. The aim here is to consider in which circumstances hypertension may itself cause significant renal impairment.

Renal function in hypertension

As well as a rightward resetting of the pressure natriuresis relationship (Fig. 1) (see OTM3, pp. 1347–8), a number of alterations in renal haemodynamics also take place in established uncomplicated essential hypertension. Renal blood flow is reduced and renal vascular resistance is increased. Glomerular filtration rate remains normal, and consequently filtration fraction (the ratio of glomerular filtration rate to renal plasma flow) is increased. Although increased vascular resistance in all tissue beds is general in hypertension, in the case of the kidney it assumes particular significance. The glomerulus is unique in having a portal arterial circulation, with a balanced increase in resistance of both the afferent and efferent arterioles in hypertension, so that glomerular capillary hydraulic pressure (P_{GC}), the major determinant of glomerular filtration rate, is maintained at a normal level (Fig. 2). The rarity of significant renal impairment in essential hypertension (see below) suggests that an increase in afferent arteriolar resistance shields the kidney from the damaging effects of high systemic arterial

*It is with regret that we report the death of Professor A.E.G. Raine. His chapter in OTM3 has been abbreviated by Professor J.G.G. Ledingham.

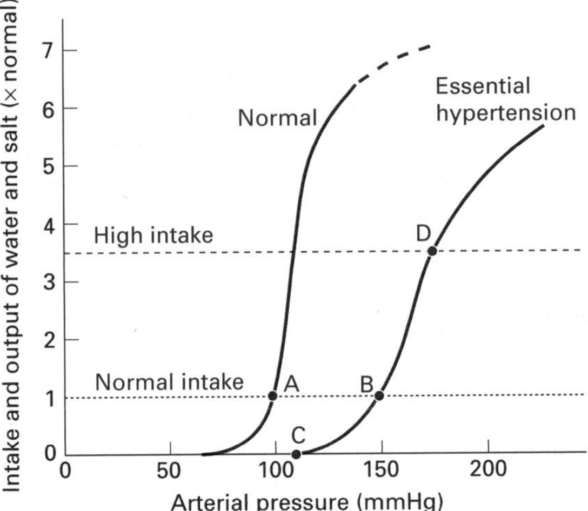

Fig. 1 Renal function curves illustrating the normal pressure natriuresis relationship and resetting of the relationship in essential hypertension. (A) Arterial pressure at which sodium balance is maintained in a normal subject. (B) Corresponding arterial pressure in hypertension.
(Reproduced from Guyton et al. 1972, with permission.)

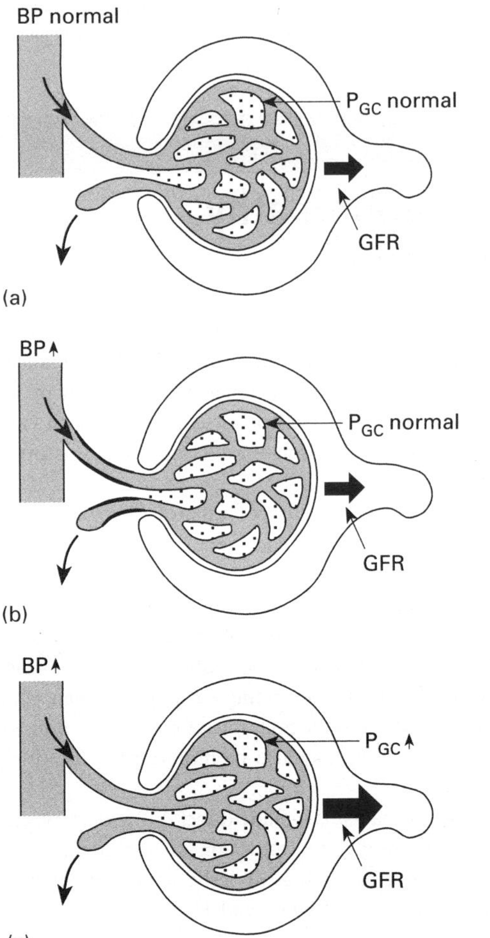

Fig. 2 Representation of glomerular haemodynamics: (a) normal; (b) essential hypertension, afferent and efferent arteriolar resistances are increased, P_{GC} (glomerular capillary hydraulic pressure) and GFR (glomerular filtration rate) remain normal; and (c) chronic renal failure (surviving nephron), systemic hypertension is transmitted to the glomerulus, P_{GC} and GFR are increased.

pressure, while a simultaneous increase in efferent arteriolar resistance enables maintenance of normal glomerular filtration pressure.

Hypertension as a cause of renal failure

Essential hypertension

Significant renal dysfunction is very rare in uncomplicated essential hypertension. Estimates in Caucasian populations have suggested that the relative risk of developing renal failure in primary hypertension is of the order of 1 in 6000 cases. The true incidence is probably even lower; many patients who present with severe renal failure and hypertension and are given a diagnosis of 'hypertensive nephrosclerosis' do not undergo histological examination by renal biopsy to exclude an underlying primary renal disease such as glomerulonephritis.

Hypertension appears to lead to progressive renal impairment much more frequently in patients of African or Afro-Caribbean origin. Some American surveys suggest that the relative risk of end-stage renal failure due to hypertension in these patients is 18 times that of Caucasians. This racial difference in morbidity persists even when equal and adequate blood pressure control is achieved, implying the existence of genetic or environmental factors to account for it.

Both hypertension and a gradual and relatively modest decline in renal function due to glomerulosclerosis are common accompaniments of ageing. The microscopic appearances of the kidney in the elderly are very similar to those of 'hypertensive' nephrosclerosis, with renal vascular changes including medial hypertrophy and reduplication of the internal elastic lamina. Hypertension is a major risk factor for both large-vessel and microvascular atherosclerotic disease. It appears likely that, in the elderly, essential hypertension sustained over many years results in significant atherosclerotic narrowing of intrarenal small vessels, and an ischaemic nephropathy with an increased rate of glomerulosclerosis. Bilateral renal artery stenosis is another cause of renal failure in essential hypertension.

Accelerated hypertension

In accelerated phase (malignant) hypertension, renal involvement is very common. Seventy-three of a series of 89 patients documented in the 1950s had impaired renal function at presentation, and uraemia was by far the commonest cause of death. The changes in the optic fundi in accelerated hypertension are due to loss of retinal vessel autoregulation, and resultant overperfusion and increase in transmural pressure. Endothelial integrity is lost in dilated segments of arterioles, with leakage of plasma constituents and fibrin deposition in vessel walls, forming the characteristic 'fibrinoid necrosis'. Such changes result in ischaemic and hyperperfusion damage in the territory served by affected vessels. Similar changes are likely to occur in the renal vasculature, leading to the fibrinoid necrosis seen in afferent arterioles and the glomerular tuft in accelerated hypertension. The other characteristic pathological change observed is a proliferative endarteritis of interlobular arteries (Fig. 3). The resulting narrowing or obliteration of the arterial lumen causes both glomerular and tubulointerstitial ischaemia and fibrosis, with resulting loss of renal function.

Effective treatment combined with dialysis if required, has transformed the previously bleak outlook for this condition. The goal is a gradual reduction in blood pressure to a level of 160 to 170/100 to 110 mmHg over a 24-h period, to avoid the risk of cerebral ischaemia. This is often best achieved with an intravenous infusion of sodium nitroprusside (0.5–3.0 μg/kg per min) or of labetalol (2 mg/min),

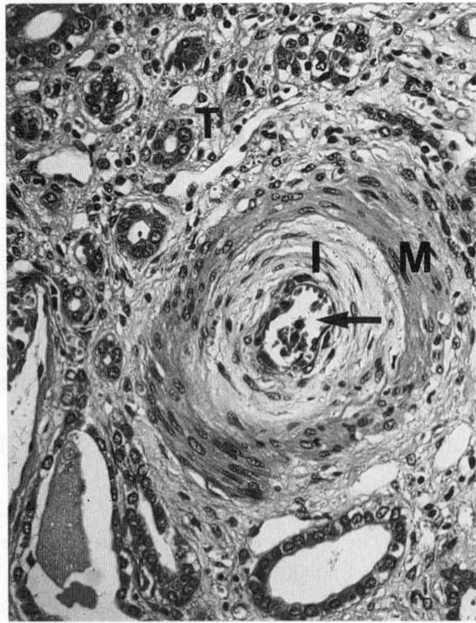

Fig. 3 Proliferative endarteritis of an interlobular artery in malignant hypertension. The arrow shows a severely narrowed arterial lumen: I, arterial intima with gross proliferative change and 'onion-skin' appearance; M, arterial media; T, tubulointerstitial fibrosis.
(By courtesy of Dr A.J. d'Ardenne.)

although oral agents such as calcium-channel blockers have proved equally safe and effective. The long-term outlook for recovery of renal function is good if serum creatinine is 300 µmol/l or less at presentation, but patients with more marked initial renal impairment often progress to end-stage renal failure, despite adequate blood pressure control.

Hypertension and progressive renal impairment

Uncontrolled hypertension in chronic renal failure accelerates the rate of loss of renal function. Reduction in the number of functioning nephrons, by whatever disease process, is suggested to lead to adaptive alterations in renal vascular resistance, resulting in increased blood flow and transmission of systemic hypertension to the glomerulus in surviving nephrons. The resulting glomerular capillary hypertension and hyperperfusion might then lead to increased proteinuria and ultimately to glomerular scarring. Micropuncture studies in animal models of diabetic nephropathy and renal ablation nephropathy have shown that increases in systemic blood pressure are transmitted to the glomerulus and result in increased transcapillary hydraulic pressure and glomerular hyperfiltration.

Other changes, such as glomerular hypertrophy and elaboration of growth factors within the glomerular mesangium, may play a part as important as glomerular hypertension. Large-scale, controlled studies of mild and moderate hypertension have not been able to demonstrate any beneficial effect of treatment on renal function, as there is such a low incidence of renal dysfunction in essential hypertension other than in the malignant phase. The most convincing clinical evidence has come from trials of antihypertensive therapy in patients with diabetic nephropathy. In patients with type 1 diabetes, the worsening of both incipient nephropathy with 'microalbuminuria' and of established diabetic nephropathy with renal impairment appear to be retarded by effective antihypertensive therapy.

Benefit has been particularly suggested (but not proven) for converting enzyme inhibitors, relating to the ability of these agents to blunt angiotensin II-mediated efferent arteriolar constriction, thus reducing glomerular capillary pressure. There are now sufficient grounds to recommend that in all patients with progressive renal dysfunction, the aim should be to reduce arterial pressure to less than 140/90 mmHg. Converting enzyme inhibitors may confer a particular benefit, although this is by no means proven, and caution with these agents is required in the presence of known or suspected renovascular disease.

Further reading

Brazy, P.C., Stead, W.W., and Fitzwilliam, J.F. (1989). Progression of renal insufficiency, role of blood pressure. *Kidney International*, **35**, 670–4.

Case records of the Massachusetts General Hospital. (1996). A 60-year-old man with progressive renal failure and the abrupt onset of dyspnoea. *New England Journal of Medicine*, **374**, 973–9.

Isles, C.G., Robertson, S., and Hill, D. (1999). Management of renovascular disease: a review of renal artery stenting in 10 studies. *Quarterly Journal of Medicine*, **92**, 159–67.

Mann, J.F.E., Allenberg, J., and Luft, F.C. (1998). In: *Oxford textbook of clinical nephrology*, (2nd edn) (ed. A.M. Davison, J.S. Cameron, J.-P. Grünfeld, D. Kerr, E. Ritz, and C.G. Winearls), pp. 1467–88. Oxford University Press, Oxford.

Wilcox, C.S. (1993). Angiotensin converting enzyme inhibitors for diagnosing renovascular hypertension. *Kidney International*, **44**, 1379–90.

Chapter 12.25

Toxic nephropathy

B. T. Emmerson

This term refers to any adverse alteration in renal structure or function caused by an exogenous agent. Conventionally excluded are renal damage due to agents causing renal hypoperfusion or intratubular obstruction. Analgesic nephropathy, together with renal manifestations of toxicity of non-steroid anti-inflammatory drugs are discussed in Chapter 12.20.

Many cases of renal failure of unknown origin may have been caused by a drug or other toxic agent, but detection is difficult and precise prevalence is, therefore, unknown; in developed countries, toxic renal damage may be seen in up to 3 per cent of hospital inpatients, and up to 20 per cent of those undergoing intensive care.

The kidney is particularly susceptible to the ill effects of toxins because of its function in excreting such agents, their concentration in the renal medulla and the high rate of renal blood flow. Glomerular structure and function may also be important in localising immune complexes (Fig. 1).

Pathogenic mechanisms include direct cytotoxicity where the effect is proportional to the concentration of the toxin and immuno-mediated mechanisms, such as underlie acute interstitial nephritis or glomerulonephritis (see Table 1 and Fig. 1)

Renal tubular dysfunction

This results from toxic damage mild enough only to impair function rather than cause tubular cell death. The effects include: (a) the Fanconi syndrome, showing as glycosuria, aminoaciduria, and phosphaturia, seen most frequently in some acute metal nephropathies;

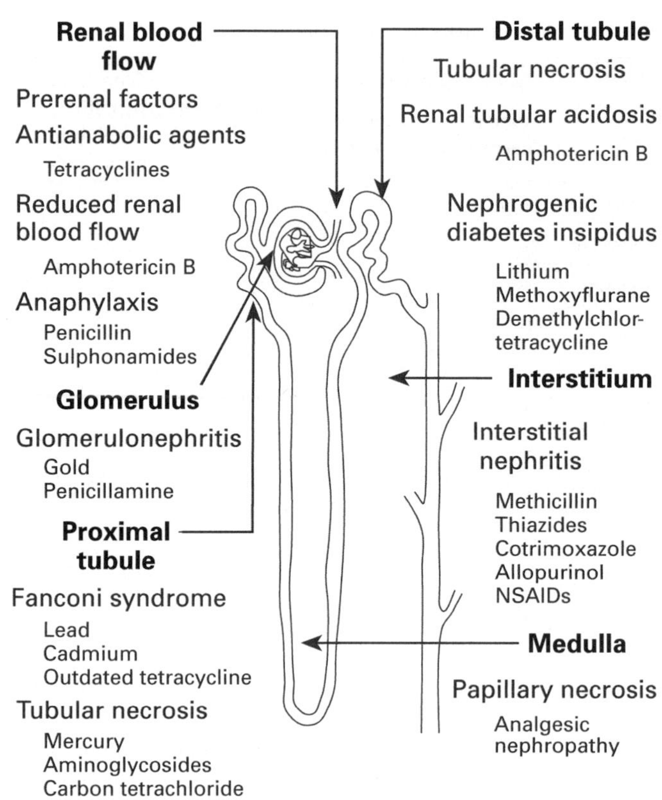

Fig. 1 Mechanisms of nephrotoxicity and representative factors involved in the pathogenesis of toxic renal damage affecting various parts of the nephron.

Table 1 Pathogenetic mechanisms of toxic renal damage

	Syndrome	Example
Direct cytotoxin mediated		
Tubular dysfunction	Proximal: Fanconi syndrome	Acute lead
	Distal: Nephrogenic diabetes insipidus	Lithium
	Renal tubular acidosis	Amphotericin B
Acute tubular necrosis	Acute renal failure	Mercury
Chronic nephron damage	Chronic renal failure	Lead
Immunologically mediated		
Immunoallergic	Acute interstitial nephritis	Methicillin
Immune complex	Membranous glomerulopathy	Penicillamine
Cell-mediated	Minimal change nephropathy with nephrotic syndrome	Non-steroidal anti-inflammatory drugs
Hypersensitivity	Vasculitis	Sulphonamides

(b) impairment of concentrating capacity leading in severe cases to nephrogenic diabetes insipidus, which can result from toxicity from lithium, fluoride, and demethylchlortetracyline; (c) renal tubular acidosis, typically resulting from treatment with amphotericin B.

Table 2 Some major drugs causing immune-mediated acute interstitial nephritis (This list is not comprehensive and a large number of drugs can infrequently cause this response)

• Analgesics	• Antibacterial agents
• Non-steroidal anti-inflammatory agents (especially fenoprofen)	• β-Lactams
	• Methicillin
	• Ampicillin
	• Penicillin
• Others	• Cephalothin
• Allopurinol	• Sulphonamides
• Sulphinpyrazone	• Co-trimoxazole
• Phenindione	• Rifampicin and ethambutol
• Cimetidine	• Diuretics
• Captopril	• Thiazides
• Phenytoin	• Furosemide
• Glafenine	

Acute renal toxicity

In its mildest form, only slight proteinuria with increased cell excretion in the urine may be found, associated with some degree of nitrogen retention and possibly oliguria. In its most severe form, the pattern will be that of acute tubular necrosis with the early development of oliguria and cessation of renal excretory function. Such tubular necrosis is potentially reversible after removal of the causative agent unless the damage has been extreme. A typical example is that seen with the aminoglycoside antimicrobials.

Acute interstitial nephritis

This syndrome presents with deterioration of renal function which develops some days or weeks after exposure to the causative agent. The renal failure is usually non-oliguric. Haematuria and proteinuria are usual, together with systemic manifestations, including fever, arthralgia, rash, eosinophilia, elevated IgE concentrations, and sometimes abnormal liver function. The diagnosis is supported by the demonstration of eosinophilic leucocytes in the urine, but a renal biopsy may be needed to establish the diagnosis. Mostly, the renal insufficiency is of moderate degree and remission occurs when the causative agent is withdrawn. However, continuing exposure can cause the acute insufficiency to develop into chronic renal impairment. If the renal insufficiency has not begun to reverse within a week of withdrawal of the cause, steroid therapy should be considered and has usually appeared to hasten remission. Over 50 drugs have been associated, including penicillins, diuretics, antiepileptic drugs, allopurinol, and non-steroidal anti-inflammatory drugs (Table 2).

Chronic renal failure

Chronic renal failure of toxic origin has few clinical features to distinguish it from other causes of renal damage. Lead is a model and, in this case, there is a slowly progressive deterioration of renal function over many years, even in the absence of continuing exposure to the underlying toxin. In other cases, hypertension with associated vascular disease may be an important contributor to progression.

Glomerulonephritis

An immune-mediated response to an exogenous toxin may be clinically indistinguishable from other varieties of glomerulonephritis, with insidious proteinuria, haematuria, and nitrogen retention. Sufficient proteinuria may lead to a nephrotic syndrome, usually due to a membranous or minimal change nephropathy. Sometimes an autoimmune process is operating and in others a hypersensitivity vasculitis may be seen. Typical examples of this type of nephrotoxicity occur with penicillamine, gold, and trimethadione, and with certain exogenous poisons, including some snake venoms.

Detection

It is difficult to define early markers of nephrotoxicity. Nitrogen retention may be a relatively late manifestation and abnormalities appearing on microscopy with haematuria and/or proteinuria are relatively non-specific. Increased urinary eosinophils may be found in at least 50 per cent of cases of acute interstitial nephritis. Determination of whether proteinuria is glomerular or tubular (low molecular weight) may prove useful in localizing the site of injury. Urinary excretion of *N*-acetylglucosaminidase as a marker of lysosomal enzyme loss from tubular epithelial cells shows potential as an indicator of tubular cell damage, but its clinical value as a predictor has yet to be established. Acutely affected kidneys are usually enlarged radiologically.

Specific syndromes

Metal nephropathies

The spectrum of renal responses to metal intoxication depends upon the acuteness, severity, and duration of exposure, upon the mechanism of toxicity of the particular metal or its salt, and the responses of the host, particularly the immune mechanisms. Any of the clinical syndromes can occur, although acute interstitial nephritis is less common (Table 3). Demonstrating an aetiological association between the metal toxicity and the later development of chronic renal disease may require extensive epidemiological studies.

Table 3 Features of metal nephrotoxicity

Metal	Acute nephropathy		Chronic interstitial nephropathy	Glomerulo-nephritis /nephrotic syndrome
	Tubular necrosis	Fanconi syndrome		
Lead	+	+		+0
Cadmium	+	+		+0
Mercury	+	0		?+
Gold	0	0		++
Lithium	+	−		++
Platinum	+	+		+−
Germanium	+	−		+−
Uranium	+	+		+0
Copper	+	+		+0
Bismuth	+	+		+0
Thallium	+	0		0+

Lead (see also Chapter 18.1)

Acute toxicity usually interferes principally with proximal tubular function, leading to glycosuria and aminoaciduria. This probably reflects damage to brush-border membranes and may be associated with enzyme loss in the urine. Nitrogen retention can occur but it is rarely severe enough to cause acute renal failure. Intranuclear eosinophilic inclusion bodies (which consist of a lead–protein complex) are seen in proximal tubular cells which can often be demonstrated in the urine. Mitochondrial function is also affected. This nephrotoxicity is potentially reversible, either with removal from exposure or following treatment with a chelating agent such as calcium ethylene diaminetetraacetic acid (EDTA) in a dose of 1 g/day in 5-day courses until the toxicity has remitted. The symptoms of acute lead intoxication are often vague and may include intestinal colic, peripheral neuritis, and anaemia. Porphyrin synthesis will usually be disordered and will result in coproporphyrinuria and an increased urinary excretion of δ-aminolaevulinic acid. *Chronic* lead nephropathy leads to a reduced number of functioning nephrons and the pattern of a granular contracted kidney, principally with tubulointerstitial disease.

In Queensland, Australia, acute childhood lead poisoning, from the ingestion of powdered and flaking paint, was common until lead paint was made illegal in 1930. Follow-up revealed a high prevalence of granular contracted kidneys. The criteria for diagnosis included the presence of uniform and equal contraction of both kidneys; long-standing chronic renal disease; exclusion of an alternative cause; and evidence of excessive past lead absorption, usually provided by increased lead stores in bone or by the presence of an increased excretion of lead in urine after a standardized dose of calcium-EDTA. Affected patients showed disproportionate hyperuricaemia, and half developed gouty arthritis, resulting from excessive reabsorption or urate in the proximal tubule. Moderate hypertension was also a feature.

A similar pattern was seen in 'moonshine' drinkers in the southern United States using illicit stills with lead condensers but they also showed features of continuing lead intoxication with raised tissue lead concentrations and abnormal porphyrin metabolism.

Prolonged industrial exposure to lead with resultant intoxication is still seen in developing countries. Clear proof of an aetiology for renal disease is difficult, because of the varying degrees of exposure and absorption, and of the variety of individual responses. Exposure needs to be fairly heavy and to continue for years.

The management of chronic lead nephropathy is that of chronic renal failure from whatever cause. The rate of progression is normally slow and proteinuria is never severe. Unless there are signs of acute lead intoxication, no benefit to renal function can be obtained at this time from therapy with EDTA.

Cadmium (see OTM3, Section 8)

Exposure to cadmium induces the production of a cysteine-rich protein, metallothionein, which binds the metal in a non-toxic form. The toxic unbound cadmium initially affects renal cell membrane function and later intracellular organelles, resulting in cell necrosis.

Cadmium can be absorbed from either the respiratory or the alimentary tract. Although *acute* nephrotoxicity is rare because absorption is usually limited by the acute respiratory toxicity, renal tubular and cortical necrosis can occur. *Chronic* cadmium nephrotoxicity can result from prolonged low-grade exposure both in cadmium workers and in a population whose food and water has a high cadmium content because of environmental contamination. The early adverse effects on the kidney show principally as tubular dysfunction, with generalized aminoaciduria, glycosuria, and phosphaturia, as well as by a reduction in concentrating ability and acid excretion. A distinctive feature is the excretion of 'tubular' proteins of low molecular weight ranging between 20 000 and 40 000. These consist principally of β_2-microglobulin and retinol-binding proteins but can also include mucoproteins and enzyme proteins. Albuminuria of glomerular origin may also be present. This type of renal damage appears to be progressive and not reversible, even after removal from further exposure.

Another feature of chronic cadmium nephropathy is the association with hypercalciuria and hyperphosphaturia, which increase the risk of renal calculi and also of osteomalacia. This type of painful osteomalacia is the basis for '*itai-itai*' or 'ouch-ouch' disease which occurs in Japanese populations who live in regions heavily contaminated with cadmium. The pathology is that of a chronic tubulointerstitial nephritis, somewhat similar to that due to lead, but associated with hypercalciuria and tubular proteinuria without disproportionate hyperuricaemia and gout.

Chelating agents have not been shown to be of value in this situation and removal from further exposure as soon as possible after toxicity is detected is the only course of action. The effects of the renal tubular acidosis and altered tubular functions can be corrected by appropriate specific supplements (for example, sodium bicarbonate).

Mercury (see OTM3, pp. 1105–15)

Nephrotoxicity involves an inhibition of membrane function, particularly of the brush-border membrane of the renal tubules, by interfering with reactive sulphydryl groups. High tissue concentrations of sulphydryl-containing compounds such as glutathione and cysteine may be protective against toxicity. Ultimately, mercury can interfere with the functions of the mitochondrial membrane and of sulphhydryl-containing enzyme systems.

Mercury can be absorbed by inhalation, via the mucous membrane, or skin. Most exposure is now either accidental or industrial, although Minamata disease (from eating mercury-contaminated fish) once common in Japan has now re-emerged in the Amazon region. Acute mercurial poisoning usually causes acute oliguric renal failure. Early manifestations include proteinuria with cellular casts. Regeneration of tubules may occur if damage is not too severe, but calcification of necrotic proximal tubules occurs more frequently with mercury than in other metal nephropathies. Although there are claims that mercury can produce a chronic interstitial nephropathy, most evidence suggests that this reflects residual damage after the acute tubular necrosis.

There is increasing evidence that mercury can produce an immune-complex type of glomerulonephritis, a reaction to a self-antigen modified by metal toxicity. The histological picture is usually a membranous glomerulonephritis. The level of proteinuria may vary widely and a full nephrotic syndrome may develop. Removal from exposure may allow a lessening of this proteinuria. Heavy environmental contamination with organic mercurials at Minimata Bay in Japan, although causing principally neurological features, was associated with a low molecular weight proteinuria, thought to reflect early renal damage.

Gold

Most toxic reactions to gold occur during the therapeutic administration of gold salts to patients with rheumatoid arthritis. Gold accumulates in the kidneys, initially in the proximal tubular cells and later in the distal tubule and interstitial macrophages, where it may persist for up to 30 years. Toxic reactions may involve the skin, the bone marrow, or the kidney in varying combinations, and the kidneys are not always involved. Acute tubular necrosis is rarely, if ever, seen with therapeutic doses and the first manifestation is usually mild proteinuria or microhaematuria, which may occur in up to 30 per cent of treated patients and may be severe enough to induce the nephrotic syndrome in about 2 per cent. Proteinuria and glomerulopathy may develop at any stage of gold treatment, even as late as 2 years.

Within a few months of stopping gold therapy, the proteinuria begins to remit and has usually subsided completely within 2–3 years. Steroid therapy is indicated only rarely. After remission, there has usually been no further deterioration of renal glomerular function. There is an increased association of renal damage in patients with HLA-B8 and DR3 antigens. Renal histopathology has usually shown a membranous glomerulonephritis with subepithelial deposits of immune complexes, sometimes containing IgG and complement. Gold is usually absent from the glomerular lesions. In a few cases the lesions may be of a minimal change, with mesangial-dense deposits, or without any morphological glomerular change.

Lithium

Lithium is eliminated from the body almost entirely by the kidney, being filtered at the glomerulus and reabsorbed in the proximal tubule, resulting in a clearance of one-third of that of creatinine. Its principal toxicity relates to distal tubular function by inhibition of adenylate cyclase and generation of cyclic adenosine monophosphate, leading to polyuria and, if sufficiently severe, to nephrogenic diabetes insipidus. Ultimately this can lead to tubular loss with scarring. Sufficiently severe acute toxicity can affect the proximal tubule to cause acute tubular necrosis.

Even during careful control of dosage and of serum concentrations, a number of patients show defective renal concentrating capacity with polyuria and polydipsia unresponsive to vasopressin. This effect is concentration dependent and reversible. Patients who develop polyuria should not be allowed to become salt depleted because this results in increased proximal tubular reabsorption of lithium. Acute toxicity is most commonly precipitated by diarrhoea or vomiting, or the unwise use of diuretic agents which should only be prescribed in those taking lithium with the greatest circumspection. The addition of indomethacin, or the withdrawal of phenothiazines, may also increase the serum lithium concentration. Occasional patients with serum lithium concentrations in the normal range may develop a nephrotic syndrome with minimal glomerular changes which remits on cessation of the lithium. Chronic low-grade intoxication appears to be associated with chronic renal impairment with focal atrophy of nephrons, tubular dilatation, and interstitial fibrosis. Haemodialysis is the most effective means of removing lithium during intoxication, particularly if there is associated oliguria.

Platinum

Cisplatin causes a characteristic dose-related nephrotoxic reaction. Doses of 20 mg/m^2 per day for 5 days usually produce no nephrotoxicity, while high-dose therapy at twice this level usually causes depression of renal function, sometimes for up to 2 years. Minor renal dysfunction can show as aminoaciduria and tubular proteinuria. The distal parts of the proximal tubule and the distal nephron are principally affected. Reversible azotaemia occurs in up to one-third of patients, and occasionally renal failure is irreversible. Sodium and water reabsorption in both proximal and distal tubules may be depressed for up to 6 months after a course of treatment. Increased renal losses of potassium may also occur as can chronic renal disease of the tubulointerstitial type.

Partial protection against the nephrotoxic effect of cisplatin is provided by a mannitol and saline diuresis, attributable to a reduced duration of exposure of the tubules to toxic concentrations. There is some evidence that sodium thiosulphate and other SH-containing compounds may be protective. The newer platinum compounds, such as carboplatin, appear to be less nephrotoxic.

Germanium

Inorganic germanium is increasingly consumed in high doses as a tonic, particularly in Japan. Sufficient rapid accumulation can lead to acute renal failure, while prolonged low-grade intake can result in chronic impairment of renal function without proteinuria or haematuria. The histological pattern is of vacuolar degeneration, particularly affecting the distal tubules, with interstitial fibrosis and minor glomerular abnormalities. When consumption is stopped, there may be a gradual improvement in renal function.

Antimicrobial and chemotherapeutic agents

Aminoglycosides

Gentamicin produces dose-related acute renal failure in a significant percentage (average 10 per cent) of all subjects to whom it is administered. It is cationic and hydrophilic and is accumulated within the proximal tubular cells by endocytosis. Its potential to bind anionic phospholipids in the liposomal membrane can then lead to necrosis of the proximal convoluted tubules. One of the first clinical manifestations is the presence of non-oliguric renal failure with elevation of the serum creatinine concentration. Impaired urine concentrating ability will be present and enzymuria with *N*-acetylglucosaminidase, proteinuria with β_2-microglobulin, and lysozymuria may be observed. However, these do not invariably precede or predict the later development of renal failure. The associated renal failure is potentially reversible, depending upon the extent of the tubular damage and other complicating factors. In some cases, recovery may be slow and incomplete. The risk of renal damage may be increased by associated treatment with diuretics or cephalosporins, and any toxicity is potentiated by increasing age, pre-existing cardiac or renal failure or ischaemia, and the presence of endotoxinaemia.

Tobramycin has less potential for nephrotoxicity. Other more toxic aminoglycosides, neomycin and kanamycin, are no longer used.

Penicillins

Almost all of the penicillin group have the potential to induce an acute interstitial nephritis. This occurred in up to 20 per cent of patients during methicillin therapy. Nephropathy usually presents with a steadily developing renal insufficiency, coming on some days after the beginning of treatment, usually associated with haematuria, and sometimes with fever, eosinophilia, and a rash. Eosinophils can often be found in the urine and the histological picture is typical of an acute interstitial nephritis. The mechanism is thought to involve an immune response to an antigen–protein complex, caused either by the coupling of the penicilloyl hapten to an intrinsic renal protein or by the development of antibodies to tubular basement membrane. Subsequent exposure to another penicillin derivative often results in a recurrence of the syndrome. With removal of the cause the condition usually settles. If there is delay in resolution, or if the patient becomes severely ill, prednisone seems to speed resolution significantly.

Cephalosporins

The cephalosporins are rapidly excreted by secretory mechanisms within the proximal convoluted tubule. Accumulation in the cortex and any associated toxicity can be inhibited by probenecid and other inhibitors of tubular transport. Cephaloridine has dose-dependent nephrotoxicity and should no longer be used. The second- and third-generation cephalosporins have minimal nephrotoxicity, although there are a few reports of acute interstitial nephritis associated with their use. Nephrotoxicity is frequently reported during combined therapy with cephalosporins and the aminoglycosides. Seriously ill patients with pre-existing renal disease who are dehydrated with a contracted plasma volume are particularly susceptible, especially if exposed to high concentrations of antimicrobials for more than a few days.

Sulphonamides

Crystal nephropathy is now rare and the main renal complications from these drugs are allergic. These usually manifest either as an acute interstitial nephritis, as an immune-complex glomerulonephritis, or as a necrotizing angiitis. Such reactions are particularly likely to be associated with the long-acting sulphonamides. Co-trimoxazole (trimethoprim–sulphamethoxazole) can also cause these reactions but they are uncommon in patients with normal renal function. The dose should be reduced in the presence of renal insufficiency.

Tetracycline

Tetracycline increases urea production by inhibiting the utilization of amino acids for protein synthesis. This becomes a problem only in patients with pre-existing renal insufficiency in whom the excretion of tetracycline is delayed and its protein catabolic effect intensified. Its use is also associated with an increase in salt and water excretion which, in patients with pre-existing renal insufficiency, can lead to weight loss, acidosis, and deterioration of renal function. Doxycycline, which has only a slight antianabolic effect, does not have such adverse effects.

Outdated or deteriorated tetracycline has caused toxic tubular damage with a reversible Fanconi syndrome and a marked renal tubular acidosis with hypocalcaemia and hypouricaemia. Proteinuria, glycosuria, phosphaturia, and aminoaciduria have also been reported.

Demethylchlortetracycline (demeclocycline) can impair renal concentrating ability and induce nephrogenic diabetes insipidus. This is reversible and dose related and is sometimes used in the treatment of the chronic syndrome of inappropriate secretion of antidiuretic hormone.

Antituberculous agents

Rifampicin may induce immune-mediated renal insufficiency, with associated influenza-like symptoms of chills, malaise, vomiting, and fever. This syndrome has often developed when recommencing therapy after a prior course of the drug. Anti-rifampicin antibodies have been found in the serum of many affected patients but not in all and similar antibodies have been demonstrated in the serum of patients who do not have such complications. It seems likely that a critical level of antigen–antibody complex is needed to induce the syndrome, and this tends particularly to occur when therapy is intermittent. Some patients have shown immunoglobulin deposits around the renal tubules, while some have had a positive Coombs test and others a positive macrophage migration inhibition reaction. The usual lesion is an acute interstitial nephritis, although it has a number of unusual features.

Ethambutol may be associated with acute renal failure which subsides after withdrawal of the drug, only to leave persistent impairment of renal function in some patients. The pattern is that of an acute interstitial nephritis. Rarely, *p*-aminosalicylate may also be associated with an acute interstitial nephritis with allergic skin lesions.

Amphotericin B

This drug affects the permeability of cellular membranes, particularly the luminal membrane of the tubular epithelium, resulting in a failure of hydrogen ion excretion and an increased urinary loss of potassium. Proximal tubular damage may be reflected by phosphaturia and uricosuria, and impairment of renal concentrating power which may be sufficient to give a nephrogenic diabetes insipidus. The glomerular filtration rate falls, roughly in proportion to the dose of amphotericin B, and some renal vasoconstriction has been postulated. The associated renal failure is potentially reversible at low dosage, and withdrawal of the drug will usually lead to a slow recovery of renal function. However, a sufficiently high dose can produce acute tubular necrosis with irreversible renal failure. Necrosis of the proximal and distal tubules may be sufficient to produce calcium deposits in both tubules and interstitium.

The risk of nephrotoxicity must be weighed against the risk of the untreated disease. The early administration of potassium and magnesium salts and alkali in the form of sodium citrate or bicarbonate may ameliorate toxic effects and a good urine volume should be maintained throughout, but there is no clear evidence that a mannitol diuresis reduces nephrotoxicity.

Cyclosporin

Nephrotoxicity has two components. The first is an effect upon the renal vasculature which, in the acute situation, leads to renal vasoconstriction and is reversible by dopamine. It results in a 30–40 per cent reduction in renal blood flow and glomerular filtration, and an increase in the filtration fraction. There is also increased reabsorption of sodium and urate from the proximal convoluted tubule. The second is a dose-dependent cytotoxicity affecting the proximal convoluted tubule, potentially reversible but occasionally leading to necrosis, interstitial fibrosis, and chronic renal disease. This dose-dependent cytotoxicity can be minimized by the careful control of plasma cyclosporin concentrations. The drug is metabolized by the hepatic cytochrome P450 system, and drugs that inhibit this system, such as erythromycin, ketoconazole, and diltiazem, may increase blood cyclosporin concentrations and increase nephrotoxicity. The clinical pattern of a gradual deterioration of renal function with increasing concentrations of creatinine, potassium, and urate. Usually, this will stabilize and not progress. A metabolic acidosis may develop together with fluid retention. Hyperuricaemia is found in over 70 per cent of patients and an accelerated form of gout in up to 20 per cent.

D-Penicillamine

Nephrotoxicity with mild proteinuria occurs frequently, and initially may settle with dosage reduction. Less commonly, proteinuria may become severe. This usually occurs during the first 12 months of therapy and may cause a nephrotic syndrome. The condition usually settles on withdrawal of treatment and steroid treatment is not necessary. Although remission may be delayed, most cases resolve within 2 years, although incompletely in some. There is minimal deterioration of glomerular filtration.

The histology is usually that of a membranous glomerulonephritis. A few patients show mesangial-dense deposits or minimal glomerular changes. Patient susceptibility, as reflected by HLA-B8 and/or DR3 tissue antigens, and/or by an abnormal sulphoxidation status, is an important contributory factor. Penicillamine inhibits the covalent binding of C4 and may thereby interfere with the handling of immune complexes.

Anticonvulsants

Phenytoin may rarely cause a hypersensitivity reaction with multi-system involvement, including dermatitis, hepatitis, myositis, and fever, in which acute renal failure may occur. It should be managed as for an acute interstitial nephritis.

The oxazolidinediones, particularly trimethadione and paramethadione, occasionally cause proteinuria which may be severe enough to induce a nephrotic syndrome, which usually settles on withdrawal of the drug, but the rate of recovery and the completeness of the remission vary and chronic renal failure may develop. The pathology has varied widely, sometimes suggesting an acute interstitial nephritis and in others an immune-complex glomerulonephritis. It is difficult to advise on specific therapy because some patients have remitted, albeit slowly, on withdrawal of the drug, whereas others appear to have needed steroid and immunosuppressive drugs.

Diuretics

Both frusemide and the thiazide diuretics have occasionally caused an acute interstitial nephritis. Some patients have shown the features of a hypersensitivity vasculitis. In other cases, diuretics appear to have augmented the nephrotoxicity of other agents.

Drugs altering urate concentrations

Allopurinol may cause an acute interstitial nephritis which can vary in severity up to the full syndrome with fever, exfoliative dermatitis, eosinophilia, eosinophiluria, and abnormal liver function. These reactions are more likely in patients with pre-existing renal disease, especially if the dose of allopurinol has not been reduced in proportion to the glomerular filtration rate. Sulphinpyrazone has been implicated in a similar syndrome. Unless improvement is apparent within a week, steroid therapy is indicated and usually promotes rapid subsidence. High doses are usually used, either as intravenous methylprednisolone (500 mg daily for 4 days) or oral prednisolone (60 mg/day) until the creatinine begins to fall or a diuresis occurs. The dose is then reduced at a rate depending on the response, but usually over at least 2 weeks. If any relapse occurs following withdrawal of steroids, an increase in dose is needed and prolonged therapy may be justified. Occasionally, despite steroid treatment, the renal insufficiency has been severe, prolonged, and occasionally fatal.

Radiographic contrast media

The true incidence of this reaction is difficult to ascertain because of variation between patients in susceptibility and because it may pass unnoticed. The most important risk factor is pre-existing renal disease, especially myeloma and diabetic nephropathy; those over 60 years of age are also at greater risk, as are those given repeated large doses of contrast over short periods. The result is an increase in plasma creatinine within 24 h of the procedure, reaching a maximum at 4 days and usually reverting to the original value by 7–10 days. The higher the initial serum creatinine concentration, the longer does the renal insufficiency take to subside. Sometimes it may be prolonged, even to requiring dialysis, and in some cases, the serum creatinine may never return to the previous level.

There appear to be two elements in causation. The first is a reversible renal vasoconstriction. The second a direct tubule-cell cytotoxic response, which is largely dependent on the concentration of medium achieved within the cell.

Prevention consists first in recognizing patients at risk and using an alternative radiographic procedure if possible. Doses of contrast should be adjusted in accordance with the degree of nitrogen retention, and repeated procedures avoided. Patients should be well hydrated before the procedure and given a saline infusion of up to 500 ml/h throughout, provided they can tolerate this without overhydration. Mannitol may be added for its diuretic effect, or frusemide if there is volume overload. The simultaneous use of prostaglandin synthetase inhibitors is particularly contraindicated. Use of the newer non-ionic contrast agents has not shown a reduction in nephrotoxicity in the higher risk patients.

Hydrocarbons and organic solvents (see also Chapter 18.1)

Carbon tetrachloride and the halogenated hydrocarbons can induce a range of damage to the tubule up to, and including, acute tubular necrosis. Tubular disorders, such as the Fanconi syndrome and renal tubular acidosis, have been reported following glue-sniffing. An immune-complex type of glomerulonephritis can follow relatively low-grade exposure to a wide variety of hydrocarbons. Studies in patients with glomerulonephritis, and of renal disease in persons with chronic industrial exposure to hydrocarbons, have suggested that such hydrocarbon exposure may be causal in the development of glomerular disease. Limitations of study design reduce the certainty with which causality can be established, but the accumulating data are increasingly supportive of such a relationship, particularly in Goodpasture's syndrome.

The clinical presentation is either as a membranous glomerulonephritis or arising as a response to toxic injury of mesangial cells. In some exposed industrially to hydrocarbons, features of coexisting tubular damage, in the form of a tubular proteinuria and increased excretion of *N*-acetylglucosaminidase, may be found in those with features of glomerulonephritis.

Ethylene glycol

Nephrotoxicity is part of a more generalized toxic reaction often involving encephalitis, myocarditis, and myositis. The ethylene glycol is metabolized by alcohol dehydrogenase to oxalate and other toxic intermediates, and the crystals of calcium oxalate may be found within the lumina of the proximal tubules, many of which demonstrate necrosis. The clinical pattern is of acute oliguric renal failure which is potentially reversible, but which may pass into chronic renal failure if damage has been sufficiently severe.

The key points in management are maintenance of a diuresis using frusemide and mannitol, early haemodialysis, correction of acidosis and the administration of alcohol. As the ethylene glycol is metabolized by alcohol dehydrogenase, its metabolism to toxic compounds can be delayed considerably by the simultaneous administration of ethanol at a dose of 10 g/h.

Further reading

DeBroe, M.E., Porter, G.A., Bennett, W.M., and Verpooten, G.A. (ed.) (1988). *Clinical nephrotoxins, renal injury from drugs and chemicals.* Kluwer Academic Publishers, Dordrecht.

Hoitsma, A.J., Wetzels, J.F.M., Koene, R.A.P. (1991). Drug-induced nephrotoxicity, aetiology, clinical features and management. *Drug Safety,* **6**, 131–47.

Nuyts, G.D., Van Vlem E., Thys, J., De Leersnijder, D., Haese, P.C.D. Elseviers, M.M., and DeBroe, M.E. (1995). New occupational risk factors for chronic renal failure. *Lancet*, **346**, 7–10.

Chapter 12.26

Prescription drugs and renal function

D. J. S. Carmichael

The kidney is the major route of elimination of many drugs and their metabolites. This may be by glomerular filtration, tubular secretion, or both. In practice, a minority of drugs need dose adjustment (dosage and/or interval) and it is those with a narrow therapeutic range or whose adverse effects are related to the concentration of the drug or its metabolites which cause the major problems.

Excretion is affected most by renal impairment, but absorption, distribution (including protein binding), metabolism, and renal haemodynamics, as well as pharmacodynamics, may be altered. The major determinant of alteration in dosage is the change in drug clearance which can be broadly estimated by measurement of glomerular filtration rate (GFR). Guidelines for the adjustment of dosage are derived from measurement or estimation of changes in clearance, half-life ($t_{1/2}$) and volume of distribution (V_d). These measurements should be regarded only as approximations. Many of the adverse effects of drugs in kidney disease occur because there is often ignorance of renal impairment before a drug is prescribed, ignorance of how a drug is cleared from the body, and failure to monitor therapeutic and adverse effects.

Pharmacokinetics

Distribution

Protein binding may be reduced by accumulation in the plasma of a number of acidic compounds that compete for binding sites on albumin and other plasma proteins. *Phenytoin* therapy is one of the few instances where these changes may be clinically significant. Binding of phenytoin to plasma protein is reduced in direct proportion to the fall in GFR and, consequently, the proportion of free drug increases for a given total plasma concentration. The therapeutic range, estimated by total plasma concentration, has therefore to be adjusted to a lower level. *Digoxin* is an example of a drug whose

Table 1 Parent drugs, metabolites, and possible adverse effects in renal failure

Drug	Metabolite	Effect of metabolite
Allopurinol	Oxypurinol	? Cause of rashes—interstitial nephritis
Clofibrate	Chlorophen-oxyisobutyric acid	Muscle damage, neuropathy
Nitroprusside	Thiocyanate	Toxic symptoms
Primidone	Phenobarbitone	Active drug
Procainamide	*N*-Acetyl procainamide	Anti-arrhythmic
Sulphonamides	Acetyl sulphonamides	Rashes—interstitial nephritis
Pethidine	Norpethidine	Causes seizures
Morphine	Morphine-6-glucuronide	Prolongs analgesia/ respiratory
Codeine	Morphine	depression
Propoxyphene	Norpropoxy-phene	Cardiotoxic
Acebutolol	*N*-Acetyl analogue	Confers selectivity
Nitrofurantoin	Metabolite	Peripheral neuropathy

Table 2 Examples of drugs actively secreted into tubular fluid

Organic acids	Organic bases
Penicillins	Amiloride
Cephalosporins	Procainamide
Sulphonamides	Quinidine
Frusemide	
Thiazides	
Salicylates	
Probenecid	

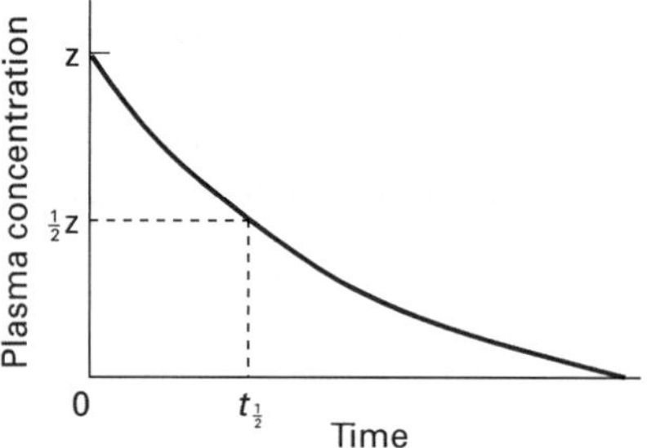

Fig. 1 Plot of log concentration of a drug against time, to demonstrate the half-life of a drug.

tissue binding (and consequently volume of distribution) falls in renal failure, and a smaller loading dose is needed.

Metabolism

The majority of drugs are excreted by the kidney either as the original compound or after metabolism in the liver to more polar (water-soluble) substances. There may be reduced clearance of metabolites which have therapeutic or adverse effects (see Table 1). Accumulation of inactive or relatively inactive metabolites may also confound interpretation of plasma concentration measurements of some drugs.

Renal excretion

Although renal clearance of drugs can be expressed as a function of GFR, this is often not a linear relationship because of the confounding effects of tubular reabsorption secretion and passive diffusion.

Compounds with a molecular weight below 60 000 Da are filtered to a variable extent depending on molecular size and degree of protein binding. Non-polar (lipid-soluble) drugs diffuse readily across tubular cells, whereas polar (water-soluble) compounds do not. The latter generally remain in the tubular fluid and are excreted in the urine, while the former are reabsorbed by passive diffusion down their concentration gradient. Some polar drugs are eliminated in the urine as a result of active or facilitated transport mechanisms (Table 2).

In addition, some agents interact to inhibit tubular secretion of others (for example, probenecid with penicillin, with cephalosporins, and with frusemide). Elimination of organic acids or bases is affected by the H^+ ion concentration of tubular fluid. In the non-ionized state these agents diffuse readily through the tubules, whereas ionization prevents such diffusion. The amount of ionized drug at any particular pH is determined by its pK (is the pH at which 50 per cent of the drug is ionized). If an organic acid has a pK_A <7.5, increasing urinary pH increases the amount ionized and therefore excretion. The converse is true for organic bases with a pK_B >7.5. The excretions of salicylates (weak acids) and amphetamines (weak bases) exemplify these principles, which underlie the reason, for instance, of considering alkaline diuresis in the treatment of salicylate poisoning.

Drugs present in tubular fluid may affect the excretion of other compounds; for example, aspirin and paracetamol reduce methotrexate excretion. Although it is a simplification to disregard the tubular handling of drugs, in renal impairment both filtration and secretion of drugs appear to fall in parallel. The most important aspect of prescribing in renal disease is therefore awareness of the existence of renal impairment and of changes in GFR.

Drug kinetics

Most drugs that are eliminated by the kidney display first-order kinetics, so that the rate of removal is proportional to the concentration. The elimination rate constant, k_e, is the proportion of total amount of drug removed per unit time. This produces a simple exponential decline in concentration (Fig. 1). The half-life ($t_{1/2}$) of a drug is the time for its plasma concentration to fall by half after absorption and distribution are complete. It is useful in determining dosage interval, drug accumulation, and persistence of drug after dosing is stopped. It is inversely related to k_e.

The clearance of a drug depends upon $t_{1/2}$ (k_e) and volume of distribution (V_d) (an apparent volume in which the drug would have distributed to produce the measured plasma concentration). This volume may be affected by protein and tissue binding of drugs, changes in intravascular and extravascular fluid volumes, and lean body mass.

Clearance can be used to calculate the steady-state concentration of a drug (C_{ss}) that can be anticipated in response to any particular dosage regimen. This concentration is proportional to the dose and $t_{1/2}$ of the drug and inversely proportional to the V_d and dosage interval. From these relationships it can be seen that C_{ss} will increase with a longer $t_{1/2}$ and a smaller V_d; the C_{ss} can be reduced either by lowering the dose or by increasing the dose interval.

Dialysis and haemofiltration

The clearance of a drug depends on molecular weight (and size) and protein binding. Haemofilter membranes have a pore size of 0.01 μm and those for haemodialysis 0.001 μm. In haemofiltration, drugs with a molecular weight below that of inulin (5200 Da) will pass through, whereas in haemodialysis most of those with a molecular weight below 500 Da (which includes many antibiotics) will be cleared excepting, for instance, drugs such as vancomycin (1800 Da), amphotericin (960 Da), and erythromycin (734 Da) Heavily protein-bound agents, even with a lower molecular weight (for example, propranolol, 259 Da), will not be filtered, but drugs which are displaced from binding sites in renal impairment will become available for filtration. Water-soluble drugs pass through filters more readily than those that are fat soluble. A list of some commonly used drugs and their clearance by haemodialysis or peritoneal dialysis is shown in Table 3. Differences resulting from the use of the different techniques for haemodialysis, haemodiafiltration, and intermittent and continuous haemofiltration are dealt with in other texts. Peritoneal dialysis clears drugs very much less efficiently than do haemodialysis or haemofiltration.

Drug prescribing

When a drug, known to be cleared largely by the kidney, is to be given to a patient with impaired renal function, either the size of each dose or the frequency of administration can be reduced. Plasma concentrations should be used to confirm that the initial adjustment of dosage was correct. Steady-state concentrations of anticonvulsants, digoxin, and theophylline can be measured after the equivalent of five half-lives of the drug. For antibiotics such as gentamicin it is essential to measure the peak-and-trough level after the first day's administration and thereafter if renal function is impaired or changing.

A combination of reduction in dosage and less frequent administration is suitable for most drugs. Adjustments must be kept simple as unfamiliar dosages and administration at unusual times make for error. It is best to use a limited number of drugs so that those responsible develop familiarity with regimens used in renal failure.

Patients with multisystem failure

Neuromuscular blocking agents

Succinylcholine is rapidly hydrolysed by plasma cholinesterase; no dose adjustment is needed. For more prolonged paralysis atracurium, which is degraded independent of renal or hepatic function is preferable. It is removed by dialysis and haemofiltration and the dose is titrated to produce a therapeutic effect. Tubocurarine, gallamine, alcuronium, pancuronium, and vercuronium should be avoided.

Anaesthetic and sedating agents

Propofol, fentanyl, and alfentanil require no dose adjustment but the last two may have prolonged effects if there is concomitant hepatic dysfunction. Diazepam has metabolites that accumulate and midazolam is preferable with dosage reduction if the GFR falls below 10 ml/min. Phenothiazines, butyrophenones, and Heminevrin® can be given in usual doses.

Table 3 Effectiveness or otherwise of clearance of drugs by dialysis

Dialysed	Slightly dialysed	Not dialysed
Haemodialysis		
Acyclovir	Amantadine	Acebutolol
Allopurinol	Cilastatin	Amphotericin B
Amikacin	Ciprofloxacin	Bretylium
Amoxycillin	Co-trimoxazole	Chloroquine
Ampicillin	Enalapril	Clonidine
Atenolol	Erythromycin	Cyclosporin
Aztreonam	Ethambutol	Diazoxide
Carbenicillin	Ethosuximide	Digoxin
Cefotaxime	Lorazepam	Disopyramide
Ceftazidime	Methylprednisolone	Flecamide
Cefuroxime	Nadolol	Glutethamide
Cephalexin	Procainamide	Heparin
Cephradine	Tetracyclines	Methicillin
Flucytosine	Vancomycin	Methotrexate
Gentamicin		Metoprolol
Isoniazid		Miconazole
Lithium		Oxazepam
Mecillinam		Pethidine
Metronidazole		Phenytoin
Moxolactam		Prednisone
Netilmicin		Procainamide
Penicillin		Propoxyphen
Ranitidine		Propranolol
Streptomycin		Valproic acid
Theophylline		Vancomycin
Ticarcillin		Warfarin
Tobramycin		
Trimethoprim		
Peritoneal dialysis		
Aztreonam	Aminoglycosides	Isoniazid
Ceftazidime	Aspirin	Phenobarbitone
Ethambutol	Cephalexin	Quinidine
Gallamine	Flucytosine	Theophylline
Ranitidine	Lithium	

Narcotic analgesics

Diamorphine and morphine metabolites accumulate in renal failure and can prolong both analgesia and respiratory depression. Pethidine is converted to norpethidine which also accumulates and can cause seizures. Reduced intermittent doses, epidural administration or low-dose continuous infusions are the best approach. Papaveretum should be avoided.

Cardiac drugs

Adrenaline, dobutamine, dopamine, and noradrenaline should be used in the minimum possible doses in order to avoid renal vasoconstriction. Low-dose dopamine (2 μg/kg per min) is often used to preserve renal blood flow. Intravenous nitrates can be given in normal dosage. Sodium nitroprusside is metabolized in the liver to sodium thiocyanate which is eliminated by the kidney, and so may accumulate in renal failure to cause toxicity. It is removed by haemodialysis or peritoneal dialysis.

Antiarrhythmics

Most antiarrhythmic drugs are used without dose modification (for example, lignocaine, flecainide, mexiletine, and verapamil). Digoxin is a notable exception with a lower loading and much lower maintenance dose than usual. The maintenance dose of amiodarone should be reduced to 100 mg daily when the GFR falls below 20 ml/min.

Antimicrobials

With the exception of aminoglycosides and vancomycin, little or no dose adjustment is usually made until the GFR is less than 20 ml/min. Antimicrobials that are removed by dialysis should be administered after dialysis, or a supplemental dose should be given at that time. Adjustments are shown in Table 4.

Penicillins

All should be given in reduced dose. Carbenicillin and ticarcillin solutions contain approximately 5 mmol Na^+/g, and caution is needed in the presence of salt and water retention. Mezlocillin, unlike other penicillins, is not dialysed.

Intravenous cephalosporins and other β-lactams

Cephalosporins should be given in lower doses in renal impairment.

Aminoglycosides

There are many nomograms and other guidelines for dose adjustment of aminoglycosides for patients with renal impairment, but each has drawbacks. As their volume of distribution is not materially affected by renal impairment, an adequate loading dose (1–1.5 mg/kg of gentamicin) is required. Reduced doses given at the usual intervals may increase the likelihood of subtherapeutic peak plasma levels. If only the dose interval is prolonged, there is also the risk of subtherapeutic plasma concentrations when the drug is given over long periods. A combination of both methods with frequent peak and trough measurements is optimal. Such measurements should be made daily when alterations in renal function are anticipated and two to three times a week under other circumstances. Doses and therapeutic concentrations are shown in Table 5.

Vancomycin and teicoplanin

Vancomycin excreted by the kidney is not dialysed. In patients with endstage renal failure on dialysis, therapeutic concentrations can be maintained for 5 days or more after a single intravenous dose; the target steady-state plasma concentration is approximately 15 mg/l. Following a loading dose of 15 mg/kg, further doses are given on the basis of plasma concentration. Teicoplanin, behaves rather differently. The half-life is prolonged in renal failure (approximately three times) and after a loading dose of 400 mg the maintenance dose of 200 mg/day should be reduced after 3 days even in mild renal failure. It is not cleared by dialysis.

Ciprofloxacin

Renal excretion exceeds GFR, and in patients with normal renal function approximately 60 per cent is cleared by the kidneys. It is recommended that the dose should be reduced in renal impairment but the proportion that is cleared by the liver and gut is increased in renal failure. Ciprofloxacin is not significantly removed by haemodialysis but may be removed by haemofiltration.

Tetracyclines

All the tetracyclines except minocycline and doxycycline are renally excreted. Plasma half-lives are markedly prolonged (up to 100 h) in

Table 4 Guidelines for adjustment of doses of antimicrobials in renal failure (GFR, ml/min)

Drug	Renal function	Dose reduction	Comments
Ampicillin			Seldom needed
Flucloxacillin		Nil	
Amoxycillin+ clavulanic acid	<20	By 50%	Half dose postdialysis
Benzyl penicillin	<20		Daily dose should not exceed 20 mU
Piperacillin	20–50 <20	By 50% By 66%	Half dose postdialysis
Cefotaxime } Ceftazidime }	20–50 <20	By 66% By 75%	Half dose postdialysis
Aztreonam	<10	By 75%	Half dose postdialysis
Imipenem/cilastatin	<20	By 50%	Half dose postdialysis
Erythromycin		Nil	
Trimethoprim	<20	By half	Half dose postdialysis
Ciprofloxacin	<10		500–750 mg/day maximum
Rifampicin		Nil	Avoid with cyclosporin
Flucytosine	20–50 <20	By half By three-quarters	Half dose postdialysis
Fluconazole	<50	By half	After 2 days
Acyclovir	Stepwise reduction from 800 mg five times a day with GFR 50 ml/min to 10 ml/min		

GFR, glomerular filtration rate

Table 5 Doses and therapeutic plasma concentrations of aminoglycosides

	Usual daily	Therapeutic concentration	
Drug	dose	Peak (mg/l)	Trough (mg/l)
Gentamicin	2–5 mg/kg	5–10	<2.5
Tobramycin	2–5 mg/kg	5–10	<2.5
Netilmicin	2–5 mg/kg	5–10	<2.5
Amikacin	10–30 μg/kg	20–30	<10
Kanamycin	10–30 μg/kg	20–30	<10

Peak concentration is measured 1 h postinjection.

Trough concentration is measured immediately before next dose.

Usual daily dose is administered 8 hourly.

The netilmicin dose can be increased to 7.5 mg/kg per day in severe infections, but requires careful therapeutic monitoring.

renal impairment. Doxycycline or minocycline can be used cautiously in patients with renal impairment, but the other tetracyclines are always contraindicated.

Sulphonamides, co-trimoxazole, and trimethoprim

Sulphonamides are eliminated by acetylation followed by renal excretion. High doses of co-trimoxazole are needed in the treatment of *Pneumocystis carinii* infection, the risk of adverse effects being balanced against the seriousness of the condition in patients who often have impaired renal function. The initial dose of trimethoprim is 20 mg/kg body weight per day and of sulphamethoxazole, 100 mg/kg per day divided in two or more doses. The plasma concentration should be maintained at approximately 5–8 μg/l measured after five doses, and can sometimes be achieved by lower maintenance doses.

Pentamidine

The usual dose is 4 mg/kg, given by slow intravenous infusion over 90 min. There is considerable tissue binding and the drug is excreted in the urine over long periods. The dose should be reduced in patients with renal impairment and by 30–50 per cent if the serum creatinine increases by 80–100 μmol/l (about 1 mg/100 ml).

Antiviral agents

Acyclovir and gancyclovir are both eliminated by the kidney and are dialysed. Lower doses of both drugs are required in the presence of renal failure.

Antifungal agents

Amphotericin is nephrotoxic, and should only be used with great caution in patients who already have renal impairment. Toxicity may be ameliorated by sodium supplementation provided the kidney can excrete the extra load. Both flucytosine and fluconazole are excreted in the urine. Ketoconazole is less well absorbed in renal failure and interferes with cyclosporin metabolism.

Antiprotozoal agents and malaria

Quinine is given in usual doses unless acute renal failure develops, when the dose should be reduced after 2–3 days. The dose of chloroquine is reduced by half if the GFR is less than 50 ml/min, and to a quarter if the GFR is less than 10 ml/min; primaquine is given in usual doses. Prophylactic chloroquine can be given in the usual dose of 300 mg/week in patients with renal impairment. Proguanil (usual dose 200 mg daily) should be given in half the usual dose if the GFR is less than 10 ml/min.

Drugs acting on the central nervous system

Antidepressants

All can be given at the usual dosage.

Lithium

The dose should be reduced in renal impairment, after the introduction of diuretics, in sodium depletion, and perhaps also if non-steroidal anti-inflammatory drugs (**NSAIDs**) are added.

Tranquillizers

No dose change is required for phenothiazines or butyrophenones. Benzodiazepines can also be prescribed in usual dosage, but diazepam and chlordiazepoxide have active metabolites that may accumulate. It is preferable, to use nitrazepam and temazepam.

Anticonvulsants

Phenytoin, carbamazepine, and valproic acid are given in usual dosages with the proviso concerning therapeutic concentrations of phenytoin (see above).

Weaker analgesics

Codeine and dihydrocodeine may cause severe respiratory depression in some patients, as does dextropropoxyphene. Its metabolite, norproxyphene, accumulates in renal failure and sometimes causes cardiac toxicity. Buprenorphine can be given in normal dosage. Paracetamol is also used in normal doses. Aspirin has the disadvantage of increasing the bleeding diathesis of patients with uraemia.

Antihistamines

Both terfenadine and prochlorperazine can be used at the usual dosage.

Cardiac failure and oedema

Diuretics

Spironolactone, triamterene, amiloride, and combinations such as moduretic or dyazide should be avoided in renal impairment because of the danger of hyperkalaemia. Thiazides apart from metolazone become less effective if the GFR is below 25 ml/min. Higher doses of loop diuretics are needed.

Angiotensin-converting enzyme inhibitors

Starting doses should be low and increased slowly with careful monitoring of serum creatinine and potassium. Particular caution is necessary if these drugs are used in combination with diuretics or in other high-renin states (such as volume depletion), when marked hypotension (first-dose effect) may be anticipated. Caution is also necessary when there is (or may be) a possibility of renal artery stenosis, both because of the risk of hypotension and also because of reduced GFR in the affected kidney(s). They should generally not be used with potassium-sparing diuretics because of the added risk of hyperkalaemia. All are eliminated by the kidney, which accounts for the reduced dose often required in the elderly. They are all dialysed.

Hypertension

β-Blockers

Atenolol, bisoprolol, pindolol, nadolol, and sotalol are all excreted by the kidney and reduced doses may be needed. The metabolites of acebutolol may accumulate. Other β-blockers can be prescribed unchanged.

Vasodilators, calcium-channel blockers, and a-blockers

No dose adjustment is needed for any of these drugs.

Centrally acting agents

α-Methyldopa and clonidine are given in usual doses.

Diabetes mellitus

Insulin

Insulin requirements fall with declining renal function, as a consequence of its reduced renal metabolism. In patients on haemodialysis it is often necessary to give supplemental insulin during treatment. The same situation applies in patients on haemofiltration in acute renal failure, particularly if they are being fed parenterally. Non-diabetic patients may require insulin temporarily under these circumstances. Patients on continuous ambulatory peritoneal dialysis may need a change in insulin preparation and adjustment in the frequency and route of administration. The intraperitoneal requirement is approximately 50 per cent of intravenous requirements.

Oral hypoglycaemic agents

Gliclazide and glipizide are the safest drugs to use in renal failure, although dose reduction may be needed if the GFR is below 10 ml/min. Other sulphonylureas, particularly chlorpropamide, have a prolonged half-life. The biguanides should not be used if the GFR is below 20 ml/min.

Asthma

Doses of β-agonists administered by inhalation, oral, or parenteral routes need no adjustment in patients with renal impairment. Aminophylline and theophylline can also be given in usual doses.

Gastrointestinal drugs

H_2-antagonists and antiulcer drugs

Cimetidine metabolites accumulate if the GFR is less than 20 ml/min. Ranitidine is preferable in this situation; but it may interfere with creatinine secretion and raises plasma creatinine. It is partly cleared by the kidneys and the dose should be halved when the GFR is less than 10 ml/min. It is dialysed, and a supplemental dose is needed after dialysis but not after haemofiltration. Omeprazole and misoprostol are given in usual doses. Misoprostol may cause reductions in GFR through haemodynamic changes in the kidney.

Antacids

Alginates, magnesium trisilicate mixture (but not magnesium trisilicate powder), and sodium bicarbonate all have a high sodium content. The use of aluminium hydroxide or sulcralfate in patients with severe renal impairment or those on dialysis is controversial because of the potential risks of aluminium retention. Calcium carbonate should not be used as an antacid but only as a phosphate binder.

Hyperuricaemia

Allopurinol

The dose should be reduced to 100 mg/day when the GFR is less than 20 ml/min, and in haemodialysis patients this drug should be given at the end of treatment. Allopurinol interferes with the metabolism of 6-mercaptopurine, which is an active metabolite of azathioprine. When the two drugs are given together, therefore, it is often necessary to reduce the dose of azathioprine.

Probenecid

Probenecid prolongs the effect of penicillins, cephalosporins, naproxen, indomethacin, methotrexate, and sulphonylurea, causing accumulation and the potential for toxicity. It also inhibits tubular secretion (and hence activity) of frusemide and bumetanide.

Colchicine

Colchicine remains valuable in patients in whom NSAIDs are undesirable and can be given in the usual doses.

Anti-inflammatory agents

In patients with cardiac failure, nephrotic syndrome, liver disease, glomerulonephritis, and other renal disease cyclo-oxygenase inhibitors predictably cause a reversible fall in GFR, which can be severe. They also cause fluid retention, blunt the effects of antihypertensive drugs, and may also cause hyperkalaemia. Any of this class of drugs should only be given to patients with renal failure with circumspection. The NSAIDs are highly protein bound and are not removed by dialysis.

Anticoagulants

Warfarin is used in normal dosage. It is highly protein bound and there may be slight displacement and consequent reduction in the volume of distribution in renal failure. In nephrotic patients hypoalbuminaemia leads to increased sensitivity to warfarin. It is not dialysed. Heparin can be used in normal dosage.

Corticosteroids and immunosuppressive agents

Prednisone and prednisolone are not eliminated by the kidney. Methylprednisolone is cleared by haemodialysis, and should therefore be given after dialysis. Azathioprine accumulates in renal impairment and the dose should be reduced from a maximum of 3 mg/kg per day to 1 mg/kg per day if the GFR falls below 10 ml/min.

Cyclosporin is extensively bound to plasma proteins and has a large volume of distribution. Only minor amounts are excreted as parent drug or metabolites in the urine. Renal impairment does not affect its metabolism.

Lipid-lowering agents

The anion-exchange resins (for example, colestipol) and 3-hydroxy-3-methylglutaryl coenzyme A reductase inhibitors (simvastatin, pravastatin) are given at their usual dose. The fibrates (gemfibrozil, bezafibrate) can be used with dose reduction at GFRs of less than 20 ml/min. It is probably best to avoid clofibrate altogether as myopathy is more likely to occur in the presence of renal dysfunction.

Further reading

Bennet, W.M., Plamp, C., and Poter, G.A. (1977). Drug-related syndromes in clinical nephrology. *Annals of Internal Medicine*, **87**, 582–90.

Fillastre, J.-P. and Godin, M. (1998). Drug-induced nephropathies. In: *Oxford textbook of clinical nephrology*, (2nd edn) (ed. A.M. Davison, J.S. Cameron, J.-P. Grünfeld, D. Kerr, E. Ritz, and C.G. Winearls), pp. 2645–57. Oxford University Press, Oxford.

Humes, H.D. (1988). Aminoglycoside nephrotoxicity. *Kidney International*, **33**, 900–11.

Neilson, E.G. (1989). Pathogenesis and therapy of interstitial nephritis. *Kidney International*, **35**, 1257–70.

Chapter 12.27

Genitourinary tuberculosis

L. R. I. Baker

Genitourinary tuberculosis is typically a late manifestation of previous pulmonary infection. It probably develops in 4–5 per cent of cases of pulmonary tuberculosis.

Pathogenesis

The tubercle bacillus invades the urogenital tract by haematogenous spread from the lungs or less often from the gut. Such dissemination of mycobacteria most often affects the renal cortices. Small granulomas develop in the glomerular or adjacent capillaries. Subsequent rupture of capillaries spreads mycobacteria to the tubules. The immune response in the medullary region is weak, so that medullary granulomas may enlarge and often rupture with consequent spread to infect the renal pelves, ureters, bladder, and the genital organs. Direct seeding via the bloodstream and lymphatics to adjacent organs may also occur.

Pathology

Tubercle bacilli may be found in caseating granulomas which tend to remain small in the cortex, but medullary lesions enlarge and cavitate. Healing leads to fibrosis with parenchymal atrophy, calyceal infundibular stenosis, obstruction of the ureter (most commonly of the vesicoureteric junction), and bladder fibrosis with wall thickening and loss of volume. Obstruction from strictures may cause renal atrophy. Calcification may involve the renal parenchyma, pelvicalyceal system, ureter, or bladder. Cystoscopic appearances vary from a region of inflammation or superficial granulation at one or other ureteric orifice to a generalized cystitis with oedema and widespread granulations. Healed bladder lesions have a stellate appearance caused by bands of fibrous tissue meeting at a central point. Severe fibrotic change may cause the ureteric orifice to become withdrawn and widely patent ('golf-hole ureter').

Presentation

The male/female ratio is 2:1 and the large majority of patients are aged between 20 and 40 years. A previous personal or family history of tuberculosis is not uncommon.

Urinary tract tuberculosis often produces little in the way of symptoms until the bladder is involved. The most common presenting symptom is urinary frequency followed by dysuria. Macroscopic haematuria and renal pain, usually mild, are present in less than 30 per cent of patients. Ureteric colic is rare. Constitutional symptoms (malaise, tiredness, weight loss, night sweats, fever, and anorexia) are seen in less than one-fifth of patients. Much less commonly, patients present with polyuria, renal salt-wasting, hypertension, or chronic renal failure. Patients may also present with chronic epididymitis or other symptoms of infection of the genital tract. In many instances the diagnosis is unsuspected but revealed by standard laboratory or imaging examinations.

Investigation

Urine examination

Pyuria may or may not be present. 'Sterile pyuria' should raise the suspicion of urinary tract tuberculosis, although many other causes exist. Conversely, the finding of significant bacteriuria does not exclude the diagnosis of tuberculosis, as superimposed secondary infection may be present in advanced cases.

The isolation of *Mycobacterium tuberculosis* by urine culture is the definitive diagnostic test. Three to five early morning urine specimens should be provided and should reach the laboratory at the earliest opportunity, as the longer the urine remains in contact with the organism the less likely is the mycobacterium to grow. *Mycobacterium tuberculosis* is present only intermittently in the urine and in low count, and grows poorly on culture media. It is important that drugs inhibiting mycobacterial growth, such as aminoglycosides and tetracyclines, be stopped for 1 week or more before urine is cultured. The Ziehl–Neelsen (ZN) stain performed on concentrated urine sediment may reveal the presence of mycobacteria, although the yield of this approach is not high. Confusion may arise in the not infrequent presence of saprophytic *Mycobacterium smegmatis*. Guinea-pig inoculation is now seldom used in diagnosis.

Almost all patients have a positive reaction to 5 IU of tuberculin, except for the immunosuppressed. Other methods of diagnosis include culture of material aspirated from abscesses, histological examination of biopsy specimens with ZN staining (the only method of diagnosis in some cases of diffuse interstitial tuberculosis with normal urinary tract anatomy and negative culture findings), and culture of such material.

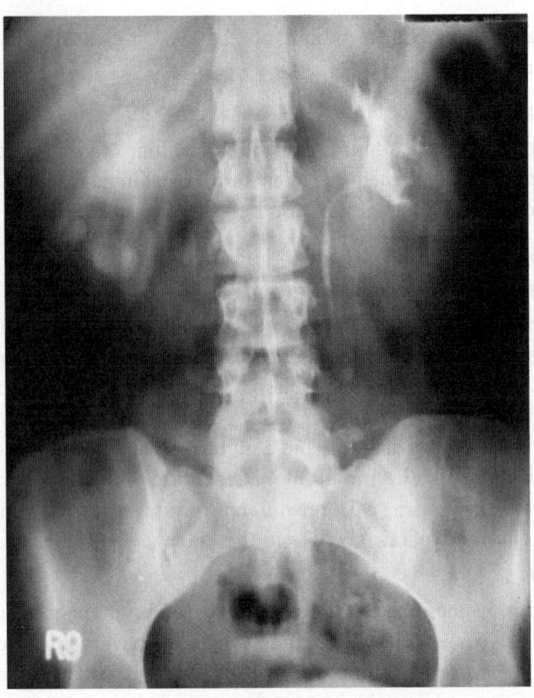

Fig. 1 Bilateral renal tuberculosis showing right hydronephrosis secondary to obstruction of the lower ureter and a closed cavity. Note the absence of normal calyces in the lower pole of the left kidney.

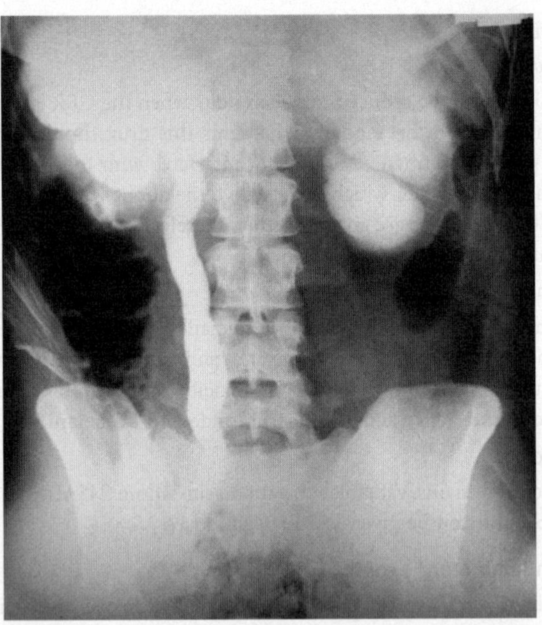

Fig. 2 Shows clearer detail outlined by right antegrade (percutaneous) pyelogram and left cyst puncture.

Imaging

Plain radiographs of the chest and abdomen are essential to exclude an active pulmonary lesion and calcific deposits in the kidneys or elsewhere in the genitourinary tract.

Intravenous urography

A high-dose intravenous urogram will detect destructive renal lesions and urinary tract obstruction (Figs 1, 2, and 3). Tomograms define the presence of faint calcification. If urinary tract obstruction is absent

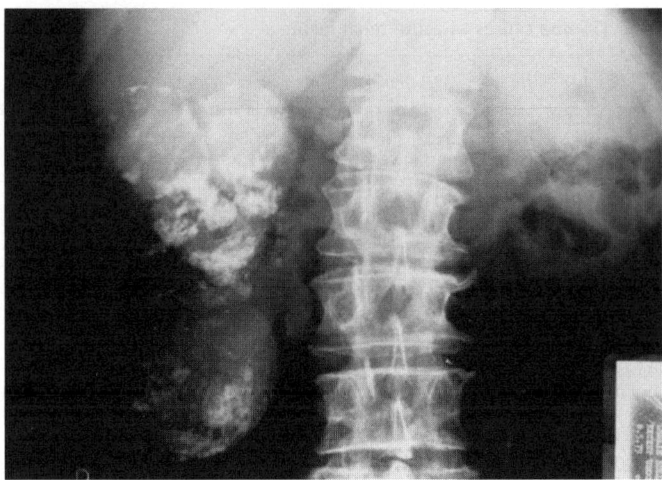

Fig. 3 Calcified tuberculous pyonephrosis.

at the time of diagnosis, intravenous urography should be repeated 4–6 weeks after commencement of treatment, as healing by fibrosis may produce strictures leading to obstruction.

The differential diagnosis of calyceal abnormality due to tuberculosis includes renal papillary necrosis from other causes, calyceal diverticulae, and medullary sponge kidney. Tuberculous granulomatous disease in renal parenchyma may be mimicked by lobar nephronia (the nephrological equivalent of lobar pneumonia), xanthogranulomatous pyelonephritis, and malignant renal tumours.

Retrograde ureterography and pyelography

This examination has now largely been replaced by computed tomography (Fig. 4) or antegrade pyelography (Fig. 2).

Renal ultrasonography

Ultrasonography has a role in the follow-up of hydronephrosis secondary to an obstructive lesion and in the differential diagnosis of a renal mass.

Cystoscopy

Biopsy of bladder mucosa may allow a rapid histological diagnosis of tuberculosis but in such cases *Mycobacterium tuberculosis* is almost invariably grown from urine and it has been claimed that tuberculous meningitis may follow biopsy in acute tuberculous cystitis.

Indications for treatment

Treatment should usually be withheld until a positive culture of the organism has been obtained. However, when classical radiological appearances are accompanied by acid-fast bacilli on ZN staining, there has been a positive bladder biopsy, or the patient is ill, treatment may be begun immediately.

Medical treatment

Principles of drug treatment and the management of difficult cases is discussed in Section 16. A reasonable regimen in urogenital tuberculosis comprises isoniazid (300 mg daily as a single oral dose), rifampicin (600 mg daily before breakfast), and pyrazinamide (1 g daily). Drug doses need not be changed unless renal function is severely impaired. After 4 months the treatment regimen may be reduced to two drugs (rifampicin and isoniazid) unless the results of *in vitro* sensitivity tests dictate otherwise. Treatment is continued for a total of 9 months.

Follow-up

Three early morning urines are cultured on completion of the course of treatment and at 6 and 12 months thereafter. If negative results are obtained, the patient may be discharged but those with renal calcification or impaired renal function need long-term follow-up.

Corticosteroid administration

The addition of corticosteroids to antituberculous drugs has been advocated to prevent or reduce healing by fibrosis and hence the development of urinary tract obstruction, but controlled trials are lacking and the consensus is that such prophylaxis is not to be recommended. In tuberculous interstitial nephritis with renal impairment, anecdotal evidence suggests a protective effect of concomitant corticosteroids upon renal function, but again no controlled studies are available.

Surgical treatment

Nephrectomy may be indicated in the presence of: (a) non-functioning kidney with or without calcification; (b) extensive disease involving

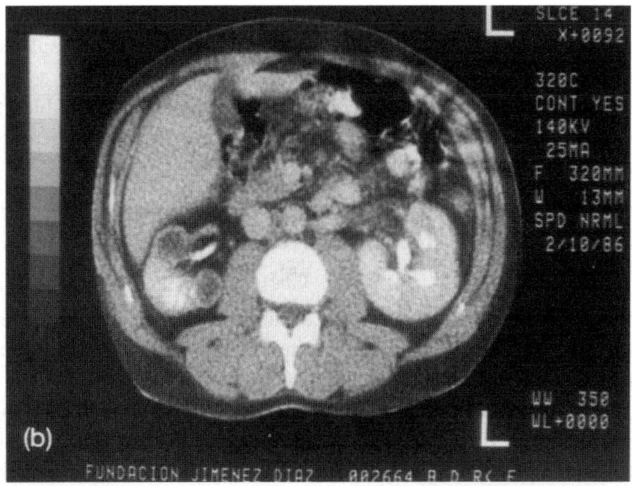

Fig. 4 Computed tomography after administration of intravenous contrast. (a) The upper pole shows calcified parenchyma. (b) In the lower pole, low-density areas represent obstructed calyces with cortical thinning.
(Reproduced from Cameron, J.S. et al. (ed.) (1992). Oxford textbook of clinical nephrology p. 1724. University Press, Oxford, with permission.)

the whole kidney associated with superimposed secondary infection or haemorrhage; (c) small, very poorly functioning kidney with extensive calcification and pelviureteric obstruction causing pain; (d) coexisting renal cancer. Partial nephrectomy is now very seldom required. The two main indications are: (a) a localized, calcified lesion which has failed to respond to chemotherapy, and (b) an area of calcification which is increasing in size and threatens to destroy the entire kidney. Cavernostomy still has a place in management, although imaging techniques allow the contents of a tuberculous abscess to be aspirated and antituberculous drugs inoculated. Epididymectomy is required when a caseating abscess has failed to respond to drug therapy. Involvement of the testes is common, but orchidectomy is required in only 5 per cent of cases.

Reconstructive surgery

If obstruction persists or increases despite medical treatment, surgery will be needed to correct pelviureteric junction or ureterovesical junction obstruction. Ileo-, colo-, or caecocystoplasty is necessary when healing results in a contracted bladder with resultant severe daytime frequency and nocturia. It should rarely be performed early in the course of treatment, for sometimes surprising improvement follows the use of antituberculous drugs.

Further reading

Christensen, W.I. (1974). Genitourinary tuberculosis. A review of 102 cases. *Medicine* (Baltimore), 53, 377–90.

Lattimer, J.K. (1975). Renal tuberculosis. *New England Journal of Medicine*, 273, 208–11.

Leitch, A.G. and Horne, N.W. (1998). In: *Oxford textbook of clinical nephrology*, (2nd edn) (ed. A.M. Davison, J.S. Cameron, J.-P. Grünfeld, D. Kerr, E. Ritz, and C.G. Winearls), pp. 1277–85. Oxford University Press, Oxford.

Chapter 12.28

Acute renal failure

J. D. Firth and C. G. Winearls

Acute renal failure is defined as a significant decline in renal excretory function occurring over hours or days. It may arise as an isolated problem, but much more commonly occurs in the setting of severe illness, trauma, or surgery. There are many possible causes (Table 1), but in any given clinical context very few of these are likely to require consideration.

Table 1 Some causes of acute renal failure

Some causes of acute renal failure
Prerenal uraemia
'Acute tubular necrosis'
Following haemodynamic compromise, commonly with sepsis
Following exposure to nephrotoxins: including drugs, chemicals, rhabdomyolysis (see Table 7), snake bite
Vascular causes
Acute cortical necrosis
Large vessel obstruction
Small vessel obstruction: accelerated-phase hypertension and systemic sclerosis
Glomerulonephritis and vasculitis (see Table 8)
Interstitial nephritis (see Table 9)
'Haematological' causes
Haemolytic uraemic syndrome/thrombotic thrombocytopenic purpura
Myeloma
Hepatorenal syndrome
Urinary obstruction
Intrarenal: crystalluria
Postrenal; renal stones, papillary necrosis, retroperitoneal fibrosis, bladder/prostate/cervical lesions

Diagnosis of the presence of acute renal failure

Symptoms and signs are often not apparent until the condition is far advanced. Hyperkalaemia is the greatest danger, as this may produce no symptoms before inducing cardiac arrest.

All patients admitted to hospital with acute illness should be considered at risk of developing acute renal failure. Those who have some pre-existing impairment of renal function are particularly susceptible. This group includes all elderly patients, in whom a combination of low muscle mass and low dietary meat consumption may maintain an apparently 'normal' plasma creatinine, despite a reduction in glomerular filtration rate to as little as 25 per cent of that of a healthy young adult.

Care of all acutely ill patients should include careful monitoring of fluid input and output, daily weighing, lying and standing blood pressure, and regular estimation of plasma creatinine, urea, and electrolytes. The estimation of urinary output and of gastrointestinal losses is usually not difficult. Precise determination of fluid input is more problematic, except in those who are only receiving fluids parenterally. Fluid balance charts are often difficult to interpret because recording of intake is erroneous. Daily weighing provides a much more reliable picture of net overall fluid balance. Patients who are acutely ill invariably lose flesh weight, commonly at a rate of up to a few hundred grams per day. If weight falls at a rate faster than this, negative fluid balance is likely; greatly increased 'insensible' losses through the skin and lungs during fever being the commonest explanation. If weight rises, this must be due to positive fluid balance, whatever the input/output charts may suggest. It may not be obvious from clinical examination where the fluid has gone: the possibilities of sequestration in the peritoneal cavity or in the tissue interstitium should be recognized.

Diagnosis of the cause of acute renal failure

In the initial assessment three questions should be asked.

Is the renal failure really acute?

There may be records of previous indices of renal function. The finding of two small kidneys on ultrasound examination indicates

Table 2 Causes of acute renal failure requiring renal replacement therapy at a single centre between 1956 and 1988

	No. of patients (% total)	Diagnoses present (% patients)	
Surgical	638 (47.5)	General surgery	445 (33.1)
		Surgical sepsis	126 (9.4)
		Urinary obstruction	116 (8.6)
		Trauma	94 (7.0)
		Cardiovascular surgery	81 (6.0)
		Malignancy	52 (3.9)
		Pancreatitis	24 (1.8)
		Burns	17 (1.3)
General medical	285 (21.2)	Sepsis	112 (8.3)
		Acute liver disease	44 (3.3)
		Salt and water depletion	43 (3.2)
		Ischaemic heart disease	36 (2.7)
		Diabetes mellitus	30 (2.2)
		Others	53 (3.9)
Renal parenchymal disease	166 (12.4)	Polyarteritis	31 (2.3)
		Crescentic nephritis	25 (1.9)
		Haemolytic uraemic syndrome	21 (1.6)
		Proliferative glomerulonephritis	19 (1.4)
		Histology unknown	19 (1.4)
		Systemic lupus erythematosus	15 (1.1)
		Others	36 (2.7)
Obstetric	142 (10.6)		
Poisoning	112 (8.3)		
Total	1343 (100)		

Modified from Turney *et al.* (1990)

Some patients fell into more than one diagnostic category.

During the period of study there were significant changes in case-mix. Between 1980 and 1988, the following categories were more frequent: general medical (33.2% of all cases) and cardiovascular surgery (15.1%); and the following categories were less frequent: general surgery (26.4%), trauma (2.8%), and obstetric (1.3%).

the presence of chronic disease. Other features are poor discriminators between acute and chronic renal impairment. A history of vague ill-health of some months' duration, of nocturia, of pruritus, or the findings of skin pigmentation or anaemia would all suggest chronicity, although anaemia is not invariable in chronic renal failure and it can develop over a few days in acute renal failure, as may hypocalcaemia and hyperphosphataemia. Radiological evidence of renal osteodystrophy is only found in patients with long-standing renal failure but rarely aids the clinical distinction between acute and chronic disease.

Is urinary obstruction a possibility?

This diagnosis should not be missed, as it is readily treatable and delay may cause permanent renal damage. Anuria, or alternating polyuria and oligoanuria are helpful clues; but patients may pass normal or elevated volumes of urine despite significant obstruction. Three factors present in obstruction tend to impair urinary concentrating ability and thereby lead to preservation of urinary volume despite obstructive depression of filtration rate. These are structural damage to the inner medulla and papilla, functional changes in the distal nephron resulting from increased intraluminal or interstitial pressure, and loss of medullary hypertonicity at low filtration rates.

Ultrasound examination is the usual first method of investigation but it detects calyceal dilatation, not obstruction, and cases of obstruction are not infrequently missed either because the calyces fail to dilate or do so minimally. Furthermore, the quality of the image obtained by renal ultrasonography is highly variable—depending on the patient, the equipment, and on the operator. If doubt persists the examination should be repeated, and if uncertainty still remains diethylenetriamine pentaacetic acid (DTPA) renography with frusemide injection and/or cystoscopy with retrograde ureteric catheterization should be undertaken. Obstruction, once diagnosed, must be relieved urgently (see Chapter 12.22).

Are glomerulonephritis, interstitial nephritis, vasculitis, or other rarities possible?

Stick testing of the urine for protein and blood, followed by microscopy of the urinary sediment is an essential part of the assessment of any patient with unexplained acute renal failure. Red cell casts are present in acute glomerulonephritis, renal vasculitis, accelerated-phase hypertension, and (sometimes) in interstitial nephritis, but not in other conditions. Their presence indicates the need for urgent specialist referral.

Prerenal failure and acute tubular necrosis

The vast majority of cases of acute renal failure will fall into this category. The term 'prerenal failure' is used when renal dysfunction is entirely attributable to hypoperfusion, when restoration of renal perfusion leads to rapid recovery. The term 'ATN' is not a good one. Although necrosis of tubular cells can usually be found by diligent examination, the lesion maybe inconspicuous and the pathophysiologic remains uncertain. The glomeruli and vessels are usually normal. In common usage 'acute tubular necrosis' (**ATN**) describes a clinical entity comprising acute renal failure with three main characteristics: (a) it is seen in specific clinical contexts, frequently involving circulatory compromise and/or nephrotoxins; (b) urinary abnormalities usually suggest tubular dysfunction; and (c) essentially complete recovery of renal function is expected within days or weeks if the patient survives the precipitating insult, with a period of polyuria commonly following oliguria.

The syndrome can be seen after any episode of severe circulatory compromise, but not all causes of circulatory derangement are equally devastating to renal function. Primary impairment of cardiac performance, for example following myocardial infarction, may cause plasma creatinine to rise somewhat, but rarely causes renal failure of sufficient severity to require renal replacement therapy. By contrast an apparently similar haemodynamic upset caused by sepsis frequently does. Table 2 shows the causes of acute renal failure requiring renal replacement therapy in over 1000 cases treated at a single centre between 1956 and 1988. Circumstances associated with a particularly high risk include repair of ruptured aortic aneurysm (20 per cent, as opposed to 3 per cent for elective repair), hepatobiliary surgery (10 per cent), pancreatitis (10 per cent), and burns.

Pathophysiology

When the circulation is compromised, perfusion of the kidney is reduced before that of any other organ. In the face of modest underperfusion, the glomerular filtration rate is relatively preserved by a compensatory increase in filtration fraction. This, along with other factors, leads to increased tubular reabsorption of sodium, water, and urea—a situation rapidly reversed by restoration of renal perfusion. However, following prolonged circulatory shock, renal function frequently deteriorates in a manner which is not immediately reversible (ATN). It is not obvious why this should be. Normally the kidney enjoys high blood flow, and oxygen tension in the renal venous effluent is high, suggesting that oxygen supply exceeds demand. Such a situation might be expected to confer protection from the effects of circulatory compromise, but in fact the kidney is more susceptible to damage than other organs. Acute renal failure resembling ATN can be produced in animal models by ischaemia. This, coupled with the setting of profound haemodynamic disturbance in which clinical acute renal failure is frequently seen, has led to the supposition that renal ischaemia is the cause of renal failure in such circumstances. Two main hypotheses, not necessarily mutually exclusive, have been proposed to explain this. The first stresses that arteriovenous shunting of oxygen, resulting from the specialized anatomical relationships between intrarenal arteries and veins, leads to the presence of areas of profound hypoxia within the normal kidney, perhaps susceptible to ischaemic damage in response to modest compromise of whole-organ blood flow. The second is based on evidence of intense constriction of renal vessels during shock, and suggests that very severe reduction in renal blood flow (perhaps only transient) may be responsible for the initiation of ischaemic damage. The justification for many of the interventions used in the management of incipient or established acute renal failure, is that they might preserve renal blood flow and/or reduce renal oxygen consumption, thus rendering the development of ischaemic injury less likely.

Table 3 Urinary biochemical indices in prerenal failure and acute tubular necrosis

Indices	'Typical' prerenal failure	'Typical' acute tubular necrosis
Urinary sodium (mmol/l)	<20	>40
Urine osmolarity (mosmol/l)	>500	<350
Urine/plasma urea	>8	<3
Urine/plasma creatinine	>40	<20
Fractional sodium excretion (%)	<1	>2

Reasons why urinary biochemical indices are of very limited clinical use:

(1) Intermediate values are common.

(2) 'Typical' values do not reliably predict renal prognosis. It is increasingly recognized that cases which are otherwise indistinguishable from 'typical' acute tubular necrosis can have low urinary sodium.

(3) Diuretics and pre-existing tubular disease will impair tubules' ability to retain sodium in prerenal failure.

(4) In hepatorenal syndrome indices are prerenal.

(5) Treatment is not dictated by urinary indices.

Once damage has been sustained, a variety of factors may be responsible for the persistence of excretory failure. Renal blood flow may remain low, the glomerular ultrafiltration coefficient may be reduced, renal tubules may be obstructed, and backleakage of filtrate from damaged tubules may occur. It is impossible to determine which of these factors is most important at any given time, but, many of these abnormalities have a structural, rather than functional basis; hence, rapid reversal cannot be expected.

Diagnosis

In prerenal failure the urinary biochemical composition reflects the response of normal tubules to impaired renal perfusion. There is avid retention of sodium and water, leading to low urinary sodium and high urinary urea and creatinine concentrations, together with a high urinary osmolarity. Restoration of renal perfusion leads to rapid improvement in renal function. By contrast, in the 'typical' case of ATN the urinary sodium concentration is elevated and the urinary urea and creatinine concentrations and urinary osmolarity are relatively low (Table 3); in such instances, whatever the treatment, renal function rarely improves rapidly. However, for reasons listed in Table 3 there are so many exceptions to the 'typical' findings described that such analysis is rarely of value. In practice, treatment is begun on the same lines whether the expected diagnosis is of prerenal failure or of ATN. The response to initial treatment retrospectively defines the diagnosis and determines further management.

Table 4 Evaluation of intravascular volume

Clinical signs of volume depletion
• Jugular venous pressure low
• Hypotension, postural drop in blood pressure of >10 mmHg and rise in pulse rate of >10 b.p.m (lying and sitting, if lying and standing not possible)
• Collapsed peripheral veins and cool peripheries (nose, fingers, toes)
• Fast, thready pulse
Clinical signs of volume overload
• Jugular venous pressure high
• Gallop rhythm
• Hypertension, peripheral oedema, liver congestion, basal crepitations
Directly measurable indices of intravascular volume
• Central venous pressure
• Pulmonary capillary wedge pressure
Therapeutic tests of volume depletion or excess
• Trial of fluid infusion
• Trial of fluid removal (diuretic, haemofiltration/haemodialysis, venesection (exceptionally))

Circumstances predisposing to prerenal failure are almost invariably associated with raised plasma levels of antidiuretic hormone. This acts on the collecting duct to increase tubular reabsorption of both water and urea; hence plasma levels of urea rise out of proportion to creatinine in prerenal failure. Plasma urea may also appear to be disproportionately raised with sepsis, steroids, tetracycline (catabolic effect), and gastrointestinal haemorrhage (protein meal).

Avoidance

Acute renal failure can arise despite exemplary treatment, but poor care increases the likelihood. The cornerstones of good management are: the maintenance of optimal intravascular volume, and the avoidance of, or reduction of, exposure to nephrotoxic agents.

Maintenance of optimal intravascular volume

The features listed in Table 4 are indicators of depletion or excess of intravascular volume, and the presence of any one of these should lead to consideration of whether the patient would benefit from increasing or decreasing that volume. Reduced skin turgor, reduced ocular tension, and dry mouth and tongue, are poor guides and may be misleading, particularly in the elderly.

A central venous pressure line provides more precise measurement of right atrial pressure than can be gained from inspection of the jugular venous pulse, and the pulmonary capillary wedge pressure line provides information on left-sided filling pressure. However, the advantages of inserting these lines must be weighed against the disadvantages. There are some patients, in whom the jugular venous pulse cannot be seen at all. In them a central venous pressure line is invaluable. By contrast, in the majority of patients the jugular venous pulse can be seen. In these cases the benefits of a central venous pressure line may not outweigh the risks. It is dangerous to try and insert a central venous pressure line into someone whose intravascular volume is clearly low. With constricted central veins the procedure is likely to be technically difficult, with greatly increased likelihood of complications. In most patients central venous pressure should be maintained at a level of 5–8 cm of water but even with accurate measurement it is not always easy to decide whether intravascular volume is optimal. When in doubt, the renal response to the challenge of an infusion of saline or colloid can be very helpful, albeit with particular attention to the risk of inducing pulmonary oedema. The administration of 250 ml of colloid or 0.9 per cent saline should be rapid, and the patient should be observed closely for the next 5 min. If there is no perceptible deterioration, the process can be repeated.

In the specific case of repair of an abdominal aortic aneurysm, the risk of postoperative acute renal failure is much reduced by preoperative infusion of crystalloids and meticulous attention to fluid balance. Maintenance of a diuresis appears to be protective. Some advocate the use of mannitol, but the massive diuresis resulting can add to difficulties in volume and electrolyte control and mannitol has no clear advantage over simple saline diuresis.

Avoidance/reduction of exposure to nephrotoxins

These problems are addressed in Chapters 12.25 and 12.26.

Clinical findings

The clinical picture is likely to be dominated by the primary condition of which acute renal failure is a consequence. Oliguria may alert nursing staff, but it is not invariable and polyuria may confuse. Unsuspected and potentially fatal hyperkalaemia is the greatest danger. In the later stages of acute renal failure there are manifestations of uraemia with anorexia, nausea, and vomiting (only occasionally diarrhoea); muscular cramps; and signs of encephalopathy—including a 'metabolic' flapping tremor (asterixis) progressing only rarely to depressed consciousness and *grand mal* convulsions. Skin bruising and gastrointestinal bleeding may occur. Uraemic haemorrhagic pericarditis occurs much less frequently in acute than in chronic renal failure.

Renal recovery occurs in the vast majority of those who survive the precipitating insult. Only a few suffer acute cortical necrosis with little or no recovery of renal function. Recovery may begin at any time from a few days to a few months (median 10–14 days) after the onset, with a progressive increase in urinary volume typically preceding improvement in plasma levels of creatinine and urea. A period of polyuria may ensue, placing the patient at risk of sodium and water depletion. Young patients can be expected to recover clinically normal renal function, but in those over 70 years recovery may be delayed, incomplete, and not infrequently, does not occur at all.

Biochemical changes

Apart from rises in urea and creatinine concentrations, important changes include hyperkalaemia, metabolic acidosis, hypocalcaemia, and hyperphosphataemia. Hyperkalaemia is due not only to reduced urinary excretion, but also to potassium release from cells—either as a consequence of cell death or as a result of metabolic acidosis. Particularly rapid rises are to be expected when there is extensive tissue damage or hypercatabolism, as in rhabdomyolysis, burns, and sepsis. Transfusion of stored blood is sometimes said to cause dangerous rises in plasma potassium concentration in oliguric patients. Loss of blood into the gastrointestinal tract or body tissues is followed by red cell lysis and the absorption of a considerable potassium load.

Acidosis due to retention of sulphuric and phosphoric acids, is usually modest in degree (plasma pH 7.2–7.35), but can be more severe, manifesting as sighing Kussmaul respiration and/or with circulatory compromise.

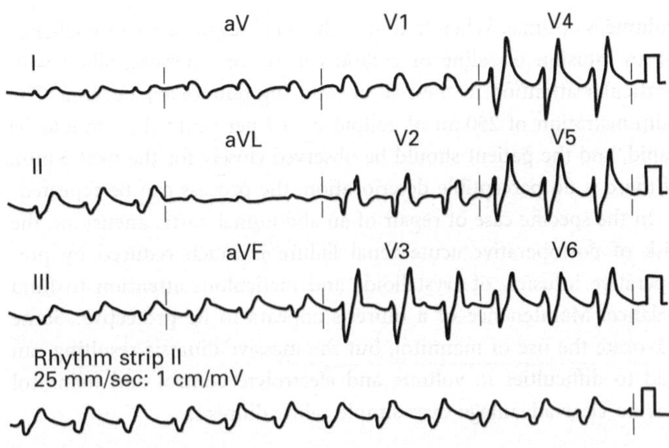

Fig. 1 An electrocardiogram showing severe hyperkalaemia changes in a patient with a serum potassium level of 8.6 mmol/l.

Calcium malabsorption occurs early in acute renal failure and is probably secondary to disordered vitamin D metabolism. Hypocalcaemia can develop with surprising rapidity. It is usually asymptomatic, but tetany and fits may be provoked by injudicious over-rapid correction of acidosis with resultant depression of ionized calcium. Profound hypocalcaemia and marked hyperphosphataemia, together with hyperuricaemia, is to be expected in rhabdomyolysis; during the recovery phase transient hypercalcaemia is frequently seen; probably caused by secondary hyperparathyroidism. This phase may be prolonged and accompanied by metastatic calcification in patients in whom there has been extensive muscle injury.

Plasma sodium concentration is usually normal. On occasion, however, intake of water may exceed the rate of excretion, and hyponatraemia results.

Medical management

There are three goals: (a) treatment of life-threatening complications of acute renal failure; (b) prompt diagnosis and treatment of hypovolaemia; and (c) specific treatment of the underlying condition.

Life-threatening complications

Hyperkalaemia

All doctors who work with acutely ill patients should be able to recognize the characteristic electrocardiogram (ECG) appearances, which are a better indicator of cardiac toxicity than the serum potassium level. As serum potassium rises, the following changes progressively occur (Fig. 1): (a)'tenting' of the T-wave; (b) reduction in size of P-waves, increase in PR interval, widening of QRS complex; (c) disappearance of P-wave, further widening of QRS complex; (d) irregular 'sinusoidal' ECG; and (e) asystole. Any change more severe than tenting of the T-waves demands immediate treatment, as described in Table 5 and Chapter 12.4.

Pulmonary oedema

Severe cases are dramatic. The patient is terrified, restless, and confused. Examination reveals cyanosis, tachypnoea, tachycardia, widespread wheeze or crepitations in the chest, and a gallop rhythm. Investigation demonstrates arterial hypoxaemia and widespread interstitial shadowing on the chest radiograph. The patient should be sat up, supported, and given oxygen by face mask in as high a concentration as possible. Frusemide is of little value in renal failure but morphine relieves symptoms rapidly. The definitive treatment is removal of fluid by haemodialysis, haemofiltration, or, less satisfactorily, peritoneal dialysis, but the immediate beneficial effects of venesection of 500 ml blood from the patient *in extremis* should not be forgotten.

Recognition and treatment of volume depletion

If features suggestive of intravascular volume depletion (Table 4) are present, the deficit should be corrected rapidly. Large-bore intravenous access should be established and fluid (normal saline or colloid) infused at maximum rate. The patient should be continuously observed and the infusion stopped when features of volume depletion have disappeared, but before volume overload has been induced. There has been debate about the best type of replacement fluid, but little evidence on which to base firm recommendations. It seems sensible to include blood in replacement when blood has obviously been lost, or the haemoglobin concentration is less than 10 g/dl. Dextrose saline (containing 0.15 per cent saline) or 5 per cent dextrose infusions have no place, as these solutions distribute throughout the total body water and only a small fraction remains within the vascular compartment.

Other measures alleged to improve renal function

There is no compelling evidence of benefit of any of the remedies often prescribed in an endeavour to protect or to improve renal function. Modest doses of diuretics (frusemide 40–120 mg, mannitol 25 g) given intravenously to a volume-replete patient undergoing a procedure such as bile duct surgery, resection of aortic aneurysm or cardiac bypass, may afford protection. In established acute renal failure large doses of frusemide (0.5–2 g/day) may substantially increase urinary volume, and this can ease the management of fluid balance and reduce the degree of hyperkalaemia but will probably not greatly alter the requirement for renal replacement therapy, and there is no evidence that they reduce mortality. The evidence in favour of 'renal dose' dopamine (1–3 μg/kg per min) is even weaker and, it may well be that the effects that are sometimes observed relate to the diuretic effects of dopamine and to improvements in cardiac output rather than to any direct effect on renal vasculature. All other treatments should be regarded as experimental.

Fluid and electrolyte requirements in established acute renal failure

In the absence of normal renal function the greatest care must be taken to regulate the intake of fluids and electrolytes to match losses in the urine, from the gastrointestinal tract, and from other 'insensible' sources. Fluid intake is limited to the volume of the previous day's urine output and gastrointestinal losses plus 500 ml; but this allocation may need to be substantially increased in the presence of fever or in hot environments, when insensible losses may be much increased. Fluid balance charts are frequently inaccurate and unthinking adherence to the 'output plus 500 ml' rule can lead to grief. There is no substitute for careful, twice-daily clinical examination for signs of intravascular volume depletion or excess, supplemented by accurate daily weighing.

The intake of sodium must also be matched to output. In oliguric patients, requirements are usually very small, perhaps only 15–30 mmol/day. In polyuric patients, however, the requirements can be considerable, with a danger of volume depletion if these are not met. The urine will usually contain sodium at a concentration of 50–70 mmol/l: hence if urine output is 3 litres/day then over 200 mmol of sodium may be required. On occasion, the urine output in polyuric

Table 5 Treatment of hyperkalaemia

Treatment	Comment
1. Intravenous calcium (10 ml of 10% calcium gluconate, over 60 s, repeated until ECG improves)	Acts instantly to 'stabilize' cardiac membranes (mechanism unknown). Does not alter serum potassium
2. Intravenous insulin and glucose (10 units rapidly acting insulin + 50 ml 50% glucose, over 10 min)	Insulin stimulates Na-K-ATPase in muscle and liver, thus driving potassium into cells. Serum potassium falls by 1–2 mmol/l over 30–60 min
3. Intravenous sodium bicarbonate (50–100 ml of 4.2% solution over 10 min)	Traditionally thought to increase blood pH, inducing exchange of intracellular protons for extracellular potassium. May not work in this manner as hypertonic saline has been shown to be effective
4. Cation exchange resins, e.g. sodium or calcium polystyrene sulphonate (15 g by mouth 6 hourly or 15–30 g per rectum 6 hourly)	Exchanges sodium or calcium for potassium in the gut lumen and thus induces loss of potassium from body (unlike 1–3 above). Takes 4 h to produce an effect. Precautions against severe constipation are necessary
5. Haemodialysis/filtration	Except in those rare cases where renal function can rapidly be restored, e.g. relief of obstruction, it is likely that hyperkalaemia will recur and haemodialysis or high-volume haemofiltration will be required

acute renal failure can be even higher and, if the response is to administer an even greater quantity of fluid (output plus insensible losses), it is possible to contrive a vicious cycle whereby ever increasing urinary output is met by ever increasing fluid infusion. In that situation, limiting input to urinary output alone and allowing other fluid losses to establish a mild overall negative balance is often helpful. For reasons that are not known, excess of sodium and water in patients with tubular necrosis leads to peripheral or pulmonary oedema, whereas in those with glomerulonephritis it tends to produce hypertension.

It is essential to check plasma potassium at least daily; and in those with hypercatabolism or gastrointestinal bleeding, or who require surgery, more frequently. In oliguric cases, dietary potassium consumption should be limited to the minimum compatible with an adequate intake of protein and amino acids (20–30 mmol/day).

Potassium-retaining diuretics, such as spironolactone, amiloride, and triamterene, should never be used in renal failure. Antimicrobial agents containing potassium should also be avoided whenever possible. In oliguric patients, excretion of potassium can sometimes be enhanced by the use of high doses of frusemide (0.5–1 g daily). By contrast, in polyuric acute renal failure substantial losses of potassium can occur and need to be replaced.

Renal replacement therapy

Mandatory indications for immediate instigation of renal replacement therapy are: (a) encephalopathy, pericarditis, or uraemic bleeding; (b) refractory hyperkalaemia; (c) intractable fluid overload; and (d) acidosis producing circulatory compromise. Other than in these situations there is no hard and fast rule as to when renal replacement therapy should be initiated. Modern practice is to begin when the blood urea reaches 25–30 mmol/l and the serum creatinine 500–700 µmol/l, unless there is clear evidence that spontaneous recovery is occurring.

Peritoneal dialysis is the method most commonly used worldwide. The principle is the same as that described for treatment of chronic renal failure (see Chapter 12.29), the major differences being: (a) catheters can be inserted percutaneously using a metal stylet, and (b) smaller volume exchanges with shorter dwell-times are the norm. The technique is precluded in the many patients whose renal failure is associated with abdominal surgery. Other problems include difficulties in maintaining dialysate flow, leakage, peritoneal infection, protein losses, and restricted ability to clear fluid and uraemic wastes. Particularly in the hypercatabolic patient, peritoneal dialysis is frequently unable to provide good dialysis as judged by the best standards. *Haemodialysis*, performed daily or on alternate days, can provide much better control of uraemia. Major disadvantages arise from the fact that it is an intermittent treatment. In each 4 h treatment at least 2–3 litres of fluid must be removed to make 'space' either for infusion of drugs/parenteral fluids or for oral fluid intake in the 24–48-h period before the next dialysis. Such a procedure can impose substantial haemodynamic stress and so is frequently not tolerated by those with impaired cardiovascular function. This is the main reason why *continuous haemofiltration* techniques have largely replaced haemodialysis in intensive care units. This process is tolerated well, even by patients who are very ill.

Indications for renal biopsy

In probable ATN renal biopsy should not be performed, as the information gained is unlikely to influence management, and the risks of the procedure are not warranted. Biopsy should be considered: (a) when the history, examination, or laboratory tests suggest a systemic disorder that could cause acute renal failure and could be diagnosed by renal biopsy; (b) when the urine sediment contains red cell casts; (c) when the case history is atypical; and (d) when renal failure is unusually prolonged (say beyond 6 weeks), although cortical necrosis (see below) is better diagnosed by angiography.

Nutrition

Patients with acute renal failure are invariably catabolic. If nutrition is neglected, patients lose weight very rapidly, and those that lose most have the highest mortality. Early institution of nutritional support probably improves prognosis. The diet for the undialysed patient with acute renal failure should provide all essential amino acids in a total protein intake of 0.3–0.5 g/kg body weight daily, with fat and carbohydrate to bring up the energy intake to at least 2000 cal, or 4000 cal in hypercatabolic cases. In patients too unwell to take adequate food by mouth, tube feeding or parenteral nutrition should be started early. Protein restriction is no longer appropriate once a decision has been made to initiate dialysis.

Bleeding

In uraemia the bleeding time is prolonged. Better control of uraemia and the routine use of H_2-receptor antagonists has been associated

Table 6 Practical strategies for the management of bleeding in acute renal failure

1. Exclude the possibility of a heparin effect
2. Blood transfusion to obtain haematocrit >30% (occasionally erythropoietin is of value)
3. Cryoprecipitate (10 bags) has its maximal effect between 1 and 2 h after administration. Its effect disappears at 24–36 h
4. Desmopressin (0.3 μg/kg intravenously) acts by increasing factor VIII coagulant activity. Shown in acute renal failure to shorten prolonged bleeding time. Repeated doses have a lesser effect
5. Conjugated oestrogen: 0.6 mg/kg per day for 5 days. Shown to reduce bleeding time (for at least 14 days) in patients with chronic renal impairment and haemorrhagic tendency

with a greatly reduced risk of upper gastrointestinal bleeding, a previously frequent and grave occurrence. There are some patients who bleed from anywhere and everywhere. Guidelines for the management of such cases are given in Table 6.

Sepsis

Overwhelming septicaemia is a common (and sometimes occult) cause of acute renal failure. It is the commonest cause of death in those with acute renal failure. If a patient with acute renal failure appears to be deteriorating in any way, sepsis must be suspected. Unused intravenous lines and urinary catheters should be removed, and those that are necessary but in any way 'suspicious' should be replaced. The patient should be examined regularly for signs of a septic focus. There should be a low threshold for repeated, thorough microbiological investigation. Proven infection should be treated promptly with modified doses of appropriate antimicrobials. In many cases, it will be necessary to start treatment 'blind', having taken specimens for culture and made an educated guess at the likely pathogen, with the possibility of Gram-negative septicaemia high on the list. In the patient who appears 'septic', but in whom no cause can be found, computed tomography (CT) scanning, to search for abdominal sepsis should be performed but not be relied upon too faithfully; surgical exploration should be undertaken if there is any doubt.

Prescription of drugs in acute renal failure

This matter is discussed in Chapter 12.26.

Other specific causes of acute renal failure

Nephrotoxic causes of acute renal failure

Exogenous nephrotoxins

A wide variety of exogenous agents, including therapeutically prescribed drugs, can cause or exacerbate acute renal failure (see Chapter 12.25).

Endogenous nephrotoxins

Myoglobin-rhabdomyolysis

Myoglobinuric acute renal failure is associated with crush injury or other trauma to muscle, but the mechanism of renal failure remains unclear. There are also a large number of causes of non-traumatic rhabdomyolysis (Table 7) which are easily missed, as muscular pain, swelling, and tenderness may not be prominent features, and may even be absent. The combination of dark-brown urine, positive for 'blood' on a reagent strip but without red cells on microscopy, indicates myoglobinuria and confirms the diagnosis. The findings of a very high plasma urate (>750 μmol/l) and phosphate (>2.5 mmol/l) and of unusually low plasma calcium (<1.5 mmol/l) in any patient with acute renal failure should lead to consideration of the condition. Gross elevation of plasma uric acid may conceivably contribute to the mechanism of renal damage. Extremely high levels of plasma myoglobin, aldolase, creatine phosphokinase, and lactic dehydrogenase—all released from damaged muscle—are to be expected.

If the diagnosis of rhabdomyolysis is made, the question of whether to initiate an alkaline diuresis arises, as on theoretical grounds alkalinization of the urine should lead to enhanced excretion of the putative toxin and protect against acute renal failure. Victims of a crush injury have been treated with infusion of very large volumes of fluid (12 litres/day) and big doses of mannitol (160 g/day) and bicarbonate (240 mmol/day). In comparison with historical (volume-depleted) controls the incidence of renal failure was impressively reduced; but the difficulties of controlling potassium balance in the face of such a massive diuresis should not be underestimated. Avoidance of hypovolaemia using a less aggressive and more easily managed fluid regimen may be equally efficacious and is the more usual treatment given.

Table 7 Some causes of rhabdomyolysis

Direct muscle injury
Ischaemic muscle injury
Compression
Vascular occlusion
Any cause of coma (e.g. opiate overdose, diabetes mellitus, cerebrovascular accident) or of prolonged immobility (e.g. following a fall in the elderly) can be associated with rhabdomyolysis due to a pressure effect.
Excessive muscular activity
Seizures
Sporting, e.g. marathon running
Inflammatory myositis
Immunological, e.g. dermatomyositis, polymyositis
Infection, e.g. viral (influenza, coxsackie)
Metabolic
Hypokalaemia, hypophosphataemia
Genetic abnormalities of carbohydrate metabolism, e.g. myophosphorylase deficiency (McArdle's syndrome), phosphofructokinase deficiency
Toxins/drugs
Snake bite, carbon monoxide, alcohol, hemlock, paint/glue sniffing
Clofibrate, aminocaproic acid, HMG-CoA reductase inhibitors
Others
Malignant hyperpyrexia
Neuroleptic malignant syndrome
Phaeochromocytoma 'storm'

Haemoglobin

Acute renal failure is seen in association with massive haemolysis in malaria, glucose 6-phosphate dehydrogenase deficiency, mismatched blood transfusion, arsine poisoning, copper sulphate poisoning, burns, and as a complication of bladder irrigation with hypotonic solutions. In each circumstance it is possible, but not proven, that the development of acute renal failure might be attributable to, or exacerbated by, the presence of large amounts of free haemoglobin within the circulation.

Urate and phosphate

A rapid rise in plasma uric acid concentration complicating treatment of lymphoma, leukaemia, myeloma, or other 'high-turnover' tumours may result in the deposition of urate crystals in the distal tubule. Hyperuricaemia and renal failure have been described on rare occasions after recurrent epileptic seizures.

In the context of the treatment of malignancy the risk of hyperuricaemic acute renal failure is predictable, and preventable. Dehydration should be avoided. Before the initiation of chemotherapy, a brisk saline or alkaline diuresis should be initiated, and allopurinol treatment started. In those with normal renal function a dose of 900 mg/day may be preferred to the conventional dose of 300 mg/day. If hyperuricaemic acute renal failure does develop, administration of alkali may be contraindicated if plasma phosphate is raised concurrently. Prompt improvement usually follows reduction in plasma uric acid levels, which can be accomplished much more effectively by haemodialysis than by peritoneal dialysis. On very rare occasions the ureters can become obstructed by urate crystals and ureteral catheterization and washout may be required. Similar obstruction by phosphate is also rarely seen in the context of massive cell destruction in the treatment of malignant disease. Urinary alkalinization should then be avoided because it may promote intratubular phosphate precipitation.

Vascular causes of acute renal failure

Acute cortical necrosis

Acute cortical necrosis accounts for perhaps less than 1 per cent of all cases of suspected ATN. Most cases used to be the result of obstetric disaster, but this is now very rare in the 'developed world'. In the non-obstetric population, patients with pancreatitis, endotoxaemia, and disseminated intravascular coagulation are at risk. The pathological findings are of microvascular thrombosis, mainly affecting interlobular arteries, arterioles, and glomeruli, with complete infarction of affected areas of cortex. The medulla and a rim of juxtamedullary tissue are spared. The diagnosis is usually first suspected when renal function fails to recover in a patient thought to be suffering from ATN. Renal angiography reveals attenuation of interlobular arteries, an increase in the subcapsular vessels, and a negative outer cortical nephrogram. Biopsy, which samples only a very small piece of tissue, may mislead because of the patchy nature of renal damage. Dimercaptosuccinic acid scans are sometimes advocated, but are frequently difficult to interpret in patients with poor renal function. Return of renal function in cases of acute cortical necrosis occurs very slowly, if at all, and is attributable to the survival of islands of intact cortical tissue. About 50 per cent of cases recover function sufficiently to get off dialysis, but the glomerular filtration rate rarely exceeds 10–20 ml/min; hypertension (including accelerated phase) may be a major problem, and a subsequent decline in renal function with the necessity for a return to dialysis/transplantation is not uncommon. The kidneys tend to contract, and cortical calcification, producing an eggshell or tramline appearance on the abdominal radiograph, is a characteristic sequel.

Large vessel obstruction

Occlusion of the main renal arteries—or of the artery of a solitary functioning kidney—by trauma, dissection, thrombosis, or embolism may rarely be the reason for acute renal failure. Loin pain sometimes occurs, and fever would be expected, but symptoms can be notable by their absence. Proteinuria and haematuria may occur. Diagnosis is important, because renovascular surgery can be surprisingly effective in restoring function, even when undertaken 24 h or more after onset. Symptoms may mimic acute pyelonephritis, and suspicion should be aroused by complete, sudden anuria in the absence of urinary obstruction in an appropriate clinical setting. DTPA renography and angiography are the appropriate diagnostic tests, but CT scanning can also reveal the characteristic wedge-shaped infarcts when occlusion is incomplete. Renal vein thrombosis may also cause acute renal failure (see Chapter 12.5).

Small vessel obstruction

Accelerated-phase hypertension

So-called malignant hypertension can lead rapidly to acute renal failure related to the changes of necrosis in renal arterioles. The higher the creatinine at diagnosis, the poorer the renal prognosis. In one study, only 9 per cent of those with an initial plasma creatinine below 300 mmol/l progressed to endstage renal failure, compared with two-thirds of those with figures above this level. This is one of the conditions in which renal function sometimes recovers after a long period on dialysis. A similar situation arises in the so called 'scleroderma renal crisis' (see Chapter 10.12), but arterial pressure in that situation is not always increased.

Glomerulonephritic and vasculitic causes of acute renal failure

A large number of glomerulonephritic and vasculitic diseases can cause acute renal failure, sometimes in association with pulmonary haemorrhage. These are listed in Table 8, and are discussed in detail elsewhere.

Interstitial nephritis as a cause of acute renal failure

Acute interstitial nephritis caused by drugs or due to other rarer causes must always be considered (see Table 9). The individual causes and management are discussed elsewhere.

Leptospirosis (see also Chapter 16.67)

Acute renal failure due to an interstitial nephritis may appear within a few days of the onset of disease, but more commonly occurs in the second week. It is frequently mild, but may be severe, with plasma urea rising rapidly due to hypercatabolism. The diagnosis should be considered in any patient with unexplained acute renal failure who has myalgias/muscle tenderness, conjunctival infection, and/or haemorrhage or jaundice.

Hantavirus disease (see also Chapter 16.29)

Several serotypes of Hantavirus produce a disease similar in many respects to leptospirosis. In both the European and Asian (more severe) forms, myalgias, conjunctival haemorrhage, and thrombocytopenia may be observed, but jaundice is rare. The diagnosis

Table 8 Glomerulonephritides and vasculitides causing acute renal failure

Antiglomerular basement membrane disease
Primary glomerulonephritis
Mesangial IgA nephropathy
Mesangiocapillary glomerulonephritis
Primary systemic vasculitis
Microscopic polyarteritis/idiopathic rapidly progressive (crescentic) glomerulonephritis
Wegener's granulomatosis
Churg–Strauss syndrome, polyarteritis nodosa, giant-cell arteritis, Takayasu's arteritis (all rarely cause renal failure)
Other causes
Cryoglobulinaemia
Systemic lupus erythematosus
Infection—post-streptococcal, infective endocarditis, ventriculoatrial shunt, visceral abscess

Table 9 Some causes of interstitial nephritis causing acute renal failure

Drugs	
β-Lactam antibiotics	Penicillin G, methicillin, ampicillin, cephalothin
Other antibiotics	Sulphonamides (co-trimoxazole), rifampicin
Anti-inflammatory agents	Fenoprofen, naproxen, ibuprofen, glafenin, mefenamic acid
Diuretics	Thiazides, frusemide, chlorthalidone, triamterene
Others	Cimetidine, phenindione, diphenylhydantoin, allopurinol
Note: Many other drugs have been incriminated on the basis of occasional association	
Infections	
Septicaemia	Direct invasion by Gram-negative organisms, Staphylococcus, *Candida albicans*
Direct/indirect effects	Commonly in leptospirosis and Hantavirus disease. Less commonly in scarlet fever and diphtheria. Occasionally in infectious mononucleosis and HIV disease. Many other infections have been incriminated on the basis of occasional association
Infiltration	
Lymphoma, leukaemia, plasma cell dyscrasia (multiple pathogenic mechanisms)	
Other	
Sarcoidosis	
Idiopathic: no plausible cause found, diagnosed by exclusion. Occasionally associated with uveitis or iritis, chronic active hepatitis, primary biliary cirrhosis, ulcerative colitis	

depends on serological evidence of infection. There is no specific treatment.

'Haematological' causes of acute renal failure

Haemolytic uraemic syndrome, thrombotic thrombocytopenia purpura, idiopathic post-partum renal failure, and acute renal failure in myeloma are discussed elsewhere.

Hepatorenal syndrome

The hepatorenal syndrome consists of the association of severe and usually progressive liver disease with acute renal failure. The renal failure is characterized by: (a) no evidence of renal parenchymal damage—if the kidney is transplanted it functions normally in the recipient; (b) characteristic 'prerenal' urine biochemistry (Table 3); (c) no sustained response to volume expansion; and (d) exclusion of other causes of acute renal failure. The mechanism of renal failure is not known, but it is associated with markedly reduced renal perfusion.

The most important consideration in management is avoidance of known precipitants (drugs, excessive diuresis, delay in treatment of sepsis). Nevertheless, the syndrome develops in up to 20 per cent of cirrhotics admitted to hospital. There is no specific treatment and the prognosis is extremely poor. In the presence of potentially reversible liver disease, or with the prospect of liver transplantation, intensive therapy and renal replacement therapy are justified.

Tropical

The spectrum of diseases which causes ATN is in the tropics is substantially different from that encountered in the 'developed' world. Medical causes account for 65 per cent of cases, surgical causes 25 per cent, and obstetric causes 15 per cent. Common tropical infections causing acute renal failure include falciparum malaria, leptospirosis, melioidosis, salmonellosis, and shigellosis. Snake bite is the cause of 2–3 per cent of cases, and a much higher proportion in some centres at some times of the year. Acute renal failure develops in two-thirds of those bitten by Russell's viper. Heat stroke can cause acute renal failure.

Prognosis

Acute renal failure of sufficient severity to require renal replacement therapy has a high mortality. In a series of over 1300 cases the actuarial 1-year survival of all medical and surgical cases rose from 39 per cent to 58 per cent between 1956 and 1988, despite an increase in the median patient age from 41 to 61 years over this period. The prognosis varies according to the cause: it is best in obstetric and poisoning cases (80–90 per cent survival) and worst in burns (15–20 per cent survival). Death is nowadays rarely attributable to renal failure *per se*, and the incidence of life-threatening gastrointestinal haemorrhage is much reduced: sepsis is the major killer. The patients die *with* but not directly *of* renal failure. If they survive the precipitating insult, largely complete recovery of renal function can be anticipated, except in the elderly (over 70 years) in whom there is a substantial chance (10–20 per cent) that dependence on dialysis will be lifelong.

Further reading

Firth, J.D. (1998). The clinical approach to the patient with acute renal failure. In *Oxford textbook of clinical nephrology*, (2nd edn) (ed. A.M. Davison and J.S. Cameron), pp. 1557–82. Oxford University Press.

Lieberthal, W. (1997). Biology of acute renal failure: therapeutic implications. *Kidney International*, **52**, 1102–15.

Mason, P.D. (1998). Special acute renal failure problems. Glomerulonephritis, vasculitis, and the nephrotic syndrome. In *Oxford textbook of clinical nephrology*, (2nd edn) (ed. A.M. Davison and J.S. Cameron), pp. 1625–34. Oxford University Press.

Shilliday, I.R., Quinn, K. J., Allison, M.E. (1997). Loop diuretics in the management of acute renal failure: a prospective, double-blind, placebo-controlled, randomized study. *Nephrology, Dialysis Transplantation*, **12**, 2592–6.

Turney, J. H., Marshall, D.H., Brownjohn, A.M., Ellis, C.M., Parsons, F.M. (1990). The evolution of acute renal failure, 1956–1988. *Quarterly Journal of Medicine*, 74: 83–104.

Chapter 12.29

Chronic renal failure

A. M. El Nahas and C. G. Winearls with contributions from P. J. Ratcliffe, D. W. R. Gray, and R. Gokal

The severity of chronic renal failure (CRF) can be classified as mild, moderate, severe and end-stage (see Table 1), but there is poor correlation between glomerular filtration rate (GFR) and symptoms or signs. Progression can be slow, and symptoms can then be attributed to age or other illness, only presenting near to a need for replacement therapy. Function is often assessed in practice by measurement of plasma creatinine concentration. The relationship between this criterion and GFR is not precise and is discussed in Chapter 12.1

Prevalence and incidence

The true prevalence is unknown but a prospective study in the UK found plasma creatinine concentrations more than 150 μmol/litre in 2058 per million adults from whom samples had been sent to hospital laboratories. This included patients with transient acute renal impairment. The figure for renal failure short of endstage was 600 per million and an annual incidence of endstage of 78 per million population (p.m.p.). Since this study, the annual incidence of endstage renal failure in England has been re-evaluated and found to be nearer 110 p.m.p./year. National registers give more precise information about the provision of replacement therapy (Table 2). The prevalence of treated endstage renal failure will vary from country to country,

Table 1 Severity of renal failure

	GFR (ml/min)	Symptoms and signs
Mild	30–50	None: ±hypertension; early secondary hyperparathyroidism
Moderate	10–29	Few: anaemia, hypertension, early osteodystrophy, lassitude
Severe	<10	Fluid retention, anorexia, vomiting, pruritus, poor intellectual performance
Endstage	<5	Pulmonary oedema, fits and coma, pericarditis, hyperkalaemia, death

GFR, glomerular filtration rate.

Table 2 Acceptance rates on to renal replacement programmes international comparisons (1996)

Country	Patients (p.m.p./year)
USA	276
Austria	136
France	123
Sweden	110
UK	78
Australia	77

United States Renal Data System 1998 Annual Data Report. International comparisons of ESRD therapy. *American Journal of Kidney Diseases*, 1998; **32**, (Suppl. 1), S136–S141. p.m.p., per million population.

Table 3 Prevalence of patients on renal replacement treatment: international comparisons (1996)

Country	Patients (p.m.p.)
USA	1041
Japan	1328
Austria	590
France	634
Sweden	615
UK	482
Australia	507

United States Renal Data System (1998). Annual Data Report. International comparisons of ESRD therapy. *American Journal of Kidney Diseases*, **32** (Suppl. 1), S136–S141. p.m.p., per million population.

and depends on the incidence of particular diseases and the availability and capacity of dialysis and transplant programmes (Table 3).

There appear to be real differences in the incidence of endstage renal failure according to age, gender, and race. In Western countries the incidence is lowest in children (10 p.m.p./year), and highest in those aged over 75 (> 400 p.m.p./year), reaching > 1000 p.m.p in the USA). In Caucasians, 30–60 years of age, the incidence ranges between 50 and 150 p.m.p./year and is slightly higher in males than females. In the USA the annual incidence of endstage renal failure in those of African or native American descent is nearly four times higher (424 p.m.p.) than in Caucasian subjects (114 p.m.p.). This difference cannot be explained solely by the higher prevalence of diabetes mellitus and hypertension within these ethnic groups. It may reflect genetic and environmental predisposition to some forms of renal disease and socio-economic factors including diet, and access to medical care. The incidence of endstage renal failure in the UK is higher in Asian immigrants and their descendants than in the native British population.

Causes

There are many causes of CRF (Tables 4 and 5), but worldwide, glomerulonephritis is the most common. Diabetic nephropathy now accounts for some 30 per cent of patients on dialysis programmes in the USA. Hypertension is frequently given as the cause of renal failure when no specific pathological entity has been identified. Many such patients probably have an undiagnosed causes, others present very

Table 4 Comparison of aetiology of endstage renal failure: estimates from the European and national registries

	Percentage of cases				
	Europe[a]		USA[b]		Australia[c]
	(1985–1993)		(1987–1996)		(1992)
Glomerulonephritis	26	20	25	11	38
Diabetes	9.5	18	14	39	14
Cystic disease	8	7.5	3	7	8
Hypertension[d]	10		29	28	9
Analgesic nephropathy	2		1	0.1	9
Pyelonephritis/interstitial nephritis	18	13	3	4.5	5
Misc[e]	11		9	2.6	12

[a] EDTA Registry 1985–1993, from A.J. Wing (1992 and personal communication).

[b] United States Renal Data System (1998). Annual Data Report. Incidence and prevalence of ESRD. *American Journal of Kidney Diseases* **32**, (Suppl. 1), S38–49.

Table 5 Some rare causes of chronic renal failure (<1% of cases)

Medullary cystic disease	Scleroderma
Hereditary nephritis with deafness (Alport's syndrome)	Haemolytic-uraemic syndrome Kidney tumour
Cystinosis	Nephrocalcinosis
Oxalosis	Gouty nephropathy
Systemic vasculitis (Wegener's granulomatosis and polyarteritis)	Fabry's disease Sickle-cell disease
Systemic lupus erythematosus	Tuberculosis
Myeloma	Balkan nephropathy
Amyloidosis	Irradiation nephropathy

late with small, shrunken kidneys from which no informative renal tissue can be obtained by biopsy and so are classified as 'aetiology unknown'.

There is an higher prevalence of obstructive uropathy and renovascular disease in the elderly among whom amyloidosis and myeloma are also more common.

There is a higher prevalence of reflux and analgesic nephropathies in women, and there is evidence of a faster rate of deterioration in male patients with polycystic disease and some forms of glomerulonephritis, for instance IgA nephropathy.

Apparent geographical variations within Europe have also been reported. More than 80 per cent of patients with endstage renal failure in Finland are thought to have chronic glomerulonephritis; the equivalent figure in the UK is less than 50 per cent, and in Greece only 5 per cent. It is unclear whether these reported differences are genuine or are accounted for by diagnostic approach or referral pattern. Diabetic nephropathy appears to be commoner in Scandinavia and analgesic nephropathy more prevalent in Belgium, Switzerland, and Australia, the latter decreasing with declining consumption and restrictions on the sale of combination analgesics. Amyloidosis is very common in the Mediterranean basin and in Turkey, where it is the cause of 30 per cent of endstage renal failure. Balkan nephropathy is confined to the former Yugoslavia and Bulgaria (see OTM3, pp. 3228–31). Glomerulonephritis appears commoner China, India, South-east Asia, Africa, and South America, when compared with Europe or the USA. In some parts of the Middle-East, schistosomiasis and its associated nephropathy are endemic.

In the USA, significant racial differences have been reported in the causes of chronic kidney disease. Diabetes mellitus (particularly type II), is 1.35-fold more prevalent in Afro-Americans than Caucasians, and a higher prevalence among native and Hispanic-Americans is also well established. Likewise, there is a higher prevalence and incidence of renal failure due to hypertension in Afro-Americans and Hispanic-Americans compared with Caucasians.

Pathophysiology of chronic renal failure

Adaptive mechanisms maintain acceptable health until the GFR is about 10–15 ml/min, and life-sustaining functions continue until the GFR is less than 5 ml/min. The 'intact nephron hypothesis' suggests that most nephrons are non-functioning, while the remaining few function normally. These later produce an increased volume of filtrate and their tubules respond appropriately by excreting fluid and solutes in amounts which maintain external balance. For sodium and potassium, some balance exists at a GFR of 5 ml/min and plasma values are commonly normal. For phosphate and urate, adaptation is less precise and plasma concentrations are increased in many patients at a GFR of 20 ml/min and in almost all at 5–10 ml/min.

The 'trade-off' hypothesis involves the concept that adaptations arising in CRF may control one abnormality, but at the expense of producing other changes. The best example is increase of parathormone secretion to increase fractional excretion of phosphate; as the GFR falls, plasma phosphate rises, parathormone secretion increases, and plasma phosphate is lowered by decreased tubular reabsorption. The cost of normal plasma phosphate is then secondary hyperparathyroidism.

Water

Inability to concentrate urine is often the first manifestation of CRF, resulting in polyuria, nocturia, and thirst when the GFR is about 30 ml/min or less. Diluting capacity is preserved until renal failure is advanced, the asymmetrical narrowing of the range of urinary osmolality eventually producing the fixed osmolality of CRF with its obligatory polyuria. Diseases that affect predominantly the medulla, such as pyelonephritis, interstitial nephritis, and medullary cystic disease, may present with a concentration defect at an earlier stage. Defective urine concentration is due to increased solute load in surviving nephrons, with minor contributions from decreased tubular function and increased GFR per nephron. Thirst maintains water balance provided there is free access to fluid but there is need for careful attention to fluid balance in the presence of anorexia, fever, surgery, and other sources of extrarenal loss. Urinary dilution is maintained until late in CRF, but large water loads are excreted more slowly than in normal subjects and excessive fluid results in hyponatraemia, mental disturbances, and convulsions.

Sodium

As renal function decreases, hormonal mechanisms increase the fraction of filtered sodium excreted so that sodium balance and extracellular fluid volume are often maintained until the GFR is less than 10 ml/min. The extent is such that the 1 per cent or less of filtered sodium excreted by normal subjects increases to 30 per cent in late CRF. Increased total body sodium, with water to maintain osmotic equilibrium, presents in most patients with hypertension without oedema. Later there is often leg oedema, elevated jugular venous pressure, pulmonary congestion, and functional incompetence of mitral and aortic valves. Precisely how sodium retention and increased extracellular fluid volume lead to hypertension is still uncertain.

In the presence of excessive dietary sodium restriction or of loss of sodium, functioning nephrons cannot retain sodium promptly so that extracellular fluid, plasma volume, and GFR all decrease. A small number of patients, usually with disease affecting the renal medulla, present with a urinary sodium leak and sodium depletion on a normal sodium diet. In them blood pressure is normal or low, and sodium supplements may be needed.

Potassium (see Chapter 12.4)

Most patients maintain close to normal external potassium balance until the GFR is less than 5 ml/min, but severe hyperkalaemia may follow a sudden reduction in residual GFR, excess dietary potassium, potassium-sparing diuretics, medication with high potassium content, surgery, acidosis and hypercatabolic states. In some patients, hyperkalaemia may be due to selective aldosterone deficiency (hyporeninaemic hypoaldosteronism) or the use of angiotensin-converting enzyme (ACE) inhibitors.

Acid–base

Acid–base disturbance is common and is discussed in Chapter 6.17.

Calcium phosphate and magnesium

Disturbances in CRF are described in Chapter 12.30. Magnesium concentrations are usually high and care must be exercised with the use of magnesium-containing drugs.

Clinical presentation and assessment

The symptoms and signs of uraemia develop insidiously and late (Fig. 1). The most common symptoms are fatigue, dyspnoea, ankle swelling, anorexia, vomiting, pruritus, and inability to concentrate. Patients are often present as 'uraemic emergencies' requiring immediate dialysis or its institution within a month. Such patients may be comatose, may have fitted, and have asterixis. The skin shows excoriation from pruritus, purpura, and bruising on a sallow yellow–brown background. The blood pressure is raised and the fundi may show haemorrhages and exudates. The left ventricular impulse is displaced and there is often a pericardial friction rub. There are basal crepitations and oedema of the face, sacrum, and ankles. Investigations show a urea of greater than 50 mmol/l, a creatinine of greater than 1000 μmol/l, hypocalcaemia, hyperphosphataemia, hyperkalaemia, and a partially compensated metabolic acidosis. There is a normochromic normocytic anaemia, a normal white blood count, and a platelet count in the low normal range. The morbidity in such patients is high but most patients present with a much milder picture. The approach to every new case of CRF should resolve the following issues:

1. Is there any life-threatening complication requiring urgent treatment? These include pulmonary oedema, hyperkalaemia, severe acidosis, encephalopathy, or accelerated-phase hypertension.
2. What factors may have caused an acute reduction in chronically impaired renal function? Can they be reversed? (Table 6).
3. What is the cause of renal failure? A specific diagnosis is needed for several reasons:
   (i) To consider specific measures to arrest the pathology. Examples include: obstructive uropathy, analgesic nephropathy, drug-related interstitial nephritis, rapidly progressive glomerulonephritis, systemic lupus erythematosus, vasculitic syndromes, accelerated phase hypertension, tuberculosis, myeloma, amyloid secondary to chronic infection or inflammation, ischaemic renal disease, and familial hyperuricaemic nephropathy.
   (ii) To anticipate potential complications and coincident disease, for example diabetes mellitus.
   (iii) To advise the family in inherited renal disease.
   (iv) To take into account when considering renal transplantation conditions that may recur, for example focal glomerulosclerosis, antiglomerular basement membrane disease, mesangiocapillary glomerulonephritis (especially 'dense deposit disease').
4. What measures are needed to delay progression?
5. Are there complications that require specific treatment? For instance hypertension, renal osteodystrophy, and anaemia.

History

Nocturia is a useful and reliable indicator of chronicity. An obstetric history may suggest the presence of renal disease during or preceding the pregnancy. A history of urinary tract infections, enuresis, and failure to thrive will point to reflux nephropathy; a heavy intake of pain killers to analgesic nephropathy. Symptoms and signs of systemic diseases, such as diabetes mellitus, hypertension, and systemic vasculitis, should be sought. A family history of renal disease may raise the possibility of adult polycystic kidney disease or Alport's syndrome. Careful enquiry about any drugs consumed regularly or irregularly is essential. An occupational history may reveal exposure to lead, analgesics, or hydrocarbons.

Physical signs (Fig. 1)

Signs of chronicity include pallor, yellow–brown skin discoloration, and nail dystrophy. Other manifestations include hypertension, cardiomegaly, congestive cardiac failure, and pericarditis. Retinal examination may reveal hypertensive changes, diabetic lesions, and, rarely, evidence of cholesterol emboli or retinitis pigmentosa. It is particularly important to detect potentially reversible cause of renal insufficiency such as dehydration, overhydration, heart failure, and urinary tract obstruction. In elderly hypertensive patient, the presence of bruits, particularly in the abdomen, suggest the possibility of underlying renal artery stenosis, the relief of which by angioplasty or vascular surgery may, in rare cases, restore sufficient renal function to delay or avoid dialysis.

Investigations

Laboratory

A full blood count is likely to reveal a normocytic normochromic anaemia but this can occur quite quickly in acute renal failure. Severe hypocalcaemia and hyperphosphataemia are suggestive of chronicity, although they too can also be observed in acute renal failure, particularly after rhabdomyolysis. High levels of bone alkaline phosphatase imply chronicity. Large casts imply tubular dilatation and

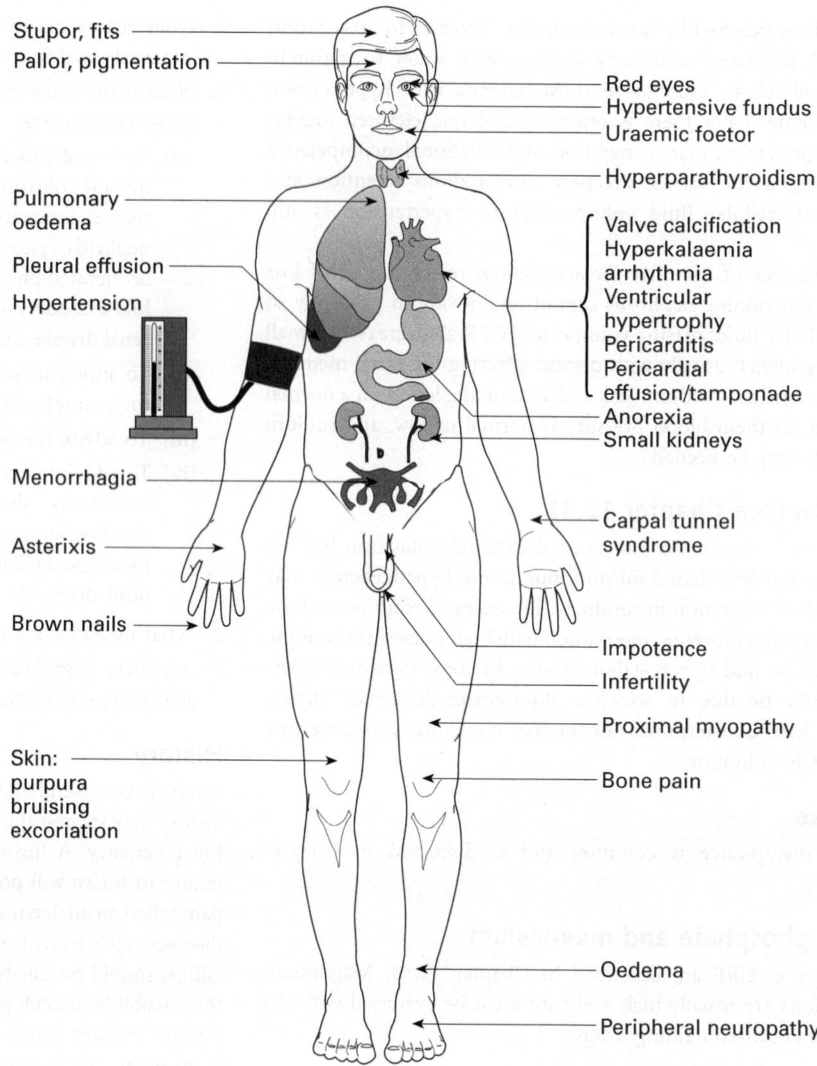

Fig. 1 Symptoms and signs of uraemia.

chronicity and white cell casts pyelonephritis or analgesic nephropathy. Sterile pyuria is a clue to analgesic nephropathy and renal tuberculosis. Crenated red cells in profusion and red cells casts suggest acute glomerulonephritis, and eosinophiluria, an acute drug-induced interstitial nephritis. When the GFR is less than 15 ml/min and plasma creatinine in excess of 600 μmol/l, proteinuria seldom exceeds 1 g/24 h. Heavy proteinuria, despite such severe CRF, suggests diabetic nephropathy, renal amyloidosis, or focal glomerulosclerosis. Tests for antinuclear antibody, ANCA, antiglomerular basement membrane antibodies, and complement are rarely helpful in the absence of clinical clues. It is always worth looking for myeloma and other causes of hypercalcaemia. Hepatitis B surface antigen is sought to alert laboratories and those who will be exposed to the patient's blood during diagnostic manoeuvres and treatment.

Radiological

Imaging, preferably by ultrasonography, is required to exclude obstruction and to determine kidney size. Chronicity is often, but not always, associated with shrunken kidneys; but size may be preserved in diabetic nephropathy, polycystic disease, amyloidosis, myeloma, and systemic sclerosis. Renal osteodystrophy may be revealed by radiography of the hands, clavicles, pelvis, and spine. A chest radiograph may raise the possibility of previously unsuspected pericardial effusion or pulmonary oedema. The presence of scars suggestive of tuberculosis should alert the clinician to possible reactivation.

Histological

Renal biopsy should not be undertaken in patients with small kidneys but, in patients with normal-sized kidneys, a biopsy is justified to rule out acute causes. Prognosis is difficult to equate with glomerular changes in chronic disease, but the presence of severe tubulointerstitial infiltrate or fibrosis usually indicates a poor outlook.

Measurement of renal function

Serum creatinine and creatinine clearance measurements, together with a plot of the reciprocal of serum creatinine (1/Cr) against time, are used to determine the degree of renal failure and its rate of progression. Creatinine clearance overestimates GFR as tubular secretion contributes to its elimination; the discrepancy between creatinine clearance and GFR is more marked at low levels. More accurate methods for the assessment of GFR include the measurement of the clearance of inulin, ^{51}Cr-EDTA, ^{99}Tc-DTPA and radiocontrast materials such as iothalamate and iohexol.

Table 6 Causes of acute on chronic renal failure

Renal hypoperfusion
Dehydration from diarrhoea, diuretics, surgery
Cardiac failure
Pericardial tamponade (rare)
Renal vascular disease
Drugs especially ACE inhibitors + NSAIDs
Systemic infection
Obstruction and infection of the urinary tract
Papillary necrosis and sloughing
Stones
Bladder cancer
Polycystic cysts
Clot in the ureter
Metabolic and toxic
Hypercalcaemia
Hyperuricaemia
Contrast media (especially in diabetes)
Drugs, especially aminoglycosides
Progression of underlying diseases
Relapse of nephritis
Development of accelerated phase hypertension
Renal vein thrombosis
Usually in chronically nephrotic patients
Pregnancy
At the end or after delivery, e.g. in patients with reflux nephropathy

ACE, angiotensin-converting enzyme; NSAIDs, non-steroidal anti-inflammatory drugs.

Electrocardiogram and echocardiogram

The electrocardiogram may reveal the presence of left ventricular hypertrophy and previous ischaemic events, and is a sensitive index of the cardiac effects of hyperkalaemia. More accurate assessment of left ventricular function and hypertrophy requires echocardiography.

Organ and metabolic dysfunction in chronic renal failure

The 'uraemic' syndrome is a consequence of a combination of effects. The potentially toxic substances that accumulate include purine metabolites, amines, indoles, phenols, myoinositol, and acid polyols. Retained 'middle molecules' of molecular weight 500–5000 Da are also suspected to contribute to uraemic toxicity. β_2-microglobulin, has been shown to cause a form of amyloid that occurs only in patients with CRF (see Chapter 6.15).

The cardiovascular system

Arterial pressure rises as renal function deteriorates and itself causes a further decline in renal function, maintaining a vicious cycle leading to hypertensive tissue damage and end-stage renal failure. There are many contributory causes to the rise in arterial blood pressure, but the major one is the retention of sodium and water.

Cardiac dysfunction may simply arise because of the combined effects of chronic hypertension with associated left ventricular hypertrophy together with chronic anaemia and coronary artery disease. Whether or not there is a specific 'uraemic cardiomyopathy' is debated; certainly there is evidence of myocardial fibrosis and valvular calcification in uraemic patients. Uraemic hypertensive patients are at much increased risk of heart failure, myocardial infarction, stroke, arrhythmia, and sudden death.

Uraemic pericarditis is a feature of advanced uraemia. The associated pericardial effusion can be either sero-fibrinous or haemorrhagic and can lead to cardiac tamponade.

Accelerated atherosclerosis is a feature of CRF, probably due to the combined effects of chronic hypertension, hyperlipidaemia, and vascular calcification.

The skeleton

The important complications of CRF relating to calcium metabolism and related bone disease are described in Chapter 12.30.

Gastrointestinal system

Anorexia, nausea, vomiting, but rarely diarrhoea are commonly observed in severe uraemia. Peptic ulcer as well as atrophic gastritis are known complications. Similarly, angiodysplasia of the gastrointestinal tract is relatively common and can cause severe and protracted bleeding, exacerbated by the underlying bleeding diathesis when uraemia is advanced.

The nervous system

Encephalopathy is characterized by confusion, loss of memory, apathy, and irritability. These are often accompanied by myoclonic jerks, flapping tremor (asterixis), and seizures. Uraemic peripheral neuropathy is mixed motor and sensory in nature. It causes paraesthesiae, including restless or burning feet. Autonomic nervous system dysfunction has also been described.

Uraemic patients accumulate the metabolites of opioid drugs and their effects are easily mistaken for encephalopathy. Reversal with opioid antagonists reveals the diagnosis. The burden of illness frequently leads to severe depression which can be mistaken for dementia.

The skin

Cutaneous manifestations include pruritus, dry flaky skin, as well as darkening and yellow pigmentation, made more obvious by the pallor of anaemia. Bullous lesions in sun-exposed areas (pseudoporphyria cutanea) are occasionally seen in patients on dialysis. Proximal skin necrosis (thighs and trunk) is a consequence of ischaemia resulting from calcification and occlusion of arterioles. Trophic nail changes are frequent, including brown nail arcs ('half-and-half nails').

Endocrine system

The major derangements are in reduced production of erythropoietin and 1,25-dihydroxy cholecalciferol. Other disturbances include dysfunction of the hypothalamopituitary axis as well as the retention of many polypeptide hormones. End-organ resistance to the action of some hormones is observed in uraemia, explaining, in part, glucose intolerance (insulin resistance), anaemia, and stunting of growth in children (growth hormone resistance).

In males, low testosterone levels are associated with loss of libido and impotence, but vascular insufficiency, drugs, and neurogenic and psychological factors also contribute. Gynaecomastia is rare nowadays and its cause was never explained. In females, there is reduced libido, irregular menstruation, or amenorrhoea. Patients with severe renal failure are usually infertile and it is rare for those on dialysis to have successful pregnancies.

Haematological effects

The normochromic normocytic anaemia is caused by a failure of the kidneys to produce sufficient erythropoietin to stimulate the erythroid marrow to a level of red cell production to compensate for a shorter than normal red cell survival. The uraemic bone marrow is responsive to erythropoietin, but it remains a matter of debate whether this response is normal or blunted. Serum erythropoietin concentrations are usually above the normal range for non-anaemic subjects and yet ferrokinetic measurements suggest that the rate of erythropoiesis is subnormal. Nevertheless, exogenous erythropoietin in supraphysiological doses can reverse the anaemia completely. Other factors to aggravate anaemia include blood loss from the gastrointestinal tract or menstrual loss. Marrow fibrosis due to hyperparathyroidism is a rare factor in those with very chronic and severe renal failure. Aluminium overload was a problem in some dialysis patients, but is now rare.

The anaemia is well tolerated until the haemoglobin falls below 10 g/dl. This tolerance may be explained by the shift in the haemoglobin–oxygen dissociation curve resulting from the increased red cell content of 2,3-diphosphoglycerate.

Platelet counts are usually normal in uraemia but function is not. Bleeding times, are prolonged. Platelet function is adversely affected; uraemic plasma and adherence to endothelium is then poor. Anaemia appears to contribute to this defect, for raising the haematocrit by transfusion shortens the bleeding time.

Polymorph function is depressed by mechanisms which remain unexplained. T-cell immunity is significantly impaired, which explains the higher risk of reactivation of tuberculosis and herpes zoster, the failure to respond to hepatitis B vaccine and to clear hepatitis B infection.

Metabolic effects

Lipids

Two-thirds of uraemic individuals have hypertriglyceridaemia and several lipoprotein abnormalities—increased very low-density lipoprotein (VLDL) with cholesterol enrichment; prevalence of VLDL subclass late pre-β-lipoprotein; an increase in particle size and triglyceride content of low-density lipoprotein, and reduced concentration of high-density lipoprotein cholesterol. Depressed lipoprotein lipase activity suggests impaired peripheral metabolism as a likely cause for dyslipoproteinaemia. Carnitine, which plays a part in the oxidation of fatty acids, may be deficient, due to poor nutrition, diminished renal synthesis, and loss in the dialysate. Its administration as a dietary supplement may reduce cholesterol and triglyceride levels but is not yet routinely recommended because of unpredictable results and side-effects.

Carbohydrate

Glucose intolerance is explained by a post-receptor block to the action of insulin in peripheral tissues. It is partially reversed by dialysis. Insulin clearance is delayed, so the development of renal failure can have contrasting effects on insulin requirements in diabetics.

Protein

Uraemia favours protein breakdown and inhibits anabolism related to chronic metabolic acidosis, malnutrition, and the production of inflammatory mediators. Protein synthesis is impaired partly because of resistance to the action of insulin. Patients frequently have reduced muscle bulk, and low concentrations of albumin and transferrin.

Natural history

The natural history of most nephropathies is of a progressive decline in renal function, although the rate of progression varies considerably between patients, with some displaying stable function over many years. Progression of chronic glomerulonephritides is generally faster than that of tubulointerstitial nephritides. Proteinuria is the most reliable prognostic factor, as its severity correlates with the rate of progression of the underlying nephropathy. The onset of proteinuria also indicates a higher morbidity and mortality from cardiovascular complications, perhaps because of associated hyperlipidaemia. The mechanism(s) by which heavy proteinuria might adversely affect the rate of loss of renal function is not known. It may be a marker rather than a directly causative factor. However, recent experimental evidence points to the stimulation by reabsorbed proteins of proximal tubular release of inflammatory and fibrogenic mediators, thus implicating proteinuria in the pathogenesis of tubulointerstitial inflammation and fibrosis.

The other important factor influencing the natural history is hypertension, which appears early and often precedes the onset of uraemia. It is associated with an accelerated decline in renal function and, although it is difficult to distinguish primary deterioration of renal function and secondary worsening of hypertension from vice versa, there is now sound evidence that uncontrolled hypertension can accelerate the loss of renal function (see Chapter 12.24).

Other factors modulating progression

Genetic racial factors

Certain antigens of the major histocompatibility complex have been associated with a poor outcome in some forms of glomerulonephritis; for instance HLA DR2, and B7 in Goodpasture's syndrome. Associations have also been described in patients with IgA and membranous nephropathies. In the latter, carriers of the haplotype B8-DR3-BfF1 may be associated with a worse prognosis. Associations have been described between polymorphism of certain genes such as that coding for ACE and the susceptibility to progressive CRF. In adult polycystic disease, patients carrying the PKD1 gene on the short arm of chromosome 16 have an earlier onset and a faster rate of decline compared with those whose abnormal gene is on chromosome 4. Genetic factors may also explain some race-related differences in susceptibility and outcome. Afro-Americans and, to a lesser extent, Hispanic-Americans suffer a faster rate of progression when compared with Caucasians. Afro-Americans and native Americans also have a faster rate of progression of diabetic nephropathy.

Gender

Function deteriorates faster in males than in females in adult polycystic kidney disease, Alport's syndrome, mesangial IgA, and membranous nephropathies.

Mechanisms of progression

Progression is marked by increasing glomerulosclerosis, tubulointerstitial fibrosis and vascular sclerosis.

Glomerulosclerosis

Common mechanisms of scarring probably affect the kidneys regardless of the initial cause and well after the initiating events have subsided. Glomerulosclerosis has been attributed to immunological (glomerulonephritis), haemodynamic (hypertension), or metabolic (diabetes mellitus) insults leading to glomerular endothelial injury. Glomerular capillary wall injury may also affect the glomeruli spared the initial insult. The current views depend on animal experiments. In these, glomeruli undergo adaptive morphological and functional changes, characterized by hypertrophy and hyperfunction (hyperperfusion and hyperfiltration). A compensatory increase in intraglomerular capillary pressure results from a disproportionate afferent arteriolar vasodilatation and the loss of autoregulation exposing remnant glomeruli to systemic hypertension. Injury to the glomerular endothelial lining favours platelet adhesion, aggregation, and the formation of glomerular microthrombi as well as the transudation of macromolecules, including lipids and growth factors, into the glomerular mesangium. These may stimulate mesangial proliferation and increased synthesis of extracellular collagenous matrix.

Comparisons have been drawn between glomerulosclerosis and atherosclerosis. In both platelets, monocytes/macrophages, and lipids infiltrate the vascular/glomerular wall. Interactions between infiltrating and resident cells through the release of autacoids and growth factors lead to mesangial proliferation and expansion of the glomerular extracellular matrix of collagen. Platelet-derived growth factor and transforming growth factor-β are likely candidates for the stimulation of the synthesis of glomerular collagen, and ultimately the development of fibrosis. The inability of scarred glomeruli to clear excessive collagen deposition may be due to loss of collagenase activity by scarred glomeruli and/or qualitative changes in glomerular collagen, making it resistant to degradation.

Tubulointerstitial scarring

Good correlations have been observed between the severity of tubulointerstitial scarring and GFR. Tubulointerstitial fibrosis bears some similarities to glomerulosclerosis. It is characterized by inadequate healing with excessive collagen deposition, involving interactions between renal tubular cells, inflammatory cells, and resident fibroblasts through the release of cytokines and peptide growth-promoting factors. Apoptosis has been implicated in the progressive loss of tubular cells leading to atrophy and functional loss.

Vascular sclerosis

In elderly patients, atherosclerosis of renal arteries has been implicated in the acceleration of renal scarring through renal ischaemia and cholesterol embolization. Hyalinosis of smaller renal vessels is also common in patients of all ages with chronic renal disease and can often be seen even when systemic hypertension is mild. The severity of these lesions often exceeds that observed in patients with essential hypertension.

Management

Conservation of renal function

There are a few causes of renal failure the pathology of which can be arrested, but most forms of glomerulonephritis, diabetic nephropathy, and adult polycystic kidney disease are all 'unstoppable'. In them a variety of measures are used to delay progression, based on both experimental and clinical evidence.

Experimental data

Animal experiments support dietary restriction of protein, calories, phosphate, sodium, and sucrose, as well as lipids. Dietary supplementation with various polyunsaturated fatty acids, such as linoleic acid and eicosapentaenoic acid (fish oil), has also proved beneficial. Pharmacological interventions to reduce systemic as well as glomerular hypertension, hyperlipidaemia, or the prevention of platelet aggregation have also proved effective as has manipulation of fibrogenic cytokines and growth factors with neutralizing antibodies and/or antagonists.

Clinical data

The heterogeneity of renal diseases makes the evaluation of the approaches suggested by animal data difficult. With the exception of the control of hypertension none of them has so far proved convincingly effective. This is also the case for dietary protein restriction, as careful review of most published literature shows its effects to be inconclusive or of marginal benefit. A reasonable approach in the light of current knowledge is to recommend the avoidance of a high-protein diet and the limitation of the intake of protein to 0.8 g/kg per day. Dietary supplementation with eicosapentaenoic acid has in five major studies failed to show protection. Other interventions, including immunosuppression, antiplatelet therapy, and anticoagulation, as well as lipid reduction, seem to have little impact on progression and are not without side-effects. Patients should be spared the potential side-effects of unproven therapies. The avoidance of potentially nephrotoxic drugs in patients with chronic renal diseases is especially important.

Compensation for the effects of chronic renal insufficiency

Control of blood pressure

The relationship between high arterial pressure and progression of chronic renal disease is discussed in Chapter 12.24. Before drugs are prescribed, simple measures of treatment include modest dietary sodium restriction ($\pm$60 mmol/day), weight loss, and regular exercise. Increasing evidence suggest that tight blood pressure control slows the progression of diabetic and non-diabetic renal disease. In non-diabetic nephropathies, it has been suggested that hypertension control should be more stringent in proteinuric patients with a target mean arterial blood pressure of 92 mmHg compared with 98 mmHg or even higher in those with mild or absent proteinuria. ACE inhibitors may be particularly effective in reducing proteinuria and slowing the progression of CRF.

Dietary and fluid intake and excretory capacity

An intake of 0.6 g/kg per day of high-quality protein will often reduce the blood urea and uraemic toxins significantly. More severe protein restriction requires special caloric supplements and carries the risk of inducing malnutrition. Restriction should be started when symptom relief is needed. This is very variable in terms of blood

Table 7 Techniques of peritoneal dialysis (home or hospital)

	Number of exchanges (21)	Duration of exchanges (hours)		Type/duration
		Day	Night	
CAPD	3–5	4	8	Continuous
CCPD	3–5	16	1–2	Continuous
IPD	40	1/2–1	1/2–1	24 h
NIPD	8–10	–	1/2–1	Nightly
TIPD	25–30	–	1/2	Nightly

CAPD, continuous ambulatory peritoneal dialysis; CCPD, continuous cyclic peritoneal dialysis; IPD, intermittent peritoneal dialysis; NIPD, night intermittent peritoneal dialysis; TIPD, tidal intermittent peritoneal dialysis.

All these peritoneal techniques (except CAPD) are automated, using a cycler to perform the exchanges.

urea. Symptoms may arise at levels as low as 25 mmol/l but can be absent at 40 mmol/l or more. Controlled trials have shown little advantage in the early introduction of a low-protein diet. Phosphate restriction (1000 mg/day) will counter one of the stimuli to parathyroid hormone oversecretion and lower the calcium phosphate product, thus limiting vascular and other soft-tissue calcification. Modest sodium restriction to 60 mmol/day will contribute to the control of arterial pressure. Some patients are 'salt losers' and require supplements, most often in patients with interstitial nephropathy, such as medullary cystic disease. Potassium restriction is only needed when CRF is severe, unless bicarbonate loss leads to early acidosis; hyperkalaemia may then be corrected by bicarbonate supplements. Fluid restriction is not usually necessary until late in renal failure. Dehydration is more common.

The mild chronic metabolic acidosis which develops when the GFR falls below 30 ml/min usually causes few problems, but when the plasma bicarbonate falls below 20 mmol/l correction by bicarbonate supplements should be considered.

Prevention and treatment of abnormalities of calcium homeostasis

See Chapter 12.30.

Treatment of renal anaemia

Significant symptoms of anaemia start to appear when the haemoglobin falls below 10 g/dl and are disabling below 6 g/dl. Before instituting erythropoietin treatment the common aggravating causes should be sought and treated. These include blood loss from the gastrointestinal tract, iron deficiency, and chronic infection. Recombinant human erythropoietin (epoetin) is given at a dose of approximately 100 U/kg per week by subcutaneous injection as two or three injections. The target haemoglobin should be 10–12 g/dl, or higher if symptoms such as angina persist. The response should be monitored monthly and the dose adjusted down if the rise in haemoglobin is more than 2 g/month. The dose can be adjusted up to more than 300 U/kg per week, but these high doses should prompt a search for confounding factors. Blood pressure tends to rise as anaemia is reversed. It is prudent then to stop the erythropoietin until blood pressure control is adequate.

Bleeding diathesis

This is usually only a problem when patients with renal failure undergo surgery. The first measure is to raise the haematocrit to

Table 8 Complications of dialysis

Acute complications of haemodialysis	Vascular access complications of haemodialysis

• Disequilibration syndrome
• Bleeding
• First use syndrome
• Technical faults
• Hypotension
• Haemorrhagic
  • membrane
  • bloodline
  • vascular access
• Air embolus
• Hypo/hypernatraemia
• Cramps
• Complement and cytokine reactions
• Hardwater syndrome
• Haemolysis
	• Inadequate flow
	• Recirculation
	• Infection
	  • cellulitis
	  • septicaemia
	• Thrombosis
	• Stenosis
	• Haemorrhage
	• Aneurysm
	• Increased cardiac output
	• Vascular steal syndrome
	• Ischaemia
	• Fistula thumb

Peritoneal dialysis	**Disorders common to all dialysis**

• Infection
  • peritonitis
  • exit/tunnel infection
• Catheter malfunction
  • migration
  • outflow/inflow
  • obstruction
  • fluid leakage
  • biofilm formation
  • cracking catheter material
• Loss of ultrafiltration
• Obesity
• Hernias
• Low back pain
• Patient dislike and 'burn out'
• Peritoneal membrane failure
	• Cardiovascular disease (cardiac failure, cerebrovascular accident)
	• Anaemia
	• Abnormal bleeding
	• Hypertension
	• Hyperlipidaemia
	• Atherosclerosis
	• Renal bone disease
	• Infections
	• Malignancy
	• Malnutrition
	• Underdialysis
	• β_2-Microglobulin amyloidosis
	• Acquired renal cysts
	• Aluminium toxicity

improve platelet function. Vasopressin (DDAVP®) 0.3 μ/kg in 100 ml NaCl in 30 min, administered before surgery, will reduce the risk of haemorrhage and can be given for bleeding, for example uncontrolled epistaxis. The next measure is administration of cryoprecipitate which shortens bleeding time for 24–36 h after infusion. A longer effect is obtained by a total dose infusion of 3 mg/kg conjugated oestrogen over 5 days. The onset of effect is delayed but lasts about 2 weeks.

Hyperlipidaemia

It is reasonable to advise patients to stay at their ideal weight, take regular exercise, and to avoid excess animal fats. If the cholesterol remains, above 6.5 mmol/l, an HMG CoA reductase inhibitor should be prescribed in preference to the fibrate drugs, which accumulate and can cause muscle damage.

Use of drugs

Because many drugs and their metabolites are excreted via the kidney, care must be taken with the selection of agent and dose in patients with renal failure (see Chapter 12.26).

Psychological

Patients with renal failure are under stress. Their general health affects their employment, social and sexual life, and recreation. Responses range from anger to depression and even suicide, but

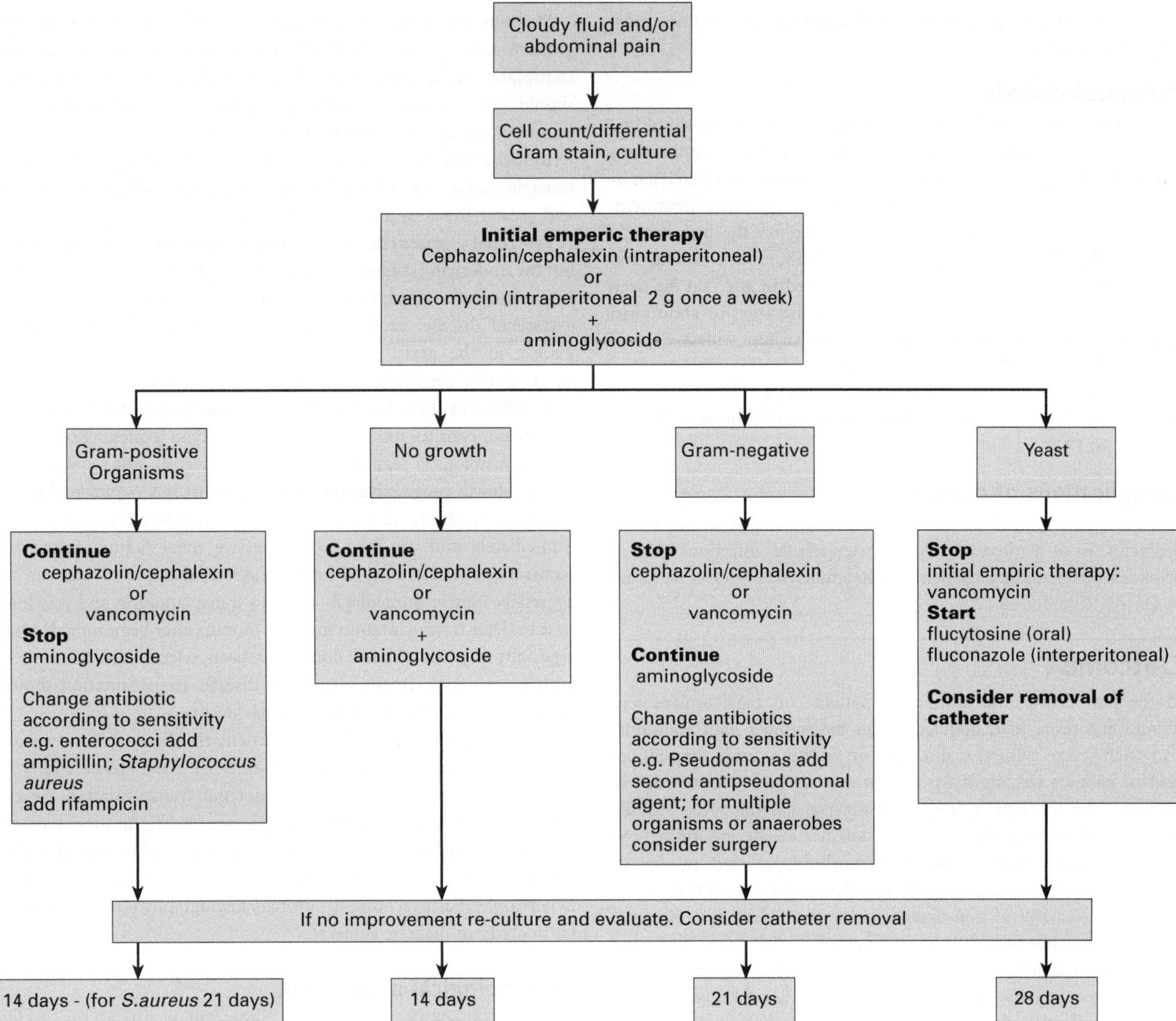

Fig. 2 Treatment of peritonitis in peritoneal dialysis patients.

it is unusual for these patients to require formal psychiatric assessment. Sedatives should be used sparingly but antidepressants prescribed appropriately.

Preparation for dialysis and transplantation

Once endstage renal failure seems inevitable, the patient must be prepared physically and psychologically for renal replacement treatment. Reciprocal plots of plasma creatinine against time can predict roughly when endstage will be reached, useful for the patient and helpful in giving guidance for the timing of the provision of vascular access for haemodialysis or placing the catheter for peritoneal dialysis.

The decision of when to begin dialysis depends on clinical features, biochemical abnormalities and resources. Uraemic symptoms that do not respond to conservative measures are the usual indication; these rarely appear before the creatinine clearance has fallen below 5 ml/min, but an earlier start may be needed in the presence of cardiovascular problems and in the case of diabetics who fare better with earlier treatment. Blood tests of urea and creatinine do not provide a sound guide when to start but it is advisable to do so (even in the absence of symptoms) in those with a small frame when the urea is some 30–40 mmol/l or creatinine 650–800 μmol/l.

The choice between haemodialysis, peritoneal dialysis or transplantation depends on many factors, not least the availability of dialysis and the patient's preference (see OTM3, p. 3307).

Haemodialysis

If haemodialysis is the choice, vascular access should be created some 2 or 3 months before the beginning of treatment. This is usually in the form of an arteriovenous fistula at the wrist. If this is not possible, vein grafts or synthetic material may be used; permanent internal jugular catheters can also provide adequate access in difficult cases. The important arm (cephalic and antecubital) and leg veins are easily destroyed or damaged by infusions or repeated venepunctures and use of them in any patient at risk of endstage renal failure must always be avoided.

Peritoneal dialysis

If peritoneal dialysis is the choice, the peritoneal catheter should be placed 2 or 3 weeks before treatment. Catheter-related complications impart significant morbidity resulting in permanent change to haemodialysis in 20 per cent of cases failing to maintain peritoneal treatment. A variety of catheters are available, all based on the one initially introduced by Tenckhoff. Implantation techniques vary but there is agreement that the insertion should be paramedian and that the deep cuff must be placed in the musculature of the anterior abdominal wall and the subcutaneous cuff near the skin surface with 2–3 cm of the exit which should is caudally directed.

The various techniques of peritoneal dialysis are summarized in Table 7 (OTM3, p. 3307) and a fuller account can be found in OTM3, Chapter 20.17.2.

Complications of dialysis

These are summarized in Table 8. In peritoneal dialysis the major problems is of peritonitis and catheter-related infections; Fig. 2 provides a guide to management. Again a fuller account can be found in OTM3, Chapter 20.17.2.

Outcome

In the past decade the number of patients on renal replacement therapy has more than doubled as has the number with additional and often severe extrarenal disorders. In addition, more than 50 per cent of patients starting dialysis treatment are now over the age of 65 years. The medium to long-term survival has improved steadily over the last two decades but these statistics are heavily influenced by age, diabetes, and associated co-morbidity at start of dialysis therapy. Data from the European Renal Registry (34 countries) show that 6-year survival of non-diabetic patients on dialysis (>60 years) is 40 per cent but only 20 per cent in diabetics; it is nearly 85 per cent for non-diabetic for 45 years. These data relate to patients taken on for dialysis in 1985–90. The Canadian Organ Renal Registry reports on an overall survival (all patients taken on for dialysis 1990–94) of 40 per cent at 5 years. There was a marginally better survival for peritoneal dialysis than in haemodialysis patients in the first 2 years. Cardiovascular complications are a major cause of mortality and cardiac causes account for about 40 per cent of all deaths, with vascular diseases accounting for another 15 per cent. Malignant disease is about three times more common in patients on dialysis than in age- and sex-matched controls. Multiple renal adenocarcinomas also occur in acquired cystic disease of endstage renal disease.

Quality of life

It is all too difficult to define and measure quality of life, but successful renal transplantation undoubtedly achieves the best rehabilitation , which is complete in less than half the patients on dialysis among which those on chronic ambulatory peritoneal fare better than those given in-hospital haemodialysis.

Renal transplantation

Only a brief account is given here. Further discussion can be found in OTM3, Chapter 20.17.3.

Planning for renal transplantation should begin as soon as progressive and irreversible renal failure seems likely, so that, on occasion, transplantation can be performed before dialysis is necessary. Patients should enter a pool of waiting recipients from which the most immunologically appropriate matches with cadaver grafts are determined and balanced against clinical urgency. Living related donor transplantation is an alternative, providing immunological advantage and greater freedom in planning the exact time of surgery.

Few renal diseases constitute a contraindication to transplantation, but the underlying diagnosis should be determined whenever possible. Implications for transplantation include the likelihood of associated extrarenal disease, urological problems, and the risk of recurrent disease in the graft. Many types of glomerulonephritis, diabetic nephropathy, amyloidosis, and oxalosis recur in renal allografts, yet graft failure in these from recurrent disease is unusual. The type of glomerulonephritis influences the risk. In type 2 mesangiocapillary disease histological recurrence is almost universal, but renal damage is only slowly progressive; the same is true of IgA nephropathy, but nephrotic syndrome in focal segmental glomerulosclerosis may recur immediately and can lead to progressive renal failure. Important recurrence is most likely if primary glomerulonephritis has run an aggressive course immediately prior to transplantation and it is then wise to defer transplantation for 6–12 months after beginning dialysis, especially if a live related donor has been selected. In the case of antiglomerular basement membrane disease, transplantation should be deferred until the antibody titre has declined.

Atheromatous vascular disease, particularly affecting the coronary arteries, is common in patients with endstage renal failure and is an important consideration in planning renal transplantation. Severe coronary disease is not uncommonly asymptomatic in these patients and the accuracy of exercise testing may be impaired by poor mobility and electrocardiogram abnormalities arising from left ventricular hypertrophy. Early recourse to coronary angiography is recommended, particularly in diabetic subjects.

Immunological assessment

ABO incompatibility is associated with a high risk of hyperacute rejection; incompatibility in the HLA system is less easy to analyse. In living related donor transplantation a major effect of HLA matching has long been evident. In patients receiving prednisolone and azathioprine, 1-year graft survival has been greater than 90 per cent for HLA identical siblings; 70–80 per cent one haplotype was shared and some 60 per cent if neither were. These results have improved since the introduction of cyclosporin, but the differences in relation to typing remain clear. More important 'half-life' estimates are 25 years, 15 years, and 10 years for living related donors sharing two, one or no haplotypes. Even so, some HLA identical grafts are still rejected despite immunosuppression; equally, graft survival can commonly be seen even with a complete mismatch of HLA antigens.

The advantage of matching at a particular locus has been more difficult to show in cadaver transplantation, but a consistent advantage is known for matching at the DR locus. Improved graft survival, fewer rejection episodes and more stable long-term function are reported with increasing benefit from two versus one versus no matches. There are also independent and additive effects for matching at HLA-B and HLA-A loci, although such matches are rare in unrelated individuals.

Sensitization to HLA antigens

Sensitization may follow blood transfusion, pregnancy, and previous allografts. Preformed complement fixing antibodies against graft HLA can destroy grafts in minutes or hours by hyperacute rejection. To monitor sensitization, sera are obtained from potential recipients and tested regularly for such antibodies and, immediately prior to transplantation, a cross-match between donor lymphocytes and recipient serum is performed. A positive reaction involving IgG antibody directed against HLA is a contradiction to transplantation. However, not all antibodies reacting with donor lymphocytes cause hyperacute rejection; some which react with non-HLA epitopes are benign so that accurate characterization of the antibody is important.

Although blood transfusion can cause sensitization against allo-HLA antigens, it can also reduce subsequent immune responses. Many units once had a policy of elective transfusion in preparation for transplantation, but recent surveys suggest too small an advantage from such a procedure so that this policy is now less often followed. The mechanism(s) by which blood transfusion improves graft survival is not known.

Cadaveric organ donation

The commonest cause of death leading to organ donation is head injury, followed by primary intracerebral haemorrhage. All age groups are potentially suitable for donation and the only firm contra-indications are serious infections (human immunodeficiency virus, hepatitis B and C, and severe bacterial infection) and past or present extra-cranial malignancy.

Brainstem death

Brain stem death defines a state in which there is irreversible loss of the capacity for consciousness combined with irreversible loss of the capacity to breathe. Clinical tests can reliably indicate brain stem death, but it is absolutely necessary to establish a set of preconditions. Unless there are fulfilled and certain exclusions met, a diagnosis of brain stem death cannot even be considered. The UK code of practice is summarized as follows:

(1) Preconditions
- (a) Comatose and on a ventilator
- (b) Establishment of an unequivocal diagnosis of the cause of coma

(2) Exclusions
- (a) Hypothermia
- (b) All depressant drugs
- (c) Severe metabolic disturbances

(3) Test for brain stem function
- (a) No pupillary response
- (b) Absent corneal reflex
- (c) Absent vestibulo-ocular reflexes
- (d) No cranial nerve motor response to painful stimuli
- (e) No gag reflex
- (f) No respiratory movement with $PaCO_2$ above 6.65 kPa (50 mmHg)

Most countries specify that tests should be performed on two occasions to exclude the possibility of error.

Further reading

Gokal, R. (1998). Peritoneal dialysis and complications of technique. In *Oxford textbook of clinical nephrology* (ed. A.D. Davison, J.S. Cameron, J.-P. Grünfeld, D. Kerr, E. Ritz, and C.G. Winearls), pp. 2049–74. Oxford University Press, Oxford.

Morris, P.J. (2000). *Kidney transplantation: principles and practice*, (5th edn). Saunders, Eastbourne.

Olbricht, C. *et al.* (1998). Haemodialysis, haemofiltration, and complications of technique. In *Oxford textbook of clinical nephrology* (ed. A.D. Davison, J.S. Cameron, J.-P. Grünfeld, D. Kerr, E. Ritz, and C.G. Winearls), pp. 2025–47. Oxford University Press, Oxford.

Peterson, J.C., Adler, S., Burkart, J.M., *et al.* (1995). Blood pressure control, proteinuria, and the progression of renal disease. *Annals of Internal Medicine*, **123**, 754–62.

Remuzzi, G., Ruggenenti, P., and Benigni, A. (1997). Understanding the nature of renal disease progression. *Kidney International*, **51**, 2–15.

Walker, R. (1997). General management of end-stage renal disease. *British Medical Journal*, **315**, 1429-32.

Weir, M.R. and Dworkin, L.D. (1998). Antihypertensive drugs, dietary salt, and renal protection: how low should we go and with which therapy? *American Journal of Kidney Diseases*, 1998, **32**, 1–22.

Chapter 12.30

Renal bone disease

J. A. Kanis

The skeletal disorders found in chronic renal failure (Table 1) are collectively termed renal osteodystrophy, and may occur singly or in various combinations. None of these is unique to renal failure nor to particular populations of patients with renal disease. The variable

Table 1 Features of renal bone disease and some clinical manifestations of disturbed calcium and phosphate metabolism in chronic renal failure

Feature	Clinical consequence
Hyperparathyroidism and osteitis fibrosa	Skeletal deformity, bone pain, pruritus, anaemia, impotence, neuropathy
Osteomalacia and decreased availability of vitamin D, calcium, and phosphate	Skeletal deformity, bone pain and tenderness, pathological fracture[a]
	Proximal myopathy, encephalopathy, microcytic anaemia,[a] haemolytic anaemia
Adynamic bone disease	Pain, pathological fracture, hypercalcaemia
Osteoporosis	Pathological fracture, skeletal deformity
Osteonecrosis	Joint pain
Osteosclerosis and periosteal new bone formation	None known
Extraskeletal calcification	Depends on site—skin ulcers, pruritus, vascular disease, cardiac failure, pseudogout

[a] More characteristic of aluminium toxicity

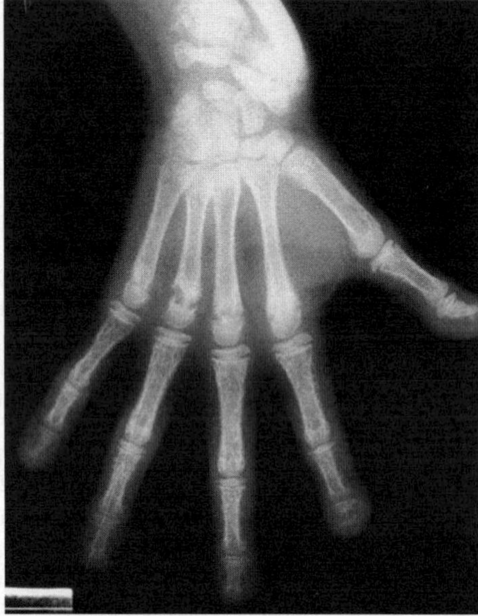

Fig. 1 Radiographic features of hyperparathyroid bone disease in an adolescent with chronic renal failure. Note the marked subperiosteal erosions of the phalanges. Erosion of the terminal, phalanges has resulted in the collapse of soft tissue, giving a drum-stick appearance of the fingers. Severe osteitis fibrosa at the wrist is indicated by the marked metaphyseal resorption, giving rise to skeletal deformity. Less marked hyperparathyroid bone disease may give rise to radiographic features resembling rickets.

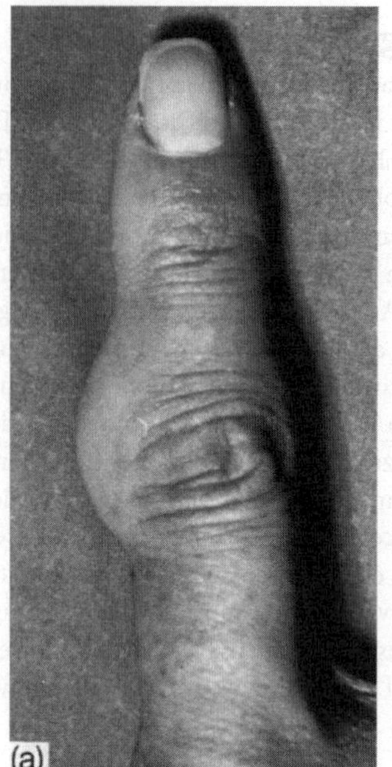

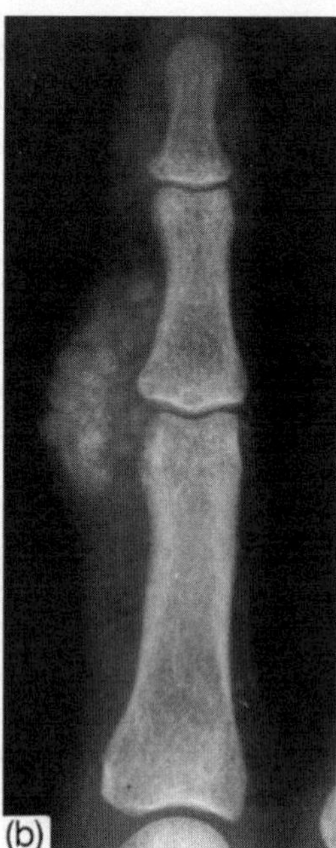

Fig. 2 Radiographic and clinical photographs of periarticular calcification due to hyperphosphataemia in a patient treated by intermittent haemodialysis.

apparent prevalence of bone disease reflects in part the use of differing histological and radiographic criteria for diagnosis, but other important factors include age, the nature and duration of renal disease, and the treatment given. By the time patients start dialysis, the majority have histological abnormalities of bone but skeletal symptoms are found in a minority (less than 10 per cent). However, the incidence of symptomatic bone disease increases thereafter as do the extraskeletal manifestations (Table 1).

Hyperparathyroidism

Secondary hyperparathyroidism increases the activity and the numbers of bone cells, so increasing bone turnover. Rapid rates of turnover are associated with deposition of fibrous tissue in the marrow spaces (osteitis fibrosa) and the formation of new bone matrix which is not lamellar but disorganized in structure (woven bone). This impairs its strength and occasionally gives rise to serious mechanical consequences (Fig. 1), particularly in the young. If hyperparathyroid bone disease is severe, an imbalance between bone formation and resorption occurs and skeletal mass diminishes, particularly that of cortical bone. In adolescents, severe hyperparathyroid bone disease may resemble rickets on skeletal radiographs. Bone loss is not invariable and patchy osteosclerosis of cancellous bone (for example vertebral bodies) is also found. Concentrations of serum parathyroid hormone (PTH), alkaline phosphatase, osteocalcin, and hydroxyproline are increased in patients with osteitis fibrosa.

Osteomalacia

Osteomalacia arises because of an abnormal delay between the onset of bone matrix formation and its subsequent mineralization. Osteomalacia and hyperparathyroidism commonly coexist and are distinguished by histological measurements on bone biopsy which estimate the rate of mineralization.

Adynamic bone disease

In contrast to hyperparathyroid bone disease, in adynamic bone disease all the elements of bone turnover are decreased—resorption, formation, and mineralization. This impairs the ability of bone to self-repair fatigue damage and gives rise to pain and fractures.

Changes in bone mass are common in renal failure. There is commonly a redistribution of skeletal mass so that osteosclerosis and osteoporosis may coexist in the same patient. Severe osteoporosis is rarely found in patients not yet requiring dialysis treatment, but is common in the dialysis-treated population and after transplantation.

Clinical features

Disturbed mineral and skeletal metabolism in renal failure has consequences other than those affecting bone (see Table 1). Both osteomalacia and osteitis fibrosa may be associated with bone pain, tenderness, and muscle weakness. Pain in the lower limbs, pelvis, and back are particularly common and may be worse on exercise. Muscle weakness is frequently proximal. Symptoms are unusual in patients not yet requiring dialysis, except in children and in those in whom renal failure has been present for many years. In patients receiving dialysis there was once great variability in the prevalence of symptoms between dialysis units, probably related to aluminium toxicity. The latter is associated with indolent fractures, particularly of the ribs, spine, pelvis, and femoral neck. Multiple rib fractures may result in respiratory failure. The manifestations of adynamic bone disease are similar when associated with aluminium toxicity. The clinical significance of low bone turnover alone is uncertain.

Osteosclerosis and periosteal new bone formation are not associated with symptoms. Osteoporosis is asymptomatic unless fractures occur.

Extraskeletal calcification is characteristically found in the vascular tree and periarticular soft tissues (Fig. 2). A predisposing factor is an increase in the plasma calcium × phosphate product. Calcification occurs commonly in the eye, as band keratopathy or in the conjunctiva.

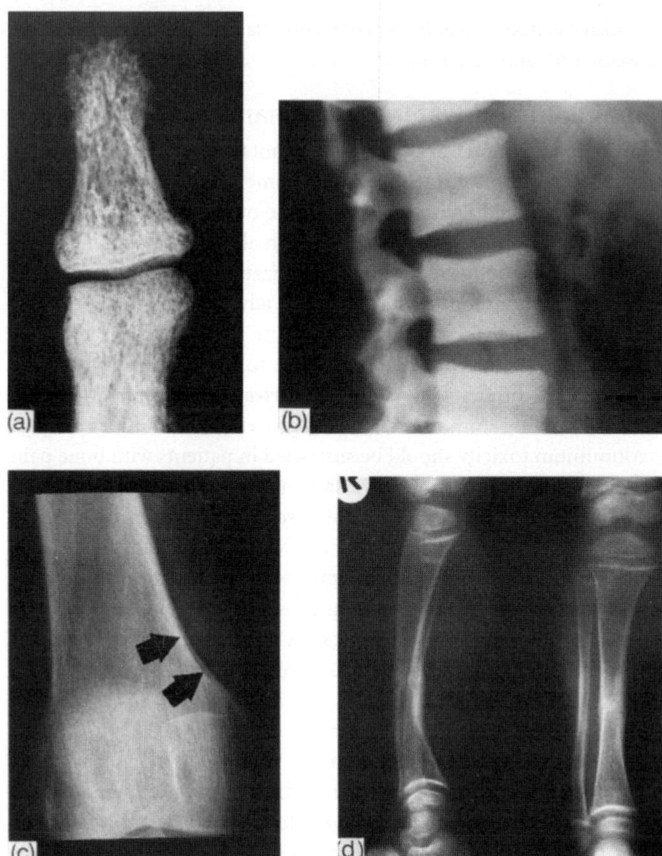

Fig. 3 Some of the radiographic features of renal bone disease. (a) Subperiosteal bone resorption of the terminal phalanx due to secondary hyperparathyroidism. (b) Changes in the lumbar spine manifest as alternate bands of increased and reduced radiodensity ('rugger jersey spine'). (c) Periosteal new bone formation—the periosteal separation from the mineralized cortex of the femur is shown by the arrows. (d) Radiographic characteristics of osteomalacia. A Looser's zone is present in the midshaft of the tibia. There is widening of both the epiphyseal plate and metaphysis.

Acute conjunctival precipitation may cause, the 'red-eye' of renal failure. Deposition in the skin may contribute to pruritus. Ischaemic necrosis of the skin is unusual.

The abdominal aorta and the femoral and digital arteries are the most common sites of vascular calcification visible on radiographs.

Avascular necrosis occurs rarely in chronic renal failure but is a significant cause of morbidity in transplant recipients.

Radiographic features

The characteristic radiographic feature of hyperparathyroid bone disease is subperiosteal erosion of bone (Fig. 3), most commonly found at the radial aspect of the middle phalanges of the hand, the tufts of the terminal phalanges, and the distal ends of the clavicles. Gross erosion may result in collapse of soft tissue normally supported by bone. In the terminal phalanges this may give rise to the appearance of pseudoclubbing (see Fig. 1).

A negative radiographic survey is not helpful in excluding osteomalacia. There may be a generalized radiolucency of bone. Looser's zones (Fig. 3) are characteristic and are most frequently seen in the pelvis. Coarse trabecular markings, osteosclerosis, and periosteal new bone formation (Fig. 3) have been attributed to hyperparathyroidism, but their appearance appears to be more consistently associated with osteomalacia. The radiographic features of osteosclerosis bear only a superficial resemblance to those of avascular necrosis.

Methods of assessing bone mass include measurement of cortical width, single photon absorptiometry, and dual-energy X-ray absorptiometry. Bone biopsy is the only certain way to exclude the presence of osteomalacia and aluminium-related bone disease.

Children are particularly prone to renal bone disease and some may show radiographic features that resemble rickets.

Biochemical features

The classical findings include a low serum calcium, hyperphosphataemia, diminished intestinal absorption of calcium, raised plasma activity of alkaline phosphatase, and increased serum values of immuno-assayable PTH. Hypercalcaemia is less common but is found in dialysis-treated patients with severe hyperparathyroidism (so called tertiary hyperparathyroidism), in vitamin D toxicity, and in some patients with aluminium retention or aplastic bone disease. The occurrence of renal failure with hypercalcaemia strongly suggests primary hyperparathyroidism and secondary renal failure.

Hyperphosphataemia occurs when the glomerular filtration rate falls below approximately 30 ml/min. Patients with osteomalacia tend to have lower values, but neither the serum calcium nor phosphate is sufficiently different from patients without osteomalacia for clinical diagnosis. Serum activity of alkaline phosphatase is commonly increased. The newer assays for intact PTH show raised values in proportion to the degree of secondary hyperparathyroidism prevailing.

Pathophysiology (Table 2)

Metabolism of vitamin D

The bone disease is 'vitamin D resistant' in the sense that the doses required to heal osteodystrophy are greater than physiological. This is due to defective renal metabolism of vitamin D. The development of bone disease and its resistance to vitamin D and to calcidiol (25-OHD_3) results from impaired production of calcitriol ($1.25(OH)_2D_3$) due to loss of renal tissue and to the inhibitory effects of hyperphosphataemia on renal 1α-hydroxylase. Serum values of calcitriol decrease when the glomerular filtration rate is less than 40 ml/min and are very low in endstage renal failure.

Deficiency of calcitriol retards skeletal growth and results in defective mineralization of matrix produced both by chondrocytes and osteoblasts. It also induces malabsorption of calcium and aggravates hypocalcaemia and secondary hyperparathyroidism. Calcitriol may also affect PTH secretion by a direct action on the gland, so that deficiency exacerbates hyperparathyroidism.

Not all patients with osteomalacia respond to treatment with 1α-hydroxylated metabolites, and healing is commonly incomplete when histological indices of response are used, suggesting that other factors may contribute to renal osteodystrophy.

The production of secalciferol ($24,25(OH)_2D_3$) is also impaired in renal failure, but its administration alone does not heal bone disease, but there is some evidence that both calcitriol and secalciferol are required for the actions of vitamin D on bone to be complete.

In most patients with chronic renal failure, serum calcidiol (25-OHD_3) is normal. Low values, are usually due to inadequate diet, reduced exposure to sunlight, or losses during chronic peritoneal

Table 2 Factors of possible importance in the pathogenesis of renal bone disease

Disturbances in endocrine function

- Defective production of dihydroxymetabolites of vitamin D_3
- Impaired metabolism, peritoneal or urinary losses of 25-hydroxyvitamin D_3 (CAPD, nephrotic syndrome)
- Secondary hyperparathyroidism
- PTH resistance
- Secretion, degradation, or action of other hormones, e.g. calcitonin, thyroxine, gonadal steroids, prolactin, and others

Accumulation of toxic products

- Aluminium, magnesium, and possibly other metals, e.g. iron cadmium, beryllium, manganese
- Products of metabolism such as hydrogen ions, middle molecules, etc.

Drugs

- Phosphate-binding agents
- Anticonvulsants and barbiturates
- Corticosteroids and cytotoxic agents
- Vitamins A, C, D
- Heparin

Deficiency states

- Phosphate
- Availability of calcium (diet, dialysis, malabsorption)
- Dietary protein
- Vitamin C, pyridoxine, vitamin D

Other

- Age (adolescence), female sex
- Duration and nature of renal disease

dialysis. Anticonvulsants induce hepatic microsomal enzymes, and might, therefore, increase the metabolism of calcidiol to inert products. A more important effect may be to block the action of vitamin D metabolites on gut and bone. Low values of calcidiol may contribute to osteomalacia, particularly when the degree of renal failure is modest.

Phosphate metabolism

During the course of progressive renal failure, serum values of calcium and phosphate may be kept relatively normal, but at the expense of an ever-increasing secretion rate of PTH. When the decrement in glomerular filtration rate is too great, hyperphosphataemia and hypocalcaemia ensue.

Calcium metabolism

It is probable that the skeletal effects of vitamin D are not solely dependent upon direct actions on bone but are also due to consequent changes in extracellular concentrations of calcium, phosphate, and PTH.

Dialysis membranes provide a site for the loss or addition of calcium into the body. Net transfer is dependent on shifts in extracellular pH and serum protein concentrations, and on the respective calcium concentrations of serum and dialysis fluid. A low dialysate calcium (for example 1.25 mmol/l) induces osteoporosis, but calcium-rich dialysis fluids (for example 2.0 mmol/l) are not advised; extraskeletal calcification may be accentuated and, despite transient effects on the secretion of PTH, the long-term skeletal response is disappointing. The ideal calcium concentration of haemodialysis fluid lies somewhere between 1.63 and 1.75 mmol/l.

Aluminium and water contaminants

Aluminium retention was once an important factor in the pathogenesis of an unusual form of osteomalacia in some dialysis-treated patients. This was associated with a high incidence of bone pain and fracture and was common in locations with a high aluminium content in the water. Its incidence decreased with deionization of the water. Skeletal retention of aluminium also gives rise to adynamic bone disease and low rates of bone formation, which cause pathological fracture. A similar syndrome has been described due to iron retention. Both are refractory to treatment with vitamin D derivatives. Phosphate-binding agents containing aluminium salts may give rise to aluminium toxicity.

Aluminium toxicity should be suspected in patients with bone pain and muscle weakness who have little radiographic or biochemical evidence for hyperparathyroid bone disease. The presence of hypercalcaemia or pathological fracture are additional features. The diagnosis can be confirmed by bone biopsy which shows focal aluminium accumulation by specific histochemical stains, and low rates of bone formation. Osteomalacia, when present, is characterized by a paucity of active-looking osteoblasts—aplastic osteomalacia.

Acidosis

The role of acidosis in contributing to renal bone disease has been advocated for many years. The acute administration of acid loads to normal subjects results in a negative calcium balance and it has been noted that the rate of mineralization increases acutely when alkalis are administered to acidotic patients with osteomalacia. The correction of acidosis appears to influence uraemic bone disease in only a minority of patients.

Parathyroid hormone metabolism

Hyperparathyroidism in chronic renal failure is dependent not only on the tendency towards phosphate retention and hypocalcaemia, but also on reduced catabolism of PTH by the diseased kidneys and the lack of the normal inhibitory effect on PTH secretion by some metabolites of Vitamin D. Aluminium also affects PTH secretion directly and excess contributes to suppression of bone turnover in adynamic bone disease. There is also evidence of skeletal resistance to the effects of PTH on bone in chronic renal failure.

Treatment of renal bone disease

It is important to ensure that the dietary intake of calcium (1 g daily) and vitamin D is at least normal with the use of appropriate dietary supplements. Plasma values of vitamin A are high in renal failure, due to increased binding by retinol-binding protein. Vitamin A increases bone resorption and may augment PTH secretion, so supplements containing this vitamin should be avoided.

Phosphate metabolism

Control of serum phosphate concentrations contributes to the prevention of hyperparathyroid bone disease and is also important in the prevention of extraskeletal calcification. It is impractical to limit the dietary intake of phosphate, but decreased availability for absorption can be achieved with the use of phosphate-binding agents. The most commonly used one is aluminium hydroxide, prescribed as a gel, in biscuits, or in capsules. Calcium carbonate also binds phosphate in the gut and has potential advantages in correcting acidosis, increasing dietary calcium, and avoiding the ingestion of aluminium; but in practice the amounts of calcium carbonate required are large and they limit the use of vitamin D analogues. It is advisable to withdraw aluminium-containing drugs when aluminium toxicity is suspected.

Phosphate-binding agents should be given before meals and the dose regulated according to effects on serum phosphate. Predialysis values of serum phosphate should be between 1.4 and 2.2 mmol/l. Factors which influence the dose required include the dietary intake of phosphate, concurrent treatment with vitamin D and its analogues or metabolites, and the dialysis treatment schedule. Profound hypophosphataemia should be avoided as it is associated with osteomalacia.

Calcium metabolism

The net absorption of calcium is critically dependent on the presence of calcitriol, but can be augmented by large amounts of calcium carbonate (5–20 g daily) and this may improve osteomalacia. It is often more practicable to give vitamin D or one of its metabolites but net intestinal absorption of calcium cannot be greatly augmented if the diet is severely deficient in calcium. The dialysate calcium which best balances the risks of osteoporosis and extraskeletal calcification lies between 1.6 and 1.75 mmol/l in patients treated by haemodialysis.

Vitamin D and related compounds

A variety of vitamin D compounds are available for use in chronic renal failure. These include vitamin D_2 (calciferol), D_3 (cholecalciferol), dihydrotachysterol (**DHT**), calcitriol, and alfacalcidol (1α-hydroxyvitamin D_3). Calcitriol and its synthetic analogue, alfacalcidol, bypass the metabolic block caused by uraemia: but DHT is also biologically active without the necessity for 1α-hydroxylation by the kidney. DHT and alfacalcidol undergo hepatic hydroxylation, and the 25-OHDHT or calcitriol so formed are the major circulating forms of these agents.

All vitamin D-like compounds are effective in augmenting calcium absorption, relieving symptoms of bone pain and muscle weakness, in increasing serum calcium, and in the majority of patients they suppress elevated serum values of alkaline phosphatase and correct radiographic abnormalities (Fig. 4).

The histological response to treatment is often less marked than the clinical, biochemical, or radiographic responses, particularly in patients maintained on intermittent haemodialysis. Both osteitis fibrosa and osteomalacia appear to respond more readily when associated with each other.

Doses of the various agents required to maintain serum calcium within the normal range and to reverse bone disease are indicated in Table 3. In general, the dose tolerated in order to avoid hypercalcaemia decreases with time (Fig. 4). The greatest risks of hypercalcaemia occur at the start of treatment in patients who ultimately respond poorly to treatment, particularly those with aluminium-related disorders; and, in others, later when biochemical responses are nearing completion. Serum calcium should be monitored frequently during these risk periods. It is also important to note that these agents increase the absorption of phosphate and the requirements for phosphate-binding agents may be increased.

The advantages of the 1α-hydroxylated derivatives of vitamin D and DHT lie in the ease with which doses are titrated according to requirements and the rapidity with which toxic effects are reversed on stopping treatment.

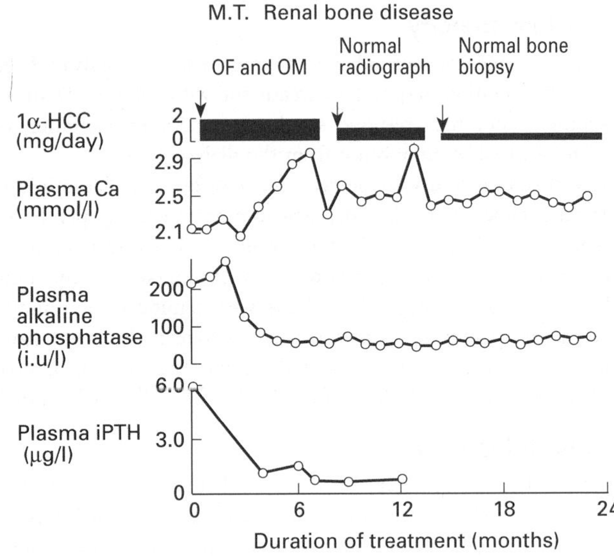

Fig. 4 Long-term treatment of renal bone disease with alfacalcidol (1α-HCC) in a dialysis-treated patient. Healing of osteomalacia and osteitis fibrosa (OM and OF) occurred within 15 months. Episodes of hypercalcaemia occurred suddenly and the dose of alfacalcidol tolerated decreased progressively once plasma alkaline phosphatase had fallen to normal values. Remission from bone disease was maintained using a dose of 1α-HCC of 1 μg thrice weekly.

Table 3 Usual dose requirements of vitamin D, dihydrotachysterol (DHT), alfacalcidol, and calcitriol in dietary deficiency rickets and in vitamin D resistance due to chronic renal failure

	D_3	DHT	Alfa-calcidol	Calcitriol
Approximate daily dose required to treat or prevent rickets (μg)	2.5–25	up to 200	up to 1.0	up to 0.5
Potency relative to vitamin D_3	100	10	250	500
Approximate daily dose required to treat renal bone disease (μg)	750–10 000	200–1000	0.5–2.0	0.25–2.0
Potency relative to vitamin D_3	100	1000	500 000	500 000

Potencies are shown relative to that of vitamin D (=100%). Note that although larger amounts of DHT than vitamin D are required to treat simple rickets, only slightly higher doses are required to treat renal bone disease with DHT (or with alfacalcidol or calcitriol—up to four times), whereas much larger doses of vitamin D (up to 400 times) are required to treat renal bone disease. Note 1 microgram D_3 or calcitriol is equivalent to approximately 40 IU.

Treatment with vitamin D or its metabolites is not without risk. Prolonged increases in plasma calcium and phosphate give rise to extraskeletal calcification. Patients with pre-existing hypercalcaemia should be treated cautiously, if at all, as such patients often respond poorly. Close control of serum calcium and phosphate, and serial assessment of renal function in patients not yet established on dialysis treatment are particularly important when any form of vitamin D is prescribed.

Aluminium toxicity

Neither osteomalacia nor adynamic bone disease resulting from aluminium retention respond to treatment with vitamin D or its metabolites. They may respond slowly to renal transplantation or adequate removal of aluminium from the dialysis fluid.

Desferrioxamine is used to decrease the body burden of aluminium. A typical regimen is to give desferrioxamine (15 mg/kg per h) by intravenous infusion during the first 2 h of each haemodialysis treatment, or to add a similar weekly dose (85 mg/kg) to the fluid used for peritoneal dialysis. In patients with significant aluminium retention, serum aluminium rises acutely due to its mobilization from tissues and chelation in the extracellular fluid. The rise can be used as a diagnostic test and to judge the duration of treatment required.

Parathyroidectomy

This is an effective treatment of hyperparathyroid bone disease and improves extraskeletal calcification, but vascular calcification improves less readily. It should be considered in patients who fail to respond to medical treatment, particularly those with tertiary hyperparathyroidism. Other indications include ischaemic necrosis of skin and intractable pruritus.

Recurrence of hyperparathyroidism is common following subtotal parathyroidectomy. Total parathyroidectomy should be considered in patients who are unlikely to receive renal transplants.

The main management problem is the immediate postoperative control of serum calcium when severe bone disease is present. Large intravenous doses of calcium (up to 6 g daily) may be required to avoid postoperative tetany. Prior treatment of patients with 1α-hydroxylated derivatives of vitamin D appears to diminish the degree and duration of hypocalcaemia.

Renal transplantation

Successful renal transplantation rapidly restores the capacity to form calcitriol. Osteomalacia is often slow to reverse, particularly when associated with aluminium retention. Bone disease, including osteomalacia and avascular necrosis, may arise *de novo* in the transplanted population. There is a high incidence of hypercalcaemia and hypophosphataemia in the transplant population and this may be in part related to phosphate depletion by the use of antacids, the persistence of hyperparathyroidism, which is slow to regress after transplantation, and the effects of corticosteroids to decrease renal tubular reabsorption of phosphate.

Experimental approaches

High intravenous doses of calcitriol or alfacalcidol suppress the secretion of PTH without raising serum calcium concentrations but the long-term effects of intravenous regimens are not known. It is also possible other metabolites of vitamin D have effects either directly on the parathyroids to suppress secretion, or on bone to increase bone formation. One such candidate is secalciferol, and its combination with calcitriol appears to have more complete effects on hyperparathyroid bone disease than the use of calcitriol alone.

Further reading

Bickle, D.D. and Negro-Vilar, A. (ed.) (1992). *Hormonal regulation of bone mineral metabolism.* Endocrine Reviews Monographs. The Endocrine Society Press.

Favus, J.J. (1996). *Primer on the metabolic bone diseases and disorders of mineral metabolism,* (3rd edn). Lippincott–Raven, Philadelphia.

Kanis, J.A. and Hamdy, N.A.T. (1998). Hypo-hypercalcaemia. In: *Oxford textbook of clinical nephrology,* (2nd edn) (ed. A.M. Davison, J.S. Cameron, J.-P. Grünfeld, D. Kerr, E. Ritz, and C.G. Winearls), pp. 225–248. Oxford University Press, Oxford.

Mundy, G.R. (1989). *Calcium homeostasis: hypercalcaemia and hypocalcaemia.* Martin Dunitz, London.

Ritz, E. and Slatopolsky, E. (1992). Renal osteodystrophy. In: *Frontiers in renal disease* (ed. L.W. Henderson and C. Jacobs). Kidney International Supplement, 38, S37–S67.

Chapter 12.31

Renal tubular disorders

J. Cunningham

Defects of water handling—nephrogenic diabetes insipidus

Nephrogenic diabetes insidius may rarely be the result of a defective gene at the tip of the long arm of the X chromosome, but various acquired forms are more common. The subject is addressed further in Chapter 12.2(and see also OTM3, p. 3120).

Aminoaciduria and Fanconi syndrome

Large amounts of amino acids appear in the glomerular filtrate and in health at least 95 per cent of these are reabsorbed by the proximal tubule. The appearance of excessive quantities in the final urine is the result of defective proximal tubular transport.

Organic solute transport in the proximal tubule is a two-step process that is carrier mediated and sodium coupled; the amino acid must first enter the proximal tubule cell via the brush border membrane against an electrochemical gradient, and exit via another transporter across the basolateral membrane. Movement of amino acids is accomplished by secondary active mechanisms whereby coupling to Na^+ transport allows the movement of amino acids to be driven indirectly by the basolateral membrane Na^+-K^+ ATPase. This enzyme lowers the intracellular sodium to about 10 per cent of that in the extracellular fluid or proximal tubular fluid, so providing the energy source for any transport system linked to the downhill movement of sodium.

Although each amino acid has a unique structure, not all have specific carriers in the proximal nephron. Instead, the amino acids segregate into four groups, based on loose structural similarities each with a group-specific carrier system (Table 1). Common to many defects of amino acid transport is a reduction of the electrochemical sodium gradient across the proximal tubular cells. This leads to impairment of linked transport of glucose, amino acids, phosphate, and a range of other solutes. Because some of the tubular amino acid transporters are expressed in the intestine also, defects may be evident at both sites. In these the clinical disease can result from the intestinal defect, the renal defect, or both.

The Fanconi syndrome

This term implies a disturbance of proximal tubular function with resulting generalized aminoaciduria, phosphate wasting, metabolic bone disease (rickets in children and osteomalacia in adults), renal

Table 1 Aminoacidurias

Type	Diseases	Amino acid	Clinical
Neutral	Hartnup disease	Alanine, asparagine, glutamine, histidine, isoleucine, phenylalanine, serine, threonine, tryptophan, tyrosine, valine.	'Pellagra' rash, ataxia, mental retardation, diarrhoea (all resulting from defective gut tryptophan absorption)
Dibasic	Cystinuria	Cystine, lysine, arginine, ornithine	Cystine stones
Imino acids and glycine	Iminoglycinuria	Proline, hydroxyproline, glycine	No sequelae
Acidic	Acidic aminoaciduria	Glutamate, aspartate	No sequelae

Table 2 Classification of Fanconi syndrome

Inherited

- Primary idiopathic
  - sporadic
  - familial
- Secondary to inborn error of metabolism
  - cystinosis (intralysosomal cystine)
  - tyrosinaemia (fumarylacetoacetate)
  - Wilson's disease (copper)
  - Lowe's syndrome
  - galactosaemia (galactose 1-phosphate)
  - hereditary fructose intolerance (fructose 1-phosphate)

Acquired

- Intrinsic renal disease
  - acute tubular necrosis
  - hypokalaemic nephropathy
  - myeloma
  - Sjögren's syndrome
  - transplant rejection
- Hormonal
  - primary hyperparathyroidism
  - secondary hyperparathyroidism (vitamin D/calcium deficiency)
- Nutritional
  - kwashiorkor
- Exogenous toxins
  - heavy metals (mercury, lead, cadmium, uranium)
  - outdated tetracycline
  - 6-mercaptopurine
  - maleic acid (in experimental animals)

tubular acidosis type 2 (proximal RTA), and renal glycosuria. Juvenile and adult Fanconi syndrome are expressions referring simply to the age of onset. The causes are numerous and it is helpful to classify them on the basis of aetiology and pathogenesis as far as possible (Table 2).

The clinical presentation usually depends more on the associated underlying abnormality than on the renal tubular defect *per se*. Nevertheless, the diagnosis ultimately depends on the demonstration of characteristic multiple proximal tubular defects. These may not all be present in all patients and may fluctuate in individual patients. Because of this variability it is best to define the specific defects existing in a patient, rather than to use the 'catch all' eponym.

Management

Treatment focuses on the cause (fructose avoidance in hereditary fructose intolerance, galactose avoidance in galactosaemia, copper chelation therapy in Wilson's disease) where this is feasible, and also on the consequences of the Fanconi syndrome (alkali and potassium for renal tubular acidosis type 2, oral phosphate and calcitriol for phosphate wasting).

Specific aminoacidurias

These are classified according to the four group-specific carrier defects (Table 1).

Neutral aminoacidurias

Hartnup disease

This is a rare (1:16 000 births) autosomal recessive disorder comprising: (a) intestinal tryptophan malabsorption; (b) a pellegra-like syndrome with photosensitive skin lesions, ataxia, and neuro-psychiatric disturbances; and (c) neutral aminoaciduria with increased renal clearance of alanine, asparagine, glutamine, histidine, isoleucine, leucine, phenylalanine, serine, threonine, tyrosine, valine, and tryptophan. The clinical manifestations flow from the tryptophan malabsorption which leads to nutritional deficiency, exacerbated by the further loss of tryptophan in the urine. Presentation is much like that of pellagra, although usually is less severe and tends to fluctuate. Analysis of the urine distinguishes the two disorders and Hartnup disease responds well to oral nicotinamide (40–200 mg daily).

Basic aminoacidurias

These comprise cystinuria, lysinuric protein intolerance, and lysinuria.

Cystinuria

This autosomally recessive disorder is the most common inherited abnormality of amino acid metabolism, affecting between 1 in 700 and 1 in 1500 births. The basic defect lies in abnormal transport of the dibasic amino acids, cystine, arginine, lysine, and ornithine across the mucosa of the small bowel and of the proximal renal tubules. The intestinal defect is not of clinical importance as all four amino acids are adequately absorbed as dipeptides. However, the failure of renal tubular reabsorption of these amino acids (which are freely filtered) results in hugely increased concentrations in the urine. For lysine, arginine, and ornithine this is not a problem, but cystine is only very poorly soluble with a threshold at 300–400 mg/l (1200–1600 mol/l) at the physiological pH of urine. Homozygotes may excrete 3000–7000 mol/l (750–1750 mg/l) of cystine, so that urine volumes must range from 3 to 6 litres/24 h to prevent deposition of cystine stones.

Biochemistry and genetics The defect in membrane transport in the kidney lies in the lack of a normal group-specific protein in the apical brush border of the proximal convoluted tubular cells with a similar abnormality in the mucosal cells of the small bowel. The carrier protein is thought to be the product of a single pair of allelic genes. Cystinuria results from three mutant genes at a single locus, perhaps on chromosome 2.

Various combinations of these alleles results in three different phenotypes, distinguished by studies of gut and renal tubular transport analyses. Stone formation is only a problem for those in the homozygous state for any two of them. Some heterozygotes have normal urinary amino acid excretion, but most excrete increased amounts of relevant amino acids, albeit in insufficient concentrations to cause cystine stones.

Diagnosis The urinary nitroprusside test is sensitive and may detect heterozygotes as well as homozygotes. The critical investigation is the quantitative measurement of the four amino acids in 24-h samples. This can also be used to assess the efficacy of treatment as well as to distinguish heterozygotes from homozygotes.

Clinical features and management Cystinuria is the cause of renal calculi in some 1–2 per cent of cases in adults but is a more common cause in children. Cystine stones may be symptomless even when they have grown to staghorn size, but most commonly patients present with pain, haematuria, infection, obstructive nephropathy or, more rarely, hypertension. The stones are radio-opaque (although less so than calcium containing stones) and are smooth and exceptionally hard, so relatively resistant to treatment by lithtripsy.

The aim of treatment must be to reduce the urinary concentration of cystine to below 1000 mol (250 mg) per litre of urine. This requires a minimum fluid intake of 4 litres and 6–8 litres is often necessary. It is important to emphasize the need to drink last thing before going to bed and again during the night, as the greatest risk of supersaturated urine is in the nocturnal oliguric period. The efficacy of treatment should be regularly monitored by 24-h measurements of cystine concentrations. Should this high fluid intake fail to reduce concentrations below 1000 mol/1itre the risk of calculus formation can be reduced but the use of sodium bicarbonate or acetozolamide to increase the urine pH above 7.5. The effect is marginal, however, and the large dose of bicarbonate required (often more than 6 g/day) brings its own problems, particularly to those in renal failure or with hypertension, as well as decreasing the solubility of calcium phosphate, thereby increasing the risk of incorporating calcium into any existing stones. It is better therefore, when high fluid intake alone is insufficient, to turn to penicillamine which reacts with cystine to form the much more soluble penicillamine-cysteine disulphide. The starting dose should be 125 g/day, increasing over weeks to the full dose of 1–2 g daily, the precise dose depending on the response in terms of urinary cystine concentrations. Penicillamine is a potentially toxic drug with a risk of blood dyscrasias, skin rashes, arthralgia, fever, lymphadenopathy, and glomerulonephropathy. Patients who are prescribed it must therefore be seen regularly, initially every 2 weeks and monthly in the longer term. Effective treatment either with high fluid intake alone or with the addition of penicillamine should prevent the formation of new stones and can dissolve existing ones.

Lysinuric protein intolerance

See Chapter 6.5.

Renal glycosuria

Glucose reabsorption occurs in the proximal tubule and is a two-step process, coupling secondary active transport by carrier-mediated Na^+-glucose cotransport across the brush border (apical) membrane, with facilitated diffusion linked with active sodium extrusion across the basolateral membrane.

Patients with renal glycosuria exhibit glycosuria at normal blood glucose concentrations. The condition is seen most frequently in normal pregnant women, in whom an increased glomerular filtration rate is associated with a high filtered glucose load which may exceed the renal tubular maximum capacity for reabsorption. The isolated form is familial with a mixed inheritance pattern. This is consistent with the notion that the condition comprises any one of a number of mutations affecting the proximal tubular glucose transporter, in turn associated with subtle differences in the transport defect. The functional basis for these defects is either reduction of tubular maximum capacity for glucose reabsorption or reduction of the tubular threshold alone.

Abnormalities of glucose transport can also arise from defective linked mechanisms. For example, reduction of the electrochemical sodium gradient leads to a generalized proximal tubular transport defect with renal glycosuria, aminoaciduria, bicarbonaturia, and phosphaturia (Fanconi syndrome—see above).

Renal glycosuria *per se* has no clinical sequelae. The isolated form must be distinguished from more complex defects, including Fanconi syndrome, that are associated with tubulointerstitial damage in children with focal and segmental glomerulosclerosis, and a rare autosomal recessive form with associated intestinal malabsorption of glucose and galactose.

Disorders of renal phosphate handling

The renal handling of inorganic phosphate is the major determinant of extracellular phosphate concentration and, in health, shows an adaptive capacity capable of maintaining normal phosphate concentrations in the face of wide fluctuations of phosphate intake. Parathyroid hormone (**PTH**) and metabolic need in relation to dietary intake separately control the handling of phosphate at its major reabsorption site, the proximal tubule. About 20 per cent of tubular phosphate transport occurs in the distal convoluted tubule and collecting duct. PTH is phosphaturic and acts on the proximal nephron via an adenylate cyclase and cyclic adenosine monophosphate, and possibly also by activation of protein kinase C. In addition, the renal tubules can respond to dietary phosphate intake, even when plasma phosphate changes little or not at all. The precise nature of the dietary phosphate signal is uncertain, and, like PTH, it operates on the proximal tubule. In parallel with the antiphosphaturic effect of reduced dietary phosphate, there is an increase in bone resorption leading to mobilization of phosphate (and calcium) from the skeleton. Both the renal and skeletal responses are unimpaired by parathyroidectomy and are therefore not mediated by PTH. A humoral message from gut to kidney and skeleton is possible, but its existence is unproven.

Tubular phosphate wasting

Phosphate transport defects are of several types and all cause hypophosphataemia, with inappropriate phosphaturia. The fractional excretion of phosphate is increased and the tubular transport maximum for phosphate (**TmP/GFR**) is decreased. The resulting clinical disturbances include rickets (in children) and osteomalacia (in adults),

Table 3 The kidney and phosphate metabolism

Disturbance	Comments
Hypophosphataemia	
• X-linked hypophosphataemic rickets	• The most common
• sporadic	• Rare
• acquired	
• oncogenous rickets • primary hyperparathyroidism • secondary • hyperparathyroidism due to vitamin D deficiency	• Increased PTH-dependent phosphaturia
Hyperphosphataemia	
• renal failure	• Reduced filtered P_i load
• hypoparathyroidism	• Reduced PTH-dependent phosphaturia
• pseudohypoparathyroidism	• Renal PTH resistance
• type I	• Absent cAMP and phosphaturic responses to PTH (G-protein defect)
• type II	• Normal cAMP and absent phosphaturic response to PTH (cAMP-dependent protein kinase C defect)

cAMP, cyclic adenosine monophosphate; PTH, parathyroid hormone.

and depend on severity, chronicity, and associated non-renal abnormalities (Table 3).

X-linked hypophosphataemic rickets

This is the most important type and usually presents with poor growth and rickets in early childhood. Inheritance is X-linked dominant. Plasma calcium and PTH are usually normal but there is a subtle disturbance of vitamin D metabolism—plasma calcitriol concentration does not show the increase expected during hypophosphataemia and is normal in most cases. Females (heterozygotes) are less severely affected than males (hemizygotes). The defect probably lies in the proximal tubular brush border membrane Na^+-P_i transporter. Diagnosis is made on the basis of the characteristic clinical features coupled with persistent hypophosphataemia and a reduced TmP/GFR.

Treatment is aimed at increasing plasma phosphate to a normal concentration—a difficult task. As phosphate rises towards normal levels during therapy, so also does the filtered load and total urinary loss of phosphate, necessitating large and frequent dosing with oral phosphate. This is usually combined with calcitriol to promote intestinal phosphorus absorption. The results are usually good, but the compliance of children with frequent dosing of oral phosphate therapy is often poor.

Oncogenous rickets

Rarely, a similar renal disturbance is acquired in association with certain mesenchymal tumours, especially giant-cell tumours of bone, neurofibromas, and cavernous haemangiomas. This condition is termed oncogenous rickets, and is almost certainly mediated by a humoral factor, as yet unidentified. The functional disturbance is indistinguishable from that of the X-linked form and successful removal of the tumour leads to complete recovery of renal phosphate handling.

Other phosphate-wasting disorders

In addition to X-linked inheritance, sporadic cases exist and present at any age, although most often in childhood. In addition, both autosomal recessive and autosomal dominant inheritance has been encountered. Although some heterogeneity of presentation and functional disturbance is found among these, common to all is impaired proximal tubular phosphate transport (low TmP/GFR), resulting in phosphate wasting and in most cases metabolic bone disease also (Table 3).

Tubular phosphate retention

Excessive tubular phosphate reabsorption (high TmP/GFR), with resulting hyperphosphataemia is seen in conditions of PTH lack or renal resistance to PTH (Table 3). All these patients have hypocalcaemia and hyperphosphataemia, the former largely the result of failure of calcitriol production by the PTH-deprived kidney and the latter the result of an inappropriately raised TmP/GFR.

Disorders of the renal tubular handling of calcium and magnesium

Idiopathic hypercalciuria

In some of these cases (a minority) a defect of tubular calcium reabsorption is the prime mover ('renal leak' hypercalciuria), with secondary increase of PTH, calcitriol, and intestinal calcium absorption. In the majority, however, calcium hyperabsorption by the intestine drives the hypercalciuria which is thus of 'overspill' type. In most of these there is a primary reduction of TmP/GFR (renal phosphate leak) stimulating calcitriol production (see also Chapter 12.23).

Familial hypocalciuric hypercalcaemia

This is a rare dominantly inherited condition, in which an intrinsic acceleration of tubular calcium reabsorption coupled with an increase in the parathyroid 'set point' for calcium act synergistically to elevate blood calcium concentration. The condition is usually benign and the diagnosis depends on exclusion of other hypercalcaemic conditions and confirmation of the dominant inheritance by assessment of family members. Children of affected patients may suffer from neonatal hyperparathyroidism and severe hypercalcaemia.

Tubular magnesium handling: hypermagnesaemia and hypomagnesaemia

Tubular magnesium handling can be varied over a wide range and, although normally only about 3 per cent of the filtered magnesium appears in the urine (most of the remaining 97 per cent is reabsorbed in the proximal tubule and the thin limb of Henle's loop), this can rise dramatically in conditions of hypermagnesaemia and also as a result of tubular injury. Because of this high potential excretory capacity, hypermagnesaemia is rare in the presence of good renal function, unless inordinately large quantities of magnesium are given parenterally. In contrast, patients with renal failure are more prone to hypermagnesaemia, particularly when magnesium intake is high, as may be the case if magnesium containing antacids are used.

Table 4 Renal magnesium wasting

Diuretics
Tubular toxins
aminoglycosides (gentamicin, tobramycin)
cisplatin
cyclosporin
Hypercalcaemia
Bartter's syndrome
Tubulointerstitial nephropathies
Obstruction

Hypomagnesaemia, on the other hand, is much more common and frequently results from renal magnesium wasting (Table 4). Iatrogenic causes are the most common, especially aminoglycoside and cisplatin toxicity. The diagnosis is easy—inappropriately high magnesium excretion (>1.5 mmol/day in a hypomagnesaemic patient) is conclusive. Symptoms are rare, but when present are similar to those of hypokalaemia and should be treated with parenteral magnesium chloride or sulphate (35–50 mmol given in 5 per cent dextrose or saline over 24 h). Smaller maintenance doses can be given by mouth but often provoke diarrhoea. In that case repeated intravenous replacement is required on rare occasions.

Disorders of tubular potassium handling

Renal potassium wasting is most commonly caused by diuretic therapy, metabolic alkalosis, mineralocorticoid or glucocorticoid excess, while Bartter's syndrome, Liddle's syndrome, and hypomagnesaemic hypokalaemia are much rarer. These disorders and those resulting in impaired renal excretion of potassium are discussed elsewhere (Chapters 7.6 and 12.4).

Further reading

Davison, A.M., Cameron, J.S., Grünfeld, J.-P., Kerr, D., Ritz, E., and Winearls, C.G. (1998). *Oxford textbook of clinical nephrology*, (2nd edn), Section 5, pp. 1019–95. Oxford University Press, Oxford.

Chapter 12.32

The renal tubular acidoses

R. D. Cohen

Renal tubular acidosis (RTA) is the term used to describe metabolic acidoses whose cause is a disorder of the renal tubules. The designation distinguishes this type of acidosis from that accompanying generalized glomerulotubular failure (uraemic acidosis). An account of the normal acid-base function of the kidney (Fig. 1(a)) can be found in OTM3, pp. 1534-5 and 3338. In the following account RTA is classified according to identifiable differences in pathogenesis.

Distal renal tubular acidosis ('classical' RTA, 'gradient RTA', RTA-1)

This form is characterized by an inability to generate a normal minimum urinary pH (4.4–5.3) even in the presence of severe systemic acidosis. It may present in infancy, childhood, or adult life, most typically with acute acidosis and hyperventilation, often accompanied by muscular weakness due to hypokalaemia. In most patients the attacks of acute acidosis represent a worsening of a mild chronic hyperchloraemic metabolic acidosis which may have been fully compensated until presentation. About 70 per cent of patients are found to have either nephrocalcinosis or calcium-containing renal calculi. Rickets and growth stunting in childhood are frequent features, and osteomalacia may be seen in adults. Although the glomerular filtration rate is characteristically normal, or nearly so, at the outset, progressive nephrocalcinosis, obstructive uropathy related to calculi, and recurrent urinary tract infections may eventually result in glomerular failure.

The diagnosis in the acute state depends on the observation of a urinary pH greater than 5.5 (and usually greater than 6) in the presence of a normal anion gap metabolic acidosis, hyperchloraemia, and normal or nearly normal plasma urea and creatinine. Severe hypokalaemia, hypercalciuria, evidence of renal calcification, and the presence of clinical features related to one of the aetiologies discussed below may provide further evidence. The failure to acidify the urine maximally in the presence of severe acidosis (plasma bicarbonate <12 mmol/l) serves to distinguish the condition from RTA-2 and RTA-4. Nephrocalcinosis is virtually confined to RTA-1. In the chronic non-acute state, which often presents with renal stones, incidental discovery of nephrocalcinosis, failure of growth, anorexia, or lethargy, the diagnosis may be confirmed by a short acid load test revealing failure to achieve normal minimum urinary pH after ingestion of a standard body-weight-related dose of ammonium chloride. There is also a group of patients with nephrocalcinosis and failure to acidify the urine normally on ammonium chloride challenge, but without systemic acidosis ('incomplete syndrome of RTA'). It is not safe to administer the acid load test if the plasma bicarbonate is below 19 mmol/l. Under such conditions, comparison of urinary pH with plasma bicarbonate is helpful (Table 1).

Pathophysiology

RTA-1 is due to a failure of the α-intercalated cells of the collecting duct to generate the 800–900:1 H^+ gradient between tubular lumen and blood that a normal subject can achieve under acidifying conditions. Except in rare patients with mixed syndromes, proximal tubular function is normal in terms of H^+ secretion and bicarbonate reabsorption. The distal nephron defect is variable in severity, but if the urine pH cannot be lowered below 6 to 6.5, increasingly large quantities of bicarbonate may appear in the urine. This represents that proportion of the 10–15 per cent of filtered bicarbonate which has reached the distal nephron, but has not been reabsorbed because of failure of distal H^+ secretion. The defect also results in the failure of titration of phosphate buffer. Because NH_4^+ excretion is lessened in alkaline urine, it may be lower than appropriate for systemic pH. All these factors, which are direct consequences of the distal tubular defect, lead to acidosis (see Fig. 1(b)). In children in particular, loss of bicarbonate may be a major contributor. The precise nature of the defect which results in failure to establish the normal H^+ gradient is, in most instances, unknown. In familial RTA-1, mutations in the anion exchanger gene have been implicated.

Table 1 Distal renal tubular acidosis—diagnostic criteria

	RTA-1	RTA-2	RTA-4
Urine pH when plasma HCO_3^- <13 mmol/l	>6	<5.4	<5.4
Plasma potassium	Low	Low	Raised
Nephrocalcinosis or renal lithiasis	+	–	–
Therapeutic requirement For bicarbonate	Modest	Large	Modest
For mineralocorticoid	–	–	+

Hypokalaemia has two origins. First, lack of H^+ flux out of the tubular cell into the lumen encourages K^+ exchange for luminal Na^+ in the distal nephron; even so, overall distal Na^+ reabsorption is impaired, leading to secondary aldosteronism, which provides the second reason for renal K^+ wasting. Correction of the acidosis, which raises distal luminal pH and therefore permits more H^+ secretion, results in amelioration of Na^+ and K^+ wasting (in contrast to RTA-2, see below).

Renal lithiasis is generally attributed to hypercalciuria and hypocitraturia. Citrate complexes with calcium ions to form the $CaCit^-$ ion, which is partly responsible for maintaining calcium ions in solution in the urine, and a situation in which there is both lack of citrate and increased calcium is likely to be lithogenic. The pathogenesis of the nephrocalcinosis is unclear. So is that of osteomalacia or rickets, which can be corrected by treatment of the chronic acidosis without vitamin D therapy.

Causes of RTA-1

RTA-1 may occur as a primary disorder, or secondary to a whole range of conditions which, in one way or another, affect distal nephron function.

The primary disorder may be hereditary, or sporadic. The hereditary form behaves as an autosomal dominant and may present in childhood or in adult life. There is, however, an infantile form of the condition which is transient and may occur in siblings without other family history. It is not clear whether this is a recessive disorder, or due to environmental factors.

In the acquired category, RTA-1 associated with autoimmune disorders accounts for a significant proportion of cases. Sjögren's syndrome is the most prominent association in this group, but other dysglobulinaemic or hypergammaglobulinaemic conditions also give rise to RTA-1. It does not appear, however, that the raised plasma globulin itself is the determining factor. RTA-1 is occasionally seen in primary biliary cirrhosis and, rarely, in fibrosing alveolitis. Although RTA-1 is a cause of nephrocalcinosis, it seems fairly clear that nephrocalcinosis itself can, by causing medullary damage, give rise to RTA-1. Thus, for instance, hyperparathyroidism and chronic vitamin D poisoning may cause RTA-1 because of nephrocalcinosis. Conditions directly damaging the renal medulla, such as pyelonephritis, papillary necrosis, chronic obstructive uropathy, medullary sponge kidney, and sickle-cell anaemia may also give rise to varying degrees of RTA-1. Among drug-related causes, analgesic nephropathy presumably acts through papillary damage. Amphotericin B causes RTA by inserting itself into luminal cell membranes of the distal nephron, thus allowing back leakage of H^+ into cells, or HCO_3^- into the tubular lumen.

Treatment

The acutely acidotic patient will often have moderate to marked hypokalaemia, which must be corrected before the acidosis. If, the acidosis is dealt with first, movement of K^+ into cells will further lower plasma K^+ and cardiac arrest may occur. Potassium, and then isotonic sodium bicarbonate, are administered intravenously, aiming to restore the abnormalities over a few hours.

In the chronic condition, therapy with oral sodium bicarbonate has markedly beneficial effects. Not only will it prevent recurrent exacerbations of acidosis, but renal potassium loss will be curtailed, hypercalciuria will be diminished, and hypocitraturia improved, osteomalacia or rickets healed, and growth restored in children. In addition, progression of nephrocalcinosis and nephrolithiasis and consequent renal damage may be halted. The daily bicarbonate requirement is usually in the range 1–3 mmol/kg body weight, but often more in children. Not infrequently, potassium supplements are required in addition to sodium bicarbonate.

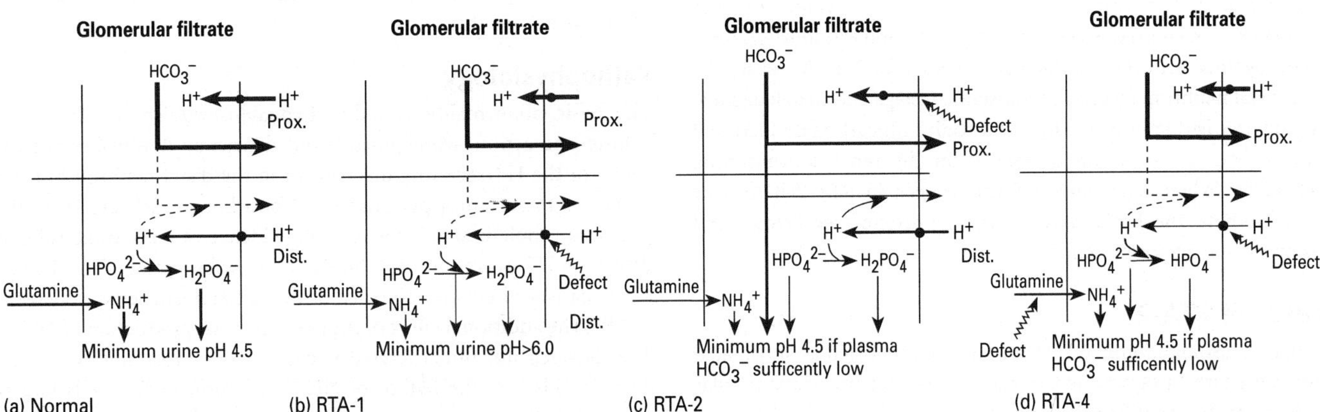

Fig. 1 Diagrams to indicate the site of the defects in different types of RTA. (a) Normal; (b) RTA-1, gradient defect in distal nephron; (c) RTA-2, proximal HCO_3^- reabsorption defect due to reduced H^+ secretion; (d) RTA-4, defects in NH_4^+ production and in capacity of H^+ pump in distal nephron due to hypoaldosteronism. The thickness of the arrows indicates semiquantitatively the magnitude of the ionic fluxes. See text for further explanation.

Proximal renal tubular acidosis (RTA-2; bicarbonate wasting RTA)

This form of RTA (Fig. 1(c)) is superficially clinically similar to RTA-1, but there are notable distinguishing features. It is rare as an isolated defect and, in the great majority of patients, is associated with multiple abnormalities of proximal tubular functions, e.g. glycosuria, aminoaciduria, hyperphosphaturia, and uricosuria (the Fanconi syndrome). Provided the patient is sufficiently acidotic, the urine pH falls to the normal minimum. Nephrocalcinosis and renal calculi are virtually never present. Bicarbonate leakage into the urine is much greater than in RTA-1 and, in consequence, very large quantities of sodium bicarbonate may be required for therapy. There may be marked polyuria and polydipsia, especially in those patients in whom the acidosis has been fully controlled by bicarbonate therapy. Proximal myopathy, osteomalacia, or rickets are common associations, probably largely because of the frequent involvement of disorders of vitamin D supply or metabolism. RTA-2 resembles RTA-1 in that it presents with a chronic (or acute exacerbation of) normal anion gap hyperchloraemic acidosis, with a marked tendency to potassium deficiency due to renal potassium loss.

Pathophysiology

The basic lesion in RTA-2 is a depression of the capacity of the proximal tubule to secrete H^+ and thus to reabsorb bicarbonate. In a normal individual or in a patient with RTA-1, the plasma bicarbonate above which bicarbonate appears in the urine is 25–28 mmol/l. In RTA-2 this bicarbonate 'threshold' is lowered, often markedly so, due to the proximal tubular defect. The result is that the distal nephron is flooded with bicarbonate which has escaped proximal reabsorption, and the low capacity (but high gradient) distal H^+ secreting mechanism cannot produce enough H^+ to reabsorb this bicarbonate, which therefore spills over into the urine. However, when, in consequence of the bicarbonate leak, plasma bicarbonate falls to a level which reduces the filtered bicarbonate load to one with which the defective proximal tubule can cope, then the distal nephron is fully capable of producing a normally minimal urinary pH of 4.5–5.3 (Fig. 1(c)). The acidosis in RTA-2 is predominantly due to the bicarbonate leak, but it is, to a lesser extent, related to failure of titration of phosphate and failure of appropriate NH_4^+ excretion due to the inappropriately high urine pH—at least while plasma bicarbonate remains above the renal threshold. The high distal load of sodium bicarbonate is also responsible for sodium wastage. This leads to secondary aldosteronism, which, together with the high demand created for Na^+/K^+ exchange in the distal nephron, results in potassium wastage and hypokalaemia. The polyuria is due both to the distal sodium bicarbonate load and to the effects of potassium deficiency on the renal concentrating mechanism. When osteomalacia/rickets is seen in RTA-2 it may be related both to the basic cause of the syndrome (see below) and possibly to the acidosis itself.

Causes of RTA-2

Familial autosomal dominant RTA-2 has been reported as an isolated lesion but nearly always some factor which damages proximal tubular function can be identified. Isolated damage to the proximal tubular H^+ secretion mechanism occurs during treatment with the carbonic anhydrase inhibitor acetazolamide and in carbonic anhydrase II deficiency, in which there is also an element of RTA-1.

More usually, RTA-2 occurs as part of more generalized proximal tubular damage, with reabsorption defects for glucose, amino acids, and phosphate. There are many causes of this Fanconi syndrome; in the genetic category are included cystinosis, Wilson's disease, and hereditary fructose intolerance, as well as the isolated hereditary variety. Among acquired causes are vitamin D deficiency, lead poisoning, multiple myeloma, therapy with outdated tetracycline, hyperparathyroidism, and the nephrotic syndrome. The precise mechanisms of damage are not usually clear but, in hereditary fructose intolerance the absence of fructose-1-phosphate aldolase in the proximal tubular cells results in the accumulation of fructose-1-phosphate during fructose ingestion. Fructose phosphorylation depletes adenosine triphosphate stores markedly and the generalized tubular malfunction may be due to this perturbation of energy metabolism. In vitamin D deficiency, the lesion is probably contributed to both by the deficiency itself and by the accompanying secondary hyperparathyroidism.

Therapy

The bicarbonate leak is much more severe in RTA-2 than in RTA-1, and the daily dose of sodium bicarbonate needed to prevent acidosis may be very large (3–20 mmol/kg body weight). In contrast to RTA-1, effective treatment of the acidosis in RTA-2 does not help, and may worsen the potassium deficiency and polyuria, by providing a greater sodium bicarbonate load to the distal tubule. If glomerular failure ensues, as for example in cystinosis, then the bicarbonate requirement may lessen. Potassium supplements in the form of oral bicarbonate will be required. If the amount of oral bicarbonate needed is intolerable, hydrochlorothiazide may be added. This agent appears to diminish the bicarbonate requirement by decreasing the filtered load of bicarbonate, but may necessitate an increase in potassium supplementation.

Hyperkalaemic renal tubular acidosis (RTA-4)

RTA-4 is characterized by hyperkalaemia rather than hypokalaemia. As in RTA-1 and RTA-2, patients present with metabolic acidosis in which the anion gap is normal or nearly so and there is a similar tendency to hyperchloraemia. As in RTA-2, if the plasma bicarbonate falls sufficiently, the distal tubule is able to mount a normal blood/urine pH gradient. These patients frequently have slight or moderate glomerular impairment, but the degree of hyperkalaemia is quite out of proportion to this.

Pathophysiology

The basic abnormality is either hypoaldosteronism or failure of aldosterone action. Mineralocorticoid deficiency diminishes the capacity of the H^+ secreting mechanism in the distal nephron but not its power to sustain a pH gradient if bicarbonate delivery from the proximal tubule is small. There is no evidence of a proximal tubular defect in H^+ secretion and bicarbonate reabsorption. The hyperkalaemia is a direct consequence of the mineralocorticoid deficiency and has the additional effect of suppressing renal production of NH_4^+. The nitrogen not thus excreted is converted to urea and H^+ in the liver. In this way the failure of NH_4^+ excretion in RTA-4 is largely responsible for the acidosis (Fig. 1(d)). A second mechanism of RTA-4 is illustrated by its induction by amiloride, which inhibits sodium reabsorption in the cortical collecting duct and thereby reduces the negative luminal potential required for K^+ and H^+ secretion.

Causes

Aldosterone deficiency leading to RTA-4 may be due to Addison's disease or certain inborn errors of steroid synthesis. Much more commonly it is related to deficient renin production, most notably in diabetes and chronic tubulointerstitial disease, such as pyelonephritis. Renin production is, to some extent, dependent on prostaglandin synthesis and, increasingly commonly, RTA-4 is being seen in patients receiving prostaglandin synthetase inhibitors in the form of non-steroidal anti-inflammatory agents. It also may occur in association with the administration of angiotensin-converting enzyme inhibitors, β-blockers, and potassium sparing diuretics. RTA-4 is also seen in patients receiving aldosterone antagonists and in infants with pseudo-hypoaldosteronism.

Treatment

Significant acidosis or hyperkalaemia, should be treated with a mineralocorticoid. Fludrocortisone (0.05–0.15 mg daily) improves NH_4^+ excretion, and restores hyperkalaemia and acidosis towards normal.

Further reading

Davison, A.M., Cameron, J.S., Grünfeld, J.-P., Kerr, D., Ritz, E., and Winearls, C.G. (1998). *Oxford textbook of clinical nephrology*, (2nd edn), Section 5, pp. 1019–95. Oxford University Press, Oxford.

Section 13
Neurology

Contents

Chapter 13.1

Introduction

M. Donaghy and J. Newsom-Davis

Clinical diagnosis

Some 75 per cent of neurological consultations are concerned with headache, black-outs, peripheral and cranial nerve lesions, cerebrovascular disease, giddiness, spinal disorders, multiple sclerosis, parkinsonism, and dementia.

History taking is still the cornerstone of diagnosis. Eye-witness accounts may be crucial for differentiating fits from other black-outs, for diagnosing early dementia, and for highlighting the inconsistencies so characteristic of psychologically determined disability. Often, specific symptoms must be sought, but enquiry must be couched in terms that do not prejudice the patient's response.

The examination usually only provides information anticipated from the history, but is particularly rewarding in determining the anatomical origin of muscle weakness. Unexpected discovery of abnormal physical signs, such as extensor plantar responses or papilloedema, will crucially alter such provisional diagnoses as psychologically determined weakness or benign tension headache. Patients with psychologically determined disorders may respond inconsistently during somatosensory testing, or show discrepant motor abilities during formal examination compared to other activities such as walking or dressing.

Sensitive issues may arise that can distress patients during a consultation. For instance, recommending a brain scan may reassure many patients, but in others it may engender anxiety that the neurologist is anticipating serious disease. Enquiries about family history of disease cause apprehension in those with descendants or incomplete families. Telling patients of progressively disabling or fatal neurological diseases is always difficult and must combine honesty with compassion. Conspiracies of secrecy with relatives should be avoided. Open confrontation rarely cures psychologically determined disorders; it is often more productive to reassure that there is no evidence of serious disease, to treat depression if present, and to offer 'face saving' escape routes.

Recent advances

Developments in imaging techniques have revolutionized the diagnosis of structural and demyelinating diseases of the central nervous system. MRI now complements CT radiography in neurological diagnosis. MRI has largely replaced spinal myelography and allows detailed imaging of the brainstem. Gadolinium-enhanced MRI reveals defects in the blood–brain barrier in multiple sclerosis. Magnetic brain stimulation can establish the site and nature of lesions in central motor pathways in a manner analogous to nerve conduction studies in the periphery. Developments in single-fibre electromyography, notably the stimulated single-fibre electromyogram, have provided the most sensitive means yet available for detecting disorders of neuromuscular transmission.

Molecular genetic detection of mutations or deletions can aid diagnosis. These include some forms of familial Alzheimer's disease (a point of mutation in the gene for amyloid precursor protein), the spongiform encephalopathies such as Creutzfeldt–Jakob disease (mutations in the prion protein gene), familial amyotrophic lateral sclerosis (abnormalities of the superoxide dismutase gene), Charcot–Marie–Tooth disease (reduplication of a chromosome 17 gene), and Duchenne and Becker muscular dystrophies (deletions in the dystrophin gene). Abnormal amplification of particular trinucleotide repeats occurs in X-linked bulbospinal muscular atrophy, fragile X syndrome, Friedreich's ataxia, and myotonic dystrophy. Mitochondrial DNA deletions underlie Leber's optic atrophy, Leigh's necrotizing encephalopathy of childhood, and the mitochondrial myopathies. Autoantibodies aid diagnosis of peripheral neuropathies, myasthenia, and paraneoplastic disorders affecting the peripheral and central nervous systems.

New therapies for neurological diseases are appearing thick and fast. Plasma exchange has significantly shortened recovery time in the Guillain–Barré syndrome, and provides valuable short-term improvement in a number of other autoantibody-mediated disorders. Intravenous immunoglobulin has a dramatic effect upon motor neuropathies. Immunosuppression has improved the prognosis in patients severely affected by chronic autoimmune disorders such as myasthenia gravis, chronic inflammatory demyelinating neuropathy, vasculitis of the nervous system, and polymyositis. The treatment of movement disorders has been advanced by localized injection of botulinum toxin in conditions such as blepharospasm and spasmodic torticollis. Interferons reduce the relapse rate in multiple sclerosis and may delay progression. The 5-hydroxytryptamine agonists are effective remedies for many patients with migraine attacks, one of the most common disorders referred to neurological clinics.

Organization and features of dysfunction

Chapter 13.2

Disturbances of higher cerebral function

J. M. Oxbury and S. M. Oxbury

The pathology underlying disturbances of higher cerebral function may be diffuse, as in Alzheimer's disease, or focal, as in cerebral infarction and small tumours. Diffuse pathology produces dementia with a global impairment of intellect, personality, memory, concentration, and attention. The associated mood change may be apathy, depression, or euphoria. Forgetfulness is particularly common, and indeed a diagnosis of dementia should be questioned if memory function is normal.

Focal pathology produces more restricted cognitive impairment. The nature of the impairment depends upon the situation of the pathology in the brain. Often there is no change of personality or loss of memory.

Localization of cognitive function

The introduction of radiological, structural and functional imaging techniques, initially computed tomography and more recently positron-emission tomography and magnetic resonance, has been a further stimulus to the increased attention to issues of localization in neuropsychology.

A special emphasis in research has been to explore both the differential function of the left and right hemispheres, demonstrating asymmetries, and functional interconnections within the hemispheres; this is in addition to the time-honoured separation of function in parallel with anatomical division of the brain into lobes (frontal, temporal, parietal, occipital). These anatomical divisions are somewhat arbitrary, but a simplified list of the major cognitive deficits that have traditionally been associated with the different regions of the brain (Table 1) may be helpful as an introduction to the field of behavioural neurology.

Table 1 Relationship between behavioural impairment and the site of brain pathology

Lobe and behavioural deficit	Main hemisphere involved			
	Left	Right	Left= Right	Bilateral
Frontal				
Language-aphasia, verbal fluency↓	+			
Speech-dysarthria			+	
Recent memory impaired			+	
Movement control↓			+	
Planning ability↓			+ <	++
Disinhibition-social and motor			+ <	++
Temporal				
Memory-verbal aspects↓	+			
Non-verbal aspects↓		+		
Severe amnesia				+
Music perception↓		+		
Language comprehension↓	+			
Kluver-Bucy syndrome				+
Aggression, rage, depression	+			
Indifference, euphoria		+		
Parietal and occipital				
Primary visual-tactile sensation↓			+	
Visual discrimination↓		+		
Gaze deviation	+	< +		
Gaze apraxia				+
Visual disorientation				+
Visual agnosia				+
Prosopagnosia				+
Heminegiect-visuospatial and body		+		
Topographical disorientation—				
Major				+
Minor		+		
Dressing apraxia		+		
Constructional apraxia			+	
Ideomotor apraxia	+			
Acalculia—				
Spatial		+		
Anarithmia	+			+
Finger agnosia	+			
Right-left disorientation	+			
Alexia and agraphia				

Aphasia

Aphasia is an acquired defect of language function due to brain damage. It is usually manifest in all four language 'modalities'—speech production, speech comprehension, reading, and writing. Aphasia must be distinguished from motor disturbances of voice production such as dysarthria and stuttering (defined below), from poverty of speech due to intellectual impairment, from language abnormalities as in schizophrenia, and from hysterical mutism.

Dysarthria is a disorder of speech production arising from dysfunction of the muscles of articulation. The dysfunction can be secondary to damage in the motor system at any point from the cerebral cortex (and then the dysarthria may be associated with aphasia) to the muscles themselves. The precise quality of the dysarthria depends on the site of the pathology and various forms are recognized, for example spastic dysarthria and ataxic dysarthria.

More than 90 per cent of normal, right-handed people have language represented on the left in the sense that damage to the left hemisphere could make them overtly aphasic but right-sided damage would not do so.

Early concepts of cerebral dominance held that the dominant hemisphere is contralateral to the preferred hand. This applies to 95 to 98 per cent of right-handers without early childhood cerebral pathology. However, the left hemisphere is also dominant in about 70 per cent of left-handers without such cerebral pathology; about 20 per cent of left-handers have right hemisphere dominance, and in 10 per cent language function is more or less equally distributed between the two hemispheres (bilateral representation).

The areas most important for language are shown in Fig. 1. They include the posterior part of the inferior frontal gyrus (Broca's area), located immediately anterior to the primary motor cortical representation for the face, mouth, and tongue, the posterior part of the superior temporal gyrus (Wernicke's area), the inferior parietal lobule including the supramarginal and angular gyri, and the cortex of the frontoparietal operculum.

Characteristics

Spontaneous speech

Difficulty in word finding is a major deficit underlying aphasia and is responsible for many of the characteristic hesitancies and/or circumlocutions. The patient's spontaneous speech may be described as 'fluent' or 'non-fluent'.

Non-fluent aphasia

At its most severe, non-fluent aphasia consists of complete loss of speech and phonation; this is nearly always associated with inability to comprehend anything but the simplest spoken language and with complete inability to read or write. Often there is an associated buccofacial apraxia (a defect of voluntary tongue and palatal movements and of voluntary facial movements, as in whistling or imitating actions such as laughing or blowing, even though all these movements are normal when performed automatically); in the acute phase there may also be an impairment of voluntary swallowing. After some recovery the patient may make phonated but inarticulate utterances or may develop a recurring utterance that is recognizable.

When the aphasia is less severe, the non-fluent speech is characterized by effortful articulation, a slow rate of word production,

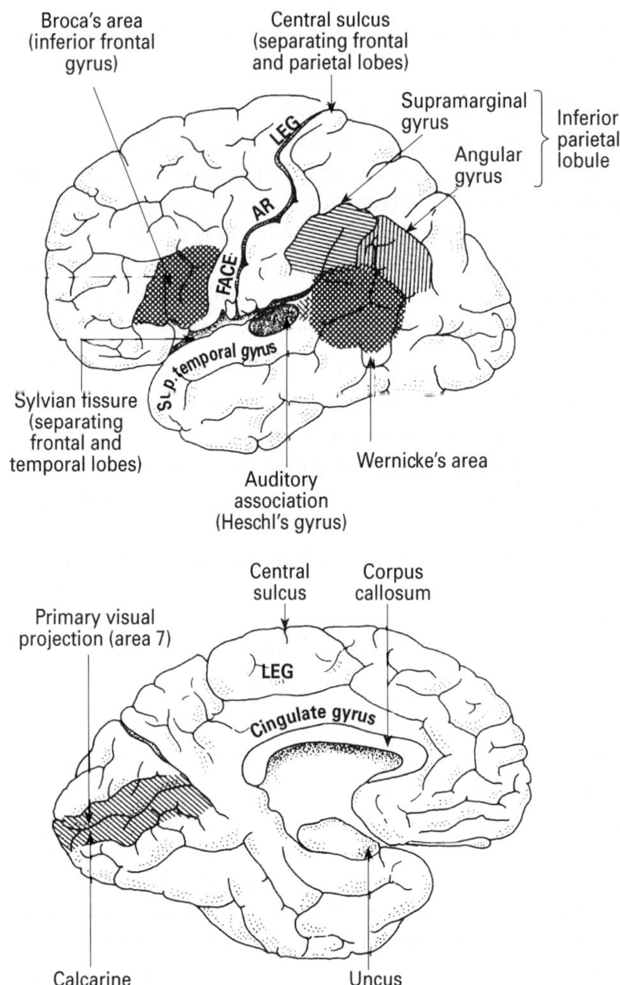

Fig. 1 A lateral view of the left cerebral hemisphere (a) to show the areas important for language functions and the motor area, with a medial view (b) to show the corpus callosum and the primary visual area.

and short phrase length. The style is agrammatic, having a telegraphic quality. The quality of writing is similar to that of the spoken language.

Fluent aphasia

This is characterized by spontaneous speech that is abnormal or even completely incomprehensible, not because it is reduced in amount—indeed the rate of word production may be higher than normal—or because it is articulated badly, but because it contains wrong words, non-words, and words arranged in an inappropriate order so that meaning is lost. It is usually accompanied by impaired comprehension. Jargon aphasia is the condition where the abnormal characteristics are present to such a degree that speech has very little meaning; the rate of word production, articulation, and prosody (pattern or melody) remain normal. Insight is often lacking, and patients with jargon aphasia may be misdiagnosed as suffering from confusion or an acute psychosis. Echolalia is a seemingly compulsive repetition of words spoken by others without any apparent understanding of their meaning. Palilalia is repetition reiterated with increasing frequency. Echolalia and palilalia are usually manifestations of diffuse brain disease such as Alzheimer's or encephalitis.

Object naming

Most aphasics have some defect of the ability to name objects, although mild aphasia may cause difficulty only with less common objects. This anomia is sometimes the first manifestation of aphasia. Aphasic anomia is usually independent of the sensory modality through which the object to be named is perceived.

Speech comprehension

Impaired ability to comprehend speech is a very important functional defect in aphasia. The bedside analysis of comprehension disturbances is difficult, and a common error is to overestimate the extent to which an aphasic patient can understand what is said.

Writing

Disturbances of writing (agraphia) can be due to a number of causes including aphasia, apraxia, and spatial disorder secondary to parietal lobe damage. Occasionally agraphia occurs in isolation, but this is rare. The writing of aphasics usually contains the same linguistic abnormalities as their speech. Copying is usually least impaired, writing to dictation more so, and spontaneous writing most of all.

Reading

As with writing, abnormalities of reading are usually proportional to other aspects of the aphasia. There are hesitations, word substitutions, omissions, and impaired comprehension. The ability to read aloud is sometimes better preserved than the ability to comprehend the material, but the reverse may happen.

Examination of the aphasic patient

A full history must be taken from the patient in so far as the aphasia allows; this provides an excellent opportunity to assess the patient's spontaneous speech, particularly if the aphasia is only mild when it may provide the only abnormalities detectable on clinical as opposed to laboratory examination. It is also essential to take a history from a relative or close friend, particularly if the aphasia is more than mild.

Even a mild aphasia will cripple some, such as barristers, whereas in other occupations people may function well despite quite marked aphasia. Hand preferences must be noted, remembering that some people write with the right hand but nevertheless prefer the left, or are ambidextrous, for other activities. A family history of left-handedness should be noted.

A scheme for examination is given in Table 2. Much of this consists of looking for abnormalities of the type described in the preceding section. Comprehension is particularly difficult to determine at the bedside. Some measure can be obtained by assessing the ability to respond correctly to commands of increasing complexity. Thus, with a collection of common objects on a table, the patient may be instructed to carry out commands such as 'close the book' (very simple) and 'close the book, touch the cup, and give me the button' (more complex).

Classification and localization of aphasic syndromes

It is generally accepted that aphasic syndromes can be broadly related to the occurrence of lesions involving relatively circumscribed regions in the cerebral cortex and their connections. At present the most widely used classification of aphasia is that proposed by Geschwind (Table 3). He classified disorders of language into two main groups:

Table 2 Examination of the aphasic patient

History: obtain in full including from a relative/friend (essential if the aphasia is more than minimal)
Spontaneous speech: assess in conversation if possible; note articulation and rhythm, hesitancies and word-finding difficulties, circumlocutions, grammatical errors, paraphasias, and neologisms
Examine patient's ability to:
1. **Name objects** and note frequency/nature of errors (visual presentation as standard, but also auditory/tactile presentation if there is a possibility of agnosia); use clearly identifiable pictures or three dimensional objects; ask patient to indicate use by words or gesture to establish that the object is recognized
2. **Recite series** (e.g. days of week/months or year) forwards and backwards—errors tend to occur particularly on backward series
3. **Generate words** by saying as many words of a defined character (e.g. beginning with C or names of towns) in a limited time (e.g. 1 minute)
4. **Repeat** sentences of varying complexity
5. **Write** name and address and sentences spontaneously and to dictation—note spelling errors, word omissions, calligraphy
6. **Read** a prose passage-note nature and frequency of errors; carry out a written command such as 'close your eyes'
Comprehension: ask patient to point to named objects and to carry out commands (see text)
Other cognitive abilities such as visuospatial, praxis, and memory should be examined at least briefly
Physical examination of other aspects of neurological dysfunction (particularly visual field defect, hemiparesis, and localized sensory change) is very important because aphasia is often associated with other features of left hemisphere pathology.

Table 3 Geschwind's classification of aphasic syndromes

Anterior aphasia (non-fluent)	*Global aphasia*
Broca's aphasia	*Disturbances closely allied to aphasia*
Aphemia	Pure alexia
Transcortical motor aphasia	Pure agraphia
Posterior aphasia (fluent)	Alexia with agraphia
Wernicke's aphasia	Colour anomia
Nominal aphasia	Acalculia
Transcortical sensory aphasia	
Conduction aphasia	
Pure word deafness	

those resulting from lesions anterior to the Rolandic (central) fissure, and those related to lesions posterior to this fissure.

Broca's aphasia (motor/expressive)

This is the most common type of aphasia other than global aphasia. Typically, the patients lose verbal fluency, and there is cortical dysarthria and agrammatism. The speech has a telegraphic quality, and connecting words such as articles, prepositions, and conjunctions are missing. The patient's verbal comprehension is adequate, although not completely normal. The aphasia may be accompanied by a right facial weakness or hemiplegia but there is usually no visual-field defect.

Wernicke's asphasia (sensory/receptive)

This is characterized by a profound loss of the ability to comprehend language. The patients usually have a fluent speech, with a marked logorrhoea or press of speech and numerous paraphasias. Reading and writing are usually impaired. The lesion is usually found in the posterior aspect of the superior temporal gyrus. The aphasia is often accompanied by a right homonomous visual-field defect and right-sided somatosensory changes without hemiparesis.

Nominal aphasia (amnestic/anomic)

The main feature of this disorder is the inability to find the correct name for objects, colours, letters, and numbers. The naming errors are of three main types: circumlocutions (e.g. 'use in door', instead of key), phonemic errors, and semantic errors. Spontaneous speech is fluent, although there are frequent word-finding difficulties. There are no comprehension deficits. Most frequently the site of the lesion is in the region of the posterior–superior temporal gyrus bordering on the angular gyrus whose involvement may add other deficits, such as reading and spelling difficulties, to the basic pattern.

Global aphasia (central)

Many moderately severe aphasics cannot be easily classified as either Broca's or Wernicke's in type. They have the expressive disturbance characteristic of Broca's aphasia with the comprehension loss characteristic of Wernicke's aphasia without disproportion between the two. When the aphasia is severe, speech may be limited to phonated inarticulate or recurrent utterances. There is almost always a marked disturbance of comprehension and inability to read or write. This is the characteristic situation after infarction of the territory supplied by the left middle cerebral artery such that there is involvement of both the cortical area whose damage causes Broca's aphasia and that responsible for Wernicke's aphasia. The aphasia is usually accompanied by a right hemiplegia with sensory loss and there is often a right homonymous hemianopia. The outlook for adequate recovery is poor.

Disturbances closely allied to aphasia

A number of disturbances, some of them rare, are usually regarded as features of damage to the posterior part of the left hemisphere. They are allied to aphasia either because of common underlying neuropsychological mechanisms or because of close overlap between their anatomical substrates.

Alexia with agraphia (cortical, parietal)

The underlying brain damage involves the left angular gyrus. The alexia is severe, so that only an occasional word can be read and the patient makes many errors identifying single letters. The ability to read numbers and music is sometimes preserved.

Pure alexia (pure word-blindness)

This syndrome is believed to be due to pathology of the pathway between the primary visual cortex and the left angular gyrus, which is of major importance for reading, such that there is a 'disconnection' between the two areas. The characteristics of the alexia are the same as in alexia with agraphia except that the letters can usually be recognized if traced with a finger (i.e., using somatosensory rather than visual sensory information). The ability to read numbers and music may or may not be preserved. Oral spelling and the recognition of words spelt aloud are normal. Similarly, writing is normal.

Pure agraphia (motor)

Agraphia more or less uncontaminated by other features of aphasia has been reported as a manifestation of damage in the parasagittal portion of the left parietal lobe.

Gerstmann syndrome

This consists of finger agnosia, right–left disorientation, agraphia, and acalculia. With finger agnosia the patients are unable to name their fingers and can neither indicate nor identify their own or other people's fingers or fingers demonstrated on models. The abnormality is almost invariably bilateral and due to damage in the left hemisphere involving the supramarginal gyrus. The right–left disorientation applies to body parts (of both patient and other people) more than to inanimate objects in extracorporeal space. The features can be found in various combinations, with or without other disturbances such as constructional apraxia, aphasia, and alexia.

Apraxia

Apraxia is defined as a condition where there is a high level disturbance of voluntary purposeful movements, not attributable to weakness or to incoordination or sensory loss, as usually understood, and not attributable to an aphasic comprehension disorder. Learned skilled movements are performed incorrectly. A rather large number of apraxias have been described. Only ideomotor apraxia and constructional apraxia will be considered here. Buccofacial apraxia has been mentioned above, and dressing apraxia will be mentioned below.

Ideomotor apraxia

Ideomotor apraxia is a defect of the ability to mime actions, to imitate how a tool or object would be used, and to make symbolic gestures. The disorder is almost invariably due to pathology of the posterior left hemisphere, and many apraxic patients are also aphasic.

Ideational apraxia is a more severe disorder in that actual use of objects and tools is markedly disturbed, but it is probably not qualitatively distinct from ideomotor apraxia.

Constructional apraxia

Constructional apraxia is manifest in activities such as building, arranging, and drawing. There is difficulty in assembling parts to make a whole where a spatial component is involved. Patients may complain of symptoms arising from their constructional apraxia. Thus they may no longer be able to perform tasks such as assembling an electric plug, dress-making, or laying the dinner table. More often the disorder is demonstrated only on clinical examination. Spontaneous drawing and copying is poor. Drawings tend to be smaller than the model and may be crowded into one corner of the page. One dimension of the drawing may be unduly prolonged and large parts may be omitted, particularly by patients with damage to the right hemisphere, who ignore the left side.

Unlike ideomotor apraxia, constructional apraxia can arise from damage to either the right or left cerebral hemispheres.

Disorders of visual, spatial, and bodily perception

These disorders arise very predominantly in association with damage to cortex in the parieto–temporo–occipital junction area of the right hemisphere, or bilaterally, and only rarely with unilateral pathology

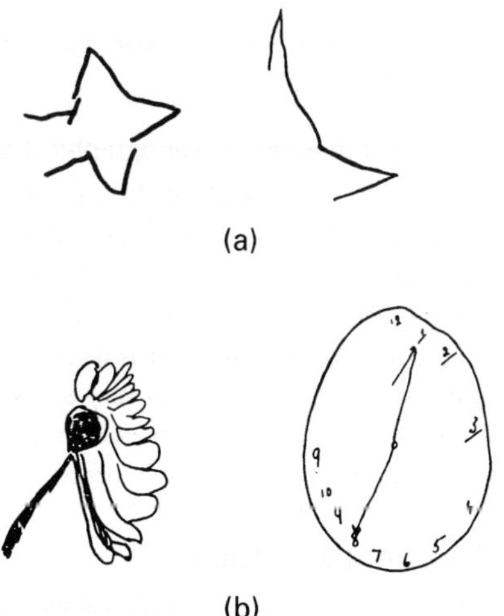

Fig. 2 Unilateral neglect. Examples of drawings by patients with right hemisphere pathology and left visuospatial neglect: (a) copies of four-pointed star; (b) freehand drawings of daisy and clock face.

of the left hemisphere (finger agnosia and right–left disorientation as part of the Gerstmann syndrome).

Disorders of visuospatial perception and space exploration

The extent of 'dominance' by the right hemisphere in the control of behaviour concerned with visuospatial perception and space exploration at least approaches that of the left hemisphere in relation to language.

Unilateral visuospatial neglect

This is a disregard of, and a failure to attend to, one half of external space, almost invariably the left. Patients tend to collide with objects situated on the left and have a marked preference for taking right rather than left turns, so that they may become lost when taking routes from one place to another. They tend to neglect the left side when copying or making free-hand drawings (Fig. 2), although the right side can be drawn very well. Writing may be crowded over on the right-hand side of the page, with the left remaining blank. They may have great difficulty in reading because they neglect the left side of lines or individual words. The disorder is usually associated with a left hemianopia and left-sided sensory loss. The patients may be aware of their disability but nevertheless be unable to overcome it. Damage to the right inferior parietal lobule seems to be the common anatomical substrate.

Gaze apraxia

This is an inability to direct the eyes towards, and then maintain fixation upon, an object appearing in an intact visual field even though there is no oculomotor palsy and both random eye movements and oculocephalic reflexes seem normal. It is usually associated with biparietal damage and most patients also have visual disorientation.

Visual disorientation

Visual disorientation is an inability to orient towards and accurately locate objects in space, using vision alone, even though the visual acuity and field seem adequate. It is usually associated with gaze apraxia and damage to both parietal lobes. Judgements of distance, length, and size are faulty, and the patients misreach. Their groping and inability to fixate an object gives the impression that they are blind, but they may recognize objects correctly and may point accurately at sources of sound.

Defective topographical memory or topographical disorientation

This is usually due to bilateral cerebral damage that may not be restricted to the parietal cortex. The patients are unable to remember or describe routes even though they may be very familiar. For instance they may lose themselves in their own homes or in villages where they have spent all their lives. The disorder is usually associated with other features of cognitive impairment, but very occasionally it exists in relative isolation, in which case it may be due to damage restricted to the right posterior parietal and occipital cortex.

Disorders of visual perception

The majority of patients with clinically recognizable, visual perceptual disorders have either focal damage in both hemispheres or diffuse damage.

Visual agnosia

Visual agnosia is a failure to identify objects by sight alone, although sufficient acuity of vision and cerebral function are present and the patient is still able to recognize the objects in question through some other sensory modality such as touch or hearing.

Prosopagnosia

Prosopagnosia is the inability to recognize people from their facial appearance or from photographs. The condition is rare. It may be so severe that even close relatives and old acquaintances are not recognized until they speak or until some characteristic item of their clothing is seen. In many patients with prosopagnosia, pathology is located more or less symmetrically in the posterior temporal and inferior parietal regions of both hemispheres.

Disorders of body perception

The higher-order disturbances of body perception, except for the Gerstmann syndrome, affect predominantly the left limbs, just as visuospatial neglect is a predominantly left-sided phenomenon.

Neglect

In its most exaggerated form, there appears to be an almost complete unawareness and occasionally even denial of the existence of one side of the body. It almost invariably affects the left and is due to extensive damage to the right hemisphere, with superadded confusion. The disturbance is usually combined with a dense hemiplegia. There may be anosognosia, which is a denial that there is any paralysis of the affected limbs. Patients seem convinced that they can and do move these limbs normally and may even seem to think that they had just demonstrated this capacity. The lack of awareness is one factor making rehabilitation of some left hemiplegics very difficult. Severe somatosensory loss, hemianopia, constructional and dressing apraxias, and unilateral visuospatial neglect are often associated with unilateral somatic neglect and anosognosia.

Dressing apraxia

This is a severe and bizarre disturbance of the ability to put on clothes. It almost always arises from damage to the right parietal lobe. Many patients also have constructional apraxia, left visuospatial neglect, and left hemiasomatagnosia.

Table 4 Categories of memory

Explicit (declarative)	Implicit (procedural)
Short-term (working)	Motor and perceptual skills
Intermediate	Classical conditioning
Long-term	
Episodic	
Semantic	

Frontal lobe damage

Damage to the frontal lobes classically produces a combination of personality change and intellectual deterioration. However, it is not unusual for even extensive damage to be present without detectable symptoms or signs, and this is why slow-growing frontal tumours may remain silent until they have reached a very considerable size. Changes in mood and character include euphoria, impulsiveness, and facetiousness, with apparently decreased anxiety and little concern about the consequences of any actions that are undertaken. Such disinhibition may occur without any evidence of other cognitive impairment. The patient may be fully aware of the disinhibition but nevertheless unable to control it. In contrast, the personality change may produce a depression-like state with decreased initiative and spontaneity.

There seems to be a decreased ability for abstract thought and for planning behaviour taking into account past experience and future consequences. Perseveration of various types is common. The patients may be very distractible and unable to concentrate or keep their attention focused on one topic for more than a short time.

Amnesia

Memory is not a unitary function and various categories are recognized. A useful classification for clinical purposes is given in Table 4.

Explicit memory systems store information that can be consciously accessed and include a major component of a person's knowledge base; the material can be verbalized and discussed. The short-term system retains material for periods measured in seconds or a few minutes at most; for instance this system holds a telephone number from the time that it has been found in a directory until it has been dialled and can be forgotten. The long-term system holds material for periods up to the remainder of the person's life. It is convenient to divide the long-term store into semantic and episodic memory. By semantic is meant knowledge of, for instance, objects, places, words, concepts, etc. Episodic memory is memory for events, including autobiographical events. Clearly, episodic and semantic memory must be closely related.

Implicit memory is the information store that enables activities to be carried out more or less automatically without conscious awareness and without the person necessarily being able to explain how they have been achieved. Implicit memory systems include those holding information that determines conditioned reflex responses and allows complex motor acts, such as riding a surf board, to be performed. It may be possible to some extent to verbalize how such complex motor acts are achieved and to subject them to conscious analysis, but it is often impossible to do so fully.

Table 5 Causes of severe amnesia

Alcohol (Korsakoff psychosis) and other causes of thiamine deficiency (including inadequate feeding, hyperemesis gravidarum, stomach cancer) leading to cell loss in the thalamic dorsomedial nuclei and the mammillary bodies
Bilateral medial temporal lobe damage including herpes simplex encephalitis and other limbic encephalitides (including non-metastatic carcinomatous), neuronal loss secondary to anoxia/hypoglycaemia/ severe convulsions, surgical
Degenerative: Alzheimer's and Pick's diseases may present with very severe memory failure with only minor general deterioration
Vascular: bilateral thalamic infarction, hippocampal infarction secondary to posterior cerebral artery territory ischaemia, bilateral cingulate cortex infarction secondary to anterior communicating artery aneurysm rupture
Pathology around ventricle III: tumours (particularly colloid cysts), chronic meningitis (particularly tubercular), neurosarcoidosis

These memory systems depend upon the proper working of multiple cerebral structures, and memory impairment of one sort or another is a common early feature of many brain diseases. The medial temporal-lobe structures—including the hippocampus, amygdala, parahippocampal gyrus, and rhinal cortex—together with the fornix system, the mamillary bodies, the thalamus, particularly the dorsomedial nucleus, and the cingulate gyri, contribute to a neuronal circuit that is of major importance for establishing new semantic and episodic memories, although the actual stores are probably in other parts of the neocortex. Damage to any part of this circuit can cause an anterograde memory disturbance, i.e., defective establishment of new memories commencing at the time of the onset of the pathological process. It may also cause a retrograde memory disturbance manifested by failure to access previously established memories on a temporal gradient, with recent memories being more susceptible to loss than longer established memories.

Bilateral damage to any part of the neuronal circuit can cause a severe amnesic syndrome. In this condition the anterograde memory disturbance is such that new material can be remembered for only a few seconds, or a few minutes at most, and then only if there is no distraction (i.e., short-term memory is preserved). Beyond this short span, new material cannot be learnt nor events remembered, with the exception that new motor and perceptual skills may be learnt (implicit memory) without the amnesic being able to recall any exposure to the activity. For example the patient may not remember ever having seen a person who has left the room for 2 or 3 min. There is usually an associated retrograde amnesia, but other aspects of cognition may be entirely preserved. Common causes of severe amnesia are shown in Table 5.

Traumatic amnesia

Amnesia is common after head injuries that are severe enough to cause unconsciousness. The duration of post-traumatic amnesia (i.e., the period of severe anterograde memory impairment) is the period between the injury and the resumption of 'normal' continuous memory. It includes the period of unconsciousness and the subsequent period of confusion; it can also include a further period in which the behaviour seems to be normal, but which cannot be remembered in detail afterwards. The duration of post-traumatic amnesia is one of the better indices of the severity of a head injury. When it lasts for more than 24 h, the injury is classified as severe and there may be permanent brain damage. The duration of the retrograde amnesia is the period between the injury and the last clear memory before it happened. Characteristically it shrinks slowly, becoming shorter as the time since the injury increases. The process of shrinking may take several months, but most cases have a final retrograde amnesia of no more than a few seconds and it is only longer in those with very severe injuries.

Transient global amnesia

This is a condition of dense amnesia usually lasting for several hours, during which the patient behaves like somebody with severe amnesia. New memories cannot be laid down and, as in severe amnesia, new material can only be retained for a few seconds or, at the most, minutes, provided that there are no distractions. The attack is usually followed by an apparently complete recovery of memory function, except that events which occurred during it cannot be recalled. At the onset of an attack there is a retrograde amnesia that may cover a period as long as several years; this shrinks during the course of the attack and is said to be only short immediately before recovery. Patients are fully conscious throughout and may carry out complex acts, such as driving long distances, quite normally. They usually seem mildly confused and agitated, frequently repeating the same questions. Most patients have no further neurological abnormality, but sometimes there are signs suggestive of ischaemia in the territory supplied by the vertebrobasilar system. These transient global amnesic attacks must be differentiated from the automatisms of temporal lobe epilepsy and from psychologically induced amnesia; an almost identical phenomenon is sometimes seen as part of a migraine attack.

Further reading

Albert, M.L. (1998). Treatment of aphasia. *Archives of Neurology*, **55**, 1417–9.

Castro Caldas, A., Peterson, K.M., Reis, A., Stone-Elander, S., and Ingvar, M. (1998). The illiterate brain: learning to read and write during childhood influences the functional organization of the adult brain. *Brain*, **121**, 1053–63.

Dalla Barba, G. and Boller, F. (1998). Memory and language in neurodegenerative diseases. *Current Opinion in Neurology*, **11**, 429–33.

Zeman, A.Z. and Hodges, J.R. (1997). Transient global amnesia. *British Journal of Hospital Medicine*, **58**, 257–60.

Chapter 13.3

The motor and sensory systems, midbrain, and brainstem

W. B. Matthews

The motor system

The lower motor neurone

The motor unit consists of a number of muscle fibres, ranging from 100 in the facial muscles to 2000 in the quadriceps, supplied by a single, fast-conducting, α-motor fibre. These originate from large cells in the anterior horns of the grey matter of the spinal cord and in the somatic motor nuclei of the cranial nerves, and are known as the lower motor neurones. Loss of function of the anterior horn cells, or interruption of their axons, causes weakness or paralysis of the muscles they supply, with loss of stretch reflexes, shown by flaccidity and loss of tendon jerks, and, if paralysis persists, wasting of the muscle due to loss of excitable tissue.

The upper motor neurone

The main descending motor pathway is derived from neurones in the precentral gyrus. Movements of the foot are controlled by neurones on the medial surface of the hemisphere, and on the lateral surface from above downwards are the areas for the leg, trunk, arm, hand, face, and tongue, although these are not rigidly demarcated centres. Descending axons converge in the posterior limb of the internal capsule and then occupy the middle third of the cerebral peduncle. In the pons the fibres are more dispersed and become concentrated again in the prominent pyramid, from which the name of the pyramidal tract is derived, on the anterior surface of the medulla. Most of the fibres cross at the lower end of the medulla and descend in the lateral columns of the spinal cord. Only a small proportion of the corticospinal fibres synapse directly on lower motor neurones and most terminate on interneurones.

An acute complete lesion of the corticospinal tract causes flaccid paralysis with loss of tendon reflexes. With the passage of time or with a partial or progressive lesion the characteristic effect is spastic weakness or paralysis. Loss of power is accompanied by an increase in stretch-reflex activity. In the upper limb the weakness is usually most evident in distal muscles, but movements of the hip joint may be affected when no other loss of power can be found in the lower limb. Loss of fine movements, particularly of the fingers, is often much more prominent than loss of strength. In many complex movements, such as walking, the normal precise sequence of contraction and relaxation of opposing muscles is lost.

The increased resistance to passive movement is more marked in the flexor muscles of the arm and the extensor muscles of the leg. It often has a 'clasp knife' character, in that the resistance suddenly lapses due to reflex lengthening. The tendon reflexes are exaggerated and reflex contractions can often be elicited in muscles other than those usually examined.

The normal plantar reflex consists of flexion of all the digits on firm stroking of the lateral side of the sole. In the extensor, or Babinski, reflex the big toe dorsiflexes and the other toes fan. This response is reliably found when an upper motor-neurone lesion or loss of function is undeniably present, but is far less useful in cases of doubt, when it is often recorded as 'equivocal'.

A curious feature of upper motor-neurone lesions is loss of certain cutaneous reflexes. The superficial abdominal reflexes, elicited by stroking the skin in each quadrant, are the best known, although a variable, finding, particularly after middle age, but unilateral loss is occasionally a valuable sign.

In the distribution of the cranial nerves an acute upper motor-neurone lesion usually causes dysphagia and dysarthria for a few days only. Bilateral lesions cause persistent symptoms, with slow tongue movements and often an exaggerated jaw jerk, elicited by a tap on the chin with the mouth half open. This condition is known as pseudobulbar palsy (the 'bulb' being the medulla) to distinguish it from the lower motor-neurone bulbar palsy. It is often accompanied by mild limb spasticity, a shuffling gait, and great lability of emotional expression.

An upper motor-neurone facial-nerve palsy differs in a number of respects from a nuclear or peripheral palsy. The muscles of the upper face are relatively or entirely spared, apparently because of bilateral cortical control.

The sensory system

The afferent inflow from skin, muscles, tendons, and joints arises from end-organs specifically adapted to respond to appropriate stimuli and also from a non-specific network of cutaneous nerve endings. In the clinical context it is the anatomy of the sensory pathways that is of obvious relevance.

The afferent fibres from the limbs are formed by one branch of the axons of the neurones of the posterior root ganglia, the other branch of which enters the spinal cord. The posterior spinal-root fibres enter the grey matter where many, apparently concerned with reflex activity, form synapses with interneurones or anterior horn cells. The main afferent stream divides: axons concerned mainly with postural sense and with some aspects of touch, and probably with vibration sense, proceed in the posterior columns of the same side of the spinal cord to the dorsal-column nuclei in the medulla, from which arise the secondary sensory axons, which decussate and ascend in the medial lemniscus to the thalamus. Fibres concerned with pain and thermal sensation synapse in the posterior horns and the axons of the secondary relay pass upwards for a few segments on the same side before decussating in the centre of the cord and passing up in the lateral columns as the spinothalamic tracts. These lie laterally in the medulla but eventually join the medial lemniscus and enter the thalamus. The sensory relay is continued to the postcentral gyrus and to a wide area of the posterior part of the cerebral hemisphere. Many afferent fibres convey information that does not enter consciousness but is concerned with reflex activity or with the afferent flow to the cerebellum.

Sensory loss from interruption of a peripheral nerve or posterior root affects all modalities. However, cutting a single posterior root may result in no detectable sensory loss, because of overlap from neighbouring roots. Similarly, the area of sensory loss resulting from a peripheral nerve lesion will be much less extensive than the full distribution of the nerve. Within the central nervous system the separation of the sensory tracts in the spinal cord allows selective loss of different sensory modalities. Pain and thermal sense will be impaired when the spinothalamic tracts are damaged, while lesions of the posterior columns result in loss of postural sense. Sense of touch is distributed between both pathways, the element involved in tickle passing through the spinothalamic tracts.

Lesions of the parietal cortex may result in loss of all forms of sensation, including that of pain, but sometimes there is severe loss of discriminatory forms of sensation with retention of appreciation of cruder modalities.

Symptoms

Patients' complaints arising from disorders of the sensory system are often difficult to interpret. Loss of cutaneous sensation may be sufficiently obvious, as with the complaint of being unable to feel the feet on the floor or to judge the temperature of the bath water, but other sensory symptoms are less easy to attribute to disturbance of a particular modality and the distinction of positive from negative symptoms is also difficult. The familiar paraesthesias, 'pins and needles', may apparently result from lesions of the sensory pathways at any level. A sensation as of a tight bandage round the leg is commonly complained of by patients with a lesion of the posterior columns of the spinal cord.

Loss of proprioceptive sensation results in sensory ataxia. Difficulty in maintaining balance is greatly increased when information derived from vision is also lost, leading, on examination, to Romberg's sign, consisting of falling when standing with feet together and eyes closed, and to the complaint of being unable to walk outside after dusk.

Pain may result from disease of the peripheral and, less commonly, of the central nervous system. Compression of a peripheral nerve, or more particularly of a dorsal root, may cause paraesthesias and pain in the distribution of the sensory fibres. Pain of a peculiarly distressing, burning character can arise from lesions of the spinothalamic tract in the spinal cord and brainstem, and similar and even more persistent pain and dysaesthesia, or unpleasantly altered cutaneous sensation on stimulation, from thalamic lesions.

Subcortical lesions: internal capsule, midbrain, and brainstem

The internal capsule

In the internal capsule the descending motor fibres are condensed into a small space immediately anterior to the similarly narrowly localized ascending fibres. Even relatively small lesions in this area can therefore cause severe hemiplegia of the opposite limbs, the degree of sensory loss depending on the extent of the lesion.

The midbrain

Among the crowded tracts and nuclei of the midbrain those that can most readily be identified as contributing to the symptomatology of lesions in this area are the descending corticospinal and corticobulbar tracts, the nuclei of the third and fourth cranial nerves, the reticular formation, and, more speculatively, the red nucleus. The contiguous superior cerebellar peduncles may also be involved.

Weber's syndrome of a third-nerve palsy and crossed hemiplegia is the result of a lesion of the cerebral peduncle involving the third nerve as it leaves the brain. Benedikt's syndrome of a third-nerve palsy with involuntary movements of the opposite limbs is thought to result from a lesion of the red nucleus.

A characteristic sign of involvement of the upper midbrain is Parinaud's syndrome, which, in its complete form, consists of paralysis of vertical gaze and of convergence.

Lesions involving the reticular formation have been held responsible for disturbances of conscious level and also for the condition of akinetic mutism in which the patient makes no voluntary movement except of the eyes.

The pons and medulla

The pons and medulla contain nuclei of the fifth to the twelfth cranial nerves, important cerebellar connections, and motor, sensory, and autonomic pathways.

The lateral medullary syndrome of Wallenberg is relatively common. It includes dysphagia and dysarthria (ninth and tenth nerve nuclei), vomiting and hiccup (nucleus ambiguus), and vertigo (vestibular nuclei) combined with cerebellar ataxia of the limbs on the side of the lesion (inferior cerebellar peduncle), ipsilateral Horner's syndrome (descending autonomic fibres), loss of pain and thermal sensation on the face on the side of the lesion (fifth nerve nucleus) and in the opposite limbs (lateral lemniscus). There is no weakness as the pyramidal tracts are spared.

The rare medial medullary syndrome consists of weakness and loss of postural sense in the limbs on the side opposite to the lesion (pyramidal tract and medial lemniscus) and ipsilateral paralysis of the tongue (twelfth nerve nucleus).

Certain signs of brainstem pathology may be encountered in isolation or combined with evidence of widespread disease. An internuclear ophthalmoplegia of the form commonly seen consists of failure of adduction of the eye in conjugate gaze to one or both sides, but with preservation of convergence, indicating that the medial rectus is not paralysed but cannot act in conjunction with the opposite lateral rectus. This results from a lesion of the medial longitudinal bundle connecting the nuclei of the third and sixth nerves.

The locked-in syndrome results from interruption of the descending and ascending long tracts in the brainstem. As no speech or movement of the limbs is possible, it is easy to assume that consciousness is lost, but this is not so and such patients readily learn to communicate by using eye-movement signals. This syndrome differs from akinetic mutism where, although the eyes are moved, no communication is possible.

Further reading

Bickerstaff, E.R. and Spillane, J.A. (1989). *Neurological examination in clinical practice*, 5th edn. Blackwell Scientific, Oxford.

Brodal, A. (1981). *Neurological anatomy in relation to clinical medicine*, 3rd edn. Oxford University Press.

Chapter 13.4

Subcortical structures—the cerebellum, thalamus, and basal ganglia

N. P. Quinn

The human brain is both proactive and reactive, not only to external stimuli but, via feedback mechanisms, to its own actions. The complexity of these operations calls for subspecialization within the nervous system, so that a deluge of inputs can be integrated semi-automatically and largely subconsciously, freeing consciousness for other things. Such are the tasks of the cerebellum and of the major subcortical nuclei that constitute the thalamus and the basal ganglia.

The cerebellum

Structure and function

The cerebellum occupies the greater part of the posterior fossa, reaching from the tentorium rostrally to the foramen magnum caudally, and lying dorsal to the lower pons and medulla, from which it is separated by the fourth ventricle. Its blood supply is derived from posterior circulation via the superior, anterior inferior, and posterior inferior cerebellar arteries.

The cerebellum can be divided into: (1) archicerebellum (flocculonodular lobe), with largely vestibular inputs; (2) palaeocerebellum (anterior lobe), with largely spinal cord inputs; and (3) neocerebellum (posterior, largest, lobe), with largely pontine inputs from cerebral cortex.

The integrating function of the cerebellum is evident from the fact that afferent fibres heavily outnumber efferent ones by about 40 to 1. Connections travel in three cerebellar peduncles, the lower two mainly afferent and the upper one efferent.

Clinical aspects

Midline vermal lesions cause truncal ataxia, often in the absence of limb ataxia. The gait is wide based and particularly precarious on turning or on heel/toe walking. Unilateral cerebellar hemispheric lesions cause deviation or falling to the ipsilateral side. Unlike a sensory ataxia, cerebellar ataxia is not made particularly worse by shutting the eyes. Generally, ataxic patients have more problem going down, and those with weakness going up, stairs.

Disease of cerebellar hemispheres or outflow tracts often causes limb ataxia, which is in fact an amalgam of several components. First, there may be dysmetria (misreaching, or past-pointing) evident in the arms on the finger–nose test or in the legs when the heel is first brought to the opposite kneecap. Secondly, there is the breakdown in force, rate, and rhythm known as dysdiadochokinesia; this can best be sought by asking the patient to tap your hand or a table gently, regularly, and rapidly with his or her fingers. The third element is intention tremor, which should augment throughout a movement from inception to completion. Many individuals claimed to have this tremor do not actually have a cerebellar syndrome. Thus, many postural tremors are positionally dependent, and may worsen or appear at the termination of a movement when the hands are either outstretched or held in front of the nose. Other non-cerebellar tremors may be present, or appear only, during action (action or kinetic tremor). Only if additional signs of cerebellar dysfunction considered above are also present is it reasonable to use the term intention tremor.

Cerebellar dysarthria may often simply manifest as slurred speech, as if intoxicated. However, in addition, some patients may have either scanning or explosive speech, due to an inability to modulate its rate, rhythm, and force appropriately. Dysarthria is usually present with lesions of the vermis, whole cerebellum, or its connections, but may be absent if one lateral hemisphere alone is involved. Cerebellar lesions may also cause the 'rebound phenomenon', resulting from impaired damping of limbs when suddenly a load is removed or a displacement applied.

Eye movements are frequently abnormal in disease of the cerebellum or its connections. The following may be seen: gaze-evoked, rebound, downbeat, or positional nystagmus; dysmetric voluntary saccades and jerky pursuit; square-wave jerks (macrosaccadic oscillations); impaired vestibulo-ocular reflex suppression; and skew deviation. The presence of diplopia usually implies additional pathology outside the cerebellum proper.

The thalamus

Structure and function

The two thalami sit at the head of the brainstem, their medial borders largely separated by the third ventricle. Their blood supply derives from the posterior circulation via the posterior cerebral arteries and perforators from the terminal part of the basilar. They constitute the largest nuclear mass in the diencephalon (the others being the hypothalamus and subthalamus), and occupy a strategic position, both anatomically and functionally.

The thalamus receives inputs from cerebral cortex, sensory tracts, basal ganglia, and cerebellum. Almost all of its output is to the cerebral cortex, either in the form of reciprocal circuits or of more complex loops from cortex through other subcortical structures to thalamus and back to cortex again, but there is a small output to the striatum.

Clinical aspects

Depending on the nuclei involved, thalamic lesions might influence either sensation or motor function, or sometimes both. Most commonly an infarct or haemorrhage (10–15 per cent of all intracerebral haemorrhages) causes contralateral sensory loss or impairment. A small lacunar infarct in the ventral posterolateral nucleus may give rise to a pure sensory stroke, sometimes sparing the face. A larger lesion may cause the thalamic syndrome of Dejerine and Roussy, in which an initial mild and transient hemiplegia is accompanied by persisting superficial and deep sensory impairment, mild hemiataxia, and astereognosis. These are commonly accompanied by choreoathetoid movements and severe, persistent, paroxysmal, often intolerable, pains on the hemiplegic side. When mild, the movements may be pseudoathetotic due to deafferentation; when severe, they suggest that the lesion may extend beyond the thalamus to involve basal ganglia connections. A significant, persisting hemiplegia implies either a large thalamic lesion also involving the internal capsule, or the possibility that the stroke is primarily capsular and not thalamic. A particular form of subcortical aphasia has been described in thalamic lesions.

Surgical lesions or deep brain stimulators stereotactically placed in the ventral intermediate nucleus relieve tremor in Parkinson's disease and benign essential tremor, and also sometimes rigidity (but not akinesia) in the former.

The basal ganglia

Structure and function

There is no uniform agreement on how many of the subcortical nuclei one should include under the terms basal ganglia and extrapyramidal motor system. However, there is agreement that they at least include the neostriatum (caudate nucleus and putamen, often together called simply the striatum) and the palaeostriatum (the external and internal globus pallidus with the latter's homologue, the substantia nigra pars reticulata).

The putamen lies lateral to the thalamus, separated from it (and from most of the caudate nucleus, except anteriorly) by the internal capsule. The caudate nucleus, whose head lies anterodorsomedial to the putamen, describes most of a circle as it follows, and progressively tapers with, the lateral ventricles through its body posteriorly, its tail swinging forward until its anteriorly pointing tip terminates in the amygdaloid nucleus. The pallidum lies medial to the putamen but still lateral to the internal capsule, and is divided into external and internal segments. The substantia nigra lies in the midbrain, transversely above the cerebral peduncles. Its pars reticulata, the termination of the striatonigral pathway, is homologous with the medial globus pallidus, and its pars compacta contains the dopaminergic neurones that form the nigrostriatal pathway. Below the thalamus, medial to the internal capsule and rostral to the midbrain, is the subthalamic nucleus. Most of the caudate, putamen, and the globus pallidus derive their arterial supply from anterior circulation via the lateral lenticulostriate arteries and the branches of the anterior choroidal and anterior cerebral arteries. Like the thalamus, the subthalamic region, and also the substantia nigra, are supplied by posterior circulation.

The basal ganglia and their (inter) connections, rich in neurotransmitters, have been extensively studied. The 'striopallidal complex' receives a wide variety of inputs from cerebral cortex. Its principal output is to the thalamus, which in turn projects back to the cortex to complete a basal ganglia–thalamocortical circuit. However, it is important to note the existence of additional output to the brainstem in the pallidotegmental tract, which terminates in the pedunculopontine nucleus. This structure is believed to play an important part in the control of balance and locomotion, and in the maintenance of rigidity. The caudate and putamen are the afferent, and the globus pallidus and substantia nigra pars reticulata the efferent, parts of the striopallidal complex. The subthalamic nucleus appears to be the most critical structure in this pathway. In Parkinson's disease the loss of neurones in the pars compacta of the substantia nigra results in overactivity of the internal segment of the pallidum and the subthalamic nucleus.

Clinical aspects (see also Chapter 13.20)

Pathology of the basal ganglia produces more than simply motor symptoms and signs. Thus, in patients with Parkinson's disease, Huntington's disease, and progressive supranuclear palsy, all of which principally (but not exclusively) involve basal ganglia, affective disorder, 'subcortical dementia', or 'frontal lobe deficits' may be seen.

Nevertheless, it is a fact that the most striking clinical features of basal ganglia disease remain those in the motor sphere, comprising tremor, rigidity, akinesia, and postural abnormality, as evidenced by Parkinson's disease, and hyperkinetic movement disorders such as chorea and dystonia seen, for example in Huntington's disease and in levodopa-treated patients with Parkinson's disease.

The classical tremor of Parkinson's disease is slow (4–6 Hz), pill-rolling, and disappears and diminishes on movement, to reappear once a new posture has been adopted. In traditional animal lesion studies a nigral lesion seems necessary, but not sufficient, to cause this tremor.

Akinesia is a symptom complex comprising slowness of movement (bradykinesia), poverty of movement, progressive diminution and fatigue of rapid alternating movements, and difficulty in initiating and sequencing movements and in accomplishing simultaneous motor acts.

Rigidity almost always accompanies akinesia. Resistance to passive movement is broadly similar throughout the range of flexion and extension ('lead pipe'), although somewhat greater in flexion to account for the commonly flexed, or simian, posture. Tremor (visible or invisible) may cause cog-wheeling, either in the presence or absence of underlying rigidity. In the akinesia of Parkinson's disease, tremor and rigidity all respond to levodopa. Lesions or deep brain stimulators in the overactive internal segment of the pallidum mainly improve levodopa-induced dyskinesias but also, to a lesser degree, all three cardinal features of Parkinson's disease. Lesions or deep brain stimulators in the overactive subthalamic nucleus greatly improve all features, and also enable substantial reductions in antiparkinsonian medication to be made.

Of the hyperkinetic movement disorders, chorea (in the case of Huntington's disease) and dystonia (when secondary to discernible brain pathology) can be related to basal ganglia disease (see Chapter 13.20).

Further reading

Albin, R.L., Young A.B., and Penney, J.B. (1989). The functional anatomy of basal ganglia disorders. *Trends in Neurosciences*, **12**, 366–75. [An excellent synthesis of anatomical and functional aspects of the basal ganglia.]

Alexander, G.E., DeLong, M.R., and Strick, P.L. (1986). Parallel organisation of functionally segregated circuits linking basal ganglia and cortex. *Annual Review of Neuroscience*, **9**, 357–81.

Marsden, C.D. (1990). Neurophysiology. In *Parkinson's disease* (ed. G.M. Stern), pp. 57–98. Chapman and Hall, London.

Marsden, C.D. and Obeso, J.A. (1994). The functions of the basal ganglia and the paradox of stereotaxic surgery in Parkinson's disease. *Brain*, **117**, 877–97.

Quinn, N.P. and Bhatia, K.B. (1998). Functional neurosurgery for Parkinson's disease. *British Medical Journal*, **316**, 1259–60.

Chapter 13.5

Visual pathways

R. W. Ross Russell

Structure and function

Each optic nerve has four regions: (1) the optic disc and nerve head within the globe; (2) the orbital portion; (3) the canalicular portion traversing the optic foramen in the sphenoid bone; and (4) the intracranial portion joining the optic chiasm.

Eighty per cent of the medullated nerve fibres in the optic nerve are axons of small, retinal ganglion cells that project to the parvocellular layer of the lateral geniculate nucleus. The remainder are axons of larger ganglion cells that project either to the magnocellular layer of the geniculate nucleus or via small fibres directly to the midbrain. Retinal ganglion cell density is greatest at the central retina and the majority of nerve fibres of all types subserve central vision. Both large and small ganglion cells receive input from cone photoreceptors but only the small ganglion cells subserve colour vision. Each optic nerve is enclosed in a tough dural sheath and the pia arachnoid is continuous with the intracranial subarachnoid space.

As the optic nerve approaches the chiasm the axons from the nasal retina (comprising 60 per cent of the total) separate from the remainder and cross to the other side to join the optic tract. Upper and lower fibres in the optic nerve take a slightly different course (see Fig. 1). Axons subserving the central parts of the visual field, which occupy the centre of the optic nerve, cross in the posterior portion of the chiasm. The position of the chiasm is variable but it usually lies just above the sella; its most important relations are the pituitary gland below and the cavernous sinuses and carotid arteries on each side.

The optic tracts extend from the chiasm to the lateral geniculate nuclei, encircling the cerebral peduncles. In the anterior tract, macular fibres lie medially, but further back they occupy a dorsal position. In the lateral geniculate nucleus, axons from corresponding parts of the

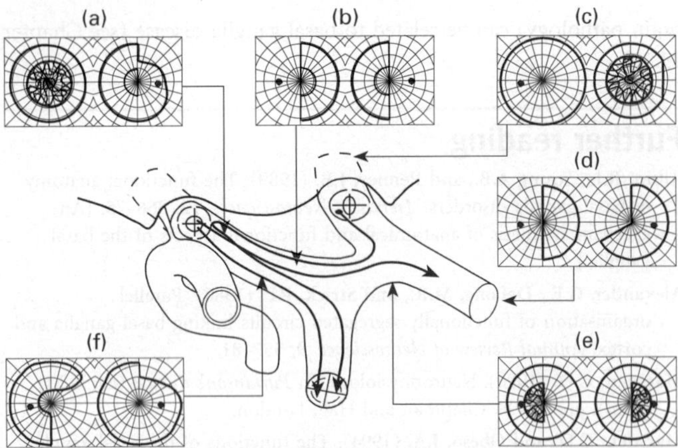

Fig. 1 Optic chiasm and left internal carotid artery viewed from behind to show the arrangement of nerve fibres and the visual-field defects produced by lesions at various points. (a) Lesion at junction of optic nerve and chiasm: central scotoma, left eye; upper temporal defect, right eye (note route taken by lower crossing fibres from right optic nerve). (b) Central chiasmal lesion interrupting all crossing fibres: complete bitemporal hemianopia. (c) Right optic-nerve lesion: general depression of field with central scotoma. (d) Lesion of right optic tract: left homonymous hemianopia (incongruous). (e) Lesion affecting posterior aspect of chiasm (crossing fibres from central field): scotomatous bitemporal hemianopia. (f) Lesion affecting left side of chiasm: central and nasal field defect, left eye; early upper temporal quadrantanopia, right eye.

two retinas terminate in vertical columns of cells. The majority of axons in the optic tracts synapse at this point, but some bypass the nucleus and proceed to the superior colliculus and midbrain tectum; these bypassing axons are concerned with the pupillary light reflex and with reflex eye movements that orientate the eyes towards the object of interest.

The optic radiation begins in the geniculate nucleus, spreads out to form a wide white-matter tract, and ends in the striate cortex. The upper fibres pass through the parietal lobe on their way to the upper bank of the calcarine fissure; the lower fibres take a longer course through the temporal lobe to end in the lower bank.

The primary visual (striate) cortex occupies the medial aspect of the posterior part of each occipital lobe. Much of it is buried in the calcarine fissure. Projections from corresponding half-retinas terminate in a point-to-point fashion in columns of cells precisely arranged in a retinotopic map. Some cortical neurones respond to stimulation from either eye, some from one eye only. Central parts of the visual field have a relatively large cortical representation compared with more peripheral parts. This larger projection is situated at or near the posterior pole, while more peripheral parts of the field project more anteriorly.

Lesions of the visual pathways

Optic nerve

A wide variety of disease processes may affect one or both optic nerves at any point in their course. Anterior lesions within the orbit tend to cause proptosis and ophthalmoplegia in addition to visual loss. Charting of the visual field usually shows a general depression of the field with a relative or absolute central scotoma, but arcuate (fibre-bundle) defects may occur with lesions near the optic disc. Visual acuity is normally depressed and colour vision is affected early. In acute cases the optic disc may be swollen, and in long-standing cases it becomes atrophic.

Swelling of the optic disc has a number of causes (Table 1). The term papilloedema is reserved by convention for swelling caused by raised intracranial pressure, which is usually bilateral, causes little interference with vision, and is accompanied by other features of raised pressure, such as headache, vomiting, and diminished conscious level. Visual fields show enlarged blind spots and usually slight peripheral constriction. Brief bilateral obscurations of vision are a feature of severe papilloedema and may herald permanent visual loss.

Pseudopapilloedema refers to congenital abnormalities that resemble papilloedema but occur without raised intracranial pressure.

Swelling of the disc from demyelination, inflammation, or ischaemia is referred to as papillitis. The characteristics are similar to those of papilloedema but the loss of acuity and visual field is much greater.

Optic atrophy may follow a variety of disorders of the optic disc; the disc becomes waxy or white from gliosis, loss of axons, and reduced vascularity. The edges of the disc remain clear cut and the retinal vessels are normal.

Demyelinating disease

This is one of the most common lesions of the optic nerve and usually affects young patients; it is frequently the first sign of multiple sclerosis. Demyelination is patchy, may involve any part of the nerve, and in acute cases the disc may be swollen (papillitis). Atrophy follows at a later stage. Ocular pain is a common accompaniment and is characteristically worse on eye movement. Any degree of visual loss may occur, even of light perception, and the usual visual-field deficit is a central scotoma, with particular loss of colour vision. Nerve conduction through demyelinated segments of optic nerve is very sensitive to small changes in temperature and patients often notice a marked deterioration in vision on exercise or external heating (Uthoff's phenomenon). Despite the severity of the initial symptoms, most patients make a good functional recovery over a few weeks. Within 5 years, however, two-thirds will have developed other signs of multiple sclerosis. The cortical-evoked potential to a patterned stimulus is markedly delayed.

Compressive and infiltrating lesions

Compression of the optic nerve by tumour is usually extrinsic and involves the posterior part of the nerve near the optic foramen. Proptosis and ophthalmoplegia may also be present. Meningiomas arising from the nerve sheath or from the margins of the optic canal, lymphomas, plasmocytomas, nasopharyngeal carcinomas, or metastases are the most common types. In dysthyroid eye disease, compression of the nerve may result from grossly enlarged extraocular muscles. Within the skull the optic nerve may be directly compressed or indirectly displaced against the rigid margins of the dura by such lesions as meningioma, pituitary adenoma, carotid aneurysm, or ectatic carotid arteries. Intrinsic compression occurs in glioma of the optic nerve, a rare tumour of childhood often associated with neurofibromatosis.

Inflammatory lesions

Acute or chronic inflammation or granulomas in the ethmoid or sphenoid sinuses may extend into the orbit and are a rare cause of optic neuritis (e.g. fungal infections or Wegener's granuloma). Within the cranial cavity one or both optic nerves may be involved by chronic basal meningitis caused by conditions such as tuberculosis, syphilis, sarcoidosis, or cryptococcosis.

Table 1 Swelling of the optic disc; causes and features

	Congenital	Papilloedema	Papillitis	Ischaemia
Laterality	Either or both	Bilateral	Unilateral	Unilateral
Acuity	Usually normal	Normal until late	Early loss	Usually affected
Colour vision	Usually normal	Normal	Early loss	Early loss
Pupils	Normal	Normal	RAPD[a]	RAPD[a]
Visual fields	Normal/variable loss	Blind spot enlarged	Central scotoma	Altitudinal defect
Disc	Abnormal size, shape vessels	Swollen	Swollen	Swollen, pale
Fundus	May have choroidal pigment	Normal	Normal	Vascular changes
Common causes		Intracerebral, intraorbital tumour, haematoma, venous sinus occlusion, retinal vein thrombosis, CO_2 retention	Optic neuritis	Hypertension, diabetes, arteritis

[a] RAPD, relative afferent pupillary defect.

Vascular lesions (ischaemic optic neuropathy)

This common condition usually affects elderly patients with degenerative arterial disease or with cranial arteritis. The head of the optic nerve is a vulnerable area because of its tenuous blood supply from the posterior ciliary arteries. Loss of vision is rapid and painless, and the optic disc appears swollen and pale. In the non-arteritic variety, visual-field loss is altitudinal and partial, and central acuity may be preserved. In the arteritic type, vision is often lost entirely. Both types show a tendency to involve the other eye after a short interval. High-dose steroid treatment appears to suppress the arteritic process and may prevent spread to the second eye, but has little effect in the non-arteritic group.

Toxic and nutritional amblyopias

These disorders are characterized by painless, slowly progressive, bilateral visual loss, showing diminished acuity, central or centrocaecal scotomas, and a variable degree of optic atrophy. They may occur in a setting of generalized malnutrition or with specific deficiency states (e.g. vitamin B_1, B_{12}, or folate deficiency). The syndrome may also follow chronic exposure to a number of toxic substances or drugs, such as alcohol (often in combination with heavy tobacco abuse), ethambutol, isoniazid, halogenated hydroxyquinolines, chlorpropamide, chloramphenicol, streptomycin, D-penicillamine, ergotamine, digitalis, and heavy metals.

Hereditary optic atrophy

There are a number of varieties of inherited optic atrophy, of which the best characterized is Leber's optic neuropathy. This causes severe visual loss in otherwise healthy young patients, beginning in the second decade. About 85 per cent of patients are male and 18 per cent of female carriers are affected. The onset may be acute and unilateral. The disease is inherited through the female line and the inheritance is consistent, with a mutation of mitochondrial DNA. Three such mutations have been identified in affected families. The disease progresses to severe loss of central vision but seldom causes complete blindness. No treatment has been shown to modify the progress of the condition.

Optic chiasm

Axons from the nasal retinas, which decussate in the chiasm, are at particular risk in compressive lesions. The classical field defect in chiasmal lesions is a bitemporal hemianopia with a sharp demarcation at the vertical meridian. Most patients have optic atrophy.

Central lesions produce a symmetrical field loss affecting both eyes to an equal extent, but there are two important variations in eccentrically placed lesions: (1) a lesion at the junction of optic nerve and chiasm may cause a central scotoma in the ipsilateral eye and an upper temporal quadrantanopia in the contralateral eye; (2) a lesion affecting the lateral side of the chiasm may cause nasal and central field loss in the ipsilateral eye and upper temporal quadrantanopia in the contralateral eye. Most of the important lesions affecting the chiasm are compressive, and the main features are shown in Table 2.

Modern CT with enhancement or MRI reliably demonstrate and distinguish adenomas, meningiomas, and craniopharyngiomas. Angiography may be necessary to confirm an aneurysm.

Optic tract

Lesions of the optic tract are rare, the most common causes being craniopharyngioma, an unusually placed pituitary adenoma, or following pituitary surgery. The visual-field defect is homonymous but incongruous, i.e., it affects the two eyes to a different extent. Optic atrophy is often present and helps to distinguish this from a hemisphere lesion.

Optic radiation

Parietal lobe

Cerebral tumours are the most common type of lesion in this area. They are usually malignant gliomas but metastases and meningiomas may also occur. Vascular lesions include spontaneous cerebral haemorrhage and 'watershed' infarction affecting the border zone between the territories of the three main cerebral arteries. All these lesions tend to damage the upper fibres of the radiation, causing a homonymous lower quadrantanopia (Fig. 2(b)).

Temporal lobe

Lesions of the posterior temporal lobe may interrupt the lower fibres of the visual radiation, giving rise to an upper homonymous quadrantanopia (Fig. 2(b)). In the dominant hemisphere dysphasia and memory loss may also be present.

Table 2 Lesions of the optic chiasm

	Occurrence	Visual field	Optic disc	Associated features	Treatment
Pituitary	Adults	Bitemporal hemianopia	Atrophy	Endocrine, prolactin GH[a], ACTH[b]	Surgery, bromocriptine, radiotherapy
Parasellar meningioma	Adults, F>M	Asymmetric bitemporal hemianopia	Atrophy	None	Surgery
Craniopharyngioma	Any age	Bitemporal, homonymous hemianopia	Atrophy, papilloedema (children)	Retarded growth, sexual development	Surgery, radical or palliative, ?radiotherapy
Optic nerve, chiasmal glioma	Children	Variable	Atrophy	Neurofibroma	Very slow-growing, possibly radiosensitive
Carotid aneurysm	Elderly, F>M	Lateral chiasm syndrome	Atrophy (late)	Pain, rarely SAH[c]	Usually conservative ?carotid ligation

[a] GH, growth hormone.
[b] ACTH, adrenocorticotrophic hormone.
[c] SAH, subarachnoid haemorrhage.

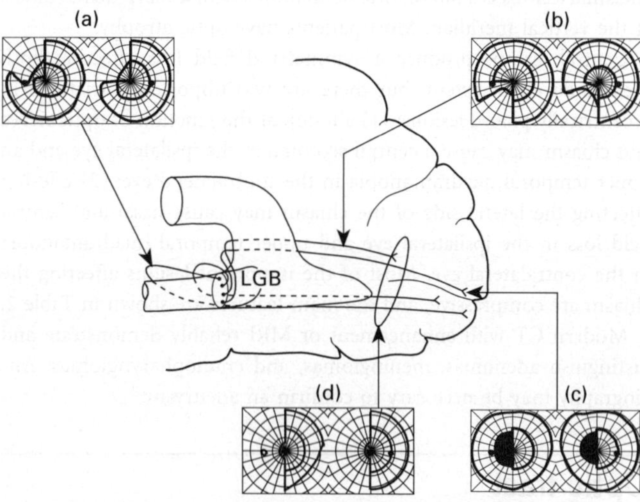

Fig. 2 Right cerebral hemisphere viewed from its medial aspect to show the geniculocalcarine pathway and the visual-field defects produced by lesions at various points. (a) Lesion involving the lower fibres of the right optic radiation looping around the temporal horn of the lateral ventricle: left upper quadrantanopia. (b) Lesion involving the upper fibres of visual radiation in the posterior parietal lobe: left lower quadrantanopia. (c) Localized lesion of the calcarine cortex: left homonymous hemianopic scotomas. (d) Subcortical lesion involving the posterior visual radiation: complete left homonymous hemianopia.

Visual cortex: occipital lobe

Lesions of the calcarine (visual) cortex give rise to a homonymous hemianopia, often complete, but with preserved central visual acuity (Fig. 2(c)). Usually this is an isolated defect without motor or sensory loss. Pupillary reactions to light are preserved and optokinetic nystagmus is normal to each side. Small lesions may produce congruous scotomatous defects (i.e., exactly the same in each eye). The great majority of lesions in this area are ischaemic (Fig. 3); the blood supply is from the posterior cerebral artery but the border zone between this territory and that of the middle cerebral artery runs close to the posterior pole. The 'macular sparing', which is a feature of vascular lesions, is probably explained by this alternative source of blood supply to the posterior pole where the central visual field is represented.

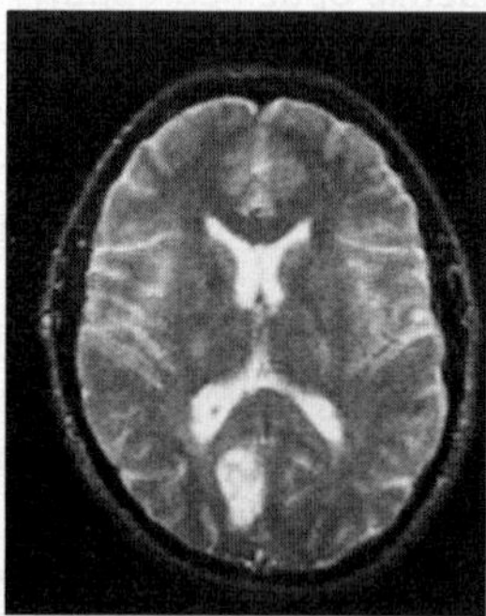

Fig. 3 Infarction: MRI axial scan of a 56-year-old woman with sudden onset of right homonynous hemianopia; there is infarction in the territory of the left posterior cerebral artery caused by embolism from the left atrium.

Simultaneous or successive occlusion of both posterior cerebral arteries causes a bilateral homonymous hemianopia or cortical blindness. Vision may be lost entirely, but more commonly a small central island of visual field is retained. Pupillary light reactions remain normal. These patients frequently show evidence of damage to other adjacent areas of cerebral cortex in the form of visual hallucinations and amnesia. Some may deny that they are blind (anosagnosia).

Further reading

Glaser, J.S. (1990). *Neuro-ophthalmology.* Harper and Row, Maryland.
Walsh, F.B. and Hoyt, W.F. (1969). *Clinical neuro-ophthalmology.* Williams and Wilkins, Baltimore.
Zeki, S. (1993). *A vision of the brain.* Blackwell Scientific, Oxford.

Chapter 13.6

The cranial nerves

P. K. Thomas and P. Rudge

The olfactory nerve

Loss of the sense of smell (anosmia) is most commonly encountered as a sequel to head injury and is probably related to severance of the central processes of the neurones of the olfactory mucosa as they pass through the cribriform plate to the olfactory bulb. It is usually permanent. Distortion of olfaction (parosmia) may occur and may be persistent. The sense of smell is occasionally congenitally absent or may be acutely and permanently lost after a coryzal infection. Hyposmia is also a feature of Kallman's syndrome (see OTM3, p. 1620). Bilateral anosmia is frequently accompanied by impairment of taste related to reduced detection of the volatile substances that impart flavours to foods. Unilateral anosmia may occur in meningiomas of the olfactory groove or other subfrontal tumours; this is usually not detected by the patient.

The central connections of the olfactory pathways are complex and include projections to the temporal lobes, hypothalamus, the septal region, and the amygdaloid nuclei. Olfactory hallucinations are well known to occur as a manifestation of temporal lobe epilepsy. Identification of odours may be impaired after bilateral medial temporal lesions and may be defective in multiple sclerosis, possibly as the result of demyelination in the olfactory tracts.

Third, fourth, and sixth cranial nerves

The third, or oculomotor, nerve supplies all the external ocular muscles with the exception of the superior oblique and lateral rectus. It also carries the parasympathetic innervation of the pupilloconstrictor fibres of the iris. A complete third-nerve lesion produces a dilated and unreactive pupil, complete ptosis, and loss of upward, downward, and medial movement of the eye. The eye becomes deviated downwards and laterally. Diplopia is only experienced when the lid is held up.

The fourth or trochlear nerve supplies the superior oblique muscle. Following a lesion of this nerve, there is extorsion of the eye when the patient looks outwards. When the patient looks downwards and medially, diplopia is experienced, which is particularly disturbing because of its occurrence on looking downwards, and produces difficulty in walking and in descending stairs. The patient may compensate for this by tilting the head to the opposite side.

The sixth or abducens nerve supplies the lateral rectus. A lesion of this nerve causes convergent strabismus and inability to abduct the affected eye, and diplopia, which is maximal on lateral gaze to the affected side.

The third, fourth, and sixth nerves may be affected singly or in combination; the paralysis may be complete or partial. In some instances, the lesion is within the brainstem, where it may affect either the nuclei or intramedullary portion of the nerve fibres. In older patients, the most common causes are brainstem vascular disease and neoplasms.

Extramedullary lesions of the third, fourth, and sixth nerves are more frequent, and may occur at any point along their course, either intracranially or within the orbit. A third-nerve palsy may develop in the region of the tentorial hiatus as a false localizing sign related to brainstem displacement produced by supratentorial, space-occupying conditions. Unilateral or bilateral sixth-nerve palsies may also arise as a consequence of raised intracranial pressure, probably caused by traction, again secondary to brainstem displacement. These nerves can be involved singly or together in conditions such as chronic basal meningitis or carcinomas of the skull base.

The third, fourth, and sixth nerves traverse the cavernous sinus, as do the first and second divisions of the trigeminal nerve. In this situation, they are most commonly damaged by an intracavernous aneurysm of the internal carotid artery. The third nerve is affected more often than the fourth and sixth. The consequent internal and external ophthalmoplegia is frequently accompanied by pain, and sometimes sensory loss and paraesthesias, in the corresponding frontal region related to compression of the first division of the trigeminal nerve, and occasionally in the cheek from damage to the maxillary division. In the superior orbital fissure syndrome, caused for example by a tumour invading the fissure, a total ophthalmoplegia may result, associated with pain and sensory loss in the distribution of the first division of the trigeminal nerve. The eye is often proptosed because of obstruction of the ophthalmic vein. The Tolosa–Hunt syndrome consists of a painful external ophthalmoplegia related to a granulomatous angiitis. Within the orbit, the third, fourth, and sixth nerves may be affected by conditions such as tumours and granulomas. They may be damaged as a result of trauma at any point along their course, and may be affected singly or in combination as part of a cranial neuropathy, of which diabetes, the Miller–Fisher syndrome, Lyme borreliosis, and sarcoidosis are the most important examples.

Pupillary abnormalities

Constriction of the pupil (miosis) occurs as a result of paralysis of the sympathetic innervation of the pupillodilator fibres of the iris and may be accompanied by the other features of Horner's syndrome—a mild ptosis, and vasodilatation and anhidrosis of the face on the same side. The ocular manifestations may be encountered alone if the damage is restricted to the intracranial portion of the sympathetic plexus around the carotid artery.

Pupillary dilatation may be caused by lesions of the third nerve, although it is of interest that the isolated third-nerve palsies of presumed vascular origin that may occur in diabetes mellitus, in contradistinction to compressive lesions of the nerve, characteristically spare the pupil. Anticholinergic drugs such as atropine and related substances give rise to pupillary dilatation, as does cocaine.

The Argyll Robertson pupil is small, fails to react to light, but constricts on ocular convergence, and, if bilateral, the pupils are frequently unequal in size (anisocoria). The pupil may be irregular in outline and it does not dilate fully in response to mydriatics. Argyll Robertson pupils are almost always related to neurosyphilis but somewhat similar pupils are occasionally encountered in diabetic neuropathy and in some hereditary neuropathies.

The myotonic pupil (Holmes–Adie syndrome) reacts abnormally slowly both to light and on convergence, but particularly so for the response to illumination. A very bright light may be required to demonstrate any pupillary constriction, or if the patient remains in a dark room for some minutes the pupil slowly dilates. The condition may be unilateral or bilateral and is more common in women than men. Myotonic pupils may be associated with absence or depression of the tendon reflexes and occasionally with anhidrosis in the limbs.

Trigeminal nerve

The fifth cranial nerve is predominantly sensory in function, but also innervates the muscles of mastication. It emerges from the pons and runs forward to the Gasserian ganglion, which is situated in Meckel's cave near the apex of the petrous temporal bone. The three sensory divisions of the nerve run anteriorly from the ganglion. The first or frontal division passes through the cavernous sinus and the superior orbital fissure. Its branches supply sensation to the anterior part of the scalp, the forehead, and the eye, including the conjunctiva and cornea. The second or maxillary division leaves the skull through the foramen rotundum, traverses the infraorbital canal, and supplies the cheek. The mandibular division emerges from the skull through the foramen ovale to reach the infratemporal fossa with the motor root, with which it unites to form a single trunk. It is distributed to the lower lip, chin, and the lower part of the cheek, and its auriculotemporal branch supplies part of the ear and temporal area. It also supplies the inner aspect of the cheek and the anterior two-thirds of the tongue, and its lingual branch carries taste fibres from the anterior two-thirds of the tongue, which leave it in the chorda tympani to join the facial nerve. The motor root innervates the temporalis muscle, the masseter, the pterygoids, mylohyoid, the anterior belly of the digastric, and also tensor tympani and tensor palati.

Trigeminal neuralgia

Symptoms

This condition is characterized by paroxysms of intense pain strictly confined to the distribution of the trigeminal nerve. In most cases the cause is unknown. It is generally encountered in individuals over the age of 50 years. Rarely, compression of the nerve, for example by tumours in the cerebellopontine angle, is responsible.

The salient feature of the disorder is pain, which is usually unilateral. The pain occurs in brief, searing paroxysms, each attack lasting only a matter of seconds. The pain is often described as piercing or knife-like. The paroxysms may be spontaneous or provoked by movements of the face and jaw, by touching the skin, or by draughts of cold air on the face. Eating and speaking may become extremely difficult. 'Trigger spots' on the skin of the face may be present, the touching of which provokes the paroxysms. The attacks may be followed by less severe pain of a dull, boring character and by tenderness of the skin in the affected area. Fortunately the attacks usually cease at night.

The quality of the pain is characteristic, and when trigeminal neuralgia is present the diagnosis is not usually missed, especially if a paroxysm is witnessed. The usual mistake is to regard as trigeminal neuralgia pain that is due to some other cause, and since there are many conditions that give rise to facial pain, the opportunities for error are numerous. Pain that is of a continuous character is not trigeminal neuralgia and some other cause must be sought. Absence of provocation by eating, talking, or the touching of trigger spots also makes the diagnosis unlikely. Once the diagnosis is accepted, it is essential to exclude compressive lesions affecting the nerve.

In the early stages, remissions lasting for months or years are usual, but in older patients remissions, if they occur, are likely to be brief. In all cases the remissions tend to become shorter as time goes on, and without treatment the condition persists for the rest of the patient's life.

The distribution of the pain is usually in one or two divisions of the nerve. The first division is rarely affected primarily, but pain may spread into it from the second division. If the pain begins in the second division it may, after a time, affect the third, and vice versa.

Treatment

The introduction of carbamazepine revolutionized treatment of this distressing condition. In a high proportion of cases, the paroxysms can be abolished or reduced. A dosage of 200 mg three to five times per day is employed.

If carbamazepine is not successful, or if the patients fail to tolerate it, other drugs such as phenytoin or clonazepam can be tried, but they are rarely effective. In this event, thermocoagulation of the ganglion may have to be considered; this should be undertaken only if the disorder is established so that a prolonged natural remission is unlikely to occur. The persistent analgesia and sometimes dysaesthesias may subsequently be troublesome, and when the first division is made anaesthetic, damage to the conjunctiva leading to corneal scarring has to be avoided. If thermocoagulation fails, section of the sensory root by a posterior fossa approach employing a microsurgical technique is indicated.

Ophthalmic herpes zoster

In elderly individuals, the fifth nerve is prone to involvement in herpes zoster, the first division being most vulnerable, giving rise to the distressing condition of ophthalmic herpes. An unfortunate sequel may be visual impairment from residual corneal scarring. Particularly in older individuals, postherpetic neuralgia may also be a sequel: this gives rise to persistent and unremitting spontaneous pain associated with cutaneous hyperaesthesia in the affected area. Treatment is difficult. Analgesics, sedation, and antidepressive preparations to combat the secondary depression that is frequently present may be of some assistance.

Isolated trigeminal neuropathy

Rarely, a chronic, isolated, unilateral or bilateral affection of the trigeminal nerve may occur as a manifestation of Sjögren's syndrome or systemic lupus erythematosus, although most cases are idiopathic. Extensive nasal scarring and tissue loss may occur secondary to repeated injury from picking and scratching.

Facial nerve

The seventh cranial nerve is largely motor. The nerve traverses the facial canal in the petrous temporal bone in close relation to the middle ear and emerges at the stylomastoid foramen. Its branches pass forward through the parotid gland to be distributed to the muscles of the face, including the platysma. Within the petrous bone, a branch is given to the stapedius muscle. The chorda tympani, carrying the taste fibres from the anterior two-thirds of the tongue, joins the nerve within the facial canal and a small branch supplies cutaneous sensation to the region of the external auditory meatus. The nerve also carries preganglionic parasympathetic fibres destined for the lachrymal gland.

The distinction between upper and lower motor-neurone lesions of the facial muscles is usually easy. In general, with upper motor-neurone lesions there is a relative preservation of power in the upper facial muscles, because these have a bilateral innervation from the cerebral hemispheres. There is no loss of tone with upper motor-neurone lesions, so that the sagging of the face that is an unsightly feature of lower motor-neurone palsy does not occur.

In common with the trigeminal nerve, the facial nerve may be affected by tumours in the cerebellopontine angle. In the past, it was often involved from middle-ear infections. It may be involved in meningeal carcinomatosis, fractures and tumours of the skull base, in a variety of cranial neuropathies, and cephalic herpes zoster, but the most common lesion by far is Bell's palsy. More peripherally, the nerve may be implicated in tumours of the parotid gland.

Bell's palsy

This term describes a usually unilateral facial paralysis of relatively rapid onset related to a lesion of the nerve within the facial canal. It may develop at any age, most commonly between 20 and 50 years, and affects both sexes equally. Its causation is unknown. In the acute stage, the nerve is swollen and compression within the facial canal may contribute to the damage to nerve fibres.

The onset is rapid and is frequently heralded or accompanied by aching pain below the ear or in the mastoid region; this clears within a few days and is not present in every case. The paralysis usually reaches its maximum severity after 1 or 2 days but occasionally progresses over the course of several days. Complete paralysis may occur. In the lower face, this may cause a mild dysarthria and some difficulty in eating because of food collecting between the gums and the inner sides of the cheek and the escape of fluid when drinking. Paralysis of orbicularis oculi renders voluntary eye closure impossible and, particularly in the older individual, ectropion develops, which can result in conjunctival injury from foreign bodies or conjunctivitis.

In the more severe cases, loss of taste over the anterior two-thirds of the tongue is often present, and paralysis of the stapedius muscle may result in a lack of tolerance for high-pitched or loud sounds.

Bell's palsy has to be distinguished from selective lesions of the facial nerve within the brainstem, in which instance taste will not be affected. Facial paralysis related to cephalic herpes zoster is discussed below. A lesion of the facial nerve may represent a mononeuropathy from some generalized disorder of which diabetes, Lyme borreliosis, and sarcoidosis are the most important. Bell's palsy is rarely bilateral and the occurrence of bilateral facial paralysis would raise the possibility of the Guillain–Barré syndrome: this may begin with facial weakness, or the weakness may remain restricted to the facial musculature. The occurrence of bilateral facial weakness would also raise the possibility of sarcoidosis.

In the early stages, the main endeavour of treatment should be to prevent either a partial lesion, or complete paralysis related to a conduction block, progressing to a degenerative lesion. There is some evidence that corticosteroids may be advantageous by reducing oedema in the nerve. Thus it is justifiable to treat all cases with corticosteroids if seen within a few days of onset, providing no contraindication to such treatment exists. A course of a week's duration with an initially high dosage is recommended.

Surgical decompression of the nerve has been advised. To be effective, this would have to be performed at the outset, which is not justifiable as 85 per cent of cases will recover satisfactorily without treatment. So far there are no means of predicting which cases will progress to a degenerative lesion.

In those cases in which regeneration fails to occur, operation may be desirable for cosmetic reasons to counteract the facial deformity.

Facial paralysis related to 'geniculate' herpes zoster (Ramsay Hunt syndrome)

Facial paralysis of rapid onset accompanied by severe pain in and around the external auditory meatus and in the throat may accompany 'cephalic zoster'. Vesicles may be detectable in the ear and ulceration in the fauces, or anywhere on the head. Occasionally there is concomitant vertigo, tinnitus, and some deafness with involvement of the eighth nerve ('otic herpes zoster'). Prognosis for recovery of the facial paralysis is less good than in Bell's palsy.

Hemifacial spasm

See Chapter 13.20.

The eighth cranial nerve

The eighth nerve has both auditory and vestibular parts. The auditory part innervates the cochlear sensory receptors; all the nerve fibres are myelinated and the myelin surrounds the cell bodies as well as the axons. The central auditory pathways are complex with multiple decussations; synapses occur in the cochlear nuclei, superior olivary complex, lateral lemnisci, inferior colliculi, and medial geniculate bodies. There are several cortical areas associated with hearing, including Heschl's gyrus, and a precise tonotopic organization is maintained to this level.

The vestibular part innervates two types of receptor, the semicircular canals and the otolith organs (saccule and utricle). Angular acceleration in the three cardinal planes is detected by the semicircular canals, which partially integrate the signal to one of velocity. Linear acceleration (gravity) is detected in the sagittal and coronal planes by the otolith-bearing structures. Exceedingly complex connections between the second-order neurones of the vestibular nuclei pass to the somatic musculature, extraocular muscles, cerebellum, and cerebral cortex. In clinical practice, connections to the extraocular muscles are the most important as they are concerned with the vestibulo-ocular reflex, which maintains the eye position relative to the ground and derangement of which gives clues to the site of pathology.

Symptoms and signs due to dysfunction of the eighth nerve

Auditory system

Symptoms

Deafness is the cardinal feature of damage to the cochlea or its afferent pathways. Loss of hearing can be unilateral only if the disease process affects the end organ, eighth nerve, or cochlear nucleus. More central lesions cause symmetrical hearing loss, but significant deafness from such lesions is rare. Distortion of hearing is a frequent accompaniment of cochlear loss, as is tinnitus, but neither symptom is confined to such lesions.

Tests of auditory function

Confirmation of hearing loss is done by means of pure-tone air-conduction audiometry. The Rinne test determines whether the deafness is conductive or sensorineural. In the normal person the cochlear hair cells can be stimulated via two routes: air conduction or bone conduction. The first can be tested by placing a tuning fork of 256 or 512 Hz adjacent to the external auditory meatus. The pressure waves set up in the air contained within the external auditory canal cause the tympanic membrane and ossicles to vibrate and transmit the sound waves to the cochlea. Bone conduction can be tested by placing the vibrating fork against the mastoid process, which then transmits the signal directly to the hair cells. Since air conduction is much more efficient than bone conduction in normal individuals, a vibrating tuning fork placed adjacent to the external meatus until the sound is no longer detected cannot be heard if it is then placed on the mastoid. A similar situation exists if a sensorineural hearing loss is present; the abnormality involves the cochlea or its nerve fibres and this does not alter the relative efficiency of transduction of sound waves via the two routes to the cochlea. Conversely, if there is an abnormality of the external canal, such as the presence of wax, or of the ossicles, for example otosclerosis, the efficiency of only the air-conduction route will be impaired. In these circumstances, sound will be transmitted more efficiently by bone conduction.

If a vibrating fork is placed on the teeth or forehead in a normal person, the sound is located at the midline. On the other hand, in a unilateral sensorineural hearing loss the sound is appreciated towards the unimpaired side and with a conductive loss to the impaired side. This is the Weber test.

Conductive deafness will not be discussed further, as this is the province of the otologist. If sensorineural hearing loss is present, tests of loudness function, adaptation, and speech audiometry will help to differentiate that due to hair cell loss, for example Menière's disease, from that due to retrocochlear lesions such as eighth-nerve tumours.

Vestibular system

Symptoms

Damage to the vestibular receptors or their neural connections results in a mismatch of input between them (so-called tonus imbalance) and also with the other receptors signalling orientation in space, such as vision, proprioception, and joint position. This results in an unpleasant sensation of imbalance and vertigo, which, in extreme cases, causes nausea and vomiting; the patient is reluctant to move and prefers to be in bed. Lesions are usually destructive and their effects are rapidly compensated centrally so that the patient becomes asymptomatic over a period of a few weeks. Exceptionally, compensation, which depends upon brainstem structures including the olivary nuclei and cerebellum, is incomplete and symptoms persist.

Nystagmus

Spontaneous nystagmus, which comes in many forms, is an extremely useful sign of vestibular dysfunction. Conventionally, the direction of nystagmus is specified by the fast phase.

Vestibular nystagmus

The vestibular apparatus and nuclei are paired, one set on each side of the head. The horizontal canals, and the vestibular nuclei with which they connect, drive the eyes as a slow movement towards the opposite side. Thus in the normal person equal and opposite forces act on the eye muscles, and the eyes remain central. Destruction of one set of vestibular end-organs, their nerves or nuclei results in the eyes drifting towards that side as a slow movement (Fig. 1). This phenomenon arises because of the unopposed activity of the intact vestibular apparatus. It is rapidly detected and a counter-movement is generated by another system, the saccadic (fast) generator lying in the paramedian pontine reticular formation. This saccadic movement to one side is generated by the ipsilateral paramedian pontine reticular formation. Thus in a right-sided vestibular lesion the eyes are pushed slowly to the right by the intact left vestibular system and then are rapidly returned towards the midline under the influence of the left paramedian pontine reticular formation. Repetition of this results in vestibular nystagmus, with its characteristic saw-toothed wave form and fast phase to the side opposite the lesion.

Gaze-evoked nystagmus

Gaze-evoked nystagmus results in the eyes returning exponentially to the midline after each attempted eccentric fixation. Such gaze-evoked nystagmus is found in a wide variety of conditions, including pontine and cerebellar lesions, and after ingestion of drugs, particularly anticonvulsants.

Significance of horizontal nystagmus

Unilateral horizontal nystagmus, especially if its magnitude increases as the eyes are deviated in the direction of the fast phase (Alexander's law), is most commonly due to a peripheral lesion, but can occur

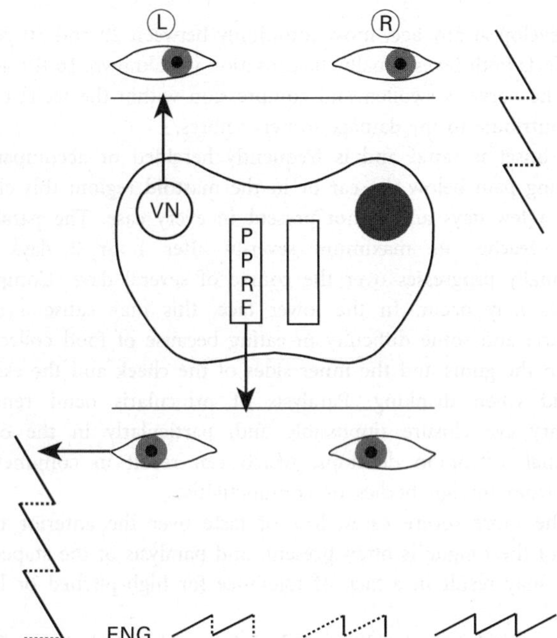

Fig. 1 Diagrammatic explanation of vestibular nystagmus due to destruction of the right vestibular apparatus, nerve, or nucleus. The slow phase is represented on the right, the fast phase on the left, and summation of the two is revealed in the electronystagmogram below. VN, vestibular nucleus; PPRF, paramedian pontine reticular formation.

with lesions of the eighth nerve or vestibular nucleus. On the other hand, horizontal nystagmus that occurs to both sides at the same time is invariably due to a central lesion.

Removal of optic fixation and recording the eye movements, either with electronystagmography or by observing the eyes with an infrared viewer, also helps to differentiate between peripheral and central lesions. Characteristically, nystagmus due to a lesion of the end-organ is enhanced by removal of fixation, whereas that due to a central lesion, including vestibular nuclear lesions, is not.

Vertical nystagmus

Although acquired spontaneous nystagmus in the vertical plane is virtually never due to an eighth-nerve disturbance, brief mention of it will be made here.

Up-beat nystagmus The fast phase is upwards. It occurs in patients with lesions in the floor of the fourth ventricle, pontine tegmentum, and perhaps the anterior cerebellum. It rarely occurs in isolation, but is not infrequent in patients with an internuclear ophthalmoplegia.

Down-beat nystagmus The fast phase is downwards. This is also uncommon. It indicates either a structural abnormality at the level of the foramen magnum, for example cerebellar tonsillar herniation or cerebellar dysfunction, especially an atrophic process.

Torsional clockwise or counter-clockwise nystagmus Rotation about the sagittal meridian is rare, but occurs in central lesions, especially those involving the medial vestibular nucleus, and in patients with cerebellar ectopia associated with syringomyelia.

Positional and positioning nystagmus

Benign positional nystagmus In this form there is a rotatory nystagmus with the fast phase towards the dependent ear—counter-clockwise if the right ear is dependent, clockwise if the left ear is dependent. This nystagmus occurs after a latent interval of a few

Table 1 Characteristics of positional nystagmus

	Benign	Central
Direction	Towards lower ear	Any
Vertigo	++	±
Latent interval	+	0
Adaptation	+	0
Fatigue	+	0

++, severe; +, moderate; ±, slight; 0, absent.

seconds and lasts for 10 to 20 s. It is accompanied by vertigo (Table 1) On returning to the upright position a lesser nystagmus of opposite sense occurs. Repetition of the test results in an attenuation of the response, this adaptation lasting a number of hours. Classically, there is no nystagmus when the other ear is dependent.

In most cases, conservative therapy with vestibular sedatives or a course of head exercises and advice about head positioning are all that is necessary for this self-limiting condition.

Central positional nystagmus This differs from the above in that its direction is not towards the dependent ear; it may be in any direction and is persistent and often unassociated with vertigo. It is frequently produced by positioning on either side. It is thought that this form of nystagmus signifies a central lesion, especially one involving the vestibulocerebellum.

In practice, the vast majority of patients with benign positional nystagmus of classical type have a peripheral and benign lesion (often following head injury, or associated with hypertension or cervical spondylosis), while central positional nystagmus requires investigation to exclude a disorder of the central nervous system (for example, multiple sclerosis, tumour), although in a substantial proportion of cases no cause will be found.

Gait and stance

Damage to the vestibular apparatus results in an abnormality of stance and gait. The patient tends to fall towards the side of the lesion if it is destructive, and veers to that side when walking. These abnormalities are most marked if the eyes are closed and if the lesion is peripheral.

Specific disorders of the eighth-nerve system

Cerebellopontine angle tumours

Although all tumours of the cerebellopontine angle are rare, early diagnosis is important since the majority are benign, and morbidity of surgical removal is less if attempted when the tumours are small. About 70 per cent of the tumours are schwannomas, the remainder being meningiomas, epidermoids, neuromas of nerves other than the eighth, and a host of other rare lesions.

Acoustic schwannomas and neurofibromas

Acoustic schwannomas usually arise on the vestibular nerves, especially the superior component. They are sporadic. Exceptionally, tumours are bilateral; this only occurs in neurofibromatosis type II (central neurofibromatosis). No age is exempt.

The presenting symptom is typically a progressive hearing loss with unsteadiness. When the tumour protrudes beyond the internal acoustic porus, or arises more centrally, other cranial nerves are involved. The fifth nerve is particularly vulnerable; its involvement causes numbness of the face on the appropriate side. Larger tumours, which compress the brainstem, cause increasing unsteadiness and, ultimately, in untreated cases, hydrocephalus. Occipital headache is a frequent symptom of acoustic tumours, even before hydrocephalus develops.

Fifth-nerve signs, especially loss of the corneal reflex, are found with large tumours, but, surprisingly, facial weakness is not a prominent sign in many cases. Long-tract signs, especially mild ipsilateral pyramidal features such as hyper-reflexia, are found when the tumours impinge upon the brainstem.

Other tumours

Meningiomas (which are more common in females) and epidermoids are much rarer than acoustic schwannomas, but can mimic the latter. Hearing loss is, in general, less severe and the caloric responses are more frequently normal. The brainstem-evoked potentials from the unimpaired ear are usually normal, even with large tumours.

Imaging and treatment

Nuclear magnetic resonance scanning is the best way to demonstrate cerebellopontine angle tumours, especially intracanalicular acoustic tumours. Gadolinium enhancement is essential.

Surgical removal is the only curative therapy. Morbidity is directly related to the size of the tumour. It is very rare to save hearing, although the seventh nerve can be preserved with modern techniques. Morbidity in terms of hearing loss may be lessened if interoperative brainstem-evoked recording is undertaken.

Menière's disease

The triad of episodic vertigo, tinnitus, and fluctuating hearing loss are the classical features of Menière's disease, in which the peak incidence of onset of vertigo is in the fourth and fifth decades. There is often a premonitory symptom of fullness of the appropriate ear. Initially the hearing loss recovers between the attacks, but later it becomes permanent and progressive. Tinnitus is a constant feature that typically increases during the attacks. Vertigo is the most distressing symptom and the patient is usually prostrated with nausea and vomiting. It lasts less than 24 h. The attacks occur in clusters with weeks or months free; the remissions are longer as the disease progresses.

Characteristically, the hearing loss is initially of low frequency, but later severe loss (about 60 dB) at all frequencies occurs. The hearing loss becomes bilateral in 10 to 25 per cent of patients.

Loss of vestibular function is frequently bilateral. Nystagmus is seen in all patients during the acute episode and tends to be towards the affected ear at the time of an attack.

A low-salt diet and administration of diuretics is of value in reducing the severity and frequency of attacks of vertigo. Betahistine (8–16 mg, three times daily) may also reduce attacks.

Other vestibular disturbances

Episodic vertigo

Episodic vertigo not usually accompanied by deafness is a common and difficult problem. Not all patients with these symptoms have Menière's disease. Indeed, the majority do not. An occasional patient has syphilis, which can mimic Menière's disease completely; the deafness then is often progressive in spite of treatment with penicillin. It is mandatory to do treponemal antibody tests in anyone presenting with a Menière's syndrome. Migraine is a disorder that profoundly affects the vestibular system and, to a lesser extent, hearing. Acute attacks of migraine are frequently associated with vestibular abnormalities (vertigo, nausea, and vomiting) and auditory dysfunction (phonophobia), both in the basilar-artery form as well as in classical migraine. In addition, patients who have had migraine in the past occasionally develop sporadic vertigo unaccompanied by headache; the cause is unknown.

Vestibular neuronitis is a syndrome of paroxysmal vertigo. The syndrome is common and found particularly in patients with hypertension and following systemic viral infections, where the term 'neuronitis' implies an unwarranted precision of diagnosis. The symptoms result from an episode of vestibular failure, of which neuronitis is but one cause.

Treatment of the vertiginous patient

During an episode of acute vestibular failure, patients are understandably terrified and fear that they are about to die. They require reassurance that they will recover, and should be put to bed and told not to move their heads. Vestibular sedatives such as prochlorperazine (12.5 mg intramuscularly) will be required if the patient is vomiting. Oral therapy can be given as soon as vomiting ceases. A wide variety of such sedatives is available, none of which is ideal; in general, a combination of sympathomimetic and antiparasympathomimetic drugs is the most efficient way of lessening symptoms, although in practice anticholinergic drugs alone are usually given. Cinnarizine (15 mg, three times a day) or prochlorperazine (5 mg, three times a day) are the most commonly prescribed agents and are moderately effective. Usually, the drugs can be discontinued after 2 to 4 weeks, by which time most patients will have recovered.

Occasionally symptoms persist. Sometimes this may take the form of benign positional vertigo, for which vestibular sedatives, head exercises, and advice about lying down are all that is required. Other patients are frightened to walk and need vestibular exercises to retrain their vestibular system, using input from other sensory modalities. Some patients are helped by clonazepam, partly because of its sedative properties, but also by its central action on the vestibular system. Such patients may require psychiatric help even though they have a good organic cause for their vertigo.

Glossopharyngeal nerve

The ninth cranial nerve leaves the skull through the jugular foramen, closely related to the tenth nerve. It supplies the stylopharyngeus muscle and the constrictor muscles of the pharynx. Parasympathetic fibres are supplied to the parotid gland. Sensory fibres are carried from the posterior third of the tongue, the ear, the fauces, and the nasopharynx, and chemoreceptor and baroreceptor afferents from the carotid sinus.

The glossopharyngeal nerve is rarely affected in isolation. Lesions usually occur in conjunction with involvement of the vagus and give rise to some dysphagia, impaired pharyngeal sensation, and loss of taste over the posterior third of the tongue. It may be affected in the jugular foramen syndrome along with the tenth and eleventh nerves, of which glomus tumours or metastatic carcinoma are the most common causes. The nerve may also be involved in diphtheritic neuropathy and in a polyneuritis cranialis.

Glossopharyngeal neuralgia is a rare form of neuralgia within the distribution of the glossopharyngeal nerve. Its features are otherwise strictly comparable to those of trigeminal neuralgia in the quality and severity of the pain, its occurrence in brief paroxysms, its provocation by actions such as speaking or swallowing, and the remissions in its course.

Vagus nerve

The tenth cranial nerve is structurally complex. Within the skull it is joined by the cranial division of the eleventh nerve. It leaves the skull through the jugular foramen. Cutaneous sensory fibres are carried from the external ear and visceral afferent fibres are carried from the pharynx, larynx, trachea, oesophagus, and the thoracic and abdominal viscera. Motor fibres are supplied to the striated musculature of the palate and pharynx, and, through the external and recurrent laryngeal nerves, to the muscles of the larynx. Parasympathetic fibres are provided to innervate the parotid gland (through the glossopharyngeal nerve), the heart, and the abdominal viscera.

The important symptoms of vagal damage are those relating to pharyngeal and laryngeal innervation. The cells of origin in the nucleus ambiguus of the medulla may be damaged in the lateral medullary syndrome, in motor neurone disease, and in acute bulbar poliomyelitis, leading to dysphagia and dysphonia. Involvement along with the glossopharyngeal nerve in the jugular foramen syndrome has already been mentioned. The recurrent laryngeal nerve may be damaged during operations on the thyroid gland or by tumours within the neck, or within the thorax, usually by carcinoma of the bronchus. The nerve on the left is vulnerable to damage from aneurysm of the aortic arch. Isolated and unexplained lesions of the recurrent laryngeal nerve are not uncommon.

Nuclear or high vagal lesions, as well as involving the larynx, cause palatal and pharyngeal paralysis. If unilateral, there are no symptoms from palatopharyngeal paralysis. The uvula is pulled up to the opposite side on phonation and pharyngeal sensation is impaired on the affected side. With bilateral paralysis, the palate is paretic leading to nasality of the voice and nasal regurgitation of liquids on attempts at swallowing. Bilateral palatopharyngeal paralysis may be encountered in motor neurone disease, bulbar poliomyelitis, diphtheritic neuropathy, and polyneuritis cranialis.

Unilateral intrinsic laryngeal paralysis from lesions of the recurrent nerve may be asymptomatic or give rise to hoarseness of the voice.

Spinal accessory nerve

The spinal accessory portion of the eleventh cranial nerve arises from the upper cervical cord and the lower medulla. The nerve passes through the foramen magnum and joins the cranial portion of the nerve before emerging from the skull through the jugular foramen. The spinal accessory nerve then separates and supplies the sternomastoid and trapezius muscles, the latter also receiving an innervation from the cervical plexus.

The nerve may be affected by lesions in the region of the jugular foramen, but more commonly it is damaged by injuries to the neck or by operations for removal of cervical glands, particularly as it crosses the posterior triangle of the neck. Isolated and unexplained lesions of the nerve are occasionally encountered.

The hypoglossal nerve

The twelfth cranial nerve supplies all the muscles of the tongue, both intrinsic and extrinsic. It leaves the skull through the anterior condyloid foramen. A unilateral lesion of the hypoglossal nerve causes weakness and atrophy of the tongue on the affected side. When protruded, the tongue deviates to the affected side. Articulation is unaffected. The nerve may be affected by tumours in the region of the anterior condyloid foramen, or by tumours or penetrating injuries in the neck. If the lesion is the result of a unilateral lower brainstem lesion, it may be combined with a crossed hemiplegia.

Bilateral lesions give rise to generalized atrophy of the tongue. Protrusion becomes impossible and articulation is disturbed. The most common cause is motor neurone disease (progressive bulbar palsy). The wasting of the tongue is usually accompanied by fasciculation.

Further reading

Baloh, R.W. (1998). Vertigo. *Lancet*, **352**, 1841-6.

Hughes, T.A. and Wiles, C.M. (1998). Neurogenic dysphagia: the role of the neurologist. *Journal of Neurology, Neurosurgery and Psychiatry*, **64**, 569-72.

Roob, G., Fazekas, F., and Hartung, H.O. (1999). Peripheral facial palsy: etiology, diagnosis and treatment. *European Neurology*, **41**, 3-9.

Tenser, R.B. (1998). Trigeminal neuralgia: mechanisms of treatment. *Neurology*, **51**, 17-9.

Chapter 13.7

The autonomic nervous system

R. Bannister

Anatomy and physiology

The peripheral autonomic nervous system, an efferent system, is made up of neurones that lie outside the central nervous system and are concerned with visceral innervation. Both sympathetic and parasympathetic systems have preganglionic neurones in the brain and spinal cord arranged as shown in Fig. 1.

The transmitter at all preganglionic terminals is acetylcholine, which is not paralysed by atropine (the nicotinic effect), whereas the action of acetylcholine at the distal end of the cholinergic postganglionic fibres is paralysed by atropine (the muscarinic effect). Noradrenaline (norepinephrine) is the principal transmitter for postganglionic sympathetic nerves, the exceptions being sudomotor nerves, which are cholinergic in humans, some vasodilator fibres to muscle, and the adrenal medulla, which is innervated by preganglionic (cholinergic) fibres and itself secretes mainly adrenaline (epinephrine). Noradrenaline is stored in the terminals and is released by nerve activity or by sympathomimetic drugs, which may act partly indirectly on the ganglia or more centrally (such as ephedrine and amphetamine) or on the terminals (such as phenylephrine or tyramine). The different actions of noradrenaline and adrenaline are caused by relative effects on different receptors. The α-receptors may be either postsynaptic (α_1) or presynaptic (α_2), which, when stimulated, decrease the release of the transmitter. The β-receptors mediate vasodilation, especially in muscles, increase the rate and force of the heart with a tendency to arrhythmias, and cause bronchial relaxation. They are further subdivided into β_1-receptors, mediating the chronotropic cardiac action of isoprenaline, and β_2-receptors, which are responsible for most of the peripheral effects of β-adrenergic stimulation.

Classification of autonomic disorders (Table 1)

Pure autonomic failure occurs alone or as an additional feature in two distinct and well-recognized types of primary neurological degenerative disease, multiple system atrophy and Parkinson's disease. Shy and Drager described the complex neurological syndrome that bears their name, now called autonomic failure with multiple system atrophy, in which postural hypotension may be accompanied by pyramidal, extrapyramidal, and cerebellar signs. Later a rare variant was recognized in which autonomic failure was associated with apparently typical Parkinson's disease. Cases of clinically pure autonomic failure examined at autopsy show either Lewy intranuclear inclusion bodies, linking these cases to Parkinson's disease, or minor changes of multiple system atrophy. The rare cases of autonomic failure with Parkinson's disease are distinct from cases of multiple system atrophy in which striatonigral degeneration or olivopontocerebellar atrophy, or both, may be present.

Clinical features of primary autonomic failure syndromes

The clinical features of primary autonomic failure are similar whether this is pure autonomic failure or autonomic failure with multiple system atrophy. When the effects of drugs and adrenal insufficiency have been excluded, persistent postural hypotension is almost certainly due to a neurological lesion, where the most common presenting symptoms are postural dizziness and fatigue, or attacks of loss of consciousness on exercise or after meals. However, the first symptoms of autonomic failure are mild, insidious, and frequently overlooked or misdiagnosed. The patients are all middle aged or elderly, and males are affected about twice as often as females. In men, impotence

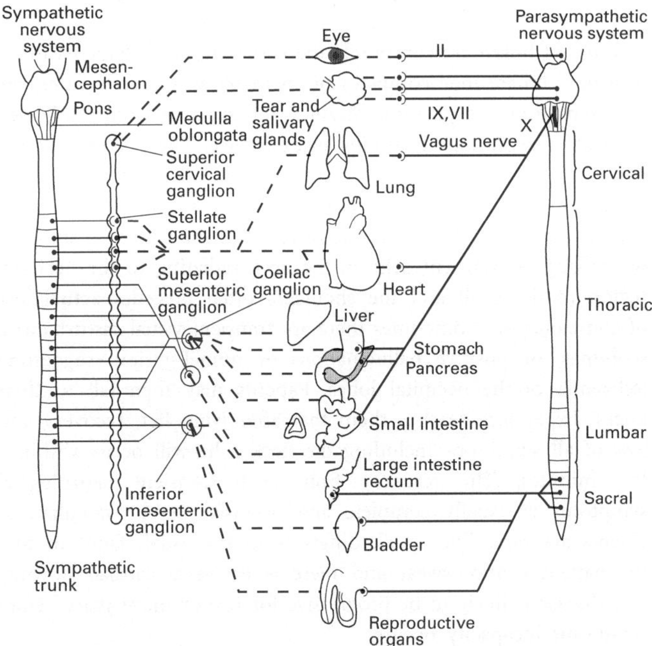

Fig. 1 Peripheral autonomic nervous system: the sympathetic innervation of vessels, sweat glands, and piloerector muscles is not shown (solid lines, preganglionic axons; dashed lines, postganglionic axons) *(reproduced from Bannister 1992, with permission).*

Table 1 Classification of autonomic disorders (adapted from Bannister and Mathias 1992, with permission)

Central, primary
• Pure autonomic failure
• Autonomic failure with multiple system atrophy
• Autonomic failure with Parkinson's disease
Central, secondary
• Central brain lesions: craniopharyngioma, vascular lesions
• Infections of the nervous system: tabes dorsalis, Chagas' disease, HIV
• Spinal cord lesions
• Familial dysautonomia
***Genetic: dopamine* β-hydroxylase deficiency**
Distal autonomic neuropathies
• General medical disorders: diabetes, amyloid, porphyria, Tangier disease, Fabry's disease, HIV
• Autoimmune disease: acute and subacute pandysautonomia; Guillain–Barré syndrome; myasthenia; rheumatoid arthritis
Drugs
• Selective neurotoxic drugs: alcoholism, Wernicke's encephalopathy
• Tranquillizers; phenothiazines, barbiturates
• Antidepressants; tricyclics; monoamine oxidase inhibitors
• Vasodilator hypotensive drugs: prazosin, hydralazine
• Centrally acting hypotensive drugs; methyldopa, clonidine
• Adrenergic neurone blocking drugs; guanethidine, bethanidine, debrisoquine
• α-Adrenergic blocking drugs; phenoxybenzamine, labetalol
• Ganglion-blocking drugs; hexamethonium, mecamylamine
• Angiotensin-converting enzyme inhibitors. Captopril

and loss of libido are commonly the first symptoms. Patients living in a hot climate may complain of an inability to sweat. Later, the first symptoms of postural dizziness or syncope occur, followed by bladder symptoms including incontinence. The postural attacks may be 'drop' attacks, resembling sudden brainstem vascular dysfunction, but more commonly there is a gradual fading of consciousness over half a minute or so while the patient is standing or walking. A transient ache in the neck radiating to the occipital region of the skull and the shoulders often precedes actual loss of consciousness. Sometimes there are transient visual disturbances, scotomas, or positive hallucinations or tunnel vision, suggesting ischaemia of the occipital lobes. Patients may then fall to their knees. Experience teaches them that after lying flat, recovery and loss of all symptoms including the neck ache will occur within a few minutes. The recovery from such transient neurological symptoms is usually complete and occlusive cerebrovascular incidents are rare. The attack differs from the usual 'faint' in that the patient cannot sweat and there is no vagal cardiac slowing. The disease is likely to be progressive for five or more years before significant incapacity occurs.

In patients with autonomic failure, the ingestion of food results in a number of hormonal, neural, and regional haemodynamic changes that may be linked to a substantial lowering of blood pressure, even in the supine position; this can present a considerable clinical problem. After ingestion of foods, splanchnic vasodilatation occurs, due to vasoactive peptides (possibly somatostatin), which is not counteracted by appropriate haemodynamic adjustments in other parts of the circulation.

Testing autonomic function

When a fall of more than some 20 mmHg of systolic pressure on standing is found in a patient with symptoms, further investigation is justified and a battery of tests is now available, summarized in Table 2. The finger arterial blood pressure can now be measured non-invasively by an inflatable cuff with a built-in infrared emitter and sensor (Finapres). On tilt the blood pressure falls due to lack of constriction in resistance and capacity vessels in muscles and in the splanchnic area. There is also a lack of the overshoot in phase IV of the Valsalva, which normally occurs as a result of reflex peripheral vasoconstriction. The instability of blood pressure in autonomic failure is due partly to lack of baroreflex control but also to supersensitivity of partially denervated vessels to the transmitter noradrenaline, and this may cause recumbent hypertension.

Neuropathology of primary autonomic failure

In almost all patients with autonomic failure and multiple system atrophy carefully studied there has been a reduction by up to 80 per cent in the number of sympathetic preganglionic neurones in the intermediolateral columns of the spinal cord. In patients with autonomic failure with Parkinson's disease, Lewy bodies are found. There have been few complete pathological studies of pure autonomic failure, but some reports show loss of intermediolateral column cells as well as definite ganglionic lesions; this suggests the existence of a more distal process in pure autonomic failure than in multiple system atrophy. In all patients with autonomic failure there is, as might be expected, a reduction of the catecholamine fluorescence of sympathetic nerve endings on muscle blood vessels, and electron microscopy of the endings shows that there is a reduction in the number of small, dense-core, noradrenergic vesicles.

Distal autonomic neuropathies

In contrast to autonomic failure there are also true distal autonomic neuropathies (see Table 1) in which the clinical features resulting from interruption of the efferent autonomic pathways produce certain symptoms and signs that resemble those of autonomic failure. The onset may be more acute, however, and partial or complete recovery may occur. Some of the distal generalized neuropathies secondary to a variety of causes, but with minor autonomic involvement, are described elsewhere in this book, but the methods of investigation and treatment of autonomic features are similar to those described previously for the primary autonomic failure syndromes. There is, however, one distal neuropathy that requires special mention, the rare acute or subacute pandysautonomia, which may involve either sympathetic or parasympathetic fibres, or both. The autonomic defects can be identified as in primary autonomic failure. This disease appears to have an autoimmune basis with a tendency to gradual recovery, which may be incomplete. It may be thought of as a variant of the type of autonomic neuropathy that occurs as a feature of the Guillain–Barré syndrome, where autonomic features are often present but rather obscured by the somatic neuropathy.

Table 2 Some useful clinical tests of autonomic failure (adapted from Bannister and Mathias 1992, with permission)

Cardiovascular reflexes
Tests performed and responses:
1. Change of posture: blood pressure and pulse rate monitored while subject is supine and then repeated measurements are made at 60° head-up tilt position. Pulse rate and plasma noradrenaline responses to standing. Lower body negative pressure is an alternative to standing
2. Deep breathing: presence or absence of sinus arrhythmia; test of vagal efferent pathway
3. Carotid sinus massage: right and left sides, in turn monitoring cardiac rate and blood pressure; test of vagal efferent pathway. Caution in case of supersensitivity
4. Hyperventilation: for 30 s, causing hypocapnia and fall in blood pressure; response suggests afferent lesion, if baroreflex block
5. Inspiratory gasp: causing reflex vasoconstriction of hands; spinal-cord reflex
6. Stress: causing hypertension and tachycardia; tests of sympathetic efferent pathway.
(a) handgrip, submaximal sustained for 90 s;
(b) sudden cortical arousal by unexpected noise;
(c) mental arithmetic (rapid serial subtraction of 7 from 100);
(d) cold pressor test—hand immersed in water at 4°C for 90 s
7. Breath-holding: test of central breathing control; prolonged if vagal afferent dysfunction
8. Valsalva manoeuvre: after a deep inspiration the patient performs a forced expiration for 12 s through a tube connected to a mercury manometer. Most subjects can maintain a pressure of 30 mmHg. In normal subjects there is an increasing tachycardia for the 10 s of sustained forced expiration. Blood pressure falls initially but should cease to fall after the first few seconds if peripheral sympathetic vasoconstriction is normal. On release from blowing there is normally a blood pressure overshoot and a compensatory reflex bradycardia
9. Pharmacological tests:
(a) plasma noradrenaline at rest and after 30 min standing or tilt;
(b) pressor response and cardiac slowing to infusion of noradrenaline (or phenylephrine) test of baroreflex sensitivity;
(c) pressor response and noradrenaline response to infusion of tyramine; test of cytoplasmic stores of noradrenaline;
(d) cardiac slowing to atropine; test of vagal function
Sweating
1. Response to body heating in order to cause a rise of 1°C oral or rectal temperature in the course of 90 min. Record sweating and measure hand blood-flow. Test of sympathetic pathway from hypothalamus to periphery
2. Response to brief trunk heating with electric lamp source for 90 s; a reflex response, without involving change of blood temperature, utilizing same efferent pathway as response to body heating
3. Responses to intramuscular pilocarpine; acts directly on sweat glands
4. Pilomotor and sudomotor response to intradermal methacholine; absent with complete postganglionic lesion
Pupillary responses
1. Instillation of 1:1000 adrenaline. Response: dilation after sympathetic postganglionic denervation; no effect on normal pupil
2. Instillation of fresh 2.5 per cent cocaine. Response: dilation of normal pupil; no effect after sympathetic denervation
3. Instillation of fresh 2.5 per cent methacholine. Response: constriction after parasympathetic denervation; no effect on normal pupil
Skin response
Intracutaneous injection of 0.05 ml of 1 1000 histamine phosphate causes a wheal surrounded by erythema and erythematous flare. The flare of this triple response is an axon reflex mediated by antidromic transmission along sensory fibres

Treatment of primary autonomic failure syndromes

Orthostatic hypotension

On lying flat overnight, patients with autonomic failure lose more sodium and fluid than does a normal individual. Almost all patients with postural hypotension due to any form of autonomic failure can be helped by the head-up bed tilt at night. Once patients have experienced the benefits they will usually be ready to tolerate the degree of discomfort this may entail. Intranasal insufflation of deamino-D-arginine vasopressin (**DDAVP**) can be used to prevent nocturnal fluid loss in these patients, as an alternative to head-up tilt, but as the patients are very sensitive to DDAVP a low dose must be given (from 5 to 40 μg at bedtime), initially in hospital, in order to ensure that hyponatraemia does not occur.

A second line of treatment that is usually helpful is the use of fludrocortisone. In a smaller dose (0.1 mg) than necessary to increase blood volume, fludrocortisone appears to increase the sensitivity of blood vessels to very small amounts of noradrenaline, which may still be capable of being released in autonomic failure. The use of external support of the leg and trunk with elastic garments or an 'antigravity suit' is unphysiological in that it reduces intrinsic myogenic tone and is rarely of much long-term benefit.

There have been many pressor drugs studied in autonomic failure, but they rarely improve the patient's standing blood pressure.

Postprandial hypotension

The therapeutic approaches to this disabling symptom include taking smaller meals, more frequent meals, less carbohydrate, and avoiding alcohol. A drug effective in preventing postcibal hypotension in autonomic failure is the somatostatin analogue, octreotide. For practical management an orally acting analogue is needed.

Further reading

Bannister, R. and Mathias, C.J. (ed.) (1992). *Autonomic failure: a textbook of clinical disorders of the autonomic nervous system*, 3rd edn. Oxford University Press, Oxford.

Ecberg, D.L. (1997). Baroreflexes and the failing human heart. *Circulation*, **96**, 4133–7.

Kaufmann, H. (1998). Multiple system atrophy. *Current Opinion in Neurology*, **11**, 351–5.

Low, P.A. (1998). Autonomic neuropathies. *Current Opinion in Neurology*, **11**, 531–7.

Polinsky, R.J. (1996). Biochemical and pharmacologic assessment of autonomic function. *Advances in Neurology*, **69**, 373–6.

Chapter 13.8

Spinal cord

W. B. Matthews

Anatomy

The spinal cord extends from the foramen magnum to the lower border of the first lumbar vertebra, being enclosed by the arachnoid membrane and the dura mater, both of which extend below the termination of the cord into the sacral canal. The blood supply consists of a posterior system supplying the posterior columns and posterior grey matter, and an anterior system supplying the remainder, including the corticospinal tracts, spinothalamic tracts, and anterior horns of grey matter, separate branches supplying the right and left sides. The most constant contributions to the anterior spinal artery are from the vertebral arteries and the arteria magna of Adamkiewicz that arises from the tenth left intercostal artery, but even these are subject to much variation and radicular arteries may enter the spinal system at any level.

The main motor and sensory pathways in the spinal cord are described in Chapter 13.10.

Knowledge of the spinal segments concerned in the reflex arcs of the tendon jerks and cutaneous reflexes commonly elicited in clinical practice is of some assistance in the localization of spinal cord lesions. Some individual variation and spread beyond a single segment must be expected, but in general the pattern is as detailed in Chapter 13.10. A reflex cannot be obtained if the arc is interrupted by disease of the relevant segment of the spinal cord.

From such anatomical approximations it is possible to identify the level and extent of spinal cord lesions. A lesion of the conus medullaris will cause weakness and wasting only of the muscles supplied by the lower sacral segments, mainly the glutei. Sensory loss involves the buttocks and perineum. The anus is patulous and the reflex contraction of the sphincter normally induced by pricking the neighbouring skin is absent. There is no sensation of fullness of the bladder or desire to empty the rectum, and reflex evacuation is also impaired, resulting in a large, atonic bladder with overflow incontinence. Sexual function in the male is lost.

A complete transverse lesion of the dorsal cord results in spastic paralysis and loss of all forms of sensation below the level of the segment involved. With partial lesions both motor and sensory deficits are incomplete and, in particular, it is sometimes possible to detect that the major impact is on one side of the cord, producing some elements of the Brown–Séquard syndrome of hemisection of the cord; this consists of spastic weakness on the side of the lesion and loss of pain and thermal sensation on the opposite side, while light touch is little disturbed. A unilateral level, below which some modes of sensation are lost, is often several segments below the level of cord injury.

A lesion of the lower part of the cervical enlargement causes wasting of the hand muscles; a discrete lesion at the sixth cervical segment results in lower motor paralysis of flexion at the elbow and abolition of the biceps and supinator tendon jerks, with spastic weakness below this level. A complete lesion of the lower cervical cord causes respiratory embarrassment from paralysis of the muscles of the chest wall, while a similar lesion above the fourth cervical segment, the main origin of the phrenic nerves, is incompatible with life without artificial ventilation.

A complete lesion of the cord at any level causes retention of urine with eventual overflow. Incomplete lesions may cause loss of the normal synergy between contraction of the bladder detrusor and relaxation of the sphincter, with resulting urgency and incontinence.

Non-traumatic paraplegia

Acute and subacute

The patient with sudden or rapidly advancing weakness of the lower limbs presents an urgent problem of diagnosis and management. The presumption is that there is a focal lesion of the spinal cord but other causes such as poliomyelitis and acute polyneuritis, the Guillain–Barré syndrome, must not be forgotten. Confusion is possible, as with an acute lesion of the spinal cord the paralysis may be flaccid, the tendon reflexes absent, and the plantar reflexes unobtainable. A sensory level on the trunk is strong evidence of a spinal cord lesion. Localized back pain is common in all forms of acute paraplegia but less so in multiple sclerosis.

Intrinsic lesions

Non-compressive causes of acute myelopathy include multiple sclerosis, acute disseminated encephalomyelitis, viral infection, systemic lupus, Behçet's disease, sarcoidosis, paraneoplastic syndrome, and infarction.

All except multiple sclerosis and acute postinfective demyelinating or necrotic transverse myelitis are extremely rare causes of acute paraplegia. A complete transverse lesion of the cord is more likely to be due to an isolated episode of myelitis than multiple sclerosis, where the lesion is usually incomplete.

Spinal cord compression

In acute paraplegia the following causes of cord compression must be considered: epidural abscess, epidural haemorrhage, cervical spondylotic myelopathy, spontaneous dislocation of the cervical vertebrae in rheumatoid arthritis, arachnoiditis, benign tumour, metastatic tumour, and arteriovenous malformation. Benign tumours and cervical spondylotic myelopathy much more commonly cause chronic progressive paraplegia but may cause acute paralysis following quite minor trauma.

Management

Urinary retention must be relieved. The level of the lesion must be determined by clinical means. The examination must naturally include a search for possible sources of metastatic lesions or infection.

Lumbar puncture solely for the purpose of examining the cerebrospinal fluid should not be done, as any changes found will not be specific and altering the intrathecal pressure below a tumour of the spinal cord may precipitate severe paralysis. If the responsible lesion cannot be shown by radiography, CT scanning, or MRI, and compression of the cord is still suspected, then the risk must be taken and a myelogram carried out.

Chronic progressive paraparesis

Here again the important distinction is between compression of the spinal cord and intrinsic lesions. Among the latter, the progressive spinal form of multiple sclerosis is by far the most frequent cause in geographical areas where this disease is common. Other intrinsic diseases that may present in this way include motor neurone disease, hereditary spastic paraplegia, tropical spastic paraplegia, and AIDS myelopathy. The distinctive features of subacute combined degeneration and syringomyelia should prevent diagnostic confusion.

Chronic compression of the spinal cord is commonly due to benign causes: cervical spondylotic myelopathy, prolapsed dorsal disc, neurofibroma, meningioma, and arteriovenous malformations. Malignant causes include myeloma, chordoma, and glioma.

Clinical features of progressive cord compression

Sensory symptoms usually precede weakness and may be misinterpreted. Root pain is easily recognizable in the cervical region, but when thoracic roots are involved visceral pain may be mimicked. Cutaneous sensory loss due to involvement of the spinothalamic tracts may show 'sacral sparing' as lamination of fibres in the tract allows those from lower segments to escape, but this sign is not diagnostic of cord compression.

Motor involvement is usually asymmetrical and, with a cervical cord lesion, classically affects the arm on the side of the lesion, then the ipsilateral leg, the other leg, and eventually the contralateral arm. The degree of sphincter involvement is highly variable.

Investigation

To misdiagnose a benign cause of cord compression as multiple sclerosis is a potentially disastrous error. Abnormal visual-evoked potentials provide strong, but not wholly conclusive, evidence of relevant lesions beyond the spinal cord, which may be more decisively shown by MRI of the head. Plain radiographs should not be neglected, including oblique views of the cervical spine where relevant. MRI of the spinal cord is replacing the need for myelography in many cases. Any cerebrospinal fluid obtained should be sent for analysis, including examination for oligoclonal banding of IgG, characteristically present in multiple sclerosis.

Subacute combined degeneration of the spinal cord

This is the most common and most serious neurological complication of the deficiency of vitamin B_{12}. The patients are predominantly middle aged or older. The first symptom is always symmetrical paraesthesias in the extremities, usually initially in the feet but occasionally confined to the hands. The sensations are often extremely unpleasant. Loss of postural sense causes ataxia in walking and, unless forestalled by treatment, the legs become weak. Examination in the early stages shows distal cutaneous sensory blunting but often severe loss of postural sense in the lower limbs. The ankle jerks may be absent and, at a later stage, the plantar reflexes are extensor.

Other neurological effects of vitamin B_{12} deficiency may be present, most commonly moderate loss of mental acuity. Visual impairment, the result of bilateral centrocaecal scotomas, is rare.

Clinical evidence of anaemia may be obvious or entirely lacking. The peripheral blood may be normal and the bone marrow is not always megaloblastic. The serum vitamin B_{12} is, however, almost always significantly reduced.

Hydroxocobalamin, 1 mg, should be injected immediately, and 1 mg repeated daily for a week and thereafter weekly for several weeks before adopting a monthly schedule that must be continued indefinitely to avoid relapse. The response to treatment is, in general, excellent. Even bedridden patients can be restored to normal walking, and extensor plantar reflexes revert to flexor. Beyond a certain point of disability, however, treatment is unavailing, presumably because of axonal degeneration, but this should now never be allowed to occur.

Syringomyelia

The essential lesion implied by this name is the presence of a cavity within the spinal cord. The spinal cord contains an irregular asymmetrical cavity, filled with cerebrospinal fluid, extending over many segments, or even its entire length, although usually most extensive in the cervical enlargement. Contiguous structures are destroyed, in particular the anterior horn cells, the sensory fibres decussating within the cord concerned with pain and thermal sensation, and the lateral corticospinal tracts. The syrinx may extend into the medulla.

The abnormality in the spinal cord is frequently accompanied by a congenital abnormality known as type I Chiari malformation, in which aberrant cerebellar tissue extends into the cervical spinal canal. Some degree of hydrocephalus is also often present.

The onset of symptoms is usually in early adult life. The first symptoms usually involve one upper limb, with a combination of wasting of the hand muscles, weakness, and sensory loss, often resulting in painless burns, either from cigarettes or from cooking. Wasting is more extensive than could be accounted for by any single, peripheral nerve lesion and is accompanied by loss of tendon reflexes in the arm. Sensory loss, classically of 'dissociated' type with preservation of light touch and proprioception but loss of pain and thermal sensation, often extends over the whole arm and upper thorax or may be bilateral over the 'cape area'. Scars of painless injuries may provide a diagnostic clue. A Horner's syndrome, or excessive sweating over one side of the face, may indicate involvement of the cervical sympathetic nerve. A mild dorsal scoliosis is almost invariable.

Although the onset is usually insidious, sudden exacerbations are common, particularly after exertion, coughing, or sneezing. The symptoms and signs may sometimes remain unchanged for many years but syringomyelia is usually progressive.

Involvement of the medulla, syringobulbia, may occur without evidence of disease of the spinal cord or, more commonly, as an extension of syringomyelia. The usual pattern of sensory loss includes the peripheral areas of the face, with sparing of the nose and mouth. Damage to the motor nuclei of the lower cranial nerves causes wasting of the tongue, dysphagia, and paralysis of the vocal cords. Rotatory nystagmus is common.

The diagnosis of syringomyelia, its extent, and causation can now be fully displayed by MRI or, less easily, by myelography and CT scanning. Such investigations are essential for the planning of surgical treatment directed to the relief of obstruction to the flow of cerebrospinal fluid or the draining of the syrinx. The former involves decompression of the posterior fossa and cervical canal. Many ingenious operations have been devised to relieve pressure within the cyst. Surgery is not always indicated and is not always successful, but should certainly be considered when disease is progressive but not yet severely disabling, or when pain is severe. Syringomyelia secondary to arachnoiditis is particularly intractable.

Vascular disease

The arteries that supply the spinal cord are not subject to atherosclerosis and ischaemic disease results from more remote causes. Infarction of the spinal cord may result from atheroma or dissecting aneurysm of the aorta, aortic or cardiac surgery, and severe hypotension following cardiac arrest or infarction. A main feeding vessel commonly arises from the tenth left intercostal artery and surgery in this area can be hazardous. Acute pain at the site of the lesion often occurs at the onset. Paraplegia develops very rapidly and, as the infarct is usually confined to the distribution of the anterior spinal artery, sensory loss is confined to those modalities conveyed in the spinothalamic tracts, pain and thermal sensibility, with sparing of postural sense. A unilateral infarct results in the Brown–Séquard syndrome and occasionally the entire cord is infarcted below a segmental level.

Recovery from incomplete lesions is often unexpectedly good, but severe residual disability may also occur. Transient ischaemic attacks affecting the spinal cord occur rarely in arteriopathic individuals and cause paraplegia for an hour or less.

Radiation myelopathy

The spinal cord is vulnerable to damage from X-irradiation directed to structures in the neck. The incidence is low and is clearly dose related. Sensory symptoms in the limbs, often accompanied by Lhermitte's symptom of an electric-shock sensation down the spine on flexing the neck, occur soon after exposure and eventually remit.

Much more serious is delayed myelopathy, developing from 6 months to 5 years after treatment and resulting in severely disabling, progressive paraplegia. The prolonged latent period has not been adequately explained.

Myelitis

An acute transverse cord lesion may occur as an isolated event following viral infection or inoculation, or for no detectable reason. Investigation must exclude compression of the cord. The outcome varies from complete recovery to permanent paraplegia. A short course of high-dosage intravenous steroids should be given, but this is not always followed by recovery.

Apart from poliomyelitis, direct viral invasion of the spinal cord is uncommon, but myelitis from infection by the Epstein–Barr and herpes zoster viruses has been reported.

Spinal arachnoiditis

Chronic spinal arachnoiditis may present many years after acute meningitis, and other identifiable causes include subarachnoid haemorrhage, intrathecal steroids, and non-water-soluble contrast media previously used in myelography but now discarded. The presentation is that of slowly progressive paraplegia or the picture of syringomyelia. Surgical treatment is not effective as the arachnoiditis is usually diffuse.

Epidural haemorrhage

Haemorrhage into the epidural space is a complication of anticoagulant therapy. The cervical spine is the usual site and haemorrhage should be suspected as the cause of rapidly advancing tetraplegia in a patient on such treatment. Recovery following evacuation of the blood is usually complete.

Epidural abscess

An acute abscess in the spinal epidural space is usually the result of staphylococcal infection, either metastatic or by spread from some contiguous site. Progression of paraplegia is rapid and pain in the back is a constant feature. Fever and a raised white-cell count are common. The cerebrospinal fluid may contain an excess of cells but may be normal, and lumbar puncture does not assist diagnosis. Predisposing factors, apart from infection elsewhere, include diabetes, alcoholism, and any cause of immunodeficiency. MRI is the essential diagnostic procedure.

Unfortunately, even with rapid diagnosis and evacuation of the abscess, the prognosis for full recovery must be guarded. Non-surgical management with antibiotics alone has sometimes been successful.

Spinal cord tumours

In contrast to the brain, the majority of tumours of the spinal cord are extrinsic, and many are benign. The neurofibroma arises from the Schwann cells of the spinal roots at any level. It may be part of generalized neurofibromatosis but is usually single. Because of its site of origin, pain of root distribution is a common early symptom. The results of surgical removal, even when damage to the spinal cord appears to be severe, are remarkably successful and complete recovery is often achieved. The spinal meningioma cannot be distinguished on clinical grounds from a neurofibroma and the results of removal are equally good.

The most common malignant tumour compressing the cord is metastatic carcinoma, either involving the vertebral body or forming a dense band of meningeal infiltration. The best hope of mitigating the effects of this disaster lie with the immediate intravenous injection of large doses of dexamethasone, precise localization of the tumour, and radiotherapy. Laminectomy is seldom helpful but more radical attempts at removing the tumour may achieve temporary success.

Arteriovenous malformations

At the time of diagnosis these lesions consist of a tangled mass of veins containing arterial blood, nearly always on the dorsal surface of the cord, but sometimes involving the dura. The essential lesion, however, is of one or more arteriovenous shunts, presumably of congenital origin.

The clinical presentation is varied. A spinal subarachnoid haemorrhage causes sudden severe pain in the back with signs of meningeal irritation and even loss of consciousness.

More commonly the onset is with paraparesis, often progressive in a stepwise manner, or fluctuating with considerable remissions. Diagnostic confusion may arise, particularly as the symptoms may relapse in pregnancy with subsequent remission, in a pattern shared by meningiomas and often erroneously thought to be typical of multiple sclerosis.

Confirmation of the diagnosis and localization of the vascular shunts prior to treatment by surgery or embolization require expert and elaborate neuroradiology.

Cervical spondylotic myelopathy

Spondylosis and cord damage due to disc prolapse are discussed in Chapter 13.10.

Further reading

Berman, M., Feldmann, S., Alter M., Zilber, N., and Kahana, E. (1981). Acute transverse myelitis: incidence and aetiologic considerations. *Neurology*, **31**, 966–71.

Bindal, A.K., Dunsker, S.B., and Tew, J.M. (1995). Chiari I malformation: classification and management. *Neurosurgery*, **37**, 1069–74.

Byrne, T.N. (1992). Spinal cord compression from epidural metastases. *New England Journal of Medicine*, **327**, 614–19.

Esses, S.I. and Morley, T.P. (1983). Spinal arachnoiditis. *Canadian Journal of Neurological Sciences*, **10**, 2–10.

Mariani, C., *et al.* (1991) The natural history and results of surgery in 50 cases of syringomyelia. *Journal of Neurology*, **238**, 433–8.

Sandson, T.A. and Friedman, J.H. (1989). Spinal cord infarction: report of 8 cases and review of the literature. *Medicine*, **68**, 282–92.

Chapter 13.9

The management of spinal cord injury

D. J. Grundy

Traumatic spinal cord injury

Eighty per cent of spinal cord injuries occur in males. Approximately 40 per cent are due to road-traffic accidents and 35 per cent to domestic and industrial injuries, particularly falls down stairs and from ladders or scaffolding. Sporting accidents, such as those occurring from diving into shallow water, rugby, horse riding, and gymnastics, account for about 20 per cent of injuries.

One study has shown that the median survival time following traumatic injury to the spinal cord for all patients surviving the first year of injury was 32 years. It was greater for those with incomplete lesions and those with low injuries. The causes of death, particularly in incomplete lesions, have moved away from the traditional causes related to spinal cord injury, such as renal failure, and have begun to approximate to those in the general population. The figures showed that 24 per cent of patients died of urinary-tract complications, 23 per cent of cardiovascular causes, and there were 14 per cent respiratory deaths, the last being more prevalent in tetraplegic patients.

Initial management at the scene of injury

A casualty with suspected injury to the spinal cord must be correctly handled if further neurological damage is not to occur. Unfortunately, some patients (5 to 19 per cent in different series) deteriorate neurologically from the time of injury to the time of admission to a spinal injuries unit because of missed or delayed diagnosis, or inadequate spinal immobilization.

Spinal injury will be suggested by local marking, bruising, or deformity. For example, grazes or lacerations to the face infer that the head was forced backwards, resulting in a cervical hyperextension injury.

The conscious patient with cord damage may complain of neck or back pain, disturbance or loss of sensation, and weakness or flaccid paralysis below a neurological level. In high lesions, diaphragmatic respiration due to intercostal paralysis occurs; in ultrahigh lesions with involvement of the phrenic nerve, assisted ventilation may be necessary from the outset. Sympathetic paralysis in the tetraplegic or high-paraplegic patient results in hypotension, bradycardia, and, commonly, priapism.

Having confirmed that the airway is secure, intravenous access is established in case cardiopulmonary support is required. Clearing the airways of secretions may cause intense bradycardia and, occasionally, cardiac arrest owing to unopposed vagal action, particularly in hypoxic patients. To minimize this risk, the heart rate must be monitored, and atropine and additional oxygen administered prior to pharyngeal suction.

If the casualty is unconscious, it must be assumed, until radiographs of the whole cervical spine are obtained, that the force rendering them unconscious has also injured the cervical spine. The head and neck are stabilized in neutral with a rigid collar, and the trunk must not be flexed or rotated in case a thoracolumbar injury is present.

The unconscious patient is at risk of aspirating vomit. Orotracheal intubation is relatively safe if an assistant holds the head and minimizes neck movement. The other method of protecting the airway is to 'log-roll' the patient into a modified lateral position, about 70–80° from prone, with the head supported in neutral, taking great care not to rotate the spine.

Associated injuries

Almost 50 per cent of patients have other injuries, particularly to the head, chest, and limbs. Thoracic spinal injuries are often associated with multiple rib fractures, haemothorax, pneumothorax, and lung contusion, which further compromise respiration and require urgent treatment.

Spinal shock

The stage of flaccidity with absent reflexes below the level of the lesion—the period of spinal shock—persists for a few hours to several weeks after injury. If the injury has been above the sacral segments of the cord, the end of spinal shock is denoted by a return of reflex activity below the level of the lesion. The anal and bulbocavernosus reflexes usually return first, followed by the lower limb reflexes. In injuries to the conus medullaris or cauda equina, the reflexes do not return. The plantar response is not always reliable in the diagnosis of acute injury to the spinal cord.

Transfer to hospital

A spinal immobilizer and extrication devices help to protect the spine during evacuation and transportation to the nearest major accident and emergency department.

Tetraplegic and high-paraplegic patients are poikilothermic because sympathetic paralysis results in loss of the usual vasomotor responses to temperature change. Blankets and thermal reflector sheets should therefore be used in cold weather to prevent hypothermia.

Most casualties will be taken to the nearest accident and emergency department but the regional spinal injuries unit should also be contacted.

Initial management at hospital (Table 1)

Respiratory function is assessed urgently to detect paralysis of respiratory muscles and complications of chest injury, such as a pneumothorax or haemothorax, which may require an intercostal drain.

Arterial blood gases and vital capacity are measured, and measurements repeated as necessary. The diagnosis of intra-abdominal injury is difficult in high lesions because of absent abdominal sensation and loss of the usual signs of peritoneal irritation—tenderness, guarding, or rigidity. If necessary, diagnostic peritoneal lavage should be performed. Intravenous fluids are continued, but oral fluids are withheld for at least 48 h after injury until normal bowel sounds return. A proton-pump inhibitor given for 3 weeks minimizes the risk of stress ulceration. High-dose methylprednisolone probably has some neuroprotective benefit if given early enough after the injury.

Radiology

After initial clinical assessment and appropriate resuscitative measures to stabilize the patient, spinal radiographs and a chest radiograph are taken under medical supervision. In injuries of the cervical spine, lateral, anteroposterior, and an open-mouth view of the odontoid process are necessary. The lateral view is the most important and does not involve moving the patient. The shoulders often obscure the lower cervical spine but careful traction on the arms to depress the shoulders should demonstrate the cervicothoracic junction.

In children, injury to the spinal cord often occurs without radiological signs of bony damage. Similarly, in older people with cervical spondylosis, a relatively minor hyperextension injury such as a fall on to the face or forehead may produce tetraplegia without evidence of bony injury.

In the thoracic and lumbar spine, anteroposterior and lateral radiographs are taken, but satisfactory views of the upper thoracic spine may be impossible without CT, which gives excellent detail of the vertebral column, and demonstrates bony fragments in the spinal canal. MRI is the investigation of choice to visualize the spinal cord and demonstrate soft-tissue causes of cord compression, such as disc prolapse or haematoma.

Table 1 Initial assessment of a patient with a suspected spinal cord injury

Resuscitation	1. Secure airway and ensure adequate oxygenation	Signs of chest injury: rib fractures haemothorax, pneumothorax, lung contusion
	2. Assess breathing	Diaphragmatic respiration in tetraplegia Variable intercostal muscle paralysis, according to level, in thoracic lesions
	3. Provide circulatory support if necessary	Signs of autonomic paralysis (hypotension, bradycardia) Blood loss from associated injuries
History		
Details of accident		
Neck or back pain		
Numbness or paralysis		
If unconscious, assume spinal cord injury until proved otherwise		
Examination		
Inspect for grazes or lacerations (suggesting mode of injury)		
Inspect for defomiity or bruising over spine		
Palpate for tenderness and irregularity over spine		
Determine sensory and motor levels, muscle tone and reflexes		
Exclude other injuries		
head, chest, limbs (common)		
intra-abdominal (uncommon)		
Investigations		
Vital signs		
Vital capacity		
Arterial blood gases and oxygen saturation by pulse oximetry		
Chest and spinal radiographs		
Urine testing		

Management of the spinal injury

The cervical spine

Dislocations can usually be reduced by applying skull callipers and gradually increasing the traction force under radiographic control with the neck in flexion until the facets are disengaged, at which stage the neck is extended and the weights reduced to a maintenance level to splint the spine. Skull traction is continued for 6 to 8 weeks, depending on radiographic evidence of healing. However, if there are no contraindications to early mobilization, halo traction followed by conversion to a halo brace is more appropriate. Spinal fusion is particularly indicated in unstable injuries, or if the lesion of the spinal cord is incomplete.

Thoracic and lumbar injuries

Thoracic and lumbar spine injuries can often be treated conservatively by 'postural reduction', placing a pillow under the lumbar spine to restore and maintain the normal lumbar lordosis. Usually after 8 weeks' bed rest, the patient is mobilized in a spinal brace. However, early surgical stabilization is often performed in lower thoracic and lumbar injuries to allow early mobilization.

Patterns of incomplete spinal cord injury

Neurological recovery is more likely in an incomplete lesion of the spinal cord. The most common incomplete pattern is the anterior cord syndrome, which follows a flexion–rotation or compression force to the spine with dislocation or compression fracture of the vertebral body and damage to the anterior part of the spinal cord, and also often to the anterior spinal artery. The resulting injury to the corticospinal and spinothalamic tracts produces loss of power, pain, and temperature sensation below the lesion.

Respiratory complications

Respiratory complications are common, particularly in tetraplegic patients who have paralysed abdominal and intercostal muscles with diaphragmatic respiration. As the phrenic nerve nucleus arises from the C3 to C5 segments there may be varying degrees of diaphragmatic function, depending on the level of tetraplegia. Furthermore, the neurological level often rises by a spinal segment within the first 48 h of injury, due to oedema of the cord; this can result in an early deterioration in respiratory function and the need for respiratory support. The reduced respiratory muscle reserve also makes respiratory failure due to muscle fatigue more likely. Abdominal distension due to paralytic ileus must be avoided, otherwise the diaphragm is splinted and respiratory failure may be precipitated.

The inability to cough effectively can quickly result in sputum retention and atelectasis, followed by chest infection. Ventilation–perfusion mismatch occurs, with further respiratory impairment.

Assisted ventilation

The use of a biphasic ventilatory-support system, providing preset positive pressures in inspiration and expiration, reduces the work of breathing and increases the functional residual capacity. It provides respiratory support and may prevent the need for full ventilation, particularly in patients with weak inspiratory muscles, who have a tendency to atelectasis.

Long-term ventilation

An increasing proportion of people with ultrahigh cord lesions are being successfully resuscitated at the scene of accident. Some will have complete paralysis of the phrenic nerve and require long-term ventilation. A battery-driven ventilator may be attached to an electrically driven wheelchair to enable the patient to have a degree of independence and mobility during the day. Domiciliary ventilation is being increasingly practised. Diaphragmatic pacing is also possible if the phrenic nerve nucleus is intact and the phrenic nerve is stimulable.

Cardiovascular complications

Paralysis of the sympathetic thoracolumbar (T1–L2) outflow, seen in high cord injuries, results in hypotension. It also results in unopposed vagal action and the risks of bradycardia and cardiac arrest previously mentioned.

Postural hypotension is often a problem when first mobilizing a tetraplegic patient. Graduated elastic stockings and an abdominal binder help to reduce peripheral pooling. If postural hypotension still occurs, 15 to 30 mg ephedrine, administered 20 min before mobilizing, is helpful.

The use of a depolarizing muscle relaxant such as suxamethonium must be avoided from 3 days to 9 months after spinal cord injury, as it can produce sudden hyperkalaemia with a risk of cardiac arrest. If muscle relaxation is required for endotracheal intubation, the non-depolarizing muscle relaxant pancuronium is safe.

Autonomic dysreflexia

Following spinal shock, patients with cord lesions at T6 and above may develop autonomic dysreflexia, a condition caused by uncontrolled reflex sympathetic activity below the level of the lesion. The precipitating factor is usually bladder distension, due to a blocked catheter or poor bladder emptying. The response via the vasomotor centre increases vagal tone with bradycardia, but peripheral vasodilation is not possible because stimuli cannot pass distally through the injured cord. The hypertension is, therefore, unrelieved. The patient complains of headache, sweating, and flushing above the level of the spinal cord lesion. Without urgent treatment, intracranial haemorrhage may occur. The patient is sat up, the precipitating cause treated, and 5 to 10 mg nifedipine given sublingually if necessary. In rare instances parenteral therapy, for example 5 to 10 mg phentolamine intravenously, is required.

Thromboembolic complications

The incidence of deep venous thrombosis following severe injury to the spinal cord is over 90 per cent, and pulmonary embolism is the most common cause of death in patients who survive the period immediately following cord injury. Anticoagulants should, therefore, be commenced within 24 to 36 h of the accident, initially using low molecular-weight heparin, followed by full anticoagulation with warfarin, unless there are contraindications such as head and chest injuries.

Management of the urinary tract

The acute stage

During the stage of spinal shock the bladder is acontractile; without treatment, retention with overflow occurs. Most patients with upper motor-neurone cord lesions subsequently develop reflex detrusor activity, but in patients with lower motor-neurone lesions, the bladder will remain acontractile.

In patients with multiple injuries, indwelling urethral catheterization is essential for accurate monitoring of the urinary output. Suprapubic catheterization has the advantages of indwelling urethral catheterization without the risk of urethral damage, and with less risk of prostatitis and epididymo-orchitis. In addition, the catheter can be clamped at intervals to see whether voiding occurs. However, intermittent urethral catheterization is the standard method of early bladder management in many spinal injuries units.

Renal ultrasonography, plain abdominal radiography, and video urodynamic investigations are normally performed about 3 months after injury. Video urodynamics (a study of the pressure–volume relations in the bladder during slow filling and voiding) will detect early detrusor–sphincter dyssynergia before renal damage occurs. Further urological follow-up is done with renal ultrasound and plain abdominal radiography.

Long-term bladder management

Several options are available. Although achieving continence may be desired, the main aim is always to preserve renal function.

Most male patients with reflex bladder emptying manage their bladders by condom drainage, but one-third require an endoscopic distal urethral sphincterotomy to achieve satisfactory bladder emptying.

Patients with a non-contractile detrusor are particularly suitable for intermittent self-catheterization, usually performed 6 hourly once the patient is able to sit up. The ideal is to attain continence between catheterizations. In patients with reflex detrusor activity, anticholinergic drugs such as oxybutynin may be required to achieve this by reducing detrusor activity; tricyclic antidepressants such as imipramine also help by increasing bladder-outlet resistance, as well as by reducing detrusor activity. Long-term results of intermittent self-catheterization compare favourably with other methods of bladder management.

Suprapubic urethral catheterization is convenient in tetraplegic women unable to perform self-catheterization, and in elderly or frail individuals.

Some patients with reflex detrusor activity are suitable for a sacral anterior nerve-root stimulator. This is a radiolinked implant attached to the anterior nerve roots of S2, S3, and S4. Division of the posterior sacral nerve roots as part of the procedure increases bladder compliance, and abolishes reflex detrusor activity and detrusor–sphincter dyssynergia. Bladder emptying using the implant is usually efficient, with a diminished risk of urinary-tract infections and a likelihood of achieving continence.

Bowel care

Immediately after injury to the spinal cord the lower bowel is flaccid, but a gentle manual evacuation is usually performed after 48 to 72 h and continued daily or on alternate days during the period of bed rest. In upper motor-neurone cord lesions, reflex bowel emptying usually occurs following the insertion of glycerine suppositories or digital stimulation. Management of patients with lower motor-neurone lesions is usually more problematical; suppositories are ineffective and manual evacuation, possibly associated with straining using the abdominal muscles, will be required. A high-fibre diet is advisable.

Care of the joints and limbs

The paralysed joints must be passively moved daily to maintain a full range of movement and prevent contractures, and paralysed hands should be splinted in the position of function. To prevent shoulder pain and stiffness in tetraplegic patients, the arm positions should be changed when the patient is turned.

Care of the pressure areas

An understanding of safe methods of relieving pressure is essential if further neurological damage, pressure sores, and joint contractures are to be avoided. Initially, the patient should be turned 2 hourly, usually increasing to 3 hourly after a few days if the skin has not marked on 2-hourly turns.

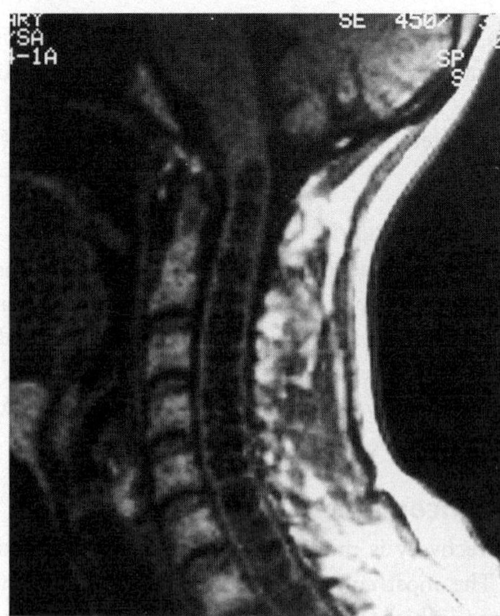

Fig. 1 Multilocular syrinx extending from the site of fracture at T4 to the foramen magnum. The patient had loss of pin-prick over the left C3 to T1 dermatomes, but no upper limb weakness.

Patients must be warned of the risks of sensory loss and, once mobilized into a wheelchair, they need to inspect their skin regularly, particularly over bony prominences such as the ischial, trochanteric, and sacral regions, the heels, and malleoli. In patients with established paralysis of the spinal cord, ischial sores may occur due to excessive interface pressures between the ischial tuberosities and the wheelchair cushion. Patients must be taught to lift in the wheelchair every 15 min, if possible. If patients cannot lift, a specialized cushion should be supplied that allows them to sit in the wheelchair, ideally all day, without producing a red mark on the skin. Trochanteric sores are particularly seen in people who sleep on their side and are not adequately turned at night.

Spasticity

Spasticity in upper motor-neurone cord injuries is often more pronounced in incomplete lesions, and in the presence of irritative foci, such as pressure sores, urinary-tract infections, and calculi. Although spasticity maintains muscle bulk, an excessive degree can reduce mobility.

Regular use of a standing frame relieves spasticity and prevents contractures. Spasticity can also be relieved by baclofen and dantrolene sodium, or in resistant cases by motor-point injections, local nerve blocks, or neurectomy, for example by obturator neurectomy in severe spasticity of hip abductors. Intrathecal baclofen administered by an implanted reservoir and pump is effective.

Post-traumatic syringomyelia (Fig. 1)

Occurring in at least 4 per cent of patients following spinal cord injury, the common presenting symptoms are unilateral pain and numbness in the arm with a dissociated sensory loss. Although symptoms may appear a few weeks after injury, they can be delayed for several years. Diagnosis is confirmed by MRI. Surgical treatment by decompression and/or shunting usually relieves the pain, but relief of sensory and motor loss is less predictable.

Psychological and social factors

The psychological trauma of spinal cord injury is huge. In high cord lesions, fear and anxiety is exacerbated by sensory deprivation. Wide mood swings, including anger, depression, and behaviour identifiable with the normal grieving process, are common. Long-term decisions must be taken with full participation of the patient if successful rehabilitation is to be achieved. Most patients wish to return home and many severely disabled people achieve this goal.

Pain

Pain at or below the level of the neurological lesion is distressingly common, particularly in lesions of the cauda equina. It often begins a few weeks after injury, is frequently described as burning or stabbing, and may be continuous or intermittent.

Most patients respond to the distraction of a busy rehabilitation programme and treatment with tricyclic antidepressants or anticonvulsants. Transcutaneous nerve stimulation, acupuncture, hypnotherapy, and relaxation techniques may also help.

Sexual function

This is generally disturbed unless the cord lesion is very incomplete. Most men with upper motor-neurone lesions experience reflex erections, as the parasympathetic connections from S2 to S4 segments of the cord to the corpora cavernosa remain intact. The majority, however, will only ejaculate using artificial methods—by the application of a vibrator to the penis or by rectal electroejaculation.

As the S2 to S4 reflex arc is no longer intact in patients with lower motor-neurone lesions, reflex erections are lost, but psychogenic erections and emissions sometimes occur if the pelvic sympathetic fibres from the T11 to L2 segments (which form the hypogastric nerves) remain connected to higher centres.

In men who cannot otherwise attain erections sufficient for intercourse, sildenafil, intracavernous alprostadil, vacuum erection aids, and, rarely, penile implants are useful. The place of Viagra is yet to be determined. In women, fertility remains normal, but in lesions above T10 labour may be painless and forceps delivery may be required. In high lesions there is a risk of autonomic dysreflexia both during ejaculation and labour.

Non-traumatic causes of spinal cord paralysis

Infection of the vertebrae

Vertebral osteomyelitis

The onset of this relatively rare cause of spinal cord paralysis is often insidious, with low-grade fever, malaise, weight loss, and spinal pain. Radiographic changes of end-plate erosion followed by destruction of vertebral bodies may not be detected for 1–2 months after the onset of infection. It is therefore not surprising that diagnosis is often delayed.

Vertebral osteomyelitis is more common in males, and in patients with diabetes mellitus and rheumatoid arthritis. In recent years, intravenous drug abuse has become increasingly associated with the condition.

The source of infection is mainly the urinary and respiratory tracts, and soft-tissue infections; *Staphylococcus aureus* is the most common pathogen.

Needle aspiration or biopsy are performed to identify the causative organism and 6 to 8 weeks' parenteral antibiotic therapy given, but surgical decompression may also be required.

Tuberculous disease of the spine

This condition, 'Pott's paraplegia', is still a major cause of spinal cord paralysis in many parts of the world, but is now uncommon in Western countries, except in immigrant populations. Prompt administration of antituberculous drugs often results in a major degree of neurological recovery, and urgent surgical intervention is not often required. The condition is discussed in detail in Section 16.

Conclusions

Patients require lifelong follow-up, and continuing care and support in the community. Although their injuries have profound physical and emotional effects, it appears that learning to cope with disability gives them special qualities, and an increasing number are achieving independence, working, having children, and integrating back into society.

Further reading

Bracken, M.B., *et al.* (1997). Administration of methylprednisolone for 24 or 48 hours or tirolazad mesylate for 48 hours in the treatment of acute spinal cord injury: results of the Third National Acute Spinal Cord Injury Randomized Controlled Trial. *Journal of the American Medical Association*, 277, 1597–604.

Grundy, D. and Swain, A. (1993). *ABC of spinal injury*, 2nd edn. British Medical Journal, London.

Ravichandran, G. and Silver, J.R. (1982). Missed injuries of the spinal cord. *British Medical Journal*, **284**, 953–6.

Stover, S.L., DeLisa, J.A., and Whiteneck, G.G. (1995). *Spinal cord injury. Clinical outcomes from the model systems.* Aspen Publishers, Gaithersburg MD.

Chapter 13.10

Disorders of the spinal nerve roots

R. S. Maurice-Williams

Anatomy

Each segment of the spinal cord gives off a ventral (motor) and dorsal (sensory) root on each side. These unite in the intervertebral foramina to leave the spinal canal as mixed spinal roots. As the spinal cord ends at the lower border of the L1 vertebra, the lower spinal roots originate from the cord above their corresponding skeletal levels and run an increasingly oblique course before they reach their foramina. The spinal dura, enclosing the spinal subarachnoid space, extends to the middle of the sacral canal, and the leash of roots within it, together with the fibrous band (the filum terminale), which is the continuation of the tip of the cord, form the cauda equina.

There are eight cervical, twelve dorsal, five sacral, and one coccygeal pairs of roots. Each root has motor and sensory fibres, which at some levels subserve clinically important tendon reflexes. The roots supplying these are shown in Table 1. The sympathetic outflow leaves the cord via roots D1 to L1, while the caudal parasympathetic outflow is via roots S2 to S4. The area of skin whose sensation is supplied by

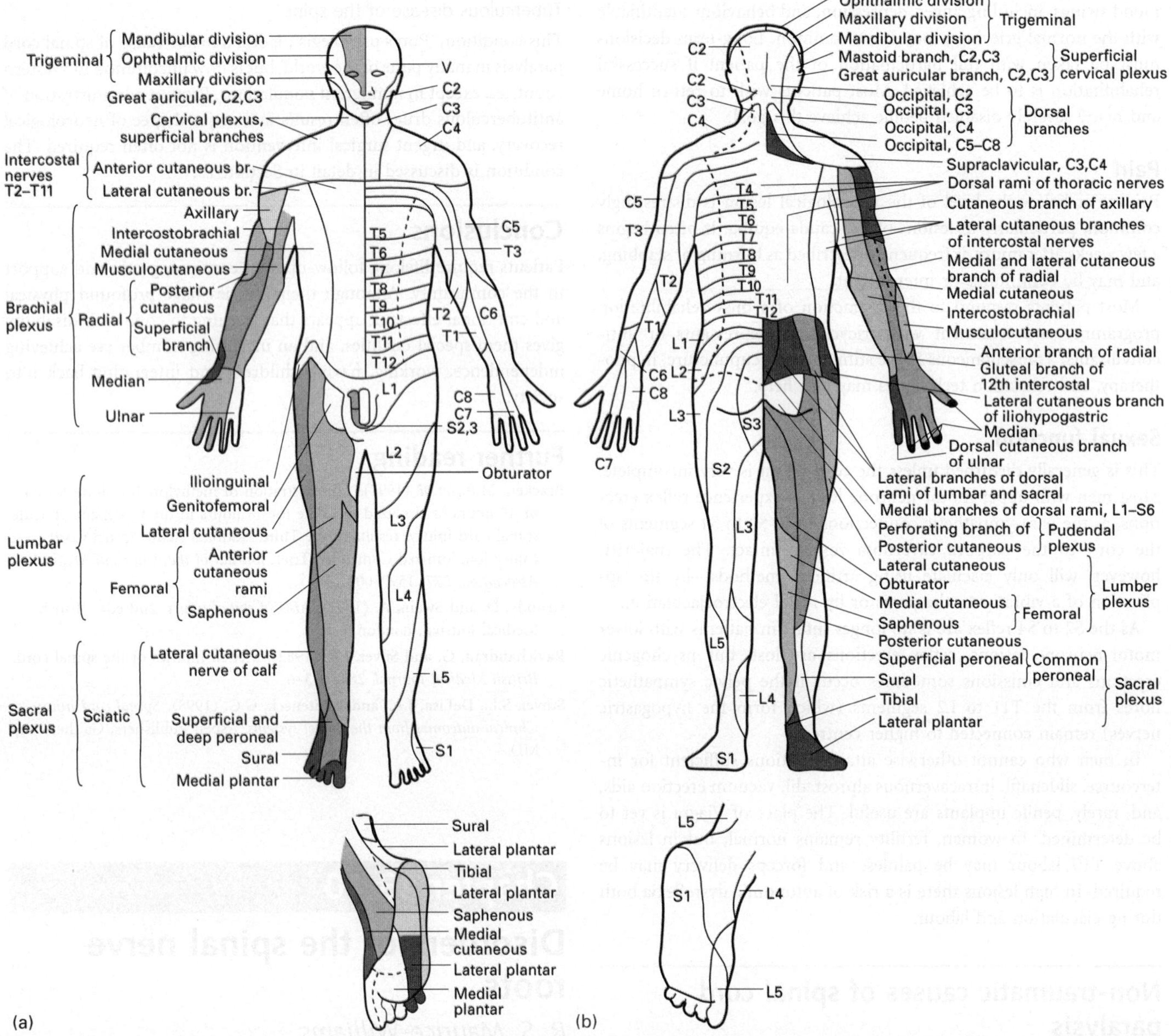

Fig. 1 (a) Cutaneous areas of distribution of spinal segments and the peripheral nerves: (a) anterior aspect; (b) posterior aspect *(reproduced from Bannister, R. (1992). Brain's clinical neurology, Oxford University Press, Oxford, with permission).*

a single root is known as a dermatome and the corresponding block of deep tissues is called a sclerotome. Figure 1 shows a dermatome map of the body. The first cervical root contains no cutaneous sensory fibres, so the C2 dermatome adjoins the area of skin supplied by the trigeminal nerve. The overlap of dermatomes and anatomical variation between individuals means that loss of a single root may give rise to a variable sensory loss that may not be detectable clinically. The main motor supply of the different roots is given in Table 2 in terms of movements. Again, there is some variation in anatomy between individuals so that precise localization of a root lesion on the basis of the pattern of motor loss may be difficult; this is especially so for roots C5–8.

Table 1 Roots involved in tendon reflexes

Reflex	Roots
Biceps jerk	Cervical 5–6
Supinator jerk	Cervical 5–6
Triceps jerk	Cervical 6–7
Finger jerk	Cervical 7–8
Knee jerk	Lumbar 2–4
Ankle jerk	Sacral 1–2

Root lesions

Effects

In addition to motor, sensory, and reflex loss, irritation or compression of a root may give rise to pain and paraesthesias in the sensory

Table 2 Main motor supply of roots

Root	Muscles
C1–4	Neck muscles (apart from spinal accessory supply to sternomastoid and trapezius) Longitudinal spinal muscles Diaphragm (C3–5, mainly C4)
C5	Shoulder abductors
C6	Elbow flexors
C7	Elbow extensors Wrist flexors/extensors
C8	Finger flexors and extensors
D1	Small hand muscles
D2–D12	Trunk muscles Longitudinal spinal muscles
L1	Hip flexors
L2	Hip flexors Hip abductors Knee extensors
L3	Knee extensors Hip flexors
L4	Knee extensors Ankle dorsiflexors Knee flexors Hip extensors
L5	Ankle dorsiflexors Dorsiflexor or hallux Hip extensors Knee flexors
S1	Ankle plantar flexors Hip extensors Knee flexors

distribution of that root. Root pain is characteristically made worse by movement of the spine and by actions that cause sudden pulses of pressure in the spinal subarachnoid space, such as coughing or sneezing. Root pain in a limb often has two components: a dull, deep, ill-defined ache thought to correspond to the sensory supply to muscle and bone (the sclerotome) and a sharp, superficial, better-defined pain related to the dermatome of the root.

Causes

Spinal degenerative disease

This is the most common cause of a root lesion, usually in the lower lumbar or lower cervical region. It is discussed in detail below.

Tumours

Spinal extradural tumours, such as metastatic carcinoma or lymphomas, lying either in the bone of a vertebra or in the fibrofatty epidural space, often produce root compression and root pain. Of the spinal intradural tumours, root pain is most often associated with a neurofibroma, which usually originates from a dorsal root. Carcinoma of the lung apex may involve the first dorsal root, producing pain and numbness down the inner surface of the arm, weakness of the small muscles of the hand, and a Horner's syndrome. This clinical picture is known as a Pancoast syndrome. Pelvic or retroperitoneal tumours may involve roots after they have left the spinal canal.

Trauma, cervical rib syndrome, neuralgic amyotrophy

See Chapter 13.30.

Arachnoiditis

See Chapter 13.8.

Herpes zoster (see Chapter 16.11)

The inflammatory process of herpes zoster is based in the dorsal root ganglion and the first symptoms are pain and hyperalgesia in the area supplied by the affected root(s), to be followed a few days later by a skin rash in the corresponding dermatomes. Spread of infection into the anterior horn cells of the cord may produce motor loss in the same segments.

Degenerative disease of the spine

Pathogenesis

This condition is the principal cause of lesions of the spinal nerve roots. The pathological basis of the condition lies in degeneration of the intervertebral discs. Collapse of the disc space leads to a number of secondary phenomena. The annulus of the disc bulges outwards, lifting the periosteum off the vertebral bodies and giving rise to the deposition of marginal osteophytes. The narrowing of the disc space leads to a misalignment of the posterior facet joints, which may accordingly show hypertrophic, osteoarthritic change. As the vertebral bodies come closer to each other, the posterior longitudinal ligament and the ligamenta flava buckle up. Finally, the disc narrowing and facet joint misalignment may permit some degree of forward or backwards subluxation of one vertebra upon another. This happens most often at the L4/5 level, where the axes of the facet joints in some individuals may permit the development of a forward spondylolisthesis.

All the above changes, osteophytic ridges, swollen facet joints, and concertina-ed ligaments, may intrude into the spinal canal and intervertebral foramina and cause cord or root compression. Collectively these chronic degenerative changes are known as spinal spondylosis. Cervical spondylosis is most marked at the C4/5, C5/6, and C6/7 levels. It may be associated with the development of a myelopathy (see below) or with root compression. The latter occurs in the intervertebral foramina, which may be narrowed anteriorly by osteophytes originating from the sides of the intervertebral disc and uncovertebral joints, and posteriorly by hypertrophied facet joints. Lumbar spondylosis may lead to narrowing of the lumbar canal and compression of the cauda equina, or to compression of individual nerve roots where they lie in the lateral recesses of the spinal canal before they reach their foramina. This so-called lateral recess stenosis results from bulging of the discs in front and the facet joints and yellow ligament behind.

Disc protrusions

In addition to the insidious neural compression caused by spondylosis, a more sudden root or cord compression may follow protrusion of an intervertebral disc. A disc protrusion consists of an acute or subacute backwards dislocation of disc substance. It may take the form of a bulge of disc material within an intact annulus or the annulus may tear at one point, permitting extrusion of a free fragment of nuclear material into the spinal canal. Disc protrusions often follow an episode of sudden or unusual exertion, but the underlying degeneration and fissuring of the disc will have been developing silently for some time as a result of normal wear-and-tear strains.

Cervical

These disc protrusions are most common at the C4/5, C5/6, and C6/7 levels, compressing the C5, C6, and C7 roots, respectively. A symptomatic protrusion occurs most often between the ages of 25 and 50 years. The onset of symptoms is generally over the course of a few days and may occur spontaneously or follow some unusual strain. The first symptom is pain and stiffness in the neck, usually extending into the shoulder or proximal arm on one side in a rather ill-defined fashion. This may be referred pain resulting from stretching of the annulus. As root compression develops there appears a better-defined, severe, lancinating pain in the territory of that root. With worsening root compression there may be paraesthesias and numbness in the dermatome of the root and reduction or loss of any tendon reflexes subserved by the root. Marked motor loss is unusual and usually indicates very severe root compression. Painful limitation of some neck movements is almost invariably found.

In the great majority of cases the symptoms abate within a few weeks with conservative measures—a collar, bed rest if necessary, and mild analgesia. Recurrent attacks are much less common than in the case of lumbar disc protrusions. Surgery is reserved for the small number of patients with an incapacitating degree of pain that persists or recurs, or where severe root compression has led to disabling motor or sensory loss. Recent advances in imaging techniques have led to some changes in the investigations preferred by individual clinicians. High-definition MRI is now the most satisfactory investigation. It not only serves to exclude unexpected pathology causing root compression, such as a tumour, but also, in the axial views, gives the maximum information about the degree of nerve root compression, for example whether this is caused by a soft disc protrusion or a bony bar. If the pathology is very marked, plain CT scanning may be sufficient before surgery.

A central cervical disc protrusion may give rise to acute or subacute compression of the spinal cord. Young adults are usually affected and an onset after trauma is common. Urgent removal by the anterior route is indicated. A posterior approach via laminectomy is usually more hazardous as it requires mobilization and retraction of the compressed cord.

Dorsal

As the dorsal spine is relatively immobile and is splinted by the rib cage, symptomatic disc protrusions are extremely rare. Root compression is relatively unusual. In most cases a dorsal disc protrusion presents as cord compression. This may be of insidious onset, and without pain.

Lumbar

Most symptomatic disc protrusions are lumbar and 95 per cent of these occur at the two lowest levels, L4/5 and L5/S1. Lumbar disc protrusions are thought to account for many and perhaps most attacks of acute low back pain and sciatica, although in only a small proportion of cases is the diagnosis confirmed by imaging and surgery. The characteristic course of a lumbar disc protrusion is of recurrent attacks of low back pain radiating into one or other leg. The peak incidence is between the ages of 25 and 50 years. Relapses often follow exertion but heavy manual workers are no more liable to the condition than are those in sedentary occupations. Relapses often occur abruptly and protective spasm of the erector spinae muscles may cause 'locking' of the lumbar spine with severe pain. Initial attacks consist of low back pain spreading into the region of the sacroiliac joint and buttock in an ill-defined fashion. These symptoms are thought to reflect distension of the sensitive posterior annulus and posterior longitudinal ligament. Many patients never progress beyond this stage, but in some patients root compression occurs. If this happens, the low back pain lessens and is replaced by severe, well-localized pain in the territory of the root, made worse by coughing or straining. An L4/5 disc protrusion compresses the L5 root some way above its intervertebral foramen, causing pain down the outside of the leg and radiating to the top of the foot, which may become numb. An L5/S1 disc protrusion compresses the S1 root, causing posterior leg pain radiating to the sole. The outer edge of the foot may become numb. A more lateral protrusion may compress the root in its foramen. In this case, an L5/S1 protrusion will compress the L5 root, and so on.

On examination, signs of root compression will be found. In the case of the lower three lumbar discs, affecting roots L4 to S1, there will be limited straight-leg raising with a positive stretch test (Lasègue's test). Compression of roots L1 to L3, which run anterior to the hip joint, gives rise to a positive femoral stretch test. The neurological changes correspond to the root affected and vary according to how severely it is compressed. L5 root involvement leads to weakness of dorsiflexion and eversion of the ankle, numbness on the dorsum of the foot and lateral shin, but no reflex loss. S1 root involvement causes numbness of the outer border of the foot and little toe, weakness of plantar flexion at the ankle, and a reduced or absent ankle jerk.

Most patients recover within a matter of 2–3 weeks with bed rest alone. Surgery is only indicated if there is prolonged or recurrent incapacitating root compression or in those cases where serious motor loss appears, especially if an L4/5 disc protrusion leads to marked weakness of dorsiflexion of the ankle. The one absolute indication for surgery is a central protrusion compressing the cauda equina (see below). Patients with clear signs of root compression do well after operation. Those with back pain as the dominant symptom fare much less well.

Plain radiographs of the lumbar spine and pelvis serve to make sure that an unsuspected tumour or inflammatory lesion is not producing bone destruction, but they are of little value in predicting the level of a symptomatic protrusion. The radiological investigation that gives the maximum information about what is going on in the lumbar canal is high-definition MRI. CT myelography may be useful for patients who have already undergone spinal surgery or for those in whom the pathological changes are not especially marked.

At operation the root is exposed from behind by laminectomy or by a more limited excision of the yellow ligament and the adjacent bone (fenestration) on one side. A full laminectomy is usually advisable if the main spinal canal is narrow at the point of the disc protrusion, or if there is a large central protrusion, particularly if this is causing compression of the cauda equina. The outcome of surgery depends on case selection, but in approximately 80 per cent of cases the patient is able to resume a normal life with little disability. The outcome of surgery is less satisfactory if there has been previous surgery to the lumbar spine, if back pain rather than sciatica is the predominant symptom, or if the patient is involved in litigation over an accident that has led to the disc protrusion.

Cauda equina lesions

Compression of the cauda equina produces bilateral leg weakness and numbness, loss of sphincter control, and loss of sexual potency. The upper level of the motor and sensory disturbance will be determined by the level of the compressing lesion, but weakness is usually most marked at the ankles and sensory loss is generally most prominent over the sacral dermatomes—the 'saddle' area of the buttocks and perineum. The ankle jerks and anal reflexes are almost always lost, and, depending on the level of the compression, the knee jerks may also be reduced. Any sphincter disturbance is of a lower motor neurone type with a patulous anus and an 'atonic' bladder that dribbles urine.

The common causes of cauda equina compression are a central lumbar disc protrusion, degenerative spondylolisthesis (most often at the L4/5 level), and a tumour. A mild, intermittent compression caused by degenerative stenosis of the lumbar canal leads to a syndrome known as claudication of the cauda equina (see below). Neoplastic compression of the cauda equina is most often due to an extradural malignant tumour such as a metastasis or a lymphoma. Intradural tumours are much rarer but are important clinically because they are often benign. They include neurofibromas, meningiomas, and ependymomas.

The compression of the cauda equina produced by a lumbar disc protrusion is often fairly abrupt in onset. The sudden onset usually reflects complete extrusion of a nuclear fragment through a tear in the annulus into the spinal canal. A past history of attacks of low back pain or sciatica may give a clue to the diagnosis. The compression is generally accompanied by excruciating bilateral sciatica in addition to motor and sensory loss below the affected level. Surgery is matter of great urgency if there is to be any chance of neurological recovery.

Claudication of the cauda equina and lumbar canal stenosis

In this condition, symptoms of dysfunction of the cauda equina appear on walking or prolonged standing and are relieved by rest. The underlying cause is almost always a congenital stenosis of the lumbar canal. Stenosis may be over several segments of the lumbar spine or at a single level. If the latter, the L4/5 level is most commonly involved. This is normally the narrowest part of the lumbar canal and is also the level most often affected by spondylolisthesis caused by degenerative arthritis of the facet joints.

Symptoms are generally absent at rest and only appear on walking or prolonged standing. The irritation of the cauda equina gives rise to pain that spreads from the lumbar spine to the buttocks and down the back of the legs to the feet. Often the pain is accompanied by paraesthesia and numbness that 'marches' over the sacral dermatomes if the patient continues walking or standing. Motor impairment may become manifest as floppiness of the ankles. The differential diagnosis from vascular claudication may be difficult. Both conditions afflict middle-aged and elderly people, and may coexist in the same person. Features suggesting claudication of the cauda equina are the 'march' of the pain, its paraesthetic quality, and the fact that on the rest the symptoms may take 5–10 min to go away, a much longer period than is required for the symptoms of vascular claudication to evaporate. Sometimes the symptoms disappear more quickly if the patient adopts a position that flexes the lumbar spine, such as crouching down on the heels or sitting forward in a chair. The reason for this is that flexion tends to widen the lumbar canal.

There are few physical signs at rest. Signs of root tension, such as limited straight-leg raising or a positive femoral stretch test, are absent and usually the only neurological deficit to be found is absence of the ankle jerks. However, if the patient exercises until symptoms are produced, root tension signs and a more extensive neurological disturbance may appear. The only treatment is surgery, which should be advised if the symptoms are incapacitating. A complete laminectomy with thorough posterior decompression of the compressed neural structures relieves symptoms in the great majority of cases.

Cervical spondylotic myelopathy

In some elderly people the features of a cervical cord disturbance are found to be associated with the changes of cervical spondylosis. The myelopathy is caused by chronic compression of the spinal cord, especially as the affected patients tend to have rather narrow cervical canals in addition to superimposed spondylotic changes. However, factors other than compression may be involved. At operation the degree of spinal cord compression is often found to be relatively slight in relation to the neurological disturbance, and even a thorough surgical decompression seldom leads to full neurological recovery.

Two related conditions, in both of which there is an undoubted relation between degenerative change of the spine and cord damage, must be differentiated from cervical spondylotic myelopathy. One is acute compression of the cervical cord by a soft disc protrusion. Here compression is indisputably the mechanism involved and surgical removal of the protrusion may lead to a gratifying degree of neurological recovery. The other condition is focal damage to the spinal cord caused by a combination of cervical spondylosis and a hyperextension injury. Extension of the neck, as may happen with a fall forwards on to the face or intubation for anaesthesia, leads to a narrowing of the cervical spinal canal. If the canal is already narrowed by cervical spondylosis, sudden hyperextension may lead to a focal contusion of the cord. An apparently mild hyperextension injury in an elderly person with cervical spondylosis may lead to severe cord damage in the absence of any cervical fracture or dislocation.

The natural course of cervical spondylotic myelopathy is variable. In a few patients there is progression to severe disability over the course of 2–3 years, while in others the disorder advances more insidiously, sometimes with episodes of sudden worsening. The most common course is for an initial period of progression, over a matter of a few months or so, followed by a plateau phase of stabilization that may last indefinitely or even be followed by a phase of spontaneous improvement. These fluctuations may reflect the enlargement and regression of soft protrusions.

The predominant symptoms are tingling and weakness of the hands, and stiffness and clumsiness of the legs. Any sphincter disturbance is usually slight and sphincter control may be preserved, even in advanced cases. Physical examination reveals spasticity of the legs, with brisk reflexes and extensor plantar responses. There may be slight weakness of hip flexion and ankle dorsiflexion but interference with gait seems to be caused more by spasticity than by weakness. The arm tendon reflexes are brisk below the level of the spondylosis and are lost at the level of the apparent cord involvement, either from interruption of the reflex arc within the cord itself or from associated root compression by osteophytes.

The first treatment to be offered the patient is a cervical collar. It is doubtful whether this alters the course of the condition, but at least it can do no harm. Most neurosurgeons reserve surgery for those patients in whom serious progression occurs despite a collar. Even for these patients, caution should be exercised when surgery is offered. Neurological worsening after operation is by no means uncommon and there can be few neurosurgeons who have not experienced catastrophes in treating this condition. Two surgical approaches are available. Where the disorder of the cord appears to be related to spondylosis at multiple levels, and if there is evidence of some generalized stenosis of the spinal canal, then laminectomy over as many segments as is necessary to decompress the cord is carried out. If the spondylotic change impinging on the cord is confined to anterior osteophytes at one or two levels, then an anterior decompression is best. Some surgeons combine the decompression with a fusion at the same levels (Cloward's operation). For posterior operations, a laminoplasty as opposed to a laminectomy may help by reducing frictional injury to the cord as well as decompressing it.

Further reading

Beggs, I. and Addison, J. (1998). Posterior vertebral rim fractures. *British Journal of Radiology*, 71, 67–72.

Herzog, R.J. (1996). The radiologic assessment for a lumbar disc herniation. *Spine*, 21, 19S–38S.

Koffman, B., Junck, L., Elias, S.B., *et al.* (1999). Polyradiculopathy in sarcoidosis. *Muscle and Nerve*, 22, 608–13.

Nadelman, R.B. and Wormser, G.P. (1998). Lyme borreliosis. *Lancet*, 352, 557–65.

Disorders of consciousness

Chapter 13.11

Epilepsy in later childhood and adult life

A. P. Hopkins

Definitions

An epileptic seizure

The basic event common to all seizures is a paroxysmal discharge of cerebral neurones. Not all paroxysmal discharges result in overt events. For example, the EEG of a man with epilepsy between seizures may well show spikes over one temporal lobe that represent the paroxysmal discharges of neurones. Such events, unaccompanied by any clinical phenomenon, are not generally considered to be seizures. For the definition of a seizure, therefore, it is necessary to add that the paroxysmal discharge of cerebral neurones must be apparent—either to an external observer, as for example in the case of a *grand mal* seizure, or as an abnormal perceptual experience suffered by the individual, as may occur in a seizure arising, and remaining confined to, one temporal lobe (see below).

It is with regret that we must report the death of Dr A. P. Hopkins.

Table 1 Classification of epileptic seizures

I. Partial seizures: seizures which start by activation of a group of neurones limited to one part of one hemisphere
A. Simple, without impairment of consciousness. Depending upon anatomical site of origin of seizure discharge, initial symptom may be motor, sensory, aphasic, cognitive, affective, dysmnesic, illusional, olfactory, or psychic. Synonyms include Jacksonian, temporal lobe, or psychomotor seizures according to type
B. Complex partial, with impairment of consciousness
(a) simple partial onset, followed by impairment of consciousness
(b) impairment of consciousness at onset: symptoms as in simple, above
C. Partial seizures, either simple or complex, evolving to generalized tonic–clonic seizures; synonym: secondarily generalized seizures. Sometimes seizures become so rapidly secondarily generalized that there is no clinical evidence of partial onset, the only evidence being electroencephalographic
II. Generalized seizures: more or less symmetrical, no evidence of focal onset
A. Absence seizures
(1) Typical absences: abrupt onset and cessation of impairment of consciousness with or without automatisms, myoclonic jerks, tonic, or autonomic components. A 3 Hz spike-and-wave discharge is the usual EEG abnormality for this diagnosis
(2) Atypical absences: less abrupt onset and/or cessation of consciousness, more prolonged changes in tone, EEG abnormality other than 3 Hz spike-and-wave discharge
B. Myoclonic seizures. Myoclonic jerks, single or multiple
C. Clonic seizures
D. Tonic seizures
E. Tonic–clonic seizures: synonyms: grand mal, major convulsion
F. Atonic or astatic seizures
III. Unclassified seizures—as yet undefined

Epilepsy

For practical purposes, epilepsy may be defined as a continuing tendency to epileptic seizures. For epidemiological purposes, an operational definition of epilepsy is more than one non-febrile seizure of any type. The diagnosis can usefully be expanded to a short diagnostic formulation, describing the patient's present age, the age of onset of seizures, the types of seizures suffered, the present frequency of seizures of each type, the presumed causation, the associated features such as mental retardation, and the patient's present social and economic position.

The different types of epileptic seizure

An International Classification of Epileptic Seizures was agreed by a commission of the International League against Epilepsy in 1981, and revised in 1989 (Table 1). Classification of seizure types depends upon an analysis of clinical phenomena observed during the seizure, the changes in the EEG between the seizures, the presumed anatomical substrate and aetiology, and the age of onset. A more detailed description of each type is given below.

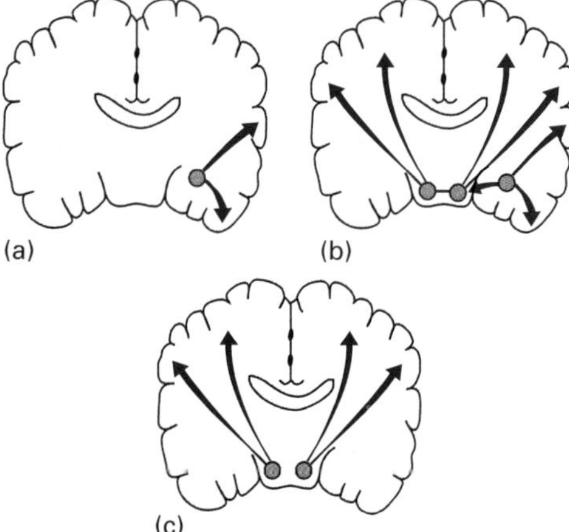

Fig. 1 Origins of different types of epileptic seizure (see text for details).

Figure 1 illustrates the two main classes of origin of seizure. In the top part of the figure, the hatched area indicates a number of neurones that are in some way abnormal, tending to discharge in paroxysms. They have the facility of driving other neurones to follow their abnormal patterns of discharge. The paths of influence of these abnormal neurones are indicated by the arrows. As long as the discharge remains in one part of the brain, the seizure is said to be a partial one. What happens during such a seizure depends upon the site and pattern of discharge of abnormal neurones. In Fig. 1(a), the abnormal focus is shown in the temporal lobe, by far the most common site of origin of partial seizures. Clinically observed features of these and other types of partial seizures are described below.

The abnormal discharge may spread, as is shown in Fig. 1(b), through connections linking the two halves of the brain, or, by affecting poorly identified central collections of cells, initiate a generalized seizure discharge. In this case the seizure is said to be a partial one that has become secondarily generalized. Some tonic–clonic (*grand mal*) seizures are of this type.

Figure 1(c) illustrates the second main class of seizure. In this, central collections of cells are themselves in some way abnormal in their behaviour, even though they may seem structurally sound by histological examination. Because of their central position, and the direction and power of their transmissions, a seizure discharge generated within them spreads more or less simultaneously to all parts of the brain. Such a seizure, generalized at onset, is a primary generalized one. Typical absences (*petit mal*) and some tonic–clonic seizures (*grand mal*) are of this type.

Tonic–clonic seizures (*grand mal* seizures, generalized convulsions)

Whether the paroxysmal discharge be primary, or secondarily generalized from a cortical focus, the hallmark of a *grand mal* seizure is disordered muscular contraction. The first phase is known as the tonic phase. The body becomes rigid, and, as it is incapable of maintaining a normal co-ordinated posture, the sufferer will, if standing, fall to the ground. The chest muscles also contract, forcing the air out through the larynx in an involuntary grunt or cry. The jaw muscles also contract, and the tongue may be bitten. The absence of ventilatory movements and the high oxygen consumption of the vigorously contracting muscles result in the rapid onset of cyanosis. The face becomes suffused by desaturated blood, which is prevented from draining into the thorax by the raised intrathoracic pressure. The normal movements of swallowing are lost, so that saliva may dribble from the mouth. The disordered contraction of abdominal and sphincter muscles may result in incontinence of urine and, occasionally, faeces.

After a brief time in the tonic phase, which may vary from a few seconds to a minute, the seizure passes into a clonic or convulsive phase, with rhythmic contractions of limbs and trunk muscles. The amplitude of these contractions is variable. They continue for a few seconds to a few minutes, after which the individual lies in a deep stupor, which gradually lightens through a stage of confusion into full consciousness. After the seizure they may have a headache, and feel generally bruised and battered by the vigorous muscular contractions. Postictal confusion must be distinguished from the automatic behaviour of a seizure arising in the temporal lobe (see below).

Once on the ground the subject should be turned into the 'coma position'—that is to say into a semiprone position—so that secretions drain from their mouth, rather than into the larynx. Any vomiting that occurs will also find easy egress this way. There is no point in trying to force an object between tightly clenched teeth. The tongue is usually bitten at the onset of the seizure, the airway is not significantly improved by opening the mouth, and damage to the teeth may result from misguided attempts to force a passage. It is useful to give them a sharp clap on the back, to drive the tongue forwards.

Typical absences (*petit mal* seizures)

This description should only be given to absence attacks associated with classical, 3-Hz spike-and-wave activity in the EEG. *Petit mal* is a disorder with onset in childhood, and attacks continuing into adult life are rare. A typical absence attack is very brief, lasting only a few seconds. The onset and termination are abrupt. The child ceases what he or she is doing, stares, looks a little pale, and may flutter the eyelids. Sometimes more extensive bodily movements occur, such as dropping the head forwards, and there may be a few clonic movements of the arms. Attacks are very commonly provoked by hyperventilation for 3 min or so, and this is well worth testing in the outpatient clinic or during electroencephalography.

About one-third of all children with *petit mal* will have one or more tonic–clonic convulsions.

Partial seizures (focal seizures)

If these are in the motor cortex, the initial manifestation will be a contraction of the muscles in the opposite side of the body. Partial motor seizures are most likely to begin at the angle of the mouth, the index finger and thumb, or the big toe. If the seizure discharge then spreads through contiguous layers of cortex, the clinical manifestations march into the homologous parts of the body. A seizure of this type is called a Jacksonian seizure.

Another type of partial seizure associated with movement is the versive seizure. Version is usually away from the hemisphere in which the abnormal cells lie, so these seizures are often called adversive. In such an attack the eyes are deviated, followed by the head, and sometimes the whole body may turn on its own axis, often with elevation and abduction of the arm. The site of origin of such seizures is in the posterior frontal region.

However, by far the most common type of partial seizure is that arising from a discharge of abnormal neurones in the temporal lobe. Such seizures are often called temporal lobe seizures, but more recently have become called complex partial seizures. The classification refers to them as partial seizures with psychic symptoms, or with autonomic symptoms, or with special-sensory symptoms.

The seizure discharge in complex partial seizures is manifested by distortions of consciousness that range from partial loss of awareness, such that the subject is dimly aware of what is going on around them, although they may be unable to reply, through to complete inaccessibility, with amnesia for events occurring during the seizure. Even in these, it may be possible to superimpose normal behaviour on the seizure; for example, the individual may be led passively to a chair, so that they can complete the seizure sitting down.

Partial seizures arising in the temporal lobe are often accompanied by stereotyped motor behaviour involving the lower part of the face. Grimacing and sucking movements are quite common, and there may be rotation of the head and eyes as the seizure discharge spreads forwards. Sometimes complex stereotyped behaviour such as undressing may occur, or the patient may be able to continue walking along the road, and indeed cross streets making appropriate judgements about oncoming traffic, even though in the midst of a seizure.

Distorted perceptions during a partial seizure arising in the temporal lobe may give the clue to the correct diagnosis. The subject may report a sense of unreality, even if partially aware of their surroundings. The phrase *déjà vu* is used to describe a sensation that what is happening around them has already occurred at some previous time. The phrase *jamais vu* is used to describe a perception that what is seen is so unreal that it bears no relation to the subject's previous life events. There may be a pervasive feeling of fear, and dizziness; olfactory and visual hallucinations are not uncommon. The visual hallucinations are sometimes well formed, so that the subject may recount complex scenes, almost analogous to a film.

The seizure discharge of any partial seizure may become generalized. For example, a brief olfactory hallucination may be an initial symptom immediately preceding a generalized seizure. This indicates that the seizure discharge was briefly confined to one or other temporal lobe before becoming generalized. All patterns may occur. For example, on some days the patient may have a partial seizure alone, on other days a generalized tonic–clonic convulsion preceded by a partial seizure, and yet on other days the secondary generalization may be so rapid that the initial symptom is not experienced.

Rare types of seizures

Atypical absences occur. They may be clinically indistinguishable from a typical absence, but show EEG discharges that are different from the classical, 3-Hz spike-and-wave discharge. A common associated feature with an atypical absence is known as a 'recruiting epileptic rhythm', which is initially rapid and of low amplitude, but then gradually becomes slower and of higher amplitude. Another variant is disordered spike-and-wave complexes at a rate slower than the classical frequency of 3 Hz. Such variant absences are often associated with mental retardation and evidence of cerebral dysgenesis, and have a much worse prognosis for seizure control. This is sometimes known as the Lennox–Gastaut syndrome.

Sometimes tonic seizures occur. In these there is a tonic posturing of all limbs, or just the limbs on one side of the body. Such seizures occur in multiple sclerosis on rare occasions, and in some of the lipidoses of childhood.

In infantile spasms, there is a brief sudden flexion of the head, trunk, and limbs, as if the infant is bowing a *salaam*. These are, therefore, sometimes known as *salaam* seizures. These seizures are often accompanied by failure of development and progressive retardation (West's syndrome). The EEG is characteristic, distinguished by irregular, high-voltage, diffuse, slow spike-and-wave complexes that are repeated at brief intervals on high-voltage, slow background rhythms. Myoclonic epilepsy is considered below.

Relation between seizure type and types of epilepsy

The term 'idiopathic' epilepsy is often used when there is no apparent cause for the seizure. More prolonged EEG recordings, using various activating techniques (see below), and the advent in particular of MRI, have shown that many tonic–clonic seizures previously considered to be idiopathic arise from a structural lesion. Partial seizures always arise from some focal area of structural abnormality in the brain, and if such exists, the epilepsy is clearly symptomatic of such a structural lesion, even though the lesion may be pathologically unimportant, such as a small area of atrophy in one temporal lobe.

There is one exception to this rule. Some older children may have partial or generalized seizures, the interictal EEG record being characterized by large spike discharges over the Rolandic area of one hemisphere. Such 'benign childhood epilepsy with centrotemporal spikes' is not associated with any structural lesion and has an excellent prognosis. It does not fit easily into an understanding of seizures as set out in the foregoing paragraphs.

True idiopathic epilepsy is now known as primary generalized epilepsy. In this type of epilepsy, the seizures are generalized from the onset, either taking the form of tonic–clonic seizures, or typical absences, or just the myoclonus associated with absences.

Sometimes it is not possible to be certain whether generalized tonic–clonic seizures arise on the basis of primary generalized epilepsy, in which the EEG happens not to have shown any seizure discharge at the time of the recording, or whether, alternatively, the seizures are very rapidly generalized from a focus that is clinically silent. Such 'cryptogenic' cases should not, however, be called idiopathic.

Causes and differential diagnosis of epilepsy

Inheritance

There is good evidence that genetic factors are an important aetiological factor in certain forms of epilepsy. These inherited forms have been estimated to account for at least 20 per cent of all epilepsies. It is useful to distinguish between those conditions in which recurrent seizures are merely one component of a more complex phenotype, and those in which they are an essentially isolated phenomenon. The former are 'single-gene' disorders that display a mendelian pattern of inheritance, whereas the latter nearly all display a 'complex' non-mendelian pattern, indicating the interaction of several genes and environmental factors.

Over 120 mendelian disorders are recognized in which epilepsy occurs in a proportion of patients as a component of the phenotype. They include inborn errors of amino acid metabolism, neurocutaneous disorders such as neurofibromatosis and tuberous sclerosis, and the progressive neurodegenerative conditions such as the ceroid lipofuscinoses and Unverricht–Lundborg disease or Baltic myoclonus.

At least two mitochondrial diseases, myoclonic epilepsy with ragged-red fibres and the mitochondrial encephalomyopathy and lactic acidosis syndrome, are complicated by epilepsy. In some of these conditions the mutated gene and its product are known, and the pathophysiology of seizure generation is at least partially understood. These mendelian disorders collectively amount for a tiny fraction, perhaps 1 per cent, of all patients with familial epilepsy.

Most epilepsy syndromes in which recurrent seizures occur in isolation in neurologically and cognitively intact individuals, and which display familial aggregation, have a 'complex' pattern of inheritance. These include idiopathic generalized epilepsies such as juvenile myoclonic epilepsy, and the absence epilepsies and idiopathic partial epilepsies, in particular benign childhood epilepsy with centrotemporal spikes. Genetic factors are also clearly important in the causation of febrile convulsions, although some authors would not classify this disorder with the epilepsies. One epilepsy syndrome—benign familial neonatal convulsions—displays mendelian inheritance, segregating in an autosomal-dominant manner.

Trauma

Penetrating injuries such as those caused by shrapnel or rifle bullets are a potent cause of epilepsy. However, in civilian life most head injuries are caused by road-traffic and industrial accidents, and result from some deceleration injury to the brain transmitted through the skull without any penetration of the skull itself. In general, head injuries resulting in a long duration of post-traumatic amnesia are not particularly likely to be followed by the development of epilepsy unless there is cortical damage, caused either by a depressed fracture or haemorrhage.

The occurrence of a seizure in the first week after a head injury has proved to be a potent predictor of late post-traumatic epilepsy. Unfortunately, the evidence is that prophylactic anticonvulsant treatment does not suppress the incidence of late post-traumatic epilepsy.

Cerebral dysgenesis

Cerebral palsy and epilepsy are often associated. Antenatal factors resulting in varying degrees of cerebral dysgenesis are responsible for most cases of cerebral palsy. With regard to mental retardation, without overt palsy, the prevalence of epilepsy increases progressively with the degree of retardation. In those with severe learning difficulties (IQ below 50), the lifetime cumulative incidence is at least 30 per cent. Both the seizures and the retardation are common manifestations of an underlying brain dysfunction, due either to metabolic abnormalities such as lipidoses or metachromatic dystrophies, or to dysplastic conditions in which neuronal embryonic migration is impaired, such as areas of cortical dysplasia or heterotopias or tuberous sclerosis. The Sturge–Weber syndrome and arteriovenous malformations of various types are also prominently associated with epilepsy.

Tumours

Tumours play only a comparatively small part (see Table 2). However, the proportion of cases in which tumours are the cause does rise with increasing age, reaching 19 per cent between the ages of 50 and 59 years in the UK general practice study. The introduction of MRI and the wide employment of surgery in the management of intractable epilepsy has shown that small areas of focal dysgenesis (hamartomas) may be responsible for seizures. The distinction between an indolent 'tumour' and 'hamartoma' is sometimes extremely difficult.

Table 2 Identified causes of epilepsy in two studies

Cause	Study 1 (%)	Study 2 (%)
Perinatal causes/congenital	8.0	n/i
Cranial injury: postoperative	5.5	3
Infections	2.5	2
Vascular	10.9	15
Tumours	4.1	6
Alcohol		7
'Other causes' e.g. Alzheimer's	3.5	6
Total	34.5	39
Idiopathic/cryptogenic	65.5	61

For sources, see OTM3, p.3917.

n/i, no information.

Infectious diseases

Bacterial meningitis may scar the cortical mantle, resulting in the subsequent development of seizures. A cerebral abscess may also cause seizures; even if the abscess is drained and heals, the thick-walled gliotic scar may well be associated with seizures subsequently.

Viral encephalitis may cause seizures during the acute illness, and subsequent seizures after the initial infection has passed. In the UK the most common identified cause is the herpes simplex virus. Persistent viral infection, such as occurs in subacute sclerosing panencephalitis, in which the measles virus persists after an initial infection, may also be accompanied by generalized seizures and myoclonus.

Echinococcal cysts, cysticercosis, toxocariasis, and toxoplasmosis are, in the UK, rarer causes of seizures, although some consider that widespread contamination of children's playing fields by *Toxocara canis* is an important cause of epilepsy in childhood. Parasitic infections, particularly cysticercosis, are common causes of epilepsy in Third World countries.

Degenerative disorders

The incidence of seizures increases in old age. They occur in Alzheimer's disease, although usually they are overshadowed by the social and intellectual deterioration.

Vascular disease

Imaging studies show a considerable excess of infarcts in the brains of those in whom epilepsy starts later in life, compared to scans of controls matched for age. These infarcts are often deep-seated lacunes, sometimes clinically silent except for the epilepsy. Deep lacunar infarction probably does not in itself cause the seizures, but is merely a marker of more widespread vascular disease.

Alcohol

Chronic abuse of alcohol may result in seizures that then continue even if the subject abstains. Seizures also occur sometimes in acute alcohol intoxication and often after abrupt withdrawal of alcohol, as part of the syndrome of delirium tremens.

Acute symptomatic seizures

Apart from the example of acute alcohol intoxication noted above, it is well recognized that some drugs may precipitate seizures. The drugs in everyday use that have been most often incriminated include phenothiazines, tricyclic antidepressants, lignocaine (lidocaine), penicillin, and isoniazid. Other metabolic causes of seizures include hypoglycaemia, most usually induced by exogenous insulin used in the treatment of diabetes; hypocalcaemia, particularly in neonates; and uraemia. Hyperglycaemia has also been reported as a cause of partial seizures. Withdrawal from barbiturates, benzodiazepines, and above all from alcohol, may be associated with seizures.

Other acute symptomatic seizures arise as the result of an acute brain illness, such as meningitis, or herpes simplex encephalitis.

Precipitants of seizures

Distinct from the causes of a continuing tendency to seizures are those factors that may precipitate an attack. For example, many patients with epilepsy say that they have more seizures when they are upset or worried; conversely some, particularly those with complex seizures, more if they are relaxed, and if their mind is not concentrating on any particular task. Other precipitants include alcohol and drugs, as mentioned above, menstruation, lack of sleep, and intercurrent illness.

Although lack of sleep may precipitate seizures the following day, drowsiness and sleep may allow seizures to 'escape'. Indeed drowsiness is such a potent activator of abnormal discharges in the EEG that the recordist will often encourage the subject to try to go to sleep during the recording. In some patients with epilepsy, seizures are virtually confined to the hours of sleep.

In some individuals, precipitants of the seizures are so potent and so stereotyped as to warrant the name 'reflex epilepsy'. Many such cases are amongst the curiosities of medicine: for example, the person who has a seizure only on hearing church bells, or on reading, or on looking at repetitive patterns such as squares of floor tiling. The most common type of reflex epilepsy is television epilepsy. Seizures may be induced in susceptible children by the normal traverse of the spot down the face of the tube. Such children are most at risk when the screen occupies a considerable proportion of the visual field, as will occur if the size of the screen is large and the child sits close to it. It has been shown that observing the set with one eye covered prevents the occurrence of these seizures.

Differential diagnosis of seizures

Before embarking upon antiepileptic treatment, it is essential to ensure that complaints such as 'funny turns' or 'black-outs' are due to a paroxysmal discharge of cerebral neurones—an epileptic seizure—and not some other event. The major conditions to be considered in the differential diagnosis include vasovagal attacks, cardiac syncope (see Chapter 2.1), transient ischaemic attacks, drop attacks, migraine and hyperventilation. Rarer conditions to consider are:

1. *Night terrors* in children may sometimes be mistaken for epileptic attacks. These affect children aged between about 6 and 8 years, who suddenly awaken from a sound sleep, wide eyed, screaming, and inconsolable. They are amnesic for the events the following morning. They seem to occur just as often in happy children as in children who are not doing well at school or in the family. Fortunately they, too, pass quickly, and once thought of, the diagnosis is quite straightforward.
2. *Tics, habits, and ritualistic movements* These usually begin at about the age of 7 or 8 years, and affect principally the upper part of the face, are bilateral, and are not associated with any disturbance of consciousness. Although the child has a compulsion to undertake such movements, they can be controlled, at least for a brief interval, by command.
3. *Vertigo*, especially if profound, as may be experienced in the course of a paroxysm of Menière's disease, may be mistaken for a seizure. It is true that vertigo may rarely be an initial symptom in a seizure arising from the posterior temporal lobe, but a far more usual cause is peripheral labyrinthine dysfunction.

Simulated seizures

Simulated seizures are often a problem in differential diagnosis, especially in those who undoubtedly have some true seizures. Simulated attacks may be used as an attention-seeking device by those with epilepsy, or by siblings or school friends of those with epilepsy. It can be surprisingly difficult to distinguish true from simulated seizures. Perhaps the best guide is that the simulator tends to overplay the seizure, and the temporal coincidence of seizures whenever there is a suitable observer. Features such as injury, tongue biting, and incontinence can be, and often are, simulated. Serum prolactin concentrations rise four- or five-fold some 20 min after a true tonic–clonic seizure or after a complex partial seizure. No such rise occurs after simulated attacks, nor after the partial seizures arising in parts of the brain other than the temporal lobe.

The investigation of seizures

There are three principal reasons for such investigation:

(1) to improve the certainty with which the diagnosis of a seizure is correct;

(2) to ascertain the type of seizure, which is important when considering appropriate medication;

(3) to ascertain a detectable cause, in case such cause is itself treatable.

Electroencephalography is a useful tool for distinguishing the various types of seizure. For example, sometimes there may be confusion between disturbances of consciousness due to typical absences, and disturbances due to complex partial seizures. The distinction, if it can be made, is important not only for the correct choice of therapy (see below) but also for prognosis (see below).

It must be clearly understood that the EEG does not prove or disprove the diagnosis of epilepsy. The record can be normal in someone with undoubted epilepsy. There is always the danger that a doctor, hovering on the brink of making a diagnosis of epilepsy, may be tipped into making a 'definite' diagnosis of epilepsy by the presence of marginal abnormalities on the EEG. If the record does show clear-cut paroxysmal activity, this does lend considerable support to the diagnosis, but a record showing only a minor excess of slower rhythms, 'compatible with epilepsy', does not contribute usefully.

There is seldom any indication for serial EEG records. Improvement in seizure control is not necessarily accompanied by improvement in any underlying abnormality in the EEG. Furthermore, abnormalities on the EEG in adults have proved to be no predictor of subsequent relapse on stopping anticonvulsant therapy, although in children relapse is somewhat more likely if the EEG is abnormal when the anticonvulsants are discontinued.

MRI is the best method of detecting abnormalities of cerebral structure. CT scanning is more widely available, and will show many structural causes of epilepsy—tumours or infarcts for instance.

Table 3 The seven principles of antiepileptic drug therapy

1. Consider the decision: should antiepileptic drugs be given anyway
2. Choose a drug, considering the following factors: age the possibility of pregnancy interaction with other drugs price
3. Give only one drug, except in unusual circumstances
4. Begin the chosen drug in modest dosage
5. Give full information to the patient about: the names and alternative names of the drug supplied the initial dosage schedule with dates of planned changes in dosage the need for compliance with instructions adverse effects of the drugs
6. Monitor progress: inform subject of date and place of next review monitor seizure frequency monitor unwanted side-effects of drugs monitor blood level of drug
7. Determine policy for termination of treatment

However, the sensitivity of MRI in detecting small lesions means that there can be no justification for choosing CT if both techniques are available. This is particularly true in the investigation of complex partial seizures arising from a temporal lobe.

It is unusual for any blood test to be helpful in elucidating the cause of epilepsy in adults. Occasionally, a blood alcohol estimation without warning (but of course with informed consent) may be fruitful, or a serological test for syphilis. However, abnormalities of glucose, calcium, magnesium, or amine metabolism in young children may be revealed by appropriate tests.

Treatment of epilepsy

Prescription of antiepileptic drugs

Seven useful principles of antiepileptic therapy are listed in Table 3. The first point is to reconsider the decision as to whether antiepileptic drugs should be given. It is not unusual to meet individuals with rare seizures occurring at intervals of 3–7 years, and in these circumstances many quite reasonably prefer to take no medication at all. Clearly, the likely social effects of subsequent seizures on employment and on eligibility to hold a driving licence may influence them in this regard.

Most sufferers will go to their doctor after their first tonic–clonic seizure, and the doctor will then have to decide whether it is worth advising antiepileptic treatment at this stage. Many studies have now shown that most of those who have a first epileptic seizure will have a second one within a year or two (Fig. 2). The greatest risk is within the first few weeks, as indicated by the initial steep part of the curve in Fig. 2.

Choice of antiepileptic drug

The first factor to consider is the type of seizure. Table 4 shows the antiepileptic drugs of choice for seizures of different types, typical

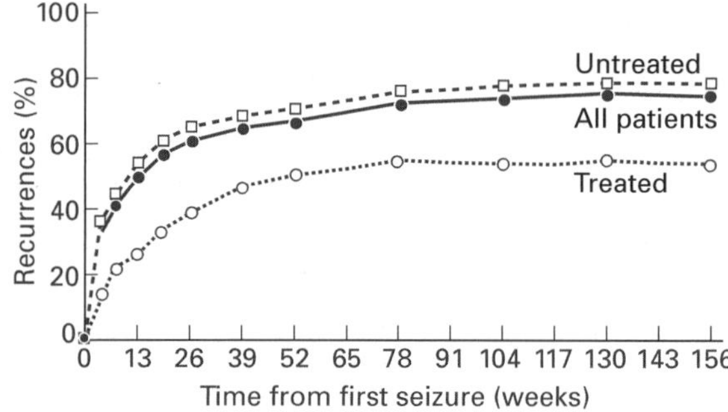

Fig. 2 Probability of seizure recurrence after a first epileptic seizure *(data from the National General Practice Study of Epilepsy, reproduced by kind permission).*

adult dosage per day, and therapeutic concentrations that represent a reasonable target.

First-line drugs

Carbamazepine

This drug has gained increasingly wide acceptance for the treatment of partial seizures, and for tonic–clonic seizures with partial onset. It is reasonably free of side-effects. A few patients develop a skin rash within a few days of starting the drug. Very rare cases of marrow depression have occurred. Sedation is relatively slight. There is a roughly linear correlation between oral dose and serum concentration. This means that it is a comparatively simple matter to increase the oral dose based upon a knowledge of past serum concentrations, without significant danger of intoxication.

Sodium valproate

This has become the drug of choice for primary generalized epilepsy (typical absences and tonic–clonic seizures associated with typical absences). It is probably as effective as carbamazepine and phenytoin in the management of partial seizures and secondarily generalized tonic–clonic seizures of partial onset.

The drug should be introduced, like all antiepileptic drugs, in a relatively low dosage and increased to a maximum of 2.5 g daily. Many patients are controlled on less than this. There is now good evidence that the clinical effect does not bear any relation to the serum concentration, which in any event fluctuates markedly after the ingestion of each tablet.

Sodium valproate is usually relatively trouble-free, but a small number of patients develop an acute hepatitic insufficiency. It is impossible to predict who will develop this, but it is clear that the drug should be avoided in those with a history of liver disease, and the manufacturers recommend that tests of liver function should be carried out as the dosage is increased. Unwanted gain in weight may also occur. In high dosage the drug may cause tremor, but this is rapidly relieved by reducing the dose. Even at average doses, however, a significant side-effect is some thinning of the hair. Fortunately the hair regrows even if the drug is continued, but newly produced hair may be unusually curly.

Phenytoin

This is a successful drug for the treatment of tonic–clonic seizures, and to a lesser extent for partial seizures. Because the enzymes responsible for hydroxylating phenytoin may become saturated, a small increment in phenytoin dosage may result in a large increase in the serum concentration.

Table 4 Antiepileptic drugs of choice for seizure types

Seizure type	Anticonvulsant drugs of choice	Therapeutic serum levels (μmol/l)[a]	Typical adult dose per day (mg)
Typical absences (petit mal)	Sodium valproate (ethosuximide clonazepam)		1500
		285–700	1000
			2
Myoclonic and akinetic seizures	Sodium valproate (nitrazepam clonazepam)		1500
			10
			2
Tonic–clonic seizures (grand mal) in association with typical absences (petit mal)	Sodium valproate (phenytoin phenobarbitone)		1500
		30–80	300
		65–170	90
	Carbamazepine	17–42	600
Tonic–clonic seizures (grand mal) in association with partial seizures, or partial seizures alone	Sodium valproate		300
	Phenytoin	30–80	
	Vigabatrin		3000
	Lamotrigine		300
	Gabapentin		1200
Infantile spasms	ACTH/prednisone		
	Nitrazepam		
	Vigabatrin		

[a] The level below which therapeutic effects are unlikely to occur and above which toxic effects are likely to occur. Measurement of benzodiazapines and valproate is probably not useful as there is no clear relationship between antiepileptic effect and blood levels. Serum monitoring for lamotrigine, vigabatrin, and gabapentin is not yet routinely available.

Phenytoin has significant drawbacks in young people. It causes hirsutism, coarsening of the facies, hypertrophy of the gums, and acne. More unusual side-effects result from the increased hepatic levels of hydroxylating enzymes induced by phenytoin. These enzymes not only hydroxylate phenytoin, but also steroid hormones, including vitamin D. Osteomalacia and rickets may result in rare circumstances, if the patient has a relatively low exposure to sunlight, or a pigmented skin. Oestrogens in contraceptive pills may also be hydroxylated in excess, resulting in inadequate contraceptive protection.

Skin rashes may also occur with phenytoin. Overdosage may result in marked sedation, but sometimes a cerebellar syndrome is seen before significant sedation occurs. Tremor, ataxia, and nystagmus are features of this. Another unusual manifestation of intoxication is chorea. Prolonged phenytoin medication may result in a neuropathy, a cerebellar degeneration, and induction of Dupuytren's contracture.

Other drugs

Phenobarbitone This is undoubtedly an effective antiepileptic drug, and may be worth a trial if other drugs have failed to control seizures. However, it is certainly not a drug of first choice, as older people may become depressed and confused, and children excitable and irritable, on this drug. Those in middle-age often state that they feel unpleasantly sedated even on moderate dosage.

Lamotrigine When added to other regimens where the older drugs are being used to maximum effect, this will result in a useful reduction in seizure frequency (greater than 50 per cent) in about 25 per cent of patients. However, some patients, particularly those with frequent myoclonus, may deteriorate when they begin this drug. A suitable initial dose for an adult is 100 mg/day, increasing to 500 mg/day (less if the patient is on sodium valproate). Adverse events include skin eruptions, sedation, and unexpected exacerbation of seizures, particularly myoclonic seizures.

Vigabatrin This is another, more recent drug that has a useful effect upon those with intractable epilepsy. About 50 per cent of patients will have their seizure frequency reduced by about 50 per cent. A usual maintenance dose is 1500 mg twice daily. Adverse effects include drowsiness, agitation, and sometimes confusion.

Gabapentin This drug also has a useful effect on the frequency of partial seizures only partly responsive to the older drugs. Adverse effects include sedation, dizziness, tremor, and unsteadiness.

Primidone This is an effective antiepileptic, probably largely because it is metabolized to phenobarbitone, although another metabolite (phenylethyl malonamide) also has antiepileptic activity. If primidone is chosen, it should be commenced at a low dosage, and increased gradually, or else sedation may be severe. Even a quarter of a 250-mg tablet twice a day is not too cautious a beginning for an adult.

Ethosuximide This is a useful drug for absence epilepsy; it may precipitate tonic–clonic seizures in some. It has largely been replaced by sodium valproate.

Clobazam This is a benzodiazepine that has had some reported success in complex partial seizures. Unfortunately, any effect appears often to be relatively short lived.

Clonazepam A benzodiazepine that is sometimes used in the management of severe childhood epilepsy, although it is unpleasantly sedative. It may be effective in myoclonic epilepsy when other drugs have failed.

Nitrazepam This benzodiazepine may be effective in controlling myoclonic jerks if these are the only remaining epileptic manifestation of primary generalized epilepsy.

Diazepam Although effective in the treatment of status epilepticus (see below), this is not an effective antiepileptic for daily use.

Using antiepileptic drugs

Price is not, in general, a significant problem with any of the older drugs, although of these sodium valproate is by far the most expensive: a year's treatment with 1500 mg/day will cost £170, compared to about £3 for phenytoin given at a dosage of 300 mg/day. The three recently introduced drugs (lamotrigine, vigabatrin, and gabapentin) are substantially more expensive than the older drugs, but in responsive patients may produce a marked improvement in quality of life.

The possibility of pregnancy must certainly be considered when prescribing an antiepileptic drug. Sodium valproate causes teratogenic effects in animals, and valproate should be used only if the likely benefits in severe epilepsy resistant to other drugs outweigh the risks of teratogenicity. However, it has also been shown that epileptic women taking phenytoin are between two or three times more likely to have an abnormal baby than other women. The risk of congenital heart disease is increased by a factor of about four, and of harelip and cleft palate by a factor of about eight. The risks of fetal maldevelopment must be weighed against the risks to the fetus and to the mother of uncontrolled epilepsy. As any fetal damage due to drugs occurs in the first few weeks of pregnancy, perhaps even before the mother realizes that she is pregnant, the decision whether to stop drugs or not has, by default, often already been taken. In this case the mother might as well continue antiepileptic therapy in modest dosage, and protect herself and the baby against the risks of epilepsy.

One question that patients will undoubtedly want answered is when they will be able to stop treatment. Clearly this depends upon seizure control, but even if immediate control of seizures results, most clinicians will advise continuing antiepileptic medication for approximately 3 years thereafter. Unfortunately, even after this long period of freedom, some patients will relapse on continued treatment, but even more will have further seizures if the drugs are withdrawn, even if a period of 2 years is spent in tailing down the dosage. Absence seizures in childhood generally have a good prognosis if drugs are withdrawn in the late teens after a 3-year period of freedom from seizures. Conversely, those who have juvenile myoclonic epilepsy may continue to experience sporadic seizures, sometimes separated by many years, throughout life. In general, the length of the history of seizures and of treatment (with the exception of absence epilepsy), the occurrence of some seizures since starting treatment, and taking more than one antiepileptic drug when withdrawal commences are all unfavourable factors. Conversely, the length of the remission on drugs before withdrawal is attempted is a favourable factor. The role of the EEG in predicting relapse is more controversial, but, at least in childhood, an abnormal EEG before withdrawal appears to predict a higher probability of relapse. Most of those relapsing do so within the first year.

Status epilepticus

Occasionally, seizures may follow each other without remission. If they are generalized tonic–clonic seizures, with major convulsions occurring in sequence without remission, the patient is at risk from death through cardiorespiratory failure. Immediate control of the seizures is necessary. Diazepam is a highly effective treatment for the management of status epilepticus. It, or the similar drugs lorazepam or clonazepam, should be given as a bolus intravenous injection as soon as it is clear that the individual is having continuous seizures without remission. A suitable dose of diazepam is 10 mg in 2 ml given over 2 to 5 min. If given more rapidly than this, respiratory depression may occur. Alternatively, a bolus of lorazepam, 4 mg intravenously, may be given. If seizures occur again shortly after treatment then one or two further boluses may be given. If these fail, there are several alternative regimens. Phenytoin may be infused intravenously at a dose of 18 mg/kg at a rate of no more than 50 mg/min. This may be done even if the status occurs in a patient already on phenytoin therapy. Alternatively, a diazepam, lorazepam, or chlormethiazole infusion may be used. If seizures continue, then the patient should be anaesthetized with propofol or thiopentone, and ventilated until 12 to 24 h after the last clinical or electrically recorded seizure, the dose then being tapered. A cerebral function monitor—a sort of compressed, slow-moving EEG—is extremely useful in the management of these patients.

Absence status or temporal lobe status may also occur, in which the presentation is not with convulsive seizures but with a confusional state, the origin of which may not be readily recognized. The principles of treatment are much the same as recorded above, and again EEG control is useful. Continual focal motor epilepsy is known as epilepsia partialis continua, and is often exceedingly difficult to control, continuing for many days without a significant disturbance of consciousness.

Surgery

Surgery may benefit refractory cases of epilepsy. It is most usually undertaken for refractory temporal lobe epilepsy, and the current view is that more patients would benefit than are being referred for operation. Prolonged and repeated EEG recordings are necessary to show that the epileptogenic lesion is confined to one or other temporal lobe, as bilateral temporal lobectomy is not possible because of the severe amnesic syndrome that results. In the original operation, the anterior 5 cm of the temporal lobe was amputated as a single block containing the uncus, amygdala, and anterior hippocampus. Mesial temporal sclerosis is the most common lesion found, but occasionally small, previously unidentified tumours or hamartomas or aggregates of abnormal-looking giant neurones are found. The increasing recognition of such dysplastic areas, together with more refined preoperative and intraoperative electrophysiological recordings, has led surgeons to undertake more limited operations confined to the amygdala and hippocampus.

Focal epilepsy can arise from other parts of the brain, and occasionally cortical excision of an epileptogenic focus, such as an angioma or scar following a penetrating head injury, may result in control of previously refractory seizures.

Prognosis and complications of epilepsy

Prognosis

The prognosis, as judged by community studies, is shown in Fig. 3. The top curve indicates the probability of completing a period of five consecutive years without seizures. For example, in 6 years after diagnosis 42 per cent of subjects have been seizure-free for 5 years. If remission of seizures is not accomplished within the first few years of the onset, subsequent worthwhile remission becomes less likely. For example, although the net probability of achieving a 5-year remission within 10 years after diagnosis was 65 per cent, for patients

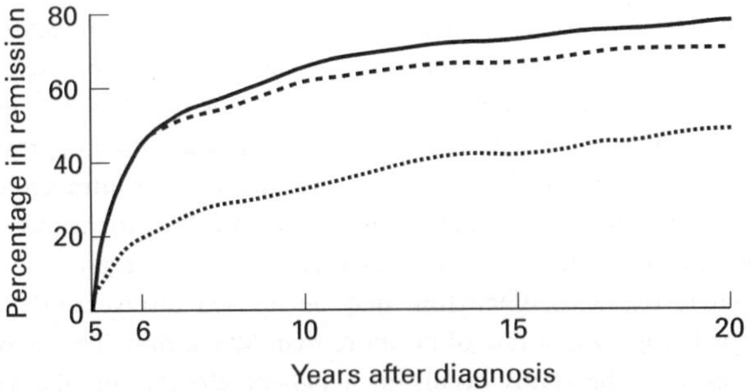

Fig. 3 Remission of epilepsy. Top curve: probability of completing a period of 5 consecutive years without seizure. For example, 6 years after diagnosis 42 per cent of subjects have been seizure-free for 5 years. Middle curve: the probability of being in remission, at any time, for at least the past 5 years. The difference between the top and middle curve is due to relapse after achievement of a 5-year remission. For example, at 20 years after diagnosis 70 per cent are currently free from seizures and have been for 5 years and a further 6 per cent have had at least one seizure-free period of at least 5 years duration but have subsequently relapsed. Lowest curve: the probability of being free of seizures for at least 5 years whilst not taking anticonvulsant drugs. In summary, 20 years after diagnosis 50 per cent have been free from seizures without anticonvulsant drugs for at least 5 years. A further 20 per cent continue to take anticonvulsant medication and are also free from sizures. Seizures continue, in spite of medication, in 30 per cent. *(Redrawn from Anneger, J.F., Hauser, W.H., and Elveback, L.R. (1979). Epilepsia,* **29**, *729.)*

not in remission 5 years after diagnosis the probability of achieving remission within the next 10 years was only 33 per cent.

Some factors are known to be particularly unfavourable: the combination of complex partial seizures with tonic–clonic seizures, clustering of seizures, injury occurring during tonic–clonic seizures, associated physical signs, and associated learning difficulties are all factors known to be associated with failure to remit.

Social aspects of epilepsy

Restrictions on adults with epilepsy should be few. Mothers with epilepsy who have very young children should not bath infants alone, in case they have a seizure during bath time and the baby drowns.

The question of eligibility to hold a driving licence is particularly important. In the UK a period free from all seizures for 1 year is required, or to have had an epileptic attack whilst asleep more than 3 years before the date when the licence is granted and shall have had attacks only whilst asleep between the date of that attack and the date when the license is granted. Stricter regulations in the United Kingdom apply to Public Service and Heavy Goods Vehicle Drivers.

Problems concerning employment will certainly arise. Obviously it is not safe to work with heavy moving machinery or at heights.

Further reading

Feely, M. (1999). Drug treatment of epilepsy. *British Medical Journal*, **318**, 106–9.

Fisher, P.D., Sperber, E.F., and Moshe, S.L. (1998). Hippocampal sclerosis revisited. *Brain and Development*, **20**, 563–73.

Mattson, R.H. (1998). Medical management of epilepsy in adults. *Neurology*, **51**, S15–20.

Chapter 13.12

Narcolepsy and related sleep disorders

C. D. Marsden

Narcolepsy

Narcolepsy is defined as 'a syndrome of unknown origin that is characterized by abnormal sleep tendencies, including excessive daytime sleepiness and often disturbed nocturnal sleep, and pathological manifestations of REM (rapid eye movement) sleep. The REM sleep abnormalities include sleep-onset REM periods and the dissociated REM sleep inhibitory processes, cataplexy, and sleep paralysis. Excessive daytime sleepiness, cataplexy, and less often sleep paralysis and hypnagogic hallucinations, are the major symptoms of the disease.

Aetiology

The cause of narcolepsy is unknown. Symptomatic narcolepsy is very rare; occasional cases have been attributed to encephalitis lethargica or multiple sclerosis. Idiopathic narcolepsy occurs in between 20 and 50/100 000 of the population. Between 10 and 40 per cent of patients give a history of a similar disorder amongst other family members, and about a quarter describe a parent as affected. The most likely mode of inheritance is autosomal dominant with variable penetrance. Virtually all patients with narcolepsy express the major histocompatibility antigens HLA-DR2 and -DQw1, compared with about a quarter of normal controls. This confirms the genetic origin of this disease and links it with the short arm of chromosome 6.

Clinical symptoms

The narcoleptic tetrad consists of excessive daytime sleepiness with sleep attacks (narcolepsy), episodes of sudden falling associated with emotion (cataplexy), sleep paralysis, and hypnagogic hallucinations. Virtually every patient develops excessive daytime sleepiness and sleep attacks, about two-thirds experience cataplexy, about a third suffer hypnagogic hallucinations, and about a sixth have sleep paralysis. Approximately one-third of patients experience all four symptoms.

Excessive daytime sleepiness and sleep attacks

These are the hallmark of narcolepsy. On average, patients will report between two and six attacks of falling asleep each day, but some may experience up to 20 or 30 episodes. Each attack lasts, on average, around 10 to 30 min, but sometimes they may be as brief as a minutes or as long as 2 h. The hallmark of narcolepsy is the bizarrerie of the situations in which the patient may drop off to sleep. Thus, narcoleptics may fall asleep over their meals, dropping into the soup, may nod off while standing, during intercourse, and even while driving the car or flying an aeroplane. Patients describe such episodes as 'irresistible'.

Cataplexy

This describes an abrupt but reversible paralysis into which a narcoleptic patient may be precipitated by emotional events. The severity of cataplectic attacks can vary from total paralysis with collapse to the ground, to lesser degrees in which the jaw sags and the head drops. Consciousness is preserved throughout the attack, but the

It is with regret that we must report the death of Professor C. D. Marsden.

patient may see double. Attacks usually last for a few seconds, but may be prolonged for as much as 10 min. They occur more frequently at times of stress, fatigue, or after heavy meals. Laughter and anger are the most common triggers, but elation or any other intense emotion may be sufficient to precipitate an episode. The frequency of cataplectic attacks is very variable, but some patients may have many attacks each day. Cataplexy tends to improve in adult life.

Sleep paralysis

In sleep paralysis the patient becomes totally unable to perform a voluntary movement despite remaining alert and aware. It may occur either on falling asleep (hypnagogic) or on awakening (hypnapomic). During an episode the patient is powerless to move, speak or even open their eyes, although they are fully aware of their condition and can recall it completely afterwards. Naturally, such episodes may cause extreme terror, particularly if they are accompanied by vivid and frightening hallucinations. An episode rarely lasts more than 10 min, and usually much less. Episodes tend to be infrequent and to improve with age.

Hypnagogic hallucinations

These almost always involve visions, which may consist merely of simple coloured forms, still or in motion, or may take the shape of animals or persons. Frightening or erotic scenes are quite common. Noises, voices, or melodies occur less frequently.

Course

Narcolepsy begins in adolescence or in early adulthood, and is lifelong; remissions are very uncommon. Around 60 per cent of cases commence between 15 and 30 years of age, but a few start before the age of 10 years or up to the age of about 50 years. Sleep attacks are the first symptom in 90 per cent of cases, but a few patients begin with cataplexy or hypnagogic hallucinations. Once established, excessive daytime sleepiness and sleep attacks never cease completely during the patient's lifetime, but cataplexy tends to become less of a problem as the patient becomes older.

Differential diagnosis

The excessive daytime sleepiness and sleep attacks characteristic of narcolepsy are difficult, on occasion, to distinguish from the range of normal. The best index of pathological sleepiness is an unambiguous history of inappropriate daytime sleep episodes. The bizarre situations in which narcoleptics fall asleep are diagnostic, and most patients will give a history of black-outs and automatic behaviour if questioned carefully. If there is any doubt, a history of cataplexy settles the issue.

Problems in diagnosis arise in separating narcolepsy and its associated features from epilepsy, in distinguishing cataplexy from other causes of drop attacks, and in separating excessive daytime sleepiness and sleep attacks from other causes of pathological sleep.

Symptomatic hypersomnia

This occurs in a range of organic brain diseases, including encephalitis, toxic or metabolic encephalopathies, tumour, vascular or traumatic brain damage. Sleep, as distinct from coma from which the patient cannot be awakened, frequently is more or less continuous in these conditions.

Functional hypersomnias

These are periodic. The sleep attacks may last one to several hours, with attacks occurring most days (short cycle), or may last a day to several weeks, with attacks occurring at intervals of a month to several years (long cycle). Patients with either short-cycle or long-cycle hypersomnias are normal between attacks. Other functional hypersomnias are associated with sleep apnoea (see below). Four short-cycle periodic functional hypersomnias are recognized.

1. *Idiopathic hypersomnia* is characterized by excessive prolonged night-time sleep, extreme difficulty in awakening, signs of 'sleep drunkenness' on awakening, and prolonged periods of sleep during the day. Such patients may sleep 15 or even 20 h a day if not disturbed. The condition is hereditary in as many as one-third to one-half of patients.
2. *Neurotic hypersomnia* may occur in some hysterics or 'faint hearted' neuraesthenic individuals, and a complaint of excessive tiredness is common in depression
3. *Nocturnal myoclonus syndrome* is characterized by short bouts of muscle jerking at night, which disturb sleep. This is accompanied by extreme restlessness of the legs, and is often associated with daytime sleepiness. A nocturnal dose of clonazepam may help.
4. *Sleep apnoea* is characterized by cessation of breathing during sleep, which causes extreme restlessness with frequent respiratory pauses and snoring during night sleep, and by daytime drowsiness and irritability (see Chapter 4.44). The diagnosis is established by polygraphic recording of sleep, which shows periods (at least 30 of 10 or more seconds' duration in 7 h of sleep) of apnoea, associated with a fall in arterial oxygen saturation. Such patients are chronically tired during the day, complain of headache and irritability, and have excessive daytime sleep and automatic behaviour.
5. *Long-cycle periodic functional hypersomnia* is rare, and may or may not be accompanied by excessive eating (Kleine–Levin syndrome). Such patients, most commonly young adult males, begin to overeat prodigiously (bulimia), become irritable, restless, and hypersexual, and then fall into a deep sleep for a day to a few weeks, during which time they awake to attend to toilet needs and can be aroused to eat. On awakening they are amnesic for that period, but rapidly return to normal behaviour and sleep patterns, and remain free of attacks for months or years

Treatment

Narcoleptic sleep attacks and excessive daytime sleepiness are, in many cases, greatly improved by the regular use of amphetamines (5–40 mg daily), or mazindol (2–8 mg daily). These drugs do not affect cataplexy, but tricyclic antidepressants such as chlormipramine (10–150 mg nightly) may abolish both cataplexy and sleep paralysis. Chlormipramine can be used safely with amphetamines or other stimulants, but blood pressure should be monitored.

Further reading

Aldrich, M.S. (1998). Diagnostic aspects of narcolepsy. *Neurology*, 50(Suppl, 1), 52–7.

Gibson, G.J., Douglas, N.J., Stradling, J.R., London, D.R., and Semple, S.J. (1998). Sleep apnoea: clinical importance and facilities for investigation and treatment in the UK. Addendum to the 1993 Royal College of Physicians Sleep Apnoea report. *Journal of the Royal College of Physicians of London*, 32, 540–4.

Wetter, T.C. (1997). Restless legs and periodic leg movement in sleep syndromes. *Journal of Neurology*, 244(4 Suppl. 1), S37–45.

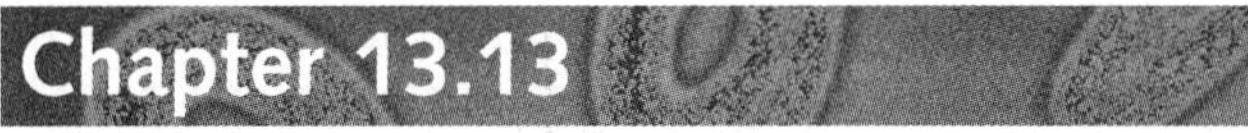

Chapter 13.13

Coma

M. J. G. Harrison

Pathophysiology

Consciousness is maintained by activity of the reticular formation of the brainstem. It follows that coma may be due to the global suppression of neuronal function or to the presence of a focal lesion in the brainstem. The latter may be an intrinsic lesion such as an infarct, or may be secondary to the compressive effects of an enlarging mass (Fig. 1).

History and examination

History taking and examination must be geared to the task of distinguishing global and 'metabolic' causes of coma from those of brainstem origin. It is particularly important to detect those patients whose declining conscious level is due to secondary compression of the brainstem, since they may need urgent neurosurgical relief of an expanding mass.

The history may provide important clues. A fit may have been witnessed and the coma prove to be only that seen transiently after a *grand mal* attack, or the patient may have fallen to the ground holding their head as though struck down by severe headache, suggesting subarachnoid haemorrhage. An empty pill bottle or a history of depression may suggest a drug overdose; a history of diabetes prompts consideration of ketotic or hypoglycaemic coma. A telephone call to relatives and medical attendants can be highly revealing.

The general examination may provide useful clues to the cause of coma. Fever suggests meningitis or other nervous system infection. Hypothermia suggests hypothyroidism or primary hypothermic coma. Cyanosis, pallor, or the cherry-red colour of carboxyhaemoglobin will suggest specific diagnoses; trauma may be obvious from bruises and lacerations, a black eye, or blood behind the eardrum. Hypotension can be the clue to septicaemia or loss of left ventricular function.

Level of coma

Documentation of the level of coma is important since progressive deterioration suggests brainstem compression. By contrast, most patients with metabolic causes of coma or an intrinsic brainstem lesion have a stable or improving level of awareness. Careful description of the patient's response to specific stimuli is required to detect subtle changes in the level of consciousness. The Glasgow coma scale is in general use (Table 1). It records the best level of response of eyelids, speech, and limb movement to verbal request, shouts, and painful stimuli. Deterioration can be detected readily, even when different observers are responsible for the sequential examination.

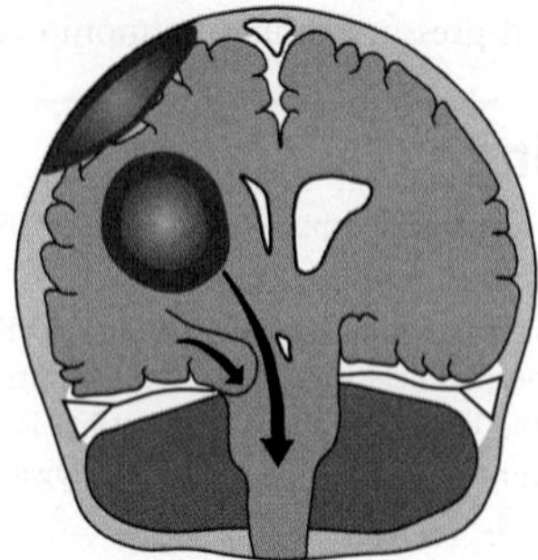

Fig. 1 Illustration of herniation of the temporal lobe (small arrow) and displacement of the upper brainstem (large arrow) resulting from an intracranial mass whether extra- or intracerebral.

Table 1 Glasgow coma scale

Eyes open	Spontaneously	4
	To speech	3
	To pain	2
	Never	1
Best verbal response	Orientated	5
	Confused	4
	Inappropriate words	3
	Incomprehensible sounds	2
	None	1
Best motor response	Obeys commands	6
	Localizes pain	5
	Withdrawal	4
	Flexion to pain	3
	Extension to pain	2
	None	1

Focal signs

The presence of a hemiparesis suggests a mass lesion of a cerebral hemisphere as the cause of the coma. Its presence must be inferred in the unconscious patient from observation of asymmetries: of the face during expiration, of spontaneous limb movements or tone, and of responses to painful stimuli. If a decorticate or decerebrate posture develops symmetrically in response to painful stimuli, no localizing significance is implied. If, however, the responses are asymmetrical, for example flexion of one arm and extension of the other, then the latter side showing the more primitive reaction is 'hemiparetic'. Rarely, asymmetries result from hypoglycaemia, hyponatraemia, or hepatic failure. Most will prove to reflect structural lesions in the cerebral hemisphere, or the brainstem.

Eye signs

A key part of the examination concerns the assessment of the pupillary responses and eye movements. If these brainstem functions are normal, the cause of coma is likely to be metabolic or a diffuse disease. Structural damage to the brainstem, on the other hand, whether local or secondarily provoked, manifests itself by loss of pupil reflexes and abnormalities of eye movement. Herniation of the temporal lobe over the free edge of the tentorial opening causes compression of the IIIrd cranial nerve, so a unilaterally dilated fixed pupil is indicative of the presence of a compressing mass lesion. Central herniation of the brainstem through the tentorial hiatus reflects a pressure gradient between a supratentorial mass-containing compartment and the posterior fossa. Such a pressure gradient is

Table 2 Diagnosis of coma

Diagnostic category	Diagnostic features
A. 'Metabolic'	Normal pupil responses
	Normal or absent eye movements depending on depth of coma
	Suppressed, Cheyne–Stokes, or ketotic respiration
	Symmetrical limb signs usually hypotonic
B. Brain-stem: intrinsic	From outset:
	Abnormal pupil responses
	Abnormal eye movements
	Abnormal respiratory pattern
	Cranial nerve signs
	Bilateral long tract signs
C. Brain-stem: compression	Papilloedema
	Hemiparesis
	Progressive:
	Loss of pupillary responses
	Loss of eye movements
	Abnormal respiratory pattern
	and/or
	Long-tract signs
	Appearance of 3rd nerve palsy

Table 3 Causes of coma

Metabolic	*Diffuse intracranial disease (cont.)*
Drug overdose	Encephalitis
Ischaemia/hypoxia	Epilepsy
Diabetic	Hypertensive encephalopathy
Hypoglycaemia	Cerebral malaria
Cardiac failure	
Respiratory failure	*Cerebral hemisphere lesions (with brain-stem compression)*
Renal failure	
Hepatic failure	Cerebral infarct
Hyponatraemia	Cerebral haemorrhage
Hypercalcaemia	Subdural haematoma
Sepsis	Extradural haematoma
Alcohol	Abscess
Wernicke's encephalopathy	Tumour
Carbon monoxide poisoning	
	Brainstem lesion
Diffuse intracranial disease	Brainstem infarct
Head injury	Brainstem haemorrhage
Meningitis	Tumour/abscess
Subarachnoid haemorrhage	Cerebellar infarct/haemorrhage

dramatically and dangerously increased by ill-advised lumbar puncture. Central herniation causes progressive brainstem compression, with sequential loss of pupil responses and abnormalities of eye movement passing from a stage of readily elicited, symmetrical, horizontal movements to one of disconjugate movements or unilateral paralysis of gaze, and finally to total immobility of the eyes. Eye movements in the unconscious patient are tested by counter-rolling of the head or by cold-water syringing of the external auditory meatuses to cause a unilateral suppression of tonic vestibular input to brainstem gaze centres. Patients in deep metabolic coma may show total loss of eye movement but will retain the pupil reflexes. With central herniation, pupil reflexes are lost as the eye movements become abnormal or are lost. Anoxia may cause large, fixed pupils with coma due to diffuse neuronal damage.

Respiration

Respiratory patterns are of limited diagnostic value. Deep breathing suggests acidosis, as in diabetic coma, regular but shallow breathing suggests depression by drug overdose, and Cheyne–Stokes breathing has no diagnostic significance. All other departures from a normal pattern, if not due to respiratory disease, suggest some brainstem compromise.

Diagnosis of type of coma and cause

The distinction between the three broad categories of coma can thus be made by bedside observations (Table 2). Associated clinical features, and special investigations such EEG and CT scans are then needed to make specific diagnoses (Table 3). If the coma appears to be metabolic in type but no systemic disorder or drug overdose has been diagnosed, the cerebrospinal fluid should be examined. Both meningitis and subarachnoid haemorrhage may cause coma, and neck stiffness is often missing when conscious level is depressed. If there are focal signs, or if papilloedema is detected, a lumbar puncture is contraindicated until after CT, MRI or EEG, and angiography, have excluded a mass lesion. Other investigations that may be needed when the diagnosis is in doubt include arterial blood gases, urea, electrolytes, liver function tests, osmolarity, cortisol, and thyroid studies. The blood sugar should always be measured urgently as delayed correction of hypoglycaemia can cause severe permanent neurological disability. The EEG can be helpful in detecting encephalitis, especially that due to human herpesvirus, some kinds of metabolic coma such as that due to hepatic encephalopathy, and status epilepticus.

If a focal lesion is suspected, a CT scan or MRI are needed to see if there is a surgically accessible problem such as a subdural haematoma or meningioma. A cerebellar haemorrhage may cause a rapidly evolving coma due to local pontine compression. It is vital to make this diagnosis quickly since surgical decompression can be life-saving. The classical presentation is with headache, nausea/vomiting, and ataxia, often unilateral, but in the unconscious patient the diagnosis is suggested by unilateral paralysis of horizontal eye movement, in the absence of a matching hemiparesis, in a patient whose conscious level is declining. Surgery is indicated for all but the smallest haematomas (see Chapter 13.15). Pontine haemorrhage causes coma with loss of horizontal eye movements and pin-point pupils that may still just react to a bright light. There are bilateral long-tract signs and the patients often develop hyperpyrexia. Surgery is rarely possible. Massive cerebral haemorrhage causing coma is also usually inoperable.

Related conditions

Confusional state

Patients suffering from an acute confusional state have a short attention span and are distractible. They often appear perplexed or bewildered, and have difficulty in following questions and commands. Their memory is poor and they have some problems with orientation. They tend to misinterpret what they see. The acute onset of such a state, with some variable drowsiness and inattentiveness, is usually due to toxic metabolic conditions; the diagnosis depends on defining the underlying physical condition. Purely psychiatric causes of confusion, and dementia in its early stages, do not affect the level of awareness, so identification of drowsiness is all important in the distinction.

Delirium

This, too, is usually due to toxic/metabolic problems such as alcohol or barbiturate withdrawal and hepatic failure, or encephalitis. It may be seen during recovery from head injury. There is disorientation, confusion, and reduced attention as in confusion but the picture is more florid, with agitation, irritability, and fear, and the disorientation is more profound. Complex delusions are often seen, with prominent visual hallucinations (auditory hallucinations are more often seen in psychoses).

Locked-in syndrome

If patients have a paralysis of vocalization and speech, and of movement of the face and limbs, they may appear unconscious when in fact they are not. They may be able to feel pain. Often they have had damage to the ventral pons or medulla, for example due to multiple sclerosis or a stroke. Communication can usually be established. They can blink or perhaps make some vertical eye movement that can be coded as 'yes' and 'no' in order that they may signal their wishes and converse in a limited way. A similar incapacity may occur with myasthenia gravis or the Guillain–Barré syndrome but its evolution does not give rise to the same problems of knowing that the patient is alert and of undiminished intellect. An EEG can help to show an alert state, reactive to external stimuli.

Akinetic mutism

This superficially resembles the locked-in state, with a patient who is mute and immobile, although apparently alert. No communication can be established, however, and the patient is doubly incontinent. The usual cause is bilateral damage to the frontal lobes or diffuse anoxic damage, or a small lesion in the reticular formation.

Psychogenic unresponsiveness

Mutism and a lack of response to the environment may also be seen in primary psychiatric conditions such as catatonia, depression, and hysteria. In these the pupil responses are normal, and caloric stimulation of the ears provokes nystagmus as in the normal person. The EEG shows a responsive, wakeful pattern. (By contrast, patients with akinetic mutism of organic origin have an EEG dominated by slow-wave activity.)

Chronic vegetative state (see Chapter 13.14)

Prolonged survival after severe head injury or anoxic insult may lead to the development of this state. There is no evidence of recovery of higher function but cycles of wakefulness appear. Some patients are akinetic but some are not. Their eyes may open to verbal stimuli. Spontaneous respiration and maintenance of blood pressure ensure continuation of life, until death from complications such as bronchopneumonia. At autopsy the brainstem is relatively spared, the forebrain showing extensive damage. The cortex usually shows laminar necrosis.

Predicting outcome in non-traumatic coma

The prognosis is poor if the coma persists for more than 6 h. Recovery is unlikely if pupil responses and cranial reflexes are still lost at 24 h, if the best motor response at 3 days is worse than withdrawal to pain, and if spontaneous roving eye movements do not return by 7 days. The severity of coma as judged by the Glasgow coma scale is predictive, as is its cause. Drug-induced coma has the best outlook, anoxia, ischaemia, and stroke the worst, with other metabolic causes occupying an intermediate position. Unfortunately, in individual cases prediction is less than precise and caution has to be exercised.

Further reading

Bates, D. (1993). The management of medical coma. *Journal of Neurology, Neurosurgery and Psychiatry*, **56**, 589–98.

Edgren E., Hedstrand U., Kelsey, S., *et al.* (1994). Assessment of neurological progress in comatose survivors of cardiac arrest. *Lancet*, **343**, 1055–9.

Multi-Society Task Force on Persistent Vegetative State (1994). Medical aspects of the persistent vegetative state. *New England Journal of Medicine*, **330**, 1499–508.

Plum, F. and Posner, J.B. (1980). *Diagnosis of stupor and coma*, 3rd edn. F.A. Davis, Philadelphia.

Young, G.B., Ropper, A.H., and Bolton C.F. (1998). *Coma and impaired consciousness: a clinical perspective.* McGraw Hill, New York.

Chapter 13.14

Brainstem death

B. Jennett

Cardiopulmonary resuscitation and intensive care are now commonplace in the developed world, so that life-threatening brain insults may now be followed by complete recovery. Sometimes, however, these interventions do not more than extend the process of dying for hours or days because the patient is brain dead. In others they are too late to save the cerebral cortex, which is more vulnerable to hypoxia than the brainstem, or the cortical connections are irretrievably damaged by head injury, and the patient then survives for a long period in the vegetative state.

Brain death

The crucial lesion is irreversible loss of function of the brainstem, with subsequent lack of downward drive to maintain respiration and of upward activation of the cerebral cortex by the ascending reticular pathways. Except when systemic hypoxia has been the initial insult the cerebral cortex may be structurally intact and islands of electrical activity may be detected on EEG. However, this makes no difference to the inevitability of spontaneous cardiac asystole within a few days of death of the brainstem. Early definitions of brain death implied that the whole nervous system was dead, with a flat EEG and absence of all motor activity. But the spinal cord is more resistant to hypoxia and is unaffected by intracranial catastrophes that wreck the brainstem—so spinal reflexes often persist after brain death. Indeed, reflex limb movements frequently become more active if ventilation is maintained for more than 24 h after the brainstem has ceased to function. To resolve this confusion the term brainstem death is now preferred in the UK.

About half the cases of brain death result from head injury, after hours or days of intensive treatment following initial resuscitation. About a third have suffered a severe, non-traumatic intracranial haemorrhage, and the rest a variety of catastrophic intracranial events, including systemic hypoxia associated with cardiac arrest.

Criteria for diagnosis

Undue emphasis on the final confirmation that no residual brainstem function persists has sometimes distracted attention from the stepwise process of diagnosing brainstem death, in which such tests are only the last stage. Indeed the most important step is the first one, satisfying the preconditions. These require that the patient be apnoeic and in deep coma due to irreversible structural damage to the brain, and this implies that reversible causes of brainstem depression have been adequately excluded. It is usually obvious that structural brain damage has occurred: there has been a recent head injury, or a classical history of spontaneous intracranial haemorrhage or of some less acute intracranial condition. Establishing the irreversibility of such brain damage depends on failure to improve with the passage of time and after the correction of factors such as systemic hypotension and hypoxia, and raised intracranial pressure. Other factors that can cause temporary absence of brainstem function are depressant drugs (including alcohol), neuromuscular relaxant drugs, and physiological factors such as hypothermia and gross metabolic imbalance. The first two of these may complicate cases of structural brain damage but it is only in a minority of cases that serious doubts arise about confusing factors. For example, when a patient is found unconscious and no satisfactory history can be discovered it may be necessary to undertake formal screening for drugs. In all cases the diagnosis of brainstem death should be delayed until sufficient time has passed for the exclusion of all temporary causes of brainstem depression.

The tests applied to indicate lack of brainstem function are simple to carry out and to interpret. There should be no response of the pupils to light, of the eyelids to corneal touching, of the facial muscles to pain, of the throat muscles to movement of the endotracheal tube, or of the eyes to syringing of each external auditory meatus with ice-cold water (the caloric or vestibulo-ocular reflex). Only when there has been a negative response to all of these is the final crucial test applied—to verify that there is still apnoea. There must be no respiratory movement after disconnection from the ventilator for long enough to allow the $Paco_2$ to rise to 6.65 kPa (50 mmHg), oxygenation being maintained by delivering 6 l/min of oxygen down the endotracheal tube. It is usual to require that all these tests be repeated to exclude any possibility of observer error; the interval before repeating the two tests need be no more than half an hour, provided that the preconditions were fully satisfied before undertaking tests for the first time. No confirmatory EEG or radiological tests are recommended in the UK, and their use is optional in the United States of America.

Action after diagnosis of brain death

There is now wide acceptance of the concept that when the brain is dead the person is dead. In the UK the legal time of death is when the first tests confirm brainstem death, and not some later time when the heart stops. It can help to clarify the situation for nurses and relatives if a death certificate can be issued before discontinuing the ventilator. Some doctors are still reluctant to make this diagnosis explicitly and then to act logically and legally by disconnecting the ventilator. The useless ventilation of brain-dead patients deprives them of death with dignity, needlessly prolongs the distress of relatives, wastes resources for intensive care, and is bad for the morale of nursing staff. Moreover, the opportunity to offer organs for transplantation is lost because gradual circulatory failure makes such organs useless for donation. It would be of benefit to bereaved families, nurses, and other patients if doctors shared a greater readiness to recognize brain death and then to act appropriately.

The persistent vegetative state

This term was introduced in 1972 by Jennett and Plum to describe the clinical condition resulting from loss of function in the cerebral cortex with a functioning brainstem. Because of the latter, vegetative patients breathe spontaneously and are not ventilator-dependent; another difference from brain death is that they can survive for many years, if adequately fed and nursed. The most common cause of vegetative survival after acute brain damage is severe head injury, the mechanism being severe diffuse axonal injury severing the subcortical connections over a wide area. In some traumatic cases, however, secondary hypoxic brain damage is a contributing factor. Most non-traumatic cases result from severe hypoxia/ischaemia of the brain following cardiac arrest, near drowning, or strangulation, while a few result from severe hypoglycaemia in diabetics. In adults the vegetative state can also evolve gradually during the late stage of chronic dementing conditions, and in children can result from severe congenital malformations of the brain or from progressive metabolic or chromosomal diseases affecting the brain. At autopsy, after acute metabolic insults, neocortical necrosis is found with widespread loss of cortical neurones. After acute traumatic and non-traumatic damage leading to vegetative survival there is commonly severe, bilateral thalamic damage. There is also progressive degeneration over many months of nerve fibres remote from the site of initial damage, demonstrable by special stains at autopsy, and reflected during life in progressive enlargement of the ventricles and subarachnoid spaces as visualized by CT or MRI. EEG findings are variable but there is often loss of evoked cortical responses to somatic stimuli. Positron-emission tomography shows severe depression of glucose metabolism in cortical grey matter, to levels found only in experimental deep barbiturate narcosis.

In practice, however, the diagnosis depends on characteristic clinical features recorded by skilled observers over a period of time. The patient has long periods of spontaneous eye opening (hence the inappropriateness of calling this condition irreversible or prolonged coma). The eyes may briefly follow a moving object and the head turn reflexly to a sudden noise that produces a startle reaction. All four limbs are paralysed and spastic, with only reflex posturing and withdrawal from a painful stimulus, and often there is a grasp reflex. The face may grimace and groans be heard, but never words. There is no psychologically meaningful response to external stimuli or any learned behaviour—no evidence of a working mind. It is concluded that, although awake, these patients are not aware and do not suffer distress or pain. Misdiagnosis by non-experts is common, and care is needed to exclude the minimally conscious state when there are very limited responses indicating some cognitive activity, and also the locked-in syndrome. The latter is due to brainstem damage resulting in a patient who is fully aware but who can communicate only by code, using their sole remaining motor power, blinking the eyelids or moving the eyes.

Patients in a vegetative state for some time can still make some recovery, and 'persistent' does not mean permanent. Of patients in the vegetative state 1 month after an acute insult, about half of the head-injured will regain some consciousness, but few of the non-traumatic cases do. Many who recover consciousness remain very severely disabled and dependent, particularly if they have been vegetative for several months. After non-traumatic insults, permanence can be declared after 6 months, but after head injury, not until 12 months. There is a high mortality in the first year after becoming vegetative but once this period is survived patients can live for several years if tube feeding and good nursing care is maintained and infective complications are treated.

There is now a wide consensus in many countries that survival for years in a permanent vegetative state is of no benefit to the patient, and that it is therefore appropriate to withdraw life-sustaining treatment once permanence is declared. Many courts in the United States and the UK have agreed that artificial nutrition and hydration is medical treatment that can be withdrawn if judged to be of no benefit to the patient. Once this is done a peaceful death occurs in 8 to 12 days, and the cause of death is regarded as the original brain damage. Only in the UK is it a legal requirement to seek approval before withdrawing such treatment, although this situation is under review.

Several groups have declared that it is appropriate to let such patients die by withdrawing tube feeding. In the United States many cases have been brought before the courts, including one to the Supreme Court, seeking permission to withdraw tube feeding. These courts have all agreed to this and have indicated that judicial review should no longer be necessary before such action, unless there is some dispute between the involved parties. At the end of 1992 the first case legally tested in Britain came before the High Court, the Court of Appeal, and the House of Lords, and withdrawal of life support was unanimously declared to be lawful.

Further reading

Brain death

Conference of the Medical Royal Colleges and their Faculties in the United Kingdom (1979). Diagnosis of death. *British Medical Journal*, **1**, 322.

Jennett, B. (1981). Brain death. *British Journal of Anaesthesia*, **53**, 1111–19.

Pallis, C. (1983). *ABC of brain death.* British Medical Journal, London.

President's Commission for the Studies of Ethical Problems in Medicine (1981). Guidelines for the determination of death. *Journal of the American Medical Association*, **246**, 2184–6.

Vegetative state

British Medical Association (1993). *Guidelines on treatment decisions for patients in the persistent vegetative state.* Appendix 7, *Annual Report.* British Medical Association, London.

Council on Ethical and Judicial Affairs of the American Medical Association (1990). Persistent vegetative state and the decision to withdraw or withhold life support. *Journal of the American Medical Association*, **263**, 426–30.

Institute of Medical Ethics (1991). Working Party Report on withdrawing life supporting treatment from patients in a vegetative state after acute brain damage. *Lancet*, **337**, 96–8.

Jennett, B. (1997). A quarter century of the vegetative state: an international perspective. *Journal of Head Trauma Rehabilitation*, **12**, 1–12.

Royal College of Physicians Working Group (1996). The permanent vegetative state. *Journal of the Royal College of Physicians of London*, **30**, 119–21.

The Multi-Society Task Force on the Persistent Vegetative State (1994). Medical aspects of the persistent vegetative state. *New England Journal of Medicine*, **330**, 1499–508; 1572–9.

Chapter 13.15

Cerebrovascular disease

C. P. Warlow

Cerebrovascular disease comprises disorders of the vascular system that cause ischaemia, infarction, or haemorrhage in the brain. This is the third most common cause of death worldwide, after coronary heart disease and cancer.

Definitions

Many terms used to describe cerebrovascular disease are confusing but two are generally accepted. (1) A transient ischaemic attack is an acute loss of focal cerebral or monocular function with symptoms lasting less than 24 h, and which, after adequate investigation, is assumed to be due to embolic or thrombotic vascular disease. (2) A stroke (or cerebrovascular accident) is a rapidly developing episode of focal, and at times global (applied to patients in deep coma and to those with subarachnoid haemorrhage), loss of cerebral function, with symptoms lasting more than 24 h or leading to death, with no apparent cause other than that of vascular origin; the main pathological types of stroke are ischaemic stroke, primary intracerebral haemorrhage, and subarachnoid haemorrhage.

Epidemiology

The annual incidence of stroke in Caucasian (white) populations is about 2 per 1000 population, but the exact figure depends on their age structure because the incidence rises steeply with increasing age (Fig. 1). The annual incidence of transient ischaemic attacks is about 0.5 per 1000 population, and there are some 25 000 new cases per annum in the UK.

About 80 per cent of strokes are due to cerebral infarction, 10 per cent to primary intracerebral haemorrhage, and 10 per cent to subarachnoid haemorrhage. In Japan and China, the proportion due to primary intracerebral haemorrhage is rather higher.

The risk factors for stroke are similar to those for coronary heart disease. Hypertension is the most important, both for ischaemic stroke and primary intracerebral haemorrhage. The risk of stroke increases with increasing blood pressure in both sexes and at all ages; this risk about doubles with each 7.5 mmHg rise in diastolic blood pressure. Interestingly, there is much less difference in the incidence of stroke between males and females (Fig. 1) than there is for myocardial infarction. Other risk factors for ischaemic stroke include heart disease of any kind, atrial fibrillation, transient ischaemic attacks,

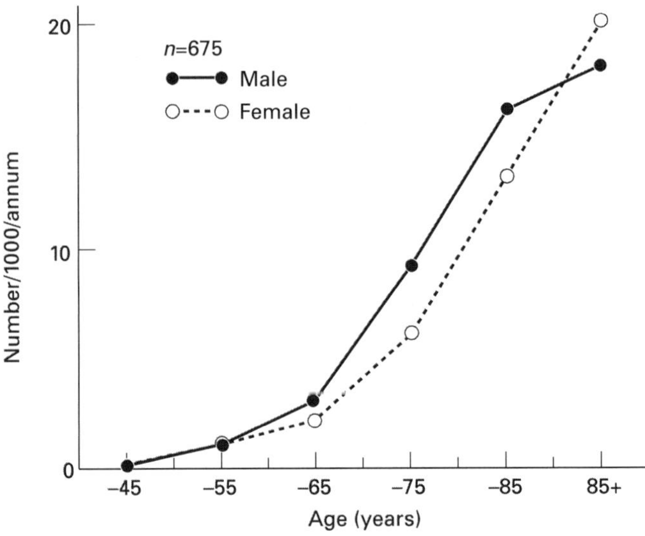

Fig. 1 Age- and sex-specific incidence of first-ever-in-a-lifetime stroke in Oxfordshire, 1981–6. About 25 per cent occur under the age of 65, 50 per cent below the age of 75, and 50 per cent above the age of 75 years.

Table 1 Some causes of 'familial' stroke

Vascular anomalies
Vascular malformation
Saccular aneurysm
Hereditary haemorrhagic telangiectasia
Connective tissue anomalies
Ehlers–Danlos syndrome
Pseudoxanthoma elasticum
Marfan's syndrome
Polycystic kidney disease
Mitral leaflet prolapse
Haematological diseases
Haemophilia and other coagulation factor deficiencies
Sickle-cell disease
Antithrombin III deficiency
Protein C deficiency
Protein S deficiency
Others
Familial hypercholesterolaemia
Cerebral amyloid angiopathy (Icelandic and Dutch forms)
Neurofibromatosis
Tuberous sclerosis
Homocystinaemia
Fabry's disease
Migraine
Cardiac myxoma
Von Hippel–Lindau syndrome
Mitochondrial cytopathy

peripheral vascular disease, diabetes mellitus, smoking, high blood cholesterol, high blood fibrinogen, factor VII coagulant activity, heavy alcohol consumption, cervical arterial bruit, poor maternal and infant health, and social deprivation. The contraceptive pill increases the risk of stroke by about three times.

Although the effect of racial and genetic factors is not fully known, there are some well-known but rare familial causes of stroke (Table 1)

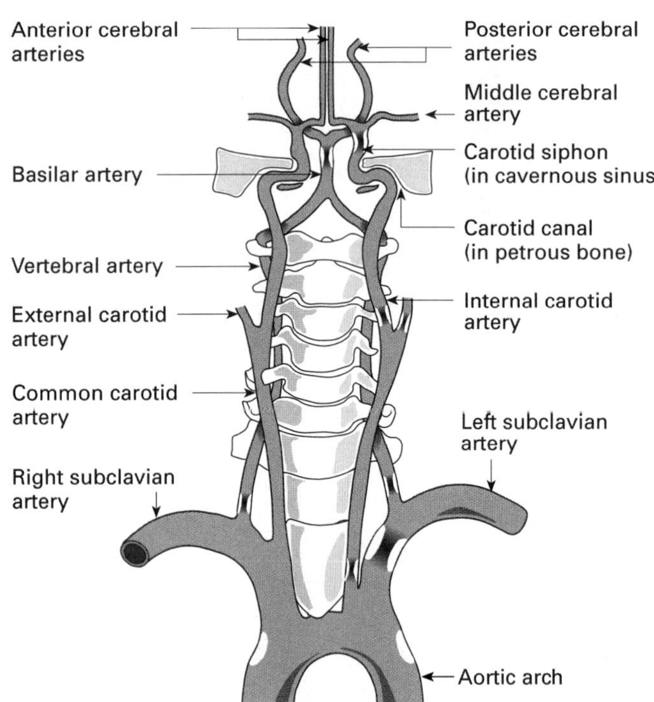

Fig. 2 The arterial blood supply to the brain and eye; places most often affected by atherothrombosis are shown as white indentations into the arterial lumen.

The blood supply to the brain

Because most strokes are the result of cerebral infarction it is important to be familiar with the anatomy of the cerebral arterial supply and the way in which it is affected by atheroma. The brain has a particularly rich blood supply that is derived from four main arteries, the left and right internal carotid and vertebral arteries (Fig. 2). The internal carotid artery supplies the eye through the ophthalmic artery and then divides into the anterior and middle cerebral arteries, which supply the anterior two-thirds of the cerebral hemisphere, the basal ganglia, and the internal capsule regions (Fig. 3). The vertebral arteries unite to form the basilar artery, whose branches supply the brainstem and cerebellum, which then divides into the two posterior cerebral arteries supplying the posterior one-third of the cerebral hemispheres (Fig. 3). The carotid arterial systems are interconnected by the anterior communicating artery and are linked with the vertebrobasilar system by the posterior communicating arteries, so forming the circle of Willis at the base of the brain (Fig. 4). In many individuals, parts of this arterial ring are hypoplastic and fewer than half are of the standard pattern. None the less, it can form, unless affected by disease, an excellent collateral channel for blood to the brain if one or more of the four main extracranial arteries is occluded.

The pattern of atheroma

Atheroma tends to occur at points of arterial branching and tortuosity, which are sites of haemodynamic stress on the arterial wall, turbulent blood flow, and blood stasis. It is more extensive in hypertensive than normotensive individuals. The common sites of atheroma in the arteries supplying the brain are shown in Fig. 2.

Thrombosis occurs on atheromatous plaques that have ulcerated as a result of plaque fracture, necrosis, or intraplaque haemorrhage,

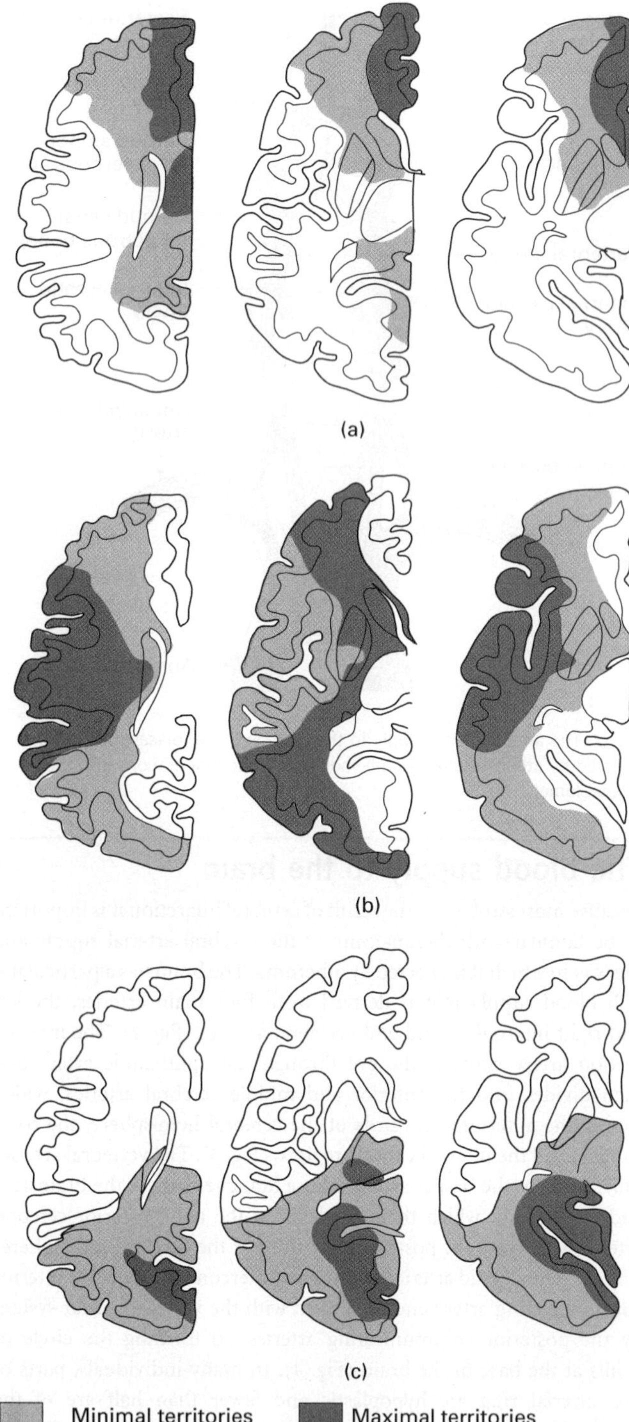

Fig. 3 The areas supplied by the anterior cerebral artery (a), middle cerebral artery (b), and the posterior cerebral artery (c) in horizontal slices through the brain. The dark shadowing represents the minimal territories and the light shadowing the maximal territories.
(Adapted, with permission, from the work of Dr Albert van der Zwan.)

and also in areas of turbulent or sluggish blood flow in relation to atheromatous stenotic areas that are severe enough to have an important haemodynamic effect. Thrombi may occlude arteries, embolize to distal sites, be lysed, become incorporated into the plaques themselves, or propagate proximally and/or distally. It is this underlying pathology that is the single most common cause of cerebral

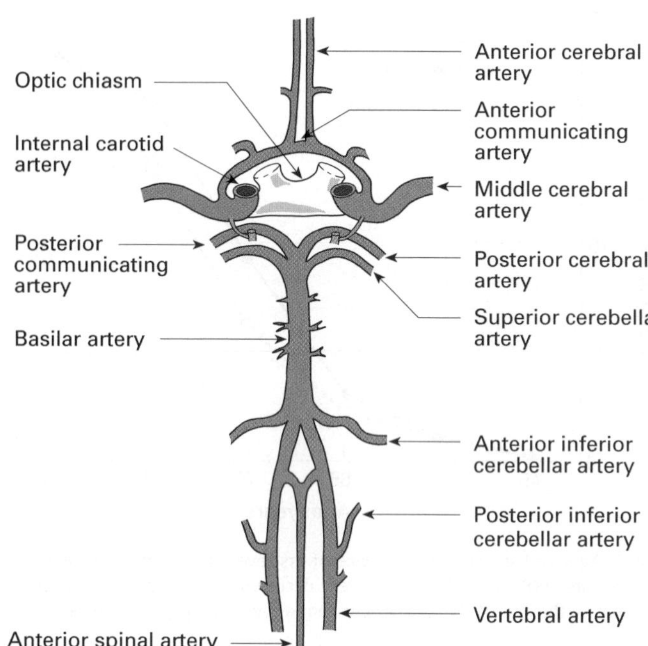

Fig. 4 The circle of Willis as seen at the base of the brain in relation to the optic chiasm.

ischaemia and infarction. It is important to stress the close correlation between atheroma in arteries supplying the brain, coronary arterial atheroma, and arterial disease in the periphery; a patient with clinically manifest disease in one area will almost certainly have subclinical, or clinically manifest, disease in other areas.

Transient ischaemic attacks

Transient ischaemic attacks are due to atherothromboembolism more often than anything else, and in patients with episodes in the distribution of the internal carotid artery the prevalence of angiographically demonstrated disease of the artery is about 50 per cent. However, the heart (Table 2) is also a particularly potent source of emboli to the brain, eye, and elsewhere: about 30 per cent of patients with a transient ischaemic attack have a potential, if not a definite, cardiac source of embolism, the most common being non-rheumatic atrial fibrillation; in perhaps 20 per cent of patients with a transient ischaemic attack, embolism from the heart is the actual cause of the attack. Like lacunar ischaemic stroke (see below), some transient ischaemic attacks are due to small-vessel disease within the brain. Others may be due to embolism from atherothrombosis affecting the aortic arch. A transient fall in blood pressure (e.g. due to postural hypotension, vasodilators or other hypotensive drugs, cardiac arrhythmia, hot bath, heavy meal, etc.) can cause transient ischaemic attacks but only if one or more arteries to the brain (or eye) are extremely stenotic or occluded, or there is a focal area of defective autoregulation as a result of previous ischaemic damage. In general, a fall in blood pressure causes non-focal neurological symptoms such as faintness, bilateral dimming of vision, and generalized weakness.

About 5 per cent of patients with a transient ischaemic attack have rare forms of arterial disease (Table 3) or a haematological disorder (Table 4).

Table 2 Cardiac sources of embolism (in anatomical sequence)

Paradoxical embolism from the venous system
Atrial septal defect
Ventricular septal defect
Patent foramen ovale
Pulmonary arteriovenous fistula
Left atrium
Atrial fibrillation
Sinoatrial disease
Myxoma
Interatrial septal aneurysm
Mitral valve
Rheumatic stenosis or regurgitation
Infective endocarditis
Non-bacterial thrombotic (marantic) endocarditis
Prosthetic valve
Mitral annulus calcification
Mitral leaflet prolapse
Libman–Sacks endocarditis
Left ventricular mural thrombus
Acute myocardial infarction
Left ventricular aneurysm
Cardiomyopathy
Myxoma
Blunt chest injury
Aortic valve
Rheumatic stenosis or regurgitation
Infective endocarditis
Non-bacterial thrombotic (marantic) endocarditis
Prosthetic valve
Calcification and/or sclerosis
Syphilis
Congenital cardiac disorders
(particularly with right to left shunt)
Cardiac surgery

Clinical features

A transient ischaemic attack starts abruptly and is not normally related to any particular activity. The attack may be single, recurrent but infrequent, or repetitive, and involve one or more parts of the brain or eye. On occasion, attacks can be remarkably stereotyped. The symptoms usually all appear within a matter of seconds, with no spread from one part of the body to another, and depend on which part of the brain or eye is ischaemic. It can be difficult to elucidate the exact location of ischaemia in an individual patient, depending as it almost always does on a history taken after recovery. However, it is important to try to divide transient ischaemic attacks into carotid and vertebrobasilar distribution events if carotid surgery is a consideration (see below).

Ischaemia in the carotid territory may cause weakness in the contralateral face, arm, hand, or leg in isolation or in various combinations; numbness or paraesthesias in a similar distribution; language disturbance if the dominant hemisphere is affected; dysarthria, but usually only in association with facial weakness; and transient monocular blindness (amaurosis fugax) in the ipsilateral eye. Ischaemic amaurosis fugax may involve the whole visual field of one eye or only the top or bottom half of the field; it is often described like a blind, curtain, or shutter obscuring vision over a matter of seconds. It is important to realize that amaurosis fugax is a symptom, not a disease, and has several causes (Table 5).

Table 3 Causes of arterial disease

Atheroma	*Dissection*
	Trauma
Intracerebral small-vessel disease	Cystic medial necrosis
(lipohyalinosis, microatheroma)	Fibromuscular dysplasia
	Inflammatory arterial disease
Inflammatory vascular disease	Marfan's syndrome
Giant-cell arteritis	Pseudoxanthoma elasticum
Systemic lupus erythematosus	Ehlers–Danlos syndrome
Systemic vasculitis	Infective arterial disease (e.g.
Sarcoid angiitis	syphilis)
Behçet's disease	
Progressive systemic sclerosis	*Congenital*
Rheumatoid disease	Fibromuscular dysplasia
Sjögren's syndrome	Loops, coils, etc.
Relapsing polychondritis	Aneurysms
Takayasu's disease	
Isolated granulomatous angiitis of	*Infections*
the nervous system	Tonsillitis, pharyngitis
Malignant atrophic papulosis	Cervical lymphadenitis
(Kohlmeier–Degos disease)	Endarteritis obliterans etc.
Buerger's disease	due to tuberculosis, syphilis,
	bacterial or fungal meningitis
Trauma	Herpes zoster
Penetrating injuries of the neck	Mucormycosis
Blow to the neck	
Cervical manipulation	*Miscellaneous*
Yoga	Homocystinaemia
Cervical rib	Angioendotheliosis
'Whiplash' injury	Neoplastic invasion
Tonsillectomy	of the arterial wall
Strangulation	Irradiation
Atlantoaxial dislocation/instability	Embolism from extra- or
Fractured clavicle	intracranial aneurysm sacs
Fractured base of skull	Fabry's disease
Angiography	Inflammatory bowel disease
	Migraine
	Drug abuse
	Mitochondrial cytopathy
	Binswanger's disease
	Nephrotic syndrome
	Fat embolism
	Fibrocartilagenous embolism

Table 4 Haematological causes of ischaemic stroke or infarction

Sickle-cell disease	'Hyperviscosity' syndromes
Polycythaemia rubra vera	Multiple myeloma
Essential thrombocythaemia	Waldenström's
Acute or chronic leukaemia	macroglobulinaemia
Thrombotic thrombocytopenic	Severe anaemia (probably causes
purpura	only transient cerebral symptoms)
Paroxysmal nocturnal	
haemoglobinuria	

Table 5 Causes of transient monocular blindness (i.e. amaurosis fugax)

Retinal ischaemia (i.e. transient ischaemic attack)	Retinal venous thrombosis
Papilloedema	Intraorbital tumour
Glaucoma	Macular degeneration
Uhthoff's phenomenon in retrobulbar neuritis	Caroticocavernous fistula
Retinal haemorrhage	Intracranial arteriovenous malformation
Retinal detachment	Reversible diabetic cataract
	Retinal migraine?

Ischaemia in the vertebrobasilar territory may cause hemiparesis or hemisensory disturbance, bilateral blindness or a homonymous hemianopia, diplopia, vertigo, vomiting, dysarthria, dysphagia, ataxia, a bilateral motor deficit, or a bilateral sensory deficit. Thus, in patients with only unilateral motor or sensory symptoms it is impossible to be sure which arterial distribution has been affected unless there is some other symptom that definitely suggests carotid or vertebrobasilar ischaemia (such as dysphasia or diplopia, respectively).

Symptoms during a transient ischaemic attack may, by definition, last up to 24 h but are normally over in a matter of minutes, or perhaps an hours, and ischaemic amaurosis fugax rarely lasts more than 5 min. The rate of recovery is usually slower than the onset of the symptoms.

It is extremely unusual to lose consciousness and then, to make the diagnosis of transient ischaemic attack, there must be some additional focal neurological feature. Vertigo, dizziness, diplopia, faintness, dysarthria, unsteadiness, or confusion as isolated symptoms can be to due to thromboembolism in the vertebrobasilar territory, but are often caused by something else, such as a drop in systemic blood pressure, sudden head movement, or labyrinthine disorders. Therefore, transient ischaemic attack should never be diagnosed if there is only one such symptom in isolation.

Drop attacks

The patient, typically a middle-aged or elderly woman, suddenly falls to the ground, usually while walking, sometimes while standing. Consciousness may be lost for a fraction of a second so that the patient does not remember the actual fall. Considerable injury can result. In most patients no cause is found, there is no particular evidence of vascular disease, the attacks resolve and there are no long-term consequences.

Transient global amnesia

For a matter of a few hours there is profound loss of ability to remember any new information (anterograde amnesia) and there is usually retrograde amnesia as well, sometimes stretching back many years. The patient is fully conscious, knows his or her name, and is able to continue normal activities such as eating, walking, or even driving. He or she cannot recall what they have just done or what has just been said and so often repetitively ask the same question about such matters. Recovery is normally complete, but memory for the duration of the attack itself is not regained. This syndrome of transient global amnesia is very rarely caused by vertebrobasilar ischaemia affecting the temporal lobes or thalamus bilaterally through their posterior cerebral arterial supply. Occasional cases are epileptic, particularly if the attacks are frequently repeated and last less than an hour. In the vast majority of patients, however, no cause at all is found and the prognosis is very good, certainly much better than after a transient ischaemic attack, although sometimes the attacks do recur.

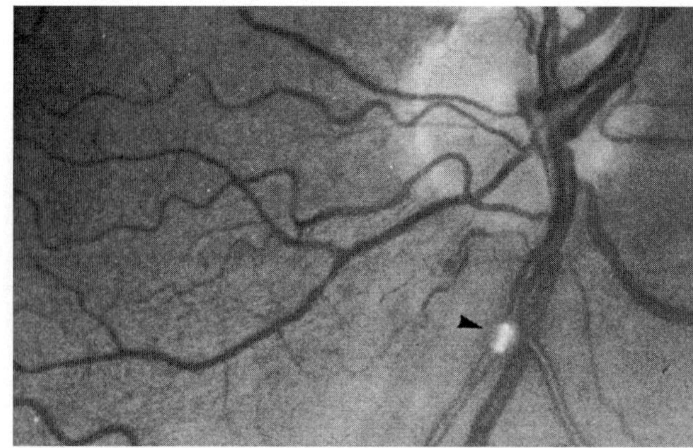

Fig. 5 A cholesterol embolus (black arrow) at the bifurcation of a retinal arteriole. Cholesterol emboli are yellow, refractile bodies that usually impact at arteriolar branching points without necessarily obstructing blood flow.

Subclavian steal

Subclavian steal is a very rare syndrome in which, as a result of stenosis or occlusion of the subclavian artery proximal to the origin of the vertebral artery, any increased metabolic demand of the arm musculature during ipsilateral arm exercise is met by retrograde blood flow down the vertebral artery to cause symptoms of brainstem ischaemia, particularly 'dizziness'. There is always a difference between the two radial pulses and unequal systolic blood pressures between the two arms, usually greater than 30 mmHg. Often there is a bruit in the supraclavicular fossa over the affected subclavian artery.

Differential diagnosis

Transient ischaemic attacks may be caused by any kind of arterial (Table 3), cardiac embolic (Table 2), haematological (Table 4), or other disease leading to transient ischaemia of the brain or eye. They must be differentiated from migraine and focal epileptic seizures on the basis of an adequate history, if necessary from a witness as well as the patient. The aura of migraine is a spreading and slowly intensifying phenomenon and the symptoms are usually positive (e.g. scintillating scotomas). The aura characteristically reaches a maximum within about 5 min, lasts 20 to 30 min, and is usually, but not always, followed by severe headache, often with nausea and vomiting. Focal seizures normally cause positive symptoms, particularly twitching, jerking, or dysaesthesias, which spread or march up one limb and from one limb to another on the same side, over a minute or so.

Physical signs

If the patient happens to be examined during an attack, then the signs appropriate to the ischaemic part of the nervous system will be found. But usually the patient is examined after the attack, when there should be no abnormal neurological signs. It is important to examine carefully the arterioles in the retina for any evidence of embolization (Fig. 5). Of considerable importance is examination of the vascular system, with a search for bruits over the carotid and subclavian arteries, absent or diminished foot pulses, femoral bruits, the pulses and blood pressure in both arms, and any signs of ischaemic or valvular heart disease.

Table 6 Investigations recommended in cases of transient ischaemic attack (TIA)

Investigation	Treatable disorder detected
Baseline tests for most TIA patients	
Full blood count	Anaemia, polycythaemia, leukaemia, thrombocythaemia
Erythrocyte sedimentation rate	Vasculitis, infective endocarditis, hyperviscosity
Plasma glucose	Diabetes, hypoglycaemia
Plasma cholesterol	Hypercholesterolaemia
Syphilis serology	Syphilis, anticardiolipin antibody syndrome
Urine analysis	Diabetes, renal disease
Electrocardiogram	Left ventricular hypertrophy, arrhythmia, conduction block, myocardial ischaemia or infarction
Non-routine investigations	
Electrolytes (if on diuretics)	Hyponatraemia or hypokalaemia
Urea (if hypertensive)	Renal impairment
Thyroid function (if in atrial fibrillation)	Thyrotoxicosis
Chest radiography	Enlarged heart, calcified valve, pulmonary arteriovenous malformation
Cranial CT/MRI	Structural brain lesion
Carotid ultrasound	Carotid stenosis
Echocardiography	Cardiac source of embolism
24-h ECG	Cardiac arrhythmia
Activated thromboplastin time, dilute Russell viper venom time, anticardiolipin antibody	Antiphospholipid antibody syndrome
Antinuclear antibodies	Systemic lupus erythematosus
Serum protein electrophoresis	Myeloma
Haemoglobin electrophoresis	Sickle-cell trait/disease
Electroencephalogram	Epileptic seizures
Protein C, protein S, antithrombin III	Deficiency
Plasma/urine amino acids	Homocystinaemia
Cerebrospinal fluid	Neurosyphilis, multiple sclerosis, infective endocarditis
Temporal artery biopsy	Giant-cell arteritis
Blood cultures	Infective endocarditis
Cardiac enzymes	Acute myocardial infarction

Investigations

Investigations are directed towards confirming the diagnosis of transient ischaemic attacks and excluding other causes of transient focal neurological events; finding the cause of the attack; defining risk factors for vascular disease in general; and the management of any associated vascular disease (Table 6).

CT or MRI exclude most structural intracranial disorders, but these are found unexpectedly in very few cases (well under 5 per cent). On CT about 25 per cent of patients have an area of infarction relevant to the transient ischaemic attack, even though clinically the symptoms lasted less than 24 h, but this does not alter management. If there is any reason to believe that there is a relevant cardiac source of embolism, then chest radiography and echocardiography, followed by further appropriate cardiological investigation, are required.

Imaging the cerebral circulation

Arterial imaging is used to delineate the anatomy of arterial lesions that are appropriate to the symptoms and potentially amenable to carotid surgery, and then only in patients who are fit enough and willing to consider such surgery. The first step is real-time ultrasound imaging of the carotid bifurcation, combined with Doppler analysis of blood flow, to eliminate patients with little or no stenosis from the dangers of carotid angiography (about 1 per cent permanent stroke risk). For patients with carotid stenosis or possible occlusion, selective intra-arterial carotid angiography (by conventional or digital techniques) is then usually performed to demonstrate the symptomatic internal carotid artery in the neck and the intracranial circulation. Tightly stenosing lesions at the origin of the internal carotid artery (Fig. 6) are operable (see below). The presence of a carotid bruit makes the likelihood of stenosis of the internal carotid artery high but, even without a bruit, there can be extreme stenosis with very low blood flow. Conversely, there can be a bruit, even in the presence of a relatively normal or occluded internal carotid artery, due to stenosis of the external carotid artery, or transmitted from the aortic valve or aortic arch. The absence of a carotid bruit should not, therefore, discourage one from Duplex if subsequent surgical intervention for carotid disease might be indicated.

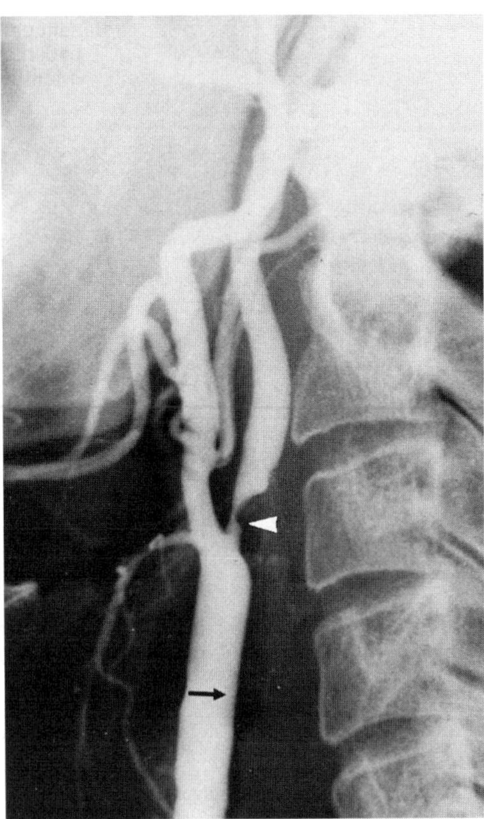

Fig. 6 Lateral view of a selective carotid angiogram to show stenosis at the origin of the internal carotid artery (white arrow) just past the bifurcation of the common carotid artery (black arrow).

Medical treatment

The risk of stroke after a transient ischaemic attack is about 12 per cent in the first year and then 7 per cent per annum, that of myocardial infarction or cardiac death is also about 7 per cent per annum, and of 'stroke, myocardial infarction, or vascular death' about 10 per cent per annum. The excess risk of stroke in these patients is seven times that of the background population. Individual patients at highest risk are those with frequent transient ischaemic attacks, the elderly,

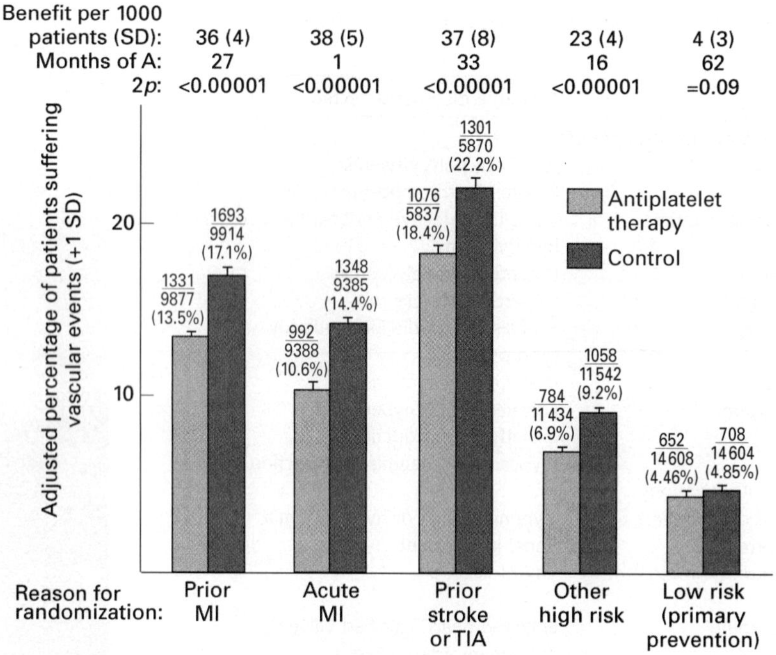

Benefit per 1000 patients (SD): 36 (4) | 38 (5) | 37 (8) | 23 (4) | 4 (3)
Months of A: 27 | 1 | 33 | 16 | 62
2*p*: <0.00001 | <0.00001 | <0.00001 | <0.00001 | =0.09

Adjusted percentage of patients suffering vascular events (+1 SD)

Antiplatelet therapy
Control

Prior MI: 1331/9877 (13.5%); 1693/9914 (17.1%)
Acute MI: 992/9388 (10.6%); 1348/9385 (14.4%)
Prior stroke or TIA: 1076/5837 (18.4%); 1301/5870 (22.2%)
Other high risk: 784/11 434 (6.9%); 1058/11 542 (9.2%)
Low risk (primary prevention): 652/14 608 (4.46%); 708/14 604 (4.85%)

Reason for randomization: Prior MI | Acute MI | Prior stroke or TIA | Other high risk | Low risk (primary prevention)

Fig. 7 Absolute effects of antiplatelet drugs on serious vascular events (myocardial infarction, stroke, or vascular death) in all main high-risk categories of patient and in low-risk (primary prevention). Months of A = means of scheduled antiplatelet duration. No trial lasted under 1 month.
(Figure reproduced by permission of the British Medical Journal and the Antiplatelet Trialist's Collaboration.).

claudicants, those with severe carotid stenosis, or with left ventricular hypertrophy.

The most important issue in the management of transient ischaemic attacks is, therefore, reduction in the risk of stroke and coronary events, which can occur within hours, days, weeks, or years of the transient ischaemic attack. It is, therefore, logical to start any treatment as soon as the diagnosis is made, even if there has only been one attack. It is important to control hypertension and cigarette smoking. A 'statin' is probably indicated in those who have the clinical manifestations of coronary artery disease.

Long-term aspirin reduces the odds of serious vascular events by about one-fifth, similar to the reduction in other patients with high-risk vascular disease (Fig. 7). The dose is 75 mg daily, provided there are no contraindications such as peptic ulceration, but if there is indigestion then enteric-coated preparations are available. The second-choice antiplatelet drug is clopidosrel (75 mg daily) but this very much more expensive. Adding dipyridamole to aspirin may be more effective than aspirin alone, although there is some uncertainly about this. It is conceivable that antiplatelet drugs increase the risk of intracranial haemorrhage, which counteracts some of their beneficial effect in reducing the risk of ischaemic stroke. If, as is sometimes the case, aspirin does not control very frequent transient ischaemic attacks, then it is reasonable to try formal oral anticoagulation, which can be tailed off and replaced by aspirin a few weeks after the attacks stop. If the transient ischaemic attacks do not stop, either the diagnosis is wrong or the treatment is ineffective, in which case it should be reconsidered and perhaps stopped.

Patients with a definite major cardiac valvular source of embolism (such as mitral stenosis, a prosthetic valve, or dilating cardiomyopathy) should be anticoagulated indefinitely to prevent further intracardiac fibrin formation, particularly if atrial fibrillation is also present; the INR should be kept at about 3.0. If transient ischaemic attacks occur within days or weeks of an acute myocardial infarction, anticoagulation is only required for a matter of 3 to 6 months. Patients with non-rheumatic atrial fibrillation should also be anticoagulated, but if this is not practical or too risky they should be given aspirin.

Surgery

For patients who have recovered from a carotid ischaemic event, the removal of any tightly stenosing atherothrombotic lesion at the origin of the symptomatic internal carotid artery by carotid endarterectomy is logical because such a lesion is likely to cause stroke by embolism to the brain, or a reduction in cerebral blood flow if the stenosis is extreme. This logic has the unambiguous backing of randomized trials, which have shown that the more severe the stenosis is (above about 80 per cent diameter reduction of the arterial lumen) the greater the probability of ipsilateral ischaemic stroke without surgery and, therefore, the more worthwhile is the inevitable risk of surgery, which is about 7 per cent stroke and/or death. However, carotid endarterectomy should only be done in centres with adequate experience and where the risk is kept under continuous review. Carotid occlusion is inoperable.

Cerebral infarction

The underlying pathogenesis is, like that of transient ischaemic attack, mostly atherothromboembolism, or embolism from the heart, and any difference between ischaemia and infarction is one of degree. Prolonged hypotension or anoxia normally causes widespread cerebral infarction and, if the patient survives the circulatory catastrophe, this infarction is often found to have occurred in the boundary zones between arterial territories (see below).

Clinical features

The symptoms, signs, duration, and severity of stroke due to cerebral infarction are very varied and depend on the location and extent of the lesion (Table 7). The onset of symptoms is normally quite sudden, or occurs during sleep, but there may be worsening in a subacute or stepwise fashion over a few hours; occasionally the clinical picture develops over a matter of several days but very rarely over a few weeks. An increase in the neurological deficit over a few hours or days is sometimes referred to as stroke-in-evolution, but the cause may not only be propagating thrombosis but also further embolization,

Table 7 The distribution of the subtypes of ischaemic stroke in the Oxfordshire Community Stroke Project

Total anterior circulation infarction		15%
Partial anterior circulation infarction		35%
Lacunar infarction	25%	
Pure motor stroke	50%	
Pure sensory stroke	5%	
Sensory motor stroke	35%	
Ataxic hemiparesis	10%	
Posterior circulation infarction		25%

haemorrhage into infarcted brain, or cerebral oedema, and these possibilities are difficult, if not impossible, to distinguish with any degree of certainty.

Cerebral hemisphere infarcts

Infarction in one cerebral hemisphere may cause contralateral hemiparesis or hemiplegia, hemisensory loss, or homonymous hemianopia. The motor and/or sensory disturbance may involve the entire side of the body, the upper limb, the face and the upper limb, both limbs, occasionally the leg alone, and rarely just the face. A small cortical infarct may cause clumsiness of the hand, or only of some of the fingers of one hand. To begin with, any hemiplegia tends to be flaccid with diminished deep tendon reflexes, albeit with an extensor plantar response, but within days or weeks spasticity and increased reflexes gradually appear. Lesions in the dominant hemisphere are likely to impair language function (speaking, reading, or writing) while in the non-dominant hemisphere may cause visuospatial problems, such as constructional or dressing apraxia. If the parietal lobe is affected, there is a tendency for the patient to ignore the contralateral side of the body; astereognosis; sensory inattention; sensory loss to all modalities; or just isolated loss of joint-position sense. To begin with the head and eyes may be turned towards the side of the lesion but this usually resolves in a few days. Dysarthria tends to be in proportion to the extent of any facial weakness. Initially there is often some contralateral palatal weakness and dysphagia. Headache is quite common, but not usually very severe. Epileptic seizures are unusual but can be an early, or more often late, complication of cerebral infarction (less than 5 per cent of patients). If the infarct is extensive, and particularly if transtentorial herniation occurs, consciousness is impaired and Cheyne–Stokes or some other abnormality of the respiratory pattern develops.

It is helpful to identify patients who have infarcted the whole of their middle cerebral arterial territory, usually because of occlusion of the middle cerebral artery as a result of embolism from the heart or a proximal site of atherothrombosis. Total anterior circulation infarction is recognized by a combination of weakness, with or without a sensory deficit, of two out of three body areas (arm, leg, face) plus a homonymous hemianopia plus new higher cerebral dysfunction (e.g. dysphasia, apraxia). If the patient is drowsy, then one has to assume the hemianopia and cognitive deficit. On the other hand, patients with partial anterior circulation infarction, likely due to embolic occlusion of a branch of the middle or the anterior cerebral artery, are recognized by having only two of the three features of total anterior circulation infarction or new higher cerebral dysfunction alone, or a motor/sensory deficit restricted to one body area or part of one body area, or a predominantly proprioceptive deficit.

Lacunar infarction

Small, deep infarcts (usually less than 1.5 cm in diameter) in the basal ganglia, thalamus, internal capsule, cerebral peduncle, and pons are called lacunes. Higher cortical function is normal and the patient is conscious. Such patients can usually be recognized by a number of characteristic clinical syndromes as follows.

Pure motor stroke. Complete or incomplete weakness of one side of the body, involving the whole of two out of the three body areas (face, upper limb, leg). Sensory symptoms, but not signs, may be present, and there may be dysarthria and sometimes dysphagia.

Pure sensory stroke. Sensory symptoms and/or sensory signs (but not impaired joint-position sense alone) in the same distribution as pure motor stroke.

Sensory motor stroke. A combination of pure motor and pure sensory stroke.

Ataxic hemiparesis. A combination of hemiparesis and ipsilateral cerebellar ataxia, often with marked dysarthria, clumsiness of the hand, and unsteadiness.

Most lacunar infarcts are thought to be caused by disease of the small perforating vessels within the brain substance. There is tortuosity, thickening, and disorganization of the vessel wall. It is these damaged vessels that may form microaneurysms (Charcot–Bouchard aneurysms), which rupture to produce either small, localized haematomas or massive intracerebral haematomas (see below). Therefore, lacunar syndromes are usually caused by small-vessel disease leading to a small, deep infarct, but they can occasionally be caused by embolism to the same vessels, and certainly to small intracerebral haematomas in the same part of the brain.

Brainstem infarction

Infarction in the brainstem tends to cause a rather complicated neurological deficit. Hemiparesis, hemiplegia, tetraparesis, tetraplegia, and unilateral or bilateral sensory loss can all occur. In addition, there may be a disturbance of gaze or palsies of extraocular muscles, dysphagia, dysarthria, hiccups, ataxia, Horner's syndrome due to a lesion involving the descending sympathetic pathways, deafness, vertigo, vomiting, periodic breathing, and respiratory arrest particularly during sleep. An extensive brainstem infarct can result in the locked-in syndrome in which, despite being conscious, the patient is unable to move anything except perhaps the eyelids, or the eyes in the vertical plane, and can neither speak nor swallow.

Boundary zone (or watershed) infarction

A profound but transient fall in systemic blood pressure usually causes syncope (i.e., faintness or unconsciousness) or generalized weakness; if it continues for some minutes, an epileptic seizure can occur. More prolonged hypotension can cause massive cerebral infarction, leading to the persistent vegetative state or death, or, sometimes, to infarction between arterial territories, particularly in the parieto-occipital region, which is the boundary zone between the middle, anterior, and posterior cerebral arteries. Boundary-zone infarction in this area is commonly bilateral, and the symptoms include cortical blindness or visual disorientation, associated with a visual-field defect and often memory impairment.

Boundary-zone infarction can be recognized partly by the distribution on CT and partly by the circumstances of the stroke (i.e., when a fall in blood pressure is likely).

Table 8 Causes of intracranial venous thrombosis

Local conditions affecting the cerebral veins and sinuses directly
• Head injury (with or without fracture)
• Intracranial surgery
• Local sepsis (sinuses, ears, scalp, mastoids, nasopharynx)
• Subdural empyema
• Bacterial meningitis
• Tumour invasion of dural sinuses
• Dural or cerebral arteriovenous malformation
• Catheterization of jugular veins for parenteral nutrition, etc.
Systemic disorders
• Dehydration, hypernatraemia
• Septicaemia
• Pregnancy and the puerperium
• Oral contraceptives
• Haematological disorders (Table 4)
• Inflammatory vascular disease (Table 3)
• Diabetes mellitus
• Congestive cardiac failure
• Inflammatory bowel disease
• Androgen therapy
• Antifibrinolytic drugs
• Non-metastatic effect of extracranial malignancy
• Nephrotic syndrome

Migrainous stroke

Occasionally ischaemic stroke with a persistent neurological deficit occurs during a migrainous episode. This is possibly due to arterial narrowing caused by oedema of the vessel wall rather than vasospasm. It probably only occurs in patients with migraine with aura, and the neurological deficit has a similar clinical pattern to the transient neurological symptoms during the previously experienced auras.

Stroke and pregnancy

Stroke occurs most often in the last trimester of pregnancy, or in the puerperium. However, this is rare; about 30 cases/100 000 deliveries in the UK. The middle cerebral artery is the most frequently occluded vessel, but the cause is unknown since there appears to be no underlying arterial disease. Some cases could be due to paradoxical embolism from thrombosis in the venous system of the legs or pelvis. Intracranial venous thrombosis is another cause.

Cortical venous and/or dural sinus thrombosis (i.e., intracranial venous thrombosis)

Thrombosis of the cortical veins and/or dural sinuses is a much less common cause of cerebral infarction than arterial disease, and occurs as a result of local conditions affecting the cortical veins or dural sinus, or systemic disorders (Table 8). Venous infarcts are commonly haemorrhagic. The clinical picture can be like infarction of a cerebral hemisphere caused by arterial occlusion, but epileptic seizures headache and impaired consciousness are more common and raised intracranial pressure develops rapidly if the dural sinuses become obstructed. Cortical venous and sinus thrombosis may propagate widely to produce a catastrophic encephalopathic illness with similar features to severe viral encephalitis. Isolated thrombosis of the sagittal or transverse dural sinus is one cause of the benign intracranial hypertension syndrome. The diagnosis is increasingly being made by MRI rather than conventional angiography. Treatment with anticoagulation seems to be both effective and surprisingly safe, even if there are haemorrhagic venous infarcts. Thrombosis of the cavernous sinus is rare but is usually due to pyogenic or fungal infection spreading from the face, sinuses, or nasal space; the symptoms include unilateral orbital pain and swelling, proptosis, visual loss, papilloedema, and often palsies of the IIIrd, IVth, Vth, and VIth cranial nerves.

Differential diagnosis

The clinical picture of stroke, either due to cerebral infarction or indeed to primary intracerebral haemorrhage, is characteristic and the diagnosis depends not so much on where the lesion is thought to be, but on the sudden onset. Usually the patient is over the age of 50 years and has one or more vascular risk factors or diseases (such as hypertension or angina). It is important to consider the possibility of a chronic subdural haematoma, or drug overdose, in an unconscious patient with few or no focal signs, and without a good history of a sudden onset. Encephalitis, cerebral abscess, sudden deterioration in a patient with a cerebral tumour, multiple sclerosis, peripheral nerve lesion, hypoglycaemia, and somatization can all usually be excluded after an adequate history, clinical examination, and straightforward investigations. In acute stroke, as in other severe acute illnesses, there is often transient hypertension, fever, hyperglycaemia, glycosuria, and a neutrophil leucocytosis. Sometimes there are arrhythmias and ischaemic changes on the electrocardiogram (but not the classical development of Q waves as in myocardial infarction), making it difficult to know if cerebral infarction has occurred as a result of embolism from left ventricular mural thrombus overlying an acute myocardial infarct. In any stroke patient it is important to remember that there are rare but often treatable underlying causes (Tables 2, 3 and 4).

Complications

The most important brain complication of ischaemic stroke is the development of cerebral oedema, which impairs, possibly only temporarily, local blood flow and neuronal function over a wider area than just the infarct and, if extensive, causes transtentorial herniation. There are also a number of general complications of acute paralysis: these include bronchopneumonia, particularly if consciousness or swallowing are impaired; venous thromboembolism; pressure sores and septicaemia; urinary infection, particularly if catheterization is necessary, and eventually uraemia; contractures in spastic limbs; frozen shoulder; disturbances of cardiac rhythm; and mood disorder (Table 9). Death in the first week is almost always due to the infarct itself and the effects of cerebral oedema, but later it is more often due to one of the general complications, particularly pneumonia.

Investigations

These are the same as in patients with transient ischaemic attacks, but tempered by the age of the patient, the likelihood of recovery, and the chance that they will influence the immediate and long-term management. The most reliable way in which primary intracerebral haemorrhage can be differentiated from ischaemic stroke is by an unenhanced CT scan within hours of stroke onset; neither the clinical picture nor the absence of blood in the cerebrospinal fluid rules out primary intracerebral haemorrhage. The high density of an intracerebral haematoma appears at once, although after it has resolved (in a matter of weeks and only days if the haematoma is small) the scan may become normal or show only a low-density area very similar to that after cerebral infarction. The characteristic low-density appearance of infarction usually takes a day or two to appear clearly,

Table 9 General complications of stroke

Respiratory	*Mechanical*
• Pneumonia • Inhalation • Pulmonary embolism	• Spasticity • Contractures • Malalignment/subluxation/ frozen shoulder
Cardiovascular • Myocardial infarction • Cardiac failure • Cardiac arrhythmia • Neurogenic pulmonary oedema	• Falls and fractures • Osteoporosis • Ankle swelling • Peripheral nerve pressure palsies
Infections • Pneumonia • Urinary • Skin • Septicaemia	*Others* • Pressure sores • Depression, anxiety, apathy • Epileptic seizures • Deep venous thrombosis
Metabolic • Vomiting • Dehydration • Electrolyte imbalance • Hyperglycaemia • Renal failure	• Acute gastric ulceration • Incontinence of urine/faeces

Table 10 Indications for CT scan in acute stroke

Uncertain diagnosis with the possibility of non-stroke intracranial pathology, particularly cerebral tumour or subdural haematoma. This situation usually only arises if there is uncertainty over the details of the symptom onset and the time course of the neurological deficit
The patient is taking, or may need to take, antihaemostatic drugs (anticoagulants, antiplatelet drugs, thrombolytics). To distinguish reliably between primary intracerebral haemorrhage and cerebral infarction, the scan should be performed as soon as possible, preferably within h of stroke onset. A normal scan or hypodense lesion more than 2 or 3 weeks poststroke does not exclude a haemorrhagic origin
Cerebellar stroke
Subarachnoid haemorrhage
Uncharacteristic deterioration after the first 24 h, making non-stroke intracranial pathology rather more likely
Mild carotid distribution stroke possibly suitable for carotid endarterectomy
Young patient

although subtle loss of brain density can be apparent within hours of onset. Small infarcts less than about 0.5 cm in diameter, particularly in the posterior fossa, are not visible on CT but are much more readily seen by MRI. MRI is not, however, so good as CT at reliably detecting primary intracerebral haemorrhage immediately after stroke onset and, in any event, it is not very practical in restless and confused patients, even when it is available. Ideally, stroke patients should never be anticoagulated nor even exposed to antiplatelet drugs unless a CT scan has been done first to exclude primary intracerebral haemorrhage. Indications for CT scanning are summarized in Table 10.

Cerebral angiography is not usually indicated during the acute phase of ischaemic stroke since the result is unlikely to influence the immediate management, and the procedure itself can make the patient worse. In a young patient there is an argument for urgent angiography, particularly if there is a possibility of traumatic arterial dissection with medicolegal implications, but usually it is best left until any recovery is well under way when it will be easier to decide whether carotid surgery is likely to be indicated. There are no reliable angiographic criteria for distinguishing between arterial embolism and thrombosis.

The cerebrospinal fluid may need to be examined if there is a possibility of encephalitis, neurosyphilis, or multiple sclerosis. It is not helpful in ruling out primary intracerebral haemorrhage, which can, if small, be confined within the brain without any blood leaking into the cerebrospinal fluid. After stroke there are no more than 100 white blood cells/mm^3 unless there have been septic emboli to the brain.

Prognosis

Recovery, to some extent, is the rule after ischaemic stroke unless it is severe enough to cause death. Sudden death (i.e., within an hours of the onset of symptoms) is very rarely due to ischaemic stroke or any other form of cerebrovascular disease except spontaneous subarachnoid haemorrhage. Most of any recovery occurs in the first 3 months but may not be absolutely complete for something like 1 or 2 years. The immediate prognosis is particularly poor if there is any impairment of consciousness. Case fatality is about 20 per cent at 1 month for stroke in general, but much higher after primary intracerebral haemorrhage than ischaemic stroke. Of the survivors from stroke, about a half recover completely, or more or less completely, while the rest are disabled to some degree. Good prognostic factors for recovery of function include young age, urinary continence, rapid improvement, mild stroke, and no perceptual or cognitive disorder.

Treatment

There is little that medical treatment and nothing that vascular surgery can do to alter the immediate outcome after ischaemic stroke. In theory the reduction of cerebral oedema by mannitol, glycerol, or dexamethasone should be useful, but there have been no adequate clinical trials. Thrombolysis causes intracerebral haemorrhage but this risk may be outweighed by the potential benefit and further trials need to be done. Immediate aspirin, 300 mg daily, is safe and reduces the risk of very early recurrences. Routine heparin seems to cause as many haemorrhagic strokes as ischaemic stroke recurrences and has no overall beneficial effect, notwithstanding some reduction in the risk of deep venous thrombosis. It is important to remember that there are many reasons for stroke patients to deteriorate, and some are potentially reversible (Table 11).

If there is a definite cardiac source of embolism the patient should be anticoagulated long term provided that there is no CT evidence of intracerebral haemorrhage (see discussion of anticoagulation in patients with transient ischaemic attacks above). Anticoagulants are contraindicated in infective endocarditis because of the risk of haemorrhage from mycotic aneurysms, which form when the arterial wall is weakened by bacterial infection spreading from an infected embolus. Anticoagulation in acute embolic stroke always carries some risk because of the possibility of haemorrhage into infarcted brain, so there is a dilemma between anticoagulating too early and causing

Table 11 Causes of neurological deterioration after stroke

Local	General
Recurrent embolism	Hypoxia (pneumonia, pulmonary embolism, cardiac failure)
Recurrent haemorrhage	Infection (chest, urine, septicaemia)
Haemorrhagic transformation of the infarct	Dehydration, hyponatraemia
Cerebral oedema	Hyper- or hypoglycaemia
Brain shift and herniation	Sedatives/hypnotics
Hydrocephalus	Depression
Epileptic seizures	

haemorrhagic transformation of the infarct and too late after further embolization has occurred. It is perhaps advisable to start an oral anticoagulant after a week or two and achieve full anticoagulation over a matter of a few days.

Ischaemic stroke often causes transient hypertension, which settles without treatment. If the patient is taking antihypertensive drugs, they should normally be continued. If the systolic blood pressure is greater than about 240 mmHg, it is probably best to reduce it, but slowly over a matter of days, and with extreme caution, because not only is there loss of normal cerebral autoregulation in and around infarcts, but in chronic hypertension autoregulation is set higher so that rapid and extreme reduction of blood pressure can lead to a catastrophic fall in cerebral blood flow and more extensive cerebral infarction. Surprisingly, no adequate trials of the speed and extent to which the blood pressure should be manipulated have yet been done.

The complications of ischaemic stroke are often preventable and treatable (Table 9). Chest physiotherapy and care of the airway, particularly in unconscious patients and those with difficulty swallowing, will reduce the risk of pneumonia, which, if it occurs, can be treated with antibiotics. Nasogastric tube feeding is used for adequate hydration and electrolyte balance in patients who cannot swallow, and later for feeding if necessary. Good nursing should prevent pressure sores. Early physiotherapy will reduce the risk of contractures, pain, and stiffness in hemiplegic limbs and leads naturally on to active physical rehabilitation. Urinary catheterization is often avoidable in men, for whom an appliance is a better alternative, but in women it may be necessary so that the skin can be kept dry to reduce the chance of pressure sores. Compression stockings should reduce the risk of venous thromboembolism. Epilepsy, if it occurs, should be treated in the normal way.

For secondary prevention, risk factors for vascular disease should be minimized as in patients with transient ischaemic attacks and aspirin given, 75 mg daily. There is little doubt that adequate treatment of hypertension after stroke will reduce the risk of recurrence, and fears that any such treatment will, by causing low pressure, lead to cerebral infarction are unfounded, provided drugs are used carefully and overt postural hypotension avoided.

In the UK up to 50 per cent of stroke patients are treated at home by their general practitioners and it is uncertain whether hospital treatment in a non-specialist unit confers any particular benefit unless the domestic circumstances make home nursing impossible. However, units specifically for the acute care and subsequent rehabilitation of stroke patients reduce both case fatality and morbidity.

Multi-infarct (or vascular) dementia

Multi-infarct dementia is defined as a deterioration in previously normal mental function due to cerebral ischaemia and infarction. It is a less common cause of dementia than Alzheimer's disease. The main distinction between the two conditions is that in multi-infarct dementia the progression tends to be in a series of more or less sudden 'steps', because it is due to repeated episodes of ischaemia or infarction, some of which may cause overt strokes. It is a more likely cause of dementia than Alzheimer's disease if there are hypertension, focal neurological symptoms or signs, focal or lateralizing features on the electroencephalogram, vascular bruits, and reduced regional cerebral blood flow.

Table 12 Causes of spontaneous intracranial haemorrhage

Hypertension (chronic, acute) *Aneurysms* saccular atheromatous mycotic myxomatous dissecting *Vascular malformations* arteriovenous venous cavernous telangiectasis *Cerebral amyloid angiopathy* *Haemostatic failure* haemophilia and other coagulation disorders thrombocytopenia thrombotic thrombo-cytopenic purpura anticoagulation therapeutic thrombolysis antiplatelet drugs polycythaemia rubra vera essential thrombocythaemia sickle-cell disease paraproteinaemias disseminated intravascular coagulation renal failure liver failure snake bite	*Inflammatory vascular disease* (Table 3) *Haemorrhagic transformation of cerebral infarction* *Intracranial venous thrombosis* (Table 8) *Moyamoya syndrome* *Carotid endarterectomy* *Posterior fossa surgery* *Alcoholic binge* *Vascular tumours* melanoma malignant astrocytoma oligodendroglioma medulloblastoma choroid plexus papilloma hypernephroma endometrial carcinoma bronchogenic carcinoma choriocarcinoma *Drug abuse* *Infections* Herpes simplex leptospirosis anthrax *Scorpion bite*

Spontaneous intracranial haemorrhage

About 20 per cent of strokes in caucasians are due to intracranial haemorrhage, which usually occurs as a result of rupture of a saccular aneurysm or an arteriovenous malformation, or hypertensive vascular disease. Rarer causes are listed in Table 12. The site of bleeding may be destroyed by haemorrhage, which is usually into the subarachnoid space from a saccular aneurysm and directly into the brain (primary intracerebral haemorrhage) from hypertensive vascular disease or a vascular malformation. There can be blood in both sites after intracranial haemorrhage from any cause.

Primary intracerebral haemorrhage

Haemorrhage is most common in the basal ganglia, thalamus, cerebellar hemisphere, pons, and subcortical areas. Haemorrhage in the

Table 13 Causes of nearly simultaneous and multiple intracerebral haemorrhages

Cerebral amyloid angiopathy	Vascular malformations
Metastases (Table 12)	Malignant hypertension
Haemostatic defect	Multiple haemorrhagic infarcts
Intracranial venous thrombosis	Head injury
Inflammatory vascular disease	Drug abuse

cerebral hemispheres outside the basal ganglia region (so-called lobar haemorrhage) is less likely to be due to hypertensive vascular disease than to one of the other causes mentioned above. Sometimes primary intracerebral haemorrhage is multiple (Table 13). A haematoma may cause transtentorial herniation in the same way as does a large cerebral infarct.

Clinical features

Clinically, it is difficult, if not impossible, to distinguish reliably between primary intracerebral haemorrhage and ischaemic stroke. However, severe headache and coma within a few hours of onset is unusual in ischaemic stroke. The symptoms, signs, investigations, differential diagnosis, and general management of infarction and haemorrhage are similar, but with some important exceptions, which need to be discussed separately below.

Cerebellar haematoma

This condition, although rare, is important because surgical treatment can be life-saving and survivors may have remarkably little neurological disability. The patient presents with sudden occipital headache, dizziness, truncal ataxia, rapid reduction in consciousness, a gaze palsy to the side of the lesion, ipsilateral facial weakness, and often raised intracranial pressure due to acute obstruction of the flow of cerebrospinal fluid. Cerebellar signs cannot normally be elicited unless the patient is conscious. Any hemiparesis is mild, although bilateral extensor plantars are common. Sensory signs are unusual. The diagnosis is confirmed by CT scan.

Angiography

Cerebral angiography is unnecessary if a haematoma has been demonstrated by CT scanning and the patient is extremely ill or seriously disabled. However, if the patient has recovered useful function, is normotensive, and not particularly elderly or compromised by some other disease, angiography may reveal a cause for the haemorrhage that is potentially treatable, for example an arteriovenous malformation or an aneurysm that has bled directly into the brain substance rather than into the subarachnoid space.

Medical treatment

Naturally, anticoagulants are contraindicated. If a patient's course is complicated by pulmonary embolism, it is unclear whether the benefits of anticoagulation are outweighed by the risks of making the cerebral haemorrhage worse. Medical treatment and rehabilitation are otherwise the same as for patients with ischaemic stroke (see above). If a patient survives, the recovery and long-term prognosis are often remarkably good.

Surgical treatment

The evacuation of a haematoma, particularly if it is superficial, is a tempting surgical possibility, but whether this increases the chance of recovery is uncertain. Some surgeons operate on haematomas acutely but there have been no clinical trials to support such a policy. A more widely accepted indication is in the patient whose conscious level is deteriorating, usually because of brain shift and transtentorial herniation.

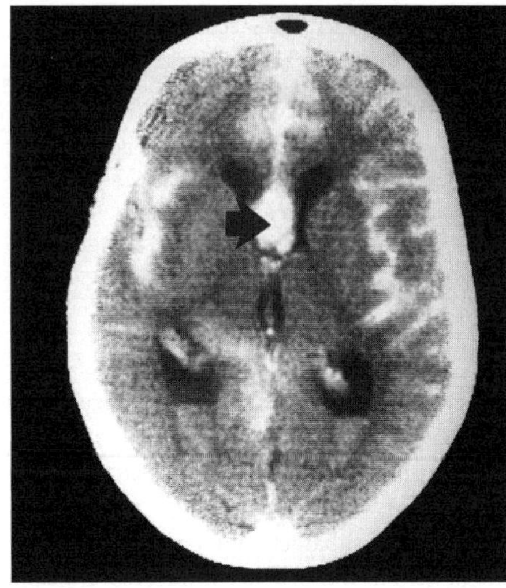

Fig. 8 Unenhanced CT scan showing blood (white areas) in the subarachnoid space and between the frontal horns of the lateral ventricles (arrow) where an aneurysm of the anterior communicating artery has ruptured.

Spontaneous subarachnoid haemorrhage

Most patients have ruptured an intracranial saccular aneurysm; about 5 per cent have bled from an arteriovenous malformation, and a few have rare causes of intracranial haemorrhage (Table 12). In about 15 per cent of patients no cause can be identified, particularly in those with a restricted haemorrhage around the midbrain (perimesencephalic subarachnoid haemorrhage), and in this group the prognosis is particularly good.

The clinical picture is distinctive and not easily confused with stroke due to cerebral infarction or primary intracerebral haemorrhage. The onset is with sudden headache, usually but not always severe, which is often occipital and radiates over the head and down the neck, sometimes down as far as the back or legs as blood tracks down the spinal canal. Consciousness is often impaired or lost transiently at the onset and if the haemorrhage is extensive the patient remains comatose. Vomiting is common and occasionally epileptic seizures are an early feature. Meningism develops, but sometimes not for several hours, and there are no signs of focal neurological damage unless bleeding has also occurred into the brain substance, or unless there is an oculomotor palsy due to pressure from a posterior communicating artery/distal internal carotid artery aneurysm. The patient is very often irritable, confused, photophobic, and drowsy for several days, and the headache may persist for weeks.

The diagnosis can be most easily confirmed by early CT scan, which almost always shows blood in the cerebrospinal fluid pathways (Fig. 8) and perhaps a collection of blood in relation to the ruptured aneurysm or arteriovenous malformations. If a CT scan is not easily available or is normal, then lumbar puncture is mandatory and the cerebrospinal fluid will be bloodstained. If the haemorrhage is more than about 12 h old, the cerebrospinal fluid becomes xanthochromic due to altered blood pigment. Clearly, if there is any clinical difficulty

Table 14 Associations of intracranial saccular aneurysms

Polycystic kidney disease*	Ehlers–Danlos syndrome*
Fibromuscular dysplasia	Pseudoxanthoma elasticum*
Cervical artery dissection*	Hereditary haemorrhagic telangiectasia*
Coarctation of the aorta	Moyamoya syndrome
Intracranial vascular malformations*	Klinefelter's syndrome
Marfan's syndrome*	Progeria

*Can be familial.

distinguishing between subarachnoid haemorrhage and acute meningitis, then the cerebrospinal fluid should be examine at once. The CT scan and cerebrospinal fluid become normal within days or weeks of the onset.

The complications of subarachnoid haemorrhage are similar to those of ischaemic stroke and primary intracerebral haemorrhage. In addition, organized blood clot in the subarachnoid space may cause obstruction to the flow of cerebrospinal fluid and thus acute hydrocephalus. This is common and often asymptomatic, but it may lead to a deterioration in the patient's conscious level a few days or weeks after the onset of the haemorrhage, when progress has otherwise been satisfactory. This complication can be easily diagnosed by CT and then treated with a ventricular drainage procedure. Delayed cerebral ischaemia, said to be due to vasospasm, is discussed below.

Intracranial saccular aneurysms

These develop on the medium-sized arteries at the base of the brain and the common sites are at the distal internal carotid/posterior communicating artery origin (30 per cent), the anterior communicating artery complex (40 per cent), and at the bifurcation of the middle cerebral artery (25 per cent). The basilar artery is a less common site (5 per cent). About 25 per cent of cases have multiple aneurysms. The aneurysms vary from a few millimetres to several centimetres in diameter. A few aneurysms may be congenital but most develop in adult life, probably as a result of atherosclerosis and hypertension. Various associated conditions may be present (Table 14). Aneurysmal rupture can be caused by sudden increases in blood pressure during strenuous exercise, lifting, defaecation, and coitus. Many aneurysms remain asymptomatic and are found in 2 per cent of routine autopsies. A few grow to a large size and present as a space-occupying lesion.

Vascular malformations

Arteriovenous malformations

These are congenital vascular anomalies that vary greatly in size from a few millimetres to several centimetres in diameter. They consist of convoluted masses of blood vessels that are fed by large arteries and drained by increasingly large veins as time goes by. They may present with epilepsy, primary intracerebral haemorrhage, subarachnoid haemorrhage, and rarely as a space-occupying lesion or with headache. Early death (about 10 per cent) and risk of rebleeding is much less than after rupture of a saccular aneurysm, but the neurological damage is usually more extensive. However, even after several recurrent haemorrhages, patients may survive for many years with remarkably little disability.

There are other, less common vascular malformations involving the brain. Telangiectases are made up of groups of dilated capillaries. They may be associated with the Osler–Rendu–Weber syndrome and occasionally rupture, although this is very unusual. Cavernous malformations form circumscribed collections of blood-filled spaces. They may be associated with similar lesions elsewhere in the body and can be familial. They may present with epilepsy, but rarely rupture. Haemangioblastomas are tumours of angioblastic origin that consist of vascular channels and spaces, and tend to form cysts. They can be multiple and are usually found subtentorially, often in the cerebellum, medulla, or even the spinal cord, and present as a space-occupying lesion. Bleeding is unusual, although polycythaemia may occur. They are often associated with anomalies elsewhere in the body: haemangioblastoma of the retina, cysts of the pancreas and kidneys, hypernephromas and tumours of the suprarenal glands together comprise the von Hippel–Lindau syndrome, which is autosomal dominant in many cases. Finally, in the Sturge–Weber syndrome there may be extensive capillary–venous malformations affecting one hemisphere, particularly the parieto-occipital region, associated with a characteristic wavy pattern of subcortical calcification. There is usually an associated port-wine stain on the ipsilateral face and there may be associated glaucoma. Epilepsy is the main clinical manifestation.

Management of subarachnoid haemorrhage

About 25 per cent of patients die within 24 h of aneurysmal subarachnoid haemorrhage. Another 25 per cent die in the first month (usually due to recurrent haemorrhage, or infarction perhaps as a consequence of vasospasm) and 50 per cent survive for longer, but still with a risk of rebleeding (about 2 per cent per annum). The first week is the time of maximum risk of rebleeding so, if possible, neurosurgical intervention to clip the aneurysm or insertion of a coil into the aneurysm by a neuroradiologist should be done as soon as possible. Increasingly, interventional neuroradiological techniques to insert platinum coils into the aneursym are being used, and tested in randomized trials. The risk of surgery is unacceptably high if the patient is unconscious or has a severe neurological deficit. If the patient is conscious with little or no deficit, then four-vessel angiography should be undertaken to delineate the site of the bleeding and surgery carried out soon afterwards.

'Vasospasm' and delayed cerebral ischaemia may occur in relation to, and even at a distance from, the aneurysm-bearing artery and is one explanation for the high risks of surgery in ill patients. The cause of vasospasm is unknown but is probably to do with some constituent of the blood in the subarachnoid space.

If an arteriovenous malformation has bled and is surgically accessible, it should probably be removed. Ligation of the feeding vessels has little or nothing to offer since the arteriovenous malformation will be revascularized by vessels too small to be seen on the preoperative angiogram. Embolization and radiotherapy have been suggested but, like surgical removal, there have been no adequate clinical trials.

From the medical point of view, cautious control of severe hypertension is wise, and occasionally disturbances of cardiac rhythm or even acute neurogenic pulmonary oedema require appropriate treatment. Analgesia for the headache and sedation if the patient is very irritable are useful. Antifibrinolytic drugs reduce the risk of rebleeding by inhibiting the lysis of the fibrin clot plugging the ruptured aneurysm, but do not improve the overall prognosis, probably because the risk of vasospasm is increased. Prophylactic nimodipine reduces the risk of delayed cerebral ischaemia after aneurysmal subarachnoid haemorrhage. Bed rest for a few weeks is usually recommended, but there is an increasing tendency gently to mobilize patients when the headache has resolved.

Further reading

Barnett, H.J.M., Mohr, J.P., Stein, B.M., and Yatsu, F.M. (1992). *Stroke: pathophysiology, diagnosis and management*, 3rd edn. Churchill Livingstone, New York.

Caplan, L.R. and Stein, R.W. (1993). *Stroke: a clinical approach*, 2nd edn. Butterworth, Boston.

Ebrahim, S. (1999). *Stroke*, (2nd edn). Oxford University Press, Oxford.

Hankey, G. and Warlow, C.P. (1994). *Transient ischaemic attacks*. W.B. Saunders, London.

Vermuelen, M., Lindsey, K.W., and van Gijn, J. (1992). *Major problems in neurology: subarachnoid haemorrhage*. W.B. Saunders, London.

Warlow, C.P. (1993). Disorders of the cerebral circulation. In *Brain's diseases of the nervous system*, 10th edn (ed. J.W. Walton), pp. 197–268. Oxford University Press.

Warlow, C., Sandercock, P., Wardlaw, J., *et al.* (1996). *The practical management of stroke*. Blackwell, Oxford.

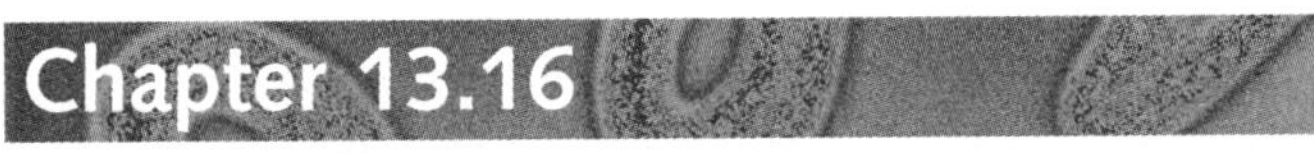

Dementia

J. R. Hodges

Definition

Dementia is defined as 'a syndrome consisting of progressive impairment in two or more areas of cognition (i.e., memory, language, visuospatial and perceptual ability, thinking and problem-solving, and behaviour) sufficient to interfere with work, social function, or relationships, in the absence of delirium or major non-organic psychiatric disorders (e.g. depression, schizophrenia)'.

Although a global or diffuse loss of higher cerebral function is the eventual fate of patients with dementing illnesses, the vast majority of cases begin with more circumscribed deficits. The requirement of impairment in two or more cognitive domains excludes patients with isolated cognitive deficits such as aphasia, or amnesia (e.g. Korsakoff's syndrome), but allows a diagnosis of dementia to be made before the patient reaches a state of gross, generalized mental decay. The contrasting features of dementia and delirium, and the patterns of deficit associated with various types of dementia, will be discussed here.

Epidemiology and causes

Dementia is, predominantly, a disorder of later life. The prevalence and incidence of mild dementia have not been fully established since there have been few comprehensive community-based studies, but some 5 to 8 per cent of all people above the age of 65 years suffer from moderate or severe dementia. This figure hides the dramatic increase with advancing age: the prevalence doubles every 5 years about the age of 65, reaching over 20 per cent in 80-year-olds.

A very large number of neurological diseases can cause dementia, as shown in Table 1, but most of these are very rare. In many of the conditions listed, such as multiple sclerosis, systemic lupus erythematosus, and the inherited metabolic disorders, the dementia is almost invariably in the setting of other neurological symptoms or signs. Alzheimer's disease is by far the most common cause of dementia, comprising between 50 and 70 per cent of cases in most epidemiological surveys. Recent studies indicate that two other primary degenerative conditions which previously would have been subsumed within the rubric of Alzheimer's disease—dementia with Lewy bodies and frontotemporal dementia (or Pick's disease)—appear to be relatively common, perhaps accounting for up to 25 per cent of cases previously diagnosed as Alzheimer's, and an even greater proportion of early-onset cases (under 65 years of age). Vascular dementia remains the second most common cause, accounting for 20 to 30 per cent of cases, although its prevalence appears to be falling. The term vascular dementia encompasses a number of separate disorders, the most common being multi-infarct disease secondary to atherosclerosis of the extra- and intracranial arteries. Of the inherited disorders that may present as dementia, Huntington's disease is the most common. Unfortunately, curable disease still accounts for only a small minority of cases—around 10 to 20 per cent in hospital-based series, but a much smaller proportion of unselected, community-based cases.

Patterns of cognitive impairment: cortical versus subcortical dementia

The division between those diseases that affect primarily the cerebral cortex and those that have their major pathological impact on subcortical structures (i.e., the basal ganglia, thalamus, and deep white matter) has proved useful. Table 2 contrasts the major features of cortical and subcortical dementias.

Cortical dementias: Alzheimer's disease

Alzheimer's disease is the prototypical example of a cortical dementia, in which disturbances of memory, language, praxis, and visuospatial and perceptual abilities predominate. Marked impairment in memory is virtually always the earliest feature: this amnesic deficit results from a failure to lay down (encode) new memories and, to a lesser extent, to recall older memories, which reflects that the focus of the pathology is in the medial temporal lobe. Within the domain of language, aphasia occurs fairly early in the course of the disease: the semantic, 'word meaning' component of language is selectively affected, causing word-finding difficulty in spontaneous conversation, impaired object naming on formal tests, and difficulty understanding the meaning of less common words. Impairment in attentional ability and visuospatial deficits, apparent on constructional tests, are also common. The general slowing of cognitive processes that characterizes the subcortical dementias is not seen, at least early in the course of the disease. Likewise, personality and social conduct are well preserved in the initial stages.

Although largely a disorder of elderly people, Alzheimer's disease can present in individuals as young as 30 years. Autosomal-dominant pedigrees account for only 5 to 10 per cent of cases, in a small proportion of which mutations in the presenilin or amyloid precursor protein (**APP**) genes can be found. Individuals with Down's syndrome may develop the histological changes of Alzheimer's disease in their third or fourth decades, attributable to an extra copy of the *APP* gene.

Cortical atrophy affects particularly the medial temporal lobes (hippocampus), which be demonstrated on MRI, especially using coronal views (see Fig. 1). Histopathologically the hallmarks of

Table 1 Causes of dementia

Primary degenerative diseases
Alzheimer's disease
Frontotemporal dementia (Pick's disease)
Huntingdon's disease
Parkinson's disease
Dementia with Lewy bodies (diffuse cortical Lewy body disease)
Progressive supranuclear palsy (Steele-Richardson-Olszewski syndrome)
Corticobasal degeneration
Vascular diseases
Multi-infarct disease secondary to atherosclerotic disease of extracranial vessels or cardiac emboli
Hypertensive encephalopathy
Binswanger's disease (subcortical arteriosclerotic encephalopathy)
Vasculitides: systemic lupus erythematosus, polyarteritis nodosa, Behçet's disease, giant-cell arteritis, isolated CNS angiitis
Primary cerebral amyloid (congophilic) angiopathy
CADASIL (congenital autosomal dominant angiopathy with subcortical infarcts and leukocephalopathy)

Infections
AIDS dementia complex
Progressive multifocal leucoencephalopathy
Cerebral toxoplasmosis ⎫
Cyptococcal meningitis ⎬ associated with immune compromise
Creutzfeldt-Jakob and other prion-related diseases ⎭
Syphilis
Subacute sclerosing panencephalitis and progressive rubella panencephalitis
Whipple's disease

Neoplastic causes
Primary intracerebral tumours: frontal gliomas crossing the corpus callosum butterfly glioma), posterior corpus (callosal or midline (thalamic, pineal, third ventricle) tumours, cerebral lymphoma, etc.
Extracerebral tumours: frontal meningiomas, posterior fossa tumours (acoustic neuroma) causing hydrocephalus
Multiple cerebral metastases
Malignant meningitis
Non-metastatic (limbic) encephalitis

Other non-neoplastic space-occupying disorders
Chronic subdural haematoma
Normal pressure hydrocephalus
Chronic intoxications
Alcoholic dementia
Heavy metals: leads, mercury, manganese
Carbon monoxide poisoning
Drugs: lithium, anticholinergics, barbiturates, digitalis, neuroleptics, cimetidine, propranolol

Acquired metabolic disorders and deficiency states
Cerebral anoxia
Chronic renal failure
Portosystemic encephalopathy
Hypothyroidism
Cushing's disease
Panhypopituitism
Hypoglycaemia (chronic or recurrent)
Hypoparathyroidism
Vitamins B_{12}, B_1, folic acid deficiency

Inherited metabolic diseases which may present with dementia in early adult life
Wilson's disease
Porphyria
Leucodystrophies; adrenoleucodystrophy, metachromatic leucodystrophy, globoid cell leucodystrophy
Gangliosidoses
Niemann-Pick disease
Cerebrotendinous xanthomatosis
Adult onset neuronal ceroid-lipofusceinosis (Kufs' disease)
Mitochondrial cytopathies
Subacute necrotizing encephalopathy (Leigh's disease)

Miscellaneous
Multiple sclerosis
Sarcoidosis
Sickle-cell disease
Macroglobulinaemia
Recurrent head injury, dementia pugilistica
Hashimoto's encephalopathy

Table 2 Contrasting features of cortical and subcortical dementia

Characteristic	Cortical dementia	Subcortical dementia
Speed of cognitive processing	Normal	Slowed down (bradyphenic)
Frontal 'executive' abilities*	Preserved in early stages	Disproportionately impaired from onset
Memory	Severe amnesia Recall and recognition	Forgetfulness Recognition better affected
Language	Aphasic features	Normal except dysarthria and reduced output
Visuospatial and perceptual abilities	Impaired (late)	Impaired (late)
Personality	Intact until late	Typically apathetic and inert
Mood	Usually normal	Depression common

*Planning, problem-solving, initiation, etc.

Alzheimer's disease are neurofibrillary tangles and senile plaques (see OTM3, p. 3972).

There are no specific diagnostic tests for Alzheimer's disease and the antemortem diagnosis remains a clinical one, with supportive evidence from structural and/or functional brain imaging and neuropsychological assessment.

Creutzfeldt–Jakob disease (see Chapter 13.17) is another form of cortical disease that causes a rapidly progressive dementia, often resulting in death within months of presentation. Its cognitive features have not been well characterized, but severe memory impairment and aphasia are usually present, and some patients develop cortical blindness. Myoclonus is present in 80 per cent of cases.

Subcortical dementias (Table 3)

In subcortical dementia, such as Huntington's disease and progressive supranuclear palsy (Steele–Richardson–Olszewski syndrome), impairment in frontal 'executive' function (i.e., planning, problem-solving, self-initiated activity) predominates. Patients appear mentally slowed down (or bradyphrenic). Changes in mood, personality, and social conduct are very common, resulting often in an indifferent, withdrawn state. Spontaneous speech is reduced; answers to questions

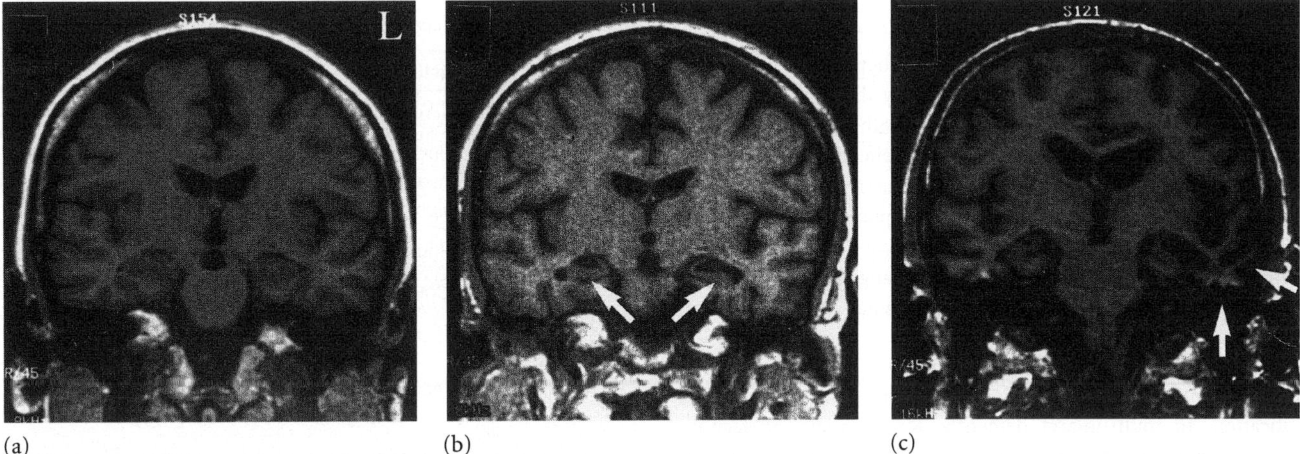

Fig. 1(a)–(c) MRI scans showing the different patterns of damage due to semantic dementia and Alzheimer's disease. Panel (a) shows the brain of a healthy control individual. Panel (b) shows the scan of a patient in the early amnestic stages of presumed Alzheimer's disease, with bilateral shrinkage of the hippocampal complex and compensatory enlargement of the temporal horns of the lateral ventricles (arrows). Panel (c) displays the brain scan of a patient with semantic dementia (the temporal-lobe variant of frontotemporal dementia), with striking atrophy of inferior and lateral regions of the left temporal lobe (arrows).

Table 3 Major causes of subcortical dementia

Degeneration	**Metabolic**
Progressive supranuclear palsy	Wilson's disease
Huntingdon's disease	Demyelinating disease
Parkinson's disease	Multiple sclerosis
Striatonigral degeneration	Leucodystrophies
Corticobasal degeneration	AIDS dementia complex
Vascular disorders	**Miscellaneous**
Multi-infarct dementia (lacunar state)	Normal pressure hydrocephalus
Binswager's disease	Cortical features often coexist
CADASIL	

are slow and laconic. Memory is moderately impaired due to reduced attention with poor registration for new material, but the severe amnesia that typifies Alzheimer's disease is not seen in the early stages. Features of focal cortical dysfunction, such as aphasia and agnosia, are characteristically absent, but visuospatial deficits develop in the later stages.

Frontotemporal dementia

The term frontotemporal dementia is now preferred to the older label Pick's disease to describe patients presenting with features of focal atrophy of the frontal and/or anterior temporal lobes.

Only a minority of such patients have specific, intraneuronal, tau-positive inclusions (Pick bodies); most show severe neuronal loss, spongiform changes, and gliosis without identifiable inclusions.

When the frontal lobes are selectively involved, often called dementia of frontal-lobe type, patients present with an insidious change in personality and social conduct. Disinhibition, stereotypic or ritualized behaviours, and a change in food preference with craving for sweet foods are particularly common. Cognitive testing shows deficits in frontal 'executive' functions. Within the cortical–subcortical dichotomy, these features epitomize subcortical dementia. This apparent contradiction can be resolved if it is remembered that the subcortical dementias make their impact by deactivating the frontal cortex. Hence it is entirely consistent that subcortical and frontal pathologies should present with similar clinical syndromes; indeed, some have used the term frontostriatal dementia to encompass both.

Patients with focal temporal-lobe atrophy present with a progressive aphasic syndrome characterized by fluent, empty speech, and with severe anomia and impaired word comprehension. Since the central feature of the syndrome is a breakdown in the conceptual database underlying the use of language, the term semantic dementia has been applied. The left temporal lobe is more frequently involved than the right. Behavioural changes develop as the disease progresses.

The age of onset of frontotemporal dementia is almost always below 65 years, most typically 45 to 60 years. In a quarter to a third of cases there is a positive family history. In a small proportion of familial cases, a gene mutation involving the region coding the microtubule-associated protein tau on chromosome 17 has been identified. There is also an association between frontotemporal dementia and motor neurone disease: patients typically present with the former then rapidly develop bulbar symptoms, amyotrophy and fasiculations, which can be confirmed by EMG.

The diagnosis is suggested by the clinical features. CT may show frontal- or temporal-lobe atrophy, but MRI is considerably more sensitive in detecting shrinkage of the anterior and lateral temporal lobe (see Fig. 1). In contrast to Alzheimer's disease, the hippocampus is relatively spared.

Dementia with Lewy bodies

Lewy bodies are the pathological hallmark of Parkinson's disease, but there they are confined, very largely, to the substantia nigra. In dementia with Lewy bodies (also referred to as diffuse or cortical Lewy body disease) these same intraneuronal inclusions are widely distributed in cortical and subcortical structures, causing a mixture of parkinsonian and Alzheimer-like signs. The behavioural features are also in keeping with mixed cortical and subcortical pathology: attentional and frontal 'executive' deficits are prominent, but there are also marked visuoperceptual and memory impairments. Visual hallucinations and fluctuations in cognitive performance also characterize this disorder. Patients are exquisitely sensitive to the extra-pyramidal and cognitive side-effects of neuroleptic drugs and may develop the malignant neuroleptic syndrome.

Corticobasal degeneration

This recently recognized syndrome results in progressive degeneration of basal ganglia and cortical areas, particularly the superior parietal and prefrontal regions. Patients present with asymmetric parkinsonism, severe limb apraxia causing a loss of effective limb function, and gait disturbance. The 'alien or anarchic hand sign' is common, in which the hand appears to act semipurposefully without the patient's conscious control. Myoclonus and bulbar features may occur, and many patients develop behavioural and language abnormalities that overlap with those seen in vascular dementia.

Vascular dementia

Not all dementing disorders fit neatly into the cortical–subcortical classification. In multi-infarct dementia, for instance, the lacunar lesions that are largely responsible for the cognitive impairment preferentially involve the basal ganglia, thalamus, and adjacent white matter, resulting in a subcortical syndrome. Larger-vessel strokes that cause cortical features (aphasia, apraxia, etc.) frequently coexist. The syndrome of cerebral autosomal-dominant arteriopathy with subcortical infarcts and leucoencephalopathy (CADASIL) should also be considered.

Differential diagnosis

Pseudodementia

This term has been used to describe two distinct disorders, depressive pseudodementia and hysterical pseudodementia. Of these, the former is more common and represents the most important treatable cause of memory failure. Depressive pseudodementia is almost invariably a condition of elderly people. The patient presents with complaints of poor memory and concentration but usually denies overt symptoms of depression. Clues to the diagnosis are biological features of depression (particularly a disturbed sleep pattern and loss of appetite), low energy, pessimistic and ruminative thoughts, and a lack of interest in work or hobbies. The onset is usually relatively acute or subacute over weeks or months. A past or family history of affective disorder can be an important marker. On bedside cognitive assessment, attention is impaired and performance on tests of memory and of frontal 'executive' function is patchy and often inconsistent. Language output may be sparse but paraphasic errors are not seen. Responses to questions are often 'don't' knows', and performance improves with encouragement.

Patients with hysterical pseudodementia present with a fairly abrupt onset of memory and/or intellectual impairment. They typically appear unconcerned. Unlike organic amnesic disorders, the memory loss is worse for salient personal and early life-events. Loss of personal identity is very common. There is usually an identifiable precipitant (such as bereavement, marital or financial problems, or recent offending) as well as a past psychiatric history. Patients may show features of the so-called Ganser syndrome, the core symptom of which is the giving of bizarre approximate answers. For instance, when asked 'How many legs does a cow have?', they reply 'three' or 'five'. As in other hysterical conversion states, there may be an underlying organic disorder that has been grossly exaggerated at a conscious or subconscious level.

Delirium (acute confusional state)

This clinical syndrome is characterized by the abrupt onset of marked attentional abnormalities, clouding of consciousness, disorders of perception, thinking, memory, psychomotor activity, and the sleep–wakefulness cycle, and a marked tendency to fluctuations in cognitive performance and behaviour. The features of dementia and delirium are contrasted in Table 4. It should be noted that a disturbance in attention is the most consistent abnormality: patients are unable to sustain attention to external stimuli, are distractible, and easily lose the thread of conversations. Severe disorientation in time is invariable. Thinking ability is drastically affected and delusions are common. Illusions and hallucinations are also a frequent feature, particularly in the visual domain. Patients may be restless, excitable, and hypervigilant. Alternatively, they may be excessively sleepy, but most commonly they oscillate between these extremes, with a tendency to be more aroused and restless at might. Delirium occurs most frequently in elderly people. Those with the beginnings of dementia are particularly vulnerable. The potential causes are legion and include any form of metabolic disturbance, intoxication by drugs and poisons, drug and alcohol withdrawal states, infections both intra- and extracranial, head trauma, epilepsy (postictal states and non-convulsive status), raised intracranial pressure, subarachnoid haemorrhage, and focal brain lesions, particularly if the right hemisphere is involved. The prognosis clearly depends on the aetiology, but if the underlying cause is cured then a return to baseline performance can be expected.

Table 4 Differential diagnosis of delirium and dementia

Characteristic	Delirium	Dementia
Onset	Acute or subacute	Insidious and chronic
Course	Fluctuating with lucid intervals, often worse at night	Stable over the course of the day
Duration	Hours to weeks	Months to years
Consciousness (response to environment)	Clouded	Clear
Attention	Impaired with marked distractibility	Relatively normal
Orientation	Almost always impaired for time; tendency to mistakes on place and person	Impaired in later stages
Memory	Impaired	Impaired
Thinking	Disorganized, delusional	Impoverished
Perception	Illusions and hallucinations common, usually visual	Absent in early stages, common later
Speech	Incoherent, hesitant, slow or rapid	Aphasic features common
Sleep-wake cycle	Always disrupted	Usually normal

Isolated disorders of higher cerebral function

Occasionally, patients with focal cognitive deficits are mistakenly diagnosed as demented. This is perhaps most common in those with fluent Wernicke's-type aphasia, who often have no other signs and are erroneously thought to be confused. Occasionally, patients with visual agnosia resulting from posterior cerebral lesions may be misdiagnosed, as may those with the amnesic syndrome, in which memory is severely impaired but other aspects of cognitive function are relatively unaffected. Causes include alcoholic Korsakoff's syndrome, diencephalic damage from bilateral paramedian thalamic infarction or tumours of the third ventricle, and medial temporal-lobe damage following herpes simplex virus encephalitis, surgical resection, head injury, cerebral anoxia, or strokes in the territory of a posterior cerebral artery.

Assessment of suspected dementia

There are two questions to be asked when assessing patients with suspected dementia. First, does the patient fulfil the criteria for a diagnosis of dementia and can other potential causes of cognitive impairment (discussed above) be confidently excluded? Secondly, if so, what is the likely cause of the dementia? Since Alzheimer's disease is responsible for the majority of cases of dementia, one of the fundamental goals is to decide whether there are any symptoms or signs that are not typical of Alzheimer's. Some of the more common clinical features that should alert one to alternative diagnoses are listed in Table 5.

History

A careful history is the key to diagnosis. The earliest observed problems (e.g. memory loss, personality change, etc.) should be established, as well as the subsequent course of the illness. The pattern and rate of decline (insidious, stepwise, fluctuating, rapidly progressive, etc.) are important, as is the need to probe both the patient and the informant for any symptoms suggestive of focal neurological deficits or raised intracranial pressure. A particular note should be made of any symptoms suggestive of past cerebrovascular events (transient ischaemic attacks or stroke) and of risk factors for thromboembolic disease. Alcohol intake, tobacco usage, and all medications must be documented. In younger patients, or those with other unusual features, the possibility of immunocompromise from AIDS must be considered. In all patients, the state of health, or cause and age of death of first-degree relatives should be recorded, and specific enquiries made about any family history of neurological or psychiatric disease.

Cognitive functions: suggested areas of enquiry

Memory

Anterograde: recall of new information in day-to-day life (e.g. messages, appointments, family news, etc.), repetitiveness

Retrograde: past personal and public events

Language

Output: word finding, grammar, word errors (paraphasias)

Comprehension

Reading and writing ability

Numerical skills

Handling money, shopping, dealing with bills

Visuospatial and perceptual abilities

Dressing

Spatial orientation and route finding

Recognition of objects, colours, and people

Thinking and problem-solving

Personality and social conduct

Disinhibition, impulsivity

Stereotypic or ritualistic behaviours

Motivation

Eating habits, manners, and food preference

Self-care

Symptoms of depression

Delusions and hallucinations

Table 5 Clinical features which suggest diagnoses other than Alzheimer's disease

Young age (<65 years)	Huntingdon's disease, infections (e.g. AIDS, SSPE), inherited metabolic disorders (e.g. Wilson's disease), vasculitudes, neoplasia
Rapid progression (weeks or months)	Neoplasia, infections, Creutzfeldt-Jakob disease
Personality change early in course	Pick's disease, subcortical dementias, frontal tumours
Early onset incontinence	Tumours, normal pressure hydrocephalus
Cardiac disease, past TIA or stroke	Cerebral vascular disease (multi-infarct dementia), CADASIL
Symptoms of raised intracranial pressure	Tumours, subdural haematoma
Fluctuating performance	Subdural haematoma, vascular dementia, dementia with Lewy bodies
Immunocompromise	Infections (e.g. PML, toxoplasmosis), primary intracerebral lymphoma
Systemic illness	Metabolic disorders, neoplasia, infections, vasculitudes
Family history of dementia or involuntary movements	Huntingdon's disease, inherited metabolic diseases
Anosmia	Frontal meningioma
Eye movement abnormalities	Progressive supranuclear palsy, multiple sclerosis, mitochondrial cytopathies
Ocular signs	Syphilis, Wilson's disease, raised pressure
Myoclonus	Creutzfeldt-Jakob disease, SSPE, postanoxia, myoclonic epilepsies
Gait disturbance	Normal pressure hydrocephalus, tumours, progressive supranuclear palsy, Huntingdon's disease

Abbreviations: AIDS, acquired immunodeficiency syndrome; SSPE, subacute sclerosing panencephalitis; PML, progressive mulitfocal leucoencephalopathy; TIA, transient ischaemic attack.

Examination

All patients presenting with dementia require a full neurological examination. Clues to possible diagnoses are listed in Table 5. Cognitive evaluation is also mandatory, and should include assessment of orientation, concentration/attention, reasoning, memory, language, numerical skills, praxis, and visuospatial ability. This qualitative assessment of cognition should be supplemented with a quantitative score. Of the many available brief assessment instruments, the Mini-Mental

Table 6 The Mini-Mental State Examination

	Score
Orientation	
Year, month, day, date, season	/5
Country, county, town, hospital, ward (clinic)	/5
Registration	
Examiner names three objects (e.g. orange, key, ball)	
Patient asked to repeat the three names.	
Score one for each correct answer	/3
Then ask the patient to repeat all three names three times	
Attention	
Subtract 7 from 100, then repeat from result, stop after 5: 93, 86, 79, 72, 65	
Alternative if patient makes errors on serial subtraction: spell 'world' backwards: DLROW	
Score best performances on either task	/5
Recall	
Ask for the names of the three objects learned earlier.	/3
Language	
Name a pencil and a watch	/2
Repeat 'No ifs, and, no buts'	/1
Give a three-stage command. Score one for each stage (e.g. 'Take this piece of paper in your right hand, fold it in half, and place it on the chair next to you.')	/3
Ask patient to write a sentence. Score correct if it is sensible and has a subject and a verb.	/1
Copying	
Ask patient to copy intersecting pentagons	
Score as correct if they overlap and if each has five sides	/1
Total score	/30

State Examination (Table 6) is the most widely standardized and validated. A score of 24 out of 30 was originally suggested as the lower limit of normal, but it has been repeatedly shown that performance on even this simple test is influenced very considerably by age and by educational attainment. Hence, a young adult with university-level education should perform flawlessly, whereas a normal elderly person who left school at the age of 14 may score as low as 22 or 23. With this proviso, the Mini-Mental State Examination provides a reasonable screening instrument and is particularly useful for grading and monitoring the severity of dementia, although it should be noted that patients with the early amnesic stage of Alzheimer's, as well as those with frontal pathology, often score above the cut-off of 24.

Investigations

The minimum investigations for a newly presenting patient with dementia are shown in Table 7. The main indication for performing a CT scan is to exclude hydrocephalus and benign tumours; where resources are limited, scanning should be reserved for cases with atypical features. The extent of further investigations will depend on the patient's age, the presence of specific features in the history and examination, and the results of preliminary screening investigations. Examination of the cerebrospinal fluid is recommended in young patients, and in those in whom there is any doubt about the diagnosis. Electroencephalography is particularly valuable in cases of suspected Creutzfeldt–Jakob disease.

Treatable causes of dementia

Normal-pressure hydrocephalus

The classical presentation of normal-pressure hydrocephalus is a triad of cognitive impairment, gait disturbance, and incontinence. The cognitive profile is that of subcortical dementia with prominent psychomotor slowing. The gait disorder is best described as an apraxia and patients may show the pathognomonic 'glued-to-the-floor' sign when they stand and first attempt to walk. Despite these abnormalities of gait, there are usually few, if any, pyramidal or extrapyramidal signs when examined on the bed. Urinary incontinence is a late and more variable feature of the condition.

These patients show periods of intermittently raised pressure due to raised resistance to cerebrospinal fluid outflow, usually at the level of arachnoid villi. The known causes include prior head injury, subarachnoid haemorrhage, and meningitis. Despite full investigation, however, in many cases there is no identifiable cause. The screening investigation of choice is the CT scan, which shows ventricular enlargement out of proportion to the degree of cortical atrophy, sometimes accompanied by periventricular, low-density changes.

Patients with ventricular enlargement should be referred to a neurosurgeon for consideration of insertion of a ventricular shunt.

Chronic subdural haematoma

This treatable complication of head injury can present with subacute dementia, often associated with symptoms of raised intracranial pressure. Focal signs may be present. Fluctuations in conscious level or in cognitive performance are characteristic. It commonly occurs in individuals prone to recurrent head trauma (alcoholics, the elderly, epileptics). Those with coagulation defects are also at high risk. On CT scan a chronic subdural haematoma is seen as a peripheral mass lesion of varying signal intensity. Treatment is by surgical evacuation except in cases with very small collections without significant mass effect. Recurrence is fairly common (10 to 40 per cent of cases) and patients may require further drainage procedures, but the long-term outcome is usually excellent.

Benign tumours

Patients with subfrontal meningiomas typically present with an insidious change in personality and other features of a frontal-lobe syndrome. Examination may reveal anosmia or unilateral visual failure with optic atrophy.

Metabolic and endocrine disorders

Virtually any acquired metabolic derangement (e.g. hyponatraemia, uraemia, hepatic failure) can cause cognitive impairment, but the features are almost invariably those of delirium (acute confusional state) rather than dementia. Chronic hypocalcaemia and recurrent hypoglycaemia sometimes cause dementia, although overt psychiatric symptoms often coexist. Hypothyroidism sometimes presents with prominent complaints of mental slowing, apathy, and poor memory. The psychological symptoms of Addison's disease and hypopituitarism are very similar, and in all of these disorders the overall picture is more like that seen in subcortical than in cortical dementias (see above). Cushing's syndrome is frequently associated with psychiatric symptoms (depression, paranoid delusions) and may rarely present with a dementia. An encephalopathic state with episodic seizures and focal neurological signs has been identified in association with very

Table 7 Recommended investigations in dementia

Routine	Other tests which may be indicated in certain cases
Full blood count and ESR	MRI (especially in presenile cases to look at pattern of atrophy)
Biochemical profile: urea or creatinine, electrolytes, calcium, liver function	EEG (e.g. Creutzfeldt-Jakob disease and SSPE)
Serum vitamin B_{12}, and folate	Functional brain imaging: SPECT
Thyroid function	CSF examination (e.g. infections, malignant meningitis, etc.)
Serological tests for syphilis	Screening for cardiac sources of emboli
Chest radiograph	Immunological tests for vasculitides (e.g. SLE)
CT scan	Slit-lamp examination for Kayser-
	Fleischer rings and caeruloplasmin estimation (Wilson's disease)
	Specific blood and/or urine tests for inherited metabolic disorders
	Cerebral biopsy

Abbreviations: CSF, cerebrospinal fluid; CT, computed tomography, EEG, electroencephalography, ESR, erythrocyte sedimentation rate; SLE, systemic lupus erythematosus; SPECT, single photon emission tomography; SSPE, subacute sclerosing panencephalitis.

high concentrations of antithyroid antibodies but normal thyroid function, and is referred to as Hashimoto's encephalopathy.

Deficiency states

In vitamin B_{12} deficiency the classical features of subacute degeneration of the spinal cord and peripheral nerves are accompanied by a progressive, low-grade dementia. It is, however, extremely unusual for the cognitive features to predominate; cases of dementia without the other neurological manifestations are even rarer. Folic acid deficiency may cause mild cognitive dysfunction but this hardly ever amounts to a true dementia. Severe thiamine (vitamin B_1) deficiency results in the Wernicke–Korsakoff syndrome. In the acute stages, there is delirium. If it is not promptly treated, a chronic amnesic syndrome may ensue.

Infections

Primary infection of the central nervous system by human immunodeficiency virus is now the most common cause of early-onset dementia in some parts of the world. The encephalopathy (the AIDS–dementia complex), which develops early in the course of the disease, may be the sole manifestation. It is characterized by poor concentration, psychomotor slowing, personality change, and other features of a subcortical dementia.

Investigations reveal increased protein, pleocytosis, and oligoclonal bands in cerebrospinal fluid. White-matter changes may be seen on CT and are more obvious on MRI. Combination treatment with antiretroviral agents can improve the cognitive deficits. Patients with AIDS are also at risk from a number of opportunistic infections, including cerebral toxoplasmosis, cryptococcal meningitis, and progressive leucoencephalopathy, which can all present with rapidly progressive dementia. Neurosyphilis is now a rare cause of dementia but should be considered in patients with other neurological features (seizures, dysarthria, ptosis, pupillary abnormalities, tremor, pyramidal signs, ataxia, etc.). Specific serological tests are positive and the cerebrospinal fluid shows an increase in protein and pleocytosis. Treatment with penicillin may result in some improvement.

Further reading

Bendixen, B. (1993). Vascular dementia: a concept in flux. *Current Opinions in Neurology and Neurosurgery*, **6**, 107–12.

Galton, C.J. and Hodges, J.R. (1999). The spectrum of dementia and its treatment. *Journal of the Royal College of Physicians*, **33**, 234–9.

Hodges, J.R. (1994). *Cognitive assessment for clinicians.* Oxford University Press.

McKeith, I.G., Galasko, D., Kosaka, K., *et al.* (1996). Consensus guidelines for the clinical and pathologic diagnosis of dementia with Lewy bodies (DLB): report of the Consortium on DLB International Workshop. *Neurology*, **47**, 1113–24.

Neary, D., Snowden, J.S., Gustafson, L., *et al.* (1998). Frontotemporal lobar degeneration: a consensus on clinical diagnostic criteria. *Neurology*, **51**, 1546–54.

Smith, A.D. and Jobst, K.A. (1996). Use of structural imaging to study the progression of Alzheimer's disease. *British Medical Bulletin*, **52**, 575–86.

Chapter 13.17

Prion diseases

J. Collinge

The prion diseases are neurodegenerative conditions that affect both humans and animals and that have been known as the spongiform encephalopathies, slow virus diseases, or transmissible dementias. Creutzfeldt–Jakob disease, Gerstmann–Sträussler–Scheinker syndrome, and *kuru* represent the traditionally recognized human conditions. These diseases are transmissible to experimental animals by inoculation and are, in the case of the familial forms of the human prion diseases, also transmitted in an autosomal-dominant fashion. The prion diseases are biologically unique in this regard. For many years these diseases have been an intense and controversial area of research interest because of the unique properties of the transmissible agent, or prion. The need for a clearer understanding of these rare human diseases has been highlighted by the epidemic of a prion disease amongst cattle herds in the UK and elsewhere (bovine spongiform encephalopathy) and the potential threat posed to the public health.

Aetiology

The nature of the transmissible agent in these diseases has been a subject of debate for many years. The initial assumption that the agent must be some form of virus was challenged both by the failure to demonstrate such a virus directly (or indeed any immunological response to it) and by evidence indicating that the transmissible agent showed remarkable resistance to treatment expected to inactivate nucleic acids (such as ultraviolet radiation or treatment with nucleases). Such findings led to the suggestion in 1967 that the transmissible agent might be a protein. Progressive enrichment of brain homogenates for infectivity resulted in the isolation of a protease-resistant sialoglycoprotein, designated the prion protein (**PrP**). The term prion (from *pro*teinaceous *in*fectious particle) was proposed by Prusiner in 1982 to distinguish the infectious pathogen from viruses or viroids. Remarkably, PrP turned out to be a host- rather than infectious pathogen-encoded protein. The PrP gene (designated *PRNP* in humans) is highly conserved in mammals and is expressed in many tissues, but at its highest concentrations in the central nervous system. The normal cellular function of PrP remains unclear.

Prion diseases of both humans and animals are associated with the accumulation in the brain of an abnormal, partially protease-resistant, isoform of PrP, designated PrP^{Sc}. PrP^{Sc} is derived from its normal cellular precursor, PrP^{C}, by a post-translational process that involves a conformational change. PrP^{C} is rich in α-helical structure while PrP^{Sc} appears to be predominantly composed of β-sheet. According to the 'protein-only' hypothesis, an abnormal PrP isoform is the principal, and possibly the sole, constituent of the transmissible agent or prion. PrP^{Sc} is hypothesized to act as a conformational template, promoting the conversion of PrP^{C} to further PrP^{Sc}. According to such a model, prion replication, with recruitment of PrP^{C} into the aggregated PrP^{Sc} isoform, may be initiated by a pathogenic mutation (resulting in a PrP^{C} predisposed to form PrP^{Sc}) in inherited prion diseases, by exposure to a 'seed' of PrP^{Sc} in acquired cases, or as a result of the spontaneous conversion of PrP^{C} to PrP^{Sc} as a rare stochastic event in sporadic prion disease.

The human prion diseases can be divided into three aetiological categories: sporadic, acquired, and inherited. The acquired prion diseases include iatrogenic Creutzfeldt–Jakob disease and *kuru*, and arise from accidental exposure to human prions through medical or surgical procedures or participation in cannibalistic feasts. Variant Creutzfeldt–Jakob disease is a newly recognized, acquired prion disease discussed below. Epidemiological studies do not provide any evidence for an association between sheep scrapie and the occurrence of Creutzfeldt–Jakob disease in humans. Sporadic Creutzfeldt–Jakob disease occurs in all countries, with a random case distribution and an annual incidence of 1 per million. Around 15 per cent of human prion disease is inherited and all cases to date have been associated with coding mutations in the prion protein gene (*PRNP*), of which over 20 distinct types are recognized. No such pathogenic *PRNP* mutations are present in sporadic and acquired prion disease. However, a common PrP polymorphism at residue 129, where either methionine or valine can be encoded, is a key determinant of genetic susceptibility to acquired and sporadic prion diseases, the large majority of which occur in homozygous individuals. This protective effect of *PRNP* codon 129 heterozygosity is also seen in some of the inherited prion diseases, heterozygotes having a later age at onset than codon 129 homozygotes.

Multiple strains or isolates of prions with distinct biological properties are recognized, a finding that has provided a challenge to the 'protein only' model of prion replication. However, it is now clear that prion strains can be distinguished by differences in the biochemical properties of PrP^{Sc} and prion strain diversity may be encoded by differences in PrP conformation and pattern of glycosylation. Molecular strain typing has allowed the identification of four main types amongst cases of Creutzfeldt–Jakob disease, sporadic and iatrogenic Creutzfeldt–Jakob disease being of PrP^{Sc} types 1 to 3, while all cases of variant Creutzfeldt–Jakob disease are associated with a distinctive type 4 PrP^{Sc}.

An increasing number of animal prion diseases are recognized. Scrapie, a naturally occurring disease of sheep and goats, has been recognized in Europe for over 200 years. Its transmissibility between sheep (and goats) was demonstrated in 1936 by experimental inoculation. Transmissible mink encephalopathy and chronic wasting disease of mule deer and elk were described from the 1940s onwards. The appearance of bovine spongiform encephalopathy in UK cattle from 1986 onwards was widely attributed to transmission of sheep scrapie, endemic in the UK and many other countries, to cattle via contaminated feed prepared from rendered carcasses. However, an alternative hypothesis is that epidemic bovine spongiform encephalopathy resulted from recycling of rare cases of sporadic bovine spongiform encephalopathy, as cattle were also rendered to produce cattle feed. Whether or not bovine spongiform encephalopathy originated from sheep scrapie, it was, however, clear from 1990 onwards, with the occurrence of novel spongiform encephalopathies amongst domestic and captive wild cats, that its host range was different from that of scrapie. Many new species have developed spongiform encephalopathies coincident with, or following the arrival of, bovine spongiform encephalopathy, including greater kudu, nyala, Arabian oryx, scimitar-horned oryx, eland, gemsbok, bison, ankole, tiger, cheetah, ocelot, puma, and domestic cats. Several have been confirmed to be caused by a bovine spongiform encephalopathy-like prion strain, and it is likely that most or all are bovine spongiform encephalopathy-related.

In late 1995, cases of what appeared to be sporadic Creutzfeldt–Jakob disease began to be reported in unusually young people in the UK, most with ages at onset in their twenties and some were teenagers. Sporadic Creutzfeldt–Jakob disease is exceedingly rare, with onset at ages under 40 years, and only four cases had previously been recorded in teenagers; none of these cases had occurred in the UK. Review of the histology of these cases showed a remarkably consistent and unique pattern. These cases were named 'new variant' Creutzfeldt–Jakob disease, although it was clear that they were also rather atypical in their clinical presentation. Extensive studies of archival cases of Creutzfeldt–Jakob disease or other prion diseases failed to show this picture and it seemed that it did represent the arrival of a new form of prion disease in the UK. The statistical probability of such cases occurring by chance was vanishingly small and ascertainment bias seemed most unlikely as an explanation. It was clear that a new risk factor for Creutzfeldt–Jakob disease had emerged and appeared to be specific to the UK. A case of variant Creutzfeldt–Jakob disease was soon after reported in France. Direct experimental evidence that variant Creutzfeldt–Jakob disease is caused by bovine spongiform encephalopathy was provided by molecular analysis of human prion strains and transmission studies in transgenic and wild-type mice (see under Aetiology). While it appears clear that prions of bovine spongiform encephalopathy have infected humans, the extremely prolonged incubation periods of prion diseases in humans (which with *kuru* may reach decades), allied with effect of crossing a 'species barrier' (which limits transmission of prion strains between different species and usually results in a marked prolongation of mean incubation periods) means that it may be some years before the scale of any human epidemic can be predicted with any degree of confidence.

It is still unclear why young people should be particularity affected by variant Creutzfeldt–Jakob disease and why none had a pattern of unusual occupational or dietary exposure to bovine spongiform

Table 1 Human prion diseases

Type	Clinical syndromes	Aetiology
Acquired	Kuru	Exposure to human prions during cannibalistic feasts
	Iatrogenic CJD	Accidental inoculation with human prions
	Variant CJD	Exposure to BSE-like prion strain
Sporadic	CJD	May represent somatic PrP mutation or spontaneous PrPC to PrPSc
	Atypical CJD	
Inherited	Familial CJD	Germline *PRNP* mutation
	GSS Fatal familial insomnia	
	Various atypical dementias	

CJD, Creutzfeldt–Jakob disease; GSS, Gerstmann–Sträussler–Scheinker syndrome; *PRNP*, human prion protein gene; BSE, bovine spongiform encephalopathy.

encephalopathy. However, very little is known of which foodstuffs contained high-titre bovine offal. It is possible that certain foods containing particularly high titres were eaten predominately by younger people. An alternative is that young people are more susceptible to bovine spongiform encephalopathy following dietary exposure or that they have shorter incubation periods. It is important to appreciate that bovine spongiform encephalopathy-contaminated feed was fed to sheep, pigs, and poultry and that, although there is no evidence of natural transmission to these species, it would be prudent to remain open minded about other dietary exposure to novel animal prions.

Clinical features

With the advances in our understanding of their aetiology it now seems more appropriate to divide the human prion diseases into inherited, sporadic, and acquired forms (see Table 1), with Creutzfeldt–Jakob disease, Gerstmann–Sträussler–Scheinker syndrome, and *kuru* being clinicopathological syndromes within a wider spectrum of disease.

Sporadic (classical) Creutzfeldt–Jakob disease

The core clinical syndrome of Creutzfeldt–Jakob disease is of a rapidly progressive, multifocal dementia, usually with myoclonus. The onset is usually in the 45- to 75-year age group, with peak onset between 60 and 65 years. The clinical progression is typically over weeks, progressing to akinetic mutism and death, often in 2 to 3 months. Around 70 per cent of cases die in under 6 months. Prodromal features, present in around one-third of cases, include fatigue, insomnia, depression, weight loss, headaches, general malaise, and ill-defined pain sensations. In addition to mental deterioration and myoclonus, frequent additional neurological features include extrapyramidal signs, cerebellar ataxia, pyramidal signs, and cortical blindness. Routine haematological and biochemical investigations are normal, although occasional cases have raised serum transaminases or alkaline phosphatase. There are no immunological markers and acute-phase proteins are not elevated. Routine examination of the cerebrospinal fluid is normal, although 14–3–3 protein, neuronal-specific enolase, and S-100 are usually elevated. However, these are not specific for Creutzfeldt–Jakob disease. Neuroimaging with CT or MRI is useful to exclude other causes of subacute neurological illness, but there are no specific diagnostic features; cerebral and cerebellar atrophy and abnormal signal in the basal ganglia on MRI may be present. The most useful investigation is the EEG, which shows characteristic pseudoperiodic sharp-wave activity in most cases. Serial recordings may be necessary to demonstrate this feature. Prospective epidemiological studies have demonstrated that cases with a progressive dementia, and two or more of the following—myoclonus; cortical blindness; pyramidal, cerebellar, or extrapyramidal signs; or akinetic mutism in the setting of a typical EEG—nearly always turn out to be confirmed as histologically definite Creutzfeldt–Jakob disease if neuropathological examination is performed. Neuropathological confirmation of the disease is classically by demonstration of the triad of spongiform change, neuronal loss, and astrocytosis. However, PrP immunocytochemistry is more sensitive, demonstrating various types of abnormal PrP immunoreactivity. PrP amyloid plaques are present in only a small proportion of cases. PrP^{Sc}, specific to prion disease, can almost always be demonstrated by Western blot analysis, which also allows PrP^{Sc} typing (see under Aetiology). Brain biopsy may be considered in highly selected cases to exclude treatable alternative diagnoses. False negatives are seen, due to the sometimes localized distribution of pathology. Genetic susceptibility to Creutzfeldt–Jakob disease has been demonstrated in that most classical cases of this disease are homozygous at *PRNP* codon 129. Atypical forms of Creutzfeldt–Jakob disease are well recognized. Around 10 per cent of cases have a much more prolonged clinical course, lasting over 2 years, although such prolonged durations are suggestive of *PRNP* mutations. *PRNP* analysis should be performed in all apparently sporadic cases: the inherited prion diseases can mimic other neurological (or psychiatric) disease, and both non-paternity and the late onset of some of these diseases may account for lack of a relevant family history.

Iatrogenic Creutzfeldt–Jakob disease

While prion diseases can be transmitted to experimental animals by inoculation, it is important to appreciate that they are not contagious in humans. Documented case-to-case spread has only occurred by cannibalism (*kuru*) or following accidental inoculation with prions. Such iatrogenic routes include the use of inadequately sterilized intracerebral electrodes, dura mater, and corneal grafting, and from the use of human cadaveric pituitary-derived growth hormone or gonadotrophin. These cases are rare, but a careful history of such exposure should be sought in suspected cases. Interestingly, cases arising from intracerebral or optic inoculation manifest clinically as classical Creutzfeldt–Jakob disease, with a rapidly progressive dementia, while those resulting from peripheral inoculation present frequently with a progressive cerebellar ataxia initially, reminiscent of *kuru*. Unsurprisingly, the incubation period in intracerebral cases is short (19–46 months for dura mater grafts) as compared to peripheral cases (mean estimated at around 15 years).

Variant Creutzfeldt–Jakob disease

The clinical presentation is with behavioural and psychiatric disturbances, and in some cases with sensory phenomena. Initial referral is often to a psychiatrist and the most prominent feature is depression, but anxiety, withdrawal, and behavioural change are also frequent. Suicidal ideation is infrequent and response to antidepressants poor.

Delusions, which are complex and unsustained, are common. Other features include emotional lability, aggression, insomnia, and auditory and visual hallucinations. A prominent early feature in some was dysaesthesias or pain in the limbs or face, which was persistent rather than intermittent and unrelated to anxiety levels. A minority of cases have been noted to have forgetfulness or mild gait ataxia from an early stage but in most cases overt neurological features are not apparent until some months into the clinical course. In most patients a progressive cerebellar syndrome develops, with gait and limb ataxia. Dementia usually develops later in the clinical course, with progression to akinetic mutism in the majority of cases. Myoclonus is seen in most patients, in some cases preceded by chorea. Cortical blindness develops in a minority of patients in the late stages of disease. Upgaze paresis, an uncommon feature of classical Creutzfeldt–Jakob disease, has been noted in some patients. The age at onset to date ranges from 16 to 51 years (mean 29 years) and the clinical course is unusually prolonged (9–35 months, median 14 months). The EEG is abnormal, most frequently showing generalized slow-wave activity, but without the pseudoperiodic pattern seen in most cases of sporadic Creutzfeldt–Jakob disease. Neuroimaging by CT is either normal or shows only mild atrophy. However, a high signal in the posterior thalamus on T_2-weighted MRI is seen in a proportion of cases. The sensitivity and specificity of this sign is unclear at present. 14–3–3 protein may be elevated in cerebrospinal fluid. All cases to date are homozygous for methionine at *PRNP* codon 129. Variant Creutzfeldt–Jakob disease can be diagnosed by detection of characteristic PrP immunostaining and PrP^{Sc} on tonsil biopsy. Importantly, tonsillar PrP^{Sc} is only detectable in variant Creutzfeldt–Jakob disease, and not other forms of human prion disease. The PrP^{Sc} type detected on Western blot in tonsil from variant Creutzfeldt–Jakob disease has a characteristic pattern designated type 4t. A positive tonsil biopsy obviates the need for brain biopsy, which may otherwise be considered in such a clinical context to exclude alternative, potentially treatable, diagnoses.

The neuropathological appearances of variant Creutzfeldt–Jakob disease are striking and consistent. While there is widespread spongiform change, gliosis and neuronal loss, most severe in the basal ganglia and thalamus, the most remarkable feature was the abundant PrP amyloid plaques in cerebral and cerebellar cortex. These consist of *kuru*-like, 'florid' (surrounded by spongiform vacuoles), and multicentric plaque types. The 'florid' plaques, seen previously only in scrapie, are a particularly unusual but highly consistent feature. There is also abundant pericellular PrP deposition in the cerebral and cerebellar cortex, and PrP deposition in the molecular layer of the cerebellum.

Some of the features of variant Creutzfeldt–Jakob disease are reminiscent of *kuru*, in which behavioural changes and progressive ataxia predominate. In addition, peripheral sensory disturbances are well recognized in the *kuru* prodrome. *Kuru* plaques are seen in around 70 per cent of cases and are especially abundant in younger *kuru* cases. The observation that iatrogenic prion disease related to peripheral exposure to human prions has a more *kuru*-like than Creutzfeldt–Jakob disease-like clinical picture may well be relevant and would be consistent with a peripheral prion exposure.

The relatively stereotyped clinical presentation and neuropathology of variant Creutzfeldt–Jakob disease contrasts sharply with that of sporadic Creutzfeldt–Jakob disease. This may be because variant Creutzfeldt–Jakob disease is caused by a single prion strain and may also suggest that a relatively homogeneous, genetically susceptible, subgroup of the population with short incubation periods to bovine spongiform encephalopathy has been selected to date.

Gerstmann–Sträussler–Scheinker syndrome

This is an autosomal-dominant disorder that presents classically as a chronic cerebellar ataxia with pyramidal features, with dementia occurring later in a much more prolonged clinical course than that seen in Creutzfeldt–Jakob disease. The mean duration is around 5 years, with onset usually in either the third or fourth decades. Histologically, the hallmark is the presence of multicentric, PrP–amyloid plaques. While first associated with the P102L *PRNP* mutation, Gerstmann–Sträussler–Scheinker syndrome is now recognized as a pathological syndrome associated with several different *PRNP* mutations and forms a part of the phenotypic spectrum of inherited prion disease.

Inherited prion diseases

The identification of one of the pathogenic *PRNP* mutations in a case with neurodegenerative disease allows diagnosis of an inherited prion disease and subclassification according to mutation. Over 20 pathogenic mutations have been described in two groups: (1) point mutations resulting in amino acid substitutions in PrP or, in one case, production of a stop codon resulting in expression of a truncated PrP; (2) insertions encoding additional integral copies of an octapeptide repeat present in a tandem array of five copies in the normal protein. A suggested notation for these diseases is 'inherited prion disease (PrP mutation)', for instance: inherited prion disease (PrP 144 bp insertion) or inherited prion disease (PrP P102L). They are all autosomal dominantly inherited conditions.

Kindreds with inherited prion disease have been described with phenotypes of classical Creutzfeldt–Jakob disease, Gerstmann–Sträussler–Scheinker, and also with a range of other neurodegenerative syndromes. Some families show remarkable phenotypic variability, which can encompass both Creutzfeldt–Jakob disease- and Gerstmann–Sträussler–Scheinker-like cases as well as other cases that do not conform to either Creutzfeldt–Jakob disease or Gerstmann–Sträussler–Scheinker phenotypes. Such atypical prion diseases may lack the classical histological features of a spongiform encephalopathy entirely, although PrP immunohistochemistry is usually positive. Progressive dementia, cerebellar ataxia, pyramidal signs, chorea, myoclonus, extrapyramidal features, pseudobulbar signs, seizures, and amyotrophic features are seen in variable combinations. The most frequently seen forms include *PRNP* E200K, which most frequently presents as a Creutzfeldt–Jakob disease-like syndrome (and which, unlike most inherited prion disease, often has a typical EEG), *PRNP* P102L, which often presents as a progressive cerebellar ataxia, and insertional mutations, which have a particularly variable clinical presentation, often with a long duration mimicking Alzheimer's disease. Fatal familial insomnia, usually associated with the D178N *PRNP* mutation, is characterized clinically by untreatable insomnia, dysautonomia, and motor signs, and neuropathologically by selective atrophy of the anterior–ventral and mediodorsal thalamic nuclei. One variant, *PRNP* P105L, presents as a progressive spastic paraparesis. Age at onset varies from the early twenties (seen often with insert mutations) to seventies in some cases. The duration varies from less than a year in some variants to over 20 years. Penetrance appears to be full in most forms of inherited prion disease, although experience is limited with many variants. Elderly unaffected gene carriers are seen with *PRNP* E200K, although penetrance is probably full by the age of 80 years. Significant clinical overlap exists with familial Alzheimer's disease, Pick's disease, frontal lobe degeneration of non-Alzheimer type, and amyotrophic lateral sclerosis with dementia. In view of the ability of inherited prion disease to mimic many other neurodegenerative conditions, *PRNP* analysis should be considered in all presenile dementing or ataxic conditions.

PRNP analysis allows presymptomatic testing of unaffected but at-risk family members, as well as antenatal testing. Testing of asymptomatic individuals should only follow adequate counselling of individuals and requires their full informed consent. Because of the effect of codon 129 genotype on the age of onset of disease associated with some mutations, it is possible to determine within a family whether a carrier of a mutation will have an early or late onset of disease. Genetic counselling in prion disease resembles that of Huntington's disease in many respects and those protocols established for Huntington's disease have been adapted for counselling of prion disease.

Prognosis

All the prion diseases currently recognized are relentlessly progressive and invariably fatal. No current treatment affects outcome. General supportive care for the patient and family is all that can currently be offered. The rapid advances in the molecular biology of these diseases are leading to realistic possibilities of specific therapies. Such approaches may include agents with selective binding properties for PrP isoforms to inhibit the interactions between PrP^{C} and PrP^{Sc} thought to underlie prion propagation.

Prophylaxis and control of infection

Certain occupational groups are at risk of exposure to human prions, for instance neurosurgeons and other operating theatre staff, pathologists and morticians, histology technicians, as well as an increasing number of laboratory workers. Because of the prolonged incubation periods to prions following administration to sites other than the central nervous system, which is associated with clinically silent prion replication in the lymphoreticular tissue, treatments inhibiting prion replication in lymphoid organs may represent a viable strategy for rational secondary prophylaxis after accidental exposure. A provisional suggested regimen is a 2-week course of high-dose oral corticosteroids in individuals with significant accidental exposure to human prions.

As prions resist normal hospital sterilization procedures there is concern that prion diseases, particularly variant Creutzfeldt–Jakob disease with its extensive involvement of lymphoreticular tissues, may be transmitted iatrogenically via surgical instruments. For this reason, instruments used on patients with suspected prion disease should be disposable where possible; other instruments should be quarantined and not reused unless a non-prion diagnosis is confirmed. Patients with, or at risk of, developing prion disease should not be blood or other tissue donors and should be advised to inform surgeons and dentists of their condition.

Further reading

Alpers, M. (1996). Kuru. In *Oxford textbook of medicine*, 3rd edn (ed. D.J. Weatherall, J.G.G. Ledingham, and D.A. Warrell). Oxford University Press, Oxford.

Collinge J. (1998). Human prion diseases: aetiology and clinical features. In *The dementias* (ed. J.H. Growdon and M. Rossor). Butterworth-Heinemann, Newton MA.

Collinge, J. (1999). Prion disease. In *New Oxford textbook of psychiatry*, 2nd edn (ed. M.G. Gelder, J.J. Lopez-Ibor Jr, and N.C. Andreasen). Oxford University Press.

Collinge, J. (1999). Variant Creutzfeldt–Jakob disease. *Lancet*, **354**, 317–23.

Collinge, J., Sidle, K.C.L., Meads, J., Ironside, J., and Hill, A.F. (1996). Molecular analysis of prion strain variation and the aetiology of 'new variant' CJD. *Nature*, **383**, 685–90.

Hill, A.F., Butterworth, R.J., Joiner, S., *et al.* (1999). Investigation of variant Creutzfeldt Jakob disease and other human prion disease with tonsil biopsy samples. *Lancet*, **353**, 183–9.

Chapter 13.18

Inherited disorders of the nervous system

P. K. Thomas

There are many genetically determined neurological disorders, and others in which a genetic predisposition can be detected. Inherited disorders of the extrapyramidal system, peripheral nerves, and muscle, and those aminoacidurias that are associated with neurological involvement, are considered elsewhere, as is the question of genetic predisposition in the aetiology of conditions such as developmental abnormalities of the nervous system, epilepsy, migraine, Alzheimer's disease, and multiple sclerosis.

Hereditary ataxias

The classification of the hereditary ataxias remains a matter of controversy. Spinocerebellar degeneration may develop in disorders with a known metabolic basis, for instance abetalipoproteinaemia, ataxia telangiectasia, and xeroderma pigmentosum. The majority of the inherited cerebellar and spinocerebellar degenerations are at present of unknown cause. In general these can be divided into examples of early onset (under the age of 20 years), which are usually of autosomal-recessive inheritance and of which Friedreich's ataxia is the most common example, and the later-onset cases of cerebellar degeneration, which are most often dominantly inherited.

Early-onset hereditary ataxias

Friedreich's ataxia

This disorder is an example of a spinocerebellar degeneration and is dominated by progressive ataxia with an onset in childhood or adolescence. The condition is inherited as an autosomal-recessive trait and affects males and females approximately equally. The responsible gene has been mapped to the long arm of chromosome 9 in the region of q13–q21. Degeneration of the larger dorsal-root ganglion cells occurs, with consequent loss of the larger myelinated fibres in the peripheral nerves and degeneration of the dorsal columns. There is variable loss of Purkinje cells in the cerebellum.

The average age of onset is 11 to 12 years. The initial symptom is almost invariably ataxia of gait, although foot or spinal deformity may antedate this. Involvement of the upper limbs develops later, at first giving rise to clumsiness of fine movements, subsequently for all movements. A coarse intention tremor becomes obvious. The trunk is also affected. Dysarthria of cerebellar type develops and may become severe enough to make speech almost unintelligible.

Weakness develops as the disease advances, beginning in the legs and later involving the upper limbs. It results from degeneration in the corticospinal pathways and tends to vary in severity between cases. The plantar responses become extensor, but tone is not usually increased. Bladder and bowel function is usually unaffected.

Loss of the larger dorsal-root ganglion cells leads to impairment of joint position sense, vibration sense, and to some extent of touch–pressure sensibility, initially distally in the legs. The impairment of proprioception superimposes a sensory element in the cerebellar ataxia. The tendon reflexes are depressed or absent.

Apart from occasional nystagmus, the ocular movements are usually intact. The pupils are unaffected. Optic atrophy is present in about one-third of cases and 10 per cent develop sensorineural deafness.

Associated skeletal deformities are common, in particular foot deformities (pes cavus and pes equinovarus) and kyphoscoliosis. Contractures of the knees may develop in the later stages. Electrocardiography demonstrates widespread T-wave inversion and ventricular hypertrophy in nearly 70 per cent of patients. Cardiac failure occurs late and is usually precipitated by supraventricular arrhythmias. There is an increased incidence of diabetes mellitus in Friedreich's ataxia (10 per cent).

The disease is slowly progressive, the average age of death being in the latter part of the fourth decade. Ultimately patients become bedridden. Death is usually from an intercurrent infection with associated cardiac failure.

Other early-onset hereditary ataxias

A genetically distinct disorder that resembles Friedreich's ataxia is recognizable but has a more benign prognosis. The condition has a similar age of onset, is also of autosomal-recessive inheritance, but exhibits preserved tendon reflexes and is not associated with cardiac abnormalities or diabetes. Further rare disorders in this category include progressive myoclonic ataxia (Ramsay Hunt syndrome), in which a spinocerebellar degeneration is associated with myoclonic epilepsy, and a cerebellar degeneration that is accompanied by hypogonadism.

Later-onset hereditary ataxias

Autosomal-dominant cerebellar ataxia

This comprises the main group of disorders within the adult-onset hereditary ataxias. The age of onset ranges from the third to the fifth decades. In type I spinocerebellar ataxia, linkage analysis has located the gene to 6p22–p23. A trinucleotide-repeat expansion has been identified in this region in affected individuals, the longest abnormal allele being observed in cases of juvenile onset. In other families the disorder maps to chromosome 12q23–q24.1 (type 2 spinocerebellar ataxia) and 14q24.3–q31 (type 3), and in further families linkage to all three of these loci has been excluded. Progressive cerebellar ataxia with dysarthria, intention tremor in the upper limbs, and an ataxic gait are the salient clinical features. However, many of these patients show additional clinical manifestations that include dementia, optic atrophy, ophthalmoplegia, and extrapyramidal rigidity, which occur in varying combinations. Pathologically these dominantly inherited cerebellar ataxias have been equated with olivopontocerebellar atrophy, although it is clear that the neuropathological changes are more widespread than this, and that the pattern of the neuropathological change also varies between individuals within the same family.

Hereditary spastic paraplegia

Hereditary spastic paraplegia can be subdivided into a 'pure' form (Strümpell's disease) and others in which a variety of other features coexist. Strümpell's disease may display either an autosomal-dominant or autosomal-recessive inheritance. It may present during childhood or even with delayed motor development in infancy; in other cases the onset is retarded until adult life. It gives rise to difficulty in walking because of weakness and spasticity in the legs. The tendon reflexes are exaggerated and the plantar responses are extensor. In cases of early onset, foot deformity may be present. Some patients show a mild degree of cerebellar ataxia and sensory impairment in the legs of posterior-column type. The disease progresses slowly and may later affect the upper limbs. Precipitancy of micturition or urinary incontinence may occur. Pathologically there is degeneration of the corticospinal pathways in the lateral columns of the spinal cord and some fibre loss in the gracile fasciculi.

If there is severe spasticity, this may be alleviated to some extent by baclofen or dantrolene orally. Continuous intrathecal administration of baclofen by an infusion pump is helpful in selected cases. The precipitancy of micturition may be improved by propantheline. Surgical correction of foot deformities is sometimes required.

Disorders of lipid metabolism (see also Chapter 6.11)

Neurolipidoses

The lipidoses constitute a group of disorders characterized by the intracellular accumulation of a variety of different lipids. Some predominantly involve the nervous system; others primarily affect the reticuloendothelial system, but may also involve nervous tissue. They may be classified in terms of the particular lipid that is stored.

Niemann–Pick disease

This consists of a group of four recessively inherited disorders in which there is an accumulation of lipid in 'foam cells' in the reticuloendothelial system. In type B, progressive mental deterioration and hypotonic paralysis in association with hepatosplenomegaly appear in the first 6 months of life, leading to death before the age of 3 years. Cherry-red spots are present at the macula in 50 per cent. Type B does not affect the nervous system. Types C and D resemble type A but the storage material consists of cholesterol and neutral lipids.

Glucosyl ceramide lipidosis (Gaucher's disease)

Three variants exist, all recessively inherited, characterized by hepatosplenomegaly related to the accumulation of glucosyl ceramide in histiocytes as a consequence of a deficiency of the enzyme glucocerebrosidase. The type 1, adult-onset form does not affect the nervous system but types 2 and 3, with an infantile and juvenile onset, respectively, and a more rapid progression, display widespread cerebral involvement.

Gangliosidoses

These comprise a group of recessively inherited disorders in which there is a combination of progressive dementia, epilepsy, and visual failure. They are related to defective ganglioside degradation. Several GM_1 gangliosidoses exist and are the result of an inherited deficiency of acid β-galactosidase. In the infantile form, onset is at birth or in early infancy, and initially is manifested by a failure to thrive and by hepatosplenomegaly. Later, mental and motor deterioration becomes evident, and a cherry-red spot may be present at the macula, related to retinal degeneration. Death takes place before the age of 3 years. A juvenile-onset variant also exists.

The GM_2 gangliosidoses involve the storage of GM_2 gangliosides, which are largely confined to the nervous system. In the type 1 variety (Tay–Sachs disease), the disorder usually begins within the first 6 months of life. It is encountered most frequently in Ashkenazim Jews. Initially there is retardation of development, which is followed by progressive dementia, hypotonic weakness, and blindness. There is a cherry-red spot at the macula. Later, seizures occur and terminally generalized spasticity develops. Death generally takes place in the fourth year of life. The disorder is related to an inherited deficiency of hexosaminidase A and the gene has been localized to chromosome 15q23–q24. Carrier detection is possible by a serum assay, and mass screening programmes have been undertaken in some countries. Antenatal diagnosis by amniocentesis is also possible.

Neuronal ceroid lipofuscinosis

Under this heading are grouped a number of rare disorders in which retinal degeneration, progressive dementia, epilepsy, spasticity, and ataxia occur in various combinations. The age of onset may be infantile (Santavuori), late infantile (Jansky–Bielschowsky), juvenile (Spielmeyer–Vogt), or adult (Kufs). Eponyms abound: the late infantile and juvenile cases are often collectively termed Batten's disease. There is neuronal storage of lipopigment, but the molecular basis for these disorders has not been established. The gene for the juvenile form has been localized to chromosome 16p12.1.

Leucodystrophies

These disorders are characterized by a diffuse disintegration of white matter in the central nervous system and sometimes also by segmental demyelination in the peripheral nerves.

Metachromatic leucodystrophy (sulphatide lipidosis)

The most common variant is the late infantile type, which usually begins in the third year of life with weakness and ataxia in the limbs. Subsequently a progressive dementia supervenes, seizures may occur, and in some instances optic atrophy develops. The tendon reflexes may be depressed or absent in those patients in whom peripheral nerve involvement is prominent. Nerve conduction velocity is reduced. Death sometimes occurs after a course of a few months, sometimes of as much as 5 or 6 years. Terminally the affected children are demented, with a spastic tetraplegia, and are often blind.

The disorder, which maps to chromosome 22q13–13qter, is inherited in an autosomal-recessive manner, and is due to a deficiency of aryl sulphatase A. This can be demonstrated by assay on leucocytes. Juvenile- and adult-onset forms of metachromatic leucodystrophy are also encountered, but are rare.

Globoid-cell leucodystrophy (Krabbe's disease)

This derives its title from the presence of large, multinucleate cells containing galactosylceramide in areas of white-matter damage. The condition begins at the age of 3 or 4 months as a failure to thrive. Developmental regression then becomes evident and the tendon reflexes are lost. As the disease advances, generalized hypertonus appears, together with various types of seizure, and optic atrophy. Death often occurs in the first year of life or may be delayed into the second year. There are also rare late-onset cases.

The disorder is inherited in an autosomal-recessive manner and is due to a deficiency of galactosylceramide β-galactosidase. It maps to chromosome 14q21–q31. This may be demonstrated by assays in leucocytes or serum.

Adrenoleucodystrophy and adrenomyeloneuropathy (see Chapter 13.20)

Amongst a group of conditions that give rise to widespread demyelination in the brain with an onset during childhood, cases of adrenoleucodystrophy can be separated by virtue of X-linked inheritance and associated adrenal insufficiency. The disorder maps to chromosome Xq28. The affected boys exhibit a progressive illness characterized by the development of dementia, cortical blindness, ataxia, and spastic weakness in the limbs. A myeloneuropathy is sometimes the presenting deficit, as well as other phenotypes. Manifesting female carriers may show a mild spastic paraparesis or adrenal insufficiency.

Fabry's disease (α-galactosidase A deficiency) (see also Chapter 6.8)

This condition is an inborn error of glycosphingolipid metabolism. Neutral glycosphingolipids are deposited in various tissues as a consequence of a deficiency of the enzyme α-galactosidase A. The disorder is inherited in an X-linked recessive manner and maps to chromosome Xq21.33–q22. Affected hemizygous males develop a mild peripheral neuropathy, which is manifested by the occurrence of severe pains in the extremities, often beginning in childhood. Cerebrovascular lesions also occur, either cerebral infarction or haemorrhage. Non-neurological features include corneal opacification, punctate angiectatic lesions over the lower trunk, buttocks, and upper legs, and cardiac and renal lesions. Heterozygous females may display mild manifestations, most usually corneal opacification.

Hereditary lipoprotein deficiency

The occurrence of peripheral neuropathy in hereditary high-density lipoprotein deficiency (Tangier disease) is discussed in Chapter 6.11. Hereditary abetalipoproteinaemia (Bassen–Kornzweig disease) is a recessively inherited disorder in which a spinocerebellar degeneration may develop with features that bear some resemblance to Friedreich's ataxia. Other manifestations of this uncommon disorder include intestinal malabsorption, pigmentary retinal degeneration, and the presence of acanthocytes in the peripheral blood. In addition to the absence of serum low-density lipoproteins, the serum cholesterol is substantially reduced. There is evidence that the development of the neurological lesions may be prevented by the administration of vitamin E, the absorption of which from the gut is impaired.

Isolated vitamin E deficiency

A spinocerebellar syndrome resembling Friedreich's ataxia has been described due to vitamin E deficiency in the absence of generalized fat malabsorption. Its precise mechanism has not yet been established. The disorder is of autosomal-recessive inheritance and maps to chromosome 8q. Treatment is by vitamin E replacement.

Neurocutaneous syndromes

Neurofibromatosis

Two major forms of this disorder exist. Both are of autosomal-dominant inheritance. The gene for type 1 neurofibromatosis (von Recklinghausen's disease) is on the proximal long arm of chromosome 17 at q11.2. The gene product, neurofibromin, is a member of the GTPase-activating family of proteins. The disorder has a wide range of manifestations, the most constant of which are focal areas of hyperpigmentation (*café-au-lait* spots), multiple neurofibromas, and Lisch nodules on the iris. Six or more *café-au-lait* spots are necessary for them to be considered abnormal. Axillary and inguinal freckling is frequent. The cutaneous fibromas are of varying dimensions and can be extremely numerous. At times, giant plexiform neuromas develop, in which there is extensive subcutaneous overgrowth of neurofibromatous tissue. Massive mediastinal, pelvic, or retro-abdominal plexiform neurofibromas can occur, as well as cervical paraspinal tumours and astrocytomas of the optic nerve, cerebellum, or brainstem. Malignant change occurs in a small proportion of peripheral neurofibromas. Mental retardation due to diffuse cortical dysgenesis is encountered in at least 10 per cent of patients. Other manifestations include congenital glaucoma, phaeochromocytoma, spinal deformity, pathological fractures of limb bones with malunion and pseudoarthrosis, and local gigantism of a limb.

The gene for type 2 neurofibromatosis (central neurofibromatosis) has been mapped to chromosome 22q12.2. This disorder is characterized in particular by bilateral acoustic neurinomas but tumours may occur on other cranial nerves or spinal roots and also paraspinally. Meningiomas and gliomas may develop. A further feature is the occurrence of juvenile posterior subcapsular lenticular opacities.

Tuberous sclerosis

The features of this condition are mental retardation, epilepsy, and the occurrence of characteristic skin lesions. The disorder is dominantly inherited, but may be transmitted by individuals who are asymptomatic and who show only minimal clinical evidence of the disease. Isolated cases are frequent, comprising as many as 80 or 90 per cent of index cases. Many of them probably represent new mutations; others are transmitted by gene carriers with trivial manifestations. Genetic heterogeneity has now been established, with separate loci on chromosomes 9 (*TSC1*) and 16p13.3 (*TSC2*). The gene *TSC2* has been identified and its product, called tuberin, has the structure of a GTPase-activating protein.

The earliest cutaneous lesions are irregular, foliate areas of depigmentation over the trunk. These patches are readily identified when viewed under ultraviolet illumination using a Wood's lamp. Adenoma sebaceum is a second type of skin lesion, which develops over the cheeks in a 'butterfly' distribution and on the forehead (Fig. 1). Multiple, small warty elevations appear, which histologically are fibromatous and not adenomatous. Finally, a 'shagreen patch' may be present over the lower back. This consists of an area of elevated roughened skin with a yellowish tinge, which has been likened to shark skin.

The cerebral changes give rise to mental retardation, evident in early life, which may be static or involve a slowly progressive cognitive decline, often complicated by behaviour disorder. Epilepsy with recurrent generalized or focal seizures may occur in association with mental retardation or in individuals of normal intelligence. The cerebral lesions, which are demonstrable by CT scanning or MRI, are

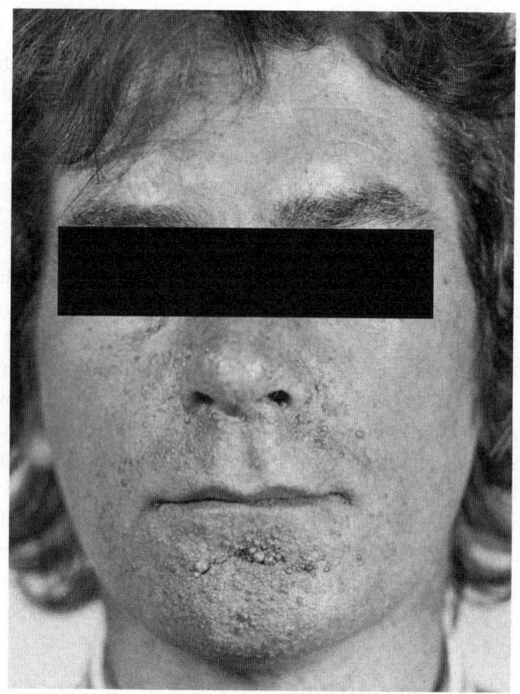

Fig. 1 Adenoma sebaceum in a patient with tuberous sclerosis.

typified by nodular or tuberous masses composed of proliferated glial cells and enlarged distorted neurones. They may become calcified. They are found scattered throughout the cerebral cortex and also extend into the ventricles. Gliomas sometimes arise in these lesions.

Retinal tumours, termed phakomas, may be present, and cardiac rhabdomyomas occasionally arise as well as hamartomas of the lungs and kidneys. Polycystic disease of the kidneys may also be associated.

Treatment consists of control of the epilepsy and the management of the mental retardation and behaviour disorder. Many of the more severe cases require admission to appropriate institutions.

Cerebelloretinal haemangioblastosis (von Hippel–Lindau disease)

This condition comprises the occurrence of vascular tumours in the retina and within the central nervous system, most commonly in the cerebellum and spinal cord. The inheritance is autosomal dominant in pattern. The disorder maps to chromosome 3p26–25.

The retinal lesions consist of angiomatous vascular malformations. The cerebellar lesion is a haemangioblastoma, often cystic, which may slowly expand and present with features of a cerebellar tumour. It may require surgical treatment. Such tumours may be associated with polycythaemia, related to the production of erythropoietin or similar substance by the tumour. Haemangioblastomas may occur in the spinal cord and rarely in the cerebral hemispheres.

It should be emphasized that the majority of cerebellar haemangioblastomas are non-genetic.

Ataxia telangiectasia (Louis–Bar syndrome)

The inclusion of this disorder with the neurocutaneous syndromes depends upon the coincidence of a progressive cerebellar degeneration with cutaneous vascular lesions. The inheritance is of autosomal-recessive type and the gene is localized on chromosome 11q22.3–q23.1. Ataxia begins in early childhood; choreoathetosis and oculomotor apraxia appear later. Telangiectasia of the conjunctiva is present as a relatively early feature and later becomes evident in the pinnas, over the face, and in the limb flexures. Some patients show an immunoglobulin deficiency and recurrent infections, or the development of malignancies may complicate the clinical picture. Defective DNA repair after X-irradiation is demonstrable in cultured skin fibroblasts. Affected children usually become unable to walk by the age of 12 years and death occurs during the second or sometimes third decade of life.

Hereditary myoclonic epilepsies

A number of conditions exist in which generalized epileptic seizures and myoclonus are associated with a progressive degenerative neurological disorder occurring on a genetic basis.

Lafora-body disease

This is the most clearly defined form of progressive myoclonic epilepsy. It consists of a combination of major seizures, myoclonus, and progressive dementia, with an onset in late childhood or early adolescence, and death usually before adult life is reached. Cerebellar signs may appear later in the illness. The condition is characterized by the presence of intracellular inclusion bodies found most consistently in neurones of the cerebral cortex and in the cerebellar dentate nuclei. They are also detectable in the liver and in skeletal muscles, both of which are convenient sites for biopsy in order to establish the diagnosis. These Lafora bodies are composed of a polyglucosan. The disorder is caused by an autosomal-recessive gene. Treatment is directed towards control of the epilepsy.

Sialidosis

The cherry-red spot–myoclonus syndrome is an autosomal-recessive disorder with an onset in late childhood, adolescence, or early adult life that combines action myoclonus with ataxia, cherry-red spots at the macula, and cataracts. This condition is related to a deficiency of sialidase.

The myoclonus may respond to treatment with clonazepam or to piracetam in high dosage. 5-hydroxytryptophan is less effective than in postanoxic action myoclonus.

Other miscellaneous disorders

A wide variety of other rare inherited conditions exist, of which the following deserve brief mention.

Hereditary optic neuropathy

Dominantly inherited juvenile optic neuropathy

This disorder gives rise to the insidious bilateral onset of optic atrophy during childhood, with either mild or severe loss of vision. A central or centrocaecal scotoma may be detected. There are no associated neurological abnormalities.

Leber's hereditary optic neuropathy

This disorder typically gives rise to acute or subacute bilateral visual loss in males between the ages of 18 and 30 years, although earlier and later ages of onset may be encountered. It may remain monocular for months or years. Initially there is enlargement of the blind spot and later this increases to involve central vision, producing a large centrocaecal scotoma. In the acute phase there is swelling in the nerve-fibre layer around the optic disc, with tortuous retinal arterioles and peripapillary telangiectases. Later the disc becomes atrophic. In affected females the age of onset tends to be later and a multiple sclerosis-like syndrome may develop. The disease is only transmitted by females and is due to mitochondrial DNA mutations.

Mucopolysaccharidoses (see also Chapter 6.8)

The mucopolysaccharidoses constitute a group of disorders related to deficiencies of specific lysosomal enzymes, involving an accumulation in various tissues of acid mucopolysaccharides and gangliosides, and the presence of mucopolysaccharides in the urine. In both the recessively inherited Hurler's syndrome and the X-linked recessive Hunter's syndrome, the skeletal and other manifestations may be accompanied by mental retardation and pigmentary retinal degeneration. A spastic weakness in the limbs may develop in Hurler's syndrome. Mental retardation is also seen in the recessively inherited Sanfilippo's syndrome.

Subacute necrotizing encephalopathy (Leigh's syndrome)

Typically this label is applicable to a fatal encephalopathy that develops during the first 2 years of life with variable combinations of mental retardation, seizures, optic atrophy, cerebellar ataxia, and central respiratory failure associated with lactic acidosis. Later-onset cases with similar pathological changes occur. The disorder is genetically heterogeneous.

Lesch–Nyhan syndrome

This is an X-linked recessive disorder related to the absence of an enzyme of purine metabolism (see also Chapter 6.6). The salient features are overproduction of uric acid and consequent hyperuricaemia, which are associated with various behavioural and neurological manifestations, including mental retardation, self-mutilation, choreoathetosis, pyramidal signs, and spasticity in the limbs. The neurological abnormalities develop in childhood and death usually occurs in the second or third decade from renal failure. Allopurinol may reduce some of the non-neurological consequences of the hyperuricaemia, but no treatment influences the neurological abnormalities. Prenatal diagnosis and carrier detection are available.

Further reading

Barchi, R.L. (1998). Ion channel mutations affecting muscle and brain. *Current Opinion in Neurology*, **11**, 461–8.

Brice, A. (1998). Unstable mutations and neurodegenerative disorders. *Journal of Neurology*, **245**, 505–10.

Moser, H.W. (1998). Neurometabolic disease. *Current Opinion in Neurology*, **11**, 91–5.

Rosenberg, R.N., Prusiner, S.B., DiMauro, S., Barchi, R.L., and Kunkel, L.M. (ed.) (1993). *The molecular and genetic basis of neurological disease.* Butterworth-Heinemann, Oxford.

Chapter 13.19

Demyelinating disorders of the central nervous system

D. A. S. Compston

Clinicians usually suspect demyelination when symptoms and signs arising from damage to white-matter tracts within the central nervous system develop subacutely in young adults; the diagnosis of multiple sclerosis—by far the most common demyelinating disease in man—becomes probable when these episodes recur and affect different parts of the brain and spinal cord. Demyelinating disease is also the basis for many of the neurological syndromes triggered by infectious illness and vaccination. The clinical manifestations of demyelination are not specific and identical symptoms are seen in other disorders affecting the same parts of the nervous system. For discussion and full references see Compston *et al.* (1998).

Isolated demyelinating syndromes

Multiple sclerosis is characterized by demyelinating events that recur and are disseminated throughout the nervous system. In other situations, demyelination is focal and monophasic, but even in these cases imaging studies show that a high proportion of patients have more than one lesion. The distinction between multiple sclerosis and the various isolated demyelinating disorders can therefore reliably be made only when more than one episode has occurred, affecting two or more sites, and not merely on the basis of anatomical dissemination of lesions.

Acute disseminated encephalomyelitis

Typically, acute disseminated encephalomyelitis follows 14 days after an infectious illness. The disorder is usually cerebral, resulting in focal neurological deficits, fits, and drowsiness. In some cases, the manifestations are confined to the brainstem, optic nerves, or spinal cord. A proportion of patients recovering from the initial attack subsequently relapse and their illness cannot then be distinguished from the encephalitic presentation of multiple sclerosis. In some patients, although the presenting illness remains monophasic, separate sites are involved sequentially over several weeks but the disorder does not recur and differs from multiple sclerosis in this important respect.

Formerly, acute disseminated encephalomyelitis affected 1:1000 children with exanthematous illnesses, the risk being slightly higher following pertussis and scarlet fever than measles and rubella; with vaccination, these illnesses are less common, as is acute disseminated encephalomyelitis, and a high proportion of cases now occur without identification of the provocative agent. About 50 per cent of post-varicella cases present with a pure cerebellar syndrome. A greater variety of causative organisms has been implicated in adult-onset acute disseminated encephalomyelitis, but in both groups a presumptive diagnosis often has to be made in the absence of preceding infection; recently identified causes include echovirus, coxsackie and herpes viridae, mycoplasma, borreliosis, and cases associated with AIDS.

Headache, drowsiness, meningeal irritation, signs of systemic infection, focal or generalized fits, and combinations of lesions indicating damage to the cerebrum, optic nerves, brainstem, or spinal cord evolve over the course of a few days; the cerebrospinal fluid contains a mixture of polymorphonuclear cells and lymphocytes, with raised protein and a slight reduction in glucose; oligoclonal bands may be present. Although there is an appreciable mortality, especially in acute haemorrhagic encephalomyelitis (Huest's disease), the majority of patients survive, albeit with persistent neurological deficits; the outcome probably is influenced by the early use of high-dose steroids. MRI shows changes similar to those occurring in multiple sclerosis, but the lesions are more extensive and symmetrical; they persist long after recovery of the clinical illness. Some patients develop new lesions after evolution of the presenting episode, indicating continuing disease activity, and the diagnosis of multiple sclerosis then becomes more likely.

Optic neuritis

Optic neuritis presents with pain on eye movement, followed by blurred vision that evolves over hours or days, sometimes to complete blindness; there may be selective loss of colour vision and flashes of light (phosphenes) on eye movement. The pain disappears within a few days; vision improves in 90 per cent of patients over months but defects of colour perception frequently persist. Optic neuritis may present with progressive visual failure but in this situation care must be taken to exclude compression of the anterior visual pathway. Transient visual loss, mimicking optic neuritis, also occurs in ischaemic optic neuropathy and sarcoidosis, and a family history should be taken since the presentation of visual failure in Leber's hereditary optic neuropathy is similar to bilateral sequential optic neuritis in men.

The frequency with which the optic nerve is involved in multiple sclerosis leads to anxiety in the informed patient that an episode of optic neuritis is likely to be the first manifestation of multiple sclerosis. The risk is highest in the first 5 years but the proportion of cases having recurrent demyelination increases thereafter and life-table analysis suggests that up to 80 per cent of cases eventually develop multiple sclerosis. In children, optic neuritis is commonly bilateral, and recurrent demyelination affecting other parts of the nervous system rarely occurs; bilateral simultaneous optic neuritis in adults, although less common than in children, also carries a low risk of conversion to multiple sclerosis. Periventricular white-matter abnormalities demonstrated by MRI are found in more than 60 per cent of patients with optic neuritis, and the risk of developing multiple sclerosis is substantially increased for those having two or more such lesions at presentation; the presence of oligoclonal bands on cerebrospinal fluid electrophoresis during the acute phase is also a significant risk factor.

Transverse myelitis

Acute necrotizing myelitis causes rapidly progressive, flaccid, areflexic paraplegia with anaesthesia and loss of sphincter control. The intensity of inflammation results in severe pain with meningism, pyrexia, and systemic symptoms. The condition mimics cord compression; the changes in cerebrospinal fluid resemble those in pyogenic or tuberculous infection of the central nervous system. Acute necrotizing myelitis has recently been described in association with herpesvirus infection, and as a complication of acute lymphocytic leukaemias, lymphoma, carcinoma, and AIDS.

Transverse myelitis presents with pain at the site of the lesion, followed by weakness in the legs, sensory symptoms, and sphincter involvement. The weakness increases and the clinical picture is that of spinal shock, features that are rarely seen in acute cord lesions due to multiple sclerosis; sphincter control is lost but, unlike patients with multiple sclerosis, there is usually difficulty in emptying rather than filling the bladder. The need to exclude a structural abnormality in patients with transverse myelitis means that many patients undergo radiological investigation, which may demonstrate cord swelling. The spinal fluid shows an increased mononuclear cell count, numerically intermediate between the marked pleocytosis of acute necrotizing myelitis and the marginal abnormalities seen in multiple sclerosis; total protein is raised and oligoclonal bands may be present on electrophoresis, but the glucose is usually normal. Transverse myelitis is more common in adults than in children; there is a high frequency of persistent disability but a much lower conversion to multiple sclerosis than following optic neuritis.

Devic's disease

Devic's disease is characterized by massive, confluent demyelination in the anterior visual pathway, together with equally severe damage in the spinal cord, occurring simultaneously or sequentially and in either order, the episodes usually separated by weeks or months. Demyelinating disease often follows the Devic pattern in Japanese, where multiple sclerosis is otherwise rare, and findings in some series of patients with Devic's disease in northern Europe have emphasized the low conversion rate to multiple sclerosis.

Multiple sclerosis

Aetiology

The aetiology of multiple sclerosis involves an interplay between genetic and environmental factors. The lifetime risk of multiple sclerosis in northern Europeans—about 1:800—increases to 1:50, 1:20, and 1:3 for the offspring, siblings, and monozygotic twin partners of affected individuals, respectively.

Susceptibility to multiple sclerosis is polygenic. Population studies demonstrate an association between the class II MHC alleles DR15 and DQ6 and their corresponding genotypes. Regions of interest emerging from three systematic genome screens are 1p, 3p, 5cen, 6p, 6q, 7q, 17q, 18q, 19q and X. Conditioning the UK genome screen DR15 shows that the regions of interest on 1p, 17p, 17q, and X cluster in families that are linked to DR15 whereas the DR15 non-sharing group associates with 1cen, 3p, 5cen, 7p, 14q and 22q.

The distribution of multiple sclerosis cannot be explained only on the basis of population genetics. In white South Africans and in Australia, prevalence rates are half those documented for many parts of northern Europe, and there is a gradient in frequency, both in Australia and in New Zealand, that does not follow genetic clines. Multiple sclerosis occurs at a low frequency in Caribbeans but the risk increases substantially in their first-generation descendants raised in the UK. Conversely, the risk is higher for English-speaking whites migrating into South Africa as adults than in childhood.

Prospective studies have demonstrated that new episodes of demyelination are more likely to occur following viral exposure, but no one triggering agent has been identified. The risk of developing multiple sclerosis is increased for individuals who are exposed to measles, mumps, rubella, and Epstein–Barr virus infection relatively late in childhood or adolescence. These studies do not implicate any one of these agents as the exclusive cause of multiple sclerosis but suggest that a narrow and age-linked period of susceptibility to viral exposure exists in those who are constitutionally at risk of developing the disease.

Pathophysiology

Myelin injury blocks saltatory conduction through myelinated axons. Partially demyelinated pathways cannot transmit fast trains of impulse; depolarization may cross the lesion but at reduced velocity, accounting for the characteristic delay in the arrival of evoked potentials. Partially demyelinated axons discharge spontaneously, causing unpleasant distortions of sensation and facial myokymia; and increased mechanical sensitivity results in movement-induced phosphenes and the electric sensation provoked by neck flexion (Lhermitte's symptom). Increased temperature sensitivity explains the temporary increase in symptoms after exercise or immersion in hot water; and ephaptic transmission between neighbouring, partially demyelinated axons results in paroxysmal symptoms of demyelination such as trigeminal neuralgia or tonic brainstem seizures.

Clinical symptomatology

Special senses

Involvement of the visual pathways is almost invariable and most commonly affects the optic nerve (see above); the postchiasmal visual pathway is occasionally involved, resulting in hemianopic field defects. Deafness occurs in multiple sclerosis, occasionally at presentation. Feelings of unsteadiness are common; and acute brainstem demyelination causes severe positional vertigo, vomiting, ataxia, and headache. Taste may be subjectively abnormal but aguesia is rarely described.

Motor symptoms and signs

Impaired mobility affects the majority of patients with multiple sclerosis, usually as a result of spinal disease; movements are slow, weakness differentially affects extensors in the arms and flexors in the legs, and there are the expected signs of upper motor-neurone lesions. Spasticity may be more problematic than weakness and all aspects of immobility are frequently complicated by fatigue. Cerebellar involvement causes incoordination of speech, bulbar control, eye movements, the individual limbs or balance, usually in combination with corticospinal damage.

Sensory symptoms and signs

Altered sensation occurs at some stage in nearly every patient with multiple sclerosis. Damage to the posterior columns in the cervical cord produces tight, burning, twisting, tearing, or pulling sensations, which are usually painful; associated loss of proprioception severely compromises function. Involvement of the spinothalamic tract leads to loss of thermal and pain sensation. Non-specific tingling without accompanying signs is often described; the most common physical sign found in the absence of symptoms is impaired vibration sense in the legs.

Autonomic involvement

Autonomic symptoms occur in many patients with multiple sclerosis. Bladder symptoms are most common in women whereas impotence occurs frequently in males. Loss of inhibition of reflex bladder emptying, normally mediated by cholinergic neurones that contract the detrusor and relax the internal sphincter, results in urgency and frequency, with incontinence when combined with immobility. Impaired control of the rectal sphincter is much less of a problem than failure of emptying.

Eye movements

Abnormalities of eye movement are extremely common in multiple sclerosis and often occur in the absence of symptoms. Weakness of the lateral rectus, or an internuclear ophthalmoplegia, produces double vision. Visual instability (oscillopsia) occurs most commonly in the context of bilateral internuclear ophthalmoplegia or downbeating nystagmus, and with ocular flutter and opsoclonus.

Cognitive and affective symptoms

Defects of visual and auditory attention occur in multiple sclerosis, sometimes at an early stage, and these are also detectable in patients with isolated demyelinating lesions; an overall impairment in intelligence quotient relates more to duration of disease, and onset of the progressive phase, affecting memory by comparison with language skills. Psychotic behaviour is rare but depression occurs more frequently than in patients with comparable neurological disability; hypomania is occasionally seen but should not be confused with pathological laughter and crying, arising from loss of central inhibition of facial and bulbar reflexes in association with extensive brainstem disease.

Clinical course and prognosis

Eighty per cent of patients present with relapsing/remitting disease, episodes occurring at random frequency and for an unpredictable period, but averaging about one per year and decreasing with time. Later, a high proportion of patients enter a slowly progressive phase of the disease, but in 20 per cent the illness is progressive from onset. Life expectancy is at least 25 years, and a high proportion of patients die from unrelated causes. Recovery from each attack is invariably slower than onset, and may be incomplete.

The spinal cord bears the brunt of progressive multiple sclerosis, but optic-nerve, cerebral, and brainstem disease may also deteriorate slowly. Primary progressive spinal disease is the usual mode of presentation when multiple sclerosis develops beyond the fifth decade. Secondary progressive multiple sclerosis tends to affect whichever system has been involved during the relapsing phase. Progression may follow directly upon a severe relapse and be interrupted by further episodes.

About 25 per cent of patients have multiple sclerosis in a form that is not disabling. In about 5 per cent of patients, a latent period of more than 20 years occurs between the presenting and the next episode. Benign disease usually occurs in young females with predominantly sensory symptoms and complete recovery from individual episodes. Conversely, in 5 per cent relapses occur frequently and do not recover, leading rapidly to disability and early death; and up to 15 per cent become severely disabled within a short time. Occasionally, patients die acutely from respiratory failure when the medulla is affected and from massive cerebral demyelination.

Two per cent of patients with multiple sclerosis present before the age of 10 years, and 5 per cent before 16 years of age; even so, there is reluctance to make the diagnosis in children. The presentation is often similar to that seen in adults, although an encephalitic onset mimicking acute disseminated encephalomyelitis is well recognized.

Investigation

Investigations are required in patients suspected of having multiple sclerosis when the clinical findings are insufficient for establishing the diagnosis; they are used to demonstrate anatomical dissemination of lesions and provide evidence for intrathecal inflammation. Conditions that mimic demyelinating disease may also need to be excluded.

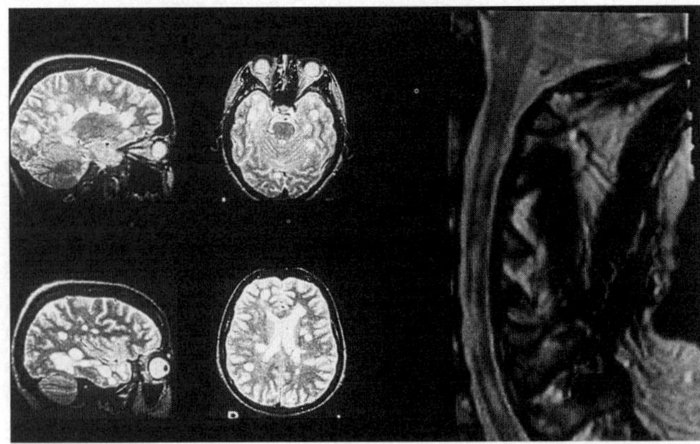

Fig. 1 MRI in a patient with multiple sclerosis showing white-matter, T_2-weighted signals in the cerebrum and spinal cord.

Electrophysiology

Demyelination can be detected in clinically unaffected pathways using visual-, auditory-, somatosensory-, central motor-, and event-related potentials; their latencies are characteristically delayed, whereas, except in acute lesions, the amplitude is unaffected. Evoked potentials add little diagnostic information in situations where the pathway under investigation is clinically affected but do provide evidence for the process of demyelination.

Imaging

Low-density lesions, corresponding to areas of demyelination, may be seen using contrast-enhanced CT, and these occasionally have the appearances of cerebral tumour or abscess, but this technique is insensitive compared with MRI (Fig. 1). More than 95 per cent of patients with clinically definite multiple sclerosis have periventricular lesions, and more than 90 per cent also show discrete white-matter abnormalities, each corresponding to areas of histological damage. Gadolinium enhancement of these lesions signifies altered permeability of the blood–brain barrier and indicates that they are of recent origin. The lesions are not specific; similar changes occur with inflammatory or vascular lesions and with advancing age. Focal lesions can be imaged in the optic nerve, brainstem, and spinal cord.

Imaging is not necessary for diagnostic purposes in patients with a history of relapsing disease and signs indicating involvement of multiple sites within the central nervous system. The major practical use is in the investigation of individuals with isolated demyelinating lesions, recurrent episodes at a single site, or progressive disease affecting the spinal cord. In all these situations the requirement is to exclude a structural lesion, especially since these can present with relapsing symptoms. Once the clinically affected part has been negatively screened for a structural lesion, the diagnosis of multiple sclerosis also requires the demonstration of cerebral periventricular lesions.

Cerebrospinal fluid

Analysis of cerebrospinal fluid provides information, which is complementary to imaging abnormalities, in patients suspected of having multiple sclerosis. The cell count rarely exceeds 50 lymphocytes/mm^3, even during periods of clinical activity, and is normal in more than 50 per cent of patients. There is a rise in total protein, with a specific increase in the immunoglobulin concentration and the presence of oligoclonal bands on protein electrophoresis in more than 90 per cent of cases, after correction for leakage of serum proteins through the blood–brain barrier, providing evidence for synthesis of immunoglobulin within the central nervous system.

Differential diagnosis

The most common error in clinical practice is to make the diagnosis of multiple sclerosis in patients with progressive spinal disease in whom a structural lesion has not been adequately excluded. Lesions at the foramen magnum are particularly well placed to cause confusion through appearing to produce evidence for independent spinal and brainstem lesions. Errors also arise with progressive or relapsing manifestations of brainstem or spinal arteriovenous malformations.

Care must be taken in the diagnosis of multiple sclerosis when several members are affected within one family. Hereditary spastic paraplegia mimics familial multiple sclerosis, and this should also be considered in isolated cases of progressive spastic paraplegia when pyramidal manifestations occur in isolation and with disproportionate spasticity. Other familial disorders that are confused with multiple sclerosis include the hereditary ataxias and adult-onset leucodystrophies.

Clinical, immunological, and imaging abnormalities indistinguishable from multiple sclerosis occur with granulomatous and vasculitic diseases of the brain, especially the cerebral variant of systemic lupus erythematosus, which usually occurs in the absence of systemic manifestations or informative serology. Sarcoidosis may present with clinical involvement of the central nervous system, and typical abnormalities on MRI and in cerebrospinal fluid. Orogenital ulceration in a patient with the clinical manifestations of multiple sclerosis suggests the diagnosis of Behçet's disease.

Direct infections of the nervous system can mimic the isolated demyelinating syndromes and multiple sclerosis; these include tuberculous and other chronic meningitides, and the neurological manifestations of AIDS. Borreliosis can also cause a chronic or relapsing disorder of the central nervous system, but this is usually preceded by the characteristic painful polyradiculitis and facial palsy that epitomizes Lyme disease. Similarities between multiple sclerosis and neurosyphilis should not be forgotten in the context of opportunistic infection complicating infection with human immunodeficiency virus.

Treatment of demyelinating disease

Caution is usually observed in recommending treatment in patients with multiple sclerosis since no agent has yet proved effective in altering the long-term course of the disease, and a significant proportion of affected individuals remain free from disability over several decades. However, treatments that modify existing symptoms and accelerate the rate of recovery from relapse are often used in the management of individual patients.

The treatment of acute relapse

Since the natural history of relapse is for spontaneous recovery, treatment is not required for every exacerbation. Corticosteroids shorten the duration of relapse and have few complications, even when multiple courses have been administered. They abbreviate acute episodes in multiple sclerosis. For many years, neurologists have used high-dose intravenous methyl prednisolone but a comparison of oral [daily over 3 weeks (costing £2.80)] and intravenous methylprednisolone (1 g daily for three days by slow infusion in dextrose) showed equivalence and many now use an oral regimen on the basis of cost-effectiveness.

The treatment of symptoms

Many manifestations of multiple sclerosis can be improved symptomatically. Patients with urinary symptoms due to involvement of the spinal cord often achieve reasonable bladder emptying by abdominal pressure or perineal stimulation, and tolerate mild incontinence; urgency or frequency respond well to drugs that include anticholinergic activity (oxybutynin or propantheline), but when detrusor and sphincter function become uncoupled, causing impaired bladder emptying with failure to fill, the preferred treatment is clean intermittent self catheterization, which is easily adopted by motivated patients with adequate vision and arm function, and ensures complete bladder emptying, often with unimagined advantages to social activities and sleep. Permanent use of a catheter is preferable to dribbling incontinence, with its attendant risks of skin excoriation. Constipation should be managed by dietary alteration and the use of bulk laxatives, avoiding agents that act directly on the bowel wall.

Sexual function is frequently impaired in males with spinal demyelination. Potency can be restored by pharmacological treatments including yomhibine (an α_2-agonist), self-administered cavernous injection of papaverine, and prostaglandin E_1 or phentolamine, which can be applied through the urethra. Sildenafil (Viagra), a phosphodiesterase inhibitor that acts by increasing local production of nitric oxide in response to sexual stimulation, offers an easier method for restoring potency in males including those with demyelination of the spinal cord. More complicated techniques for stimulating ejaculation can be used to ensure fertility in impotent males who wish to have children.

Weakness and spasticity contribute differentially to immobility in patients with multiple sclerosis, depending on which spinal pathways are most affected. The relief of spasticity can aggravate weakness and paradoxically reduce mobility, since patients may depend on increased muscle tone in order to stand. High-dose intravenous methylprednisolone, baclofen, dantrolene sodium, or tizanidine each have some effect on spasticity: they are indicated in individuals with preserved muscle strength, or those with painful spasms who no longer attempt to stand or walk; these agents can be used in combination since many act at different sites involved in the maintenance of muscle tone. Spasticity can be relieved by intrathecal baclofen, using a delivery pump, local injection of botulinum toxin, or, ultimately, by surgical interruption of the reflex pathways or tenotomy, but these techniques must be regarded as irreversible.

The paroxysmal manifestations of multiple sclerosis are usually very responsive to treatment; tonic brainstem seizures stop abruptly with the use of carbamazepine or other anticonvulsants that increase membrane stability, and these also help in patients with trigeminal neuralgia and more refractory forms of pain due to spinal demyelination. These unpleasant sensations are influenced by alterations in mood and respond to antidepressants.

Influencing the course of multiple sclerosis

Attempts to influence the course of multiple sclerosis are based on the logic that tissue injury is immunologically mediated. Non-specific immune stimulation with interferon-γ is known to increase disease activity. Immune suppression stabilizes the clinical course in rapidly progressive multiple sclerosis, but adverse effects are common, the benefits are rarely maintained, and are of a magnitude that is not necessarily useful for the individual patient. A meta-analysis of trials using azathioprine confirms the statistically significant but individually limited role of this well-tolerated immunosuppressive agent.

The main therapeutic development in multiple sclerosis has been introduction of the β-interferons. Most would now accept that Betaferon™, Avonex™, and Rebif™ reduce the relapse rate by around 30 per cent and achieve an even more substantial reduction in the accumulation of new lesions. Betaferon™ may also delay progression in patients with secondary progressive multiple sclerosis whether or not they continue to have superimposed relapses. Whether there are useful differences in efficacy or immunogenicity between the three products, dose–response effects, and additive effects of other immunological agents remains to be resolved. The main adverse effects of interferon-β are flu-like symptoms, pyrexia, and injection-site reactions; the long-term adverse effects are still not known, although anecdotal reports of autoimmunity are starting to appear. Up to 45 per cent of patients on high-dose interferon-β_{1b} (Betaferon™) develop neutralizing activity; this usually occurs in the first year. The reported rate is lower in a secondary progressive study (28 per cent) and with the two interferon-β_{1a} products (Avonex™ and Rebif™). Antibodies to interferon-β_{1a} and -β_{1b} are immunologically and biologically cross-reactive.

Pulsed treatment with the humanized monoclonal antilymphocyte antibody (CAMPATH-1H) suppresses disease activity for at least 18 months but does not inhibit progression from deficits acquired prior to treatment; these can be explained by brain atrophy due to axon degeneration, which is conditioned by the amount of initial inflammation.

Central pontine myelinolysis (see also Chapter 12.2)

Central pontine myelinolysis is not rare. A high proportion of cases first described had metabolic disturbances resulting from alcohol abuse, but the condition occurs in association with Wernicke's encephalopathy, non-alcoholic cirrhosis, Wilson's disease, after hepatic transplantation, as a complication of uraemia and haemodialysis, after prolonged vomiting, and following diuretic therapy. In each of these situations, affected individuals are usually hyponatraemic before the onset of neurological symptoms. This observation has led to the hypothesis that central pontine myelinolysis results from over zealous correction of a low serum sodium. Pontine damage correlates both with the degree of hyponatraemia and the rate at which this is corrected: starting concentrations of less than 110 mmol/l or rates of correction of greater than 2 mmol/l/h substantially increase the risk of central pontine myelinolysis. Rapid changes in sodium are better tolerated in acute than chronic hyponatraemia; pontine myelinolysis is occasionally seen as a result of rapidly corrected hypernatraemia.

The illness affects pathways placed centrally within the pons and spreads centrifugally. The fully evolved clinical picture is of flaccid paralysis with facial and bulbar weakness, disordered eye movements, loss of balance, and altered consciousness.

Further reading

Compston, D.A.S., Ebers, G.C., Lassmann, H., *et al.* (1998). *McAlpine's multiple sclerosis.* Churchill Livingstone, London.

European Study Group on Interferon β-1b in Secondary Progressive MS (1998). Placebo-controlled multicentre randomised trial of interferon β-1b in treatment of secondary progressive multiple sclerosis. *Lancet*, **352**, 1491–7.

IFNB Multiple Sclerosis Study Group and the University of British Columbia MS/MRI Analysis Group (1995). Interferon beta-1b in the treatment of multiple sclerosis: final outcome of the randomised controlled trial. *Neurology*, **45**, 1277–85.

Jacobs, L.D., Cookfair, D., Rudick, R.A. *et al.* (1996). Intramuscular interferon beta-1a for disease progression in relapsing multiple sclerosis. *Annals of Neurology*, **39**, 285–94.

PRISMS Study Group (1998). Randomised double-blind placebo-controlled study of interferon β-1a in relapsing/remitting multiple sclerosis. *Lancet*, **352**, 1498–504.

Chapter 13.20

Movement disorders

C. D. Marsden

Diseases of the extrapyramidal motor systems cause either a loss of movement (akinesia) accompanied by an increase in muscle tone (rigidity), or abnormal involuntary movements (dyskinesias) often accompanied by a reduction in muscle tone. The akinetic–rigid syndrome, called parkinsonism, and the dyskinesias represent opposite ends of the spectrum of movement disorders.

Akinetic–rigid syndromes

Parkinson's disease

Definition

A disease with insidious onset, usually in the second half of life, characterized by slowly progressive akinesia, rigidity, postural abnormality, and tremor. The symptoms of Parkinson's disease have now been established as due to striatal dopamine deficiency consequent to death of the substantia nigra. The pathology in the substantia nigra consists of loss of pigmented neurones in the zona compacta, with eosinophilic inclusions, called Lewy bodies, in remaining neurones.

Aetiology

The cause of Parkinson's disease is unknown. A similar akinetic–rigid syndrome with characteristic tremor was a common aftermath of the worldwide epidemic of encephalitis lethargica that occurred 60 years ago (1918–1930) (postencephalitic parkinsonism). Neuroleptic drugs (such as reserpine, phenothiazines, and butyrophenones) also may produce the same clinical picture (drug-induced parkinsonism) by blockade of striatal dopamine receptors.

Parkinsonism may also be the main feature of a number of other degenerative diseases of the central nervous system, but other abnormalities point to the diagnosis of these various syndromes of 'parkinsonism-plus' (Table 1): they include progressive supranuclear palsy, multiple-system atrophy, and corticobasal degeneration, which are discussed later.

Parkinson's disease is a common disorder with a prevalence of about 1 in 1000, rising to 1 in 200 in elderly people. It occurs worldwide in all ethnic groups (although perhaps less frequently in

It is with regret that we report the death of Professor C. D. Marsden.

Table 1 Causes of akinetic–rigid syndrome in adults

Pure parkinsonism	Parkinsonism-plus
Parkinson's disease	Progressive supranuclear palsy
Drug-induced parkinsonism	Multiple system atrophy, olivopontocerebellar degeneration, striatonigral degeneration, autonomic failure
Postencephalitic parkinsonism	Corticobasal degeneration
MPTP toxicity	Parkinsonism-dementia-ALS syndrome (Guam)
Other toxins (e.g. manganese carbon monoxide)	Basal ganglia calcification

Abbreviations: ALS, amyotrophic lateral sclerosis; MPTP, 1-methyl-4-phenyl-1,2,3, 6-tetrahydropyridine.

China and Africa), in all social classes, and is slightly more common in men than in women. Hereditary factors are not evident in the majority of cases, but about 5 to 10 per cent of patients give a history of the same illness in other family members. Evidence of dominant inheritance occurs in some rare families, and the genetic data have been taken to suggest the influence of a dominant gene with poor penetrance. However, recent studies of identical twins have failed to find high concordance when one twin is affected with Parkinson's disease, which suggests that heredity alone is not responsible for the condition.

Extensive studies have failed to identify any viral agent responsible for Parkinson's disease. Toxins can cause human parkinsonism. Certain drug addicts in California, in the course of synthesizing a heroin substitute, meperidine, inadvertently produced a contaminant, 1-methyl-4-phenyl-1,2,3,6-tetrahydropyridine (MPTP). Within a few days of intravenous injection of this compound, they developed acute severe parkinsonism, similar in nearly all respects to the idiopathic disease. This event has led to an intensive search for similar environmental toxins, but none has been identified as yet.

Pathology

Anatomical

The essential pathological abnormality is loss of pigmented neurones in the pars compacta of the substantia nigra. These neurones, which contain neuromelanin, project to the caudate nucleus and putamen (neostriatum), and employ dopamine as their neurotransmitter.

In all cases of Parkinson's disease the degenerating pigmented brainstem neurones contain eosinophilic inclusion bodies, Lewy bodies, which are characteristic of the disease. Lewy bodies are found also in about 4 per cent of brains from patients without parkinsonism dying of other causes; these may be patients with subclinical Parkinson's disease, for 80 per cent of the zona compacta must degenerate before clinical symptoms appear. Lewy bodies are found not only in pigmented neurones, but also in other areas, including the cerebral cortex. Their origin is unexplained.

Biochemical

There is profound loss of dopamine in the striatum (putamen more than caudate) and substantia nigra of patients dying with Parkinson's disease. Loss of dopamine in the caudate nucleus and putamen correlates with the extensive cell loss, atrophy, and glial scarring in the substantia nigra. It is necessary to lose something of the order of 50 to 60 per cent of nigral neurones, and to deplete the striatum of about 80 to 85 per cent of its dopamine content, for frank symptoms of Parkinson's disease to appear.

Symptoms

The onset is insidious and in 70 per cent of patients the presenting feature is tremor, which usually commences unilaterally. Parkinsonian tremor is present at rest, is decreased by action, is increased by emotion or stress, and disappears during sleep. The arms are most often affected initially, but tremor may spread to involve the face, jaw, and legs. It is due to rhythmical alternating contraction in opposing muscles at a frequency of 4 to 6 Hz. In the arm it characteristically causes rhythmic pronation/supination and 'pill rolling' of the opposed thumb and fingers. Occasionally, tremor may be more evident on posture and movement. Rigidity is appreciated by the patient as stiff muscles, and by the examiner as a plastic resistance to passive movement, equal in opposing muscle groups and constant throughout the range of manipulation. Rigidity affects all muscles, but is most marked in the neck and trunk, and in proximal muscles at the shoulder or hip. When tremor coexists the smooth, plastic nature of rigidity may be broken up by rhythmic catches (cogwheel phenomenon). Akinesia refers to the poverty (hypokinesia) and slowness (bradykinesia) of movement so characteristic of Parkinson's disease. There is a delay in initiation of movement, a slowness in execution of voluntary movement, and a loss of normal automatic movements, such as those of emotional expression and blinking. Postural changes include generalized flexion of the limbs, neck, and trunk, and postural instability causing falls.

These four cardinal signs of Parkinson's disease—tremor, rigidity, akinesia, and postural changes—contribute to the many typical features and disabilities of the illness. The face is strikingly bland and mask-like. The voice loses volume and normal modulation of tone to become soft and monotonous. The bent, flexed patient walks with slow, small steps, without swinging their arms; it may be difficult to start walking ('freezing'), but once in motion the pace may quicken and the patient may be unable to stop ('festination'). They may 'freeze' into immobility when passing through a door or around furniture. While standing, a push may lead to falling or tottering in the direction of displacement until the patient falls, or comes into contact with a solid object. They sit immobile and flexed like a statue. Getting out of a chair and turning over in bed may be impossible. The handwriting becomes small (micrographia), tremulous, and untidy (Fig. 1). Rapid movements of the hands and feet are impaired. Eating, washing, and toilet demands become increasingly difficult.

While objective sensibility is unimpaired, patients often complain of fatigue, pain, and discomfort, and of hot or cold sensations. Vision, hearing, taste, and smell are normal. Eye movements are unaffected, except for paralysis of convergence, some limitation of up-gaze, and loss of speed of voluntary saccades. The pupils are normal. The eyelids may be tremulous (blepharoclonus) and spasms of eye closure (blepharospasm) may occur. Drooling of saliva is common, due to failure to swallow, and dysphagia may occur. Constipation is universal; urinary frequency and urgency are frequent complaints. Excessive sweating and a greasy skin (seborrhoea) contribute to the facial appearance. Some patients develop postural hypotension. The tendon reflexes and plantar responses are normal.

Most patients have normal intellectual function initially, although some defects of cognitive abilities attributable to frontal-lobe functions may be detectable; slowness of thought processes (bradyphrenia), and slight difficulties with memory and word retrieval ('tip of the tongue'

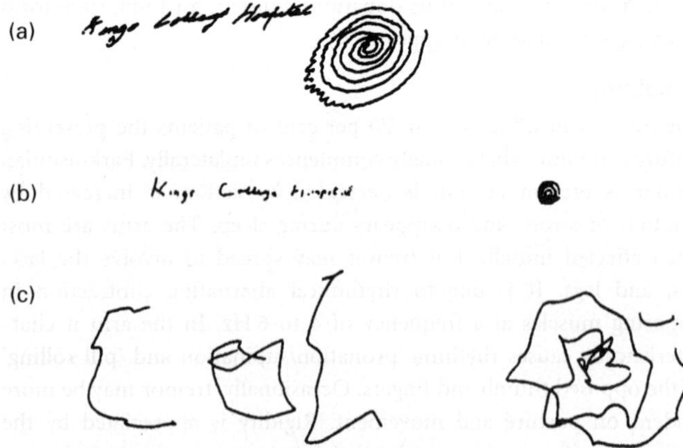

Fig. 1 Samples of handwriting and spiral drawings from (a) a 50-year-old woman with benign essential tremor, (b) a 38-year-old man with Parkinson's disease, and (c) a 20-year-old boy with torsion dystonia (who attempts to write COLLEGE).

phenomenon) may be evident. Subsequent drug therapy may provoke mental disturbances and, with the passage of time and progression of the disease, a proportion of patients develop organic mental changes. Depression is very common, affecting 30 per cent or more, and often antedating the appearance of obvious physical symptoms. The most common mental consequence of drug therapy is a toxic confusional state, but other behavioural disturbances, such as a schizophreniform psychosis or isolated hallucinosis with insight, can occur. Many patients complain of more severe slowness of thought and defects of memory in the later stages of the illness, and a proportion (perhaps 20 per cent) finally develop a frank global dementia. The latter may be due to the coexistence of Alzheimer's disease in this elderly population, or to diffuse Lewy-body disease. The appearance of dementia in a patient with Parkinson's disease warrants full investigation to exclude other treatable causes.

Natural history

The mean age of onset of Parkinson's disease is about 55 years. Onset under 40 years is rare, but thereafter the incidence rises exponentially with increasing age. Most patients localize the onset of symptoms to one or other side, but progression to bilateral signs and disability is the rule. In most patients the disease progresses inexorably, with increasing difficulty in speaking, eating, washing, dressing, standing, and walking. Eventually, in those most severely affected, the patient becomes chair- or bed-bound and anarthric. Many patients, however, remain reasonably active, but with increasing restrictions, until they die from other causes. The rate of progression is very variable. Prior to the advent of levodopa therapy, death occurred on average about 9 years after the onset of symptoms; the range varied from benign parkinsonism with little or no progression over 30 years or more, to malignant parkinsonism with death in 1 or 2 years from onset. Mortality was some three times that expected in a general population of the same age and sex. Death was usually from vascular diseases, bronchopneumonia, or intercurrent neoplasia. Older treatments did not influence the prognosis of idiopathic Parkinson's disease, but it is likely that levodopa therapy has prolonged life expectancy. Indeed, a number of studies have now shown that with present-day treatment the patient with Parkinson's disease is likely, on average, to live as long as unaffected people of the same age.

Diagnosis

The combination of tremor, rigidity, akinesia, and postural abnormality constitutes the syndrome of parkinsonism. A history of intake of neuroleptic drugs indicates drug-induced parkinsonism, which remits in 95 per cent of cases slowly over weeks or months when the offending drug is withdrawn. Drugs that may cause parkinsonism include not only the antipsychotic neuroleptic agents used to treat schizophrenia, but also antiemetics such as phenothiazines and metoclopramide, and some calcium-blocking agents. All these drugs are dopamine-receptor antagonists.

A number of other degenerative diseases affecting the basal ganglia may produce a parkinsonian syndrome, but other distinctive features give the clue to the true diagnosis. In general, these conditions show little or no response to treatment with levodopa or dopamine agonists. A gaze palsy for voluntary and following eye movements, particularly when down-gaze is affected, with preserved vestibulo-ocular reflex eye movements, indicates progressive supranuclear palsy. A cerebellar ataxia or cerebellar atrophy on CT scan, and orthostatic hypotension with other features of an autonomic neuropathy, point to multiple-system atrophy. Severe rigidity of a limb, with apraxia and myoclonus, suggests corticobasal degeneration.

The presence of frank dementia and pyramidal signs indicates a widespread disease such as diffuse Lewy-body disease, Alzheimer's disease, or cerebrovascular disease such as multi-infarct dementia. The last most commonly occurs in long-standing sufferers of poorly controlled hypertension and often is characterized by the additional presence of a pseudobulbar palsy with emotional incontinence and a distinctive gait that is upright, short-stepped, and military (*marche à petit pas*).

Parkinson's disease is the diagnosis when the syndrome appears in middle or late life without other evidence of neurological damage, and in the absence of any history of provoking drugs or encephalitis lethargica.

The condition of benign essential tremor is commonly mistaken for Parkinson's disease. However, in benign essential tremor, which is often inherited, the tremor is postural and other signs of parkinsonism are absent, for there is no true rigidity or akinesia.

Depression may pose diagnostic problems. Patients with profound psychomotor retardation due to severe depression often exhibit a superficial resemblance to those with Parkinson's disease, particularly with their sad, expressionless face, bowed posture, and immobility. Many patients with the earliest symptoms of Parkinson's disease are misdiagnosed as depressed, which indeed they may well be.

Treatment

The treatment of Parkinson's disease involves the use of drugs, physical therapy, and occasionally surgery.

Drug treatment

Until 1967, when oral levodopa was introduced, treatment was with anticholinergic drugs and stereotaxic surgery. Levodopa is now the best therapy available, and stereotaxic surgery is only rarely indicated. Levodopa is converted into dopamine in the brain by the enzyme dopa decarboxylase, thereby restoring striatal dopamine action. Less than 5 per cent of an oral dose of levodopa reaches the brain; the rest is metabolized by dopa decarboxylase in gut wall, liver, kidney, and cerebral capillaries. This peripheral decarboxylation can be prevented by the addition of a selective extracerebral decarboxylase inhibitor, such as carbidopa or benserazide, which themselves do not penetrate into the brain. Levodopa combined with carbidopa

(Sinemet) or benserazide (Madopar) is now the treatment of choice when levodopa is indicated. Such combined therapy requires a lower dose of levodopa for optimal benefit, and results in a quicker therapeutic response and a lower incidence of those side-effects that are due to the formation of levodopa metabolites outside the brain; these include nausea and vomiting, cardiac dysrhythmias, and, at least in part, postural hypotension. The main side-effects of combined therapy are dyskinesias and psychiatric disturbances. Both are dose-dependent and remit when the drug dosage is reduced.

Initiation Sinemet or Madopar, which appear similar in potency and side-effects, do not affect the underlying pathology or cause of Parkinson's disease; they are equivalent to a substitution therapy for striatal dopamine deficiency. It is not necessary to use such drugs in every patient on diagnosis. Either drug is indicated if disability is severe, or if it fails to respond to simple therapy. In the mild case, the monoamine oxidase B inhibitor selegiline (Eldepryl), 5 mg twice daily, has been shown to delay the need for levodopa.

An anticholinergic such as benzhexol, 2 or 5 mg tablets or orphenadrine, 50 mg tablets, three to eight times daily, may be beneficial initially. Anticholinergics cause peripheral parasympathetic blockade with a dry mouth, blurred vision, and constipation. They may also precipitate glaucoma and urinary retention, and a toxic confusional state, so generally should be avoided in elderly people. Small doses should be used initially and gradually increased. Alternatively, in a mild case, amantadine hydrochloride, 100 mg twice or three times daily, may be effective. Amantadine, originally introduced as an antiviral agent, is slightly more powerful than anticholinergics, but less effective than levodopa. However, it causes few side-effects, mainly ankle oedema and the skin rash, livedo reticularis. In high dosage it can provoke a toxic confusional state or fits.

If disability warrants levodopa therapy, Sinemet or Madopar should be started in small dosage and gradually increased over a period of weeks to the maximum tolerated, or until adequate therapeutic benefit has been obtained. Nausea and vomiting are less common with these combined preparations than with plain levodopa, and if vomiting occurs it can usually be prevented by taking the drug after meals, prefaced by an antiemetic such as domperidone. The most common dose-limiting side-effects are dyskinesias and mental disturbances and the aim should be to keep the patient free of these complications. The usual starting dose of Sinemet (each tablet of Sinemet-275 contains 250 mg levodopa and 25 mg carbidopa) is half a tablet twice or three times daily. The average optimum dose is three to four tablets daily. Elderly individuals are particularly sensitive to levodopa, and Sinemet-110 (containing 100 mg levodopa and 10 mg carbidopa) may be used. Sinemet-plus (containing 100 mg levodopa and 25 mg carbidopa) has also been introduced to provide adequate carbidopa intake for those on low doses of levodopa. For Madopar the starting dose is one Madopar-125 capsule (which contains 100 mg levodopa and 25 mg benserazide) twice or three times daily. The average optimum dose is two to four capsules daily of Madopar-250 (which contains 200 mg levodopa and 50 mg benserazide). Maximum dosage of Sinemet-275 is about six to eight tablets daily, and of Madopar-250 about five to eight capsules daily, but some patients require even more than this. Other formulations of Sinemet and Madopar include Sinemet LS (containing 50 mg of levodopa and 12.5 mg of carbidopa) and Madopar-62.5 (containing 50 mg of levodopa and 12.5 mg of benserazide), which may be useful in those who are very sensitive to these drugs. Recently, longer-acting delayed-release formulations of both drugs have been introduced (Sinemet CR and Madopar CR), which may prove valuable.

Maintenance The response to levodopa therapy usually is obvious. In those who do respond, approximately two-thirds will experience some loss of benefit after 2 to 5 years of treatment. Those patients who deteriorate while on long-term levodopa therapy do so in one of two ways. Some experience a progressive recurrence of their parkinsonian disability, particularly akinesia and postural instability with freezing and falls. Such patients usually are elderly and frequently show signs of dementia as well. Such a progressive loss of benefit and deterioration is very difficult to reverse. Increasing the daily dose of levodopa often causes toxic confusional states without the added benefit. A few such patients may gain renewed relief by switching to a directly acting dopamine agonist such as bromocriptine (see below), but mental side-effects are common with these drugs.

Other patients on long-term levodopa therapy, particularly the younger individuals, develop fluctuations in mobility throughout the day associated with the appearance of levodopa-induced dyskinesias. Such fluctuations initially take the form of end-of-dose deterioration or the 'wearing-off' effect. When levodopa is first started, each dose usually lasts for a matter of 4 h or so. With the passage of years, the duration of action of each dose of the drug shortens to as little as 1 or 2 h. On the usual three or four times daily regimen, this means that patients begin to experience a recurrence of disability, particularly immobility, before the next dose. At this stage, the correct management is to take an adequate dose of levodopa at more frequent intervals. Such patients may require to take levodopa every 2 h or so, or may benefit from the longer-acting forms of Sinemet CR and Madopar CR.

Unfortunately, many of those with end-of-dose deterioration cannot be controlled adequately by such dose adjustments, or go on to develop other types of fluctuation in response. Typically, levodopa-induced dyskinesias become more severe, either at the peak time of levodopa action or biphasically before, and at the end of action of, each dose. In addition, the swings from mobility (with dyskinesias) to immobility (with distress, and sometimes tremor and rigidity) become more frequent and abrupt, hence the description of this problem as the 'on–off' effect, for it can be like switching a light on and off. Such swings also become increasingly unpredictable and variable, quite unrelated to the timing of levodopa dosage, so that the patient may 'yo-yo' from mobility to immobility many times a day.

The management of severe 'on–off' problems, which usually occur in the younger patient with preserved intellect, is exceedingly difficult. Once stabilized on optimum timing of levodopa dosage, consideration should be given to adding a directly acting dopamine agonist such as bromocriptine (Parlodel).

Unfortunately, some patients who develop severe 'on–off' phenomena during chronic levodopa therapy eventually become resistant to all conventional forms of treatment. Such patients may benefit from the use of apomorphine injections to rescue them from severe 'off' periods, or continuous apomorphine infusions subcutaneously to maintain mobility.

Surgery

In the 1950s and early 1960s, stereotaxic surgery was employed widely to treat Parkinson's disease. The initial target was the globus pallidus, but subsequent experience showed that the most favourable site was in the ventrolateral nucleus of the thalamus. A small lesion at that site was created mechanically, electrolytically, or thermally. Such a stereotaxic thalamotomy could abolish rigidity and tremor in the opposite limbs, but unfortunately did not relieve the disabling akinesia and postural instability. Both were found subsequently to respond to levodopa, at least initially, so by the early 1970s most centres were doing few or no stereotaxic operations for Parkinson's disease. Today, the operation is reserved for the uncommon patient with early Parkinson's disease, whose tremor is severe, resistant to drug therapy, and so disabling as to prevent work. However, new surgical techniques, such as continuous thalamic stimulation, are being reconsidered.

Physical therapy and aids

Parkinson's disease produces a wide range of functional locomotor disabilities, many of which can be helped by sensible aids. An initial assessment by the physiotherapist and occupational therapist will identify each individual patient's particular problems. Special training can then be given to help eating, washing, dressing, and walking. Advice on shoes ('slip-on' with sliding soles, not rubber), the use of Velcro rather than zips, feeding utensils with built-up handles, and other aids are invaluable. A visit to the patient's home will allow assessment of the need for structural alterations such as hand rails in the bathroom and lavatory, raising the toilet seat, removal of door sills, provision of high chairs (patients with Parkinson's disease find great difficulty in getting out of the usual low, soft chair or sofa), removal of scatter rugs that slip, and provision of rubber mats.

Management of specific problems

Psychiatric illness

Toxic confusional states are common in Parkinson's disease, and may be due to drug overdosage or intercurrent acute illness, such as infection with fever. In practice, if no obvious other condition is apparent, it is wise to assume that drugs are the cause, for any of those employed to treat Parkinson's disease may provoke delirium. For reasons that are not clear, it may take some days or even weeks for such a patient to regain mental clarity. Some never do, and it is apparent that this acute toxic confusional state was superimposed upon an underlying dementia, which should be investigated in its own right.

Psychotic behaviour, disrupting home life or ward routine, is common in such patients. Conventional neuroleptic drugs are best avoided in Parkinson's disease, because they antagonize dopamine action, but they may have to be used. In fact, the noisy disruptive parkinsonian may be calmed without deterioration in their mobility by a judiciously chosen dose of thioridazine (Melleril) or other neuroleptic. Such drugs also may be of value for night sedation of those with reversed sleep rhythm.

Depression has been noted as very common in Parkinson's disease, often demanding treatment. Conventional monoamine oxidase inhibitors are quite contraindicated for they interact with levodopa to cause severe hypertension. However, tricyclics such as amitriptyline (Tryptizol) can be used in the usual way, and their anticholinergic properties may add a little antiparkinsonian action.

Drug interaction

Patients with Parkinson's disease often require other drugs to control other illnesses. No interactions between antiparkinsonian drugs and the following have been noted: anticoagulants, benzodiazepines, tricyclic antidepressants, digoxin, diuretics, trinitrin, propranolol, antiarrhythmic drugs, antibiotics, thyroxine, and hypoglycaemic agents.

Diabetic control is not altered usually. Antihypertensive therapy with α-methyldopa (Aldomet) leads to an increase in levodopa-induced side-effects, for α-methyldopa inhibits dopa decarboxylase. Propranolol or other β-adrenergic antagonists probably are the drugs of choice to treat hypertension for they also slightly benefit parkinsonian tremor.

Levodopa should never be given with a conventional monoamine oxidase inhibitor, and the directly acting sympathomimetic amines contained in bronchodilators and some cold remedies are best avoided due to the risks of paroxysmal hypertension.

Surgery

Patients with Parkinson's disease may require surgery for other illnesses, but the need should always be balanced against the risks. Some patients deteriorate severely after anaesthesia and enforced bed rest, and may never make up the lost ground. If surgery is essential, then levodopa therapy should be continued up to the night of the operation. The morning dose is omitted, but treatment is restarted as soon as the patient can swallow. In those with prolonged postoperative difficulties, levodopa can be given via a nasogastric tube, or apomorphine by injection.

Other akinetic–rigid syndromes in adults

Progressive supranuclear palsy

This syndrome has similarities to parkinsonism, but with an additional characteristic and diagnostic abnormality of voluntary eye movement. The illness is progressive and is characterized by akinesia, axial rigidity, postural imbalance, dysarthria, a supranuclear paralysis of voluntary vertical eye movements, and mental changes, with onset in middle or late life. The cause is not known. It is a rare sporadic disease. Males are affected more than females, and no familial cases have been described. There is widespread neuronal loss and gliosis in the brainstem, affecting particularly the globus pallidus, substantia nigra, subthalamus, red nucleus, tectum and periaqueductal grey matter, and dentate nucleus. Such affected nerve cells contain neurofibrillary tangles. The cerebral cortex, however, is unaffected and senile plaques do not occur.

The illness most commonly presents either with imbalance or visual symptoms. The latter consist of difficulty with reading or coming down stairs, because both demand voluntary downward gaze, and vertical gaze characteristically is impaired. The patient cannot voluntarily look up and down, nor follow an object moved in the vertical plane. But a full range of vertical eye movements can be elicited reflexly by rapid posturing of the head (the doll's eye manoeuvre). Horizontal eye movement is similarly affected, but usually later than vertical eye movement.

Unexplained falls are a common early complaint. At this stage the patient also will exhibit characteristic axial rigidity of neck, trunk, and proximal limb muscles, and poverty of movement, particularly of whole-body movement. Speech is dysarthric, as in a pseudobulbar palsy, and swallowing may be impaired. Power is preserved, as is sensation; the tendon reflexes are brisk and the plantar responses may be extensor. The disease is relentlessly progressive, the patient becoming bedridden and anarthric, leading to death in 5 to 7 years.

The crucial diagnostic feature is the supranuclear gaze palsy. However, eye movements may also be abnormal in patients with other types of parkinsonism. Progressive supranuclear palsy is diagnosed with confidence only when down-gaze is affected, but this may occur late in the illness.

There is no effective treatment for this condition, although levodopa or other dopamine agonists are worth trying.

Multiple-system atrophy (see also Chapter 13.7)

Definition

Three separate conditions are included in this category: cerebellar ataxia due to olivopontocerebellar degeneration, parkinsonism due to striatonigral degeneration, and autonomic failure overlap. The cause of this disease, which may account for 10 per cent of those with parkinsonism, is unknown. Nearly all cases are sporadic. Both sexes are affected and symptoms usually begin in middle age.

The most striking abnormality to the naked eye in olivopontocerebellar degeneration is gross shrinkage of the pons and middle cerebellar peduncles due to loss of pontine nuclei and of their transverse fibres.

In striatonigral degeneration there is gliosis and extensive loss of neurones in the caudate, and especially in the putamen, and in the substantia nigra.

In autonomic failure there is widespread neuronal loss in caudate nucleus, substantia nigra, locus coeruleus, inferior olives, Purkinje cells, dorsal vagal nucleus, Onuf's nucleus, and intermediolateral column of the thoracic cord, the last being held responsible for the sympathetic failure.

Clinical features

Olivopontocerebellar degeneration presents as a progressive cerebellar ataxia of gait and arms, accompanied by dysarthria and, often, nystagmus. In addition, there may be pyramidal signs, akinesia, and rigidity.

Striatonigral degeneration presents as a parkinsonian syndrome indistinguishable from that of Parkinson's disease, although cerebellar atrophy may be evident on CT or MRI brain scans.

Autonomic failure presents as postural hypotension, urinary incontinence, loss of sweating, sexual impotence, akinesia and rigidity, and sometimes tremor and severe dysarthria. Serious respiratory stridor and sleep apnoea may develop.

With time and progression of the disease, patients become increasingly disabled by an akinetic–rigid syndrome with profound postural imbalance, and by severe postural hypotension and urinary incontinence. The intellect is usually spared. Death occurs within some 10 years.

Diagnosis

Multiple-system atrophy may be confused with any of the other causes of a progressive cerebellar syndrome, including cerebellar tumour, other spinocerebellar degenerations, multiple sclerosis, and the cerebellar ataxia that may be associated with myxoedema, a remote neoplasm, or alcoholism.

Striatonigral degeneration is usually misdiagnosed as Parkinson's disease, but does not respond to treatment.

Orthostatic hypotension may be due to drugs, diabetes, or other causes of an autonomic neuropathy, including amyloid and Parkinson's disease due to Lewy-body degeneration.

Treatment

There is no effective therapy for multiple-system atrophy. The akinetic–rigid parkinsonian features do not usually respond to levodopa or anticholinergic drugs as well as they do in Parkinson's disease but amantadine may be of benefit.

Corticobasal degeneration

This condition, which occurs sporadically in middle or late life, has only been recognized recently. It is characterized pathologically by atrophy of the frontal and parietal cortex, and of the striatum, globus pallidus, subthalamus, substantia nigra, and other brainstem nuclei. The cause is unknown.

The onset is insidious and the course progressive. Common early features are clumsiness of one limb, usually the arm, due to a mixture of rigidity, akinesia, and apraxia. The affected limb may exhibit uncontrollable wandering (the alien limb), spontaneous and reflex myoclonic jerks, dystonia or a jerky tremor, and sensory loss. This motor deficit spreads to involve other limbs, balance and gait become impaired, speech becomes dysarthric, and a supranuclear palsy of gaze appears. Frontal release and pyramidal signs are common. The intellect and language usually remain intact until the later stages of the illness, which leads to death within some 7 to 10 years. There is no effective treatment.

Cerebral anoxia

Severe cerebral anoxia of whatever cause may cause disproportionate damage to the basal ganglia, leading to bilateral necrosis of the striatum or globus pallidus. While the effects of damage to the cerebral cortex are apparent immediately, those resulting from the destruction of basal ganglia may appear days or up to about a month after the insult, and thereafter, for reasons that are not clear, the syndrome may progress.

After the episode of cerebral anoxia, the patient may recover from the initial coma, only to relapse over the next few weeks into an increasingly severe akinetic–rigid state with profound dysarthria and dysphagia. The arms characteristically are flexed while the legs are extended, all limbs showing dystonic posturing and athetoid movements of the fingers and toes. Progression to death may occur, but the condition can arrest or even improve, and levodopa sometimes helps.

Wilson's disease

This disorder is described in Chapter 6.10. Its neurological manifestations are caused by copper deposition in the brain. The globus pallidus and especially the putamen are strikingly affected, but the cerebral cortex and other basal ganglia structures are also damaged. The liver shows portal cirrhosis.

Symptoms

Wilson's disease presents to neurologists as a behaviour disturbance, an akinetic–rigid syndrome, and with a variety of dyskinesias. Onset is usually in childhood or adolescence, but may be delayed as late as the fifth decade of life. The first symptoms of the disease frequently lead to psychiatric referral with conduct disorders, personality change, or frank psychotic disturbance. Common initial neurological symptoms include tremor of any type, dysarthria and drooling, chorea, dystonic spasms and posturing, or akinesia and rigidity. Without treatment, progression is inevitable, with dementia, increasingly severe dysarthria and dysphagia, and increasing akinesia, rigidity, and dystonia, leading to contractures and immobility. Vision, hearing, and sensation are not affected, and the tendon reflexes and plantar responses are usually normal. Fits may occur in a minority of cases.

A Kayser–Fleischer ring may be seen in the cornea with the naked eye and is always present in those with neurological symptoms when looked for with a slit-lamp (Plate 1, Chapter 6.10). A 'sunflower' cataract, due to copper deposition in the lens, may also be seen.

Table 2 Causes of tremor

Rest tremor	Postural tremor
Parkinson's disease	Physiological tremor
Postencephalitic parkinsonism	Exaggerated physiological tremor, as in:
Drug-induced parkinsonism	Thyrotoxicosis
Other extrapyramidal diseases	Anxiety states
Intention tremor	Alcohol
Brainstem or cerebellar disease, as in:	Drugs (e.g. sympathomimetics, antidepressants, valproic acid, lithium)
Multiple sclerosis	Heavy metal poisoning (i.e. mercury—'hatter's shakes')
Spinocerebellar degenerations	Structural neurological disease, as in:
Vascular disease	Severe cerebellar lesions ('red nucleus tremor')
Tumour	Wilson's disease
	Neurosyphilis
	Peripheral neuropathies
	Benign essential (familial) tremor
	Orthostatic tremor

In some patients with neurological deficit, there may be no clinical evidence of liver damage, although liver function tests will be abnormal.

Investigation

Any child or young adult presenting with any form of dyskinesia or akinetic–rigid syndrome, or with unexplained liver disease, should be investigated to exclude Wilson's disease (see Chapter 6.10). Brain CT or MRI often shows cerebral atrophy and degenerative changes in the basal ganglia.

Treatment

This is described in Chapter 6.10.

The dyskinesias

Most abnormal involuntary movements may be classified into one of five main categories: tremor, chorea, myoclonus, tics, and dystonia. Each type of dyskinesia may be caused by a variety of diseases. In some patients the dyskinesia is accompanied by other neurological deficits or some other clue as to the cause; in others, the involuntary movements occur in isolation and constitute the illness. Nearly all dyskinesias disappear in sleep, are made worse by anxiety and stress, and are improved by relaxation.

Tremor is a rhythmic sinusoidal movement of a body part, due to regular rhythmic muscle contractions. The common causes of tremor are shown in Table 2.

Chorea consists of a continuous flow of irregular, jerky, and explosive movements, that flit from one portion of the body to another in random sequence. Each muscle contraction is brief, often appearing as a fragment of what might have been a normal movement, and quite unpredictable in timing or site. The common causes of chorea are shown in Table 3.

Myoclonus consists of rapid, shock-like muscle jerks, often repetitive and sometimes rhythmic. The common causes of myoclonus are shown in Table 4.

Tics are similar to myoclonic jerks in appearance, but are repetitive, stereotyped movements that can be mimicked voluntarily and can be held in check by an effort of will at the expense of mounting inner tension. Simple tics are confined to a few muscles; complex tics may involve more coordinated quasi-purposeful movements. The common causes of tics are shown in Table 5.

Table 3 Causes of chorea

Sydenham's chorea	Drug-induced chorea
Variants include: chorea gravidarum, chorea caused by contraceptive pill	Neuroleptic drugs
Huntington's disease	Anticonvulsants
Variants include: senile chorea, juvenile chorea, Westphal variant	Contraceptive pill
Benign hereditary chorea	Alcohol
Neuroacanthocytosis	Hemiballism (hemichorea)
Symptomatic chorea	Stroke
Thyrotoxicosis	Tumour
Systemic lupus erythematosus	Trauma
Polycythaemia rubra vera	Post-thalamotomy
Encephalitis lethargica	
Hypernatraemia	
Hypoparathyroidism	
Subdural haematoma	

Dystonia consists of sustained spasms of muscle contraction that distort the limbs and trunk into characteristic dystonic postures—the twisted (torticollis), flexed (antecollis), or extended (retrocollis) neck, the arched (lordosis) or twisted (scoliosis) back, the hyperpronated arm, and plantar-flexed inverted foot. Such dystonic spasms typically occur on willed action (action dystonia). Dystonic spasms may be intermittent, producing dystonic movements, which may be repetitive to give a rhythmic character, or sustained to hold a fixed dystonic posture. The common causes of torsion dystonia are shown in Table 6.

Many of the diseases known to cause these various dyskinesias are discussed elsewhere. However, a number of conditions in which the dyskinesia is the major feature of the illness will be described here.

Tremor

Benign essential (familial) tremor

This is an illness characterized by postural tremor of the arms and head, often inherited as an autosomal-dominant trait, which presents at any age and is usually only slowly progressive, causing mild disability.

The cause is unknown. A positive family history is obtained in over half the patients. No pathological or biochemical abnormality has been identified, but few cases have come to autopsy.

Tremor is present in one or both hands on maintaining a posture, as when holding a cup or glass. Handwriting becomes untidy and tremulous (see Fig. 1). There is no tremor at rest, but a rhythmic oscillation develops when the patient holds the arms outstretched. On movement, as in finger–nose testing, the tremor continues but does not get strikingly worse, as is the case with cerebellar intention tremor. Tremor of the head (titubation) and jaw is present at about 50 per cent of cases, and tremor of the legs occurs in about a third. Despite the tremor, tests of coordination usually are performed normally, walking is unaffected, and there are no other neurological abnormalities.

Two other factors are characteristic of this disorder. First, a family history (see above) and, secondly, the observation that small or moderate doses of alcohol may suppress the tremor. The illness is static or only slowly progressive in most patients, causing predominantly a

Table 4 Causes of myoclonus

Causes of myoclonus
Generalized myoclonus
Progressive myoclonic encephalopathies*
With demonstrable metabolic cause:
Lafora body disease
GM_2 gangliosidosis (Tay–Sachs disease)
Gaucher's disease
Ceroid-lipofuscinosis (Batten's disease)
Sialidosis (cherry-red spot—myoclonus syndrome)
Mitochondrial encephalomyopathy
Hereditary myoclonus with no known metabolic cause:
Familial myoclonic epilepsy (Unverricht–Lundborg disease)
Myoclonus associated with spinocerebellar degenerations
Myoclonus, ataxia, and deafness syndrome
Juvenile neuroaxonal dystrophy
Infantile poliodystrophies (Alpers' disease)
Other sporadic diseases:
Encephalitic lethargica
Subacute sclerosing leucoencephalitis
Creutzfeldt–Jacob disease
Alzheimer's disease
Metabolic myoclonus
Uraemia
Hyponatraemia
Hypocalcaemia
Hepatic failure
CO_2 narcosis
Drug-induced myoclonus
Alcohol and drug withdrawal
Static myoclonic encephalopathies[d]
Infantile perinatal myoclonic encephalopathy
Postanoxic action myoclonus (Lance–Adams syndrome)
Post-traumatic myoclonus
Myoclonic epilepsies[‡]
First year of life
Infantile spasms
Benign infantile myoclonus
'Dancing eyes' syndrome
2 to 6 years
Lennox–Gastaut syndrome
Cryptogenic myoclonic epilepsy (Aicardi)
Other children and adolescents (and adults)
Photosensitive epileptic myoclonus
Myoclonic absences
Juvenile myoclonic epilepsy
Benign essential (familial) myoclonus
Focal myoclonus
Spinal myoclonus
Tumour
Infarct
Demyelination
Trauma
Palatal myoclonus
Hemifacial spasm
Cortical myoclonus
Epilepsia partialis continua

*Obvious myoclonus (with or without seizures) clearly as part of a progressive encephalopathy.

[d] Obvious myoclonus after some acute and now static cerebral insult.

[‡]Obvious epilepsy as the main problem, with myoclonus.

social disability, but individuals whose occupations dependent upon manual skill may be severely disabled.

Table 5 Causes of tics

Simple tics	Symptomatic tics
Transient tic of childhood	Encephalitis lethargica
Chronic simple tic	Drug-induced tics
Multiple tics	Neuroacanthocytosis
Chronic multiple tics	
Gilles de la Tourette syndrome	

Although alcohol may suppress the tremor effectively, and can be of value if used wisely, there is a risk of patients with benign essential tremor becoming alcoholics. Benzodiazepines, such as diazepam, may give some relief at times of stress, but have no major effect on the tremor. A proportion of patients, perhaps 30 to 40 per cent, respond satisfactorily to a β-adrenergic-receptor antagonist such as propranolol. Primidone, in standard anticonvulsant dosages, also helps some patients. Stereotaxic thalamotomy may be required in the very small number of patients whose tremor is so severe that it warrants the risks of such surgery.

Chorea

Sydenham's chorea

Sydenham's chorea is now a rare disease, for the incidence of rheumatic fever has declined dramatically. It affects children and adolescents between the ages of 3 and 20 years, most often in spring months. In about a third of cases it appears up to 3 months after a bout of rheumatic fever due to group A streptococcal infection, but the remainder give no such history. It may recur in adult life, particularly in pregnant women (chorea gravidarum) or in those taking the contraceptive pill. Pathologically the brain shows a diffuse inflammatory encephalitis. Vascular changes are not conspicuous, and the cerebral complications of rheumatic fever may be due to deposition of immune complexes, as in disseminated systemic erythematosus, although this is not proven.

The onset is usually gradual, but may be abrupt. The initial symptoms are often psychological, with irritability, agitation, disobedience, and inattentiveness. A frank organic confusional state occurs in about 10 per cent of patients. Generalized chorea then appears and may get worse for a few weeks, causing difficulty in holding objects and walking. Speech is impaired in about a third of patients, but headaches, fits, and sensory changes are not features of the illness.

The chorea and psychological disturbance slowly recover over 1 to 3 months, rarely up to 6 months, but recurrences occur in about a quarter of patients in the next 2 years. About a third of patients will show evidence of rheumatic cardiac involvement at the time of the illness, and about the same proportion later develop chronic rheumatic heart disease.

The chorea may be controlled with diazepam, a phenothiazine or haloperidol, or tetrabenazine. A course of penicillin should be given, and prophylactic oral penicillin should be continued until about the age of 20 years to prevent further streptococcal infection.

Huntington's disease

This rare, dominantly inherited, relentlessly progressive disease, usually of middle life, is characterized by chorea and dementia. The prevalence of the disease is about 1 in 20 000; it occurs worldwide and in all ethnic groups. The cause is unknown. The autosomal-dominant trait has full penetrance, so that the children of an affected

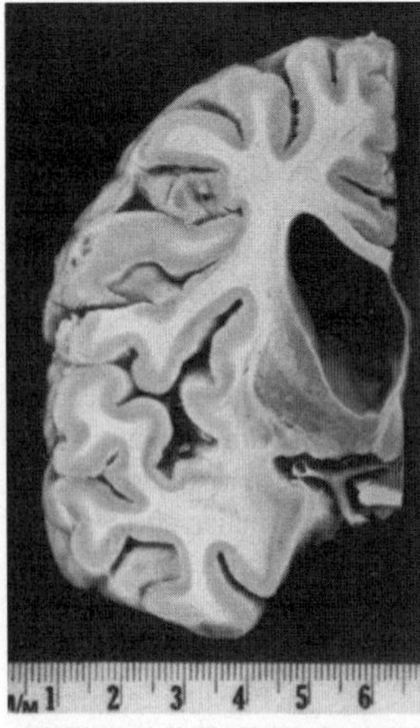
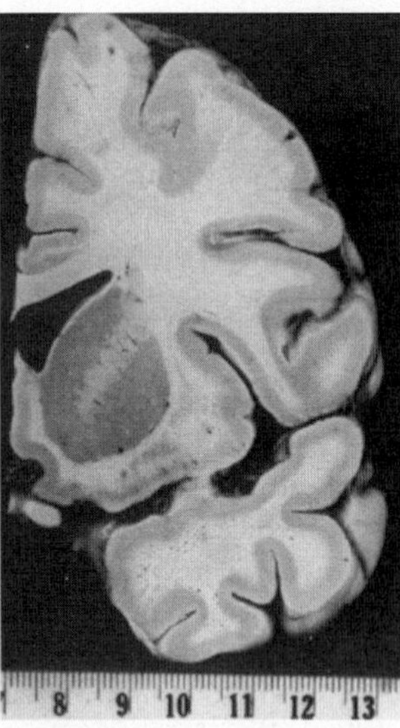

Fig. 2 Coronal section of the brain, on the left, of a patient with Huntington's disease (a woman aged 49 years; brain weight 1065 g) compared, on the right, with a normal brain (a woman aged 69 years; brain weight 1415 g). Note (a) the gross loss of substance in the caudate nucleus and putamen, and (b) the thinning of the cortical mantle and widening of the sulci.
(Reproduced from: Corsellis (1976). In Greenfield's neuropathology, 3rd edn. Arnold, London, with permission.)

parent have a 50 per cent risk of the disease, which never skips a generation. The risk to a grandchild of a sufferer, when the child's parent is free of symptoms, is roughly half the parent's risk. The father is more likely to transmit the disease than the mother in those in whom symptoms begin in childhood. New mutations are almost unknown, but relatives frequently conceal the family history.

Linkage studies have shown the abnormal gene to lie on the short arm of the fourth chromosome.

The characteristic feature on a coronal section of the brain is dilation of the lateral ventricle, whose floor becomes concave rather than convex, due to marked caudate atrophy (Fig. 2); commonly, a degree of cortical atrophy is also evident.

The chorea of Huntington's disease appears to result from relative overactivity of dopamine mechanisms in the brain, perhaps because the intact dopaminergic nigrostriatal pathway is releasing approximately normal quantities of dopamine on to only a few remaining striatal neurones.

Symptoms

The onset is insidious in middle life, usually between the ages of 30 and 50 years. The initial symptoms are frequently those of a change in personality and behaviour, but chorea may be the first sign of the illness. The initial mental disturbances are often subtle: a change in personality, a coarsening of sensitivities, a blunting of drive and depth of feeling, an irritability and truculence, and a tendency to uncontrolled aggressive or sexual behaviour. At this stage the patient often retains distressing insight, fully aware of what is in store. Serious depression is common and suicide is a risk. Erratic behaviour at work or in society may lead to psychiatric referral, or a frank schizophreniform psychosis may develop. As the disease progresses, dementia becomes more pronounced and chorea more severe and grotesque. Walking, speech, and use of the hands become impaired. As the disease progresses, many patients develop increasing rigidity and akinesia, leading to slowing and reduction of the chorea. Finally the patient becomes bed-ridden and emaciated. Death occurs on average about 14 years from the onset.

Diagnosis

The diagnosis is not difficult if the family history is available. Problems arise when no family history is known, or is hidden. In children, Huntington's disease must be differentiated from Sydenham's chorea, from 'juvenile parkinsonism', and athetoid cerebral palsy, and from the many other degenerative conditions affecting the basal ganglia in childhood.

There is another rare form of chorea, known as benign hereditary chorea, which is also inherited as an autosomal-dominant trait. This illness presents in childhood, but without intellectual change, and such patients have only mild disability and show little progression throughout life. Other causes of hereditary chorea include neuroacanthocytosis (see below) and rare degenerations such as dentatorubropallido-Luysian atrophy.

In adults, it is important to exclude thyrotoxicosis, drugs (including neuroleptics and the contraceptive pill), polycythaemia rubra vera, and systemic lupus erythematosus as causes of sporadic chorea. Senile chorea must be differentiated from hemiplegic chorea that may follow stroke.

Treatment

There is no cure for the disease. The chorea may be controlled by a phenothiazine such as chlorpromazine, or perphenazine, or by drugs such as haloperidol, pimozide, flupenthixol, reserpine, or tetrabenazine. Such drugs are administered in increasing dosage until chorea is controlled or drug-induced parkinsonism causes disabling symptoms. Sooner or later, chronic hospital care is required.

Genetic counselling

The spouse or close relative bears the brunt of the patient's anger, frustration, and mental disintegration, and the hereditary nature of the illness raises agonizing issues. Children of a parent with Huntington's disease inevitably have a 1 in 2 risk of developing the illness themselves, and their children have a 1 in 4 risk. Inevitably, those at risk, once aware of the facts, ask whether there is some means of predicting whether they have inherited the disease, and effective diagnostic tests using molecular genetics are now available. Blood DNA samples are required from as many family members as possible. Exclusion testing can also be done *in utero*.

Hemiballism (hemichorea)

Hemiballism refers to wild flinging or throwing movements of one arm and leg. These movements, like those of chorea, are irregular in timing and force, but predominantly involve the large, proximal muscles of the shoulder and pelvic girdle.

The syndrome is usually seen in elderly hypertensive diabetic patients as a result of a stroke. Hemiballism may appear as the hemiplegic weakness improves, when it is often accompanied by thalamic pain. In other patients the hemiballism appears abruptly without weakness or sensory deficit. The intensity of the movements varies from mild to such a severity as to cause injury and to require treatment. Acute hemiballism usually, but not always, is due to a vascular lesion in the contralateral subthalamic nucleus or its connections. Tumour at the same site rarely may produce progressive hemiballism.

Usually, hemiballism due to stroke gradually remits spontaneously over 3 to 6 months. Treatment with a phenothiazine, haloperidol, or tetrabenazine will usually control hemiballism until recovery occurs, but occasionally stereotaxic surgery is required.

Neuroacanthocytosis

This inherited condition (the exact mode of inheritance is uncertain) causes a brain degeneration, with chorea, tics, myoclonus or dystonia and mental change, a peripheral neuropathy, and acanthocytes (without malabsorption or vitamin E deficiency). It can be confused with Huntington's disease and a variety of other movement disorders.

Myoclonus

Unexpected, involuntary muscle jerks may be caused by many neurological diseases (Table 4). Generalized myoclonus occurs in four clinical settings:

(1) as a dominant feature of a progressive brain disease (progressive myoclonic encephalopathy);

(2) as a residual feature of some transient brain insult (static myoclonic encephalopathy);

(3) as a feature of obvious epilepsy (myoclonic epilepsy); or

(4) as the solitary feature of the illness (essential myoclonus).

Myoclonic encephalopathies

Most of the diseases causing a progressive myoclonic encephalopathy are described in detail elsewhere, particularly the lysosomal storage enzyme defects and the spinocerebellar degeneration.

Familial myoclonic epilepsy

This disorder is inherited as an autosomal-recessive trait. Fits and myoclonus commence in childhood, accompanied by slowly progressive ataxia and dysarthria. Spasticity eventually develops and the affected individual eventually becomes chair-bound, but progression is slow and dementia is mild or absent. The myoclonus is strikingly stimulus-sensitive and occurs also on willed movement (action myoclonus). At necropsy the brain shows Purkinje cell loss but no inclusion bodies.

Lafora body disease

This disease, in which the brain at necropsy is found to contain mucopolysaccharide inclusions in nerve cells, also commences with myoclonus and fits in childhood or adolescence, and frequently is familial with autosomal-recessive inheritance. However, there is a progressive dementia, blindness, ataxia, and spasticity so that death occurs within 5 to 10 years of onset. Lafora bodies also are found outside the brain, for example in liver and intestinal mucosa.

Postanoxic action myoclonus

This is a distinct entity that may appear after a period of cerebral anoxia. After recovery of consciousness, such patients exhibit muscle jerks affecting face, trunk, and limbs, often provoked by sensory stimuli, and strikingly elicited by willed voluntary action. A cerebellar ataxia also may be evident, as may dementia, spasticity, and incontinence. Treatment with clonazepam, piracetam, and sodium valproate may be dramatically effective in some cases.

Myoclonic epilepsies

In the myoclonic epilepsies, epileptic seizures are the dominant feature of the illness. There is some confusion in separating the many conditions that may cause this syndrome, which occurs particularly in children. A convenient, if arbitrary, distinction is based on the age of onset.

In the first year of life, infantile spasms (West's syndrome) pose a particular problem. The peculiar seizures characteristic of infantile spasms (*salaam* attacks) commence usually between the ages of 3 and 9 months. Many hereditary, antenatal, and postnatal brain insults may cause infantile spasms, which are associated with mental retardation in over 80 per cent of cases.

Older children, up to the age of about 6 years, may develop an epileptic syndrome of multiple seizures including absences, atonic and tonic fits, head nods ('cornflakes fits'), and falls. These unfortunate children may repeatedly damage themselves due to unexpected drop attacks and may need to wear protective helmets. Many are found to show atypical spike-and-wave activity in the EEG, reminiscent of the classical 3-s spike and wave seen in true *petit mal*, but at a slower frequency. Unfortunately, the outlook for those with the Lennox–Gastaut syndrome may be gloomy, with a large proportion of such children (90 per cent or more) suffering from severe, uncontrolled epilepsy with many falls, and mental deterioration. Such children show irregular spike–wave complexes at 1.5 to 2.5 Hz in the EEG. This syndrome, like infantile spasms at a younger age, indicates a severe disorder of cerebral function.

In children over the age of 7 years, and in adolescents, myoclonus takes different forms in epilepsy. Many such children with idiopathic epilepsy experience early morning myoclonic jerks of the arms. This form of juvenile myoclonic epilepsy, which often is inherited, can be successfully controlled by treatment with sodium valproate. Also there is the syndrome of photosensitive myoclonus and epilepsy, in which children are provoked to periocular and facial myoclonus, often progressing to a generalized seizure, by a flickering television set.

Benign essential myoclonus

This condition produces widespread, random muscle jerks affecting all four limbs, trunk, neck, and face, occurring at about 10 to 50/min, enhanced by action and sensory stimuli. Many families inherit the condition as an autosomal-dominant trait. Onset is usually in childhood or adolescence, but disability is strikingly mild, there is no progression, intellect is normal, fits do not occur, and no other deficit appears. Some patients report that alcohol helps their jerks, and many respond to a β-adrenergic antagonist such as propranolol.

Focal myoclonus

There are a number of conditions in which myoclonic muscle jerking may be restricted to one part of the body. Some pathological processes may cause focal myoclonus limited to those segments innervated by the part of brainstem or spinal cord affected (segmental myoclonus). Similar pathologies causing cerebral damage, particularly to the cerebral cortex, may cause rhythmic, repetitive, focal muscle jerking associated with electrical evidence of epileptic cortical discharge in the EEG (epilepsia partialis continua).

Hemifacial spasm

Hemifacial spasm most commonly affects middle-aged or elderly women, and usually appears without obvious cause. Rarely, it may be symptomatic of obvious facial-nerve compression due to a cerebellopontine angle tumour or angioma, when it can be accompanied by trigeminal neuralgia. However, in most cases the cause is thought to be aberrant blood vessels in the posterior fossa compressing the facial nerve at its exit from the brainstem.

The condition consists of irregular, but repetitive, clonic twitching of the muscles of one side of the face. Usually those around the eyes are first involved, producing a feeling identical to the benign myokymia of the lower eyelid that occurs in normal people when fatigued. However, the repetitive twitching spreads slowly to involve the whole face, each spasm closing the eye and drawing up the corner of the mouth. At this stage, a mild facial weakness and contraction becomes evident, but a frank facial palsy never develops. Facial sensation is normal and there are no other physical signs.

Treatment with drugs is usually unrewarding. Exploration of the posterior fossa, with separation of blood vessels from the seventh nerve, gives long-lasting relief. However, injection of botulinum toxin into the facial muscles, repeated every 3 to 4 months, is a simpler and effective treatment.

Tics

A simple tic is a sudden, rapid, twitch-like movement, always of the same nature and at the same site. Such tics are part of our motor personality, such as an eye twitch, a grimace, a sniff, or a hand gesture. Simple motor tics occur in about a quarter of all children and often disappear within a year or so (transient tic of childhood). Sometimes, however, they persist into adult life, but are rarely considered as abnormal (chronic simple tic). Simple tics in a minority of people become so marked as to lead to a request for medical help. Frequently the request is for psychiatric assistance, for the tics are an expression of an underlying psychological disorder.

Sometimes tics are more widespread and severe, and take the form of complicated stereotyped patterns of motor action (complex tics). Characteristically, complex and simple tics can be suppressed voluntarily. However, this causes mounting inner tension, which is relieved by letting the tics come out. Complex multiple tics may be accompanied by vocal utterances, particularly swear-words (coprolalia), and compulsive thoughts. This constitutes the syndrome of Gilles de la Tourette.

Gilles de la Tourette syndrome

Aetiology

The cause of this bizarre illness is unknown, and no pathological or pathophysiological abnormality has been identified. The condition appears to be inherited as an autosomal-dominant trait, with variable penetrance. In affected families the genetic abnormality may be expressed as the full syndrome, as chronic multiple tics alone, or as an obsessive compulsive neurosis (see below).

Symptoms

The illness usually begins between the ages of 5 and 15 years with multiple, involuntary, repetitive muscular tics. Typical initial symptoms are eye blinking, head nodding, sniffing, or stuttering. With time other more complex tics appear affecting other parts of the body. The individual tics are brief and variable, but are repetitive and reproducible.

Sooner or later, many patients with multiple tics begin to make involuntary noises, such as grunting, squealing, yelping, sniffing, or barking. Indeed, the coexistence of such noises with multiple tics is essential for the diagnosis of Gilles de la Tourette's syndrome. In about 60 per cent of cases, such noises become transformed into swear-words.

A large proportion of those with Gilles de la Tourette syndrome also exhibit typical features of an obsessive–compulsive nature. These psychic manifestations of the illness may be even more disabling than the tics. Repeated touching, hitting, or self-injury may occur. A hyperactive attentional disorder is common in children.

Table 6 Causes of torsion dystonia

Generalized dystonia	**Generalized dystonia (cont.)**
Idiopathic dystonia	Symptomatic dystonia (cont.)
Inherited	Progressive pallidal atrophy
Autosomal dominant	Pelizaeus–Merzbacher disease
X-linked recessive	Spinocerebellar degenerations
Dopa-responsive dystonia–parkinsonism	Postencephalitic
	Postanoxic
Sporadic	Paroxysmal dystonia (paroxysmal choreoathetosis)
Drug-induced dystonia	
Acute dystonic reactions	Paroxysmal kinesigenic choreoathetosis
Chronic tardive dystonia	
Symptomatic dystonia	Paroxysmal dystonic choreoathetosis
Athetoid cerebral palsy	
Encephalitis lethargica	**Focal dystonia**
Wilson's disease	Blepharospasm
Mitochondrial encephalomyopathy	Oromandibular dystonia
Dystonic lipidosis	Spasmodic dysphonia
GM_1 gangliosidosis	Spasmodic torticollis
GM_2 gangliosidosis	Axial dystonia
Metachromatic leucodystrophy	Dystonic writer's cramp (and other occupational cramps)
Organic acidurias	
Homocystinuria	Hemiplegic dystonia
Ceroid lipofuscinosis	Stroke
Lesch–Nyhan disease	Tumour
Ataxia telangiectasia	Arteriovenous malformation
Juvenile Huntington's disease	Trauma
Hallervorden–Spatz disease	Post-thalamotomy

Once established, Gilles de la Tourette's syndrome usually is lifelong, although its severity waxes and wanes. No other neurological abnormality develops; intellect and motor coordination are normal.

Treatment

Neuroleptic drugs such as haloperidol or pimozide may satisfactorily control tics, noises, and coprolalia. The obsessive–compulsive symptoms of the illness may benefit from treatment with drugs such as clomipramine or fluoxetine.

The dystonias

Definition

This is a group of illnesses characterized by dyskinesias consisting of prolonged spasms of muscle contraction affecting various parts of the body, causing dystonic movements and postures. Dystonia may affect the whole body (generalized dystonia), may affect adjacent parts such as an arm and the neck (segmental dystonia), or may be restricted to one part (focal dystonia) as in spasmodic torticollis, dystonic writer's cramp, blepharospasm, oromandibular dystonia, and laryngeal dystonia.

Aetiology

Dystonia may be caused by a variety of cerebral insults or by drugs (symptomatic dystonia). The many metabolic and other inherited or sporadic diseases that can cause dystonia (Table 6) usually produce other neurological symptoms and signs, including cognitive impairment, fits, disorders of eye movement, ataxia and pyramidal signs, and a peripheral neuropathy. A symptomatic cause for dystonia is found in about 50 per cent of children with the illness, but is rare in those presenting in adult life. When no symptomatic cause for dystonia can be discovered, the syndrome is described as idiopathic or primary dystonia. Since the characteristic feature of the symptomatic dystonias is damage to the basal ganglia, it is assumed, by inference, that idiopathic torsion dystonia is due to some unidentified functional abnormality of the basal ganglia.

Idiopathic dystonia often is inherited (see below), but the focal dystonias of spasmodic torticollis, writer's cramp, blepharospasm, and oromandibular dystonia usually occur as sporadic cases with onset in middle life.

Idiopathic dystonia

Symptoms

The illness may present in childhood, when it is frequently inherited as an autosomal-dominant trait, or in adult life, when a family history is unusual. In many families, genetic linkage studies have localized the abnormal gene to chromosome 9. Ashkenazim Jews are particularly prone to the illness, which usually presents in children with dystonia spasms of the legs on walking, or sometimes of the arms, trunk, or neck. The affected child often begins to walk on the toes with the foot plantar flexed and inverted.

The illness is usually progressive when it commences in childhood; the spasms spread to all body parts, leading to severe disability within about 10 years. Intellect is preserved and there are no signs of pyramidal or sensory deficit. Speech is often spared, allowing such patients to pursue intellectual employment despite severe physical disability.

In adults, the condition usually presents as a focal dystonia (blepharospasm, oromandibular dystonia, spasmodic dysphonia, torticollis, axial dystonia, or dystonic writer's cramp). The legs tend to be spared, and progression is slow, with the dystonia remaining confined to its site of origin.

Treatment

Dystonia is distressing and difficult to treat. Every child and young adult with dystonia should receive a trial of levodopa (Sinemet-Plus up to two tablets three times a day for 3 months), for they may have the condition of dopa-responsive dystonia–parkinsonism (see below). The drugs that most patients find helpful are a benzodiazepine such as diazepam, often in a large dose of 20 to 50 mg daily, and an anticholinergic such as benzhexol, again in large doses.

When advanced, the disease may be so disabling that stereotaxic surgery seems warranted. A unilateral thalamotomy may suppress dystonia of the contralateral limbs, with a risk of hemiplegia of about 1 per cent. Unfortunately, however, severe dystonia is usually bilateral and involves axial structures. Bilateral thalamotomy is required in such cases, with the additional risk of severe impairment of speech in 15 per cent or more patients, and cranial and neck axial dystonia respond far less favourably to thalamotomy than does limb dystonia.

Dopa-responsive dystonia–parkinsonism

This is an uncommon but important familial condition, inherited as an autosomal-dominant trait, and characterized by the onset of typical dystonic posturing and torsion spasms of the legs in childhood and adolescence, but usually with marked diurnal variation in the severity of symptoms. Such patients may have little or no dystonia on waking from sleep, but as the day goes on, dystonia gets worse, particularly with exercise, so that by the afternoon or evening these patients exhibit their worst symptoms. Rest without sleep does not help, but sleep relieves their dystonia. Many of these patients also exhibit features of parkinsonism. Other features include postural imbalance with falls, and pseudopyramidal signs (brisk reflexes with dystonic extensor plantar responses). Some of these patients are thought to have an unexplained 'spastic paraparesis' or diplegic cerebral palsy, athetoid cerebral palsy, or a curious ataxic syndrome.

The other feature characteristic of this curious syndrome is its dramatic response to treatment with levodopa, which may completely abolish all signs of the illness. Small doses are effective, and a stable therapeutic response continues for decades.

Spasmodic torticollis

Spasmodic torticollis may be the presenting feature of dystonia in childhood, but isolated spasmodic torticollis usually occurs in middle-aged or elderly individuals. The onset is usually insidious, often with initial pain, and sometimes appears to be precipitated by trauma. The dystonic spasms affect sternomastoid, splenius, and other neck muscles to cause the head to turn to one side (torticollis), or occasionally to extend (retrocollis) or to flex (antecollis).

The illness usually is lifelong, but remissions of a year or more occur in about a fifth of cases. Most patients are otherwise normal. As with all types of dystonia, the frequency and intensity of the muscle spasms vary considerably, being particularly worse in conditions of mental or emotional stress. A feature characteristic of spasmodic torticollis is the *geste antagonistique*, in which the patient discovers some particular manual act that controls the deviation of the head. A touch of the forefinger to the jaw may suffice, but other more complex and bizarre actions are common.

Spasmodic torticollis, like other types of adult-onset focal dystonia, usually does not benefit from drug therapy. A benzodiazepine such as diazepam or an anticholinergic such as benzhexol may be of value.

The best treatment now is injection of botulinum toxin A into the most affected muscles. Botulinum toxin prevents the release of acetylcholine and causes functional denervation with localized muscle weakness. Recovery, by terminal sprouting, occurs within a matter of 2 to 4 months. Botulinum is injected into the sternomastoid and splenius muscles for simple torticollis. The injections need to be repeated 3 or 4 times a year.

Dystonic writer's cramp

A specific complaint of inability to write (or to type, to play a musical instrument, or to wield any manual instrument) may be due to a variety of causes, including joint disease, a carpal tunnel syndrome, a spastic or ataxic hand, Parkinson's disease, or benign essential tremor. However, no objective neurological deficit is found in many patients, other than abnormal posturing of the hand and arm on writing. Typically, the pen is gripped with great force and driven into the paper. However, in some patients the arm adopts a typical dystonic posture and in such cases of dystonic writer's cramp, other manual acts such as wielding a knife or screwdriver are similarly affected. Dystonic writer's cramp may be the initial symptom of generalized torsion dystonia, but in adults it often remains as an isolated disability.

The same considerations apply to other occupational cramps, such as pianist's cramp, drummer's cramp, violinist's cramp, typist's cramp, Morse-code operator's (telegraphist's) cramp, and the wide range of other such disabilities described in association with specific repetitive manual activities.

Writer's cramp, and other similar conditions, are usually permanent disabilities that do not respond satisfactorily to psychiatric, behavioural, or drug therapy. Benzhexol and diazepam are worth a try, but more potent drugs rarely are indicated. Advice to employ different writing instruments and to adjust to the disability is often the best that can be offered. Botulinum toxin injections into the affected forearm muscles may help some patients.

Table 7 Drug-induced extrapyramidal disease

Disorder	Drugs responsible	Susceptible age group	Incidence	Onset after initiation of therapy	Effect of withdrawal of drug	Treatment
Tremor	Bronchodilators Tricyclics Lithium carbonate Caffeine	Any	Dose-dependent about 35 per cent	Rapid	Disappears	Withdraw drug
Parkinsonism	Reserpine Tetrabenazine Neuroleptics	Any but increases with age	Dose-dependent about 50 per cent	Gradual, within first months	Disappears slowly, may take a year	Anticholinergics
Acute dystonia	Neuroleptics Diazoxide	Children, young adults	2–5 per cent	Acute, within first few hours or days	Disappears	Anticholinergics Diazepam
Akathisia	Neuroleptics	Any	About 30 per cent	Gradual, within first months	Disappears	Anticholinergics
Tardive dyskinesia	Neuroleptics	Increases with age	20–40 per cent	Delayed, but increases	May get worse; persists in about 40 per cent	Withdraw drug Tetrabenazine

Blepharospasm and oromandibular dystonia (cranial dystonia)

Blepharospasm refers to recurrent spasms of eye closure. The orbicularis oculi forcibly contracts for seconds or minutes, often repetitively and sometimes so frequently as to render the patient functionally blind. Spasms of eye closure commonly occur while reading or watching television, or in bright light; they often decrease or disappear when the sufferer is alerted or under scrutiny. Oromandibular dystonia refers to recurrent spasms of muscle contraction affecting the mouth, tongue, jaw, larynx, and pharynx, causing spasms of lip protrusion or retraction, jaw closure or opening, and difficulty in speech and swallowing. Such patients may lacerate their lips and tongue or even dislocate their jaw, and usually are unable to cope with dentures. Speech may take on a characteristic, forced/strained quality, and chewing and swallowing may be impaired.

These two conditions are closely related, for the patient with blepharospasm may develop oromandibular dystonia and vice versa. Both conditions may occur in generalized torsion dystonia, or be produced by drugs, but also appear in isolation in late life without evident cause.

Treatment

Both blepharospasm and oromandibular dystonia are notoriously difficult to control with drugs. Some patients may be helped by agents such as benzhexol, and may take a benzodiazepine such as diazepam to relieve anxiety. The best treatment is to inject botulinum toxin into the orbicularis oculi. This gives relief from blepharospasm in about 70 to 80 per cent of cases, thereby restoring normal vision for about 3 months. The injections can be repeated as necessary. Botulinum toxin injections can be used to control some jaw spasms.

Spasmodic dysphonia

Dystonic spasms of the muscles controlling the vocal cords causes spasmodic dysphonia, which impairs speech and singing, and may be severe enough to prevent communication. The most common type involves the adductor muscles, leading to a strangled speech with pitch breaks and stops. Less common is abductor dysphonia, which produces a breathy, low-volume voice. The diagnosis can be established by direct, non-invasive visualization of the vocal cords during talking. Speech can be restored by injection of botulinum toxin into the overactive vocal muscles, identified by electromyography.

Drug-induced extrapyramidal disease

The extensive use of antipsychotic neuroleptic drugs (which include the phenothiazines, butyrophenones, thioxanthenes, and dibutylpiperidines) has led to much iatrogenic extrapyramidal disease. These drugs, all of which block dopamine receptors in the basal ganglia and elsewhere, are used widely to control acute psychotic behaviour, whatever its cause, and to prevent relapse of schizophrenia. They also are employed as antiemetics, as are other similar drugs such as metoclopramide, and to treat vertigo. The major neurological complications of these drug therapies are summarized in Table 7.

Akathisia refers to an irresistible and unpleasant sensation of motor restlessness, and the inability to sit or stand still, all of which may be mistaken for a recurrence of psychotic behaviour. Such patients not only complain of motor restlessness but also exhibit repetitive, stereotyped, akathitic movements, particularly of the legs. Akathisia remits if the offending neuroleptic is withdrawn, or if the dose can be reduced sufficiently. Akathisia usually does not respond to anticholinergic drugs, but may be helped by a benzodiazepine or propranolol.

Acute dystonic reactions commonly consist of oculogyric crises, trismus, neck retraction, or torticollis, and may be mistake for tetanus or meningitis. Although uncommon, acute dystonic reactions pose a repeated diagnostic problem in casualty departments. Those unfamiliar with their bizarre characteristics often dismiss such behaviour as 'hysterical'. The acute dystonia rapidly disappears after an intravenous injection of an anticholinergic drug or a benzodiazepine.

Chronic tardive dyskinesias are the most serious complications, for they may be permanent despite drug withdrawal. About 20 per cent of those on chronic neuroleptic therapy will exhibit a tardive dyskinesia. The characteristic syndrome is one of orofacial mouthing, with lip smacking and tongue protrusion (orobuccolingual dyskinesia), accompanied by trunk rocking and distal chorea of hands and feet. Tardive dyskinesias usually appear after at least 6 months' neuroleptic drug therapy, and their incidence increases with exposure to the drugs and also with the age of the patients. They often get worse in the weeks immediately after stopping the offending drug, or may appear then for the first time. After drug withdrawal, they disappear in about 60 per cent or more of patients over the next

3 years, but continue unaltered in the remainder. Tardive dyskinesias are difficult to treat. The indication for administration of neuroleptic drugs should be reviewed, and the offending agent withdrawn if at all possible. However, many psychiatric patients, particularly those with chronic schizophrenia, benefit from long-term neuroleptic therapy to prevent relapses of their psychiatric illness.

That many other drugs may cause dyskinesias has been noted, and the fact that levodopa may provoke any form of dyskinesia in patients with Parkinson's disease has been discussed. It seems likely that most such drug-induced dyskinesias are due to pharmacological effects on dopamine mechanisms in the basal ganglia, resulting in dopaminergic overactivity, in contrast to the akinetic–rigid syndrome produced by dopamine depletion or blockade.

Further reading

Arzimanoglou, A.A. (1998). Gilles de la Tourette syndrome. *Journal of Neurology*, **245**, 761–5.

Brin, M.F. and Koller, W. (1998). Epidemiology and genetics of essential tremor. *Movement disorders*, **13**(Suppl. 3), 55–63.

Hartmann, A., Pogarell, O., and Oertel, W.H. (1998). Secondary dystonias. *Journal of Neurology*, **245**, 511–8.

Quinn, N.P. (1998). Classification of fluctuations in patients with Parkinsons disease. *Neurology*, **51**(Suppl. 2), S25–9.

Chapter 13.21

Headache

J. M. S. Pearce

The clinical approach to headache rests on a detailed analysis of symptoms and a thorough examination. Investigations are applicable to only a small number of patients, prompted by typical symptoms and signs suggesting a particular pathology.

Headaches may be acute, usually signifying meningeal irritation or, rarely, raised intracranial pressure; recurrent as in migraine; or chronic as in tension headaches.

Table 1 compares the more common causes of chronic or recurrent headaches in different age groups.

Migraine

Classic migraine with an aura is a paroxysmal disorder, with headache, often unilateral at onset, associated with nausea, anorexia and often vomiting. It is preceded or accompanied by visual, sensory, motor, or mood disturbances and is often familial. This classic syndrome accounts for some 20 per cent of migraine cases. More commonly (in some 75 per cent of cases) there is no aura (common migraine). Migraine variants occur in 5 per cent of patients.

It is common for patients to have tension headaches between their migraines: these should be identified to prevent misdirected treatment.

Migraine is common, affecting approximately 20 per cent of women and 15 per cent of men at some time in their lives. However, many attacks are not incapacitating, and half the sufferers may never seek medical attention. The frequency of attacks varies from one to two per week to a few sparsely scattered over a lifetime. Daily headaches are never migrainous.

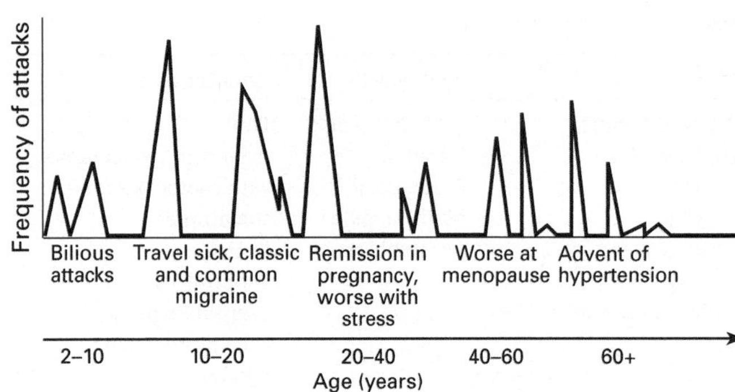

Fig. 1 Scheme of life pattern of attacks of migraine.

Clinical features

Over 80 per cent of migraineurs have their first attacks before the age of 30 years, and the diagnosis should be viewed with suspicion in anyone over 40 years of age. Some people have only a few attacks in a lifetime; most have several attacks each year. Attacks tend to lessen after the age of 50 years, when headache may disappear, leaving attacks of aura alone (Fig. 1). Remission occurs in 70 per cent of pregnancies. Exacerbation, rarely resulting in cerebral infarction, may result from the use of oral contraceptives.

The prodrome is probably of hypothalamic origin. It comprises vague yawning, euphoria, unbridled energy, or depression and lethargy, sometimes with craving or distaste for various foods, in the 24 h before the headache.

The aura is usually visual. Flashing lights, zigzag castellations, balls, or filaments of light may start peripherally and spread centripetally, or centrally spreading centrifugally. Fragmentation, jigsaw appearances, with or without central scotomas (like frosted glass), micropsia, and metamorphopsia (Alice in Wonderland syndrome) are common. Vague blurring is not migrainous. Auras typically last 30 min and are succeeded by headache. Attacks may start with numbness and tingling of one or both hands, or of the face, lips, and tongue. The spread of paraesthesias is slow over many minutes and should not be confused with the more rapid march of jacksonian epilepsy. Weakness, clumsiness, and occasionally a hemiparesis with or without dysphasia may occur (hemiplegic migraine).

Headache is commonly, but not always, unilateral. It is typically described as throbbing or pulsating, but there is often a non-specific, dull ache, and not infrequently patients complain of a tight band or pressure.

Table 1 Chronic and recurrent headaches in different age groups

Children (3–16)	Adults (17–65)	Elderly (65+)
Migraine	Tension headache	Cervicogenic
Psychogenic/fatigue	Migraine	Cranial arteritis
Post-traumatic	Post-traumatic	Persisting tension headache
Tumour (rare, except posterior fossa)	Cluster headache	Persisting migraine
	Tumour/subdural haematoma	Rare cluster headache
	Cervicogenic	Tumour/subdural haematoma
	Paget's disease	Paget's disease
	Glaucoma	Glaucoma
		Hypnic headaches

Table 2 Treatment of migraine

Avoid	Prophylactic*	Symptomatic
Physical factors	Cyproheptadine	**Oral**
Bright light	Pizotifen	Aspirin or paracetamol
Fasting	Propranolol	with metoclopramide,
Fatigue	Methysergide	sumatriptan
Irregular sleep	Amitryptiline	**Rectal**
Dietary		Suppository
Individual precipitants		ergotamine or chlorpromazine
?Tyramine (e.g. cheese)		**Inhalation**
?Phenylethylamine (e.g. chocolate)		'Medihaler' ergotamine
Alcohol		**Intramuscular**[d]
Sodium nitrate		Codeine,
Monosodium glutamate		chlorpromazine, or prochlorperazine

*If migraine frequency is greater than twice a month.

[d] Very rarely needed.

Nausea and vomiting often occur at the height of pain. Headache may be relieved by vomiting, and sleep often terminates headache and is an integral part of the attack. Diarrhoea, chills, pallor, faintness, fluid retention, and, rarely, facial bruising may complicate the picture. All vigorous activities are shunned; light and sound aggravate the symptoms, hence the retreat to bed in a dark room. Many attacks end gradually after 24 to 48 h, but attacks in children often last only 2 to 6 h.

Aetiology

The phasic pattern and diversity of precipitating agents support the notion of a cerebral rather than a primary vascular disorder. Genetic factors operate in 70 per cent of patients, but there is no simple mendelian pattern. Cerebral symptoms of the aura may be initiated by depression of neuronal activity (theory of Leão) with secondary spreading regional oligaemia. Food idiosyncrasies or allergies, red wines, and missing a meal are precipitants but not causes. Serotonin derived from platelets is depleted in the aura; other anomalies in opioid, prostaglandin, and peptide metabolism are reported but provide no general explanation.

Treatment

Assessment of the patient's habits, work, personality, and stresses is important. Known precipitants should be sought, if necessary with the aid of a diary, and should be eliminated when possible.

Symptomatic treatment is offered for individual attacks (Table 2). Rest, dark, and quiet, where practicable, are supplemented by simple analgesics (paracetamol 1 g, or aspirin 0.6 g) or non-steroidal anti-inflammatory drugs, such as naproxen, 500 mg. The addition of caffeine and spasmolytics add to expense but not to benefit. Codeine, 15 to 30 mg, may enhance pain relief. Analgesics should be taken immediately the attack begins, then repeated 4- to 6-hourly as needed. Absorption is improved by taking aspirin or paracetamol with, or 10 min after, metoclopramide (10 mg) or domperidone (10–20 mg). These drugs are useful both in relieving gastric stasis and as anti-emetics. If vomiting is severe, suppositories of domperidone, prochlorperazine, or chlorpromazine are valuable. Ergotamine is effective in 50 per cent of cases, but is badly absorbed orally and should be given by suppository or by inhalation (Medihaler-Ergotamine®, 0.36 mg/puff). If a single dose does not work, it should not be repeated. Ergotamine has no place as a prophylactic and when overused leads to habituation with ergotamine-induced headache.

Sumatriptan is a selective agonist of 5-hydroxytryptamine-1 (similar to ergotamine) causing vasoconstriction and reduced plasma extravasation in dural vessels. A dose of 6 mg subcutaneously or 100 mg orally provides prompt and effective relief of all symptoms in 60 to 70 per cent of patients, but headache rebounds in one-third of patients. This expensive treatment can be repeated.

Prophylaxis

Prophylaxis should be attempted if attacks occur more often than twice each month. In patients with exacerbations related to stress or anxiety, amitriptyline, 50 to 100 mg at night introduced gradually, is often effective. Propranolol, atenolol, and metoprolol give adequate reduction in about 60 per cent of cases.

Serotonin (5-hydroxytryptamine) inhibitors are valuable in 60 to 70 per cent of patients. Cyproheptadine, 4 mg three times a day, inhibits calcium channels and serotonin and histamine activity. Pizotifen, 0.5 mg three times a day or 1.5 mg at night, is moderately effective and free of hazards other than sedation and weight gain. Methysergide, 1 to 2 mg three times a day, is the most potent of this group but should be used only under hospital supervision in courses not exceeding 3 to 4 months. Pleural, pericardial, and retroperitoneal fibrosis are rare but serious side-effects that may result from more prolonged use; they usually regress when the drug is stopped. Calcium antagonists [Flunnarizine (not marketed in the UK but available in Europe and USA), verapamil] and sodium valproate have been established as useful prophylactics in recent trials.

Menstrual migraine

Migraine occurring exclusively with menstruation is uncommon, but may be relieved by oestrogen patches or implants. Migraine, between menstrual periods, but worse with menstruation, is common but usually resistant to diuretics and hormonal manipulation.

Cluster headache

This is a distinctive clinical syndrome separable from migraine, which predominantly affects men (M:F 10:1). It begins at any age, most often between 20 and 50 years, and is characterized by daily bouts of unilateral headache of great severity lasting 30 to 120 min. The brevity, severity, lack of aura and vomiting, occurring daily in clusters lasting usually for 4 to 16 weeks clearly separate it from migraine. The pain is boring, aching, or stabbing and is centred on one orbit with radiation to the forehead, temple or cheek, and jaw ('lower-half headache'). It characteristically strikes at night, an hour or so after sleep, and may recur during the day, often at the same time ('alarm-clock headache').

In many cases the ipsilateral eye becomes red and bloodshot, watering profusely. The nostril may be blocked or may run. A transient Horner's syndrome is seen in 25 per cent of cases and occasionally this persists. Alcohol and other vasodilators are important precipitating factors: nitroglycerine has been used as a provocative test—a typical attack following within an hour of a sublingual 0.5-mg tablet. Clusters last for 1 to 4 months, although occasionally the condition continues for a year or more—chronic migrainous neuralgia. Remissions are complete but the clusters usually recur every year or two. The cause of this syndrome is unknown. The diagnosis is made on the classical symptoms and investigation is rarely warranted.

Treatment

The essence of treatment is prevention. During clusters, ergotamine is given 1 h before anticipated daytime attacks, and just before getting into bed for nocturnal attacks. Suppositories are the most useful preparation. Control is excellent in 75 per cent of patients and the drug is stopped each Sunday to see if the cluster recurs; if so, ergotamine is continued for a further week, until the cluster ends. If ergot is unsuccessful, sumatriptan 100 mg orally, methysergide 1 to 2 mg three times a day, or verapamil 40 to 80 mg three times a day are useful alternatives. Oxygen, 5 to 10 l/min for 10 min at the onset, is effective, but β-blockers and pizotifen are not. Lithium can be used in the chronic variant if other methods fail. In intractable cases, a 'crash course' of corticosteroids may provide dramatic relief of symptoms.

Tension headache (synonym: muscle contraction headache)

Tension headache is common. It constitutes 70 per cent of referrals to a 'headache clinic' and in random samples of healthy individuals over 90 per cent volunteer one or more previous attacks of recognizable tension headache. In most instances it is a short-lived complaint with obvious preceding cause: overwork, lack of sleep, or an emotional crisis. This is entirely benign and is recognized by patients as 'normal headaches'.

Chronic tension headache

The chronic syndrome is encountered by physicians in all branches of clinical practice. The pain is diffusely felt all over the head. It is, however, often located on the vertex, or may start in the forehead or in the neck. Some patients describe several points of pain, which they point to with a single finger, usually in both temples or over the crown. It may radiate over the glabella on to the bridge of the nose, or from the temples into the jaws. It is commonly bilateral, but there are cases where the pain is unilateral.

The quality of the pain is characteristic. Patients complain of a sense of pressure, a feeling of tightness, or as if a heavy weight were pressing down on the crown. 'A tight band like a skullcap' or 'as if a clamp or vice was squeezing my head' are common descriptions. Some are at pains to relate 'it is not really a pain, but a pressure'. The symptoms may also seem to originate from inside the cranium: 'as if my head is bursting' or 'about to explode'. A 'creeping' sensation (formication) may be felt under the scalp, or a sense of sharp knives or needles driven in, burning hot, may be related by other patients.

Tension headache is a daily occurrence, in contrast to the periodic and paroxysmal attacks of migraine. It is worse as the day goes by, whereas migraine commonly presents on waking. Visual disturbance and vomiting do not occur, although nausea may accompany the pain. Most patients continue their normal work during tension headache. Patients are not photophobic and confined to bed in a darkened room—as in migraine.

Clinical examination may appear to be superfluous in the face of such distinctive symptoms, but it is of great importance. Most patients are frightened, emotional, and anxious. They harbour fears of brain tumours, hypertension, and of 'clots in the brain'. A thorough examination is of the utmost therapeutic value and provides a rational basis for effective reassurance.

Treatment is most effective when the history is short. To cure such headaches after 10 or more years is a daunting and often unsuccessful task. The main step is to try to identify the events that determined the onset. No amount of superficial reassurance will eradicate tension headache if its origins are obscure and the complex psychological mechanisms deriving from the source are untreated. In the common situation where daily pain has persisted for years, the prognosis is less predictable, but short courses of benzodiazepines for 4 weeks or amitriptyline may be helpful and will secure the occasional 'cure'.

Headaches as a symptom of intracranial disease

Confronted by a patient with headaches, the major clinical responsibility is to exclude a cause requiring specific investigation or treatment.

Characteristics of raised-pressure headache

Its location is non-specific, though when a progressive headache starts to involve the neck, tonsilar coning is imminent. The headache is:

(a) worse in the morning;

(b) aggravated by sitting up or standing, and relieved by lying down;

(c) aggravated by coughing, straining, and vomiting;

(d) relieved by aspirin or paracetamol in the early stages (in contrast to psychogenic headache);

(e) associated with vomiting, and eventually with papilloedema and progressing focal signs.

Acute headache

Headaches of abrupt onset may signify trauma, spontaneous intracranial haemorrhage, hydrocephalus, or acute meningeal irritation. The most common cause is acute meningeal irritation due to subarachnoid haemorrhage or to meningitis. An abrupt onset, fever, neck stiffness, and Kernig's sign accompany the obvious severe pain, vomiting, and photophobia. Examination of the cerebrospinal fluid is mandatory if infection is considered, provided that an abscess mass or haematoma have been first excluded.

CT or MRI is usually the first investigation to exclude a mass lesion, haematoma, or hydrocephalus, each of which precludes lumbar puncture. Subarachnoid haemorrhage may be shown, but can be missed by CT in up to 20 per cent of patients on admission. When a mass lesion is excluded, lumbar puncture may be necessary to examine the cerebrospinal fluid for subarachnoid bleeding and meningitis. Acute migraine and tension headache can rarely produce a meningitic picture, diagnosable by exclusion.

Acute headache should be distinguished from the common and totally benign 'exploding head syndrome' in which patients are alarmed by a sudden, momentary, very loud noise in the twilight stage of sleep. Acute headache, sometimes severe, and lasting between 30 min and 24 h, may occur with sexual orgasm—'coital cephalgia'. It recurs with intercourse for several months. Propranolol (40–80 mg) before intercourse is effective, and can be withdrawn after a month's freedom from the symptom.

Atypical facial pain

This label conceals a number of cases with chronic face ache whose cause we do not understand. They are often mistaken for the distinctive trigeminal neuralgia. Patients present a characteristic and clinically recognizable pattern. They are mostly women aged between 30 and 50 years, with a dull, constant, aching pain in one or both cheeks. It has no trigger factors, but is worse with fatigue and under mental duress. It is continuous, although often sparing sleep, and may radiate into the ear, forehead, and jaw. With reassurance and a prolonged course of tricyclic drugs or monoamine oxidase inhibitors many patients obtain lasting relief.

Temporomandibular pain

Although patients with rheumatoid and osteoarthritic changes on radiographs of their temporomandibular joints commonly have no pain, myofascial pain dysfunction is a common cause of complaint in young adults. The syndrome is of aching in front of the ear, worse with jaw opening and accompanied by clicks and clunks—signs not uncommon in asymptomatic people. The quality and relation of pain to chewing and jaw opening distinguish it from trigeminal neuralgia; radiographs exclude sinus disease and neoplasm. Correction of a gross disorder of dental bite (occlusion) may be worthwhile; a trial injection of steroids and lignocaine (lidocaine), 2 per cent, into the joint will afford striking relief in some patients. A course of tricyclics such as amitriptyline can provide substantial benefit in some sufferers.

Headache in elderly people

In addition to the causes of headache already discussed, certain syndromes feature more prominently in middle-aged and elderly people, although age is not a diagnostic barrier.

Cervicogenic headache

Cervicogenic headache refers to head pain referred from cervical spondylosis. It is undoubtedly common, with pain on one or both sides of the neck radiating to the occiput, but also to the temples and frontal region. It is probable that the pain arises from the posterior zygapophyseal joints and related ligaments as the result of osteophytes; irritation of the C2 nerve root or of the greater occipital nerves are important contributory factors that may respond well to local injection of lignocaine and hydrocortisone. Immobilization in a collar is often used but seldom very effective. Manipulation endangers the vertebral arteries and is contraindicated.

Giant-cell arteritis (synonyms: cranial or temporal arteritis)

This common condition, rarely seen under the age of 60 years, is described in Chapter 10.15.

Hypnic headache

This is a curious headache, seen mainly in the over 60s. Patients are woken by pulsating headache, sometimes accompanied by nausea one to three times each night. This occurs most nights, lasts about 30 min, and may coincide with rapid eye-movement sleep. But it differs from chronic cluster headache in the respect of age, generalized location, and absence of autonomic features. There are no physical signs and the disorder is benign. The response to lithium, 300 mg at night, is often spectacular.

Further reading

Antonaci, F. (1998). Drug abuse headache: recognition and management. *Cephalalgia*, **18**(Suppl. 22), 47–52.

Ferrari, M.D. (1998). Migraine. *Lancet*, **351**, 1043–51.

Silberstein, S.D. (1998). Comprehensive management of headache and depression. *Cephalalgia*, **18**(Suppl. 21), 50–5.

van Gign, J. (1999). Pitfalls in the diagnosis of sudden headache. *Proceedings of the Royal College of Physicians of Edinburgh*, **29**, 21–31.

Chapter 13.22

Intracranial tumours

P. J. Teddy

Intracranial tumours as those elsewhere may be benign or malignant, primary or secondary. However, perhaps more than at any other site, management of tumours within the cranial cavity is influenced as much by their exact location and by the potential adverse effects of treatment on surrounding normal tissue as by the degree of malignancy of the neoplasm itself. Most primary tumours of the brain in adults occur above the tentorium cerebelli and must be considered generally to be malignant.

Incidence and distribution

Autopsy findings suggest that intracranial tumours comprise approximately 8 per cent of all primary neoplasms. Metastatic lesions account for about 25 per cent of all those found at autopsy. Intracranial tumours represent the sixth most common form of neoplasm in adults, of which 70 per cent occur above the tentorium.

Pathology

Primary intracranial tumours may be derived from the skull itself, from any of the structures lying within it, or from their tissue precursors. They may be divided into tumours of neurectodermal origin (derived from the neural tube, neural crest, and ectoderm) and those of other cell types (see Table 1). It is better to avoid assessing malignancy of primary intracranial tumours on histological grounds alone or on their propensity to metastasize outside the central nervous system. Primary tumours may involve almost all parts of the brain, are not limited by sulci, and may cross the midline in corpus callosum, hypothalamic, or thalamic regions. Equally, however, histologically benign lesions may involve vital structures, rendering tumour management much more difficult than for some of their more malignant counterparts. Histologically low-grade gliomas may undergo rapid and frank malignant change after many years of slow progression. Metastases outside the central nervous system from primary tumours are rare but do occur, particularly with medulloblastoma. Widespread dissemination through the brain and spinal cord is seen in cases of medulloblastoma, ependymoma, and pineal germinoma. The spread occurs along the pial or ependymal surfaces or through the cerebrospinal fluid. Leukaemic or carcinomatous deposits on the meninges may also disseminate widely through the cerebrospinal fluid pathways.

A comprehensive list of intracranial tumours, together with their cells of origin, is given in Table 1, and the classification and frequency of occurrence of the more common intracranial tumours in Table 2. Note that, although the term 'glioma' may be used loosely to describe all tumours derived from neural tube, and particularly those of glial

Table 1 Classification of intracranial tumours

Tumour type	Cells/site of origin (cellular precursor)	Site of predilection
Astrocytoma	Astrocytes (neural tube)	Cerebral hemisphere, cerebellum, brain-stem, optic pathways
Glioblastoma	Astrocytes	Cerebral hemisphere
Oligodendroglioma	Oligodendrocytes	Cerebral hemisphere
Ependymoma	Ependymal cells (neural tube)	Lateral and IV ventricle
Colloid cyst		III ventricle
Choroid plexus papilloma		Lateral and IV ventricle
Medulloblastoma	Neurones (neural tube)	IV ventricle, cerebellar vermis
Ganglioneuroma		
Ganglioglioma		
Pinealoma	Pinealcytes (neural tube)	Pineal gland
Pineoblastoma		
Neurofibroma	(neural crest)	Cranial nerves
Schwannoma	Schwanna cells	VIII and V nerves
Meningioma	Arachnoid cap cells	Dural surface, ventricles
Craniopharyngioma	Epithelial cells (ectoderm)	Hypothalamus, III ventricle
Cholesteatoma		
Chordoma	(notochord)	Clivus
Germinoma	Germ cells	Pineal gland
Teratoma	(germinal layers)	Pineal gland
Microglia	Uncertain	Cerebral hemisphere
Sarcoma	Connective tissue	Meninges
Glomus tumour	Glomus jugulare	Glomus jugulare
Pituitary adenoma	Adenohypophyseal cells	Pituitary gland
Haemangioblastoma	Uncertain (?vascular)	Cerebellum
Secondary tumours	Bronchus, breast, kidney, thyroid, melanoma, large bowel, leukaemia, lymphoma	Cerebral hemisphere, cerebellum, meninges
Tumours of the skull	Cholesteatoma, osteoma, chordoma, osteoblastoma, bone cysts, myeloma, osteosarcoma Secondary tumours (nasopharynx, breast, prostate, bronchus, thyroid)	

Table 2 Incidence of commoner intracranial tumours

Tumour	Overall percentage incidence	Most common ages of presentation
Astrocytoma and glioblastoma (adults)	38	40–60 years
Astrocytoma (childhood)	Approximately 50 per cent of childhood primary intracranial tumours	6–12 years
Oligodendroglioma	3	30–60 years
Ependymoma	3	6–12 years, occasional in adults
Medulloblastoma	3	5–15 years, occasional in adults
Schwannoma	8	40–70 years
Meningioma	18.5	40–60 years
Craniopharyngioma	2	5–60 years, above half in children
Haemangioblastoma	9	10–20 years
Pituitary adenoma	10	Adult life
Metastatic	4, but 25 per cent of all intracranial tumours at autopsy	
Miscellaneous	1.5	

cell, origin (astrocytes, oligodendrocytes, and ependyma), its everyday use is usually confined to tumours of astrocytic origin, i.e., astrocytoma and glioblastoma.

Astrocytomas

These are the most common primary intracranial tumours. They are derived from the supportive astrocytic framework of the brain. They are classified as being either astrocytoma, anaplastic astrocytoma, or glioblastoma, on a scale of increasing malignant tendency. The benign astrocytomas of childhood arise in either the optic nerve or chiasm, the hypothalamus, or the cerebellum. Within the cerebellum they are generally cystic and the cyst wall contains a well-circumscribed, solid component of variable size. The solid part of the tumour secretes a yellowish, glairy (like egg white) cyst fluid. Such lesions are usually very slow growing and curable by complete removal, although some are frankly malignant and show a tendency to recur. The so-called piloid astrocytomas, which involve the optic pathways and hypothalamus, are slowly growing but, because of their position, are difficult to remove.

Low-grade astrocytomas in the cerebral hemispheres in both adults and children may remain well circumscribed for many years or show only slowly progressive infiltration accompanied by few clinical symptoms. Some undergo patchy calcification but others undergo change to a more malignant form after long periods of apparent quiescence.

Malignant astrocytomas are seen in the brainstem, usually of children and adolescents, and produce enlargement of the brainstem itself. Disturbances of gait, conjugate gaze, and lower cranial nerves are common but, interestingly, obstructive hydrocephalus is usually a late complication.

In adults, malignant astrocytomas are found most frequently in the cerebral hemispheres. They are rapidly growing, diffusely infiltrating, and commonly undergo central necrosis. The most malignant forms are often designated glioblastoma multiforme. Malignant gliomas commonly induce considerable oedema in the surrounding 'reactive' brain.

Oligodendroglioma

These are usually slow-growing tumours with a very long history (10–15 years) and occur almost invariably in adults. They may show patchy calcification. Eventually they tend to undergo differentiation to become indistinguishable from malignant astrocytoma.

Ependymomas

These are predominantly tumours of children or young adults and arise in the walls of the fourth or, less commonly, the lateral ventricle. They are occasionally malignant, when they may disseminate widely through cerebrospinal fluid pathways.

Medulloblastomas

These are highly malignant tumours, usually arising in the roof of the fourth ventricle and infiltrating locally into the cerebellar vermis. They occur most commonly in the first decade of life and rarely beyond the mid-teens. They have a tendency to metastasize, not only through the cerebrospinal fluid pathways but also outside the central nervous system to involve bone, bone marrow, and lymph nodes.

Pineal tumours

Pineal and parapineal tumours are a mixed group and the natural history of the individual components is uncertain since surgical access to them is often limited or hazardous and many have therefore been treated by a shunt procedure and irradiation without biopsy.

Schwannomas

These lesions are derived from Schwann cells of the neural sheaths and are known as neurilemmomas and neurinomas as well as by the common misnomer of neuroma. They are benign and usually arise on the vestibular branch of the VIIIth nerve or less commonly on the trigeminal nerve, and rarely on the vagal group. They are usually very slow-growing but can reach an enormous size with consequent pressure effects on surrounding structures. Bilateral VIIIth-nerve schwannomas have been found in association with von Recklinghausen's neurofibromatosis.

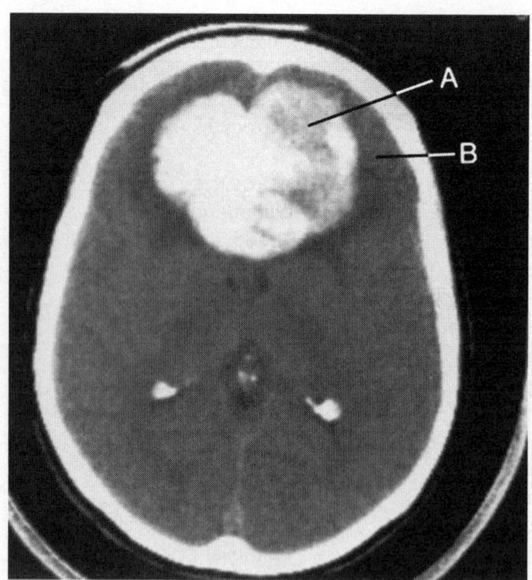

Fig. 1 Contrast CT scan: large bifrontal meningioma (A) with surrounding oedema (B).

Meningiomas

These tumours arise from the arachnoid covering the brain, particularly from the arachnoid villi, and are thus commonly found close to the major dural venous sinuses. They arise most often from the dura of the falx (parasagittal), the sphenoid wing, the convexity of the cerebral hemispheres, and from the olfactory nerve in the anterior fossa. However, they derive from any dural compartment and may be found on the tentorium, in the suprasellar region, and even within the lateral ventricle. They are mainly adult tumours, occurring between the ages of 40 and 50 years, and are occasionally multiple. Most are benign but, incompletely removed, have a tendency to recur. Some are frankly malignant and recur rapidly even after apparently complete removal.

Meningiomas tend to involve the skull close to the site of dural origin, invoking a focal endostosis or occasionally an exostosis. Sometimes there will be osteal hypertrophy and sclerosis overlying the tumour and this is generally seen in the meningioma *en plaque* of the sphenoid wing. Meningiomas are usually benign and slow growing but may reach an enormous size before presentation, particularly when adjacent to relatively silent parts of the brain (Fig. 1). They tend to form a nest in the brain, and have a relatively clear arachnoid plane between tumour capsule and surrounding cortex. The more indolent lesions may calcify or even ossify. Even when entirely benign, the position of some meningiomas makes them either inoperable or amenable only to partial excision; this is particularly true of those that involve the cavernous and sagittal sinuses or surround the proximal part of the internal carotid artery.

Craniopharyngiomas

These tumours, which are found both in adults and children, are formed of epithelial cell remnants in the region of the pituitary stalk. Although considered to be a congenital anomaly, they may grow extensively, causing compression of the optic nerves and chiasm, obstruction of the third ventricle with subsequent hydrocephalus, and may expand into the pituitary fossa with resultant hypopituitarism. About 50 per cent of craniopharyngiomas are calcified and may be identified on skull radiographs as speckled areas of calcification above the posterior clinoid process. A few tumours may be confined within the pituitary fossa itself. They may be wholly or partially cystic.

Pituitary adenomas

These are the most common neoplasm of the pituitary gland and, although usually benign, they range in size from small growths entirely limited to the adenohypophysis to giant forms. They may have large suprasellar components, or extend laterally to involve the cavernous sinus or beyond into the basal cisterns and under the frontal and temporal lobes (invasive adenoma). Adenocarcinomas of the pituitary are extremely rare and resemble metastatic lesions.

Both non-secretory and secretory tumours may also produce effects through space occupation, the most common sequel being compression of the optic chiasm from below. Occasionally the tumours can become big enough to occlude the third ventricle and produce an obstructive hydrocephalus.

Colloid cysts

Colloid cysts occur in the third ventricle, always at its anterior end. They are rare tumours and occur predominantly in young adults. They are benign, probably arising from ependyma in the region of the tela choroidea. Although these masses may present slowly with evidence of progressive dementia or mental changes, they more often present with acute episodes of loss of consciousness, thought to be related to their acting intermittently as a ball valve with obstruction of the foramen of Munro. Occasionally they may be large enough to completely fill the third ventricle and even obstruct the entrance to the aqueduct.

Choroid plexus papillomas

These frond-like tumours are usually benign and arise, predominantly in the first decade of life, in the lateral and fourth ventricles. They may reach an enormous size and produce symptoms by mass effect through obstructive hydrocephalus or by excessive secretion of cerebrospinal fluid. Occasionally they are malignant and may seed through the cerebrospinal fluid pathways.

Ganglioneuromas and gangliogliomas

These are rare, well-circumscribed tumours occurring mainly in children and found predominantly in the floor of the third ventricle. They are fairly indolent and tend not to recur if removal is complete.

Cholesteatomas

These are developmental inclusion lesions in which epithelial remnants are incorporated into deeper layers. They include epidermoid and dermoid cysts. These rare tumours are found predominantly in the cerebellopontine angle and in the parasellar region. They have a tendency to recur, for whereas the contents of the cyst (pearly-white degenerative material) is easy enough to remove, the capsule is thin and adherent to many of the surrounding structures.

Chordomas

Chordomas arise from remnants of the primitive notochord. Intracranial chordomas arise therefore from the clivus and sella turcica. They may be locally invasive, with bony erosion despite usually being benign. One of the chief problems in their treatment is their inaccessibility.

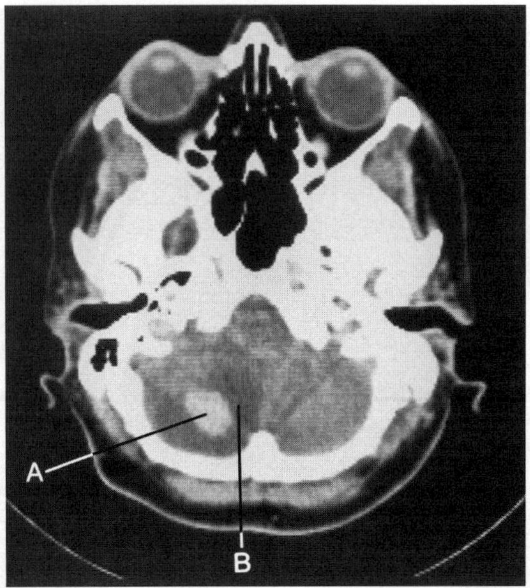

Fig. 2 Contrast CT scan of posterior fossa: solid nodule (A) within typical cyst cavity (B) of haemangioblastoma.

Haemangioblastomas

These tumours are seen in older children and young adults and are most commonly found in the cerebellum. They constitute about 2 per cent of all intracranial tumours. Most are single but they may be associated with retinal and renal or pancreatic cysts, and occur in families—von Hippel–Lindau disease. Haemangioblastomas are occasionally solid but much more commonly cystic, containing a small mural nodule attached to the inner wall of the cyst (see Fig. 2). They are usually benign and the solitary lesions generally do not recur if complete removal is effected. Occasionally, they are associated with ectopic erythropoietin production and polycythaemia.

Glomus jugulare tumours

These are very rare neoplasms arising from the jugular body in the adventitia of the jugular bulb. The mass grows into the middle ear and may present as a pulsating vascular lesion at the external auditory meatus. In about half the cases, growth is into the posterior fossa and presents as a mass at the cerebellopontine angle.

Cerebral lymphomas

Lymphomas of the central nervous system may be primary or secondary. They are being identified more frequently and may occur in immunosuppressed patients. They may be indistinguishable from other forms of intracranial tumour on CT scan or MRI. This provides one very good reason for obtaining a histological diagnosis of tumours recognized on scans, even in cases where the prognosis seems gloomy.

Intracranial metastases

Although the incidence of secondary intracranial neoplasm is only about 4.5 per cent of all intracranial tumours in neurosurgical practice, these secondary tumours represent about 25 per cent of the total in autopsy studies. They may occur in the skull or involve any structure within the cranium. Although they most commonly occur in the cerebral hemispheres or cerebellum, the brainstem, meninges, or cranial nerves may be involved. They are usually multiple (see Fig. 3), variable in size, and well circumscribed, but the differentiation between

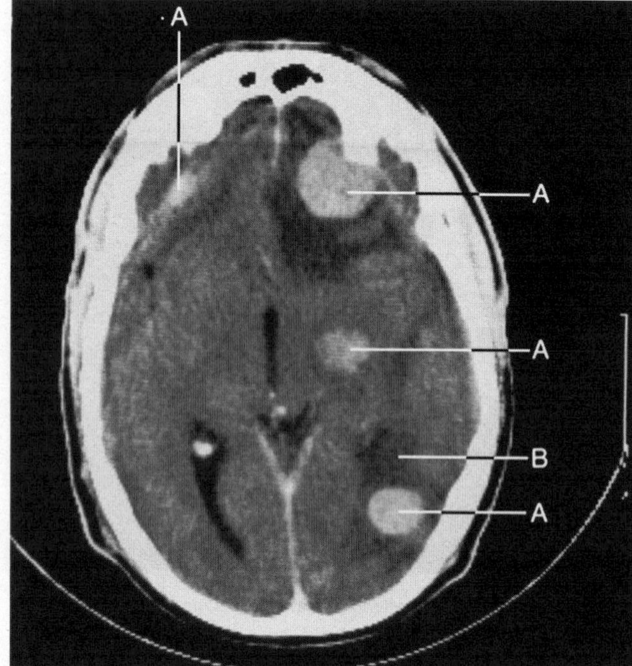

Fig. 3 Contrast CT scan: multiple metastatic deposits (arrows A), each surrounded by an area of cerebral oedema (B).

tumour and surrounding brain is not always clear. The most common primary tumours are those of bronchus and breast, followed by malignant melanoma, renal carcinoma, and various carcinomas of the alimentary tract. Malignant lymphoma and melanoma may be seen as primary neoplasms within the intracranial cavity. Infiltration of the meninges by carcinoma, leukaemia, and lymphoma may produce a malignant meningitis, often associated with palsies of lower cranial nerves owing to infiltration around the brainstem.

Pathophysiology

By infiltrating or compressing normal structures close to the site of the mass, tumours produce focal neurological deficits. Irritation of the cerebral hemisphere may result in epilepsy, and infiltration of the dura may lead to local pain and to meningeal irritation. Increase in the size of the mass within the effectively fixed volume of the skull will lead to a rise in intracranial pressure. Of all these effects the increase in pressure is usually the most important in terms of precipitating rapid, irreversible deterioration.

As intracranial masses increase in size, other phenomena occur that are of great significance in terms of brain function and may prelude rapid clinical deterioration (see Figs 4 and 5). Axial displacement of the brain at the foramen magnum, when the cerebellar tonsils are driven through this aperture, is commonly seen with masses in the posterior fossa. This cerebellar tonsillar herniation is known as coning. The term has been extended to include axial and lateral displacement of the brain at the level of the hiatus. A unilateral hemisphere mass may displace towards the unaffected side, causing the medial part of the temporal lobe (the uncus) to be pushed into the tentorial hiatus. Lateral displacement of the brain combines with the uncal herniation to force the contralateral cerebral peduncle against the free edge of the tentorium. Conduction in the fibres traversing the compressed peduncle becomes impaired, leading to a false localizing sign with ipsilateral hemiparesis (Kernohan's notch

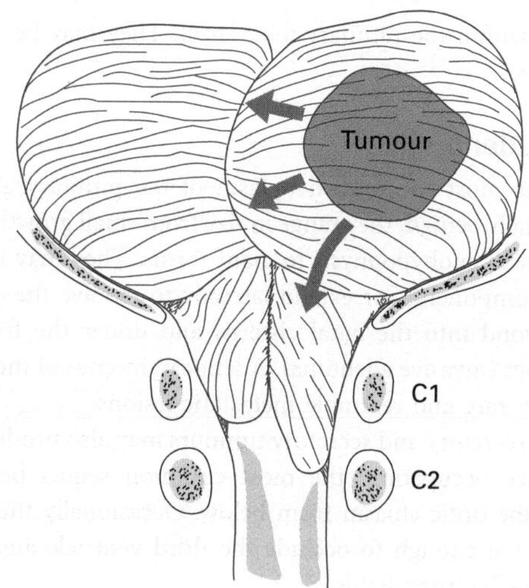

Fig. 4 Herniation of cerebellar tonsils.

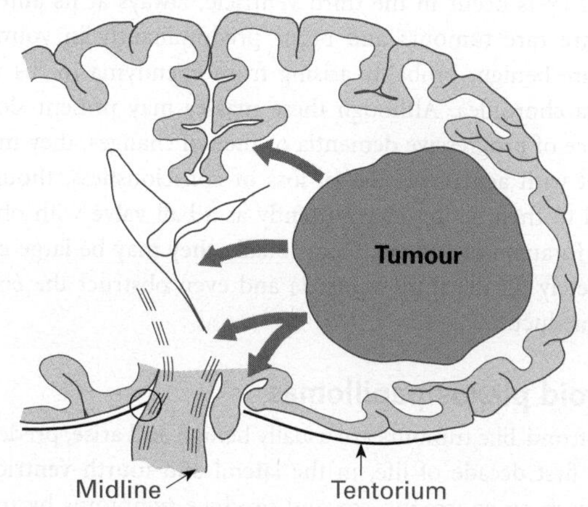

Fig. 5 Diagram of inferior aspect of the brain with a left temporal tumour: the arrow shows the uncus compressing the oculomotor nerve; note also how descent of the posterior cerebral artery stretches the nerve.

phenomenon). Lateral displacement producing tentorial herniation may also press the oculomotor nerve against the petroclinoid ligament and stretch it by virtue of downward displacement of the posterior cerebral artery, around which it hooks; this will result in pupillary dilatation and fixation that may be reversible in the early stages but may become irreversible if the blood supply to the nerve is impaired.

Supratentorial masses may also depress the tentorium and displace the contents of the posterior fossa downwards so that the cerebellar tonsils herniate through the foramen magnum. Deformation of the brainstem distorts arteries that penetrate it; with severe brainstem distortion, infarcts and haemorrhages may occur, which may be fatal. With incipient tentorial and tonsillar herniation a further change in pressure differential between the supratentorial and infratentorial or infratentorial and spinal compartments may be catastrophic. Lumbar puncture must therefore be strictly avoided until a suspected intracranial mass lesion has been excluded.

Papilloedema is most probably caused by the effects of increased intracranial pressure transmitted to the cerebrospinal fluid in the optic nerve sheath. However, even very large, slowly growing intracranial masses can present without demonstrable papilloedema; this may relate anatomically to differing degrees of patency of the optic nerve sheaths. Papilloedema will be absent in cases in which optic atrophy has already supervened.

Clinical features

All intracranial tumours will present in one of (or in a combination of) three ways: raised intracranial pressure, focal neurological deficits, or epilepsy.

Raised intracranial pressure

Evidence of raised intracranial pressure is, perhaps, the most ominous feature of intracranial mass lesions and should prompt urgent investigation. The cardinal symptoms are those of headache, vomiting, and drowsiness. Headaches are seldom of localizing value, although tumours of the posterior fossa may produce occipital and upper cervical pain. Evidence of neck stiffness in conjunction with nuchal pain in the patient with a suspected intracranial mass lesion requires immediate investigation.

Vomiting sometimes occurs as an isolated symptom or precedes headache by many months, particularly in cases of fourth ventricular tumour.

Two sinister symptoms of raised intracranial pressure are failing vision and deterioration of the level of consciousness. Papilloedema is present in only about half of all patients with intracranial tumours. However, chronic papilloedema may result in enlargement of the blind spot and defects of central vision, and ultimately leads to episodes of transient blindness (visual obscurations). These attacks are often exacerbated by coughing, straining, or stooping. Prolonged raised intracranial pressure may produce complete visual failure when optic atrophy supervenes.

Focal neurological deficits

These are legion owing to the variability of type and site of intracranial tumours and only a few specific syndromes associated with the more common tumours can be described here.

Tumours of the non-dominant frontal and anterior temporal lobe and those within the anterior one-third of the corpus callosum or within a ventricle may be manifest purely by symptoms and signs of raised intracranial pressure without focal deficit. Bifrontal lesions may result in intellectual deterioration with memory loss and urinary incontinence, and those involving the third ventricle and hypothalamus can cause hormonal and metabolic changes together with raised intracranial pressure through obstructive hydrocephalus.

Two facets of neurological examination are frequently overlooked or improperly performed by inexperienced clinicians—testing the sense of smell and assessing visual fields. There are probably many patients who have been diagnosed as having simple dementia whose large meningiomas of the olfactory groove have been missed for want of simple tests of sense of smell. Smell may also be lost in cases of extrinsic tumours invading through the floor of the anterior cranial fossa.

Chiasmal lesions are classically regarded as producing a bitemporal hemianopia, and while this is very commonly the case, the deficit is often asymmetric, producing obvious symptoms in one eye whereas the other eye shows changes demonstrable only by refined field testing.

Tumours of the midbrain may produce complex disorders of eye movement (internuclear ocular palsies). Tumours in the pineal region compress the dorsal midbrain, resulting in failure of upward gaze and abnormal pupillary reactions (Parinaud's syndrome).

Disorders of Vth nerve function are usually manifest as either numbness or pain in the face in one or more divisions of the sensory root. The most common site for tumours to affect Vth nerve function is in the region of the pons, most particularly meningiomas or schwannomas in the cerebellopontine angle. Occasionally both sensory and motor impairment of the trigeminal nerve is seen with intrinsic pontine lesions.

Epilepsy (see also Chapter 13.11)

Only some 10 per cent of adults presenting with late-onset epilepsy (after age 25 years) will prove to have an intracranial supratentorial neoplasm. However, the diagnosis should at least be suspected, particularly in cases of focal epilepsy in which the character of the attacks changes. Epilepsy occurs in about 30 per cent of cases of supratentorial tumour and the type of fit may give some idea as to the site and nature of the tumour.

Differential diagnosis

The symptoms associated with intracranial tumours are usually of gradual onset so that the major differential diagnoses are other causes of raised intracranial pressure or progressive neurological signs and fits rather than causes of abrupt deterioration such as stroke. However, one catch is that of meningioma presenting in a stuttering fashion suggestive of transient ischaemic attacks or incomplete stroke. The differential diagnosis of intracranial neoplasm includes chronic subdural haematoma, which is not always associated with known head injury and is often attended by a fluctuating level of consciousness; cerebral infarction; cortical venous thrombosis; benign intracranial hypertension; cerebral abscess, which is usually associated with infection of the sinuses and middle ear or with congenital heart disease; herpes simplex encephalitis; granulomatous disease, including syphylitic gumma and tuberculoma; and causes of hydrocephalus other than those associated with neoplasm (e.g. aqueduct stenosis).

Investigations

Non-radiological investigation may include formal plotting of visual fields in cases of suspected optic nerve or chiasmal compression, caloric testing, audiometry, and measurement of brainstem-evoked potentials in cases of possible acoustic tumour, full endocrine assessment for cases of suspected pituitary adenoma, and serological and haematological investigation to help exclude syphilis and other bacterial infection.

Chest radiography is mandatory in all cases of suspected intracranial tumour to exclude primary neoplasm or tuberculosis.

Plain radiographs of the skull may show evidence of raised intracranial pressure in both adults and children (erosion of the dorsum sellae, 'copper beating' of the skull vault, and separation of the sutures). Calcification is commonly seen in oligodendrogliomas, in virtually all cases of craniopharyngioma of childhood, and in about half the adult cases with this particular neoplasm. Calcification of the pineal in children is highly suggestive of pineal tumour. Unilateral tumours of the cerebral hemispheres may displace a calcified pineal gland.

Hyperostosis or bony erosion of the skull can occur immediately adjacent to meningiomas, and acoustic schwannomas commonly erode the internal auditory meatus. In such cases tomography of the petrous bones or an MRI scan is indicated.

MRI and CT

Although MRI is unlikely to replace CT scanning completely in the investigation of intracranial mass lesions, it is of great value in demonstrating small, multiple metastases, basal intracranial tumours, differentiating tumour from demyelination, and defining tumour masses within an area of cerebral oedema. Contrast enhancement with gadolinium is particularly useful in diagnosing malignant meningitis.

Even if MRI is available, some patients are unable to undergo this investigation because of claustrophobia, previous intracranial surgery involving the insertion of ferrous materials (usually older-type aneurysm clips), or because they have cardiac pacemakers. MRI is also less useful in calcified lesions, but it is particularly good for distinguishing bleeds into tumours as opposed to primary intracerebral haematomas.

With contrast-enhancement CT, over 95 per cent of intracranial tumours may be demonstrated with a resolution of around 2 mm, depending on the density of the tumour compared with that of the surrounding brain. CT scanning will also show whether the tumour is solid or partially cystic, and will show the amount of lateral shift produced by the tumour mass and surrounding oedema. Finally, both CT and MRI will demonstrate the presence of obstructive hydrocephalus associated with intracranial masses.

Management

Except for cases in which age or general medical condition preclude operation, most intracranial tumours will require some form of surgery, either to obtain a histological diagnosis, to palliate and help to control fits or neurological symptoms, or to achieve total removal. With malignant tumours, radiotherapy is often used in conjunction with a surgical procedure (see Table 3). Medical treatment is largely supportive and symptomatic in the absence of any specific antitumour agent.

Immediate treatment

The principal features associated with intracranial neoplasms that require urgent investigation and treatment are raised intracranial pressure, particularly when associated with deteriorating level of consciousness and/or failing vision, and epileptic fits. Raised pressure associated with tumour mass and surrounding reactive oedema may be reduced by giving intravenous frusemide (furosemide) or 20 per cent w/v solution of mannitol (200 ml over about 15 min). Intravenous dexamethasone (12–16 mg) may also be used in extreme cases.

Corticosteroids may also be used in rather less urgent cases. Dexamethasone (4 mg 6-hourly) may produce symptomatic relief by reducing brain swelling and may make subsequent surgery safer. If there is doubt about whether a mass lesion is an abscess or neoplasm, steroids should be avoided until a diagnosis has been firmly established.

Raised intracranial pressure from obstructive hydrocephalus requires some form of ventricular drainage procedure or ventricular shunting. Once this has been done, fuller investigation may be undertaken rather less urgently and elective surgery planned as required.

Severe headaches should be treated with codeine or dihydrocodeine but other opiate analgesics are generally contraindicated because of their tendency to depress respiration, conscious level, and pupillary responses. Vomiting may be controlled with metaclopramide or cyclizine.

Surgical treatment

Surgery is aimed, whenever possible, at obtaining as complete a removal as is feasible without producing neurological deficit. Benign tumours that are surgically accessible and not involving important structures such as brainstem, basal ganglia, or major vessels are curable by complete surgical excision. Tumours in which complete excision is most commonly attempted include meningiomas, colloid cysts, neurofibromas, schwannomas, and pituitary adenomas. Most supratentorial tumours are removed at craniotomy, the exact approach being dictated by the site of the tumour. Pituitary adenomas are removed trans-sphenoidally, transethmoidally, or transcranially.

Gliomas of the frontal, temporal, and occipital poles might seem curable by lobectomy with a line of excision well behind the apparent limits of the tumour as judged on the CT scan or, more accurately, MRI. However, even in these circumstances, histological examination often shows tumour cells to be present right up to the line of excision, implying that removal has not been complete. The benefit of this procedure is a good internal decompression and, with the more slowly growing neoplasms, a considerable remission of symptoms. Lobectomy is most appropriate to polar tumours in patients with evidence of raised intracranial pressure but few focal neurological signs.

Complete removal of single metastatic lesions is often well worth while. Even in those cases in which prolongation of life cannot be achieved, the quality of the survival time is often improved, sometimes remarkably so. For instance, patients who are completely incapacitated by vomiting and ataxia related to a metastasis in the cerebellum can achieve almost complete alleviation of these symptoms by excision of the mass.

Malignant gliomas infiltrate diffusely and it is rarely possible to excise them completely. The aim of surgery is to remove the maximum amount of tumour possible without producing or adding to neurological deficit.

With the advent of CT scanning and MRI it was thought that sufficient definition could be achieved to recognize with total confidence intracranial neoplasms and to distinguish them from other pathology. Despite advances in scan technology, there may still be difficulty in differentiating abscess, benign tumour, or malignant neoplasm. For these reasons it is preferable in almost all cases to obtain a tissue diagnosis by biopsy. This may be carried out through a burr-hole with needle biopsy, by stereotactic procedures, or by craniotomy. However, the mass may be lying in the basal ganglia, thalamus, or brainstem, in which case even needle biopsy could be detrimental.

Radiotherapy

The usual method of irradiating intracranial tumours is to give external irradiation to the site of the tumour in fractionated doses over a period of about 6 weeks. Improved techniques over the past few years have reduced many of the unwanted side-effects of cranial irradiation, although lethargy, hair loss, and minor radiation damage to the scalp are seen almost invariably.

The tumours showing the greatest sensitivity to radiotherapy are medulloblastoma and pineal germinoma. Ependymomas and cystic

Table 3 Treatment and prognosis of the more common intracranial tumours

Tumour	Commonest surgical procedure	Effect of radiotherapy	Prognosis
Glioblastoma	Biopsy or partial removal	Minimal	Less than 20 per cent 1-year survival rate
Astrocytoma	Biopsy or subtotal removal, decompression	Variable, average of 10 per cent increase in survival	Up to 50 per cent 5-year survival rate reported
Oligodendroglioma	Biopsy or subtotal removal	Given for 'recurrent' tumour; marginal effect	55 per cent 10-year survival rate; tend to undergo malignant change
Cerebellar cystic astrocytoma	Complete removal	Not generally used	Over 70 per cent recurrence-free
Ependymoma	Radical removal, possibly with shunt	Variable, probably sensitive	30–40 per cent 5-year survival rate
Medulloblastoma	Radical removal, possibly with shunt	Whole neuraxis irradiation improves survival	Average survival about 1 year, recent reports much more favourable
Haemangioblastoma	Complete removal, possibly with shunt	Not generally used	15 per cent recurrence; excellent prognosis if totally removed
Meningioma	Complete removal	Minimal effect	10 per cent recurrence after 'total' removal; occasionally frankly malignant
Acoustic schwannoma (neuroma)	Complete removal	Not used	Excellent prognosis if totally removed; high rate of recurrence with subcapsular removal
Craniopharyngioma	Complete removal or subtotal removal	Given after subtotal removal; claims of less than 10 per cent 5-year recurrence	10 per cent 5-year recurrence after total removal, but high risk of endocrine dysfunction
Pituitary adenoma	Transnasal microadenectomy; transfrontal craniotomy for mainly suprasellar tumours; total removal by trans-sphenoidal or transethmoidal routes	Given for invasive or recurrent tumour Variable response, probably beneficial	About 12 per cent recurrence after surgery and radiotherapy

Tables 2 and 3 are derived from tables published in *Medicine International* and reproduced with kind permission of Medical Education (International) Ltd.

astrocytomas of the cerebellum show variable sensitivity but postoperative radiotherapy is generally advised, particularly if surgical excision is judged not to have been complete.

Craniopharyngioma, optic glioma, and hypothalamic gliomas are usually irradiated, most frequently following some form of surgery. Potential radiation damage due to the visual pathways, pituitary, and hypothalamus, however, has to be balanced against a low risk of recurrence in cases in which there has been complete surgical excision. Cases of pituitary invasive adenoma that have been treated by partial surgical excision are generally given postoperative radiotherapy. Similarly, certain forms of metastatic tumour may be given postoperative irradiation when the primary tumour is known to be radiosensitive.

The role of radiotherapy in the treatment of malignant gliomas is uncertain.

Chemotherapy

Various forms of chemotherapy may have a place in the treatment of secondary deposits within the brain (e.g. *cis*-platinum in the treatment of seminoma; the nitrosoureas, vincristine, and procarbazine in secondary lymphoma) but there is no real evidence as yet to suggest that chemotherapy has any large part to play in the treatment of primary intracranial tumours. The management of cerebral leukaemia and lymphoma is considered further in Section 3.

Prognosis and long-term management

The prognosis relating to most of the common intracranial tumours is given in Table 3. Patients with glioblastomas have a mean survival time of only 6 to 12 weeks from presentation. Patients with low-grade tumours have a mean survival of about 9 months following surgery and radiotherapy, although there have been reports of up to 50 per cent 5-year survival in grade I cases.

Meningiomas, apparently completely resected, are still associated with a 5 to 10 per cent recurrence rate within 10 years, and this rises to over 20 per cent symptomatic recurrence if fragments of tumour are known to have been left behind. Cerebellar astrocytomas and haemangioblastomas are associated with a good prognosis after complete removal, although occasionally cerebellar astrocytoma may act in a more malignant fashion.

Patients with intracranial tumours, particularly those associated with large amounts of cerebral oedema, are generally kept on steroid medication throughout their course of surgery and on a lower dose during their course of radiotherapy. They will need to be warned about the potential side-effects of steroids. Some patients with malignant gliomas or with inoperable recurrent tumour who have some evidence of raised intracranial pressure but without rapidly progressive focal deficit may also be treated with dexamethasone. However, the long-term use of steroids in these instances should be avoided as they certainly become less effective after a few weeks.

Patients should also be warned of the possible social consequences of their tumour and its treatment, with particular reference to driving. Patients with benign supratentorial lesions who have undergone major surgery will normally be banned from driving in the UK for 1 year following operation even if they have suffered no fits. Drivers of heavy goods vehicles may well have their licences withdrawn permanently.

Further reading

Darling, J.L. and Wan, T.J. (1998). Biology and genetics of malignant brain tumours. *Current Opinion in Neurology*, 11,619–25.

Lagerwaard, F.J., Levendag, P.C,, Nowak, P.J., *et al.* (1999). Identification of prognostic factors in patients with brain metastases: a review of 1292 patients. *International Journal of Radiation Oncology, Biology, Physics*, 43, 795–803.

Shapiro, W.R. (1999). Current therapy for brain tumours: back to the future. *Archives of Neurology*, 56, 429–32.

Chapter 13.23

Benign intracranial hypertension

N. F. Lawton

Benign intracranial hypertension is a syndrome of raised intracranial pressure occurring in the absence an intracranial mass lesion or enlargement of the cerebral ventricles due to hydrocephalus. Synonyms include idiopathic intracranial hypertension and pseudotumour cerebri. Although rarely life threatening, the rise in intracranial pressure may result in permanent visual loss due to optic nerve damage.

Incidence

Benign intracranial hypertension is a rare disease. It is more common in females, the preponderance over males ranging from 3:1 to 8:1. Although it may occur in infants and elderly people, it is primarily a disease of young women between the ages of 17 and 44 years.

Clinical features

The presenting symptoms and signs are those of raised intracranial pressure alone. The diagnosis should not be entertained in the presence of neurological features that suggest a focal lesion. Furthermore, there is a remarkable preservation of consciousness and intellectual function rarely encountered in patients with mass lesions or hydrocephalus. Preservation of cerebral function also distinguishes this disorder from viral or bacterial meningoencephalitis. Patients with benign intracranial hypertension are unlikely to present as medical emergencies.

Headache is the most common symptom, usually having been present for weeks or months. Characteristically it is typical of raised intracranial pressure. Obesity is sufficiently common to be a characteristic feature.

Papilloedema is a virtually universal finding and the importance of fundus examination in every patient with headache cannot be overemphasized. The classical symptom of papilloedema, which is not specific to benign intracranial hypertension, is a transient obscuration of vision. Obscurations may be provoked by straining or a change in posture, but may also occur spontaneously. Occasionally, sudden and permanent loss of vision results from infarction of the optic nerve.

Visual-field analysis is the essential investigation in the diagnosis and follow up of patients with benign intracranial hypertension. The most common defects are enlargement of the blind spots, generalized constriction of the fields, and scotomas caused by damage to the optic nerve.

About 30 per cent of patients complain of horizontal diplopia due to VIth nerve palsy, which may be bilateral. The cause is a false localizing sign of raised intracranial pressure.

Aetiology

In the majority of patients with benign intracranial hypertension no cause can be identified. Known associations are rare, with the exception of obesity in up to 90 per cent of patients. Both vitamin A deficiency and excessive vitamin A intake are well documented, though rare, causes. Treatment for acne with combined tetracycline and retinoids, which are vitamin A derivatives, is an important iatrogenic cause. Occasionally the condition is familial.

Dural sinus thrombosis

A syndrome resembling benign intracranial hypertension may occur following venous thrombosis in dural sinuses or in the extracranial jugular system. Sinus thrombosis may complicate pregnancy, the use of oral contraceptives, venous occlusive disease due to hypercoagulability states, or mediastinal obstruction. Sinus thrombosis should be suspected clinically when the onset of headache is sudden and accompanied by focal signs, seizures, or impaired consciousness. In classical benign intracranial hypertension, venous obstruction is not the predisposing cause and the cerebral venous system is patent at angiography.

Pathogenesis

The mechanism by which intracranial pressure rises is poorly understood and the contribution of various factors controversial. Since the intracranial contents are housed in a rigid container, an increase in cerebrospinal fluid pressure may result from an increase in blood volume, swelling of the brain parenchyma, or an increase in the volume of cerebrospinal fluid due to overproduction or malabsorption. A failure of absorption of cerebrospinal fluid via the arachnoid villi is the favoured hypothesis.

Investigations

The diagnosis can only be confirmed by measurement of cerebrospinal fluid pressure, but in suspected cases it is essential to exclude a mass lesion or hydrocephalus before proceeding to lumbar puncture. Characteristically, CT scanning shows small and slit-like cerebral ventricles, which may increase in volume as the intracranial hypertension resolves. A similar appearance is seen on MRI. Angiography is usually required, however, if sinus thrombosis is suspected. Currently the preferred technique is by digital-subtraction angiography following intravenous contrast injection, but MR angiography promises to avoid the need for contrast injection.

At lumbar puncture the opening pressure is greater than 200 mm cerebrospinal fluid but it is important to note that in simple obesity the cerebrospinal fluid pressure may be as high as 250 mm. The diagnostic significance of cerebrospinal fluid pressure must therefore be correlated with the clinical picture. In the few patients whose cerebrospinal fluid pressure is equivocal, continuous monitoring may demonstrate intermittent peaks of raised pressure.

The composition of the cerebrospinal fluid is entirely normal, and the presence of white cells or a raised protein concentration casts serious doubt on the diagnosis. An exception to this rule is the rare syndrome resembling benign intracranial hypertension that occurs in association with postinfective polyneuropathy and with spinal tumours. Both conditions may lead to raised intracranial pressure with papilloedema and normal-sized ventricles but a marked rise in protein in the cerebrospinal fluid.

Management

This is aimed at the reduction of intracranial pressure to protect vision and relieve headache. The methods available are difficult to evaluate because of the high rate of spontaneous remission and the lack of controlled trials. Choice of treatment is further complicated by the absence of reliable risk factors for visual loss. In particular, the height of the cerebrospinal fluid pressure at diagnosis is of no prognostic significance.

In the past, repeated therapeutic lumbar puncture every 2 to 5 days was shown to reduce cerebrospinal fluid pressure temporarily and could occasionally lead to spontaneous remission. When acute medical treatment is indicated, prednisolone (40–60 mg daily) is effective in relieving headache and visual obscuration due to papilloedema. However, steroids are unsatisfactory as long-term treatment because of their complications, especially in obese young females. For this reason, diuretics are widely used in patients with mild symptoms. Acetazolamide or a thiazide diuretic may relieve headache, but the efficacy of diuretics in preventing slowly progressive visual loss is unproved.

Because of the limitations of medical treatment, an increasing number of patients are treated surgically, progressive loss of visual field and unrelieved headache being the indications for operation. Because of the difficulty of tapping small cerebral ventricles, a lumboperitoneal shunt is usually favoured. Unfortunately, the technical failure rate of these shunts is high and surgical revision may be required in up to 20 per cent of patients. For this reason the alternative surgical procedure in which the optic nerve is decompressed by fenestration of the nerve sheath has recently been revived.

Currently it would seem reasonable to begin treatment with diuretics, reserving steroids as a temporary medical treatment in patients with severe symptoms. If surgery becomes necessary, lumpoperitoneal shunting is the logical procedure, with resort to fenestration of the optic nerve sheath in the event of repeated shunt failure.

Although the efficacy of weight loss *per se* has not yet been established, a weight-reducing diet is recommended in obese patients.

Prognosis

Benign intracranial hypertension is a chronic condition in most patients but spontaneous relapse and remission of symptoms is common. There is evidence that raised intracranial pressure may be found at follow-up lumbar puncture in patients whose symptoms have been in remission for several years. Permanent visual loss occurs in up to 50 per cent of patients and is a significant disability in 10 per cent.

Further reading

Johnson, L.N., Krohel, G.B., Madsen, R.W., *et al.* (1998). The role of weight loss and acetazolamide in the treatment of idiopathic intracranial hypertension (pseudotumour cerebri). *Ophthalmology*, **105**, 2313–7.

Soler, D., Cox, T., Bullock, P., *et al.* (1998). Diagnosis and management of benign intracranial hypertension. *Archives of Disease in Childhood*, **78**, 89–94.

Chapter 13.24

Head injuries

G. M. Teasdale

Each year in the UK one million head-injured patients attend hospital. Fortunately most injuries prove to be mild: 80 per cent of patients have not even been 'knocked out', only 1 in 5 is admitted to hospital and most of these stay for less than 48 h. Nevertheless, some 5000 patients die each year and many others survive with mental disability.

The pathology of head injury

Scalp and skull injury

A scalp laceration is present in about 40 per cent of patients who attend hospital but a skull fracture is found in only 1.5 per cent. Although each feature can indicate the location and severity of impact on the head, this is less important diagnostically than the contribution they make to establishing that a head injury has occurred—if a history is not available—and the clue they provide to the risk of subsequent complications. The excellent healing of the scalp after surgical toilet and closure reflects its generous blood supply, but this can sometimes result in a laceration bleeding so profusely that shock ensues. This risk is highest in children or elderly people with extensive scalp injuries.

A skull fracture is described by several features: (1) location—the vault of the cranial cavity, the posterior fossa, or the base of the skull; (2) shape—linear (fissure) or comminuted into fragments; (3) if the fragments are depressed inwards; (4) if it is open or compound, i.e., associated with a local wound that creates a passage between the exterior and the interior of the cranial cavity.

Traumatic brain damage (Table 1)

A certain amount of brain damage is sustained at the time of injury and in a closed, non-missile injury is the result of shear strains

Table 1 Traumatic brain damage

Primary (impact) damage
Diffuse: axonal injury
Focal: cortical contusion and lacerations
Secondary complications
Extracranial: hypoxia, hypotension
Intracranial: haematoma, infection
Consequences of complications
Brain swelling, raised intracranial pressure
Brain shift
Hypoxic/ischaemic brain damage

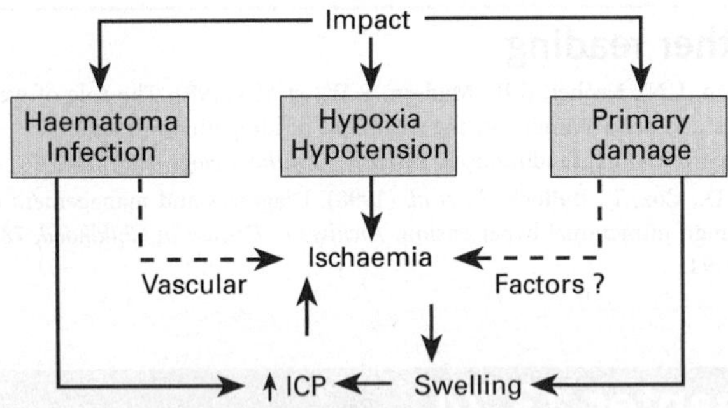

Fig. 1 Interactions between impact brain damage and the complications leading to secondary ischaemic brain damage. ICP, intracranial pressure.

occurring within the head at the moment of impact. More important than such primary damage, at least from the point of view of early management, are the complications that lead to secondary brain damage. In a severe injury it is common for more than one disorder to be present; indeed the interactions between the various pathophysiological processes illustrated in Fig. 1 can pose the greatest threat to the brain, with ischaemia being the most important final mechanism in most cases.

Primary

Diffuse axonal injury

This results when the shear strains between different parts of the brain cause distortion, stretching, and even tearing of the axons in the white matter of the cerebral hemispheres and brainstem. The tiny neuronal lesions that result are distributed widely and diffusely, and it is now believed that the number of these lesions and whether or not they are reversible or permanent are the main determinants of the initial severity of a head injury. Clinically their characteristic feature is an immediate impairment of consciousness. In its most mild form, this may be restricted to a transient loss of awareness and memory for a few minutes, classically referred to as 'concussion'. At the other extreme the patient may be in profound and prolonged coma. Diffuse white-matter lesions are also thought to underlie many of the symptoms and much of the disability that follows when consciousness is ultimately recovered.

Contusions and lacerations

These are found focally, predominantly in the cerebral cortex. Whatever the site of a blow on the head, the subsequent contusions are located maximally on the undersurfaces of the frontal and temporal lobes, and are due to displacement of the brain and contact with the sharp bony ridges at the base of the skull.

Secondary

Secondary brain damage develops after a delay and should be treatable or preventable. The damage to the brain is ultimately the result of ischaemia, usually either a consequence of impaired oxygenation of the blood or an inadequate cerebral blood flow.

Intracranial complications

Traumatic intracranial haematoma

An extradural haematoma is usually associated with a skull fracture and is the result of bleeding between the site of the fracture and the underlying dura.

Intradural haematomas are more common (three out of four cases). The bleed may be into the subdural space or within the brain itself (intracerebral haematoma); in a third of cases there is a combination of subdural bleeding, cortical laceration, and intracerebral haemorrhage, the so-called burst frontal or temporal lobes. Many patients have a skull fracture but intradural clots often are not closely related to the fracture as are the extradural clots.

Table 2 Risk of an operable intracranial haematoma in head injured patients

GCS	Risk	Other features	Risk
15	1 in 3615	None	1 in : 31 300
		PTA	6700
		Skull fracture	81
		Skull fracture and PTA	29
9–14	1 in 51	No fracture	1 in :180
		Skull fracture	: 5
3–8	1 in 7	No fracture	1 in : 27
		Skull fracture	: 4

GCS, Glasgow Coma Scale. PTA, post-traumatic amnesia.

Blood vessels giving rise to a traumatic intracranial haematoma probably are damaged at the time of injury, but some time is needed before the size of the haematoma is sufficient to exhaust the brain's capacity to compensate for a space-occupying lesion. There then ensues a combination of shift and mechanical distortion of the brain, and also an impairment of cerebral blood flow secondary to the rise in intracranial pressure. The most important clinical characteristic of the resulting cerebral ischaemia is a deteriorating level of consciousness.

The interval between injury and deterioration is usually measured in hours or days, but may be as short as a few minutes or occasionally as long as a few weeks. During this period the patient is rarely completely well, most have persisting confusion or altered consciousness as a result of a degree of primary damage.

Risk of a haematoma

During this 'silent' interval, information about the presence or absence of a skull fracture and whether or not the patient is fully conscious can be used to estimate the risk of their later developing a haematoma. (The data for an adult are shown in Table 2.) More profound degrees of impairment of consciousness carry much greater risks. Even without a fracture, persisting coma carries a risk of a haematoma of 1 in 4.

Infection

Meningitis and brain abscess are complications of either a compound depressed fracture of the vault of the skull or an open fracture of the base of the skull. Infection may develop several days, weeks, or sometimes years after the injury.

Other neurological complications

The damaged brain around a contusion or underneath a blood clot may become progressively swollen; this can also occur diffusely in one or both cerebral hemispheres. Other structures that may be damaged in a head injury include the cranial nerves (especially the olfactory, optic, oculomotor, facial, and auditory nerves), and, in severe injuries, the pituitary gland and hypothalamus. Deafness and dizziness may also be caused by damage to the structures of the middle and inner ear, either as a result of the initial forces of the injury or a fracture of the base of the skull.

Management in the acute stage

Resuscitation

The ABC of resuscitation is the priority in those patients who arrive at hospital in coma, or who have multiple injuries. The *a*irway must be cleared and maintained free from the earliest possible moment. As a temporary measure this may be achieved by placing the patient in the semiprone position; later the use of oropharyngeal or endotracheal tubes may be necessary. If *b*reathing proves inadequate, particularly as judged by abnormal blood-gas values, mechanical ventilation may be necessary. Restoration of an adequate *c*irculation is essential; hypotension is rarely the result of a head injury alone and should be a signal to search for serious extracranial injuries.

Diagnosis

In a patient with impaired consciousness an accurate initial diagnosis can be difficult but it is important to discover the answers to two questions. Has the patient had a head injury? Has the patient had only a head injury? Common errors include the misdiagnosis of a head-injured patient as being 'drunk' or suffering from a stroke, or the overlooking of major injuries elsewhere in the body in a patient with an obvious head injury.

Assessing brain damage and its evolution

Changes in the level of consciousness are more important than focal neurological signs and provide an overall index of brain dysfunction and damage. Repeated assessments of the degree of altered consciousness provide a guide to the initial severity of brain damage and to the pattern of recovery. When a patient has suffered only primary damage, a steady improvement can be anticipated; if the patient's consciousness does not improve, and particularly if there is deterioration, the occurrence of secondary damage should be suspected.

It is therefore important to learn as much as possible about the immediate effects of the injury on conscious level and to reassess consciousness frequently. Communication of such information is made simpler by the use of the Glasgow coma scale (see Chapter 13.13). Comparisons of the movements and power of the limbs can be useful clues to focal damage, but tendon and plantar reflexes are rarely helpful. Changes in the response of the pupil to light are an important sign of dysfunction of the IIIrd cranial nerve, and of developing intracranial shift and brainstem compression.

Radiological investigations

A skull radiograph can provide helpful information because the finding of a fracture greatly increases the risk of intracranial complications. Fractures of the vault are readily shown in radiographs but fractures in the base of the skull can be difficult to detect because some bones are paper thin and others extremely thick and dense. Suspicion should be raised by the finding of intracranial air or fluid levels in the paranasal air sinuses.

A skull radiograph is not needed for all head injuries; clinical criteria that help to select patients for radiography are shown in Table 3. Whenever there is a question of multiple injuries, additional plain radiographs of the cervical spine, chest, and pelvis should be taken.

CT scanning

CT scanning (Fig. 2) can detect only the more severe forms of primary brain damage but its ability to show very clearly the presence of a haematoma has transformed the management of head injuries. Selection of patients for CT scanning is discussed below.

Table 3 Indications for skull radiograph after recent head injury

A. Orientated patient • History of loss of consciousness or amnesia • Suspected penetrating injury • CSF or blood loss from nose or ear • Scalp laceration (to bone or > 5 cm long) bruise or swelling • Violent mechanism of injury • Persisting headache and/or vomiting • In a child, fall from a significant height (which depends in part on the age of the child) • and/or on to a hard surface; tense fontanelle; suspected non-accidental injury,
B. Patient with impaired consciousness or neurological signs • All patients unless urgent CT is performed or transfer to neurosurgery is arranged

Note: Skull radiograph is not necessary if CT is to be performed.

Table 4 Guidelines for patients in coma or with possible multiple injuries

1. Assess for respiratory insufficiency, for shock, and for internal injuries, especially after a high-velocity injury, e.g. a road traffic accident
2. Perform: (a) chest radiograph; (b) blood gas estimation; (c) cervical spine radiograph; (d) other investigations as relevant
3. Appropriate treatment may include: Intubate (e.g. if airway obstructed or threatened) Ventilate (e.g. cyanosis, Pa_{O_2} <60 mmHg, Pa_{CO_2} >45 mmHg Commence IV infusion (1500 ml/24 h) Mannitol, only after consultation with neurosurgeon Application of cervical collar or cervical traction Immobilization of fractures, treatment of internal injuries
4. If accepted for transfer the patient should be accompanied by personnel able to insert or to reposition an endotracheal tube, and to initiate or to maintain ventilation

Management of intracranial complications

Intracranial haematoma

Until recently the diagnosis of an intracranial haemorrhage rested mainly upon finding evidence of deteriorating responsiveness. The capacity of CT scanning to enable diagnosis before deterioration becomes advanced and before cerebral compression becomes irreversible has provided the opportunity for more effective intervention.

The data about a skull fracture, the patient's initial conscious level, and the risk of a haematoma (Table 2) provide a basis for guidelines about which patients may merit admission for observation, which can be sent home, and those for whom CT scanning should be arranged without delay.

The outcome of operation for an extradural haematoma is usually good, but with a mortality of 10 to 15 per cent. Although an intradural clot is more often associated with primary brain damage and mortality is 30 to 40 per cent, prompt evacuation is also usually followed by recovery.

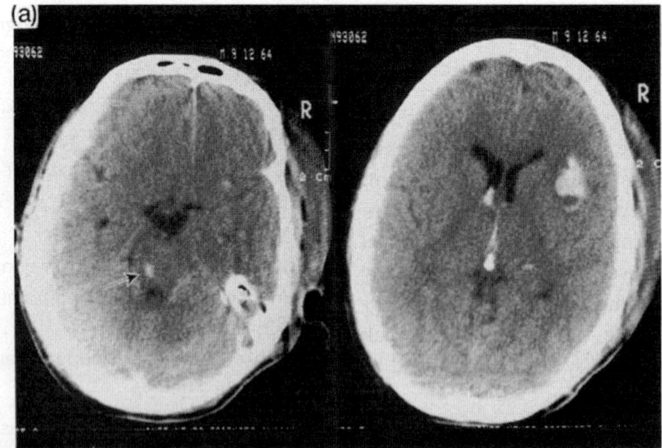

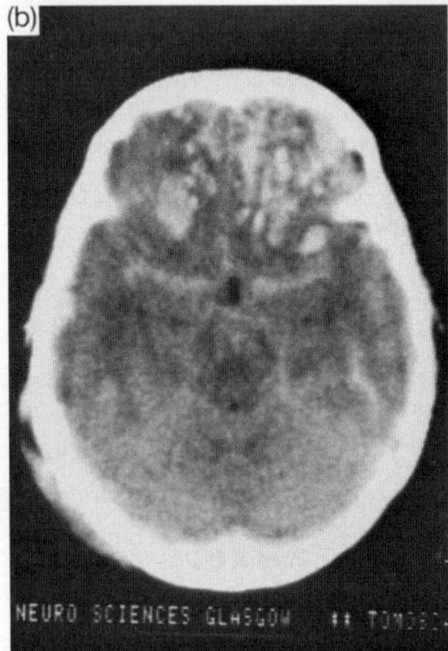

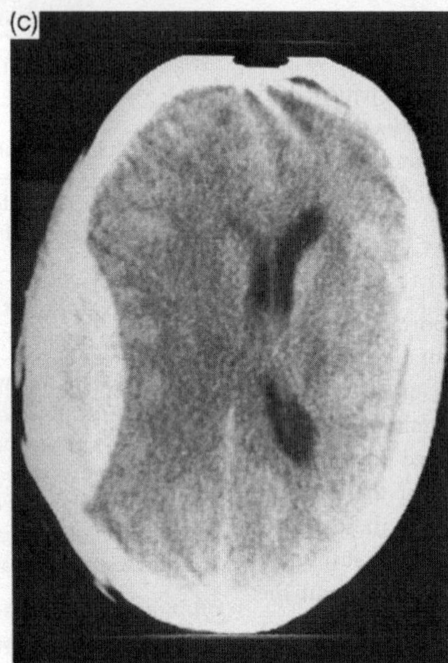

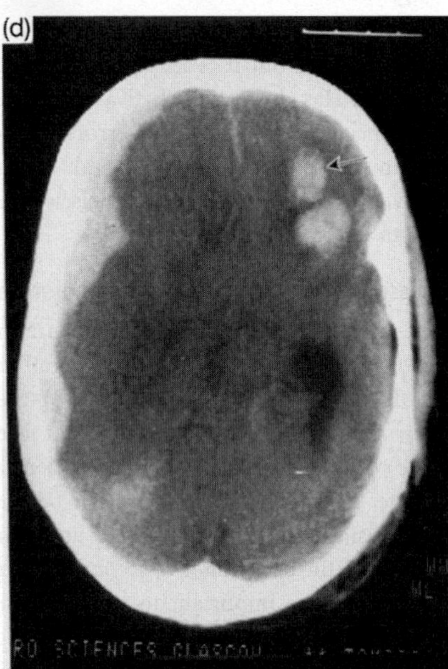

Fig. 2 CT images of head injury: (a) small areas of bleeding (white lesions) in the basal ganglia and brainstem (arrowed) of a patient with severe diffuse axonal injury; (b) contusions in the cortex of frontal and temporal lobes; (c) an extradural haematoma; (d) subdural and intracerebral (arrowed) bleeding.

Depressed skull fracture

Open fractures of the vault of the skull require surgical debridement and closure both of the skin and of the dura. The dura forms a very good barrier to subsequent infection. If the operation is carried out within the first 24 h the risk of infection is minimal, but heavily contaminated wounds are treated with prophylactic antibiotics.

Cerebrospinal fluid leakage and basal fracture

Such injuries are often associated with substantial primary damage to the brain but many of these fractures heal spontaneously. Therefore it is usual to delay operation and to close the fistula only in patients whose cerebrospinal fluid leak persists for more than a week. Most British neurosurgeons recommend prophylactic antibiotic treatment during this period.

Multiple injuries

It is vital to diagnose and treat these injuries in order to stabilize the general condition of the head-injured patient; this takes priority over investigation and operation on intracranial injuries, and is particularly important in victims of high-speed road traffic accidents. Table 4 shows the recommendations given to hospitals in the West of Scotland for the assessment and management of patients in coma or with multiple injuries prior to transfer to the neurosurgical unit.

Ventilation

This is necessary in patients whose respiratory dysfunction threatens adequate oxygenation; this may be the result of inadequate ventilation, due to airway obstruction or thoracic injury, for example, or of inadequate gas exchange—atelectasis from aspiration of blood or gastric contents. Hyperventilation lowers cerebral blood volume and hence intracranial pressure, but can also reduce cerebral blood flow so that ischaemia develops; it is now used selectively and as briefly as possible.

Osmotic agents

Agents such as mannitol or frusemide (furosemide) are given intravenously to remove water from the brain and effectively lower intracranial pressure. They can be useful in producing a temporary improvement, for example to buy sufficient time to allow definitive intracranial investigation, but repeated doses lose efficacy and may result in hypovolaemia with reduced cerebral perfusion pressure, as well as leading to electrolyte imbalance.

Late sequelae and disability after head injury

Amnesia

Recovery from altered consciousness is usually followed by a period of confusion and loss of memory. The time from the injury to the restoration of continuing memory is referred to as post-traumatic amnesia and its duration provides a good index, albeit in retrospect, of the severity of brain damage. Some loss of memory for events immediately prior to the injury is common, but such retrograde amnesia is usually relatively brief and shrinks as time passes.

Postconcussional symptoms

Even an apparently mild injury can be followed by a variety of symptoms, including headache, dizziness, failure of concentration, and impairment of memory. Because physical signs may be lacking, and any abnormalities are often subtle, the basis of these symptoms has been in debate. There is now evidence that periods of loss of consciousness of even as little as 5 min can result in diffuse axonal brain damage. In many patients the symptoms resolve spontaneously, if sometimes slowly, but they can be perpetuated by premature return to 'stressful' work or by other causes of anxiety or depression.

Disability after severe injury

Prolonged loss of consciousness in the early stage increases the risk of persisting disabilities, and these are almost invariable when post-traumatic amnesia has been longer than a month. Obvious physical deficits, such as hemiparesis and ataxia, are less common and much less important than changes in mental function, and particularly in memory and personality.

Post-traumatic epilepsy (see also Chapter 13.11)

Epilepsy occurring within 1 week of a head injury is distinguished from that developing later, which is more likely to recur. The main pointers to the risk of late epilepsy are the presence, in the acute stage, of an intracranial haematoma, a compound depressed skull fracture, particularly with dural laceration, and amnesia for more than 24 h. If any of these are present, the patient should be advised to seek the approval of the Department of Transport before re-commencing driving.

Chronic subdural haematoma

A fluid collection of blood between the dura and the brain can follow even a relatively mild head injury, particularly in elderly people, alcoholics, or those with impaired coagulation function. In about half of cases no injury is recalled. Symptoms may occur hours or even months after the injury. Particularly in the elderly individual, however, the trivial injury is frequently forgotten. The most common symptom is headache and, as the condition worsens, vomiting. The most common neurological signs are pupillary inequality, and long-tract signs with motor limb asymmetry and, occasionally, an extensor plantar response. Dysphasia occurs in about a fifth of patients. Fits are less common, although they occurred in approximately 5 to 10 per cent of cases in one large series.

In the majority of cases, the condition can be diagnosed by CT scanning, although, because the subdural collection may be isodense at some stage during its evolution, the interpretation can be difficult. The treatment of choice is to evacuate the haematoma through burr holes. It is possible that very small collections can be allowed to resolve under careful surveillance. Importantly, the prognosis is not related to age and therefore this condition should be sought and treated actively in all age groups.

Hydrocephalus

Hydrocephalus very occasionally results from an obstruction of the cerebrospinal fluid pathways and should not be confused with the passive, *ex vacuo* ventricular enlargement that occurs with cerebral atrophy after a severe head injury. This can be brought about by fibrosis, a sequel to bleeding in the early stages, and such patients may be greatly benefited by insertion of a ventriculoperitoneal shunt in order to divert the cerebrospinal fluid flow.

Further reading

Bartlett, J., Kett-White, R., Mendelow, A.D., Miller, J.D., Pickard, J.D., and Teasdale, G.M. (1998). Guidelines for the initial management of head injuries. Recommendations from the Society of British Neurological Surgeons. *British Journal of Neurosurgery*, **12**(4), 349–52.

Maas A.I.R., *et al.* (1997). EBIC Guidelines for management of severe head injury in adults. *Acta Neurochirugica*, **139**, 286–94.

Teasdale, G.M. (1995). Head injury. *Journal of Neurology, Neurosurgery and Psychiatry*, **58**(5), 526–39.

Clinical presentation of infections of the nervous system

Chapter 13.25

Bacterial meningitis

*D. A. Warrell, D. W. M. Crook, and Prida Phuapradit**

Bacterial, pyogenic, purulent, or cerebrospinal meningitis is an inflammation of the leptomeninges with infection of the cerebrospinal fluid within the subarachnoid space of the brain and spinal cord, and the ventricular system.

Acute bacterial meningitis

Classification

Spontaneous meningitis differs from post-traumatic meningitis following neurosurgery or fracture of the skull, and from meningitis associated with cerebrospinal fluid shunts and drains, in the pattern of its causative organisms, clinical presentation, management, and outcome.

Aetiological agents and epidemiology

Bacteria causing meningitis vary by geographical region and according to the categories mentioned above. Age and local social conditions affect the incidence and mortality of spontaneous meningitis.

Meningitis in neonates and infants up to 3 months old is usually caused by group B streptococci (*Streptococcus agalactiae*), K1 capsulate

*We regret to report the death of Dr Prida Phuapradit in a road traffic accident in 1998.

Escherichia coli, and *Listeria monocytogenes*. Less common causes are *Neisseria meningitidis*, *Strep. pneumoniae*, and *Haemophilus influenzae*.

Spontaneous community-acquired meningitis in children (under 14 years of age) is usually caused by these three. However, the introduction of *H. influenzae* type b (hib) capsular vaccine has dramatically reduced the incidence of meningitis caused by that organism. The highest attack rate of all three bacterial species is in children under 1 year of age and falls off rapidly with increasing age. The decrease in susceptibility to infection by these organisms with increasing age results from the acquisition of protective immunity, mainly through nasopharyngeal carriage.

In adults, 70 to 80 per cent of spontaneous community-acquired meningitis is caused by *N. meningitidis* and *Strep. pneumoniae*. *Listeria monocytogenes*, aerobic Gram-negative bacilli (such as *E. coli*), *H. influenzae*, and *Staphylococcus aureus* cause most of the remaining cases. The attack rate of meningococcal meningitis is usually low (1–5 cases/10^5 persons per year) but may reach epidemic proportions (for example, more than 300 cases/10^5 persons per year). Crowding plays a part in the epidemics occurring in military recruits, South African miners, and other crowded together in closed environments. The incidence of meningococcal infection may increase secondarily to epidemics of influenza A.

The attack rate of *Strep. pneumoniae* meningitis (1–2 cases/10^5 persons per year) is remarkably constant around the world. It increases in patients of advanced age (over 70 years old). Many patients with pneumococcal meningitis have an associated infected focus, such as otitis media or sinusitis (30 per cent) and pneumonia (25 per cent). Hypogammaglobulinaemia (primary or secondary; for example in nephrotic syndrome and chronic lymphocytic leukaemia), sickle-cell disease, and skull trauma (see below) are risk factors.

Streptococcus suis (group R haemolytic streptococcus) is an important cause of meningitis (and rarely infective endocarditis) in the Far East (Hong Kong, Thailand) and in other countries, related to occupational contact with pigs or pork.

Listeria monocytogenes meningitis (attack rate approximately 0.2 to 0.4 cases/10^5 persons per year) is responsible for 1 to 5 per cent of the cases of meningitis. Unpasteurized soft cheeses, pâté, and poorly refrigerated precooked chicken have been implicated. People at the extremes of age, pregnant women, and those on prolonged immunosuppression with corticosteroids or azathioprine are at increased risk. *Staphylococcus aureus* causes 1 to 5 per cent of cases of spontaneous meningitis, usually associated with infective endocarditis. Spontaneous cases of *H. influenzae* meningitis, both capsulate type b and non-capsulate strains, account for up to 5 per cent of adult cases of meningitis. Aerobic Gram-negative (for example *E. coli*) meningitis occurs especially in the aged, debilitated, and diabetic. The source in these infections is probably the renal tract.

Post-traumatic meningitis follows skull fracture and head, neck, or spinal surgery. It is usually associated with a cerebrospinal fluid leak and arises soon after the injury, but may occur many years later. Clinically apparent leakage of cerebrospinal fluid carries a 25 per cent risk of meningitis. Hospital-acquired infections are caused by aerobic Gram-negative bacilli, such as *E. coli*, *Klebsiella pneumoniae*, other Enterobacteriaceae, *Acinetobacter* spp., or *Pseudomonas* spp. Less commonly, *Strep. pneumoniae*, *H. influenzae*, *Staph. aureus*, and other members of the normal flora of the upper respiratory tract cause meningitis in patients in hospital. Community-acquired post-traumatic meningitis is caused by *Strep. pneumoniae* (more than 90 per cent of cases) and *H. influenzae*.

Device-associated meningitis may occur in patients with cerebrospinal fluid drains and shunts. Nosocomial infections are caused by coagulase-negative staphylococci (50–60 per cent) and *Staph. aureus* (15–30 per cent). Aerobic Gram-negative bacilli, *Streptococcus* spp., *Corynebacteria* spp., *Strep. pneumoniae*, *N. meningitidis*, and *H. influenzae* are less commonly implicated.

Recurrent meningitis occurs in patients with an underlying anatomical defect (for example, cerebrospinal fluid leak or spina bifida) or an immunological defect such as hypogammaglobulinaemia and complement deficiencies.

Pathogenesis

The neonate is infected from the vagina and perineum during delivery, or from the environment soon after birth. An unusual feature of *E. coli* K1 and many *Strep. agalactiae* III strains is their polysialic acid capsules.

Organisms causing spontaneous meningitis are acquired by person-to-person spread. Colonization is followed by invasion. Asymptomatic carriage is sufficient to produce immunity and resistance to disease. The greatest risk of disease, therefore, is in the first few years of life, at a time when the non-immune host first encounters these pathogens. In animal models of *H. influenzae* meningitis the nasopharynx is the probable site of systemic invasion resulting in bacteraemic spread to the cerebrospinal fluid. Invasion of the cerebrospinal fluid is probably dependent on the concentration of organisms in the blood and on the species causing the bacteraemia. Enterococci can cause intense bacteraemia but seldom enter the cerebrospinal fluid, whereas *N. meningitidis*, *H. influenzae*, and *Strep. pneumoniae* frequently invade it. The highly vascular choroid is probably the site of invasion.

Once in the subarachnoid space, bacteria multiply in the cerebrospinal fluid, relatively uninhibited by host defences. Neutrophils rapidly accumulate in the infected fluid but have little inhibitory effect on the growth of the infecting bacteria in experimental animals. The concentration of complement in cerebrospinal fluid is too low to have much antibacterial effect. The pneumococcal cell wall is a potent inducer of inflammation, which can be attenuated by cyclo-oxygenase inhibitors, suggesting that prostaglandins are involved. The role of cytokines in the cerebrospinal fluid is not clear, but the pneumococcal cell wall is a potent inducer of systemic interleukin 1, but not of tumour necrosis factor. The main bacterial component responsible for inducing inflammation in *H. influenzae* type b meningitis is lipopolysaccharide (endotoxin), a potent inducer of interleukin 1 and tumour necrosis factor in cerebrospinal fluid. Certain antibiotics that enhance the release of lipopolysaccharides may temporarily exaggerate the inflammatory reaction in a type of Jarisch–Herxheimer reaction.

The permeability of the blood–brain barrier and antibiotic penetration of the cerebrospinal fluid are increased. Increased intracranial pressure results from cerebral oedema secondary to the accumulation of interstitial fluid. Communicating hydrocephalus results from decreased reabsorption of cerebrospinal fluid and cellular swelling secondary to injury. A vasculitis may affect mainly the large vessels traversing the subarachnoid space, disrupting autoregulation of cerebral blood flow. Vessels may become obstructed with thrombus, causing a cerebral infarct. Increased intracranial pressure and vasculitis decrease cerebral perfusion, causing hypoxic brain injury.

Pathology

There is diffuse acute inflammation of the pia arachnoid, with migration of neutrophil leucocytes and exudation of fibrin into the cerebrospinal fluid. Pus accumulates over the surface of the brain, especially around its base, the emerging cranial nerves, and around the spinal cord. The meningeal vessels are dilated and congested, and may be surrounded by pus. Pus and fibrin are found in the ventricles, and there is ventriculitis with subependymal gliosis and loss of ependymal lining. The ventricular system dilates in obstructive or communicating hydrocephalus. Other abnormalities include subdural effusion or empyema, septic thrombosis of the cerebral venous sinuses, subarachnoid haematomas, compression of intracranial structures as a result of intracranial hypertension, and herniation of the temporal lobes or cerebellum. However, pressure coning is rarely found. Death may be attributable to septicaemia. Bilateral adrenal haemorrhage (Waterhouse–Friderichsen syndrome) may be a terminal phenomenon rather than a cause of fatal adrenal insufficiency. Patients with meningococcal septicaemia may develop myocarditis and acute pulmonary oedema. Pericarditis and pericardial effusion occur, particularly in group C meningococcal infections.

Clinical features

Acute bacterial meningitis carries an untreated mortality of 70 to 100 per cent. Early diagnosis and treatment reduces mortality and the incidence of complications. When meningitis is secondary to infection elsewhere, such as pneumococcal pneumonia or *H. influenzae* otitis media, the presenting symptoms may be those of the original infection. The incubation period is only a few days. Progression may be so rapid (*N. meningitidis*) that the patient becomes comatose within a few hours of the first symptoms. Early manifestations include malaise, irritability, fever, usually without rigors, headache, myalgias, vomiting, and diarrhoea. Convulsions occur in infants and children. Headache quickly becomes more severe and is the dominant symptom; photophobia and drowsiness develop later. Diarrhoea, and pain in the calves, are features of meningococcal infection.

Meningism is best elicited by gentle passive flexion or rotation of the neck with the patient lying supine. To elicit Kernig's sign the lower limb is flexed at the hip. The patient with meningism will resist extension of the knee by contracting the hamstring muscles. Patients with marked meningism, especially children, lie with their neck and back fully extended (Fig. 1) as in tetanic opisthotonos. The differential diagnosis of neck stiffness includes cervical adenitis, cervical spondylitis, temporomandibular arthritis, dental problems, and pharyngeal lesions. Patients with other febrile conditions, such as pyelonephritis, may exhibit meningism. The optic fundi must be examined before attempting lumbar puncture. Papilloedema suggests cerebral oedema, cerebral abscess, or a sub- or epidural empyema. The absence of papilloedema does not exclude cerebral oedema, and CT scanning is increasingly performed before proceeding to lumbar puncture. Pulsation of retinal veins excludes intracranial hypertension. Hypertensive retinopathy will suggest hypertensive encephalopathy, and subhyaloid haemorrhages a subarachnoid haemorrhage. The rash of meningococcal infections is petechial, often appearing first on the shins or volar surface of the forearms. Petechiae may be visible on the bulbar and tarsal conjunctiva, and in the palate. An identical rash may occur with echovirus type 9, leptospirosis, *Staph. aureus, Strep. pneumoniae, Strep. suis, H. influenzae, Salmonella typhi*, and other infections, especially in those associated with infective endocarditis. The brownish or reddish, geometrical, vasculitic rash of fulminant meningococcaemia is unmistakable. There is associated profound hypotension, shock with peripheral cyanosis, gangrene of the extremities, and spontaneous systemic bleeding. Herpes labialis is associated with all forms of bacterial meningitis (Fig. 1). Otitis media, sinusitis, mastoiditis, and nasopharyngeal and other possible sites of sepsis must be excluded. Patients with recurrent bacterial meningitis may have a congenital dermal sinus in the midline between head and coccyx, marked by a tuft of long hairs. Watery discharge from the nose or ears may be cerebrospinal fluid: it should be tested for glucose; a basal skull fracture should be excluded.

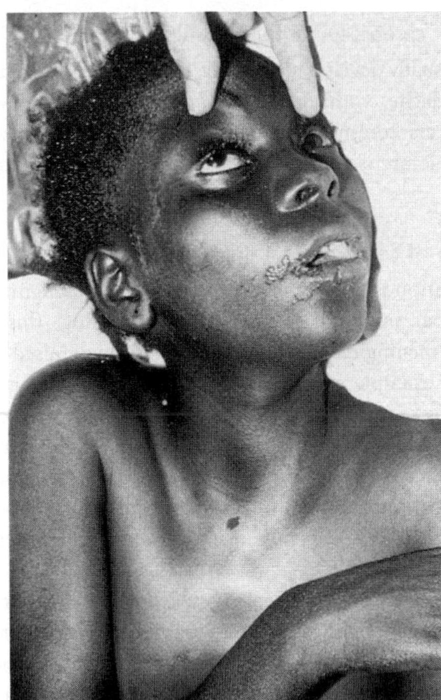

Fig. 1 Nigerian girl in coma with severe meningococcal meningoencephalitis: note head retraction, dysconjugate gaze, and herpes labialis
(copyright D.A. Warrell.)

The most common lesions of cranial nerves are of VI, III, VII, VIII, and II. Patients who become unconscious (meningoencephalomyelitis) may lose all signs of meningism and develop focal neurological signs, focal epileptiform convulsions, dysconjugate gaze, upper motor-neurone signs, and involuntary movements. Vascular lesions may produce hemiparesis or quadriparesis, speech disorders, and visual-field defects. Bilateral sensorineural deafness may develop 2 to 9 days after the start of symptoms; this may be associated with tinnitus and vertigo, and progress to complete deafness within 24 h.

Subdural effusion or empyema is a common complication of *H. influenzae* meningitis in children under 2 years old.

Neonates and infants

Diagnosis is difficult. Infants may become irritable or lethargic, stop feeding, and are found to have a bulging fontanelle, separation of the cranial sutures, meningism, and opisthotonos, and they may develop convulsions. Neonates may present with respiratory distress, diarrhoea, or jaundice.

Post-traumatic meningitis

Fever and a deterioration in the level of consciousness or loss of vital functions may be the only signs of meningitis. A cerebrospinal fluid leak supports a diagnosis of meningitis.

Infections of cerebrospinal fluid shunts

Symptoms usually develop insidiously, with features of shunt blockage such as headache, vomiting, fever, and a decreasing level of consciousness. Less commonly, especially if virulent organisms are involved, the picture is that of acute spontaneous meningitis

Diagnosis

Examination of cerebrospinal fluid

This examination is crucial for the diagnosis of meningitis. The main risk of lumbar puncture is fatal pressure coning; this is rare in spontaneous meningitis. If there is any suggestion of raised intracranial pressure (for example, papilloedema, loss of retinal venous pulsation, focal neurology especially cranial-nerve or brainstem lesions, hypertension, bradycardia, opisthotonos, and coma), CT scanning is indicated to exclude space-occupying lesions or oedema. Contraindications to lumbar puncture include local skin sepsis at the site of puncture, clinical suspicion of spinal-cord compression, and a bleeding diathesis.

A raised white-cell count (pleocytosis) in cerebrospinal fluid is typical of bacterial meningitis. Rarely, the count may be normal (fewer than six lymphocytes/μl). More than 80 per cent of the cells are neutrophils. A predominantly lymphocytic pleocytosis may be found in early bacterial meningitis or *L. monocytogenes* infection. Red blood cells and xanthochromia are sometimes present. Other conditions associated with pleocytosis include early viral meningitis, parameningeal septic foci, meningeal or cerebral tumours, cerebral infarction, chemical meningitis, aseptic meningitis complicating immunoglobulin replacement, cerebral vasculitis, and demyelination.

Gram staining of cerebrospinal fluid reveals organisms in 50 to 80 per cent of cases.

A glucose concentration of less than 40 mg per cent in cerebrospinal fluid is considered low. Since the glucose concentration is related to the serum glucose, a more reliable measure of hypoglycorrhachia (low cerebrospinal fluid glucose) is the ratio of serum to cerebrospinal fluid glucose concentration. A ratio below 0.31 for glucose concentrations of simultaneously obtained serum and cerebrospinal fluid indicates hypoglycorrhachia. Other conditions associated with reduced cerebrospinal fluid glucose are tuberculous, syphilitic, parasitic, fungal, or mumps meningitis, herpes simplex encephalitis, carcinomatous meningitis, meningeal sarcoidosis, postsubarachnoid haemorrhage, severe systemic hypoglycaemia, and rare forms of central nervous vasculitis.

Protein concentration and lactate dehydrogenase activity in cerebrospinal fluid are often raised. Bacterial capsular polysaccharide antigens of pneumococci, meningococci, *H. influenzae*, and group B streptococci may be detected.

Acute viral meningitis is the most common differential diagnosis of bacterial meningitis. The cerebrospinal fluid in viral meningitis typically contains a preponderance of lymphocytes, fewer than 1000 white cells/μl, and a normal glucose.

Other tests

Blood cultures should be taken. CT scanning can reveal shunt obstruction, skull fractures, or parameningeal septic foci such as sinusitis, spinal epidural abscess, or brain abscess.

Differential diagnosis

Meningeal irritation is seen in many acute febrile conditions, especially in children. Tetanus is easily confused with meningitis if the persisting rigidity and recurrent spasms pass unnoticed. In all these conditions the cerebrospinal fluid will be normal. Subarachnoid haemorrhage presents with sudden headache. Intracranial tumours and tuberculous, cryptococcal, and other fungal meningitides usually develop more slowly. Cryptococci and free-living amoebae may be mistaken for lymphocytes in the cerebrospinal fluid unless an India ink preparation is examined. Meningism of aseptic meningitis is associated with abnormalities of the cerebrospinal fluid but no organism is culturable; causes include partially treated bacterial meningitis and chemical meningitides resulting from the introduction of irritants into the subarachnoid space (contrast media, antimicrobial agents, and contaminants of lumbar puncture and spinal anaesthesia). The glucose concentration in cerebrospinal fluid may be very low. Lead encephalopathy may present with meningism, lymphocyte pleocytosis, and an increase in protein in cerebrospinal fluid.

Mollaret's meningitis (benign recurrent aseptic meningitis or benign recurrent lymphocytic meningitis) is an important differential diagnosis of recurrent bacterial meningitis. Herpes simplex viruses type 1 and 2 may be detected by polymerase chain reaction.

Table 1 Recommended immediate antimicrobial treatment by general practitioners in cases of suspected meningococcus meningitis/septicaemia

Antimicrobial	Route	(1)	(2)	(3)
Benzylpenicillin	IV/IM	1.2 g	600 mg	300 mg
Cefotaxime	IV/IM	1.0 g	500 mg	250 mg
Chloramphenicol	IV	1.0 g	500 mg	250 mg

(1) Adults and children 10 years and over; (2) Children 1–9 years; (3) Infants less than 12 months.

Management

Antibiotic treatment must be started immediately the diagnosis is suspected clinically; this is specially important in meningococcal meningitis/septicaemia. The patient should be given benzylpenicillin (intravenous or intramuscular), ceftriaxone or cefotaxime (intravenous or intramuscular), or chloramphenicol (intravenous), preferably after a blood culture has been taken (Table 1). These drugs should be carried by general practitioners in their emergency bags. In hospitals, a lumbar puncture should be performed once a space-occupying lesion has been excluded. Antimicrobial treatment should then be started, based on clinical assessment, before the results of the examination of cerebrospinal fluid are known.

Antimicrobial treatment

Empirical treatment is dictated by the clinical circumstances, the likely causative agents, and their antibiotic susceptibilities (Table 2).

In the community, children are at risk of meningitis caused by *N. meningitidis*, *Strep. pneumoniae*, and, rarely in type b (hib)-vaccinated children, *H. influenzae*. The following three empirical regimens are accepted as effective: ceftriaxone or cefotaxime, plus vancomycin if pneumococcal infection seems likely. Spontaneous meningitis in adults is usually caused by *Strep. pneumoniae* or *N. meningitidis*, but in older (more than 50 years) and chronically immunosuppressed patients, there is an increased risk of *L. monocytogenes* and infection caused by Enterobacteriaceae (for example *E. coli*). In younger adults, ceftriaxone or cefotaxime (plus vancomycin if pneumococcal infection is suspected) can be used. In older and immunosuppressed patients,

Table 2 Empirical treatment of meningitis

Type	Drug	Dose	Frequency	Duration
SPONTANEOUS MENINGITIS				
Childhood	Cefotaxime Ceftriaxone	200mg/kg/day divided IVI 100mg/kg/day given IVI	6 hourly 1 daily	Until organism is isolated OR 2 weeks
Adult	**Prevalence of intermediate penicillin-resistant organisms low and *S. aureus* unlikely**			Until organism is isolated OR 2 weeks
	Penicillin	2.4 g IVI	4 hourly	
	Prevalence of intermediate penicillin-resistant organisms > 5% and *S. aureus* unlikely			
	Cefotaxime or ceftriaxone	2 g IVI 2 g IVI	4 hourly 12 hourly	
	High prevalence of penicillin-resistant pneumococci (MIC > 1 mg/ml)			
	Cefotaxime or ceftriaxone plus vancomycin	1 g IVI	12 hourly (measure levels)	
	Underlying immunosuppression, pregnancy or age > 65 years			
	Ampicillin plus cefotaxime or ceftriaxone	2 g IVI 2 g IVI 2 g IVI	4–4 hourly 4 hourly 12 hourly†	Until organism is isolated OR 3 weeks
POST-TRAUMATIC MENINGITIS				
Community acquired	Treat as for spontaneous meningitis in adults		Until organism is isolated OR 2 weeks	
Nosocomial	**Probability of *Pseudomonas* spp. high**			Until organism is isolated OR 3 weeks
	Ceftazidime	2 g IVI	8 hourly	
	Probability of *Pseudomonas* spp. low	Until organism is		
	Cefotaxime or ceftriaxone	2 g IVI 2 g IVI	4 hourly 12 hourly†	
SHUNT-ASSOCIATED MENINGITIS				
Insidious onset	Vancomycin	1 g IVI and 5–10 g intrathecally	12 hourly 48–72 hourly	Until organism is isolated OR 2 weeks
Acute onset	Treat as for nosocomial post-traumatic meningitis			

Empirical treatment should be started immediately the diagnosis is made, and in this table does not take into account Gram stain of antigen test results. Cultures of blood can usually be obtained before antibiotics are given. If CSF has not already been sample, it should be obtained as soon as possible after starting treatment.

†Once the patient is improving and stable, 2 g IVI may be given once a day.

ampicillin or co-trimoxazole or gentamicin should be added if listeriosis seems possible. Ceftriaxone should be used.

Community-acquired post-traumatic meningitis is caused mainly by *Strep. pneumoniae*, *H. influenzae*, and a wide range of other bacterial species. Cefotaxime or ceftriaxone (plus vancomycin if pneumococcal infection is suspected) plus ampicillin (if listeriosis is suspected) should be given. Nosocomial post-traumatic meningitis is mainly caused by multiresistant hospital-acquired organisms such as *K. pneumoniae*, *E. coli*, *Pseudomonas aeruginosa*, and *Staph. aureus*. Depending on the pattern of susceptibility in a given hospital, ceftazidime (2 g intravenously 8-hourly), cefotaxime, or ceftriaxone should be chosen. If *Ps. aeruginosa* infection seems likely, ceftazidime is preferred.

Device- and shunt-associated meningitis is caused by a wide range of organisms, including methicillin-resistant staphylococci (mostly coagulase-negative) and multiresistant aerobic bacilli. Vancomycin should be given intravenously (1 g 12-hourly) and via the shunt (10 mg), and serum concentrations measured, together with a third-generation cephalosporin such as cefotaxime, ceftazidime (which has antipseudomonal activity), or ceftriaxone in acute cases. The infected shunt or drain should be removed immediately.

Once the aetiological agent has been isolated and its susceptibilities determined, the empirical treatment should be changed, if necessary, to an agent or agents specific for the isolate (Table 3).

General management and treatment of complications

General treatment

Severe headache and pyrexia may require appropriate treatment. In unconscious patients, the airway should be maintained.

Septicaemic patients require careful monitoring and treatment of shock: a combination of fluid administration to expand the intravascular volume, pressors, and inotropic support. Multiple organ failures may require intensive medical support, including ventilation and dialysis.

Treatment of complications

Raised intracranial pressure: raising the head of the bed to 30°, administration of mannitol or dexamethasone, and mechanical hyperventilation may lower intracranial pressure.

Table 3 Specific treatment of meningitis

Type and drug	Dose	Frequency	Duration
Pneumococcal (choice of drug depends on susceptibility tests)			
Penicillin	2.4 g IVI	4 hourly	2 weeks
or			
ceftriaxone	2 g IVI	12 hourly	
or			
cefotaxime	2 g IVI	4 hourly	
or			
vancomycin	1 g IVI	12 hourly	
Meningococcal			
Penicillin	1.4 g IVI	4 hourly	7 days
or			
ampicillin	2 g IVI	4 hourly	
or			
ceftriaxone	2 g IVI	12 hourly	
or			
cefotaxime	2 g IVI	4 hourly	
Haemophilus influenzae			
Ampicillin	2 g IVI	4 hourly	14 days
or			
ceftriaxone	2 g IVI	12 hourly	
or			
cefotaxime	2 g IVI	4 hourly	
Gram-negative bacillary (e.g. *E. coli*)			
Ceftriaxone	2 g IVI	12 hourly	3–4 weeks
or			
cefotaxime	2 g IVI	4 hourly	
Pseudomonas aeruginosa			
Ceftazidime	2 g IVI	8 hourly	3–4 weeks
Listeria monocytogenes			
Ampicillin	2 g IVI	4 hourly	3 weeks
plus			
gentamicin	1 mg/kg IVI	3 hourly	2 weeks
or			
trimethoprim/ sulphamethoxazole*	5 mg/kg trimetho-prim IVI	12 hourly	3 weeks
Staphylococcus aureus			
Flucloxacillin	2 mg IVI	4 hourly	4 weeks
or			
nafcillin	2 mg IVI	4 hourly	

*Trimethoprim/suphamethoxazole is formulated in a fixed ratio of one part trimethoprim and five parts sulphamethoxazole.

Dexamethasone (0.4 mg/kg 12-hourly for 2 days intravenously starting 10 min before the first dose of antibiotic) may reduce the incidence of neurological and audiological sequelae of *H. influenzae* meningitis in children. Some studies have suggested that dexamethasone may reduce the mortality and incidence of permanent sequelae in adult patients with pneumococcal meningitis.

Seizures occur in up to 40 per cent of patients with meningitis. Subclinical fitting should be considered in patients with persisting coma. Seizures can be rapidly controlled using intravenous diazepam or lorazepam. Phenytoin should be used for the longer-term control of seizure activity. Severe cases that fail treatment with these antiepileptic agents should undergo endotracheal intubation and receive high-dose phenobarbitone.

Hyponatraemia may develop as a result of the syndrome of inappropriate antidiuretic hormone secretion. Such cases may require fluid restriction.

Prognosis

In Europe and North America the overall mortality of meningitis caused by *N. meningitidis* is about 7 to 14 per cent; for *H. influenzae*, 3 to 10 per cent; for *Strep. pneumoniae*, 15 to 60 per cent; and for group B streptococci and *L. monocytogenes* meningitis, above 20 per cent. The level of consciousness at presentation has prognostic significance. Other features of bad prognosis are hypertension, seizures, and delay in treatment.

Permanent neurological complications include mental retardation, deafness and other cranial-nerve deficits, and hydrocephalus. The reported incidence of sensorinueural deafness after meningitis ranges from 5 to 40 per cent.

Prevention

Vaccination

Vaccines are available for the three major pathogens causing community-acquired meningitis (see Chapters 16.39, 16.41, and 16.47). Surprisingly, pneumococcal vaccine proved deleterious in human immunodeficiency virus (**HIV**)-seropositive Ugandan adults.

Chemoprophylaxis

Immediate contacts of index cases and of meningococcal *H. influenzae* type b meningitis are at 500- to 1000-fold higher risk of meningitis than the population at large. Rifampicin, ceftriaxone, or ciprofloxacin eliminate the carrier state and presumably the risk of secondary cases of meningitis (see Chapters 16.39, 16.41, and 16.47). In those countries where type b (hib) vaccination has been implemented, the need for chemoprophylaxis is under review. Doctors, nurses, and other health-care workers need not receive chemoprophylaxis unless they have given mouth-to-mouth resuscitation.

Chemoprophylaxis has not proved beneficial in patients with skull fracture and cerebrospinal fluid leak.

Tuberculous meningitis

Most cases of tuberculous meningitis are in young children but primary infection can be acquired at a later age and, in recent years, a larger proportion of patients with tuberculous meningitis have been adults. The disease is uncommon, but severe, in pregnant women.

HIV-infected patients with tuberculosis are at increased risk of meningeal involvement.

Pathogenesis

Small, caseous microtubercles develop in the brain, meninges, skull or vertebrae close to the meninges as a result of seeding through the bloodstream from the primary lesion or a site of chronic infection. Miliary tuberculosis is often associated . Tuberculous meningitis results from rupture of a microtubercle discharging tuberculoprotein and mycobacteria into the subarachnoid space. In sensitized (tuberculin-positive) patients, this causes fever and meningeal irritation. Subacute inflammation, especially of the basal meninges, then develops, producing cranial-nerve lesions, cerebral arteritis causing infarction, impairment of cerebrospinal fluid absorption, or obstruction to the cerebrospinal fluid circulation causing hydrocephalus, and, in the spinal cord, spinal arachnoiditis, producing radiculopathy or myelopathy.

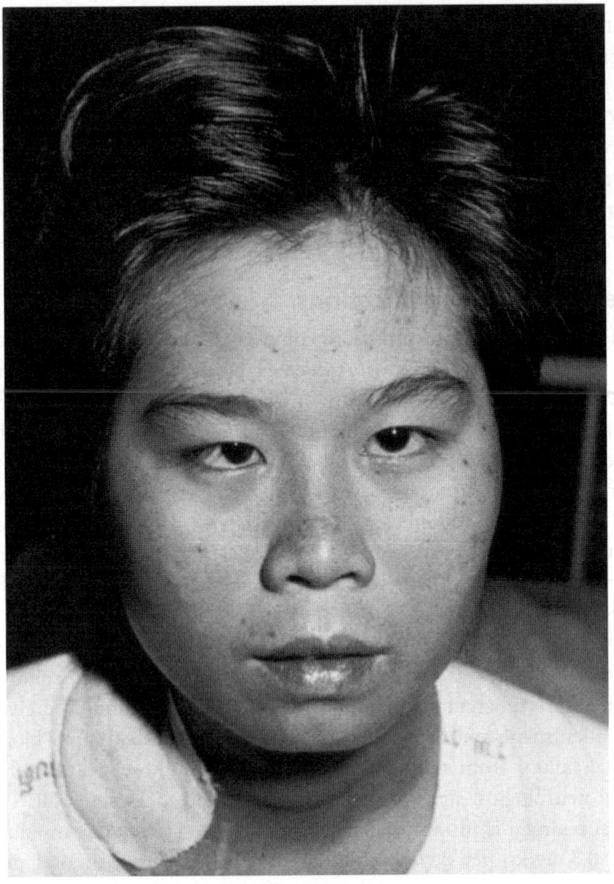

Fig. 2 Bilateral VIth nerve palsies in a Thai girl with tuberculous meningitis; the cervical node biopsy was positive for acid-fast bacilli (copyright Prida Phuapradit.)

Pathology

There are meningeal miliary tubercles on the brain surfaces, especially at the sylvian fissure. There may be larger caseous plaques deeper in the sulci. In fatal cases the brain is oedematous. Thick, greyish exudate encases the base of the brain, filling the basal cisterns and ventricular system and choking the choroid plexus, damaging cranial nerves and obliterating the internal carotid artery and its branches. This exudate contains lymphocytes, plasma cells, giant cells, and foci of caseation, but mycobacteria are usually scanty. Communicating or obstructive hydrocephalus develops in most cases. The exudate may extend into the spinal cord, enveloping the nerve roots, and spinal cord and producing spinal arachnoiditis and spinal block.

Clinical features

Clinical and laboratory features and prognosis in HIV seronegative and seropositive patients with tuberculous meningitis are similar. Symptoms of meningitis are preceded by 2 to 8 weeks of non-specific malaise, irritability, insomnia, lethargy, anorexia, headache, abdominal pain, vomiting, and behavioural changes. Low-grade fever is usual. Half of the patients will have symptoms and signs of tuberculosis in the lungs or elsewhere.

During the second stage there is meningeal irritation (headache, vomiting, neck stiffness), cranial-nerve damage, developing hydrocephalus, and cerebral endarteritis. Infants exhibit irritability, opisthotonos, and a tense fontanelle. In 25 per cent of cases there are lesions of cranial nerves II, III, IV (Fig. 2), VI, VII, and VIII. Pupils may be dilated, unequal, and unresponsive. Papilloedema is observed in 40 per cent and there is sometimes evidence of optic atrophy. Choroid tubercles are occasionally seen. Hydrocephalus often presents with severe headache, ocular palsy, pyramidal signs in the lower limbs, and urinary incontinence. Untreated, patients become stuporose or comatose and develop signs of brainstem damage, such as decerebrate rigidity, irregular breathing, and impairment of brainstem reflexes. About 20 per cent of patients develop focal neurological signs such as hemiparesis, hemianaesthesia, aphasia, and hemianopia resulting from cerebral infarction caused by the endarteritis. Convulsions are common in children but rare in adults. About 10 per cent of patients develop symptoms and signs of spinal arachnoiditis: radicular pain, radicular weakness of the lower limbs, and urinary retention, or paraplegia with sensory loss on the trunk. The syndrome of inappropriate secretion of antidiuretic hormone is common in patients with severe tuberculous meningitis.

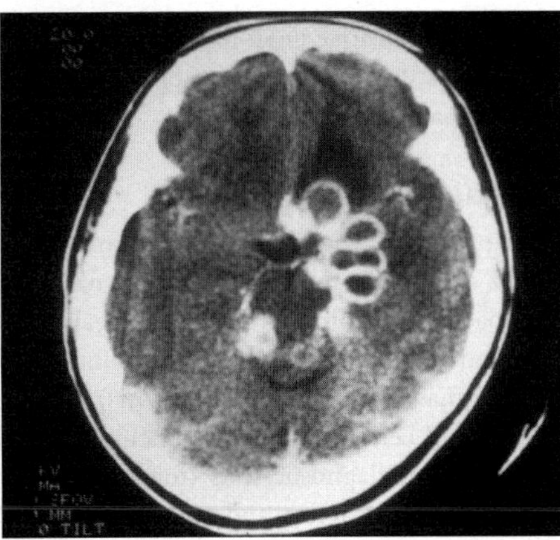

Fig. 3 CT scan with enhancement of a patient with tuberculous meningitis, showing multiple tuberculomas developing near the basal cisterns (copyright Prida Phuapradit.)

Diagnosis

Blood leucocytosis (more than 20 000/μl) or leucopenia is sometimes seen. Examination of cerebrospinal fluid is crucial: its opening pressure is raised in most patients, but may be low in those developing block from spinal arachnoiditis. The cerebrospinal fluid appears clear or slightly turbid but may form a spider's web clot on standing. In patients with spinal block the fluid may be xanthochromic and has a very high protein concentration (Froin's syndrome). Pleocytosis ranges from 10 to more than 1000/μl. Lymphocytes and neutrophils are present. The glucose concentration in cerebrospinal fluid is low in about 90 per cent of patients. Tubercle bacilli can be detected in cerebrospinal fluid by acid-fast, auramine, or fluorescent staining in 10 to 20 per cent of cases. Culture of mycobacteria is successful in 10 to 90 per cent of cases. Specimens other than cerebrospinal fluid (for example sputum, gastric washings in children, urine, etc.) should also be cultured. The genome of *Mycobacterium tuberculosis* can be detected in the cerebrospinal fluid by polymerase chain reaction. A search for evidence of tuberculosis elsewhere in the body is useful. Chest radiographs are normal in about half of the patients, and miliary mottling is seen in only a minority. CT scans are useful in detecting the complications of tuberculous meningitis: communicating hydrocephalus and enhanced basal exudates can be demonstrated in about 80 per cent of the patients (Fig. 3).

The tuberculin test is positive in 50 to 95 per cent of patients with tuberculous meningitis, but reactivity is suppressed in debilitated or immunosuppressed patients.

Differential diagnosis

This includes cryptococcal, coccidioidal, histoplasmal, and candidal meningitides and other subacute or chronic meningitides, such as partially treated bacterial meningitis, parameningeal infections, neoplastic and granulomatous infiltrations of the meninges (for example, carcinomas, leukaemias, lymphomas, sarcoidosis), and cerebral tumours. Examination of cerebrospinal fluid, including cytology, India ink preparation, immunodiagnostic tests (for example, cryptococcal latex agglutination), serological tests and microbial cultures, will allow differentiation.

Treatment

The untreated mortality of tuberculous meningitis is close to 100 per cent. Full treatment must be started when the diagnosis is suspected on clinical grounds. Isoniazid, pyrazinamide, ethionamide, and cycloserine are freely distributed into the cerebrospinal fluid. Penetration is limited, but still adequate during the first few months of the meningitis, in the case of rifampicin, ethambutol, and streptomycin. *p*-Aminosalicylic acid should not be used because it does not enter the cerebrospinal fluid. During the first 2 months, three or four antituberculosis drugs should be given. During this active phase of meningitis, most antituberculosis drugs achieve therapeutic concentrations in the cerebrospinal fluid. The combination of isoniazid and rifampicin for 12 months, with pyrazinamide and streptomycin during the first 2 months, is an effective regimen that has been widely used. In adults, daily single doses of 300 mg isoniazid, 600 mg rifampicin, and 1500 mg pyrazinamide provide adequate concentrations in the serum and cerebrospinal fluid of patients with active tuberculous meningitis.

Intensive short-course chemotherapy with isoniazid, rifampicin, ethionamide, and pyrazinamide for 6 months has also proved successful. Where rifampicin cannot be afforded, triple therapy with isoniazid, pyrazinamide, and streptomycin should be tried. Responses to treatment and the outcome of tuberculous meningitis are similar in HIV seropositive and HIV seronegative patients. Ethionamide, kanamycin or amikacin, and cycloserine should be considered when isolates prove drug resistant.

Response to antituberculosis chemotherapy is slow, particularly in patients who are not given corticosteroids. There may be an increase in temperature and in the protein concentration in cerebrospinal fluid and transient neutrophil pleocytosis during the first 2 months after starting optimal chemotherapy. However, some signs of clinical improvement are usually seen within the first few weeks. Early clinical evidence of response is an improvement of the headache, sense of general well-being, and a decrease in the elevated intracranial pressure. It usually takes weeks or months for the cerebrospinal fluid to return to normal. In some patients the high protein concentration persists. A rapid return to cerebrospinal fluid of normal composition within a few days virtually excludes the diagnosis of tuberculous meningitis, in which case antituberculosis treatment should be stopped.

'Trial' of chemotherapy is justified when there is clinical suspicion of tuberculous meningitis, particularly when diagnostic facilities are limited. Treatment should be continued for 12 months unless there is rapid improvement in the patient's condition and the composition of the cerebrospinal fluid, suggesting another cause for aseptic meningitis. In some severely ill patients who present acutely with features of acute bacterial meningitis (for example, neutrophil pleocytosis) but in whom initial laboratory results are not helpful, it may be necessary to initiate 'blind' treatment for acute bacterial and tuberculous meningitis simultaneously. In these, fortunately rare, cases, isoniazid, rifampicin, and streptomycin or ethambutol, together with penicillin or a third-generation cephalosporin, can be given.

Treatment of complications

Raised intracranial pressure from communicating hydrocephalus can be treated conservatively with repeated lumbar punctures in combination with acetazolamide, with or without frusemide (furosemide), and corticosteroids. Within the first 4 to 6 weeks of treatment, the cerebrospinal fluid pressures of the majority of the patients return to normal and the transependymal oedema (periventricular lucency on the CT scan) disappears. Intrathecal hyaluronidase has proved beneficial in the treatment of communicating hydrocephalus and spinal arachnoiditis. If these measures fail, surgical shunting will be needed.

A recent, large, controlled trial has demonstrated that dexamethasone increases survival and decreases complications in children with severe tuberculous meningitis. Corticosteroids should be given to patients with hydrocephalus, threatened or established spinal block, visual failure from optochiasmic arachnoiditis, those who develop focal neurological signs caused by arteritis, and the severely ill. The usual regimen is intramuscular dexamethasone (16 mg/day in adults and 0.5 mg/kg per day in children) in divided doses, or oral prednisolone 60 mg/day for adults, 2 mg/kg per day for children, given in a tapering course over 3–6 weeks. There is no evidence that corticosteroids interfere with the penetration of antituberculosis drugs into the cerebrospinal fluid. Intrathecal injection of corticosteroids is unnecessary.

Fluid, electrolyte, and acid–base disturbances are common, the result of vomiting, inadequate fluid intake, and the syndrome of inappropriate secretion of antidiuretic hormone. Cerebral tuberculomas may occasionally develop during the course of the treatment of tuberculous meningitis (Fig. 3); they should be treated conservatively and the response to antituberculosis treatment assessed by CT scan. Biopsy or surgical intervention is not necessary and may be harmful. Tuberculomas usually respond very slowly to antituberculosis drugs and it usually takes at least 24 months or longer for the lesions to disappear.

Prognosis

Mortality is about 15–30 per cent in Western countries, and between 30 and 50 per cent in developing countries. The prognosis is worst and the risk of complications highest in those admitted in coma with signs of brainstem damage, in the very young and very old, in pregnant women, and in those with malnutrition or other diseases. There are permanent complications in 10 to 30 per cent of survivors: intellectual impairment, recurrent seizures, blindness, deafness, squints, residual weakness, and persistent spinal block of cerebrospinal fluid.

Prevention (see also Chapter 16.59)

Vaccination with bacillus Calmette–Guérin at birth reduces the risk of infection by at least 80 per cent in some populations. It is recommended for all infants born into communities where tuberculosis is prevalent, including Asians living in Britain and expatriates living in tropical countries. To prevent the development of tuberculous meningitis in household contacts of newly diagnosed cases of pulmonary tuberculosis, prophylaxis with isoniazid 10 mg/kg daily for 6–12 months is recommended for all Mantoux-positive children under the age of 5 years.

Further reading

Acute bacterial meningitis

Bisno, A.L. (1989). Infections of central nervous system shunts. In *Infections associated with indwelling medical devices* (ed. A.L. Bisno and F.A. Waldvogel), pp. 93–109. Washington.

Gray, L.D. and Fedorko, D.P. (1992). Laboratory diagnosis of bacterial meningitis. *Clinical Microbiological Reviews*, **5**(2), 130–45.

Pruitt, A. A. (1998). Infections of the nervous system. *Neurology Clinics*, **16**, 419–47.

Roos, K. L. (1998). Pearls and pitfalls in the diagnosis and management of central nervous system infectious diseases. *Seminars in Neurology*, **18**, 185–96

Schaad, U.B., *et al.* (1993). Dexamethasone therapy for bacterial meningitis in children. *Lancet*, **342**, 457–61.

Scheld, W.M., Whitley, R.J., and Durack, D.T. (1997). *Infections of the central nervous system*, 2nd edn. Lippincott-Raven, Philadelphia.

Townsend, G.C. and Scheld, W. M. (1998). Infections of the central nervous system. *Advances in Internal Medicine*, **43**, 403–47.

Tuberculous meningitis

Alarcon, F., Escalante, L., Perez, Y., Banda, H., Chacon, G., and Duenas, G. (1990). Tuberculous meningitis: short course chemotherapy. *Archives of Neurology*, **47**, 1313–17.

Berenguer, J., *et al.* (1992). Tuberculous meningitis in patients infected with the human immunodeficiency virus. *New England Journal of Medicine*, **327**, 668–72.

Dooley, D.P., Carpenter, J.L., and Rademacher, S. (1997). Adjunctive corticosteroid therapy for tuberculosis: a critical reappraisal of the literature. *Clinics in Infectious Disease*, **25**, 872–87.

Girgis, N.I., *et al.* (1998). Tuberculous meningitis, Abbasia Fenet Hospital – Naval Medical Research Unit No. 3 – Cairo, Egypt from 1976 to 1996. *American Journal of Tropical Medicine Therapy.* 58: 28–34

Parsons, M. (1988). *Tuberculous meningitis. A handbook for clinicians*, 2nd edn. Oxford University Press.

Schoeman, J.F., Donald, P., van Zyl, L., Keet, M., and Wait, J. (1991). Tuberculous hydrocephalus: comparison of different treatments with regard to intracranial pressure, ventricular size and clinical outcome. *Developmental Medicine and Child Neurology*, **33**, 396–405.

Shankar, P., Manijunath, N., Mohan, K.K., Prasad, K., Shriniwas, M.B., and Ahaja, G.K. (1991). Rapid diagnosis of tuberculous meningitis by polymerase chain reaction. *Lancet*, **337**, 5–7.

Chapter 13.26

Viral infections of the central nervous system

D. A. Warrell and P. G. E. Kennedy

Virology

There is considerable geographical and seasonal variation in the incidence of meningitis, myelitis, and encephalitis caused by different viruses.

Enteroviruses cause 80 to 90 per cent of diagnosed cases of viral meningitis. Outbreaks have been associated with coxsackieviruses A7 and 9, all the coxsackie B types, and many echoviruses, especially 4, 6, 9, 11, 14, 16, and 30. Mumps causes about 10 to 20 per cent of cases of viral meningitis. Less common are herpes zoster, herpes simplex (predominantly HSV-2), measles, adenoviruses, Epstein–Barr virus and, in the United States, togaviruses, such as St Louis, eastern and western equine encephalitides, and bunyaviruses, such as California (La Crosse) encephalitis viruses.

Polioviruses remain the leading cause of viral 'paralytic' myelitis outside the Americas, but coxsackie A7 (AB IV) has caused small outbreaks. Other coxsackie A and B viruses, echoviruses, and enterovirus 70 cause sporadic cases. Herpes zoster, paralytic rabies, Epstein–Barr, and *Herpes simiae* B viruses can cause myelitis or ascending paralysis, and HSV-2 can cause lumbosacral myeloradiculitis.

Viruses causing encephalitis vary from country to country. Japanese (B) encephalitis virus is the most widespread human togavirus infection in the world but is confined to Asia, New Guinea, and adjacent islands. In North America, herpes simplex virus is the most common cause of sporadic fatal viral encephalitis, followed by the California encephalitis group, St Louis encephalitis virus, herpes zoster, enteroviruses, mumps, and measles. In the United States, herpes simplex encephalitis has an estimated annual incidence of 2.3/million population. HSV-1 accounts for 95 per cent of cases; HSV-2 causes encephalitis mainly in neonates and those who are immunosuppressed, such as transplant patients and those with AIDS. In the UK, mumps is the most frequently diagnosed viral cause of encephalitis, followed by echoviruses, coxsackieviruses, measles, herpes simplex virus, herpes zoster virus, Epstein–Barr virus, and adenoviruses (especially adenovirus 7). In many developing countries, rabies is an important cause of viral encephalitis.

Postinfectious encephalomyelitis follows measles, vaccinia, varicella, rubella, mumps, and influenza, and nervous-tissue antirabies vaccine. Guillain–Barré syndrome, a sensorimotor polyneuropathy (Chapter 13.30), has complicated infections by Epstein–Barr virus, cytomegalovirus, coxsackie B, and herpes zoster virus, and nervous-tissue antirabies vaccination and vaccination against influenza and smallpox.

Immunodeficient patients with depressed cell-mediated immunity (Hodgkin's disease) may develop herpes zoster encephalitis; those with AIDS may get progressive multifocal leucoencephalopathy, a chronic and fatal papovavirus infection and a subacute encephalitis. In patients with hypogammaglobulinaemia, enteroviruses, including live attenuated polio vaccine, may produce a progressive and fatal meningoencephalitis. Human immunodeficiency virus itself can cause acute meningoencephalitis at the time of seroconversion and subacute chronic encephalomyelopathies and dementia in patients with AIDS.

Epidemiology

Many viral infections of the central nervous system are seasonal or occur as epidemics. Others, such as herpes simplex encephalitis, are sporadic. Epidemics of Japanese encephalitis occur in the summer or rainy season when the vector mosquitoes are abundant. Tick-borne encephalitides occur in spring and early summer when the ticks are most active. Mumps encephalitis is most common in the late winter or early spring; enterovirus infections occur most often in the summer and early autumn.

Invasion of the central nervous system seems to be exceptional in most viral infections. In the case of Japanese encephalitis, there may be only one case of encephalitis for every 500 to 1000 asymptomatic infections.

Pathogenesis

Most viral infections reach the central nervous system from the primary site of infection and multiplication via the bloodstream. Viruses that enter through the respiratory tract (for example measles, mumps, varicella) or gut (enteroviruses) multiply in local lymphoid tissue before they enter the bloodstream. Viraemia is a feature of most viral infections, yet invasion of the central nervous system is rare in most of them. In the case of rabies, herpes simplex and herpes zoster viruses, the virus enters the central nervous system through the peripheral nerves. Virus has been inoculated directly into the central nervous system by infected corneal transplant grafts (rabies) and infected brain surface electrodes. Herpes simplex encephalitis may complicate primary herpes simplex virus infection in children and young adults, but in most cases of herpes simplex encephalitis the cause is thought to be reactivation of latent virus (HSV-1) in the trigeminal nerve, autonomic nerve roots, or brain.

Some viruses, such as the enteroviruses and mumps, usually infect the meninges rather than the parenchyma of the central nervous system, whereas others, such as the togaviruses, usually cause encephalitis. Some neural cells show selective vulnerability to different neurotropic viruses. Polioviruses have a predilection for motor neurones of the anterior horns of the spinal cord and rabies for neurones of the limbic system and cerebellar Purkinje cells. The pathological effects of viral infections on the central nervous system include:

(1) the destruction and phagocytosis of neurones (neuronophagia) as a result of either viral invasion or immune lysis;

(2) demyelination;

(3) inflammatory oedema with the compressive effects of raised intracranial pressure;

(4) vascular lesions.

Postinfectious encephalitis and Guillain–Barré syndrome are thought to result from sensitization to central and peripheral myelin, respectively.

Host humoral or cell-mediated immune responses to viruses may be directed against the virus itself or the virus-infected cell. An important local immune response at infected surfaces is provided by IgA antibody, present in secretions in the gut, saliva, and respiratory tract. Systemic viral infection may be limited of circulating IgG and IgM neutralizing antibodies. Immune responses may also occur locally within the central nervous system, where local synthesis of immunoglobulins, sometimes in oligoclonal pattern, may be of diagnostic value. Immune responses to viruses may become pathogenetic when there is deposition of immune complexes in blood vessels. In lymphocytic choriomeningitis virus infection, the induction of virus-specific, cytotoxic T lymphocytes is itself responsible for the production of encephalitis.

Pathology

Most viral encephalitides are characterized by infiltration of the meninges and perivascular cuffing (Virchow–Robin spaces) in the cortex and underlying white matter by lymphocytes, plasma cells, histiocytes, and some neutrophils. There is proliferation of microglia-forming glial nodules. Neuronolysis and demyelination vary in their degree and location. Infected neurones may show characteristic inclusion bodies in their nuclei (measles, herpes simplex virus, and adenoviruses) or cytoplasm (Negri bodies in rabies). Microhaemorrhages and foci of necrosis may be found.

Herpes simplex encephalitis

There is gross cerebral oedema, and severe haemorrhagic and necrotizing encephalitis, which is often asymmetrically localized to the inferior and medial parts of the temporal lobe, the insula, and the orbital part of the frontal lobe; this may be the result of viral spread along specific neural pathways rather than differential susceptibility of particular cell populations. HSV-1 is latent in the trigeminal, superior cervical, and vagal ganglia of many normal individuals, whether or not they have a history of cold sores.

Clinical features

Meningitis

Symptoms start suddenly with fever, headache, a stiff neck, and vomiting, especially in children. Headache is less severe than in bacterial meningitis and tends to be frontal or retrobulbar (eye movements may be painful). Neck stiffness is less marked. Nausea, anorexia, abdominal pain, myalgias, and sore throat are particularly common in enteroviral meningitis. Myalgia is particularly severe with coxsackie B infections. Infants usually present with vague irritability and a tense fontanelle, and young children with fever and irritability or lethargy. Conjunctival injection, pharyngitis, and cervical lymphadenopathy may be found. Macular or petechial exanthems or enanthems are seen with coxsackie A and B and echovirus infections (especially echo 9); vesicles are found on the hands, feet, and mouth with coxsackie A16 and enterovirus 71 infections. Neurological features include vertigo, nystagmus, cerebellar ataxia, facial spasms, and involuntary movements.

The specific cause of viral meningitis may be suggested by characteristic signs outside the nervous system, such as genital or rectal vesicles in the sexually active age group (HSV-2), herpes zoster skin lesions, swelling in the parotid region (mumps and occasionally coxsackie, lymphocytic choriomeningitis, and Epstein–Barr viruses), orchitis (mumps and lymphocytic choriomeningitis virus), and arthritis (lymphocytic choriomeningitis virus).

Paralytic poliomyelitis

Infection (see Chapter 16.22) is by droplet spread from the respiratory tract or faecal–oral. The 'minor illness', coinciding with viraemia, consists of influenza-like symptoms: fever, headache, sore throat, malaise, and mild gastrointestinal symptoms, which resolve in a few days. In a minority, the 'major illness' follows, sometimes after a few days' remission of symptoms. Muscle pain, spasms, and sensory disturbances may precede or accompany the development of lower motor-neurone (flaccid) paralysis. Respiratory and bulbar paralysis is life threatening. Encephalitis is rare. Common causes of death are aspiration and airway obstruction, resulting from bulbar respiration paralysis.

Encephalitis

Patients present with symptoms of meningitis (fever, headache, neck stiffness, vomiting) but with altered consciousness, convulsions, focal neurological signs, signs of raised intracranial pressure, or psychiatric symptoms.

Herpes simplex encephalitis

Symptoms suggestive of herpes simplex encephalitis are behavioural abnormalities, olfactory and gustatory hallucinations, anosmia, amnesia, expressive aphasia, and temporal-lobe seizures. Herpetic skin or mucosal lesions are rarely found, except in the case of acute genital HSV-2, or proctitis, and a past history of 'cold sores' is not significant. Cerebral oedema may be severe. Patients usually lapse into coma towards the end of the first week and most deaths occur within the first 2 weeks.

Postinfectious encephalomyelitis

Sudden convulsions, coma, fever, or pareses appear 10 to 14 days after the start of nervous-tissue rabies vaccination or after infection with measles, varicella, rubella, mumps, or influenza. Measles, varicella, and rubella encephalitides develop 2 to 12 days after the rash has appeared, and mumps encephalitis before or after parotid swelling. Involuntary movements, cranial-nerve lesions (VII, III), pupillary abnormalities, nystagmus, ataxia, and upper motor-neurone signs are common

Diagnosis

Clinical and epidemiological details

The time of year, known current epidemics, the patient's age, occupation, and countries or states visited recently may help to narrow down the possibilities. The diagnosis may be suggested by distinctive clinical features of the encephalitis itself (for example, hydrophobia in rabies, temporal-lobe features in herpes simplex encephalitis) or of the associated infection (for example, mumps parotitis; measles rash; skin and mucosal lesions of herpes viruses; and gastrointestinal symptoms associated with enteroviral infections).

Laboratory investigations

The most important investigation is examination of the cerebrospinal fluid. Contraindications to lumbar puncture are the same as in acute bacterial meningitis (see Chapter 13.25). Pleocytosis ranges from tens to thousands of cells/µl. Lymphocytes and other mononuclear cells predominate, except in the early stages of infection. The cerebrospinal fluid contains erythrocytes or is xanthochromic in haemorrhagic encephalitides such as herpes simplex encephalitis and acute necrotic leucoencephalitis. Its protein concentration is usually increased (to 50–150 mg/dl). Its glucose concentration is usually normal or increased towards that in a blood sample taken simultaneously; low concentrations are occasionally reported, especially in mumps and lymphocytic choriomeningitis virus infections. Initially, the cerebrospinal fluid may be normal in 10 to 15 per cent of patients with herpes simplex encephalitis.

Virology

In 70 to 75 per cent of cases of lymphocytic meningitis and 30 to 40 per cent of patients with meningoencephalitis a virological diagnosis can be expected (Table 1). Direct immunofluorescence may reveal herpes simplex virus (skin and brain), herpes zoster virus (skin lesion scrapings), rabies (skin sections and brain), and measles (nasopharyngeal aspirate). Electron microscopy of skin lesions will identify a herpes virus. Some viruses can be isolated from the cerebrospinal fluid (for example, mumps, enteroviruses, lymphocytic chorio meningitis virus, Central European encephalitides, louping-ill, and human immunodeficiency virus). Polio and other enteroviruses can be cultured from stool; arthropod-borne viruses from blood culture. Specific viral IgM can be detected in serum for mumps, Epstein–Barr virus, cytomegalovirus, or measles, or, using a microcapture technique, in the cerebrospinal fluid for Japanese encephalitis virus. A viral diagnosis is often delayed until a rising convalescent antibody titre is found.

The polymerase chain reaction allows identification of herpes simplex virus in the cerebrospinal fluid of suspected cases of herpes simplex encephalitis within a short time of the onset of symptoms. This technique is being used for the early diagnosis of a wide variety of central nervous viral infections.

Brain biopsy

Electroencephalography, CT or MRI scans, angiography, or technetium scans can help to direct the surgeon towards the affected area of brain. Failing this, a biopsy of the medial or inferior surface of the temporal lobe is most likely to yield the diagnosis; opinion is divided about the safety and importance of this procedure.

Imaging of the brain and spinal cord

CT and MRI scans of the brain and spinal cord are extremely useful for the diagnosis of the site, nature, and extent of mass lesions and associated oedema, sub- and epidural empyemas, meningitis, cerebritis, and ventriculitis, the presence of intracranial hypertension, hydrocephalus, cerebral and brainstem herniation, demyelination, and other anatomical abnormalities.

CT scans are superior for bony details and calcifications, are quicker to perform, and are less dependent on the patient being able to lie motionless. The resolution of MRI is greater for parenchymal lesions but MRI cannot be used in patients with pacemakers and may be dangerous in those with metal clips in cerebral blood vessels.

Differential diagnosis

This includes the other causes of aseptic meningitis, such as partially treated bacterial meningitis, tuberculous meningitis, spirochaetal infections (leptospirosis, borreliosis, Lyme disease, and syphilis), and fungal, amoebic, neoplastic, granulomatous, and idiopathic meningitides. Viral myelitides must be distinguished from other causes of transverse myelitis and the Brown–Séquard syndrome; these include spinal compression by tumours, abscesses, helminths or their ova, or vertebral disease.

The differential diagnosis of paralytic poliomyelitis includes postinfectious and other immunopathic polyneuroradiculopathies, such as

Table 1 Specimens for the virological diagnosis of acute meningitis or meningo-encephalomyelitis (after Johnson 1982; Jackson and Johnson 1989)

	Specimens for virus isolation/identification						Serology	
	Throat swab	Stool	CSF	Blood	Other specimens	PCR CSF	Acute	Convalescent
Adenovirus	++[a]	+	−		?[b]	?[b]	+	
Arenavirus								
Lymphocytic choriomeningitis	−	−	+++	+		?[b]	+	+ 2–3 months
Enteroviruses								
Polioviruses	+	+++	−	−		++[c,d]	+	+
Coxsackie and echoviruses[f]	+	+++	+++	−		+	+	+
Herpesviruses								
Cytomegalovirus	−	−	−	−	Urine[a]	+	+[a]	+
Epstein–Barr	+[a]	−	−	−		+	+[a]	+
Herpes simplex								
type 1	+[a]	−	+	−	Brain	+++	+[a]	+
type 2	−	−	+	−	Vesicular fluid	+	+[a]	+
Herpes simiae (B)	−	−	−	−	Vesicular fluid	−	+[a]	+
Herpes varicella/zoster	−	−	+	−	Vesicular fluid	+[b]	+[a]	+
Mumps	+++	−	++	−	Saliva, urine	?[b]	+	+
Rhabdoviruses								
Rabies	−	−	+	−	Skin biopsy, saliva, brain	?[b]	+	+
Retroviruses								
HIV-1	−	−	+	+++		+++[e]	+++	−
HIV-2	−	−	+	+++		?	+++	−
HTLV-1	−	−	+	−		+	+++	−
Togaviruses	−	−	+	++		+[e]	+	+

[a] Isolations or antibody responses may represent non-specific activation.

[b] Too few data to indicate general usefulness in diagnosis.

[c] Also serum/blood.

[d] Also stool.

[e] Also brain tissue.

[f] Some Coxsackie A serotypes (especially A1–6) cannot be grown on cells.

Guillain–Barré syndrome and Landry's ascending paralysis; and metabolic neuropathies such as acute porphyria. The lack of objective sensory loss in poliomyelitis usually distinguishes it from these other entities.

The differential diagnosis of viral encephalitis includes other infective encephalopathies—bacterial, fungal, protozoal, and parasitic; intracranial abscesses and neoplasms; toxic and metabolic encephalopathies; and heat stroke.

Reye's syndrome

Reye's syndrome is an acute encephalopathy affecting children between the ages of 2 and 16 years. It is rapidly fatal in 10 to 40 per cent of cases. The defining characteristics are sudden impairment of consciousness, increase in serum aminotransferase concentrations (or, if a biopsy is done, a fatty liver), and the exclusion of other diseases. There is an association between Reye's syndrome and the use of salicylates, but not of paracetamol.

Treatment

Antiviral chemotherapy

Acyclovir (Zovirax®) has proved effective in treating herpes simplex encephalitis. This nucleoside analogue is only taken up by cells infected by herpes simplex virus and is therefore non-toxic to normal, uninfected cells. Treatment should be started as soon as herpes simplex encephalitis is suspected clinically. Acyclovir has been used for herpes zoster virus encephalitis. Gancyclovir has been used in cytomegalovirus infections of the central nervous system. The rare but very dangerous encephalomyelitis caused by *Herpes simiae* B virus should be treated with acyclovir (see Chapter 16.13). Ribavirin is effective against some RNA viruses, such as those causing Lassa fever, haemorrhagic fever with renal syndrome, and possibly Argentine haemorrhagic fever, Rift Valley fever, and Congo Crimean haemorrhagic fever.

Supportive treatment

Corticosteroids have been used in most of the viral, postinfection, and postvaccine encephalomyelitides but convincing evidence of benefit, from controlled trials, is lacking. The immunosuppressive effects of corticosteroids have not led to obvious clinical deterioration, except perhaps in some cases of diffuse myelitis. Severe intracranial hypertension should be treated with intravenous mannitol or mechanical hyperventilation. Seizures must be controlled with prophylactic phenytoin, fever lowered by cooling, respiratory failure treated by mechanical ventilation, and attention given to fluid, electrolyte, and acid–base balance. Hyponatraemia is attributable to inappropriate secretion of antidiuretic hormone in some cases.

Prognosis

Viral meningitis has an excellent prognosis, but some patients with HSV-2 infection have recurrent attacks with involvement of the spinal cord or nerve roots. Case fatality rates of some viral encephalomyelitides are as follows: rabies, 100 per cent; herpes simplex encephalitis (untreated), 40 to more than 75 per cent (highest in neonates and those over 30 years old); eastern equine encephalitis, 50 per cent; Japanese encephalitis, 10 to 40 per cent; measles, 10 to 20 per cent; varicella, 10 to 30 per cent; western equine encephalitis, 8 per cent; St Louis encephalitis, 3 per cent; California encephalitis, Venezuelan encephalitis, and mumps, less than 1 per cent.

Neurological complications are found in 5 to 75 per cent of survivors of Japanese encephalitis and herpes simplex encephalitis, and are especially common in infants; they include mental retardation, loss of memory, speech abnormalities (including subtle expressive aphasias), hemiparesis, ataxia, dystonic brainstem and cranial-nerve lesions, recurrent convulsions, and various behavioural and personality disturbances. Complications are common with postinfectious encephalomyelitis. An unusual sequel to paralytic poliomyelitis developing after an interval of many years is a condition characterized by progressive muscle weakness and wasting, which has some similarities to motor neurone disease.

Prevention

Prophylactic vaccination against poliomyelitis and measles has virtually eradicated encephalitides caused by these viruses in many communities. Post- and pre-exposure rabies vaccination has also proved effective. A formalin-inactivated, adult mouse brain vaccine is manufactured in Osaka for Japanese encephalitis; it appears to be effective and carries a very low risk of objective neurological complications (one in a million courses).

Hyperimmune immunoglobulin has been used for prophylaxis (and in some cases attempted treatment) of measles, herpes zoster virus, HSV-2, vaccinia, rabies, and some other infections in high-risk groups. Immunocompromised patients, such as those with leukaemia, who are household contacts of a case of herpes zoster virus infection, should be given prophylactic hyperimmune globulin and, if they develop skin lesions, they should be treated with acyclovir to prevent development of severe disease.

Control of animal vectors and reservoirs

Arthropod-borne viral encephalitides can be prevented by avoiding or controlling the arthropod vectors (for example, by the use of mosquito nets, insect repellents, insecticides, etc.), by attempting to control the numbers of wild vertebrate reservoir species, or by immunizing domestic animals, such as horses (eastern and western equine encephalitides) and pigs (Japanese encephalitis). Control of rabies is discussed in Chapter 16.24.

Other viral infections or disorders in which viruses may play a part in the pathogenesis of neurological disease

Subacute sclerosing panencephalitis

Children and young adults may become persistently infected with the measles virus. The condition is also known as subacute sclerosing leucoencephalitis and inclusion-body encephalitis.

Aetiology

Measles virus antibody titres are extremely high in blood and cerebrospinal fluid, measles antigen has been demonstrated in the brain, and the virus has sometimes been isolated. Most affected children have had measles at an unusually early age. There is a mean interval of some 6 years between infection and the onset of encephalitis. The disease can occur in children vaccinated with live measles virus, but the risk is much lower than that following the natural disease.

Clinical features

The onset is usually in the first two decades. The disease is twice as common in boys as in girls. Incidence has fallen sharply in countries where measles vaccination is at a high level.

There is usually a prolonged period of altered behaviour, mild intellectual deterioration, and loss of energy and interest, often misinterpreted as sloth or neurosis. After some weeks or months increasing clumsiness or the appearance of focal neurological symptoms draw attention to the organic nature of the disease. Periodic involuntary movements then appear, the most common form being myoclonus, consisting of a stereotyped jerk or lapse of posture involving the limbs, often asymmetrically, occurring every 3 to 6 s. The myoclonus may result in sudden falls, which are occasionally the presenting symptom. Eye signs may be prominent, with papilloedema, retinitis, optic atrophy, or cortical blindness. Choroidoretinal scarring is present in 30 per cent of cases.

Further progression is marked by intellectual deterioration, rigidity and spasticity, and increasing helplessness. Some 40 per cent die within a year but a similar proportion survive for more than 2 years. A period of apparent arrest is common; in some patients, particularly at the upper end of the age range, substantial remission and prolonged survival occur.

Investigation

The cerebrospinal fluid is normal apart from oligoclonal bands of IgG. The measles antibody titres in blood and cerebrospinal fluid are usually raised. In established disease, the EEG shows highly characteristic periodic discharges, synchronous with the myoclonus, but persisting in the absence of the movements. CT scanning shows low-density white-matter lesions and cerebral atrophy.

Treatment

There is no effective treatment for subacute sclerosing panencephalitis.

Progressive multifocal leucoencephalopathy

This disease is caused by opportunistic infection by papovaviruses, most commonly JC virus and SV40 (see Chapter 16.32). A high proportion of normal adults have antibodies to the former and the agent appears to be ubiquitous. The reservoir of SV40 is in monkeys and the agent was apparently transmitted in early types of poliomyelitis vaccine, without evident ill effects. These viruses are potentially oncogenic but non-pathogenic for humans unless the immune system has been compromised.

Progressive multifocal leucoencephalopathy occurs in patients with lympho- or myeloproliferative diseases, sarcoidosis, and other chronic granulomatous diseases or AIDS, and also in those therapeutically immunosuppressed.

Clinical features

There are progressive signs of a focal lesion of one cerebral hemisphere: limb weakness, aphasia, or a visual-field defect such as homonymous hemianopia. More widespread signs gradually develop, leading to personality changes, intellectual deterioration, dysarthria or fluent aphasia, and bilateral weakness. Fits are rare. There is no systemic evidence of infection. Spontaneous temporary arrest or partial remission are common but eventual progression causes death in 6–12 months, although much more chronic cases are on record, with survival, exceptionally, to 5 years.

Investigation

The cerebrospinal fluid is normal apart from occasionally mild elevation of protein and slight pleocytosis, and is not under increased pressure. The EEG shows a bilateral excess of slow activity. The CT scan may at first show little abnormality, but eventually large, non-enhancing, low-density lesions appear in the cerebral white matter. MRI is more sensitive. Serum antibodies are of no diagnostic help but the response in the cerebrospinal fluid has not been fully evaluated. The diagnosis can be confirmed only by cerebral biopsy, but it is essential that white matter be included in the specimen. This may be important to distinguish lymphoma and, rarely, herpes simplex encephalitis involving white matter.

Treatment

No treatment is of proven value.

Progressive rubella panencephalitis

This is an extremely rare disorder (see also Chapter 16.27) that follows congenital rubella or rubella in early childhood. It evolves insidiously some 10 years after the original illness and is characterized by progressive mental retardation with behaviour changes, fits, ataxia, spasticity, optic atrophy, and macular degeneration (see OTM3, p. 4074).

Vogt–Koyanagi–Harada syndrome

This rare syndrome is thought to be due to an inflammatory autoimmune reaction to an unidentified viral infection. It affects tissues having a common embryological origin in the neural crest. There is patchy whitening of eyelashes, eyebrows, and scalp hair, alopecia, and vitiligo, meningoencephalitis, raised intracranial pressure, neurosensory deafness, tinnitus, nystagmus, ataxia, ocular palsies, focal cerebral deficits, uveitis with pain and photophobia, more generalized inflammation of the eye, retinopathy, and impaired visual acuity. The condition tends to be self-limiting but may result in serious permanent ocular and neurological deficits. Steroids and immunosuppressive drugs have been used and are said to arrest the progression of at least some features of the disorder.

Further reading

Boos, J. and Esiri, M.M. (1986). *Viral encephalitis: pathology, diagnosis and management.* Blackwell Scientific, Oxford.

Jackson, A.C. and Johnson, R.T. (1989). Aseptic meningitis and acute viral encephalitis. In *Handbook of clinical neurology*, Vol. 12 (56), *Viral diseases* (ed. P.J. Vinken, G.W. Bruyn, H.L. Klawans, and R.R. McKendall), pp. 125–48. Elsevier, Amsterdam.

Kennedy, P.G.E. and Johnson, R.T. (1987). *Infections of the nervous system.* Butterworths, London.

Krupp, L.B., Lipton, R.B., Swerdlow, M.L., Leeds, N.E., and Llena, J. (1985). Progressively multifocal leukoencephalopathy: clinical and radiological features. *Annals of Neurology*, **17**, 344–9.

Mims, C.A. and White, D.O. (1984). *Viral pathogenesis and immunology.* Blackwell Scientific, Oxford.

Pattison, E.M. (1965). Uveomeningoencephalitic syndrome (Vogt–Koyanagi–Harada). *Archives of Neurology*, **12**, 197–205.

Price, R.W. and Plum, F. (1978). Poliomyelitis. In *Handbook of clinical neurology*, Vol. 34 (ed. P.J. Vinken, G.W. Bruyn, and H.L. Klawans), pp. 93–132. North Holland, Amsterdam.

Scheld, W.M., Whitley, R.J., and Durack, D.T. (ed.) (1997). *Infections of the central nervous system.* Lippincott-Raven, Philadelphia.

Townsend, J.J., *et al.* (1975). Progressive rubella panencephalitis—late onset after congenital rubella. *New England Journal of Medicine*, **292**, 990–3.

Whitley, R.J., *et al.* (1986). Vidarabine versus acyclovir therapy in herpes simplex encephalitis. *New England Journal of Medicine*, **314**, 149.

Chapter 13.27

Intracranial abscess

P. J. Teddy

Intracranial abscesses may occur within the extradural or subdural space, or may be intracerebral. Occasionally, abscesses exist in more than one tissue plane. Intracerebral and subdural abscesses may rupture into the subarachnoid space and be accompanied by meningitis; intracerebral pus may rupture into the ventricular system and produce ventriculitis.

Aetiology

Extradural abscesses are usually related to focal osteomyelitis of the skull, mastoiditis and nasal sinusitis, penetrating injuries of the skull, and are a rare complication of craniotomy.

Subdural empyema is related most commonly to infection of the paranasal sinuses and middle ear. Other causes include septicaemia related to cyanotic congenital heart disease, lung abscess, trauma, and intracranial surgery.

The most common intracranial abscess is found within the intracerebral compartment, with about 60 per cent related to middle-ear infection and 20 per cent to frontal sinusitis. Other established causes are septicaemia related to congenital heart disease with a right-to-left shunt, lung abscess, bronchiectasis, penetrating injuries of the head, and bacteraemia following tooth extraction. In about 10 per cent of cases no primary source of infection can be identified. Owing to their strong connection with sinus and middle-ear disease, most intracerebral abscesses are found within the frontal or temporal lobes, or within the cerebellum. Infection disseminated through the bloodstream from more distant sites may result in multiple abscesses in any part of the brain.

Microbiology

The most common organisms associated with subdural empyema are aerobic, anaerobic, and micro-aerophilic streptococci, *Staphylococcus aureus*, and *Bacteroides* spp.

Cerebral abscesses associated with otitis media, mastoiditis, and nasal sinusitis usually show a mixed growth of anaerobes and aerobic organisms including anaerobic and micro-aerophilic streptococci and *Bacteroides. Streptococcus viridans and Staph. aureus* are frequently seen. *Listeria* spp. tend to produce areas of focal cerebritis rather than true abscess.

Pathology

Infection within an accessory air sinus or the petrous bone may cause an area of localized osteitis just above the dura, which can then spread intracranially. Initially it may be entirely confined to the extradural space, but will eventually penetrate the dura and spread subdurally or, if the adjacent arachnoid is stuck to the inflamed patch of dura, then it will spread into the subarachnoid space to give meningitis. If the subarachnoid space has been obliterated, it may penetrate the brain to produce initially a focal cerebritis. Usually after about 10 days the area of cerebritis becomes enclosed within an area of gliotic brain, and after about 3 weeks a firm capsule forms around the pus. Large intracerebral abscesses may rupture into the ventricular system, producing a ventriculitis.

Cerebral abscesses are usually surrounded by areas of oedematous brain, which may exert a considerable mass effect.

Clinical features

These will depend upon the site, size, and number of lesions, and the involvement of neighbouring structures such as the cerebral ventricles and the venous sinuses. The signs are therefore legion, but the diagnosis should be considered in any case where there is an obvious primary source of infection associated with evidence of raised intracranial pressure, focal neurological signs, epileptic seizures or meningeal irritation, or any combination of these.

Extradural abscess may be difficult to detect clinically, but is sometimes manifest by severe, unremitting, localized headache in association with sinusitis or mastoiditis. Patients with subdural empyema frequently appear toxic, with a swinging pyrexia, severe headache, a depressed level of consciousness, contralateral hemiparesis, papilloedema, meningeal irritation, and seizures. There is usually an accompanying frontal sinusitis with tenderness of the forehead and redness and swelling of the eyelids, or mastoiditis or scalp infection.

Diagnosis

If a brain abscess is suspected, predisposing sources of infection, including possible distant sites, should be carefully sought, as intracranial abscesses derived by haematogenous spread are often more fulminating in their course than those associated with local cranial disease. If CT is available, scans of the skull base, including views of the mastoids and other skull sinuses, should be performed. Otherwise, skull radiography with sinus views is necessary. Chest radiographs should be obtained.

The investigations of choice for all forms of suspected intracranial abscess are either CT scanning, with and without contrast, or MRI. CT will normally demonstrate both extradural and subdural empyema, may demonstrate diffuse cerebritis in early cases, and will normally show intracerebral abscesses as ring-enhancing lesions with low-attenuation centres (see Fig. 1). Nevertheless, there are pitfalls, particularly in the early stages both of subdural empyema and of cerebral abscess. Subdural empyema may initially be fairly thinly spread over

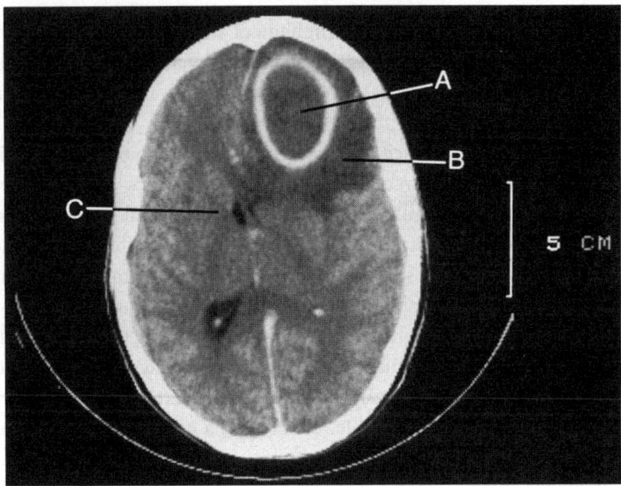

Fig. 1 Contrast CT scan showing large right frontal cerebral abscess (A) with surrounding oedema (B) and ventricular compression (C).

the cerebral cortex, producing relatively little midline shift, and may be virtually isodense with brain on CT. Under such circumstances, contrast-enhanced MRI (particularly with coronal views) is of great value.

The principal differential diagnoses in an intracranial abscess are meningitis, subdural haematoma, and intracranial tumour. It is not always possible to differentiate between intracerebral abscess and tumour on CT scan, particularly when there is an appearance of ring enhancement, and it is largely for this reason that the biopsy of suspected cerebral tumour is advocated in nearly all such cases. MRI, however, tends to show a low-signal capsule on T_2-weighted images and may be helpful in making this differentiation.

One obvious concern is to differentiate between bacterial meningitis and intracerebral abscess. Both may present with pyrexia, neck stiffness, and with some focal signs, but if there is any evidence whatsoever of raised intracranial pressure, or any other supportive evidence of cerebral abscess, a lumbar puncture should be strictly avoided until a neurosurgical opinion has been sought. Lumbar puncture in the presence of cerebral abscess can lead to tonsillar or tentorial herniation, and in any event, the cerebrospinal fluid can be entirely normal.

Management

Except in a few cases of multiple or inaccessible abscess, and the occasional patient whose general medical condition is such that surgery is precluded, treatment of the intracranial infection requires evacuation of pus and high-dose intravenous antibiotic therapy.

The single, main factor in securing a good outcome is early diagnosis. Early management includes taking specimens for blood culture and culture of any extracranial infective lesion, setting up an intravenous infusion, administration of anticonvulsant agents, and, in cases of grossly depressed level of consciousness and massive cerebral oedema seen on CT scan, giving intravenous dexamethasone.

Pus from the suspected primary site of infection should be collected immediately and both aerobic and anaerobic cultures obtained. The intracranial pus must be similarly cultured. Antimicrobial treatment, using massive intravenous doses, should be commenced immediately without waiting for the culture report, and subsequently changed in the light of the sensitivity findings. The antimicrobial regimen should include penicillin (4 mega units 4-hourly), metronidazole, ampicillin, and either gentamicin or chloramphenicol depending on the likely source of infection and the infective agent. Intravenous antimicrobials should be continued for at least 1 week before reverting to oral medication.

Most supratentorial abscesses can be sterilized by aspiration through a burr hole, and the direct instillation of antibiotics is sometimes employed. Aspiration must usually be repeated several times, but in about 30 per cent of cases a single aspiration will suffice. Once the abscess is sterile, the capsule will shrink and finally form an irregular gliotic scar within the brain. Shrinkage of the abscess must be checked by serial CT scan. Subdural empyema should be evacuated through a craniotomy rather than burr holes, as very often the pus can spread widely, and particularly alongside the falx cerebri. Extradural empyema is evacuated through a burr hole, or through a craniotomy for larger collections.

Cerebellar abscess, when diagnosed early, may be aspirated through a burr hole, but immediate total excision is often recommended because the small volume of the posterior cranial fossa leaves little latitude in terms of tonsillar herniation and death.

Prognosis

The mortality is around 10 per cent, but the main problems remain those of late diagnosis and resistant bacteria. Even with an otherwise good outcome, epilepsy may continue in about 30 per cent of cases, particularly in patients with temporal-lobe abscess and subdural empyema.

Further reading

Lorber, B. (1997). Listeriosis. *Clinical Infectious Diseases*, 24,1–9.

Mathisen,, G.E and Johnson, J.P. (1997). Brain abscess. *Clinical Infectious Diseases*, 25, 763–79.

Report of the Quality Standards Subcommittee of the American Academy of Neurology. (1998). Evaluation and management of intracranial mass lesions in AIDS. *Neurology*, 50, 21–6.

Chapter 13.28

Neurosyphilis

R. J. Greenwood

Despite the current rarity of neurosyphilis, early recognition remains of paramount importance, since treatment with penicillin before the onset of irreversible neurological damage so effectively produces a cure. An expectation that patients will present with textbook features of neurosyphilis is seldom rewarded; diagnosis should be established before the classic features of tabes dorsalis, general paresis, or meningovascular syphilis are apparent. Concurrent human immunodeficiency virus (HIV) infection produces an increased frequency of accelerated or resistant disease, particularly in immunocompromised individuals, with more frequent ocular changes.

Clinical features and natural history (see also Chapter 16.69)

Invasion of the central nervous system by *Treponema pallidum* occurs within the first few weeks or months of primary infection. During this period the majority of patients are neurologically normal. In many patients with untreated primary or secondary syphilis, 41 per cent in one recent study, there are minor abnormalities in the cerebrospinal fluid comprising a slight elevation of cells or protein, or positive serology, usually specific rather than non-treponemal. This is asymptomatic neurosyphilis.

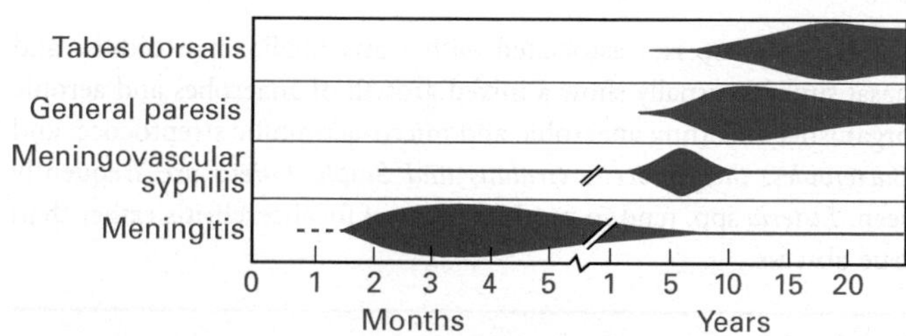

Fig. 1 Approximate interval between primary infection and symptomatic neurosyphilis by type
(for source see OTM3, p. 4084).

If untreated, by the end of the secondary stage of syphilis these cerebrospinal abnormalities have resolved in the majority of patients. One to 2 per cent of patients develop an acute meningitis, while only 5 to 10 per cent go on to develop tertiary (meningovascular) or late (general paresis or tabes dorsalis) neurosyphilis (Fig. 1).

The disease, whether acquired congenitally or later in life, can be regarded as a meningovasculitis, which may occasionally be acute but is usually more or less chronic.

Meningeal and vascular neurosyphilis

Within the first 10 to 12 years of infection a sequence of histopathological change can be seen. Various combinations of a subacute or chronic diffuse leptomeningitis, subpial parenchymal degeneration in the brainstem and cord, and inflammation of the media and adventitia of large and medium-sized vessel walls with intimal fibroblastic proliferation (Heubner's endarteritis obliterans) develop, and may lead to vascular occlusion with infarction. Thus serological tests are essential in young patients presenting with meningitis, stroke, isolated cranial-nerve palsies, papilloedema of uncertain cause, acute vertigo, or recent sensorineural deafness. The onset of symptoms may be gradual rather than abrupt, sometimes preceded by several weeks of headache or personality change.

Acute syphilitic meningitis usually occurs within 2 years of infection. Patients are usually afebrile, and meningeal irritation may be obvious clinically or evident only upon lumbar puncture. There may be a considerable lymphocytosis of the cerebrospinal fluid, although in the acute stage polymorphs may predominate and occasionally a low sugar is found. Other features of secondary syphilis should be sought, especially the rash and hepatomegaly or evidence of disordered liver function. Characteristically, cranial-nerve palsies occur, especially of nerves III, VI, VII, and VIII, sometimes bilaterally; swelling of the optic disc or fits may be seen. Treatment is usually successful, provided it is begun early.

Chronic meningovascular neurosyphilitic syndromes result from pathological emphasis upon leptomeningeal fibrosis. Thus chronic basal meningitis may result in hydrocephalus and involvement of a variety of cranial nerves, including the optic nerves and chiasm. Hypothalamic disturbances may occur. Syphilitic meningomyelitis is accompanied by symptoms of patchy root irritation and appropriate radicular wasting and weakness, for example, sciatica and foot drop. Localization of the leptomeningitis to the cervical region produces an amyotrophic meningomyelitis in which there is obvious wasting, usually asymmetrical, of arm muscles and neck extensors, often with few sensory symptoms and little pain. These cord syndromes may be confused with motor neurone disease but generally do not produce the widespread fasciculation and wasting usually seen in that condition.

Large and medium-sized arteritic occlusions may occur independently or may accompany leptomeningeal disease. Any vessel may be involved, especially the middle and posterior cerebral arteries, producing results similar to those seen after arteriosclerotic occlusion, although often in younger patients. Angiography reveals multifocal narrowing of the intradural vessels resembling that seen in other forms of cerebral vasculitis.

General paralysis of the insane

General paralysis of the insane is a subacute, progressive meningo-encephalitis that occurs 5 to 20 years after infection. Presenting symptoms are often vague, as in any dementing illness, consisting of ill-defined personality changes with irritability and forgetfulness, headaches, weight loss, and poor concentration and work record. Behaviour gradually deteriorates as memory, insight, and judgement are progressively impaired. Dress, personal appearance, and social behaviour become inappropriate. Alcohol excess, vagrancy, sexual aberration, and various psychotic delusions may occur, although a simple dementia is most often seen. Classic grandiose delusions are uncommon. Fits, sometimes with transient focal neurological deficits, may accompany deterioration, or occasionally herald it. Motor signs gradually appear until the 'insane' patient becomes 'generally paralysed', mute, and incontinent. Death usually occurs from intercurrent infection.

Physical signs usually appear after at least some degree of mental deterioration. Commonly seen signs are a relaxed and expressionless face; tremor of the face, tongue, and lips, and often of the whole body; a slurred and tremulous dysarthria; pupillary abnormalities, often of Argyll Robertson type (see below); and, with time, an increasingly severe quadriparesis. Tabes dorsalis may coexist (taboparesis).

Tabes dorsalis

Presentation of tabes dorsalis 10 to 25 years after infection is usual, although the interval may be much longer. Presentation with the triad of lightning pains, ataxia in the lower limbs, and sphincter dysfunction due to bladder hypotonia is common. These symptoms are often accompanied by pupillary abnormalities, of Argyll Robertson type (see below), loss of knee and ankle jerks, and of vibration, position, and deep pain sensation in the legs. Similar symptoms and signs in the arms are much less common. The gait is broad-based, slapping, and worsened by eye closure. Lightning pains strike at right angles to the limb like a needle stab. Crises of pain and dysfunction in various viscera may occur; gastric crises, the most common, may cause epigastric or shoulder-tip pain with or without vomiting, or vomiting without pain. Charcot joints, usually in the legs or lumbar spine, perforating foot ulcers, muscular hypotonia, ptosis, optic atrophy, colonic distension as well as a large bladder and impairment of genital sensation, or coexisting general paralysis of the insane (taboparesis) may also be present.

Neuro-ophthalmological features

Neuro-ophthalmological features may be seen in any form of the disease but most commonly occur in tabes and often provide confirmation of the diagnosis. When fully developed, the pupils are completely unreactive to light but constrict briskly to accommodation–convergence. They are small and irregular, and there is often a poor response to sympathetic stimulation or mydriatics (Argyll Robertson pupils).

Involvement of the optic nerve may result from inflammation and arteritis of the nerve itself in meningovascular disease, either secondary or tertiary, and may subacutely produce a central scotoma with significant visual loss (optic neuritis).

Laboratory diagnosis

Serological tests for syphilis divide into those that detect antibodies against lipoidal antigens secondary to treponema–host interaction (reagins) and those detecting antigens derived from *T. pallidum*. They are described and analysed in Chapter 16.69.

Treatment

Treatment in the early stages of any form of neurosyphilis often fully reverses the disease. If it is delayed, progressive changes may be only partially reversible. Patients with signs of neurosyphilis but with an unreactive cerebrospinal fluid, as is seen in late tabes, will not improve with treatment and may deteriorate. Antimicrobial treatment and possible complications are discussed in Chapter 16.69.

The cell count in cerebrospinal fluid should return to normal within 3 months, the protein within 6 months. This response should be checked, particularly after treatment that does not include penicillin, by repeat lumbar puncture at 6 weeks and 3 months after completion of therapy, and thereafter at 6-monthly intervals until cells and protein have been normal on two consecutive occasions. In HIV-positive patients, the cerebrospinal fluid and VDRL, if initially positive, may remain abnormal despite adequate treatment; relapse, needing retreatment, may occur more than 12 months later, and protracted follow up is necessary.

Symptomatic treatment may be required for confusion, ataxia, Charcot joints, or urinary retention. Lightning pains may be treated with carbamazepine or phenytoin, gastric crises with subcutaneous adrenaline (epinephrine) solution BP (0.5 ml of 1:1000).

Further reading

Editorial (1978). Modified neurosyphilis. *British Medical Journal*, **2**, 647–8.

Feraru, E.R., Aronow, H.A., and Lipton, R.B. (1990). Neurosyphilis in AIDS's patients: initial CSF VDRL may be negative. *Neurology*, **40**, 531–3.

Holmes, M.D., Brant-Zawadski, M.M., and Simon, R.P. (1984). Clinical features of meningovascular syphilis. *Neurology*, **34**, 553–6.

Johns, D.R., Tierney, M., and Feisensten, D. (1987). Alteration in the natural history of neurosyphilis by concurrent infection with the human immunodeficiency virus. *New England Journal of Medicine*, **316**, 1569–72.

Marra, C.M., Longstreath, W.T., Jr, Maxwell, C.L., and Lukehart, J.A. (1996). Resolution of serum and cerebrospinal fluid abnormalities after treatment of neurosyphilis. Influence of concomitant human immunodeficiency virus infection. *Sexually Transmitted Diseases*, **23**, 184–9.

Chapter 13.29

The motor neurone diseases

M. Donaghy

These diseases result from selective loss of function of the lower and/or upper motor neurones controlling the voluntary muscles of the limbs or bulbar region. Precise diagnosis is essential for advising patients about prognosis, for identifying those diseases with genetic implications, and to offer immunosuppressant therapy to some patients with some acquired lower motor-neurone syndromes.

In practice, differential diagnosis requires clinical and electrophysiological classification to discern whether the disease involves the upper or the lower motor neurones, or both. This anatomical differentiation is augmented by the age of onset, the rate of deterioration, and familial occurrence (Table 1).

The clinical signs of lower motor-neurone involvement consist of muscle wasting, fasciculations, and flaccid weakness. Sensation and cognition are normal. The tendon reflexes are often retained until profound denervation or fibrous replacement have affected the muscle. Fasciculations are visible flickerings within the muscle belly, insufficient to produce joint movement; electromyography shows that they correspond to simultaneous discharge of all the muscle fibres within a diseased motor unit. Nerve-conduction studies will exclude peripheral neuropathy. Electromyography helps to distinguish denervation from myopathy. Muscle biopsy is often required to exclude myopathy, particularly in syndromes causing slowly progressive proximal weakness.

Table 1 Classification of the motor neurone diseases

Combined upper and lower motor neurone syndromes
Amyotrophic lateral sclerosis
sporadic (AE)
familial adult onset (*D) (A)
familial juvenile onset (*R) (C)
Lower motor neurone syndromes
Proximal hereditary motor neuronopathy:
acute infantile form (Werdnig-Hoffinann) (*R) (1)
chronic childhood form (Kugelberg-Welander) (*R) (1, C)
adult onset (*R) (A)
adult onset (*D) (C,A)
Hereditary bulbar palsy
with deafness (Brown-Violetto-van Lacre) (*) (C,A)
without deafness (Fazio–Londe) (*R) (C)
X-linked bulbospinal neuronopathy (*) (A,E)
Hexosaminidase deficiency (*R) (C,A)
Multifocal motor neuropathies (A,E)
Postpolio syndrome
Postirradiation lumbosacral radiculopathy
Monomelic, focal, or segmental spinal muscular atrophy (A)
Upper motor neurone syndromes
Primary lateral sclerosis (AE)
Hereditary spastic paraplegia (*D) (AE)
Lathyrism (A)

*, inherited disorder: D, dominant; R, recessive.

Age of onset: 1, infantile; C, childhood; A, adult (15–50 years); E, elderly (more than 50 years).

Upper motor-neurone involvement produces spasticity, clonus, extensor plantar responses, and weakness. Sphincter control and sexual function are usually preserved in motor neurone disease, although weakness of the trunk and abdominal wall may make excretion slow and awkward.

Motor neurone diseases are incurable for the most part, and therefore treatment must aim to overcome, or minimize, the various sources of disability. Malnutrition due to dysphagia can be circumvented by nasogastric tube feeding or gastrostomy. Various forms of assisted respiration offset respiratory muscle weakness, including continuous positive airways pressure via a facial mask. Limb spasticity can be reduced by baclofen, dantrolene, or diazepam. Wheelchairs and arm appliances may overcome inadequate limb function. Electronic communication devices should be supplied to those whose speech is incomprehensible. Amitriptyline may help contain the embarrassing emotional lability of pseudobulbar palsy. Housing and workplace modifications can allow patients to maintain independence despite their disability.

Combined upper and lower motor-neurone syndromes

Amyotrophic lateral sclerosis

Amyotrophic lateral sclerosis occurs worldwide and the incidence increases with advancing age; it is unusual before the fifth decade of life. The cause of the common sporadic form is unknown. Autosomal-dominant inheritance is evident in approximately 5 per cent of patients with the adult-onset form and is associated with superoxide dismutase gene mutations in some.

Pathology

Lower motor neurones are lost from clinically affected areas of the spinal cord and brainstem.

Clinical features

At presentation, patients either have bulbar or spinal symptoms, although both usually become evident as the disease progresses.

The bulbar form causes dysphagia, dysphonia, and inhalation of foodstuffs due to weakness of the tongue, pharynx, and larynx. The tongue is wasted, weak, and fasciculating, palatal movements are reduced, and the ability to cough explosively is lost due to paralysis of the vocal cords. This bulbar palsy is usually accompanied, or even preceded, by varying degrees of pseudobulbar involvement. The tongue is spastic and immobile, with 'hot potato' speech and difficulty in containing emotional responses such as laughing or crying. Ventilatory respiratory failure may develop due to weakness of diaphragm and intercostal muscles. Occasionally, amyotrophic lateral sclerosis can present with dyspnoea.

The spinal form usually presents with wasting and weakness of one limb, usually as wasting of intrinsic hand muscles or foot drop. Asymptomatic involvement of other limbs is often evident on examination. It is diagnostically important to demonstrate combined upper and lower motor-neurone signs in at least two limbs. Wasted, fasciculating muscles also exhibiting clonus or hyper-reflexia are a helpful finding. With time, the limbs become useless due to progressive denervation. Patients become wheelchair- or bed-bound, or are unable to use their arms for grooming or feeding. Sphincter control is not affected, although practical difficulties in excretion may result from immobility, and because weakness of the abdominal wall prevents intra-abdominal pressure being raised to aid excretion.

Prognosis

Amytrophic lateral sclerosis progresses relentlessly, both in severity and the extent of muscular involvement. Death commonly results from ventilatory respiratory failure, from choking, or from inhalational pneumonia; malnutrition often contributes. The median survival from first symptoms in those with bulbar onset is approximately 20 months, with only 5 per cent surviving 5 years. The alternative diagnosis of X-linked bulbospinal neuronopathy should be considered in these long survivors. The median survival for those with spinal onset is approximately 29 months, with nearly 15 per cent surviving 5 years.

Differential diagnosis and investigation

A diagnosis of amyotrophic lateral sclerosis is usually depressingly obvious on simple clinical grounds. Often only electrophysiological investigation is necessary to confirm denervation and to exclude a potentially treatable myopathy or demyelinating neuropathy. If patients present with the combination of arm denervation and upper motor-neurone signs in the legs, the cervical spinal canal should be imaged with magnetic resonance or myelography in order to exclude a compressive lesion, most often spondylitic radiculomyelopathy.

The usual diagnostic problem lies in differentiating amyotrophic lateral sclerosis from other motor neurone diseases, e.g. the postpolio syndrome, X-linked bulbospinal neuronopathy, multifocal motor neuropathy, or adult-onset proximal hereditary motor neuronopathy.

Treatment

No treatment is known to cure amyotrophic lateral sclerosis. Yet much can be done to overcome disability and alleviate distress by the care team of speech therapist, physiotherapist, occupational therapist, social worker, and physician. The Motor Neurone Disease Association is often able to provide equipment promptly. Severe dysphagia is most effectively treated by percutaneous endoscopic gastrostomy. Speech failure can be circumvented by computer-assisted communication devices operated through an appropriate modality, such as pressure, blowing, head-nodding, or blinking, depending upon which muscles remain strong. Decisions on the advisability of instituting assisted respiration pose complex practical and ethical dilemmas. Patients with diaphragmatic weakness and nocturnal dyspnoea may be helped by continuous positive airways pressure delivered by a facial mask. Endotracheal intubation and ventilation are rarely recommendable in a disease causing such ubiquitous irreversible weakness.

Lower motor-neurone syndromes

These forms of motor neurone disease generally follow a much more benign course than amyotrophic lateral sclerosis. They include syndromes previously described as spinal muscular atrophy and progressive muscular atrophy.

Proximal hereditary motor neuronopathy

Early-onset forms

Acute infantile form (Werdnig–Hoffmann disease)

This autosomal-recessive disease has a frequency of approximately 1:25 000 in England and results from a gene frequency of 1:160. Half the infants die by 6 months and almost all have succumbed by 18 months, usually because of respiratory complications.

Chronic childhood form (Kugelberg–Welander disease)

This form develops at any time from infancy to the early teens. It is also autosomal recessive and follows a comparatively benign course. More than 90 per cent of patients are able to walk or to sit unsupported at some time, although these abilities are often lost eventually. Tongue involvement occurs in only half the patients, and significant dysphagia is unusual. Some patients develop respiratory insufficiency as a result of intercostal muscle involvement. The proximal limb weakness and wasting is only slowly progressive and may stabilize spontaneously. The prognosis varies, although survival into middle age is usual.

Adult-onset forms

The autosomal-recessive adult form starts from 15 to 60 years of age. Autosomal-dominant forms are rare. Slowly progressive proximal limb weakness ensues, but significant disability for walking usually does not occur until the sixth or seventh decade. Life expectancy is only slightly reduced. Distal muscles can be involved too; the tendon reflexes are usually lost, but bulbar involvement is uncommon. The lack of upper motor neurone signs or of bulbar involvement, and the rather indolent progression, distinguish this from sclerosis.

X-linked recessive bulbospinal neuronopathy (Kennedy syndrome)

This disorder occurs only in men, with onset in the third to fifth decades of life. It is due to a mutation causing increased-length CAG repeat sequences within the androgen receptor gene. Molecular genetic analysis now forms the basis of a diagnostic test. Weakness usually first affects hand or pelvic girdle muscles and the bulbar symptoms may not be evident until 20 years later, if at all. Fasciculations are usually visible in the limb, tongue, and facial muscles. The disorder is only slowly progressive. Most patients survive into their seventh or eight decades, except when bulbar involvement is unusually severe. Unlike amyotrophic lateral sclerosis, there are no upper motor-neurone signs and patients commonly show gynaecomastia, diabetes mellitus, and absent action potentials in sensory nerves.

Hexosaminidase deficiency

Autosomal recessive GM_1 gangliosidosis presents a variable neurological picture, occasionally as a pure motor-neurone syndrome due to lower and, rarely, upper motor-neurone involvement. More usually these are combined with other neurological abnormalities, such as cerebellar ataxia or dementia.

Hexosaminidase assays should be reserved for those patients with early onset of unusual motor-neurone disorders, particularly Ashkenazim Jews.

Hereditary bulbar palsy

The Brown–Vialetto–van Laere syndrome presents in the teens with bilateral sensorineural deafness, followed some years later by bulbar, facial, limb, and sometimes respiratory muscle, weakness. Fazio–Londe disease is a bulbar palsy of childhood, without deafness, and respiratory muscle involvement may lead to death within a few years. It is usually inherited as an autosomal-recessive trait.

Monomelic, focal, or segmental motor neuronopathies

This condition usually occurs sporadically and most patients are young adult males. It presents with distal wasting and weakness of one hand or forearm; this progresses steadily for the first 2 years before either stabilizing, or settling to a slow rate of subsequent progression. Nerve-conduction studies are necessary to exclude focal entrapment neuropathies, or multifocal motor neuropathy with conduction block. MRI of the cervical spine will detect syringomyelia or other spinal-cord disease.

Postirradiation lumbosacral radiculopathy

This may follow months or years after the lower thoracic and upper lumbar spine are included in irradiation fields. It usually affects both legs, and some patients eventually develop involvement of sphincters and sensation. It is painless, and electrophysiology does not reveal the myokymic discharges, or abnormal sensory nerve action potentials, of irradiation plexopathy. The normal imaging of the lumbosacral plexus and cauda equina, and the absence of pain, exclude tumour recurrence.

Postpolio syndrome

After two or more decades, very slowly progressive weakness may affect muscles previously involved by acute paralytic poliomyelitis. Although this predominantly affects the limbs, approximately half the patients also have mild choking or dysphagia. The sluggish deterioration, lack of upper motor-neurone involvement, and previous history serve to distinguish postpolio syndrome from amyotrophic lateral sclerosis.

Multifocal motor neuropathy and neuronopathy

Patients with these conditions may present at any stage of adult life with multifocal and slowly progressive muscle weakness for as long as 20 years. The clinical picture is immensely variable. Distal limb muscles are mainly involved, often notably asymmetrically. The first symptoms and most severe weakness usually affect the arms. Reflex loss is generally restricted to affected muscles. Serum antibodies to GM_1 gangliosides are detectable in at least half the patients, but are not of proven pathogenetic significance. Paraproteinaemia may occur, particularly IgG. These motor neuropathies usually progress insidiously, sometimes in a stepwise manner, and occasionally spontaneous remissions occur. It is important to detect the subgroup of patients with multifocal motor conduction block, or with diffuse demyelinating neuropathy, because improvement may follow immunosuppressant therapy. High-dose intravenous human immunoglobulin therapy can produce dramatic temporary improvement. Unfortunately, steroid therapy does not improve multifocal motor neuropathy, and may precipitate further deterioration.

Upper motor-neurone syndromes

The pure upper motor-neurone syndromes are the rarest forms of motor neurone disease. They should be considered only after MRI has excluded structural or demyelinating disease of the spinal cord, foramen magnum, or brain. Spasticity is often severe but unfortunately antispasticity medications are often relatively ineffective. Rarely, similar upper motor-neurone syndromes may be seen with syphilis, Lyme disease, and human T-cell leukaemia virus type 1 infection.

Primary lateral sclerosis

This rare, sporadic form of motor neurone disease has an average age of onset of 50 years, usually starts in the legs, and slowly progresses thereafter for an average of 15 years.

Autosomal-dominant 'pure' familial spastic paraplegia

See Chapter 13.18.

Lathyrism

Neurolathyrism is a spastic paraparesis caused by regular consumption of the chickling pea vetch (*Lathyrus sativus*) for some months. It is endemic in parts of India and may be epidemic in times of famine. Patients present either subacutely or chronically with a spastic paraparesis. Once it has developed, neurolathyrism is usually not progressive, but little or no recovery occurs even after consumption of chickling pea ceases.

Further reading

Bowen, J., Gregory, R., Squier, M., and Donaghy, M. (1996). The post-irradiation lower motor neurone syndrome: neuropathy or radiculopathy? *Brain*, **119**, 1429–40.

Cochrane, G. and Donaghy, M. (1993). Motor neuron disease. In *Neurological rehabilitation* (ed. R.J. Greenwood, M.P. Barnes, T.M. MacMillan, and C.D. Ward), pp. 571–85. Churchill Livingstone, Edinburgh.

Harding, A.E. (1993). Inherited neuronal atrophy and degeneration predominantly of lower motor neurons. In *Peripheral neuropathy*, 3rd edn (ed. P.J. Dyck, P.K. Thomas, J.W. Griffin, P.A. Low, and J.F. Poduslo), Ch. 55. W.B. Saunders, Philadelphia.

Howard, R.S., Wiles, C.M., and Loh, L. (1989). Respiratory complications and their management in motor neuron disease. *Brain*, **112**, 1155–70.

Pringle, C.E., Hudson, A.J., Munoz, D.G., *et al.* (1992). Primary lateral sclerosis. Clinical features, neuropathology and diagnostic criteria. *Brain*, **115**, 495–520.

Sonies, B.C. and Dalakas, M.C. (1991). Dysphagia in patients with the post-polio syndrome. *New England Journal of Medicine*, **324**, 1162–7.

Chapter 13.30

Peripheral neuropathy

P. K. Thomas

Pathophysiological considerations

Disorders of peripheral nerve function can be categorized by the site of the primary disturbance. Conditions that lead to the death of the neurone as a whole, with the loss of the cell body and the axon, are categorized as neuronopathies. Conditions that have a selective effect on axons are termed axonopathies. Axonopathies may be focal or generalized. Focal axonopathies occur as a result of insults such as trauma or ischaemia. Axonal interruption leads to Wallerian degeneration below the site of the injury. Recovery has to take place by axonal regeneration, which is a slow process with a rate of about 1 to 2 mm/day.

Other neuropathies primarily affect the myelin, either directly or through an interference with Schwann-cell function. The consequence is a selective demyelination with relative preservation of axonal integrity; this may be restricted to the region of the nodes of Ranvier (paranodal demyelination) or involve whole internodal segments (segmental demyelination) with consequent conduction block.

Recovery after paranodal or segmental demyelination occurs by remyelination. Initially, the newly formed myelin is thin, which results in abnormally slow conduction velocity. Reductions in conduction velocity may be focal, for example in relation to localized myelin damage in entrapment neuropathies, or widespread, as in the Guillain–

Barré syndrome or the inherited demyelinating neuropathies. In the last, conduction velocity in motor nerves is sometimes reduced to 10 m/s or less.

Finally, in other neuropathies the nerve fibres may be secondarily damaged by processes that primarily affect the connective tissues of the nerve or the vasa nervorum. Usually a combination of demyelination and axonal loss occurs.

Clinical categories of neuropathy

Mononeuropathy, multifocal neuropathy, and polyneuropathy

Peripheral neuropathies may be divided into two broad categories depending upon the distribution of the involvement. The first category comprises lesions of isolated peripheral nerves or nerve roots, termed mononeuropathy, or multiple isolated lesions, termed multifocal neuropathy (multiple mononeuropathy or 'mononeuritis multiplex'). The lesions in a widespread multifocal neuropathy may summate to produce a symmetrical disturbance, but the history or a careful examination may indicate the involvement of individual nerves. Isolated or multiple isolated lesions of peripheral nerves arise from conditions that produce localized damage, such as mechanical injury, nerve entrapment, thermal, electrical, or radiation injury, vascular causes, granulomatous, neoplastic, or other infiltrations, and nerve tumours.

Secondly, there may be a diffuse and bilaterally symmetrical disturbance of function, which can be designated polyneuropathy. When such a process affects the spinal roots, or affects the roots and the peripheral nerve trunks, the terms polyradiculopathy and polyradiculoneuropathy are sometimes employed. In general, polyneuropathies result from causes that act diffusely on the peripheral nervous system, such as metabolic disturbances, toxic agents, deficiency states, and certain instances of immune reaction.

Symptomatology

Weakness or paralysis may be due either to conduction block in the motor nerve fibres or to axonal degeneration. Recovery may occur by remyelination, and may be rapid and complete as in localized nerve lesions, for example 'Saturday night' paralysis of the radial nerve (see below), or in more widespread polyneuropathies, such as acute idiopathic polyneuropathy (Guillain–Barré syndrome). If there is axonal interruption, axonal degeneration occurs below it. The muscle weakness is accompanied by denervation atrophy and electromyographic signs of denervation. In a reversible process, recovery has to take place by axonal regeneration, which is often slow and incomplete.

In generalized symmetrical polyneuropathies, the muscle weakness and wasting are commonly peripheral in distribution with an onset in the lower limbs. At times, a symmetrical involvement of the proximal musculature in the limbs occurs in polyneuropathies, for example in the Guillain–Barré syndrome or porphyric neuropathy. Fasciculation due to spontaneous contraction of isolated motor units is most often a feature of anterior horn-cell disease but may be encountered in peripheral neuropathies, as may muscle cramps. Loss of the tendon reflexes is a frequent accompaniment of a peripheral neuropathy, and usually first affects the ankle jerks.

Sensory symptoms and sensory loss in symmetrical polyneuropathies are usually distal in distribution, giving rise to the 'glove and stocking' pattern of involvement. The sensory loss may affect all modalities or be restricted to certain forms of sensation. If the loss is restricted, two broad patterns are discernible. In the first, the impairment chiefly affects joint position sense, and vibration and touch–pressure sensibility, corresponding to a predominant loss of function in the larger, myelinated nerve fibres. In the second pattern of selective sensory loss, pain and temperature sensibility are chiefly affected, often associated with loss of autonomic function, corresponding to a predominant loss of small, myelinated and unmyelinated axons.

Paraesthesias are a frequent feature in peripheral neuropathy; these are usually of a tingling nature ('pins and needles'), but may involve thermal sensations, most often with a burning quality.

Spontaneous pains of an aching or lancinating character may complicate a number of generalized polyneuropathies.

Diagnosis and investigation

The history and physical examination frequently indicate that the disturbance has affected the peripheral nerves. If confirmation is required, this may usually be obtained by nerve-conduction studies. Examination of the cerebrospinal fluid is not commonly of value in the diagnosis of peripheral neuropathies. Nerve biopsy may be of value in establishing the cause of the neuropathy, particularly in conditions that affect the vasa nervorum or neural connective tissues, or in 'storage' disorders.

Individual nerves

Phrenic nerve (C2–C4)

Paralysis may be detected by unilateral or bilateral elevation of the diaphragm in a chest radiograph and its failure to descend on inspiration. The phrenic nerve may be involved in its course through the neck or thorax by wounds, or tumours such as bronchial carcinoma, and it is sometimes affected in idiopathic brachial plexus neuropathy (neuralgic amyotrophy).

Nerve to serratus anterior (C5–C7)

The serratus anterior acts as a fixator of the scapula, holding it against the chest wall when forward pressure is exerted by the arm. When serratus anterior is paralysed in isolation, the position of the scapula is normal at rest but if the extended arm is pushed forwards against resistance, 'winging' of the scapula becomes evident. The nerve to serratus anterior may be involved in penetrating wounds, but usually in association with damage to the brachial plexus. Weakness of the serratus anterior is a common component of idiopathic brachial plexus neuropathy (neuralgic amyotrophy) and it is not infrequently encountered as an isolated and unexplained lesion.

Brachial plexus

The brachial plexus may be affected by penetrating wounds of the neck, in fractures and dislocations of the shoulder and clavicle, as a result of traction on the arm, by pressure from an aneurysm or a cervical rib, and by neoplastic involvement.

Traction lesions

Traction on the arm may result in damage to the plexus itself or may lead to avulsion of the spinal roots from the cord.

In severe traction lesions, commonly encountered as a result of motorcycle accidents, the whole of the plexus may be damaged. With forcible downward displacement of the shoulder, only the upper part of the plexus, involving the contribution from the fifth and sixth cervical nerve roots, may be damaged. Selective injury to the lower part of the plexus involving the contributions from the eighth cervical and first thoracic nerve roots occurs as a result of traction with the arm extended, as when an someone falls from a height and tries to save themselves by hanging on to a ledge.

Selective damage to the upper portion of the plexus (C5 and C6 roots or upper trunk) results in paralysis of deltoid, biceps, brachialis, brachioradialis, and sometimes supraspinatus, infraspinatus, and subscapularis. The arm hangs at the side, internally rotated at the shoulder, with the elbow extended and the forearm pronated in the 'waiter's tip' position. Abduction at the shoulder and flexion at the elbow are not possible. The biceps and brachioradialis jerks are lost. Selective paralysis of the lower brachial plexus (C8, T1) results in paralysis of all the intrinsic hand muscles and a consequent claw-hand deformity, weakness of the medial finger and wrist flexors, and sensory loss along the medial border of the forearm and hand and over the medial two fingers. Cervical sympathetic paralysis, giving rise to Horner's syndrome, is frequently associated.

When the spinal roots are avulsed from the cord, regeneration is impossible and intractable spontaneous pain may be a highly troublesome sequel. Where the injury is distal to the dorsal root ganglia, lesions of the upper portion of the brachial plexus recover more satisfactorily than lesions of the lower plexus.

Thoracic outlet syndromes

The contribution of the eighth cervical and first thoracic roots to the brachial plexus may be damaged by angulation over an abnormal rib or, more usually, a fibrous band arising from the seventh cervical vertebra and attached to the first rib. The subclavian artery may be affected by cervical ribs giving rise to aneurysmal dilatation and vascular symptoms such as Raynaud's syndrome and embolic phenomena.

Damage to the lower part of the brachial plexus leads to weakness and wasting of the small hand muscles, and of the medial forearm wrist and finger flexors. Numbness, pain, and paraesthesias occur along the inner border of the forearm and hand, extending into the medial two fingers. The pain tends to be provoked by carrying heavy articles in the hand on the affected side. Horner's syndrome may be a feature. Surgical removal of the rib or fibrous band often leads to abolition of the pain and paraesthesias, but recovery of power in the small hand muscles is frequently disappointing.

Neoplastic involvement

Tumours may arise locally in the brachial plexus, such as neurofibromas in von Recklinghausen's disease (type I neurofibromatosis) or a solitary neurinoma; or the plexus may be invaded by tumours arising in other structures, most commonly the involvement of the lower part of the plexus by an apical carcinoma of the lung (Pancoast syndrome), which gives rise to wasting and weakness of the small hand muscles and of the medial forearm wrist and finger flexors, pain and sensory loss affecting the medial border of the forearm and hand, and cervical sympathetic paralysis. Other tumours that may invade the brachial plexus include carcinoma of the breast and malignant lymphomas affecting the lymph glands in the root of the neck.

Neuralgic amyotrophy

This condition may follow immunizing procedures, in particular the administration of antitetanus serum, or operations, or occur without recognizable antecedent event.

The disorder develops acutely with intense pain in the shoulder region that ceases after a few days. Paralysis of the muscles of the shoulder girdle becomes evident within a day or two of the onset of the pain, sometimes also of the arms or of the diaphragm. It may be unilateral or bilateral and may be associated with sensory loss. The cerebrospinal fluid is consistently normal. The affected muscles show electromyographic evidence of denervation, but recovery is usually ultimately satisfactory. Not all cases recover fully and there may be recurrences. Corticosteroids do not influence either the initial pain or the ultimate outcome.

Postirradiation brachial plexus neuropathy

The brachial plexus may be damaged by radiotherapy for breast carcinoma or other tumours in the neck. The onset of symptoms is usually several years after treatment, but may be within months. It can be difficult to distinguish from tumour recurrence but is less likely to be painful; MRI may be helpful.

Radial nerve (C5–C8)

The long course of the radial nerve and its position in relation to the humerus make it unusually susceptible to external compression. It may be injured in wounds of the axilla so that the paralysis includes triceps, resulting in loss of extension at the elbow. The most frequent type of injury is compression of the nerve in the middle third of the arm against the humerus; this is encountered as 'Saturday night paralysis' in which an individual falls asleep when intoxicated with their upper arm over the arm of a chair. Triceps is spared, but brachioradialis, supinator, and all the forearm extensor muscles are paralysed. Sensory impairment is limited to the dorsum of the hand. Commonly the lesion consists of a localized conduction block (neurapraxia) so that muscle wasting does not occur and a muscle response can be obtained on stimulation of the nerve below the level of the lesion. Recovery is complete within a matter of weeks.

The deep branch of the nerve may be injured distal to the supinator muscle. This muscle is, of course, spared, together with brachioradialis and the radial wrist extensors, and there is no sensory loss. A lesion of the posterior interosseus nerve gives rise to weakness confined to abduction and extension of the thumb and extension of the index finger.

Axillary nerve (C5–C6)

This is a branch of the posterior cord of the brachial plexus. It supplies deltoid and teres minor, and the skin over deltoid through the upper lateral brachial cutaneous nerve. It may be damaged in injuries to the shoulder and the chief symptom is an almost complete inability to raise the arm at the shoulder. In the past, it was sometimes injured by pressure from a crutch ('crutch palsy').

Median nerve (C6–C8, T1)

The median nerve has no muscular branches above the elbow. It supplies all the muscles in the anterior aspect of the forearm except flexor carpi ulnaris and the medial half of flexor digitorum profundus. The main trunk passes deep to the flexor retinaculum of the wrist and its recurrent muscular branch supplies abductor pollicis brevis, opponens pollicis, and contributes to the innervation of flexor pollicis brevis. It also supplies the lateral two lumbrical muscles and the skin of the lateral aspect of the palm, and the lateral three-and-a-half digits over their palmar aspects and terminal parts of their dorsal aspects.

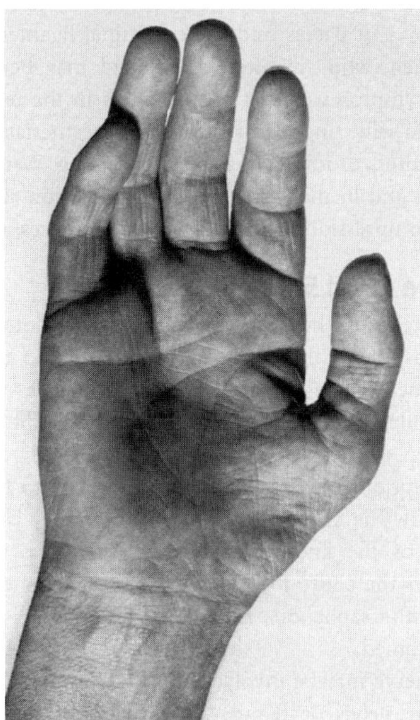

Fig. 1 Thenar wasting in a patient with the carpal tunnel syndrome.

Lesions of the forearm

The median nerve may be injured in the region of the elbow or compressed at the level of the pronator teres muscle. Entrapment neuropathies in the upper forearm, however, are uncommon. Occasionally the anterior interosseus branch is involved in isolation.

Lesions at the wrist

The superficial situation of the median nerve at the wrist renders it liable to injury in lacerations sustained by falling against a window with the hand outstretched, or in suicidal attempts. It may also be damaged as an occupational hazard by individuals who exert repeated pressure on the butt of the hand.

Much the most common lesion at this site is the carpal tunnel syndrome, in which the median nerve is compressed as it passes deep to the flexor retinaculum. The usual presentation is with numbness, tingling, and burning sensations felt in the hand and fingers, the pain sometimes radiating up the forearm as far as the elbow or even as high as the shoulder or root of the neck. The paraesthesias are sometimes restricted to the radial fingers, but may affect all the digits. The attacks of pain and paraesthesia are most common at night and often wake the patient from sleep. They are then relieved by shaking the hand. The hand tends to feel numb and useless on waking in the morning but recovers after it has been used for some minutes. The symptoms may recur during the day following use, or at times if the patient sits with the hands immobile. Such symptoms of acroparaesthesia may persist for many years without the appearance of symptoms of median-nerve damage. In other patients, weakness of the thenar muscles develops (Fig. 1), particularly of abduction of the thumb, and is associated with atrophy of the lateral aspect of the thenar eminence. Sensory loss may appear over the tips of the median-innervated fingers.

The symptoms are usually characteristic. If confirmation is required in atypical cases, this can generally be obtained by nerve-conduction studies.

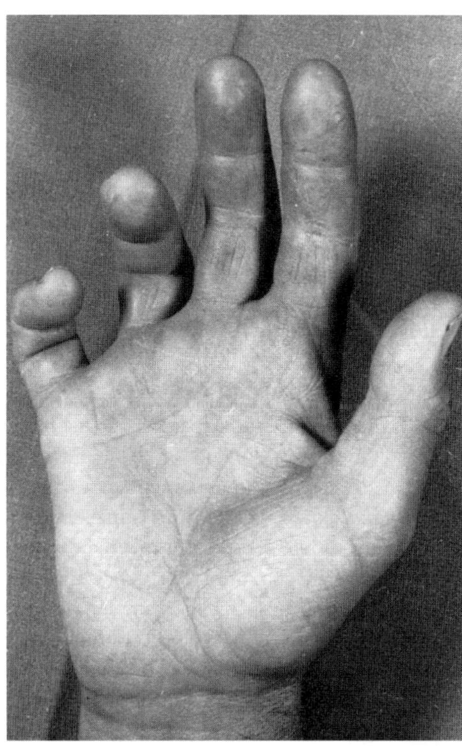

Fig. 2 Claw-hand deformity in a patient with an ulnar-nerve lesion.

It may develop as a consequence of osteoarthritis of the carpus, perhaps related to an old fracture. Other predisposing causes are pregnancy, myxoedema, acromegaly, and infiltration of the flexor retinaculum in primary and hereditary amyloidosis.

In cases in which muscle weakness and wasting, or sensory loss, are present when the patient is first seen, treatment should be decompression of the nerve by section of the flexor retinaculum. Injection of the carpal tunnel with a long-acting corticosteroid preparation may give temporary relief Splinting of the wrist to reduce movement during the day may also be useful. If the symptoms persist despite conservative measures, decompression is then advisable.

Ulnar nerve (C7, C8, and T1)

This nerve arises from the medial cord of the plexus, usually with a contribution from the lateral cord. In the upper arm, branches arise that supply flexor carpi ulnaris and the medial part of flexor digitorum profundus. In the forearm, the dorsal branch arises that winds around the ulna and supplies the skin over the dorsal aspect of the hand and the medial one-and-a-half fingers. In the hand, a superficial branch supplies palmaris brevis, and the skin over the medial aspect of the palm and the medial one- and-a-half fingers. The deep branch, after supplying the hypothenar muscles, innervates the interossei, the third and fourth lumbricals, the adductor pollicis, and part of flexor pollicis brevis.

Lesions at the elbow

Total paralysis from lesions at this level, including the branches to flexor carpi ulnaris and flexor digitorum profundus, gives rise to wasting along the medial side of the forearm flexor mass. There is weakness of flexion of the fourth and fifth fingers. Paralysis of the hypothenar muscles abolishes abduction of the fifth finger. Paralysis of the interossei and the medial two lumbricals gives rise to the 'claw-hand' deformity (Fig. 2).

In the hand, there is wasting of the hypothenar muscles, of the interossei, and the medial part of the thenar eminence. Movements of abduction and adduction of the fingers are weak, as is adduction to the extended thumb against the palm.

The ulnar nerve may be damaged by dislocations or fracture dislocations at the elbow and is sometimes compressed in individuals who habitually lean on their elbows. When it is suspected that the nerve has been subjected to repeated compression at the elbow, surgical transposition to the front of the medial epicondyle should be considered. If the nerve is compressed in the cubital tunnel, decompression by slitting the aponeurosis may suffice.

Lesions at the wrist or in the hand

Damage to the nerve at the wrist will spare the dorsal branch, so that cutaneous sensation over the dorsum of the hand and fingers is spared. Damage to the deep palmar branch spares the hypothenar muscles, but causes weakness of the other ulnar-innervated, small hand muscles. Lesions at the wrist or in the hand are usually the result of compression by ganglia or by repeated occupational trauma. Damage to the deep palmar branch, for example, may be caused by firm pressure from a screwdriver or drill. If occupational pressure is the cause, recovery follows cessation of the precipitating cause. Should improvement fail to occur after an appropriate interval, surgical exploration to establish whether a ganglion is present is merited.

Lumbosacral plexus

Lesions of the lumbosacral plexus are not common. The plexus may be involved in pelvic malignancy or be the site of a local neural tumour. It may be compressed by a haematoma in patients receiving anticoagulant therapy or suffering from haemophilia, or be involved in fractures of the pelvis. The lumbosacral cord may be compressed against the rim of the pelvis by the fetal head during parturition, with consequent weakness of the anterior tibial and peroneal muscles, and sensory impairment in the distribution of the fourth and fifth lumbar dermatomes. The superior gluteal nerve may also be affected. Recovery is initially good but may not be complete.

Femoral nerve (L2–L4)

Damage to the femoral nerve causes weakness of knee extension, wasting of the quadriceps, loss of the knee jerk, and sensory impairment over the front of the thigh and in the distribution of the saphenous nerve. With a proximal lesion, there may also be weakness of hip flexion from paralysis of iliacus.

The femoral nerve may be injured in fractures of the pelvis or femur, in dislocations of the hip, and at times during operations on the hip. It may be involved by psoas abscesses, tumours, or implicated in wounds of the thigh. It is commonly involved in large haematomas of the psoas muscle in haemophiliacs.

Obturator nerve (L2–L4)

Damage to the obturator nerve results in weakness of adduction and internal rotation at the hip, pain in the groin, and sensory impairment on the medial part of the thigh. The nerve may be involved in neoplastic infiltration in the pelvis and can be damaged by the fetal head or by forceps during parturition.

Lateral cutaneous nerve of the thigh (L2–L3)

This nerve supplies the skin over the anterolateral aspect of the thigh. Meralgia paraesthetica is an entrapment neuropathy resulting from its compression as it passes under the inguinal ligament. It is more common in men, who are often obese, and may be unilateral or bilateral. The symptoms consist of numbness in the territory of the nerve combined with tingling or burning paraesthesias provoked by prolonged standing, or following excessive walking. Weight reduction may be helpful and in many instances the condition subsides spontaneously. Decompression of the nerve is rarely necessary.

Sciatic nerve (L4–L5; S1–S3)

The sciatic nerve enters the thigh through the sciatic notch. It descends the posterior aspect of the thigh and separates into the tibial and common peroneal nerves in the lower thigh, which supply all the muscles below the knee; both nerves contribute to the formation of the sural nerve.

Total interruption of the sciatic nerve gives rise to foot drop. All movement below the knee is paralysed. If the injury is in the upper thigh, flexion of the knee is also weak. The skin is completely anaesthetic over the entire foot except for the medial border, which is supplied by the saphenous nerve. The ankle jerk is lost but the knee jerk is retained.

The sciatic nerve may be involved in pelvic tumours or injured by fractures of the pelvis or femur. After the radial and ulnar, it is implicated in gunshot wounds more frequently than any other nerve. Partial injury of the tibial division may be followed by causalgia. Incomplete lesions of the nerve may be caused by pressure of the nerve against the hard edge of a chair in individuals who fall asleep while intoxicated. Similar lesions may occur in diabetic persons, in whom the peripheral nerves are more susceptible to pressure neuropathy.

The syndrome of root pain and sciatica is considered in Chapter 13.10.

Tibial nerve (L4–L5; S1–S3)

After separating from the peroneal division of the sciatic nerve in the lower thigh, this nerve supplies the popliteus, all the muscles of the calf, and, through the plantar nerves, the small muscles of the sole of the foot and sensation to the sole. When the nerve is interrupted, the patient is unable to plantarflex or invert the foot, or flex the toes, and cannot stand on the ball of the foot. Paralysis of the interossei leads to a claw-like deformity of the toes. Sensation is lost over the sole.

The tibial nerve is occasionally compressed under the flexor retinaculum (tarsal tunnel syndrome), usually precipitated by osteoarthritis or post-traumatic deformities at the ankle, or by tenosynovitis. Burning pain and tingling paraesthesias occur in the sole, usually following prolonged standing or walking. The condition is generally unilateral. Careful examination may demonstrate wasting of the intrinsic muscles in the medial aspect of the foot, and sensory impairment over the sole. Nerve-conduction studies may be helpful. Treatment is by surgical section of the flexor retinaculum.

Painful neuromas sometimes develop on the digital branches of the plantar nerves; these give rise to the syndrome of Morton's metatarsalgia in which pain occurs in the anterior part of the foot on standing. A localized area of tenderness is detectable on palpation. The condition is relieved by excision of the neuroma.

Common peroneal nerve (L4–L5; S1–S2)

After separating from the tibial division of the sciatic nerve in the lower part of the thigh, this nerve descends through the popliteal fossa, winds around the neck of the fibula, and divides into its superficial and deep branches.

Damage to the common peroneal nerve is more frequent than injury to its two branches because of its vulnerable superficial position at the neck of the fibula. It gives rise to foot drop with paralysis of dorsiflexion and eversion at the ankle, and of toe extension. Cutaneous sensation is impaired over the lateral aspect of the lower leg and ankle, and on the dorsum of the foot.

Paralysis caused by external pressure frequently gives rise to a local conduction block (neurapraxia) with satisfactory recovery within a few weeks. If electromyography indicates that nerve degeneration has taken place, a foot-drop support should be provided while axonal regeneration is awaited.

Generalized neuropathies

Neuropathies related to metabolic and endocrine disorders

Diabetes mellitus

A significant degree of peripheral neuropathy develops in about 15 per cent of patients with diabetes. In general, the neuropathies that appear can be divided into symmetrical sensory polyneuropathies and autonomic neuropathies on the one hand, and isolated lesions of peripheral nerves or multifocal neuropathies on the other. Mixed syndromes are common.

The most common form is a mild symmetrical sensory polyneuropathy, giving rise to numbness and tingling paraesthesias in the toes and feet, and less often in the fingers. Aching or lancinating pains in the feet and legs, particularly at night, may be a troublesome feature. Examination reveals loss of vibration sense in the feet, depression of the ankle jerks, and mild distal cutaneous sensory impairment. More rarely a more severe sensory neuropathy develops, sometimes referred to as 'diabetic pseudotabes'.

Autonomic neuropathy frequently accompanies the sensory neuropathy and may be the salient manifestation. It rarely occurs in isolation. Pupillary disturbances usually take the form of a reduced response to light. Anhidrosis may occur distally in the limbs; if it is extensive and also affects the trunk, heat intolerance may result. Symptoms referable to the alimentary tract include dysphagia from oesophageal involvement, episodes of vomiting related to gastric atony, and episodic nocturnal diarrhoea, often alternating with periods of constipation. Those related to the genitourinary system include impotence, retrograde ejaculation, and bladder atony with difficulty in voiding and urinary retention with overflow. Vascular denervation sometimes results in postural hypotension, and cardiac denervation may be demonstrable by an elevated resting heart rate and the absence of beat-to-beat variation with respiration.

Isolated nerve lesions tend to occur more commonly in diabetic elderly people. At times they develop insidiously, at others they have an abrupt onset with pain. Of the cranial nerves, the nerves to the external ocular muscles, particularly the IIIrd, and also the facial nerve, are the most often affected. In contradistinction to the effects of compression of the IIIrd nerve by a carotid aneurysm, the pupillary innervation is often spared. In the limbs, the lesions tend to occur at the common sites of compression or entrapment. It seems likely that diabetic nerve exhibits an excessive vulnerability to damage from pressure.

Diabetic amyotrophy represents a particular example of a multifocal neuropathy that develops usually in elderly obese diabetics. It consists of an asymmetrical proximal motor syndrome that affects the anterior thigh muscles and hip flexors, and sometimes also the anterolateral muscles of the lower leg. Less commonly it is symmetrical. Its onset may be acute or insidious and is often accompanied by pain, particularly at night. There is generally little or no associated sensory loss. The knee jerks are usually depressed or absent.

Focal peripheral nerve lesions and diabetic amyotrophy, if of acute onset, often recover adequately, as does acute painful diabetic neuropathy when satisfactory control is achieved. The symmetrical sensory and autonomic neuropathy, once established, recovers less satisfactorily, even with good diabetic control.

Amyloidosis

The peripheral nerves may be involved in both AA and AL amyloidosis. There are also several dominantly inherited forms of amyloid neuropathy. Isolated lesions may occur from the infiltration of amyloid into nerves. More strikingly, a generalized neuropathy may develop. It begins with selective loss of pain and temperature sensation in the feet and later in the hands. Motor involvement, loss of tendon reflexes, and impairment of other sensory modalities occur later. Autonomic involvement is an early feature. Amyloid deposits are present in the peripheral nerve trunks, which may be enlarged, and in the dorsal root and sympathetic ganglia.

No treatment influences the progress of the neuropathy, except possibly in the inherited form. The spontaneous pains are sometimes improved by carbamazepine.

Uraemia

Uraemic neuropathy occurs in patients with severe chronic renal failure. The symptoms are usually predominantly sensory, with numbness and tingling paraesthesias in the feet. A distal motor neuropathy may be associated and occasional cases are purely motor. The condition is improved by increased haemodialysis and more dramatically by renal transplantation.

Myxoedema

Compression of the median nerve in the carpal tunnel in myxoedema has already been discussed. Rarely, a generalized mixed motor and sensory neuropathy develops; this improves on treatment of the hypothyroidism.

Acromegaly

The occurrence of the carpal tunnel syndrome in acromegaly has also been mentioned. A rare manifestation of this condition is a sensorimotor polyneuropathy in which the peripheral nerves are thickened because of an overgrowth of the neural connective tissues.

Critical-illness polyneuropathy

A generalized polyneuropathy involving widespread axonal degeneration may be encountered in patients in intensive care units with sepsis and multiple organ failure. The neuropathy is discovered when attempts are made to wean them from the ventilator. Slow recovery occurs.

Toxic neuropathies

Industrial and environmental substances (see also Section 18)

Acrylamide

This substance is now widely employed industrially. The monomer is neurotoxic and causes peripheral neuropathy with mixed motor and sensory features. Ataxia is prominent and is possibly the result of concomitant cerebellar damage. Slow recovery takes place on cessation of exposure.

Arsenic

Arsenical poisoning is occasionally seen as a result of accidental or homicidal ingestion of insecticides containing arsenic, or from indigenous medicines in India. Gastrointestinal symptoms develop after acute ingestion, followed by a mixed sensory and motor neuropathy after 1 to 3 weeks. Desquamation of the skin of the feet and hands takes place after about 6 weeks and white lines (Mees' lines) appear in the nails. With chronic ingestion of smaller quantities, gastrointestinal symptoms are less obtrusive and a slowly progressive neuropathy makes its appearance. The skin may become generally pigmented or show focal 'raindrop' pigmentation, and hyperkeratosis of the palms of the hands and soles of the feet may appear.

Slow recovery in the neuropathy occurs with removal from exposure. Chelating agents are of value in treating the non-neurological complications, but it is uncertain whether they are effective for the neuropathy.

Lead (see also Chapters 12.25 and 18.1)

Lead neuropathy is now a rare occurrence in Britain, although it was encountered as a consequence of the contamination of drinking water by lead pipes in old buildings. Lead neuropathy is predominantly motor, typically giving rise to wrist and foot drop. Other features of lead poisoning that may be associated include a sideroblastic anaemia and a 'lead line' on carious teeth. The neuropathy improves on cessation of lead intake; the utility of treatment with dimercaprol (BAL), edetate, or penicillamine is uncertain.

Mercury

Exposure to inorganic mercury salts and to organic mercurial compounds may lead to neurological damage. Dementia, cortical blindness, and ataxia occur, together with sensory changes in the limbs attributed to a sensory neuropathy, although how far these have a peripheral origin is uncertain.

Thallium

This is present in certain pesticides and rodent poisons. Accidental or homicidal poisoning is occasionally encountered. Abdominal pain and diarrhoea are followed after 2 or 5 days by the development of a mixed motor and sensory neuropathy, which is often painful. Evidence of damage to the central nervous system may be present, with behaviour disorder, optic neuropathy, and choreiform movements. Alopecia develops later, after about 2 or 3 weeks, and renal damage may be produced. Diethyldithiocarbamate, which binds thallium, has been employed in treatment.

Iatrogenic

Cisplatin

This platinum derivative is used in the chemotherapy of malignancy. A predominantly sensory neuropathy that recovers poorly may develop after the administration of several courses. Ototoxicity is more frequent, causing high-tone deafness and tinnitus.

Isoniazid

A mixed motor and sensory neuropathy may be produced by isoniazid and is more likely to occur in individuals who acetylate the drug slowly. The neuropathy is related to an interference with pyridoxine metabolism.

Nitrofurantoin

Excessively high blood concentrations of this preparation, as may occur in patients with reduced renal function, can cause a mixed motor and sensory neuropathy.

Vincristine

A neuropathy will occur in everyone given sufficient amounts of this cytotoxic agent. Mild sensory symptoms and loss of tendon reflexes may have to be accepted if a satisfactory therapeutic effect of the drug is to be achieved. If the neuropathy advances, bilateral weakness of the extensors of the wrist and fingers develops, followed by more widespread weakness. The neuropathy improves satisfactorily if the drug is withdrawn or if the dosage is reduced.

Other substances

Less important drugs that may give rise to neuropathy are almitrine, amiodarone, dapsone, disulfiram, gold, metronidazole, rnisonidazole, nitrous oxide (with a myelopathy), perhexilene, suramin, and zimeldine. A mild sensory neuropathy may develop after prolonged administration of phenytoin, and neuropathy was one of the complications produced by thalidomide. Pyridoxine, if taken in large doses, as 'megavitamin therapy', causes a sensory neuropathy.

Deficiency neuropathies

Beri beri neuropathy

Thiamine deficiency is probably involved, but a deficiency of other vitamins of the B group may also be implicated. A distal motor and sensory neuropathy develops, frequently accompanied by spontaneous aching pain in the extremities, cutaneous hyperaesthesia, and tenderness of the soles of the feet and calves. Thiamine deficiency is established by the finding of reduced erythrocyte transketolase activity; this enzyme requires thiamine as a cofactor.

Axonal degeneration occurs in the peripheral nerves and slow recovery ensues with vitamin replacement.

Alcoholic neuropathy

This always occurs on a background of nutritional deficiency. The dietary intake of the alcoholic individual is high in carbohydrates and low in vitamins. Moreover, alcoholics are known to have a reduced capacity to absorb thiamine. A direct toxic effect of alcohol on peripheral nerves may also be involved. The clinical features of alcoholic neuropathy are similar to those of *beri beri*.

Vitamin B_{12} deficiency

Vitamin B_{12} deficiency from whatever cause may be responsible for the development of a distal sensory neuropathy, with 'glove and stocking' sensory loss and paraesthesias, and areflexia, either in isolation or in association with a myelopathy or other central nervous manifestations. Haematological changes are not always present. The peripheral neuropathy improves more satisfactorily with treatment than the central disturbances. This condition is considered in detail in Section 3.

Vitamin E deficiency

Chronic severe vitamin E deficiency has recently been established as a cause for peripheral neuropathy in combination with a spinocerebellar degeneration. This disorder may occur in abetalipoproteinaemia, and isolated vitamin E deficiency, both of autosomal-recessive inheritance, and in congenital biliary atresia, cystic fibrosis, and occasional adults with chronic intestinal malabsorption.

Inflammatory and postinfective neuropathies

Leprous neuropathy

Peripheral nerve involvement in leprosy is considered in Chapter 16.61.

Guillain–Barré syndrome (acute idiopathic inflammatory polyneuropathy)

The syndrome is characterized by a polyneuropathy that develops over the course of a few days up to maximum of 4 weeks. Cases that progress for up to 8 weeks (subacute) are probably distinct. An identifiable infection may precede the onset of the neuropathy by 1 to 3 weeks. This is commonly an upper respiratory-tract infection or an infection with an enterovirus, Epstein–Barr virus, or mycoplasma. More recently, *Campylobacter jejuni* has been recognized as an important cause, as has human immunodeficiency virus (**HIV**) infection. In approximately 40 per cent of cases no antecedent event is identifiable.

The neuropathy may be ushered in by severe lumbar or interscapular pain. Motor involvement usually predominates over sensory loss and may be of a proximal, distal, or generalized distribution, and in severe cases affects the respiratory musculature. Distal paraesthesias in the limbs are common. The cranial nerves may be affected, in particular the facial nerves, but bulbar involvement also occurs sometimes. Autonomic disturbances may be associated, including bladder atony, ileus, hypertension and orthostatic hypotension. Further variants are a combination of an external ophthalmoplegia, ataxia, and tendon areflexia (Miller Fisher syndrome), or diffuse cranial-nerve involvement (polyneuritis cranialis), as possibly are instances of acute sensory neuropathy or pandysautonomia.

Nerve-conduction studies reveal evidence of demyelination in most cases. The cerebrospinal fluid protein is usually raised, often to a substantial degree, but it may be normal, particularly in the early stages. The cell content of the is usually normal, but there may be a mild lymphocytic pleocytosis; this is more likely to occur in cases related to HIV infection or infectious mononucleosis. Histologically, abnormalities are maximal in the spinal roots. In the demyelinating form, accumulations of inflammatory cells surround demyelinated nerve fibres.

Most cases of the Guillain–Barré syndrome recover satisfactorily within weeks or months. Severely affected patients, particularly those that require assisted respiration and in whom extensive axonal degeneration occurs, recover slowly and often show residual muscle weakness. Occasional patients have recurrences, which are sometimes multiple.

Plasma exchange and high-dose intravenous human immunoglobulin have both been shown to improve the rate of recovery if given before the nadir of the disease. Because of significant morbidity, particularly with plasma exchange, and cost, these forms of treatment are best reserved for more severe cases. Such patients may require support in an intensive care unit because of respiratory failure and autonomic dysfunction.

Chronic inflammatory demyelinating polyneuropathy

Instances of peripheral neuropathy occur that resemble the Guillain–Barré syndrome in that the neurological involvement is predominantly motor and the cerebrospinal fluid protein is elevated, but which pursue either a chronic relapsing or chronic progressive course. They are also associated with widespread demyelination in the spinal roots and peripheral nerves, and with inflammatory infiltrates. Nerve conduction velocity is usually markedly reduced and multifocal conduction block may be evident. Cases may respond to treatment with corticosteroids, plasma exchange, high-dose intravenous human immunoglobulin, or cytotoxic drugs. The response is less satisfactory in the chronic progressive cases.

Lyme borreliosis

Lyme borreliosis is a multisystem disease caused by a tick-borne spirochaete *Borrelia burgdorferi.* The peripheral nervous system is frequently affected both during the phase of early disseminated infection and during the late stage. Cranial neuropathies or an acute or subacute radiculoneuritis characterize involvement in the early stages, and a mild, predominantly distal, neuropathy characterizes the late stage.

HIV infection

A variety of neuropathies may be related to HIV-1 infection, particular types tending to occur in different phases of the disease. Characteristically, the Guillain–Barré syndrome or chronic inflammatory demyelinating polyneuropathy occur at the time of seroconversion, when the patient is otherwise well, and a multifocal vasculitic neuropathy occurs in the early symptomatic stage. A distal, often predominantly sensory and painful, neuropathy occurs mainly in the later AIDS phase, and an aggressive lumbosacral polyradiculoneuropathy from cytomegalovirus infection is encountered in advanced cases.

Sarcoid neuropathy

Sarcoidosis may give rise to a multifocal neuropathy with a particular tendency to involve the facial nerves, or to a generalized neuropathy. Evidence of involvement of other systems is not always present.

Diphtheritic neuropathy

The neuropathy of diphtheria is caused by exotoxin. Palatal weakness tends to develop after 2 to 3 weeks following pharyngeal diphtheria, and local muscle paralysis after a similar interval following cutaneous diphtheria. Paralysis of accommodation and sometimes of the external ocular muscles appears after an interval of 4 to 5 weeks. A generalized, predominantly motor, neuropathy of distal distribution may develop after 5 to 7 weeks. In severe cases the respiratory muscles are affected, but if death occurs it is usually as a result of an associated myocarditis.

Neuropathy in autoimmune connective-tissue disorders

Peripheral nerve involvement may be encountered in a wide range of the 'collagen–vascular' disorders. Polyarteritis nodosa characteristically gives rise to a multifocal neuropathy, often with considerable pain. Wegener's granulomatosis and rheumatoid arthritis may similarly be associated with a florid neuropathy. An ataxic sensory neuropathy related to a sensory ganglionitis can complicate Sjögren's syndrome.

The neuropathy of polyarteritis nodosa or rheumatoid arthritis may respond to corticosteroids or cyclophosphamide. The neuropathy of Sjögren's syndrome is largely refractory to treatment.

Neoplastic and paraneoplastic neuropathy

Peripheral neuropathy may develop as a non-metastatic complication of carcinoma, most often bronchial or gastric, or of lymphoreticular proliferative disorders. The neuropathy may antedate the discovery of the carcinoma by as much as 2 or 3 years. The Guillain–Barré syndrome may be encountered in Hodgkin's disease and in chronic lymphocytic leukaemia, and a subacute, mainly motor, neuropathy in relation to lymphoma. Non-metastatic carcinomatous neuropathies may regress following removal of the underlying tumour, or may remain unaffected.

Direct invasion of cranial nerves or spinal roots may occur in malignant infiltration of the meninges, and of the cervical and lumbosacral plexuses from local malignancies. Infiltration of peripheral nerve trunks happens most commonly in malignant lymphomas.

Paraproteinaemic neuropathy (see Chapter 13.31)

A sensory or sensorimotor polyneuropathy related to benign monoclonal paraproteins (monoclonal gammopathies of undetermined significance) has emerged in recent years as an important cause of late-onset neuropathy. The neuropathy is usually demyelinating, with features similar or identical to chronic inflammatory demyelinating polyneuropathy. A postural tremor of the upper limbs is often a prominent feature. The paraprotein is most commonly an IgM, less frequently IgG or IgA. Neuropathies associated with IgG or IgA paraproteins may respond to corticosteroids, immunosuppressive drugs, or plasma exchange; the response in IgM paraproteinaemic neuropathy is disappointing. Although a distal sensorimotor and often painful axonal neuropathy may be associated with myeloma, a demyelinating neuropathy accompanied by a dermato-endocrine syndrome may be encountered, referred to as the POEMS syndrome (*p*olyneuropathy, *o*rganomegaly, *o*edema, *M* protein, *s*kin changes; or *p*eripheral neuropathy, *o*rganomegaly, *e*ndocrinopathy, *m*onoclonal gammopathy, and *s*kin changes). Neuropathies are most often related to osteosclerotic myeloma.

Multifocal, predominantly lower limb, neuropathy may be caused by single or mixed cryoglobulins in myeloma, lymphoma, systemic lupus erythematosus, rheumatoid arthritis, or Waldenström's macroglobulinaemia.

Genetic neuropathies

Porphyria

A predominantly motor neuropathy may complicate acute attacks in the autosomal-dominant disorders of acute intermittent and variegate porphyria and hereditary coproporphyria, and in the recessively inherited δ-aminolaevulinic acid dehydratase deficiency. It tends to affect the proximal muscles to a greater extent. There may be associated sensory loss, which, although sometimes distal in distribution, can affect the trunk and the proximal portions of the limbs. Accompanying autonomic features include abdominal pain and vomiting, tachycardia and hypertension; mental confusion, psychotic behaviour, and epilepsy may be associated.

Axonal degeneration occurs in the peripheral nerves, so that recovery is slow and often incomplete.

Familial amyloid polyneuropathy

A number of inherited amyloid neuropathies have been recognized, related to point mutations in the gene for transthyretin, formerly known as prealbumin, which is on chromosome 18.

Hereditary motor and sensory neuropathy, types I and II, and X-linked (Charcot–Marie–Tooth disease, peroneal muscular atrophy)

Hereditary motor and sensory neuropathy (**HMSN**) types I and II usually present during childhood or adolescence with difficulty in walking or because of foot deformity. The deformity is most commonly pes cavus associated with clawing of the toes and sometimes with an equinovarus position of the foot. Muscle weakness tends to affect the lower leg muscles and may give rise to a bilateral foot drop with a 'steppage' gait. The muscle wasting is often restricted to below the knees, producing a 'stork leg' appearance. Weakness and wasting of the small hand muscles may appear later. The tendon reflexes become depressed or lost, and there is a variable degree of distal sensory loss. Progress of the disease is slow and cases with little disability or who are asymptomatic are common.

In the more common, type I families, there is a diffuse demyelinating neuropathy. The onset is most frequently in the first decade. Foot deformity and scoliosis occur more often than in type II HMSN. Sensory loss and ataxia tend to be greater and generalized tendon areflexia is usual. Weakness in the hands appears earlier. The peripheral nerves may be thickened. Cases with ataxia and upper-limb tremor are sometimes referred to as the Roussy–Lévy syndrome. They are not genetically distinct. The onset in the type II form, which is an axonal neuropathy, is most often in the second decade but it may be delayed until middle or even late adult life. Inheritance in both types I and II HMSN is usually autosomal dominant. In most families the disorder (HMSN Ia) is caused by a segmental duplication of chromosome 17, which includes the gene for peripheral myelin protein 22. X-linked dominant HMSN is uncommon. The clinical features resemble those of HMSN I but female carriers are asymptomatic or only mildly affected.

Nerve conduction velocity is severely reduced in type I cases, moderately reduced in the X-linked form, and either normal or only slightly reduced in HMSN II.

HMSN type III (Dejerine–Sottas disease)

This condition produces a slowly progressive, mixed motor and sensory polyneuropathy with an onset in childhood, often accompanied by ataxia. Inheritance is usually autosomal recessive. Striking enlargement of the peripheral nerve trunks is detectable on palpation, or may even be visibly evident.

Refsum's disease (see also Chapter 6.8)

This is an autosomal-recessive disorder that gives rise to a mixed motor and sensory polyneuropathy accompanied by a variety of other clinical features, including ataxia, anosmia, pigmentary retinal degeneration, pupillary abnormalities, deafness, cardiomyopathy, and ichthyosis. The presentation is usually during adolescence or early adult life, and the course may be steadily progressive or relapsing.

The disorder is due to an inability to metabolize phytanic acid, a long-chain fatty acid, which accumulates in the blood and tissues. It is largely of dietary origin and clinical improvement may be achieved with diets low in phytanic acid. For acute episodes of deterioration, plasma exchange is effective.

Hereditary sensory neuropathies

Predominantly sensory neuropathies may occur with either an autosomal dominant or recessive inheritance. The symptoms in the latter instance are usually present from birth; in the former they generally develop during the second or third decades. In both, the sensory loss often leads to a mutilating acropathy, with neuropathic joint degeneration and chronic cutaneous ulceration, particularly of the feet.

Other hereditary neuropathies

Peripheral nerve involvement occurs in metachromatic and globoid-cell leucodystrophy and adrenomyeloneuropathy, in Fabry's disease, and in hereditary lipoprotein deficiency (Tangier disease and hereditary abetalipoproteinaemia). Certain families show an inherited liability to pressure palsies with autosomal-dominant inheritance. Nerve fibres show focal regions of myelin thickening (tomacula) and are related to deletions on chromosome 17 affecting the gene for peripheral myelin protein 22.

Further reading

Coelho, T. (1996). Familial amyloid polyneuropathy: new developments in genetics and treatment. *Current Opinion in Neurology*, **11**, 311–8.

Gomi, G. and Corbo, M. (1998). Metabolic neuropathies. *Current Opinion in Neurology*, **11**, 523–9.

Hahn, A.F. (1998). Guillain-Barré syndrome. *Lancet*, **352**, 635–41.

Reilly, M.M. (1998). Genetically determined neuropathies. *Journal of Neurology*, **245**, 6–13.

Steck, A.J., Schaeren-Wiemers, N., and Hartung, H.P. (1998). Demyelinating inflammatory neuropathies, including Guillain-Barré syndrome. *Current Opinion in Neurology*, **11**, 311–8.

Thomas, P.K. (1997). Tropical neuropathies. *Journal of Neurology*, **244**, 475–82.

Chapter 13.31

The POEMS syndrome

J. G. G. Ledingham

Introduction

The acronym POEMS was first suggested by Bardwick and his colleagues in 1980 as an appropriate label to describe a syndrome variably combining *p*eripheral neuropathy, *o*rganomegaly, *e*ndocrinopathy, *m*onoclonal gammopathy, and *s*kin changes. The term is now widely used but synonyms include the Crow–Fukase syndrome, Takatsukis syndrome, and PEP (*p*olyneuropathy, *e*ndocrinopathy, and *p*lasma-cell dyscrasia).

The cause(s) of this rare syndrome is quite obscure and the major features are not all present in individual cases. It is probably more common in Japanese people, but this perception may be a reflection of the frequency of reporting the disease from Japan. The most common and earliest manifestation is undoubtedly the characteristic neuropathy, and most would agree that the diagnosis should not be made in its absence. A number of disorders not included in the acronym have now been reported to coincide with the syndrome more often than can be attributed to chance (see below).

Peripheral neuropathy

A progressive sensorimotor polyneuropathy is found in nearly all cases of the syndrome and is the most common presenting feature. Beginning distally, it characteristically spreads proximally; involvement of respiratory muscles has been described, but pain is unusual and cranial-nerve or autonomic dysfunction are not features. There is usually an increase in the protein content of the cerebrospinal fluid, sometimes exceeding 200 mg/100 ml, without abnormality in cell counts. Motor and sensory nerve conduction velocities are much reduced, and biopsy of nerve tissue shows segmental demyelination and axonal degeneration. Antibodies to myelin-associated glycoproteins have been detected in some cases in the presence of an IgM paraprotein, and the presence of complement-mediated damage to nerves has been postulated. Papilloedema, usually with increases in cerebrospinal fluid pressure, is common and has been reported in 40 to 60 per cent of cases.

Organomegaly

The organ most commonly found to be enlarged is the liver (in some 80 per cent); splenomegaly has been detected in around a quarter of cases. Lymphadenopathy is common (60 per cent) and in many cases the pathology is that of Castleman's disease (angiofollicular lymph node hyperplasia (see Chapters 3.27, 3.28)); this can be either of the hyaline vascular or plasma-cell type, in the latter case associated with systemic symptoms and often a poor prognosis. The enlarged nodes are found most commonly in the mediastinum and abdomen.

Endocrinopathy

Gonadal dysfunction is the most common endocrine association in the POEMS syndrome, with amenorrhoea a feature in nearly every case reported in women of child-bearing age. In men, gynaecomastia, impotence, or both affect some 70 per cent of patients. Hypothyroidism, with or without increased plasma concentrations of thyroid-stimulating hormone, has also been a common association; more rarely there have been reports of adrenocortical insufficiency, glucose intolerance, and hyperprolactinaemia.

Monoclonal gammopathy

Monoclonal increases in immunoglobulins, more commonly IgG than IgA, have been reported in 60 to 75 per cent of patients with other manifestations of the POEMS syndrome. In contrast to the pattern characteristic of myeloma, when κ light chains predominates over λ in a ratio of 2:1, excess of λ is more common in the POEMS syndrome and has been reported in some 80 per cent of cases. These immunoglobulin abnormalities have been associated with a variety of myelomatous lesions in bone. These may consist of solitary, usually painless, sclerotic lesions, which have been reported in some 60 per cent of cases. So-called ring lesions, with areas of peripheral sclerosis surrounding a central lucency, have also been reported, but the classical lucent areas of multiple myeloma are less common. Biopsy of affected areas of bone often shows an excess of monoclonal plasma cells, but routine examination of bone marrow shows such increases in plasma cells in only about 40 per cent of cases.

There have also been a few examples of polyclonal increases in immunoglobulins associated with other manifestations of the POEMS syndrome in patients who have apparently been exposed to organic solvents or other chemicals.

Other features

A number of much less frequent associations have now been described and are listed in Table 1. Some combinations of these features may coincide with the finding of high titres of antinuclear antibodies and/ or rheumatoid factor. Given the multisystem involvement in most

Table 1 Recognized associations with the POEMS syndrome

Oedema, pleural effusions, and ascites
Polycythaemia, leucocytosis, and thrombocythaemia
Fever and malaise
Raynaud's phenomenon
Hyperpigmentation, hirsutism, hyperhidrosis
Clubbing of the fingers
Dilated cardiomyopathy
Proteinuria and microangiopathic changes in renal glomeruli
Flushing resembling the carcinoid syndrome
Otherwise unexplained premature peripheral vascular calcification

cases of the POEMS syndrome, the differential diagnosis from systemic lupus erythematosus can sometimes be particularly difficult.

Treatment

Case reports of remission following removal or irradiation of local bone lesions suggest that at least in some cases a product(s) of abnormal plasma cells may play a central part in causing the syndrome. Interleukin 6 has been a suggested, but not proven, mediator in some cases.

More commonly there is a need for drug therapy and a large variety of agents are reported to have been used successfully. There are many reports of moderate to excellent responses to high-dose steroid therapy. Other agents used include azathioprine, cyclophosphamide, chlorambucil, cytosinarabinoside, thioguanine, and even tamoxifen and recombinant interferon. Given a large number of anecdotal case reports of the value or otherwise of these individual agents, it is probably sensible to start treatment with a combination of prednisolone (40–60 mg/day) and azathioprine (2–2.5 mg/kg per day) or a similar dose of cyclophosphamide. The response to treatment has been very variable. Many cases do very well for a number of years. Others do not, and this is perhaps a reflection of the heterogeneity of the disease, which we can only recognize at the moment by description, with almost no understanding of its pathogenesis.

Further reading

Miralles, G.D., O'Fallon, J.R., and Talley N.J. (1992). Plasma cell dyscrasia with polyneuropathy. The spectrum of POEMS syndrome. *New England Journal of Medicine*, 327, 1919–23.

Disorders of voluntary muscles

Chapter 13.32

An introduction

J. Walton

The anatomy and physiology of muscle

Voluntary muscle is made up of muscle fibres, each of which is a multinucleate cell containing myofibrils, sarcoplasm, and discrete intracellular organelles including mitochondria, ribosomes, and the sarcotubular system. Each fibre is enclosed within a sarcolemmal sheath beneath which muscle nuclei are situated and each has a motor endplate in which the nerve fibre terminates.

Under normal conditions, muscle fibres never contract singly; the functional unit of activity is the motor unit, which comprises the group of fibres supplied by a single anterior horn cell and its axon. Discharge of an anterior horn cell causes simultaneous contraction of all of its muscle fibres. The individual muscle fibres that make up a motor unit are often widely separated within the muscle.

Synaptic vesicles in the motor nerve terminal contain packets of acetylcholine, which is released continuously to give small depolarizations (miniature endplate potentials) in the nerve terminal. When an action potential reaches the nerve terminal, calcium ions (Ca^{2+}) enter it from the extracellular space and many packets of acetylcholine are released synchronously. Once released, the acetylcholine diffuses through the synaptic clefts to combine with receptors on the fibre membrane. The arrival of the nerve action potential causes a localized depolarization of the muscle-fibre membrane, giving rise to an endplate potential. When the endplate potential reaches a critical size, an action potential is induced, which travels from the endplate along the fibre surface membrane. At rest, the inside of the membrane is some 80 mV negative with respect to the outside, but as the action potential passes, the polarization of the membrane reverses, so that the inside of the fibre becomes positive. This reversal of polarity is caused by increased sodium permeability. The wave of excitation spreads into the fibre substance via a transverse system of tubules (the T-system); the resulting release of calcium ions in the sarcoplasmic reticulum initiates contraction of the fibrils.

The unit of structure of the myofibril is the sarcomere, extending from one Z-line (situated in the midst of the I-band) to the next (Fig. 1). Attached to each Z-line are thin filaments of actin, which interdigitate with thicker myosin filaments, the latter corresponding to the dark (birefringent) A-bands (Fig. 2). In cross-section, each myosin filament is surrounded by a hexagonal array of actin filaments; the actin and myosin filaments are joined by molecular cross-bridges. During contraction, these cross-bridges repeatedly disengage and re-engage at successive sites, and the actin and myosin filaments slide upon one another so that the myofibril shortens. The biochemical changes accompanying this process are complex, but creatine phosphate is broken down in the presence of calcium to creatine and phosphate, and ATP is broken down to ADP. The release of high-energy phosphate bonds provides energy.

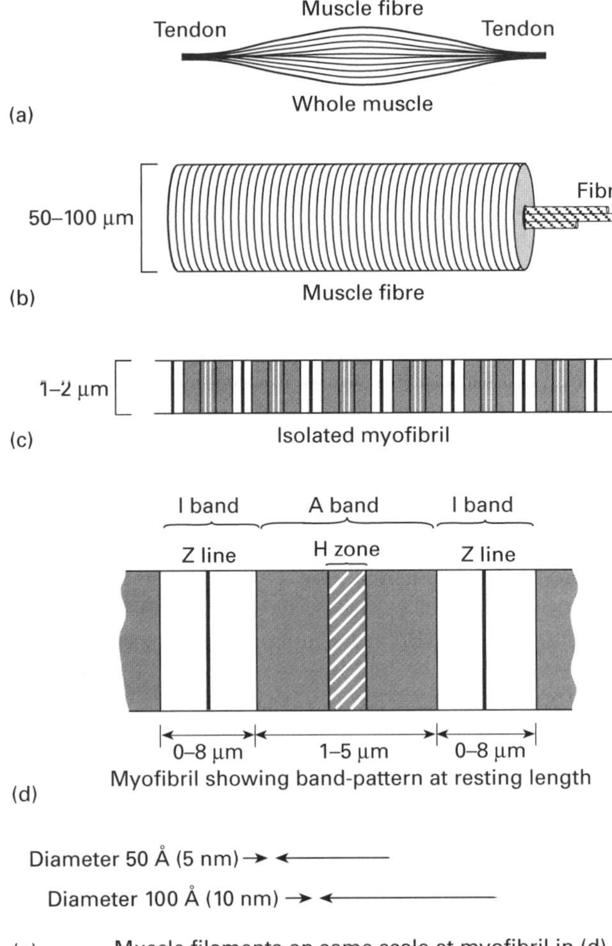

Fig. 1 The dimensions and arrangement of the contractile components in a muscle. The whole muscle (a) is made up of fibres (b), which contain cross-striated myofibrils (c, d). These are constructed of two types of protein filaments (e), put together as shown in Fig. 2.
(Reproduced from Huxley and Hanson 1960, with permission.)

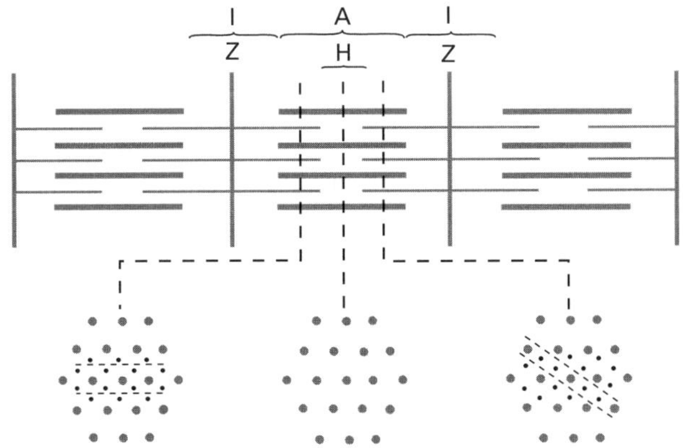

Fig. 2 Diagram illustrating the arrangement of the kinds of protein filaments (thick filaments, myosin; thin filaments, actin) in a myofibril. At the top are three sarcomeres drawn as they would appear in longitudinal section. Below are transverse sections taken through the H-zone and through the other parts of the A-band where the thick and thin filaments interdigitate. The plane of section determines whether, in electron micrographs, there seem to be one or two thin (actin) filaments between two thick (myosin) ones.
(Reproduced from Huxley and Hanson 1960, with permission.)

Skeletal muscles are not homogeneous but contain at least two main types of muscle fibre, which are morphologically and histochemically distinct. The type 1 fibre is slightly smaller than the type 2; it contains myofibrils that are more slender, and many mitochondria. These fibres contain a high concentration of oxidative enzymes and more fat than do the second type. The larger type 2 have slightly coarser and broader myofibrils; they contain fewer mitochondria than the type 1 fibres and less fat is present, although there is a higher concentration of glycogen and of enzymes, such as phosphorylase, that are concerned with anaerobic metabolism. In man, all skeletal muscles contain an admixture of type 1 and type 2 fibres, so that in sections stained histochemically a checkerboard pattern is seen. Physiologically, the type 1 fibres are concerned largely with the maintenance of posture, and contract and relax relatively slowly. Type 2 fibres, by contrast, contract more rapidly (fast-twitch fibres). All muscle fibres being supplied by a single motor neurone are of the same histochemical type and, in a sense, therefore, we can talk of type 1 and type 2 neurones. For a more detailed discussion, see OTM3, pp. 4139–44.

General comments on muscle disorders

The term 'myopathy' can be used to define any disease or syndrome in which the patient's symptoms and/or physical signs can be attributed to pathological, biochemical, or electrophysiological changes involving the muscle fibres or the muscular interstitial tissues, and in which there is no evidence that the symptoms are secondary to disordered function of the central or peripheral nervous systems. This group includes many genetically determined diseases, others of metabolic origin, and yet others in which the disease process is inflammatory.

Pain, muscular weakness, and fatiguability are the most important symptoms of muscle disease. Muscle weakness is the predominant symptom of most forms of myopathy. It is important to judge its distribution and tempo of development. Proximal muscle weakness in the upper limbs results in difficulty in lifting the arms above the head, and in the lower limbs difficulty in climbing stairs and in rising from the floor or a low chair. In most genetically determined disorders of muscle, weakness develops gradually over months or years; a more rapid onset suggests that the patient more probably has an inflammatory or metabolic myopathy. Periodic attacks of weakness with complete recovery in between strongly suggest one of the periodic paralyses. Fatiguability is characteristic of myasthenia gravis and myasthenic syndromes.

On physical examination, general examination is important as there may be changes in the eyes, skin, lymph nodes, or viscera indicating that the patient's muscular weakness is but one manifestation of a systemic multisystem disease. On examining the muscular system, the presence of atrophy, hypertrophy, or fasciculation may be of diagnostic value, as may the presence of muscular contractures and skeletal deformity. Fibrillation (the spontaneous contraction of single muscle fibres) is an electrical phenomenon that can be recorded electromyographically from denervated muscle, but cannot be seen through the skin. Fasciculation (the spontaneous contraction of individual muscle fasciculi) is seen most often in patients with anterior horn-cell disease; it is uncommon in primary muscle disease but occurs rarely in polymyositis or thyrotoxic myopathy. Coarse fasciculation, particularly in the calf muscles, is a benign phenomenon and may occur in normal individuals.

Further reading

Cullen, M.J. and Lander, D.N. (1994). The normal ultrastructure of skeletal muscle. In *Disorders of voluntary muscle* (ed. Lord Walton of Detchant, G. Karpati, and D. Hilton-Jones), pp 87–137. Churchill Livingstone, Edinburgh.

Dale, H. (1934). Chemical transmission of the effects of nerve impulses. *British Medical Journal*, **ii**, 835–7.

Landon, D.N. (1992). Skeletal muscle—normal morphology, development and innervation. In *Skeletal muscle pathology*, 2nd edn (ed. F.L. Mastaglia and Lord Walton of Detchant), pp. 1–94. Churchill Livingstone, Edinburgh.

Walsh, F.S. and Doherty, P. (1994). Cell biology of muscle. In *Disorders of voluntary muscle* (ed. Lord Walton of Detchant, G. Karpati, and D. Hilton-Jones), pp. 33–61. Churchill Livingstone, Edinburgh.

Walton, J.N., *et al.* (1993). Disorders of function in the light of anatomy and physiology. In *Brain's diseases of the nervous system*, 10th edn, pp. 28–32. Oxford University Press.

Wray, D. (1994). Neuromuscular transmission. In *Disorders of voluntary muscle*, 6th edn (ed. Lord Walton of Detchant, G. Karpati, and D. Hilton-Jones), pp. 139–78. Churchill Livingstone, Edinburgh.

Chapter 13.33

The muscular dystrophies

J. Walton

Muscular dystrophy can be defined as genetically determined, primary degenerative myopathy. Classification is the only safe guide to prognosis and genetic counselling; the most satisfactory clinicogenetic classification of the 'pure' muscular dystrophies based upon current knowledge is as follows.

1. *X-linked muscular dystrophy*:
   - (a) severe (Meryon–Duchenne);
   - (b) benign (Becker);
   - (c) benign with early contractures (Emery–Dreifuss) (rarely autosomal dominant);
   - (d) benign with acanthocytes (McLeod syndrome);
   - (e) scapuloperoneal (rare).
2. *Autosomal-recessive muscular dystrophy*:
   - (a) limb girdle (usually scapulohumeral, rarely pelvifemoral);
   - (b) childhood type, resembling Duchenne;
   - (c) distal type;
   - (d) congenital muscular dystrophy.
3. *Autosomal-dominant muscular dystrophy*:
   - (a) facioscapulohumeral;
   - (b) scapuloperoneal;
   - (c) late-onset proximal (limb girdle);
   - (d) benign early onset with contractures (?Bethlem, ?Emery–Dreifuss type);
   - (e) distal;
   - (f) ocular;
   - (g) oculopharyngeal.

Although this classification is comprehensive, some cases that are difficult to fit into any of the groups described still emerge.

Aetiology

Powerful evidence now suggests that in Duchenne dystrophy (this name is generally accepted even though the condition was described earlier by Meryon) there is a defect in the plasma membrane of the muscle fibre, and that this allows the uncontrolled entry of calcium. This in turn causes areas of hypercontraction of myofibrils and activation of calcium-activated neutral proteases, leading to necrosis of the muscle fibre. The gene responsible for Duchenne dystrophy is located in the Xp21 region of the X chromosome. The genes for Duchenne and Becker dystrophy are allelic. Their clinical expression depends, at least in part, upon the number and extent of deletions within the gene. However, some patients with Duchenne dystrophy do not have deletions and in them the disease is assumed to result from a point mutation. The missing gene product is a protein named dystrophin, which is totally absent in almost all cases of Duchenne dystrophy and much reduced in those of the Becker variety. Dystrophin forms a vital structural component of the skeletal muscle fibre membrane. The gene responsible for X-linked Emery–Dreifuss muscular dystrophy has been located on the distal part of the long arm of the X chromosome (Xq28), that for facioscapulohumeral dystrophy on chromosome 4, and that for myotonic dystrophy on chromosome 19. Limb-girdle dystrophy has proved to be heterogeneous: 10 per cent of cases are due to an autosomal-dominant gene (type 1); type 1B may be allelic to autosomal-dominant Emery–Dreifuss dystrophy. Three dominant and eight recessive subtypes have been identified, with gene locations on chromosomes 2, 4, 5, 13, 15, and 17. In type 2A a specific muscle protease (calpain 3) is deficient and in several recessive subtypes there are deficiencies of specific sarcoglycans (dystrophin-associated glycoproteins). The missing protein in the Emery–Dreifuss variety has been called emerin.

Pathology

The histological features of muscular dystrophy are similar in all varieties of the disease, though differing in severity. The most common are marked variation in fibre size, fibre splitting, central migration of sarcolemmal nuclei, patchy atrophy of muscle fibres, nuclear chains, segmental areas of necrosis within fibres with phagocytosis of necrotic sarcoplasm, and basophilia with enlargement of sarcolemmal nuclei showing prominent nucleoli. There is also infiltration by fat cells and connective tissue. Immunocytochemical techniques using monoclonal antibody stains show total absence of dystrophin in Duchenne, and partial absence in Becker and in carriers of the Duchenne gene. In Duchenne dystrophy, and to a greater extent in the Fukuyama variety of congenital dystrophy, various forms of cerebral dysgenesis are often found, while some degree of cortical atrophy with cerebral ventricular dilation is common in myotonic dystrophy.

Electromyography

Electromyography reveals volitional activity characteristic of any form of myopathy, and spontaneous activity is usually absent on recording from relaxed, resting muscle, although spontaneous fibrillation and positive sharp waves are occasionally recorded, especially in more rapidly progressive cases.

Symptoms and signs

The symptoms and signs of the disease depend upon the muscles first involved by the disease and upon its rate of progression. Weakness of pelvic-girdle muscles gives slowness in walking, inability to run, frequent falling, difficulty in climbing stairs or in rising from the floor, and eventually accentuation of the lumbar lordosis with a characteristic waddling gait. Climbing up the legs on rising from the floor (Gowers' sign) is characteristic but not specific. Involvement of the shoulder girdles gives a sloping appearance with a tendency for the scapulae to rise prominently when the patient abducts the arms. Facial weakness, as in facioscapulohumeral dystrophy, causes inability to whistle, difficulty in pouting the lips or in closing the eyes, while distal weakness in the extremities (as seen in the distal variety) causes weakness of grip and of fine finger movement, and foot drop. Contractures are common in all forms of dystrophy in the later stages, but are seen especially in the Duchenne and Emery–Dreifuss types. The most important clinical feature of all forms of dystrophy is that muscles are picked out selectively. Although there are differences in the patterns of weakness and wasting seen in the various subvarieties, it is common in the upper limbs to find that the serrati and pectorals are weak and atrophic, as are biceps and brachioradialis, while deltoid and triceps remain relatively unaffected. In the lower limbs, quadriceps and anterior tibials are usually involved first, and the calf muscles are spared, but in limb-girdle cases the hamstrings and quadriceps are often affected equally. In facioscapulohumeral dystrophy, the first leg muscles involved are usually the anterior tibials.

The severe X-linked Duchenne type

Although this condition is due to an X-linked recessive gene, about half of the affected boys are isolated cases, and in about one-third the disease is assumed to have resulted from a new mutation occurring in the ovarian cells of the mother or maternal grandmother.

Although many affected children are late in beginning to walk, the condition usually first becomes overt towards the end of the third year, with slowness in walking, frequent falling, and difficulty in climbing stairs. Enlargement of the calf muscles, and sometimes of quadriceps and deltoids, occurs in about 90 per cent of cases at some stage, but later disappears. Most patients deteriorate steadily and become unable to walk by about the age of 10 years, but apparent improvement may occur between the ages of 5 and 8 years, when the rate of deterioration is outstripped by the processes of normal development. When the boy is confined to a wheelchair, progressive deformity with skeletal distortion and atrophy occur. Death usually results from inanition, respiratory infection, or cardiac failure. With improved management, including the prevention of scoliosis and early treatment of complications (including assisted ventilation to control chronic alveolar hypoventilation, in appropriate cases), many sufferers now survive into their late twenties. Involvement of cardiac muscle is invariable, though not clinically detectable at first; the ECG typically shows tall R waves in the right precordial leads and deep Q waves in the limb and left precordial leads.

The benign X-linked (Becker) type

In this disorder the onset of the disease is usually between 5 and 25 years of age. There is often an initial phase of generalized muscular hypertrophy before weakness and wasting of pelvic, and later of shoulder girdle, muscles develops; most patients become unable to walk 25 years or more after the onset. Cardiac involvement is usually absent, contractures and skeletal deformity occur late, and many patients, though severely disabled, survive to a normal age.

The Emery–Dreifuss type

This uncommon, X-linked dystrophy usually is due to a gene lying on the Xq28 region of the long arm of the X chromosome but rare cases of dominant inheritance have been described. Muscular weakness and wasting is most prominent in a humeroperoneal distribution; the onset is between 5 and 15 years of age; there is slow progression with the early development of contractures (especially in the neck, knees, and ankles) and of cardiac involvement, causing conduction abnormalities (many patients eventually require a pacemaker).

The X-linked scapuloperoneal type

While scapuloperoneal muscular atrophy is usually neurogenic rather than myopathic, and more often dominant than X-linked, families in which the condition was clearly myopathic and X-linked have been described. The condition resembles the Emery–Dreifuss variety.

Limb-girdle muscular dystrophy

This form of the disease is very heterogeneous; most varieties occur equally in the two sexes and usually begin in the second or third decade of life, although they occasionally first appear in middle life.

In about half the cases muscle weakness begins in the shoulder girdle muscles and may not involve the pelvic girdle for many years, but in the remainder, pelvic-girdle muscles are first involved and weakness affects the shoulders within about 10 years. Enlargement of calf muscles is not uncommon. Sometimes muscular weakness and wasting are asymmetrical initially and occasionally the disease process arrests temporarily, but most patients are severely disabled within 20 years of the onset.

Childhood muscular dystrophy with autosomal-recessive inheritance

The existence of this comparatively rare variety, now equated with limb-girdle muscular dystrophy due to α-sarcoglycan deficiency, has been confirmed by the occasional occurrence of muscular dystrophy superficially resembling the Duchenne type in young girls and sometimes occurring in families with parental consanguinity. The onset may be in the second year or as late as the fourteenth, but is most often in the second half of the first decade of life. Progression is comparatively slow and patients usually become unable to walk in their early twenties, but sometimes as early as 15 years or as late as 40 years. The pattern of weakness is similar to that found in typical Duchenne dystrophy and most patients die in middle life.

Congenital muscular dystrophy

This rare disorder presents with severe, generalized muscular hypotonia, which is noted from birth and is accompanied by relatively non-progressive muscular wasting and weakness. Many affected children have widespread contractures suggesting arthrogryposis multiplex congenita. Occasionally the weakness increases rapidly after birth and the disease terminates fatally within the first year of life, but in most cases it seems relatively non-progressive. Few affected patients are ever able, however, to sit or stand unsupported and the prognosis is uniformly unfavourable. Diagnosis from spinal muscular atrophy of infancy can only be made with confidence by EMG, serum enzyme studies, and muscle biopsy. In about half of all cases the responsible gene has been localized to chromosome 6q.2 and there is a deficiency of laminin-α_2 (merosin). In the Fukuyama type, more common in Japan, there is also severe mental handicap and the gene is at chromosome 9q31–33.

Facioscapulohumeral muscular dystrophy

This variety, inherited as an autosomal-dominant trait and due to a gene at chromosome 4q35, occurs equally in the two sexes and can begin at any age from childhood until adult life but is usually first recognized in adolescence. Facial involvement, with a typical pouting appearance of the lips and difficulty in closing the eyes, is apparent early and is accompanied by weakness of shoulder-girdle muscles, with bilateral scapular winging and wasting of the pectorals. Muscular enlargement is uncommon; in the lower limbs the anterior tibial muscles are often first involved, causing bilateral foot drop. In many patients the disease runs a prolonged course with periods of apparent arrest, so that contractures and skeletal deformity develop late. Most affected individuals survive and remain active to a normal age. Heart muscle is not involved and the range of intelligence is usually normal, but some patients develop retinal vascular disease, others sensorineural deafness.

Diagnosis depends upon serum enzyme and EMG studies but especially upon muscle biopsy; the localization of the gene means that restriction fragment length polymorphisms now enable precise diagnosis; presymptomatic and antenatal diagnosis are now possible.

Distal muscular dystrophy

Distal muscular dystrophy is rare in Britain and in the USA, but is not uncommon in Sweden. It is generally inherited as an autosomal-dominant trait due to a gene located on chromosome 14, and usually begins between the ages of 40 and 60 years, involving both sexes. Weakness begins in small hand muscles and in the anterior tibials and calves, but eventually spreads to proximal muscles, unlike the pattern seen in peroneal muscular atrophy, with which it is most often confused. In occasional cases, inclusion bodies, skeletin filaments, and sarcoplasmic bodies are found in muscle, causing difficulty in differentiation from inclusion-body myositis (see Chapter 13.36).

The ocular and oculopharyngeal varieties

Involvement of the external ocular muscles is uncommon in most varieties of muscular dystrophy but can occur in dystrophia myotonica (see Chapter 13.35).

It is now evident that a mitochondrial myopathy is responsible for many, but not all, cases of progressive external ophthalmoplegia. A few such patients have spinal muscular atrophy with loss of neurones from the oculomotor nuclei, and others peripheral neuropathy. While the term ocular myopathy, or muscular dystrophy, is losing popularity, it remains the most satisfactory description for a few otherwise unexplained cases of progressive external ophthalmoplegia.

The oculopharyngeal variety, however, is due to a gene lying on chromosome 14. The external ophthalmoplegia commonly develops at between 40 and 50 years of age but is rarely symptomatic, whereas the dysphagia becomes progressively more troublesome, and mild weakness of facial, neck, and proximal limb muscles is usually present.

Developments in molecular genetics, carrier detection, prenatal diagnosis, and embryo research

In a family in which the gene for Duchenne or Becker dystrophy is known to have been transmitted, any sister of a dystrophic boy will have a 50:50 chance of being a carrier; if she is, half her sons will be affected and half her daughters will also be carriers. In families in which an isolated case is assumed to have resulted from a new mutation, the probability of carrier status in the sister of a dystrophic boy is much less and will depend upon whether the mutation arose in his mother's or his grandmother's ovary (in the latter case his mother would be a carrier). Some carrier females do show minor (and some more severe) clinical, biochemical, and histological evidence of muscular dystrophy (manifesting carriers) due to uneven lyonization of the X chromosome.

The use of DNA restriction fragment length polymorphisms linked to the gene has made accurate detection of carriers possible in many families; the method is about 98 per cent accurate in informative families. However, the use of complementary DNA probes and the polymerase chain reaction still detects only about 65 per cent of mutations. Antenatal diagnosis with elective abortion of affected males is now possible through chorionic-cell biopsy in informative families. Preimplantation diagnosis following *in vitro* fertilization and blastocyst biopsy is now becoming feasible.

Neonatal screening

Using the luciferase technique for the estimation of serum creatine kinase on a single drop of blood on a filter paper, it is possible to identify at birth (with subsequent confirmation from a venous blood sample) those newborn male infants who will subsequently develop Duchenne muscular dystrophy.

Treatment

Complications such as respiratory infection may require antibiotics, physiotherapy, and even suction. Hope for the future rests in gene therapy, with the objective of replacing a missing gene product, such as dystrophin, within diseased muscle either in early infancy in affected individuals identified as neonates (or even *in utero*) or at least as early as possible in the course of the disease. Upregulation of another membrane protein, utrophen, normal in muscular dystrophy, may prove to be another alternative.

Moderate physical exercise can help delay the march of weakness and the development of contractures. A regular exercise programme should be started soon after diagnosis under the supervision of a physiotherapist and subsequently continued at home. Passive stretching of tendons (such as the Achilles), which tend to shorten, is also useful, but night splints are even better. Light spinal supports are helpful in delaying scoliosis but it is now clear that in many cases spinal fusion (the Luque operation) is much more effective in the long term and should be undertaken prophylactically when there is a high risk of a rapidly evolving curve and of a restrictive lung syndrome. Callipers and standing frames can help many patients walk for longer than they would otherwise be able to do.

In some obese patients with Duchenne dystrophy, obstructive sleep apnoea may occur and in patients with other neuromuscular disorders, including various congenital myopathies, cases of myotonic dystrophy, and motor neurone disease, severe respiratory insufficiency due to diaphragmatic weakness may develop while the patient is still ambulant. When the vital capacity falls below 700 ml, the patient's life is in danger. Often hypoventilation is at its worst during sleep. In most cases of Duchenne dystrophy, and in those with similar respiratory difficulties due to neuromuscular disease, overnight intermittent positive-pressure ventilation via the mouth using a face mask may produce a dramatic improvement in alertness, and in the quality of life and longevity. In Duchenne dystrophy, steroid treatment has been shown to produce marginal improvement, but the complications associated with long-term treatment are such that these drugs are little used.

Further reading

Cullen, M.J., Johnson, M.A., and Mastaglia, F.L. (1992). Pathological reactions of skeletal muscle. In *Skeletal muscle pathology*, 2nd edn (ed. F.L. Mastaglia and Lord Walton of Detchant), pp. 123–84. Churchill Livingstone, Edinburgh.

Dubocvitz, V. (1996). New developments in congenital muscular dystrophy. *Neuromuscular Disorders*, **6**, 228.

Emery, A.E.H. (1992). *Duchenne muscular dystrophy*, 2nd edn. Oxford University Press, Oxford.

Emery, A.E.H. (1998). The muscular dystrophies. *British Medical Journal*, **317**, 991–5.

Galasko, C.S.B. (1994). The orthopaedic management of neuromuscular disease. In *Disorders of voluntary muscle*, 6th edn (ed. Lord Walton of Detchant), pp. 851–77. Churchill Livingstone, Edinburgh.

Gardner-Medwin, D. and Walton, J.N. (1994). The muscular dystrophies. In *Disorders of voluntary muscle*, 6th edn. (ed. Lord Walton of Detchant, G. Kaspati, and D. Hilton-Jones), pp. 543–94. Churchill Livingstone, Edinburgh.

Greenberg, C.R., *et al.* (1998). Gene studies in newborn males with Duchenne muscular dystrophy detected by neonatal screening. *Lancet*, **ii**, 425–7.

Mastaglia, F.L. and Walton, J.N. (Lord Walton of Detchant), ed. (1992). *Skeletal muscle pathology*, 2nd edn. Churchill Livingstone, Edinburgh.

Nicholson, L.V.B., Johnson, M.A., Gardner-Medwin, D., Bhattacharya, S., and Harris, J.B. (1990). Heterogeneity of dystrophin expression in patients with Duchenne and Becker muscular dystrophies. *Acta Neuropathologica*, **80**, 239–50.

Neuromuscular disorders: gene location (Table) (1996). *Neuromuscular Disorders*, **6**, I–X.

Chapter 13.34

The floppy infant syndrome

J. Walton

Generalized muscular hypotonia in infancy can be due to many causes, including cerebral palsy, mental retardation, various metabolic disorders, cerebral degenerative disease, and a number of neuromuscular conditions. Spinal muscular atrophy (Werdnig–Hoffmann disease) is an important cause and in such cases the hypotonia is usually profound and widespread, there is generalized areflexia, weakness of respiratory muscles, and often fasciculation of the tongue. The diagnosis can be confirmed by EMG and muscle biopsy. This condition, of grave prognosis, may be mimicked by congenital muscular dystrophy.

Benign congenital or infantile hypotonia

This term is often used to identify those floppy infants in whom hypotonia is not shown to be the result of any specific metabolic disorder, nor secondary to mental handicap or disease in the central or peripheral nervous system; in such cases full investigation, including EMG and muscle biopsy, may fail to demonstrate any specific abnormality of the muscle fibres other than, in some cases, an overall decrease in their diameter. Sometimes all the muscle fibres seem to be of one uniform histochemical type, suggesting a disorder of muscle differentiation, but these cases are rare. In yet others there is a marked disproportion in number and size between the fibres of different histochemical types (congenital fibre-type disproportion); the cause of that condition is unknown but it usually improves progressively with increasing age.

Undoubtedly, the syndrome of benign congenital or infantile hypotonia is one of multiple causes. Some patients demonstrating similar diffuse hypotonia in early infancy show improvement later, although the muscles remain weak, slender, and hypotonic throughout life, and these cases have been regarded as examples of 'benign congenital myopathy', even though the EMG and muscle biopsy findings in such individuals are often non-specific. Some such patients, however, are found to be suffering from apparently specific, though benign, disorders of muscle, three of which will now be mentioned. Other rare causes include fingerprint body myopathy.

Central core disease

The condition is sometimes due to an autosomal-recessive gene and runs a benign course, but its pathogenesis is obscure and X-linked recessive inheritance has also been described. There is widespread muscular hypotonia and biopsy reveals large muscle fibres, most of which show one or sometimes two central cores, that have different staining properties from the other fibrils. The central core is devoid of oxidative enzymes and of phosphorylase activity, and seems to be non-functioning. The gene for central core disease lies on chromosome 19q and is linked to that for malignant hyperpyrexia; the ryanodine receptor is deficient. A rare variant called multicore or minicore disease has been described

Nemaline myopathy

This is another congenital and relatively non-progressive myopathy due to a gene located on chromosome 1q21–23, causing α-tropomyosin deficiency; collections of rod-shaped bodies are found within the muscle fibres, usually lying beneath the sarcolemma. These patients often show evidence of diffuse myopathy, but also facial weakness, a high-arched palate, mandibular prognathism, and skeletal changes resembling those of arachnodactyly, although none of the other stigmata of Marfan's syndrome are present. Even though the condition runs a benign course in most patients, there are rare severe cases causing death in infancy, and progressive respiratory insufficiency is not uncommon. No specific treatment is available.

Myotubular or centronuclear myopathy

A syndrome characterized by facial diplegia, external ocular palsies, a decrease in muscle mass, moderate symmetrical muscle weakness, and poor development of all limb muscles. It is usually due to an X-linked recessive gene located at Xq28. Dominant inheritance rarely occurs. Most muscle fibres contain central nuclei, often lying in chains; the appearances in the muscle are similar to those of the myotubes seen in normal fetal muscle in the early months of intrauterine life. These fibres differ, however, in several respects from fetal myotubes; nevertheless the condition seems to represent an example of cellular developmental arrest. It is usually benign, with progressive improvement.

Further reading

Fardeau, M. (1991). Congenital myopathies. In *Skeletal muscle pathology*, 2nd edn (ed. F.L. Mastaglia and Lord Walton of Detchant), pp. 781–836. Churchill Livingstone, Edinburgh.

Gardner-Medwin, D. (1994). Neuromuscular disorders in infancy and childhood. In *Disorders of voluntary muscle*, 6th edn (ed. Lord Walton of Detchant, G. Karpati, and D. Hilton-Jones) pp. 781–836. Churchill-Livingstone, Edinburgh.

Mastaglia, F.L. and Walton, J.N. (Lord Walton of Detchant), ed. (1992). *Skeletal muscle pathology*, 2nd edn. Churchill-Livingstone, Edinburgh.

Neuromuscular disorders: gene location (Table) (1996). *Neuromuscular Disorders*, **6**, I–X.

Chapter 13.35

Myotonic disorders

J. Walton

Myotonia is the continued active contraction of a muscle after the cessation of voluntary effort or stimulation; an electrical after-discharge accompanies the phenomenon in the EMG. Clinically it is best demonstrated as slowness in relaxation of the grip or by persistent dimpling after a sharp blow on a muscle belly, for example in the thenar eminence or tongue.

Myotonia appears in four hereditary syndromes, three of autosomal-dominant inheritance, one recessive: myotonia congenita, dystrophia myotonica, the rare proximal myotonia myopathy, and paramyotonia. While dystrophic changes occur in certain muscles in dystrophia myotonica, these disorders are more closely related to each other than to the muscular dystrophies.

In a rare syndrome variously called one form of myokymia, pseudomyotonia, or neuromyotonia, a phenomenon similar clinically but electrically different from myotonia is associated with myokymia (benign coarse fasciculation), cramps, hyperhidrosis, and sometimes muscle wasting. Its nature is little understood, though recent evidence strongly suggests an autoimmune aetiology.

Myotonia can also be produced experimentally by drugs and it may rarely be a symptomatic phenomenon in polyneuropathy, polymyositis, and motor neurone diseases.

Myotonia congenita

The classic, dominantly inherited variant of myotonia congenita (Thomsen's disease) is usually present from birth. Myotonia is generalized, accentuated by rest and by cold, and gradually relieved by exercise. In infancy, these children are often difficult to feed and have a peculiarly strangled cry. Later, myotonia of the tongue may cause difficulty in speaking. Diffuse hypertrophy of muscles usually persists throughout life, though the myotonia tends to improve with increasing age. The gene responsible for Thomsen's disease is linked to the *TCRB* gene locus on chromosome 7q35, at the site of a human muscle chloride channel gene.

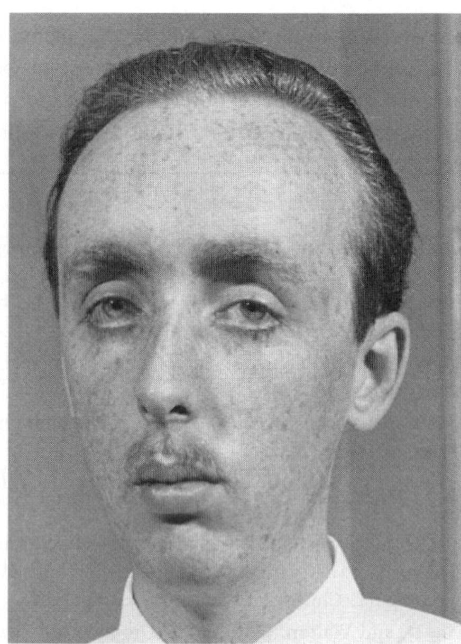

Fig. 1 The typical facial appearance of myotonic dystrophy (dystrophia myotonica).

A recessively inherited variant of myotonia congenita, clinically milder and significantly more common than Thomsen's disease, first becomes apparent later in childhood, usually during the first decade. It, too, is linked to the 7q35 locus.

Dystrophia myotonica

Dystrophia myotonica is a diffuse systemic disorder in which myotonia, facial myopathy and distal muscular atrophy are accompanied by cataracts, frontal baldness in the male (Fig. 1), gonadal atrophy, cardiomyopathy, impaired pulmonary ventilation, mild endocrine anomalies, bone changes, mental defect or dementia, and abnormalities of the serum immunoglobulins. The gene responsible for this disease segregates as a single locus at chromosome 19q13.3 where an abnormal CTG triplet repeat is almost invariably found. The size of this fragment varies between affected siblings and increases in size through generations in parallel with increasing severity of the disease; this explains the well-known phenomenon of anticipation (i.e., the fact that the disease is of earlier onset and greater severity in successive generations). Identification of this gene has now made possible accurate preclinical and antenatal diagnosis, so that selective therapeutic abortion of affected fetuses is now possible.

The presenting symptoms are usually weakness of the hands and difficulty in walking, and myotonia is rarely obtrusive. Poor vision, weight loss, impotence, ptosis, and increased sweating are common. The condition may present in infancy and childhood with severe muscular weakness, hypotonia, and physical and mental developmental delay; when it does so the affected parent is almost always the mother. More often the condition becomes clinically overt between the ages of 20 and 50 years.

The facial appearance of the affected adolescent or adult is typically long and haggard; ptosis is usual and rarely there is external ophthalmoplegia. Wasting of the masseters, temporal muscles, and sternomastoids is invariable; in the extremities, weakness and wasting involves particularly forearm muscles (sparing the small muscles of the hands), the anterior tibial group, and the calves and peronei.

Sensorineural hearing loss is common. Slit-lamp examination reveals posterior cortical cataracts in most cases. Cardiac conduction defects and/or cardiomyopathy are common; the pulmonary vital capacity and maximum expiratory pressure are often impaired. Drowsiness and hypersomnolence are frequent. Dysphagia is due to disordered oesophageal contraction. The testes are usually small and, histologically, the changes are like those of Klinefelter syndrome. Females often show irregular menstruation, infertility, and prolonged parturition. Progressive dementia, once thought to be common, is rare. There is a high incidence of abnormal EEGs; CT or MRI scanning may demonstrate cerebral cortical atrophy, or more often progressive ventricular enlargement.

Proximal myotonic myopathy

A rare variant, involving proximal limb muscles (but with myotonia in the periphery), and not associated with CTG repeats has been described recently, linked to a locus on the long arm of chromosome 3.

Paramyotonia

This rare condition is characterized by myotonia appearing only on exposure to cold. In addition, cold precipitates attacks of generalized muscular weakness like those of periodic paralysis. In some patients the myotonia is accentuated, rather than being relieved, by exercise and muscle hypertrophy is common, but there are none of the stigmata of myotonic dystrophy. The diagnosis is best made by testing the objective response of muscles to cooling, as by immersing the hand and forearm in iced water. With cooling, stiffness increases, to be followed by weakness and occasionally total paralysis but with a persistent after-contraction, the latter persisting for a few minutes; the weakness often passes off in about half an hour. Most patients also show myotonic lid lag. The condition is closely related to hyperkalaemic periodic paralysis, being due to an abnormal sodium channel α-subunit gene, localized to chromosome 17q13.1–13.3.

Diagnosis

Myotonia must be distinguished from the slowness of muscular contraction and relaxation that can occur in hypothyroidism (Hoffmann's syndrome). The painful physiological (and reversible) contracture that may follow exertion in patients with myophosphorylase deficiency (McArdle's disease) and related diseases can also give diagnostic difficulty, but these disorders can be distinguished electromyographically. In dystrophia myotonica, the EMG shows not only myotonic discharges evoked by movement of the exploring electrode, but myopathic potentials are recorded from weakened and wasted muscles during contraction. The serum creatine kinase activity is normal in myotonia congenita and paramyotonia, but may be raised to between two and ten times the normal upper limit in myotonic dystrophy. In biopsy samples, cases of myotonia congenita and paramyotonia may show only hypertrophy of muscle fibres and perhaps occasional ringbinden, but in myotonic dystrophy changes similar to those of muscular dystrophy are seen in addition to frequent long chains of nuclei in the centre of muscle fibres, combined sometimes with ringed annulets and peripheral sarcoplasmic masses.

Treatment

No treatment influences the progressive muscular wasting and weakness that eventually develop in dystrophia myotonica; principles of management include moderate regular exercise and the prevention of contractures and deformity, as well as occupational therapy and the provision of appropriate appliances. Cardiac conduction defects, if symptomatic, will require appropriate drugs and, if respiratory insufficiency becomes severe, nocturnal nasal ventilation (as in other forms of muscular dystrophy) may be needed. Hypersomnolence is more often due to central dysfunction than respiratory insufficiency, and may respond to methylphenidate. Testosterone may increase the lean body mass but does not improve strength.

While paramyotonic symptoms may respond to treatment with lidocaine (lignocaine) and its derivatives, tocainide, a drug normally prescribed to control cardiac ventricular arrhythmia, has been found to be effective in a dose of 400 to 1200 mg daily in both paramyotonia and recessive generalized myotonia. Drugs used in the past to control myotonia in cases of myotonia congenita, whether dominantly or recessively inherited, have included quinine, steroids, procainamide, and phenytoin, the last often proving effective in a dosage of 100 mg three times daily. Others have found acetazolamide to be more effective in myotonia congenita than the other standard agents.

Course and prognosis

Myotonia congenita is essentially a benign disorder that does not shorten life, and the same is true of paramyotonia. Most patients with dystrophia myotonica, however, show progressive deterioration and become severely disabled and unable to walk within 15 to 20 years of the onset. Death from respiratory infection or cardiac failure usually occurs well before the normal age.

Further reading

Abdalla, J.A., Casley, W.L., Cousin, H.E., *et al.* (1992). Linkage of autosomal dominant myotonia congenita to TCRB gene locus on chromosome 7Q35. *Neurology*, **42**, 1426 (Abstract).

Buxton, J., *et al.* (1992). Detection of an unstable fragment of DNA specific to individuals with myotonic dystrophy. *Nature*, **35**, 547–8.

Harper, P.S. (1989). *Myotonic dystrophy*, 2nd edn. Saunders, London.

Howeler, C.J., Busch, H.F.M., Geraedts, J.P.M., Niermeijer, M.F., and Staal, A. (1989). Anticipation in myotonic dystrophy; fact or fiction? *Brain*, **112**, 779–97.

Malloy, P., Mishra, S.K., and Adler, S.H. (1990). Neuropsychological deficits in myotonic muscular dystrophy. *Journal of Neurology, Neurosurgery, and Psychiatry*, **53**, 1011–13.

Neuromuscular disorders: gene location (Table) (1996). *Neuromuscular Disorders*, **6**, I–X.

Thornton, C.A. and Ashzawa, T. (1999). Getting a grip on the myotonic dystrophies. *Neurology*, **52**, 12–13.

Chapter 13.36

Inflammatory myopathies

J. Walton

The inflammatory myopathies constitute the largest group of acquired myopathies of adult life and also occur in infancy and childhood. They have in common the presence of inflammatory cellular infiltrates in skeletal muscle, usually with evidence of muscle fibre destruction. Some are due to known viral, bacterial, or other microbial agents, while in others no infective agent can be identified and immunological mechanisms have been implicated. An outline classification is given in Table 1: Table 2 lists causes of acute viral myositis, while parasitic and fungal infections are listed in Table 3.

Myopathies due to microbial agents and parasites

Viral myositis (Table 2)

Several DNA and RNA viruses can cause acute myopathy (Table 1).The clinical syndromes range from a localized, self-limiting myositis to a more generalized, necrotizing myopathy associated with myoglobinuria (acute rhabdomyolysis).

Postinfluenzal myositis is well documented. This syndrome is seen in the week after an attack of influenza and is characterized by severe pain, tenderness, and sometimes swelling, usually of calf muscles but sometimes also involving those of the thigh; it usually resolves spontaneously within about a week. The serum creatine kinase activity is usually increased.

Table 1 Classification of the inflammatory myopathies

Due to an infective agent	*Idiopathic (cont.)*
viral	eosinophilic myositis
bacterial	focal
fungal	focal interstitial myositis
protozoal	focal eosinophilic myositis
helminthic	localized nodular myositis
	monomelic myositis
Idiopathic	orbital myositis
generalized	inflammatory pseudotumour
polymyositis	proliferative myositis
dermatomyositis	
inclusion-body myositis	
granulomatous myositis	

Reproduced, with permission, from Mastaglia and Walton (1992).

Table 2 Syndromes of acute viral myositis and causative agents

Benign acute myositis	*Acute myoglobinuric myositis*
influenza A and B	influenza A and B
parainfluenza	parainfluenza 3
adenovirus 2	Coxsackie A9, B2, B3, B5
	echovirus 9
Epidemic pleurodynia	adenovirus 21
Coxsackie B1, B3, B4, B5	herpes simplex 2
	Epstein–Barr virus

Reproduced, with permission, from Mastaglia and Walton (1992).

Table 3 Parasitic and fungal infections of muscle

Protozoal	*Fungal*
toxoplasmosis	candidiasis
sarcosporidiosis	actinomycosis
trypanosomiasis	coccidioidomycosis
microsporidiosis	sporotrichosis
amoebiasis	
	Helminthic
	trichinosis
	cysticercosis
	echinococcosis

Reproduced, with permission, from Mastaglia and Walton (1992).

The coxsackie B virus, particularly B1, B3, B4, and B5, is typically associated with epidemic pleurodynia (Bornholm disease), a self-limiting disorder occurring usually in childhood and characterized by acute and severe pain, with tenderness of the chest, back, shoulders, or abdomen. Fulminant acute myositis with myoglobinuria has also been linked with coxsackie, echo, and other viral infections (Table 2).

It is now well recognized that many neuromuscular syndromes may develop in patients with human immunodeficiency virus infection and more especially in AIDS. Numerous neuropathies and myopathies have been described. The latter include non-specific myositis, giant-cell myositis, rod-body (nemaline) myopathy, necrotizing myopathy with myoglobinuria, and a myopathy that is probably due to zidovudine treatment.

Bacterial myositis

Suppurative staphylococcal pyomyositis is discussed in Chapter 13.41.

Clostridium welchii produces a toxin and enzymes, such as collagenase and hyaluronidase, that cause necrosis of muscle fibres and interstitial tissues. This condition (gas gangrene) usually follows extensive septic wounds of skeletal muscle; if the infection is controlled by antibiotics and necrotic tissue is entirely removed, regeneration may be effective, but marked fibrosis and muscular atrophy usually result.

Other bacterial forms include tuberculous, syphilitic, and leprous myositis.

Parasitic myositis (Table 3)

Helminth infections

Trichinosis

This is the most common parasitic infection of muscle. The causative agent, *Trichinella spiralis*, is a nematode, usually acquired by man through eating incompletely cooked pork, bear, or horse meat. There is severe myalgia and tenderness, often with weakness, which may be generalized or limited to certain groups, such as the ocular muscles. Periorbital and conjunctival oedema, and a skin eruption, often occur. Eosinophilia is usual; muscle biopsy may demonstrate the parasites in various stages of development and encystment. Except in very severe infestations, recovery is usual.

Cysticercosis

This condition, common in India and Eastern Europe but less so in other parts of the world, results from infestation with the encysted larval stage of the pork tapeworm, *Taenia solium*. In the acute stage there may be muscle tenderness, fever, and eosinophilia, but often evidence of involvement of muscle and of the central nervous system is only found many years later, when the patient presents with a hypertrophic myopathy or with epilepsy. Nodules may be palpable in the tongue and other muscles, but, in the hypertrophic form, gross enlargement of limb muscles may occur. Spindle-shaped cysts may be found in the interstitial connective tissue in muscle biopsy specimens.

Protozoal infections

Toxoplasma gondii can give a multifocal, disseminated myositis; the organism may be revealed by muscle biopsy.

Sarcocystis lindemanni rarely invades skeletal muscles in man; when it does, the condition is usually asymptomatic and the parasite may be found unexpectedly in a muscle biopsy.

Trypanosomiasis cruzi (Chagas' disease), indigenous to South America, is characterized by disseminated focal polymyositis, myocarditis, and encephalomyelitis.

Fungal myositis

Actinomycosis may involve skeletal muscle through direct extension from an infective focus in pleura or skin, when abscesses and fistulas discharging purulent material containing characteristic yellow granules, composed of colonies of the fungus, are often seen. Coccidioidomycosis and sporotrichosis are other rare causes of granulomas in muscle, while fever, a skin rash, and diffuse muscle pain and tenderness may occur in disseminated candidiasis.

Muscular involvement in collagen or connective-tissue diseases, sarcoidosis, and Sjögren's syndrome

In rheumatoid arthritis, sections of a muscle biopsy may demonstrate foci of inflammatory cell infiltration, but this focal nodular myositis is not usually accompanied by muscular wasting and weakness, save for that resulting secondarily from joint disease. Only rarely does a diffuse inflammatory myopathy (polymyositis or dermatomyositis) complicate rheumatoid disease; polyneuropathy is a much more common complication.

In sarcoidosis, muscle involvement may cause a subacute weakness and wasting of proximal muscles, and typical sarcoid granulomas may be observed on muscle biopsy. Localized muscle pain, subcutaneous oedema, and tenderness can also occur as a result of muscle infarction in polyarteritis nodosa and in Wegener's granulomatosis. In systemic lupus erythematosus, muscular involvement is sometimes severe and diffuse, and is then indistinguishable from polymyositis. Polymyositis is an uncommon accompaniment of Sjögren's syndrome and may also complicate chronic graft-versus-host disease. It occurs more often in mixed connective-tissue disease in which features of systemic sclerosis, systemic lupus, and arthritis may coexist. Localized changes resembling those of polymyositis may be found in muscles underlying areas of linear morphoea or scleroderma.

Polymyositis and dermatomyositis

These terms are generally used to identify a group of cases in which muscular weakness and wasting may be associated with muscle pain and tenderness or with evidence of some form of connective-tissue or collagen disease. A classification of polymyositis and dermatomyositis based upon current knowledge is given in Table 4.

Aetiology

In polymyositis the autoimmune process is primarily cell-mediated through killer T cells; in dermatomyositis it is largely, if not exclusively, a humoral vasculopathy. Polymyositis occurs worldwide in many ethnic groups and in both sexes. About 15 per cent of cases occur under the age of 15 years, another 15 per cent between the ages of 16 and 30 years, about 25 per cent between 31 and 45 years, and 33 per cent between the ages of 45 and 60 years. It usually develops spontaneously but can follow febrile illness or the administration of various drugs, such as sulphonamides or penicillamine.

Table 4 Classification of polymyositis (PM) and dermatomyositis (DM)

Childhood
infantile myositis
juvenile DM
Adult life
isolated PM
isolated DM
PM or DM associated with malignancy
PM or DM associated with connective tissue diseases
PM or DM associated with immune deficiency states
PM or DM associated with other systemic disorders
drug-induced PM or DM
inclusion body myositis
localized nodular myositis
neuromyositis
eosinophilic myositis
granulomatous myositis

Modified, with permission, from Mastaglia and Walton (1992).

Symptoms and signs

Apart from occasional acute cases in which widespread muscle pain, fever, constitutional upset, and rapidly progressive paralysis, often with respiratory weakness, may develop, the condition usually runs a subacute or chronic course. Muscle pain and tenderness occur in approximately 50 per cent of cases, as does dysphagia. Cutaneous manifestations are seen in about two-thirds of all patients, and may take the form of widespread erythema with desquamation, particularly on the face and on other exposed areas of the trunk, but occasionally involving the whole body. Heliotrope periorbital erythema and oedema are particularly characteristic and so, too, is congestion of the nail beds. Sometimes the skin changes are slight, with a faint butterfly-type rash on the face; in others, particularly in childhood, there may be ulceration over bony prominences with subcutaneous calcification.

Joint pain and stiffness occur at some stage in about one-quarter of all patients. Proximal limb muscles are almost invariably involved and the neck muscles are characteristically affected in about one-third of cases. Involvement of distal limb muscles is less common, but weakness may be generalized in about one-third of cases; when the condition runs a subacute or chronic course, contractures sometimes develop (chronic fibrosing myositis). Facial weakness and involvement of the external ocular muscles are rare. The deep tendon reflexes may be depressed in affected muscles but are often surprisingly brisk despite the weakness.

Diagnosis

In many cases the clinical picture is characteristic, but when involvement of the skin and joints is unobtrusive and the course of the illness is subacute, it may be mistaken for muscular dystrophy or for various forms of metabolic myopathy. In patients over 55 years of age, polymyalgia rheumatica, often associated with giant-cell arteritis, may cause difficulty, but in the latter condition it is pain and stiffness rather than weakness that restricts movement.

The serum creatine kinase activity is often greatly raised in polymyositis; the erythrocyte sedimentation rate is often, though not invariably, increased. Electromyography demonstrates a myopathic pattern of volitional activity, but there may also be spontaneous fibrillation, positive sharp waves, and occasional pseudomyotonic discharges recorded from resting muscle. Biopsy specimens often demonstrate widespread necrosis and phagocytosis of muscle fibres, and interstitial and perivascular infiltrations of inflammatory cells, mainly lymphocytes and plasma cells.

Treatment

The condition should usually be treated with 60 mg of prednisone daily, given for 4 or 5 days and subsequently regulating the maintenance dose according to the serum creatine kinase activity and the clinical response. Maintenance therapy may have to be continued for many years before the drug can eventually be withdrawn. Most authorities now give an additional immunosuppressive drug, such as azathioprine, methotrexate, or cyclophosphamide, in an appropriate level of dosage depending upon age and body weight, along with prednisone from the beginning. Total body or total lymphoid irradiation may be effective if all else fails, while intravenous immunoglobulin can also have a strikingly beneficial effect. Plasmapheresis is useful in severe cases of dermatomyositis but probably does no more than to produce temporary remission while steroids and immunosuppressive agents are being given time to act.

Clinical variants

Sarcoid myopathy, polymyalgia rheumatica, and focal nodular myositis have been mentioned above. Other related disorders include the following.

Localized nodular myositis

This is a rare condition in which localized, painful, and tender swellings may develop in one or more skeletal muscles and are shown on biopsy to demonstrate massive necrosis and cellular infiltration of muscle fibres. Many patients go on to develop signs and symptoms of diffuse polymyositis.

Infantile myositis

This rare condition, with typical inflammatory changes in muscle biopsy sections, can cause muscular weakness and atrophy with hypotonia in the neonatal period or early infancy.

Inclusion-body myositis

This is a distinctive variety of idiopathic inflammatory myopathy. It is a relatively chronic myopathy not associated with connective-tissue or malignant disease. It occurs particularly in men in their sixties, and is seen occasionally in younger patients. Slowly progressive, painless weakness involves distal as well as proximal muscle groups and there is often dysphagia. The rate of progression is variable and some patients are severely handicapped even within 2 years; treatment with corticosteroids and other immunosuppressive agents is usually ineffective. Muscle biopsy specimens show inclusion bodies and rimmed vacuoles; amyloid, prion-related protein, phosphorylated tau, β-amyloid protein, α-antichymotrypsin, and apo-E4 immunoreactive deposits, as found in the brain in Alzheimer's disease, are also present in most cases.

Eosinophilic polymyositis

This rare inflammatory myopathy occurs as a part of the systemic hypereosinophilic syndrome characterized by eosinophilia, anaemia, hypergammaglobulinaemia, cardiac and pulmonary involvement, skin changes, peripheral neuropathy, and encephalopathy. The myositis usually presents with a localized tender swelling in a muscle in one calf or thigh, like localized nodular myositis. The serum creatine kinase is raised and often a more extensive proximal myopathy develops.

Granulomatous myositis

Granulomatous lesions similar to those of sarcoid, developing in the absence of any other evidence of sarcoidosis elsewhere and giving a clinical picture suggesting polymyositis, identify the syndrome of granulomatous myositis. These patients show a response to steroid therapy that is generally as satisfactory as that seen in subacute polymyositis.

Course and prognosis

Even without treatment, the course of the illness is variable. Sometimes it runs a fluctuating course with spontaneous exacerbations and remissions. Progressive deterioration with a fatal termination within a few weeks or months is seen, particularly in acute dermatomyositis, but spontaneous arrest occurs occasionally. Slow, insidious progression is common in middle age, but spontaneous recovery occurs rarely in childhood. With aggressive modern treatment, up to 50 per cent of patients can ultimately be cured, and in about 25 per cent the disease process is arrested.

The high incidence of malignant disease indicates that all patients developing this syndrome in middle or late life (especially those with dermatomyositis) should be investigated with the possibility of occult neoplasia in mind.

Further reading

Chou, S.M. (1988). Viral myositis. In *Inflammatory diseases of muscle* (ed. F.L. Mastaglia), pp. 125–53. Blackwell, Oxford.

Emslie-Smith, A.M. and Engel, A.G. (1990). Microvascular changes in early and advanced dermatomyositis: a quantitative study. *Annals of Neurology*, 27, 343–56.

Engel, A.G. and Emslie-Smith, A.M. (1989). Inflammatory myopathies. *Current Opinion in Neurology and Neurosurgery*, 2, 695–700.

Mastaglia, F.L. and Walton, J.N. (1992). Inflammatory myopathies. In *Skeletal muscle pathology*, 2nd edn (ed. F.L. Mastaglia and Lord Walton of Detchant), pp. 453–91. Churchill Livingstone, Edinburgh.

Ojeda, V.J. and Mastaglia, F.L. (1988). Miscellaneous conditions. In *Inflammatory diseases of muscle* (ed. F.L. Mastaglia), pp. 185–95. Blackwell, Oxford.

Walton, J.N. (1991). The idiopathic inflammatory myopathies and their treatment. *Journal of Neurology, Neurosurgery and Psychiatry*, 54, 285–7.

Chapter 13.37

Miscellaneous disorders

J. Walton

Restless legs (Ekbom's syndrome)

This syndrome gives unpleasant aching in the muscles of the lower limbs when the patient rests in a chair or lying in bed. This aching, accompanied by a sense of intolerable restlessness, can be accompanied by muscular cramps, which interfere with sleep. Sometimes the condition develops in pregnancy, and in patients with chronic renal disease. There are no abnormal physical signs and the EMG, nerve conduction-velocity measurements, and muscle biopsy are usually normal. Recent research suggests that the disorder is due central dopaminergic dysfunction. Levodopa, pramipexole, and pergolide are each effective in treatment in many cases.

Tibialis anterior syndrome

Severe, boring pain in the tibialis anterior muscle may occur on one or both sides after unaccustomed exercise; the condition is due to ischaemic swelling of the muscle within its tight fascial compartment. Occasionally, the pain is intense, and widespread necrosis of the muscles occurs. In mild, chronic cases, recurrent pain occurs after any exertion and relief can only then be obtained by surgical decompression of the anterior crural compartment.

Progressive myositis ossificans

Progressive myositis ossificans is a genetically determined disorder (usually autosomal dominant) in which there is widespread ossification of muscles, usually preceded by sclerosis of intramuscular connective tissue. Most cases present in childhood and affected individuals often have associated anomalies of their great toes or other digits. The condition usually begins with swelling or swellings in the neck, mimicking congenital torticollis; eventually the muscles of the back, shoulder, and in particular, the pelvic girdles, become ossified. The overlying skin may ulcerate and terminal aspiration pneumonia is common, but the condition may run a benign course over many decades. Diphosphonate treatment can promote resorption of bone in some cases.

The stiff-man syndrome

This syndrome of so-called progressive fluctuating muscular rigidity and spasm predominantly affects adult men, who, after a prodromal phase of aching and tightness of the axial muscles, go on to develop a symmetrical, continuous stiffness of the skeletal muscles upon which painful muscular spasms are superimposed and may be precipitated by movement. The condition is of neuronal rather than muscular origin, and the finding that antibodies against cell bodies and axon terminals of GABA-ergic neurones may be present in the serum and cerebrospinal fluid indicates an autoimmune cause. The condition, which is sometimes dominantly inherited, may be difficult to distinguish from neuromyotonia. Diazepam, baclofen, clonazepam, and sodium valproate have all relieved the symptoms in individual cases.

Further reading

Brodeur, C., Montplasir, J., Godbout, R., and Marinier, R. (1988). Treatment of restless legs syndrome and periodic movements during sleep with L-dopa: a double-blind, controlled study. *Neurology*, **38**, 1845–8.

Gorin, F., Baldwin, B., Tait, R., *et al.* (1990). Stiff-man syndrome: a GABAergic autoimmune disorder with autoantigenic heterogeneity. *Annals of Neurology*, **28**, 711–14.

Hilton-Jones, D. (1994). The clinical features of some miscellaneous muscular disorders. In *Disorders of Voluntary Muscle*, 6th edn (ed. Lord Walton of Detchant, G. Karpati, and D. Hilton-Jones), pp. 967–82. Churchill Livingstone, Edinburgh.

Pitt, P. and Hamilton, E.B.D. (1984). Myositis ossificans progressiva. *Journal of the Royal Society of Medicine*, **77**, 68–70.

Turjanski, N., Lees, A.J., and Brooks, D.J. (1999). Striatal dopaminergic function in restless legs syndrome. *Neurology*, **52**, 932–7.

Chapter 13.38

Disorders of neuromuscular transmission

J. Newsom-Davis

Myasthenia gravis

Myasthenia gravis is an antibody-mediated, postsynaptic disorder of the neuromuscular junction, characterized by fatiguable muscle weakness. It can present from early childhood to extreme old age. The antigen (acetylcholine receptor) has been identified, the causative antibodies can be detected in the serum in the majority of patients, and the way in which they lead to loss of acetylcholine receptors has been established. Recognition of the immunological nature of myasthenia gravis has helped to explain the long-standing observation that thymectomy is often beneficial, and has led to the increasing use of immunological treatments and a greatly improved prognosis.

Pathogenesis

Neuromuscular transmission depends on the opening of acetylcholine-gated ion channels (acetylcholine receptors) in muscle by the nerve-evoked, quantal release of neurotransmitter from the nerve terminal. The resulting endplate potential triggers the muscle action potential, leading to muscle contraction. The primary abnormality in myasthenia gravis is loss of acetylcholine receptors, which is caused by heterogeneous IgG antibodies that can be detected in the serum by radioimmunoassay in about 85 per cent of patients. Evidence for the pathogenetic role of these autoantibodies includes the clinical response to plasma exchange, the transfer to experimental animals of similar physiological changes by injection of plasma or IgG from myasthenia gravis, and the production of an animal model of myasthenia gravis by immunizing with affinity-purified acetylcholine receptor. In the 15 per cent of patients with typical myasthenia gravis who are 'seronegative' for these antibodies by the standard radioimmunoassay, humoral factors nevertheless appear also to underlie the disorder.

The thymus is often abnormal in myasthenia gravis. The most striking change is present in the 60 per cent of patients who have early-onset disease (age under 40 years); this is characterized by the presence in the thymic medulla of many lymphoid follicles with germinal centres, which look very similar to those found in peripheral lymph nodes. Acetylcholine receptor is present in thymic myoid cells in myasthenia gravis and in non-myasthenia gravis thymus. However, only in patients with myasthenia gravis are acetylcholine receptor-reactive T cells enriched and their thymic cells able spontaneously to synthesize antiacetylcholine receptor antibodies.

A small group of patients (10 per cent) have a thymoma. Some tumours invade locally, and may seed in the pleural cavity but rarely metastasize further. Curiously, removal of thymoma does not usually improve the myasthenia gravis, which occasionally will develop after removal of thymoma.

The late-onset group of patients (age over 40 years) usually have a normal or atrophic thymus, as do those who are seronegative.

Classification

Acquired myasthenia gravis needs to be distinguished from the non-immunological, hereditary/congenital forms of the disease (see below). But acquired myasthenia gravis itself appears to be heterogeneous as indicated by differences in thymic pathology, age at onset, anti-acetylcholine receptor antibody titre, and immune-response gene associations, which may imply differences in triggering factors.

The different subgroups of acquired myasthenia gravis also have implications for treatment (see below). The early-onset cases often respond to thymectomy, in contrast to the late-onset and seronegative cases; the late-onset or seronegative ocular patients seem particularly responsive to prednisolone. Penicillamine-induced myasthenia gravis recovers within a few months of withdrawing the drug.

Neonatal myasthenia gravis is due to the placental transfer of antiacetylcholine receptor antibodies that leads to a transient myasthenic illness in the new-born. Arthrogryposis can occasionally occur, as in other conditions, causing reduced fetal movement.

Clinical features

The hallmark of myasthenia gravis is weakness of skeletal muscle that increases with exercise. Infection, emotional stress, and the use of muscle relaxants during general anaesthesia can precipitate the first clinical evidence of the disease.

The most common presenting symptoms are double vision and ptosis, accounting for about two-thirds of cases; ocular symptoms occur in almost all patients at some time. In some patients, symptoms remain confined to the eye muscles (ocular myasthenia) and antibody titres are then usually low or absent. More commonly, the symptoms are generalized. Myasthenic weakness causes a characteristic nasal speech, difficulty in chewing and swallowing that increases during a meal, nasal regurgitation, and a 'snarling' smile. There may be difficulty in holding the head up. Weakness in the limbs particularly affects the arms and the proximal muscles in the legs, which sometimes results in the patient falling. Respiratory muscle weakness is rarely a presenting feature but can be a serious complicating factor in those with bulbar weakness.

The signs of myasthenia gravis are confined to the motor system and, in mild cases, may be evident only after testing for fatigue. Double vision may increase with sustained gaze, and signs of ocular weakness may be asymmetrical. Weakness of eye closure, facial expression, jaw opening, or neck flexion or extension may be present. In the limbs, fatiguable weakness is common in proximal muscle groups, but also particularly in triceps (elbow extension) and the small muscles of the hand. Wasting can occur but is rare and usually only in long-standing cases. Reflexes are characteristically brisk; indeed, depressed or absent reflexes raise the possibility of an alternative diagnosis, for example the Lambert–Eaton myasthenic syndrome. Cardiac arrhythmias may occur, usually associated with anticardiac muscle antibodies, and other autoimmune syndromes coexist more frequently than would be expected by chance.

The natural history of myasthenia gravis is characterized by a period of between 5 and 7 years when the disease is active and may be progressive, followed by relative quiescence, although late relapses can occur. The spontaneous remission rate appears to be about 1 per cent per year, and is more common in children and in those who are seronegative.

Diagnosis

The presence of a raised serum titre of antiacetylcholine receptor antibody (more than 5×10^{-10} mol/l) is specific for myasthenia gravis, and definitively establishes the diagnosis. Titres of $2–5 \times 10^{-10}$ mol/l are equivocal and are particularly common in ocular cases. Where the assay is unavailable or the titre is normal, an intravenous edrophonium (Camsilon, formerly Tensilon) test can be done. Adverse effects occur occasionally, and it is therefore sensible to have resuscitation equipment available and to premedicate with atropine 0.6 mg intravenously. A test dose of edrophonium, 2 mg intravenously, should be given and in some instances evokes a clear-cut improvement. If so, a further dose is unnecessary. Otherwise, a further 6 to 8 mg may be given, if necessary flushed through with saline to avoid dispersion of the pharmacological effect. A response will be evident after about 30 s and will have subsided by 5 min.

The most sensitive electromyographic index of a defect in neuromuscular transmission is an increase in jitter. In seronegative myasthenia gravis, which includes many of those with ocular myasthenia gravis, the diagnosis will depend on clinical features, edrophonium response, and electromyographic abnormalities.

Thymoma is best diagnosed by CT of the mediastinum, although large tumours may be evident on plain radiographs. Most patients with thymoma will have detectable serum antistriated muscle antibody; this antibody is also sometimes present in non-thymoma cases.

Management

Anticholinesterase treatment

All patients will obtain some symptomatic improvement with anticholinesterase medication, but it is of greatest value in those with mild disease. Pyridostigmine is the drug of choice, usually taken three to five times daily. A starting dose of 30 mg (in adults) may need to be increased to 60 or 90 mg, but caution should be exercised in using higher doses because of the increasing risk of cholinergic side-effects (intestinal colic, excess secretions), which can be ameliorated by propantheline bromide, 15 mg.

Thymoma

Thymoma requires surgical removal because of the risk of local infiltration. Where removal is incomplete, local radiotherapy may be required, or chemotherapy if there has been pleural seeding.

Ocular myasthenia

Ocular symptoms responding inadequately to anticholinesterase medication will nearly always improve with alternate-day prednisolone therapy. Indeed, if they do not, the diagnosis should be questioned. Many patients will develop a complete remission. An initial dose of prednisolone 5 mg on alternate days, taken as a single morning dose, can be increased by 5 mg at weekly intervals until either a full remission occurs or an acceptable maximal dose is reached. This dose should then be maintained for 2 to 3 months before being reduced slowly (5 mg per month) and adjusted to define the minimal effective dose. Symptoms will usually recur if corticosteroids are fully withdrawn.

Early-onset, generalized seropositive myasthenia gravis

Patients with early-onset, seropositive, generalized symptoms typically show thymic hyperplasia and usually benefit from thymectomy. Results from several large clinical series indicate that 30 per cent will develop a remission and 40 to 50 per cent will improve substantially over a 1- to 3-year period postoperatively; the effect in the remainder appears to be neutral. Thymectomy is thus the treatment of choice in this group who are still symptomatic despite optimal anticholinesterase therapy.

Seronegative, and late-onset seropositive myasthenia gravis

Evidence that these two groups of patients benefit from thymectomy is unconvincing. Most of them, however, will respond to immunosuppressive drug treatment (see below), which, on present evidence, is the treatment of choice for those with generalized symptoms not adequately controlled by pyridostigmine.

Myasthenic crisis

Crisis in patients with established myasthenia gravis should be managed initially by control of the airway, which usually means intubation, rather than by attempting to adjust the anticholinesterase dose. Immunological treatment (plasma exchange or intravenous immunoglobulin, and immunosuppressive drugs) will then almost always be needed to control the disease process.

Plasma exchange and intravenous immunoglobulin

These are valuable means of obtaining short-term control of symptoms. Maximum improvement usually develops at 10 to 14 days after starting treatment, and will subside over the subsequent 2 to 4 weeks. They are probably of equal efficacy. The indications include:

(1) myasthenic crisis;

(2) control of symptoms pre- and post-thymectomy in those with severe weakness;

(3) initiation of corticosteroid treatment in patients with generalized or bulbar weakness, that can otherwise often be accompanied by deterioration;

(4) those with long-standing severe disease who may need repeated courses, together with immunosuppressive drugs, while their disease is brought under control.

Immunosuppressive drug treatment

This therapy is valuable in those whose symptoms are inadequately controlled by anticholinesterase medication or by thymectomy in appropriate cases. Prednisolone, either alone or with azathioprine, forms the mainstay of treatment; a recent randomized, controlled trial favoured the combined treatment. Initiating prednisolone therapy at high dosage can acutely increase myasthenic symptoms. This risk is reduced by an incrementing (10 mg per dose) alternate-day regimen, aiming for a maximum dose of 1 to 1.5 mg/kg body wt. Improvement may take up to 2 months to become evident, usually first manifest as an alternate-day increase in strength.

Azathioprine is very slow in its action and for that reason is not usually prescribed alone. Maximum tolerated dosage should be continued until full remission has developed or improvement has reached a plateau, which may take many months. The dose should then be slowly reduced, aiming to define the minimal dose at which symptoms are fully or adequately controlled.

For patients who are unable to tolerate corticosteroids and/or azathioprine at maximum dosage, or who are unresponsive after an adequate duration of treatment (minimum of 1 year), methotrexate or cyclosporin A are alternatives.

Prognosis

Immunological treatment has greatly improved the outlook for patients with myasthenia. Plasma exchange or intravenous immunoglobulin, together with improved intensive care techniques, has been valuable in acute cases. Prednisolone treatment induces a remission or substantial improvement in the majority of patients with ocular myasthenia, while combination treatment with prednisolone and azathioprine will bring substantial improvement or remission to many previously poorly controlled cases.

Lambert–Eaton myasthenic syndrome

The Lambert–Eaton myasthenic syndrome (**LEMS**) is an autoantibody-mediated, presynaptic disorder of the neuromuscular junction causing predominantly proximal muscle weakness and autonomic symptoms. The antigenic target is the voltage-gated calcium channel at the nerve terminal on which acetylcholine release depends. It associates specifically with small-cell lung cancer in the majority of cases.

Although first recognized in association with lung cancer (C-LEMS), it later became clear that LEMS could occur alone (NC-LEMS). The latter form accounts for the cases of childhood onset as well as some in the adult age group.

Pathogenesis

The primary defect in LEMS is a reduced number of voltage-gated Ca^{2+} channels at the nerve terminal leading to a decreased number of vesicles (quanta) released by the nerve action potential, and consequent conduction block.

IgG anti-P/Q type calcium-channel antibodies are responsible for the loss of calcium channels. Membrane voltage-gated calcium channels are expressed by cells of small-cell lung cancer, and potassium-stimulated (voltage-gated) Ca^{2+} influx can be demonstrated in cell lines from that cancer. These antibodies also account for the autonomic dysfunction.

Clinical features

LEMS can occur with or without small-cell lung cancer. In the former, the neurological disorder typically precedes radiological evidence of the tumour by up to 5 years. The presenting symptom is usually difficulty with walking, the legs being described as heavy, stiff, or weak. Autonomic symptoms of dry mouth, constipation, and, in males, sexual impotence are often already present. Bulbar weakness is rare, but double vision occurs in some patients. Fatigue is not a dominant feature as it is in myasthenia gravis. Symptoms may be mild in some, but in others may render them bed-bound. Onset is usually gradual but in some patients it is subacute, developing over 2 or 3 weeks.

Mild bilateral ptosis may be present, and sometimes weakness of the face or neck muscles. Limb weakness may be generalized, although affecting proximal muscles most severely. Tone is normal and there is no wasting. The diagnostic features are an augmentation of strength during the first few seconds of a maximal effort, and the reappearance of initially depressed or absent tendon reflexes following a brief (e.g. 10 s) maximum voluntary contraction of the muscle being tested. In advanced cases, however, this may not be demonstrable clinically. There is no sensory disturbance.

Diagnosis

The diagnosis is made by the characteristic electromyographic findings of a reduced amplitude of the compound muscle action potential and the presence of a more than 100 per cent increment following maximum voluntary contraction of the muscle being tested. Detection of a clearly raised titre of anticalcium-channel antibodies provides strong evidence for LEMS in patients with electrophysiological evidence of myasthenia.

Management

An underlying small-cell lung cancer needs to be sought and, if found, treated. Successful treatment will improve the neurological disorder and may allow remission in some 3 to 6 months.

Most patients will benefit from oral 3,4-diaminopyridine. The drug acts by blocking K^+ conductance at the nerve terminal, thereby prolonging the nerve action potential and increasing transmitter release. Guanidine may also be beneficial but risks of toxicity are higher.

Plasma exchange or intravenous immunoglobulin can produce short-term benefits in severe cases, with either form of LEMS. Prednisolone (up to 100 mg on alternate days) may be helpful in C-LEMS. In NC-LEMS, a combination of prednisolone and azathioprine (2.5 mg/kg body weight) appears optimal, and a proportion of patients will develop full remission on this regimen. The thymus in LEMS is normal and thymectomy is not indicated.

In NC-LEMS, the prognosis is substantially improved with the introduction of immunosuppressive drugs, although some patients are very resistant to therapy.

Congenital/hereditary myasthenia

This comprises a rare, heterogeneous, and genetically diverse group of disorders in which there are no immunological abnormalities. The defect in neuromuscular transmission is usually postsynaptic acetylcholine-receptor deficiency or prolonged opening (slow channel syndrome). In many families these have now been shown to be due to mutation of the acetylcholine receptor gene. Rarely, acetylcholinesterase deficiency is the cause, also due to genetic mutation.

A diagnosis of congenital/hereditary myasthenia should be suspected in children of a consanguineous marriage who have developed symptoms in early life, or where there is a family history of myasthenia. Absence of detectable antiacetylcholine receptor antibody is an essential diagnostic criterion, and very early onset will also make myasthenia gravis very unlikely. Electromyography may reveal increased decrement, and jitter is increased in single-fibre studies. Screening for the acetylcholine receptor gene may establish the diagnosis. Some patients show a positive response to intravenous edrophonium, and are helped by oral pyridostigmine, but this therapy is not effective in all forms of the disorder.

Acquired neuromyotonia

Neuromyotonia describes a state of spontaneous and continuous muscle fibre contraction caused by the hyperexcitability of peripheral motor nerves. The patient is aware of spontaneous muscle twitching, and of muscle stiffness and cramps on attempted exercise. Sweating may be excessive. Acquired neuromyotonia is a rare disorder that develops spontaneously and is distinguished from the neuromyotonia that may associate with hereditary motor–sensory neuropathies. Examination reveals myokymia (muscle twitching), which can be widespread. Muscles sometimes show hypertrophy. Reflexes may be normal or reduced, and some weakness may be evident.

Recent evidence indicates that some cases of acquired neuromyotonia are antibody-mediated. The disorder has been reported to associate with thymoma and myasthenia gravis. Present evidence suggests the antigenic target is the voltage-gated K^+ channel at the nerve terminal that normally controls nerve excitability.

The diagnosis is made by the presence of the characteristic electromyographic discharges. Antipotassium channel antibodies can be detected in about 50 per cent of patients. In many patients, the abnormal discharges are controlled by phenytoin or carbamazepine. In resistant cases, treatment with plasma exchange and with immunosuppressive drugs should be considered.

Further reading

Newsom-Davis, J. (1996). Myasthenia gravis. *Medicine* (Baltimore), **24**(6), 110–13.

Newsom-Davis, J. (1998). Autoimmune and genetic disorders at the neuromuscular junction. *Developmental Medicine and Child Neurology*, **40**, 199–206.

Chapter 13.39

Metabolic and endocrine myopathies

D. Hilton-Jones

The term metabolic myopathy is applied most frequently to those disorders in which there is a primary defect, usually an enzyme deficiency, in the biochemical pathways associated with energy generation (ATP synthesis). This group includes the extremely important mitochondrial disorders (see Chapter 13.40).

Endocrine myopathies, and nutritional and toxic myopathies, including drug-induced myopathies, can be considered as secondary metabolic myopathies. Inherited defects of muscle ion channels have been shown to underlie several myopathic disorders: hyperkalaemic periodic paralysis (sodium channel), hypokalaemic periodic paralysis (calcium), myotonia congenita (chloride), and malignant hyperthermia (ryanodine).

Primary metabolic myopathies

The major energy currency of living cells is adenosine triphosphate (ATP) (Fig. 1). Whereas in most organs the rate of ATP utilization is fairly constant, in voluntary muscle the change from rest to strenuous activity may increase the demand on ATP generation several

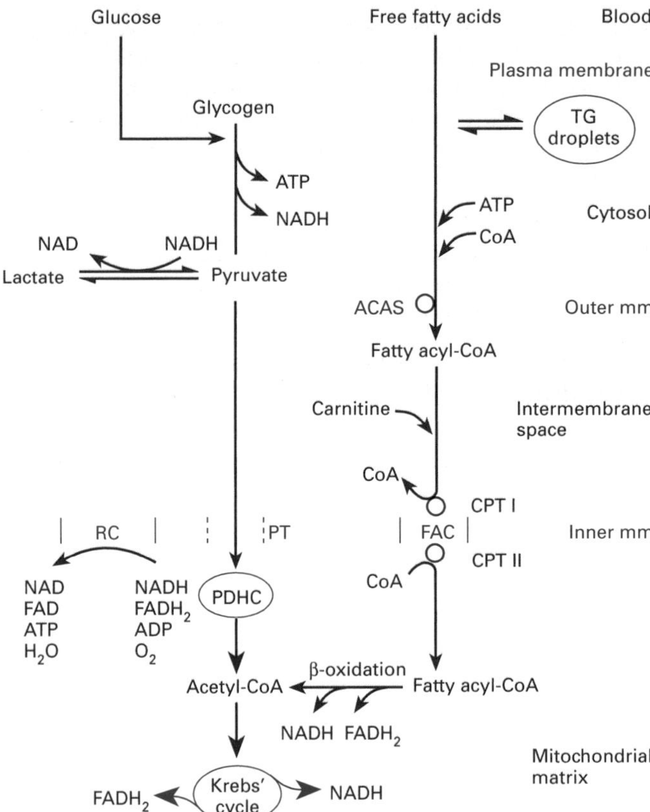

Fig. 1 Major pathways associated with energy production in skeletal muscle. ACAS, acyl-CoA synthetase; ADP, adenosine diphosphate; ATP, adenosine triphosphate; CoA, coenzyme A; CPT, carnitine palmityl transferase; FAC, fatty acyl-carnitine; FAD, flavin adenine dinucleotide; FADH, reduced FAD; mm, mitochondrial membrane; NAD, nicotinamide adenine dinucleotide; NADH, reduced NAD; PDH, pyruvate dehydrogenase complex; PT, pyruvate translocase; RC, respiratory chain; TG, triglyceride.

thousand-fold. If that demand is not met, contractile failure (i.e., fatigue or weakness) will develop and may be accompanied by destruction of muscle fibres.

Disorders of glycogen and glucose metabolism (see also Chapter 6.2)

Several of the glycogenoses show significant involvement of skeletal muscle. They are autosomal-recessive disorders, except for phosphoglycerate kinase deficiency, which is X-linked recessive. In most of these disorders the serum creatine kinase is elevated, massively so after exercise-induced muscle damage.

Acid maltase deficiency (type II glycogenosis)

Acid maltase is a lysosomal enzyme not directly involved in energetic pathways, and exercise-induced symptoms are absent. The adult form is of considerable importance and has probably been underdiagnosed. The most obvious feature is a slowly progressive, painless, proximal myopathy. Diaphragmatic involvement is very common and one-third of patients first present with symptoms of respiratory failure. Nocturnal assisted ventilation alleviates symptoms and may prolong survival for many years. Muscle biopsy is usually suggestive but the definitive diagnosis is established by enzyme assay in muscle, fibroblasts or leucocytes, or by demonstrating glycogen granules by periodic acid– Schiff staining in lymphocytes on a peripheral blood film.

Myophosphorylase deficiency (type V glycogenosis; McArdle's disease)

Onset of symptoms is usually in childhood and the cardinal features are pain, weakness, and stiffness of muscles early in exercise, relieved by rest. Strenuous exercise may induce painful, electrically silent muscle contractures. Muscle fibre breakdown is reflected in myalgia and myoglobinuria, which, if severe, may cause renal failure. Progressive proximal weakness frequently develops and is sometimes the mode of presentation in late-onset cases.

Failure of lactate generation during ischaemic forearm exercise is consistent with the diagnosis, but not specific, and may give a misleading result if the enzyme deficiency is partial. The definitive diagnosis is established by demonstrating absence of phosphorylase staining, or by enzyme assay, on muscle biopsy.

Debrancher enzyme deficiency (type III glycogenosis; Cori–Forbes disease)

In infancy and childhood the main features of this disorder are hepatomegaly, hypoglycaemia, and failure to thrive. During adolescence, muscle symptoms become more prominent. A small group of patients first presents in adult life with muscle symptoms, but may give a history of a protuberant abdomen in childhood. Both exercise intolerance and a slowly progressive proximal myopathy are present. It has recently been recognized that most patients develop a potentially fatal cardiomyopathy.

The ischaemic forearm test shows impaired lactate generation, muscle biopsy shows glycogen accumulation, and administration of glucagon fails to produce a hyperglycaemic response. Enzyme assay can be performed on muscle, liver, erythrocytes, and leucocytes.

Phosphofructokinase deficiency (type VII glycogenosis; Tarui's disease)

The clinical picture is very similar to that of myophosphorylase deficiency, but deficiency of phosphofructokinase in erythrocytes leads to the additional features of haemolytic anaemia and gout. Diagnosis is established by enzyme assay in muscle.

Defects of distal glycolysis

Deficiencies of phosphoglycerate kinase, phosphoglycerate mutase, and lactate dehydrogenase have been described recently. All three are associated with exercise intolerance and myoglobinuria. It is highly likely that other defects of glycolysis causing similar symptoms remain to be discovered.

Treatment

There is as yet no specific treatment for any of the disorders described above. Attempts at dietary manipulation have generally proved unsuccessful. Patients must be aware of the risk to renal function from myoglobinuria, and try to avoid intense exercise.

Disorders of lipid metabolism

Unlike glycolysis, lipid metabolism is entirely dependent upon oxidative processes, and there is a close relation between the disorders described below and defects of the mitochondrial respiratory chain (see Chapter 13.40).

Carnitine deficiency

Muscle carnitine deficiency, causing fluctuating weakness and lipid storage, and systemic carnitine deficiency causing weakness and recurrent, often fatal, Reye-like episodes, have been described. The carnitine deficiency may be secondary to another metabolic disorder, most commonly defects of β-oxidation or of the mitochondrial respiratory chain.

Defects of β-oxidation

Many enzyme deficiencies have been described, but clinical features are limited. They may present in the neonatal period with hypotonia, hypoglycaemia, cardiomyopathy, failure to thrive, and early death. Later-onset cases develop Reye-like crises, muscle weakness, and cardiomyopathy. A high-carbohydrate, low-fat diet may help.

Carnitine palmityl transferase deficiency

This rare disorder shows male predominance. Symptoms are precipitated by sustained exercise (e.g. a route march) or prolonged fasting, and consist of muscle pain followed by myoglobinuria, which may cause renal failure. A high-carbohydrate, low-fat diet may reduce the frequency of attacks.

Endocrine myopathies

Weakness is a common symptom in many endocrine disorders. The mechanisms are generally poorly understood, the myopathy responds to treatment of the underlying hormonal disorder, and extensive investigation of the myopathic component is rarely required. The most common pattern is limb-girdle weakness.

Thyroid disorders

Thyrotoxicosis

Typically, weakness develops shortly after the onset of other thyrotoxic symptoms. The shoulder-girdle muscles tend to be involved before the pelvic musculature. Serum creatine kinase is usually normal. Electromyography shows features consistent with muscle disease. The myopathy responds to treatment of the thyrotoxicosis.

Thyrotoxic periodic paralysis

Most cases have been reported in individuals from the Orient, with a strong male predominance. The clinical features closely mimic those of familial hypokalaemic periodic paralysis, and the attacks cease when the patient is rendered euthyroid.

Hypothyroidism

Hypothyroid myopathy may be asymptomatic, but mild weakness is probably present in most patients. Even in the absence of weakness the serum creatine kinase is often markedly elevated. Slow relaxation of the tendon jerks may be present in isolation. Muscle pain and cramps are common. All hypothyroid myopathic symptoms respond to thyroxine replacement.

Disorders of the pituitary–adrenal axis

Acromegaly

Proximal weakness, pelvic more than shoulder girdle, is present in about one-half of patients. Serum creatine kinase is normal or slightly elevated. Normalizing the amount of growth hormone improves the myopathy, but recovery may be incomplete.

ACTH or glucocorticoid excess

In the myopathy associated with cortisol excess the most common picture is of a slowly progressive limb-girdle weakness, pelvic more than shoulder girdle, often accompanied by myalgia. The clinical features are similar whether the cause is Cushing's syndrome or iatrogenic. The 9α-fluorinated steroids, including dexamethasone, triamcinalone, and betamethasone, appear to have the greatest myopathic potential. Topical steroids can also cause myopathy.

The serum creatine kinase is usually normal and muscle biopsy shows non-specific atrophy of type II fibres. Steroid withdrawal or cure of Cushing's syndrome is followed by recovery over several months.

Addison's disease

Weakness, fatigue, and myalgia occur in up to one-half of patients. The serum creatine kinase is normal or slightly increased. Glucocorticoid replacement therapy is curative.

Disorders of calcium, vitamin D, and parathormone metabolism (see also Chapter 7.5 and Section 9)

In osteomalacia, one-third of patients have weakness as the presenting symptom. Bone pain is also prominent. The serum creatine kinase is usually normal. The pain responds fairly rapidly to vitamin D treatment, but the weakness recovers more slowly.

In primary hyperparathyroidism, myalgia, stiffness, and complaints of fatigue are common, but overt weakness is rare. Symptoms resolve after successful parathyroidectomy.

Endstage renal failure is frequently accompanied by a predominantly pelvic-girdle myopathy, sometimes with buttock and thigh pain. Symptoms of renal osteodystrophy respond to dialysis, transplantation, and/or vitamin D.

Rarely, a painful ischaemic myopathy with arterial narrowing due to calcium deposition complicates renal failure. Skin ulceration and bowel infarction may also occur.

Nutritional and toxic myopathies

Alcoholic myopathies

Chronic alcoholics may develop subacute or slowly progressive proximal muscle weakness with mild wasting, mainly affecting the lower limbs. Much more dramatic is acute alcoholic myopathy, which usually occurs during a drinking 'binge'. There may be widespread cramps, pain, and weakness, but the most striking feature is the development of extremely painful muscle swelling, which may be localized or generalized. Myoglobinuria presents a threat to renal function and hyperkalaemia may be present in severe cases. The serum creatine kinase is elevated and muscle biopsy shows acute necrosis. Recovery, which may be incomplete, occurs over several weeks.

Vitamin E deficiency

Vitamin E deficiency probably causes a myopathy, but interpretation is confused by the presence of additional neurological problems including neuropathy and ataxia.

Drug-induced myopathies

Drug-induced neuromuscular disorders are common, under-recognized, and under-reported. Numerous drugs have been implicated, several mechanisms are responsible (Table 1), and some drugs can affect both muscle and peripheral nerve (e.g. vincristine, D-penicillamine, perhexiline).

Ion-channel disorders

Periodic paralysis

Marked hypokalaemia and hyperkalaemia from whatever cause may produce weakness or paralysis (secondary periodic paralysis). The

Table 1 Drug-induced myopathies

Focal damage/fibrosis	Inflammatory myopathy
Intramuscular	Procainamide
opiates	D-Penicillamine
antibiotics	L-Dopa
paraldehyde	Hypokalaemic weakness
Necrosis	Diuretics
Heroin	Carbenoxolone
Clofibrate	Liquorice
ω-Aminocaproic acid	Purgatives
Myoglobinuria/	Subacute or chronic painless
rhabdomyolysis	proximal myopathy
Heroin	Corticosteroids
Methadone	Chloroquine
Amphetamines	β-Blockers
Barbiturates	Myasthenic syndrome
Diazepam	D-Penicillamine
Isoniazid	Aminoglycoside antibiotics
Carbenoxolone	Malignant hyperthermia
Phenformin	Suxamethonium
Amphotericin B	Cyclopropane
	Halothane
	Enflurane
	Ketamine

primary periodic paralyses are familial, dominantly inherited disorders characterized by recurrent attacks of paralysis, and which have previously been subdivided into hyperkalaemic, hypokalaemic, and normokalaemic forms on the basis of changes in the serum potassium during attacks. Hyperkalaemic and normokalaemic periodic paralysis, and paramyotonia congenita, are caused by mutations affecting in the muscle sodium channel, whereas hyperkalaemic periodic paralysis, which is clinically very similar to the hyperkalaemic form, is related to calcium-channel mutations.

Hypokalaemic

Attacks usually start in the second decade of life and then vary in frequency from daily to years between episodes. Weakness may be present on waking or develop during the day, typically in response to a heavy carbohydrate meal or during rest after strenuous exercise. The weakness involves legs more than arms, proximal muscles more than distal, and may be asymmetrical. Attacks last from hours to several days. The tendon reflexes may be depressed or lost during an attack. Permanent and progressive proximal weakness often develops by middle age.

The serum potassium typically falls during an attack, but not necessarily outwith the normal range. If diagnostic doubt remains, an attack may be precipitated by administration of glucose and insulin.

Acetazolamide (up to 1.5 g daily) is the treatment of choice to prevent attacks. Acute attacks respond to oral potassium.

Hyperkalaemic

Attacks tend to start at an earlier age than in the hypokalaemic form, and do not last as long. Precipitants include cold, fasting, rest after exercise, pregnancy, alcohol intake, and potassium loading. Readily utilized carbohydrate sources, such as a sweet drink, may abort an attack. A progressive proximal myopathy may also develop.

The serum potassium may rise during an attack, but the change is often slight.

Mild attacks respond to carbohydrate ingestion. Kaliuretic diuretics usually prevent attacks.

Paramyotonia congenita

Paramyotonia congenita describes a dominantly inherited condition characterized by cold-induced weakness and muscle stiffness (paramyotonia), and which is sometimes accompanied by periodic paralysis. Hyperkalaemic periodic paralysis, hyperkalaemic periodic paralysis with myotonia, paramyotonia congenita, and paramyotonia congenita with periodic paralysis are allelic disorders involving the tetrodotoxin-sensitive sodium channel of adult skeletal muscle.

Myotonia congenita

This condition is caused by mutations in the skeletal muscle chloride gene. Different mutations in the same gene are associated with autosomal-dominant and recessive patterns of inheritance. They are clinically very similar, but with the recessive type tending to be more severe. The characteristic feature is generalized myotonia, first evident in childhood, without persistent weakness. The myotonia eases with repetitive contractions ('warm up'). Myotonia is easily demonstrated on muscle percussion. Mexiletine offers symptomatic relief.

Malignant hyperthermia

The main features are a rapidly rising body temperature and generalized muscular rigidity during anaesthesia. Additional features include skin mottling, cyanosis, tachypnoea, tachycardia, cardiac dysrhythmias, and autonomic instability. Attacks in susceptible individuals may be triggered by suxamethonium and anaesthetic agents (halothane, cyclopropane, enflurane, ketamine). A similar, but probably different, disorder may be associated with heat stroke.

Attacks are life threatening. Treatment consists of withdrawal of the offending agent, general supportive measures. and intravenous dantrolene (2 mg/kg body weight).

Disturbed calcium homeostasis underlies the attacks, with excessive influx of calcium ions into the sarcoplasmic reticulum.

The disorder is inherited as an autosomal-dominant trait. Screening for susceptibility involves muscle biopsy and *in vitro* testing for a reduced contractile threshold to halothane and caffeine.

Further reading

Argov, Z. and Mastaglia, F.L. (1994). Drug-induced neuromuscular disorders in man. In *Disorders of voluntary muscle*, 6th edn (ed. J. Walton, G. Karpati, and D. Hilton-Jones). Churchill Livingstone, Edinburgh.

Hilton-Jones, D., Squier, M., Taylor, D., and Mathews, P., ed. (1995). *Metabolic myopathies.* W.B. Saunders, London.

Hudson, A.J., Ebers, G.C., and Bulman, D.E. (1995). The skeletal muscle sodium and chloride channel diseases. *Brain*, **118**, 547–63.

Chapter 13.40

Mitochondrial myopathies and encephalomyopathies

A. E. Harding

The term mitochondrial myopathy or encephalomyopathy is applied to a clinically and biochemically heterogeneous group of diseases that often exhibits major structural abnormalities of mitochondria in skeletal muscle. Ragged red fibres are the morphological hallmark of these disorders, which present with psychomotor retardation, dementia, pigmentary retinopathy, ataxia, seizures, movement disorders, stroke-like episodes, deafness, and peripheral neuropathy in various combinations. Involvement of other systems, such as the heart, endocrine glands, and haemopoietic tissues, also occurs.

Aetiology

Biochemistry

Many patients with mitochondrial encephalomyopathy have a pathological increase in serum lactate concentration during and after exercise, suggesting a defect of aerobic metabolism in muscle mitochondria, and defects of the mitochondrial respiratory chain have been demonstrated in the majority of cases investigated.

Studies of respiratory-chain function and oxidative phosphorylation in muscle have identified a variety of defects in patients with mitochondrial encephalomyopathy, involving single or multiple respiratory-chain complexes, all of which are associated with a wide range of clinical syndromes.

Genetics

The mitochondrial respiratory chain has the special characteristic of being encoded by two genetic systems, mitochondrial DNA as well as nuclear genes. The coding function of mitochondrial DNA and its mode of transmission led to the hypothesis that the defects of this genome could cause mitochondrial encephalomyopathy. As a constituent of the ovum's cytoplasm, mitochondrial DNA is exclusively maternally transmitted. The majority of patients with mitochondrial encephalomyopathies do not have a history of affected relatives, but when individuals are affected in more than one generation, maternal transmission to offspring is far more frequent than paternal transmission.

Several different types of mitochondrial DNA defects have been reported in patients with mitochondrial encephalomyopathy (Table 1). The most common is a single, large deletion, varying between about 1.5 and 9 kb in length. Deleted mitochondrial DNAs coexist with normal molecules in the muscle and, sometimes, other tissues of patients; they are rarely detectable in blood. Patients with such deletions do not have affected relatives and it seems most likely that deletions originate during oogenesis in the patients' mothers. In contrast to patients with deletions, those with point mutations of mitochondrial DNA commonly have affected relatives with either a similar or less severe phenotype.

Table 1 Mitochondrial DNA defects in mitochondrial encephalomyopathies

Defect	Disease
Primary mitochondrial DNA defects	
Large single deletions/duplications (sporadic)	PEO, Kearns–Sayre syndrome
Point mutations (may be maternal FH)	
in tRNA genes (bp):	
8344, 8356	MERRF*
3243, 3250, 3271	MELAS/other encephalomyopathies*
3260	Myopathy/cardiomyopathy*
in reading frame:	
8993	Neurogenic weakness, ataxia, RP*
Mitochondrial DNA defects secondary to presumed nuclear mutations	
Multiple deletions (AD)	PEO, myopathy, deafness, neuropathy
Depletion (varies between tissues) (AR)	Myopathy/encephalopathy/renal/hepatic failure

*Detectable in blood samples and hence a useful screening test; there are other less common mutations.

AD, autosomal dominant; AR, autosomal recessive; bp, base pair; FH, family history; MELAS, mitochondrial encephalopathy, lactic acid, and stroke-like episodes; MERRF, myoclonic epilepsy with ragged red fibres; PEO, progressive external ophthalmoplegia; RP, retinitis pigmentosa;

Clinical features

The clinical presentations of mitochondrial encephalomyopathy are diverse, but can be divided into four broad categories.

Infantile lactic acidosis

This is the most severe phenotype and characteristically comprises a floppy baby with failure to thrive and developmental delay. Lactic acidosis is the clue to diagnosis, although respiratory-chain deficiencies are not the only cause of this syndrome; others include pyruvate dehydrogenase deficiency and β-oxidation defects. There may be non-neurological features, including defective haemopoiesis, renal tubular acidosis, and cardiac failure.

Progressive external ophthalmoplegia and the Kearns–Sayre syndrome

Progressive external ophthalmoplegia has an insidious onset and usually develops during childhood or adolescence, giving rise to ptosis and limitation of eye movements in all directions of gaze. Fatigue, a 'salt and pepper' type of retinopathy, and proximal limb weakness are common associated features, and the presence of retinopathy points to a diagnosis of mitochondrial encephalomyopathy.

The Kearns–Sayre syndrome is defined by progressive external ophthalmoplegia and pigmentary retinopathy with onset before the age of 20 years, with one or more of the following features: ataxia, an increased protein concentration in cerebrospinal fluid (more than 1 g/l), and cardiac conduction defects. Other features may occur, such as diabetes, hypoparathyroidism, short stature, and deafness. Deletions of mitochondrial DNA in muscle are observed in 80 to 90 per cent of patients with Kearns–Sayre syndrome, a similar proportion of those with progressive external ophthalmoplegia and retinopathy, and about half of those with progressive external ophthalmoplegia alone. All patients with Kearns–Sayre syndrome and the majority of those with progressive external ophthalmoplegia are sporadic cases, which reflects the association with a mitochondrial DNA deletion in many cases.

Myopathies

A relatively small proportion (about 15 per cent) of patients with mitochondrial encephalomyopathy have limb and facial weakness alone, sometimes with accompanying ptosis but no restriction of extraocular movements. Such patients sometimes have retinopathy.

The muscle weakness is usually enhanced by exertion and associated with elevation of serum lactate concentrations which increases after exercise.

Encephalomyopathies

Within mitochondrial encephalomyopathy syndromes are two that are clinically very distinctive, namely myoclonic epilepsy with ragged red fibres (**MERRF**) and mitochondrial encephalopathy, lactic acidosis, and stroke-like episodes (**MELAS**). However, these account for less than one-half of patients with encephalomyopathies and there is substantial overlap between them in some cases. The cardinal features of MERRF are myoclonus, epilepsy, and ataxia. Onset is most commonly in the second and third decades of life. Associated features include deafness, muscle weakness, dementia, optic atrophy, neuropathy, and multiple lipomas. Seizures are often photosensitive and include absences or drop attacks, as well as generalized tonic–clonic seizures. This syndrome is particularly commonly maternally inherited and this reflects the presence of a point mutation of mitochondrial DNA at position 8344 in approximately 80 per cent of cases.

Patients with the MELAS syndrome classically present in childhood or early adult life with recurrent stroke-like episodes. These often have migrainous elements, with headache, vomiting, and visual disturbance, and the neurological deficit is frequently heralded by a focal seizure. Hemiparesis or hemianopia persist for days to months and usually leave minor residual disability; after numerous episodes the cumulative effects are disabling, leading to dementia, quadriparesis, cortical blindness, and ataxia. Other features such as short stature, peripheral neuropathy, deafness, and progressive external ophthalmoplegia are common. About half of patients have affected maternal relatives, and 80 per cent of patients with this syndrome have a point mutation of mitochondrial DNA, again in a tRNA gene at position 3243. Muscle weakness does not occur in some patients, and not all have ragged red fibres. Stroke-like episodes occur in only about 50 per cent of patients with this mutation, and some have progressive external ophthalmoplegia and/or myopathy alone, or deafness, ataxia, and dementia of adult onset, or diabetes.

Diagnosis

The differential diagnosis of mitochondrial encephalomyopathy syndromes is wide, particularly in those with involvement of the central nervous system. This diagnosis should be considered in children and adults with multisystem central nervous disease of unclear origin. In possible encephalomyopathy syndromes it is logical to perform mitochondrial DNA analysis of blood samples as a screening investigation, as this is relatively non-invasive. In the vast majority of symptomatic patients with the 3243 and 8344 base-pair mutations these are detectable in blood, although the proportion in muscle is usually higher. If these analyses are negative, histochemical analysis of a muscle biopsy is the most useful investigation.

An increase in lactate concentrations in blood and cerebrospinal fluid, particularly after exercise, is common in mitochondrial encephalomyopathy, but this is not always the case and the controlled exercise required is difficult for disabled patients. Plasma creatine kinase is often normal or only mildly elevated, and electromyography may be normal in patients with encephalopathies. In such cases, CT and MRI show a wide range of abnormalities, including multifocal low-density lesions, cerebral and cerebellar atrophy, and calcification of the basal ganglia. Such abnormalities are particularly frequent in the MELAS syndrome. More widespread tissue involvement may be demonstrated by the ECG, echocardiography, and renal, endocrine, and liver function tests.

Prognosis

Prognosis is determined largely by age of onset and degree of central nervous involvement. It is worst in patients with infantile lactic acidosis, who may not survive infancy, and encephalopathies such as MELAS developing in childhood. In those with progressive external ophthalmoplegia alone, disability may be minimal and life expectancy normal. On the whole, treatment of these disorders is disappointing.

Further reading

Howell, N. (1999). Human mitochondrial diseases: answering questions and questioning answers. *International Review of Cytology*, **186**, 49–116.

Shoffner, J.M. (1996). Maternal inheritance and the evaluation of oxidative phosphorylation diseases. *Lancet*, **348**, 1283–8.

Shoubridge, E.A. (1998). Mitochondrial encephalomyopathies. *Current Opinion in Neurology*, **11**, 491–6.

Chapter 13.41

Pyomyositis, tropical pyomyositis, or tropical myositis

D. A. Warrell

Pyomyositis is a condition, virtually confined to tropical countries until the advent of AIDS, in which abscesses develop within skeletal muscles. Abscesses extending secondarily into muscle from adjacent structures are excluded from this definition.

Pyomyositis has been reported from most parts of the tropical world. In some places (e.g. in Uganda and Ecuador) it accounts for up to 4 per cent of hospital admissions. In temperate climates, pyomyositis has been very rare, but increasing numbers of are now being described in patients with human immunodeficiency virus (HIV) infection (especially in males with CD4 counts below 30) and other kinds of immunosuppression.

Aetiology

Staphylococcus aureus is the organism most commonly cultured from the abscesses. *Streptococcus pyogenes* (usually group A), *Strep. pneumoniae*, *Haemophilus influenzae*, *Escherichia coli*, *Proteus* and *Pseudomonas* spp., and mycobacteria have also been implicated. There is a history of preceding trauma to the affected muscle in more than 20 per cent of patients. Perhaps a muscle haematoma provides a nidus for blood-borne infection. HIV-1 and HIV-2 immunosuppression has become the major predisposing cause in tropical and temperate regions. Other predisposing factors may include general debilitation, sickle-cell disease, arboviral infection, *Toxocara*, *Lagochilascaris minor*, and filariasis. Most helminth-associated abscesses (e.g. Guinea-worm abscesses) are inter- rather than intramuscular.

Pathology

Pyomyositic abscesses are usually large, loculated, and situated beneath the deep fascia within skeletal muscles. There is focal muscle necrosis, mononuclear cell infiltration, and inflammatory oedema.

Clinical features

Pyomyositis is most common in young males. Pain and tenderness of the affected muscle may develop over a few days. A single muscle in the trunk or lower limbs is most commonly affected, but multiple abscesses in distantly separated muscles can occur. Initially, there is an ill-defined tender and thickened area, which later becomes localized, very tender, hot, and swollen. Overlying skin may be red and oedematous. The swelling is usually non-fluctuant and there is no local lymphadenopathy. Peripheral leucocytosis is not invariable. Eosinophilia is frequently associated but is usually prevalent in the populations most affected by tropical pyomyositis. Despite local muscle destruction, serum concentrations of muscle enzymes may remain normal, but myoglobinaemia, myoglobinuria, and acute renal failure may develop. Infection may spread to adjacent structures (e.g. joints, pleural cavity) or via the bloodstream to the heart valves. The case fatality of those admitted to hospital in the pre-AIDS era was less than 1.5 per cent but it is now high (approximately 25 per cent) in HIV-seropositive patients in Africa.

Diagnosis

Depending on the muscle involved, pyomyositis can simulate other conditions such as acute abdomen, deep venous thrombosis, and meningitis. The differential diagnosis includes muscle haematomas, torn muscles, vascular or necrotic tumours of connective tissue or muscle (e.g. rhabdomyosarcoma), and swellings caused by migratory helminths (e.g. *Loa loa*, *Gnathostoma*, *Paragonimus*, and *Sparganum*). *Staphylococcus aureus* is usually cultured from the pus, but blood cultures are positive in less than 5 per cent of cases. Ultrasound, CT, and MRI imaging are useful for localizing abscesses and guiding diagnostic and therapeutic needle aspiration.

Treatment

Surgical exploration, debridement, and drainage is essential. Because the abscesses are usually loculated, needle aspiration is inadequate. Parenteral flucloxacillin should be started immediately. Benzyl penicillin can be substituted if a group A streptococcus is isolated.

Further reading

Marcus, R.T. and Foster, W.D. (1968). Observations on the clinical features, aetiology and geographical distribution of pyomyositis in East Africa. *East African Medical Journal*, **45**, 167–76.

Harbarth S.J. and Lew, D.P. (1997). Pyomyositis as a nontropical disease. *Current Clinical Topics in Infectious Diseases*, **17**, 37–50.

Vassilopoulos, D., Chalasani, P., Jurado, R.L., Workowski, K., and Agudelo, C.A. (1997). Musculoskeletal infections in patients with human immunodeficiency virus infection. *Medicine, Baltimore*, **76**(4), 284–94.

Section 14
Psychiatry

Contents

Chapter 14.1

Psychiatry in medicine

M. G. Gelder

This section gives an account of adult psychiatric disorders that commonly present to physicians. It is selective because psychiatry deals with many issues that seldom arise in medical wards, for example the care of patients with chronic schizophrenia. The account focuses on practical issues of diagnosis and management. The topic of dependence on drugs and alcohol is presented in Chapters 14.9 14.18. For a more comprehensive account of psychiatry readers are referred to the *New Oxford Textbook of Psychiatry* or a similar postgraduate text for psychiatrists.

The detection of psychiatric disorder in physically ill patients

Psychiatric disorder is common among the physically ill, but frequently goes undetected. When reliable standardized interviews and strict diagnostic criteria are used, about 20 per cent of medical inpatients are found to have psychiatric disorders, but only half are detected by their physicians. Most of these disorders are emotional or complications of alcohol abuse.

It is important to detect psychiatric disorders in the physically ill for several reasons: severe psychiatric disorders may worsen if not treated promptly, some may carry a risk of suicide; moderately severe disorders reduce compliance with medical treatment and so delay recovery from physical illness; mild disorders may increase the distress of physical illness; finally, psychiatric conditions need to be considered in the differential diagnosis of physical symptoms.

Psychiatric symptoms may go unnoticed because they are more difficult to detect in physically ill than in physically healthy patients, and because some physicians do not enquire about them in a systematic and routine way. There are several reasons why psychiatric symptoms are more difficult to detect in patients who have a physical illness. First, the symptoms may be mistaken for a normal emotional reaction to physical illness—patients may be thought to be understandably despondent when in fact they are suffering from a depressive disorder. Second, some of the symptoms characteristic of psychiatric disorder are also symptoms of physical disorder, for example insomnia, lack of energy, and weight loss. Third, psychiatric patients who are depressed or apathetic may remain unnoticed because they are quiet and compliant.

Some physicians do not ask routinely about psychiatric symptoms because they believe that questioning will upset the patient. These reservations are usually greatest when asking patients with malignant disease about hopelessness and tearfulness, and also when asking patients about suicidal ideas. Such enquiries are not distressing if made sensitively, and if the physician leaves enough time to listen sympathetically to the answers. Questions about feelings may induce an immediate reaction of weeping and other signs of distress, but if the physician responds in a sympathetic and unhurried way, patients generally are relieved to express feelings and share concerns. Questions about suicide do not increase the risk of suicide; on the contrary they make patients feel that their distress has been understood, which in turn makes them less hopeless and less likely to attempt suicide.

Mental state examination in medical work

The full mental state examination used in psychiatry is too detailed for the non-psychiatrist who may use a shorter interview focusing on disorders of mood and cognition. This can be expanded to include disorders of thinking and perception when appropriate (for example when delirium or acute schizophrenia is a possibility). If the brief examination suggests a major mental disorder, it is important to interview another informant who knows the patient well because some patients have limited insight into the nature or extent of their abnormal behaviour.

A useful routine is to ask all patients about mood disorder, starting with difficulty in sleeping as this is a natural route into discussion of worries that may be keeping a patient awake and may also elicit a key symptom in diagnosing endogenous depression (early morning wakening); particular reference should be made to worry, tension, low spirits, and hopelessness. Questions about orientation and memory may be resented by patients with a normal mental state; it is usually evident when such questions must be asked, because the possibility of impairment of orientation or memory has been suggested by the patient's responses during the medical history. If necessary, the questions can be introduced by explaining that such enquiries are routine.

Reactions and disorders

There is a useful diagnostic convention that normal emotional responses to adverse circumstances (including those associated with physical illness) are called emotional reactions, and that abnormal responses are called psychiatric disorders. The distinction between normal and abnormal responses is made on two criteria. The first is a commonsense judgement about the amount of distress that most patients experience in similar circumstances. A degree of depression or anxiety is a normal response to physical illness, to pain or to other kinds of physical discomfort, to the unfamiliar surroundings of hospital life, and to uncertainty about the future. Physicians who see many patients within their specialty are usually better placed than a psychiatrist to judge whether a psychological reaction to a particular physical illness is normal or abnormal. The second criterion is that an abnormal reaction can be identified as a clinical syndrome with a specific pattern of symptoms. Psychiatric syndromes are usually not difficult to recognize. Physicians should be able to detect the majority of syndromes, but psychiatric advice should be sought in doubtful cases.

When to obtain psychiatric advice

For certain conditions, the physician should always seek specialist advice; these include schizophrenia, mania and severe depression. In most other conditions, if a diagnosis is certain and the disorder is not severe, the physician may initiate treatment or ask the family doctor to do so. For more severe cases, or if in doubt, he may refer the patient to a psychiatrist. This will be easier where a specialist liaison psychiatric service exists. The main indications for referral are: uncertainty about the psychiatric diagnosis; the psychiatric disorder not responding to treatment prescribed by the physician; a disorder of great severity, particularly when there may be a risk of suicide or of harm to other people; and behaviour that is disruptive and not controlled by simple measures. These points are taken up in subsequent sections.

Reactions to stressful events

Physicians see many patients who have emotional and physical symptoms as reactions to stressful events. Some of these reactions are abnormal and are classifiable as psychiatric disorders. Most are normal reactions and specialist help is not indicated.

Acute stress reactions

An acute stress reaction is the immediate normal emotional response to a major stress. The symptoms are anxiety, depression, irritability, poor sleep, difficulty in concentration, restlessness, and symptoms of autonomic arousal such as palpitation and tremor. Physicians see these reactions in people admitted to hospital in stressful circumstances, or in the relatives of the seriously ill. Usually acute stress reactions resolve within a few days as the stress subsides or the person adjusts to it. The emotional response can usually be reduced by encouraging the person to talk about the stressful experience and by supportive empathic listening. If the reaction is severe, an anxiolytic or hypnotic drug could be prescribed for 2 or 3 days. If the stressful event was very distressing it may be necessary to help the patient to talk about it several times to release emotions.

Adjustment reactions

An adjustment reaction is the emotional response to prolonged stressful circumstances such as a serious illness or a major loss. The symptoms of an adjustment reaction resemble those of an acute reaction to stress, but the response lasts longer because the stress is more prolonged. Patients may avoid stressful situations, or may deny knowledge of the seriousness of their situation even though it has been explained clearly. Such responses may protect from high levels of anxiety or depression and may be adaptive in the early stages, but if persistent, avoidance and denial may prevent the making of a healthy adjustment and the adjustment may become morbid, warranting treatment. Treatment is directed to helping the normal processes of adjustment. Problem-solving counselling may be used to reduce avoidance and denial, and to encourage resolution and acceptance of the new situation. Drugs are seldom indicated, but occasionally benzodiazepines are helpful for a few days to improve sleep and to reduce anxiety.

Post-traumatic stress disorder (PTSD)

Post-traumatic stress disorder is an intense, prolonged, and sometimes delayed reaction to an exceptionally stressful event such as a major road accident, rape, or other severe trauma The diagnosis is not applicable until symptoms have persisted for at least 1 month. This kind of reaction may affect anyone, but the risk is greater if the stressful experience is extremely severe, if the person under stress is a child or elderly, or if the person has a past history of psychiatric disorder. The clinical features include anxiety, depression, irritability, poor concentration, and insomnia, often with panic attacks and sometimes episodes of aggression; intrusive daytime images ('flashbacks') and nightmares of the stressful events, together with difficulty in recalling the events at will; detachment, diminished interest, and inability to feel normal emotions. Symptoms usually resolve within a few months but occasionally persist for years. Specialist treatments involving exposure therapy, cognitive behavioural strategies, and brief focal psychotherapy are helpful in PTSD. Antidepressants may also be indicated.

Table 1 Physical symptoms of anxiety

Cardiovascular	**Genitourinary**
Palpitation	Frequent or urgent micturition
Awareness of missed beats	Failure of erection
Discomfort in the chest	Amenorrhoea
	Menstrual discomfort
Respiratory	
Overbreathing	**Neuromuscular**
Sense of dyspnoea	Tremor
	Aching muscles
Gastrointestinal	Pricking sensations
Dry mouth	Headache
Difficulty in swallowing	Dizziness, tinnitus
Epigastric discomfort	
Excessive wind	
Frequent or loose motions	

Anxiety and obsessional disorders

Anxiety disorders

Anxiety is a normal reaction to stressful events, but in a few cases, the severity and duration of the anxiety are out of proportion to the stressful circumstances. Such anxiety disorders are common and present to physicians in most clinical settings because the symptoms, which may be very severe, can resemble those of physical illness. It is important, therefore, that physicians should be able to recognize and arrange appropriate treatment for anxiety states. These are of three kinds: generalized anxiety disorders, in which anxiety is continuous; panic disorder, in which anxiety is episodic without any consistent relationship to external stimuli; and phobic anxiety disorders, in which anxiety is episodic and occurs in relation to specific stimuli. The symptoms are the same in all three and will be described in relation to generalized anxiety disorder.

Generalized anxiety disorder

Clinical picture

The patient often complains of one or more physical symptoms that result from autonomic arousal and increased tension in skeletal muscles. Such symptoms are numerous but can be grouped conveniently into cardiovascular, respiratory, gastrointestinal, genitourinary, and neuromuscular symptoms (see Table 1). Anxious patients often overbreathe without realizing it and thereby get faintness, tinnitus, palpitation, precordial discomfort, tingling in the extremities and, (in severe cases) carpopedal spasm. When patients are very anxious they may exhibit tremor and pace up and down.

In medical settings, the patient may not volunteer psychological symptoms because of a belief that they are normal reactions to a worrying physical symptom such as palpitation. It is often difficult for the patient or their doctor to know which comes first. These psychological symptoms include fearful anticipation, inner restlessness, irritability, and poor concentration. The latter may lead to complaints of poor memory, as poor concentration leads to poor registration. Not surprisingly, many patients have persistent worrying thoughts that they are seriously ill and will nto be reassured by normal medical tests in the face of their own experience of marked physical symptoms. Other features are difficulty in falling asleep, and wakening during the night. These sleep disturbances contrast with the early morning wakening which is characteristic of depressive disorder, but depression and anxiety frequently coexist.

Differential diagnosis

Generalized anxiety disorder has to be distinguished from physical illness and from other psychiatric disorders. Anxiety disorder can present with symptoms resembling physical illness (somatization), whilst some physical illnesses are accompanied by marked anxiety symptoms. When a patient complains of physical symptoms of anxiety such as palpitation or epigastric discomfort, the correct diagnosis can usually be reached by enquiring about other symptoms of the syndrome of generalized anxiety disorder; in a medical setting it is most appropriate to ask first about the other symptoms listed in Table 1, then go on to ask about sleep disturbance which can lead into a discussion about worries and fears. As the physical syndrome is presented basically one of overactivity of the sympathetic nervous system, sometimes with hyperventilation, appropriate investigations may be required to exclude thyrotoxicosis, phaeochromocytoma, and hypoglycaemia.

Any physical illness may be accompanied by an anxiety disorder or depression; this could appear to add to the symptoms of the physical illness unresponsive to specific treatments for the physical disorder, e.g. hyperventilation in pre-existing asthma would not respond to increased steroids. A patient who has a special reason to fear a particular type of physical illness, for example if a relative died after developing similar symptoms is likely to develop anxiety symptoms.

Several psychiatric disorders can present with anxiety symptoms. Depressive disorder is the most frequent, and patient with personality disorder may have coexisting severe anxiety, but senile dementia and schizophrenia may also come to notice in this way. Alcohol withdrawal is another important cause of symptoms resembling anxiety disorder.

Prognosis

Without treatment about three-quarters of generalized anxiety disorders persist up to 3 years. The outcome is worse when the history is long, stressful circumstances are persistent, and the personality is abnormal. If somatized anxiety is not correctly diagnosed and treated, patients may seek repeated medical consultation with a variety of specialists, and over many years.

Treatment

Treatment in the medical setting should begin with an explanation that the physical symptoms are a severe exaggeration of the normal response to fear and not evidence of physical disease. Patients find helpful an explanation about the physiological effects of anxiety and overbreathing, demonstrating, as it does, an understanding of their problem and not dismissing it as something they have imagined. The patient should be encouraged to make connections between their physical symptoms and their emotional state. They should be encouraged to deal with stressful problems if they can, or helped to come to terms with any that cannot be resolved. If symptoms persist, anxiety management is indicated. If patients continue to hyperventilate when anxious, they should be shown how to terminate the acute episode by rebreathing expired air from a paper bag to restore normal alveolar concentrations of carbon dioxide. To prevent further episodes patients can practise slow, controlled, diaphragmatic breathing which is timed by tape-recorded instructions.

If the patient does not respond to these simple measures, or if the symptoms are very severe, drug treatment may be needed. Antidepressants have both anxiolytic and antidepressant actions. They do not cause dependency and are often effective for treatment of anxiety in doses lower than those needed for depression. Patients presenting with somatized anxiety are vigilant about physical symptoms and readily attribute symptoms of their disorder to side-effects of medication; extra care is needed in explaining about side-effects and it may be necessary to begin with very small doses which are built up gradually until a therapeutic response is obtained. β-Adrenergic agonists are useful to control severe palpitation and tremor, but do not have a direct anxiolytic effect. Care should be taken to observe the contraindications to their use (notably heart block, a history of bronchospasm, metabolic alkalosis, and prolonged fasting), and to follow the manufacturer's guides to usage. Benzodiazepines can produce rapid relief of anxiety, but may cause dependence. They are are best avoided except for short-term use when symptoms are severe.

Antidepressants have both anxiolytic and antidepressant actions. They do not cause dependency and the anticholinergic side-effects of tricyclics are seldom troublesome in the doses required to control generalized anxiety (about 75 mg per day of amitriptyline). These drugs are useful for chronic generalized anxiety disorders that have not responded to anxiety management.

Panic disorder

This comprises sudden attacks of symptoms of severe anxiety which are not provoked by external stimuli. Patients with panic disorder have an abnormally reactive adrenergic system. They also have fears that anxiety symptoms will be followed by a medical emergency such as a heart attack and it is not unusual for them to attend accident and emergency departments and cardiologists. The fears and the overactive central adrenergic activity interact to set up a vicious circle. Anxiety leads to physical symptoms, which activate fear of physical illness, which leads to more anxiety , and so on. In the past cardiologists who saw these patients referred to the condition as disorderly action of the heart, or effort syndrome. It is clear now that the causes are psychological and the heart is normal.

Prognosis

When the condition is of recent onset, patients often recover if the benign nature of the symptoms is explained and the fears of physical illness are dispelled. When the condition has lasted more than 6 months, it is likely to persist for years unless treated.

Treatment

Imipramine, a tricyclic antidepressant drug with anxiolytic properties, is effective and does not cause dependency. When first prescribed for panic disorder, it may cause apprehension and sleeplessness. For this reason a small starting dose should be used; for example 10 mg per day for 3 days, increased by 10 mg every 3 days to a dose of 50 mg per day, and then by increments of 25 mg per week to the final dose. Some patients with very severe symptoms may need very high final doses and in these cases, specialist advice should be sought. Imipramine should be continued for 6 months and then withdrawn gradually. About one-third of patients relapse and need further treatment with imipramine or with cognitive therapy. Selective serotonin reuptake inhibitors are also effective, safe in overdose, and have fewer side-effects than imipramine (see Chapter 14.6).

Cognitive therapy requires a specialist therapist. It is designed to change the fears of physical symptoms that contribute to the panic attacks. The patient is helped to recognize the irrational basis of the fears and to control them. The results of cognitive therapy are similar to those of imipramine, and the relapse rate may be lower. In some countries the preferred treatment for panic attacks is with high doses of benzodiazepines. Prolonged treatment may lead to dependency and should be supervised by a specialist.

β-Blockers have been widely prescribed for this condition despite evidence that they are not effective in panic disorder.

Phobic anxiety disorder

The symptoms of phobic anxiety disorder resemble those of generalized anxiety disorder, the difference being that the symptoms occur in relation only to specific situations. For example agoraphobic patients become severely anxious when they leave home, enter crowded places or are in situations that they cannot leave easily. Phobic patients tend to avoid situations that provoke symptoms, and this avoidance may limit their ability to have necessary medical treatment, for example fear of injections or enclosed spaces (as in scanning procedures). Treatment with behaviour therapy is usually successful.

Obsessive compulsive disorder

The main features of obsessive compulsive disorder are thoughts that intrude repeatedly and insistently into the patient's awareness and are recognized by the patient as irrational. The thoughts are usually associated with repetitive behaviours (rituals). Patients feel ashamed of the symptoms and may not reveal them to a physician. A common theme is that of spreading disease by touching objects and thereby contaminating them. Other obsessional thoughts are fearful preoccupations about illness ('disease phobias'), often cancer or venereal disease. Admission to hospital or an investigation may reveal the condition by provoking the patient's obsessional symptoms (for example fears of contamination), and consequent anxiety.

Obsessional symptoms are common in other psychiatric disorders, notably depression, but primary obsessive compulsive disorder is a relatively rare syndrome. When obsessional disorders are mild and of recent onset, the treatment is with supportive encouragement to resist rituals. Exacerbations of symptoms are often caused by an associated depressive disorder which should be treated with an antidepressant drug. Persistent obsessional disorders should be assessed by a psychiatrist. Treatments include 5-HT uptake blocking drugs and a form of behaviour therapy known as response prevention.

Psychiatric conditions with physical complaints

The term somatization describes the presentation of psychological distress as bodily complaints and the seeking of medical help for these complaints. Somatization in its acute form is a common process. Amongst patients who attend general practitioners with stress reactions, anxiety disorders or depressive disorders, more complain of physical than of psychological symptoms. Headache, insomnia, and tiredness are common complaints related to stress. The conditions in which somatization operates are classified as somatoform disorders. Most cases are readily treatable somatized forms of stress reactions, anxiety states and or depressive disorders. Persistent somatization disorders are much less frequent in the general population. They are of four main kinds: somatization disorder, hypochondriasis, dysmorphophobia, and psychogenic pain. In the US National Classification conversion disorder is included in the somatoform disorders but in the International Classification of Diseases it is classified separately.

Somatization disorder

This is a chronic condition in which patients complain of multiple, recurrent, and often changing physical symptoms for which no physical cause can be found and where long-standing, but perhaps unrecognized, treatable conditions such as anxiety states and depressive disorders have been excluded. The patient is not satisfied with appropriate investigation and reassurance and their complaints continue or change to another symptom, which can be of any kind. Patients with somatization disorder are extremely persistent in seeking further help and investigation. Many are referred to rehabilitation services that provide care for chronic illnesses. Some give a clear history of emotional deprivation or abuse in childhood, and have long-standing difficulties in personal relationships, indicating that their disorder and illness behaviour are but one manifestation of a more pervasive personality disorder.

There is no specific psychological treatment for somatization disorder. It is important that the correct diagnosis is made and access of patients to medical advice and to investigations should be kept within reasonable limits, which are agreed and adhered to by the physician and general practitioner. Psychiatrists can help in formulating this plan of management, and in making sure that a primary depressive disorder or a chronic state of anxiety has been excluded as a cause for the symptoms, but they can seldom provide more specific and effective treatment.

Hypochondriasis

Hypochondriasis is a preoccupation with illness that persists despite reassurance based on appropriate medical investigation. In medical practice hypochondriacal concerns are met frequently in patients who have no psychiatric disorder. Severe and persistent hypochondriasis is usually associated with psychiatric disorder or personality disorder.

Clinical features

Hypochondriacal concerns take many forms, but they usually relate to physical disease or to the appearance of the face or body. Concerns about disease are often associated with awareness of a normal bodily sensation such as a forceful heart action, flatulence, or minor aches and pains, which are interpreted as symptoms of undetected disease. Other concerns relate to normal variations in appearance such as pigmented areas in the skin or benign lumps. Preoccupations with cancer or AIDS are common. These preoccupaitons persist despite repeated reassurance based on appropriate and thorough investigation. They often cause great distress. Some patients are concerned with a single symptom and a single disease, others have a series of changing concerns.

Aetiology

Hypochondriasis may be provoked by stressful events. In mild cases there may be no associated psychiatric disorder, but in some severe and persistent cases there is a depressive, anxiety, or obsessional disorder.

Occasionally, hypochondriacal complaints are the first evidence of schizophrenia or dementia. Most other cases of severe persistent hopochondriasis are associated with a personality disorder. There is not single personality type, but obsessional and paranoid traits occur frequently.

Treatment

When hypochondriasis is mild and related to stress, it usually subsides when the stressful circumstances pass and the patient is given reassurance. When hypochondriasis is secondary to a psychiatric disorder, it usually improves when the primary disorder has been treated successfully. If the personality is abnormal, treatment is difficult. Review by a psychiatrist can be helpful in identifying patients with a depressive or other psychiatric disorder. The psychiatrist may be able to suggest ways of managing some patients, but there is no established treatment for primary hypochondriasis. As hypochondriasis confers no protection against physical illness, some hypochondrical patients eventually develop a serious medical condition. For this reason, new symptoms should be investigated as carefully in these patients as in any others.

Table 2 Principal dissociative symptoms*

Motor symptoms	Sensory symptoms
Seizures	Anaesthesia
Paralysis	Paraesthesia
Aphonia and mutism	Pain
Tremor	Deafness
Tics	Blindness
Disorders of gait	
	Mental symptoms
	Amnesia
	Pseudodementia
	Fugue
	Stupor

*Motor and sensory symptoms are called conversion symptoms in the American National Classification.

Dysmophophobia

Dysmorphophobia is a persistent and inappropriate concern about the appearance of the body, for example the shape of the nose or ears. The intensity of the conviction varies, but in some people it is delusional. In these cases it is important to search for signs of schizophrenia, which is an occasional cause of this symptom. In most cases, however, no associated psychiatric disorder is present. The condition is seen mainly by plastic surgeons and dermatologists. Psychological treatment seldom lessens the concerns of patients who receive plastic surgery. It is not easy to predict the outcome of surgery, but a joint assessment by a psychiatrist and a surgeon is often helpful.

Psychogenic pain

Psychogenic pain may be experienced in any part of the body, but the head, neck, and lower back are the common sites. Psychogenic pain is most often associated with depressive disorders and anxiety disorders (in the latter pain may be associated with increased muscle tension). Pain may also be a symptom of dissociative disorder. Whenever psychogenic pain has been diagnosed, there should be careful follow-up to exclude an organic disorder.

Diagnosis depends on taking a careful history of the quality, site, and timing of the pain; these features can then be compared with the features of pain with organic causes. At the same time an enquiry should be made to elicit any symptoms of the relevant psychiatric disorders. Although descriptions of pyschogenic pain are often vague and dramatic, such descriptions should not influence the diagnosis because they depend more on the patient's personality than on the cause of the pain. If there is a psychiatric disorder, it should be treated in the usual way. Otherwise, the patient should be helped to reduce any stressors or internal conflicts, and should be encouraged to live as normal a life as possible despite the pain. The prognosis of psychogenic pain is that of the associated psychiatric disorder.

Dissociative disorder (hysteria)

Dissociative disorder is the term used in the International Classification of Diseases to refer to the syndrome previously called hysteria. In dissociative disorder, signs and symptoms resembling organic disease occur in the absence of corresponding physical pathology. These signs and symptoms are caused not by malingering but by psychological processes of which the patient is not completely aware. The symptoms may resemble those of physical disease or mental disorder. In the International Classification of Diseases both types of symptom are called dissociative disorder. In the US National Classification, however, it is the convention to restrict the term dissociative disorder to symptoms resembling mental disorder, such as sudden total memory loss, while the term conversion disorder is applied to symptoms resembling physical disorder. The term dissociative denotes failure to integrate different aspects of mental activity, for example to integrate the intention to move a limb with the processes that initiate movement. The term conversion derives from the notion of mental distress being converted into physical symptoms. In addition to unexplained physical symptoms, three features characterize dissociative disorder: it begins in stressful circumstances; there is 'secondary gain', that is, the symptoms enable the patient to avoid stressful circumstances; and there is 'belle indifference', that is, an apparent lack of distress about the physical symptoms.

It is often extremely difficult to be certain that organic disease has been excluded as a cause of symptoms that may be dissociative. For this reason, the diagnosis of dissociative (or conversion) disorder should be made with great caution, and should be regarded as provisional until appropriate follow-up has confirmed the absence of physical pathology.

Clinical features

Dissociative symptoms are of many kinds (Table 2). The most frequent symptoms resemble disease of the nervous system as they involve loss of voluntary functions. Despite the resemblance, they differ from the features of organic disease of the nervous system in important ways. Sometimes the differences are gross; for example a patient may report inability to move a limb, but examination reveals active but opposed contraction of extensor and flexor muscles. Sometimes the difference is less obvious; for example there may be a discrepancy between the distribution of the patient's sensory impairment and the distribution of sensory impairment associated with any possible neurological lesion.

These disorders can occur in people with a normal personality who are under very extreme stress. Patients with highly abnormal personality can develop these disorders under lesser degrees of objective stress, albeit the stress is subjectively intolerable for that individual.

Some dissociative symptoms require special comment. *Dissociative seizures* differ from epileptic seizures in that the patient may appear inaccessible, but does not lose consciousness; convulsive movements lack the regular, stereotyped form seen in epilepsy; and there is no incontinence, cyanosis, injury, or biting of the tongue. It is sometimes difficult to distinguish between complex partial seizures and dissociative seizures. In these cases ambulatory monitoring of the EEG during a seizure helps to decide the diagnosis, but even then, surface EEG recordings can fail to demonstrate unequivocal seizure activity in deep structures within the brain.

Difficulty in swallowing without an identified organic cause is occasionally due to a dissociative disorder ('globus hystericus'), but it is more often due to an undetected organic lesion. For this reason, physical investigation should be particularly thorough before the diagnosis of dissociative disorder is made, and follow-up should be especially careful. Difficulty in swallowing can also occur in somatized anxiety or panic where the patient experiences a dry mouth and a choking feeling along with other autonomic symptoms of arousal and fearful thoughts.

Amnesia is the most frequent dissociative mental symptom. It differs from amnesia caused by organic disease in affecting the recall of distant memories as much as the recall of recent ones. In dissociative memory disorder, there may be denial of awareness of personal identity (in memory disorder due to organic causes, personal amnesia occurs only as part of a severe general intellectual deterioration). Diagnosis can be difficult because dissociative memory disorder may occasionally be provoked (for unknown reasons) by organic brain disease at a stage when there are no localizing neurological signs. Dissociative memory disorder may also follow a head injury, and may occur in epilepsy and multiple sclerosis.

The term *dissociative pseudodementia* is applied to a syndrome in which patients respond to tests of general intellectual functions with answers that are wrong but systematically related to the question (e.g. $7+3 = 11$; $8+5 = 14$). The syndrome is rare, but has been described in patients with parietal lobe lesions; hence the diagnosis of dissociative pseudodementia should be made cautiously. Systematic wrong answering can also be due to malingering.

The term *compensation neurosis* refers to psychologically determined physical or mental symptoms occurring when there is an unsettled claim for compensation. Although the condition has been grouped with hysteria in the past, few cases are due to dissociative disorder. Most are prolongations of physical disability induced by psychological and social factors. These factors include but are not restricted to the unsettled claim.

The term *epidemic hysteria* refers to the spread of dissociative symptoms among a group of people, usually members of a closed social group such as a school or hostel, often at a time of stress for the group. Usually the epidemic begins when a member of the group has a definite or suspected physical illness which alarms the others. A few vulnerable people then develop dissociative symptoms resembling those of the primary case. Other members of the group become anxious, and progressively more people become affected.

Differential diagnosis

Many of the important points have been mentioned above. The difficulties in distinguishing dissociative disorder from undiagnosed organic disease are so great that the diagnosis of dissociative disorder should generally be regarded as provisional until adequate follow-up has been carried out. When in doubt it is helpful to consider four points. First, dissociative disorder occurs in response to stress; if no stressors can be identified the diagnosis of dissociative disorder is less likely. The finding of stressful circumstances, however, does not add to the evidence for dissociative disorder because such circumstances are often associated with organic disease by chance. Second, secondary gain is invariable in hysteria and its absence is against the diagnosis. The presence of secondary gain, however, does not add to the evidence for dissociative disorder because the limitations imposed by physical illness sometimes result in patients avoiding stressful situations. Third, 'belle indifference' (apparent lack of distress) is a non-specific symptom not restricted to dissociative disorder. Fourth, dissociative disorder seldom occurs for the first time in patients over the age of 40 years. By paying attention to these four points many errors of diagnosis can be avoided.

Dissociative disorder has to be distinguished particularly from malingering and factitious disorder which are considered below.

Prognosis

Most dissociative disorders of recent onset recover quickly, and these usually occur in people with a normal personality under very severe acute stress. When symptoms have lasted for a year they usually persist for several more. As explained already, physical disease is often missed in patients who are thought to have dissociative symptoms. In one series from a specialist neurological hospital, one-third of patients diagnosed as having 'hysteria' developed an organic disease during 7 to 11 years of follow-up.

Treatment

Treatment is along simple practical lines. First, information should be given to the patient about the steps that have been taken to exclude physical pathology. Second, an unhurried explanation should be given of the nature and origins of the condition. It is not enough to leave the patient with a list of conditions that have been ruled out; the patient should understand that the symptoms have arisen in response to stress, by a dissociation of psychological functions. This process can be explained as a difficulty in exerting voluntary control over movement, or in integrating sensory input. This explanation requires time and can seldom be given effectively in the course of a busy ward round.

After this explanation, the focus of concern should be directed away from the symptoms to the stressful problems that provoked them. In helping the patient to resolve these problems, the form of counselling known as problem-solving may be used. The patient should be assured that the physical symptoms will improve. It is often useful to arrange physiotherapy to encourage mobility or restore sensory awareness. Further psychological treatment should focus on ways of dealing with stressful problems more effectively in the future. As explained above, it is important to confirm the diagnosis by follow-up; for this purpose observations should be as unobtrusive as possible to ensure that the patient is not made more anxious by them.

More complex psychological treatment is seldom more effective than these simple measures. In dynamic psychotherapy patients with dissociative disorder readily produce memories of traumatic experiences in earlier life, but few show lasting benefit from such treatment.

Malingering and factitious disorders

Malingering is the deliberate and fraudulent production of physical or psychological symptoms with the motive of financial gain or other reward. Malingering is seen most often in prisoners or members of the armed forces who wish to avoid some duty, or in people who are attempting to obtain financial compensation for supposed injury or illness. Malingering should be diagnosed only after full investigation.

The term *factitious disorder* refers to the deliberate production of physical or psychological symptoms when there is no obvious material gain of the kind seen in malingering. Instead the gain is psychological, and often related to complex abnormalities of personality. Both malingering and factitious disorder need to be distinguished from dissociative disorder. The distinctions between the three disorders depend on judgements by the physician as to whether there is clear benefit to the patient, and whether or not the patient has deliberately produced the symptoms. Often these judgements can be made without difficulty, but sometimes they are very difficult. Some factitious disorders consist of a single symptom, for example recurring skin lesions (dermatitis artefacta), bruising, or self-induced fever. Some patients deliberately aggravate a true physical illness, for example by preventing the healing of varicose ulcers. These conditions are usually episodes in a long history of emotional difficulties arising from a disorder of personality.

The most extreme form of factitious disorder is *Munchausen's syndrome*, a rare disorder in which patients present repeatedly with dramatic symptoms that suggest the need for urgent medical or surgical treatment. Munchausen's syndrome was described first by Asher in 1951, and was named after Baron Munchausen whose extravagant fabrications and restless wanderings had been described by Rudolph Raspe in 1787.

Munchausen's syndrome is more common in men than women, and usually begins before middle age. The patient feigns an acute and urgent illness and gives a plausible and often dramatic history, which is subsequently found to be false. A false identity is also usually used and the patient finds excuses to prevent staff from speaking to another informant. There may be spurious physical signs, for example self-induced bleeding from the urinary or gastrointestinal tract, or haematemesis caused by ingested blood. When a full history has been compiled, it is usually found that the patient has been admitted many times to different hospitals, often far apart, and that the patient has usually discharged himself before investigations could be completed, or once confronted. Some patients have the scars of multiple operations, including laparotomies and sometimes craniotomies. These patients often have detailed medical knowledge and give histories which, although false, are extremely convincing.

The personality is often characterized by failure to make close relationships, aggressive behaviour, restlessness, and extreme forms of lying. These features strongly suggest a profound disorder of personality. The nature and origins of this disorder can seldom be determined because patients avoid giving accurate information about their past. Although some patients attempt to get powerful analgesics, most are not addicted to drugs. Those who obtain opiates by simulated illness could usually have done so in other ways. When an accurate history can be obtained, it often reveals a severely disrupted childhood with parental abuse or neglect and sometimes prolonged hospital treatment.

The management of these patients is difficult. Psychiatric treatment is rarely effective, and the patients seldom remain in hospital long enough to receive it. After physical disease has been excluded, the immediate treatment is to tell the patient of the findings, though not in a confrontational way which would only increase hostility and lack of co-operation. Help should be offered for any social problems that can be identified, but most patients refuse it. If the patient agrees, a psychiatric opinion can be obtained; this may throw more light on the complex motivation for the behaviour, but is unlikely to result in effective treatment that the patient will accept. Such people may be dangerous to others if employed as a health care professional.

Personality and its disorders

The term personality refers to the enduring characteristics manifest as ways of behaving in a wide variety of circumstances. When the personality is so abnormal as to cause suffering to the person or to other people, the person is said to have a personality disorder.

Clinical features

There are many different kinds of personality disorder and only those of special interest to the physician will be described here (a comprehensive account is given in the *New Oxford textbook of psychiatry*).

Obsessional personality

People with obsessional personality have rigid views, adapt poorly to change, and expect high standards of performance from themselves and others. They readily feel guilt, are often moralistic, and do not enjoy themselves easily. Some obsessional people are indecisive, seek more and more advice, and worry about a decision once made. Although outwardly courteous and eager to please, obsessional people often harbour unexpressed feelings of irritation or anger. They do not respond well to the changes imposed by illness, and they may find it difficult to make choices about treatment.

Histrionic (hysterical) personality

This personality is characterized by self-dramatization and a shallow, self-centred approach to relationships. When ill, histrionic people may appear demanding, selfish, and inconsiderate. They may describe symptoms in a demonstrative way and may show extremes of emotion.

Paranoid personality

People with this kind of personality are markedly sensitive, touchy, and suspicious. They distrust other people, and are secretive, argumentative, and ungrateful. Such people take offence easily and yet behave in ways that invite rebuffs. People of this kind make difficult patients. They seem constantly ungrateful for efforts to help them, and they may complain about their treatment unreasonably and for a long time.

Schizoid personality

People with schizoid personalities are emotionally cold, introspective, and unduly self-sufficient. They appear aloof and ill at ease in company, and do not make friends easily. When ill, schizoid people underplay their suffering and confide little in their doctors. Their lack of warmth and their social awkwardness make it difficult for doctors to discover their real concerns.

Antisocial personality disorder

This disorder is also called psychopathic personality. There are four important features of this kind of personality: impulsive actions, lack of guilt, failure to make loving relationships, and failure to learn from experience. Antisocial people are heartless and aggressive, and may be cruel and violent. They are often inadequate parents, and may neglect or abuse their children,usually having received the same treatment themselves. These qualities may be obvious, or masked by superficial and deceptive charm. Antisocial people lack consistent goals, and seek immediate gratification rather than long-term achievement. They often break the law. Their behaviour is often made worse by overindulgence in alcohol or drugs. When ill, antisocial people are difficult and demanding patients. They often expect immediate help, but generally avoid taking responsibility for themselves, and fail to comply with long-term plans for treatment. When frustrated they may become angry and at times dangerous.

Differential diagnosis

Personality disorder is diagnosed when there is a continuous history of abnormal behaviour from the teenage years. In contrast, mental disorders start after a period of normal psychological functioning. Two circumstances may give rise to difficulty in diagnosis. First, in adolescence abnormal behaviour may occasionally be due to a mental disorder. Second, in response to stressful circumstances people with abnormal personalities may exhibit behaviour suggestive of mental disorder. This problem arises mainly when people with paranoid or antisocial personalities respond with behaviour resembling that of schizophrenia. In doubtful cases a psychiatric opinion should be sought.

Treatment

Even with intensive psychological treatment only small changes occur in most personality disorders. It is usually realistic to help the patient to find a way of living that leads to fewer problems. This adaptation may take several years. The requirement is for a commonsense approach provided by whichever doctor the patient trusts most. A psychiatric assessment may help to determine whether the patient is one of the few patients who could benefit from psychotherapy.

Further reading

Adshead, G. (1995). Treatment of victims of trauma. *Advances in Psychiatric Treatment*, 1(6):161–9.

Bass, C.M. (1990). *Somatization: physical symptoms and psychological illness* (ed. C. Bass), Blackwells, Oxford.

Gelder, M.G., Lopez-Iber, J.J., and Andreasen, N. (eds.) (2000). *New Oxford textbook of psychiatry.* Oxford University Press, Oxford.

Goldberg, D., Benjamin, S., and Creed, F. (1994). *Psychiatry in medical practice.* (2nd edn). Routledge, London.

Kennerley, H. (1990). *Managing anxiety: a training manual.* Oxford University Press, Oxford.

Nutt, D. and Lawson, C. (1992). Panic attacks: A neurochemical overview of models and mechanisms. *British Journal of Psychiatry*, 160, 165–78.

Sussman, N. and Hyler, S.E. (1985). Factitious disorders. In *Comprehensive textbook of psychiatry*, (5th edn). (ed. H.I. Kaplan and B.J. Saddock). Williams and Wilkins, Baltimore.

Toone, B.K. (1990). Disorders of hysterical conversion. In *Somatization: physical symptoms and psychological illness*, (ed. C. Bass). pp. 207–34. Blackwells, Oxford.

Chapter 14.2

Mood disorders

D. H. Gath

Mood disorders are those in which a change of mood is the central feature. The change may be of depression, elation, or rarely a combination of the two.

Depressive disorders

Physically ill patients are often unhappy and sorrow may be a normal reaction to the illness. Sometimes, however, it is a symptom of a depressive disorder which can complicate the management of physical illness, cause suffering and, in severe cases, threaten life. Physicians also encounter patients with depressive disorders who are somatizing. For these reasons, it is important that physicians should be able to detect and treat depressive disorders.

Depressive illness is common in the general population: the 1-month prevalence for major depression is about 1–2 per cent for men and about 3 per cent for women, with an overall lifetime prevalence of about 5 per cent. Among physically ill patients the rates are higher, and much of the depression seen will be mild to moderate, rather than severe.

Clinical features

The central features of a depressive disorder are low mood and impaired capacity for enjoyment shown in social withdrawal and loss of interest in work and hobbies (Table 1). These features are accompanied by two other groups of symptoms. The first group, known as biological symptoms, are reduced energy, sleep disturbance with early morning waking, a worsening of symptoms in the first part of the day ('diurnal variation'), loss of appetite and weight, constipation, low libido, and amenorrhoea. Some patients seek medical help for one or more of these physical symptoms rather than the low mood itself. The second group, known as cognitive symptoms, are hopelessness and pessimistic thoughts about the future, ruminations about death as a release from suffering and suicidal ideas, and guilty preoccupations. Other symptoms, which are common but less specific include irritability, anxiety, and poor concentration with consequent poor recall. True memory disorder does not occur in depressive disorder. Hypochondriachal preoccupations are common.

The patient's facial appearance is of sadness, and the posture may be bowed. Movements and speech are slow and the tone of the voice is monotonous. Occasionally these outward signs of depression are lacking and in these cases it is easy to miss the depressive disorder unless systematic enquiries are made about all the symptoms that make up the syndrome. Other atypical features include restlessness instead of retardation, overeating instead of weight loss, and excessive somnolence instead of insomnia. Delusions and hallucinations may be present in a severe depressive disorder and, when this happens, the condition is called a psychotic depression. Depressive delusions are concerned with guilt, worthlessness, serious illness, and poverty. Sometimes the delusions are persecutory and in this case patients generally regard the supposed persecution as something they have brought upon themselves; an attitude that contrasts with that of schizophrenic patients who are resentful or angry. Hallucinations are

Table 1 Principal features of depressive disorders

Depressed mood to a degree that is definitely abnormal for the subject, present for most of the day and almost every day
Fearful or depressed appearance
Mood is non-reactive to environmental events: cannot be cheered up
Diurnal mood variation, worse in the morning
Marked loss of interest or pleasure in activities that are normally pleasurable
Loss of confidence and self-esteem
Social withdrawal or decreased talkativeness
Unreasonable feelings of self-reproach, with excessive and inappropriate guilt
Brooding self-pity or pessimism
Recurrent thoughts of death or suicide, or any suicidal behaviour
Somatic symptoms (can be confounded by presence of physical illness)
Decreased energy or increased fatigability
Complaints or evidence of diminished ability to think or concentrate
Sleep disturbance of any type but particularly early morning wakening
Change in psychomotor activity, with agitation or retardation
Change in appetite (decrease or increase) with corresponding weight change

usually of words or phrases that confirm the ideas of guilt and worthlessness (for example a voice saying that the patient is wicked). When delusions and hallucinations are present, suicide risk should be assessed most carefully because it is usually increased, and psychiatric advice should be obtained promptly.

Variations of the clinical picture

Anxiety symptoms

In depressive disorders of mild to moderate intensity anxiety symptoms are often present in the form of generalized anxiety by day, early onset insomnia, and phobias. Panic attacks may also occur.

Somatic symptoms

Somatic presentations of depression are particularly common in general hospital patients. Patients complain of tiredness, malaise, poor appetite, constipation, or aches and pains, rather than depressed mood. There are often coexisting physical symptoms of anxiety (autonomic arousal and hyperventilation).

Worsening of physical complaints

Depressed patients will worry more and are less able to tolerate discomfort that they endured previously and may seek fresh help for long-standing problems of back pain, osteoarthritis, or bronchitis. If the physical condition is unchanged, the possibility of depression should be considered.

Failure to comply with medical treatment

Depressed patients who lack energy and feel hopeless may neglect the treatment of concurrent physical illness such as diabetes or hypertension. Failure to comply with treatment in a patient who has previously complied well, suggests the possibility of a depressive disorder.

Brief depressive episode

Usually a depressive disorder persists for several months but a few patients have repeated episodes of severe depression lasting for a few days with normal mood between. These brief depressive episodes are difficult to control. Specialist advice should be obtained.

Excessive use of alcohol

Some depressed patients try to improve their mood by taking alcohol. Although there may be a brief lessening of distress, the longer-term effect of alcohol is to deepen the depression and patients will often improve with abstinence.

Differential diagnosis

For the physician there are four main issues: (1) to distinguish depressive disorder from normal feelings of sadness; (2) to detect depressive disorder in patients with unexplained physical symptoms; (3) to distinguish depressive disorder from other psychiatric disorders; and (4) to identify depressive disorder as a cause of excessive use of alcohol.

From normal sadness

This distinction is made by enquiring about other symptoms of a depressive disorder (see Table 1). Biological symptoms are particularly significant if not accounted for by the physical condition, and, although uncommon, psychotic symptoms are even more important. When there is uncertainty, another person who knows the patient may describe features that the patient has not revealed.

As a cause of unexplained physical symptoms

The first step is to identify the symptoms of the syndrome of depressive disorder. The second step is to establish whether the physical symptoms preceded or followed the depressive symptoms. If the physical symptoms came first it is likely that depressive disorder is secondary to a physical illness rather than the primary problem. Physical problems of anxiety often coexist.

From other psychiatric disorders

When anxiety symptoms are prominent the other symptoms of a depressive disorder may be overlooked. It is important, therefore, to enquire about depressive symptoms when patients complain of anxiety. Some depressed patients complain of poor memory and usually this is secondary to poor concentration, but the possibility of dementia should be considered. If mood changes and psychotic symptoms of acute onset are present in a medical inpatient, delirium is the most likely diagnosis. Despite careful observations it is often difficult to be certain of the correct diagnosis and, if in doubt, specialist advice may be needed.

As a cause of alcohol abuse

Some patients with depressive disorder take excessive alcohol to obtain temporary relief of their symptoms. Diagnosis can be difficult because excessive use of alcohol leads to depressed mood, and disturbs sleep. The correct diagnosis may be reached by finding out whether depressed mood preceded or followed the excessive use of alcohol, and systematic examination for other symptoms of a depressive disorder (see Table 1). Often, diagnosis is not certain until the patient has been persuaded to abstain from alcohol for several days.

Prognosis

Most untreated depressive disorders last for 3 to 9 months, although a few persist for several years. Younger patients usually recover completely but in old age residual symptoms are more frequent. Recurrence is common, the risk increasing with the number of previous episodes. A careful history of previous episodes of depression, not all of which may have been treated, is an essential guide to prognosis. Patients with depressive disorder have an increased risk of suicide: 10–15 per cent of patients with severe and recurrent depressive disorder eventually die by suicide.

Treatment

Most depressive disorders can be managed successfully by physicians and general practitioners but it is important to identify those who require psychiatric treatment. The principal indications for referral to a specialist are: (1) severe depressive disorder especially with hallucinations or delusions, and severe biological symptoms including failure to eat and drink adequately; (2) high suicide risk, or difficulty in assessing suicide risk; (3) failure to respond to first line treatment; and (4) relapsing or recurring disorder.

All patients require simple psychological management starting with an explanation that the condition is an illness, not a sign of personal failure. Easily understood information should be given about the nature of the illness and the good prospect of recovery. Patients should be helped to deal with current problems but exploration of past problems is not appropriate during the acute state of the illness. The more severe the depressive disorder, the more the patient should be relieved temporarily of responsibilities and encouraged to live from day to day rather than worry about future difficulties.

If the depressive disorder is mild, these simple measures may be all that is required until spontaneous recovery takes place. However, in most cases of depressive disorder an antidepressant drug should be prescribed. There are many such drugs, which differ in their side-effects but not their therapeutic effects. A commonly used drug is the tricyclic antidepressant amitriptyline, which is well tried and inexpensive. Basic drug management is described in Chapter 14.6.

Mania and manic depressive disorder

Mania is characterized by elevated mood, increased activity, and self-important ideas. When these features are severe, the condition is called mania, when mild to moderate it is called hypomania. People who experience mania at one time in their lives usually have a depressive disorder at another time. This sequence is called manic depressive disorder or bipolar affective disorder (bipolar referring to the opposite 'poles' of mania and depression). Surprisingly, a few patients show features of both mania and depression at the same time (e.g. increased activity with depressive ideas); such patients are said to have a mixed affective disorder.

Mania is much less common than depression. The estimated 1-month prevalence rate for bipolar disorder is 0.4 per cent with rates for men and women about equal.

Differential diagnosis

When a physically ill patient becomes acutely psychotic with a gross disturbance of mood, an important differential diagnosis is between functional psychosis and delirium, the latter being much more likely. The correct diagnosis can usually be made by examining for the cognitive impairments characteristic of delirium.

Prognosis

Without treatment, moderate and severe mania lasts usually for a few months, although mild cases may recover more quickly. Although patients recover eventually recurrence is frequent, in the form either of a manic or a depressive episode.

Treatment

Treatment of mania is with drugs and psychological management. It is important to avoid responding to uninhibited behaviour or irritable mood as if it were directed deliberately at the doctor, rather than a symptom of illness because such a response is likely to increase the abnormal behaviour. An antipsychotic drug such as haloperidol will usually control symptoms within a few days. The advice of a psychiatrist should be obtained at an early stage because further treatment of the mania may be difficult and mania may be followed by severe depression. Further information is given in Chapters 14.6 and 14.7.

Further reading

Gelder, M.G., Lopez-Iber, J.J., and Andreason, N. (eds). (2000). *New Oxford textbook of psychiatry.* Oxford University Press, Oxford.

Edicott, J. (1994). Measurement of depression in out-patients with cancer. *Cancer,* 53, 2243–8.

Chapter 14.3

Schizophrenia

M. G. Gelder and E. J. Feldman

Schizophrenia is the most severe form of functional mental disorder affecting mainly thinking and perception. Most patients have recurrent episodes or chronic illness. The care of schizophrenic patients is a major part of the work of psychiatrists. Schizophrenia presents to physicians less often. It may do so in several ways, for example: (1) a patient with chronic schizophrenia may present with a physical disorder; (2) occasionally a schizophrenic patient has the delusion that they are physically ill; (3) very rarely the disorder may be provoked by a physical illness. Because the involvement of physicians with schizophrenia is small, the present account is brief. (For more comprehensive accounts see *New Oxford textbook of psychiatry.)*

Clinical features

The clinical picture of schizophrenia is varied, but two well-recognized syndromes can be described: (1) an acute syndrome with delusions, hallucinations, and disordered thinking ('positive'symptoms'); and (2) a chronic syndrome with apathy, slowness, and social withdrawal ('negative'symptoms).

Acute syndrome

Delusions in schizophrenia are commonly persecutory ('paranoid') or grandiose. These kinds of delusion, although frequent in schizophrenia, are found in other psychiatric disorders and are not valuable in diagnosis. Certain other delusions are less common, but seldom seen in other psychiatric disorders and therefore more valuable in diagnosis. These diagnostic delusions (often called 'first rank' symptoms) are as follows: the delusion that the patient's thoughts are being transmitted to other people ('thought broadcasting'), the delusion that thoughts are being taken out of the patient's head ('thought withdrawal'), the delusion that some of the patient's thoughts have been implanted by an outside agency ('thought insertion'), and the delusion that the patient's actions are being controlled by an outside agency. Another first rank symptom, delusional perception, is the attribution of a very odd significance to a normal percept; for example, a schizophrenic patient may believe that the positioning of a chair indicates that they are about to be harmed by persecutors.

Hallucinations are of several kinds. Auditory hallucinations are among the most frequent symptoms of schizophrenia. They may be experienced as noises, or voices uttering words, phrases or conversation. The voices may seem to speak to the patient. Two or more voices may seem to discuss the patient; this kind of hallucination is known as a 'third person' hallucination because the voices refer to the patient as 'he' or 'she'. Third person hallucinations differ from other auditory hallucinations in that they seldom occur in disorders other than schizophrenia. They therefore have the most diagnostic value. Other kinds of hallucination particularly characteristic of schizophrenia (although found infrequently) are hearing one's own thoughts spoken aloud as if by another person, and hallucinations of bodily sensations. Visual hallucinations and those of taste, smell, and bodily sensations also occur in schizophrenia, but they are less common than auditory hallucinations.

Disorders of thinking in schizophrenia cannot be detected reliably and are therefore not a good guide to diagnosis. The main feature is lack of logical connection between ideas. The disorder of thought is reflected in the patient's speech, which is vague and difficult to follow, and which becomes more obscure as the interviewer seeks to clarify the reasoning. *Abnormal emotional responses* may be of several kinds: lack of emotional response ('flattened affect'), depressed or elevated mood, or inappropriate emotional responses ('incongruity of affect'). *Behavioural disorders* in acute schizophrenia include social withdrawal, oddity of manner, or noisy or disruptive acts. Memory and consciousness are not impaired, and therefore disorder of these functions (other than apparent memory problems due entirely to poor concentration) should prompt a search for an organic cause of the patient's symptoms.

Occasionally the first evidence of schizophrenia is a concern about physical health. A few schizophrenic patients experience somatic hallucinations of uncomfortable feelings in the chest, abdomen, or genital regions, and they may seek the advice of physicians about these sensations. Often the true nature of the problem is revealed by eliciting the patient's ideas about the cause of the symptoms. This question may reveal that hallucinatory sensations are being interpreted in a delusional way. For example, sensations in the vagina may be ascribed to the actions of unknown people who are having intercourse with the patient during sleep; or hallucinatory sensations in the abdomen may be ascribed to malefactors. If available, a relative or other informant should be interviewed and asked about the patient's abnormal behaviour or ideas. For cases of this kind the opinion of a psychiatrist will be required.

Chronic schizophrenia

The main features are apathy, slowness, and social withdrawal. Delusions, hallucinations, and disordered thinking also occur; they are similar to those of acute schizophrenia, but generally less prominent. Depressive symptoms are frequent in chronic schizophrenia.

As in acute schizophrenia, memory and consciousness are not impaired in the chronic syndrome (except difficulty in remembering age and past dates); if impairment is found, an organic cause should be considered, which may be either primary or superimposed on pre-existing schizophrenia.

Differential diagnosis

For the physician the issue of diagnosing schizophrenia is likely to arise when a physically ill patient develops abnormal behaviour; it is then particularly important to distinguish schizophrenia from an acute organic psychiatric disorder such as an agitated delirium with prominent delusions and hallucinations, drug induced states, complex partial seizures, or encephalitis, and (rarely) cerebral syphilis (see Chapter 16.69). Of the drug-induced states, the condition caused by excessive use of amphetamine most closely resembles schizophrenia, but the effects of taking LSD or very large amounts of cannabis can present diagnostic problems. Alcoholic hallucinosis (see Chapters 14.9–14.18) may also resemble schizophrenia. When long-standing and frequent complex partial seizures arise in the temporal lobe, some patients develop a mental disorder with persecutory delusions, which is very difficult to distinguish from schizophrenia. In psychiatric practice, the commonest differential diagnoses are mania, psychotic depression, and some forms of personality disorder. A physician should seek the advice of a psychiatrist in making any of these diagnostic distinctions.

Treatment

The physician is likely to be concerned with two specific aspects of treatment: the control of symptoms in an emergency and the continuation of drug treatment for chronic schizophrenic patients admitted to hospital for treatment of a medical illness. The treatment of acute symptoms is described in Chapter 14.7, and only maintenance drug treatment will be considered here.

Clinical trials have shown that symptoms can be kept under control and relapse can be prevented if patients with chronic schizophrenia receive long-term treatment with an antipsychotic drug. Many schizophrenic patients fail to take oral medication regularly; therefore the drugs are often given by intramuscular injection of a long-acting preparation, every 2 to 4 weeks, in a schedule and dosage established for each patient. A physician should continue this treatment while the patient is in hospital. If there is reason to do otherwise the advice of a psychiatrist should be obtained.

Frequently, schizophrenic symptoms cannot be controlled without provoking extrapyramidal side effects. Antiparkinsonian drugs will usually reduce these side-effects but anticholinergic drugs should not be given to every patient because they may increase the risk of tardive dyskinesia (a late and sometimes irreversible effect of prolonged treatment with antipsychotic drugs). Some new antipsychotic drugs are relatively free from extrapyramidal side effects.

If physical illness is associated with an increase of schizophrenic symptoms it is usually better to give additional oral rather than intramuscular medication. Suitable drugs include chlorpromazine if a sedating effect is required, and trifluoperazine if not (see Chapter 14.6 for further information about antipsychotic drugs).

Further reading

Gelder, M.G., Lopez-Iber, J.J., and Andreasen, N. (eds.) (2000). *New Oxford textbook of psychiatry.* Oxford University Press, Oxford.

Chapter 14.4

Organic (cognitive) mental disorders

R. A. Mayou

Table 1 lists the main general and specific organic, or cognitive, syndromes. This chapter reviews all of these with the important exception of dementia, which is discussed elsewhere. Whilst dementia is especially common in the elderly, it is an important differential for younger patients.

Delirium

Delirium may occur at any age but is especially common in the elderly. Because it occurs in association with severe illness, it is extremely common amongst general hospital inpatients, especially those aged over 60 and those recovering from acute illness or major surgery.

The cardinal characteristic disturbance is reduced consciousness and this is accompanied by widespread cognitive symptoms and behavioural changes including disturbances of attention, perception, thinking, memory, and behaviour, as well as effects on emotion and sleep. Delirium is often transient and is characteristically fluctuating. The symptoms are likely to be particularly severe at night, when sensory input is reduced and orientation more difficult to maintain. Agitated and overactive delirious patients are more conspicuous but less common than those who are quietly confused and whose management usually causes little difficulty (Table 2).

Delirium does not have a specific medical cause, but indicates generally disturbed cerebral function. In an elderly person it could be triggered by a minor illness such as a urinary tract infection but in a young person, it is usually an indication of a very serious physical illness. Alcohol withdrawal is a frequent cause of delirium developing during a hospital admission.

Differential diagnosis

Delirium needs to be distinguished from dementia and from acute psychotic illnesses. It may be difficult to distinguish complaints of subjective confusion occurring in psychotic illnesses from the clouding of consciousness of delirium and a specialist opinion may be necessary.

Table 1 Classification of organic mental states

Global syndromes
Delirium
Dementia
Specific syndromes
Amnesic syndrome
Organic mood disorder
Organic delusional state
Organic personality disorder

Table 2 Clinical features symtoms of delirium

Impaired consciousness	*Mood*
disorientation	anxious, irritable
poor concentration	depressed
Behaviour	perplexed
overactive	
under	*Perception*
	misinterpretations
Thinking	illusions
muddled (confused)	hallucinations (mainly visual)
ideas of reference	
delusions	*Memory*
	impaired
	Fluctuating course, worse in the evening

Management

Diagnosis is based upon the clinical features and on the history. Patients are often unable to give any coherent account and it is essential to obtain information from relatives and, if in hospital, the ward staff. The diagnosis does not depend upon identifying a specific physical cause, but treatment does and appropriate physical investigations should proceed in parallel. Occasionally no physical cause is ever found but this should not cause doubt about the diagnosis if there are clear clinical features. Assessment of predisposing factors in the patient's situation is essential.

If delirium is not associated with significant distress or with management problems, there is little need to consider specific treatment. However, it is always necessary to make special efforts to explain to the patient what is going on, to repeat information as frequently as is necessary, and also to explain the nature of the disorder to relatives.

Delirium is an acute reversible condition, dementia is a chronic disorder. The two syndromes may occur together, especially in the elderly. When this happens the underlying dementia may be overlooked or, alternatively, the reversible acute stage may not be detected or treated. Sometimes the long-standing dementia becomes apparent only after successful treatment of the more recent delirium. Delirium can usually be diagnosed correctly by an acute onset, fluctuating course, impaired consciousness, and disorganized thinking. Perceptual disturbance is more frequent and alertness more often impaired in delirium.

In more severe delirium, the emphasis should be on general measures rather than psychotropic drug treatment, although this is indicated if the patient is acutely distressed or is behaving in a manner that is causing difficulties for carers. The minimum effective amount of medication should be used and doses should be reviewed regularly over a period of days, so as to avoid erratic drug regimes in which the patient varies from being oversedated to being distressed and disturbed.

Management of an acutely disturbed patient is described in Chapter 14.7. Further drug treatment is usually with a regular regime of oral (tablet or syrup) haloperidol, an effective antipsychotic drug that does not have the cardiovascular side-effects of phenothiazines. However, the latter are a useful more sedating alternative for agitated patients when haloperidol is ineffective. Once the acute episode has been treated, it is necessary to institute a regular regimen of oral medication which is reviewed daily and is progressively reduced. An antiparkinsonian agent , such as procyclidine, is advisable to prevent the side-effects of rigidity and dystonia. Treatment regimes for patients with alcohol withdrawal and other substance abuse syndromes are described in Chapters 14.9–14.18.

Specific organic syndromes

A number of specific syndromes do not cause global psychological severe impairment, which may or may not be associated with evidence of neurological deficit.

Amnesic disorder

This uncommon disorder (also known as amnestic or Korsakov's syndrome) is characterized by impairment of short-term memory without altered consciousness, general intellectual deterioration, or perceptual abnormality. It is commonly accompanied by confabulation. The clinical picture is characteristic in that the patient appears articulate and aware but gradually reveals an inability to remember information for more than a few seconds. The most frequent cause of organic memory disorder is thiamine deficiency, most often due to chronic alcoholism but occasionally to prolonged vomiting or starvation. The neuropathological basis is usually a lesion in the posterior hypothalamus or nearby midline structures, the common factor to all pathologies being damage to the limbic system.

Organic personality disorder

Localized cerebral damage may lead to changes in personality without evidence of cognitive damage. Occasionally personality change is the first sign of a cerebral lesion and uncharacteristic behaviour should suggest the possibility of an organic mental state.

Organic mood disorder

Depression may be a direct result of a number of physical disorders, such as some primary brain diseases (for example, multiple sclerosis and Parkinson's disease) and endocrine disorders. However, it is often very difficult to distinguish organic mood disorder from depression arising as either a psychological reaction to physical illness or coincidentally. Treatment of the underlying physical cause can be expected to relieve the depression. Antidepressants are often effective, whatever the aetiology.

Organic anxiety disorder

Several conditions can cause organic anxiety disorder, including hyperthyroidism, hypoglycaemia, and phaeochromocytoma. The treatment is that of the underlying cause.

Delusional disorder

A schizophrenia-like delusional disorder is a rare complication of complex partial seizures (temporal lobe epilepsy) and other brain diseases. Management is often difficult but follows the general principles for psychotic disorder.

Aspects of differential diagnosis

Organic or functional?

It may be difficult to distinguish between functional and organic psychiatric disorder, especially when an organic disorder presents in the emergency department with disturbances of behaviour and thinking in the absence of obvious neurological symptoms or signs. It is sensible to consider a possible organic cause in every case of psychological or behavioural disturbance, and especially when there are atypical features. Psychiatric causes are not identified solely by exclusion of organic causes but on positive evidence of psychological aetiology since organic causes may be undetectable in the early stages of illness.

The points in favour of an organic cause of disturbed behaviour are: cognitive disorder preceding mood or other disorder, specific cognitive defects, neurological signs, and symptoms not typical of functional disorder.

In affective disorder and schizophrenia there may be an impression of impairment of cognitive functions. A common diagnostic problem is presented by so-called depressive pseudodementia. In this syndrome, a depressed patient complains of poor memory and performs poorly on cognitive tests, thus giving the appearance of dementia. The patient's difficulty in remembering occurs because poor concentration leads to inadequate registration. A history from another informant may show that the depressed mood preceded the cognitive problems. Careful memory testing may show that the poor performance on tests is due to lack of interest and motivation rather than impaired intellectual functions. These patients are retarded and usually unwilling to co-operate in the interview; in contrast, patients with dementia are usually willing to reply to questions but make mistakes.

Further reading

Gelder, M.G., Lopez-Iber, J.J., and Andreasen, N. (eds.) (2000). *New Oxford textbook of psychiatry*. Oxford University Press, Oxford.

Chapter 14.5

Non-pharmacological management of mental disorders

M. G. Gelder

Psychological treatment varies in complexity from simple support and explanation, which is part of good medical care, to specialist psychotherapy. The present account is restricted to an outline of the kinds of psychological treatment most likely to be of value for patients encountered by physicians. These treatments comprise supportive therapy, problem solving counselling and crisis intervention, and certain cognitive and behaviour therapies. Brief mention will be made also of dynamic psychotherapies. The simplest of these psychological measures can be carried out by the physician, some of the others can be given by another member of the medical team—often a social worker or nurse specialist—while the rest require referral to a psychiatrist, a clinical psychologist, or a psychiatric nurse-specialist. A fuller account will be found in the *New Oxford textbook of psychiatry*.

The value of listening and giving information

There is often considerable value in allowing patients to express their worries and to find out about the illness and its effects. Many mildly anxious or depressed patients need no more help than a simple interview of this kind. Surveys of patients have shown that most wish to receive a fuller explanation of the nature of the illness, the results of tests, the purpose of medication, the length of time they may be off work, and whether any lasting disability is to be expected. Although physicians try to provide this information, they do not always allow enough time to find out what patients want to know and whether they have understood what they have been told.

Information should be in simple language, avoiding technical terms, but complete; doctors often underestimate patients' capacity for understanding medical matters. Extra care is needed when giving information to a person from another culture who may hold different views about illness or treatment. Because anxious people remember little of what they have been told, important points should be repeated or put in writing to be read later.

Reassurance should be offered only after finding out the patient's concerns in some detail and it should be realistic and truthful. It is important, of course, to find out what others may have told the patient so that the advice does not appear contradictory or, if it is different, that the reasons for the alternative view are explained. Relatives as well as patients, may need advice and reassurance and it is not uncommon to find that a patient's excessive anxiety does not subside until the relatives have been reassured.

Supportive counselling

Some patients require more than one interview to talk over their concerns about the illness and its effects. This supportive counselling can be carried out by the physician or may be delegated to a nurse counsellor who has experience of the problems associated with physical illness: this arrangement is sometimes adopted for example for patients after myocardial infarction, or for patients requiring a colostomy.

Problem solving counselling and crisis intervention

Problem solving counselling is a more structured treatment designed to help patients to find solutions to problems that are causing distress. The aim is to help patients deal with problems themselves, not to do this for them; in this way they are more likely to deal effectively with future problems without help. Problem solving counselling can be learnt quickly and used by physicians, or carried out by nurses or social workers. There are four stages. First, patients are encouraged to list and define their current problems. This alone often helps people who feel overwhelmed by their illness and other problems. Second, patients select a problem to work on, are helped to consider possible ways of dealing with this problem, and are encouraged to choose a solution likely to succeed. Third, patients are encouraged to carry out the first part of the chosen plan and to report the result. These activities are presented as experiments in which an attempt that proves unsuccessful is not viewed as a failure but as a source of information leading to a more effective plan. This approach is important for patients who are demoralized as a result of persistent ill health and social difficulties. Fourth, when the first problem has been solved, another is chosen and the process is repeated. This simple but systematic counselling has been shown in randomized clinical trials to be as effective as drug treatment for patients with anxiety and the less severe cases of depression treated in primary care and it is equally suitable for use in hospital practice.

When problem solving counselling is used for patients whose life problems have suddenly become overwhelming it is called crisis intervention. Suitable patients include those who have taken a drug overdose as a form of deliberate self-harm. These patients are usually in a state of high emotional arousal when first interviewed, and before problem solving counselling can be started it is usually necessary to reduce arousal by allowing the patient to talk about their feelings. As in the treatment of patients who are not in crisis, it is important to emphasize that the patient is not just resolving the present crisis but also learning a general approach that can be used should there be future problems.

Cognitive behaviour therapy

This type of psychological treatment corrects ways of thinking and behaving that delay recovery from certain psychiatric disorders. There are many different cognitive-behavioural treatments, each designed for a specific disorder or group of disorders. These specific treatment procedures are based on research showing which ways of thinking and behaviour prolong each of the several kinds of disorder that are treated in this way. The techniques most relevant to patients treated by physicians are for anxiety disorders, bulimia nervosa, and for chronic fatigue syndrome. Cognitive behavioural treatments are provided by clinical psychologists, some clinical nurse specialists, and some psychiatrists. Readers requiring a more comprehensive account should consult the book by Hawton *et al.* (see Further reading).

Brief dynamic psychotherapy

This term describes a group of treatments for emotional disorders and difficulties in relationships which seek to discover the connections between the current problems and events in earlier life and to help the patient gain more control of feelings. Although it usually lasts for about 6 months the treatment is described as 'brief' to distinguish it from longer methods of psychotherapy such as psychoanalysis. There are several ways of carrying out dynamic psychotherapy (originating in the work of Freud, Jung, Klein, and others) but these variations of technique have not been shown to affect the outcome.

Brief dynamic psychotherapy is most useful for patients with recurrent anxiety or depression or relationship difficulties, associated with feelings of worthlessness or other problems resulting from disturbed family relationships in childhood. Dynamic psychotherapy has been used for some medical disorders when these are exacerbated by the emotional problems mentioned above. Two randomized controlled trials have shown that dynamic psychotherapy has positive results with two conditions in which psychological factors appear to exacerbate the disorder in some cases, namely asthma and irritable bowel syndrome, but further studies are needed to confirm these findings.

It is reasonable to consider brief dynamic psychotherapy for patients whose medical condition appears to be exacerbated repeatedly by anxiety, depression, or suppressed anger and when these emotions arise mainly from the patient's psychological make-up rather than from the circumstances of life. The advice of a psychiatrist should be obtained on the suitability for this treatment which may be carried out by a psychiatrist, or a specialist psychotherapist.

Further reading

Gelder, M.G., Lopez-Iber, J.J., and Andreasen, N. (eds.) (2000). *New Oxford textbook of psychiatry.* Oxford University Press, Oxford.

Hawton, K., Salkovskis, P.M., Kirk, J., and Clark, D.M. (1999). *Cognitive behaviour therapy for psychiatric problems; a practical guide.* (2nd edn.). Oxford University Press, Oxford.

Butler, G. and Hope, T. (1995). *Manage your mind: the mental fitness guide.* Oxford University Press, Oxford.

Chalder, T (1995). *Coping with chronic fatigue.* Sheldon Press, London.

Chapter 14.6

Psychopharmacology in medical practice

P. J. Cowen

All clinicians need to have understanding of the uses and side-effects of psychotropic drugs, particularly how such medication can interact with drugs used to treat other medical disorders. Table 1 lists the main groups of drugs discussed below. Most psychotropic drugs are prescribed for depression and anxiety disorders, reflecting the frequency of these conditions in both primary care and general hospital settings; accordingly, drug treatment for anxiety and depression is often started by general practitioners and hospital clinicians. Antipsychotic drugs are used frequently in general hospitals in the management of organic psychoses, and patients receiving long-term therapy may require treatment for coexisting medical disorders where a knowledge of the effects of lithium on different body systems and its liability to produce adverse drug interactions will be required.

Table 1 Classification of clinical psychotropic drugs

Name	Examples of classes	Indications
Antipsychotic	Phenothiazines Butyrophenones Substituted benzamindes	Acute treatment of schizophrenia and mania, prophylaxis of schizophrenia
Antidepressant	Tricyclic antidepressants Monoamine oxidase inhibitors Selective 5-HT uptake blockers	Major depression (acute treatment and prophylaxis), anxiety disorders, obsessive compulsive disorder (5-HT uptake blockers)
Mood stabilizer	Lithium Carbamazepine	Acute treatment of mania Prophylaxis of recurrent affective disorder
Anxiolytic	Benzodiazepines Azapirones (buspirone)	Generalized anxiety disorder
Hypnotic	Benzodiazepines Cyclopyrrolones (zopiclone)	Insomnia

Drug overdose

When prescribing psychotropic drugs, particularly for depressed patients, the risk of overdose should always be considered. If such a risk is present the practitioner should: (1) ensure that medication is dispensed in small amounts; (2) consider asking a close relative to supervise the medication; (3) use a relatively non-toxic drug, if possible.

Pharmacokinetic factors

Most psychotropic drugs are highly lipophilic and are well absorbed from the gastrointestinal tract. They are metabolized by the liver to water-soluble derivatives, which are eliminated by the kidney. The half-life of psychotropic drugs will be prolonged in patients with hepatic or renal impairment. Where psychotropic medication is added to other drug treatment the possibility of drug interaction must be considered. Alcohol potentiates the sedative effects of many psychotropic agents and should be avoided during treatment. Sudden discontinuation of psychotropic drugs, particularly tranquillizers, antidepressants, and perhaps lithium, can cause withdrawal symptoms such as insomnia, anxiety, and affective disturbance. Where possible, therefore, the dose of medication should be tapered under supervision.

Compliance with treatment

Compliance is an even greater problem than it is in general therapeutics. Psychoactive drugs frequently have unpleasant side-effects which are experienced early in treatment whilst several days may elapse before a therapeutic response is evident. In addition, patients may not see the need for treatment, or do not believe that it can help them. Careful explanation, supplemented by written instructions, can help ensure that necessary medication is taken.

Antidepressant drugs

Tricyclic antidepressants

Pharmacology

Tricyclic antidepressants inhibit the neuronal uptake of 5-hydroxytryptamine (5-HT) and noradrenaline. These acute pharmacological actions are followed by a cascade of secondary changes in monoamine and other neurotransmitter receptors. It is believed that the antidepressant effects of drug treatment are caused by these secondary adaptive changes which produce an overall facilitation of both 5-HT and norarenaline neurotransmission.

Principal drugs

These are amitriptyline, clomipramine, desmethylimipramine, dothiepin, doxepin, imipramine, nortriptyline, and protriptyline.

Indications and use

Tricyclic antidepressants are still the most widely prescribed agents for the management of depressive illness, but their use, particularly in less severe depressive states, is giving way to newer compounds that are better tolerated at therapeutic doses (see below). However, none of the newer antidepressants is more efficacious than the tricyclics and their therapeutic activity in more severely ill patients is not as well established. For this reason, unless there are specific contraindications, tricyclic antidepressants should be considered for

Table 2 Some adverse effects of tricyclic antidepressants

Pharmacological action	Adverse effect
Muscarinic receptor blockade (anticholinergic)	Dry mouth, tachycardia, blurred vision, glaucoma, constipation, urinary retention, sexual dysfunction, cognitive impairment
α-Adrenoceptor blockade	Drowsiness, postural hypotension, sexual dysfunction, cognitive impairment
Histamine H_1-receptor blockade	Drowsiness, weight gain
Membrane stabilizing properties	Cardiac conduction defects, cardiac arrhythmias, epileptic seizures
Other	Rash, oedema, leucopenia, elevated liver enzymes

depressed inpatients or in those with marked melancholic features.

Depressed patients with prominent sleep disturbance and anxiety should be treated with a sedating antidepressant such as amitriptyline; for other patients, less sedating compounds such as imipramine or desipramine can be used. In order to obtain tolerance to side-effects it is usual to begin treatment at a low dose, for example 50 mg of amitriptyline at night, and to increase the amount over about 1–2 weeks to the usual therapeutic dose, which ranges between 75 and 200 mg daily for amitriptyline and imipramine. Tricyclic antidepressants have long half-lives and a single daily dose taken at night is usually appropriate. Patients should be warned about side-effects (see below) because this helps ensure compliance in the early stages of treatment. They should also be advised that a clear therapeutic response may not appear for up to 2–4 weeks. If treatment is successful it is usual to continue the antidepressant for 4–6 months at the original dose if tolerance allows. This reduces the risk of early relapse. Some patients with recurrent depressive illness require long-term prophylactic treatment.

Side-effects

As well as inhibiting the uptake of noradrenaline and 5-HT, tricyclic antidepressants possess antagonist properties at a variety of neurotransmitter receptors, including muscarinic cholinergic receptors, α_1-adrenoceptors and H_1-histamine receptors. These receptor antagonist effects account for much of the adverse effect profile of tricyclics, particularly, of course, their anticholinergic properties (Table 2). Tricyclics also possess membrane stabilizing effects that underlie their most serious side-effect of cardiotoxicity. This can be particularly problematic in tricyclic overdose, where ingestion of less than 1 g may sometimes prove fatal. Tricyclics lower seizure threshold and can cause fits in predisposed subjects.

Drug interactions

Tricyclic antidepressants antagonize the antihypertensive effects of adrenergic neurone blockers and clonidine but can be safely combined with thiazides, β-blockers (except sotalol), and angiotensin converting enzyme (ACE) inhibitors. The ability of tricyclics to block noradrenaline uptake can lead to hypertension with systemically administered noradrenaline and adrenaline. Plasma concentrations of tricyclics may be increased by cimetidine and calcium-channel blockers.

Newer antidepressants

Principal drugs

These can be classified as follows: (1) selective 5-HT uptake inhibitors (SSRIs), citalopram, fluoxetine, fluvoxamine, paroxetine, sertraline; (2) selective noradrenaline re-uptake inhibitor, reboxetine; (3) selective serotonin and noradrenaline re-uptake inhibitor (SNRI), venlafaxine; (4) modified tricyclic, lofepramine; (5) monoamine receptor antagonists, mianserin, mirtazepine, nefazodone, trazodone.

Pharmacology

The actions of selective 5-HT re-uptake inhibitors are essentially confined to inhibition of 5-HT re-uptake. Their use is associated with a sustained increase in brain 5-HT neurotransmission. In contrast, the tricyclic compound lofepramine mainly inhibits noradrenaline re-uptake. It also possesses anticholinergic properties, but to a lesser extent than amitriptyline. Reboxetine is a highly selective noradrenaline re-uptake inhibitor that also lacks anticholinergic properties. Venlafazine inhibits re-uptake of both 5-HT and noradrenaline but again lacks the receptor antagonist effects of tricyclic antidepressants. Mianserin and trazodone probably act via blockade of presynaptic α_2-adrenoceptors which facilitates noradrenaline release. They are also effective antihistamines and mianserin is a potent α_1-adrenoceptor antagonist. The mode of action of trazodone and nefazodone is uncertain. They are 5-HT_2 receptor antagonists but are also metabolized to *m*-chlorophenylpiperazine, a drug with 5-HT agonist properties. All these compounds, including lofepramine, lack the cardiotoxicity of conventional tricyclic antidepressants. They are, therefore, much safer in overdose.

Indications and use

The newer antidepressants should be used in patients where the use of tricyclic antidepressants is contraindicated because of their anticholinergic and cardiotoxic effects. In addition, some patients unable to tolerate a clinically effective dose of a tricyclic may find one of the newer drugs causes fewer side-effects. The lack of sedation associated with the selective 5-HT uptake inhibitors venlafazine and lofepramine can be beneficial in outpatients striving to carry out their usual activities. Unlike tricyclics, selective 5-HT uptake inhibitors venlafazne and lofepramine do not stimulate appetite and may therefore be appropriate in patients in whom weight gain would be undesirable. Finally, in patients where the risk of overdose cannot be minimized, the newer drugs may be preferred because of their lower acute toxicity. Perhaps because of its combined facilitation of 5-HT and noradrenergic neurotransmission, venlafaxine may be somewhat more effective than SSRIs in severely depressed patients and may be used as an alternative to tricyclic antidepressants in this patient group. Trazodone, mianserin, and mirtazepine have sedating properties and can be used in patients with significant agitation and insomnia where the adverse effects of tricyclics contraindicate their use. Nefazodone is less sedating than trazodone.

Side-effects

The clinical profiles of the newer antidepressants are shown in Table 3. The major distinction between compounds is whether or not they are sedating. The sedating antidepressants have the advantage of improving sleep at an early stage but may impair cognitive function, while the reverse is true for selective 5-HT uptake inhibitors, venlafaxine and lofepramine. Like tricyclic antidepressants, the newer compounds appear to lower seizure threshold to some extent, though

Table 3 Pharmacological actions and adverse effects of some newer antidepressants

	Dose (daily) (mg)	Adverse effects
5-HT uptake inhibitors		
Fluoxetine	20–60	Nausea, vomiting, anxiety,
Fluvoxamine	100–300	insomnia, headache, reduced
Sertraline	50–200	appetite, sweating, skin rash,
Paroxetine	20–50	extrapyramidal movement disorders (rare), generalized allergic reaction (rare), seizures (rare)
Noradrenaline re-uptake inhibitor		
Reboxetine	8	Dry mouth, constipation, anxiety, sweating
Serotonin and noradrenaline re-uptake inhibitor (SNRI)		
Venlafaxine.	75–225	Nausea, headache, insomnia, somnolence, sexual dysfunction, seizures (rare), hypertension (high doses)
Modified tricyclic		
lofepramine	140–210	Anxiety, insomnia, dry mouth, constipation, seizures (rare)
Receptor antagonists		
Trazodone	150–300	Cognitive impairment, postural hypotension, priapism (rare), cardiac arrhythmias (rare).
Nefazodone	400	Asthenia, dry mouth, nausea, somnolence, dizziness
Mianserin	30–120	Cognitive impairment, weight gain, postural hypotension, bone marrow depression (rare), seizures (rare)
Mirtazepine	30–45	Drowsiness, weight gain (reversible white cell disorders (rare))

this effect may be lower with SSRIs and trazodone. The SSRIs have rarely been implicated in the development of extrapyramidal disorders such as akathisia and parkinsonism. SSRIs have also been associated with low sodium states, particularly in the elderly.

Drug interactions

With the exception of citalopram, the selective 5-HT uptake inhibitors slow the metabolism of numerous other drugs including warfarin, antipsychotic agents, and tricyclic antidepressants. Nefazodone also inhibits hepatic enzymes and should not be prescribed with terfenadine or astemizole. Dangerous interactions, characterized by 5-HT neurotoxicity, have been reported between SSRIs and monoamine oxidase inhibitors (MAOIs) and venlafaxine and MAOIs. This may be particularly problematic with fluoxetine, whose active metabolite norfluoxetine has a half-life of 7–10 days. At least 5 weeks should therefore elapse between stopping fluoxetine and prescribing monoamine oxidase inhibitor. Selective 5-HT uptake inhibitors may also produce neurotoxicity in combination with lithium. Trazodone, mianserin, and mirtazepine may increase the sedative effects of other centrally acting drugs. The interactions of lofepramine are similar to those of other tricyclic antidepressants.

Monoamine oxidase inhibitors (MAOIs)

Pharmacology

Monoamine oxidase inhibitors block the enzyme monoamine oxidase, which deaminates the neurotransmitters 5-HT, noradrenaline, and dopamine. Monoamine oxidase exists in two forms, known as type A (which deaminate noradrenaline and 5-HT) and type B (which preferentially deaminate dopamine and tyramine). Conventional monoamine oxidase inhibitors irreversibly deactivate both type A and type B monoamine oxidase. This has two main consequences of importance: (1) there is a potential for serious food and drug interactions; and (2) the consequent drug and food restrictions need to be continued for 2 weeks after cessation of monoamine oxidase inhibitor treatment so that new monoamine oxidase can be synthesized.

The new monoamine oxidase inhibitor, moclobemide differs from conventional monoamine oxidase inhibitors in that its inhibition is reversible and it selectively inhibits type A monoamine oxidase only. This leads to an increase in brain noradrenaline and 5-HT but other amines such as tyramine are much less affected. These factors make moclobemide much less likely than the older monoamine oxidase inhibitors to produce adverse food interactions, which gives it a significant safety advantage. However, current clinical experience with moclobemide is still somewhat limited and accordingly the discussion below will focus on the conventional monoamine oxidase inhibitors.

Principal drugs

These are isocarboxazid, phenelzine, tranylcypromine, and moclobemide.

Indications and use

Conventional monoamine oxidase inhibitors are rarely used as a first choice of antidepressant except where a patient is known to have responded to them in the past. They are accordingly usually reserved for subjects who have failed to respond to tricyclic antidepressants or electroconvulsive therapy, where a very useful antidepressant effect can often be achieved. Monoamine oxidase inhibitors may also be more effective than tricyclics in atypical depressive states characterized by mood reactivity, hypersomnia, hyperphagia, and excessive sensitivity to real or imagined rejection. In addition, some forms of bipolar depression, with features of anergia and hypersomnia respond better to monoamine oxidase inhibitors than to tricyclics.

Phenelzine and tranylcypromine are the two most commonly prescribed monoamine oxidase inhibitors. The usual therapeutic dose for phenelzine is between 30 and 90 mg daily. As with tricyclic antidepressants, patients should be informed about side-effects and advised that a therapeutic response from monoamine oxidase inhibitors may not be apparent for 3–4 weeks. Once a response is obtained, it is usually necessary to continue treatment for several months.

Side-effects

Monoamine oxidase inhibitors may cause the following side-effects. *Central nervous system*: dizziness, muscular twitching, insomnia, confusion, mania. *Cardiovascular*: tachycardia, postural hypotension, hypertension. *Other*: dry mouth, blurred vision, impotence, peripheral oedema, hepatocellular damage, leucopenia.

Food and drug interactions

The major hazard of conventional monoamine oxidase inhibitor treatment is through interaction with indirect sympathomimetics, that is, agents that release noradrenaline from nerve endings. The usual source of the interaction is tyramine in certain foodstuffs, especially cheese and meat extracts. Tyramine is usually metabolized by monoamine oxidase in the gut wall and liver but in patients taking monoamine oxidase inhibitors large amounts may enter the systemic circulation, resulting in hypertension and even cerebrovascular accidents. Similar adverse effects have been reported when sympathomimetic drugs, such as amphetamine or ephedrine, are administered to patients taking monoamine oxidase inhibitors. As the latter drug, or its derivatives, are frequently present in cold cures, patients must be warned against self-medication. Hypertensive episodes resulting from interaction of sympathomimetic drugs and monoamine oxidase inhibitors are best treated with an α_1-adrenoceptor antagonist, such as phentolamine. If this is unavailable, intramuscular chlorpromazine is an alternative. Monoamine oxidase inhibitors also produce important interactions with other commonly used drugs including opiates, insulin, and oral hypoglycaemics. Except in special circumstances, combination with tricyclic antidepressants is best avoided. Combination with clomipramine and selective 5-HT uptake inhibitors can cause a 5-HT neurotoxicity syndrome and is contraindicated.

From the foregoing it will apparent that conventional monoamine oxidase inhibitors should only be prescribed to patients capable of adhering to the necessary dietary restrictions. Written instructions listing prohibited foods should be provided. No additional medication should be given until the possibility of adverse drug interaction has been excluded.

Moclobemide

Controlled studies have shown that the reversible type A monoamine oxidase inhibitor, moclobemide, is effective in the treatment of major depression. Moclobemide is well tolerated, although insomnia and nausea may occur. Unlike conventional monoamine oxidase inhibitors, moclobemide does not cause significant interaction with tyramine; adverse drug interactions also seem to be less likely. However, caution is recommended when prescribing with opiates and, until further data is available, combined use with selective 5-HT uptake inhibitors and sympathomimetic agents should be avoided. Because of the reversible nature of moclobemide's interaction with monoamine oxidase and its short half-life (about 3 h), normal monoamine oxidase activity is restored within a day of stopping treatment.

While moclobemide appears to be effective in the treatment of uncomplicated major depression, it is not yet clear whether its antidepressant effect matches that of phenelzine and tranylcypromine in patients resistant to tricyclic antidepressants. Similarly it is not yet known whether moclobemide is effective in the treatment of patients with atypical depression.

Mood stabilizing drugs

Lithium

Pharmacology

Lithium salts have effects on receptor transduction systems, particularly the turnover of phosphoinositols, that may prevent excessive intracellular signalling. Lithium also produces marked increases in some aspects of brain 5-HT function.

Indications and use

The main use of lithium is in the prophylaxis of recurrent affective disorders, especially manic depressive illness. Lithium is also used in the acute treatment of mania but is less immediately effective than antipsychotic medication, particularly in the presence of psychotic symptoms. Depressed patients unresponsive to antidepressant drugs often show benefit when lithium is added to their antidepressant drug treatment.

The excretion of lithium is critically dependent on the kidney and since there is little margin between therapeutic plasma levels of lithium (0.5–1.0 mmol/l) and those causing toxicity (> 1.5 mmol/l) the introduction of lithium therapy should be preceded by a clinical and laboratory assessment of renal function. Renal function tests should include urine analysis and estimations of plasma creatinine and electrolytes. A creatinine clearance test should be performed if there is any suggestion of impaired renal function.

Patients should initially be treated with 400–800 mg daily of lithium carbonate. It is usually preferable to administer the whole daily dose at night. Slow release preparations of lithium are available but their pharmacokinetics *in vivo* are very similar to those of the standard preparation. Dosage should be adjusted every 5–7 days on the basis of plasma lithium determinations obtained approximately 12 h after the last dose. For prophylaxis of recurrent mood disorders plasma levels of 0.5–0.8 mmol/l are usually satisfactory; however, some patients, particularly those with an acute manic episode may require higher levels (0.8–1.0 mmol/l). Most patients achieve adequate plasma levels on dosages of lithium carbonate between 800 and 1600 mg daily, and following this the lithium requirement is usually remarkably stable. In the absence of clinical indications it is usually sufficient to check lithium levels every 2–to 3 months and repeat renal function tests every 6 months. Lithium can also cause hypothyroidism, so thyroid function tests should be performed prior to treatment and at 6-monthly intervals thereafter. If necessary lithium can be combined with thyroxine replacement therapy.

Side-effects

Many patients suffer from a fine tremor and nausea; diarrhoea may occur, especially at the start of treatment (Table 4). Some degree of thirst and polyuria is often present and a few patients develop nephrogenic diabetes insipidus. These last effects are caused by lithium blocking the effect of antidiuretic hormone (ADH) on the renal tubule. Most patients taking lithium have a demonstrable impairment of tubular concentrating ability, although this is rarely of clinical significance. Glomerular function is not usually affected by lithium, although, following lithium toxicity, glomerular damage and interstitial fibrosis have been reported. From current evidence it seems unlikely that long-term use of lithium within therapeutic plasma concentrations results in irreversible renal damage except in very rare situations.

Up to 80 per cent of the lithium filtered by the renal glomerulus is reabsorbed by the proximal tubule, the amount linked closely to sodium reabsorption. . Conditions such as diarrhoea and excessive sweating, which decrease body sodium, result in increased lithium reabsorption by the renal tubule leading to elevated plasma lithium levels.

Table 4 Some adverse effects and interactions of lithium

Central nervous system	Drowsiness, lethargy, headache, memory impairment, fine tremor
Cardiovascular system	Conduction defects (rare)
Gastrointestinal system	Nausea, vomiting, diarrhoea
Genitourinary system	Polydipsia, polyuria, nephrogenic diabetes insipidus
Endocrine system	Hypothyroidism (T4 ↓ TSH ↑), hyperglycaemia, hyperparathyroidism
Other	Leuococytosis, skin rash, weight gain
Drug interaction (lithium level ↑)	Diuretics, non-steroidal anti-inflammatory drugs, metronidazole, erythromycin
Signs of toxicity (plasma level >1.5 mmol/l)	Nausea, vomiting, coarse tremor, drowsiness, dysarthria, seizures, coma, renal failure, cardiovascular collapse

T_4, thyroxine; TSH, thyroid stimulating hormone.

Drug interactions

Thiazide diuretics, through their effect on sodium excretion, increase lithium reabsorption and can produce lithium toxicity unless the dose of lithium is reduced and plasma concentrations carefully monitored. It is said that loop and potassium sparing diuretics are unlikely to alter lithium clearance but it is prudent, nevertheless, to monitor lithium levels when using these drugs. Plasma lithium levels may also be increased by concomitant administration of non-steroidal anti-inflammatory drugs, and a similar effect may be produced by metronidazole, erythromycin, and ACE inhibitors. While the effects of lithium on cardiac conduction are usually considered benign, the effects of cardiac glycosides on conduction may be potentiated. Lithium may increase the liability of antipsychotic drugs to cause extrapyramidal movement disorders and can potentiate the effects of SSRIs, occasionally causing 5-HT neurotoxicity.

Lithium toxicity (see also Chapter 12.25)

Acute lithium toxicity usually appears at plasma levels above 1.5 mmol/l. Early signs are coarse tremor, drowsiness, and dysarthria. Higher plasma concentrations (> 2.5 mmol/l) can lead to seizures, coma, and death. Lithium toxicity is therefore a potentially fatal disorder and any suspicion of intoxication should lead to immediate withdrawal of lithium treatment and close monitoring of serum lithium and plasma electrolyte and creatinine concentrations. Severely ill patients with high serum lithium levels may require dialysis.

Carbamazepine

Pharmacology

Like certain other anticonvulsant drugs, carbamazepine blocks neuronal sodium channels. The relation of this effect to its therapeutic actions in affective disorder is uncertain. Similarly to lithium, carbamazepine facilitates some aspects of brain 5-HT neurotransmission.

Indications and use

Carbamazepine is effective in the acute treatment of mania and in the prophylaxis of bipolar affective disorder. It is used in patients who have difficulty tolerating or who do not respond to lithium therapy. It is possible in the latter patients for carbamazepine to be combined with lithium.

The dose range of carbamazepine employed to treat affective illness is similar to that used in the treatment of seizure disorders, although it is advisable to titrate the dose according to clinical response. Plasma level monitoring may be used to help avoid toxicity. Initial treatment should be with 100 mg of carbamazepine twice daily and the dose increased according to tolerance over the next 2–4 weeks. The effective dose range in the treatment of bipolar disorder is generally between 600 and 1200 mg daily, although some patients may require higher doses.

Side-effects

Dizziness, drowsiness, and nausea are common early in treatment, particularly with rapid dose titration, but tolerance to these effects usually occurs. Persistent ataxia and diplopia may indicate toxic plasma levels. A moderate degree of leucopenia is often seen during carbamazepine treatment and agranulocytosis may develop occasionally. For this reason it is prudent to monitor white cell counts well as carbamazepine levels during treatment. Skin rashes are also quite common. Other rarer adverse effects include low plasma sodium concentrations and liver cell damage. Circulating thyroid levels may be lowered by carbamazepine treatment but thyroid stimulating hormone (TSH) levels generally remain in the normal range and clinical hypothyroidism is unusual. Carbamazepine can impair cardiac conduction and should be used with caution in patients with cardiovascular disease.

Drug interactions

Carbamazepine increases the metabolism of a number of other drugs including tricyclic antidepressants, haloperidol, oral contraceptive agents, warfarin, and other anticonvulsants. A similar mechanism may underlie the decline in plasma carbamazepine levels sometimes seen during continued treatment. Carbamazepine levels may be increased by erythromycin, and some calcium-channel blockers such as diltiazem and verapamil. Reversible neurotoxicity has been reported when carbamazepine has been combined with lithium.

Antipsychotic drugs

Pharmacology

Antipsychotic drugs, also known as major tranquillizers or neuroleptics, are a group of agents of varied structure that have in common the ability to block dopamine receptors in the central nervous system. It is likely that the antipsychotic effect of major tranquillizers is caused by blockade of dopamine receptors in mesolimbic and mesocortical brain regions. However, while the dopamine receptor blockade occurs within hours of drug administration, a useful clinical response may not occur for days and sometimes weeks after the start of treatment.

Principal drugs

These are chlorpromazine, haloperidol, flupenthixol, fluphenazine, loxapine, pimozide, thioridazine, and trifluoperazine. Another group of drugs are referred to as 'atypical' antipsychotics because of their decreased liability to cause extrapyramidal movement disorders. Some of these drugs are highly selective dopamine receptor antagonists which may produce a preferential blockade of dopamine D_2 receptors in the mesolimbic regions (amisulpiride and sulpiride). Others produce powerful blockade of 5-HT_2 receptors which exceeds their ability to antagonize dopamine D_2 receptors (clozapine, olanzepine, qetiapeine, risperidone, sertindole).

Table 5 Extrapyramidal disorders and antipsychotic drugs

Disorder	Description	Treatments employed
Dystonic reaction	Involuntary muscle contraction, especially face and jaw, occulogyric crisis	1. Benztropine (1–2 mg intramuscular or IV)
		2. Diazepam (10 mg IV)
Akathisia	Sense of subjective motor restlessness, continual pacing	1. Reduce dose of antipsychotic drug
		2. Benztropine (1–6 mg daily)
		3. Propranolol (40–120 mg daily)
		4. Diazepam (10–30 mg daily)
Parkinsonism	Rigidity, bradykinesia, tremor	1. Reduce dose of neuroleptic
		2. Benztropine (1–6 mg daily)
Tardive dyskinesia (late onset)	Choreoathetoid movements, especially tongue, lips and jaw	1. Withdraw antipsychotic drug
		2. Sulpiride
		3. Calcium channel blocker
Neuroleptic malignant syndrome (rare)	Fever, muscular rigidity, coma, death	1. Discontinue neuroleptic
		2. Intensive care support
		3. Bromocriptine
		4. Dantrolene

Indications and use

Antipsychotic drugs are used mainly in the management of schizophrenia. They are also used to treat mania and sometimes given to depressed patients who have psychotic symptoms or who are particularly agitated. Antipsychotic drugs are also used in the management of disturbed behaviour arising from other causes, for example, confusional states, but their use as non-specific tranquillizing agents should be limited to short-term use if possible because of potentially serious side-effects.

In the treatment of acute confusional states, haloperidol, in doses of 1.0–5.0 mg is often helpful. This can be administered either orally or parenterally and the dose repeated after an hour if the patient remains disturbed. Cardiovascular and respiratory side-effects are unlikely with haloperidol but acute dystonias can occur and should be treated appropriately (Table 5). Thioridazine is popular for the treatment of confused elderly patients but its anticholinergic properties may worsen orientation and memory. Certain groups of demented patients (particularly those with Lewy body type dementia) may suffer severe extrapyramidal effects from comparatively low doses of antipsychotic drugs.

The treatment of patients with schizophrenia or mania with antipsychotic drugs requires careful monitoring and persistence because the full therapeutic response may be delayed for some weeks and the dose of antipsychotic drug required may vary considerably from patient to patient and also within the same patient at different stages of the illness. Generally for a young person with an acute psychosis, up to 500 mg a day of chlorpromazine may be necessary, this dose being achieved gradually over several days, while sedative and hypotensive side-effects decrease. In patients with cardiovascular disease, treatment with haloperidol in doses from 5–20 mg daily is safer. All antipsychotic drugs are subject to first-pass metabolism so parenterally administered medication produces a proportionally greater effect. If a patient has responded to an antipsychotic drug it is usual to continue the medication for a number of months into remission. Frequently it is necessary to administer medication on a long-term basis to prevent relapse, in which case the use of long-acting intramuscular preparations will improve compliance. The decanoates of fluphenazine, flupenthixol, and haloperidol are most commonly used.

Side-effects

Movement disorders

Through their blockade of brain dopamine receptors, antipsychotic drugs produce a variety of movement disorders that can mimic signs of basal ganglia disease (Table 5). Many patients, for example, may exhibit symptoms of parkinsonism very similar to those of the idiopathic disorder (although tremor is less prominent). A side-effect that appears early in treatment is acute dystonia, which can present with abnormal postures or dramatic muscular spasms involving the face and limbs. Laryngeal spasm with respiratory distress can also occur. A history of recent antipsychotic drug use can help avoid misdiagnoses (it is not unusual, for example, for such reactions to be viewed as 'hysterical'). Another movement disorder that patients find very distressing is akathisia, which is a state of motor restlessness often with agitation and dysphoria. Distinguishing this reaction from symptoms arising from the underlying psychiatric disorder may not be easy.

All these movement disorders may be treated by a reduction in dosage of the antipsychotic drug or by the introduction of anticholinergic medication such as benzotropine. However, anticholinergic drugs should not be prescribed routinely with antipsychotic medication because of the risk of abuse for their euphoriant effects. Later in treatment tardive dyskinesia may develop. This consists of involuntary repetitive movements usually involving the tongue and lips though other parts of the body may be involved. Tardive dyskinesia may be associated with supersensitivity of postsynaptic dopamine receptors in the basal ganglia; at present this disorder cannot be treated easily and anticholinergic medication may make it worse. If possible the antipsychotic drug should be stopped but this decision is often difficult because of the risk of relapse of the psychiatric disorder. Of the available antipsychotic drugs, the atypical agents (see below) are less likely to cause movement disorders.

Neuroleptic malignant syndrome

A rare but potentially very serious reaction to antipsychotic drugs is the neuroleptic malignant syndrome (Table 5). This is characterized by fever, rigidity, and altered consciousness, together with tachycardia and labile blood pressure. Laboratory investigations usually reveal a leucocytosis together with markedly raised levels of creatinine phosphokinase. Antipsychotic drug treatment should be withdrawn immediately if the neuroleptic malignant syndrome is suspected. Management in an intensive care facility may be needed to deal with cardiovascular, respiratory, and renal complications. Treatment with dopamine receptor agonist, bromocriptine, and the antispasticity agent, dantrolene, appears to be beneficial.

Other side-effects

Antipsychotic drugs, especially chlorpromazine and thioridazine, can produce a variety of side-effects due to blockade of muscarinic receptors and α-adrenoceptors. These include drowsiness, psychomotor impairment, confusion, tachycardia, postural hypotension, blurring of vision, precipitation of glaucoma, dry mouth, constipation, urinary hesitancy, and impaired sexual function. Other side-effects include *endocrine*: elevated prolactin levels, amenorrhoea, and galactorrhoea; *skin*: rashes, pigmentation, and photosensitivity (especially phenothiazines); *other*: precipitation of seizures, hypothermia (especially chlorpromazine), cardiac arrhythmias (pimozide), weight gain, cholestatic hepatitis, leucopenia, and retinitis pigmentosa (thioridazine in doses > 800 mg daily).

Drug interactions

Antipsychotic drugs potentiate the effects of other central sedatives. They may delay the hepatic metabolism of tricyclic antidepressants and antiepileptic drugs leading to increased plasma levels of these latter agents. The hypotensive properties of chlorpromazine and thioridazine may enhance the effects of antihypertensive drugs.

Atypical antipsychotic drugs

Clozapine

Clozapine is a weak dopamine D_2 receptor antagonist but binds strongly to the 5-HT_2 receptor subtype. A significant proportion (perhaps about 50 per cent) of patients refractory to conventional antipsychotic drugs may derive clinical benefit from clozapine treatment. Interestingly, negative symptoms of schizophrenia, such as apathy and amotivation, which are frequently refractory to conventional antipsychotic drugs, may also respond. However, the use of clozapine is associated with a significant risk of leucopenia (about 2–3 per cent), which can progress to agranulocytosis. Weekly white cell counts during treatment are mandatory and with this intensive monitoring the early detection of leucopenia can be followed by immediate clozapine withdrawal and reversal of the low white cell count. While this procedure makes progression to agranulocytosis very unlikely, rare fatalities due to clozapine-induced agranulocytosis have been reported. In severe and intractable schizophrenia, however, the use of clozapine may be justified.

Clozapine is less likely than other neuroleptics to cause extrapyramidal movement disorders and does not increase plasma prolactin. However, its use is associated with hypersalivation, drowsiness, postural hypotension, weight gain, and hyperthermia. Seizures may occur at higher doses. It is usually recommended that clozapine be used as the sole antipsychotic agent in a treatment regime and clearly it is wise to avoid concomitant use of drugs, such as carbamazepine, which may also lower white cell count.

5-HT_2/D_2 receptor antagonists (olanzepine, quetiapine, risperidone, sertindole)

These drugs resemble clozapine in that their abilty to block 5-HT_2 receptors is greater than their ability to antagonize dopamine D_2 receptors. All these drugs are less likely than conventional antipsychotic drugs to cause extrapyramidal movement disorders. In this respect it is worth noting that riperidone has a rather narrow dose–response curve and loses its advantage over conventional antipsychotic drugs at doses of greater than 6 mg daily. All these drugs are at least as effective as haloperidol against positive symptoms but may be more effective against negative symptoms. With the exception of clozapine there is not yet compelling evidence that they are effective in treatment resistant patients. With the exception of risperidone the 5-HT_2/D_2 receptor antagonists are less likely to increase plasma prolactin and therefore to cause menstrual and other adverse effects related to hyperprolactinaemia.

Substituted benzamides

These drugs are selective D_2 receptor antagonists which may have preferential effects in mesolimbic and mesocortical brain regions thus sparing the basal ganglia and the associated extrapyramidal movement disorders. At lower doses amisulpiride and sulpiride may selectively antagonize presynaptic dopamine D_2 receptors and thereby increase dopamine release in certain brain regions. This has been postulated to account for their ability to decrease negative symptoms reported in some studies. Such effects are better established for amisulpiride.

Antianxiety agents

Benzodiazepines

Pharmacology

Benzodiazepines enhance the action of the neurotransmitter γ-aminobutyric acid (GABA) in the central nervous system, by binding to a specific benzodiazepine receptor located in a complex with a GABA receptor and a chloride ion channel. The pharmacological effects of benzodiazepines are attributed to facilitation of GABA neurotransmission.

Principal drugs

These are alprazolam, chlorazepate, diazepam, flurazepam, lorazepam, lormetazepam, nitrazepam, and temazepam.

Indications and use

The prescription of benzodiazepines is now decreasing following concern about their liability to produce dependence. For most anxiety-related disorders, alternative therapies are available and it is recommended that the drug treatment of anxiety and insomnia should be limited to a few weeks duration. The major indication for the use of benzodiazepines is to help patients in a crisis when anxiety and insomnia are causing functional impairment and reducing ability to cope. Patients should be advised that drug treatment will be of short duration to help them manage their immediate difficulties. All benzodiazepines have hypnotic and anxiolytic properties. The major distinction of clinical importance is their length of action. Derivatives with a 3-hydroxy group such as temazepam are metabolized by the liver to inactive glucuronides and have shorter half-lives; such drugs are suitable hypnotics because of their lack of hangover effect. Other benzodiazepines, for example diazepam, have long half-lives and are metabolized to active compounds. These drugs may used for the treatment of anxiety, either in the form of regular dosing, or on the now preferred 'as required' basis with an agreed maximum daily dose.

Side-effects and interactions

Benzodiazepines have a low acute toxicity. Their adverse effects are extensions of their clinical effects and include the following: drowsiness, psychomotor impairment, dizziness, ataxia, and paradoxical aggression (rare). Benzodiazepines potentiate other central sedatives, particularly alcohol. The effects of benzodiazepines are potentiated by cimetidine.

Patients who have taken clinical doses of a benzodiazepine for more than a few months may show a withdrawal syndrome when the medication is stopped. In many respects this syndrome resembles an anxiety state but perceptual disturbances and dysphoria may also occur. It is thus apparent that benzodiazepines can cause physical dependence and although the withdrawal syndrome is less severe than that seen following cessation of barbiturates, patients frequently find it extremely difficult to stop their medication. A gradual reduction is usually best. Generally, withdrawal from a long-acting benzodiazepine is easier than from a short-acting preparation. If patients taking short-acting benzodiazepines have difficulties withdrawing, a switch to a long-acting preparation may be helpful.

Other drugs that increase brain GABA function

Zopiclone and Zolpidem

Zopiclone and zolpidem are non-benzodiazepine hypnotics that bind to a site close to benzodiazepine receptors and thereby facilitate brain GABA function. They are both indicated for the short-term treatment of insomnia and are claimed to be less likely than benzodiazepine hypnotics to produce tolerance and withdrawal effects. These proposals, however, have yet to be fully evaluated.

Chlormethiazole

Chlormethiazole also binds at the GABA receptor complex but its clinical effects resembles barbiturates rather more than benzodiazepines in that it can cause serious respiratory depression in overdose, particularly in combination with alcohol. Chlormethiazole is a popular treatment to ameliorate the symptoms of alcohol withdrawal but should be used in short courses to prevent the development of dependence. Because of its short half-life (4–5 h), chlormethiazole is also used as a hypnotic in the elderly; dependence in this age group has not been reported.

Drugs altering monoamine function

Buspirone

Buspirone is a 5-HT receptor agonist, structurally unrelated to benzodiazepines. It is effective in the treatment of generalized anxiety disorder (less so in patients previously exposed to benzodiazepines) but has a slow onset of action (1–3 weeks). Unlike benzodiazepines buspirone does not cause significant sedation or cognitive impairment and at present appears unlikely to cause dependence. It does not have hypnotic properties. Side-effects include nervousness, dizziness, and headache.

Other drugs

Tricyclic antidepressants, selective 5-HT uptake inhibitors and monoamine oxidase inhibitors are effective in the management of patients with anxiety syndromes characterized by frequent panic attacks. Alprazolam is also used for this purpose but carries the general disadvantages of benzodiazepine treatment. Obsessive compulsive disorder is also classified as an anxiety disorder, although benzodiazepines are not an effective treatment. In fact, the drug treatment response of patients with obsessive compulsive disorder is rather specific in that clear superiority over placebo has been demonstrated only for drugs such as the selective 5-HT uptake inhibitors and clomipramine that potently inhibit the uptake of 5-HT.

Further reading

Nutt, D.J. and Bell, C. (1997). Practical pharmacotherapy for anxiety. *Advances in Psychiatric Treatment* , 3, 79–85.

Spigset, O. and Martenssen, B. (1999). Drug treatment of depression. *British Medical Journal*, 318, 1188–91.

Thomas, C.S. and Lewis, S. (1998). Which atypical antipsychotic? *British Journal of Psychiatry*, 172,106–9.

Chapter 14.7

Psychiatric emergencies and problems arising in accident and emergency departments

R. A. Mayou

Some urgent psychiatric problems may require immediate action by the physician. They include acute psychiatric and behavioural disturbance, in which there is insufficient time to obtain specialist help, and also less dramatic problems, encountered in emergency departments or elsewhere in the general hospital, that require immediate decisions about management, for example severe anxiety. The management of alcohol withdrawal, intoxication and substance abuse is dealt with in Chapters 14.9–14.18 and the medicolegal aspect of behavioural disturbance are covered in Chapter 14.19.

Whatever the problem, the patient should be interviewed calmly so that a good relationship is established and information obtained about symptoms, past history, personality, and observations made of behaviour and mental state. In an emergency a systematic approach may be difficult but time can be saved and mistakes avoided if this can be achieved. Many emergencies become less urgent and bewildering if dealt with in a calm and deliberate way. It is not always necessary to make an accurate diagnosis since the treatment of disturbed behaviour is similar whatever the cause.

General considerations

The disturbed patient

Before seeing a disturbed patient as much information as possible should be obtained from medical notes and from informants such as relatives, nursing staff, and police. Table 1 lists some of the psychological and physical causes of disturbed behaviour. The list includes several important physical causes that are easily missed, especially if there is a history of psychiatric, alcohol, or drug problems that might deflect attention from organic causes.

Whenever possible disturbed patients should be interviewed in a room that is private and has a telephone and emergency bell with other staff available close by. Having obtained as much information as possible from the case notes and from others, the doctor should try to take a history, observe behaviour, and perform a physical examination. Many disturbed patients are frightened or angry: when these feelings are understood and taken seriously the disturbed behaviour often becomes less. The approach to the patient should be friendly and time should be spent at the beginning of the interview listening, explaining, and reassuring. Occasionally medication is necessary to calm the patient (see below). When the disturbed behaviour

Table 1 Some causes of disturbed behaviour

Anxiety, fear
Alcohol or drug abuse and withdrawal
Personality disorder
Delirium (acute organic stage, confusional state)
Side-effects of treatment
Hypoglycaemia
Epilepsy
Head injury
Encephalitis and meningitis
Dementia
Schizophrenia and paranoid psychoses
Affective disorder: depression and mania

Table 2 Management of violence

Ensure adequate help and medication is immediately available
Make sure you can retreat rapidly. Do not take risks
Do not let the patient feel trapped
Listen to the patient, talk calmly, and do not argue
Do not try to restrain patient in any way unless you have adequate support
If there are medical indications for restraint, act quickly and effectively but with minimum force.

has settled a full physical examination and appropriate investigation should be carried out.

The violent patient

The causes of aggressive behaviour and the assessment are the same as those for other disturbed behaviour. Whenever there is the threat of violence, the doctor should be sure that adequate but unobtrusive support is available before approaching the patient (Table 2). The doctor should always be ready to listen, sympathize, and, if necessary, make sensible compromises. Extreme caution is, of course, required with any patient thought to possess any kind of offensive weapon and in such cases it is often best to ask the police to intervene. Staff should always avoid single-handed restraint or actions, such as a physical examination suggesting that physical contact is intended, unless the purpose has been clearly understood and agreed by the patient.

If restraint cannot be avoided, it should be accomplished quickly by an adequate number of people using the minimum of force. Medication, such as parenteral haloperidol or chlorpromazine, should always be available. The use of such medication may provide the only way to calm the patient so as to carry out a physical examination or obtain further information.

Emergency drug treatment of disturbed or violent patients

This section is concerned with immediate management. For a patient who is moderately frightened, diazepam (5–10 mg) may be useful. For a more disturbed patient, rapid calming is best achieved with 2–5 mg of haloperidol intramuscularly, repeated if necessary every 30 min or every hour up to 20 mg in 24 h. Occasionally larger doses are required, but it is desirable to obtain a specialist opinion from a psychiatrist.

When the patient has become calmer, regular oral doses of haloperidol, probably three to four times a day, should be started, preferably as syrup or tablets. The exact dosage requires regular review and depends on the patient's weight and general physical state, and on the initial response to the drug. Regular nursing observations of behaviour, conscious level, and blood pressure are necessary during tranquillization. Chlorpromazine (75–150 mg intramuscularly) is a useful alternative to haloperidol but more likely to cause hypotension. Extrapyramidal side-effects may require treatment with an antiparkinsonian drug.

Stupor

In psychiatry the term stupor denotes a condition in which the patient is immobile, mute, and unresponsive but appears to be fully conscious, usually because the eyes are open and following external objects. (The term is also sometimes used by physicians to refer to impaired consciousness.) It may be due either to neurological or psychiatric conditions. The most common psychiatric causes of stupor are severe depressive disorder, hysteria, and schizophrenia (catatonia). As a patient in stupor stops eating and drinking, energetic management is necessary and the opinion of the psychiatrist should be obtained.

Thorough neurological examination and assessment is always necessary, even if the patient has a history of psychiatric disorder. A psychiatric diagnosis should be made only when tests of cerebral hemisphere and brainstem function have been found to be normal. Information from other informants is essential to establish the onset, nature, and cause of the condition.

Psychiatric syndromes as causes of emergencies

Organic mental disorders

Acute and chronic organic mental disorders may cause agitation, aggressive, or erratic behaviour. The characteristic behavioural and cognitive symptoms are usually easily recognized, but in the absence of a clear history or obvious physical signs, a functional psychiatric illness may be diagnosed in error. Doctors should always be suspicious that odd, out-of-character behaviour is a sign of an organic mental disorder, and they should be prepared to undertake full physical examination and assessment.

It is wise to assume that any patient who is exhibiting disturbed behaviour and is elderly or has physical illness, may have an organic mental disorder until proved otherwise. Careful psychiatric assessment that may reveal fluctuating disorientation or cognitive functions that seem impaired is judged by what is known of the patient's normal functioning.

Treatment is primarily medical. Confused patients require consistent nursing care, with repeated reassurance and explanation from a few familiar nurses. It may be useful to nurse the patient in a single room with some light at night. Regular visits from close family and friends are helpful. Modest dosages of a benzodiazepine hypnotic or a tranquillizer (such as haloperidol or a phenothiazine) are valuable in the management of agitation, restlessness, and disturbed behaviour.

Regular but flexible dosage regimes are preferable to the intermittent treatment of crises.

Victims of trauma

Survivors of major accidents and other trauma and people who have suffered bereavement or other emotional shocks may be dazed, numbed, or distressed, and present as emergencies. They may also describe unpleasant intrusive memories of the trauma, which may be severe enough to be diagnosed as post-traumatic stress disorder. They require sympathy, reassurance, and assistance with immediate practical problems. It is useful to talk through distressing thoughts and fears and also give the patient and relatives advice leaflets to read when they return home. An anxiolytic hypnotic can be helpful. Patients should be advised to seek further help from their doctor if they continue to suffer intrusive memories or anxiety.

Victims of violence may find it difficult to discuss the distressing event and particular sensitivity is needed to help them do this and to express their feelings. The risk of further violence (for example in the home) should be reviewed; immediate referral to a social worker may be necessary. After the emergency, further help may be needed from the general practitioner or from a self help group.

A particular problem is the management of victims of rape or other sexual assault. Apart from treating injuries, doctors should record any evidence that may be needed for subsequent legal proceedings. They should give the victim advice about possible venereal disease or pregnancy and, with the victim's permission, they should talk to his or her relatives or close friends. The victim should be given the opportunity to talk about the experience and their feelings with an experienced and sensitive member of staff and also encouraged to talk to relatives or friends. Follow-up advice should be offered. Some hospitals have special services for rape victims and many hospitals are able to refer to a local rape crisis organization with special expertise in providing help.

The emergency department should be prepared to offer psychological and social help to victims and to staff as a part of disaster planning. This means identifying experienced staff who can be called upon to provide immediate help and to organize follow-up care.

Somatic symptoms without physical cause

Somatic symptoms for example abdominal pain, chronic fatigue, chest pain, without significant physical cause are very common in medical practice and may present as emergencies. Some of these patients also have an undoubted physical illness and are often said to have 'functional overlay'. Such complaints should always be taken seriously as 'real' medical problems. Mild cases usually respond to authoritative reassurance after thorough history taking and examination. It is important not only to reassure that there is no serious physical cause but also to explain the cause of the symptoms and allow the patient to ask questions. It is sensible to encourage follow-up assessment for further advice, discussion, and reassurance.

A small proportion of patients present repeatedly with recurrent functional physical complaints. Although proper history taking and examination is necessary on each occasion, it is a mistake to order further investigations or specialist advice unless there are clear medical indications.

Conversion and dissociative disorder

Patients with acute onset of symptoms such as paralyses, sensory impairments, and amnesias are occasionally seen as emergencies. Such symptoms of conversion and dissociative disorder (hysteria) require full medical examination and appropriate special investigations. The doctor should always bear in mind that some cases originally diagnosed as conversion or dissociative disorder are later found to have physical illness, and that physical illness can occur in patients with a history of recurrent hysterical symptoms. Once conversion or dissociative disorder is suspected, the exclusion of organic disorder must be accompanied by a search for a psychological explanation of the patient's symptoms. Admission to hospital may be necessary for further assessment and for treatment.

Symptoms of acute onset often recover quickly. Resolution is helped by thorough assessment and sympathetic and authoritative reassurance, and by avoiding anything that might reinforce the symptoms. The patient should not be confronted but rather given face-saving opportunities for improvement. As with other forms of emotional disorder, psychological treatment directed to underlying emotional difficulties is important and patients should be offered outpatient follow-up.

Table 3 Somatic symptoms without physical cause

Simulated symptoms
• malingering
• factitious disorder
• specific simulated symptoms
• Munchausen syndrome
'Functional' symptoms
• transient fear of illness responding to reassurance
• misinterpretation of physiological processes or minor pathology
• somatic symptoms of a primary psychiatric disorder
• hypochondriacal personality

Simulated illness (Table 3)

Malingering is the faking of illness for obvious rewards (e.g. to obtain narcotics, taking time off work, or to gain compensation). Suspicions should be raised by inconsistencies in the patient's account of the symptoms and of previous medical treatment and vagueness about addresses and the names of doctors and other informants. The diagnosis can be confirmed only by the patient's confession, and careful history taking and gentle confrontation are often effective in securing this.

Factitious disorder covers the dramatic but rare Munchausen syndrome seen in emergency departments, and the much more frequent simulation of particular symptoms such as bleeding skin lesions and pyrexia. It differs from malingering in bringing no obvious external reward for the fabrication of symptoms. Although the grosser syndromes of recurrent faking and pathological lying are notably resistant to all forms of psychological treatment, patients exhibiting them should be confronted tactfully and offered referral to a psychiatrist. Patients with less extreme and more specific forms of simulated illness are somewhat more likely to respond to psychological treatment. It is essential to avoid angry confrontations but the patient should gently be made aware of the doctor's suspicions and offered the opportunity to discuss them. Even though patients are often unwilling to admit to their behaviour it may be possible to agree on an appropriate management plan.

Chapter 14.8

The patient who has attempted suicide

H. G. Morgan

Episodes of self-harm, usually in the form of drug overdosage, constitute the most common cause of acute hospital medical admission in females and are second only to ischaemic heart disease in males. The term 'deliberate self-harm', is used here rather than 'attempted suicide' because a true wish to die is present in only a minority of these patients.

Epidemiology

Deliberate self-harm is most frequent in young adults. For some 10 years beginning in the early 1960s its incidence increased rapidly in countries throughout the Western hemisphere. During the 1970s the incidence continued to rise but much more slowly. The incidence in each sex stabilized in the 1980s but more recently there has been an increase, much more marked in males. The early preponderance of teenage females has become less striking and in the UK the female–male ratio is now about 1.2:1. It is more prevalent in social classes 4 and 5, tending to be concentrated in those parts of urban areas where social problems abound, particularly in local authority housing estates.

Methods

The most frequent method is some kind of drug overdosage (about 90 per cent of episodes). Psychotropic drugs (minor tranquillizers and sedatives about one-fifth, antidepressants about one-fifth) feature prominently and these are usually obtained through medical prescription. In contrast, non-opioid analgesics such as salicylates and paracetamol are commonly obtained without prescription at retail chemists although in the UK amounts available are now restricted. Poisons and gassing are each used in less than 1 per cent of cases. Self-injury, usually in the form of skin laceration with or without drug overdosage, occurs in about 10 per cent of deliberate self harm presenting to hospitals. Concomitant alcohol intake within the previous six hours has been reported in 50 to 66 per cent of men and in 25 to 45 per cent of women.

Causes

Many episodes of deliberate self-harm appear to be impulsive acts by vulnerable persons who have become emotionally upset in response to some kind of disturbing event; the intention being either to seek temporary oblivion or to achieve some change in the situation. Factors such as imitation and availability of agent are also important. Conscious suicidal intent, though it may be absent or transient in such cases, should always be given serious consideration in clinical assessment. Overall, about two-thirds of patients have a major psychiatric disorder. An important minority who survive are truly failed suicides. In these patients, who are more likely than the others to be suffering from some form of mental illness, the suicide risk is particularly likely to continue after the event: its reliable identification is an important part of clinical assessment. It should always be considered seriously in elderly patients. Florid mental illness most commonly takes the form of depression. Personality disorder is seen in 15 per cent overall, and misuse of alcohol in 55 per cent of males and 35 per cent of females. Drug abuse is more common in males (14 per cent) than females (5 per cent).

Some kind of upsetting life event appears to be important in about two-thirds of cases. Most commonly this takes the form of disharmony with a person who is important to the patient (46 per cent). Other factors that are seen less frequently include problems concerned with work, financial matters, or physical health..

Assessment

Adequate assessment of deliberate self-harm depends upon full and reliable information and, whenever possible, other relevant informants should be interviewed as well as the patient. A detailed evaluation of social and interpersonal factors is necessary, as well as a clinical assessment. Some patients are unwilling to discuss personal matters and suicidal ideas openly, a few are suspicious because of psychotic ideas, and aggressive behaviour may have arisen from a toxic confusional state due to the overdose of drugs.

The main immediate risks are physical complications, a further episode of non-fatal self-harm, or suicide, and hazards concerning dependent children or other family members. These should all be evaluated and dealt with urgently where necessary.

Suicide risk

Most deliberate self-harm patients are interviewed in the hospital ward as soon as they are able to discuss matters fully and clearly, usually a day or so after the event. The detection of the minority who are true failed suicides is an important immediate objective. This is a difficult and uncertain task, but it is helped by the fact that the social and clinical correlates of completed suicide tend to be different from those of patients whose deliberate self-harm does not have a fatal outcome. Factors associated with increased risk of suicide are listed in Table 1.

Assessment of risk involves the compilation of an overall picture of individual and environmental/relationship factors, both current and from the past. The factors listed in Table 1 are not necessary for suicide to occur, but merely represent an important checklist of those that have been shown to have a positive association with increased suicide risk. They are particularly useful as indicators of caution whenever assessment otherwise may suggest that such risk is not significant. The essential element of suicide risk assessment must be the precise clinical picture and weighting of individual risk factors, which will vary from one patient to another.

Interviewing the suicidal

There is no evidence that open discussion will in any way increase the risk of suicide, and indeed a common error is failure to enquire about such risk adequately. However, the enquiry must be made appropriately: a brusque, challenging, and unsympathetic approach is hazardous, particularly in tense angry patients who are liable to react with dangerous impulsive behaviour.

Continued suicidal motivation may not be easy to assess by interview, and it is necessary to be aware of the potential pitfalls as well as ways of circumventing them. Assessment should ideally be performed without interruption in a quiet situation where it is possible

Table 1 Clinical and social factors associated with increase risk of suicide

Massive drug overdosage posing major physical risk
Extensive deep lacerations
Use of potentially lethal agent (e.g. firearm)
Precautions to avoid discovery and to succeed in killing self
Detailed planning
Increased age
Male sex
Recent bereavement, separation, or divorce
Unemployment
Social isolation, alienation
Incapacitating physical disability and illness
Depressive illness
Other mental illness (organic brain disorder, schizophrenia, drug addiction)
Personality difficulties (especially poor impulse control and social difficulties)
Epilepsy complicated by mood disorder

to talk in private and without hurry. The patient usually shows varying amounts of depression, despair, anger, or frustration and may express an unwillingness to talk about personal feelings. There may also be reluctance to discuss the act of self-harm because this provokes, guilt, shame, and the fear of adverse consequences. Assessment of the mental state should be directed particularly to the detection of the characteristic clinical features of depressive illness. These include overt depression of mood, tearfulness, disorders of thinking such as poor concentration, ideas of futility, and morbid self-blame. Biological changes such as insomnia, reduced libido, poor appetite, and weight loss are important features of a severe depressive illness, although suicide risk can be significant even in their absence.

If the patient appears despairing and hopeless, it is appropriate to signify recognition of this in a sympathetic and reassuring way at an early stage in the interview. Such an approach can be an important first step in overcoming the feelings of isolation and alienation which are so characteristic of suicidal persons. Discussion of suicidal ideas should be entered upon carefully. A useful sequence of questions, which leads gradually up to discussion of suicidal ideas, their severity, and associated risks is listed in Table 2. Continuing suicidal ideas must of course always be taken seriously.

A suicidal person may exhibit marked hour to hour fluctuation in the degree of overt distress, and some who are at risk may at times appear to be free from symptoms. This is particularly likely in those who are admitted to hospital and thereby removed from the life problems which led to despair. Those with continued suicidal intent often show anger and resentment towards either their situation or other people, and they may appear unco-operative or unreasonable as well as depressed and despairing. When the clinical picture is of this mixed kind it is important not to underestimate suicide risk.

More than half of those who actually commit suicide turn to others for help in the weeks preceding their death, and they communicate their suicidal ideas openly before killing themselves. It is therefore wrong to believe that people who talk about suicidal ideas never end

Table 2 Interview sequence of topics in assessing suicidal motivation

Hope that things will turn out well
Get pleasure out of life
Feel hopeful from day to day
Able to face each day
See point in it all
Ever despair about things
Feel that it is impossible to face next day
Feel life a burden
Wish it would all end
Wish self dead
Why feel this way (e.g. be with a dead person, life bleak morbid guilt)
Thoughts of ending life. If so, how persistently
Thought specifically about method of suicide (means readily available)
Ever acted on them
Feel able to resist them, anything make them disappear
How likely to kill self
Ability to give reassurance about safety, e.g. until next appointment
Circumstances likely to make things worse
Willingness to turn for help if crisis occurs
Risk to others

their lives. It is also rash to dismiss such comments as mere threats or manipulation, unless the patient is well known to the doctor and such an interpretation is wholly consistent with previous behaviour. Even then such a judgement can be mistaken. A high proportion of individuals who have severe suicidal intent are ambivalent about ending their lives and may temporarily recover hope. This may lead an unsuspecting interviewer into a false sense of optimism. Occasionally a person at serious risk of suicide conceals the fact because of the belief that no help is likely to be effective. When a person who denies suicidal ideas has behaved in an inconsistent manner, such as having left a suicide note, or having engaged in serious life-endangering behaviour, particular care should be taken not to accept this denial too readily.

Non-fatal repetition

Another risk which requires immediate assessment is that of a further non-fatal act of self-harm. The patient may talk openly about wishing to repeat the act and such statements should never be dismissed lightly, particularly when upsetting life events that led up to the episode remain unresolved or are even made worse by it, for example by increasing the hostility of other people. Other correlates of non-fatal repetition include abuse of alcohol or drugs, a previous history of deliberate self-poisoning or injury, a history of violence, having a criminal record, unemployment, social class V, civil status single, divorced, or married but separated, and age 25–54 years.

Others at risk

The welfare of dependants such as children should always be assessed carefully. There is some evidence of an increased incidence of child abuse in persons who carry out acts of deliberate self-harm.

Management

During the initial period the emphasis of treatment must be upon physical risk and complications. Nevertheless, from the beginning the hazard of suicide and non-fatal repetition should not be forgotten. The degree of risk should be decided in every case and if any doubt exists psychiatric advice should be obtained immediately. It has long been recognized that the degree of physical risk correlates poorly, if at all, with the severity of suicidal ideation. In view of this, inpatient overnight admission to allow thorough assessment next day has been commended as the ideal practice in the management of all deliberate self-harm patients. Discharge home from the accident and emergency department should always be a matter of great caution, although it seems that considerable numbers have in recent years been managed in this way. It should be remembered that adolescents in particular may be difficult to assess thoroughly in an accident and emergency department. Once the degree of risk is decided it should be clearly understood by all those concerned with the patient's care. Particular attention should be given to prevent any access to hazards such as open stairs and windows. It is the hospital's responsibility to ensure that such patients are nursed only in situations where their safety can be reasonably assured. The number of nursing staff available is important and the need should be reviewed frequently. Patients who have taken drug overdoses may be noisy and unco-operative as a result of confusion induced by drugs or disinhibition due to concomitant alcohol intake, often compounded by personality difficulties. Such patients are not always those most welcome in medical wards. Each hospital ward should have a clear code of practice concerning the levels of supportive observation required according to the degree of perceived suicide risk. These may vary from one or more nurses remaining with the patient at all times in the case of severe risk (nurses may need to be appropriately skilled if impulsive behaviour is a possibility), through graded levels of care to unrestricted movement within the ward when risk is judged to be minimal. It is useful initially to nurse in bed all patients who are admitted to medical wards following deliberate self-poisoning or injury, no matter how trivial the physical risk may be, at least until thorough psychiatric assessment has provided a full evaluation of the immediate risk of suicide or non-fatal repetition. Physical hazards in the ward itself should always be kept in mind in order to ensure that the environment is sufficiently safe when suicide risk is high.

About 10 per cent of patients admitted to a general hospital after deliberate self-harm require admission to psychiatric inpatient care, usually because of florid mental illness, continuing risk of self-harm, or a worsening social situation. A very small proportion may have to be admitted under a compulsory legislative provision when the immediate risk of suicide is very serious, the patient is mentally ill, and unwilling to accept help. In the England and Wales, this situation most commonly involves a Section 2 Assessment Order of the 1983 Mental Health Act. This requires an application by (or on behalf of) the nearest relative together with two medical recommendations, one of which must be made by an approved specialist in psychiatry. Medicolegal issues are further discussed in Chapter 14.19. About a quarter of patients are returned directly to and remain in the care of their general practitioners. Approximately a half are given appointments in psychiatric outpatient clinics but only a half of these attend. Such low compliance with treatment is a major problem: it has many possible causes, which may include a reluctance to look at underlying causes once symptoms have settled and the crisis has blown over, or simply an unwillingness to become a psychiatric patient. Young males are more difficult than females to engage in treatment and are more likely to discharge themselves from hospital. The treatment that is offered needs to be perceived by the patient as valid, relevant, and feasible if it is to be accepted readily. A problem-solving approach is a good example: this clarifies the principal difficulties faced by the patient, and identifies mutually agreed steps in resolving them. The use of contract techniques in achieving the goals can be particularly helpful. Poor communication with key other persons may require conjoint work, and it may be necessary to involve other agencies, such as social services, particularly when the welfare of dependants such as children or elderly persons is relevant.

Ongoing suicide risk

When a serious depressive disorder is the underlying cause of the suicidal behaviour, antidepressant medication may be needed, or even physical treatment such as electroconvulsive therapy. However, psychotropic drugs alone are never an adequate safeguard against the risk of suicide. There is evidence that persons who later proceed to commit suicide have often been prescribed such drugs for long periods in dosages too low to be effective. Sometimes it is necessary to support a suicidal person as an outpatient over a long period, especially when intensive treatment in hospital has not produced a complete resolution of the problems, for example when there are intractable social or interpersonal difficulties. Interview techniques should include appropriate concern, sympathy, and non-judgemental attitudes from the therapist and a refusal to share the patient's feeling of despair. Provision of 'hotline' contact for vulnerable individuals can be useful, either with the medical services or one of the voluntary agencies such as the Samaritans.

Prevention of non-fatal repetition

During the subsequent year about a quarter of patients repeat one or more non-fatal acts of self-harm, particularly within the first 3 months. There may merely be a further single episode, or a chronic pattern of repeated episodes is resumed, and this may cluster around acute episodes of stress. The likelihood of repetition is greater when the person has made one or more previous attempts. In planning treatment, it is advisable to take into account the style of help the patients prefer: some wish to attend their general practitioner, others think psychiatric help more relevant to their problems. There is now some evidence to suggest that after a first episode of deliberate self-harm open access to help as opposed to fixed appointments may reduce the incidence of non-fatal repetition. Paradoxically, however, such an approach may increase repetition in those who already have a history of deliberate self-harm. This suggests that treatment strategies need to differ from one patient subgroup to another. For example, in patients who already have an established pattern of deliberate self-harm it may be particularly important to address any secondary gain resulting from it. Recent regulations limiting packsize of paracetamol products are a welcome development though their effects on the incidence of deliberate self-harm remain to be evaluated.

Further reading

Hawton, K. and Catalan, J. (1987). *Attempted suicide. A practical guide to its nature and management*, (2nd edn). Oxford University Press, Oxford.

Substance abuse

Chapter 14.9

Introduction

M. Farrell and J. Strang

Up to 25 per cent of patients admitted to a general hospital have an alcohol related problem and approximately 6 per cent of the general population are alcohol dependent. Some 30 per cent of the adult population smoke tobacco. Half of the young people who start to smoke will become lifelong smokers, half of whom will die of tobacco related diseases. Over half of the young adult population have tried illegal drugs including cannabis. More than 2 per cent of the adult population may be regular cannabis smokers. One per cent of the population have injected drugs at some time in their lives and about half of those have continued to do so.

It is important that every clinician has the ability to assess how tobacco, alcohol and consumption of other drugs is affecting a patient's life. Dependence is a learned habit that becomes self-perpetuating and difficult to eradicate. It is a psychophysiological state that can result from the direct reinforcing effect of the drug or from relief or avoidance of withdrawal.

Confidentiality of consultation

When examining and treating a patient who is using illicit drugs and who may have been involved in prohibited activities in order to fund the illicit drug use, the doctor must be particularly careful about confidentiality. This must not only be observed, but must be seen to be observed. As in other areas of medical practice, the doctor must attempt to respond simultaneously to the different expectations of the patient, family, community and professional organization. Only in the most extreme circumstances, where there a threat to the life of another person, is the doctor justified in breaching the essential confidentiality of a clinical consultation.

It is appropriate and necessary for the doctor to express concern about the patient's continuing criminal or other deviant activity, or their insistance on continuing to work, or to drive a motor vehicle. However, while the doctor may strongly urge the patient to stop doing something or to notify the relevant authorities of their alcohol/drug abuse, these authorities should not be informed by the doctor without the consent of the patient, except in exceptional circumstances where doctors' duty to the public outweighs their duty of confidentiality to the individual patient.

Notification of diseases and addiction

There is no longer need for notification of addiction but doctors dealing with drug abusers should complete a regional drug misuse database form as part of initial assessment and treatment. Infections are common among drug injectors; some must be notified as part of epidemiological surveillance. The precise regulations vary between countries, but statutory obligations or professional responsibility cover the notification of HIV, hepatitis B, and other recent hepatitis viruses.

Chapter 14.10

Assessing drug abuse and use of 'Brief interventions'

M. Farrell, I. Crome, P. Anderson, and J. Strang

The assessment of alcohol, drug, and smoking behaviour requires attention and time that doctors often feel unable to give. A thorough and detailed history will usually allow a comprehensive assessment of the impact of drug abuse on overall physical, psychological, and social well being.

Cigarette smokers are usually dependent on nicotine, while less than 10 per cent of all alcohol drinkers, but 35 per cent of heavy drinkers may be dependent. The detection of dependence upon alcohol, opiate, or benzodiazepines is important for appropriate ward management of the affected individuals so that acute withdrawal syndromes can be anticipated and detoxification carried out when necessary.

Screening

The checklist of questions about alcohol and drug taking provided below should be used in anyone identified as having a problem with these substances.

Alcohol and drug history

1. *Personal, developmental and family history:* childhood disruption, educational achievements, employment, marital, sexual, and forensic histories. Are any of them influenced by the patient's alcohol or drug consumption?
2. *Recent drinking and drug taking behaviours:* alcohol (units*) or other drug use in the past 24 hours, past month, and past 6 months.
3. *Drinking and drug use history:* age of first use, first regular use, first daily use. Routes of drug use for each drug. Withdrawal symptoms; tremor, night sweats or morning nausea, convulsions, and delirium tremens. Other features of dependence; tolerance, compulsion to drink, prominence of drink-seeking behaviour, rapid reinstatement after abstinence. Inquire about periods of abstinence. Inquire if the patient ever injected, shared needles, and the pattern of injecting and risk-taking behaviour.
4. *Previous treatment history*; Any consultation with a general practitioner or a specialist alcohol or drug treatment service?
5. Related problems:
   (i) Physical: e.g. gastritis, hepatitis, cirrhosis, abscess, trauma, neuropathy, pancreatitis.
   (ii) Psychological: e.g. anxiety, depression, phobias, delusions, suicidal ideation or suicide attempts, hallucinations.
   (iii) Social: e.g. marital, occupational, or financial problems.

Smoking history

Patients are usually able to give an accurate account of how much and what they smoke. It is important to find out:

IN THE LAST MONTH: have you had an alcoholic drink at all? YES NO If YES: Please answer A and B

(A) About how often have you had any of the following types of drink over the last month

Beer, lager, cider, etc. :	NOT AT ALL	LESS THAN ONCE A WEEK	1–2 TIMES A WEEK	3–4 TIMES A WEEK	5–6 TIMES A WEEK	EVERY DAY
Wine, sherry, vermouth etc. :	NOT AT ALL	LESS THAN ONCE A WEEK	1–2 TIMES A WEEK	3–4 TIMES A WEEK	5–6 TIMES A WEEK	EVERY DAY
Gin, vodka, rum, brandy, whisky, etc. :	NOT AT ALL	LESS THAN ONCE A WEEK	1–2 TIMES A WEEK	3–4 TIMES A WEEK	5–6 TIMES A WEEK	EVERY DAY

(B) When you've had a drink over the last month how much of the following types of drink have you usually had a day (i.e. 24-h period)

Pints of beer, lager cider, etc. :	NONE	$\frac{1}{2}$–1	1–2	3	4–5	6–7	8 or more
Glasses of wine, sherry vermouth, etc. :	NONE	1–2	3–4	5–6	7–9	11–14	15 or more
Measures of spirits (gin, vodka rum, brandy, whisky, etc.) :	NONE	1–2	3–4	5–6	7–9	11–14	15 or more

Fig. 1 Quantity frequency questionaire to measure alcohol consumption.

1. Average daily cigarette consumption.
2. Time from waking to smoking first cigarette as indicator of nicotine dependence.
3. Description of previous attempts to stop smoking (use of nicotine patches).
4. Motivation to stop smoking.
5. Related problems, such as respiratory, cardiovascular complications.

Screening and the use of 'Brief interventions'

Quantity Frequency Questionnaires

Standard questions provide a simple, and often reliable method of finding out how much a patient drinks. Simply asking patients, 'How much do you drink?' tends to elicit responses, such as 'not a lot', 'just occasionally'.

In order to assess the true amount of alcohol that a patient drinks each week in units, ask the following questions:

- 'On average, how many days a week do you have an alcoholic drink?'
- 'On average, on a day when you have had an alcoholic drink, how much do you usually have? (half-pints of beer, lager, cider, glasses of wine, sherry or vermouth, and singles of spirits).'

A written record of the declared alcohol intake for a typical week and the patient's total weekly alcohol consumption should be entered in the medical notes (Fig. 1).

Alcohol-Use-Disorders Identification Test

The World Health Organization (WHO) has developed a simple instrument for use with people with early signs of alcohol related problems. The WHO core screening instrument consists of ten simple questions (Fig. 2).

Table 1 Menu of strategies for 'Brief Motivational Interviewing'

1.	Opening strategy: lifestyle, stresses, alcohol and drug abuse
2.	Opening strategy: health and substance abuse
3.	A typical day/session
4.	The good things and the less good things
5.	Providing information
6.	The future and the present
7.	Exploring concerns
8.	Helping with decision making

Other measures of psychosocial consequences of drinking

These include the 25-item Michigan Alcoholism Screening Test (MAST) and its shortened 10-item version and the 4-item CAGE questionnaire (see OTM3, p. 17). The CAGE is a more sensitive instrument than the MAST questionnaire for identifying the individual with drinking problems in general hospital and general practice populations. Two or more positive replies to the CAGE questionnaire are said to identify the problem drinker. Although it is reported in general hospital settings to have a high sensitivity (85 per cent) and specificity (89 per cent), the CAGE instrument provides less

*1 unit (10g alcohol) = 1 glass of table wine = half-pint of beer, lager, or cider = 1 measure of spirits = 1 measure of sherry or vermouth. Standard bottle of spirits = 32 units; standard bottle of wine = 8 units; can of extra-strong lager = 4 units)

Tick the number that comes closest to the patient's answer.

1. How often do you have a drink containing alcohol?

(0) NEVER	(1) MONTHLY OR LESS	(2) TWO TO FOUR TIMES A MONTH	(3) FOUR OR MORE TIMES A WEEK	(4) FOUR OR MORE TIMES A WEEK

2.* How many drinks containing alcohol do you have on a typical day when you are drinking? [CODE NUMBER OF STANDARD DRINKS]

(0) 1 OR 2	(1) 3 OR 4	(2) 5 OR 6	(3) 7 OR 8	(4) 10 OR MORE

3. How often do you have six or more drinks on one occasion?

(0) NEVER	(1) LESS THAN MONTHLY	(2) MONTHLY	(3) WEEKLY	(4) DAILY OR ALMOST DAILY

4. How often during the last year have you found that you were not able to stop drinking once you had started?

(0) NEVER	(1) LESS THAN MONTHLY	(2) MONTHLY	(3) WEEKLY	(4) DAILY OR ALMOST DAILY

5. How often during the last year have you failed to do what was normally expected from you because of drinking?

(0) NEVER	(1) LESS THAN MONTHLY	(2) TWO TO FOUR TIMES A MONTH	(3) FOUR OR MORE TIMES A WEEK	(4) FOUR OR MORE TIMES A WEEK

6. How often during the last year have you needed a first drink in the morning to get yourself going after a heavy drinking session?

(0) NEVER	(1) LESS THAN MONTHLY	(2) MONTHLY	(3) WEEKLY	(4) DAILY OR ALMOST DAILY

7. How often during the last year have you had a feeling of guilt or remorse after drinking?

(0) NEVER	(1) LESS THAN MONTHLY	(2) MONTHLY	(3) WEEKLY	(4) DAILY OR ALMOST DAILY

8. How often during the last year have you been unable to remember what happened the night before because you had been drinking?

(0) NEVER	(1) LESS THAN MONTHLY	(2) MONTHLY	(3) WEEKLY	(4) DAILY OR ALMOST DAILY

9. Have you or someone else been injured as a result of your drinking?

(0) NO	(2) YES, BUT NOT IN THE LAST YEAR	(4) YES, DURING THE LAST YEAR

10. Has a relative or friend or a doctor or other health worker, been concerned about your drinking or suggested you cut down?

(0) NO	(2) YES, BUT NOT IN THE LAST YEAR	(4) YES, DURING THE LAST YEAR

* In determining the response categories it has been assumed that one 'drink' contains 10 g alcohol. In countries where the alcohol content of a standard drink differs by more than 25 per cent and 10 g, the response category should be modified accordingly.

Record sum of individual item scores here ______.

Fig. 2 World Health Organization Core Screening Instrument.

information for intervention than the longer AUDIT instrument (Fig. 2).

Biological markers

The most commonly used biological markers of excessive alcohol consumption are Mean Cell Volume (MCV) and δ-glutamyl transpeptidase (γ-GT). Of these, γ-GT is a better predictor than MCV. Although the MCV is related to alcohol consumption, a raised MCV is very unreliable as a screening instrument. The proportion of heavy drinkers who have an MCV over 98 ranges somewhere between 20 and 30 per cent and the false-positive rate is between 4 and 6 per cent.

Increased γ-GT activity in the serum can be observed after a few weeks of high alcohol intake but may also be raised by single high dose binges. Following reduction in drinking, serum γ-GT levels rapidly fall, returning to normal levels within 2 to 4 weeks. The rise of the enzyme in the serum is primarily due to hepatic enzyme inductions. Nevertheless, γ-GT is not good as a screening instrument. Only about 50 per cent of heavy drinkers have a level above 50 iu/l. The false-positive rate is between 10 and 20 per cent. Other causes of a raised γ-GT include other diseases of the liver, biliary tract, and pancreas.

Carbohydrate deficient transferrin (CDT)

A newer test measures the proportion of transferrin in serum deficient in one of its carbohydrate chains. The specificity of CDT as a marker of heavy drinking may exceed that of γ-GT because other inflammatory diseases of the liver are less likely to cause a raised CDT. However, this test is currently more costly and requires more evaluation.

Drugs can be detected in body fluids. Urine is usually preferred for drug screening because of the ease and safety of collection and the wider window of coverage than blood for cannabis and also for opiates and stimulants. Recently hair analysis has been developed to determine exposure to opiates and stimulants over longer periods.

Detectability is influenced by the pharmacokinetics of the drug. Heroin and cocaine with short half-lives will be detectable in urine for a shorter period than more slowly eliminated drugs such as methadone. Cannabis may be excreted in the urine for at least a week, particularly when it has been consumed in high doses over prolonged periods. Recently, plasma assays of methadone have been used to assess adequacy of dosage. Anticonvulsants and anti-tuberculosis drugs may accelerate the metabolism of methadone, and dosage adjustment may also be required during pregnancy.

'Brief intervention' for potentially hazardous alcohol consumption

Potentially hazardous alcohol consumption has been defined as a consumption of 350 g (35 units) or more per week for men and 210 g (21 units) or more per week for women. Firm but friendly advice should be given to cut down. The patient should be reassured that they are not thought to be an 'alcoholic', but that if they go on drinking as much, health damage, and work and personal problems, might develop.

A patient's target should be to keep below a weekly limit of 210 g (21 units) of alcohol for men and 140 g (14 units) of alcohol for women. Some people will want or need to abstain altogether. It is important that the patient agrees that the target is realistic; for someone drinking very heavily, a higher interim target might be set with a longer term aim to cut down further.

The patient's motivation will be strengthened if they know that their progress will be followed. Self-help booklets (Health Education Authority) are available in many counties, which can supplement the doctor's advice. These booklets give the patient some advice on preparing to cut down on alcohol and some tips on how this can be achieved.

'Brief intervention' for harmful alcohol consumption

Alcohol consumption can result in physical, social, or psychological harm. Abnormal liver function tests confirm this. 'Brief motivational interviewing' recognizes the fact that most patients are ambivalent about changing their alcohol consumption. Those who are not ready to change may become defensive if pressed directly.

Ambivalence is a common and normal experience. For people with a drinking problem, there is a conflict between indulgence and restraint, which appears to increase as they approach the moment of decision-making. The most effective way to help them is to explore this conflict and to encourage them to express their reasons for concern and the arguments for change. In a recent study of excessive drinkers in hospital, 29 per cent were not ready to change, 26 per cent were ready, and 45 per cent were ambivalent. The doctor's task is to establish the patient's degree of readiness for change and then to select a strategy appropriate to this level of motivation.

There is a menu of eight strategies (Table 1), each of which takes 5–15 minuts to work through. Successive strategies demand greater willingness to change on the part of the patient. This patient-centred approach to negotiating behavioural change may be new to many doctors. Although more time consuming, it is more effective than simply giving advice, and will ultimately be of more benefit to the patient.

Patients who show signs of dependence on, or serious physical illness from, alcohol consumption will require a different approach, such as abstinence and referral to a more specialized service.

Further reading

Anderson, P. (1991). *Management of drinking problems.* WHO Regional Publications, European Series, No 32. World Health Organization Regional Office for Europe, Copenhagen.

Bush, B., Shaw, S., Cleary, P., Delbanco, T.L., and Aronson, M.D. (1987). Screening for alcohol abuse using the CAGE questionnaire. *American Journal of Medicine*, **82**, 231–5.

Institute of Medicine. (1990). *Broadening the base of treatment for alcohol problems.* Washington, National Academy Press.

Miller, W.R.and Rollnick, S. (1991). *Motivational interviewing. Preparing people to change addictive behaviour.* New York, The Guilford Press.

Watson, R.R. (ed.). (1989). *Diagnosis of alcohol abuse.* Florida, CRC Press.

World Health Organization.(1992). *AUDIT, The Alcohol Use Disorders Identification Test. Guidelines for use in primary health care.* (WHO/PSA/92.4). Geneva, World Health Organization.

Chapter 14.11

Reducing the harm resulting from drug abuse

J. Strang

Harm reduction has been brought to the fore by HIV and the need to prevent the spread of blood-borne pathogens. Strategies must be identified and promoted that will lead to the reduction in specific harmful effects of drug abuse to the individual and to the public in general. This approach requires consideration of the broader population of drug takers. The general practitioner or hospital doctor who identifies alcohol or drug abuse only when it is the presenting feature will miss many opportunities to benefit the health of individuals and the public at an early stage. Only a minority of problem drinkers or drug takers are identified and put in contact with specialist treatment services. It is up the clinical acumen of doctors working in a general medical setting to suspect and detect alcohol or drug problems in patients who are referred for other reasons.

'Brief intervention': advice on smoking and other drug use

The model of 'brief interventions' for alcohol (see Chapter 14.10) can also be applied with equal effect to other areas of substance abuse. Doctors are used to giving advice about reducing or stopping smoking. This is based on emphasizing the risk to health and the benefits from changing. In the case of other drugs, different advice is offered for different patterns of behaviour. The 'never user' should be warned about the risks of starting, the occasional user should be warned about the risks and associated health and social complications of moving to regular use, and the regular user should be warned about the risks, and urged to stop or, if not wishing to stop, to reduce to a level at which the complications were less serious.

The drug injector should be warned about the risks of this practice, the need for hepatitis B vaccination, and scrupulous hygienic injecting technique.

Chapter 14.12

Physical complications of drug abuse

M. Farrell, D. Hawkins, and R. Brettle

Drug abuse is associated with great morbidity. A full understanding of the nature and extent of this should facilitate appropriate responses. Access to medical care should be promoted. There may be acute complications of intoxication (see Section 18) or chronic complications as a result of end-organ damage or as a result of the complications of the method by which the drug is taken (technique specific hazards) such as infection by HIV and hepatitis viruses from injecting drugs.

Technique specific hazards

Lung cancer from tobacco smoking is probably the commonest technique specific hazard globally. Hazards of injecting are usually related to poor sterile and injecting technique, or, despite careful aseptic precautions, from normal skin flora or contamination of the drug itself. Guidelines have been issued for cleaning injecting equipment 'works', should sterile equipment not be available. However, no technique other than perhaps autoclaving is guaranteed to be effective against all possible pathogens and so harm reduction rather than harm elimination is the best that can be achieved.

Infections

Soft tissues

Commensal skin bacteria such as *Staphylococcus aureus* and *Streptococcus pyogenes* may infect an injection site leading to cellulitis and thrombophlebitis. Antibiotics are needed together with incision and drainage of an abscess. Large abscesses may lead to extensive skin ulceration requiring debridement and even skin grafting. Muscle abscesses can lead to the serious complications of necrotzing fasciitis and pyomyositis.

Septicaemia

It is likely that bacteraemia commonly accompanies injecting episodes but this is usually contained by the immune system. However, septicaemia may develop leading to endocarditis. Septicaemia should be suspected in any drug injector who develops a fever. Appropriate cultures should be set up before starting parenteral broad spectrum antibiotics. Systemic fungal infection, especially with Candida, may result from the use of contaminated heroin or from the lemon juice used to dissolve the drug. Candidal ophthalmitis is a serious complication; early systemic antifungal therapy (e.g. with amphotericin) should be instituted if this is suspected.

Endocarditis (see Chapter 2.25)

Endocarditis is a relatively uncommon but very serious illness among injecting drug users. HIV positive users may have a wider variety of, often multiple, infecting organisms. *Staphylococcus aureus* is found in about two-thirds of cases, *Streptococcus viridans* in 20 per cent, and a variety of Gram- negative bacilli, and fungi. Tricuspid involvement with shedding of emboli into the pulmonary circulation may lead to dyspnoea, cough, haemoptysis, and pleuritic chest pain. Mortality is usually less than 5 per cent if the causative organism(s) are identified early and treated but among HIV positive individuals it is 24 per cent.

Hepatitis (see Chapter 5.31)

This is becoming the commonest and most serious complication of injecting drug use. The most important causes are hepatitis viruses B, D, and C. There may be no history of acute hepatitis. Markers of hepatitis B infection show that some 50–80 per cent of injecting drug users have been exposed worldwide. Chronic carriers make up about 5–10 per cent and further transmission, both sexually and parenterally, is a common event as the virus is often present in very high copy numbers in blood and other body fluids. Immunosuppression by HIV increases the proportion of chronic carriers. In view of the risk of chronic liver disease, cirrhosis, and liver cell carcinoma, immunization should be offered to all susceptible drug users.

Hepatitis C is even more seroprevalent than hepatitis B among injectors. Possibly 20–30 per cent of carriers will go on to develop chronic liver disease, including hepatocellular carcinoma, although this may take several decades.

Continuing alcohol consumption speeds progression of liver disease.

Pulmonary problems

The commonest lung problem in drug abusers is bacterial pneumonia, probably related to heavy cigarette smoking and general debilitation associated with their lifestyle. Pulmonary tuberculosis is also common. Recurrent bacterial pneumonia and pulmonary tuberculosis contribute to morbidity and mortality in HIV positive patients and are now classified as AIDS diagnoses by CDC.

Inadvertent penetration of the lung when injecting into neck veins may cause pneumothorax. Injection of inert particulate matter such as talc may cause pulmonary hypertension or granulomatosis.

Orthopaedic problems

Septic arthritis and osteomyelitis may result from septicaemia or from direct infection or extension from an adjacent abscess. Osteomyelitis may be caused by emboli from a distant infected focus; common sites of involvement are thoracic and lumbar vertebrae.

Renal problems

Glomerulonephritis in long-term injectors is attributable to staphylococcal and other bacterial infections or chronic hepatitis B or hepatitis C (cryoglobulinaemia and membranoproliferative glomerulonephritis).

Other injecting complications

Vascular complications

Long-standing injecting drug abusers frequently have problems with venous access and may become quite ingenious in their search for veins. Injecting into the femoral vein risks deep venous thrombosis complicated by pulmonary embolism or venous gangrene. Anticoagulation is indicated. Expanding abscesses must be decompressed if contributing to venous occlusion.

Inadvertent arterial injection may damage the vessel wall at the needle entry point leading to arterial occlusion or cause local vasospasm from irritant materials or peripheral embolism of injected particular matter. Mycotic (infected) aneurysms may develop some distance from the injection site. In cases of vasospasm or peripheral embolism initial treatment is with heparin, low molecular weight dextran, or sympathetic nerve blockade. However, surgical intervention may be needed. Analgesia for intensely painful ischaemic lesions in dependent drug abusers can be difficult. For this reason, decisions about pain relief are best made by close collaboration between medical and surgical teams and the substance abuse service.

Repeated episodes of lymphangitis associated with 'skin popping' may result in lymphatic obstruction and chronic lymphoedema, characteristically on the back of the hand. This may persist long after stopping the abuse of drugs.

Substance specific complications

Opiate overdose

Opiate overdose may be deliberate or accidental, in combination with alcohol and benzodiazepam or following the use of heroin of unexpected purity or when a period of abstinence had led to reduced tolerance. This often arises when prisoners with a history of drug dependence are released from custody. They should be warned as part of their prison education and rehabilitation.

Opiates may cause coma, respiratory depression, and pinpoint pupils. Reversal with naloxone may be dramatic (see Chapter 18.1) but toxicity may recur if they have taken a longer-acting opiate such as methadone and continuous infusion of naloxone should be considered in the presence of methadone users.

Poor response to naloxone suggests other CNS-depressant drugs. Patients should be supported in intensive care as long as necessary.

Stimulants (amphetamines, ecstasy, and cocaine)

Ecstasy (3,4-methylene-dideoxymethamphetamine), a synthetic amphetamine derivative, can cause anorexia, tachycardia, paranoia, irritability, depression, and bruxism (see Section 18). However, severe reactions are unpredictable and may be precipitated by physical exertion as in dances or 'raves' when fatal convulsions, collapse, hyperpyrexia, disseminated intravascular coagulation, rhabdomyolysis, and acute renal failure have occurred. The risk of hyperthermia is well recognized by drug agencies. The advice given to those who use the drug is to wear loose clothing, to drink liquids, and to stop dancing when they feel exhausted. Some clubs provide 'chill-out' rooms with seats and non-alcoholic liquids. Urgent management includes control of convulsions, measurement of core temperature, rapid rehydration, and cooling.

Cocaine has many dangerous effects (see Chapter 18.1).

Sedatives

Benzodiazepines and barbiturate abusers commonly present for management of intoxication or withdrawal (see Section 18). Injection of some benzodiazepines (e.g. temazepam) can cause arterial occlusion or compartment syndromes, sometimes requiring limb amputation. Use of high doses of intravenous benzodiazepines is associated with other injecting and risk taking behaviour associated with transmission of vital hepatitis and HIV.

Respiratory effects

Opiate overdose can cause acute pulmonary oedema or respiratory depression. Heroin can precipitate asthma and bronchospasm. Sedative hypnotics may depress respiration, while hallucinogens may cause hyperventilation ('bad trips' and 'flashbacks')

Volatile substance abuse (see Section 18)

These include butane gas (lighter fluid, aerosols), solvents, toluene, dry cleaning fluid, typewriter correction fluid, glues, and fire extinguisher contents. Users, often children, risk sudden death from cardiac arrhythmias during an episode of 'sniffing'. Other dangers are asphyxia when using a plastic bag over the face, inhalation of vomit, or traumatic falls and fatal accidents while intoxicated. Laryngospasm may occur as a result of spraying aerosols into the back of the pharynx. Many deaths have been caused by aerosol and butane abuse. Many agents are highly inflammable and severe burning injuries occur. In the UK, up to 140 young people die from volatile solvent abuse each year.

Other types of behaviour that may lead to physical harm

The lifestyle associated with the acquisition of illicit drugs increases the risk of trauma and contact with the criminal justice system. Sexual activity may be disinhibited by almost any drug and less attention paid to 'safer sex' practices to prevent HIV, viral hepatitis and other sexually transmitted infections. Sex may be exchanged for drugs. In the USA, female crack cocaine users have a particularly high HIV seroprevalence. To minimize the risks of these additional sources of infection-related morbidity, it is important for those looking after drug abusers to maintain close links with family planning services and sexually transmitted disease clinics. Obstetric and neonatal morbidity is increased in drug abusers and early attendance at antenatal clinics should be encouraged, to allow stabilization of drug use.

Further reading

Banks, A. and Waller, T.A. (1988). *Drug misuse: a practical handbook for GPs.* Blackwell Scientific Publications, Oxford.

Brettle, R., Farrell, M., and Strang, J.S. (1990). The clinical manifestations of HIV in drug users. In: *AIDs and drug misuse* (ed. J.S. Strang and G. Stimson). Routledge, London.

Farrell, M. (1991). Physical complications of drug misuse. In: *International handbook of addiction behaviour* (ed. I. Glass). Routledge, London.

Chapter 14.13

Nutritional deficiency syndromes complicating alcohol abuse

T. J. Peters

Although the application of multiple biochemical and haematological tests to alcohol abusers will show evidence of deficiency of one or more nutrients in 25–50 per cent of cases, it is only in a small proportion that this becomes a clinical problem. The *Wernicke-Korsakoff syndrome* is the most important. It may be subdivided into neurological disorder, Wernicke's disease, and the psychiatric Korsakoff syndrome. Although one or other clinical pictures may predominate, there is frequently considerable overlap and progression between these two disorders. They have a common pathology, with severe neuronal loss in the mammillary bodies and associated lesions around the aqueduct and fourth ventricle. Lesions of the vermis and anterior cerebellar lobules are common.

The biochemical basis is thiamine deficiency. Patients with Wernicke's disease display the triad of ophthalmoplegia, most commonly nystagmus and impaired occular abduction, ataxia most predominantly of cerebellar type, and a confusional state. The last predominates in the Korsakoff syndrome, and is characterized by disorders of behaviour and mental function. The patient shows apathy for mental and physical activity and impaired awareness and concentration with deranged perceptual functions. Some patients show a clinical picture complicated by features of withdrawal syndrome. The classical Korsakov amnesic syndrome, which may persist after vitamin replacement and prolonged abstinence, comprises severe antegrade and retrograde amnesia with confabulation and lack of insight and is a serious condition, with a poor long-term prognosis.

The clinical findings may be complex or dominated by a single clinical feature. Clinical evidence of vitamin deficiency (e.g. oral or labial inflammation), cardiovascular disorder (e.g. hypotension), high output cardiac failure (e.g. beriberi), and peripheral neuropathy may assist in alerting to the diagnosis. Diagnosis is confirmed by assays of the thiamine-dependent erythrocyte enzyme transketolase, whose activity is often reduced to half normal values. Restoration of enzyme activity by prior incubation of the red homogenate with thiamine pyrophosphate is more discriminating. The classical test in which an abnormal rise in venous pyruvate followed a glucose load is obsolete and dangerous. Treatment with thiamine, both oral and parenteral, should not be delayed while awaiting the results of the biochemical investigations (see below). Intravenous glucose can precipitate the acute syndrome.

Alcoholic cerebellar degeneration

This is an important, but rare, complication of chronic alcohol abuse caused mainly by prolonged spirit drinking accompanied by a poor nutritional intake. There is gross ataxia, particularly of the lower limbs, due to atrophy of the anterosuperior lobules and vermis of the cerebellum. Histopathologically, there is Purkinje cell loss. Modern imaging techniques, particularly MRI, may demonstrate cerebellar atrophy. The syndrome is probably part of the clinical spectrum of the Wernicke-Korsakov syndrome and may, at least in the early stages, before the degeneration is apparent macroscopically, respond well to thiamine treatment.

A common finding in alcohol abusers, peripheral neuropathy ranges from purely subjective symptoms of paraesthesiae to a severe distal combined sensory–motor neuropathy. The neuropathy is due to a variable combination of vitamin deficiency and chronic alcohol toxicity. The lower limbs are usually involved more severely and more frequently than upper limbs: cranial nerves are rarely involved. Tendon reflexes are lost in approximately half the patients. Foot and wrist drop, distal muscle weakness and wasting, and positive signs on detailed sensory testing may be found. It is useful to distinguish the neuropathy with secondary muscle wasting from the common proximal muscle metabolic myopathy.

Assessment of vitamin deficiency by erythrocyte enzyme assays, (transketolase (thiamine), aspartate aminotransferase (pyridoxine), and glutathione reductase (riboflavin)) will usually show a multiple deficiency, particularly if the more sensitive *in vitro* activation studies are performed.

Treatment by immediate parenteral vitamin supplements and a successful abstinence programme with physical rehabilitation will usually lead to considerable, if not complete, recovery, but this may take many months. Alcohol abusers are candidates for other forms of neuropathy (eg, carcinomatous, viral, traumatic, and vascular nerve damage).

Pellagra is an unusual complication of alcohol abuse with inadequate vitamin intake, particularly of niacin and tryptophan-containing proteins. It is not uncommon among raw spirit drinkers in third-world countries, who have combined vitamin and protein deficiency. Diagnosis is supported by assays of urinary nicotinic acid and its metabolites and demonstration of amino acid deficiencies, most notably tryptophan. Treatment is by multiple vitamin replacement, principally oral nicotinic acid or, if necessary, parenteral nicotinamide, in addition to a high protein diet, particularly of animal derived proteins.

Alcohol–tobacco amblyopia is a rare, but important, complication of alcohol misuse, combined with nutritional deficiencies, including vitamin B_{12}. It is most likely a complication of optic neuritis with impaired visual acuity and visual field defects, and usually improves with multiple vitamin therapy.

Miscellaneous disorders

Cerebral dementia is a frequent finding in chronic alcohol abusers: this may be only discernible on detailed psychological testing or may progress to severe dementia with dilated ventricles and marked cortical atrophy, most strikingly demonstrated by CT and MRI scanning. It is claimed that alcohol abuse is one of the commonest causes of presenile dementia. The pathogenic mechanism appears to be an alcohol-mediated neuronal loss. Interestingly, abstinence can be accompanied by both cognitive and neuroradiographic improvement.

Central pontine myelinolysis is a rare, but often fatal, disorder associated with alcohol abuse, in which there is extensive demyelination of the pons. The patient has quadriplegia with psuedobulbar palsy and often other features of CNS damage. The lesions may be strikingly demonstrated by MRI scanning. The pathogenic mechanism is unclear, but several cases have been reported in patients with hyponatraemia, particularly with rapid changes in electrolyte levels (see Chapter 12.2).

Marchiafava-Bignami syndrome is due to alcohol-associated demyelination of the corpus callosum, and occurs in adult male alcoholics with a varied clinical picture indicating multiple cortical dysfunction. Neuroradiographic imaging can demonstrate the lesions in life which are often associated with other features of alcohol-related CNS damage.

Fetal alcohol syndrome is considered to be the commonest single cause of mental handicap. Maternal alcohol abuse within the first 4 weeks of conception is associated with craniofacial abnormalities, including microphthalmia, elongated mid-face, long upper lip with poorly developed philtrum, and CNS involvement with intellectual impairment and development delay. Alcohol abuse at other stages of pregnancy may result in intellectual auditory and visual deficits, specific learning difficulties, and hyperkinetic syndromes in infancy. Maternal alcohol abuse can also be associated with a variety of cardiovascular, hepatic, and musculoskeletal defects in the infant. The pathogenic mechanism is unclear. Acetaldehyde formed in the placenta, protein-calorie malnutrition, associated vitamin and zinc deficiency, and a synergism with heavy tobacco usage have been implicated. Clinical studies indicate that up to a half of women drinking heavily during pregnancy have affected offspring. Even social drinking has been associated with fetal abnormalities, including an increased risk of abortion. Clearly prevention is a major public-health challenge.

Further reading

Charness, M.E., Simon, R.P., and Greenberg, D.A. (1989). Ethanol and the nervous system. *New England Journal of Medicine.* **321**, 442–54.

Peters, T.J. and Edwards, G. (eds.) (1994). Alcohol misuse. *British Medical Bulletin*, **50**, no. 1.

Chapter 14.14

Management of withdrawal syndromes

A. R. Johns

Psychological and pharmacological interventions are used to relieve withdrawal symptoms and prevent complications, including relapses. The general principles are as follows.

As a first step, every patient should be thoroughly assessed; relevant history, mental state examination and physical examination should be completed. Diagnostic tests are essential, either to identify complications such as liver disease and infection, or to confirm the recent history of consumption of drugs or alcohol. It is very important to appreciate the hopes and fears of the patient. Ambivalence is common. This may be due not only to reluctance to abstain, but also to fear of withdrawal symptoms and anxiety about coping when drug-free. Withdrawal symptoms may be more prominent in those who are anxious or depressed.

Psychological interventions are important. Brief counselling may cover support and practical issues. Relapse-prevention is an approach which aims to equip the patient to deal with situations, moods, and thoughts which could lead to relapse. The patient may be asked to keep a daily record of withdrawal symptoms, predominant mood, and activities undertaken. Self-support groups such as Alcoholics Anonymous, and Narcotics Anonymous, can be invaluable. The patient's family or partner can also be enlisted to give support.

The doctor's approach and attitude is important. Moralizing will only undermine the patient's self-esteem. There should be early agreement about the prescribing regime, frequency of contact, and the consequences of the abuse of drugs or alcohol. A written treatment plan can serve as a reminder of what was agreed.

Many of the drugs used in the management of withdrawal states can also induce dependence. In the UK, doctors should be aware of *Drug Misuse and Dependence: Guidelines on Clinical Management* (DoH 1999) and requirements for prescribing controlled drugs as summarised in the most recent edition of the *British National Formulary.*

Clinical management of withdrawal syndromes

Alcohol

The withdrawal syndrome

The initial symptoms are tremors, nausea, sweating, and mood changes such as anxiety, agitation or depression. Vomiting, diarrhoea and tachycardia may be present. These symptoms usually appear within 6 h of stopping alcohol, peak at 48 h, and subside over a week. Grand-mal type seizures ('rum fits') may appear in the first 12 to 24 h of withdrawal. Risk factors include severe alcohol dependence, concomitant abuse of sedative drugs, or previous experience of withdrawal fits. About 5 per cent of patients show delirium tremens ('the DTs') characterized by delirium, hallucinations, and tremor with tachycardia, sweating, and hypertension. The symptoms fluctuate but peak on the third to the fourth day of withdrawal.

Management

Patients with mild withdrawal symptoms usually respond to reassurance and practical advice. However, a reducing course of sedative medication is indicated if the recent consumption was more than 15 units a day for more than 10 days, or if withdrawal symptoms are more marked or if there is a previous history of convulsions or delirium. Most patients can be managed in their home or in a clinic, provided that social and medical support is adequate. Daily review by the patient's partner or a health worker allows for support and monitoring. Sedatives should be withheld if alcohol has been taken. Indications for admission include severe withdrawal symptoms or associated illness, a previous history of convulsions or delirium tremens.

Benzodiazepines are the treatment of choice. For outpatients, use chlordiazepoxide 20–30 mg four times daily or diazepam 10 mg four times daily in the first 36 hours, reducing to nil over 5 days. For inpatients, a higher starting dose may be titrated against symptoms such as agitation or tremors, reducing over 7 days.

Chlormethiazole is as effective, but dangerous in patients who continue to misuse alcohol. It is not recommended for unsupervised use by outpatients or in the community. As a guide, the starting dose is three capsules (each containing 192 mg chlormethiazole base) four times a day, reducing over not more than 9 days.

Carbamazepine has no abuse potential and is as effective as benzodiazepines, but 10 per cent of patients show side-effects limiting its use. A suggested schedule is 200 mg/day in divided doses, increasing to 400 mg/day by day 3 and tapering off by day 8.

Management of complications

Severe alcohol dependence carries a risk of Wernicke's encephalopathy. A high-potency multivitamin preparation such as Pabrinex® should be given (a pair of Pabrinex I/V high potency ampoules contain thiamine, 250 mg, and other vitamins). A pair of ampoules may be given by slow intravenous injection, daily for 5 days. There is a low risk of anaphylaxis. For less severely dependent individuals, 200 mg thiamine hydrochloride should be given daily for a week.

Patients at risk of withdrawal seizures require a loading dose of chlordiazepoxide on admission. Phenytoin may be added if there is a previous history of epilepsy or recurrent multiple fits. Seizures that are not self-limiting usually respond to diazepam (as Diazemuls®), 10 mg intravenously over 5 min, repeated if needed after 5 min.

Delirium tremens requires energetic intervention. Chlormethiazole infusion (0.8 per cent) may be given intravenously at a rate of 40–100 ml (320–800 mg) over 5 to 10 min, continued as necessary at a reduced rate, depending on the patient's response. Close observation is needed to ensure that an accumulation of the drug does not lead to respiratory depression or coma. Alternatively, use oral chlordiazepoxide 100–200 mg/day or diazepam 50—100 mg/day. For severe agitation give doperidol or haloperidol, 10 mg intramuscularly. Fluids should be given sparingly and electrolyte imbalance may require correction. The patient should be nursed in a well-illuminated room to prevent disorientation.

Medication to prevent relapse

Disulfiram causes nausea, dyspnoea, and headache 15–20 minutes after drinking alcohol. Awareness or actual experience of these effects is aversive. When combined with specialist advice and community support, it can be an effective adjunctive therapy. Start with daily loading doses of 800 mg, 600 mg, 400 mg, and then continue with 200 mg/day for up to 6 months. Alcohol challenge can be fatal and must be avoided. The patient must be warned to avoid alcohol in foods or medicines.

Opiates

The opiate withdrawal syndrome

Withdrawal symptoms start with anxiety, restlessness, irritability, insomnia, and a craving for opiates. Yawning becomes frequent, with increased saliva, tears, and nasal and bronchial secretions. Sweating may be profuse. Piloerection leads to the appearance of 'goose-flesh'. Nausea and vomiting may be accompanied by anorexia, abdominal pain, and diarrhoea. The pupils are dilated. Sensations of diffuse bodily pains and of feeling cold occur. Mild elevations of blood pressure, body temperature, and respiratory rate may be observed. Symptoms may be expected to start within 8–16 hours for heroin, and within 24 hours for methadone. Acute symptoms may last a week, followed by fluctuating insomnia and craving which can persist for many weeks.

Management

Most opiate addicts will have attempted self-detoxification, but few succeed. Symptomatic medication is indicated for patients with mild dependency or those for whom an opiate prescription would be inappropriate, such as the younger patient.

Thioridazine and diphenoxylate/loperamide

Phenothiazines have useful antiemetic, sedative, and anticholinergic effects without addictive potential. Thioridazine is preferred because it carries a low risk of extrapyramidal side-effects. A dose of 25 mg twice a day and 50–75 mg at night for no more than 1–2 weeks should be prescribed, with a tapering of dose towards the end of this time. This may be combined with Lomotil® (diphenoxylate hydrochloride 2.5 mg, atropine sulphate 25 μg) or loperamide (loperamide hydrochloride 2 mg) for symptomatic relief of diarrhoea and colicky pain. The dose of each is two tablets four times daily for 3 to 4 days, reduced over two further days.

α-Adrenergic agonists

Clonidine (clonidine hydrochloride 0.1 mg) can suppress some of the autonomic signs of opiate withdrawal, but is less effective in providing subjective relief and has no effect on the duration of symptoms. Side-effects such as hypotension and sedation limit its use to supervised outpatient settings. Treatment starts with 0.2–0.4 mg/day in divided doses, increasing gradually to a maximum of 1.2 mg/day for up to 10 days, and is then tailed off. Many patients may not tolerate this dose and the medication should be withheld if the diastolic blood pressure falls below 60 mmHg.

Lofexidine (lofexidine hydrochloride, 0.2 mg) reduces opiate withdrawal symptoms without adverse sedative or hypotensive side-effects. The initial dose is 0.4 mg/day, increased to a maximum of 2.4 mg/day for 7 to 10 days, and then tapered off over 2–4 days.

α-Adrenergic agonists combined with opiate antagonists

Opiate antagonists precipitate severe withdrawal symptoms in dependent individuals. Clonidine ameliorates this response and, in combination with naltrexone, shortens withdrawal without worsening the symptoms. Following a naloxone challenge test (0.8 mg naloxone intramuscularly), give clonidine 0.1–0.3 mg. Naltrexone, 12.5 mg, is given later on the first day, followed by daily doses of 25 mg, 50 mg, 100 mg, and 100 mg on day 5. Clonidine is given in divided doses of up to 0.9 mg/day for 2 days, reducing to 0.3 mg/day on days 4 and 5; the dose is adjusted according to the intensity of withdrawal symptoms and signs of hypotension. This schedule should be initiated only by clinicians experienced in its use.

Sedative medication

Severe withdrawal symptoms can be eased by benzodiazepines, but these drugs have no specific effect on the opiate withdrawal syndrome and their misuse leads to dependence. However, anxiety, agitation, and insomnia will be reduced. Benzodiazepines may be useful when opiate prescribing is neither advisable nor permissible. A suggested regime is an 8-day reduction from diazepam 40–80 mg/day, the starting dose being adjusted in response to the severity of withdrawal symptoms.

Opiate detoxification

This involves the progressive reduction in dose of a drug such as methadone that has cross-tolerance with the opiate of misuse. The choice of medication is influenced by the needs of the patient, treatment setting, and by legal constraints on prescribing opiates. The prescriber has a duty to minimize the potential for misuse of pharmaceutical opiates by ensuring that the patient is not obtaining drugs from any other illicit or licit source, such as another doctor. Although most patients can be managed in the community or clinic, contact should be frequent enough to allow for close monitoring of progress, including the use of urinary drug tests. The possibility of misuse is further reduced by dispensing opiates for no more than a few days at a time.

Dihydrocodeine

Dihydrocodeine is effective in the management of mild to moderate opiate withdrawal symptoms. Generally, the starting dose should not exceed 8–12 (30 mg) tablets of dihydrocodeine a day. If withdrawal symptoms remain uncontrolled on such a dose, then alternative medication should be considered. The period of withdrawal may last for 2–6 weeks in the clinic or community, or for a week in inpatients.

Buprenorphine

Buprenorphine is a partial opiate agonist/antagonist with a long duration of action. Following dose assessment, opiate addicts may be stabilized on sublingual daily divided doses of 2–8 mg which may be tapered over 8 or more weeks. However there is concern about misuse of this drug among addicts.

Methadone

Methadone is a synthetic opiate with an action lasting longer than 24 hours. In the UK, methadone can be prescribed by any registered doctor, provided that the regulations on prescribing controlled drugs are adhered to. As an oral preparation ('Methadone mixture 1 mg/ml BNF') it is available as a coloured syrup which cannot readily be injected. Tablet and ampoule forms should generally not be prescribed without specialist advice.

Dose-assessment is recommended. This involves the witnessed consumption of a test dose of 10–20 mg methadone mixture when opiate withdrawal symptoms are apparent and the repeated administration of doses of 10 mg when symptoms recur, while the patient is observed for signs of intoxication. The 24-hour dose then becomes the baseline or stabilization dose. Most patients will be found to require a daily stabilization dose of less than 60 mg methadone.

The duration and effectiveness of the subsequent withdrawal is dependent on setting. As an inpatient, the dose may be reduced over 5–10 days. In an outpatient setting, dose reduction may occur over 2–4 weeks, but it is not advisable to prescribe for much longer without specialist advice. Withdrawal symptoms often peak when the last dose is given, and symptoms such as insomnia, episodic craving, and discomfort may last for weeks. Symptoms such as severe insomnia or anxiety may require medication such as thioridazine. Inpatient detoxification may be needed following repeated failure of outpatient interventions—other indications include associated physical or psychological problems, severity of withdrawal symptoms, or polydrug dependency.

Medication to prevent relapse

Naltrexone has a high affinity for the μ-opiate receptor and competitively prevents opiate-induced euphoria. Taking opiates is therefore unrewarding and craving for these drugs is reduced. Naltrexone administration may be a continuation of the rapid clonidine–naltrexone withdrawal schedule already referred to. Otherwise, naltrexone should not be given within 5–7 days after the last use of heroin, or 10–14 days after the last use of methadone. A challenge test involves giving 12.5 mg naltrexone orally. If there are no opiate withdrawal symptoms, prescribe naltrexone 25 mg twice a day for the first day followed by 50 mg/day. An alternative regime is to give 100 mg on Mondays and Wednesdays, and 150 mg on Fridays. Naltrexone should be avoided if liver function tests are abnormal.

Benzodiazepines

Benzodiazepines are not only the most commonly prescribed minor sedatives but are also widely misused by those taking alcohol, opiates, and other drugs.

The benzodiazepine withdrawal syndrome

There is a risk of withdrawal symptoms after use of benzodiazepines for more than a few weeks, after high-dose consumption, or prolonged use of a short half-life drug, such as lorazepam or temazepam. Tiredness, lassitude, impaired memory, and concentration are common. Perceptual changes include hypersensitivity to sound, light and touch, depersonalization, and derealization. The mood may be labile with depression and anxiety. Gastrointestinal upsets, anorexia, tremor, sleep disturbance with vivid dreams, and confusion are reported. Withdrawal convulsions may occur. Symptoms often fluctuate and usually last 1–6 weeks, but some may persist for months.

Management of benzodiazepine withdrawal

Abrupt discontinuation is dangerous. Most patients taking prescribed benzodiazepines may undergo withdrawal in the clinic or community. Any day-to-day variation in dose should be stabilized. Diazepam may be substituted if previous attempts to discontinue the shorter-acting benzodiazepines have failed; for example 10 mg of diazepam should be prescribed for every 1 mg of lorazepam. A 6-week withdrawal schedule is appropriate for most outpatients, although up to 12 weeks may be needed in difficult cases. Antidepressants may be needed in the later stages of the withdrawal. Psychological measures such as anxiety-management training and self-help group support are valuable.

Patients who are dependent on high doses of benzodiazepines and those with a history of severe withdrawal symptoms usually require inpatient management. Start by giving 10–20 mg of diazepam at 6-hourly intervals to achieve a daily dose which achieves stability without signs of intoxication. Reduction can then proceed over the next 14–21 days, or longer if there is a risk of severe symptoms, including convulsions. Ideally, the patient should be encouraged to remain in hospital for a further week when drug-free as, rarely, convulsions may occur in this period.

Barbiturates and other general sedatives

These include barbiturates, chlormethiazole, glutethamide, mepbromate, and methaqualone. Withdrawal features include tremor, agitation, delirium, and convulsions and inpatient detoxification is generally necessary. Specialist advice should be sought. Patients may be stabilized on phenobarbitone, 120 mg orally repeated after 1 hour if necessary, and then 6 hourly over the first day. A similar approach is suitable for the management of chlormethiazole withdrawal. The stabilization dose is 2–3 capsules (each containing 192 mg of the base), repeated after an hour if necessary and then 6 hourly as indicated. Once stabilization on any of these drugs has been continued for a few days, withdrawal may then proceed over 14–21 days.

Cocaine and other stimulants

Heavy use of cocaine may lead to depression, anxiety, and craving on withdrawal. Counselling with psychological and social support is the mainstay of treatment. Severe depressive symptoms may respond to fluoxetrine, but this may take nearly 2 weeks to have an effect. Amphetamine withdrawal leads to lethargy and low mood, which does not usually require symptomatic medication.

Tobacco

Withdrawal symptoms are seen within a day of stopping cigarette smoking. These are craving for nicotine, irritability, anxiety, poor concentration, restlessness, bradycardia, and increased appetite. Most symptoms resolve within 1 month, but craving, increased appetite, and weight gain may continue for 6 months.

Management of nicotine withdrawal and prevention of relapse

Simple advice from medical practitioners induces a small proportion of smokers to give up. The best treatment currently seems to be a combination of group support and nicotine chewing gum. A 4-week course of this sort helps up to 70 per cent of patients to stop smoking by the end of treatment, and up to 30 per cent to abstain for 1 year. Transdermal delivery of nicotine is now possible by use of a self-adhesive skin-patch. Daily patches of decreasing strength are applied over 3 to 4 weeks.

Further reading

Department of Health. (1999). *Drug misuse and dependence: guidelines on clinical management.* HMSO, London.

Chapter 14.15

The legal aspects of controlled drug prescribing

J. Strang

Drug prescribing—restrictions and regulations

(i) **Restrictions and regulations relating to the drug:** all Controlled Drugs (distinguished by the suffix CD in their entry in the British National Formulary) must be written in the doctor's own handwriting (except for phenobarbitone, or with doctors who have a special handwriting exemption*), must state the form and strength of the preparation, the dose, and the total quantity of the prescription in both words and figures. 'Repeat prescriptions' cannot be issued for Controlled Drugs.

For NHS practice in hospitals, a special form is available for prescribing most opiates and cocaine in the treatment of drug addiction. These include the facility for instructing the pharmacist to dispense in instalments. Since the late 1980s, equivalent prescription forms have been introduced for general practitioners, who may now also issue instructions for daily dispensing of these drugs when treating drug users.

(ii) **Restrictions and regulations relating to the particular patient:** diamorphine (heroin), cocaine, and the synthetic opiate dipipanone (which with cyclizine is available as Diconal) are prohibited drugs in the treatment of drug dependence. A doctor may use these drugs for other therapeutic purposes, although in a patient known to be a drug addict this might be ill-considered. For example, if analgesia is required in an opiate addict, it may be wiser and more appropriate to consider non-opiate drugs, an opiate other than heroin or dipipanone, or another approach to the problem.

(iii) **Restrictions and regulations relating to the doctor:** there are currently no special restrictions on the prescribing powers of doctors in the UK in their treatment of the drug dependence, apart from the barring of the prescribing of heroin, cocaine, or dipipanone (see above). Nevertheless, the doctor should be specially careful about prescribing drugs with a high-abuse potential, high black market value (especially the pharmaceutical opiates and synthetic opioids), and, in particular, drugs which may be injected despite being prescribed in an oral form, such as tablets of dextromoraminde (Palfium), buprenorphine (Temgesic), and capsules of temazepam. In the case of drug dependence where the use of injectable drugs is considered justifiable (either in the management of the drug dependence or for another reason) the general doctor should seek an opinion from a colleague specializing in the treatment of drug addiction.

*Doctors whose practice involves a large amount of prescribing of Controlled Drugs may apply for an exemption from this handwriting requirement.

Chapter 14.16

Strategies for managing drug and alcohol problems

M. Farrell and J. Strang

Community based interventions

After conducting a full assessment, the key initial task is to develop a coherent treatment plan that is realistic and appropriate to the needs of the patient. Why has the patient come for treatment and what can be achieved? What previous attempts have been made and what problems were encountered that could be anticipated this time? How well formed is the patient's resolution to change? What is required to achieve withdrawal, and once achieved what will be required to maintain abstinence? What support is available? What are the risk areas for relapse? Most doctors should establish good links with local community drug and alcohol teams who should be able to provide support and backup if difficulties occur.

Goal setting, relapse prevention, and other supports

Identifying the patient's willingness to change can help clinicians to set appropriate goals (see Chapter 14.10). The maintenance of abstinence can be achieved through a combination of psychosocial and/or pharmacological approaches. Cognitive behavioural strategies are often used to prevent relapses. Alternative coping strategies can be rehearsed, such as practising ways of refusing a drink, other drug, or cigarette

Substitute prescribing for drug dependent individuals

Heroin addiction and smoking are frequently tackled by substitute prescribing—with methadone or nicotine respectively (see Chapter 14.14). The goals of treatment are improvement in physical, psychological, and social well being. These are best achieved through complete drug withdrawal. Many people will present at a time when they are newly resolved to change their lives. In those with long histories, more is achieved by adopting a gradual and realistic action plan over a defined period, with specific goals and milestones to work towards.

Maintenance to abstinence

In the case of heroin addiction, the usual plan is to start a methadone replacement aiming for a gradual reduction over 8–12 weeks and to stop heroin and other illegal drugs immediately. The maximum initial dose of methadone should be 30 mg for 50 mg can be fatal in a non-tolerant individual. Compliance should be monitored with both urine testing and physical examination. Usually there is a fairly rapid improvement in health and well being, but probably less than 20 per cent of those who embark on such treatment will achieve a drug free state. Many will want to try this approach many times before considering inpatient detoxification or residential rehabilitation or methadone maintenance treatment.

Maintenance

Drug substitution treatment for opiate dependence with a long-acting opiate such as methadone hydrochloride has proved effective in reducing levels of illicit opiate use and criminal behaviour and in improving general social stability in over half of those treated. The standard dose of methadone for maintenance treatment ranges from 60–120 mg, but there is a wide range of individual variation in patterns of methadone metabolism, and in the naive or non-tolerant individual 50 mg may be a fatal dose. The mode of dispensing may vary from supervised on-site consumption, to supervised community pharmacy consumption, to pharmacy-dispensed take-home medication. The dangers of diversion of these controlled drugs to other people makes it important that dispensing, and compliance progress should be carefully monitored.

Residential rehabilitation

For individuals who cannot achieve their goals in the community there is a large network of residential rehabilitation programmes for those addicted to drugs or alcohol. The original programmes, imported from the US, are termed 'Concept houses' based on a structured hierarchical model. More recently the Twelve Step model based on the Alcoholics Anonymous and Narcotics Anonymous models, has been developed and there is an extensive network of Christian rehabilitation houses. The outcome from such treatment is good but is related to the length of stay.

Self help groups

Self help groups such as Alcoholics Anonymous and Narcotics Anonymous are important in the treatment of addictions. These are now international organizations with branches in most parts of the world. Not everybody is keen to attend such groups, but those who do can derive immense benefit from the fellowship and support in their struggle to maintain an abstinence. The key tenet of these groups is that alcohol and other drugs undermine personal autonomy.

Chapter 14.17

Drug dependence in pregnancy

C. Gerada

Drugs have direct and indirect effects on both mother and fetus. The fetal alcohol syndrome is described in Chapter 14.14.

Gestation of pregnancy

The fetus is most susceptible to structural damage (teratogenicity) early in development while drugs taken in the later stages of pregnancy (day 55 until full term) are more likely to affect growth or cause neonatal addiction and subsequent withdrawal. Cocaine may be excreted by the newborn for 5 days and methadone may persist for a week or more.

Maternal well being

Complications of drug dependence are compounded by social adversity such as homelessness and poverty. General neglect and late

Table 1 Complications of long-term drug use

Obstetric complications	Fetal complications
• Abruptio placentae • Amnionitis • Eclampsia • Placental insufficiency • Postpartum haemorrhage • Premature labour	• HIV/AIDS • Intrauterine addition • Intrauterine growth retardation • Neonatal addiction and withdrawal • Neonatal death • Prematurity • Stillbirth
Medical complications	
• Anaemia • Chronic bronchitis (especially if the drug is inhaled) • Malnutrition • Sexually transmitted diseases • Urinary tract infections	

presentation for health care, poor nutrition, intercurrent infections, cigarette smoking, complications of dirty and shared needles, together with erratic and chaotic lifestyles predispose the drug-using pregnant woman to a wide variety of health problems and increases the risk of complications of pregnancy. Encouraging women to attend for treatment can reduce some of these complications.

Complications of drug use (Table 1)

Obstetric and medical complications

Drug using women and their fetuses are at higher risk of obstetric and medical complications and perinatal morbidity and mortality. Cocaine is particularly hazardous in pregnancy as its vasoconstrictor action decreases blood flow to the placenta and increases uterine contractibility resulting in an increased rate of spontaneous abortion, abruptio placentae, and premature labour. A single intravenous injection of cocaine may stimulate the onset of labour.

Fetal and infant complications

General

The commonest fetal complications are prematurity (20–33 per cent in the UK) and intrauterine growth retardation. Sudden intrauterine withdrawal from heroin can result in premature delivery or intrauterine death. Opiates also have a direct effect on intrauterine growth, resulting in small-for-dates babies even after controlling for factors such as infrequent antenatal care and smoking. Cerebral infarction, possibly related to excessive vasoconstriction, occurs with increased frequency in babies born to cocaine-abusing mothers.

Neonatal dependence and withdrawal

Neonates regularly exposed to drugs *in utero* may become physically dependent and may suffer if the drug is suddenly withdrawn. The severity of the withdrawal syndrome will be determined by the specific drug/s involved, dosage used, timing of the last dose before delivery, and the maturity of the infant. Before birth, withdrawal is characterized by increased fetal movement starting approximately 30 minutes to 1 hour before the mother experiences withdrawal symptoms. Within 24–48 hours after delivery the infant may develop a withdrawal reaction. The infant may become jittery and irritable, with sneezing, feeding disorders, vomiting, and diarrhoea. Severe withdrawal may prove fatal from generalized seizures or electrolyte disturbances. Symptoms may persist for up to 10 weeks, especially in babies born to crack/cocaine-using mothers.

Management of the pregnant drug abuser

General principles of treatment

(1) Identify women possibly involved in drug abuse

(2) Provide antenatal and health care

(3) Recommend reduction of all illicit drugs and replace with prescribed substitutes if relevant (see below)

(4) Co-ordinate management with a multidisciplinary team.

Maintaining contact with the women by prescribing low doses of the drug(s) is sometimes more realistic than total withdrawal and decreases additional illicit drug use, increases stability, and enables closer monitoring of the pregnancy. Women enrolled in treatment programmes usually have better antenatal care, less anaemia, and better general health, even if they continue to use illicit drugs.

Opiates

Methadone Mixture BNF 1 mg/ml is the substitute drug of choice for opiate users (see Chapter 14.14). An initial dose of 20–40 mg issued depending on the patient's drug history, in particular the length of habit and recent use of heroin. After stabilization, a programme of slow reduction should be devised, usually involving 2.5–5 mg reductions in the methadone per week. Reduction can be started at any time, but ideally should be in the second trimester (14–28 weeks). If carried out in the first trimester a spontaneous abortion may erroneously be attributed to the reduction. If the woman presents after 30 weeks of pregnancy it may be impossible to implement a stabilization and withdrawal programme in the time available. These women should receive a stable dose of methadone till delivery.

Stimulants

Stimulants such as 'Ecstasy' and cocaine do not produce serious physical dependence. It may be more appropriate to recommend gradual daily reduction of the drug rather than substitute other stimulants.

Benzodiazepines

Long-acting diazepam should be substituted for other benzodiazepines. Withdrawal can then be achieved by small weekly reductions. Temazepam capsules must never be prescribed as their contents may be injected.

Labour

Women who have received antenatal care should undergo routine assessment and management of their labour and delivery. There is no indication for withholding analgesia, in addition to a daily methadone dose. Epidural anaesthesia is not contraindicated. The opiate dependent drug user presenting in labour is an obstetric emergency because of the increased risks of low birth weight babies, premature delivery, and severe withdrawal symptoms in the baby. Methadone is the drug of choice for the management of opiate dependent women.

Naloxone must not be given to the newborn baby as it may induce severe withdrawal symptoms. Infants should be observed for signs of withdrawal during their first 72 hours after birth.

Postnatal period

Breastfeeding

Methadone and heroin are excreted into breast milk, but in quantities to small to be harmful to the infant. Methadone in the breast milk may prevent withdrawal symptoms in addicted infants.

Despite the risk of transmission of infection from HIV seropositive women to their babies by breast feeding, this should not be discouraged in parts of the world where infectious diseases and malnutrition are the main causes of infant deaths. In other areas HIV positive mothers should be advised to feed their babies with formula milk.

Contraception

Detoxification from illicit drugs increases sense of well being, weight, and libido and restores normal menstrual functions—all of which increase fertility. Pre-existing liver damage may contraindicate the combined oral contraceptive pill. However, injectable long-acting progestogen (Depo Provera) that bypasses the liver is safe. Barrier methods of contraception should be encouraged in addition to other methods. Intrauterine devices can be used unless the woman is HIV positive or has pelvic inflammatory disease.

Follow-up

As many as 25 per cent of the infants born to drug abusing women will be adopted, emphasizing the need for continuing support for the mother and child.

Further reading

Chasnoff, I. J. (ed). (1986). *Drug use in pregnancy: mother and child.* MTP Press, Lancaster, UK

van Baar, A. (1991). *The development of infants of drug dependent mothers.* Swets and Zeitlinger BV, Amsterdam.

Chapter 14.18

Particular problems in special settings

M. Farrell, J. Strang, H. Ghodse, and A. Maden

In general hospital wards

Possibly about 10 per cent of general hospital admissions are alcohol dependent, 1 per cent are dependent on non-prescribed drugs, and up to 40 per cent are smokers. Tobacco, alcohol, and illicit drugs present particular problems in hospital wards. It may be difficult to prohibit or limit their consumption. Most wards now have clear no-smoking policies and do not permit the use of illicit drugs on hospital premises but some wards allow the consumption of alcohol. The maintenance of a tobacco smoke free environment has become reasonably well established in hospitals and provides a useful framework for the implementation of policies on cannabis and other illicit drugs. In some hospitals substance misuse liaison teams have been set up with skills in the management of substance related problems. They can work to enhance the skills of the general ward staff. Some of their work with injecting drug users may take place in units providing treatment and care for HIV-related conditions.

Ward staff should make clear that the use of non-prescribed drugs is not acceptable. It is sometimes helpful to make an analogy with prohibition of smoking tobacco on the ward. Traditionally, the policy has been to discharge anyone who continues to use drugs in the ward but this may be difficult with people with life-threatening conditions. In this situation it may be best to prescribe in order to discourage further drug use. The opportunity to inform patients about local services and to refer them should be taken wherever possible. The stigma attached to being identified as a drug addict on a hospital ward results in concealment and underdetection of the problem. Explicit prejudice against such patients may result in ethically unacceptable practices by medical staff, including withholding of treatment. Many difficult and potentially violent situations can arise with some drug users but as hospital wards become more experienced in handling drug users most will pass through experiencing high standards of care and humane thoughtful treatment.

Occasionally patients may be admitted who are being prescribed injectable opiates. Those should be administered by the ward staff and the opportunity taken to instruct the patient on hygienic technique, the value of rotating injection sites, and the use of the subcutaneous route for ease and safety of access.

The prescribing of strong analgesics to control pain may result in drug dependence. Like many other drug users, these patients are distressed to be regarded as drug abusers or addicts. They view their drug use as being primarily for the control of pain and staff need to be aware of this sensitivity. The timing of dispensing of drugs to individuals who are dependent on them requires planning. It is generally advisable to use longer-acting opiates in the management of opiate dependence as this can reduce tension and can be used to disentangle drug dependence from pain control. Conditions such as sickle cell crisis may result in frequent hospital admissions. Diagnostic confusion may develop between the crisis and opiate dependence.

A variety of strategies is available for pain control in those with chronic pain conditions (see Section 1).

Accident and emergency departments

Doctors in accident and emergency departments are extremely busy and often feel ill-equipped to deal with alcohol and drug problems. Guidelines should be drawn up for the management of intoxication and withdrawal and the prescribing of controlled drugs for those who are dependent. Such guidelines provide support for junior doctors when they are under pressure and in difficult situations. The commonest presentations are for complications as outlined above. Opiate overdose is usually dealt with in the province of the accident and emergency department, where leaflets about overdose prevention should be available and information about local services should be given to all patients who require resuscitation or antagonist treatment. Many will leave the department against medical advice so printed information about further sources of help is important. Assessment is important where there is evidence of associated depression and a full psychiatric assessment is highly desirable. All alcohol and drug users should be given some printed information about local support services before they leave the department.

In custodial settings

The principles of assessing and treating drug or alcohol users in custody are much the same as in other situations but must take account of the custodial environment and legal concerns.

On reception into custody

For all prisoners, this is the time of highest risk for psychiatric morbidity and mortality, usually from suicide. The transition from freedom to imprisonment brings isolation from social supports. Anxiety is increased by impending legal proceedings and the fear of victimization within prison. The substance abuser has the added fear of withdrawal symptoms.

The clinical and medicolegal components of the doctor's task can never be entirely separated. The immediate clinical priorities are the assessment and treatment of withdrawal symptoms, and other complications of substance abuse. The medicolegal priorities are the assessment of fitness to be detained and fitness to be interviewed by police. These assessments depend on the degree of intoxication or the severity of withdrawal symptoms and the extent to which they can be treated without impairing cognitive function. There are no generally accepted criteria for fitness to be detained or interviewed.

This work is complicated by the circumstances in which it is carried out, often within a police station. All actions may be scrutinized by a court, sometimes after a delay of years, so scrupulous record keeping is essential. The time for interview and examination may be limited, the premises unsuitable because of noise or lack of privacy, and the patient may be unco-operative and threatening. It is the doctor's responsibility to ensure that conditions allow him to carry out his work adequately and safely. Any difficulties should be noted, along with the steps taken in an attempt to resolve them.

The doctor should begin all interviews by introducing himself, explaining his role and the purpose of the interview. If the doctor is likely to prepare reports for the court, the defendant should be informed of this, and warned that the interview is not confidential and that he or she is not obliged to answer any questions.

Physical and mental state examination

General physical inspection may reveal systemic or localized complications of substance abuse. Offenders, especially heavy drinkers, are often the victims of violence and may also have sustained injuries while being arrested, including head injury.

Mental state examination aims to confirm the diagnosis of substance dependence or abuse, detect withdrawal symptoms, and exclude other psychiatric disorders. Severe alcohol withdrawal or drug intoxication must be distinguished from other acute organic syndromes. Depression may be a consequence of stimulant withdrawal or the adverse circumstances, so questions about suicidal thoughts and intent are essential; negative and positive findings must be adequately recorded. Personality disorder is commonly associated with substance abuse but its presence should not be assumed, nor should it be disregarded when present. Chronic low self-esteem, self-mutilation, uncontrolled anger, and unsatisfactory or violent relationships will influence the possibilities for treatment. Psychosis may accompany drug intoxication or withdrawal and may be indistinguishable from functional psychosis. Substance abuse complicates some cases of chronic schizophrenia and increases the chances that the patient will come into conflict with the law.

Special investigations

Blood or urine samples confirm drug use. Quantitative measures of alcohol can be of great medicolegal importance.

Management

The management of withdrawal syndromes is determined by the particular characteristics of the drug but the custodial setting can create additional problems. Doctors may face demands to prescribe excessive quantities of drugs or there may be an institutional ethos which resists all demands for medication. Neither attitude is justified. Institutions should develop a policy on prescribing and drug withdrawal regimes, which can be implemented with minimal variation and reduce confrontation. Occasionally, the complications of drug withdrawal can be life-threatening, in which case the aim is to secure urgent transfer to hospital.

Many problem drug users will be released on bail after a short period in custody. Further treatment should be offered through liaison with other agencies. The impact of being arrested will lead some users to consider stopping taking drugs. It is important that they are made aware of the available types of treatment.

The court report

The report should give a diagnosis where appropriate and discuss possible treatments. Questions of retribution and punishment should be left to the court. The Criminal Justice Act 1991 allows for the treatment of drug or alcohol problems as a condition of a probation order. Treatment need not be in hospital, so a knowledge of local treatment agencies is essential, as is liaison with the probation service.

Serving a sentence

Substance abuse within prison

The extent of drug use and sexual behaviour within prisons is a matter of debate and speculation but with little hard evidence. Doctors working in prison must be aware of the possibility of drug intoxication and the need for HIV counselling. It has been suggested that the risk of HIV transmission within prison might be reduced by providing condoms, syringes or cleaning materials, or by maintenance prescribing. So far, none of these approaches has been widely adopted in English prisons.

Release from prison presents a high risk of relapse. The stress of rebuilding a life in the outside world is combined with a return to the setting of previous drug use and the loss of supports established within prison. Fatal overdoses are common and former drug users should be warned of the dangers of their reduced tolerance. The vulnerability of this population requires that far greater work be done to prepare them for release and to prevent their ending up homeless.

Further reading

Singleton, N., Meletzer, H., Coid, J., and Deasy, D. (1998). *Prison psychiatric morbidity survey.* Office of National Statistics. HMSO, London.

Chapter 14.19

The use of the Mental Health Act and common law in mentally disordered general hospital patients

E. J. Feldman

This chapter covers the application of the Mental Health Act (1983) and common law principles in England and Wales with respect to the management of mentally disordered patients in NHS general hospitals.

Mental Health Acts

Unlike other aspects of clinical care, medicolegal issues do not necessarily cross national boundaries. In the UK alone, there are three Mental Health Acts (MHAs) currently in force, one for Scotland (1984), one for Northern Ireland (1986), and one for England and Wales (1983). Eire also has its own Act (1945). This chapter focuses on the common law and Mental Health Act in England and Wales.

The remit of the Act

The MHA allows for the legal detention and treatment of adults with mental illness, mental impairment, and psychopathic disorder where admission is considered necessary in the interest of their health and safety, or for the protection of others, and where they are unable or unwilling to consent to such admission. The MHA does not apply to the detention and treatment of patients for physical illness, for which they must give informed consent, or be treated under common law. In legal terms it is an enabling Act which means it does not have to be used in all possible instances of the above, but its use provides certain legal safeguards for patients and for staff responsible for the patients subject to the MHA. Whilst any mental disorder can fall within the remit of the MHA, in practice there are common circumstances where restraint and treatment are applied without recourse to the Act. In these situations, the actions performed (if carried out without the real consent of the patient) can only be defended if within the scope of the common law.

In section 1 of the MHA, mental disorder is defined very broadly: s.1(2) states: 'mental disorder' means mental illness, arrested or incomplete development of the mind, psychopathic disorder *and any other disorder or disability of the mind* and 'mentally disordered' shall be construed accordingly' (my italics), and hence this may include temporary states of mental disturbance such as delirium and intoxication (subject to exclusion under s.1(3) of the Act – see below), as well as more prolonged conditions such as dementia and brain damage. Use of the MHA would be unusual in these conditions in general acute psychiatric practice with the exception of drug induced psychosis. In general psychiatry, the MHA is usually applied to functional psychoses and little else. In general hospital psychiatric practice, the MHA is more likely to be temporarily applied to patients with organic brain disorders in circumstances of risk to self or others. It should be noted in particular that someone who is intoxicated with alcohol or drugs, and who is judged to have the capacity to refuse essential intervention other than alcohol or drug addiction alone [s.1(3) states that the Act cannot be applied to persons by 'reasons only of promiscuity or other immoral conduct, sexual deviancy or dependence on alcohol or drugs'].

Although not appropriate for the treatment of physical disorder *per se*, the MHA may apply where physical disorder contributes to mental disorder or is otherwise inextricably linked with the mental disorder, e.g. feeding in anorexia nervosa, or use of thyroxine in mental disorder caused by hypothyroidism. It does not apply in situations where the treatment of the physical illness will not impact upon the mental disturbance; this area falls within the scope of the common law.

The use of holding orders

Sections 5(2) and 5(4), the emergency medial and nursing holding orders for those that are already voluntary inpatients, are not applicable in the accident and emergency department which is regarded as an outpatient setting. Detention of an outpatient would require an admission or treatment order, viz. section 2, 3 or 4. Patients cannot be conveyed on an admission or treatment order. Where different NHS hospital Trusts operate on the same site, it is advisable for the respective Trust Managers formally to agree to act on each other's behalf with respect to the MHA.

Any consultant in charge of a patient's care is the Responsible Medical Officer (RMO) with respect to the MHA; therefore, according to the law, consultant physicians and surgeons may detain their own inpatients using section 5(2). In general hospitals, the initials RMO are frequently applied to the resident medical officer who is usually only of senior house officer grade; it is therefore very important to be clear that, where the term RMO is applied in respect of the Mental Health Act, it always refers to the consultant with medical responsibility for the case. The MHA allows for the nomination of a deputy by any RMO and this deputy must be a registered medical practitioner (**not** a preregistration house officer). Under the current MHA, consultant physicians and surgeons may therefore nominate their own juniors, who are senior house officer grade or above, to act as their deputies. Whether or not this is a good practice is another matter. The Code of Practice on the use of the MHA (Department of Health and Welsh Office, 1993) has advised that only consultant psychiatrists should nominate a deputy, and that where an RMO of another speciality wishes to detain their own patient, they should make immediate contact with a psychiatrist. Problems can arise if junior physicians are left to invoke the powers of section 5(2) because they and their seniors are often unclear about the precise nature and scope of the powers, the powers may not be administered correctly, and the patient may not be assessed by an approved psychiatrist with a view to an admission order, treatment order, or discharge of holding order.

The use of the place of safety order and the role of the police

Section 136 empowers the police to detain and take to a place of safety an individual who falls within its remit. It is not an emergency admission section. Its purpose is to enable the police to take a patient somewhere where they can safely be assessed by two doctors and an approved social worker with a view to detention under the MHA. There is no official documentation for section 136.

Police may legitimately escort to hospital patients who request their help, or those who require hospital treatment but are incapable of consenting. However, they should not bring patients **against their will** to a hospital unless under section 136 of the MHA and where, by local agreement, the hospital is the designated place of safety. In many districts, hospitals are not the designated place of safety, but the police cells are. Accident and emergency departments, far from being safe places for severely mentally disturbed individuals, are often ill equipped to deal wit the kind of people that the police pick up, and hospital staff and other ill patients in the vicinity may be placed at risk.

Managerial arrangements for the MHA

Managers of general hospitals need to make arrangements for the receipt and holding of section papers and need to liaise with relevant officers in the psychiatric hospitals for staff training, audit, and general administrative purposes. If the general hospital is in a different Trust to the psychiatric hospital, there either needs to be a designated person within the general hospital who is properly trained in the administration of the Mental Health Act, or there needs to be a written agreement whereby clinical staff of the general hospital will have access to the relevant Mental Health Act officer in the psychiatric Trust.

Clarifying the common law for use in the general hospital

What is the common law?

The common law refers to the body of rights, duties, obligations, and liabilities recognized by the courts over the years and is made up of principles identified by judges which are adapted and changed to meet the needs of particular cases and, hence, particular developments in society. This judge-made law is to be distinguished from statute law which comprises the rules and regulations agreed by Parliament. When the common law principles have been identified, their application to novel circumstances should follow. Common law should ideally reflect good judgement in tune with modern society: Lord Donaldson referred to the common law as 'common sense under a wig'.

When does common law apply?

Common law principles may assist where there are no statutory protections or mechanisms in play. In England and Wales, the Mental Health Act 1983 is the relevant codifying statute, and where its provisions apply there is little room for the common law principles. On issues where the statute law is silent, the lawfulness of any act or omission is tested by the application of the common law.

What common law principles may be applicable to the treatment of mentally disturbed individuals?

Assumption of capacity in adults

The starting point is the recognition in common law that every adult has the right and capacity to decide whether or not he/she will accept medical treatment, even if a refusal may risk permanent damage to his/her physical or mental health, or even lead to premature death. The reasons for the refusal are irrelevant. Capacity is a legal concept and concerns an individual's ability to understand what is being proposed to them and the consequences of either refusing or accepting the advice given. In law, pre-registration house officers are not qualified to assess a patient's capacity to accept or refuse treatment but all registered medical practitioners are (British Medical Association and Law Society, 1995). Where mental disorder is present or likely, psychiatric involvement is necessary for a proper assessment of capacity, for example in a patient who has made a suicide attempt.

Necessity

The courts have recognized the existence of a common law principle of 'necessity', and extend it to cover situations where action is required to assist another person without his or her consent. Although such a situation will usually be some form of emergency (or 'urgency necessity'), the power to intervene is not created by that urgency, but derived from the principle of necessity. In Black v. Forsey (House of Lords, *The Times*, 31 May 1988), Lord Griffiths, when dealing with the common law power to restrain a dangerous lunatic, said that the power was 'confined to imposing temporary restraint on a lunatic who has run amok and is a manifest danger either to himself or to others – a state of affairs as obvious to a layman as to a doctor. Such a common law power is confined to the short period necessary before the lunatic can be handed over to the proper authority.'. In common language, the judge is pointing out that it is appropriate to act to restrain a patient believed to be suffering from mental disorder and who is exhibiting behaviour which suggests they are a risk to themselves or others, but where they have not yet been detained under the MHA. In practice, there is usually a period of time when patients who are about to be made subject to the Mental Health Act will have to be restrained before the formalities of the Act can be completed. It is also quite common for such patients to require some sedation prior to the completion of formalities. Such actions will be defensible if carried out as a necessity and using the minimal intervention required.

Actions performed out of necessity should not continue for an unreasonable length of time, but progress should be made either to a situation of consent or to the use of power under the Mental Health Act. It is not possible precisely to define what is a reasonable or unreasonable length of time as this would vary with the particular circumstances of each case.

Duty of care

Common law imposes a duty of care on all professional staff to all persons within a hospital; by assuming the responsibility of a particular clinical staff appointment, and claiming professional expertise, an individual undertakes to provide proper care to those needing it. Staff may be negligent by omission. Actions involving the use of reasonable restraint and driven by professional responsibility in circumstances of necessity are supported by common law.

As well as individual staff, hospitals also have duties, for example to provide back-up staff who are properly trained to assist with aggressive unco-operative patients in a casualty department, and the hospital must ensure that such staff are authorized to act if necessary. Many hospitals experience problems with fulfilling this duty because they fail to train the security staff in this role, and commonly such staff are disinclined to assist in necessary restraint as they believe that they will be exposed to the risk of litigation for assault or battery. This is a key area for improved staff training and the involvement of the hospital's risk management advisers.

The Bolam test

Where clinical decisions are being made, an individual clinician's competence will be judged against what is considered reasonable and proper by a body of responsible doctors at that time, as ascertained in court from expert testimony, i.e. the Bolam test (Bolam v. Friern Hospital Management Committee [1957] 2 All ER 118–128 at 122).

The law applied to clinical situations

A few vignettes illustrate the practical application of the law in the clinical context. All the cases have been invented for illustrative purposes. The advice given is not intended to be prescriptive, but to provide an illustration of how principles discussed in the chapter may be applied in practice. In the law, as in medicine, there is always a place for considered judgement according to the particular circumstances in each case.

(1) Acute organic brain syndrome

A 54-year- old male on the high dependency unit is recovering from a cardiac arrest which required prolonged resuscitation. As he emerges from several days of coma, he becomes acutely distressed, disorientated, and paranoid. He requires heparin for his prosthetic heart valves, and antiarrhythmic drugs, but refuses to have either and is walking about, dressed and demanding to leave. He has already tried to push past you and the nursing staff. You assess that the only way to help him is to restrain and sedate him against his will, keeping him on the high dependency medical unit.

This man's refusal is not based on any real understanding of his circumstances and, in delirium, he has no grasp of his risk; it is very clearly in his best interests for him to be detained and sedated so that he can have life-saving treatments. Any reasonable lay person would not dispute this man's need for treatment and would consider hospital staff negligent if they knowingly allowed him to leave and failed to do whatever was necessary to help him.

The MHA could be applied for detention and sedation to treat the delirium (a form of mental illness), but delirium is not a situation in which the MHA is commonly used. Such patients are more often detained and treated without recourse to the MHA in view of the transient nature of the disturbance, the (so far) undisputed need for intervention, and the evident lack of capacity to give meaningful consent or refusal. However, if strong measures are required, such as the use of psychiatric nursing staff to pin this man to his bed whilst he is forcibly injected with haloperidol, or if the situation persists over a prolonged period, it may be advisable to use the MHA. The Section should be cancelled as soon as the patient recovers mentally.

Treatments other than sedation in this case are not authorized by the MHA, but are justifiably given in a legal sense if the post-registration physician directing the treatment has judged that the patient does not have the capacity to make a meaningful refusal. The same legal decision **could** also apply to the use of sedation, in which case a psychiatrist need not be involved as, in law, any registered medical practitioner is considered able to judge a patient's capacity to consent (British Medical Association and Law Society, 1995). This does not apply to patients under the MHA after the first 3 months of treatment; only the RMO is then judged to be able to determine a patient's capacity to consent.

(2) Patient refusing medical intervention after deliberate self harm

A 30-year-old male is brought to the accident and emergency department following an overdose of 70 paracetamol taken 4 hours prior to arrival at hospital. There is no history available and the patient refuses to say anything about himself other than he wants to be left alone to die. He refuses to give blood for a paracetamol level and refuses any medical intervention. Can treatment be given without his consent?

This illustrates a fairly common scenario. The patient presents the medical staff with the dilemma of whether they should assume he has full capacity to refuse medical treatment, in which case they might leave him to suffer the consequences of liver failure, possibly death, or whether they should act out of necessity and as part of their duty of care to treat someone in whom capacity may reasonably be in doubt and where the patient could be mentally ill. A psychiatrist will not be in a position to assess the patient for mental disorder before the harmful effects of paracetamol become irreversible and the Mental Health Act does not assist with respect to treatment for the poisoning. Even where there is no formal mental illness, a patient in the state of emotional crisis surrounding attempted suicide may not be said to be in a position to make a fully reasoned decision, and many who refuse treatment on admission are grateful for their rescue the morning after. A reasonable approach in such cases is to take it that there is reasonable doubt with respect to the patient's capacity to make a fully informed and reasoned choice and proceed with whatever action is needed, as a matter of urgent necessity, to save his life. This is defensible under the common law. At the end of the day, is it better for a clinician to have a living patient who may sue for assault and battery for saving the life they said they did not want in a highly emotional state, or to have a dead patient with grieving relatives who may sue for negligence? There are currently no precedents either way.

(3) Intoxicated patient refusing to co-operate with assessment following deliberate self harm

A young adult male is brought to the accident and emergency department by paramedics who found him lying in a doorway with a suicide note and an empty bottle of paracetamol. He is intoxicated with alcohol, belligerent, refuses to talk to any staff, and is making moves to leave. You have no other information and have to make a decision whether or not to let him go.

This case typifies a common clinical problem faced by accident and emergency staff and psychiatrists covering accident and emergency departments. If there is sufficient concern to warrant detaining this patient for further assessment of a possible underlying mental disorder, then the use of the MHA is certainly justified. The fact that the patient is intoxicated is not an obstacle to use of the MHA, as the Act is not being used to detain or treat someone because of alcohol abuse or dependence alone [a use of the MHA excluded under section 1(3)], but because the concern that there may be an underlying mental disorder which is temporarily obscured by intoxification and lack of co-operation.

(4) Anorexia nervosa patient *in extremis* and refusing food

A 19-year-old female weighing only 26 kg has been admitted to the acute medical unit. She consents to a saline drip, but not to any dextrose or parenteral feeding. She is close to death from starvation.

The MHA is frequently used in relation to patients with anorexia who are close to death to authorize feeding as part of the psychiatric as well as part of the physical treatment of these patients. Experts in eating disorders regard refeeding as an essential first step in the psychiatric treatment, as starvation itself produces distorted thinking. There are legal precedents to support this view. The Mental Health Act Commission has issued guidance on this particular topic which discusses the legal issues in more detail.

(5) Anorexia nervosa patient with diabetes, refusing insulin

The same patient as in case 4 above now also has insulin dependent diabetes; this time she agrees to feeding, but refuses insulin, since she knows she will not gain weight without it. She would die if you followed this plan and so the hospital staff must feed her and give her insulin if her death is to be prevented.

A reasonable view is that there is no difference between this case and the preceding situation. Insulin is as essential for healthy weight gain as is food; hence, its administration would also form part of the psychiatric treatment plan under Section 3 of the MHA. There is currently no legal precedent on this precise point.

(6) Patient with schizophrenia refuses surgery, but is accepting other medical care

A 59-year-old male with chronic schizophrenia is a long-stay patient under Section 3. He develops a gangrenous foot and the surgeon's advice is to proceed to amputation. The patient refuses surgery on the grounds that he does not want an amputation, but he agrees to antibiotics and all other forms of treatment. The surgeon asks if the operation can be carried out as part of treatment under Section 3 and he impresses upon you his conviction that the patient is likely to die without the amputation.

The MHA does not apply unless the treatment of physical disorder would improve the patient's mental disorder. Precedent on this [In re C (Adult: Refusal of Treatment) [1994] 1 WLR 290] found that a patient's gangrenous leg could not be amputated as the patient's refusal of surgery was unrelated to his chronic schizophrenia (i.e. he had the capacity to refuse and this refusal was not part of his psychotic thinking) and surgery would not improve his mental condition.

As a general rule, where physical illness and mental disorder coexist, and the issue of the treatment under the MHA arises, the clinician must establish:

(1) whether treatment of the physical illness would make a difference to the mental disorder

(2) whether or not the refusal is a valid one in a patient with the capacity to make a decision on this issue.

Where the treatment of physical illness dos ameliorate the mental disorder, then it is also the case that this is treatment of the mental disorder (as in the cases with anorexia) and use of the MHA is justified. If refusal of physical treatment is not the result of the mental disorder, and the treatment is unlikely to make any difference to the mental disorder, then use of the MHA would not be justified (as in the case of the patient with schizophrenia and a gangrenous foot). If refusal is the result of the mental disorder, but treatment would not ameliorate the mental disorder, then the MHA cannot be used to justify the treatment either, although treatment for physical illness may be justifiable under common law where the patient's capacity to either consent or refuse may reasonably be in doubt.

Further reading

British Medical Association and Law Society. (1995). *Assessment of mental capacity: for guidance for doctors and lawyers.* British Medical Association, London.

Department of Health and Welsh Office. (1993). *Code of Practice Mental Health Act (1983).* HMSO, London.

The Mental Health Act. (1983). HMSO, London.

Chapter 14.20

Eating disorders

C. G. Fairburn

Anorexia nervosa and bulimia nervosa share many features and together they are a major source of psychiatric morbidity amongst young women. Anorexia nervosa has long been recognized, with particularly good descriptions being published in the last century. In contrast, the first series of patients with bulimia nervosa was described as recently as 1979.

Anorexia nervosa

Definition

Three features are required to make a diagnosis of anorexia nervosa.

1. The active maintenance of an unduly low weight, usually defined as 15 per cent below the expected weight for the person's age, height, and sex. This is achieved by a variety of means, including strict dieting or fasting, excessive exercising, laxative and diuretic misuse, and, in some, self-induced vomiting. Patients with diabetes mellitus may underuse or omit insulin giving rise to 'brittle diabetes'.
2. The presence of certain characteristic attitudes to shape and weight which are pathognomonic of anorexia nervosa and bulimia nervosa. These include a 'relentless pursuit of thinness' and a 'morbid fear of fatness'. Such concerns are far more intense than the dissatisfaction with shape and weight experienced by many young women today.
3. Amenorrhoea.

Distribution

Anorexia nervosa is largely confined to women aged between 10 and 30 years and to Western countries in which thinness for women is considered attractive. Estimates of the incidence range from 0.24 to 14.6 per 100 000 female population per annum, increasing in recent decades. In adolescent girls, the group most at risk, estimates of prevalence range from 0.2 to 1.1 per cent. The disorder is rarely encountered in men (less than 10 per cent of cases are male) and it is also uncommon among non-Caucasians. The social class distribution seems to be uneven, with an over-representation of cases from the upper socio-economic groups.

Development of the disorder

The onset of anorexia nervosa is usually in adolescence, often starting as normal adolescent dieting, which then gets out of control. As the dieting intensifies, weight falls and physiological and psychological features characteristic of semistarvation develop. Additional methods of controlling shape and weight may be adopted at any stage. The characteristic attitudes to shape and weight usually develop slightly later on.

General clinical features

Weight loss is mainly achieved through a severe reduction in food intake. The amount consumed may be very small and some patients fast at times. Typically the range of foods eaten is restricted, with those viewed as fattening being avoided. Except in long-standing cases, appetite persists and for this reason the term 'anorexia' is not appropriate. Frequent intense exercising is common and adds to the weight loss. Laxative and diuretic misuse and self-induced vomiting may also be practised.

Accompanying disturbed eating habits is the so-called body image disturbance. This may include a perceptual component such that all, or parts, of the body are seen as larger than their true size, and an attitudinal component characterized by an intense dislike of the body or parts of it. Neither feature improves as weight is lost: indeed, both tend to get worse.

Depressed mood, lability of mood, irritability, anxiety, and obsessional symptoms related to eating are all common features. In more chronic cases there may be hopelessness and thoughts of suicide.

Symptoms and signs

Many patients with anorexia nervosa have no physical complaints. However, enquiry often reveals heightened sensitivity to cold and a variety of gastrointestinal symptoms such as constipation, fullness after eating, bloatedness, and vague abdominal pains. Other symptoms include restlessness, lack of energy, low sexual appetite, and early morning wakening. In females who are not taking an oral contraceptive, amenorrhoea is by definition present. Occasionally patients complain of infertility.

The degree of emaciation may be striking. Growth may be stunted in those with a prepubertal onset and there may be failure of breast development. Unlike patients with hypopituitarism, axillary and pubic hair is preserved and there is no breast atrophy. A fine downy lanugo hair may be present on the back, arms and side of face. Typically the skin is dry and the hands and feet are cold. Blood pressure and pulse are low. There may be dependent oedema.

Endocrine abnormalities

Luteinizing hormone releasing hormone (LHRH) secretion is impaired, and as a result levels of luteinizing hormone (LH), follicle stimulating hormone (FSH) and oestradiol are low. There is an immature pattern of luteinizing hormone release. The luteinizing hormone response to LHRH is reduced, but the follicle stimulating hormone response is normal or exaggerated.

Hypothalamic disturbance is also evident in the delayed thyrotrophin (thyroid stimulating hormone; TSH) response to thyrotrophin releasing hormone (TRH). In addition, there is reduced peripheral conversion of thyroxine (T_4) to tri-iodothyronine (T_3), and an increased conversion of thyroxine to inactive reverse tri-iodothyronine. These changes are seen in other chronic illnesses. Thyroxine levels are in the low normal range, whereas tri-iodothyronine levels are depressed. Clinical evidence of hypothyroidism includes sensitivity to cold, constipation, dry skin, and bradycardia.

Plasma cortisol levels are raised and the normal diurnal variation is lost. These changes are due in part to the increased half-life of cortisol seen in starvation and in part to a relative increase in cortisol production. Growth hormone levels are also increased, another secondary effect of starvation. Prolactin secretion is normal.

Haematological changes

A normocytic normochromic anaemia is found in a minority of patients and is sometimes attributable to a low intake of iron or folate. Mild neutropenia is common. The erythrocyte sedimentation rate is often low.

Other metabolic abnormalities

Hypercholesterolaemia is frequently present. The mechanism is not understood. Increased serum β-carotene may also be found and reflects increased dietary intake. Life-threatening hypoglycaemia occurs very occasionally, and may not present typically due to an impaired sympathetic response. Hypokalaemic alkalosis is found in those who vomit frequently or misuse large quantities of laxatives or diuretics.

Other abnormalities

Cranial computed tomography (CT) has revealed enlargement of the cortical sulci and cisternes and ventricular dilatation. This appears to be reversible and has been termed 'pseudoatrophy'.

In long-standing cases, osteopenia and osteoporotic fractures are common and thought to be secondary to the oestrogen deficiency and low weight. The extent to which the bone loss is reversible has yet to be established.

Delayed gastric emptying and a prolonged gastrointestinal transit time are common and may account for the complaints of fullness after eating, bloatedness, and constipation. Acute gastric dilatation is a rare complication that can be provoked by episodes of overeating or over-vigorous attempts at refeeding.

Aetiology

Predisposing factors

Dieting appears to be a general vulnerability factor for both anorexia nervosa and bulimia nervosa. It is a common precursor, and the two disorders are largely confined to countries in which dieting amongst young women is common. However, whilst many young women diet, few develop an eating disorder: other aetiological factors must therefore operate. These include a family history of an eating disorder, obesity, and depression. Anorexia nervosa is about eight times more common in the female first degree relatives of anorectic probands than in the general population. Twin studies suggest that this vulnerability may be partly genetic. These patients often report low self-esteem and extreme perfectionism. The role of disturbed family communication is difficult to evaluate as it has not been established whether or not it predates the onset of the eating disorder or is in response to it.

Maintaining factors

As food intake decreases and weight is lost, there are secondary physical and psychological changes, some of which perpetuate the disorder: for example, delayed gastric emptying gives a feeling of fullness even when small amounts are consumed. Those who have been overweight are understandably pleased with the weight loss and may be complimented on it. Many patients report that exerting strict control over their behaviour is rewarding in its own right. Sometimes, refusing to eat also has gratifying effects within the family.

Assessment

Few patients with anorexia nervosa refer themselves for treatment. Usually they are persuaded to seek help by concerned relatives or friends, and as a consequence they attend somewhat reluctantly.

A careful history from both the patient and, if possible, from an informant will make the diagnosis clear. It will be evident that the low weight has been achieved through the patient's own efforts and is associated with the characteristic core psychopathology. Unless there are good reasons to suspect another physical condition, no tests are required to exclude other medical disorders. Excluding the presence of coexisting depressive disorder can be difficult, as many depressive symptoms are a known consequence of semistarvation. It may be necessary to wait until body weight has been restored to a healthy level, before the presence or absence of comorbid depression can be assessed. It is more straightforward to exclude the possibility of a depressive disorder as the sole diagnosis because the core psychopathology of anorexia nervosa is not present in depression and the weight loss is rarely self-induced.

Some patients present with features associated with anorexia nervosa rather than the disorder itself: for example, gastrointestinal symptoms, amenorrhoea or infertility, or with depressive or obsessional symptoms. However, once the weight loss has been identified and the core psycho-pathology elicited, the diagnosis becomes clear.

The plasma electrolytes should be checked, especially in those who admit to vomiting, or misuse laxatives or diuretics.

Management

There are two aspects to treatment. One is establishing healthy eating habits and a normal weight, and the second is the removal of those factors that are maintaining the disorder. Both are essential. The normalization of eating habits and weight is mainly achieved through a combination of commonsense advice and nutritional counselling. This may be achieved on an inpatient, daypatient, or outpatient basis. Addressing the maintaining factors generally requires the use of more specialized treatments such as family therapy and cognitive behaviour therapy. Both these treatments are best conducted on an outpatient basis.

Drugs have a limited role. Short-acting minor tranquillizers may occasionally be used to lessen the anxiety some patients experience prior to eating and, if depressive symptoms persist following weight restoration, antidepressant drugs should be prescribed. Tube feeding and intravenous hyperalimentation are rarely indicated.

Occasionally it is appropriate to use drugs to stimulate the resumption of regular menstruation. Most patients whose weight has reached a reasonable level and who are eating healthily restart menstruating within 6–12 months. If this does not happen, either clomiphene or LHRH is usually effective in inducing menstruation. It is not appropriate to use these drugs with patients who are underweight or who are eating abnormally.

Most patients with anorexia nervosa may be managed on an outpatient basis by a specialist with experience of managing eating disorders, but the outpatient department is not appropriate if the patient's physical health is a cause for concern, or if the patient is depressed and at risk of suicide. Physical indications for admission include a weight below 70 per cent of the expected weight for the person's age, height, and sex, rapid weight loss, and the presence of medical complications such as massive oedema, severe electrolyte disturbance, significant symptomatic hypotension, or significant intercurrent infection. Under these circumstances admission should be to a general medical ward or a psychiatric unit with immediate access to emergency general medical help. A small number of patients refuse admission even though their life is in danger. In such cases compulsory hospitalization and a treatment order may be indicated.

Inpatient treatment

Admission may be to a general or psychiatric hospital. It is a great advantage if the ward staff is experienced in the management of these patients. Weight restoration may be achieved in either setting, but with a psychiatric admission it is easier to make arrangements for the other forms of treatment needed to maximize the chance that progress will be maintained following discharge.

Within a few days of admission, patients should be introduced to the consumption of regular meals and snacks of between 1000 and 1500 kcal a day; and, if possible, by the end of 2 weeks these should be of a normal quantity and composition, consisting of about 2000 kcal a day. Over-rapid refeeding can be dangerous because it may result in severe fluid retention, cardiac failure, or acute gastric dilatation. A target weight gain of about 1 kg per week should be set with the patient and staff monitoring the weight gain each morning. As between 3000 and 5000 kcal a day are likely to be required to achieve this rate of weight gain, average-sized meals and snacks will not be sufficient. The best solution is to supplement the patient's diet with energy-rich drinks; this is preferable to encouraging them to overeat, which does little to help establish healthy eating habits and may increase the risk that they develop bulimia nervosa.

The target weight range should be one at which the patient is eating healthily and not dieting, and one at which normal physiological functioning is restored. Once patients enter the target range, the energy-rich drinks should be phased out, leaving them with a diet sufficient to maintain their weight. At this stage patients should be given full control over their eating and they should be encouraged to shop, cook, and eat out with friends and family. Unless considerable effort is put into this phase of treatment, the risk of relapse after discharge is considerable.

Running concurrently with weight restoration should be other forms of therapy. At first, straightforward support is often best, but once the patient's mental state begins to improve, more specific treatments may be introduced including family therapy and cognitive behavioural procedures.

With an inpatient regime of this type, body weight is usually restored to a healthy range within 2–3 months and the patient discharged 2–4 weeks later. The transition from inpatient to outpatient care should be carefully planned.

Course and outcome

For some, anorexia nervosa is a relatively benign self-limiting disorder; for others, up to one-quarter of sufferers, it may lead to death or chronic disability. The presence of a long history and late onset, a low body weight, bulimic episodes, self-induced vomiting or laxative abuse, and a history of premorbid psychosocial problems, is also associated with a poor outcome.

Although at least half of patients recover weight and menstrual function, disturbed attitudes to shape and weight often persist and eating habits may remain disturbed. Up to a quarter develop bulimia nervosa. Standardized mortality ratios have been reported between 1.36 and 6.01, the deaths being either a direct result of medical complications or suicide. The most recent data indicate lower mortality on follow-up. The outcome in males appears to be essentially the same as that in females.

Bulimia nervosa

Definition

Three features are required to make a diagnosis of bulimia nervosa.

1. The presence of frequent bulimic episodes. These 'binges' involve the consumption of unusually large amounts of food and a sense of loss of control at the time.
2. The use of extreme behaviour to control body shape and weight. This behaviour resembles that used by patients with anorexia nervosa, although self-induced vomiting and laxative or diuretic misuse are much more common.
3. The presence of attitudes to shape and weight similar to those found in anorexia nervosa.

There are some patients with anorexia nervosa who have bulimic episodes and are therefore potentially eligible for both diagnoses. In practice, the diagnosis of anorexia nervosa is given precedence over that of bulimia nervosa.

Distribution

People with bulimia nervosa are somewhat older than those with anorexia nervosa, most presenting in their twenties, and they have a broader social class distribution. The disorder is rarely seen in men.

The prevalence amongst young women in Britain and North America is between 1 and 2 per cent, with the great majority of cases not having come to medical attention. Although there are no satisfactory data on incidence, it seems that the disorder has become more common over the last 25 years. In all countries in which anorexia nervosa is found, there has been a dramatic increase in the number of cases of bulimia and now it is the most common eating disorder encountered in psychiatric practice.

General clinical features

There are close similarities between the clinical features of bulimia and those of anorexia nervosa. Patients share the same extreme concerns about shape and weight and engage in the same methods of weight control, but there are two features which are distinguishing: first, the body weight of most bulimic patients is in the healthy range; second, bulimic episodes are much more frequent. The binges are a source of great shame and are kept secret and, in the majority of cases, are followed by self-induced vomiting or the taking of laxatives. A distinctive feature is the overall amount of food consumed, on average about 3000 kcal per episode. Some bulimic episodes are extremely large and carry the risk, albeit remote, of acute gastric dilatation or rupture. Between episodes, the patients restrict their food intake in much the same way as patients with anorexia nervosa.

Depressive and anxiety symptoms are also a more prominent feature than in anorexia nervosa. A significant minority have problems with alcohol or drugs and other self-destructive behaviours.

Physical features

Symptoms and signs

The majority of patients have few physical complaints. Those most commonly encountered are irregular or absent menstruation, weakness and lethargy, vague abdominal pains, and toothache. Appearance is usually unremarkable, but salivary gland enlargement may be present: typically, this involves the parotids and gives the patient's face a slightly rounded appearance. Sometimes it is associated with a raised serum amylase level, the increase being in the salivary isoenzyme. The underlying pathophysiology is not understood. In those who vomit there may be calluses on the dorsum of the dominant hand (Russell's sign) due to the fingers being used to stimulate the gag reflex. There may be significant erosion of the dental enamel particularly on the lingual surface of the upper front teeth. A minority of patients, particularly those who take large quantities of laxatives or diuretics, have intermittent peripheral or facial oedema.

Abnormalities on investigation

Metabolic alkalosis, hypochloraemia, and hypokalaemia are the most common abnormalities and they may account for the weakness and tiredness (and on rare occasions hypokalaemic paralysis). The picture has been termed 'pseudoBartter's syndrome', as it is self-inflicted and usually reversible. Hypokalaemia may be severe and persistent but with few if any symptoms. Despites concern about possible cardiac arrhythmias, nephrogenic diabetes insipidus, and the suggestion that chronic hypokalaemia may induce changes in the renal proximal tubular cells, aggressive treatment of this type is rarely appropriate: instead, it should be monitored and the focus kept on the treatment of the eating disorder itself.

Endocrine abnormalities resemble those in anorexia nervosa, but they are not as severe. There have been recent reports that ovarian morphology is abnormal in a high proportion of cases. This is also likely to be reversible.

Aetiology

Many patients give a history of disturbed eating from adolescence, and about one-third have previously fulfilled diagnostic criteria for anorexia nervosa. Most of the remainder started with an anorexia-like picture, although the weight loss was not great enough to reach the diagnostic threshold. It may be assumed that most factors relevant to the aetiology of anorexia also operate in bulimia.

Assessment

Most people with bulimia nervosa are ashamed of their eating habits and keep them secret for many years. When they present for help they may complain of features associated with the disorder rather than the disorder itself, for example, gastrointestinal or gynaecological symptoms, depression, or substance abuse. Under these circumstances making the correct diagnosis may be difficult because there are rarely any clear pointers to the eating disorder.

Those patients who complain of loss of control of their eating are generally referred to psychiatrists, and, unlike those with anorexia nervosa, they are usually eager for help. No physical tests are needed to make the diagnosis but the electrolytes should be checked.

Treatment

The great majority of patients may be managed on an outpatient basis. Full or partial hospitalization is indicated under four unusual circumstances: first, if the patient is either too depressed to be managed as an outpatient or there is a risk of suicide; second, if the patient's physical health is a cause for concern; third, if the patient is in the first trimester of pregnancy, because there is some evidence that the spontaneous abortion rate may be high; and fourth, if the eating disorder proves refractory to outpatient care. If hospitalization is indicated, it should be brief and serve as a preliminary to outpatient care.

The most effective treatment for bulimia nervosa is a specific form of cognitive behaviour therapy. This is a specialized psychological treatment that aims to modify not only the disturbed eating habits but also the disturbed attitudes to shape and weight. It usually involves about 20 sessions over 5 months and results in substantial improvement in all aspects of the psychopathology. Some patients respond to brief educational treatments and self-help manuals probably have a role.

Antidepressant drugs are the only pharmacological treatment to have shown promise. They result in a decline in the frequency of overeating and an improvement in mood, but the effect is not as great as that seen with cognitive behaviour therapy and, more importantly, it is often not maintained. These drugs cannot be recommended as a first line treatment. Appetite suppressants have no beneficial effect.

Course and outcome

Some of the cases identified in community surveys appear to be relatively benign in that they are short lived. In contrast, patients who are referred for specialist treatment often have long histories and previous unsuccessful attempts at treatment. Most respond well to cognitive behaviour therapy with the changes being maintained for at least the following 12 months. There have been no studies of long-term outcome.

Pregnancy and child rearing

There is growing concern about the effects of eating disorders on pregnancy and child rearing. Eating disorders tend to improve during pregnancy, but the amount of weight gained may be abnormal. The impact on the fetus has yet to be established, although there have been reports of intrauterine growth retardation and low birth weight. Child rearing is influenced in some cases with adverse effects on both infant feeding and growth.

Atypical eating disorders

In addition to anorexia nervosa and bulimia nervosa, various atypical eating disorders are encountered: indeed, they make up over one-third of all referrals. They have not been well characterized. Most common are disorders resembling anorexia nervosa or bulimia nervosa but not quite meeting their diagnostic criteria, either because one or more features is absent or because the features are not of sufficient severity, or both. In addition, there are people with eating problems distinct from anorexia nervosa and bulimia nervosa, for example, those who vomit when anxious, and people who have difficulty eating or swallowing in public. Both these groups should be classed as having an anxiety disorder and treated accordingly. There is another group who stop eating as a way of bringing attention to themselves. Such people generally have major personality difficulties. In common with those with anxiety disorders, they do not show the attitudes to shape and weight that are characteristic of patients with anorexia nervosa and bulimia nervosa.

Further reading

Brownell, K.D. and Fairburn, C.G. (1995). *Eating disorders and obesity: a comprehensive handbook.* Guildford Press, New York.

Garner, D.M. and Garfinkel, P.E. (1997). *Handbook of treatment for eating disorders.* Guildford Press, New York.

Walsh, B.T. and Devlin, M.J. (1998). Eating disorders: progress and problems. *Science*, 280, 1387–90.

Section 15
Palliative medicine

Contents

Section 15

Palliative medicine

M. J. Baines and N. Sykes

> *'I conceive it the office of the physician not only to restore the health but to mitigate pains and dolours; and not only when such mitigation may conduce to recovery but when it may serve to make a fair and easy passage'*
>
> Francis Bacon (1561–1626)

Modern scientific medicine is involved with the diagnosis and treatment of disease. Such a view regards death as a disaster, the doctor's ultimate failure. Yet this attitude ignores the physician's responsibility to manage the process of dying by 'mitigating pains and dolours' and by giving appropriate support to the dying patient, the family and the professional carers.

In the 1960s, the suffering of the dying was increasingly recognized; the modern hospice movement was born and Palliative Medicine has been established as a medical discipline.

The diagnosis of dying

The decision that active treatment, aimed at prolongation of life, is no longer appropriate must always be difficult. Yet such decisions must be made. To continue in an attempt to cure the incurable adds to the patient's distress and makes good symptom control and psychological support much more difficult.

The decision to abandon active treatment is most commonly made in patients with advanced malignant disease, in the expectation of steady deterioration. It is partly for this reason that palliative medicine has concentrated on cancer patients and most writing, including this chapter, is based on experience with this group. However, many cancer patients die with pneumonia, renal failure, or organic brain disease and much of the symptom control and psychosocial care which has been developed will have wider application.

In other branches of medicine, criteria have been described for stopping active treatment. In most of the common respiratory or cardiovascular diseases the diagnosis of dying is made by exclusion, after a failure to respond to treatment and rehabilitation.

Symptom control in terminal illness

The patient dying of a chronic illness usually presents a complex clinical picture and will develop a multiplicity of symptoms in the last weeks or months of life. The foundation of good palliative care is meticulous attention to these symptoms, so that the necessary emotional support can be given to the patient and family.

Studies of dying patients with and without cancer and also those with motor neurone disease and AIDS have revealed a considerable level of suffering during the last months of life. The prevalence of pain was between 57 and 69 per cent of patients in all groups. Palliative treatment involves diagnosing the cause, or causes, of each symptom. This will usually be based on a careful history and physical examination with the minimum of investigations.

Principles of treatment

Although a patient has an advanced or terminal illness it is often possible to reverse a cause of a particular symptom with resulting improvement. Even if the cause proves irreversible, a knowledge of the mechanism involved will point to the correct symptomatic treatment. For example, vomiting from renal failure requires different management from the vomiting caused by gastric outlet obstruction.

Symptoms in terminal illness are usually persistent but are amenable to regular medication, the dose interval depending on the plasma half-life of the drug used. The oral route is preferred and can often be used until shortly before death. Good symptom control requires regular and frequent review as the situation changes and new symptoms develop.

Psychological factors can exacerbate the physical symptoms of terminal illness. A sympathetic explanation of the disease, its symptoms, treatment, and future course will often allay the fears of a patient and family, help them to talk together and so reduce tension and pain.

The following sections discuss the major symptoms associated with terminal illness, their common causes, and suggested treatment.

Anorexia

A diminished appetite is common, and expected, as the patient's health deteriorates. However, appetite and the ability to eat continue to rate highly in quality of life studies and treatment is requested to improve the problem. Causative factors such as infection, depression, and nausea should be treated appropriately. Helpful dietary measures include the serving of small portions and the imaginative use of nutritional supplements.

Corticosteroids, either prednisolone 30 mg daily or dexamethasone 4 mg daily, normally lead to an improvement in appetite within a week. However, the side-effects of corticosteroids make them less suitable for long-term use and megestrol acetate 320 mg daily is preferred for patients with a prognosis of over 2 months.

Cancer pain (see also Section 1)

Pain is the symptom most expected and most feared by cancer patients and their families. Sadly, this fear has often been justified for, in the past, cancer pain has been poorly understood and inadequately treated. Fortunately, the situation has now improved and most patients with cancer should be guaranteed good pain relief throughout their illness.

For effective treatment, a diagnosis of the cause of pain is important. Most patients with advanced cancer have more than one pain, some caused directly by the tumour, others resulting from treatment, debility, or concurrent illness. Most cancer pain is nociceptive, in that it is caused by mechanical or chemical stimuli, in bone, viscera, or soft tissue and is conducted along intact somatosensory pathways. However, there is an important neuropathic component, caused by damage to the central or peripheral nervous system. Neuropathic pain is felt in the appropriate dermatome, is often described as 'burning' or 'shooting', and is associated with motor, sensory, or autonomic changes.

Treatment for pain should be started immediately, based on the presumptive diagnosis of the cause. For most patients a combination of the following methods will be required:

Analgesic drugs

Adjuvant analgesic drugs

Psychological and emotional support

Palliative radiotherapy

Anaesthetic techniques.

The last two methods should always be considered but in most terminally ill patients the correct treatment is with the skilled use of drugs and the support of patient and family.

Analgesic drugs

Analgesic drugs should be given as soon as pain develops, regularly and if possible, by mouth. The dose should be individually determined, being the lowest compatible with pain control.

Paracetamol (acetominophen) 1000 mg 4-hourly is recommended for the treatment of mild pain. If this proves ineffective, the choice is between adding a weak opioid such as codeine with paracetamol (co-codamol) or a low dose of a strong opioid. With escalating pain or a very sick patient it is advisable to change directly from paracetamol to morphine.

Morphine

Morphine is well absorbed when given by mouth and is rapidly distributed throughout the body. It is metabolized mainly in the liver, to glucuronides, which are excreted in the urine. The plasma half-life of morphine and its active metabolites is about 3 hours.

If pain has escaped control with regular paracetamol, morphine 5 mg 4-hourly (MST 15 mg 12-hourly) is suggested. Morphine 10 mg 4-hourly is usually needed if the patient has been receiving co-proxamol or a similar weak opioid. This dose should be increased by 50 per cent increments every 24 hours until the pain is relieved, using top-up doses for breakthrough pain as often as necessary. Most patients require less than 150 mg daily but occasionally 1000 mg daily, or even higher, is needed. Adjusting the dose of morphine according to the patient's pain, allows for individual variation in age, weight, and renal function.

Preparations of morphine

- Morphine sulphate solution or tablet given 4-hourly, e.g. Oramorph, Sevredol.
- Slow release morphine sulphate tablet given 12-hourly, e.g. MST, Oramorph SR or 24-hourly e.g. MXL, Morcap.
- Morphine injections given 4-hourly. Parenteral to oral potency ratio is about 3:1 in patients receiving regular morphine. Diamorphine is identical in action to morphine; if it is available (as in the UK) it is preferred for injection because of its greater solubility. Diamorphine, or morphine, is given by injection or subcutaneous infusion only if the patient is unable to take oral drugs. There is no evidence that these routes improve pain control except for rapidity of action, in an emergency.
- Epidural morphine is given 12-hourly or by infusion. The ratio of epidural dose–oral dose is 1:10.

Problems with morphine

A few patients feel nauseated on starting morphine. Metoclopramide will prevent or relieve this. Constipation should be anticipated and laxatives prescribed routinely. Respiratory depression is not usually a clinical problem. A dry mouth is common and requires regular mouth care.

Tolerance, although widely feared, is a minor problem. When an increasing dose of morphine is needed, this is usually due to increased pain from an enlarging malignancy. Addiction—an overpowering drive to take a drug for its psychological effects—does not appear to occur in patients with pain. Physical dependence does develop but if the pain lessens, for example, after radiotherapy, it is possible to reduce the dose of morphine slowly without producing withdrawal symptoms.

Myoclonic jerks are a sign of opioid toxicity and may occur with a stable dose of morphine if renal function is deteriorating. A reduction in morphine dose usually lessens the problem. Drowsiness may occur when morphine is started or the dose increased but patients on a stable dose have unaltered cognitive function and are allowed to drive.

Alternative strong analgesics are shown in Table 1.

Adjuvant analgesic drugs and other treatments

The correct use of adjuvant treatment may mean that morphine is not required or it may be possible to give it in a lower dose. The use of such treatments in various types of cancer pain is summarized in Table 2.

Chronic non-malignant pain

Two-thirds of non-cancer patients experience chronic pain in the last year of life. The many causes include osteoarthritis and rheumatoid arthritis, trigeminal and post-herpetic neuralgia, back problems, bedsores, and the pain of immobility from stroke or severe disability.

Non-opioids, weak opioids, and NSAIDs are the preferred treatment. However, some patients gain partial or good sustained analgesia with morphine, without major side-effects. With severe pain, such as from gangrene, it is essential that adequate doses of morphine are given without delay.

Tricyclic antidepressants and anticonvulsants are used for post-herpetic and trigeminal neuralgia and diabetic neuropathy. Epidural steroids are used for root irritation, sympathetic blocks for ischaemia, and epidural infusions with bupivacaine for severe pain in the lower part of the body, for example with an inoperable fractured femur. Physical methods such as local anaesthetic sprays, TENS, and acupuncture seem of greater value in chronic non-malignant pain than in the pain caused by cancer (see Section 1).

Confusion

Most people nearing death develop some alteration of consciousness, often only in the last few hours of life but sometimes for weeks or more. 'Confusion' is used here to describe the symptoms of both the acute confusional state and dementia. It includes memory loss, inappropriate behaviour, aggression, disorientation, and paranoia.

Causes of confusion

A diagnosis of the cause (or causes) of confusion should be attempted, as even if no reversible factor is found the patient and family will be relieved to know that the altered behaviour is due to physical disease rather than impending insanity.

Potentially reversible causes include medication, especially opioids, and psychotropic drugs. Corticosteroid psychosis is rare. Infections and biochemical changes are often treatable and cerebral oedema associated with tumours can be reduced with dexamethasone. Elderly patients with pre-existing mild dementia may become acutely confused when admitted to hospital.

Table 1 Alternatives to oral morphine

Name	Preparation	Dose interval (hours)	Dose required to give equianalgesic effect to morphine 10 mg/4-hourly	Comment
Buprenorphine	200 μg, 400 μg	6–8	300 μg 8-hourly	Given sublingually
Dextromoramide	5 mg, 10 mg	2	5 mg (short lived peak effect)	Too short-acting for regular use
Fentanyl patch	25 μg/h, 50 μg/h, 75 μg/h, 100 μg/h	72	25 μg/h every 72 h	Titration difficult. Expensive
Hydromorphone	1.3 mg, 2.6 mg, normal release. 2, 4, 8, 16 mg: slow release	4 normal release 12 slow release	1.3 mg 4 hourly	Similar properties to morphine
Methadone	5 mg	12	10 mg (single dose). About 2 mg with repeated administration	Long plasma half-life thus accumulation occurs
Pethidine	50 mg	2–3	100 mg 2–3 hourly	Weak oral analgesic. Short acting
Phenazocine	5 mg	8	2.5 mg 8-hourly	Useful alternative to morphine.
Tramadol	50 mg	4–6	50 mg 4-hourly	Should be considered an alternative to codeine

Table 2 Adjuvant therapy in cancer pain

Type of pain	Adjuvant drug	Other treatment
Bone pain	Diclofenac 150 mg daily or other NSAID	Palliative radiotherapy Immobilization, e.g. surgical fixation
Refractory bone pain	Bisphosphonates, e.g. pamidronate 30–60 mg by intravenous infusion	
Neuropathic pain	Amitriptyline 25 mg at night, with increasing dose for dysaesthetic pain Carbamazepine 200 mg daily, with increasing dose for lancinating pain Flecainide 100–200 mg daily	Epidural steroids Epidural bupivacaine (in lumbar region) TENS
Pancreatic or liver pain	NSAID	Coeliac plexus block
Intestinal colic (from inoperable obstruction)	Hyoscine butylbromide 60–200 mg daily	
Headaches (from raised intracranial pressure)	Dexamethasone 16 mg daily, reducing dose as possible	Cranial irradiation
Chest wall pain	NSAID	Intercostal or thoracic paravertebral block
Lymphoedema		Compression bandaging

Symptomatic management of confusion

Staff should try to understand the patient's experience without agreeing with the underlying misconceptions. A familiar routine is helpful, preferably in home surroundings.

The 'quietly muddled' person may be worsened by sedative drugs. Psychotropic drugs are used to reduce agitation, hallucinations, or paranoia; trifluoperazine and haloperidol sedate relatively little; thioridazine or chlorpromazine rather more.

Constipation

Constipation in terminal illness is usually attributable to inactivity, a low fibre diet, general weakness, confusion, and drugs such as opioids, phenothiazines, and tricyclic antidepressants.

Assessment

The history should include the patient's previous bowel habit, as well as the recent stool frequency and characteristics. Abdominal and rectal examinations avoid misdiagnosis.

Management

Some exercises and added dietary fibre are impossible in the very ill and laxatives are usually required. Faecal softeners, e.g. magnesium sulphate or hydroxide, lactulose and poloxamer, retain water in the bowel by osmosis or increase water penetration of faeces. Stimulant laxatives, e.g. senna, bisacodyl, and danthron, increase colonic muscle activity. This division is not pharmacologically tenable as increased stool size itself causes increased peristalsis, but it remains clinically useful.

A combination of both types of laxative e.g. lactulose and bisacodyl, magnesium hydroxide, and liquid paraffin emulsion with senna, and codanthramer (danthron and poloxamer) avoids either painful colic or a rectum loaded with soft faeces. The dose should be gradually increased until a regular soft bowel action results.

Suppositories, enemas, or manual removal may be needed if the rectum is loaded or the laxative regimen is ineffective. Their use can be minimized by adequate titration of the laxative doses.

Cough

Common causes of cough include bacterial or viral infections, primary or secondary respiratory tract tumours, cardiac failure, asthma, or chronic obstructive airways disease and smoking.

Specific treatments are antibiotics, diuretics, bronchodilators, corticosteroids, and radiotherapy as appropriate. Symptomatic treatments include:

Simple linctus—soothes the pharynx and reduces coughing. Proprietary preparations offer no advantages.

Steam inhalations or nebulized saline—aid the expectoration of viscid sputum, especially if followed by physiotherapy.

Opioids—codeine, morphine, and methadone suppress the cough reflex centrally. They should be reserved for those with a dry cough, those too weak to expectorate or occasionally at night if cough disturbs sleep. If codeine 30–60 mg 4-hourly is ineffective morphine 5mg 4-hourly should be started and the dose titrated until relief is obtained.

Nebulized local anaesthetic—5 ml of 2 per cent lignocaine or 0.5 per cent bupivicaine 4-hourly may be effective but poorly tolerated.

Dysphagia

Causes include malignant or benign obstructive lesions of the pharynx or oesophagus, cerebrovascular disease, cerebral tumours, and motor neurone disease. Dysphagia can be caused, or exacerbated, by pain on swallowing, a dry mouth, and anxiety.

Specific treatments include nystatin or fluconazole for oropharyngeal candida, and radiotherapy, laser therapy, bouginage, or stenting for oesophageal tumour. If a patient with mediastinal lymphadenopathy is unfit for radiotherapy, corticosteroids (dexamethasone 8 mg/day) may produce temporary relief.

General measures comprise dietary modification, correct positioning, and unhurried eating. Patients with obstructive lesions usually find it easier to swallow a nourishing, fluid diet. Those with neurological problems prefer semisolid food. Use of a nasogastric tube, parenteral nutrition, or a gastrostomy in patients with advanced, irreversible disease may simply prolong the process of dying.

Drugs for relief of symptoms may have to be given by subcutaneous infusion or rectally. Aspiration pneumonia should usually be treated symptomatically.

Dyspnoea

Dyspnoea-like pain is subjective. Its severity may be poorly related to tachypnoea or pulmonary pathology. Causes of breathlessness include infection, primary or secondary lung tumour, chronic obstructive airways disease, cardiac failure, pleural effusion, pulmonary embolus, and anxiety. Specific treatment should be combined with symptomatic measures. Low dose oral morphine eases dyspnoea and pain from a chest infection and can be withdrawn if the infection resolves with antibiotics and physiotherapy.

As the disease progresses there is less justification for specific treatment, either because it is ineffective or the patient declines it. Dyspnoea and pain must be palliated even if, for example, antibiotics are not prescribed.

Symptomatic treatment of dyspnoea

Explanation and adjustment. Severe dyspnoea is frightening and is exacerbated by the resultant anxiety. Patients' fears, usually of choking or suffocating, demand explanation and reassurance. An open window, a fan, or a backrest in bed may help, as can relaxation techniques and breathing exercises.

Morphine is an effective symptomatic treatment for dyspnoea in advanced cancer, chronic obstructive airways disease, and motor neurone disease. The mechanism of action involves reduction of the sensitivity of the respiratory centre and peripheral vasodilatation (helpful when there is pulmonary oedema). The sensation of dyspnoea appears to be reduced more than the level of ventilation. Regular oral morphine, starting with 2.5–5 mg 4-hourly and increasing slowly according to symptoms, is safe and effective.

Bronchodilators may help even when wheeze is not obvious, especially in patients with a history of smoking or chronic bronchitis.

Benzodiazepines. Lorazepam 0.5–1 mg given sublingually, is used for the rapid relief of dyspnoea associated with anxiety. Diazepam 2–10 mg at night will give a prolonged effect.

Hyoscine (scopolamine) and glycopyrronium are used, in combination with diamorphine or morphine, to lessen the 'death rattle' which can occur in the last hour of life. The dose of hyoscine is 0.2–0.4 mg 4-hourly by injection, or up to 2.4 mg over 24 hours by subcutaneous infusion. Glycopyrronium is more potent so that dose is half that of hyoscine.

Oxygen. Dyspnoea in terminal illness does not reflect the level of hypoxia. Morphine may be preferable to an oxygen mask or nasal cannulae, which are barriers between the patient and family.

Respiratory emergencies

These include major haemoptysis, pulmonary embolus, or acute tracheal compression. Intravenous midazolam or diazepam 10–20 mg should be given slowly, or diazepam rectal solution 10–20 mg. An alternative is an injection of diamorphine 5 mg with hyoscine 0.4 mg.

Nausea and vomiting

Vomiting results from impulses reaching the vomiting centre in the medulla from a variety of sites in the body. These include the chemoreceptor trigger zone, gastrointestinal tract, vestibular apparatus, intracranial pressure receptors, and cerebral cortex. The cause, or causes, of vomiting can usually be determined from a careful history and clinical examination. Note should be taken of the volume, content, and timing of vomits. A biochemical profile may be needed but other investigations are often inappropriate.

Nausea can be treated with oral medication but alternative routes are needed for the patient with severe vomiting. An antiemetic injection is suitable to control a single episode but, with a persistent problem, it is preferable to give drugs by subcutaneous infusion using a syringe driver. Antiemetics can also be given rectally.

Suggested treatment for some common causes of vomiting is as follows:

Renal failure. Haloperidol 1.5–10 mg/24 h is usually effective. Methotrimeprazine 12.5–50 mg/24 h may be needed for intractable symptoms.

Hypercalcaemia. Most patients are treated with bisphosphonates. If this is ineffective or inappropriate, treatment is similar to that that for renal failure.

Cytotoxic chemotherapy. The use of 5-HT_3 antagonists such as ondansetron has greatly improved the control of emesis, even with cisplatinum. The effect is enhanced by combining them with dexamethasone.

Inoperable gastric outlet obstruction. Metoclopramide 30–80 mg/24 h may be effective if the obstruction is partial. Dexamethasone 8 mg daily, by injection, can shrink inflammatory oedema around an obstructive lesion. Octreotide, a somatostatin analogue, 0.3–0.6 mg/24 h by subcutaneous infusion, reduces gastrointestinal secretions and motility. It may reduce the volume and frequency of vomits, otherwise intubation will be required.

Inoperable intestinal obstruction. Treatment is started with haloperidol 3–5 mg/24 h or cyclizine 150 mg/24 h. The antiemetic will usually be given with diamorphine (for pain) and hyoscine butylbromide 60–200 mg/24 h (for colic). Octreotide is expensive but effective in the majority of patients. Methotrimeprazine 12.5–100 mg/24 h is sometimes needed but the higher doses cause considerable sedation.

Raised intracranial pressure. If dexamethasone is contraindicated or ineffective, cyclizine is the antiemetic of choice.

The last days

The correct management of the last few days of life involves the care of both patient and family. The way in which the death is handled will influence the family's grief, bereavement, and their ability to cope with the future.

As death approaches there is usually a gradual increase in drowsiness and weakness. Experienced staff will recognize that this is not a temporary deterioration but represents the imminence of death. This 'diagnosis of dying' must be confirmed and medication reviewed; all drugs should be stopped except those for symptom relief.

Studies have shown that two-thirds of patients continue to take some oral medication until the last day of life, but essential drugs must be charted so that if swallowing becomes impossible, they can be given by subcutaneous infusion or by regular injection or suppository. The essential drugs are as follows:

Morphine or diamorphine. The oral dose should be converted to the dose for injection and given either by subcutaneous infusion or 4-hourly (see above).

Anticonvulsants should be replaced by diazepam suppositories 10–20 mg twice daily or by midazolam by subcutaneous infusion.

Hyoscine hydrobromide or glycopyrronium may be needed for the 'death rattle' (see above).

Psychotropic drugs While most patients become more drowsy and lapse into coma, some become restless and agitated. This may be due to unrelieved pain, a distended bladder or rectum, or morphine toxicity, especially if renal function is deteriorating. However, usually no cause can be identified. The following drugs are used:

Midazolam 30–100 mg/24 h by subcutaneous infusion.

Methotrimeprazine 25–100 mg/24 h by subcutaneous infusion.

Diazepam suppositories 10 mg as needed.

Phenobarbitone 400–1000 mg/24 h by subcutaneous infusion in separate syringe driver.

Care for the family

It is essential that the close family are informed that death is approaching. They will usually understand that the question 'How long?' cannot be accurately answered and accept 'Just a few hours (or days)'. They should have been involved already in discussions about the illness and its outcome but many will wish to ask specific questions about the process of dying and the continuing need for medication and nursing care at this stage.

The natural urge of families to 'do something' for someone who is dying can be harnessed in practical tasks such as mouth care, washing, and turning. They should be reminded that hearing and touch are the last senses to go, so their physical contact and speech can continue to bring comfort.

Staff should help the family to be present at the death, if this is what they want. But many people have not witnessed a death and need help about what to expect, for example, the changing pattern of breathing.

However much the death has been expected, the actual moment comes as a profound emotional and physical shock. Families therefore need a time of quiet privacy to absorb what has happened and to express their emotions in their own way. After this is the time for staff to show their sympathy. Some family members will wish to help with washing and dressing the body; all will value assurance that this will be done with care and respect, taking into account their wishes and their cultural or religious practices.

Psychological aspects of terminal illness

An understanding of the main psychological and social aspects of terminal illness is as essential to the physician as a knowledge of the methods of pain control. Patients and their families place considerable emphasis on their doctor's ability to communicate effectively and to understand their emotions as well as their physical condition. Yet studies have shown that many doctors have received minimal training in this area and lack the necessary skills.

Talking about death

Most cancer patients now know their diagnosis and are informed about the progress of their illness. This change, over the last 30 years, has come about because of the wishes of patients for information and because it has been shown that anxiety and depression are reduced when open discussion is welcomed.

As the disease progresses and death approaches, open communication remains important. Most dying patients are aware of what is happening and value the opportunity to share their thoughts and fears with the doctor they have come to know. Commonly expressed fears include the possibility of uncontrolled pain, choking, and confusion. Many elderly people dread the prospect of the final stage being prolonged 'artificially' and can be reassured that this will not be done.

Anxiety and depression

It is inevitable that everyone facing death should, at times, feel anxious and depressed. Patients may find themselves unable to concentrate, irritable, unable to sleep, and fearful of the future. These are normal responses to a crisis and, in most cases, resolve with short-term psychological help, giving information, helping the patient find practical steps in adjusting to the circumstances, and emphasizing past strengths and coping mechanisms.

About 10 per cent of terminally ill cancer patients become clinically depressed; this level tends to fall as death approaches. Diagnosis is difficult as biological indicators, such as poor appetite and loss of energy, are of little value. There is a loss of interest and enjoyment in almost all activities.

Treatment is with a combination of antidepressants and psychological measures. Tricyclics and selective serotonin reuptake inhibitors (SSRIs) are equally effective so the choice will depend on their differing side-effects. Since many patients suffer with a dry mouth, drowsiness, and constipation, an SSRI such as paroxetine may be preferred.

For anxiety, diazepam 2–10 mg may be given at night or trifluoperazine 2–4 mg daily in divided doses. Lorazepam 1 mg, given sublingually, is used in panic attacks.

Support for the family

The news that someone is dying has a profound effect on all members of the family and so, in palliative medicine, care must embrace the whole family group. A simple family tree can be made when the patient is first seen, to indicate the size of the family, the previous losses by death or separation, the elderly dependent, and the children who are closely involved. This should enable staff to be aware of some of the family stresses which have been caused by the impending death and they should gently encourage an open discussion of these changes.

Whenever possible, children need preparation before the death; they need to be given information in a form that they can understand and have the chance to ask questions and to express and share their feelings. Parents often value professional help in this immensely difficult task.

Spiritual pain

Faced with serious illness or impending death, many patients will begin to think more deeply about their life and its meaning. Some will have a profound sense of guilt and failure about the past, things left undone, or failed relationships. Others feel deeply that life is meaningless, that there is no point or purpose in it. A few are troubled by the fear of what happens after death.

These, and other considerations, are aspects of spiritual pain and are very real to many dying patients. Doctors need to be aware of these issues, to have thought out their own beliefs and to be able to offer spiritual help if this is asked for. They should be aware of the patient's religious beliefs so that the specific practices of different groups can be adhered to.

Bereavement

Bereavement is something which all people go through at some time in their lives; it remains a bewildering and frightening experience. The bereaved may be overwhelmed by physical or psychological symptoms which they do not understand and suspect that they are seriously ill or going mad.

Immediately after the death there is usually a period of numbness lasting some days but this is followed by a long period when the bereaved person may feel exhausted, eat and sleep poorly, and often feel depressed, guilty, or angry—even with the dead person. Slowly, over many months, these feelings fade, though the 'pangs of grief' may continue, especially at anniversaries. Doctors need to be familiar with the stages of normal grief and mourning so that they can recognize when grief is delayed, inhibited, or becomes chronic and professional help is needed.

Ethical issues in terminal illness

Ethical decisions about treatment are particularly common in the care of the terminally ill. British law provides the following framework:

1. Patients who are conscious and lucid and refuse treatment must have their wish respected. If patients are incompetent, their parent(s) or legal guardian can speak for them, but only if they act in their best interests.
2. When a patient is near death, a doctor is not obliged to embark on or continue extraordinary treatment, including artificial nutrition and hydration, which has no prospect of benefiting the patient.
3. There is an obligation to relieve pain and restore comfort. If, to ease pain, measures must be taken which may hasten death, this is permissible, provided pain relief is the principal aim.
4. Acts with the primary intention of causing the patient's death, or the facilitation of suicide, are forbidden.

Do opioids shorten life?

Appropriate doses of morphine probably lengthen life through the resumption of activity enabled by relief of pain. Two uncommon situations exist in which medication for symptom control may shorten life. The first is when a patient presents with severe malignant dyspnoea associated with pain and the appropriate treatment is with oral morphine, carefully titrating the dose until relief is obtained. The second dilemma is with a patient in a severe, agitated delirium when benzodiazepines or other psychotropic drugs are needed to relieve intolerable distress. The resultant respiratory depression or sedation in these cases may sometimes shorten life, but the aim of treatment in each situation is to relieve suffering.

Nutrition and hydration in terminal illness

Dehydration, in terminal illness, is not painful and patients rarely complain of thirst. Continuing hydration may actually increase the distress of dying as a result of pulmonary oedema, incontinence, and the retained respiratory secretions. Increasing numbers of people have stated that they do not wish their death to be prolonged by artificial means. Hence intravenous fluids are given only if the cause of dehydration is reversible, e.g. hypercalcaemia. The only distressing symptom of terminal dehydration, a dry mouth, is readily treatable with local measures. This approach must be explained to the family: 'He won't drink and therefore he will die' needs to be turned into 'He is dying and therefore does not need to drink'.

Voluntary euthanasia

There is persistent pressure, for a change in the law to allow doctors to prescribe or administer a lethal injection at the patient's request. In The Netherlands euthanasia, although illegal, is tolerated if certain safeguards are met. It appears that 1.8 per cent of deaths in The Netherlands result from euthanasia, although considerable underreporting persists. There continue to be well reported cases where terminal pain has not been controlled, but the major motivation for euthanasia is not poor symptom control but a desire for personal control. Many fear that 'voluntary' euthanasia would not remain voluntary for long. There are major economic forces at work with an ageing population and unspoken pressures on the elderly and dependent who often feel that they are a burden on their families.

Further reading

Doyle, D., Hanks, G.W.C., and MacDonald, N. (eds).(1997). *Oxford textbook of palliative medicine* (2nd edn). Oxford University Press, Oxford.

Kaye, P. (1994). *A-Z of hospice and palliative care* (revised reprint). E.P.L. Publications, Northampton.

Randall, F. and Downie, R.S. (1996). *Palliative care ethics—a good companion.* Oxford University Press, Oxford.

Saunders, C. and Sykes, N. (eds). (1993). *The management of terminal malignant disease* (3rd edn). Edward Arnold, London.

Worden, J.W. (1991). *Grief counselling and grief therapy* (2nd edn). Routledge, London.

Section 16
Infectious disease

Contents

(continued overleaf)

Contents *(continued)*

Fungal infections and mycoses

Protozoa

Nematodes (roundworms)

Cestodes (tapeworms)

Trematodes (flukes)

Infectious disease syndromes

Chapter 16.1

An approach to the patient with suspected infection

H. P. Lambert

Some points are especially important in taking the history when infection is suspected. A careful 'systems inquiry' must be included, since minor system-related clues in a patient with obscure febrile illness may provide the only localizing evidence. But remember that words in common use such as fever have surprisingly different connotations for different people. Thus, 'gastroenteritis', used to equate with diarrhoea, may lead the unwary to assume an infective illness, whereas diarrhoea and vomiting can, of course, have a host of non-infectious causes. The timing and duration of symptoms is especially helpful. For example, viral infection is often postulated in patients with prolonged fever, but acute fevers of viral origin rarely last longer than a few weeks. Prolonged fever is certainly often microbial in origin, but its cause is rarely viral. Travel is another important element of the history, especially when malaria is possible; the dates of travel and possible exposure are often well known and can be related to known incubation periods. Travellers may also acquire infections which are not specifically tropical, notably sexually transmitted and respiratory infections. The travel history may have implications for public health as well as for the individual patient, as when diseases such as tuberculosis, typhoid, or Lassa fever are in question. Occupation provides occasional leads, and health care personnel must be included in those at special risk. Previous medication is sometimes relevant, especially in patients developing fever during treatment.

Physical examination

Fever is not always caused by infection and not all infections produce fever, but infection is the most frequent cause of fever. Oral or skin temperature measurements are unreliable in severely ill or shocked patients, and core temperature must then be measured. At the other extreme, pathological fever has to be differentiated from normal cyclical variations of body temperature in minor fevers of long standing.

Patterns of fever are in practice seldom helpful, chiefly because 'classical' fever charts are of low sensitivity for the relevant diagnosis, and because patterns are easily altered by antibiotics or antipyretics. The most dangerous misconception is associated with malaria. Regular tertian or quartan cycles are not found in the early days of the illness and often not at all in the most dangerous, *P. falciparum* infections; the temperature pattern is often quite erratic and malaria must be considered in all febrile (and some non-febrile) patients in or from a malarial area. Hectic fever, with large variations in the body temperature accompanied by chills and even rigors, is a feature of pyogenic infections such as acute pyelonephritis or pyogenic abscesses, but can be seen in many other conditions, for example, with lymphoma, sometimes in tuberculosis, and even in drug fever.

As with the history, some features of the full physical examination are especially useful in fever. Rashes may be pathognomonic, as in measles, varicella, herpesvirus 6, parvovirus, and Lyme disease (see OTM3, p. 267). The haemorrhagic rash of meningococcal sepsis is a vitally important sign, but the early rash in this infection may be non-specific. Of travellers' infections, rickettsial disease, leptospirosis, and the viral haemorrhagic fevers such as Lassa fever are notable. Other signs worth special notice include: oral signs, e.g. of HIV-associated infections and the raw red tongue of scarlet fever, toxic shock syndrome, and Kawasaki disease: murmurs suggesting endocarditis: the fundi, lymph nodes, and spleen. Patients with meningitis, encephalitis, or brain abscess usually have initial clinical features such as neck stiffness or changes in cerebration which indicate central nervous system involvement, but meningitis may be difficult to diagnose in babies and the elderly, and the onset of cryptococcal meningitis may be very insidious. Whatever signs are or are not found, however, an important rule is to make repeated and detailed examinations. A changing heart murmur, a new skin lesion, or the finding of an abdominal mass may immediately redefine the diagnostic possibilities.

Many infectious illnesses have no specific clinical features; their elucidation relies entirely on laboratory study. Since most infectious disease worldwide afflicts patients with minimal or no access to laboratory tests, diagnosis is often therefore a best guess. But even a modest number of laboratory tests, some of them inexpensive and not requiring much training, greatly enlarges the diagnostic range. Microscopy of blood films is essential for the diagnosis of malaria, and may reveal trypanosomiasis, some forms of filariasis, leptospirosis, relapsing fever, and bartonellosis. The differential leucocyte count is an important staging post in the diagnosis of febrile patients. Neutrophilia is found in pyogenic bacterial infections, amoebiasis, leptospirosis, thromboembolism, various forms of connective tissue disease, rheumatic fever, Still's disease, in exacerbations of chronic hepatitis, and in mechanical tissue damage. Neutropenia is common in malaria, visceral leishmaniasis, typhoid, brucellosis, rickettsial disease, and in many viral infections including HIV. Eosinophilia, especially if substantial, can be an invaluable lead, so too can a high proportion of atypical mononuclear cells or the presence of primitive precursors. Microscopy of a fresh urine specimen reveals pus cells and bacteria, important since focal symptoms may be entirely absent in urinary infection. At a somewhat more elaborate level, diagnostic possibilities are further increased by the ability to culture urine, blood, pus, stools, and occasionally other specimens, while the addition of a chest radiograph makes another big inroad into the diagnosis. These investigations are often the most readily available tests, but are all of high diagnostic yield in suspected infection.

Where more sophisticated laboratory and imaging facilities are available, investigation of suspected infection is, of course, much more extensive, and often includes initial serology and antigen detection tests for suspected pathogens, and relevant imaging methods. In particular, modern imaging and radionucleide techniques have greatly aided diagnosis of the more elusive and prolonged illnesses. Biopsy and culture of a suspect site, often with ultrasound guidance, has also been especially productive in establishing the diagnosis when the situation is obscure. Decisions about further investigation call for fine judgement of costs and benefits; unnecessary multiplication of investigations, often repeated because of poor organization rather than medical necessity, should be avoided.

Further reading

Farrar, W. E., Wood, M. J., and Innes, J. A. (1992). *Infectious diseases—text and color atlas.* 2nd edn. Gower Medical, London.

Mandell, G. L., Douglas, R. G., and Bennett, J. E. (1990). *Principles and practice of infectious diseases.* 3rd edn. Churchill Livingstone, Edinburgh.

Chapter 16.2

The host's response to infection

B. M. Greenwood

Introduction

Man is exposed constantly to potentially pathogenic micro-organisms, yet clinical infections are rare events and fatal infections even rarer. Why does one individual exposed to an organism such as the meningococcus develop an asymptomatic infection while another exposed to the same bacterium succumb to an illness that kills within a few hours of the first appearance of symptoms? 'Why me, not him?' is a question that the unfortunate victim could reasonably have asked. Occasionally there is an obvious answer, for example the patient with fulminating meningococcal disease might have had a complement deficiency, but in many cases there is no obvious explanation. In many traditional societies the power of supernatural forces may be invoked, and in societies where this kind of explanation is no longer accepted there is a tendency to fall back on the concept of 'chance' or 'bad luck'. While random selection of victims must occur, the invocation of chance is usually an expression of our ignorance about the many complex variables that influence the course of an infection in a particular individual.

The outcome of the contact between a potential pathogen and its host can be influenced by the virulence or infecting dose of the pathogen or the host's genetic characteristics, immunity (naturally acquired or induced), hormonal or nutritional status, the presence of an underlying infection, or use of drugs.

The pathogen

Virulence

The ability of an organism to cause disease requires colonization of its host. In tetanus, this is all that is required, but in pneumococcal infection, disease occurs only if tissue invasion is achieved. Pathogens may, therefore, require both adhesins and invasins. Different strains of the same organism may vary in their ability to colonize or invade, an important variable influencing the outcome of a pathogen–host encounter. Once colonization or invasion has been achieved, tissue damage may result from the production of either powerful exotoxins, such as tetanus toxin, or endotoxins which cause local tissue destruction. Strains may vary in their ability to produce toxins and thus in their ability to cause disease.

In the case of some infections, tissue damage depends not upon the direct effect of products of the invading organism but upon the ability of these to induce a damaging immune response by the host. Different strains may vary in their ability to do this, for example there has recently been some suggestion that different strains of *Plasmodium falciparum* vary in their ability to induce the production by the host of tumour necrosis factor, a cytokine that probably plays an important part in the pathogenesis of cerebral malaria.

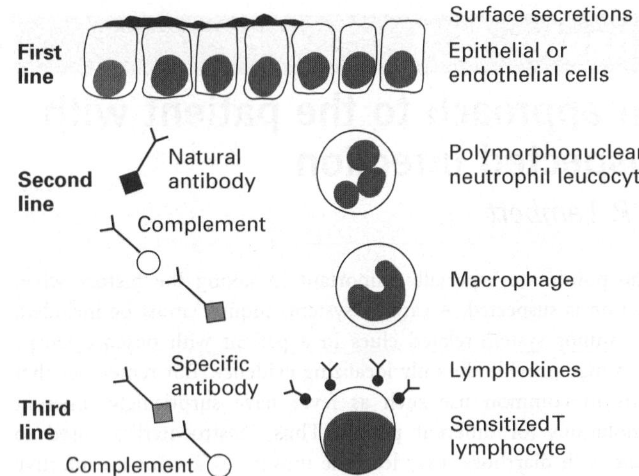

Fig. 1 Three lines of defence against infection.

Dose

The importance of infecting dose as a determinant of the outcome of infection has probably been underestimated. However, studies in animals and in human volunteers have clearly shown the importance of dose in determining the severity of gastrointestinal infections. Cleaning one's teeth in contaminated water may be relatively safe while to drink it would be disastrous. Infective dose is probably also an important factor in determining the outcome of infections spread by respiratory droplets. The high mortality of measles seen in secondary cases infected by an older sibling is probably a reflection of the large dose of virus to which these children have been exposed.

Host defences

Man has a complex set of defences against potentially pathogenic organisms (Fig. 1). These include mechanical barriers such as the skin and mucosae, whose efficacy is enhanced by the secretion of non-specific bactericidal substances such as lysozyme and gastric acid. Action of respiratory cilia helps to protect the lower respiratory tract.

If pathogens succeed in breaching the host's local defences they may be countered by a variety of non-specific and specific immune mechanisms. Fever, acute phase proteins such as C-reactive protein, and polymorphonuclear neutrophil leucocytes may provide some immediate partial protection while specific humoral and cellular immune responses are being generated. The speed with which the latter are brought into play will be influenced strongly by whether or not the host's immune response has been primed by previous exposure to a relevant antigen through natural exposure or through vaccination. Antibodies may protect by neutralization of toxins, opsonization, or by causing complement mediated membrane damage. Cellular responses may involve direct T lymphocyte mediated membrane damage or activation of macrophages which kill directly or with the aid of antibody.

Factors that can influence the host's response to infection

A large number of factors can influence the host's response to infection.

Genetic factors and susceptibility to infection

Studies with inbred strains of experimental animals have indicated clearly that genetic factors influence susceptibility to infectious diseases and their clinical outcome. Differentiation of the role of genetic and environmental factors in determining susceptibility to infection in man has proved to be more difficult. However, studies conducted in identical twins have provided strong evidence for the role of genetic factors in some infectious diseases. Thus, the twin of a patient with tuberculosis or leprosy has a higher risk of contracting the infection than a control, even when the twin is brought up in a different environment from his/her sibling. The relationship between the HLA system and susceptibility to infection has been investigated in several ways. At a population level it has been shown that the distribution of certain HLA antigens is related to the geographical distribution of widespread infections such as malaria. At the individual level it has been demonstrated that patients with some infections, for example tuberculosis or leprosy, possess certain HLA haplotypes significantly more frequently than carefully matched controls. Finally, it has been shown that in families with more than one case of infection, affected siblings carry the same haplotype as the index cases significantly more frequently than non-affected siblings, although the haplotype involved may vary from family to family.

Histocompatibility-related factors may influence the clinical outcome of an infection as well as its incidence. HLA-determined factors may influence whether a patient infected with *Mycobacterium leprae* develops the lepromatous or tuberculoid form of the disease. The likelihood that hepatitis B infection will progress to chronic liver disease is HLA-related as is the development of hepatic fibrosis in patients with schistosomiasis. Possession of the HLA antigen B27 increases the likelihood that arthritis will develop after gastrointestinal infection with yersinia, salmonella, or shigella.

Immune responsiveness is related to the possession of certain genetically determined allotypes of immunoglobulin molecules. In man, immune responsiveness to meningococcal and *H. influenzae* polysaccharides is related to the presence of a specific κ_m allotype of IgG and some studies have shown a decreased incidence of bacterial meningitis in κ_mI-positive subjects.

Possession of specific blood-group antigens also influences susceptibility to some infections. Severe schistosomiasis mansoni and giardiasis are encountered more frequently in blood group A individuals than in subjects with other ABO blood groups, and non-secretors of blood-group antigens have an increased risk of becoming meningococcal nasopharyngeal carriers.

Mechanisms by which genetic factors increase susceptibility to infection

Influence on surface receptors

Genetic factors may influence the function of cell-membrane receptors involved in invasion. Thus, red cells can be infected with *P. vivax* only if they possess a surface receptor closely related to the Duffy red-cell antigen. Most West Africans lack Duffy antigens, thus offering the probable explanation for the infrequent occurrence of *P. vivax* malaria in West Africa. Recently, it has been shown that subjects with a genetic variant of the CCR5 receptor of CD4 T lymphocytes are protected against HIV infection.

Influence on the specific immune response

A number of clearly defined, genetically determined, primary immunodeficiency syndromes have been described which are associated with an increased susceptibility to infection, but these are responsible for only a small fraction of all severe infections. It is possible that more subtle genetically determined defects of the immune system contribute to the pathogenesis of a much larger proportion of cases of infectious disease but that these have not yet been defined.

Processed antigens are presented to T lymphocytes as peptides in association with HLA class I or class II antigens and it is, therefore, not surprising that HLA type can influence susceptibility to infection. Binding of microbe-derived peptides to some but not to other HLA class II antigens may facilitate the ability of some individuals to mount an effective immune response. Presentation of peptides in association with HLA class I antigens may induce a T cell mediated cytotoxic attack. This may help to eliminate the infection but only at the cost of extensive cell damage. Thus, individuals may vary in their susceptibility to immunopathology according to their HLA type.

Constitutional factors and susceptibility to infection

Age

Many infectious diseases show a characteristic age distribution. Infants are often protected against infection with ubiquitous organisms by antibody transmitted across the placenta. Susceptibility to infection increases in the old in association with a decline in immune responsiveness. The age distribution of many infectious diseases is determined by age-dependent occupational or social activities. Thus, in some areas malaria is primarily a disease of adult males who work in the forest where they are exposed to infection.

Age influences not only susceptibility to infection but also its clinical severity. Poliomyelitis, yellow fever, infectious hepatitis, EBV infection, and mumps are all milder infections in children than in adults. Why this should be the case has never been explained satisfactorily. It is possible that immunopathological reactions are more marked in adults than in children because of maturation of the immune system or because of previous exposure to cross-reacting antigens, but this is unlikely to be the only explanation for this phenomenon.

Sex and hormonal factors

Variation in the sex distribution of infectious diseases may be brought about by both social and hormonal factors. Some infections are commoner in men than in women because men come into close contact with the source of the infection more frequently than women as a result of their occupation, as mentioned above. However, for reasons that are not obvious, young women are more susceptible to tuberculosis than young men. Certain infections, e.g. hepatitis, pneumococcal infection, amoebiasis, and malaria, are more severe when they occur during pregnancy than when they occur at other times.

An excess of glucocorticosteroids, resulting from adrenal hyperplasia, an adrenal tumour, or steroid therapy, increases susceptibility to many infections and increases their severity. Herpes simplex and herpes zoster can cause severe, and sometimes fatal, infections in patients who are receiving large doses of corticosteroids. Tuberculosis, amoebiasis, and strongyloidiasis can all be activated by these drugs and strongyloidiasis may be particularly severe in patients receiving corticosteroids.

Patients with diabetes, show an increased susceptibility to several infections. Boils, abscesses, and urinary tract infections are common.

Table 1 Some common infections seen more frequently, or with increased severity, in the malnourished

Protozoa	Bacteria	Viruses	Yeasts
Amoebiasis	Cholera	Viruses	Yeasts
Giardiasis	Gram-negative sepsis	Herpes simplex	Candidiasis
Pneumocystis	Infectious diarrhoea Tuberculosis	Infectious hepatitis Measles	

Tuberculosis may be activated, and pulmonary infections with yeasts or fungi may occur.

Trauma

Trauma predisposes to infection in several ways. Damage to the surface defences, for example by a severe burn, opens the way to systemic invasion by organisms which are normally confined to the surface of the body. Severe burns also have a depressive effect on the immune system. Tissue destruction as a result of mechanical trauma or vascular damage can create an environment in which anaerobic organisms, such as *Clostridium tetani* and *C. perfringens*, can thrive. Salmonellae may invade bone infarcts in patients with sickle cell disease. Tonsillectomy and intramuscular injections predispose to paralytic poliomyelitis but the mechanism of this association is uncertain.

Malnutrition

Numerous studies in experimental animals have shown that dietary deficiency of protein, of individual vitamins, and of trace elements increases susceptibility to infection with a wide variety of organisms. Likewise, in man clinical studies have shown that certain infections are more frequent or more severe in malnourished subjects than in healthy controls (Table 1). Children with kwashiorkor are much more susceptible to infection than those with marasmus. The pathogenesis of the enhanced susceptibility to infection shown by subjects with protein energy malnutrition is complex, for this form of malnutrition affects adversely nearly all host defence mechanisms.

In man, severe isolated deficiencies of metals and vitamins are rarely encountered, but it has been shown that iron deficiency increases susceptibility to certain bacterial infections. Deficiency of vitamin A predisposes to infection at epithelial surfaces and increases the severity of measles.

Studies in severely malnourished refugees have shown that refeeding may be associated with an increased prevalence of tuberculosis, brucellosis, amoebiasis, malaria, and herpes. Furthermore, some studies have shown that treatment of iron-deficient subjects with iron increases their susceptibility to malaria. Thus, dietary deprivation may under some circumstances protect against infection.

Infection

The fact that one infection frequently follows hard upon the heels of another is well known. Some examples of this phenomenon are shown in Table 2. The mechanisms underlying these associations vary from infection to infection and they are, in some instances, very complex. Tissues damaged by one organism may provide a favourable environment for invasion by another. Thus, *C. tetani* can colonize infected wounds and tetanus may follow a guinea-worm infection. Old tuberculous cavities may be colonized by moulds such as Aspergillus. Damage to the epithelium of the respiratory tract by viruses may predispose to subsequent pulmonary infection with bacteria. Some degree of immunosuppression accompanies most infections; it is the rule rather than the exception. In some cases immunodepression produced in this way is of interest to the immunologist but of little importance to the patient. However, in a few cases, suppression of the immune response of the host regularly leads to a secondary infection which has a major influence on the outcome of the patient's illness. Measles is an important example of this phenomenon. Children with this infection frequently develop secondary bacterial infections, such as pneumonia and severe gastroenteritis. Tuberculosis may be activated and activation of herpes simplex may result in severe ulceration of the mucosa of the mouth and the cornea or, occasionally, an overwhelming viraemia. HIV infection provides another striking example of the ability of one infection to increase susceptibility to another by an effect on the immune response, in this case destruction of CD4 cells. A surprising feature of the enhanced susceptibility of HIV infected subjects to secondary infections is its selectivity. Thus, HIV-infected subjects are greatly at risk from tuberculosis but HIV appears to have little effect on leprosy. HIV-infected subjects have a greatly increased risk of pneumococcal and salmonella infections but this is not the case for some other bacterial infections. CD4 cells are believed to play an important part in the development of immunity to malaria and yet there is little evidence that the HIV epidemic in Africa has had any effect on this infection.

Drugs

The problem of infection in patients receiving cytotoxic or immunosuppressive drugs is considered in Chapter 16.117. Alcohol in excess increases susceptibility to many infections, especially when cirrhosis of the liver has supervened. Septicaemia is a common terminal event in intravenous drug addicts who neglect simple hygienic precautions. Smoking, by damaging the epithelium of the respiratory tract, predisposes to respiratory infections.

Malignant disease

Immune responsiveness is impaired in patients with widespread malignant disease, and such patients have an increased risk of infection, sometimes with organisms of low virulence. The risk of infection may be increased further by extensive radiotherapy or by treatment with cytotoxic drugs.

Modulation of the host response to infection

Suppression of the immune response to infection

When an immunopathological response dominates the clinical features of an infection, it may be necessary to depress the immune response of the host, even if this carries the risk of allowing enhanced growth of the causative organism. The drugs used most frequently to prevent or control immunopathological complications of infection are corticosteroids. Some examples of the use of corticosteroids to diminish an immunopathological complication of infection are given in Table 3.

Enhancement of the host's response to infection

There are a number of ways in which the resistance to an infection of an individual, or of a community, can be enhanced.

Table 2 Examples of situations in which one infection predisposes to another

Primary infection	Secondary infection	Likely mechanism of susceptibility
Bartonellosis	Salmonella septicaemia	Haemolysis
HIV	Pneumocystis, tuberculosis, and many other infections	↓ Cell-mediated immunity and other immune functions
Influenza	Bacterial pneumonia	Damage to epithelium
Malaria	Salmonella septicaemia	↓ PMN function ↓ Humoral immunity Haemolysis
Measles	Bacterial pneumonia, gastroenteritis, herpes simplex, tuberculosis	Severe impairment of cellular and humoral immunity
Meningococcal disease	Herpes simplex	↓ Cell-mediated immunity
Pneumococcal disease	Herpes simplex	↓ Cell-mediated immunity
Schistosomiasis	Salmonella septicaemia	Adult worm acts as a focus
Septic abortion	Tetanus, gas gangrene	Tissue damage
Tuberculosis	Aspergillosis	Tissue damage
Trypanosomiasis	Pneumococcal pneumonia	↓ Humoral immunity

Table 3 Some examples of the use of corticosteroids to diminish the immunopathological response to an infection

Condition	Comments
Acute rheumatic carditis	Short-term beneficial effect; no protection against valve damage
Chronic hepatitis B infection (chronic active hepatitis)	Corticosterois given with azathioprine increase survival
Mumps orchitis	Symptomatic relief; no protection against sterility
Onchocerciasis	Diminish reaction to treatment with diethylcarbamazine
Acute schistosomiasis (Katayama fever)	Reported to be effective
Tuberculous meningitis and pericarditis	Probably reduces late sequelae

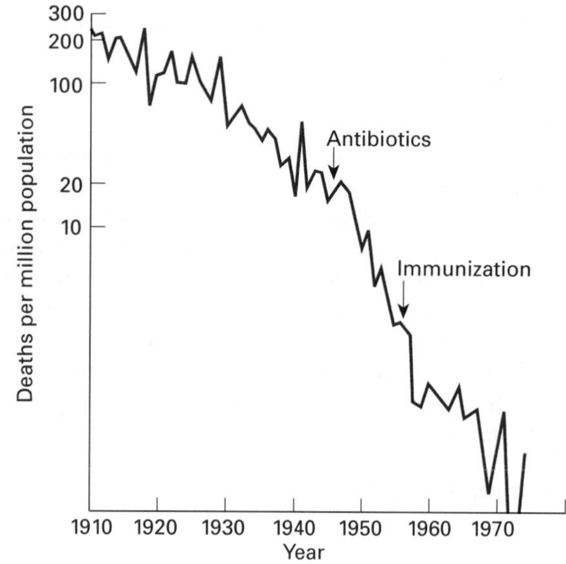

Fig. 2 Whooping-cough deaths per million population in England and Wales in relation to the introduction of antibiotics and whooping-cough immunization
(modified from Dick (1978). In New trends and developments in vaccines (ed. A. Voller and H. Friedman). MTP Press, Lancaster).

Correction of predisposing factors to infection

Improvement in general living standards is sometimes as important a factor in controlling an infectious disease as specific immunoprophylaxis. This point is clearly illustrated by studying the incidence of major infectious diseases in industrialized countries throughout the twentieth century. In many cases, for example, whooping cough, the incidence of the infection and the mortality that it caused, fell considerably before the discovery of antibiotics and before the introduction of vaccination (Fig. 2). The importance of correcting underlying nutritional deficiencies has recently been demonstrated by trials of vitamin A supplementation, which have led to reductions in overall mortality and morbidity from gastrointestinal and respiratory diseases in several, although not all, studies.

Chemoprophylaxis

Chemoprophylaxis has a valuable role to play in increasing host resistance to infection in specific circumstance (Chapter 16.7). A decision as to whether to embark upon chemoprophylaxis in a particular situation requires careful balancing of potential benefits and risks as nearly all drugs used for chemoprophylaxis have the potential to cause serious side-effects. Furthermore, widespread use of antimicrobials for chemoprophylaxis encourages the emergence of resistant organisms. Chemoprophylaxis is most effective when used in a subject of high risk of infection for a short period.

Passive immunoprophylaxis

Polyvalent gamma globulin

Polyvalent gamma globulin, given by regular intramuscular or by less painful intravenous injections, is of proven value in protecting patients with agammaglobulinaemia or severe hypogammaglobulinaemia from a variety of infections.

Specific antisera

Specific antisera are still used to provide protection against a limited number of infections. Antisera with a high titre of antibodies to tetanus toxin effectively prevent tetanus, although not infection with *C. tetani.* Antitetanus serum is used less widely than in the past now that a high proportion of the population of areas where tetanus is prevalent has been actively immunized against tetanus in infancy. Hyperimmune rabies immunoglobulin (RIG) is recommended for patients with a high risk of infection; administration of RIG in the correct dose not interfere significantly with the response to active immunization provided that vaccine is given first. Gamma globulin has been used extensively in the past to provide short-term protection against hepatitis A infection but it is likely to be used less frequently for this purpose in the future now that a hepatitis A vaccine is commercially available.

Antisera with high titres of antibody against specific micro-organisms have been used to provide short-term protection for immunocompromised children exposed to a potentially dangerous infection such as herpes zoster.

Polymorphonuclear neutrophil leucocytes

Transfusions of granulocytes can help to provide short-term protection against infection in patients with severe leucopenia resulting from cytotoxic drug therapy, malignant disease, or infection. However, this is an expensive and not very effective form of prophylaxis.

Cytokines

As the complex nature of the cytokine networks becomes better defined it may be possible to modulate the immune system in a particular direction through cytokine therapy. For example, in some infections a Th1 immune response may be associated with a protective immune response while a Th2 response is not. Cytokine therapy might help to drive the immune response in the direction required. Cytokines are used already in the management of some infections, for example the use of gamma interferon to treat chronic hepatitis C infection, but immunomodulatory therapy is still only at an early stage of development.

Active immunization

The best and most successful approach to enhancing an individual's resistance to infection lies through active immunization, one of the greatest successes of modern medicine. This topic is considered in Chapter 16.6.

Conclusion

In this chapter some of the numerous factors that can influence susceptibility to infection have been considered. This list must be borne in mind whenever a patient with a serious infection is seen. In such a situation the first task of the physician is to identify correctly the causative organism and to start an appropriate form of treatment. However, he or she must also try to establish how and why the patient became infected. Failure to recognize an underlying systemic illness may lead to failure of an apparently appropriate course of chemotherapy.

Further reading

Hill, A.V.S. (1999). Immunogenetics of human infectious diseases. *Annual Review of Immunology*, in press.

Liu, C.-C., Young, L.H.Y., and Young, D.-E. (1996). Lymphocyte mediated cytolysis and disease. *New England Journal of Medicine* **335**, 1651–8.

Saper, C.B. and Breder, C.D. (1994). The neurologic basis of fever. *New England Journal of Medicine* **330**, 1880–6.

Chapter 16.3

Epidemiology and public health

R. T. Mayon-White

Introduction

Epidemiology began as the investigation of large outbreaks of disease (epidemics) and has evolved into the study of the factors related to disease in populations. Public health is the application of epidemiological knowledge to the health of populations. Practical epidemiology follows a course that resembles clinical practice, identifying the presenting problem, collecting facts about the disease in a population (history taking), looking for more information (clinical examination), using epidemiological methods to test explanations for the outbreak (diagnostic investigations), and applying preventive measures (treatment).

Host, environment, and agent (see also Chapter 16.2)

To become infected, a person must be exposed to an infective dose of a micro-organism to which they are susceptible and the host and micro-organism must be brought together by environmental factors. Severe infections are relatively uncommon considering the ubiquity of many pathogenic micro-organisms, but pathogens survive better if they do not incapacitate or kill their hosts.

Variation in the occurrence of disease

The public's interest is excited by epidemics, when the incidence of disease is abnormally high. The term 'outbreak' is used for small, confined epidemics—two or more associated cases of any disease. When it is uncertain whether the cases are linked, the expected incidence is the measure of whether there is an outbreak. Seasonal variation in incidence is predictable, and well illustrated by respiratory infections, like influenza, which occur more often in winters of both the Northern and Southern hemispheres. The peaks in influenza are demonstrated by increased deaths and hospital admissions from pneumonia, absence from work, general practice consultations for 'flu', and the laboratory detection of influenza viruses.

Interactions between different organisms play a part in seasonal and geographical variation. Influenza is associated with the winter increase of meningococcal disease. Viral damage to the pharyngeal mucosa may facilitate the invasion of meningococci, resulting in bacteraemia and meningitis instead of a non-pathogenic colonization. In the 'meningitis belt' of subSaharan Africa, meningococcal disease has a marked seasonal incidence, with epidemics coming at the end of the dry season, possibly because dust acts as the preliminary irritant to the nasal mucosa. Malaria, with its dependence on the Anopheles mosquito, has a marked geographical and seasonal variation. Within tropical areas, high altitude reduces the number of mosquito vectors.

Table 1 The transmissibility of infectious diseases

Route of spread	Examples	Comment
Airborne respiratory droplets	Colds, measles, chickenpox, meningitis	Droplets are expelled by coughing, sneezing, and speech
Direct contact	Streptococcal skin infections, scabies, gonorrhoea	Close or intimate contact is required
Indirect contact via hands of nurses and doctors	Staphylococcal infection; bladder infections in catheterized patients	Hospital infection is sometimes called nosocomial
Faecal–oral	Poliomyelitis, Giardia, Shigella	Organisms on unwashed hands may reach food
Food or water borne	Salmonella, Cryptosporidium	Food offers the bacteria an opportunity to multiply
Blood borne	Hepatitis B, HIV	Transfusions, needle-stick injuries
Congenital and perinatal	Rubella, toxoplasmosis, group B streptococci	Infections that cross the placenta, or are acquired in the birth canal
Mammal bites	Rabies	
Insect borne	Malaria, yellow fever	

In the subtropics, malaria is much less common in winter months when insect activity is reduced. In temperate regions, the summer conditions are too short to sustain the necessary pool of infected mosquitoes and people to make malaria an endemic disease.

In addition to the regular variations caused by climate, there are unexpected fluctuations in the incidence of infection. Often these are the result of either the arrival of a new infection in a susceptible population or a fault in the normal control mechanisms. In a way that is parallel to the individual susceptibility, populations vary in their susceptibility, through past exposure, vaccination, education, and the environments that they inhabit and modify.

The spread of infection

The transmissibility of infectious diseases makes the methods of spread fundamental to their control (Table 1). Often the course of an epidemic suggests the means of spread. A food-borne outbreak is typically short and sharp following a single meal. A water-borne outbreak has a lower but more persistent incidence, because of the smaller chances of consuming an infected dose in a single drink of water, but the exposure is frequent. Person-to-person faecal–oral spread will produce the classical epidemic curve, with the numbers of cases starting low, rising exponentially as the infection spreads from case to case, and finally falling sharply when most of the susceptible people have been infected and recovered.

Surveillance

Surveillance is the systematic collection and analysis of information about disease. Public interest in epidemics depends on, and itself determines, which diseases are monitored. Most surveillance methods are based on medical events: consultations with a doctor, hospital admissions, deaths, laboratory diagnoses. For surveillance, these events must be recorded routinely, and reported to a local or central office for analysis. The results should be reported back to the recorders and to the public.

In the notification of infectious diseases and the certification of deaths, doctors are legally required to give medical information on named individuals to officials in the public interest. Mortality statistics are a long-standing method of surveillance. In practice, notifications of infections are incomplete, but the trends have epidemiological significance.

The incompleteness of notifications has promoted alternatives. Sentinel or 'spotter' practices are doctors who record all new cases of selected conditions. This is a sensitive, rapid way of detecting influenza epidemics. It has a well-defined denominator (the population registered with the general practitioner), and confidentiality because patients' names are not required. Another system is based on laboratory reports to a central agency, the Communicable Disease Surveillance Centre for England, Wales, and Northern Ireland, or to the Scottish Centre for Infection and Environmental Health (SCIEH). Special surveys can directly study the population from which information is required. As an example, a cross-section of the population of children at school and women at antenatal clinics may be sampled and blood specimens taken for rubella virus antibodies to see how well the combined effects of natural infection and vaccination are protecting girls against rubella in pregnancy.

Investigation of outbreaks

One of the key functions of surveillance is to detect outbreaks in time to investigate their causes and to apply preventive measures. Once an outbreak is suspected, the first step is to check the diagnosis on the index (first reported) case. If the diagnosis or the incidence is doubtful, more definite evidence of an outbreak will be needed before a full investigation is justified. Knowledge of the incubation period (the time between the moment of infection and the onset of disease) will indicate the time when infection could have occurred. Interviews with early cases will often reveal several leads to the possible causes, and show where there may be further cases to study. With a case definition to determine who is counted as part of the outbreak, more information is collected covering age, sex, home and work address, occupation, recent travel, and factors that are pertinent to the disease in question, especially on features that may be shared with other cases. The information can be collected by interview or written questionnaires. An analytical epidemiological method (a case-control or a cohort study) can test the strength of the association between the disease and the presumed source. Once complete, the investigation should be written up with recommendations on how similar problems could be prevented. In an outbreak, the press will take a very active interest, so that public relations are an important part of the outbreak management.

Methods of infectious disease control

Hygiene

One of the simplest methods of infection control is hygiene. Hygiene rules are conventional modes of behaviour, like hand-washing after defaecation or avoiding coughing directly into somebody's face, which are taught in childhood. Their purpose is commonly understood and they fit with what is known about the spread of infection. However, inadequate facilities, such as a shortage of soap or water, and poor discipline can make the rules difficult to observe.

Codes of good practice are used to prevent hospital infection, food poisoning, and occupational diseases, and are referred to if a complaint is made against the hospital, caterer, or employer. They incur costs, not only for the materials required, but also by consuming time and restricting activities.

The removal of pathogenic organisms is a key part of good hygiene. The complete removal of pathogens is sterilization. Often it is sufficient to reduce the pathogens to below a harmful dose (disinfection or decontamination), by cleaning to dilute or wash off the pathogen, chemical inactivation, by lesser degrees of heat, or by filtration.

Vaccination is discussed in Chapter 16.6.

Chemotherapy and chemoprophylaxis

Antimicrobial chemotherapy has a small but significant role in public health. The treatment of tuberculosis, sexually transmitted infections, typhoid fever, and diphtheria reduces the risk of further cases. The contacts of newly diagnosed cases should be followed up and offered treatment. Regular penicillin prophylaxis for patients who have rheumatic fever, antimalarial drugs for travellers to warmer climates, and rifampicin for the close contacts of patients with meningococcal meningitis (see Chapter 16.41) are three generally recommended preventive uses of chemotherapy.

Isolation

When there are no other methods of infection control, isolation of the infected individual is useful, typically by putting the infected patients in single-bedded hospital rooms. This is irksome to isolated patients when they are recovering; elderly or mentally ill patients may become confused. The ultimate isolation is plastic tents with controlled ventilation in high-security infectious disease units for patients with viral haemorrhagic fevers. This may be unnecessary, because patients with Lassa fever have been nursed in ordinary single rooms without secondary cases. British law provides for the compulsory admission to hospital of patients with notifiable infectious diseases to prevent the spread of infection, but this power is very rarely used and can be applied only for short periods. Therefore it is not possible to control the risk of infection from someone who is persistently infectious (e.g. HIV infection or untreated tuberculosis) by enforced admission. Attempts to control infection by reverse isolation, that is, by the exclusion of infected people, are also prone to failure. Quarantine at seaports failed to exclude plague or cholera from European countries, and health screening at immigration desks in airports fails to exclude tuberculosis or HIV today. Infected schoolchildren may provoke demands that they be excluded from school, despite the higher risk of transmission from the children who have not had their infections recognized. Food handlers who have become convalescent carriers of non-typhoid salmonellae do not need to be excluded from work if good hygiene is observed. The threat of isolation and exclusion tends to make people frightened and hide their infections.

Further reading

Bassett, W. H. (ed.) (1995). *Clay's handbook of environmental health.* Chapman and Hall, London.

Beneson, A. S. (1995). *The control of communicable diseases in man.* 16th edn. American Public Health Association, Washington DC.

Committee of Inquiry into the Future of the Public Health Function (1988). *Public health in England.* HMSO, London.

Salisbury, D.M. and Begg, N.T. (1996). *Immunisation against infectious disease.* HMSO, London.

Chapter 16.4

Physiological changes in infected patients

P. A. Murphy

Both systemic and local inflammation are due to mediators of host origin whose initial effects are on vascular endothelium and on phagocytic cells.

Clinical sepsis is most commonly caused by bacterial infection, but may also result from non-bacterial infections, or from major trauma without evidence of infection. Since inflammation progresses through multiple cascades of host-mediated reactions, removal of the bacteria after inflammation has been initiated may not affect the outcome. This is why patients still die of pneumococcal pneumonia even if the pneumococcus is exquisitely sensitive to penicillin. If we understood how inflammation progressed, we might be able to interfere with some crucial mediator, and save patients who are too far gone to respond to antibiotics alone.

Triggers for inflammation

Bacteria and fungi

All bacteria are recognized as foreign and cause inflammation immediately on entry into tissue. The mechanisms are multiple and primitive, and do not require previous exposure to the organism. They include recognition of bacterial carbohydrates by the alternative pathway of complement fixation; this depends on the fact that most mammalian carbohydrates terminate in sialic acid residues whereas bacterial ones do not. Bacterial proteins are recognized as foreign because the initial amino acid is *N*-formyl methionine. Bacterial cell-wall polymers, endotoxin or peptidoglycan depending on Gram stain reaction, cause inflammation because they are recognized by receptors on macrophages. Fungi are recognized as foreign because of the carbohydrates in the cell wall, but are less phlogistic than bacteria because they do not contain endotoxin or peptidoglycan.

Immunological

Immunological responses, mediated either by antigen–antibody complexes, or by sensitized T cells, contribute in varying degrees to the inflammation caused by bacteria, viruses, fungi, parasites, and tumours. There are infectious conditions in which the mere presence of the parasite in tissue is inconsequential, but tissue destruction results from the immune response to parasite antigens. Immune responses are particularly important in chronic infections with the tubercle bacillus, *Histoplasma capsulatum* and similar fungi, and tissue helminths such as schistosomes. These are all characterized by little local reaction at first, followed by chronic, fibrosing, destructive lesions. Especially in tuberculosis, patients may die even when the local lesions have not compromised respiration or some other vital function. This 'toxicity' is generally unexplained, but may be a response to widespread T cell-mediated macrophage activation.

Tissue damage

Tissue damage and cell death are also important inflammatory stimuli. Burns, fractures, and myocardial infarcts are examples of conditions which cause local and systemic inflammation in the absence of infection. Most viruses do not contain components which are directly inflammatory, and signs of disease only arise after extensive cell death has occurred, or as a consequence of immunological reactions. Obviously, severe inflammation of any type may be enhanced by cell death. A small minority of cases do not fit into any of these three categories; thus, fever in Hodgkin's disease is attributable to the production of pyrogens by the tumour cells.

Changes caused by particular organisms

There are a few infections where the symptoms and signs are mostly attributable to specific properties of the causative organism. The production of toxin by the diphtheria bacillus or the binding of poliovirus to receptors on spinal motoneurons determine the course of those diseases. Infectious diseases such as these, and others such as measles, tetanus, leptospirosis, and whooping cough have unique and characteristic symptoms and signs, and can be diagnosed simply on the basis of the history, the physical examination, and a thorough knowledge of epidemiology. However, even when there are distinctive features, some aspects of the illness are shared in common with other infections. Almost always there is fever; generally, inflamed areas hurt.

Infection without specific features

Most of the infections met with in ordinary clinical practice do not have symptoms and signs which enable one to make an organism-specific diagnosis. Rather, the features suggest acute or chronic inflammation in a particular organ or organs. One diagnoses pneumonia, meningitis, urinary tract infection, or endocarditis. The species of organism responsible may be guessed at, but the only safe method of diagnosis is through the laboratory. Competent clinicians cannot diagnose streptococcal sore throat, and experienced radiologists shown only a radiograph have great difficulty in deciding whether a pneumonia is due to a bacterium or a virus. The fact is that the lung or the pharynx can react to infection in a rather limited number of ways, and that the symptoms, signs, and pathological appearances are very similar whatever the causative organism.

Importance of bacterial numbers

Both locally and systemically, the crucial variable in determining outcome is the number of micro-organisms present. Numbers are important because the reactions of bacterial and viral components with host enzymes and cells follow log dose-response laws. A minimum weight of endotoxin or peptidoglycan of the order of 1 to 10 μg is required to elicit an inflammatory response. A minimum weight of antigen is required to elicit any immunological response: this varies from a few milligrams for an Arthus reaction to a few nanograms for an IgE-mediated, mast-cell degranulation. In all cases, the required weight greatly exceeds that of one organism (about one picogram for a bacterium). Weights which exceed the minimum produce graded responses: in the case of serum components, more molecules are activated; in the case of cells, the response of each cell is proportional to log concentration, and in addition more cells may become activated.

All bacteria produce very similar inflammatory responses because they have very similar cell-wall constituents. The major irritant of Gram negative organisms is endotoxin; Gram positive organisms have peptidoglycan and teichoic acid. Endotoxin proves to be more toxic than peptidoglycan by one to three orders of magnitude depending on the test used. In humans dead Gram negative bacteria caused a standardized inflammatory response in the skin when injected in a dose of 10^6 organisms. The species of bacteria was not important, and pathogens produced no more inflammation than non-pathogens. Gram-positive organisms were less effective; they had to be injected in a dose of 10^7 organisms to produce the same histological response. This kind of evidence strongly suggests that the main difference between 'pathogens' and 'non-pathogens' is that pathogens have devices such as capsules and leucocidins which frequently enable them to multiply to a titre which will cause clinically obvious infections. It also accounts for the fact that almost any organism can cause pneumonia, endocarditis, or meningitis on occasion, and that people with grossly compromised defences frequently develop serious or fatal infections with 'non-pathogens'.

The features of bacterial infection are responses to large numbers of organisms, and species is of little consequence, provided a critical population is attained. Fluids accidentally infected with Gram-negative organisms frequently cause severe shock and sometimes death; fluids infected with Gram-positive organisms cause high fever, but deaths are rare. This observation corresponds to the measured difference in toxicity between endotoxin and peptidoglycan. Many of the bacteria causing these accidents are of unusual, or even unnamed species, which are incapable of causing any kind of spontaneous disease. Furthermore, antibiotics do not ameliorate the symptoms, and if the patient dies there is generally no evidence of bacterial multiplication in the tissues at autopsy. The only important variable is the number of bacteria given to the patient before the situation is recognized and the infusion stopped. If that number is high enough, death will result. A local example of the same phenomenon is respirator-associated pneumonia. If organisms are allowed to multiply in the nebulizer reservoir and large numbers are subsequently blown straight down the trachea, pneumonia will develop even though the organism may be ordinarily non-pathogenic.

Inflammatory reactions of endotoxin

Endotoxin fixes complement by the alternative pathway, causes activation of Factor XII of the plasma clotting system, and binds to a specific receptor on the cell membrane of macrophages. However, there is now general agreement that activation of clotting, fibrinolysis, the kinin system, and the complement system are of relatively minor importance. The key cell in inflammatory responses, both local and systemic, is the macrophage. The key mediators which initiate the inflammatory cascade are interleukin I (IL-1), interleukin 6 (IL-6), and tumour necrosis factor (TNF)-α which are proteins secreted by macrophages (monokines).

IL-1 and TNF separately produce effects on vascular endothelium, but relatively large quantities are required. However, minute amounts of these monokines synergize to induce large effects. Activated endothelium displays adhesion molecules for phagocytic cells. They include E selectin, which is synthesized; and P selectin, which is mobilized from Weibel–Palade bodies.

IL-1 and TNF also induce soluble inflammatory mediators. Both cause activation of phospholipase A2 in many tissues and cells. This enzyme liberates arachidonic acid from cell membrane lipids. Arachidonic acid supply is rate-limiting for prostaglandin, thromboxane, and leukotriene synthesis. Another important soluble mediator is platelet activating factor (PAF). Both enzymes on the PAF synthetic pathway are indirectly activated by IL-1 and TNF, probably through phosphorylation. Finally, both IL-1 and TNF induce synthesis of the highly chemotactic protein, IL-8.

The ligands for selectins are integrins; membrane proteins expressed on the membranes of phagocytic cells. Phagocytic cells, especially neutrophils, adhere to each other and to activated endothelium. In mild inflammation, most of the adherent cells migrate through the endothelium without inducing major increases in permeability. In severe inflammation, the endothelial cells are damaged or destroyed by activated polymorphonuclear neutrophils (PMN). The final destructive agents are proteases and various free radicals and activated forms of oxygen which are ultimately derived from superoxide. The most important may be the hydroxyl radical, .OH, which peroxidates cell membrane lipids. Hydroxyl radical can be generated either from superoxide and hydrogen peroxide, or through an interaction between superoxide and nitric oxide. It is of some interest that endothelium contains nitric oxide synthetase, and that the activity of that enzyme is up-regulated by IL-1 and TNF.

All of the multitudinous actions of endotoxin, including the sepsis syndrome, can be understood as the consequence of activation of this series of host-mediated reactions. At the local level, these reactions are protective. They allow antibodies, complement, and phagocytic cells to gain access to infected tissue and set about eliminating the invading organism. If the organism escapes local control, and invades the bloodstream, small vessels all over the body become inflamed, and the peripheral circulatory failure is likely to induce a downward spiral to death.

Inflammatory reactions provoked by Gram-positive bacteria components

The major irritative components of Gram-positive bacteria are peptidoglycan and teichoic acid. Peptidoglycan is quite efficient at causing abscesses: 10 μg in the skin of a man is an adequate dose. Peptidoglycan is a powerful activating stimulus for macrophages, but concentrations of 10–100 ng/ml are required (compare endotoxin). The active group appears to be *N*-acetyl muramyl-l ala-D isoglutamine (MDP). Macrophages activated by MDP secrete the same substances as do macrophages stimulated with endotoxin. Teichoic acids are efficient activators of complement via the alternate pathway. In addition, antibodies to teichoic acids are present in all normal sera after infancy, sometimes in large quantities.

Table 1 Typical haemodynamic measurement in shock states

	Left atrial pressure (mmHg)	Cardiac output (l/min)	Systemic vascular resistance (dyn/s/cm^5)
Normal	10	5	1200
Left ventricular failure	25	2	3000
Bleeding	0	3	3000
Sepsis	2	12	400

Note: Left atrial pressure is only available if the patient has been fitted with an indwelling pulmonary arterial catheter.

Inflammation in non-bacterial infections

It is common clinical experience that the local inflammation of viral infections, and the consequences of viraemia, are much less dramatic than those of bacterial infections. The reason appears to be that most of the damage is due to cell death: few viruses contain components which promote inflammation directly. Large particles such as myxoviruses can activate macrophages, but the concentrations required are huge, and the degree of activation achieved is modest. Later in disease, virus components may be demonstrable in antigen–antibody complexes. However, very large quantities of antigen–antibody complexes are required to produce clinically evident inflammatory changes, and as soon as large quantities of antibody are synthesized, viral infections tend to be suppressed, cutting off the supply of antigen. Dengue haemorrhagic fever is thought to be produced by the effects of antigen–antibody–complement complexes on neutrophils. Focal glomerulonephritis appears to be an immune complex disease in which the antigen is often viral. Some cases of periarteritis nodosa are caused by complexes containing hepatitis B antigens. None of these conditions are common compared to the total incidence of infection with those viruses.

The most serious acute viral infections, such as measles and smallpox, are those in which there is widespread activation of cell-mediated immunity.

Shock

Shock is a condition in which vital tissues are inadequately perfused with blood. Tissue ischaemia leads to further changes which cause progressive deterioration of the circulation, with steadily falling blood pressure. Unless something happens to break this vicious circle, death is inevitable. Death is most usually due to a cardiac arrhythmia, but it is only apparently sudden, and attempts at resuscitating septic patients who have sustained cardiac arrest almost invariably fail.

Shock may be caused by pump failure, as in myocardial infarction; or by severe loss of intravascular volume, as in haemorrhage or dehydration. These conditions are characterized by low cardiac output and high systemic vascular resistance. Apart from anaphylaxis, which is rare, the sepsis syndrome is the only important cause of peripheral circulatory failure, with high cardiac output and low systemic vascular resistance. This is so reliable that sepsis is often diagnosed from the haemodynamic parameters, in the absence of any other evidence of infection (Table 1).

As previously discussed, bacteria can cause hypotension in several ways, initially by activating the complement and kinin cascades. Other soluble mediators of hypotension which have been demonstrated in

Table 2 A simplified pathogenesis of sepsis

Bacteria
Macrophages and endothelial cells
TNF-α, IL-1, IL-6
Arachidonate metabolites and PAF
Leaky, sticky, small-vessel walls lined with activated PMN
Endothelium destroyed by PMN proteases and reactive oxygen derivatives
Vessel-wall destruction causes adult respiratory distress syndrome and multiple organ failure

septic patients and may be important include products derived from arachidonic acid such as prostaglandins, thromboxane A_2 and leukotrienes, endogenous opioids, and nitric oxide.

A simplified pathogenesis of sepsis is shown in Table 2, which was derived from experiments in animals. It shows that the crucial reaction in sepsis is the secretion of TNF, IL-1, IL-6, and IL-8 by macrophages. All of the subsequent reactions can be induced by these mediators, although in a whole animal activation of plasma-protein cascades and activation of other cell types add details to the picture. But the evidence that the macrophage is the key cell is overwhelming. In septic people, circulating levels of TNF-α, IL-1, and IL-6 are generally elevated, although correlation is not precise. Furthermore, patients with extremely high serum levels of these mediators do not survive. Although experiments in man cannot be carried to the lengths they are in animals, intravenous infusions of small doses of IL-1, Il-6, and TNF have made it clear that all three of these mediators can induce features of sepsis in humans.

The most important cyclo-oxygenase product seems to be thromboxane A_2 (TXA_2), which is usually measured as its stable metabolite TXB_2. Non-survivors of sepsis had plasma TXB_2 levels ten times higher than those who did survive. TXB_2 levels were particularly high in patients with adult respiratory distress syndrome (ARDS) and multiple organ failure. As regards leukotrienes, they are certainly liberated in septic animals and man, and there is evidence in animals that inhibitors of 5 lipoxygenase, or leukotriene receptor antagonists attenuate some of the hypotensive and pulmonary features of sepsis.

PAF is not an arachidonic acid derivative, but it is liberated from cell membranes by the action of two enzymes which are both up-regulated by IL-1 and TNF-α. The first enzyme is phospholipase A_2; the second is a specific PAF synthetase. PAF is a major mediator of PMN adhesion to vessel walls, and of subsequent PMN activation to secrete proteolytic enzymes and activated forms of oxygen. PAF antagonists have ameliorated the pathology in several models of local and systemic infection in animals. In addition, PAF antagonists have attenuated vascular damage in several non-infectious conditions such as reperfusion injury.

The end stages of sepsis

The earliest event in septic shock is generalized peripheral vasodilation. But most of the increased flow seems to occur in arteriovenous anastomoses, with stagnation in the true capillaries. If shock is long continued, blood is readmitted to the capillaries but flow remains stagnant. The capillary walls leak fluid and protein, and there is a progressive loss of intravascular volume. Shocked patients usually, though not always, have evidence of disseminated intravascular coagulation, and small vessels all over the body may be obstructed by fibrin thrombi as well as by masses of agglutinated platelets and PMN.

In the lungs, alveoli steadily fill with fluid exuding from leaky capillaries. Hypoxaemia and tachypnoea are early symptoms of sepsis; advanced stages of the same process cause the ARDS.

Myocardial failure supervenes quite early, probably because the heart normally extracts almost all oxygen from the blood supplied to it. There is some evidence suggesting that left ventricular failure in sepsis is due to a circulating myocardial toxin rather than directly caused by ischaemia. In any event, myocardial function is depressed from the outset of sepsis. The high initial cardiac output is supported mostly by tachycardia rather than by increased stroke volume. With continuing sepsis, left-ventricular stroke output declines, and cardiac output falls into the normal range, or below.

Major organs such as the brain, kidneys, intestine, and liver are subjected to progressive anoxia because of small vessel obstructions, and because of edema related to their leaky capillaries. Added to this is low oxygen delivery related to worsening pulmonary and cardiac function. Clinically, one sees various degrees of clouding of consciousness, ranging from lethargy to stupor, and from slight disorientation to frank delirium. Urine flow first diminishes and then ceases. Jaundice may occur if the patient survives long enough. Chemically, there is evidence of progressive liver and renal failure. Lactic acid accumulates in the blood because of glycolysis in the anoxic tissues. The serum pH is lowered, and the heart is even further compromised. Lysosomes are destabilized and their enzymes released in many tissues. This vicious circle soon leads to death. It is thought that the final event may be massive endotoxin influx from the ischaemic bowel.

The end stage is referred to as multiple organ failure (MOF), and is seen in the terminal stages of all forms of shock, although sepsis is the most common cause. It is generally lethal, with mortalities of about 50 per cent for sepsis plus ARDS, and over 80 per cent for sepsis with failure of three or more organs. It is apparent that patients in this state are unlikely to be helped by antagonists of early mediators of sepsis.

Fever

The cause of fever in infectious illnesses can now be regarded as settled. Fever is due to a resetting of the anterior hypothalamic thermostat so that the body temperature is regulated with the same exquisite sensitivity as in the normal person, but the regulation is at a higher level. Fever in infectious illness is a purposeful reaction which evolved because it potentiated the immune and inflammatory responses to infection. If the nervous system is intact, fever in infectious illness never exceeds about 41°C, and is usually lower.

The resetting of the thermostat is due to synthesis of prostaglandin(s), probably PGE_2, in the brain. There are no presynthesized stores of prostaglandins, in the brain or elsewhere. The site of synthesis is probably the organum vasculosum laminae terminalis. This area has permeable blood vessels which would allow stimuli to enter from the bloodstream, it is exquisitely sensitive to PGE_2, and it projects to the anterior hypothalamus.

It would be expected that if PGE_2, or another arachidonic acid derivative, were an essential part of the development of fever, then cyclo-oxygenase inhibitors would antagonize fever. And indeed aspirin and similar drugs have been well known antipyretics for more than a century, long before we knew how they worked.

The stimuli for prostaglandin synthesis are the three monokines IL-1, TNF-α, and IL-6, which have been discussed above. Each of these mediators alone is pyrogenic, and each has been shown to stimulate prostaglandin synthesis in the anterior hypothalamus. TNF-α is doubly pyrogenic because it also induces synthesis and secretion of IL-1 and IL-6. These three proteins are secreted by macrophages stimulated by bacteria and by a variety of other substances.

The list of substances which cause macrophages to secrete IL-1, TNF-α, and IL-6 is very long. It includes whole bacteria, both Gram-positive and Gram-negative, as well as bacterial cell-wall components such as endotoxin and peptidoglycan. Certain bacterial toxins such as the toxic shock toxin of *Staph. aureus* can activate macrophages at very low concentration. In the toxic shock syndrome, the patient shows all the features of sepsis, but blood cultures are negative. Macrophages are activated to secrete proteins by intact fungi, fungal cell walls, and by certain large viruses. Macrophages are also activated by T cells that have responded to antigen displayed on the macrophage surface, and by antigen–antibody complexes and complement components.

Fever, like sepsis, is therefore another manifestation of the leakage of inflammatory mediators into the bloodstream from a local site of infection. If the organism is in the bloodstream, mediators are released directly into blood by circulating monocytes and by tissue macrophages such as Kupffer cells which line blood sinusoids. Virtually all clinical fevers can be so explained. The exceptions are fever seen in neurological diseases which in one way or another damage the temperature-regulating centres; heat stroke, which is caused by inability to cool the body fast enough to compensate for the existing heat load; and certain fevers accompanying leukaemias or lymphomas, in which IL-1 and other pyrogens are synthesized by the tumour cells.

Other systemic changes associated with fever

Changes in plasma proteins

Infected people usually show a stereotyped array of changes in their plasma proteins. The erythrocyte sedimentation rate is raised because of increased synthesis of fibrinogen by the liver. Several other proteins present in normal plasma or serum are also synthesized in increased quantity during infection; they include the haptoglobins and caeruloplasmin. In addition, some proteins which are not present at all in normal serum are synthesized in very large quantities by the liver; the best examples are C-reactive protein and serum amyloid-associated protein. Proteins whose concentration increases during infection are known as the 'acute phase reactants'; most have α_2-globulin mobility, and they are responsible for the increased density of this area in serum electrophoretic strips from infected people.

The obverse of increased synthesis of some proteins by the liver is a lessened synthesis of other proteins normally made by the liver, especially albumin. In severely infected animals, synthesis of albumin mRNA in hepatocytes essentially stops within a few hours. Since the half-life of serum albumin is about 5 days, there is no immediate fall in serum albumin level. However, as sepsis continues, albumin is lost into the tissues and is not replaced. The consequence is severe hypoalbuminaemia. The main cause for the shift in liver protein synthesis is IL-6. IL-1 serves a synergic function, but is relatively ineffective by itself, and may in fact work by stimulating IL-6 synthesis by hepatocytes.

Changes in serum iron

Sick people also show a marked fall in serum iron and serum zinc. The fall in serum iron is clearly adaptive, because all organisms need iron to grow, and the virulence of several pathogenic bacteria can be enhanced by many orders of magnitude if enough ferric iron to saturate serum transferrin is given intravenously. As regards zinc, no evidence is available. Finally, sick people generally show a neutrophil leucocytosis, which again is obviously adaptive. These changes appear to be primarily mediated by IL-1.

Changes during prolonged infection

A prolonged infection always results in major nutritional problems. Sick people have an elevated energy requirement: fever raises the metabolic rate approximately 15 per cent for each 1°C of temperature elevation. In addition, there is an increased metabolic rate, out of proportion to fever, in serious infections such as peritonitis. Sick people seldom have good appetites, and they tend to eat mostly fluid and carbohydrate. Rarely is the caloric intake sufficient to balance the increased metabolic load, and the protein intake is almost always subnormal.

However, the nutritional changes of prolonged infection are not just due to starvation. There is an apparently obligatory breakdown of protein in muscle and bone, mainly mediated by adrenal corticosteroids. The amino acids are deaminated and the skeletons are used for gluconeogenesis in the liver. The ammonia is converted to urea and excreted in the urine. Normal urea nitrogen is 6–15 g/day, but may rise to 30 g/day during severe systemic infection, in the absence of any protein intake. Muscular wasting and loss of bone matrix is always seen in prolonged infections. Loss of calcium from bone may cause semi-spontaneous fractures or renal calculi.

Fat is also broken down at an increased rate. The glycerol is used for liver gluconeogenesis and the fatty acid portions are mostly burned in muscle. The respiratory quotient during prolonged sepsis is 0.7–0.8, indicating a major use of fat as fuel. Fat synthesis essentially stops because TNF-α down-regulates transcription of the gene for lipoprotein lipase.

The nutritional response to prolonged infection is identical with the response to major trauma, major surgery, or burns. The response is so stereotyped that it must have adaptive value. However, during prolonged infections some clearly maladaptive changes occur. The changes can be partially overcome by aggressive feeding, and unless one can clearly see that the infection will be controlled within a week or so, that should be considered. It is especially important if the patient was malnourished before the infection developed. Exactly what should be repleted is still being determined. Most people would agree with providing calories and protein, and correcting severe anaemia or hypoalbuminaemia. However, there may be specific nutritional defects which are worth correcting. There is evidence from animal experiments that glutamine deficiency causes increased intestinal permeability, and that enteral glutamine repletion may reduce the frequency and severity of the multiple organ failure syndrome.

Summary

It is easy to forget that mediators of inflammation have the primary function of protecting the host. What we see as clinical disease always represents a failure of local control of infection. The most important functions of TNF-α , IL-1, and IL-6 are to initiate the local inflammatory reaction, and attract phagocytes to the area to dispose of the invading organisms. IL-1 is also fundamentally important in mediating the activation of T cells and, indirectly, B cells which underlie the specific immune responses to infection. These processes go on in everyone every day and are normally so efficient that they never rise to the level of clinical notice.

What happens in a clinical infection is a function of how far the invading organism succeeds in multiplying. Single organisms are disposed of by phagocytosis without any other response, and even a few thousand bacteria cause only microscopic inflammation. A few million organisms incite the generation of substances which cause enough vasodilation, increased capillary permeability, and chemotaxis to be clinically visible as inflammation. Many millions of organisms are required to cause local abscesses; the tissue destruction is actually caused by proteolytic enzymes liberated from dead and dying PMN. In chronic bacterial infections such as tuberculosis, local tissue destruction is a result of gross overstimulation of macrophages.

If the local lesion is extensive, then IL-1, TNF-α, IL-6, and other mediators leak into the bloodstream. This induces systemic changes such as fever, the acute phase serum protein changes, and neutrophil leucocytosis. Septicaemia occurs when large numbers of organisms enter the bloodstream, and there is systemic activation of the plasma enzyme cascades and macrophages. The clinical hallmark of sepsis is peripheral circulatory failure, with raised cardiac output, low systemic vascular resistance, and generalized capillary leakage. The damage to vessel walls is initially pharmacologically mediated by substances such as kinins, histamine, and anaphylatoxins derived from complement. However, the lethal endothelial damage which leads to ARDS and multiple organ failure is initiated by the action of bacterial products on macrophages. Major macrophage-derived mediators of endothelial damage are TNF-α, IL-1, and IL-6. Although these proteins have multiple effects, the most important appears to result in adhesion of PMN to vessel walls. One important intermediate step is IL-1/TNF-directed synthesis of PAF by endothelial cells. Vessel walls are finally destroyed by polymorph enzymes and activated forms of oxygen. Knowledge of these reaction sequences can be expected in the near future to lead to better management of infected patients.

Further reading

General

Gallin, J.I., Goldstein, I.M., and Snyderman, R. (1992). *Inflammation: basic principles and clinical correlates.* 2nd edn. Raven Press, New York.

Mackowiak, P.A. (1991). *Fever: basic mechanisms and management.* Raven Press, New York.

Neugebauer, E.A. and Holaday, J.W. (1993). *Handbook of mediators in septic shock.* CRC Press, Boca Raton, FL.

Detailed topics

Abraham, E., Glauser, M.P., Butler, T., *et al.* (1997). P55 tumor necrosis factor receptor fusion protein in the treatment of patients with severe sepsis and septic shock. *Journal of the American Medical Association* **277**, 1531–8.

Beasley, D., Schwartz, J.H., and Brenner, B.M. (1991). Interleukin 1 induces prolonged L arginine dependent cGMP and nitrite production in rat vascular smooth muscle. *Journal of Clinical Investigation* **87**, 602–8.

Cannon, J.G., Tompkins, R.G., Gelfand, J.A., *et al.* (1990). Circulating IL-1 and TNF in septic shock and experimental endotoxin fever. *Journal of Infectious Diseases* **161**, 79–84.

Ohllsson, K., Bjork, P., Bergenfeldt, M., *et al.* (1990). Interleukin 1 receptor antagonist reduces mortality from endotoxin shock. *Nature* **348**, 550–2.

Wakabayashi, G., Gelfand, J.A., Jung, W.K., *et al.* (1991). Staphylococcus epidermidis induces complement activation, TNF and IL-1, a shock-like state, and tissue injury in rabbits without endotoxemia. *Journal of Clinical Investigation* **87**, 1925–35.

Chapter 16.5

Antimicrobial chemotherapy

P. G. Davey

Introduction

Infectious diseases kill more people than either cardiovascular diseases or cancer. Among infectious diseases, the single organism responsible for most deaths is *Mycobacterium tuberculosis.* Globally, there are 8 million new cases and 2.9 million deaths from tuberculosis per year, almost twice as many deaths as caused by AIDS (1.5 million/year). Antimicrobials are unique among drugs in that overuse may lead to development of drug resistance. The failure of antimicrobial chemotherapy to control infectious diseases is due in part to the emergence of drug-resistant microbes. However, it is also due to inadequacies of prevention through public health systems and the failure of individual prescribers to use drugs in the most effective manner.

Pharmacology of antimicrobial drugs

Mechanisms of action

The term 'antibiotic' was introduced by Waksman in 1942 to describe substances which are produced by micro-organisms and which are antagonistic to the growth of others in high dilution. The last clause is necessary to exclude substances like gastric juices, hydrogen peroxide, and alcohol, which are naturally occurring antiseptics. More recently improved molecular techniques have led to the synthesis of drugs which have been specifically designed to attack identified targets in micro-organisms. Strictly speaking, synthetic antimicrobial drugs are not antibiotics.

Antibacterial drugs

Bacteria have a cell wall as well as a cell membrane. This fundamental difference from mammalian cells is the principal target for penicillins and cephalosporins (Table 1). The other principal targets for antibacterial drugs are intracellular (Table 1). It is increasingly common to see examples of drugs which have been designed from an understanding of some of the important relationships between structure and activity. However, new drugs bring new problems: temafloxacin was withdrawn from clinical practice only 6 months after its introduction in 1992. Although carefully designed to take advantage of existing knowledge linking structure with antibacterial activity, its clinical use was associated with rare reports of haemolysis and renal failure which had not been associated with other flouroquinolones. This occurrence serves as a reminder that knowledge about the structure and activity of a new drug is limited to what is already known about existing drugs of the same class. While this knowledge may help in the design of drugs with improved antimicrobial activity, there is always the risk that the new drug will have completely new adverse effects which are impossible to predict with existing experimental techniques.

Table 1 Mechanism of action of antibacterial, antifungal, and antiprotozoal drugs

Mechanism of action	Antibacterial drugs	Antifungal drugs	Antiprotozoal drugs
Inhibition of synthesis or damage to cell wall	Penicillins, cephalosporins and other β-lactams; vancomycin	Fungi do not have a cell wall	Protozoa do not have a cell wall
Inhibition of synthesis or damage to cytoplasmic membrane	Polymyxin	Amphotericin, nystatin; clotrimazole; fluconazole; terbinafine; amorolfine	Amphotericin; ketoconazole; fluconazole
Inhibition of synthesis or metabolism or function of nucleic acids	Ciprofloxacin; rifampicin; nitrofurantoin; metronidazole	Griseofulvin	Metronidazole
Protein biosynthesis	Gentamicin; tetracycline; chloramphenicol; erythromycin; fusidic acid	Flucytosine	Tetracyclines; azithromycin; clarithromycin
Modification of energy metabolism	Sulfonamides; trimethoprim; isoniazid	No example	Dapsone; sulfonamides; pentamidine; pyrimethamine

Antifungal and antiprotozoal drugs

Fungi and protozoa are nucleated, eukaryotic cells. Although, like mammalian cells, they do not have a cell wall, there are a number of drugs which do have selective toxicity for these organisms, including folate antagonists and other antibacterial drugs which act by modification of energy metabolism (Table 1). Many of the drugs used to treat protozoal infections are antibacterial antibiotics (Table 1) or have similar mechanisms of action to these drugs. Some of the most useful antiprotozoal agents (e.g. quinine) are derived from ancient herbal remedies and their mechanism of action remains unclear.

Antiviral drugs

Development of drugs with selective toxicity against host cells that have been infected by viruses is analogous to the problems of development of cytotoxic drugs for cancer chemotherapy. Nonetheless, there is an increasing range of safe, effective antiviral drugs. The targets for available antivirals are only expressed in cells in which viral replication is taking place.

Mechanisms of resistance

The three most common mechanisms are production of drug-inactivating enzymes, alteration of the target site, and mechanisms which prevent access of the drug to the target site. It is important to distinguish between intrinsic and acquired resistance. Intrinsic resistance means that a bacterial species is inherently resistant to the effects of the antibacterial drug (e.g. streptococci have always been resistant to aminoglycosides). Acquired resistance means that a bacterial species has acquired a mechanism of resistance since the introduction of antibacterial drugs into clinical medicine (e.g. penicillinase-producing staphylococci). Acquisition of resistance can occur either by mutation or by transfer of genetic information between bacteria on plasmids.

Prescribers should be aware of which bacteria are intrinsically resistant to the antibacterial drugs they use regularly. However, knowledge of acquired resistance requires collaboration between laboratories and clinicians. By definition the situation is constantly changing and may show quite marked geographical differences, even within one hospital. The information presented in Fig. 1 is only a guide. The most important point to note is that, with the single exception of β-haemolytic streptococci, all bacterial species have acquired resistance to a wide variety of drugs.

Interpretation of tests for resistance

Testing for resistance in the laboratory involves measurement of the minimum drug concentration required to inhibit bacterial growth. The term resistance implies a clearer distinction than is usually present in clinical practice; it is more realistic to think of reduced sensitivity, for bacteria with reduced sensitivity may still respond to treatment with a drug if it achieves sufficiently high concentrations at the site of infection. Moreover, it may be necessary to test bacteria with drugs other than the one that the patient is receiving. A common example is methicillin resistant *Staphylococcus aureus.* Methicillin is not used in clinical practice but it is the best substrate to use in the laboratory to identify *S. aureus* which have changes in their penicillin-binding proteins that make them less sensitive to treatment with any β-lactam drug (penicillin or cephalosporin). The experienced microbiologist knows that a *S. aureus* with reduced sensitivity to methicillin in the laboratory will also have reduced sensitivity to all other β-lactams (e.g. cefuroxime) in the patient, even though the *S. aureus* may appear (misleadingly) to be sensitive to cefuroxime in the laboratory. It is likely that the interpretation of laboratory testing of antimicrobial susceptibility will become increasingly complex with increasing ranges of drugs and mechanisms of resistance. It is important that prescribers of antibacterial drugs and people responsible for antibiotic policies are aware of these problems. It is no longer a simple process of testing one organism against the drug which the patient is receiving; indeed that approach may give dangerously misleading results. Failure to invest in good quality testing could be a very short sighted economy if it leads to increased treatment failure through failure to identify drug resistant strains correctly.

Pharmacokinetics

Dosing of antimicrobials is based in part on a knowledge of their absorption, distribution, and elimination from the body. Information about intestinal elimination and distribution into tissues is especially important.

Intestinal elimination

The human body contains a large number of bacteria which have important functions, particularly in the gut. The adverse effects of antibiotics on the normal flora include emergence of resistant strains from among the normal flora and replacement of the normal flora by more harmful organisms such as pathogenic fungi or *Clostridium difficile.* The term bioavailability is used to describe the amount of drug

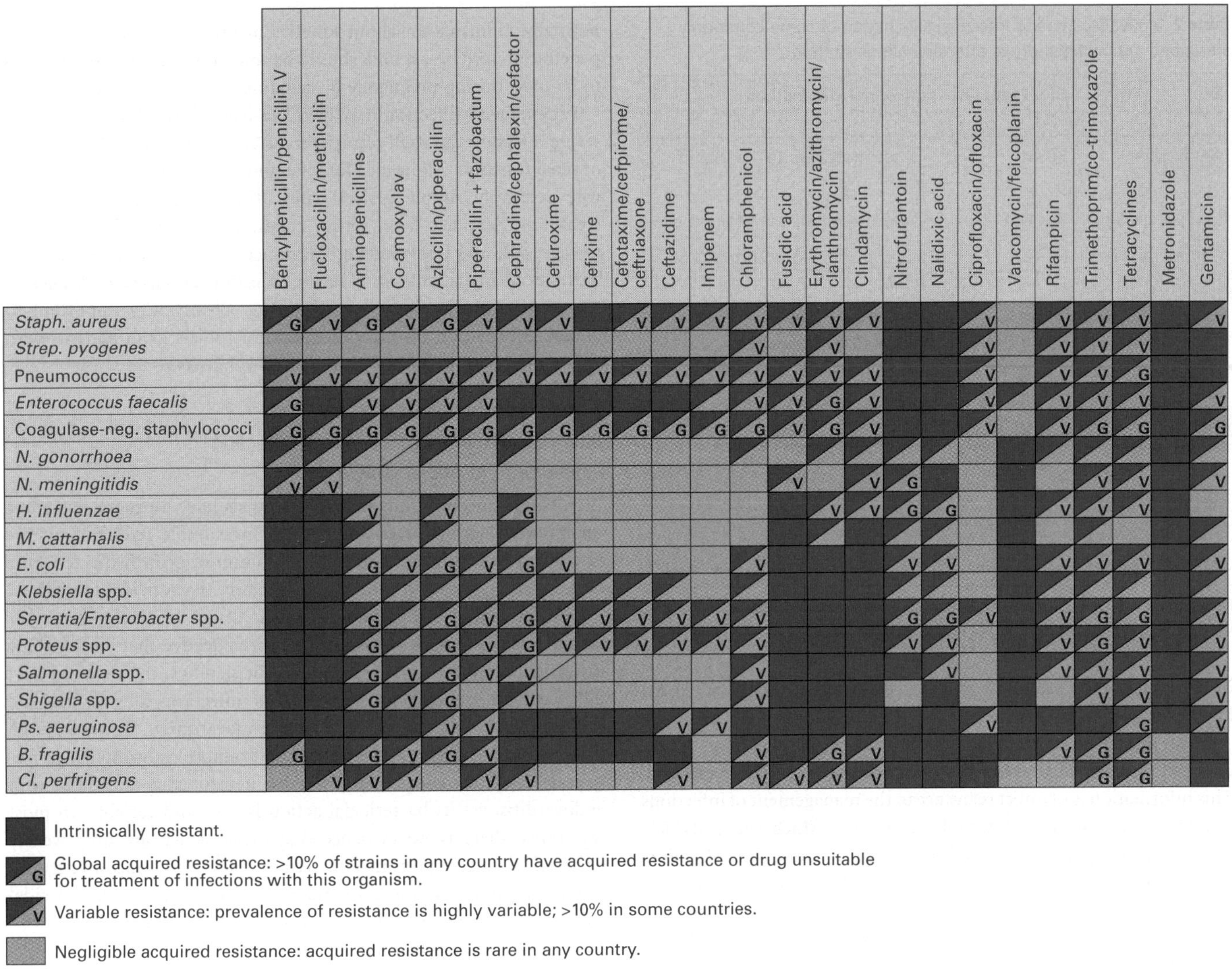

	Benzylpenicillin/penicillin V	Flucloxacillin/methicillin	Aminopenicillins	Co-amoxyclav	Azlocillin/piperacillin	Piperacillin + fazobactum	Cephradine/cephalexin/cefactor	Cefuroxime	Cefixime	Cefotaxime/cefpirome/ ceftriaxone	Ceftazidime	Imipenem	Chloramphenicol	Fusidic acid	Erythromycin/azithromycin/ clanthromycin	Clindamycin	Nitrofurantoin	Nalidixic acid	Ciprofloxacin/ofloxacin	Vancomycin/feicoplanin	Rifampicin	Trimethoprim/co-trimoxazole	Tetracyclines	Metronidazole	Gentamicin
Staph. aureus	G	V	G	V	G	V	V	V		V	V	V	V	V	V	V			V		V	V	V		V
Strep. pyogenes													V		V				V		V	V	V		
Pneumococcus	V	V	V	V	V	V	V	V	V	V	V	V	V	V	V	V			V		V	V	G		
Enterococcus faecalis	G		V	V	V	V							V	V	G	V			V		V	V	V		V
Coagulase-neg. staphylococci	G	G	G	G	G	G	G	G	G	G	G	G	G	V	G	V			V		V	G	G		G
N. gonorrhoea																									
N. meningitidis	V	V												V		V	G					V	V		V
H. influenzae			V		V		G								V	V	G	G			V	V	V		
M. cattarhalis																									
E. coli			G	V	G	V	G	V					V				V	V			V	V	V		V
Klebsiella spp.																									
Serratia/Enterobacter spp.			G		G	V	G	V	V	V	V	V	V				G	G	V		V	G	G		V
Proteus spp.			G		G	V	G	V	V	V	V	V	V				V	V			V	G	V		V
Salmonella spp.			G	V	G	V	V						V					V			V	V	V		V
Shigella spp.			G	V	G		V						V									V	V		V
Ps. aeruginosa					V	V					V	V							V				G		V
B. fragilis	G		G	V	G	V							V		G	V					V	G	G		
Cl. perfringens		V	V	V		V	V				V		V	V	V	V						G	G		

Intrinsically resistant.

G Global acquired resistance: >10% of strains in any country have acquired resistance or drug unsuitable for treatment of infections with this organism.

V Variable resistance: prevalence of resistance is highly variable; >10% in some countries.

Negligible acquired resistance: acquired resistance is rare in any country.

Fig. 1 Development of resistance to antimicrobials.

absorbed after ingestion and varies quite widely among commonly prescribed antibacterials (Table 2). Drugs with low bioavailability have a more profound effect on the normal flora of the colon. However, after absorption of an antimicrobial from the gut it may be eliminated from the body by secretion into bile or by secretion by enterocytes. Thus even intravenously administered antimicrobials reach the gut in sufficient quantities to cause harmful effects on the normal flora.

Tissue distribution

Infections can occur in any tissue, but most bacteria are located in the extracellular fluid (Table 3). However, some bacteria (e.g. *M. tuberculosis* and *Legionella pneumophila*) survive within cells. Drugs which are used to treat these infections must be capable of entering into and functioning within mammalian cells. Viruses and the malaria parasites are essentially intracellular organisms.

Distribution in extracellular fluid of non-specialized tissues

Most tissues are supplied by fenestrated capillaries which allow the free diffusion of antimicrobial drugs from plasma to the extracellular fluid. In this case the average drug concentration in plasma is the same as in the extracellular fluid.

Distribution of drugs into extracellular fluid of specialized tissues

The capillaries supplying the central nervous system, the posterior chamber of the eye, and the prostate are non-fenestrated. The tight junctions between the endothelial cells of these capillaries can only be crossed by lipid soluble drugs which are capable of passage through the cells. Concentrations of antimicrobials within these specialized sites cannot be predicted from a knowledge of plasma concentrations. Infection may also occur in sites with impaired blood supply because of trauma or because of collection of fibrin, as in the cardiac vegetations of bacterial endocarditis.

Intracellular fluid

Penetration of drugs into intracellular fluid depends on the lipid solubility of the drug. β-lactams and aminoglycosides have poor lipid solubility and do not achieve high concentrations in cells. In contrast, lipid-soluble drugs like macrolides and quinolones may achieve higher concentrations within cells than in the plasma or extracellular fluid.

Interpreting data about drug concentrations in tissue fluid

For extracellular bacterial infections it can be assumed that the average concentration in the plasma is a reasonable indication of the average

Table 2 Bioavailability and intestinal elimination of some commonly prescribed antibacterial drugs after oral administration

Drug	Bioavailability (%)	Intestinal elimination
Amoxicillin	80–90	Concentrated up to 10-fold in bile
Cephalexin	80–100	Concentrated up to 3-fold in bile
Cefuroxime axetil	30–40	Bile concentrations up to 80 of serum
Ciprofloxacin	70–85	Concentrated up to 10-fold in bile; additional enteral secretion
Erythromycin	18–45	Concentrated up to 300-fold in bile
Metronidazole	80–95	Concentrations in bile similar to serum
Rifampicin	90–100	Concentrated up to 1000-fold in bile
Trimethoprim	80–90	Concentrated up to 2-fold in bile

Drugs which are well absorbed may still achieve high concentrations in the faeces because of secretion into bile or other enteral secretions

drug concentration at the site of infection and a knowledge of plasma kinetics is all that is required.

Most intracellular bacterial infections occur in the lung, where distribution of antibacterials has been relatively well characterized. This information is of direct relevance to the management of infections caused by the obligate intracellular pathogens which cause atypical pneumonia (*L. pneumophila, Chlamydia pneumoniae*) or *M. tuberculosis.* Ability to penetrate eukaryotic cells is a prerequisite for drugs aimed at infections by these organisms. However, high lung-tissue concentrations are of less certain relevance in the majority of lung infections, which are caused by extracellular pathogens.

Effects of individual patient characteristics on pharmacokinetics

Pharmacokinetics are profoundly affected by age and pregnancy. In the very young, systems for drug binding or metabolism are poorly developed, whereas in the very old, they may no longer function normally. Information about kinetics in pregnancy and about drug penetration into breast milk should be sought when considering drugs to be used during pregnancy or lactation.

Patients with infection may have pre-existing renal failure but any severe infection can itself result in transient or permanent impairment of renal function. Allowance for changing renal function can be made with relatively simple general rules, the key being estimation of creatinine clearance from serum creatinine concentrations adjusted for age, sex, and body weight. Clearance of antimicrobials may also be reduced in patients with severe infection because of changes in the volume of distribution of the drug. Clearly it is important to obtain information on kinetics of antimicrobials from patients with severe infection, in addition to normal volunteers.

Pharmacodynamics

Pharmacodynamics of antimicrobial action

Inhibition of microbial growth

Increasing concentrations of antimicrobials have a progressive effect on microbial growth, starting from a measurable reduction in the rate of growth, through complete inhibition of growth (bacteristatic effects) to reduction in numbers of bacteria (bactericidal effects).

The few clinical situations in which drugs which are primarily bactericidal have been shown to be more effective than bacteristatic drugs include infections in patients with significantly impaired host defences (e.g. neutropenic patients), or infections at sites that are inaccessible to phagocytic cells (e.g. endocarditis). However, even these situations are not clear-cut. For example, vancomycin is frequently used to treat patients who are neutropenic, and those with endocarditis, yet its bactericidal action is slow and variable. In most infections, there is no evidence that drugs which are only weakly bactericidal (e.g. erythromycin, tetracyclines, and vancomycin) are inferior to those which have more rapid or complete bactericidal effects (e.g. aminoglycosides, β-lactams, and quinolones).

Importance of microbial growth phase

In vitro, bacterial numbers in a culture increase exponentially for 6–12 h depending on the growth conditions. The exponential growth phase is followed by a stationary growth phase during which bacterial numbers remain constant, but there may be some limited growth to replace bacteria which die. The same is observed *in vivo* when bacteria

Table 3 Kinetic requirements for treatment of bacterial infections at different anatomical sites

Anatomical site of infection	Relevance of blood levels?	Natural barrier from blood to interstitial fluid?	Intracellular penetration desirable?	Penetration into luminal secretions required?
Meningitis	Yes	Yes, all infections	Only for listeria meningitis	Effective CSF concentrations crucial
Biliary tract	Yes	No	None proven, causative organisms do not survive in cells	High biliary concentrations probably not necessary
Respiratory tract	Bacteraemia common for pneumonia only	No	Essential for atypical pneumonia and tuberculosis but unnecessary for most common pathogens (*Strep. pneumoniae* and *H. influenzae*)	High concentrations in bronchial secretions may be desirable when part of the aim of treatment is reduction of bacterial load in sputum (e.g. cystic fibrosis)
Urinary tract	Bacteraemia common with pyelonephritis	Only for prostatitis	Only for *Chlamydia trachomatis* (prostatitis/epididymo-orchitis); unnecessary for common causes of urinary tract infection	Effective urinary concentrations essential; drugs which achieve low concentrations in interstitial fluid (nitrofurantoin) are relatively ineffective in pyelonephritis

Table 4 Examples of dose-related adverse effects of commonly prescribed antimicrobials

Drug	Adverse effect	Comment
Antibacterial drugs	Superinfection by yeasts or *C. difficile*; selection of drug-resistant bacteria from the normal flora	These are universal adverse effects of antibacterial drugs and are related to the duration of exposure
β-Lactams (e.g. penicillins)	Myelosuppression; Drug fever	Neutropenia or fever may occur after 1–2 weeks high dose IV therapy
Aminoglycosides (e.g. gentamcin)	Nephrotoxicity; ototoxicity	Monitoring of serum concentrations minimizes, but does not avoid, toxicity, which is primarily related to the duration of treatment
Glycopeptides (e.g. vancomycin, teicoplanin)	Histamine release ('Red man syndrome')	Related to the rate of infusion of vancomycin; does not occur with teicoplanin
Macrolides (e.g. erythromycin)	Gastrointestinal stimulation	This is a pharmacological effect which occurs with IV or oral administration
Quinolones (e.g. ciprofloxacin)	CNS stimulation	Quinolones are weak GABA antagonists; this effect is potentiated by coadministration with NSAIDs
Amphotericin	Rigors/hyperthermia/hypotension	Related to the rate of infusion
Acyclovir	CNS adverse effects; crystalluria	Rare except with high-dose IV therapy
Zidovudine	Gastrointestinal; myelosuppression; myopathy	All related to unit dose and to duration of treatment

are growing in a confined space. Both *in vitro* and *in vivo*, all antimicrobials have relatively little bactericidal effect on bacteria in the stationary phase of growth.

In vivo, microbes tend to attach to surfaces and to form biofilms. The biofilm probably acts as a physical barrier to antimicrobials. Organisms within the biofilm are in the stationary phase of growth and therefore inherently less susceptible to the actions of antimicrobials.

Relevance of pharmacodynamics to in vitro susceptibility testing

Many factors affect the relationship between drug concentration and antimicrobial effect *in vivo*, and so it is difficult to predict the sensitivity of microbes to treatment from the results of *in vitro* tests alone.

Pharmacodynamics of adverse effects on the patient

All antimicrobials have some dose-related adverse pharmacological effects (Table 4), but, fortunately, these are rare at clinical doses. Exceptions include aminoglycosides, amphotericin, quinine, and zidovudine. For other antimicrobials, such as β-lactams, the most common adverse events are idiosyncratic. By definition these are unpredictable from a knowledge of the basic pharmacology of the drug and do not show any simple dose–response relationship.

Patients should always be asked about previous exposure to antimicrobials and about any adverse effects that they experienced. If a patient reports that they are allergic to penicillin or another antimicrobial it is important to obtain as much information as possible from them or their medical records. Rashes may be attributable to the infection rather than to drug allergy. Fewer than 10 per cent of children with a history of rashes associated with penicillin therapy have any obvious rash after re-exposure. In contrast, a history of anaphylaxis suggests immediate hypersensitivity. If a patient has a history suggesting an anaphylactic reaction to penicillin they should avoid all β-lactam drugs (i.e. penicillins, cephalosporins, carbapenems and monobactams). If β-lactam drugs must be given, full resuscitation facilities should be available. Fortunately there is a wide range of alternative drugs.

Design of dosing regimens for antimicrobials

Ideally dosing should be based on a thorough understanding of pharmacokinetics and pharmacodynamics. However, for older antimicrobials there may be very little information about kinetics in normal volunteers, let alone in patients with infection. Traditional recommended dosing regimens for some of these drugs are difficult to justify. For example, both sodium fusidate and metronidazole have long half-lives (8–10 h) and are likely to accumulate at the currently recommended dosing interval of 8 h. Fortunately, deficiencies in understanding the pharmacology of older antimicrobials are being addressed and used to produce more effective dosing strategies. In particular, the application of clinical pharmacology to antiprotozoal therapy has led to clinically significant improvements in dosing strategies.

The importance of outcome measures in designing dosing regimens

Infections for which dose–response relationships are clear

Information about dose responses of antimicrobials *in vitro* and in experimental infections form a sound basis for design of dosing regimens for clinical practice. For some infections there are clear biological measures of outcome. In general these infections are fatal if untreated and there is a clear relationship between the biological outcome measure and mortality (e.g. clearance of malaria parasites from the blood).

It follows that it should be relatively easy to establish dosing regimens for infections for which unsuccessful treatment carries a high risk of serious consequences, particularly when treatment also has serious, dose-related side-effects. Examples include use of aminoglycosides for treatment of endocarditis, quinine for treatment of falciparum malaria, and zidovudine for treatment of HIV infection. The components which need to be determined are the daily dose and the duration of treatment. Increase in either of these may increase the probability of successful outcome but will also inevitably increase the probability of adverse effects.

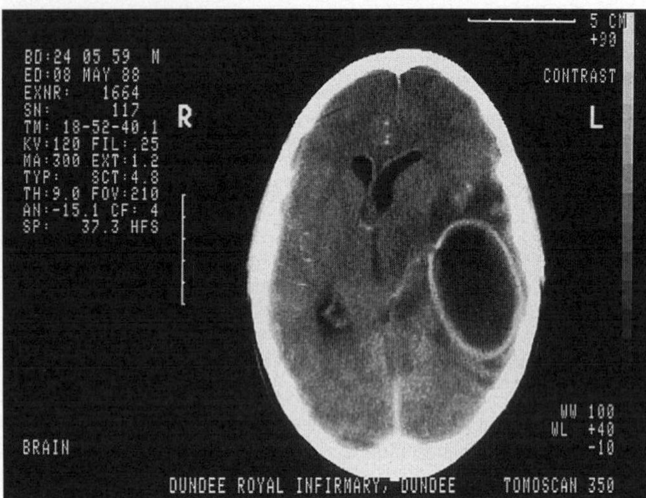

Fig. 2 CT scan showing a large cerebral abscess in a 24-year-old man who had a 6-week history of discharge from the right ear. Note that the mastoid process is opaque on the right side.

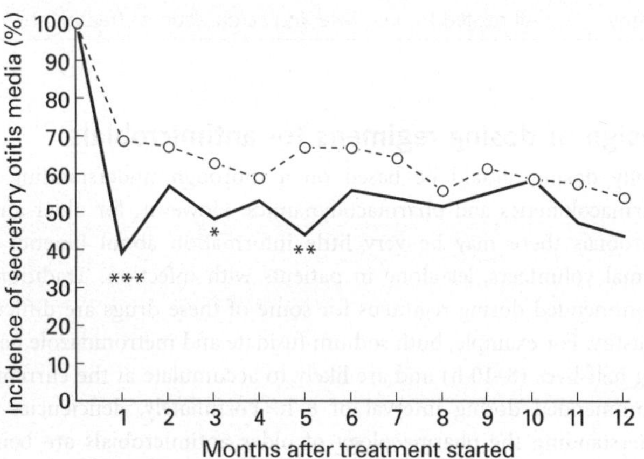

Fig. 3 Incidence of secretory otitis media in 131 children treated for 1 month with co-amoxyclav (—) versus 133 children who received placebo (----). There is a statistically significant difference between the co-amoxyclav and placebo groups at one, three, and five months after initiation of treatment.

Infections for which dose–response relationships are unclear

Many infections which are commonly treated with antimicrobials would resolve spontaneously if they were not treated, which makes it very difficult to establish optimum doses. Even today, the consequences of inadequately treated otitis media can be severe (Fig. 2) but mastoiditis is now estimated to occur in only 0.04 per cent of cases. For most patients antibiotic treatment produces measurable, but short-lived benefits (Fig. 3). In this example of secretory otitis media, 50 per cent of the treated children still have middle-ear effusions after treatment and after a few months there was no difference in outcome between the children who did or did not receive antibiotics.

Clinical aspects of antimicrobial use

Control of resistance to antimicrobials

Epidemiology of antimicrobial resistance

Every common bacterial pathogen has developed resistance to at least one commonly prescribed antibacterial drug (Fig. 1) and resistance to antiviral, antiprotozoal, and antifungal drugs is also increasing. There is no doubt that development of resistance is linked to use of antimicrobials. There are quite marked international differences in the prevalence of resistance (Table 5) and these can be explained in part by the relative consumption of drugs in these countries. Development of resistance is particularly common in developing countries in which antibiotics are freely available without prescription.

What factors determine the emergence of resistance? Clearly characteristics of the bacteria themselves are important. *Pseudomonas* spp. have always been relatively resistant to antibacterial drugs and have been successful in acquiring mechanisms of resistance to all of the antipseudomonal drugs which have been developed (Fig. 1). In contrast, strains of *Streptococcus pyogenes* have acquired resistance to erythromycin but remain sensitive to the other drugs which have been used to treat streptococcal infections. In particular, *S. pyogenes* have not acquired β-lactamases. The likely sequence of events is that a minority of strains of a bacterial species either possess a resistance mechanism or acquire it by plasmid transfer from another species. The prevalence of the resistance mechanism within the species is then determined by the selective pressure exerted by antimicrobial use.

Reservoirs of resistance, animate or inanimate

Examples of animate reservoirs of resistance include countries, hospitals, individual clinical units, individual patients, and animals. Examples of inanimate reservoirs include surfaces, clothing, and even the apparatus used to dispense antiseptics. Patients may acquire infection with drug-resistant bacteria simply by contact with animate or inanimate reservoirs of resistance.

Principles of antimicrobial chemotherapy

Emergence of drug resistance is related to the number of patients exposed to antimicrobials and to the duration of treatment of individual patients. It follows that spread of resistance may be reduced by treating as few patients as possible with as few drugs as possible for as short a time as possible.

Chemoprophylaxis

In general chemoprophylaxis should be considered if there is a well-defined high risk of infection (e.g. wound infection after colonic surgery) or if the risk is low but the consequences are dire (e.g. infection of a prosthetic joint). It is not possible to review all of the indications for chemoprophylaxis in this chapter. However, two important general principles will be discussed.

Timing of chemoprophylaxis

It should be self evident that prophylaxis is likely to be most effective if it is administered when the risk of infection is maximal. The aim of surgical prophylaxis should be to ensure that effective drug concentrations are present at the time of surgery. For most drugs this means that intravenous administration should occur within two hours of the incision being made (Fig. 4). Earlier administration means that most of the dose is in the urine at the time of surgery, whereas delay in administration clearly diminishes effectiveness (Fig. 4).

Duration of chemoprophylaxis

Continuation of prophylaxis beyond the period of likely exposure is, with few exceptions, unnecessary. An obvious exception is the chemoprophylaxis of malaria, which should be continued for 4 weeks after leaving the area where malaria is prevalent. However, for surgical prophylaxis there is very little evidence that continuing prophylaxis beyond the end of the operation is beneficial. Despite this, audit of

Table 5 Variation in resistance of *S. aureus* and *Pseudomonas* spp. to selected antibiotics in Europe

		Mean (range) resistance		
Organism	**Antibiotic**	**Northern Europe**	**Central Europe**	**Southern Europe**
S. aureus	Cefazolin and other β-lactams	2 (0–4)	3 (0–18)	16 (1–24)
	Ciprofloxacin	1 (0–13)	2 (0–5)	8 (0–18)
	Gentamicin	2 (0–4)	3 (3–23)	14 (4–58)
Pseudomonas spp.	Ceftazidime	6 (0–15)	13 (8–29)	14 (0–29)
	Ciprofloxacin	4 (0–10)	7 (4–8)	16 (0–25)
	Ceftazidime	6 (0–15)	14 (8–29)	14 (0–29)
	Imipenem	10 (0–15)	13 (0–15)	10 (3–14)
	Piperacillin	18 (0–30)	29 (13–43)	34 (19–56)

Susceptibility tests were performed on consecutive blood culture isolates by 37 laboratories in Northern, Central, and Southern Europe. Northern Europe: Sweden, Finland, Denmark, United Kingdom; Central Europe: Belgium, Netherlands, West Germany, Austria; Southern Europe: France, Spain, Portugal, Italy, Greece.

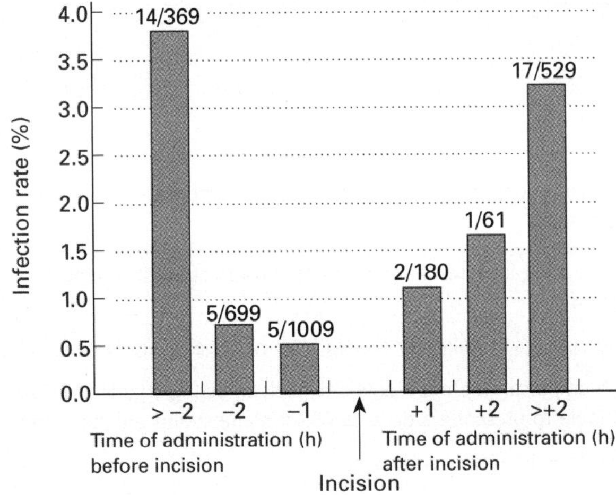

Fig. 4 Wound infection rate corresponding to the timing of administration of prophylaxis in relation to the time of incision. Data from 2487 patients undergoing elective clean or clean–contaminated surgical procedures. *(Redrawn with permission from Classen et al. (1992). New England Journal of Medicine,* ***326****, 281–6.)*

antibiotic use consistently reveals so-called prophylaxis being continued for days after surgery. It is truly alarming that a recent European survey showed that the average duration of 'surgical prevention' was from 4.4–6.5 days (Table 6). As well as being wasteful, this unnecessary prolongation of surgical prophylaxis must be increasing the risk of drug resistance.

Chemotherapy

The general principles can be drawn together into a series of questions which the prescriber should answer before initiating chemotherapy. *Does the clinical presentation warrant consideration of a treatable infection?* Acute respiratory symptoms are the commonest reason for acute consultations in community practice but the majority are caused by viruses for which there is effective treatment. Systematic recording of symptoms and signs has been used to help doctors to assess the probability that the patient has bacterial infection and may benefit from antimicrobial treatment.

Should cultures be taken or should treatment be given empirically? The answer to this question depends on the facilities for storage and transport to the laboratory and the evidence that the information obtained affects clinical decision making. With respect to decision making, it is important to recognize that the information obtained may have epidemiological importance, in addition to its relevance to the person from whom the sample was obtained.

Should empirical treatment cover all likely infecting strains or is it reasonable to prescribe a drug to which some strains are resistant? If the probability of bacterial infection is high and the consequences of failure to eradicate bacteria are severe then it is relatively easy to show that it is important to start appropriate antibacterial treatment as soon as possible. Surgical peritonitis is an example of such an infection. Even if the patient survives a period of inappropriate treatment, appropriate treatment may not be effective if it is delayed until abscesses have formed. Other examples for which prompt appropriate treatment is essential include meningitis, septicaemia, infections in the neutropenic patient, herpes encephalitis, and falciparum malaria. Another potential consequence of ineffective treatment is the spread of infection to other people, for example with drug resistant strains of *Neisseria gonorrhoeae.*

Is parenteral treatment necessary? Parenteral administration certainly improves the bioavailability of a drug, that is, the proportion of the dose administered which reaches the blood stream. However, parenteral therapy is more expensive than oral therapy and increases the risk of adverse effects. Parenteral therapy should be reserved for initial therapy of patients who are severely ill and in whom there is reason to doubt the adequacy of oral absorption. With very few exceptions, oral therapy should be substituted as soon as clinical signs have stabilized (temperature, pulse rate, blood pressure) and the patient is taking normal diet and/or other oral medication. Possible exceptions include infections at specialized sites at which average drug concentrations are below average serum concentrations (endophthalmitis, endocarditis, meningitis).

Should serum concentrations be monitored? The answer is only if serious, dose-related adverse effects occur at concentrations similar to those required to treat infection (e.g. aminoglycosides).

How long should treatment be continued? In general, the longer treatment continues, the more likely it is that the original infection will be eradicated. However, for every infection there must be a maximum effective length of treatment and prolonging treatment also increases the risk of selecting resistant strains, of encouraging superinfection by other microbes, and of dose-related, pharmacological adverse effects. The duration of treatment should be

Table 6 International variation (%) in prescribing antibacterial drugs in hospitals based on records completed by doctors for between 1000 and 1900 patients per country

	France	Germany	Italy	Spain	UK
Route of administration (all infections)					
Oral	50	45	12	30	60
i.m. injection	5	1	48	10	2
i.v. injection	45	54	40	60	38
Mean duration of therapy (days, all infections)					
Therapeutic	9.8	10.7	11.4	10.7	7.1
Surgical prevention	4.8	5.8	6.5	6.3	4.4
Use of individual drugs for lower respiratory tract infection					
Aminopenicillins	50	25	26	20	55
Cephalosporins	10	25	40	22	10
Macrolides	22	5	2	12	25
Quinolones	2	8	4	2	2
Tetracyclines	2	15	1	1	0
Other drugs	14	22	27	43	8

Data from Mr G. Halls, Medical Market Studies Ltd., UK, with permission.

planned at the outset, either as a fixed duration or dependent on response (e.g. for 2 days after the temperature is normal). Overall, the duration of treatment of many common infections is probably unnecessarily long

What should be done if the clinical response is not satisfactory? The answer is emphatically not an empirical change in chemotherapy, or even worse the prescription of one or more additional drugs. Instead, the prescriber should work systematically through a checklist of possible reasons for poor response:

(1) Is the clinical diagnosis wrong? The patient may be receiving an antibacterial drug for a viral infection, or may not have an infection at all (most fevers in hospital are caused by trauma or inflammation, not infection).

(2) Does the patient have an abscess which requires surgical or percutaneous drainage?

(3) Is the prescribed drug likely to reach the anatomical site of infection?

(4) Are the dose and route of administration appropriate?

(5) If the answer to all of the above is yes, is it possible that the patient's infection is caused by a drug-resistant organism?

If the possibility of drug resistance remains then it would be advisable to discuss the patient with a microbiologist or infectious diseases physician to consider the need for further samples for culture as well as the most appropriate alternative treatment.

Proposals for improvement of current practice

Prescribers should address a few simple questions whenever they plan to initiate chemotherapy (Table 7). Unfortunately, the extreme variations in current practice both in the community and in hospitals (Table 6) suggests that there is little consensus about the answers to them. It is vital that doctors, pharmacists, and administrators resist the temptation to resolve these differences through hasty imposition of consensus documents which are in reality spurious endorsements of essentially arbitrary current practice. Instead, the questions posed in Table 7 should be addressed through audit of current practice and randomized controlled trials to assess the relative cost-effectiveness of the many alternatives which exist. There is an extensive literature about methods for influencing prescribing of antimicrobials. In general, peer review of prescribing and feedback of information to prescribers are highly effective and there are data which show that continued review of prescribing reduces overall use of antimicrobials and the prevalence of drug-resistant bacteria.

Table 7 Questions to be answered before prescribing antimicrobial chemotherapy

Does the clinical presentation warrant consideration of treatable infections?
Should cultures be taken or should treatment be given empirically?
Should empirical treatment cover all likely infecting strains or is it reasonable to prescribe a drug to which some strains are resistant?
Is parenteral treatment necessary?
Should serum concentrations be monitored?
How long should treatment be continued?
What should be done if the clinical response is not satisfactory?

Further reading

Cohen, M.L. (1992). Epidemiology of drug resistance: implications for a post-antimicrobial era. *Science* 257, 1050–5.

Davey, P. and Nathwani, D. (1996). Antibiotic policies. In *Antibiotic and chemotherapy* (ed. F. O'Grady, H. Lambert, R. G. Finch, and D. Greenwood). London, Churchill Livingstone.

De Santis, G., Harvey, K.J., Howard, D., *et al.* (1994). Improving the quality of antibiotic prescription patterns in general practice—the role of educational intervention. *Medical Journal of Australia* **160**, 502–5.

Dornbusch, K. and European Study Group on Antibiotic Resistance (1990). Resistance to β-lactam antibiotics and ciprofloxacin in Gram-negative bacilli and staphylococci isolated from blood: a European collaborative study. *Journal of Antimicrobial Chemotherapy* **26**, 269–78.

Dornbusch, K., Miller, G.H., Hare, R.S., *et al.* (1990). Resistance to aminoglycoside antibiotics in Gram-negative bacilli and staphylococci isolated from blood. Report from a European collaborative study. *Journal of Antimicrobial Chemotherapy* **26**, 131–44.

Goldmann, D.A., Weinstein, R.A., Wenzel, R.P., *et al.* (1996). Strategies to prevent and control the emergence and spread of antimicrobial-resistant microorganisms in hospitals. A challenge to hospital leadership. *Journal of the American Medical Association* **275**, 234–40.

Halls, G.A. (1993). The management of infections and antibiotic therapy: a European survey. *Journal of Antimicrobial Chemotherapy* **31**, 985–1000.

Winstanley, P.A. and Watkins, W.M. (1992). Pharmacology and parasitology: integrating experimental methods and approaches to falciparum malaria. *British Journal of Clinical Pharmacology* **33**, 575–81.

Working party of the British Society of Antimicrobial Chemotherapy (1994). Working Party Report—Hospital antibiotic control measures in the UK. *Journal of Antimicrobial Chemotherapy* **34**, 21–42.

Young, L.S. (1993). The Garrod Lecture: mycobacterial diseases in the 1990s. *Journal of Antimicrobial Chemotherapy* **32**, 179–94.

Chapter 16.6

Immunization

D. Isaacs and E. R. Moxon

Introduction

Although improved socio-economic circumstances, especially clean water and sanitation, resulted in drastic reductions in mortality from many infectious diseases, vaccination has been decisive in the control of at least nine major microbial diseases—smallpox, diphtheria, tetanus, yellow fever, pertussis, polio, measles, mumps, and rubella. These successes must be tempered by an appreciation of the enormous unfulfilled potential for preventing microbial diseases.

There is a dual challenge. First, the development of safe, effective, and inexpensive vaccines; secondly, their successful implementation. There can be many impediments to overcome in developing a successful vaccine. The rapid generation (doubling times) of many microbes, together with their capacity to generate genetic and epigenetic variation, facilitates their ability to avoid host defences. Despite the relatively small size of the genome of many of the most virulent microbes, for example viruses, their capacity to vary surface structures has made the task of developing effective vaccines extremely difficult, a problem that has been long appreciated for influenza virus and has been more recently emphasized by HIV.

Immune mechanisms

Immunity from disease may result from different mechanisms, adaptive and non-adaptive. Adaptive mechanisms involve two classes of lymphocytes, B cells and T cells. B cells produce antibodies, proteins that are capable of preventing infection. Antibodies can be produced naturally, actively induced, passively acquired by injection, or transferred from mother to fetus/infant via the placenta or breast milk. Antibodies can neutralize, facilitate removal of, or kill, microbes when they are outside host cells. Alternatively, antibodies can eliminate infected cells (antibody-mediated cellular cytotoxicity) directly or in conjunction with lysis by complement. This radical function of antibodies is achieved through the specific recognition of conformational structures (i.e. the three-dimensional shape) on the surface of microbes. In contrast to B cells, neither T cells nor their products, acting alone, can prevent infection. Their role is most prominent in facilitating the quality and quantity of antibody production through regulating the ability to make antibodies ('helper' and 'suppressor' functions) and through effector functions that include delayed-type hypersensitivity, cytotoxicity, and augmentation of non-adaptive immune responses (interferons and cytokines). In contrast to B cells, T cells can recognize a wide variety of microbial structures irrespective of their location (e.g. surface, internal), thereby overcoming to an extent the constraints imposed by the genetic variations of microbes. Although the T-cell repertoire and function are genetically restricted for each individual, allelic variation (polymorphisms) helps to ensure that at least some individuals within the population are favourably endowed to resist lethal infection with any particular microbe. Crucial to the adaptive function of B and T cells in immune function is the concept of biological memory. Lymphocytes acquire and 'fine tune' their affinity for particular microbial determinants through an evolutionary process that involves genetic rearrangements, somatic mutation, and subpopulation selection. Biological memory resides in the prior selection (priming) of lymphocyte clones with specific receptors so that persistence of the relevant microbial antigen or re-exposure to it maintains, mobilizes, and expands the availability of the relevant immune-effector functions.

Passive immunization

Passive immunization is the administration of preformed antibodies in an immune serum, human or animal, and is used to prevent or modify disease following exposure to an organism or toxin. Passive immunization is used where there is exposure of an immunocompromised individual to an organism that is normally relatively benign (e.g. varicella-zoster immune globulin to prevent or modify chickenpox) or following exposure of a normal host to a particularly virulent organism such as rabies. Passive can be combined with active immunization, particularly if the incubation period is long; for example, hepatitis B immunoglobulin and vaccine are both given to neonates or after accidental exposure to virus. Passive immunization may also be used to neutralize toxins, such as those of diphtheria and tetanus.

There are three main types of sera used for passive immunization. First, normal human immunoglobulin, which is purified, pooled serum from normal individuals; this can be given intramuscularly or intravenously. It is used intravenously as replacement therapy in congenital immunodeficiency, but also intramuscularly following some exposures to infection e.g. hepatitis A, measles. Secondly, hyperimmune serum, which is serum pooled from humans known to have a high titre of antibodies to a given organism, e.g. varicella-zoster immune globulin (VZIG). Thirdly, animal sera, which are generally used as antitoxins to neutralize potent toxins. Examples of the use of these three types of sera are given in Table 1.

Normal human immunoglobulin

Normal human immunoglobulin is prepared by Cohn alcohol fractionation of pooled human serum, which is known to kill HIV-1 and -2, and hepatitis B viruses. The use of early intravenous preparations to treat immune-deficient patients was associated with inadvertent transmission of hepatitis C.

Both intramuscular and intravenous immunoglobulins are over 95 per cent γG, with traces of γA, γM, and other serum proteins.

Table 1 Vaccines in common use in primary immunization schedules

Vaccine	Nature	Route[1]	Age[2]	Indications
Bacille Calmette–Guérin (BCG)	Live bacteria	ID, SC	Birth or 12–13 years	Neonatal period in developing countries
Diphtheria–tetanus–pertussis (DTP)	Toxoids of diphtheria and tetanus; inactivated pertussis	IM	2,3,4 months or 2,4,6 months	Boosters at 18 months, 5 years
Hepatitis B	Surface antigen (yeast or plasma derived)	IM	0,1,6 months or starting later	Booster every 5 years
Haemophilus influenzae type b (Hib) conjugate vaccines	Hib polysaccharide conjugated to protein	IM	2,3,4 months or 2,4,6 months	Booster at 18 months
Measles–mumps–rubella (MMR)	All live, attenuated viruses	SC	12 months	One or two doses
Poliovirus	Live, attenuated, oral (OPV)	Inactivated, injected (IPV) SC	2,3,4 months or 2,4,6 months	Booster at 5 years

[1] ID, intradermal; IM, intramuscular; SC, subcutaneous.

[2] The ages at which these vaccines are given and the exact schedules vary from country to country.

They may cause reactions resembling serum sickness, and very rarely can cause anaphylactic reactions. The half-life of immunoglobulin is 3–4 weeks.

Hyperimmune globulin

The efficacy of different types of hyperimmune globulin, administered as soon as possible after exposure, has been known for nearly a century. In 1907, Cenci prevented measles in children by the prophylactic administration of convalescent serum. Since then, early administration of normal human immunoglobulin has been shown to prevent measles and, if given late, to reduce its severity. Therefore, normal human immunoglobulin rather than a hyperimmune preparation is used for measles.

The use of hyperimmune preparations will prevent or modify varicella-zoster infections and prevent cytomegalovirus infections. Treatment of established infections such as cytomegalovirus or respiratory syncytial virus with hyperimmune globin is more controversial.

Animal sera

Animal sera are much more likely to cause anaphylaxis, and human sera are preferable, if available. It has been estimated that equine tetanus antitoxin causes fatal anaphylaxis at a rate of 1 in 100 000 doses. Adrenaline (1 : 1000) should always be available for immediate administration in case of anaphylaxis.

Active immunization

It is important that, as diseases become rare through effective immunization programmes, the side-effects of immunizations do not become overemphasized and the severity of the diseases forgotten. Evidence of the efficacy of immunizations and their continued need, despite improvements in living standards, which it has been argued by some have made the diseases less severe, comes from two main sources. One is the recurrence of whooping cough in the late 1970s in the UK and Japan when the numbers of individuals immunized against pertussis had fallen: the resultant severe epidemics resulted in hundreds of infant deaths and many more children were left handicapped as a result of whooping cough with encephalopathy. The second source of evidence is from communities or sects that do not immunize themselves for religious or other reasons, such as the Amish, who are at high risk for outbreaks of measles, pertussis, and poliomyelitis.

Primary vaccination schedules

The vaccines commonly used in the primary immunization schedule in many developed and developing countries are shown in Table 1. In 1974, as the global smallpox eradication programme neared successful completion, the Expanded Programme on Immunization (EPI) was launched by the World Health Organization (WHO). The goal of EPI was global immunization of children against tuberculosis, diphtheria, tetanus, pertussis, polio, and measles. Within 20 years, 80 per cent of the world's children had been immunized against these six diseases, through the efforts of the WHO, the United Nations, and local governments. It is estimated that 3.2 million children's lives are saved each year by this increased level of immunization. In the US the incidence of all these vaccine-preventable diseases has been reduced by over 95 per cent since immunization was introduced. Hepatitis B vaccine has since been added to the EPI schedule.

Toxoids

Diphtheria and tetanus are toxin-mediated diseases, caused by exotoxins released by *Corynebacterium diphtheriae* and *Clostridium tetani*. The toxoid vaccines against these diseases are prepared by treating a cell-free preparation of the respective toxin with formaldehyde. Immunization with toxoid protects against the disease, but does not prevent colonization. A primary course of three doses of diphtheria and tetanus toxoids, with two boosters, provides long-lasting protection.

Pertussis vaccines

The most commonly used pertussis vaccines are whole-cell suspensions of killed *Bordetella pertussis* organisms. These cause a relatively high incidence of local side-effects, fever, and rarely, even neurological events. Whether pertussis vaccine causes encephalopathy (or possibly merely uncovers underlying brain damage) is controversial, but it is clear that the risk of brain damage from the disease is many hundreds of times greater than any risk from the vaccine.

Acellular pertussis vaccines, which contain various combinations of *B. pertussis* enzymes, have been used in Japan since 1981 and are being introduced in many other countries. They are less reactogenic than whole-cell vaccines. It is likely that acellular pertussis vaccines will replace whole-cell vaccines in future.

Polio vaccines (see also Chapter 16.22)

There are two types of vaccine against poliomyelitis, live attenuated oral polio vaccine (OPV), first developed by Albert Sabin, and inactivated polio vaccine (IPV), first developed by Jonas Salk. These vaccines contain the three serotypes of poliovirus that can cause paralytic poliomyelitis. An enhanced-potency inactivated polio vaccine is now available.

OPV induces a secretory immune (IgA) response to polio not seen with IPV. OPV spreads readily within families, boosting levels of immunity. It is also considerably cheaper than IPV, a factor of major importance in developing countries, where OPV is the vaccine of choice. On the other hand, OPV causes vaccine-induced paralytic poliomyelitis at a rate of approximately 1 in 2.5 million doses. IPV does not cause vaccine-induced polio. Some developed countries use OPV, some use IPV, and there is a growing interest in the option, used in France and the USA, to start immunization with IPV and then change to oral. Poliomyelitis has been eradicated from the Americas, the last case occurring in Peru in 1991.

Hepatitis B vaccines

Hepatitis B vaccines consist of hepatitis B surface antigen (HBs) purified from plasma or derived by genetic engineering. In the US, universal immunization of all children from birth is recommended. Most other Western countries screen pregnant women for hepatitis B and immunize the babies of hepatitis B antigen-positive mothers and babies from ethnic groups with a high prevalence of hepatitis B infection. Universal hepatitis B immunization, recommended by the WHO, will have most impact in countries in, for example, South-East Asia and Africa where the prevalence is extremely high.

Haemophilus influenzae type B conjugate vaccines

Protection against *Haemophilus influenzae* type b (Hib) infection is mediated primarily by antibody to the polysaccharide capsule of the organism, the type b antigen. However, this polysaccharide is poorly immunogenic in children under 2 years of age, and the maximum age for infection is the first year of life. The Hib conjugate vaccines are the first effective example of vaccines using the hapten principle, whereby a poorly immunogenic molecule is bound to an immunogenic protein, thus converting the poor immunogen to a good one. The different Hib conjugate proteins used include diphtheria toxoids, tetanus toxoid, or outer-membrane proteins of *Neisseria meningitidis*. This is an important advance in vaccine development and conjugate vaccines are being developed for other weak immunogens such as pneumococcal and meningococcal polysaccharides.

Measles–mumps–rubella vaccine

Measles–mumps–rubella (MMR) vaccine is now the most common formulation used for childhood measles immunization, although previously each of these viral vaccines was used on its own. All are live, attenuated viruses. A single dose given at 12 months gives long-term protection, although some countries such as Sweden, the US, and Australia recommend a second dose, which is given either at 5 years or 12–13 years of age.

Hepatitis A

Inactivated hepatitis A virus vaccines have been developed, and are immunogenic in children and adults. They are mainly used for health care workers and travellers to endemic countries.

Influenza vaccines

Influenza vaccines are inactivated virus vaccines containing A and B strains. Because of antigenic drift and occasional shift of wild influenza virus, the vaccines are revised each year in the light of prevailing epidemic strains. They provide about 70 per cent protection for a year and are recommended for high-risk individuals. Examples are adults over 65 years old; adults and children with chronic debilitating disease, especially cardiac, pulmonary, renal, and metabolic disorders; residents of nursing homes; and immunocompromised patients.

Meningococcal vaccines

Meningococcal polysaccharide vaccines contain polysaccharides from serogroups A and C, and sometimes groups W and Y, but not serogroup B, which is non-immunogenic. The vaccines are poorly immunogenic in children under 2 years of age. They are indicated for travellers to endemic areas where the prevalent strain is included in the vaccine (usually serogroup A). They can be useful to prevent transmission of meningococcal infection in outbreaks due to serogroups A or C in closed communities. They are also indicated for patients with immune deficiency with an increased risk of meningococcal sepsis, such as those with defects in one of the terminal components of the complement pathway and patients with congenital or acquired asplenia.

Pneumococcal vaccines

Pneumococcal polysaccharide vaccines contain polysaccharides from the most common of the many pathogenic pneumococcal serotypes. Response is poor in children under 2 years of age. The main indication for pneumococcal vaccine is for children with congenital asplenia, functional asplenia as in sickle-cell disease, and for children and adults who have had a splenectomy. Where splenectomy is elective, pneumococcal vaccine should be given before surgery, but the immune response is only marginally better than if given after. Other indications for pneumococcal vaccine are elderly people in chronic care; chronic diseases, particularly cardiac, renal or pulmonary disease; diabetes; alcoholism; patients with cerebrospinal fluid leaks (at risk of pneumococcal meningitis); and immunocompromised patients such as those with nephrotic syndrome, lymphoma, Hodgkin's disease, multiple myeloma, HIV infection, and immunosuppressed post-organ transplant. The vaccine is not completely protective and penicillin prophylaxis may also be indicated.

Varicella vaccine

The OKA strain of live attenuated varicella vaccine was first used in clinical trials in Japan in 1973. It is immunogenic in normal children and in children with leukaemia. Its routine use has been recommended in the USA.

Vaccines with special indications

A number of vaccines are available for travel to endemic areas or to protect laboratory workers (see Chapter 16.7).

Vaccines being developed

There are some infections for which new or improved vaccines have already been developed and are undergoing clinical trials of safety, immunogenicity, and efficacy. Rotavirus vaccine is one such new vaccine, while acellular pertussis vaccines are examples of improved vaccines.

For other infections, effective vaccines are desperately needed, but their development has so far been unsuccessful. Perhaps the outstanding infections to fall into this category are malaria, HIV, and respiratory syncytial virus infections.

There is a third group of infections for which vaccines are available, but where problems with safety or efficacy of the existing vaccine mean that new vaccines urgently need to be developed. Examples are cholera and tuberculosis.

A comprehensive list of infections for which vaccines are being, or need to be, developed is given in OTM3, p. 320, Table 4.

Combination vaccines

Vaccines already in regular use which are combinations of two or more vaccines include diphtheria/pertussis/tetanus (DPT) and MMR vaccines. Combination vaccines containing DPT, Hib conjugate vaccines, hepatitis B vaccines, and IPV are being developed, and the development of further combination vaccines is anticipated.

Immunization in developed countries

Most developed countries employ a primary immunization schedule similar to that shown in Table 1, with the exception that neonatal BCG is given only to babies whose ethnic background or family history puts them at high risk of tuberculosis, and universal hepatitis B vaccination from birth is only used in a small number of developed countries. The exact extent of immunization coverage required to achieve 'herd immunity', that is, the inability of an organism to cause epidemic spread to susceptibles because of the high number of immunes, varies for different diseases. For example, outbreaks of measles in highly immunized populations (over 95 per cent) in the US suggest that almost 100 per cent immunization may be needed to prevent spread of measles. In contrast, because immunization with Hib conjugate vaccines decreases colonization with Hib, much lower levels of immunization produce substantial herd immunity.

In most developed countries, immunization is provided by the government as part of a comprehensive health-care system. Measures that appear to increase immunization rates are computerized notification of appointments for immunizations, easy access to and ready availability of immunization clinics, and an encouraging approach to immunization by health-care professionals. Parent-held child health records have been successfully used in some regions. Rapid knowledge of local immunization rates and the delineation of community health staff responsible for immunization in areas of a manageable size have been highly successful in raising immunization levels in the UK.

Legislation, either requiring immunization before entry to child-care facilities or school, as in parts of the US, or requiring evidence of immunization status at child care or school entry with exclusion of susceptibles during outbreaks, as in parts of Australia, is controversial. Education of parents and health-care professionals about the continued importance of immunizing against vaccine-preventable diseases is vital. Many children have gaps or delays in immunization because of false contraindications, perpetuated by family, friends, or health professionals.

Opportunistic immunization is one way in which immunization levels can be improved. This requires all health-care personnel to ask about immunization status at any health-care visit, and either to immunize or arrange appointments for children whose immunizations are not up to date. In the US, up to 30 per cent of unimmunized children who developed measles had been seen previously by a health-care professional and could have been immunized, while 57 per cent of women who delivered a baby with congenital rubella syndrome had one or more missed opportunities for rubella vaccination.

Immunization in developing countries

Priorities in developing countries differ from those in developed countries. Tuberculosis kills over 3 million people annually in the world. Neonatal BCG provides about 50 per cent protection against disease and 60–70 per cent protection against severe manifestations such as tuberculous meningitis and death from TB. Exposure to poliovirus may occur early, and polio immunization is commenced at birth. Neonatal tetanus kills about 800 000 babies annually in developing countries, but does not occur if the mother is immune to tetanus. Therefore, immunization of women of child-bearing age against tetanus is incorporated in the EPI. Measles occurs at younger age than in developed countries, and maternal antibody interferes less with immunization. Children in cities in developing countries are at particular risk of early measles. Measles immunization is recommended at 9 months of age.

There are problems with delivering immunization in developing countries. The first problem is the obvious one of cost, not just of the vaccines themselves, but of delivering them to children in remote areas. The organizational structure needs to be there for vaccine delivery. A further problem is maintenance of the 'cold chain', so that vaccines are not damaged by excessive heat. It has been shown, using special thermometers, that the cold chain generally can be maintained, and modern vaccines have been made more heat stable. War is extremely disruptive of health services, and immunization levels are lowest, often disastrously low, in countries ravaged by long wars.

Further reading

Colditz, G.A., Brewer, T.F., Berkey, J.S., *et al.* (1994). Efficacy of BCG vaccine in the prevention of tuberculosis. *Journal of the American Medical Association* 271, 698–702.

Edwards, K.M. (1993). Acellular pertussis vaccines—a solution to the pertussis problem? *Journal of Infectious Diseases* **168**, 15–20.

Gardner, P. and Schaffner, W. (1993). Immunization of adults. *New England Journal of Medicine* 328, 1252–8.

Moxon, E.R. (1990). *Modern vaccines.* Edward Arnold, London.

Peter, G. (1992). Childhood immunizations. *New England Journal of Medicine* 327, 1794–800.

Robbins, A., Freeman, P., and Powell, K.R. (1993). International childhood vaccine initiative. *Pediatric Infectious Diseases Journal* 12, 523–7.

Chapter 16.7

Travel and expedition medicine

C. P. Conlon and D. A. Warrell

Pretravel advice

This can be obtained from medical practitioners interested in travel medicine, embassies of the countries to be visited, travel agencies, organizations, and specialist clinics. To enter some countries, a certificate of vaccination against yellow fever may be needed. Details of other immunizations, allergies, blood group, and regular medications should also be carried. Adequate insurance is essential. The geographical area to be visited, the age and health of the traveller, and any special risks of the journey (e.g. mountain climbing) are taken into account. In remote areas or those with inadequate health facilities the policy must cover repatriation.

General advice about health

The *first-aid kit* should include an antiseptic solution, bandages, plasters, proprietary drugs for pain, diarrhoea, dyspepsia, allergy and itch, sunscreen preparations, water purification tablets, and insect repellents.

For motion sickness, antiemetic drugs such as cyclizine are useful but may cause sedation and a dry mouth. Long-acting transdermal skin patches containing scopolamine are preferable. Long-haul air flights lead to jet lag: sleep disturbance, fatigue, and poor concentration. A short-acting benzodiazepine, such as temazepam, taken for the first couple of nights after flying, helps to re-establish a regular sleeping pattern. There is insufficient evidence to support the use of melatonin. Diabetics may need advice on adjusting their insulin regimen or diet for changes in time zones.

Climatic and environmental extremes. At high altitudes snow blindness and severe sunburn can occur even at very low ambient temperatures under clear skies. Those going to high altitudes should acclimatize slowly and build up their level of physical activity gradually (see p 8.5.5(d)). They should be aware of the symptoms and signs of altitude sickness. Acetazolamide is effective prophylaxis for mild mountain sickness but there is no substitute for rapid descent if severe symptoms develop. In the tropics, heat, dehydration, and salt depletion may cause problems.

Strict food and water hygiene are important in countries with relatively poor sanitation. 'Boil it, peel it, or forget it'; but tomatoes may be infective even if peeled. Water purification tablets and many types of portable water filters are available. Beverages made with boiled water are generally safe, whereas bottled water and, particularly, ice cubes are unreliable. Treated water should be used even for tooth cleaning.

In many developing countries, blood-borne pathogens, such as hepatitis B and C viruses, HIV, HTLV-1 and in some areas malaria, trypanosomiasis, and other infections are prevalent. Screening of donated blood may not be rigorous and needles are commonly reused, sometimes without adequate sterilization. As a result, travellers have been advised to take 'AIDS kits', usually containing needles, cannulae, intravenous giving sets, syringes, and artificial plasma expanders. These are too bulky and expensive for most travellers, but it is worth taking a few 21-gauge needles and 10-ml syringes in case blood must be taken for a laboratory test. A covering letter from a doctor may allay the suspicion of customs officials that they are to be used for drug abuse.

Travellers seem particularly likely to engage in promiscuous sexual activity especially if they are taking alcohol or other recreational drugs. Since sexually transmitted diseases, including HIV, are highly prevalent in many holiday resorts, good-quality condoms, often not available when travelling, should be carried and used.

Patients with chronic illnesses, such as diabetes or asthma, should take plenty of their current medications as these may not be available abroad.

Immunizations

The record of routine childhood immunizations should be reviewed. Many adults will require booster doses for tetanus, polio, and diphtheria.

Yellow fever is endemic only in tropical Africa and South America, not in Asia. Cholera vaccine is no longer recommended by the World Health Organization as its adverse effects outweigh its usefulness but a new oral vaccine is promising. Other immunizations may be recommended after considering the travel itinerary and risk of exposure (Table 1).

The risk of hepatitis A in developing countries is 300–2000/100 000 unprotected travellers/month of stay. Active immunization is safe, effective, and durable (see Chapter 16.34).

In the 'meningitis belt' of subSahelian Africa and in some other areas, dry season meningococcal meningitis outbreaks are so common that immunization is recommended.

Pre-exposure rabies vaccination is being used increasingly. Although the risk of transmission is fairly low, the lack of effective treatment for rabies encephalitis and the fear engendered by a dog bite justifies considering immunization (see Chapter 16.24).

Plague vaccine is effective but may give rise to serious side-effects. An alternative in endemic areas is prophylactic or postexposure doxycycline treatment (see Chapter 16.51). Japanese (B) encephalitis vaccine is safe but the risk of infection is low unless travellers spend more than 3 months in certain rural parts of Asia in the rainy season (see Chapter 16.28). Hepatitis B is a risk for medical staff, whose work involves contact with human blood (see Chapter 16.34).

Prevention of malaria

Both travellers and non-specialist physicians must be educated about prevention and recognition of malaria (see Chapter 16.84).

Travellers' diarrhoea

This is the most common health problem of travellers. Symptoms are usually mild, lasting only about 3–5 days, but holiday and business plans may be disrupted. The most common cause is enterotoxigenic *Escherichia coli* (ETEC). *Salmonella* spp., *Campylobacter* spp., *Shigella* spp., and other pathogenic *E. coli* are also common. Protozoan pathogens, such as *Giardia lamblia*, *Entamoeba histolytica*, *Cryptosporidium parvum*, and viruses are less common causes.

Strict food and water hygiene reduces the risk of gastroenteritis. Heating water to 100°C will kill most pathogens, as will chemical treatment with chlorine or iodine. Water filters are useful additions. Antimicrobials such as co-trimoxazole, doxycycline, and the 4-fluoroquinolones are protective to some extent but are not cheap, may cause side-effects, cannot be taken for prolonged periods, and may encourage antimicrobial resistance. Colloidal bismuth salts are cheaper, safer, and reasonably effective but the large volumes are inconvenient. An effective vaccine may soon be available.

Treatment is by maintaining an adequate fluid intake and using sachets of oral rehydration salts that can be made up with boiled water. Antidiarrhoeal agents, such as codeine phosphate or loperamide, often relieve symptoms sufficiently for normal activities to be continued. Short courses of empirical antimicrobials, for example ciprofloxacin, can be useful, particularly for patients with underlying diseases. Localized abdominal pain or bloody diarrhoea are indications for seeking medical help immediately.

Table 1 Immunizations

Vaccine	Type	Route	Primary course	Booster
Routine				
Polio (Sabin)	Live virus (attenuated)	PO	3 doses at monthly intervals	10 years
Polio (Salk)	Killed virus	IM	As above	10 years
Tetanus	Adsorbed toxoid	IM	3 doses at monthly intervals	10 years (maximum 5 doses)
Diphtheria	Adsorbed toxoid	IM	3 doses at monthly intervals	Single low dose if > 10 years
Haemophilus influenzae **b**	Conjugated polysaccharide	IM	2–3 doses 2 monthly	Single dose
Pneumococcal	23-valent polysaccharide	IM	Single dose	Repeat in those at high risk
Influenza	Killed virus	IM	Single dose	Yearly
Travel				
Yellow fever	Live virus (attenuated)	IM	Single dose	10 yearly
Typhoid	Killed bacteria	IM	2 doses a month apart	3 yearly
Typhoid	Live Ty21a strain (attenuated)	PO	4 doses on alternate days	5 yearly
Typhoid	Capsular Vi polysaccharide	IM	Single dose	3 yearly
Meningo-coccal	Polysaccharide types A,C,(Y,W)	IM or SC	Single dose	3 yearly
Rabies[1,2]	Killed virus	IM or ID	3 doses on days 0, 7, and 28	2–3 yearly
Japanese (B) encephalitis	Killed virus	IM	3 doses on days 0, 7, and 28	1 year, then 4 yearly
Hepatitis A	Killed virus	IM	2 doses 2–4 weeks apart	6–12 months, then ? 5 yearly
Hepatitis B[1]	Adsorbed	IM	0, 1, and 6 months	3–5 yearly
BCG	Attenuated	ID	Single dose	None
Gamma-globulin	Pooled immunoglobulins (mainly IgG)	IM	Single dose	6 monthly (while at risk)

[1] Should not be given into buttock; deltoid or anterior thigh preferred.

[2] Efficacy reduced if given with chloroquine antimalarial prophylaxis.

Immunocompromised travellers

Except for asplenic patients, immunocompromised travellers should not be given live vaccines such as yellow fever, oral polio, and oral typhoid. Killed or synthetic vaccines are safe. Those patients with little to moderate immune suppression, including those with early HIV infection, will probably make a reasonable response to immunization; those with more severe immunosuppression may still make a useful, though less durable response. Influenza, pneumococcal, and *Haemophilus influenzae* b (Hib) conjugate vaccines are recommended, as the risk of respiratory infection and bacteraemia is increased. Gammaglobulin is the preferred prophylaxis against hepatitis A in these patients, as the response to hepatitis A vaccine may be unreliable. Asplenic individuals should be on prophylactic antibiotics, such as amoxycillin, particularly if travelling, and should be dissuaded from travelling to areas with high rates of malaria transmission.

Immunocompromised patients should carry antimicrobials with them for treating respiratory or gastrointestinal infections, should seek medical help when abroad, and should carry a letter from their physician outlining their condition and medication.

Pregnant travellers

Commercial airlines will not normally convey a woman who is 36 weeks or more pregnant without a covering letter from her physician. Insurance to cover the costs of delivery abroad should be considered.

The risk–benefit assessment of immunizations and chemoprophylaxis is of particular importance for the pregnant woman and the fetus. Live vaccines should be avoided, but if there is a genuine risk of yellow fever the vaccine should be given as there is no recognized associated teratogenicity. Inactivated polio vaccine may be given parenterally and tetanus immunization is safe. Heat-killed typhoid vaccine is best avoided as it might cause a febrile reaction, stimulating premature labour. Pneumococcal, meningococcal, and hepatitis B vaccines are safe in pregnancy, as is gammaglobulin.

Malaria is specially dangerous in pregnant women (see Chapter 16.84). Chloroquine and proguanil are safe chemoprophylactic drugs and quinine, in normal therapeutic doses, is safe for treatment. Pregnant women should take special care with food and drink when abroad, as dehydration may threaten the fetus. There are concerns about congenital goitre when pregnant women use iodine to purify water. The maximum recommended daily intake is 175 μg. Loperamide as an antidiarrhoeal agent is safe but antimicrobials such as tetracyclines and quinolones should be avoided.

Extremes of age

Young children should have completed their routine immunizations before travelling. Malaria chemoprophylaxis is recommended for all

Table 2 Causes of fever in returned travellers

Tropical (short incubation; < 3 weeks)	*Tropical (long incubation; > 3 weeks)*
• African trypanosomiasis	• Amoebic abscess
• Brucellosis	• Brucellosis
• Dengue	• Filariasis
• Haemorrhagic fevers (Lassa)	• Hepatitis A, B, or C
• Hepatitis A	• HIV
• Leptospirosis	• Leishmaniasis
• Malaria	• Malaria
• Relapsing fevers	• Tuberculosis
• Tick/scrub typhus	• Typhoid
• Typhoid	***Non-infective causes of fever***
Other infections	• Connective tissue disease
• Endocarditis	• Drug reaction
• Pneumonia	• Factitious
• Prostatitis	• Inflammatory bowel disease
• Sexually transmitted disease	• Malignancy
• Sinusitis	
• UTI[1]	

[1] UTI, urinary-tract infection.

Table 3 Causes of rash in returning travellers

Infective	Non-infective
Cutaneous larva migrans, myiasis	Drug reaction
Cutaneous leishmaniasis	Erythema multiforme
Dengue	Insect bites
Dermatophytes	Sunburn
Lyme disease	
Meningococcus	
Mycobacterial	
Scabies/lice	
STDs[1]	
Tick/scrub typhus	
Tinea versicolor	
Typhoid (Enterovirus, mycoplasma, streptococcal infection, etc.)	

[1] STD, sexually transmitted disease

Table 4 Infective causes of eosinophilia in travellers

Ascariasis	Trichinosis
Echinococcus	*Trichuris*
Filaria	Visceral larva migrans
Hookworm	Angiostrongylus, Gnathostoma (and other gut nematodes)
Schistosomiasis	
Strongyloides	

ages. Yellow fever vaccine should be given only to children older than 9 months as a few cases of vaccine-associated encephalitis have occurred in younger children. Most other vaccines, including rabies, are safe. Hepatitis A is rarely symptomatic in children under 5 years old. Families planning to live in developing countries should be offered BCG vaccination for their children to reduce the risk of tuberculous meningitis.

The elderly should have the same immunizations as younger adults and should take antimalarial drugs. They are more prone to respiratory infection and should, therefore, be given influenza, pneumococcal, and *Haemophilus influenzae* vaccines. Jet lag and changes in time zones may be very disturbing. Older people are more likely to have an underlying medical condition requiring medication. It is important that sufficient supplies of medicines are taken abroad and that the patient has a detailed list of these medicines and their dosages in case the tablets are lost or stolen and the name and contact address of their physician at home in case of emergency.

Explorers and expeditions

Expeditions involve exposure to greater environmental extremes and hazards than other types of travel and are usually to areas remote from medical care, so greater responsibility falls on the members. Most mortality in recent years has been from road traffic accidents, mountaineering disasters, drowning, and homicidal attacks. Pre-expedition advice and information can be obtained from books (see below), organizations such as the Expedition Advisory Centre of the Royal Geographical Society in London (Tel: 0207–581–2057; Fax: 0208–584–4447), and from clubs specializing in mountaineering, cave exploring, diving, and other activities. All expeditions should have a designated medical officer and as many members as possible should receive first-aid training. Medical kits should be more comprehensive than those carried by ordinary tourists. Lightweight emergency insulation, an adequate water supply, and a lightweight collapsible stretcher may be needed. A covering letter on official notepaper, signed by a doctor, is helpful in getting medications through customs. Local medical facilities must be identified and contacted in advance. Emergency plans must be drawn up for evacuation of the severely ill or injured. In East Africa, 'Flying Doctor' (AMREF) will evacuate casualties. Insurance cover must include medical care and repatriation of the injured. Before leaving home, expedition members should have a dental check and treatment for any unresolved medical or surgical problems. Expedition members should be chosen for their experience, technical skills, physical fitness, and a reputation for psychological stability under stress. A reliable local agent should be appointed.

Illness in returning travellers

Details are needed about the countries visited, activities while travelling, immunizations, and antimalarials taken. Common problems are fever, rash, diarrhoea, and eosinophilia (Tables 2, 3, and 4).

In travellers with acute diarrhoea, a dietary history, assessment of hydration state, stool microscopy and culture, abdominal films, and sigmoidoscopy may be needed. Patients with chronic diarrhoea may be infected with Giardia, Cryptosporidium, *Entamoeba histolytica*, shigellae, or salmonellae. Investigations should include a search for

Clostridium difficile and its toxin, especially if the patient had antimicrobials while abroad. A minority of patients may develop a postinfective enteropathy, with the most common problem being a secondary lactose intolerance. Rarely, bacterial overgrowth or tropical sprue develop.

The commonest causes of eosinophilia are allergy and helminths (Table 4).

Further reading

Auerbach, P.S. (1995). *Wilderness medicine. Management of wilderness and environmental emergencies*, 3rd edn. Mosby, St Louis.

Behrens, R.H. and McAdam, K.P.W.J. (ed.) (1993). Travel medicine. *British Medical Bulletin* **49**, 257–478.

Journal of Wilderness Medicine (1990–). Published for the Wilderness Medical Society by Chapman and Hall Medical, 11 New Fetter Lane, London EC4P 4EE.

Potter, S.A. (ed.) (1992). *Anare Antarctic field manual*, 4th edn. Australian Antarctic Division, Kingston, Tasmania.

Salisbury, D.M. and Begg, N.T. (ed.) (1996). *Immunisation against infectious disease.* HMSO, London.

Ward, M.P., Milledge, J.S., and West, J.B. (1989). *High altitude medicine and physiology.* Chapman and Hall Medical, London.

Warrell, D. and Anderson, S. (ed.) (1998). *The Royal Geographical Society expedition medicine.* Profile Books, London.

Chapter 16.8

Nosocomial infections

I. C. J. W. Bowler and D. W. M. Crook

Definitions

Hospital-acquired or nosocomial (Gk. *νοσοκομειον*, hospital) infections are distinct from community-acquired infections. They may affect patients and hospital staff. Most are readily recognized because they develop while a patient is in hospital, but others are not so clearly seen as hospital acquired; for example, hepatitis B infection may be acquired in hospital but, because of the prolonged incubation period, may not become clinically apparent until months after the patient has been discharged. Endogenous infections are produced by the patient's normal flora, while exogenous infections result from transmission of organisms to the patient from elsewhere. In practice, it may not always be possible to distinguish endogenous from exogenous infections. However, it is important to attempt differentiation between these two sources of infection as it has significant implications for deciding how to control them.

Scale of nosocomial infection

On a national scale, the number, severity, and cost of nosocomial infections have been difficult to measure. Rates of between 5.7 and 8.2 infections per 100 admissions have been reported. The urinary tract, surgical wounds, and the lower respiratory tract are the first, second, and third most common sites for these nosocomial infections (see Table 1).

Host

The principal factor contributing to the risk of nosocomial infection is the severity of the underlying disease (e.g. neutropenia, organ system failure). To a lesser extent, extremes of age, male sex, previous community-acquired infection, and length of preoperative hospital admission are associated with an increased risk of infection.

Micro-organisms

The main aetiological agents are bacteria. Viruses, fungi, and protozoa play a minor part. The five leading bacterial groups or species associated with nosocomial infections, in decreasing order of frequency are *Escherichia coli*, *Staphylococcus aureus*, *Enterococcus* spp., *Pseudomonas* spp., and coagulase-negative staphylococci.

Whether endogenously or exogenously acquired, the organisms that cause nosocomial infection are usually part of a patient's colonizing flora. Therefore, it may be difficult to distinguish, by bacteriological tests alone, organisms causing infection from those merely colonizing a surface. A shift towards a more resistant colonizing flora occurs during admission to hospital, particularly in burns and intensive-care units. Empirical antibiotic therapy must therefore accommodate the likely antibiotic-resistance patterns of the infecting flora. For example, *Pseudomonas aeruginosa*, methicillin-resistant *Staph. aureus* (MRSA), and enterococci are organisms that exhibit multiresistance to antimicrobials and require the use of alternative and expensive antibiotics.

Principles of hospital infection control

The main goal of hospital infection control is to prevent nosocomial infection. The first step is to identify hospital-acquired infections and determine if they are endemic or epidemic by clinical recognition and careful epidemiological investigation of the relation between cases. The identification and typing of isolates causing nosocomial infection provides an additional powerful tool for recognizing organisms that are epidemiologically linked. Invasive and multiresistant organisms, for example MRSA, often require application of infection control measures to prevent their spread.

Epidemic nosocomial infections and their control frequently receive greater attention because they involve the obvious spread of an infectious disease. They often involve person to person spread or a common point source and are usually amenable to measures that

Table 1 Rates and sites of nosocomial infection reported from three countries

	Canada (1976)	UK (1981)	USA (1986)
Rates (cases/100 admissions)			
	8.2[1]	9.2[1]	5.7[2]
Sites (% of all infections)			
UTI	39	30	42
SWI	24	19	24
LRI	26	16	11
Other	11	35	23

[1] Cases/100 admissions (prevalence).

[2] Cases/100 admissions/year (incidence).

UTI, urinary-tract infection; SWI, surgical wound infection; LRI, lower respiratory-tract infection.

Table 2 Micro-organisms causing nosocomial urinary tract infections (%)

	UK	USA
Escherichia coli	43	32
Proteus spp.	13	7
Klebsiella spp.	8	9
Enterococci	7	14
Pseudomonas aeruginosa	5	11
Coagulase-negative staphylococci	3	3
Enterobacter spp.	1	4
Other	14	22

interrupt the spread of infection. Control of the former includes the use of gowns and gloves by those attending patients, and careful hand washing after patient contact. Transfer of colonized or infected patients to a single room or an isolation ward is a physical means of preventing spread. Patients infected with the same organism can be grouped together and be attended by a cohort of nurses who do not care for uninfected patients. Identification of additional carriers and elimination of colonization may be necessary for some epidemic outbreaks. Controlled trials demonstrating the efficacy of such measures have not been made, but many observational studies support their use. Control of point-source outbreaks involves thorough microbiological and epidemiologial investigations to identify the hazard, which may be food or airborne, and the rapid implementation of corrective measures.

Control and reduction of endemic nosocomial infections is a less tractable, but not insurmountable, problem. It is important that such infections are documented by careful surveillance since they are often less obvious to health care workers. Control measures include the use of prophylactic antimicrobials for some types of surgery and meticulous sterile technique for invasive procedures (e.g. placement of intravenous devices and all forms of surgery).

Nosocomial infections by site

Nosocomial urinary-tract infection

Identification is by urine culture. Most patients remain asymptomatic, but 20–30 per cent develop the symptoms of urinary-tract infection, of which a small proportion, about 1 in 100, develops bacteraemia. The types of organisms that cause nosocomial urinary-tract infections are listed in Table 2.

Indwelling urinary catheters account for 80 per cent of nosocomial urinary-tract infections, which is scarcely surprising as 50 per cent of patients catheterized for longer than 7–10 days develop bacteriuria. Most of the other urinary-tract infections are accounted for by instrumentation of the urinary tract. The main source of organisms is the periurethral flora. Bacteria gain access to the bladder, usually by spreading up the outside of the lumen of the catheter. Occasionally, the infecting organisms are acquired from an exogenous source, as part of an epidemic nosocomial infection. Most symptomatic or bacteraemic urinary-tract infections occur within 24 h of the organisms gaining access to the bladder.

Clinically, symptomatic cases present with dysuria, frequency, lower abdominal discomfort, loin pain, fever, and sometimes features of septic shock. Treatment of a symptomatic patient requires broad-spectrum antimicrobials administered empirically after obtaining appropriate cultures. Treatment should later be adjusted according to the results of bacteriological studies. There is no need to treat asymptomatic patients.

Prevention of nosocomial urinary-tract infections has received much attention. Prophylactic antimicrobial treatment does not have a significant role, but it is important to avoid urinary catheterization or reduce the period of catheterization. Catheters should be inserted aseptically, and closed sterile drainage systems, uninterrupted gravity drainage, or intermittent or suprapubic catheterization used.

Surgical wound infection

As there is no objective test for the diagnosis of a surgical wound infection, no precise definition is available. One acceptable definition requires the presence of a purulent discharge in, or exuding from, a wound. The two leading causes of this infection are *Staph. aureus* (15–33 per cent of all wound infections) and *E. coli* (12–19 per cent). A wide range of other aerobic and anaerobic bacterial species can also be implicated.

There are a number of risk factors for surgical wound infection. The main risk is the degree of wound contamination at operation. Operations can be classified as 'clean' (e.g. herniorrhaphy), 'clean contaminated' (e.g. appendicectomy which requires incision of bowel) and 'contaminated' (e.g. gross spillage from the gastrointestinal tract during surgery). The risk of wound infection obviously increases from 'clean' to 'contaminated'. Other risk factors include the length of the operation, obesity, a remote infection, and underlying disease. Most wound infections follow the direct inoculation of organisms into the wound at the time of surgery or spread of bacteria to open wounds such as burns.

Clinically, wound infections present with erythema, pain, swelling, or pus at the site of the wound and produce general features of infection such as fever. Management consists first of taking appropriate cultures, including blood cultures, draining pus if it is present, and empirically giving broad-spectrum antimicrobials effective against the likely flora. Treatment can subsequently be changed according to the bacteriological results. Prevention of wound infection depends largely on meticulous aseptic technique, good surgical technique, and the use of prophylactic antimicrobials given within 2 h of the induction of anaesthesia.

Nosocomial pneumonia

Pneumonia is defined clinically. Features include the production of purulent sputum, chest signs, a fall in arterial Po_2 and the appearance of infiltrates on the chest radiograph not ascribable to pulmonary emboli, atelactasis, or pulmonary oedema. Between 0.55 and 1.5 per cent of patients admitted to hospital are estimated to develop lower respiratory-tract infections. The mortality attributable to pneumonia has not been reliably determined because many of the patients with pneumonia have serious underlying illnesses that are independently associated with death. Crude case fatalities of between 20 and 30 per cent are quoted. Intubated and ventilated patients have the highest risk of acquiring pneumonia. The source of the organisms is the bacteria colonizing the gastrointestinal and upper respiratory tracts. They probably gain access to the lung by aspiration. This infecting flora is frequently acquired by the patient after admission to hospital. The types of organisms cultured from bronchoscopic samples are listed in Table 3.

Table 3 Causative organisms identified in samples drained at bronchoscopy by protected specimen brush (% of all pneumonias)

	France	Spain
Pseudomonas aeruginosa	31	35
Acinetobacter spp.	15	30
Proteus spp.	15	
Moraxella catarrhalis	10	
Haemophilus spp.	10	
Staphylococcus aureus	33	25
Streptococci	15	20
Other species	37	60
Polymicrobial	21	50

Clinically, these patients will present with general signs and symptoms of infection and new physical signs typical of pneumonia or bronchopneumonia. Chest radiography should reveal a new infiltrate and blood gases show evidence of an increasing arterial alveolar oxygen gradient (a–A gradient). Culture of expectorated sputum or tracheal aspirate is poorly predictive of the bacterial cause of nosocomial pneumonia, which is best determined by quantitative culture of specimens obtained by sampling the terminal airways (e.g. by bronchoalveolar lavage). Initially, broad-spectrum antimicrobials appropriate for the likely infecting flora should be given empirically. Once the susceptibility of the causative pathogen has been determined, specific antimicrobial treatment can be applied. Prevention of endemic nosocomial infections has attracted considerable attention. However, despite reducing the occurrence of these infections using measures such as selective decontamination of the digestive tract, no reduction in the mortality of ventilated patients has been seen. Epidemic nosocomial infections that usually result from bacterial contamination of respiratory equipment such as nebulizers, ventilators, or bronchoscopes can be prevented by meticulous control measures.

Intravascular device-associated infections

The most important clinical outcome of intravascular device-associated infection is bacteraemia, which varies in its incidence from a low of about 0.04 per cent for subcutaneous central venous ports to about 0.2 per cent for peripheral intravenous cannulae to a high of approximately 10 per cent for central venous haemodialysis catheters.

Bacteria usually gain access to the blood by direct spread from the skin surface along the subcutaneous catheter tunnel to its tip in the blood vessel. Bacteraemia from intraluminal bacteria results from contamination of connecting devices. This is particularly important in catheters with subcutaneous cuffs, such as Hickman catheters, where the periluminal route of infection is less likely. The leading organisms causing intravenous device-related sepsis are *Staph. aureus*, *Pseudomonas* spp., and *Candida* spp. In patients with haematological malignancies, coagulase-negative staphylococci and enterococci are, in addition, frequently implicated.

Line-related sepsis can present with local inflammation around the catheter or occasionally with signs of thrombophlebitis. Usually, it presents with features of bacteraemia. Management involves obtaining blood cultures, removing and culturing the affected catheter, and giving empirical antimicrobials. In some circumstances, long-term intravenous catheters, such as Hickman lines, can be 'sterilized' by giving parenteral antibiotics down the line. Intravascular catheter sepsis is prevented by using aseptic technique when inserting catheters, maintaining a high standard of line care, and removing catheters as soon as possible. The insertion site should be disinfected with a reliable disinfectant such as 70 per cent alcohol containing chlorhexidine. At the time of insertion the operators should wash their hands, and for long-line insertion, wear sterile gloves, gown, a mask, and use large sterile drapes to cover the patient. Peripheral intravenous cannulae should not be left in for more than 3 days. Replacing the entire intravenous delivery set every 72 h is sufficient to reduce sepsis secondary to the intraluminal contamination of 'giving' sets.

Further reading

Ayliffe, G.A.J., Lowbury, E.J.L., Geddes, A.M., and Williams, J.D. (ed.) (1992). *Control of hospital infection: a practical handbook*, 3rd edn. Chapman and Hall, London.

Meers, P., Jacobsen, W., and McPherson, M. (1992). *Hospital infection control for nurses*. Chapman and Hall, London.

Wenzel, R.P. (ed.) (1997). *Prevention and control of nosocomial infections*, 3rd edn. Williams and Wilkins, Baltimore.

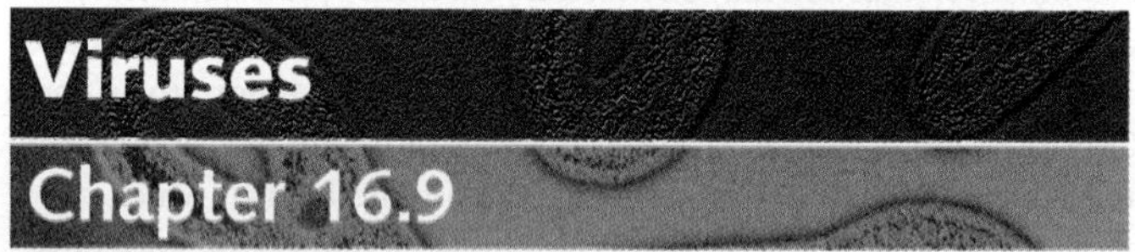

Respiratory tract viruses

D. Isaacs

Introduction

Acute respiratory infections (Table 1) are estimated to cause 4 million childhood deaths in the world each year and viruses cause a large proportion of these infections. In developed countries, respiratory virus infections are responsible for significant childhood morbidity and absence from work.

Epidemiology

Respiratory viruses are ubiquitous. Most preschool children in developed countries experience about six to eight respiratory viral infections per year, predominantly with rhinoviruses. Determinants of the number of infections include age (maximum 6 months to 4 years), day-care or kindergarten attendance, having school-age siblings, living in an urban area, maternal smoking, and psychological stress. Breast-feeding protects against respiratory virus infections. The popular belief that getting cold or wet causes colds has not been borne out by experiment. Lowering the body temperature of volunteers by immersion in cold water does not increase their susceptibility to infection. However, many respiratory viruses cause more infections in the colder months of the year.

Modes of transmission

Respiratory viruses are transmitted mainly by respiratory droplet spread. Infections may also be spread on hands, either by direct contact with a child's nose, or by contact with intermediate objects

Table 1 Features of respiratory virus infections

Virus	DNA or RNA	Incubation period (days)	Modes of transmission	Main diseases	Comments
Rhinoviruses	RNA	1–3	Secretions on hands Large droplets Infect nasal mucosa or conjunctiva	Colds, URTIs, sinusitis, otitis media, wheeze, pneumonia	More than 100 serotypes
Coronaviruses	RNA	2–4	Large droplets Aerosols (small droplets)	Colds, URTIs, wheeze, pneumonia	Two main serotypes Reinfections common
Adenoviruses	DNA	3–7	Small droplets Large droplets Nose, pharynx, or conjunctiva		Over 40 serotypes Asymptomatic shedding can persist for months
Parainfluenza	RNA	1–4	Large droplets Secretions on hands	Type 1 croup, pneumonia Type 2 croup Type 3 croup, bronchiolitis, pneumonia Type 4 cold, URTI	Autumn epidemics every 2nd year Autumn every 1–2 years Summer epidemic Sporadic Reinfections common
Influenza viruses	RNA	1–6	Large droplets Small droplets Secretions on hand	Influenza, croup, pneumonia	Types A, B, C Type A can cause pandemics Amantidine only effective against type A
Respiratory syncytial virus	RNA	2–8	Secretions on hands Fomites	Bronchiolitis, pneumonia, otitis media, wheeze	Two major groups, A and B Reinfections common

URTI, upper respiratory-tract infection.

or fomite spread. Viruses can then be inoculated by fingering the nasal mucosa or conjunctiva.

Pathogenesis

Respiratory viruses infect cells by taking advantage of natural host-cell receptors. For example, almost all rhinoviruses bind to the intercellular adhesion molecule receptor, ICAM-1, to gain entry to fibroblasts and other cells. Most respiratory viruses replicate locally in the respiratory tract and cause relatively little viraemia. In contrast, influenza A virus infection can cause viraemia, which results in interferon-α appearing in the serum, and probably causing many of the symptoms of 'flu', since interferon alone can cause fever, headaches, myalgia, and malaise.

The local symptoms of respiratory viral infections are caused largely by inflammatory mediators, particularly bradykinins. Rhinoviruses cause very little destruction of the nasal mucosal epithelium, but respiratory syncytial virus (RSV) is more destructive and can cause necrosis of respiratory epithelium.

Immunity

Immunity against reinfection with a respiratory virus depends mainly on specific serum IgG and/or secretory IgA antibody. Immunity against one serotype of a virus (e.g. rhinovirus) does not confer cross-protection against other serotypes. The vast number of serotypes (over 100 rhinovirus serotypes alone) explains the large number of infections suffered by children.

Antibody is usually produced too slowly to be effective in recovery from acute infection. In general, cellular immunity is more important. Children with isolated antibody deficiency recover normally from respiratory viral infections whereas children with pure T-cell deficiency are at increased risk of life-threatening infections with RSV, parainfluenza, and measles viruses. Interferon-α is produced locally, appearing in nasal secretions as viral titres fall, and is probably another important factor in recovery from most acute respiratory viral infections.

Diagnosis

Inoculation of respiratory secretions on to tissue culture has long been the mainstay of the diagnosis of respiratory virus infections, but rapid diagnosis is now possible by detection of selected viral antigens in respiratory secretions, either by immunofluorescence using a fluorescein-labelled specific antibody, or by enzyme immunoassay. Viral nucleic acid can be detected by polymerase chain reaction.

Secretions aspirated by gentle suction from the back of the nose (nasopharyngeal aspirates) are the preferred specimens for respiratory viral detection. Nose and throat swabs give a lower yield.

Serology is useful for diagnosing many infections, but generally not in babies and infants. Acute and convalescent sera taken at least 10–14 days apart are needed for detection of at least a fourfold rise in IgG antibody titre. Virus specific IgM tests are available for a few viruses.

Rhinoviruses

Rhinoviruses, together with the enteroviruses (coxsackie, echo, and polio), comprise the picornaviruses (pico (= small) RNA viruses).

The RNA is infectious and can act as mRNA, so that replication is entirely cytoplasmic.

Epidemiology

Rhinoviruses exhibit great antigenic diversity and there are over 100 serotypes. Infection with one strain does not generally confer cross-protection against other strains. Several serotypes usually circulate simultaneously in a community, and infections occur throughout the year, but particularly from late autumn to spring. The infection rate is highest in preschool children. They are the most important cause of colds, and of episodes of wheeze in asthma.

Transmission

Transmission depends on prolonged close contact, and is by droplet spread, or via contaminated nasal secretions hand-to-hand or fomite-to-hand and thence to nasal mucosa or conjunctiva. It has been estimated that a susceptible adult has a 50 per cent chance of being infected by 100 h of close exposure to someone with a moderately severe cold.

Immunity

Rhinoviruses stimulate nasal production of interferon-α and specific nasal IgA, both of which appear within about 24 h of infection, and probably contribute to recovery. Protection against reinfection correlates best with the presence of serotype-specific nasal IgA antibody, and to a lesser extent with serum IgG antibody.

Pathogenesis

Rhinoviruses replicate mainly in the upper respiratory tract in ciliated epithelial cells. They generally elicit little local mucosal damage, and cause rhinorrhoea with mucus production through the action of local inflammatory mediators such as bradykinins, which are potent endogenous vasoactive peptides. Histamine is not involved.

Clinical manifestations

Rhinoviruses usually cause the common cold, but they have also been detected in the middle-ear fluid of children with acute otitis media, and in sinuses during acute sinusitis. They are an occasional cause of infantile bronchiolitis, producing a clinical syndrome indistinguishable from RSV bronchiolitis. They are a common cause of wheezing in asthmatics. Rhinoviruses can cause pneumonia in children and the elderly, occasionally severe, and rarely fatal. They can also cause exacerbations of cystic fibrosis.

Treatment

There is no effective specific therapy for rhinoviruses, and so treatment is symptomatic. Controlled trials of vitamin C have shown no clear-cut benefit, while aspirin actually enhances viral shedding.

Coronaviruses

Coronaviruses, so-called because of the sun-like crown appearance seen under the electron microscope, are even more fastidious in their growth than rhinoviruses. Antigens from the two prototype strains 229E and OC4 have been used to develop serological assays, and serosurveys have contributed greatly to understanding coronavirus epidemiology.

Diagnosis

Human coronavirus infections have usually been diagnosed serologically, but antigens can be detected in nasopharyngeal secretions by enzyme immunoassay, or nucleic acid by polymerase chain reaction (PCR).

Epidemiology

Human coronaviruses are found worldwide and cause midwinter outbreaks of respiratory infection. Reinfections are common and are demonstrated by a rise in antibody titre in adults with prior antibody.

Transmission

Human coronaviruses are infectious by the respiratory route, and volunteers can be infected by intranasal inoculation. Both aerosol and large-droplet spread are thought to be important routes of transmission.

Immunity and pathogenesis

Nasal production of secretory IgA and interferon-α are probably important in recovery from acute coronavirus infection. Immunity against reinfection is transient but has been shown to last at least 1 year.

The virus causes quite marked destruction of the ciliated epithelium of the nasal mucosa and trachea.

Clinical manifestations and treatment

The most frequent manifestation of human coronavirus infection is the common cold: coryza, nasal soreness and congestion, and sneezing. In adults, the OC43 strain can cause sore throat and cough. Pharyngitis is frequent in children, and cervical adenitis, coryza, and low-grade fever are also common. Human coronaviruses can cause childhood pneumonia, wheezing in asthmatic children, and exacerbations of chronic bronchitis in adults.

There is no specific therapy.

Adenoviruses

Adenoviruses are non-enveloped DNA viruses. Most adenoviruses grow readily in tissue culture. Enteric adenoviruses are not cultivable but are seen on electron microscopy of faeces. Over 40 different adenoviral serotypes have been described. Diagnosis of respiratory adenovirus infection is by culture, antigen detection, or serology.

Epidemiology

Adenovirus infections can occur at any age but are most common in infants and preschool children. Epidemics can occur, primarily in institutions such as day-care centres and orphanages, but also in association with swimming pools, schools, and military barracks.

Infections with adenoviruses occur worldwide. Epidemics are most frequent from winter through to early summer, but sporadic cases occur throughout the year.

Transmission

Transmission is by small droplets, which infect the nose, throat, or conjunctiva. In swimming-pool epidemics of pharyngoconjunctival fever, the virus survives in the water and can infect conjunctivae. Adenoviruses may be carried asymptomatically in the nasopharynx of children for several months following acute infection, and may act as a source of spread.

Immunity

Local secretory IgA is produced in the nasopharynx from about 3 days after adenovirus infection, followed by specific nasal IgG at 7 days and then serum neutralizing antibody.

Adenovirus early protein can bind major histocompatibility complex class I molecules, and thus evade immune surveillance by T cells.

Pathogenesis

Respiratory adenoviruses invade the ciliated epithelium of the respiratory tract. Viraemia may occur early, resulting in rashes. Lung and pleural involvement could be due to local or viraemic spread. In severe pneumonia there is necrotizing bronchiolitis with necrosis and hyaline membrane formation.

Clinical manifestations

Adenoviruses can cause various respiratory syndromes. Tonsillitis is frequently follicular or exudative, with high fever, and may mimic group A streptococcal infection. Epidemic conjunctivitis, either alone or in conjunction with pharyngitis, is frequently due to adenoviruses. Pneumonia is less frequently due to adenovirus than to RSV, rhinoviruses, or parainfluenza viruses, but severe and often fatal cases in children under 18 months have been attributed to types 3, 7, and 21. Severe infantile adenovirus pneumonia may result in bronchiectasis, bronchiolitis obliterans, or unilateral hypertranslucent lung (McLeod's syndrome). Acute respiratory disease was described in the Second World War, occurring in epidemics in military recruits, and characterized by fever, dry cough, sometimes paroxysmal, pharyngitis, laryngotracheitis, and often wheezing. The disease may progress to pneumonia.

Adenovirus type 7 is the strain most likely to cause disseminated disease, with hepatitis, myocarditis, nephritis, and meningoencephalitis.

Treatment

There is no proven specific treatment for systemic adenovirus infections. Topical interferon-β was effective against adenovirus keratoconjunctivitis in a comparative trial. There are anecdotal reports of the successful use of nebulized ribavirin to treat adenovirus pneumonia in children.

Parainfluenza viruses

The parainfluenza viruses are RNA paramyxoviruses. There are three main serotypes, parainfluenza viruses 1, 2, and 3, which show little antigenic variation. Type 4 is subdivided into 4A and 4B.

Epidemiology

Parainfluenza virus infections occur worldwide. Type 3 infections occur early, so that 60 per cent of infants are seropositive by 12 months of age. Type 1 and 2 infections occur later in childhood.

Parainfluenza 1 virus tends to cause autumn outbreaks of laryngotracheitis (croup) in alternate years in the Northern Hemisphere, or sporadic cases for a few years. In the Southern Hemisphere the biennial epidemic nature is not always so clear-cut. Parainfluenza 2 virus causes less well-defined autumn or winter epidemics of croup every 1–2 years. Parainfluenza 3 virus is endemic or causes annual summer epidemics of croup and bronchiolitis.

Transmission

Person-to-person contact is the main route of transmission, with spread by large droplets or infected secretions. Parainfluenza viruses can survive for prolonged periods in the environment.

Immunity

Immunity is at best partial, and reinfections occur. Children with impaired cellular immunity suffer prolonged, symptomatic infections, suggesting that T cells are important in recovery from acute infection. Local nasal interferon-α is produced in acute infection and may contribute to recovery. Maternal antibody is partially protective, but after recovery from acute infection, secretory antibody appears to be more important than serum antibody in protecting against reinfection.

Pathogenesis

Parainfluenza viruses infect the respiratory epithelium by attaching to specific receptors. Local respiratory-tract spread is mainly by cell-to-cell transfer but viraemic spread may also occur. In severe infections there is extensive epithelial necrosis and inflammation throughout the respiratory tract, even involving the alveoli.

Clinical manifestations

Laryngotracheitis or croup is the most commonly recognized clinical manifestation of parainfluenza virus infection, mainly due to types 1 and 2. Infection may also involve the large airways, causing wheezing and producing laryngotracheobronchitis. Febrile, upper respiratory-tract infections, often with rhinitis and sore throat, are actually more common than croup. Other important manifestations are infantile bronchiolitis and pneumonia, usually due to type 3 and occurring throughout the year but often in summer (unlike RSV). Type 4 may cause colds. Parainfluenza viruses can precipitate wheezing in asthmatics, exacerbate cystic fibrosis and chronic bronchitis, and are a rare cause of pneumonia in military recruits. Reinfections are common and are usually successively milder.

Treatment

Nebulized ribavirin can suppress chronic parainfluenza virus infection in children with severe combined immunodeficiency, long enough to allow curative bone-marrow transplantation.

Influenza viruses

Influenza was once attributed to divine influence, hence its name, which is said to have come from Florence in the fifteenth century. Influenza A viruses are renowned for causing pandemics with a very high mortality: the pandemic of 1918–19 killed an estimated 20 million, more people than both world wars combined.

The influenza viruses are RNA orthomyxoviruses, with three main types, A, B, and C, and multiple subtypes. Influenza surface proteins include haemagglutinin (H) and neuraminidase (N). Viruses are described by the type, origin, strain, year, and H and N subtypes: hence, influenza virus A/Shanghai/6/90 (H3N2).

Epidemiology

Influenza viruses are renowned for their ability to escape host immune surveillance by antigenic changes. These are either minor changes in H or N, called antigenic drift, which occur with influenza A and B, or major changes in the H and/or N proteins to a new subtype, antigenic shift, which is confined to influenza A.

Influenza viruses cause winter epidemics of varying degree. These may be small local outbreaks, nationwide epidemics, or global pandemics. A possible epidemic was described by Hippocrates and Livy in 412 BC. Recently there have been pandemics every 10–20 years, the largest being in 1918–19.

The highest attack rate for influenza is in young children, but the highest mortality is in the elderly. Mortality is higher in the immunocompromised and those with heart disease, chronic lung disease, diabetes, and chronic renal disease.

Transmission

Large-droplet spread from coughs and sneezes is probably the main mode of spread. Experimentally, a fine aerosol reaching the alveoli is more infectious than nasal deposition. Virus may also spread via nasal secretions on hands.

High titres of virus are found in respiratory secretions. Shedding is for 1–2 weeks, but the incubation period is only 2–3 days. These factors contribute to rapid epidemic spread. Closed communities such as schools, military barracks, residential homes, and even hospitals are likely to suffer dramatic outbreaks.

Immunity

In recovery from acute infection, cellular immunity (specific cytotoxic T cells), nasal interferon-α production, and nasal IgA all appear to be important. Protection against reinfection correlates with pre-existing specific ('memory') cytotoxic T cells, specific serum IgG antibody, and specific nasal IgA antibody.

Natural immunity following acute infection lasts for about 4–6 years, but depends in part on the degree of antigenic variation. Vaccine-induced immunity, using an inactivated influenza vaccine, lasts for only one influenza season, but the vaccines contain the strains that the WHO predicts are likely to circulate in the coming winter.

Pathogenesis

The principal site of influenza virus infection is the ciliated columnar epithelial cell. Necrosis of nasal and tracheal ciliated cells occurs early, often within the first day, and impairment of the mucociliary escalator predisposes to bacterial superinfection. Influenza pneumonia is characterized by bronchiolar epithelial necrosis with haemorrhagic alveolar exudate and lymphocytic infiltration of the alveoli, peribronchial areas, and interstitium. Secondary bacterial pneumonia is an important contributor to illness and death.

Clinical manifestations

Influenza A virus is unusual in causing a similar febrile illness in children and adults, with sudden fever, chills, headache, myalgia, and dry cough. Sore throat and rhinitis or nasal stuffiness are common. In children, it is the second most common cause of viral croup, and influenza viruses can cause febrile convulsions in preschool children. Influenza B may be milder and is more likely to cause ocular symptoms: conjunctivitis, eye pain, or photophobia. In children, abdominal pain and vomiting are common. The illness usually lasts 2–3 days, rarely up to 1 week.

Primary pneumonia due to influenza viruses is found particularly in immunocompromised patients or those with pre-existing heart disease, and this may be progressive. Bacterial superinfection can occur, usually with pneumococci or *Staphylococcus aureus*. The latter is particularly fulminant, with haemoptysis and dyspnoea, pneumatoceles and empyema, and often a rapid demise.

Cardiac complications of influenza virus may be asymptomatic. Myocarditis and pericarditis are well described. Sudden deaths from influenza have occurred, either spontaneously during exercise, or merely on getting out of bed, due to subclinical myocarditis.

Myalgia is normal in influenza, but if severe may indicate true myositis. The serum levels of muscle enzymes are usually grossly elevated in myositis. Rhabdomyolysis with myoglobinuria occurs rarely. Influenza B is a more common cause of myositis than influenza A.

Rare complications of influenza virus infection include Reye syndrome (fatty liver, hypoglycaemia, and encephalopathy) and neurological conditions, such as Guillain–Barré syndrome and transverse myelitis. Glomerulonephritis rash and parotitis have been described.

Prevention and treatment

Current influenza vaccines are formalin inactivated, usually contain two influenza A strains and one B strain, and are chemically treated to reduce pyrogens ('split' vaccines) or untreated ('whole' vaccines) (see Chapter 16.6). Annual immunization is recommended for the elderly and for adults and children with chronic respiratory, heart, or renal disease, diabetes or immuno-suppression.

Chemoprophylaxis using amantidine (or the related drug rimantidine) reduces the incidence of influenza A infection, but is ineffective against B. Amantidine has been used in boarding schools and geriatric homes for routine winter prophylaxis; to limit spread during outbreaks; and for winter prophylaxis of children with cystic fibrosis. Amantidine can cause central nervous system side-effects, such as difficulty in concentrating, while both amantidine and rimantidine can result in gastrointestinal effects, nausea, and anorexia.

Specific treatment of severe influenza A infections is possible using oral amantidine or rimantidine, both of which have been shown to be effective. The adult dose of amantidine is 200 mg once, followed by 100 mg once daily for 5–7 days. The child dose is scaled down proportionately.

Nebulized ribavirin is effective against both influenza A and B virus infections in adults.

Respiratory syncytial virus (RSV)

RSV kills about a million children a year in developing countries. RSV was isolated in 1955 from a chimpanzee with a cold. The name derives from the tendency to cause syncytia, or multinucleate giant cells, in tissue culture. RSV is an enveloped RNA virus of the paramyxovirus group. There are two major groups of RSV, A and B, or 1 and 2.

One of the earliest successes of rapid viral diagnosis was the detection of RSV antigen in nasopharyngeal secretions using fluorescein-labelled antisera, either specific for RSV (direct immunofluorescence) or directed against an antibody to RSV (indirect). ELISA and PCR are now available.

Epidemiology

Infection occurs worldwide. In temperate climates there are epidemics every winter, lasting about 4 months, while in equatorial climates RSV epidemics usually occur in the rainy season. Group A or B may predominate in different years, or a group A and a group B strain may circulate concurrently.

The peak incidence is at 2–6 months of age, when it might be expected that passively acquired maternal IgG would be protective. In fact, serum IgG is at best only partially protective, and reinfections with RSV are extremely common. Adults can readily be reinfected, and can act as a source of infection for spread to children at home and in hospitals. The incidence of RSV infection increases with exposure to other children (urban environment, overcrowding, day care) and with passive exposure to tobacco smoke, particularly maternal smoking. The incidence is lower in breast-fed than in bottle-fed babies.

There is an association between RSV infection and recurrent wheezing, but it is not known whether RSV bronchiolitis causes asthma, or whether the virus merely causes bronchiolitis in atopic children who were destined to be asthmatic.

RSV infection can be very severe in the elderly.

Transmission

Close contact is necessary for efficient spread of RSV, which is carried in large droplets and secretions, and survives for some hours on metal or plastic surfaces. RSV infection can occur by inoculation of the nasal mucosa or conjunctiva. The incubation period is 2–8 days (median 5 days). Infants with RSV infection usually shed virus for up to 10 days although sometimes for 3–4 weeks, or even longer, particularly if immunocompromised.

Pathogenesis

RSV infects the respiratory epithelium. Viraemia is unusual. Severe infection causes necrosis of the bronchiolar epithelium, and RSV antigen can be demonstrated in epithelial cells throughout the respiratory tract. The alveoli are spared, unless there is RSV pneumonia. Obstruction of small airways by cell debris results in hyperinflation.

It has long been felt that the host immune response may contribute to pathogenesis of the infection. Nasopharyngeal cells from some infected infants have RSV-specific IgE bound to their surface, and this correlates with subsequent wheezing. Alveolar macrophages produce tumour necrosis factor and mononuclear cells produce platelet-activating factor when stimulated with RSV, both of which may contribute to disease.

Immunity

Children and adults with impaired T-cell immunity, including those with HIV infection, are susceptible to more severe RSV infection; infection can be prolonged and symptomatic with wheezing, and may be fatal. Reinfections are common and most adults can be readily infected. Cytotoxic T cells appear in the peripheral blood early in infection, even in babies, and correlate with milder disease and with recovery. In a mouse model of RSV, moderate numbers of cytotoxic T cells will clear RSV infection whereas large numbers potentiate disease, suggesting that there may be a critical level of T-cell response.

Secretory IgA appears in the nasopharynx early and may contribute to recovery, and to resistance to further infections. Serum IgA is only partially protective.

Clinical manifestations

Almost all children (90–95 per cent) have been infected with RSV by the age of 2 years. Initial infections are nearly always symptomatic, and about 40 per cent cause clinical bronchiolitis, with wheeze, cough, rhinorrhoea, and fever. RSV is by far the most important cause of bronchiolitis.

RSV bronchiolitis is particularly severe in immunocompromised children, those with underlying cardiopulmonary disease including congenital heart disease, bronchopulmonary dysplasia and cystic fibrosis, and babies born prematurely.

The virus is an important precipitant of asthma attacks in older children and can cause pneumonia, particularly in infancy. Infections with RSV otherwise tend to become progressively milder. Children under 5 years may develop otitis media. School-age children and adults are likely to have a febrile upper respiratory infection with pharyngitis and cough. The elderly may develop pneumonia, which can be fatal.

Prevention

There is no effective vaccine against RSV. It is an important cause of nosocomial infection in children's hospitals, neonatal units, and homes for the elderly. Spread may be reduced by cohorting (isolating) RSV-positive patients, and improved hand washing.

Treatment

Nebulized ribavirin results in modest improvements in the clinical severity and oxygen saturation, and sometimes in viral shedding. The morbidity is slightly reduced in children with congenital heart disease or bronchopulmonary dysplasia, but mortality has not been affected. Ribavirin can precipitate in ventilator tubing and cause fluctuations in pressure. It is expensive and is not indicated for previously healthy babies with RSV infection, but might be considered for children or adults with underlying immune deficiency or cardiopulmonary disease.

Treatment of RSV infection is otherwise supportive. The need for supplemental oxygen is best assessed by pulse oximetry.

Further reading

Dick, E.C., Hossain, S.U., and Mink, K.A. (1986). Interruption of transmission of rhinovirus colds among human volunteers using virucidal paper handkerchiefs. *Journal of Infectious Diseases* **153**, 352–6.

Dick, E.C., Jennings, L.C., Mink, K.A., *et al.* (1987). Aerosol transmission of rhinovirus colds. *Journal of Infectious Diseases* **156**, 442–8.

Hall, C.B. and Douglas, R.G., Jr (1981). Modes of transmission of respiratory syncytial virus. *Journal of Pediatrics* **99**, 100–3.

Johnston, S.L., Pattemore, P.K., Sanderson, G., *et al.* (1995). Community study of role of viral infections in exacerbations of asthma in 9–11 year old children. *British Medical Journal* **310**, 1225–8.

Ruuskanen, O., Meurman, O., and Sarkkinen, J. (1985). Adenoviral diseases in children: a study of 105 hospital cases. *Pediatrics* **76**, 79–83.

Chapter 16.10

Herpes simplex virus infections

*J. B. Kurtz**

There are two types of herpes simplex virus—HSV-1 and HSV-2. Both can cause a primary infection in the non-immune; subsequently the virus persists in that person for life. Intermittent reactivation of the virus from its latent state causes asymptomatic virus shedding and vesicular skin lesions, e.g. cold sores.

* Includes some material from Chapter 7.10.2, *Oxford textbook of medicine*, 3rd edition (Herpes simplex virus infections by T.E.A. Peto and B.E. Juel-Jensen).

Epidemiology

Humans are the only natural reservoir for HSV. Transmission is through direct contact with infected secretions via mucocutaneous sites or traumatized or diseased skin. HSV is relatively labile and there is no evidence that transmission can occur from inanimate objects or by aerosols. Spread of HSV-1 is predominantly by contact with oral secretions and HSV-2 by genital secretions. Spread from oral secretions to other areas of skin is an occupational hazard of dentists, medical health workers, and in certain contact sports (wrestlers, exponents of judo, and rugby football players). The virus can be transmitted from the genital tract sexually, during birth to the neonate, and by autoinoculation to hands, thighs, and buttocks.

Transmission occurs both from people with active herpetic lesions and from asymptomatic excretors. Surveys have shown that between 0.65 and 15 per cent of adults are excreting herpes simplex virus at any one time. The majority of new HSV infections (1 and 2) are acquired from asymptomatic people who are shedding the virus. Because more than 80 per cent of primary infections are asymptomatic the prevalence of the disease is best assessed by serological surveys. The prevalence of infection is changing. Until the 1950s, sero-epidemiological studies showed a seroprevalence of about 90 per cent by the fourth decade of life. Since then, rates in the higher socioeconomic groups have shown a slow decline. For instance, in 1953 in the UK, 85 per cent of a sample of children aged between 3 and 15 years had antibodies compared to only 41 per cent when the survey was repeated in 1965, and 24 per cent in 10–14-year-olds in 1996. In the period 1964–68, 33 per cent of 181 British-born Oxford clinical students had antibodies, contrasting with 62 per cent of 42 students born in Third World countries. The age of primary infection has shifted upwards.

In contrast to HSV-1, HSV-2 is the predominant cause of genital herpes. The highest rate of infection occurs between the ages of 15 and 25 years. The prevalence of HSV-2 antibodies is rising and is dependent on sexual activity, ranging from 0 per cent in celibate adults to over 80 per cent in prostitutes. The seroprevalence of HSV-2 was 22 per cent in adults in the US in a 1989–91 survey but under 5 per cent in a similar 1994 UK population survey.

Pathogenesis

HSV-1 and -2 are members of the herpes virus group. The virus has an internal core containing double-stranded DNA of about 150 kbp encoding about 33 virion proteins; a further 30 proteins are expressed during cellular infection. HSV-1 and -2 share about half their nucleotide sequence and express functionally equivalent proteins. The two strains differ antigenically and biologically.

On entry into skin sites, HSV replicates locally in parabasal and intermediate epithelial cells, causing cell lysis resulting in a local inflammatory response. The early papules are associated with multinucleated giant cells formed by the fusion of infected and uninfected neighbouring cells. Typical vesicles are caused by cell degeneration and oedema fluid, which elevates the stratum corneum. The vesicle fluid contains degenerating cells, multinucleated giant cells, and cell-free virus. Evolution of vesicles into pustules is associated with invasion by inflammatory cells.

After the primary infection, HSV tracks up sensory nerves and becomes latent within their ganglia. The exact mechanism of latency remains unclear as does that of reactivation. The latter can be triggered by fever, trauma, stress, sunlight, and menstruation.

Clinical manifestations

The clinical manifestations of HSV-1 and -2 overlap. Both types can cause primary orofacial and genital infections, and these infections are clinically indistinguishable. However, the frequency of future reactivations is influenced by the anatomical site and the type of virus. Recurrence of genital HSV-2 infection is more common than genital HSV-1 infection. Orofacial HSV-1 infection recurrence rates range from frequent to rare whereas orofacial HSV-2 recurrences hardly ever occur.

Primary infections are frequently asymptomatic but, especially in adults, may be serious. Any skin site may be involved, although perioral and genital areas are most commonly affected.

Orofacial infection

Primary infection

The incubation period ranges from 2–12 days and in symptomatic cases is followed by high fever, sore throat, and pharyngeal oedema. The disease can be trivial, especially in children, but painful vesicles may appear on the pharyngeal and oral mucosa, spreading to an extensive gingivostomatitis (Plate 1). Hypersalivation and drooling often occur. Lesions may extend to the lips and cheeks. In adults the disease is sometimes confined to the pharynx and tonsils. The high fever, toxicity, and severe mouth pain can persist for several days. There is cervical lymphadenopathy and sometimes splenomegaly. In some cases, patients cannot eat or drink. Without treatment the illness subsides after about 10–14 days and the vesicles heal slowly. Occasionally, autoinoculation occurs to other sites, especially the fingers.

The diagnosis is usually made clinically from the widespread oral lesions together with a severe systemic disease. The main differential diagnosis is severe Stevens–Johnson syndrome or severe, non-specific, aphthous ulceration. A good many cases of so-called 'Vincent's angina' are probably examples of herpetic gingivostomatitis. Zoster of the second branch of the trigeminal nerve confined to the mouth may be confusing but it is unilateral. Infectious mononucleosis may give an identical picture, as may cytomegalovirus infection. Coxsackie and echoviruses must also be excluded, and bacterial infections, particularly β-haemolytic streptococcal infection and diphtheria, should be considered.

Recurrent infections (cold sore; herpes labialis, fever blisters)

Recurrent herpes labialis usually starts with localized prodromal symptoms (pain, burning, tingling, or itching) lasting from 6–48 h. Vesicles most commonly occur on the lips or skin around the mouth, and in the nostrils, and are often painful. Multiple recurrences usually recur in the same site for each person. There are usually no systemic symptoms associated with recurrences. After several days the lesions crust; complete healing takes about 10 days. Sometimes the lesions become secondarily infected, typically with *Staphylococcus aureus*. The frequency of recurrences varies greatly. Fewer than 10 per cent of the seropositive population have more than one attack per month, while about 50 per cent have fewer than two attacks per year. There appears to be a decrease in the frequency of recurrences with time. Diagnosis is usually easy. The main differential diagnosis includes zoster, which rarely recurs in the same site.

Herpetic whitlow

This is an occupational disease of medical personnel, dentists, nurses, and physiotherapists. Patients with a high fever or those with a tracheostomy are particularly likely to excrete virus in their secretions. In children, whitlows can result from autoinoculation. The skin of the hand is rarely intact, allowing the virus to invade. Usually only one finger is infected, although infection may spread to an adjoining finger (Plate 2).

The whitlow is extremely painful. The digit swells, becomes red, and may be accompanied by painful lymphadenopathy, high fever, and systemic disease. A day or two later the typical vesicle develops, with clear fluid evolving into a cloudy fluid and then into a yellow, crusty lesion. Without treatment, recovery from the systemic illness takes about 2 weeks. The main differential diagnosis is a bacterial infection and it can also be confused with orf. Recurrent whitlows are less common than recurrent cold sores. They are often heralded and accompanied by severe neuralgic pain in the hand and arm.

Traumatic herpes; herpes gladiatorum; scrum pox

Primary herpes can occur in any part of the skin if it is traumatized. The clinical course is similar to that of the herpetic whitlow. Herpes gladiatorum occurs in contact sports such as wrestling, judo, or rugby football in participants whose faces come into close contact with other parts of the body. If the cheek is affected the differential diagnosis includes cellulitis, impetigo, and trigeminal zoster. There may be recurrence at the site of the primary infection.

Genital herpes

HSV is the commonest cause of genital ulceration. Primary genital herpes occurs after sexual contact. The illness is similar to other primary infections. Non-primary first episodes of genital herpes tend to be less severe. In women there is often a vaginal discharge with severe genital pain, dysuria, and urinary retention. Herpetic lesions involve the vulva, perineum, cervix, and vagina. Extragenital lesions on the buttocks and thigh are common (Plate 3). An accompanying sacroradiculomyelitis can cause urinary retention, neuralgia, and constipation. Whereas women often have severe systemic illness, men usually have a milder primary attack. In men the vesicles occur on the shaft of the penis (Fig. 1) or the glans, together with an associated urethritis. Herpes simplex proctitis occurs after anorectal intercourse: symptoms include anorectal pain and discharge, tenesmus, constipation, sacral paraesthesiae, impotence, and urinary retention. Sigmoidoscopy reveals ulcerative lesions up to 10 cm. HSV meningitis is a well-recognized complication of primary genital herpes; the virus can occasionally be isolated from the cerebrospinal fluid or be detected by polymerase chain reaction. It is a benign infection, symptoms resolving in about a week.

About 70 per cent of cases will have recurrent skin and mucosal lesions and periods of asymptomatic shedding within the first year of primary infection. The rate of recurrence is about 0.33 attacks per month for HSV-2 and less than 0.1 attacks per month for HSV-1. Recurrence rates tend to decrease with time. Recurrent attacks are less severe than the primary attack but may be more severe in women than in men. Prodromal symptoms of local or radiating pain may precede the lesions by 12–24 h and there may also be irritability, malaise, and fever.

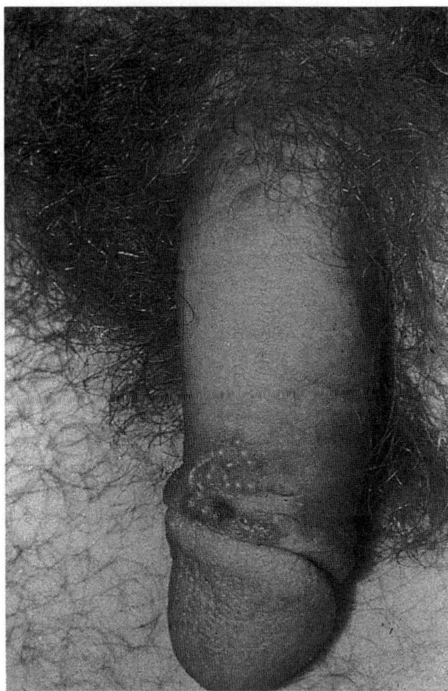

Fig. 1 Herpetic vesicles on the shaft of the penis.

Ocular herpes

Primary infections present with fever and constitutional symptoms, together with a unilateral follicular conjunctivitis, or a blepharitis with vesicles on the lids, and preauricular lymphadenopathy. There is associated photophobia, chemosis, excessive lacrimation, and oedema of the eyelids. In uncomplicated cases, the symptoms spontaneously resolve completely within 2–3 weeks. However, in some cases there is involvement of the cornea, producing acute herpetic keratoconjunctivitis to form the characteristic branching ('dendritic') lesions. There is pain and a foreign-body sensation. Occasionally the underlying stroma is affected, which can lead to corneal ulceration or corneal scarring. The use of topical corticosteroids may exacerbate the symptoms and make permanent corneal damage more likely.

Recurrences happen in about 25 per cent of cases and are a serious ophthalmological problem. They usually present as a keratitis with dendritic ulceration, seen with fluorescein stains, or stromal involvement. Repeated attacks can lead to corneal scarring and neovascularization, with eventual loss of vision.

Ophthalmic herpes should be managed and treated by specialist ophthalmologists.

Infections of the central nervous system (see also Chapter 13.26)

Herpes simplex encephalitis

This is an acute necrotizing viral encephalitis with a mortality, untreated, of over 70 per cent, and a high incidence of neurological sequelae in survivors. Except in newborns, the infection is usually caused by HSV-1. It is a rare disease with an estimated frequency in the US of about 1 in 400 000 per year. It can occur at any age and does not appear to be more frequent in the immunosuppressed host.

Presentation is with high fever, headache, nausea, and vomiting, followed by reduced consciousness and seizures. Sometimes there are signs of meningeal irritation. Focal neurological signs typically involve the temporal, orbitofrontal cortex, and limbic systems. Patients have dysphasia, hallucinations, peculiar behaviour, and memory loss. In some cases there is rapid progression to coma and death. In other cases, progression is slower, with several days of lethargy and bizarre behaviour, which can be confused with acute psychosis or delirium tremens. There are usually no skin manifestations of herpes simplex infection. The differential diagnosis includes other cases of viral encephalitidis, cerebral abscess, and bacterial meningitis. CT scanning or MRI of the brain will show typical features of changes in the temporal lobes. Lumbar puncture should only be attempted if the clinician is certain there is not significant cerebral oedema. Examination of the cerebrospinal fluid (CSF) shows a moderate pleocytosis, mildly elevated protein concentration, and normal glucose concentration. The diagnosis is made by detecting HSV-DNA by polymerase chain reaction in the CSF or by demonstrating virus in a brain biopsy, but the latter is rarely indicated clinically. Characteristically, there is a greater than fourfold rise in serum and CSF antibody titres.

Herpes simplex meningitis

Apart from the meningitis associated with a primary attack of genital herpes, HSV can cause benign aseptic meningitis at times following the first attack, sometimes in association with vesicles but frequently without skin lesions. This meningitis may be recurrent (Mollaret's meningitis). Diagnosis is made by detecting HSV-DNA in the CSF by polymerase chain reaction. Serum antibody titres do not change following herpes simplex meningitis.

Idiopathic neurological syndromes

Herpes simplex has been implicated in the aetiology of Bell's palsy, trigeminal neuralgia, atypical pain syndromes, ascending myelitis, and temporal-lobe epilepsy. These associations depend mainly on serological evidence and the precise role of herpes simplex virus in the aetiology of these syndromes has not been definitely established.

Visceral and disseminated infections

Infection of visceral organs occurs only rarely. Oropharyngeal herpes can extend into the oesophagus, especially in the presence of nasogastric tubes, causing dysphagia, substernal pain, and weight loss. Ulcers are seen on endoscopy. Similarly extension can occur, following endotracheal intubation, to the bronchial tree and lungs, causing pneumonia. Very rarely, herpes simplex virus is a cause of hepatitis and, in a few cases, especially in pregnant women in the third trimester or transplant recipients, can be part of a fulminating, disseminated infection. There is associated leucopenia, thrombocytopenia, and disseminated intravascular coagulation.

Neonatal infections

Infection in the newborn ranges from a mild disease to a fatal disseminated infection. In the US the incidence is about 1 in 2500 to 1 in 10 000, while in the UK the disease is less common. Most infections are caused by spread of herpes simplex virus from the maternal genital tract or sometimes postnatally from health care workers or relatives with oral herpes or herpetic whitlows. It is unclear to what extent infection occurs either before the onset of labour or during passage of the fetus through the birth canal. The use of fetal scalp monitoring increases the risk of transmission. The risk of neonatal infection is about 40 per cent with active primary infection but less than 8 per cent with recurrent infections at the time of delivery and rare with asymptomatic shedding.

Neonatal infection appears several days or even weeks after birth. It presents as a neonatal sepsis syndrome, sometimes with vesicles or conjunctivitis but often with no skin manifestations. In babies with no passively transferred maternal antibodies to herpes simplex, visceral dissemination is present and there is an overall mortality of 65 per cent. Neonatal herpes encephalitis presents more incidiously and on MRI gives a picture of multiple frontal lobe haemorrhages. Lethargy, seizures, and cranial nerve palsies may occur. Neurological sequelae usually persist.

Congenital infection, a consequence of primary infection early in pregnancy, can cause severe abnormalities, which, in the absence of vesicles, are difficult to distinguish from similar syndromes caused by rubella, toxoplasmosis, or cytomegalovirus.

Herpes simplex virus in the immunocompromised host

Patients with impaired cellular immunity are at risk from severe disease. They include organ transplant recipients on immunosuppressive chemotherapy, patients with lymphoreticular malignancies, haematological malignancies and AIDS, and children with congenital immunodeficiencies or malnutrition.

Immunosuppressed patients are at risk from disseminated disease following primary infection. Recurrences are also more frequent in these patients. Although recurrent herpes often resolves spontaneously, the vesicles sometimes enlarge slowly, ulcerate, and become necrotic, extending to deeper tissues. The lesions spread slowly both on the skin and into the oesophagus and trachea. In spite of this spread, dissemination following recurrent infections is rare. In these patients, failure to respond to antiviral treatment may indicate the development of resistant HSV.

Herpes simplex in skin disorders

Eczema herpeticum; Juliusberg's pustolosis acuta varioliformis; Kaposi's varicelliform eruption

Herpes simplex infections are much more severe and extensive in patients with underlying skin disorders. Patients with eczema, burns, pemphigus, Darier's disease, and Sezary's syndrome are unable to contain the infection, which causes widespread cutaneous dissemination. As these patients are often on corticosteroid treatment, the spread of the herpes simplex lesions is further facilitated. There are usually systemic symptoms: fever, rigors, general adenopathy, and enlargement of the liver and spleen. Untreated the condition is likely to recur, although the systemic symptoms may be less severe.

Herpes simplex and erythema multiforme

Recurrent herpes simplex infections may be associated with erythema multiforme. About 15 per cent of all cases of erythema multiforme are preceded by a symptomatic attack of recurrent herpes simplex. In susceptible individuals, the skin rash can be induced by the intradermal inoculation of inactivated herpes simplex virus antigen. The rash starts several days after the onset of the herpetic vesicles. In severe cases the rash can involve the mucous membranes (Stevens–Johnson syndrome). The frequency of these attacks can be reduced by antiviral prophylaxis.

Diagnosis

Most cases of herpes simplex infection can be made on clinical grounds alone. Confirmation is best made by the isolation of the virus from vesicles in cell culture where a typical cytopathic effect appears within 48–96 h. Direct examination of the fluid by electron microscopy may demonstrate herpesvirus particles. A variety of other methods are available for rapid and specific identification of the virus including monoclonal antibodies specific to HSV-1 and -2 antigens, and DNA amplification. Serological tests that demonstrate rising titres of HSV antibody in paired sera can only be used for the retrospective diagnosis of primary infection. Conventional serology cannot differentiate between HSV-1 and HSV-2, but for epidemiological surveys the two can be distinquished by using HSV type-specific glycoprotein G as the antigen.

Treatment

Treatment of primary HSV is both symptomatic and with an antiviral drug. Analgesia and, in women with genital infection causing urinary retention, assistance with passing urine (urinating in the bath or catheterization) may be necessary. In general, the newer antivirals, famciclovir (250 mg thrice daily for 5 days) or valaciclovir (500 mg twice daily for 5 days), should be used in preference to aciclovir (200 mg 5 times per day for 5 days) where administration is by the oral route because they are much better absorbed and therefore give higher tissue levels of the active drug. The dosage for recurrent infection is for aciclovir 200 mg 5 times per day, for famciclovir 125 mg twice daily, and for valaciclovir 500 mg twice daily, all for 5 days. These drugs, like aciclovir, reduce the severity of infection and the duration of both symptoms and virus shedding. In addition, in the mouse model famciclovir, but not valaciclovir, has been shown to reduce the number of latently infected brain stem cells if the drug is commenced up to 3 days after an experimental infection. Once latency has developed, antiviral treatment will not clear the virus. Aciclovir should still be used to treat HSV infection in pregnancy and in the neonate as its safety profile in these groups is proven.

All primary infections should be treated as soon as possible, preferably within a day of onset. In immunosuppressed patients and those unable to swallow, intravenous aciclovir (5mg/kg, 8-hourly) should be given.

Treatment of recurrent infections in the immunocompetent host is often unnecessary as the condition is usually mild and self-limiting; however, in some patients, when recurrences are associated with neuralgia, irritability, lassitude, or depression, treatment should be given. In these cases treatment should again be given as soon as possible and if given at the onset of symptoms, before lesions appear, an attack may be aborted. Sufferers of very frequent recurrences (more than six episodes per year, and accompanied by systemic symptoms) should be considered for long-term prophylaxis, the dose of the antiviral being tailored to the minimum required to prevent breakthroughs; the few that do occur are usually minor and short-lived. Topical preparations may be helpful for recurrences of labial herpes but are unsatisfactory for genital herpes which may be at multiple sites and inaccessible. Many patients with recurrent herpes have profound sexual and psychological dysfunction and may require professional advice and help, or assistance from self-help groups.

In immunocompromised patients recurrences may be severe and prolonged. If long-term treatment is given there is a possibility that resistance to the antiviral may develop and the lesions progress. An alternative antiviral, foscarnet, which has a different method of action, should be substituted.

HSV encephalitis must be treated with intravenous aciclovir (10–15 mg/kg, three times daily) as soon as it is suspected. Following laboratory confirmation of the diagnosis treatment should continue for 14 days. It is also recommended that a repeat cerebrospinal fluid is examined after the course of treatment and if the polymerase chain reaction is still positive for HSV-DNA a second course of treatment should be given in order to prevent a relapse. Again, several experts recommend a few months of oral antiviral prophylaxis following treatment, for this purpose.

Prevention

Avoidance of exposure to HSV is difficult because many carriers are asymptomatic shedders of virus. Medical and nursing staff should wear gloves if they are likely to come into contact with lesions or bodily secretions. Likewise medical personnel who have herpetic whitlows should not handle patients. Perinatal exposure from the mother who has a primary infection near the time of delivery is associated with a high incidence of severe neonatal herpes. Primary HSV in the first and second trimesters of pregnancy, with a good antibody response before labour begins, or a history of previous genital herpes, is not associated with an increase in neonatal morbidity. Caesarean section is recommended for any woman with active lesions in the birth canal at the beginning of labour and it is advisable to give antiviral prophylaxis to the neonate. Antiviral prophylaxis for the last 10 days of pregnancy, to reduce viral shedding of a mother who is known to have recurrences of genital herpes, offers an alternative course of action. The risk to the baby during delivery from an asymptomatic mother who is shedding HSV is very low.

A number of HSV vaccines are currently under trial. In addition to preventing primary HSV infections, it is hoped these vaccines will prove useful therapeutically, by boosting normal immunity, in reducing the severity and frequency of clinical disease in people who suffer frequent recurrences.

Further reading

Brown, Z.A., Selke, S., Zeh, J., *et al.* (1997). The acquisition of herpes simplex virus during pregnancy. *New England Journal of Medicine*, **337**, 509–15.

Cinque, P., Cleator, G.M., Weber, T., *et al.* (1996). The role of laboratory investigation in the diagnosis and management of patients with suspected herpes simplex encephalitis: a consensus report. The EU Concerted Action on Virus Meningitis and Encephalitis. *Journal of Neurology, Neurosurgery, and Psychiatry*, **61**, 339–45.

Thackray, A.M. and Field, H.J. (1996). Comparison of effects of famciclovir and valaciclovir on pathogenesis of herpes simplex virus type 2 in a murine infection model. *Antimicrobial Agents and Chemotherapy*, **40**, 846–51.

White, C. and Wardropper, A.G. (1997). Genital herpes simplex infection in women. *Clinical Dermatology (United States)*, **15** (1), 81–91.

Chapter 16.11

Varicella-zoster virus infections: chickenpox and zoster

*M. J. Warrell**

Varicella-zoster virus causes two distinct clinical entities, chickenpox (varicella) and zoster (shingles). The primary infection in the non-immune host is chickenpox. After the acute, often trivial, primary infection, the virus becomes latent in nerve cells. In the 'immune' host, reactivation of the virus results in zoster, a predominantly dermatomal infection.

Epidemiology

Humans are the only known reservoir of infection. Varicella-zoster virus is the most infectious of the human herpesviruses. Transmission is by droplets from nasopharyngeal secretions (chickenpox) or from vesicular fluid (chickenpox or zoster). Patients are infectious for 2 days before the onset of the rash until the skin lesions are crusted. The incubation period is about 15 days (range 10–21 days). The attack rate within household non-immune contacts is about 90 per cent after chickenpox but only 15 per cent after zoster. In temperate countries about 90 per cent of the population are seropositive by early adulthood, but in tropical countries only 50 per cent of young adults are seropositive.

Following the primary infection there is a relatively increased risk of zoster in the first year of life and in elderly people. Outbreaks of zoster are sporadic and do not occur in clusters. Trauma may be responsible for reactivation. The chance of young, seropositive adults acquiring zoster is about 0.7/1000 per year, rising to 10/1000 per year in people over 80 years old. Overall, at least 20 per cent of all adults suffer from zoster at some time and about 1 per cent suffer two attacks. The risk of zoster is greatly enhanced by immunosuppression.

Pathogenesis

Varicella-zoster virus is an alphaherpes virus, with icosahedral symmetry containing double-stranded DNA, surrounded by an envelope which is essential for infection. The envelope is sensitive to air drying, detergents, and ether. The virus can infect a variety of cell cultures, but does not readily infect animals.

During primary infection the virus spreads locally in the upper respiratory tract, and there is thought to be a primary viraemia in the first week spreading to the reticuloendothelial system. Shortly before the clinical illness, a secondary viraemic phase results in spread to the skin and the mucosal surfaces with vesicle formation. Multinucleation of infected cells with condensation of viral proteins within the nuclei results in intranuclear inclusions. The infection is contained by the development of both humoral and cell-mediated immune responses.

Following the primary infection, the virus becomes latent in the sensory ganglia and in motor neurones in perineuronal and neuronal cells. The molecular basis for latency and the trigger for the reactivation of the virus are unknown. The ganglion is the site of intense inflammation in zoster. There is degeneration of axons and myelin, and virus particles occur in epidermal and perineural cells. Repeated exposures to virus in immune individuals can sometimes enhance the immune status of the host and delay reactivation as clinical zoster.

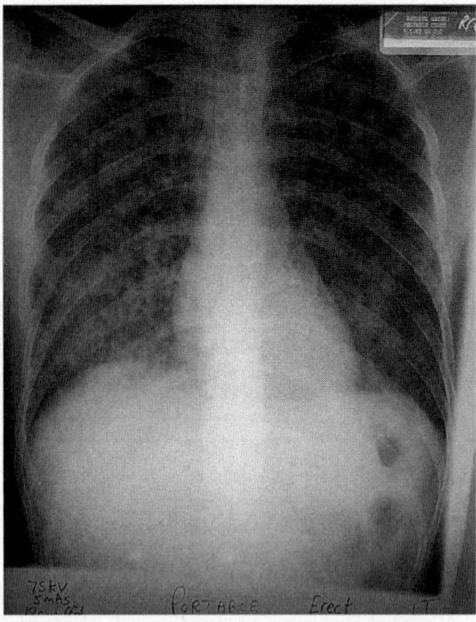

Fig. 1 Chest radiograph of a young man who had severe chickenpox infection also involving the lungs. There are scattered infiltrates, which, in the course of the next few days, coalesced, giving a clinical picture of adult respiratory distress syndrome. The patient survived.

Chickenpox

In children prodromal symptoms are minimal or absent, and the characteristic centripetal rash is the first manifestation of the illness. It may be so slight—like a few drops of water on the skin—that it is missed. In adults, prodromal symptoms are common and occasionally severe. Headaches, aches and pains, fever, and extreme malaise are typical. There may be a transient pink rash before the vesicles erupt. The vesicles tend to be irregular (Plate 1). Within 12 h the itchy vesicles become papular and then progress to pustules and subsequently to scabs, which last about 10 days. No scar is left unless the scabs have been scratched. Characteristically, different crops of vesicles appear over 3–4 days, starting with the head and progressing to the trunk and limbs. All stages of the exanthem are seen in the same region of the skin. The infection is not limited to the skin and can lead to serious complications. Recurrent chickenpox in otherwise healthy individuals is extremely rare and may be familial.

Complications in the immunocompetent host

The mortality of chickenpox in immunocompetent individuals is age dependent. Neonates are at highest risk, while the mortality in children aged 1–14 years is only about 1 in 70 000 cases. In adults the mortality rises to 1 in 3000 and is higher in older patients.

Pneumonitis

The incidence of pneumonitis is about 0.3 per cent in immunocompetent adults. Smokers are particularly susceptible. Patients present with breathlessness, cough, hypoxia, and bilateral chest infiltrates on the chest radiograph a few days after the onset of the chickenpox (Fig. 1). The disease can progress rapidly, with increasing

*Includes some material from Chapter 7.10.3, *Oxford textbook of medicine*, 3rd edition (Herpes simplex virus infections by T.E.A. Peto and B.E. Juel-Jensen).

shortness of breath, pulmonary oedema, cyanosis, and chest pain, and can be fatal. The long-term pulmonary prognosis of survivors is excellent. Minor chest radiographic changes occur asymptomatically in about 16 per cent of young adults, with occasional progression to benign nodular calcification.

Encephalitis

Mild encephalitis can occur within 10 days before to several days after the onset of the rash. Cerebellar signs or encephalopathy are associated with a pleocytosis and elevated protein in the cerebrospinal fluid. Severe encephalitis is uncommon, and the overall mortality is about 5 per cent. Cerebellar ataxia has an excellent prognosis.

Thrombocytopenia and bleeding disorders: purpura fulminans

Both disseminated intravascular coagulation and idiopathic thrombocytopenia are rare but potentially life-threatening disorders in chickenpox. Following typical chickenpox, ecchymoses appear symmetrically in the lower extremities, and occasionally on the arms, from 5–18 days after the rash began. Large areas of skin slough, with extensive tissue necrosis and mortality from renal failure, shock, or sepsis. There is a low prothrombin and reduced factors V, VII, VIII, and X. Intravascular coagulation occurs in the peripheral vessels and the picture is one of thrombotic purpura. Treatments have included fresh-frozen plasma combined with heparin.

Secondary bacterial infection

Secondary infection with staphylococci and streptococci is common if the lesions are scratched, but secondary bacterial infections of the respiratory tract are infrequent.

Chickenpox in the immunocompromised host

Patients on corticosteroids, other immunosuppressive drugs, or with late HIV disease are at greater risk from severe chickenpox. The skin lesions can continue cropping for much longer. The mortality in children on treatment for leukaemias reaches 18 per cent.

Maternal, congenital, and perinatal infection

Pregnancy increases the risk of chickenpox with a mortality of 1 per cent and an incidence of pneumonitis of 10 per cent. Chickenpox in the first and second trimester is associated with a rare fetal varicella syndrome of skin scarring, hypoplastic extremities, eye abnormalities, and evidence of central nervous impairment. The risk of congenital abnormalities is about 1 per cent, but higher before 20 weeks. Chickenpox in the newborn following maternal infection in the third trimester is serious; about 10 per cent have severe disease. Delivery should be delayed to allow time for antibodies to appear in the maternal plasma, thereby protecting the newborn.

Zoster

Shingles and zoster both mean 'a belt'; the Danes aptly call it 'hellfire'. Paraesthesia over the affected dermatome, and perhaps shooting pains, precede the eruption, by 2–3 days usually, but by up to 3 weeks. A few patients remain pain free. Erythematous, maculopapular lesions appear on skin and mucosae and rapidly evolve into a vesicular rash, forming new lesions over a period of 3–5 days (Fig. 2) often accompanied by a mild systemic illness with a low-grade fever. The vesicles normally scab after 3–7 days, and all dry scabs have separated at the end of a fortnight, but there is a risk of secondary bacterial infection.

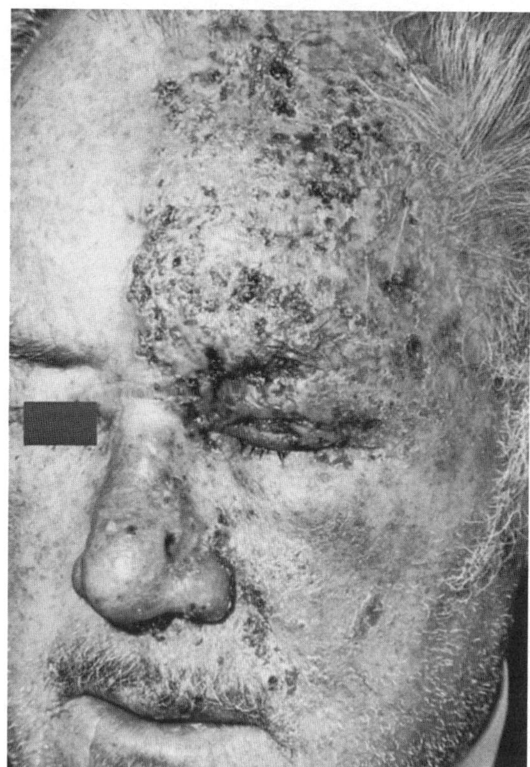

Fig. 2 Frontal and maxillary zoster.

The characteristically unilateral eruption varies greatly. In young people it is often trivial (Plate 2), and it may be mistaken for herpes simplex. In severe cases several dermatomes may be involved, with an oedematous base and a dense rash covering the entire segment. Bilateral zoster is very rare. There are often some outlying lesions, varying from a few to a dense eruption, but dissemination is not necessarily serious in immunocompetent patients. Rarely, reactivation occurs without a rash: zoster sine herpete. Patients can present with pain that has a dermatomal distribution. There are case reports implicating zoster as the cause of polyneuropathy, myelitis, aseptic meningitis, and severe hepatic necrosis.

Complications

Ophthalmic zoster

Eye involvement is common when zoster affects the first division of the trigeminal nerve, causing conjunctivitis, keratitis, and rarely sight-threatening complications such as glaucoma secondary to uveitis or cataract. Widespread periorbital oedema sometimes spreads bilaterally, but is not a sign of dissemination of infection.

Motor zoster

Zoster is not confined to the sensory nerves and often associated motor nerves are affected; for example in ophthalmic zoster, involvement of the cranial nerves III, IV, and VI is not uncommon. Zoster of C5 and C6 may lead to diaphragmatic palsy, and motor zoster of the upper limb (usually of the deltoid) and lower limbs is occasionally a complication of sensory zoster at that level. A facial-nerve paralysis is more dramatic, although the accompanying pain, vesicles in the external auditory meatus, and loss of taste in the anterior two-thirds of the tongue can easily be missed. It is associated with zoster of adjacent sensory branches of the trigeminal, glosspharyngeal, or vagus nerves, or of the cervical plexus. Apart from facial nerve palsy, where the outcome is variable, the prognosis of motor zoster is good.

Autonomic zoster

Bladder involvement in sacral zoster results in acute retention of urine, or haemorrhagic cystitis due to zoster vesicles on the bladder wall. Lumbar zoster can be associated with bowel atony, and can be confused with an acute abdomen.

Zoster encephalomyelitis

A mild encephalitis is not uncommon and is similar to that found in chickenpox. It can occur both before or up to 6 weeks after the onset of the illness and is probably due to an immune-mediated mechanism. The prognosis is good. Very rarely, the encephalomyelitis can be severe, sometimes with cerebellar involvement.

Purpura fulminans

This very rare condition can lead to alarming tissue loss. It follows a similar course to the condition in chickenpox.

Immunocompromised host and disseminated zoster

In the immunocompromised host, zoster is more likely to occur and to disseminate, uncontrolled by the usual redevelopment of immunity. The disease is normally self-limiting, but dissemination can be fulminating and the disease life-threatening. A chronic verrucous form of zoster rarely occurs in patients with impaired immunity.

Acute retinal necrosis

Patients present with blurring of the vision and pain in the affected eye. The progressive necrotizing retinitis can lead to permanent visual impairment and retinal detachment, without any other manifestation of zoster reactivation. In contrast, acute retinal necrosis in HIV-infected patients occurs following cutaneous zoster infection. Specific antiviral treatment can prevent the progression of the disease; retinal complications may require surgery.

Postherpetic neuralgia

One month after the onset of zoster, pain is still present in at least 10 per cent of all untreated patients. The proportion of patients experiencing pain rises with age, to 73 per cent in those over 70 years of age, lasting over 1 year in more than 40 per cent. The pain may be either (a) a steady burning, ache, or (b) paroxysmal and jabbing, sometimes with an associated area of hypoaesthesia.

Diagnosis

The diagnosis of chickenpox is usually made by a history of exposure and physical examination. A unilateral segmental rash suggests shingles. The differential diagnoses include: animal poxviruses; impetigo due to streptococci which can cause vesicles; eczema herpeticum caused by herpes simplex, but the vesicles tend to be all at the same stage of development; and disseminated coxsackievirus infections ('hand, foot, and mouth disease').

If necessary, the diagnosis of chickenpox can be confirmed serologically, by a greater than fourfold rise in paired sera. A serological boost follows shingles. Using vesicular fluid, the diagnosis can be established by isolation of the virus, or more rapidly by antigen detection by polymerase chain reaction, and electron microscopy will show herpesvirus particles. Varicella-zoster antigen can also be shown in cells from the base of skin lesions by immunofluorescence.

Management and treatment

Symptomatic treatment

Patients with chickenpox can be given calamine lotion or antihistamines to ease the itch and warned not to scratch to avoid secondary infection and scarring.

Patients with zoster require careful skin care to avoid infection and usually need pain relief during the acute attack. The treatment of postherpetic neuralgia demands adequate analgesia, including opiates if necessary, but non-steroidal anti-inflammatory drugs are not effective. Additional remedies include topical anaesthetic, tricylic antidepressants, anticonvulsants, vibration, transcutaneous electrical nerve stimulation, and stellate ganglion blockade. Patients appreciate continual support and sympathy.

All patients with zoster of the first division of the trigeminal nerve should be examined ophthalmologically with the aid of a slit lamp and the complications treated appropriately with topical steroids, antimicrobials, and mydriatics. Steroids given in the active phase of the infection must be accompanied by antiviral therapy.

Antiviral therapy

Three nucleoside analogues are effective in some VZ virus infections. They are aciclovir, and the newer famciclovir and valaciclovir (a prodrug of aciclovir) which are more bioavailable given orally, but there is no evidence of their superiority over aciclovir. This drug is excreted in the urine and the dose must be reduced in severe renal failure (plasma creatinine > 300 μmol/l). The oral dose of aciclovir is 800 mg five times a day, and the intravenous dose is 5 mg/kg 8-hourly. Treatment should be continued until 48 h after the last new skin/mucosal eruption. Topical antivirals are ineffective.

Antiviral treatment in chickenpox is indicated in neonates, adults, in severe disease with systemic complications, in immunocompromised patients, and in pregnancy. In patients with zoster, 7 days' antiviral therapy, begun within 72 h of appearance of the rash, reduces acute pain and accelerates the healing of lesions. Antiviral therapy is recommended in ophthalmic zoster, disseminated or complicated zoster, and infection in immunosuppressed patients. The analysis of several drug trials provides evidence that antiviral treatment reduces the duration of postherpetic neuralgia, and so is most beneficial in older patients and those with more severe pain at presentation, who are more likely to develop this complication. Side-effects are minimal. These drugs are expensive.

Prevention

Prevention of spread of varicella-zoster in hospital

Patients with varicella infections are highly infectious and it is essential that non-immune, immunocompromised patients be protected. Infectious patients should be isolated and nursed by immune staff. Non-immune staff who are accidentally exposed should, in turn, avoid contact with non-immune, immunocompromised patients.

Varicella immune globulin

There is some evidence that varicella-zoster immune globulin, if given early after exposure to non-immune individuals, can attenuate the infection. Because it is in short supply, therapy is usually restricted to immunosuppressed or pregnant patients, and neonates born to mothers with chickenpox 7 days before to 28 days postpartum, to non-immune pregnant women, and to immunodeficient patients.

Vaccination

A live, attenuated varicella vaccine (Oka strain) has been available since 1974 in Japan and is used routinely in the USA. It is not yet licensed in the UK but is available for individual patients. Protection from severe clinical disease is excellent. Mild chickenpox may follow vaccination. The incidence of zoster in vaccinated, immunocompromised children is lower than in unvaccinated children who have had natural infection. Vaccination of healthy older patients with a history of chickenpox boosts the response to varicella skin tests, indicating an increase in cell-mediated immunity, and preliminary trial results suggest attenuation of clinical zoster.

Further reading

Christie, A.B. (1988). Chickenpox (varicella). In *Infectious diseases*, 4th edn. Churchill Livingstone, Edinburgh.

Enders, G., Miller, E., Cradock-Watson, J., *et al.* (1994). Consequences of varicella and herpes zoster in pregnancy: prospective study of 1739 cases. *Lancet*, **343**, 1547–51.

Harding, S.P. (1993). Management of ophthalmic zoster. *Journal of Medical Virology* (Suppl. 1), 97–101.

Juel-Jensen, B.E. and MacCallum, F.O. (1972). *Herpes simplex, varicella and zoster.* Heinemann, London.

Kost, R.G. and Straus, S.E. (1996). Postherpetic neuralgia-pathogenesis, treatment, and prevention. *New England Journal of Medicine*, **333**, 32–42.

Pastuszak, A.L. *et al.* (1994). Outcome after varicella infection in the first 20 weeks of pregnancy. *New England Journal of Medicine*, **330**, 901–5.

Wood, M.J., Kay, R., Dworkin, R.H., *et al.* (1996). Oral acyclovir therapy accelerates pain resolution in patients with herpes zoster: a meta-analysis of placebo-controlled trials. *Clinical Infectious Diseases*, **22**, 341–7.

Chapter 16.12

The Epstein–Barr virus

M. A. Epstein and D. H. Crawford

Background

The virus

Epstein–Barr virus (EBV), discovered in 1964, is one of the eight herpesviruses of man. It consists of an outer envelope, a protein capsid, and an inner double-stranded linear DNA genome.

Viral infectious cycle

Natural infection is limited to man and susceptible target cells are circulating B lymphocytes and squamous epithelial cells of the oral cavity, pharynx, and genital tract. Infection of epithelial cells leads to a lytic infection with production of viral progeny and cell death. The virus causes a latent infection of B cells *in vivo* and can transform normal B lymphocytes *in vitro* into continuously growing, latently infected, immortalized lymphoblastoid lines. Specific virus-coded proteins are expressed in each type of infection.

Virus-coded proteins

EBV-coded proteins are categorized according to the time of their appearance during the infectious cycle as latent, early, or late antigens. Most elicit both cytotoxic T-cell responses and serum antibodies; the latter are important in diagnosis.

General epidemiology

The virus is widespread in all human populations. Primary infection usually occurs in early childhood, at which age it is clinically silent, but leads to the generation of antibodies to the virus-determined antigens, and of specific cytotoxic T lymphocytes. A lifelong carrier state ensues, in which both humoral and cellular immune responses are maintained continuously. The virus persists as a latent infection in a few circulating B lymphocytes and as a productive, lytic infection in cells of the mouth, pharynx, urogenital tract, and perhaps the salivary glands; the exact nature of these lytically infected cells is still controverisal. EBV is shed into the buccal fluid in considerable amounts in about 20 per cent of those who have been infected and in small amounts in the remainder; the virus has also been detected in genital secretions. Virus in the buccal fluid provides the main source for transmission of the infection, by droplets and casually contaminated objects in children, and by salivary transfer during kissing amongst the sexually active. In developing countries, 99.9 per cent of children are infected by the second to fourth year of life but in industrialized countries with high standards of hygiene many do not meet the virus as young children. The percentage of teenagers or young adults remaining free of infection in Western societies depends on socioeconomic group—the higher the standard of living, the greater the percentage; 50 per cent of very affluent young adults may escape childhood infection.

Infectious mononucleosis

Infectious mononucleosis (IM) occurs in about 50 per cent of those who miss the EBV infection in childhood when, sooner or later, they undergo delayed primary infection; the other 50 per cent of delayed infections are symptom free. Because teenagers and young adults in the affluent classes of Western countries escape infection as children IM is a disease of upper socioeconomic groups; conversely it is exceptionally rare in developing countries. Although most cases occur in adolescents and young adults, children and the middle aged may sometimes develop the disease, and rarely also the elderly. IM is associated with kissing and is acquired when a healthy carrier, who is shedding virus in his/her saliva, passes this during close buccal contact directly into the oropharynx of a partner who has not been primarily infected in the usual way as a child. This explains why case-to-case infection and epidemics are not seen and why the incubation period, perhaps 30–50 days, is difficult to calculate. Primary EBV infection giving IM-like symptoms may also be transmitted by blood transfusion or organ grafting from an infected donor.

Symptoms

Classical IM may follow some days of vague indisposition or may start abruptly. It presents with sore throat, fever with sweating, anorexia, headache, and fatigue, together with malaise quite out of proportion to the other complaints. Dysphagia may be noticed and also brief orbital oedema. An erythematous rash occurs in a small number of patients but affects most of those taking ampicillin. Tonsillar and pharyngeal oedema can rarely cause pharyngeal obstruction.

Signs

The fever may rise to 40°C but high levels and swings are not seen. There is redness and oedema of the pharynx, fauces, soft palate, and uvula, and about half the patients develop a greyish exudate. Generalized lymphadenopathy is almost always present, most marked in the cervical region; the glands are symmetrical, discrete, and slightly tender, and are accompanied by splenomegaly in about 60 per cent of cases and an enlarged liver in 10 per cent. There is usually a moderate bradycardia. Besides the rash, characteristic palatal enanthematous crops of reddish petechiae are found in about one-third of patients, and jaundice occurs in about 8 per cent.

Clinical course

Mild cases may resolve in days, but 1–2 weeks is more usual, followed by a period of lethargy. The duration of this convalescence is influenced by psychological factors, particularly the speed with which patients are encouraged to resume full activity. About 1 case in 2000 may continue in a truly chronic or recurrent form for several months or years, and here exhaustive investigations have shown immunological defects. Most other cases of so-called chronic IM are in reality manifestations of 'chronic fatigue syndrome' but it is highly controversial as to whether this is a true entity rather than belief disorder; credible connections with EBV have not been established. In contrast, there is an extremely rare, genetically determined, X-linked, lymphoproliferative condition (XLP disease, or Duncan syndrome after the first family to be recognized) in which the affected young males of certain kindred die from IM owing to a specific inability to respond normally to EBV during primary infection; the disease progresses inexorably, with necrotic destruction of vital organs and multisystem failure. There is evidence that an aberrant immune response to EBV in XLP disease results in unregulated natural killer-cell and cytotoxic T-cell activity being directed against the normal cells of vital organs instead of concentrating solely on EBV-infected cells displaying EBV antigens.

Complications

Minor non-specific complications may occur; rare, more serious complications, include secondary bacterial throat infections, traumatic rupture of the enlarged spleen, asphyxia from pharyngeal oedema, massive hepatic necrosis, Guillain–Barré syndrome, and autoimmune manifestations such as thrombocytopenia and haemolytic anaemia.

Differential diagnosis

Classical IM is diagnosed on the basis of the clinical picture considered in conjunction with serological and haematological laboratory investigations (see below). An IM-like disease can occur in primary cytomegalovirus infection and in toxoplasmosis, but in both conditions the sore throat is much less severe and with cytomegalovirus the lymphadenopathy may be minimal or absent.

Laboratory diagnosis

A rapid screening test (Monospot test) can be used to detect the presence of heterophil antibodies in the patient's serum. Although these heterophil antibodies are not directed against viral-coded proteins they are present in up to 85 per cent of acute IM sera. Cases of Monospot-negative IM tend to be those outside the classical 15–25-year age range, and false-positive tests may occur in pregnancy and autoimmune disease. However, the presence of serum IgM antibodies to EB virus capsid antigen (VCA) are diagnostic of IM. An additional important feature of IM is the presence of lymphocytosis of up to 15×10^9/l, with the majority of cells having an 'atypical' morphology.

Treatment

Bedrest and aspirin for headache and pharyngeal discomfort are the only treatments required. When the fever resolves the patient should be encouraged to get up and resume some activities as fast as is practicable, but violent exercise should be avoided for 3 weeks after an enlarged spleen resolves. Only complications need active therapy: splenic rupture requires surgery, bacterial infections call for appropriate antibiotics, airway obstruction must be relieved by tracheostomy, and corticosteroids should be given for life-threatening pharyngeal oedema and neurological and haematological complications.

Pathogenesis

Why children do not have symptoms during primary EBV infection whereas adolescents and young adults frequently react by developing IM is not fully understood. The immunological reactions of young adults on first encountering EBV are more exuberant than those of children reflecting physiological differences in responsiveness. The mode of infection and consequent size of infecting dose also play an important part; children come into contact with small amounts of virus in saliva from a shedder in droplets or casually contaminating some sucked object, whereas a young person may take in large amounts of virus-containing saliva from a carrier during kissing. An exaggerated immunological response to a large infecting dose of EBV underlies the changes seen in IM and it appears that large numbers of reactive T cells are stimulated by a virus-coded superantigen on infected B cells. These T cells, which present in the circulation, in lymph nodes, in tonsils, in lymphoid tissue of the mouth and pharynx, in spleen, and in other organs such as liver, are responsible for causing the sore throat, fever, malaise, lymphadenopathy, and hepatosplenomegaly by immunopathological mechanisms.

Endemic (or 'African') Burkitt lymphoma

The classic form of this B-cell tumour, first described by Burkitt in 1958, is found in certain parts of Africa and Papua New Guinea where the temperature does not fall below 16°C or the rainfall below 55 cm. Endemic Burkitt lymphoma (BL) is distinct from the 'Burkitt-like' tumours that occur sporadically everywhere in the world (sometimes called 'American' Burkitt lymphoma) and that have a different age incidence, anatomical distribution, and response to therapy, and arise from B cells with different phenotypic characteristics.

The association between EBV and endemic BL is so close that it is generally accepted that the virus is a necessary but not sufficient element in the aetiology of the disease, an essential link along with cofactors in a complicated chain of events which leads to the malignancy. Hyperendemic malaria has been identified as the important cofactor, and its spread by anopheline mosquitoes requiring warmth and moisture explains the climate dependence of BL. There are now credible explanations as to how EBV gene products combine with cofactors to cause the tumour.

BL is a disease of childhood, is extremely rare over the age of 14 years, and in the endemic areas it is more common than all other childhood tumours added together. Full accounts may be found in OTM3, pp. 354–5, and in texts on paediatric oncology or tropical medicine.

Lymphomas in immunosuppressed states

In primary and secondary suppression of cellular immunity there is a loss of immune control of persisting EBV infection which leads to increased virus replication in the oral cavity, increased numbers of circulating, virus-carrying B lymphocytes, and increased levels of serum antibodies to EBV antigens. This is sometimes described as a 'reactivated infection' although the condition is clinically silent. However, on occasions the loss of control leads to the development of EBV-associated lymphomas.

In organ graft recipients

Organ graft recipients who receive lifelong immunosuppressive drugs to prevent graft rejection have a 28–100 times increased risk of developing lymphoproliferative disease and lymphoma compared to normal controls; most of these conditions are of B-cell origin, and contain the EBV genome and viral antigens in their cells. Lymphoproliferative disease has two forms: in about 50 per cent of cases it is associated with primary EBV infection in patients who were seronegative at the time of grafting, occurs within the first year after transplantation in a young age group, and has IM-like symptoms. The second type occurs in older patients late after transplantation as a localized mass, commonly in the gut, central nervous system, or transplanted organ; biopsy shows large-cell lymphoma, which is usually monoclonal.

Reduction of immunosuppressive therapy, with or without acyclovir therapy, is the first line of treatment, with cytotoxic drugs and/or radiotherapy being used only where there is no response or after recurrence.

In acquired immunodeficiency syndrome (AIDS)

Two types of lymphoma are seen in AIDS patients: large-cell lymphoma and BL, and both may be associated with EBV.

Large-cell lymphomas similar to those found in organ-graft recipients (see above) occur in severely immunocompromised AIDS patients; their distribution is extranodal involving many unusual sites, most commonly the central nervous system. These lymphomas show a strong association with EBV, which reaches 100 per cent in cerebral tumours; the progress is rapid, with a mean survival time from diagnosis of 3–4 months. Treatment (radiotherapy) is disappointing because terminal AIDS patients are in such poor condition.

BL occurs earlier in the course of human immunodeficiency virus (HIV) disease while the immune system is still relatively intact and is therefore more amenable to treatment. About 50 per cent of these lymphomas contain EBV DNA.

Hodgkin disease and T-cell lymphomas

There has long been a suspicion that EBV is involved in the induction of Hodgkin disease because of the similar socioeconomic epidemiology of Hodgkin disease and IM, and because within 5 years of IM there is a four- to sixfold increase in the likelihood of developing Hodgkin disease. Evidence has recently has been obtained that, in Hodgkin's lymphomas, EBV DNA is carried and expressed in both Reed–Sternberg and the tumour reticulum cells. These findings are as yet insufficient to implicate EBV in the aetiology of Hodgkin disease, but point to the need for further investigation of a possible relationship. A similar situation exists with oral T-cell lymphoma in AIDS patients and nasal T-cell lymphomas.

Nasopharyngeal carcinoma

This tumour is restricted to the postnasal space where it arises from squamous epithelial cells. The tumour is seen rarely throughout the world but has a remarkably high incidence in southern Chinese and in the Inuit and related circum-Arctic races. In high incidence areas, nasopharyngeal carcinoma (NPC) is the most common cancer of men and the second most common of women. A rather high incidence of NPC is seen amongst Malays, Dyaks, Indonesians, Filipinos, and Vietnamese, and a medium-high incidence belt stretches across North Africa, through the Sudan, to the Kenya highlands. The tumour usually occurs in middle or old age, but in North Africa it has bimodal age peaks, one involving young people up to 20 years of age and a second much later in life. Irrespective of geographical region, NPC cells always carry the EBV genome.

Symptoms

NPC causes nasal obstruction, discharge, or bleeding; deafness, tinnitus, or earache; headache; ocular paresis from tumour spread to involve cranial nerves. Patients may present with a single symptom caused locally by the tumour or with several symptoms, and about one-third complain only of cervical lymph-node enlargement due to metastatic spread from an occult primary tumour.

Signs and clinical course

Direct spread from the primary tumour may involve soft tissues, bone, parotid gland, buccal cavity, and oropharynx. The neoplasm may extend into the nasal fossae, the paranasal sinuses, or the orbit, and can invade the eustachian canal or the parapharyngeal space where cranial nerves IX, X, XI, and XII can be involved. Invasion of the skull or cranial foramina may damage cranial nerves II, IV, V, and VI.

Lymphatic spread causes enlarged cervical lymph nodes and subsequently extends to the supraclavicular glands. If blood-borne metastases occur they are most frequent in bones, liver, and lungs, but may be in any organ.

Untreated NPC progresses inexorably to death.

Differential diagnosis

NPC must be distinguished from other tumours of the nasal cavities, namely adenocarcinomas, sarcomas, malignant lymphomas, and rare malignancies such as chordoma, teratoma, and melanoma.

Laboratory diagnosis

The diagnosis of NPC is made histologically on a biopsy sample either from the primary tumour or from an enlarged cervical lymph node. In addition, serum antibody titres to EBV antigens show a characteristic reaction pattern—IgG and IgA antibodies to VCA and diffuse early antigen (EA-D) are raised, with the titre correlating with the tumour burden. Uniquely, IgA antibodies to VCA and EA are also found in the saliva from patients.

Treatment

NPC responds well to radiotherapy, the treatment of choice. In the earliest stages of the disease, radiotherapy gives 5-year survival rates of 50 per cent or more, and of those surviving 5 years 70 per cent remain permanently free of relapse. More advanced stages of NPC have correspondingly worse prognoses.

Pathogenesis

The role of EBV in NPC is now widely accepted as a necessary agent that is not sufficient on its own. Besides the racial predisposition, southern Chinese with an A2BW36 haplotype are 4–6 times more likely to have NPC than those without.

Epidemiological studies suggest important environmental cofactors associated with the Chinese way of life; two likely candidates are traditional herbal medicines, taken as snuff, and containing tumour-promoting substances of phorbol ester type; and traditional salt fish which has been shown to contain carcinogenic nitrosamines.

Hairy leukoplakia in AIDS

This lesion occurs in HIV-positive homosexual men and in other immunosuppressed individuals; it usually presents as painless white patches on the tongue or on the lateral buccal mucosa. The lesions are slightly raised, poorly demarcated, and have a 'hairy' or corrugated surface; the patches are usually multiple and measure up to 3 cm in diameter.

The squamous epithelial cells of this condition contain large amounts of actively replicating EBV. Treatment with acyclovir arrests the EBV replication and the lesions regress, but only for as long as the drug is continued.

Smooth muscle tumours and gastric carcinoma

Recently EBV has been implicated in various types of gastric carcinoma and in leiomyomas and leiomyosarcomas in children immunosuppressed by AIDS or after organ transplantation. Much further study of these relationships is required.

Further reading

Epstein, M.A. and Achong, B.G. (ed.) (1979). *The Epstein–Barr virus*, pp. 1–459. Springer Verlag, Berlin, Heidelberg, and New York.

Kieff, E. (1996). Epstein–Barr virus and its replication. In *Virology* (ed. B.N. Fields, D.M. Knipe, and P.M. Howley), pp. 2343–96. Raven Press, New York.

Rickinson, A.B. and Kieff, E. (1996). Epstein–Barr virus. In *Virology* (ed. B.N. Fields, D.M. Knipe, and P.M. Howley), pp. 2397–446. Raven Press, New York.

Rickinson, A.B., Murray, R.J., Brooks, J., *et al.* (1992). T-cell recognition of Epstein–Barr virus associated lymphomas. *Cancer Surveys*, 13, 53–80.

Shanmugaratnam, K. (1971). Studies on the etiology of nasopharyngeal carcinoma. In *International review of experimental pathology* (ed. G.W. Richter and M.A. Epstein), Vol. 10, pp. 361–413. Academic Press, New York and London.

Thomas, J.A., Allday, M.J., and Crawford, D.H. (1991). Epstein–Barr virus-associated lymphoproliferative disorders in immunocompromised individuals. *Advances in Cancer Research*, 57, 329–80.

Chapter 16.13

Human infections caused by simian herpesviruses

L. E. Chapman and C. J. Peters

Among the herpesviruses isolated from non-human primates, only the alpha herpesvirus Cercopithecine herpesvirus 1 is clearly recognized to have human pathogenicity. Cercopithecine herpesvirus 2 (simian agent 8, or SA8), a closely related alpha herpesvirus of baboons and African green monkeys, has been possibly implicated in one human case of encephalitis.

Cercopithecine herpesvirus 1 (formerly Herpesvirus simiae, commonly known as B virus) is closely related to herpes simplex virus (HSV), and in many ways is an analogous virus in its natural host, monkeys of the genus *Macaca*.

Epidemiology

B virus is enzootic among Old World *Macaca* monkeys, in which it cases minimal morbidity. No other monkeys have been reported as harbouring B virus naturally. Fatal disease associated with B-virus infections has been reported among several non-macaque species of primates in addition to humans.

The prevalence of B-virus infections among macaques approaches 80 per cent or higher in adult populations. The vesicular oral lesions seen in some cases are thought to represent acute infections. Chronically infected monkeys shed virus intermittently, particularly when they are ill, under stress, or during the breeding season. Virus can be cultured with equal frequency from the conjunctivae, buccal mucosa, and genital areas even though vesicular lesions are not usually present. *Macaca* monkeys, native to Asia and northern Africa, have been transported throughout the world. Humans who have contact with these animals or their products may be exposed to B virus through bites, scratches, mucosal exposures, and other routes.

Human B-virus infections usually occur as single cases, but two clusters have been described. The only reported human-to-human transmission of B-virus infection occurred through direct, repeated inoculation of drainage from active primary B-virus herpetiform lesions onto the skin disrupted by contact dermatitis. Humans have most frequently been infected through injuries sustained while working in the biomedical research industry.

Clinical features

Fewer than 30 human B-virus infections have been reported in detail. Symptoms developed 3–30 days after exposure.

The most common presentation is with rapidly ascending encephalomyelitis following a prodrome characterized by non-specific febrile malaise, variably accompanied by herpetic blisters and/or peripheral nequraesthesia near the site of injury and infection. Neurological features may include paraesthesia of the limbs, followed by weakness or loss of reflexes. Neck stiffness, facial paralysis, dysphagia, or diplopia are ominous signs, rapidly followed by respiratory arrest and coma.

Without treatment the case fatality is approximately 70 per cent. However, the clinical symptoms and signs of at least five laboratory-confirmed human B-virus infections have resolved following high-dose intravenous therapy with acyclovir or ganciclovir.

Diagnosis

Viral culture, serology, and a recently developed polymerase chain reaction are complicated by the extensive cross-reactivity between antibodies to HSV and B virus, and biosafety requirements for propagation of B virus. Any apparent human seroconversion should be confirmed by testing a third serum specimen.

Paralytic rabies must be considered in the differential diagnosis of anyone who presents with neurological disease following bites from free-living primates or primates housed in outdoor facilities.

Prevention

All macaques should be presumed to be shedding B virus and handled accordingly. Adequate and timely wound decontamination is important. The eyes, mouth, nose, or other exposed mucosal surfaces should be irrigated for at least 15 min with sterile saline solution or rapidly flowing water only. For injuries in other locations, concentrated solutions of any detergent may be used.

Further reading

Holmes, G.P., *et al.* (1995). Guidelines for preventing and treating B virus infections in exposed persons. *Clinical Infectious Diseases*, **20**, 421–39.

Weigler, B.J. (1992). Biology of B virus in macaques and human hosts: a review. *Clinical Infectious Diseases*, **14**, 555–67.

Chapter 16.14

Cytomegalovirus

S. Stagno

Most cytomegalovirus (CMV) infections are subclinical. Occasionally it causes a syndrome of cytomegalic inclusion disease in newborns and a mononucleosis-like syndrome in immunocompetent adults. In contrast, among immunosuppressed individuals, recipients of organ transplants, premature infants, and patients with AIDS, it can cause severe disease. The infection that occurs in a seronegative, virgin host is referred to as primary infection while recurrent infection represents reactivation of latent infection or reinfection in a seropositive, immune host. Disease may result from primary or recurrent infection but the former usually causes more severe symptoms. Following a primary infection, viral excretion from one or multiple sites persists for weeks, months, or even years before it becomes latent. As with other herpesvirus infections, episodes of recurrent infection with renewed viral shedding are common even years after the primary infection.

Epidemiology–transmission

Seroepidemiological surveys have found evidence of CMV infection in every population examined. The prevalence of antibody increases with age and varies in different areas of the world. Transmission occurs by direct person-to-person contact. Sources of CMV include saliva, milk, cervical and vaginal secretions, urine, semen, tears, stools, and blood. Indirect transmission is possible through contaminated fomites, such as children's toys. Spread requires very close or intimate contact. The incidence of congenital infection ranges from 0.2–2.2 per cent. Transmission occurs *in utero* as a consequence of viraemia during primary or recurrent infections. Transmission during the perinatal period is common, reaching 10–60 per cent by 6 months of age. After the first year of life the rate of infection is highly dependent upon child-rearing practices. Day-care centres, where infection rates of 50–80 per cent are common, and similar facilities contribute to the rapid spread of CMV. For children who are not exposed to other toddlers the rate of infection increases very slowly throughout the first decade of life. During adolescence a second spurt may be noticed. This is partly the result of sexual transmission.

Seronegative parents of young children shedding CMV and seronegative day-care workers exposed to infected children have a 20 per cent annual risk of acquiring CMV, compared with a 1–3 per cent annual risk for the general population. Health-care workers such as nurses working with patients with AIDS, recipients of organ transplants, or with children and infants with documented congenital CMV infection are not at increased risk.

Nosocomial CMV infection is a hazard of transfusion of blood and blood products. Infection is usually asymptomatic but there is a definite risk of disease in seronegative patients. In immunosuppressed patients and seronegative premature infants the hazard of significant disease is 10–30 per cent. The risk of infection can be eliminated or significantly reduced by selecting seronegative donors, or using leucocyte-depleted, filtered, or cryopreserved blood.

After organ transplantation many patients excrete CMV. Sources for primary infection are transplanted organs and, to a lesser degree, blood or blood products. Recurrent infections are more likely to result from reactivation of latent infection although the above sources may also contribute.

Clinical manifestations

The clinical manifestations of CMV infection vary with age, route of transmission, and the immune competence of the subject. In most cases, including those with congenital infection, CMV infection is subclinical.

Congenital infection

Only 5 per cent of all congenitally infected infants have severe cytomegalic inclusion disease, another 5 per cent have mild involvement, and 90 per cent are born with subclinical but chronic infection. The signs and symptoms are given in Table 1. With cytomegalic inclusion disease, the outlook for normal development is poor. More than 90 per cent of all symptomatic patients develop central nervous and hearing defects in later years. In infants with subclinical infection the outlook is much better, but 5–15 per cent will develop some sequelae such as sensorineural hearing loss, developmental abnormalities, microcephaly, chorioretinitis, and neurological defects that are generally less severe than in infants with symptomatic infection at birth. Most symptomatic congenital infections and those resulting in sequelae are the result of primary infection acquired during gestation (10–25 per cent) rather than recurrent (0.5–2 per cent) infections in pregnant women.

Table 1 Clinical and laboratory findings in 106 infants with symptomatic congenital cytomegalovirus infection in the neonatal period

Abnormality	Positive/total examined (%)
Prematurity (< 38 weeks)	36/106 (34)
Small for gestational age	53/106 (50)
Petechiae	80/106 (76)
Jaundice	69/103 (67)
Hepatosplenomegaly	63/105 (60)
Purpura	14/105 (13)
Neurological findings	
One or more of the following:	72/106 (68)
Microcephaly	54/102 (53)
Lethargy/hypotonia	28/104 (27)
Poor suck	20/103 (19)
Seizures	7/105 (7)
Elevated ALT (> 80 u/l)	46/58 (83)
Thrombocytopenia: $< 100 \times 10^3/\text{mm}^3$	62/81 (77)
$< 50 \times 10^3/\text{mm}^3$	43/81 (53)
Conjugated hyperbilirubinaemia: direct serum bilirubin, 4 mg/dl	47/68 (69)
Haemolysis	37/72 (51)
Increased CSF protein (120 mg/dl)*	24/52 (46)

*Determinations in the first week of life.

ALT, alanine aminotransferase; CSF, cerebrospinal fluid.

Perinatal infections

Infections resulting from exposure to CMV in the maternal genital tract at delivery or to breast milk occur in the presence of maternally derived, passively acquired antibody. The majority of infants remain asymptomatic and do not suffer long-term complications. Occasionally, perinatally acquired CMV infection is associated with pneumonitis. Premature and sick full-term infants may have neurological sequelae and psychomotor retardation. However, the risk of hearing loss, chorioretinitis, and microcephaly does not appear to be increased.

Transfusion-acquired infection can cause significant illness and death, particularly in premature infants (birth weight < 1500 g) born to mothers seronegative for the virus.

Young children

Most CMV infections acquired in childhood are asymptomatic. Occasionally they cause hepatosplenomegaly with abnormal liver function tests or respiratory illnesses.

Adolescents and adults

Serologically proven CMV infection increases with age, with a burst in adolescence. While CMV has been implicated in disease of virtually every organ system, well-established clinical syndromes are few. A

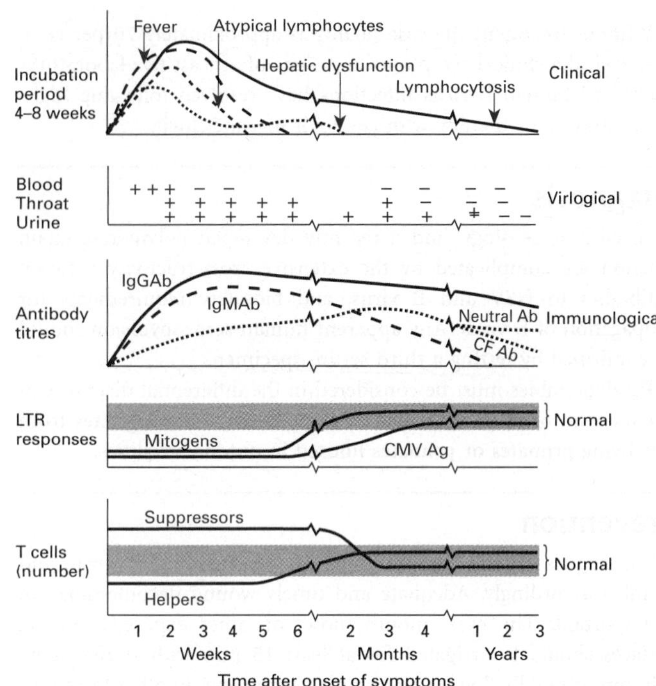

Fig. 1 Findings with symptomatic primary CMV infection (mononucleosis syndrome) in normal hosts (see OTM3, p.362 for source).

heterophile antibody-negative mononucleosis syndrome occurs spontaneously in adults and can develop following infection acquired by blood transfusion at any age (Fig. 1). In contrast to the Epstein–Barr virus-induced syndrome, tonsillopharyngitis, lymphadenopathy, and splenomegaly are less common. There is malaise, myalgia, fever, abnormal liver function, and lymphocytosis with a significant increase in the proportion of atypical lymphocytes. The course of cytomegalovirus mononucleosis is generally mild, but occasionally patients may present with high persistent fever, or with clinically apparent hepatitis, generalized lymphadenopathies, and/or morbilliform rashes. Rare complications of acute primary cytomegalovirus infection include pneumonitis, myocarditis, pericarditis, neuritis, and myelitis (Guillain–Barré syndrome), encephalitis, aseptic meningitis, thrombocytopenic purpura, haemolytic anaemia, and retinitis. In normal hosts, recurrent infections are asymptomatic. In immunocompromised individuals the risk of illness and death is increased, especially in primary but also in recurrent infections. Clinically, pneumonitis is most common, but hepatitis, chorioretinitis, gastrointestinal disease, and fever with leucopenia occur individually or in combination (see Plates 12, 13, The eye and disease).

The greatest risk is in patients undergoing transplantation and those with AIDS. As with other populations, primary infections are clearly more virulent. Pneumonitis is a hallmark of CMV disease in this group, particularly in bone-marrow transplant patients. Hepatic dysfunction is common but frank hepatitis is rare. In liver transplant recipients, hepatitis must be distinguished from rejection episodes. Gastrointestinal complications are difficult to evaluate. Submucosal ulcerations can occur anywhere in the gastrointestinal tract from oesophagus to rectum. Haemorrhage and perforation are known complications, so are pancreatitis and cholecystitis. CMV retinitis is a serious complication that may occur at any time after transplantation or during immunosuppression.

Laboratory diagnosis

The diagnosis of CMV infection requires laboratory confirmation. Infection can be demonstrated by direct methods such as viral cultures, polymerase chain reaction (PCR), or antigen detection. Preferred specimens include: urine, saliva, milk, cervical secretions, buffy coat, or other tissues obtained by biopsies or at autopsy. Rapid viral diagnosis is now possible. Direct methods cannot distinguish between primary and recurrent (reactivation/reinfection) infections.

A primary infection is confirmed by seroconversion (*de novo* appearance of IgG antibodies), or the simultaneous detection of IgG and IgM antibodies. Rising IgG antibody titres may follow primary or recurrent infections. IgG antibodies persist for life. IgM antibodies can be demonstrated transiently (4–16 weeks) during the acute phase of symptomatic or asymptomatic primary infection in adults. Radioimmunoassay, enzyme immunoassay, and an IgM-capture radioimmunoassay have acceptable specificity and sensitivity. With these assays IgM antibodies are not found, or are only transiently detected in patients with recurrent infection.

A recurrent infection is defined by the reappearance of viral excretion in a patient known to have been seropositive in the past. The distinction between reactivation of endogenous virus and re-infection with a different strain of CMV requires restriction enzyme analysis of viral DNA.

In immunocompromised patients, excretion of cytomegalovirus, rises in IgG titres, and even the presence of IgM antibodies is common, making the distinction between primary and recurrent infections more difficult. Determining the serological status of patients before transplantation and immunosuppressive treatment helps future management. Viraemia (positive culture, PCR, or antigenaemia) implies active disease and a worse prognosis whether the type of infection is primary, recurrent, or unknown.

The decisive way of distinguishing congenital from perinatal CMV infection is by isolating virus during the first 2 weeks of life from urine or saliva. A negative IgG antibody result excludes the diagnosis but a positive result generally reflects maternal immunity. Demonstration of stable or rising titres during the first year of life does not help because perinatal infections are common. In general, IgM tests lack sensitivity and specificity, and are technically demanding. No reliable test is commercially available.

Treatment

Ganciclovir and foscarnet have been used with encouraging results in life-threatening CMV infections in immunocompromised hosts. Both agents are toxic, with significant renal toxicity with foscarnet and myelosuppression with ganciclovir. A regimen of 10 mg/kg per day of ganciclovir given at 12-h intervals for 2–3 weeks, followed by a once-a-day maintenance of 5 mg/kg given until regression of clinical manifestations, has proved to have some efficacy. The usual foscarnet regimen is 180 mg/kg per day, with individual doses given at 8-h intervals for 14–21 days followed by chronic maintenance at 90–120 mg/kg per day. Combination therapy has been used in refractory patients. CMV retinitis and gastrointestinal disease appear to be clinically responsive to therapy but, like viral excretion, recur upon cessation of therapy. Drug toxicity is extensive with both antivirals. Recent trials indicate a beneficial effect of prophylactic ganciclovir in some immunosuppressed transplant patients. No results of controlled studies of treatment for congenital CMV infection are yet available.

Prevention

Passive immunoprophylaxis

The use of prophylactic hyperimmune plasma or globulin in recipients of transplants has resulted in a significant reduction of symptomatic disease but not in prevention of infection. The efficacy of immunoglobulin is more striking in situations in which the risk of primary CMV infection carries a high risk of morbidity such as in bone marrow transplantation. One recommended regimen is 1.0 g/kg of immunoglobulin given as a single intravenous dose beginning within 72 h of transplantation and once weekly thereafter until day 120 after transplantation.

Active immunization

Vaccines would be most useful for seronegative women of childbearing age and seronegative transplant recipients. Vaccine trials with live attenuated vaccines have been disappointing. Subunit and recombinant vaccines are being developed and tested.

Other preventive measures

The use of CMV-free blood and blood products, and when possible, the use of organs from CMV-free donors, represent important measures to prevent CMV infection and disease in non-immune patients.

Further reading

Britt, W.J. and Alford, C.A. (1996). Cytomegalovirus. In *Virology*, 3rd edn (ed. B.N. Fields *et al.*), pp. 2493–523. Lippincott-Raven, Philadelphia, 1996.

Gold, E. and Nankervis, G.A. (1989). Cytomegalovirus. In *Viral infections of humans: epidemiology and control*, 3rd edn (ed. A.S. Evans), pp. 169–89. Plenum, New York.

Ho, M. (1995). Cytomegalovirus. In *Principles and practice of infectious diseases*, 4th edn (ed. G.L. Mandell, *et al.*), pp. 1351–64. Churchill Livingstone, Edinburgh.

Stagno, S. (1999). Cytomegalovirus. In *Infectious diseases of the fetus and newborn infant*, 5th edn (ed. J.S. Emington and J.O. Klein), Chapter 7. W.B. Saunders, Philadelphia. (In press.)

Chapter 16.15

Human herpesviruses 6, 7, and 8

P. E. Pellett and J. A. Stewart

Human herpesviruses 6A, 6B, 7, and 8 (HHV-6A, HHV-6B, HHV-7, and HHV-8 (also known as Kaposi's sarcoma-associated herpesvirus or KSHV)) were discovered within the past 15 years. These are not 'new' viruses, rather, they are viruses that have had a role in human biology over an evolutionary time scale.

HHV-6

HHV-6 is is predominantly tropic for T cells both *in vitro* and *in vivo*, although it can grow in other cell types. HHV-6 isolates form two groups: HHV-6 variants A and B (HHV-6A and HHV-6B). HHV-6A has not been specifically associated with human disease. HHV-6B causes roseola (exanthem subitum or sixth disease) and other febrile illnesses in children. HHV-6 infections are easily misdiagnosed, for example as antibiotic sensitivity, measles or rubella, or post-transplant graft-versus-host disease.

Primary infection with HHV-6 generally occurs 6 months to 2 years after birth. In most populations, over 90 per cent of people over 2 years of age are seropositive for at least one HHV-6 variant. Transmission is probably via saliva. The most common clinical manifestation of primary HHV-6B infection is roseola. Roseola is characterized by a 3–4-day febrile phase (frequently over 40°C) followed by rapid defeverescence and then the onset of a rash that persists for 1–3 days. Diarrhoea, bulging fontanelle, and bronchopneumonia are frequently observed, while convulsions, hepatocellular dysfunction, and intussusception are less frequent. Roseola generally resolves untreated without complication. Primary HHV-6 infection can also lead to a variety of other conditions, including subclinical infections and variations on the febrile phase followed by rash theme, such as rash without fever and fever without rash. Other examples of diseases occasionally associated with primary HHV-6 infection include liver dysfunction, fatal fulminant hepatitis, fatal haemophagocytic syndrome, hepatosplenomegaly, heterophile negative mononucleosis, induction of spontaneous abortion, meningoencephalitis, encephalitis, and fatal disseminated infection. About 20 per cent of febrile admissions to emergency departments for children between 6 and 12 months of age are due to primary HHV-6 infections.

HHV-6 can be active in immunocompromised patients, including organ transplant recipients and AIDS patients. Symptoms associated with HHV-6 reactivation or reinfection include fever, severe interstitial pneumonitis, sinusitis, and rashes that can be mistaken for acute graft-versus-host disease. Although its role in the progression of AIDS is uncertain, late in AIDS, HHV-6 is frequently disseminated into many tissues and organs.

In addition to peripheral blood T cells, HHV-6 is present in most normal brains. In patients with multiple sclerosis, HHV-6 is present in the plaque regions, with a cellular distribution different from that seen in normal brains; the significance of this is being studied.

There is no clear aetiological link between HHV-6 and malignancy, although HHV-6 has been isolated, or its DNA detected, in tissues from patients with various lymphoproliferative disorders. There is also no clear evidence for an association between HHV-6 and chronic fatigue syndrome. Determining HHV-6 antibody status in chronic fatigue syndrome patients is pointless, because most people are positive for the virus and there is no diagnostically useful antibody titre.

HHV-6 can be detected by culture of patient's lymphocytes either alone or by cocultivation with activated human cord blood lymphocytes, with confirmation by using commercially available HHV-6-specific monoclonal antibodies. Because of its speed, polymerase chain reaction (PCR) detection may be of particular value in monitoring transplant recipients. Interpretation of virus culture and PCR results is complicated by the occasional positive culture and the more frequent detection of viral DNA by PCR in healthy people. HHV-6 antibodies can be detected in standard serological assays, including indirect immunofluorescence, anticomplement immunofluorescence, and microplate enzyme-based immunoassays. HHV-6-specific IgG can be detected frequently within two weeks of primary infection, and titres can rise significantly in response to reactivation or re-infection. The most useful diagnostic results are obtained from sequential specimens, so that changes in status can be detected.

The most effective agents for inhibiting HHV-6 growth *in vitro* are gancyclovir, phosphonoacetic acid, and phosphonoformate. Clinical efficacy has not been studied.

HHV-7

HHV-7 is genetically and biologically closely related to the HHV-6 variants. HHV-7 is highly prevalent (>85 per cent) in adults, is acquired early in life, usually after primary HHV-6 infection, and is likely to be transmitted via saliva. The clinical spectrum of HHV-7 is poorly defined. Primary HHV-7 infection is associated with some cases of roseola infantum, febrile rashes that can be mistaken for either measles or rubella, fever of unknown origin, 'cytomegalovirus' disease following organ transplants, and pityriasis rosea. Diagnostic methods and considerations are similar to those for HHV-6.

HHV-8

HHV-8 was first identified in Kaposi's sarcoma (KS) tissues (Plates 1, 2) and probably causes the disease. The virus has also been detected in primary effusion (or body cavity-based) lymphomas and lymphoid hyperplasias including multicentric Castleman's disease and angio-immunoblastic lymphadenopathy.

HHV-8 seroprevalence may be less than 10 per cent in the US and UK, but it is over 50 per cent in areas of Italy where KS is endemic, as well as in some African countries. The primary route of transmission has not been identified, but is probably sexual in some populations. Primary HHV-8 infection has been associated with a febrile rash illness in Ugandan children.

Further reading

Black, J.B. and Pellett, P.E. (2000). Human herpesvirus 7. *Reviews in Medical Virology*, in press.

Braun, D.K., Dominguez, G., and Pellett, P.E. (1997). Human herpesvirus 6. *Clinical Microbiology Reviews*, **10**, 521–67.

Moore, P.S. and Chang, Y. (1997). Kaposi's sarcoma-associated herpesvirus. In *Clinical virology* (ed. D.D. Richman, R.J. Whitley, and F.G. Hayden), pp. 509–24. Churchill Livingstone, New York.

Chapter 16.16

Poxviruses

G. L. Smith

Introduction

Poxviruses are a family of large, complex DNA viruses that replicate in the cytoplasm of infected cells. The family is subdivided into entomopoxviruses (which infect insects) and chordopoxviruses (which infect chordates). The chordopoxviruses are divided into eight genera of which the orthopoxvirus genus has been of greatest importance to human health. The most infamous orthopoxvirus, variola virus, was the aetiological agent of smallpox, a devastating disease that caused up to 40 per cent mortality in non-immune populations but which has been eradicated by vaccination. Cowpox virus was the vaccine used by Jenner in 1796 to vaccinate against smallpox, but vaccinia virus was the virus used for this purpose throughout this century.

Vaccinia is a distinct virus from cowpox virus and has an uncertain origin. Monkeypox virus causes sporadic zoonotic infections of man and has a pathology similar to that of smallpox, but is less easily transmitted.

Much of our knowledge of poxviruses comes from studies with vaccinia virus, but many features are likely to be very similar in other poxviruses. There are two structurally distinct infectious forms of vaccinia virus which have different biological properties. Historically, most work concentrated on the intracellular mature virus (IMV) since this represents the great majority of infectious progeny and could easily be purified. IMV is released by cell lysis and probably is responsible for spreading infection between hosts. Extracellular enveloped virus (EEV) is shed from infected cells before cell death and contains an additional lipid envelope and associated proteins (of virus and cellular origin), which are absent from IMV. EEV and IMV bind to different cell receptors and enter cells by low pH dependent or independent mechanisms, respectively. EEV is responsible for virus dissemination within the body and is neither neutralized by antibody nor destroyed by complement.

An emerging feature of poxviruses is the extraordinary repertoire of genes which are not essential for virus replication in culture but which enable the virus to escape the host response to infection. Specifically, vaccinia virus expresses proteins that oppose apoptosis, synthesize steroids, capture chemokines, counteract complement, interfere with interferon and intercept interleukins. The study of these virus immunomodulatory proteins is increasing our understanding of virus pathogenesis and the immune system, indicating how these viruses might be engineered as safer and more immunogenic live vaccines, and may provide novel immunotherapeutics for intervention in immunological disorders or infections.

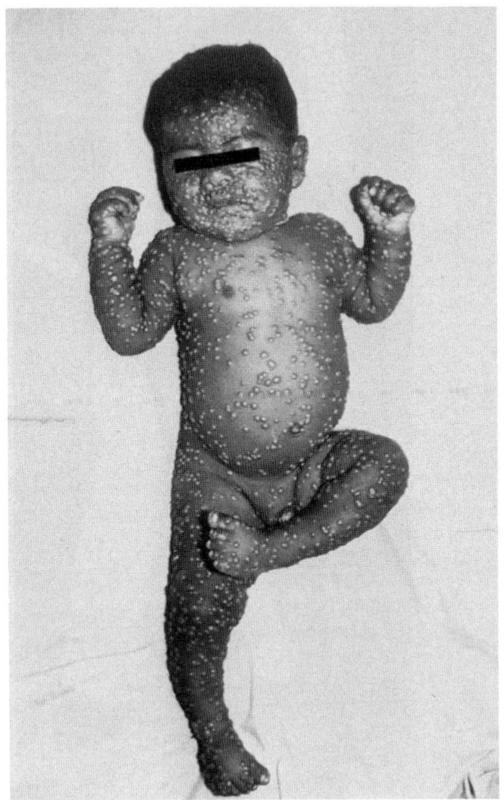

Fig. 1 Smallpox in a 9-month-old boy in Pakistan, photographed on the eighth day of the rash
(by courtesy of the WHO).

Smallpox

Smallpox (Fig. 1) was eradicated by vaccination with the immunologically related orthopoxviruses, cowpox and vaccinia. The eradication was completed in 1977, certified by the WHO two years later, and remains the most complete triumph for human medicine. For vaccinologists it is worth remembering that the eradication was achieved without knowing which antigens the vaccine induced immunity against, nor how similar were the corresponding target antigens of variola viruses. It was used because it was effective.

Now that smallpox is eradicated, the WHO have agreed that the remaining stocks of variola virus, held in Russia and the USA, should be destroyed in 1999. Destruction will take place only after the complete nucleotide sequences of several representative variola virus strains (major and minor) have been determined and will not include the cloned (non-infectious) DNA fragments of the genomes. This proposal has prompted fierce debate. Advocates of destruction state that this is natural completion of the eradication programme, the virus can never again escape from a laboratory, it will no longer be necessary to maintain virus in high security freezers, and it removes any threat of the virus being used as a terrorist weapon. Opponents of the policy state that destruction will prevent valuable information being gained about why variola virus, but not closely related orthopoxviruses, caused such devastating disease, and that learning how variola virus overcame the host immune system will aid our understanding of how other viruses cause disease that may ultimately lead to their treatment or prevention. Opponents argue that keeping only the cloned virus DNA is insufficient because studying a gene in isolation from its natural host does not enable a full understanding of its function. For example, the interleukin (IL)-1β receptor from vaccinia virus prevents fever during virus infection; this observation could only have been made after virus infection, and was not predicted because there are many other endogenous pyrogens (e.g. tumour necrosis factor) in addition to IL-1β. Lastly, some of the immunomodulatory proteins from variola virus may prove useful therapeutic reagents.

Monkeypox virus

Monkeypox virus (Fig. 2) was recognized in captive monkeys in Europe and the USA from 1958 onwards, but from 1970 onwards infections in man were recognized in countries of Western and Central Africa. The disease resembled smallpox in its incubation period and distribution of lesions but had an important difference in that it was less easily transmitted from the index case so that outbreaks were sporadic and isolated. Nonetheless, the ability of a poxvirus, closely related to variola virus, to cause a similar disease was of concern to the WHO during the later stages of the smallpox eradication campaign. Although the virus is called monkeypox virus, the natural reservoir for the virus is probably arboreal squirrels.

From February 1996 to February 1997 the largest ever outbreak of human monkeypox occurred in Zaire (now Democratic Republic of Congo). This outbreak had several important differences from previous monkeypox virus infections of humans. The proportion of infected patients aged 15 years or more (27 per cent) was higher than for other outbreaks (8 per cent), as was the proportion of secondary cases (73 per cent) (compared to 30 per cent in previous reports).

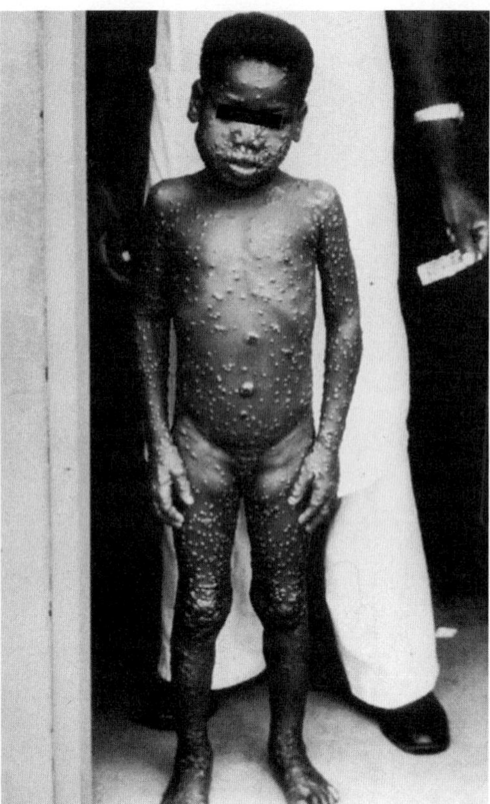

Fig. 2 Moderately severe monkeypox in a girl of 7 years from Equateur Province, Zaire
(by courtesy of the WHO).

Transmission of the virus between people therefore accounted for the majority of the outbreak. However, the mortality rate (3 per cent) was lower than in earlier outbreaks (10 per cent) and all deaths were in patients less than 3 years old. Factors that might have affected this and possible future outbreaks are the diminishing immunity of the population to orthopoxviruses now that vaccination against smallpox is discontinued, virus variation leading to adaptation in man, and the increasing burden of immunosuppression due to HIV infection.

An antiviral drug, cidofovir, has proved effective against monkey pox in animals.

Further reading

Fenner, F., Anderson, D.A., Arita, I., *et al.* (1988). *Smallpox and its eradication.* World Health Organization, Geneva.

Jezek, Z. and Fenner, F. (1988). *Human monkeypox.* Monographs in Virology (ed. J. L. Melnick). Karger, Basel.

Smith, G.L., Symons, J.A., Khanna, A., *et al.* (1997). Vaccinia virus immune evasion. *Immunological Reviews,* 159, 137–54.

Chapter 16.17

Orf

N. Jones

Aetiology

Orf virus, a member of the *Parapox* genus, normally causes a disease in sheep. Orf virions are ovoid (approximate size, 260 × 160 nm), with tubular threadlike structures criss-crossing the surface of the virions, visible by negatively stained electron microscopy. The orf virus genome is double stranded DNA of 135 kbp.

Epidemiology

The disease affects mainly young lambs, who contract the infection from one to another, or possibly from persistence of the virus in the pastures (the virus can remain viable for long periods in dried scabs from lesions). Human disease is usually occupational, following contact with infected sheep. It is not uncommon in shepherds, veterinary surgeons, and farmers (Plate 1). One attack normally confers immunity and human to human spread has not been recorded.

Clinical features

Synonyms for orf are contagious pustular dermatitis, contagious ecthyma, and scabby mouth. In sheep, papules and vesicles appear on the lips of sheep (scabby mouth) and gradually heal with no scarring over 4 weeks. In humans, after an incubation period of 5–6 days, a small, red, firm papule enlarges to form a flat-topped haemorrhagic pustule or bulla; the centre may be crusted. The lesion is usually 2–3 cm in diameter, but may be as large as 5 cm. Lesions are solitary or few in number and commonly occur on the hands and forearms, occasionally the face. Lymphangitis or regional lymphadenopathy are not uncommon. Slight fever and malaise can occur. Recovery is usually complete in 6 weeks and is spontaneous.

Large fungating granuloma or tumour-like lesions have been reported, especially in association with haematological malignancy.

Erythema multiforme occasionally develops, typically 10–14 days after the onset of orf. Rarely, bullous pemphigoid has been reported in association with orf.

Diagnosis

The characteristic lesion in a person exposed to sheep and lambs allows a clinical diagnosis. This can be confirmed in the laboratory by electron microscopy of a biopsy of the orf lesion. The virus can also be isolated in cell culture, but this is rarely performed. Histopathological examination of biopsy specimens shows a proliferation of keratinocytes with cellular swelling and balloon degeneration and B type cytoplasmic inclusion bodies.

Treatment

No specific treatment is available. Secondary infection should be treated if it occurs. Large lesions can be removed surgically, but recurrence can occur in the immunocompromised. Occasionally lesions have been treated with idoxuridine.

Further reading

Gill, M.J., Arlette, J., Buchan, K.A., *et al.* (1990). Human orf. *Archives of Dermatology*, **126**, 356–8.

Groves, R.W., Wilson-Jones, E., and MacDonald, D.M. (1991). Human orf and milkers nodule: a clinicopathological study. *Journal of the American Academy of Dermatology*, **25**, 706–11.

Chapter 16.18

Molluscum contagiosum

N. Jones

Molluscum contagiosum is a benign skin tumour, caused by a poxvirus, which mostly affects children and young adults. It is exclusively a human disease.

Aetiology

Molluscum contagiosum virus (MCV) is a member of the Poxviridae, genus *Molluscipox*. MCV has not been transmitted to laboratory animals and there is no *in vitro* cultivation system currently available. Restriction endonuclease analysis of the genome has identified three types, MCV I, MCV II, and MCV III. The majority of infections seem to be due to MCV 1.

Epidemiology

Molluscum contagiosum is common and disease usually follows contact with an infected individual or contaminated object. In tropical countries, the infection tends to occur in younger children (1–4 years) than in temperate climates (10–12 years). Sexual transmission accounts for a second incidence peak in young adults. Unusually widespread lesions have been reported in HIV disease, sarcoidosis, and those taking immunosuppressive therapy.

Clinical features

The incubation varies from 14 days to 6 months. The individual lesion is a shining, pearly, hemispherical, umbilical papule with a central pore. Lesions can occur singly but are commonly multiple (Fig. 1). The lesions gradually grow to a diameter of 5–10 mm over 6–12 weeks. Occasionally one very large lesion can develop (> 10 mm), or a plaque of very small lesions (agimate form). Most cases persist for 6– 9 months, occasionally as long as 5 years, following which spontaneous resolution occurs.

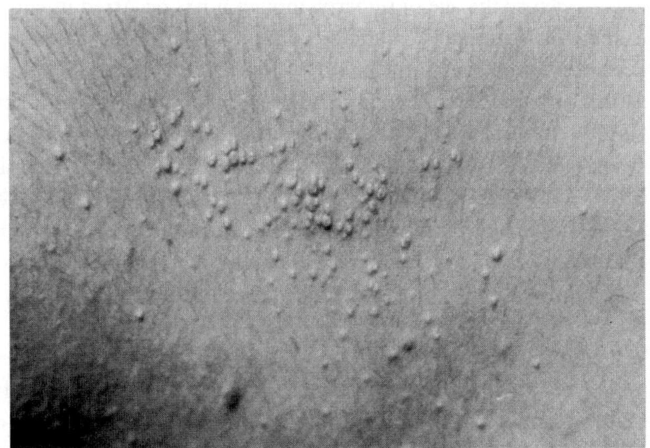

Fig. 1 Molluscum contagiosum on skin.

Lesions are commonly seen on the neck, trunk, or axilla, although any part of the skin can be affected. Lesions are rare on the palms, soles, and mucous membranes. Sexually acquired infections normally result in anogenital lesions. In about 10 per cent of cases, especially where there is a history of atopy, a patchy dermatitis develops around the lesions. In the HIV patient molluscum can be widespread, affecting the face and upper body particularly. Lesions may become large and atypical, and are mistaken for basal cell carcinomas or other skin tumours. The disease is often unremitting with increasing severity, especially when HIV is advanced.

Diagnosis

The diagnosis is usually clinical, but histological and electron microscopic examination of a curetted lesion establishes the diagnosis.

Treatment

Advice on prevention of spread of the infection to others should be given, such as avoidance of swimming pools, contact sports, or shared towels, until the lesions have resolved. Treatment may not be necessary, and depends on the site and number of the lesions and the age of the patient.

Cryotherapy (with liquid nitrogen) is effective and should be repeated at 3–4-weekly intervals. Other techniques include diathermy or curettage. In children the application of local anaesthetic cream prior to the procedure may be necessary.

Topical agents such as phenol (10–20 per cent solution), salicylic acid (15–20 per cent), trichloroacetic acid, lactic acid, tretinoin, and cantharidin are used. The agent can be delivered to the inside of the lesion using the sharpened end of a wooden applicator stick.

In severe cases associated with HIV, therapy is similar. Recently, the antiviral agent, cidofovir (intravenously or topically), has been successfully used to treat molluscum contagiosum.

Further reading

Birthistle, K. and Carrington, D. (1997). Molluscum contagiosum virus. *Journal of Infection*, **34**, 21–8.

Meadows, K.P., Tyring, S.K., Pavia, A.T., and Rallis, T.M. (1997). Resolution of recalcitrant molluscum contagiosum virus lesions in human immunodeficiency virus infected patients treated with cidofovir. *Archives of Dermatology*, **133** (8), 987–90.

Schwartz, J.J. and Myskowski, P.L. (1992). Molluscum contagiosum in patients with human immunodeficiency virus infection. A review of twenty seven patients. *Journal of the American Academy of Dermatology*, **27**, 583–8.

Thompson, C.H. (1999). Molluscum contagiosum; new perspectives on an old virus. *Current Opinion in Infectious Disease*, **12**, 185–9.

Chapter 16.19

Mumps: epidemic parotitis

*B. K. Rima and A. B. Christie**

Aetiology

Mumps is an acute, generalized virus infection of children and young adults, caused by a paramyxovirus that can infect almost any organ: salivary glands, pancreas, testes or ovary, brain, mammary gland, liver, kidney, joints, and heart. Swelling of the face is the most familiar symptom (see OTM3, p. 372).

Epidemiology

The incubation period lies between 14 and 18 days. In any outbreak, 30–40 per cent of those infected have subclinical illness. Mumps is highly infectious. Transmission depends on close personal contact with a patient who is excreting virus in the saliva and spreads the virus in droplets. In the prevaccine era, the peak incidence was in the late winter or early spring months, in 3- to 7-year cycles. The major morbidity is associated with meningitis and orchitis. The case fatality is about 2 per 10 000.

Pathogenesis and pathology

Mumps virus causes an infection of the upper respiratory tract which spreads to the draining lymph nodes. The subsequent transient viraemia and infection of the lymphocytes and macrophages causes spread to many organs, but because mumps is not often lethal, there is little information about the changes caused. Lymphocytic infiltration and destruction of periductal cells lead to blockage of the ducts both in salivary glands and in the seminiferous tubules of the testes. Lymphatics in the tissues surrounding and lying over the parotid glands become obstructed, producing a gel-like oedema that may spread down over the chest wall, especially when swelling of the salivary glands is severe.

Mumps virus frequently invades the nervous system: changes can be detected by electroencephalography or by examination of the cerebrospinal fluid in at least half the patients. However, in most of these cases there are no nervous symptoms or signs. Mumps virus is one of the most common known causes of lymphocytic meningitis. Neuronal damage probably does occur and explains the occurrence of quadriplegia or single-nerve paralysis in some patients. Apart from transient weakness of the facial nerve, which may be due to pressure of a swollen gland or damage by mumps virus, these complications are all very rare.

Mumps encephalitis is a different entity; cerebrospinal fluid is normal and contains no virus. At autopsy there is perivascular demyelination exactly the same as in other forms of postinfectious encephalitis (see Chapter 16.117).

Clinical features and diagnosis

Parotitis

A patient with mumps parotitis may have a fever (40–40.5°C) without rigors and pain near the angle of the jaw. The face and neck become distorted with swelling. The skin over the gland is hot and flushed but there is no rash, unlike erysipelas. If the swelling is severe, the mouth cannot be opened for pain and tightness, and is dry because the flow of saliva is blocked. This discomfort lasts for 3–4 days. Sometimes, as one side clears the parotid on the other side swells. When there is bilateral parotitis, clinical diagnosis is usually obvious. One condition that must be excluded is bull-neck diphtheria (see Chapter 16.37), which can look very like mumps.

The submaxillary and sublingual salivary glands may also be affected in mumps, but this occurs rarely. The symptoms are similar to those in parotitic mumps, but it is difficult or impossible to distinguish the swelling from other forms of submaxillary swellings, especially inflammation of various groups of lymph nodes. In mumps, the neck swelling is ill-defined and the angle of the jaw is impalpable. To determine if cervical lymph nodes are swollen from some other cause, one must examine the pharynx carefully. One must also examine the fauces for signs of tonsilitis that might cause cervical adenitis. The lymph nodes in contact with the submaxillary and sublingual salivary glands drain the corner of the eye, the side of the nose, the cheeks, the lips, and the floor of the mouth. One must look for lesions there, for otherwise diagnosis from submaxillary or sublingual mumps is difficult. Laboratory tests are needed for definite diagnosis.

In infectious mononucleosis the glands stand out distinctly and the parotid is not affected. In septic parotitis there is more parotid tenderness; there may be fluctuation, and pus exudes from the orifice of Stensen's duct. Calculus causes spasmodic pain and swelling and may be detected radiographically. Recurrent parotitis and Mikulicz's syndrome are unlikely to be confused with mumps except in the earliest stages, nor are uveoparotid fever and tumours of the gland, for they are chronic conditions. Serum amylase may be elevated for several weeks in mumps parotitic and pancreatitis. Inflammation of the two organs may be distinguished by measuring isoenzymes and serum pancreatic lipase.

Orchitis

Orchitis may occur 4–5 days after the onset of parotitis. Quite often it occurs without preceding parotitis. It is an acute condition, with chills, sweats, headache, and backache, and a swinging temperature as well as severe local testicular pain and tenderness. The scrotum is swollen and oedematous, and the testicles are impalpable. Most often only one testicle is affected but sometimes both: the second testicle may become affected just as the swelling of the first is subsiding. The illness lasts 3–4 days before the swelling begins to subside. Orchitis is unusual before the age of puberty, though it has occurred in young boys and even in infants. In adolescent and young males it develops in 1:5 cases. Some degree of atrophy of the testicle occurs in at least one-third of patients with orchitis. Azoospermia after mumps is rare and only temporary. The fear of sterility after mumps orchitis has been exaggerated, so the doctor can reassure the patient. Orchitis, when it occurs without parotitis, is difficult to diagnose from gonococcal epididymo-orchitis unless there has been contact with mumps. The rare case of orchitis in infancy may resemble torsion of the testis and perhaps it is safer to operate than risk a serious misdiagnosis.

Meningitis and encephalitis

Lymphocytic or viral meningitis may develop a few days after the start of parotitis, but almost as often it occurs in the absence of parotitis. In the cerebrospinal fluid, protein and lymphocytes are both increased and mumps virus can be isolated in the first few days. The

*Dr A.B. Christie died in 1987. Much of his second edition chapter was retained in OTM3.

meningitis is usually mild and self-limiting. Occasionally the patient develops transient paralysis of limbs. Polyneuritis, neuritis of the trigeminal or facial nerve, and retrobulbar optic neuritis have been described in mumps but all are rare.

In encephalitis the outlook is different. The patient is mentally disturbed and may lapse into coma and remain comatose for days, weeks, or months. Almost 2 per cent of the encephalitis cases are fatal.

Other complications

Deafness is sometimes reported after mumps; but it is rarely permanent. Women sometimes complain of ovarian pain during an attack of mumps, but it is rarely as severe as in men with orchitis. There is no evidence that it affects fertility. Mastitis occurs in 15 per cent of the cases, both in females and males, but it is usually mild and fleeting. Mild upper abdominal pain in about 50 per cent of the cases may be related to viral changes in the pancreas. The amount of amylase in duodenal fluid may be less than normal, but levels of the pancreatic isoenzyme of amylase are increased in serum. This is probably caused by blocking of the ducts in the pancreas. Although there are anecdotal reports of diabetes occurring after an attack of mumps, there is no virological or immunological evidence for a direct link.

Mumps in the fetus and infant

Abortion may occur in women with mumps in the first trimester of pregnancy. It is not common and probably not caused by virus damage to the fetus. The connection between primary endocardial fibroelastosis and mumps is rather vague. Mumps virus has not been isolated from heart tissue at autopsy and these infants have no mumps antibody in their blood. They may show a delayed hypersensitivity response to the skin test. This has not been explained, but may reflect some immune defect in the fetus which could cause myocarditis and fibroelastosis.

Normally, maternal IgG passes to the fetus and seems to protect the infant against mumps during the first year of life. The typical disease of mumps in infants is a rare clinical finding even in populations with no previous experience of the disease. Orchitis has been reported in infants, and mumps virus may be isolated in vague respiratory infections in infants.

Laboratory diagnosis

In cases without parotitis, especially meningitis, and in the absence of contact history, serological tests and virus isolation are the only means of reaching a firm diagnosis. Mumps virus can be grown during the acute illness from saliva, throat washings, or a swab of the Stensen's duct orifice. Virus can be isolated from the cerebrospinal fluid for the first 3–4 days of the meningeal illness.

Mumps virus contains several different antigenic components, which provoke distinct antibodies. The most important are haemagglutinin-neuraminidase protein (V antigen) and the nucleocapsid protein (S antigen). S antibody rises in the first 2 weeks of infection but then declines rapidly. V antibody appears at the end of the first week, usually in high titre; it may persist for years and is an index of past infection. Neutralizing antibodies also develop. Nowadays, sensitive enzyme-linked immunosorbent assays allow early diagnosis by detection of mumps-specific IgM and IgA. IgA can be detected in saliva or mouth washings on about the fourth day after infection, and in the serum early in the disease.

Treatment

There is no specific treatment. Symptomatic treatment includes simple analgesics, but for the severe pain of orchitis, morphia (15–30 mg) may be required for a day or two. Corticosteroids are worth trying in severe cases of parotitis, more especially in orchitis. A dose of 300 mg cortisone or its equivalent daily for 2–3 days sometimes give dramatic relief from pain though it may not reduce the swelling.

Prevention and control

Isolation is not effective as the patient has been infectious for days before parotitis occurs and inapparent cases are frequent, but attenuated live vaccine, gives 95 per cent seroconversion, and protects for at least 15 years. In developed countries, mumps vaccine is given between 14 and 16 months of age as one component of a trivalent mumps–measles–rubella (MMR) vaccine with live attenuated strains of all three viruses. This has succeeded in suppressing the incidence of mumps by > 98 per cent in the US and UK. This is contraindicated in patients with immunodeficiency due to immunosuppressive therapy or disease, but HIV seropositive children should be vaccinated with the MMR vaccine.

Further reading

Christie, A.B. (1980). *Infectious diseases: epidemiology and clinical practice*, 3rd edn. Churchill Livingstone, Edinburgh.

Feldman, H.A. (1989). Mumps. In *Viral infections of humans*, 3rd edn (ed. A.J. Evans), pp. 471–91. Plenum Medical, New York.

Rima, B.K. (1994). Mumps virus. In *Encyclopedia of virology* (ed. R.G. Webster and A. Granoff), pp. 876–83. Academic Press, London.

Wolinsky, J.S. (1996). Mumps virus. In *Virology*, 3rd edn (ed. B.N. Fields, D.M. Knipe, P.M. Howley), pp. 1243–65. Lipincott-Raven, Philadelphia.

Chapter 16.20

Measles

H. C. Whittle and P. Aaby

Measles is an acute, highly transmissible, human viral infection causing much death and suffering, especially among children of the developing world. Its severity varies according to host and socioeconomic factors, not to antigenic variation or alteration in virulence of the virus. There is no reservoir of infection other than man and no evidence of a carrier state. The virus causes a generalized infection coupled with severe immunosuppression. The chief clinical features result from infection of the skin, mucous membranes, and respiratory tract. Global coverage by measles immunization has now increased to 80 per cent, with a corresponding drop in deaths to 900 000 annually which is still unacceptably high.

Aetiology

Measles, a paramyxovirus that contains a single strand of RNA, is highly pleomorphic, with diameter 100–300 nm. The virus propagates by budding from the cell membrane, from which it acquires an envelope. The membrane of infected cells and the virion envelope contain two surface glycoproteins, the haemagglutinin (**H**) and fusion

(F) proteins, and a non-glycosylated matrix (M) protein, which forms the inner layer. The H protein, which allows attachment of the virus to cells, is the main target for neutralizing antibodies; the F protein is responsible for fusion and syncytium formation of infected cells. The internal components or nucleocapsid consist of RNA, the nucleoprotein (N), which is the major protein, the phosphoprotein (P), and the large protein (L).

Epidemiology

The epidemiology of this global infection varies markedly between developed and developing countries. In the developed world most children are infected between 3 and 6 years of age, when in nursery or primary schools. Mortality is low (<0.05 per cent) with most cases occurring in the winter and spring. Recently the biannual epidemicity has been influenced by widespread immunization which has dramatically reduced both the number of cases and the frequency of complications.

In the developing world, measles is severe and different: it kills between 3 and 15 per cent of children in the community and some 10–20 per cent of those admitted to hospital. Mortality from measles is considerably higher among rural than urban populations, particularly in isolated villages. Measles also has a higher fatality rate in children with chronic disease, including kwashiorkor, tuberculosis, and HIV infection.

There are many reasons for the greater in severity in the developing world, including young age at infection, severe malnutrition, and overcrowding. Exposure to a large dose of the virus when in close contact with the index case may be an important factor, as secondary and tertiary cases in large families are at high risk of dying. Severity and mortality of secondary cases depends on the severity of the infecting case. The much higher mortality found in West Africa is likely to be a result of the very large polygynous and extended families which increase the risk of intensive exposure.

Acute measles is often less severe among children under 6 months of age, among previously immunized children, and among those who have received immunoglobulin when exposed. The course of infection in these subjects, which is modified by antibody, is characterized by a prolonged incubation period, a short prodrome, mild symptoms, and a favourable outcome.

Pathogenesis and the immune response

The course of infection and the immune response to this invasion are shown in Fig. 1. The measles virus, which is thermolabile and survives best at low humidities, is spread to susceptible contacts in droplets during sneezing and coughing. First it infects and multiplies in the epithelium of the upper respiratory tract or the conjunctivae. Some 4–6 days later the virus is found in the reticuloendothelial tissue of the liver and the spleen after passage through lymph nodes and spread by the blood. Here it multiplies. Around day 8 the measles virus is carried by the blood, either free or in mononuclear cells, to the target tissues which are the epithelia of the eye, lung, and gut. Again, the agent multiplies to cause bright redness of the mucosa and Koplik's spots which are the foci of viral multiplication.

The rash, appearing around days 14–16, is in fact the sign of a strong and complicated allergic reaction to the virus in the epithelia. The extent and severity of the rash, which is a good index of the clinical severity of the disease, is determined by the number of cells

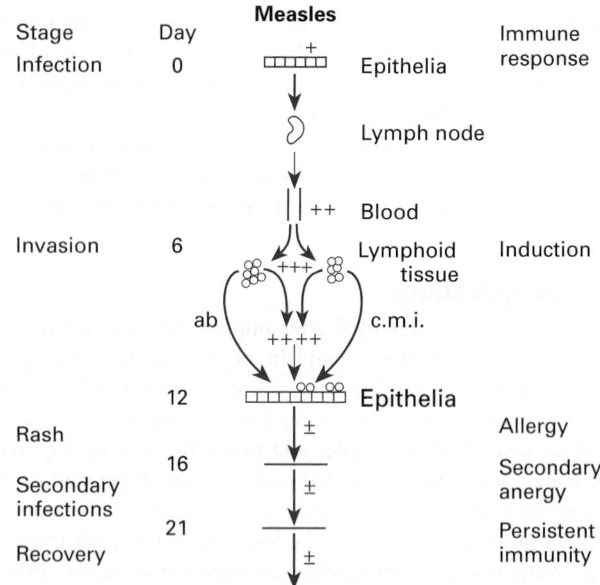

Fig. 1 Pathogenesis of measles. + Denotes amount of virus, ab = antibody.
(Reproduced from Parry (1984). Principles of medicine in Africa, (2nd edn). Oxford University Press, Oxford.)

infected. An intact cell-mediated immune response is essential to generate the rash and clear the virus, for if impaired, as in the case of children with leukaemia, or occasionally in severe kwashiokor, the virus multiplies unchecked and no rash appears. Two or three days after the start of the rash, around day 17 or 18, the virus can no longer be cultured in the epithelia, for infected cells have been disrupted and the free virus neutralized by antibody. There is a switch towards a type 2 helper T lymphocyte response with consequent loss of delayed hypersensitivity reactions and potential reactivation of viruses such as Herpes simplex or intracellular bacteria such as *M. tuberculosis* which are held in check by cellular immune responses. These changes are particularly marked in malnourished children or those with advanced HIV infection who already have marked defects in cell mediated immunity.

By the third week, day 21, as the patient recovers, antibody is in full production. Levels remain elevated for the rest of the patient's life, either because of repeated subclinical infections or because the virus persists in latent form in the spleen and other organs, so stimulating antibody. A study from Guinea-Bissau has suggested that measles may have a long-term impact on the immune system as young adults who had had clinical measles were less likely to be atopic compared to vaccinated children who had not had the disease.

Clinical features and complications

The clinical features of measles and some complications are shown in Fig. 2.

Prodrome (days 10–14)

Diagnosis is often missed at this stage, when fever coupled with a runny nose and sometimes complicated by convulsions is the main feature. Other signs are mild conjunctivitis, red mucosa, Koplik's spots, and diarrhoea. Koplik's spots are found in the buccal mucosa. They are small irregular spots of bright red colour; in the centre of each is seen a bluish-white speck.

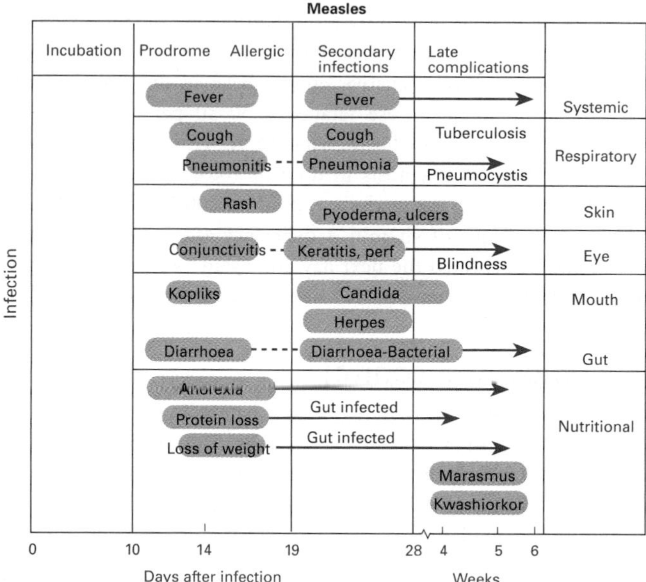

Fig. 2 Clinical features of measles and some of its complications. *(Reproduced from Parry (1984). Principles of medicine in Africa, (2nd edn). Oxford University Press, Oxford.)*

Rash (days 14–18)

The morbilliform rash first appears on the forehead and neck and then spreads, over a period of 3–4 days, to involve trunk and finally limbs. In Africa and other parts of the developing world, the rash is often red, confluent, raised, very extensive, and sometimes accompanied by bleeding into the skin and gut. Later the rash blackens, then the skin peels causing extensive desquamation. Other epithelial surfaces are inflamed, the severity matching that of the rash. Cough, a cardinal sign, may be hoarse, and coupled with difficulty of inspiration if the larynx and trachea are inflamed. Signs of pneumonitis are apparent, which in severe cases may cause cyanosis or be complicated by mediastinal and subcutaneous emphysema. Conjunctivitis, especially in those who are vitamin A deficient, can be severe; enteritis may cause profuse diarrhoea with resulting loss of protein, and malabsorption of food and water. The mouth is painful and red, which adds to the misery of the child, who becomes anorexic and may even refuse to suck the breast. In the uncomplicated case, as is usual in the West, the convalescent period is short, usually lasting less than a week. If fever persists, while the rash is fading or desqamating, complications should be suspected.

Early complications (day 18–30)

As a result of the widespread severe allergic reaction to the measles virus signified by the rash, the patient is left severely immunosuppressed and is susceptible to infection.

Pneumonia causes most deaths and is heralded by a rise in fever, leucocytosis, and respiratory difficulties. Lobar pneumonia is usually caused by *Strep. pneumoniae* but bronchopneumonia, which is more common, results from other bacteria, such as *Staphylococcus aureus*, or secondary viral infections such as with Herpes simplex or adenovirus. A variety of other organisms such as Gram-negative bacteria, cytomegalovirus, fungi, *M. tuberculosis*, and *Pneumocystitis carinii* should be considered as potential pathogens of the lung in the malnourished or immunocompromised child.

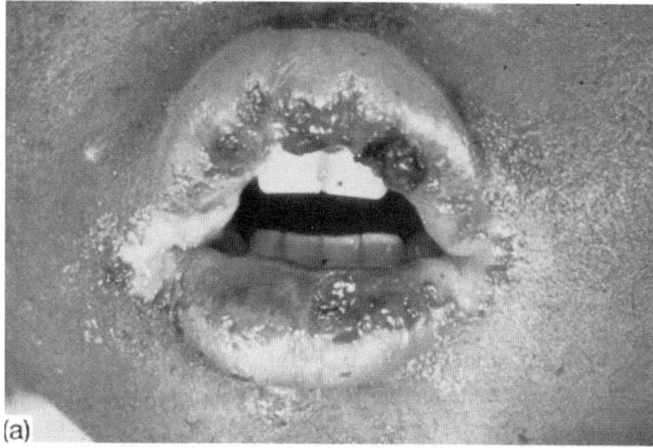

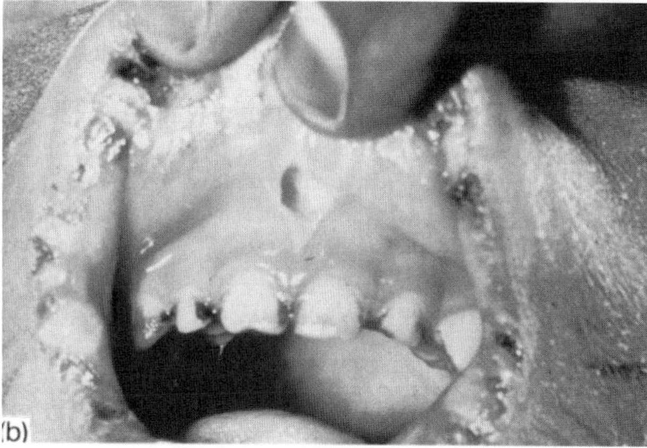

Fig. 3 Herpes simplex ulceration of lips and gingiva following measles.

Chronic diarrhoea and a sore mouth caused by Candida infection are common complications of measles in children in the developing world. The gut is often superinfected with Bacteroides, *Escherichia coli*, Pseudomonas, and *Staph. aureus*, which results in malabsorption and protein loss. Deep ulcers caused by Herpes simplex virus erode the corners of the mouth, gums, and inner surface of the lips causing much misery, illness, and pain (Fig. 3).

Corneal ulceration leading to impaired vision or blindness is common after measles, especially in malnourished and vitamin A-deficient children. Several studies from Africa have shown that more than half of childhood blindness is related to measles. The causes are multiple: measles itself can erode the cornea as does Herpes simplex which is reactivated during measles, and bacterial superinfection is common especially in vitamin A deficient children.

Pyoderma is common after measles. In the malnourished, deep eroding ulcers may bore through the skin even into bone (cancrum oris, noma). Otitis media is also common.

Encephalitis

This is a rare but much feared complication found in approximately 1–2 per 1000 cases. The onset is usually between 4 and 7 days after the start of the rash but rarely it may occur within 48 hours or up to 2 weeks from the onset. In addition to seizures there is often fever, irritability, headache, and a disturbance in consciousness that may progress to profound coma.

Late complications

Malnutrition is the most frequent complication, for children of the developing world often lose much weight during measles and may take many weeks to regain it. Those originally underweight who have had severe measles are at greatest risk, for in these children anorexia is prolonged, much protein is lost from the gut, and secondary infections, which lead to marasmus or marasmic kwashiorkor, are frequent. Measles has been shown to persist in the epithelia and lymphocytes of the severely malnourished for 30 or more days after the rash.

Giant-cell pneumonia is found in patients with defects in cell-mediated immunity: children with leukaemia or kwashiorkor are particularly vulnerable. The lung disease may develop weeks after measles, and in most cases the rash of measles has been absent and thus the diagnosis may not be suspected. The diagnosis is made by virological and histological examination of lung tissue. Most of these children die.

Subacute sclerosing panencephalitis (SSPE) is a rare complication caused by persistent measles virus infection of the brain. The child with SSPE has usually experienced normal measles, albeit at a young age, 5–10 years earlier. The first indication is a disturbance in intellect and personality. There then follows seizures akin to myoclonus, signs of extrapyramidal and pyramidal disease, and finally a state of decerebrate rigidity followed by death.

Laboratory diagnosis

In the prodromal phase, and within 3 days of the onset of the rash, measles virus or its antigens can be detected in scrapings from buccal mucosa or in the cells from a nasophyngeal aspirate. The simplest test is to stain cells from these specimens with Leishmann's stain and examine for giant cells under a microscope. Immunofluorescent staining, which is more sensitive, can also be used. The diagnosis can also be made by demonstrating a fourfold or greater rise in antibody titre between the acute and convalescent phase of measles 4–6 weeks later. A variety of tests including the plaque reduction neutralizing test, the most sensitive, and ELISA kits which measure either IgM or IgG antibody are available. A single acute phase blood sample with a high level of measles IgM antibody suggests the diagnosis.

Treatment of measles and its complications

No effective antimeasles drug exists, yet some children do benefit from treatment in hospital. The following criteria indicate severe measles and a need for admission: a widespread, confluent rash darkening to deep red or purple; signs of laryngeal obstruction of subcutaneous emphysema; marked dehydration; blood in the stool or more than five stools a day; convulsions or loss of consciousness; severe secondary pneumonia; corneal ulceration or severe ulceration of the mouth and skin. These signs should be taken particularly seriously when the child in underweight or frankly malnourished.

Hydrate the child orally or intravenously. Treat lobar pneumonia with benzylpenicillin, and bronchopneumonia with combined antibiotics such as gentamicin and cloxacillin, or with co-trimoxazole or amoxycillin. Antibiotic eye ointments relieve discomfort and possibly prevent secondary infections of measles conjunctivitis. Antibiotics, topical and systemic, and vitamin A should be given routinely for eye ulcers. If Herpes simplex virus is the cause, use acyclovir topically or, when severe, systemically. Candida infections of the mouth or gut often respond dramatically to nystatin. Feeding, by tube if necessary, needs careful planning and presentation, for the anorexic infected child will be in severe negative energy balance due to a greatly increased catabolic rate. Case fatality is 30–50 per cent lower in children in hospital treated with vitamin A. This should be given orally at the time of diagnosis in dose of 100 000 i.u. for children below 12 months of age and in a dose of 200 000 i.u. for older children. If eye signs of vitamin A deficiency are present the initial dose should be repeated the next day and again 1–4 weeks later. No specific effective treatment exists for encephalitis or SSPE.

Prevention and control

Passive immunization with human immunoglobulin is highly effective if given within 2 or 3 days of exposure, in a dose for children of 0.2 ml/kg. Immunoglobulin should be given to those for whom vaccination is contraindicated: children immunosuppressed by kwashiorkor, by malignancies such as leukaemia or lymphoma, or by steroids or cytotoxic drugs. Passive immunization is also used to protect the pregnant and those with active tuberculosis.

The currently used vaccines are live strains, attenuated by culture in chick fibroblasts. The complications of vaccination are few and generally mild. Fever of moderate severity is infrequent, and a mild rash with some signs of upper respiratory tract infection occurs rarely. Underweight children respond normally to the vaccine as do ill children in the outpatient department and on the ward. As clinics and hospitals are major sites of transmission of the virus in the developing world, all susceptible children in these places, unless seriously immunocompromised as in leukaemia or kwashiorkor, should be vaccinated.

The optimal age for vaccination in the developed world is 14–16 months, when maternal antibody, which neutralizes the virus to cause vaccine failure, has disappeared. This counsel does not apply to children in the developing world, because there measles infects at an early age. WHO recommends one measles vaccination at 9 months of age. However, in the future it may be necessary to immunize earlier because mothers who were immunized in childhood transfer fewer antibodies to their children who will therefore become susceptible at an earlier age. With improvements in measles control and reduction in exposure to the natural virus, antibody levels will decrease more rapidly in the future. It may become necessary to introduce multiple dose schedules to prevent the re-emergence of measles outbreaks.

Some have argued that measles vaccines will have a limited impact on childhood survival, for disadvantaged children, saved from measles by vaccination, will only die at a later date from other infections or malnutrition. However, a variety of epidemiological studies has documented remarkable reductions in mortality after standard measles vaccine. In Bangladesh, measles vaccination was associated with a 36 per cent reduction in all-cause mortality from the age of 9 months despite the fact that acute measles only accounted for 4 per cent of deaths in the community. The reason for this unexpected benefit is unknown.

New vaccines, which can be given in infancy, or new double-dose strategies using the standard vaccine at 6 and 9 months will be necessary to contain measles in the developing world. Eradication, which has nearly been achieved in the USA by insistence that children be immunized before going to school, will be difficult on a global scale because measles is highly infectious. One-dose schedules with current vaccines are inadequate because too few get immunized and vaccine efficacy is often low. New vaccines which could be given earlier and have a better efficacy may be necessary for measles eradication but Latin America has accomplished a high degree of measles control by immunization of all children in national immunization days. The future of measles may well depend on whether the current drive to eradicate polio is successful thus demonstrating to the international community that eradication can be accomplished.

Further reading

Aaby P., *et al.* (1995). Non specific beneficial effects of measles immunization: analysis of mortality studies from developing countries. *British Medical Journal,* **311**, 481–5.

Fenner, F. (1948). The pathogenesis of the acute exanthems. An interpretation based on experimental investigations with mouse-pox (infectious ectromelia of mice). *Lancet,* **ii**, 915–20.

Hussey, G.D. and Klein, M. (1990). A randomized, controlled trial of vitamin A in children wih severe measles. *New England Journal of Medicine,* **323**, 160–4.

Morley, D. (1969). Severe measles in the tropics. *British Medical Journal,* **1**, 297–300: 363–5.

Whittle, H.C., Dossetor, J., Oduluju, A., Bryceson, A.D.M., and Greenwood, B.M. (1978). Cell-mediated immunity during natural measles infection. *Journal of Clinical Investigation,* **62**, 678–84.

Chapter 16.21

Nipah virus

M. J. Warrell

Nipah virus was discovered as the cause of an outbreak of febrile encephalitis and respiratory infection in peninsular Malaysia in 1998–99. Among 257 cases of febrile encephalitis, 100 deaths were attributed to the infection, of which 65 were confirmed serologically. Infection was related to contact with pigs, and nearly 1 000 000 animals were slaughtered to control the outbreak. No human-to-human transmission was reported.

The clinical features may be confused with Japanese encephalitis, occurring in the same area, and also transmitted from pigs. Dual infection has been suspected. Nipah virus is a paramyxovirus, related to Hendra virus, an Australian encephalitic equine morbillivirus, which also causes human disease. The natural host may be fruit bats (*Pteropus* spp.).

Further reading

Centers for Disease Control Update (1999). Outbreak of Nipah virus—Malaysia and Singapore, 1999. *Mortality and Morbidity Weekly Reports,* **48**(6), 335–7.

Chapter 16.22

Enteroviruses

N. R. Grist

Enteroviruses are common infectious agents which cause a variety of clinical syndromes (Table 1). They are typical picornaviruses, stable, resistant to treatment with deoxycholate, ether, and other fat solvents, and acid (pH 3 for 1 h). They survive for long periods in water at low temperature but are inactivated by drying or exposure to heat (50°C for 1 h) or free residual chlorine (0.3–0.5 ppm). The numerous enterovirus types affecting humans are classified as polioviruses (causing paralytic disease in primates); coxsackieviruses, which cause paralysis in newborn mice with severe myositis (Group A) or damage to brain and viscera (Group B); echoviruses (not usually pathogenic for mice but grown in cell cultures); and more recently discovered enterovirus types, which may share some of these properties (Table 1). Enterovirus Type 72 (hepatitis A) is not considered here (see Chapter 16.34).

Epidemiology

Antibody responses to first infections in life are typespecific. Serological cross-reactions are common in older children and adults because some antigens are shared by different enteroviruses. Post-infectious immunity to the same serotype of enterovirus is good. Transient reinfections of the gut by poliovirus of a type to which the individual already has antibody are not uncommon, showing that 'gut immunity' is neither absolute nor permanent. Vaccination alters the situation for poliomyelitis. Circulation of 'wild' polioviruses in crowded tropical populations may continue, with unvaccinated individuals or groups vulnerable to infection. In incompletely, though well-vaccinated, populations, pockets of unvaccinated, non-immune persons may support sporadic outbreaks of poliomyelitis. Urbanization of populations from isolated rural areas of developing countries

Table 1 The enteroviruses

Group	Major disease
Poliovirus types 1–3	Paralytic poliomyelitis Viral ('aseptic') meningitis
Coxsackievirus types A1–24*	Viral ('aseptic') meningitis Herpangina Hand, foot, and mouth disease Conjunctivitis (type A24)
Coxsackievirus types B1–B6	Viral ('aseptic') meningitis Pleurodynia (Bornholm disease) Myo/pericarditis Fatal neonatal disease
Echovirus types 1–34*	Viral ('aseptic') meningitis Skin rashes Febrile illness
Enterovirus types 68–72*	Conjunctivitis (type 70) Poliomyelitis-like disease (type 71) Hepatitis (type 72)

*Coxsackie A23 = echovirus 9; coxsackie A24 = echovirus 34; echovirus 10 = reovirus 1; echovirus 28 = reovirus 1; enterovirus 72 = hepatitis A.

Table 2 Main pattern of infection by a typical enterovirus

Portals of entry

- Oral
- Respiratory

Primary site of multiplication

- Pharynx
- Alimentary tract
- Viraemia—in some cases

Secondary sites of viral multiplication and damage

- CNS (meningitis, poliomyelitis, encephalitis)
- Heart (myocarditis, pericarditis)
- Muscles (Bornholm disease)
- Skin and mucosae (exanthem; enanthem)
- Respiratory tract (upper; lower)
- Liver (hepatitis A)
- Liver, pancreas, and other viscera in generalized infections—mainly in infants

Portals of exit

- Faeces
- Pharyngeal and respiratory secretions

provides opportunities for epidemic spread among persons not previously exposed to the particular poliovirus (or other enterovirus). Thus the epidemiological situation of the world is complex and unstable, requiring constant surveillance and efficient use of polioviral vaccines.

Pathogenesis (Table 2)

After infection by the oral or respiratory route, usually silent, viraemic spread to other organs may lead to their infection and damage, directly by cytolytic and/or immune mechanisms. Most infections are acute, terminated by the immune response but often with residual damage (e.g. anterior horn motoneurone deaths in acute anterior poliomyelitis). Immunological reactions may contribute to the damage, for example to the myocardium, and there is growing interest in possible chronic viral persistence in some diseases.

Clinical features

Many infections are silent, trivial, and transient in effect, causing a small proportion of febrile sore throats, with or without rhinitis, mainly in children, especially in summer and autumn. During outbreaks, some of these may show more specific and serious features.

Mucocutaneous syndromes

These are not uncommon in young children. Enteroviral enanthems include *herpangina* (with fever, headache, sore throat, and painful aphthous ulcers on reddened fauces and soft palate, mainly due to coxsackie A viruses), and *hand, foot, and mouth disease* (mainly in children infected with coxsackievirus A16 or enterovirus 71, similar to herpangina but small maculopapular or vesicular lesions appear on palms, soles, and sometimes other skin areas). Various transient erythematous skin rashes may accompany enteroviral infections of young children, usually with fever, sometimes in outbreaks, often with aseptic meningitis, especially in adults. Echovirus 9 can cause such outbreaks, fever, and rash in children, often resembling rubella.

Neurological diseases (see also Chapter 13.26)

Acute paralytic poliomyelitis was the first enteroviral disease to be recognized, caused by polioviruses but also occasionally by coxsackie A7, enterovirus Type 71, or rarely other enteroviruses. Typically, a minor febrile illness with sore throat is followed by abrupt onset of more serious neurological disease—viral meningitis—which may resolve or be complicated by development of flaccid (lower motoneurone) paralysis, usually asymmetrical, of some or many muscles in one or more limbs and the trunk (perhaps including intercostals and diaphragm) sometimes with life-threatening respiratory paralysis. The most severe and dangerous form involves the brainstem, cranial nerve nuclei, respiratory, and circulatory centres. Death may result from respiratory or circulatory failure, or obstruction of airways by saliva and mucus if swallowing and clearing the pharynx become difficult.

Aseptic meningitis (benign lymphocytic meningitis; viral meningitis). This condition, which outnumbers bacterial meningitis, is most often due to enteroviruses. During outbreaks, some associated cases show features varying according to the enterovirus concerned—for instance, acute flaccid paralysis in poliovirus outbreaks, skin rash (echovirus 9 and echovirus infections in young children), myalgia, or myocarditis (especially in coxsackie B infections of adults). A brief febrile prodrome may precede sudden onset of fever, headache, sore throat, and stiff neck with lymphocytic pleocytosis of spinal fluid (maybe transient polymorph preponderance in the earliest stage, especially in echovirus 9 infection). Illness usually subsides within a week with complete recovery.

Encephalitis. This, with or without neurological sequelae, is a rare complication mainly of severe neonatal infections with coxsackieviruses, and is also seen in enterovirus 71 and polioviral epidemics.

Myalgic encephalomyelitis ('ME'); postviral fatigue syndrome (see also Chapter 16.118). Suggestions of a viral cause for some cases of this controversial syndrome are supported by reports of coxsackie B infection in some outbreaks, of persistent enterovirus excretion, and of enteroviral RNA sequences in some muscle biopsies.

Diseases of heart and muscle

Coxsackieviruses, especially type B, can damage muscles in humans as well as in newborn mice. *Myocarditis and pericarditis.* Acute 'myopericarditis', usually due to Type B coxsackievirus infection, presents mainly as myocarditis in young children, or pericarditis in older children and adults. In early childhood, prodromal fever and throat congestion may precede major illness, with dyspnoea and weakness, tachycardia, and sometimes heart block. Myocarditis may be fatal in the acute stage or after some months of persisting failure but most children recover completely, sometimes with constrictive pericarditis as a late sequel in older children.

Carditis in older children and adults. Pericarditis may be associated with Bornholm disease. Its onset may be sudden, with fever, precordial pain and dyspnoea, irregular pulse, and pericardial effusion (sometimes recurrent). Constrictive pericarditis is a rare late sequel. Associated myocarditis may be severe and febrile with congestive failure, slow to recover or with relapses for months or years, sometimes fatal. Chronic congestive cardiomyopathy may be a late complication, with or without a history of the acute infective disease.

Myositis: Bornholm disease; epidemic pleurodynia/myalgia. This affects mainly children or young adults, sporadically or in outbreaks with sudden onset of severe localized pain in abdomen or chest, with muscle tenderness, usually unilateral and possibly suggesting appendicitis in children, pneumothorax or cardiac infarction. Fever, headache, and sore throat are common, but nausea and vomiting are unusual. Myocarditis may be associated. Full recovery is usual in a week or two, sometimes with relapses.

Disease of gastrointestinal tract and associated organs

Enteroviruses do not appear to cause *diarrhoea*, but are often detectable as 'passengers' in such conditions. *Hepatitis* can be a feature of acute generalized coxsackie B infections of infants, but otherwise only type 72 enterovirus ('hepatitis A' virus; see Chapter 16.34) is a significant cause of liver disease. *Pancreatitis is* a rare complication of coxsackievirus B infections, but there is growing evidence of *insulin-dependent diabetes mellitus* as a late consequence of infection in persons with certain HLA serotypes.

Picornavirus epidemic conjunctivitis

Epidemic conjunctivitis due to coxsackievirus A24 and the more severe *acute haemorrhagic conjunctivitis* caused by coxsackievirus type 70 have produced epidemics in Africa, South-East Asia, and elsewhere. Spread by eye–hand–fomite routes, these diseases are temporarily incapacitating but complete recovery is usual. Occasional neurological complications of enterovirus 70 have been reported.

Other enteroviral diseases

Perinatal and neonatal infections

Viraemic infections in pregnancy may reach the fetus, with effects ranging from absence of obvious disease to severe generalized infection, usually by coxsackie B viruses, affecting particularly the liver, nervous system, and heart. Presentation with fever, gastrointestinal disturbances, lethargy or irritability, or even convulsions, often with skin rash, sometimes with disseminated intravascular coagulation and haemorrhages, can resemble bacterial sepsis; polymorph leucocytosis is common. Heart, brain, liver, lungs, and other organs may be affected. Later in infancy meningitis and acute carditis are the main manifestations of enterovirus infection, which more often cause only minor or respiratory illness. *Orchitis* and *parotitis* are occasional complications of coxsackievirus B infections.

Pathology

Most enteroviral infections are non-fatal. Pathological studies are therefore limited to fatal cases. In these, necrosis of infected cells in target organs (Table 2) with inflammatory infiltrates are characteristic. In fatal paralytic poliomyelitis, the acute stage shows death of neurones in grey matter, especially motoneurones of the anterior horn of the spinal cord. Loss of corresponding axons and atrophy of related muscle fibres correspond to partial or complete paralysis. Degeneration and death of myocardial cells is seen in carditis, with prominent infiltration by chronic inflammatory cells.

Laboratory diagnosis

Virus may be detected in faeces, cerebrospinal fluid (rarely poliovirus), throat swab (in virus transport medium), or tissue biopsy, by isolation in cell culture (or inoculation of newborn mice for many coxsackie A viruses), or by the polymerase chain reaction (which can detect those enteroviruses not identified by current isolation methods). Specific neutralizing antibody may be detected in blood serum (preferably two samples at a 10-day interval); specific IgM may be detected in acute-phase serum. In cases of acute flaccid paralysis possibly due to poliovirus, full investigation should be undertaken to distinguish infection by viruses other than enterovirus, enteroviruses other than poliovirus, type of poliovirus, and whether vaccine-derived, or unrelated disease such as Guillain–Barré syndrome. The local virus laboratory should be asked for advice on available tests.

Treatment

This is supportive and symptomatic in most cases but supplemented by special measures in acute flaccid paralysis (usually paralytic poliovirus disease) and life-threatening bulbar paralysis which can require intensive life-supporting measures to sustain respiration and maintain clear airways. Subsequent paralysis of muscle groups can cripple and requires prolonged rehabilitation and orthopaedic measures.

Myocardial damage may occur during these severe illnesses, needing careful monitoring, rest, and cautious convalescence. Myopericarditis in other cases also requires care, appropriate support, sometimes pericardial tap in the event of tamponade, and follow-up in case constrictive paricarditis develops and requires surgical relief.

Prognosis

This is generally good. After acute paralytic poliomyelitis, considerable recovery of weak muscles is usual with slow improvement over several months after acute illness. Crippling may be severe and lasting, however, and weakness of affected muscles may recur in later life. Orthopaedic management can be essential. Some severe cases of bulbar paralysis may permanently require life-support systems to maintain breathing and some other functions in patients who survive the acute illness. Non-paralytic 'aseptic meningitis' usually improves completely after one or more weeks, sometimes with residual headaches for a while. Acute myositis generally resolves in a few weeks, occasionally with relapses. In young children recovery from acute myocarditis is usually complete without sequels, but more lasting and chronic heart disease sometimes affects adults.

Prevention and control

In general, good hygiene and sanitation, avoiding consumption of faecally polluted food and drink, and avoiding contagion from likely excreters (e.g. young and sick children) reduce the chance of infection, but may be difficult to achieve in many developing or deprived communities.

Vaccines against poliovirus infection can both protect individuals and eradicate this crippling disease from communities, as already achieved in the Americas. All three serotypes of poliovirus are present in the vaccines which are of two types: live, attenuated vaccine (OPV) and (enhanced) inactivated vaccine (eIPV) (see also Chapter 16.6). OPV is given by mouth in 3 monthly doses from 2 months of age (plus a preliminary dose at birth in endemic areas), with follow-up doses at school entry and in adult life if exposed to risk. It is effective in temperate climates, but variably so in the tropics. It is also safe, with rare cases where limited virulence has been regained during infection of the vaccinee which may cause disease in close non-immune contacts. OPV has been the type recommended (for price, simplicity, and effectiveness) by the WHO in its eradication campaigns. eIPV is given in 2 doses at 2-month intervals (with later doses at school entry and if exposed to infection). It is more expensive, requires injection, and gives less mucosal immunity, but is preferred by some industrialized countries where infection has been controlled to low level or eradicated (protection is still necessary until global eradication has been achieved). Thus the USA now recommends sequential vaccination by eIPV at ages 2 months and 4 months followed by OPV at ages 12–18 months and 4–6 years. eIPV can be given at the same time as routine inactivated antibacterial vaccines (DPT). Combined schedules of inactivated and oral attenuated poliovirus vaccine have given safe, effective protection in high-risk areas, overcoming limitations of either type alone in high-risk, tropical areas. Careful surveillance remains essential until the eradication programme has succeeded, reporting all cases of 'AFP' (acute flaccid paralysis) and subjecting these to virological testing to confirm the identity of the infecting virus (polio or other; 'wild' virulent or vaccine-derived poliovirus). Antibody surveys of populations show their immune status and may reveal vulnerable, non-immune groups requiring immunization.

Further reading

Riding, M.H., Stewart, J., Clements, G.B., and Galbraith, D.N. (1996). Enteroviral polymerase chain reaction in the investigation of aseptic meningitis. *Journal of Medical Virology*, **50**, 204–6.

WHO Collaborative Study Group on Oral and Inactivated Vaccines (1996). Combined immunization of infants with oral and inactivated poliovirus vaccines: results of a randomized trial in the Gambia, Oman, and Thailand. *Bulletin of the World Health Organization*, **74**, 253–68.

Chapter 16.23

Viruses causing diarrhoea and vomiting

C. R. Madeley

Introduction

Viruses probably account for nearly half the episodes of diarrhoea in infants and young children, particularly in the poorer, overcrowded parts of the world. The list of new viruses has gradually lengthened, helped by finding similar viruses in the faeces of domestic animals with diarrhoea, all of which have been shown to be infected by their own rotaviruses.

These gastroenteropathy viruses are responsible for considerable morbidity throughout the world and mortality in poor tropical areas where malnutrition is common and sanitation poor.

Epidemiology

Gastroenteropathy viruses have been found throughout the world and, in temperate climes, are more common in winter, but what triggers their activity is unknown. A wave of rotavirus infection has been charted across the US, usually from west to east, and probably represents person-to-person spread. During the season, any of the viruses (see OTM, p. 391, Table 1) may be found but, in general, rotaviruses outnumber the others by about 4:1. Adenoviruses are often the second most common but there are variations between one country and another for reasons which are also unknown.

Outbreaks of vomiting and diarrhoea, which are often shellfish- or water-borne (see also Chapter 18.2), are common throughout the world but are better documented in the developed world. Such outbreaks are usually associated with schools, old people's homes, social events, or cruise liners. Endemic activity has also been noted. They are usually self-limiting, severe only in those with pre-existing disease, and rarely fatal.

Disease associated with stool viruses

These viruses have been found in stools of babies and young children suffering from a range of symptoms; very mild with 'normal' stool to severe watery diarrhoea with vomiting. With such variation in severity, it is not possible to define a syndrome peculiar to each virus. There is now some evidence that severity due to rotaviruses varies according to whether a virus-coded protein is expressed. Strains found in newborn nurseries frequently lack this protein and appear to be less virulent as a result.

The associated disease consists of passive loose or watery stools of abrupt onset, often but not invariably associated with vomiting. Usually self-limiting with a peak incidence in children between 12 and 18 months, it affects both sexes equally. Loss of fluid may induce dehydration particularly in tropical climates where most deaths occur. There may be a low-grade pyrexia. Transmission is mostly faecal–oral but droplet and fomite spread may also occur. These infections are difficult to contain even with barrier nursing, and carriage by asymptomatic adults cannot be ruled out. A lack of sensitivity in diagnostic methods makes epidemiological tracing difficult.

Viruses involved

Rotavirus

This is a comparatively large virus (see Table 1, OTM3, p. 391) with a characteristic structure recognized readily by electron microscopy. It has been found to be endemic in every country in which it has been sought and similar viruses have been found to infect every investigated animal species, both domestic and wild. Its ease of detection has tended to concentrate attention on it possibly to the exclusion of other viruses which are smaller and more difficult to recognize.

Although associated with diarrhoea, rotaviruses have also been found in asymptomatic babies and newborn animals. Recent evidence incriminating a virus 'toxin' suggests that different strains vary in their virulence. If so, serological surveys suggest that avirulent strains are probably very common as antibody to the virus is acquired by 80–100 per cent of the population by the age of 3 years wherever serosurveys have been done. This suggests that virulent strains may be in the minority.

Rotaviruses of humans and animals can be classified into six groups (A–F), and Group A can be divided into two subgroups (I and II). At least 9 serotypes exist in Group A but only Groups A–C have been found in man. Rotaviruses can be further subdivided on the basis of additional tests and it is becoming clear that their antigenic structure is complex. This becomes important when a vaccine is being considered (see below).

Astrovirus

These are spherical particles with a 5–6-point surface star visible on about 10 per cent. They are identified less frequently (about 10 per cent of that of rotaviruses), but their capacity for causing disease and high seroprevalence parallels that of rotaviruses. Animal strains have also been noted (lamb, pig, calf, etc.). It is probably underdiagnosed.

Calicivirus

Initial reports linked this virus with outbreaks of winter and summer vomiting. Prevalence is probably seasonal and serosurveys also show that it is more common than the comparatively few positive identifications suggest.

Other small spherical viruses

Stool samples may also contain other virus-like particles which appear to be spherical. Some are featureless spheres (small round viruses, SRVs) and others have a rough or 'hairy' surface (small round structured viruses, SRSVs).

SRSVs

Norwalk was first identified in a school outbreak in Ohio in 1970. Other viruses similar in appearance, but antigenically distinct, have been found associated with outbreaks of vomiting and diarrhoea throughout the world. They probably represent different serotypes of essentially the same virus but show differences in genome sequences and cannot yet be classified together.

SRSVs are mostly associated with outbreaks although endemic cases occur (possibly 'seeding' outbreaks). They affect adults as well as children and serosurveys suggest that antibody is acquired later in life, allowing wider susceptibility into adulthood. Because they lack clear identifying features they are probably underreported, particularly in endemic situations. There are superficial resemblances to caliciviruses but the two are probably separate.

SRVs

These are found less frequently than the other viruses and because they, too, fail to grow in cell culture are probably underreported and underassessed. Where they have been associated with outbreaks their possible pathogenic role has been clearer.

Adenovirus

These illustrate the paradox of this topic well. Adenoviruses have been regularly isolated from stool specimens since the advent of cell cultures but these cultivable strains are rarely implicated in diarrhoea. Occasionally they have been the only virus in common source outbreaks but the evidence of causation is not convincing. Nonetheless, large numbers of typical adenovirus particles were found in some diarrhoeal stools by electron microscopy and later identified as types 40 and 41. Why these types are involved in diarrhoea is not known but they would appear to be more pathogenic for the gut than the common 'respiratory' adenoviruses (mostly types 1–7).

Pathology

Since infected patients rarely die, the pathology has been inferred from animal experiments. Most of these gut viruses damage the intestinal villi and cause the distal structure to slough. The residual stump then regenerates from the crypts and, because the damage is repaired quickly, the resultant malabsorption of both fluid and nutrients is rarely severe. It is not clear whether the damage is widespread at one time throughout the small bowel or progresses as a wave down the gut.

Laboratory diagnosis

The only method capable of detecting all known types of virus in a stool is electron microscopy and its use is essential in the investigation of any outbreaks of vomiting or diarrhoea. This technique suffers from the disadvantages of being both insensitive and labour-intensive in screening large numbers. Other methods based on antibodies have therefore been developed for some of these viruses, including detection of partial growth in cell culture by immunofluorescence, enzyme immunoassay, and latex agglutination. Commercial kits based on the last two are now available for rotaviruses and, to a lesser extent, adenoviruses. Antibody-based tests for some of the other viruses (Norwalk, astrovirus) have been developed but are not yet available commercially. Few laboratories can afford to repeat tests for each possible virus; many concentrate on rotaviruses alone. A stool specimen is always necessary for the detection of virus and attempts have been made to find virus in other body fluids and secretions, such as Norwalk and rotaviruses in vomitus.

Tests for antibody, including those for the different classes (IgG, IgM, and IgA), are available in some laboratories and seroconversion has been demonstrated. Whether this adds to the recognition of virus in the stool is debatable. It is certainly slower than EM.

It is difficult to interpret the results from one stool or one patient, so it is important to contact the laboratory before deciding to send specimens.

Treatment

There is no specific treatment of virus infection to the gut. Management of the diarrhoea depends on restoring hydration and electrolyte balance. This may be either by the use of oral fluids (solutions of glucose or sucrose plus electrolytes) or intravenous fluids if necessary as outlined elsewhere (see Chapter 5.1).

Prognosis

Provided hydration and calorie intake is maintained, these virus infections are unlikely to be fatal even in the face of substantial fluid loss. The duration, if any, of immunity is unclear and reinfections can occur.

Prevention and control

Considerable efforts, particularly in the US, to develop an adequate vaccine against rotavirus as the commonest cause have produced some evidence for protection but this has to be related to the severity of the challenge. In poorer parts of the world, these vaccines have worked less well but it is likely that one will be marketed in the US shortly. A variety of different serotypes must be covered. There are some doubts about whether circulating antibody is protective. So far, no vaccines against the other viruses have been developed and the demand is unlikely to justify them. Nevertheless, a small trial of oral pooled normal gammaglobulin showed evidence of protection against symptoms due to rotavirus but did not prevent virus excretion.

Prevention of spread in children's wards has proved difficult even with barrier nursing. As with other infectious agents, the best precaution is adequate hand-washing. The value of disinfectants is unpredictable, largely because of the amount of protein in faeces.

Further reading

Barnes, G.L., *et al.* (1982). A randomised trial of oral gammaglobulin in low birth-weight infants infected with rotavirus. *Lancet*, **i**, 1371–3.

Estes, M.K. (1996). Rotaviruses and their replication. In *Fundamental virology* (ed. B.M. Fields, D.M. Knipe, and P.M. Howley), pp. 731–61. Lippincott-Raven, Philadelphia.

Madeley, C.R. (1994). Viruses associated with acute diarrhoeal disease. In *Principles and practice of clinical virology*, 3rd edn (ed. A.J. Zuckerman, J.E. Banatvala, and J.R. Pattison), pp. 189–227. Wiley, Chichester.

Midthun, K. and Kapikian, A.Z. (1996). Rotavirus vaccines: an overview. *Clinical Microbiology Reviews*, **9**, 423–34.

Parrino, J.A., *et al.* (1977). Clinical immunity in acute gastroenteritis caused by Norwalk agent. *New England Journal of Medicine*, **297**, 86–9.

Chapter 16.24

Rhabdoviruses: rabies and rabies-related viruses

M. J. Warrell and D. A. Warrell

Virology

The Rhabdoviridae are rod- or bullet-shaped RNA viruses. Two genera infect animals: Vesiculovirus (vesicular stomatitis virus of cattle and horses, which occasionally causes an influenza-like illness in farmers or laboratory workers) and Lyssavirus (comprising 7 genotypes) (Table 1). The core of the rabies virion is a helical ribonucleoprotein complex, enveloped by a coat of glycoprotein (G) bearing numerous spikes. The virus is readily inactivated by drying, heating, 45 per cent ethanol, soap solution, detergents, proteolytic enzymes, hypochlorite, and glutaraldehyde solutions. Virus isolated from naturally infected animals is known as 'street' virus. Strains of rabies and rabies-related viruses can be identified using monoclonal antibodies or genetic sequencing, revealing the geographical and vector-related diversity of the virus.

Rabies-related viruses known to infect man are: Mokola, Duvenhage, European bat lyssaviruses, and an Australian bat lyssavirus (Table 1). Infections may be missed because the diagnosis of rabies encephalitis is usually made on clinical evidence alone. A routine diagnostic immunofluorescence test is unreliable for these genotypes.

Epidemiology

Rabies, a zoonosis, is endemic in most parts of the world (Fig. 1). The British Isles, Iceland, Norway (but not Svalbard islands), Sweden, Finland, Spain (except Ceuta in North Africa), Portugal, Cyprus and other Mediterranean islands, New Guinea, Bali, New Zealand, Antarctica, Oceania, peninsular Malaysia, Singapore, Japan, Taiwan, Hong Kong islands (but not the New Territories), Uruguay, and Caribbean islands (but not Cuba, the Dominican Republic, Grenada, Haiti, Trinidad and Tobago) are currently free of rabies.

Primarily an infection of wild mammals, rabies is spread by bites, by inhalation of aerosols in bat caves, and by ingestion of infected prey. Urban and sylvatic cycles overlap to varying degrees in different countries. Urban rabies in domestic dogs and cats, which is important throughout Asia and parts of Africa, causes more than 90 per cent of human cases worldwide. The sylvatic phase has different wild-mammal reservoir species in different geographical areas: in the US, striped skunks, foxes, raccoons, and insectivorous bats, are the main vector species. Elsewhere, reservoirs include: mongooses in the Caribbean and South Africa; vampire bats in Latin America; wolves, jackals, and small carnivores in Africa and in Asia; and foxes, wolves, raccoon dogs, and insectivorous bats in Europe.

Vampire bat-transmitted bovine paralytic rabies is costly in Latin America. Non-haematophagous bats are now the main cause of rabies deaths in the USA, causing 1–2 cases a year. In Australia, a lyssavirus has recently been identified in flying foxes (Pteropus and other bat species) and has caused a fatal human rabies-like encephalitis.

Cyclical epizootics of rabies, such as the current fox epizootic in Europe, result from an uncontrolled increase in the population of the key reservoir species. About 3 per cent of foxes survive the infection and become immune. The European and African bat viruses are all rabies-related genotypes 4–6. European bat lyssavirus was isolated from a single bat in an English port in 1996.

Incidence of human rabies

The true incidence of human rabies throughout the world is not reflected in official figures, and in many countries cases are not recorded. India now reports a mortality of 30 000, and in Bangladesh in 1992 it was 2000 (1.8/100 000 population). In the same year in Nepal, 200 deaths (1.1/100 000) and in Sri Lanka, 112 (0.64/100 000) deaths were reported. The true mortalities were probably considerably higher. Unofficial annual estimates include 6500 in Pakistan and 2000 in North Vietnam. In the US there have been about 2 cases per year since 1980. Rabies was eradicated from Britain by 1903. In the last 20 years, 9 people have died of rabies in England. Eight were infected in the Indian subcontinent, and one in Africa. In continental Europe very few cases are now reported.

Transmission

Virus can penetrate broken skin and intact mucosae. Humans are usually infected when virus-laden saliva is inoculated through the skin by the bite of a rabid dog or other mammal (Fig. 2). Rare modes of infection are by inhalation of infected bat secretions in caves or of aerosolized virus in laboratory accidents. Ten patients developed rabies after receiving infected corneal grafts. The saliva, respiratory

Table 1 Lyssaviruses that have infected humans

Genotype	Virus	Source	Known geographical area	Human disease
1	Rabies	Mammals	Widespread (see Fig. 1)	Encephalomyelitis
3	Mokola	Shrews, rodents, cat, dog	Africa	Fatal encephalitis (no hydrophobia), pharyngitis
4	Duvenhage	Insectivorous bat	Southern Africa	Furious rabies-like encephalitis
5	European bat lyssavirus (biotype 1)	Insectivorous bat	Denmark, Netherlands, Germany, Russia, Poland, Spain, France	Furious rabies-like encephalitis
6	European bat lyssavirus (biotype 2)	Insectivorous bat	Netherlands, Switzerland	Fatal encephalitis with paralytic and furious signs
7	Australian bat lyssavirus	Flying foxes and insectivorous bats	Australia	Rabies-like encephalitis

Genotype 2, Lagos bat virus, has not been detected in man.

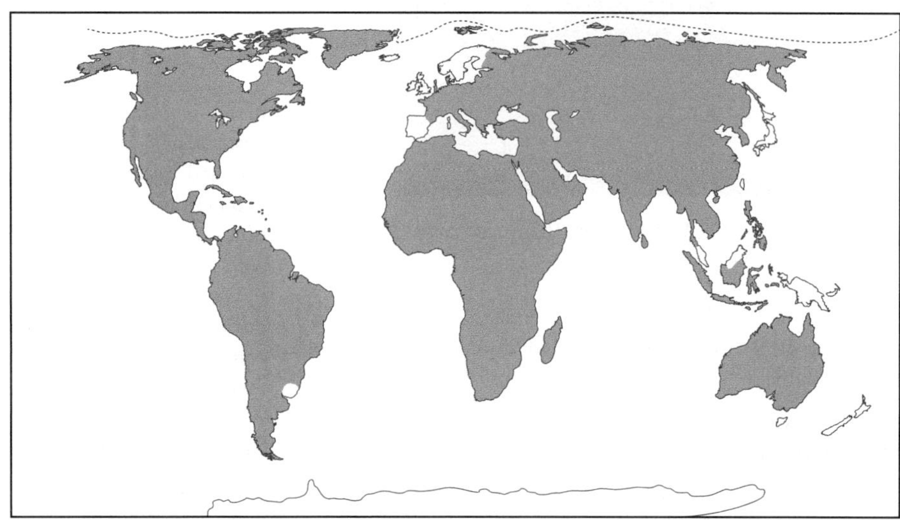

Fig. 1 Global distribution of rabies. Rabies-free areas in white.

secretions, tears, and urine of humans with rabies contain virus but there have been no virologically proven cases of person-to-person transmission. Transplacental infection must be exceptionally rare and several women with rabies encephalitis have been delivered of healthy babies.

Pathogenesis

Rabies virus may replicate locally in muscle cells or it attaches directly to motor or sensory nerve endings and travels centripetally within the axoplasm. On reaching the central nervous system, there is massive viral replication on membranes within neurones and direct viral transmission across synaptic junctions. Centrifugal spread from the central nervous system in the axoplasm of many efferent nerves deposits virus in tissues such as skeletal and cardiac muscle, adrenal medulla, kidney, retina, cornea, pancreas, and nerve twiglets in hair follicles. Viral replication and shedding, especially in the salivary glands, allows transmission of rabies by bites to other mammals.

Immunology

There is no detectable immune response until encephalitic symptoms develop, suggesting immune evasion. Neutralizing antibodies (induced by viral glycoprotein) become detectable in serum after about 7 days, and in cerebrospinal fluid a little later. They may rise to high levels in patients whose lives are prolonged by intensive care. A lymphocyte pleocytosis appears in only 60 per cent of patients. In animals, latent infections can be reactivated by corticosteroids and stress. This provides a possible explanation for occasional reports of long incubation periods.

Vaccine-induced rabies-neutralizing antibody is detectable as early as 7 days after the start of primary immunization.

Rabies in animals

In dogs the incubation period is usually between 3 and 12 weeks (range 5 days to 14 months). The first symptom may be intense irritation at the site of the infection. Despite the popular idea of the 'mad' rabid dog, only 25 per cent develop furious rabies. There is an early and marked change in behaviour. Clinical features include dysphagia, ptosis, altered bark, paralysis of the jaw, neck and hind limbs, hypersalivation, congested conjunctivae, pruritus, shivering, trembling, snapping at imaginary objects, pica, and extreme restlessness, causing the animal to wander miles from home. Virus may be excreted in the saliva 3 days before symptoms appear, and the animal usually dies within the next 7 days. There are rare reports from India, Ethiopia, and elsewhere, of chronic excretion of virus in the saliva of apparently healthy dogs.

Rabid foxes lose their fear of man and most show paralytic signs. Furious rabies develops in 75 per cent of infected cats. Dysphagia

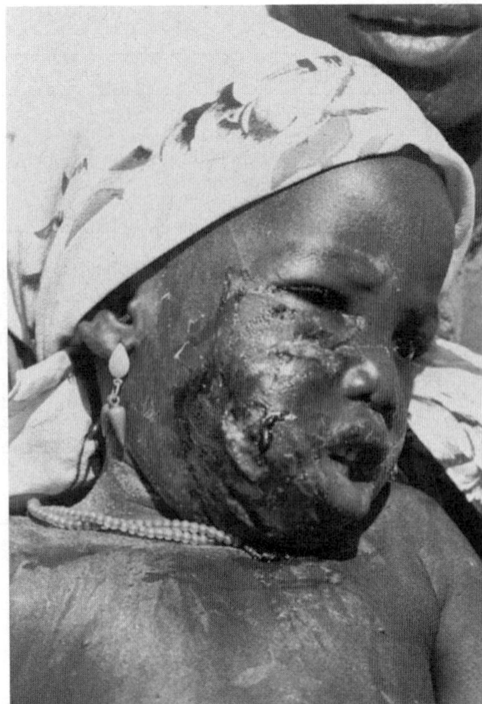

Fig. 2 Child bitten on the face by rabid dogs. This wound carries a high risk of rabies with a short incubation period.
(Copyright D.A. Warrell.)

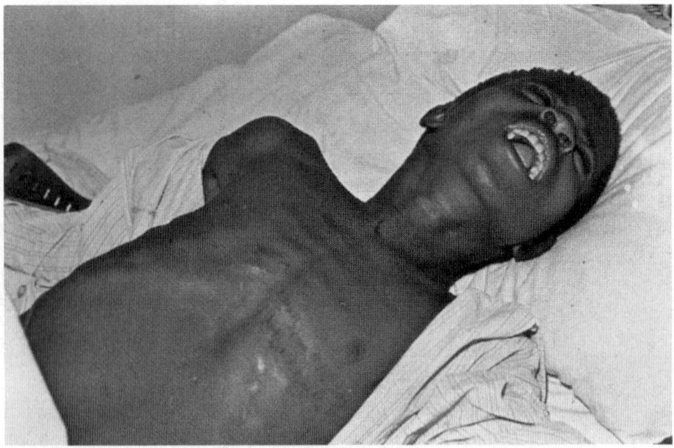

Fig. 3 Hydrophobic spasm in a 14-year-old Nigerian boy with furious rabies. Note the violent contraction of inspiratory muscles: sternomastoids and diaphragm (depressing xiphisternum).
(Copyright D.A. Warrell.)

and inability to drink are common in rabid animals, but they not exhibit hydrophobia.

Rabies in man

The incubation period is usually between 20 and 90 days (range 4 days to many years). It tends to be shorter after bites on the face (average 35 days) than after those on the limbs (average 52 days).

Prodromal symptoms

The first symptom is usually itching, pain, or paraesthesia at the site of the healed bite wound. Other symptoms include fever, chills, malaise, weakness, tiredness, headache, photophobia, myalgia, anxiety, depression, irritability, and symptoms of upper respiratory-tract and gastrointestinal infections. Subsequently, symptoms of either furious or paralytic rabies will develop, depending on whether the spinal cord or brain are predominantly infected.

Furious rabies

Furious rabies is the more common presentation. The diagnostic symptom is hydrophobia: a combination of jerky, violent inspiratory muscle spasms, associated with terror (Fig. 3). This reflex can be excited by a variety of stimuli: attempts to drink water, a draught of air ('aerophobia'), water splashed on the skin, irritation of the respiratory tract and ultimately, the sight, sound, or even mention of water. The neck and back are extended, the arms thrown up, and the episode may end in generalized convulsions precipitating cardiac or respiratory arrest.

Patients experience periods of generalized arousal, during which they become wild, hallucinated, fugitive, and sometimes aggressive, alternating with lucid intervals. Signs include meningism, cranial-nerve lesions (especially III, VI, VII, IX, X, XI, and XII), upper motor-neurone lesions, fasciculation, and involuntary movements. Disturbances of the hypothalamus or autonomic nervous system are reflected by hypersalivation, lacrimation, sweating, hypertension or hypotension, hyperthermia or hypothermia, inappropriate secretion of antidiuretic hormone, or diabetes insipidus and, rarely, priapism with spontaneous orgasms.

Without supportive treatment, about one-third of patients will die during a hydrophobic spasm in the first few days. The rest lapse into coma and generalized flaccid paralysis, and rarely survive for more than a week without intensive care.

Paralytic or dumb rabies

After the usual prodromal symptoms, especially fever, headache, and local paraesthesiae, flaccid paralysis develops, usually in the bitten limb, and ascends, with pain and fasciculation in the affected muscles and mild sensory disturbances, resulting in paraplegia, sphincter involvement and, finally, fatal paralysis of deglutitive and respiratory muscles. Hydrophobia is unusual. Even without intensive care, patients with paralytic rabies have survived for up to 30 days.

Other manifestations and complications

In patients whose lives have been prolonged by intensive care complications include bronchopneumonia, primary rabies pneumonitis, pneumothorax, cardiac arrhythmias (supraventricular tachycardias, sinus bradycardia, atrioventricular block, and sinus arrest), hypotension, pulmonary oedema, congestive cardiac failure, raised intracranial pressure resulting from cerebral oedema or internal hydrocephalus, and haematemesis.

Differential diagnosis

Rabies should be suspected whenever a patient develops severe neurological symptoms after being bitten by a mammal in a rabies endemic area. Some patients forget that they have been bitten. Hydrophobia is pathognomonic of rabies. Tetanus, which can also follow an animal bite, is distinguished by its shorter incubation period (usually less than 15 days), the presence of trismus, the persistence of muscle rigidity between spasms, the absence of meningoencephalitis (cerebrospinal fluid is universally normal), and the better prognosis. Delirium tremens and plant poisoning (e.g. *Datura fastuosa*) and

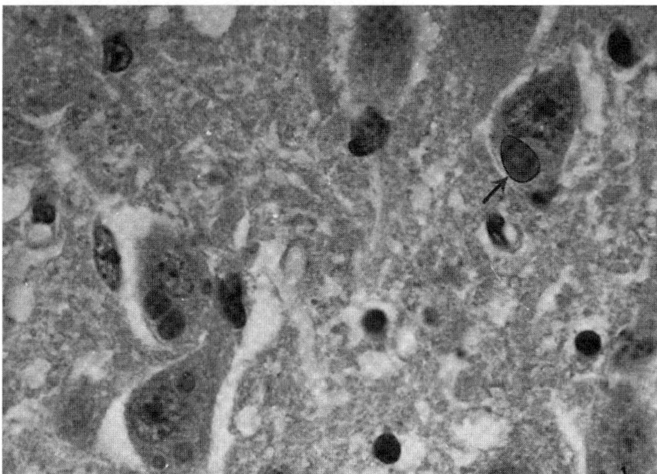

Fig. 4 Street virus in human brain as seen with the light microscope. Many Negri bodies can be seen (one is arrowed). The section is from Ammon's horn of the hippocampus, stained with haematoxylin and eosin (× 1000). *(Reproduced by courtesy of Professor P. Atanasiu, Institut Pasteur, Paris.)*

drugs (phenothiazines and amphetamines) may cause some of the features of rabies.

Paralytic rabies can be confused with other causes of ascending (Landry-type) paralysis. Postvaccinal encephalomyelitis usually develops within 2 weeks of the first dose of the older types of rabies vaccines. In poliomyelitis, objective sensory disturbances are absent. Cerebrospinal fluid examination may help to distinguish acute inflammatory polyneuropathy (Guillain–Barré syndrome). Herpes simiae (B virus) encephalomyelitis is transmitted by monkey bites, but the incubation period (3–4 days) is usually shorter than in rabies.

Pathology

The brain, spinal cord, and peripheral nerves show ganglion-cell degeneration, perineural and perivascular mononuclear cell infiltration, neuronophagia, and glial nodules. Inflammatory changes are most marked in the midbrain and medulla in furious rabies and in the spinal cord in paralytic rabies. The diagnostic Negri bodies (Fig. 4), which are eosinophilic intracytoplasmic inclusions, predominantly consisting of masses of viral ribonucleoprotein, are found especially in hippocampal pyramidal cells and cerebellar Purkinje cells. Neuronolysis is often surprisingly mild and patchy, and death can occur without any inflammatory response.

Laboratory diagnosis

In animals, rabies can be confirmed within a few hours by a direct immunofluorescent antibody test on acetone-fixed, brain impression smears or by using a rapid enzyme immunodiagnosis kit if a fluorescent microscope is not available. Virus isolation takes about 4 days in tissue culture.

In humans, rabies can be confirmed early in the illness by demonstration of viral antigen by immunofluorescence in nerve twiglets in skin (Fig. 5) or in brain biopsies. Corneal impression smears are often falsely negative. The use of the polymerase chain reaction is being evaluated.

During the first week of illness virus may be isolated from saliva, brain, cerebrospinal fluid, and rarely urine. Rabies antibodies are not usually detectable in serum or cerebrospinal fluid before the eighth day of illness in unvaccinated patients. Rabies neutralizing antibody may leak into the cerebrospinal fluid in patients with postvaccinal encephalomyelitis, but a very high titre suggests a diagnosis of rabies. The cerebrospinal fluid is normal in 40 per cent of patients in the first week of illness; a mild lymphocytic pleocytosis is usual. A peripheral neutrophil leucocytosis is common in the early stages of the disease.

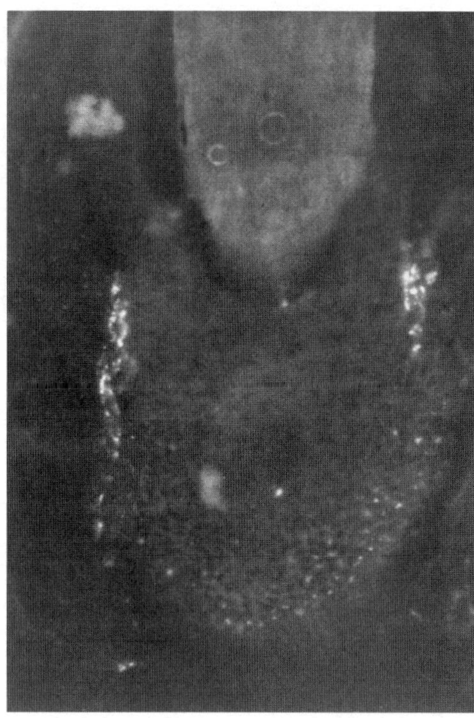

Fig. 5 Diagnosis of human rabies during life. Vertical section through a hair follicle and shaft showing brilliant fluorescence of nerve cells around the follicle indicating the presence of rabies antigen (× 250). *(Copyright M.J. Warrell.)*

Treatment

Patients with rabies must be sedated heavily and given adequate analgesia to relieve their pain and terror. Rabies is regarded as a fatal disease. Only 2 patients have recovered and 4 have survived with severe neurological deficit. Intensive care of rabies victims can prolong life by correcting cardiac arrhythmias, cardiac and respiratory failure, raised intracranial pressure, convulsions, fluid and electrolyte disturbances, and hyperpyrexia. Antiserum, antiviral agents, interferon-α, corticosteroid, and other immunosuppressants have proved useless.

Prevention and control

In countries where rabies is endemic

Information is needed about the prevalence and host range of rabies in wild and domestic animals. Domestic animals can be protected by yearly vaccination. People should be discouraged from keeping wild carnivores as pets. Vaccination of key reservoir species by using live oral vaccines distributed in bait has been successful in foxes in Europe. Rabies is most likely to be controlled or eradicated where the principal reservoir is the domestic dog. Humans who are particularly at risk, such as veterinarians and dog catchers, can be given pre-exposure vaccination.

Table 2 Specific postexposure prophylaxis for use in a rabies endemic area* following contact with a domestic or wild rabies vector species, whether or not the animal is available for observation or diagnostic tests

Minor exposure (including licks of broken skin, scratches, or abrasions without bleeding)
• Start vaccine immediately
• Stop treatment if animal remains healthy for 10 days
• Stop treatment if animal's brain proves negative for rabies by appropriate laboratory tests
Major exposure (including licks of mucosa, minor bites on arms, trunk, or legs, or major bites—multiple or on face, head, fingers, or neck)
• Immediate rabies immune globulin and vaccine
• Stop treatment if domestic cat or dog remains healthy for 10 days
• Stop treatment if animal's brain proves negative for rabies by appropriate laboratory tests

*This scheme is a simplification of the WHO recommendations on rabies postexposure treatment (1997).

In countries where rabies is not endemic

Importation of domestic dogs and cats, wild bats, and carnivores should be strictly controlled. Pre-exposure vaccination is needed only by those who handle imported animals in quarantine kennels, stables, farms, zoos, and laboratories; those who work with rabies virus in laboratories; and travellers to rabies-endemic areas who are specially at risk (e.g. veterinarians, cave explorers, naturalists, and animal collectors).

Pre-exposure immunization regimens

Tissue culture rabies vaccine is given on days 0, 3, and 28 (or 21). The dose is one vial intramuscularly into the deltoid (or the anterolateral thigh in children), or 0.1 ml intradermally. The neutralizing antibody response need not be checked unless immunosuppression is suspected. Chloroquine taken for malaria prophylaxis suppresses the immune response to intradermal vaccine. Rabies laboratory staff at continuous risk should be tested every 6 months and those at frequent risk every 2 years. A booster dose, 6–24 months after the primary course, results in persistence of neutralizing antibody levels for 5 years or more.

Postexposure prophylaxis (Table 2)

Wound cleaning

As soon as possible after the bite, the wound must be scrubbed with soap or detergents under a running tap for at least 5 min. A virucidal agent such as 40–70 per cent alcohol, povidone iodine, or 0.01 per cent aqueous iodine should be applied liberally. In hospital, wounds should be explored, debrided, and irrigated. Suturing should be avoided or delayed and occlusive dressings should not be used. Attention should be given to tetanus prophylaxis and the range of bacterial and other pathogens particularly associated with mammal bites (Table 2). Most of the bacteria are sensitive to amoxicillin/clavulanic acid, cephoxitin, or tetracycline.

Active immunization

Cell-culture vaccines

Human diploid cell vaccine (HDCV) (Pasteur–Mérieux), purified chick embryo cell vaccine (PCEC) (Behring), and purified vero cell vaccine (PVRV) (Pasteur–Mérieux) are recommended vaccines. The manufacturers advise 5 intramuscular doses: on days 0, 3, 7, 14, and 30. Two economical multiple-site intradermal postexposure regimens have proved effective and are now approved by the WHO. The 8-site regimen uses vaccines in ampoules containing 1 ml (HDCV, PCEC), and requires eight intradermal injections of 0.1 ml (deltoids, suprascapular, lower-quadrant abdominal wall, and thighs) on day 0, four intradermal injections of 0.1 ml (deltoids and thighs) on day 7, and a single intradermal dose of 0.1 ml on days 28 and 91. The 2-site regimen with PVRV (0.5 ml per ampoule) requires 0.1 ml intradermal injection at 2 sites (deltoid areas) on days 0, 3, and 7, and single intradermal 0.1 doses on days 28 and 91.

A highly purified Swiss duck embryo vaccine is of similar potency to, and as safe as, cell-culture vaccines, and is given by the same regimens. Side-effects of cell-culture vaccines are mild and transient.

Nervous-tissue vaccines

These vaccines, initially introduced by Pasteur 100 years ago and developed by Semple, Hempt, and Fuenzalida, are still widely used in Africa, Asia, and Latin America. Neurological reactions occur in up to 1 in 220 courses of sheep brain Semple type vaccine, with a 3 per cent case fatality and in 1:7865 to 1:27 000 courses of suckling mouse brain vaccine with a 22 per cent case fatality. Most reactions to Semple vaccine affect the central nervous system, whereas at least 70 per cent of those following suckling mouse brain vaccine involved the peripheral nervous system.

The incubation period is usually between 7 and 14 days but can be several weeks after the first injection of vaccine. Prednisolone, 40–60 mg/day, is thought to be helpful. Vaccination should be stopped as soon as symptoms appear and the course continued with a cell-culture vaccine.

Passive immunization

Rabies immune globulin (RIG) is recommended after the first dose of vaccine, and is specially important for severe bites (on the head, neck, hands, and for multiple or deep bites). The dose of equine RIG is 40 IU/kg bodyweight. Serum sickness occurs in 1–6 per cent of cases. Hypersensitivity tests do not predict the majority of reactions; adrenaline must always be available to treat anaphalyxis. The dose of human rabies immune globulin (HRIG) is 20 IU/kg bodyweight.

The RIG is infiltrated into the tissues around the bite wound, and any remaining is injected intramuscularly into the thigh, not the buttock. If RIG is given hours or days before the first dose of vaccine, the immune response to vaccination will be impaired. RIG is very expensive and not available for 99 per cent of postexposure courses in Africa and Asia.

Postexposure prophylaxis in people who have received previous vaccination

If a complete pre- or postexposure course of cell-culture vaccine has been given in the past, or if the neutralizing antibody level has been over 0.5 IU/ml, only two doses of cell-culture vaccine need be given (on days 0 and 3), with a third dose on day 7 for severe bites. RIG is not required.

Further reading

Baer, G.M. (ed.) (1991). *The natural history of rabies*, 2nd edn. CRC Press, Boca Raton.

Centres for Disease Control and Prevention (1999). Human rabies prevention—United States, 1999: recommendations of the Advisory Committee on Immunization Practices. *Morbidity and Mortality Weekly Report*, **48**, No. RR-1.

Rupprecht, C.E., Dietzschold, B., and Koprowski, H. (ed.) (1994). *Lyssaviruses*. Springer-Verlag, Berlin.

Warrell, M.J. and Warrell D.A. (1995). Rhabdovirus infections of man. In *Handbook of infectious diseases*. Vol. 3, Exotic viral infections (ed. J.S. Porterfield and D.A.J. Tyrrell), pp. 343–83. Chapman and Hall, London..

World Health Organization (1997). *WHO recommendations on rabies post-exposure treatment and the correct technique of intradermal immunization against rabies.* (WHO/EMC/ZOO.96.6). WHO, Geneva.

Chapter 16.25

Colorado tick fever and other arthropod-borne reoviruses

M. J. Warrell and D. A. Warrell

Colorado tick fever

The reovirus (genus *Coltivirus*) responsible for Colorado tick fever or 'mountain fever' is an 80-nm, RNA-containing particle, covered with capsomeres. It has the unique ability to infect human erythrocytes.

Colorado tick fever is a zoonosis involving adult hard (ixodid) ticks (principally *Dermacentor andersoni*), and wild mammals including porcupines and other rodents, coyotes and deer.

Epidemiology

Colorado tick fever is acquired from tick bites in western and northwestern parts of the US (including California), British Columbia, and Alberta. Very rarely, it has been caused by an infected blood transfusion. Several hundred cases are reported each year in the US, but the true incidence is thought to be at least 10 times higher than that. Hikers and campers are at special risk, particularly from May to July when ticks are most active.

Clinical features

In adults, the infection is nearly always mild, but in children it is occasionally severe or even fatal. A sudden fever occurs 1–19 (usually 3–6) days after the tick bite, with rigors, generalized aches, myalgia, headache, and backache. In half the patients there is a biphasic fever. A maculopapular or petechial rash appears in about 10 per cent of cases and gastrointestinal symptoms in 20 per cent. Laboratory findings include leucopenia with relative lymphocytosis, thrombocytopenia, and mild lymphocyte pleocytosis. The illness usually resolves in about 10–14 days, but convalescence may be prolonged. Severe manifestations include meningism and drowsiness, spontaneous bleeding, thrombocytopenia, and disseminated intravascular coagulation. Late, possibly immunological, effects include myocarditis, pericarditis, pleurisy, arthritis, and epididymitis. Colorado tick fever may precipitate abortion.

Diagnosis

Viral antigen may be detected in erythrocytes by immunofluorescence 1–120 days after the start of symptoms, and a reverse transcriptase polymerase chain reaction (PCR) method can detect virus after 1–8 days. An indirect fluorescent antibody test can provide early serodiagnosis. Neutralizing antibody and specific IgM enzyme immunoassays become positive after 14–21 days and the IgM disappears after 45 days.

Differential diagnosis

Many other tick-borne acute febrile illnesses, some with rashes and nervous-system involvement, can be acquired in the endemic area for Colorado tick fever. These include Rocky Mountain spotted fever, tularaemia, Lyme disease, erlichiosis and relapsing fever. Tick paralysis caused by *D. andersoni* and other ixodid ticks presents as a poliomyelitis-like, ascending, flaccid paralysis unlikely to be mistaken for the meningitic or encephalitic syndromes of Colorado tick fever.

Treatment

Salicylates should not be used for the symptomatic treatment of fever and pain because of the thrombocytopenia.

Other arthropod-borne reoviruses

These include Kemerovo in Europe, Changuinola in Panama, and Orungo and Lebombo viruses in Africa (see OTM3, p. 406).

Further reading

Monath, T.P. and Guirakhoo, F. (1996). Orbiviruses and coliviruses. In *Fields virology*, 3rd edn (ed. B.N. Fields, D.M. Knipe, P.M. Howley, *et al.*), pp. 1735–66. Lippincott-Raven, Philadelphia.

Chapter 16.26

Alphaviruses

D. I. H. Simpson, S. P. Fisher-Hoch, and J. B. McCormick

There are more than 36 members of the genus *Alphavirus*, all transmitted by mosquitoes. Nine are capable of causing human epidemics. Alphaviruses have a diameter of 60–70 nm and contain a single strand of positive-sense RNA enclosed in an icosahedral nucleocapsid, surrounded by a lipid membrane. Illnesses caused by alphaviruses range from mild fever, often with a rash, myalgia, and arthralgia, to frank encephalitis. A mild fever, often unrecognized, occurs during the initial viraemic stage. Occasionally a second, more severe encephalitic phase develops. Most infections are asymptomatic. Most can be diagnosed by isolation of virus in the first few days of illness. Virus-specific IgM enzyme immunoassays have proved useful. Most other serological tests are plagued by cross-reactions with other alphaviruses. Reverse transcriptase polymerase chain reaction (RT-PCR) systems for detecting viral genome in blood or other fluids or tissues are available.

Chikungunya

Chikungunya (meaning 'that which bends up', in a Tanzanian language) has been frequently isolated during epidemics in Asia and throughout Africa. Large urban epidemics have been seen in India. The virus is transmitted by *Aedes* mosquitoes, and man appears to be the only natural reservoir. The incubation period of 2–12 days is followed by sudden fever, incapacitating joint pains that may persist for months, and mild headache. Fever subsides, only to return with a maculopapular, pruritic rash on the trunk and extensor surfaces of the limbs in most patients. Recovery is rapid and complete. Haemorrhagic chikungunya virus disease is rare. No vaccine is produced commercially.

O'nyong nyong virus

This virus caused a major epidemic that began in Uganda during 1959 and quickly spread to Kenya, Tanzania, and Malawi, involving an estimated 2 million people. There have been no recent epidemics. The disease is like chikungunya, except that lymph nodes may be enlarged. It is transmitted to man by *Anopheles* mosquitoes. The mammal reservoir is unknown. After an incubation period of up to 8 days, there is sudden fever, rigors, and sometimes epistaxis, followed by backache, severe joint pains, headache, pain in the eyes, generalized lymphadenopathy, and a pruritic rash beginning on the face and spreading to the trunk and limbs. Joint pains and malaise may be protracted. No sequelae or deaths are reported.

Mayaro virus

This virus is transmitted by *Haemagogus* mosquitoes in rain forest areas of Central and South America, where there are periodic outbreaks of fever, headache, conjunctivitis, prostration, joint and muscle pains, and a rash. The arthralgia can last for 2 months.

Ross River virus

This virus has caused 'epidemic polyarthritis' in Australia and the Pacific Islands, sometimes involving several thousand cases. It has been isolated from *Aedes* mosquitoes and wild mammals. The main symptom is arthralgia, which may be accompanied by a mild fever, or no fever. The arthralgia is apparently a cell mediated response induced by viral antigen, and the exudate is almost entirely mononuclear leukocytes. Fever is often accompanied by a sore throat and generalized maculopapular rash, occasionally with small vesicles, petechiae, and enanthem. The arthralgia is of the small joints of the hands and feet with paresthesiae of the palms and soles of the feet. Arthritis lasts from a few days to months.

Sindbis and related viruses

These viruses are widely distributed in Africa, India, tropical Asia, and Australia, but they have only occasionally been associated with disease. The clinical features include fever, rash, arthralgia, myalgia, malaise, and headache. The maculopapular rash progresses from trunk to extremities and vesicles can occur on the palms and soles. In Northern Europe, Ockelbo virus is responsible for outbreaks across central Sweden and Finland (Pogosta virus). Karelian fever is similar.

Eastern equine encephalitis (EEE) virus

EEE occurs in small outbreaks along the eastern seaboard states of North, Central, and South America. Wild birds and *Culiseta* mosquitoes maintain the virus. The most virulent of the two closely related variants of EEE occurs in the US, where sporadic and sometimes clusters of severe equine infections occur each summer in coastal regions. Human infections are generally sporadic with only a small number of severe cases. The incubation period is more than a week, and onset is abrupt with high fever. About 2 per cent of infected adults and 6 per cent of children develop encephalitis. There is neck stiffness, spasticity, and, in infants, bulging fontanelles, and oedema of the legs and face with cyanosis. Cerebrospinal fluid pressure may be raised, with slightly increased protein, normal sugar, and up to 2000 cells/mm. Case fatality of the encephalitis is 50–75 per cent. Death can occur within 3–5 days of onset. Sequelae, common in non-fatal encephalitis, include convulsions, paralyses, and mental retardation. IgG antibody is usually present at onset of illness, so that serological diagnosis is possible. Vaccines have been used successfully in horses and an inactivated vaccine is available for laboratory staff.

Western equine encephalitis (WEE) virus

This is a complex of closely related viruses isolated in North and South America. The epidemic potential of certain US viral strains appears the most significant. Flooding, which increases breeding of *Culex* mosquitoes, precipitates summer epidemics of encephalitis. The virus has been isolated from a variety of wild birds. Equine epizootics generally precede the appearance of human cases, but horses play no part in the transmission cycle. The incubation period is about 7 days, and illness to infection ratios for encephalitis are over 1 : 1000. About 2 per cent of infected children develop encephalitis. There is typically headache, vomiting, stiff neck, and backache. Restlessness and irritability are often seen in children. Convulsions occur in 90 per cent of affected infants and in 40 per cent of children between 1 and 4 years old, but are rare in adults. Drowsiness, severe occipital headache, mental confusion, and coma are seen in up to 40 per cent of adults. Recovery in 5–10 days is common, but convalescence may be protracted. Sequelae are rare in adults and older children, but more common in infants, with half of those with encephalitis left with convulsions, and/or severe motor or intellectual deficits. Neurological sequelae were reported in three of five infants of women infected in pregnancy. Mortality is about 3–7 per cent. As with EEE, IgG antibody may be present at the onset of illness. Inactivated vaccine is available for laboratory staff and horses.

Venezuelan equine encephalitis (VEE) virus

This is another complex of closely related viruses, which can cause large epizootics of encephalitis in equines in Northern, Southern, and Central America, sometimes reaching the southern US. Encephalitis occurs in a small proportion of patients. Epizootics in 1971 killed 200 000 horses and caused several thousand human infections. The viruses are maintained by rodent–mosquito cycles. The incubation period is 1–6 days. About 60 per cent of infected persons develop a brief febrile illness with nausea or vomiting, headache, which may be severe, and myalgia. Fever lasts about 4 days and convalescence may take 3 weeks. Encephalitis develops in less than 1 per cent of adults, but in up to 4 per cent of children. Case fatality in hospitalized cases is 10–15 per cent, but sequelae are uncommon. Transmission between humans has not been documented, although there have been several laboratory-acquired infections. Horses do not play a role in human epidemiology, except that equine epidemics may alert physicians to the possibility of concurrent human epidemic disease. Live attentuated and inactivated vaccines have been used in laboratory workers. Equine immunization has been effective in controlling epizootic disease.

Further reading

Eldridge, B.F. (1987). Strategies for surveillance, prevention and control of arbovirus diseases in western North America. *American Journal of Tropical Medicine and Hygiene*, 37 (Suppl.), 797–855.

Calisher, C.H. (1995). Alphavirus Infections. In *Exotic infections. Kass handbook of infectious diseases* (ed. J.S. Porterfield), pp. 1–18. Chapman and Hall Medical, London.

Monath, T.P. (ed.) (1988, 1989). *The arboviruses: epidemiology and ecology.* Vols I–III (1988); IV–V (1989). CRC Press, Boca Raton.

Chapter 16.27

Rubella

S. Logan and P. Tookey

Introduction

Rubella infection usually causes a mild exanthematous disease but infection in early pregnancy may result in multiple congenital abnormalities.

The enveloped RNA virus of rubella is classified in a separate genus, *Rubivirus*, within the family Togaviridae. There are a number of strains of rubella which differ in virulence but are serologically indistinguishable.

Epidemiology

Humans are the only known host. Before the introduction of a vaccine, rubella epidemics were superimposed on endemic infection every 4–9 years, and pandemics every 10–30 years. In most unvaccinated populations around 10 per cent of women reach childbearing age still susceptible to rubella infection.

Infection is rare in infancy. The incidence rises slowly during the first 4 years and then rapidly, with a peak between 5 and 9 years of age.

Postnatally acquired infection

The rash usually begins on the face and spreads to the trunk and then the extremities; the pink maculopapular lesions are initially discrete but later coalesce. The suboccipital and posterior cervical lymph nodes are characteristically enlarged. Mild fever, sore throat, coryza, cough, and conjunctivitis may be present; symptoms are usually mild and last 3–7 days. There may be a prodrome with malaise and fever, especially in adults. There is no specific treatment.

Arthralgia is a common complication in older patients but frank arthritis is unusual; both are normally transient but recurrent or persistent symptoms have been reported, mainly in older women. Less common complications include purpura, thrombocytopenia, postinfectious encephalitis, transverse myelitis, and the Guillain–Barré syndrome.

Table 1 Defects associated with congenital rubella

Classic triad	Other defects

• Sensorineural deafness
• Abnormalities of the cardiovascular system:
  • Persistent ductus arteriosus
  • Pulmonary stenosis
  • Aortic and renal artery stenosis
  • Tetralogy of Fallot
  • Ventricular septal defect
  • Myocarditis
• Abnormalities of the eye
  • Retinopathy
  • Cataracts
  • Microphthalmos
  • Glaucoma
	• Growth retardation
	• Microcephaly
	• Mental retardation
	Other signs in infancy and the neonatal period
	• Hepatosplenomegaly Jaundice
	• Rash
	• Purpura
	• Thrombocytopenia
	• Osteopathy
	• Hypogammaglobulinaemia
	• Pneumonitis

Rubella is clinically indistinguishable from several other infections and as at least half of all infections may be clinically inapparent or non-specific, a history of clinically diagnosed rubella infection is unreliable.

The incubation period is 14–21 days. Patients are infectious from 5–7 days before to 3–5 days after symptoms appear, but infectivity is highest immediately before, and on the first day of, symptoms. Congenitally infected infants shed large amounts of virus from the oropharynx and may be a source of infection for many months.

Infection usually produces lifelong immunity but reinfection is occasionally reported.

Congenital infection

Congenital rubella is typically associated with cataracts, cardiac anomalies, and, most commonly, sensorineural hearing loss (SNHL). The teratogenic effects may result in a wide range of defects (Table 1). The earlier the infection the more likely the child will have severe, multiple problems. The risk of damage to a child infected in the first 10 weeks of pregnancy is around 90 per cent; this drops rapidly thereafter, and after 16 weeks' gestation abnormalities are rare; no abnormalities have been demonstrated after 18 weeks' gestation.

Some defects, particularly SNHL, may not develop or reveal themselves until later in childhood. Other late-onset problems reported include diabetes mellitus, thyroid dysfunction, and possibly autism. A progressive rubella panencephalitis has been reported but is rare.

Not all maternal rubella infection results in transmission to the fetus. Inapparent maternal infection is thought to carry a similar risk to symptomatic infection. The risk following maternal reinfection is thought to be extremely low although there are a few case reports of subsequent damage.

Diagnosis of congenital rubella infection is by culture or serology. Virus can be isolated from multiple sites including the oropharynx, urine, and conjunctival fluid during the first months of life; viral shedding may occasionally persist for years. The presence of IgG antibody is not diagnostic, but the persistence of high levels is suspicious. Rubella IgM antibody in early infancy is virtually diagnostic because postnatal infection is rare at this age. When abnormalities present late, a presumptive diagnosis can be made on the basis of a compatible clinical picture and the persistence of rubella IgG antibodies in young unvaccinated children.

Management of possible rubella during pregnancy

A woman with suspected rubella infection or exposure during the first 4 months of pregnancy must be offered investigation; even women previously reported to be immune should be investigated in case of laboratory error or reinfection. A blood sample should be tested for IgG and IgM antibodies, with a repeat test after 2 weeks if results are equivocal. Rising IgG or the presence of IgM antibody is diagnostic of recent infection.

Vaccination

Live virus vaccines, first licensed in 1969, produce protective levels of antibody in around 95 per cent of recipients; protection is probably lifelong in most individuals. Reinfection can occur both naturally and after vaccine challenge, and there are occasional reports of loss of immunity. A few cases of congenital rubella have been reported in infants of women in whom rubella antibody had been demonstrated after vaccination.

Vaccine strategies include mass immunization of all children between 12 and 15 months of age, sometimes combined with a booster at a later age, or selective immunization of schoolgirls after the age of peak incidence and susceptible women. The UK switched from a selective strategy to universal immunization of toddlers in 1988, supplemented by a booster at four since 1996. Health personnel should be screened and susceptibles immunized.

Vaccination has led to dramatic declines in the number of susceptible pregnant women, in rubella-associated terminations, and in congenital rubella births. In the UK only 6 congenitally infected infants have been reported on average each year between 1990 and 1996, compared with 58.5 per year in the 1970s (when case ascertainment was less efficient).

In children, rubella vaccine causes few side-effects. Low-grade fever and rash are occasionally reported, and transient arthralgia has been seen in about 3 per cent of vaccinees; there have also been rare reports of myositis and vasculitis. Joint symptoms are common in adult women though less frequent and severe than following naturally acquired rubella. Symptoms are generally mild and transient but a handful of cases of apparently recurrent or persistent arthritis after rubella immunization have been described.

There have been concerns that the vaccine virus might be teratogenic if given during pregnancy. Although vaccinees cannot infect other susceptible individuals, the virus can cross the placenta. Studies of children born to women inadvertently vaccinated up to 3 months before conception or during pregnancy show less than 3 per cent with serological evidence of congenital infection, and no reported case of attributable abnormalities; the likely maximum theoretical risk is less than 5 per cent.

Further reading

Banatvala, J.E. and Best, J. (1990). Rubella. In *Topley and Wilson's principles of bacteriology, virology and immunity,* 8th edn (ed. L. Collier and M. Timbury), pp. 501–31. Arnold, London.

Department of Health (1996). *1996 Immunisation against infectious disease,* pp. 193–202. HMSO, London.

Miller, E. (1990). Rubella infection in pregnancy. In *Modern antenatal care of the fetus* (ed. G. Chamberlain), pp. 247–70. Blackwell Scientific, Oxford.

O'Shea, S., Best, J.M., Banatvala, J.E., *et al.* (1984). Persistence of rubella antibody 8–18 years after vaccination. *British Medical Journal,* **288,** 1043.

Tookey, P.A., Jones, G., Miller, B.H.R., and Peckham C.S. (1991). Rubella vaccination in pregnancy. *Communicable Disease Report,* **1,** R86–8.

Chapter 16.28

Flaviviruses

T. P. Monath

Introduction

The family Flaviviridae comprises 69 viruses, of which 38 cause human illness and are transmitted by mosquitoes or ticks. Humans serve as viraemic hosts in the transmission cycles of dengue and yellow fever, but other flaviviruses circulate between wild or domestic animals, and humans do not contribute to transmission. Flavivirus infections are not communicable.

Disease syndromes include non-specific febrile illness, fever with arthralgia and rash, haemorrhagic fever, and central nervous system infections. Pathogenesis is mediated by direct viral injury to infected cells or, in some cases (e.g. dengue haemorrhagic fever) indirectly by cytokines released from cells during the process of immune clearance. Because the clinical illness is rarely pathognomonic (except in an epidemic), epidemiological information and specific laboratory tests are required for an accurate diagnosis. Vaccines are available for prevention of several flavivirus infections; no effective antiviral drugs have been discovered, so treatment is symptomatic.

Flaviviruses are small (37–50 nm) spherical particles consisting of a lipid–protein bilayer envelope surrounding a nucleoprotein core containing the single-stranded, positive-polarity RNA genome 11 kilobases in size. Virus replication occurs in the cytoplasm. The viral envelope glycoprotein subserves virus attachment and contains the principal antigens stimulating protective immunity.

Dengue and dengue haemorrhagic fever

Epidemiology

Dengue fever is the most prevalent flavivirus infection of humans, and has a worldwide distribution in tropical regions. Fifty to 100 million infections occur annually. Dengue is transmitted principally by *Aedes aegypti* mosquitoes, an abundant species in human habitations. Viraemic humans are the source of virus for mosquito infection. Air travel is a factor in epidemic emergences, as passengers often travel during the incubation period (2–7 days) of the disease. Many cases are imported annually into the US and Europe.

Clinical features

Onset is sudden, with fever, headache, retro-orbital pain, and lumbosacral pain, followed by severe malaise, myalgia, and bone pain. The pulse is slow in relation to the fever, which may reach 41°C. A transient macular rash or mottling of the skin is often seen during the early illness. Between the second and sixth day, patients experience anorexia, nausea, vomiting, upper respiratory symptoms, cutaneous hypersensitivity, and altered taste sensation. Defervescence occurs between days 3 and 6, followed by the appearance of a morbilliform, non-pruritic rash on the trunk, spreading to limbs and face, sparing palms and soles, lasting 1–5 days, and sometimes resolving with desquamation. The fever may rise again after the appearance of the rash, producing a 'saddle-back' fever curve. Other findings may include generalized lymphadenopathy and haemorrhagic phenomena (e.g. petechiae, purpura, epistaxis), neutropenia, thrombocytopenia, and slightly elevated serum transaminase levels. There are no fatalities; the disease resolves in the second week, but patients often experience generalized asthenia and depression lasting several weeks. Persistent or recurrent musculoskeletal complaints or arthritis are not observed.

Diagnosis and differential diagnosis

The differential diagnosis includes influenza, measles, rubella, and other arboviral infections with rash (e.g. chikungunya and Ross River fever). Specific diagnosis is made by virus isolation or polymerase chain reaction on blood or serum (during the first few days of illness), or by serological tests, especially IgM enzyme immunoassay; commercial kits are available. Advice on the availability of these tests and on handling and transport of specimens should be sought from local or national health authorities.

Treatment

Treatment is symptomatic. Salicylates should be avoided because of the bleeding diathesis and rare association with Reye's syndrome.

Prevention

In areas infested with *Ae. aegypti*, patients should be safeguarded from mosquito bite. An intensive effort is underway to develop vaccines. Live, attenuated vaccines against all four serotypes have been tested clinically, but none is licensed yet.

Dengue haemorrhagic fever (DHF)

Over 3 million cases of DHF with 45 000 deaths have been reported to the WHO since 1956. The annual incidence exceeds 100 000 cases and is increasing. In South-East Asia, DHF is a major cause of pediatric hospitalization. The disease appeared in the Americas in 1981 (Cuba), caused recent epidemics in Brazil and Venezuela, and is predicted to increase in incidence with cocirculation of multiple dengue serotypes. DHF is caused by all four dengue serotypes; however, certain serotypes and strains of individual serotypes are more frequently associated with the DHF syndrome, suggesting that viral factors may influence disease expression.

The case-definition of DHF established by the WHO includes a dengue-like illness with thrombocytopenia $(100 \times 10^9/L)$ and a haemoconcentration (haematocrit elevated by (20 per cent). This reflects diffuse capillary leakage of plasma, manifested by pleural effusion and hypoalbuminaemia. Haemorrhage varies from minor (petechiae, epistaxis, gingival bleeding) to major gastrointestinal bleeding. In its most severe form (designated dengue shock syndrome (DSS) occurring in up to one-third of individuals with DHF), patients experience hypotension, narrowing of the pulse pressure (20 mmHg), and circulatory failure/shock. The case-fatality rate of DHF/DSS is 10 per cent or more if untreated. With supportive treatment (see below), fewer than 1 per cent of such cases succumb.

DHF/DSS is an immunopathological process, dependent on prior sensitization by a heterotypic dengue infection ('immune enhancement'). Enhanced infection of Fc-bearing monocytes mediated by immune complexes, T cell activation, clearance of infected cells, and release of mediators causing capillary leakage and disseminated intravasular coagulopathy are the essential elements of the pathogenic process. Persons of the black race appear to be less susceptible to DHF/DSS. Children are more frequently affected than adults.

The early symptoms are similar to dengue fever. Mild DHF cases exhibit only the laboratory abnormalities noted above or spontaneous haemorrahages, without physiologically relevant signs of capillary leak. In cases of DSS, however, between 2 and 5 days after onset the patient rapidly worsens, complains of epigastric pain, is restless and irritable, and has signs of hypotension, clammy extremities, cyanosis, diaphoresis, and oliguria. Examination reveals non-tender hepatic enlargement, shallow pulse, and rapid respiratory rate. Jaundice occurs rarely but may lead to confusion with yellow fever. Spontaneous haemorrhages are common. Dyspnoea and rapid respiration rate reflect pulmonary oedema, hypoxemia, and metabolic acidosis. Chest radiograph and ultrasound studies typically reveal pleural effusion. A variety of neurologic manifestations are described, particularly encephalopathy, possibly due to cerebral oedema. Although most patients respond to treatment, those with profound shock or severe GI haemorrhage have a poor prognosis.

Early supportive treatment is critical. Intensive monitoring of vital signs and haematocrit, replacement of intravascular volume with lactated Ringer's or isotonic saline, correction of metabolic acidosis, and O_2 therapy are life-saving steps. Once the patient is stabilized, capillary leakage ceases and resorption of extravasated fluid begins, care must be taken not to induce pulmonary oedema with continued intravenous fluids. Heparin and corticosteroids are not effective and should not be used. No antiviral agents are available; interferon-α is of uncertain benefit.

The differential diagnosis includes septic shock, leptospirosis, rickettsial infection, meningococcaemia, and other viral haemorrhagic fevers. Specific laboratory diagnosis is as described for dengue fever.

Japanese encephalitis

This encephalitic disease was described clinically in 1871. The virus was isolated from brain tissue in 1935, and mosquito transmission was proven in 1938. The virus exists as a single serotype, but geographic strains differ by RNA sequencing. The virus is closely linked antigenically to St Louis encephalitis, Murray Valley encephalitis, and West Nile viruses.

Epidemiology

Japanese encephalitis virus causes disease throughout Asia. The annual morbidity exceeds 50 000 cases, with highest incidence in temperate and subtropical regions of China, northern Thailand, Nepal, and India, where epidemics occur in the summer coincident with abundance of the principal vector, *Culex tritaeniorhynchus*. The vector breeds in irrigated rice fields, and humans are infected in this ecological setting. Cases have occurred in expatriates visiting or living in endemic areas. Pigs and wild birds are the viraemic hosts in the transmission cycle, and man and horses are 'dead-end' hosts. Children suffer the highest attack rates, because of cumulative immunity with age. Infection in pigs results in abortion and stillbirth, whereas horses develop encephalitis.

Clinical features

Most infections are asymptomatic or escape medical detection. Approximately 1 in 300 infections results in encephalitis. After an incubation period of 6–16 days, illness begins with a non-specific prodrome lasting several days, followed by fever, chills, headache, meningism, photophobia, nausea, vomiting, and seizures. Variable neurological signs appear, including cranial-nerve palsies, tremors, ataxia, abnormal reflexes, paralysis, delirium and, ultimately, coma. The cerebrospinal fluid contains under 1000/mm^3 cells (polymorphonuclear initially, followed by lymphocytic), mildly elevated protein, and normal glucose levels. Respiratory dysregulation, coma, abnormal plantar reflexes, and prolonged convulsions are associated with poor prognosis. The case-fatality rate exceeds 25 per cent. Sequelae including parkinsonism, paralysis, and retardation occur in 30–70 per cent of survivors. In pregnant women infected during the first or second trimester, spontaneous abortion, and fetal death are reported. Data are insufficient to determine the quantitative risk of congenital infection or the risk of infection in the third trimester. There are reports of recurrent encephalitis in children, with intervals of up 6–12 months between occurrences.

Treatment

Treatment is supportive, and includes attention to fluid management, respiratory support, avoidance of infection and bed sores, and use of anticonvulsants. Cerebral oedema may require prompt diagnostic evaluation and intervention (see Chapter 13.26).

Diagnosis and differential diagnosis

The differential diagnosis includes encephalitides treatable with antiviral drugs (herpes and enterovirus infections), cerebral malaria, and bacterial infections. Epidemiological features (place of travel or residence, season of the year, and occurrence of other cases in the community) provide clues to the diagnosis. Specific diagnosis is by serological tests, particularly IgM enzyme immunoassay, which should be done on acute and convalescent sera and cerebrospinal fluid. From fatal cases, virus may be isolated from brain tissue or demonstrated by immunofluorescence. Virus is rarely recoverable from blood during acute illness.

Prevention

Formalin-inactivated vaccine derived from mouse brain is used for childhood immunization in Japan and some other Asian countries and is licensed in the US (JE-Vax™, Pasteur–Merieux–Connaught, Swiftwater, PA) and Britain (Cambridge Selfcare Diagnostics Ltd), and is used in other developed countries to protect travellers. The vaccine has recently been associated with a variety of allergic complications (generalized urticaria, angio-oedema) at a rate of 0.1–1 per cent. Use of the vaccine should be restricted to travellers at highest risk (travel to an epidemic area, residence in an endemic area for more than 30 days, or extensive outdoor exposure in rural areas.) In endemic areas, it is estimated that the risk of acquiring encephalitis may approach 1 in 5000 per month of exposure. Tissue culture-based vaccines (inactivated and live, attenuated vaccines) are widely used in China, and second-generation genetically engineered vaccines are under development.

Kyasanur Forest disease

Epidemiology

In 1957 this virus was isolated during an outbreak in Karnataka (then Mysore) State, India of haemorrhagic fever affecting monkeys and humans. The virus is a member of the tick-borne encephalitis antigenic complex (see below). Several hundred cases are recognized annually among persons with forest exposure in Karnataka State, with a case-fatality rate of 10–15 per cent. In 1983 a record 1555 cases and 150 deaths occurred. The peak seasonal incidence is between February and May. The virus is transmitted between immature ixodid ticks (*Haemaphysalis spinigera*) and small mammals (rodents, porcupines), passes to the adult tick stage during moulting, and is spread to man and wild monkeys by adult ticks. In 1995, a closely related virus was responsible for typical clinical cases and deaths among butchers in Saudi Arabia.

Clinical features

After an incubation period of 2–7 days there is an abrupt onset of fever, chills, headache, myalgia, abdominal pain, nausea, vomiting, and diarrhoea; physical signs include bradycardia, lymphadenopathy, and haemorrhagic manifestations. Hypotension is frequently noted towards the end of the acute stage. Fatal cases develop shock and pulmonary oedema. A biphasic illness is not uncommon, with resolution of the first phase in 5–12 days, and return of fever and signs of meningoencephalitis after an interval of 1–3 weeks. Localizing neurological signs are infrequent, and residual deficits rare. Convalescence is prolonged. Laboratory abnormalities include leucopenia, thrombocytopenia, and elevated serum transaminases during the acute phase. Diagnosis is by virus isolation from blood collected during the first week after onset or by serological tests. The best source of information about the disease is the Virus Research Institute, Pune, India. Outside India, laboratories with biocontainment level-4 facilities (Public Health Laboratories, Porton Down, Salisbury; Centers for Disease Control, Atlanta) are able to provide diagnostic assistance.

Treatment and prevention

No specific treatment is available; general supportive care, oxygen fluid replacement, and management of hypotension are appropriate.

A formalized tissue culture vaccine developed in India is in limited use.

Louping ill

This is a disease of veterinary importance, causing encephalitic illness in sheep and to a lesser extent in cows, horses, farmed deer, sheepdogs, and pigs. The virus, isolated in 1931, is a member of the tick-borne encephalitis complex, and is transmitted by *Ixodes ricinus*. Louping ill occurs in the hill country along the western coast of Scotland and northern England, Ireland and Norway. Natural infections resulting in human disease have been rare, but laboratory infections are not uncommon. Ten naturally occurring cases are documented, including a veterinarian, abattoir workers, and farmers. Some of these cases were attributable to contact with sheep blood. The human disease is characterized by aseptic meningitis or encephalitis; no fatal infections have occurred. Avoidance of tick bite in enzootic areas is recommended. The licensed tick-borne encephalitis vaccine may be protective.

Omsk haemorrhagic fever

This disease was first recognized in 1945 in western Siberia. Cases were frequent between 1945 and 1949, with morbidity rates of 500 to 1400/100 000, but subsequently have been rare. The virus is a member of the tick-borne encephalitis complex. Human infections are acquired by tick bite or contact with infected muskrats. The disease is characterized by abrupt onset of fever, headache, myalgia, facial flushing, conjunctival suffusion, minor haemorrhagic manifestations, and leucopenia. Recovery occurs in the second week, and the case-fatality rate is low (0.5–3 per cent). The differential diagnosis includes tularaemia, rickettsial infection, and leptospirosis. Specific diagnosis is made by virus isolation from blood during the acute phase or by serological tests. Only a few laboratories outside Russia with biocontainment level-4 facilities are capable of providing laboratory assistance (see Kyasanur Forest disease). Tick-borne encephalitis vaccines may cross-protect against Omsk haemorrhagic fever.

Murray Valley encephalitis

This disease, originally labelled 'Australia X disease', was recognized during an epidemic of encephalitis in New South Wales, Queensland, and the Murray Valley of Victoria in 1917–18. The virus was isolated in 1951 and belongs to the Japanese encephalitis virus complex. Another outbreak occurred in 1974, and sporadic cases have been recorded in other years in NSW and in Western Australia. The total recorded number of cases is only approximately 300, but with a case-fatality rate of 40 per cent. Children and elderly people are at highest risk. The virus is transmitted by *Culex annulirostris* mosquitoes, with wild birds the principal amplifier hosts. Asymptomatic infection is the rule, with serosurvey data suggesting one clinical case per 800–1000 infections. Those who become ill, however, experience severe disease similar to Japanese encephalitis. Diagnosis is by serological tests; the diagnostic assays must distinguish Murray Valley virus infection from that due to a closely related sympatric virus (Kunjin), which also causes encephalitis illness. Virus isolation from brain affords a postmortem diagnosis. Treatment is supportive. No vaccine is available.

Powassan encephalitis

The virus was first isolated from the brain of a fatal case in Powassan, Ontario in 1958. Since then, approximately 20 human cases have been recognized in eastern Canada and the eastern US, primarily in children, with a case-fatality rate of 10 per cent and a high incidence of residual neurological dysfunction. Serological surveys indicate an antibody prevalence of 1–3 per cent. The distribution of the virus in North America is considerably wider than indicated by human cases, and the diagnosis should be suspected in any case of summer–fall encephalitis. Asymptomatic infection occurs in Russia, and one human fatality has been reported. The virus is transmitted between *Ixodes* ticks and rodents. The clinical features are those of viral encephalitis, with localizing neurological signs and convulsions. Diagnosis is by serological tests, which should include analysis of local (IgM) responses in cerebrospinal fluid. There is no specific treatment or vaccine.

Rocio encephalitis

The virus was first isolated in 1975 during an epidemic of human encephalitis affecting the Ribeira Valley south-east of São Paulo, Brazil. The virus is more closely related to members of the Japanese encephalitis complex than to other flaviviruses. Epidemics in 1975–76 caused 871 cases (incidence 3.8 per cent), principally young adult male agricultural workers and fishermen. Since then, only rare sporadic infections have occurred. The probable vector is *Aedes scapularis* and wild birds are amplifying hosts. The clinical disease is characteristic of viral encephalitis; 4 per cent of the cases died and 20 per cent had neuropsychiatric sequelae. Diagnosis is by IgM enzyme immunoassay on serum or cerebrospinal fluid. Virus is not recoverable from blood, but postmortem diagnosis is made by virus isolation from brain tissue. Treatment is supportive; there is no vaccine.

St Louis encephalitis

Epidemiology

The virus, antigenically related to Japanese encephalitis, was isolated from human brain during an epidemic in Illinois and Missouri in 1932–33. Since 1955, 5000 cases have been reported, representing 30 per cent of all cases of viral encephalitis diagnosed in the US and 70 per cent of all cases of arboviral encephalitis. The case-fatality rate is 8 per cent overall, but 20 per cent in persons over 60 years. The ratio of infection to clinical illness is high, ranging from 800:1 in children under 10 years to 85:1 in persons over 60 years. The disease occurs throughout the US. Outbreaks have also occurred in southern Canada and northern Mexico. The virus has a wide distribution in tropical America, but few human cases are recorded. In North America, the virus is transmitted between *Culex* mosquitoes and wild birds.

Clinical features

Three clinical syndromes are recognized, with increasing severity: fever with headache, aseptic meningitis, and encephalitis. After an incubation period of 4–21 days, the typical case of encephalitis presents with fever, headache, chilliness, nausea, and urinary-tract symptoms (frequency, urgency, dysuria). Within 1–4 days, central nervous signs appear with meningism, tremor, abnormal reflexes, ataxia, and cranial-nerve palsies, convulsions (especially in children), stupor, and coma. The cerebrospinal fluid contains fewer than 500 cells/mm^3, principally lymphocytes. The peripheral leucocyte count, serum transaminase, and creatine phosphokinase levels may be raised. The syndrome of inappropriate antidiuresis has been noted in up to one-third of patients. Deaths occur within 2 weeks of onset. Complications include bronchopneumonia, sepsis, stress ulcer, and pulmonary embolism. Underlying diseases (hypertension, diabetes, alcoholism) adversely affect outcome. Pathological study reveals inflammation and neuronal degeneration principally in the thalamus, midbrain, and brain-stem. Up to 50 per cent of patients who recover may have a prolonged convalescence (irritability, memory deficits, asthenia, ataxia) lasting several months, and some of these patients seem never to recover fully.

Diagnosis and differential diagnosis

The differential diagnosis includes other viral encephalitides, and bacterial and fungal infections of the central nervous system. Some elderly patients have initially been diagnosed as having had a stroke. Epidemiological features (residence, season of the year, and occurrence of other cases in the community) provide diagnostic clues. Specific diagnosis is by serological tests, particularly IgM enzyme immunoassay, on sera and cerebrospinal fluid. From fatal cases, virus may be isolated from brain tissue or demonstrated by immunofluorescence. Virus is rarely recoverable from blood during the acute phase.

Treatment and prevention

Treatment is supportive. Inappropriate antidiuresis is managed by water restriction. If signs of cerebral oedema are present, this condition should be treated. No antiviral agents are available.

There is no vaccine. Prevention is aimed at surveillance and mosquito abatement.

Tick-borne encephalitis

Epidemiology

The disease was described in 1932 in the far east of the former Soviet Union, and a virus (now called Russian spring–summer encephalitis, RSSE) isolated from blood of patients and from ixodid ticks in 1934. RSSE virus, Central European encephalitis (CEE) virus, louping ill, Powassan, Kyasanur Forest disease, and Omsk haemorrhagic fever viruses belong to the tick-borne encephalitis antigenic complex.

The distribution of RSSE and CEE viruses is determined by that of their vectors, *Ixodes persulcatus* and *I. ricinus*, respectively. RSSE causes human disease principally in the Far East, the Urals, and western Siberia, whereas CEE occurs at highest incidence in Eastern and Central Europe, Moldavia, the Ukraine, and Byelorus, with smaller numbers of cases from Western Europe, the Balkans, and Scandinavia. Infections occur during the period of tick activity. Hundreds to thousands of cases occur annually, with morbidity rates approaching 20/100 000 in some areas. Occupational and vocational pursuits favouring tick exposure are risk factors. The transmission cycle involves immature ticks, insectivores, and rodents; the virus is passed to the adult ticks through the moulting process, and then by tick bite to man and domestic animals, which do not contribute to virus transmission. Human infection may also be acquired by consumption of raw milk or cheese from goats, or more rarely, sheep or cows. Domestic livestock do not have observable symptoms; however, dogs may occasionally acquire clinical infections.

Clinical features

The incubation period is 7–14 days. The onset of RSSE virus is acute, with fever, headache, photophobia, chilliness, nausea, and vomiting, followed by meningism, and evolution of the encephalits syndrome over several days. Paralysis of the upper extremities, shoulder girdle, face, and neck are typical. The case-fatality rate is approximately 20 per cent, and up to 60 per cent of survivors are left with neurological sequelae, including flaccid paralysis. CEE is milder and typically has a biphasic course. The first phase is a non-specific influenza-like illness lasting a week. After a period of remission of a few days, fever returns, with aseptic meningitis or encephalomyelitis. The case-fatality rate is 1–5 per cent; about 20 per cent of survivors have neurological effects.

Diagnosis and differential diagnosis

The differential diagnosis is similar to Japanese encephalitis; the pattern of flaccid paralysis may be confused with poliomyelitis. A history of bite by small ixodid ticks is elicited in fewer than half the cases. Specific diagnosis is made by virus isolation from blood or cerebrospinal fluid during the first week of illness, or by serological tests, including IgM enzyme immunoassay.

Treatment and prevention

Treatment is supportive.

Effective inactivated vaccines prepared in tissue culture are produced in Russia, Austria, and Germany. The vaccine produced against the CEE virus by Immuno AG, Vienna has been used to immunize the entire Austrian population, with a dramatic decline in disease incidence. Cross-protection is probable (but not clinically established) between the CEE and RSSE vaccines. Use of a licensed vaccine (in Britain, obtainable from Immuno Ltd) should be seriously considered for tourists planning camping or extensive outdoor activities during the tick transmission season in endemic areas, particularly as Russia and Central Europe open up to tourism. In addition to the vaccine, commercial hyperimmune globulin preparations are available (in Britain, also from Immuno Ltd) for use after tick exposure or to provide short-term pre-exposure prophylaxis.

West Nile fever

Epidemiology

This virus, recovered from a fever patient in Uganda in 1937, is a member of the Japanese encephalitis antigenic complex. Despite its wide distribution in Africa, the Middle East, Southern Europe, and Asia, human disease is relatively infrequent. Epidemics have occurred in Israel in the 1950s and 1960s, in South Africa in the 1970s, and in Romania in 1996 (with over 600 cases of central nervous system disease), and in New York in 1999. Sporadic cases and small clusters of cases have been reported from India, Egypt, and subSaharan Africa. Encephalitis in horses has been described in southern France and Egypt. The transmission cycle involves mosquitoes (*Culex* spp.) and wild birds. Humans are incidental hosts.

Clinical features

Human infections are usually asymptomatic or so mild as to escape attention. The incubation period is 1–6 days. Disease may present as a dengue-like illness, lasting up to a week. The accompanying rash is maculopapular or roseolar and non-pruritic; unlike dengue, desquamation does not occur. In its more severe form, West Nile virus infection causes aseptic meningitis or encephalitis. The latter appears to be more frequent and severe in elderly people (like St Louis and Japanese encephalitis), but severe and fatal cases are also described in children. The case-fatality rate in cases of encephalitis approaches 5 per cent. Unusual clinical presentations include myocarditis, pancreatitis, and hepatitis.

Diagnosis and differential diagnosis

The differential diagnosis includes influenza, sandfly fever, dengue, chikungunya, Sindbis, and other viral infections. Cases with meningitis or encephalitis must be distinguished from enteroviral infections, herpes, and Japanese and tick-borne encephalitis. Specific diagnosis is by virus isolation from blood during the first few days of fever. Serologic diagnosis may be complicated by cross-reactivity with other flaviviruses.

Treatment and prevention

There is no specific treatment or vaccine. Experimental and epidemiological studies suggest that Japanese encephalitis vaccine might protect against West Nile disease.

Yellow fever

History and epidemiology

The disease was described in the seventeenth century and was one of the great plagues of mankind for over 200 years. In 1900, mosquito transmission and viral aetiology were proven. The virus was isolated in 1927 and vaccines developed in the 1930s. Epidemics still occur, especially in West Africa. Between 1986 and 1991, a series of outbreaks in Nigeria caused over 100 000 cases (although only about 5000 were officially reported), with attack rates in affected areas of 30/1000 and case-fatality rates exceeding 20 per cent. Cases among unvaccinated travellers are rare; however, in 1996 two travellers died in the US and Europe of infection acquired in Brazil.

The virus is present in tropical America and Africa, but does not occur in Asia. In South America the disease affects up to 300 persons/year, principally young adult males engaged in forest work exposed to tree-hole breeding *Haemagogus* mosquitoes (jungle yellow fever). The virus transmission cycle involves these mosquitoes and monkeys. In the past 15 years the domestic mosquito and historical yellow-fever vector, *Ae. aegypti*, has reinvaded South America, resulting in the re-emergence of urban yellow fever in Bolivia in 1998, in which humans serve as viraemic hosts in the transmission cycle. In Africa, monkeys and a variety of tree-hole breeding *Aedes* spp. sustain transmission. Epidemics occur in moist savanna regions, involving these vectors and humans as viraemic hosts. In dry areas and urban centres, where water-storage practices breed domestic *Ae. aegypti*, this mosquito is responsible for epidemic transmission.

Clinical features

Approximately 1 in 20 infections results in clinical disease with jaundice. In its classical form, disease occurs abruptly after an incubation period of 3–6 days. The initial phase ('period of infection'), during which time viraemia is present, is characterized by fever, chilliness, headache, lumbosacral pain, myalgia, nausea, and prostration. On examination, the patient is febrile, with a relative bradycardia, and conjunctival injection. Within several days, the patient may recover transiently ('period of remission'), only to relapse ('period of intoxication') with jaundice, albuminuria, oliguria, haemorrhagic manifestations (especially 'black vomit' haematemesis), delirium, stupor, metabolic acidosis, and shock. The prognosis is such cases is poor, and 20–50 per cent die during the second week. Laboratory tests reveal leucopenia, hepatic dysfunction, and renal failure. The bleeding diathesis is caused by decreased synthesis of clotting factors and may be complicated by disseminated intravascular coagulation. Pathological findings include midzonal hepatic necrosis and eosinophilic degeneration of hepatocytes (Councilman bodies), possibly representing apoptosis, and acute renal tubular necrosis. Focal myocarditis, and brain swelling and petechial haemorrhages contribute to pathogenesis. Recovery is complete, without postnecrotic hepatic cirrhosis.

Diagnosis and differential diagnosis

Exposure and travel history provide important clues to aetiology. The differential diagnosis includes viral hepatitis, leptospirosis, DHF, Rift Valley fever, Ebola, and Crimean–Congo haemorrhagic fever. Specific diagnosis is accomplished by testing serum obtained during the period of infection by virus isolation, polymerase chain reaction, or antigen. Serological methods (especially IgM enzyme immunoassay) are useful, but cross-reactions with other flaviviruses may complicate interpretation. Postmortem histopathological examination of the liver is diagnostic, with or without immunocytochemical staining for viral antigen. Liver biopsy should never be performed on living patients, as it may precipitate lethal haemorrhage.

Treatment and prevention

Treatment is symptomatic. Intensive care and countermeasures to acidosis, shock, and other pathophysiological disturbances should be instituted. Patients with renal failure may require dialysis.

The live, attenuated 17D vaccine, delivered as a single 0.5 ml subcutaneous dose, is highly effective. Immunity is probably lifelong, but for travel certification revaccination is recommended every 10 years. Reactogenicity is minimal. Persons with documented egg allergy should not be immunized or should be skin tested with the vaccine. The vaccine must not be given to children under 6 months of age, in whom there is a risk of postvaccinal encephalitis, and it is best to delay vaccination until 12 months of age if possible. On theoretical grounds, persons with immunosuppression (including those with clinical AIDS) should not be immunized; the immune response in HIV infected subjects is impaired. No evidence of clinical congenital infection was found. Immunization during pregnancy is contraindicated, but, if inadvertently performed, mothers should be reassured and followed. The immune response in pregnancy was found to be impaired.

Other flaviviral infections

Sporadic cases of illness caused by other flaviviruses have been reported.

Viruses causing febrile illness with myalgia/arthralgia, with or without rash: **Apoi** (Asia, no vector known); **Banzi** (Africa, mosquito-borne); **Bussuquara** (South America, mosquito-borne); **Cacipacore** (South America. no vector known); **Dakar bat** (Africa, a bat virus, no arthropod vector); **Edge Hill** (Australia, mosquito-borne); **Kokobera** (Australia, mosquito-borne); **Koutango** (Africa, mosquito-borne); **Sepik** (New Guinea, mosquito-borne); **Spondweni** (Africa, mosquito-borne); **Usutu** (Africa, mosquito-borne); **Wesselsbron** (Africa, Asia, mosquito-borne); **Zika** (Africa, Asia, mosquito-borne).

Viruses causing febrile illness, aseptic meningitis, or encephalitis: **Ilheus** (South America, mosquito-borne); **Kunjin** (Australia, mosquito-borne); **Langat** (Asia, tick-borne); **Modoc** (North America, no vector known); **Negishi** (China, Japan, tick-borne); **Rio Bravo** (North America, a bat virus, no arthropod vector).

Further reading

Centers for Disease Control (1993). Inactivated Japanese encephalitis virus vaccine. Recommendations of the Advisory Committee on Immunization Practices (ACIP). *Morbidity and Mortality Weekly Reports*, 42, 1–15.

Halstead, S.B. (1989). Antibody, macrophages, dengue virus infection, shock, and hemorrhage: a pathologic cascade. *Reviews of Infectious Diseases*, **11**, S830–9.

Kurane, I., *et al.* (1991). Activation of T lymphocytes in dengue virus infections. High levels of soluble interleukin 2 receptor, soluble CD4, soluble CD8, interleukin 2, and interferon-γ in sera of children with dengue. *Journal of Clinical Investigation*, **88**, 1473–80.

Monath, T.P. (ed.) (1989). *The arboviruses: epidemiology and ecology*, Vols I–V. CRC Press, Boca Raton, FL.

Monath, T.P. and Tsai, T.F. (1997). The flaviviruses. In *Clinical virology* (ed. D.D. Richman, R.J. Whitley, and F.G. Hayden). Churchill Livingstone, New York.

Robertson, S.E., Hull, B.P., Tomori, O., *et al.* (1996). Yellow fever. A decade of resurgence. *Journal of the American Medical Association*, **276**, 1157–62.

Chapter 16.29
Bunyaviridae

J. S. Porterfield and J. W. LeDuc

The family Bunyaviridae contains over 300 viruses, divided between five genera, *Bunyavirus*, *Hantavirus*, *Nairovirus*, *Phlebovirus*, and *Tospovirus*, with some unassigned viruses; the larger genera are further subdivided into serogroups. Over 60 family members infect humans, about 20 causing important and sometimes fatal diseases (see Table 1). All members share basic structural, biochemical and genetic properties like a spherical, enveloped virion 80–120 nm in diameter, and a genome of single-stranded, negative sense RNA divided into three segments. Significant biochemical and biological differences exist between the genera. Bunyaviruses, nairoviruses, and phleboviruses are all arboviruses, their principal vectors being, respectively, mosquitoes, ticks, and phlebotomines, whereas hantaviruses are zoonotic agents infecting primarily rodents, which may spread to humans by close contact. Tospoviruses are arthropod-transmitted plant viruses of no known medical importance.

Bunyaviridae occur worldwide, some in several continents, others having a more limited range. Their distribution is largely dependent upon that of their associated vector (bunyaviruses, nairoviruses, and phleboviruses), or relevant murine host (hantaviruses). The epidemiology of some, such as La Crosse virus (genus *Bunyavirus*)

Table 1 The family Bunyaviridae: genera, serogroups, vectors, and viruses infecting humans

Genus and serogroup	Vector	Viruses infecting humans
Bunyavirus(over 150)		
Anopheles A (12)	Mosquito	Tacaiuma
Anopheles B (2)	Mosquito	
Bakau (5)	Mosquito	
Bunyamwera (32)	Mosquito	**Bunyamwera1**, Calovo, Fort Sherman, Germiston, Ilesha, Maguari, Shokwe, Tensaw, Wyeomyia
Bwamba (2)	Mosquito	Bwamba, Pongola
C group (14)	Mosquito	Apeu, Caraparu, Itaqui, Madrid, Marituba, Murutucu, Nepuyo, Oriboca, Ossa, Restan
California (14)	Mosquito	**California encephalitis**, Guaroa, **La Crosse**, **Inkoo**, **Jamestown Canyon**, **snow-shoe hare**,**Tahyna**, trivittatus
Capim (10)	Mosquito	
Gamboa (8)	Mosquito	
Guama (12)	Mosquito	Catu, Guama
Koongol (2)	Mosquito	
Minatitlan (2)	Mosquito	
Nyando (2)	Mosquito	Nyando
Olifanstsvlei (5)	Mosquito	
Patois (7)	Mosquito	
Simbu (24)	Mosquito	**Oropouche**, Shuni
Tete (5)	Mosquito	
Turlock (5)	Mosquito	
Unassigned (3)	Mosquito	
Hantavirus (8)		
Hantaan (8)	Rodent	**Hantaan**, **Sin Nombre**, Prospect Hill, **Puumala**, **Seoul**, **Dobrava/Belgrade**
Nairovirus (34)		
Crimean-Congo (3)	Tick	**Crimean–Congo haemorrhagic fever**, Hazara
Dera Ghazi Khan (6)	Tick	
Hughes (10)	Tick	Soldado
Nairobi S.D. (3)	Tick	Dugbe, Ganjam, Nairobi sheep disease
Qalyub (3)	Tick	
Sakhalin (7)	Tick	Avalon
Thiafora (2)	Tick	Thiafora
Phlebovirus (57)		
Phlebotomus (44)	Sandfly[1]	Alenquer, Candiru, **Chagres**, Corfu, **Punta Toro**, **Rift Valley fever**, **sandfly fever**, **Naples**, and **Sicilian**, **Toscana**
Uukuniemi (13)	Tick	Uukuniemi, Zalev-Terpeniya
Unassigned (53)	Mosquito	Bangui, Kasokero, Tataguine
	Tick	Bhanja, Keterah, Tamdy, Wanowrie
Tospovirus (1)	Thrip	

Numbers in parentheses indicate the approximate number of viruses in the genus or serogroup.

Bold type indicates the type species and viruses causing major disease in humans.

[1] Mosquito vector for Rift Valley fever virus.

or Rift Valley fever virus (genus *Phlebovirus*) is fairly well understood, but for the majority details are incompletely known.

After entry by vector bite or other routes, the virus replicates and a viraemia follows. Symptoms develop when virus undergoes further replication cycles leading to fever, sometimes with haemorrhages or encephalitis, or in some hantavirus infections to profound renal or pulmonary involvement leading to shock and death.

Laboratory diagnosis relies upon virus isolation or detection of a specific antibody response. Enzyme-linked immunosorbent assay and polymerase chain reaction techniques now assist classical diagnostic approaches, but awareness of what viruses are active in any area is essential. Some viruses require containment facilities at biohazard category 3 (hantaviruses) or 4 (Crimean–Congo haemorrhagic fever virus).

Specific treatment was limited to the use of virus-specific immunoglobulin in a very few instances, but recently there have been encouraging reports of successful application of ribavirin therapy to patients infected with some nairoviruses or hantaviruses.

Bed nets, protective screening, and other antivector procedures can reduce the danger of infection with arthropod-borne members of the family, and appropriate steps to avoid exposure to small animals limit the risks of infection with hantaviruses. Specific vaccines are available against some viruses causing animal diseases, but few are for use in humans.

Genus *Bunyavirus*

Bunyamwera virus is the type species of the genus and family. It is widespread in subSaharan Africa, but most infections are unrecognized. Most medically important viruses are in the California and Simbu serogroups. In the former, Jamestown Canyon, La Crosse, snowshoe hare, and California encephalitis viruses occur in many parts of the US, causing the clinical syndrome, California encephalitis. Most cases occur in children, more often males than females, although Jamestown Canyon virus is unusual in that more adults are involved. There is nearly always a history of outdoor exposure in areas where woodland mosquitoes are prevalent. Incubation period is 5–10 days, and is followed by gradual onset of symptoms, with fever, mild at first, and becoming more severe and frontal, leading to mental confusion and convulsions. Neck rigidity is common, as is nausea and vomiting. General lethargy may progress to coma, and although there may be meningeal signs, paralysis or permanent damage to the central nervous system is rare and mortality is less than 1 per cent. Other California serogroup viruses occur in Europe, Africa, and Asia. Tahyna virus is widely distributed in Europe and the former USSR, with antibody rates exceeding 95 per cent in parts of former Czechoslovakia and around 50 per cent in the Rhone valley in France and the Danube basin near Vienna; however, overt disease is seldom recognized. Inkoo virus is prevalent in Finland and neighbouring regions of Russia, with the great majority of adult Lapps having antibodies; emerging information suggests that small children may have signs of central nervous involvement during acute infection. Antibodies reactive with California serogroup viruses were found in human sera in Sri Lanka, China, and the far northern latitudes of Eurasia, where viruses related to Inkoo, Tahyna, and snowshoe hare viruses were isolated from mosquitoes.

In 1961 Oropouche virus (Simbu serogroup) caused a substantial epidemic in Belem, northern Brazil. Over the ensuing decades, massive Oropouche epidemics were recorded throughout the Amazon Basin, with as many as 200 000 persons infected. Symptoms include headache, generalized body and back pains, prostration, and moderately high fever (40°C). Rash occasionally accompanies infection, as does meningitis or meningismus. Illness lasts from 2–5 days, occasionally with protracted convalescence. No fatalities have been reported.

Genus *Hantavirus* (see also Chapter 12.11)

This takes its name from Hantaan virus, the cause of Korean haemorrhagic fever, which was isolated in 1976 from its rodent host, *Apodemus agrarius*. The clinical diseases it and related hantaviruses cause have been known under many different synonyms, including epidemic haemorrhagic fever, Korean haemorrhagic fever, nephropathia epidemica, and haemorrhagic fever with renal syndrome; the last was adopted by the WHO to serve as a common name for hantaviral disease which may be caused by three distinct viruses: Hantaan virus, found primarily in Asia, with an enclave of disease in the Balkan region of Europe; Puumala virus, found in Scandinavia, western Russia, and recently in much of Europe; and Seoul virus, probably globally distributed wherever *Rattus norvegicus* populations exist uncontrolled. Recently another hantavirus, Sin Nombre virus, was shown to cause a severe and often fatal condition, hantavirus pulmonary syndrome, in North and South America.

Hantaan virus causes a severe, life-threatening disease with mortality of about 5 per cent, reaching as high as 30 per cent in select populations. Puumala virus infections are less severe, although patients still require hospitalization, with death in less than 1 per cent of admitted cases. Seoul virus is thought to be the least severe of the pathogenic strains, although it too has been associated with human deaths. Sin Nombre virus has a mortality of around 50 per cent, affecting mainly adults, and is unusual in that symptoms are primarily those of acute unexplained adult respiratory distress syndrome, rather than renal disease.

Each hantavirus is specifically associated with a particular rodent host in nature: Hantaan virus with the striped field mouse, *Apodemus agrarius*; Puumala virus with the bank vole, *Clethrionomys glareolus*; Seoul virus with the Norway rat, *Rattus norvegicus*, and Sin Nombre virus with the deer mouse, *Peromyscus maniculatus*. Additional hantaviruses causing pulmonary disease have recently been discovered.

Genus *Nairovirus*

This is named after Nairobi sheep disease, an acute, haemorrhagic gastroenteritis affecting sheep and goats in East Africa, which was recognized as a viral disease associated with the sheep tick, *Rhipicephalus appendiculatus*, in 1917. In addition to the type species, which has caused laboratory infections, the genus also includes several other viruses known to infect humans, the most important being Crimean–Congo haemorrhagic fever (CCHF) virus. Crimean haemorrhagic fever was described in 1946 as an acute, febrile, haemorrhagic disease affecting humans in the Crimean region of the former USSR, transmitted by ticks and carrying a mortality of 15–30 per cent. In Africa, Congo virus was first isolated in the then Belgian Congo (now Zaire) from the blood of a child, and it caused a moderately severe laboratory infection in a European; Crimean haemorrhagic fever virus is serologically indistinguishable from Congo virus, hence the name. Different strains of CCHF virus have been associated with outbreaks of severe and sometimes fatal disease in the Crimea, Rostov, and

Astrakhan regions of the former USSR; Albania, Bulgaria, and Yugoslavia; East, West, and South Africa; Iran, Iraq, and western Pakistan; and China. Most infections are acquired by tick bites, but airborne infections have occurred in both hospital and laboratory environments. Mortality is about 15–30 per cent, but may reach 40–80 per cent in hospital or nosocomial outbreaks.

Genus *Phlebovirus*

At least nine different phleboviruses are known to infect humans. Pappataci fever, sandfly fever, or Phlebotomus fever was recognized as a clinical entity in the Mediterranean area during the nineteenth century, and the association with *Phlebotomus papatasi* sandflies was clearly demonstrated. Naples virus was isolated from human serum collected during an outbreak of sandfly fever in Naples, and Sicilian virus was isolated from troops with a similar fever in Palermo, Sicily. The two viruses have many common properties, but are serologically quite distinct. Sandfly fever is widespread throughout the Mediterranean area and occurs in Egypt, Greece, Iran, Turkey, the former Yugoslavia, Bangladesh, India, Pakistan, and the southern states of the former USSR. Toscana virus, serologically related to Naples virus, was isolated in Italy, Portugal, and Cyprus; it is notable for its ability to infect the central nervous system. The viruses that cause classical sandfly fever do not occur in the New World, but in South and Central America a similar clinical condition follows infection with Alenquer, Candiru, Chagres, and Punta Toro viruses.

The most important phlebovirus is Rift Valley fever virus, which has long been known as a disease of domestic animals, mainly sheep, in East Africa, and occasionally spreads to farm workers and others handling infected animals. The infection is endemic, but seldom recognized, in many wild game animals in Africa. Rift Valley fever virus differs from sandfly fever viruses, and most other members of the genus, in being normally transmitted by mosquitoes rather than sandflies. In East and Central Africa the virus was isolated from various mosquito species (*Aedes, Culex, Eratmopodites*) and recent studies found that it is capable of persisting in mosquito eggs during the dry season, emerging with the next generation of mosquitoes the following rainy season. In 1977 the virus spread, apparently for the first time, into Egypt, producing a major epizootic in cattle and some 600 human deaths within a period of 3 months. In Egypt, the principal vector seems to have been *Culex pipiens.* The Egyptian and later Mauritanian epidemics appear to be linked to major ecological changes following the construction of the Aswan Dam on the Nile and dams on the Senegal River.

Further reading

Calisher, C.H. and Nathanson, N. (1995). *Bunyavirus* infections. In *Exotic viral infections* (ed. J.S. Porterfield), pp. 246–60. Chapman and Hall Medical, London.

LeDuc, J.W. (1995). *Hantavirus* infections. In *Exotic viral infections* (ed. J.S. Porterfield), pp. 261–84. Chapman and Hall Medical, London.

Swanepoel, R. (1995). *Nairovirus* infections. In *Exotic viral infections* (ed. J.S. Porterfield), pp. 285–93. Chapman and Hall Medical, London.

Verani, P. and Nicolett, L. (1995). *Phlebovirus* infections. In *Exotic viral infections* (ed. J.S. Porterfield), pp. 295–317. Chapman and Hall Medical, London.

Chapter 16.30

Arenaviruses

S. Fisher-Hoch and J. B. McCormick

Rodent arenaviruses associated with human disease include Lassa virus in West Africa; Junin, Machupo, Guanarito, Sabia, and possible other viruses in South America; and lymphocytic choriomeningitis virus (LCMV) world-wide. Rodents experience silent, lifelong viraemia with high titre viruria, the primary source of environmental contamination. Human infection is primarily through cuts and scratches, and possibly the mucosae. Many mild or inapparent infections occur as well as severe (haemorrhagic) disease. Person-to-person spread is reported for Lassa fever, but is apparently rare with other arenaviruses.

Virology

The viruses are enveloped, pleomorphic viruses ranging in diameter from 50–300 nm, with a mean diameter of 110–130 nm. They contain two ambisense segments of single-stranded RNA, tightly associated with nucleocapsid protein of 65 000–72 000 molecular weight. The large strand of RNA encodes the viral polymerase and a zinc-finger protein, and the small RNA the glycoprotein precursor and the nucleoprotein. Two glycoproteins are produced by post-translational cleavage.

Lassa fever

Epidemiology

Lassa virus is found from Northern Nigeria to Guinea. The reservoir is *Mastomys natalensis*, a common peridomestic rodent. Lassa fever, although endemic and sometimes epidemic, tends to be focal, varying from village to village depending on Mastomys populations. An estimated 100 000 infections occur annually with several thousand deaths, affecting all age groups and sexes. In Sierra Leone 9–26 per cent of those infected develop symptoms, and 5–14 per cent of all febrile illness are caused by Lassa virus infection. 5–8 per cent of infections result in hospital admission, and about 17 per cent of the patients die if untreated. Lassa fever in Sierra Leone accounts for 10–16 per cent of all adult medical admissions and 30 per cent of deaths on adult medical wards. Direct contact between virus-contaminated articles and surfaces and cuts and scratches on bare hands and feet may be the most important and consistent mode of transmission in endemic areas. Rodent-to-human infection is highly associated with indiscriminate food storage, and catching, cooking, and eating rodents. In villages, risk of human-to-human spread is associated with direct contact, nursing care, or sexual contact with someone during the incubation, acute, or early convalescent phases of illness. Nosocomial spread in hospitals is associated with inadequate disinfection and direct contact with infected blood and contaminated needles.

Clinical features

The incubation period is 7–18 days. There is insidious fever, weakness, malaise, severe headache, usually frontal, and a very painful sore throat. Joint and lumbar pain and non-productive cough are common. Many patients develop a severe retrosternal chest pain, and about half will have nausea with vomiting or diarrhoea and abdominal pain.

Respiratory rate, temperature, and pulse rate are elevated and blood pressure may be low. There is no characteristic skin rash and petechiae and ecchymoses are not seen (except in conjunctivae of a few patients). Also common are conjunctivitis and pharyngitis, often with exudates, diffusely inflamed and swollen posterior pharynx and tonsils, but few ulcers. The abdomen is tender. Neurological signs in the early stages are limited to a fine tremor, most marked in the lips and tongue.

About 30 per cent of hospitalized patients progress to a prostrating illness 6–8 days after onset of fever. Persistent vomiting and diarrhoea are a poor prognostic sign. Patients are often dehydrated with elevated haematocrit. Proteinuria is common, and blood urea may be moderately elevated. There is diffuse abdominal tenderness without localizing signs or loss of bowel sounds. The severe retrosternal or epigastric pain with abnormal electrocardiograms seen in many patients may be due to pleural or pericardial involvement. Pneumonitis, and pleural and pericardial rubs develop in early convalescence in about 20 per cent of patients in hospital, occasionally in association with congestive cardiac failure. Myocarditis is not seen. Neurological signs are infrequent, but carry a poor prognosis, with progression from tremors and confusion to severe encephalopathy with or without general seizures, but without focal signs. Cerebrospinal fluid is usually normal, with a few lymphocytes. Bleeding is seen in only 15–20 per cent of patients, limited primarily to the mucosal surfaces or, occasionally, conjunctival haemorrhage or gastrointestinal or vaginal bleeding. Severe pulmonary oedema or adult respiratory distress syndrome is common in fatal cases with gross head and neck oedema, pharyngeal stridor, and hypovolemic shock.

Early lymphopenia is followed by relative or absolute neutrophilia, as high as 30×10^9/l. Though thrombocytopenia is moderate, even in severely ill patients, platelet function is markedly depressed or even absent. A serum aspartate aminotransferase (AST) level in excess of 150 u/l is associated with a case fatality of 50 per cent, and there is a correlation between an increasing AST level and a higher risk of fatal outcome. Alanine aminotransferase (ALT) is only marginally raised. Prothrombin times, and glucose and bilirubin levels are normal. Viraemia in excess of 3 $\log_{10}$ tissue culture ID_{50}/ml is associated with increasing case fatality. High virus titres are found in liver, ovary, pancreas, uterus, and placenta, but organ failure is not observed. Elevated viraemia and AST together carry a risk of death of nearly 80 per cent.

Complications and sequelae

Uveitis, pericarditis, orchitis, pleural effusion, ascites, and acute adrenal insufficiency are rare; renal and hepatic failure are not seen. A complex of haemorrhagic pericarditis and cardiac tamponade with pleural effusions and ascites 6 months after acute Lassa fever has been described. Mortality is 30–50 per cent in the third trimester of pregnancy depending on the level of obstetric care, and is a common cause of maternal mortality in West Africa. Fetal loss is more than 87 per cent. Virus is present in breast milk. Lassa fever is common in children, but may be difficult to diagnose because manifestations are so general. In very young babies, marked oedema has been reported.

Nearly 30 per cent of patients with Lassa fever infection suffer an acute loss of hearing in one or both ears, developing in early convalescence. About half of them recover within 3–4 months. Cerebellar signs are common during convalescence from severe disease, particularly tremors and ataxia, which usually resolve in a matter of weeks or months.

Pathogenesis and immunology

There is focal necrosis of the liver, adrenal glands, and spleen, with concomitant hepatic regeneration. Lassa virus depends primarily on cytotoxic T-cell responses for clearance. By the 6th day of illness, IgG antibodies are found in 46 per cent of patients and IgM antibody in 59 per cent, reaching 100 per cent by the 16th day. However, high viraemia and high IgG and IgM titres often coexist, and may persist for several months. Neutralizing antibodies to Lassa virus are absent in the serum of patients at the beginning of convalescence, and in most people are never detectable. Hyperimmune human convalescent plasma is not protective. Similarly, killed vaccine, and vaccinia-vectored vaccines expressing the nucleoprotein elicited high-level antibodies to Lassa virus, but no protection, while vaccinia-vectored glycoprotein vaccine elicited little antibody, but nevertheless provided protection. Reinfection does not lead to clinical disease.

Laboratory diagnosis

Specimens should preferably be drawn into a vacuum tube system to minimize risk of contamination and infection, and gloves must be worn. The laboratory diagnosis of arenavirus infections is by isolation of virus from serum, demonstration of a four-fold rise in antibody titre—IgG antibody with virus-specific IgM antibody in association with compatible clinical disease. The reverse transcriptase-polymerase chain reaction (RT-PCR) for detection of viral RNA is now the method of choice for diagnosis of acute disease.

Patient management and treatment

Fluid, electrolyte, respiratory, and osmotic imbalances should be corrected, and full intensive-care support, including mechanical ventilation, should be provided where possible. Care must be taken to avoid fluid overload. Pregnant women often present with absent fetal movements, and their survival depends on removal of the fetus and placenta. Ribavirin is most effective in treating acute Lassa fever when given early in disease, preferably intravenously as a 2-g loading dose followed by 1 g every 6 h for 4 days, then 0.5 g every 8 h for 6 more days. Toxicity is confined to mild reversible anaemia. Ribavirin should also be used for postexposure prophylaxis of high-risk contacts, 600 mg orally four times a day for 10 days.

Prevention and control

Lassa virus withstands drying, but can be inactivated by heat, detergents, chlorine, formalin, and ultraviolet radiation (including sunshine). The key to prevention of transmission is good hospital and laboratory practice, with simple isolation of febrile patients and rigorous use of gloves and disinfection. Lassa fever is by far the most prevalent of the haemorrhage fever viruses associated with person-to-person and nosocomial transmission. The possibility of Lassa fever must be considered in patients in or from endemic areas. Patient isolators should not be used, since they interfere with optimal care, and provide little, if any, extra protection.

Prevention

A candidate Lassa fever vaccine expressing the glycoprotein in vaccinia virus was successful in protecting monkeys challenged with a lethal inoculum of Lassa virus. Elimination of contact with rodents was effective in reducing the rate of infection in Sierra Leone.

Lymphocytic choriomeningitis virus (LCMV)

LCMV persistently infects the house mouse, *Mus musculis.* Its distribution is world-wide. Transmission to humans is sporadic, apparently because frequency of contact between humans and rodent urine is low in endemic areas, nevertheless it is likely that the majority of infections are undiagnosed.

Epidemiology

Prevalence of antibody to LCMV is between 1 and 5 per cent and in urban centres. Sporadic rural disease occurs mostly during colder months when rodents are driven indoors. Human infections are usually attributable to pet or laboratory rodents, particularly hamsters, white mice, or nude mice, especially when an aerosol of highly infectious material, such as blood, is generated.

Clinical features

The incubation period is about 1–3 weeks. The illness begins with fever, malaise, weakness, myalgia, marked in the lumbar region, and headache, often severe, retro-orbital, and associated with photophobia. Anorexia, nausea, and dizziness are common. There may be sore throat, vomiting, and arthralgias, with chest pain and pneumonitis. Only two deaths have been reported. Signs include pharyngeal inflammation, usually without exudate, and meningism.

Laboratory findings

The initial white blood-cell count is often 3^9/1 or less with a mild thrombocytopenia. There is a pleocytosis of several hundred/ml, predominantly lymphocytes, with mildly increased protein and occasionally reduced glucose.

Complications and sequelae

These include encephalopathy, aseptic meningitis, interstitial pneumonia, alopecia, orchitis, transient arthritis of the hands, and deafness. Convalescence is prolonged.

Laboratory diagnosis

Antibody to LCMV appears as early as the first week of illness, and peaks at 40–60 days. Virus may readily be cultured from cerebrospinal fluid during the acute phase of disease. IgG and IgM antibody may be detected in serum by immunofluorescent assay. RT-PCR assays are available.

Patient management

Ribavirin is known to be effective *in vitro*, and might reasonably be used; however, its penetration into the cerebrospinal fluid is poor.

New World arenaviruses

The New World arenaviruses causing human disease include Junin (Argentine haemorrhagic fever, AHF), Machupo (Bolivian haemorrhagic fever, BHF), Guanarito (Venezuelan haemorrhagic fever, VHF), and Sabia (Brazil). All are endemic in geographically limited areas. The major rodent hosts are the common *Calomys* spp.

Epidemiology

AHF was first recognized in the 1950s in northwestern Buenos Aires Province. About 21 000 cases have been reported over 30 years with seasonal peaks each May. Antibody prevalence is 12 per cent in endemic areas. Men working in rodent-infested grain fields are mainly affected. The largest known epidemic of BHF, involving several hundred cases, occurred in San Joaquin in 1963–64.

Transmission to humans is through dust and grain contaminated with virus-laden rodent urine. Person-to-person transmission is not a feature of South American haemorrhagic fever viruses.

Clinical features

After an incubation period of about 12 days there is insidious onset of malaise, high fever, severe myalgia, anorexia, lumbar pain, epigastric pain, and abdominal tenderness, conjunctivitis and retro-orbital pain, often with photophobia and constipation. Nausea and vomiting frequently follow. There is marked erythema of the face, neck, and thorax, and conjunctivitis. Patients appear toxic and there are petechiae in the axillae. Relative bradycardia is often observed.

A second stage of illness may follow with epistaxis and/or haematemesis or acute neurological disease. Haemorrhage manifestations are seen in nearly half of the patients in the form of gingival haemorrhages, epistaxis, metrorrhagia, petechiae, ecchymoses, purpura, melaena, and haematuria. Severe cases have nausea, vomiting, intense proteinuria, microscopical haematuria, oliguria, and uraemia. Fatal cases develop hypotensive shock, hypothermia, and pulmonary oedema. Renal failure has been reported. There is some electrocardiographic evidence of myocarditis. Up to 50 per cent of patients have neurological symptoms, including tremors of the hands and tongue, delirium, oculogyrus, and strabismus. Meningeal signs and abnormalities of the cerebrospinal fluid are rare. Case fatality is 22 per cent in BHF and 16 per cent for AHF.

VHF resembles AHF and Lassa fever. There is fever, prostration, headache, arthralgia, cough, sore throat, nausea/vomiting, and diarrhea with marked epistaxis, bleeding gums, menorrhagia and melaena. On physical examination, there is pharyngitis, conjunctivitis, cervicial lymphadenopathy, facial oedema, and petechiae. Thrombocytopenia and neutropenia are common. Case fatality was over 60 per cent in a small hospital series.

Laboratory findings

A white blood-cell count under 10^9/1, and a platelet count under 100^9/1 are invariable. Coagulation is mild. Proteinuria and microscopical haematuria are common. Liver and renal function tests are mildly abnormal.

Laboratory diagnosis

Immunofluorescent and EIA antibody tests may be positive by the end of the second week of illness. Neutralizing and complement-fixing antibodies to Junin are usually detectable 3–4 weeks after onset. Virus may also be cultured from serum. RT-PCR for the detection of viral RNA is becoming more widely available.

Patient management

Hyperimmune plasma reduced the mortality of AHF from 16 per cent to 1 per cent in patients treated in the first 8 days of illness. Late treatment is less successful. Plasma with high neutralizing antibody titre is more effective but may induce a late cerebellar syndrome. Ribavirin is effective in experimentally infected non-human primates, and therapeutic use of ribavirin late in disease (when plasma is not effective) is recommended for all South American arenavirus infections.

Prevention

A live attenuated vaccine against the virus has virtually eliminated AHF in endemic areas. The key to prevention and control is rodent control.

Further reading

Cummins, D. *et al.* (1990). Acute sensorineural deafness in Lassa fever. *Journal of the American Medical Association*, **264**, 2093–6.

Dykewicz, C.A. *et al.* (1992). Lymphocytic Choriomeningitis outbreak associated with nude mice in a research institute. *Journal of the American Medical Association*, **267**, 1349–53.

Helmick, G.G., Webb, P.A., Scribner, C.L., *et al.* (1986). No evidence for increased risk of Lassa fever infection in hospital staff. *Lancet*, **ii**, 1202–5.

Holmes, G.P. *et al.* (1990). Lassa fever in the United States. Investigation of a case and new guidelines for management. *New England Journal of Medicine*, **323**, 1120–3.

Maiztegui, J.I., Mckee, K.T., Barrera-Ovo, J.G., *et al.* (1998). Protective efficacy of a live attenuated vaccine against Argentine hemorrhagic fever. AHF Study Group. *Journal of Infectious Diseases*, **117**, 277–83.

Chapter 16.31

Filoviruses: Marburg and Ebola fevers

S. P. Fisher-Hoch and J. B. McCormick

Filoviruses

Ebola and Marburg are filoviruses from Africa which cause severe infections in man. There are several Ebola strains. Ebola (Zaire) causes the highest mortality. Other strains are from Sudan and Gabon and Côte d'Ivoire. There is only one known strain of Marburg virus, which apparently exists in Kenya and Uganda. African filovirus disease is characterized by acute onset, severe febrile illness with frequent haemorrhagic manifestations, and high mortality. Human infections are fortunately rare, but fulminating outbreaks have had a high profile, engendering considerable fear. The reservoir, presumably in the rain forests of equatorial Africa, is unknown, but bats are suspected. There is no evidence for insect vectors, and monkeys when infected develop a disease as fulminating as that in man, and like man are most probably accidental, dead-end hosts. Dead monkeys, however, may be a source of infection for man, but human to human transmission in conditions of poor medical care has been by far the most common cause of human infection. Transmission in these circumstances has been associated with misuse of needles and syringes, direct blood contact, and inappropriate surgery. A closely related filovirus, Reston virus, from the Philippines, causes disease in monkeys but is apparently not pathogenic in man.

Epidemiology

There have been a number of outbreaks:

- 1967, Marburg and Frankfurt, Germany and Belgrade, Yugoslavia—31 cases with seven deaths acquired from imported African green monkeys. Mostly laboratory acquired.
- 1976, equatorial Zaire and Sudan—318 cases with 280 deaths. Unsterilized needles in hospitals were largely responsible for the spread. Two new, separate filoviruses were isolated: Ebola (Zaire) and Ebola (Sudan).
- 1989–90, Reston, Virginia, US—a new Ebola-like 'Reston virus' was isolated from cynomolgus monkeys from the Philippines (Setocannersion), but no illness was found in humans.
- 1994, Kikwit, Zaire—315 cases with 244 deaths due to Ebola, amplified in a hospital.
- 1996, Gabon—February, 17 cases, originating from a single infected patient; most were hospital acquired. July, 27 cases with 18 deaths due to another strain of Ebola; 12 of the cases had been in contact with a dead chimpanzee.

Clinical spectrum of Ebola and Marburg

The incubation is 3–12 days depending on the virus strain. The onset is abrupt with fever, severe headache (usually periorbital and frontal), myalgia, arthragia, conjunctivitis, and extreme malaise. Sore throat is a common symptom, often associated with severe swelling and dysphagia, but no exudative pharyngitis. A papular, eventually desquamating, rash may occur in some patients, especially on the trunk and back; morbilliform rash has been observed on white skins. In non-human primates, petechiae are striking. Gastrointestinal symptoms develop in most patients on the second or third day of illness, with abdominal pain and cramping followed by diarrhoea and vomiting. Jaundice is not a feature of Marburg or Ebola disease. The bleeding begins about the fifth day of illness and is most commonly from the mucous membranes; gastrointestinal tract, gingiva, nasopharynx, and vagina. Death occurs in a large proportion of patients, and is associated with hypovolaemic shock and severe bleeding. Infection in pregnancy results in high maternal fatality and virtually 100 per cent fetal death. The persistence of vomiting and the onset of any signs of mucosal bleeding carry a high risk of fatal outcome. CNS involvement has led to hemiplegia and disorientation, blindness, and sometimes frank psychosis. Even in convalescence patients show prolonged weakness, severe weight loss, and in a few survivors, serious, but reversible, personality changes including confusion, anxiety, and aggressive behaviour. Mortality ranges from 35 per cent for Marburg disease, affecting patients in Europe-afforded good medical care to 90 per cent in Ebola disease in remote regions of Africa. Reduction in case fatality with human transmission has also been documented.

Pathogenesis

High titres of virus are found in serum and tissues taken at autopsy. Severe, acute fluid loss, often with frank bleeding into the tissue and into the gut, results in dehydration and electrolyte and acid–base imbalance. Bleeding is prominent, with thrombocytopenia invariable, but bleeding is not usually of sufficient volume to account for the shock. Disseminated intravascular coagulation (DIC) is not documented except in the terminal phases. Tumour necrosis factor (TNF) may play an important role. Platelet dysfunction is described in experimentally-infected primates. Profound lymphopenia early in disease is followed by marked neutrophilia. Liver enzymes aspartate aminotransferase and alanine aminotransferase (AST and ALT) are raised, but the rise in AST is disproportionately higher than ALT, and the ratio may be as great as 11:1, a feature which usefully distinguishes viral haemorrhagic fevers from fulminant viral hepatitis.

Autopsy shows widespread haemorrhagic diathesis involving skin, membranes, and soft tissue. There is focal necrosis in liver, lymph nodes, ovaries, and testes, with Councilman-like eosinophilic inclusion bodes in hepatocytes, without much inflammatory response.

Laboratory diagnosis

Care should be taken in both drawing and handling blood specimens since virus titre may be extremely high, and the virus is stable for long periods, even at room temperature. Gloves should be worn at all times, and discarded into disinfectant. All sharp instruments (needles, syringes, etc.) should be discarded. A blood specimen should be taken without anticoagulant and the serum separated by the most experienced staff under the most stringent safety facilities available at the admitting hospital or clinic (BSL 3 if possible). Serum should be transferred to a leak-proof plastic container and double-wrapped in leak-proof containers in which it may be transported to a suitable reference laboratory. Virus may be inactivated by heating at 60°C for 30 min.

High or rising titre filovirus-specific IgG is diagnostic as is the presence of IgM by IFA, but the disease evolves so rapidly that many patients die without developing antibody. Virus may be isolated and identified within 2–3 days if suitable facilities are available. Polymerase chain reaction (PCR) assays are widely available and are now the method of choice. Antigen capture EIA techniques are available in some centres.

Control of filovirus disease

No specific precautions can be identified which would avoid infections since the natural source is uncertain. Potentially-infected monkeys should be handled with extreme care to avoid direct blood contact. Prompt identification of active cases is mainly dependent on an accurate and detailed history. Early institution of safe and orderly care of the ill, along the lines currently used for AIDS patients, can be set up with effective surveillance of high-risk contacts and prompt isolation of further cases. This has been shown to ensure rapid control of an epidemic. Patient isolators are not recommended since the documented hazard to contacts is not aerosol, but direct inoculation of virus in blood or other material. Isolators induce loss of manual dexterity and fatigue, inhibit intensive care procedures and communication, do not protect against sharp instrument injury, and have no provision for resuscitation.

High-risk contacts who have had direct contact with blood or body fluids from acutely-infected humans or animals, or sexual contact with a convalescent case, should be placed under surveillance for 17 days. Laboratory accidents must be treated seriously with careful review of level of risk. Tracing and surveillance of any further potential contacts such as family members is essential. If the risk is low, simple surveillance of the individual by daily telephone contact for fever during the incubation period suffices. There is currently no prophylaxis treatment and vaccines are not available. Filoviruses do not induce classical neutralizing antibodies.

Patient management

Fluid, electrolyte, respiratory, and osmotic imbalances should be managed carefully. Patients may require full intensive care support, including mechanical ventilation, along with blood, plasma, or platelet replacement. Since the loss of fluids and macromolecules is widespread and severe, with a marked capillary leak syndrome, the maintenance of intravascular volume is a particular challenge. Nevertheless, complete recovery can be expected in survivors. Pregnant patients may present with absent fetal movements, and their survival may depend on aggressive obstetric intervention. Ribavirin and related compounds are ineffective. Early optimism that convalescent plasma might be effective is unsupported by experimental data, and, in any event, neutralizing antibodies cannot be demonstrated. Heparin is contraindicated and interferon has demonstrated no action *in vitro*.

Further reading

Feldman, H., Klenk, H-D., and Sanchez, A. (1993). Molecular biology and evolution of filoviruses. *Archives of Virology*, 7 (suppl.), 81–100.

Georges-Courbot, M.C., Lu, C.Y., Lansoud-Soukate, J., Leroy, E., and Baize S. (1997). Isolation and partial molecular characterisation of a strain of Ebola virus during a recent epidemic of viral haemorrhagic fever in Gabon [letter]. *Lancet*, **349**, 181.

World Health Organization (1978). Ebola haemorrhagic fever in Sudan, 1976. Report of a WHO/international study team. *Bulletin of the World Health Organization*, **56**, 247–70.

World Health Organization (1978). Ebola haemorrhagic fever in Zaire, 1976. Report of an international commission. *Bulletin of the World Health Organization*, **56**, 271–93.

Chapter 16.32

Papovaviruses

K. V. Shah

Papovaviruses are small, spherical, non-enveloped, doubled-stranded DNA viruses that multiply in the nucleus. Viruses of the papovavirus family fall naturally into two subfamilies: papillomaviruses (wart viruses) and polyomaviruses. They infect a wide variety of species including man and are largely host-specific. Within each subfamily the viruses are immunologically related and share nucleotide sequences but there are no such similarities between the two subfamilies.

Two polyomaviruses infect man: BK virus, associated with haemorrhagic cystitis in recipients of bone marrow transplants, and JC virus, the aetiological agent of progressive multifocal leucoencephalopathy, a fatal demyelinating disease that occurs in people who are immunodeficient, notably with AIDS.

Human papillomaviruses

So far, more than 80 human papillomaviruses have been recognized, of which about 30 infect mucous membranes (the genital tract, the respiratory tract, and the oral cavity) and the rest infect the skin.

Human papillomaviruses cannot be propagated in tissue culture and require nucleic acid hybridization assays for their identification.

The most important disease associations and characteristics of mucosal human papillomaviruses are listed in Table 1; the genital tract is the reservoir for all but a few. Genital human papillomavirus infections constitute the most common, viral, sexually transmitted disease and may sometimes infect non-genital mucosal sites, for example, the respiratory tract, the mouth, and the conjunctiva. Transmission of genital-tract human papillomavirus (HPV) types 6 and 11 from an infected mother to the baby at birth may result in

Table 1 Mucosal human papillomaviruses: chief clinical associations

Clinical association	Viral type(s)
Exophytic condyloma; respiratory papillomas; oral and conjunctival papillomas.	HPV-6,-11
Cervical cancer 'High-risk' infections	HPV-16,-18,-45,-56
'Intermediate-risk' infections	HPV-31,-33,-35,-39,-51,-52,-58
'Low-risk' infections	HPV-6,-11,-42,-43,-44
Focal epithelial hyperplasia of the oral cavity	HPV-13,-32

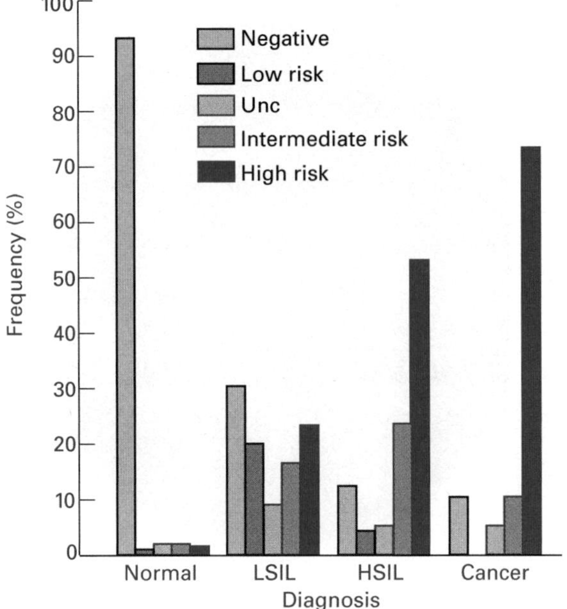

Fig. 1 Distribution of human papillomavirus (HPV) types in normal women and in preinvasive (low-grade and high-grade squamous intraepithelial lesions (SILs)) and invasive cancer. In each diagnostic category, specimens are grouped as containing high-risk, intermediate-risk, and low-risk HPV types (see Table 1), or as containing unclassified HPVs (Unc), or as negative (Neg).
(Modified and reproduced from Lörincz et al. (1992), with permission.)

juvenile-onset recurrent respiratory papillomatosis. Infection with two types, HPV-13 and -32, appears to be confined to the mouth.

Cervical cancer (see Chapter 17.6)

Human papillomavirus DNAs are recovered from over 90 per cent of cases of invasive cervical cancer, and certain virus types are preferentially associated with malignancy. From their distribution in normal individuals and in preinvasive and invasive cervical disease, genital-tract human papillomaviruses have been categorized as 'high-risk', 'intermediate-risk', and 'low-risk' types (Fig. 1; Table 1). HPV-16 and -18 are the predominant viruses in invasive cancers and account for 40–60 per cent and 5–20 per cent, respectively, of cervical cancers in different studies. About a dozen additional types of human papillomavirus are found in small proportions of invasive cancers. The 'low-risk' human papillomaviruses are almost never detected in invasive cervical cancers. Comparisons of different human papillomavirus types for their ability to transform human keratinocytes *in vitro* show that HPV-16 and -18, those most clearly associated with naturally occurring cervical cancers, also have the greatest oncogenic potential in laboratory studies. The transforming human papillomavirus proteins E6 and E7 interact with cellular tumour-suppressor proteins p53 and Rb, respectively, and distort the cell cycle, leading to genetic instability and accumulation of cellular mutations which underlie cervical cancer.

The possibility that diagnosis of human papillomavirus may be a useful adjunct to Pap smears in screening for cervical cancer and for clinical management of women with Pap smear abnormalities is a subject of extensive, ongoing investigations. In addition, HPV-specific immunotherapy of established cervical cancers and prophylactic vaccination to prevent cervical cancer are expected to be tried in the near future.

Cancers at other lower anogenital tract sites

Synchronous neoplasia at multiple sites in the female lower genital tract is almost always associated with human papillomaviruses, especially HPV-16. Carcinoma of the vulva is aetiologically heterogeneous. Vulvar cancers occurring in younger women are associated with human papillomaviruses but the typical squamous-cell carcinoma of the vulva in older women is not. Neoplasia of the anal canal, seen frequently in homosexual men seropositive for human immunodeficiency virus, is strongly associated with human papillomaviruses.

Anogenital warts*

Anogenital warts (condylomas) are the most commonly recognized, clinical manifestations of genital human papillomavirus infections. More than 90 per cent of condylomas result from infections with HPV-6 and HPV-11. It is estimated that in the USA there are more than a million annual consultations with private physicians for anogenital warts.

Epidemiology

Genital and anal warts are most common between the ages of 16 and 24 years. They are transmitted by direct sexual contact to 60 per cent of sexual partners of people with genital warts. Rarely, genital lesions are secondary to common warts on non-genital areas. Both anogenital warts and laryngeal papillomatosis may occur in children whose mothers had vulval warts at the time of delivery. Anogenital warts in children can also be due to close but non-sexual contact within a family or can be secondary to common skin warts, but in many cases sexual abuse by an infected adult is responsible.

Clinical features

The incubation period is between 3 weeks and 8 months (mean 2.8 months). In men, condylomata acuminata (exophytic condylomas) most often appear on areas exposed to coital trauma—the glans penis, coronal sulcus, prepuce, and terminal urethra. The soft, fleshy vascular tumours are usually multiple and may coalese into large masses (Fig. 2). Sessile or papular warts are more likely to occur on dry areas such as the shaft of the penis (Fig. 3). The raised pink or grey lesions, 0.5–3 mm in diameter, may occur alone or with exophytic condylomas. Subclinical HPV lesions (flat condylomas) are identified by examining the genitalia with magnification after the application of 5 per cent aqueous acetic acid solution. The affected areas are slightly raised

*Based on OTM3, pp. 3366–9 (Chapter 21.7 Genital warts. J.D. Oriel).

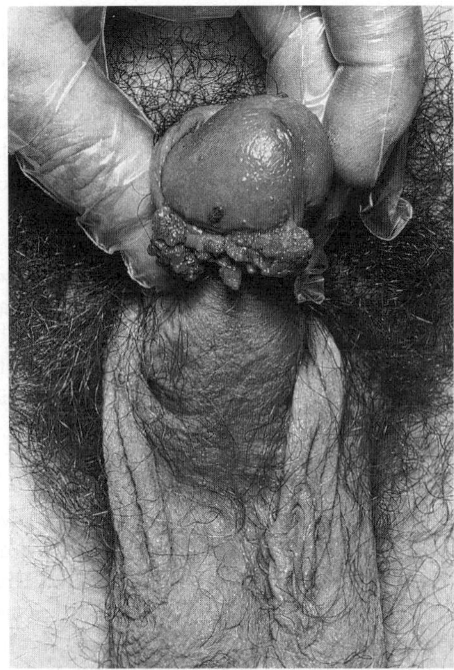

Fig. 2 Condylomata acuminata (exophytic condylomas) of penis.

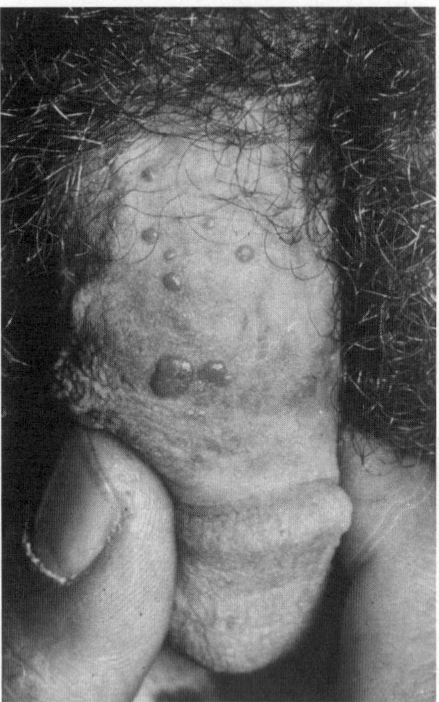

Fig. 3 Sessile (papular) warts of penis.

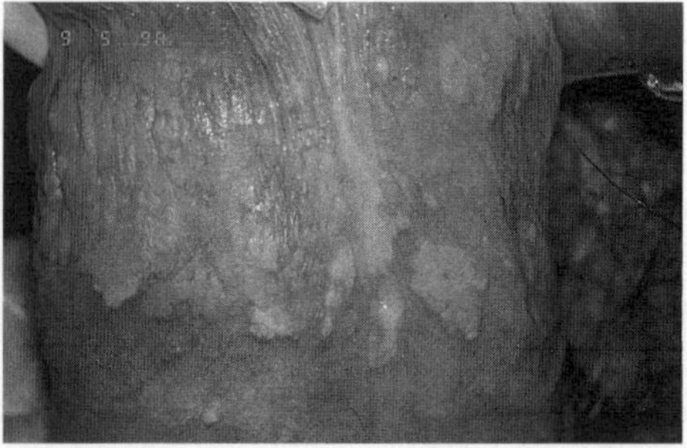

Fig. 4 Subclinical human papillomavirus lesions (flat condylomas) of penis after application of 5 per cent aqueous acetic acid.

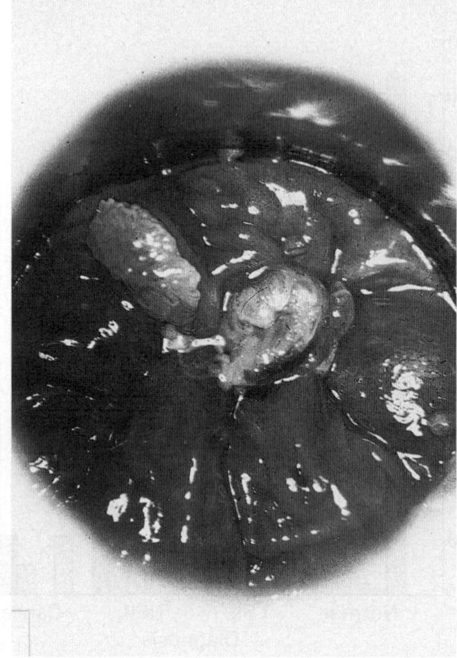

Fig. 5 Condylomata acynubate of anal canal in an anoreceptive homosexual man.

and shiny white (acetowhite), with a rough surface (Fig. 4). Flat condylomas affect the same areas as exophytic condylomas.

Perianal warts are usually exophytic and in moist conditions around the anus may reach a large size. In 50 per cent of cases, condylomas also appear in the anal canal (Fig. 5). Areas of acetowhite epithelium indicative of subclinical HPV infection may be associated with perianal warts or occur alone.

In women, exophytic condylomas are the most common HPV lesions (Fig. 6). They appear at the fourchette and adjacent areas and may spread to the rest of the vulva, the perineum, anus, vagina, and cervix. Multiple sessile warts may affect the labia and perineum. Subclinical HPV infection presents as slightly raised acetowhite lesions: the fissuring of these may cause dyspareunia. About 15 per cent of women with vulval warts have exophytic condylomas on the cervix. Subclinical infection is more common, and consists of acetowhite lesions with punctation due to capillary loops, which can be identified by colposcopy (Fig. 7). Large, exophytic vulval condylomas may develop during pregnancy and may become so large that they compromise delivery. Most regress postpartum.

Intraepithelial neoplasia comprises Bowen's disease, Bowenoid papulosis, and carcinoma *in situ*. They may be associated with genital warts but contain sequences of HPV-16 or -18 and may become malignant.

Diagnosis and management

Genital warts must be distinguished from Fordyce's spots, fibroepithelial polyps, molluscum contagiosum, and the papullar lesions of secondary syphilis. Intraepithelial neoplasia may be difficult to distinguish; lesions that appear atypical or respond poorly to treatment must be biopsied early.

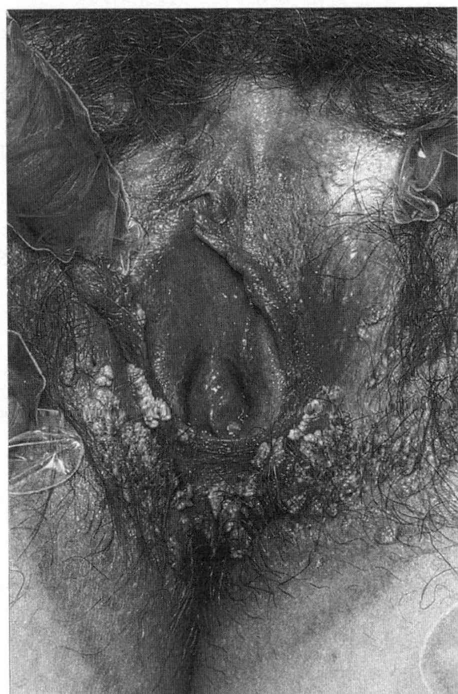

Fig. 6 Condylomata acuminata of vulva.

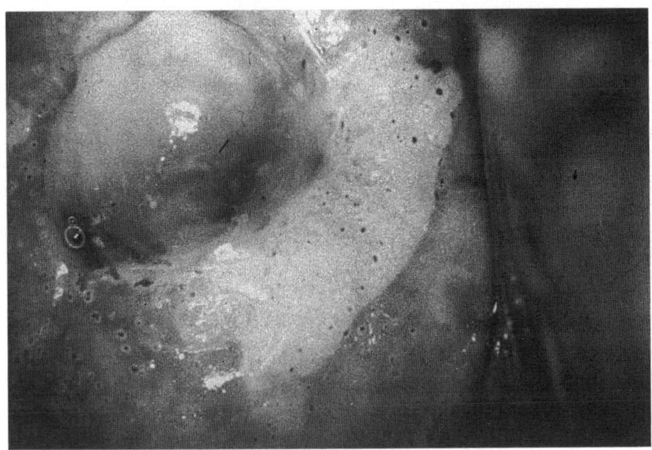

Fig. 7 Subclinical human papillomavirus infection of cervix.

Associated sexually transmitted diseases must be excluded. Sexual partners should be examined. Intraepithelial neoplasia must be excluded. Cervical cytological examination should always be done on women with vulval warts and on female partners of men with penile warts.

No specific antiviral treatment is available. The application of podophyllin or other cytotoxic agents, such as 5-fluorouracil and tricloracetic acid, is often unsuccessful. Warts may be destroyed with cryotherapy by liquid nitrogen or a nitrous oxide cryoprobe, electrocautery, electrodessication, and scissor excision. Interferons have been used in the treatment of persistent anogenital warts. A topical cream, which can be self-administered and is immunomodulatory, has become available recently in the treatment of genital warts.

Respiratory papillomatosis

This is a rare disease that may occur at any age but is most common in children under the age of 5 years. It may become life threatening if it obstructs the airways. The most common site of papillomatosis is the vocal cords and the usual presenting symptoms are hoarseness or voice change. Respiratory papillomas tend to recur after surgical removal.

Most are caused by HPV-6 and-11, genital-tract human papillomaviruses. In juvenile patients, transmission occurs from mother to offspring during passage through an infected birth canal, and in adults the transmission may occur by sexual contact. Respiratory papillomas very rarely progress to invasive cancer.

Caesarean delivery for mothers who are found to have genital warts or are infected with HPV-6 or -11 would reduce the risk of juvenile-onset respiratory papillomatosis, but many caesarean deliveries would be required to prevent a case. Interferon therapy is not very effective.

Skin warts (see Section 11)

Skin warts and verrucas may occur at any location on the skin and have diverse morphological features. They are most common in older children and young adults. Except in the rare condition known as epidermodysplasia verruciformis (see below), they almost never become malignant, and most regress within 2 years. Some human papillomavirus types are strongly associated with specific types of warts; for example HPV-1 with deep plantar warts, HPV-2 and -4 with common warts, and HPV-3 and -10 with flat skin warts.

Epidermodysplasia verruciformis

This is a rare, life-long disease in which a patient has extensive warty involvement of the skin that cannot be resolved. Many HPV types are recovered from these lesions. In about a third of the cases, foci of malignant transformation occur in the lesions located in areas of the skin exposed to sunlight. The tumours are slow growing and they rarely metastasize. The disease is often familial and patients sometimes have a history of parental consanguinity. The pattern of inheritance is suggestive of an X-linked recessive defect resulting in an immunological inability to resolve the warty infection. Carcinomas in these patients are associated with infection by specific human papillomavirus genotypes, for example HPV-5 and -8. Thus the factors that contribute to the occurrence of carcinoma in these patients include a genetic defect, infection with specific human papillomaviruses, and exposure of the affected area to sunlight.

Human polyomaviruses

BK virus and JC virus, the two polyomaviruses that infect man, were both recognized in 1971. BK and JC viruses have 75 per cent nucleotide sequence homology, but the two infections are readily distinguishable from one another by conventional tests.

Infections with both viruses occur in childhood and are largely subclinical. Most of the children affected have antibodies to BK virus by the age of 10; infection with JC virus occurs at a somewhat later age. Both viruses establish latent, often life-long infection in the kidney and are occasionally excreted in the urine of normal individuals. Reactivation of the viruses in immunodeficient patients is responsible for most associated illnesses. The viruses are reactivated in pregnancy but without any apparent harm to the mother or the newborn.

BK virus-associated illnesses

Reactivation of BK virus in renal transplant recipients is associated with some cases of ureteral obstruction, which is a late and uncommon complication of transplantation. Reactivation does not increase the risk of death or of loss of renal function. In bone marrow transplant

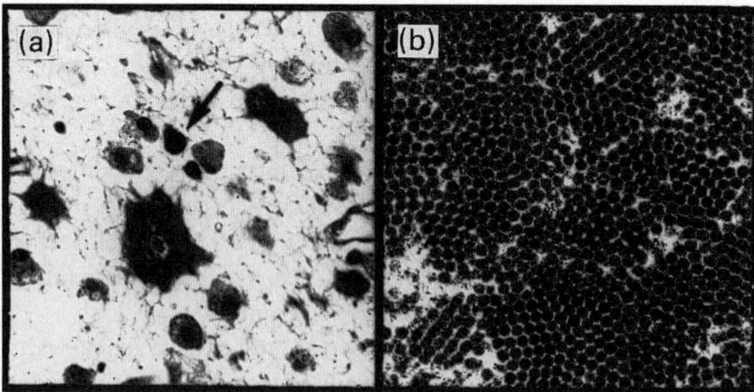

Fig. 8 A lesion of progressive multifocal leucoencephalopathy showing oligodendrocytes with enlarged, deeply staining nuclei (arrow) and giant astrocytes (left). Crystalloid array of JC virus particles in an infected oligodendrocyte nucleus (right).
(Reproduced from Shah (1992), with permission.)

recipients receiving allogeneic marrow, late-onset haemorrhagic cystitis and BK viruria are strongly correlated. Primary infection with BK virus may be responsible for an occasional case of cystitis in normal children and for rare cases of tubulointerstitial nephritis in immunodeficient individuals.

Progressive multifocal leucoencephalopathy (see also Chapter 16.35 and Section 13)

JC virus is the aetiological agent of progressive multifocal leucoencephalopathy, a subacute demyelinating disease of the central nervous system that occurs as a complication of illnesses known to impair cell-mediated immunity. It was a previously rare disease found mainly in patients in the fifth or sixth decades of life who were suffering from lymphoproliferative disorders or chronic diseases. In the past decade, this encephalopathy has been seen much more frequently and in younger patients because it occurs in 1 to 2 per cent of AIDS cases, who are now the majority of all patients with this disease. The encephalopathy has also been recognized in children who have inherited immunodeficiency diseases or AIDS.

The key pathogenetic event in the leucoencephalopathy is the cytocidal JC virus infection of oligodendrocytes, which are responsible for the production and maintenance of myelin. Destruction of the oligodendrocytes by JC virus leads to foci of demyelination that tend to coalesce over time and involve large areas of the brain. Infected oligodendrocytes, containing large inclusion-bearing nuclei filled with abundant numbers of virus particles, surround the foci of demyelination (Fig. 8). Enlarged astrocytes, which often show bizarre nuclear changes but are mostly virus negative, are found within the foci of demyelination. JC virus is disseminated haematogenously to the central nervous system, probably through virus-infected B lymphocytes. (Clinical aspects are discussed in Chapter 16.35.)

Further reading

Brown, D.R. and Fife, K.H. (1990). Human papilloma virus infections of the genital tract. *Medical Clinics of North America*, 74, 1455–85.

Crawford, L. (1993). Prospects for cervical cancer vaccines. *Cancer Surveys*, 16, 215–29.

Gross, G., Jablonska, S., Fister, H., and Stegner, H.E. (ed.) (1990). *Genital papilloma virus infections*. Springer-Verlag, Berlin.

Lörincz, A.T., Reid, R., Jenson, A.B., Greenberg, M.D., Lancaster, W., and Kurman, R.J. (1992). Human papillomavirus infection of the cervix: relative risk associations of 15 common anogenital types. *Obstetrics and Gynecology*, 79, 328–7.

Shah, K.V. (1992). Polyomavirus, infection and immunity. In *Encyclopedia of immunology* (ed. I.M. Roitt), pp. 1256–8. Academic Press, New York.

Shah, K.V. and Howley, P.M. (1996). Papillomaviruses. In *Virology* (ed. B.N. Fields *et al.*), pp. 2077–109. Lippincott-Raven, Philadelphia.

zur Hausen, H. (1994). Molecular pathogenesis of cancer of the cervix and its causation by specific human papillomavirus types. In *Human pathogenic papillomaviruses* (ed. H. zur Hausen), pp. 131–56. Springer Verlag, Heidelberg.

Chapter 16.33

Parvoviruses

B. J. Cohen

Members of the family Parvoviridae are small (23 nm), non-enveloped, single-stranded DNA viruses with icosahedral symmetry. The genus Erythrovirus includes parvovirus B19 (B19 virus), the only member of Paroviridae known to cause disease in human. Initially described in healthy blood donors, B19 is now known to cause a spectrum of disease (see below).

Clinical features of parvovirus B19 infection

B19 infection is most common in children aged between 6 and 10 years. It is asymptomatic or presents as a non-specific, febrile illness in about 50 per cent of children.

Erythema infectiosum

The most common specific clinical manifestation is erythema infectiosum, an erythematous rash illness (fifth disease) of childhood. Classically, this begins with facial erythema ('slapped-cheek disease') (Plate 1) and subsequently involves the trunk and limbs where the rash has a lacy or reticular appearance and tends to fade and recrudesce for a week or so after its initial appearance. School outbreaks are common during winter and spring. One or two epidemic years are followed by several with a low incidence. Sporadic cases also occur in children and adults; they may be misdiagnosed as rubella, streptococcal infection, or allergy. Occasionally, B19 infection presents as a purpuric rash, sometimes with thrombocytopenia.

Acute arthropathy

Joint involvement occurs in less than 10 per cent of children with B19 infection but approximately 80 per cent of adult cases (especially in females) are complicated by arthropathy. The typical presentation is an acute-onset, symmetrical, polyarthritis affecting mainly the small joints of the hands and resolving within a few weeks. Occasionally, the arthropathy persists for months or years and resembles rheumatoid arthritis. In such cases, however, rheumatoid factor is usually negative and there is no erosive joint disease, so an association between rheumatoid arthritis and B19 infection cannot be confirmed.

Embryopathy

About 10 per cent of B19 infections in pregnancy end in spontaneous abortion in the second trimester, a rate of fetal loss 10 to 20 times

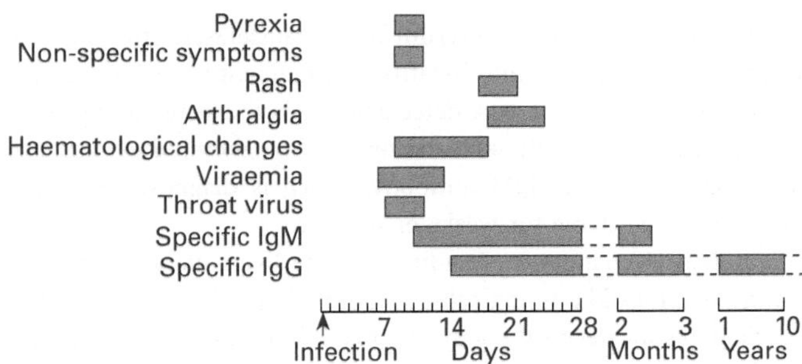

Fig. 1 Sequence of events in human volunteers experimentally infected with parvovirus B19 by intra-nasal inoculation of a dilution of a blood donor plasma containing B19 virus.

greater than that in unaffected pregnancies. Embryopathy is usually detected 4–6 weeks after a symptomatic or asymptomatic maternal infection and typically presents as fetal hydrops. Fetal B19 may be treaded with *in utero* blood transfusions. Surviving infants have no evidence of congenital disease.

Transient aplastic crisis

The transient interruption of erythropoiesis caused by B19 infection is insufficient to cause anaemia in individuals with normal red cells. In those with a shortened red cell lifespan, such as patients with sickle cell anaemia, B19 infection rapidly leads to a more profound anaemia. The event is termed an aplastic crisis and has also been recorded in patients with hereditary spherocytosis, β-thalassaemia intermedia, pyruvate kinase deficiency, and other red cell disorders.

B19 infection in immunocompromised patients

Patients with underlying immunodeficiency (Nezerlof's syndrome, organ transplantation, acute lymphatic leukaemia, human immunodeficiency virus infection) fail to produce neutralizing antibody to B19 virus and infection becomes chronic. This results in persistent anaemia and patients may become transfusion dependent.

Prevention and therapy

A recombinant DNA-derived B19 vaccine is under development but is not yet available. To help minimize the risk of spread by infected blood components, blood donor screening has been proposed but it is not yet known whether this is cost-beneficial. Early recognition of B19 infection in hospitalized cases is important for the prevention of nosocomial transmission. Severe infections in immunocompromised patients are treated with high doses of intravenous normal immunoglobulin.

Laboratory diagnosis

B19 infection is commonly confirmed by specific IgM serology since, in most cases, the rash and joint symptoms are postviraemic phenomena (Fig. 1). Detection of virus is important for the diagnosis of fetal B19, aplastic crisis, and infection in immunocompromised patients.

Further reading

Brown, K.E., Young, N.S., and Liu, J.M. (1994). Molecular, cellular and clinical aspects of pervovirus B19 infection. *Critical Reviews in Oncology/Hematology*, **16**, 1–31.

Hall, S.M. (1990). Parvovirus B19 and pregnancy. *Reviews in Medical Microbiology*, **1**, 160–7.

Pattison, J.R. (1987). B19 virus—a pathogenic human parvovirus. *Blood Reviews*, **1**, 58–64.

Chapter 16.34

Hepatitis viruses and TT virus

J. N. Zuckerman and A. J. Zuckerman

Introduction

The last three decades have witnessed an explosion in knowledge of viral hepatitis, a major public health problem throughout the world affecting several hundreds of millions of people. Viral hepatitis is an important cause of morbidity and mortality, both from acute infection and chronic sequelae which include, with hepatitis B and hepatitis C infection, chronic active hepatitis, cirrhosis, and primary liver cancer.

The hepatitis viruses include a range of unrelated human pathogens:

- Hepatitis A virus (HAV) is a small, unenveloped, symmetrical RNA virus which shares many of the characteristics of the picornavirus family. Classified as a hepatovirus within the heparnavirus genus, it is the cause of infectious or epidemic hepatitis transmitted by the faecal–oral route.
- Hepatitis B virus (HBV) is one of the hepadnavirus group of double-stranded DNA viruses that replicate by reverse transcription. Hepatitis B virus is endemic in the human population and hyperendemic in many parts of the world. It is transmitted by blood-to-blood contact and by the sexual route. Mutations of the surface coat protein of the virus and of the core and other proteins have been identified in recent years.
- Hepatitis C virus (HCV) is an enveloped, single-stranded, RNA virus, distantly related to flaviviruses, but not transmitted by arthropod vectors. Seroprevalence studies confirm the importance of the parenteral route of transmission and transmission by blood and blood products, but in as many as 50 per cent of patients the origin of the infection remains unknown. Several genotypes have been described. Infection is common; it is associated with chronic liver disease and, at least in some countries, with primary liver cancer.
- Hepatitis D virus (HDV) is an unusual, single-stranded, circular, RNA virus, resembling plant viral satellites and viroids. This virus requires hepadnavirus helper functions for propagation in hepatocytes, and is an important cause of acute and severe chronic liver damage in some regions of the world. The modes of transmission are similar to the parenteral transmission of hepatitis B.
- Hepatitis E virus (HEV) is an enterically-transmitted, non-enveloped, single-stranded, RNA virus which shares many biophysical and biochemical features with caliciviruses. It has caused large epidemics of acute hepatitis in the Indian subcontinent, Central and South-East Asia, the Middle East, parts of Africa, and elsewhere; it is responsible for high mortality during the third trimester of pregnancy.
- GB viruses and hepatitis G virus—in 1995 two independent viruses, GBV-A and GBV-B, were identified in infectious plasma of tamarin monkeys inoculated with serum from a surgeon (GB) with jaundice. A third virus, GBV-C, was later isolated from a human specimen

that was immunoreactive with a GBV-B protein. GBV-C RNA was found in several patients with clinical hepatitis. GBV-A/C, GBV-B and the hepatitis C viruses are members of distinct viral groups whose genomes show local regions of sequence identity with various flaviviruses. A virus described in 1996 as hepatitis G (HGV) is an independent isolate of GBV-C.

TT virus

TT stands for the initials of a patient in Japan with post-transfusion hepatitis. TT virus DNA has been detected in up to 97 per cent of the healthy population in some countries. Preliminary evidence indicates that this virus is similar to Circoviridae, viruses which infect plants and farm animals. The pathogenic role, if any, of this virus in human disease remains to be established.

Hepatitis A

For centuries, frequent outbreaks of jaundice have been described. The term infectious hepatitis was coined in 1912 to describe these epidemics. Hepatitis A virus (HAV) is spread by the faecal–oral route. It remains endemic throughout the world and is hyperendemic in areas with poor standards of sanitation and hygiene. Since the Second World War, the seroprevalence of antibodies to HAV has declined in many countries. Infection results most commonly from person-to-person contact, but large epidemics do occur. For example in 1988 an outbreak of hepatitis A associated with the consumption of clams in Shanghai resulted in almost 300 000 cases.

Classification

In 1983, HAV was classified in the genus enterovirus (as enterovirus 72) of the family Picornaviridae, on the basis of its biophysical and biochemical characteristics, including stability at low pH. This preempted the isolation and analysis of complementary DNA (cDNA) clones that led to the determination of the entire nucleotide sequence of the viral genome. There is limited sequence homology with the enteroviruses and rhinoviruses, although the structure and genome organization are typical of the Picornaviridae. Four genotypes of HAV have now been classified as hepatoviruses within the heparnavirus genus.

Clinical features and epidemiology

The incubation period of hepatitis A is 3–5 weeks, with a mean of 28 days. In areas of high prevalence, most children are infected early in life and such infections are generally asymptomatic. Infections acquired later in life are of increasing clinical severity. Less than 10 per cent of cases of acute hepatitis A in children up to the age of six are icteric but this increases to 40–50 per cent in the 6–14 age group and to 70–80 per cent in adults.

Non-specific, prodromal symptoms are followed by jaundice with malaise. Patients may be incapacitated for many weeks. Acute liver failure with a high mortality is very rare, as is progression to cholestatic relapsing hepatitis. Vasculitis, haemolysis, and cryoglobulinaemia have been reported. The prognosis is good and there is no evidence of subsequent chronic liver damage. Treatment is symptomatic; alcohol is forbidden, but no antiviral therapy is available.

Hepatitis A virus enters the body by ingestion. The virus then spreads, probably by the bloodstream, to the liver, a target organ. Large numbers of virus particles are detectable in faeces during the incubation period, as early as 10–14 days after exposure and persisting usually until peak elevation of serum aminotransferases. After jaundice is apparent, virus is found relatively infrequently. Persisting IgG antibody to hepatitis A virus is detectable late in the incubation period, coinciding approximately with the onset of biochemical evidence of liver damage. Specific IgM antibody, which is diagnostic of acute infection, is detectable for weeks or months.

Pathological changes are confined to the liver: marked focal activation of sinusoidal lining cells; accumulations of lymphocytes and especially histiocytes in the parenchyma, often replacing hepatocytes lost by cytolytic necrosis predominantly in the periportal areas; occasional coagulative necrosis resulting in the formation of acidophilic bodies; and focal degeneration.

Outbreaks with a common source are initiated most frequently by faecal contamination of water and food, but waterborne transmission is not a major factor in maintaining this infection in industrialized communities. Foodborne outbreaks can be attributed to the shedding of large quantities of virus in the faeces during the incubation period of the illness in infected food handlers; the source of the outbreak can often be traced to uncooked food or food that has been handled after cooking. Although hepatitis A remains endemic and common in the developed countries, the infection occurs mainly in small clusters, often with only a few identified cases. The infection is rarely transmitted by blood although transmission by blood coagulation products has been reported. Chronic excretion of the virus does not occur.

Various serological tests are available for hepatitis A, including immune adherence haemagglutination, radioimmunoassay, and sensitive enzyme immunoassay.

Control and prevention of hepatitis A

Control of hepatitis A infection is difficult. Strict isolation of cases is not a useful control measure because faecal shedding of the virus is at its highest during the late incubation period and the prodromal phase of the illness. Spread of hepatitis A is reduced by simple hygiene measures and the sanitary disposal of excreta.

Passive immunization against hepatitis A

Normal human immunoglobulin, containing at least 100 international units (IU)/ml of antihepatitis A antibody, given intramuscularly before exposure to the virus or early during the incubation period, will prevent or attenuate a clinical illness temporarily. Whenever possible, active immunization should be deployed.

The dosage should be at least 2 IU of antihepatitis A antibody/kg body weight, but in special cases such as pregnancy or in patients with liver disease that dosage may be doubled. Immunoglobulin does not always prevent infection and excretion of hepatitis A virus, and inapparent or subclinical hepatitis may develop. The efficacy of passive immunization is based on the presence of hepatitis A antibody in the immunoglobulin, and the minimum titre of antibody required for protection is believed to be about 10 IU/l.

Immunoglobulin is usually used as postexposure prophylaxis for close personal contacts of patients with hepatitis A and for those exposed to contaminated food. Immunoglobulin has also been used effectively for controlling outbreaks in institutions such as homes for the mentally handicapped and in nursery schools.

Active immunization against hepatitis A

Two doses of killed hepatitis A vaccine, given 6 months apart, induce long-lasting protective immunity. It is used to protect those at risk of infection because of personal contact or because of travel to highly endemic areas. Other groups at risk of hepatitis A infection include staff and residents of institutions for the mentally handicapped, day-care centres for children, sexually active male homosexuals, intravenous drug abusers, sewage workers, some laboratory and health-care personnel, military personnel, and certain low socio-economic groups in defined community settings.

Patients with blood coagulation defects and patients with chronic liver disease should be immunized against hepatitis A. In some developing countries, the incidence of clinical hepatitis A is increasing as improvements in socioeconomic conditions result in infection later in life and strategies for immunization are yet to be developed.

Hepatitis E

Retrospective testing of serum samples from patients involved in various epidemics of hepatitis associated with contamination of water supplies with human faeces indicated that an agent other than HAV (or HBV) was involved.

Properties of the virus

Physicochemical studies have shown that hepatitis E virus is very labile and sensitive to freeze–thawing. Morphologically the virus is spherical and unenveloped, measuring 32–34 nm in diameter with spikes and indentations visible on the surface of the particle. Confirmation that the virus has been propagated in cell culture is awaited. HEV resembles most closely the sequences of rubella virus and a plant virus, beet necrotic yellow vein virus.

Hepatitis E virus was cloned in 1991 and the entire 7.5 kb sequence is known. The genome is a single-stranded, positive sense, polyadenylated RNA molecule, with three overlapping open reading frames. New and distinct variants have been described recently in the US and Italy.

Clinical features and epidemiology

The average incubation period is slightly longer than for hepatitis A, with a mean of 6 weeks. Individual cases cannot be differentiated on the basis of clinical features from other cases of hepatitis. In epidemics, most clinical cases will have anorexia, jaundice, and hepatomegaly. Serological tests indicate that clinically inapparent cases occur. The severity of the infection and a mortality rate of 20–39 per cent during the third trimester of pregnancy are notable. Hepatitis E does not become chronic.

The epidemiological features of the infection resemble those of hepatitis A. The highest attack rates are found in young adults.

All epidemics of hepatitis E reported to date have been associated with faecal contamination of water, with the exception of a number of foodborne outbreaks in China. Sporadic hepatitis E has been associated with the consumption of uncooked shellfish and in travellers returning from endemic areas. Epidemics of hepatitis E and a high prevalence of antibody have occurred in the subcontinent of India, South-East and Central Asia, the Middle East, North and West Africa, and outbreaks have occurred in East Africa and Mexico. Infection has been reported in returning travellers.

Diagnosis

Serological tests for diagnosis detect anti-HEV IgM in up to 90 per cent of acute infections if serum is obtained 1–4 weeks after the onset of illness, and IgM remains detectable for about 12 weeks. Anti-HEV IgG appears early and reaches a maximum titre 4 weeks after the onset of illness, falling rapidly thereafter.

Tests for HEV RNA by the polymerase chain reaction are available in specialized laboratories.

Prevention

The provision of safe public water supplies, public sanitation and hygiene, safe disposal of faeces and raw sewage, and personal hygiene are essential measures. Passive immunization with immune globulin derived from endemic areas has not been successful. Vaccines are under development.

Hepatitis B

Hepatitis B virus was recognized originally as the agent responsible for 'serum hepatitis'. The incubation period is variable, ranging from 1–6 months. Clinical features of acute infection resemble those of the other viral hepatitides. Acute hepatitis B is frequently anicteric and asymptomatic although a severe illness with jaundice can occur and occasionally acute liver failure may develop.

More than a third of the world's population had been infected with hepatitis B virus, and the World Health Organization estimates that hepatitis B virus results in 1–2 million deaths every year.

The virus persists in approximately 5–10 per cent of immunocompetent adults, and in as many as 90 per cent of infants infected perinatally. Persistent carriage of hepatitis B, defined by the presence of hepatitis B surface antigen (HBsAg) in the serum for more than 6 months, has been estimated to affect about 350 million people world-wide. The pathology is mediated by the responses of the cellular immune system of the host to the infected hepatocytes. Long-term, continuing virus replication may lead to progressive chronic liver disease, cirrhosis, and hepatocellular carcinoma.

Structure and organization of the virus

The hepatitis B virion is a 42-nm particle comprising an electron-dense core (nucleocapsid) 27 nm in diameter surrounded by an outer envelope of the surface protein (HBsAg) embedded in membranous lipid derived from the host cell. The surface antigen, originally referred to as Australia antigen, is produced in excess by the infected hepatocytes and is secreted in the form of 22-nm particles and tubular structures of the same diameter.

The nucleocapsid of the virion contains the viral genome which is approximately 3.2 kb in length, and is composed of two linear strands of DNA held in a circular configuration by base pairing at the 5′ ends. Surrounding the genome is the core antigen (HBcAg) and an associated soluble *e* antigen (HBeAg). The presence of these in the serum indicates active viral replication. A DNA-dependent polymerase is also present in the nucleocapsid.

Immune responses and serological diagnosis

Antibody and cell-mediated immune responses to various types of antigens are induced during the infection; however, not all these are protective and, in some instances, may cause autoimmune phenomena that contribute to disease pathogenesis. The immune response to infection with hepatitis B virus is directed toward at least three antigens: hepatitis B surface antigen, the core antigen, and the *e* antigen.

The surface antigen (HBsAg) appears in the sera of most patients during the incubation period, 2–8 weeks before biochemical evidence of liver damage or onset of jaundice. It persists during the acute illness and usually clears from the circulation during convalescence. Next to appear in the circulation is virus-associated DNA polymerase activity, which correlates in time with damage to liver cells as indicated by elevated serum transaminases. The polymerase activity persists for days or weeks in acute cases and for months or years in some persistent carriers. HBeAg may be detectable during the same period. Antibody of the IgM class to the core antigen is found in the serum 2–10 weeks after the surface antigen appears and persists during replication of the virus. Core antibody of the IgG class is detectable for many years after recovery. Finally, antibody to the surface antigen component, anti-HBs, appears, and may be accompanied by antibody to HBeAg.

During the incubation period and during the acute phase of the illness, surface antigen–antibody complexes may be found in the sera of some patients. Immune complexes have been found in the sera of all patients with fulminant hepatitis, but are seen only infrequently in non-fulminant infection.

Immune complexes are also important in the pathogenesis of chronic liver disease and of other disease syndromes characterized by severe damage of blood vessels (for example polyarteritis nodosa, some forms of chronic glomerulonephritis, and infantile papular acrodermatitis).

Epidemiology

Although various body fluids (blood, saliva, menstrual and vaginal discharges, serous exudates, seminal fluid, and breast milk) have been implicated in the spread of infection, infectivity appears to be especially related to blood and to body fluids contaminated with blood. The epidemiological propensities of this infection are therefore wide; they include infection by inadequately-sterilized syringes and instruments, transmission by unscreened blood transfusion and blood products, by close contact, and by sexual contact. Antenatal (rarely) and perinatal (frequently) transmission of hepatitis B infection from mother to child may take place; in some parts of the world (south-east Asia and Japan), perinatal transmission is very common.

Protection against hepatitis B

The discovery of variation in the epitopes presented on the surface of the virions and subviral particles identified several subtypes of HBV which differ in their geographical distribution. All isolates of the virus share a common epitope, *a*, which is a domain of the major surface protein and is believed to protrude as a double loop from the surface of the particle. Two other pairs of mutually exclusive antigenic determinants, *d* or *y* and *w* or *r*, are also present on the major surface protein. Four principal subtypes of HBV are recognized: *adw*, *adr*, *ayw*, and *ayr*. Subtype *adw* predominates in northern Europe, the Americas, and Australasia and is also found in Africa and Asia. Subtype *ayw* is found in the Mediterranean region, eastern Europe, northern and western Africa, the Near East, and the Indian subcontinent. In the Far East, *adr* predominates but the rarer *ayr* occasionally may be found in Japan and Papua New Guinea.

Passive immunization

Hepatitis B immunoglobulin (HBIG) is prepared specifically from pooled plasma with high titre of hepatitis B surface antibody and may confer temporary passive immunity under certain defined conditions. The major indication for the administration of hepatitis B immunoglobulin is a single acute exposure to hepatitis B virus, such as occurs when blood containing surface antigen is inoculated, ingested, or splashed onto mucous membranes and the conjunctiva. Doses of 250–500 IU have proved effective. In adults, 3 ml (containing 200 IU of anti-HBs per ml) is usually given. It should be administered immediately after exposure, preferably within 48 h, not after 7 days. It is generally recommended that two doses of hepatitis B immunoglobulin should be given 30 days apart.

Results with the use of hepatitis B immunoglobulin for prophylaxis in neonates at risk of infection with hepatitis B virus are good if it is given as soon as possible, or within 12 h of birth. In this case, the number of the babies developing the persistent carrier state is reduced by about 70 per cent. Studies using combined passive and active immunization indicate an efficacy approaching 90 per cent. The dose of hepatitis B immunoglobulin recommended in the newborn is 1–2 ml (200 IU of anti-HBs per ml).

Active immunization

The major response of recipients of hepatitis B vaccine is to the common *a* epitope with consequent protection against all subtypes of the virus. First generation vaccines were prepared from 22-nm HBsAg particles purified from plasma donations from chronic carriers. These preparations are safe and immunogenic but have been superseded in some countries by recombinant vaccines produced by the expression of HBsAg in yeast cells. The expression plasmid contains only the 3' portion of the HBV surface open reading frame and only the major surface protein, without adjacent pre-S epitopes, is produced. Vaccines containing pre-S2 and pre-S1 as well as the major surface proteins expressed by recombinant DNA technology are undergoing clinical trial.

In many areas of the world with a high prevalence of HBsAg carriage, such as China and South-East Asia, the predominant route of transmission is perinatal. Although HBV does not usually cross the placenta, the infants of viraemic mothers have a very high risk of perinatal infection. Transmission from an HBeAg-positive mother can be prevented by giving the first dose of a course of vaccine immediately after birth. The protective efficacy of vaccination may be increased from approximately 70 per cent of cases to greater than 90 per cent by the simultaneous administration of hepatitis B immune globulin (HBIG).

Immunization against hepatitis B is now recognized as a high priority in preventive medicine in all countries and strategies for immunization are being revised. Universal vaccination of infants and adolescents is a possible future strategy to control transmission. More than 100 countries now offer hepatitis B vaccine to all children, including the US, Canada, and most western European countries.

In some countries with a low prevalence of hepatitis B, immunization is recommended only to groups which are at an increased risk of acquiring the infection, including people receiving repeated transfusions of blood or blood products; prolonged inpatient treatment; patients who require frequent tissue penetration or need repeated circulatory access; patients with natural or acquired immune deficiency, and patients with malignant diseases. Viral hepatitis is an occupational hazard among health-care personnel and the staff of institutions for the mentally-retarded, and in some semiclosed institutions. High rates of infection with hepatitis B occur in narcotic drug addicts and intravenous drug abusers, sexually active male homosexuals, and prostitutes. Individuals working in highly endemic areas are at an increased risk of infections and should be immunized.

Young infants, children, and susceptible people visiting or living in certain tropical and subtropical areas where present socio-economic conditions are poor and the prevalence of hepatitis B is high should also be immunized. As the mode of infection of hepatitis B is not known in about 30 per cent of patients there is a powerful argument for universal immunization.

Hepatitis B vaccine should be given intramuscularly in the upper arm or the anterolateral aspect of the thigh and not in the buttock. Several factors are associated with a poor or undetectable antibody response to currently licensed vaccines including inoculation into the buttocks, intradermal injection, sex, age, overweight, and immunosuppression. In addition, the antibody response to plasma-derived hepatitis B vaccines and recombinant DNA vaccines is inadequate in at least 5 per cent and 10 per cent of healthy immunocompetent subjects ('non-responders' and 'hyporesponders'). Definitions vary, but non-responders or hyporesponders generally have less than 10 IU/l or 100 IU/l of anti-HBs, respectively, against an international standard.

Hepatitis B surface antibody escape mutants

Production of antibodies to the group antigenic determinant *a* mediates cross-protection against all subtypes. The epitope *a* is located in the region of amino acids 124–148 of the major surface protein.

During a study of the immunogenicity and efficacy of hepatitis B vaccines in Italy, Singapore, and elsewhere, people who had apparently mounted a successful immune response producing anti-HBs, later became infected with HBV. In these patients, non-complexed anti-HBs and HbsAg coexisted, and a point mutation had occurred in the nucleotide sequence encoding the *a* epitope.

Variants of HBV with altered antigenicity of the envelope protein show that HBV is not as antigenically singular as believed previously and that humoral escape mutation can occur *in vivo*. This finding gives rise to two causes for concern: failure to detect HBsAg may lead to transmission through donated blood or organs; and HBV may infect individuals who are anti-HBs positive after immunization.

HBV precore mutants

A mutation of the penultimate codon of the precore region to a termination codon was found in some anti-HBe positive patients who were positive for HBV DNA in serum by hybridization. In most cases there was an additional mutation in the preceding codon. Precore variants have been described in many patients with severe chronic liver disease and some failed to respond to therapy with interferon. Whether the mutants are more pathogenic than the wild-type virus is unknown.

HBV and primary liver cancer

Regions of the world where the chronic carrier state is common are coincident with those where there is a high prevalence of primary liver cancer, and patients with this tumour are almost invariably seropositive for HBsAg. Case-control and cohort studies have shown a specific causal association between hepatitis B virus and hepatocellular carcinoma (HCC) and that up to 80 per cent of such cancers are attributable to this virus. Hepatitis B is thus second only to tobacco (cigarette smoking) among the known human carcinogens.

Southern hybridization of tumour DNA yields evidence of chromosomal integration of viral sequences in at least 80 per cent of HCCs from HBsAg carriers. There is no similarity in the pattern of integration between different tumours, and variation is seen both in the integration site(s) and in the number of copies or partial copies of the viral genome. Sequence analysis of the integrants reveals that the direct repeats in the viral genome often lie close to the virus–cell junctions, suggesting that sequences around the ends of the viral genome may be involved in recombination with host DNA.

The mechanisms of oncogenesis by HBV remain uncertain. HBV may act non-specifically by stimulating active regeneration and cirrhosis which may be associated with long-term chronicity. However, HBV-associated tumours occasionally arise in the absence of cirrhosis and such hypotheses do not explain the frequent finding of integrated viral DNA in tumours. In rare instances, the viral genome has been found to be integrated into cellular genes such as cyclin A and a retinoic acid receptor. Translocations and other chromosomal rearrangements also have been observed. Although insertional mutagenesis of HBV remains an attractive hypothesis to explain its oncogenicity, there is insufficient supportive evidence.

Like many other cancers, development of hepatocellular carcinoma is likely to be a multifactorial process. The clonal expansion of cells with integrated viral DNA seems to occur early and clones may accumulate in the liver throughout the period of active virus replication. In areas where the prevalence of primary liver cancer is high, virus infection usually occurs in the young and the virus replicates for many years before a tumour is detected.

Hepatitis D

Delta hepatitis was first recognized following detection of a novel protein, delta antigen (HDAg), by immunofluorescent staining in the nuclei of hepatocytes from patients with chronic active hepatitis B. Hepatitis delta virus (HDV) is now known to require a helper function of HBV for its transmission. HDV is coated with HBsAg which is needed for release from the host hepatocyte and for entry in the next round of infection.

Two forms of delta hepatitis infection are known. In the first, a susceptible individual is coinfected with HBV and HDV, often leading to a more severe form of acute hepatitis caused by HBV. In the second, an individual chronically infected with HBV becomes superinfected with HDV. This may cause a second episode of clinical hepatitis and accelerate the course of the chronic liver disease, or cause overt disease in asymptomatic HBsAg carriers. HDV itself seems to be cytopathic and HDAg may be directly cytotoxic.

Delta hepatitis is common in some areas of the world with a high prevalence of HBV infection, particularly the Mediterranean region, parts of Eastern Europe, the Middle East, Africa, and South America. It has been estimated that 5 per cent of HBsAg carriers world-wide (approximately 18 million people) are infected with HDV. In areas of low prevalence of HBV, those at risk of hepatitis B, particularly intravenous drug abusers, are also at risk of HDV infection.

Structural organization of HDV

The HDV particle is approximately 36 nm in diameter and composed of an RNA genome associated with HDAg, surrounded by an envelope of HBsAg. The genome is a closed circular RNA molecule of 1679 nucleotides and resembles those of the satellite viroids and virusoids of plants and similarly seems to be replicated by the host RNA polymerase II with autocatalytic cleavage and circularization of the progeny genomes via *trans*-esterification reactions. Unlike the plant viroids, HDV codes for a protein, HDAg.

Pathology and diagnosis

Pathological changes in HDV infection are limited to the liver and histological changes are those of acute and chronic hepatitis with no particular distinguishing features apart from severity and, in tropical areas in particular, microvesicular steatosis. Hepatitis D antigen is localized by specific nuclear fluorescence in hepatocytes of patients with chronic hepatitis B.

Laboratory diagnosis in acute infection is based on specific serological tests for anti-HDV IgM or HDV RNA or hepatitis delta antigen in serum. Acute infection is usually self-limited and markers of HDV infection often disappear within a few weeks.

Superinfection with HDV in chronic hepatitis B may lead to suppression of HBV markers during the acute phase. Chronic infection with HDV (and HBV) is the usual outcome in non-fulminant disease.

Epidemiology of HDV

Antibody to delta hepatitis has been found in most countries, commonly among intravenous drug abusers, patients with haemophilia, and those requiring treatment by blood and blood products. A high prevalence of infection has been found in: Italy and the countries bordering the Mediterranean; eastern Europe, particularly Romania; the former Soviet Union; South America, particularly the Amazon basin, Venezuela, Columbia (hepatitis de Sierra Nevada de Santa Marta), Brazil (Labrea black fever), and Peru; and parts of Africa, particularly West Africa.

The ratio of clinical to subclinical cases of HDV and superinfection is not known. However, the general severity of both forms of infection suggests that most cases are clinically significant. A low persistence of infection occurs in 1–3 per cent of acute infections and about 80 per cent or higher in superinfection of chronic HBV carriers. The mortality rate is high, particularly in the case of superinfection, ranging from 2–20 per cent.

Prevention and control

Prevention and control for HDV are similar to those for hepatitis B. Immunization against hepatitis B protects against HDV. The difficulty is protection against superinfection of the many millions of established carriers of hepatitis B and studies are in progress to determine whether specific immunization against HDV based on hepatitis D antigen is feasible.

Hepatitis C

Transmission studies in chimpanzees established that the main agent of parenterally acquired non-A, non-B hepatitis was likely to be an enveloped virus some 30–60 nm in diameter. The hepatitis C virus, obtained from plasma samples, was cloned in 1989, but it has still not been satisfactorily cultivated *in vitro*. The genome of HCV resembles those of the pestiviruses and flaviviruses.

Hepatitis C virus consists of a family of six highly related, but nevertheless distinct, genotypes, and various subtypes with differing geographical ranges. Diversity within the viral envelope proteins of different groups makes a broad, cross-neutralizing antibody response to infection unlikely.

Diagnosis of HCV infection

Cloning of portions of the viral genome permitted the development of diagnostic tests. First, the 5-1-1 antigen was detected by antibodies in the serum of an infected patient. Then, a larger clone, C100, was assembled from a number of overlapping clones and expressed in yeast as a fusion protein, which formed the basis of first generation ELISA tests for HCV infection. Unfortunately, these were associated with a high rate of false positive reactions when applied to low incidence populations.

Second and third generation tests include antigens from the nucleocapsid and further non-structural regions of the genome, and are more sensitive and specific. Positive reactions by ELISA require confirmation by supplementary testing using, for example a recombinant immunoblot assay (RIBA). Nevertheless, indeterminate results obtained by ELISA represent a significant problem which need resolution. It should also be noted that the time for seroconversion is variable and where it can be measured more precisely, for example after transfusion, it is generally 7–31 weeks.

The presence of antibodies to specific antigen components is variable and may or may not reflect viraemia. Detection and monitoring of viraemia are important for management and treatment. Sensitive techniques are available for the measurement of HCV RNA based on reverse-transcribed PCR amplification, nested-PCR, signal amplification using branched DNA analytes, and others.

Epidemiology and clinical features

Infection with hepatitis C virus occurs throughout the world. Much of the seroprevalence data are based on blood donors, who represent a carefully selected population in many countries. The prevalence of antibodies to HCV in blood donors varies from 0.02–1.25 per cent in different countries. Higher rates have been found in southern Italy, Spain, central Europe, Japan, and parts of the Middle East, with as many as 19 per cent in Egyptian blood donors. Until screening of blood donors was introduced, hepatitis C accounted for the vast majority of non-A, non-B post-transfusion hepatitis. However, it is clear that while blood transfusion and the transfusion of blood products are efficient routes of transmission of HCV, these represent a small proportion of cases of acute clinical hepatitis in a number of countries—the source of infection cannot be identified in 50 per cent of patients in industralized countries; 35 per cent of patients have a history of intravenous drug misuse; household contact and sexual exposure do not appear to be major factors in the epidemiology of this common infection; and occupational exposure in the health-care setting accounts for about 2 per cent of cases. Transmission of HCV from mother to infant occurs in about 10 per cent of viraemic mothers and the risk appears to be related to the level of viraemia.

Most acute infections are asymptomatic, with about 20 per cent of acute infections associated with jaundice. Fulminant hepatitis has been described. Extrahepatic manifestations include mixed cryoglobulinaemia, membranous proliferative glomerulonephritis, and porphyria cutanea tarda.

About 80 per cent of infections with HCV progress to chronicity. Histological examination of liver biopsies from asymptomatic HCV-carriers (blood donors) revealed that none have normal histology and that up to 70 per cent have chronic, active hepatitis and/or cirrhosis. Whether the virus is cytopathic or whether there is an immunopathological element remains unclear. HCV infection is also associated with progression to primary liver cancer. For example in Japan, where the incidence of hepatocellular carcinoma has been increasing despite a decrease in the prevalence of HBsAg, HCV is now the major risk factor.

Vaccine development

Difficulties in vaccine development include the sequence diversity between viral groups and the substantial sequence heterogeneity among isolates. Inability to culture the virus prevents the development of inactivated or attenuated vaccines (compare with Yellow fever vaccines, Chapter 16.28). Neutralizing antibodies have not been clearly defined.

GB viruses and hepatitis G virus

A serum which was obtained on the third day of jaundice from a surgeon (GB) with jaundice induced hepatitis in each of four inoculated South American tamarins or marmosets, and the agent was passaged serially in these animals. With the application of modern molecular virological techniques, two independent viruses, GBV-A and GBV-B, were identified in the infectious plasma of tamarins inoculated with GB.

GBV-A does not replicate in the liver of tamarins whereas GBV-B causes hepatitis. Cross-challenge experiments showed that infection with the original infectious tamarin inoculum conferred protection from reinfection with GBV-B but not GBV-A. A third virus, GBV-C, was isolated subsequently from a human specimen which was immunoreactive with a GBV-B protein. GBV-C RNA was found in several patients with clinical hepatitis and was shown to have substantial sequence identity to GBV-A.

A series of studies, including phylogenetic analysis of genomic sequences, showed that GBV-A, B, and C are not genotypes of hepatitis C virus, and that GBV-A and GBV-C are closely related. GBV-A/C and GBV-B and the hepatitis C viruses are members of distinct viral groups. The organization of the genes of the GBV-A, B, and C genomes shows that they are related to other positive-strand RNA viruses with local regions of sequence identity with various flaviviruses. The three GB viruses and HCV share only limited overall amino acid sequence identity.

Serological tests, using recombinant antigens and RT-PCR for specific RNA, in blood donors and other populations with a high incidence of viral hepatitis indicated the presence of antibody to each of the GB viruses in 3 per cent to as many as 14 per cent.

The virus identified as hepatitis G (HGV) is an independent isolate identical to GBV-C. The blood-borne nature of GBV-C/HGV has been clearly demonstrated and there is evidence that it persists. The association of the virus with liver damage is illustrated by raised alanine transaminase levels (ALT) and detectable GBV-C/HGV RNA in a number of patients. However, between 40 and 90 per cent of viraemic subjects have normal ALT. In some patients, there is co-infection with HBV and/or HCV. The primary manifestations, if any, of GBV-C/HGV infection may be extrahepatic and liver damage may be the result of coinfection with the hepatitis viruses—or an as yet unidentified hepatotropic agent. GBV-C/HGV infection may cause hepatitis, but data from transfusion recipients show that the rate of infection with this virus are similar among those who do and do not develop hepatitis. Although persistent infection with GBV-C/HGV is common, the role of the virus in chronic liver disease has not been established.

Treatment of viral hepatitis

Specific antiviral therapy is not available for the treatment of acute viral hepatitis but significant developments have been reported with antiviral drugs for chronic infection associated with hepatitis B, C, and D.

While a substantial number of antiviral compounds have been evaluated for the treatment of chronic hepatitis B, only interferon-α remains the mainstay of treatment. Under optimal conditions and careful selection of patients 30–50 per cent respond at least transiently, and about 20 per cent clear the virus accompanied by improvement in liver function. Combination therapy with nucleoside analogues and other drugs have shown a variable response. Lamivudine and famciclovir are effective and have just been licensed. A comparison of prednisolone withdrawal followed by interferon versus treatment with interferon only does not provide added benefit for the combined regimen.

Interferon-α is the only drug approved at present for the treatment of chronic hepatitis C and its efficacy is limited in selected patients. Combination therapy with ribavirin is under evaluation and appears to be promising.

Further reading

Carman, W.F., Thomas, H.C., Zuckerman, A.J., and Harrison, T.J. (1998). Molecular variants of Hepatitas B virus. In *Viral hepatitis*, (ed. A.J. Zuckerman and H.C. Thomas), (2nd edn), pp.141–72. Churchill Livingstone, Edinburgh.

Jenny-Avital, E.R. (1998). Hepatitis C. *Current Opinions in Infectious Disease*, **11**, 293–9.

Koff, R.S. (1998). Hepatitis A. *Lancet*, **351**, 1643–9.

Lai, M.M.C. (1995). The molecular biology of hepatitis delta virus. *Annual Review of Biochemistry*, **64**, 259–86.

McGarvey, M.J., Houghton, M., Weiner, A.J., *et al.* (1998). Hepatitis C virus. In *Viral hepatitis*, (ed. A.J. Zuckerman and H.C. Thomas), (2nd edn), pp. 253–358. Churchill Livingstone, Edinburgh.

Mushahwan, I.K. and Zuckerman, J.N. (1998). Clinical implication of GB virus C. *Journal of Medical Virology*, **56**, 1–3.

Schalm, S.W., de Man, R.A., Heytink, R.A., and Nieters, H.G.M. (1995). New nucleoside analogues for chronic hepatitis B. *Journal of Hepatology*, **22**, 52–6.

Vidor, E., Fritzell, B., and Plotkin, S. (1996). Clinical development of a new inactivated hepatitis A vaccine. *Infection*, **24**, 447–58.

World Health Organization (1983). Prevention of liver cancer. *Technical Report Series*, No. 691. Geneva.

Zuckerman, J.N. (1996). Non-response to hepatitis B vaccines and the kinetics of anti-HBs production. *Journal of Medical Virology*, **50**, 283–8.

Zuckerman, J.N., Sabin, C., Craig, F.M., Williams, A., and Zuckerman, A.J. (1997). Immune response to a new hepatitis B vaccine in healthcare workers who had not responded to standard vaccine: randomised double blind dose-response study. *British Medical Journal*, **314**, 329–33.

Chapter 16.35
HIV infection and AIDS

G. A. Luzzi, R. A. Weiss, and C. P. Conlon

Introduction

The acquired immunodeficiency syndrome (AIDS) was first recognized in 1981 in the US, when several cases of *Pneumocystis carinii*

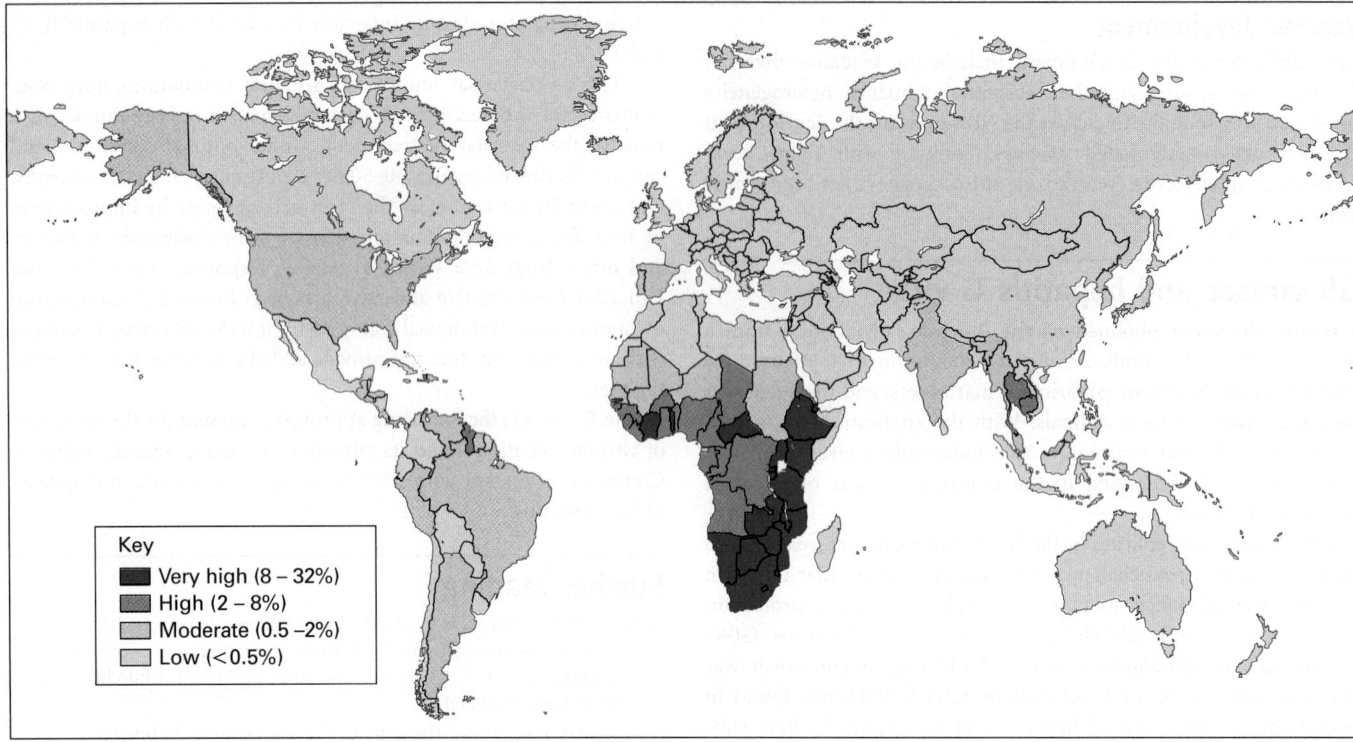

Fig. 1 World distribution of HIV (UNAIDS/WHO, 1998)
(Reproduced from Report on the global HIV/AIDS epidemic, June 1998.(1998). UNAIDS/WHO, with permission).

pneumonia and Kaposi's sarcoma were reported in homosexual men in New York and California. The variety of unusual infections and other conditions signified a new form of cellular immunodeficiency. Soon after, the syndrome was reported in injecting drug users, haemophiliacs, and recipients of blood transfusions. Early epidemiological data suggested that the cause was a blood-borne infective agent that was sexually transmissible. In 1983, a new retrovirus was isolated from a patient with persistent, generalized lymphadenopathy in France. Initially referred to as lymphadenopathy associated virus (LAV) or human T-lymphotropic virus III (HTLV-III), it was renamed human immunodeficiency virus (HIV) in 1986.

At the time of its discovery, HIV was already globally widespread, the earliest infections having probably occurred before the 1950s. The recognition of heterosexual intercourse as the most common means of HIV transmission world-wide followed the investigation of epidemics in Africa and the Caribbean. Infected mothers could pass the virus on to their fetus or neonate, establishing vertical transmission as another important route of HIV infection.

In 1986, a second retrovirus causing AIDS, HIV-2, was identified in West Africa. It is largely confined to this region, while HIV-1 is the cause of the world pandemic of AIDS. Over the past 5 years, our understanding of the pathogenesis of HIV, its clinical monitoring, and therapy has greatly increased.

Epidemiology

The global HIV-1 pandemic has particularly affected developing countries. Despite under-reporting, the WHO estimated that by the end of 1997 over 30 million people were living with HIV worldwide. Over 90 per cent of them live in sub-Saharan Africa, South and South-East Asia, and Central and South America (Fig. 1).

The numbers of people infected with HIV must be distinguished from cases of AIDS, which follows an asymptomatic period of about 10 years and may be influenced by interventions such as combination antiretroviral therapy. World-wide, the WHO estimated a 9 per cent increase in new infections in 1997 compared to 1996.

In North America, western Europe, and Australasia the epidemic began in the late 1970s and early 1980s among homosexual men and injecting drug users. However, in these regions the proportion attributable to heterosexual transmission is increasing. The estimated incidence of AIDS in western Europe rose every year between 1985 and 1994, stabilized in 1995, and fell by 10 per cent in 1996 and by over 20 per cent in 1997. A similar trend has been observed in North America. Cases attributed to injecting drug use form the largest proportion of diagnosed cases of AIDS in Europe. Emerging epidemics of HIV have been reported in injecting drug users in several countries of the former Soviet Union.

Two-thirds of the global total live in sub-Saharan Africa, where HIV transmission is predominantly heterosexual and perinatal. The estimated overall prevalence there is 7–8 per cent, rising to 20–30 per cent in some countries such as Zambia and Zimbabwe, where AIDS has greatly reduced population growth. Because of the predominant heterosexual transmission, the overall male-to-female ratio in Africa is approximately 1:1 compared to 9:1 in North America and western Europe.

In Africa, rates of AIDS and new HIV infection are predicted to plateau by 2000 and then to fall, whereas trends suggest a continuing rise in South and South-East Asia, where the emergence of epidemic HIV occurred later and opportunities for prevention were missed. A rapid rise in incidence occurred in Thailand and India in the late 1980s, initially among intravenous drug users and prostitutes and then through heterosexual spread; the WHO now estimates that 3–5

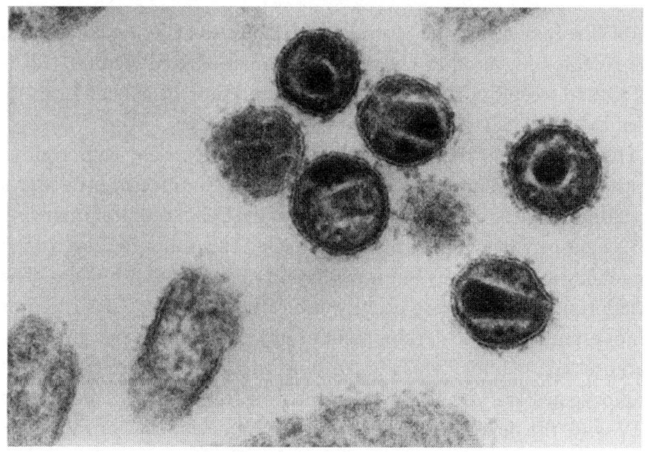

Fig. 2 Electron micrograph of HIV-1
(reproduced by courtesy of H. Gelderblom.)

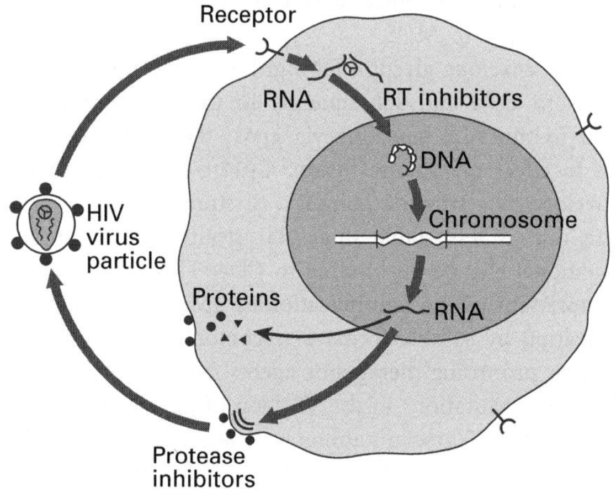

Fig. 3 Replicative cycle of HIV.

million people are infected in India alone. Rapid spread and major epidemics of HIV are also reported in China, Cambodia, Myanmar, and Vietnam.

High rates of transmission of HIV continue in developing countries because of ignorance, poverty, high rates of other sexually transmitted infections, and risky behaviour such as use of prostitutes and, increasingly, injecting drug use.

HIV-2 is endemic in parts of West Africa and is increasingly prevalent in Angola, Mozambique, France, and Portugal. In other parts of the world the prevalence is very low, although it is present in India. The clinical features of HIV-2 are similar to those of HIV-1, but some patients with HIV-2 appear to progress much more slowly, if at all: the reasons for this are unclear.

Cellular biology of HIV

The viral replication cycle

HIV-1 (Fig. 2) and HIV-2 belong to the lentivirus subfamily of retroviruses. Retrovirus implies a 'backwards' step in biological information during viral replication attributable to its enzyme, reverse transcriptase. As with all retroviruses, the viral genes in infectious particles are carried as RNA but upon infection of the host cell, reverse transcriptase catalyses the synthesis of a double-stranded DNA viral genome (Fig. 3). Insertion of the DNA genome into the chromosomal DNA of the infected cell is effected by viral integrase. The integrated provirus may remain latent, particularly in resting lymphocytes. In actively infected cells, however, RNA transcripts and proteins are synthesized, leading to the formation of new virus particles.

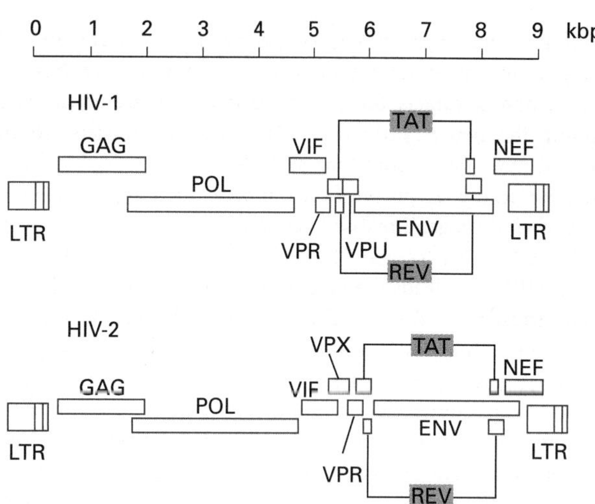

Fig. 4 The HIV genome.

The core proteins derived from the *gag* and *pol* genes are made as large polypeptides that are then cleaved into smaller components representing the enzymes and building blocks of the virus. This cleavage is achieved by the viral protease. The unique reverse transcriptase and protease are targets of antiretroviral therapy. The integrase may become a target in the future, and agents may be developed to block viral entry and viral RNA processing. Compounds that inhibit any stage of HIV replication, without being too toxic to the infected person, might be developed as antiviral drugs. Reverse transcriptase inhibitors, such as zidovudine and lamivudine, affect an early step in HIV replication, whereas the protease inhibitors, such as saquinavir or indinavir, block a late stage of virus assembly (Fig. 3).

HIV genes and proteins

Although regarded as a complex retrovirus, HIV has only nine genes (Fig. 4). The three structural genes are *gag*, *pol*, and *env*, encoding the core proteins (p19, p24, and p17), the enzymes (protease, reverse transcriptase, and integrase), and the envelope glycoproteins (gp120 and gp41) respectively. The major regulatory genes *tat* and *rev* encode proteins that are not assembled into the virus but are essential for replication in the cell. The Tat protein acts in positive feedback to enhance transcription of viral RNA from the DNA provirus, while Rev protein helps the efficient transport of viral RNA from the nucleus to the cytoplasm. Either of these proteins could be a suitable target for antiviral therapy, particularly Tat, because the synthesis of all the other viral proteins depends on its activity.

The functions of the four accessory genes of HIV are less well understood. *Vif* encodes a protein assembled in virus particles that appears necessary for infectivity at a stage soon after entry, possibly by facilitating disassembly of the virion to allow reverse transcription. *Nef* also effects an early postentry function; it is not needed by laboratory-adapted HIV strains or if virus enters via endosomal vesicles rather than fusing with the outer cell membrane. It also downregulates surface expression of the primary cell surface receptor for HIV, the CD4 antigen, by drawing CD4 into clathrin-coated pits.

Vpu similarly interacts with CD4, promoting its degradation by directing it to the ubiquitin–proteasome pathway. *Vpr* has dual functions; first it directs the preintegration complex of the virus, containing the newly-synthesized DNA, into the nucleus so that it can integrate into chromosomal DNA; secondly it blocks cell proliferation in the G2 phase of the cell cycle, thereby enhancing the amount of viral progeny released per cell.

Unlike HIV-1, HIV-2 and SIV lack *vpu* but have an alternative gene *vpx*. HIV-2 *vpr* leads the viral genome into the cell nucleus but does not arrest the cell cycle. These proteins presumably recognize cellular proteins and some of these interactions are species-specific. Thus the *vpr* and *vif* proteins in SIV of African green monkeys do not function in human cells while the equivalent proteins of SIV from sooty mangabey monkeys work well in human cells. This could explain why sooty mangabey SIV crossed host species to infect humans and became HIV-2, whereas the more widespread African green monkey SIV has not led to a zoonosis. Another difference is that HIV-1 incorporates the cellular protein cyclophylin A (the target of the drug cyclosporin A) into virus particles, where it may co-operate with *vif* and is required for steps early in the infection. In contrast, HIV-2 does not contain cyclophylin A and replicates well without it.

HIV receptors and cellular tropism

CD4 is the cell surface receptor for HIV; it is expressed on T-helper lymphocytes, the cells that become depleted in AIDS. CD4 is also expressed (to a lesser extent but sufficient to permit infection) on macrophages, Langerhans dendritic cells in mucous membranes, and brain microglial cells. These are the other target cells for HIV infection. CD4 is necessary to initiate HIV infection but is not sufficient to allow the virus to fuse with host cell membranes: another cellular component or coreceptor is required.

Different substrains of HIV, even those isolated from the same patient, exhibit specific tropisms for different cell types in culture. All isolates can infect primary CD4 lymphocytes, but only some infect macrophages while others can infect cell lines established from $CD4^+$ leukaemic cells. Macrophage-tropic strains predominate early in the course of HIV infection, and may be more transmissible from person to person. They do not cause CD4 lymphocytes to fuse together in culture and hence are referred to as non-syncytium inducing (NSI) strains. In contrast, many HIV isolates established from late-stage infection rapidly adapt in culture to infect T-cell lines and are syncytium inducing (SI). Approximately 50 per cent of AIDS patients develop SI strains in addition to NSI strains. It had been suggested that subtype E virus from Thailand infected Langerhans cells more readily than the virus subtype B prevalent in western countries and that this tropism related to a heterosexual mode of transmission. However, this claim has not been confirmed on examining more isolates from many subtypes. Indeed, the differences in cellular tropism and SI/NSI phenotype occur in all HIV subtypes or clades, which appear to reflect geographical variation of HIV rather than specific biological properties of the virus.

A partial explanation of the complex cellular tropism of HIV has been provided by the recent discovery that different members of the chemokine receptor family act as coreceptors for HIV entry into cells. Chemokines are chemoattractant, locally-acting hormones or cytokines that bind to one or more receptors which are structurally related to olfactory and neurotransmitter receptors. Following binding to the CD4 receptor, primary NSI strains use CCR5, the chemokine receptor for macrophage inhibitory proteins (MIP-1α, MIP-1β) and RANTES. In contrast, the SI strains of HIV use the CXCR4 coreceptor, the receptor for another chemokine, stromal-derived factor-1 (SDF-1). Other receptors such as CCR3 (the receptor of eotaxin) can be used by some NSI strains.

High levels of MIP-1α or β in the blood correlate with relative resistance to HIV infection. Some exposed yet uninfected individuals are homozygous for an inherited defect of the CCR5 receptor involving a 32 base-pair deletion in the CCR5 gene. This mutation has a high frequency in Caucasians but is not found in Africans and Asians. The deletion homozygotes are healthy, indicating that the CCR5 receptor is not essential for the development of immune competence, probably because MIP-1 and RANTES can bind to alternative receptors. But homozygotes are genetically resistant to infection by NSI strains of HIV and the few homozygotes with A32 deletions who are HIV positive appear to have been infected with SI strains that utilize CXCR4 instead. Other, more subtle, mutations in the promoter region of the CCR5 gene allowing only low levels of coreceptor expression may confer relative resistance to HIV infection and also, if infected, slower progression to AIDS.

The outer envelope glycoprotein, gp120, is the molecule on HIV that binds to CD4 and subsequently to the coreceptor. Gp120 is anchored to the viral envelope via gp41, the viral protein that is thought to effect membrane fusion. Gp120–gp41 is present in the viral envelope as a trimeric complex. SI strains have a gp120–gp41 structure that is less stable than NSI strains, readily undergoing conformational change on binding to CD4. This property makes SI strains more sensitive to neutralization by gp120 antibodies and also to inactivation by soluble forms of recombinant CD4, which were once seen as promising therapeutic agents. NSI strains, however, are more resistant. Mutations in the V3 loop of gp120 can convert NSI strains to SI strains. These mutations arise naturally during progression to AIDS and may allow HIV to switch to infect different cell types via new coreceptors.

The discovery that chemokine receptors serve together with CD4 to let HIV into cells promises to provide a new target for antiviral therapy. The natural chemokines themselves act as competitive inhibitors of HIV entry; certain chemically modified chemokines act as strong HIV inhibitors without triggering the downstream signalling of the receptor. This may lead to a new class of anti-HIV drugs.

Diagnosis of HIV infection

Acute infection is accompanied by the development of serum antibodies to the core and surface proteins of the virus, usually in 2–6 weeks. Over 90 per cent of seroconversions occur within 3 months of infection, but in a minority of cases seroconversion may be delayed to 6 months or longer. Diagnostic tests, if negative, therefore need to be repeated 3 months after possible exposure and after 6–9 months where there has been a high risk of transmission.

Following seroconversion, antibody to envelope protein persists indefinitely in the serum and forms a highly specific test for HIV infection. In general, one or more sensitive enzyme immunoassay (EIA) tests directed towards HIV-1 and HIV-2 are used as the initial screening tests. Positive screening tests are confirmed by second line tests, usually a western blot or immunofluorescence assay.

Where possible, patients should understand the implications of being tested for HIV and should give informed consent before the test is done. This is especially true for asymptomatic individuals. The benefits of awareness of being HIV-positive relate to the availability of effective prophylaxis against the major opportunistic infections, and the advent of highly active antiretroviral drugs. Knowledge of HIV status also allows behavioural change to reduce the risk of transmission to sexual partners, and may benefit children exposed to perinatal infection. The disadvantage of early diagnosis is that it may cause distress, with disruption of domestic, social, and professional lives although they may be free from symptoms for many years. HIV-positive people may still experience difficulties in obtaining life or medical insurance, finding work, buying houses, and travelling abroad.

Where HIV is relevant to the investigation of a patient's symptoms, it is in their interests to undergo HIV testing so that appropriate treatment for an opportunistic condition, antiretroviral therapy, and prophylaxis can be provided. Where the patient is too ill to give consent, testing may be justifiable on these grounds. In all circumstances a high level of confidentiality is required; disclosure of HIV-positive status should generally be allowed only in the medical interests of the patient and with their knowledge and consent.

Primary infection in the neonatal period poses special difficulties in the laboratory diagnosis of HIV. During primary infection, tests for HIV antibodies may be absent or weakly positive and need to be repeated at intervals. Over subsequent weeks or months, anti-HIV IgG and IgM antibodies may show changes in titre characteristic of primary infection. However, rapid diagnosis during the early stages of primary infection, when anti-HIV antibodies may be absent, may be provided by detecting HIV viraemia using tests for HIV RNA or DNA (by PCR), p24 antigen, or viral culture assays.

In children younger than 18 months, false positive anti-HIV antibody results may arise because of passive transfer of maternal antibodies to the fetus. Techniques for virus detection (HIV DNA by PCR, viral culture, or p24 antigen) allow confirmation of HIV infection in 95 per cent of infected infants by 1 month of age.

Clinical presentation and features

Primary infection

Two to 6 weeks after exposure to HIV, 50–70 per cent of those infected develop a transient, non-specific illness (sometimes called seroconversion illness) similar to infectious mononucleosis, with fever, malaise, myalgia, lymphadenopathy, and pharyngitis. However, unlike infectious mononucleosis over 50 per cent develop a rash, typically erythematous, maculopapular, and affecting the face and trunk. Other rashes and patterns of distribution, and oral and genital ulcers have also been reported. The illness begins abruptly and usually lasts for 1–2 weeks but may be more protracted. Neurological complications may occur, especially acute encephalitis, lymphocytic meningitis, and peripheral neuropathy. Severe or long-lasting illness and neurological involvement are associated with accelerated progression to AIDS and a bad prognosis, which may be influenced by early treatment with antiretroviral therapy (see below).

Diagnosis requires a high index of suspicion. Primary infection is a time of high viraemia (typically 10^5–10^6 viral particles/ml) during which antibodies to HIV may initially be absent. Serological tests often need to be repeated at intervals to establish the diagnosis (Fig. 5; see below). A transient decrease in CD4 lymphocytes is usual during primary illness. Occasionally, this may be substantial and associated with opportunistic infections such as oral or oesophageal candidiasis, and rarely *Pneumocystis* pneumonia.

A number of theoretical considerations support the treatment of primary HIV infection with a highly active antiretroviral regimen (see below). Following acute HIV infection, a relatively stable level of viral load is attained after 6–9 months (Fig. 5). The plasma HIV RNA level at this 'set point' is of prognostic importance; treatment of the initial viraemic illness may theoretically allow establishment of a very low set point and therefore lower the risk of subsequent progression. A placebo-controlled trial of zidovudine monotherapy during primary HIV infection and continued for 6 months showed improvement in the subsequent clinical course. Consequently, it is conventional to use a highly active triple combination, such as zidovudine and lamivudine with a protease inhibitor, but the optimal duration of therapy is unknown.

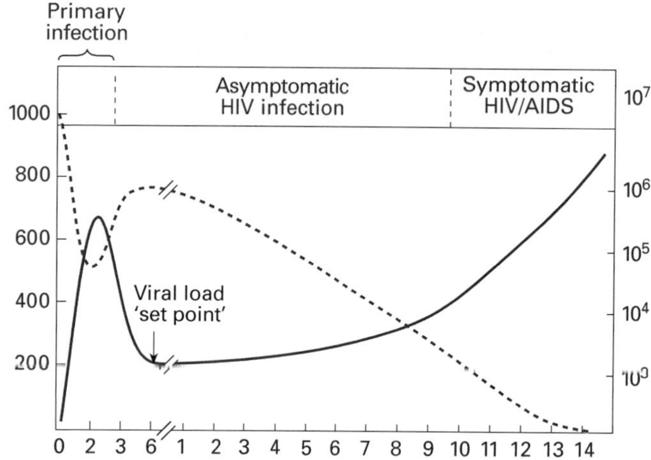

Fig. 5 Schematic representation of typical changes in CD4 lymphocyte count and plasma HIV-1 RNA with time during the natural history of HIV infection.

Early HIV infection

Following the primary syndrome or subclinical seroconversion, there usually follows an asymptomatic period lasting on average 10 years without antiretroviral therapy. Although a time of clinical latency, there is intense viral and lymphocyte turnover: up to 10^9–10^{10} viral particles and over 10^7 circulating CD4 lymphocytes are replaced daily.

During the asymptomatic period, physical examination may be normal, but about one-third of patients have persistent generalized lymphadenopathy (PGL). The enlarged nodes, caused by a non-specific follicular hyperplasia, are usually symmetrical, mobile, and non-tender. The cervical and axillary nodes are most commonly affected. Nodes that are markedly asymmetrical, painful, or rapidly enlarging should be biopsied to exclude tumours such as lymphoma and opportunistic infections such as tuberculosis.

Patients are frequently affected by minor opportunistic conditions affecting skin and mucous membranes. These are also common throughout the later stages of HIV disease. They include a range of infections: fungal (e.g. tinea, Pityrosporum), viral (e.g. warts, molluscum contagiosum, herpes simplex, herpes zoster), and bacterial (e.g. folliculitis, impetigo); and also eczema, seborrhoeic dermatitis, and psoriasis.

Drug rashes may occur at all stages of HIV, and particularly in late disease. Reactions to co-trimoxazole occur in about 30 per cent. They are most common when high doses are used in the treatment of *Pneumocystis* pneumonia. Dapsone, clindamycin, β-lactam antibiotics, pentamidine, and nevirapine are commonly associated with drug rash.

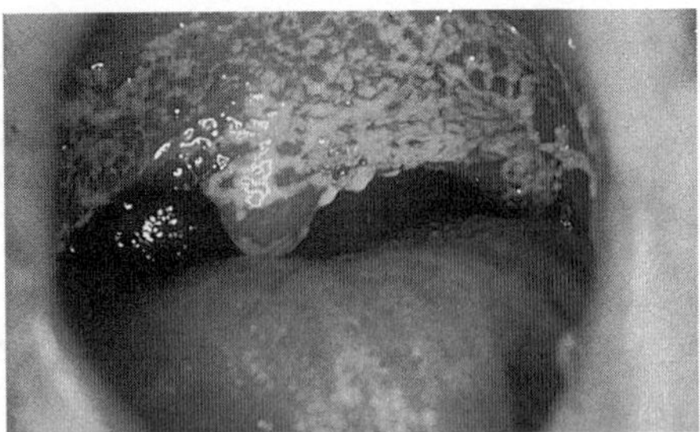

Fig. 6 Oral candidiasis.

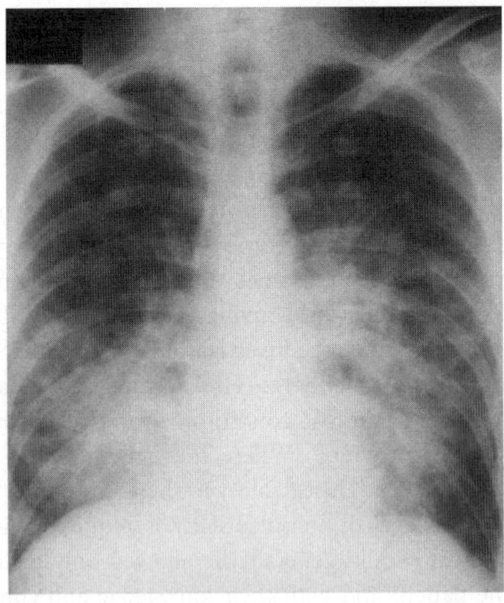

Fig. 7 Chest radiograph: *Pneumocystis carinii* pneumonia.

Oral hairy leucoplakia usually appears as corrugated greyish-white lesions on the lateral borders of the tongue in homosexual men. The condition is symptomless and non-progressive, but acts as a useful clue to HIV seropositivity. Epstein–Barr virus DNA has been demonstrated in these lesions.

One of the characteristic clinical presentations of HIV disease is a sore mouth and throat due to oropharyngeal candidiasis (oral thrush) (Fig. 6). This sign of worsening immunodeficiency may be recurrent. Topical antifungals (amphotericin lozenges or nystatin suspension) are usually effective in the early stages, but later oral azole antifungals (ketoconazole, fluconazole, or itraconazole) are needed. Most cases are caused by *Candida albicans*, but other species (e.g. *C. glabrata*) may be responsible.

There is an increased incidence of periodontal disease in those with HIV. Necrotizing (ulcerative) gingivitis and periodontitis may require extensive debridement and antimicrobials. Recurrent oropharyngeal aphthous ulceration is common and may be painful. Recurrent ulcers may also occur in the oesophagus and other parts of the gastrointestinal tract. They usually respond to local or systemic corticosteroid therapy. Resistant cases may respond to thalidomide.

Later in the course of infection, intermittent or persistent, non-specific, constitutional symptoms may develop including lethargy, anorexia, diarrhoea, weight loss, fever, and night sweats. These symptoms may presage severe opportunistic infections or tumours.

Progression to AIDS

Various staging systems for HIV infection and case definitions of AIDS have been used since 1982 and modified by increased understanding of the pathogenesis and natural history. The 1987 Centers for Disease Control (CDC) definition listed a range of specific diseases indicative of AIDS. In 1993, an expanded definition was introduced in the US that included additional AIDS indicator diseases and, in addition, individuals with proved HIV infection and a CD4 lymphocyte count of less than $200/mm^3$ ($0.2 \times 10^9/l$), irrespective of clinical manifestations. So far, this last criterion has not been adopted in Europe.

The value of making a distinction between AIDS (as defined) and HIV infection at other stages is increasingly questionable, especially in industrialized countries. AIDS-defining illnesses were essential for surveillance when HIV status was frequently unknown, the natural history of HIV infection was poorly understood (the proportion developing opportunistic complications was uncertain) and disease-modifying drugs were not available. However, effective prevention of many of the opportunistic infections has led to an increase in the proportion of symptomatic patients who do not fulfil the criteria for AIDS. Combination antiretroviral therapy may improve clinical condition and survival even when started after progression to AIDS.

These factors have undermined the epidemiological value and prognostic importance of a strict AIDS case definition. It is, perhaps, more useful to consider HIV disease as a continuous spectrum.

However, clinical criteria to identify symptomatic HIV disease and AIDS are needed in developing countries, where laboratory confirmation of HIV seropositivity and AIDS-defining diseases is not possible. WHO has, therefore, adopted clinical case definitions for AIDS surveillance in resource-poor countries, based on clinical manifestations with or without laboratory confirmation of HIV infection.

Non-progression

While the average time between infection with HIV and the development of AIDS is about 10 years, approximately 20 per cent of patients progress rapidly to AIDS within 5 years and 10–15 per cent remain clinically well for 15–20 years. Long-term, healthy survivors are often called non-progressors, and to an extent this subgroup represents simply the tail end of a normal distribution of progression rates. Cohort studies have demonstrated that most apparent non-progressors are slow progressers in whom gradual decline in CD4 lymphocyte count and increments in HIV viral load can be demonstrated. Although several investigators have reported virological, genetic, and cellular, and humoral immunological factors that may be associated with non-progression, limitations in study design have made it difficult to identify what was responsible. A mutation in the gene for the macrophage chemokine receptor CCR5 is associated with non-progression in the heterozygous state; homozygotes have high level resistance to HIV infection.

Late complications and their management

Pneumocystis carinii pneumonia

P. carinii pneumonia, one of the hallmarks of AIDS, is now less common because of primary prophylaxis and antiretroviral therapy; 85 per cent of cases occur in patients with CD4 lymphocyte counts below $200/mm^3$. Symptoms, typically increasing shortness of breath, dry cough, and fever, usually develop subacutely over a few weeks. Malaise, fatigue, weight loss, and chest pains or tightness may occur. Chest signs are usually minor (crackles) or absent on chest examination. The characteristic chest radiograph shows bilateral perihilar interstitial shadowing (Fig. 7) but may be normal. Other

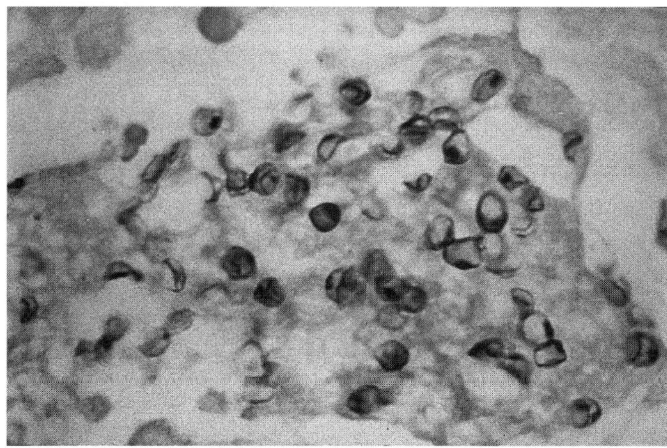

Fig. 8 *P. carinii* cysts in bronchoalveolar lavage aspirate.

appearances include localized infiltrates or consolidation, upper lobe shadows resembling tuberculosis (TB), nodular lesions, and pneumothorax; effusions are very rare. The arterial oxygen saturation is less than 95 per cent at rest or falls after exercise.

P. carinii was originally thought to be protozoan, but ribosomal RNA analysis indicates that it is a fungus. The foamy intra-alveolar exudate contains abundant *P. carinii* and is associated with an interstitial inflammatory infiltrate and progressive impairment of lung function. The diagnosis is usually confirmed by microscopy of sputum induced by nebulized saline in isolated, properly ventilated rooms to reduce the risk of TB transmission. *P. carinii* cysts and trophozoites are visualized by use of special stains. If this is negative, fibreoptic bronchoscopy with bronchial lavage may be indicated (Fig. 8); other causes of lung disease or coexistent infection may also be diagnosed by this technique, including TB, fungal infections, and Kaposi's sarcoma. Immunofluorescence using monoclonal antibodies or DNA amplification by PCR may improve diagnostic sensitivity when compared with conventional staining techniques but these methods are not used routinely.

High-dose co-trimoxazole (120 mg/kg per day) for 3 weeks is the first-line treatment for *Pneumocystis* pneumonia. Oral therapy is often adequate, but in moderate and severe cases the drug should be given intravenously. The drug can be given orally if fever, symptoms, and oxygenation have improved after 10 days. Adverse reactions to co-trimoxazole, especially neutropenia, anaemia, rash, and fever, occur in up to 40 per cent of patients, usually after 6–14 days. Intravenous pentamidine (4 mg/kg per day) is the second-line choice for patients who do not tolerate co-trimoxazole.

Patients intolerant of co-trimoxazole and pentamidine may be treated with clindamycin plus primaquine or dapsone plus trimethoprim. These regimens have been evaluated only in patients with mild to moderate *Pneumocystis* pneumonia, as has atovaquone, an antiprotozoal drug that is active against *P. carinii.* Although slightly less effective than co-trimoxazole, atovaquone causes fewer adverse effects.

In patients with moderate or severe *Pneumocystis* pneumonia, clinical trials have shown reductions in morbidity and mortality by addition of high dose corticosteroids. If the arterial oxygen tension (PaO_2) is less than 9.3 kPa or the alveolar–arterial oxygen gradient is greater than 4.7 kPa, oxygen and intravenous methylprednisolone or oral prednisolone should be given for 5–10 days. Patients who develop respiratory failure may require ventilatory support. After treatment for *Pneumocystis* pneumonia has been completed, secondary prophylaxis should be given to prevent recurrence. This may become unnecessary if antiretroviral therapy establishes very low viral load and improvement in immune status (see below).

Bacterial pneumonia

The risk of bacterial pneumonia is increased in HIV, especially if the CD4 lymphocyte count is below 200/mm^3. The most common cause is *Streptococcus pneumoniae*; *Haemophilus influenzae* and *Moraxella catarrhalis* are relatively common, and *Staphylococcus aureus*, *Klebsiella*, and other Gram-negative rods are important causes in advanced HIV disease. Rarer causes include *Nocardia* spp. and *Rhodococcus equi*. The presentation may be atypical, and radiological appearances frequently include diffuse infiltrates that resemble *Pneumocystis* pneumonia, as well as more typical segmental or lobar patterns. Cavitation with abscess formation, pleural effusion, and empyema may occur. HIV predisposes to recurrent invasive pneumococcal infections with bacteraemia; recurrent bacterial pneumonia in a 12-month period is an AIDS-defining condition. Chronic lung damage with bronchiectasis and colonization by *Pseudomonas aeruginosa* have been reported.

Other pulmonary complications

Disseminated fungal infections, including *Cryptococcus*, may involve the lungs. In endemic areas, histoplasmosis, coccidioidomycosis, and disseminated *Penicillium marneffei* infection need to be considered. Invasive *Aspergillus fumigatus* infections may occur in patients with advanced HIV disease who have additional risk factors such as severe neutropenia. Patients usually have severe, systemic illness. The radiographic appearances in all these fungal infections are usually non-specific. Bronchoalveolar lavage may be needed for diagnosis. HIV-associated lymphocytic interstitial pneumonitis (LIP) causes diffuse abnormalities, usually in children but occasionally in adults.

Tuberculosis

The interaction between HIV and TB was recognized early in the HIV epidemic. Studies in Central Africa in the mid-1980s showed that more than 60 per cent of newly-diagnosed TB patients were HIV-positive at a time when the background seroprevalence of HIV in the population was much lower. Intravenous drug users were shown to have an increased risk of developing active TB if they were HIV-positive. After decades of progressive decline in the incidence of TB in the US, notifications increased in the mid-1980s, soon after the emergence of the HIV epidemic. A similar trend has been observed more recently in western Europe. Overall, TB is the most frequent life-threatening, opportunistic infection in AIDS.

Most cases of TB in HIV-positive individuals represent reactivation of dormant bacilli. However, molecular typing of isolates of *M. tuberculosis* by restriction fragment length polymorphism (RFLP) analysis suggests that up to 40 per cent are new infections. The WHO estimates that one-third of the world's HIV-positive population is coinfected with TB. In communities where *M. tuberculosis* is a common endemic organism, those who are immunosuppressed by HIV have an increased risk of relapsing or new infections. Where the background prevalence of TB is low, the disease is uncommon in HIV-positive patients unless they become exposed, for instance through travel. Testing for HIV should be considered in patients presenting with active TB, and TB should be considered as a cause of unexplained symptoms in HIV patients.

Active TB may occur at any time in the course of HIV infection. In early-stage HIV, it is more likely to present with the typical clinical features: subacute history of cough, fever, and weight loss, upper lobe cavitary disease and/or pleural disease on chest radiographs, and a positive skin test to tuberculin. In late-stage HIV infection, patients are more likely to have atypical presentations with unusual chest findings, extrapulmonary involvement, and anergy. The chest radiograph may be normal in up to 40 per cent of cases. Sputum smears should be examined for acid-fast bacilli, and blood cultures may be positive for *M. tuberculosis.* Patients with advanced HIV infection are more likely to develop extrapulmonary TB involving lymph nodes, pericardium, liver, bone marrow, or meninges.

The standard 6-month regimen of three or four anti-TB drugs (isoniazid, rifampicin, pyrazinamide, and ethambutol) is generally effective in HIV patients, unless there is resistance to one or more of these first-line drugs. The drug regimen may need to be adjusted when *in vitro* sensitivity results are known. For fully sensitive organisms, after 2 months on three or four drugs, isoniazid and rifampicin should be continued for a further 4 months. Life-long isoniazid is recommended to prevent relapse. Patients with pulmonary TB should be isolated initially. Contact tracing is important; HIV-positive contacts are at particular risk. Tuberculin testing is used to determine whether contacts should take isoniazid chemoprophylaxis.

Up to 20 per cent of HIV patients experience adverse reactions to TB drugs. In HIV-positive patients with TB in Africa, the sulfa-based drug thiacetazone has been associated with serious skin reactions, including toxic epidermal necrolysis and fatal cases of Stevens–Johnson syndrome. Whereas response rates for conventional, short-course TB treatment in industrialized countries are similar to those achieved in HIV-negative patients, in resource-poor countries, and where compliance is less easily achieved, lower cure rates are observed and there is a risk that resistance will develop. Several countries have adopted 'directly observed therapy' (DOT) to address this problem.

Multidrug-resistant tuberculosis

Over 15 outbreaks of multidrug-resistant tuberculosis (MDRTB) have been reported since the late 1980s. MDRTB isolates are resistant to at least two first-line anti-TB drugs, most commonly isoniazid and rifampicin, and often resistant to several agents. Most have occurred in HIV units in hospitals but outbreaks have also occurred in prisons, drug treatment centres, and nursing homes. Most documented outbreaks have been in the US, but they have also occurred in other parts of the world. One involved over 200 people in Buenos Aires, Argentina and another affected over 100 people in Lisbon, Portugal. In these MDRTB outbreaks, health-care workers may also become infected. Initially, the mortality among HIV-positive patients was very high (up to 93 per cent), but in recent years the outcome has improved because of reduced diagnostic delay and appropriate treatment with at least four drugs to which the *M. tuberculosis* isolate is sensitive *in vitro.* To prevent outbreaks of MDRTB, special precautions are required when HIV-positive patients with possible TB are admitted to hospitals, including isolation in negative-pressure rooms, respiratory protection for staff, and special precautions during certain procedures such as bronchoscopy or nebulized pentamidine administration. With effective treatment, patients rapidly become non-infectious but precautions need to be continued until the sputum is repeatedly smear negative.

Mycobacterium avium complex (MAC)

Patients with advanced HIV infection and CD4 lymphocyte counts below 50/mm^3 are at high risk of disseminated *M. avium* complex infection, particularly in industrialized countries where it is reported to develop in up to 40 per cent of patients with AIDS. *M. avium* is an ubiquitous environmental organism of low pathogenicity that can be isolated from domestic water supplies. Infection is likely to be through the gastrointestinal tract. MAC becomes widely disseminated in those with advanced HIV and causes fever, night sweats, weight loss, diarrhoea, abdominal pain, anaemia, disturbed liver function, and reduced overall survival. The organism can usually be cultured from blood or bone marrow, or may be recognized as acid-fast bacilli in tissue biopsies (e.g. from lymph node, small bowel, or liver). It is not clear why the diagnosis is uncommon in underdeveloped countries; high mortality from other opportunistic infections at earlier stages of immunosuppression may be partly responsible.

MAC is intrinsically resistant to most first-line anti-TB drugs. The most effective and best tolerated regimen has not been determined, and although clinical benefit and microbiological response is often achieved, survival benefit has been difficult to prove. Comparative trials suggest that initial therapy should be with two or three drugs: a macrolide (clarithromycin or azithromycin) and ethambutol should be used, and additional rifabutin or a quinolone (e.g. ciprofloxacin) can be considered. In severely ill patients, intravenous amikacin may be useful as the third agent. Lifelong treatment may be required to prevent relapse; but if immune restoration can be achieved with combination antiretroviral therapy, this may no longer be necessary and it may prove possible to cure MAC.

Other non-tuberculous mycobacteria

Other mycobacteria, notably *M. kansasii, M. genavense,* and *M. celatum,* may cause opportunistic infections in HIV. *M. genavense,* which colonizes pet birds, was discovered in European HIV patients and causes fever, diarrhoea, and severe weight loss. HIV does not seem to affect the incidence or natural history of leprosy (*M. leprae*).

Oesophageal candidiasis

Oesophagitis presents with restrosternal pain on swallowing, and in patients with HIV is most commonly caused by *Candida albicans*; other *Candida* species may be identified. Oesophageal candidiasis indicates advanced immunosuppression and is an AIDS-defining condition. The diagnosis should be suspected in a patient with oral candida and dysphagia, and may be supported by barium swallow or confirmed by endoscopy and biopsy. Treatment is with oral azole antifungals. Fluconazole may be more effective than ketoconazole. Oesophageal candidiasis may recur and in a minority of patients with marked immunosuppression the *Candida* may become resistant to azole treatment. This tends to develop gradually and can be monitored by *in vitro* sensitivity testing. Such patients require treatment or continuous suppression with high doses of fluconazole (which is better tolerated than high doses of ketoconazole or itraconazole) or intermittent treatment with intravenous amphotericin. Azole-resistant oro-oesophageal candidiasis has become less common since the advent of combination antiretroviral therapy.

The differential diagnosis of oesophageal candidiasis includes oesophagitis caused by cytomegalovirus or herpes simplex virus, which require specific antiviral therapy, and aphthous ulceration which may respond to oral prednisolone or thalidomide.

HIV and the nervous system

Cerebral toxoplasmosis

Cerebral infection with the intracellular protozoan *Toxoplasma gondii* is the most frequent infection of the central nervous system in AIDS when the CD4 lymphocyte count is below 200/mm^3. It usually results

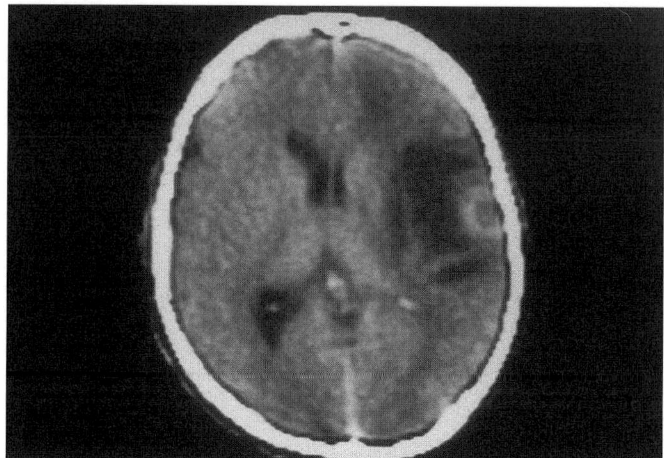

Fig. 9 Cerebral toxoplasmosis: ring enhancement and surrounding cerebral oedema (CT scan with contrast).

from reactivation of *Toxoplasma* cysts in the brain, leading to the formation of focal lesions that are typically multiple but may be single. Symptoms develop subacutely and include focal neurological disturbance, headache, confusion, fever, and convulsions. On CT scanning the lesions appear as ring-enhancing masses with surrounding oedema (Fig. 9). MRI is more sensitive and frequently detects lesions not visible on the CT scan. Serum antibodies to *Toxoplasma* are usually detectable; their absence makes the diagnosis unlikely but does not exclude it. Detection of *Toxoplasma* DNA in cerebrospinal fluid by PCR is being evaluated as a diagnostic test. The principal differential diagnosis is cerebral lymphoma; other causes of focal brain lesions in AIDS include cryptococcoma, cerebral abscess (including *Nocardia* infection), tuberculoma, progressive multifocal leucoencephalopathy, and neurosyphilis. Brain biopsy is necessary for a definitive diagnosis, but as toxoplasmosis is by far the most common treatable cause of focal cerebral lesions in HIV, it is standard practice to treat for toxoplasmosis and only consider biopsy if there is no clinical improvement in 7–10 days.

The condition responds well if treatment is started early; and a combination of sulfadiazine 4–6 g/day and pyrimethamine 50–75 mg/day is the treatment of choice. More than 40 per cent of patients experience adverse effects, especially rash and nephrotoxicity caused by sulfadiazine. The haematological toxicity of pyrimethamine may be reduced by adding folinic acid (10 mg/day). If sulfa drugs are not tolerated, clindamycin with pyrimethamine has been shown to be an effective alternative.

Treatment is usually given for 3–6 weeks, but relapse of cerebral toxoplasmosis is common after stopping, and life-long maintenance therapy is required using pyrimethamine (25–50 mg/day) with a sulfa drug or clindamycin.

Cryptococcal meningitis

Although infection of the central nervous system with *Cryptococcus neoformans* can occur in the absence of immunodeficiency, it most commonly arises in association with HIV infection. Before widespread use of azole antifungals for mucosal candidiasis, it accounted for 5–10 per cent of opportunistic infections in AIDS. The presentation is usually subacute and may be subtle and non-specific with headache, vomiting, and mild fever and few neurological signs. Less frequently, psychiatric disturbance, convulsions, cranial nerve palsies, truncal ataxia, or focal intracerebral lesions may occur. Neck stiffness is unusual. The diagnosis is made by identifying cryptococci in the cerebrospinal fluid (CSF) by India ink staining, detection of cryptococcal antigen in the CSF (uniformly positive), and culture. Cryptococcal antigen is also usually detectable in serum. *C. neoformans* causes minimal inflammation in AIDS so the CSF white cell count is often only mildly raised and the CSF protein and glucose may be normal.

Cryptococcal meningitis is treated with either fluconazole or amphotericin B, with or without flucytosine. A large comparative study showed that the overall mortality (17 per cent) was similar in both treatment groups. However, there were more early deaths in the fluconazole group. Amphotericin sterilized the cerebrospinal fluid more rapidly, but fluconazole was better tolerated. Factors predictive of death included abnormal mental status, high CSF cryptococcal antigen titre (1:1024 or greater), and less than 20 white cells/mm^3 in the CSF. Therefore, patients with severe cryptococcal meningitis and poor prognostic features should be treated with amphotericin initially; mild to moderate presentations can be treated with oral fluconazole. Addition of flucytosine improves outcome but increases haematological toxicity. Adverse reactions to amphotericin occur frequently, especially fever, myalgia, renal impairment, and electrolyte disturbances. Close monitoring is required. Lipid formulations of amphotericin are better tolerated but much more costly, and are generally used in patients who cannot tolerate the conventional formulation. Raised intracranial pressure is associated with clinical deterioration and the risk of blindness: repeated lumbar punctures, ventricular shunting, or acetazolamide therapy may be required.

Without secondary prophylaxis after treatment, relapse of cryptococcal meningitis occurs in 50–80 per cent of HIV patients. Oral fluconazole (200 mg/day) is effective for lifelong maintenance. Whether this can be discontinued following response to combination antiretrovirals remains to be demonstrated. Resistance of *Cryptococcus* to fluconazole has been described but is very rare.

Progressive multifocal leucoencephalopathy (PML)

PML is a progressive demyelinating condition of advanced HIV disease caused by JC virus, a polyomavirus that is cytopathic for oligodendroglia. It presents with focal neurological deficits, personality changes, or ataxia; headache and mass effects are absent. Brain MRI scan is the investigation of choice and usually shows multiple, white matter lesions; JC virus may be detected in the CSF by PCR but this is not usually necessary for the diagnosis. There is no specific treatment. Survival of less than 6 months is usual, but progression may be halted or reversed by combination antiretroviral therapy.

HIV encephalopathy

HIV can infect the nervous system directly, leading to a variety of clinical problems. Most patients dying of AIDS show histological evidence of brain involvement including neurone loss. A smaller number (up to 10 per cent) develop the cognitive, behavioural, and motor abnormalities of dementia. In the early stages, there is impairment of concentration and memory and mood changes mimicking depression; gradual progression leads to intellectual incapacity and motor disability so that patients cannot care for themselves. Neurological signs include slow movement, inco-ordination, motor weakness, hyper-reflexia, and extensor plantar responses; brain imaging shows reduced grey matter volume in the cortex and basal ganglia. Ultimately, a nearly vegetative condition develops with virtual mutism, inability to walk, and incontinence. These patients die within

2 years. Antiretroviral treatment can prevent, and in the earlier stages reverse, AIDS dementia.

Other psychological/psychiatric problems include anxiety, panic attacks, and depression. Psychotherapy may be helpful. Antidepressants may be needed in severe cases. Acute psychosis is rare.

In the late stages of HIV disease, the differential diagnosis of HIV dementia includes cytomegalovirus encephalitis. This usually presents with rapidly progressive confusion and dementia, impaired consciousness, fever, cranial nerve lesions, and convulsions. MRI shows necrotizing periventriculitis; CSF protein may be elevated and CMV DNA is detectable in the CSF by PCR. Ganciclovir and other anti-CMV agents may be helpful.

Myelopathy and neuropathies

HIV may involve the spinal cord directly causing a vacuolar myelopathy. This usually presents with bilateral leg weakness and sensory symptoms, usually paraesthesiae, and may progress to spastic paraparesis, ataxia, and incontinence. Peripheral neuropathy can occur at any stage of HIV infection, even at seroconversion, but is commonest in advanced disease, when 10–15 per cent of patients have a distal, symmetrical sensorimotor neuropathy of axonal type causing pain and paraesthesiae that may limit walking and, less often, distal weakness and atrophy. Mononeuritis multiplex and acute inflammatory demyelinating polyneuropathy resembling Guillain–Barré syndrome are described, generally at an earlier stage. Drugs used in HIV patients, including stavudine, didanosine, and vincristine, may cause or exacerbate peripheral neuropathy. HIV-related autonomic neuropathy may cause postural hypotension, diarrhoea, impotence, impaired sweating, and bladder symptoms. Cytomegalovirus infection in AIDS presents with a lumbosacral polyradiculopathy causing sacral paraesthesiae and numbness, lower limb weakness, and urinary retention that may progress to flaccid paraparesis if untreated.

Ocular disease

Cytomegalovirus retinitis

Without combination antiretroviral therapy, up to 30 per cent of patients with AIDS (and CD4 lymphocyte count below 50/mm^3) develop reactivation of cytomegalovirus (CMV) in the form of a destructive and blinding retinitis. This is rare in other types of immunosuppression. It usually presents with blurring of vision, scotomata, floaters, or flashing lights. The characteristic retinal changes are patches of irregular retinal pallor, caused by oedema and necrosis, and haemorrhages in a perivascular distribution (Fig. 10). The retinitis usually starts peripherally and progresses rapidly to involve the macula and whole retina, leading to blindness. Complications include retinal detachment, branch retinal artery occlusion, persistent iritis, and cataract. CMV retinitis should not be confused with cotton-wool spots (HIV retinopathy) small pale retinal lesions without haemorrhages that commonly occur in HIV patients. The common, benign, cotton-wool spots often come and go. (See Plates 12, 13, The eye and disease.)

The diagnosis of CMV retinitis is clinical, based on the characteristic retinal appearance. Serum CMV IgG antibodies are detectable as evidence of previous exposure; CMV viraemia may be detectable by PCR and high or rising CMV viral load is associated with increased risk of developing retinitis and other CMV disease. Anti-CMV drugs (ganciclovir, foscarnet, cidofovir) are virustatic and before the availability of highly-active antiretroviral drug combinations, the aim of treatment was to stop progression rather than to cure disease.

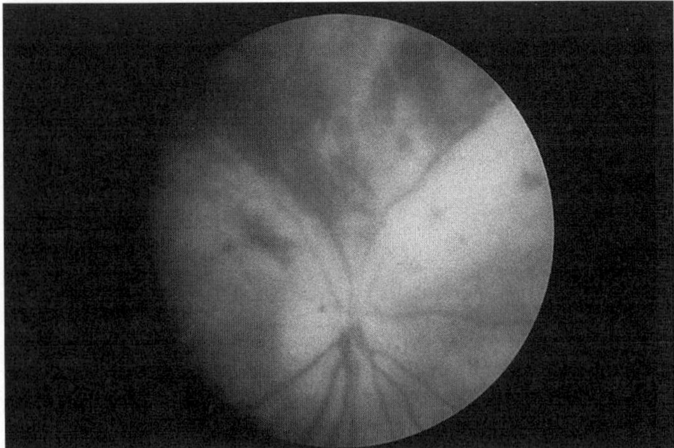

Fig. 10 Cytomegalovirus retinitis.

First-line treatment is with intravenous ganciclovir, which may cause severe neutropenia and thrombocytopenia that are dose-limiting in about 10 per cent of patients. Foscarnet (phosphonoformate) is a relatively toxic, second-line agent that causes dose-limiting, reversible renal impairment and symptoms of hypocalcaemia in about 20 per cent of patients. Ganciclovir can also be given as a slow release intraocular implant, but this may allow CMV to develop at other sites including the other eye.

For maintenance therapy, oral ganciclovir may be adequate, convenient and well tolerated, although there is a greater risk of disease progression than with daily intravenous infusions of ganciclovir or foscarnet, and the eyes must be examined frequently. Cidofovir is more active against CMV than the other anti-CMV drugs. It can be given by intermittent intravenous infusion, initially weekly and then every 2 weeks. Whereas ganciclovir and foscarnet require a central venous catheter, cidofovir may be given in short infusions through a peripheral vein because of its prolonged antiviral effect. However, cidofovir is relatively toxic, causing irreversible nephrotoxicity, neutropenia, and peripheral neuropathy in over a third of patients. It is uncertain whether sustained suppression of HIV viral load and improvement in immune status may make lifelong treatment for CMV retinitis unnecessary. New manifestations of ocular CMV, such as vitritis, have been reported in patients treated with antiretroviral drugs.

Other ocular syndromes

Acute retinal necrosis is a rare condition originally reported in varicella zoster virus reactivation in otherwise healthy adults. In patients with advanced HIV infection, it is usually preceded by dermatomal herpes zoster and typically presents with blurring of vision and pain in the affected eye. Progressive necrotizing retinitis leads to visual deterioration that may be associated with uveitis. In AIDS patients an outer retinal necrosis syndrome with little ocular inflammation also occurs. There is a high risk of visual loss and retinal detachment. Both eyes may be affected. Suspected acute retinal necrosis should be treated with intravenous aciclovir.

Acute toxoplasma choroidoretinitis may resemble CMV retinitis, but the retinal scarring that follows treatment looks quite different. The disease is more common in countries such as Brazil and France where the background prevalence of toxoplasmosis is much higher than in the UK. Choroidoretinitis is a rare complication of histoplasmosis and cryptococcosis.

HIV-related tumours

Kaposi's sarcoma

Kaposi's sarcoma (KS) characteristically presents as multiple, purplish, nodular skin lesions (Plate 1). Lesions start as small pink, deep purple, or brown macules, and develop into nodules or plaques that may ulcerate. They also occur on mucosal surfaces, commonly on the hard palate (Plate 2). Local or regional oedema and lymph node enlargement may occur. Mucocutaneous lesions are cosmetically and psychologically important but are rarely of clinical importance. However, visceral disease, which most commonly affects the lungs and gastrointestinal tract, is an important cause of morbidity and even mortality. Lung lesions cause dyspnoea, cough, or haemoptysis, and gut involvement may cause abdominal pain, bleeding, or a rare protein-losing enteropathy. Extensive visceral involvement can cause constitutional symptoms such as fevers, night sweats, and weight loss. KS rarely affects the central nervous system.

In industrialized countries, KS is over 2000 times more common in HIV-infected individuals than in the general population. Classic KS in HIV-negative individuals occurs in middle-aged and elderly men of eastern European or Mediterranean origin. Endemic KS in Africa has been known for decades. It is predominantly a disease of older men that has a fairly indolent course. HIV-related KS, on the other hand, is a more aggressive disease and occurs largely in those people who have acquired HIV via a sexual route, namely homosexual and bisexual men and in younger African men and women. There is currently an epidemic of KS in Central and East Africa that exactly mirrors the HIV epidemic in these regions. KS is rare in intravenous drug users and very rare in recipients of blood products, including haemophiliacs. These epidemiological features suggested a sexually transmissible aetiological agent. In 1994, a new herpes virus, human herpesvirus-8 (HHV-8), was found in HIV-related KS and was soon detected in the lesions of all forms of KS. HHV-8 is detectable in semen and sexual transmission is likely, but in Africa, where serological surveys show that HHV-8 infection is common, it is also transmitted by other routes including from mother to child.

KS lesions are characterized by proliferating spindle cells, possibly of endothelial origin, thin-walled slit-like vascular spaces, infiltration by lymphocytes and plasma cells, and extravasated red cells. Multiple lesions appear synchronously in widely dispersed areas. Recent work has suggested a monoclonal origin for KS lesions, but they may be reactive proliferative rather than truly cancerous. HHV-8 is detectable in spindle cells and flat endothelial cells lining the vascular spaces of KS lesions. The virus may trigger the release of cellular and virus-encoded cytokines that promote the proliferation of spindle cells.

Cutaneous lesions may be left untreated or treated with local radiotherapy, cryotherapy, or intralesional vinblastine. Widespread skin or visceral disease is usually treated by systemic chemotherapy, with single or multiple-agent regimens of vincristine, vinblastine, bleomycin, etoposide, and anthracyclines. The combination of vincristine and bleomycin is effective in 50 per cent of patients and well tolerated, but responses are usually short-lived. Regimens including etoposide and daunorubicin may be useful when the disease becomes resistant to the first-line agents. Liposomal preparations of anthracyclines (e.g. daunorubicin) may be effective and better tolerated. KS is not yet curable, and apart from chemotherapy for pulmonary KS, treatment does not prolong survival. The impact of combination antiretroviral therapy on the natural history of KS remains to be assessed, and in the future antiherpesvirus therapy using new antivirals may control HHV-8 and KS.

Non-Hodgkin's lymphoma

Non-Hodgkin's lymphoma develops in 3–10 per cent of HIV patients, an incidence 60–100 times higher than in the general population. Most tumours are extranodal and, histologically, 60 per cent are large cell B-cell lymphomas; 30 per cent are Burkitt's type, and the rest are of T-cell or non-B, non-T cell origin. The 50 per cent are associated with Epstein–Barr virus infection, and are more aggressive with shorter survival. Recently, a minority of HIV-related lymphomas have been associated with HHV-8. They present as body-cavity lymphomas, causing pleural or peritoneal effusions ('primary effusion lymphoma').

AIDS-related lymphoma outside the central nervous system may respond well to standard lymphoma chemotherapy regimens. Response is better in the less immunosuppressed (CD4 above 200/mm^3 and no previous AIDS diagnosis) and is generally poor in those who have advanced HIV disease. Opportunistic infections cause many deaths during chemotherapy. Lower-dose or less toxic chemotherapy protocols are sometimes advocated for patients with more advanced HIV disease.

The central nervous system is a common site of AIDS-related non-Hodgkin's lymphoma, which is nearly always associated with EBV and sometimes with HHV-8 as well. Patients usually present with the symptoms and signs of a space-occupying cerebral tumour. Detection of EBV DNA in the CSF may help to distinguish these lymphomas from cerebral toxoplasmosis. Neither chemotherapy nor radiotherapy have much impact, and median survival after diagnosis is about 3 months.

Other tumours in AIDS

Some studies have reported an increased frequency of Hodgkin's disease in HIV patients, particularly of the mixed cellularity type. Disseminated disease with a poor prognosis seems to be more frequent than for HIV-negative Hodgkin's disease. Castleman's disease (angiofollicular lymph node hyperplasia) is an HHV-8-associated lymphoproliferative condition which, in the multicentric form, is also associated with HIV. The incidence of squamous cell anal carcinoma is increased in homosexual men, but the risk does not seem to be greatly magnified by HIV; however, the risk of anal intraepithelial neoplasia (AIN), a precursor of anal carcinoma, is significantly increased. HIV-infected women suffer a higher incidence of cervical intraepithelial neoplasia (CIN) but predisposition to cervical carcinoma by HIV infection has not been proved, even though cervical cancer has been designated an AIDS-defining condition. The development of AIN and CIN may be related to coinfection with oncogenic types of human papillomavirus (HPV), especially type 16. It is not clear why HIV should predispose to premalignant epithelial conditions without increasing the risk of invasive cancer.

Miscellaneous conditions

Bacillary angiomatosis

Disseminated infection with *Bartonella henselae*, the principal agent of cat scratch disease, is the cause of bacillary angiomatosis, an HIV-associated condition that typically causes multiple subcutaneous vascular lesions, fever, liver lesions (bacillary peliosis hepatis), and osteolytic bone lesions. The skin lesions are usually purplish nodules that may be mistaken for KS, but the histology is distinct—acute neutrophilic inflammation and capillary proliferation, and clusters of bacilli revealed by modified silver staining. The organism may be cultured from blood. A similar syndrome in HIV patients can be caused by the agent of trench fever, *B. quintana*. Bacillary angiomatosis usually responds to treatment with a macrolide antibiotic. Cats and cat fleas form a reservoir for *B. henselae*, and patients who develop bacillary angiomatosis frequently have a history of contact with cats.

Other disseminated infections

In regions where invasive fungal infections are endemic (e.g. *Histoplasma capsulatum* in the Mississippi river region, *Coccidioides immitis* in the southern US, *Penicillium marneffei* in South-East Asia) or where there is a relevant travel history, disseminated fungal infection should be considered in HIV patients presenting with fever, weight loss, anaemia, pulmonary infiltrates, lymphadenopathy, and hepatosplenomegaly. Papular skin lesions may be seen in disseminated histoplasmosis and *P. marneffei* infection. Similar lesions resembling giant molluscum may occur with disseminated cryptococcosis. Blood or bone marrow cultures or direct identification by use of special stains on tissue obtained from skin lesions, bone marrow, or liver are required for diagnosis. Initial therapy is generally with intravenous amphotericin; itraconazole (for histoplasmosis and *P. marneffei*) or fluconazole (for coccidioidomycosis) may be adequate for subsequent maintenance treatment. HIV-associated disseminated leishmaniasis is mostly reported from the Mediterranean littoral, South America, and Africa. It is caused by dissemination of *Leishmania* spp, protozoan parasites transmitted by sandflies. A high index of clinical suspicion is required because although the classical features are fever, weight loss, anaemia, and hepatosplenomegaly, a high proportion of patients have fever alone. Most cases can be diagnosed by bone marrow examination. Treatment is usually with the organic antimonial compound sodium stibogluconate, given parenterally.

Other visceral disease

Cryptosporidium (see Chapter 16.87) and CMV may cause a sclerosing cholangitis-like syndrome with irregular dilatations and stenoses of the biliary tree (demonstrable by endoscopic retrograde cholangiography), abnormal liver blood tests, and occasionally jaundice. CMV is frequently identified histologically in the pancreas at autopsy but its role in the development of clinical pancreatitis is unproved. A characteristic nephropathy (HIV-related glomerulosclerosis), primary pulmonary hypertension, and cardiomyopathy are well described in AIDS.

Haematological conditions

Anaemia is common in HIV patients with advanced infection, and is frequently related to medications (e.g. zidovudine). Human (B19) parvovirus infection is an important reversible cause of chronic anaemia in HIV. Bone marrow biopsy typically shows isolated erythroid hypoplasia and B19 parvovirus may be detected by DNA hybridization. The anaemia may respond to treatment with intravenous immunoglobulin.

Mild neutropenia is common in HIV patients at all stages of infection, and may be partly responsible for the increased risk of pyogenic bacterial infections; however profound neutropenia (below 0.5×10^9/l) is rare. Antineutrophil antibodies may be present. Drugs (e.g. co-trimoxazole, ganciclovir, antiretrovirals) may increase the incidence and severity of neutropenia. In selected HIV patients with refractory or life-threatening bacterial or fungal infection and severe neutropenia, addition of recombinant human granulocyte colony-stimulating factor to the treatment regimen may improve the outcome.

Thrombocytopenia is relatively common (5–15 per cent) in HIV infection and associated with antiplatelet antibodies; symptomatic thrombocytopenia is uncommon but more likely in the later stages of HIV. Life-threatening bleeding is rare. Thrombocytopenia is not a marker for HIV progression and spontaneous remissions are frequent. When treatment is required, the principles and response are similar to those that apply in the treatment of HIV-negative immune thrombocytopenia, and include the use of prednisolone, intravenous immunoglobulin, and splenectomy. Thrombocytopenia also frequently responds to antiretroviral therapy using combinations that include zidovudine, which improves platelet production.

Skin conditions in advanced HIV

In the later stages of HIV infection, a number infections have atypical cutaneous manifestations. These include giant molluscum contagiosum, characterized by large, flesh-coloured, non-tender umbilicated lesions often affecting the face in homosexual men. In advanced HIV disease, genital herpes simplex infection may cause painful, chronic genital or anal ulcers that can become resistant to aciclovir and related compounds; intravenous foscarnet or cidofovir are effective. Aciclovir-resistant varicella zoster virus (VZV) also occurs in AIDS; and VZV reactivation can take an unusual form, with a subacute course and dissemination causing scattered vesicular lesions in the absence of dermatomal zoster. CMV is a cause of chronic perianal ulceration that can be treated with ganciclovir. Atypical cutaneous presentations of syphilis may occur at any stage of HIV infection.

Common syndromes

Fever of unknown cause

Fever is rarely attributable to HIV infection *per se*, and patients should be fully investigated. There is increased susceptibility to pyogenic infections as well as opportunistic infections and tumours. Unlike fever of unknown origin (FUO) in other patients, most cases of FUO in HIV patients are caused by an infection. A detailed history should be taken and full physical examination performed. Cultures of blood, urine, and faeces should be obtained, and chest radiography done. If sputum is available it should be stained and cultured for TB. In patients with intravenous lines and devices, catheter-related bacteraemia is an important cause. Occult infections (including sinusitis and dental sepsis) and drug-related fever should always be considered. Rarely, *Pneumocystis* and *Cryptococcus* can present as fever without their typical focal signs, and dissemination to other sites (e.g. skin, fundi) may occur. Disseminated leishmaniasis is an important cause in those who have visited an endemic area (see Chapter 16.94).

In advanced disease, the most common causes of persistent high swinging fevers are disseminated MAC infection and non-Hodgkin's lymphoma (see Chapter 3.29). MAC may be isolated from faeces or sputum but this is not diagnostic of dissemination. Definitive diagnosis is made by isolation from blood or bone marrow using special culture media. Acid-fast staining of bone marrow or lymph node aspirate may give the diagnosis before the culture result. Imaging techniques, in particular CT scanning of the abdomen, are essential to find a suitable site for biopsy to diagnose lymphoma.

In some cases, the cause of fever is not found; in early disease the fever may resolve spontaneously. In advanced disease fever and sweats may continue intermittently for many months. Symptomatic treatment includes non-steroidal anti-inflammatory drugs and low dose prednisolone; therapeutic trials of anti-MAC treatment may be justified.

Breathlessness

Appropriate management of breathlessness is important because the commonest cause, *Pneumocystis* pneumonia, can be rapidly progressive. The differential diagnosis is broad and includes bacterial pneumonia, pneumothorax, pulmonary Kaposi's sarcoma, other tumours, fungal infections, asthma, and heart failure. Routine investigations should include chest radiography and blood oxygen saturation and peak flow measurement. Blood cultures should be sent in febrile patients. Sputum should be obtained, if necessary by induction with nebulized saline, and stained for *Pneumocystis*, TB, and fungi. Bronchoalveolar lavage should be considered early as patients sometimes progress quickly and become too ill for bronchoscopy without the support of mechanical ventilation.

Empirical treatment should cover *Pneumocystis*, *S. pneumoniae*, and *H. influenzae* by combining high-dose co-trimoxazole with a suitable broad spectrum antimicrobial such as cefotaxime. A macrolide such as erythromycin or clarithromycin may be added if atypical pneumonia (e.g. *Mycoplasma*) is suspected. If clinical suspicion of *Pneumocystis* is high, corticosteroids should be included if the patient is hypoxaemic. Continuous positive airway pressure (CPAP) or mechanical ventilation may be needed in severe cases to allow diagnosis and time for patients to respond to treatment. If the chest radiograph shows diffuse bilateral infiltration and bronchoalveolar lavage fails to reveal any pathogen, presumptive treatment for *Pneumocystis* pneumonia should be continued. If no diagnosis is made and deterioration occurs despite empirical treatment, open lung biopsy should be considered to establish the diagnosis but the prognosis is generally poor.

Diarrhoea

Chronic diarrhoea is a common problem in advanced HIV infection, particularly in the tropics, and may be associated with weight loss and malabsorption. No cause other than HIV can be identified in at least half of cases; an HIV enteropathy characterized by partial villous atrophy has been described. The most common opportunistic cause is infection by the protozoan *Cryptosporidium parvum*, which causes a self-limiting gastroenteritis in the non-immunosuppressed. In HIV patients, diarrhoea may be protracted and severe, with marked fluid and electrolyte losses. The diagnosis is made by finding cryptosporidial oocysts in the stool using a modified acid-fast stain. Symptoms of cryptosporidiosis are often intermittent, as is excretion of the oocysts, so multiple stool specimens may need to be examined. No effective treatment has been found; the aminoglycoside paromomycin (aminosidine) orally has been useful anecdotally, but controlled trials showed no benefit. Symptomatic treatment with antidiarrhoeal drugs (such as loperamide), fluid and electrolyte replacement, and nutritional support are required. Octreotide may be useful in the most severe cases.

The coccidian protozoa *Isospora belli* and *Cyclospora* are important, but less common, causes of HIV-related chronic diarrhoea, diagnosed by the presence of sporocysts in the stool. Isosporiasis may respond to treatment with co-trimoxazole but the relapse rate after stopping treatment is 50 per cent, and similar experience is reported for cyclosporiasis. Microsporidia such as *Enterocytozoon bieneusi* and *Encephalitozoon* (formerly *Septata*) *intestinalis* are intracellular pathogens that may cause diarrhoea in advanced HIV disease. Special diagnostic staining methods applied to stool samples or electron microscopy of a rectal biopsy are needed to make the diagnosis. Albendazole may be effective, and treatment with highly-active antiretroviral therapy may induce remission of intestinal microsporidiosis.

Giardia lamblia and *Entamoeba histolytica* cysts are more commonly found in the faeces of homosexual men than heterosexual men, but these protozoa usually respond to conventional treatment with metronidazole and do not cause special problems in those with HIV. Bacterial infections with enteric pathogens such as *Salmonella*, *Shigella*, *Campylobacter*, and *Clostridium difficile* do not lead to chronic diarrhoea but may take longer to clear. *Salmonella* infections may cause disseminated infection with recurrent bacteraemia that recurs even after prolonged antimicrobial therapy.

With advanced disease, MAC infection may cause diarrhoea among other symptoms. CMV causes a colitis that typically presents with abdominal pain and tenderness, fever, and bloody diarrhoea. Rectal or colonic biopsy may confirm the diagnosis by identifying the characteristic nuclear inclusion bodies. HIV-related autonomic neuropathy is a rare cause of diarrhoea that is often most troublesome at night; anticholinergic drugs may help in addition to antidiarrhoeals. Diarrhoea in HIV patients is a frequent side-effect of medications such as antibiotics and antiretrovirals.

HIV wasting syndrome

Weight loss is one of the most distressing features of progressive HIV infection. Its course fluctuates even in advanced disease; frequently it is attributable to specific complications such as diarrhoeal diseases, lymphoma, or disseminated MAC infection. It may also progress with no cause identified other than advanced HIV infection. In developing countries such as sub-Saharan Africa the wasting syndrome is characteristic evidence of AIDS and has been called 'slim disease'. Despite severe weight loss, patients may remain well for many months or even years. Numerous therapeutic approaches have been tried, mostly with disappointing results, including oral nutritional support, enteral feeding, total parenteral nutrition, and trials of growth hormone and thalidomide. Controlled trials of treatment with the anabolic steroid megestrol acetate demonstrated weight gain and good tolerability, but its use has not been widely adopted and careful selection of patients is needed. Highly active antiretroviral therapy is important in the prevention of and, to some extent, reversal of HIV-related cachexia; but the fat redistribution associated with protease inhibitors may cause face and limb wasting.

Children and HIV

Most paediatric infections result from vertical transmission of HIV, although some children may be infected by blood products. The risk of vertical transmission is increased during advanced maternal HIV disease, if delivery is by the vaginal route, and if the baby is breastfed. Diagnosis is important in the first year of life because about 20 per cent of HIV-infected children progress rapidly to AIDS during that time; however a special diagnostic approach is needed before 18 months of age, because over this period uninfected children may have maternal HIV antibody.

HIV-infected children should be managed by paediatricians with experience in HIV care, usually in specialized units. About 10 per cent die in infancy, and progression to AIDS subsequently occurs at the rate of about 5 per cent per year. In recent European series, 40 per cent of children had developed AIDS before the age of 5 years and 25 per cent had died. The commonest AIDS diagnosis in infancy is *Pneumocystis* pneumonia. The CD4 lymphocyte count is of less value in monitoring than in adults, particularly in very young children; consequently it is conventional to give prophylaxis against *Pneumocystis* regardless of the CD4 count during the first year. In older children the principles of monitoring are similar to those in adults, using clinical status, CD4 counts, and viral load estimation by plasma HIV-1 RNA measurement. The CD4 per cent (percentage of total lymphocytes) and CD4:CD8 cell ratio vary less with age and are more useful than absolute CD4 counts in children under the age of 5 years.

Clinical conditions in children that are reasonably predictive of HIV infection include persistent oral candida, parotid swelling, and recurrent or frequent serious bacterial infections including pneumonia. Failure to thrive, diarrhoea, fever, lymphadenopathy, and hepatosplenomegaly are also more common in HIV-infected infants but are non-specific and less predictive. HIV dementia and other neurological and developmental problems are associated with a poor prognosis. HIV-related lymphocytic interstitial pneumonitis (LIP) is almost confined to children and characterized by progressive widespread reticulonodular shadowing on chest radiography. LIP develops gradually and may be asymptomatic; however cough, breathlessness, clubbing, secondary bacterial infections, and bronchiectasis occur in severe cases; these may be treated with oral prednisolone.

The principles for using antiretroviral therapy in children with HIV are similar to those for adults. Clinical trials are in progress to determine optimal antiretroviral combinations, when to start treatment, and the tolerability of the newer drugs, especially the protease inhibitors and new nucleoside drugs. Zidovudine, stavudine, ritonavir, and nelfinavir are already in use, although data for children are limited.

Management of HIV and prevention of complications

General management

Ideally, HIV infection should be identified at the asymptomatic stage. Clinical and laboratory monitoring can aid early detection of waning immunity and the risk of disease progression, so that appropriate antiretroviral therapy and prophylaxis against infections such as *Pneumocystis* pneumonia can be started. Serological screening detects past or current infections such as *Toxoplasma*, CMV, hepatitis C, and syphilis, which may reactivate or progress during immunosuppression. Clinic visits provide an opportunity for discussions with the physician or a trained counsellor of such issues as healthy lifestyles and safer sex. Throughout the course of HIV infection, many of the problems that develop can be managed by a primary care physician. Routine dental services are also needed. However, clinical and laboratory monitoring, the management of late complications of HIV, and the prescription and monitoring of antiretroviral drugs require specialist supervision.

Monitoring

Monitoring is a crucial component of the management of HIV-positive patients and involves regular clinical assessment and use of prognostic laboratory tests. Development of HIV-related symptoms, such as oral candidiasis, or physical signs, such as asymptomatic cutaneous Kaposi's sarcoma, are of prognostic importance. From the range of potential laboratory markers examined in prospective studies, the two markers that have the best prognostic value are the CD4 lymphocyte count and quantitative estimation of HIV RNA in the blood plasma (viral load).

The CD4 lymphocyte (T-helper cell) count is a reliable indicator of HIV-related immune impairment. Normal CD4 counts are at or above 600/mm^3 but in a given individual there is considerable variability, even in the absence of HIV infection. When the CD4 lymphocyte count has fallen to about 200/mm^3, the risk of opportunistic

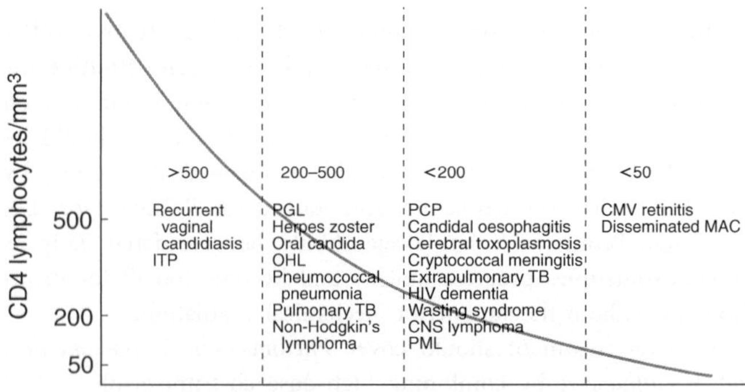

Fig. 11 Ranges of CD4 lymphocyte counts at which the principal opportunistic infections and other complications of HIV typically begin to occur.

infections and other manifestations of AIDS is increased, to about 80 per cent over 3 years. However, progression is variable and a minority remain well for several years with stable, low CD4 counts. This variability is partly explained by differences in HIV viral load. The level of CD4 lymphopenia also broadly determines the spectrum of infections that may arise (Fig. 11). For instance, whereas oral and oesophageal candidiasis and *Pneumocystis* pneumonia are frequent at CD4 counts of 100–200/mm^3, disseminated MAC infection and CMV retinitis are rarely seen until the CD4 count is below 50/mm^3.

The prognostic value of measurement of HIV RNA in plasma was reported in the US in 1996. In HIV-positive men in a subgroup of the Multicenter AIDS Cohort Study (MACS), only 8 per cent with less than about 5000 copies of HIV RNA/ml progressed to AIDS over 5 years, whereas 62 per cent with viral loads above about 35 000 developed AIDS. Viral load estimation was shown to be a better predictor of progression to AIDS than the CD4 lymphocyte count. For a given level of CD4 lymphocytes, variations in viral load predict the risk of progression. Consequently, in the monitoring of HIV patients the most useful prognostic information is derived from the CD4 count and viral load taken together (Fig. 12).

In industrialized countries, HIV viral load testing by detection of HIV-1 RNA in plasma, for instance by reverse transcription followed by amplification by polymerase chain reaction (RT-PCR), has become widely available. Highly sensitive tests with very low detection limits (about 20 copies/ml) have been developed, and are increasingly used in monitoring the effects of antiretroviral therapy.

Antiretroviral therapy

Nucleoside analogues

Knowledge of the viral life cycle (Fig. 3) has led to the development of a number of antiretroviral compounds with clinically useful activity against HIV. The forerunner of these was zidovudine (AZT or ZDV), first shown to be active against HIV *in vitro* in 1985. Zidovudine, a nucleoside analogue that inhibits the reverse transcriptase enzyme of HIV, slowed down the rate of disease progression over a 12-month period in patients with AIDS, with short-term improvements in survival and in patients' well being, body weight, and neurological features. However, the duration of response to zidovudine monotherapy was limited. Clinical progression was observed a year or two into therapy and this was correlated with viral resistance to the drug. The Anglo-French Concorde study, which compared early treatment with zidovudine to deferred zidovudine, showed no difference in survival or disease progression in asymptomatic patients with HIV over a 3-year period.

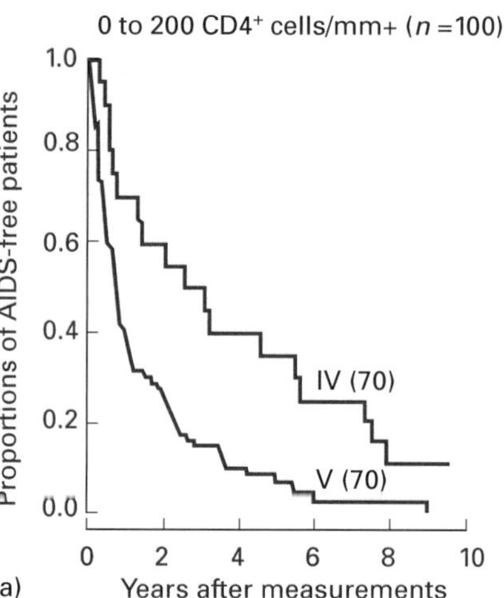

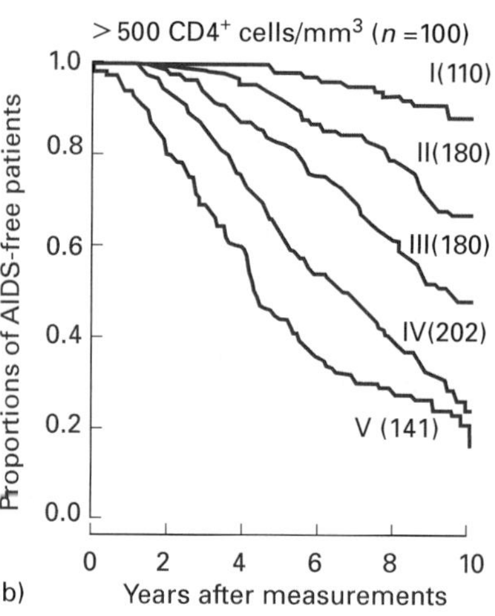

Fig. 12 Curves showing AIDS-free survival with time among groups with different baseline CD4 lymphocyte counts, according to HIV-1 RNA category (copies/ml): I, 500 or less; II, 501 to 3000; III, 3001 to 10 000; IV, 10 001 to 30 000; and V, >30 000.
(Adapted from Mellers, J.W., Munoz, A., Giorgi, J.V., et al. Plasma viral load and CD4+ lymphocytes as prognostic markers of HIV-1 infection. Annals of Internal Medicine, **126***(12), 946–54.)*

The clinical failure of monotherapy prompted the evaluation of combinations of anti-HIV drugs in attempts to reduce the development of drug resistance. Randomized trials demonstrated that double nucleoside combinations (zidovudine plus didanosine (ddI) or zalcitabine (ddC)) were superior to zidovudine monotherapy, especially in patients without prior exposure to zidovudine. For instance in the Delta study the mortality over a median duration of 30 months was reduced from 21 per cent for zidovudine alone to 13 per cent for zidovudine/didanosine in AZT-naive patients with CD4 counts below 350/mm^3 or symptomatic HIV disease. Other double nucleoside combinations, such as zidovudine/lamivudine (3TC) and lamivudine/stavudine (d4T), were also shown to be superior to monotherapy.

Protease inhibitors

The HIV-encoded protease (or proteinase) is required for the production of mature, infectious viral particles. This enzyme cleaves a number of structural proteins and enzymes from the polyprotein precursors produced by translation of the *gag* and *gag–pol* genes. Inhibitors of HIV protease act synergistically with nucleoside drugs and are potent inhibitors of HIV replication. Several have been developed for therapeutic use.

The effects of protease inhibitors on HIV viral load and CD4 counts are greater than those seen with nucleoside reverse transcriptase inhibitors, especially when they are used in a triple therapy combinations. This was first shown for saquinavir: using viral load reduction and increased CD4 counts as end points, triple therapy with zidovudine, zalcitabine, and saquinavir was superior to double therapy (zidovudine/saquinavir or zidovudine/zalcitabine) over 48 weeks (AIDS Clinical Trials Group (ACTG) trial 229). In the original formulation, saquinavir was poorly absorbed, leading to low bioavailability. A new soft-gel formulation was developed to address this.

The protease inhibitor indinavir, in combination with two nucleoside analogues (zidovudine/lamivudine or stavudine/lamivudine) produced excellent results in a large, controlled trial with clinical primary end points (ACTG 320). Compared with double therapy (two nucleosides), the triple combination reduced the proportion of patients who progressed to AIDS or death from 11 per cent to 6 per cent over about 38 weeks. The responses of CD4 cells and plasma HIV RNA paralleled the clinical results. Similar results were reported for combinations that included the other protease inhibitors, ritonavir, and nelfinavir.

Non-nucleoside reverse transcriptase inhibitors

The prototype of the class was nevirapine, a potent and selective inhibitor of HIV reverse transcriptase. When administered as monotherapy, resistance to nevirapine develops rapidly—nevirapine is of limited effectiveness in double therapy combinations or when added to existing, failing regimens. However, in antiretroviral-naive patients without AIDS (CD4 200–600/mm^3) over a half of patients treated with nevirapine plus two nucleosides (zidovudine/didanosine) had undetectable plasma HIV RNA after 1 year of therapy, compared with 12 per cent for zidovudine/didanosine. Delavirdine and efavirenz are other non-nucleoside reverse transcriptase inhibitors with similar properties to nevirapine. Combinations of non-nucleoside drugs and protease inhibitors, such as indinavir with efavirenz, are being studied in clinical trials.

Other compounds being investigated include: agents that inhibit HIV integrase and prevent proviral DNA integration into the host cell genome; hydroxyurea, which acts synergistically with nucleoside reverse transcriptase inhibitors *in vitro* and is an inexpensive compound that may prove valuable in resource-poor settings; and interleukin-2, which can induce impressive elevations of CD4 lymphocyte counts in HIV patients.

General points on HIV therapy

Since the first clinical studies on zidovudine, the identification of a range of antiretroviral compounds with good tolerability has led to a plethora of clinical trials and results for analysis. The search for effective combinations of drugs and great number of potential combinations and regimens have led to a high degree of complexity.

It is clear that monotherapy with any of the known antiretroviral drugs promotes viral resistance that leads to treatment failure. Combinations of at least three antiretroviral agents reduce the risk of viral resistance and have greater clinical effectiveness in reducing progression of HIV disease or death. Reductions in HIV viral load during treatment correlate with risk of disease progression or death. Combinations using three antiretroviral drugs (two nucleoside drugs plus protease inhibitor or non-nucleoside reverse transcriptase inhibitor) are more potent than double drug combinations at reducing viral load, and show greater clinical effectiveness than double drug regimens over a 1 to 2-year time period.

In general, there is agreement that treatment should be started at CD4 counts of around 350/mm^3 or below, or when clinical manifestations of HIV arise regardless of CD4 count, but the optimal point at which to start antiretroviral therapy has not been determined. Circumstantial evidence and certain theoretical assumptions form the basis of the argument for treatment at an earlier stage, but evidence for long-term benefit is not yet available from clinical trials. Viral resistance is ultimately responsible for treatment failure; there is evidence that resistant mutants arise spontaneously even in the absence of antiretroviral therapy. This tendency is greatest when HIV viraemia is high, and lowest when HIV replication is completely suppressed by a potent drug combination.

The optimal drug combination or regimen is not known, and the optimal strategy for sequencing treatment has not been determined. Expert panels, for instance in the US and UK, have summarized the available evidence and defined by consensus the broad limits within which treatment choices should be made. Such guidelines have to be updated regularly in the light of new knowledge.

With existing drug combinations, treatment fails to control viraemia in up to 40 to 50 per cent of patients. It is unknown whether viral suppression can be maintained indefinitely in a subgroup of patients if an appropriate treatment strategy is used, or whether resistance to multiple drugs inevitably appears.

At present, it is also unknown if antiretroviral drugs will ever eradicate HIV and bring about a 'cure'. Early studies using triple therapy (two reverse transcriptase inhibitors and a protease inhibitor) showed dramatic reductions in viral load and rises in circulating CD4 lymphocytes. However, even in patients treated soon after primary infection where drugs lead to an inability to detect circulating virus in the plasma, low levels of viral RNA and proviral DNA can be found in lymphoid tissue and, in some cases, virus can be grown from the tissue.

Drug resistance

Extensive genotypic variation of HIV occurs because of very high viral turnover and transcription errors by the reverse transcriptase enzyme, so that all possible single point mutations spontaneously arise. Numerous codon mutations in reverse transcriptase that confer resistance to nucleoside and non-nucleoside reverse transcriptase inhibitor drugs, when used as monotherapy, have been characterized. For instance, zidovudine resistance is most commonly conferred by a mutation in codon 215 of reverse transcriptase, and codon 184 for lamivudine resistance (cross-resistant to didanosine and zalcitabine). Resistance to protease inhibitors and non-nucleoside reverse transcriptase inhibitors confers cross-resistance to other members of each class. Controlling viral replication with a highly potent treatment regimen may limit the appearance of resistant HIV mutants.

Zidovudine-resistant HIV can be transmitted horizontally and vertically. Resistance mutations to antiretrovirals are identifiable in 7–14 per cent of recent seroconverters in the US. Laboratory assays are being developed to identify codon mutations that correlate with *in vivo* resistance to antiretrovirals; these are likely to play an increasing role in the selection of drug regimens and monitoring of HIV treatment in the future.

Drug toxicity and interactions

Adverse reactions to antiretroviral agents are relatively common and may be require discontinuation of treatment. They are mostly minor gastrointestinal disturbances (nausea, vomiting, diarrhoea), rashes, and headache but serious adverse reactions occur. The possibility of drug interaction is an important consideration when prescribing antiretroviral drugs, especially in late HIV disease when the likelihood of treatment with other medications is higher. Antiretroviral agents may interact with each other and with other drugs. Ritonavir, because of potent inhibition of cytochrome P-450, is especially prone to raising blood levels of other drugs and should not be coadministered with several antiarrhythmics, anxiolytics, and antihistamines; caution is required with several analgesics, anticonvulsants, and other categories of medication.

Protease inhibitors have a number of important adverse effects including hyperglycaemia, lipodystrophy, fat redistribution, and hyperlipidaemia. Whether the effects on lipid metabolism increase the risk of ischaemic vascular diseases is uncertain. Indinavir may induce renal calculus formation (on average 5 per cent within 1 year) or flank pain caused by precipitated indinavir; the risk is reduced if a high fluid throughput is maintained.

Patient compliance

The impact of combination antiretroviral therapy on the lives of HIV patients should not be underestimated. In common with all chronic diseases a significant proportion, possibly 30 per cent of patients, are not fully compliant with treatment recommendations. The behavioural and psychological factors underlying this are complex; adherence to treatment requires a high level of understanding and motivation in the patient. This is of particular concern in HIV therapy because of the risk of developing drug resistance mutations during suboptimal therapy.

Prevention of opportunistic infections

The risk of developing an opportunistic infection rises greatly once the peripheral CD4 lymphocyte count consistently falls below 200/mm^3. It is standard practice to introduce low dose co-trimoxazole prophylaxis for *Pneumocystis* pneumonia at this stage. This also reduces the risk of cerebral toxoplasmosis and may, in addition, prevent bacterial pneumonia.

The risk of developing active tuberculosis in HIV-positive, American, intravenous drug users with positive tuberculin skin tests has been shown to be about 8 per cent per year and can be reduced by taking isoniazid for a year. In developing countries, in particular, the risk of active tuberculosis in HIV-positive individuals is high and isoniazid alone or in combination with rifampicin can reduce the risk, but the feasibility and cost-effectiveness of this approach in resource-poor countries require further evaluation. BCG vaccination does not appear to be protective in HIV.

Primary prophylaxis may prevent other conditions, such as CMV retinitis, cryptococcal meningitis, and histoplasmosis but because of the relatively low incidence and lack of predictors of risk for these conditions, it is not cost-effective. Simple measures, other than drugs, may be able to reduce the risk of some infections. Avoiding undercooked eggs and poultry may reduce the risk of disseminated *Salmonella* infection and adequate boiling of drinking water can prevent cryptosporidiosis. Stopping cigarette smoking may reduce the risk of bacterial chest infections.

After treatment of an opportunistic infection, in general, the underlying tendency to the infection remains. Thus in early studies, following an episode of *Pneumocystis* pneumonia patients had a 50 per cent chance of a further episode within a year. Secondary prophylaxis with co-trimoxazole was found to be effective. Secondary prophylaxis is also needed for other opportunistic infections including cerebral toxoplasmosis, cryptococcosis, and histoplasmosis.

Marked reductions in morbidity and mortality have been attributed to the use of intensive antiretroviral regimens that include protease inhibitors. Among patients attending HIV clinics in eight cities in the US, mortality declined from 30 per 100 person-years in 1995 to 9 per 100 person-years in 1997. The incidence of *Pneumocystis* pneumonia, disseminated MAC infection, and CMV retinitis declined dramatically. Mortality of patients with CD4 counts below 100/mm^3 fell for the first time in 1996, and a decline in the incidence of a broad range of opportunistic infections was reported from the US and Europe.

The advent of potent antretroviral therapy has also changed the natural history of opportunistic infections in HIV patients. Preliminary reports suggest that in selected patients with disseminated MAC infection, CMV retinitis, and other infections, secondary prophylaxis can be discontinued when antiretroviral therapy has successfully established very low viral load and a rise in CD4 lymphocytes; however, current evidence suggests that it is unlikely that the full repertoire of cellular immune responses can be revived.

Prevention of HIV transmission

Sexual transmission

Sexual transmission accounts for most new cases of HIV infection. Education to alter behaviour and reduce the risk of HIV infection is an important part of HIV control programmes. The benefits of 'safer sex' should be publicised; condom promotion in Thailand has made an impact on HIV transmission rates. Other sexually transmitted infections act as cofactors in HIV transmission. Studies in Tanzania and elsewhere have demonstrated that programmes to prevent and treat sexually transmitted infections can reduce the incidence of new HIV infections.

Vertical transmission

As the number of women infected with HIV increases, the problem of vertical transmission of the virus assumes greater importance. In developed countries, the risk for transmission of HIV from a seropositive pregnant woman to her child is about 15 per cent but this figure may be as high as 30 per cent in sub-Saharan Africa and other parts of the tropics. Although infection of the fetus can occur at any time during pregnancy and has been shown to occur with breastfeeding, it is likely that most infections occur during labour. It was shown that zidovudine reduced the risk from 25 per cent to 8 per cent, when given to women during late pregnancy and labour and to the neonate for 4 weeks. Simpler, cheaper regimens have been shown to be effective. During vaginal delivery, intrapartum interventions such as fetal blood sampling and use of fetal scalp clips should be avoided. Elective caesarean section delivery further reduces vertical transmission. Breastfeeding should be avoided, if possible, but is still generally recommended in developing countries where the risks of bottle-feeding probably outweigh the risks of breastfeeding. Currently a minority of HIV-positive women are aware of their infection at the time of delivery. Increasingly, the offer of HIV testing is being incorporated into antenatal care in developed countries.

Blood products

Screening of blood products began as soon as testing for HIV became available, and heat-treatment for factor VIII concentrate was also introduced. These measures dramatically reduced the risk of virus transmission by blood and blood products in industrialized countries. However, there may still be a problem in developing countries where screening is not efficient, or where the background seroprevalence of potential donors is so high that HIV-infected blood may be screened as negative when donated by an individual in the 'window period' immediately after initial infection.

Transmission via injecting drug use

Needle-exchange programmes and the prescription of controlled drugs to registered addicts may reduce the incidence of new HIV infections in injecting drug users. Major problems still exist in countries such as India and Russia, where injecting drug use is becoming more common and education about the risk and the availability of clean needles are very limited.

Occupational exposure and postexposure prophylaxis

The average risk of HIV infection after needlestick injury or other percutaneous exposure is about 1 in 325 and is greatest for deep injuries, and if the source patient has advanced HIV disease. A small retrospective study demonstrated an 80 per cent reduction in the likelihood of seroconversion in health-care workers who took zidovudine soon after percutaneous exposure to HIV. In view of the greater activity of antiretroviral combinations, currently it is recommended that high-risk occupational exposures to HIV are treated immediately with two nucleoside inhibitors (typically zidovudine and lamivudine) and a protease inhibitor, for 1 month. The recommended regimen may change as new antiretrovirals and information on effectiveness become available. A careful risk assessment should be done and where significant risk of HIV transmission is identified, antiretroviral therapy should be offered and started promptly. There is a theoretical argument for taking antiretroviral drugs after high-risk sexual exposure to HIV; at present there is no consensus on this and no data on clinical or cost-effectiveness.

Vaccine development

The high degree of viral variation and immune escape present difficulties for the development of an effective HIV vaccine. Nonetheless, group-specific neutralizing antibodies and cross-reacting T-cell clones have been identified, and there is evidence from female prostitutes repeatedly exposed to HIV that certain individuals can develop specific T-cell responses without persistent infection. These individuals may be protected from infection when exposed to live virus.

Non-infectious, killed, whole virus or recombinant subunit vaccines have not been successful to date in protecting chimpanzees from HIV infection, or macaques from SIV infection and disease. Certain live attenuated strains of SIV, with deletion mutations in *nef* and other regulatory genes, initially appeared to protect adult monkeys from challenge with virulent SIV strains, but more recently were reported to cause AIDS. Despite this setback with monkeys, a candidate attenuated virus vaccine is being developed for evaluation in humans.

The first full scale human testing is planned for a vaccine made from tiny recombinant fragments of gp120, the surface glycoprotein of HIV that binds to host cell CD4 receptors. Similar vaccines have not been successful in animals. Several other approaches currently being examined may prove more effective in inducing protective humoral and killer T-cell mediated immunity. These include use of live vectors (such as that based on a genetically altered bird virus, canary pox) to deliver portions of the HIV envelope, and DNA vaccines, consisting of pieces of HIV DNA incorporated into harmless plasmid DNA from bacteria. Effective vaccination is likely to hold the greatest promise for controlling HIV in the future.

Further reading

Collier A.C., Coombs R.W., Schoenfeld D.A., *et al.* (1996). Treatment of human immunodeficiency virus infection with saquinavir, zidovudine, and zalcitabine. *New England Journal of Medicine*, **334**, 1011–7.

Concorde Coordinating Committee (1994). Concorde: MRC/ANRS randomised double-blind controlled trial of immediate and deferred zidovudine in symptom-free HIV infection. *Lancet*, **343**, 871–81.

Delta Coordinating Committee (1996). Delta: a randomised double-blind controlled trial comparing combinations of zidovudine plus didanosine or zalcitabine with zidovudine alone in HIV-infected individuals. *Lancet*, **348**, 283–91.

Flexner, C. (1998). Drug therapy: HIV-protease inhibitors. *New England Journal of Medicine*, **338**, 1281–92.

Hammer, S.M., Squires, K.E., Hughes M.D., *et al.* (1997). A controlled trial of two nucleoside analogues plus indinavir in persons with human immunodeficiency virus infection and CD4 cell counts of 200 per cubic millimeter or less. *New England Journal of Medicine*, **337**, 725–33.

Ho, D.D., Neumann, A.U., Perelson, A.S., *et al.* (1995). Rapid turnover of plasma virions and CD4 lymphocytes in HIV-1 infection. *Nature*, **373**, 123–6.

Letvin, N.L. (1998). Progress in the development of an HIV-1 vaccine. *Science*, **280**, 1875–80.

Levy, J.A. (1998). *HIV and the pathogenesis of AIDS*, (2nd edn). ASM Press, Washington D.C.

Lipsky, J.J. (1996). Antiretroviral drugs for AIDS. *Lancet*, **348**, 800–3.

Mellors, J.W., Rinaldo, C.R.Jr, Gupta, P., *et al.* (1996). Prognosis in HIV-1 infection predicted by the quantity of virus in plasma. *Science*, **272**, 1167–70.

Palella, F.J.Jr, Delaney, K.M., Moorman, A.C., *et al.* (1998). Declining morbidity and mortality among patients with advanced human immunodeficiency virus infection. *New England Journal of Medicine*, **338**, 853–60.

Perrin, L. and Telenti, A. (1998). HIV treatment failure: testing for HIV resistance in clinical practice. *Science*, **280**, 1871–3.

USPHS/IDSA. (1997). Guidelines for the prevention of opportunistic infections in persons infected with human immunodeficiency virus: disease-specific recommendations. *Clinics in Infectious Diseases*, **25** (Suppl. 3), S313–35.

Chapter 16.36

HTLV-I and -II and associated diseases

C. R. M. Bangham and S. Nightingale

HTLV-I

Human T cell leukaemia virus type 1 (HTLV-I) causes no disease in approximately 95 per cent of infected people. About 2 per cent develop adult T-cell leukaemia/lymphoma, and 2 to 3 per cent develop a range of subacute or chronic inflammatory conditions, of which the best recognized is tropical spastic paraparesis/HTLV-I-associated myelopathy (TSP/HAM). The factors that determine these different outcomes are unknown.

The virus infects about 10–20 million people world-wide. It has a patchy endemic distribution, with a local seroprevalence of 1–20 per cent of the population in many tropical countries, particularly the Caribbean, West Africa, South America, Papua New Guinea, and northern Australia. It is also prevalent in Hokkaido and Kyushu in Japan, and throughout the world the virus occurs in some communities of intravenous drug abusers. In the UK, HTLV-I is found in 1 to 4 per cent of people of Caribbean origin.

In endemic areas, HTLV-I is chiefly transmitted by breast feeding. Sexual contact is the main mode of transmission in adults, particularly from males to females. In the remaining cases, the virus is acquired by transfusion of infected blood or blood products that contain cells (virus is virtually absent from cell-free body fluids), or by contact with contaminated needles.

HTLV-I is closely related to leukaemia viruses of monkey and cattle; its relationship to HIV is distant. Five major proteins are produced by the virus: the core protein Gag; the receptor-binding protein Env; the polymerase (reverse transcriptase) Pol; and 2 proteins, Tax and Rex, which regulate viral transcription. The cellular receptor for the virus has not been identified. Although it can infect many cell types *in vitro*, HTLV-I replicates efficiently only in CD4+ (helper) T cells, which are the cells that are transformed in adult T cell leukaemia or lymphoma.

In addition to an antibody response directed mainly against the Env and Gag proteins, most infected individuals mount a vigorous cytotoxic T lymphocyte (CTL) response to the Tax protein of the virus; the CTL are partly responsible for restricting the virus load.

The diagnosis of HTLV-I infection depends on detection of virus-specific antibodies in a particle agglutination assay, enzyme immunoassay, or western blot.

Tropical spastic paraparesis/HTLV-I-associated myelopathy (TSP/HAM)

TSP/HAM mainly affects those living in or having emigrated from areas of endemic HTLV-1 infection, but it also occurs in others infected by maternal transmission, sexual activity, intravenous drug abuse, or blood transfusion. It is more common in women, and usually begins in the third to sixth decade. The lifetime risk of HAM/TSP in infected people is approximately 0.2 to 2 per cent. The common class I human leucocyte antigen HLA-A*02 halves the odds of TSP/HAM in HTLV-I carriers.

There is a gradually progressive spastic paraparesis with few sensory features, causing a disturbance of gait which often confines the patient to a wheelchair within 10 years. Most patients experience back or leg pain and symptoms of a spastic bladder. Less common features include spastic weakness of the arms, a sensory level on the trunk, male impotence, sensorineural deafness, and optic atrophy. Rarely, lower motor neurone signs are observed. The severity of the paraparesis may fluctuate and eventually stabilize, but in contrast to multiple sclerosis, tropical spastic paraparesis does not result in acute relapsing and remitting disease.

Patients with TSP/HAM are seropositive for HTLV-I. However, progressive paraparesis in an HTLV-I positive patient should not be assumed to be due to TSP/HAM without excluding other spinal disorders including intrinsic or extrinsic tumours, syringomyelia, B_{12} deficiency, syphilis, and Lyme disease. Familial clusters of tropical spastic paraparesis have been reported but hereditary spastic paraparesis should also be considered when there is a family history.

The cerebrospinal fluid usually shows a slight pleocytosis (5–50 cells/μl) and the protein level may be as high as two or three times normal. MRI scanning of the brain may show scattered lesions in the white matter similar to, though usually less extensive than, the lesions seen in multiple sclerosis.

The pathology of the spinal cord mainly consists of perivascular infiltration of mononuclear cells with proliferation of microglia and reactive astrocytic gliosis. There may be demyelination as well as capillary proliferation. The degree of inflammatory response is variable.

There is no specific treatment for TSP/HAM but patients will benefit from rehabilitation and management of their spasticity and bladder symptoms.

Adult T-cell leukaemia/lymphoma (ATLL)

A person infected with HTLV-I has a 1–2 per cent life-time risk of developing ATLL; the interval between infection and disease is frequently over 20 years. The disease is slightly more common in males (M:F = 1.2:1), and there is evidence of familial clustering of cases. In high endemic areas it is an important cause of malignant disease: in Kyushu, Japan, ATLL accounts for 75 per cent of all non-Hodgkin lymphomas.

The typical clinical features of ATLL are lymphadenopathy, skin infiltrates, and hepatosplenomegaly. Lytic bone lesions and hypercalcaemia are common.

The morphology of the leukaemic cells is characteristic: the nucleus is large, lobulated, and flower-like. The cells are almost invariably CD4+, and typically the interleukin-2 receptor (CD25) is strongly expressed on the cell surface. Karyotypic abnormalities are common in the leukaemic cells.

Morphologically similar cells are found in small numbers in the peripheral blood in some asymptomatic carriers of the virus. When the proportion of abnormal cells is high, and there is a lymphocytosis, there is a greatly increased risk of development of ATLL. However, in some cases the atypical cells regress spontaneously. Intermediate states between lymphocytosis and frank ATLL are often called smouldering or pre-ATLL.

The syndrome of ATLL is refractory to treatment. Sometimes remission can be obtained with cytotoxic regimens, but the disease soon relapses. The mean survival times for acute, lymphomatous, and chronic (smouldering) ATLL in Japan are 6.2, 10.2, and 24.3 months, respectively.

Other disorders associated with HTLV-I

Where HTLV-1 is endemic, many disorders may occur by chance in asymptomatic carriers of the virus. The aetiological relationship of HTLV-1 to tropical spastic paraparesis and ATLL is accepted but the range of disorders for which HTLV-1 is responsible is uncertain. A list of disorders that have been associated serologically with HTLV-1 is shown in Table 1. It is likely that over the next few years the spectrum of HTLV-1-associated disorders will widen.

Table 1 Disorders associated with HTLV-1

Adult T-cell leukaemia/lymphoma (ATLL)
Tropical spastic paraparesis or HTLV-1 associated myelopathy (TSP/HAM)
Polymyositis
Chronic arthritis
Uveitis
Motor neurone disease-like disorder
Sicca syndrome
Lymphocytic alveolitis
Chronic infective dermatitis

HTLV-II

HTLV-II, a retrovirus closely related to HTLV-I, was first isolated from a patient with hairy-cell leukaemia. The virus occurs sporadically in West Africa and is common in several native groups in both North and South America. In intravenous drug abusers in Europe and North America, infection with HTLV-II is as common as HTLV-I.

Since the early 1980s, there have been occasional reports of HTLV-II infection in patients with hairy-cell leukaemia or a paralytic syndrome similar to HAM/TSP, but no unequivocal association of any disease with HTLV-II infection has yet been demonstrated.

Further reading

Bangham, C.R.M., Hall, S.E., Jeffery, K.J.M., *et al* (1999). Genetic control and dynamics of the cellular immune response to the human T-cell leukaemia virus, HTLV-I. *Philosophical Transactions of the Royal Society, London B*, in press.

Manns, A., Hisada, M., and LaGrenade, L. (1999). Human T-lymphotropic virus type 1 infection. *Lancet*, 353, 1951–8.

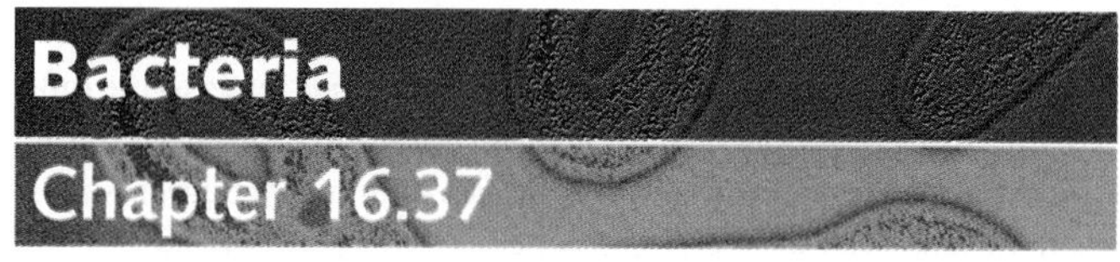

Diphtheria

A. B. Christie, Tran Tinh Hien, and D. B. Bethell*

Diphtheria is an acute infection of the upper respiratory tract and occasionally of other mucous membranes or skin, frequently occurring in children, and caused by *Corynebacterium diphtheriae*. In the eighteenth and nineteenth centuries the developed world was plagued by a series of diphtheria pandemics. Today *C. diphtheriae* and diphtheria have been virtually eliminated from most industrialized nations, but are still prevalent in many developing countries. There has been a recent increase in incidence in the Russian Federation and the Ukraine.

Bacteriology

C. diphtheriae is a Gram-positive, non-motile, non-sporulating, pleomorphic bacillus with a characteristic club shape. The presence of a lysogenic β-phage, which can pass from toxigenic to non-toxigenic

*Dr A.B. Christie died in 1987. Much of his second edition chapter was retained in OTM3.

strains, enables *C. diphtheriae* to produce toxin. The three main subtypes, *gravis, mitis,* and *intermedius,* can be differentiated by colonial morphology.

Pathogenesis

The pathological effects of diphtheria in man are caused by diphtheria exotoxin. This spreads through the body by haematogenous and lymphatic routes, and halts protein synthesis by inactivating tRNA translocase (elongation factor 2).

C. diphtheriae is non-invasive and usually stays in the respiratory mucosa and skin lesions where it induces a mild, localized inflammatory reaction. However, if the organism is toxigenic, toxin induces the formation of a pseudomembrane composed of fibrin, leucocytes, erythrocytes, necrotic cells, and organisms. The underlying tissue oedema and cervical adenitis results in the typical 'bull neck' appearance, which may be accompanied by severe respiratory embarrassment.

Within the heart, fatty degeneration of cardiac muscle and infiltration of the interstitium with leucocytes is seen. Neurological complications are caused by demyelination of peripheral nerves, affecting mainly motor but also sensory fibres. The lesions in most other organs are non-specific.

Spread of infection and host immunity

Humans are the only known reservoir for *C. diphtheria.* Diphtheria spreads via airborne droplets and direct contact with respiratory secretions or skin lesions. The organism resists drying and can be isolated from floor dust in a ward or an infected classroom. Diphtheria has been spread by milk contaminated by a human carrier. Pasteurization kills *C. diphtheriae* as does exposure to most common disinfectants.

In a highly immunized community, *C. diphtheriae* tends to die out. In parts of the world lacking an efficient immunization programme *C. diphtheriae* may be a common pathogen and many children suffer severe or fatal attacks of diphtheria before the age of 5 years.

Clinical features

Diphtheria is predominantly an infectious disease of children. After an incubation period of 2–5 days, it presents in a variety of different forms depending largely upon the location of the pseudomembrane.

Anterior nasal

The main symptom is nasal discharge, initially watery, then thick, purulent, and bloody, with soreness of the nostril and the skin above the lip, and crusting inside the nostril. Nasal diphtheria is relatively common in infancy. It is often mild except when faucial or nasopharyngeal forms coexist.

Faucial

This is the most common form of diphtheria. The onset is insidious. On the first day of illness there may be just a tiny spot of membrane on the tonsils, yellowish white, and with an irregular edge. Soon the membrane spreads over both tonsils, greyish-yellow, a millimetre thick, confluent, and edged with a rim of redness. The rest of the throat and fauces look normal. There is mild accompanying cervical adenitis. After another day or two the membrane is greenish-black, and later it sloughs off. Faucial diphtheria can easily be confused with other forms of tonsillitis.

Tracheolaryngeal

Diphtheria of the larynx is usually secondary to faucial diphtheria (85 per cent). Occasionally there is no membrane on the pharynx at all. Initial symptoms include moderate fever, with hoarseness and non-productive cough. This is followed by a gradual onset of dyspnoea which may become life-threatening. Without tracheostomy the child may soon die. Tracheostomy brings rapid relief if the membrane is confined to the larynx and upper part of the trachea. In a few cases the membrane has spread down into the bronchi and bronchioles and then tracheostomy helps very little.

Malignant

The onset is more acute, the patient soon becoming very ill with high fever, tachycardia, hypotension, and cyanosis. The membrane spreads rapidly and as it advances the earlier parts become necrotic. There is massive cervical lymphadenopathy with surrounding tissue oedema, the so-called 'bull neck' appearance. The patient may bleed from the mouth, nose, and skin. Cardiac involvement with heart block occurs early, within a few days from the onset, and acute renal failure may supervene. Such a patient has little hope of recovery.

Skin

In contrast to the severe course of some faucial infections, *C. diphtheriae* often causes chronic but mild infections of the skin. This is especially common in the tropics. Sores and ulcers are most common on the legs but may occur anywhere. The sores are indolent and slow to heal. Absorption of toxin is slow from the skin; paralysis or myocarditis may occur, but both are rare.

Other sites

Mild conjunctivitis is not uncommon. Occasionally, pseudomembrane forms in the lower conjunctiva and spreads over the cornea causing great destruction of tissue. *C. diphtheriae* may spread to the oesophagus from the fauces causing dysphagia, and there are a few reports of membrane in the stomach and the intestine. Diphtheria may be spread on a child's fingers from the throat to the vulva causing localized sores, and rarely *C. diphtheriae* invades the vagina and cervix. Diphtheria of the penis has occurred in infants after circumcision, and in men in conditions where diphtheria of the skin is spreading. Endocarditis occurs but is extremely rare.

Complications

Diphtheria is a devastating disease. Even if the patient survives the acute, destructive phase of the infection, he or she may die from delayed effects of the toxin. The most prominent toxic complications of diphtheria are myocarditis and neuritis. The risk and the severity of toxin damage correlate with the extent of the membrane and the delay in administration of antitoxin.

Myocarditis

Approximately 10 per cent of patients overall and two-thirds with severe infection will have some evidence of cardiac involvement. Cardiac complications are more frequent with laryngeal or malignant diphtheria, or if antitoxin is delayed for more than 48 h. The first evidence of cardiac toxicity usually occurs after the first week of illness. Cardiac failure can occur, and in severe cases cardiogenic shock ensues. Electrocardiographic changes are common: flattening or inversion of the T-wave, lengthening of the PR or QTc interval and, in severe cases, bundle-branch or complete heart block. Atrial or ventricular fibrillation may occur. Death is not inevitable but most deaths from diphtheria do occur at this stage. If the patient survives, cardiac recovery is usually complete.

Paralyses

Paralyses usually develop several weeks after the onset of illness. Palatal paralysis is common, and appears during the third week; it causes a nasal voice and regurgitation of fluids, and usually disappears after a week or so. Some days later the child may develop blurred vision from paralysis of accommodation or a squint from extraocular muscle paralysis; again recovery usually takes place within a couple of weeks. During the sixth or seventh week the more severe paralyses develop: pharynx, larynx, and the muscles of respiration. There may be weakness or complete paralysis of the limbs. Late paralyses are often life-threatening, but with appropriate supportive treatment full recovery should occur.

Diagnosis

In parts of the world where diphtheria is still common a clinical diagnosis may be made in a child with thick, discoloured pseudomembrane on the throat. Direct stained smears from throat swabs, if positive, can help experienced clinicians. Smears from cultures are more helpful during an outbreak and they meet most needs. In isolated cases where there is bacteriological doubt, full biochemical, immunological, and toxigenic tests must be done.

Treatment

Early administration of antitoxin is essential to neutralize toxin, and so must be given on clinical suspicion before bacteriological confirmation. The dosage depends on the site of primary infection, the extent of membrane, and the delay between the onset of illness and the antitoxin administration: 20 000 to 40 000 units for faucial diphtheria of less than 48 h duration or cutaneous infection; 40 000 to 80 000 units for faucial in excess of 48 h or laryngeal infection; 80 000 to 100 000 units for malignant diphtheria. Antitoxin is usually given intravenously in severe cases. However, because up to 10 per cent of individuals may show some hypersensitivity to horse protein, an intradermal test dose is essential.

C. diphtheriae is nearly always sensitive to penicillin, and this drug is usually given for a total of 10–14 days, parenterally, until the patient is able to swallow when oral penicillin may be used. Erythromycin (50 mg/kg) can be substituted if the patient is truly allergic to penicillin. Most throat carriage can be cleared with antibiotics.

For cardiac complications, intensive care is needed. Sedation is advisable and often the child needs additional oxygen. Digoxin may be useful when there is congestive cardiac failure. Inotropic support to counter severe hypotension may also be of some value. Temporary cardiac pacemaker insertion has been used successfully in several cases to overcome temporary conduction failure. For paralyses supportive care, with assisted ventilation if appropriate, is needed. Steroids are of no benefit for either myocarditis or neuritis.

Prevention

Diphtheria toxoid should be given as DTP vaccine to infants from 6–8 weeks of age. The usual course is of three doses separated by 4–8 weeks. A booster dose of diphtheria tetanus (DT) vaccine at school entry will ensure prolonged immunity. The recent, marked increase in numbers of cases of diphtheria in Russia and the Ukraine has prompted a recommendation in Britain that travellers to these areas should have a full primary course if they have never been vaccinated or a booster dose of low-dose vaccine if their primary vaccination course was more than 10 years previously. Patients should also be given toxoid immunization as the disease does not reliably induce protective levels of antitoxin.

Contacts of a patient may be protected for 2 or 3 weeks by 1000–2000 units of antitoxin. This may be useful when there is danger of cross-infection in a ward from a missed case, or in home contacts of a patient. However, penicillin given to close contacts may be equally effective and is also the best treatment for carriers.

Further reading

Christie, A.B. (1980). *Infectious diseases: epidemiology and clinical practice* (3rd edn). Churchill Livingstone, Edinburgh.

Farizo, K.M., Strebel, P.M., Chen, R.T., Kimbler, A., Cleary, T.J., and Cochi, S.L. (1993). Fatal respiratory disease due to *Corynebacterium diphtheriae*: case report and review of guidelines for management, investigation and control. *Clinical Infectious Diseases*, **16**, 59–68.

Wilson, S.A.K. (1954). Diphtheria. In *Neurology*, Vol. 11. Butterworth, London.

Chapter 16.38

Streptococci and enterococci

S. J. Eykyn

Classification

No single system of classification is ideal for streptococci; they are a heterogeneous group of organisms. Classification relies on several features including the degree of haemolysis on blood agar (usually α-haemolytic with green discoloration or β-haemolytic with lysis of the erythrocytes), Lancefield group antigen, growth characteristics, biochemical reactions, and, latterly, genetic analysis. Most Lancefield group D streptococci have now been assigned to a new genus, *Enterococcus*. The streptococci can conveniently be divided into the pyogenic streptococci, most of which are β-haemolytic on blood agar, and the oral streptococci, many of which are α-haemolytic on blood agar. *Streptococcus bovis* is neither a pyogenic nor an oral streptococcus and, although it bears the group D antigen and is found in the normal gut flora, it is much more antibiotic-sensitive than the enterococci and is most readily considered with the oral streptococci. The pyogenic streptococci include the major human pathogen *S. pyogenes* (Group A), group B streptococci (*S. agalactiae*), group C streptococci, group G streptococci, and the *S. milleri* group. They also include *S. pneumoniae* (see Chapter). The oral streptococci have undergone considerable taxonomic upheaval and include the *S. sanguis* group, the

S. oralis group, *S. mutans,* and *S. salivarius* as well as the newly-designated, nutritionally-exacting strains (*S. adjacens* and *S. defectivus*). The enterococci include *E. faecalis* and *E. faecium.*

The pyogenic streptococci

Streptococcus pyogenes (β-haemolytic group A)

This organism is one of the most important human pathogens. In addition to causing a wide range of infections, most commonly acute pharyngitis ('strep throat') and skin infections (pyoderma/ impetigo), it is also associated with the non-suppurative sequelae of acute rheumatic fever and acute glomerulonephritis (see Chapter 12.11). Since the mid to late 1980s there has been an increase in severe *S. pyogenes* infection with shock, bacteraemia, necrotizing fasciitis, and myositis, often in otherwise healthy people. Such cases have been reported not only in the UK but from most of the developed world. *S. pyogenes* infection is usually community-acquired but may also be acquired in hospital, when the most serious infections are post-operative.

Carriage

Although *S. pyogenes* is an invasive organism, it lives on epithelial surfaces (asymptomatic carriage), usually in the nose and throat; carriage can also be anal, vaginal, and on the scalp. Pharyngeal carriage rates are much higher in children (5–15 per cent) than adults (0.5 per cent) and also vary with season, year, and geographical location; they are higher in crowded living conditions. *S. pyogenes* can persist for months after acute pharyngitis though with decreased numbers of organisms. Survival in the environment is poor and *S. pyogenes* can only survive on skin squames and dust for a limited period and in low numbers.

Pathogenicity, virulence, and typing

S. pyogenes is an extracellular pathogen and produces a wide range of virulence factors that enable it to avoid host defences and help it to spread in tissues. The main virulence factor is the M protein and organisms rich in M protein resist phagocytosis by polymorphs. Immunity to *S. pyogenes* infection is associated with the development of opsonic antibodies to antiphagocytic epitopes of M protein; it is usually type specific and lasts for many years, perhaps indefinitely. M protein was first described in the 1920s by Rebecca Lancefield, and the M serotyping system has since differentiated over 100 M types. Lancefield also developed the supplementary T typing system which distinguishes 26 serotypes of a trypsin-resistant surface protein (T antigen), most of which can be expressed by several different M types. Certain M types also produce a serum opacity factor (OF+). These typing systems are still widely used in epidemiological studies to distinguish between strains of *S. pyogenes.* Recent studies have shown considerable genetic diversity in *S. pyogenes,* and horizontal transfer and recombination of virulent genes have played a major role in this. This finding is likely to be relevant to the emergence of new, unusually virulent clones of the organism.

In addition to M protein, lipoteichoic acid, important in the host–bacterial interaction, is expressed on the surface of the organism and is the adhesin that binds the organism to fibronectin on the surface of the oral epithelial cell membranes and initiates the colonization that precedes infection. *S. pyogenes* has a hylauronate capsule which, like M protein, is antiphagocytic, and is an additional virulence factor. The extent of encapsulation varies and colonies with prominent capsules are very mucoid on blood agar. Strains of *S. pyogenes* that are both rich in M protein and heavily encapsulated are readily transmitted from person to person, and tend to produce severe infections.

S. pyogenes produces many extracellular substances, several of which are important in the pathogenesis of infection. The most familiar are streptolysin O, deoxyribonuclease (DNase) B, and hyaluronidase, as serum antibodies to these provide retrospective confirmation of recent streptococcal infection. Other extracellular products include DNases A, C, and D, streptolysin S, proteinase, streptokinase, and the substances previously known as erythrogenic toxins. These toxins have now been designated streptococcal pyrogenic exotoxins (SPE) A, B, C, and possibly D. SPE-A, and possibly others, is coded by a phage gene. These toxins, known as superantigens, have diverse effects on the host. In addition to the rash of scarlet fever, they cause fever, changes in the blood–brain barrier, organ damage, and lethal shock in animals. They have profound effects on the immune system including increasing susceptibility to endotoxic shock, blockade of the reticuloendothelial system, and alterations in T-cell function.

When *S. pyogenes* enters the body, either through the upper respiratory tract mucosa or a break in the skin, a local lesion may occur or there may be spread along tissue planes or lymphatics. The M protein is not toxic in itself but protects the streptococcus from phagocytosis and antibodies to the M protein are opsonic. In some two-thirds of patients with serious invasive disease, who may present with fever, shock, and renal impairment, the portal of entry is the skin and infection of soft tissue is apparent, but in others the site of infection may not be evident.

Infections caused by *S. pyogenes*

S. pyogenes causes a variety of illnesses ranging from very common, usually mild conditions such as pharyngitis and impetigo to less common, very severe infections such as necrotizing fasciitis, bacteraemia, and toxic shock.

Streptococcal pharyngitis

Streptococcal pharyngitis or tonsillitis is one of the commonest bacterial infections in children from 5–15 years, but all ages are susceptible. The incubation period, at least in outbreaks, is short (1–3 days) and the onset of the infection is marked by the abrupt onset of sore throat and pain on swallowing with malaise, fever, and headache. There is redness and oedema of the pharynx and enlarged red tonsils with spots of white exudate and enlarged tender anterior cervical lymph glands. Nausea, vomiting, and abdominal pain are common in children. In infants and preschool children there may be few definite signs of pharyngitis but fever, nasal discharge, enlarged cervical lymph glands, and otitis media occur.

Suppurative complications Direct extension of streptococcal pharyngitis can give rise to acute sinusitis or otitis media and other suppurative complications include peritonsillar abscess (quinsy) and retropharyngeal abscess, which often contain oral flora including anaerobes with or without *S. pyogenes,* and suppurative cervical lymphadenitis.

Scarlet fever

Scarlet fever results from infection with a strain of *S. pyogenes* that produces SPE (erythrogenic toxin). It is usually associated with streptococcal pharyngitis but may follow streptococcal infections at other sites and occurs with invasive disease. Scarlet fever rarely follows streptococcal pyoderma. Most cases occur in school-age children and the rash must be distinguished from viral exanthems, Kawasaki disease, and staphylococcal toxic shock syndrome. The rash, which generally appears on the second day of clinical illness, is usually a diffuse erythema, symmetrical, and blanches on pressure. It is seen most often on the neck, chest, folds of the axilla, and groin. Occlusion of sweat glands gives the skin a 'sandpaper' texture, a useful sign in dark-skinned patients. The face appears flushed with circumoral pallor. There are small, red, haemorrhagic spots on the plate and the tongue is initially covered with a white fur through which red papillae appear ('strawberry tongue') and then, usually after the rash develops, the white furs peels off leaving a raw red papillate surface ('raspberry tongue'). The rash persists for several days and later (up to 3 weeks) peeling may occur, usually on the tips of the fingers, toes or ears, and, less often, over the trunk and limbs.

Streptococcal perianal infection

This is a superficial, well-demarcated rash spreading out from the anus in young children, usually boys, associated with itching, rectal pain on defaecation, and blood-stained stools. *S. pyogenes* is isolated from perianal cultures and usually also from pretreatment throat swabs.

Streptococcal vulvovaginitis

Vulvovaginitis in prepubertal girls is often caused by *S. pyogenes* and presents with serosanguinous discharge and erythema of the labia and vaginal orifice. As with perianal infections, *S. pyogenes* is usually also found in the throat.

Streptococcal skin and soft tissue infections

Pyoderma/ impetigo Almost any purulent lesion of the skin can yield *S. pyogenes*, sometimes with *Staphylococcus aureus*. Such lesions include impetigo, infected cuts and lacerations, insect bites, scabies, intertrigo, and ecthyma. *S. pyogenes* also often causes secondary infection in varicella, occasionally with resultant bacteraemia. The term pyoderma is used synonymously with impetigo for discrete, purulent, apparently primary infections of the skin that are prevalent in many parts of the world, especially in children. These lesions are initially papules, then vesicular with surrounding erythema, and finally pustules with crusting exudate; they may be localized to one part of the body or generalized. Outbreaks of impetigo can occur amongst adults subject to skin trauma such as rugger players (scrumpox) and streptococcal infection of cuts on the hands and forearms are an occupational hazard for workers in the meat trade. Ecthyma is an ulcerated form of impetigo in which ulceration extends into the dermis.

Invasive streptococcal infections of skin and soft tissues

Erysipelas This is an acute inflammation of the skin with lymphatic involvement. The streptococci are localized in the dermis and hypodermis. It usually affects the face, particularly in the elderly. There is usually a history of sore throat but the mode of spread to the skin is unknown. Erysipelas may also affect the limbs or trunk, generally at the site of a surgical incision or wound. It is usually accompanied by fever, rigors, and toxicity. The cutaneous lesion begins as a localized area of erythema and swelling and then spreads with rapidly advancing raised red margins that are well-demarcated from adjacent normal tissue. Facial erysipelas begins over the bridge of the nose and spreads over the cheeks (Plate 1). Vesicles and bullae appear which become crusted when they rupture. There is marked oedema and the eyes are often closed. When the infection resolves it is often followed by desquamation.

Streptococcal cellulitis This is an acute, spreading inflammation of the skin and subcutaneous tissues with local pain, swelling, and erythema (Plate 2). There may be fever, rigors, and malaise and associated lymphangitis. Streptococcal cellulitis differs from erysipelas in that the lesion is not raised and the demarcation between affected and unaffected skin is indistinct. It may result from infection of burns, wounds, or surgical incisions and follow mild trauma. Lymphoedema predisposes to streptococcal cellulitis and when this involves the leg often results from fungal infection of the feet. Intravenous drug users are also at risk of streptococcal cellulitis associated with skin and tissue infection and septic thrombophlebitis.

Necrotizing fasciitis (streptococcal gangrene) This infection, described by Meleney in 1924, involves the deep subcutaneous tissues and fascia (and occasionally muscle as well) with extensive, rapidly-spreading necrosis and gangrene of the skin and underlying structures. It is generally community-acquired, usually involving the arm or leg, though it may also occur postoperatively. The infection begins at the site of trivial or even inapparent trauma with redness, swelling, fever, and pain followed by purple discoloration and the development of bullae, often haemorrhagic. Bacteraemia is often present and about a week after onset, skin necrosis occurs followed by extensive sloughing. The patient is profoundly ill and the disease has a high mortality rate. The UK media memorably dubbed *S. pyogenes* the 'flesh eater' in reports of a cluster of cases of necrotizing fasciitis in 1994.

Streptococcal toxic shock syndrome

This syndrome was described in 1987 in patients with severe *S. pyogenes* infections and clinical features remarkably similar to those of the staphylococcal toxic shock syndrome described a decade earlier. Neither are likely to be new diseases. Definitions of streptococcal toxic shock syndrome (STSS) vary. Some limit the definition to cases of shock and multiorgan failure where there is a rash or desquamation whilst others include all cases of shock and its non-specific sequelae, such as coagulopathy, uraemia, or jaundice, irrespective of skin lesions. STSS is usually associated with necrotizing fasciitis or myositis. It can occur at all ages and many of those affected are young and previously healthy. Most cases have been community-acquired though it can be acquired in hospital. M1 has been the predominant serotype in many countries though others, especially 2, 3, 12, and 28 have also been implicated. Most strains produce SPE-A. Interestingly, there is an amino acid homology of 50 per cent and immunological cross-reactivity between SPE-A and staphylococcal enterotoxins B and C, which together with staphylococcal TSS toxin-1 are relevant in non-menstrual staphylococcal TSS.

Streptococcal bacteraemia

In parallel with the increase in serious *S. pyogenes* infections, there has been an increase in bacteraemic infections, both community- and hospital-acquired (usually postoperative) (Plate 3). Whilst many patients have an underlying disease, most often malignancy and immunosuppression or diabetes, others are previously healthy adults between 20 and 50 years. The portal of entry is usually the skin. The mortality is higher in patients with underlying disease.

Other streptococcal infections

Puerperal sepsis Historically, *S. pyogenes* has always been an important cause of 'childbed fever', but in the post-antibiotic era it was rarely encountered in obstetric practice until the mid 1980s when sporadic cases have occurred, some with STSS, and some women have died. These infections follow abortion or delivery when streptococci (usually colonizing the patient herself) invade the endometrium, lymphatics, and bloodstream. They can be devastatingly severe and present with non-specific signs such as restlessness and gastrointestinal upset that may not immediately suggest sepsis. Fever may be absent, resulting in further diagnostic confusion.

Other infections *S. pyogenes* can, though rarely does, cause pneumonia (usually associated with viral infection or pulmonary disease), osteomyelitis, septic arthritis, meningitis, pericarditis (Plate 4), and endocarditis.

Laboratory diagnosis of *S. pyogenes* infection

S. pyogenes is easy to culture in the laboratory and usually grows on blood agar in 24 h. Throat swabs must be taken before antibiotics are given or the chance of recovery is slim. Kits for the detection of the group A antigen directly from throat swabs are available and give few false positive reactions but they are seldom used in the UK. Even trivial skin lesions are worth swabbing (if necessary with a moistened swab) and a search for such lesions often pays dividends. Swabs from the surface of cellulitis and erysipelas seldom yield streptococci, but they may be recovered from specimens obtained by aspiration. Blood cultures should be done in any patient who is ill whether febrile or not. Serological confirmation of infection with *S. pyogenes* when the organism has not been isolated can be obtained by the detection of raised antibodies to its extracellular products. Most laboratories tend to use two or more tests. Interpretation requires knowledge of the level of titres in the community for those without a history of recent streptococcal infection. In the UK, the upper limit of titres in teenagers and young adults without such a history is antistreptolysin O (ASO) 200, antideoxyribonuclease B (ADB) 240, and antihyaluronidase (AHT) 128.

Management and antibiotic treatment of *S. pyogenes* infection

Remarkably, *S. pyogenes* remains exquisitely sensitive to penicillin, which is the antibiotic of choice for treatment, parenterally for severe infections and orally otherwise. Conventionally, 10 days treatment is recommended for pharyngeal infections to eradicate the organism and prevent acute rheumatic fever. In practice, compliance with this regimen is poor as once the symptoms abate there is a natural reluctance to continue the antibiotic. Treatment of penicillin-allergic patients is most often with erythromycin or the newer macrolides (azithromycin and clarithromycin) but some 3–5 per cent of strains are erythromycin resistant. *S. pyogenes* is also sensitive to cephalosporins. Topical agents such as mupirocin and fusidic acid are useful in addition to systemic antibiotic treatment in impetigo and other skin lesions. Patients with STSS will need intensive care and many require inotropic support, ventilation, and haemodialysis. Urgent surgical intervention is needed for necrotizing fasciitis and myositis. Clindamycin (in addition to penicillin) has been recommended for patients with established, invasive infections since this drug stops the metabolic activity of the streptococci and thus halts further production of toxin. Intravenous immunoglobulin has also been used in an attempt to neutralize the streptococcal toxins but reports of its effects are inconclusive. Lastly, it should be remembered that *S. pyogenes* is readily transmitted from person to person and thus appropriate infection control precautions should be taken until swabs show the organism has been eradicated.

β-Haemolytic groups C and G streptococci

These streptococci are most conveniently regarded as 'pyogenes like' as the infections they cause are similar to those caused by *S. pyogenes*, though groups C and G streptococci tend to be less virulent. They must be distinguished from small colony streptococci of the *S. milleri* group (see below) that can bear the same Lancefield antigens. Infections with these streptococci are less common than *S. pyogenes* infections. Although poststreptococcal glomerulonephritis has been associated with pharyngitis caused by both groups C and G streptococci, acute rheumatic fever has not.

Group C streptococci are less frequently encountered in human infections than group G. Most infections are caused by *S. equisimilis* and those caused by *S. zooepidemicus* have an animal source. Group G streptococci are frequently isolated from leg ulcers and pressure sores, usually with other bacteria. In such patients, cellulitis and systemic upset are very rare and the organisms are just colonizing the lesions. They, like *S. pyogenes*, can cause cellulitis in lymphoedematous limbs.

β-Haemolytic group B streptococci (*S. agalactiae*)

The group B streptococci have been known for over a century as a cause of bovine mastitis and in the 1930s they were recognized as a vaginal commensal, an occasional cause of puerperal fever, and an uncommon cause of invasive disease in adults. Not until the 1960s was it realized that group B streptococci were important neonatal pathogens, and they later replaced *Escherichia coli* as the predominant neonatal pathogens.

Carriage

Group B streptococci can be recovered from various sites in healthy adults but vaginal carriage has been most extensively investigated. Swabs from the lower vagina are more often positive than cervical swabs and carriage rates of 3 to over 40 per cent have been reported. Higher rates have been obtained with selective media and enrichment techniques. Carriage also increases with sexual activity and is highest in women attending genitourinary clinics. The urethra, vagina, perineum, and anorectal region have all been suggested as the prime site of carriage. Some 5–10 per cent of normal adults carry group B streptococci in the throat and this is independent of urogenital and anorectal carriage.

Pathogenicity, virulence, and typing

The chief determinant of virulence appears to be the capsular polysaccharide, and most human strains carry one or other of six sialic acid-containing polysaccharides that surround the cell wall. In addition, a protein antigen (c, X, or R) may be carried. Certain combinations are common; serotypes III or III/R form one-quarter of all isolates from superficial sites on women but three-quarters of all group B streptococci causing meningitis in infants. They are also the commonest serotypes found in adult (non-pregnant) infections. The type polysaccharide, like the M protein of *S. pyogenes*, inhibits phagocytosis. Colonization of the mucous membranes of the neonate results from vertical transmission of the organism from the mother either *in utero* by the ascending route or at delivery. The rate of vertical transmission in neonates born to mothers colonized with group B streptococci is about 50 per cent, but the incidence of symptomatic infection in neonates born to colonized mothers is only about 1–2 per cent. It is much higher in preterm infants. Nosocomial colonization of neonates can also occur. In most cases of adult infections (other than in pregnant women) the source of the infection is unknown.

Infections caused by group B streptococci

The main infections caused by group B streptococci are those in the neonate, puerperal infections, and infections in the non-pregnant adult.

Neonatal infection

The frequency of neonatal infection (bacteraemia, meningitis, or both) has been variously quoted as between 0.3 and 5.4 cases/ 1000 live births but these figures have wide confidence limits. Two fairly distinct clinical patterns of disease predominate but the spectrum is wide, and includes impetigo neonatorum, septic arthritis, osteomyelitis, peritonitis, pyelonephritis, facial cellulitis, conjunctivitis, and endophthalmitis.

Early-onset disease Symptoms develop within the first 5 days of life with a mean of 20 h, though they can present at birth suggesting an intrauterine onset of infection. Early-onset disease is most often a bacteraemia with no identifiable focus of infection, but can also be pneumonia or, infrequently, meningitis. The presenting signs include lethargy, poor feeding, jaundice, grunting respirations, pallor, and hypotension and they are common to all types of disease. Respiratory symptoms are nearly always present. The only reliable way of detecting meningitis is by lumbar puncture. Mortality rates are high in low birth weight babies. In addition to positive blood cultures, the infecting strain can be found in the mother's vagina and at 'screening' sites on the baby; these include ear, throat, and nasogastric aspirate.

Late-onset disease This usually presents between 7 days and 3 months after birth, often in previously healthy babies, born after a normal labour who are then readmitted unwell from home. The pathogenesis is less clear than for early-onset disease and only about half the cases are associated with mucosal colonization during delivery. Most babies have meningitis and concomitant bacteraemia and present with non-specific symptoms such as lethargy, poor feeding, irritability, and fever. Neurological sequelae are common among survivors.

Puerperal infection

The commonest infections with Group B streptococci in adults occur in women within 24–48 h of delivery or abortion. The source of the organism is always the vagina and infection is more likely when there has been premature rupture of the membranes and chorioamnionitis. Most infections are endometritis with fever and uterine tenderness and infected postcaesarean section wounds, but they also occur in association with retained products of conception. Bacteraemia is common. Other bacteria, both aerobes and anaerobes, are sometimes isolated from the genital tract and wounds in addition to the group B streptococcus. Very rarely the streptococcus may spread to other sites in puerperal women.

Infections in non-pregnant adults

The prominence given to group B streptococci as neonatal and puerperal pathogens has tended to overshadow their importance in non-pregnant women and men, in whom they cause significant morbidity and mortality. Most infections are community-acquired, occur in the middle-aged and elderly, and are as common in males as females. Many, though by no means all, patients with group B streptococcal infection have underlying diseases, particularly diabetes and myeloma. Skin and soft tissue infections are especially common in diabetics. Occasional urinary tract infections occur, and not only in pregnant women. Bacteraemic infections serve to emphasize the virulence of group B streptococci, and they have increased in incidence, or perhaps have been increasingly recognized, since the early 1990s. Community-acquired group B streptococcal bacteraemia is similar in many respects to that caused by *Staphylococcus aureus* since common clinical manifestations include endocarditis, vertebral osteomyelitis, septic arthritis, endophthalmitis, and meningitis. As with staphylococcal infections, some bacteraemic patients have more than one metastatic focus of infection which can lead to diagnostic confusion.

Laboratory diagnosis of group B streptococcal infection

Group B streptococci are readily isolated from any clinical specimen in the laboratory and easily identified by Lancefield grouping. The group B antigen is not shared by any other streptococcus. Importantly, the antigen can be reliably detected in fluids such as blood, urine, or CSF by latex particle agglutination, enabling a rapid diagnosis.

Treatment

Group B streptococci are sensitive to penicillin and this is the antibiotic of choice for treatment. They are rather less sensitive to penicillin than *S. pyogenes* with minimum inhibitory concentrations some four to ten fold higher. For this reason, penicillin is sometimes combined with gentamicin for meningitis though this is not of proven benefit. Certainly, the maximum recommended dose of parenteral penicillin should be given whether combined with gentamicin or not. Penicillin allergy is not likely to be an issue in neonates; adults with meningitis can be treated with chloramphenicol. Most group B streptococci are sensitive to erythromycin and they are sensitive to cephalosporins.

Prevention of neonatal infection with group B streptococci

This is clearly a laudable objective but it is not easy to achieve. Vaginal carriage of group B streptococci during pregnancy cannot be eradicated with oral antibiotics and eradication is not worth attempting. However, chemoprophylaxis at delivery is indicated for carriers, particularly those with ruptured membranes and premature labour. In the UK at least, it is rare for labour ward staff to be aware of results of previous vaginal swabs.

S. milleri group

This heterogeneous group of streptococci has finally been allocated to three species, *S. anginosus*, *S. constellatus*, and *S. intermedius*, but, despite increasing awareness of the clinical significance of the *S. milleri* group, little is known about the association between individual species and specific sites of isolation and diseases. *S. milleri* is found in large numbers in the upper respiratory tract, gastrointestinal tract, and genital tract, and the organisms are commonly isolated from a range of pyogenic infections, sometimes in pure culture, but often with other organisms, particularly anaerobes. These infections include dental abscesses, intra-abdominal abscesses (especially liver abscesses), subphrenic abscesses, lung abscesses, and empyema and brain abscesses. Such is the propensity of these organisms to cause deep-seated abscesses that isolation of *S. milleri* from a blood culture should prompt investigations to detect such a focus. *S. milleri* is also commonly isolated from inflamed appendices and from post-appendicectomy wound infection. Unlike other viridans and non-haemolytic streptococci, *S. milleri* seldom causes endocarditis. Some *S. milleri* have Lancefield antigens A, C, G, and F. All group F streptococci are *S. milleri* whereas not all *S. milleri* are group F. Another useful clue to their identity in the laboratory is the distinct caramel smell of many strains on blood agar, the result of the diacetyl metabolite. Most strains are very sensitive to penicillin.

The oral (viridans) streptococci and *S. bovis*

These streptococci are the largest single group of bacteria causing infective endocarditis. *S. sanguis* and *S. oralis* are the species most commonly associated with endocarditis of oral or dental origin. *S. bovis* is similar to the enterococci (and may be misidentified as an enterococcus) in that it is a bowel (rather than a mouth) commensal and bears the Lancefield group D antigen, but, unlike the enterococci, it is sensitive to penicillin. *S. bovis* bacteraemia and endocarditis is often associated with colonic malignancy, and patients should be specifically investigated for this. These organisms are considered in more detail in Chapter 2.25.

The nutrientally variant streptococci

These streptococci, which occasionally cause endocarditis, require pyridoxal or thiol group supplementation for growth in the laboratory and tend to form satellite colonies round *S. aureus*. Although most blood culture media will support their growth, successful subculture will require supplementation or cross-streaking of the plates with *S. aureus* to provide the necessary growth factors. The nutrientally variant streptococci have been divided into two species, *S. adjacens* and *S. defectivus*. They are less susceptible to penicillin than other streptococci.

The enterococci

Most clinical isolates of enterococci are *E. faecalis*, but *E. faecium* is increasingly encountered in some specialist hospital units. Other species, including *E. casseliflavus*, *E. durans*, and *E. avium*, are occasionally isolated from clinical specimens. Enterococci can grow and survive in extreme cultural conditions, and are also more resistant to antibiotics than streptococci. They form part of the normal gut flora of man and animals.

Infections caused by enterococci

Enterococci are an increasingly important cause of nosocomial infections (and colonization), possibly the result of the large-scale use of antibiotics such as cephalosporins to which they are inherently resistant. They occasionally cause community-acquired urinary tract infections but the most important community-acquired infection is endocarditis, which is increasing in incidence (see Chapter 2.25). They are predominantly hospital pathogens and cause urinary infection, particularly after instrumentation, intra-abdominal infections, and wound infections (usually with other organisms) and infections associated with intravascular devices and dialysis. They present a cross infection risk and have caused outbreaks in specialist units.

Antibiotic sensitivity and treatment

Enterococci are not only intrinsically resistant to many antibiotics, they show a remarkable ability to acquire new mechanisms of resistance with important therapeutic consequences, particularly for the treatment of endocarditis and other serious infections. Fortunately, many patients from whom enterococci are isolated do not require antibiotic treatment. Even sensitive enterococci cannot be killed by ampicillin/amoxicillin alone, though combination with an aminoglycoside is bactericidal (synergy). Some strains now exhibit high-level gentamicin resistance and for these the combination of ampicillin/amoxicillin plus gentamicin is not bactericidal. Enterococci, particularly *E. faecium*, may be resistant to ampicillin/amoxicillin and in the late 1980s vancomycin resistant enterococci (VRE) were described, and some VREs are also resistant to teicoplanin. Treatment of serious infection caused by a multiresistant enterococcus is a daunting exercise and requires not only considerable laboratory expertise but sometimes also the use of new, unlicensed agents.

Further reading

Bisno, A.L. (1995). *Streptococcus pyogenes*. In *Principles and practice of infectious diseases* (ed. G.L.Mandell, J.E.Bennett, and R.Dolin), pp. 1786–99. Churchill Livingstone, New York.

Colman, G., Tanna, A., Efstratiou, A., and Gaworzewska, E.T. (1993). The serotypes of *Streptococcus pyogenes* present in Britain during 1980–1990 and their association with disease. *Journal of Medical Microbiology*, **39**, 165–78.

Edwards, M.S. and Baker, C.J. (1995). *Streptococcus agalactiae* (Group B streptococcus). In *Principles and practice of infectious diseases* (ed. G.L. Mandell, J.E.Bennett, and R.Dolin), pp 1835–45. Churchill Livingstone, New York.

Jacobs, J.A. (1997). The '*Streptococcus milleri*' group: *Streptococcus anginosus*, *Streptococcus constellatus* and *Streptococcus intermedius*. *Reviews in Medical Microbiology*, **8**, 73–80.

Katz, A.R. and Morens, D. (1992). Severe streptococcal infections in historical perspective. *Clinical Infectious Diseases*, **14**, 298–307.

Murray, B.E. (1990). The life and times of the *Enterococcus*. *Clinical Microbiological Reviews*, **3**, 46–65.

Stevens, D.L. (1992). Invasive Group A streptococcus infections. *Clinical Infectious Diseases*, **14**, 2–13.

Chapter 16.39

Pneumococcal infection

B. M. Greenwood

The organism

When grown on blood agar, *Streptococcus pneumoniae* (the 'pneumococcus') produces small, shiny colonies of Gram-positive bacteria, surrounded by a greenish area of α-haemolysis. Pneumococci differ from other α-haemolytic streptococci by their solubility in bile and sensitivity to ethyl hydrocuprein chloride (optochin).Virulent strains possess a polysaccharide capsule. About 90 structurally different capsular polysaccharides have been identified and these form the basis for a pneumococcal typing system. Pneumococcal surface protein A (PspA), pneumolysin, and a 37-kDa antigen are proteins of interest for vaccine development. Until 25 years ago, nearly all pneumococci were sensitive to penicillin. However, pneumococci that are resistant to penicillin (MIC >1.0 g) have now been isolated in many parts of the world, especially in Spain and parts of eastern Europe. They are still relatively infrequent in the UK and the US (<5 per cent of isolates) but clustering of resistant isolates has been found. Penicillin resistance is probably acquired in a step-wise fashion as a result of several mutations and is associated with changes in the penicillin-binding proteins 1 and 2.

Epidemiology

Incidence of pneumococcal infection

Four to five million children die from acute respiratory infections each year, over 90 per cent in the developing world. At least a million

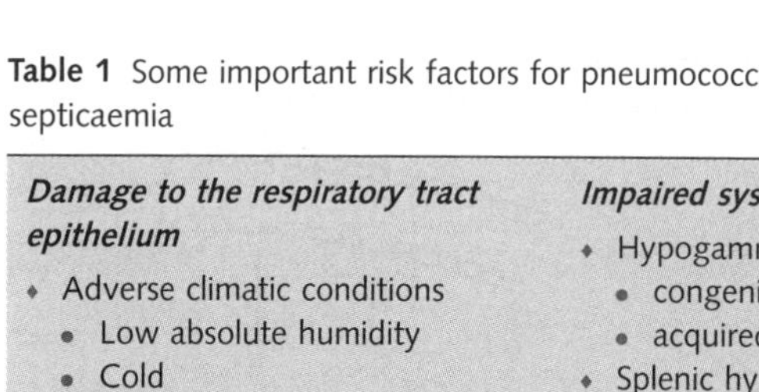

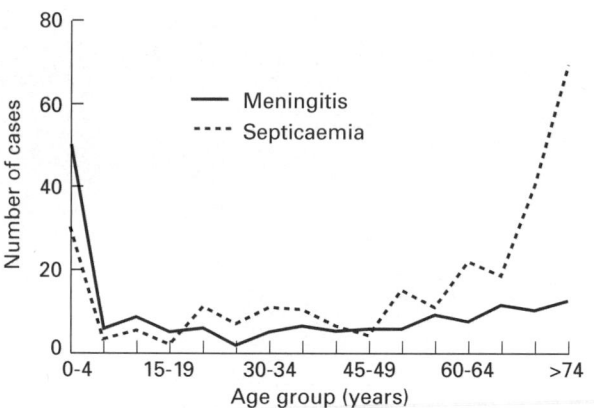

Fig. 1 The age distribution of cases of pneumococcal meningitis and pneumococcal septicaemia in the Netherlands, 1990.
(Annual report, Netherlands Reference Laboratory for Bacterial Meningitis.)

of these are attributable to pneumococci. In industrialized countries, the pneumococcus is the most frequent cause of community-acquired pneumonia. Between 150 000 and 500 000 cases of pneumococcal pneumonia occur in the US each year, with 10 000–25 000 deaths. About 20 per cent of American children experience at least one attack of pneumococcal otitis media during the first few years of life. Pneumococcal disease is global in distribution, being most prevalent in communities where crowding and poor living conditions prevail.

Seasonality

In temperate climates, pneumococcal pneumonia, like other respiratory tract infections, occurs more frequently in winter than in summer.

Age and sex distribution of cases

In industrialized countries, pneumococcal infections are seen mainly in the very young and in the old (Fig. 1). In developing countries, the incidence of pneumococcal pneumonia and meningitis peaks during the first 2 years of life but invasive pneumococcal disease is seen more frequently in older children and in young adults than in industrialized societies.

Predisposing factors

Diabetes, congestive cardiac failure, nephrotic syndrome, HIV, alcoholism, and drug addiction predispose to invasive pneumococcal infections (Table 1). Patients with congenital or acquired hypogammaglobulinaemia and with no functioning spleen (e.g. sickle cell disease) are more vulnerable.

Pathogenesis and immunity

Spread of infection

Pneumococci spread by droplet infection. In industrialized societies, around 25–50 per cent of healthy subjects carry pneumococci in their nasopharynx as do nearly 100 per cent of children in developing countries. Local spread of pneumococci from the nasopharynx may cause otitis media and its complications (Fig. 2). Most cases of pneumococcal pneumonia result from aspiration of nasopharyngeal secretions containing pneumococci into alveoli; blood-borne spread from the nasopharynx is also possible. Pneumococci may spread directly from the lung to adjacent pleura or pericardium and through

Table 1 Some important risk factors for pneumococcal pneumonia and septicaemia

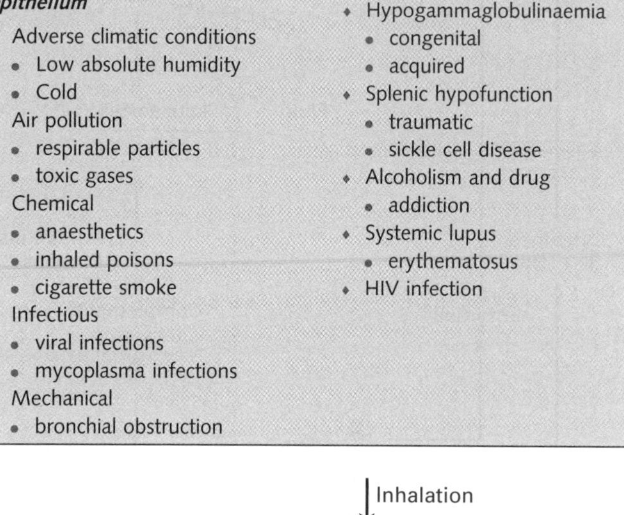

Damage to the respiratory tract epithelium	*Impaired systemic immunity*
• Adverse climatic conditions	• Hypogammaglobulinaemia
• Low absolute humidity	• congenital
• Cold	• acquired
• Air pollution	• Splenic hypofunction
• respirable particles	• traumatic
• toxic gases	• sickle cell disease
• Chemical	• Alcoholism and drug
• anaesthetics	• addiction
• inhaled poisons	• Systemic lupus
• cigarette smoke	• erythematosus
• Infectious	• HIV infection
• viral infections	
• mycoplasma infections	
• Mechanical	
• bronchial obstruction	

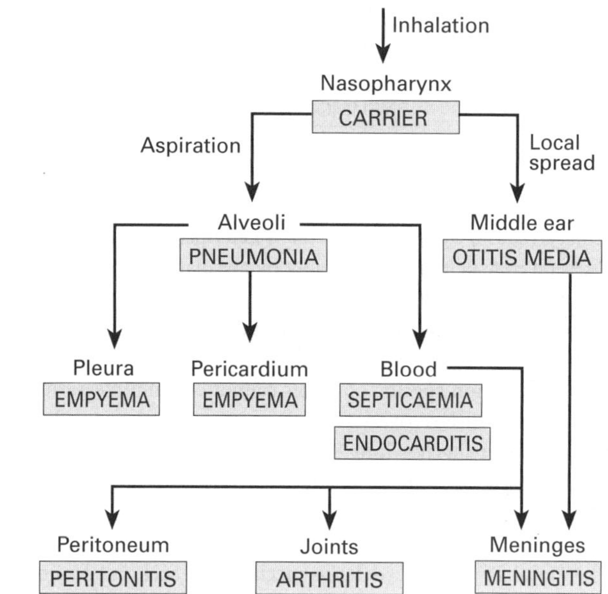

Fig. 2 The pathway of pneumococcal infection.

the systemic circulation to reach the meninges, joints, eyes, or other distant sites.

Pathogenesis

Pneumococci produce an acute inflammatory reaction characterized by an increase in vascular permeability, oedema, and an accumulation of polymorphonuclear neutrophil leucocytes at the affected site (Fig. 3). Pneumococcal cell wall components, especially techoic acid and peptidoglycan, stimulate the production by mononuclear cells of the cytokines IL-1 and TNF which upregulate endothelial receptors such as ICAM-1. Some pneumococcal capsular polysaccharides activate the alternative complement pathway with production of C3a and C5a which are chemotactic for neutrophils.

Immunity

Both local and systemic defence mechanisms are involved in protection against pneumococcal disease. Pneumococci are prevented from reaching the alveoli by the epiglottis, the sticky mucus that lines the

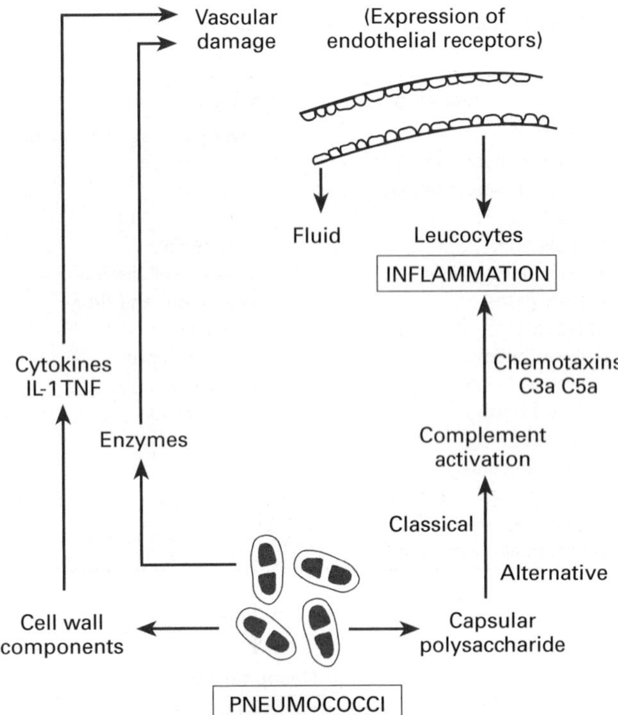

Fig. 3 The pathogenesis of pneumococcal infection.

bronchial tree, and by respiratory cilia. Pneumococci that manage to reach alveoli may be destroyed rapidly by alveolar macrophages. The small amounts of antibody and complement present in alveolar secretions may facilitate phagocytosis. Neutrophils are brought to the site of infection in large numbers and attempt to ingest pneumococci. Neutrophils and non-specific opsonins cannot contain infection with some virulent strains; recovery from these infections can be achieved only if the patient survives long enough to form specific anticapsular antibodies which agglutinate pneumococci and which are powerful opsonins.

Vulnerability to pneumococcal infection may result from defects in either local or systemic defence mechanisms such as alcoholism and asplenia (Table 1).

Pathology

Initially, there is an exudation of oedema fluid which helps to carry bacteria into adjacent parts of the lung. Neutrophils and erythrocytes then accumulate in affected alveoli. Finally, the affected part of the lung becomes consolidated with a dense accumulation of leucocytes. A consolidated lobe can recover completely, but invasion of pleura or pericardium frequently results in the formation of pus and subsequent fibrous scaring may result in constrictive pericarditis.

Clinical features

Pneumonia

Symptoms

Typically, the illness starts suddenly, although there may be a history of a recent upper respiratory tract infection. Fever is usually the first symptom, frequently accompanied by rigors. The patient feels ill, anorexic, and weak. Headache and myalgia may be severe.

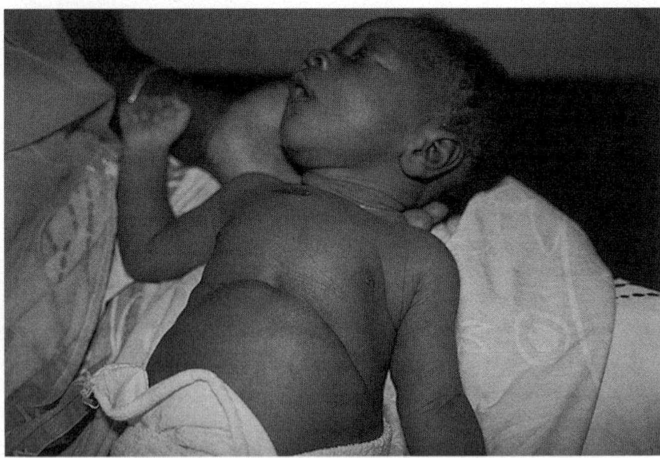

Fig. 4 Severe lower chest in-drawing in a child with pneumococcal pneumonia
(by courtesy of Dr Alice Greenwood).

Pleuritic chest pain usually appears in the course of illness. The patient may try to obtain relief by splinting the affected side of his chest with his hands or lying on the affected side. If the diaphragmatic pleura is involved, pain may be referred to the shoulder or to the abdomen.

Cough may be absent at the onset of the illness but it becomes a prominent symptom in most patients. Initially non-productive and painful, it becomes productive of a blood-tinged 'rusty' sputum. Finally, the sputum becomes frankly purulent.

In young children and the elderly, pneumococcal pneumonia may present less dramatically. The mothers of young children with pneumonia usually mention fever, cough, and rapid respiration. Old patients and the immunocompromised may have little or no fever and few respiratory symptoms. Prior antibiotic treatment can modify the symptoms.

Physical signs

Adult patients with lobar pneumonia are usually febrile and toxaemic. At first, no abnormal physical signs may be detected in the respiratory system. Later the classical signs of lobar consolidation may appear. The patient's breathing becomes rapid and distressed and the nostrils may dilate on inspiration. Cyanosis may be present. On the affected side, chest movements are diminished and there are signs of consolidation, fine crepitations, and a pleural rub. Tachycardia is usual. The abdomen may be distended or, if the diaphragmatic pleura is involved, there may be upper abdominal tenderness and guarding. Jaundice may be present. The patient, especially if elderly, may be confused.

Lobar consolidation is found infrequently in infants with pneumococcal pneumonia although some auscultatory abnormalities, such as crepitations, can usually be detected. In young children, the most prominent features of pneumococcal pneumonia are usually a raised respiratory rate, chest wall indrawing (Fig. 4), and nasal flaring.

Laboratory findings

A neutrophil leucocytosis is usually present; a low white cell count carries a poor prognosis. In jaundiced patients, conjugated and unconjugated bilirubin levels are raised and serum aminotransferases may be elevated. The PO_2 is often diminished; the PCO_2 is normal except in terminal respiratory failure.

Table 2 WHO criteria for the diagnosis of pneumonia in young children who present with cough or difficulty in breathing

Cough or difficulty with breathing plus Rapid respiration/in-drawing
< 2 months > 60 per min
2–11 months > 50 per min
12–59 months > 40 per min
Pneumonia is considered to be severe if there is chest wall in-drawing and very severe if the child has cyanosis or stops feeding.

The sputum of untreated patients usually shows large numbers of Gram-positive diplococci, together with neutrophil leucocytes, and culture is frequently positive for pneumococci. Blood culture is positive in 10–30 per cent of patients.

The chest radiograph usually shows homogeneous opacification of the affected part of the lung with a small pleural effusion in some patients. Pneumococci can cause either segmental or lobar consolidation or patchy shadowing. The latter is encountered most frequently in children. The lower lobes are affected more frequently than the upper. In about one-third of patients, more than one lobe is involved.

Differential diagnosis

The World Health Organization has devised a simple diagnostic scheme to help primary health care workers determine which children with acute respiratory tract infections probably have pneumonia and require antibiotic treatment (Table 2).

In adults, acute bacterial pneumonia may be confused with pulmonary infarction. Lower lobe pneumonia, by producing abdominal pain and guarding, may suggest an acute abdominal condition such as a perforated peptic ulcer.

Pneumococcal pneumonia can usually be differentiated from viral pneumonia or *Mycoplasma pneumoniae* pneumonias by its sudden onset, associated severe toxaemia, and neutrophil leucocytosis. Differentiation from other forms of acute bacterial pneumonia requires microbiological investigations. Confusion, signs of multisystem damage, lymphopenia, or a low serum sodium suggests legionnaire's disease (see Chapter 16.71).

Course and prognosis

Overall case fatality is about 5 per cent but it may be as high as 30 per cent in patients with bacteraemia. Mortality is highest among the old, the very young, and those with an associated underlying illness. Complications result from local, lymphatic, or bacteraemic spread.

Pleural effusion and empyema (see also Chapter 4.37)

In a small percentage of patients, pleural effusion or an empyema may develop despite treatment. Other patients present with a pleural effusion without preceding symptoms of pneumonia.

Symptoms

Fever, malaise, anorexia, and marked weight loss may have developed over days or weeks. Fever may be hectic with rigors and episodes of profuse sweating. Patients with a large pleural effusion are breathless and they may complain of dull chest pain on the affected side. A productive cough is unusual unless a bronchopleural fistula is present.

Physical signs

There is persistent fever and tachycardia. The patient may look toxaemic and there may be signs of recent weight loss. There are signs of a pleural effusion. The chest wall overlying an empyema may be tender.

Investigations

A persistent neutrophil leucocytosis is nearly always present. Radiographs or ultrasound may be very helpful in localizing a loculated effusion. On aspiration, turbid fluid or thick pus is obtained which contains pneumococci and degenerate white cells.

Differential diagnosis

Absence of copious purulent sputum differentiates an empyema from a lung abscess. Differentiation from tuberculosis may be difficult on clinical grounds alone. Diagnosis of an empyema is confirmed by the aspiration of pus from the pleural cavity. Repeated needling with a wide-bored needle, preferably under ultrasound control, may be needed to find a loculated empyema.

Course and prognosis

Empyema may rupture through the chest wall (empyema necessitatis) or rupture into a bronchus causing a bronchopleural fistula. Even when pus is aspirated and healing achieved, subsequent fibrosis and calcification may seriously restrict expansion of the underlying lung.

Pericardial effusion and empyema (see also Section 2)

Pneumococci may spread from an infected lower lobe to produce pericarditis that may be clinically silent in some patients but is, occasionally, the dominant feature of a pneumococcal infection.

Symptoms

Usually there is a history of several days, or even weeks, of persistent fever, malaise, anorexia, and weight loss. There may be dull central chest pain and swelling of the ankles or abdomen.

Physical signs

Many patients with a pneumococcal pericaridal empyema are critically ill by the time that they reach hospital. There may be signs of severe pericardial tamponade—a rapid, small volume pulse, pulsus paradoxus, a low blood pressure, elevation of the jugular venous pressure that increases an inspiration, and peripheral oedema and ascites. Percussion of the chest may show some enlargement of the area of cardiac dullness but this is an unreliable clinical sign. The heart sounds are usually faint and a pericardial rub may be heard.

Laboratory findings

A blood neutrophil leucocytosis is present. Blood culture may be positive for pneumococci. A chest radiograph may show globular enlargement of the heart, an unusually sharp cardiac outline, and evidence of an associated lung infection. Ultrasound may define the best site for drainage. Turbid fluid or thick pus may be aspirated from which pneumococci can be isolated or in which pneumococcal antigen can be detected. The electrocardiogram shows low voltage potentials and S–T elevation or depression may be present.

Differential diagnosis

Signs of pericardial tamponade in a patient who is febrile and toxaemic suggests pericardial empyema. Staphylococci and, rarely, other pyogenic bacteria can produce a similar clinical picture. Diagnosis is confirmed by ultrasound and pericardial aspiration.

Course and prognosis

This is a serious condition with a high mortality, even in treated patients. Patients who survive the initial episode may develop constrictive pericarditis within weeks or months.

Otitis media

This is probably the commonest form of pneumococcal infection. It is seen most frequently in young children.

Symptoms

The onset is sudden, although there may be a history of a recent, upper respiratory tract infection. Fever and severe pain in the ear are usual in adults and older children, associated with deafness and tinnitus. Fever, crying, extreme irritability and febrile convulsions are observed in young children.

Physical signs

The tympanic membrane is red, swollen, and bulging. If perforation has occurred, the external ear may be full of pus and a ragged hole may be seen in the tympanic membrane. The affected ear is usually partially deaf. In children meningism may be present.

Laboratory findings

A neutrophil leucocytosis is usual. If the drum has ruptured, pneumococci may be found in the purulent discharge but contaminants are likely to be present also.

Differential diagnosis

The diagnosis is not difficult provided that the ears of all febrile and irritable children are examined carefully. Specific aetiology can be established by examining fluid obtained from the middle ear with a fine needle.

Course and prognosis

Prompt treatment usually results in rapid and complete resolution of the infection. However, some patients, especially those in whom the drum has ruptured, are left with partial conductive deafness. Untreated, pneumococcal otitis media can give rise to a chronic discharging ear requiring prolonged and complicated treatment. Posterior spread may result in acute mastoiditis, upward spread in pneumococcal meningitis and/or a cerebral abscess.

Pneumococcal meningitis (see also Chapter 13.25)

This may follow damage to the base of the skull, or as a complication of pneumococcal otitis media or pneumococcal pneumonia. Many patients have no obvious primary focus infection.

Symptoms

Fever and headache is followed by nausea, backache, photophobia, and convulsions. Confusion is prominent in the elderly. Failure to feed is the first symptom in infants.

Physical signs

Patients are febrile and toxaemic with neck stiffness and a positive Kernig's sign. Consciousness is often impaired. Bradycardia and

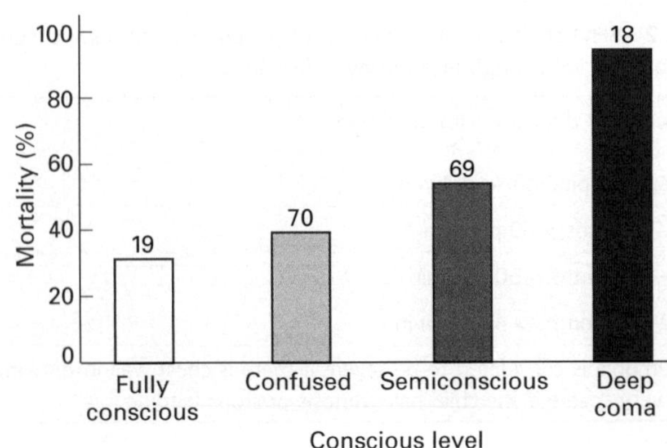

Fig. 5 Mortality from pneumococcal meningitis by conscious level at the time of presentation. Numbers of patients are shown above the bars. *(For source see OTM3, p.518.)*

hypertension may indicate raised intracranial pressure but papilloedema is rarely seen. Bulging of the anterior fontanelle may be present in infants. Cranial nerve palsies, most frequently of the sixth or third cranial nerves, may be found.

Signs of otitis media or pneumonia, may be found. Petechiae are seen occasionally. Herpes labialis may be present.

Laboratory findings

A blood neutrophil leucocytosis is usual. Blood culture may be positive. The cerebrospinal fluid (CSF) is turbid, containing cells and bacteria. CSF protein is increased and CSF glucose decreased. Gram stain and culture of CSF are usually positive.

Differential diagnosis

Problems may arise in the very young and in the very old in whom signs of meningeal irritation may be absent. The diagnosis is confirmed by examination of the CSF.

Course and prognosis

Many patients die within the first 24–48 h after their admission to hospital. Over one-half of all survivors are left with some intellectual impairment or other sequelae such as deafness or hemiplegia.

Case fatality varies from around 30 per cent in industrialized countries to over 50 per cent in the developing world. Impairment of consciousness on admission to hospital, associated pneumonia, a low CSF white cell count, and a high CSF bacterial count are poor prognostic features (Fig. 5).

Other clinical syndromes

Acute, fulminating pneumococcal septicaemia is rare. It is encountered most frequently in asplenic or immunocompromised patients. A milder form of bacteraemia is sometimes encountered in children who present with fever or febrile convulsions without any obvious focus of pneumococcal infection. Acute endocarditis may complicate pneumococcal septicaemia. Pneumococci can cause arthritis, ophthalmitis, or orchitis.

Pneumococcal peritonitis may occur in patients with the nephrotic syndrome or alcoholic cirrhosis of the liver. It has also been described in healthy young girls, perhaps as a complication of pelvic infection, and occasionally in neonates.

Pneumococci may be cultured from blood, pus, or from pleural, pericardial, peritoneal, middle ear, or cerebrospinal fluid. However, blood culture is positive in only 10–30 per cent of cases of pneumococcal pneumonia. Sputum culture is not diagnostic—pneumococci frequently occur in the upper respiratory tract of healthy individuals. Transtracheal aspiration, lung aspiration, and bronchoscopy may be employed. These relatively invasive investigations may be indicated in patients who are very ill, clinically atypical cases, and in those who have failed to respond to treatment. Per cutaneous lung aspiration gives a much higher yield of pneumococci than blood culture but may occasionally cause a small haemoptysis or a pneumothorax.

Treatment

Antibiotics

Penicillin is the first choice for proven invasive pneumococcal infections in areas of the world where the prevalence of penicillin insensitive strains is still less than 5 per cent. However, as pneumococcal meningitis is such a serious condition it is probably unwise to take even a small risk that a penicillin resistant organism is the cause of a meningeal infection and an alternative drug should be given. Where the prevalence of penicillin resistance is known to be high, alternative therapy (e.g. ceftiaxone plus vanomycin) should be given for all suspected invasive pneumococcal infections.

Patients with otitis media and pneumococcal pneumonia respond well to a 5–7-day course of treatment, patients with meningitis require treatment for 14 days, and those with empyema or endocarditis require 4–6 weeks of treatment. An effective regimen for adults with uncomplicated pneumonia is parenteral crystalline penicillin, 2 million units 6-hourly for 24 h, followed by an aminopenicillin, such as oral amoxicillin, for a further 6 days. For patients with pneumococcal meningitis, to ensure adequate CSF concentrations, crystalline penicillin should be given in an initial adult dose of 16 million units per day, administered intravenously.

Chloramphenicol can be used as an alternative in patients with penicillin-sensitive infections where chloramphenicol-insensitive pneumococci are infrequent. Chloramphenicol has the advantage that it diffuses well into the CSF. Patients with penicillin-resistant pneumococcal infection do not respond well to treatment with chloramphenicol even if *in vitro* disc tests suggest sensitivity. Penicillin and chloramphenicol combined are no more effective than chloramphenicol given alone.

The antibiotic of choice for a patient with suspected penicillin-resistant pneumococcal infection is a third generation cephalosporin such as ceftriaxone or cefotaxime (adult doses 2 g per day and 2 g 6-hourly respectively). Some penicillin-resistant pneumococci are also resistant to cephalosporins and so the administration of a cephalosporin with vancomycin is recommended for a patient with pneumococcal meningitis until the results of sensitivity tests are available. Dexamethasone interferes with the entry of vancomycin into the CSF so if dexamethasone is given (see below) rifampicin is preferred.

The emergence of resistant pneumococci poses major problems for the management of pneumonia in developing countries, where many cases are treated in health centres and dispensaries. Cephalosporins are beyond the budget of most developing countries (approximately £50 to treat an adult patient with pneumonia compared with £5 for penicillin) and there is no obvious alternative; penicillin-resistant strains are usually resistant to other cheap antibiotics such as chloramphenicol and co-trimoxazole.

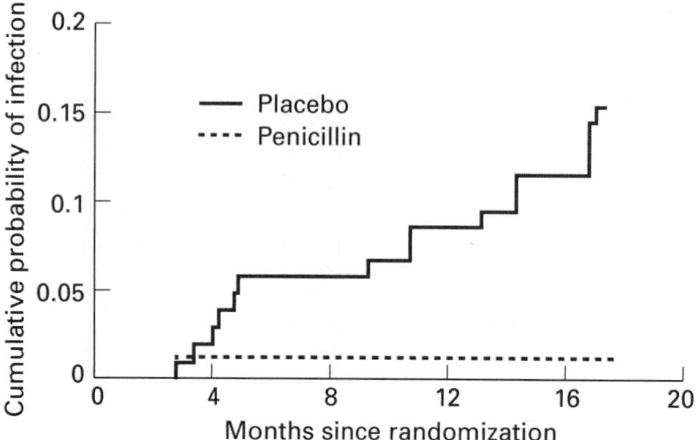

Fig. 6 Protection of children with sickle cell disease from pneumococcal infection by chemoprophylaxis with oral penicillin.
(For source see OTM3, p. 521.)

Supportive measures

General nursing care

Isolation is necessary for patients with an infection caused by a multiple-antibiotic-resistant strain.

Fluid therapy

Patients are often dehydrated by the time that they reach hospital and intravenous fluid therapy may be required.

Oxygen and physiotherapy

Patients with pneumonia, especially those with more than one lobe of the lung involved, are often hypoxic and require oxygen therapy. Physiotherapy is important in helping the patient to clear tenacious sputum during the recovery phase of the infection.

Analgesics

Local pain may be severe in patients with pneumococcal infections and sufficient analgesics should be given to control this symptom. Analgesics with a central depressant action should be avoided whenever possible.

Corticosteroids

The role for dexamethasone in the management of patients with pneumococcal meningitis is still uncertain.

Subdural empyema

Local collections of pus should be removed by needle aspiration or by surgical drainage.

Prophylaxis

Chemoprophylaxis

Chemoprophylaxis has been little used in the control of pneumococcal disease because of difficulties in identifying those who are at risk from the infection. Secondary cases are seen only rarely among those who have been in close contact with a patient. Children with sickle cell disease have an increased incidence of pneumococcal infection and should be given regular chemoprophylaxis with oral penicillin from the age of 3 months until they have reached at least the age of 2 years, when they should be vaccinated (Fig. 6). Some paediatricians also advise penicillin chemoprophylaxis for children with the nephrotic syndrome. Chemoprophylaxis is also recommended for patients who have been splenectomized, especially in childhood, but hard evidence is lacking for need and efficacy.

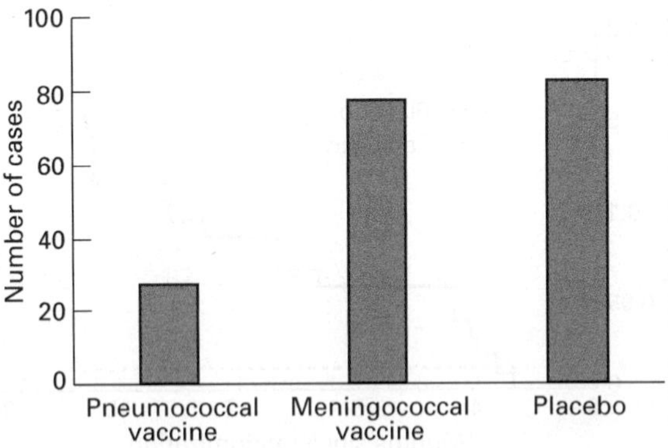

Fig. 7 Protection of South African miners from pneumococcal pneumonia or bacteraemia. The number of cases of infection caused by pneumococci of serotypes represented in the vaccine are shown. There were approximately equal numbers of subjects in each group.
(For source see OTM3, p. 522.)

Table 3 Indications for immunization with pneumococcal capsular polysaccharide vaccine recommended in the USA

Children > 2 years old
Hyposplenia including sickle cell disease
Nephrotic syndrome
Cerebrospinal fluid leak
Immunosuppressive disorders including HIV
Other at-risk groups such as the Inuit
Adults
Those over the age of 65 years
Immunocompetent adults with an increased risk of pneumococcal disease such as those with chronic cardiovascular or pulmonary disease, diabetes, alcoholism and cirrhosis
Immunocompromised subjects with hyposplenia, lymphoma, chronic renal failure or nephrotic syndrome and those on immunosuppressive drugs
Subjects with HIV infection

Vaccination

Purified pneumococcal capsular polysaccharides have been commercially available since the late 1970s. Current vaccines contain 23 capsular polysaccharides, representing 80–90 per cent of the serotypes responsible for invasive pneumococcal disease in the US and western Europe. The effectiveness of pneumococcal capsular polysaccharide vaccines in preventing pneumococcal lobar pneumonia has been demonstrated clearly in controlled trials undertaken in adults in South Africa (Fig. 7) and in Papua New Guinea. In the US, pneumococcal vaccines give about 60 per cent protection against systemic pneumococcal infection in healthy elderly subjects but are less effective in immunocompromised people.

Pneumococcal capsular polysaccharide vaccines are recommended in industrialized countries for several groups of subjects (Table 3), especially those with absent or poorly functioning spleen.

In common with other polysaccharide vaccines, pneumococcal polysaccharides are T-cell independent antigens which are poorly immunogenic in infants and poor at inducing immunological memory. Immunogenicity can be enhanced by conjugating the polysaccharide to a protein such as tetanus or diphtheria toxoid. This approach has led to the successful development of *H. influenzae* type b vaccines (see Chapter 16.47). Several pneumococcal conjugate vaccines are being developed commercially. Because invasive pneumococcal disease may be caused by bacteria of many different serotypes a complex vaccine containing 10 or more conjugates is required which is likely to be expensive and beyond the means of poorer countries where it is most needed.

Further reading

Anderson, E.L., Kennedy, D.J., Geldmacher, K.M., Donnelly, J., and Mendelman, P.M. (1996). Immunogenicity of a heptavalent pneumococcal conjugate vaccine in infants. *Journal of Pediatrics*, **128**, 649–53.

Austrian, R. (1999). The pneumococcus at the millennium: not down, not out. *Journal of Infectious Diseases*, **179** (suppl. 2), 5338–41.

Bruyn, G.A., Zegers, B.J., and van Furth, R. (1992). Mechanisms of host defence against infection with *Streptococcus pneumoniae. Clinical Infectious Diseases*, **14**, 251–62.

Poland, G. A. (1999). The burden of pneumococcal disease: the role of carrying out vaccines. *Vaccine*, **17**, 1674–9.

Quagliarello, V. and Scheld, M.W. (1992). Bacterial meningitis: pathogenesis, pathophysiology and progress. *New England Journal of Medicine*, **327**, 864–72.

Shann, F. (1986). Etiology of severe pneumonia in children in developing countries. *Pediatric Infectious Disease Journal*, **5**, 247–52.

Shapiro, E.D., Berg, A.T., Austrian, R., *et al.* (1991). The protective efficacy of polyvalent pneumococcal polysaccharide vaccine. *New England Journal of Medicine*, **325**, 1453–60.

Chapter 16.40

Staphylococci

S. J. Eykyn

Taxonomy

In the laboratory, *Staphylococcus aureus* is distinguished from other staphylococci by its ability to coagulate plasma. The slide coagulase test detects cell-associated clumping factor (bound coagulase), which reacts with fibrinogen to cause aggregation of the organisms. Commercial kits are now used for this test and some also detect protein A, present in most strains of *S. aureus.* Occasional strains do not produce clumping factor or protein A, and certain other species of staphylococci produce clumping factor, hence the gold standard for the identification of *S. aureus* in the laboratory is the tube coagulase test in which staphylococci are mixed with rabbit or human plasma in a test tube. This detects extracellular coagulase (free coagulase), which activates prothrombin and initiates clot formation. The slide coagulase test is used to screen organisms whereas the tube test is confirmatory and of more taxonomic significance. Other useful screening tests for *S. aureus* are the detection of DNA-ase activity and fermentation of mannitol, but neither is as reliable as the tube coagulase test.

Until recently, coagulase-negative staphylococci tended to be classified in many laboratories as *S. epidermidis (sensu lato)* or *S. saprophyticus* or even, in more traditional quarters, as 'Staph. albus'.

Availability of commercial identification kits has enabled speciation of some (but not all) coagulase-negative staphylococci in the routine laboratory, and it is clear that although most clinical isolates are *S. epidermidis (sensu stricto)* or *S. saprophyticus*, other species can occasionally be important pathogens.

Typing

For epidemiological purposes, it may be necessary to differentiate strains of the same species of staphylococci, and the principle typing method involves bacteriophages. The current international phage set consists of 23 phages with four major phage groups, I, II, III, and V, and strains may be lysed by a single phage from one group, more than one phage from a single group, or by phages from more than one group. There are additional phages for typing methicillin-resistant strains of *S. aureus* (MRSA). Phage typing of coagulase-negative staphylococci is not organized internationally and interpretation of results is often difficult. Molecular typing methods are sometimes useful both for *S. aureus* and coagulase-negative staphylococci.

Staphylococcus aureus

Pathogenicity

S. aureus produces extracellular substances including general toxic agents (such as catalase, hyaluronidase, lipase, haemolytic toxins, and leucocidin) that may be involved in the pathogenesis of local or systemic inflammation, and specific toxins (such as enterotoxins and epidermolytic toxins) that mediate particular non-suppurative diseases.

Enterotoxins

There are seven staphylococcal enterotoxins and about 40 per cent of *S. aureus* produce enterotoxin, sometimes of more than one type. Staphylococcal food poisoning results from the ingestion of foods containing preformed enterotoxin. Enterotoxins have a range of biological activities in addition to their ability to induce vomiting; they are pyrogenic, mitogenic, and can produce thrombocytopenia and hypotension.

Epidermolytic toxins

These cause intraepidermal splitting and are responsible for the scalded skin syndrome (SSSS) and the blistering of impetigo. The production of epidermolytic toxin is particularly associated with *S. aureus* of phage group II. There are two epidermolytic toxins, ETA which is heat stable and under chromosomal control and ETB which is heat labile and plasmid-mediated; most phage group II staphylococci produce ETA or both ETA and ETB.

Toxic shock syndrome toxin (TSST-1)

This toxin is responsible for the toxic shock syndrome (TSS). Most cases of menstrually-associated TSS are mediated by TSST-1 produced by phage group I strains of *S. aureus*; TSS not associated with menstruation can occur with strains producing TSST-1 but also with phage group V strains that produce enterotoxin B.

Carriage

S. aureus is part of the normal flora in some individuals; about 25 per cent 'carry' the organism permanently, a similar proportion never do, and the rest do so intermittently. Common carriage sites are the nose, axilla, perineum, and toewebs. Nasal carriage rates vary from 10 per cent to 40 per cent in normal adults outside hospital, but higher rates are often found in patients in hospital. High carriage rates are also found in individuals with skin diseases such as eczema, in insulin-dependent diabetics, patients on chronic haemodialysis, and intravenous drug abusers.

Host factors in *S. aureus* infection

Intact skin and mucous membranes are important defences against staphylococcal infection. Wounds frequently become colonized which may result in localized infection or in dissemination via the blood to distant sites. Sometimes trivial, even unrecognized, skin trauma precedes such haematogenous spread. Burns and skin diseases are important portals of entry for staphylococci. Certain viral infections such as influenza damage the respiratory epithelium and allow secondary staphylococcal invasion. Foreign material, including intravascular catheters, arteriovenous shunts, and vascular and orthopaedic prostheses, is also relevant to the pathogenesis and perpetuation of staphylococcal infection. Once *S. aureus* has gained access to the tissues, then polymorphs are the most important line of defence. Phagocytosis involves chemotaxis, opsonization, and intracellular killing. Chemotactic defects occur, for example, in Job syndrome in which patients with recurrent eczema suffer from repeated skin infections and cold abscesses with *S. aureus.* Opsonic defects tend to predispose to a variety of pyogenic infections, including, but not specifically, *S. aureus* infection. However, *S. aureus* is a major pathogen in chronic granulomatous disease producing local and metastatic abscesses. In this disease, intracellular killing by the polymorphs is defective.

Susceptibility of *S. aureus* to antibiotics and antiseptics

Resistance to antibiotics is not an indicator of particular virulence in *S. aureus.* Strains sensitive to all antistaphylococcal antibiotics occasionally cause severe community-acquired infections. The majority of isolates however, whether community- or hospital-acquired, produce β-lactamase and are resistant to penicillin itself and a number of related compounds including ampicillin and amoxycillin. Methicillin-resistant strains of *S. aureus* (MRSA) were detected soon after the introduction of methicillin in 1960, and reports of their isolation increased until 1971 when they accounted for some 5 per cent of strains submitted to the Staphylococcus Reference Laboratory of the Central Public Health Laboratory in the UK. MRSA then diminished in frequency in the UK, but there was a resurgence in the early 1980s. MRSA are usually resistant to a variety of other antibiotics in addition to methicillin, and are resistant to all cephalosporins. MRSA have caused hospital outbreaks in many countries, and although in many outbreaks they have caused colonization rather than infection, severe infection has also occurred. Colonization with MRSA is a notoriously recalcitrant problem on geriatric wards and spread of the organism difficult to avoid. Worldwide, most MRSAs have been of phage group III or non-typable. Several distinct strains of MRSA have caused epidemics and they are designated E(epidemic) MRSA-1 etc.; type 16 is currently most common. *S. aureus* (though not MRSA) is sensitive to many cephalosporins, though the newer 'third generation' cephalosporins, such as ceftazidime, are much less active than cefuroxime and cefradine. The incidence of erythromycin resistance is related to use of the antibiotic and varies from about 5 to 20 per cent. Gentamicin resistance is unusual, except in MRSA. Resistance of *S. aureus* to fusidic acid is uncommon, but most cultures contain small numbers of resistant mutants and a fully resistant population can emerge particularly after topical use. Resistance of *S. aureus* to vancomycin or teicoplanin has not been reported. Rifampicin is highly active against *S. aureus* but, as with fusidic acid, minority populations of resistant cells are found and resistance may emerge during treatment. The topical antibiotic mupirocin is very active against most strains of *S. aureus* and is invaluable in the eradication of staphylococci (especially MRSA) from the nose and other superficial sites. Most disinfectants and antiseptics inhibit or kill *S. aureus.* Chlorhexidine, hexachlorophane, and iodine-containing compounds such as povidone iodine are all used for skin disinfection and when used correctly are highly effective in removing staphylococci from the skin.

Clinical manifestations

S. aureus usually causes localized infection sometimes with local spread, but this may result in bacteraemia and dissemination of the infection. Certain staphylococcal syndromes are produced by extracellular toxins rather than local invasion and will be considered separately.

Localized infections

Infection of the skin and its appendages

These infections often arise in association with hair follicles, and minor trauma, maceration, and skin diseases predispose to them. Folliculitis is a superficial infection of the hair follicle commonly caused by *S. aureus.* Boils are deep-seated infections around a hair follicle usually on the neck, axillae, buttocks, and thighs, often recurrent, and sometimes involving more than one member of a family. When several adjacent hair follicles are involved a carbuncle develops, usually on the back of the neck, with multiple draining sinuses and systemic disturbance. Although boils are very common, carbuncles are now rarely seen. Impetigo is a blistering skin lesion with crusting exudate affecting exposed areas (often the face), usually in children. Epidermolytic toxin is associated with these infections. Most acute paronychias are caused by *S. aureus.* Mastitis and breast abscess in the puerperium are also caused by *S. aureus.* Newborn babies commonly suffer from staphylococcal infection, with septic spots, 'sticky umbilicus', 'sticky eye', and occasionally breast abscess, as well as the much rarer toxin-mediated staphylococcal diseases. Styes are also caused by *S. aureus.*

ENT infections

Staphylococcal infection of the hair follicles or sebaceous glands in the outer external auditory canal causes acute localized otitis externa with severe pain and itching. Acute otitis media is seldom caused by *S. aureus* and staphylococci are seldom isolated in sinusitis. Although *S. aureus* is commonly grown from throat swabs, it behaves as a commensal at this site, and such patients have usually been taking antibiotics.

Wound infection

S. aureus is the commonest cause of wound infection following surgery or trauma that does not involve the mucous membranes with their rich anaerobic commensal flora. The clinical presentation of staphylococcal wound infection varies from minimal erythema and serous discharge, through small abscesses often in relation to sutures, to marked cellulitis, deep pus, and wound dehiscence with considerable pain and systemic disturbance. *S. aureus* is an important cause of infection associated with intravascular devices. These infections, which may present as obvious local sepsis or more insidiously, as a pyrexia, often severe, without overt localizing signs, can occur as early as 48 h after insertion of the catheter, but more usually after a longer period. It is also an important pathogen in infections associated with other prosthetic material.

Pleuropulmonary infection

Staphylococcal pneumonia arises from aspiration or haematogenous spread with metastatic seeding of the lung. Aspiration pneumonia generally complicates pre-existing lung disease or viral respiratory disease, usually influenza. In children, other viral infections of the respiratory tract, including severe measles in developing countries, may be followed by secondary bacterial infection with staphylococci. *S. aureus* from carriage sites reach the damaged lung tissue via the trachea and bronchi. In contrast to aspiration pneumonia, haematogenous staphylococcal pneumonia characteristically affects a previously normal lung. In some cases there may be an identifiable local infection, often of the skin and usually trivial, that has resulted in haematogenous seeding, or there may be evidence of release of infected thrombi via the venous system as in tricuspid endocarditis or occasionally when there is an infected intravascular device. Staphylococci can readily be isolated from the blood in haematogenous pneumonia, though seldom in aspiration pneumonia. Whatever its pathogenesis, *S. aureus* pneumonia is a severe disease with high fever and cyanosis. When secondary to influenza, it may occur without an obvious flu-like prodromal illness and with alarming suddenness. It is usually complicated by abscess formation, empyema, and, in children, by pneumatoceles and pyopneumothorax, but the radiological findings at presentation vary from local consolidation to multiple patchy infiltrates, and abscess formation may or may not be detected.

Urinary tract infection

S. aureus urinary tract infection is uncommon and unlikely in patients with a normal urinary tract except in staphylococcal septicaemia when the organism can often be recovered from the urine, presumably the result of microabscesses in the kidney. It sometimes occurs in patients with abnormal bladder function, usually in association with instrumentation or catheterization presumably from previous urethral colonization with the strain.

Bacteraemia and septicaemia

Bacteraemia means bacteria in the blood, that is a positive blood culture; it may or may not be symptomatic in the patient. A symptomatic bacteraemia is usually referred to as a septicaemia. In fact, *S. aureus* in the blood is almost always symptomatic and thus strictly a septicaemia, but the terms tend to be used interchangeably. Most staphylococcal bacteraemias, particularly those acquired in hospital, are secondary to a local site of infection but *S. aureus* can also enter the blood from carrier sites or trivial, unnoticed abrasions that become colonized, and these bacteraemias can then result in serious, deep-seated infection involving bones, joints, lungs, and heart valves. Such bacteraemias have been called 'primary' and are usually much more severe than those secondary to a defined focus of infection. Primary bacteraemia can occur at any age, and often in a previously healthy individual. Occasionally, patients with community-acquired *S. aureus* bacteraemia present with profound toxaemia, shock, and disseminated intravascular coagulation (DIC). Such patients often have signs of meningitis and their cerebrospinal fluid (CSF) contains polymorphs, often in large numbers, though staphylococci are rarely detected. The infection is often thought to be meningococcal. Figure 1(a, b) shows just such a meningococcaemic-like infection in a 22-year-old man

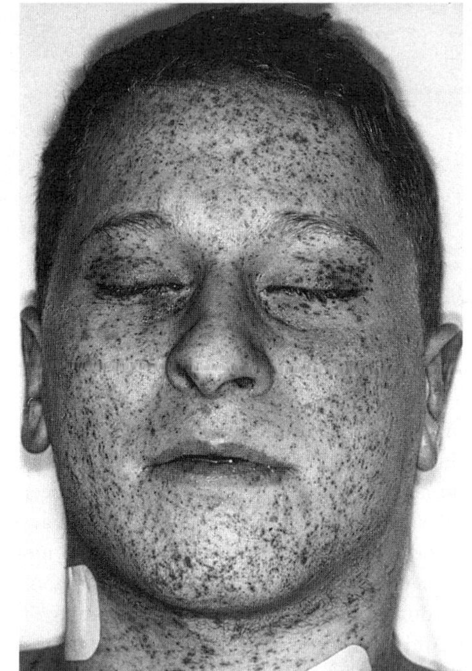

(a)

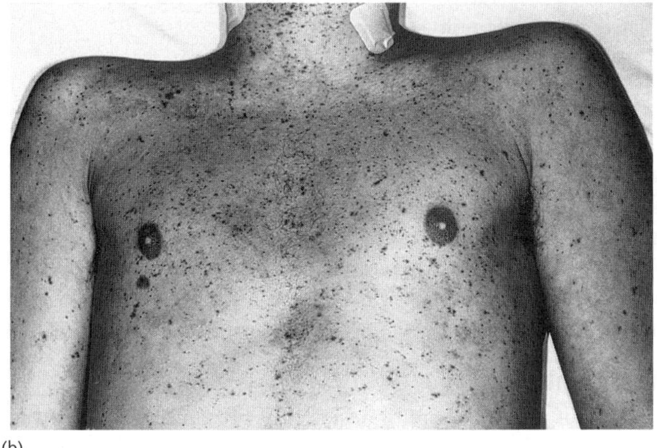

(b)

Fig. 1(a, b) Meningococcaemic-like infection in a 22-year-old man who died from an aortic-root abscess from *S. aureus* endocarditis on a bicuspid aortic valve. A false-positive meningococcal latex agglutination test on the cerebrospinal fluid (which contained 1500 polymorphs, but no organisms) taken on admission further increased the clinical confusion.

who died with an aortic root abscess from *S. aureus* endocarditis on a bicuspid aortic valve. Figure 2(a, b) shows another fatal case of *S. aureus* septicaemia with DIC: this previously healthy, 54-year-old man was febrile and confused and became hemiplegic within 48 h of admission. Both blood cultures and CSF (which contained 5000 polymorphs) grew *S. aureus*. Postmortem was refused, but he too most probably had (undiagnosed) endocarditis.

Metastatic (haematogenous) infection

Endocarditis

S. aureus endocarditis usually results from a 'primary' community-acquired bacteraemia and is a devastating illness, often in a previously healthy individual. An asymptomatic left sided valvular abnormality such as a bicuspid aortic valve or mitral leaflet prolapse is sometimes, though not invariably, present. The infection presents as a flu-like illness often with initial gastrointestinal disturbance. Meningism is seen in about 25 per cent of cases and polymorphs, though seldom organisms, are detected in the CSF. The patient develops systemic emboli and valvular insufficiency within days, sometimes hours, of admission. Acute staphylococcal endocarditis is a rapidly destructive disease, justifiably called malignant endocarditis by Osler. Emergency valve replacement may be required and should never be delayed; it is this and not further antibiotics that will save the patient's life. Staphylococcal endocarditis is occasionally complicated by splenic abscess for which splenectomy may be required. *S. aureus* endocarditis may also be acquired in hospital from infected intravascular devices or from sternal wound infection after valve replacement surgery.

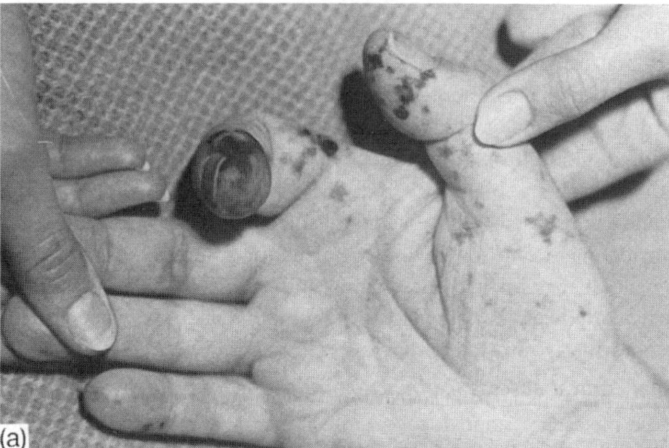

(a)

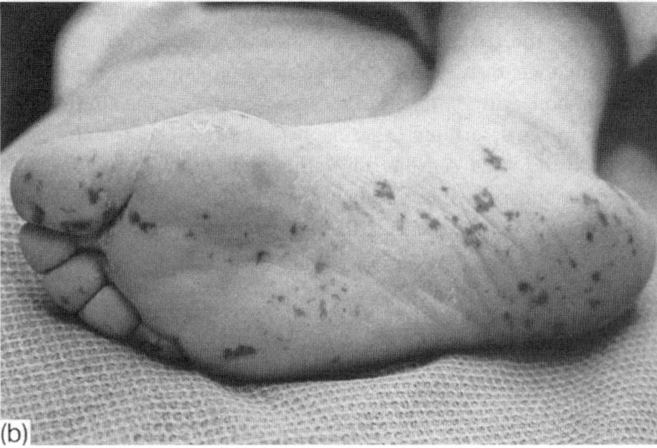

(b)

Fig. 2 Meningococcaemia-like disease. (1) Hand and (b) foot of a man with primary staphylococcal bacteraemia and meningitis, who had DIC.

Intravenous drug abusers are at particular risk of staphylococcal endocarditis but unless the affected individual has a previous valvular abnormality, the infection involves the tricuspid valve and presents as a quite different and often less acute illness. There is fever, malaise, and respiratory signs that result from septic pulmonary emboli.

Bone and joint infections

S. aureus remains the commonest cause of acute bone and joint infection. These infections can result from a 'primary' bacteraemia but also from a contiguous focus of infection after trauma or surgery especially that involving prosthetic implants. The incidence of acute haematogenous osteomyelitis has decreased, and there has also been a change in its localization. Osteomyelitis of the long bones, an infection seen primarily in children particularly boys, has decreased, and the vertebral column is now the commonest site. Most patients with staphylococcal vertebral osteomyelitis are middle aged or elderly. Vertebral osteomyelitis can be a notoriously difficult diagnosis, and pain, not always persistently localized to the spine, the only consistent feature. Fever is not always present, but at least should lead to the taking of blood for culture which is likely to be positive. Any patient with backache, a high CRP and ESR, and *S. aureus* in the blood should be assumed to have vertebral infection. Staphylococcal septic arthritis may occur in previously normal or abnormal joints and at any age. It may involve one or more joints and multiple infection is particularly likely in patients with rheumatoid arthritis, when it may be notoriously difficult to diagnose.

Renal cortical abscess (carbuncle) and perinephric abscess

These metastatic staphylococcal infections are rare and usually lead to considerable diagnostic confusion. A renal cortical abscess, also known as a carbuncle, is a multilocular abscess involving the renal parenchyma, the result of the coalescence of cortical microabscesses from haematogenous seeding of the kidney from a previous infection, typically a boil, with *S. aureus*. Although *S. aureus* is the commonest pathogen in renal carbuncle, perinephric abscesses, that is abscesses external to the renal capsule but within the perinephric fascia, are more commonly caused by Gram-negative aerobes. A renal carbuncle may rupture into the perinephric space producing a perinephric abscess.

Pyomyositis

Pyomyositis is an acute inflammation of skeletal muscle that is almost unique to the tropics and subtropics, it is rarely encountered in temperate climates. Usually a single large muscle is affected, most commonly the gluteal and quadriceps, but multiple muscle involvement may occur. The infection predominantly affects males and presents with muscular pain followed by fever, localized pain, induration, and swelling. Its pathogenesis remains obscure. Treatment consists of drainage and antibiotics.

Infections mediated by toxins of *S. aureus*

Staphylococcal food poisoning

This syndrome, characterised by severe vomiting, nausea, abdominal cramps, and diarrhoea, is caused by the ingestion of staphylococcal enterotoxin preformed in the food. The onset occurs within hours of ingestion of food contaminated during its preparation by an individual infected with, or shedding, an enterotoxin-producing staphylococcus. Only about 5 per cent of outbreaks of bacterial food poisoning reported to the Communicable Disease Surveillance Centre for which an aetiological agent is identified are caused by *S. aureus*. The diagnosis can be confirmed by culturing samples from the incriminated food, any skin lesions and the nose of food handlers, and stools of the victims. In most outbreaks, both the organism and its toxin can be defined, but occasionally enterotoxin alone is demonstrated in the food.

Staphylococcal scalded skin syndrome (SSSS)

This rare disease, more commonly seen in children than adults (Fig. 3), is characterized by the sudden onset of extensive erythema followed by bullous desquamation of large areas of skin. It is caused by the epidermolytic toxins of *S. aureus*.

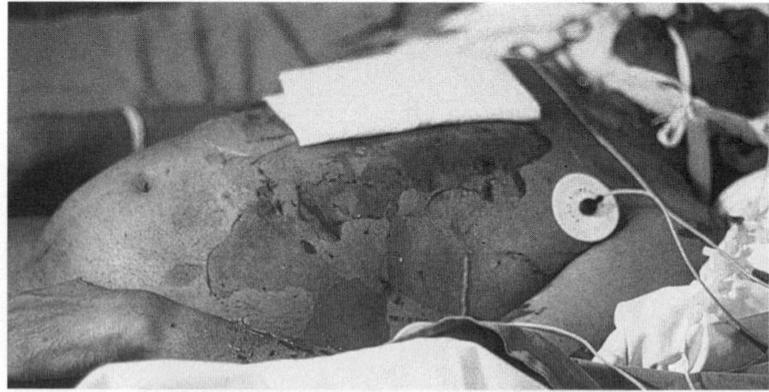

Fig. 3 Staphylococcal scalded-skin syndrome (SSSS) in an adult.

Toxic shock syndrome (TSS)

This syndrome, consisting of high fever, mental confusion, erythroderma, diarrhoea, hypotension, and renal failure, was first defined in children in 1978 but had been recognized 50 years earlier and thought to be staphylococcal scarlet fever. In the late 1970s, there was an epidemic of TSS in women associated with menstruation and tampon use, initially, and predominantly, in the US, but later, though in far fewer numbers, in other countries. TSS has also been described in women who were not menstruating and in men with a wide variety of conditions and operations. TSS may be fatal and a mortality rate of around 5 per cent was reported during the 'tampon epidemic'. Since the syndrome is mediated by toxin, the mainstay of treatment is supportive. Antistaphylococcal antibiotics should be given to eradicate *S. aureus* from the local site and any tampon should be removed. Bacteraemia has rarely been reported in TSS. The staphylococci isolated are usually resistant only to penicillin.

Laboratory diagnosis of *S. aureus* infection

S. aureus is readily isolated in the laboratory and a Gram-stained film will often enable a rapid diagnosis of a staphylococcal aetiology to be made. The diagnosis can be confirmed by culture within 24 h. Staphylococcal bacteraemia is detected by routine blood culture methods. The isolation of *S. aureus* from blood is almost always indicative of a genuine bacteraemia and the organism should only be dismissed as a contaminant if the patient has extensive skin disease such as eczema.

Treatment

Drainage of pus, if present, is an essential prerequisite of the management of infection with *S. aureus*. This may occur spontaneously or with only minor surgical intervention in most superficial infections such as boils, paronychias, styes, stitch abscesses, etc. Deep abscesses in wounds or organs and osteomyelitis that has progressed to the point of pus formation require definitive surgical drainage. Infections associated with an intravascular device or other prosthetic material seldom resolve with antibiotics and removal of the foreign material is nearly always required. Antibiotics are of no benefit in staphylococcal food poisoning but should be given in SSSS and TSS to eradicate toxin-producing *S. aureus*. The initial choice of agent for staphylococcal infection (before sensitivities become available) depends on the patterns of susceptibility of *S. aureus* in the community from which the patient comes. Penicillin itself is suitable only if the strain does not produce β-lactamase, and should never be used for the initial 'blind' treatment. For most strains there is a wide choice of effective antibiotics. In most instances, a β-lactamase resistant penicillin such as flucloxacillin or a cephalosporin such as cefuroxime will be appropriate. Alternative agents to β-lactams, particularly where the patient is hypersensitive to penicillin, include the macrolides erythromycin, clarithromycin, and azithromycin. Fusidic acid is an excellent antistaphylococcal agent although resistance may arise during treatment especially when the organism cannot readily be eradicated.

The only agents with reliable activity against MRSA are vancomycin and teicoplanin. Most staphylococcal infection is satisfactorily treated with a single antibiotic but combination therapy is often used for serious infections, particularly endocarditis and bone or joint infection. The length of antibiotic treatment required to treat staphylococcal infection is unknown but for serious community-acquired infections such as endocarditis, bone and joint infections, and pneumonia several weeks treatment are needed. For most other infections, antibiotics should be given until there is clinical improvement or for about 48 h after fever has resolved. Persistent positive blood cultures with *S. aureus* despite appropriate antibiotic therapy is seldom an indication for changing the antibiotics, but rather for an assessment of the need for intervention, for example to remove an infected intravascular device, excise an infected heart valve, or aspirate and washout a joint. Topical antibiotics and antiseptics are useful for the treatment of skin infections.

Coagulase-negative staphylococci

Although coagulase-negative staphylococci are the commonest contaminants in the laboratory (particularly in blood cultures), they can also be important pathogens whose incidence continues to increase. The availability of kits for their speciation has served to emphasize that they cannot be regarded as a homogeneous entity; the different species vary not only in their incidence in clinical infections but also in the type and severity of disease produced. Most infections are hospital acquired, but certain species cause severe community-acquired infection.

Pathogenicity

Those coagulase-negative staphylococci (usually *S. epidermidis*) that cause infections associated with prosthetic devices and intravascular catheters produce an exopolysaccharide ('slime') which is an important factor in enabling the adherence of these organisms to plastic material and probably also in their resistance to phagocytosis and other host defences and to antimicrobial action. Coagulase-negative staphylococci isolated from clinical infections also produce a variety of potential toxins, including haemolysins, cytotoxins, deoxyribonuclease, fibrinolysin, proteinase, and lipase-esterase, similar to those produced by *S. aureus*, and infections caused by *S. lugdunensis* and *S. simulans* and possibly others mimic that caused by *S. aureus*.

Carriage

Coagulase-negative staphylococci form the greater part of the human skin flora. Although many different species are found on the skin, the commonest is *S. epidermidis*. Distribution of species varies on different skin areas and there are also geographical variations.

Host factors in coagulase-negative staphylococcal infection

Most infection with coagulase-negative staphylococci is associated with prosthetic material. Infection of intravascular catheters can arise via the catheter access site or the catheter hub from frequent disconnections. Prosthetic material can also become infected at the time of percutaneous or surgical implantation.

Antibiotic susceptibility

Hospital-acquired coagulase-negative staphylococci are usually multiply resistant. Most are resistant to methicillin (and thus to cephalosporins), and many to gentamicin and erythromycin. Thus the usual nosocomial strain of coagulase-negative staphylococcus has an antibiotic susceptibility pattern comparable to many MRSAs. Rare resistance to vancomycin and teicoplanin has been reported. Community-acquired infections are usually caused by very sensitive strains.

Infections caused by coagulase-negative staphylococci

Most infections are acquired in hospital in association with a prosthetic device or implant. Community-acquired infections though rare are probably increasing, and are usually severe. In many infections, isolation of the organism from the blood is essential for the diagnosis, and true bacteraemia must be distinguished from contamination. Repeated cultures should always be taken and only organisms of similar sensitivity and biochemical profile considered the same. Infection with more than one strain is not unusual in nosocomial infections.

Intravascular devices

There has been a marked increase in infection of intravascular devices with coagulase-negative staphylococci, particularly in neonates and immunocompromised patients, and they are now the commonest bacteria involved in such infections. The degree of systemic disturbance varies, and this should determine the approach to treatment. In contrast to infections of intravascular devices caused by *S. aureus*, with those caused by coagulase-negative staphylococci it may be possible to leave the catheter *in situ* and give appropriate antibiotics, usually vancomycin or teicoplanin. If this fails then the catheter must be removed. Very occasionally, as with *S. aureus*, persistent bacteraemia can result in metastatic seeding of a heart valve or vertebral body.

Cerebrospinal fluid shunts

Coagulase-negative staphylococci, predominantly *S. epidermidis*, are the commonest cause of infection of CSF shunts. They also cause infection of CSF reservoirs used for chemotherapy. Signs of meningitis may be absent and usual findings include low grade fever, malaise, and shunt malfunction. Serum antibodies to *S. epidermidis* can be used to monitor treatment and detect relapse. Treatment may require removal of the shunt and antibiotics, usually vancomycin with rifampicin, are best given intraventricularly. Occasionally, glomerulonephritis ('shunt nephritis') occurs in patients with colonized shunts.

Peritonitis associated with continuous ambulatory peritoneal dialysis (CAPD)

Coagulase-negative staphylococci are the commonest cause of CAPD peritonitis. Patients have abdominal pain, occasionally nausea, diarrhoea and fever, and abundant polymorphs in the dialysate in which Gram-positive cocci (usually scanty and intracellular) may be detected. The antibiotic sensitivities of infecting strains vary and since treatment must always be started before this information is available, vancomycin (preferably intraperitoneally) is the drug of choice.

Endocarditis

Coagulase-negative staphylococci can infect native or prosthetic heart valves. Nosocomial native valve infections with coagulase-negative staphylococci (usually *S. epidermidis*) generally result from infected intravascular devices; the affected valve may or may not have been previously abnormal. Nosocomial prosthetic valve endocarditis can be acquired in the theatre (or shortly thereafter) at the time of the original valve replacement and presents within weeks or more often months of surgery ('early onset'). In many series, coagulase-negative staphylococci are the commonest cause of early-onset prosthetic valve endocarditis. Prosthetic infection can also be acquired from an infected intravascular device. Nosocomial staphylococci tend to be multiply resistant. Community-acquired endocarditis, which may involve native (usually) or prosthetic valves, is increasingly recognized. Most patients with native valve infection have a pre-existing cardiac abnormality. The organisms must derive from the patient's skin but predisposing skin lesions are seldom detected. The infection often mimics *S. aureus* endocarditis with rapidly destructive valvular disease, neurological manifestations, and concomitant vertebral osteomyelitis. The commonest pathogen is *S. epidermidis*, but there are increasing reports of other species, particularly *S. lugdunensis* which seems to be especially virulent. These community-acquired strains are frequently penicillin sensitive.

Urinary tract infection

Coagulase-negative staphylococci are urinary pathogens both in the community and in hospital. *S. saprophyticus* is an important urinary pathogen in sexually active women, second only to *Escherichia coli*. It commonly produces cystitis, but may cause upper urinary tract infection and has been isolated from infected calculi. Most strains are readily recognized in the laboratory by their resistance to novobiocin. They are sensitive to a wide range of antibiotics. Some nosocomial urinary tract infections are also caused by coagulase-negative staphylococci, predominantly *S. epidermidis*. These infections, usually occurring after urological surgery, are seldom accompanied by pyuria, and may clear spontaneously on removal of the catheter. Sometimes they are of clinical significance and require treatment. Nosocomial urinary isolates of coagulase-negative staphylococci are often multiply resistant.

Other infections

Coagulase-negative staphylococci are increasingly isolated from the blood of neonates and immunocompromised, neutropenic patients. Distinguishing true bacteraemia from contamination can be difficult. In many cases bacteraemia is related to the presence of an intravascular catheter. In premature neonates, colonization of the respiratory tract occurs and respiratory infection can result. Infection of prosthetic joints and vascular prostheses is sometimes caused by coagulase-negative staphylococci. The organisms are introduced at the time of the surgery, although the clinical signs of infection may not become evident for weeks or months. Attempts to treat such infections with antibiotics generally fail and removal of the prosthesis is required. Coagulase-negative staphylococci are the commonest cause of post-operative endophthalmitis after intraocular surgery.

Laboratory diagnosis

The laboratory diagnosis of much infection with coagulase-negative staphylococci poses greater difficulties than the diagnosis of *S. aureus* infection. A further problem with these organisms is the use of broth enrichment cultures for specimens such as excised tissue when a single contaminating staphylococcus will multiply in liquid media, thereby misleading unwary clinicians.

Treatment

An integral part of the successful treatment of infections with coagulase-negative staphylococci is a critical clinical assessment of the need for removal of any prosthetic material with which so many infections are associated. That said, most patients will be treated with antibiotics, and often before sensitivity results are available. So many nosocomial infections are caused by resistant strains that the only reliable initial therapy is vancomycin or teicoplanin. The length of treatment in most instances is somewhat arbitrary and the same principles apply to infections with these organisms as to those with *S. aureus*. Community-acquired infections, usually endocarditis, can often be treated with β-lactam antibiotics, often with penicillin. As with serious *S. aureus* infections, combination therapy is often used.

Further reading

Archer, G.L. (1995). Staphylococcus epidermidis and other coagulase-negative staphylococci. In *Principles and practice of infectious diseases* (ed. G.L.Mandell, J.E.Bennett, and R. Dolin), pp.1777–84. Churchill Livingstone, New York.

Chesney, P.J., Bergdoll, M.S., Davis, J.P., and Vergeront, J.M. (1984). The disease spectrum, epidemiology, and etiology of toxic-shock syndrome. *Annual Review of Microbiology*, **38**, 315–38.

Espersen, F., Fromodt-Moller, N., Rosdahl, V.T., Skinhoj, P., and Bentzon, M.W. (1991). Changing pattern of bone and joint infections due to Staphylococcus aureus: study of cases of bacteraemia in Denmark, 1959–1988. *Reviews of Infectious Diseases*, **13**, 347–58.

Etienne, J. and Eykyn, S.J. (1990). Increase in native valve endocarditis caused by coagulase negative staphylococci: an Anglo-French clinical and microbiological study. *British Heart Journal*, **64**, 381–4.

Marples, R.R. and Reith, S. (1992). Methicillin-resistant *Staphylococcus aureus* in England and Wales. *Communicable Disease Report*, **3**, R25–9.

Vandenesch, F., Etienne, J., Reverdy, M.E., and Eykyn, S.J. (1993). Endocarditis due to Staphylococcus lugdunensis: report of 11 cases and review. *Clinical Infectious Diseases*, **17**, 871–6.

Waldvogel, F.A. (1995). Staphylococcus aureus (including toxic shock syndrome). In *Principles and practice of infectious diseases* (ed.G.L.Mandell, J.E.Bennett, and R.Dolin), pp.1754–77. Churchill Livingstone, New York.

Chapter 16.41

Meningococcal infection

B. M. Greenwood

The organism

Meningococci are bean-shaped, Gram-negative diplococci. Since they are sensitive to chilling or drying, samples must be inoculated and cultured as soon as possible after collection. They possess an outer polysaccharide capsule, outer membrane, cytoplasmic membrane, and underlying peptidoglycan layer. Currently, the system of typing used most widely is based upon the antigenic characteristics of: (a) the capsular polysaccharide; (b) the class 2/3 outer membrane protein; (c) the class 1 outer membrane protein; and (d) the organism's sensitivity to sulphonamides. B:2a:P1.1:R indicates a strain with a group B capsular polysaccharide, a type 2a class 2 protein and a type 1 class 1 protein which is resistant to sulphonamides. The basis of the antigenic characteristics of the lipopolysaccharides, the isoenzyme profile, or the electrophoretic pattern of the DNA produced by digestion with restriction enzymes can also be used for typing.

Typing is useful as an indication of virulence (e.g. group A capsule), for identification of 'clones' responsible for individual outbreaks or epidemics, and to study the relationship between epidemics (Fig. 1).

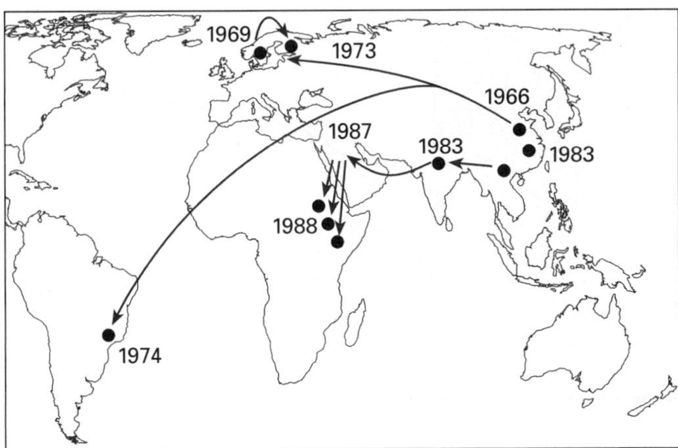

Fig. 1 The spread of the group A meningococcus clone III-I as indicated by molecular epidemiological techniques. From Saudi Arabia the clone was carried to many other countries by pilgrims returning from Mecca..
(From Achtman 1990, Review of Medical Microbiology, **1**, *29, with permission.)*

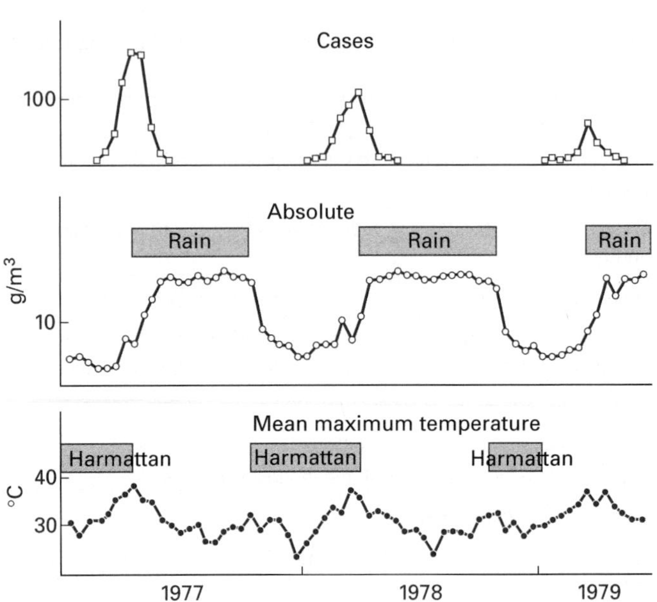

Fig. 2 The seasonality of meningococcal disease in sub-Saharan Africa. The harmattan is a hot, dusty wind that blows from the Sahara.
(From Greenwood, B.M., et al. 1984, Lancet, **1**, *1339.)*

Sulphonamide resistance, from mutation in the chromosomal dihydropterate synthetase gene, is common. There is high level resistance to rifampicin through mutations in the *rpoB* gene and low level resistance through decreased membrane permeability. Resistance to tetracyclines among genital and anorectal isolates of *Neisseria meningitidis* results from the plasmid *tet(M)* gene. Low level resistance to penicillin has resulted from changes in penicillin-binding protein-2 but high level resistance though α-lactomase production is very rare. Meningococci with reduced sensitivity to penicillin (MICs 0.1–1.0 mg/l) are reported. Recently, high level resistance to chloramphenicol has been demonstrated, due to a transposon from *Chlostridium perfringens* at its *catP* gene site.

Meningococci are sensitive to most antibiotics but are no longer sensitive to sulphonamides. Recently there have been reports from Southern Africa and from various countries in Europe, particularly Spain, of the emergence of meningococci with a reduced sensitivity to penicillin (MIC in the range of 0.1–1.0 mg/l).

Epidemiology

Geographical distribution

Meningococcal disease occurs globally. In temperate climes, the infection is usually endemic but numbers fluctuate in cycles extending over several years and focal clusters of cases may occur. Most endemic meningococcal disease is caused by serogroups B or C.

Within the African 'meningitis belt', extending across sub-Saharan Africa from Ethiopia to the Gambia, there are major epidemics of meningococcal disease every 5–10 years. The last was in 1996. These epidemics usually start in the middle of the dry season, when it is hot, dry, and dusty, and end a few months later with the coming of the rains (Fig. 2). Most African epidemics are caused by group A meningococci, Group C epidemics are much less common.

Age and sex

When meningococcal infection is endemic, most cases of clinical disease are seen among the young; older children and adults are affected more frequently during epidemics. The sexes are equally susceptible.

Nasopharyngeal carriers

Most people infected with meningococci become asymptomatic nasopharyngeal carriers. The ratio of carriers to cases may be as high as 10 000:1 in endemic situations or as low as 100:1 during epidemics. Nasopharyngeal carriage rates do not predict the likelihood of an epidemic.

Risk factors for meningococcal disease

See Table 1 and Fig. 3.

Pathogenesis and immunity

Spread of infection

Meningococci are usually spread by respiratory droplets; occasionally sexual transmission occurs. To become established in the nasopharynx meningococci must adhere to nasopharyngeal cells, and then pass through them to reach the circulation where most are destroyed rapidly by antibody and phagocytic cells before causing tissue damage. In a few unfortunate individuals, bacteraemia results in the clinical syndrome of acute meningococcaemia. In others, meningococci are cleared from the circulation but lodge in the meninges where they induce an inflammatory response.

Pathogenesis

Endotoxin released by meningococci activates various biological pathways including the complement and cytokine systems. High levels of inflammatory cytokines such as tumour necrosis factor (TNF) are found in the plasma of patients with acute meningococcaemia and in the cerebrospinal fluid (CSF) of patients with meningococcal meningitis.

Some patients develop arthritis, cutaneous vasculitis, episcleritis, or pericarditis several days after the start of their illness, at a time when other features of their infection are improving. These lesions are attributable to immune complexes formed at sites where antigen is trapped during the bacteraemic phase of the infection.

Table 1 Risk factors predisposing to the development of meningococcal disease

Socio-economic
Poor living conditions attack rates are highest in deprived sections of a community.
Overcrowding outbreaks are frequent in military camps, doss houses and hostels.
Household contact
Subjects in close contact with a case are at risk, especially during epidemics. The risk may be as high as 1:20 for siblings of a patient.
Damage to respiratory mucosa
Adverse environmental conditions low absolute humidity may be important in Africa (dry season) and in Europe (winter).
Antecedent viral infections
Several studies suggest that preceeding influenza is a risk factor for meningococcal disease (Fig. 3)
Smoking—both active and passive smoking have been implicated as risk factors in separate studies
Immunological
Deficient levels of IgG or IgM bactericidal antibodies
High levels of blocking IgA antibody
Hereditary or acquired complement deficiencies, especially late components
ABO non-secretor status perhaps induced by intestinal infection with a cross-reactive organismmay account for up to 10 per cent of cases in conditions of low endemicity

Note: So far no evidence has been found that HIV infection predisposes to invasive meningococcal disease.

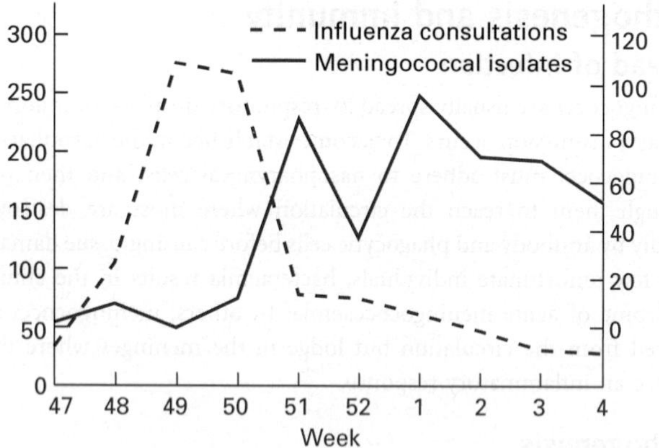

Fig. 3 The relationship between consultations with general practitioners for influenza (per 100 000 population) and the isolation rate for meningococci among samples submitted to a reference laboratory.
(From Cartwright et al. 1991, Lancet, ***338****, 354.)*

Local immunity

Locally produced secretory IgA antibodies may have a protective role, perhaps by preventing bacterial adherence to epithelial cells, but this has not been proved. Adverse climatic conditions and viral infections may damage local defences predisposing to invasion.

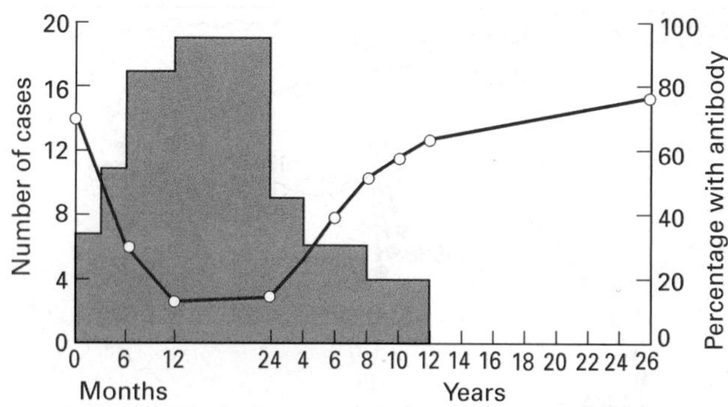

Fig. 4 The relationship between the age at onset of meningococcal disease and the prevalence of group C meningococcal antibodies in American subjects of different ages.
(From Goldschneider et al., 1969, Journal of Experimental Medicine, ***129****, 1307.)*

Systemic immunity

It has been clearly demonstrated that bactericidal antibodies directed against the capsular polysaccharide or the outer membrane proteins protect against meningococcal disease (Fig. 4). Bactericidal antibody production can be induced by asymptomatic nasopharyngeal infection with a meningococcus or with a cross-reacting bacterium such as *N. lactamica*. Complement is required for antibody-mediated killing of meningococci; patients with congenital or acquired complement deficiencies have an increased susceptibility to meningococcal disease.

Clinical features

Meningococci can cause a variety of clinical syndromes, varying in severity from a mild sore throat to rapidly fatal, acute meningococcaemia.

Nasopharyngeal infection

Most infections are asymptomatic but some subjects develop a mild sore throat.

Acute meningococcaemia

Symptoms

Acute meningococcaemia can strike with frightening rapidity; a victim may be well at breakfast time but dead by the same afternoon. The early symptoms of acute meningococcaemia—fever, general malaise, headache, and diarrhoea—are quite non-specific.

Physical signs (Plates 1–3)

Initially there is fever and tachycardia. Careful examination may reveal small petechiae in the skin or in the conjunctivae (Plate 1) or an erythematous rash. Within hours, more extensive haemorrhagic lesions may appear and there may be bleeding from mucosae. The blood pressure is often normal initially, but then begins a remorseless fall. The central venous pressure is low and small vessels are usually constricted, giving cold extremities. There may be a gallop rhythm and some patients develop cardiac arrhythmias. Patients with acute meningococcaemia are often drowsy and may rapidly become comatose.

Laboratory findings

A blood neutrophil leucocytosis is usual but leucopenia is found occasionally. Thrombocytopenia is usual and there may be other signs of disseminated intravascular coagulation. Blood culture is frequently positive and meningococcal polysaccharide antigen can often be detected in the serum. The CSF is clear and contains a normal, or only slightly elevated, number of white cells.

Course and prognosis

Patients with acute meningococcaemia may die within a few hours of the start of their illness from peripheral circulatory collapse, haemorrhage, cardiac arrhythmia, or a combination of all three. Peripheral circulatory collapse and impairment of consciousness at the time of presentation are poor prognostic signs. Those who survive the first few hours of their illness may remain unconscious. Some survivors develop severe pulmonary oedema which may be complicated by a secondary chest infection. Others develop acute renal failure. Ulceration may occur at the site of haemorrhage into the skin and gangrene of extremities has been recorded. Vascular damage may lead to bone infarction.

About 5 per cent develop arthritis attributable to direct invasion of a synovial joint during the initial phase of septicaemia. However, arthritis develops most frequently about 6 days after the start of illness, associated with a secondary rise in fever and cutaneous vasculitis (Plate 2), episcleritis, or pericarditis. Allergic skin lesions usually start as blisters that may rupture leaving extensive, superficial ulcers. Pericarditis is usually asymptomatic but a pericardial effusion can develop and occasionally causes tamponade.

Rarely, meningococcaemia follows a subacute benign course characterized by mild fever and petechiae only. Unsuspected meningococcaemia may be revealed by a routine blood culture.

Meningitis (see also Chapter 13.25)

Symptoms

Severe headache, fever, and general malaise are the usual presenting symptoms. Backache, photophobia, nausea, and vomiting are common complaints. Convulsions are especially in young children.

Physical signs

In older children and in adults, signs of meningeal irritation are usually present. Focal neurological signs such as sixth or third cranial nerve palsies long tract signs may be detected. Bradycardia and hypertension suggest raised intracranial pressure; papilloedema is rarely seen. Petecchiae may be present in the skin, conjunctivae, or on the palatal mucosa. Cardiac enlargement, gallop rhythm, and mild ECG abnormalities on the electrocardiogram are sometimes present, indicating associated myocarditis, but heart failure is rare. In infants, fever, convulsions, or feeding difficulties may be the only abnormal clinical features; there may be bulging of the anterior fontanelle.

Laboratory findings

A blood neutrophil leucocytosis is usual. Blood culture is positive in a few patients. CSF is usually turbid with marked pleocytosis. Nearly all the cells are neutrophils. CSF protein is increased, CSF sugar is usually decreased. Meningococci can often be seen within CSF leucocytes and free within the CSF, and usually a positive culture can be obtained. Meningococcal polysaccharide antigen can usually be detected in the CSF.

Course and prognosis

Patients sometimes die suddenly during their first few hours in hospital, death is rare in those who survive their first 24 h. Case fatality is usually between 5 and 10 per cent.

Some patients develop a secondary spike of fever, due to a local collection of pus, such as subdural empyema, or to immunological complications. Herpes simplex, sometimes extensive, may appear during the course of recovery.

Some patients are left with neurological deficits, in particular deafness. The incidence of permanent deafness varies with the strain of meningococcus and the quality of treatment. On average 5 per cent of patients remain deaf in one or both ears.

Chronic meningococcaemia

This is a rare condition characterized by persistent meningococcaemia. Episodes of fever, urticarial rashes, arthritis, and splenomegaly are the usual clinical features.

Other clinical syndromes

Pyogenic arthritis, pericarditis, and panophthalmitis may result from dissemination of meningococci through the circulation. Meningococci have been isolated from patients with urethritis, proctitis, or conjunctivitis. Rarely meningococci, particularly those belonging to serogroup Y, cause pneumonia.

Diagnosis

Acute meningococcaemia

Meningococcaemia should enter into the differential diagnosis of all patients with fever and petechiae but many other organisms can produce a similar clinical picture. The diagnosis is confirmed by blood culture or detection of meningococcal polysaccharide antigen in serum.

Meningitis

A clinical diagnosis of acute meningitis is usually made readily in adults and older children from the characteristic history and abnormal physical signs. Meningitis must be considered as a possible diagnosis in all irritable, febrile infants, especially in those with convulsions.

Confirmation of diagnosis is by lumbar puncture which should be performed in all suspected cases of meningitis unless there are definite contraindications such as signs of raised intracranial pressure.

Meningococci can be demonstrated in the CSF by Gram stain or culture in up to 80 per cent of patients investigated before the start of treatment. Culture is often negative in patients who have received antibiotics; in such cases bacterial antigens may still be present. Group A or C polysaccharides are readily detected by simple assays such as latex agglutination tests but detecting group B polysaccharide is more difficult. Culture of nasopharyngeal swab is useful in patients with suspected meningococcal meningitis or meningococcaemia as this may yield a meningococcus, even in partially treated patients.

Treatment

Acute meningococcaemia

Antibiotics

Penicillin remains the antibiotic of choice for the treatment of acute meningococcaemia; 4 mega units of crystalline penicillin should be given 6-hourly by intravenous injection in adults. This is effective even in infections caused by meningococci that are relatively insensitive to penicillin. Chloramphenicol is an alternative treatment for patients who are known to be sensitive to penicillin or who are at risk of infection with a penicillin insensitive strain.

Because meningococcal infections can progress so rapidly, it is recommended that penicillin or acephalosporin should be injected immediately meningococcal infection is suspected (fever with neck stiffness or rash) even before referral to hospital.

Supportive

Whenever possible patients with acute meningococcaemia should be nursed in an intensive care unit. Fluid balance, acid–base status, central venous pressure, and the electrocardiogram should be monitored. Assisted ventilation may be required. Circulatory volume is usually reduced, requiring infusion with a plasma expander. Pressor agents such as epinephrine (adrenalin) may be needed. Dopamine increases tissue perfusion and reduces the afterload on the heart. If a vasodilator is used, further colloid infusion may be required to maintain the circulation.

The value of corticosteroids in the management of shocked patients with acute meningococcaemia has never been established by a controlled trial and, at present, there is insufficient evidence to recommend high dose steroids as routine therapy. Cardiac arrhythmias should be treated conventionally.

Bleeding may be an important feature of acute meningococcaemia. A beneficial response to therapy with heparin has been reported in individual cases but a controlled trial showed no overall benefit. If bleeding is severe, blood and platelet transfusions may be required.

Attempts have been made to remove endotoxin by plasmapheresis or to neutralize endotoxin/cytokines with more clonal or polyclonal antibodies. No large scale controlled trials have yet been reported.

Meningitis

Antibiotics

Crystalline penicillin, 3–5 mega units, should be given intravenously or intramuscularly every 6 h for 5–7 days. The emergence of penicillin insensitive strains has encouraged the use of cephalosporins such as ceftriaxone in some countries. Chloramphenicol, given to adults in a dosage of 750 mg 6-hourly, is an effective alternative to penicillin.

During large epidemics medical resources may be swamped. Under such circumstances, a single injection of an oily preparation of chloramphenicol (Tifomycine) (adult dose 3 g) has saved many lives.

Penicillin and chloramphenicol suppress, but do not usually eradicate, nasopharyngeal carriage of meningococci and a patient could infect contacts after leaving hospital. Thus, it has been suggested that patients should be given treatment to eradicate carriage (see below) before discharge from hospital.

Supportive

Unconscious patients require careful nursing, particular attention being paid to their airway. They are often dehydrated, especially in hot countries and intravenous rehydration may be required. Headache may be very severe and may be an important cause of restlessness. If it cannot be controlled with simple analgesics, pethidine may be needed. Diazepam is of value in quietening restless and violent patients, and in controlling convulsions. If signs of severe raised intracranial pressure are present, dexamethasone should be considered.

The development of arthritis or cutaneous vasculitis during the recovery phase of the infection is not an indication for the continuation of antibiotic therapy. Arthritis responds well to aspirin.

Dexamethasone reduces the incidence of late complications, especially deafness in children with *Haemophilus influenzae* meningitis but, at present, no firm recommendations can be made about the efficacy of dexamethasone in preventing neurological sequelae in patients with meningococcal meningitis.

Table 2 Recommended doses of antibiotics for chemoprophylaxis against meningococcal disease

	Rifampicin (2 days)	Ceftriaxone (1 day)	Ciprofloxacin (1 day)
Adults	600 mg twice/day	250 mg single dose	500 mg single dose
Children >1 year	10 mg/kg twice/day	125 mg single dose	125/250 mg single dose

Prophylaxis

Chemoprophylaxis

Rifampicin is the antibiotic most widely used for chemoprophylaxis in household and intimate contacts of cases of meningococcal disease. This has resulted in the rapid appearance of rifampicin-resistant meningococci. Recently, studies have shown that a single injection of ceftriaxone or a single dose of oral ciprofloxacin can eradicate carriage (Table 2).

Vaccination

Introduction

Bivalent (A+C) and tetravalent (A, C, Y, and W135) capsular polysaccharide vaccines are widely available. Several large trials, mostly conducted in Africa, showed that group A and group C capsular polysaccharide vaccines could control epidemics very effectively but protection was only temporary in young children. Thus, polysaccharide protein conjugate vaccines are being developed, which are immunogenic in young children, which induce immunological memory and which should provide prolonged protection. Several trials of such vaccines are now in progress.

The group B capsular polysaccharide is poorly immunogenic and, in its native form, cannot be used as a vaccine. Attempts have been made to improve its immunogenicity by modifying the structure of the polysaccharide in various ways but clinical vaccines based on this approach have not yet been developed. More success has been achieved with group B vaccines based on outer membrane proteins and two experimental vaccines, developed in Cuba and Norway, have been tested in clinical trials with some success. However, no group B vaccines are currently available commercially.

Management of endemic meningococcal disease or small outbreaks

When a single case or a small cluster of cases of meningococcal disease are detected preventive measures should be taken to stop further spread (Fig. 5). Those most at risk of contracting meningococcal disease are close household contacts of a patient. If the organism is known to belong to group A, C, W135, or Y, contacts should be vaccinated immediately with an appropriate polysaccharide vaccine. However, as many secondary, or perhaps coprimary cases, occur within a few days of the onset of illness in the index case, chemoprophylaxis should also be given.

When a case of meningococcal disease occurs in a residential school, doss house, or barracks, further cases can be expected. Subjects in close contact with the patient, for example those sleeping in the same small dormitory, should be managed in the same way as household contacts. People with less contact with the patient should be vaccinated if the causative meningococcus belongs to serogroup A, C, W135, or Y. Whether such contacts should be given chemoprophylaxis will depend upon the nature of the outbreak—this may be impractical and unnecessary if the number of contacts is very

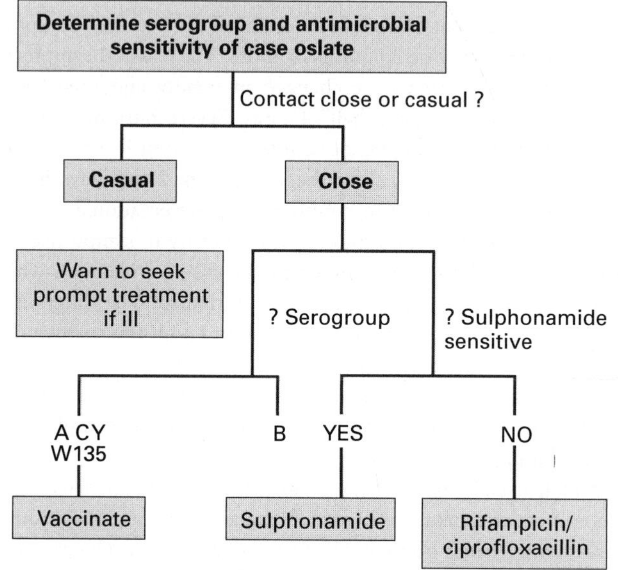

Fig. 5 A scheme for the management of a contact of a patient with meningococcal disease.

large. Recently, there have been a few reports of spread of the infection in day schools, so vaccination and/or chemoprophylaxis for the class mates of a case is probably a wise precaution. Clinical staff who come into regular contact with patients with meningococcal disease or with their laboratory samples should also be vaccinated.

Management of an epidemic

The first essential in the management of an epidemic of meningococcal disease is to establish as soon as possible that an epidemic has started. In Africa, an epidemic is likely when the incidence of cases is a defined area exceeds 15 per 100 000 population per week averaged over a period of 2 weeks. The next essential is to determine as quickly as possible the serogroup and antimicrobial sensitivity pattern of the causative meningococcus. A sound management team must be built up rapidly and, in areas where outbreaks are frequent, an action plan should be in existence that can be activated at short notice. Epidemics of meningococcal meningitis may swamp the routine medical services, a hundred new cases a day is not unusual, so it may be necessary to establish temporary treatment centres. Long-acting chloramphenicol is invaluable for treatment in such circumstances. Chemoprophylaxis is of little or no value in the management of epidemics but the effects of vaccination may be dramatic, stopping an epidemic of group A or group C meningococcal meningitis in its tracks. Vaccination must be done as soon as possible after an epidemic has been identified if it is to achieve its maximum effect and limited supplies of vaccine should be maintained in areas where epidemics are likely. The whole population should be vaccinated unless vaccine is in short supply, when targeted vaccination may be indicated. Too often unnecessary lives have been lost when vaccination was delayed until an epidemic was already past its peak.

Further reading

Cassio de Moraes, J., Perkins, B.A., Camargo, M.C.C., *et al.* (1992). Protective efficacy of a serogroup B meningococcal vaccine in São Paulo, Brazil. *Lancet*, **340**, 1074–8.

Galmand, M. *et al.* (1998). High level chloramphenicol resistance in *Neissena meningitidis. New England Journal of Medicine*, **339**, 868–74.

Gedde-Dahl, T.W., Bjark, P., Hoiby, E.A., Host, J.H., and Brun, J.N. (1990). Severity of meningococcal disease: assessment by factors and scores and implications for patient management. *Reviews of Infectious Diseases*, **12**, 973–92.

Moore, P.S. (1992). Meningococcal meningitis in sub-Saharan Africa: a model for the epidemic process. *Clinical Infectious Diseases*, **14**, 515–25.

Quagliarello, V. and Scheld, W.M. (1992). Bacterial meningitis: pathogenesis, pathophysiology and progress. *New England Journal of Medicine*, **327**, 864–72.

Quagliarello, V.J. and Scheld, W.M. (1997). Treatment of bacterial meningitis. *New England Journal of Medicine*, **336**, 708–16.

Riedo, F.X., Plikaytis, B.D., and Broome, C.V. (1995). Epidemiology and prevention of meningococcal disease. *Pediatric Infectious Disease Journal*, **14**, 643–57.

Westendorp, R.G.J., Langermans, J.A.M., Huizinga, T.W.J., *et al.* (1997). Genetic influence on cytokine production and fatal meningococcal disease. *Lancet*, **349**, 170–3.

Chapter 16.42

Neisseria gonorrhoeae

D. Barlow

Pathogenesis

Neisseria gonorrhoeae, first observed by Albert Neisser in 1879, colonizes the mucosa of the anogenital tract but can invade other sites (oropharynx, eyes), and cause systemic disease. For successful colonization, the gonococcus must adhere to an epithelial cell, attaching preferentially to columnar rather than to squamous epithelium.

After attachment, the organism enters the cell and has evolved mechanisms to evade host defences and to cause repeated infection. The main antigens of the outer membrane of the gonococcus that are exposed to the immune response are pili, lipo-oligosaccharide, and three major outer membrane proteins, Por, Opa, and Rmp.

Pili, Opa, and lipo-oligosaccharide can alter their antigens thus presenting a range of immunologically distinct proteins not recognized by the host. Secretory IgA in mucosal secretions may be cleaved by extracellular gonococcal IgA1 protease. Gonococci that are piliated and express some Opa proteins can survive in phagocytes. The balance between the ability of phagocytes to kill gonococci and survival of bacteria within these cells is probably the major determinant in the pathogenesis of gonorrhoea.

Vaccination against gonorrhoea is unsuccessful, probably due to antigenic variation.

Epidemiology

Figure 1 details cases of gonorrhoea notified between 1918 and 1997 in England. Although the sharp decline from 1946 coincided with a more widespread availability of penicillin, suggesting a causal relationship, the subsequent increase between the mid-1950s and mid-1970s accompanied a proliferation of antimicrobial agents with activity against the gonococcus. Behaviour is probably at least as important as effective treatment in determining levels of infection, although antimicrobials have reduced the incidence of complications in the Western world.

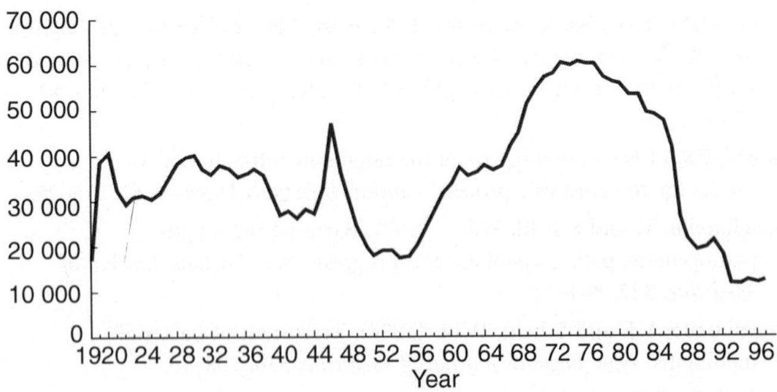

Fig. 1 Reported cases of gonorrhoea in England between 1918 and 1997 (Department of Health, UK).

Table 1 Historical incubation period (IP) of gonorrhoea in men

Year of study	No. of patients	Mean IP (days)	Treatment
1932	115	4.9	Topical
1942	220	4.6	Sulphonamides
1952	193	6.0	Penicillin
1954/5	145	6.1	Penicillin
1978	242	6.2	Penicillin
1989	113	7.9	Penicillin
1990/2	228	8.3	Penicillin

Like other STDs, including HIV, gonorrhoea is not evenly distributed through the sexually active population. The same behaviour (unprotected penetrative sexual intercourse) may carry different risks depending on the context. Sporadic cases of gonorrhoea are seen in rural areas and small towns but the highest incidence in the UK and US is found in larger conurbations, among the young, the socioeconomically deprived, and ethnic minorities. Differential incidence of gonorrhoea between subpopulations reflects relative lack of sexual mixing.

Populations with high incidences of gonorrhoea have a higher risk of HIV and gonorrhoea is an independent cofactor for HIV transmission. HIV-positive men with gonococcal urethritis are more likely to have virus particles in urethral secretions than those without gonorrhoea, successful treatment abolishing this difference.

The incidence of neonatal gonococcal ophthalmia and the prevalence of gonorrhoea in antenatal populations reflect the comparative success of control programmes. By both of these criteria gonorrhoea is not a significant problem at present in the UK.

Changes since the Second World War include decreasing sensitivity to antimicrobials, lengthening of the incubation period, and diminution in symptoms. These changes have coincided with (and may well have resulted from) widespread and, in some parts of the world, indiscriminate use of antimicrobials. The infectivity of the gonococcus is probably higher for male-to-female transmission than in the opposite direction. Condoms, if used properly and invariably, reduce transmission of gonorrhoea.

Incubation period, symptoms, and signs

The incubation period of gonorrhoea in men is increasing—a recent study giving a mean of 8.3 days with a median of 5.8 days (Table 1). By 14 days, 86 per cent of men had developed symptoms. The upper limit of the range may be 3 months or more. The classical symptoms of discharge and dysuria have changed in quality and prevalence, occurring in only perhaps a half of cases. Severe burning is rarely reported. Asymptomatic gonococcal infection is seen in up to 5 per cent of cases. An increase, since the 1930s from 2 to 6 days in the delay between development of symptoms and presentation at a clinic for treatment may reflect a diminution in severity of symptoms.

Gonorrhoea progresses from mucoid to profuse, purulent, off-white discharge, eventually becoming scanty if untreated. The differential diagnosis includes foreign body in the urethra and, unusually, non-gonococcal urethritis.

Oropharyngeal and rectal gonorrhoea in either sex are usually not associated with symptoms, apart from the occasional complaint of rectal discharge.

Although usually asymptomatic, 40 per cent of women with gonorrhoea note an increase in vaginal discharge (without distinguishing features) with dysuria occurring in perhaps 12 per cent. The presence of another sexually transmitted disease such as *Trichomonas vaginalis* may prompt attendance.

Signs of uncomplicated gonorrhoea in women are unreliable, a purulent exudate from the cervical os being found in other conditions.

Complications

In the UK, epididymo-orchitis associated with urethral gonorrhoea (usually unilateral) occurs in fewer than 2 per cent of cases and other local complications are of only anecdotal occurrence. Urethral stricture is rarely seen today.

Complications of gonorrhoea in women amount to less than 5 per cent of cases in the UK. They include bartholinitis, skenitis, and periurethral abscess (all rare). Infection may spread to the endometrium, fallopian tubes, and pelvic organs. Commonly, symptomatic pelvic infection first appears towards the end of, or soon after, a menstrual period. Lower abdominal pain and tenderness (often unilateral) and deep dyspareunia occur, with some constitutional upset. Reduced fertility and increased risk of ectopic pregnancy are later sequelae.

The FitzHugh–Curtis syndrome, perihepatitis, is today more often associated with chlamydial than gonococcal infection and occurs predominantly in women without genital symptoms. The right hypochondrial pain, sometimes referred to the shoulder and sometimes associated with a sympathetic pleural effusion with rub, leads the patient to a surgeon or a general, rather than genitourinary, physician.

Gonoccocal bacterial endocarditis and meningitis are rare today. Gonococcal septicaemia occurs in 1 to 2 per cent of cases and affects predominantly skin and joints. Certain auxotypes (AHU) are associated with disseminated gonococcal infection and are uniformly sensitive to penicillin. This is a surprisingly benign condition although penicillinase-producing *N. gonorrhoeae* (PPNG) may produce a destructive monoarthritis

The skin lesions, found mainly on the extremities, have a reddened areola and evolve through macular (1–2 mm in diameter), vesiculopustular, haemorrhagic, and necrotic stages. They are virtually pathognomonic of disseminated gonococcal infection. There are usually between four and ten lesions, not particularly painful, and the gonococcus can be cultured from these. Frankly haemorrhagic bullae and erythema nodosum-like lesions have been described.

Joint involvement may simply be a flitting polyarthralgia, although effusions in larger joints are seen. The shoulder, knee, wrist, and ankle, followed by the small joints of the hands and feet, are commonly involved often with an associated tenosynovitis. Blood culture or examination of effusion are less helpful than culture of samples from anogenital sites.

Patients with disseminated infection tend not to have had genital symptoms, women outnumbering men by 5 to 1. The systemic manifestations lead patients to present more often to dermatologists, rheumatologists, or general physicians rather than genitourinary physicians.

Prepubertal gonococcal vulvovaginitis should raise the possibility of sexual abuse but undoubtedly infection can be transmitted by fomites such as flannels and towels. Gonococcal ophthalmia neonatorum presents with a purulent conjunctival exudate within 48 h of birth and remains important in developing countries and 1 per cent aqueous silver nitrate, applied to the eyes of newborn babies, may be used prophylactically. In the UK, neonatal sticky eye is more likely to be due to *Chlamydia trachomatis*.

Diagnosis

More time and effort is spent excluding rather than diagnosing gonorrhoea. Investigations therefore need high sensitivity (and specificity). The diagnosis of gonococcal infection in men is easier than in women.

In men, uncomplicated infection affects the anterior urethra. Rectal infection results from insertive anal intercourse or occasionally from digital insertion. Oropharyngeal infection is found in 5 to 20 per cent of cases (the higher figure in homosexual men). Transmission from throat to penis can occur during fellatio and in both sexes the throat may be the source of disseminated gonococcal infection.

In infected women, the organism is found in the cervix (90 per cent), the urethra (75 per cent), rectum (40 per cent), and oropharynx (15 per cent). In about 5 per cent of cases each, the organism will be found only in the rectum or urethra—both sites should be free from infection to exclude gonorrhoea.

A diagnosis of gonorrhoea should prompt search for other sexually transmitted diseases and the initiation of contact tracing.

Microscopy, culture, and identification

Microscopy is the first line in diagnosis. The organisms must be Gram-negative, intracellular diplococci. In samples from the male urethra, microscopy will identify 95 per cent of symptomatic cases but only 80 per cent of asymptomatic ones. Less than 1 per cent will be found on culture to be *N. meningitidis*.

Microscopy of stained samples from female sites identifies less than 55 per cent of true positives. Laboratory culture is therefore essential in women. The presence of other neisseriae negates the usefulness of microscopy from the oropharynx.

Culture remains the 'gold standard' for the diagnosis of gonorrhoea. Highest isolation rates are obtained by inoculating the specimen directly on fresh medium in the clinic, incubating at 37°C until transported to the laboratory. Alternatively, the swab can be transported in Stuart's or Amies' medium. Speed is of the essence.

Culture media should be selective but non-inhibitory, containing antibiotics and an antifungal. It is advisable to repeat full tests at least once when negative results are obtained from gonorrhoea contacts.

Successful incubation requires freshly prepared media with high humidity and carbon dioxide for at least 48 h (OTM3, p. 547). Culture for *N. gonorrhoeae* has a sensitivity approaching 100 per cent in clinics and laboratories with the appropriate experience and skill but the isolation rate may be lower in general practice and smaller clinics.

Routine culture of samples from the male urethra provides an important means of quality control of the laboratory service. Serological tests lack specificity and sensitivity and should not be used in the diagnosis or exclusion of gonorrhoea.

Other means of detecting gonococci include enzyme-linked assays, immunofluorescence, and DNA probes. None is as rapid, simple, or economical as the Gram stain for presumptive diagnosis and culture remains necessary for antimicrobial susceptibility testing. Correct identification as *N. gonorrhoeae*, by carbohydrate utilization tests and monoclonal antibodies, is important in cases of possible sexual or child abuse. Two techniques have been used extensively: auxotyping (determination of nutritional requirement) and serotyping (identifying patterns of reactivity with a panel of monoclonal antibodies (see OTM3, p. 548).

Treatment

The ideal management of gonorrhoea—diagnosis before treatment—is not universally applied. The 'epidemiological' approach—treatment before (or without) diagnosis—may be without alternative if proper diagnostic facilities are not available.

Gonococci with plasmid-mediated resistance to penicillin pose serious therapeutic dilemmas in Third World countries. In the UK, PPNG remains largely imported and can often be predicted by means of travel history or geographical family background.

Uncomplicated gonorrhoea is ideally treated with a single dose of antimicrobial, orally or by intramuscular injection. In London, in 1998, 2 g of amoxicillin with 1 g of probenecid gives a cure rate of over 95 per cent, provided cases of PPNG are predicted and treated appropriately. The Centers for Disease Control (CDC) in Atlanta advise 3.5 g of amoxycillin with 1 g of probenecid for uncomplicated gonorrhoea (reflecting reduced sensitivity of organisms in the US).

Most of the 4-quinolones, for instance ciprofloxacin 500 mg orally, are highly effective against gonorrhoea, including PPNG.

Single intramuscular treatments for uncomplicated gonorrhoea include procaine benzylpenicillin 2.4 g, with 1 g of probenecid, third-generation cephalosporins (cefotaxime 1 g or ceftriaxone 0.5 g) and spectinomycin 2–4 g. The last three are effective against PPNG.

Oropharyngeal infection responds to a single 500 mg dose of ciprofloxacin or ceftriaxone 250 mg, intramuscular.

Pregnant women have been successfully treated in London with two doses of amoxycillin 3 g, given 24 h apart. Ceftriaxone 0.25 g, intramuscularly, gives good cure rates in the US.

Disseminated gonococcal infection will require 2 g of amoxycillin with 1 g of probenecid daily, in divided doses, for 5 to 7 days. Response to treatment is rapid.

The eye may not be the only site infected in the newborn and systemic treatment is advised for ophthalmia neonatorum. Ceftriaxone, recommended by the CDC, is not licensed during the first 6 weeks of life in the UK but single-dose cefotaxime 100 mg/kg intramuscular has been recommended. Alternatives include benzylpenicillin 30 mg/kg (50 000 IU/kg) intramuscularly in two divided doses daily for 2 days, or procaine benzylpenicillin 50 000 IU intramuscularly daily for 3 days.

Pelvic infection associated with gonorrhoea is likely to be complicated by *Chlamydia trachomatis* and antigonococcal therapy should be changed after 1 or 2 days to oxytetracycline or erythromycin stearate, 2 g daily in divided doses for 2 weeks. A similar regimen may be used for gonococcal epididymo-orchitis. Rest in bed is advised for both conditions.

Following treatment of gonorrhoea, investigations should be made at 1 to 2 and, say, 10 days to identify relapse and reinfection. Contact tracing reduces the rate of reinfection.

Antimicrobial resistance (see OTM3, pp. 548–9) is found mostly among imported strains.

Further reading

Barlow, D. and Phillips, I. (1978). Gonorrhoea in women—diagnostic, clinical and therapeutic aspects. *Lancet*, i, 761–4.

Bignell, C. (1996). Antibiotic treatment of gonorrhoea—clinical evidence for choice. *Genitourinary Medicine*, 72, 315–20.

Bignell, C. (1999). *National guidelines on the management of gonorrhoea in adults.* www.mssvd.org.uk

Ison, C.A. (1996). Antimicrobial agents and gonorrhoea: therapeutic choice, resistance and susceptibility testing. *Genitourinary Medicine*, 72, 253–7.

Ross, J.D.C. (1996). Systemic gonococcal infection. *Genitourinary Medicine*, 72, 404–7.

Sherrard, J. and Barlow, D. (1996). Gonorrhoea in men—clinical and diagnostic aspects. *Genitourinary Medicine*, 72, 422–6.

Chapter 16.43

Enterobacteria, Campylobacter, and miscellaneous food-poisoning bacteria

M. B. Skirrow

In this chapter is described the main groups of bacteria (other than cholera vibrios) that cause acute intestinal infection and diarrhoea. The impact of these infections is immense. In developing countries they are a major cause of childhood morbidity and mortality, and in industrialized countries they are a severe burden on economic and health resources. But before describing these infections, a word must be said on the role of enterobacteria and similar Gram-negative bacilli in infections elsewhere in the body, particularly as a cause of hospital infection.

Extraintestinal infections caused by enterobacteria and related organisms

Enterobacteria thrive under a variety of wet conditions and readily colonize hospital environments. They are a potent source of nosocomial infection (see Chapter 16.8). Among the groups most likely to be encountered are *Escherichia, Klebsiella, Enterobacter, Citrobacter,* and *Proteus.* A commonly used all-embracing term for these organisms is 'coliform bacteria'. Other groups of Gram-negative bacilli that behave in a similar way to enterobacteria and are often found in mixed infections with them are *Pseudomonas, Alcaligenes,* and *Acinetobacter.* Many of these show natural resistance to commonly used antimicrobial agents and to many antiseptics.

The widespread use and misuse of antibiotics encourages these bacteria to become established in the hospital environment. Such organisms often replace the normal sensitive bowel flora of patients within a few days of admission, particularly if antibiotics are being given. The patient's anus then becomes the gateway to infection elsewhere in the body—the urinary and respiratory tracts, wounds, catheter sites, ulcers, or wherever the body integument is broken. In most cases this is simple colonization for which specific treatment is neither necessary nor feasible, but sometimes these infections can be a nidus for septicaemia. These infections are described in the relevant sections elsewhere in the book.

Salmonella infections

Clinically, it is convenient to divide salmonellae into two groups: those that cause typhoid and paratyphoid fever (*S. typhi*; *S. paratyphi* A, B, and C), and those associated with food poisoning and acute enteritis. The latter group include *S. enteritidis* and *S. typhimurium*, which account for 75 per cent of all human salmonella infections, but there are well over 2000 other serotypes, usually named after the place they were first isolated, for example *S. indiana, S. newport.* Only a small proportion of these 2000 serotypes regularly cause human infection. Individual strains within these serotypes are recognized by phage typing.

Epidemiology

In Europe and North America, the incidence of salmonella enteritis is 50–70 per 100 000 of the population per year, according to laboratory diagnosed infections, but the true incidence is probably at least ten times higher. In the US, the socio-economic cost is estimated to be $1.4 billion per annum. In temperate zones there is a seasonal peak of infection in late summer.

Salmonella enteritis is essentially a food-borne infection originating from food producing animals in which salmonellae are enzootic. This is in sharp contrast to *S. typhi* and *S. paratyphi,* which are confined to man. Raw meats, especially poultry, eggs, and raw dairy products are foods that are regularly contaminated. This is not as bad as it might appear, for the dose of salmonellae required to cause clinical infection is usually large and only likely to be reached if multiplication of bacteria is allowed to occur in the food before consumption.

Processed foods can occasionally become contaminated during manufacture and cause outbreaks on a wide scale. Examples of foods implicated in such outbreaks are dried egg, dried milk infant food, desiccated coconut, bean sprouts, cheese, and chocolate.

The prevalence of serotypes causing human infection is constantly changing according to the pattern of infection in food-producing animals. For example since 1985 the incidence of *S. enteritidis* phage type 4 infection in Europe rose to unprecedented heights as a result of its establishment in poultry, for which these strains became unusually invasive. In particular, oviduct infection led to the contamination of eggs, which was a new and unexpected development.

Person-to-person spread of salmonellae is only likely to occur among infants, old people, and patients living in closed communities such as nursing homes and asylums. Salmonellae can be especially troublesome in hospital maternity units. The importance of a salmonella-excreting food handler as a source of infection has been exaggerated. Such a person is more likely to be the victim of handling contaminated animal products at work than a source of infection.

Pathology

Although the infective dose of salmonellae is usually high, there are important exceptions. As few as 50 bacteria contained in certain high-fat foods, notably chocolate, cheese, and salami, can cause illness.

Anything that reduces gastric acidity, such as atrophic gastritis, treatment with H2 receptor blocking agents, or previous gastric surgery, also lowers the infective dose. Broad spectrum antibiotics increase susceptibility by suppressing the normal competitive microflora of the gut.

The small intestine is the main site of infection, but the colon may also be affected. Salmonellae are invasive in the bowel mucosa and they can penetrate deep to the lamina propria. Invasion is accompanied by an acute inflammatory response with polymorphonuclear cell infiltration of the submucosa. Flattening or loss of secretory epithelium occurs adjacent to these inflamed areas. Inflammatory cells are usually present in faeces.

Bacteraemia has been reported in 1.5 per cent of all laboratory diagnosed infections, but at much higher rates in patients with *S. cholerae-suls* (75 per cent) and *S. dublin* (40 per cent) infections.

Clinical features

Not everyone with salmonella infection becomes ill, in every food-poisoning outbreak there are unaffected persons who excrete salmonellae in their faeces. Others suffer a typical attack of acute enteritis lasting 2 or 3 days, and there are usually a few who suffer a more severe, prolonged attack. The proportion of people who become ill is determined by the extent of contamination of the food and the properties of the infecting strain.

The incubation period is usually 12 to 24 h (range 6 to 48 h). The onset is abrupt, with malaise, nausea, abdominal cramps, diarrhoea, headache, and sometimes vomiting. Fever is common. Severe, even fatal illness, with dehydration, oliguria, and uraemia may affect infants or elderly patients.

Reactive arthritis is an occasional late sequel of infection. Estimates of its incidence range from 1.2 to 7.3 per cent of all infections. Patients with HLA B27 haplotype have a strong predisposition for this troublesome but, usually benign, complication.

Most patients continue to excrete salmonellae in their faeces for 4 to 8 weeks after infection. Carriage of salmonellae (other than *S. typhi* or *S. paratyphi*) for more than 6 months is rare.

Focal infection

Focal infections may be difficult to diagnose because they may only manifest themselves long after an episode of enteritis—or the original bowel infection may even have been silent. They have a tendency to chronicity and can mimic tuberculosis, particularly in cases of osteomyelitis of a vertebra or paravertebral abscess. Salmonella osteomyelitis and arthritis are strongly associated with sickle-cell anaemia (see Chapter 3.19). Salmonella abscess may develop in the liver, gall bladder, spleen, psoas muscle, uterus (after septic abortion), and in the peritoneal cavity (e.g. subphrenic, pelvic). Patients with deep-seated salmonella infection who go untreated suffer high mortality.

Laboratory diagnosis

Diagnosis depends on isolation of the salmonella. In most clinical laboratories, recognition of an organism as a salmonella is straightforward, but identification of the serotype or phagetype is a task for a reference laboratory.

Treatment

Supportive treatment is all that is required for patients with uncomplicated salmonella enteritis. Antimicrobial therapy shows little or no clinical benefit in these patients, but it is advisable for severely ill patients. It is essential for invasive and focal disease, which may require intensive treatment for several weeks. Laboratory control is necessary owing to the increasing rates of antimicrobial resistance among salmonellae. For this reason, ampicillin and co-trimoxazole have largely been superseded by fluoroquinolones, which are at least as effective, although resistance is emerging even to this group. Ciprofloxacin has been used successfully to eradicate salmonellae from chronic carriers.

Prevention and control

The ultimate aim in the prevention of salmonella enteritis is to control infection in food-producing animals, but there are many problems to this approach and currently control is only partial. Thus prevention relies heavily on the correct handling, preparation, and storage of food.

All milk sold to the public should be pasteurized, and dishes incorporating raw eggs should not be served to the public. The terminal disinfection of poultry carcasses by irradiation would do much to reduce infection.

Shigella infections: bacillary dysentery

There are four groups of dysentery bacilli. *Sh. dysenteriae* is the classical organism described by Kiyoshi Shiga in 1897 and is the most highly pathogenic species. There are 10 serotypes, but only type 1 ('*Sh. shigae*') and type 2 ('*Sh. schmitzi*') are important human pathogens. *Sh. flexneri* (13 serotypes) and *Sh. boydii* (15 serotypes) are of intermediate pathogenicity. The least pathogenic is *Sh. sonnel*, which is serologically homogenous, but strains can be differentiated by phage and colicine typing.

Epidemiology

Sh. dysenteriae type 1 causes epidemics of classical dysentery, such as those that ravaged the soldiers of the Crimean and American civil wars. It thrives under conditions of poverty, overcrowding, and squalor. After a period of quiescence, it re-emerged in the late 1960s to cause epidemic dysentery in central America, Mexico, and the Indian subcontinent. It is not endemic in industrialized countries. *Sh. flexneri* occurs world-wide but it is most prevalent in developing countries, as is the less common *Sh. boydii.*

Sh. sonnei is the prevalent species in industrialized countries. It particularly affects children in infant and primary schools, but outbreaks in residential institutions such as military barracks also occur.

Sources and transmission

Unlike salmonellae, shigellae are only found naturally in man and certain primates. With an unusually small infective dose, shigellosis is the most communicable of all bacterial infections of the gut. The principal route of transmission is from person to person by the direct faecal–oral spread of bacteria, mainly via the fingers, on which the bacteria can survive for several hours. Patients are most infectious when their stools are fluid, for not only are shigellae present in abundance but there is greater opportunity for droplet spread. Food and drink can easily become contaminated via the fingers and the bacteria do not have to multiply in food to cause infection. Flies can transmit infection from exposed human faeces and the incidence of dysentery tends to parallel fly activity. Large outbreaks of shigellosis have occasionally arisen through the faecal pollution of water supplies.

Pathology

The cardinal pathogenic feature of shigellae is their ability to invade and multiply in epithelial cells. *Sh. dysenteriae* type 1 produces a powerful exotoxin (Shiga toxin), which is associated with the haemolytic uraemic syndrome.

Colonization initially takes place in the jejunum and upper ileum, but the characteristic pathology produced by shigellae is an acute, locally invasive colitis. This ranges from mild catarrhal inflammation of the mucous membrane of the rectum and sigmoid colon, typical of *Sh. sonnei* infections, to severe necrotizing lesions affecting the whole colon and sometimes the terminal ileum, such as are seen in the worst forms of *Sh. dysenteriae* type 1 infection. Shigellae penetrate and multiply in the epithelial cells of the colon, invade the mucosa, and may penetrate deep to the lamina propria or even the muscularis mucosae. In the most severe forms of the disease, areas of mucosa undergo coagulation necrosis, which appear as thickened, semirigid, greyish patches. These eventually separate to leave raw, ulcerated areas that may ultimately fibrose and cause stenosis. Haemorrhage and perforation may also result from such lesions. Much protein is lost, which adds to the severe debility that accompanies these infections.

Clinical features

The incubation period is short, usually 2–3 days, but exceptionally it may be as long as a week. The illness usually starts with abdominal colic and watery diarrhoea, which may be the only manifestation of infection with *Sh. sonnel.* In the more severe forms of shigellosis, diarrhoea is accompanied by fever, headache, and malaise. After 1–3 days the diarrhoea gives way to the passage of small amounts of blood-stained mucus ('red-current jelly') and pus, with abdominal cramps and tenesmus—the classic dysenteric syndrome. The patient becomes toxic and restless, the pulse rapid and feeble, and there is a risk of death from circulatory failure or haemolytic uraemic syndrome (HUS). Recovery in such cases is invariably slow and some patients continue with chronic or relapsing infection resembling ulcerative colitis. Exacerbation of haemorrhoids and rectal prolapse may result from rectal oedema and straining at stool.

Reactive arthritis, Reiter's syndrome, purulent keratoconjuctivitis, and neuritis are uncommon, late complications of shigellosis. Shigellae are usually excreted in the faeces for a few weeks after the illness; about 10 per cent of patients excrete them for more than 10 weeks.

Laboratory diagnosis

Culture remains the standard method for detecting shigellae. They are delicate bacteria that perish in acid conditions, so it is necessary to refrigerate specimens or place them in buffered transport medium if there is to be a delay of more than a few hours before they are delivered to the laboratory.

Antimicrobial chemotherapy

Antimicrobial therapy is seldom needed for *Sh. sonnet* and other mild forms of shigellosis, but it is the mainstay of treatment for severe shigellosis. Laboratory control should always be sought, as strains showing multiple antimicrobial resistance are common, especially in developing countries.

Co-trimoxazole and ampicillin have been the drugs of choice for shigellosis, but most strains are now resistant. Nalidixic acid is effective and cheap, but high resistance rates have arisen where the drug has been used intensively. Resistance to ciprofloxacin, which is 100 times more active against shigellae than nalidixic acid, is less frequent. A single dose of 1 g is effective in adults infected with shigellae other than *Sh. dysenteriae* type 1, but up to 10 doses are required for infections with the latter type.

Prevention and control

The safe disposal of excreta, provision of purified water, and control of flies are fundamental to the control of shigellosis. Where these are lacking, incidence can be reduced by the promotion of personal and domestic hygiene, notably hand washing after defecation and before handling food. Breast feeding substantially increases resistance to infection in children, and oral vaccines for use in developing countries are being developed.

Infected food handlers and health-care workers nursing high risk patients should be excluded from work until they have produced at least three consecutive negative stool samples taken not less than 24 h apart and at least 2 days after cessation of any antimicrobial treatment.

Escherichia coli infections

E.coli bacteria are normally harmless inhabitants of the human intestinal tract, but certain strains possess virulence factors that make them potentially dangerous pathogens.

Enteroadherent *E. coli* (EAEC)

The characteristic feature of EAEC strains is that they produce an 'attaching and effacing' lesion in the brush border of enterocytes and the destruction of microvilli. This interferes with fluid reabsorption, which results in diarrhoea. EAEC strains are divided into three subgroups according to the manner in which they adhere to HEp-2 cells—locally, diffusely, or aggregatively. The former group contains most of the classical enteropathogenic *E. coli* (EPEC) strains that caused major outbreaks of infantile gastroenteritis in the late 1940s and 1950s, since when their importance in developed countries has declined.

Diffusely adherent *E. coli* (DEAC) and enteroaggregative *E. coli* (EAggEC) cause diarrhoea in children in developing countries, and there is mounting evidence that they cause traveller's diarrhoea in adults. Their study is hindered by the lack of easily applied methods of detection.

Enterotoxigenic *E. coli* (ETEC)

ETEC are a leading cause of childhood diarrhoea in developing countries and they are the commonest cause of traveller's diarrhoea or 'turista'. They are uncommon in temperate regions, but they have sometimes caused outbreaks of infection from contaminated water supplies, including outbreaks on cruise ships. ETEC are non-invasive, but produce diarrhoea through the action of one or both of two enterotoxins: a heat-labile (LT) cholera-like toxin and a heat-stable

(ST) toxin. These toxins can only exert their effect after the bacteria have adhered to the bowel epithelium by means of host-specific adhesins. For this reason strains that cause disease in, say, pigs do not do so in man. The dose of bacteria needed to cause disease is large—about 10^8–10^{10}. The incubation period ranges from 1–3 days depending on the size of infecting dose. The illness consists of watery diarrhoea with abdominal cramps, nausea, and sometimes vomiting, seldom lasting for more than 3 days.

There is no easy way to detect ETEC in faeces. The ideal approach is to detect the genes encoding LT or ST production directly in faeces by means of genetic probes, but such methods are not generally available. Immunological tests (ELISA, radioimmunoassay) are more widely available, but are not employed routinely, so it is vital that clinicians inform the laboratory if a patient's circumstances suggest ETEC infection.

Fluid and electrolyte replacement is usually all that is required for ETEC diarrhoea. Several antimicrobial agents, for example co-trimoxazole or trimethoprim, when taken prophylactically, reduce the incidence of ETEC diarrhoea in travellers to endemic areas, but drug toxicity and promotion of drug resistance in other pathogenic organisms are disadvantages (see Chapter 16.7).

Vero cytotoxin-producing *E. coli* (VTEC)

These strains, also known as enterohaemorrhagic *E. coli* (EHEC), get their name from the irreversible cytopathic changes they produce in African vervet monkey kidney (Vero) cells. They are the most dangerous of the pathogenic *E. coli* as they can cause haemorrhagic colitis and haemolytic uraemic syndrome (HUS) (see Chapter 12.10). Their virulence is due to the production of two Shiga-like toxins. Most VTEC strains belong to serogroup 0157.

The incidence of human VTEC infection is highest in late summer, but outbreaks may arise at any time of year. Dangerous though it is, the infection remains generally rare, with an annual incidence of 1–8 per 100 000. The source of VTEC strains is mainly beef cattle, but VTEC are also found in pigs and sheep. Undercooked minced beef is the food most often implicated in infection, but the range of food sources is potentially wide and largely undetermined. Outbreaks have been caused by the consumption of raw milk and untreated water. Infection can be passed from person to person.

The classical picture of VTEC infection is one of severe cramping abdominal pain and bloody diarrhoea with little or no fever. The diarrhoea is usually watery at first and in mild cases remains so. HUS may set in anything from 2–14 days (mean 7 days) after the onset of illness, particularly in children and old patients.

The diagnosis is usually made by detecting 0157 strains by culture on sorbitol MacConkey agar, but tests to detect the genes encoding for Shiga-like toxin production directly in faecal samples are more sensitive, and they detect toxigenic strains that belong to serogroups other than 0157. Such tests are currently available only in specialist laboratories. Serological tests that detect antibody to toxin or the 0157 group antigen are valuable for retrospective diagnosis in patients who present with HUS after the acute infection has resolved.

The most important element in treatment is to watch for signs of HUS, so that the patient can be given the necessary supportive treatment at the earliest opportunity. There is no clear evidence of the efficacy of antimicrobial agents, either to reduce acute symptoms or reduce the risk of HUS.

Enteroinvasive *E. coli* (EIEC)

EIEC are shigella-like bacteria that mainly cause dysentery in developing countries. Occasionally they have caused food-borne outbreaks in industrialized countries, mainly in residential institutions.

Campylobacter infections

Campylobacters are small, highly motile, curved or spiral vibrio-like organisms belonging to a distinct group of bacteria that includes *Helicobacter pylori.* The type species, *Campylobacter fetus,* causes infectious abortion in cattle and sheep, and it occasionally causes systemic infection in patients with immune deficiency or underlying disease. Here we more are concerned with the two species *C. jejuni* and *C. coli,* which cause campylobacter enteritis. Several other organisms of this group cause intestinal infection (e.g. *C. upsallensis, C. hyointestinalis,* and *Arcobacter butzleri*), but they are much less common. *Helicobacter cinaedi* and *H. fennelliae* are associated with proctitis in homosexual men.

Epidemiology

Campylobacters are the most frequent cause of acute infective diarrhoea in industrialized countries. The incidence of infection, according to laboratory reports, is about 100/100 000 per year, with a peak in early summer, but the true incidence is likely to be at least ten times this figure. Campylobacter enteritis affects people of all ages, especially young adults, but in developing countries it is almost entirely confined to young children, who become immune from repeated exposure early in life.

Sources and transmission

Like salmonellosis, campylobacter enteritis is a zoonosis. Campylobacters are found in a wide variety of warm-blooded animals, especially birds. Pigs are the main host of *C. coli.* Infection may be acquired by direct contact with infected animals, but more usually it is transmitted indirectly via contaminated meat, milk, and water, either through inadequate cooking or the crosscontamination of other foods from raw meats.

Contamination rates of 50–60 per cent are usual among retailed broiler chickens. Campylobacters do not multiply in food like salmonellae; the infective dose is small enough for the food to act as a passive vehicle. Cases of food-borne infection therefore tend to be sporadic, or in small family outbreaks, rather than as explosive outbreaks. However, major outbreaks affecting as many as 3000 people have been caused by the distribution of raw milk and untreated water.

The infectivity of campylobacters is low because they cannot withstand drying. Food handlers who are healthy excreters are a negligible risk to others provided they wash their hands after defecation.

Pathology

Infection starts in the upper ileum and progresses distally to affect the terminal ileum and colon. There is an acute inflammatory response with crypt abscess formation in the mucosa indistinguishable from that caused by salmonellae. This, and the presence of mesenteric adenitis, suggest that campylobacters invade the mucosa, although bacteraemia is detected in only 0.1–0.2 per cent of infections.

Many strains produce a cholera-like enterotoxin and/or cytotoxins *in vitro,* but their role in the pathogenesis of the disease is unclear.

Table 1 Principal microbial causes of food-poisoning outbreaks

Organism and mechanism	IP (h) (extreme range)	Main symptom
Salmonella Infection	12–24 (6–48)	Diarrhoea, 1–7 days
Staphylococcus aureus Toxin, preformed in food	2–6	Vomiting, 6–24 h
Clostridium perfringens Toxin, preformed in food, also in gut	6–22	Diarrhoea, 1–2 days
Clostridium botulinum Toxin, preformed in food	12–36 (2–12)	Neurological
Vibrio parahaemolyticus Infection	12–18 (2–48)	Diarrhoea, 1–2 days
Bacillus cereus Toxin, preformed in food Toxin, preformed in food also in gut	1–5 8–16	Vomiting, 6–24 h Diarrhoea, 12~24 h
Norwalk and small round-structured viruses (SRSV) Infection	15–50	Vomiting and diarrhoea, 12–72 h
Campylobacter Infection	72 (1–7 days)	Diarrhoea, 1–7 days
Escherichia coli 0157 Infection	3–4 days (1–8 days)	Diarrhoea (often bloody), 1–7 days

IP, incubation period.

Clinical features

After an incubation period of 2–7 days (mean 3 days) the illness starts either with abdominal pain and diarrhoea, or with a prodromal period of fever, headache, and other influenza-like symptoms which precedes the diarrhoea by a few hours to a few days. Some patients may present with the symptoms and sigmoidoscopic appearances of acute ulcerative colitis. A fever of 40°C or more is not unusual and it may be associated with convulsions in children and delirium in adults. Nausea is common but vomiting is not. Abdominal pain tends to be particularly severe and it can mimic acute appendicitis. The faeces usually contains inflammatory cells, and frank blood may appear after a day or two. Most patients are culture negative after about 5 weeks.

Complications

Acute complications are rare. They include gastrointestinal haemorrhage, glomerulonephritis, HUS, and rashes in the form of urticaria and erythema nodosum. Cholecystitis and pancreatitis have also been reported. Two late complications may arise 1–3 weeks after the onset of illness. The first is a troublesome but ultimately benign reactive arthritis that affects about 1 per cent of patients. The second is the uncommon but more serious Guillain-Barré syndrome (GBS), or acute polyneuropathy (see Section 13). Indeed campylobacter enteritis is the most frequently identified antecedent event in this condition (26–41 per cent of cases). Moreover, campylobacter-associated cases have a worse prognosis than average.

Laboratory diagnosis

Diagnosis depends on the isolation of campylobacters from faeces, as the disease cannot be distinguished clinically from other forms of bacterial diarrhoea. Faecal samples held for more than a few hours should be refrigerated. A retrospective diagnosis can be made serologically in culture-negative patients who have a suspected late complication such as reactive arthritis.

Antimicrobial therapy

Antimicrobials are of limited value because patients are usually recovering by the time a bacteriological diagnosis is made. They are effective if given early in the disease when patients are acutely ill. Erythromycin is the drug of first choice (e.g. erythromycin stearate 500 mg twice daily for 5 days). Resistance rates seldom exceed 5 per cent in most countries. Ciprofloxacin and other fluoroquinolones are effective, but resistant strains are common in some countries. Gentamicin is recommended for rare, life-threatening septicaemic infections. It should be noted that campylobacters are naturally resistant or partially resistant to almost all cephalosporins and ampicillin.

Prevention and control

As campylobacters and salmonellae share the same food-producing animal hosts, the measures taken to control salmonellosis also apply to campylobacters, in particular the application of good hygienic practice in the preparation and handling of food. A longer-term but much needed measure is the control of infection in broiler flocks and poultry processing plants.

Non-cholera vibrios and vibrio-like organisms

Vibrio parahaemolyticus

This marine bacterium causes a disease like that produced by enterotoxigenic *E. coli*, namely watery diarrhoea lasting for about 3 days.

The infection is acquired from eating raw seafood. It is the most common form of food poisoning in Japan, but is uncommon in most temperate countries. The incubation period is usually about 20 h (range 4–96 h).

Several other aquatic vibrios associated with shellfish (*V. fluvialls, V. hollisae, V. mimicus*) can cause watery diarrhoea and vomiting. *V. vulnificus* is a rare cause of severe septicaemia arising from intestinal infection acquired by eating raw oysters. Some vibrios, notably *V. alginolyticus*, cause external otitis and wound infection in swimmers in brackish or sea water.

It is essential to inform the laboratory if infection with any of these vibrios is suspected, as several of them are halophilic and require culture media supplemented with extra salt.

Aeromonas and *Plesiomonas*

Aeromonads are ubiquitous in water, soil, and cold-blooded animals. Their status as human pathogens is unclear, but it seems that some strains, mainly *Aeromonas hydrophila*, are capable of causing diarrhoea. Aeromonads are more frequent in hot climates, so most aeromonas infections are encountered in travellers visiting tropical and subtropical regions. Persistent aeromonas-associated diarrhoea with blood and mucus mimicking ulcerative colitis has been described in western Australia. These patients were treated successfully with trimethoprim.

Plesiomonas shigelloides is another aquatic, vibrio-like organism that is occasionally associated with diarrhoea, usually of a mild nature. It has been implicated in outbreaks of diarrhoea in the Far East and has been isolated from sporadic cases throughout the world.

Bacillus cereus and other food-poisoning bacteria

B. cereus is a member of a large group of Gram-positive, aerobic, spore-forming bacilli which includes the anthrax bacillus. It sometimes causes wound sepsis, but here we are concerned with its ability to form toxins if allowed to multiply in food. Two sorts of toxin may be produced: an emetic toxin that causes vomiting, and an enterotoxin that causes diarrhoea (Table 1). The former is almost exclusively associated with Chinese restaurants that prepare boiled rice in bulk for repeated reheating and serving. As a spore-forming bacterium it is able to survive this treatment and multiply to enormous numbers. Diagnosis depends on finding counts of *B. cereus* in excess of 105 per g in the suspect food and its detection in vomitus or faeces of victims.

The main microbial causes of food poisoning and their principal features are summarized in Table 1.

Further reading

Bennish, M.L. and Salam, M.A. (1992). Rethinking options for the treatment of shigellosis. *Journal of Antimicrobial Chemotherapy*, **30**, 243–7.

Blaser, M.J., Smith P.D., Radvin J.I., Greenberg H.B., and Guerrant R.L. (eds) (1995). *Infections of the intestinal tract.* Raven Press, New York.

Lang, D.R., Blaser, M.J., and Mishu Allos, B. (eds). (1997). Development of Guillain–Barré syndrome following *Campylobacter infection. Journal of Infectious Diseases*, **176**, (Suppl 2).

Law, D. (1994). Adhesion and its role in the virulence of enteropathogenic *Escherichia coli. Clinical Microbiology Reviews*, 7, 152–73.

Mead, P.S. and Griffin, P.M. (1998). *Escherichia coli* 0157:H7. *Lancet*, **352**, 1207–12.

Mishu Allos, B. and Blaser, M.J. (1995). *Campylobacter jejuni* and the expanding spectrum of related infections. *Clinical Infectious Diseases*, **20**, 1092–9.

Chapter 16.44

Typhoid and paratyphoid fevers

J. Richens

Typhoid

Introduction

Typhoid and paratyphoid, types A, B, and C (often referred to collectively as enteric fever) make up the small group of salmonelloses whose main host is human. The clinical features of these four infections show much overlap and similarity to those observed in other forms of salmonellosis, ranging from a simple gastroenteritis (more common with paratyphoid) to the life-threatening septicaemic illness characteristic of severe typhoid.

Aetiology

The agents of enteric fever (*Salmonella typhi* and *paratyphi*) are robust, Gram-negative bacilli capable of surviving in harsh environments such as ice and able to reach high concentrations in dairy products, processed meats, and shellfish. The three antigens which have been traditionally exploited for purposes of serodiagnosis are the somatic oligosaccharide O antigen, the protein flagellar H antigen, and the polysaccharide envelope Vi antigen which appears to confer virulence by masking the O antigen from immunological attack. Extensive research on *S. typhimurium*, which serves as a good animal model of typhoid in mice, has led to the identification of many genes which enable invasive salmonellas to survive ingestion and even induce apoptosis in phagocytic cells.

Epidemiology

Typhoid is endemic in many parts of the tropics, notably South America, sub-Saharan Africa, Indonesia, and the Indian subcontinent. In areas of high transmission, annual incidence rates can reach 120 per 100 000 population (Papua New Guinea) and up to 1 per cent of the population may be carriers. In the tropics, case-fatality rates among hospitalized patients of 10 per cent are not unusual. In affluent countries, typhoid is mainly encountered in returned travellers and with prompt diagnosis and treatment well under 1 per cent of patients succumb to infection.

The sources of typhoid transmission are mainly excreting chronic or convalescent carriers and occasionally the acutely infected. Most transmission occurs indirectly through contamination by carriers of food or by contamination of water supplies by raw effluents containing infected urine or faeces from carriers.

Pathogenesis

Studies have shown that 10 million organisms (Quailes strain of *S. typhi*) are sufficient to infect 50 per cent of healthy experimental subjects. From the gut the bacteria pass through the cytoplasm of both normal enterocytes and M cells that overlie lymphoid tissue (Peyer's patches) of the small intestine to reach the lamina propria from which they are conveyed to the mesenteric nodes, eventually reaching the blood stream via the thoracic duct. During a transient primary bacteraemia the organism is seeded to reticuloendothelial sites where silent intracellular multiplication occurs throughout the usual 7–14 day incubation period. A second bacteraemia then follows, accompanied by the onset of symptoms and the infection spreads extensively throughout liver, gallbladder, spleen, Peyer's patches, and bone marrow. Concentrated sites of infection in these tissues, known as typhoid nodules, are characterized by an infiltrate of lymphocytes and macrophages followed by the development of ischaemia and necrosis. Explanations for the symptomatology and pathology of typhoid have, in the past, focused on the role of endotoxin. Experimental work on human volunteers has shown that, although administration of endotoxin can provoke typhoid-like symptoms, it is possible to desensitize subjects to endotoxin without affecting their susceptibility to symptomatic typhoid. Recent advances in our understanding of mechanisms of sepsis suggest that its is highly likely that in typhoid, as in other types of sepsis, endotoxin plays a central role in pathogenesis, by stimulating the release of cytokines such as TNF-α and interleukins 1 and 6 from macrophages and neutrophils, by activation of the complement cascade and upregulation of the adhesive capacity of neutrophils and endothelial cells.

Specific, cell-mediated, mucosal and humoral immune responses can be observed in typhoid. Circulating antibodies can remain detectable for 2 years following infection. Prolonged elevation of Vi antibody occurs in chronic carriers. Susceptibility to reinfection with typhoid was reduced by 75 per cent in volunteers re-exposed 20 months after initial infection. Immunodeficiency has been associated with recurrent salmonellosis and fulminating colitis in typhoid patients.

Clinical features

Typhoid is predominantly an infection of children and young adults, affecting both sexes equally. It usually develops after 7–14 days of incubation. Although the main focus of typhoid is in the small bowel, systemic symptoms often overshadow local abdominal symptoms. The most prominent feature is a high fever which is notable for its gradual onset and its tendency to remain on a high plateau of 39–40°C with relatively little diurnal variation. Nearly all patients complain of headache and malaise with the fever. Deafness is a frequent complaint. Cough is often present. The principal abdominal symptoms are diffuse abdominal pain and altered bowel habit. Constipation is common with early typhoid. Many but not all patients will experience diarrhoea, usually without blood, at some stage. Diarrhoea is occurs more frequently in younger patients and can be very severe in immunocompromised patients.

In developing countries, many typhoid patients present with late features and complications. Neuropsychiatric symptoms, particularly mental torpor, delirium, confusion, and psychosis are frequently seen and carry a high risk of fatal outcome. Other patients may present with intestinal haemorrhage, acute abdomen from ileal perforation, septic shock, or with pneumonic or nephritic complications.

Physical examination is often unremarkable apart from the presence of fever. The frequency with which well-known relative bradycardia (temperature–pulse dissociation) is noted in typhoid shows great variability around the world and between young and old. It has weak specificity as a clinical sign. The most suggestive sign of typhoid is the presence of rose spots. These are usually pink macular or maculopapular blanching lesions found in small numbers, mostly on abdominal skin. The frequency with which they are observed varies from 5 per cent or less in some series to 90 per cent (Osler). Much more florid versions of the rash are associated with paratyphoid. The abdomen is likely to be tender and enlargement of the liver and spleen may be noted. A coated tongue is commonly observed. Wheezes and crackles may be heard when the chest is examined. The patient with advanced typhoid often displays a dull, apathetic appearance (typhoid facies), tremor, and gait ataxia.

In young children, typhoid is more likely to present with diarrhoea, convulsions, or a meningitic picture. Blood culture studies of children under the age of two, presenting with mild fever and respiratory symptoms in Chile showed unexpectedly high isolation rates of *S. typhi* and *paratyphi.*

Early typhoid can resemble many other acute infections, notably malaria, hepatitis, pneumonia, and a variety of gastrointestinal infections. Differentiation from falciparum malaria should always be given high priority.

Pathology

The hallmark of typhoid at autopsy is the presence of ulcers of gut-associated lymphoid tissue of the ileum (Peyer's patches) with associated mesenteric lymphadenitis. Typhoid nodules, as described above, may be observed in liver, spleen, and other reticuloendothelial sites. Lesions of lymphoid tissue commence with hypertrophy and progress to necrosis, seen in the ileum as black necrotic slough. Non-specific changes associated with sepsis are seen in heart, brain, lungs, and kidneys.

Laboratory diagnosis

A secure diagnosis of typhoid rests on the isolation of *S. typhi* from a patient with typical symptoms. Isolation is possible from blood, bone marrow, stool, urine, bile, and even rose spots. Bone marrow, while giving the highest yield, including those patients already exposed to antibiotics, is somewhat inconvenient though the use a fine needle technique can be recommended (see Hedley *et al.* (1982) *Lancet*, ii, 415–6). Most clinicians culture blood, stool, and sometimes urine. There is a long tradition of serodiagnosis (especially the Widal test) for typhoid but there are many pitfalls. Elevated levels of antibody occur in healthy individuals in endemic areas, vaccinated persons, in those previously infected or infected with cross-reacting bacteria, whilst some individuals fail to mount certain types of response. To be of value, serological tests for typhoid results should only be used where up-to-date data on predictive values for the population in which it is to be used are available. With this information, recently developed slide agglutination techniques can be very helpful for rapid confirmation of a clinical diagnosis of typhoid. Promising rapid tests for *S. typhi* antigens in blood or urine have been described.

Additional laboratory findings in typhoid commonly include normochromic anaemia, mild thrombocytopenia, and a low white cell count. Liver enzymes are often mildly elevated and white cells and protein may be observed in the urine.

Treatment

The aims of management are to eliminate the infection swiftly with antibiotics, to restore fluid and nutritional deficits, and to monitor the patient for dangerous complications.

The management of typhoid in recent years has undergone radical changes. The world-wide dissemination of strains of *S. typhi* multiply resistant to chloramphenicol, co-trimoxazole, and amoxicillin has led

Table 1 Randomized trials comparing fluorinated quinolones with ceftriaxone in the treatment of uncomplicated typhoid fever.

Drug	Dosage	No. of patients	Clinical cure (%)	Mean days to defervescence (SD)	Relapse (%)
Ciprofloxacin	500 mg twice daily 7 days	20	100	6.0	0
Ceftriaxone	3 g daily 7 days	22	73	7.8	5
Fleroxacin	400 mg daily 7 days	15	100	3.4 (1.7)	0
Ceftriaxone	2 g daily 5 days	15	87	6.7 (3.1)	0
Ofloxacin	200 mg twice daily, 5 days	22	100	3.4 (1.0)	0
Ceftriaxone	3 g daily 3 days	25	78	8.2 (3.6)	1

Source: White, N.J. and Parry, C.M. (1996). The treatment of typhoid fever. *Current Opinion in Infectious Diseases*, **9**, 298–302.

to abandonment of these antibiotics in many areas. The impressive results reported in trials of fluorinated quinolones for typhoid indicate that this class of antibiotics is not only effective in most cases of resistant typhoid but leads to more rapid resolution of symptoms, lower rates of long-term carriage and relapse, and requires shorter periods of administration than older antibiotics. Drawbacks to the use of quinolones are continuing concerns over safety in children and pregnant women and early signs of resistance to quinolones emerging in areas of heavy usage. Effective alternatives to quinolones in multiply resistant typhoid include cephalosporins (ceftriaxone, cefixime) and furazolidone which is the cheapest drug available for the treatment of resistant typhoid. Randomized comparisons of typhoid treatments (Table 1) have indicated the following:

(i) quinolones produce more rapid defervescence than alternative antibiotics and the best rates of clinical and microbiological cure;

(ii) the duration of therapy for quinolones can be reduced to as little as 3 days (data from Vietnam) without significantly reducing efficacy.

Dosage recommendations for typhoid are listed in Table 2. Where patients continue to be treated with chloramphenicol they should be monitored for reversible, dose-related, bone marrow suppression. Follow-up data on large numbers of Vietnamese children treated for typhoid indicated no evidence of toxicity from short-course quinolones.

Supportive care

Cooling measures are to be preferred to antipyretic drugs for managing high fever. Simple analgesia may be used to help headache but paracetamol should be used with care as it has been reported to increase the half-life of chloramphenicol five-fold. Most patients can eat and drink normally and there is no respectable evidence that bland diets or starvation diets are needed to protect the bowel from perforation. The emphasis should be on meeting the greatly increased caloric needs of these febrile patients.

Severely ill patients may require management in an intensive care unit with parenteral fluids, intravenous steroids (see below), inotropic support, and sedation.

Complications

Table 3 lists some of the many complications that have been reported in typhoid patients. Most of them are rare and seen mostly in patients with untreated infections of over 2 weeks duration. Important complications are discussed below.

Severe typhoid

Typhoid is one of the few forms of sepsis where, in contrast to other Gram-negative septicaemias, high-dose steroids have been shown in a well-conducted, randomized, controlled trial to lower mortality. In a study from Indonesia patients with marked mental confusion or shock given 3 mg/kg of dexamethasone infused over half an hour, followed by eight doses of 1 mg/kg at 6-hourly intervals showed a 10 per cent case-fatality rate compared with a rate of 55.6 per cent in controls.

Intestinal perforation and haemorrhage

Ileal perforation should be considered in typhoid patients developing acute abdominal signs. When perforation occurs the outcome is much better in patients diagnosed promptly and operated on after full resuscitation. Excellent results have been reported with simple closure of perforations, although more experience surgeons report less post-operative morbidity when procedures designed to by-pass and rest damaged sections of bowel are carried out. Closure of the perforation should be accompanied by peritoneal toilet and adjunctive therapy with metronidazole. In the best hands survival following prompt surgery for perforation exceeds 90 per cent, whereas survival following non-operative management of perforation is substantially lower. Conservative and operative approaches to perforation have not been assessed in randomized trials.

Bleeding from ileal ulcers will occasionally be severe enough to require blood transfusion. Surgical intervention is seldom indicated.

Relapse

In about 10 per cent of patients with untreated or chloramphenicol-treated typhoid the illness returns in milder form a week or two after recovery from the initial episode. Isolates generally show the same antibiotic sensitivity as the initial episode and the illness can be managed with a similar or abbreviated course of the same therapy used in the initial episode.

Typhoid carriers

The number of organisms present in stool (or urine) generally declines at a steady rate as the patient recovers. Many patients convalescing from illness continue to excrete organisms for a week or two and pose a potential infectious hazard. The 3 per cent or so of patients found to be still excreting at 3 months are likely to become long-term carriers. The presence of gall bladder disease, opisthorchiasis, or renal pathology predisposes to long-term carriage. Long-term carriers generally remain well but an increased risk of carcinoma of the gall bladder has been reported. Persistently elevated titres of Vi antibody are associated with carriage and this offers a useful screening tool. Eradication of carriage with norfloxacin or ciprofloxacin is possible and these antibiotics appear to work better than high-dose ampinopenicillins or co-trimoxazole. Cholecystectomy is now rarely justifiable.

Table 2 Guidelines for drug dosages in typhoid

1. Drugs for typhoid with reported 100% clinical and microbiological cure in recent trials[a]				
Antibiotic	**Daily dose**	**Route[b]**	**Doses/day**	**Duration**
Ciprofloxacin	0.5g	O/IV	2	7 days
Ceftriaxone	3 g	IM	1	7 days
Fleroxacin	400 mg	O/IV	1	3 days
Ofloxacin	15 mg/kg	O	1	3 days
2. Other drugs useful in management of typhoid				
Antibiotic	**Daily dose**	**Route[b]**	**Doses/day**	**Duration**
Chloramphenicol	50–75 mg/kg	O/IM/IVc	4	14 days
Co-trimoxazole	6.5–10 mg/kg TMP; 40 mg/kg SMO	O/IM/IV	2–3	14 days
Amoxycillin	75–100 mg/kg	O/IM/IV	3	14 days
Furazolidone	7.5 mg/kg	O	4	14 days
Cefoperazone	100 mg/kg until defervescence, then 50 mg/kg	IM	2	14 days
Cefixime	20 mg/kg	O	2	14 days
Norfloxacin, ofloxacin	800 mg	O/IV	2	10 days
Pefloxacin	800 mg	O/IV	2	14 days
Enoxacin	400 mg	O/IV	2	14 days
3. Treatment of carriers				
Antibiotic	**Daily dose**	**Route**	**Doses/day**	**Duration**
Ampicillin or amoxycillin with probenecid	100 mg/kg 30 mg/kg	O	3–4	3 months[d]
Co-trimoxazole	6.5–10 mg TMP	O	2	3 months
Ciprofloxacin	1500 mg	O	2	28 days
Norfloxacin	800 mg	O	2	28 days

TMP, trimethoprim; SMO, sulphamethoxazole. O, oral; IM, intramuscular; IV, intravenous.

[a] Source: White, N.J. and Parry, C.M. (1996). The treatment of typhoid fever. *Current Opinion in Infectious Disease*, **9**, 298–302.

[b] Oral therapy is satisfactory for most patients. Parenteral therapy is generally reserved for severely ill patients.

[c] The oral route is preferred; there are reports of lower blood levels of chloramphenicol in patients given parenteral therapy.

[d] The duration of treatment can be shortened if parenteral therapy is given, e.g. 8-hourly intravenous ampicillin for 2 weeks.

Prevention and control

Typhoid was brought under control in industrialized countries long before the introduction of antibiotics by the provision of clean drinking water, safe disposal of human sewage, legislation to ensure high standards of food hygiene, and programmes to detect and monitor chronic carriers. Phage typing of isolates plays an important role in the investigation of the occasional outbreaks that occur when one of these measures fails.

Measures for individual protection include boiling, iodination, or chlorination of drinking water, special care with food prepared outside the home and vaccination for travellers to endemic areas. Patients and convalescents should wash their hands after using the toilet, avoid handling food for others, and use separate towels.

Vaccines

A recently published meta-analysis of typhoid vaccine trials reported 3-year cumulative efficiencies of 73 per cent for two doses of parenteral whole cell vaccine, 55 per cent for a single dose of parenteral Vi vaccine, and 51 per cent for three doses of oral Ty21a vaccine. The whole cell vaccine commonly causes fever, malaise, and local pain and the oral Ty21a vaccine can cause gastrointestinal upset. None of the currently available vaccines afford cross-protection against paratyphoid.

Paratyphoid

Paratyphoid, of which three types have been described (A, B, and C), bears a close clinical resemblance to typhoid and is managed in the same way. The principal points of difference are in transmission (more often food-borne), incubation (generally shorter, 4–5 days), clinical features (more florid rash, gastroenteritic features more common, severity and complications less than typhoid), and sequelae (less relapse and long-term carriage). Isolates of *S. paratyphi* show similar antibiotic susceptibilities to *S. typhi.*

Table 3 Complications of typhoid

Abdominal	*Neuropsychiatric*
Intestinal perforation	Delirium
Intestinal haemorrhage	Psychosis
Hepatitis	Depression
Cholecystitis	Deafness
Spontaneous splenic rupture	Meningitis
Rupture and haemorrhage of mesenteric nodes	Encephalomyelitis
	Transverse myelitis
Pancreatitis	Upper motor neurone signs
	Extrapyramidal disorders
Genitourinary	Impairment of co-ordination
Retention of urine	Optic neuritis
Glomerulonephritis	Peripheral and cranial neuropathy
Pyelonephritis	Guillain-Barré syndrome
Cystitis	Pseudotumor cerebri
Orchitis	
	Haematological
Cardiovascular	Anaemia, leucopenia, thrombocytopenia, pancytopenia
Myocarditis	
Pericarditis	Disseminated intravascular coagulation
Endocarditis	
ECG abnormalities	Haemoloysis
Phlebitis and arteritis	Haemolytic uraemic syndrome
Deep venous thrombosis	
Gangrene	*Focal infections*
Shock	Abscesses of brain, liver, spleen, breast, thyroid, muscle, lymph nodes
Sudden death	
	Parotitis
Respiratory	Osteitis
Bronchitis	Pharyngitis
Pneumonia	Arthritis
Laryngeal ulceration	
Glottal oedema	*Other*
	Myopathy
	Hypercalcaemia
	Decubitus ulceration
	Abortion
	Development of chronic carrier state
	Relapse

Further reading

Engels, E.A. *et al.* (1998). Typhoid fever vaccines: a meta-analysis of studies of efficacy and toxicity. *British Medical Journal*, **316**, 110–16.

White, N.J. and Parry, C.M. (1996). The treatment of typhoid fever. *Current Opinion in Infectious Diseases*, **9**, 298–302.

Chapter 16.45

Anaerobic bacteria

S. J. Eykyn

Anaerobic infections are common and may affect any tissue or organ. Anaerobic bacteria were seldom isolated in clinical laboratories until the mid-1970s when they were 'rediscovered' as common and important pathogens. Since then enormous advances have been made in the isolation, taxonomy, clinical diagnosis, management, and prevention of anaerobic infection.

Taxonomy

The classification of many anaerobic bacteria presents difficulties and only dedicated anaerobists can hope to be abreast of current taxonomy. The genus *Bacteroides* is now limited to the *B. fragilis* group. Saccharolytic species have been assigned to the new genus *Prevotella*, which includes pigmented and non-pigmented species, and asaccharolytic pigmented Gram-negative rods are now *Porphyromonas*. Other taxonomic changes have affected the anaerobic Gram-positive cocci which have almost all become *Peptostreptococcus* spp.

Anaerobic commensal flora of man

The commensal flora of man is largely anaerobic.

Skin

The skin supports a considerable anaerobic microflora, predominantly 'anaerobic diphtheroids' (propionibacteria).

Mouth

Anaerobes are found in the tonsillar crypts, tongue crypts, gingival crevices, and dental plaque and includes *Prevotella*, fusobacteria, and peptostreptococci.

Intestine

The stomach and upper small intestine are normally sterile or contain small numbers of transient organisms. The flora of the terminal ileum is similar to the colon with a vast anaerobic flora. *Bacteroides* account for about 25 per cent of the species isolated. Clostridia are also found in large numbers and most of the other anaerobic genera occur in the colon.

Genitourinary tract

The normal flora of the vagina is predominantly anaerobic, mostly lactobacilli, but also small numbers of *Prevotella*, fusobacteria, and peptostreptococci. The urethra contains small numbers of peptostreptococci.

Pathogenesis

Anaerobic bacteria usually derive from the host's commensal flora and most anaerobic infections are polymicrobial with aerobes also involved. The anaerobic component seems to be the more important. Predisposing factors include disruption of normally intact cutaneous or mucosal barriers, tissue injury and necrosis, impaired blood supply, and obstruction. Virulence factors are also involved and include adhesins, capsules, lipopolysaccharide, hydrolytic and other enzymes, soluble metabolites, etc. Precise virulence determinants for most anaerobic infections have not been established.

Diagnosis of anaerobic infection

Clinical

Much anaerobic infection arises in association with the anaerobic commensal flora. Putrid discharge characterizes some infections and results from the metabolic products of the anaerobes. Anaerobic infections, particularly necrotizing infections, are sometimes associated with cellulitis and gas formation. Another useful clue to the presence of anaerobes is a report of 'sterile pus' despite the presence of organisms on a Gram-stained film. Lastly, in any patient on antibiotics inactive against anaerobes such as aminoglycosides, and still appearing septic, an anaerobic infection should be considered.

Collection and transport of specimens for anaerobic bacteriology

All anaerobic bacteria are sensitive to oxygen but they vary in their aerotolerance. *B. fragilis* and *Cl. perfringens* will tolerate 2–4 per cent oxygen but fusobacteria and some peptostreptococci are much more sensitive to oxygen and more difficult to grow in the laboratory and less likely to survive the journey from patient to culture medium. The best specimens for the isolation of anaerobes are aspirates, pus (in a universal container), or excised tissue and although rapid delivery of specimens to the laboratory is desirable, in practice, anaerobes (even fastidious species) survive well in pus and tissue. Swabs are less satisfactory, and for them a transport medium should be used. Complex commercial systems for the collection and transport of specimens for anaerobic bacteriology have been devised but are unlikely to appeal to clinicians.

Laboratory

The putrid smell of the pus in many anaerobic infections has been mentioned, and in such cases even swabs will be noticeably foul when processed. The Gram-stained smear of anaerobic discharge is often diagnostic to the experienced microscopist as it characteristically contains a variety of different bacteria. Successful culture of anaerobes requires fresh media and a reliable anaerobic atmosphere with 10 per cent carbon dioxide. Most laboratories now have special anaerobic cabinets. Relatively aerotolerant species will usually grow in 24 h but many anaerobes take much longer. Fastidious anaerobes require undisturbed anaerobiosis and leaving inoculated culture plates out on the bench is likely to result in failure. The definitive identification of many anaerobes is a lengthy and technically demanding process and taxonomic exactitude has minimal appeal to clinicians. Commercially available identification kits enable rapid identification of the commonly isolated species but they require practice in setting up and interpretation.

Clinical spectrum of anaerobic infection

Infections of the head and neck

Acute necrotizing ulcerative gingivitis (Vincent's disease)

This affects the gingiva and buccal mucosa with painful bleeding gums, sometimes with a pseudomembrane and foul breath. The diagnosis can be confirmed with a Gram-stained smear on which large numbers of spirochaetes, fusiforms, and other bacteria are seen.

Dental sepsis

The oral commensal flora is found (with aerobic and microaerophilic oral commensal bacteria) in periodontal infection and dental abscesses and in postoperative infections associated with maxillofacial surgery.

Infections of the neck and jaw

These unusual necrotizing infections are frequently anaerobic and may be accompanied by marked cellulitis and oedema and cause respiratory embarrassment. Ludwig's angina is infection involving the main anterior compartment of the neck, the submandibular space. The source of the infection is usually the lower molar teeth, but it can arise from tonsillar infection as in the patient shown in Fig. 1. It may involve the chest with mediastinal abscess and empyema formation.

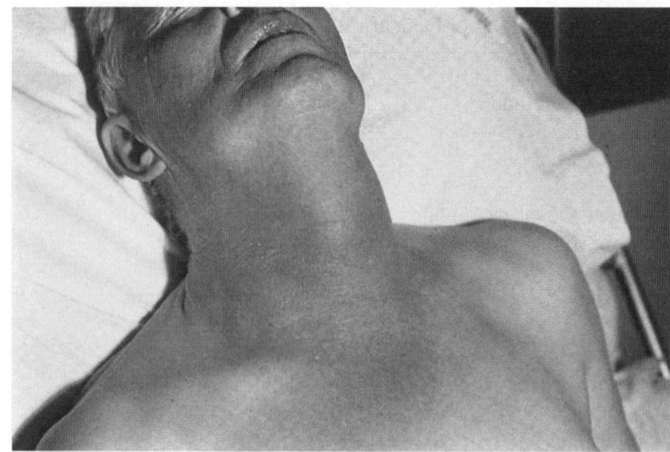

Fig. 1 Spreading cellulitis of the neck resulting from tonsillar sepsis (fatal) 'anaerobic neck'.

ENT infections

Anaerobes are frequently isolated from tonsillar tissue in recurrent streptococcal tonsillitis and are also involved in peritonsillar abscesses (quinsy). They are commonly found in chronic infection of the sinuses, middle ear, and mastoid. Chronic sinus infection occasionally results in acute orbital cellulitis.

Infections of the central nervous system

Anaerobic bacteria are the major pathogens in cerebral abscesses other than those that follow surgery or trauma. Otogenic cerebral abscesses are most common and involve the temporal lobe or cerebellum. *B. fragilis* is usually isolated and aerobes, particularly *Proteus* spp. are often present. Frontal lobe abscesses of sinusitic or dental origin are usually caused by *Str. milleri* group, although oral anaerobes may also be found.

Pleuropulmonary infection

Anaerobic pleuropulmonary infection usually results from oropharyngeal aspiration but also occasionally from haematogenous seeding, particularly by fusobacteria (see necrobacillosis below). Anaerobic pleuropulmonary infections include aspiration pneumonia, necrotizing pneumonitis, lung abscess and empyema, as well as secondary infection in bronchiectasis and bronchial carcinoma. The anaerobes are the oral commensals. Patients with an anaerobic lung abscess will usually admit to the revolting taste (as well as smell) of their sputum. Definitive bacteriological diagnosis of anaerobic pleuropulmonary infection requires culture of an invasive specimen—expectorated sputum is rarely suitable.

Intra-abdominal infections

These infections are usually associated with intra-abdominal pathology such as perforated gastric or duodenal ulcers, appendicitis, diverticulitis, inflammatory bowel disease, or malignancy and produce peritonitis or abscesses. Most are polymicrobial and the predominant anaerobes those of the *B. fragilis* group.

Hepatic and biliary tract infection

Hepatic abscesses are rare but likely to be caused by anaerobic bacteria (usually fusobacteria and *B. fragilis*) as well as by *Str. milleri* group. They result from biliary tract infection, haematogenous spread from an intestinal source, or direct extension of contiguous infection.

Anaerobes are found in the bile in obstructive disease and stasis, and may cause cholangitis in patients who have had previous enterobiliary anastomoses.

Infections of the female genital tract and neonatal infection

Anaerobic bacteria cause bacterial vaginosis, tubo-ovarian sepsis, Bartholin's abscess, endometritis, septic abortion, and infection associated with intrauterine contraceptive devices. Vaginal hysterectomy carries a high risk of postoperative anaerobic infection, but wound infection after abdominal hysterectomy is likely to be caused by *S. aureus*. Prolonged rupture of the membranes is associated with anaerobic infection and foul smelling liquor is often noted. Anaerobes, of vaginal origin, can be cultured from the liquor, the placenta, and the nasogastric aspirate, ear, and other surface swabs of the baby, which may develop anaerobic pneumonitis.

Infections of the male genitalia and prostate

The commensal anaerobic flora of the urethra is found in balanoposthitis, whose foul odour is well known to genitourinary physicians. Anaerobes also cause secondary infection of penile lesions. Scrotal abscesses are usually caused by anaerobes unless they follow acute epididymo-orchitis. Anaerobic scrotal abscesses, which are often recurrent, arise either *de novo*, and probably result from secondary infection of blocked apocrine glands, or after surgery to the genitalia or urethra.

Fournier's gangrene is a necrotizing infection involving the scrotum, and often extending into the perineum, thighs, and abdominal wall. It is characterized by the sudden onset of intense pain and swelling with foul discharge and gas in the tissues as well as marked systemic disturbance. It occurs in middle-aged or elderly men, particularly diabetics and alcoholics, and there is a cutaneous, anorectal, or genitourinary source for the anaerobes.

Acute prostatic abscesses are rare but are sometimes caused by anaerobes. Anaerobes may also be relevant in chronic prostatitis, and can sometimes be cultured from prostatic secretions.

Infection of the urinary tract

Anaerobic urinary infection is very rare, so much so that urine is not routinely cultured anaerobically. Anaerobes can be recovered from the urine when there are abnormalities within the urinary tract such as vesicocolic fistulae, tumours, pyonephrosis, or perinephric abscess, and sometimes from ileal conduit specimens.

Bone and joint infection

Anaerobes are uncommon pathogens in acute osteomyelitis and septic arthritis. Acute anaerobic osteomyelitis affecting long bones is likely to be caused by fusobacteria, whereas acute vertebral osteomyelitis, a infection occurring mainly in elderly patients, is likely to be caused by *B. fragilis*. Acute anaerobic septic arthritis usually occurs in patients with rheumatoid arthritis or other joint pathology and is also likely to be caused by *B. fragilis*. Anaerobes are sometimes isolated in chronic osteomyelitis.

Skin and soft tissue infection

Diabetic foot ulcers Diabetic foot ulcers often grow anaerobes, and these infections may be associated with underlying chronic osteomyelitis and sometimes with cellulitis, necrotizing fasciitis, and gas formation.

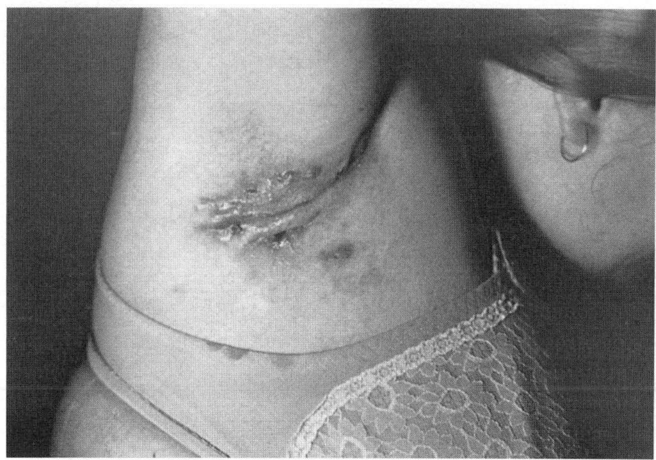

Fig. 2 Hidradenitis suppurativa of axilla.

Venous ulcers Anaerobes are often isolated from venous ulcers but are secondary invaders and are not relevant to the aetiology or perpetuation of the ulcer.

Decubitus ulcers These are frequently infected with anaerobes and anaerobic bacteraemia may occasionally result.

Sebaceous cysts Anaerobes, notably peptostreptococci, are often isolated from infected sebaceous cysts.

Axillary abscess and hidradenitis suppurativa Most axillary abscesses are caused by *S. aureus* but some are anaerobic. These abscesses are recurrent and more indolent than staphylococcal abscesses. Recurrences can result in hidradenitis suppurativa (Fig. 2). Anaerobic axillary abscesses and hidradenitis suppurativa result from apocrine blockage and infection is secondary. Hidradenitis suppurativa is not confined to the axilla but can occur in the perineum, groins, buttocks, and back.

Perirectal abscess These abscesses are frequently caused by anaerobes and when associated with an underlying fistula yield gut-specific anaerobes of the *B. fragilis* group and coliforms. Perirectal abscesses without a fistula are usually anaerobic but are not infected with gut-specific organisms, and may result from infection of blocked apocrine glands.

Breast abscess Breast abscesses are usually assumed to be staphylococcal but are as likely to be anaerobic in the non-puerperal woman. Anaerobic breast abscesses are secondary infections of an underlying blocked duct, and are usually recurrent, subareolar, and associated with inverted nipples.

Human and animal bites Human bites have been mentioned with reference to infection of the joints of the hand, but they may involve other parts of the body. Animal bites can also give rise to anaerobic infection but are more likely to become infected with *Pasteurella* spp.

Paronychia Paronychia can be caused by anaerobes, usually with aerobes. The anaerobes are oral commensals and are probably transferred to the fingers by licking or biting. Anaerobic paronychias are usually less acute than those caused by *S. aureus* or *Str. pyogenes*.

Synergistic necrotizing infections

Anaerobic bacteria, usually with aerobes, cause a range of 'synergistic' infections. These infections can involve skin, fascia, and sometimes muscle, and affect many areas of the body, occurring either spontaneously or after trauma or surgery (Fig. 3).

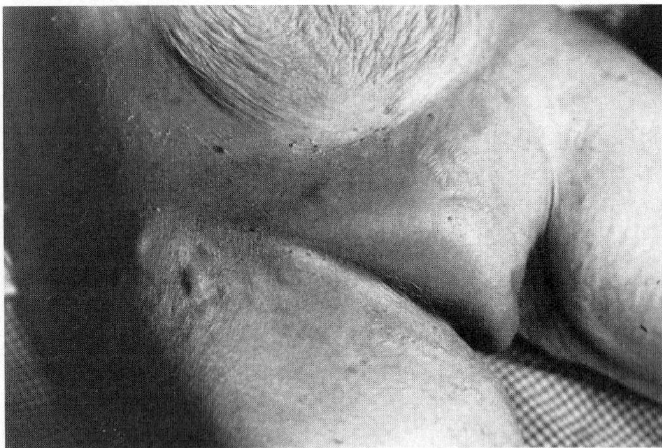

Fig. 3 Necrotizing fasciitis involving perineum, buttock, and thigh, 3 weeks after gastrectomy for carcinoma.

Bacteraemia and endocarditis

Anaerobic infection at any site, but particularly intra-abdominal infection, can cause bacteraemia, sometimes with shock. Anaerobes account for only around 5 per cent of positive blood cultures, with the *B. fragilis* group most common. Anaerobes are also found in polymicrobial bacteraemia.

Fusobacterial bacteraemia, necrobacillosis, and Lemierre's postanginal septicaemia

Most anaerobic infections are polymicrobial, with not only several anaerobic species but also several aerobic species frequently isolated. Fusobacteria, however, can be sole pathogens and produce severe infections. Their virulence is probably attributable to their lipopolysaccharide which is similar to that of Gram-negative aerobic bacteria. Although these serious infections are rare, they were well described in the preantibiotic era. The species most often isolated from septicaemic disease is *F. necrophorum* and it is to this species that the term necrobacillosis refers.

Necrobacillosis

The earliest reports of necrobacillosis in man were of zoonotic skin infections acquired from animals with local infection with *F. necrophorum*, usually in mixed culture, but in 1930, two fatal cases that presented 'hitherto undescribed clinical and pathological features of systemic infection' were described: a girl of 19 who died of lung abscesses, septic arthritis of the hip, and jaundice six days after a sore throat with rigors; and a man of 64 who died of a retropharyngeal abscess with gangrene and extension into the peritracheal and subcutaneous tissues. The former case is the 'postanginal septicaemia' later described by Lemierre (see below). The latter sounds like necrotizing fasciitis. Further clarification of the entity of necrobacillosis was provided in 1955 by Alston who recognized four different types of infection caused by *F. necrophorum*: those involving the skin and subcutaneous tissues; a large group where the infection started with a sore throat or otitis media; a third group associated with the female genital tract, the alimentary tract, or the urinary tract; and a fourth with empyema. Pyaemia and abscesses were very common in the last three groups. Alston's second group corresponds to Lemierre's postanginal septicaemia although Lemierre considered septicaemias arising from otitis media and mastoiditis to be a separate group. Since Alston's study, there have been sporadic case reports of necrobacillosis and in 1989 a large UK series was published. The term necrobacillosis is best used for septicaemic infection with *F. necrophorum*, and postanginal septicaemic infection designated as Lemierre's disease since this is a distinct entity.

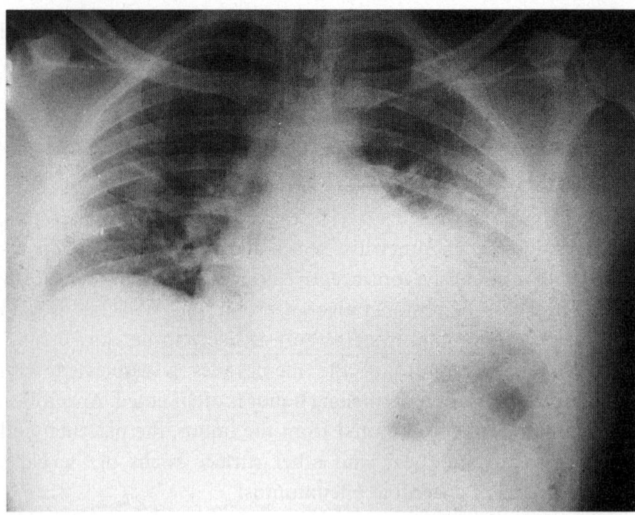

Fig. 4 Chest radiograph taken on admission to hospital of a 21-year-old heating engineer who had developed rigors and severe shortness of breath about a week after a sore throat. He was thought to have possible legionnaire's disease, hence given erythromycin (to which fusobacteria are usually resistant); *F. necrophorum* was isolated from blood cultures.

Lemierre's postanginal septicaemia (Lemierre's disease)

This unique manifestation of necrobacillosis occurs in previously healthy, young people. Lemierre suggested that it affected both sexes equally but the recent UK series found a male predominance. There is an antecedent sore throat, often severe, and sometimes acute tonsillitis. Painful cervical lymphadenopathy is usual and septic jugular thrombophlebitis can occur. Within days, sometimes only hours, of the onset of sore throat, rigors develop with marked systemic upset and often impaired renal and hepatic function. Metastatic spread is characteristic, most commonly involving the lung, but also bone, joint, liver, brain, and heart valves. The 'pneumonia' is often severe and extensive, and cavitation of the septic infarcts and empyema may occur. Unless the relevance of an antecedent sore throat is appreciated, the diagnosis will be missed (Fig. 4). Although *F. necrophorum* is very sensitive to both penicillin and metronidazole the infection responds only very slowly to antibiotic treatment, a reflection of the innate virulence of the organism.

Sensitivity of anaerobic bacteria to antimicrobial agents

The susceptibility of most anaerobic bacteria to antimicrobial agents is remarkably uniform. Intrinsic resistance is often predictable and acquired resistance uncommon.

Metronidazole

Metronidazole is unique amongst the antimicrobial agents that are active against anaerobic bacteria as it is only active against anaerobes with no activity against aerobes. Although it has been used to treat anaerobic infections for nearly 30 years, most clinically important anaerobes remain sensitive and resistance is very rare.

β-Lactam antibiotics

Many anaerobes are still very sensitive to penicillin including many strains of *Prevotella*, *Porphyromonas*, and fusobacteria as well as clostridia, peptostreptococci, and spirochaetes. The *B. fragilis* group are almost uniformly resistant to penicillin, and resistance is also increasing amongst *Prevotella* and *Porphyromonas*. These penicillin-resistant anaerobes are also resistant to ampicillin, amoxicillin, acylureidopenicillins, carboxypenicillins, and most cephalosporins. The addition of the β-lactam inhibitor clavulanic acid in the antimicrobial co-amoxiclav renders the *B. fragilis* group susceptible to the amoxicillin in the combination. Carbapenems are active against most anaerobes.

Other agents

Most anaerobes are sensitive to clindamycin, and its antianaerobic activity is similar to that of metronidazole. Chloramphenicol is also highly active against anaerobes. Other agents with useful activity include erythromycin, co-trimoxazole, and tetracyclines. The glycopeptides vancomycin and teicoplanin, whilst inactive against most Gram-negative anaerobes, possess useful activity against clostridia and peptostreptococci.

Treatment of anaerobic infection

Surgical intervention, particularly drainage of pus and excision of necrotic tissue, is important in anaerobic infections. Since most anaerobic infections are mixed with aerobes, it may be necessary to treat both groups of organisms. For anaerobic infections other than those of the *B. fragilis* group there is a wide choice of agent, but few clinicians think of anaerobes in distinct groups and it is easier to recommend overall anaerobic cover, which is best provided by metronidazole.

Prevention of anaerobic infection

Antibiotic prophylaxis for operations likely to be followed by postoperative anaerobic wound infection did not become routine until the mid 1970s but since then many trials bear witness to the efficacy of such prophylaxis in surgery involving sites with an anaerobic commensal flora and the putrid wound infections so familiar to gastrointestinal surgeons in the past are rarely seen today. Most regimens include cover for both aerobes and anaerobes. Antianaerobic prophylaxis is given for many different types of surgery, but particularly for that involving the gastrointestinal tract, genital tract, and upper respiratory tract. Such prophylaxis should be perioperative, intravenous, and of short duration (usually three doses). There are many possible regimens but cefuroxime and metronidazole are widely used.

Further reading

Alston, J.M. (1955). Necrobacillosis in Great Britain. *British Medical Journal*, **ii**, 1524–28. [Old paper providing insight into various clinical presentations of fusobacterial septicaemia.]

Eykyn, S.J. (1989). Necrobacillosis. *Scandinavian Journal of Infectious Diseases*, (suppl. 62), 41–6.

Finegold, S.M. and George, W.L. (eds) (1989). *Anaerobic infections in humans.* Academic Press, New York.

Lemierre, A. (1936). On certain septicaemias due to anaerobic organisms. *Lancet*, **i**, 701–3. [This paper contains the classic description of postanginal septicaemia.]

Unattributed. (1984). International symposium on anaerobic bacteria and their role in disease. *Reviews of Infectious Diseases*, **6** (suppl. 1).

Chapter 16.46

Cholera

C .C .J. Carpenter

Cholera is an acute illness caused by *Vibrio cholerae*. In severe cases, fluid and electrolytes are rapidly lost from the gut, resulting in hypovolaemic shock and, if untreated, death.

Aetiology and epidemiology

V. cholerae are short, motile, halophilic, Gram-negative rods. Past cholera epidemics have been attributable to *V. cholerae* 01 strains. However, in 1992–93, a non-01 strain, *V. cholerae* 0139 Bengal, was responsible for epidemic disease in India, Bangladesh, and Thailand; the 0139 Bengal strain remains endemic in the Gangetic delta.

There have been seven global pandemics of cholera since 1830. The seventh began in 1961, and extended throughout Asia, Africa, and mediterranean Europe. In 1991, the epidemic extended to South America. Cases were first observed in Peru in January of 1991 and within 1 year over 300 000 cases were recognized. By 1997, cholera cases had occurred in all North and South American nations.

Man is the only mammalian host of *V. cholerae*. Most major epidemics have been waterborne, but direct contamination of food is also important in transmission. Shellfish, which can harbour *V. cholerae* for long periods, were important vectors in Peru. People with mild or asymptomatic infections may also spread the disease. The clinical case: infection ratio with the *V. cholerae* is usually about 1:10. In endemic areas attack rates are 10 times greater in children under 6 than in older age groups. When the disease spreads to previously uninvolved areas, attack rates are initially as high in adults as in children. When cholera persists, the endemic pattern develops, with young children predominantly affected.

Pathogenesis

V. cholerae cause disease when the bacteria colonize the small bowel and produce enterotoxin. The incubation period varies from 12 h to several days. Because of susceptibility of *V. cholerae* to gastric acid, an enormous number of bacteria must generally be ingested to cause illness. Those with achlorhydria are abnormally susceptible to cholera.

The cholera enterotoxin binds rapidly to the small bowel epithelial cells, where it stimulates intracellular adenylate cyclase activity. The resultant increase in intracellular cyclic adenosine 3′,5′-monophosphate (cyclic AMP) leads to rapid secretion of electrolytes into the bowel lumen.

The secretion of fluid by gut mucosal cells reflects effects on two intestinal ion transport sites. The net result is rapid outpouring of isotonic fluid into the gut at a rate which exceeds the absorptive capacity of the colon, resulting in rapid loss of isotonic fluid. In adults with voluminous diarrhoea the electrolyte pattern in cholera stool is remarkably consistent, with sodium and chloride concentrations slightly less than those of plasma, bicarbonate concentration roughly twice that of plasma, and potassium concentration three to five times that of plasma.

All signs and symptoms in cholera result directly from the gut fluid loss.

Clinical features

Symptoms usually appear abruptly, with painless, watery diarrhoea. Stool volumes vary greatly, and the majority of cases do not require hospitalization. In more severe cases, the initial stool volume may exceed 1500 ml. At variable intervals after the onset of diarrhoea, vomiting ensues; this is productive of rice-watery material. Painful muscle cramps, commonly involving the calf muscles, usually develop. Prostration occurs at varying intervals after onset, in direct relationship to the magnitude of the fluid loss.

Severely ill cholera patients present a characteristic appearance (Fig. 1(a)). They are collapsed, cyanotic, with no palpable peripheral pulses, pinched facies, and scaphoid abdomen. The skin turgor is remarkably diminished. The voice is weak and high-pitched. Vital signs include tachycardia, tachypnoea, and hypotension, often with no obtainable blood pressure. Heart sounds are faint or inaudible, and bowel sounds are hypoactive. Major alterations in mental status are not common in adults. As many as 10 per cent of small children may have central nervous system abnormalities that range from stupor to convulsions.

Laboratory abnormalities result from the gastrointestinal loss of isotonic, alkaline, virtually protein-free fluid (Table 1). Plasma findings include increased specific gravity, elevated protein, decreased bicarbonate, normal sodium, slightly increased chloride, and moderately elevated potassium. Abnormal blood chemical findings are rapidly corrected with appropriate fluid therapy (Table 1).

The illness may last from 12 h to 7 days. Later clinical manifestations depend on the adequacy of therapy. With adequate fluid repletion, recovery is remarkably rapid (Fig. 1(b, c)). If therapy is inadequate, the case mortality rate may exceed 50 per cent. Important causes of death are hypovolaemic shock, uncompensated metabolic acidosis, and renal failure.

Diagnosis

The working diagnosis of cholera should be made on the basis of the clinical picture; fluid replacement therapy should be initiated immediately. Although cholera-like illness may be caused by organisms other than *V. cholerae*, most frequently enterotoxigenic *Escherichia coli*, the resulting pathophysiological abnormalities are the same, so that identical fluid replacement therapy may be used in all such cases.

Stool examination characteristically shows neither leucocytes nor erythrocytes. With dark-field microscopy, rapid tentative diagnosis can be made by direct observation of the characteristic rapid motility of the comma-shaped bacilli in fresh stool. *V. cholerae* grow rapidly on a number of selective media. Thiosulphate–citrate–bile salt–sucrose (TCBS) agar has the distinct advantage of not requiring sterilization before use. On TCBS agar, *V. cholerae* can be distinguished from other enteric micro-organisms by a distinct, opaque yellow colonial appearance.

Management

Successful therapy demands only prompt oral and/or intravenous replacement of gastrointestinal losses of fluid and electrolytes.

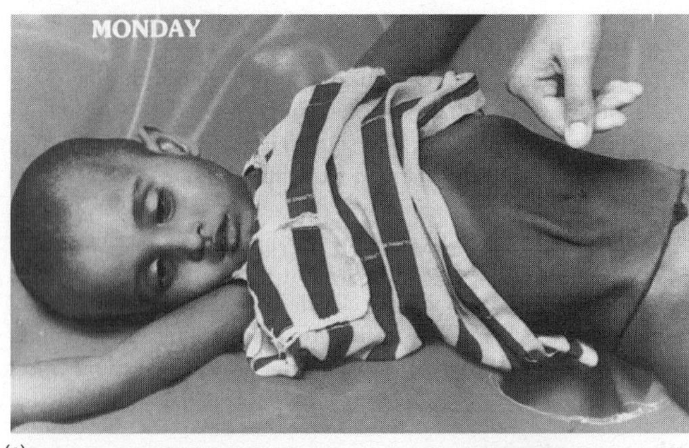

(a)

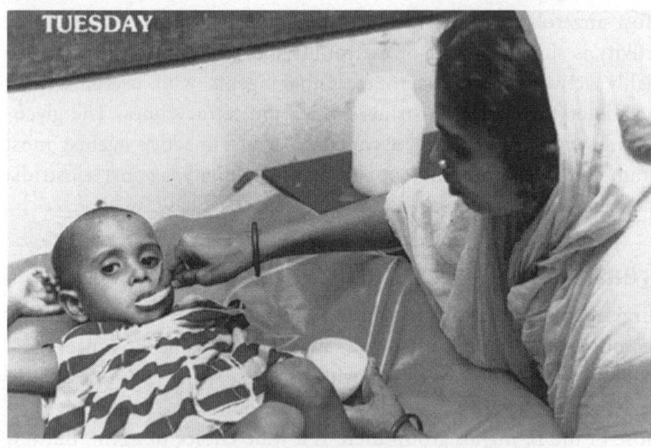

(b)

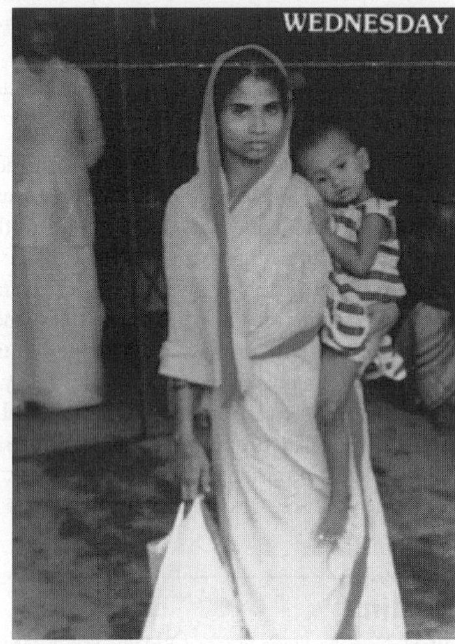

(c)

Fig. 1(a)–(c) Oral rehydration therapy (ORT) in cholera. (a) Before treatment. (b) After 24 h of ORT. (c) Asymptomatic after 48 h of ORT.

Intravenous fluids

An effective treatment solution may simply be prepared by adding 4 g sodium chloride, 6.5 g sodium acetate, and 1 g potassium chloride to a litre of water. Alternatively, lactated Ringer's solution may be administered. Either of these intravenous fluid preparations should

Table 1 Blood chemical determinations in 38 adult cholera patients before and 4 hours after intravenous fluid therapy

	Mean values	
	Admission	4 hours after admission
Arterial blood pH	7.17	7.40
Plasma bicarbonate (mmol/l)	7.0	20.0
Plasma potassium (mmol/l)	5.6	3.2
Total plasma protein (g/dl)	14.2	7.5

be infused intravenously and rapidly, 50–100 ml/min in adults, until a strong radial pulse has been restored. Subsequently, the same fluid should be infused in quantities equal to gastrointestinal losses. Intravenous fluid should be given at a rate sufficient to maintain a normal pulse volume and normal skin turgor. Overhydration can be avoided by careful observation of the neck veins and auscultation of the lungs. Close observation is mandatory during the early phase of the illness; an adult can lose as much as one litre of isotonic fluid per hour during the first 24 h of the disease. Inadequate fluid replacement results in a high incidence of acute renal insufficiency.

In children, complications can be avoided by careful administration of appropriate fluids designed to replace the faecal electrolyte losses. The above diarrhoea treatment solution has been used successfully in children as well as adults. If lactated Ringer's solution is used in the paediatric patient, peroral supplementation of potassium and glucose is needed. The outcome in paediatric cholera should be essentially as favourable as that in the adult disease, with a mortality rate less than 1 per cent.

Oral replacement fluids

Oral replacement of electrolytes is remarkably effective in both adults and children, especially if initiated shortly after onset of diarrhoea. An oral glucose–electrolyte solution (prepared by the addition of 20 g glucose, 3.5 g sodium chloride, 2.5 g sodium bicarbonate, and 1.5 g potassium chloride to one litre of drinking water) can be given in mild cholera cases throughout the course of illness, and is also satisfactory in more severe cases once the shock has been corrected by initial rapid intravenous therapy. With oral therapy, about 1.5 volumes of oral solution must be given to replace each volume of stool loss. Glucose is essential in this solution, as the success of oral therapy in cholera depends upon glucose enhancement of sodium absorption. Although cholera enterotoxin alters electrolyte movement across intestinal mucosa, it does not impair the glucose-facilitated sodium absorption by the gut. Sucrose may be substituted for glucose in the oral solutions; if sucrose is used, 40 g sucrose must be added to each litre, as sucrose is rapidly broken down into glucose and fructose and only the glucose enhances sodium absorption. In addition, precooked rice, 50–80 g per litre, may replace glucose in oral solutions. The starch is rapidly broken down in the gut, providing both glucose and amino acids to facilitate sodium absorption.

Antimicrobials

Adjunctive antimicrobial therapy dramatically reduces the volume of diarrhoea and results in rapid eradication of vibrios. Tetracycline (40–50 mg/kg body weight, daily) given in four equal portions perorally every 6 h for 2 days, was uniformly successful until 1980, when tetracycline-resistant *V. cholerae* strains were first isolated. Furazolidone and trimethoprim/sulfamethoxazole are effective in the case of tetracycline resistance. Fortunately, most *V. cholerae* strains remain highly sensitive to tetracycline.

Results with current management

When the current cholera pandemic reached Peru in January of 1991, the medical community was quickly mobilized. With the early use of oral rehydration therapy, supplemented by intravenous fluids in the most seriously ill patients, a survival rate greater than 99 per cent was achieved in over 300 000 cholera patients. This magnificent achievement was unprecedented, and provided a convincing demonstration of the effectiveness of oral rehydration therapy properly administered by well prepared medical and paramedical personnel.

Immunization and prevention

Immunization using standard commercial vaccine provides only 60–80 per cent protection for 3–6 months to adults. An oral vaccine that combines killed whole vibrios with the B subunit of choleratoxin provides roughly 60 per cent protection for at least 3 years. Recently, a live attenuated oral vaccine with genetic deletions of the active subunit of choleratoxin has also proved about 60 per cent effective in early field trials. At the present time careful hygiene provides the only certain protection against cholera.

Since immunization with currently available cholera vaccines are not effective in altering transmission, vaccine is not recommended by the World Health Organization for travellers who visit endemic areas.

Further reading

Barua, D. and Greenough, W.B. (eds) (1992). *Cholera*. Plenum Medical Book Co., London.

Carpenter, C.C.J. (1992). The treatment of cholera: Clinical science at the bedside. *Journal of Infectious Diseases*, **166**, 2–14.

Clemens, J.D., Sack, D.A., Harris, J.R., *et al.* (1990). Field trial of oral cholera vaccines in Bangladesh: results from three-year follow-up. *Lancet*, **335**, 270–3.

Field, M. (1970). Intestinal secretion: effect of cyclic AMP and its role in cholera. *New England Journal of Medicine*, **284**, 1137–45.

Levine, M.M. and Kaper, J. (1993). Live vaccines against cholera: an update. *Vaccine*, **11**, 207–12.

Chapter 16.47

Haemophilus influenzae

E. R. Moxon

General

Haemophili (Gram-negative bacilli) are commensals found in the mouth or nasopharynx, the mucosae of the conjunctiva, and, occasionally, the genital tract of humans. The most important species is *Haemophilus influenzae*. Transmission occurs by airborne droplets or by direct contagion with secretions; carriage of one or more strains for periods of days to months is common. Most people are colonized with unencapsulated organisms, but in 3–5 per cent of people, the

Table 1 Carriage and pathogenicity of *Haemophilus influenzae*

Strains and principal manifestations of pathogenicity	Common upper respiratory carriage rates (%)
Non-encapsulated Exacerabations of chronic bronchitis, otitis media, sinusitis, conjunctivitis; bacteraemic infections rare, patients commonly adults	50–80
Encapsulated, type b Meningitis, epiglottitis, pneumonia and empyema, septic arthritis, cellulitis, osteomyelitis, pericarditis, bacteraemia; rarer manifestations include glossitis, tenosynovitis, peritonitis, endocarditis, ventriculitis, associated with infected shunt-tubing	2–4
Encapsulated types a, c–f Rarely incriminated as pathogens	1–2

strains express one of six antigenically distinct, polysaccharide capsules, designated a to f; this is the basis of the major typing system. Most carriers are healthy, but two patterns of disease occur (Table 1). First, invasive bacteraemic infections, such as meningitis, are usually caused by type b strains and characteristically occur in young children. Second, less serious but numerically more common infections occur as a result of contiguous spread of *H. influenzae* within the respiratory tract, for example otitis media and pneumonia, usually, but not invariably, caused by unencapsulated strains.

Epidemiology, pathogenesis, and immunology

The importance of type b capsule in the pathogenesis of systemic infections has been well established in animal models. Lipopolysaccharide plays a dual role; it facilitates survival in the blood, and is a key molecule in the pathophysiology of damage to tissues such as the blood–brain barrier. Attachment to epithelial cells is facilitated by inhibition of ciliary clearance mechanisms by cell wall glycopeptides and by specific bacterial adhesins, such as pili. Prior virus infections (e.g. influenza) potentiate infection and appear to facilitate both contiguous spread within the respiratory tract, as in otitis media or sinusitis, and the probability of dissemination into the blood.

Serum antibodies to type b capsule mediate protective immunity against systemic infections in humans. The serum of newborns and young infants, up until 3 months, generally has sufficient amounts of passively acquired maternal antibodies to afford protection. Thereafter, the natural decline of maternally derived antibodies is followed by a period lasting until the age of 2–4 years when the levels of antibody are absent or inadequate to provide protection.

In contrast to systemic type b infections where deficiencies in opsonophagocytic mechanisms are paramount, impairment of non-specific host defence mechanisms (e.g. impaired ciliary clearance) is the most obvious feature of individuals who have disease caused by unencapsulated *H. influenzae.* Predisposing factors include smoking, virus infections, immunodeficiency, or chronic lung disease (e.g. cystic fibrosis).

Haemophilus influenzae type b

Meningitis

Despite the availability of antibiotics and more recently an effective vaccine, type b meningitis is the commonest cause of purulent meningitis in childhood world-wide, and the cause of substantial deaths and permanent CNS damage in survivors. The majority of the cases occur in young children aged <5 years, the peak incidence being from about age 3 months to 2 years. Reported risk factors include male sex, black rather than white race, absence of breast feeding, socioeconomic deprivation, winter months, siblings (often asymptomatic carriers), and attendance at daycare or preschool nurseries.

A typical presentation of meningitis is of a few days' antecedent symptoms of upper respiratory tract infection in a young child; an associated or preceding otitis media is common. The most common signs are fever and altered nervous system function ranging from irritability to coma, but young babies may be afebrile and have few specific symptoms and signs. Raised intracranial pressure produces headache and vomiting and may cause a bulging fontanelle in young infants. Seizures are a common feature in children; subdural effusions are present in about 33 per cent of children and occur most frequently in the younger babies. The key to diagnosis is examination of the cerebral spinal fluid.

The outlook for *H. influenzae* meningitis in the UK is that about 95 per cent will survive but about 8 per cent of survivors have serious CNS sequelae, the commonest being sensorineural deafness.

Epiglottitis

Acute respiratory obstruction, caused by a cellulitis of the epiglottis and aryepiglottic folds, typically occurs as a fulminating, life-threatening infection. Sore throat, fever, and dyspnoea progress rapidly to dysphagia, pooling of oral secretions, and drooling of saliva from the mouth. The child is restless and anxious and adopts a sitting position with neck extended and chin protruding in order to reduce airway obstruction. In the absence of adequate treatment, death commonly occurs within a few hours. The course may be less dramatic with a prodromal illness of sore throat and hoarseness from one to several days preceding the onset of acute symptoms. The characteristic findings are that the epiglottis is red and swollen, obstructing the pharynx at the base of the tongue. Examination of the larynx should be done only in a setting in which an airway can be placed since fatal respiratory obstruction may occur abruptly. Indeed, the most important aspect of management of acute epiglottitis is the provision of an adequate airway and ventilation.

Pneumonia and empyema

Lower respiratory tract infections occur most often in children aged less than 5 years and presents as lobar pneumonia, often with pleural involvement. *H. influenzae* pneumonia in adults with primary lung disease or alcoholism has been recognized increasingly in recent years.

Cellulitis

This important infection occurs in young children who present with fever and a raised, warm, tender area of distinctive reddish–blue hue, most often located on one cheek or in the periorbital region, that evolves over a few hours.

Septic arthritis

H. influenzae type b is one of the commonest causes of septic arthritis in children <2 years of age. Typically, there is involvement of a single large, weight-bearing joint, usually without osteomyelitis. Response to drainage and appropriate systemic antibiotics is usually dramatic and apparently curative, but long-term follow-up is important since residual joint dysfunction occurs in a proportion of children.

Treatment of diseases caused by type b strains

Chloramphenicol remains an excellent drug for treating *H. influenzae* meningitis, but isolates showing resistance have emerged. There is a dose-related, reversible bone marrow toxicity, but this is rarely a problem and can be completely avoided if blood levels are monitored. Idiosyncratic bone marrow aplasia has been reported but is extremely rare. Ampicillin, formerly considered an ideal treatment for *H. influenzae* meningitis, is no longer favoured because of the relatively high prevalence of resistant (β-lactamase producing) strains. There is now a trend to use parenteral third generation cephalosporins (cefotaxime or ceftriaxone); these have been shown to be highly effective as initial treatment of suspected bacterial meningitis. Cefuroxime is less effective.

Young children in the same household as a case of invasive type b disease are at significantly increased risk of secondary invasive infection by *H. influenzae* type b. Rifampicin given orally once daily for four days is effective in eradicating nasopharyngeal carriage, and is recommended for all household contacts (children and adults).

Active immunization

In the late 1960s, it was recognized that stimulation of serum antibodies specific for the type b capsule could prevent infection. Use of purified type b polysaccharide as a vaccine did not protect infants and children aged <2 years. Further research was directed towards developing vaccines whose immunogenicity for young children was much improved. Conjugate vaccines involve chemical linking of capsule to a carrier protein, such as tetanus toxoid. Several conjugate vaccines have been developed commercially and all have proved to be very safe and capable of affording high levels (>90 per cent) of protection to children immunised as early as 2 months. Although the vaccines have been in routine use for only a short time, the number of cases of serious type b disease among immunized populations has fallen dramatically.

Diseases caused by non-typeable *H. Influenzae*

Pneumonia

Unencapsulated *H. influenzae* (ntHi) is an important cause of pneumonia in children and adults, especially the elderly, and in individuals with established lung disease, such as chronic bronchitis. In many countries where adverse socioeconomic circumstances are prevalent, acute pneumonia in infants caused by ntHi represents a major cause of morbidity and mortality.

It has been recognized for many years that exacerbations of chronic bronchitis correlate with an increase in the production of purulent sputum from which ntHi are cultured. Such episodes are often precipitated by prior viral infection. A current view holds that the progressive damage in chronic lung disease of individuals with conditions such as chronic bronchitis, cystic fibrosis, and hypogammaglobulinaemia, occurs through the heightened and protracted inflammatory response to a variety of bacteria, including ntHi, in individuals whose respiratory tract lacks the appropriate clearance mechanisms.

Maternal and neonatal sepsis

ntHi are a well documented cause of tubo-ovarian abscess or chronic salpingitis. More ominously, the infant born to such mothers, often prematurely, may develop life-threatening neonatal septicaemia, meningitis, and a form of acute respiratory distress syndrome that is indistinguishable from that caused by group B streptococci.

Acute otitis media and sinusitis

H. influenzae accounts for about one-fifth of all cases of acute bacterial otitis media and more than 90 per cent of the strains isolated from middle ear fluid are non-typeable. Although such episodes occur at any age, they are most common in children aged 6 months to 5 years. Since more than two-thirds of children have one or more episodes of otitis media by age 3 years, a conservative estimate would indicate that more 100 000 cases of ntHi otitis media occur each year in the UK. ntHi is also a common cause of sinusitis in both adults and children.

Conjunctivitis

H. influenzae is an important cause of purulent conjunctivitis. Most of the strains are non-typeable and were formerly considered to be sufficiently distinctive in phenotype as to be referred to as *H. aegyptius*. Interest in these strains was heightened when, in 1984, an apparently new and serious disease was described in Brazilian children who developed life-threatening infections known as Brazilian purpuric fever (BPF). Its peak age incidence is 1–4 years; purulent conjunctivitis, high fever, vomiting, purpura, vascular collapse, and a high mortality are characteristic.

Other infections

All of the diseases that are commonly caused by type b strains are, on rare occasions, caused by strains of capsular serotypes a, c, d, e, and f as well as ntHi. In addition, there are a number of unusual infections documented in small series and case reports; these include: endocarditis, pericarditis, peritonitis, and epidydimo-orchitis. Two other species, *H. parainfluenzae* and *H. aphrophilus*, are also causes of disease, such as endocarditis.

Treatment

Serious infections caused by ntHi, such as meningitis, lower respiratory tract infections, tubal abscess, and neonatal sepsis require systemic treatment with a third generation β-lactam (e.g. ceftriaxone) or co-trimoxazole. Chloramphenicol is also highly effective but blood levels would need to be monitored carefully, especially in premature infants. Sinusitis and otitis media caused by ntHi are often treated effectively with oral amoxicillin, but augmentin would be preferable given the relatively high incidence of strains producing β-lactamase. Oral co-trimoxazole would be an equally sound or alternative choice for trimethoprim-susceptible strains. The use of antibiotics as prophylaxis or treatment of exacerbations of chronic bronchitis is controversial but many advocate their use either to reduce the number of haemophili in the lower respiratory tract or to eradicate them. Drugs of the tetracycline group are effective, but are contraindicated in pregnancy, impaired renal function, or children less than age 10 years; amoxicillin and co-trimoxazole have also proved useful.

Passive immunization

An important group of individuals with increased susceptibility to infection with *H. influenzae*, but particularly non-typeable strains, is that of immunodeficiency, especially primary deficiency of antibody synthesis. These persons benefit from passive infusion of immunoglobulin preparations administered either intramuscularly or intravenously. This form of immunoglobulin replacement undoubtedly decreases the incidence of both systemic infections in these individuals and the number of episodes of both upper and lower respiratory tract infections caused by ntHi.

Further reading

Booy, R. and Moxon, E.R. (1991). Immunisation of infants against *Haemophilus influenzae* type b in the UK. *Archives of Disease in Childhood*, **66**, 1251–4.

Hoiseth, S.K. (1991). The genus *Haemophilus*. In *The Prokaryotes, a handbook on the biology of bacteria: ecophysiology, isolation, identification, applications* (eds. A. Balows, H.G. Trüper, M. Dworkin, W. Harder, and K.H. Schleifer). Springer-Verlag, New York.

Moxon, E.R. (1986). The carrier state: *Haemophilus influenzae*. *Journal of Antimicrobial Chemotherapy*, **18**, S17–24.

Murphy, T.F. and Apicella, M.A. (1987). Non-typeable *Haemophilus influenzae*: A review of clinical aspects, surface antigens, and the human immune response to infection. *Reviews of Infectious Diseases*, **9**, 1–15.

Chapter 16.48

Haemophilus ducreyi and chancroid

A. Ronald

Introduction

Genital ulcer disease (GUD) is the presenting feature of 5 per cent of patients with sexually transmitted diseases (STD) in industrialized societies and of 10–50 per cent in developing countries. *Hemophilus ducreyi* accounts for most ulcers in many developing countries.

Aetiology

Hemophilus ducreyi is a small, bipolar, faintly staining, Gram-negative, non-motile, coccobacillary organism that on initial Gram stain classically is arranged in a 'school of fish' appearance. The organism is fastidious and requires haemin, CO_2, and a temperature of 33°C for optimal growth and produces colonies after 48–72 h of incubation. These are yellow–grey in colour, very cohesive, and vary in size and opacity. The colonies are unique in that they can be nudged intact with a straight wire.

Epidemiology

The estimated global prevalence of chancroid is 7 million. In eastern and southern Africa, Thailand, India, and the Caribbean, the annual incidence in men exceeds 1 per 1000. At least 20 separate recorded introductions and subsequent outbreaks have occurred in industrialized countries during the last two decades. Prostitutes who continue to exchange sex for drugs, money, or other favours despite having active ulcers are the source of most infections. Uncircumcised men are three times as susceptible and continuing epidemics do not occur in populations where most men are circumcised. *H. ducreyi* is rarely present on the genital mucosa without ulceration and no large asymptomatic reservoir exists. Following unprotected sex with an infected individual, 50 per cent or more will become infected. Occasionally *H. ducreyi* can cause urethritis.

Chancroid is a significant risk factor for the heterosexual spread of both HIV-1 and HIV-2. Genital ulcers in women increase two to eight fold their probability of acquiring HIV-1 infection, presumably due to the presence of macrophages and CD4 lymphocytes in the ulcer. In both men and women, ulcers increase markedly HIV excretion in genital secretions and dramatically enhance the risk of partners becoming HIV infected.

Pathogenesis and pathology

H. ducreyi attaches to and invades epithelial cells and produces a cytotoxin and a haemolysin. These are necessary for virulence and presumably produce the tissue necrosis and ulceration characteristic of chancroid. Although humoral and cell-mediated immune response to *H. ducreyi* occur, their role in preventing or modifying infection is unknown. The predominant cellular response to *H. ducreyi* infection is a mononuclear cell infiltrate, predominantly T-lymphocytes and macrophages. *H. ducreyi* can be seen extracellularly and also within neutrophils and histiocytes.

Clinical features

The chancroid ulcer begins with a tender papule which rapidly ulcerates and enlarges. It is painful, irregular, and sharply demarcated. Induration and surrounding erythema are usually not present. The base of the ulcer is uneven with a yellow-greyish purulent exudate that bleeds readily. Most women and about 50 per cent of men have multiple ulcers. 'Kissing' lesions on contiguous skin surfaces are common. Many variants of chancroid have been described including giant ulcers, dwarf chancroid resembling herpes, follicular chancroid mimicking pyogenic infection, transient ulceration with acute regional lymphadenitis similar to lymphogranuloma venereum, and a painless single ulcer resembling syphilis. Due to the capacity of chancroid to mimic all other aetiologic agents, the clinical diagnosis is fraught with error. Also, about 10 per cent of ulcers with *H. ducreyi* also have a second GUD pathogen, usually *T. pallidum* or *H. simplex*. Although chancroid lesions occur anywhere on the genitalia, over 50 per cent are present on the prepuce. In women, most lesions occur on the fourchette, the labia majora and minora, and perianal area with ulcers rarely present on the cervix or vaginal wall. Inguinal lymphadenitis occurs in about 40 per cent of men and 20 per cent of women. Initially the nodes are discrete but, if untreated, they quickly progress to a suppurative buboe that may rupture and form an inguinal abscess.

Laboratory diagnosis

Definitive diagnosis of chancroid requires culture of *H. ducreyi* or demonstration by PCR technology of its presence. The Gram stain is inadequate for diagnosis. No serological tests are available.

Transport media for *H. ducreyi* has been described and the organism will survive on swabs for up to 24 h at 4°C. Gonococcal agar supplemented with vitamins, vancomycin (3 mg/l), and 0.25 per cent activated charcoal supports the growth of *H. ducreyi*. Cultures should be incubated at 31–33°C in a candle extinction jar with a moist paper towel to provide CO_2 and maximum humidity. Colonies appear in

48–72 h and can be further identified by Gram stain, a positive oxidase test, and a requirement for haemin.

Plasmids mediating antimicrobial resistance are present in most *H. ducreyi* and resistance to penicillin, tetracycline, chloramphenicol, sulfonamides, trimethoprim, kanamycin, and streptomycin are widely disseminated. Many of these plasmids are closely related to those in *N. gonorrhoeae* and in *H. influenzae.* All isolates remain susceptible to the macrolides, third-generation cephalosporins, and the fluoroquinolones.

Treatment

Trimethoprim/sulfamethoxazole is no longer effective in most countries. Single-dose therapy with a number of regimens has been very effective but recent studies suggest that concomitant infection with HIV results in recurrences in some individuals treated with single-dose therapy. As a result, current recommendations suggest that most regimens should be prescribed for 3–7 days. Erythromycin, 250 mg three times a day for 7 days, azithromycin as a single 1 g dose, ciprofloxacin 500 mg once daily for 3 days, and fleroxacin as a single dose of 400 mg daily for 3 days will each cure over 95 per cent of patients. A single dose of ceftriaxone was initially very effective but with the rapid spread of HIV infection in this population, failure is now commonplace.

All patients with genital ulcers should be treated for both chancroid and syphilis. Clinical diagnosis is inadequate to select specific treatment for either aetiological agent.

Prognosis

With adequate treatment, the ulcer becomes less painful within 1–2 days and begins to resolve. Most ulcers are healed by 10 days. Persistence past 14 days requires further investigation.

Buboes should be incised or aspirated in order to relieve discomfort and prevent rupture.

Prevention and control

Chancroid can be eliminated with limited resources. Men and women who present with genital ulcers need to be treated at first contact with the health system using a 'Syndromic WHO Approved Approach' that will treat both chancroid and syphilis with effective regimens. Contacts need to be found and treated epidemiologically regardless of whether ulcers are present. Women who sell sex must encourage their partners to use condoms and must have routine monthly examinations for diagnosis and treatment of ulcers. With the very substantial evidence that STD control, particularly eradication of chancroid, will markedly reduce HIV transmission, interventions to do this must be a priority in all societies.

Further reading

Bogaerts, J., Vuylsteke, B., Tello, W.M., Mukantabana, V., Akingeneye, J., Laga, M., and Piot, P. (1995). Simple algorithms for the management of genital ulcers: evaluation in a primary health care centre in Kigali, Rwanda. *Bulletin of the World Health Organization*, **73**, 761–7.

Trees, D.L. and Morse, S.A. (1995). Chancroid and *Haemophilus ducreyi*: an update. *Clinical Microbiology Reviews*, **8**, 357–75.

Chapter 16.49

Bordetella

C. C. Linnemann, Jr

The bacteria of the genus *Bordetella* are primarily pathogens of the respiratory tract because of their propensity for adhering to ciliated epithelial cells. The only distinctive presentation of *Bordetella* infections is the whooping cough syndrome or pertussis, which is characterized by paroxysmal coughing, an inspiratory whoop, and lymphocytosis. This syndrome is usually caused by *B. pertussis,* although *B. parapertussis* and *B. bronchiseptica* occasionally produce the same syndrome. In the past, some pertussis was mistakenly attributed to viral infections

Bordetella infections should be suspected whenever a persistent lower respiratory tract infection is associated with paroxysmal coughing, with or without an inspiratory whoop; or when respiratory symptoms develop after close contact with a documented infection. Most *Bordetella* infections go unrecognized because the symptoms are indistinguishable from other respiratory tract infections and diagnostic tests are seldom done. *B. bronchiseptica* is a pathogen in animals and should be considered in animal handlers with respiratory tract infections. However, most *B. bronchiseptica* infections will be diagnosed from routine cultures collected to evaluate infections in immunosuppressed patients.

The causative agent

Bordetella are small, aerobic, Gram-negative, coccobacillary organisms. *B. pertussis* is a fastidious bacterium requiring special media for culture and grows slowly, requiring 2–5 days to produce recognizable colonies. *B. parapertussis* and *B. bronchiseptica* are less fastidious and will grow on a simple infusion agar or blood agar within 1 or 2 days.

Bordetella pertussis adheres to ciliated epithelial cells in the respiratory tract, producing ciliostasis and subsequent loss of ciliated cells. These organisms are not invasive and usually remain on the surface of the respiratory tract. There are isolated reports of bacteraemia with *B. parapertussis* and *B. bronchiseptica.*

Epidemiology

Man is the only known reservoir of *B. pertussis* and *B. parapertussis,* in contrast to *B. bronchiseptica,* which is found in dogs, rabbits, guinea pigs, swine, and other mammals. *B. pertussis* is transmitted by droplets from symptomatic patients. Asymptomatic infections have been identified but are not important in the spread of disease, and there are no chronic carriers. The transmission of *B. parapertussis* is probably similar to *B. pertussis. B. bronchiseptica* infections may be acquired from contact with animals, but infections have occurred in hospital patients without exposure to animals, suggesting that man is also a reservoir.

Before vaccine was available, epidemics of *B. pertussis* spread through schools and children carried the infection into their homes. The secondary attack rates were 25 to 50 per cent in schools, and 70 to 100 per cent in homes. The high secondary attack rates at home reflected the intense and prolonged exposure to the organism. Most children developed clinically recognizable disease. Mild infections or reinfections occurred in adults caring for sick children.

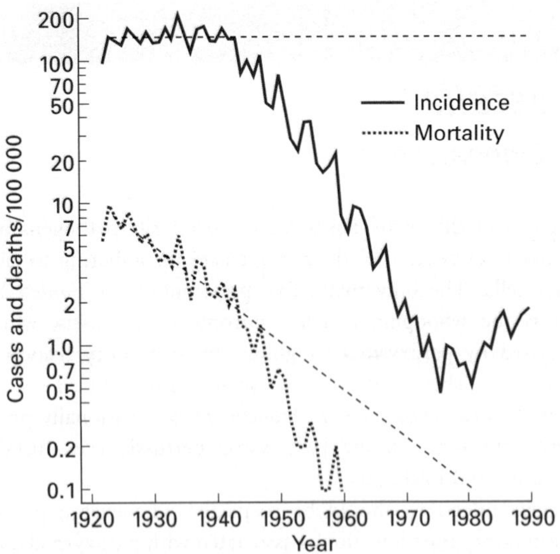

Fig. 1 The effect of pertussis vaccine and the mortality of pertussis in the US. The lines superimposed on the graph indicate the trends prior to the vaccine and as projected if vaccine had not been introduced.

In the vaccine era, major epidemics have disappeared in most developed countries (Fig. 1). In a highly vaccinated population, adults may be important in the transmission of disease. Before vaccine was available, the source of infection could be identified in most cases as another child. Now it is more difficult to trace the source, and, in very young infants, an adult family member frequently appears to be the source. Physicians or nurses may acquire infection from patients and transmit it to other hospital staff and patients.

The epidemiology of *B. parapertussis* is similar to *B. pertussis* except that it has not been modified by vaccine usage. It is widespread in many countries but is seldom recognized because of the mildness of the disease.

Clinical manifestations

After an incubation period of 7–10 days, the illness develops with non-specific upper respiratory symptoms, malaise, anorexia, and sometimes a low-grade fever. This 'catarrhal stage' is indistinguishable from other mild respiratory infections. A dry hacking cough then appears and becomes progressively worse. Older, and presumably partially immune, patients may not progress beyond the catarrhal stage. After 1 or 2 weeks, the paroxysmal stage begins and continues for several weeks. Prolonged coughing episodes may be followed by the characteristic 'whoop', which is produced by forced inspiration through a partially closed glottis. In severe cases, the paroxysms of coughing may be followed by vomiting, and may be associated with epistaxis, petechiae, conjunctival or scleral haemorrhages, haemorrhagic myringitis, or periorbital oedema. Young infants may not have the whoop, and their paroxysms of coughing may be followed by cyanosis and apnoea. Fever is uncommon at this stage in uncomplicated infections. The convalescent stage begins after 2–4 weeks, with gradually resolving paroxysms of coughing. The coughing may persist for weeks to months, and exacerbations with whooping may occur with subsequent respiratory viral infections.

The most characteristic laboratory finding is lymphocytosis appearing towards the end of the catarrhal stage and continuing into the paroxysmal stage. The lymphocytosis is most marked at the time of the most severe coughing but may not occur in very young infants or older children and adults.

Fever suggests a secondary bacterial infection such as otitis media or pneumonia. Atelectasis occurs as a result of bronchial obstruction by the thick mucus, but bronchiectasis is uncommon. The pressures developed during the paroxysmal coughing probably contribute to complications such as mediastinal and subcutaneous emphysema, pneumothorax, inguinal hernias, and rectal prolapse. The most serious non-infectious complications are neurological, including convulsions, paralysis, coma, blindness, deafness, and movement disorders. These are extremely rare.

B. parapertussis produces a milder respiratory illness. Twenty per cent or less of infected children will develop whooping cough. A nondescript bronchitis is probably the most common clinical presentation of *B. bronchiseptica* infections. It can cause sinusitis, tracheobronchitis, and pneumonia in immunosuppressed patients. Bacteraemia, endocarditis, peritonitis, and meningitis have been reported.

Diagnosis

B. pertussis infections are diagnosed by isolation of the organism from nasopharyngeal swabs plated on Bordet–Gengou agar. Fluorescent antibody staining of the swab specimen will provide a presumptive diagnosis. Polymerase chain reaction assays have been used for diagnosis, but are not standardized and are expensive. Infections can be diagnosed by antibody responses in acute and convalescent sera as measured by enzyme immunoassay.

B. parapertussis and *B. bronchiseptica* grow on a routine media used for recovery of Gram-negative bacteria. There are case reports of both these organisms being recovered in blood cultures, and *B. bronchiseptica* has been cultured from urine.

Treatment

Most patients can be managed at home, but infants may need to be in hospital to ensure good nursing care. Cough medicines are of no value, nor is passive immunization. Salbutamol and steroids have been suggested but not proven to be of use. Some physicians sedate young children, but this should be done carefully, if at all.

Early antibiotic treatment during the catarrhal stage will shorten the course of the illness, but if treatment is not started until the paroxysmal stage, antimicrobials will have only a limited effect. Even though there is little clinical benefit, patients in paroxymal stage should receive antimicrobials to render them non-infectious. Erythromycin is the drug of choice. Children should receive 40–50 mg/kg per day, and adults 1.5–2 g per day, for 14 days. Nasopharyngeal cultures will become negative in the first few days of treatment but the erythromycin should be continued to prevent bacteriological relapse (Fig. 2). *B. pertussis* is also sensitive to the newer macrolides, clarithromycin and azithromycin, and treatment with these antibiotics may prove to be effective. Trimethoprim–sulfamethoxazole has been used in children who do not tolerate erythromycin, although its efficacy has not been proven.

B. bronchiseptica is not sensitive to erythromycin. Antipseudomonal penicillins and aminoglycosides have been used successfully to treat serious infections, although the optimal treatment regimen has not been determined.

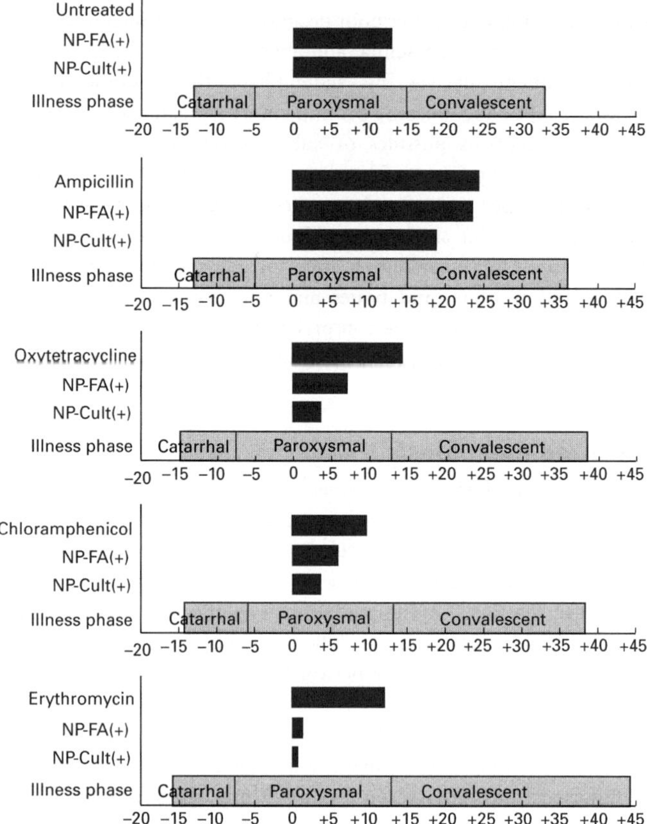

Fig. 2 Duration of excretion of *B. pertussis* as detected by fluorescent antibody staining and culture, and the effect of antimicrobial treatment. The graphs show group means of patients treated with antimicrobial agents compared with untreated control patients.
(Reproduced from Bass, J.W., et al. (1969). Journal of Pediatrics, **75**, *768, with permission.)*

Prevention

Infected patients should avoid contact with susceptible individuals to prevent droplet transmission. The untreated patient will remain infectious for weeks, but communicability will decrease rapidly after the initiation of erythromycin therapy, with cultures becoming negative with 48–72 h. Patients admitted to hospital are usually isolated for the first 5 days of treatment.

Chemoprophylaxis of close contact of patients with *B. pertussis* infection with erythromycin may be effective. If unimmunized, vaccination should continue according to routine schedules. Some recommend a booster dose of vaccine for preschool children who have not received a booster within 6 months. For exposures with a lower risk of transmission, such as those that occur outside the home or day-care centre, contacts should be treated with erythromycin only if they develop respiratory symptoms.

Prevention of *B. pertussis* infections relies on the use of vaccine. Older, whole-cell pertussis vaccines prevent disease, but are associated with frequent reactions. These are being replaced with acellular pertussis vaccines with high efficacy and low reaction rates. An effective immunizing schedule includes three injections at 1 to 2-month intervals beginning at 6–12 weeks of age, and a fourth dose given 1 year after the third. A booster dose is given before entry to school.

Pertussis vaccines have not been given after 6 years of age because of the local reactions even though immunity is neither complete nor lifelong. However, re-exposure to *B. pertussis* may induce continuing immunity in previously vaccinated patients. There are no vaccines available for *B. parapertussis* or *B. bronchiseptica.*

Further reading

Aoyama, T., Sunakawa, K., Iwata, S., Takeuchi, Y., and Fujii, R. (1996). Efficacy of short-term treatment of pertussis with clarithromycin and azithromycin. *Journal of Paediatrics*, **125**, 761–4.

Bass, J.W., Klenk, E.L., Kotheimer, J.B., Linneman, C.C., and Smith, M.H.D. (1969). Antimicrobial treatment of pertussis. *Journal of Pediatrics*, 73, 768–81.

Linnemann, C.C., Jr, (1979). Host-parasite interactions with pertussis. In *International symposium on pertussis* (ed. C. Manclark and J. Hill), pp. 3–18. US Government Printing Office, Washington, DC.

Thomas, M.G. (1989). Epidemiology of pertussis. *Review of Infectious Diseases*, **11**, 255–62.

Woolfrey, B.F. and Moody, J.A. (1991). Human infections associated with *Bordetella bronchiseptica. Clinical Microbiology Reviews*, **4**, 243–55.

Chapter 16.50

Melioidosis and glanders

D. A. B. Dance

Introduction

Melioidosis is infection of humans or animals by the bacterium *Burkholderia* (*Pseudomonas*) *pseudomallei.* (For the history of the disease and its causative organism, see OTM3, p. 590.)

Aetiology

B. pseudomallei is an ovoid, oxidase-positive, motile, bipolar, Gram-negative bacillus. It is closely related to *Burkholderia* (*Pseudomonas*) *mallei*, and to *Burkholderia cepacia*, with which it may be confused in culture. It grows well on most standard culture media, often producing wrinkled colonies and a sweet, earthy smell. Intrinsic resistance to aminoglycosides and polymyxins are characteristic.

Epidemiology

In north-east Thailand, melioidosis accounts for nearly 20 per cent of community-acquired septicaemia, and in the Northern Territory of Australia it is the commonest cause of fatal community-acquired sepsis. It is estimated that 2000–5000 cases occur each year in Thailand, whilst up to 50 cases are diagnosed annually in Singapore and Australia. The disease is also common, but probably under-diagnosed, in Malaysia and elsewhere in south and east Asia including China and the Indian subcontinent. Sporadic cases have also been reported from the Pacific Islands, the Middle East, central Africa, central and south America, and the Caribbean, and an epizootic occurred in France during the 1970s.

B. pseudomallei is an environmental saprophyte found in soil and surface water, particularly rice paddy, in endemic areas. Man and a wide range of other animals are infected by inoculation, inhalation, or ingestion of environmental bacteria, although a specific episode of exposure is rarely identified. Iatrogenic and laboratory-acquired infections have been described occasionally, but person-to-person spread is rare.

Melioidosis is a disease of people in regular contact with soil and water, such as rice farmers in south-east Asia and aboriginals in Australia. All age groups may be affected, although the peak incidence occurs from 40–60 years. Male cases generally outnumber females. There is underlying diseases in 50–70 per cent of cases, such as diabetes mellitus (which may increase the relative risk of infection by up to 100-fold), chronic renal impairment, or other forms of immunocompromise. Perhaps surprisingly there is little evidence that HIV infection predisposes to melioidosis. The disease is markedly seasonal, with a peak occurring during the rainy season. Although most cases are probably recently acquired, the disease may remain latent for more than 20 years before becoming apparent, usually at times of intercurrent illness. The proportion of seropositive persons who are latently infected is unknown.

Pathogenesis and pathology

The outcome of infection with *B. pseudomallei* depends on a balance between the virulence of the organism, the size of inoculum, and the resistance of the host. Little is known about the specific immunological mechanisms responsible for protection, although cell-mediated immunity is probably important. Potential *B. pseudomallei* virulence factors include lipopolysaccharide, a lethal exotoxin, various enzymes (lecithinase, lipase, proteases, acid phosphatase), extracellular polysaccharides, and a siderophore. Intracellular survival of *B. pseudomallei* probably contributes to the recalcitrant nature of melioidosis.

B. pseudomallei causes localized abscesses or granulomata at the site of primary infection, depending on the duration of the lesion. Invasion of the bloodstream leads to septicaemia, which may in turn lead to metastatic foci of infection in other tissues. A high level of bacteraemia (>50 cfu/ml) is associated with a fatal outcome. The host response may also contribute to pathogenesis, since serum levels of several cytokines, including interferon-α, TNF, interleukin-6, and interleukin-8 are also correlated with mortality.

Clinical features

Infections may be acute or chronic, localized, or disseminated. One form of the disease may progress to another. Most infections are presumably mild or asymptomatic. A flu-like illness associated with seroconversion has been reported from Australia.

Septicaemic melioidosis

Sixty per cent of cases of culture-positive melioidosis have positive blood cultures. The majority of these are clinically septicaemic, although some may have a milder, typhoidal illness. There is usually a short history (median 6 days; range 1 day to 2 months) of high fever and rigors. Approximately half have evidence of a primary focus of infection, usually pulmonary or cutaneous. Confusion and stupor, jaundice, and diarrhoea may also be prominent features. Initial investigations usually reveal anaemia, a neutrophil leucocytosis, coagulopathy, and evidence of renal and hepatic impairment. Patients often deteriorate rapidly, developing widespread metastatic abscesses, particularly in the lungs, liver, and spleen, and metabolic acidosis with Kussmaul's breathing. Once septic shock has supervened the mortality approaches 95 per cent, many patients dying within 48 h of hospital admission. Other poor prognostic features include absence of fever, leucopenia, azotaemia, and abnormal liver function tests.

If the patient survives this acute phase, the manifestations of metastatic septic foci become prominent. The organism may seed to any site. Cutaneous pustules or subcutaneous abscesses occur in approximately 10 per cent of cases and an abnormal chest radiograph is found in 80 per cent of patients, the most common pattern being widespread, nodular shadowing ('blood-borne pneumonia'). Other common sites for secondary lesions include the liver and spleen, kidneys and prostate, and bones and joints. Brain abscesses, or a recently described syndrome comprising peripheral motor weakness, brainstem encephalitis, aseptic meningitis, and respiratory failure, may also occur.

Localized melioidosis

Localized melioidosis is commonest in the lung, usually causing a subacute cavitating pneumonia accompanied by profound weight loss. This may be confused with tuberculosis, although relative sparing of the apices and the infrequency of hilar adenopathy may help to distinguish the two. Any lung zone may be affected, although there is a predilection for the upper lobes. Complications include pneumothorax, empyema, purulent pericarditis, and ultimately progression to septicaemia.

Acute suppurative parotitis is a characteristic manifestation of melioidosis in children in Thailand, although it has not been described in imported cases. The reason for this strong age–site association is obscure. Most cases are unilateral and result in parotid abscesses which require surgical drainage, although they may rupture spontaneously into the auditory canal. Facial nerve palsy and septicaemia are rare complications.

Other manifestations of localized melioidosis include cutaneous and subcutaneous abscesses, lymphadenitis, osteomyelitis and septic arthritis, liver and/or splenic abscesses, cystitis, pyelonephritis, prostatic abscesses, epididymo-orchitis, keratitis, and brain abscesses.

Laboratory diagnosis

Melioidosis should be considered in any patient with septicaemia or abscesses who has ever visited an endemic area, particularly if they have underlying diseases such as diabetes mellitus. Microscopy of a Gram-stained smear of pus or sputum is neither specific nor sensitive. Definitive diagnosis depends on isolation and identification of *B. pseudomallei* from cultures of blood or clinically affected sites (e.g. pus, sputum). It is important to alert the laboratory to the suspicion of melioidosis, both to enable appropriate methods and media to be employed and to warn them of the risk of infection (containment level 3 organism). Preliminary culture results should be available within 48 h, although identification may be missed or delayed in non-endemic areas because microbiologists are not familiar with the organism. Several rapid diagnostic techniques for the detection of *B. pseudomallei* antigens or nucleic acids have been developed, but these are not yet widely available.

The serological test most widely used in endemic areas is an indirect haemagglutination (IHA) test, although other assays which detect IgG antibodies give similar results. High background seropositivity means that false positive reactions are common in people from endemic areas, but a single high IHA titre (>1:40) in someone from a non-endemic area, or a rising titre, may be diagnostically useful.

Tests for specific IgM (e.g. indirect immunofluorescence, ELISA) correlate better with disease activity.

Treatment and prognosis

Treatment—general

Patients with septicaemic melioidosis usually require aggressive supportive treatment, including correction of volume depletion and septic shock, respiratory and renal failure, and hyperglycaemia or ketoacidosis. Abscesses should be drained whenever possible.

Treatment—specific

B. pseudomallei is intrinsically resistant to many antibiotics, including aminoglycosides and early β-lactams, and a failure to respond to these agents is characteristic of melioidosis. The fluoroquinolones are also relatively inactive. Several recent studies have shown that the mortality of acute severe melioidosis can be substantially reduced by newer β-lactam agents such as ceftazidime or co-amoxiclav, with or without co-trimoxazole. Ceftazidime is currently the treatment of choice and should be given in full doses (120 mg/kg per day or a dose appropriately adjusted for renal function) for 2–4 weeks according to the clinical response. Carbapenems such as imipenem have some theoretical advantages over ceftazidime, but await prospective evaluation in melioidosis. If these agents are not available, and for β-lactam-allergic patients, chloramphenicol 100 mg/kg per day and doxycycline 4 mg/kg per day, with or without co-trimoxazole 10/50 mg/kg per day, should be used

Following parenteral treatment, prolonged oral antibiotics are needed to prevent relapse, which occurs in up to 23 per cent of patients, and is commoner in patients with more severe disease. This can be reduced to less than 10 per cent if antibiotics are given for 20 weeks. The combination of chloramphenicol (40 mg/kg per day), doxycycline (4 mg/kg per day), and co-trimoxazole (10 mg trimethoprim + 50 mg sulfamethoxazole/kg per day) has been associated with a lower relapse rate than co-amoxiclav (60 mg amoxycillin + 15 mg clavulanic acid/kg per day), although either regimen is probably adequate. Co-amoxiclav is preferable in children and pregnant or lactating women. In patients with mild localized disease, either of the oral regimens described above may be used.

Prognosis

Even with optimal treatment, the mortality from acute severe melioidosis is high (25–40 per cent). In patients who survive, there is often chronic morbidity resulting both from the disease itself and the underlying conditions, and there is an ever-present risk of relapse. Long-term follow-up should therefore be arranged. Monitoring of IgM titres or C-reactive protein may assist in the early detection of relapse. Patients should also be carefully monitored bacteriologically in order to detect the development of antibiotic resistance, which occurs in 5–10 per cent of cases.

Prevention

No *B. pseudomallei* vaccine has been developed for human use, although experimental vaccines have been used in animals. Prevention is thus limited to the avoidance of contact with *B. pseudomallei* in the environment, particularly by 'at-risk' individuals such as diabetics. Whilst this is feasible in developed countries, it is often impractical for the inhabitants of regions where melioidosis is most prevalent. The organism should be handled in a containment level 3 laboratory. Patients should ideally be nursed in standard isolation.

Glanders

Glanders, a rare infection of equines, humans, and other animals, is caused by *B. mallei*. Like *B. pseudomallei*, *B. mallei* may cause granulomatous or pyogenic lesions depending on the duration of infection.

Further reading

Chaowagul, W., White, N.J., Dance, D.A.B., *et al.* (1989). Melioidosis: a major cause of community-acquired septicemia in Northeastern Thailand. *Journal of Infectious Diseases*, **159**, 890–9.

Dance, D.A.B. (1991). Melioidosis: the tip of the iceberg? *Clinical Microbiology Reviews*, **4**, 52–60.

Suputtamongkol, Y., Hall, A.J., Dance, D.A.B., *et al.* (1994). The epidemiology of melioidosis in Ubon Ratchatani, northeast Thailand. *International Journal of Epidemiology*, **23**, 1082–90.

Chapter 16.51

Plague

T. Butler

Introduction

Plague may have caused more deaths than most other diseases and warfare combined; it was estimated to have killed a fourth of Europe's population in the Middle Ages. The present pandemic of plague began in China in the 1860s and spread from Hong Kong by ship's rats to the rest of the world. In the 1960s and 1970s, Vietnam during its war became the leading country for plague, reporting more than 10 000 cases a year. In the last two decades, more cases have been reported from African countries than from Asia and the Americas.

Bacteriology

Y. pestis (formerly *Pasteurella pestis*) is an aerobic Gram-negative, bacillus of the family Enterobacteriaceae. It is readily identified by its failure to ferment lactose on MacConkey agar, an alkaline slant and acid butt in triple–sugar–iron agar and negative reactions for citrate utilization, urease, and indole. *Y. pestis* is virulent because it carries a 45 MDa plasmid that encodes for V and W antigens, which confer a requirement for calcium to grow at 37°C. Additionally, it produces lipopolysaccharide endotoxin and a capsular envelope containing the antiphagocytic principle fraction I antigen.

Epidemiology

During the 1980s there were 8554 cases with 981 deaths reported to the World Health Organization. The countries with more than 100 cases were, in decreasing order: Tanzania, Vietnam, Zaire, Brazil, Madagascar, Peru, Uganda, Burma, Bolivia, US (mostly New Mexico and Arizona), and Botswana. Most of the American cases occur during the months of May to October, when people are outdoors coming into contact with rodents and their fleas. Each endemic region has a specific season for plague.

Table 1 Plague syndromes

Syndrome	Features
Bubonic	Fever, painful lymphadenopathy (bubo)
Septicaemic	Fever, hypotension without bubo
Pneumonic	Cough, haemoptysis, with or without bubo
Cutaneous	Pustule, eschar, carbuncle, or ecthyma gangrenosum, usually with bubo
Meningitis	Fever, nuchal rigidity, usually with bubo

Plague is a zoonotic infection transmitted among the natural animal reservoirs, which are predominantly urban rats and sylvatic rodents, by flea bites, or by ingestion of contaminated animal tissues. Throughout the world, the urban and domestic rats *Rattus rattus* and *R. norvegicus* are the most important reservoirs. During epizootics, when human cases are likely to be reported, intensity of infection in susceptible rodents is increased, leading to 'die-offs' of sometimes massive numbers of rodents. The most efficient vector for transmission is the oriental rat flea *Xenopsylla cheopis.* In sylvatic foci of plague, such as occur in the US, the important reservoirs are the ground squirrel, rock squirrel, and prairie dog. Man is an accidental host in the natural cycle of plague when he is bitten by an infected rodent flea, and plays no part in the maintenance of plague in nature. Only rarely, during epidemics of pneumonic plague, is the infection passed directly from person to person. Rarely, hunters can develop infection by handling contaminated animal tissues. Males and females are equally susceptible and 60 per cent of cases occur in persons less than 20 years old. Within endemic areas, risk factors associated with acquiring plague include direct contact with rodents or carnivores and the presence of refuges and food sources for wild rodents in the vicinity of the home.

Pathogenesis and pathology

Bacteria are inoculated into the skin by a flea bite and migrate to regional lymph nodes, where they multiply during an incubation period of 2–8 days. Inflamed lymph nodes show polymorphonuclear leucocytes, destruction of normal architecture, haemorrhagic necrosis, and dense concentrations of extracellular plague bacilli. Bacteraemia occurs and results in purulent, necrotic, and haemorrhagic lesions in many organs.

Clinical manifestations

Bubonic plague

The most common presentation is bubonic plague (Table 1). Typically, patients develop sudden fever, chills, weakness, and headache. Later they notice the bubo, signalled by intense pain, usually in the groin, axilla, or neck. A swelling evolves in this area, which is so tender that the patients typically avoid any motion that might provoke discomfort. For example if the bubo is in the femoral area, the patient will characteristically flex, abduct, and externally rotate the hip to relieve pressure on the area and will walk with a limp. When the bubo is in an axilla, the patient will abduct the shoulder or hold the arm in a splint.

The buboes are oval swellings that vary from 1–10 cm in length and elevate the overlying skin, which may appear stretched or erythematous. They may appear either as a smooth ovoid mass or as an irregular cluster of several nodes with intervening and surrounding oedema. Palpation elicits extreme tenderness. There is warmth of the overlying skin and an underlying, firm, non-fluctuant mass. Around the lymph nodes there is usually considerable oedema, which can be either gelatinous or pitting in nature. Although often infections other than plague can produce acute lymphadenitis, plague is unique for the suddenness of onset of the fever and bubo, the rapid development of intense inflammation in the bubo, and the fulminant clinical course that can produce death as quickly as 2–4 days after the onset of symptoms. The bubo of plague is also distinctive for the usual absence of a detectable skin lesion in the anatomical region where it is located as well as for the absence of an ascending lymphangitis near it (Fig. 1).

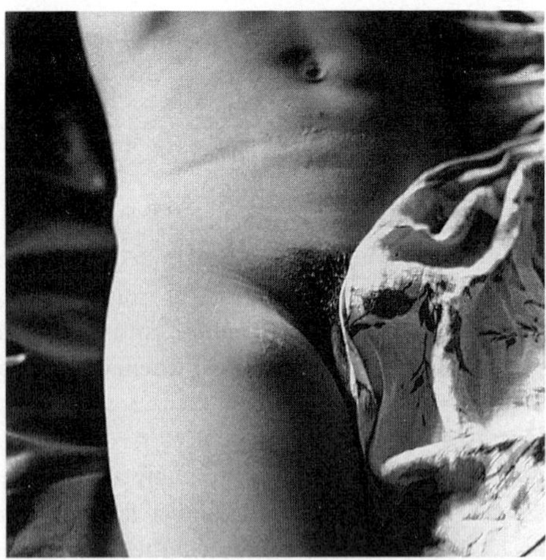

Fig. 1 A right femoral bubo consists of an enlarged, tender lymph node with surrounding oedema.

Patients are typically prostrate and lethargic, or restless and agitated. Occasionally, they are delirious with high fever, and seizures are common in children. Temperatures are usually elevated in the range 38.5 to 40.0°C, and the pulse rates are increased to 110–140/min. Blood pressures are characteristically low, in the range of 100/60 mmHg. Lower pressures that are unobtainable may occur if shock ensues. The liver and spleen are often palpable and tender.

About one-quarter of patients show varied skin findings including pustules, vesicles, eschars, or papules near the bubo or in the anatomical region of skin that is lymphatically drained by the affected lymph nodes, and they presumably represent sites of the flea bites (Fig. 2). Ulceration rarely leads to a larger plague carbuncle. Purpuric lesions may become necrotic, resulting in gangrene of distal extremities, the probable basis of the epithet 'Black Death' attributed to plague through the ages.

Septicaemic plague

In the early stages of bubonic plague, all patients probably have intermittent bacteraemia. Single blood cultures are positive in about a quarter of patients. A blood smear revealing characteristic bacilli has been used as a prognostic indicator in this disease. Occasionally, bacteria proliferate in the body without producing a bubo. This syndrome, 'septicaemic plague', carries a higher case fatality rate than bubonic plague because of delays in diagnosis and treatment.

Pneumonic plague

Secondary pneumonia develops in about 10 per cent of patients with bubonic plague. Infection reaches the lungs by haematogenous spread

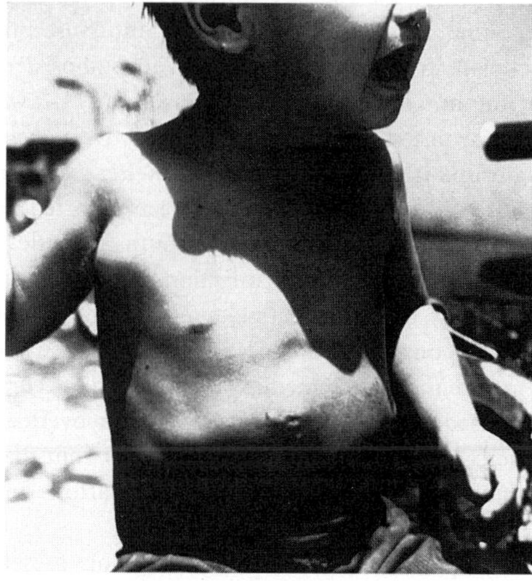

Fig. 2 A right axillary bubo was accompanied by a purulent ulcer on the abdomen, which was the presumed site of the flea bite.

and causes cough, chest pain, and often haemoptysis. Radiographically, there is patchy bronchopneumonia, cavities, or confluent consolidation. The sputum is usually purulent and contains plague bacilli. Primary inhalation pneumonia is rare now but is a potential threat following exposure to a patient with plague who has a cough.

Other syndromes

Plague meningitis is a rare complication that develops more than a week after inadequately treated bubonic plague. It results from haematogenous spread and carries a higher mortality rate than uncomplicated bubonic plague. It presents with typical meningitis symptoms and a polymorphonuclear pleocytosis with Gram-negative bacteria.

Plague pharyngitis may resemble acute tonsillitis. The anterior cervical lymph nodes are usually inflamed, and *Y. pestis* may be recovered from a throat culture or by aspiration of a cervical bubo. It is presumed to follow the inhalation or ingestion of plague bacilli.

Prominent gastrointestinal symptoms such as nausea, vomiting, diarrhoea, and abdominal pain, may precede the bubo or, in septicaemic plague, occur without a bubo; they commonly result in diagnostic delay.

Laboratory findings

The white blood cell count is typically elevated in the range of 10 000 to 20 000 cells/mm^3, with a predominance of immature and mature neutrophils. Severely ill patients tend to have the higher white blood cell counts. Platelets may be normal or low in the early stages of bubonic plague. Although patients with plague rarely develop a generalized bleeding tendency from profound thrombocytopenia, disseminated intravascular coagulation is common in this infection. 'Liver function tests', including serum aminotransferases and bilirubin, are frequently abnormally high. Renal function tests may be abnormal in hypotensive patients.

Diagnosis

Plague should be suspected in febrile patients in endemic areas. A bacteriological diagnosis is made by smear and culture of a bubo aspirate. The aspirate is obtained by inserting a 20-guage needle on a 10-ml syringe containing 1 ml of sterile saline into the bubo and withdrawing it several times until the saline becomes blood-tinged. Because the bubo does not contain liquid pus, it may be necessary to inject some of the saline and immediately reaspirate it. Drops of the aspirate are placed on to microscopic slides. The Gram stain will reveal polymorphonuclear leucocytes and Gram-negative coccobacilli and bipolar-staining bacilli ranging from 1–2 μm in length. Smears of blood, sputum, or spinal fluid can be treated similarly.

The aspirate, blood, and other appropriate fluids should be inoculated on to blood and MacConkey agar plates and into broth for bacteriological identification. At reference laboratories, a serological test, the passive haemagglutination test utilizing fraction I of *Y. pestis*, is available for testing acute- and convalescent-phase serum. A fourfold or greater increase in titre or a single titre of 1:16 or higher is evidence of plague infection.

Treatment and prevention

Antimicrobials

Untreated plague has a mortality rate of greater than 50 per cent and early antibiotic is life-saving. In 1948, streptomycin was identified as the drug of choice by reducing the mortality rate to less than 5 per cent. Streptomycin should be given intramuscularly in two divided doses daily, totalling 30 mg/kg body weight per day for 10 days. Gentamicin 3–5 mg/kg per day may be substituted for streptomycin and given intramuscularly or intravenously.

A satisfactory alternative for ambulatory patients is tetracycline given orally in a dose of 2–4 g/day in four divided doses for 10 days. For patients with meningitis, chloramphenicol should be given intravenously with a loading dose of 25 mg/kg followed by 60 mg/kg per day in four divided doses.

For correction of dehydration and hypotension, intravenous 0.9 per cent saline solution should be given for the first few days. The buboes usually recede without local therapy. Occasionally, however, they may enlarge or become fluctuant during the first week of treatment, requiring incision and drainage.

Precautions

All patients with suspected plague should be reported to the appropriate health department and to the World Health Organization. Patients with uncomplicated infections who are promptly treated present no health hazards to other people. Those with cough or other signs of pneumonia must be placed in respiratory isolation for at least 48 h after starting antimicrobial therapy or until the sputum culture is negative. The bubo aspirate and blood must be handled with gloves and with care to avoid aerosolization in the clinic and laboratory.

Vaccine and prevention

A formalin-killed vaccine, Plague Vaccine USP is available for travellers to endemic areas. A primary series of two injections is recommended with a 1- to 3-month interval between them. Booster injections are given every 6 months for as long as exposure continues. In Britain, vaccine is obtainable, for named patients only, from Greer Laboratories, PO Box 800, Lenoir, North Carolina 28643, US. People living in endemic areas should provide themselves with as much personal protection against rodents and fleas as possible, including living in rat-proof houses, wearing shoes and garments to cover the legs, and dusting houses with insecticide.

Further reading

Bonacorsi, S.P., Scavizzi, M.R., Guiyoule, A., Amouroux, J.H., and Carniel, E. (1994). Assessment of a fluoroquinolone, three B-Lactams, two aminoglycosides and a cycline in treatment of murine *Yersinia pestis* infection. *Antimicrobial Agents Chemotherapy*, 38, 481-6.

Butler, T. (1994). Yersinia infections: centennial of the discovery of the plague bacillus. *Clinical Infectious Diseases*, 19, 655–63.

Campbell, G.L. and Hughes, J.M. (1995). Plague in India: a new warning from an old nemesis. *Annals of Internal Medicine*, 122, 151–3.

McClean, K.L. (1995). An outbreak of plague in Northwestern province, Zambia. *Clinical Infectious Diseases*, 21, 650–2.

Russell, P., Eley, S.M., Bell, D.L., Manchee, R.J., and Titball, R.W. (1996). Doxycycline or ciprofloxacin prophylaxis and therapy against experimental *Yersinia pestis* infection in mice. *Journal of Antimicrobial Chemotherapy*, 37, 769–74.

Chapter 16.52

Yersiniosis*

D. G. Lalloo

Definition

Yersiniosis is caused by two Gram-negative enteric bacteria, *Y. enterocolitica* and *Y. pseudotuberculosis*. These cause a wide spectrum of clinical manifestations, including acute watery diarrhoea, acute mesenteric adenitis, extraintestinal infection, and bacteraemia. Post-infectious sequelae such as arthritis or erythema nodosum are well recognized.

Aetiology and epidemiology

Y. enterocolitica causes infection throughout the world, but appears to be most common in northern Europe and the US. Both sporadic infections and outbreaks occur. Although *Y. enterocolitica* occurs in many hosts, the most important source of infection for man is the pig; however, contact with household pets may also be important. Infection normally occurs after eating or drinking contaminated pork, food, or water and children appear to be more susceptible than adults. A limited number of specific serotypes are associated with infection.

Y. pseudotuberculosis causes zoonotic disease of wild and domestic mammals and human cases are far less common than with *Y. enterolitica*. Infection results from contact with animals and birds and normally affects patients aged between 5 and 20 years.

Clinical features

The incubation period for yersiniosis is 3–7 days. An acute presentation may be followed by secondary immunological complications. An acute enteritis due to *Y. enterocolitica* is most common; this is indistinguishable from *Salmonella* or *Campylobacter* infection with diarrhoea, abdominal pain, nausea, and vomiting. Mesenteric adenitis and terminal ileitis can occur, mimicking acute appendicitis. Ultrasound may be helpful in distinguishing between appendicitis and infectious ileocaecitis. Rare complications include diffuse ulceration of the small intestine and colon, perforation, intussusception, toxic megacolon, cholangitis, and mesenteric vein thrombosis.

Secondary immunological manifestations occur 1–2 weeks after the onset of gastrointestinal symptoms. A reactive polyarthritis or erythema nodosum is most common, but Reiter's syndrome, glomerulonephritis, and myocarditis have all been reported. Symptoms of reactive polyarthritis may take several months to settle.

Y. enterocolitica may cause focal infection in the absence of bacteraemia in a variety of extraintestinal sites, including the pharynx, skin and subcutaneous tissues, bones, conjunctiva, renal tract, and lungs. *Y. enterocolitica* bacteraemia most often occurs in immunocompromised people or patients with iron overload; in this population the case fatality rate may reach 50 per cent. Bacteraemia may lead to metastatic infections including endocarditis, intravenous line infection, meningitis, and septic arthritis.

Mesenteric lymphadenitis is the most common presentation of infection with *Y. pseudotuberculosis*. This mimics acute or subacute appendicitis with abdominal pain and pyrexia. The infection is usually self limited. At laparotomy, enlarged mysenteric lymph nodes are found in the ileocaecal angle and there may be swelling of the terminal ileum or caecum. These presentations must be distinguished from Crohn's disease, tuberculosis, and neoplasia.

Diagnosis

A definitive diagnosis of yersiniosis may be made by culture of the organism from stool, lymph nodes, or blood depending upon the clinical presentation. Serology may be helpful; a serum agglutinin titre of 1: 128 or greater in a previously healthy individual is suggestive of infection. However, negative or minimal titres do not rule out yersiniosis in infants or immunocompromised patients.

Treatment

Antimicrobal therapy is not indicated in uncomplicated disease and treatment does not shorten the course of enterocolitis. Localized infection, bacteraemia, or enterocolitis in an immunocompromised patient should be treated. *Y. enterocolitica* is resistant to most penicillins (including amoxicillin/clavulanate), and first generation cephalosporins. Aminoglycosides, fluoroquinolones, chloramphenicol, tetracycline, and co-trimoxazole are all effective; therapeutic failures have been reported with third generation cephalosporins. *Y. pseudotuberculosis* is also sensitive to ampicillin and cephalosporins.

Further reading

Gayraud, M., Scavizzi, M.R., Mollaret, H.H., Guillevin, L., and Nornstein, M.J. (1993). Antibiotic treatment of *Yersinia enterocolitica*. *Clinical Infectious Diseases*, 17, 405–10.

*Based on the chapter by A. D. Pearson in OTM3, pp. 608–12.

Chapter 16.53

Pasteurellosis*

D. G. Lalloo

Pasteurella species are small, Gram-negative coccobacillae which cause a wide range of diseases from local infection and abscesses to severe systemic infection. The majority of human infections are caused by *Pasteurella multocida* subspecies *multocida*, and subspecies *septica*. They are most often acquired from contact with domestic animals.

Epidemiology

P. multocida is widely distributed as a nasopharyngeal or gastro-intestinal commensal of animals and birds. The organism is carried by 70–90 per cent of domestic cats and 50–70 per cent of dogs. *P. multocida* is usually transferred to man by bites, scratches, or licks from dogs and cats, but in up to 15 per cent of cases no known animal contact occurs. *Pasteurella* spp. can be isolated from 20–30 per cent of dog bite wounds and 50 per cent of cat bite wounds although only a small proportion will become clinically infected. Person-to-person spread has not been recorded, although *P. multocida* can occasionally be found in the nasopharynx of healthy humans exposed to animals.

Clinical features

The most common presentation is local tissue infection following an animal bite. Symptoms such as local erythema, swelling, purulent discharge, and local lymphadenopathy may start within several hours of the bite. Localized infections can also involve deeper tissues, causing abscesses, tenosynovitis, septic arthritis, or osteomyelitis.

P. multocida may be isolated from patients with respiratory tract infection who have no history of animal contact. Most of these patients have chronic respiratory tract disease and isolation may represent long-term colonization. However, *P. multocida* has been implicated in acute upper and lower respiratory tract infection, including acute pneumonia. Local spread may cause tonsillitis, sinusitis, pharyngitis, and epiglotitis.

Bacteraemia may occur from localized infections in many different sites, but endocarditis appears to be relatively rare. However, invasive infection does occur at other sites and *P. multocida* may cause meningitis and other CNS infections, intra-abdominal infections, and urinary tract infections (Table 1).

Diagnosis and treatment

Pasteurella species can be identified as small, Gram-negative rods in stains and can be isolated from sputum, pus, blood, or CSF. Penicillin is the treatment of choice for established infections, tetracycline is a good oral alternative. Third generation cephalosporins and chloramphenicol have been used successfully in more severely ill, hospitalized patients.

*Based on the chapter by A. D. Pearson in OTM3, pp. 606–8.

Table 1 Infections caused by *Pasteurella multocida*: presentations and complications

Skin and soft tissue infections
Cellulitis; subcutaneous abscess; infected decubitus or stasis ulcer; wound infection
Oral and respiratory infections
Tonsillitis or peritonsillar abscess; sinusitis, pharyngitis, epiglottitis; otitis media, mastoiditis and submandibular abscess; lung abscess; tracheobronchitis, pneumonia and empyema
Serious invasive infections
Cardiovascular: endocarditis; bacteraemia; mycotic aneurysm; purulent pericarditis; infected vascular graft
Bone and joint: septic arthritis; osteomyelitis; septic arthritis with osteomyelitis; bursitis; prosthetic joints
Central nervous system: meningitis; brain abscess; subdural empyema
Gastrointestinal tract: liver abscess; spontaneous bacterial peritonitis; omental or appendiceal abscess; peritonitis due to ruptured viscus; gastroenteritis
Genitourinary tract: cystitis or pyelonephritis; infected ileal loop and renal abscess; uterine infection; vaginitis, cervicitis; bartholin gland abscess; chorioamnionitis; epididymitis
Eyes: conjunctivitis; corneal ulcer; endophthalmitis

Treatment of domestic animal bites

The most important factor in avoiding *Pasteurella* infections is the adequate treatment of bites. Thorough cleaning, debridement, and tetanus prophylaxis is crucial. Approximately 5–15 per cent of dog bites and up to 50 per cent of cat bites become infected; the role of prophylactic antibiotics is controversial. Most advocate prophylactic antibiotics for 'high-risk' bites, crush injuries, deep puncture wounds, and wounds to the hands. Many units use prophylactic antibiotics routinely; patients who are immunosuppressed, who have no spleen, or have alcoholic liver disease should certainly be treated. Although small studies have shown no clear benefit from prophylactic antibiotics, a meta-analysis suggested that routine (NNT) antibiotics reduced the incidence of infection with a number needed to treat of 14 to prevent one infection.

Although penicillin has good activity against *Pasteurella* species, prophylactic antibiotics need to cover other organisms commonly found in the oral flora of dogs and cats, for example *Staphylococcus aureus*, other *staphylococcal* species, anaerobes, and *Capnocytophaga canimorsus*. Amoxicillin/clavulanic acid is the prophylactic drug of choice; tetracycline is a good alternative in penicillin-hypersensitive patients. Erythromycin has been used for prophylaxis, but is less effective.

Further reading

Cummings, P. (1994). Antibiotics to prevent infection in patients with dog bite wounds: a meta-analysis of randomized trials. *Annals of Emergency Medicine*, **17**, 405–10.

Goldstein, E.J.C. (1991). Bite wounds and infection. *Clinical Infectious Diseases*, **14**, 633–40.

Talan, D.A., Citron, D.M., Abrahamian, F.M., Moran, G.J., Goldstein, E.J.C. (1999). Bacteriologic analysis of infected dog and cat bites. *New England Journal of Medicine*, **340**, 85–92.

Weber, D.J., Wolfson, J.S., Swartz, M.N., and Hooper, D.C. (1984). *Pasteurella multocida* infections. Report of 34 cases and review of the literature. *Medicine*, **63**, 133–53.

Chapter 16.54

Tularaemia*

D. G. Lalloo

Tularaemia is a zoonotic, arthropod- and water-borne disease caused by *Francisella tularensis*, a small, Gram-negative bacterium that has a complex maintenance system in ticks, wildlife, and aquatic ecosystems. Human infections occur predominantly in the northern hemisphere. Within the species *F. tularensis*, there are several subspecies distinguished by their virulence, epidemiology, and ecology.

Epidemiology

Tularaemia foci occur throughout the world but the majority of cases have been diagnosed in the northern hemisphere (Figs 1,2). Published reports from the former USSR, Europe, and North America describe more than a million cases of human tularaemia during the last 70 years. However, the recognition of occupational hazards and mass vaccination has reduced the incidence.

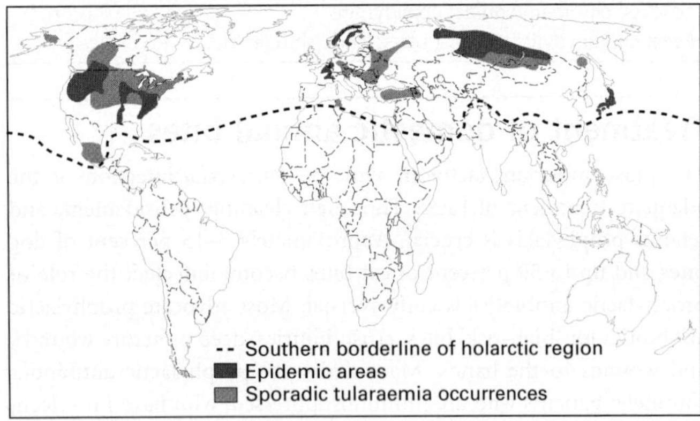

Fig. 1 Tularaemia foci around the world.

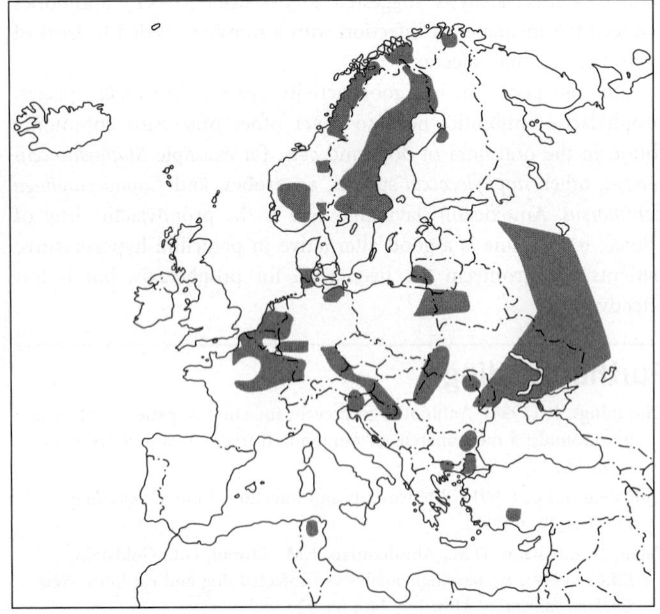

Fig. 2 Tularaemia foci in Europe.

Two types of infection have been described in man: *F. tularensis* subspecies *tularensis* (type A) and *F. tularensis* subspecies *holarctica* (type B). Subsp. *tularensis* primarily affects ticks and lagomorphs (hares and rabbits) and is more virulent for man and rabbits than subsp. *holarctica.* In North America, 95 per cent of human infections are due to subsp. *tularensis.* In Europe, infection is by the less virulent subsp. *holarctica*, which has a greater variety of reservoirs and vectors.

In the US, subsp. *tularensis* is carried by ground squirrels, cottontail rabbits, hares, and jack-rabbits, and can be found from time to time in other wild and domestic animals. Human infections are usually sporadic but with a summer peak, associated with tick or fly bites, and a winter peak attributed to hunting. Ticks of the genera *Dermacentor, Amblyomma, Haemaphysalis,* and *Ixodes* transmit the organism; infections have also been attributed to dog ticks and contact with sick dogs.

Subsp. *holarctica* is less common in the US; strains of this type have been isolated from muskrats, in which they cause epizootics. In the former USSR, subsp. *holarctica* strains are harboured in a wide variety of ecological situations and in a variety of mammals, mainly rodents, as well as hares. The main tick vectors are of the genera *Dermacentor, Ixodes,* and *Rhipicephalus.* Epidemics in Europe have arisen by a number of different mechanisms: hunters and butchers touching infected animals; from the bites of arthropods, ticks, and mosquitoes; from water or foodborne-water contaminated by the dead bodies or excreta of infected animals; and from airborne dissemination of infection acquired by the inhalation of contaminated particles, such as dust from rodent-infested hay.

Clinical presentations of tularaemia (rabbit fever, deerfly fever, Ohara disease)

This depends on the route of transmission and virulence of the organism. The incubation period is usually between 3 and 5 days. Most patients have fever, chills, and prostration, with a relapsing, protracted illness unless they are treated or vaccinated. A number of discrete and mixed clinical syndromes have been described (Fig. 3).

Clinical infections with *F. tularensis* subsp. *tularensis* (type a)

Ulceroglandular tularaemia

Most North American cases are ulceroglandular. Patients present with sudden chills, fever, and often severe headache. At the site of the initial entry of the organism there is an indurated and ragged ulcer or ulcers, often quite small and usually causing little pain, with local tender lymphadenopathy that may steadily increase in size and frequently suppurates. Lymphadenopathy may occur without a visible skin ulcer. The nodes may persist for weeks before the diagnosis is made. Pharyngeal tularaemia may occur if there has been entry of the organism due to oral contact with infected material, but pharyngitis and enlarged local lymph nodes may also occur in patents with ulceroglandular tularaemia who have no history of oral contact with infected material.

Oculoglandular tularaemia is relatively rare. The primary lesion is in the conjunctiva or cornea; conjunctivitis with congestion and

*Based on the chapter by A.D. Pearson in OTM3, pp. 599–605.

Clinical presentations
subsp. *tularensis* (type A, *nearctica*)

American classification
Ulceroglandular
Pulmonary
Typhoidal (enteric or cryptogenic)
Oculoglandular

Classification of clinical forms,
subsp. *holarctica* (type B, *palaearctica*)

Primary stage with primary complex	Generalized infection with septicaemia
External Ulcero-oculo-oral-tonsillar glandular forms	**Internal** Influenzal/pulmonary forms

Secondary generalization
Erythema nodosum
General glandular swelling
Multiple lung infiltrations
Abdominal organs
Central nervous system

Fig. 3 Clinical presentations of human tularaemia caused by *F. tularensis* subsp. *tularensis* (type a) and classification of clinical forms caused by subsp. *holarctica* (type b).

oedema, and a characteristic unilateral preauricular lymphadenopathy occur. This form of tularaemia is usually associated with a history of splashing the face while cleaning infected animals, swimming in contaminated water, or from laboratory accidents.

Typhoidal tularaemia

This form of tularaemia may occur following any mode of acquisition of infection. It is not associated with significant lymphadenopathy. A febrile illness is associated with systemic symptoms which include fevers, chills, pharyngitis, myalgia, and gastrointestinal symptoms including watery diarrhoea. Patients may become severely ill and secondary pneumonic involvement is common.

Pulmonary tularaemia

Pulmonary disease may be primary, resulting from the inhalation of infected aerosols, or secondary from haematogenous spread. Pneumonia is commonly associated with typhoidal disease. Asymptomatic radiological changes are not uncommon but some patients have marked respiratory symptoms and signs of pneumonia. Radiologically, there are multiple parenchymal infiltrates which may be confined to one lobe; these may coalesce and hilar lymphadenopathy may occur. Most infiltrates clear rapidly on therapy, but severe disease with marked toxaemia does occur.

Complications

Suppuration of lymph nodes is common in glandular forms, even following appropriate treatment. Some patients may be unwell with fatigue for several months. In severe disease, impaired renal function, elevated creatine kinase levels, and abnormal liver function may occur; severe disease may be more common in patients with pre-existing illness. Case fatality rates since treatment with streptomycin started are approximately 2–3 per cent.

Clinical infections with *F. tularensis* subsp. *holarctica* (type b)

This subsp. appears to be less virulent than subsp. *tularensis*. Similar forms of infection have been described: the commonly used classification system in the former USSR distinguishes primary and internal complexes from secondary spread of infection (Fig. 3).

Ulcero-cutano-oculo-oral-tonsillar glandular forms

Ulceroglandular tularaemia presents in European cases with either induration or an ulcer at the site of a mosquito bite or single or multiple lesions (Plate 1) after skinning an infected animal. The lymphadenopathy in the drainage area of the primary ulcer or indurated area will be accompanied by sudden chills, fever, and, frequently, severe headache. Later in the course of ulceroglandular disease, hypersensitivity reactions, such as erythema nodosum, may develop.

Other forms

Pulmonary forms of disease occur; in one Swedish epidemic, due to airborne dissemination of crop dust contaminated with vole faeces, 405 patients presented with fevers, chills, and malaise associated with respiratory symptoms. Occasionally, bacteraemic forms with severe disease have been reported.

Diagnosis

In a region where *F. tularensis* is endemic, a provisional diagnosis can often be made on clinical grounds supported by information about the patient's possible exposure, occupation, and recent activities, particularly when a primary lesion is present. When there is no local ulcer, and if the patient has left the area in which the infection was acquired, the illness presents simply as persistent, debilitating fever, pneumonitis, or tonsillitis in which a detailed travel and epidemiological history and laboratory investigations are essential for diagnosis. Routine laboratory investigations are rarely helpful, although sterile pyuria has been noted in up to 20 per cent of cases.

A definitive diagnosis can be made by isolation of the organism, but *F. tularensis* will not grow on routine plating and samples require inoculation on to supportive media. It is important for clinicians to inform the laboratory if tularaemia is suspected; laboratory aerosols cause serious, and occasionally fatal, laboratory-acquired infection. Swabs or aspirates from local lesions and lymph glands should be transported in approved containers. Risks to laboratory personnel may be reduced by using an immunofluorescence method to identify organisms in smears and tissues.

Most diagnoses are made by serology, usually by various agglutination assays. A four-fold rise in titre, or a titre of 1:320 in a single sample by the end of the third week of illness, are diagnostic of tularaemia. Antibody may persist for years after infection. Enzyme-linked immunosorbent assay techniques are more sensitive for the early detection of tularaemia, with the advantage that class-specific immunoglobulins can be detected. Delayed hypersensitivity can be detected by means of an intradermal test, but these tests have not been standardized. Diagnosis of the infecting subspecies cannot be made morphologically or by serology.

Treatment

Aminoglycosides are bactericidal for *F. tularensis* and should be used for the treatment of subsp. *tularensis* (type a) and severe infections with subsp. *holarctica* (type b). Streptomycin is considered to be the drug of choice by many physicians experienced in treating tularaemia, and usually produces a dramatic clinical response. Gentamicin is an effective alternative, although relapses occur more commonly. Tetracycline and chloramphenicol have been used successfully, although relapse rates of 12 per cent and 21 per cent respectively have been reported; tetracyclines may be adequate for mild infections with subsp. *holarctica* if given in an oral dose of 2 g/day for 2 weeks.

In vitro, the organism is also sensitive to erythromycin, second and third generation cephalosporins, and quinolones; their role in treatment of disease is not clear and treatment with ceftriaxone has been unsuccessful in a number of cases.

Prevention

Avoiding human contact with animals and other principal vectors in endemic areas is the most important factor. Immunization may be considered when contact with potentially infected material is inevitable. Vaccines developed from live attenuated strains of subsp. *holarctica* are effective and should be considered for laboratory workers who regularly handle *F. tularensis* or for others with repeated occupational exposure.

Further reading

Evans, M.E., Gregory, D.W., Schaffner, W., and Mcgee, Z.A. (1985). Tularemia: A 30 year experience with 88 cases. *Medicine*, **64**, 251–69.

Penn, R.L. and Kinasewitz, G.T. (1987). Factors associated with a poor outcome in tularemia. *Archives of Internal Medicine*, **147**, 265–8.

Chapter 16.55

Anthrax

A. B. Christie and P. C. B. Turnbull*

Anthrax is primarily a disease of herbivores, although few mammals or birds are thought to be totally resistant to it. Man generally acquires anthrax directly or indirectly from animals. Human anthrax remains common in anthrax endemic countries, principally in Africa and Asia. In non-endemic regions, occasional cases still occur as a result of the handling of contaminated wool, hair, hides, or bones imported from endemic areas.

Aetiology

The causative agent of anthrax is *Bacillus anthracis*, a Gram-positive, aerobic, spore-forming, rod-shaped, non-motile bacterium of approximate dimensions 3–8 μm by 1–2 μm. In the presence of oxygen, spores are formed, one per bacillary (vegetative) cell, centrally or subterminally, and not causing the cell to swell.

In the animal body, the bacilli occur in pairs or short chains, but in laboratory culture they form long filamentous chains. In the absence of oxygen and in the presence of HCO_3^-, conditions met in the body, the bacilli surround themselves with a polypeptide capsule. They compete poorly with putrefactive organisms and die out in the unopened carcass.

The spores are resistant to levels of heat, cold, pH, desiccation, chemicals, etc. that would kill most other living things.

Epidemiology

Herbivores are the most susceptible species and generally acquire anthrax when grazing from contaminated ground. An animal dying of anthrax excretes anthrax bacilli in enormous numbers in bloody discharges from the nose, mouth, and anus (10^7–10^9 bacilli/ml). A proportion of these will sporulate to produce persisting contamination from which subsequent animals may become infected a few hours to many decades later. This is exacerbated if the carcass is opened with spillage of more blood. Infection in livestock normally occurs by uptake of the organism from the environment and is not transmitted directly from animal to animal. Occasionally, wild animals may acquire it more directly by osteophagia and carnivores through feeding on anthrax carcasses.

Humans acquire the disease directly or indirectly from animals. Recorded incidents of human-to-human transmission are exceedingly rare. Human anthrax is traditionally classified as either non-industrial or industrial depending on whether the disease is acquired directly from animals or indirectly during handling and processing of contaminated animal products. Non-industrial anthrax usually affects people who work with animals or animal carcasses and is almost always cutaneous. Industrial anthrax, from handling contaminated animal products, is usually cutaneous but has a higher chance of being pulmonary through inhalation of spore-laden dust.

Most industrial processes kill anthrax spores, so final products such as processed wool and woollen goods, leather, charcoal, etc. are free of spores. However, effluent from early stages of processing such as the initial wash may carry spores into the environment where they may infect livestock.

Biting flies are believed, in some countries, to transmit anthrax in both animals and man.

Pathogenesis

B. anthracis is not invasive and requires a lesion through which to establish its infection. In herbivores, such lesions probably result from uptake of sharp soil particles or thorns, spiky leaves, grass, etc.

On entry into a lesion, the spores germinate to set up a local infection or get carried to the regional lymph nodes where the systemic infection is initiated with involvement of the spleen soon after. In the lymph nodes and spleen the bacteria multiply and produce toxin without the appearance of symptoms until the organs break down releasing the toxin and large numbers of the bacilli in a burst. This leads to sudden onset of hyperacute illness with fever followed within a few hours by disorientation and shock, coma, and death. The course of the disease is generally slower in the more resistant omnivorous or carnivorous species with lower mortality rates. Local oedemas and swollen lymph nodes are early pathognomonic signs. Oedema in the neck, if severe enough, may result in death from asphyxiation.

By far the most common form of the disease in humans is cutaneous anthrax acquired from handling carcasses or products from animals that have died of the disease. The organism gains entry through cuts or abrasions in the skin. Pulmonary anthrax may result from breathing spore-laden dust in industries which process contaminated animal

*Dr A. B. Christie died in 1987. Much of his second edition chapter was retained in OTM3.

products. Circumstantial evidence, however, indicates that humans are relatively resistant to infection.

In the cutaneous form, the infection usually remains localized producing the characteristic eschar and oedema at the site of infection but occasionally it becomes generalized. Experimental studies have shown that inhaled spores can persist for several weeks in the alveoli, being slowly taken up by the alveolar macrophages and carried to the lymph nodes where they germinate and multiply with subsequent events as already described.

The two known virulence factors of *B. anthracis* are the polypeptide capsule which protects it from phagocytosis by the host's defence cells and the toxin produced in the exponential phase of growth. The toxin consists of three synergistic but separable proteins produced simultaneously in the log phase of growth and termed protective antigen (PA), lethal factor (LF), and oedema factor (EF). EF is an adenylate cyclase and PA + EF as a complex produces the altered water and ion movements that lead to the characteristic oedema of anthrax which prevents mobilization of the polymorphonuclear leucocytes. LF is also an enzyme and LF + PA as a complex is the major cause of tissue damage and death.

The genes for PA, LF, and EF are located on a 170–185 kbp plasmid, pXO1. Similarly, the genes involved in capsule synthesis reside on a 90–95 kbp plasmid, pXO2, and code for three enzymes mediating the polymerization of D-glutamic acid.

As the only readily obtainable entities truly specific to *B. anthracis*, the toxin components, make the best antigens for enzyme immunoassays and other diagnostic systems. Similarly, molecular detection systems are based on sequences within the genes encoding the toxin antigens or the capsule precursors.

Clinical manifestations and diagnosis

Cutaneous anthrax

The anthrax sore begins as a pimple which grows rapidly in 2–3 days. Its centre ulcerates, but by about day 4 or 5 becomes a dry, black, firmly adherent scab surrounded by a circle of purplish vesicles (Fig. 1). There is little local pain. Pus and pain only develop if the lesion is secondarily infected. Substantial to massive, non-pitting oedema is a primary characteristic of anthrax (Fig. 2). It should not be incised as this will lead only to an intractable sinus and scarring. Lymph nodes usually enlarge and may be tender.

In uncomplicated cases, the eschar begins to resolve about 10 days after the appearance of the initial pimple. Resolution is slow—2 to 6 weeks regardless of treatment—but usually complete leaving little trace; over the jaw or the eyelid scarring may be more serious. The oedema and lymphadenitis are often very slow to resolve.

The amount of illness varies. Occasionally, the patient continues to feel well but chills, headache, anorexia, and nausea are common. The temperature may be normal, but more often is around 38.3–38.8°C. However, if the infection becomes generalized, the patient may have rigors and the temperature reaches 40°C.

When the lesion is on the face or neck, the oedema may encircle the neck and press on the trachea or affect the larynx making breathing difficult. Tracheotomy must be done without delay.

Considerations in differential diagnosis should include boil, orf, plague, primary syphilitic chancre, erysipelas, glanders, and tropical ulcer.

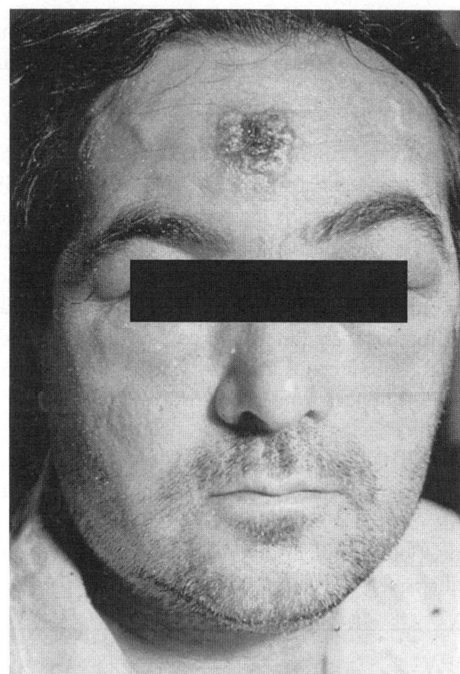

Fig. 1 Anthrax sore showing central eschar and ring of vesicles.

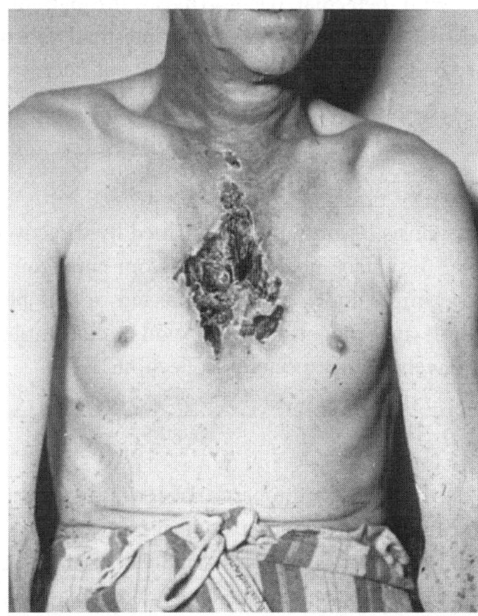

Fig. 2 Anthrax: healing eschar of chest wall. The primary sore was on the back of the patient's neck. Oedema spread from the neck over the chest and abdomen into the scrotum.

Pulmonary anthrax

Illness begins insidiously with no symptoms or with mild, non-specific symptoms of slight fever and malaise. This phase (2 to a few days after exposure) ends with the abrupt onset of chills. In an hour or two the patient is dsypnoeic, cyanosed, and acutely ill with soaring temperature and pronounced rales, rapid heart beat, and feeble pulse. The spleen may be enlarged and tender, there may be some tender lymph nodes in the axilla, but there is nothing else to point to the diagnosis except perhaps the patient's occupation. Untreated, death occurs within hours. Milder cases probably occur as bronchitis in which the diagnosis of anthrax is not considered or recognized.

Intestinal anthrax

This is analogous to cutaneous anthrax with the anthrax lesion developing on the intestinal mucosa instead of the skin. Symptoms of mild to acute gastroenteritis may occur but are sometimes absent. Sudden onset of severe malaise follows the benign incubation period of 2 to a few days with fever, shock, collapse, and death all occurring within a few hours. Effective treatment is likely to depend on awareness of the possibility that it could be anthrax. Subclinical or undiagnosed mild cases with spontaneous recovery occur. Intestinal anthrax in temperate regions appears to be unrecorded.

Anthrax meningitis

Anthrax meningitis is a rare and dangerous complication, usually of the cutaneous form. The meninges are inflamed and in some parts haemorrhagic. Cerebrospinal fluid may be bloodstained and contain anthrax bacilli.

Pathology

Postmortem is forbidden in most countries. Inadvertent postmortems and postmortems of experimentally-infected animals reveal dark, unclotted blood, markedly enlarged haemorrhagic spleen, and affected lymph nodes, with petechial haemorrhages throughout the other visceral organs. In intestinal anthrax, the intestinal mucosa is dark red with glassy oedema and one or more areas of necrosis at the site of the eschar.

Laboratory diagnosis

The clinical diagnosis of anthrax is confirmed by directly visualizing and/or isolating the infecting *B. anthracis* from cutaneous lesions or from blood or lymph nodes or other affected organs postmortem. These procedures are straightforward provided that antibiotic treatment was not given before specimen collection.

Treatment

Penicillin or its relatives are the best antibiotics. Isolates resistant to penicillin have only been reported on three or four occasions and there is no evidence that resistance, when it does occur, is transmissible. In severely toxic or late cases, the first doses may be given intravenously. *B. anthracis* is sensitive to numerous other broad spectrum antibiotics.

The lesion becomes sterile within 24–48 h of antibiotic administration, but the eschar still takes 2–3 weeks to pass through its cycle of development and resolution. It should not be incised or dressed in a way that interferes with repair and there is no need to keep the patient isolated or in hospital. On resolution, there is usually a pale scar left on the skin. Very occasionally there is damage to the underlying tissue sufficient to require surgical repair, especially where the eyelid has been affected.

In pulmonary, intestinal, or hypertoxic cases, the patient needs intensive care. Plasmaphoresed serum or gammaglobulin from a vaccinated person could well be of life-saving value in an emergency. If breathing is threatened by oedema around the neck, early tracheotomy is advised.

Prevention

Control of anthrax depends on control in livestock. Well-supervised disposal of carcasses and of materials contaminated from these carcasses and disinfection of affected premises backed up by immediate vaccination of other members of the affected herd ensure good containment of the disease.

In less developed countries, the only realistic approach is mass vaccination of the livestock. However, in many such regions, the herds are beyond easy reach and the limited resources of the owners and veterinary services make it hard to achieve the ideal.

Vaccines

The livestock vaccine consists of approximately 10^7 spores/ml of the Sterne strain $34F_2$ in 50 per cent glycerine–saline with ± 0.5 per cent saponin as adjuvant. Although theoretically avirulent in being acapsular, this strain does retain a residual virulence and occasional casualties occur with its use. As a result, an analogous live vaccine is not considered suitable for human use in western countries and acellular vaccines for administration to humans have been formulated. Administration of vaccines to humans is only indicated for persons in at-risk occupations such as wool, hides, meat, and bonemeal processing, certain veterinarians and laboratory workers, etc.

The decline in the incidence of human anthrax in Britain since the early part of this century is attributable to effective vaccination programmes in both endemic countries a from which animal products are imported and in Britain itself, together with improved industrial hygiene, particularly good ventilation, dust control measures, suitable clothing and washing facilities, and pretreatment of imported materials. In addition, animal products are frequently pretreated in the country of origin nowadays. There has also been a marked reduction in the number of tanneries in recent years, presumably from the increased use of man-made alternatives. Finally, many manufacturers regard sterilization as good practice thereby again reducing the likelihood of transmission of the disease.

Further reading

Dixon, T.C., Meselson, M., Guillemin, J., and Hanna, P.C. (1999). Medical progress: anthrax. *New England Journal of Medicine*, **341**, 815–26.

Logan, N.A. and Turnbull, P.C.B. (1999). *Baccilus*. In *Manual of clinical microbiology*, (eds P.R. Murry, E.J. Baron, M.A. Pfaller, F.C. Tenover, and R.H. Yolken), 7th edn, pp. 357–69. AMS Press, Washington, D.C.

Quinn, C.P. and Turnbull, P.C.B. (1998). Anthrax. In *Topley and Wilson's microbiology and microbial infections*, (eds L. Collier, A. Balows, and M. Sussman), 9th edn, pp. 799–818. Arnold, London.

Chapter 16.56

Brucellosis

M. M. Madkour

Brucellosis is a common, classical zoonotic disease of world-wide distribution. It is transmitted to man from infected animal reservoirs. Human brucellosis may be caused by one of four species: *Brucella melitensis* (the most common cause worldwide) from goats, sheep, and camels; *B. abortus* from cattle; *B. suis* from hogs; and *B. canis* from dogs. Brucella organisms are small, non-encapsulated, non-motile, non-sporing, Gram-negative, aerobic bacilli, which are facultative intracellular parasites.

Epidemiology

The overall incidence of brucellosis in the world is increasing. Childhood brucellosis indicates the endemicity of the disease in an area. In non-endemic areas, human brucellosis is mostly an occupational disease particularly among workers in meat processing industries and in farmers, veterinarians, and laboratory workers. The disease is transmitted by ingestion of untreated milk or its products, raw meat, liver, or bone marrow. Animal contact and inhalation of the organisms is a frequent cause of infection particularly among children, herdsmen, dairy farm workers, and laboratory workers. Penetration of intact or abraded skin is a common route of infection among abattoir workers. Accidental autoinoculation or conjunctival splashing of live brucella vaccine during animal vaccination may occur among veterinarians. Transplacental transmission of infection from mother to fetus may occur. Brucella organisms have been isolated from human breast mild and nursing mothers may infect their infants through breast feeding. Sexual transmission in human, similar to that in animals, has been reported, with isolation of the organisms from human semen. Rarely, transmission may occur through blood transfusion or bone marrow transplants.

Pathogenesis

Polymorphonuclear leucocytes migrate to the site of entry and phagocytosis of the organism occurs. Activated macrophages play a similar role. The interaction between the host and bacteria determines the outcome of the infection. Intracellular multiplication of the organisms may occur. They then pass through lymphatics to regional lymph nodes and organs rich in reticuloendothelial tissue. Other organs and tissue may be invaded through the blood stream. Cell-mediated immunity plays an important role against infection with non-specific inflammatory cell infiltrates or granulomas. Caseation, necrosis, and even abscess formation may occur. Production of specific antibodies is important. IgM is the first to appear, followed a few days later by IgG. After a few months, the IgM levels tend to fall while IgG remains high.

Clinical features

The incubation period is 1–3 weeks but may extend up to several months. The clinical features of brucellosis are not specific. *B. melitensis* has a high pathogenicity producing more intense symptoms. The onset may be sudden (1–2 days) or gradual (1 week or more). It presents as a febrile illness, with or without localization to particular organs. Brucellosis has been arbitrarily classified into acute, subacute, chronic, bacteraemic, serologic, localized, or mixed type, which does not serve any purpose. The term 'active brucellosis with or without localization' may be more useful for the purpose of diagnosis and treatment. Clinical history, symptoms, and signs of brucellosis are given in Tables 1 and 2.

Table 1 History and symptoms in 500 patients with brucellosis due to *B. melitensis*

History/symptoms	No. (%)	History/symptoms	No. (%)
Animal contact	368 (73.6)	Headaches	403 (80.6)
Raw milk/cheese	350 (70.0)	Loss of appetite	388 (77.6)
Raw liver ingestion	147 (29.4)	Weight loss	326 (65.2)
Family history	188 (37.6)	Constipation	234 (46.9)
Fever	464 (92.8)	Abdominal pain	225 (45.0)
Chills	410 (82.0)	Diarrhoea	34 (6.8)
Sweating	437 (87.4)	Cough	122 (24.4)
Body aches	457 (91.4)	Testicular pain (of 290 males)	62 (21.3)
Lack of energy	473 (94.6)		
Joint pain	431 (86.2)	Skin rash	72 (14.4)
Back pain	431 (86.2)	Sleep disturbances	185 (37.0)

Table 2 Signs in 500 patients with brucellosis due to *B. melitensis*

Signs	No. (%)	Signs	No. (%)
Looks ill	127 (25.4)	Epididymo-orchitis	62 (21.3)
Pallor	110 (22.0)	Skin rash	72 (14.4)
Lymphadenopathy	160 (32.0)	Jaundice	6 (1.2)
Splenomegaly	125 (25.0)	CNS abnormalities	20 (4.0)
Hepatomegaly	97 (19.4)	Cardiac murmur	17 (3.4)
Arthritis	202 (40.4)	Pneumonia	7 (1.4)
Spinal tenderness	241 (48.0)		

Bone and joints

Reactive migratory polyarthritis is common and affects mainly large joints. Septic monoarthritis may be a presenting feature. The spine may be affected and brucella spondylitis occurs mostly in adults and is extremely rare during childhood. The lumbar spine, particularly L4, is the most frequent site. Extraspinal osteomyelitis is rare and affects mainly long bones. Bursitis, tenosynovitis, and subcutaneous nodules may also occur. Unlike with septic arthritis and osteomyelitis due to other organisms, the peripheral white cell count is normal and the erythrocyte sedimentation rate is normal or accelerated.

Cardiovascular

Cardiovascular complications may include endocarditis, myocarditis, pericarditis, aortic root abscess, mycotic aneurysms, thrombophlebitis, and pulmonary embolism. Brucella endocarditis may occur on a previously damaged valve or a congenital malformation but can occur even on normal valves. Blood culture should be extended up to 6 weeks in suspected patients.

Respiratory

Respiratory complications are common but mild. A 'flu-like' illness with sore throat, tonsillitis, and mild dry cough is common. Hilar and paratracheal lymphadenopathy, pneumonia, solitary or multiple nodular or miliary lung shadowing, pleural effusion, or emphysema may occur.

Gastrointestinal

Gastrointestinal complications are usually mild. Hepatitis with mild jaundice may be present. Rarely, mesenteric lymphadenitis, cholecystitis, peritonitis, and pancreatitis may be a presenting feature. The liver transaminases, alkaline phosphatase, and serum bilirubin may be mildly raised. Liver biopsy may show non-specific reactive hepatitis, micro-, or macrogranuloma formations.

Genitourinary

Genitourinary complications may be the presentation of brucellosis including unilateral or, rarely, bilateral epididymo-orchitis, prostatitis, seminal vesiculitis, dysmenorrhoea, and amenorrhoea. Pregnant women may develop abortion, intrauterine fetal death, retention of products of conception, premature delivery, or normal delivery.

Neurobrucellosis

Neurobrucellosis is an uncommon but serious complication. It includes meningoencephalitis, multiple cerebral or cerebellar abscesses, ruptured mycotic aneurysm, cranial nerve lesions, transient ischaemic attacks, hemiplegia, myelitis, radiculoneuropathy, Guillain–Barré syndrome, multiple sclerosis-like picture, sciatica, granulomatous myositis, and rhabdomyolysis. The psychological features of brucellosis are no greater than those cause by other infections. The cerebrospinal fluid (CSF) pressure is usually elevated and the fluid may look turbid or rarely haemorrhagic. The CSF protein, cells (predominantly lymphocytes), and oligoclonal immunoglobulin are raised, while glucose may be reduced or normal. Brucella organisms may be cultured from CSF.

Dermatological complications may include maculopapular eruption, contact dermatitis, erythema nodosum, purpura, abscess formation, superficial thrombophlebitis, or rarely discharging sinuses.

The eyes may be involved through direct splashing of live vaccine or by neuro-ophthalmic complications. This may lead to conjunctivitis, keratitis, uveitis, retinopathy, retinal detachment, endogenous endophthalmitis, papilloedema, papillitis, optic atrophy, or ophthalmoplegia.

Thyroiditis, adrenal insufficiency, and the syndrome of inappropriate secretion of antidiuretic hormones have been reported.

Diagnosis

The diagnosis depends on the detection of raised serum brucella agglutinins with or without positive blood (or other body fluids or tissues) culture in a symptomatic patient. An agglutinin titre of 1/160–1/320 or higher is considered as significant. Brucella antibodies can be detected by the standard tube test (STT), rose bengal plate test, 2-mercaptoethanol test (2-ME), antihuman globulin (AHG-Coombs) test, radioimmunoassay, and enzymeimmunoassay. A false-negative standard tube test (Prozone phenomenon) may occur due to the presence of blocking antibodies which can be avoided by screening sera at low and high titres. An elevated IgG antibody indicates recent infection, while low titre indicates previous contact with the organisms. An elevated IgM antibody indicates active disease. The total peripheral blood white cell count is usually normal and leucopenia with relative lymphocytosis does not always occur. Thrombocytopenia and features of disseminated intravascular coagulation may occur. In the great majority, joint, bone, and spine will have normal plain radiographs and occasionally show soft tissue swelling or subarticular demineralization. Destructive arthropathy is rare. Bone destruction at a discovertebral junction with anterior osteophytes and reduction in disc space can be seen on plain radiographs. Bone scintigraphy is more sensitive (for early screening and accurate localization of affected areas) than plain radiography. Computed tomography (CT) scanning is useful for further evaluation of bone, disc, paraspinal soft tissue, and extension of infection into spinal canal and neural foramina. Magnetic resonance imaging (MRI) is more sensitive than CT for showing the extent of brucella spondylitis.

Treatment

A combination of a tetracycline and an aminoglycoside remains the most effective regimen because of its synergistic effect. Oral doxycycline (100 mg, twice daily) is preferred to other tetracyclines (500 mg, 6-hourly). Streptomycin is given intramuscularly in a dose of 1 g/day for patients under 45 years of age and 0.5–0.75 g/day for older patients; the plasma trough concentration should be 1–2 μg/ml. Netilmicin, 4–6 mg/kg per day, is given intramuscularly in two divided doses or intravenously in divided doses, 8-hourly; the plasma trough concentration should be 2–4 μg/ml. Gentamicin, 2–5 mg/kg daily, is given intravenously in divided doses, 8-hourly; the plasma trough concentration should be 1–2 μg/ml. Combination therapy should be given for 1 month, followed by tetracycline and rifampicin (600–900 mg/day as a single oral dose) for a further 1–2 months.

Children aged 7 years or more should be treated with the above regimen after adjusting the doses. Infants and children under 7 years of age should be treated with a combination of rifampicin and co-trimoxazole for 2–3 months. Rifampicin is given as a single dose either orally or intravenously, 10–20 mg/kg. Co-trimoxazole is given in infancy up to 6 months of age, 8–10 mg/kg per day in two to four divided doses intravenously or 240 mg/day in two divided doses orally. Children under 40 kg in weight should be given 8 mg/kg every 12 h. In endemic areas, for infants and children up to 7 years of age with serious complications, discoloration of the teeth is of secondary importance. Doxycycline and an aminoglycoside combination should be used—doxycycline 50–100 mg/day orally; gentamicin, infants aged up to 2 weeks, 3 mg/kg every 12 h, aged 2 weeks–12 years, 2 mg/kg every 8 h intramuscularly or by slow intravenous injection; netilmicin, infants aged up to 1 week, 3 mg/kg every 12 h, aged over 1 week, 2.5–3 mg/kg every 8 h intramuscularly or intravenous infusions.

Pregnant women should be treated with the combination of co-trimoxazole and rifampicin for 2–3 months. Patients with renal impairment can be treated with doxycycline and an aminoglycoside if plasma drug concentration and renal function testing are available. Otherwise the combination doxycycline and rifampicin should be used. Patients with brucella endocarditis and meningitis, rifampicin 600–900 mg/day should be added to the combination therapy for the whole duration of treatment. Urgent cardiac surgery may be required of the patient develops cardiac failure or aortic root abscess.

Further reading

Madkour, M.M. (1989). *Brucellosis.* Butterworth, London.

Chapter 16.57

Tetanus

F. E. Udwadia

Tetanus is an acute, often fatal, disease, resulting from contamination of wounds by *Clostridium tetani.* This is a spore-forming, Gram-positive, motile, rod-shaped organism. It can only grow under anaerobic conditions, when the vegetative forms secrete a powerful exotoxin which on reaching the central nervous system produces the increased muscle tone and spasms that characterize the disease.

Epidemiology

Spores of *Cl. tetani* are ubiquitous. The natural habitat is manure and cultivated soil. Spores are also present in animal and human faeces, and have been recovered from house dust and from the air of buildings, slums, and even of hospitals and operating theatres.

Tetanus chiefly afflicts the poor, uneducated, and underprivileged people of the world. It is widely prevalent in India, Pakistan, Bangladesh, parts of South-East Asia, Africa, and South America, where the disease is commoner in the young and newborns. World-wide, about 800 000 neonates die of tetanus each year. The disease is increasingly rare in the West, because of improved economy, better health care, and good immunization programmes. In the West it is commoner in adults older than 50 years, when the effects of immunization have worn off, in the unimmunized, in the impoverished, and in drug addicts.

Physiopathology

Under anaerobic conditions the tetanus bacillus within a wound produces the toxin tetanospasmin which spreads to underlying muscles and is bound to the ganglioside membrane receptors of presynapic motor nerve endings. It then travels retrogradely, intra-axonally, to reach the motor horn cells of the segments of the cord supplying these muscles. The toxin within the wound also enters the bloodstream and is distributed via the blood to the peripheral nerve endings of all muscles in the body. It ascends intra-axonally through numerous peripheral nerves to reach motor cells of the whole spinal cord and brainstem, and also sympathetic neurones in the lateral horns and parasympathetic centres. After reaching cell bodies in the spinal cord and brainstem, the toxin retrogradely crosses the presynaptic cleft and binds to presynaptic nerve terminals of inhibitory neurones, blocking the release of inhibitory neurotransmitters (chiefly glycine and γ-aminobutyric acid). This blockage releases motor and autonomic neurones from inhibitory control (Fig. 1). The uncontrolled, disinhibited efferent discharge from motor neurones in the cord and brainstem leads to widespread muscle rigidity and reflex spasms characteristic of the disease. Disinhibited autonomic discharge leads to disturbances in autonomic control, involving both the sympathetic and parasympathetic systems.

Medullary and hypothalamic centres can be affected by the toxin. Myocardial dysfunction and disturbances in impulse conduction may occur. Tetanus toxin can also produce peripheral neuromuscular blockade by preventing the release of acetylcholine. This paralytic effect is observed in cephalic tetanus.

Clinical features

In 15–25 per cent of patients with tetanus there is no evidence of a recent wound. This is because tetanus can result from the most trivial of wounds. Wounds contaminated by manure, garden soil, or injury by rusty metals are particularly dangerous. Tetanus can complicate burns, ulcers, discharging middle ear infections, septic abortions, childbirth, and can also occur following surgery or after intramuscular injections. Tetanus neonatorum is almost always due to non-sterile obstetric techniques, and in India to the dreadful practice of applying cowdung to the cut end of the umbilical cord.

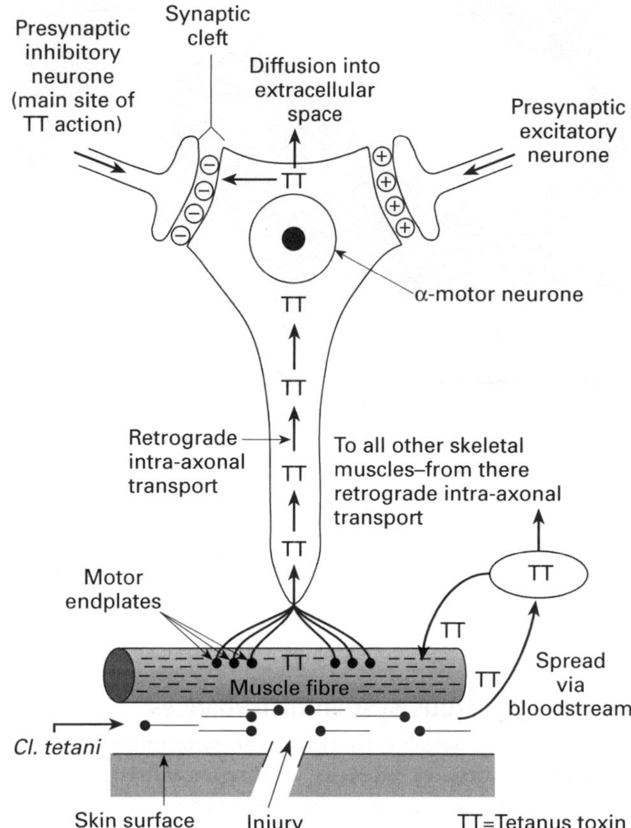

Fig. 1 Retrograde intra-axonal transport of tetanospasmin and its main site of action in the CNS.

The incubation period averages 7–10 days but may range from 1–2 days to a couple of months. The period of onset is the interval between the first symptom and the onset of spasms.

The clinical features of tetanus are rigidity and muscle spasms or seizures. Severe tetanus is also invariably associated with autonomic disturbances.

Rigidity

Stiffness of the masseters is often the first manifestation of the disease resulting in difficulty in opening the mouth—trismus or lockjaw. Typically, rigidity then spreads to involve the face, all skeletal muscles, and muscles of the pharynx resulting in dysphagia. The tetanus facies is diagnostic. The eyes appear partially closed and the forehead furrowed, corrugators contracted, nasolabial folds prominent, the angles of the mouth being stretched outwards and slightly downwards to produce a 'risus sardonicus' (Fig. 2). The expression suggests pathetic anguish, anxiety, and fear. Stiffness of thoracic muscles impairs respiration, and stiffness of abdominal muscles often causes a board-like abdominal rigidity. Rigidity of the neck and back may lead to opisthotonos, particularly in children.

Muscle spasms

Mild tetanus is characterized solely by rigidity without spasms. Spasms or seizures consist of reflex tonic contractions of stiff muscles. They may be transient and mild, or protracted and severe. Spasms are frequently brought on by touch, but can also be triggered by visual, auditory, or emotional stimuli. In severe cases, seizures are almost continuous, rendering breathing impossible or shallow, so that the

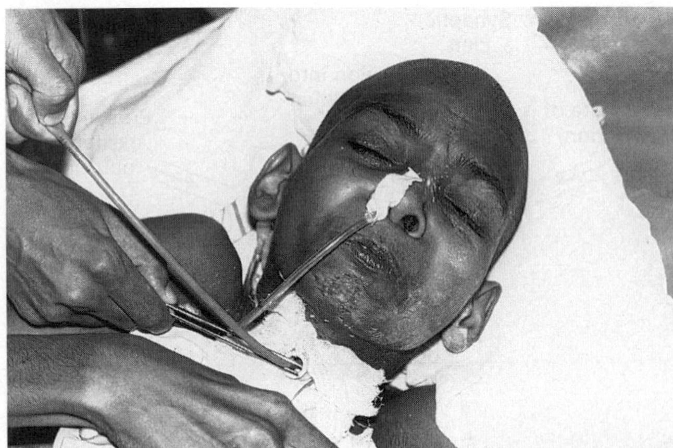

Fig. 2 Facies in tetanus.

patient is hypoxic and cyanosed. Pharyngeal spasms prevent swallowing and result in pooling of saliva in the mouth and throat. Protracted, unrelieved laryngeal spasm can cause death from asphyxia. In the poorly-managed patient death chiefly occurs from respiratory failure or cardiovascular complications.

Autonomic nervous system disturbances

Severe tetanus is invariably associated with sympathetic and parasympathetic disturbances. These include marked tachycardia, severe drenching sweats, modest elevations in systemic blood pressure, increase in salivary and tracheabronchial secretions, and evidence of increased vagal tone.

The disease peaks over 7–10 days, reaches a plateau for the next 1–3 weeks, and then subsides over the next 10–15 days. Muscle stiffness my persist for months after recovery.

Severity of tetanus

Grading the severity of tetanus is important for prognosis and management. The following criteria, though subjective and arbitrary, have stood the test of time in our unit.

Grade I (mild)—generalized rigidity; no spasms.

Grade II (moderate)—marked rigidity; short-lasting spasms; mild dysphagia; moderate respiratory embarrassment.

Grade III (severe)—severe spasms; marked dysphagia; tachycardia >120/min; respiratory rate >40/min; apnoeic spells.

Grade IV (very severe)—grade III plus violent autonomic disturbances. These include severe, persistent hypotension, severe persistent hypertension or episodes of severe hypertension and tachycardia alternating with hypotension and bradycardia.

Cephalic tetanus

This occurs after injury to the head and is confined to muscles innervated by the cranial nerves. It is characterized by unilateral facial palsy with associated stiffness of other muscles of the face. Rarely, bilateral facial palsy and paresis of the glossopharyngeal and vagus nerves may occur. Cephalic tetanus often progresses to generalized tetanus.

Tetanus neonatorum

The earliest symptom is difficulty in suckling and swallowing due to stiffness of muscles of the jaw and pharynx. Risus sardonicus, muscle stiffness, and frequent spasms with opisthotonos occur. Autonomic disturbances are common and death results from cardiorespiratory failure.

Local tetanus

Rarely muscle rigidity and spasms may be localized to muscles adjacent to the wound or be confined to a limb.

Complications

Complications in tetanus are frequent and numerous, chiefly involving the respiratory and cardiovascular systems.

Respiratory complications

These include: (a) atelectasis and aspiration pneumonia; (b) pneumonia, bronchopneumonia, mainly due to Gram-negative organisms; (c) laryngeal spasms; (d) severe hypoxia and respiratory failure due to uncontrolled spasms; (e) episodes of respiratory distress with tachypnoea, probably central in origin; (f) acute lung injury due to the disease per se, or to complicating sepsis; (g) complications related to tracheostomy and to prolonged ventilator support.

Cardiovascular and autonomic complications

These include: (a) sustained tachycardia >170–180/min; (b) persistent hypotension; (c) autonomic storms—episodes of hypertension and tachycardia alternating with hypotension and bradycardia; (d) increased vagal tone causing bradycardia or even cardiac arrest; (e) supraventricular and ventricular arrhythmias; (f) hyperthermia and rarely hypothermia suggestive of hypothalamic involvement.

Sudden death

Sudden cardiac arrest causing death remains the single most dreaded complication of moderate and severe tetanus. It may be related to: (a) cardiovascular instability due to fluctuating autonomic tone; (b) excessive vagal activity; (c) severe hypoxia; (d) sudden hyperpyrexia; (e) impaired infranodal conduction; (f) pulmonary embolism.

Other complications

These are generally incidental to the prolonged management of critically ill patients on ventilator support. These include: (a) iatrogenic sepsis with multiple organ failure; (b) gastrointestinal bleeds, ileus, or diarrhoea; (c) renal insufficiency; (d) fluid, electrolyte, and acid–base disturbances; (e) fractures, generally of one or more mid-thoracic vertebrae during severe spasms; (f) miscellaneous complications, for example bedsores, thrombophlebitis, peripheral neuritis, corneal ulcers, anaemia, hypoproteinaemia.

Diagnosis

Diagnosis is based solely on clinical features. Absence of a wound does not exclude tetanus. Trismus produced by tetanus should be distinguished from masseter spasm due to alveolar or peritonsillar abscesses. Dystonic reactions caused by phenothiazines and metoclopramide, spasms due to hypocalcaemic tetany, and seizures due to strychnine poisoning may superficially mimic tetanus. Meningitis or meningoencephalitis can also produce trismus, rigidity, seizures, and opisthotonus, but can be differentiated by CSF examination which is normal in tetanus. Cephalic tetanus can be mistaken for rabies because of severe dysphagia—however, hydrophobia never occurs in tetanus.

Mortality

Tetanus neonatorum carries a mortality of 60–80 per cent. Mortality in adult tetanus ranges from 20–60 per cent. It is higher in the older age group and in those with a short incubation period (<4 days). A short period of onset (<2 days), more reliably prognosticates severe disease. The introduction of critical care and ventilator support in severe tetanus has lead to a drop in overall mortality from 30 per cent to 12 per cent and the mortality in fulminant tetanus from near 100 per cent to 23 per cent, in our unit. In a good, well-equipped, critical care unit in Bombay, the mortality in severe tetanus in adults was as low as 6 per cent.

Management

All patients with tetanus should be admitted to an intensive care unit. Unfortunately, this is not always possible in poor, developing countries. Motivation and training for better patient care, coupled with basic equipment for respiratory care and support can, however, work wonders in reducing mortality even in the absence of full intensive care facilities.

The use of antiserum

Equine antiserum is generally available even in poor countries; 10 000 units are given intravenously on admission, skin test do not reliably predict hypersensitivity to the equine serum and fatal anaphylaxis has occurred even when the skin tests show negative. Human immunoglobulin is superior to equine antiserum, produces no hypersensitivity reactions, and if available should be given in preference to the latter in a dose of 5000 units, intravenously. The intrathecal use of tetanus antiserum is best avoided as claims of its efficacy remain unproven. Antiserum should be given before local manipulation of the wound, which is treated according to the usual surgical principles with debridement of necrotic tissue.

Antibiotics

Crystalline penicillin, 2 mega units, are administered intravenously, 6-hourly for 8 days. Metronidazole, 500 mg intravenously 8-hourly for 8 days, may be even more effective.

Management strategies

Mild (Grade I) tetanus should be treated conservatively with the use of sedatives and muscle relaxants. Grade II (moderate) tetanus in addition to the use of sedative and muscle relaxants, should have a tracheostomy. Grades III and IV (severe forms) tetanus require sedation, tracheostomy, and continuous ventilator support following induced paralysis with curare-like drugs until spasms relent and recovery ensues.

Use of sedatives and muscle relaxants

Sedatives and muscle relaxants (to reduce rigidity and control spasms) form the cornerstone of management in Grade I and Grade II tetanus.

Diazepam is the drug of choice in most units. The dose is 5–20 mg thrice daily in children and adults, and 2 mg thrice daily in neonates. In mild tetanus it is given orally; in moderate tetanus it is given intravenously as a slow drip over 24 h. It is best not to exceed the dose of 80–120 mg over 24 h in adults, as respiration is otherwise invariably depressed.

Chlorpromazine continues to be used in a few units—50 mg 6-hourly intramuscularly in adults, 25 mg in children, and 12.5 mg in neonates. It can be used in combination with diazepam or with diazepam and phenobarbitone.

The ideal dosage schedule should ensure relaxation and sleep, but allow the patient to be aroused and obey commands. An objective guide to adequate dosage is relaxation of the abdominal muscles which feel much less rigid on palpatation.

Induced paralysis with ventilator support

This is mandatory in Grades III and IV tetanus, as management restricted to the use of high doses of sedatives and muscle relaxants results in a forbidding mortality.

Gallamine or pancuronium are the drugs generally available to induce paralysis in poor countries. Pancuronium is to be preferred as it has less effect on the cardiovascular system. Vecuronium is, however, the drug of choice; it is now available in India but is still far too expensive. The principle in using curare-like drugs is to induce paralysis and allow efficient ventilator support. The dose of gallamine is 20–40 mg intravenously, and of pancuronium 2–4 mg intravenously every half to two hours. The dose of vecuronium is 0.1 mg/kg. Pancuronium or vecuronium can also be given in a slow intravenous drip and the dose titrated to produce the desired effect. As the patient improves, pancuronium or vecuronium are given at longer intervals or the infusion rate is reduced. Patients with severe tetanus generally require 3–8 weeks of ventilator support.

It is inadvisable and harmful in our opinion to use large doses of intravenous diazepam in paralysed patients on ventilator support—30 to 40 mg diazepam over 24 h suffices to counter anxiety in these patients.

Treatment of autonomic circulatory disturbances

Intravenous β-blockers, heavy sedation, intravenous morphine sulphate, labetalol, magnesium sulphate infusion, and intravenous clonidine have all been used to control autonomic storms in severe tetanus. These drugs do not alter overall mortality. We prefer to avoid drugs that strongly depress the central or autonomic nervous systems.

1. Hypotensive spells are best treated with a volume load; if this is ineffective or contraindicated, a titrated dose of dopamine is used to keep the systolic pressure between 100 and 120 mmHg.
2. Hypertensive spells are best treated by titrated dose of oral propranolol or nifedipine. Intravenous propranolol is dangerous and should not be used.
3. Bradyrhythmias are treaded with atropine, and bursts of sinus tachycardia with verapamil or oral propranolol.

Sedatives and drugs used in doses that strongly depress the central or autonomic nervous systems probably contribute to a high mortality by predisposing to cardiac arrest (particularly following hypotensive spells and sudden bradyrhythms), and by preventing successful resuscitation.

Management principles outlined above have been shown to result in a very low mortality in severe tetanus (6 per cent).

Treatment of other complications

These should be promptly diagnosed and treated. All organ systems may need support.

Critical care and nursing

Critical care and good nursing are essential for survival. Particular stress should be laid on (a) adequate arterial PaO_2, O_2 saturation, and O_2 transport; (b) fluid–electrolyte balance; (c) prevention, detection, and control of infection and sepsis; and (d) good nutrition.

Tetanus is a dreadfully catabolic disease—a diet of 3000–3500 calories with 100 g of proteins should be administrated through the nasogastric tube.

Use of tetanus toxoid

Tetanus does not confer immunity. Active immunization is achieved by giving the first dose of tetanus toxoid during convalescence and the next two doses at the recommended intervals.

Prevention

Tetanus is a preventable disease through active immunization with adsorbed tetanus toxoid (ATT) and by proper management of wounds.

Active immunization

The following regime is advocated:

- in infancy and childhood—three doses of triple vaccine (tetanus, diphtheria, pertussis) are given at monthly intervals, and a booster dose is given at 4–6 years of age.
- unimmunized individuals above 7 years—triple vaccine in three doses, the first and second, 6 weeks apart, and the third dose 6 months after the second.

Subsequent immunization

Booster doses of tetanus toxoid should be given every 10 years—a practical impossibility in poor countries.

Immunization after minor, uninfected wounds

Passive immunization with equine or human tetanus antitoxin is not indicated for minor, clean wounds. Active immunization (with 0.5 ml ATT) is indicated if: (a) immunization status is unknown; or (b) more than 10 years have elapsed after the last dose of ATT. Under the above circumstances, especially in poor countries, ATT is also administered prior to emergency surgery, deliveries, obstetric procedures.

Immunization after infected or major wounds

Passive immunization (250–500 units human tetanus immunoglobulin or 5000 units equine antitoxin intramuscularly) is recommend in all individuals who are not immunized, partially immunized, or whose immunization status is unknown. Indication for administration of ATT is the same as for minor, uninfected wounds. It would, however, be safer to use a booster dose of ATT even in a well-immunized individual if more than 5 years have elapsed since the last dose of ATT.

Prevention of tetanus neonatorum

Primary immunization of pregnant women with two injections of ATT at monthly intervals, preferably in the last two trimesters, together with education of nurses and midwives on sterile obstetric techniques, would significantly reduce the incidence of tetanus neonatorum in developing countries.

Further reading

Adams, E.B., Laurence, D.R., and Smith, J.W.G. (1969). *Tetanus.* Blackwell Scientific, Oxford.

Sutton, D.N., Trenlitt, M.B., Woodcock, T.E., and Nielsen, N.S. (1990). Management of autonomic dysfunction in severe tetanus: the use of magnesium sulphate and clonidine. *Intensive Care Medicine*, **16**, 75–80.

Udwadia, F.E. (1994). *Tetanus.* Oxford University Press, Bombay.

Udwadia, F.E., Lall, A., Udwadia, Z.F., Sekhar, M., and Vora, A. (1987). Tetanus and its complications: intensive care and management experience in 150 Indian patients. *Epidemiology and Infection*, **99**, 675–84.

Udwadia, F.E. *et al.* (1992). Haemodynamic studies during the management of severe tetanus. *Quarterly Journal of Medicine*, **83**, 449–60.

Chapter 16.58

Botulism, gas gangrene, and clostridial gastrointestinal infections

H. E. Larson

Botulism

Botulism is an acute, symmetrical, descending paralysis of cranial and autonomic nerves caused by the exotoxin of *Clostridium botulinum.* Intoxication results from ingestion of canned, smoked, or fermented food containing toxin or rarely from wound infection or intestinal colonization.

Occurrence

C. botulinum spores contaminate food from soil and mud, survive brief periods of heating at 100°C, and multiply and release toxin in the anaerobic conditions required for food preservation. Outbreaks typically involve small groups. Botulinum toxin is rapidly inactivated by ordinary cooking temperatures.

Ingested toxin crosses mucous membranes and binds irreversibly and preferentially to nerves with frequent depolarization cycles. Impulse transmission mediated by acetylcholine is blocked at myoneural junctions, autonomic ganglia, and parasympathetic nerve terminals.

History

Symptoms begin 12–72 h after eating poisoned food. Patients with short incubation periods are likely to have ingested large amounts of toxin. However, but the clinical attack rates varies. Initial complaints include dizziness, unsteadiness, diplopia, and blurred vision; these progress to difficulty with speech or swallowing, limb paralysis, and generalized weakness. Parasympathetic blockade may produce nausea, vomiting, abdominal bloating, mouth dryness, and pain in the throat. Further symptoms are difficulty holding up the head and breathing, constipation, and urinary hesitancy. Death can occur within a day of the first symptoms.

Physical examination

Clinical signs reflect autonomic and motor nervous system dysfunction. Mucous membranes are dry and the tongue is furrowed. Lateral rectus weakness produces internal strabismus. Accommodation fails and the pupils fix in mid position or dilate and fail to respond to light. Ptosis, weakness of other extraocular muscles, and inability to protrude the tongue or to raise the shoulders are other early findings. Weakness in the limbs is of the flaccid, lower motor neurone type and deep tendon reflexes are initially preserved. Facial muscles, gag, and corneal reflexes may be spared. Respiratory muscle weakness can develop rapidly. Autonomic paralysis causes hypotension without compensatory tachycardia, intestinal ileus, and urinary retention.

Diagnosis

The differential diagnosis includes the descending form of acute inflammatory polyneuropathy or Guillain–Barré syndrome, diphtheria, intoxication with atropine or organophosphorus compounds, myasthenia gravis, cerebrovascular disease involving the brainstem producing bulbar palsy, paralytic rabies, tick paralysis, and neurotoxic snake bite. Carbon monoxide poisoning invariably produces headaches; mushroom poisoning causes severe abdominal pain. Symptoms begin soon after poisoning from chemicals or fish. Botulism is confirmed by detecting toxin in serum, urine, or stomach contents. Electromyography shows reduced amplitude muscle action potentials that enhance after tetanic stimulus. Nerve conduction velocities are normal; this result differentiates botulism from Guillain–Barré syndrome.

Treatment

Respiratory effort should be monitored closely with vital capacity or peak flow measurements. Some aminoglycosides potentiate neuromuscular blockade. Hypotension can be consequent to hypoxaemia, acidosis, hypovolaemia, or autonomic paralysis.

Trivalent (types A, B, and E) antitoxin reduces case fatality and shortens the course of the illness. Treatment is initiated on clinical grounds, before the diagnosis can be confirmed. The toxin type cannot be specified from the clinical history. Antitoxin is available from designated regional hospitals in the UK: half the dose is given intramuscularly and half intravenously. It is customary to give 0.1 ml of the antiserum intradermally, but most serum reactions are not predicted by this. Human botulism immune plasma can be obtained from the Center for Disease Control, Atlanta, Georgia, US.

Drug treatments have not improved respiratory muscle weakness or tidal volume. Gastric lavage, repeated high enemas, and cathartics may remove unabsorbed toxin and antibiotic treatment may prevent endogenous toxin formation. Ileus and urinary retention are treated supportively. Mortality from botulism was 60–70 per cent but has improved to 23 per cent with respiratory support. In 1977, there were no deaths among 59 cases. Recovery from botulism depends upon the formation of new neuromuscular junctions; clinical improvement thus takes weeks to months. One severe case recovered after being ventilated for 173 days.

Wound botulism

Rarely, botulism may develop 4–17 (average 7) days after injury. Recognition may be delayed by the presence of fever, by gas gangrene, or by the absence of gastrointestinal symptoms. Respiratory failure may occur in a patient receiving aminoglycosides. The diagnosis is confirmed by electromyography; botulinum toxin is detected in serum in about half of the reported cases. *C. botulinum* can be recovered from wounds in the absence of clinical botulism.

Gas gangrene

Gas gangrene is a rapidly-spreading infection of muscle by toxin-producing clostridial species. It occasions profound constitutional toxicity and is invariably fatal if untreated. Gas gangrene occurs after battlefield, civilian, and iatrogenic trauma. Antibiotic prophylaxis virtually eliminates the risk after elective surgery. Rapid evacuation and treatment by well organized surgical teams reduced the incidence to a very few cases during the Vietnam and Falklands conflicts.

Gas gangrene is caused by anaerobic, Gram-positive, spore-forming bacilli, usually *C. perfringens* type A, sometimes *C. novii* and *C. septicum*, and rarely *C. histolyticum*, *C. sordellii*, and *C. fallax*. Clostridia occur naturally in the soil and in the gastrointestinal tracts of man and animals. Oxygen inhibits their growth and prevents toxin production. Necrotic tissue, foreign bodies, and ischaemia in a wound all reduce the locally available oxygen. Gas gangrene can be a primary infection of the perineum or scrotum, or present in a limb seeded from colonic neoplasm colonized with the relatively aerotolerant *C. septicum*.

History

The incubation period of gas gangrene is usually less than 4 days, often less than 24 h, and occasionally as short as 1–6 h. The most characteristic symptom is sudden, severe or excruciating pain at the site of the wound.

Physical examination

Early in the disease it can be difficult to account for the patient's pain. Swelling, bluish discoloration, or darkening of the skin at the affected site then develops. The wound becomes oedematous and a thin, serous ooze emerges. Pain increases in severity; the overlying skin becomes stretched and develops a brown or 'bronzed' discoloration. Haemorrhagic vesicles and areas of frank necrosis then appear. A sweet odour from the wound has been described. Gas is not invariably present. Crepitus may be felt and the wound becomes exquisitely tender. Patients become sweaty and febrile, and though alert and oriented, are very distressed. The pulse rate is elevated out of proportion to the fever, which is not necessarily high. Death may occur within 48 h. At operation, infected muscle appears dark red with purple discoloration; necrosis and liquefaction may occur.

Clostridial myonecrosis must be distinguished from anaerobic cellulitis and anaerobic streptococcal myositis (see Chapters 16.45, 16.38). Diabetic patients develop gas gangrene due to their predisposition to ischaemic vascular disease. Numerous micro-organisms, both aerobic and anaerobic, can produce gas in tissues.

Diagnosis

The diagnosis is clinical. Sudden deterioration in a postoperative patient or following trauma requires examination of the wound and surrounding tissue. Gram stain of the wound discharge, aspirate, or needle biopsy specimen may show many large, plump, Gram-positive bacilli, usually without spores and few, if any, polymorphonuclear leucocytes. In anaerobic streptococcal myositis and anaerobic cellulitis, many leucocytes are found and in the former, long chains of Gram-positive cocci. Imaging may detect small amounts of intramuscular gas in early lesions, but the absence of gas does not exclude the diagnosis.

Treatment

All affected muscle must be surgically removed. Antimicrobials, hyperbaric oxygen, and antitoxin are adjunctive. Penicillin in doses 20–30 million units daily, clindamycin at a dose of 900 mg every 6 h, and metronidazole are used. Clindamycin and metronidazole may reduce toxin production.

Administration of gas-gangrene antitoxin is controversial, but its use during the Second World War was said to have reduced mortality.

Shock, blood loss, dehydration, other infections and acute renal failure may complicate management. The mortality of established disease, even in specialized centres, still ranges between 11 and 31 per cent.

Prevention

Antimicrobial prophylaxis is essential for elective operations associated with an increased risk, such as amputation for ischaemic vascular disease. Penicillin, a first generation cephalosporin, or metronidazole is given intravenously prior to surgery. Wounds should be excised widely followed by antibiotic treatment with delayed closure. Both passive and active immunization can confer protection.

Clostridial infections of the gastrointestinal tract

Pseudomembranous colitis

Pseudomembranous colitis is an acute, exudative infection of the colon caused by *Clostridium difficile*.

Aetiology

C. difficile is an anaerobic, spore-forming, Gram-positive bacillus that can colonize the large intestine where it produces toxins that inflame the mucous membrane. Healthy adults rarely carry *C. difficile*. Antimicrobial treatment impairs native resistance to colonization with *C. difficile*.

Clinical history

Direct questioning may elicit a history; antimicrobials self-administered, taken for trivial complaints, or used as long as 3 or 4 weeks before the start of diarrhoea. Pseudomembranous colitis is most strongly associated with clindamycin, ampicillin, and the cephalosporins, but is not exclusive to them. It occasionally occurs in individuals with no previous antibiotic treatment. The disease is more common in older patients but has been described in infants. Diarrhoea may be self-limiting or debilitating and prolonged; occasionally an acute megacolon presentation may be difficult to distinguish from acute obstruction or peritonitis. Patients may develop sudden chills, fever, and signs of an acute abdomen. Severe abdominal pain is not common and finding of frank blood in the stools suggests a different type of colitis.

Physical examination

Elderly patients appear tired, toxic, and ill. Low fever, a dry furred tongue, and abdominal tenderness, sometimes with peritonism, are the most common clinical signs. Signs of dehydration may be present, but hypotension attributable to hypovolaemia is not common. Spiking temperatures may also be seen and a distended, tense abdomen suggests obstruction.

Diagnosis

Most patients have a polymorphonuclear leucocytosis, sometimes exceeding 30 000/µl. Leucocytes are present in the faeces. Patients with prolonged diarrhoea develop azotaemia out of proportion to their dehydration. Hypoalbuminaemia reflects faecal protein loss. Faeces should be examined for the presence of *C. difficile* toxin. For immediate diagnosis sigmoidoscopy may reveal raised, mucoid to opaque yellow plaques (0.2–2 mm across). If the mucosa appears normal, lesions may be present on rectal biopsy. Pseudomembranes can be distributed unevenly in the colon or may be absent in mild cases.

The differential diagnosis of pseudomembranous colitis includes other forms of antimicrobial-associated colitis, diarrhoea due to *Salmonella*, *Shigella*, and *Campylobacter* series, intestinal amoebiasis, Crohn's disease, and non-specific ulcerative colitis. Two-thirds or more of patients with simple antimicrobial-associated diarrhoea do not have infection with *C. difficile*. Often they complain of sudden abdominal pain and bloody diarrhoea that subsides within a day or two of stopping antimicrobial treatment. Occasionally, patients may be infected with *C. difficile* in addition to another micro-organism capable of causing diarrhoea. *C. difficile* may exacerbate in some patients with inflammatory bowel disease.

Treatment

Stopping the causative antimicrobial may allow *C. difficile* colitis to resolve spontaneously. More seriously ill patients benefit from enteral vancomycin 125 mg or metronidazole 250 mg four times a day. Severe cases usually show improvement after 48 h of treatment. Some physicians regard metronidazole as less effective. Failure to respond to vancomycin suggests that the diagnosis is incorrect or that an additional condition or complication may be present. Parenteral administration of either vancomycin or metronidazole may fail to cure the infection. Patients who are dehydrated need fluid resuscitation; constitutional toxicity and peritonism resolve with treatment. Cholestyramine resins have no effect on the clinical course of colitis. Surgery is appropriately reserved for indications such as free abdominal air or obstruction. In patients who are unable to take vancomycin orally, some physicians have attempted to instil it into the colon via a caecostomy tube; others combine intragastic vancomycin, intermittent clamping of the nasogastric tube, and parenteral metronidazole. *C. difficile* antitoxin is not available in the UK.

Antimicrobial treatment may be followed by relapse. Relapse is not due to antimicrobial resistance and patients continue to respond to treatment with the original or an alternative drug. Patients relapse either because treatment did not clear them of *C. difficile* or because a new exposure to environmental strains has occurred. Vancomycin and metronidazole themselves can induce susceptibility to the disease and prolonged treatment may prolong susceptibility. Patients whose *C. difficile* colitis resolves without antibiotic treatment do not relapse.

Regimens suggested for the treatment of multiple relapses include tapering doses of vancomycin, a *Lactobacillus* preparation three times a day, or cholestyramine three times a day after a therapeutic course of vancomycin. Cholestyramine combined with tapering vancomycin doses to once daily when diarrhoea stops, then to alternate days, then to progressively longer dosing intervals, can prevent early relapse. Some patients with severe colitis or multiple relapses may continue to have diarrhoea due to lingering mucosal injury. Bowel rest with total parenteral nutrition can allow healing and recovery; continued treatment against *C. difficile* is not required. Normal flora may be reconstituted by giving a suspension of normal faeces as an enema.

It may be necessary under certain circumstances to continue an antimicrobial when a patient has developed pseudomembranous colitis. Concurrent therapy with vancomycin can be successful, although some physicians believe that clinical improvement occurs more slowly. If antimicrobial therapy has to be continued after recovery from colitis, administration of vancomycin 125 mg once a day has prevented immediate relapse. It would be reasonable to replace a drug commonly associated with pseudomembranous colitis by one which is not, such as a quinolone, aminoglycoside, tetracycline, or sulphonamide. Repeat treatment with an inducing antimicrobial at some later time is not contraindicated in a patient who has recovered from pseudomembranous colitis.

Prevention

Pseudomembranous colitis can be nosocomial. Patients with diarrhoea and incontinence are the most important sources of cross-contamination. The chain of infection for isolated cases may be difficult to trace because spores persist for weeks to months. Physical cleanliness, enteric precautions, confinement to a single room, and reduced use of the most frequent inducing antimicrobials reduce the incidence. There is no value in retesting patients until they are free of toxin nor in treating asymptomatic toxin excretors.

Necrotizing enterocolitis

Definition

Necrotizing enterocolitis is characterized by necrosis of the intestinal mucosa and the gut wall. Outbreaks in different circumstances have produced variant terms: darmbrand (Germany), pig bel (Papua New Guinea), enteritis necroticans, or gas gangrene of the bowel. Cases can be sporadic or epidemic.

C. perfringens (*C. welchii*) is the cause of adult and epidemic cases of necrotizing enterocolitis. Sporadic adult cases usually yield *C. perfringens* type A, but there is evidence implicating *C. perfringens* type C in German and Papua New Guinea outbreaks. This type produces large amounts of β-toxin. Patients with pig bel show rising β-antitoxin titres, and specific passive or active immunization prevents the disease. Patients with severe persistent neutropenia may develop caecal infection with *C. septicum* which progresses to a fulminant and fatal colitis. Necrotizing enterocolitis in infants has not been shown to be caused by clostridia.

History and physical examination

Isolated cases are usually in people over 50 years of age or in an individual recovering from surgery. Epidemics follow ingestion of contaminated food or dramatic change in eating habits, such as pig feasting among New Guinea highlanders. Symptoms develop suddenly with colicky abdominal pain becoming severe and continuous. Bloody diarrhoea and vomiting may occur. The patient may be extremely toxic. On examination there is a fever, with abdominal distension, localized or diffuse tenderness, and reduced bowel sounds. A tender mass may be palpated. The clinical and laboratory findings of septic shock may be present. If there is recovery from acute illness, intestinal scarring can produce malabsorption or chronic partial obstruction.

Treatment and prevention

Patients with suspected pig bel should be treated by aspirating gastric contents though a large nasogastric tube and by administering intravenous fluids. Pyrantel is given by mouth and the bowel rested by fasting. Penicillin is given intravenously, 1 million units every 4 h, and the patient observed for surgical complications. *C. perfringens* type C toxoid vaccine is useful in local areas where pig bel continues to be common. Two doses spaced 3–4 months apart are given.

Clostridium perfringens food poisoning

Occurrence and clinical findings

In the UK and the US, food poisoning caused by *C. perfringens* is the third most common type of food-borne illness. Meat and poultry are responsible for 90 per cent of the outbreaks, which occur in schools, hospitals, factories, or catering establishments. The circumstances surrounding an outbreak repeat themselves with monotonous regularity. A meat dish prepared by stewing, braising, boiling, or steaming is allowed to stand at ambient temperatures for a period of 4 to 24 h. The food is served cold or after desultory rewarming. Six to 12 h after eating, victims complain of crampy abdominal pain and diarrhoea. Vomiting and fever are unusual. Twelve to 24 h later the diarrhoea and pain have subsided. Many cases of *C. perfringens* food poisoning are not reported because symptoms are self-limiting. Antibodies to the toxin mediating the symptoms are highly prevalent.

Aetiology

C. perfringens is an ubiquitous, sporulating anaerobe. Strains associated with food poisoning are type A, are heat resistant, and produce heat-labile enterotoxin associated with sporulation. *C. perfringens* often contaminates the surface of raw meat and rolling and grinding distributes it throughout. Heat-resistant strains survive cooking methods with maximum temperatures of 100°C. The spores germinate and multiply to 10^6 to 10^7 cells/g in the nutrient rich, anaerobic environment created when meat cools slowly or stands at ambient temperature. If re-heating does not kill these cells, they multiply again when ingested, sporulate, and release toxin. Enterotoxin-producing strains of *C. perfringens* may overgrow in the gut and cause diarrhoea in elderly patients without known contact with contaminated food. Diarrhoea is associated with colony counts of 10^8 to 10^{10}/g of faeces and high titres of free toxin. Previous antimicrobial treatment may encourage the overgrowth and the same strain has been found to cross infect patients.

Further reading

Bartlett, J.G. (1992). The 10 most common questions about *Clostridium difficile*-associated diarrhoea/colitis. *Infectious Diseases in Clinical Practice*, 1, 254–9.

Case records of Massachusetts General Hospital No. 48 (1980). *New England Journal of Medicine*, **303**, 1347–55.

Critchley, E.M.R., Hayes, P.J., and Isaacs P.E.T. (1989). Outbreak of botulism in north west England and Wales, June 1989. *Lancet*, **ii**, 849–53.

Darke, S.G., King, A.M., and Slack, W.K. (1977). Gas gangrene and related infection: classification, clinical features and aetiology, management and mortality. A report of 88 cases. *British Journal of Surgery*, **64**, 104–12.

Larson, H.E., Price, A.B., Honour, P., and Borriello, S.P. (1978). *Clostridium difficile* and the aetiology of pseudomembranous colitis. *Lancet*, **1**, 106–34.

Lawrence, G.W., Murrell, T.G.C., and Walker, P.D. (1979). Pigbel. *Papua New Guinea Medical Journal*, **22**.

Shouler, P.J. (1983). The management of missile injuries. *Journal of the Royal Navy Medical Service*, **69**, 80–4.

Stevens, D.L. *et al.* (1990). Spontaneous, nontraumatic gangrene due to *Clostridium septicum*. *Reviews of Infectious Diseases*, **12**, 28–96.

Chapter 16.59

Tuberculosis

P. D. O. Davies, D. J. Girling, and J. M. Grange

The causative organism

Tuberculosis is a chronic granulomatous disease of humans and other mammals caused by a group of closely related obligate pathogens, the *Mycobacterium tuberculosis* complex, comprising *M. tuberculosis*—the human tubercle bacillus, *M. bovis*—the bovine tubercle bacillus, *M. africanum*—a heterogeneous type found principally in equatorial Africa with properties intermediate between the former two species, and *M. microti*—a rare cause of disease in voles and other small mammals but attenuated for humans. The vaccine strain, Bacille Calmette–Guérin (BCG), though derived from a strain of *M. bovis*, has distinctive properties.

Humans are the usual, but not unique, host of *M. tuberculosis*. *M. bovis* causes disease in cattle and also in badgers, deer, and other mammals. Humans are incidental hosts, usually acquiring infection by drinking contaminated milk although infection of farm workers may occur by the aerogenous route. Humans may transmit *M. bovis* to cattle but human-to-human transmission is rarely reported.

Morphology and staining

Tubercle bacilli are slightly curved rods, about 4 μm long and 0.5 μm in diameter. In clinical specimens they often occur in small clumps and in early cultures they usually appear as rope-like microcolonies termed 'serpentine cords'. Mycobacteria are Gram positive, although they are not easily stained by this method, and they are resistant to decolorization by mineral acids after staining with arylmethane dyes, hence the term 'acid-fast bacilli'.

Virulence

Determinants of virulence in the *M. tuberculosis* complex have proved elusive. Virulence is almost certainly multifactorial. Mycobacteria can resist innate, non-specific defence mechanisms and induce inappropriate immune reactions.

Immunology and pathology

Immune responses in tuberculosis are either protective, leading to resolution, or tissue-destroying, leading to the pathological characteristics of active disease. Both responses are cell mediated and the actual type is determined by the balance between the two maturation types of T cells: Thl and Th2. A Thl response leads to protective immunity whereas a Th2, or mixed Thl/Th2, response mediates tissue-necrotizing hypersensitivity.

There are two components of protective immunity—activation of macrophages by cytokines from Thl helper T cells and the generation of cytotoxic cells that destroy immunologically effete cells that are laden with tubercle bacilli. Activated macrophages aggregated to form the granuloma (Fig. 1), which has an anoxic and acidic centre, leading to tissue necrosis which, from its cheese-like appearance, is termed caseation. The environment within this necrotic caseous material does not favour mycobacterial growth or survival. Most of the bacteria therefore die, the lesions become quiescent and are sealed off by fibrous scar tissue. A few bacilli may, however, survive in a dormant form and cause reactivation of tuberculosis months or years later.

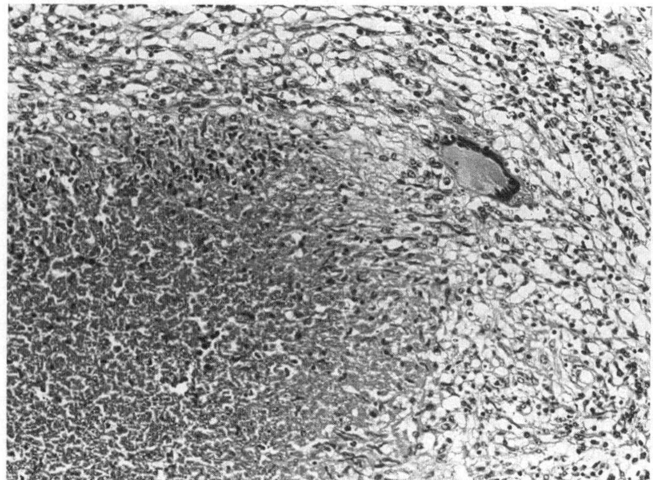

Fig. 1 A granuloma of tuberculosis, showing a central area of caseation, epithelioid cells, lymphocytes, and multinucleate giant cells *(by courtesy of Dr William Taylor).*

The initial lesion of tuberculosis occurs at the site of implantation of the bacillus, usually the lung but occasionally the skin or alimentary tract, including the tonsil. Implanted bacilli are ingested by phagocytic cells, some of which remain at the site of implantation while others migrate to the draining lymph nodes where secondary lesions develop, causing enlargement of the affected nodes. In the lung, the initial lesion is termed a Ghon focus and this, together with the hilar lymphadenopathy, forms the primary complex. Further dissemination leads to non-pulmonary manifestations of primary disease, notably meningeal, bone, and renal tuberculosis.

Delayed hypersensitivity

Three to eight weeks after the primary infection, delayed hypersensitivity develops. Injected mycobacterial antigen, usually purified protein derivative of tuberculin (PPD), leads to oedema and induration of the overlying skin.

A positive tuberculin test indicates previous exposure to mycobacterial antigens, either infection with a tubercle bacillus or BCG vaccination. Exposure to environmental mycobacteria may, in some instances, lead to cross-reactivity. Tuberculin reactivity does not correlate with protective immunity.

Postprimary tuberculosis

Postprimary tuberculosis follows endogenous reactivation of quiescent primary infection or exogenous reinfection. It usually involves the upper lobes of the lung. In contrast to primary disease, extensive caseous necrosis occurs in the lesions which may develop into large tumour-like masses termed tuberculomas (Fig. 2). This is, at least in part, due to the release of tumour necrosis factor (TNF-α) from activated macrophages. Factors derived from, or induced by, the Th2-mediated responses render cells within the lesion exquisitely sensitive to killing by TNF-α and thereby facilitate the extensive tissue necrosis.

Being anoxic and acidic, the tuberculoma contains few acid-fast bacilli. Proteases derived from macrophages liquefy the caseous material so that if the lesion erodes into a bronchus, this is discharged and a cavity is formed. Oxygen and carbon dioxide enter the cavity, facilitating replication of the bacilli so that enormous numbers are

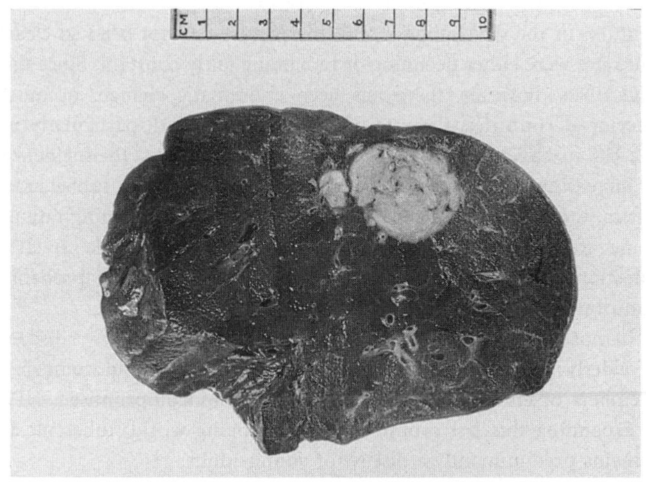

Fig. 2 A tuberculoma in the excised right upper pulmonary lobe of a 34-year-old woman.

found in the cavity wall. Bacilli enter the sputum and the patient is said to have open or infectious tuberculosis.

The lymphatic and haematogenous dissemination characteristic of primary tuberculosis is uncommon in postprimary disease. Instead, bacilli spread directly via the air passages from cavities to other parts of the lungs and to the larynx. Bacilli in swallowed sputum may cause indurating lesions in the alimentary tract.

Tuberculosis and immunosuppression

A degree of non-specific immunosuppression is found in active tuberculosis but it is rectified by effective antituberculosis therapy. The tuberculin test may be negative in advanced tuberculosis: in early studies this led to the false assumption that tuberculin reactivity was a correlate of protective immunity.

Patients with congenital or acquired immunosuppression are particularly prone to tuberculosis. World-wide, the most important immunosuppressive disorder leading to tuberculosis is HIV infection. As cavity formation is the result of an active immune response, many immunosuppressed patients do not have cavities but develop spreading lesions of rather indeterminate radiological appearance. Non-pulmonary lesions and disseminated disease are frequently encountered.

Infection by HIV enhances the reactivation rate of tuberculosis in the infected (tuberculin-positive) person: about 10 per cent per year. Although HIV-related tuberculosis usually responds to standard antituberculosis therapy, TNF-α and other immunological mediators generated by the immune response to tuberculosis trigger the replication of the HIV. Thus, active tuberculosis, even if effectively treated, may result in an earlier onset of AIDS. Accordingly, preventive antituberculosis therapy of dually infected persons is indicated whenever possible.

Clinical bacteriology

The bacteriology laboratory plays a key role in the diagnosis of tuberculosis and management of chemotherapy. Although sensitive and specific, conventional cultivation on egg-based media (e.g. Löwenstein Jensen) requires 3–6 weeks before growth is visible. Radiometric techniques reduce this time to less than 2 weeks and nucleic acid-based methods, some of which are commercially available, hold promise for even more rapid results.

Collection of specimens

The collection of adequate specimens is essential. Specimen containers must be sterilized to avoid 'pseudoepidemics' of mycobacterial disease due to environmental mycobacteria. For diagnosis of pulmonary tuberculosis, the usual specimen is sputum, 2–5 ml of which should be collected into wide-mouthed, screw-capped glass or plastic pots, and placed in plastic bags for transport to the laboratory. At least three sputum samples, preferably early morning samples, should be collected.

When sputum is not produced, induction of sputum, laryngeal swabbing, gastric aspiration (to harvest bacilli swallowed overnight), and fibreoptic bronchoscopy may be used.

Specimens for diagnosis of non-pulmonary tuberculosis include urine (three early morning specimens), pleural, peritoneal, and pericardial fluids (collected into bottles containing citrate to prevent clotting or added directly to double-strength liquid culture medium) and biopsies of lymph nodes and pleural, peritoneal, and pericardial membranes.

Microscopical examination

Microscopical detection of acid-fast bacilli is simple and rapid, but relatively insensitive. Bacilli are only seen in about half the patients with active pulmonary tuberculosis. Sputum must contain at least 5000 bacilli/ml for them to be detectable by microscopy. There is a close correlation between sputum smear positivity and the infectiousness of the patients. Individual species cannot be identified by microscopy and laboratory reports merely state that acid-fast bacilli have been seen.

Culture

Cultural techniques are more sensitive than microscopy and facilitate identification and drug susceptibility tests but they are time-consuming and costly and require a high standard of technical competence. Specimens must be treated to destroy any fungi or other bacteria that might overgrow the more slowly growing mycobacteria; a process termed decontamination.

Acid-fast isolates are examined to determine whether they are members of the *M. tuberculosis* complex or environmental mycobacteria. Identification to species level, usually undertaken by reference laboratories, is based on cultural and biochemical characteristics. Nucleic acid-based methods are increasingly used.

Drug susceptibility tests

There is no absolute definition of drug resistance. Cultures of 'susceptible' tubercle bacilli contain bacteria with a range of drug susceptibilities. Tests are thus designed to determine whether a patient infected with a given strain is likely to respond to treatment with a drug at its usual therapeutic concentration. This usually involves observation of growth on solid media containing various concentrations of drugs. In the UK, the result is expressed as the ratio of the concentration of the drug that inhibits growth of the test strain to that inhibiting growth of a set of control strains. The test requires several weeks incubation on conventional media but radiometric tests require less time. Methods for the rapid detection of mutations conferring resistance to rifampicin are available in some reference centres.

Susceptibility tests require careful standardization and quality control and should only be undertaken if consistently reliable results can be guaranteed. Even in good centres, errors occur and results should always be interpreted in the light of clinical information.

Drug resistance and its clinical significance

Clinically, drug resistance is divisible into 'initial' and 'acquired'. The former is seen in patients who claim that they have never received antituberculosis chemotherapy. The latter occurs during the course of chemotherapy and is due to the selection of drug-resistant mutants.

The commonest form of initial resistance is to isoniazid, the incidence of which varies greatly from country to country. Initial resistance to rifampicin, pyrazinamide, and ethambutol is uncommon but a high incidence of rifampicin resistance occurs in certain regions. Standard chemotherapy is usually successful in patients with resistance to a single drug and a change of regimen should only be considered if the patient is not responding to treatment. The most important reason for treatment failure is poor compliance of the patient with the therapy, in which case relapses are usually due to drug-susceptible organisms. Multidrug resistance (that is resistance to rifampicin and isoniazid and, sometimes, other drugs) is much more serious and requires the use of alternative drug combinations selected on the basis of susceptibility tests.

Emergence of drug resistance may occur if the patient has been prescribed an inadequate regimen or fails to take all the drugs regularly, thereby allowing the number of viable resistant mutants to rise while that of the susceptible organisms falls. The regimen must be changed if acquired resistance emerges and drug susceptibility testing enables suitable retreatment regimens to be selected. Single drugs should never be added blindly to a failing regimen.

Molecular techniques

Molecular biology is providing new approaches to the diagnosis and epidemiology of tuberculosis and holds promise for rapid drug susceptibility testing. Amplification of DNA specific for *M. tuberculosis* by the polymerase chain reaction (PCR) enables a diagnosis to be made within a few hours of receipt of the specimen. Use of the standard PCR technique has met with problems of sensitivity, specificity, and cross-contamination, but closed, simpler, isothermal systems based on amplification of ribosomal RNA represent a major advance. Nucleic acid probes are increasingly used to identify mycobacteria obtained by standard and radiometric culture methods.

Detection of resistance-determining mutants in genes coding for the targets of antimicrobial drugs provides a rapid means of determining such resistance. Methods for detection of such mutants in the *RpoB* gene determining rifampicin resistance have been described.

Restriction fragment length polymorphism analysis (RFLP; 'DNA fingerprinting') enables the *M. tuberculosis* complex to be divided into a large number of relatively stable types that facilitate epidemiological studies. The standard method utilizes the insertion sequence IS6110, of which from one to over 20 copies are present in almost all strains within this complex. Other typing techniques, including those applicable to PCR products, are also available.

Epidemiology

The global pattern of tuberculosis was radically transformed during the 1980s. Up until about 1985, global patterns of tuberculosis had been steady and almost predictable. In the industrialized world, where reliable records are available, case rates had declined progressively, except during the war years, from the first half of the nineteenth century. In the developing world, the picture has not been so clear, but rates were either declining or remaining fairly constant. Since the mid-1980s, however, there has been a dramatic change. In most developed countries, the rate of decline slowed and, particularly in the US, in Great Britain, and in some other countries, the incidence is increasing. In the developing world, particularly in subSaharan Africa, the number of cases has begun to rise, at an alarming rate in some areas. This change seems to be largely attributable to HIV infection, though migration and social deprivation have probably contributed.

In most developed countries, tuberculosis is predominantly a disease of elderly people, recent immigrants from Third World countries, members of ethnic minorities, and the immunocompromised. HIV is expanding this last group. In the developing world, tuberculosis remains predominantly a disease of young adults.

The relation between disease and infection

An estimated one-third of the world's population is infected with the tubercle bacillus. Every year approximately 8 million cases of tuberculosis arise from this infected pool and 3 million die. Those with disease infect approximately 100 million each year. Once infected, the likelihood of developing tuberculosis is 10 per cent in a lifetime.

The impact of HIV on disease

In an individual infected with *M. tuberculosis*, HIV increases substantially the risk and shortens the time of developing disease. Those with dual infection have an estimated 10 per cent risk of developing active tuberculosis each year, and those with HIV infection alone are at a greatly increased risk of contracting tuberculosis. In 1994, the World Health Organization estimated that there were 30 million HIV-positive people world-wide, of whom 10 million were also infected with *M. tuberculosis*: 78 per cent of those with double infection live in sub-Saharan Africa.

Methods of assessing the impact of tuberculosis in a population

Epidemiological studies are used to monitor both infection by the tubercle bacillus and overt tuberculosis. Infection is a state in which the tubercle bacillus is present in the body without producing symptoms or detectable evidence of disease. In overt tuberculosis, one or more organs shows evidence of an active pathological process by symptoms, signs, bacteriologically, or radiographically. There are four main epidemiological methods for assessing the impact of infection or disease on a population: mortality, morbidity, prevalence of sputum smear-positive cases, and annual risk of infection.

Mortality

Historically, mortality has been the most reliable method of assessing the impact of tuberculosis in a population, but it has become less accurate since the introduction of effective chemotherapy.

Morbidity notification

Notification by a clinician 'who believes a patient is suffering from tuberculosis' has been compulsory in Great Britain since 1912. Any clinician diagnosing a case of tuberculosis, whether infectious or not, must complete a notification form and send it to the proper officer for the district in which the patient is normally resident. Contact tracing can then be instigated. Notification is the basis for national statistics. Most other developed countries have similar systems but they were stopped during the 1970s in some. Notification, where efficiently applied, indicates the number of new cases over a period of time. If the total population is known, the rate or incidence can be derived.

Prevalence

The point prevalence of tuberculosis is defined as the number of cases in a numerically-defined population at a specified point in time. As tuberculosis is a chronic disease, the prevalence of the disease is higher than the annual incidence of new cases. The prevalence may be determined by conducting a survey of an indicator of active tuberculosis, such as sputum smear positivity or characteristic radiological abnormalities. Prevalence surveys are of the greatest value in developing countries where notification schemes may be difficult to set up and operate efficiently. Estimates of changes in the prevalence of tuberculosis can be made by surveys of a random sample of a population at two points in time.

Annual risk of infection

The tuberculin test is the standard method for detecting infected people. It aids tuberculosis control programmes by allowing those infected by a source case to be traced.

The annual risk of infection is calculated by skin testing members of an appropriate age group, such as schoolchildren or military recruits, over several years. The annual risk of infection gives an indirect measurement of the number of open or infectious cases of tuberculosis in the community and provides one of the best means of estimating the efficacy of tuberculosis control measures.

Tuberculin testing

The two principal methods for tuberculin testing are the Mantoux and Heaf tests.

Mantoux test

In the Mantoux test, 0.1 ml of solution containing a known number of international units (IU) of purified protein derivative (PPD) of tuberculin is injected intradermally. The diameter of the induration is read 48–72 h later. In the UK, a test using 10 IU is normally used. In other countries, 2 or 5 IU is usually used for standard Mantoux testing.

Heaf test

The Heaf test is made on the volar surface of the forearm using a spring-loaded, six-needled gun, which introduces a drop of undiluted PPD (100 00 IU/ml) into the dermis. The reaction is read 3–10 days later:

- Grade I: four or more discrete papules;
- Grade II: confluent papules forming a ring;
- Grade III: a disc of induration;
- Grade IV: a disc of induration greater than 10 mm in diameter or vesiculation of the disc.

Interpretation of the tuberculin test

Approximate equivalence of the Heaf test to 10 IU PPD by the Mantoux test is shown in Table 1. BCG will convert 80 per cent of individuals to grade I or II. Those with grade III or IV should still be regarded as having infection by *M. tuberculosis* but 10 per cent of reactions in these categories may be attributable to BCG.

The cut-off point for a positive test (i.e. indicating infection with *M. tuberculosis*) may vary from country to country as tuberculin reactions are affected by exposure to environmental mycobacteria. A grade III or IV Heaf test probably denotes infection and should be followed up. Grade II reactions require follow-up only if they come from a high-risk group (see below).

Table 1 Equivalence of Heaf test to Mantoux (10 TU PPD)

Heaf grade	Mantoux (mm induration)
0	0–4
I	5–9
II	10–14
III	15–19
IV	20+

Table 2 Method and action in tuberculosis control

Method	Action
Case finding: Passive: patient presents to clinic Active: survey high-risk groups	Treatment of patient with disease
Detection of infected individuals at risk of developing disease	Chemoprophylaxis
Prevention of established infection in individuals not yet infected	BCG or chemoprophylaxis

Tuberculosis control

Successful control of tuberculosis demands correct assessment of disease, infection and risk of infection, and appropriate action. The principal methods and actions are as shown in Table 2.

Case finding (active)

Contacts

Close contacts of patients with smear-positive tuberculosis should be screened, particularly those in the same household, as about 10 per cent will develop the disease. Screening of casual contacts of sputum smear-positive cases will yield less than 1 per cent of further cases. Contacts of adults with smear-negative or extrapulmonary disease need not be screened but close contacts of children with primary tuberculosis (pulmonary, pleural, meningeal, or erythema nodosum) should be screened, as infection is likely to be recent, and a source case should be identified and treated to prevent further spread of disease to the community.

Immigrants

Recent immigrants from countries with an annual incidence of tuberculosis of 40 or more per 100 000 should be screened. In the absence of radiological evidence of tuberculosis, a tuberculin test should be made. If this is strongly positive, preventive chemotherapy should be recommended for children and young adults (up to 35 years of age). If it is negative, BCG vaccination is recommended.

HIV positivity

At least 30 per cent of those with concurrent HIV and *M. tuberculosis* infections will develop overt tuberculosis. Preventive chemotherapy is recommended where it can be properly supervised.

Health workers

Health and hospital workers vary in their risk of contracting and disseminating tuberculosis. Staff caring for patients with tuberculosis should have a history or scar evidence of previous BCG. If not a tuberculosis test should be carried out and those who are tuberculin negative given BCG. Routine chest radiography during employment is not recommended.

Chemoprophylaxis

There are two types: primary prophylaxis is given to uninfected people at high risk of infection (e.g. small children in close household contact with a smear-positive patient); and secondary prophylaxis, more properly termed preventive therapy, is given to healthy but infected people to prevent overt tuberculosis. The usual regimens are isoniazid alone for 6–12 months or isoniazid with rifampicin for 3 months. Preventive therapy (secondary prophylaxis) is recommended for the following:

(1) recent tuberculin converters (i.e. those recently infected);

(2) tuberculin-positive children under the age of 5 years;

(3) strongly positive reactors (Heaf grade III or IV) in high-risk groups such as immigrants from countries with a high prevalence of tuberculosis;

(4) children found to have strong tuberculin reactions (grade III or IV) on routine school testing, even though the risk of disease is low;

(5) patients with evidence of old, healed tuberculosis who are about to be treated with corticosteroids or other immunosuppressive agents;

(6) HIV-positive people with positive tuberculin reactions;

(7) close contacts of smear-positive cases with a Heaf grade III or IV reaction and who are under 16 years, or under 35 if they are in a high-risk group. Prophylaxis is indicated for some close contacts who are grade II, and have not had previous BCG (Fig. 3).

BCG vaccination

The efficacy of BCG vaccination shows wide geographical variation, as revealed by a number of major BCG trials. In Great Britain, the protective efficacy, irrespective of the incidence of the disease, is about 75 per cent when given to children aged 13 years.

Vaccination policies vary considerably from country to country. In Great Britain, the national policy is still that schoolchildren should be vaccinated routinely at the age of 11–13 years. Vaccination should also be offered to infants born into communities where the risk of infection is high (e.g. immigrants from the Indian subcontinent). Those exposed to occupational risk (e.g. health workers), those about to travel to high-incidence countries, and tuberculin-negative contacts of smear-positive patients should also be vaccinated (Fig. 3).

Mass BCG vaccination of neonates may be valuable. There is evidence that vaccination at a very early age is beneficial even in those countries where later vaccination seems to confer little or no protection.

Technique

Only those negative on tuberculin testing (under 10 mm of induration to 10 IU by the Mantoux or grade 0 or I by the Heaf method) should be vaccinated; 0.1 ml (0.05 ml for neonates) of freeze-dried vaccine

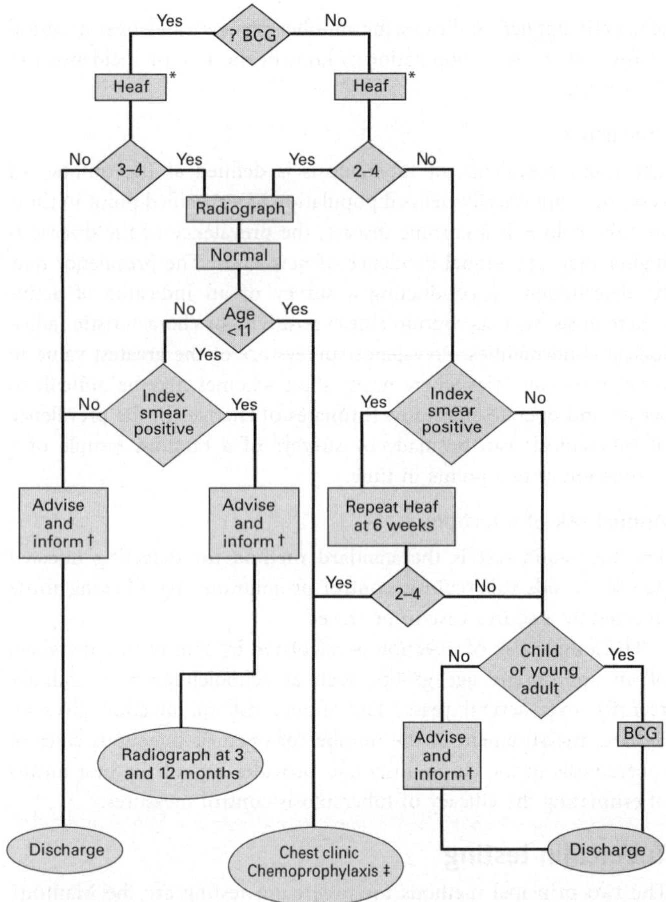

* Negative test result in immunosuppressed does not exclude tuberculous infection.
† Advise patient of tuberculosis symptoms, inform GP of contact.
‡ Persons eligible for but not given chemoprophylaxis should have a chest radiograph at 3 and 12 monthss

Fig. 3 Examination of close contacts of tuberculosis. *Note*: children under 2 years who are close contacts of an adult index patient with positive sputum smears should be given chemoprophylaxis irrespective of tuberculin status, plus BCG later if applicable.
(Reproduced from Thorax, with permission.).

suspended in a dilutent is injected intradermally over the lower insertion of the deltoid in the left arm.

Adverse reactions are rare and are usually caused by faulty technique. They include local abscess formation with, occasionally, enlargement or suppuration of the regional lymph nodes. Generalized infection is extremely rare and usually occurs only in the immunosuppressed. Isoniazid or erythromycin may hasten recovery.

BCG vaccination and HIV infection

The World Health Organization recommends that, in high-prevalence countries, children with clinical signs of AIDS should not be given BCG vaccine but asymptomatic HIV-positive children should be vaccinated. In low-prevalence countries, BCG is not recommended for children born to HIV-positive mothers unless, after the age of 12–15 months (when maternal antibodies have been eliminated) they are found to be HIV-negative. HIV-positive adults should not be given BCG but may be given primary chemoprophylaxis if they are at high risk of infection.

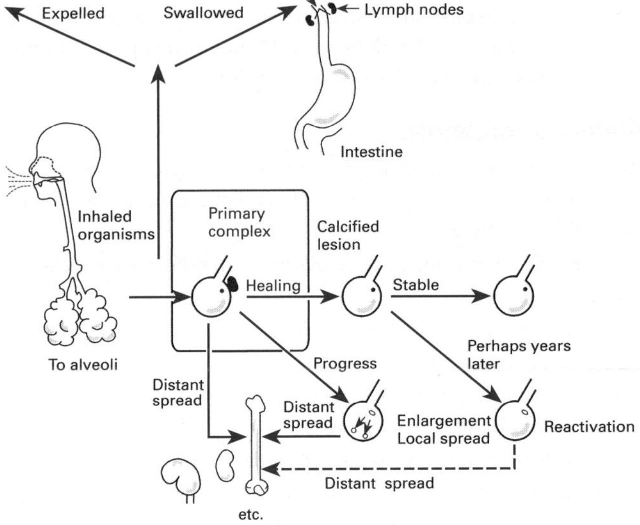

Fig. 4 Diagrammatic representation of the ways in which tuberculosis may spread through the body.

The clinical course of tuberculosis

Tuberculosis is spread principally by inhalation of expectorated droplet nuclei containing bacilli. Rarely, infection is acquired by drinking milk containing *M. bovis* or by traumatic inoculation into the skin. Only a small proportion of those infected develop overt tuberculosis. Determinants of the outcome of primary infection are poorly understood but probably include various non-specific immune defence mechanisms, the size of the infecting dose, priming of the specific immune defences by contact with environmental mycobacteria, and the patient's general state of health and nutrition.

The initial infection may resolve completely or may merely be contained, with progression to postprimary disease in the future (Fig. 4).

Primary tuberculosis

The initial lesions of tuberculosis develop before specific cell-mediated immune reactions contain the infection. Dissemination to the regional lymph nodes causes the primary complex and there is further haematogenous spread to all parts of the body. Necrosis is inconspicuous or absent and, except in rare cases of progressive primary disease, pulmonary cavitation is not seen.

Asymptomatic cases may be found on routine examination. In other cases the symptoms include cough, sometimes with haemoptysis, fever, decreased appetite, and, in children, failure to thrive. Signs include wheezes due to bronchial compression by enlarged lymph nodes and those of pneumonia secondary to lobar collapse.

Immediate complications include bronchopneumonia, pleural effusion, and disseminated (miliary) disease. Intermediate complications include the various non-pulmonary forms of primary disease and late complications include bronchiectasis and postprimary tuberculosis.

Diagnosis

A peripheral lesion with enlarged hilar lymph nodes on chest radiography in a child is virtually diagnostic of a primary complex. Tuberculin conversion usually occurs 3–8 weeks from the time of infection. Bacteriological confirmation is unusual because sputum is difficult to obtain in children, but material obtained by gastric washing, laryngeal swabs, or bronchoscopy may yield the diagnosis.

Allergic manifestations

The two main types are erythema nodosum and phlyctenular conjunctivitis.

Treatment and outcome

Standard chemotherapy is used. Most primary infections pass unnoticed and may be detected only by tuberculin conversion or if a subsequent radiological examination reveals a calcified focus. Nonpulmonary disease, such as tuberculous meningitis or miliary tuberculosis, may result from haematogenous dissemination.

Postprimary tuberculosis

The course of postprimary tuberculosis is very variable. In the prechemotherapeutic era, about one-third of patients died, one-third apparently achieved a spontaneous cure, and one-third developed chronic disease with gradual healing by fibrosis over many years.

Presentation

Postprimary tuberculosis can range clinically from absence of symptoms to extreme prostration. Patients may be slightly unwell for several months before seeking medical attention, during which time extensive disease may develop. Most cases are pulmonary (about 85 per cent of cases among white patients in Great Britain) but involvement of non-respiratory sites is common in immigrants and in the immunocompromised.

Some symptom-free patients are detected on routine screening; others present with malaise, weight loss, fever, night sweats, and anorexia. Those with pulmonary disease may present with cough (worse in the morning and sometimes with haemoptysis), chest pain, breathlessness, and signs of pneumonia. On examination, the lung signs are variable and usually less evident than the radiological signs would suggest. They include crackles, diminished breath sounds, and bronchial breathing. Patients with chronic disease may have tracheal deviation and coarse crackles over the area of disease due to fibrosis.

Diagnosis

Occasionally, diagnosis may prove very difficult and is made retrospectively after a successful trial of chemotherapy. The most important diagnostic tools are bacteriological and radiological examinations but some cases are diagnosed by histological appearances and tuberculin reactivity.

Sputum (and other specimens) for bacteriological examination should be obtained as outlined above. Microscopical demonstration of acid-fast bacilli in sputum smears provides a rapid presumptive diagnosis, although the technique is not very sensitive and fails to distinguish between tubercle bacilli and environmental mycobacteria. The more sensitive cultural methods, including rapid radiometric ones, prove the diagnosis. The polymerase chain reaction may give rapid diagnosis.

Radiological changes, though sensitive, are rather non-specific. Tuberculosis may cause virtually any radiological abnormality and atypical pictures are frequent, especially in HIV-positive and other immunocompromised persons. Thus bacteriological confirmation should always be sought. The following radiological features are characteristic of postprimary pulmonary tuberculosis:

(1) soft, floccular, unilateral or bilateral, nodular shadowing in the upper lobes, particularly in the posterior and apical segments (Fig. 5);

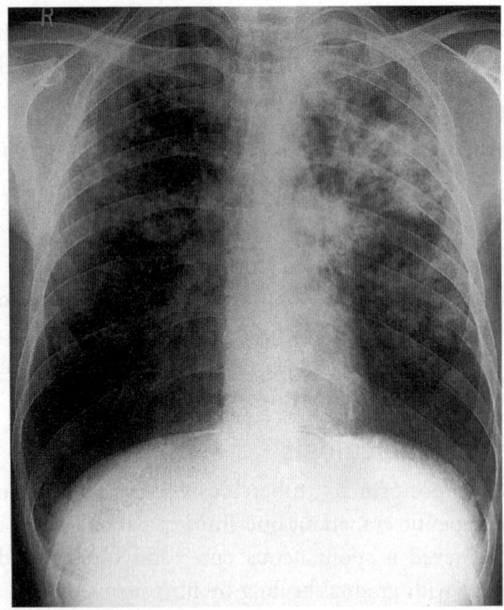

Fig. 5 Anteroposterior chest radiograph of a 43-year-old man showing extensive bilateral tuberculosis.

(2) cavitation, usually in the upper posterior parts of the lung;
(3) calcification due to old, healed disease;
(4) linear shadowing indicative of fibrosis in the upper zones;
(5) a combination of (3) and (4) and soft shadowing—this is highly suggestive of reactivation of old, healed, postprimary disease;
(6) small (<1 cm diameter) nodules throughout the lung fields, indicative of miliary disease;
(7) pleural effusion or mediastinal enlargement;
(8) extensive patchy shadowing throughout the lung fields indicative of widespread tuberculous bronchopneumonia.

Granulomas, with caseation and giant cells, in lung biopsies obtained by fibreoptic bronchoscopy or in non-pulmonary lesions, are virtually diagnostic of tuberculosis. If caseation is not present, the differential diagnosis includes sarcoidosis, lymphomas, and foreign-body granulomas.

A strongly positive Mantoux test (>15 mm induration to 10 IU PPD) in a patient with other evidence of active tuberculosis strongly supports the diagnosis. Strong reactions may, however, occur in healthy people with repeated occupational exposure to infectious tuberculosis patients and in those with old, healed disease.

The results of other laboratory tests are not specific. There is no reliable serological test.

Complications

Postprimary pulmonary tuberculosis may present with a complication due to the direct spread of bacilli or with an indirect complication. Direct complications include:

(1) pleural effusion—diagnosis may be made by biopsy;
(2) empyema—surgical drainage may be required towards the end of a course of chemotherapy;
(3) laryngeal disease: leading to pain and dysphonia;
(4) more distant spread of disease.

Indirect complications include:

(1) airflow obstruction due to a swelling of bronchial lymphatics;
(2) aspergilloma due to the colonization of old cavities resulting in a ball of fungal hyphae;
(3) haemoptysis, which may occur during active disease or many years later due to a breakdown of fibrous scarring or invasion by an aspergilloma and which may be fatal.

Differential diagnosis

Tuberculosis has been called the great mimic as its signs and symptoms are extremely variable. It must be differentiated from a wide range of other diseases including:

(1) carcinoma of the lung, particularly in middle-aged or elderly smokers;
(2) pneumonia—unresolved pneumonia, especially if due to staphylococci or *Klebsiella* spp.;
(3) allergic bronchopulmonary aspergillosis—this is confirmed by tests for antibody to *Aspergillus*;
(4) fibrotic lung disease due to sarcoidosis, extrinsic allergic alveolitis, pneumoconiosis, and silicosis—silicosis predisposes to tuberculosis so the two diseases may coexist;
(5) the chronic malaise and cachexia of tuberculosis resembles that due to anorexia nervosa, diabetes mellitus, and hyperthyroidism;
(6) tuberculosis may present as pyrexia of unknown origin—other causes, particularly malignancies, must be considered;
(7) lymphoma—biopsies should be obtained whenever possible.

Outcome

The overall mortality for all forms of tuberculosis in Great Britain is about 8 per cent, varying from under 1 per cent for children and young adults to over 30 per cent in those aged 75 years or more. Mortality is higher for patients with extensive disease, smear positivity, and cavitation. Mortality appears to be the same in both sexes, even though males are twice as likely to develop pulmonary disease. Most deaths occur early in treatment. Even when chemotherapy is successful, long-term sequelae due to scarring may occur.

Tuberculosis in the HIV-positive patient

HIV testing should be considered in all cases of tuberculosis. HIV considerably accelerates the progression of infection to overt disease by reducing the host's cell-mediated immunity. In Africa and Asia, tuberculosis is common in HIV-infected people and is often the earliest sign of immunosuppression. Non-respiratory disease, particularly lymph-node disease, is much more common in the HIV-infected host. Pulmonary disease is less likely to be cavitating and smear-positive and so more difficult to diagnose. Chemotherapy is usually effective but relapse, perhaps due to a subsequent infection, is more common than in HIV-negative patients.

Multidrug-resistant tuberculosis

There have been a number of reports of outbreaks of multidrug-resistant tuberculosis. This is defined as resistance to isoniazid and rifampicin only, or in combination with resistance to other drugs. These differ from previously described outbreaks in that they have spread rapidly, involved larger numbers of patients, and occurred in institutions.

Multidrug-resistance is associated with a history of previous treatment, HIV-seropositivity, homelessness, and drug abuse. Patients who are homeless and/or drug abusers are more likely to have been in contact with source cases who may have been poorly compliant with therapy, thus increasing the chance that they will develop secondary resistance and infect others with drug-resistant strains.

The emergence of multidrug resistance has brought with it enormous ethical and administrative problems. These include the social consequences of isolating and treating patients against their wishes, the cost of therapy with alternative drugs, amounting to US $200 000 or more per patient in order to achieve a 50 per cent cure rate, and the problem of long-term isolation of those who do not respond to such therapy. Surgical procedures may be required as an adjunct to chemotherapy.

Identification of the bacterial gene causing rifampicin resistance provides a quick way of showing drug resistance.

Non-respiratory tuberculosis

A substantial minority of cases of tuberculosis, particularly in immigrants, ethnic minorities, and immunocompromised patients, occur at sites other than the lung.

Lymph node tuberculosis

Cervical nodes are the most frequently involved extrathoracic lymph nodes. In countries with a high prevalence of tuberculosis, children and young adults are most frequently affected whereas in low-prevalence countries the disease is more common in older adults, particularly women.

Lymph node swelling is usually slow and insidious. A single node or a number in a particular chain may be affected. They feel rubbery or hard and may be tender. They may suppurate to form abscesses and sinuses that result in a chronic discharge of pus. Spread of disease from the sinuses may cause chronic skin tuberculosis (scrofuloderma). One- to two-thirds of patients have fever, night sweats, weight loss, and malaise.

Histological and microscopical confirmation of the diagnosis should be attempted. Surgical intervention may lead to chronically discharging sinuses, which may take months to heal.

Standard chemotherapy is effective. The nodes may enlarge during or after chemotherapy, perhaps as a result of hypersensitivity reactions. Corticosteroids are often used to reduce such enlargement but are of unproven efficacy. Surgery may, on rare occasions, be required for cosmetic reasons.

Lymphadenitis in children and, to an increasing extent, young adults may be caused by environmental mycobacteria (see Chapter 16.60).

The differential diagnosis includes sarcoidosis, lymphoma, and carcinoma.

Genitourinary tuberculosis

Urinary tract disease

Clinical features include frequency and dysuria, ureteric colic, loin pain, backache, loin swelling due to a cold abscess, and symptoms of renal failure. Constitutional symptoms are uncommon unless other organs are affected.

Tuberculosis should be suspected in the presence of 'sterile' pyuria. At least three early-morning urine specimens should be taken for culture, as environmental mycobacteria often contaminate the genital tract. Acid-fast bacilli are rarely seen on direct smear.

It is important to assess renal function and to watch for the development of anatomical abnormalities during and after treatment.

Standard chemotherapy is used. Drugs excreted unchanged by the kidney, such as streptomycin and ethambutol, should be avoided when there is renal impairment. Ureteric obstruction may be avoided by giving corticosteroids at a dose of 20–40 mg daily for the initial 3 months of chemotherapy. Surgical intervention may be required for ureteric obstruction.

Genital tuberculosis

In males the epididymis is the most common site of genital tuberculosis, causing scrotal pain and swelling. Nodularity of the epididymis, vas deferens, and seminal vesicles may be felt. Sinus formation with skin involvement may occur.

In the female the fallopian tubes and endometrium are the usual sites of disease. Pain, menstrual disorder, dyspareunia, and vaginal discharge may occur. Infertility is usual. Diagnosis may be made by histological or bacteriological examination of appropriate biopsies and endometrial curettings.

Bone and joint disease

The spine is involved in about half the cases. The knee, hip, ankle, wrist, and elbow are involved in decreasing frequency, but any bony site may be affected and involvement of multiple sites is frequent. Infection of long bones tends to begin at the ends. The lesion may rupture through bone into the soft tissues causing a cold abscess. This is common in spinal disease and a paravertebral abscess may develop. Such abscesses may track along fascial planes in soft tissue and present at distant sites.

Spinal tuberculosis (Pott's disease)

The usual presenting symptom is back pain. A tracking abscess may present as a fluctuant mass on the chest wall or, in the case of a psoas abscess, in the groin. Late cases may present with kyphosis, paraesthesia, or paraplegia. Examination may show local tenderness, muscular spasm, or kyphosis.

Disease usually starts in the anterior aspect of the intervertebral disc and spreads to adjacent vertebrae along the anterior longitudinal ligaments, resulting in erosion of the anterior edges of the superior and inferior vertebral borders. Progressive destruction results in loss of volume of vertebral bodies anteriorly, with loss of height and kyphosis. Lower thoracic and lumbar vertebrae are those most commonly affected.

Lateral radiography and CT scan often show a characteristic appearance (Figs 6 and 7) with loss of volume anteriorly. An attempt to obtain tissue for culture should be made, but a wide excision is required to ensure adequate specimens. The differential diagnosis includes pyogenic infections and malignant metastases; the latter more commonly involve the pedicles and spinal bodies leaving the discs intact.

Treatment is by standard chemotherapy. In the absence of severe deformity and spinal-cord compression, operative procedures afford little benefit, although in skilled hands radical excision and bone grafting ('Hong Kong operation') results in more rapid bony fusion and less residual spinal deformity.

Tuberculous meningitis

See Chapter 13.25.

Abdominal tuberculosis

Tuberculosis of the gastrointestinal tract may be a manifestation of primary tuberculosis caused by consuming milk containing *M. bovis*. More commonly it occurs in patients with postprimary pulmonary tuberculosis who have swallowed infected sputum. Tuberculous peritonitis, however, is rarely associated with pulmonary disease. The usual symptoms are those of subacute intestinal obstruction—recurrent

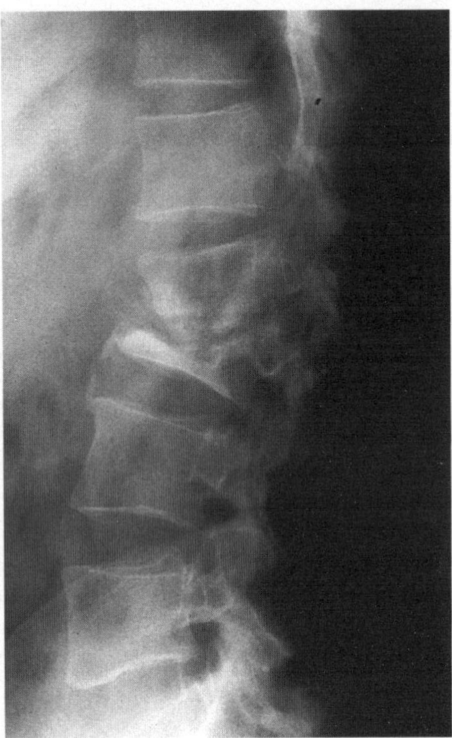

Fig. 6 Lateral radiograph of tuberculosis of the spine (Pott's disease) showing collapse of the L2 and L3 vertebrae and of the intervertebral disc *(by courtesy of Professor Alan Scher, University of Stellenbosch, South Africa).*

abdominal pain and constipation—together with constitutional symptoms and weight loss. A plain abdominal radiograph may show fluid levels. The 'doughy abdomen', said to be characteristic of tuberculous peritonitis, is an uncommon late manifestation.

The diagnosis is made by histological and bacteriological examination of specimens.

Standard chemotherapy is used. The use of corticosteroids to prevent obstructions and adhesions due to scarring remains controversial.

Tuberculous pericarditis

Disease is usually due to the erosion of adjacent infected lymph nodes into the pericardial space. It presents as pericardial effusion, subacute or chronic constrictive pericarditis, or a combination of the two. Subacute constriction is typically associated with the presence of fibrocaseous material within the pericardial space, chronic constriction with fibrosis, and calcification.

The onset of effusion or subacute constriction is usually insidious, with fever, malaise, substernal pain, and dyspnoea on exertion. The signs include sinus tachycardia, arterial pulsus paradoxus, raised jugular venous pressure, hepatomegaly, and ascites, the last three being particularly prominent in the presence of constriction. A pericardial rub may be heard. Effusion, especially if it develops rapidly, may cause tamponade. The electrocardiogram commonly shows non-specific but widespread T-wave abnormalities and low-voltage QRS complexes. On radiography, the heart shadow is enlarged, particularly when an effusion is present.

Chronic constriction may develop weeks to years after the subacute stage, despite therapy. The cardiac silhouette may be normal in size but a ring of pericardial calcification may be seen.

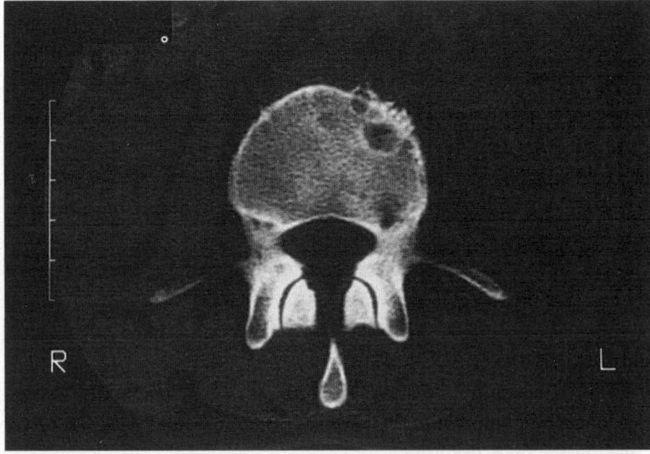

(a)

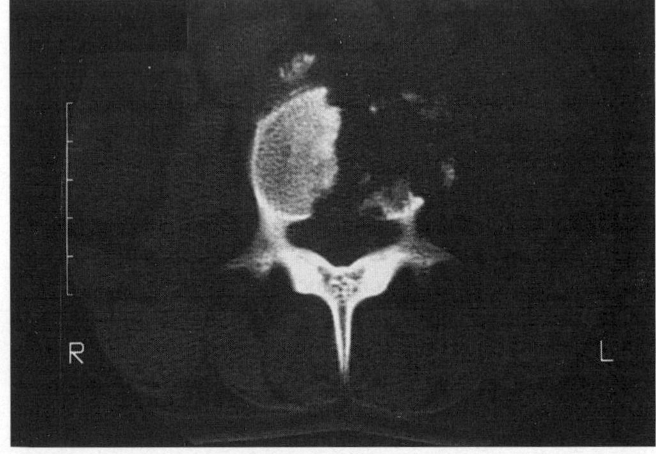

(b)

Fig. 7(a)(b) Two consecutive CT scans of a vertebra taken at an interval of several months showing progressive erosion. Note the body of the vertebra is affected from anterior backwards.

The diagnosis of tuberculous pericarditis may be confirmed by histological examination of a pericardial biopsy. Conventional cultures of pericardial aspirates are positive in about 60 per cent of cases of effusion but the yield may be improved to 75 per cent by direct 'bedside' inoculation of pericardial fluid into double-strength liquid Kirschner medium.

Treatment is with standard antituberculosis chemotherapy. Pericardiectomy may be required for the relief of constriction. The addition to antituberculosis chemotherapy of prednisolone, 60 mg daily then in tapering doses over 11 weeks, has been shown to increase the rate of clinical improvement and reduce the risk of death.

Lupus vulgaris

Lupus vulgaris is a manifestation of tuberculosis of the skin, usually of the head and neck. Jelly-like nodules first appear, which may go on to ulcerate and cause extensive scarring. Standard chemotherapy is usually effective.

Management of the patient with tuberculosis

Most patients with tuberculosis, whether pulmonary or extra-pulmonary, are well enough to be managed as outpatients. Hospital

Table 3 The relative efficacy of antituberculosis drugs in prevention of emergence of resistance, early bacterial activity and sterilizing activity.*

Extent of activity	Prevention of emergence of resistance	Early bacterial activity	Sterilizing activity
High	Isoniazid	Isoniazid	Rifampicin
	Rifampicin		Pyrazinamide
		Ethambutol	
	Ethambutol	Rifampicin	Isoniazid
	Streptomycin		
		Streptomycin	Streptomycin
	Pyrazinamide	Pyrazinamide	Thiacetazone
Low	Thiacetazone	Thiacetazone	Ethambutol

*From Mitchison, D.A.(1985). The action of antituberculosis drugs in short course chemotherapy. *Tubercle*, **66**, 219–25.

admission to obtain specimens such as bronchoalveolar washings to confirm the diagnosis for sputum smear-negative pulmonary tuberculosis may be required.

For the particularly ill patient or the elderly, admission for observation during the first days of treatment may be advisable as adverse reactions to treatment are more common and severe in these groups. Mortality tends to be highest in the few weeks immediately after treatment has started. The strongly smear-positive patient is rendered rapidly non-infectious so that isolation is not necessary beyond 2 weeks of treatment. Segregation may be necessary where HIV-positive patients are being nursed on the same ward. Often bacilli can be detected microscopically in sputum for some months after treatment has begun because dead bacilli may continue to be expectorated. After 2–3 months of treatment, cultures are almost always negative. A full 6 months of treatment is required to prevent relapse.

An intermittent supervised form of chemotherapy, in which the patient attends an outpatient clinic two or three times a week, is now recommended by WHO. This is called Directly Observed Therapy (DOT). If DOT is not employed after treatment has started, initial follow-up should be monthly for two visits. Sputum may be obtained for culture to ensure there is conversion. Follow-up chest radiographs are usually unnecessary. Jaundice, sickness, and cutaneous side-effects usually occur in the first month, forcing the patient to stop therapy, which is why an early appointment is essential.

The antituberculosis drugs

The four key first-line drugs used for previously untreated patients are isoniazid, rifampicin, pyrazinamide, and ethambutol. Streptomycin is a valuable additional drug. Reserve drugs, which may be used when first-line treatment has failed, are ethionamide or prothionamide, kanamycin, capreomycin, viomycin, cycloserine, and quinolones such as ofloxacin and the newer macrolides such as azithromycin.

All strains of *M. tuberculosis* contain drug-resistant mutants; thus active tuberculosis should never be treated with a single drug because of the risk that acquired resistance will emerge (Table 3). The dosages are shown in Table 4.

Isoniazid

Isoniazid (isonicotinic acid hydrazide) is the main drug used in the treatment of all forms of tuberculosis. After a single oral dose, similar peak serum concentrations are seen in all patients, but 4–6 h after administration the serum concentrations differ according to the rate at which individuals metabolize the drug. There is a genetically determined bimodal distribution of slow and rapid acetylators, giving mean serum half-lives of about 3 and 1.4 h, respectively. The half-life may be prolonged in those with grossly impaired hepatic function.

Rifampicin

Rifampicin is an excellent combination drug for isoniazid. Rifampicin induces hepatic microsomal enzymes, and hence reduces the serum half-lives and clinical efficacy of a number of drugs, including corticosteroids, digitoxin, coumarin anticoagulants, oral contraceptives, the antidiabetic sulphonylureas and biguanides, and dapsone, if given concurrently. Patients should be told that it may turn their urine, and occasionally other body fluids, red.

Pyrazinamide

The main metabolite of pyrazinamide, pyrazinoic acid, inhibits the renal tubular secretion of uric acid, causing the serum uric acid concentration to rise.

Ethambutol

Ethambutol is bacteriostatic for *M. tuberculosis* in the dosages that can safely be given, and is used to prevent the emergence of strains resistant to other drugs. It should be avoided in the treatment of patients with impaired renal function as it may accumulate and cause serious ocular toxicity. It should not be given to young children or any patient unable to report early symptoms of ocular toxicity.

Streptomycin

After parenteral administration, the serum half-life of streptomycin, an aminoglycoside, may be greatly prolonged if renal function is impaired. Its half-life is considerably longer in newborn babies and in adults over about 40 years of age than in older children and young adults, thereby increasing the risks of toxicity. The drug should be avoided in patients with conditions affecting the VIIIth cranial nerve because of its ototoxicity, in pregnant women because it crosses the placenta and can damage the fetal VIIIth nerve, in patients with myasthenia because it is a weak neuromuscular blocker, and in those known to be hypersensitive to the drug because of the risk of a severe reaction. Transmission of HIV and other blood-borne pathogens may occur with poor needle sterilization. Replacement of streptomycin with ethambutol is now recommended.

Thiacetazone

Thiacetazone, a thiosemicarbazone, is bacteriostatic for *M. tuberculosis*. Because of adverse reactions in the presence of HIV, it is being phased out of regimens.

p-Aminosalicylic acid (PAS)

PAS (*p*-aminosalicylic acid and its salts) is bacteriostatic for *M. tuberculosis* and is used as a reserve drug when it has not already been used. Because it frequently causes gastrointestinal reactions and is bulky and unpleasant to take, it has now largely been replaced by other drugs.

Ethionamide and prothionamide

The use of ethionamide or prothionamide (propyl ethionamide) is limited by their adverse effects, notably gastrointestinal irritation.

Other aminoglycosides

Kanamycin, capreomycin, and viomycin can be used either as alternatives to the more active streptomycin in patients hypersensitive

Table 4 Dosage of the main antituberculosis drugs

Drug	Daily dosage			Intermittent dosage		
	Adults and children (mg/kg)	Adults Weight	Dose	Adults and children (mg/kg)	Adults Weight	Dose
Isoniazid	5	–	300 mg	15	–	–
Rifampicin	10	<50 kg ≥50 kg	450 mg 600 mg	15	–	600–900 mg
Streptomycin	15–20	<50 kg ≥50 kg	750 mg 1 g	15–20	<50 kg ≥50 kg	750 mg 1 g
Pyrazinamide		<50 kg ≥50 kg	1.5 g 2.0 g	50 3 times/week 75 twice/week	<50 kg ≥50 kg <50 kg –	2.0 g 2.5 g 3.0 g
Ethambutol[1]	25 for 2 months then 15*			30 3 times/week		
Thiacetazone	4 (for children)	–	150 mg			
Rifater		per 10 kg >60 kg	1 tablet 6 tablets			
Ethionamide and prothionamide	15–20 (adults)	<50 kg ≥50 kg	750 mg 1 g			
Cycloserine	15 (adults)	<50 kg ≥50 kg	750 mg 1 g			

[1] It is important to calculate the dose accurately to ensure efficacy and avoid toxicity.

[2] Adults only.

*Most clinicians use 15 mg/kg for the initial 2 months.

to that drug, or as reserve drugs. There is cross-resistance between the three, and between kanamycin, viomycin, and streptomycin.

Cycloserine

Cycloserine has a low level of activity and is only used as a reserve drug. Its use is limited by the mental disturbances it not infrequently causes. It should not be given to patients with a history of epilepsy or psychiatric disturbance.

Ofloxacin/ ciprofloxacin/ sparfloxacin

A number of the quinolone antibiotics have antimycobacterial activity. Ofloxacin, one such drug, is a valuable reserve antituberculosis drug. If possible, it should be avoided in patients with renal failure, and it should not be given to those with known allergy to quinolones.

Other drugs

In vitro tests show some efficacy of the amoxicillin/clavulanic acid combination and also clofazimine. Though used in drug resistant disease, no clinical evidence exists for their efficacy.

Adverse effects of the antituberculosis drugs

Principal adverse reactions are listed in Table 5. The standard recommended combination of isoniazid, rifampicin, and pyrazinamide is usually well tolerated and rarely causes serious toxicity.

Cutaneous and generalized hypersensitivity reactions

Mild cutaneous reactions to an antituberculosis regimen may be self-limiting and require only symptomatic treatment without interrupting or altering the regimen.

Generalized reactions usually occur during the first 1 or 2 months of chemotherapy. They consist of a rash, fever, malaise, vomiting, aching limbs, headache, generalized lymphadenopathy, hepatosplenomegaly, and occasionally jaundice.

The principles of management are:

(1) stop all chemotherapy until the reaction has subsided;

(2) identify the drug or drugs responsible (Table 6);

(3) resume adequate chemotherapy as soon as possible, using at least two drugs to which the patient is not hypersensitive.

Hepatitis

It is unnecessary to test for liver-cell damage routinely during antituberculosis chemotherapy, unless the patient has liver disease. Small, transient, and symptomless increases in serum hepatic enzyme concentrations are usual during the early weeks of treatment, which should not therefore be interrupted or altered because of them. If clinically evident hepatitis occurs, all drugs should be stopped while liver damage is confirmed by appropriate tests. If the hepatitis has been caused by the drug regimen, it usually resolves rapidly. Treatment with the same drugs can often be resumed uneventfully, but tests for liver-cell damage should be made regularly. The aim should be to resume treatment, with either the original or an alternative regimen, as soon as possible.

The risk of drug-induced hepatitis is about 1 per cent, but increases with age. Deaths from presumed drug-induced hepatitis are rare.

Combined drug action

The combination of isoniazid, rifampicin, and pyrazinamide has proved to be highly effective, containing as it does the most powerful

Table 5 Adverse reactions to the antituberculosis drugs

Drug	Reactions: Common	Uncommon	Rare
Isoniazid		Hepatitis Cutaneous hyper-sensitivity Peripheral neuropathy	Giddiness Convulsion Optic neuritis Mental symptoms Haemolytic anaemia Aplastic anaemia Agranulocytosis Lupoid reactions Arthralgia Gynaecomastia
Rifampicin		Hepatitis Cutaneous reactions Gastrointestinal reactions Thrombocyto-penic purpura Febrile reactions 'Flu syndrome'	Shortness of breath Shock Haemolytic anaemia Acute renal failure
Pyrazinamide	Anorexia Nausea Flushing	Hepatitis Vomiting Arthralgia Cutaneous hyper-sensitivity	Sideroblastic anaemia Photosensitization
Ethambutol		Retrobulbar optic neuritis Arthralgia	Hepatitis Cutaneous hypersensitivity Peripheral neuropathy
Streptomycin	Cutaneous hyper-sensitivity Giddiness Numbness Tinnitus	Vertigo Ataxia Deafness	Renal damage Aplastic anaemia Agranulocytosis
Thiacetazone	Gastrointestinal reactions Cutaneous hyper-sensitivity Vertigo Conjunctivitis	Hepatitis Erythema multiforme Exfoliative dermatitis Haemolytic anaemia	Agranulocytosis

Table 6 Challenge doses for detecting cutaneous or generalized hypersensitivity

Drug	Challenge doses: Day 1	Day 2
Isoniazid	50 mg	300 mg
Rifampicin	75 mg	300 mg
Pyrazinamide	250 mg	1.0 g
Ethionamide, prothionamide	125 mg	375 mg
Cycloserine	125 mg	250 mg
Ethambutol	100 mg	500 mg
PAS	1.0 g	5.0 g
Thiacetazone	25 mg	50 mg
Streptomycin or other aminoglycoside	125 mg	500 mg

Challenge doses of the drugs of the regimen should be given in the sequence in which they are shown. The drugs near the bottom of the list are the ones most likely to cause a reaction. If the reaction was a severe one, smaller initial challenge doses should be given (approximately one-tenth the doses shown for day 1).

bactericidal drug, isoniazid, the two uniquely active sterilizing drugs, rifampicin and pyrazinamide, and the two drugs most effective in preventing the emergence of acquired resistance, isoniazid and rifampicin.

Suitability for intermittent use

Isoniazid, rifampicin, pyrazinamide, streptomycin, and ethambutol are all effective when given intermittently in the dosages shown in Table 4. The dose size of intermittent streptomycin cannot be raised above the daily dose size because of the risk of acute toxicity. The effective dose size of rifampicin is similar whether it is given daily or intermittently.

Antituberculosis regimens

Recommended regimen for newly diagnosed patients

The regimen recommended for newly diagnosed patients (Table 7) is a 6-month regimen of isoniazid (H), rifampicin (R), pyrazinamide (Z), and ethambutol (E) given daily for 2 months or 8 weeks (2HRZE), followed by isoniazid and rifampicin for 4 months (4HR); the standard abbreviation for this regimen is 2HRZE/4HR.

Fixed-dose combination preparations of proven drugs and bioavailability should be used when available to aid compliance and to reduce the risk of incorrect dosage. Alternatively, directly observed

Table 7 Regimen of chemotherapy (P659)

Category no.	Patients	Initial phase	Continuation phase
Standard 6-month regimen 2HRZ/4HR When there is a high level of initial resistance add S and/or E to initial phase			
Variants: When fully supervised intermittent chemotherapy can be organized 2 HRZ/$4H_3R_3$ 2 HRZ/$4H_2R_2$ 2 $H_3R_3Z_3E_3/4H_3R_3$ 2 $S_3H_3R_3Z_3/4H_3R_3$			
WHO recommended regimens (where sensitivity results are not available)			
1	New smear +ve or PTB seriously-ill extrapulmonary by: e.g. TB meningitis	2 SHRZ or 2 HRZE	6 HE or 4 HR or 4 H3 R3
2	Smear +ve, relapse treatment failure, return after default	2 SHRZE/I HRZE	5 H3R3E3 or 5 HRE
3	Smear –ve, PTB extra-pulmonary TB	2 HRZ or 2 $H_3R_3Z_3$	6 HE or 2HR/ 4H or 2 H_3R_34H
Alternative best active regimens of longer duration 2 SHRZ/6HT 2 SHRZ/6 S2H2Z2 2 SHR/7HR 2 HRE/7HR 9HR 2SHT/10HT 2SHE/10HE			

therapy (DOT) should be used. WHO and IUATLD now stress the use of DOTS in all circumstances and advocate intermittent regimes if this makes direct observation more practical.

This standard regimen should be used in the treatment of pulmonary and extrapulmonary disease in adults and children. It has the ability (i) to cure patients rapidly, even the majority of those who default after 2 to 3 months of treatment; (ii) to cure the great majority of patients with bacilli initially resistant to isoniazid; and (iii) to prevent therapeutic failure due to the emergence of acquired resistance. There are variants of this regimen that have advantages in some circumstances, as follows.

Intermittent administration

The continuation phase may be given three times or twice a week: 2HRZE/$4H_3R_3$ or 2HRZE/$4H_2R_2$. Every dose of the continuation phase can then be given under the direct observation of outpatient health staff, paramedical staff, or lay people taught to supervise chemotherapy. In this way the level of compliance is known and a high level can be encouraged.

In programmes in which chemotherapy is administered throughout under full supervision to outpatients, the regimen may be given three times a week from the start. When this is done, either ethambutol (E) or streptomycin (S) should be added to the initial phase: $2E_3H_3R_3Z_3$ or $2S_3H_3R_3Z_3/4H_3R_3$.

Populations with a high level of initial drug resistance

When there is a high level of initial drug resistance, or if the patient's strain is suspected to be resistant to isoniazid, a fourth drug, ethambutol or streptomycin, should be added to the initial phase. This regimen is now recommended as standard by WHO, the British Thoracic Society, and other authorities.

WHO drug regimens for poorly resourced countries

Different regimens are recommended by the WHO according to sputum smear and/or relapse status (Table 7).

Category 1—newly diagnosed sputum smear positive pulmonary tuberculosis or serious extrapulmonary tuberculosis, e.g. tuberculous meningitis.

Category 2—relapsed sputum smear, positive pulmonary disease.

Category 3—sputum smear negative, pulmonary disease or extrapulmonary disease (excluding category 1).

Patients whose primary chemotherapy has failed

When there is no response to chemotherapy in a patient who has been fully compliant it is probable that the initial strain was multidrug resistant. When there is bacteriological response at first, followed by bacteriological failure while chemotherapy is still being given, this is probably because acquired drug resistance or additional resistance has emerged. In either case the regimen must be changed but it is first necessary to try to establish whether apparent failure was really due to the patient's failure to take chemotherapy. A detailed drug history should be compiled, including the compliance of the patient in treatment. Susceptibility tests on cultures taken after treatment failure may be helpful, but only if they have been done by a laboratory practising good quality control.

Whenever possible, the patient should be retreated for at least 12 months from the time the sputum smears become negative, using a regimen containing, for the first 3–4 months, at least three drugs to which the organisms are likely to be susceptible; preferably three that have not been used before and for which there is no cross-resistance with any that have. Chemotherapy should then be continued with at least two drugs. A single drug should not be added to a regimen that has failed.

Retreatment should be fully supervised, in hospital if necessary, especially if the patient has been unco-operative in the past. Careful bacteriological monitoring is essential.

Patients in whom relapse has occurred after chemotherapy

Relapse after chemotherapy is rare if the recommended regimen or one of its variants has been administered regularly by an efficient service and the patient has complied and responded well during treatment. If relapse occurs in these circumstances, or in a patient who defaulted after only a short period of regular chemotherapy, resistance is unlikely to have emerged, and the patient should be retreated with the same drug combination, but for 9 rather than 6 months and under stricter supervision.

If an inferior regimen has been used, or if relapse has occurred in a patient whose chemotherapy was poorly supervised and who has taken the drugs irregularly for much of the time, resistance is much more likely to have emerged and the patient should be managed as one whose primary chemotherapy has failed.

Patients with impaired renal function

In patients with impaired renal function, drugs such as isoniazid, rifampicin, pyrazinamide, and ethionamide or prothionamide, which are eliminated by metabolism or biliary excretion, should be given in their usual dosage, whatever the degree of renal impairment. Such patients should be treated with the recommended regimen (2HRZ/4HR) without modification. If possible, drugs such as ethambutol, aminoglycosides, and ofloxacin, which are excreted unchanged in the urine, should be avoided.

Patients with impaired hepatic function

It should not be assumed that patients with impaired hepatic function are more at risk than others for hepatic toxicity, although this may be so. The rate of metabolism of both isoniazid and rifampicin is reduced when liver function is grossly impaired. In treating such patients, many clinicians prefer to use daily isoniazid and ethambutol for 12 months, giving streptomycin as well for the first 2 months. Whatever regimen is used, tests for liver-cell damage should be made regularly during treatment.

Pregnant women

None of the antituberculosis drugs has been shown to have teratogenic effects in the human fetus. If a woman is known to be pregnant when tuberculosis is diagnosed, the pregnancy is likely to have advanced beyond 12 weeks, by which time there is little risk.

Streptomycin should never be given at any stage of the pregnancy because of the risk of damaging the VIIIth cranial nerve of the fetus.

Breast-feeding women

Women receiving antituberculosis drugs can safely breast feed their infants. Such an infant ingests at most 20 per cent of the usual therapeutic dose of isoniazid daily from the milk, and a much lower proportion of the other drugs. The risk of toxic reactions in the infant is thus very low.

Patients with HIV infection or AIDS

Response to the recommended antituberculosis regimen (2HRZ/4HR) is usually good in tuberculous patients with HIV infection or AIDS, and this is the regimen that should be used, being given for the standard 6-month duration. Nevertheless, successful antituberculosis treatment should be followed by lifelong prophylaxis with daily isoniazid because relapse or infection is more likely to occur than in patients with an intact cell-mediated immune mechanism and because there is evidence that recurrence of tuberculosis can itself accelerate the progression of HIV disease.

Compliance is likely to be poor in some groups of patients, particularly intravenous drug users; treatment should be given to such patients under full supervision. Adverse reactions to the antituberculosis drugs are common in HIV-positive patients, particularly cutaneous and hypersensitivity reactions (particularly to thracetazone, which should be avoided), haematological reactions, and hepatic toxicity. Anaphylactic reactions to rifampicin may occur. Rifampicin and isoniazid may interact with ketoconazole and fluconazole, making antifungal treatment ineffective. Also, ketoconazole can inhibit the gastrointestinal absorption of rifampicin, thereby reducing the efficacy of the antituberculosis regimen. Whenever possible, these drugs should not be given together. Rifampicin also interferes with antiretrovival drugs and care is required in HIV-positive persons receiving these drugs. CDC recommendations should be consulted.

Further reading

Centers for Disease Control (1998). Prevention and treatment of tuberculosis among patients infected with human immunodeficiency virus: principles of therapy and revised recommendations. *Morbidity and Mortality Weekly Report*, **47** (RR-20), 1–58.

Collins, C.H., Grange, J.M., Yates, M.D. (1997). *Tuberculosis bacteriology—organization and practice*, (2nd edn). Butterworth–Heinemann, Oxford.

Crofton, J., Horne, N., and Miller, F. (1998). *Clinical tuberculosis*, (2nd edn). Macmillan, London.

Davies, P.D.O. (ed.) (1998). *Clinical tuberculosis*, (2nd edn). Chapman and Hall, London.

Department of Health (1992). *Immunisation against infectious disease*, pp. 76–94. HMSO, London.

Girling, D.J. (1989). The chemotherapy of tuberculosis. In *The biology of the mycobacteria*, Vol. 3: Clinical aspects of mycobacterial disease, (ed. C. Ratledge, J.L. Stanford, and J.M. Grange), pp. 285–323. Academic Press, London.

Harries, A.D. and Maher, D. (1996). *Tuberculosis/HIV—a clinical manual.* World Health Organization, Geneva.

Humphries, M. (1992). The management of tuberculous meningitis. *Thorax*, **47**, 577–81.

Mitchell, D.M. and Miller, R.F. (1992). Recent developments in the management of the pulmonary complications of HIV disease. *Thorax*, **47**, 381–90.

Porter, J.D.A. and Grange, J.M. (1999). *Tuberculosis—an interdisciplinary perspective.* Imperial College Press, London.

World Health Organization (1997). *Treatment of tuberculosis. Guidelines for national programmes.* WHO, Geneva.

World Health Organization (1997). *Guidelines for the management of drug-resistant tuberculosis.* WHO, Geneva.

Chapter 16.60

Disease caused by environmental mycobacteria

J. M. Grange, D. J. Girling, and P. D. O. Davies

The genus *Mycobacterium* includes over 60 species that are environmental saprophytes, some of which occasionally cause opportunistic disease. These environmental mycobacteria (EM) are divisible into two main groups according to their growth rate on subculture (Table 1).

Types of human EM disease

EM causes two named diseases—swimming pool granuloma caused by *M. marinum* and Buruli ulcer caused by *M. ulcerans.* Other diseases are less specific, often resembling tuberculosis, and require identification of the causative organism for diagnosis. There are four main types of such disease: pulmonary, lymphadenitis, post-inoculation, and disseminated.

Chronic pulmonary disease

This principally occurs in middle-aged or elderly patients with predisposing pulmonary disease, but may also occur in otherwise healthy persons. Common causes are the *M. avium* complex (MAC) and *M. kansasii.* Less frequent causes include *M. xenopi*, *M. scrofulaceum*, *M. szulgai*, *M. malmoense*, and *M. chelonae.*

Disease due to EM is likely if several sputum specimens from symptomatic patients, with acute or chronic illness, whose chest radiographs show abnormalities consistent with mycobacterial disease

Table 1 The principal environmental mycobacteria causing opportunistic disease in man

Slow growers	
M. avium[a]	The 'avian tubercle bacillus'
M. intracellulare[a]	
M. genevense	A very poorly growing species causing AIDS-related disease
M. gordonae	Common in the environment but a rare cause of disease.
M. haemophilum	A rare cause of skin granulomas in transplant recipients.
M. kansasii	
M. xenopi	
M. szulgai	
M. malmoense	
M. marinum	The cause of swimming pool granuloma
M. scrofulaceum	The 'scrofula scotochromogen'[b]
M. simiae	
M. terrae	An uncommon cause of wounds contaminated by soil.
M. ulcerans	The cause of Buruli ulcer
Rapid growers	
M. chelonae	Previously spelt *M.chelonei*
M. fortuitum	

[a] Usually grouped together as *M. avium* complex (MAC).

[b] Scotochromogens form yellow pigments in the dark.

yield the same strain of mycobacterium. Single isolates from sputum are unlikely to be of significance as EM may easily contaminate specimens or cultures.

Lymphadenitis

This is most common in otherwise healthy children under the age of 5 years and usually affects a single cervical node. Total excision, if possible, is curative. In the absence of immunosuppression, disseminated disease is rare. Several species of EM cause such lymphadenitis, the most frequent being MAC. Cases in older patients may be HIV-related.

Postinoculation mycobacterioses

Buruli ulcer (*M. ulcerans* infection) (see OTM3, p. 679). This disease was first described in the Bairnsdale district of Australia and occurs in parts of Africa, Mexico, Malaysia, and Papua New Guinea. *M. ulcerans* is inoculated into the skin by spiky vegetation or by other injuries.

The disease commences as a firm skin nodule which may either resolve or spread through the subdermal tissue causing necrosis of the overlying skin and the formation of deeply undermined ulcers (Plate 1). Lesions are usually single and occur mainly on the limbs and other exposed parts of the body. Occasionally, the ends of long bones are affected with sinus formation. Ulcerating lesions are initially progressive but after a few months or years an effective immune response develops and healing ensues, though often with deforming

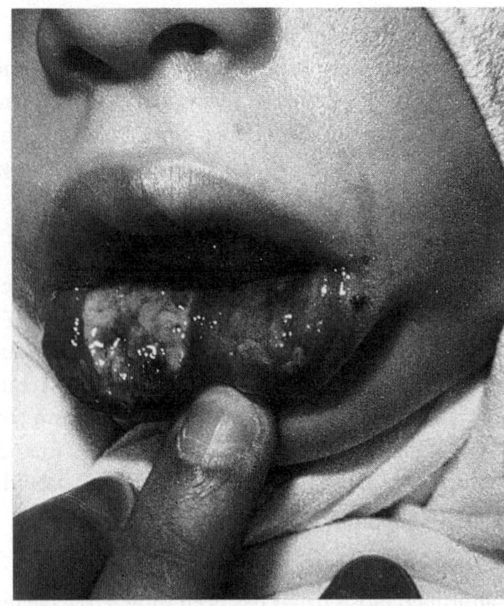

Fig. 1 Ulcers of the lower lip as the initial manifestation of disseminated *Mycobacterium chelonae* infection in a 4-year-old girl with autosomal IgA deficiency
(by courtesy of Dr K. Schopfer).

and disfiguring contractures. Chemotherapy is generally ineffective and radical excision is therefore required.

Swimming pool granuloma (fish tank granuloma)

The causative organism, *M. marinum*, enters cuts and abrasions acquired whilst swimming or tending tropical fish tanks. The cutaneous lesions are usually warty although pustules and ulcers may develop, as may 'sporotrichoid' spread of lesions along the draining lymphatics (Fig. 1). Tenosynovitis, carpal tunnel syndrome, osteomyelitis, and disseminated disease are rare complications. Lesions heal spontaneously after a few months although treatment (see below) accelerates resolution.

Other postinoculation EM disease

Postinjection abscesses, usually caused by *M. chelonae* and *M. fortuitum*, occur sporadically or in miniepidemics due to use of contaminated injectable materials. They appear from 1–12 months after injection and may enlarge to 7 cm or more in diameter. Localized abscesses usually respond well to excision or curettage but multiple or spreading lesions with cellulitis (seen, for example, in insulin-dependent diabetes) require chemotherapy (see below). Serious infections have followed accidental inoculation during surgical operations, especially when contaminated materials, including heart valve xenografts, have been inserted.

Corneal trauma predisposes to infection by *M. chelonae* and *M. fortuitum*. Although topical therapy by amikacin and erythromycin may lead to a temporary resolution, relapse is common and corneal grafting is usually required.

Disseminated disease

This was rare before the advent of the HIV pandemic and occurred in young people with congenital immune deficiencies and in renal transplant recipients. The cause in such patients is usually MAC or, less often, *M. chelonae* or *M. haemophilum*. Disseminated disease, principally due to MAC but occasionally to other species including *M. genevense*, is a common AIDS-related condition, almost always occurring after the patient has developed other AIDS-defining infections (see also Chapter 16.35). Diagnosis is made by culture of sputum and blood or of biopsies of liver, lymph nodes, or bone marrow. The bacilli may be isolated from faeces but they may also be present in the intestinal tract of healthy persons. Treatment is not curative but it improves the quality of life.

Treatment

Treatment is dictated by the site and severity of the disease, presence of predisposing conditions, the species of EM involved, and results of *in vitro* drug susceptibility tests.

Skin lesions may resolve on excision, curettage, or drainage and isolated lymph node involvement is usually curable by excision. Lesions due to *M. marinum* respond to minocycline, trimethoprim with sulfamethoxazole, or a combination of rifampicin and ethambutol.

Pulmonary disease often responds to a three-drug regimen based on rifampicin, ethambutol, and isoniazid. Regimens of 18 or 24 months' duration lead to up to an 80 per cent cure rate in disease due to MAC, *M. xenopi*, and *M. malmoense*. A 9-month course of rifampicin and ethambutol is usually adequate for *M. kansasii* infections. Regimens containing quinolones and the newer macrolides are under evaluation. Surgery is also used for localized pulmonary lesions.

Various multidrug regimens have been described for MAC infection in AIDS patients. Clarithromycin and azithromycin are highly effective and one of these should always be used. Companion drugs include quinolones, rifabutin, and ethambutol. It is usually necessary to continue therapy for the remainder of the patient's life.

Treatment of disease due to *M. chelonae* and *M. fortuitum* is based on anecdotal experience and the results of *in vitro* susceptibility tests. Duration of therapy depends on clinical response. Localized disease often responds to erythromycin with trimethoprim and/or doxycycline while spreading or disseminated disease may require the addition of amikacin, gentamicin, a cephalopsporin, a quinolone (for *M. fortuitum*), or imipenem (for *M. chelonae*).

Further reading

Banks, J. and Campbell, I.A. (1998). Environmental mycobacteria. In *Clinical tuberculosis*, (ed. Davies PDO), (2nd edn), pp. 521–33. Chapman and Hall, London.

Collins, C.H., Grange, J.M., Noble, W.C., and Yates, M.D. (1985). *Mycobacterium marinum* infections in man. *Journal of Hygiene*, **94**, 135–49.

Grange, J.M., Noble, W.C., Yates, M.D., and Collins, C.H. (1988). Inoculation mycobacterioses. *Clinical and Experimental Dermatology*, **13**, 211–20.

Khooshabeh, R., Grange, J.M., Yates, M.D., McCartney, A.C.E., and Casey, T.A. (1994). A case report of *Mycobacterium chelonae* keratitis and a review of mycobacterial infections of the eye. *Tubercle and Lung Disease*, **75**, 377–82.

van der Wef, van der Graaf, W.T.A., Tappero, J.W., and Asiedu, K. (1999). *Mycobacterium ulcerans* infection. *Lancet*, **354**, 1013–18.

Waters, M.F.R. (1996). *Mycobacterium ulcerans* infection. In *Oxford textbook of medicine*, (3rd edn), (ed. D.J. Weatherall, J.G.G. Ledingham, and D.A. Warrell), pp. 679–80. Oxford University Press, Oxford.

Chapter 16.61

Leprosy (Hansen's disease, hanseniasis)

M. F. R. Waters

Definition

Leprosy is a chronic, inflammatory disease of man caused by *Mycobacterium leprae*, which displays a wide clinical 'spectrum' related to the host's ability to develop and maintain specific cell-mediated immunity. In high-resistant 'tuberculoid' leprosy, localized signs are restricted to skin and peripheral nerve, whereas low-resistant 'lepromatous' leprosy is a generalized bacteraemic disease involving many systems, with widespread lesions of the skin, peripheral nerves, upper respiratory tract, the reticuloendothelial system, eyes, bone, and testes. Common complications include immunologically mediated inflammatory episodes ('reactions'), secondary inflammation in the anaesthetic areas that result from nerve damage, and deformity of face, hands, and feet.

Aetiology

M. leprae, discovered by Hansen in 1873, is an intracellular, rod-shaped organism, more acid- and less alcohol-fast than *M. tuberculosis*, which it resembles. No claim to have grown *M. leprae in vitro* has been confirmed to date. Successful experimental transmission was not achieved until 1960, when Shepard reported limited infection in mouse foot-pads, an inoculation of 5000 bacilli yielding 10^6 after 6–8 months, the generation time being 12 days, the longest of any known bacterium. In normal mice no subsequent increase occurs, but in nude mice multiplication continues, yielding 10^9 per foot-pad with lepromatous histology, and systemic spread occurs. Lepromatous leprosy may also be obtained in about three-quarters of normal, nine-banded armadillos inoculated intravenously with leprosy bacilli, thereby providing *M. leprae* for research.

M. leprae is detected in the skin lesions of patients by Wade's 'scraped incision' method (see OTM3, p. 668). Leprosy bacilli are very scanty in tuberculoid lesions and are often not detected routinely. They become more numerous as the spectrum is crossed, being present in huge numbers in lepromatous lesions. The density of bacilli in smears or tissues is termed the bacterial index (BI), which is best scored on Ridley's logarithmic scale (see OTM3, p. 668).

In lepromatous tissues, the bacilli are characteristically in 'cigar-bundle' groups, and in large 'globi' situated in multinucleate Virchow giant cells. The cytoplasm of many bacilli is fragmented; such bacilli are dead, only very slowly breaking down, and remaining in tissues for many months or years.

A standardized, autoclaved suspension of *M. leprae* is used as an intradermal skin test, the 'lepromin' test. The late (Mitsuda) reaction is read at 4 weeks and gives an accurate assessment of specific cell-mediated immunity, being negative in lepromatous and strongly positive in tuberculoid patients. The test is not, however, diagnostic of infection, and shows some cross-reactivity with tuberculin.

There is no significant animal reservoir of leprosy.

Although *M. leprae* cannot yet be grown *in vitro*, mapping of its genome is far advanced, and a complete gene 'library' is held in *Escherichia coli.*

Epidemiology

Past governmental returns submitted to the World Health Organization produced a world estimate of 10.6 million leprosy patients. Following the introduction of limited duration multidrug therapy in 1982, and a change in definition of a 'registered case', the current estimate has fallen to around 1.14 million, although the detection rate remains around 570 000 new patients per year. In addition, 2 to 3 million treated patients are left with significant deformity. Leprosy occurs in almost all tropical and warm-temperate climate regions, having this century died out in northern Europe and Canada. It is associated particularly with overcrowding, and as living standards rise, the disease becomes less common.

The main source of infection in the community consists of untreated or relapsed lepromatous patients, who may shed 10^8 leprosy bacilli in 24 h in their nasal secretions although few bacilli are excreted through intact skin. The exact mode of infection remains unknown; entry via the upper respiratory tract is the most likely route; entry through contaminated skin remains a possibility; transplacental infection is unproven, although antigen can cross the placenta.

There is no simple, specific skin test, comparable to the Mantoux test, for studying the spread of infection in the community although specific lymphocyte transformation tests have confirmed sensitization due to subclinical infection.

Opportunity for contact with the disease, especially in childhood, appears important in the spread of leprosy. Its incidence among household contacts of lepromatous leprosy is 5–10 times that of the general population. Yet only 5 per cent of spouses of lepromatous patients acquire the disease.

Studies of genetic markers, especially HLA, have produced no firm evidence that genetic factors account for individual susceptibility, although certain HLA-DR phenotypes correlate with the type of leprosy developed.

The incubation period is measured in years, being longer in lepromatous than tuberculoid leprosy. The incidence of tuberculoid is higher than that of lepromatous leprosy. In most races, at least from puberty onwards, the incidence appears higher in males than in females.

Pathology and clinical manifestations

Whatever its portal of entry, the target organ for the invading *M. leprae* is probably the endoneurium, an immunologically protected site, the type of disease that ensues being decided by the degree of resistance developed, and maintained, by the infected individual.

Indeterminate leprosy

Child contacts may develop a single hypopigmented macule, 2–5 cm in diameter, showing hypoaesthesia and decreased sweating. Most of such lesions are self-limiting, but about a quarter evolve to one of the determinate 'spectrum' types of leprosy to be described below. Histological changes are slight and non-specific.

The spectrum of leprosy

Leprosy has two special features; the invasion by *M. leprae* of certain superficial nerves, which may become thickened and firm; and the wide range of clinical and histological manifestations, reflecting the intricacies of the host–parasite relationship. This spectrum was first defined, in 1966, by Ridley and Jopling who proposed a five-group system of classification related to the cytology of the host cells of the monocyte–macrophage series (whether histiocytic or epithelioid), the degree of infiltration by lymphocytes, and the bacterial density. The five groups are, in order across the spectrum, tuberculoid (TT), borderline tuberculoid (BT), (mid-) borderline (BB), borderline lepromatous (BL), and lepromatous (LL). Most patients can be diagnosed accurately from their clinical features, although the intermediate 'borderline' BT, BB, and BL groups tend to move towards lepromatous before treatment and toward tuberculoid after commencing chemotherapy.

Skin lesions, best seen in good oblique light, occur anywhere, although they rarely involve the hairy scalp, axillae, and perineum. The palpable nerves of predilection include the ulnars above the medical epicondyle of the humerus, the superficial radials and medians at the wrist, the great auriculars in the neck, the lateral popliteals at the neck of the fibula, and the posterior tibials posterior to the medial malleolus. When nerves of predilection are affected, appropriate regional anaesthesia, muscle weakness, and wasting may occur, resulting in claw hand (ulnar and/or median), foot drop, and claw toes. Branches of the facial and trigeminal nerves, although not palpable, may also be involved, resulting in lagophthalmos and corneal anaesthesia. Wrist drop is rare. In the sensory nerves, the small-calibre fibres are principally affected, so that temperature, light touch, and superficial pain sensation, together with sweating, are routinely lost. Tendon reflexes are preserved.

Tuberculoid leprosy (TT)

When a high degree of cell-mediated immunity is developed, the infection remains very localized and asymmetrical. Only a small number of skin lesions develop, although the associated cutaneous sensory nerve is frequently thickened.

A typical lesion is large and annular, with a sharply raised outer edge and thin, erythematous rim that slopes to a hypopigmented, flattened centre, in profile, resembling a saucer the right way up. The surface is dry, sometimes scaly, and markedly anaesthetic, save for some lesions situated in the midline of the face. Sometimes the lesion is a plaque or a hypopigmented macule. The nerves of predilection are usually little involved; rarely, however, symptoms and signs may be purely neural. Histological examination reveals a tuberculoid granuloma; acid-fast bacilli are so scanty as to be seldom found, and dermal nerves within the granuloma are unrecognizable. Caseation, absent in the skin, may occur in nerve.

Borderline tuberculoid leprosy (BT)

The skin lesions, very few to moderate in number, resemble those of TT leprosy, but are usually smaller in size, or else small 'satellite' lesions may be present near their periphery (Fig. 1). Sharp-edged papules may also appear. Cutaneous sensory nerves are occasionally enlarged (Fig. 2), whereas asymmetrical enlargement of the peripheral nerves of predilection is common; (sometimes the symptoms and signs may be purely neural. Therefore BT leprosy is often associated with deformity of one or both hands and/or feet, a patient often presenting with peripheral burns, infection, or plantar ulceration. Lagophthalmos may result in exposure keratitis. Histologically, the tuberculoid granuloma tends to be more diffuse than in TT leprosy, some dermal nerves may still be seen, and small numbers of leprosy bacilli may be detected.

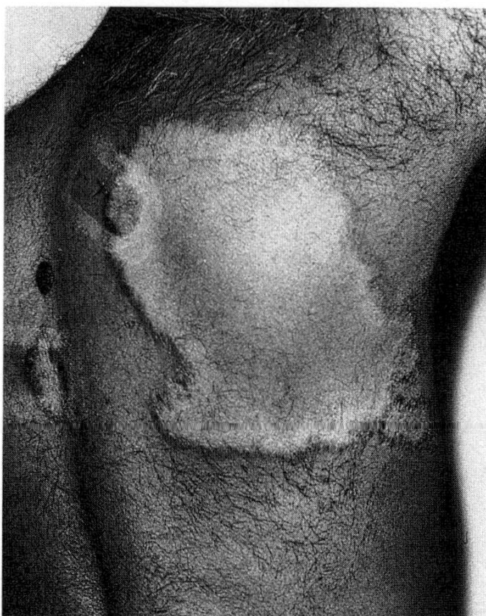

Fig. 1 Active tuberculoid annular lesions showing the sharp outer edge, thin, raised, erythematous, dry rim, and the broad, hypopigmented, dry centre with slight hair loss. The 'satellite' lesion at the lower outer edge indicates that this is borderline tuberculoid leprosy. As shown, biopsies and smears should be taken from the raised, active rim.

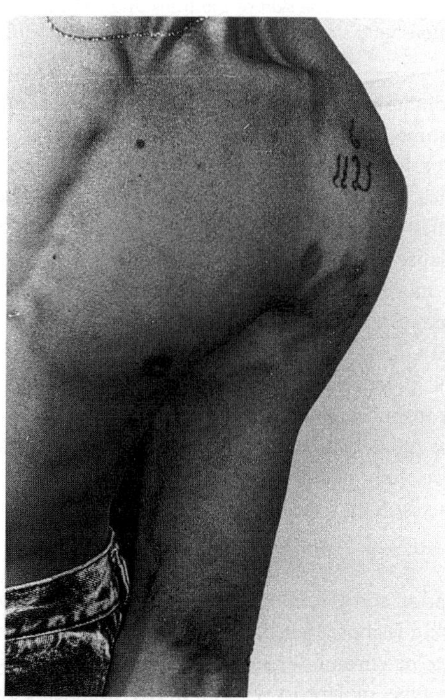

Fig. 2 The lateral supraclavicular nerve is clearly visible and enlarged as it crosses the clavicle and runs towards the proximal edge of the large, borderline tuberculoid, annular lesion. Nerve biopsy confirmed the presence of epithelioid cell granuloma.

Borderline leprosy (BB)

The asymmetrical skin lesions are rather numerous, vary markedly in size, and are erythematous or hypo- or hyperpigmented. The most characteristic lesion is annular with a broad rim (Fig. 3). The outer edge is flattish and irregular, rising to a thick inner edge overlooking a sharply 'punched-out', hypopigmented, anaesthetic centre. In profile, it resembles a saucer the wrong way up but with a deep central depression. Satellite lesions are common. Widespread, usually moderate, enlargement of the nerves of predilection may occur. Histologically, the skin lesion consists of a diffuse epithelioid infiltrate, bacilli being present in moderate numbers. The specific lymphocyte transformation and lepromin tests are usually negative.

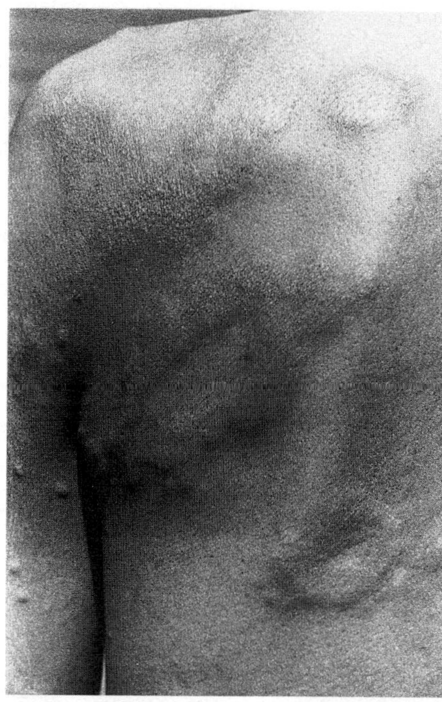

Fig. 3 Borderline annular lesions on the shoulder and back: the rim is broad, the edge irregular, and the 'punched-out' centre is hypopigmented and anaesthetized.

Borderline lepromatous leprosy (BL)

The skin lesions are moderate to many in number, although still somewhat asymmetrical in distribution. They consist of erythematous or hyperpigmented papules, often dimpled in outline, nodules or plaques that are moist and succulent, and that possess near-normal sensation, and/or hypopigmented macules, variable in size, with indefinite edges (Fig. 4). Nerves of predilection may be only slightly enlarged. Ear lobes may appear normal, or asymmetrically enlarged. Although bacilli are very numerous in the lesions, present histologically in a diffuse histiocyctic granuloma, they are often undetected in the normal-looking intervening skin.

Lepromatous leprosy (LL)

The early skin lesions consist of very numerous, small, symmetrical, vague-edged, hypopigmented macules with erythematous, smooth, shiny surfaces that are neither anaesthetic nor anhydrotic, and small papules with indefinite edges. The nerves of predilection may show little thickening, though they slowly and symmetrically enlarge. Thickening of the nasal mucosa often occurs early, causing nasal blockage and discharge; plaques and nodules develop, the skin progressively thickens, and the ear lobes enlarge. Nodules may occur on the palate, nasal septum, and sclera. The lips often swell, eyebrows and eyelashes become scanty (Figs 5 and 6), and iritis and keratitis are common. Saddle-nose deformity and lepromatous laryngitis may develop. Oedema of the extremities sometimes occurs, and the skin of the lower legs often becomes firm and shiny and ulcerates easily. Testicular involvement may lead to atrophy. The dermal nerves are gradually

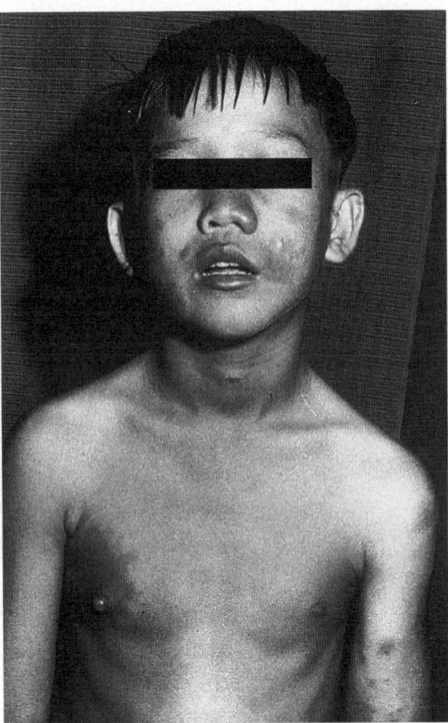

Fig. 4 Borderline lepromatous leprosy: there are numerous moist, shiny plaques on the face, neck, and over the right nipple, typical of BL leprosy, although large, broad-rimmed BB lesions were present on the limbs indicating recent 'downgrading' from BB to BL.

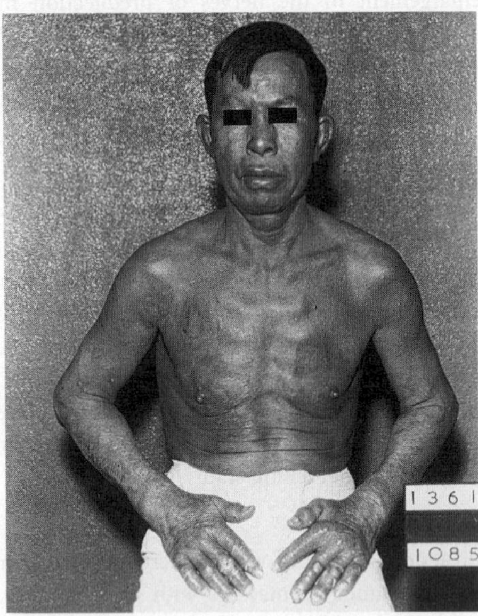

Fig. 5 Active, untreated lepromatous leprosy, showing generalized infiltration of the skin, swelling of fingers and lips, and thinning of eyebrows and eyelashes. The residual annular lesions visible in both pectoral regions indicate that this patient has 'downgraded' from borderline.

destroyed, leading to a progressive pseudo 'glove-and-stocking' anaesthesia, eventually covering most of the body except the hairy scalp, axillae, perineum, and groins, but position sense is well preserved. Some patients repeatedly traumatize their anaesthetic fingers and toes; as a result, the digits progressively shorten and secondary infection may occur.

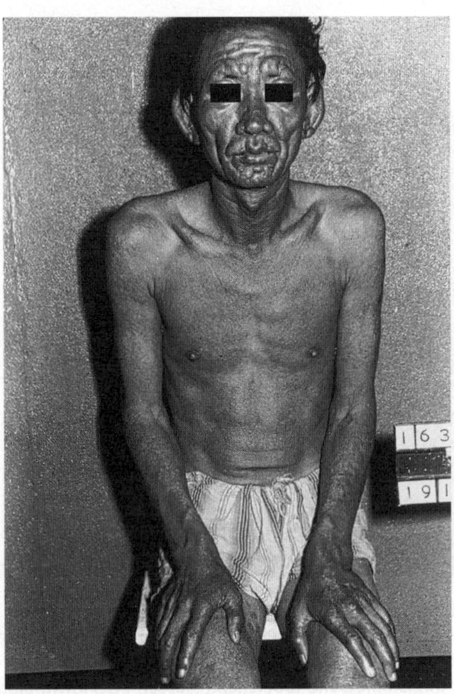

Fig. 6 Leonine facies in advanced untreated lepromatous leprosy, with gross thickening of the ear lobes. The skin of the trunk and limbs is infiltrated and mildly erythematous, and small papules are present on some knuckles.

Many lepromatous cases originate as borderline, and in these 'subpolar lepromatous' (LLs) patients, a small number of residual BB- or BT-type lesions with central anaesthesia may be found. In Central America, some lepromatous patients develop diffuse infiltrate with no nodules (primary diffuse lepromatous leprosy). Should an LL patient relapse, his new lesions are initially asymmetrical, more rounded, and more discrete from the surrounding skin than typical lepromatous papules.

Histologically, the dermis is diffusely infiltrated with foamy histiocytes full of leprosy bacilli and globi. Untreated lepromatous patients suffer from bacteraemia and bacilli are present, often in large numbers in the reticuloendothelial system, the testes, and the anterior part of the eye, although they are scanty in the kidneys, and the central nervous system, heart, and lungs appear to be unaffected.

Reactions

The multiplication and spread of *M. leprae* clinically causes only a mild erythema of skin lesions. Nevertheless, episodes of immunologically-mediated acute or chronic inflammation, known as 'reactions', may occur in any type of leprosy except indeterminate. The majority develop in patients receiving chemotherapy and, unless adequately treated, they may result in crippling deformity.

Non-lepromatous lepra reactions (reversal, upgrading, or Jopling type 1 reactions)

These occur very frequently in treated BT, BB, and BL, and more rarely in LLs leprosy, and in some untreated BT patients. Over the course of a few days or weeks, the leprous lesions themselves become swollen, erythematous, and often scaly, new skin lesions may appear, and the hands, feet, and sometimes the face may become oedematous (Fig. 7). Friable skin lesions may ulcerate. Painful (sometimes painless) neuritis may develop, with or without signs of skin reaction, and can rapidly result in functional nerve damage (Fig. 8). The reaction usually

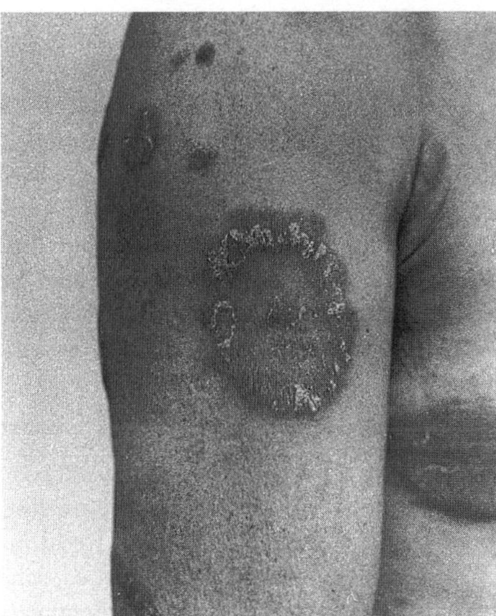

Fig. 7 Reversal or upgrading reaction: this BL patient developed new, sharp-edged, well-defined, erythematous plaques with desquamating surfaces about 6 months after changing chemotherapy for drug resistance.

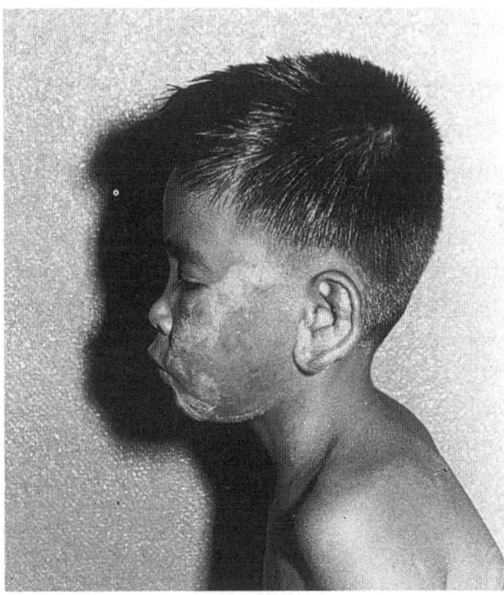

Fig. 8 Reversal-reaction plaque on the left cheek and ear: the edge of this BT lesion has become very sharply defined, more raised, and erythematous, dry, and scaly. Treatment with corticosteroids is imperative, as the patient is at grave risk of rapidly developing lagophthalmos due to associated involvement of branches of the facial nerve.

lasts for several months before gradually fading. By then, many patients have changed in classification towards tuberculoid. The histological picture is variable.

Erythema nodosum leprosum (lepromatous lepra or Jopling type 2 reactions)

Erythema nodosum leprosum (ENL) occurs only at the lepromatous end of the spectrum, in about 30 per cent of treated LL patients, and the occasional untreated LL or treated BL, suffering from one or more episodes. Over the course of a few hours, a crop of painful, erythematous papules develops, typically on the extensor surfaces of the limbs and back. The papules become more purple over 2 or 3 days and then gradually subside, leaving dark staining of the skin. The episodes are usually associated with general malaise and fever. They may be of all degrees of severity, in some patients being isolated and almost unnoticed and in others recurring continuously over years, leading, if untreated, to gross weakness and occasionally death. The most frequent complication is painful neuritis, but acute lymphadenitis, iridocyclitis, and epididymo-orchitis may also occur, and more rarely nephritis and arthritis. Episodes of ENL usually commence a few months after the start of effective treatment. Severe chronic ENL may last for years, only dying out as the BI approaches zero. Histologically, the lesions show a polymorphonuclear infiltrate.

Haematology and immunology

In LL and BL leprosy, mild normochromic anaemia may occur, worsening during episodes of ENL when a polymorphonuclear leucocytosis is usually present. Reversal of the albumin:globulin ratio occurs in many LL and some BL patients, and IgG is almost always raised. In untreated LL and BL patients, there is gross specific depression of cell-mediated immunity for *M. leprae.* There is a relative and absolute decrease in the number of circulating T lymphocytes in the blood of untreated LL patients with depression of the T-helper: T-suppressor cell ratio, and T-helper cells in lepromatous skin lesions predominantly belong to subset 2 (Th2), and secrete interleukin 4. The depression of specific cell-mediated immunity very rarely improves in LL patients in under 20–25 years after commencing chemotherapy. Reversal reactions are thought to be due to an increase in cell-mediated immunity, and may be produced experimentally in lepromatous nude mice by the administration of syngeneic lymphocytes. There is no experimental model for ENL, which is due to immune-complex formation.

Diagnosis and differential diagnosis

The diagnosis of leprosy must be considered in any patient with skin or peripheral-nerve lesions who has resided in an endemic area (especially when skin or nasal symptoms persist despite routine treatment), in idiopathic foot drop, in unusual presentations of arthritis and erythema nodosum, in chronic plantar ulceration, and in painless burns or injuries to the hands and feet. The discovery of any of the following three findings is almost pathognomonic for spectrum leprosy: (i) anaesthetic skin lesions; (ii) the thickening of one or more nerves, either of predilection or cutaneous sensory; and (iii) the presence of acid-fast bacilli in skin smears, which are positive in some BT and in all untreated BB, BL, and LL patients. Therefore skin lesions should be tested for anaesthesia, peripheral nerves systematically palpated for thickening, and skin smears taken from both ear lobes and up to four typical skin lesions. The diagnosis should be confirmed by biopsy of the skin; in pure neural leprosy, a thickened sensory nerve can be safely biopsied. The diagnosis of indeterminate leprosy is difficult, but the finding of lack of sweating in the lesion is particularly helpful.

Leprosy is the only common cause of peripheral-nerve thickening and its finding will exclude almost all other neurological conditions. The anaesthesia of TT and BT leprosy differentiates tuberculoid lesions from vitiligo, mycotic skin infections, lupus vulgaris, and sarcoidosis. Certain conditions bear a superficial resemblance to lepromatous leprosy, including diffuse cutaneous leishmaniasis and secondary syphilis, but may be easily differentiated by the absence of nerve thickening and the failure to find acid-fast bacilli.

Treatment

In leprosy it is essential to treat the 'whole patient', because of the stigma still persisting needlessly, the extreme chronicity of the infection

Table 1 Minimum inhibitory concentrations (MIC) against *M. leprae*, peak serum concentrations, durations of coverage, and bactericidal activities of standard antileprosy drugs

Drug	Human dosage (mg)	MIC in mice (ng/ml)	A	B	C
Rifampicin	600	300	30	1	++++
Dapsone	100	3	500	10	+
Clofazimine[1]	50–100	?	?	?	+
Ofloxacin	400				+++
Minocycline	100	200		10–20	+++
Clarithromycin	500				+++

A, ratio of peak serum concentrations in man after a single dose to MIC determined in the mouse.

B, serum concentrations in man after a single dose.

C, relative degrees of bactericidal activity (+, ++, ++++).

[1] Because clofazimine is deposited in cells, the significance of serum concentrations is uncertain.

Adapted from Ellard, G. A. (1980). *Leprosy Review*, **51**, 200 and WHO Study Group (1994).

and the liability to relapse after many years, the high incidence of reactions occurring during chemotherapy, and the continuing possibility of damage to anaesthetized hands and feet.

Treatment of the infection—chemotherapy

Effective chemotherapy was introduced in 1943, and dapsone, slowly effective but cheap, became the drug of choice by 1951. But relapse off treatment, after prolonged bacteriostasis or due to microbial persistence, was quickly recognized. Secondary dapsone resistance, first proven in 1964, increased steadily in incidence in LL and BL patients and, from 1977, primary dapsone resistance began to be detected in any type of leprosy. Therefore multidrug therapy of limited duration became essential, and two regimens very suitable for general use were recommended, in 1982, by the WHO Study Group on Chemotherapy of Leprosy for Control Programmes.

In the past decade over 90 per cent of all registered leprosy patients have received WHO multidrug therapy or very similar regimens. Compliance rates have been excellent, and relapse rates extraordinarily low. New drug resistances have been virtually completely prevented, although the minimum duration of treatment required to keep relapses in LL and BL leprosy to an acceptably low level is not yet fully known. The current aim of WHO is to extend multidrug therapy to all registered cases of leprosy worldwide. The principal drugs found to be bactericidal for *M. leprae* on mouse foot-pad testing are listed in Table 1.

Dapsone (4-4′-diaminodiphenyl-sulphone, DDS)

Clinical improvement is detected from about 3 months after starting dapsone in LL and BL patients; bacilli from nose and skin will then no longer infect normal mice, although the BI takes many years (2 in BB, 4–5 in BL, and 8–11 in LL) to become smear negative. The recommended standard adult dose is 100 mg/day (1–2 mg/kg body weight) by mouth. The important toxic side-effect of dapsone is allergy, which may occur 3–7 weeks after starting dapsone.

Rifampicin (rifampin)

This is so rapidly bactericidal that after a single dose of 600–1200 mg, bacilli obtained from the skin 3 days later usually fail to multiply in the foot-pads of mice. Clinical improvement begins within 7–14 days of starting rifampicin. The recommended dosage is 10–15 mg/kg body weight, that is 600 mg to those weighing 35 kg or over, preferably taken on an empty stomach. Because of the prolonged generation time of *M. leprae*, rifampicin may be given monthly. As rifampicin resistance develops relatively rapidly in lepromatous leprosy, it should always be used in combination with at least one other effective antileprosy drug.

Clofazimine

This riminophenazine dye is deposited in fat cells; therefore its MIC cannot be measured, although the minimum effective dose preventing multiplication of *M. leprae* in mice is 0.0001 per cent in the diet. It kills leprosy bacilli at about the same speed as dapsone. Standard dosage is 50 mg daily. The drug is also anti-inflammatory and has been widely used in high dosage to control ENL reactions, though several weeks elapse before its full anti-inflammatory effect is produced. Its chief disadvantage is that it causes a reddish-brown pigmentation of the skin with increased melanin production, which is objectionable to many light-skinned patients.

Recommended regimens

Multibacillary leprosy

For all LL, BL, and BB patients and those BT and indeterminate patients who are skin-smear positive for acid-fast bacilli at diagnosis (where skin smears are unreliable, WHO now includes BT patients with more than five lesions), it is essential to give a minimum of three drugs, to prevent the emergence of resistance to a second drug should dapsone resistance, whether primary or secondary, be present. The 1982 WHO Study Group designed a single regimen to cover all types of multibacillary patients, which is equally effective in both treated and untreated, and in dapsone-sensitive and dapsone-resistant patients, and provides basic supervision of the more expensive drugs, particularly rifampicin. The regimen consists of:

- rifampicin, 600 mg once monthly (or every 4 weeks), supervised;
- clofazimine, 50 mg daily, unsupervised, plus 300 mg (supervised) every month or 4 weeks;
- dapsone, 100 mg daily, unsupervised.

Where regular monthly supervision is not possible, several months' supply of blister packs of the drugs may be supplied for supervision by the village health-care worker.

It is recommended (by the WHO in 1994) that the regimen should always be given for 2 years. Relapse rates after stopping triple-drug therapy are surprisingly low to date, of the order of 0.12/100 person years, although further long-term follow-up is still required. Those few patients who have relapsed after multidrug therapy and have been investigated have not been found to have acquired any new drug resistances. In 1998, the WHO suggested that 1 year of treatment may be sufficient, especially in less bacilliferous patients, but appropriate relapse data are incomplete. According to the WHO in 1994, the alternatives of minocycline or ofloxacin are now preferred.

Paucibacillary leprosy

It is important to treat effectively and in the shortest possible time, all skin-smear negative tuberculoid and indeterminate patients, whether suffering from dapsone-sensitive or primary dapsone-resistant leprosy.

The recommended regimen consists of rifampicin 600 mg monthly for six supervised doses, plus dapsone 100 mg daily unsupervised for 6 months. WHO aims that all patients should complete the 6 months' treatment within 9 months. Patients suffering from dapsone allergy should substitute clofazimine 50 mg daily. So far, crude relapse rates have been very satisfactorily low, of the order of 0.13/100 person years of follow-up. Should a patient be unable to come every month for the supervised dose of rifampicin, blister packs may be supplied for supervision by the village health-care worker. Patients suffering from single lesion paucibacillary leprosy may respond to a single dose of rifampicin 600 mg, minocycline 100 mg, and ofloxacin 400 mg (recommended by the WHO in 1998) but no data on relapse rates are yet available.

New antileprosy drugs

Recent studies have shown than ofloxacin 400 mg daily, minocycline 100 mg daily, and clarithromycin 500 mg daily, all achieve a 99.99 per cent kill of *M. leprae* in around 4 weeks, and in 1994 the WHO recommended regimens utilizing them for patients suffering from rifampicin allergy or resistance, or who refuse clofazimine.

Treatment of reactions

It is essential to continue the course of antileprosy chemotherapy unchanged during reactions.

Erythema nodosum leprosum

Mild ENL may usually be controlled with paracetamol or soluble aspirin. ENL is graded severe if there is high or prolonged fever or if any other system apart from skin is involved. There are three alternative regimens. Prednisolone usually suppresses ENL. But often steroid therapy proves to be prolonged, and severe steroid toxicity may occur. Thalidomide is equally effective in controlling ENL and in general is safer than steroids, but its use is contraindicated in women of child-bearing age (see OTM3, p. 677). The third alternative is clofazimine, 300 mg daily for an initial period of about 3 months, the dosage being subsequently progressively lowered. It is not as powerful as thalidomide or prednisolone and it takes 4–6 weeks to achieve its full suppressive action; therefore, if a rapid effect is required, it should be combined initially with prednisolone. In iridocyclitis, local treatment with steroid and homatropine eye drops is also recommended.

Reversal reactions

Mild reactions can usually be controlled with paracetamol or soluble aspirin. In severe reactions, especially if there is peripheral oedema, or if there is nerve pain and tenderness or loss of nerve function, the signs of inflammation should be suppressed with prednisolone. The initial dose is usually 30–40 mg daily, and maintenance therapy will be required for several months before the prednisolone can be finally tailed off.

Treatment of neuritis

Untreated patients with a recent history (less than 3–6 months) of increasing nerve damage, or found to have one or more tender nerves, should be given steroids for several months, commencing with the specific chemotherapy.

Ancillary treatment

It is essential to educate patients to protect their anaesthetized limbs, which they should inspect daily. Callosities over pressure points should be regularly softened by soaking in water, and trimmed. Well-fitting shoes with microcellular rubber insoles help to prevent plantar ulceration. A plantar ulcer requires rest or the application of a below-knee walking-plaster splint and appropriate treatment of secondary infection. Injured or infected anaesthetized hands may also require splinting. Patients suffering from lagophthalmos or paralysis of hands or feet require physiotherapy and may be helped by reconstructive surgery.

Prognosis

With early diagnosis and correct treatment, the prognosis is now excellent. Death from LL leprosy is rare, although secondary amyloidosis still occasionally occurs, especially in inadequately treated ENL, where the diagnosis must be made in the prenephrotic stage to prevent renal failure. Widespread nerve damage may still develop in BT and BB patients, if reversal reactions are inadequately treated. Patients who fail to care for anaesthetic limbs may develop increasing deformity. Iridocyclitis may cause impairment of vision or blindness and cataract is common in LL patients.

Prophylaxis

The strategy of leprosy control still relies on early case finding and treatment of infectious LL and BL patients. Vaccination with BCG gives some protection. Some evidence suggests that preference should be given to vaccinate young, presumed naive subjects, and that BCG given to neonates for protection against tuberculosis may also be protective against leprosy.

Vaccination with several other culturable mycobacteria and with irradiated-killed *M. leprae* combined with live BCG is being investigated. Immunotherapy as an adjunct to chemotherapy of multibacillary leprosy is also being studied, with the objective of overcoming both specific anergy and microbial persistence.

Contact tracing, especially of child contacts of LL and BL patients, remains important. Such children could be offered (further) BCG vaccinations.

Once the protective antigens of *M. leprae* have been identified, the technology is already well advanced to produce a second-generation vaccine.

Further reading

Ridley, D.S. and Jopling, W.H. (1966). Classification of leprosy according to immunity: a five-group system. *International Journal of Leprosy*, **34**, 255–73.

Shepard, C.C. (1960). The experimental disease that follows the injection of human leprosy bacilli into foot pads of mice. *Journal of Experimental Medicine*, **112**, 445–54.

WHO Expert Committee on Leprosy (1988). Sixth Report. *World Health Organization Technical Report Series*, No. 768. WHO, Geneva.

WHO Expert Committee on Leprosy (1998). Seventh Report. *World Health Organization Technical Report Series*, WHO, Geneva.

WHO Study Group on Chemotherapy of Leprosy for Control Programmes (1982). *World Health Organization Technical Report Series*, No. 67. WHO, Geneva.

WHO Study Group on Chemotherapy of Leprosy (1994). *World Health Organization Technical Report Series*, No. 847. WHO, Geneva.

WHO (1997). Progress towards leprosy elimination. *Weekly Epidemiological Record*, 72, 165–72.

Chapter 16.62

Actinomycoses

K. P. Schaal

'Actinomycoses' are polyaetiological inflammatory syndromes characterized by slowly progressing infiltrations, formation of multiple abscesses, and a tendency to develop draining sinus tracts. Various fermentative (facultatively anaerobic, capnophilic) actinomycetes of the genera *Actinomyces*, *Propionibacterium*, and *Bifidobacterium* are implicated.

Aetiology of human actinomycoses

Actinomyces israelii and *A. gerencseriae* are by far the most frequent and most characteristic causes of human actinomycoses. *Propionibacterium propionicum*, *Actinomyces naeslundii*, *A. odontolyticus*, *A. viscosus*, *A. meyeri*, and *Bifidobacterium dentium* (formerly *Actinomyces eriksonii*) are further potential but much less common causes.

Epidemiology

Actinomycoses are not transmissible and cannot be brought under control by vaccination or measures that prevent spread. Sporadically, they occur world-wide. In Germany, the incidence of the disease was estimated to range from 1:40 000 (acute and chronic cases together) to 1:80 000 (chronic cases alone) per year.

Males are affected two to four times more frequently than are females. This disposition appears to be restricted to the cervicofacial form in mature males. Although actinomycoses may be found in patients of any age, men are predominantly seized with the disease between the twentieth and fortieth year and women in the second and third decade of their lives. Before puberty and in old age, actinomycoses occur sporadically in patients of both sexes.

Pathogenesis and pathology

Most of the fermentative actinomycetes pathogenic to man are found regularly and abundantly in the oral cavity of healthy adults. In the digestive, respiratory, and genital tracts as well as in the mouths of babies before teething and of adults after loss of all natural teeth, these microbes occur only sporadically or in low numbers. Therefore, they may be considered facultatively pathogenic commensals of the human mucous membranes, which, apart from the very rare actinomycotic wound infections after human bites or fist fights, produce disease exclusively as endogenous pathogens.

For active invasion of the tissue, the classical pathogenic fermentative actinomycetes require a negative redox potential, which may result either from insufficient blood supply (caused by circulatory or vascular diseases, crush injuries, or foreign bodies) or from the reducing and necrotizing capacity of other microbes in the lesion. Immunocompromise does not predispose to actinomycotic infections.

Synergistic polymicrobial infection

True actinomycoses are synergistic mixed infections, in which the actinomycetes act as the specific component, the so-called 'guiding organisms', determining the characteristic course and the late symptoms of the disease. 'Concomitant microbes', which may vary considerably in composition and number of species from case to case, are often responsible for the initial clinical picture and for certain complications, and they are also part of the resident or transient surface flora of the human mucous membranes (see OTM3, p. 682 for further details). Particularly pronounced synergistic interactions appear to exist between *A. israelii* or *A. gerencseriae* and *Actinobacillus* (*Haemophilus*) *actinomycetemcomitans*. The latter organism may even sustain the inflammatory process under similar clinical symptoms after chemotherapeutic elimination of the causative actinomycete.

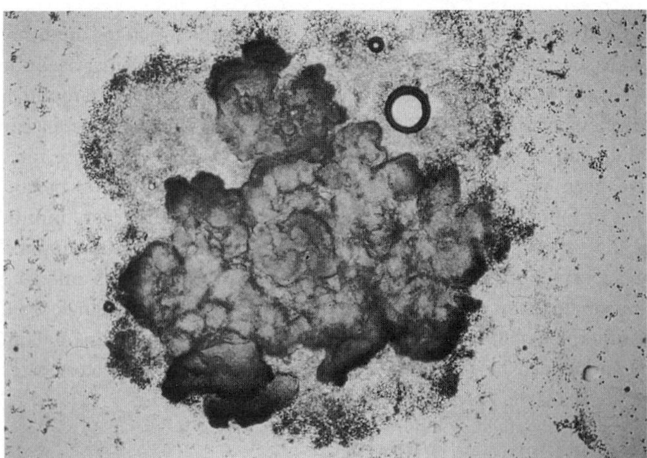

Fig. 1 Actinomycotic sulphur granule. Micrograph of a particle embedded in 1 per cent methylene blue solution, original diameter 0.8 mm. Note the cauliflower-like structure in the centre of the particle and the partially blue-stained granulocytes in the periphery.

Histopathology

Initially, an inflammatory granulation tissue develops, which usually breaks down either to form an acute abscess or chronic multiple abscesses with connective tissue proliferation. The pathagnomonic sulphur granules are formed primarily in the infected tissue, but may also appear as free structures in abscess contents or sinus discharge. They are of the highest diagnostic importance.

Sulphur granules are macroscopically visible (up to 1 mm in diameter), yellowish, reddish to brownish particles, which exhibit a cauliflower-like appearance under the microscope at low magnifications (Fig. 1). They consist of a conglomerate of filamentous actinomycete microcolonies formed *in vivo* and surrounded by tissue reaction material, especially polymorphonuclear granulocytes. At high magnification, a Gram-stained smear of the completely crushed granule reveals the presence of clusters of Gram-positive, interwoven, branching filaments with radially-arranged peripheral hyphae and of a variety of other Gram-positive and Gram-negative rods and cocci, which represent the concomitant flora. On the tips of peripheral filaments, a club-shaped layer of hyaline material may be seen, which can aid in the differentiation of actinomycotic sulphur granules from macroscopically similar particles of various other microbial and non-microbial origins.

Clinical features

The primary actinomycotic lesion usually develops in tissue adjacent to a mucous membrane at cervicofacial, thoracic, or abdominal sites.

The infection tends to progress slowly and to penetrate without regard to natural organ borders, or to spread haematogenously even to distant sites. Remission and exacerbation of symptoms with and without antimicrobial treatment is characteristic. As in other endogenous microbial diseases, the incubation period of actinomycoses is not defined.

Cervicofacial actinomycoses

In the vast majority of cases, actinomycotic lesions primarily involve the face or neck. Conditions predisposing to these cervicofacial infections include tooth extractions, fractures of the jaw, periodontal abscesses, foreign bodies penetrating the mucosal barrier (bone splinters, fish bones, awns of grains or grasses (e.g. beard of barley)), and suppurating tonsillar crypts.

Initially, the cervicofacial actinomycoses present either as an acute, usually odontogenic, abscess or cellulitis of the floor of the mouth, or as a slowly developing, chronic, hard, painless, reddish or livid swelling. Small acute actinomycotic abscesses may heal after surgical drainage alone. More often, however, the acute initial stage is followed by a subacute to chronic course if no specific antimicrobial treatment is given, thereby imitating the primarily chronic form which is characterized by regression and cicatrization of central suppurative goci while the infection progresses peripherally producing hard, painless, livid infiltrations. These may lead to multiple, new areas of liquefaction, fistulae, which often discharge pus containing sulphur granules, and multilocular cavities with poor healing and a tendency to recur after temporary regressions of the inflammatory symptoms.

With inappropriate or no treatment, cervicofacial actinomycoses extend slowly and may become life-threatening by invasion of the cranial cavity, mediastinum, or blood stream.

Thoracic actinomycoses

Thoracic manifestations, which are much less common than the cervicofacial form, usually develop after aspiration or inhalation of material from the mouth (dental plaque or calculus, tonsillar crypt contents) or a foreign body that contains or is contaminated with the causative agents. Occasionally, this may result from extension of an actinomycotic process of the neck, from an abdominal infection perforating the diaphragm, or from a distant focus by haematogenous spread.

Primary pulmonary actinomycoses present as bronchopneumonic infiltrations that may imitate tuberculosis or bronchial carcinoma radiographically, appearing as single dense or multiple spotted shadows, in which cavitations may develop. If not diagnosed and treated properly, pulmonary infections may extend through the pleural cavity producing empyema, to the pericardium, or to the chest wall; they may even become apparent as paravertebral (psoas) abscesses tracking down to the groin.

Abdominal actinomycoses

Actinomycoses of the abdomen and pelvis are rare. They originate either from acute perforating gastrointestinal diseases (appendicitis, diverticulitis, various ulcerative diseases), from surgical or accidental trauma including injuries caused by ingested bone splinters or fish bones, or from inflammations of the female internal reproductive organs.

Women who wear intrauterine contraceptive devices or vaginal pessaries for long periods often show a characteristic colonization of the cervical canal and the uterine cavity by various fermentative actinomycetes and other anaerobes resembling the synergistic actinomycotic flora. However, this colonization only rarely results in an invasive actinomycotic process, which is difficult to diagnose because it closely resembles cervical or ovarian carcinoma.

Most of the abdominal actinomycoses present as slowly growing tumours, which are difficult to differentiate from malignant neoplasms. By direct extension, any abdominal tissue or organ may be involved including muscle, liver, spleen, kidney, fallopian tubes, ovaries, testes, bladder, or rectum. Haematogenous liver abscesses have been seen, especially from genital actinomycoses.

Actinomycotic infections of the central nervous system

Actinomycoses of the brain and the spinal cord are very rare. They may arise from direct extension of cervicofacial infections. Haematogenous spread is also possible, particularly from lesions in the lungs or abdomen. The spinal canal may be directly involved from these sites. Brain abscess is much more common than meningitis.

Actinomycoses of bone

Bone involvement is also very rare. It usually develops by direct extension from soft tissue infection resulting in a periostitis with new bone formation visible upon radiography. If the bone itself is invaded, localized areas of bone destruction surrounded by increased bone density usually develop. Mandible, ribs, and spine are most frequently involved.

Cutaneous actinomycoses

Actinomycotic lesions of the skin are extremely rare. Usually, they originate from wounds that were contaminated with saliva or dental plaque following human bites or fist fights, but they may also result from haematogenous spread. Symptoms are very similar to those of cervicofacial actinomycoses.

Diagnosis

Clinical symptoms are often misleading, especially in the early stages of the disease, histopathological appearances are unreliable, and diagnosis chiefly rests on bacteriological methods.

Radiography

In cervicofacial cases, radiography is useful only for detecting bone involvement. A pulmonary infiltrate associated with a proliferative lesion or destruction of ribs is highly suggestive of either actinomycosis or a tumour. Radiography may also help to locate the abdominal processes and to identify the involvement of organs such as liver, kidney, urinary bladder, or ureter. In general, however, radiographic changes are not diagnostic.

Laboratory diagnosis

Clinical chemistry and haematology

Small, localized actinomycotic lesions are usually not associated with abnormalities. In advanced cases, however, especially those in the thoracic or the abdominal area, a raised erythrocyte sedimentation rate and pronounced leucocytosis may be found. When the central nervous system is involved, a polymorphonuclear or mononuclear pleocytosis is commonly found. The protein content of the cerebrospinal fluid is frequently elevated and the sugar content moderately depressed.

Bacteriology

Pus specimens containing sulphur granules, and occasionally looking like semolina, should prompt the clinician to ask and the bacteriologist to look specifically for actinomycetes using suitable culture techniques and other methods.

Pus, sinus discharge, bronchial secretions, granulation tissue, or biopsy materials are suitable specimens. Precautions must be taken to prevent contamination of the specimen by the indigenous mucosal flora. In cases of cervicofacial actinomycoses, pus should therefore be obtained only by transcutaneous puncture of the abscesses or by transcutaneous needle biopsy. When abscesses already have been incised, a sufficient amount of pus should be collected instead of using only a swab. Because sputum always contains oral actinomycetes, bronchial secretions should be obtained by transtracheal aspiration, or material should be collected by transthoracic percutaneous needle biopsy. Percutaneous puncture of suspected abscesses is often also the only way of obtaining suitable specimens for diagnosing abdominal actinomycoses.

The transport of specimens to the bacteriology laboratory should be as fast as possible, preferably by messenger. Alternatively, a reducing transport medium such as one of the modification of Stewart's medium should be used. The specimen should arrive in the laboratory within 24 h, although it has occasionally proved possible to isolate actinomycetes from samples that took 7 days or more to get to the diagnostic laboratory by post.

A quick and comparatively reliable diagnosis is possible microscopically when sulphur granules are present (Fig. 1). The demonstration of concomitant bacteria allows the differentiation of actinomycotic granules from similar particles produced by *Nocardia*, *Actinomadura*, or *Streptomyces* spp. in cases of actinomycetoma.

Use of transparent culture media and careful microscopic examination of the cultures after at least 2, 7, and 14 days of incubation enables a specialized laboratory to detect possible actinomycete colonies and to subculture them for identification. Isolation, subculture, and definite identification to the species level may require 1–4 weeks. Techniques such as gene probes or polymerase chain reaction (PCR) for detecting pathogenic fermentative actinomycetes are being developed.

Serology

Sensitivity and specificity are too low.

Treatment

As the aetiology of human actinomycoses is always polymicrobial, the antibacterial drugs used for treatment should cover both the causative actinomycetes and all of the concomitant bacteria. This usually requires the administration of drug combinations in which aminopenicillins currently represent the main components because they are slightly more active against the pathogenic actinomycetes than is penicillin G, and they are able to inhibit *Actinobacillus actinomycetemcomitans*, which is mostly resistant to narrow-spectrum penicillins. However, the presence of concomitant β-lactamase producers such as *Bacteroides fragilis*, *B. thetaaiiotraomicron*, or *Staphylococcus aureus* (β-lactamase producing) may impair the therapeutic efficacy of aminopenicillins, and that of most other β-lactams, so that the combination with a β-lactamase inhibitor is advisable or even necessary.

For cervicofacial actinomycoses, amoxicillin plus clavulanic acid has proved to be the treatment of choice. Three doses of 2.2 g amoxicillin plus clavulanic acid per day for 1 week and three doses of 1.1 g of the combination for an additional 7 days usually results in complete cure. Thoracic actinomycoses mostly respond to the same regimen. However, it is advisable to maintain doses of 2.2 g three times per day for 2 weeks, and to continue treatment for 3–4 weeks. Advanced pulmonary cases may require the addition of 2 g ampicillin, three times a day, in order to increase the aminopenicillin tissue concentrations and, depending on the composition of the concomitant flora, the addition of an antimicrobial specifically active against strict anaerobes (metronidazole, clindamycin) or resistant Enterobacteriaceae.

Since in abdominal actinomycoses Enterobacteriaceae and β-lactamase producing *Bacteroides* spp. are usually present, suitable antimicrobial combinations for these cases are amoxicillin, plus clavulanic acid, plus metronidazole, plus tobramycin (gentamicin) or ampicillin, plus an aminoglycoside. Imipenem could also be a good choice, but this drug has not yet been used very often for treating actinomycotic infections.

Neither clindamycin nor metronidazole should be used alone as clindamycin is virtually ineffective against *Actinobacillus actinomycetemcomitans* and metronidazole shows no activity at all against pathogenic actinomycetes. The use of other combinations, including additional aminoglycosides, cephalosporins, or β-lactamase-stable penicillins, may be necessary depending on the presence of unusual aerobic organisms. In patients allergic to penicillins, tetracyclines or possibly cephalosporins may be tried instead of aminopenicillins.

Incision of abscesses and drainage of pus may still be necessary as an adjunct to the antimicrobial chemotherapy and may help to accelerate recovery and to decrease the risk of relapses.

Prognosis

The prognosis of the cervicofacial and cutaneous actinomycoses is good provided that the diagnosis is established early and the antimicrobial treatment is adequate. However, thoracic, abdominal, and systemic manifestations remain serious conditions that require all possible diagnostic and therapeutic efforts. Without proper treatment, the prognosis is grave.

Further reading

Schaal, K. P. (1986). Genus *Actinomyces* Harz 1877, 133. In *Bergey's manual of systematic bacteriology* (eds. P.H.A. Sneath, N.S. Mair, M.E. Sharpe, and J.G. Holt), Vol. 2, pp. 1383–418. Williams and Wilkins, Baltimore.

Schaal, K P. (1992). The genera *Actinomyces, Arcanobacterium,* and *Rothia.* In *A handbook on the biology of bacteria: ecophysiology, isolation, identification, applications,* Vol. 1, The prokaryotes, (eds. A. Balows, H.G. Trüper, M. Dworkin, W. Harder, and K.H. Schleifer), (2nd edn), pp. 850–905. Springer-Verlag, New York.

Schaal, K.P. and Lee, H.-J. (1992). Actinomycete infections in humans—a review. *Gene,* **115**, 201–11.

Schaal, K.P. and Pulverer, G. (1984). Epidemiologic, etiologic, diagnostic, and therapeutic aspects of endogenous actinomycete infections. In *Biological, biochemical, and biomedical aspects of actinomycetes,* (eds. L. Ortiz-ortiz, L.F. Bojalil, and V. Yakoleff), pp. 13–32. Academic Press, Orlando FL.

Slack, J.M. and Gerencser, M.A. (1975). *Actinomyces, filamentous bacteria. Biology and pathogenicity.* Burgess Publishing Company, Minneapolis.

Chapter 16.63

Nocardiosis

R. J. Hay

Nocardiosis (nocardiasis) is a systemic or, more rarely, cutaneous infection caused by *Nocardia* species, usually *Nocardia asteroides* but less commonly *N. brasiliensis*, *N. caviae*, and *N. transvaliensis*. These organisms are also important causes of actinomycetoma (see Chapter 16.81). The nocardiae are aerobic, Gram-positive, filamentous, branching bacteria which may also break up into bacillary forms and, in some conditions, aggregate into grains typical of mycetomas.

Pathogenesis

Nocardia species are found in soil but may also be aerosolized. Most infections are respiratory although an alternative route of infection is via percutaneous inoculation. The characteristic histopathological response to infection is the production of polymorphonuclear leucocyte abscesses without extensive fibrosis; metastatic infection can occur in other organs. By contrast, in primary cutaneous infections the lesion is usually localized to an abscess containing filaments at the site of inoculation and is accompanied by local lymphadenopathy.

Epidemiology

Otherwise healthy patients may be infected by nocardia, although the frequency of subclinical exposure and sensitization in normal populations is unknown. The usual site of primary infection is the lung and the disease may remain restricted to this site. However, the majority of patients with systemic nocardiosis are immunocompromised, most commonly with a condition that affects the expression of T lymphocyte-mediated immune responses including HIV infection, cancer, lymphoma, and in recipients of high-dose corticosteroid therapy.

Clinical features

Primary cutaneous nocardiosis

This is an uncommon infection that appears to follow traumatic inoculation of organisms in a superficial abrasion. The primary lesion is a small nodule, ulcer, or abscess often accompanied by the development of a chain of secondary nodules (compare with sporotrichosis) along the course of a lymphatic and local lymphadenopathy is common. This is usually caused by *Nocardia asteroides*.

Nocardia mycetoma

Nocardia brasiliensis is the usual cause.

Pulmonary nocardiosis

Pulmonary infection is seen in about 75 per cent of cases of systemic nocardiosis, even where there are disseminated lesions elsewhere. Symptoms of pulmonary nocardiosis are variable, with cough, fever, and leucocytosis. In otherwise healthy individuals the changes and signs may be very similar to pulmonary tuberculosis, whereas in the immunocompromised patient the lesions present as rapidly developing, single or multiple lung lesions. Chest radiographs may show segmental or lobar infiltrates, cavitation, nodules, or diffuse miliary infiltrates. Most cases of pulmonary nocardiosis are caused by *N. asteroides*.

Disseminated nocardiosis

Haematogenous spread is common in the immunocompromised patient and may occur without evidence of pulmonary infection. The most common site for dissemination is the brain, where it presents with localized abscesses without meningeal involvement. The signs are those due to an intracerebral space-occupying lesion. Spread to other sites is less common, although dissemination to skin, liver, kidneys, and bone may occur.

Laboratory diagnosis

The infection is often recognized initially by Gram-stained specimens of pus, bronchial washings, or tissue. Nocardia species grow aerobically on ordinary media, including Lowenstein–Jensen medium. In histopathology, filaments stain with modified acid-fast stains using an aqueous solution of a weak acid for decolorization but they can also be highlighted with the methenamine-silver stain (Grocott modification). Serological tests (usually counterimmunoelectrophoresis or enzyme immunoassay) can be obtained in reference centres.

Management

The mainstays of therapy are sulphonamides such as sulphadiazine and sulphafurazole, given in doses of 4–6 g daily. Co-trimoxazole is also effective, particularly in pulmonary forms, although the ratio of the trimethoprim to sulphonamide components is not ideal for intracerebral infections. Much of the recommended drug therapy though is derived from the personal experiences of few cases. Other drugs that have been used include amikacin, ampicillin, impipenem, and minocycline—although testing is necessary before using these.

Clustering of cases may occur occasionally, suggesting exposure to a common source of infection such as local construction work. At present, no methods of prevention are known, although the existence of more than two cases in a single or adjacent wards should alert clinicians to the possibility of environmentally-acquired infection.

Further reading

Boiron, P., Provost, F., Chevrier, G., and Dupont, B. (1992). Review of nocardial infections in France, 1987–1990. *European Journal of Clinical Microbiology and Infectious Diseases*, **11**, 709–14.

Curry, W.A. (1980). Human nocardiosis. *Archives of Internal Medicine*, **140**, 818–24.

Javaly, K., Horowitz, H.W., and Wormser, G.P. (1992). Nocardiosis in patients with human immunodeficiency virus infection. Report of 2 cases and review of the literature. *Medicine*, **71**, 128–38.

Chapter 16.64

Rat bite fevers

D. A. Warrell

Rodent bites can transmit lymphocytic choriomeningitis and other arenaviruses, rabies, leptospirosis, melioidosis, tularaemia, plague, murine typhus, trench fever, *Pasteurella multocida*, and the two rat bite fevers—streptobacillary, caused by *Streptobacillus moniliformis*, and spirillary, caused by *Spirillum minus*.

Streptobacillus moniliformis infection (streptobacillary rat bite fever and Haverhill fever)

Streptobacillus moniliformis is a pharyngeal commensal of wild and laboratory rats, also found in mice, guinea-pigs, gerbils, squirrels, and turkeys, and also found in mammals that feed on them. *S. moniliformis*, named from the filaments and chains with yeast-like swellings seen in mature cultures on solid media, is a non-motile, pleomorphic, filamentous, Gram-negative rod that is difficult to grow. In culture, L-phase variants occur spontaneously; lacking a cell wall they are resistant to penicillin. *S. moniliformis* has been cultured from patients' bite wounds, blood, synovial and pericardial fluid, and from abscesses.

Epidemiology

The infection occurs worldwide in two forms. Rat bite fever is caused by bites or scratches by rodents or their predators, or mere contact with these mammals, living or dead. Most victims of rat bites are children of poor families living in urban areas. The bite may be inflicted during sleep and may not be suspected. Laboratory staff who work with rats are also at special risk. Haverhill fever, named after the town in Massachusetts, follows ingestion of raw milk, food, or water contaminated by rats' faeces. An outbreak in a boarding school in England in 1983 affecting 304 people, 43 per cent of the school's population, was attributed to contamination of the water supply by rats.

Clinical features

After an incubation period of 2–10 (extreme range 1–22) days, there is a sudden high fever with rigors, vomiting, severe headache, myalgia, and regional lymphadenopathy. Evidence of the bite has usually disappeared by this stage. Erythematous macules and petechiae appear symmetrically, especially on the palms, soles, and face, 1–8 days later. Half the patients will develop an asymmetrical migratory polyarthritis of large joints often with effusions. Symptoms subside in a few days in treated cases, but fever and arthritis may persist or relapse over many months in those untreated in whom the case fatality is 10–13 per cent. Severe manifestations include bronchitis, pneumonia, metastatic abscesses (including cerebral abscess), meningitis, infective endocarditis (case fatality >50 per cent), myocarditis, pericarditis with effusion, subacute glomerulonephritis, interstitial nephritis, splenitis or splenic abscess, amnionitis, and anaemia.

Haverhill fever (erythema arthriticum epidemicum) follows a similar clinical course after the patient has drunk unpasteurized milk or contaminated water. Vomiting, stomatitis, and upper respiratory-tract symptoms such as sore throat are said to be more prominent than in rat bite fever.

Diagnosis

This is confirmed by culturing the organism from blood, joint fluid, or pus. A peripheral leucocytosis of $10–30 \times 10^9$/l is usual. False-positive serological tests for syphilis are found in 15–25 per cent of cases.

Treatment

Intravenous benzylpenicillin is given for 5–7 days followed by oral penicillin for 7 days. In mild cases, oral penicillin alone may be adequate. Penicillin-resistant L-variants are susceptible to streptomycin, tetracycline, and probably erythromycin.

Spirillum minus infection (sodoku, sokosha)

Spirillum minus (*Spirillum minor*) is recoverable from the blood of healthy rodents and from eyes and mouths of rats with eye infections. It is a relatively thick, tightly coiled, Gram-negative spirillum (not a spirochaete) resembling a campylobacter. It can only be isolated by rodent inoculation.

Epidemiology

Sodoku is found world-wide but is particularly common in Japan. It results from bites, scratches, or mere contact with rodents or their predators including dogs, cats, and pigs.

Clinical features

The initial bite wound usually heals without signs of local inflammation. After an incubation period of 7 days or more (range 5–30), there is sudden fever that peaks in 3 days and resolves by crisis after a further 3 days. Other acute symptoms include rigors, myalgia, and prostration. At the start of the illness the healed bite wound becomes inflamed and swollen; it may break down to become necrotic or suppurative. Regional lymph nodes are usually enlarged and tender. The rash spreads from the site of the bite. It consists of angry, purplish or reddish-brown, indurated papules, plaques, or macules with urticaria. Arthralgia may be severe but there are no joint effusions. Severe manifestations are seen in about 10 per cent of cases; meningitis, cerebral abscess, encephalitis, endocarditis, myocarditis, myocardial abscess, pleural effusion, chorioamnionitis, subcutaneous abscesses, and involvement of liver and kidney. Fever, rash, and other symptoms may relapse for 2–12 months in untreated patients in whom the case fatality is 2–10 per cent.

Differential diagnosis

Sodoku is distinguishable from streptobacillary rat bite fever by its longer incubation period, the marked reaction at the bite site with local lymphadenopathy at the start of symptoms, the different rash (dark papular rather than morbilliform and petechial), and by the rarity of arthritis.

Diagnosis

Aspirate from the bite wound, lymph nodes, exanthem, or blood is examined by dark-field microscopy or stained with Wright's or Giemsa stains. Spirilla can be detected in the blood, peritoneal fluid, or heart muscle of inoculated rodents. False-positive serological tests for syphilis and reactions with Proteus OXK are common.

Treatment

Penicillin is the drug of choice. A Jarisch–Herxheimer reaction may be provoked.

Further reading

McEvoy, M.B., Noah, N.D., and Pilsworth, R. (1987). Outbreak of fever caused by *Streptobacillus moniliformis*. *Lancet*, ii, 1361–3.

Roughgarden, J.W. (1965). Antimicrobial therapy of rat bite fever: a review. *Archives of Internal Medicine*, **116**, 39–54.

Rupp, M.E. (1992). *Streptobacillus moniliformis* endocarditis: case report and review. *Clinics in Infectious Diseases*, **14**, 769–72.

Chapter 16.65

Lyme disease

T. G. Schwan and W. Burgdorfer

Lyme disease is a tick-borne spirochaetosis with clinical manifestations involving several organ systems, such as the skin, joints, central nervous system, and heart. It is caused by *Borrelia burgdorferi* and other closely related species of spirochaetes (*B. garinii* and *B. afzelii*) associated with various tick vectors, primarily those of the *Ixodes ricinus–I. persulcatus* complex.

Aetiology

B. burgdorferi is a helical bacterium, 0.18 to 0.25 × 4 to 30 μm. An outer membrane surrounds the protoplasmic cylinder consisting of the peptidoglycan layer, cytoplasmic membrane, and the enclosed cytoplasmic contents. Seven periplasmic flagella (axial filaments or axial fibrils) are attached subterminally at each end in a row parallel to the organism's long axis and overlap at the central region of the cell. Like certain tick-borne spirochaetes of relapsing fever, it grows well in modified Kelly's medium (also referred to as BSK-II medium) between 34 and 37°C.

Epidemiology

In the US, most cases of Lyme disease have been from three geographical areas: the north-east and midwest, where *I. scapularis* (= *I. dammini*) is the principal vector (Fig. 1); and the west where *I. pacificus* carries the spirochaete. In 1982, after the discovery of the causative agent, Lyme disease became a reportable disease. From then until 1996, nearly 98 000 human cases have been reported with the highest incidence in Connecticut, New York, Rhode Island, and New Jersey.

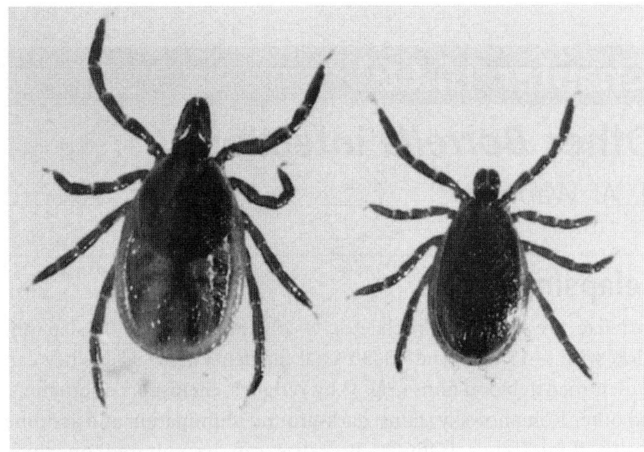

Fig. 1 *Ixodes scapularis*. Females on the left, male on the right (×15).

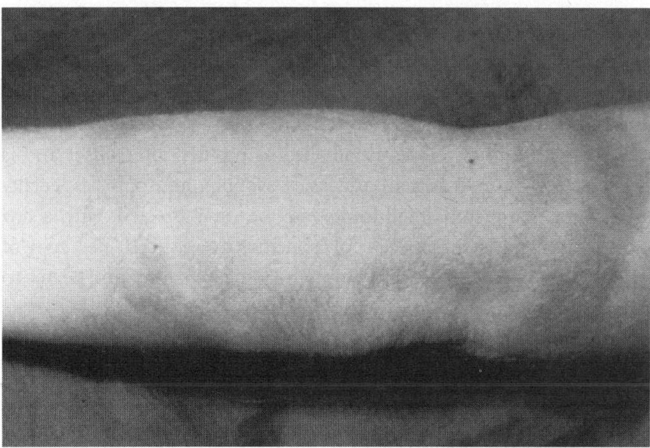

Fig. 2 Typical erythema migrans lesion on the arm of a Lyme disease patient.

In Europe, Lyme disease and related disorders have been reported from practically all countries within the distribution of *I. ricinus*, including Scandinavia, middle, eastern, and most of southern Europe, and England. Lyme disease spirochaetes have been isolated from *I. persulcatus* ticks in several parts of Asia, including Russia, China, Japan, and Korea, although the number of human cases from these areas is not known.

Clinical features

Development of the skin lesion, erythema migrans, is a unique clinical marker (Fig. 2). It is characterized by a small, red papule or macule, often considered to be the site of the tick bite, which 3–23 days later spreads centrifugally with indurated, usually flat, borders up to 2 cm wide. The centres of early lesions are usually erythematous and indurated, but may also be vesicular or necrotic. As the lesions expand, their centres clear. Common sites for these itching, burning, and often painful lesions are the thigh, groin, and axilla. In some patients, secondary annular lesions may appear within several days after onset of the initial lesions; they are generally smaller, less migratory, and lack the indurated centres. During or soon after resolution of the initial and secondary lesions new lesions may develop in the form of red circles and blotches (2–3 cm in diameter) that do not migrate but may persist for several weeks.

The early disease is usually characterized by the expanding erythema, but may be accompanied by fever, headache, stiff neck, myalgia, arthralgia, malaise, and enlargement of lymph nodes. These early clinical manifestations may last for several weeks and may be followed by recurrent or chronic arthritis and neurological and cardiac manifestations, although not necessarily in that order. Patients may experience a mild disease with erythema migrans but without other manifestations; or they may show skin, nerve, heart, and joint involvement at the same time; others lack the annular skin lesions.

Early signs of nervous involvement are meningeal and attacks of headache, neck pain, and stiffness. After several weeks to months, about 15 per cent of patients develop neurological abnormalities such as meningitis, cranial nerve lesions such as Bell's palsy, and peripheral radiculoneuropathy. In Europe, lymphocytic meningoradiculitis (Bannwarth's syndrome) is the most common manifestation of infection of the central nervous system. These manifestations may last for months but usually resolve completely.

Within a few weeks to 2 years after onset of illness, about 60 per cent of patients develop brief (a few weeks to months) but recurrent attacks of mono- or oligoarticular arthritis in the form of migratory musculoskeletal pains in joints, tendons, bursae, muscles, or bone. Arthritis with joint swelling usually begins months after onset and is characterized by intermittent attacks of swelling and pain, especially in the knee. Large and small joints may become affected, with a few patients showing symmetrical polyarthritis. In about 10 per cent of patients, involvement of large joints becomes chronic and leads to the erosion of cartilage and bone.

Approximately 4–8 per cent of patients experience fluctuating degrees of atrioventricular block and acute myopericarditis, ventricular dysfunction, and cardiomegaly. Usually preceded by erythema migrans, these cardiac complications may be accompanied by neurological manifestations, such as meningoencephalitis, cranial as well as peripheral neuropathy, and arthritis, as described above. Accompanying symptoms include syncope or dizziness, shortness of breath, and substernal chest pain lasting from 3 days to about 6 weeks.

Maternal–fetal transmissions of the Lyme disease spirochaete has been documented in a woman who contracted Lyme disease during the first trimester of pregnancy. Among another 19 patients with Lyme disease during pregnancy, 14 were completely normal but in the remainder there were cases of intrauterine fetal death, prematurity, and developmental delay with cortical blindness. It is important to diagnose and treat Lyme disease as early as possible during pregnancy.

Laboratory diagnosis

Currently, a diagnosis of Lyme disease is based primarily on the clinical picture, especially if it includes the development of erythema migrans following tick bite and exposure in an area where the disease is endemic. Histological demonstration of silver-stained spirochaetes in skin biopsy specimens, and cultivation of the organisms from blood, cerebrospinal fluid, and skin also are useful diagnostic methods but of low sensitivity and seldom used in clinical laboratories. In the absence of erythema migrans, the diagnosis may be confirmed serologically by the indirect immunofluorescence or enzyme immunoassay with cultured spirochaetes. Because of the close relationship of *B. burgdorferi* to other spirochaetes, particularly those causing relapsing fever and syphilis, cross-reactions do occur leading to false-positive serological tests when using whole spirochaetes as the antigen in the test. Patients who are treated early in the illness with appropriate antibiotics may not develop a detectable serological response to *B. burgdorferi*. Intrathecal synthesis of specific IgG antibodies to *B. burgdorferi* has been demonstrated in patients with lymphocytic meningoradiculitis. Detection of these antibodies may be helpful in diagnosing infection of the central nervous system. The polymerase chain reaction (PCR) offers the potential for detecting spirochaetes in clinical samples, but practical problems with this assay have restricted its use to relatively few laboratories to date. Recombinant DNA technology has also been used to produce specific, individual proteins of the Lyme disease spirochaete for use in serological assays with greater specificity.

Treatment

Antimicrobials are effective but dosage and duration are not yet agreed upon for more chronic forms of the disease. For early disease in adults, treatment with oral tetracycline, 250 mg four times a day, or amoxicillin, 500 mg four times a day, for 10–30 days is recommended. In children under 8 years old, amoxicillin or penicillin V, 250 mg three times a day, or 20 mg/kg body weight per day (not less than 1 g/day or more than 2 g/day) in divided doses for the same duration is effective. Erythromycin, 30 mg/kg body weight per day in divided doses for 15–20 days, may be given to patients who are allergic to penicillin. High-dose intravenous penicillin G, 20 million units/day in six divided doses, or ceftriaxone, are recommended for the treatment of neurological abnormalities and chronic arthritis. However, despite this therapy, patients may continue to have frequent arthralgias and musculoskeletal pain.. Intra-articular corticosteroids should be avoided. Regardless of the antibiotic given for Lyme disease, recurrent episodes of headache, or pain in joints, tendons, bursae, or muscles occur in about half of the patients. For some cases, treatment failure suggests that an alternative diagnosis should be considered.

Prevention and control

Currently, one of the most effective means of protection is to reduce the exposure of humans to infected ticks. This is accomplished by reducing one's activity in tick-infested areas, wearing protective clothing, using repellents, and by frequent checks while in tick-infested areas to prevent ticks from attaching and feeding. Two recombinant vaccines prepared from the spirochaete's outer-surface protein A (OspA) have now been tested and approved by the United States Food and Drug Administration for use in humans.

Further reading

Barbour, A.G. (1988). Laboratory aspects of Lyme borreliosis. *Clinical Microbiology Reviews*, **1**, 399–414.

Centers for Disease Control and Prevention (1999). Recommendations for the use of Lyme disease vaccine: recommendations of the Advisory Committee on Immunization Practices (ACIP). *Morbidity and Mortality Weekly Reports*, **48**, 1–25.

Steere, A.C. (1989). Lyme disease. *New England Journal of Medicine*, **321**, 586–96.

Steere, A.C. *et al.* (1983). The spirochetal etiology of Lyme disease. *New England Journal of Medicine*, **308**, 733–40.

Steere, A.C. *et al.* (1998). Vaccination against Lyme disease with recombinant *Borrelia burgdorferi* outer-surface lipoprotein A with adjuvant. *New England Journal of Medicine*, **329**, 209–15.

Chapter 16.66

Other *Borrelia* infections

D. A. Warrell

Relapsing fevers

Borreliae are motile spirochaetes, 8–20 mm long and 0.2–0.6 mm thick, with 3–15 coils and 15–30 axial filaments or flagella. They can be identified in blood films (Fig. 1) by Wright's, Giemsa's, Leishmann's, and other Romanowsky stains; dark-ground illumination and acridine orange fluorescence (QBC®). Borreliae can be cultured on chick chorioallantoic membrane and maintained in rodents and ticks and

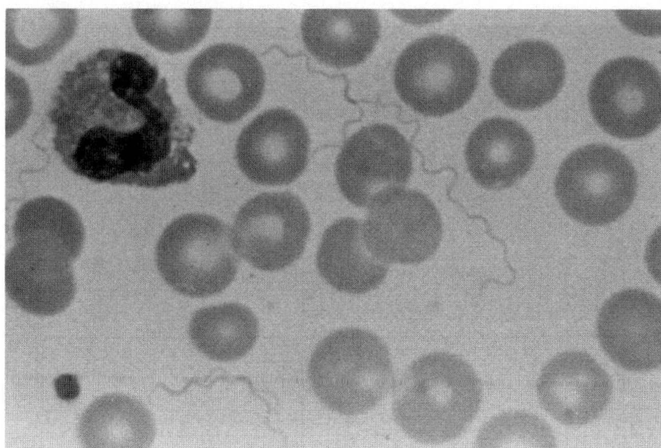

Fig. 1 *Borrelia recurrentis* spirochaetes in a Giemsa-stained, thin blood film from a patient with louse-borne relapsing fever.
(Copyright D.A. Warrell.)

several species, including *Borrelia recurrentis*, can be cultured in artificial media.

Epidemiology

Louse-borne (epidemic) relapsing fever (LBRF)

Human body and head lice (*Pediculus humanus corporis* and *P.h. capitis*), the sole vectors, are infected with *B. recurrentis* while feeding on blood from a human patient. Infected haemolymph may be inoculated through the skin when the louse is crushed by scratching. Spirochaetes can also penetrate intact skin. War, famine, and other disasters favour the spread of louse-borne infections such as LBRF and typhus. During the first half of the twentieth century there were at least 50 million cases, with a 10 per cent mortality in Europe, the Middle East, and northern Africa. Currently, the main endemic focus is in the highlands of Ethiopia, where there is an annual epidemic of some 10 000 cases in the cool, rainy season. There have been outbreaks in the Sudan and Somalia. There is no known animal reservoir. Between epidemics, *B. recurrentis* persists as mild or asymptomatic human infections.

Tick-borne (endemic) relapsing fever (TBRF)

The numerous species of *Borrelia* causing TBRF are transmitted by soft (argasid) ticks (genus *Ornithodoros*) which also act as reservoirs. Mammalian reservoir species include rodents, lagomorphs, insectivores, bats, and small carnivores. In Africa, the domestic tick *O. moubata* transmits *B. duttoni* between humans without an animal reservoir. In West and North Africa and the Middle East, small rodents living in burrows near human dwellings are reservoirs of the Borrelia Crocidurae group. Rodent ticks (*Alectrobius sonrai*—formerly *O. erraticus sonrai*) transmit the infection to humans. In the western US, *O. hermsi*, a parasite of chipmunks and other tree squirrels, transmits *B. hermsii*, especially to people who sleep in log cabins near the Grand Canyon, Arizona. Tick-borne relapsing fever is widely distributed except in Australasia and the Pacific. In western Senegal, it was found in 1 per cent of children. It is common in Rwanda, Burundi, and Tanzania (Dodoma). Spirochaetes are taken up by ticks in blood meals from infected humans or animals. They invade the ticks' salivary and coccal glands, and genital apparatus, and so can be transmitted when the tick feeds on a new host and transovarially to the tick's progeny. Ticks are reservoirs whereas lice are not. Imported TBRF is occasionally diagnosed in travellers, intravenous drug abusers, and recipients of blood transfusions.

Pathophysiology

In relapsing fevers, spontaneous crises, and the Jarisch–Herxheimer reaction (J-HR) induced by antimicrobial treatment are associated with a transient marked elevation in plasma concentrations of tumour necrosis factor, interleukin-6, and interleukin-8. In LBRF, the stimulus for cytokine release is phagocytosis of spirochaetes which release a pyrogen, a variable major protein (VMP). Benzylpenicillin attaches to penicillin-binding protein I in *B. hermsii* spirochaetes and produces large surface blebs. The damaged spirochaetes are phagocytosed rapidly by neutrophils in the blood and by the spleen.

The marked peripheral leucopenia that develops during the J-HR is the result of sequestration. The petechial rash is attributable to thrombocytopenia, not to a vasculitis.

Immunity and the relapse phenomenon

In mice experimentally infected with *B. hermsii*, there is spontaneous variation of protein antigens resulting in a mixed population of up to 26 new serotypes. Genes controlling synthesis of VMP antigens are activated by extrachromosomal DNA on linear plasmids. Between attacks, undetectable asymptomatic spirochaetaemia may persist. Spirochaetes may retreat to immunologically compromised sites such as the brain and eye. Antibody destroys the population of spirochaetes to which it is specific and selects out antigenic variants.

Pathology

Spirochaetes are usually confined to the lumen of blood vessels but tangled masses are also found in splenic miliary abscesses, infarcts, and adjacent to haemorrhages in the central nervous system. A perivascular, histiocytic, interstitial myocarditis causes conduction defects, arrhythmias, and fatal myocardial failure. Splenic rupture with massive haemorrhage, cerebral haemorrhage, and hepatic failure are other causes of death. Hepatitis is associated with patchy midzonal haemorrhages and necrosis. Other changes include meningitis, perisplenitis, petechial haemorrhages of serosal cavities, and thrombi in small vessels.

Clinical features

After an incubation period of 4–18 (average 7) days, the illness starts suddenly with rigors and high fever. Early symptoms include headache, dizziness, nightmares, generalized aches and pains especially affecting the lower back, knees, and elbows, anorexia, nausea, vomiting, and diarrhoea. Later there is upper abdominal pain, cough, and epistaxis. Patients are usually prostrated and confused. Hepatic tenderness is found in about 60 per cent of patients, hepatomegaly in about half. Splenic tenderness and enlargement are frequent. Jaundice occurs in between 10 and 80 per cent of patients. A petechial or ecchymotic rash is seen, especially on the trunk, in between 10 and 60 per cent, epistaxis (25 per cent), haemoptysis, and conjunctival and retinal bleeding are typical. Many patients have tender muscles. Neurological features include meningism (40 per cent), cranial nerve lesions, monoplegias, flaccid paraplegia, and focal convulsions.

Severe manifestations include myocarditis, which presents as acute pulmonary oedema, liver failure, and severe bleeding attributable to thrombocytopenia, liver damage, and disseminated intravascular coagulation. Dysentery, salmonellosis, typhoid, typhus, malaria, and tuberculosis can complicate relapsing fever. TBRF is usually a milder

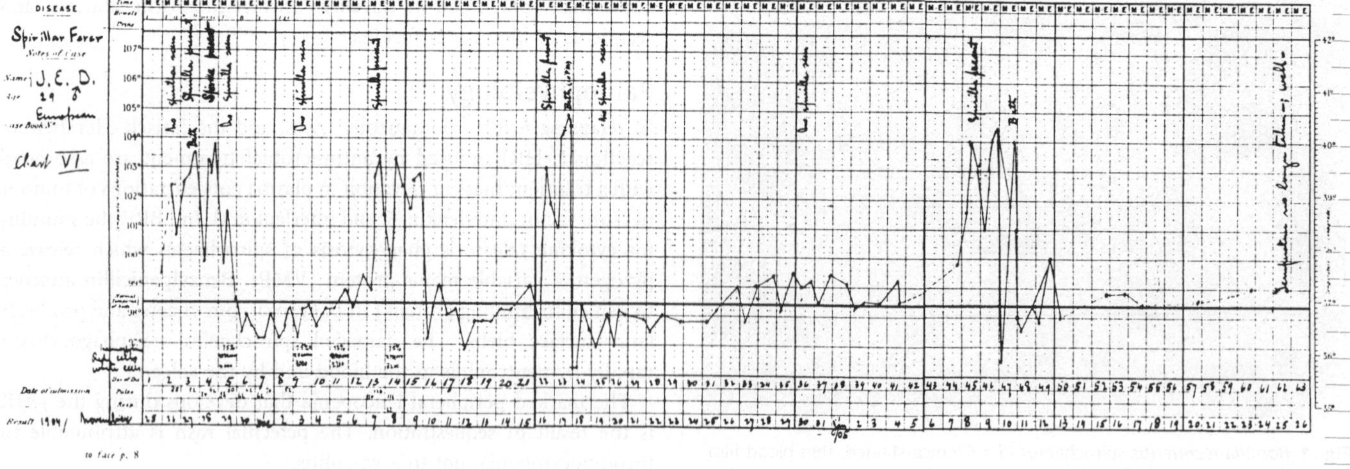

Fig. 2 Temperature chart of J. Everett Dutton, codiscoverer of the transmission of tick-borne relapsing fever. He contracted TBRF at the beginning of November 1904 and had relapses of fever and spirochaetaemia on 7 and 16 December and 8 January 1905.

and shorter illness than LBRF with a lower incidence of jaundice but a higher incidence of neurological signs.

Case fatality in treated cases is less than 5 per cent, but during major epidemics of LBRF it can reach 40 per cent or higher.

Relapses

In untreated cases of LBRF, the first attack of fever resolves by crisis in 4–10 (average 5) days. In TBRF, initial fever lasts only about 3 days. There follows an afebrile remission of 5–9 days and then a series of up to five relapses in LBRF and up to 13 in TBRF (Fig. 2). The relapses are less severe than the initial attack; there is no petechial rash but iritis or iridocyclitis and severe epistaxis may occur and deaths in relapses are reported in TBRF.

The spontaneous crisis and Jarisch–Herxheimer reaction

With or without treatment, the illness usually ends dramatically. One to two hours after antibiotic treatment, or on about the fifth day of the untreated illness, the patient becomes restless and apprehensive, and develops intense chills, lasting 10–30 min. Temperature, respiratory and pulse rates, and blood pressure rise sharply associated with gastrointestinal symptoms, cough, limb pains, and delirium. Some patients die of hyperpyrexia at the peak of fever. The flush phase, lasting several hours, is characterized by profuse sweating, vasodilatation, a fall in blood pressure, and slow decline in temperature. Fatal shock or the development of acute pulmonary oedema are attributable to myocarditis.

Diagnosis

Spirochaetes can be demonstrated in thin or thick blood films (Fig. 1), except towards the end of the attack, during remissions, and particularly in children with tick-borne disease. Serological methods are not generally used. There are false positive reactions for Proteus OXK, OX19, and OX2, and syphilis in 5–10 per cent of cases.

Differential diagnosis

In a febrile patient with jaundice, petechial rash, bleeding, and hepatosplenomegaly, the following should be considered: falciparum malaria, yellow fever, viral hepatitis, rickettsial infections (especially louse-borne typhus) and leptospirosis. There is a risk of a complicating infection, particularly typhoid.

Treatment

Antimicrobials

TBRF is more difficult to treat than LBRF because spirochaetes can persist in the central nervous system and eye to produce relapses. Oral tetracycline, 500 mg 6-hourly for 10 days, is, however, effective. Oral erythromycin stearate can be given to pregnant women (500 mg 6-hourly for 10 days) and children (125–250 mg 6-hourly for 10 days). In patients unable to swallow tablets, intravenous tetracycline hydrochloride, 250 mg, or erythromycin lactobionate, 300 mg, can be used.

LBRF is curable with a single oral dose of 500 mg of tetracycline or 500 mg of erythromycin stearate. Patients who are vomiting can be treated with a single intravenous dose of tetracycline hydrochloride, 250 mg, or for pregnant women and children, erythromycin lactobionate, 300 mg (children, 10 mg/kg body weight). In mixed epidemics of LBRF and louse-borne typhus, a single oral dose of 100 mg of doxycycline is effective.

Intramuscular benzylpenicillin (300 000 u), procaine penicillin with benzylpenicillin (600 000 u), and procaine penicillin with aluminium monostearate (600 000 u) may fail to prevent relapses; the long-acting preparations clear spirochaetaemia slowly.

Jarisch–Herxheimer reaction

Potentially fatal J-HRs complicate treatment in 30–90 per cent of cases. There is no evidence, however, that the shorter and more intense reaction following tetracycline is more dangerous than the more prolonged but apparently milder reaction following slow-release penicillin. Corticosteroids and paracetamol do not prevent the J-HR. Meptazinol, an opioid antagonist with agonist properties, decreases the intensity of the J-HR. A polyclonal, ovine, Fab, antitumour necrosis factor antibody infused for 30 min before treatment with penicillin or tetracycline reduced the incidence and severity of the J-HR.

Patients must be nursed in bed for at least 24 h after treatment to prevent postural syncope and fatal cardiac arrhythmias. Hyperpyrexia should be prevented with antipyretics, tepid sponging, and fanning. Most patients with acute LBRF are relatively hypovolaemic. Adults may need four or more litres of isotonic saline intravenously during the first 24 h. Infusion should be controlled by monitoring central venous pressure. Acute myocardial failure responds to digoxin, 1 mg intravenously over 5–10 min. Vitamin K is indicated in patients with prolonged prothrombin times. Heparin is ineffective and contraindicated. Complicating infections should be treated appropriately.

Prevention

Patients with LBRF are infectious until louse-infested hair is shaved off and they are washed, with soap or 1 per cent lysol solution, and dusted with 10 per cent DDT, 1 per cent malathion, or 0.5 per cent permethrin. Clothes can be disinfected by heat. Ticks are rarely found on patients with TBRF because they feed for only a short time and then detach. Ticks can be controlled by spraying buildings with insecticides (2 per cent benzene hexachloride or 0.5 per cent malathion).

Other spirochaetal infections

Borrelia vincenti, now renamed *Treponema vincentii*, was implicated in acute necrotizing ulcerative gingivitis and Vincent's angina but is now regarded as part of the normal flora of the mouth (see Chapter 5.2).

Further reading

Barbour, A.G. (1987). Immunobiology of relapsing fever. *Contributions to Microbiological Immunology*, **8**, 125–37.

Bryceson, A.D.M., Parry, E.H.O., Perine, P.L., Warrell, D.A., Vucotich, D., and Leithead, C.S. (1970). Louse-borne relapsing fever. A clinical and laboratory study of 62 cases in Ethiopia and a reconsideration of the literature. *Quarterly Journal of Medicine*, **39**, 129–70.

Fekade, D., Knox, K., Hussein, K., *et al.* (1996). Prevention of Jarisch-Herxheimer reactions by treatment with antibodies against tumor necrosis factor α. *New England Journal of Medicine*, **335**, 311–15.

Goubau, P.F. (1984). Relapsing fevers. A review. *Annales de la Societé Belge de Médecine Tropicale*, **40**, 335-64.

Chapter 16.67

Leptospirosis

V. Sitprija and P. Newton

Leptospirosis is a zoonotic bacterial infectious disease caused by the *Leptospira interrogans* complex. It has diverse clinical manifestations ranging from subclinical infection, fever with conjunctival suffusion and myalgia, aseptic meningitis, to renal failure and jaundice (Weil's disease) and pulmonary haemorrhage. Leptospirosis is an important cause of fever of unknown origin.

Aetiology

Leptospires are highly motile, thin, tightly coiled, 5–20 μm long spirochaetes (Order Spirochaetales) with terminal hooks. There is only one species of leptospire, *L. interrogans*, which is divided into two complexes: the pathogenic interrogans complex and the saprophytic biflexa complex. The interrogans complex has 30 serogroups and approximately 240 serotypes or serovars.

Epidemiology

Pathogenic leptospires have a global distribution. Although classically considered a rural endemic disease, urban leptospirosis also occurs—as recently reported in Baltimore, US. Epidemics, for example that which occurred in Nicaragua in 1995, are also important. Estimates of annual incidence include 0.05/100 000 in the US and 30/100 000 in New Caledonia.

Leptospires have been isolated from diverse vertebrates, but rodents, especially rats, are probably the most important reservoirs. Leptospires may persist in rodents without causing pathological damage and their alkaline urine permits prolonged renal colonization and urinary shedding of leptospires into the environment. They may survive for weeks in moist, warm soil or surface water. Transmission to man probably occurs by the entry of leptospires through abrasions in the skin or intact mucous membranes. The incidence is highest during and after the rainy season, especially amongst young men who work in an environment where there are infected hosts, soil, or water. In the Philippines, 40 per cent of rice farmers had serological evidence of past infection. Occupational, environmental, or recreational risks, such as household dogs and rodents, cutting sugar cane, rice farming, or canoeing are important but in a series from the US 36 per cent of patients had no recognized risk factor for contracting the disease. In the Seychelles, contracting leptospirosis was associated with skin wounds, having a cat at home, and rainfall. Transmission through blood and saliva also occur and leptospirosis can be transmitted by ticks experimentally but there is no evidence that this occurs outside the laboratory. Although recorded, human-to-human transmission through urine, semen, breast milk, and via the placenta is probably very unusual. Some serovars are associated with certain host species. For example *L.i. icterohaemorrhagiae* is associated with rats and *L.i. pomona* and *L.i. hardjo* with cattle.

Pathogenesis

During the initial spirochaetaemic phase leptospires spread through the blood and within 48 h they are recoverable from all tissues. After 4–7 days leptospires disappear from the blood, IgM agglutinins appear, and opsonization occurs. Leptospiruria continues for 1–4 weeks. Why some patients die of multiorgan failure whilst others develop only a self limiting fever is unknown.

A specific leptospire toxin has been hunted for many years without success. Several clinical features of leptospiral infection resemble endotoxaemia. However, endotoxin is only detectable in certain serovars and leptospire lipopolysaccharide is not pathogenic. There is evidence from animal experiments that unusual leptospire long chain fatty acids are toxic and that a glycolipoprotein toxin inhibits Na-K ATPase. In cell culture virulent, but not avirulent, leptospires are able to invade epithelial cells and induce apoptosis in macrophages. The rise in antibody titre coincides with the disappearance of leptospires from the cerebrospinal fluid, suggesting an immunological mechanism for the concurrent development of meningeal symptoms. The pathophysiology of pulmonary haemorrhage is unclear but as thrombocytopenia and clotting factor abnormalities are not severe, presumably capillary fragility is important. Antiplatelet and anticardiolipin antibodies have been found, especially in patients with severe disease. Hepatocyte apoptosis has been demonstrated in guinea pigs.

Clinical manifestations

The incubation period varies from 7–12 days (range 2–20 days) and symptoms begin suddenly (the so-called 'brutal beginning').

Ninety per cent of cases are anicteric. Classically, both anicteric and icteric cases are described as following a biphasic course but the phases frequently merge. The initial septicaemic phase is characterized by fever with chills, myalgia, headache, abdominal pain, vomiting, and conjunctival suffusion lasting from 4–7 days. Renal involvement is common with varying degrees of functional impairment associated with mild proteinuria, leucocyturia, haematuria, and granular casts. Headache, myalgia, fever, and chills occur in over 85 per cent of cases. Other symptoms and signs include diarrhoea, abdominal pain, cough, haemorrhage, pharyngitis, psychosis, arrhythmias, splenomegaly, jaundice, lymphadenopathy, and hepatomegaly.

Myalgia, either localized or generalized, and conjunctival suffusion and haemorrhage, without inflammation, are frequently observed and are clinical hallmarks of the disease. Mild macular, maculopapular, erythematous, urticarial, or haemorrhagic skin rashes can occur and are usually centripetal. A pretibial erythematous eruption has been noted in patients with *L. autumnalis* infection. Parotitis, orchitis, epididymitis, prostatitis, otitis media, erythema nodosum, and arthritis occur rarely.

The second or immune phase lasts from 4–30 days and is characterized by a decline in fever, rise in circulating antibody titres, and disappearance of leptospires from most tissues except for the kidney and aqueous humour. There may be no second clinical phase in about 35 per cent of cases or the disease may progress with hepatic and renal dysfunction, meningitis, uveitis, rash, and secondary fever. Meningeal symptoms disappear within a few days. Cerebrospinal fluid pressure and glucose are usually normal with a slightly raised protein content and initially a preponderance of polymorphonuclear cells. Later, mononuclear cells predominate. Encephalitis, focal weakness, nystagmus, seizures, peripheral neuritis, cranial nerve palsies, radiculitis, myelitis, and Guillain–Barré syndrome are rare findings. The anterior uveal tract may be affected by the third week of illness with iritis, iridocyclitis, and choroidoretinitis.

Hepatic and renal dysfunction may worsen (Weil's disease) and be associated with changes in consciousness, haemorrhage, myocarditis, and cardiovascular collapse. Any serotype can produce this syndrome although is most commonly caused by *L. i. icteroihaemorrhagiae*. Cholestatic jaundice occurs, without significant hepatocellular destruction, within 2–7 days after the start of the illness. Oliguria or anuria are surprisingly associated with hypokalaemia in about 50 per cent of patients in Brazil, possibly due to impairment of proximal tubular NaCl absorption with secondary kaliuresis. In Barbados, a urine/plasma osmolality ratio of >1.2 reliably predicted those who had prerenal failure and would respond to fluid replacement. ECG abnormalities are common with some 25 per cent having prolongation of the PR interval. In the lungs, patchy consolidation, adult respiratory distress syndrome, and massive haemorrhage may occur. Pulmonary haemorrhage has been a notable feature of leptospirosis in Korea, Nicaragua, Australia, and the Andamans and may occur without jaundice. Associated disseminated intravascular coagulation (DIC) and haemolytic uraemic syndrome are both very rare. The elevation in fibrin degradation products probably represent reduced liver clearance rather than DIC. As yet there has been no recorded exacerbation during coinfection with the human immunodeficiency virus. A recent study from French Guyana showed a 50 per cent fetal death rate in pregnant women with leptospirosis.

Pathology

Leptospires cause primarily endothelial changes. Hepatic lesions consist of focal centrilobular necrosis and lymphocytic infiltration with disorganization of liver-cell plates, proliferation of Kupffer cells, and cholestasis, although leptospires are rarely seen. In the kidneys, mesangial proliferation with neutrophil infiltration is noted early during bacterial invasion. There is focal thickening of the basement membrane with dense deposits and fusion of foot processes. In the arteriolar wall and in the glomeruli C3 is deposited with endothelial swelling and necrosis. Although tubular necrosis and interstitial nephritis are seen in renal failure, interstitial changes can be observed without tubular necrosis or renal failure. Myocardial changes are characterized by interstitial oedema and infiltration of mononuclear cells and plasma cells. Necrosis is associated with neutrophil infiltration. In skeletal muscle there is vacuolation of myofibril cytoplasm and fragmentation, with haemorrhagic hyaline necrosis but minimal neutrophil infiltration. The meninges show some thickening with perivascular infiltration of blood vessels in the brain and spinal cord. Haemorrhage can occur in the gastrointestinal tract, lungs, pleura, tracheobronchial tree, pancreas, and adrenals. Persistence of leptospires in the aqueous humour may be responsible for chronic, recurrent, and latent uveitis.

Diagnosis

The diagnosis of leptospirosis cannot reliably be made clinically. It may resemble other febrile illnesses such as malaria, viral hepatitis, enteric fever, hantavirus infection, rickettsial diseases, glandular fever, influenza, dengue fever, relapsing fever, atypical pneumonia, and aseptic meningitis. In the Far East ingestion of carp's bile may cause acute hepatic and renal dysfunction (OTM3, p. 1143).

Leucocytosis (usually $<20 \times 10^9$/l) with mild neutrophilia is usual but leucopenia can occur. The erythrocyte sedimentation rate, plasma fibrinogen, and blood viscosity are elevated. Thrombocytopenia is common and mild anaemia, increased serum fibrin degradation products, low C3, and mild intravascular haemolysis may occur. Serum amylase may be raised, secondary to renal failure, pancreatitis, and from unknown sources. In those with high plasma bilirubin, a modestly increased serum alkaline phosphatase with mild elevations of serum transaminases ($<5 \times$ normal) are important clinical clues favouring the diagnosis of leptospirosis. In addition, elevated serum creatine phosphokinase ($2–10 \times$ normal), due to muscle involvement, and neutrophilia also support the diagnosis of leptospirosis rather than viral hepatitis.

Isolation of leptospires from blood or cerebrospinal fluid can be made only during the first 10 days of clinical illness, is slow, and has low sensitivity. Urine culture becomes positive after the second week until about 1 month. Fletcher's semisolid, Stuart's, and EMJH mediums are routinely used but growth of leptospires is slow, usually requiring several weeks. Animal inoculation may be used, especially when the specimen is contaminated. Dark-field microscopy of body fluids for leptospires is complicated by false positives (pseudoleptospires). Silver, fluorescent antibody and immunoperoxidase, but not Gram, stains can be used. In muscle biopsies, leptospiral antigen and characteristic histology can be demonstrated.

Serological diagnosis is very helpful during the second week of the disease and is the mainstay of diagnosis. The macroscopic slide-agglutination test uses killed or formalinized antigens from local serogroups and can be used as a rapid serogroup screening test. The microscopic agglutination test (MAT) using live antigens determines the titre and specific serotype. A positive result requires a fourfold or greater rise in titre during the course of the disease, seroconversion, or a single titre of >1:800. Elevated titres are commonly noted by day 6–12. A single microscopic agglutination titre of 1:100 is thought sufficient to warrant a diagnosis of previous infection. Other serological tests include complement fixation, serum and salivary ELISA, rapid IgM dipstick ELISA, and gold immunoblot which may become positive earlier than MAT, allowing earlier diagnosis. Evaluation of a blood polymerase chain reaction test to detect leptospire DNA in blood in New Caledonia showed a 100 per cent agreement with conventional serology. This technique has also detected leptospires in urine in the first week of the illness, in cerebrospinal fluid, and the aqueous humour.

Treatment

Supportive therapy, including renal replacement, is of paramount importance. Cerebral oedema has developed during intermittent haemofiltration/dialysis and continuous therapy is probably preferable. Penicillin, ampicillin, streptomycin, tetracycline, and erythromycin kill leptospires. A randomized, double-blind trial showed that intravenous penicillin shortened duration of fever, renal impairment, and hospital stay. It did not support the view that antibiotics are of no use in the second, putative immune, phase of the illness. Jarisch–Herxheimer reactions are probably very rare. Parenteral benzylpenicillin 1 mega unit, 6-hourly for a period of 1 week, is recommended in adults. Alternative drugs are tetracycline 2 g daily, provided renal function is normal, or doxycycline 200 mg daily. Drug resistance has not been a problem. In a few patients, exchange transfusion and plasmapharesis have been used in severe leptospirosis, and steroids in pulmonary haemorrhage and thrombocytopenia, with some apparent success.

Prognosis

Mortality remains high in those with multiorgan failure but very low in those without. Recent, published in-hospital mortality ranges from 0–18 per cent. Risk factors predicting death include greater age, severe renal dysfunction, thrombocytopenia, ECG repolarization changes, and pulmonary haemorrhage. Iridocyclitis may persist for several years but chronic renal or liver dysfunction probably do not occur. A link between leptospirosis and the subsequent development of Moya-Moya syndrome (a cerebral vasculitis) has been suggested.

Prevention

In domestic mammals at risk of few serovars, vaccines are effective in preventing the disease but not leptospiruria. In man vaccines, are usually impracticable due to exposure to many serotypes. However, vaccination against a specific serotype prevalent in an area has been effective. Other methods include surface decontamination, the wearing of protective clothing, and the eradication of the animal reservoir. A randomized, double-blind trial in Panama demonstrated that chemoprophylaxis with doxycycline, 200 mg weekly, had an efficacy of 95 per cent in reducing the incidence of leptospirosis. It is recommended only for short-term use in high-risk individuals. The best postexposure prophylaxis is uncertain, but parental penicillin or oral doxycycline have been recommended.

Further reading

Faine, S. (1993). *Leptospira and leptospirosis.* CRC Press, Baca Raton.

Merien, F., Baranton, G., and Perolat, P. (1995). Comparison of polymerase chain reaction with microagglutination test and culture for diagnosis of leptospirosis. *Journal of Infectious Diseases,* **172**, 281–5.

Sitprija, V., Pipatanagul, V., Mertowidjojo, K., Boonpucknavig, V., and Boonpucknavig, S. (1980). Pathogenesis of renal disease in leptospirosis: clinical and experimental studies. *Kidney International,* **17**, 827–36.

Watt, G. *et al.* (1988). Placebo-controlled trial of intravenous penicillin for severe and late leptospirosis. *Lancet,* **i**, 433–5.

Zaki, S.R. *et al.* (1996). Leptospirosis associated with outbreak of acute febrile illness and pulmonary haemorrhage, Nicaragua, 1995. *Lancet,* **347**, 535–6.

Chapter 16.68

Non-venereal endemic treponematoses: yaws, endemic syphilis (bejel), and pinta

P. L. Perine

The endemic treponematoses are chronic, granulomatous diseases caused by spirochaetes belonging to the genus *Treponema.*

Aetiology

Yaws is caused by *Treponema pallidum* ssp. *pertenue,* a spirochaete that is morphologically identical to *T. pallidum* ssp. *pallidum,* the cause of venereal and non-venereal syphilis, and to *T. carateum,* the cause of pinta. These treponemes share common antigens so that infection by one species produces varying degrees of cross-immunity to the others. No serological test can differentiate the antibodies produced, and none of these organisms grows *in vitro.* The only means of differentiating yaws, syphilis, and pinta are their epidemiological characteristics and the pattern of infection produced in man and experimentally infected laboratory animals (Table 1).

The treponemes of yaws, syphilis, and pinta are fragile and readily killed by exposure to atmospheric oxygen, drying, mild detergents, or antiseptics. They prefer temperatures below 37°C, which may explain their predilection for the skin and bones of the extremities. These organisms cannot penetrate intact skin, and gain entry to the body through small abrasions and lacerations.

Epidemiology (Table 1)

Yaws is transmitted by direct contact with an infectious lesion or by fingers contaminated with lesion exudate. It is enhanced by a crowded environment with poor sanitation and personal hygiene. The disease is usually acquired in childhood between the ages of 5 and 15. In endemic areas more than 80 per cent of the population are infected. In humid, warm environments the early lesion tends to proliferate and teems with spirochaetes, thus increasing the infectious reservoir; whereas in dry, arid climates or seasons the reverse is true.

There was a precipitous decrease in cases of yaws and other endemic treponematoses following mass penicillin treatment campaigns in the 1950s and 1960s sponsored by the World Health Organization. An

Table 1 Major features of the treponematoses

Feature	Venereal syphilis	Endemic syphilis	Yaws	Pinta
Organism*	*T. pallidum*, ssp. *pallidum*	*T. pallidum*, ssp. *endemicus*	*T.pallidum*, ssp. *pertenue*	*T. carateum*
Age of infection	15–10	2–10	5–15	10–30
Occurrence	Worldwide	Africa; Middle East	Africa, South America, Oceania, Asia	Central, South America
Climate	All	Dry, arid	Warm, humid	Warm, rural
Transmission				
Direct:				
Venereal	Common	Rare	No	No
Non-venereal	Rare	Rare	Common	Common
Congenital	Yes	Unproven	No	No
Indirect:				
Contaminated utensils	Rare	Common	Rare	No
Insects	No	No	Rare	No
Reservoir of infection	Adults	Infectious and latent cases	Infectious and latent cases; ? non-human primates	
Infectious cases				
Ratio infectious: latent cases	1:3	1:2	1:3–5	?
Late complications				
Skin	+	+	+	+
Bone, cartilage	+	+	+	No
Neurological	+	Unproven	No	No
Cardiovascular	+	Unproven	No	No

estimated 152 million people were examined and 46.1 million clinical cases, latent infections, and contacts were treated. The yaws reservoir was greatly reduced in West and Central Africa, Central and South America, and Oceania. However, over the past decade, yaws has been resurgent in the rural populations of Ecuador, the Ivory Coast, Ghana, Togo, Benin, Zaire, the Central African Republic, and Ethiopia in Africa, and in the island nations in the Pacific. Several nations initiated new campaigns of mass treatment in the 1980s.

Some African nations, such as Nigeria, previously rendered yaws-free by mass treatment campaigns, have also experienced a sharp rise in the incidence of venereal syphilis, perhaps representing a decline of herd immunity to yaws, and thereby to syphilis.

Endemic syphilis is transmitted by non-venereal contact among children. In contrast to yaws, transmission of infection by contaminated drinking vessels may be more common than by direct contact with infectious lesions. The disease tends to be familial with spread of infection from children to adults rather than to the community in general. Endemic syphilis lesions are virtually indistinguishable from early yaws, and the two diseases may occur at different times in the same population but not in the same person. Venereal syphilis can be acquired by children through social contact with adults suffering from venereal syphilis and then be spread by non-venereal, person-to-person contact if the level of sanitation and personal hygiene are low.

The Sahelian nations of Mauritania, Mali, Niger, Burkina Faso, and Senegal have reported dramatic increases in the number of cases of endemic syphilis. The disease is also prevalent among the nomadic tribes of the Arabian peninsula, where late complications such as osteoperiostitis predominate.

Several variants of endemic syphilis are recognized by their geographical distribution: bejel of the Eastern Mediterranean and North Africa, njovera or dichuchwa of Africa. Bejel is the only type of endemic syphilis still prevalent. It is found in mainly seminomadic people such as the Tuareg living in the Saharan regions of Africa.. Pinta is found only in remote parts of Central and South America, principally in the semiarid region of the Tepalcatepec Basin of southern Mexico and focal areas of Colombia, Peru, Ecuador, and Venezuela.

Clinical features

Like venereal syphilis, the clinical course of yaws and endemic syphilis have primary, secondary, and tertiary or late stages, separated by quiescent or latent periods.

The initial lesion in yaws usually appears on the extremities after an incubation period of 3–5 weeks. Characteristically it is a papule; a painless lesion which appears at the site of infection, enlarges, forming a raspberry-like ('framboesia'), vegetative lesion called a papilloma. The papilloma is round to oval, elevated and not indurated, ranging in size from 1–3 cm in diameter. The surface teems with spirochaetes and is often covered by a thin yellow crust, which is easily removed. The papilloma may ulcerate as it enlarges and becomes secondarily infected with other micro-organisms. Lymph nodes draining the initial lesion may enlarge and become tender but systemic symptoms are rare.

Secondary or disseminated papillomata appear after 2–6 months, often without an intervening latent period, on the skin of moist areas such as the axillae, joint flexures, genitalia, and the gluteal cleft (Fig. 1). They also occur on the soles and palms and, because they

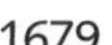

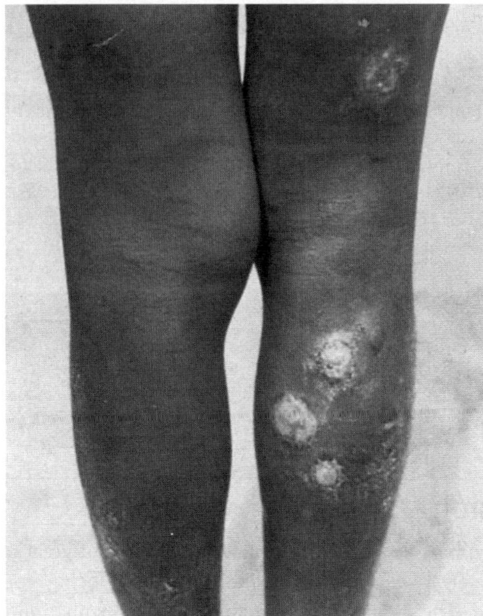

Fig. 1 Early ulceropapillomatous yaws.

are tender, may interfere with gait and use of the hands. Papillomata in different stages of development persist for 6–8 months and heal without scars unless they become secondarily infected. Despite the size and number of lesions, children with generalized papillomata experience little discomfort or other constitutional symptoms.

Slightly raised, scaly, pigmented, macular yaws lesions measuring from 1–4 cm in diameter commonly occur when the climate is dry and arid. These lesions have the same distribution as papillomata and may appear together with lesions of different morphology in the same patient (maculopapular yaws).

The periosteum and osseous tissue of the bones of the extremities are frequently inflamed during early yaws, causing swelling, night-pain, and tenderness. Painful osteoperiostitis of the legs affecting mainly the tibia and fibula is especially common. Scaly, tender, hyperkeratotic lesions of the palms and soles also occur and may be incapacitating. Hyperkeratotic and bone lesions are not contagious, and macular lesions are only minimally so.

One or more relapses of secondary-type lesions usually occur during the first 5 years of infection, each separated by a period of latency. Late yaws lesions occur thereafter in about 10 per cent of untreated cases.

Late yaws lesions are not infectious because they contain few treponemes. Cutaneous plaques produce atrophic scars; subcutaneous, granulomatous nodules erode skin and produce deep ulcers that destroy underlying tissue and disfigure. Hyperkeratotic palmar and plantar yaws are incapacitating and often prevent the use of hands, or the ability to walk normally. The weight is placed on the sides of the feet, which produces a gait much like that of a crab ('crab' yaws; Fig. 2).

The granulomas of late yaws have a histological appearance like the gummata of syphilis. These proliferative lesions may involve the palate and destroy the soft tissues of the nose, causing a terrible disfiguration called gangosa (Fig. 3). Gummatous periostitis of the skull, fingers, and long bones is erosive and often retards or stops growth. Active periostitis is occasionally found in young and middle-aged adults who had yaws in childhood.

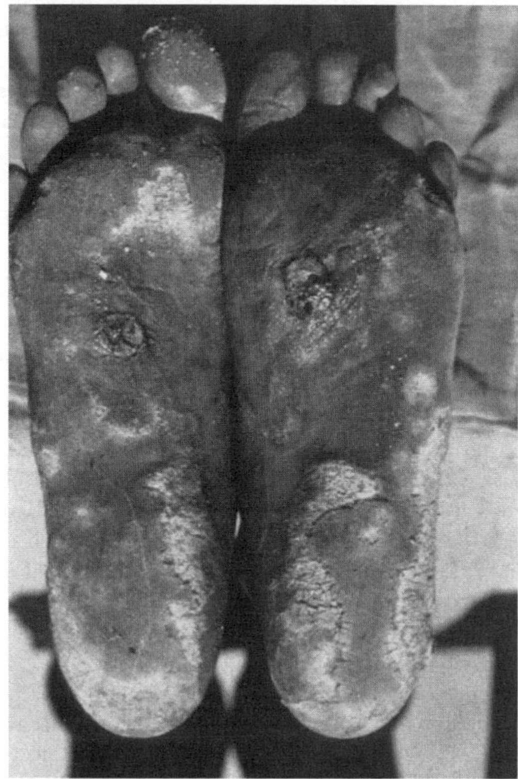

Fig. 2 Planter papillomata with hyperkeratotic, macular, early plantar yaws ('crab' yaws); these lesions are painful.

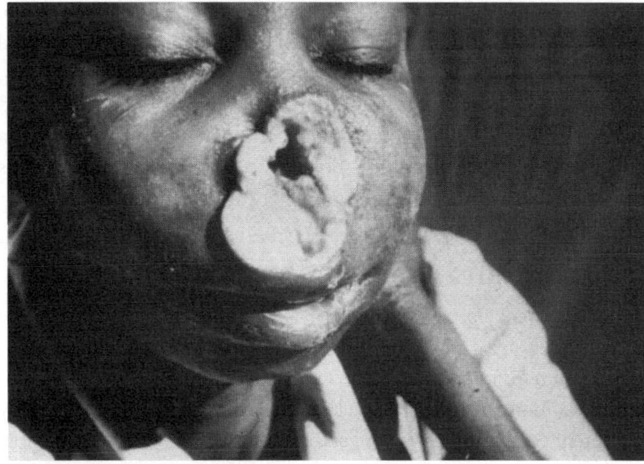

Fig. 3 Gangosa (rhinopharyngitis mutilans) of endemic syphilis and yaws in an adolescent child.

The initial lesions of endemic syphilis usually appear at the mucocutaneous borders of the mouth or on the oral mucous membranes (mucous patches) as the result of transmission by contaminated drinking vessels. Late ulceronodules and osteoperiostitis are seen in late endemic syphilis, but cardiovascular and neurological complications are extremely rare.

In pinta, the initial papule appears on the skin of the extremities and enlarges slowly over a period of several weeks or months to form an erythematous plaque. Satellite papules form at the edge of the lesion and undergo a similar type of evolution. The plaques coalesce to form violaceous, pigmented plaques that, in several years, slowly depigment from lighter shades of blue to white, leaving atrophic depigmented scars.

Ulceronodular skin lesions of yaws and endemic syphilis resemble tropical ulcers. Yaws lesions are not as painful, necrotic, nor as deep as tropical ulcers, which are usually singular and restricted to the lower one-third of the leg.

Plantar warts are frequently confused with plantar papillomata of yaws and both conditions may occur in the same patient.

Diagnosis

The diagnosis of yaws is made by a combination of clinical assessment, of positive dark-ground examination of lesions, and of reactive serological tests for syphilis.

The diagnosis of early yaws, or endemic syphilis, is not difficult in endemic areas where the disease is familiar. The most difficult diagnostic problem arises when a person who had yaws as a child emigrates to an area of the world where the disease never existed. Such a person usually has reactive serological tests for syphilis and may have a few atrophic scars suggestive of earlier infection. What are the chances that this patient has or has had venereal syphilis? Should he be treated for latent yaws or syphilis?

The patient's social and medical history should be carefully reviewed. Clinical findings suggestive of old yaws (scars, inactive tibial periostitis), and the absence of stigmata of congenital and venereal syphilis support the diagnosis of inactive or treated yaws.

If the patient has a reagin titre of less than 1:8 dilutions, he probably does not have active latent yaws or syphilis. If he received at least one therapeutic dose of long-acting penicillin in his native country during a yaws campaign, he requires no further treatment. On the other hand, if the patient is a contact of a case of infectious venereal syphilis, he should be treated as potentially infected with syphilis, because *T.p. pallidum* occasionally superinfects people who have had yaws as children. If treatment is given, the patient should receive a certificate stating the drug and dosage used and the results of his serological tests to prevent unnecessary future treatment.

Treatment and prevention

Long-acting benzylpenicillin given by intramuscular injection is the recommended treatment for all the endemic treponematoses. The preparation used in previous mass treatment campaigns was penicillin aluminium monostearate (PAM), but benzathine penicillin is currently recommended because it is longer acting and more readily available than is PAM. Active infections and non-infectious cases should be given 1.2 mega units in a single intramuscular injection; children under 10 years of age receive 0.6 mega units. Patients allergic to penicillin may be given tetracycline or erythromycin, 500 mg by mouth four times daily for 2 weeks; children under 10 years of age should be given erythromycin in dosages adjusted for their age. Treatment failures have been reported in Papua New Guinea.

Prevention of yaws in a community requires elimination of the reservoir of infection, often by treating the entire population with penicillin.

Further reading

Centurion-Lara, A., *et al.* (1998). The flanking region sequences of the 15-kDa lipoprotein gene differentiate pathogenic treponemes. *Journal of Infectious Diseases*, 177, 1036–40.

Guthe, T. (1969). Clinical, serological and epidemiological features of framboesia tropica (yaws) and its control in rural communities. *Acta Dermatologica-Venerologia*, Stockholm, **49**, 343–68.

Hackett, C.J. and Loewenthal, L.J.A. (1960). *Differential diagnosis of yaws.* World Health Organization, Geneva.

Perine, P.L., Hopkins, D.R., Niemel, P.L.A., St. John, R.K., Causse, C., and Antal, G.M. (1984). *Handbook of endemic treponematoses.* World Health Organization, Geneva.

Chapter 16.69

Syphilis

D. J. M. Wright and G. W. Csonka

Definition

Venereal syphilis is a systemic contagious disease of great chronicity caused by *Treponema pallidum* and capable of being congenitally transmitted. The natural host is man. It has an incubation period of around 3 weeks at the end of which a primary sore (chancre) develops at the site of inoculation; usually on the genitalia, associated with regional lymphadenitis. In most patients this is followed in 2–6 weeks by the secondary bacteraemic stage characterized by a symmetrical rash, generalized lymphadenopathy, and other lesions. After a latent asymptomatic period of many years this ends, in 40 per cent, in a destructive and potentially dangerous late stage which may involve the skin, mucous membranes, skeleton, central nervous system (CNS), eyes, hearing, and, above all, the aorta. Occasionally other organs are also affected.

Bacteriology

T. pallidum is a bacterium which causes venereal syphilis, non-venereal endemic childhood syphilis, bejel, and njovera. The organism is seen in the wet preparation by dark-field microscopy and shows a steady 'deliberate' linear progression (translation). *T. pallidum* is a delicate, motile, spiral organism, 6–15 µm long and 0.15 µm wide, below the level of resolution of light microscopy, hence the need for dark-field or phase contrast illumination. The pathogenic treponemes which cause syphilis, non-venereal syphilis, yaws, and pinta cannot be differentiated morphologically or molecularly. All give rise to the same serological reactions and are susceptible to penicillin but produce dissimilar lesions both in man and in laboratory animals.

The approximate infective dose of bacteria lies between 10^6 and 10^7 organisms, giving an average incubation period of 3 weeks. The cell wall contains peptidoglycan in the inner layer of the bacterial membrane accounting for the microbes susceptibility to penicillin. The phospholipids in the outer membrane, of which cardiolipin is the most prominent hapten, provide the antigenic basis for the synthetically substituted VDRL, used as a serological test for syphilis (see below). The recent sequencing of the complete genome of *T. pallidum* will lead to further insights into the organism's metabolism and pathogenic properties.

Epidemiology

Transmission

Sexual transmission is the rule in adults. The untreated patient remains infective for 4 years after acquiring the infection. Asexual transmission by close contact with an open lesion of early acquired or congenital syphilis is rare. Other unusual modes of transmission are by direct blood transfusion with blood from an infectious individual and contact with infected fomites. Congenital syphilis still remains a problem world-wide, except in northern Europe.

Incidence

There has been a steady decline in the incidence of syphilis in the West since the 1850s. Since the 1980s the UK and American rates have diverged. The appearance of AIDS and the national programmes for 'safe sex' has resulted in the annual number of infectious cases of syphilis falling to 283 in the UK in 1995, there being in the UK an estimated 34 per cent of cases of syphilis related to homosexual activity. Most of the recent infections have been acquired heterosexually abroad. In the US, however, the number of cases of syphilis has continued to rise, especially in the underprivileged Afro-American and Hispanic community and among the HIV-infected drug abusers. In the US, the number of cases of early syphilis has fallen to 11 110 in 1996. In contrast, in the Russian Federation, the tremendous social and economic upheaval in the last few years has led to the number of cases of newly diagnosed and reported syphilis rising from 7911 in 1990, to a projected 324 200 in 1996 (WHO figures). In other parts of the world, notably in the Far East, infected prostitutes may play a central role in the spread of early syphilis. Estimates by WHO suggest that each year there are 10–20 million cases of syphilis world-wide.

The changing clinical presentation of syphilis and the effect of the HIV epidemic

There is some clinical evidence that syphilis is becoming milder and less typical. This has been especially noted in neurosyphilis; the gumma has virtually disappeared. The widespread use of antibiotics for unrelated conditions may be responsible. Meningovascular syphilis has not shown the dramatic decrease of GPI and tabes dorsalis, possibly because the latter two conditions take many more years to develop giving cumulative chances of antibiotics being given. Its exclusion by serology and other tests is therefore becoming more important.

The advent of AIDS has led to a re-examination of the progression and manifestations of concomitant syphilis. Although a variety of unusual syphilitic rashes has been described in association with HIV infections, all were recorded in the older literature. However, in a German co-operative study, ulcerative skin (or mucous membrane) lesions seems to be associated, in AIDS patients, with low CD4 counts. The suggestions that there might be an increase in syphilitic meningovascular relapse in patients with HIV infections again may reflect the natural history of syphilis, since approximately 20 per cent of patients with early syphilis have a pleocytosis in the cerebrospinal fluid (CSF). If these patients are untreated, about a fifth develop neurosyphilis. The high prevalence of syphilis in HIV American patients leads to an apparent, rather than a real, increase in syphilitic complications. Syphilitic relapses do not occur despite the potential for the persistence of spirochaetes (see below). Benzathine penicillin G is less effective in eliminating spirochaetes (see below) in patients with altered immunity. CSF should be examined 18 months to 2 years after treatment of neurosyphilis in AIDS patients.

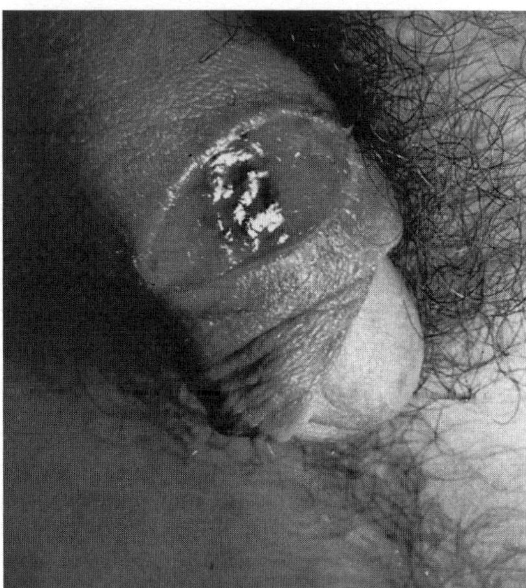

Fig. 1 Large primary sore. Note even shape and the absence of secondary infection.

The natural course of untreated syphilis

The estimated figure for infectivity varies but is commonly assumed to be around 50 per cent for both homosexual and heterosexual patients. After a single exposure the figure is nearer 25 per cent.

T. pallidum penetrates the abraded skin and intact mucous membrane. Within hours it becomes disseminated via the bloodstream and lymphatics and is beyond any effective local treatment. The incubation period is traditionally given as 9–90 days but in practice it is around 3 weeks. The primary lesion develops at the site of contact and heals in 2–6 weeks. In a proportion of patients, a secondary stage appears 6 weeks after the primary lesion has healed but there may be an overlap of the healing primary and the onset of the secondary stage. In some cases the period between these stages can be prolonged to several months. The main characteristic of the secondary stage is a generalized, symmetrical, painless, and non-irritating rash. In about 20 per cent of cases, infectious relapses occur during the following year and may continue for up to 4 years. In the rest, the latent asymptomatic period follows and may persist for life in at least 60 per cent. Historically, in 30–40 per cent a third late destructive stage develops, approximately, half the changes appear within 10 years, the remainder over the next 20 years. Its more benign form involves only the skin, mucous membranes, and bones. In the serious form the CNS, aorta, and other internal organs are affected.

Clinical features

Primary syphilis

The first sign is a small, painless papule which rapidly ulcerates. The ulcer (chancre) is usually solitary, round or oval, painless, and often indurated (Fig. 1). It is surrounded by a bright red margin. It is not usually secondarily infected, a feature of all open syphilitic lesions of any stage. *T. pallidum* can be demonstrated in exudate from the sore which is easily obtained after slightly abrading the base. In heterosexual men, the common sites are the coronal sulcus, the glans, and inner surface of the prepuce. The sore may also be found on the shaft of the penis and beyond. In homosexual men, the ulcer is usually present in the anal canal, less commonly in the genitalia and mouth. In women most chancres occur on the vulva, the labia, and, more rarely, the cervix, where they are liable to be overlooked.

Extragenital chancres may occur on other sites. The regional lymph nodes are invariably enlarged a few days after the appearance of the chancre and with genital sores, the lymph nodes are bilaterally involved. The lymph nodes are painless, discrete, firm, and not fixed to surrounding tissues. A small inoculum usually produces a small, atypical ulcer or papule and looks trivial. This may also occur in patients who had previously-treated syphilis and the lesion may be dark-field negative. If *T. pallidum* cannot be recovered from the primary sore, it may be possible to demonstrate it from the needle aspirate of the regional lymph node.

Genital lesions which must be differentiated from primary syphilis are: genital herpes, which is much more common than syphilis in either sex, traumatic sores and erosive balanitis, fixed drug eruptions, and chancroid. Other conditions which may have to be considered are scabies, Behçet's syndrome, donovanosis, and lymphogranuloma venereum.

Secondary syphilis

The lesions are numerous, variable, and affect many systems. Inevitably there is a symmetrical, non-irritating rash and generalized, painless lymphadenopathy. Constitutional symptoms are mild or absent; they include headaches (often nocturnal), malaise, slight fever, and aches in joints and muscles. The rash is commonly macular, pale red, and sometimes so faint as to be visible only in tangential light. It may be papular and sometimes squamous (Fig. 2). Pustular and necrotic rashes are rarely seen in temperate climates but still occur in tropical regions. It usually covers the trunk and proximal limbs, but when it is seen on the palms, soles, and the face, syphilis should always be high on the list of probable causes (Fig. 3). In warm and moist areas such as the perineum, external female genitalia, perianal region, axillae, and under pendulous breasts, the papules enlarge into pink or grey discs, the condylomata lata, which are highly infectious (Fig. 4). Mucous patches in the mouth and genitalia are painless greyish-white erosions forming circles and arcs ('snail-track ulcers'). They too are very infectious.

Meningism and headache, especially at night, are due to low-grade meningitis which can be confirmed by a raised cell count and raised protein in the CSF. Less common are alopecia and laryngitis; internal organs are rarely involved. All these lesions disappear spontaneously without scarring.

Latent syphilis

By definition the patient is asymptomatic with normal CSF findings but positive serology for syphilis. It is arbitrarily divided into early (<2 years) and late latent (>2 years) syphilis. Infectiousness does not stop with the advent of latency, as women may continue to give birth to congenitally-infected infants for 2 years into the late latent stage. Approximately 60 per cent of patients remain latent for the rest of their lives, the only evidence of syphilis being positive serology, usually with a low titre.

Late syphilis (tertiary syphilis)

This includes late latent syphilis already referred to, benign tertiary syphilis, involvement of viscera, the CNS, and the aorta.

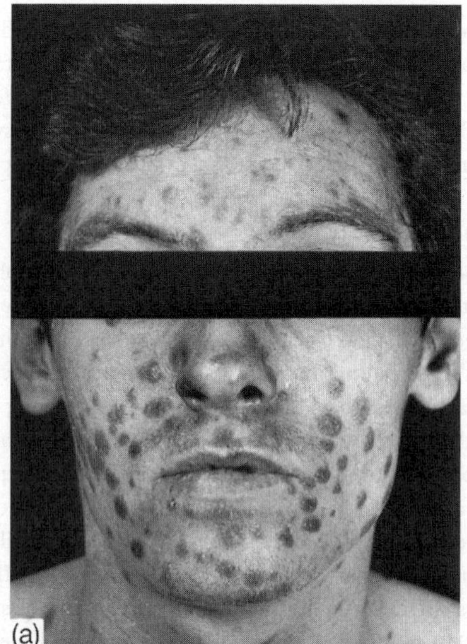

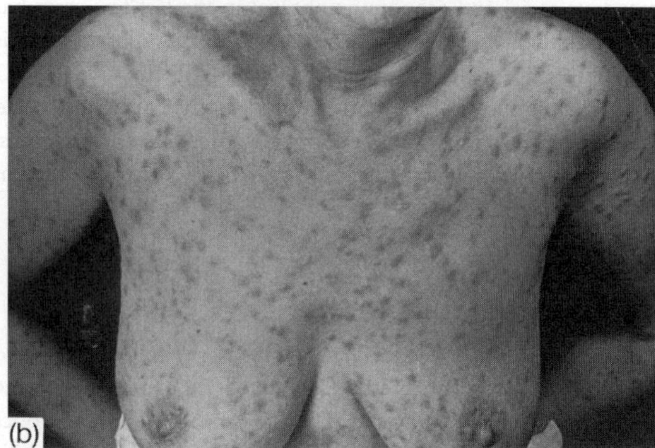

Fig. 2 Secondary papular rash of face/secondary rash of trunk.

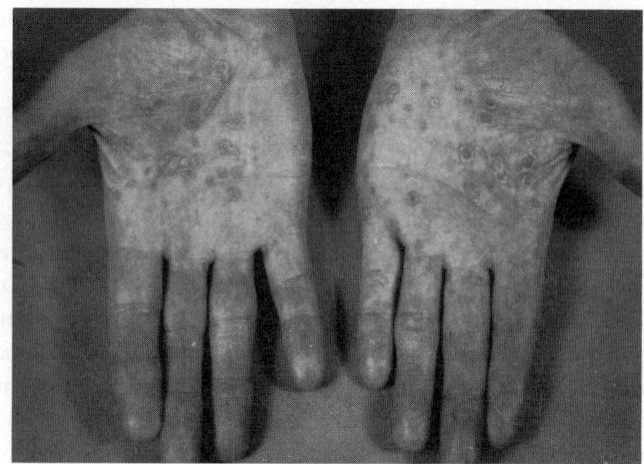

Fig. 3 Secondary rash of palms.

Pathogenesis of late benign syphilis

The gumma is a chronic granulomatous lesion which is an intense inflammatory response to a few treponemes. Histologically, there is central structured necrosis with peripheral cellular infiltration of

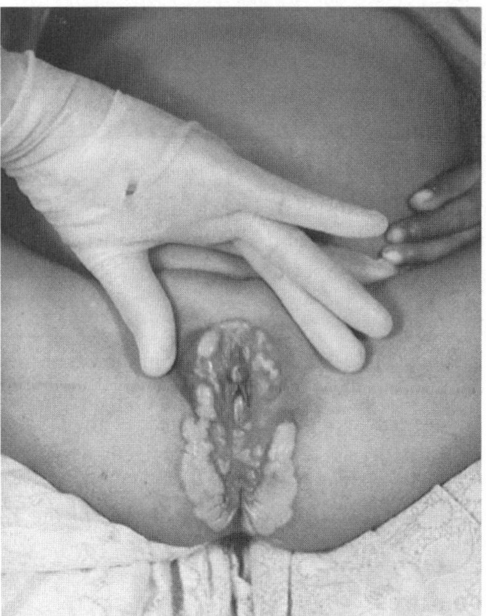

Fig. 4 Condyloma lata.

lymphocytes, mononuclear cells, and occasional giant cells with perivasculitis and obliterating endarteritis. *T. pallidum* is present and can be demonstrated by rabbit inoculation.

Clinical features

1. Cutaneous gumma are usually single but may be multiple or diffuse. Clinically, it starts as a slowly progressive, painless nodule which becomes dull red and breaks down into one or several indolent, punched-out ulcers. The base has a 'wash-leather' appearance and is remarkably free from secondary infection. It heals slowly from the centre which may become depigmented, whilst the periphery shows hyperpigmentation. Eventually a paper-thin scar forms. This combination of pigmentation, depigmentation, and atrophic scars can be of considerable retrospective diagnostic help. The sites preferentially involved are the face, legs, buttocks, upper trunk, and scalp. The process may be more superficial, producing papulosquamous lesions which include the palms and soles. It too heals with the typical scars already described.
2. Mucosal gumma are most commonly seen in the oropharynx and involve the palate, pharynx, and the nasal septum. Diffuse gummatous infiltration of the tongue may produce necrotic white patches on the dorsum of the tongue and this leucoplakia has a strong tendency to become malignant. Penicillin has no effect on the progress of syphilitic glossitis.
3. Mucocutaneous gumma may have to be differentiated from fungal skin lesions, psoriasis, and Kaposi's sarcoma. The deep gummata may resemble deep mycoses, sarcoidosis, tuberculosis, leprosy, donovanosis, lymphogranuloma venereum, reticulosis, and epithelioma of the skin. It must be borne in mind that positive serum tests for syphilis may be coincidental and misleading, since late syphilis is rare, unlike malignancy which should always be excluded.
4. Osteoperiostitis of long bones such as the tibia and fibula causes thickening and irregularities which may be diffuse, as in the 'sabre tibia', or localized and evident as a circumscribed bony swelling. Unlike most other syphilitic lesions, those of the bone are often painful, the pain being worse at night. Very rarely, lesions in the skull occur. Conditions to be considered include primary and secondary carcinoma, Paget's disease, chronic osteomyelitis, tuberculosis, and leprosy. All forms of non-venereal syphilis, except pinta, give rise to similar lesions.

Visceral syphilis

This is not common and response to treatment is variable. The patients may present with deafness and vertigo or uveitis. The liver, lungs, stomach, and testes may also be involved. Syphilis is a rare cause of paroxysmal cold haemoglobinuria.

Syphilis of the nervous system (see also Chapter 13.28)

Less than 10 per cent develop involvement of the nervous system. If the CSF is normal 2 years after untreated infection, neurosyphilis will not develop. If the serology for syphilis becomes negative, that too effectively rules out neurosyphilis. If neurosyphilis is present, the Dattner criteria of cure is a normal cell count and protein level in CSF 6 months after treatment.

Asymptomatic neurosyphilis

There are no neurological manifestations but the CSF shows abnormalities such as a raised cell count (8 or more cells/ml), raised protein (over 40 mg/ml), and commonly a positive FTA–ABS test (see below). A positive VDRL in the CSF is less reliable as a sole abnormality; it is probably a result of passive transfer of antibody rather than intrathecal production. In the absence of treatment, 20 per cent of patients with asymptomatic neurosyphilis develop clinical neurosyphilis.

Neurosyphilis

The manifestations of meningovascular syphilis, general paralysis of the insane, tabes dorsalis, and neuro-opthalmological involvement, are described in Chapter 13.28. In treatment, penicillin must be given but results are generally unsatisfactory, as by the time the diagnosis is made there is much irreversible neurone destruction.

Cardiovascular syphilis

Symptomatic lesions develop in 10 per cent of untreated syphilis some 10–40 years after initial infection. Aortic reflux is the commonest lesion, caused by dilatation of the aortic root. Coronary ostial stenosis may give rise to angina pectoris, especially at night. Gummata in the A–V node or bundle of His can cause Stokes–Adams attacks.

Syphilitic aneurysm of the aorta

The ascending aorta is the most common site for a syphilitic aneurysm, which may remain symptom-free until it gives rise to pressure on the right lung, superior vena cava, and second and third ribs. It may be seen on radiographs and felt as a pulsating mass. Pressure on the pulmonary vein may lead to right heart failure; pressure on the ribs and sternum causes erosion which is painful. Rupture of the aneurysm into the pericardium is a possibility. There is diagnostic fine linear calcification of the ascending aorta on radiography (Fig. 5). Less common is aneurysm of the arch of the aorta, which may result in unequal radial pulses, especially delayed on the right side, and complications due to retrosternal compression. Rarer still are aneurysms in the descending aorta or affecting major branches, such as the innominate.

Pathology

There is endarteritis obliterans of the vasa vasorum of this aorta and perivascular cellular infiltration with lymphocytes and plasma cells. The consequence is destruction of the muscular and elastic layers of

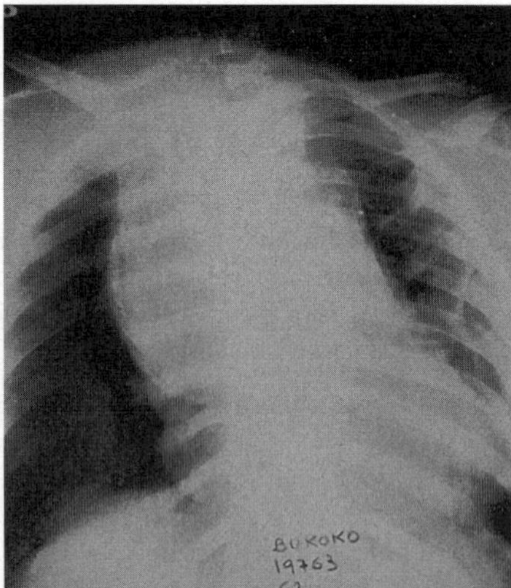

(a)

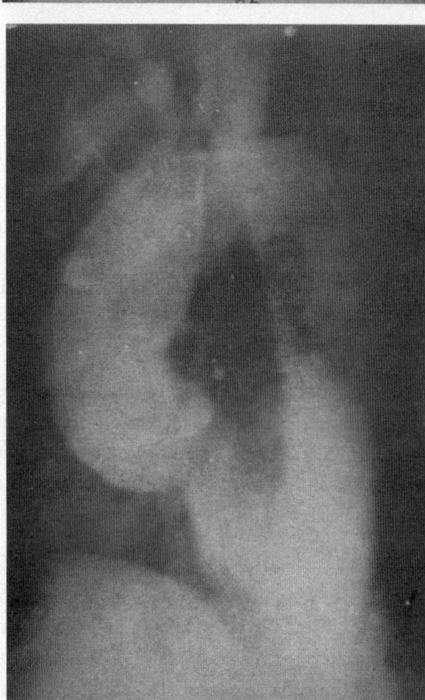

(b)

Fig. 5 Radiograph of aorta calcification with aneurysm and angiogram of coronary ostial artery stenosis.

the aortic wall and replacement with functionally inert scar tissue. The ostial stenosis of the coronary arteries appears to be due to their involvement whilst traversing the aortic wall. *T. pallidum* is believed to spread to the aorta during the early stages of the infection possibly by the lymphatics from the mediastinal nodes.

Prognosis

It is estimated that the overall mortality for cardiovascular syphilis was 30 per cent before the widespread availability of cardiac surgery. Syphilitic aortitis rarely progresses to aortic regurgitation. If syphilitic regurgitation is established, some two-thirds die within 10 years, while syphilitic aortic aneurysm, without surgery and without symptoms, has a life expectancy of 5 years. Adverse factors are heavy manual labour, angina pectoris, aortic regurgitation, congestive heart failure, aneurysmal pressure signs, and size of aneurysm over 6–7 cm. A course of penicillin is indicated if previously untreated followed by surgery, perhaps with excision of diseased aortic tissue and replacement by graft. Severe ostial stenosis can be relieved by endarterectomy of the coronary orifices or by bypass grafting.

Congenital syphilis

Syphilis may be transmitted to the fetus by the infected mother throughout pregnancy but lesions develop only after the fourth month when immunological competence becomes established.

Incidence

Congenital syphilis had all but disappeared in the western world after the 1960s. However, within the past few years there has been a sharp increase in congenital syphilis in urban areas of the US, Russia, and Australia. In underdeveloped countries, congenital syphilis remains a serious health threat. The pathological changes are similar to those found in secondary acquired syphilis but lesions of the viscera and bones are much more common.

Clinical features

There is no primary sore. In early cases there may be a bullous or papulosquamous rash involving especially the palms, soles, and lower part of the face. Healing is with scar formation such as the linear scars radiating from the nose, angle of the mouth, and anus. Weight loss may be severe with wrinkling of the skin, especially of the face, giving rise to the 'old-man' look. There may be patchy hair loss and discoloration of the skin ('cafe-au-lait'). Mucous membrane patches may develop in the mouth, pharynx and larynx ('aphonic cry') and the nasal cavity ('syphilitic snuffles'). All these lesions are highly infectious. Lymphadenopathy and hepatosplenomegaly may be prominent. With meningeal involvement there will be bulging fontanelles, meningism, and convulsions. The CSF shows increase in cells and protein. The CSF VDRL may be positive. Anaemia is a marked feature. In the first few months, osteochondritis of the long bones of both upper and lower limbs in the areas of rapid growth near the epiphyses occurs, together with periostitis which will give rise to pain and the limbs will be held immobile. Later syphilitic dactylitis, giving rise to sausage-shaped fingers, may develop. Choroidoretinitis gives rise to the 'salt and pepper' fundus.

Diagnosis

Dark-field microscopy of samples from open lesions will invariably demonstrate the presence of *T. pallidum*. A positive blood test for syphilis, in the absence of physical signs, must be evaluated to exclude passive transfer of maternal antibodies of the IgG class. In this situation, a positive VDRL test at birth usually becomes negative within 3 months. Tests for treponemal-specific 16S IgM can be interpreted as evidence of congenital infection. A rising titre of the VDRL test and/or failure of the test to become negative within 6 months is suggestive of congenital syphilis.

Differential diagnosis

Early bullous rash must be differentiated from infected scabies, bullous impetigo, herpes simplex, measles, rubella, cytomegalovirus infection, and toxoplasmosis.

Late congenital syphilis

Lesions appearing for the first time two or more years after birth characterises symptomatic late congenital syphilis. The lesions are not infectious. More commonly, the only abnormality is a positive serology in late latent congenital syphilis. Problems of diagnosis arise when, in later life, a persistent antitreponemal test is the only abnormality.

Late symptomatic congenital syphilis

Interstitial keratitis is the commonest presentation and may begin at any age between 5–30 years. Congenital neurosyphilis develops in more than 15 per cent of children. It is more resistant than the acquired form. It includes cranial nerve palsies, monoplegia or hemiplagia, general paresis with simple dementia, and deafness early in childhood. Penicillin appears to be ineffective. Epileptiform attacks are not uncommon. Juvenile tabes is very rare. Osteoperiostitis is seen between 5 and 25 years of age. The tibia is most commonly affected with thickening of the middle third giving rise to the characteristic 'sabre tibia'. The skull may show thickening of the vault. Gummatous destructive lesions may dominate involving especially the palate and nasal septum. However, the well-known saddle nose is thought to be due to poor development of the nasal bones following 'syphilitic snuffles'. Clutton's joints are caused by chronic, painless synovitis usually of the knee; the condition clears spontaneously and penicillin does not influence its course.

The stigmata

Certain scars and deformities can be characteristic of congenital syphilis and are called stigmata. The skeleton may be underdeveloped, thus stature is small and the pelvis in women may be inadequate for easy birth requiring caesarean section. The face is typically flat giving congenitally syphilitic children a 'family appearance'. Hutchinson's teeth and linear scars radiating from the mouth (rhagades) and nose are diagnostic. There may be gummatous destruction of the nasal septum and palate. Hutchinson's teeth are only found in permanent incisors with central notching and gaps between the peg-shaped teeth due to failure in development of the middle tooth buds. The dome-shaped mulberry molars of Moon are also due to poor development. The usual treatment is aqueous procaine benzylpenicillin, 50 mg/kg, twice daily for 10 days.

Currently used serological tests for syphilis

As yet no laboratory test is available to distinguish syphilis from the other treponematoses.

VDRL Test

This is the preferred test as it is used world-wide and is simple and inexpensive. The titres reflect activity, and may be of great value in providing the only evidence of reinfection in a patient with previous syphilis whose VDRL was either negative or weakly positive after treatment. A sharp sustained four-fold rise of the titre or higher, even in the absence of clinical signs, indicates active infection. False positive VDRL is usually of a low titre (1:8 or less). The VDRL test becomes positive during the primary stage and rises to its maximum during the secondary stage (1:32 or more). After successful treatment, the titre declines (1:4 or less), and if treatment was given early in the disease it often becomes negative.

Specific antitreponemal tests

1. The *T. pallidum* haemagglutination (TPHA) test. This uses an indirect haemagglutination method with red cells sensitized by sonicated *T. pallidum* extract.
2. The FTA–ABS test. This uses the indirect fluorescent technique with killed *T. pallidum* as antigen. The organisms are fixed on a slide to which the serum is added. The FTA–ABS is the most sensitive test available and is also specific. It becomes positive earlier during the primary stage of syphilis than other procedures. It is not suitable to assess activity, as it persists long after successful treatment. When the routine serology includes the VDRL and TPHA tests, the FTA–ABS test should be added in cases of problem sera.
3. The FTA–ABS–IgM test. In the search for a specific test to differentiate active infection which has to be treated from adequately treated or 'burnt out' inactive disease, the FTA–ABS–IgM is being evaluated to test for specific IgM which develops in the course of syphilis.

Diagnosis of neurosyphilis by examination of the CSF

Tests include the VDRL, cell count, and total protein globulin. The CSF VDRL is unreliable as it can be negative in up to 50 per cent of samples from patients with active neurosyphilis. Cell counts exceeding 8/mm^3, but usually not above 50/mm^3, and protein above 40 mg/ml are non-specific signs of inflammation.

The specific FTA–ABS and TPHA tests in the CSF may be positive due to passive transfer of serum IgG from adequately treated patients. If they are negative, active neurosyphilis can almost certainly be excluded. CSF specific serology is virtually always positive in active disease and frequently remains so after adequate treatment, or in burnt out tabes, whereas the VDRL often becomes negative. A positive, specific serological test is thus not a good indication of active disease.

Biological false-positive test for syphilis

They concern mainly the finding of positive cardiolipin tests (VDRL) when the confirmatory TPHA and FTA–ABS are negative. Biological false-positive tests are classified as acute if they become negative within 6 months. They are associated with a number of bacterial and viral infections including mycoplasma pneumonia and infectious mononucleosis. They are chronic if they persist for longer than 6 months and occur in about 20 per cent of drug addicts, autoimmune disease (when they may precede the symptoms by years) leprosy, and in a small proportion of people over 70. Particular mention should be made of the thrombotic antiphospholipid syndrome.

Serological tests for syphilis in HIV infection

Patients with secondary syphilis and concomitant AIDS may have a negative VDRL and FTA–ABS test. This indicates that a clinical diagnosis may have to be made without the benefit of serology. Further work showed that persistent seronegative syphilis did not exist. There seemed to be a delay in the untreated patients in developing positive tests both in the serum and CSF if HIV infection was present. The serology tended also to become negative a shorter time after treatment. The higher titres of cardiolipin antibodies in HIV infections may give a negative VDRL, because of a prozone phenomenon (i.e. the optimal proportions of the antigen: antibody reaction were not met).

The management of syphilis

As soon as a diagnosis of infectious syphilis has been made, the patient should be interviewed by the social worker regarding all sexual contacts. In the case of primary syphilis this should cover the previous 3 months, in patients with secondary syphilis this should be extended to 1 year, and in patients with early latent syphilis to 2 years because of the possibility of infectious relapses during that period. The patient is warned against intercourse during treatment and for a further 2 weeks.

If the patient gives no history of penicillin allergy, penicillin is the first choice for the treatment of all stages of the disease; aqueous procaine benzylpenicillin 1.2 mu/day given intramuscularly for 10 days in early syphilis, 15 days for late syphilis and neurosyphilis, and 20 days for cardiovascular syphilis. If there is penicillin allergy, the alternative drugs are tetracycline/doxycycline and erythromycin for 30 days. The recent finding of a wild strain of *T. pallidum* resistant to erythromycin, and tetracycline resistance in the related *T. denticola*, has led to an extensive investigation into the use of newer cephalosporins. Cephalosporins are effective but there is cross-allergy with penicillin in 5–7 per cent of patients and it is therefore not advised.

Some physicians prefer a single injection of the long-acting benzathine penicillin (2.4 million units) for the sake of simplicity, but the concentration reached is low and does not give a useful level in the CSF. In patients with neurosyphilis and HIV infections, the expected decline in VDRL CSF titres after treatment occurred less often than in those without concurrent HIV infection.

Reactions

There are a variety of idiosyncratic penicillin reactions ranging from anaphylactic episodes and bronchospasms to urticaria and arthralgia. However, the systemic Jarisch–Herxheimer reaction is believed to be due to the release of endotoxin-like substances when large numbers of *T. pallidum* are killed by antibiotics. It is mainly associated with early syphilis and is not a feature of neonatal syphilis. The reaction can be expected in 50 per cent of primary syphilis, 90 per cent of secondary syphilis, and in 25 per cent of early latent infection, but is very rare in late syphilis.

The reaction begins 4–12 h after the first injection, and is not seen with subsequent injections. There is malaise, slight to moderate pyrexia, a flush, tachycardia, leucocytosis, and existing lesions, especially the rash, become more prominent. In some patients with early syphilis, a secondary rash may become visible which was absent before treatment. Rarely, syphilis may be suspected by the appearance of the febrile Jarisch–Herxheimer reaction, perhaps with a fleeting rash, when treating another infection with a treponemocidal antimicrobial (e.g. penicillin in gonorrhoea or a gold preparation in the rheumatoid arthritic).

The patient with early syphilis should be warned about the possibility of mild indisposition on the day of the first injection. In late syphilis, the Jarisch–Herxheimer reaction can be more serious. Thus in neurosyphilis it may lead to a rapid, irreversible progression, and in general paresis it can cause exacerbation amounting to temporary psychosis. Sudden death has been reported in cardiovascular syphilis. In laryngeal gumma, local oedema may necessitate emergency tracheotomy.

It is customary to give corticosteroids in late symptomatic syphilis starting a day before the first penicillin injection and tailing it off the day after the first injection. This may ameliorate the Jarisch–Herxheimer reaction. We never withhold penicillin in late syphilis because of the remote chance of a reaction, nor do we give small initial doses as it is not dose-related.

Further reading

Fraser, C.M., Norris, S.J., Weinstock, G.M. *et al.* (1998). Complete genome sequence of *Treponema pallidum*, the syphilis spirochete. *Science*, **281**, 375–88.

Goldmeier, D. and Hay, P. (1993). A review and update on adult sexually transmitted syphilis, with particular reference to its treatment. *International Journal of Disease and AIDS*, **4**, 70–82.

Gromyko, A. (1997). *Epidemiological trends of HIV/AIDS and other sexually transmitted diseases in Eastern Europe*, pp. 1–9. WHO, Reg. Office for Europe.

Norris, S.J. (1989). Syphilis. In *Immunology of sexually transmitted diseases*, (ed. D.J.M. Wright), pp. 1–31. Kluwer, Dordrecht.

Schofer, H., Imhof M., Thoma-Gerber E., *et al.* (1996). Active syphilis in HIV infection: a multicentre retrospective survey. *Genitourinary Medicine*, 72, 176–81.

World Health Organization (1993). *Draft recommendations for the management of sexually transmitted diseases. WHO advisory group meeting*, pp. 24–31. WHO, Geneva.

Chapter 16.70

Listeria and listeriosis

P. J. Wilkinson

Listeria monocytogenes

Characteristics

Listeria monocytogenes is a non-sporing, facultatively anaerobic, Gram-positive bacillus that resembles a diphtheroid, from which it is distinguishable in a hanging-drop preparation by its characteristic 'tumbling' motility. Whereas *L. monocytogenes* is the only listeria likely to be isolated from blood, cerebrospinal fluid (CSF), pus, or tissues, other, non-pathogenic listeriae may be found in faeces, food, and specimens from the environment. Enrichment and selective methods are used to enhance the isolation of *Listeria* spp. Monoclonal antibodies, PCR, and DNA probe techniques are being developed for rapid detection.

Serological typing of *L. monocytogenes* has been used for tracing food sources, distinguishing relapse from reinfection, and investigating outbreaks. There are 11 serotypes but three (Ia, Ib, and IVb) cause most human infections. Subtyping systems currently under development include phage typing, multilocus enzyme electrophoresis, plasmid analysis, restriction fragment length polymorphism, and ribosomal DNA fingerprinting (ribotyping).

Pathogenesis

The factors that influence whether invasive disease will occur include the virulence of the infecting organism, the susceptibility of the host, and the size of the infecting dose of bacteria. Food-borne *L. monocytogenes* must penetrate the intestinal mucosa and presumably multiply in cells in the Peyer's patches. *L. monocytogenes* can invade the eye and skin of humans after direct exposure, and cross the placenta during maternal bacteraemia. The virulence of *L. monocytogenes* is related to the production of specific toxins, including listeriolysin O (a 52 kDa protein) and haemolysin. Most listeriosis occurs in people in whom cell-mediated immunity is depressed by pregnancy, disease (including AIDS), or immunosuppressive or cytotoxic therapy.

Listeriosis

Epidemiological associations

Listeriosis causes abortions and meningoencephalitis in cattle, sheep, and goats. *L. monocytogenes* from the animal gut can contaminate meat, milk, or vegetables and much human listeriosis is now known to be food-borne. An outbreak in 1981 in Nova Scotia caused 41 cases (7 adult, 34 maternofetal) and provided the first reported evidence for the transmission of listeriosis by food, namely coleslaw made from cabbages contaminated by sheep faeces. Outbreaks of food-borne listeriosis have also been associated with other vegetables, raw fish, raw hot dogs, undercooked chicken, pork rillettes, meat paté, and cheese and dairy products. The UK Department of Health now advises pregnant women and the immunocompromised to avoid eating soft ripened cheeses such as Brie, Camembert, and blue-vein types; all types of paté; and cook-chill meals and ready-to-eat poultry unless thoroughly reheated

Clusters of cases of hospital-acquired, late-onset neonatal listeriosis have been reported from a number of countries. Poor hand hygiene, close contact between infected patients and their mothers, and fomites such as rectal thermometers have all been implicated. Both person-to-person and food-borne spread have been suspected in outbreaks among adult immunosuppressed patients in hospital. Eye and skin infections without systemic involvement have also been occupationally-acquired by agricultural, veterinary, and laboratory workers who have been directly exposed to infected animals or to culture material.

Clinical features

The clinical presentation of infection with *L. monocytogenes* can vary from a mild, influenza-like illness to fatal septicaemia and meningoencephalitis. The syndromes recognized include maternofetal and neonatal listeriosis, septicaemia, meningoencephalitis, cerebritis, and localized infections.

Maternofetal listeriosis

This syndrome can occur at any time during pregnancy. The mother may develop a fever, with headache, myalgia, and low back pain, associated with the bacteraemic phase of the disease. Transplacental infection causes amnionitis and usually leads to spontaneous septic abortion or to premature labour with the delivery of an infected fetus or baby.

Neonatal listeriosis

Early-onset neonatal listeriosis results from intrauterine infection. It has a high mortality. Usually, the mother has had an influenza-like illness before starting labour. The liquor is meconium-stained and the baby septic and jaundiced, with signs of purulent conjunctivitis, bronchopneumonia, meningitis, or encephalitis. Granulomas in many organs are a unique feature of this disease, which is therefore also termed granulomatosis infantisepticum. Late-onset disease, which occurs after several days to weeks in a baby who is initially healthy, may be acquired from the mother's genital tract or through cross-infection in nurseries or labour suites.

Septicaemia

Listeria septicaemia occurs mainly in patients with malignancies, in transplant recipients, and in immunosuppressed and elderly people. Most present with fever, hypotension, and shock but a third to a half develop meningitis, which is often then the presenting feature.

Meningoencephalitis

Meningoencephalitis with *L. monocytogenes* may start abruptly but in adults it can also develop insidiously, with progressive focal neurological signs even in the absence of a brain abscess. Most patients have meningism, but fever may not be marked, particularly in elderly or immunosuppressed people. In one series, *L. monocytogenes* was the reported cause of 10 per cent of cases of community-acquired meningitis in the US, and this infection should now be considered in any patient with an acute brainstem disorder associated with fever, particularly if there are no risk factors for cerebrovascular disease.

Cerebritis

L. monocytogenes cerebritis is increasingly recognized, particularly in the immunosuppressed patient. Headache, fever, and varying degrees of paralysis can resemble a cerebrovascular accident. Rhomboencephalitis has been reported, beginning with headache, fever, nausea, and vomiting, followed in several days by symmetrical, progressive cranial nerve palsies, decreased consciousness, and cerebellar signs. Areas of uptake without ring enhancement may be shown by MRI or CT scan, and the CSF usually shows few if any cells, and normal protein and sugar levels.

Localized infections

These are rare, occur mainly in immunosuppressed people, and include osteomyelitis, septic arthritis, cholecystitis, abscesses, and peritonitis. They usually result from seeding during an initial bacteraemic phase, but focal skin and eye infection can also result from direct, occupational exposure.

Diagnosis

The microbiological diagnosis of invasive listeriosis is made by culture of the organism from meconium, nose or eye swabs, urine, CSF, blood, tracheal aspirate, placental tissue, and/or lochia. Gram-positive bacilli may be seen in a stained smear. Tests for listeria antibodies in maternal and cord blood samples are unhelpful.

Antibiotic treatment

There are no controlled trials of antibiotic treatments for listeriosis. *L. monocytogenes* is generally susceptible *in vitro* to ampicillin, benzylpenicillin, chloramphenicol, ciprofloxacin, erythromycin, gentamicin and other aminoglycosides, imipenem, mezlocillin, rifampicin, some sulphonamides, tetracyclines, trimethoprim, and vancomycin. The organism is only moderately susceptible to some cephalosporins (cefazolin, cefotaxime, ceftriaxone) and resistant to others, including the oral cephalosporins and ceftazidime. Some strains are partially resistant to penicillin, but synergy can be demonstrated *in vitro* between ampicillin and gentamicin, and between mezlocillin and gentamicin, combinations that are bactericidal, as is gentamicin alone.

A combination of ampicillin and gentamicin is considered to be the treatment of choice for listeriosis. Gentamicin is best avoided in pregnancy, when ampicillin or amoxicillin may be used alone. Successful treatment has also been reported with intravenous chloramphenicol and with co-trimoxazole. Treatment failures have been reported with penicillin alone and with cephalosporins, despite apparent *in vitro* susceptibility. Rifampicin has not been evaluated in human listeriosis, but, like chloramphenicol, is bacteriostatic against

L. monocytogenes in vitro and may be antagonistic when used with ampicillin or penicillin. Ciprofloxacin has *in vitro* activity against *Listeria* spp. but has not yet been evaluated in listeriosis.

The appropriate duration of therapy is also uncertain. Two weeks has been sufficient in some series, but 3–6 weeks of treatment is probably safer, particularly in immunosuppressed patients. Cerebritis should be treated for at least 6 weeks. Neonatal listeriosis should be treated with ampicillin or amoxicillin, 200–400 mg/kg per day in four to six divided doses given intravenously or intramuscularly for at least 3 weeks (up to 6 weeks in meningitis), and combined with gentamicin in conventional doses for the first 14 days. Adults should be given intravenous ampicillin or amoxicillin, 6–12 g daily in three or four divided doses, combined with gentamicin for the first 14 days in a dosage of 6 mg/kg per day, adjusted according to renal function with the help of plasma concentration measurement. Focal listeriosis may be treated with ampicillin or amoxicillin, 3–6 g daily or 100 mg/kg daily, until clinical resolution. In cases of genuine penicillin allergy, alternatives are co-trimoxazole, 20 mg/kg per day (trimethoprim component) or chloramphenicol, 60 mg/kg per day, both in four divided doses. Vancomycin has also been used, but treatment failures have been reported.

Prognosis

Despite antibiotic therapy, the case fatality of septicaemia and meningoencephalitis with case *L. monocytogenes* is 20–50 per cent. There is significant long-term morbidity in the survivors. Efforts should therefore continue to be focused on the prevention of this infection by improvement in the microbiological safety of methods of food production and preparation, and by education of the public so that vulnerable people can avoid high-risk foods.

Further reading

Durand, M.L., Calderwood, S.B., Weber, D.J. *et al.* (1993). Acute bacterial meningitis in adults. A review of 493 episodes. *New England Journal of Medicine*, 328, 21–8.

Jurado, R.L., Farley, M.M., Pereira, E. *et al.* (1993). Increased risk of meningitis and bacteraemia due to Listeria monocytogenes in patients with human immunodeficiency virus infection. *Clinical Infectious Diseases*, 17, 224–7.

Schlech III, W.F. (1991). Listeriosis: epidemiology, virulence and the significance of contaminated foodstuffs. *Journal of Hospital Infection*, 19, 211–24.

Chapter 16.71

Legionellosis and legionnaires' disease

J. B. Kurtz and J. T. Macfarlane

In 1976, an outbreak of pneumonia occurred among American legionnaires who had attended a convention in a Philadelphia hotel. A total of 221 people developed pneumonia, 'legionnaires' disease', of whom 34 died. It was shown by workers at the Centres for Disease Control, Atlanta, that a newly identified organism, named after this outbreak, *Legionella pneumophila*, was responsible.

Clinical illness caused by bacteria of the family Legionellaceae is called legionellosis. This can be pneumonia, Legionnaires' disease, or a non-pneumonic illness, 'Pontiac fever'. What determines the type of illness that will follow infection is unknown. Although, in a given outbreak, disease of both pneumonic and non-pneumonic types occurs, usually either one or other form predominates.

The organism

The Legionellaceae are aerobic, non-sporing, Gram-negative bacilli of variable lengths from coccal to filamentous forms, 20 μm or longer whose cell walls contain distinctive branched-chain fatty acids. In the laboratory, legionellae are fastidious in their growth requirements and will not grown on standard bacteriological media. Aces buffered charcoal yeast extract (BCYE) agar, pH 6.9, supplemented with L-cysteine, α-ketoglutarate, and iron, is a very satisfactory medium and is made semiselective by the addition of antibacterial and antifungal agents that suppress other microflora in specimens from contaminated sites. On BCYE agar, incubated at 35–37°C, typical colonies usually appear in 3–5 days; occasional slow-growing strains require the plates to be incubated for 10 days. By serological typing and other methods, more than 40 species have now been recognized in the Legionellaceae family. Some of these species can be subdivided into serogroups. *L. pneumophila* is responsible for over 80 per cent of legionellosis and of its 16 serogroups, serogroup 1 is the most frequent to cause human infection. Other *Legionella* species appear to be less pathogenic and are more frequently found as opportunistic pathogens in immunocompromised people, or have only been isolated from the environment.

Epidemiology

The natural habitat of legionellae is fresh water of streams, lakes, and thermal springs, moist soil, and mud. They have been found worldwide in waters with temperatures varying from 5–62°C and pH of 5.4–8.2. They are inhibited by sodium chloride and are not found in sea water. In natural habitats, they are found in only small numbers, forming part of the consortium of micro-organisms that makes up the biofilm. This includes amoebae and other protozoa, in certain of which it has been shown legionellae can multiply and survive. Inside these protozoa the bacteria form microcolonies, which are protected from adverse conditions (for example in amoebic cysts from desiccation and up to 50 parts/10^6 free chlorine). This association might therefore help the bacteria to disseminate widely.

Legionellae are also found in man-made water distribution systems. There, in biofilms, stagnation and temperatures of 20–45°C encourage multiplication. The most common sites in buildings in which legionellae have been found are hot-water calorifiers and storage tanks, where there are temperature strata often providing ideal conditions for growth at the bottom. Piped water, especially hot water from the calorifiers in large buildings and industrial complexes with long runs of pipework, is a potential source of infection. Other well-recognized sources include:

- recirculating water in air-conditioning and cooling systems;
- whirlpool spas and other warm-water baths;
- decorative fountains;
- nebulizers and humidifier reservoirs of hospital ventilation machines if topped up with contaminated tap water.

Potting compost was the source of several outbreaks of pneumonia caused by *L. longbeachae* serogroup 1 in Australia.

Dissemination of infection is by contaminated water droplets (aerosol), which are inhaled or aspirated. Person-to-person spread of legionellosis has never been reported.

Legionnaires' disease occurs in outbreaks, but sporadic cases account for about three-quarters of cases reported in England and Wales. A source is rarely found for the latter. Some sporadic cases can be linked by a history of visiting a common site within the incubation period of the disease. An association with overseas travel was found in one-third of the sporadic cases in England and Wales in the years 1979 to 1986. Apart from travel, an analysis of sporadic cases in Glasgow between 1978 and 1986 supported the hypothesis that cooling water towers were the source. Cases were clustered in both time and space, with a relative risk three times greater for people living within 500 m of a cooling tower compared with those living more than 1000 m away.

In temperate countries, most cases occur in the summer and autumn. A British Thoracic Society study of community-acquired pneumonia requiring hospital admission in 1982–83 showed that 2 per cent had legionnaires' disease. This suggests that about 1500 cases occur per year in Britain. The susceptibility to infection of exposed people varies. For non-pneumonic legionellosis the attack rate is very high. In the Loch Goiland Hotel outbreak caused by *L. micdadei* in the whirlpool spa, 91 per cent of those exposed were affected. In contrast, the attack rate for legionnaires' disease is about 1 per cent. Illness is more common in men than in women (2–3:1). Immunosuppression, pre-existing chronic disease, smoking, and high alcohol intake all increase vulnerability. Subclinical or mild infections can follow exposure, as indicated by serological surveys of workers (nurses, hotel staff, etc.) at sites where there have been outbreaks. For example of the staff at the Stafford District General Hospital who were tested following the outbreak in 1985, 42 per cent had an antibody titre of 1 in 16 or greater.

Hospital-acquired legionellosis is a particular problem because of the size and complexity of the buildings and the difficulty of maintaining the hot water hot enough (storage at 60°C and 50°C at the taps), either because of the length of pipework or for fear of scalding patients. Hospital patients, too, are a highly susceptible population and species other than *L. pneumophila* more frequently cause infections in these circumstances.

Table 1 Clinical features of 739 patients with legionella pneumonia

Respiratory symptoms (%)		*General symptoms (%)*	
Cough	75	Rigors	59
New sputum production	45	Headaches	32
Dyspnoea	50	Confusion	45
Chest pain	36	Diarrhoea	33
Haemoptysis	21	Fever over 39°C	70
Bronchial breathing in lung	16		
Crepitations in lung	74		

Data adapted from Table 3.2: Barlett, C.R., Macrae, A.D., and Macfarlane, J.T. (1986). *Legionella infections.* Edward Arnold, London, with permission of the publishers.

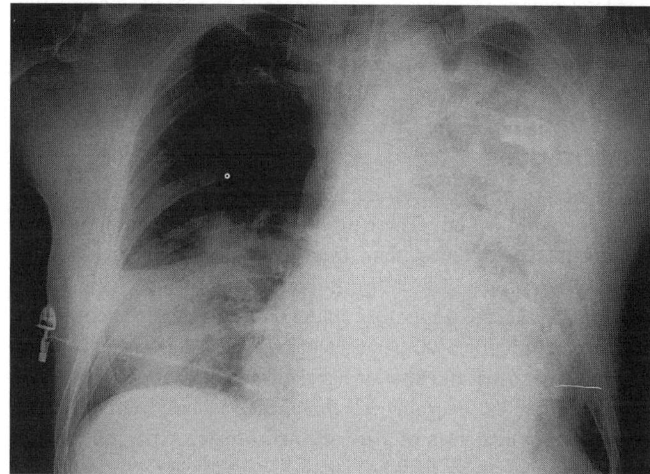

Fig. 1 The chest radiograph of a 58-year-old man who returned from a hotel holiday by the Mediterranean with legionella pneumonia. There is extensive, bilateral, homogeneous consolidation. He required assisted ventilation for worsening respiratory failure.

Legionella pneumonia

Clinical features (Table 1)

The illness typically starts fairly abruptly, following an incubation period of 2–10 days, with high fevers, shivers, bad headache, and muscle pain. Upper respiratory tract symptoms, herpes labialis, and rashes are uncommon. The cough that follows may be insignificant and dry initially but dyspnoea is common and the illness often progresses quickly. Sometimes there is a history of a recent hotel holiday abroad or a stay in hospital, which can alert the clinician to the possible diagnosis.

The patient commonly looks toxic and ill, with a high fever over 39°C in three-quarters of cases. Sometimes non-respiratory features, such as confusion and delirium or diarrhoea, which occur in more than one-half of the patients, can dominate the clinical picture, masking the true diagnosis of pneumonia, although localizing signs can usually be detected in the chest. Focal neurological signs, particularly of a cerebellar type, are well described but meningitis does not occur. Amnesia on recovery is common.

Laboratory and radiographic features

The total white count is usually only moderately raised, to $15 \times 10^9/1$ in two-thirds of cases, often with a lymphopenia. Hyponatraemia, hypoalbuminaemia, and abnormality of liver function tests are detected in over one-half of the cases. Other features may include raised blood urea and muscle enzymes, hypoxaemia, haematuria, and proteinuria but none of these is unique for legionella pneumonia.

Radiographic shadowing is usually homogeneous and commonly confined to one of the lower lobes on presentation. Characteristically, radiographic deterioration occurs with spread of shadows both within the same lung and to the opposite side (Fig. 1). A small pleural effusion can occur in one-quarter of cases; lung cavitation is rare except in immunosuppressed patients. Clearance of pulmonary shadows in survivors is particularly slow; only two-thirds of radiographs clear within 3 months and some take more than 6 months.

Therapy

There are no clinical trials on the efficacy of different antimicrobials for legionella infection and recommendations are based on retrospective case studies, as well as *in vitro* and animal experiments.

Although the organism is susceptible to a wide range of antimicrobials *in vitro*, the most relevant factor is their ability to penetrate intracellularly into alveolar macrophages where the legionellae hide and divide. Erythromycin is at present recommended as the drug of first choice, in dosages of 500–1000 mg every 6 h, being given intravenously if required. Treatment is generally recommended for up to 2–3 weeks to prevent relapse, although shorter courses are often effective.

In vitro and animal experiments support the efficacy of rifampicin, quinolones, and newer macrolides. Rifampicin is often recommended as additional therapy to erythromycin, in a dose of 600 mg once or twice a daily in patients who are deteriorating. Uncontrolled case series also support the use of doxycycline and ciprofloxacin.

General supportive measures are particularly important, with attention to adequate hydration and correction of hypoxaemia with the early use of assisted ventilation for advancing respiratory failure. Anecdotal experience suggests extra corporial membrane oxygenation (ECMO) may occasionally buy time for drug therapy to work in the presence of respiratory failure not controlled by mechanical ventilation.

Complications

A wide variety of complications has been reported, affecting nearly every system of the body. These probably arise more commonly from a multisystem toxic effect than from direct spread of the bacteria, which appears rare. The most important, immediate pulmonary complication is acute respiratory failure requiring assisted ventilation, which occurs in up to 20 per cent of cases. Cardiac complications, including pericardial and myocardial involvement, are well recognized. A wide variety of neurological complications has been reported, leading to the suggestion of a specific neurotoxin. Acute, but usually reversible, renal failure may be seen in severe disease.

Prognosis and mortality

The two most important factors affecting outcome are the prior health of the patient and appropriate early therapy. The case fatality in previously fit patients is low, in the order of 5 to 15 per cent, but in immunosuppressed individuals can approach 75 per cent.

Pathology

The lungs are usually the only organs affected in fatal cases and reveal lobar consolidation. Affected lung tissue on section characteristically shows a severe inflammatory response, with alveoli and terminal bronchioles distended by fibrin-rich debris, macrophages, and neutrophils (Fig. 2). In survivors, alveolar and interstitial fibrotic changes can result from the organization of fibrin and hyaline membranes.

Pontiac fever

This is the acute non-pneumonic form of legionella infection and presents as a short-lived, self-limiting, flu-like illness. The attack rate is extremely high, with an incubation period of usually 36–48 h. Previously healthy people are affected, with high fever, shivers, headache, myalgia, malaise, and dizziness, some dry cough but no localizing signs in the chest. Investigations and chest radiograph are normal, and illness improves spontaneously, usually within 5 days. The diagnosis is usually made retrospectively by serological testing. Treatment is symptomatic. Deaths have not been reported, although non-specific symptoms and lassitude may be experienced following recovery. It is possible that Pontiac fever is a reaction to inhaling amounts of legionella antigen from large numbers of predominantly dead bacteria.

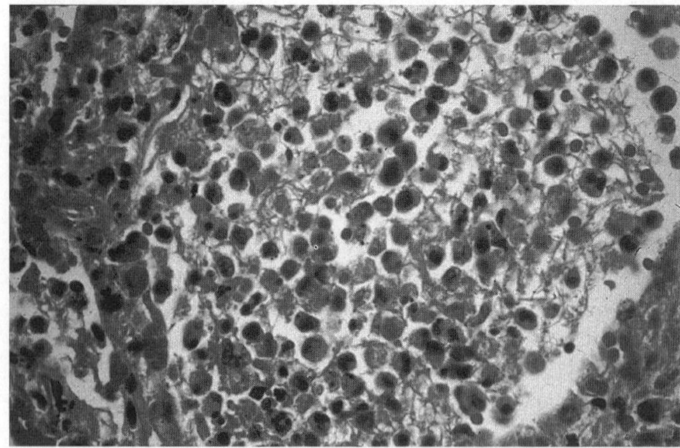

Fig. 2 Photomicrograph of an alveolus of a patient who died of legionella pneumonia. Note that the alveolar space is packed with mononuclear cells and fibrin.

(Reproduced with permission from Macfarlane, J.T., Finch, R.G., and Cotton, R.E. Colour atlas of respiratory infections, Chapman and Hall, London.)

Laboratory diagnosis

There is no distinctive clinical, biochemical, or radiographic pattern that allows the early differentiation of legionella infection from other causes of pneumonia. A range of microbiological procedures that can be used to diagnose legionellosis:

(1) culture on a permissive medium, e.g. BCYE agar;

(2) direct detection of bacteria or their nucleic acid;

(3) urinary antigen detection;

(4) serological response.

Suitable specimens from which legionellae can be isolated are expectorated sputum, endotracheal aspirates, bronchoalveolar lavage fluid, and lung. Isolation is the method of choice; it allows the causative strain to be typed and compared with those from the environment. A quicker diagnosis can be made by examining these samples directly for evidence of legionellae. With specific monoclonal antisera the bacteria can be visualized by immunofluorence or immunoperoxidase techniques. Alternatively legionella ribosomal RNA can be detect review transcription by the polymerase chain reaction (RT-PCR) directly in a specimen.

Soluble antigen is excreted in the urine for 1–3 weeks during the acute pneumonia and longer in immunocompromised infected patients. Tests to detect *L. pneumophila* serogroup 1 urinary antigen have a high specificity and sensitivity.

Serology is the most widely used diagnostic approach. The major problem with serodiagnosis is the delay due to slow production of antibodies, peak titres appearing 2–4 weeks after the onset of illness.

In Britain, the serological criteria for diagnosis of *L. pneumophila* serogroup 1 are either a four-fold rise in indirect fluorescent antibody titre to more than 64 or a single titre in excess of 128 (or microagglutination titre of greater than 32). The single titre that gives a presumptive diagnosis must be determined locally and must be higher than a cut-off level of antibody in that population. Only 20 per cent of patients with legionnaires' disease have diagnostic titres of antibody within 3 days of hospital admission, although about 40 per cent will have lesser but suggestive levels by that time. Approximately 20 per cent of those infected appear not to respond serologically.

Reference laboratories therefore use a battery of antigens to increase their ability to diagnose legionellosis caused by non-serogroups *L. pneumophila* and other species. Occasionally patients with Q fever, leptospirosis, *Citrobacter freundii*, and more commonly with campylobacter infections make antibodies that cross-react with *L. pneumophila* serogroup 1. As diarrhoea can be an early feature of legionnaires' disease as well as a major consequence of campylobacter enteritis, it is important to culture stool samples and interpret with caution the legionella serology from such patients.

Prevention

Legionellosis is acquired from environmental water sources by the aspiration or inhalation of water droplets. There are three aspects to consider in reducing the risk of legionellosis:

(1) measures to minimize colonization, growth, and the release of legionellae into the atmosphere;

(2) physical or chemical treatment of water to kill the bacteria;

(3) the protection of personnel who work on contaminated systems.

In Britain, particularly following the Stafford Hospital outbreak, a large number of publications aimed at minimizing the risk of legionellosis have appeared. In 1991 in Britain, an Approved Code of Practice, *The prevention or control of legionellosis (including legionnaires' disease)*, set out statutory requirements for dealing with this risk. Together with the Health and Safety guidance booklet HS(G)70, which was published with it and should be consulted for more details, the Code applies wherever water is stored or used in a way that may create 'a reasonably foreseeable risk of legionellosis'.

Further reading

Bhopal, R.S., Fallon, R.J., Buist, E.C., Black, R.J., and Urqhart, J.D. (1991). Proximity of the home to a cooling tower and the risk of non-outbreak legionnaires' disease. *British Medical Journal*, **302**, 378–83.

Committee of Inquiry (1986). *First report of the Committee of Inquiry into the outbreak of legionnaires' disease in Stafford in April 1985.* Cmnd 9772. HMSO, London.

Committee of Inquiry (1987). *Second report of the Committee of Inquiry into the outbreak of legionnaires' disease in Stafford in April 1985.* Cmnd 256. HMSO, London.

Health and Safety Commission (1991). *Approved code of practice—the prevention or control of legionellosis (including legionnaires' disease).* HMSO, London.

Health and Safety Executive (1991). *The control of legionellosis including legionnaires' disease*, HS(G)70. HMSO, London.

Muder, R.R. and Yu, V.L. (1994). Legionella. In *Respiratory infections; a scientific basis for management*, (eds M.S. Niederman, G.A. Sarosi, and J. Glassroth). W.B. Saunders, Philadelphia.

Woodhead, M.A. and Macfarlane, J.T. (1985). The protean manifestations of legionnaires' disease. *Journal of the Royal College Physicians (London)*, **19**, 224–30.

Chapter 16.72

Rickettsial diseases including ehrlichioses

D. H. Walker

Rickettsiae (Table 1) are obligate intracellular bacteria, which, during at least a part of their existence, occupy specific arthropods as their environmental niche. *Rickettsia* are transmitted to man by their arthropod hosts and invade the cells of the blood vessel. The target cell of *Orientia* (formerly *Rickettsia*) *tsutsugamushi* in humans with scrub typhus remains undefined, yet the vascular lesions resemble those of the rickettsioses. In contrast, organisms of the genus *Ehrlichia* invade mainly phagocytes and do not cause primary vascular injury. *Coxiella burnetii* differs from other rickettsial organism in its evolutionary relations, its ecological niche, and in its clinical manifestations. Man acquires *C. burnetii* mainly by inhalation of aerosols from birth products of infected animals. The organisms proliferate within the acidic phagolysosome of host macrophages and cause an illness that ranges from acute atypical pneumonia to chronic endocarditis.

The public health importance of rickettsioses is underestimated because of difficulties with clinical diagnosis and lack of laboratory methods in many geographical areas. Active surveillance and serological surveys suggest that there is significant, unrecognized exposure to rickettsial organisms. It is particularly important to consider a rickettsial diagnosis when caring for the neglected poor of developing countries and travellers returning from areas endemic for murine typhus, scrub typhus, boutonneuse fever, African tick bite fever, other spotted fevers, and Q fever. Rickettsiae infect previously healthy, active people, and if undiagnosed, diagnosed late, or untreated, Rocky Mountain spotted fever, epidemic typhus, scrub typhus, Q fever endocarditis, boutonneuse fever, human ehrlichioses, and murine typhus are life threatening.

Many commonly prescribed antibiotics, including the penicillins, cephalosporins, and aminoglycosides, have no effect on the course of rickettsial diseases but those antimicrobials active against rickettsial organism can reduce morbidity and mortality.

Epidemics of louse-borne typhus fever have influenced the outcome of many wars between the 1500s and the 1920s. Wherever there is war, famine, floods, or other massive disasters leading to widespread louse infestation of a population, the threat of epidemic typhus exists. Recent epidemics have occurred in Burundi, the economically-devastated former USSR, and in extremely poor populations in the Andes.

Contemporary molecular analyses reveal that the spotted fever and typhus groups of the genus *Rickettsia* are very closely related to one another and not to *O. tsutsugamushi.* They are relatively close relatives of *Ehrlichia* and the facultatively intracellular *Bartonella*, and are evolutionarily distant from *Coxiella* and *Chlamydia.*

Vasculopathic rickettsial diseases of the spotted-fever and typhus groups

Aetiological agents

These bacteria measure approximately 0.3×1.0 μm and have a cell wall typical of Gram-negative bacteria.

Table 1 Aetiology, epidemiology, and ecology of rickettsial diseases

Disease	Agent	Geographical distribution	Natural history	Transmission to man
Spotted fevers				
Rocky Mountain spotted fever	*R. rickettsii*	North, Central, and South America	Transovarial maintenance in ticks: less extensive horizontal transmission from tick to mammal to tick	Tick bite
Boutonneuse fever	*R. conorii*	Mediterranean basin, Africa, Asia	Transovarial maintenance in ticks; role of horizontal transmission is not clear	Tick bite
African tick-bite fever	*R. africae*	Southern and eastern Africa	Presumably transovarian maintenance in ticks	Tick bite
North Asian tick typhus	*R. sibirica*	Russia, China, Mongolia, Pakistan, Kazakhstan, Kirgiziya, Tadzhikistan	Transovarial maintenance in ticks; horizontal transmission from tick to mammal to tick	Tick bite
Japanese spotted fever	*R. japonica*	Japan	Presumably a transovarial tick host; the role of horizontal transmission is not clear	Tick bite
Queensland tick typhus	*R. australis*	Eastern Australia	Transovarial transmission in Ixodes ticks; the role of horizontal transmission is not clear	Tick bite
Flinders Island spotted fever	*R. honei*	Southern Australian islands, Thailand	Unknown	Presumably tick bite
Rickettsialpox	*R. akari*	USA, Ukraine, Croatia, possibly worldwide	Transovarian transmission in *Liponyssoides sanguineus* mites; horizontal transmission from mite to mouse to mite	Mite bite
Cat flea typhus	*R. felis*	North America	Transovarial transmission in *Ctenocephalides felis* fleas	Unknown
Epidemic typhus	*R. prowazekii*	South America, Africa, Asia, Central America, Mexico	Man to louse to man	Louse faeces scratched into skin
Sylvatic typhus	*R. prowazekii*	United States	Flying squirrel to louse and flea ectoparasites to flying squirrel	Presumably flea of flying squirrels to man
Recrudescent typhus	*R. prowazekii*	Worldwide	Reactivation of latent human infection years after acute illness	None
Murine typhus	*R. typhi*	Worldwide, predominantly tropical and subtropical	Rat to rat flea to rat; opossum to cat flea to opossum	Flea faeces scratched into skin, rubbed into conjunctiva, or inhaled
Scrub typhus	*O. tsutsugamushi*	Japan, southern and eastern Asia, northern Australia, islands of the western and south-western Pacific	Transovarial transmission in *Leptotrombidium* chiggers	Chigger bite
Ehrlichioses				
Human monocytotropic ehrlichiosis	*E. chaffeensis*	USA, Portugal, Spain, Mali, Thailand	Horizontal transmission between mammals (e.g., deer, dogs) and ticks	Tick bite
Human granulocytotropic ehrlichiosis	*E. phagocytophilia*-like	USA, Europe	Horizontal transmission between mammals (e.g., deer mice, red deer, sheep, cattle, horses) and *Ixodes* ticks	Tick bite
Sennetsu ehrlichiosis	*E. sennetsu*	Japan, Malaysia	Suspected maintenance in fish or snail flukes	Suspected ingestion of raw fish infected with ehrlichia-infected flukes
Q fever	*C. burnetii*	Worldwide	Mammals including sheep, goats, cattle, rabbits and cats; ticks	Aerosol of infected mammalian birth products

Table 1 *continued*

Disease	Agent	Geographical distribution	Natural history	Transmission to man
Bartonella **Infections**				
Trench fever	*B. quintana*	Worldwide	Louse to man to louse	Louse faeces
Cat-scratch disease	*B. henselae*	Worldwide	Cat-to-cat, flea-to-cat	Cat scratch or bite
Bacillary angiomatosis and peliosis	*B. henselae* and *B. quintana*	Worldwide	Cat-to-cat, flea-to-cat	Cat scratch or bite
Endocarditis	*B. quintana* *B. henselae* *B. elizabethae*	Worldwide	Cat-to-cat, flea-to-cat	Cat scratch or bite
Oroya fever, verruga peruana	*B. bacilliformis*	Peru, Ecuador, Colombia	Human to sand fly to human	Sand fly presumably via bite

Epidemiology

Seasonal incidence and geographical distribution are determined by vector activity. Spotted-fever group rickettsiae are maintained in nature principally by transovarial and transtadial transmission in their tick or mite hosts. The most virulent rickettsiae are capable of killing their arthropod hosts (e.g. *R. prowazekii* and *R. rickettsii*) and so require horizontal transmission to infect other arthropods. Reactivation of latent *R. prowazekii* infection in man is the source for infection of lice that initiates epidemics of typhus fever.

Spotted-fever group rickettsiae are transmitted to man by secretion of infected tick saliva into the blood pooled in the site of the bite and typhus-group rickettsiae by infected louse or flea faeces deposited on human skin during arthropod feeding. Fluid or faeces of infected ticks crushed between the fingers may enter a cutaneous wound or be rubbed into the conjunctiva.

Pathogenesis

Rickettsiae of some species of the spotted-fever group frequently invade endothelial cells at the cutaneous portal of entry, proliferate, and cause a focus of dermal and epidermal necrosis, an eschar. Rickettsiae spread via the bloodstream to all parts of the body, where they attach to endothelial cells lining blood vessels. Phagocytosis is induced, and rickettsiae escape from the phagosome into the cytosol, where they proliferate by binary fission. Typhus rickettsiae reach massive numbers intracellularly until the endothelial cell bursts. Spotted-fever group rickettsiae are propelled through the cytosol by stimulating F-actin polymerization at one pole and spreading from cell-to-cell. Rickettsial lipopolysaccharides are non-endotoxic in the quantities present during human infections, and there is no evidence of rickettsial exotoxin. Host immune, inflammatory, and coagulation systems are activated with apparent overall benefit to the patient.

Progressive, disseminated infection and injury to endothelial cells cause increased vascular permeability, oedema, hypovolaemia, and signs and symptoms resulting from multifocal vascular injury in affected organs (Fig. 1). Infection of the pulmonary microcirculation and the resulting increase in vascular permeability produce adult respiratory distress syndrome. Despite an interstitial myocarditis, myocardial function is preserved. Arrhythmias may result from vascular lesions affecting the conduction system. The vascular lesions in the brain are associated with coma and seizures in severe cases (Fig. 2). Multifocal infectious lesions in the dermis are the basis for the maculopapular, sometimes petechial, rash. Acute renal failure occurs in severe cases, usually as prerenal azotaemia or less frequently as acute tubular necrosis associated with severe hypotension.

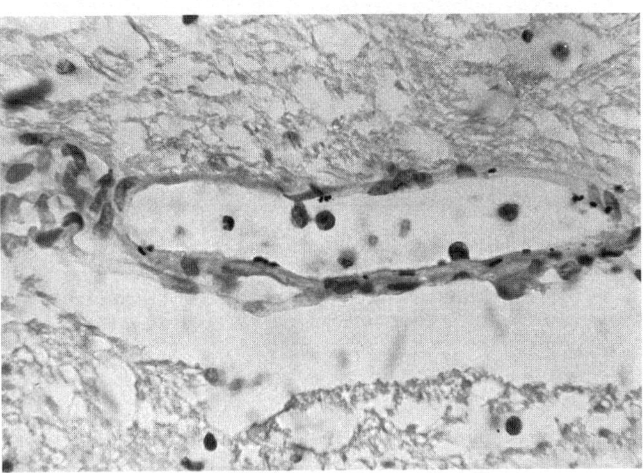

Fig. 1 Immunoperoxidase-stained *Rickettsia rickettsii* appear as dark bacilli in endothelial cells of a cerebral blood vessel with perivascular oedema but no host immune-cell infiltration.

Clinical manifestations

The incubation period averages 1 week (range 4 days to 2 weeks) after cutaneous inoculation. It is related inversely to the dose of inoculum. Symptoms start with non-specific malaise, chills, fever, myalgia, and headache that is often severe, followed by anorexia, nausea, vomiting, abdominal pain, photophobia, and cough. A rash usually appears after 3–5 days of illness. Initially, it consists of macular or maculopapular lesions, 1–5 mm in diameter, that blanch on pressure. Later, petechiae appear.

Pulmonary involvement causes cough, pulmonary oedema, radiographic infiltrates, hypoxaemia, dyspnoea, and pleural effusions in severe cases. Neurological manifestations consist of lethargy, progressing to confusion, delirium, stupor, ataxia, coma, focal neurological signs, and seizures. There may be a cerebrospinal fluid (CSF) pleocytosis of 10–100 cells/μl with variable proportions of mononuclear and polymorphonuclear leucocytes, and/or an increased protein concentration.

Although serum aminotransferases and bilirubin may be elevated, jaundice is observed in fewer than 10 per cent of patients, and hepatic failure does not occur. The white blood cell count is usually normal.

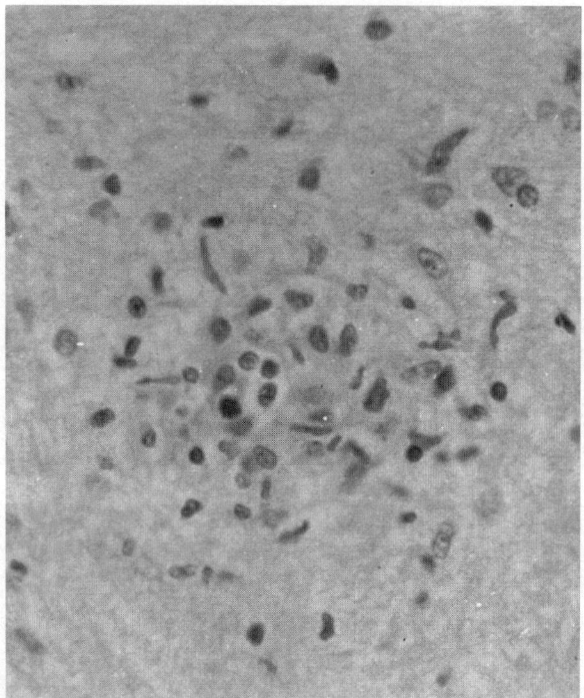

Fig. 2 Epidemic typhus fever. The typical lesion of rickettsial encephalitis is exemplified by the typhus nodule in the brain of a patient (death about 12th day) showing perivascular infiltration by macrophages and lymphocytes. *(Reproduced from Medical Clinics of North America (1959),* **43***, 1512, by permission.)*

Hypoalbuminaemia is probably the result of leakage of this plasma protein into the interstitial space because of increased permeability of the microcirculation. Hyponatraemia is most often the result of the appropriate secretion of antidiuretic hormone in response to the hypovolaemic state.

Diagnosis

Differential diagnosis

Early, before the rash has appeared, the differential diagnosis includes influenza, typhoid fever, enteroviral infection, and infectious diseases suggested by geographical exposure (e.g. malaria, Lassa fever). Nausea, vomiting, and abdominal pain may suggest infectious enterocolitis. Prominent abdominal tenderness has occasionally led to the differential diagnosis of acute surgical abdomen and to exploratory laparotomy. Cough and abnormalities of physical and radiographic examination of the chest may suggest bronchitis or pneumonia. Fever, seizures, coma, neurological signs, and abnormalities of the CSF may lead to consideration of meningitis and arboviral or herpes viral encephalitis. If an eschar is detected, the differential diagnosis may include cutaneous anthrax, tularaemia, syphilis, and chancroid. Once a rash has developed differential diagnosis includes meningococcaemia, Gram-negative bacterial sepsis, toxic shock syndrome, leptospirosis, disseminated gonococcal infection, secondary syphilis, measles, rubella, enteroviral exanthem, infectious mononucleosis, dengue, filoviral or arenaviral haemorrhagic fevers, idiopathic or thrombotic thrombocytopenic purpura, and immune complex vasculitides (e.g. systemic lupus erythematosus). It is important to enquire about exposure to ticks, fleas, mites, and lice and to consider the seasonal occurrence and the geographical exposure, but people are frequently unaware of their exposure to arthropods and cases may occur outside the seasonal peak .

Laboratory diagnosis

Serological tests are useful in confirming the diagnosis in the convalescent stage, but seldom detect specific antibodies during the first week of illness. At present, the best serological assays generally available are an indirect immunofluorescent antibody test, indirect immunoperoxidase antibody test, and latex agglutination test. These tests detect antibodies that are cross-reactive within the spotted-fever or typhus group. The Weil–Felix tests of agglutination of *Proteus* OX-19 and OX-2, although still used in some places, should be replaced because of poor sensitivity and specificity.

Isolation of the aetiological rickettia, the definitive diagnosis of an infectious disease, is seldom attempted because of the biohazard.

Identification of rickettsiae by immunohistochemistry in skin requires the presence of a rash to determine the site for biopsy and has a sensitivity of approximately 70 per cent and a specificity of 100 per cent in the hands of an experienced microscopist. A novel approach to the identification of rickettsial organisms that can be employed even during the period of illness before the onset of rash is immunofluorescent staining of rickettsiae in circulating endothelial cells captured by a monoclonal antibody fixed to immunomagnetic beads. PCR has not been very successful in diagnosing Rocky Mountain spotted fever early in the course of illness but has proved useful in murine typhus, epidemic typhus, Japanese spotted fever, boutonneuse fever, *R. felis* infection, and scrub typhus. Treatment should never be withheld while awaiting the results of tests.

Treatment

Spotted-fever and typhus group rickettsioses respond favourably to treatment with doxycycline (200 mg/day for adults and children greater than 45 kg, and 4.4 mg/kg body weight per day for smaller children), tetracycline (2 g/day in four divided doses for adults and 25 mg/kg body weight per day in four divided doses for children), or chloramphenicol (2 g/day in four divided doses for adults and 50 mg/kg body weight per day in four divided doses for children). Fluoroquinolones appear to be active against most rickettsiae, and ciprofloxacin (200 mg, intravenously every 12 h or 750 mg orally every 12 h), ofloxacin (200 mg orally every 12 h), and pefloxacin (400 mg intravenously or orally every 12 h) have been used successfully to treat boutonneuse fever. Epidemic typhus fever has been treated effectively under field conditions with a single, 200 mg dose of doxycycline. Treatment is generally continued for 2 or 3 days after defervescence to avoid relapse of the infection.

Intravenously administered doxycycline or chloramphenicol is employed when oral treatment cannot be used because of vomiting or coma. Chloramphenicol and josamycin (3 g/day for 8 days) have been used to treat rickettsioses during pregnancy when the tetracyclines are contraindicated.

Seizures should be treated with anticonvulsants. Renal failure is managed by haemodialysis, and hypoxaemia associated with interstitial pneumonitis and adult respiratory distress syndrome may require oxygen and mechanical ventilation.

Prevention

Immunization

Immunity to reinfection with spotted-fever or typhus group rickettsiae is quite strong, although some patients with epidemic typhus fever will develop recrudescence of latent *R. prowazekii* infection many years after their acute infection. There are at present no vaccines in general use against rickettsial diseases.

Vector control

Delousing reduces the spread of louse-borne epidemic typhus. Rodent control and insecticides decrease the incidence of murine typhus and rickettsialpox. Regular daily or twice-daily inspection of the entire body, especially the scalp and groin, and prompt removal of ticks prevents inoculation of rickettsiae. Ticks are best removed by grasping their anterior parts firmly with pointed forceps flush with the skin and exerting steady traction until the intact tick is removed, frequently with a bit of attached skin. Care should be taken to avoid introduction of potentially infected tick fluids into the wound or mucous membranes. The tick bite wound should be thoroughly cleaned.

Spotted fevers

Boutonneuse fever

Aetiology

The most prevalent spotted-fever rickettsiosis in Europe is boutonneuse fever, or Mediterranean spotted fever. *Rickettsia conorii* has also been isolated in Spain, South Africa, Kenya, Morocco, India, France, Croatia, Georgia, Russia, Ukraine, Pakistan, Israel, and Ethiopia. Recent investigations reveal that *R. conorii* has more antigenic diversity than the other carefully analysed spotted-fever group rickettsia, *R. rickettsii*, and that tick-borne *R. africae* is highly prevalent in southern and eastern Africa.

Epidemiology

R. conorii is maintained in *Rhipicephalus sanguineus* transovarially and is transmitted to humans by its bite. The peak incidence along the Mediterranean coast of southern Europe is in July and August when immature stages of the tick predominate. Boutonneuse fever occurs in urban, suburban, and rural environments, owing largely to the carriage of *Rh. sanguineus* by dogs. Mortality rates of 1.4–5.6 per cent have been observed in patients admitted to hospital. In those who are elderly or have underlying diseases, alcoholism, or glucose-6-phosphate dehydrogenase deficiency, case fatality may be 33 per cent.

Pathogenesis

The *tache noire* (black spot) or eschar at the site of the infective tick bite results from perivascular oedema and dermal and epidermal necrosis that is not secondary to thrombosis. Reduction in the number of rickettsiae in the eschar is associated with a perivascular influx of lymphocytes and macrophages. Autopsies of fatal cases of boutonneuse fever show systemic vascular infection and injury by *R. conorii*, with lesions in the brain, meninges, lungs, kidney, gastrointestinal tract, liver, pancreas, heart, spleen, and skin including sites of peripheral gangrene. Direct rickettsial injury of infected endothelial cells is the major pathogenic event. Hepatic biopsies show multifocal dead hepatocytes with a predominantly mononuclear cellular response.

Clinical manifestations

During the incubation period of boutonneuse fever, a red papule appears at the site of the tick bite and progresses to an eschar in approximately 70 per cent of cases, often associated with regional lymphadenopathy (Plate 1). The illness starts with fever, sometimes accompanied by headache and myalgias. The rash, which usually appears on the fourth day of illness, is maculopapular (Plates 2, 3), and petechial in 10 per cent of patients, and involves the palms and soles. Other features include nausea, vomiting, cough, dyspnoea, conjunctivitis, stupor, meningism, and hepatomegaly. Increased vascular permeability manifests as mild oedema, hypoalbuminaemia, and arterial hypotension. The white blood-cell count is usually normal. Platelet counts less than 100×10^9/l are detected in 12.5 per cent of the patients. Hyponatraemia of less than 130 mmol/l occurs in 23 per cent. Hypoproteinaemia is observed in 23 per cent of patients.

Serum urea and creatinine concentrations are elevated in 25 and 17 per cent of patients, respectively. Serum concentrations of aspartate and alanine aminotransferases are increased in 39 and 37 per cent, respectively, and serum bilirubin is greater than 20 μmol/l in 9 per cent. Severe features (6 per cent of patients) include cutaneous purpura and other haemorrhagic phenomena, neurological signs, altered mental status, respiratory symptoms and hypoxaemia, and acute renal failure.

Diagnosis

In the acute stage, diagnosis can be established by immunohistological demonstration of *R. conorii* in a biopsy of the *tache noire* or rash, or in circulating endothelial cells (see above). *R. conorii* can be isolated in guinea pigs or cell culture. Serological methods include indirect immunofluorescent antibody assay, latex agglutination test, indirect immunoperoxidase assay, dot enzyme immunoassay, and complement fixation test.

Treatment

See above.

Prevention

There is no vaccine to protect against *R. conorii.*

Rocky Mountain spotted fever

R. rickettsii is pathogenic for *Dermacentor* ticks, perhaps explaining why fewer than 1 in 1000 ticks in endemic areas contains *R. rickettsii.* There are dramatic, asynchronous, geographical fluctuations in the incidence of Rocky Mountain spotted fever over periods of 5–20 years. The annual reported occurrence has been approximately 600 cases in recent years.

R. rickettsii, the most virulent rickettsial species of the spotted-fever group, is also more invasive than other rickettsial species, causing infection not only of endothelial cells but also vascular smooth muscle cells. Host factors also play a part in severity of illness. Fatality rates are higher in older patients, males, and blacks. Fulminant Rocky Mountain spotted fever with death occurring within 5 days after onset is associated with haemolysis, particularly in black males with glucose-6-phosphate dehydrogenase deficiency.

Untreated, Rocky Mountain spotted fever has a 20 per cent case fatality rate. In recent series, the death rate has been 5 per cent, with respiratory failure in 12 per cent, acute renal failure in 14 per cent, and anaemia requiring red cell transfusion in 11 per cent. Thrombocytopenia occurs in 32–52 per cent of patients. Coma is a grave prognostic sign.

Early in the illness, nausea or vomiting occurs in 38–56 per cent of cases and abdominal pain in 30–34 per cent. The rash usually appears on the third day of illness, but may be delayed to or after day 6 in 20 per cent (Fig. 3). In 10 per cent of patients, a rash never appears. Petechiae occur in only 41–59 per cent of cases and appear late in the course, only on or after day 6 in 74 per cent. The palms

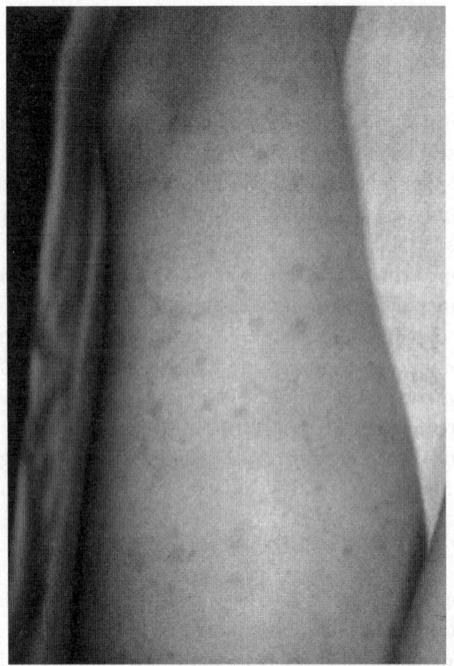

Fig. 3 The early rash of Rocky Mountain spotted fever consists of pink macules in this 4-year-old boy on the fourth day of illness.

and soles are affected by the rash in 36–82 per cent, with involvement occurring after day 5 in 43 per cent (Fig. 4).

A history of tick exposure is obtained from only 60 per cent of patients. Reagents for indirect immunofluorescent antibody assay, latex agglutination test, and dot-enzyme immunoassay for antibodies to *R. rickettsii* are commercially available.

Other tick-borne spotted-fever rickettsioses

R. sibirica, *R. australis*, *R. japonica*, *R. honei*, and *R. africae* differ antigenically in their surface proteins, DNA sequences, tick hosts, and known geographical distribution, but their clinical manifestations are similar to boutonneuse fever. The spotted-fever rickettsiosis of Flinders Island, Australia and Queensland tick typhus are clinically similar. Israeli spotted fever is a variant of boutonneuse fever in which eschar formation is usually lacking. *Rickettsia slovaca*, previously considered as non-pathogenic, was associated with clinical illness in western Europe. In Sweden, *R. helvetica*, transmitted by *Ixodes ricinus* ticks, has recently been implicated in fatal chronic perimyocarditis, *R. conorii*, *R. typhi*, and *R. rickettsii* are also known to affect the myocardium.

Rickettsialpox

R. akari has been isolated in the US, Ukraine, Croatia, and Korea. It is maintained by transovarian transmission in the gamasid mite

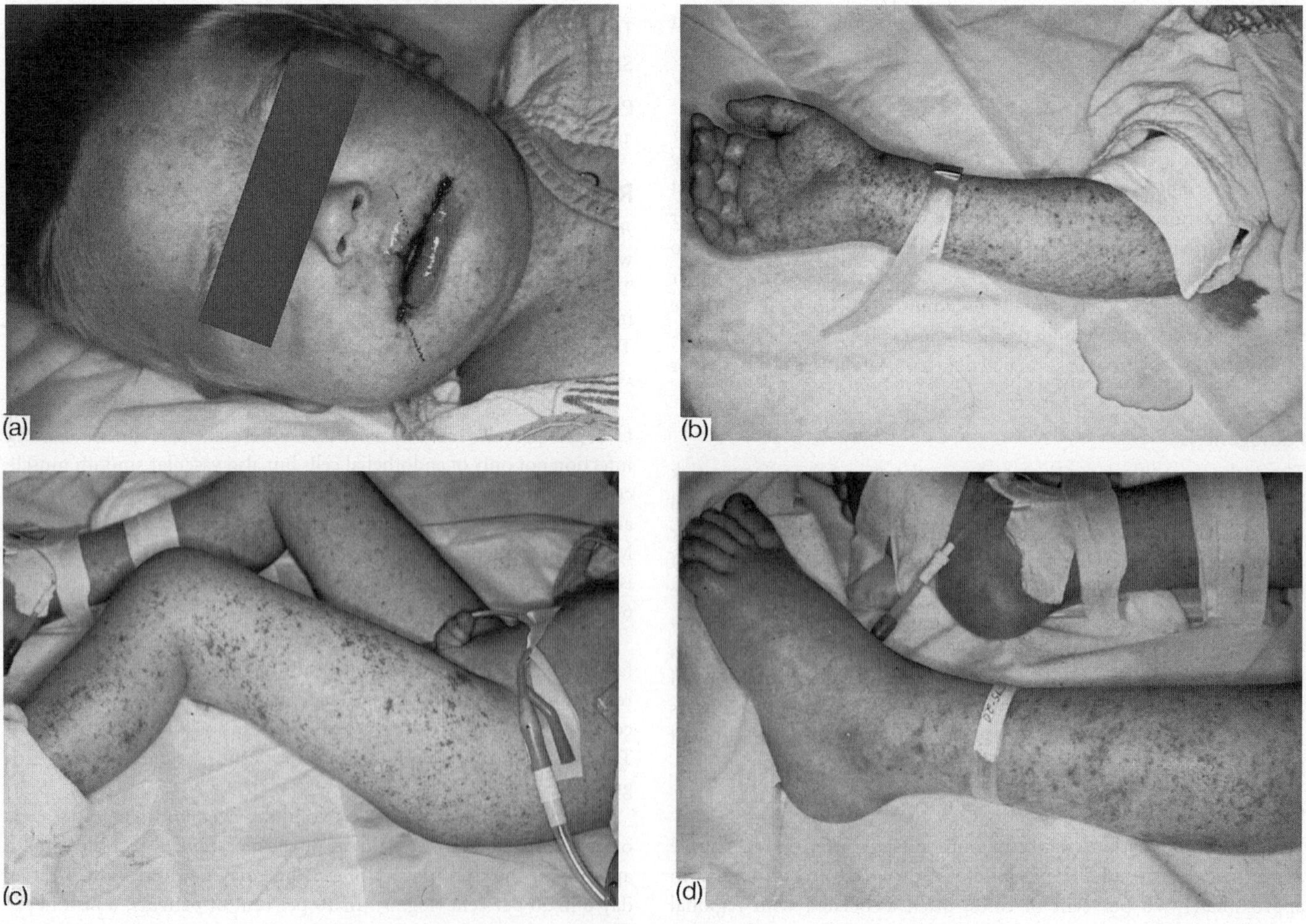

(a)

(b)

(c)

(d)

Fig. 4 Rocky Mountain spotted fever. Series showing haemorrhagic exanthem in a 4-year-old boy on about the eighth day of illness. Note oedema of face, hands, arms, and feet, and bleeding from mouth. Specific therapy with chloramphenicol resulted in complete recovery.

Liponyssoides sanguineus, whose host is the domestic mouse, *Mus musculus*.

A cutaneous papule appears during the incubation period at the site where the mite has fed and evolves into an eschar over the next 2–7 days. About 10 days later malaise, fever, chills, severe headache, and myalgia develop. A macular rash of discrete erythematous lesions, 2–3 mm in diameter, appears 2–6 days later and evolves into maculopapules some of which develop central, deep-seated vesicles.

Typhus fevers

Murine typhus

Endemic flea-borne typhus fever caused by *R. typhi* occurs in all continents except Antarctica and is more prevalent in warm, coastal ports. It is maintained in a commensal cycle involving rat fleas, *Xenopsylla cheopis*, and rats, *Rattus rattus* and *R. norvegicus*. Rats are infected by *R. typhi* in flea faeces deposited on the skin. Fleas become infected affected for life after a rickettsaemic blood meal. Other species of fleas and other mammals can also maintain an infectious cycle of *R. typhi* (see Table 1).

A rash is detected in 80 per cent of fair-skinned persons and in 20 per cent of blacks. Other features include nausea (48 per cent), vomiting (40 per cent), abdominal pain (23 per cent), diarrhoea (26 per cent), cough (35 per cent), abnormal chest radiographs (23 per cent), thrombocytopenia (48 per cent), elevated serum hepatic transaminases (90 per cent), and central nervous abnormalities (8 per cent) including confusion, stupor, and hallucinations. Case fatality is only 1 to 2 per cent, but the illness may last for 2 weeks. Nearly 10 per cent of patients admitted to hospital are severely ill with acute renal failure, respiratory failure, or severe neurological abnormalities including seizures. Older age, delayed treatment, and initial treatment with sulphonamides are risk factors for severe disease.

Epidemic typhus, recrudescent typhus, and sylvatic typhus

R. prowazekii causes epidemic louse-borne typhus fever, recrudescence of latent infection years after acute epidemic typhus, and zoonotic infection acquired from the ectoparasites of infected flying squirrels in North America. There is intense headache, prostration, continuous high fever, a macular rash usually appearing on the fourth or fifth day of illness, myalgia, and neurological abnormalities. Within 24–48 h of its appearance the rash becomes red, petechial, and does not blanch on pressure (Fig. 5). Its development is centrifugal from the trunk to the extremities. Other symptoms include cough, rales (71 per cent), nausea (30 per cent), abdominal pain (30 per cent), mental dullness (14 per cent), delirium (48 per cent), coma (6 per cent), seizures (1 per cent), and gangrene (3 per cent).

The infection is now restricted to a few foci of sporadic occurrence in eastern Europe, central Africa, Ethiopia, southern Africa, Afghanistan, northern India, China, Mexico, Central America, and the Andes Mountains of South America. However, the danger of spread still exists as occurred recently during the war in Burundi where it is estimated that 50 000 cases occurred. Recrudescent typhus (Brill–Zinsser disease) is the most important reservoir for initiation of epidemic louse-borne typhus in a susceptible population. Clinically it is milder than epidemic typhus (Fig. 6).

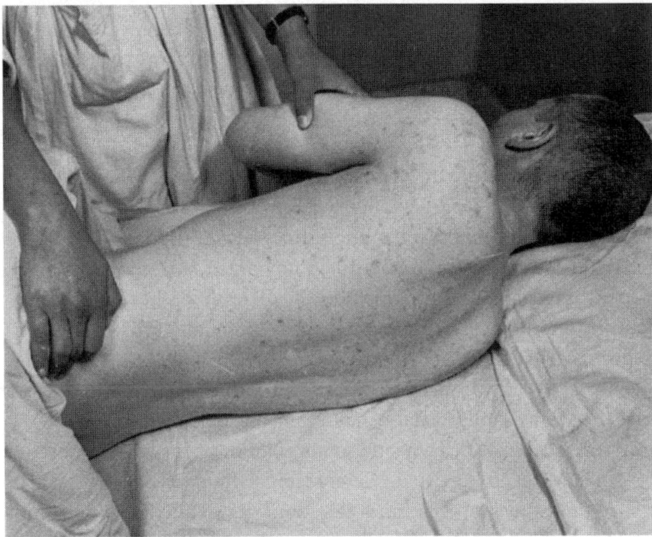

Fig. 5 Epidemic typhus fever. Typical truncal rash in louse-borne typhus on about the eighth day of illness showing many discrete haemorrhagic lesions.

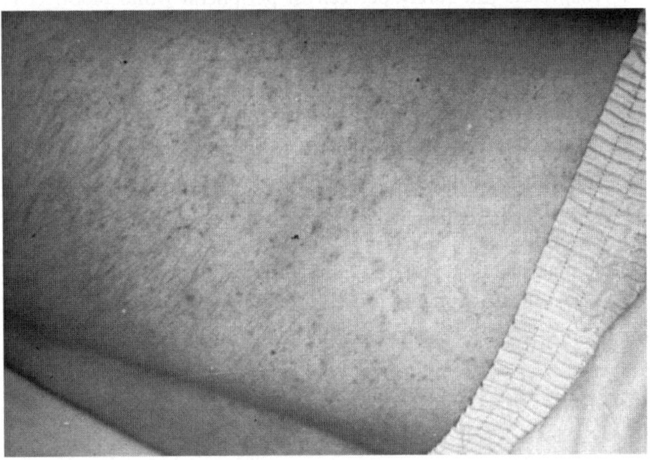

Fig. 6 Recrudescent typhus (Brill–Zinsser disease). Note the erythematous macular rash on the trunk. Illness is in an adult whose initial infection with typhus was 30 years earlier in Poland; second attack was a week after appendectomy—full recovery.

Ehrlichial diseases

Aetiological agents

Ehrlichiae are small, Gram-negative, obligately intracellular bacteria that reside in a cytoplasmic vacuole and are transmitted by ticks. The three human pathogens are *E. chaffeensis*, *E. sennetsu*, and a granulocytotropic ehrlichia, closely related to *E. phagocytophila*.

Ehrlichiae enter the host cell via phagocytosis, and they actively inhibit fusion of lysosomes with the phagosome. They undergo binary fission to form clusters within the host vacuolar membrane. When stained by the Wright–Giemsa method, the cluster of organisms appears dark violet-blue and stippled and is called a morula from the Latin word for mulberry.

Epidemiology (See Table 1)

Ehrlichioses are maintained in a cycle involving a mammalian host and a tick vector. *Ehrlichia sennetsu* is a member of a clade which resides in flukes that parasitize fish and snails and will eventually be placed in a separate genus. Most patients recall a recent tick bite. *E. chaffeensis* and human granulocytic ehrlichia infections peak between May and July, the season of greatest tick activity.

Human ehrlichioses

Haemopoietic cells are the primary targets of infection by *E. chaffeensis.* Leucopenia and thrombocytopenia are probably caused by peripheral sequestration. Perivascular lymphohistiocytic infiltrations without vascular damage are observed in virtually any organ, including meninges. Hepatic involvement may include focal death of hepatocytes. Interstitial mononuclear pneumonitis has been observed, as well as diffuse alveolar damage.

Clinical severity ranges to fatal infection. Most patients have a fever, headache, chills, malaise, nausea, myalgias, and anorexia. Respiratory or renal insufficiency and abnormalities of the central nervous system have been reported. Cerebrospinal fluid pleocytosis, leucopenia, thrombocytopenia, and elevations in serum hepatic aminotransferases are the clinical laboratory abnormalities demonstrated most often. Overwhelming, often fatal, cases occur in immunosuppressed patients, particularly those with HIV-1 infection.

E. chaffeensis can rarely be seen in peripheral white blood cells. The standard diagnostic test is indirect immunofluorescent antibody assay. A four-fold rise or fall in titre with a peak of 64 or greater is considered diagnostic. Human ehrlichiosis can also be diagnosed by detection of *E. chaffeensis* DNA amplified from the patient's peripheral blood by PCR. The *E. phagocytophilia*-like human granulocytic ehrlichial infection is diagnosed by finding of morulae in neutrophils in peripheral blood smears or by specific PCR or by serology. It has been reported as a relatively mild disease in Europe.

Human ehrlichioses respond to treatment with tetracycline (25 mg/kg body weight per day in four divided doses) or doxycycline (200 mg/day in two divided doses). Prevention is by avoiding tick bites.

Further reading

Azad, A.F. (1990). Epidemiology of murine typhus. *Annual Review of Entomology*, **35**, 553–69.

Bakken, J.S., Krueth, J., Wilson-Nordskog, C., Tilden, R.L., Asanovich, K., and Dumler, J. S. (1996). Clinical and laboratory characteristics of human granulocytic ehrlichiosis. *Journal of the American Medical Association*, **275**, 199–205.

Kass, E.M., Szqniawski, W.K., Levy, H., Leach, J., Srinivasan, K., and Rives, C. (1994). Rickettsialpox in a New York City hospital, 1980 to 1989. *New England Journal of Medicine*, **331**, 1612–7.

LaScola, B. and Raoult, D. (1997). Laboratory diagnosis of rickettsioses: current approaches to diagnosis of old and new rickettsial diseases. *Journal of Clinical Microbiology*, **35**, 2715–27.

Lotric-Furlan, S., Zupanc, T.A., Nicholson, W.L., Sumner, J.W., Child, J.E., and Strie, F. (1998). Human granulocytic ehrlichiosis in Europe: clinical and laboratory findings for four patients from Slovenia. *Clinical Infectious Diseases*, Sep 27(3), 424–8.

McDade, J.E. and Newhouse, V.F. (1986). Natural history of *Rickettsia rickettsii*. *Annual Review of Microbiology*, **40**, 287–309.

Nilsson, K., Lindqvist, O., and Pahlson, C. (1999). Association of *Rickettsia helvetica* with chromic perimyocarditis in sudden cardiac death. *Lancet*, **354**, 1169–73.

Perine, P.L., Chandler, B.P., Krause, D.K., McCardle, P., Awoke, S., Habte-Gabr, E., Wisseman, C. L. Jr, and McDade, J.E. (1992). A clinico-epidemiological study of epidemic typhus in Africa. *Clinical Infectious Diseases*, **14**, 1149–58.

Raoult, D., Weiller, P.J., Chagnon, A., Chaudet, H., Gallais, H., and Casanova, P. (1986). Mediterranean spotted fever: clinical, laboratory and epidemiological features of 199 cases. *American Journal of Tropical Medicine and Hygiene*, **35**, 845–50.

Rikihisa, Y. (1991). The tribe *Ehrlichieae* and ehrlichial diseases. *Clinical Microbiology Review*, **4**, 286–308.

Schreifer, M.D., Sacci, J.B. Jr, Dumler, J.S., Bullen, M.G., Azad, A.F. (1994). Identification of a novel rickettsial infection in a patient diagnosed with murine typhus. *Journal of Clinical Microbiology*, **32**.

Sexton, D.J., Dwyer, B., Kemp, R., and Graves, S. (1991). Spotted fever group rickettsial infections in Australia. *Reviews of Infectious Disease*, **13**, 876–86.

Walker, D.H. (1988). *Biology of rickettsial diseases*, Vols I and II. CRC Press, Boca Raton, FL.

Walker, D.H. and Gear, J.H.S. (1985). Correlation of the distribution of *Rickettsia conorii*, microscopic lesions, and clinical features in South African tick bite fever. *American Journal of Tropical Medicine and Hygiene*, **34**, 361–71.

Walker, D.H. and Fishbein, D.B. (1991). Epidemiology of rickettsial diseases. *European Journal of Epidemiology*, **7**, 237–45.

Walker, D.H. and Dumler, J.S. (1996). Emergence of ehrlichiosis as human health problems. *Emerging Infectious Diseases*, **2**, 18–29.

Walker, D.H. and Dumler, J.S. (1997). Human monocytic and granulocytic ehrlichioses. Discovery and diagnosis of emerging tick-borne infections and the critical role of the pathologist. *Archives of Pathology and Laboratory Medicine*, **121**, 785–91.

Chapter 16.73

Scrub typhus

G. Watt

Scrub typhus or Tsutsugamushi fever is an acute, febrile zoonosis of rural Asia. The causative organism, *Orientia* (formerly *Rickettsia*) *tsutsugamushi*, is transmitted to humans by bites of larval *Leptotrombidium* mites (chiggers). An eschar and regional lymphadenopathy often develop at the site of infection; this may by followed by a systemic illness ranging in severity from inapparent to fatal. Case fatality rates in untreated disease vary from 0–50 per cent. Many cases go undiagnosed, particularly those in which an eschar cannot be found. Serological confirmation is available only in specialized reference centres, but non-microscopic, rapid diagnostic tests have now been developed.

Aetiology and epidemiology

O. tsutsugamushi looks like a rickettsia under light microscopy but differs in cell wall structure and antigenic composition. There are multiple serotypes, and infection with one type confers only transient cross-immunity to another. Scrub typhus is a zoonosis. Larval mites (of the *Leptotrombidium deliense* group) usually feed on small rodents, particularly wild rats of the subgenus *Rattus.* Man becomes infected when he enters a zone where there are infected mites. These zones are often made up of secondary growth, hence the term scrub typhus. However, mite habitats as diverse as seashores, rice fields, and semideserts have been described. Infected chiggers are generally found in only very circumscribed foci within these zones. Large numbers of cases can occur when humans enter these 'mite islands'. During the Second World War, 1255 allied soldiers became ill with *O. tsutsugamushi* infection on two small islands off the coast of New

Guinea within 4 months. The endemic area forms a triangle bounded by northern Japan and south-eastern Siberia to the north, Queensland, Australia, to the south, and Pakistan to the west.

Pathology and pathogenesis

Scrub typhus is a disseminated, multiorgan vasculitis. There are great variations in clinical manifestations and severity.

Clinical features

The chigger bite can occur on any part of the body and is usually unnoticed. An eschar forms at the bite site in about 60 per cent of primary infections and in considerably fewer secondary infections. It begins as a small, painless papule which develops during the 6 to 18- (usually 9 to 12) day incubation period. It enlarges, undergoes central necrosis, and acquires a blackened scab (Plate 1). Regional lymph nodes are enlarged and tender. The eschar is generally well developed and healing at the start of symptoms. Fever and headache begin abruptly, and are frequently accompanied by myalgias, malaise, and weakness. More specific clues to the presence of scrub typhus are deafness and tinnitus, in up to a third of cases, conjunctival suffusion, and lymphadenopathy. A macular rash is a helpful sign, but is difficult to see on dark-skinned patients. The rash appears on the trunk late in the first week of illness and then spreads peripherally and becomes maculopapular.

Pulmonary involvement frequently dominates the clinical picture in mild cases and is a principal cause of death in patients with severe disease. Cough, tachypnoea, and infiltrates on chest radiographs are one of the commonest presentations of scrub typhus. In severe cases, tachypnoea progresses to dyspnoea, the patient becomes cyanosed and may develop adult respiratory distress syndrome. Apathy, confusion, and personality changes in moderate cases of scrub typhus are common and infrequently progress to stupor, convulsions, and coma. Some changes, such as deafness and personality changes, may persist for months. Eventually, however, abnormalities resolve completely in non-fatal cases.

The diagnosis can be straightforward in a patient with an eschar, rash, generalized lymphadenopathy, and a history of travel to an endemic area. The single most useful diagnostic clue is the eschar, which is pathognomonic. However, even a typical eschar can be overlooked or misdiagnosed. The differential diagnosis depends on the diseases prevalent in the area in which the illness originated. Eschars frequently occur in the genital region and often lose their crust. Thus they can be confused with the ulcers of chancroid, syphilis, or lymphogranuloma venereum. A haemorrhagic rash may suggest dengue. Typhoid rarely causes generalized lymphadenopathy or conjunctival suffusion. Marked myalgia with raised serum creatinine and serum bilirubin levels may suggest leptospirosis.

Laboratory diagnosis

Slight elevations of the total white count are typical and mild increases in liver transaminases occur. The Weil–Felix test using the *Proteus* OX-K antigen is a commercially available serodiagnostic method which has been used for many years, but is extremely insensitive. The IFA and immunoperoxidase tests are currently the serodiagnostic methods of choice but are not available outside a few reference centres. A rapid, accurate non-microscopic diagnostic kit using enzyme dotblot immunoassay has recently been developed. It is practicable in rural tropical Asia where sophisticated facilities are lacking and where most scrub typhus cases occur.

Treatment

Prompt antibiotic therapy is the single most important factor in shortening the disease, reducing mortality and speeding convalescence. It must often be presumptive, but the benefits of avoiding severe scrub typhus by early antibiotic administration outweigh the risks of a 1-week course of tetracycline—the treatment of choice. Either oral tetracycline 500 mg four times daily or oral doxycycline 100 mg twice daily for 7 days are recommended. Shorter treatment courses are often curative, but may result in relapse. Parenteral therapy should be used in patients who are vomiting or have severe disease. A 7-day course of parenteral chloramphenicol (50–75 mg/kg per day) is an effective alternative in areas where parenteral formulations of tetracyclines are unavailable. Good supportive care and early detection of complications is important in severe cases if a good outcome is to be obtained.

Scrub typhus cases which responded poorly to conventional therapy have recently been described from Chiangrai, Northern Thailand. Occasional strains of *O. tsutsugamushi* from other areas have shown antibiotic resistant *in vitro*, but clinical significance is uncertain. Azithromycin is equally effective and rifampicin is more active than doxycycline against resistant strains in mice. A controlled, blinded study demonstrated that rifampicin-treated patients in Northern Thailand became afebrile more quickly than did patients who received doxycycline. However, the optimum therapeutic regimen for the treatment of drug-resistant scrub typhus has not yet been determined. Therapy for pregnant women and children poses several problems. Chloramphenicol is best avoided during pregnancy and cannot be given to neonates; tetracycline is contraindicated in pregnancy and long courses administered to young children cause staining of the permanent teeth. Newer macrolide antibiotics appear to be effective for scrub typhus. Cases of both drug-sensitive and drug-resistant scrub typhus have been cured by azithromycin and three Japanese patients were treated successfully with clarithromycin. Macrolides would be particularly useful for the treatment of infection during pregnancy and early childhood.

Prognosis

Scrub typhus was a dreaded disease in the preantibiotic era; case fatality rates reached as high as 50 per cent. Prompt antibiotic therapy generally prevents death but up to 15 per cent of patients still die in northern Thailand. Deaths are attributable to a variety of factors including late presentation, delayed diagnosis, and drug resistance. The severity of scrub typhus does not appear to be increased in patients infected with HIV.

Prevention and control

Weekly doses of 200 mg of doxycycline can prevent *O. tsutsugamushi* infection. Non-immune populations occupationally exposed would benefit most from scrub typhus protection, but chemoprophylaxis should also be considered in high-risk travellers, such as those backpacking or trekking in endemic areas. Daily doxycycline is often recommended for the prevention of the drug-resistant strains of falciparum malaria which are particularly prevalent in parts of Asia, but it is not known whether this regimen will prevent scrub typhus.

Contact with chiggers can be reduced by not sitting or lying directly on the ground and by applying repellent to the tops of boots, socks, and on the lower trousers. Previous attempts to protect people against scrub typhus by immunization with inactive vaccines gave uniformly discouraging results; there has been little work on vaccine development for the past 50 years and there is no scrub typhus vaccine on the horizon.

Further reading

Berman, S.J. and Kundin, W.D. (1973). Scrub typhus in South Vietnam. *Annals of Internal Medicine*, **79**, 26–30.

Chayakul, P., Panich, V., and Silpapojakul, K. (1988). Scrub typhus pneumonitis: an entity which is frequently missed. *Quarterly Journal of Medicine*, **256**, 595–602.

Rosenberg, R. (1997). Drug-resistant scrub typhus—paradigm and paradox. *Parasitology Today*, **13**, 131–2.

Strickman, D. (1994). Serology of scrub typhus: new directions for an old disease. *Clinical Immunology Newsletter*, **14**, 62–5.

Watt, G., Chouriyagune, C., Ruangweerayud, R., *et al.* (1996). Scrub typhus infections poorly responsive to antibiotics in Northern Thailand. *Lancet*, **348**, 86–9.

Chapter 16.74

Coxiella burnetii infections (Q fever)

T. J. Marrie

Aetiology

Coxiella burnetii the aetiological agent of Q (Query) fever, has a Gram-negative cell wall and measures 0.3 × 1 μm. It is an obligate phagolysomal parasite of eukaryotes. In nature and laboratory animals it exists in the phase I state. Repeated passages of phase I virulent organisms in embroyonated chicken eggs lead to conversion to phase II avirulent forms. Antibodies to phase I antigens predominate in chronic Q fever while the reverse is true for acute Q fever.

C. burnetii has survived for 586 days in tick faeces at room temperature, ≥ 160 days in water, in dried cheese made from contaminated milk for 30–40 days, and for up to 150 days in soil. Spore formation by *C. burnetii* explains its ability to withstand harsh environmental conditions.

Epidemiology

Q fever is an zoonosis. There is an extensive wild life and arthropod (mainly ticks) reservoir of *C. burnetii.* Domestic animals are infected through inhalation of contaminated aerosols or by ingestion of infected material. These animals rarely become ill but abortion and stillbirths may occur. *C. burnetii* localizes in the uterus and mammary glands of infected animals. During pregnancy there is reactivation of *C. burnetii* and it multiplies in the placenta. The organisms are shed into the environment at the time of parturition. Humans becomes infected after inhaling organisms aerosolized at the time of parturition or later when organisms in dust are stirred up on a windy day. Infected cattle, sheep, and goats are the animals primarily responsible for transmitting *C. burnetii* to humans. In Atlantic Canada, infected parturient cats spread this micro-organism to humans. There have been several outbreaks of Q fever in hospitals and research institutes due to transportation of infected sheep to research laboratories. Individuals whose offices or laboratories were along the transportation route have developed Q fever as well as those involved in research. Acquisition of Q fever via the percutaneous or oral route is rare. There is a suggestion that *C. burnetii* may be sexually transmitted.

Vertical transmission from mother to child has been infrequently reported. It is likely, however, that this is much more common than we realize. It is also likely that reactivation of latent Q fever occurs during pregnancy in the human female as it does in other animals. Person-to-person transmission has been documented on a few occasions. The following countries should be considered major areas for *C. burnetii* infection: Australia, UK, France, Germany, Peoples Republic of China, Nova Scotia (Canada), Portugal, Spain, The Netherlands, Uruguay.

Clinical features

Humans are the only animals known that almost always develops illness following infection with *C. burnetii.* There is an incubation period of about 2 weeks (range 2–29 days) following inhalation of *C. burnetii.* A dose–response effect has been demonstrated experimentally and clinically. *C. burnetii* is one of the most infectious agents known to man as a single micro-organism is able to initiate infection. The resulting illness in man can be divided into acute and chronic varieties.

Acute Q fever

Self-limited febrile illness

The most common manifestation of acute Q fever is a self-limited febrile illness. In areas where Q fever is endemic, 12 per cent or more of the population have antibodies to *C. burnetii*—most of these infections are subclinical.

Pneumonia

This is the most commonly recognized manifestation of Q fever. The onset is non-specific with fever, fatigue, and headache. The headache may be very severe; on occasion so severe that it prompts a lumbar puncture. A dry cough of mild to moderate intensity is present in 24–90 per cent of patients. About one-third have pleuritic chest pain. Nausea, vomiting, and diarrhoea occur in 10–30 per cent. Most cases of *C. burnetii* pneumonia are mild; however about 10 per cent of cases are severe enough to require admission to hospital and, rarely, assisted ventilation is necessary. Mortality is rare in Q fever pneumonia and is usually due to comorbid illness. The white blood cell count is usually normal—it is elevated in 33 per cent of patients. There may be mild elevation of liver enzymes—two to three times normal. Reactive thrombocytosis is surprisingly common occurring in 60 per cent of patients and often reaching values of 700–800 × 10^9/l. Microscopic haematuria is a common finding.

The chest radiographic manifestations of Q fever pneumonia are usually indistinguishable from those due to any bacterial pneumonia, however rounded opacities are suggestive of this infection.

Hepatitis

The liver is probably involved in all patients with acute Q fever. There are three clinical pictures—(i) pyrexia of unknown origin with mild to moderate elevation of liver function tests; (ii) a hepatitis-like picture; (iii) 'incidental hepatitis'. In the latter case the major manifestation of Q fever is infection of another organ system with mild elevation of liver function tests. Liver biopsy reveals the distinctive doughnut granuloma, consisting of a granuloma with a central lipid vacuole and fibrin deposits.

Neurological manifestations

Encephalitis, encephalomyelitis, toxic confusional states, optic neuritis, and demyelinating polyradiculoneuritis are uncommon manifestations of Q fever.

Rare manifestations of acute Q fever

These include myocarditis, pericarditis, bone marrow necrosis, lymphadenopathy, pancreatitis, mesenteric panniculitis, erythema nodosum, epididymitis, orchitis, priapism, and erythema annular centrifigum.

Chronic Q fever

The usual manifestation of chronic Q fever is that of culture-negative endocarditis. Seventy per cent of these patients have fever and nearly all have abnormal native heart valves or prosthetic valves. Hepatomegaly and or splenomegaly occurs in about half of these patients and one-third have marked clubbing of the digits. A purpuric rash due to immune-complex-induced leucocytoclastic vasculitis and arterial embolism occur in about 20 per cent of patients. Hyperglobulinaemia (up to 50 g/l) is common and is a useful clue to chronic Q fever in a patient with the clinical picture of culture-negative endocarditis.

Other manifestations of chronic Q fever include osteomyelitis, infection of aortic aneurysm, and infection of vascular prosthetic grafts.

Diagnosis of Q fever

A strong clinical suspicion based on the epidemiology and clinical features as outlined above is the cornerstone of the diagnosis of Q fever. This suspicion is confirmed by determining a four-fold or greater increase in antibody titre between acute and 2 to 3-week convalescent serum samples. A variety of serological tests are available to detect antibodies to *C. burnetii* antigens—complement fixation, microimmunofluorescence (IFA), and enzyme-linked immunosorbent assay. The IFA test is easiest to use. In acute Q fever, the antibody titre to phase II antigen is higher than that to phase I while the reverse occurs in chronic Q fever. In chronic Q fever, antibody titres are extremely high, in the order of $\geq$ 1:8192 to phase I antigen. In acute Q fever, antibody titres to phase I antigen are rarely $>$ 1:512, while peak antibody titres to phase II antigen are 1:1024 to 1:2048.

Treatment

Quinolones and rifampicin are the most active agents *in vitro* against *C. burnetii*. Acute Q fever is treated with a 2-week course of tetracycline, doxycycline, or trimethoprim–sulfamethoxazole. Chronic Q fever should be treated with two antimicrobial agents for at least 3 years. Some authorities recommend life-long therapy for chronic Q fever. We use rifampicin 300 mg twice per day and ciprofloxacin 750 mg twice per day as agents of first choice. Rifampicin and doxycycline or tetracyclines and trimethoprim–sulfamethoxazole have also been used to treat chronic Q fever. The combination of doxycycline and chloroquine (chloroquine alkalinizes the phagolysosome rendering doxycycline bactericidal) has also been used with success. Doxycycline is given in a dose of 100 mg/day and hydroxychloroquine 200–600 mg/day to achieve a plasma concentration of 1 μg/ml. Antibody titres should be measured every 6 months for the first 2 years. A progressive decline in antibody titres reflects successful therapy of chronic Q fever.

Cardiac valve replacement may be necessary as part of the management of chronic Q fever. The decision to replace a valve is made for haemodynamic reasons. Prosthetic valve endocarditis due to *C. burnetii* has been successfully treated without valve replacement.

Prevention

A formalin-inactivated *C. burnetii* whole cell vaccine is protective against infection and has a low rate of side effects—1 per cent of vaccines developed an abscess at the inoculation site and another 1 per cent had a lump at this site 2 months following vaccination. Other measures to reduce Q fever infection are the use of only seronegative pregnant sheep in research facilities and control of ectoparasites on livestock.

Further reading

Brouqui, P., Dupont, H.T., Drancourt, M., *et al.* (1993). Chronic Q fever: Ninety-two cases from France; including 27 cases without endocarditis. *Archives of Internal Medicine*, **153**, 642–9.

Marrie, T.J., Durant, H., Williams, J.C., Mintz, E., Waag, D.M. (1988). Exposure to parturient cats is a risk factor for acquisition of Q fever in maritime Canada. *Journal of Infectious Diseases*, **158**, 101–8.

Turck, W.P.G., Howitt, G., Turnberg, L.A., Fox, H., Longson, M., Matthews, M.B., DasGupta, R. (1976). Chronic Q fever. *Quarterly Journal of Medicine*, **45**, 193–217.

Chapter 16.75

Bartonellosis, cat scratch disease, bacillary angiomatosis-peliosis, and trench fever

*J. G. Olson**

Background

During the last decade, the aetiology of cat scratch disease (**CSD**) was discovered, bacillary angiomatosis was recognized, and the relationship of these diseases to trench fever, an epidemic scourge of soldiers in the First World War, was demonstrated. On the basis of recent microbiological and genetic evidence, the aetiological agents of these diseases have been included in the genus *Bartonella*.

Bartonellosis

Bartonellosis (Carrión's disease, verruga peruana, Oroya fever, Guaitará fever) is a vector-borne, non-contagious, bi-phasic infectious disease, endemic to the western Andes and inter-Andean valleys of Peru, Colombia, and Ecuador.

*Includes some material from chapters by B. A. Perkins and E. A. Llanos-Cuentas, C. Maguiña-Vargas, and D. A. Warrell in OTM3.

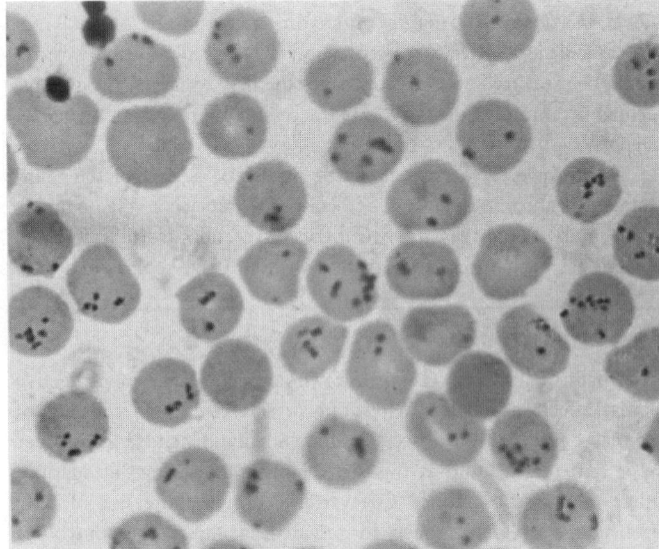

Fig. 1 Smear of peripheral blood with red blood cells parasitized by coccoid forms of *Bartonella bacilliformis* (Wright's stain: × 1048).
(Reproduced by courtesy of Professor Juan Takano Moron.)

Aetiological agent

Bartonella bacilliformis is a small, motile, aerobic, Gram-negative bacillus that stains deep red or purple with Giemsa stain (Fig. 1). The organism is flagellated and is 2–3 μm long and 0.2–2.5 μm thick. *B. bacilliformis* may occur in or on erythrocytes or in endothelial cells of infected human beings. *B. bacilliformis* and other *Bartonella* species can be cultured in blood-containing semisolid medium, or protease peptone containing rabbit serum and haemoglobin at 28°C under aerobic conditions.

Epidemiology

Bartonellosis is largely confined to narrow river valleys and canyons in the Peruvian Andes, between 500 and 3200 m above sea level. Outbreaks have been described in similar areas in Colombia and Ecuador. Transmission is greatest towards the end of the rainy season (March–May). The acute, severe form of the disease (Oroya fever) generally occurs among non-residents and epidemics have occurred when large groups of outsiders enter areas where disease is endemic. Transmission is by bites of female sandflies, *Lutzomyia verrucarum* and other anthropophilic species. Animals may also be infected. Humans may serve as a reservoir for the agent has been isolated from the blood of asymptomatic residents of endemic areas.

Clinical features

After an incubation period of about 60 days (range 10–210 days), non-specific prodromal symptoms appear: onset is usually gradual with malaise, mild chills, fever, and headache. Common symptoms include weakness, myalgias, prostration, and depression. The clinical picture is dominated by severe haemolytic anaemia; and patients rapidly become pale, dyspnoeic, and jaundiced. There may be hepatosplenomegaly, generalized lymphadenopathy, pericardial effusion, exudates, and retinal haemorrhages in the fundus, and sometimes generalized oedema, a fine vesicular or petechial rash, and exceptionally meningoencephalomyelitis. The duration of this state is variable (generally 2–4 weeks). Pregnant women are particularly at risk of a poor outcome; there may be abortion, fetal death, and transplacental transmission of the disease; maternal death is common. Patients may then become asymptomatic and take weeks to months to recover from the anaemia.

An eruptive stage (Plates 1, 2) may then develop lasting for 3–4 months and accompanied by mild arthralgia, myalgia, and sometimes fever. The skin lesions may resemble haemangioma, granuloma pyogenicum, bacillary angiomatosis, Kaposi's or fibrosarcoma, leprosy, or yaws. The mucous membranes of the mouth, conjunctiva and nose, serous cavities, and the gastrointestinal and genitourinary tracts may be involved. The eruptive phase tends to heal spontaneously. Inhabitants of endemic areas usually develop the eruptive stage as the sole manifestation of the disease.

The principal complications are secondary bacteraemias caused by *Salmonella typhi*, *S. typhimurium*, *S. dublin*, *Mycobacterium tuberculosis*, and Enterobacter and reactivation of tuberculosis, toxoplasmosis, histoplasmosis, pneumonia, and staphylococcal infections. This reflects a reversible immunosuppression.

Laboratory diagnosis

Bacteria are demonstrable in the blood film (Fig. 1) and in verrucous skin lesions and the organisms can be cultured from these sites. Serological tests, including enzyme immunoassay, indirect immunofluorescence, and Western blot and polymerase chain reaction (PCR), are useful for laboratory confirmation, but are not generally available. The haemolytic anaemia is Coombs' test negative. Reticulocytosis is marked (average 11 per cent). The marrow is hyperactive and megaloblastic with erythrophagocytosis. The white-cell count is not markedly elevated unless there is secondary infection. Thrombocytopenia is quite common.

Prognosis and treatment

Death generally occurs during the anaemic phase, Case fatality is reduced from between 20 and 95 per cent to about 8 per cent with antibiotic treatment. In the anaemic stage, chloramphenicol, penicillin, and tetracycline are dramatically effective, usually eliminating the fever in less than 48 h. Because of the common association with salmonellosis, chloramphenicol is the treatment of choice in a dose of 50 mg/kg a day for 7 days. The eruptive stages characteristically respond poorly to antibiotic therapy, although rifampicin (10 mg/kg a day for 10 days) or streptomycin (15 mg/kg a day for 10 days) may be useful.

Prevention

Sandflies can be temporarily eliminated from dwellings by spraying inside and outside with DDT or pyrethroids. Bites usually occur after dusk and can be prevented by insect repellents, sleeping inside insecticide-impregnated or fine-mesh nets, or by avoiding sleeping in highly endemic areas.

Cat scratch disease

CSD is characterized by the development of a regional lymphadenopathy followed by a cat scratch. Its first description appeared in France in 1950, and although it has long been considered an infectious disease, the aetiological agent had, until recently, remained elusive.

Epidemiology

CSD has been reported most often from North America, Europe, and Asia, but its true distribution is probably worldwide. Most epidemiological information has been based on case series, but some attempts have been made to develop population-based estimates for the incidence of CSD. In the USA, the estimated incidence of CSD in ambulatory patients is 9 cases/100 000 population. Some 0.8 cases/100 000 population are discharged from hospital with a diagnosis of CSD. These data support earlier estimates and suggest that CSD affects about 24 000 persons each year in the USA, resulting in approximately 2000 hospital admissions. Incidence in the USA is highest in humid southern states and lowest in arid western states.

Some important epidemiological aspects of CSD have been reported consistently. Most cases of CSD occur in children, but the disease is rare in infants. Estimates of the proportion of cases occurring in persons less than 18 years of age range from 55 to 87 per cent. In temperate areas, CSD has a distinct seasonal variation in occurrence with an autumn/winter peak. In the USA, 71–93 per cent of cases occur during August through January. Males and females appear to be affected equally.

The association between cats and the development of CSD was the basis for recognition of this disease. Over 90 per cent of reported cases have a history of contact with a cat, usually involving a scratch and most often by a kitten under 12 months of age. Cats implicated in transmission of CSD usually show no overt signs of illness. There have been occasional reports suggesting that injuries from other animals or inanimate objects may also result in CSD, but none has been aetiologically confirmed.

Multiple cases of CSD are often seen within a family, presumably related to exposure to the same cat. When this occurs, family members usually become unwell within a few weeks of each other, suggesting that cats may be infectious for only a short period.

In the USA, risk factors for the development of CSD include owning or being scratched or bitten by a kitten, but not by an adult cat. Compared with cat-owning controls, patients with CSD were more likely to have at least one pet kitten with fleas. This suggests that fleas may be involved in maintenance cycle of *B. henselae* in the cat.

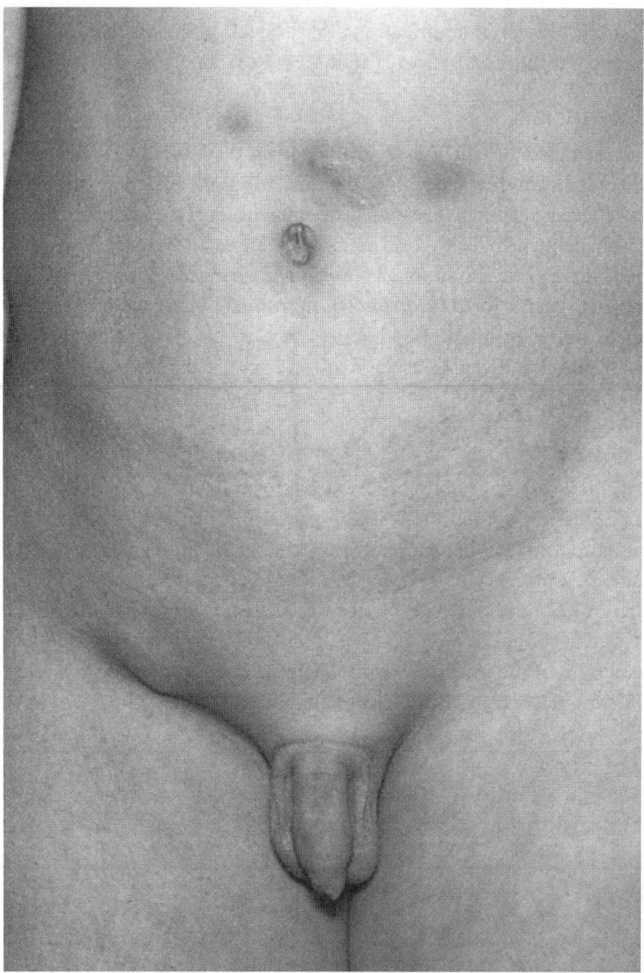

Fig. 2 Crusted erythematous papules at the site of a cat scratch above the umbilicus with bilateral inguinal lymphadenopathy, which developed 10 days later, in a 7-year-old boy.
(Copyright D. A. Warrell.)

Aetiology

Recent serological, epidemiological, and molecular findings indicate that *B. henselae* is responsible for CSD. *B. henselae* is a small, curved, pleomorphoric, Gram-negative rod that is oxidase and catalase negative, X-factor dependent, and sensitive *in vitro* to a broad range of commonly used antimicrobials including ampicillin, tetracycline, trimethoprim–sulphamethoxazole, and aminoglycosides. It is most closely related to *B. quintana*, the louse-borne agent of trench fever. There are many newly described species in the genus *Bartonella* that have been recovered from animals; but only four, *B. henselae*, *B. quintana* and two others, *B. elizabethae*, which was isolated from a single patient with endocarditis, and *B. bacilliformis* have been associated with human disease.

Clinical presentation

CSD is, by definition, a regional lymphadenopathy. Usually a single node or group of nodes is affected. The most common sites of lymphadenopathy are axillary, cervical, inguinal/femoral, and epitrochlear lymph nodes. Affected nodes are often tender and occasionally suppurate. About one-half of patients have 'primary inoculation lesions' manifested by skin papules, pustules, or other evidence of abnormal healing (Fig. 2). These lesions typically develop at the site of a cat scratch or bite 3–10 days after injury and precede the onset of lymphadenopathy by 1–2 weeks. Mild systemic complaints are common. About one-third of patients complain of fever and one-quarter have malaise or fatigue. Other non-specific clinical features associated with CSD include headache, anorexia, weight loss, vomiting, sore throat, rashes (maculopapular and rarely erythema nodusum), and splenomegaly. Although considered to be a self-limiting illness, signs and symptoms of CSD often persist for 2–4 months, and adenopathy may persist longer.

Atypical manifestations of CSD occur in less than 10 per cent of cases. Among these manifestations, Parinaud's oculoglandular syndrome is the most common. Patients present with a granuloma of the eyelid or conjunctiva and ipsilateral preauricular lymphadenitis. Recovery is usually complete without sequelae. Encephalopathy or other neurological disease, occasionally complicates CSD. Onset is sudden and usually follows the development of lymphadenopathy by 1 to 6 weeks. Although neurological signs are often dramatic and frequently include seizures and coma, patients recover completely over periods ranging from days to months. The cerebrospinal fluid is usually unremarkable. Hepatic granulomas, osteomyelitis, and pulmonary involvement have also been reported as rare complications of CSD. All parts of the respiratory tract may be affected; bilateral hilar lymphadenopathy and primary atypical pneumonia have been reported. Severe manifestations have been described in an immunocompromised patient. Fatalities are extremely rare.

Diagnosis

The diagnosis of CSD has evolved from a diagnosis of exclusion to one based on the laboratory confirmation of infection with the aetiological agent, *B. henselae.* The current case definition includes lymphadenopathy, with a serum IgG antibody titre >64 when tested by indirect immunofluorescence using *B. henselae* antigen; or PCR product specific for *B. henselae* as determined by restriction fragment length polymorphism or sequence analyses. Isolation of *B. henselae* is not practical as viable bacteria are seldom present when the patient seeks medical care.

Treatment

Antimicrobials have not yet been shown to be effective in the treatment of CSD. There are reports that Azithromycin, rifampin, ciprofloxacin, trimethoprim–sulphamethoxazole, and gentamicin may benefit some patients. Antimicrobials should be considered for severe cases of CSD but for the vast majority of uncomplicated cases of classical CSD, treatment should be directed toward relief of discomfort. Spontaneous resolution of the infected node is common, but aspiration or surgical removal may be necessary. Healing is usually rapid.

Prevention

Avoid cat scratches and bites. Cats implicated in transmission need not be destroyed.

Bacillary angiomatosis-peliosis

Bacillary angiomatosis was described in 1983 in an human immunodeficiency virus (**HIV**)-infected patient with fever and skin nodules. Since then it has been seen in many other HIV-infected patients (affecting skin and other organs) as well as in a few apparently immunocompetent individuals.

Epidemiology

Most cases of bacillary angiomatosis-peliosis have been reported from the USA but its incidence and global distribution are unknown. Epidemiological information is based on case reports, small case series and a single case–control study. In the largest reported series of cases ($n = 49$), 45 (92 per cent) were HIV infected, one was HIV negative and immunodeficient, and three (6 per cent) were HIV negative and apparently immunocompetent.

Case–control studies indicate that bacillary angiomatosis-peliosis patients whose aetiology was *B. henselae* but not *B. quintana* were more likely than controls to own cats, to be bitten or scratched by cats, to be exposed to a household cat with fleas and to be bitten by cat fleas. Case-patients with *B. quintana* infections were more likely than controls to be homeless, to have a low annual income, and to be infested with head or body lice. Neither case-patients infected with *B. henselae* or *B. quintana* were more likely than controls to be alcoholic or to use intravenous drugs.

Aetiology

Both *B. quintana* and *B. henselae* have been isolated from cutaneous lesions of bacillary angiomatosis. The aetiological role of *Bartonella* species in bacillary angiomatosis-peliosis is also supported by serological and molecular assay data. The morphological and staining characteristics, biochemical, and antimicrobial sensitivity profiles, as well as phylogenetic caveats for *B. quintana* are similar to those described for *B. henselae* in CSD.

Clinical presentation

Bacillary angiomatosis derives its name from the vascular proliferation and presence of numerous bacillary organisms in affected tissues. It has been reported to involve numerous tissues including skin, lymph node, muscle, bone, bone marrow, brain, liver, and spleen. Bacillary angiomatosis affecting the liver (also 'bacillary peliosis hepatis') and spleen has been referred to as 'bacillary peliosis'.

The most commonly recognized clinical presentation of bacillary angiomatosis is cutaneous or subcutaneous skin lesions in an HIV-infected individual, often with a low CD4 cell count. The skin lesions often mimic Kaposi's sarcoma. The presence of fever is variable and lesions may be diffuse or isolated, and slowly or rapidly progressive. Elevated liver enzymes and alkaline phosphatase are often seen in those with involvement liver or bone.

Diagnosis

Biopsy and histological examination of affected tissue is needed for the diagnosis of bacillary angiomatosis. It is not possible to distinguish bacillary angiomatosis clinically from Kaposi's sarcoma or other diseases that may affect the skin, spleen, liver, and other tissues, especially in HIV-infected or other immunocompromised persons. Histological criteria for the diagnosis of bacillary angiomatosis include characteristic vascular proliferation on routine haematoxylin and eosin staining, and of demonstration of bacillary organisms by silver staining (Warthin–Starry, Steiner, or Dieterle) or electron microscopy.

B. henselae and *B. quintana* have been isolated from cutaneous lesions of bacillary angiomatosis after cultivation of tissue homogenates with endothelial cell monolayers, followed by plating of the supernatants on to solid agar. These organisms can also be isolated from the blood using a lysis-centrifugation method.

PCR may be useful for detection of *Bartonella* species in tissue samples. Serological assays based on measurement of antibodies to *Bartonella* species may also be used to confirm aetiology.

Treatment

Erythromycin and doxycycline are the drugs of choice for patients with bacillary angiomatosis. Cutaneous and subcutaneous bacillary angiomatosis should be treated for at least 4 weeks. Treatment of parenchymal bacillary angiomatosis should be continued for a minimum of 6 weeks. Resolution of lesions is often complete but recurrence is common and longer courses of therapy may be warranted.

Prevention

Macrolide antibiotic (erythromycin, clarithromycin) prophylaxis is effective in preventing bacillary angiomatosis-peliosis. (See also under cat-scratch disease and Trench fever.)

Trench fever

Trench fever is a febrile illness first described among British soldiers in 1915. From 1915 to 1918 it was thought to account from 40 to 60 per cent of all illnesses among soldiers. There were no deaths but morbidity was significant. By 1918 it was concluded that trench fever was an infectious disease and that the aetiological agent was transmitted by the human body louse. In 1961, *B. quintana* was isolated from the blood of a patient with trench fever and Koch's postulates for the causation of trench fever by *B. quintana* were fulfilled in 1969. Since the end of the Second World War, reports of trench fever have been rare but recent data suggest that cases may have escaped recognition; clusters of cases in homeless alcoholic men have been identified in the USA and France.

Epidemiology

Endemic foci of trench fever have been identified in Poland, the former Soviet Republics, Mexico, Bolivia, North Africa, Ethiopia, and Burundi, but its true incidence and geographical distribution are unknown. *B. quintana* is transmitted by inoculation of contaminated louse faeces through a break in the skin from a louse bite or other injury. The incubation period is 7–30 days. Trench fever is not transmitted directly from person to person. The human body louse becomes infected by ingesting infected human blood.

Clinical presentation

High fever is the most common clinical feature of trench fever. Headache and myalgia are common prodromal symptoms. Onset of fever is acute or insidious and is often associated with headache, dizziness, and pains in the back, eyes, and legs, especially in the shins. Splenomegaly is common and a red macular rash (lesions 2–4 mm in diameter) may appear transiently. Complete recovery usually occurs within 5–6 weeks without antimicrobial therapy. Trench fever is not fatal but about half of the patients will have relapse of illness with fever and myalgia. Endocarditis has been described in recent reports.

Diagnosis

Blood culture using blood agar plates incubated at 37°C under 5 per cent CO_2 should yield growth of *B. quintana* within 2 weeks. Lysis-centrifugation methods for blood culture may also be useful. Serological assays may be valuable in the absence of positive cultures.

Treatment

Clinical response to tetracycline or chloramphenicol is prompt. It is not known whether extended therapy will prevent relapses.

Prevention

Control of the human body louse will prevent transmission of trench fever.

Further reading

Dalton, M.J., Robinson, L.E., Cooper, J., Regnery, R.L., Olson, J.G., and Childs, J.E. (1995). Use of *Bartonella* antigens for serologic diagnosis of cat-scratch disease at a National referral center. *Archives of Internal Medicine*, **155**, 1670–6.

Koehler, J.E., Sanchez, M.A., Garrido, C.S., Whitfield, M.J., Chen, F.M., Berger, T.G., *et al.* (1997). Molecular epidemiology of Bartonella infections in patients with bacillary angiomatosis-peliosis. *New England Journal of Medicine*, **337**, 1876–83.

Lumbreras, H. and Guerra, H. (1988). Bartonellosis. In *Tropical medicine and medical parasitology*, (ed. R. Golsmith and D. Heyneman), pp. 172–4. Lange Medical, Los Altos, CA.

Margileth, A.M. (1992). Antibiotic therapy for cat-scratch disease: clinical study of therapeutic outcome in 268 patients and a review of the literature. *Pediatric Infectious Diseases Journal*, **11**, 474–8.

Regnery, R.L. and Tappero, J. (1995). Unraveling mysteries associated with cat-scratch disease, bacillary angiomatosis, and related syndromes. *Emerging Infectious Diseases*, **1**, 17–21.

Relman, D.A. (1995). Has trench fever returned? *New England Journal of Medicine*, **332**, 463–4.

Chapter 16.76

Chlamydial infections

D. Taylor-Robinson, D. C. W. Mabey, and J. D. Treharne

Classification

The genus Chlamydia comprises at least four species of which three can infect humans. *Chlamydia trachomatis* causes ocular, genital, and systemic infections that affect millions of people world-wide. *C. pneumoniae* has been associated with outbreaks of human respiratory disease in many countries, and has also been isolated from horses. *C. psittaci* infects birds and other animals, resulting in major economic losses and is occasionally transmitted to man.

Growth cycle, serovars, and protein profile

Chlamydiae probably evolved from host-independent, Gram-negative ancestors that contained peptidoglycan in their cell wall. The chlamydial envelope, like that of Gram-negative bacteria, has inner and outer membranes. The infectious elementary bodies are electron dense, deoxyribonucleic acid rich, and approximately 300 nm in diameter. They bind to the host cell, enter by 'parasite-specified' endocytosis and after about 10 h differentiate into larger (800–1000 nm), non-infectious, metabolically active, reticulate bodies. These divide by binary fission and by 20 h begin to reorganize into a new generation of elementary bodies, which reach maturation 20 to 30 h after cell entry: their rapid accumulation forms an inclusion within the endocytic vacuole. They are released into the extracellular environment between 30 and 48 h after the start of the cycle.

All species of Chlamydia share a heat-stable, lipopolysaccharide antigen on the surface of the reticulate body, but not of the elementary body. The major outer membrane protein (MOMP) is immunodominant in the elementary body. It contains epitopes exhibiting genus, species, and serovar specificity. The serovar-specific epitope is the basis of the microimmunofluorescence test by which *C. trachomatis* has been separated into 15 serovars; A, B, Ba, and C are responsible mainly for endemic trachoma, and D to K for oculogenital infections. Serovars L1, L2, L2a and L3 of *C. trachomatis* cause the genital disease, lymphogranuloma venereum. So far, only one *C. pneumoniae* serovar has been identified. The loosely defined *C. psittaci* species is likely to contain a wide variety of host-related serovars.

Chlamydia trachomatis infections

Trachoma

Trachoma is a chronic keratoconjunctivitis believed to affect some 500 million people, of whom 7 million are blind and 10 million have visual impairment. After cataract, it is the most common cause of blindness worldwide, but is now confined largely to developing countries.

Clinical features

The active (inflammatory) stage of the disease is a follicular conjunctivitis affecting mainly the subtarsal conjunctiva, but follicles occur elsewhere on the conjunctiva and at the limbus, where on resolution they leave shallow depressions known as Herbert's pits. New vessels (pannus) (Plate 2) may be seen at this stage in the cornea, usually at the superior margin, and punctate keratitis may also be a feature. Since symptoms are mild or absent, the disease may not be suspected unless the upper eyelid is everted. Active trachoma affects mainly children in endemic areas. Among older children and adults in such areas, conjunctival fibrosis often develops as the follicles resolve (Plate 1) and, if severe, it may distort the upper lid margin, turning it inward (entropion). Lashes rubbing against the globe (trichiasis) cause continuous discomfort and sometimes blindness due to corneal damage.

Epidemiology

The reservoir of infection in endemic areas is the eye, and possibly the nasopharynx, of children with active disease. Active cases tend to cluster by household where there is the prolonged, intimate contact within the family. The higher prevalence of active disease and scarring in women than in men is due probably to the closer contact between women and children. *C. trachomatis* may be transferred from the eye of one individual to that of another, via fingers, by means of fomites, by coughing or sneezing, and by eye-seeking flies. Severe conjunctival scarring probably occurs only following repeated reinfection. The availability and use of water are important determinants of the development of trachoma. When living conditions improve trachoma tends to disappear.

Diagnosis

In endemic areas the diagnosis is generally made on clinical grounds. A number of viruses, notably adenoviruses, can cause follicular conjunctivitis. Intense cases of trachoma, in which follicles may not be visible, must be distinguished from bacterial conjunctivitis. Few conditions other than trachoma cause conjunctival scarring of the upper lid. *C. trachomatis* may be found in about 50 per cent of cases of active disease, but in only a minority where there is scarring.

Prevention

In Mexico, children who washed their faces seven or more times per week were less likely to have trachoma than those who washed less often. This simple intervention also proved effective in controlling trachoma in a study among rural villagers in Tanzania.

Genital-tract infections

Infections of the genital tract due to *C. trachomatis* (Table 1) occur worldwide and, at least in developed countries, are much more common than gonococcal infections.

Non-gonococcal urethritis

C. trachomatis is detectable in the urethra of not more than 50 per cent of patients with non-gonococcal urethritis and in up to 25 per cent of men with asymptomatic urethral infections. Chlamydiae may also cause urethritis in women but this is almost always asymptomatic. Thus, the dysuria and frequency experienced in the urethral syndrome are rarely of chlamydial origin.

Prostatitis and epididymo-orchitis

There is no evidence that *C. trachomatis* causes acute symptomatic prostatitis. In chronic abacterial prostatitis diagnosed by the Stamey

Table 1 Assessment of the extent to which *C. trachomatis*is involved in various oculogenital and associated diseases

Disease	*	Proportion of disease due to *C. trachomatis*
In men		
Acute non-gonococcal urethritis (NGU)	++++	Up to 50%
Postgonococcal urethritis	++++	Up to 50%
Persistent and recurrent NGU	+	?
Acute and chronic prostatitis	+	?
Acute epididymo-orchitis	++++	Up to 50%
Infertility	–	
In women		
Urethritis	+++	?
Bartholinitis	+	?
Vaginitis	–	
Bacterial vaginosis	–	
Cervicitis	++++	About 50%
Cervical dysplasia	+	
Endometritis	+++	?
Salpingitis	++++	40–60%
Periappendicitis	++	?
Perihepatitis	+++	?
Infertility	+++	About 10% due to chlamydial
Ectopic pregnancy	+++	?
Abortion	–	
In men or women		
Conjunctivitis	++++	?
Otitis media	++	?
Arthritis (Reiter's syndrome)	+++	About 40%
Endocarditis	++	?
Pharyngitis	–	
Proctitis	++	?
Lymphogranuloma venereum	++++	100% (by definition)
In infants		
Conjunctivitis	++++	Up to 50%
Pneumonia	++++	30%
Chronic lung disease	++	?

*Evidence that *C. trachomatis* is a cause:++++, overwhelming; +++, good; ++, moderate; +, weak; –, none.

procedure, biopsy tissues show chronic inflammation, but chlamydiae have not been detected in them by culture and direct immunofluorescence techniques, although about 10 per cent have proved positive by PCR technology. These largely negative observations, and the failure to detect chlamydial antibody, suggest that chlamydiae are not often implicated directly in the chronic disease. However, the possibility cannot be excluded that some chronic disease is chlamydial in origin, maintained possibly by immunological means.

C. trachomatis is responsible for epididymo-orchitis, especially in young men (< 35 years) in developed countries; it is detectable in at least one-third of epididymal aspirates. There is a strong correlation between IgM and IgG chlamydial immunofluorescence antibodies and chlamydia-positive disease. In patients older than 35 years, epididymo-orchitis tends to be caused by urinary-tract pathogens. There is no convincing evidence that chlamydiae cause male infertility.

Cervicitis and pelvic inflammatory disease

C. trachomatis has been associated weakly with bartholinitis, but not with bacterial vaginosis, or vaginitis. However, it causes mucopurulent/follicular cervicitis (Plate 3), which is often asymptomatic. Women younger than 25 years, unmarried, using oral contraceptives, and who have signs of cervicitis are the most likely to have a chlamydial infection. Canalicular spread of chlamydiae to the upper genital tract leads to plasma cell or lymphoid endometritis. Further spread causes salpingitis (Plate 4), perihepatitis (the Curtis Fitz-Hugh syndrome sometimes confused with acute cholecystitis in young women) and periappendicitis. Surgical termination of pregnancy or insertion or removal of an intrauterine contraceptive device may lead to dissemination.

Chlamydiae are the major cause of pelvic inflammatory disease in developed countries. Infertility complicates about 10 per cent of such disease and may be the first indication of asymptomatic tubal disease. Fertility is influenced adversely by an increasing number and severity of upper genital-tract infections and infertility may result from endometritis, blocked or damaged tubes, or perhaps abnormalities of ovum transportation. Other consequences of salpingitis are ectopic pregnancy and chronic pelvic pain.

Other diseases associated with *C. trachomatis*

Adult paratrachoma (inclusion conjunctivitis)

Adult chlamydial ophthalmia is distinguished from trachoma because it is caused by serovars D to K of *C. trachomatis* and commonly results from the accidental transfer of infected genital discharge to the eye. The acute or subacute conjunctivitis, usually unilateral, develops after an incubation period of 2 to 21 days. There is swelling of the lids, mucopurulent discharge, papillary hyperplasia due to congestion and neovascularization, and, later, follicular hypertrophy and occasionally punctate keratitis. The disease is generally benign and self-limited, but pannus formation and scarring may occur unless systemic treatment is given. One-third of patients have otitis media, complaining of blocked ears and hearing loss; *C. trachomatis* has been identified in aural discharges.

Arthritis

Arthritis occurring with or soon after non-gonococcal urethritis is termed sexually acquired reactive arthritis (SARA); in about one-third of cases, conjunctivitis and other features characteristic of Reiter's syndrome are seen. At least one-third of such disease is initiated by chlamydial infection and *C. trachomatis* elementary bodies and chlamydial DNA and antigen may be detected in the joints. *C. trachomatis* has also been associated with 'seronegative' arthritis in women. Although viable chlamydiae have not been detected in the joints, early tetracycline therapy may be indicated.

Immunocompromised states

C. trachomatis has been isolated from the lower respiratory tract of a few immunocompromised adults with pneumonia, some after renal transplantation, but its role has been obscured by the recovery of other agents from some. However, neither *C. trachomatis* nor *C. pneumoniae* are important respiratory-tract pathogens in patients with AIDS. Nor does genital chlamydial disease seem to be more widely prevalent or severe in such immunodeficient individuals and there is no evidence that hypogammaglobulinaemic patients are specially vulnerable to chlamydial infections.

Neonatal infections

Although intrauterine infection can occur, the major risk to the infant is from passing through an infected cervix. Between one-fifth and one-half of infants exposed in this way to *C. trachomatis* serovars D to K develop conjunctivitis (Table 1), usually 1–3 weeks after birth. A mucopurulent discharge and occasionally pseudomembrane formation occur, but it is usually self-limited. If complications do arise, however, they tend to be in untreated infants.

About half of the infants who develop conjunctivitis develop pneumonia, but the latter is not always preceded by conjunctivitis. Chlamydial pneumonia usually occurs between the fourth and eleventh week of life, after upper respiratory symptoms, and has an afebrile, protracted course in which there is tachypnoea and a prominent, stacatto cough. Hyperinflation of the lungs with bilateral, diffuse, and symmetrical interstitial infiltration and scattered areas of atelectasis are the radiographic findings. Children affected during infancy are more likely to develop obstructive lung disease and asthma than are those who have had pneumonia due to other causes.

Lymphogranuloma venereum

This is a systemic, sexually transmitted disease caused by serovars L1, L2, L2a and L3 of *C. trachomatis*. These chlamydiae are more invasive than the other serovars and cause disease primarily in lymphatic tissue.

Clinical features

Three stages of infection are usually recognized. After an incubation period of 3–21 days, a small, painless, papular, vesicular, or ulcerative lesion develops and disappears spontaneously within a few days without scarring. In men the lesion is on the penis, in women most commonly on the fourchette. These lesions, and especially rectal lesions in homosexual men, may go unnoticed. Extragenital primary lesions on fingers or tongue are rare.

The secondary stage is separated conventionally into inguinal and genitoanorectal syndromes. The former is more common and is usually seen in men as an acute, painful inguinal bubo. The lymphadenopathy is unilateral in two-thirds, and rarely may be so extensive that the inguinal mass is cleaved by the inelastic Poupart's ligament—the almost pathognomonic 'groove sign' of lymphogranuloma venereum. Buboes are accompanied by fever, malaise, chills, arthralgia, and headache. About 75 per cent of them suppurate and form draining cutaneous sinus tracts. In women, the external and internal iliac lymph nodes and the sacral lymphatics are involved more frequently than are the inguinal lymph nodes. Signs include a hypertrophic suppurative cervicitis, backache, and adnexal tenderness. In both sexes, but more frequently in women, a genitoanorectal syndrome characterized by a haemorrhagic proctitis or proctocolitis may occur. Inflammation is limited to the rectosigmoid colon and is accompanied by fever, a mucopurulent or bloody anal discharge, tenesmus and diarrhoea, but usually resolves spontaneously after several weeks. Rare manifestations of the secondary stage are acute meningoencephalitis, synovitis, pneumonia, cardiac involvement, and follicular conjunctivitis which is self-limited.

Lesions of the tertiary stage appear after a latent period of several years. They include genital elephantiasis, occurring predominantly in women as a sequel to the genitoanorectal syndrome and often accompanied by fistula formation, and rectal stricture which is found almost exclusively in women or homosexual men. However, such late complications are rare today because they can be prevented by broad-spectrum antibiotic therapy.

Epidemiology

Lymphogranuloma venereum is found world-wide, but its major incidence is limited to endemic foci in subSaharan Africa, South-East Asia, South America, and the Caribbean. All races are equally susceptible to infection, but the reported male: female ratio is usually greater than 5:1 because disease is recognized much more easily in men.

Diagnosis

The differential diagnosis includes genital herpes, syphilis, chancroid, donovanosis, extrapulmonary tuberculosis, cat-scratch disease, plague, filiariasis, lymphoma, and malignant diseases. Lymphadenitis of the deep iliac nodes may mimic appendicitis or pelvic inflammatory disease. Primary genital herpes causes the greatest diagnostic confusion.

The classical Frei skin test is no longer used for diagnosis. Specific detection of chlamydiae in lymphogranuloma is undertaken as for other chlamydial infections (see Laboratory diagnosis above). However, only 25–40 per cent of patients have positive cultures of bubo aspirate, endourethral, or endocervical scrapings, or of other infective material.

The complement fixation test is not specific and although the microimmunofluorescence test is not entirely specific it is the method of choice; antibody titres of more than 1:1024 are not uncommon and can be regarded as diagnostic, particularly in a patient with typical signs and symptoms.

Chlamydia pneumoniae infections

In 1989, *C. pneumoniae* was defined as the third species of the genus Chlamydia. Two isolates from conjunctival material collected in the mid-1960s from patients in trachoma endemic areas proved serologically distinct from *C. trachomatis* and *C. psittaci* and in 1983 a third *C. pneumoniae* strain was isolated, this time from the throat of a patient with acute pharyngitis. Since then, the organism has been isolated most often from respiratory infections.

Clinical features

At the outset of acute disease, pharyngitis is often present. More than 80 per cent of patients with lower respiratory-tract disease develop a sore throat. The cough comes on later. Fever is uncommon. Bronchitis is associated with some infections and in young adults, approximately 5 per cent of primary sinusitis is associated with *C. pneumoniae.* Mild respiratory infections are probably frequent but, overall, pneumonia has been the most common feature in mild cases, radiographs usually reveal a unilateral pneumonia, whereas in patients needing hospital care, bilateral pneumonia is quite common. This is often difficult to distinguish clinically from, for example, *Mycoplasma pneumoniae* infection.

Patients with chronic coronary heart disease or acute myocardial infarction were noted, first by Finnish investigators and then by others, to have antibody to *C. pneumoniae* significantly more often than age-matched controls. The topic remains contentious but the possibility that *C. pneumoniae* infection is a significant factor in the development of such disease is supported by detection of the organisms in atheromatous plaques of coronary and other major arteries by various techniques. An exaggerated synovial lymphocyte response to *C. pneumoniae* has been seen in some adults with reactive arthritis and, in addition, *C. pneumoniae* DNA and high titres of specific antibody have been detected in the joints of a few children with juvenile chronic arthritis.

Epidemiology

Serological evidence indicates that *C. pneumoniae* is widespread and endemic in many areas, and localized epidemics have been recorded in both military and civilian groups in Scandinavia, the US, and the UK. *C. pneumoniae* probably causes many mild respiratory infections that were thought previously to be viral and it is also likely that many infections attributed previously to 'human psittacosis/ ornithosis' were due to *C. pneumoniae.*

Transmission of *C. pneumoniae* appears to be from person-to-person without any intermediate host. It is quite common in families, schools, and other institutions. *C. pneumoniae* appears to be a significant cause of nosocomial pneumonia in patients in hospital with pre-existing chronic disease and may contribute to chronic obstructive pulmonary disease and asthma.

Chlamydia psittaci infections

Members of this diverse group of organisms have been isolated from mammals, frogs, and birds. Based on microimmunofluorescence serotyping and genetic analysis, 11 serovars have been proposed from mammals, seven from birds. *C. psittaci* causes a wide spectrum of animal disease and occasionally is transmitted to man, either as a result of contact with infected animals or from contact with faecal materials from an infected source. Psittacosis may be a hazard to those who keep pet birds or who work in poultry processing plants, or in animal husbandry. Many birds are known to harbour the organisms, but psittacine species (parrots), poultry, and pigeons are probably the major sources of human infection.

Clinical features

Respiratory infection with *C. psittaci* (psittacosis) is uncommon and mild in childhood and usually affects adults, particularly those in the 30 to 60-year age group. After an incubation period of 1–2 weeks, the clinical presentation can vary from a mild influenza-like illness to a fulminating toxic state with multiple organ involvement. The disease may start insidiously over a few days or start abruptly with high fever, rigors, and anorexia. Headache occurs in most, a cough, often dry, in over two-thirds, and arthralgia and myalgia in over one-third. Inspiratory crepitations are more common than classical signs of consolidation. Chest radiographs usually show patchy shadowing, most often in the lower lobes. Homogeneous lobar shadowing is less common, and miliary and nodular patterns even less so. Hilar lymphadenopathy has been reported in up to two-thirds of patients and a pleural reaction in more than half, but significant pleural effusions are infrequent. Extrapulmonary complications ascribed to *C. psittaci* are mostly rare, and include endocarditis, myocarditis, pericarditis, a toxic confusional state, encephalitis, meningitis, tender hepatomegaly, splenomegaly, pancreatitis, haemolysis, and disseminated intravascular coagulation.

Ovine *C. psittaci* strains have caused abortion in pregnant women after exposure to sheep suffering from enzootic abortion during the lambing season. The feline keratoconjunctivitis agent, isolated from the genital tract of female cats, has caused follicular conjunctivitis in man similar to that caused by *C. trachomatis* serovars D to K.

Laboratory diagnosis of chlamydial infections

Male and female 'first-catch' urine specimens, ignored for years because they were not suitable for chlamydial culture, are valuable samples, provided that the centrifuged deposits are tested by sensitive methods, notably molecular ones.

Detection tests

Isolation of *C. pneumoniae* may be facilitated by using a line of human lung cells. Culture of *C. trachomatis* involves the centrifugation of specimens (not required for *C. psittaci*) on cell cultures followed by incubation and staining with a fluorescent monoclonal antibody or with a vital dye, usually Giemsa, to detect inclusions. Direct staining of specimens with species-specific fluorescent monoclonal antibodies allows detection of elementary bodies, and is most suited to laboratories dealing with a small number of specimens and for confirming positive results obtained by other tests.

The popularity of enzyme immunoassays that detect chlamydial antigens is due to their ease of use, but it is rarely possible to detect small numbers of organisms (<10) of whatever chlamydial species. Thus, since at least 30 per cent of genital specimens contain such small numbers, many chlamydia-positive patients are misdiagnosed. However, PCR and ligase chain reactions, by enabling enormous amplification of a DNA sequence specific to the chlamydial species, have overcome the problem of poor sensitivity.

Serological tests

A good correlation has been found between IgG and/or IgA antibody, measured by microimmunofluorescence, in tears and the isolation of *C. trachomatis* from the conjunctiva of subjects with endemic trachoma or adult ocular paratrachoma. In genital infections, serum antibodies occur frequently in the absence of a current chlamydial infection of the cervix so that reliance cannot be put on a single serum or local IgA specific antibody titre to denote a current infection. In pelvic inflammatory disease, especially in the Curtis Fitz-Hugh syndrome, antibody titres tend to be higher than in uncomplicated cervical infections. A very high IgG antibody titre, for example 1:512 or greater, suggests causation in pelvic disease, but high levels do not always correlate with detection of chlamydiae and are associated more with chronic or recurrent disease. However, the detection of specific *C. trachomatis* IgM antibody in babies with pneumonia is pathognomonic of chlamydia-induced disease.

In primary respiratory infections with *C. pneumoniae*, IgM antibody develops within a few weeks and IgG antibody by 2 months. In repeat infections IgG, but not IgM, antibody develops more rapidly and to a greater titre than before. However, when only a single serum is available, it may be difficult to interpret information if there are cross-reacting antibodies to the other species. Only in children is the finding of *C. pneumoniae* antibody in a single serum sample an assurance of infection with this species. It is unwise to diagnose psittacosis or lymphorgranuloma venerum solely on the basis of the complement-fixation test as this will not distinguish between the chlamydial species.

Table 2 Susceptibility of *Chlamydia trachomatis* to various antibiotics*

Antibiotic	Minimum inhibitory concentration (μg/ml)	Minimum bactericidal concentration (μg/ml)
Rifampicin	0.005–0.25	0.015–0.25
Rosaramicin	0.015–0.25	0.05–0.25
Minocycline	0.015–0.5	
Tetracycline	0.02–0.5	0.02–2.0
Doxycycline	0.025–0.5	
Oxytetracycline	0.03–0.25	0.5
Erythromycin	0.03–0.5	0.1–4.0
Josamycin	0.03	
Roxithromycin	0.03	0.06
Miocamycin	0.06–0.125	
Chlortetracycline	0.125–2.5	0.125–2.5
Azithromycin	0.125	
Clindamycin	0.25–2.0	
Spiramycin	0.5	
Ofloxacin	0.5–1.0	0.5–1.0
Ciprofloxacin	1.0–2.0	1.0–2.0
Benzylpenicillin	0.25–50.0	1.0–>100.0
Ampicillin	0.25–50.0	>100.0
Sulphamethoxazole	0.5–50.0	
Chloramphenicol	1.0–10.0	>8.0–10.0
Augmentin	2.0	
Lomefloxacin	2.0–4.0	
Amoxycillin	2.0–>4.0	
Rosoxacin	4.0–8.0	4.0–8.0
Sulphisoxazole	2.0–200.0	2.0–500.0

*In addition, the following antibiotics with minimum inhibitory concentrations (MIC) in excess of 8 μg/ml have been tested and are shown more or less in order of increasing MIC: amifloxacin, enoxacin, pefloxacin, trospectomycin, sulphamethiazole, cloxacillin, norfloxacin, cephaloridine, trimethoprim, spectinomycin, flumequine, novobiocin, nalidixic acid, kanamycin, lincomycin, colistin, gentamicin, vancomycin, metronidazole, streptomycin.

Treatment of chlamydial infections

Chlamydiae are sensitive particularly to tetracyclines and macrolides, but also to other drugs (Table 2). Antibiotics with a MIC of 2.0 or more μg/ml are of no therapeutic value. The rifampicins are probably more active than the tetracyclines *in vitro* but are reserved usually for mycobacterial infections. Resistance to tetracyclines if it occurs, does not seem to have accounted for the occasional anecdotal report of therapeutic failure, but vigilance must be maintained for such resistance. Of the macrolides, erythromycin is used most often and

Table 3 Recommended treatment schedules for chlamydial infections and associated diseases

Disease/infection	Antibiotic	Dose schedule[a]	Duration (days)
Trachoma	Topical tetracycline or azithromycin alone	1% ointment twice daily for 5 days each month	6 months
		20mg/kg	Single dose
	For severe inflammatory trachoma		
	Tetracycline HCl or	500 mg 4 times daily	21
	doxycycline or	100 mg twice daily	21
	erythromycin sortearate	500 mg 4 times daily	21
Adult inclusion conjunctivitis	Antibiotics and regimens as for trachoma but without topical treatment		14
Non-gonococcal urethritis (NGU)	Antibiotics and regimens as for oral treatment of trachoma[b]		7
Epididymo-orchitis	Ampicillin	3.5 g	
	then antibiotics as for NGU		10
Cervicitis/urethritis	Antibiotics and regimens as for NGU		7
Pelvic inflammatory disease			
For ambulatory patient:	Ampicillin	3.5 g	
	then doxycycline	100 mg twice daily	10
For hospitalized patient:	(a) Doxycycline	100 mg twice daily (IV.)	≥4
	then doxycycline or	100 mg twice daily	10[b]
	(b) Clindamycin	600 mg 4 times daily (IV)	≥4
	and gentamicin	2 mg/kg (IV)	≥4
	and then	1.5 mg/kg 3 times daily	
	Clindamycin	450 mg 4 times daily	10[c]
Neonatal infections	Erythromycin syrup	50mg/kg daily in 4 divided doses	14
Lymphogranuloma venereum	Antibiotics and regimens as for trachoma but without topical eye treatment or		>14
	Trimethoprim-sulphamethoxazole[d]	80 mg twice daily	≥14
C. pneumoniae infections	Antibiotics and regimens as for NGU except doxycycline twice daily		7–21[e]
C. psittaci infections	Antibiotics and regimes as for NGU except doxycycline twice daily		>14

[a] All antibiotics orally unless otherwise indicated.

[b] For NGU, azithromycin given in a single 1g dose.

[c] Total duration of therapy 14 days.

[d] Less successful but does not mask concomitant syphilis.

[e] Relapse more often with short course.

is chosen for chlamydial infections in infants, young children, and pregnant and lactating women. Azithromycin in a single dose remains expensive but is gaining favour because it is effective and enhances compliance. Quinolones, particularly ofloxacin, are effective but are not used regularly.

Recommendations for dose and duration of antibiotic treatment are given in Table 3. In trachoma, because reinfection is rapid in endemic areas, treatment of individuals is ineffective and the World Health Organization has recommended regimens for mass treatment with topical 1 per cent tetracycline ointment. The principle of giving systemic treatment to eradicate nasopharyngeal carriage in severe trachoma applies also in neonatal chlamydial conjunctivitis where topical treatment provides no additional benefit. Oral erythromycin should be given to treat the conjunctivitis and to prevent the development of pneumonia. Azithromycin in a single oral dose (20 mg/kg) has been shown to be as effective as 6 weeks of topical tetracycline for active trachoma and may well be the drug of choice. In complicated genital-tract infections, such as epididymo-orchitis and pelvic inflammatory disease, treatment will almost certainly be needed before a microbiological diagnosis can be established, following which additional broad-spectrum antibiotic cover may be required. For lymphogranuloma venereum, at least 2 weeks of oral tetracycline or a sulphonamide are usually recommended (Table 3), and azithromycin is also effective. Fever and bubo pain subside rapidly but buboes may take several weeks to resolve. Suppuration and rupture of buboes are usually prevented by antibiotic treatment. Unruptured, fluctuant buboes should be aspirated using a syringe and large bore needle to prevent sinus formation. Fistulae, strictures, and elephantiasis may require plastic surgery, which should not be attempted until sufficient antibiotic treatment has been given to reduce inflammation and necrosis. In the case of *C. pneumoniae* and *C. psittaci* infections, treatment follows the same principles as for *C. trachomatis* infections, as they are susceptible to the same types of antibiotic. Treatment is likely to be most effective when given over a long rather than a short time, suboptimal doses are avoided, compliance is strict, and when, in the case of genital infections, partners of patients are also treated.

Further reading

Barron, A.L. (1988). *Microbiology of chlamydia.* CRC Press, Boca Raton FA.

Mabey, D.C.W., Bailey, R.L., and Hutin, Y.J.F. (1992). The epidemiology and pathogenesis of trachoma. *Review of Medical Microbiology,* 3, 1–8.

Mårdh, P-A., Paavonen, J., and Puolakkainen, M. (eds) (1989). *Chlamydia.* Plenum, New York.

Schachter, J., Ridgway, G.L., and Collier, L. (1998). Chlamydial diseases. In *Topley and Wilson's microbiology and microbial infections,*Vol 3 Bacterial infections (ed. L. Collier, A. Balows, and M. Sussman), pp. 977–94. Arnold, London.

Taylor-Robinson, D. (1991). Genital chlamydial infections: clinical aspects, diagnosis, treatment and prevention. In *Recent advances in sexually transmitted diseases and AIDS,* (ed. J.R.W. Harris and S.M. Forster), pp. 219–62. Churchill Livingstone, Edinburgh.

Taylor-Robinson, D. (1997). Evaluation and comparison of tests to diagnose *Chlamydia trachomatis* genital infections. *Human Reproduction,* 12 (suppl.), 113–20.

Taylor-Robinson, D. and Thomas, B.J. (1991). Laboratory techniques for the diagnosis of chlamydial infections. *Genitourinary Medicine,* 67, 256–66.

Taylor-Robinson, D. and Ward, M.E. (1989). Immunity to chlamydial infections and the outlook for vaccination. In *Vaccines for sexually transmitted diseases,* (ed. A. Meheus and R.E. Spier), pp. 67–85. Butterworth, London.

Chapter 16.77

Mycoplasmas

D. Taylor-Robinson

Mycoplasmas, originally called pleuropneumonia-like organisms, are the smallest free-living micro-organisms. Their lack of a cell wall makes them resistant to penicillins and some other antimicrobials. They are bounded by a pliable unit membrane. The mycoplasmas of human origin belong mostly to the family *Mycoplasmataceae,* comprising the genera *Mycoplasma,* organisms that metabolize glucose or arginine or both, and *Ureaplasma,* organisms that metabolize urea.

Some *Mycoplasma* species are of economic importance because of the pneumonia, arthritis, keratoconjunctivitis, and mastitis they cause among livestock and poultry in Africa, Australia, and other parts of the world, and some are a laboratory nuisance as occult contaminants of cell cultures. Sixteen *Mycoplasma* species have been isolated from humans, most often from the oropharynx. Most are constituents of the normal flora (Table 1).

Respiratory tract diseases

Mycoplasma pneumoniae infections

In the late 1930s, non-bacterial pneumonias were first recognized and brought under the heading of 'primary atypical pneumonia'. From one variety, in which cold agglutinins often developed, an infectious organism, the 'Eaton agent', was isolated in embryonated eggs in the early 1940s, and for a number of years was thought to be a virus. However, its mycoplasmal nature was established in the early 1960s and subsequently it was called *M. pneumoniae.*

Epidemiology

M. pneumoniae occurs worldwide and infection is endemic in most areas with a predilection for late summer and early autumn. Epidemic peaks have been observed about every 4–7 years in some countries. The incubation period ranges from 2 to 3 weeks. Spread from person to person is slow, fostered by continual or repeated close contact, for example within a family. It causes inapparent and mild respiratory tract infections more often than severe disease. In the USA, *M. pneumoniae* is estimated to cause 15–20 per cent of all pneumonias in general populations and in special cases, such as military recruits, it has been responsible for as much as 40 per cent of acute pneumonic illness.

M. pneumoniae affects children and adults, the consequence of infection depending upon age and immune status. In children less than 5 years of age, infections are common but usually mild and non-pneumonic. In teenagers up to 15 years old, about a quarter of infections result in pneumonia, while about 7 per cent do so in young adults. Thereafter, pneumonia is even less frequent, but generally is more severe the older the patient.

Pathogenesis

Adherence of *M. pneumoniae* organisms to respiratory mucosal epithelial cells, mediated by P1, P30, and possibly other proteins on the surface of the organisms, is a crucial factor in pathogenesis. This stimulates a humoral and a cell-mediated immune response. The pneumonic infiltrate is predominantly a peribronchiolar and perivascular cuffing by lymphocytes, most of which are thymus dependent.

Table 1 The occurrence, and disease-inducing capacity of mycoplasmas that have been isolated from humans

Mycoplasma	Frequency of isolation from the: Respiratory tract	Genitourinary tract	Cause of disease
M. buccale	Rare	–[1]	–
M. faucium	Rare	–	–
M. fermentans	Common	Moderate	++
M. genitalium	?Rare	Common	+++
M. hominis	Rare	Common	+++
M. lipophilum	Rare	–	–
M. orale	Common	–	–
M. penetrans	–	?Rare	–
M. pirum	–	?Rare	–
M. pneumoniae	Rare[2]	Very rare	++++
M. primatum	–	Rare	–
M. salivarium	Common	Rare	–
M. spermatophilum	–	?Rare	–
U. urealyticum	Rare	Common	+++
A. laidlawii	Very rare	–	–
A. oculi	–	Very rare	–

[1] No reports of isolation

[2] Except in disease outbreaks.

+++, ++,+, –, Strong, good, moderate, weak, no, respectively.

This initial lymphocyte response is followed by a change in the character of the bronchiolar exudate, with polymorphonuclear leucocytes and macrophages predominating. The rather slow development of these events on primary infection contrasts with an accelerated and often more intense host response seen on reinfection. It seems that the pneumonia which occurs in older persons is to some extent an immunopathological process, there being an immunological over-response to reinfection, the lung being infiltrated by previously sensitized lymphocytes.

Clinical features

Effects range from inapparent upper respiratory-tract infection to severe pneumonia. Clinical manifestations rarely permit an early definitive diagnosis of mycoplasmal pneumonia. Malaise and headache often precede chest symptoms by 1–5 days, and radiographic examination frequently reveals evidence of pneumonia before physical signs, such as rales, become apparent. Usually, only one of the lower lobes is involved and the radiograph most often shows patchy opacities. About one-fifth of patients develop bilateral pneumonia, but pleurisy and pleural effusions are unusual. The course of the disease is variable but often protracted and relapse is a feature. The organisms also may persist in respiratory secretions despite antibiotic therapy, particularly in hypogammaglobulinaemic patients, where excretion may continue for months or years rather than weeks. Although a few very severe infections have been reported, occurring usually in patients with immunodeficiency or sickle-cell anaemia, death has been rare.

A wide variety of extrapulmonary conditions may occur during or after the respiratory illness. These include the Stevens–Johnson syndrome and other rashes including urticaria; arthralgia; meningitis, encephalitis, and other neurological sequelae; haemolytic anaemia; myocarditis and pericarditis. Haemolytic anaemia with crisis is an autoimmune phenomenon brought about by cold agglutinins (anti-I antibodies). Some of the other complications, such as the neurological ones, may arise in a similar way, although *M. pneumoniae* has been detected in cerebrospinal fluid.

Neonatal respiratory diseases

Mycoplasmas in the vagina are transmitted to the infant rarely *in utero*, but often during birth. Ureaplasmas, in particular, may be isolated from the throats and tracheal aspirates of some newborns. Overall, ureaplasma-infected infants of very low birth-weight (under 1000 g) have died or have developed chronic lung disease twice as often as uninfected infants of similar birth-weight or those of over 1000 g. *M. hominis* has also been implicated in pneumonia soon after birth, albeit more rarely. It is uncertain whether these organisms are a cause of the disease in their own right or only together with the various bacteria that are associated with maternal bacterial vaginosis is an unresolved question.

Genitourinary and related diseases

Diseases in which mycoplasmas have been implicated are presented in Table 2.

Non-gonococcal urethritis

Most large colony-forming mycoplasmas cannot be considered as significant causes of non-gonococcal urethritis because they are isolated so rarely from the genitourinary tract either in health or disease (Table 1). However, *M. genitalium* has now been associated strongly with acute non-gonococcal urethritis, being detected in 20 per cent or more of such cases but in a significantly smaller proportion of healthy controls. In addition, it has been detected in about one-quarter of men with persistent or recurrent non-gonococcal urethritis, and may account for some of these cases.

Table 2 Genitourinary and associated diseases attributed, in part, to mycoplasmas or ureaplasmas and the strength of the association (for more details see OTM3, pp. 762–73)

Disease	*Mycoplasma or Ureaplasma* spp.	Strength of association
Non-gonococcal urethritis (acute and chronic)	*M. genitalium* *U. urealyticum*	+++ ++
Chronic abacterial prostatitis	*M. genitalium*	+
Epididymitis	*U. urealyticum*	+
Pyelonephritis	*M. hominis*	++
Infection stones	*U. urealyticum*	++
Vaginosis	*M. hominis* *U. urealyticum*	+++* ++*
Pelvic inflammatory disease	*M. genitalium* *M. hominis*	+ ++**
Postpartum and postabortal fever	*M. hominis* *U. urealyticum*	+++** +++**
Premature labour, miscarriage and low birthweight	*M. hominis* *U. urealyticum*	+++* ++*
Sexually acquired reactive arthritis	*M. genitalium* *U. urealyticum*	+ ++
Various conditions in immunocompromised patients	*M. hominis* *U. urealyticum*	+++ +++

+++,++,+, strong, moderate, weak, respectively.

*Together with other bacteria of bacterial vaginosis.

**Possibly together with other bacteria of bacterial vaginosis.

Qualitative isolation studies have failed to prove ureaplasmal pathogenicity in non-gonococcal urethritis, but quantitative data are in favour of this notion. Chimpanzee and human volunteer urethral inoculation studies and observations on immunocompromised patients indicate that ureaplasmas can cause acute non-chlamydial, non-gonococcal urethritis. Controlled antibiotic and serological studies support this contention. The frequency of ureaplasma-induced disease is not clear. The results of one volunteer experiment suggest that the organisms may cause disease the first time they gain access to the urethra but later insults result in colonization without disease, accounting for their frequent occurrence in the urethra of healthy men. They are less important than *Chlamydia trachomatis* and *M. genitalium* as causes of acute non-gonococcal urethritis and are implicated, together with *M. genitalium*, as a cause of chronic non-gonococcal urethritis.

Pyelonephritis and urinary calculi

In almost 10 per cent of patients with acute pyelonephritis, but not in controls, *M. hominis* has been isolated, sometimes in pure culture, from the upper urinary tract often in association with the development of antibody in serum and urine. These data suggest that *M. hominis* causes a few cases of acute pyelonephritis or acute exacerbations of chronic pyelonephritis, but there is no evidence for the involvement of ureaplasmas. Ureaplasmas produce calculi in animal models and have been found more frequently in the urine and in the stones of patients with infection than in patients with metabolic stones.

Pelvic inflammatory disease

Micro-organisms present in the vagina and lower cervix may ascend to the upper genital tract (normally assumed to be sterile) and cause inflammation of the fallopian tubes and adjacent pelvic structures. *M. hominis* has been isolated from the fallopian tubes of about 10 per cent of women with salpingitis but not from controls and the infection has been accompanied by a specific antibody response.

Ureaplasmas have been isolated directly from the fallopian tubes of a few patients with acute salpingitis, from pelvic fluid, and from a tubo-ovarian abscess, but their pathogenicity is uncertain.

Postpartum and postabortal fever

Like other vaginal micro-organisms, genital mycoplasmas have been found transiently in the blood after normal vaginal delivery and *M. hominis* has been isolated a day or more after delivery from the blood of 5–10 per cent of women with postpartum fever, sometimes accompanied by an antibody response. *M. hominis* has been isolated from the blood of about 10 per cent of women with post-abortion fever, together with an antibody response in about half of them. Ureaplasmas may contribute in the same way.

Joint disease

M. pneumoniae and other mycoplasma-associated arthritis

Infection with *M. pneumoniae* is often accompanied by non-specific arthralgia or myalgia during the acute phase, and occasionally it leads to migratory polyarthritis affecting middle-sized joints in adults. It is possible that this mycoplasma is implicated also in some cases of juvenile chronic arthritis, based on the occasional detection of a four-fold or greater rise in antibody titre. However, an aetiological association has not been confirmed. *M. hominis* has been isolated from septic joints, usually the hip, that have developed in mothers after childbirth and the arthritis responds to tetracycline therapy. Arthritis in immunodeficiency states is considered below.

Reiter's disease (see also Chapter 10.3)

Arthritis may occur after or concomitant with sexually transmissible, non-gonococcal urethritis (that is sexually acquired reactive arthritis: SARA) or may be associated with conjunctivitis and urethritis (Reiter's disease). *C. trachomatis* seems to be responsible for about 50 per cent of such cases in men and for an ill-defined proportion in women, who are genetically predisposed (HLA-B27 positive), and several investigators have considered a role for mycoplasmas. Ureaplasmas and *M. genitalium* should not be ignored in view of their implication in uncomplicated non-gonococcal urethritis. In this respect, arthritis has been seen to develop in untreated patients with non-gonococcal urethritis from whom ureaplasmas, but not chlamydiae, were isolated from the urethra. These organisms have not been isolated from synovial fluids or tissues but synovial lymphocytes from some patients have been shown to proliferate *in vitro* in response to ureaplasmal antigens. *M. genitalium* has been detected in the synovial fluid of a patient with SARA, but further evidence is required to establish a causal link.

Rheumatoid arthritis

Renewed interest in a possible link with mycoplasmas has been generated by polymerase chain reaction (PCR) detection of *M. fermentans* and also ureaplasmas in the joints of more than 20 per cent of patients with rheumatoid arthritis and other chronic inflammatory rheumatic disorders.

Disease in immunocompromised patients

M. pneumoniae may cause severe pneumonia in immunodeficient patients. It may persist for many months in the respiratory tract of hypogammaglobulinaemic patients, despite apparently adequate treatment. Mycoplasmal aetiology should be considered in hypogammaglobulinaemic patients who develop an abacterial septic arthritis. Thus, *M. pneumoniae,* in one instance together with *M. genitalium,* and *M. hominis, M. salivarium,* and, in particular, ureaplasmas have been isolated from synovial fluids of at least two-fifths of these patients. In some cases involving ureaplasmas, the arthritis has been associated with subcutaneous abscesses, persistent urethritis, and chronic cystitis. Although usually responding to tetracyclines or other antimicrobials to which the organisms are sensitive, they and the disease may persist for many months. Intravenous antibiotic therapy may be required and administration of antiserum prepared specifically against the organism in question may be helpful.

Haematogenous spread of *M. hominis* leading to septic arthritis, surgical wound infections, and peritonitis seems to occur more often after organ transplantation and in other patients on immunosuppressive regimens. Particularly common are sternal wound infections caused by *M. hominis* in heart and lung transplant patients.

In the late 1980s, *M. fermentans* was detected intracellularly in various tissues taken at autopsy from patients with acquired immune deficiency syndrome. Subsequently, treatment of human immunodeficiency virus (HIV)-infected cell cultures with tetracyclines or fluoroquinolones, active against mycoplasmas, was found to inhibit cell killing without affecting virus replication. In other studies, certain mycoplasmas (*M. fermentans, A. laidlawii*) enhanced cytopathic changes by HIV-1, fuelling the idea that mycoplasmas might act as a cofactor, enhancing HIV replication and accelerating disease progression. Later, *M. fermentans* was detected by PCR technology in peripheral blood mononuclear cells, throat, and urine of about 10, 20, and 5 per cent of HIV-seropositive patients, respectively, almost all of whom were homosexual men. These patients probably had the mycoplasma before they acquired the virus because the mycoplasma was detected with similar frequency in samples taken from HIV-seronegative patients, a large proportion of whom were homosexual men. The existence of mycoplasmas in the blood increases the chance of interaction with the immune system; cytokines so induced could enhance HIV replication with an increased loss of CD4+ cells, with the mycoplasma acting as a cofactor. However, no association has been found between infection by *M. fermentans* and the stage of the disease, the patients' CD4+ count or the viral load. This mycoplasma has been detected no more frequently in blood mononuclear cells of patients with fast-progressing HIV-associated disease than in such cells of patients with slow progressing disease. Thus, the importance of *M. fermentans* as a factor in the progression of HIV disease is dubious. The role of *M. penetrans,* isolated originally from the urine of a few homosexual men infected with HIV and associated serologically with HIV positivity, remains undetermined.

Laboratory diagnosis

Laboratory diagnosis of an *M. pneumoniae* infection depends usually on a serological test. While a cold agglutinin (non-specific) test may be useful, a complement-fixation test is undertaken in many laboratories and a fourfold or greater rise in antibody titre with a peak at about 3–4 weeks after the onset of disease occurs in about 80 per cent of cases and is indicative of a recent infection. An antibody titre of 1:128 or greater in a single serum is suggestive of an infection in the previous few weeks or months. Caution is required in interpretation of results because the complement-fixation test does not distinguish between *M. pneumoniae* and *M. genitalium.* Detection of antibody by microimmunofluorescence tends to be quite specific; IgM antibody in a single serum specimen provides some confidence in making an accurate diagnosis of a current infection or one within the previous few weeks.

Isolation of *M. pneumoniae* by culture is rarely attempted. The most sensitive medium is probably SP4, a modification of conventional mycoplasmal broth medium with fetal calf serum and a tissue-culture supplement. Culture and identification are slow but the PCR technique is rapid, sensitive, and specific. If an isolate is needed, the rational approach is to test specimens by both this technique and culture and then to continue to culture only those specimens that are PCR positive.

For the detection of mycoplasmas at other sites and particularly those infecting the genitourinary tract, material from urethral, cervical, or vaginal swabs or a centrifuged deposit from urine is added to separate vials of liquid medium containing phenol red and 0.1 per cent glucose, arginine, or urea. Culture of *M. genitalium* and *M. fermentans* often fails and they may be detected much more reliably by PCR technology. Commercial kits designed to isolate and identify ureaplasmas and *M. hominis* are available. Genital mycoplasmal infections stimulate antibody responses, but the various techniques available to detect them are rarely used diagnostically.

Treatment

Absence of a cell wall renders mycoplasmas indifferent to penicillins, cephalosporins, and other antimicrobials that affect cell-wall synthesis, but they are generally sensitive to those antimicrobials that inhibit protein synthesis. *M. pneumoniae*, like other mycoplasmas, is sensitive to the tetracyclines and apparently more sensitive to erythromycin than the other mycoplasmas of human origin. It is also inhibited by the newer macrolides, such as clarithromycin and azithromycin, and the newer quinolones, such as sparfloxacin. For pregnant women and children, erythromycin should be used rather than a tetracycline. Erythromycin has sometimes proved more effective than a tetracycline in adults. Successful treatment of clinical disease is not always accompanied by early eradication of the organisms from the respiratory tract, probably because most drugs are static rather than cidal. This is a possible reason for relapse in some patients and a plausible reason for recommending a 2–3-week course of antimicrobial treatment that should start as soon as possible based on clinical suspicion rather than on a confirmed laboratory diagnosis of *M. pneumoniae* infection, which may be slow.

Treatment of genitourinary infections must take into account the fact that a precise microbiological diagnosis may not be forthcoming. Patients with non-gonococcal urethritis should receive a tetracycline which inhibits *C. trachomatis, M. genitalium,* and ureaplasmas. Some ureaplasmas are tetracycline-resistant and patients who fail to respond should then be treated with erythromycin. A tetracycline should also be included for the treatment of pelvic inflammatory disease to cover *C. trachomatis* and *M. hominis.* However, some strains of *M. hominis* are tetracycline-resistant and lincomycin or clindamycin may need to be considered. Azithromycin, which is being used increasingly for chlamydial infections, is also active against a wide range of mycoplasmas.

Further reading

Cassell, G.H., *et al.* (ed.) (1993). The changing role of mycoplasmas in respiratory disease and AIDS. *Clinical Infectious Diseases,* **17** (Suppl. 1).

Maniloff, J., *et al.* (ed.) (1992). *Mycoplasmas. Molecular biology and pathogenesis.* American Society for Microbiology, Washington DC.

Taylor-Robinson, D. (1996). Infections due to species of *Mycoplasma* and *Ureaplasma*: an update. *Clinical Infectious Diseases,* **23,** 671–84.

Taylor-Robinson, D. (1996). Mycoplasmas and their role in human respiratory tract disease. In: *Viral and other infections of the human respiratory tract* (ed. S. Myint and D. Taylor-Robinson), pp. 319–39. Chapman and Hall, London.

Taylor-Robinson, D. and Furr, P.M. (1998). Update on sexually transmitted mycoplasmas. *Lancet,* **351** (Suppl. III), 12–15.

Taylor-Robinson, D. and McCormack, W.M. (1980). The genital mycoplasmas. *New England Journal of Medicine,* **302,** 1003–10; 1063–7.

Chapter 16.78

Donovanosis (granuloma inguinale)

J. Richens

Donovanosis, also known as granuloma venereum and granuloma inguinale, is a sexually transmitted infection characterized by anogenital and inguinal ulceration. It is rarely encountered outside a handful of endemic foci in the tropics. The cause is an intracellular Gram-negative bacillus called *Calymmatobacterium granulomatis* demonstrable within lesions as Donovan bodies.

Aetiology

C. granulomatis is a Gram-negative organism which will not grow on solid media. It is closely related to *Klebsiella* spp.

Epidemiology

The main endemic areas for donovanosis are currently Papua New Guinea, India, South Africa, and Brazil. The disease is particularly associated with low socio-economic status, poor hygiene, and prostitution. Transmissibility is thought to be low with reported rates of infection in partners of donovanosis patients rarely exceeding 50 per cent. In the exceptional circumstances of the donovanosis epidemic that affected Marind-Anim of Dutch New Guinea in the 1920s up to 30 per cent of adults became infected through ritual homosexual and heterosexual promiscuity. The predilection of donovanosis for the genitalia of sexually active persons and its association with other sexually transmitted diseases argue strongly for a sexual mode of

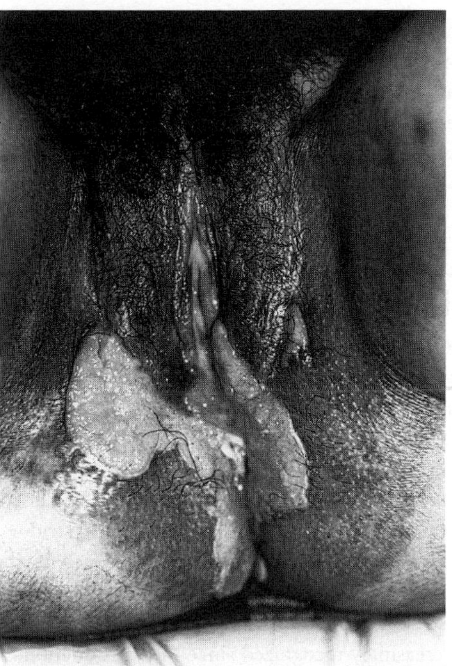

Fig. 1 Characteristic serpiginous ulcer in female patient with long-standing donovanosis.

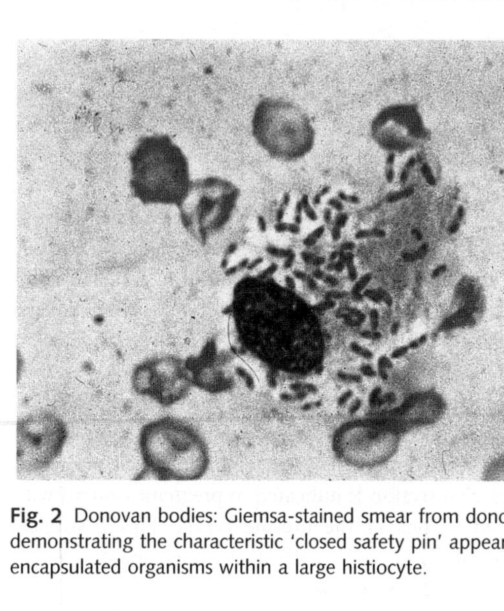

Fig. 2 Donovan bodies: Giemsa-stained smear from donovanosis lesion demonstrating the characteristic 'closed safety pin' appearance of encapsulated organisms within a large histiocyte.

transmission but rare instances of non-sexual and perinatal transmission have been recorded.

Pathogenesis

Transmission requires direct contact with an infected lesion but cannot occur through intact skin. The infection primarily affects skin and provokes a vigorous granulomatous inflammation that leads to ulceration. Extension tends to proceed along moist skin folds. The frequently observed inguinal lesions are probably seeded by lymphatic spread, although the main feature is one of ulceration of the overlying skin. Haematogenous dissemination and spread to the upper genital tract of women occur exceptionally and demonstrate the organism's ability to survive in deeper tissues. Lesions in women tend to be more extensive and may progress rapidly during pregnancy.

Clinical features

The incubation period ranges from 3 to 40 days. The first sign of infection is the development of a small papule, which then ulcerates usually on the distal penis in men and near the introitus in women. It is not easily differentiated from other types of genital ulcer. Mature lesions of donovanosis are typically non-tender, of a deep red colour, and bleed readily on contact. Hypertrophic lesions projecting above the level of the surrounding skin are common. Local oedema often accompanies lesions of the labia in women. Variants include: dry, warty lesions with a cobblestone appearance; painful, excavated ulcer; and lesions with an ill-defined edge showing diffuse subcutaneous infiltration. Chronic lesions tend to expand gradually along skin folds and across to apposed skin surfaces forming a large, continuous area of ulceration, with a characteristic serpiginous outline (Fig. 1). Inguinal lesions are common, especially in men. They start as a firm, subcutaneous swellings and often go on to ulcerate. Primary lesions of the cervix simulate carcinoma of the cervix. The uterus, fallopian tubes, ovaries, and adnexa may be involved, simulating pelvic inflammatory or malignancy with the development of a frozen pelvis, large, hard masses, or hydronephrosis. Anal lesions in women commonly spread directly from introitus; in men they are associated with anal intercourse. Involvement of the rectum seldom occurs.

Extragenital lesions occur in and around the mouth and sometimes on the neck. Haematogenous dissemination of donovanosis is associated especially with the trauma to an infected uterine cervix during pregnancy. The usual presentation is with one or more lytic bone lesions, which may break out through overlying skin. Spread to liver, spleen, and lung occurs exceptionally.

Complications of donovanosis include extensive scar formation, lymphoedema of the genitalia, penile autoamputation, and the development of squamous carcinoma in active or healed lesions. Secondary infection with fusospirochaetal organisms can cause rapid, extensive, and sometimes fatal tissue destruction.

Diagnosis

Donovan bodies are visible within large histiocytes in material taken from a lesion by biopsy or scrape (Fig. 2). Giemsa, Wright's, or Leishman stains are best for showing Donovan bodies in fresh material. For histological material, Giemsa and silver stains are the most helpful. Screening for concomitant infections, especially syphilis and human immunodeficiency virus (HIV) should be considered.

Donovanosis is readily confused with chancroid (a variant of chancroid, dubbed 'pseudogranuloma inguinale' has been described), syphilis, and anogenital cutaneous amoebiasis. The lymphoedema and inguinal lesions can resemble those seen with lymphogranuloma venereum or filariasis. The most common misdiagnoses are of squamous carcinoma of penis, vulva, or cervix, an error that may be compounded by misinterpretation of the epithelial hyperplasia as neoplastic and failure to identify Donovan bodies in haematoxylin and eosin-stained sections.

Treatment and prevention

Tetracyclines (of which doxycycline is the most convenient) are most widely recommended for the treatment of donovanosis and results are usually good, although well-documented cases of resistance have been reported. Good results has also been obtained with erythromycin, which is safe for use in pregnant women, and with co-trimoxazole. There is extensive experience with the use of chloramphenicol in Papua New Guinea and its reputedly safer relation, thiamphenicol, in South America. More recently, norfloxacin, azithromycin (500 mg daily or 1 g weekly), and ceftriaxone (1 g daily) have been shown to work well, the latter proving useful in the management of chronic resistant cases. All drugs given are given by mouth in standard doses and treatments should be continued until lesions have re-epithelialized and possibly longer, as relapse occurs quite commonly. Clinical resistance to many antibiotics has been reported; such cases may respond to a change of antibiotic. Combined antibiotic therapy should be considered in patients with HIV infection, severe disease, and resistant cases. Lesions in pregnant women may respond poorly to monotherapy. Caesarian section is indicated in pregnant woman with incompletely treated lesions of the uterine cervix. Plastic surgical procedures can do much to help patients with elephantiasis and strictures resulting from donovanosis.

Partners of patients should be examined and treated if infected. Epidemiological treatment may be appropriate for exposed contacts. The main hopes for the control of donovanosis lie in health education, condom promotion, and improving access to care for the poor in endemic areas.

Further reading

Richens, J. (1999). *Calymmatobacterium granulomatis* In: *Antimicrobial therapy and vaccines*, (ed. V.L. Yu, T.C. Merigan, S.L. Barriere), pp. 97–101. Williams and Wilkins, Baltimore.

Chapter 16.79

Rhinoscleroma

J. Richens

Rhinoscleroma or scleroma is a chronic infection that obstructs the upper respiratory tract and is caused by *Klebsiella rhinoscleromatis*. Endemic foci are found many developing countries.

Aetiology

K. rhinoscleromatis can be isolated from 60 per cent of lesions and can induce and be recovered from histologically similar lesions in the lungs of albino mice.

Pathogenesis

Transmission is believed to be from person to person in endemic areas. The incubation period is unknown. Three stages are recognized. Stage 1 resembles an atrophic rhinitis, with squamous metaplasia, hyperkeratosis, and atrophy. The nodular second stage consists of a granulomatous inflammatory reaction to the presence of *K. rhinoscleromatis* within macrophages. Bulky, soft-tissue masses develop in the respiratory mucosa and may extend into and destroy neighbouring soft tissues, cartilage, bone, and skin. Systemic spread does not occur but local spread may convey the infection to any point from the nares down to the lung hila. Histopathological examination shows a dense infiltrate of plasma cells among which are scattered the pathognomonic foam cells of Mikulicz, large histiocytes containing Gram-negative bacilli. In addition, Russell bodies, which originate from effete plasma cells, are often observed within macrophages. In the third stage of the disease, the infiltrates of early rhinoscleroma give way to increasing amounts of fibrosis and the organisms ultimately disappear.

Clinical features

Rhinoscleroma runs a very slow, fluctuating course over many years, progressing through atrophic, nodular, and fibrotic stages. Patients' general health is not affected. Most present with various combinations of nasal obstruction, nasal deformity (splaying of the lower nose, often with a visible growth extending down to the upper lip and around the alae nasi, known as Hebra nose), or bleeding (Fig. 1). An important subgroup of patients presents with stridor. Spread of nodular disease into neighbouring structures such as the paranasal sinuses, lacrimal apparatus, orbits, anterior cranial fossa, middle ear, nasopharynx, skin of the upper lip, and cervical glands may occur and has been increasingly recognized since the introduction of computed tomographic (CT) scanning and sinus endoscopy. Unusual oropharyngeal lesions of rhinoscleroma have recently been reported in a patient with human immunodeficiency virus infection.

Diagnosis

The diagnosis is best made by smear or biopsy combined with culture. Involvement of the trachea can be recognized on lateral neck radiographs or on CT scans, where concentric, irregular narrowing of the airways and crypt-like irregularities may be seen. Laryngoscopy, bronchoscopy, and endoscopy of the sinuses and nasopharynx may reveal additional sites of involvement.

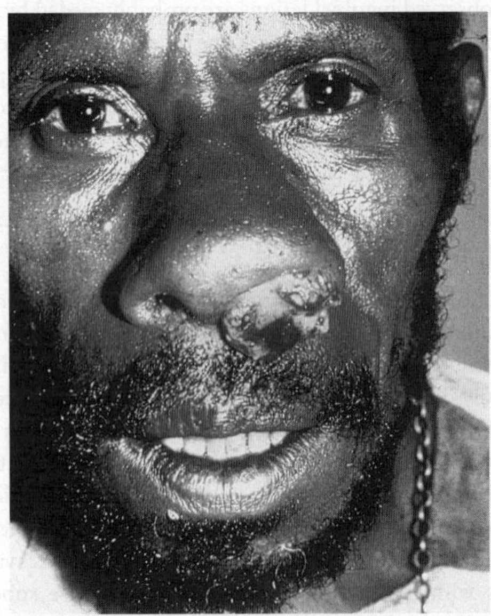

Fig. 1 Rhinoscleroma in a 30-year-old man from Papua New Guinea causing characteristic nasal splaying (Hebra nose) and obstruction of the left nostril.
(Reproduced from Cooke, R. (1987). Colour Atlas of Anatomical Pathology, p. 31. Churchill Livingstone, Edinburgh, with permission.)

Treatment

Monotherapy with tetracyclines, ampicillin, or co-trimoxazole given for 4–8 weeks may work for patients with early disease. A recent trial reported substantially better results with ciprofloxacin 250 mg twice daily for 4 weeks compared with rifampicin 300 mg twice daily and co-trimoxazole for 6 months. Patients with obstructing lesions may require referral to an ear, nose, and throat surgeon for debulking operations and occasionally temporary tracheostomy. The carbon dioxide laser has been used with encouraging results. Poor understanding of the transmission and epidemiology of rhinoscleroma has so far made it impossible to design practical interventions to prevent spread of the disease. Where the disease has declined in incidence, this has been generally attributed to improved standards of living.

Further reading

Amoils, C.P. and Shindo, M.L. (1996). Laryngotracheal manifestations of rhinoscleroma. *Annals of Otology, Rhinology and Laryngology*, **105**, 336–40.

Borgstein, J., Sada, E., and Cortes, R. (1993). Ciprofloxacin for rhinoscleroma and ozena. *Lancet*, **342**, 122.

Chapter 16.80

'Newer' and lesser known bacteria causing infection in humans

J. Paul

The range of bacteria associated with infection continues to grow and change. Correct usage of names is important in order to allow accurate communication. Clinicians need to have strategies which allow them to react appropriately when they encounter unfamiliar bacterial names during the course of their practice, such as when reading laboratory reports or when consulting the literature. Important issues include assessing the significance of an organism in a given clinical context and deciding on appropriate treatment. Part of the assessment process is the obtaining of information on the organism. It is intended that the notes presented below will act as a useful shortcut to those seeking basic information. A fuller treatment of the subject is given in OTM3, pp.778–96, which includes an alphabetical table of unusual bacteria, with a comprehensive set of references. Unfamiliar bacteria fall into a number of categories: long-known but rarely encountered pathogens, including zoonotic agents and organisms with restricted geographical distributions; long-known environmental and commensal organisms which on rare occasions cause opportunistic infection; newly characterized and described organisms associated with infection; name changes of well-known organisms. Rarely seen zoonoses include *Erysipelothrix rhusiopathiae*, the cause of erysipeloid and *Burkholderia mallei*, the cause of glanders. A number of organisms, including *Actinobacillus* spp., *Bergeyella zoohelcum* (formerly *Weeksella zoohelcum*), and *Capnocytophaga canimorsus* can be acquired from animal bites. Aeromonas infection is associated with leech bites and infections with *Streptococcus iniae*, *Edwardsiella tarda*, and *Vibrio carchariae* are associated with fish-related injuries. Organisms with restricted geographical distributions include *Burkholderia pseudomallei* associated with rice paddies in South-east Asia. A large group of environmental and commensal organisms, including *Acinetobacter* spp., *Bacillus* spp., pseudomonads, and coryneforms, may cause infection in debilitated and immunocompromised patients and in patients who have invasive or prosthetic devices. The distinction between colonist and pathogen becomes increasingly blurred, making assessment of significance more difficult. Newly described organisms, characterized as a result of advances in laboratory methods include those associated with cat-scratch disease: *Bartonella henselae* (formerly *Rochalimaea henselae*) and *Afipia felis*. Pending formal description, medically important bacteria are sometimes referred to in clinical literature by alphanumeric groups of the Centers for Disease Control, Atlanta (CDC groups). Advances in laboratory techniques allow a refined understanding of the taxonomic arrangements of groups of phenotypically similar organisms. This ongoing process necessitates taxonomic rearrangement and change of name. Recent examples include: the *Bacteroides* group, which was found to contain two new genera, *Prevotella* and *Porphyrimonas*; *Pseudomonas*, which has been split into *Pseudomonas*, *Comamonas*, *Brevundimonas*, *Burkholderia*, *Ralstonia*, and *Stenotrophomonas*; and *Flavobacterium*, which has been split into *Flavobacterium*, *Sphingobacterium*, *Empedobacter*, and *Chryseobacterium*.

The following list is intended to serve as a rough guide to some of the less familiar bacteria. It is necessarily selective and omits groups discussed elsewhere in this book, including anaerobes, chlamydias, rickettsias, mycoplasmas, spirochaetes, mycobacteria, actinomycetes, and certain genera. Generic names are listed in alphabetical order together with notes on medical importance and antibiotic susceptibilities. Caution must be exercised in interpreting the clinical significance of isolates: many are listed following published observation of association with disease, but fall short of fulfilling Koch's postulates. Antibiotics are listed as a rough guide only, many being listed on the strength of laboratory susceptibility data or usage described in single case reports; in managing individual patients, susceptibility data should be derived from the isolate causing the infection and therapeutic response monitored. Many of these obscure organisms are seen so rarely that it is difficult to establish their true clinical significance and to determine appropriate empiric treatment regimens (see OTM3, pp. 778–96).

Acinetobacter baumannii, A. calcoaceticus, A. haemolyticus, A. johnsonii, A. junii, A. lwoffi, A. radioresistens. Widespread in hospital environments. Common colonists and contaminants but also causes of infection in debilitated patients. Bacteraemia, urinary tract infection (UTI), wound infection, vascular line infection, osteomyelitis, endocarditis, meningitis. Nosocomial outbreaks may occur. Aminoglycosides, ureidopenicillins, ceftazidime, and carbapenems but may be multiresistant.

***Actinobacillus* spp.** *A. actinomycetemcomitans* occurs in human oral flora but may cause endocarditis and other infections and may be associated with actinomycosis. *A. ureae* is a respiratory tract colonist but may cause meningitis, endocarditis, and other infections. Wound infection with *A. equuli*, *A. lignieresii* or *A. suis* is associated with animal bites. Penicillin, ampicillin.

Aerococcus viridans, A. urinae. May cause bacteraemia, UTI, and endocarditis. Penicillin.

Aeromonas allosaccharophila, A. bestiarum, A. caviae, A. enteropelogenes, A. hydrophila, A. janaei, A. media, A. salmonicida, A. schubertii, A. trota, A. veronii. Wound infection, bacteraemia, meningitis, diarrhoea. Infection may be associated with exposure to water or leech bites. Aminoglycosides, ceftazidime, chloramphenicol and co-trimoxazole.

***Agrobacterium tumefaciens* (formerly *A. radiobacter*).** Endocarditis, continuous ambulatory peritoneal dialysis (**CAPD**) peritonitis and UTI.

Alcaligenes denitrificans, A. piechaudii, A. xylosoxidans. Infections in debilitated patients. Septicaemia, CAPD peritonitis, pneumonia, ear infection. Ureidopenicillins, ceftazidime.

Alloiococcus otitis. Otitis media. Role as pathogen poorly defined.

Arcanobacterium haemolyticum. Pharyngitis, cellulitis, septicaemia, osteomyelitis. Penicillin, erythromycin. *A. bernardiae* and *A. pyogenes* have been described recently from clinical material.

Bacillus. *B. anthracis* and *B. cereus* are well-known. Other *Bacillus* spp. are common contaminants and rare causes of infection, including septicaemia, meningitis, and eye infection. Species include *B. brevis, B. circulans, B. coagulans, B. licheniformis, B. sphaericus, B. thuringiensis.* Sensitivities to penicillin, carbapenems, vancomycin and clindamycin vary. Some species (of minor medical importance, including *B. alvei* have been transferred to *Paenibacillus*)

***Bergeyella zoohelcum* (formerly *Weeksella zoohelcum*).** Wound infection, septicaemia, meningitis. Dog and cat bites. β-lactams, tetracycline, quinolones.

Brevibacterium casei, B. epidermidis. Likely contaminants but possible causes of CAPD peritonitis and meningitis. Vancomycin.

***Brevundimonas diminuta, B. vesicularis* (formerly *Pseudomonas*).** Septicaemia. Opportunistic infection. Antipseudomonal antibiotics.

***Burkholderia cepacia, B. mallei, B. pseudomallei* (formerly *Pseudomonas*).** See Chapter 16.50. *B. pickettii* has been transferred to *Ralstonia.*

Capnocytophaga canimorsus, C. cynodegmi. Wound infection from dog bites. Septicaemia in splenectomized patients. Penicillin. Human species, *C. gingivalis, C. ochracea, C. sputigena* associated with septicaemia in neutropenics.

Cedecea davisae, C. lapagei, C. neterii. Rare causes of bacteraemia. Cephalosporins, aminoglycosides.

Chromobacterium violaceum. Bacteraemia, endocarditis, CAPD peritonitis. Associated with exposure to soil and water. Erythromycin, tetracycline, aminoglycosides.

***Chryseobacterium gleum, C. indologenes, C. meningosepticum* (formerly *Flavobacterium*).** Bacteraemia, meningitis, eye infection, endocarditis. Carbapenems, vancomycin, erythromycin, perfloxacin.

(***Chryseomonas luteola* has been transferred to *Pseudomonas luteola.*** Bacteraemia, endocarditis, CAPD peritonitis. Ampicillin, cefotaxime, aminoglycosides.)

Comamonas acidovorans, C. terrigena, C. testosteroni. Bacteraemia, conjunctivitis, UTI. Neutropenic sepsis. Ureidopenicillins, quinolones, carbapenems, aminoglycosides.

Corynebacterium. Generally called diphtheroids. *C. diphtheriae* is the agent of diphtheria. *C. pseudodiphtheriticum, C. ulcerans,* and *C. imitans* cause diphtheria-like infection. *C. minutissimum* is the cause of erythrasma. *C. pseudotuberculosis* causes pulmonary disease and is associated with sheep contact. Other species (*C. accolens, C. afermentans, C. argentoratense, C. auris, C. bovis, C. coryleae, C. cystitidis, C. glucuronolyticum, C. glutamicum, C. jeikeium, C. kutscheri, C. macginleyi, C. matruchotii, C. mycetoides, C. pilosum, C. propinquum, C. renale, C. seminale, C. urealyticum, C. xerosis*) may be colonists or contaminants but may cause infection in debilitated patients or under special circumstances. Empiric therapy poorly defined. Penicillin, erythromycin, or vancomycin may be appropriate.

Escherichia. *E. coli* is well-known. *E. fergusonii* is a cause of bacteraemia. *E. hermanii* and *E. vulneris* associated with wound infection. Cephalosporins, aminoglycosides.

Ewingella americana. Septicaemia, wounds, UTI. Penicillin.

(***Flavimonas oryzihabitans* has reverted to *Pseudomonas oryzihabitans.*** Septicaemia, CAPD peritonitis, eye infection. Ampicillin, gentamicin, tetracycline, cefotaxime.)

***Flavobacterium* spp.** (CDC groups IIe, IIh, IIi). From clinical material. Better known former members of *Flavobacterium* have been transferred to *Chryseobacterium*; others to *Sphingobacterium,* (*S. mizutae, S. multivorum, S. spiritivorum, S. thalpophilum, S. yabuchiae*). *Flavobacterium breve* has been transferred to *Empedobacter:* (*E. brevis*).

Hafnia alvei. Bacteraemia. Doubtful cause of diarrhoea.

Kluyvera ascorbata, K. cryocrescens. Bacteraemia, UTI, mediastinitis. Aminoglycosides, ceftazidime, quinolones, carbapenems.

Koserella trabulsii. Wounds, UTI. Chloramphenicol, gentamicin.

Myroides odoratus, M. odoratimimus. Formerly *Flavobacterium* and *Chrysobacterium.* UTI, wounds.

Ochrobactrum anthropi. Bacteraemia. Nosocomial infection in debilitated patients. Imipenem, ceftazidime.

Oligella urethralis. UTI, septicaemia. Associated with urinary catheters. Aminoglycosides, cephalosporins.

***Psychrobacter immobilis, P. phenylpyruvicus* (formerly *Moraxella phenylpyruvica*)** Meningitis, bacteraemia, eye infection. Penicillins, aminoglycosides, chloramphenicol.

Rahnella aquatilis. UTI, septicaemia. Immunocompromised patients. Quinolones.

Roseomonas gilardii, R. cervicalis, R. fauriae. Bacteraemia, wound infection, eye infection, urogenital infection. Aminoglycosides, imipenem, tetracycline.

Serratia fonticola, S. marcescens, S. plymuthica, S. proteamaculans. Septicaemia, burn sites, osteomyelitis. Nosocomial outbreaks reported. Carbapenems, ceftazidime, quinolones.

Shewanella alga, S. putrefasciens. Abdominal sepsis, meningitis, bacteraemia, UTI. Debilitated patients. Ampicillin, cefotaxime, chloramphenicol, gentamicin.

Sphingomonas paucimobilis. Septicaemia, UTI, wound infection, CAPD peritonitis. Antipseudomonal antibiotics.

Stenotrophomonas maltophilia. Bacteraemia, wound infection. Debilitated patients. Nosocomial outbreaks reported. Ureidopenicillins, cephalosporins, aminoglycosides, quinolones but may be multiresistant. *S. africana,* sensitive to ciprofloxacin, co-trimoxazole, netilmicin and colimycin, was isolated from the cerebrospinal fluid of an HIV-seropositive patient.

Further reading

Bruckner, D.A. and Colonna, P. (1997). Nomenclature for aerobic and facultative bacteria. *Clinical Infectious Diseases*, 25, 1–10.

Euzéby, J.P. (1997). List of bacterial names with standing in nomenclature: a folder available on the Internet. *International Journal of Systematic Bacteriology*, 47, 590–592.

Jousimies-Somer, H. and Summanen, P. (1997). Microbiology terminology update: clinically significant anaerobic Gram-positive and Gram-negative bacteria (excluding spirochetes). *Clinical Infectious Diseases*, 25, 11–14.

Moore, W.E.C. and Moore, L.V.H. (1992). *Index of the bacterial and yeast nomenclature changes*. American Society for Microbiology, Washington.

Skerman, V.B.D., McGowan, V., and Sneath, P.H.A. (ed.) (1989, amended edition). *Approved lists of bacterial names*. American Society for Microbiology, Washington.

Fungal infections and mycoses

Chapter 16.81

Fungal infections (mycoses)

R. J. Hay

Fungi are saprophytic or parasitic eukaryotic organisms with a subcellular organization similar to that of an animal cell but with the addition of a cell wall. Fungi form new cells either by terminal elongation to produce cell chains or hyphae (the mould fungi) or by a process of budding (the yeast fungi). Some fungi form yeasts during one phase of their life history but hyphae at another, a phenomenon known as dimorphism. Invasive fungal diseases are normally divided into three groups: the superficial, subcutaneous, and deep mycoses. In superficial infections, such as ringworm or thrush, fungi are confined to the skin and mucous membranes. Subcutaneous infections are usually tropical: the main site of involvement is within subcutaneous tissue, although secondary invasion of adjacent structures such as bone or skin may occur. In deep or systemic infections, deep sites such as lung, spleen, or brain are invaded. The fungi causing systemic mycoses are further subdivided into two groups, the opportunists and the endemic mycoses. The former cause disease in overtly compromised individuals whereas the endemic mycoses may cause infection in anyone. The geographical range of the mycoses is shown in Table 1.

Superficial fungal infections (mycoses)

The main superficial mycoses are the dermatophyte infections, superficial candidosis, and tinea versicolor. These are all common and widespread. Rare superficial infections include tinea nigra, and black or white piedra.

Dermatophyte infections (dermatophytoses)

The dermatophyte or ringworm infections are caused by a group of organisms capable of invading keratinized tissue such as stratum corneum, nail, or hair. The infections are known as ringworm or tinea.

Aetiology

Infections are caused by members of three distinct genera: *Trichophyton*, *Microsporum*, and *Epidermophyton*. Mechanisms of pathogenicity are thought to be linked to the production of extracellular enzymes, such as the three distinct keratinases produced by *Trichophyton mentagrophytes*, but other proteases may also be involved.

Epidemiology

Some dermatophyte fungi have a worldwide distribution; others are more restricted. The most common and widely distributed is *Trichophyton rubrum*. Other dermatophytes are limited to defined areas. For instance, tinea imbricata caused by *T. concentricum*, is found in hot, humid areas of the Far East, Polynesia, and South America. Scalp ringworm. tinea capitis, may occur in well-defined endemic areas where different species of dermatophytes may predominate. Thus, in North Africa, the most common cause of tinea capitis is *T. violaceum*; in southern parts of the continent, the major

Table 1 Geographic distribution of mycoses

Infection	Main geographic area
Superficial mycoses	
Dermatophytosis	Worldwide although some organisms such as those causing endothrix tinea capitis may be confined to certain countries *T. concentricum* is seen in remote areas in Oceania, Far East, and South America
Candidosis	Worldwide
Pityriasis versicolor	Worldwide
Subcutaneous mycoses	
Mycetoma	Tropics—particularly areas with low rainfall such as Sudan, Senegal, Mexico, Middle East, and Indian subcontinent
Chromoblastomycosis	Tropics—areas with higher rainfall, e.g. Central and South America, Southern Africa, and Far East
Sporotrichosis	Subtropics and tropics—southern USA, Central and South America, Africa, and Far East
Endemic systemic mycoses	
Histoplasmosis	Worldwide apart from Europe. Mostly seen in Americas, also west Africa and Far East
Blastomycosis	Mainly north and central North America—also north and central Africa. Rare elsewhere
Coccidioidomycosis	Desert and semi-desert areas of North, Central, and South America, e.g. south west USA and Mexico
Paracoccidioidomycosis	Scattered locations in Central and South America
Penicilliosis	South-east Asia, particularly northern Thailand
Opportunistic systemic mycoses	
	Worldwide. Cryptococcosis has a variable incidence in AIDS patients with high rates in some African countries and Thailand

agents may be *Microsporum audouinii*, *M. ferrugineum*, and *T. soudanense*. Not all scalp infections are endemic and dominant species may disappear to be replaced by others. *T. tonsurans*, for instance in isolated more often in US and UK cities.

Dermatophytes may be passed from person to person (anthropophilic infections), from animal to humans (zoophilic) or soil to humans (geophilic). Sources of zoophilic organisms in Europe include cats and dogs, cattle, hedgehogs, and small rodents.

Clinical features

The clinical features of dermatophyte infections are best considered in relation to the site involved. Often the term tinea, followed by the Latin name of the appropriate part (e.g. *corporis*—body) is used to describe the clinical site of infection.

Tinea pedis

Scaling or maceration between the toes particularly in the fourth interspace, is common. Itching is variable, but may be severe. Sometimes blisters may form both between the toes and on the soles of the feet. The causative organisms are commonly *T. rubrum* and *T. interdigitale*, the latter being responsible for the vesicular forms. Similar appearances can be caused by *Candida albicans*, Gram-negative bacteria and in erythrasma. *Trichophyton rubrum* infections may also affect the soles, or palms, with scaling spreading onto the sides of the foot or hands—'dry type' infections (Plate 1).

Tinea cruris

Infections of the groin, most often caused by *T. rubrum* or *Epidermophyton floccosum*, are relatively common, usually in males. An erythematous and scaly rash with a distinct margin extends from the groin to the upper thighs or scrotum. Itching may be severe.

Onychomycosis caused by dermatophytes

Invasion of the nail plate is most often seen with *T. rubrum* infections. The plate is invaded distally and becomes thickened and friable. Onycholysis may be seen. More rarely, and most often with *T. interdigitale*, the dorsal surface of the plate is invaded, causing superficial white onychomycosis.

Tinea corporis (body ringworm)

Dermatophyte or ringworm infection on the trunk or limbs may produce the characteristic annular plaque with a raised edge and central clearing (Plate 2). Scaling and itching is variable. Lesions caused by zoophilic organisms may be highly inflammatory and pustules (kerion) may develop on hairy skin. By contrast tinea of the face (tinea facei) is often difficult to recognize. Tinea imbricata is a tropical form of tinea corporis caused by *T. concentricum* which forms multiple concentric rings of scales on the body.

Tinea capitis (scalp ringworm)

Scalp ringworm is mainly a disease of childhood, with rare infections occurring in adult women. Spontaneous clearance at puberty is the rule. Certain organisms such as *M. canis* causes an ectothrix infection where spores form on the outside of the hair shaft and the scalp hair breaks above the skin surface. Scaling, itching, and loss of hair occur. Other causes of ectothrix infection include *M. audouinii*. This infection can be spread from child to child particularly in schools. By contrast, infections with *M. canis* are acquired from a primary animal source rather than by spread from human lesions.

In endothrix infections where sporulation is within the hair shaft, scaling is less pronounced and hairs break at scalp level (black dot ringworm). Examples include *T. tonsurans* and *T. violaceum*, the latter being most prevalent in the Middle East, parts of Africa, and India, although it is being recognized with increasing frequency in Europe. Infections may simply present with scaling and mimic dandruff (seborrhoeic dermatitis).

Favus, due to *T. schoenleini*, now most often seen in the tropics, is a particularly chronic form of ringworm where hair shafts become surrounded by necrotic crusts or scutula.

Table 2 Antifungal drugs

Drug	Route	Main side-effects[1]
Amphotericin B	Topical, IV	Renal failure, anaemia, hypokalaemia Fever, hypotension
Lipid associated AMB, e.g. liposomal colloidal dispersion, lipid complex	IV	Mainly fever and chills, less renal impairment than with AMB
Nystatin	Topical	–
Topical azoles (clotrimazole, miconazole, econazole, ketoconazole, etc.)		
Ketoconazole	Oral	May affect androgen biosynthesis Hepatitis
Itraconazole	Oral	Mainly nausea, headache, etc.
Fluconazole	Oral, IV	Mainly nausea, headache, etc.
Terbinafine	Oral, topical	Nausea, headache, taste disturbance
Amorolfine	Topical	–
Flucytosine	Oral, IV	Need to check plasma levels as renal excretion. Neutropenia, thrombocytopenia, hepatitis
Griseofulvin	Oral	Headache, nausea, urticaria,

[1] Side-effects after systemic use.

Laboratory diagnosis

The mainstays of diagnosis are direct microscopy of skin scales, hair, or nail clippings mounted in potassium hydroxide (20 per cent) to demonstrate hyphae, and culture. Further tests may be used to separate similar cultures. Identification of organisms is important, as it will indicate the source of infection in scalp ringworm for example. Scalp hairs may be screened with a filtered ultraviolet (Wood's light) lamp as *Microsporum* species show a green fluorescence.

Treatment

The treatment of dermatophyte infections depends to an extent on the nature and severity of infection (Table 2). Topical therapy is reserved for circumscribed infections whereas scalp and nail infections, severe or widespread ringworm, and failures of topical therapy are usually treated orally.

An old but cheap preparation is Whitfield's ointment (benzoic acid compound) usually in half-strength More specific topical antifungal drugs are at least as effective and are better tolerated than Whitfield's ointment. The important compounds in this group are miconazole, clotrimazole, ketoconazole, and econazole, which are imidazole derivatives, undecenoic acid, and tolnaftate. They are all very similar in their clinical efficacy but topical terbinafine is particularly rapid. Adverse reactions are rare.

The main oral agents are terbinafine, itraconazole, and fluconazole. Terbinafine (250 mg daily) is rapidly effective in most forms of dermatophytosis that require oral therapy and also produces rapid responses in toe-nail and sole infections, without a high rate of relapse. Itraconazole is somewhat similar in its profile. For most infections it is given in doses of 200–400 mg daily for a week and in nail infections weekly pulses of 400 mg daily are given for 2–3 months. Griseofulvin is used in some forms of dermatophytosis, like scalp ringworm. It is normally given in doses of 0.5–1.0 g daily in adults or 10 mg/kg daily in children. Treatment should be continued for at least 6 weeks in tinea capitis. It is cheaper than the alternatives, but less effective in onychomycosis.

Prognosis

Most dermatophyte infections are treatable without difficulty. Control of scalp ringworm is achieved by treating cases and their contacts.

Scytalidium infections

The organisms, *Scytalidium dimidiatum* (*Hendersonula toruloidea*), and *S. hyalinum*, can cause a superficial scaly condition that resembles a 'dry type' of dermatophyte infection on the palms or soles. Nail-plate destruction may also occur, the lateral border of the nail being the initial site of invasion. The disease has been seen in Europe, almost invariably in immigrants from the tropics, particularly the Caribbean, West Africa, and India or Pakistan. Treatment is difficult, but some improvement may follow the use of keratolytic compounds such as salicylic acid. The organisms do not respond to griseofulvin, azoles, or tolnaftate.

Miscellaneous nail infections

Occasionally, fungi other than dermatophytes or *Scytalidium* are isolated from dystrophic nails. These include *Scopulariopsis brevicaulis*, *Acremonium* species, and certain types of *Aspergillus*. These infections are usually seen in the elderly. It is often difficult, particularly with *Aspergillus* species, to establish that the organism is playing a pathogenic part.

Pityriasis versicolor (tinea versicolor)

Aetiology

Pityriasis versicolor is a superficial infection caused by species of the genus *Malassezia*. Although most common in tropical countries, it has a worldwide distribution. Dermal penetration does not occur. *Malassezia* shows dimorphism on the skin, an event which may be triggered by immunosuppression or by sun exposure.

Epidemiology

Pityriasis versicolor is very common in the tropics, where it may be widespread on the body. Its incidence in temperate climates has increased over the last 20–30 years.

Clinical features

The rash of pityriasis versicolor is asymptomatic or mildly pruritic. It presents with scaling, confluent macules on the trunk, upper arms, or neck. These may be hypopigmented or hyperpigmented. In some individuals and in the tropics, other areas including face, forearms, and thighs may be involved. The diagnosis is rarely confused with other complaints, although eczema or ringworm infections are sometimes considered. In vitiligo, depigmentation is complete and there is no scaling.

Laboratory diagnosis

The diagnosis is made by demonstration of the yeasts and hyphae of *Malassezia* in skin scales. Culture is difficult and unnecessary.

Treatment

Treatment is with antifungals such as clotrimazole or ketoconazole or antiseptics such as selenium sulphide. Oral itraconazole may be used in recalcitrant cases. Whatever the treatment, relapse is common.

Other malassezia infections

Malassezia have been implicated in the pathogenesis of a number of other skin diseases such as seborrhoeic dermatitis and a form of itchy folliculitis, malassezia folliculitis. The evidence connecting seborrhoeic dermatitis, one of the most common of skin diseases, and malassezia is largely concerned with the response of antifungal drugs and the observation that improvements in the rash mirror disappearance of organisms from the skin.

Superficial candidosis (candidiasis)

Superficial candidosis is a term used to describe infections of skin or mucous membranes caused by species of the genus *Candida*. They range in severity from oral thrush to chronic mucocutaneous candidosis, a chronic infection refractory to conventional treatment.

Aetiology and pathogenesis

Candida albicans is the species most frequently involved. It is a saprophytic yeast often found as a commensal in the mouth and gastrointestinal tract, and is commonly present in the vagina. Several factors may influence the incidence of carriage. For instance, oral colonization is more common in hospital staff than in equivalent non-hospital subjects. Vaginal carriage is more common in pregnancy. Other factors (Table 3) are known that predispose to conversion from a commensal to a parasitic role with the development of disease—candidosis. The list includes factors that influence host immunological response, such as carcinoma, acquired immune deficiency syndrome (AIDS), or cytotoxic therapy, those that disturb the population of other micro-organisms (e.g. antibiotics), and those that affect the character of the epithelium, e.g. dentures.

Other species of *Candida* may also cause superficial infections, but are less common. They include *C. tropicalis*, *C. parapsilosis*, *C. guilliermondii*, and *C. pseudotropicalis*.

Epidemiology

Superficial candida infections are seen in all countries.

Clinical features

There are a number of clinically distinct types of superficial infection caused by *Candida* species, as follows.

Oropharyngeal candidosis (thrush)

Oral infection by *Candida* is fairly common, particularly in infancy and old age, or in the immunocompromised. It is an early marker of human immunodeficiency virus (HIV) infection. The lesions present with discomfort both in the mouth and at the corners of the lips. The mouth and buccal mucosa show patchy or confluent, white adherent plaques (pseudomembranous candidosis) or areas of glazed and denuded epithelium (erythematous candidosis). Angular cheilitis

Table 3 Predisposing factors in candidosis

1. Local factors, e.g. epithelial defects, occlusion, constant immersion in water, etc. e.g. damaged nail folds, beneath dentures or intravenous lines.
2. Defects of immunity (primarily T cell or phagocytic) (a) Primary immunological disease, e.g. chronic granulomatous disease (b) Immunodefects secondary to intercurrent illness, e.g. leukaemia (c) Immunodefects secondary to therapy, e.g. cytotoxic therapy in organ transplantation
3. Drug therapy, e.g. antibiotics
4. Carcinoma or leukaemia
5. Endocrine disease (a) Diabetes mellitus (b) Hypothyroidism, hypoparathyroidism, hypoadrenalism (in chronic mucocutaneous candidosis)
6. Physiological changes, e.g. infancy, pregnancy, old age
7. Miscellaneous disorders, e.g. (a) Iron deficiency (b) Zinc deficiency (c) Malabsorption (d) Intravenous drug abuse

is often present. In AIDS patients concomitant oesophageal infection is common.

Vaginal candidosis

A similar infection can occur in the vagina with secondary spread to the vulva. This is seen in normal women, as well as in pregnancy or in association with diabetes mellitus. The presenting signs are similar and are accompanied by itching and soreness. A whitish discharge may also occur. Secondary spread of the infection to the vulva is common, with the development of a red, scaling rash. Beyond its edge, small satellite scales and pustules are seen, features typical of superficial candida infections.

Paronychia

Infection around the nail fold is seen in people whose occupations involve frequent wetting of the hands (e.g. cooks) or in those with eczema or psoriasis. In some cases, the inflammation is caused by bacterial infection, but *Candida* may also be a primary cause. The condition presents with a painful, red swelling of the nail fold. Secondary invasion of the lateral border of the nail plate by *Candida* may occur from this site.

Candida *intertrigo*

Infection of the moist folds of the skin in the groin or under the breasts causes itching and discomfort. The area becomes macerated and erythematous. *Candida* may contribute to this condition, but is certainly not the only factor. It may also superinfect the napkin area in infants. The presence of satellite pustules (see above) is a useful indicator of involvement by *Candida* in the disease process. Direct invasion of toe-web folds by *Candida* closely resembles athlete's foot caused by dermatophytes. A similar erosive infection may occur in the finger webs, and is seen most commonly in the tropics.

Chronic superficial candidosis

Chronic candida infections of the mouth, vagina, and nail present problems in management. Chronic oral candidosis, for instance, is associated with leucoplakia. Predisposing causes should be searched for. The most serious of this group of infections is chronic mucocutaneous candidosis, a rare condition in which chronic skin, nail, and mucosal infection coexist (Plate 3). A series of underlying genetic, endocrine (hypoparathyroidism, hypoadrenalism, or hypothyroidism), and immunological abnormalities has been found. Other superficial viral or fungal infections may also be present in these patients, whose condition is normally diagnosed in childhood.

Laboratory diagnosis

All these infections are diagnosed by microscopy and culture. When associated with the condition, candida cells are always evident on microscopy. Culture establishes the specific identity but as a rule, is of less value than direct microscopy.

Treatment

Two groups of drugs are effective in superficial candidosis. The polyenes such as nystatin and amphotericin B are topically active in many forms of candidosis. They are often less effective in oral candidosis in immunodeficient patients including those with AIDS. Likewise, topical azole drugs such as miconazole and clotrimazole are usually effective in superficial candidosis. For resistant cases, oral therapy with fluconazole, itraconazole, or ketoconazole may be necessary.

For vaginal infections topical creams or vaginal preparations should be used—many requiring only a single treatment. In recalcitrant cases it may be necessary to use oral therapy such as fluconazole or itraconazole. Longer courses may be necessary with these drugs.

Miscellaneous superficial mycoses

There are a few relatively rare, superficial fungal infections such as tinea nigra, and black or white piedra. They never cause invasive disease, and are mainly confined to the tropics. Tinea nigra presents with a small pigmented macule often on the palm where it must be distinguished from an early melanoma.

Subcutaneous mycoses

Subcutaneous infections caused by fungi are rare, and are mainly seen in the tropics. Most of the causative organisms have been found in environmental sources such as soil or plant debris. They are implanted through a minor injury into the skin. These infections tend to be chronic, and chemotherapy is quite lengthy and frequently unsuccessful.

Mycetoma (Madura foot)

Aetiology and pathogenesis

Mycetoma is a chronic infection involving subcutaneous tissue, bone, and skin, in which colonies of infecting fungi or actinomycetes (grains) are found within a network of burrowing abscesses and sinuses. The common actinomycete (actinomycetoma) causes are *Nocardia* species (Plate 4), *Actinomadura madurae*, and *Streptomyces somaliensis*. The most common of the fungal mycetoma (eumycetoma) agents is *Madurella mycetomatis* a pigmented fungus. All form into large hyphal aggregates or grains in tissue. Some have been found in acacia thorns in an endemic area. The infection is initiated when an infected thorn is left implanted in deep tissue. However, many years may elapse before the formation of a mycetoma.

Epidemiology

The disease is seen primarily in the tropics, although rare cases, apart from imported ones, may occur in temperate areas. Countries with the most reported cases include Sudan, India, Senegal, Mexico, and Venezuela. However, the disease is widely distributed in the tropics, particularly to the south and east of the Sahara Desert in Africa.

Clinical features

An early mycetoma may present as a hard subcutaneous swelling (Plate 5). Later, sinus tracts open on to the skin surface and visible grains may be discharged, along with serosanguinous fluid (Plate 6). Bone erosion and destruction, leading to deformity, may occur. However, severe pain is rarely a problem. Local lymph node invasion may occur, but more widespread involvement is very rare. Feet and lower legs are the most common areas involved, but the arms, buttocks, chest, and head may all be sites of infection. Mycetoma cause by *N. brasiliensis* may occur in any site, but one favoured area is the chest wall. The radiological features of mycetoma are cortical erosion, followed by the development of lytic deposits in bone. Periosteal proliferation and destruction, leading to deformity, may follow. The periosteal reaction may be pronounced in actinomycete infections.

Laboratory diagnosis

The microscopy of extracted grains and culture or histopathology is the best method of diagnosis.

Treatment

Actinomycetomas may respond to sulphones such as dapsone (50–100 mg daily) or sulphonamides such as sulphadiazine. However, eumycetomas seldom respond to antifungal therapy. On rare occasions griseofulvin, amphotericin B, ketoconazole, and itraconazole have produced remission or cure. A trial of therapy may be attempted, where the patient can be monitored closely in outpatient departments. Otherwise, radical surgery or amputation is usually necessary.

Mycetoma is slowly progressive and increasingly disabling. However, wider dissemination is very rare, and therefore cases are seldom fatal, except where the skull is involved. However, the deformity caused by the disease may be severely disabling.

Chromoblastomycosis

Chromoblastmycosis is a subcutaneous infection caused by a number of different pigmented or dematiaceous fungi. It causes verrucous or plaque-type skin lesions.

Aetiology and pathogenesis

The main causative organisms are *Fonsecaea pedrosoi* and *Cladosporium carrionii* which are environmental fungi found in association with plant debris. Other rare causes include *Phialophora verrucosa* and *Rhinocladiella acquaspersa*. Infection follows implantation through superficial injury.

Epidemiology

Chromoblastomycosis is a disease of the tropics. It is a sporadic infection seen in the humid tropical countries of central and south America, Africa, and the Far East. It is usually a disease seen in rural areas affecting otherwise healthy individuals.

Clinical features

The earliest lesion of chromoblastomycosis is a small subcutaneous nodule (Plate 7). With time this enlarges and forms a warty growth which spreads to affect a localized area usually on the extremities. Large confluent hyperkeratotic lesions may affect a large part of a limb. Other forms develop into flat plaques, sometimes with central atrophy. Complications include secondary infection, lymphoedema and in very long-standing cases squamous carcinoma.

Laboratory diagnosis

The characteristic thick-walled pigmented muriform (sclerotic) cells often divided by a cross wall can be seen in skin scrapings or biopsy where they are found in neutrophil abscesses or giant cells. The organisms are dark mould fungi which can be isolated in culture.

Treatment

The main treatments are itraconazole or terbinafine sometimes with flucytosine. In some cases lesions are also treated with heat or cryotherapy followed by chemotherapy.

Sporotrichosis

Aetiology and pathogenesis

Sporotrichosis is either a subcutaneous or systemic infection caused by the dimorphic fungus *Sporothrix schenckii* which can be found in soil, vegetation, or in association with plants or bark. People who develop the subcutaneous infection may have had contact with material that harbours the organism, such as moss or flowers (e.g. florists). It is assumed that the pathogen gains entry via an abrasion and in some endemic areas there is often a preceding history of a scratch or insect bite.

Epidemiology

Sporotrichosis is mainly seen in the tropics particularly Central and South America and southern Africa. Epidemics have been described in certain groups, such as African mine workers associated with contaminated pit props. However, normally cases are sporadic. Systemic sporotrichosis is much rarer.

Clinical features

There are two main clinical types of subcutaneous sporotrichosis. The first, the fixed type, presents with a solitary cutaneous ulcer or nodule. In the lymphangitic form, an initial nodule forms on a limb or extremity, such as a finger. This may break down and ulcerate. Subsequently, one or more secondary nodules develop along the draining lymphatic channel, which may ulcerate through the skin. Other variants include the psoriasiform or verrucous types or a superficial granuloma that resembles lupus vulgaris. The diagnosis is made by culture. Organisms are sparse in tissue and occasionally fungal yeast cells are surrounded by an eosinophilic halo, an asteroid body.

Treatment

The treatment of choice is potassium iodide administered in a saturated aqueous solution. The starting dose is 0.5–1 ml, given three times daily, and this is increased drop by drop per dose to 3–6 ml, three times daily in milk. Treatment should be given for a month after clinical resolution. Itraconazole or terbinafine are alternatives.

Other subcutaneous infections

The other subcutaneous infections, lobomycosis and subcutaneous zygomycosis are very rare.

Systemic mycoses

Endemic systemic mycoses

The systemic mycoses include some of the rare and more serious of the fungal infections. Infections caused by endemic mycoses include infections such as histoplasmosis or coccidioidomycosis. These diseases have well-defined endemic zones and the majority of those exposed remain symptomless but develop positive skin tests, without disease. In the systemic infections caused by opportunistic fungi, there is usually a serious underlying abnormality in the patient, such as carcinoma or lymphoma. Such infections are worldwide in occurrence; where tissue invasion occurs the mortality is high.

Histoplasmosis

Classical or small-form histoplasmosis (histoplasmosis capsulati)

Histoplasmosis is a systemic infection caused by the dimorphic fungus *Histoplasma capsulatum.* The main route of infection is pulmonary. The majority of those exposed are sensitized without overt signs of infection, but more rarely chronic pulmonary or disseminated forms of the disease are seen.

Aetiology

The organism, *H. capsulatum,* can be found in soil in endemic areas. Its growth is facilitated by the presence of bird excreta or bat guano. Exposure to a suitable source, such as a cave containing bats, is often recorded in acute epidemic histoplasmosis (see below). It is rarely identified in more slowly evolving cases. Slowly evolving (chronic), disseminated disease may occur in normal individuals. However, infants, elderly people, and AIDS patients are susceptible to the more rapidly progressive forms of disseminated infection.

Epidemiology

The major endemic area, as shown by skin testing, is in the central region of the USA around the Ohio and Mississippi valley basins. The disease also occurs in other parts of the USA, Mexico, Central and South America, Africa, the Far East, and Australia. The organism has been recovered from soil in central Italy, but no human cases have been diagnosed there. Outside the major endemic areas in the USA, human cases are often rare, and much of the evidence of the endemicity comes from positive skin tests or the presence of the organism in selected sites, such as caves are largely unknown.

Clinical features

The clinical forms of histoplasmosis can be placed in several clinical groups:

(1) asymptomatic;

(2) acute pulmonary

(3) chronic pulmonary;

(4) disseminated (acute, subacute, and chronic);

(5) primary cutaneous (by inoculation).

Asymptomatic infection Over 99 per cent of patients becoming infected in endemic areas record no overt symptoms but develop a positive skin test.

Acute histoplasmosis Individuals exposed to a source of infection, for instance, during cave exploration, or those who may have inhaled a large infecting dose, often develop a symptomatic illness 12–21 days after exposure. The main features are pyrexia, cough, chest pain, and malaise. Flitting arthralgia and, less commonly, erythema nodosum or multiforme may occur. The radiological appearances may be much more severe than would be supposed from the symptoms, and hilar lymph node enlargement and diffuse, patchy consolidation suggesting pneumonitis may occur. Diagnosis often depends on serological detection of antibodies. The majority of cases require no specific therapy apart from rest. Those with severe or prolonged symptoms or impaired gas exchange require intravenous amphotericin B or itraconazole. The lung lesions often heal to leave multiple scattered pulmonary calcifications.

Chronic pulmonary histoplasmosis Chronic pulmonary disease caused by *H. capsulatum* is mainly seen in the USA. It is more common in males and smokers, and there is often underlying pulmonary emphysema. Early cases may present with pyrexia and cough, but malaise and weight loss occur later. Lesions may heal initially, but relapse is common, leading to established consolidation and cavitation. The most common radiological appearance of early lesions is of unilateral, wedge-shaped, segmental shadows in the apical zones. Culture and serology are both helpful methods of diagnosis in this form of histoplasmosis. Patients may require amphotericin B therapy or itraconazole. Although chemotherapy may virtually sterilize lesions, fibrosis persists and relapse may occur. Surgical excision or lobectomy is sometimes effective. Solid lung tumours may persist after the primary infection. These may be single (coin lesions) or multiple, and have to be distinguished from carcinomas.

Disseminated histoplasmosis In rapid or acutely disseminated cases often in AIDS patients, widespread infiltration of reticuloendothelial cells of bone marrow, spleen, and liver may occur. The most prominent symptoms are fever and weight loss, with accompanying hepatosplenomegaly. Extensive purpura and bruising secondary to thrombocytopenia may occur. Skin papules and ulcers and the isolation of Histoplasma from blood has also been reported more frequently in AIDS patients. Cultures, including sputum or bone marrow, should be taken. Serology is often positive, with high titres of complement-fixing antibodies occurring in some patients; an antigen detection assay is also available. A more slowly progressive form of disseminated histoplasmosis may present with persistent oral ulcers, chronic laryngitis, or adrenal insufficiency.

The diagnosis of disseminated histoplasmosis is made on culture or biopsy of affected areas. Sera may only be positive in low titres and in all cases adrenal involvement should be looked for.

Treatment is required in all forms of disseminated histoplasmosis. Itraconazole is preferred by most physicians, although amphotericin B may be necessary in some patients. Oral ketoconazole is an alternative.

African histoplasmosis

A variant of *Histoplasma, H.capsulatum* var *duboisii* which is present in tissue are large yeasts causes a different type of disease with prominent skin (ulcers, abscesses), lymph node, or bone (lytic deposits) disease. It also responds to itraconazole.

Blastomycosis

Blastomycosis (North American blastomycosis) is caused by *Blastomyces dermatitidis,* which has been associated with damp areas prone to flooding. This infection is mainly seen in North America and more rarely in north or central Africa, the Middle East, or India. The clinical forms of blastomycosis differ from histoplasmosis in a number of important aspects. The main clinical forms are:

Chronic pulmonary blastomycosis

Chronic consolidation or cavitation of the upper or mid zones occur with chronic pulmonary infections. Fever, malaise, and cough with sputum are seen. Weight loss may be prominent.

Disseminated blastomycosis

The skin is an area that is frequently involved (chronic cutaneous blastomycosis). The face or forearms and hands are common sites for skin lesions. These are slow, spreading, verrucose plaques with central scarring. Bone or genitourinary sites of infection may also occur. The diagnosis is made by culture or demonstration of yeast cells in sputum or histology. They have a characteristic broad based bud. Treatment is with itraconazole or amphotericin B.

Coccidioidomycosis

Coccidioidomycosis is caused by the organism *Coccidioides immitis* which forms characteristic sporing structures or spherules *in vivo*. The disease is similar in pathogenesis to other endemic mycoses following inhalation to cause asymptomatic primary infection in the majority and a progressive infection in a minority. The disease is confined to the semidesert areas of the New World in the southwestern USA, Mexico, Colombia, and Argentina. The organisms can be found in soil. Epidemics of infection may follow dust storms in endemic areas.

Sensitization rates in endemic communities may exceed 70 per cent. Primary pulmonary infection is usually asymptomatic but acute pneumonia and pleural effusion with signs of arthralgia and erythema nodosum (desert bumps) may also occur. Chronic pulmonary disease with cavitation and disseminated forms of coccidioidomycosis may occur. Disseminated infections may present with meningitis, joint (Plate 8), bone or skin lesions or widespread involvement of internal organs. Pregnant women, immunocompromised including HIV-positive patients and members of certain ethnic groups (Mexican, American Indian, Black) are more susceptible to disseminated infection. The diagnosis is made by culture and serology. Histopathology or direct microscopy may show the typical spherules. Treatment is difficult in disseminated disease. For soft tissue or localized infections itraconazole or fluconazole may be used. With more widely disseminated infections amphotericin B is often used. The responses of coccidioidal meningitis are notoriously unpredictable.

Paracoccidioidomycosis

Paracoccidioides brasiliensis is a dimorphic fungus which causes a systemic infection in countries of central and south America. Areas with the largest numbers of cases are Colombia, Venezuela, Brazil, and Argentina. The natural habitat of the organism is unknown. Although sensitization rates indicating subclinical exposure are between 20 and 30 per cent in endemic areas and affect both sexes equally the disease is overwhelmingly more common in males; this is thought to be partially due to the presence of an oestrogen-binding protein in cell cytoplasm which affects the capacity or *P. brasiliensis* to transform to the pathogenic yeast phase.

The main clinical presentations are with chronic pulmonary or disseminated infections. In the lungs there are circumscribed areas of infiltration and cavitation with fibrosis. Disseminated lesions affect lymph nodes and mucocutaneous areas such as the mouth, peri-anal region, and conjunctiva. Other sites including liver and spleen may also be infected. Widespread and rapidly evolving disseminated infections may occur, sometimes in otherwise healthy individuals. This infection is not common in AIDS patients in endemic areas.

The diagnosis is made by culture and serology (complement fixation and immunodiffusion). Characteristic multipolar budding yeast cells may be seen in tissue sections or sputum smears.

The main treatment is itraconazole given in doses of 100–200 mg daily. Alternatives include amphotericin B, fluconazole, and ketoconazole. Extensive fibrosis may remain after clearance of the infection.

Infections due to *Penicillium marneffei*

Penicillium marneffei is a fungus that is a natural pathogen of the bamboo rat in South Asia. Cases in humans behave rather like disseminated histoplasmosis, with which this infection is easily confused. Infiltration of the liver, spleen, bone marrow, lungs, and skin all occur in this infection. Such cases have mainly been described from southern China and South-east Asia. The growth of a red mould and the presence of non-budding, divided, intracellular yeast-like fungi is characteristic. This infection is common in AIDS patients from the endemic areas: it is one of the most common opportunistic infections in AIDS patients in Chiang Mai, Thailand. Amphotericin B or itraconazole are the main treatments.

Systemic mycoses caused by opportunistic fungi

The opportunistic mycoses are a worldwide problem, although fortunately rare in most countries. In recent years they have been recognized more frequently with the increase in the use of transplantation of organs such as heart or bone marrow and in the wider use of immunocompromising regimens of cancer chemotherapy. Opportunistic invasion by organisms such as *Candida* or zygomycetes (*Mucor, Absidia*) may also occur in cases of malnutrition. One of the recent trends in the management of the severely immunocompromised patient has been the emergence of new pathogens such as those other than *C. albicans*, or other organisms such as *Fusarium*, *Trichosporon*, or *Bipolaris* species.

The opportunists present particular problems in diagnosis and management. Because many of the organisms are normally saprophytic, it has to be positively established that they are invasive; mere isolation may not provide sufficient evidence and in some instances low titres of antibody may be present even in normal hosts. Treatment is also difficult and it is important in most cases to attempt to reverse the process that led to the establishment of the infection. This may mean interrupting courses of cytotoxic therapy or risking loss of a transplant by reducing immunosuppressive therapy.

Systemic candidosis

In addition to their role in superficial infections, yeasts of the genus *Candida* may also cause invasive systemic disease. The clinical forms described range from a transient candidaemia to disseminated invasive disease, sometimes with involvement of a single organ, site, or body cavity (deep focal candidosis) as may occur in peritonitis or meningitis. Urinary tract infections may also be caused by *Candida* species.

Aetiology and epidemiology

The factors underlying systemic candida infections are shown in Table 3. All these factors are important in disrupting the balance by which *Candida* is maintained as a saprophyte. Intravenous or central venous pressure lines may serve as a portal of entry or as a nidus for circulating yeasts in a candidaemia. Antibiotic therapy may upset the balance by inhibiting a potentially competitive bacterial flora. *C. albicans* is the most common species involved but other species may be isolated, particularly in cases of endocarditis, for example, *C.*

parapsilosis. *C. tropicalis* has been implicated in infections of neutropenic patients. Systemic infections caused by *Candida* species are worldwide in distribution.

Clinical features

Candidaemia. The isolation of *Candida* in blood culture, candidaemia, may be linked to any of the factors listed in Table 3. Common predisposing features are the presence of intravenous lines, previous surgery (mainly gastrointestinal), antibiotic therapy or neutropenia. Patients develop a swinging fever and feel generally unwell. Clinical shock may occur. There is often an accompanying invasion of deep tissues.

Disseminated candidosis. Although multi-organ invasive candidosis may follow candidaemia, at least 50 per cent of disseminated infections develop in patients without initially positive blood cultures. Sites of infection include the skin (Plate 9), liver and spleen (hepatosplenic or chronic disseminated candidosis), thyroid, and meninges myocardium. Specific features of infections in different groups include:

Neonates—fever, meningitis, renal involvement and obstruction

Neutropenic patients—fever, widespread infection, e.g. muscles, skin. In the later stages swinging pyrexia and hepatosplenomegaly (chronic disseminated candidosis)

IV Drug abusers—fever, folliculitis, arthritis, retinitis

IV hyperalimentation—fever, retinitis

Laboratory diagnosis of disseminated candidosis. The diagnosis may be made by culture and repeated attempts to isolate should be made where cultures are initially negative. Serology is often unsatisfactory and should be repeated.

Treatment

Untreated disseminated candidosis is normally progressive and fatal. The treatment of invasive candidosis is intravenous fluconazole or amphotericin B given until there is a clinical and mycological response. This may take between 2 and 20 weeks depending on the site of infection and the underlying state of the patient.

Deep focal candidosis. Candida infections in the peritoneum or meninges most often follow direct implantation after dialysis or surgery. Alternatively, secondary invasion from the middle ear or a perforated bowel is also possible. The signs and symptoms are similar to bacterial meningitis or peritonitis but *Candida* is isolated. Sometimes these infections clear spontaneously but normally treatment is instituted with amphotericin B. Once again fluconazole is an alternative approach.

Candida endocarditis. Invasion of heart valves, mainly the mitral or aortic valves, most commonly follows homograft replacement, but it may occur also in leukaemic patients or drug addicts. Patients present with fever and weight loss with evidence of valve dysfunction or embolic phenomena. Blood cultures are usually positive at some stage in the illness but repeated sampling may be necessary. High antibody titres are usually seen in such cases and serological tests are therefore of considerable value. Treatment is valve replacement and amphotericin B.

Urinary tract candidosis. *Candida* species may be isolated from the urine particularly in conditions associated with urinary stasis such as neurogenic bladder or where there is an indwelling catheter. Maturity-onset diabetes mellitus is another predisposing factor. Treatment is normally given where there are symptoms such as dysuria or frequency or where there is a potential risk of invasion such as in immunosuppressed patients. Chemotherapy with fluconazole is usual.

Aspergillosis

Aetiology

There are a number of different disease states caused by the fungal genus *Aspergillus*. These range from allergic disorders to invasive disease. As a rule the organism affects predisposed hosts. Most diseases associated with *Aspergillus* are caused by *A. fumigatus*. *A. flavus* may cause invasive disease or an erosive paranasal granuloma in tropical countries. Both these species, together with *A. niger*, may also cause an intracavitary fungus ball or aspergilloma. On rare occasions other species are involved. They are common among the airborne spores.

Epidemiology

Aspergillus infections are sporadic but ubiquitous. Invasive disease and aspergillomas are found in all countries. The former is more common in patients receiving transplantation and intensive cytotoxic therapy. There are other regional trends in aspergillosis. The destructive paranasal granuloma normally caused by *A. flavus* is most often seen in the tropics or in patients who originate from these areas.

Clinical features

Allergic bronchopulmonary aspergillosis

Allergic bronchopulmonary aspergillosis is associated with persistent endobronchial growth of *Aspergillus*, usually *A. fumigatus*. In predisposed subjects, such as atopics, an immunological response to the organism probably involving both type I and type III hypersensitivity may contribute to the disease. The condition may start in childhood or early adult life and present with asthma followed by progressive dyspnoea and fibrosis.

In many cases the chest radiograph shows scattered linear shadows in the peripheral lung fields. In order to establish the diagnosis a positive aspergillus prick test, eosinophilia, the presence of *Aspergillus* in sputum, and weakly positive precipitins in serum are all helpful.

Treatment is difficult particularly in late cases. Attempts to remove the organism from the airways using antifungal therapy, if successful, are normally of only temporary benefit. Therapy is therefore aimed at the inflammatory response rather than the organism, and bronchodilators where appropriate, or inhaled corticosteroids are given.

Aspergilloma

The development of a fungal ball in an existing pulmonary cavity is most commonly associated with aspergilli. Frequently there are no symptoms apart from intermittent cough. However, haemoptysis of varying severity may develop. The condition is diagnosed by positive cultures and the presence of high titres of specific antibody in serum. On X-ray or computed tomogram scan a mobile opacity with surrounding halo of air can be demonstrated in a cavity. Treatment is difficult, although the mass may be expectorated. At present definitive treatment is surgery.

Invasive aspergillosis

In severely compromised individuals particularly patients with leukaemia, neutropenia, AIDS, collagen disorders, or those on immunosuppressive regimens, *A. fumigatus*, and less commonly, A. flavus, may invade tissue. The initial site is normally lung, but extrapulmonary dissemination may occur, particularly to brain, kidney, liver, and skin. Symptoms such as pyrexia and cough are often masked by the patient's poor general state and other fungal or bacterial infections often coexist. Although a variety of radiographic appearances may be seen, rapid development of a discrete focus of pulmonary consolidation, which may appear to cavitate, should arouse suspicions, particularly in the presence of a positive aspergillus culture. Often, however, both culture and serology are negative and biopsy offers the best chance of establishing the diagnosis.

Treatment should not be delayed. Intravenous amphotericin B in full dosage (1 mg/kg body weight daily) is the recommended treatment. Itraconazole is also active, although there is less information at present on its use in the neutropenic patient. Lipid associated amphotericin B (in liposomes or in colloidal dispersion or lipid complexes) is an alternative. The mortality of all invasive forms of aspergillosis, even with treatment, is high.

Cryptococcosis

Aetiology

Cryptococcosis is a systemic infection caused by *Cryptococcus neoformans*. Its most common clinical feature is meningitis, but pulmonary, cutaneous, and widely disseminated forms of the infection are also recognized. There are two varieties of *C. neoformans* called *C. neoformans neoformans* and *C. neoformans gattii*. They differ in their geographic range and ecology. The *neoformans* variety dominates in AIDS patients. *C. neoformans neoformans* can be isolated from the environment, although it is most often found in pigeon excreta. *C. neoformans* var. *gattii* has been detected in leaf and bark debris of certain *Eucalyptus* species.

Pathogenesis

The portal of entry is usually the lung, from where the organism spreads to involve other organs or sites such as the meninges. Although many isolates from natural sources have small cells, one sequel to tissue invasion is the development of a large, mucoid capsule *in vivo*, a feature that confers protection on the organism. Infections with *C. neoformans* are seen in both normal and immunocompromised hosts. The main underlying processes are AIDS, sarcoidosis, Hodgkin's lymphoma, collagen disease, carcinoma, and systemic corticosteroid therapy.

Epidemiology

Cryptococcosis has been recorded from most countries, although it is most prevalent in the USA and Australia. Exposure to appropriate sources, e.g. pigeons is only rarely recorded. It is probable that there is an asymptomatic form of cryptococcosis (cf. histoplasmosis).

Clinical features

Pulmonary cryptococcosis

Acute or subacute respiratory disease caused by *C. neoformans* presents with a chest infection with fever and cough and scattered, often well-circumscribed, areas of pulmonary infiltration seen on radiography. The laboratory diagnosis is made by biopsy or culture. Serological tests for antibody or capsular polysaccharide antigen (latex test) are often negative. Treatment is amphotericin B or fluconazole. Isolated cryptococcal granulomas (cryptococcoma) may present as coin lesions and are removed surgically to exclude carcinoma.

Disseminated cryptococcosis

The best-recognized form of extrapulmonary cryptococcosis is meningitis. This may present with signs of acute meningism. However, more usually the features are less specific. Pyrexia, headache, and mental changes such as confusion or drowsiness occur. Blurring of vision and papilloedema may also occur. Cranial nerve involvement is less common. AIDS patients present with disseminated disease. The signs of meningeal involvement may be very subtle and the infection has often spread to other sites such as liver and spleen as well as skin (Plate 10).

The cerebrospinal fluid shows pleocytosis that is highly variable. Often there are excessive numbers of lymphocytes, but sometimes polymorphonuclear leucocytes abound. In some cases only small numbers of white cells (four to 10) are seen. Characteristically, but not invariably, the glucose concentration falls and protein rises. Cryptococci can be seen in some cases in an India ink or nigrosin preparation, which is used to highlight the capsule. The latex test for antigen is usually positive for cerebrospinal fluid, but on rare occasions this is negative. Blood cultures are often positive in AIDS patients.

Other sites

Cryptococci may disseminate to other sites including liver and spleen, kidney, skin, or bone. Infection in skin and bone are most often seen in patients with sarcoidosis. In every case, underlying deep disseminated lesions (e.g. meningitis) may be found. It is important in all cases where cryptococcosis presents with lesions in an extra-meningeal site to exclude occult meningitis by lumbar puncture.

Therapy

In the non-AIDS patient the combination of flucytosine (150–180 mg/kg daily) and intravenous amphotericin B (0.3–0.6 mg/kg daily) is the most widely used treatment. In AIDS patients the object of therapy is to induce the most rapid remission possible, followed by long-term suppressive therapy. There are various regimens used for induction of remission. The use of amphotericin B with or without flucytosine is favoured by many. This is given for 2 weeks which is then followed by indefinite treatment with fluconazole or itraconazole to prevent relapse.

Invasive zygomycosis (mucormycosis, phycomycosis)

Aetiology

Invasive disease caused by zygomycete fungi is rare. In the compromised host it may lead to paranasal destruction, necrotic lung or skin lesions, and disseminated disease. The causative organisms commonly belong to one of three genera: *Absidia*, *Rhizopus*, and *Rhizomucor*. Predisposing causes include neutropenia, diabetes mellitus, and burns. The disease is worldwide in distribution.

In rhinocerebral mucormycosis the patient presents with fever and unilateral facial pain. Subsequently there may be facial swelling with nasal obstruction and proptosis. There may be invasion into the orbit leading to blindness, into the brain, and the palate. Pulmonary or disseminated forms of infection may also occur. A similar pattern of invasion of surgical wounds or burns may occur and has on occasions been associated with contamination of dressing packs. Infections are initially localized causing extensive necrosis around the original wound. The diagnosis is confirmed by histopathology and culture. Treatment should be initiated as soon as possible and extensive surgical debridement combined with conventional intravenous or lipid associated amphotericin B in maximum daily dosage offers the best chance of success.

Drugs used for the treatment of the mycoses (Table 2)

The main families of antifungal agents are the polyene (amphotericin B (AMB), lipid-associated AMB, nystatin) and azole groups, the latter consisting of two subgroups the imidazoles (e.g. clotrimazole, ketoconazole, miconazole) and the triazoles (fluconazole and itraconazole). Terbinafine, an allylamine, and amorolfine, a morpholine, are used in superficial infections. The majority of the antifungals drug work by inhibition of the biosynthesis of the cell membrane. This involves inhibition of specific stages such as demethylation of lanosterol (azoles) or epoxidation of squalene (allylamines) although the polyenes affect the structural integrity of the formed membrane. Flucytosine, by contrast, affects protein biosynthesis. Drug resistance is not common but is seen among yeast fungi treated with fluconazole and flucytosine. In general, though, antifungal susceptibility testing does not have a place in the routine management of these infections. Because of the difficulty of diagnosing opportunistic systemic infections treatment is often initiated on the basis of a reasonable suspicion in susceptible febrile patients (empiric therapy); Amphotericin B is the usual empiric treatment. Likewise the same patients may be given prophylactic treatment with fluconazole or itraconazole during periods of high susceptibility such as neutropenia.

Further reading

de Albornoz, M.C.B. (1989). Sporotrichosis. In *Tropical fungal infections*, (ed. R.J. Hay), pp. 71–96. *Baillière's Clinical Tropical Medicine and Communicable Diseases*, **4**.

Bodey, G.P., Bueltmann, B., Duguid, W., *et al.* (1992). fungal infections in cancer patients: an international autopsy survey. *European Journal of Clinical Microbiology and Infectious Diseases*, **11**, 99–109.

Denning, D.W. and Stevens, D.A. (1990). Antifungal and surgical treatment of invasive aspergillosis: review of 2,121 published cases. *Reviews of Infectious Disease*, **12**, 1187–201.

Dismukes, W.E. (1988). Cryptococcal meningitis in patients with AIDS. *Journal of Infectious Disease*, **157**, 624–28.

Dupont, B. (1992). Antifungal therapy in AIDS patients. In *New strategies in fungal disease*, (ed. J.E. Bennett, R.J. Hay, P.K. Peterson), pp. 290–300. Churchill Livingstone, Edinburgh.

Jacobs, P.H. and Nall, L. (ed.) (1997). *Fungal disease. biology, immunology and diagnosis.* Marcel Dekker, New York.

Kibbler, C.C., MacKenzie, D.W.R., and Odds, F.C. (1996). *Principles and practice of clinical mycology.* John Wiley and Sons, Chichester.

Rippon, J.W. and Fromtling, R.A. (ed.) (1993). *Cutaneous antifungal agents.* Marcel Dekker New York.

Stevens, D.A. (1990). Fungal infections in AIDS patients. *British Journal of Clinical Practice*, **44** (Suppl. 71), 11–22.

Torssander, J., *et al.* (1988). Dermatophytosis and HIV infection—study in homosexual men. *Acta Dermatologica et Venereologica*, **68**, 53–9.

Warnock, D.W. and Richardson, M.D. (ed.) (1991). *Fungal infection in the compromised patient.* Wiley, Chichester.

Chapter 16.82

Pneumocystis carinii

J. M. Hopkin

Pneumocystis carinii is a fungal organism that is the leading cause of potentially fatal opportunistic pneumonia in the immunosuppressed, e.g. marasmic institutionalized infants, patients on oncology and organ transplantation programmes, those with acquired immune deficiency syndrome (**AIDS**), and to a lesser extent those with hypogammaglobulinaemia. There is probably regular airborne exposure, but pulmonary clearance is highly effective in the normal human. Pneumonia in the immunosuppressed is the result of freshly acquired infection and may involve horizontal transmission between immunosuppressed subjects. *Pneumocystis* organisms infecting the lungs of different mammals are genetically distinct. Though disseminated infection can occur in AIDS, pneumocystis is usually confined to the lung. There, it shows two morphological forms: the trophozoite which displays close apposition to type I pneumocyte, and the cyst which lies free in the alveolar space associated with foamy debris. The number of organisms rise to 10^9/g of tissue, and cause, untreated, fatal hypoxaemia. In the interstitium of the infected lung, there is a variable degree of lymphocyte and plasma-cell infiltration.

Clinical features

The clinical features of *P. carinii* pneumonia are consistent but are mimicked by other infections—including cytomegalovirus, tuberculosis, and other fungi—and by non-infectious pulmonary disorder, including drug-induced alveolitis or pulmonary oedema.

The onset of disease may be acute or insidious (over 2–4 weeks); the latter is a more regular feature in AIDS. The main symptom is breathlessness, initially exertional but ultimately is present at rest. Mainly non-productive cough occurs in about half. Mild chilling or a sensation of fever is present in half; significant pyrexia (in excess of 38°C) is recorded in most. There is not pleuritic chest pain or wheeze. Sparse crepitations may be heard in up to a third of cases. There is tachypnoea and cyanosis dependent on the severity of disease.

In the AIDS group, rare cases of disseminated pneumocystis infection occur. Tissues involved variably include lymphoid tissues, bone marrow, and the eye causing painless lymphadenopathy and splenomegaly, anaemia, and visual disturbance.

Investigations

The plain chest radiograph and pulse oximetry are the first assessments; together with temperature recordings, they can monitor progress. The chest radiograph shows diffuse bilateral change, granular, nodular or reticular, in the great majority (Fig. 1). Cystic spaces occur in a minority. Pleural effusion is not a feature but pneumothorax is a rare complication. There are varying degrees of hypoxaemia and disease tends to be consistently more severe in the non-AIDS group.

Diagnosis is established by identification of the organism in a lung sampling obtained either as induced sputum (after inhalation of nebulized hypertonic saline) or as alveolar lavage at fibreoptic bronchoscopy. The organism cannot be cultured and is identified either on microscopy (after methenamine silver staining for the cyst phase (Fig. 2), Giemsa staining for the trophozoites and intracystic sporozoite, or fluorescence-tagged monoclonal antibody) or by DNA amplification.

Treatment

Untreated pneumocystis pneumonia is fatal. With prompt diagnosis, specific treatment results in cure 70–80 per cent. The treatment of first choice is the combination of trimethoprim and sulphamethoxazole given orally (20 mg trimethoprim, 100 mg sulphamethoxazole/kg body weight daily in divided doses) or intravenously (trimethoprim 15 mg, sulphamethoxazole 75 mg/kg daily in divided

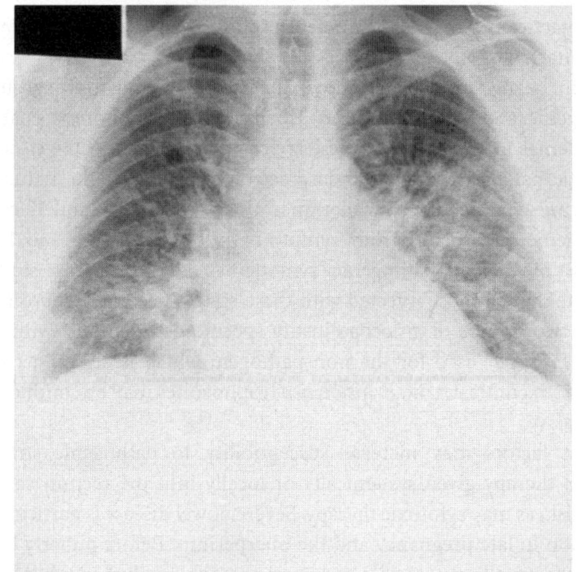

(a)

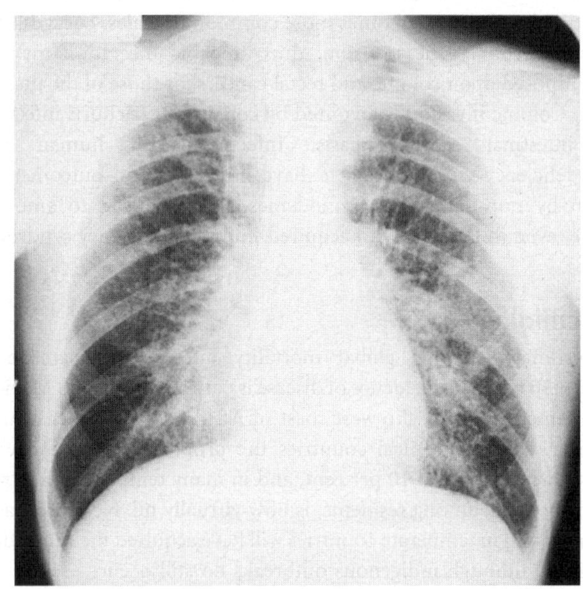

(b)

Fig. 1 Chest radiograph of two AIDS subjects with *Pneumocystis carinii* pneumonia showing (a) ground glass and (b) nodular diffuse changes.

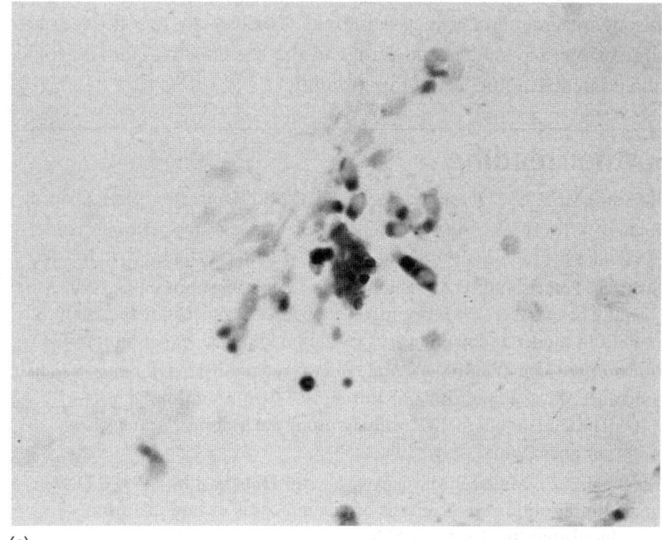

(a)

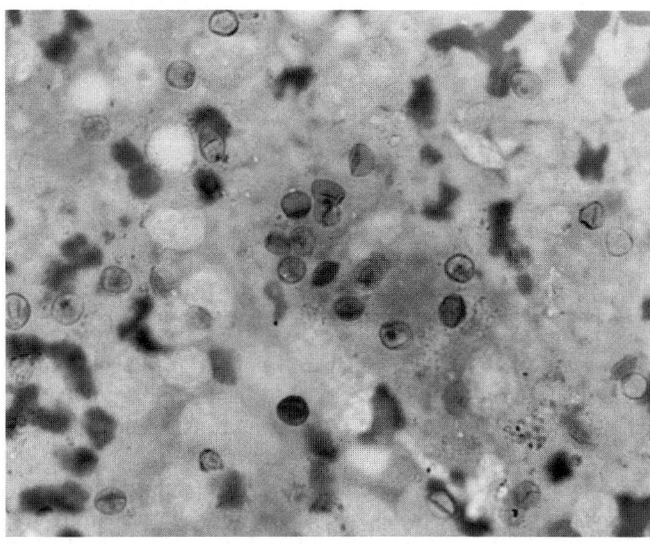

(b)

Fig. 2 The cyst phase of the organism demonstrated on microscopy of alveolar lavage after methenamine silver staining. (a) Low power, (b) higher power.

doses) over 2 weeks (3 weeks in AIDS). Doses need to be adjusted when significant renal failure is present, aiming for trimethoprim concentrations of 5–8 μg/ml at 2 h after dosage. If hypersensitivity develops, change to an alternative agent, pentamidine isethionate, is appropriate. Pentamidine is administered as 4 mg/kg daily as a slow intravenous infusion over 2 h, again over 2 or 3 weeks.

In the AIDS group adverse reactions are very common (60 per cent) to both co-trimoxazole and pentamidine—with fever, rash and pruritus, headache, vomiting, or marrow suppression. These may be tolerable with added antihistamines and antiemetics but otherwise agents such as combination trimethoprim and dapsone, combination clindamycin/primaquine, or atovaquone may be used. Pneumocystis pneumonia of mild severity may be treated with nebulized pentamidine preparation (600 mg dissolved in 6 ml water) daily; effective alveolar delivery needs a nebulizer such as the Respigard II to ensure particle size of 1.5 μm.

Adjunctive therapy with corticosteroid is useful in AIDS patients—prednisolone 40 mg daily for 5 days helps ease disease and drug-induced symptoms. In non-AIDS patients, for example the transplant population, survival from pneumocystis pneumonia may depend upon temporary withdrawal of immunosuppressive agents such as cyclosporin and azathioprine.

Prevention

Chemoprophylaxis is generally administered as periodic oral co-trimoxazole—or inhaled nebulized pentamidine. In leukaemia or organ transplant programmes, routine chemoprophylaxis with co-trimoxazole is given for at least 6 months from the initiation of immunosuppressive treatment—as trimethoprim, 5 mg/kg a day, sulphamethoxazole, 25 mg/kg a day, in two divided doses on 3 days a week. Half the dose is equally effective in renal transplant recipients.

In AIDS subjects, chemoprophylaxis may be initiated when CD4 lymphocyte counts fall to 150 and should be maintained after an episode of pneumocystis pneumonia. Toxicity to low-dosage co-trimoxazole may demand a change to the less effective but less toxic inhaled pentamidine as 300mg monthly.

Further reading

Hopkin, J.M. (1991). *Pneumocystis carinii.* Oxford University Press, Oxford.

Hughes, W.T. (1996). Recent advances in the prevention of *Pneumocystis carinii* pneumonia. *Advances in Pediatric Infectious Diseases,* **11**, 163–86.

Safrin, S., Finkelsteim, D.M., Feinberg, J., Frame P., Simpson, G., Wu, A., and Cheung, T. (1996). Comparison of three regimens for treatment of mild to moderate Pneumocystis carinii pneumonia. *Annals of Internal Medicine,* **124**, 792–802.

Saukkonen, K., Garland, R., and Koziel, H. (1996). Aerosolized pentamidine as alternative primary prophylaxis again *Pneumocystis carinii* pneumonia. *Chest,* **109**, 1250–5.

Wakefield, A.E., Miller, R.M., Guiver, L., and Hopkin, J.M. (1991). DNA amplification for the diagnosis of pneumocystis pneumonia from induced sputum. *Lancet,* **i**, 1378.

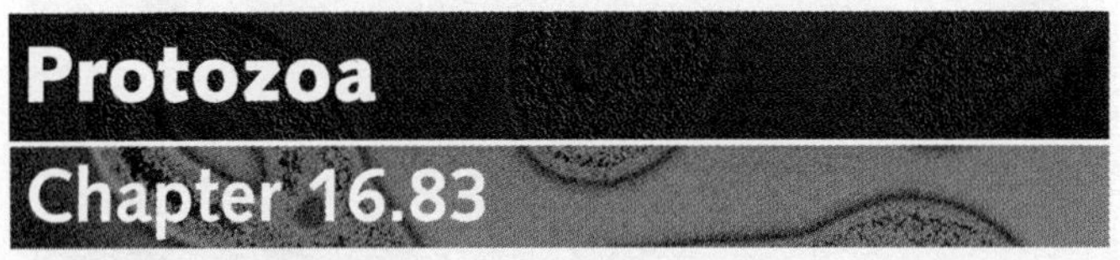

Amoebiasis

R. Knight

The amoebic species infecting humans belong to two very different groups: the obligate parasitic species of the gut, including the major pathogen *Entamoeba histolytica*; and the normally free-living, water and soil amoebae, which can become facultative tissue parasites. All motile feeding amoebae are called trophozoites; they move with pseudopodia and divide by binary fission. The hyaline external cytoplasm, the ectoplasm, is a contractile gel that surrounds the sol endoplasm containing numerous phagocytic and pinocytic vacuoles.

Entamoeba histolytica infection

Biology and pathogenicity

Within the host *E. histolytica* trophozoites occur in two forms: as an intraluminal commensal of the caecum and proximal colon; or as an invasive pathogen. Live commensal amoebae measure 10–20 μm in diameter, the endoplasm is granular and contains bacteria; the pseudopodia are blunt and movement is sluggish. The transmissive, cystic form of the parasite is derived entirely from this commensal population within the colonic lumen. Intestinal hurry from any cause, including the use of laxatives, can lead to the appearance of commensal trophozoites in the faeces.

Invasive trophozoites are derived from the commensal population of a pathogenic strain; they may reach 30–40 μm in diameter; they are very active with apparently purposeful, unidirectional movements. Their most important diagnostic characteristic is the presence of host erythrocytes within the endoplasm, which otherwise appears clear and contains no bacteria. Trophozoites containing red blood cells are described as haematophagous. Progression through tissues is by active movement, facilitated by secreted collagenase; leucocytes are drawn chemotactically towards the amoebae but most are rapidly destroyed on contact.

Strain characterization has shown that isolates belong to two groups: pathogenic and non-pathogenic. Isoenzyme electrophoresis enables zymodemes to be identified; these are populations defined by electrophoretic patterns using a standard set of enzymes. Of the naturally occurring zymodemes so far identified 10 are pathogenic and 12 non-pathogenic; all isolates from symptomatic bowel disease and liver abscess have been pathogenic zymodemes and follow-up studies indicate that all those infected with these strains become seropositive. These two groups of amoebae justify specific designations, with the name *E. dispar* used for the non-pathogen, which is always a commensal. In contrast, true *E. histolytica* trophozoites may be commensal or invasive.

Host factors may increase susceptibility to pathogenic strains. Steroid therapy given systemically or locally into the rectum carries great risk, as may cytotoxic therapy. Severe bowel disease is particularly common in late pregnancy and the puerperium. Before puberty both sexes are equally susceptible to hepatic amoebiasis but in adults this condition is at least seven times more common in males. Local disease can also favour tissue invasion; thus amoebic ulceration may be superimposed upon colonic and rectal cancers, or those of the uterine cervix. Colonic invasion is favoured by concurrent trichuris infection and intestinal schistosomiasis. Infection with human immunodeficiency-virus appears to have little effect on outcome; infection by non-pathogenic zymodemes does not lead to amoebic disease, even in patients with acquired immune deficiency syndrome (AIDS).

Epidemiology

The estimated annual global mortality due to this parasite is 40 000–110 000. The incidence of disease is particularly high in Mexico, South America, Natal, the west coast of Africa, and South-east Asia. However, even in tropical countries the proportion of pathogenic strains does not exceed 10 per cent, and in many temperate countries this proportion, among residents, is now virtually nil. Nearly all cases currently seen in temperate countries will have acquired their infection elsewhere, although indigenous outbreaks do still occur.

Symptomless or convalescent carriers are the main source of infection; patients with dysentery normally pass only trophozoites in their stool, and are therefore non-infectious. Cysts remain viable in the environment for up to 2 months. The infection is eventually self-limiting but can exceed 10 years. Tissue invasion can occur at any time during an infection with a pathogenic strain, but is much more common during the first 4 months; the incubation period may be as short as 7 days.

All the modes of faeco-oral transmission occur in amoebiasis; of special importance are the food handler and contaminated vegetables; transmission by flies and drinking water is less common. Direct spread can produce outbreaks; it occurs within institutions for children and the mentally handicapped, among male homosexuals, and with contaminated colonic irrigation equipment.

Pathology

The basic lesion is cell lysis and tissue necrosis, which, by creating locally anoxic and acidic conditions, favours further penetration of the parasite; most amoebae are seen at the advancing edge of the lesion with little inflammatory cell response. In tissue sections amoebae stain indistinctly with haematoxylin and eosin but appear bright red with periodic acid-Schiff stain; iron haematoxylin is necessary to show nuclear detail. Cysts of *E. histolytica* are never seen in tissue.

Amoebic lesions of the gut are most common in the rectosigmoid and caecum but can occur anywhere in the large bowel—involvement may be patchy or continuous; less commonly the appendix or terminal ileum are affected. The initial lesions are either small, discrete erosions of the mucosa, or minute crypt lesions. Unrestrained, the lesions extend through the mucosa, across the muscularis mucosa, and into the submucosa, where they expand laterally to produce lesions that are typically flask shaped in cross-section. Further lateral spread of the submucosal lesions leads to their coalescence, and later, to denudation of overlying mucosa. The bowel wall may become appreciably thickened. Blood vessels involved in the disease may thrombose, bleed into the gut lumen or, in the case of portal-vein radicles, provide a vehicle for the dissemination of amoebae to the liver. In very severe lesions, and usually in association with toxic megacolon, there is an irreversible coagulative necrosis of the bowel wall.

Amoebomas are tumour-like lesions of the colonic wall measuring up to several centimetres in length; they are most common in the caecum and may be multiple. Histologically there is tissue oedema, with a mixed picture of healing, and new areas of epithelial loss and tissue destruction; round-cell infiltration is patchy. Lesions may be annular and rarely an amoeboma initiates an intussusception; narrow, stricture-like amoebomas may occur in the anorectal region.

Amoebae reach the liver in the portal vein. Once initiated the amoebic lesion extends progressively in all directions to produce the liver-cell necrosis and liquefaction that constitute an 'amoebic liver abscess'. The lesions are well demarcated from surrounding liver tissue; untreated nearly all will eventually extend into adjacent structures. Secondary bacterial infection is rare and usually follows rupture or aspiration.

Clinical manifestations

Invasive intestinal amoebiasis

The clinical features show a wide spectrum from minimal changes in bowel habit to severe dysentery. Lesions may be limited to a small part of the large bowel or extend throughout its length. A relapsing course is common.

Amoebic colitis with dysentery

Dysentery, the passage of loose or diarrhoeal stools containing fresh blood, occurs when there is generalized colonic ulceration, or when more localized lesions occur in the rectum or rectosigmoid. Onset may be gradual, intermittent, or much less commonly, acute. Typically, constitutional upset is initially mild and the patient remains ambulant; mild or moderate abdominal pain is common, and is often colicky and maximal over affected parts of the gut. Tenesmus can occur but is rarely severe. Stools vary in consistency from semiformed to watery; they are foul-smelling and usually contain visible blood, even when watery, faecal matter is nearly always present. Symptoms frequently wax and wane over a period of weeks or even months and such patients can become debilitated and wasted. In a few patients the disease runs a fulminating course. The most frequent physical sign is abdominal tenderness in one or both iliac fossae; but tenderness may be generalized. Affected gut may be palpably thickened. A low fever is common, but dehydration is uncommon. Abdominal distension occurs in the more severely ill patients, who sometimes pass relatively small amounts of stool.

When stool microscopy reveals no haematophagous trophozoites a careful proctoscopy or sigmoidoscopy should be done. The endoscopic appearances may be non-specific in early, acute, or very severe colitis; the findings are hyperaemia, contact bleeding, or confluent ulceration. In more chronic cases the presence of normal-looking intervening mucosa is highly suggestive of amoebiasis; early lesions are often elevated, with a pouting opening only 1–2 mm in diameter; later, ulcers may reach 1 cm or more in diameter, with an irregular outline and often a loosely adherent, yellowish or grey exudate. Mucosal scrapings or superficial biopsies taken at endoscopy should be examined immediately by wet-preparation microscopy.

Special forms of amoebic colitis

Fulminant colitis. This may arise *de novo*, for example in pregnant women or during steroid therapy, or it may evolve during a dysenteric illness. Patients show progressive abdominal distension, vomiting, and watery diarrhoea. Bowel sounds are absent and there may be little or no abdominal tenderness, guarding, or rigidity. Plain radiographs may reveal free peritoneal gas, together with acute gaseous dilatation of the colon; affected segments of bowel may appear relatively narrow and show visible musosal pathology. Barium enema and full sigmoidoscopy are contraindicated. Stools will contain haematophagous trophozoites.

Amoebic colitis without dysentery. When ulceration is limited to the caecum or ascending colon, or early, mild, or localized lesions occur elsewhere in the colon there may be no dysenteric symptoms. Patients complain of change in bowel habit, blood-staining of the stool, flatulence, and colicky pain. Often the only physical sign is tenderness in the right iliac fossa, or elsewhere along the course of the colon. Some patients will eventually go into complete remission; others progress to a dysenteric illness.

The most important diagnostic measure is repeated stool examination for haematophagous amoebae; the finding of cysts or commensal trophozoites is of little diagnostic value, especially in endemic areas. Sigmoidoscopy is often normal when the distal bowel is not involved but colonoscopy may reveal typical lesions.

Amoeboma. These present as an abdominal mass, most frequently in the right iliac fossa. The lesion may be painful, tender, and associated with fever. Bowel habit is altered and some patients have intermittent dysentery, especially if lesions are multiple or distal. Evidence of partial or intermittent bowel obstruction may be present, particularly when lesions are distal and annular.

Localized perforation and amoebic appendicitis. Sudden perforation with peritonitis can occur from any deep amoebic ulcer; alternatively, leakage may lead to a pericolic abscess or retroperitoneal cellulitis. Amoebic appendicitis is an uncommon but important condition that occurs when amoebic lesions are confined to the appendix and caecum. The clinical presentation can resemble that of simple appendicitis, often with some clinical evidence of dysentery. If unrecognized at appendicectomy the outcome can be disastrous with gut perforation; fresh smears should be made from the resected appendix, and examined immediately.

Rectal bleeding. Some patients with amoebiasis present with rectal bleeding, with or without tenesmus; this occurs particularly in children. Massive bleeding into the gut lumen can occur in any form of amoebic colitis but is rare.

Differential diagnosis

Amoebic colitis must be differentiated from other causes of infective colitis. High-volume diarrhoea, copious mucus, and severe tenesmus

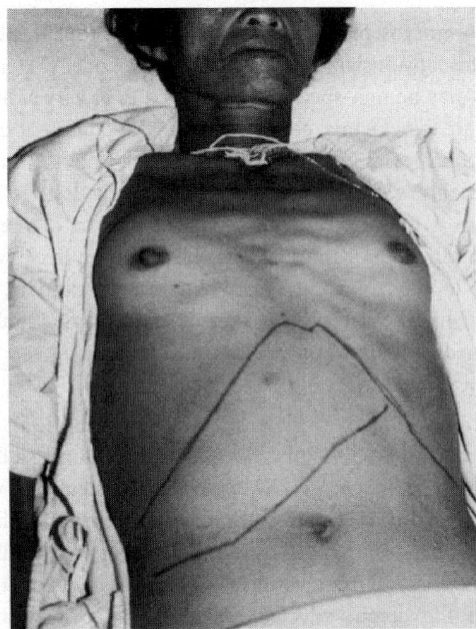

Fig. 1 Amoebic liver abscess. Hepatic enlargement with focal tenderness in a Thai woman
(by courtesy of Professor S. Looareesuwan).

are all uncommon in amoebiasis. In temperate countries, non-specific ulcerative colitis and colorectal carcinoma create the greatest diagnostic problems. Parasitic conditions to be considered are intestinal schistosomiasis, heavy trichuris infection, and balantidiasis. More chronic amoebic pathology may clinically resemble diverticulitis, Crohn's disease, ileocaecal tuberculosis, and anorectal lymphogranuloma venereum.

Hepatic amoebiasis Less than half of all patients give any convincing history of dysentery and few have concurrent dysentery. In those with no dysenteric history the interval between presumed infection and presentation may be as short as 3 weeks, or as long as 15 years; for most it is between 8 weeks and 1 year.

The dominant symptoms are fever and sweating, liver or diaphragmatic pain, and weight loss. Onset of constitutional symptoms is often insidious; but pain may begin abruptly. Most patients seek medical help within 1–4 weeks. Fever is typically remittent, with a prominent evening rise, brief rigors, and very profuse sweating. Liver pain may be poorly localized initially and later become pleuritic, referred to the right shoulder tip, or localized to the abdominal wall. Within a few weeks, patients lose much weight and often become anaemic; a painful dry cough is common.

The most important clinical finding is liver enlargement (Fig. 1) with localized tenderness, which should be searched for in the right hypochondrium, the epigastrium, and along all the intercostal spaces overlying the liver. Liver pain, on compression or heavy digital percussion, is a less useful sign. Left-lobe lesions can present as an epigastric mass. Hepatomegaly may be difficult to detect by abdominal palpation when enlargement is mainly upwards, but bulging of the right chest wall may be noted, together with a raised upper level of liver dullness on percussion. Reduced breath sounds or crepitations may be heard at the right lung base.

Important radiological findings are a raised, or locally upward-bulging, right diaphragm (Fig. 2) with immobility on screening, areas of lung collapse or consolidation, and sometimes a pleural effusion. A neutrophil leucocytosis is almost invariable, the erythrocyte sedimentation rate is raised, and normochromic normocytic anaemia is common. 'Liver function tests' are frequently completely normal, or there may be a raised alkaline phosphatase; less commonly, the serum transaminase or bilirubin is elevated. Liver scanning to demonstrate a filling defect is of great value; about 70 per cent of lesions are solitary, but multiple lesions are common in children and those with concurrent dysentery. Ultrasonographic scans and computed tomography are the most useful. Lesions appear round or oval, and are usually 4–10 cm in diameter at the time of presentation. On ultrasonography most are hypoechoic with well-defined walls without enhanced echoes. Stool microscopy is of very little diagnostic value except when there is current dysentery. Many patients show no evidence of *E. histolytica* in their stool, even after repeated examinations.

Complications

Most complications involve extension of hepatic lesions into adjacent structures: most commonly the right chest, the peritoneum, and the pericardium. Upward extension usually produces adhesions between the liver, the diaphragm, and the lung; in consequence, subphrenic rupture and amoebic empyema are rare, although a right serous pleural effusion is not uncommon. Untreated, the disease process advances upwards through lung tissue leading to hepatobronchial fistula and expectoration of brownish, necrotic liver tissue, the so-called 'anchovy sauce' sputum. Rupture into the peritoneum can occur at any time; it is sometimes the mode of presentation of an amoebic liver abscess, the cause of peritonitis being discovered only at laparotomy. Amoebic pericarditis usually results from upward extension of a left-lobe liver lesion. Initially patients have retrosternal pain, a pericardial friction rub, or a serous effusion; later rupture produces cardiac tamponade. The diagnosis is most difficult when an underlying liver abscess was not suspected.

Less commonly the lesion extends through the skin producing a sinus and cutaneous lesion. The gut, stomach, vena cava, spleen, and kidney are occasionally involved by direct spread. Blood-borne spread to the lung produces a lesion resembling an isolated pyogenic lung abscess. Amoebic brain abscesses due to *E. histolytica* are rare; most are discovered post mortem (Fig. 3). Jaundice occurs when a large lesion compresses the common bile duct or when multiple lesions compress several intrahepatic bile ducts. Portal-vein compression occasionally produces portal hypertension and congestive splenomegaly.

Differential diagnosis

Amoebic serology and scanning have now greatly simplified diagnosis. However, a few patients, generally less than 5 per cent, are initially seronegative; scanning patterns may be atypical before lesions have liquefied. Pyogenic abscess, especially when cryptogenic, may be clinically indistinguishable and this condition is quite common in some Asian countries.

Needle aspiration of the liver may be necessary for diagnostic or therapeutic purposes (see below). Suspected pyogenic abscess is the main indication for the former; blood cultures should also be taken. Whenever possible, liver scanning should precede the procedure, which should be monitored by ultrasound. A therapeutic amoebicide trial is generally preferable to diagnostic needling of the liver. Typically, the aspirate in hepatic amoebiasis is pinkish-brown, odourless, and bacteriologically sterile; a thinner, malodorous, or frothy aspirate suggests bacterial infection.

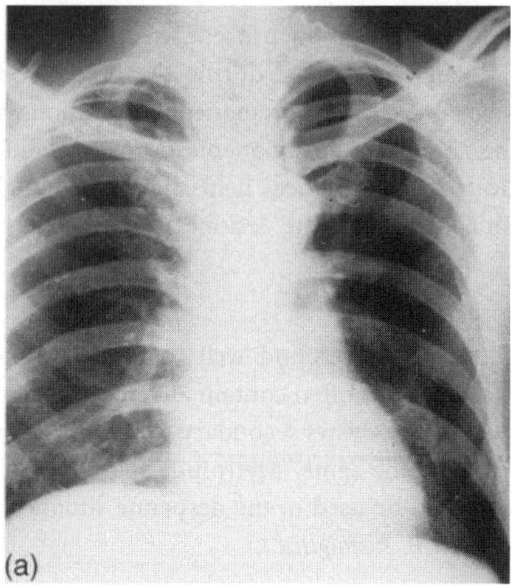

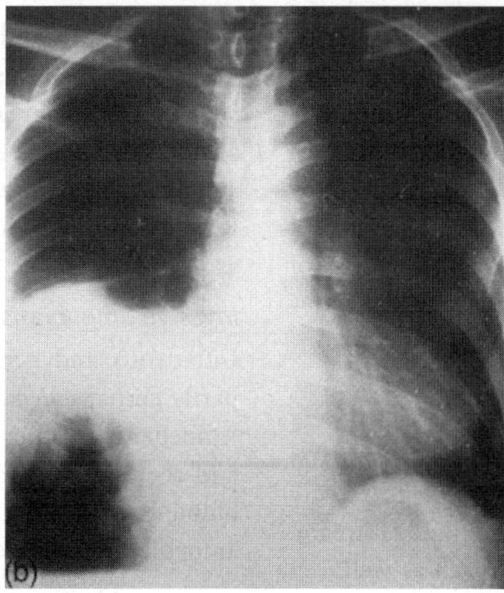

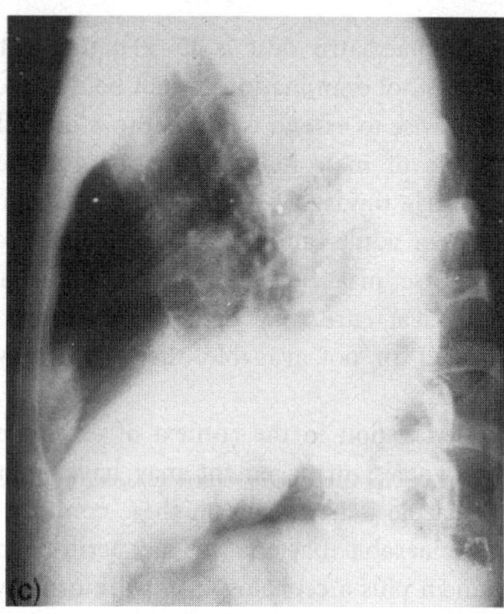

Fig. 2 Amoebic liver abscess, radiographic changes: (a) elevated right diaphragm; (b) enormous abscess in the right lobe of the liver outlined with air (fluid level) and contrast medium introduced during the aspiration of more than 1 litre of pus; (c) lateral view, same patient as (b). *(by courtesy of Professor Sornchai Loaareesuwan.)*

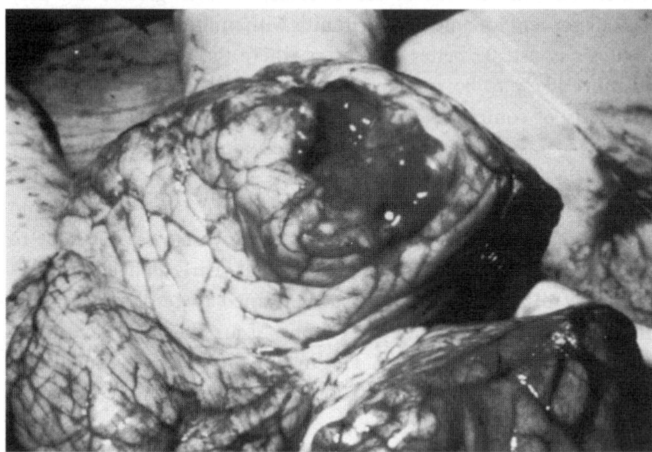

Fig. 3 Metastatic brain abscess in a patient with an amoebic liver abscess. *(By courtesy of Professor Sornchai Looareesuwan.)*

Cutaneous and genital amoebiasis Skin ulceration due to *E. histolytica* produces deep, painful, and foul-smelling lesions that spread rapidly. Secondary bacterial infection is common and may mask the amoebic pathology. Lesions are most frequent in the perianal area, but also occur at colostomy stomas, laparotomy scars, and at the site of skin rupture by a hepatic lesion. Female genital involvement results from faecal contamination, the extension of perianal lesions, or by the formation of internal fistulae from the gut, which can involve the bladder. Lesions of the vulva and uterine cervix may resemble carcinoma. Male genital lesions follow rectal coitus, the lesion beginning as a balanoposthitis and progressing rapidly.

Laboratory diagnosis

Microscopy and culture

The identification of live haematophagous trophozoites in temporary wet mounts is of prime importance because it confirms the diagnosis of invasive amoebic disease. Amoebae should be sought in dysenteric bowel-wall scrapings, the last portion of aspirate from a liver abscess, sputum, and tissue smears from skin lesions. In non-dysenteric stools, flecks of pus, blood, or mucus should be looked for and examined. The amoebae remain active for about 30 min at room temperature. Other microscopical features of faeces in amoebic colitis are scanty or absent leucocytes, clumped or degenerating red cells, and sometimes Charcot–Leyden crystals. If wet preparations are not made, or are negative, a portion of the specimen should be preserved in polyvinyl alcohol or sodium acetate-acetic acid–formalin fixative for later smear preparation; alternatively, drying faecal smears should be fixed in Schaudinn's solution.

Cysts of *E. histolytica* and non-pathogenic *E. dispar* are indistinguishable. Direct mounts are made by emulsifying a small portion of stool in 1 per cent eosin, and in Lugol's iodine; however, the diagnostic sensitivity, per specimen, is only about 30 per cent. Concentration methods such as formol–ether sedimentation give a 70 per cent sensitivity per specimen. Cultivation of intestinal amoebae with bacterial associates in Robinson's medium is relatively easy; species identification requires immunofluorescent staining. Culture lysates provide material for zymodeme assay. Positive cultures from extraintestinal sites confirm invasive *E. histolytica*; amoebae are often difficult to find microscopically in liver aspirates.

Immunological tests

Many serodiagnostic methods have been applied to amoebiasis, most detectable antibody is IgG, with some IgM in active disease. However, seropositivity does not distinguish current and past tissue invasion. The more sensitive methods are indirect haemagglutination, enzyme immunoassay, and indirect immunofluorescence. Latex agglutination and gel-diffusion precipitation are also used, the former being commercially available as a slide test, taking only minutes to perform. Using sensitive tests, over 95 per cent of patients with liver abscess are seropositive, as are about 60 per cent of those with invasive bowel disease; patients with amoeboma are nearly all seropositive. All patients with tissue invasion eventually become seropositive. Titres decline after therapy but may remain positive for 2 years or more with the more sensitive tests. Detection of faecal antigen specific for pathogenic *E. histolytica* is a new diagnostic method.

Patient management

Invasive intestinal amoebiasis

Metronidazole for 5 days will be the first choice in most patients. The usual adult dose of metronidazole is 800 mg, thrice daily for 5 or

8 days; the paediatric dose is 35–50 mg/kg in three divided doses. If follow-up stool examination cannot be done to assess parasitological cure, it is wise to extend treatment to 8 or 10 days; alternatively, a 5-day course of metronidazole can be followed by diloxanide. An alternative is tinidazole which has the advantage of a single daily dose, 2 g in adults and 50–60 mg/kg in children. A 5- or even a 3-day course may be sufficient for tissue amoebae but rates of parasitological cure may be low. When nitroimidazoles are contraindicated, or not available, then erythromycin is useful in non-severe colitis.

Gut perforation in the context of extensive colitis carries a very poor prognosis; management may have to be medical. Parenteral metronidazole is invaluable in these contexts because of its activity against anaerobic bacteria in the peritoneum and blood stream. Gentamicin plus a cephalosporin will normally be given as well.

Amoebomas respond well to metronidazole; a slow response should arouse suspicion that the amoebic lesion is superimposed upon a carcinoma. Surgical management is important in several situations. Acute colonic perforation in the absence of diffuse colitis, or ruptured amoebic appendicitis may be amenable to local repair. In the case of diffuse colitis, local repair, or end-to-end anastomosis, may not be possible because of the poor condition of the gut wall; temporary exteriorization with an ileostomy or colectomy may be necessary.

Non-invasive carrier state

Convalescent carriers should always be treated as if they carry a pathogenic zymodeme; the same applies to family contacts of cases. Infections acquired in temperate countries, including those in male homosexuals or in institutional residents or staff, need not be treated unless there are grounds for suspecting that a pathogenic strain is involved. It continues to be wise to treat people infected with *E. histolytica* who come to temperate countries from the tropics, especially when gut symptoms are present. Diloxanide is currently the drug of choice, the standard dosage in adults being 500 mg thrice daily for 10 days (paediatric dose, 20 mg/kg daily in three divided doses). Metronidazole is also effective, but an 8-day course may be necessary and side-effects troublesome; concurrent giardial infection is an indication for this drug. Unfortunately, cure rates with tinidazole are very low when followed up at 1 month.

Hepatic amoebiasis

Metronidazole or tinidazole are the drugs of choice; more data are available on the former and parenteral metronidazole can be used in patients who undergo laparotomy. A favourable response to medical treatment alone can be expected in about 85 per cent of patients. Liver abscesses may rupture before, during, or after chemotherapy. Intra-abdominal rupture will always require laparotomy. Extension into the pleural or pericardial cavities necessitates drainage of these structures, together with aspiration of the liver lesion; pericardial drainage is most urgent when tamponade is present. Hepatopulmonary lesions generally require drainage of the liver lesion but medical treatment alone has been successful in some cases. Antimicrobials will always be needed when the abscess ruptures into the peritoneum or lung.

The most common management problem is slow response to the amoebicide. Patients whose pain and fever do not subside by 72 h are at significantly greater risk of rupture or therapeutic failure, and aspiration is generally to be recommended. A likely explanation of poor initial response is a tense lesion that restricts drug entry. Regular ultrasonographic monitoring is of great value as it will indicate the risk of rupture and guide the aspiration procedure. No change in lesion size on ultrasound can be expected during the first 2 weeks, although its outline may become clearer. Percutaneous aspiration with a wide-bore needle will be possible in most patients; if unsuccessful or anatomically contraindicated, then surgical help should be sought. Resolution times for small or moderate lesions is unaffected by aspiration.

Invasive amoebiasis at other sites

Cutaneous and genital amoebiasis respond well to metronidazole, partly perhaps, because these lesions often contain anaerobic bacteria. Amoebiasis at other sites is nearly always secondary to hepatic lesions and the chemotherapy will be the same. Metronidazole crosses the blood–brain barrier and should be used in the desperate situation of amoebic brain abscess due to *E. histolytica.*

Prognosis

Uncomplicated invasive intestinal disease and uncomplicated hepatic amoebiasis should normally have a mortality rate of less than 1 per cent. In complicated disease the mortality is much greater and may reach 40 per cent for amoebic peritonitis with multiple gut perforation. Prognosis is usually better in centres where the disease is common and more likely to be recognized early. Late diagnosis increases the probability of complicated disease and mortality rises accordingly.

Unless parasitological cure is achieved, and the gut completely freed of *E. histolytica,* clinical relapse is quite common, although probably limited by immunological responses. There is so far no evidence of naturally occurring strains of *E. histolytica* resistant to normally used drugs. Hepatic scans show that nearly all liver abscesses completely disappear within 2 years; the median resolution time is 8 months. In secondarily infected lesions, bizarre hepatic calcification may be seen years afterwards. Healing of the bowel is remarkably rapid and complete; occasionally fibrous strictures persist after severe dysentery.

Prevention

Chlorination of water supplies does not destroy amoebic cysts, but adequate filtration will remove them. Boiling water for 5 min kills cysts. Other parasitic gut amoebae include four non-pathogenic Entamoeba, *Endolimax nana, Iodamoeba buetchlii,* and the probable pathogen *Dientamoeba fragilis* (see OTM3, p. 825).

Naegleria fowleri infection

Epidemiology and pathology

N. fowleri causes primary necrotizing amoebic meningoencephalitis. It is an amoeboflagellate with two trophozoite forms. The free-living amoeba moves rapidly with a single pseudopodium, it can transform into a non-feeding flagellate in hypotonic media and these free-swimming forms facilitate dispersal. Nearly all patients give a history of swimming or diving in warm fresh water, or spa water, between 2 and 14 days before the illness began. Common-source outbreaks occur during warm summer months in temperate countries. Amoebic trophozoites cross the cribriform plate from the nasal mucosa to the olfactory bulbs and subarachnoid space. At autopsy the brain shows cerebral softening and damage to the olfactory bulbs; cysts are never formed in the tissues. Although so far only about 200 cases have been documented since the first human case was reported in 1965, it is likely that some are missed. Some are discovered at autopsy, or in preserved pathological material. Specific antisera enable amoebae to be recognized by immunofluorescence staining.

Clinical features and diagnosis

Most patients are young adults and children. Initial nasal symptoms and headache are soon followed by fever, neck rigidity, coma, and later, convulsions; most patients die within a few days. Cerebrospinal fluid is often turbid, and blood-stained with high protein and low glucose levels and neutrophils. Amoebae must be urgently looked for in wet specimens using phase-contrast microscopy. Unless amoebae are seen, bacterial meningitis will be suspected; on Gram staining amoebae appear as indistinct smudges. Fixed preparations stained with iron haematoxylin will show full details of nuclear structure. Confirmation is by aerobic culture on a confluent growth of *Escherichia coli*.

Amphotericin B is the only effective drug. It should be given by daily intravenous infusion, and intrathecally, with the dosage regimens used for cryptococcal meningitis. So far, very few patients have survived but this may partly be due to diagnostic delays.

Acanthamoeba infections

Biology and epidemiology

Most patients have granulomatous amoebic encephalitis, or an amoebic keratitis. These soil amoebae have no flagellate form; the small pseudopodia are called acanthopodia, being multiple, and thin. Cysts are thick walled, angulated, and buoyant; their dispersal may be wind-borne. Humans become infected by swallowing or inhaling cysts or amoebae, or they may contaminate wounds or corneal abrasions. *Acanthamoeba* species are sometimes isolated from throat or nasal swabs, or from stool specimens.

Pathology, clinical features, and diagnosis

Many patients have predisposing factors such as craniofacial trauma, vascular brain infarct, or a systemic disorder such as lymphoma, other malignancy, or diabetes mellitus; relatively acute cerebral lesions are described in a few patients with AIDS. Cerebral lesions arise haematogenously, by direct spread, or rarely from the nasal mucosa as with *Naegleria*; clinically and pathologically they resemble chronic bacterial brain abscesses. Primary lesions have been described from the lung, orbit and other cranial structures, and the gastric wall.

Corneal lesions present as indolent ulcers unresponsive to antibiotics or corticosteroids. Infection may be by wind-borne cysts upon a damaged epithelium or from contact lenses. Solutions used to store, or wash, lenses can be contaminated by these amoebae, many of which are resistant to some antiseptics, especially as cysts.

Unless these amoebae are found in wet tissue preparations or cerebrospinal fluid, the diagnosis will be based upon histology. Cysts may be seen in tissue, but trophozoites may be missed unless stained with iron haematoxylin or immunofluorescence using specific antisera. Cultural diagnosis from fresh biopsy material is as for *Naegleria*. Most non-ocular infections are due to *A. culbertsoni*, but corneal lesions are usually due to *A. polyphaga*.

Treatment and prevention

The *in vitro* drug sensitivities of isolates should be urgently tested; a wide spectrum of resistance is common. Amphotericin B or flucytosine will be the initial choice for systemic use. Eye lesions have sometimes responded to local propamidine and neomycin, but the latter is not cysticidal; combinations of topical propamidine with chlorhexidine or polyhexamethylene have recently been successful. Corneal grafting may be necessary. Wearers of contact lenses must take especial care to avoid contamination especially when storage cases are used; raw tap water may contain *Acanthamoeba*. The most appropriate disinfectants are chlorhexidine and hydrogen peroxide.

Balamuthia mandrillaris infection

In 1990, a new cause of granulomatous amoebic encephalitis in humans and animals was described, *Balamuthia mandrillaris* (Leptomyxiidae). More than 60 human cases have been reported, in the Americas, Europe, and Australia. Immunocompetent as well as immunocompromised patients may be infected. Granulomatous facial lesions (Plate 1) may be associated with intracranial space-occupying lesions. No effective treatment has been identified. Diagnosis is made by finding amoebic trophozoites and cysts in infected tissue and by indirect immunofluorescence.

Further reading

Carter, R.F. (1972). Primary amoebic meningo-encephalitis. *Transactions of the Royal Society of Tropical Medicine and Hygiene*, **66**, 193–208.

Diamond, L.S. and Clark, C. G. (1993). A redescription of *Entamoeba histolytica* Schandinn, 1903 (emended Walker 1911) separating it from *Entamoeba dispar* Brumpt, 1925. *Journal of Eukaryote Microbiology*, **40**, 340–4.

Illingworth, C.D., Cook, S.D., Karabatsas, C.H., and Easty D.L. (1995). Acanthamoeba keratitis: risk factors and outcome. *British Journal of Ophthalmology*, **79**, 1078–82.

Martinez-Palomo, A. (ed.) (1986). *Amoebiasis*. Elsevier, New York.

Ravdin, J.I. (ed.) (1988). *Amebiasis. Human infection by* Entamoeba histolytica. Wiley, New York.

Ravdin, J.I. (1995). Amebiasis. [Review]. *Clinical Infectious Diseases*, **20**, 1453–64.

Sargeaunt, P.G. (1987). The reliability of *Entamoeba histolytica* zymodemes in clinical diagnosis. *Parasitology Today*, **3**, 40–4 and 156.

Tannick, E. (1998). *Entamrala histolytica* and *E. dispar*, comparison of molecules considered important for host tissue destruction. *Transactions of the Royal Society of Tropical Medicine and Hygiene*, **92**, 593–6.

Walsh, J.A. (1986). Problems in the recognition and diagnosis of amoebiasis: estimation of the global magnitude of morbidity and mortality. *Reviews of Infectious Diseases*, **8**, 228–38.

Chapter 16.84

Malaria

D. J. Bradley, C. I. Newbold, and D. A. Warrell

Malaria is the most important human parasitic disease, causing some 200 million clinical cases annually, of which over a million die, mostly in Africa. It has had large effects on the course of history and settlement in tropical regions, and it is currently responsible for the loss of some 35 million disability adjusted life years each year, about 2.6 per cent of the total disease burden of the world. Despite massive control efforts, there has been a resurgence of malaria over the last two decades.

Parasitology

Humans are the natural vertebrate hosts of four species of *Plasmodium*: *P. falciparum*, *P. malariae*, *P. vivax*, and *P. ovale*. Sporozoites of all species are injected into the bloodstream by female *Anopheles* mosquitoes (Fig. 1). They disappear rapidly into hepatocytes, perhaps via Kupffer cells. Schizonts develop and the liver cell nucleus may be displaced but there is no inflammation. Merozoites are released into the blood and invade erythrocytes. The development of some sporozoites of *P. vivax* and *P. ovale* becomes arrested and they remain dormant as hypnozoites, 5–6 μm in diameter, capable of causing relapses months or years later. These have been found in human liver biopsies and in hepatocytes cultured *in vitro*. *P. falciparum* and *P. malariae* have no persisting hepatic phase but may survive in the blood causing recrudescent infections. Inside erythrocytes, the parasites develop from 'ring' forms through trophozoites to multinucleated schizonts that rupture, releasing merozoites which can infect new erythrocytes but cannot reinvade the liver. Some become gametocytes which, when taken up by mosquitoes, complete a sexual cycle, producing sporozoites to infect a new human host.

Comparison of rRNA sequences of different species of *Plasmodium* shows, somewhat surprisingly, that *P. falciparum* is more closely related to avian malarias than to other mammalian species. Sequence data from extrachromosomal elements suggest that these circular DNA molecules may be of plant rather than animal origin.

In vitro culture

Since 1975, the long-term culture of asexual forms of *P. falciparum* has been possible by incubating parasitized erythrocytes in a suitable growth medium with uninfected red cells in an atmosphere of low oxygen and high carbon dioxide tension. This technique has speeded up basic research on malaria and has permitted the development of *in vitro* tests for sensitivity to certain antimalarial drugs. Cultured parasites can also be used as a source of antigen for antimalarial antibody screening tests. The complete development of the hepatic stage of *P. falciparum* has been achieved *in vitro* and gametocytes can be produced from *in vitro* culture of asexual blood forms.

Biology of the mosquito vector

Human malarial parasites are transmitted by many species of *Anopheles* mosquitoes that vary in their habits, breeding places, and their effectiveness as malaria vectors. Adult female *Anopheles* can be distinguished from other mosquitoes by the way that, during a blood feed, the whole body is inclined. Other, culicine mosquitoes have the body parallel to the skin surface (Fig. 2). Anopheline larvae have small breathing siphons and their bodies rest parallel to the surface film, whereas culicine larvae hang downwards from the tip of their longer siphons, which end at the surface film (Fig. 2).

In a particular locality only a few species of *Anopheles* are likely to be important malaria vectors. To transmit malaria they must be sufficiently abundant, must bite people, and must live long enough for ingested gametocytes to develop through to sporozoites. Most anophelines are selective in their breeding sites, so knowledge of the larval ecology may permit engineering and other measures to be directed at selective removal of the vector habitat—'species sanitation'.

Most anophelines bite in the evening and night, indoors (endophagic) or outside (exophagic). This determines whether the use of bednets and screened doors and windows will protect, or whether

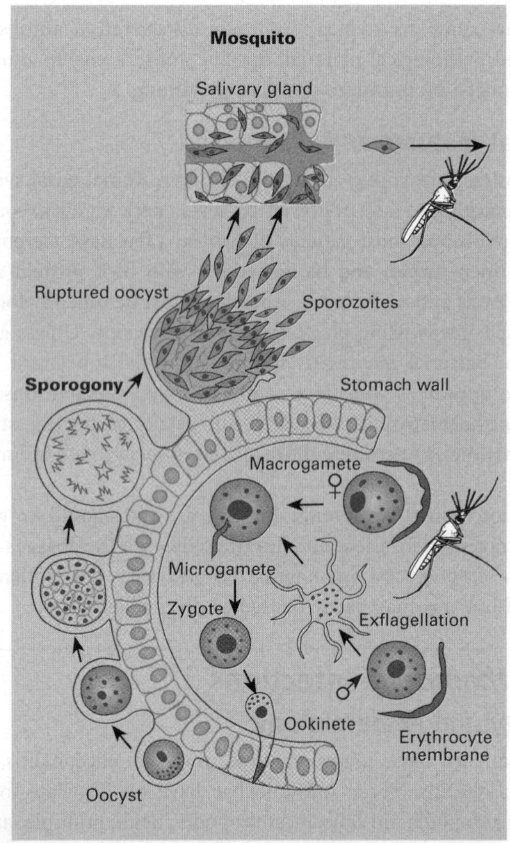

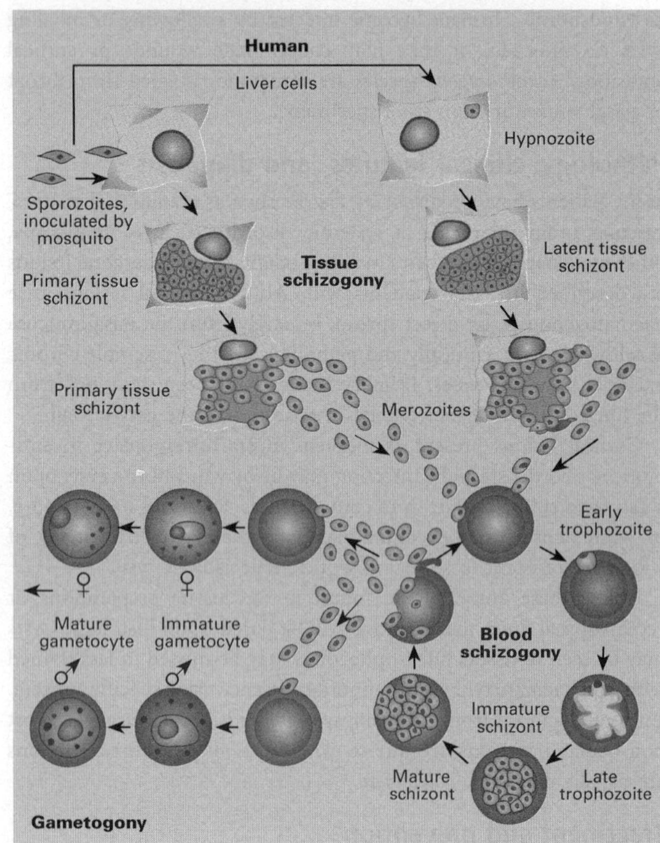

Fig. 1 Development cycle of *Plasmodium*
(redrawn by permission of F. Hoffman-la-Roche Ltd, Basel).

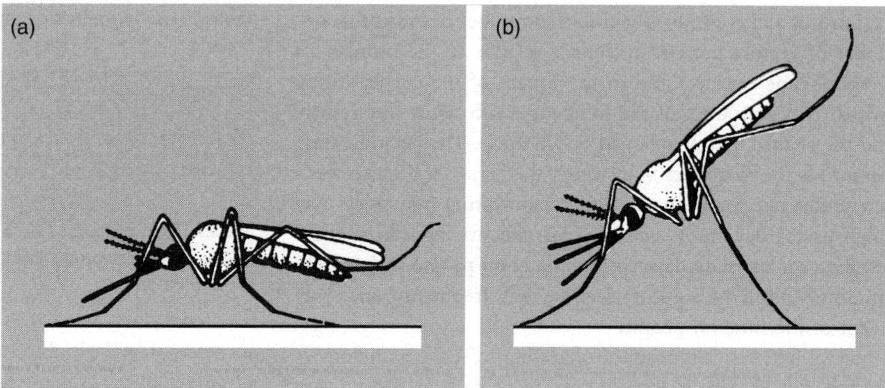

Fig. 2 Feeding postures of adult mosquitoes and resting postures of their larvae: (a) Culicine. (b) Anopheline.

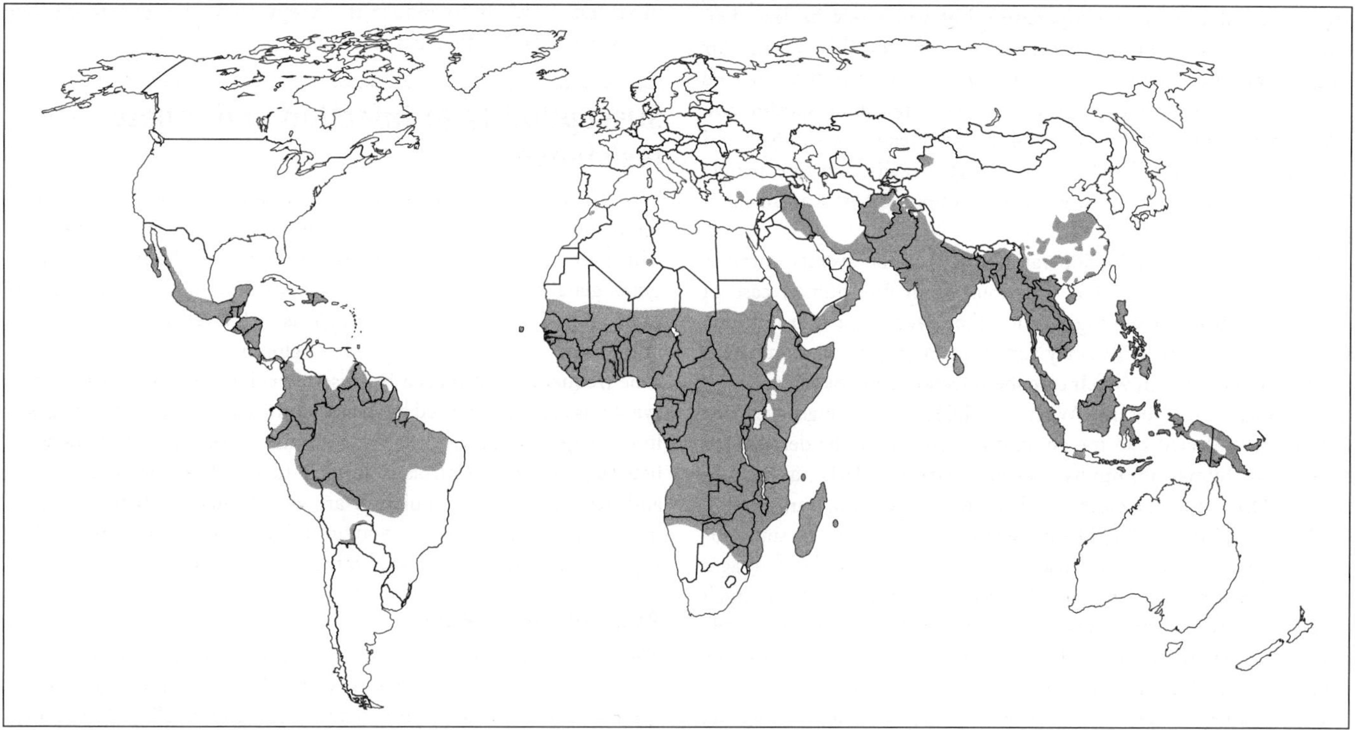

Fig. 3 Malarious areas of the world. Epidemiological assessment of the status of malaria, 1991 (WHO 93 460) *(reproduced, by permission of the World Health Organization, from World Malaria Situation in 1991. Weekly Epidemiological Record (1993).* **68,** *246).*

long sleeves, protective footwear, and repellents when outside the house are more appropriate. Endophilic mosquitoes rest on the inside walls of houses and in the roof and are thereby exposed to residual insecticides if they have previously been sprayed on the walls, whereas exophilic mosquitoes that rest outside houses, may escape the effects of insecticidal attack. The success of many antimalarial efforts has depended on the major vectors in several continents being endophilic, and failures of attempted eradication have sometimes resulted from exophilic vector species being present, as in many forested areas of South-east Asia. Anopheline mosquitoes exist in temperate countries, and in the United Kingdom several species, such as *A. atroparvus*, are capable of transmitting some imported malarial species.

Epidemiology

Malaria is widely distributed throughout the tropics (Fig. 3) except for islands of Polynesia and Micronesia. *P. falciparum* is the predominant species in the highly endemic areas of Africa, New Guinea, and Haiti, while *P. vivax* is more common in Central America, North Africa, and southern and western Asia. Both species are prevalent in South America, the rest of Asia, and Oceania. *P. malariae* is widespread but often overlooked, and in West Africa *P. ovale* largely replaces *P. vivax*, to which the indigenous inhabitants are resistant.

The epidemiological features of human malaria differ markedly even between endemic areas. At one extreme, as in West Africa, everyone is infected shortly after birth, parasitaemia is almost universal throughout childhood, and the brunt of mortality falls in early childhood; epidemics do not occur. In contrast, in parts of north India, malaria is an epidemic disease which affects all ages and causes temporary disruptive epidemics. These differences result from differing levels of malaria transmission affecting the pattern of immunity in the human population.

Climate and mosquito ecology are the primary determinants of malarial epidemiology. The density, person-biting habit, and longevity of the mosquito determines the different patterns of epidemiology.

Malaria transmission is proportional to the number of mosquitoes—the number of vectors present in a place relative to the number of people (anopheline clearity) and to the square of the person-biting habit, which is the product of the frequency with which the female feeds and the chance that people will be fed upon. The person-biting habit comprises the frequency with which the female mosquito feeds and their preference for humans. The person-biting frequency may be as high as 0.5/day in *A. gambiae*, an effective African malaria vector feeding on alternate days preferentially on people and 15-fold lower in some Asian mosquitoes feeding less frequently and only 10 per cent of the time on people.

The interval between a mosquito's ingesting infective gametocytes and the first day on which sporozoites are present in the salivary glands ready for transmission, the duration of the extrinsic cycle, depends on the ambient temperature, but will rarely be less than 10 days. Only mosquitoes that become infected and then survive for longer than the duration of the extrinsic cycle can pass on the infection. Longevity varies greatly between mosquito species and environments and affects transmission very greatly. *A. gambiae* and *A. arabiensis* are long-lived, occur at high density and bite people frequently. As a result they are the most important African malarial vectors.

The basic case reproduction rate (**BCRR**) is the average number of new cases of malaria that will result from one human case of malaria in a place, assuming all the other people are non-immune and uninfected. The BCRR may vary from over 1000 in some areas of Africa to below 1, in which case the infection will not replace itself and the disease will die out. Where the BCRR is very high everyone will become infected and the amount of malaria will be determined by acquired human immunity, so called 'stable malaria', as in sub-Saharan Africa and New Guinea. Where the BCRR is low, transmission will be intermittent and epidemics will occur from time to time, so-called 'unstable malaria'; because immunity is less, people of all ages will get ill during the epidemics, but the transmission will be much easier to control. Unstable malaria is dramatic but kills fewer people than stable malaria, in which the brunt of the mortality is borne by young children. Seasonal variation may occur even with stable malaria. The prevalence of splenic enlargement in children aged 2–9 years gives a better cumulative picture of the amount of malaria than does the parasite prevalence, which is influenced by casual chemotherapy.

Under endemic conditions there is still a great deal of variation in risk to a non-immune visitor. At one extreme, in rural Tanzania, an unprotected person is likely to be bitten on average by more than one infective mosquito nightly; while in a highly malarious part of India the corresponding rate is perhaps five times yearly or less. Yet both places will be perceived as highly malarious places by the local inhabitants.

With increasing use of chemotherapy, the acquisition of immunity is deferred and the age at which cerebral malaria is seen may increase. In West African areas of intense transmission, for example, cerebral malaria has begun to be seen in late childhood in urban areas. Malaria epidemics occur not only in areas of highly unstable malaria but also as a result of movements of refugees and migrants situations bringing susceptibles into endemic areas changes, such as those produced by the El Niño phenomenon, may produce epidemics due to increased temperature and rainfall, and long term climatic changes may also affect malaria. Increased temperatures in recent years have contributed to the transmission of malaria at higher altitudes on tropical mountains. Political instability and war may lead to the reintroduction or increase of malaria due to the breakdown of control measures and of surveillance. Water-resource development projects in developing countries may also be associated with increased transmission, while urbanization tends to reduce it, except in South Asia where one vector has adapted to urban breeding.

Table 1 Human genetic polymorphisms associated with resistance to malaria

α-Thalassaemia	Haemoglobin C	Class 1 MHC[a]
β-Thalassaemia	Ovalocytosis	Class 2 MHC
Haemoglobin S	G6PDH[b] deficiency	Duffy blood group
Haemoglobin E	ABO blood groups	S-s U blood group

[a] MHC, major histocompatibility complex; [b] G6PDH, glucose 6-phosphate dehydrogenase.

Susceptibility to infection and innate resistance

West Africans are resistant to *P. vivax* infection because they very rarely possess the Duffy blood-group antigen alleles Fy^a and Fy^b, which are receptors for penetration of the red cell by the merozoites. Other genetic determinants affect the course and outcome of infection (Table 1). The best-known example is sickle-cell disease, due to a point mutation in position 6 of the β-globin chain. Here the mutant-gene frequency is stabilized because the enhanced survival of heterozygotes is counterbalanced by the lethal consequences of homozygosity in developing countries. The relative risk of severe malaria between heterozygotes and controls is about 1 to 10. However, parasite rates and densities in the population are very similar in normal and AS individuals, except in very young children, indicating that heterozygotes are resistant to disease rather than to infection.

Acquired resistance

Those exposed to repeated malarial infection in endemic areas gradually acquire immunity that is species specific and largely strain specific. The first change observed is a reduction in clinical symptoms and signs for a given level of parasitaemia ('tolerance'). Acquired resistance to the parasites takes months to develop, first affecting the density of gametocytes in the peripheral blood and subsequently the density of trophozoites and schizonts, so that, under conditions of holoendemic transmission, the prevalence of infection in young children exceeds 80 per cent and falls to about half that by age 15 years. Infected older children and adults from highly endemic areas often have persistent, low level, asymptomatic parasitaemias.

In highly endemic areas for *P. falciparum*, several parasite strains circulate. Slow acquisition of resistance probably results from successive infection with different strains. Severe malarial anaemia in very young children is ascribed to multiple infections over a short time.

Infants born to immune mothers are partially protected against severe malaria by transplacental and breast milk antibodies for a few months, after which they suffer from severe malaria attacks with only gradual acquisition of resistance. Adult non-immunes, including visitors from non-malarious areas, are completely vulnerable, while immune women in an endemic area become more susceptible to severe disease during the second trimester of especially their first pregnancy. Splenectomy increases susceptibility to malaria.

Immunity is stage specific, in that immunity to either sporozoite challenge or to gametocyte transmission does not protect against asexual parasites. It is species, strain, and antigenic variant specific. Protection against infection by sporozoites is mediated largely by cytotoxic T cells, which can kill infected hepatocytes, but antibody to the repeat regions of the circumsporozoite protein may also have a role. Specific T and B cells as well as non-antigen-specific mechanisms are involved in the control of asexual parasitaemia. Pooled immunoglobulin from highly immune donors rapidly reduces parasitaemia. Suppressing parasitaemia below symptomatic levels involves T cells. Early in infection, Th1 cells are critical but later a Th2 phenotype is more important. High levels of cytokines such as tumour necrosis factor (**TNF-α**) during acute infection are a feature of severe malaria and are associated with a poor outcome. The acute response in non- or semi-immune individuals, while vital to the control of parasitaemia, may also contribute to the pathogenesis of disease by triggering a variety of non-specific effector mechanisms.

Effective induction of clinical immunity takes many years and several infections. It is a non-sterilizing response, for immune adults are continually reinfected. Generalized, parasite-induced immunosuppression occurs and is clinically relevant in the response to certain non-malarial antigens such as meningococcal vaccine. Some people with acute *P. falciparum* infection have impaired T-cell control of endogenous, Epstein–Barr virus-infected, B-cell proliferation and may develop Burkitt's lymphoma. The extreme polymorphism or clonal variation of immunologically relevant malarial antigens requires that the host be exposed to a variety of 'strains' before a broadly effective response can develop.

Molecular pathology

All pathological effects of malaria are consequent upon asexual parasite multiplication in the bloodstream. The characteristic bouts of fever in malaria follow the synchronous release of new merozoites into the bloodstream. Components of the infected erythrocyte, such as the lipid glycosyl phosphatidyl inositol anchor of a parasite membrane protein (perhaps MSP-1), induce the release of cytokines such as TNF-α and interleukin-1 from macrophages. The more mature stages of intra-erythrocytic parasites are more sensitive to increases in temperature, so that fever limits parasite multiplication and synchronizes parasite development.

The principal life-threatening complications of *P. falciparum* in African children are cerebral malaria and severe anaemia often associated with metabolic acidosis and respiratory distress. In non-immune adults there is single or multiple organ failure. Severe malarial anaemia is attributable to dyserythropoiesis and accelerated clearance of both parasitized and non-parasitized erythrocytes by immune and non-immune mechanisms. The central event underlying the pathology of most other manifestations of severe falciparum malaria is the cytoadherence and resulting sequestration of infected erythrocytes, which is unique to this organism. Only the younger parasites circulate; the more mature forms adhere to specific receptors on venular endothelium. Reduction in local blood flow associated with the partial occlusion of small vessels with infected erythrocytes results in reduced perfusion and tissue damage. The sequestered cells may induce local release of potentially toxic or pharmacologically active compounds (such as reactive oxygen species or nitric oxide) from macrophages, neutrophils, or endothelium.

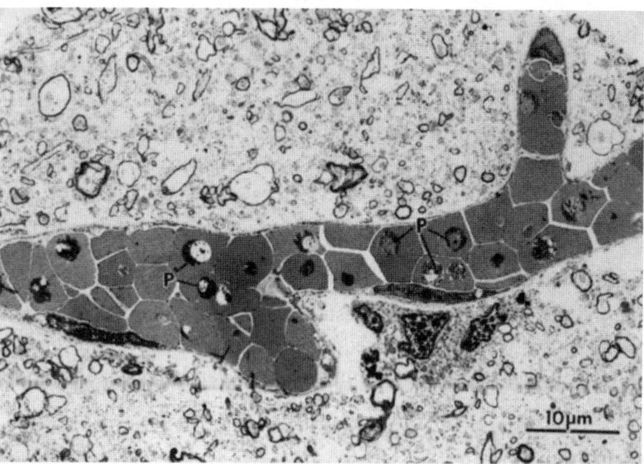

Fig. 4 Brain section of a patient who died of cerebral malaria, showing a blood vessel packed with red blood corpuscles, the majority of which were identified as being infected by the presence of parasites (P), or, at higher magnification, the presence of knobs
(by courtesy of Dr D. Ferguson, Oxford).

Several endothelial receptors have been identified, including CD36 (platelet glycoprotein IV), thrombospondin, intercellular adhesion molecule 1 (**ICAM-1**), vascular cell adhesion molecule and E-selectin. The parasite molecules involved in adhesion, $PfEMP_1$, form a family of red-cell surface proteins that undergo clonal antigenic variation during a single infection and are targets of a host-protective antibody response.

Rosetting of uninfected erythrocytes around red cells containing mature forms of the parasite has been linked to cerebral malaria in some studies. If rosettes occur *in vivo,* they may exacerbate vascular obstruction caused by cytoadherence.

Pathology

Brain

Only falciparum malaria causes cerebral pathology. At autopsy, the brain is sometimes oedematous but cerebral, cerebellar, or medullary herniation is rarely seen. Small blood vessels are congested with red blood cells containing mature parasites with pigment (Fig. 4). The brain is characteristically leaden or plum-coloured and its cut surface has a slatey-grey hue. In larger vessels, parasitized red cells line the endothelium (margination). Numerous petechial haemorrhages are seen in the white matter, resulting from haemorrhages from end arterioles, proximal to occlusive plugs of parasitized red cells and fibrin. Dürck's granulomas are small collections of microglial cells surrounding areas of demyelination at the site of these haemorrhages. An inflammatory cell response is lacking in adults but may be present in children.

Bone marrow

There is iron sequestration, erythrophagocytosis, and dyserythropoiesis that may persist for several weeks after clearance of parasitaemia. Megakaryocytes and circulating platelets are large and abnormal-looking, suggesting dysthrombopoiesis. Parasites and pigment may be present in phagocytes in the marrow, even when they are not detectable in peripheral blood.

Liver

The liver is enlarged, oedematous and brown, grey, or even black from malaria pigment. Dilated hepatic sinusoids contain hypertrophied Kupffer cells and are choked with parasitized red cells. Parasitized and uninfected red cells are phagocytosed by Kupffer cells, endothelial cells, and sinusoidal macrophages. Hepatocytes usually show only mild abnormalities.

Gastrointestinal tract

The bowel may appear congested, with mucosal ulceration and haemorrhage. Cytoadherent, sequestered, parasitized red cells may be found in capillaries of the lamina propria and larger submucosal vessels.

Kidney

Glomerular lesions range from the acute transient glomerular nephritis of falciparum malaria to the chronic lesions of quartan malarial nephrosis. Acute renal failure in falciparum malaria is associated with acute tubular necrosis. Parasitized red cells are found occasionally in glomerular and peritubular capillaries, with fibrin thrombi and pigment-laden macrophages. Tubular pigment casts occur in blackwater fever.

Lung

Pulmonary oedema is present in almost all cases. Pulmonary capillaries and venules are packed with inflammatory cells and parasitized red cells and there is interstitial oedema and hyaline-membrane formation. Secondary bronchopneumonia is common.

Spleen

The spleen is large, engorged, and dark-red or greyish-black. The red and white pulp is congested and hyperplastic, and the splenic cords and sinuses are filled with phagocytic cells containing pigment, parasitized red cells, and non-infected red cells.

Heart

There is no myocarditis. Myocardial capillaries are congested with parasitized red cells, pigment-laden macrophages, lymphocytes, and plasma cells.

Pathophysiology

Anaemia is attributable to the destruction of parasitized red cells, dyserythropoiesis and changes and immune-mediated haemolysis in some populations. There is increased splenic clearance of non-parasitized as well as parasitized red cells. In patients whose erythrocytes are congenitally deficient in enzymes such as glucose-6-phosphate dehydrogenase (G6PD), oxidant drugs, especially primaquine may provoke intravascular haemolysis. In blackwater fever, quinine-mediated haemolysis has been suspected but not proved.

Thrombocytopenia is attributable to splenic sequestration; immune-mediated lysis may also be involved.

Cerebral malaria. Some strains of *P. falciparum* express adhesive proteins such as PfEMP-1 on the surface of the parasitized erythrocyte as they develop. These bind to receptors such as ICAM-1 on cerebral venular endothelium. Expression of ICAM-1, and some other cyto-adherence receptors are increased by TNF-α and other cytokines. Obstruction to cerebral blood flow may result in stagnant anoxaemia, leading to coma. In African children with cerebral malaria, plasma concentrations of TNF-α, interleukin-1 and other cytokines correlate with parasitaemia, hypoglycaemia, case fatality, and the incidence of neurological sequelae. Cytokines may also be responsible for fever, hypoglycaemia, coagulopathy, dyserythropoiesis, and leucocytosis.

In most adults with cerebral malaria, intracranial pressure remains normal and coma is not attributable to cerebral oedema. However, in most African children with cerebral malaria, intracranial pressure is elevated and there is evidence of brain swelling. Ischaemic damage resulting from a critical reduction in cerebral perfusion pressure and other factors such as hypoglycaemia and status epilepticus are thought to be important in the mechanism of brain damage in these children.

Pulmonary oedema. This may result from iatrogenic fluid overload but adult respiratory distress syndrome is more common.

Hypoglycaemia can be caused by quinine or quinidine which release insulin from pancreatic β-cells. In malaria, glucose consumption is increased by fever, infection, anaerobic glycolysis, and the metabolic demands of the malaria parasites. Glycogen reserves may be depleted, especially in children and pregnant women. In African children with severe malaria, adult patients with severe disease, and pregnant women, hypoglycaemia can develop without quinine/quinidine treatment, possibly as a result of inhibition of hepatic gluconeogenesis by TNF-α and other cytokines.

Acute renal failure usually results from hypovolaemia. Hyperparasitaemia, jaundice, and haemoglobinuria are associated with a high risk of acute tubular necrosis. Cytoadherence of parasitized red blood cells in the renal microvasculature, deposition of fibrin microthrombi, and prolonged hypotension may contribute.

In patients with relatively normal plasma osmolalities, *hyponatraemia* has been attributed to inappropriate secretion of antidiuretic hormone (ADH) triggered by fever or reduced effective plasma volume. In patients who are hypovolaemic, ADH levels may be appropriately high. Sodium depletion may be responsible for some cases of hyponatraemia.

Hypotension and shock (algid malaria) may result from hypovolaemia but is frequently associated with a secondary Gram-negative bacteraemia.

Clinical features

The classical periodic febrile paroxysms of malaria occur every 48 or 72 h between afebrile, asymptomatic intervals. There is a tendency for recrudescence or relapse over periods of months or even years.

Falciparum malaria (malignant tertian or subtertian malaria)

The interval between an infecting mosquito bite and parasitaemia ('prepatent period') is a minimum of 5 days, but is usually 9–10 days. The interval between infection and the first symptom ('incubation period') ranges from 7 to 14 days (mean 12 days) but may be prolonged by immunity, chemoprophylaxis, or partial chemotherapy. Most patients with imported falciparum malaria present within 3 months of arriving back from the malarious area but a few present up to 1 year or later.

The illness usually starts with malaise, headache, backache, myalgia, anorexia, and mild fever. Classical tertian or subtertian periodicity (48 and 36 h between fever spikes) is rarely seen with falciparum malaria. A high irregularly spiking, continuous or remittent fever, or daily (quotidian) paroxysm, is more usual. Other common symptoms are dry cough, dizziness, postural hypotension, nausea, vomiting, abdominal discomfort, and diarrhoea. Non-immune patients are commonly prostrated. Anaemia, jaundice, and moderate tender enlargement of the spleen and liver are frequent signs. The lack of lymphadenopathy, rash (apart from herpes simplex 'cold sores'), and focal signs may be helpful in diagnosis.

Cerebral malaria and other severe manifestations and complications

Cerebral malaria develops after a few days of febrile illness, sooner in children, either with a gradual decline in the level of consciousness over several hours or with a sudden generalized convulsion without recovery of consciousness. High fever alone can cause impaired consciousness, and, in children, febrile convulsions. The term cerebral malaria (encephalopathy related to *P. falciparum* infection) should be restricted to patients with unrousable coma—no appropriate verbal response and no purposive motor response to noxious stimuli (Glasgow Coma Scale $\leq 11/15$)—and *P. falciparum* asexual parasitaemia, in whom other encephalopathies, including hypoglycaemia and transient post-ictal coma, have been excluded. Signs include dysconjugate gaze, normal brainstem reflexes (adults), brisk tendon reflexes, ankle clonus, extensor plantar responses, and absent abdominal reflexes. Abnormal posturing (decerebrate or decorticate rigidity and opisthotonos) (Plate 1) is associated with sustained upward deviation of the eyes, pouting, and stertorous breathing. Retinal haemorrhages (Plate 2) are common, exudates rare, and papilloedema very rare. About half of adult patients and more children suffer generalized convulsions. Persisting neurological sequelae are rare in adults; they include cranial nerve lesions, extrapyramidal tremor, and transient paranoid psychosis. However, some 10 per cent of African children surviving cerebral malaria have sequelae such as hemiplegia, cortical blindness, epilepsy, ataxia, and mental retardation (Plate 3). Other severe manifestations of falciparum malaria in adults are anaemia (Plate 4); spontaneous bleeding, from the gums and gastrointestinal tract; jaundice (Plate 5); hypoglycaemia; hypotension and shock (algid malaria); complicating bacterial infections (aspiration pneumonia, urinary tract infections, etc.); renal failure; blackwater fever, the association of haemoglobinuria with severe manifestations of falciparum malaria including renal failure, hypotension and coma, in a non-immune patient who is not G6PD deficient; metabolic acidosis resulting from lactic acidosis; and pulmonary oedema (Plate 6).

The symptoms and signs of hypoglycaemia—anxiety, tachycardia, breathlessness, feeling cold, confusion, sweating, lightheadedness, restlessness, fetal bradycardia, other signs of fetal distress, coma, convulsions and extensor posturing—may be misinterpreted as merely manifestations of malaria. Patients with coronary insufficiency may develop angina during febrile crises of malaria. Mild hyponatraemia with reduced plasma osmolality is often attributable to intravenous therapy with 5 per cent dextrose alone in patients who are salt depleted and dehydrated.

Delayed cerebellar ataxia has been described 3–4 weeks after an attack of otherwise uncomplicated falciparum malaria especially in Sri Lanka and India. Complete recovery is the rule.

Malarial psychosis

Acute psychiatric symptoms in patients with malaria may be caused by antimalarial drugs such as chloroquine, mefloquine, and (historically) mepacrine, or exacerbation of a pre-existing psychiatric condition. Depression, paranoia, delusions, and personality changes (brief reactive psychoses) rarely last for more than a few days.

Vivax, ovale, and malariae malarias

The prepatent and incubation periods for *P. vivax* are 8–13 and 12–17 days, respectively; for *P. ovale* 9–14 and 15–18 days; and for *P. malariae* 15–16 and 18–40 days. Only about one-third of imported cases of vivax malaria present within a month of returning from the malarious area; 5–10 per cent will present more than a year later.

The benign malarias cause paroxysmal, feverish symptoms no less severe than those of falciparum malaria. In untreated cases, the characteristic tertian (48–50 h) interval between fever spikes with vivax and ovale and the quartan (72 h) pattern in *P. malariae* infections is established after several days of irregular fever. Vivax and ovale malarias have a persistent hepatic cycle, which may give rise to relapses every 2–3 months for 5–8 years in untreated cases. *P. malariae* does not relapse but a persisting, undetectable parasitaemia may cause recrudescences for more than 50 years.

Symptoms may be severe and temporarily incapacitating, especially in non-immunes, but the acute mortality is very low. Patients suffering from vivax malaria may become anaemic, thrombocytopenic, and mildly jaundiced with tender hepatosplenomegaly. Splenomegaly may be particularly gross where *P. malariae* infection is prevalent. Splenic rupture, a very dangerous complication, is more common with vivax than falciparum malaria. It presents with abdominal pain and guarding, haemorrhagic shock (tachycardia, postural hypotension, and prostration), fever, and a rapidly falling haematocrit.

Malaria in pregnancy and the puerperium

Malaria is an important cause of maternal death and low birthweight in malaria-endemic areas. In non-immunes, cerebral and other forms of severe falciparum malaria are more common in pregnancy and carry a much higher mortality than in other patients. Fetal distress, premature labour (painless uterine contractions) and severe anaemia are common complications.

Asymptomatic hypoglycaemia may occur in pregnant women with malaria before antimalarial treatment, and pregnant women with severe or uncomplicated malaria are vulnerable to quinine-induced hypoglycaemia. There is an increased risk of pulmonary oedema precipitated by fluid overload, by the sudden increase in peripheral resistance, or by autotransfusion of hyperparasitaemic blood from the placenta, which occurs just after delivery.

Prevention

Pregnant women living in areas of malaria transmission must either be given antimalarial prophylaxis extending into the early puerperium or presumptive treatment during the pregnancy, e.g. two doses of pyrimethamine–sulfadoxine.

Congenital and neonatal malaria

Congenital malaria appears rare in malarious areas despite the high prevalence of placental infection. This confirms the adequacy of the placental barrier and the protection provided by maternal IgG, which crosses the placenta. It is much more common in infants born to non-immune mothers. All four species can produce congenital infection but, because of its very long persistence, *P. malariae* causes a disproportionate number of cases in non-endemic countries. The differential diagnosis includes rhesus incompatibility or another congenital infections such as cytomegalovirus, herpes simplex, rubella, toxoplasmosis, or syphilis.

Transfusion malaria, nosocomial malaria, and needlestick malaria

Mean incubation periods are 12 (range 7–29) days for *P. falciparum*, 12 (range 8–30) days for *P. vivax* and 35 (range 6–106) days for *P. malariae*. Whole blood, packed cells, leucocyte or platelet concentrates, fresh plasma, marrow transplants, and haemodialysis have been responsible. As patients requiring transfusion are likely to be debilitated and may be immunosuppressed, and the diagnosis may not be suspected, unusually high parasitaemias may develop, severe manifestations are common and mortality may be high.

Malaria has been transmitted between injecting drug abusers and, in a hospital through contamination of multi-use vials of saline with blood from an infected patient.

Prevention

Outside the malaria endemic area, donors who have been in the tropics during the previous 5 years should be screened for malarial antigen or antibodies. In endemic areas, recipients of blood transfusions can be given antimalarial chemotherapy, or watched carefully for evidence of infection.

Diagnosis

The diagnosis of malaria should be considered in any patient with an acute fever unless exposure can be excluded. Outside the malarious zone, patients should be asked about travel during the previous year. The possibility of malaria must not be dismissed because the patient took prophylactic drugs, for none is completely protective. Short airport stopovers, even on the runway, or working in or living near an international airport, may allow exposure to an imported, infected mosquito. Transmission by blood transfusion or needlestick should be considered. Those who grew up in an endemic area will lose their immunity after living for a few years in the temperate zone and are vulnerable when they return to their homeland on holiday. In malaria endemic regions, a large proportion of the immune population may have asymptomatic parasitaemia and it cannot be assumed that malaria is the cause of the patient's symptoms.

Differential diagnosis (Table 2)

In Europe and North America, imported malaria has been misdiagnosed as influenza, viral hepatitis, viral encephalitis, or travellers' diarrhoea, sometimes with fatal consequences. Cerebral malaria must be distinguished from other infective meningoencephalitides. Cerebrospinal fluid (CSF) examination will identify most infective causes.

Laboratory diagnosis

The diagnosis must be confirmed by examining stained thick and thin blood films on several occasions (Plate 7). Sometimes no parasites can be found in peripheral blood smears from patients with malaria, even in severe infections but parasites or malarial pigment may be found in bone marrow aspirate or in circulating neutrophils. Parasites should be counted in relation to the total white cell count (on thick films when the parasitaemia is relatively low) or erythrocytes (on thin films).

An experienced microscopist can detect as few as five parasites/μl (0.0001 per cent parasitaemia) in a thick film and 200/μl (0.004 per cent parasitaemia) in a thin film. In expert hands, the sensitivity of the quantitative buff coat method can be as good but species diagnosis is difficult, and the method is much more expensive. The Para Sight™ F dipstick antigen-capture assay employs a monoclonal antibody detecting *P. falciparum* histidine-rich protein-2 antigen. It is rapid (taking about 20 min), sensitive, and specific for *P. falciparum*. DNA probes and polymerase chain reaction now approach the sensitivity of microscopy but they are not yet rapid enough to replace microscopy for routine diagnosis. However, some could be automated for screening blood donors or for use in epidemiological surveys. Malarial antibodies can be detected by immunofluorescence or enzyme immunoassay for epidemiological surveys, for screening potential blood donors, and occasionally for providing evidence of recent infection in non-immunes.

Other laboratory investigations

Anaemia is usual, with evidence of haemolysis. Neutrophil leucocytosis is common in severe infections, but the white count can also be normal or low. Thrombocytopenia is common in *P. falciparum* and *P. vivax* infections; it does not correlate with severity. Mild abnormalities of blood coagulation are common in falciparum malaria. Total and direct (unconjugated) plasma bilirubin concentrations are usually increased, consistent with haemolysis, but in some patients with very high total bilirubin concentrations, conjugated bilirubin predominates, indicating hepatocyte dysfunction. Some patients have cholestasis. Serum albumin concentration is reduced. Serum aminotransferases, 5'-nucleotidase, and especially lactic dehydrogenase may be elevated to two or three times normal. Hyponatraemia is the most common electrolyte disturbance. Mild hypocalcaemia (after correction for hypoalbuminaemia) and hypophosphataemia have been described. Biochemical evidence of generalized rhabdomyolysis has been found in some patients. In about a third of patients with severe malaria, blood urea and serum creatinine concentrations are increased. Lactic acidosis occurs in severely ill patients, especially those with hypoglycaemia and renal failure. It may be suspected if there is a wide anion gap. Blood glucose must be checked frequently, especially in children, pregnant women, and severely ill patients. In cerebral malaria, CSF examination is important to exclude other treatable encephalopathies. The CSF may contain up to 15 lymphocytes/μl with an increased protein concentration. Blood should be cultured in patients with a high white count, shock, persistent fever, or an obvious focus of secondary bacterial infection.

Treatment

Antimalarial drugs

Chloroquine

Despite the emergence of resistant *P. falciparum* and *P. vivax*, this remains the most widely used antimalarial drug worldwide. It is the treatment of choice for *P. vivax*, *P. ovale*, and *P. malariae* infections, and for falciparum malaria acquired in Central America, Hispaniola, and parts of the Middle East. It is very rapidly absorbed after intramuscular or subcutaneous injection which can produce dangerously high plasma concentrations. Therapeutic blood concentrations persist for 6–10 days after a single dose and the terminal elimination half-time is 1–2 months. Plasma concentrations above about 250 ng/ml produce dizziness, headache, diplopia, disturbed visual accommodation, dysphagia, nausea, and malaise. Chloroquine, even in small doses, may cause pruritus of the palms, soles, and scalp in dark-skinned races and may exacerbate epilepsy and photosensitive

Table 2 Differential diagnosis of malaria

Symptom	Diagnosis
Acute fever	Other infections, heat stroke, drugs and other causes of hyperpyrexia
Fever and impaired consciousness (cerebral malaria)	Viral, bacterial, fungal, protozoal (e.g. African trypanosomiasis), or helminthic meningoencephalitis, cerebral abscess Head injury, cerebrovascular accident, intoxications (e.g. insecticides), poisonings (e.g. antimalarial drugs), metabolic (diabetes, hypoglycaemia, uraemia, hepatic failure, hyponatraemia) Septicaemias
Fever and convulsions	Encephalitides, metabolic encephalopathies, hyperpyrexia, cerebrovascular accidents, epilepsy, drug and alcohol intoxications, poisoning, eclampsia, febrile convulsions, and Reye's syndrome (children)
Fever and haemostatic disturbances	Septicaemias (e.g. meningococcaemia), viral haemorrhagic fever, rickettsial infection, relapsing fevers, leptospirosis
Fever and jaundice	Viral hepatitis, yellow fever, leptospirosis, relapsing fevers, septicaemias, haemolysis, biliary obstruction, hepatic necrosis (drugs, poisons)
Fever with gastrointestinal symptoms	Travellers' diarrhoea, dysentery, enteric fever, other bacterial infections, inflammatory bowel disease
Fever with haemoglobinuria ('blackwater fever')	Drug-induced haemolysis (e.g. oxidant antimalarials in glucose 6-phosphate-dehydrogenase-deficient patient), favism, transfusion reaction, dark urine of other causes (e.g. myoglobin, urobilinogen, porphobilinogen)
Fever with acute renal failure	Septicaemias, yellow fever, leptospirosis, drug intoxications, poisonings, prolonged hypotension
Fever with shock ('algid malaria')	Septicaemic shock, haemorrhagic shock (e.g. massive gastrointestinal bleed, ruptured spleen), perforated bowel, dehydration, hypovolaemia, myocarditis

psoriasis. Cumulative, irreversible retinal toxicity from chloroquine has been reported after lifetime prophylactic doses of 50–100 g base (i.e. after 3–6 years of taking 300 mg of base per week) (Plate 20, The eye and disease), but this is exceptionally rare when given in prophylactic doses. Chloroquine is safe during pregnancy and lactation.

Amodiaquine, a 4-aminoquinolone structurally similar to chloroquine, retains activity against chloroquine-resistant strains of *P. falciparum* in some geographical areas. It can produce hepatitis and agranulocytosis making it unsuitable for prophylaxis.

Quinine

Quinine remains the treatment of choice for falciparum malaria in many countries. It can be given safely if diluted and infused intravenously over 2–4 h. Intramuscular injection, divided between the anterior part of the thighs, is an alternative parenteral route; in this case, the stock solution of quinine dihydrochloride (300 mg/ml) should be diluted to 60 mg/ml. Strict sterile precautions should be observed. Because most deaths from severe falciparum malaria occur within the first 96 h of starting treatment, parasiticidal plasma concentrations of quinine must be achieved as quickly as possible using a loading dose of 20 mg of quinine dihydrochloride per kg, followed by a maintenance dose of 10 mg/kg every 8–12 h. The initial dose of quinine should not be reduced in patients who are severely ill with renal or hepatic impairment, but in these cases the maintenance dose should be reduced to 3–5 mg/kg if parenteral treatment is required for longer than 48 h. Quinine resistance has emerged in Thailand and Vietnam. Hypoglycaemia is the most important complication of quinine treatment. Plasma quinine concentrations above 5 mg/l cause cinchonism; transient high-tone deafness, giddiness, tinnitus, nausea, vomiting, tremors, blurred vision, and malaise. Rarely, quinine may cause haemolysis, thrombocytopenia, disseminated intravascular coagulation, hypersensitivity reactions, vasculitis, and granulomatous hepatitis. Massive overdose may result in blindness, deafness, and central nervous depression.

Quinidine

Quinidine, the *d*-diastereomer of quinine, is a more potent antimalarial than quinine but is more cardiotoxic. In the USA, it replaces quinine for the parenteral treatment of malaria. It must be infused slowly while the electrocardiogram and blood pressure are monitored. Infusion should be slowed if the blood pressure falls, the plasma concentration exceeds 22 μmol/l (7 mg/ml), or if the QT_c interval increases by more than 25 per cent.

Mefloquine

Mefloquine can only be given by mouth. It has a long elimination half-time of 14–28 days. The single dose is best divided into two halves given 6–8 h apart. Gastrointestinal symptoms occur in 10–15 per cent of patients but are usually mild and transient. Less frequent side-effects include nightmares and sleeping disturbances, dizziness, ataxia, sinus bradycardia, sinus arrhythmia, postural hypotension, seizures, and psychosis. Contraindications include β-blocker therapy and a past history of epilepsy or psychiatric disease. Resistance has been reported in South-east Asia, Africa, and South America.

Artemisinin

Artemisinin or qinghaosu comes from the Chinese medicinal herb *Artemisia annua (Compositae)* (sweet wormwood), long used to treat fevers in China. A trioxane group is responsible for activity against young trophozoites as well as other blood stages of *P. falciparum.* Parasitaemia is cleared more rapidly than by other antimalarial drugs. Intravenous or intramuscular artesunate (a water-soluble hemisuccinate), intramuscular artemether (the methyl ether suspended in peanut oil), and oral and suppository preparations of artemisinin and artesunate have proved effective in multiresistant *P. falciparum* infections. Clinical toxicity is negligible. Intramuscular artemether is given in a loading dose of 3.2 mg/kg on the first day (as a single dose or divided, 12 h apart) followed by 1.6 mg/kg per day until the patient is able to take an oral drug such as mefloquine. Artesunate is unstable in aqueous solution, but can be made up with 5 per cent bicarbonate immediately before use and injected intravenously or intramuscularly (2 mg/kg on the first day followed by 1 mg/kg until the patient can take oral treatment). Suppository formulations are particularly valuable for treating children with severe falciparum malaria at peripheral levels of the health service. Oral preparations of artemisinin and artesunate are effective for uncomplicated falciparum malaria and vivax malaria.

Primaquine

Primaquine is gametocytocidal for all *Plasmodium* species and is effective against hepatic hypnozoites, the latent stage of *P. vivax* and *P. ovale*. It may cause haemolysis in patients with congenital deficiencies of G6PD and other erythrocyte enzymes, especially in the Mediterranean (e.g. Sardinia) and Sri Lanka. As it can cross the placenta and is also excreted in breast milk, it should not be used during pregnancy or lactation where G6PD deficiency is prevalent. The dose is 15 mg base/day for 28 days but a weekly dose of 45 mg of primaquine may be better tolerated. The primaquine-resistant Chesson-type strain of *P. vivax* occurs in the Solomon Islands, Indonesia, Thailand, and Papua New Guinea. A total dose of 6 mg/kg or even more may be needed. Tafenoquine (WR238,605), a new 8-aminoquinoline, currently on clinical trial, is more than 10 times more active a hypnozoiticide than primaquine.

Sulphonamide–pyrimethamine combinations (Fansidar, Metakelfin, etc.)

These synergistic combinations are still effective for treating chloroquine-resistant falciparum infections in much of Africa and South America. The single adult dose is three Fansidar tablets (1500 mg sulfadoxine, 75 mg pyrimethamine). However, resistance has developed in many parts of South-east Asia, China, Oceania, Latin America, and East Africa. An intramuscular formulation proved effective against *P. falciparum* in southern Africa. Pyrimethamine is a folate inhibitor that may cause folic acid deficiency, especially in pregnant women, unless folinic acid supplements are given. Patients hypersensitive to sulphonamide may develop systemic vasculitis, Stevens–Johnson syndrome or toxic epidermal necrolysis. In the USA, 1 in 18 000–26 000 prophylactic courses was complicated by a fatal reaction.

These combinations are inappropriate for chemoprophylaxis; however, a fixed combination of pyrimethamine and dapsone ('Maloprim') is used in a dose of one tablet weekly in areas of moderate chloroquine resistance for those, such as sufferers from epilepsy, unable to take more usual regimens. Very long-term use, or exceeding the dose, is associated with a risk of agranulocytosis.

Hydroxynaphthoquinones

Atovaquone, an hydroxynaphthoquinone, is marketed in combination with proguanil as 'Malarone' for treatment and is undergoing trials for chemoprophylaxis.

Other antimalarial compounds

Pyronaridine, an amino-azaacridine derivative used extensively in China, has produced promising results in the treatment of chloroquine-resistant falciparum malaria in Africa. Several antimicrobial drugs, including tetracycline, doxycycline, clindamycin, azithromycin, and sulphonamides such as co-trimoxazole, have some antimalarial activity and have been used for treatment, usually in combination with a quinoline compound, or alone for chemoprophylaxis.

Antimalarial chemotherapy

In the face of the rapidly emerging resistance of *P. falciparum* to most of the available drugs, there is increasing support for the principle of combination chemotherapy using two drugs with different modes of action. Examples are lapudrine–dapsone and artemisinin combinations (e.g. artesunate-mefloquine and artemether–lumefantrine). There may be a particular advantage in combinations with an artemisinin derivative that rapidly reduces the number of infecting parasites.

Treatment of uncomplicated malaria (Table 3)

Chloroquine is the treatment of choice for *P. vivax*, *P. ovale*, *P. malariae*, and uncomplicated *P. falciparum* malarias in those geographical areas where this drug can still achieve a satisfactory clinical response. Chloroquine-resistant *P. vivax* has so far been reported only from New Guinea and adjacent islands of Indonesia but chloroquine resistant *P. falciparum* is very widespread.

Chloroquine is cheap, safe, and in the usual 3-day course well tolerated but, despite the clinical improvement following chloroquine treatment, its failure to eliminate parasitaemia and the subsequent recrudescences may eventually lead to the development of profound anaemia.

In many parts of the malaria endemic area, chloroquine is being replaced by pyrimethamine–sulphonamide combinations such as 'Fansidar' and 'Metakelfin'. These have the great advantage of being single-dose treatments that are usually well tolerated. Quinine is an effective replacement for chloroquine in most areas where multidrug-resistant strains of *P. falciparum* are prevalent. However, it has the disadvantage of producing unpleasant symptoms. In some countries a short course (3–5 days) of quinine followed by a single dose of pyrimethamine–sulphonamide is still effective. Quinine has also been combined with antibiotics such as tetracycline and clindamycin. Mefloquine, given as a single does, or in divided doses 6–8 h apart to reduce the risk of vomiting, was initially highly effective against multiresistant strains of falciparum malaria throughout the world. However, in some areas, notably in the border regions of Thailand, mefloquine resistance has developed rapidly and this drug is now used in combination with artemisinin derivatives such as artesunate.

Patients with *P. vivax* or *P. ovale* malarias who will not subsequently reside in malarious areas should be given a course of primaquine (or the new 8-aminoquinoline drug, eafenoquine) to destroy persistent exo-erythrocytic stages (see Table 3) unless they are G6PD deficient.

Treatment of severe falciparum malaria

Appropriate chemotherapy should be started as soon as possible. Dosage should be calculated according to body weight. Parenteral administration (Table 4) is the rule for patients with severe and complicated falciparum malaria. The therapeutic response must be carefully monitored by repeated clinical assessment, measurement of temperature, pulse, blood pressure, and examination of blood films. Patients should be switched to oral treatment as soon as they are able to swallow and retain tablets. They must be watched carefully for signs of drug toxicity.

General management

Patients with severe malaria should be transferred to the highest level of care available, preferably the intensive care unit. They must be

Table 3 Antimalarial chemotherapy in adults or children with uncomplicated malaria who can swallow tablets

Chloroquine-resistant *P. falciparum* or species or origin unknown	**Chloroquine-sensitive *P. falciparum* or *P. vivax, P.ovale, P. malariae* or monkey malarias**
1. *Quinine*	1. *Chloroquine*
Adults: 600 mg of a quinine salt (e.g. sulphate) 3 times each day for 7 days and, if quinine resistance is known or suspected, followed by *either* Fansidar 3 tablets (sulfadoxine 500 mg per tablet, pyrimethamine 25 mg tablet)[d] *or* tetracycline 250 mg 4 times each day for 7 days when renal function has returned to normal[c]	Adults: 600 mg of the base on the 1st and 2nd days; 300 mg on the 3rd day.
Children: approximately 10 mg of the salt/kg 3 times each day for 7 days and, if quinine resistance is known or suspected, followed by Fansidar (dose see 3 below) or clindamycin 10 mg/kg twice daily	Children: approximately 10 mg base/kg on the 1st and 2nd days; 5 mg/kg on the 3rd day
OR 2. *Mefloquine*	For radical cure of vivax/ovale add 2. *Primaquine*
Adults: 15–25 mg of the base/kg[b] (maximum 1500 mg) given as 2 doses 6–8 h apart Children: 25 mg of the base/kg given as 2 doses 6–8 h apart	Adults (except pregnant and lactating women and G6PD- deficient patients): 15 mg base/day on days 4–17 *or* 45 mg/week for 8 weeks[a] Children: 0.25 mg base/kg/day on days 4–17 *or* 0.75 mg/kg/week for 8 weeks[a]
OR 3. *Fansidar* Sulfadoxine (500 mg per tablet) plus pyrimethamine (25 mg)[d]	
Adults: 3 tablets as a single dose	
Children: <1 year $\frac{1}{4}$ tablet, <5 years $\frac{1}{2}$ tablet, <9 years 1 tablet, <15 years 2 tablets	

For salt/base equivalents see OTM3, p. 853, Table 6.

[a] For Chesson-type strains (SE Asia, W Pacific) use double dose or double duration up to a total dose of 6 mg/kg in daily doses of 15–22.5 mg in adults.

[b] Depending on geographical area and presumed immunity.

[c] Alternative to tetracycline is doxycycline 100 mg daily for 7 days or clindamycin 10 mg/kg twice daily for 3–7 days. Tetracycline and doxycycline are contraindicated in pregnancy.

[d] Sulfadoxine+pyrimethamine (Fansidar) and other sulphonamide–pyrimethamine combinations are contraindicated if the patient is hypersensitive to sulphonamide.

nursed in bed because of their postural hypotension. Body temperatures above 38.5°C are associated with febrile convulsions, especially in children, and between 39.5 and 42°C with coma and permanent neurological sequelae. In pregnant women, hyperpyrexia contributes to fetal distress. Temperature should therefore be controlled by fanning, tepid sponging, cooling blanket, or antipyretic drugs such as paracetamol (15 mg/kg in tablets by mouth, or powder washed down a nasogastric tube, or as suppositories).

Cerebral malaria

Vital signs, Glasgow coma score, and occurrence of convulsions should be recorded frequently. Convulsions can be controlled with diazepam. Stomach contents should be aspirated through a nasogastric tube to reduce the risk of aspiration pneumonia. Elective endotracheal intubation is indicated if coma deepens and the airways are jeopardized. Deepening coma is an indication for computed tomography or magnetic resonance imaging.

A number of potentially harmful remedies of unproven value have, in the past, been recommended for the treatment of cerebral malaria. Dexamethasone in adults and children did not reduce mortality but prolonged coma and increased the incidence of infection and gastrointestinal bleeding. Low-molecular-weight dextrans, osmotic agents, heparin, adrenaline, cyclosporin A, prostacyclin, and oxpentifylline have been advocated for the treatment of cerebral malaria without convincing evidence and in some cases despite obvious toxicity.

Anaemia

Transfusion with whole blood or packed cells is indicated when the haematocrit falls below 20 per cent or if there is severe bleeding and hyperparasitaemia.

Disturbances of fluid and electrolyte balance

Fluid and electrolyte requirements must be assessed individually in patients with malaria. Circulatory overload with intravenous fluids or blood transfusion may precipitate pulmonary oedema, but untreated hypovolaemia may lead to shock, lactic acidosis, and renal failure. Hypovolaemia may result from salt and water depletion through fever, diarrhoea, vomiting, insensible losses, and poor intake. The state of hydration is assessed clinically and the history of recent urine output and measurement of urine volume and specific gravity may be useful. Fluid replacement should be controlled by observations of jugular, central venous, or pulmonary artery wedge pressures.

Renal failure

Acute renal failure should be treated with haemofiltration or dialysis. Hypovolaemia is corrected by cautious infusion of isotonic saline until the central venous pressure is in the range +5 to +10 cmH_2O. If urine output remains low after rehydration, increasing doses of

Table 4 Antimalarial chemotherapy in adults or children with severe malaria or in those who cannot swallow tablets

Chloroquine-resistant *P. falciparum* or origin unknown	Chloroquine-sensitive *P. falciparum*[a] or *P. vivax, P. ovale, P. malariae* or monkey malarias
1. *Quinine*	1. *Chloroquine*[b]
Adults: 20 mg dihydrochloride salt/kg (loading dose)[c] diluted in 10 ml/kg isotonic fluid by IV infusion over 4 h, then 8 h after the start of the loading dose, 10 mg/kg over 4 h, 8 hourly until patients can swallow	10 mg base/kg (maximum 600 mg) diluted in isotonic fluid by continuous IV infusion over 8 h, followed by 15 mg base/kg (maximum 900 mg) by continuous IV infusion over 24 h
Children: 15 mg dihydrochloride salt/kg (loading dose)[c] diluted in 10 ml/kg isotonic fluid by IV infusion over 2 h, then 12 h after the start of the loading dose, 10 mg/kg over 2 h, 12-hourly until patients can swallow.	
The 7-day course should be completed with quinine tablets approximately 10 mg salt/kg 8-hourly[d,e] or give a single dose of 25 mg/kg sulfadoxine and 1.25 mg/kg pyrimethamine	
OR 2. *Quinine* (in intensive care unit)	OR 2. *Quinine* (see above, left-hand column)
7 mg dihydrochloride salt/kg (loading dose)[c] IV by infusion pump over 30 min followed immediately by 10 mg/kg (maintenance dose) diluted in 10 ml/kg isotonic fluid by IV infusion over 4 h, repeated 8–12-hourly until patient can swallow etc.[d,e]	
OR 3. *Quinidine* 15 mg of the base/kg (loading dose)[c] i.v. by infusion over 4 h, then, 8 h after the start of the loading dose, 7.5 mg base/kg over 4 h, 8 hourly until the patient can swallow, then quinine tablets to complete 7 days treatment[d] or give a single dose of 25 mg/kg sulfadoxine and 1.25 mg/kg pyrimethamine	
OR 4. *Artesunate*[f] 2.4 mg/kg by IV 'push' injection (loading dose) followed by 1.2 mg/kg at 12 and 24 h, then 1.2 mg/kg daily for 6 days	
OR 5. *Artemether* 3.2 mg/kg intramuscular (loading dose) followed by 1.6 mg/kg daily for 6 days	
OR *If it is not possible to give drugs by intravenous infusion* 1. Quinine	1. *Chloroquine*[b]
20 mg of the salt/kg (loading dose)[c] diluted to 60 mg/ml, by deep intramuscular injection (half dose into each anterior thigh) with strict sterile precautions, then 10 mg/kg 8–12-hourly until patient can swallow etc.[d,e]	Total dose 25 mg base/kg given either: (a) IM or SC 2.5 mg/kg 4-hourly; *or* (b) IM or SC 3.5 mg/kg 6-hourly
2. *Artemether, Artesunate,* or *Artemisinin* by intramuscular injection or suppository	OR 2. *Quinine* IM (see above, left-hand column)

For salt/base equivalents see OTM3, p. 853, Table 6.

[a] Currently restricted to Haiti, Dominican Republic, Central America, and parts of Middle East.

[b] Parenteral chloroquine should be used with great caution in young children.

[c] Loading dose must not be used if patient started quinine, quinidine, or mefloquine treatment within preceding 12 h.

[d] In areas of known or suspected quinine resistance add tetracycline 250 mg 4 times each day or doxycycline 200 mg daily for 7 days except for children under 8 years and pregnant women *or* add Fansidar (doses in Table 3) except in patients known to be sulphonamide hypersensitive or add clindamycin 10 mg/kg twice daily for 3–7 days.

[e] In patients requiring more than 48 h of parenteral therapy reduce the dose by one-third to a half to 5–7 mg of the salt per kg 8–12 hourly.

[f] Artesunic acid 60 mg is dissolved in 0.6 ml of 5 per cent sodium bicarbonate diluted to 3.5 ml with 5 per cent dextrose and give immediately by ('push') bolus injection.

slowly infused intravenous frusemide (up to a total dose of 1 g) and finally intravenous infusion of dopamine (2.5–5 mg/kg per min) can be tried. If these measures fail to achieve a sustained increase in urine output, strict fluid balance should be enforced. Indications for dialysis include a rapid increase in serum creatinine level, hyperkalaemia, fluid overload, metabolic acidosis, and clinical manifestations of uraemia.

Metabolic acidosis is usually caused by lactic acidosis or renal failure. It should be treated by improving perfusion and oxygenation by correcting hypovolaemia, clearing the airways, increasing the inspired oxygen concentration, and by treating septicaemia, a frequently associated complication. Severe acidosis (pH less than 7.20) can be treated by cautious infusion of sodium bicarbonate or dichloroacetate (which stimulates muscle pyruvate dehydrogenase). If the patient is uraemic, early dialysis is the treatment of choice.

Pulmonary oedema

Patients who develop pulmonary oedema should be propped upright and given oxygen to breathe. In a well-equipped intensive care unit, the judicious use of vasodilator drugs can be controlled by monitoring haemodynamic variables, fluid overload can be corrected by haemoperfusion, and oxygenation can be improved by mechanical ventilation with positive end-expiratory pressure.

Hypotension and shock (algid malaria)

Circulatory problems should be corrected with plasma expanders and dopamine. Broad-spectrum antimicrobial treatment should be started immediately. Other causes of shock in patients with malaria include dehydration, blood loss, and pulmonary oedema.

Hypoglycaemia

Blood sugar must be checked every few hours, especially in patients being treated with quinine or quinidine. A therapeutic trial of dextrose (1 ml/kg by intravenous bolus injection) should be given if hypoglycaemia is proved or suspected. This should be followed by a continuous infusion of 10 per cent dextrose but this will not always prevent recurrence. Glucose may be given by nasogastric tube to unconscious patients or by peritoneal dialysis in those undergoing this treatment for renal failure.

Hyperparasitaemia

Exchange transfusion may reduce parasitaemia more rapidly than optimal chemotherapy alone and could have the added advantages of removing harmful metabolites, toxins, cytokines, and other mediators, and replenishing erythrocytes, platelets, clotting factors, and albumin. Potential dangers of the procedure include electrolyte disturbances (for example, hypocalcaemia), cardiovascular complications, and introduction of infectious agents in the blood and through infection of intravascular lines. The use of exchange transfusion, haemopheresis, and plasmapheresis has been reported in more than 100 patients, most of whom survived. Some patients recovered consciousness or improved in other ways during the procedure. Where screening of donor blood is adequate, the procedure should be considered in non-immune patients who are severely ill, who have deteriorated on conventional treatment, and who have parasitaemias in excess of 10 per cent.

Splenic rupture

Conservative management with blood transfusion and close observation in an intensive care unit is sometimes successful but surgical help is essential in case there is a sudden deterioration.

Disseminated intravascular coagulation

Vitamin K (adult dose 10 mg by slow intravenous injection), cryoprecipitates, platelet transfusions, and fresh-frozen plasma are indicated.

Malaria in pregnancy

Quinine is safe in pregnancy. Chloroquine has been used extensively without ill effect to mother or fetus and sulphonamide–pyrimethamine has also proved an acceptable treatment in pregnancy. Tetracycline, primaquine, and aspirin (but not paracetamol) are contraindicated in late pregnancy and mefloquine should be avoided if possible, especially during the first trimester. Halofantrine is contraindicated throughout pregnancy. Total apparent volume of distribution of quinine is reduced and elimination is more rapid in pregnant women. Initial dosage is the same as in non-pregnant patients, but in severe cases requiring prolonged parenteral treatment, the dose, but not the frequency of administration, should be reduced. The main danger of quinine in pregnancy is its stimulation of insulin secretion with resulting hypoglycaemia. Blood glucose must be checked at least once a day in pregnant women with malaria, whether or not they are receiving quinine. Maternal fever should be reduced as soon as possible. Induction of labour, caesarean section, or speeding up of the second stage of labour with forceps or vacuum extractor should be considered in patients with severe falciparum malaria. Fluid balance is particularly critical in these patients. For chemoprophylaxis in pregnancy, chloroquine and proguanil, separately or together, are the most appropriate and folic acid supplements should be given. In Africa, two therapeutic doses of 'Fansidar' given during pregnancy have been found to prevent maternal and congenital infection.

Prognosis

The mortality of acute vivax, ovale, and malariae malarias is negligible. Strictly defined cerebral malaria has a mortality of about 10–15 per cent when medical facilities are good, and may be less than 5 per cent in Western intensive care units. Lack of acquired immunity or lapsed immunity, splenectomy, pregnancy, and immunosuppression predispose to severe falciparum malaria. The following carry a bad prognosis: impaired consciousness, pregnancy, renal failure, hypoglycaemia, haemoglobinuria, metabolic acidosis and pulmonary oedema, schizontaemia, leucocytosis (>12 000/μl), high cerebrospinal fluid lactate or low glucose, low plasma antithrombin III, high serum creatinine (>265 μmol/l), or blood urea nitrogen (>21.4 mmol/l), haematocrit less than 20 per cent, blood glucose less than 2.2 mmol/l, and elevated serum enzyme concentrations (for example, aspartate and alanine aminotransferases, lactate dehydrogenase).

Chronic immunological complications of malaria

Quartan malarial nephrosis

In parts of Africa, South America, India, South-east Asia, and Papua New Guinea, *P. malariae* infection causes immune-complex glomerulonephritis and nephrotic syndrome in some people. There is progressive focal and segmental glomerulosclerosis with fibrillary splitting or flaking of the capillary basement membrane, producing characteristic lacunae, with deposition of immunoglobulins and C3, and *P. malariae* antigen. Most patients present by the age of 15 years with symptoms of nephrotic syndrome. A few patients respond to corticosteroids, azathioprine, and cyclophosphamide. Antimalarial treatment is not effective but malarial nephrosis is preventable with antimalarial prophylaxis.

Tropical splenomegaly syndrome (hyper-reactive malarial splenomegaly)

Some residents of malarious areas of Africa, the Indian subcontinent, South-east Asia, South America, Papua New Guinea, and the Middle East develop progressive, sometimes massive, splenomegaly, elevated serum IgM and malarial antibody levels, and hepatic sinusoidal lymphocytosis with a clinical and immunological response to antimalarial prophylaxis. This condition is thought to result from an aberrant immunological response to repeated infection by any of the species of malaria parasite.

There are some differences between tropical splenomegaly syndrome in Africa, Flores, and Papua New Guinea. African patients have a peripheral lymphocytosis (B lymphocytes) and distinction from chronic lymphatic leukaemia may be difficult. The syndrome may evolve into a malignant lymphoproliferative disorder with villous (hairy) lymphocytes. A familial tendency in Africa and Papua New Guinea suggests a genetic factor.

Clinical features

The spleen may be enormous and the liver is usually enlarged. Episodes of severe abdominal pain with peritonism suggest perisplenitis or splenic infarction. Anaemia may be severe with acute haemolytic episodes. Most deaths are attributable to overwhelming infection. Chronic hypersplenic neutropenia or failure to mobilize neutrophils in response to acute bacterial infections may be the cause. The prognosis is poor.

Laboratory findings

Laboratory findings are of severe chronic anaemia, thrombocytopenia, neutropenia, and lymphocytosis with lymphocytic infiltration of the bone marrow. Serum IgM is greatly elevated. There is lymphocytosis of the hepatic sinusoids with Kupffer-cell hyperplasia, round-cell infiltration of the portal tracts and, in some cases, fibrosis, leading to portal hypertension. The spleen shows dilatation of the sinusoids, hyperplasia of the phagocytic cells with erythrophagocytosis, and infiltration with lymphocytes and plasma cells.

Differential diagnosis

The differential diagnosis includes leukaemias, lymphomas, myelofibrosis, thalassaemias, haemoglobinopathies, visceral leishmaniasis, and schistosomiasis.

Treatment

Prolonged antimalarial chemoprophylaxis is often effective. The dangers of splenectomy rule out this procedure in the rural tropics. Folic acid may be needed.

Endemic Burkitt's lymphoma (see Chapter 16.12)

Malaria control

Malaria control may attempt to reduce or interrupt transmission especially in areas of unstable malaria, and to ensure diagnosis and prompt treatment of those who become infected. This is predominantly the strategy in areas of stable transmission. Transmission control has been most widely carried out in the past by means of residual insecticide spraying on the entire inside walls of houses, and in some countries this was able to stop transmission for long enough to allow the parasite reservoir to die out over several years to leave a place from which malaria had been eradicated. But as insecticide resistance increases and spraying costs rise, environmental control of mosquito breeding and biological control of the larvae are being revived.

Bednets impregnated with synthetic pyrethroids such as permethrin, deltamethrin, or I-cyhalothrin give substantial malaria protection in endemic areas, even reducing the number of clinical attacks in areas of high transmission. Nets are most effective when mosquito biting is concentrated late at night, and they can give good protection to babies in cots.

Malaria control programmes contain a mixture of four component strategies. These are: (1) early diagnosis and prompt treatment of fevers and other clinical malaria, at household, primary health care facility or hospital level as appropriate; (2) selective and sustainable preventive measures which may include reducing transmission by environmental or biological control of breeding sites or residual insecticide spraying of dwellings, and by personal protection against biting by insecticide-treated bed nets; (3) early detection and containment of epidemics; and (4) chemoprophylaxis for selected vulnerable groups, particularly pregnant women. Programmes need to be flexible, and guided by a reliable surveillance system and regular reassessment of the situation. Emphasis has changed from stopping transmission to preventing death and reducing morbidity, especially in areas of stable malaria, but transmission control still has an important role elsewhere.

It is now accepted that, for much of sub-Saharan Africa, it is not technically possible, and for many other places it is not economically feasible, to stop malaria transmission completely, but that even then much can be done to limit the damage done by the parasite.

Prevention of malaria in travellers

Residents of non-malarious areas who visit endemic regions can reduce the risk of infection by: (1) awareness of risk; (2) reduction of exposure to bites by anopheline mosquitoes; and (3) chemoprophylaxis where appropriate. (1) and (2) are of the same importance as (3) in preventing malaria mortality.

No prophylactic regimen will give total protection. In the event of a fever while travelling, or afterwards, malaria must be considered as a diagnosis. Strict compliance, even with a suboptimal prophylactic regimen, is more important than vacillation over finding the optimal one. Additional ways of reducing risk include the use of bednets impregnated with a pyrethroid insecticide, sleeping in a well-screened bedroom and the use of a knock-down insecticide, wearing clothes that deter mosquito bites, repellent sprays and soaps (containing *N,N*-diethyl-*m*-toluamide or permethrin), and avoiding exposure to bites in the evenings.

Chemoprophylaxis (Tables 5 and 6)

Where chloroquine-resistant *P. falciparum* is absent (e.g. western Asia, North Africa, and Central America) chloroquine 300 mg (base), two tablets taken once a week, will give good protection. It will not prevent late attacks of *P. vivax* or *P. ovale* malaria. Proguanil, 100 mg daily, or 200 mg daily is poorly protective against *P. vivax* but carries an extremely low incidence of adverse side-effects, making it acceptable to long-term residents in endemic areas. Chloroquine can be taken for up to 6 years, after which proguanil may be substituted.

Chloroquine-resistant *P. falciparum* is a massive and increasing problem in most other parts of the malaria endemic region. Where the proportion of malaria resistant to chloroquine is low or the degree

Table 5 Recommended malaria prophylaxis (adult dose) in addition to general measures specified in text

(a) Where chloroquine-resistant *P. falciparum* is absent:
1. Chloroquine 300 mg base (2 tablets) weekly (best for short-term visitors)
or
2. Proguanil 200 mg (2 tablets) daily (best for long-term residents)
(b) Where chloroquine-resistant *P. falciparum* is not widespread and is predominantly of low degree:
1. Chloroquine 300 mg base (2 tablets) weekly *plus* proguanil 200 mg (2 tablets) daily
(c) Where highly chloroquine-resistant *P. falciparum* occurs:[a]
1. Mefloquine 250 mg (1 tablet) weekly
or
2. Chloroquine 300 mg base (2 tablets) weekly *plus* proguanil 200 mg (2 tablets) daily
or
3. Doxycycline 100 mg (1 tablet) daily
or
4. Chloroquine 300 mg base weekly *plus* Maloprim 1 tablet weekly (pyrimethamine–dapsone fixed combination)

[a] (c)1 and (c)3 are more effective in some areas of SE Asia, Africa, and South America, but there is a low but significant risk of severe side-effects. (c)2 is the safest of the four (c) regimens so far as toxic side-effects are concerned and is preferred for pregnant women and, with reduced dose, for young children (Table 6). (c)4 is still an acceptable alternative for New Guinea, the Western Pacific, and some other areas, but its efficacy is declining.

of resistance limited, the combination of chloroquine and proguanil has the advantage of low toxicity and appears effective in many areas, including India and the rest of South Asia. This combination is safe in pregnant women and in young children.

However, the efficacy of chloroquine/proguanil is now less than 70 per cent in substantial parts of sub-Saharan Africa where the malaria challenge in rural areas may exceed one infective bite per night and resistance is common, nor in South-east Asia where the transmission rate is much lower but multidrug resistant *P. falciparum* is prevalent.

Mefloquine ('Lariam') had been widely recommended as one tablet weekly gives protection of about 90 per cent in Africa. The main serious early side-effects of prophylactic mefloquine are neuropsychiatric, including anxiety, insomnia, nightmares, depression, delusions, psychotic attacks, convulsions and vertigo. They are more common in women than men and occur in between 0.1 and 1 per cent of people taking mefloquine. More than 75 per cent of adverse reactions are manifest by the third dose, so it is wise for those taking the drug for the first time to start $2\frac{1}{2}$ weeks before they intend to travel, so that there is time to change to another drug if they develop serious side-effects. Mefloquine is only slowly cleared from the body. As its safety during early pregnancy is uncertain, it is not recommended for those in the first trimester of pregnancy or likely to become pregnant during the 3 months after the end of chemoprophylaxis. It is contraindicated in people with a history of epilepsy or psychiatric disorder. Mefloquine is currently the most appropriate chemoprophylaxis for sub-Saharan Africa, the Amazon region of Brazil, Colombia, and adjacent countries, and areas of South-east Asia with high levels of malaria transmission. Sporadic cases of mefloquine resistance are already reported from Africa, and on the borders between Thailand, Burma, and Cambodia up to 40 per cent of cases of falciparum malaria are mefloquine resistant. Under these circumstances, except in pregnant or lactating women and children under 12 years old, doxycycline is an appropriate chemoprophylactic. Side-effects include photosensitization, diarrhoea, and vaginal thrush. Doxycycline is useful, in other areas of high transmission and high chloroquine resistance, for those unable or unwilling to take mefloquine. Proguanil plus choroquine has also been used for short-term tourists to Kenya, but there has been an increased incidence of malaria. An alternative for travellers to Papua New Guinea, southern Africa, and parts of South America, is 'Maloprim' (12.5 mg pyrimethamine and 100 mg dapsone per tablet). Maloprim alone gives poor protection against *P. vivax*; chloroquine may be given concurrently. The dose of Maloprim must not exceed one tablet a week or the incidence of the otherwise rare side-effect, agranulocytosis, rises. Methaemoglobinaemia occasionally occurs.

Proguanil, Maloprim, and doxycycline do not increase the risk of fits in patients with epilepsy.

Table 6 Doses of prophylactic antimalarial drugs for children[a]

Age	Weight (kg)	Fraction of adult dose		
		Chloroquine + proguanil	Maloprim (pyrimethamine + dapsone)	Mefloquine
0–5 weeks		$\frac{1}{8}$	Not recommended	Not recommended
6–52 weeks		$\frac{1}{4}$	$\frac{1}{8}$[b]	Not recommended
1–5 years	10–19	$\frac{1}{2}$	$\frac{1}{4}$	Not recommended under age 2 years or 15 kg $\frac{1}{4}$ (2–5 years)
6–11 years	20–39	$\frac{3}{4}$	$\frac{1}{2}$	$\frac{1}{2}$ (6–8 years); $\frac{3}{4}$ (9–11 years) up to 45 kg
≥12 years	>40	Adult dose	Adult dose	Adult dose

When both are available, weight is a better guide than age for children over 6 months old.

[a] For children aged under 2 years in areas of chloroquine resistance the appropriate medication is chloroquine plus proguanil. Chloroquine is available as a syrup but the proguanil has to be powdered on to jam or food. Measures against mosquito bites are specially important.

[b] Not feasible to prepare unless a paediatric formulation is available.

The following drugs are unsuitable for chemoprophylaxis: amodiaquine because of the high risk of agranulocytosis; 'Fansidar' because of the frequency of severe skin reactions; and pyrimethamine on its own, because it is ineffective in most areas.

Because no prophylactic is completely effective in chloroquine-resistant *P. falciparum* areas, travellers in remote areas away from prompt medical assistance should carry a therapeutic dose of Fansidar, quinine, or mefloquine.

All prophylactic regimens should be continued for 4 weeks after returning to a non-endemic area.

Malarial vaccines

Because immunity to the disease is specific both for the parasite species and the stage of the lifecycle, attempts have been made to develop vaccines against sporozoites, asexual blood forms, and gametocytes of *P. falciparum.* A variety of rodent or non-human primate model systems have been used. Immunization of rodents with irradiated sporozoites obtained by the irradiation of infected mosquitoes or passive transfer of a monoclonal antibody to the major protein on the sporozoite surface (the circumsporozoite protein, **CSP**) induce up to 100 per cent protection. Irradiated infected mosquitoes could also be used successfully to protect humans against challenge, but only after very large numbers of bites. This encouraged the construction of recombinant vaccines containing various regions of the CSP. Work is continuing on both protein and DNA vaccines aimed at inducing an appropriate T-cell response to CSP and another sporozoite surface protein as well as proteins made in the infected hepatocyte.

Vaccination with asexual blood stages or with purified blood-stage antigens has proved less reliable. Many different recombinant antigens have been used to vaccinate experimental rodents and non-human primates, with varied outcomes. Protection is rarely if ever complete and usually required the use of Freund's complete adjuvant (which is unacceptable in humans) for optimum results.

Patarroyo screened a wide variety of peptides derived from sequence data from numerous malarial proteins in monkeys. The most active peptides, after polymerization, were used in human trials in Latin America, Thailand, Tanzania, and the Gambia. Protection ranged from 0 to 50 per cent.

Many antigens currently under study have been identified because they were recognized by serum from endemic-area adults, who have an extremely diverse response to malarial antigens, much of which is irrelevant to protection. One of the only antigens for which a role in host protection has been suggested in field studies is $PfEMP_1$, a family of highly variable antigens. They are difficult targets for vaccines because of their enormous diversity.

Several antigens on the surface of gametocytes, zygotes, and ookinetes have been identified and cloned. Antibodies to these can significantly reduce or abolish mosquito transmission and will form an important component of an overall vaccination strategy.

Another approach is to attempt protection against disease. This could be directed either against parasite molecules that induce the release of cytokines or at those molecules involved in binding infected erythrocytes to particular endothelial receptors in cerebral malaria.

The criteria for successful vaccination will vary with different groups. Travellers or military personnel would expect close to 100 per cent protection from clinical disease, whereas in Africa a reduction in morbidity and mortality alone would be worthwhile.

In either case the vaccine would need to be stable, effective after one or two doses, provide immunity of sufficiently long duration, and be easy to administer. In Africa it would need to be effective in young infants.

Further reading

Bradley, D.J. and Warhurst, D.C. (1997). Guidelines for the prevention of malaria in travellers from the United Kingdom. *CDR Review* 7, R137–52.

Garnham, P.C.C. (1966). *Malaria parasites and other Haemosporidia.* Blackwell Scientific, Oxford.

Gilles, H.M. and Warrell, D.A. (1993). *Bruce Chwatt's essential malariology,* (3rd edn). Arnold, London.

Targett, G.A.T. (ed.) (1991). *Malaria: waiting for the vaccine.* John Wiley, Chichester.

Wernsdorfer, W.H. and McGregor, I.A. (1988). *Malaria. Principles and practice of malariology.* Churchill Livingstone, Edinburgh.

White, N.J. and Ho, M. (1992). The pathophysiology of malaria. *Advances in Parasitology,* 31, 83–173.

World Health Organization (1990). *Practical chemotherapy of malaria: report of a WHO scientific group.* Technical Report Series No. 805. WHO, Geneva.

World Health Organization (Communicable Disease Cluster). (2000). Severe falciparum malaria. *Transactions of the Royal Society of Tropical Medicine and Hygiene,* **94** (suppl.).

Chapter 16.85

Babesia

T. K. Ruebush II

Babesia are tick-borne, intra-erythrocytic protozoan parasites of wild and domestic animals that occasionally infect humans. Cases of human babesiosis have been reported from both Europe and North America. The European cases have been sporadic and widely distributed geographically. The causative organism is *Babesia divergens,* a parasite of cattle transmitted by *Ixodes ricinus* ticks; nearly all infections occurred in asplenic people. Most of the North American cases were acquired in a circumscribed area along the north-east coast of the USA. They were caused by *B. microti,* a parasite of rodents that is transmitted by *I. sapularis,* which is capable of infecting persons with functioning spleens. Sporadic cases of human babesiosis caused by unidentified species of *Babesia* have been reported from other areas of the USA.

Patients infected with *B. divergens* have a 1–3-day history of fatigue and malaise, rapidly followed by high fever, shaking chills, jaundice, and the production of small amounts of dark or blood-stained urine. Anaemia is generally severe; leucocyte counts range from normal to >40 000/mm^3. Marked elevations in levels of bilirubin, liver enzymes, blood urea nitrogen, and creatinine are common. The course of illness is generally characterized by progressive haemolytic anaemia, haemoglobinaemia, haemoglobinuria, jaundice, and renal insufficiency leading to death in most cases.

Human *B. microti* infections range from asymptomatic to prolonged severe illnesses, with symptomatic infections more common in individuals over 40 years of age. The illness usually begins with gradual onset of anorexia, fatigue, fever, chills, and generalized myalgia. Most patients have mild to moderately severe haemolytic anaemia, with low to normal leucocyte counts. Several fatal cases have been reported in asplenic patients.

Babesia parasites are most easily recognized in thin or thick blood smears stained with Giemsa, but are frequently mistaken for malaria parasites, especially *Plasmodium falciparum*, because of the very small ring forms.

No generally effective drugs are available for the treatment of human babesiosis. Therapy of *B. divergens* infections is complicated by the rapidly progressive course of the disease; most patients who have recovered have been managed with blood transfusions and renal dialysis. Combinations of pentamidine plus co-trimoxazole and quinine plus clindamycin have been reported to reduce parasitaemia, but experience with these drugs is limited.

B. microti infections in patients with intact spleens are often self-limited, although symptoms and parasitaemia may persist for several months. The best available treatment appears to be a combination of quinine plus clindamycin (25 mg/kg of each for 7–10 days). Exchange transfusions have been used successfully in several patients with very high levels of parasitaemia.

Further reading

Fernandez Villar, B., White, D.J., and Benach, J.L. (1991). Human babesiosis. *Progress in Clinical Parasitology*, 2, 129–43.

Rosner, F., Zarrabi, M.H., Benach J.L., and Habicht, G.S. (1984). Babesiosis in splenectomized adults: review of 22 reported cases. *American Journal of Medicine*, 76, 696–701.

Chapter 16.86

Toxoplasmosis

J. Couvreur and Ph. Thulliez

Parasitology, epidemiology, and transmission

Toxoplasma gondii is an obligate intracellular protozoan parasite. Its definitive host is the cat. It exists in three stages: tachyzoites (acute infection), bradyzoites in cysts (chronic infection) and oocysts which contain sporozoites and are excreted only with the faeces of the cat. Toxoplasma infection is worldwide in its extent. *T. gondii* antibody seroprevalence rates are higher in populations at risk; mostly by contact with cats or ingestion of undercooked meat. Cats infected orally by any form of the parasite shed large number of oocysts for 3 weeks. This highly infectious form can remain for months in warm moist soil. This is the source of the infection of cattle, sheep, and pigs.

Transmission in acquired toxoplasmosis is mainly related to ingestion of cysts which release sporozoites in the gut. The parasites spread through the lymphatics and bloodstream reaching every organ where they multiply intracellularly as tachyzoites. Necrosis and inflammation can occur in infected tissues. If the host is immunocompetent the parasite encysts and can persist for a lifetime in the tissues. If the host becomes immunocompromised the cysts can release bradyzoïtes and *Toxoplasma* becomes an opportunistic agent. All immunocompromising conditions, such as malignancies and their treatment, lupus erythematosus, and especially acquired immune deficiency syndrome (AIDS) must be considered. In transplantations an infected organ such as the heart can cause toxoplasmosis in a seronegative recipient (mismatched patients).

Congenital toxoplasmosis is the result of a transplacental transmission of tachyzoites following acquired infection during pregnancy in an hitherto uninfected woman.

Acute acquired toxoplasmosis

Acquired toxoplasmosis in immunocompetent hosts is usually subclinical. Lymphadenopathy, mostly posterior cervical, suboccipital, and/or retroauricular, is the commonest presentation often mimicking infectious mononucleosis. It can be protracted for months and never suppurates. Fatigue, headache, myalgias, low-grade fever, and transient rash may also occur. There is a relative neutropenia with lymphocytosis. Atypical lymphocytes similar to those of infectious mononucleosis and inversion of the CD4/CD8 ratio can occur. Histological examination of the nodes shows scattered epithelioid cells, histiocytosis, follicular hypoplasia, and monocytoid cells.

Toxoplasmosis of the central nervous system

Toxoplasma has a great affinity for brain tissue. Central nervous system involvement can occur in any form of acquired toxoplasmosis but mostly in immunocompromised hosts. Tachyzoites reach brain tissue through the bloodstream. Infection of cells leads to all intermediate patterns between disseminated foci of microglial nodules, more or less numerous large necrotic areas or granulomas and large space occupying lesions. Cysts can be seen in tissues without inflammatory reaction. Clinical patterns are protean and include:

- generalized encephalitis with meningeal involvement, and possible localizing signs progressing to coma and death within a few days and relapsing chronic encephalitis;
- space occupying mass mimicking a tumour or brain abscess;
- multiple mass lesions with clinical signs related to their localization;
- pseudo-tumor cerebri;
- miscellaneous patterns such as confusion, psychiatric features, seizures, signs of brainstem or spinal injury preceding generalized encephalitis.

Ocular toxoplasmosis

Choroidoretinitis is the most common complication of *Toxoplasma* infection. It can occur weeks, months, or even years after the onset of infection. Following vascular dissemination, trophozoites reach retinal cells where they replicate producing inflammation, necrosis with ensuing retinitis, and vitritis. Retinal destruction is self-limiting and spontaneous scarring occurs within 6–8 weeks. *Toxoplasma* persists as cysts in retinal tissue. New lesions, generally satellites of the initial scar, can occur months or years later. Clinical and pathological observations suggest that these exacerbations are associated with cyst rupture and replication of the parasite in adjacent retinal cells. An allergic reaction or an autoimmune phenomenon have also been implicated. The frequent localization of the lesions in the macular area and complications such as retinal detachment, optic atrophy, or cataracts explain the risk of visual loss. (See Plate 11, The eye and disease.)

Congenital infection is the major cause of ocular toxoplasmosis. Less often it complicates acquired toxoplasmosis. In immunocompromising conditions it can be the presenting sign of the

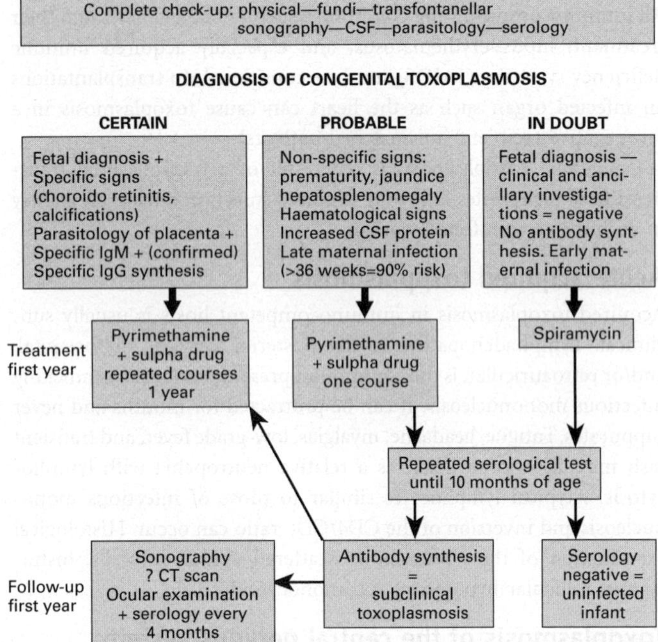

Fig. 1 Algorithm for neonates at risk of toxoplasmic fetopathy.

relapse of a formerly acquired infection. and it can be progressive, multiple, bilateral, and atypical. For unknown reasons it occurs less frequently than cerebral toxoplasmosis in AIDS patients.

Toxoplasmosis in the immunocompromised host

In more than half of the cases, cerebral toxoplasmosis occurs in patients with underlying disease and/or immunodeficiency either spontaneous or drug induced. It is generally related to the relapse of a chronic infection. Any patient with severe toxoplasmosis should be thoroughly investigated for an immune defect or an underlying disease. Any immunocompromised patient should have a prophylactic treatment against toxoplasmosis. Among malignancies the most common condition associated with cerebral toxoplasmosis is Hodgkin's disease. Others are lymphosarcoma, non-Hodgkin lymphomas, angioimmunoblastic lymphadenopathies, and all types of leukaemias. Severe toxoplasma infections have been reported in organ transplant recipients, above all in heart and heart and lung transplant recipients possibly contaminated by an infected tissue in mismatched patients transplantation (serological positive donor/negative recipient). AIDS patients are the commonest victims of cerebral toxoplasmosis: up to 30–40 per cent of them with an approximate case fatality of 20 per cent. The severity of the immune defect is a major risk factor. The probability of cerebral toxoplasmosis at 1 year is raised from 13 per cent to 20 per cent in patients with CD4 below 50/mm^3 and to 23 per cent in patients with CDC stage C manifestations. Significant abnormalities of antibody titre may be absent in immunocompromised patients. Diagnosis may require isolation of *Toxoplasma* from cerebrospinal fluid (CSF), cerebral biopsy, or broncho-alveolar lavage.

Congenital toxoplasmosis (Fig. 1)

Maternofetal transmission

Among infants born to mothers with seroconversion during pregnancy, 31 per cent are infected, 2 per cent suffer intrauterine death, and 67 per cent are uninfected. The date of maternal infection critically determines both the risk of materno-fetal transmission and the clinical pattern. The risk of fetopathy is 0 for maternal infection prior to conception (except for exceptional cases in immunocompromised patients), 1 per cent during the first month, 17 per cent during the second increasing progressively to 90 per cent for infections at the very end of pregnancy. Conversely, the clinical pattern is severe in 83 per cent of the fetuses when the mother was infected in early pregnancy vs 10 per cent only with mild patent disease when maternal infection occurred during the last month. Spiramycin given to the mother reduces by more than 50 per cent the risk of fetopathy but has no significant activity on the clinical pattern in infected babies.

Clinical patterns

(1) Systemic disease in the newborn with multivisceral involvement, neurological signs, and uveitis.

(2) Neurological signs. Hydrocephalus related to ductal stenosis (Plate 1), or microcephaly, porencephaly, cerebral calcifications, microphthalmy, choroidoretinitis.

(3) Mild disease: extramacular choroidoretinitis, mild cerebral calcification without evidence of cerebral involvement.

(4) Subclinical infection.

(5) Relapses: exacerbation of choroidoretinitis can develop in infancy, childhood and adolescence even in previously intact retinas in up to 85 per cent of the cases. Relapses in cerebral tissue associated with local synthesis of antibodies in CSF are probably frequent but subclinical.

Laboratory diagnosis

Serology is the reference method for the diagnosis but in the fetus and the immunocompromised patient the diagnosis is preferably established by demonstration of parasites in body fluids or tissues.

Serology

definitely proves the acquisition of infection. In the absence of seroconversion, the diagnosis of recent infection requires the demonstration of a significant rise in IgG antibody titre, and presence of specific IgM, in serial specimens that are obtained at 3 weeks apart and tested in parallel. A stable IgG titre is consistent with an infection acquired at least 2 months before the first specimen was obtained. As IgM antibodies may be detected for over a year after infection, the use of other methods based on acute-phase IgG antibodies is necessary to differentiate between recent and past infection, particularly in women who are evaluated late in pregnancy. This can be achieved by using the differential AC/HS agglutination test or the avidity enzyme-linked immunosorbent assay test.

In the newborn the demonstration of specific IgM after 2 days of life or specific IgA after 10 days is diagnostic of congenital infection. In some cases, the only marker of congenital infection is production of specific IgG which may be delayed for several months. Consequently in infants born to women infected during pregnancy, serological tests must be repeated until specific IgG becomes negative in order to rule out a congenital infection.

Intrathecal or intraocular production of specific antibodies can be determined by comparing the ratio of specific to total IgG in CSF or aqueous humour with that of the serum specimen.

Detection of *Toxoplasma*

Toxoplasma can be isolated from tissues or biological fluids by inoculation into mice or into cell cultures. Isolation from placenta proves the congenital infection. Isolation from blood or CSF indicates the presence of an acute infection whereas parasites can be detected in brain (Plate 2), muscle, or heart tissues in old chronic infections. Polymerase chain reaction can be used to detect *Toxoplasma* DNA in various samples. It has proved very reliable for the prenatal diagnosis of congenital infection by using the amniotic fluid only.

Treatment

Drugs

The pyrimethamine-sulphadrugs combination given orally is the mainstay of the treatment. Pyrimethamine is given in a dose of 1–2 mg/kg per day and sulphadiazine (the most commonly used sulphadrug) 50–100 mg/kg per day in two or three divided doses. Folinic acid 50 mg by oral or intramuscularly route every 2–6 days can prevent their haematological side-effects. The risk of bone marrow depression with leucopenia and/or neutropenia and thrombocytopenia requires careful monitoring of the blood every week. Other regimens include the combination pyrimethamine 25 mg-sulfadoxine 500 mg in a tablet (Fansidar) in a dose of one tablet/20 kg body weight every 7–10 days. Spiramycin is used only in pregnant women to reduce the risk of fetopathy. The difficulties encountered in treating toxoplasmosis in AIDS patients stimulated research for new drugs some of which were used in various combinations in clinical trials: macrolides (roxithromycine, azithromycin, clarithromycin), cyclines (doxycycline, minocycline), hydroxynaphthoquinones (atovaquone), folate inhibitors (trimethoprim, trimetrexate), and dapsone.

Indications

Acute infection in the immunocompetent host does not require routine therapy. Indications to treat are: pregnancy, systemic symptoms, evidence of visceral involvement, laboratory infection, or if there are severe cases in the neighbourhood.

Toxoplasmosis in the immunocompromised host and infection of the central nervous system is treated in the acute phase with pyrimethamine 200 mg/day for 2 days then 1–1.5 mg/kg per day plus sulphadiazine 100 mg/kg and folinic acid 10–20 mg/day until complete disappearance of clinical and radiological signs, i.e. 3–6 weeks. Maintenance therapy, which is lifelong in AIDS, includes pyrimethamine 50 mg/day and sulphadiazine 4 g/day. Other regimens used in cases of poor tolerance are the combinations pyrimethamine–clindamycin, pyrimethamine–clarithromycin, or azithromycin.

Acute ocular toxoplasmosis requires emergency treatment. The combination pyrimethamine–sulphadiazine is recommended. Steroids can be added to reduce quickly a devastating inflammatory process.

In congenital toxoplasmosis pyrimethamine 1 mg/kg per day for 6 months followed by 1 mg/kg three times a week for another 6 months. Pyrimethamine is combined with sulphadiazine 100 mg/kg per day for 12 months and folinic acid 5–10 mg each week.

Prevention

Patients at risk include seronegative pregnant women, immunocompromised patients, or transplant patients. Strict hygiene is essential: no contact with cats, well cooked or deep frozen meat, care in handling potentially contaminated materials such as raw meat, garden soil, and sand boxes. In AIDS patients, co-trimoxazole is considered as the drug of first choice in the prevention of cerebral toxoplasmosis.

Further reading

Couvreur, J. and Leport C. (1998). *Toxoplasmosis in antimicrobial chemotherapy and vaccines.* (ed. V.I. Yu, T. Merigan, and S. Barriere), pp. 600–12. Williams and Wilkins, Baltimore.

Dunn, D., Wallon, M., Peyron, F., Petersen, E., Peckham, C., and Gilbert, R. (1999). Mother-to-child transmission of toxoplasmosis: risk estimates for clinical counselling. *Lancet*, **353**, 1829.

Lebech, M., Andersen, O., Christensen, N.C., *et al.* (1999). Feasibility of neonatal screening for toxoplasma infection in the absence of prenatal treatment. *Lancet*, **353**, 1834.

Luft, B.J. and Remington, J.S. (1992). Toxoplasmic encephalitis in AIDS. *Clinical Infectious Diseases*, **15**, 211–12.

McAuley, J., Boyer K., Patel D., *et al.* (1994). Early and longitudinal evaluations of treated infants and children and untreated historical patients with congenital toxoplasmosis. The Chicago Collaborative Treatment Trial. *Clinical Infectious Diseases*, **18**, 38–72.

Remington, J.S., McLeod, R., and Desmonts, G. (1995). Toxoplasmosis. In *Infectious diseases of the fetus and newborn infant.* (4th edn), (ed. J.S. Remington and J.O. Klein), pp. 140–267. Saunders, Philadelphia.

Chapter 16.87

Cryptosporidium and cryptosporidiosis

D. P. Casemore

Cryptosporidia are obligate intracellular, coccidian parasites infecting a wide variety of vertebrate host species. Infection in humans is usually with one species, *Cryptosporidium parvum*. Recognized as a cause of enteritis (scours) in calves in the early 1970s and first described in humans in 1976, it has since emerged worldwide as a common cause of acute, self-limiting gastroenteritis in otherwise healthy subjects, especially children, and of severe or life-threatening infection in the severely immunocompromised, especially those with acquired immune deficiency syndrome (AIDS).

Biology

Cryptosporidia are obligate parasites with a complex life cycle, which is completed within an individual host animal. Life cycle stages include oocysts (the transmissive stage) containing four motile sporozoites (the infective stage), and asexual and sexual endogenous (tissue) forms. *C. parvum*, the species infecting humans, is readily cross-transmissible to a variety of host species. Following ingestion of oocysts, sporozoites are released and quickly attach superficially to host cells, usually in the brush border of enterocytes in the small bowel. The parasite is, however, capable of infecting mucosal cells of the entire enteric tract and other epithelial tissues such as those of the respiratory tract. Following attachment, trophozoites develop, each within a parasitophorous vacuole derived from the host cell membrane and are thus intracellular but extracytoplasmic. Oocysts are excreted fully sporulated and infective.

Molecular biology

Various antigens and enzymes have been characterized, using a variety of phenotypic and genotypic techniques. Some genes have been cloned and sequenced, and species and isolates differentiated; *C. parvum* isolates derived from livestock and humans have been shown to differ, one type being found in both animals and humans, while another appears to be restricted to humans. The serological response and seroprevalence have been studied, using molecular techniques.

Epidemiology

C. parvum has been reported worldwide and is common in humans and in livestock animals. Other cryptosporidia do not seem to be readily transmissible to humans. The epidemiology is complex, involving both direct and indirect routes of transmission, from animals to humans and from person to person. Infection is common in children attending day-care centres, where initial cases may be zoonotic in origin (for example, following visits to educational farms); domestic pets are an uncommon source of infection. Well-documented outbreaks have resulted from contamination of public drinking-water supplies, some involving thousands of cases, often amplified by transmission from person to person. Such outbreaks may involve multiple isolates including both human and animal types. Cryptosporidium is a common cause of travellers' diarrhoea.

Demography

Distribution

In some developing countries, infection is common in infants aged less than 1 year. In developed countries, infection is most common in children aged from 1 to 5 years followed by young adults; the infection is uncommon in adults over 45 years. A relative increase in adult cases is often seen in water-borne outbreaks. Seroprevalence studies indicate that the infection is common, even in developed countries, especially among those who have contact with livestock. Distribution of cases appears to be the same in both sexes.

In developed countries in particular, seasonal peaks are seen although these may vary from year to year and from district to district, and may coincide with lambing and calving and with periods of maximal rainfall. This emphasizes the importance of zoonotic sources of infection. Some waterborne outbreaks have, however, been shown to be associated with an apparently human-specific genotype and are likely to be derived from sewage effluent.

Frequency of occurrence

Cryptosporidium is one of the more common enteric pathogens. Laboratory rates of detection in faeces from non-immunocompromised subjects in developed countries average about 2 per cent of samples examined and, as expected, is more prevalent in developing countries. Marked increases in the detection rate in developed countries may indicate outbreaks likely to be associated with waterborne infection.

Cryptosporidiosis has been one of the most common causes of diarrhoea in AIDS patients, in whom prevalence has sometimes exceeded 50 per cent with high mortality. In some areas the prevalence is falling among such patients, possibly reflecting earlier detection of human immunodeficiency virus (HIV) infection and subsequent care and the effect of triple therapy. Infection rates are not generally increased for other immunocompromised groups.

Clinical aspects

Pathology

Histopathology

There is involvement of the small bowel mucosa, other parts of the gastroenteric tract, and sometimes beyond. Abnormalities of villous architecture occur and there may be evidence of mild inflammation, with cellular infiltration into the lamina propria. Rectal biopsy may reveal mild, non-specific proctitis. Extensive and chronic involvement of the bile duct and gallbladder is seen in some AIDS patients. The parasite in tissues appears, as small (2–8 μm) bodies, apparently superficially attached to the brush border, unevenly distributed over the apical cells and within the crypts, and sometimes on cells in other tissues. There is usually little intracellular change at the ultrastructural level beyond the attachment zone of the parasite.

Immunological response

An immune response has been demonstrated in each of the four main immunoglobulin classes; both humoral and cellular factors have a role in limiting or controlling infection. In AIDS patients CD4 cell counts of fewer than 200 cells/mm^3 indicate the need to take special care to avoid exposure to cryptosporidium; there is a poor prognosis if infection occurs with <100 CD4 cells/mm^3. A number of antigenic molecules have been identified, some of which are of value in seroprevalence studies and possibly for serological detection of recent cases in outbreaks. Some studies suggest a protective effect from breast feeding, although consequent protection from the environment is also a likely factor. Possible immunotherapeutic approaches are being investigated, including use of passive hyperimmune globulin, and the use of molecular techniques to identify potential therapeutic treatments.

Possible pathogenetic mechanisms

The watery diarrhoea is characteristic of non-inflammatory infection of the small bowel, although a secretagogue, neurotoxin, or other toxin, has not so far been identified. Mechanisms may include reduction in absorptive capacity for water and electrolytes, increase in secretory capacity from crypt hypertrophy, and osmotic effects from loss of brush-border enzymes resulting in malabsorption of sugars with subsequent microbial fermentation of sugars in the colon.

Clinical presentation in otherwise healthy (immunocompetent) people

Cryptosporidiosis in the immunocompetent is a self-limiting, acute gastroenteritis with a variety of presenting symptoms. The incubation period is about 5–10 days (range 2–14 days). There may be a prodrome of a few days, with malaise, abdominal pain, nausea, and loss of appetite. Gastroenteric symptoms may start suddenly, the stools often being described as watery, greenish with mucus, and 'very offensive'; blood and pus in the stool are not usually found and if present may indicate mixed infection. Patients usually open their bowels three to six times a day or more; there may be colicky, abdominal pain, especially after meals, anorexia, nausea, vomiting, abdominal distension, and marked weight loss; systemic symptoms may include malaise, headache, myalgia, and fever; respiratory symptoms occur in some cases. Gastrointestinal symptoms usually last about 7–14 days, but weakness, lethargy, mild intermittent abdominal pain (sometimes associated with biochemical evidence of pancreatitis), and occasional loose stools may persist. Oocyst excretion may be detected for 2–3 weeks after the disappearance of symptoms.

Those who have some immunity resulting from a previous infection can have very mild symptoms limited to a few loose stools and perhaps some nausea and loss of appetite, or may be asymptomatic. Mixed infections occur, particularly with campylobacters or giardia. There is no evidence of transplacental transmission but symptomatic infection during late pregnancy may cause metabolic disturbances in the mother, leading to the infant's failure to thrive. This latter has also been observed in older infants and children associated with persistent infection and enteropathy. Rare sequelae include toxic megacolon and reactive arthritis.

Clinical presentation in immunocompromised patients

Susceptibility to cryptosporidiosis and disease severity may be increased in those immunocompromised by AIDS, hypo- or agammaglobulinaemia, severe combined immunodeficiency, leukaemia, malignant disease, bullous pemphigoid, immunosuppressive treatment (cyclophosphamide, corticosteroids, etc.), and in children immunosuppressed by measles and chickenpox, especially where there is associated malnutrition. Infection in acute leukaemic patients may be unusually severe when associated with aplastic crises, and may then require modification of chemotherapy for resolution of the infection.

In AIDS patients symptoms usually develop insidiously; diarrhoea may be frequent, profuse, and watery. Associated symptoms are generally similar to those described above but may be more severe; infection of the respiratory tract may occur, possibly as a result of aspiration of vomit. The entire enteric tract and its associated organs, and sometimes also the lower respiratory tract, may be involved, often in association with other pathogens. Biliary tract involvement with right upper-quadrant abdominal pain, cholecystitis, sclerosing cholangitis, pancreatitis, and hepatitis may occur. Persistent nausea and vomiting associated with severe diarrhoea, indicate a poor prognosis.

Except in those patients whose immune suppression can be relieved by stopping immunosuppressant drugs, severe symptoms are likely to persist until death. Examination may reveal other features of HIV infection, including mixed enteric infections, particularly with cytomegalovirus and *Isospora belli*.

Nosocomial infection

Outbreaks have been reported involving transmission of cryptosporidium between staff and immunocompromised patients and between patients, for example in bone-marrow transplant units and between leukaemic children. Poor hand-washing practice and contaminated nasogastric feeding tubes have been implicated as possible vehicles. AIDS patients may have, profuse, watery diarrhoea and intractable vomiting, which together with other problems including dementia may lead to significant environmental contamination. In one such outbreak in Denmark, transmission via a ward ice-making machine was suspected.

Diagnostic investigation

Peripheral leucocytosis and eosinophilia are found rarely. Serum electrolyte abnormalities develop in patients who become severely dehydrated. In immunocompromised patients with cryptosporidial cholecystitis, serum alkaline phosphatase and γ-glutamyl transpeptidase levels are raised, while aminotransferases and bilirubin may remain normal.

Radiographic abnormalities may include dilatation of the small bowel, mucosal thickening, prominent mucosal folds and abnormal motility, and in the biliary system, dilated distal biliary ducts, stenosis with an irregular lumen, and other changes are reminiscent of primary sclerosing cholangitis.

Laboratory detection and diagnosis

Characteristic endogenous (tissue) stages may be found in histological sections but diagnosis is usually by detection of oocysts in stools (Plates 1–3). Stool consistency varies according to the time elapsed since onset that the sample is collected. Usually, the stool from patients with cryptosporidiosis does not contain blood, pus, cells, or Charcot–Leyden crystals and these may indicate mixed infection. Oocysts of *C. parvum* (4–6 μm) are difficult to identify in wet preparations; sporozoites within are difficult to distinguish even with special optical systems. Oocysts can be detected microscopically using the Ziehl–Neelsen method or phenol-auramine fluorescent stain; immunofluorescent antibody and enzyme-linked immunoassay, using monoclonal antibodies, are available; molecular techniques have been developed for detection and characterization. Concentration of stool specimens is not usually required for diagnosis in acute cases, although oocyst excretion does fluctuate and then decline as the infection progresses; detection of low-level oocyst excretion is difficult. Selection criteria have been recommended in the United Kingdom to improve standardization of approach in screening and reporting for epidemiological purposes.

Serological methods have little value in individual cases and are generally reserved for epidemiological studies.

Differential diagnosis

In immunocompetent patients, cryptosporidiosis should be considered in any acute diarrhoeal illness with abdominal pain and other gastrointestinal symptoms which may resemble those of acute giardiasis, cyclosporiasis, or isosporiasis. The diagnosis is particularly likely in patients with travellers' diarrhoea, those who work with farm animals, in children from day-care centres, and in health care personnel. In immunocompromised patients, especially those with AIDS, onset may be more insidious, the symptoms more persistent and clinical presentation confused by the effects of multiple infections.

Treatment

In immunocompetent patients, cryptosporidiosis is self-limiting, but they may become dehydrated and require intravenous fluids, electrolytes, and symptomatic treatment for vomiting and diarrhoea. Immunocompromised patients with persistent severe diarrhoea, malabsorption, and other complications may require prolonged palliative treatment. They should avoid excess milk, as lactose intolerance may develop. Parenteral feeding and fluid, electrolyte, and nutrient replacement may be needed. Anti-peristaltic agents such as loperamide, diphenoxylate, or opiates may increase abdominal pain and bloating; antiemetics may be needed but are sometimes poorly effective. Temporary relief of biliary obstruction has been achieved by endoscopic papillotomy and of cholecystitis by cholecystectomy.

Few antimicrobials have an effect on cryptosporidium, although some reports suggest some activity of paromomycin (Humatin), letrazuril/diclazuril, somatostatin, azidothymidine, diloxanide furoate, furazolidone, amprolium, and the macrolides. In some cases, there may be some amelioration of symptoms without eradication of the parasite. Apparent activity of spiramycin has not been confirmed. Immunotherapy (e.g. hyperimmune bovine colostrum or immunoglobulin and transfer factor, and interleukin-2) has been attempted, also with variable results. Zidovudine (Retrovir) therapy may also decrease symptoms. The falling incidence among some AIDS populations might possibly reflect earlier detection of HIV infection and subsequent care, including the effects of triple therapy. It is not known if this is a direct effect or the effect of improved immune function.

Infectivity, resistance, and control

Infectivity

The infectious dose is believed to be low. Human volunteer studies in the USA suggest a minimum infective dose of less than 30 oocysts and an ID_{50} of 132, for the single isolate tested. In one study using monkeys the infective dose of *C. parvum* was fewer than 10 oocysts; in gnotobiotic lambs the minimum infective dose of a lamb adapted isolate was one to five oocysts. Isolates appear to vary in their infectivity.

Resistance and disinfection

Oocyst can survive for many months in a cool, moist environment but are susceptible to desiccation, freezing, and moderate heat (e.g. pasteurization temperatures). They are remarkably resistant to many disinfectants; some disinfectants may be more effective if used at elevated temperature ($\geq 37°C$) and particular care in required in the cleaning of endoscopes. Oocysts are sensitive to 10 vol. (3 per cent) hydrogen peroxide, and to moderate levels of ozone.

Control of transmission

The multiple reservoirs and routes of transmission of cryptosporidium, the heavy output of oocysts from infected hosts, and the low infectious dose, can make control difficult. Primary control is by limiting the opportunity for faecal–oral transmission including that resulting from certain sexual practices. Symptom-free subjects not in contact with immunocompromised patients can normally be permitted to work if they use good hygiene. Contamination of water supplies is the source of some outbreaks and probably of some sporadic cases. Bottled water and water from point-of-use filters are unlikely to contain parasites but may carry an increased bacterial load, the health significance of which is uncertain for the immunocompromised. AIDS and other profoundly immunocompromised patients should be advised never to drink water that has not been boiled; water that has simply just raised to the boil is likely to be safe.

Spread via fomites is limited by the effect of desiccation on oocysts. Reduction of faecal contamination and of oocyst numbers by physical cleaning are essential for control. The adequate disinfection of instruments such as endoscopes is difficult. Prolonged immersion in glutaraldehyde at elevated temperature, after thorough cleaning, may be required.

Staff of infectious disease units, and those of other wards to which seriously immunocompromised patients may be admitted, need to be particularly vigilant in the management of patients with cryptosporidiosis. Staff should report even minor gastrointestinal symptoms and be investigated to minimize risk of spread.

Further reading

Blanshard, C., Jackson, A.M., Shanson, D.C., Francis, N., and Gazzard, B.G. (1992). Cryptosporidiosis in HIV-seropositive patients. *Quarterly Journal of Medicine*, **85**, 813–23.

Connolly, G.M. (1990). Clinical aspects of cryptosporidiosis. *Baillière's Clinical Gastroenterology*, **4**, 443–54.

Fayer, R. (ed.) (1997). *Cryptosporidium and cryptosporidiosis.* CRC Press, Boca Raton.

Meinhardt, P.L., Casemore, D.P., and Miller, K.B. (1996). Epidemiological aspects of human cryptosporidiosis and the role of waterborne transmission. *Epidemiologic Reviews*, **18**, 118–36.

Chapter 16.88

Cyclospora

D. P. Casemore

Coccidian parasite belonging to the genus *Cyclospora*, associated mainly with travellers' diarrhoea but increasingly in the USA with food-borne infection. Previously referred to as cryptosporidium-like or cyanobacterium (blue–green alga)-like bodies.

Natural history

The lifecycle is similar to cryptosporidium but oocysts sporulate only after a period in the environment, developing two inner sporocysts, each containing two sporozoites. This probably limits direct person to person transmission. The species *C. cayetanensis* n.sp. may be restricted to humans. Infection occurs at all ages; it has been detected commonly in residents of, and travellers to under-developed areas (especially Nepal, Indonesia, South and Central America), but cases have been increasingly identified in the USA in outbreaks associated with consumption of some uncooked imported food items (soft fruit, salad, etc.).

Clinical presentation

Symptoms include protracted, watery diarrhoea often lasting more than 2 weeks (range 1–8 weeks) with flatulence, bloating, dyspepsia, malaise, and marked weight loss. Asymptomatic infection has been described in indigenous people in developing countries, probably reflecting recurrent infection. The site of infection is primarily the small intestine, where the parasite has been found intracytoplasmically.

Treatment

Co-trimoxazole (1 tablet twice a day for 7 days) has proved effective in eradicating the infection.

Laboratory diagnosis

Oocysts (8–10 μm) in stools can be detected in wet preparations and by modified Ziehl–Neelsen staining (Plates 1, 2); phase-contrast microscopy of unsporulated oocysts reveals a morula (membrane-bound, spherical bodies, 1–2 μm in size) within the oocyst; fluorescence microscopy shows blue autofluorescence of the oocyst wall. Molecular techniques have been developed to confirm identity. Endogenous stages, with typical apicomplexan structures, within a parasitophorous vacuole, may be detected within the cytoplasm of enterocytes in jejunal and duodenal biopsy specimens, and possibly in other tissues (Plate 3).

Control

The source of the parasite is often unknown but transmission is probably by an indirect faecal–oral route and hence may be limited by hygienic precautions including avoidance of unboiled water, water-washed fruit, salads, uncooked vegetables, etc., in or imported from endemic areas. The increasing association with the latter indicates the importance of hygienic food production at source.

Further reading

Eberhard, M.L., Pieniazek, N.J., and Arrowood, M.J. (1997). Laboratory diagnosis of cyclospora infections. *Archives of Pathology and Laboratory Medicine*, **121**, 792–7.

Herwaldt, B.L. and Ackers, M.L. (1997). International outbreak of cyclosporiasis associated with imported berries. *New England Journal of Medicine*, **336**, 1548–56.

Soave, R. (1996). *Cyclospora*: an overview. *Clinical Infectious Diseases*, **23**, 429–37.

Chapter 16.89

Sarcocystosis

V. Zaman

Humans can act both as the final and intermediate host of the parasite belonging to the genus *Sarcocystis*. When humans act as the final host, parasites develop in the intestinal tract and oocysts or sporocysts are passed in the faeces. When humans act as an intermediate host, cysts develop in the muscles (Fig. 1).

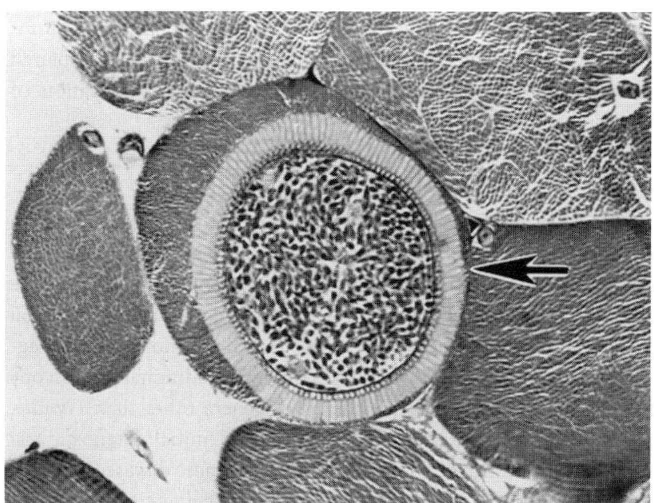

Fig. 1 Sarcocyst in muscle: the thickness of the cyst wall varies in different species; in this species a thick, striated wall is visible and the elongated structures inside the cyst are cystozoites (×400).

Sarcocystis hominis (syn. *Isospora hominis*)

The intermediate host is cattle. Human infection results from eating uncooked beef. Prevalence in human populations is not known but has been reported from many countries.

Clinical aspects

The majority of patients passing oocysts are asymptomatic and the development of the sporogonic stage in the human intestine is either non-pathogenic or only slightly pathogenic, resulting in mild gastrointestinal upset. However, the symptoms may vary, depending on the number of parasites ingested, and severe symptoms may occur after ingestion of heavily infected beef.

Diagnosis

This is based on the detection of oocysts or sporocysts in the faeces of infected individuals.

Treatment

No chemotherapeutic agents are available. Prevention consists of not eating uncooked beef.

Sarcocystis suihominis

The life cycle is similar to that of *S. hominis*, except that the intermediate host is the pig.

Clinical aspects

Human volunteers given infected tissues have experienced diarrhoea and mild fever. As in the case of *S. hominis* the intensity of symptoms probably varies with the size of the infective dose. If large amounts of heavily infected pork are ingested, symptoms could be quite severe. As this rarely happens, the majority of patients have only mild or no symptoms.

Diagnosis

This is based on the detection of oocysts or sporocysts in faeces. These are almost identical to those of *S. hominis*.

Treatment

No chemotherapeutic agents are available. Prevention consists of not eating raw pork.

Sarcocystis in muscles

There is probably more than one species involved. Infection is acquired by the ingestion of oocysts or sporocysts passed in the final hosts. The final hosts are unknown but could be carnivores, such as dogs or cats.

Clinical aspects

The majority of cases are asymptomatic. In some individuals there may be fever, chronic myositis, and eosinophilia.

Diagnosis

Diagnosis is made by muscle biopsy.

Treatment

No specific treatment is available.

Further reading

Bunyaratvej, S., Bunyawongwiroj, P., and Nitiyanant, P. (1982). Human intestinal sarcosporidiosis: report of six cases. *American Journal of Tropical Medicine and Hygiene*, **31**, 36–41.

Chapter 16.90

Giardiasis, balantidiasis, isosporiasis, and microsporidiosis

M. F. Heyworth

Giardiasis

Aetiology

Giardiasis is caused by *Giardia intestinalis* (*G. lamblia*), a protozoan parasite that colonizes the small intestinal lumen. The parasite's lifecycle comprises two stages: motile trophozoites (Fig. 1) and thick-walled cysts that are excreted in the faeces. Trophozoites absorb nutrients from the intestinal contents and generate energy by anaerobic metabolism.

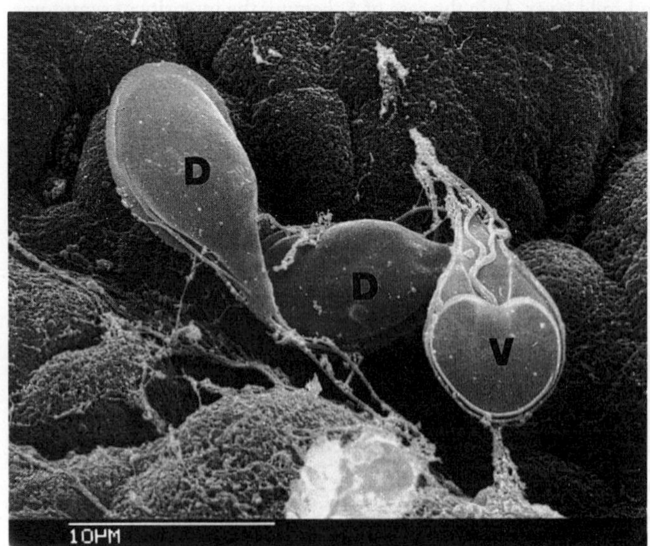

Fig. 1 Scanning electron micrograph of three *Giardia intestinalis* trophozoites on a jejunal biopsy specimen from a patient with giardiasis. The dorsal surfaces of two trophozoites are visible (D), and the ventral adhesive disc of the other trophozoite is shown (V).

Illustration by courtesy of Dr. Robert L. Owen; modified from Carlson, J.R., Heyworth, M.F., and Owen, R.L. (1984). Giardiasis: Immunology, diagnosis and treatment. Survey of Digestive Diseases, **2**, *201–13, S. Karger AG, Basel, and used by permission.*

Epidemiology

G. intestinalis infection is usually acquired by drinking water that contains cysts of the parasite. Direct faecal–oral transmission of cysts also occurs, as in day-care centres for infants and small children. Dogs, cats, and beavers can harbour infections with *Giardia* trophozoites that are similar or identical to *G. intestinalis*. Studies in North America suggest that excretion of *G. intestinalis* cysts by beavers can sustain the contamination of potential drinking water supplies by the parasite.

Antibody deficiency diseases predispose to severe and persistent giardiasis. Relevant conditions include common variable hypogammaglobulinaemia and X-linked immunoglobulin deficiency. In some patients with common variable hypogammaglobulinaemia and chronic giardiasis, there is abnormal enlargement of lymphoid follicles in the small intestine (nodular lymphoid hyperplasia). These abnormal follicles contain numerous immature B lymphocytes, whose maturation appears to be arrested at the IgM-expressing stage. The association of persistent giardiasis and antibody deficiency suggests that antibody responses contribute to protection against *G. intestinalis* infection.

Pathophysiology

The mechanisms responsible for the clinical features of giardiasis are not entirely clear. Some investigators have reported that giardiasis can lead to shortening of intestinal villi and of microvilli on intestinal epithelial cells. Reduced activity of intestinal disaccharidasaes has also been reported in individuals with giardiasis. When cultured in the presence of sodium glycocholate, *G. intestinalis* trophozoites take up this bile salt from the culture medium. Collectively, these observations suggest that the diarrhoea that occurs in giardiasis might reflect: (1) reduced epithelial surface area; (2) an osmotic effect of undigested disaccharides; and (3) fat malabsorption consequent on bile salt deficiency.

Clinical features

G. intestinalis infections can be asymptomatic (as shown by cyst excretion in the absence of symptoms) and can also lead to clinical problems. These include watery diarrhoea, steatorrhoea, weight loss, nausea, and abdominal cramps. In immunologically normal persons, untreated giardiasis typically lasts for several weeks, with symptoms of fluctuating severity. Megaloblastic anaemia resulting from impaired absorption of vitamin B_{12} or folic acid is a rare complication of giardiasis.

Laboratory diagnosis

Traditionally, giardiasis has been diagnosed by stool microscopy to look for *G. intestinalis* cysts. During the past decade, this approach has been supplemented by immunofluorescence microscopy for whole cysts, and by immunoassays for *G. intestinalis* antigens, in faecal specimens. Although there is evidence that these more recent diagnostic approaches have greater sensitivity than traditional microscopy of stools, they do not detect parasites of genera other than *Giardia*. Traditional stool microscopy is an appropriate initial diagnostic test in a patient presumed to have an intestinal parasitic disease, in whom giardiasis is not the only diagnostic possibility being considered.

For diagnosing giardiasis, microscopic examination of duodenal fluid or duodenal biopsies for trophozoites is an alternative approach to faecal examination (see OTM3, pp. 879–80).

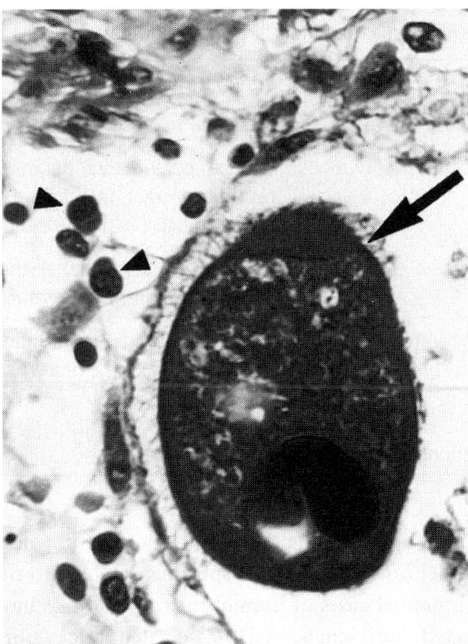

Fig. 2 Light micrograph of *Balantidium coli* trophozoite (arrow) in colonic tissue. Cilia are visible on the surface of the organism. Arrowheads indicate tissue plasma cells.×705.
Modified from Neafie, R.C. (1976). Balantidiasis. In Pathology of tropical and extraordinary diseases, Vol. 1 (ed. C.H. Binford and D.H. Connor), pp. 325–7. Armed Forces Institute of Pathology, Washington, DC, and used by permission.

Treatment

Drug regimens for treating giardiasis include a 7-day course of either mepacrine (quinacrine) or metronidazole, or three weekly single doses of tinidazole (total adult weekly dose 2 g). As indicated above, giardiasis can be difficult to eliminate in patients with antibody deficiency diseases.

Prevention and control

Filtration of municipal water supplies through sand or diatomaceous earth removes *G. intestinalis* cysts. The cysts can also be removed by membrane filters with a pore diameter of less than 5 μm. *Giardia* cysts in water are killed by boiling. Drinking water can be screened for *G. intestinalis* cysts by microscopic examination of particulate material obtained by filtration. This examination can include immunofluorescence microscopy with fluorescent antibodies directed against the cysts. Polymerase chain reaction (**PCR**) amplification of *G. intestinalis* DNA, and detection of PCR products, is a promising additional approach to screening water samples for the parasite.

Balantidiasis

Aetiology

This infection is caused by *Balantidium coli*, a ciliate protozoan that is the largest protozoan parasite of humans. *B. coli* has a two-stage lifecycle comprising motile ciliated trophozoites, which parasitize the colon (Fig. 2), and non-motile cysts. New hosts acquire the infection by ingesting the parasite.

Epidemiology

Balantidiasis occurs in temperate and tropical countries. A high prevalence of this infection has been seen in human communities that live in close proximity to *B. coli*-infected pigs. This observation suggests that pigs are a reservoir for spread of the infection to humans, although balantidiasis has also occurred in human subjects who had no known contact with pigs or other animals.

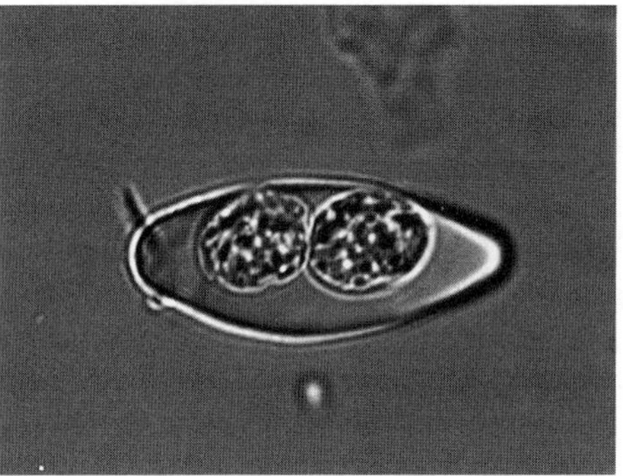

Fig. 3 Light micrograph of an *Isospora belli* oocyst containing two sporoblasts.×2500.
Illustration by courtesy of Dr. William L. Current. From Garcia, L.S. and Bruckner, D.A. (1993). Diagnostic medical parasitology (2nd edn). American Society for Microbiology, Washington, DC, and used by permission.

Pathophysiology

Balantidium coli trophozoites penetrate human tissues, such as the colonic mucosa. In the 1950s, it was reported that the trophozoites produce hyaluronidase, and there has been speculation that this enzyme contributes to tissue destruction by the parasite.

Clinical features

Human subjects with *B. coli* infection can be asymptomatic or can develop diarrhoea with stools that are either watery or that consist of blood and mucus. Patients can develop colonic ulceration, perforation of the colon, distal ileum, or appendix, and spread of the parasite to the liver or lungs. Death can occur as a result of peritonitis or bacterial septicaemia. Balantidiasis may be clinically indistinguishable from ulcerative colitis, amoebiasis, and bacillary dysentery.

Laboratory diagnosis

Balantidiasis can be diagnosed by finding trophozoites or cysts of *B. coli* in diarrhoeal stools or in colonic mucus obtained at sigmoidoscopy. Histological examination of rectal biopsies may show *B. coli* trophozoites.

Treatment

Little interpretable information about the treatment of balantidiasis is currently available, although eradication of the parasite has been reported in some individuals treated with tetracycline or metronidazole. Surgical intervention may be necessary in patients with liver abscess or clinical evidence of intestinal perforation.

Isosporiasis

Aetiology

Isospora belli, the cause of isosporiasis, is a coccidian parasite of the human intestine. It appears that infection is acquired by ingestion of *I. belli* oocysts (Fig. 3), presumably in water and/or food. The lifecycle comprises asexual and sexual phases that occur in intestinal epithelial cells (see OTM3, p. 882). The sexual phase leads to production of oocysts, which are excreted in the faeces.

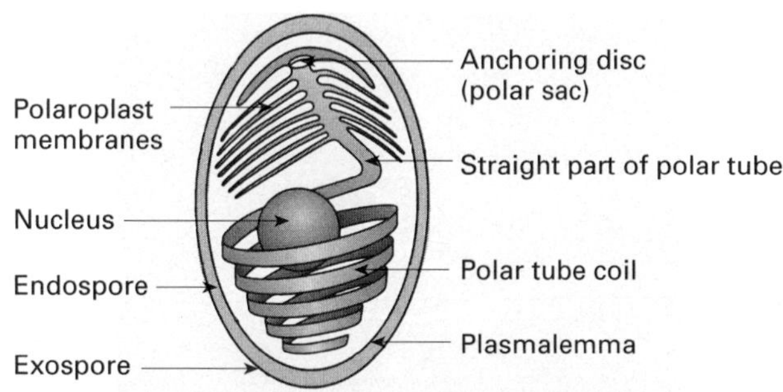

Fig. 4 Diagram of a microsporidian spore, showing internal structure. Illustration by courtesy of Professor Elizabeth U. Canning.
Modified from Canning, E.U. and Hollister, W.S. (1992). Human infections with microsporidia. Reviews in Medical Microbiology, **3**, *35–42, and used by permission.*

Epidemiology

There is evidence that *I. belli* causes diarrhoea in immunocompetent persons. The organism is, however, a particular problem in patients with human immunodeficiency virus (**HIV**) infection. Patients infected with HIV appear to have increased susceptibility to chronic isosporiasis. The prevalence of isosporiasis seems to be higher in tropical than in temperate regions. Reported prevalence rates of *I. belli* infection in patients with acquired immune deficiency syndrome (**AIDS**) have been approximately 15 per cent in Haiti and ≤1 per cent in Los Angeles.

Pathophysiology

The gastrointestinal symptoms of isosporiasis presumably reflect parasitic invasion of intestinal epithelial cells.

Clinical features

Watery diarrhoea, abdominal cramps, fat malabsorption, dehydration, and weight loss have been reported in patients with *I. belli* infection. Most of the relevant patients described in recent years had HIV infection, which is known to predispose to colonization by various opportunistic intestinal parasites in addition to *I. belli*. Evidence that *I. belli* is a cause of 'AIDS enteropathy' comes from clinical studies in which resolution of diarrhoea has accompanied treatment with a drug regimen that reportedly cures *I. belli* infection.

Laboratory diagnosis

Isosporiasis can be diagnosed by microscopic examination of faecal specimens for *I. belli* oocysts.

Treatment

Successful treatment of *I. belli* infection with trimethoprim–sulphamethoxazole has been reported. Anecdotal case reports have raised the possibility that pyrimethamine and diclazuril might also be effective in treating this infection.

Microsporidiosis

Aetiology

Microsporidia are protozoa with features that are sufficiently distinctive for the organisms to be classified as a separate phylum (Microspora). The lifecycle of microsporidia comprises an extracellular stage (spore) and stages that occur in host cells. Spores (Fig. 4) are shed into the environment by infected hosts and infect other members of the host species. *In vitro* studies have shown that spores infect host cells by extruding a hollow tube that impales a cell and forms a channel for entry of microsporidian DNA into the host cell.

Most documented cases of human microsporidiosis have occurred in HIV-infected individuals. AIDS-associated microsporidiosis has mainly been seen in patients with advanced immunodeficiency, as judged by peripheral blood CD4 (helper) T-lymphocyte counts of <100/μl.

Table 1 lists microsporidia that infect humans. (This table omits a few 'species' of doubtful taxonomic status.)

Table 1 Species of microsporidia that infect humans

Species	Site(s) of infection
Enterocytozoon bieneusi	Intestinal mucosa, bile duct epithelium
Encephalitozoon hellem	Cornea, conjunctiva, paranasal sinuses, respiratory tract, intestinal epithelium, urinary tract, prostate
Encephalitozoon cuniculi	Conjunctiva, duodenal epithelium, respiratory tract, urinary tract
Encephalitozoon (formerly *Septata*) *intestinalis*	Intestinal mucosa, nasal mucosa, biliary tract, kidney, blood
Vittaforma corneae	Cornea
Trachipleistophora hominis	Skeletal muscle

Epidemiology

The association of microsporidiosis and HIV infection strongly suggests that microsporidia are opportunistic parasites of immunodeficient patients. To date, *Enterocytozoon bieneusi* has been the most frequently described microsporidian in patients with AIDS. In addition, at least one immunocompetent individual with transient diarrhoea attributed to *E. bieneusi* has been described. *Encephalitozoon hellem* and *Encephalitozoon intestinalis* are well documented causes of opportunistic infection in AIDS. *Encephalitozoon cuniculi* has been isolated from a few HIV-infected patients with microsporidiosis. This organism infects rabbits, an observation which has led to speculation that infected rabbits might be a source for *E. cuniculi* infection of human subjects.

Because *Enterocytozoon bieneusi* and *Encephalitozoon intestinalis* infect the gastrointestinal tract, it seems reasonable to assume that the respective infections are acquired by ingestion of spores. Infection of tracheobronchial and nasal epithelium by *E. hellem* suggests inhalation of spores as a route of infection by this organism. *E. hellem* and *E. cuniculi* are morphologically very similar, but can be distinguished by staining with species-specific antibodies and by PCR and Southern blotting with specific DNA primers and probes, respectively.

Pathophysiology

Clinical features of microsporidian infections are attributable to parasitization of epithelial cells in the intestine, biliary tract, and respiratory tract, as well as parasitization of cells in the conjunctiva and cornea. Myalgia in *Trachipleistophora hominis* infection is attributable to parasitization of skeletal muscle cells.

Clinical features

In HIV-infected individuals, microsporidia cause chronic watery diarrhoea, cholangiopathy, rhinitis, sinusitis, and keratoconjunctivitis.

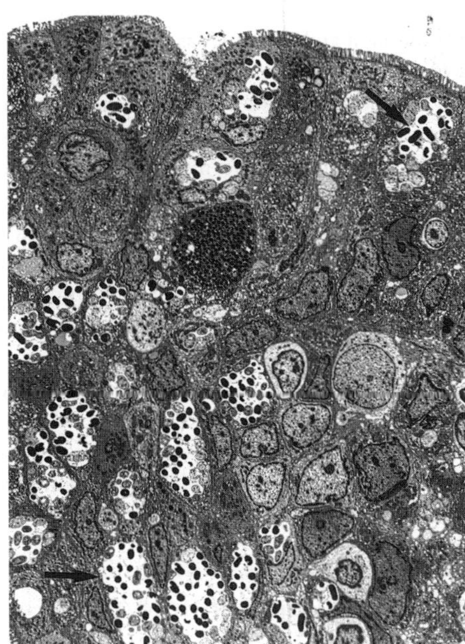

Fig. 5 Transmission electron micrograph of jejunal biopsy from a patient with AIDS and *Encephalitozoon intestinalis* infection. The microvillus border (epithelial surface) is at the top of the photograph. Epithelial cells and lamina propria leukocytes are heavily infected with *E. intestinalis* (arrows). *Illustration by courtesy of the Electron Microscopy and Histopathology Unit, London School of Hygiene and Tropical Medicine. From Croft, S.L., Williams, J., and McGowan, I. (1997). Intestinal Microsporidiosis. Seminars in Gastrointestinal Disease,* **8**, *45–55, W.B. Saunders, Philadelphia, and used by permission.*

The literature also includes occasional reports of skeletal muscle infection with *Trachipleistophora hominis* (leading to myalgia), urinary tract infection with *Encephalitozoon hellem* (with or without renal failure and/or prostatitis), and infection of the corneal stroma by *Vittaforma corneae* in immunocompetent individuals.

When it has been sought, *Enterocytozoon bieneusi* has been found in approximately one-third of patients with diarrhoea, weight loss, and HIV infection. Although it is likely that *E. bieneusi* is a cause of AIDS-associated diarrhoea, this question has not been answered unambiguously. *E. bieneusi* infection of intestinal epithelial cells has been seen in some HIV-infected individuals without diarrhoea. To date, it has not been possible to eradicate *E. bieneusi* infection from the intestine of individual HIV-infected patients. In contrast, there is evidence that encephalitozoon infections can be cured (see below); in this situation, the concurrence of parasite eradication and regression of symptoms establishes a pathogenic role for *Encephalitozoon* species in humans.

Keratoconjunctivitis attributable to *Encephalitozoon* species (most commonly *E. hellem*) is characterized by conjunctival pain and redness, photophobia, and corneal opacities that reduce visual acuity.

Laboratory diagnosis

Microsporidian infections can be documented by light microscopic and electron microscopic examination of biopsy specimens from parasitized tissues (Fig. 5). Since the late 1980s, efforts have been aimed at developing non-invasive techniques for diagnosing microsporidian infections. Microscopic examination of faecal specimens for *Enterocytozoon bieneusi* and *Encephalitozoon intestinalis* spores is a well established approach. The spores can be identified by using a number of stains, including chromotrope 2R (leading to pink staining of the spores), optical brighteners such as Uvitex 2B and Calcofluor White M2R (which lead to bright staining of spores on fluorescence microscopy), and fluorescent antibodies directed against the spores. Microsporidian spores are detectable in urine specimens from patients with urinary tract microsporidiosis.

Microsporidian infection of the nasal mucosa and paranasal sinuses can be diagnosed by microscopic examination of nasal secretions for spores. Approaches to diagnosis of microsporidian keratoconjunctivitis include examination of conjunctival/corneal scrapings or biopsies for microsporidian spores and (non-invasively) *in vivo* examination of the cornea with a scanning confocal microscope to look for spore-filled epithelial cells.

Diagnostic techniques based on demonstration of microsporidian DNA in clinical specimens have been described. In particular, there is a substantial literature on the demonstration of PCR amplification products generated using primers complementary to genes encoding microsporidian ribosomal RNA.

Treatment

Encephalitozoon infections are treatable with oral albendazole. This approach can cure diarrhoea caused by *E. intestinalis* and has reportedly led to the eradication of disseminated encephalitozoon infection in some patients. There are reports suggesting that fumagillin eye drops are effective for treating keratoconjunctivitis due to *E. hellem.*

No curative treatment for *Enterocytozoon bieneusi* infection has been developed, although a pilot study suggests that atovaquone might have some promise for treating this infection.

Further reading

Ackers, J.P. (1997). Gut coccidia—*Isospora, Cryptosporidium, Cyclospora* and *Sarcocystis. Seminars in Gastrointestinal Disease,* **8**, 33–44.

Adam, R.D. (1991). The biology of *Giardia* spp. *Microbiological Reviews,* **55**, 706–32.

Croft, S.L., Williams, J., and McGowan, I. (1997). Intestinal microsporidiosis. *Seminars in Gastrointestinal Disease,* **8**, 45–55.

Heyworth, M.F. (1996). *Giardia* infections. In *Enteric infections and immunity* (ed. L.J. Paradise, M. Bendinelli, and H. Friedman), pp. 227–38. Plenum Press, New York.

Markell, E.K., Voge, M., and John, D.T. (1992). *Medical parasitology* (7th edn.). W. B. Saunders, Philadelphia.

Chapter 16.91

Blastocystis hominis

V. Zaman

Blastocystis is a common intestinal protozoan of doubtful pathogenicity.

Morphology

They are generally spherical in shape but their size and internal contents are very variable. The size ranges from 5 to 40 μm with occasional giant cells reaching 200 μm. In cultures they can be divided into three groups: (1) vacuolated; (2) granular; and (3) amoeboid.

The vacuolated form predominates in faecal specimens and is characterized by a large central 'vacuole' with the cytoplasm lying at the periphery of the cell. Cysts have recently been identified.

Clinical aspects

According to one school of thought this parasite is a pathogen and can cause various gastrointestinal problems including diarrhoea, anorexia, flatus, and abdominal discomfort. Symptoms usually last about 3–10 days, but may persist for months. Eosinophilia occurs in some cases. There appears to be a favourable response to metronidazole therapy.

Diagnosis

This is based mainly on stool examination. It has been claimed that patients having problems attributable to *Blastocystis* pass a large number of parasites (mostly vacuolated forms) in their stools. *Blastocystis* grows easily in media used for culturing *Entamoeba histolytica.*

Treatment

Treatment is indicated only in symptomatic cases. The most widely accepted drug is metronidazole, which is given in a dose of 750 mg, three times daily for 5 days (for children 35–50 mg/kg in three divided doses for 5 days).

Further reading

Stenzel, D.J. and Boreham, P.F.L. (1996). *Blastocystis hominis* revisited. *Clinical Microbiology Reviews*, **9**, 563–84.

Chapter 16.92

Human African trypanosomiasis

D. H. Smith

Human African trypanosomiasis (sleeping sickness) is caused by a subspecies of the protozoan haemoflagellate, *Trypanosoma brucei* (subgenus *Trypanozoon*) and transmitted by tsetse flies (*Glossina*). *T. brucei* is widely distributed in wild and domestic animals, and humans in Africa between 15 N and 20 S in 36 countries extending from the sub-Saharan region in the north to the deserts of Botswana and Namibia in the south (Fig. 1). Human disease exists in more than 200 foci and occurs in two main forms known as *T. brucei gambiense* and *T.b.rhodesiense. T.b.gambiense,* usually produces a chronic infection occurring focally through areas of west and central Africa and *T.b.rhodesiense* causes more acute, severe disease occurring in east and southern Africa.

Human trypanosomiasis has caused massive epidemics in the past and in the past decade there has been a resurgence of disease notably in Zaire, Uganda, Tanzania, Mozambique, Sudan, and Angola, often associated with war, civil disturbance, and refugee groups as well as deteriorating health services.

Aetiology

In the vertebrate host trypanosomes range from 25 × 2.5 μm (long slender forms) to 19 × 3.5 μm (short stumpy forms). The undulating membrane is prominent and continues as a free flagellum. In addition to a centrally placed nucleus, trypanosomes also possess a kinetoplast, composed of DNA and sited at the base of the undulating membrane.

Trypanosomes are taken up during tsetse feeding into the mid-gut where they develop into procyclic forms and multiply. They lack the surface glycoprotein coat and are non-infective to vertebrates. Parasites migrate to the salivary glands and become non-dividing, metacyclic forms which are infective to mammalian hosts. In the human host trypanosomes are coated by variant surface glycoprotein, which by extensive and regular antigenic variation allows trypanosomes to evade host immune responses.

There are no morphological differences between *T.b.gambiense, T.b.rhodesiense,* and human non-infective *T.b.brucei.* Biochemical techniques especially isoenzyme electrophoresis have shown the diversity of *T. brucei* populations (zymodemes) and identified more clearly the role of animal reservoirs of human infection.

Transmission and epidemiology

Sleeping sickness is usually transmitted biologically from infected tsetse flies, although mechanical transmission via *Glossina* or other biting flies may occur as well as transmission from blood transfusion. Congenital transmission occurs in *T.b.gambiense.*

T.b.gambiense is transmitted by the *Glossina* '*Palpalis*' group flies, *G. palpalis, G. tachinoides,* and *G. fuscipes,* which inhabit forest, riverine, or lacustrine situations and feed on humans readily, leading to high human–fly contact notably at river margins during washing and water collection. *T.b.rhodesiense* is transmitted by the *Glossina* '*Morsitans*' group flies, *G. morsitans, G. pallidipes,* and *G. swynnertoni,* which are less dependent on shade and humidity, inhabit more open woodland savannah, and have feeding preferences for larger animals.

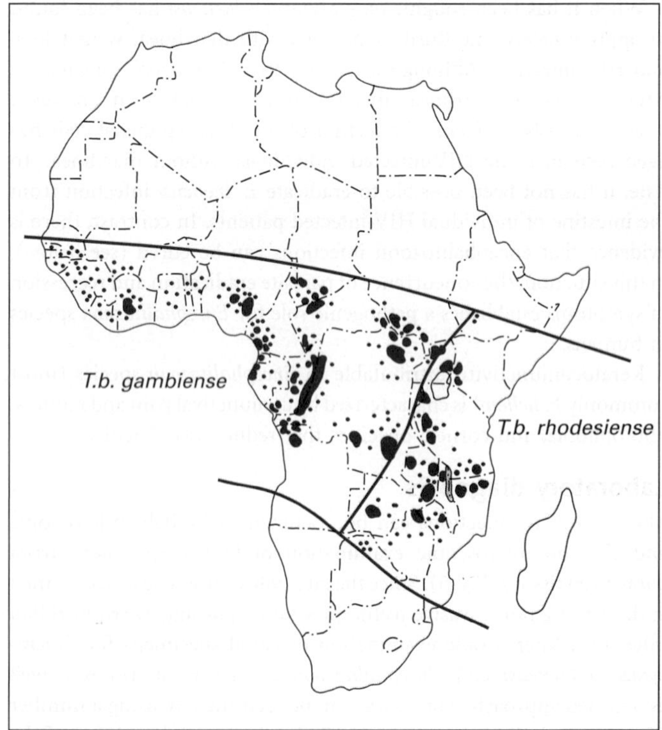

Fig. 1 The geographical distribution of African trypanosomiasis.

Table 1 The epidemiological features of human African trypanosomiasis

	Vector	Main reservoir and transmission	Animal reservoir	
			Wild	Domestic
T.b.gambiense	'Palpalis' group tsetse:	Humans	Kob	Cattle
West and Central Africa	*G. palpalis* *G. tachinoides*	High focal endemicity Riverine: water collection and washing points Forest	Hartebeest	Pig
T.b.rhodesiense	'Morsitans' group tsetse:	Wild game animals		
Endemic sporadic	*G. morsitans*	Sporadic infection	Bushbuck	Cattle
East and southern Africa	*G. pallidipes*	High-risk groups and activities	Reedbuck Waterbuck	Pig Dog
T.b.rhodesiense	'Palpalis' group tsetse	Domestic animals	Hartebeest	Sheep
Epidemic	*G. fuscipes*	Humans	Lion	Goat
East Africa, Kenya, Uganda		Outbreaks and epidemics Both sexes all age groups Peridomestic transmission	Hyena Kob	

The important vectors and animal reservoirs of human trypanosomiasis are shown in Table 1.

T.b.gambiense

In most endemic areas humans are the only important reservoir of infection. In many endemic, riverine habitats, the disease is focal and prevalence rates in foci may rise to high levels. High and rising endemicity is favoured by the prolonged relatively mild haemolymphatic stage, the feeding preferences of transmitting *Glossina* species and is highest at focal points of intense human–fly contact. Transmission in forest habitats is usually lower.

T.b.rhodesiense

Throughout most of the range infection is maintained in wild animal reservoirs, especially wild game animals such as bushbuck. Infection in domestic animals, including bovids and pigs, brings the parasite into closer contact with human populations increasing the potential for outbreaks. Both wild and domestic reservoir hosts usually develop low-grade sustained parasitaemia with few clinical manifestations, although dogs suffer severe, usually fatal infection. Humans are infected sporadically and particular occupational groups are predominantly at risk: hunters, poachers, game wardens, tourists, cattle herders, and others, such as fishermen who pass through tsetse infested areas.

Epidemic *T.b.rhodesiense* occurs in settled areas around Lake Victoria especially in South Eastern Uganda since 1976, where *T.b.rhodesiense* is transmitted by *G.f.fuscipes*, reservoir hosts include domestic animals, and epidemics affect all age groups.

Pathogenesis

Trypanosomes divide rapidly at the site of inoculation and may induce the typical 'chancre', with marked tissue response characterized by a cellular reaction; vasculitis with perivascular mononuclear cell infiltration, oedema, tissue damage, and local lymphadenopathy. Trypanosomes then circulate through the blood and lymphatic system. Frequent antigenic variation of the surface glycoproteins, with an antigen repertoire of some 1000 variants leads to fluctuating waves of parasitaemia, the predominantly IgM antibody response and the relapsing nature of the early haemolymphatic stage.

Parasites eventually invade the central nervous system from the choroid plexus, spreading throughout the cerebrospinal fluid (**CSF**) and Virchow Robins spaces producing perivascular infiltration and the characteristic menigoencephalitis. The brainstem is mainly involved, although cortical areas are also affected. The brain is oedematous and intracranial pressure elevated. The inflammatory response includes vasculitis, lymphocytic and plasma cell infiltration, and characteristic foamy IgM laden plasma cells—the 'Morular cell of Mott'. Neuronal destruction and focal demyelination occur late in the course of the meningoencephalitis. The neuropsychiatric manifestations of late-stage trypanosomiasis may in part be biochemically mediated through neurotransmitters and cytokines from activated astrocytes. Pathological lesions also occur in other organs including the heart (pancarditis), liver, kidney, serous membranes, and the endocrine system.

The immunological response is characterized by polyclonal B-lymphocyte activation accompanied by immunosuppression, disturbance of cytokines, and other mediator activity, immune complex formation, and autoantibody production all of which may contribute to the pathological processes. Antibody production is predominantly IgM. A haemolytic anaemia occurs in early trypanosomiasis but is usually mild compared with infections in animals. In endemic areas other associated causes of anaemia are also common. Thrombocytopenia is a common finding. Myocardial, renal and hepatic involvement, jaundice, and disseminated intravascular coagulation also occur in severe infections.

The clinical features

A trypanosomal chancre may develop at the site of inoculation in *T.b.rhodesiense*. Trypanosomes multiply in the extracellular tissue fluids in the chancre and rapidly invade lymphatics and gain access to the blood. A patent parasitaemia develops within days of the development of the chancre—*Haemolymphatic stage (stage I)*. After a variable period parasites invade the central nervous system and CSF leading to a meningoencephalitis—*Meningoencephalitic stage (stage II)*.

In *T.b.gambiense* infections the early symptoms are mild and meningoencephalitis develops late and runs a protracted course over months or years. In *T.b.rhodesiense* the initial stage is acute and severe, with early progress to, and rapid progression of, meningoencephalitis leading to death within 3–6 months.

The trypanosomal chancre

The chancre develops within a few days of an infected bite. It starts as a small raised oedematous papule which rapidly increases in size and is associated with a local lymphadenopathy. They increase in size during the first week and then subside during the subsequent 2 or 3 weeks leaving a scar with changes in pigmentation. In *T.b.gambiense* infection chancres are rarely seen, while in *T.b.rhodesiense* chancres may be present in 10–50 per cent of infections.

Haemolymphatic trypanosomiasis (stage I)

The clinical features of haemolymphatic trypanosomiasis are mostly non-specific. Episodes of fever occur with chills, rigors, prostration, headache, general malaise, and joint pains. In *T.b.gambiense* infections, the early stage is often mild and may be asymptomatic. Febrile episodes become less severe as the disease progresses. Lymphadenopathy is common, especially in gambiense infections where enlargement of the posterior cervical glands is characteristic (Winterbottom's sign). Hepatosplenomegaly occurs in up to 30 per cent. A transient erythematous rash 'circinate erythema' occurs on the trunk or extremities, but is visible only in fair skins. Myocarditis with cardiac arrhythmias or cardiac failure occurs in *T.b.rhodesiense* infections and may lead to early death. Patchy oedema is common especially periorbital oedema and facial puffiness. Anaemia occurs in the early stages, especially in *T.b.rhodesiense*. In severe infections there is hepatic and renal involvement and a coagulopathy with haemorrhagic features.

Meningoencephalitic trypanosomiasis (stage II)

Meningoencephalitis is an inevitable consequence of infection. In *T.b.rhodesiense* infections, cerebral involvement occurs within weeks of initial infection, while in *T.b.gambiense* meningoencephalitis is delayed months or years after infection. The onset is insidious and early central nervous system involvement cannot be determined clinically.

Headache increases and becomes more protracted and there may be neck stiffness. Changes in behaviour and personality occur early, before the objective development of meningoencephalitis. Features include apathy, loss of interest, lack of attention, agitation, and paranoid and delusional states. Individuals lose interest in their surroundings and their own well being and may exhibit inappropriate or uncharacteristic behaviour. Circadian rhythms are disturbed; abnormalities of sleep including diurnal and inappropriate somnolence are characteristic. At night there is insomnia often with agitation. The faces are blank and expressionless. Speech becomes slow, slurred, and incoherent.

Extrapyramidal and cerebellar features are the characteristic neurological features. Tremors, muscle fasciculation, and choreic and athetotic movements may all occur. The gait becomes slow, unsteady and then grossly ataxic. There may be abnormal 'parkinsonian'-like features with shuffling gait and rigidity. Primitive reflexes such as the cheiro-chin reflex occur and indicate frontal lobe involvement. Kerandel's sign refers to the delayed but intensified response to painful stimuli. Intractable pruritus is common and increases as the disease progresses. Pyramidal signs and focal cranial nerve lesions are less common. The meningoencephalitis progresses relentlessly with progressive stupor. Convulsions are common in advanced disease and indicate a poor prognosis. There is progressive wasting and cachexia and sleeping sickness usually terminates in deepening coma and death. In the later stages intercurrent infection may supervene, notably bronchopneumonia. Endocrine abnormalities include amenorrhoea, impotence, female fat distribution, gynaecomastia, and abortion.

Diagnosis

The clinical diagnosis of trypanosomiasis is difficult. The features of early disease are non-specific and resemble malaria and other common endemic febrile disease. In *T.b.gambiense* the early stages of infection may be subclinical. Routine laboratory tests show a normal total white cell count with a normal or increased lymphocyte count, elevated erythrocyte sedimentation rate, anaemia, thrombocytopenia, elevated IgM, and coagulation abnormalities but these findings are non-specific. In severe infections tests of renal and hepatic function (notably liver enzymes) may be abnormal. The serum albumin is low and there may be hypocomplementaemia, circulating immune complexes, and rheumatoid factor. Spurious hypoglycaemia occurs if blood sugar estimation is not carried out immediately.

A parasitological diagnosis provides certain proof of infection. This includes examination of blood, lymph gland needle aspirates (especially in *T.b.gambiense*), chancre aspirates, and CSF examination for trypanosomes. Repeated examination of the blood may be required especially in *T.b.gambiense* and late-stage infections. Trypanosomes may also be seen in marrow smears. Examination of material for motile trypanosomes must be carried out as soon after sample collection as possible. Animal inoculation is a very sensitive technique in *T.b.rhodesiense* infections.

Wet film examination for motile trypanosomes is simple but insensitive. Thick blood films, stained with Giemsa or Field's stain improve the sensitivity. Sensitivity is further improved with microhaematocrit centrifugation (**MHCT**) with examination of the area above the buffy coat. The quantitative buffy coat technique, a modification of the MHCT where motile trypanosomes are stained with Acridine orange and examined by fluorescent microscopy of the expanded buffy coat has recently been shown to be a very sensitive and rapid diagnostic technique

Immunological tests provide presumptive evidence of infection. Tests include, indirect immunofluorescence (**IIF**), enzyme-linked immunosorbent assay (**ELISA**), IgM levels in blood and CSF. The 'Card Agglutination Test for trypanosomiasis' (**CATT** utilizes a commonly occurring variant surface antigen of *T.b.gambiense* (LiTat 1.3) and provides a test for the preliminary screening of populations in *T.b.gambiense* areas.

Cerebrospinal fluid findings in late-stage trypanosomiasis

A confirmed infection with African trypanosomes requires examination of the CSF to determine the presence of meningoencephalitis. Meningoencephalitis is defined by the presence CSF abnormalities; CSF cell count above 5 per mm^3 (commonly between 50–500 lymphocytes per mm^3), elevated protein level, raised CSF IgM, or the presence of trypanosomes.

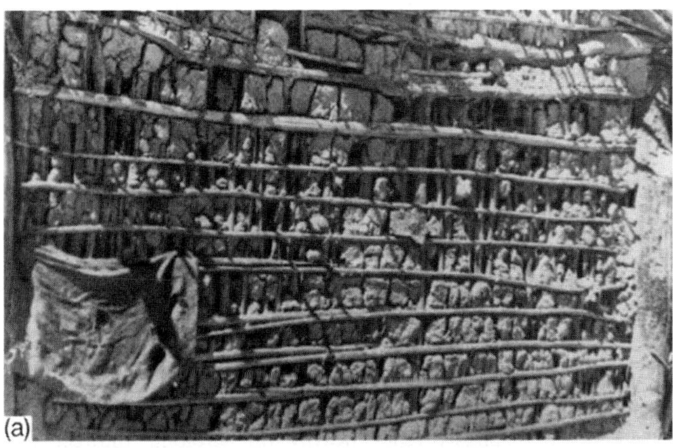

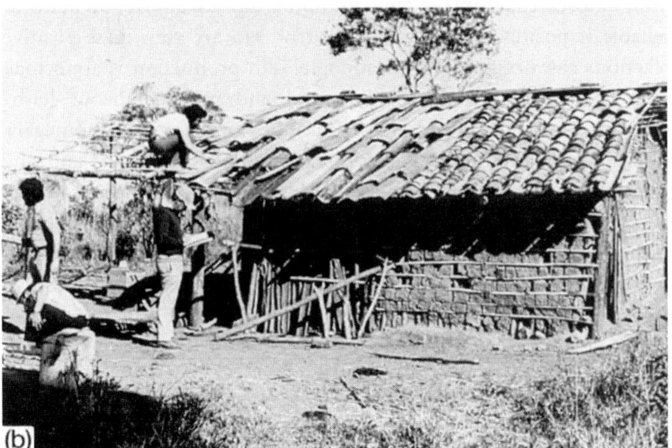

Fig. 2 Wall made of lath and mud, an ideal triatomine habitat *(by courtesy of the Wellcome Museum of Medical Science).*

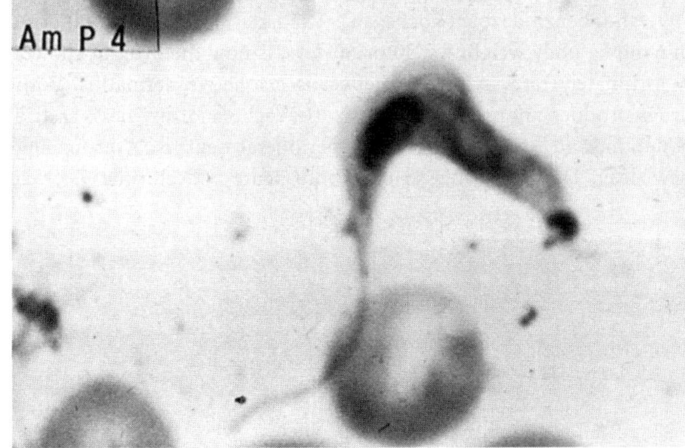

Fig. 3 *T. cruzi* in peripheral blood; note the large kinetoplast.

kinetoplast (a DNA organelle characteristic of this family). Multiplication occurs only in the amastigote phase, which grows in a variety of tissue cells especially muscle. Chronic inflammation of the heart muscle and the smooth muscle of the gut is the basis of the pathology. Early in the infection such infiltrates in the heart muscle are associated with amastigote nests but in chronic cases parasites cannot be found. Chronic chagasic cardiomyopathy may resolve either from damage to the cardiac cells associated with humoral, cell-mediated, and/or autoimmune processes, or by progressive neurotransmission blockade and subsequent denervation of the autonomic nervous system.

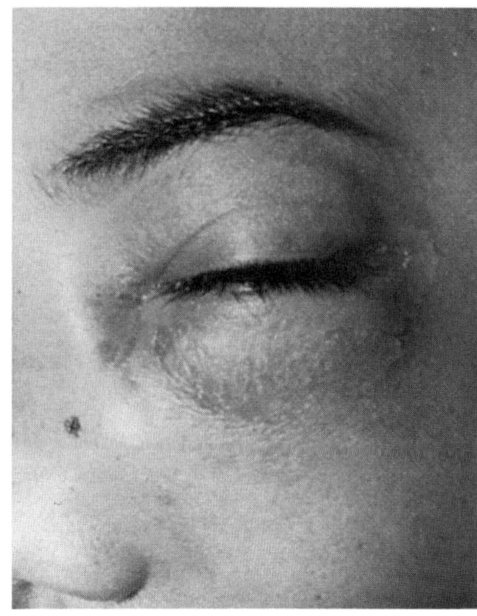

Fig. 4 Romañas sign, clinical manifestation typically observed in the acute phase of some Chagas' disease patients.

The chagasic heart at autopsy shows a thinning of the ventricular muscle and frequently an apical aneurysm. Muscle fibres appear fragmented and an infiltrate of lymphocytes and plasma cells is associated with areas of oedema, degeneration, and haemorrhage. Inflammation around parasympathetic ganglia in the smooth muscle of the gut wall leads to incoordinated peristalsis. Solid residues accumulating in the oesophagus and colon give rise to mega-syndromes.

After the initial wave of parasitaemia the number of circulating trypanosomes falls below detectable levels. IgM and IgG antibodies, however, usually appear within a month. The presence of IgM antibodies assists in confirming congenital Chagas' disease in the neonate. However, small numbers of viable organisms persist in the tissues, probably for life.

Clinical presentation and diagnosis

Patients from endemic areas are usually familiar with the triatomine bugs and it is important to ask whether they have lived in an infested house.

There are three phases of the infection. The acute phase usually passes unnoticed but there may be an inflamed swelling or chagoma at the site of entry of the trypanosomes. Romañas sign is when this swelling involves the eyelids (Fig. 4). Such clinical evidence of local parasitic multiplication occurs only in about 1–2 per cent of the cases. Reticuloendothelial activation is shown by hepatosplenomegaly and lymphadenopathy. In the acute phase, mortality is less than 5 per cent and death may result from acute heart failure or meningo-encephalitis. Congenital Chagas' disease may be aymptomatic, or there may be fever and hepatosplenomegaly. Often, infection of pregnant women results in abortion or low-birthweight neonates. *T. cruzi* trypomastigotes may be detected in fresh blood smears.

The intermediate phase is clinically asymptomatic and is detected by the presence of specific antibodies. Serodiagnosis has improved greatly due to the development of specific recombinant antigens. Fifty per cent of these patients have small numbers of circulating trypanosomes detectable by 'xenodiagnosis' (getting a clean bug to

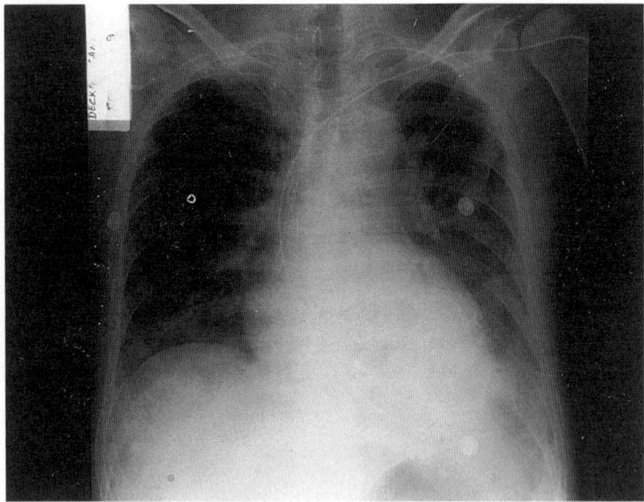

Fig. 5 Posteroanterior chest radiograph showing enlarged heart. This patient also showed megacolon and mega-oesophagus.

feed on the patient and then examining it for trypanosomes). In many patients with positive serology disease never appears.

The chronic phase of Chagas' disease appears decades after infection but a rare subacute form has been described in which heart muscle failure supervenes only months after the acute phase. Longitudinal studies in Brazil of seropositive but disease-free individuals revealed that after 10 years, 24 per cent developed electrocardiogram abnormalities and 2 per cent developed clinically apparent mega-oesophagus. Chagasic cardiomyopathy has two principal manifestations: heart muscle failure and conduction defects. Bilateral or ventricular failure tend to occur. Patients usually have pulmonary oedema. Intraventricular thrombi are common, and systemic or pulmonary emboli may be the initial sign of this disease. Heart size is variable but is frequently greatly enlarged (Fig. 5). There are no organic valvular lesions, only functional mitral or tricuspid incompetence. Complete right bundle branch block with left anterior hemiblock is a characteristic electrocardiographic finding but extrasystoles and any form of atrioventricular conduction defect may be present. Left bundle branch block and atrial fibrillation are rare. Complete heart block with Stokes–Adams attacks may cause the patient's admission to hospital. Repeated heart failure, massive embolus, or cardiac arrest are common causes of death. Severe heart disease is commoner in males 30–50 years old.

Mega-oesophagus has been classified into four degrees of severity depending mainly on oesophageal diameter on barium swallow. In the most severe grades (III and IV) difficulty in swallowing may lead to wasting and parotid gland hypertrophy (the 'cat face'). Food residue overspill may produce lung infections and bronchiectasis. The patient gives a clear history of swallowing difficulty and with each mouthful may need water to accomplish deglutition. Likewise megacolon is associated with severe constipation. Faecal impaction and sigmoid volvulus are side-effects of megacolon (Fig. 6).

Laboratory diagnosis relies heavily on serology. Indirect immunofluorescence, and enzyme immunoassay are all over 95 per cent reliable if positive and negative control sera are run. False-positive reactions can occur when immunoglobulin production is abnormal, such as lepromatous leprosy, visceral and mucocutaneous leishmaniasis, treponematoses, hyperimmune malarious splenomegaly, collagenoses, autoimmune disorders, multiple myeloma, and the hereditary macroglobulinaemias. *T. rangeli* is important as a cause of false-positive testing, especially in Amazon areas where it coexists with *T. cruzi.* The use of *T. cruzi* defined antigens (recombinant proteins or synthetic peptides) should help to eliminate false-positive reactions in endemic areas.

Treatment and prevention

The acute stage should be treated with an antitrypanocidal drug because damage to parasympathetic ganglia is thought to occur in the acute stage and theoretically the parasitaemia reduction achieved with such drugs should be advantageous. Two drugs are in common use. Nifurtimox (Lampit) production of which was discontinued in 1991 and, benznidazole (Rochagan). The latter, given in an oral dose of 6 mg/kg body weight for 30 or 60 days, is now the drug of choice. A fortunately rare serious side-effect is exfoliative dermatitis. Both drugs produce anorexia, weight loss, headache and dizziness, gastric irritation, and, in 12–30 per cent, peripheral neuritis. A promising new drug, D0870, is able to cure both acute and chronic *T. cruzi*

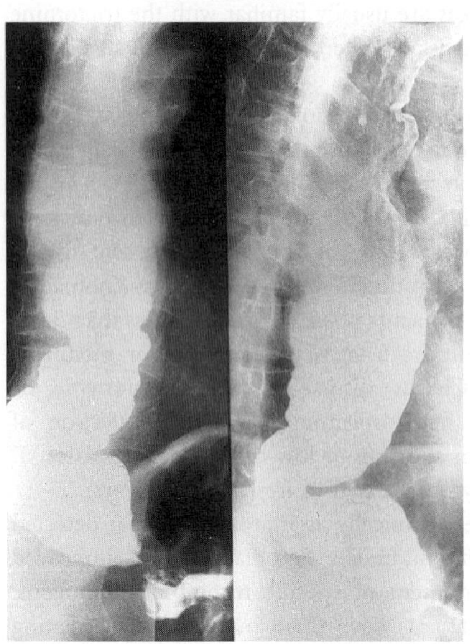

(a)

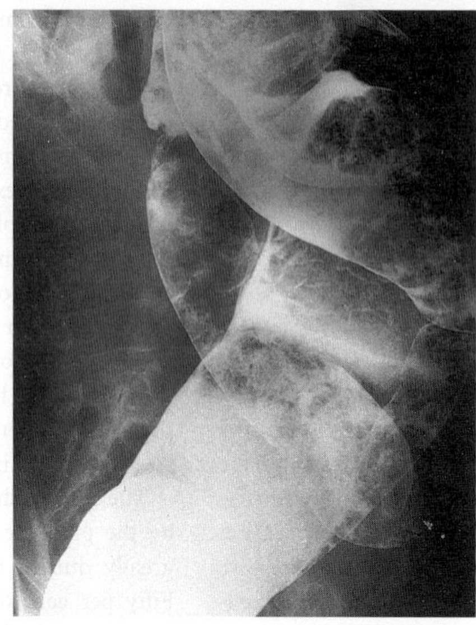

(b)

Fig. 6 (a) Chagasic mega-oesophagus showing stenosis typical of achalasia. (b) Chagasic megacolon with enlargement of the sigmoid. *(From Guevara, A.G., et al. (1997). Revista da Sociedade Brasileira de Medicina Tropical,* ***30****, by permission of the authors and publishers.)*

infection in experimental animal models and is being tested in preclinical studies.

Treatment of patients in the intermediate or chronic phase is controversial. However, chronic chagasic patients treated with benznidazole showed fewer electrocardiographic changes and a lower frequency of clinical deterioration. Control of heart failure with digitalis and diuretics may be of benefit but antiarrhythmic drugs should be used with caution. β-adrenergic blockers may produce bradycardia and shock.

Pacemaker implantation to relieve severe heart block has a better prognosis if the heart is of normal size. Early mega-oesophagus can be relieved by balloon dilatation but established, severe mega-oesophagus and megacolon require surgery. Half the patients with mega-oesophagus have abnormal electrocardiograms.

Congenital Chagas' disease and transfusion-associated acute disease require benznidazole therapy. Transfusion infection can be prevented by donor screening or, mixing the blood with gentian violet for 24 h (dilution 1:4000) to kill *T. cruzi*.

The effectiveness of residual insecticides in controlling domestic bug population was first reported in the 1940s. Recently, new efficient tools for triatomine control have been developed including fumigant canisters, insecticidal paints, and sensor boxes. In Brazil, in 1982, some 711 Brazilian municipalities reported infestation with *Triatoma infestans* but in 1993 only 83 municipalities reported the infestation after appropriate use of household insecticides. Brazilian health authorities hope to eliminate vector transmission by 1998. The same field control programmes involving insecticide spraying with modern pyrethroids and tools for delivery as well as compulsory screening of blood donors in endemic areas is being carried out in other countries in Latin America. However, despite effective control measures, a large number of patients with cardiomyopathy and megasyndromes will continue to be seen due to the long period of evolution of the disease.

Further reading

Garcia-Zapata, M.T.A. and Marsden, P.D. (1993). Chagas' disease: control and surveillance through use of insecticides and community participation in Mambai Goias Brazil. *Bulletin of The Pan American Health Organization*, **27**, 265–79.

Garcia-Zapata, M.T.A., McGreevy, P.B., and Marsden, P.D. (1991). American trypanosomiasis. In *Hunters tropical medicine*, (7th edn) (ed. T. Strickland), pp. 628–37. Saunders, Philadelphia.

Guevara, A.G., Taibi, A., Alava, J., Guderian, R.H., and Ouaissi, A. (1995). Use of a recombinant *Trypanosoma cruzi* protein antigen to monitor cure of Chagas disease. *Transactions of the Royal Society of Tropical Medicine and Hygiene*, **89**, 447–8.

Iosa, D. (1994). Chronic chagasic cardioneuropathy: pathogenesis and treatment. In: *Chagas' disease and the nervous system*, p. 99–148. Scientific Publication 547. Pan American Health Organization.

Chapter 16.94

Leishmaniasis

A. D. M. Bryceson

Leishmaniasis is caused by parasites of the genus *Leishmania*. The infection is normally zoonotic, in wild or peridomestic canines or rodents, among which it is transmitted by phlebotomine sandflies. The disease in humans is usually either cutaneous or visceral. The most important variant is mucosal leishmaniasis of South and Central America. In certain places the disease is common and important, but there are few accurate statistics.

Aetiological agent and lifecycle

In its vertebrate host the oval amastigote form of the parasite, 2–3 μm in diameter, is found in cells of the reticuloendothelial system (Fig. 1). In the sandfly or in culture medium it is in the elongated, motile, promastigote form with an anterior flagellum.

The most important species of *Leishmania* that cause disease in humans and their own reservoir hosts are shown in Table 1; isoenzyme patterns and DNA hybridization are used to distinguish species.

Sandflies require a precise microclimate that is provided in certain places in each endemic focus at particular seasons of the year. Transmission is often seasonal. Amastigotes are ingested from blood or tissues of the mammalian host by the female fly, and transform into promastigotes in the mid-gut, rendering the fly infective after about 10 days.

Cutaneous leishmaniasis

Epidemiology (see Table 1)

The vectors of *Leishmania major* live in rodent burrows. Hunters, travellers, tourists, and dwellers at oases or in new settlements are affected. The disease may be sporadic or epidemic. The vectors of *L. tropica* live in crevices in buildings and walls. The disease may be endemic or epidemic. The vector of *L. aethiopica* bites people sleeping in their huts. The disease is endemic and most people are affected by early adulthood. *L. infantum* causes simple, self-healing skin lesions in some parts of southern Europe and North Africa. *L. donovani* causes post-kala-azar dermal leishmaniasis (**PKDL**) in India.

In the New World, transmission is usually in the forest. *L. braziliensis*, the major cause of American cutaneous and mucosal leishmaniasis, is the most widely distributed of the New World species. Its vectors are highly anthropophilic and human infection is common. Periurban foci of infection are increasing. Infection with *L. peruviana* occurs in high Andean valleys, where it may be locally common.

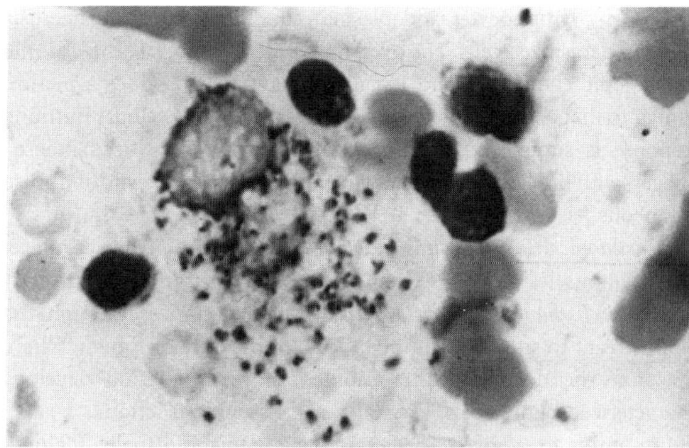

Fig. 1 Amastigotes of *L. donovani* in a reticuloendothelial cell from the splenic aspirate of a patient with visceral leishmaniasis.

Table 1 Epidemiology of leishmaniasis

Organism and geography	Reservoir	Vector
Old World		
L. donovani North-east India, Bangladesh, Burma	Humans	*Phlebotomus argentipes*
L. infantum Mediterranean basin, Middle East, China, central Asia	Dogs, foxes, jackals	*P. perniciosus, P. major, P. chinensis* etc.
L. donovani (Africa) Sudan, Kenya, Horn of Africa, ?Senegambia	?Rodents in Sudan, ?canines, ?humans	*P. orientalis, P. martini*
L. major Semideserts in Middle East, north India, Pakistan, North Africa, central Asia	Gerbils (especially *Rhombomys, Meriones* etc.)	*P. papatasi*
L. major Sub-Saharan savannah, Sudan	Rodents (especially *Arvicanthus, Tatera*)	*P. duboscqi*
L. tropica Towns in Middle East, Mediterranean basin, central Asia	Humans, ?dogs	*P. sergenti*
L. aethiopica Highlands of Kenya, Ethiopia	Hyraxes (*Procavia, Heterohyrax*)	*P. longipes, P. pedifer*
New World		
L. chagasi Central America, northern South America, especially Brazil, Venezuela	Foxes, dogs, opossums (*Didelphys*)	*Lutzomyia longipalpis*
L. mexicana Yucatan, Belize, Guatemala	Forest rodents (especially *Ototylomys*)	*Lu. olmeca*
L. amazonensis Tropical forests of South America	Forest rodents (especially *Proechimys, Oryzomys*)	*Lu. flaviscutellata*
L. brasiliensis Tropical forests throughout South and Central America	?Forest rodents, peridomestic animals	*Psychodopygus wellcomei*, etc., *Lutzomyia* spp.
L. guyanensis Guyanas, Surinam into Brazil, Colombia	Sloths (*Choleopus*), arboreal anteaters (*Tamandua*)	*Lu. umbratilis*
L. panamensis Panama, Costa Rica, Colombia	Sloths (*Choleopus*)	*Lu. trapidoi* etc.
L. peruviana West Andes of Peru, Argentine highlands	Dogs	*Lu. verrucarum, Lu. peruensis*

Pathogenesis and pathology

Leishmania inoculated by the sandfly invade and multiply in macrophages in the skin. The parasitized macrophage granuloma is infiltrated by lymphocytes and plasma cells. Piecemeal focal necrosis destroys parasitized cells. The overlying epidermis ulcerates. In chronic lesions epithelioid cells and Langhans' giant cells produce a picture similar to that of non-caseous tuberculosis. Rarely, the cellular immune response is suppressed histology slows heavily, parasitized macrophages, with little or no lymphocytic infiltrate, characteristic of diffuse cutaneous leishmaniasis (DCL).

L. aethiopica, L. mexicana, and *L. brasiliensis* may invade cartilage. Cartilaginous lesions are extremely chronic. *L. brasiliensis,* and occasionally *L. panamensis* or *L. guyanensis* metastasizes through the bloodstream to sites deep in the mucosa of the nose or mouth, where they may lie dormant. After months or years a lesion develops characterized by necrosis, vasculitis, and tissue destruction.

Immunity to a given species of *Leishmania* is usually lifelong. Second infections occur occasionally, especially in the elderly or immunosuppressed.

Clinical features

After an incubation period of a few days to several months an erythematous nodule develops at the site of the infected sandfly bite. A golden crust forms. The sore reaches its final size, usually 1–5 cm diameter, over weeks or months. The crust may fall away leaving an ulcer with a raised edge (Fig. 2). Satellite papules are common. After months or years the lesion starts to heal leaving a depressed, mottled scar. Secondary infection is unimportant. The lesion is not normally painful, but may disfigure or disable if scarring is severe or over a joint. Draining lymphatic vessels may be thickened or nodular.

There are many variations on this classical pattern. Sores due to *L. major* form and heal most rapidly and may be inflamed and exudative: the so-called wet or rural sore. Sores due to *L. tropica* tend to be less inflamed and more chronic: the so-called dry or urban sore. Lesions due to *L. infantum* have an incubation period of many months, and may persist over several years. In *L. aethiopica* infections satellite papules accumulate to produce a slowly growing, shiny tumour or plaque that may not crust nor ulcerate (Fig. 3);

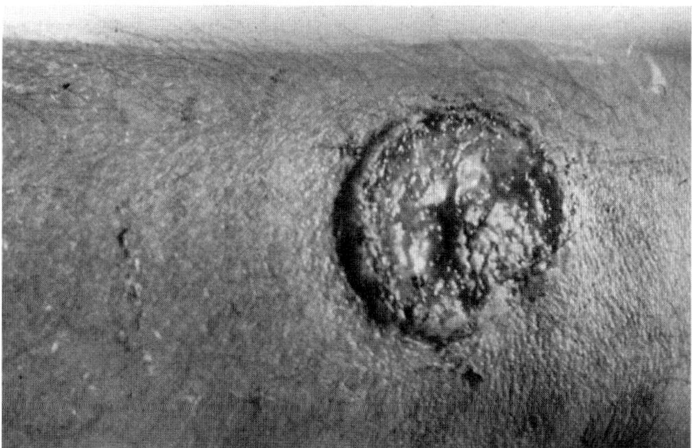

Fig. 2 Punched out' ulcer with nodular edge, characteristic of *L. brasiliensis*, Brazil
(by courtesy of Professor Alfredo Pons).

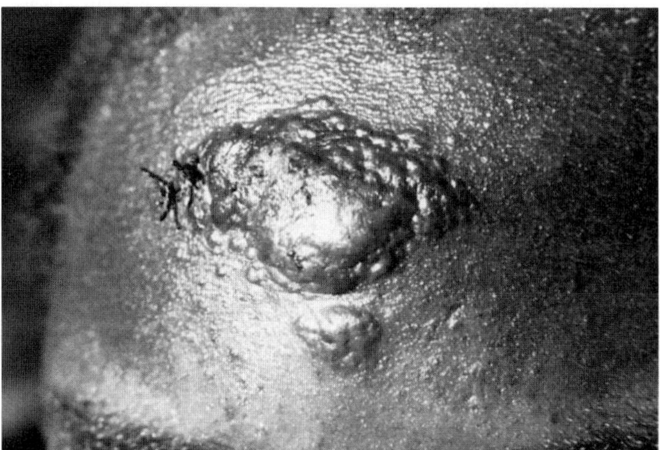

Fig. 3 Spreading nodular lesion, typical of *L. aethiopica*, Kenya.

mucocutaneous leishmaniasis may develop, producing swelling of the lips and expansion and elongation of the nose.

L. brasiliensis often causes deep, spreading ulcers. Up to 15 per cent of patients will relapse after spontaneous or therapeutic cure. *L. mexicana* lesions, 'chiclero ulcer', are commonly on the pinna of the ear. These take years to heal and may destroy the pinna.

Three forms of cutaneous leishmaniasis do not heal spontaneously: DCL, leishmaniasis recidivans, and American mucosal leishmaniasis.

Diffuse cutaneous leishmaniasis

This occurs rarely with *L. aethiopica* and *L. amazonensis* infections. The primary nodule spreads locally without ulceration, and secondary blood-borne lesions appear on other sites in the skin, affecting especially the face and the cooler extensor surfaces of the limbs (Fig. 4). The eye, mucosae, viscera, and peripheral nerves are spared. The infection proceeds gradually over many years.

Leishmaniasis recidivans or lupoid leishmaniasis

This is a rare complication of *L. tropica* infection. The sore heals, but papules recrudesce in the edge of the scar for many years.

American mucosal leishmaniasis, espundia

Up to 40 per cent of patients with untreated cutaneous ulcers due to *L. brasiliensis* may develop mucosal lesions, half of them within 2 years of the appearance of the original lesion, and 90 per cent within

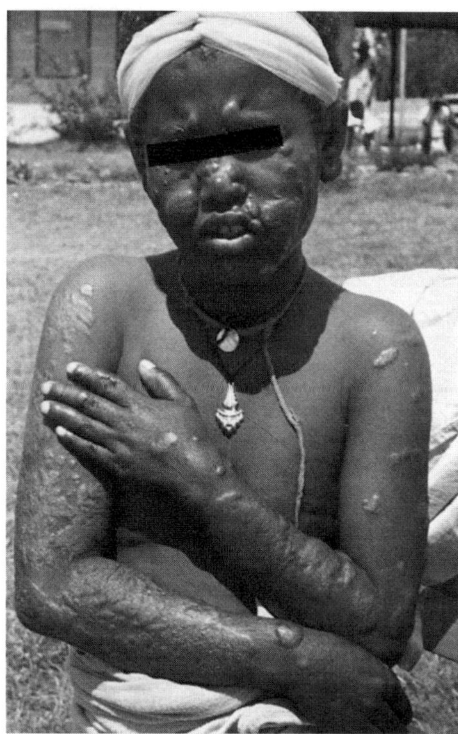

Fig. 4 Diffuse cutaneous leishmaniasis, caused by *L. aethiopica*, Ethiopia.

10 years. About one in six cases gives no history of a previous skin lesion. In most cases the nasal mucosa is affected, and in a third another site is also involved: the pharynx, palate, larynx, and upper lip, in order of frequency. The initial lesion is a nodule and the initial symptom is of nasal obstruction. Mucosal leishmaniasis is slowly destructive, the septum perforates, and eventually the whole nose and mouth may be destroyed (Fig. 5). Death may result from secondary sepsis, starvation, or laryngeal obstruction.

Laboratory findings

Parasitological diagnosis

Leishmania may normally be isolated from 80 per cent of sores during the first half of their natural course. The nodular part of the lesion is grasped firmly between the finger and thumb till it blanches. An incision is made a few millimetres long into the dermis with the point of a scalpel, which is used to scrape dermal tissue and juice. Material obtained may be used to inoculate special diphasic culture medium and to prepare smears for staining with Giemsa, Wright's, or Leishman's stain (Fig. 1). Biopsy material may be used to make impression smears, for culture and for histology. Diagnosis of mucosal leishmaniasis requires deep punch biopsy. Species diagnosis is desirable for American parasites, to assess the risk of mucosal leishmaniasis.

Immunological diagnosis

The leishmanin test is an intradermal test of delayed hypersensitivity which becomes positive in over 90 per cent of cases of self-healing forms of cutaneous leishmaniasis and mucosal leishmaniasis and is 95 per cent specific. Evaluation of a positive test must take into account naturally acquired positivity in the population at risk. Serology is unhelpful.

Treatment

Old World sores or those due to *L. mexicana*, *L. amazonensis*, and *L. peruviana* that are not troublesome may be left to heal naturally. But

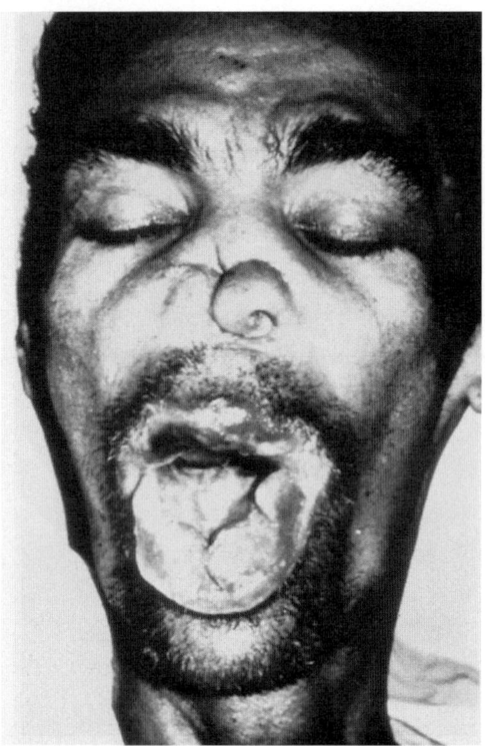

Fig. 5 Severe mutilation of mouth and nose in a Brazilian mucosal leishmaniasis due to *L. brasiliensis* *(by courtesy of Professor Philip Marsden)*.

those that are disfiguring, potentially disabling, inconvenient, or around the ankle, where they heal slowly, should be treated either locally or systemically. Systemic treatment is required when there is risk that the sore may be due to *L. brasiliensis*, *L. panamensis*, or *L. guyanensis*, when the sore is too large or badly sited for local treatment, and for mucosal leishmaniasis, DCL, and recidivans leishmaniasis.

Local treatment

Surgery, curettage, and cryotherapy are methods of removing small sores. Local infiltration of the lesion with a pentavalent antimonial, twice weekly for 2 or 3 weeks may be successful. Leishmanicidal ointments are under evaluation.

Systemic treatment (See Table 2 for dosage regimens)

All cutaneous species of *Leishmania* are sensitive to pentavalent antimonials in conventional dosage except *L. aethiopica*, when pentamidine or aminosidine may be used. Ketoconazole may be useful for *L. major* and *L. mexicana* infections. Patients with DCL should be treated for at least 2 months longer than it takes to clear parasites from the skin, and relapses should be retreated promptly. Relapsed cases of mucosal leishmaniasis have usually become unresponsive to antimonials and should be treated with amphotericin B desoxycholate for at least 4–6 weeks or liposomal amphotericin B for 3 weeks. In addition they may require antibiotics for secondary sepsis, attention to nutrition, and later plastic surgery.

Table 2 Dosage regimens for the treatment of leishmaniasis (see text for choice of regimen)

Sodium stibogluconate or meglumine antimoniate 20 mg Sb/kg body weight once daily for 21 days (visceral or cutaneous disease) or 28 days (mucosal disease)
Amimosidine 16 mg/kg body weight daily for 21 days
Pentamidine 4 mg salt/kg body weight once weekly to once monthly
Ketoconazole 600 mg/day (adult) for 4–6 weeks
Amphotericin B desoxycholate 1 mg/kg body weight on alternate days for 2 weeks (visceral disease) or 4–6 weeks (mucosal disease)
Liposomal amphotericin B (AmBisome, Nextar) ampoules of 50 mg, 2–3 mg/kg body weight daily for 7–10 doses, using whole ampoules to avoid waste, to total at least 21 mg/kg. In India a total dose of 6–9 mg/kg is sufficient

Visceral leishmaniasis

Epidemiology

Visceral leishmaniasis is found in four main zoo-geographical zones (Table 1). Around the Mediterranean littoral, across the Middle East and central Asia, and in northern and eastern China, human disease is endemic in many places. Children under 5 years of age are especially affected. In other places the disease is sporadic. Non-immune adults such as tourists, hunters, and soldiers are susceptible. The Ganges and Brahmaputra river valleys of India and Bangladesh are the home of epidemic visceral leishmaniasis, or kala-azar, which returns approximately every 15–20 years. The majority of cases are under 15 years old. In the interepidemic period the parasite survives in patients with PKDL. Visceral leishmaniasis is endemic in parts of Sudan and Kenya. Older children and teenagers are most commonly affected. Sporadic cases also occur in nomads and visitors. An epidemic that began in southern Sudan in the late 1980s is still raging, and has caused over 100 000 deaths. It has been especially severe among refugees from the civil war.

In South America the disease is most common in north-eastern Brazil, where older children are affected. Foxes bring the infection to the homesteads while raiding chicken houses.

Visceral leishmaniasis may be transmitted by blood transfusion from subclinical cases and appear unexpectedly in immunosuppressed patients, for example after renal transplantation, or as a coinfection with the human immunodeficiency virus (**HIV**).

Pathogenesis and pathology

For every case of classical visceral leishmaniasis, there are about 30 subclinical infections that cause leishmanin positivity and life-long immunity to *L. donovani*. Malnutrition predisposes to clinical disease. Established visceral infections are characterized by the failure of specific cell-mediated immunity. The leishmanin test is negative. The parasite multiplies freely in macrophages in the spleen, bone marrow, lymphoid tissues, and jejunal submucosa and Kupffer cells of the liver. Histology shows a variable degree of granuloma formation, and of interstitial inflammation that may lead to fibrosis. In the spleen especially there is massive reticuloendothelial hyperplasia and infiltration with plasma cells. Small splenic infarcts may develop.

Antibodies, polyclonal IgG, and immune complexes circulate at high concentration but rarely cause complications. About half the patients have mild malabsorption but seldom diarrhoea. Jaundice when present is usually due to intercurrent viral hepatitis. Spontaneous bleeding is unusual and is associated with hypoprothrombinaemia. Visceral leishmaniasis is characterized by anaemia, leucopenia, thrombocytopenia, and hypoalbuminaemia. The anaemia results mainly from shortened red-cell survival with destruction of cells in the spleen,

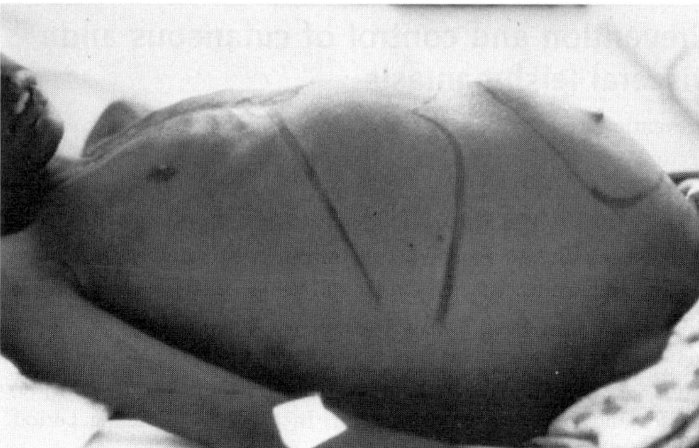

Fig. 6 Visceral leishmaniasis in a Kenyan child. Note the wasting and massive enlargement of spleen and liver.

together with splenic pooling and sequestration (hypersplenism). In young children, profound anaemia may develop rapidly as a result of severe haemolysis. Death is usually due to secondary infection.

Clinical features

The male/female ratio is 3–4:1. The incubation period is usually 2–8 months. In endemic areas the onset is usually ill defined. The patient develops fever, discomfort from an enlarged spleen, abdominal swelling, weight loss, cough, or diarrhoea. Classically the fever spikes twice daily, usually without rigors, but daily, irregular or undulant fevers are common. During an epidemic or in visitors to an epidemic area, the onset is abrupt with high fever and rapid progression of illness with toxaemia, weakness, dyspnoea, and acute anaemia.

Early cases have only symptomless splenomegaly. Late cases are wasted with hair changes and pedal oedema typical of hypoalbuminaemia. Hyperpigmentation is characteristic of visceral leishmaniasis in India (kala-azar means black sickness). The spleen is huge, smooth, and non-tender unless there has been a recent infarct. The liver is moderately enlarged in one-third of cases. In Africa generalized lymphadenopathy is common.

Over months or years the patient becomes emaciated, with a distended abdomen (Fig. 6). Intercurrent infections are common, especially pneumococcal otitis, pneumonia, and septicaemia, tuberculosis, measles, dysentery, other locally important infections, and rarely, cancrum oris. Untreated, 80–90 per cent of patients die.

Post-kala-azar dermal leishmaniasis

Twenty per cent of Indian patients and 5 per cent of African patients develop a rash on the face and extensor surfaces of the arms and legs after recovery from visceral leishmaniasis. In India the rash begins after an interval of 1 or 2 years and progresses over many years: pale macules become erythematous plaques or nodules resembling lepromatous leprosy, and almost all the body surface may be involved (Fig. 7). In Africa the rash appears while the patient is still recovering, as discrete nodules which show a tuberculoid histology. It heals spontaneously within 6 months.

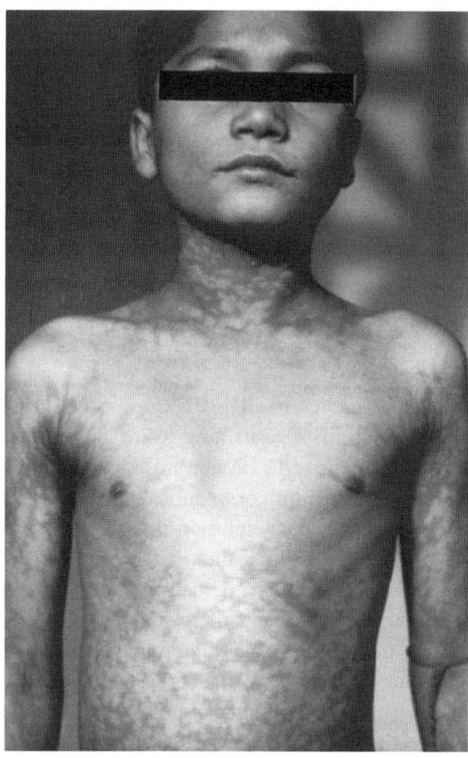

Fig. 7 Post-kala azar dermal leishmaniasis in an Indian child, showing the typical hypopigmented macular rash. Note also the nodules on the lower lip.

Visceral leishmaniasis and the acquired immune deficiency syndrome (AIDS)

Visceral leishmaniasis may be associated with HIV infection and is an AIDS-defining illness in adults in southern Europe. It may be due to reactivation of latent infection with leishmania or to a recent infection. In Spain, 50 per cent of adults with visceral leishmaniasis are HIV positive, and it is estimated that 9 per cent of HIV-infected individuals will acquire visceral leishmaniasis. The presentation may not be typical. Often the parasite is found by chance, for example in a rectal or skin biopsy taken for other purposes, or in bronchiolar lavage. The bone marrow is teeming with parasites, but two-thirds of cases have no detectable antileishmanial antibodies. In 90 per cent of cases the CD4 count is under 0.3×10^6/litre.

Laboratory diagnosis

Parasitological diagnosis

Leishmania may be isolated from reticuloendothelial tissue. Yields are of the order: spleen over 95 per cent, bone marrow or liver 85 per cent, African lymph node 65 per cent, and buffy coat 70 per cent. Bone marrow aspiration is most commonly used, but splenic aspiration is simple, painless, and safe if the prothrombin time is normal and the platelet count above 40×10^9/litre. Occasionally, the diagnosis is made accidentally on biopsy of bone marrow, liver, lymph node, or bowel mucosa. Antibodies are present in high titre. Indirect immunofluorescence is suitable for individual cases. Enzyme-linked immunosorbent assay or direct agglutination are the techniques of choice for field diagnosis. The leishmanin test is negative.

Other findings

There is normochromic, normocytic anaemia without reticulocytosis and neutropenia, eosinopenia, and thrombocytopenia. Serum albumin is low (20 g/litre) and globulin high (70 g/litre), IgG and IgM being approximately thrice and twice the normal population values. Hepatic enzymes and prothrombin and partial thromboplastin times are usually normal.

Treatment

Chemotherapy (See Table 2 for dosage regimens)

Liposomal amphotericin B (AmBisome) by intravenous infusion is the best drug for visceral leishmaniasis. It is concentrated and retained in reticuloendothelial cells and is not toxic. All patients respond promptly, but HIV-coinfected patients relapse. At the moment it is far too costly for most countries where visceral leishmaniasis is endemic. Therefore, a pentavalent antimonial remains the drug of choice in most situations.

Sodium stibogluconate containing 100 mg antimony (Sb) per ml and meglumine antimoniate containing 85 mg Sb/ml, are of equal efficacy and toxicity. The drug is administered by intramuscular injection, which may be painful, or by intravenous injection through a fine-gauge needle, slowly or by infusion in 50–100 ml of 5 per cent dextrose over 20 min to reduce the risk of venous thrombosis. Treatment is given daily for 21 days. Usually the drug is well tolerated, but towards the end of treatment there may be malaise, anorexia, nausea, vomiting, and muscle pains. Should toxic effects develop, rest for 1 day and reduce each dose by 2 mg Sb/kg. Hepatic and pancreatic enzyme levels may rise and haemoglobin levels fall, but return to normal when treatment is stopped. The electrocardiogram develops unimportant T-wave changes. At higher doses the corrected QT interval may be prolonged, heralding the development of a serious arrhythmia. If it is essential, for example during an epidemic, to give a shorter course of treatment, 10 mg Sb/kg may be safely given every 8 h for 10 days in complete safety.

The aminoglycoside antibiotic aminosidine or paromomycin (Solopak, Chicago, IL, USA) is equally effective and well tolerated. It is given by intramuscular injection or intravenous infusion over 90 min.

Conventional amphotericin B desoxycholate is particularly effective in India.

Patients who are immunoincompetent as a result of HIV coinfection or immunosuppressive drugs respond slowly, require longer treatment, and are more liable to relapse than immunocompetent patients. Ideally, treatment should be monitored by splenic aspirate counts of parasites, and continued for 2–3 weeks beyond parasitological cure. Aminosidine is the drug of choice, as it is well tolerated and not prohibitively expensive. Renal function and hearing should be monitored. Clinical pancreatitis has been reported with the antimonials. Liposomal amphotericin B, although well tolerated, does not prevent relapse.

Supportive treatment

Intercurrent infection must be sought and treated, and nutritional deficiencies corrected. Blood transfusion is rarely needed.

Response to treatment

Fever, splenic size, haemoglobin, serum albumin, and body weight are useful monitors of progress. Proof of parasitological cure is not usually necessary. Reassessment at 6 weeks and 6 months will detect over 90 per cent of relapses. Relapse rates should be almost zero in Mediterranean and Indian disease and about 2 per cent in African disease. Relapsed patients are slower to respond, and run a 40 per cent chance of further relapse(s) and of becoming unresponsive to antimony. Primary resistance is increasing in India where the first choice lies between aminosidine and amphotericin B desoxycholate.

Prevention and control of cutaneous and visceral leishmaniasis

Prevention is a matter of controlling reservoir hosts and sandfly vectors, or of avoiding bites by vectors. Successful control requires an accurate knowledge of transmission in each ecological focus.

In the Old World, urban cutaneous leishmaniasis is controlled by case-finding and treatment, better housing, and domestic spraying with residual insecticides, while rural leishmaniasis is controlled in the Middle East and North Africa by the destruction of gerbil colonies. Mediterranean visceral leishmaniasis may be controlled by the destruction or treatment of dogs. In India, mass campaigns to spray houses and cattle sheds are needed. In the inter-epidemic period, cases of PKDL should be sought and treated.

Individuals may take precautions to prevent infection during the season of transmission, by use of insect repellent creams and fine mesh bed nets impregnated with permethrin.

Further reading

Alvar, J., Cañavate, C., Gutiérrez-Solar, B., *et al.* (1997). *Leishmania* and human immunodeficiency virus coinfection: the first ten years. *Clinical Microbiology Reviews*, **10**, 298–319.

Davidson, R.N., Di Martino, L., Gradoni, L., *et al.* (1994). Liposomal amphotericin B (Ambisome) in Mediterranean visceral leishmaniasis. *Quarterly Journal of Medicine*, **87**, 75–81.

Grimaldi, G., Jr., Tesh, R.B., and McMahon-Pratt, D. (1989). A review of the distribution and epidemiology of leishmaniasis in the New World. *American Journal of Tropical Medicine and Hygiene*, **41**, 687–725.

Olliaro, P. and Bryceson, A.D.M. (1993). Practical progress and new drugs for changing patterns of leishmaniasis. *Parasitology Today*, **9**, 323–8.

Seaman, J., Mercer, A.J., and Sondorp, E. (1998). The epidemics of visceral leishmaniasis in Western Upper Nile, Southern Sudan: course and impact from 1984 to 1994. *International Journal of Epidemiology*, **25**, 862–71.

World Health Organization (1990). *Control of the leishmaniases.* Technical Report Series 793. WHO, Geneva.

Chapter 16.95

Trichomoniasis

J. P. Ackers

Trichomoniasis is caused by infection with the protozoan parasite *Trichomonas vaginalis*. *T. vaginalis* is a motile, round or oval flagellate, 10–13 μm long and 8–10 μm wide when living; fixed and stained it is about 25 per cent smaller. Diagnostic features include the jerky motility, induced by four anterior flagella and the undulating membrane, and a rigid, microtubular rod (the axostyle), which runs through the body and projects as a long thin spine from the posterior end. The life cycle is simple, multiplication being by binary fission. No resistant cysts are formed and no intermediate or reservoir hosts involved in transmission. Two other trichomonads are uncommon and probably harmless human parasites: *T. tenax*, which is normally found in the periodontal crevices but which may possibly, very rarely, spread to the respiratory tract; and *Pentatrichomonas hominis*, which is an occasional inhabitant of the large bowel. All three species appear to be site specific and urogenital trichomoniasis is not due to contamination from other sites.

Pathology

In women, *T. vaginalis* may be found in the vagina and the exterior cervix in over 95 per cent of infections, but is only recovered from the endocervix in 13 per cent. The urethra and Skene's glands are also very commonly infected. Dissemination beyond the lower urogenital tract is extremely rare and is not found even in severely immunocompromised patients. In men the urethra is the most common site of infection, but the organism has also been recovered from epididymal aspirates.

Previously regarded as unpleasant but harmless, epidemiological studies have recently linked trichomoniasis in women with a modest increase in the risk of human immune deficiency infection via sexual intercourse and with adverse pregnancy outcome and have suggested that it might be the actual cause of a few per cent of cases of cervical neoplasia.

Epidemiology

Despite the difficulty often experienced in isolating the organism from male contacts of infected women, all epidemiological evidence suggests that the vast majority of infections are sexually acquired. Few studies have been made of genuinely unselected populations, but it has recently been estimated that, world-wide, 170 million new infections occur each year. Most surveys have examined either pregnant women or those attending STD clinics; there are wide national variations, but most report 10–25 per cent infected, although the full range is 0–63 per cent. In most clinical surveys female cases outnumber male by 5 or 10 to 1. In several developed countries there has been a steady decline in the incidence of trichomoniasis in the past two decades, but this has not occurred in less-developed countries nor in deprived inner-city areas in industrialized nations.

Symptoms

A recent study tried to eliminate confounding effects due to mixed infections and showed that trichomoniasis remains associated with symptoms of yellow vaginal discharge and vulvar itching, and signs of colpitis macularis (strawberry cervix), purulent vaginal discharge, and vulval and vaginal erythema. Colpitis was seen frequently if colposcopy was undertaken, but hardly ever found by naked-eye examination. Dyspareunia, mild dysuria, and lower abdominal pain are also described and in most series 10–50 per cent of women are asymptomatic. Vaginal pH is usually elevated.

The majority of men with trichomoniasis are asymptomatic, but the parasite is clearly responsible for a small but significant proportion (5–15 per cent) of non-gonococcal urethritis.

Diagnosis

The symptoms and signs described above are in no case sufficient to establish the diagnosis, which must be made by detecting the parasite. This is most frequently (and most cheaply) done by wet-film microscopic examination of vaginal (not endocervical) secretions, urethral scrapings mixed with a drop of saline, centrifuged urine sediment or prostate fluid. The specimen should be examined as soon as possible; a motile trichomonad is unmistakable (Plate 1), while a dead one is nearly unrecognizable. This procedure will detect about half to three-quarters of infected women, but only 10–20 per cent of infected men.

Culture provides significantly greater sensitivity; media vary in efficiency but Diamond's TYM is among the best. Most will be positive within 48 h but should be kept for 7–10 days before being finally discarded. A number of new immunological, DNA probe and polymerase chain reaction-based tests have been developed; although still experimental and expensive, they can combine the speed of the wet film with the sensitivity of culture methods.

Treatment

The 5-nitroimidazole drugs provided the first and so far only group of effective chemotherapeutic agents. Doses given here are for metronidazole and should be adjusted to give the equivalent amount of other compounds. Two regimens are used—the original one of 250 mg three times a day for 7 days, or a single 1.6- or 2-g dose. Cure rates in women are similar (about 95 per cent) with both regimens if male sexual partners are also treated, but appear to be lower with the single-dose regimen if they are not. Only the 7-day regimen has been extensively evaluated in males, where it is equally effective. Treatment failures with any of the 5-nitroimidazole drugs are rare, but a small proportion is due to resistant isolates.

Further reading

Honigberg, B.M. (ed.) (1989). *Trichomonads parasitic in humans*. Springer-Verlag, New York.

Krieger, J.N. (1995). Trichomoniasis in men: old issues and new data. *Sexually Transmitted Diseases*, 22, 83–96.

Petrin, D., Delgaty, K., Bhatt, R., and Garber, G. (1998). Clinical and microbiological aspects of *Trichomonas vaginalis*. *Clinical Microbiology Reviews*, 11, 300–17.

Nematodes (roundworms)

Chapter 16.96

Filariasis

B. O. L. Duke

General principles of filarial infections and diseases

Six filarial species commonly cause disease in humans: *Wuchereria bancrofti*; *Brugia malayi* and *B. timori*; *Onchocerca volvulus*; *Loa loa*; and *Mansonella streptocerca*. Multiple infections are common in many areas, especially in Africa. Adult filarial worms live in the lymphatic vessels, the subcutaneous and deep connective tissues, or the serous cavities, according to species. Their life-spans may extend for 10–20 years. The fertilized females produce a continuous supply of living motile embryos, known as microfilariae (**mfs**), which find their way to the blood or skin according to species. The microfilariae live for some 6–24 months and most die in the body because they cannot develop further unless they are ingested by a blood-feeding female insect capable of acting as a vector. The microfilariae of some species living in the blood exhibit periodicity, i.e. they are only found in the peripheral blood at a certain period of the 24 h, which coincides with the biting activity of the vector.

Inside the vector the microfilariae develop, without multiplying, for 6–15 days to become infective larvae or L_3. When the insect bites again, the L_3 enter the human host, develop to adult worms, mate, and begin to produce microfilariae. Development from L_3 to adult worm takes place without multiplication. It follows, that repeated exposure to L_3 over many years is necessary before infections of high intensity can build up in the human host.

In areas where filarial parasites are endemic, a high proportion of the human population will be infected. Some will have asymptomatic infections, others will show signs and symptoms of filarial disease. Although control schemes may demand that whole populations are treated in order to interrupt transmission, the clinician is likely to be called upon to treat only those who have manifest disease or are at high risk of developing it.

Onchocerciasis

Geographical distribution and vectors

Transmission of *Onchocerca volvulus* occurs mainly near the fast-flowing watercourses where the *Simulium* vectors (black-flies) breed. In Africa, members of the *S. damnosum* complex are vectors across the tropical sub-Saharan belt, from west to east, in Senegal, Mali, Burkina Faso, Niger, Guinea Bissau, Guinea, Sierra Leone, Liberia, Côte d'Ivoire, Ghana, Togo, Benin, Nigeria, Cameroon, Chad, Central African Republic, Gabon, Congo, Zaire, Equatorial Guinea, Burundi, Angola, Sudan, Ethiopia, Uganda, Tanzania, and Malawi. There is also a focus in Yemen. Species of the *S. neavei* complex are important vectors locally in parts of east and central Africa. In America, *S. ochraceum* is the main vector in Guatemala and Mexico. Smaller foci occur in Venezuela (*S. metallicum* and *S. pintoi*), Brazil (*S. amazonicum/sanguineum* group), Ecuador (*S exiguum* and *S. quadrivittatum*), and Colombia (*S. exiguum*).

Lifecycle of the parasite and pathology

The pre-patent interval between the inoculation of infective larvae by *Simulium* and the first symptoms of microfilariae in the skin is usually 9–18 months. The adult worms (males 5 cm × 0.2 mm; females 50 cm × 0.4 mm) live in fibrous nodules. They have an average life-span of 9–10 years (maximum 15 years). Some nodules are subcutaneous and palpable; others, probably more numerous, lie deep and impalpable, between the muscles, and against the capsules of joints (especially the hip joint) or the periosteum of the long bones. The microfilariae are 220–350 μm × 5–9 μm. They can live for 12–24 months and cause almost all the pathology of onchocerciasis. In the skin, they provoke small granulomatous reactions infiltrated with eosinophils, which lead to itching and a rash. Prolonged and heavy infection of the skin leads to fibrosis, scarring of the papillae, replacement of dermal collagen by hyalinized scar tissue, and atrophic changes. When microfilariae invade the eye, they give rise to all the ocular lesions of the disease. The pathology of the anterior segment lesions centres on microfilariae granulomas; in the posterior segment, although microfilariae have been found in the retina and optic nerve, there may also be an autoimmune response to retinal proteins incited by the presence of parasites.

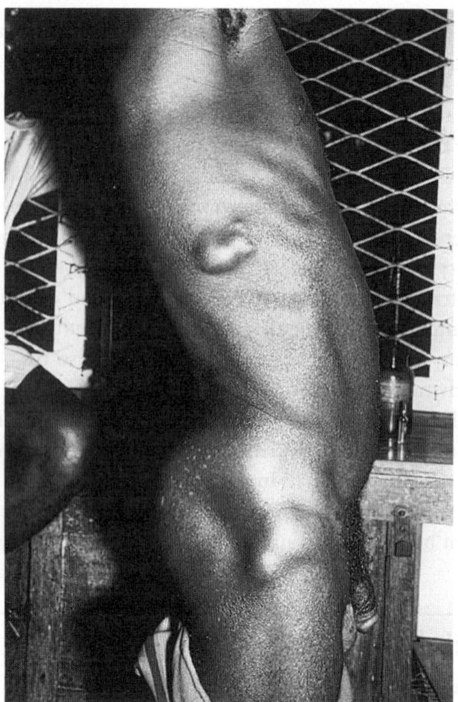

Fig. 1 Prominent subcutaneous nodules.

Clinical picture

Palpable nodules and skin lesions

Subcutaneous, palpable nodules normally lie over bony prominences (Fig. 1), especially the knees, trochanters, iliac crests, ribs, and the head.

'Acute' skin lesions

Lightly and recently infected persons, including expatriates, usually present on account of the itching cutaneous lesions of onchocerciasis (*gâle filarienne*). Typically, such cases harbour an adult worm or worms (often impalpable) in the subcutaneous or deep tissues on one side of the limb-girdle concerned. microfilariae then invade the skin, predominantly over the same anatomical quarter, and give rise to a persistent and variously itchy rash of lop-sided distribution, usually involving the buttock, thigh, and leg on one side (Fig. 2) with extensions to the opposite buttock and up the back (Fig. 3); or the shoulder and arm on one side, with extensions down the back, across to the other shoulder or up the same side of the neck. The rash comprises numerous small discrete papules, 1–3 mm in diameter, which show red on a white skin. Weals, vesicles, scratch marks, and secondary skin infection may be superimposed. The skin fold is thickened on the affected side, and the skin may be blacker than normal in black persons (a condition known as 'sowda'), or reddened in white subjects. There is some enlargement of the draining lymph nodes on the affected side. Deep-seated aches and pains may be felt in the limb concerned.

Chronic lesions of the skin and lymph glands

Chronic, disfiguring skin lesions are seen in Africans with long-standing heavy infections. The lower limbs are usually worst affected. Gross lichenification and thickening of the skin with hyper-pigmentation, give way later to atrophy and 'lizard' skin; and/or a mottled depigmentation over the shins (Fig. 4). The femoral and inguinal lymph nodes enlarge and hang in pockets of loose skin,

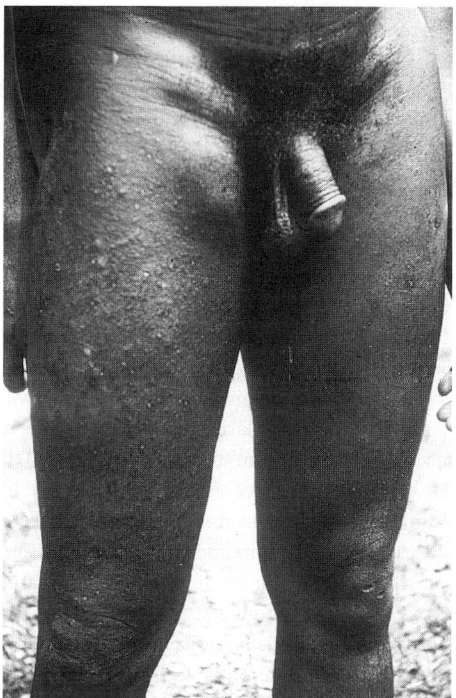

Fig. 2 Acute skin rash and groin lymphadenopathy.

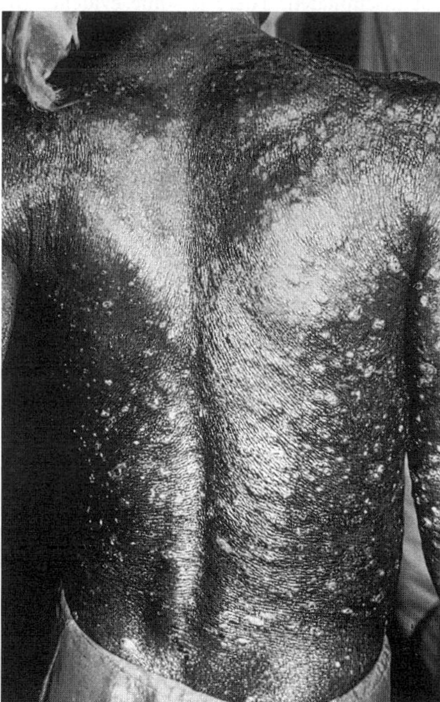

Fig. 3 Papular pruritic rash of onchocerciasis on the back.

known as 'hanging groins' (Fig. 5) and predisposing to herniae. Elephantiasis of the lower limbs or scrotum may develop.

Ocular lesions

Punctate keratitis is made up of 'snowflake' opacities—cellular aggregates around dead microfilariae in the cornea—up to 100 or more in number and each up to 0.5 mm. in diameter. Typically symptomless and occurring in light and recent infections, they resolve spontaneously but may be succeeded by further crops.

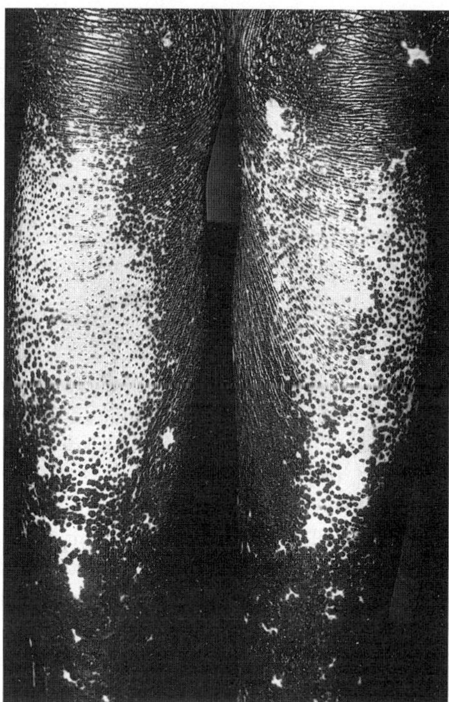

Fig. 4 Mottled depigmentation of the shins.

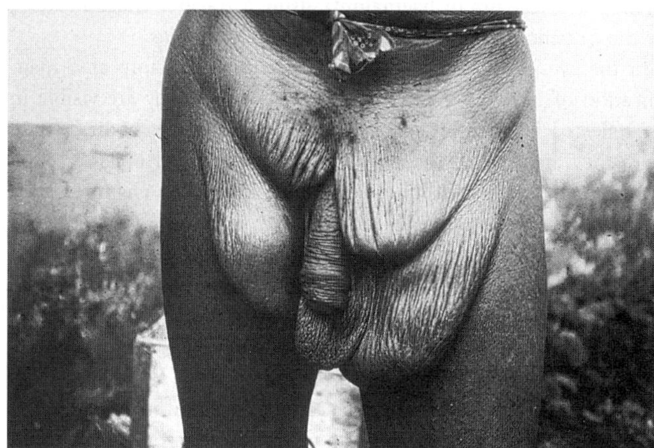

Fig. 5 'Hanging groins'

Sclerosing keratitis occurs in heavy infections with abundant microfilariae in the cornea. A chronic interstitial keratitis develops from the sides and below, headed by a slowly advancing zone of milky opacification in the corneal stroma, behind which develops a scantily vascularized and usually pigmented 'pannus'. The clear segment above may contain many hundreds of visible microfilariae both living and dead, until the cornea becomes opaque and blindness ensues.

Anterior uveitis

Acute episodes of uveitis are superimposed on a chronic inflammatory process. The pigment ruff of the pupil is lost and the pupil becomes distorted, often pear-shaped, with posterior synechiae. Secondary glaucoma and cataract may follow leading to blindness.

Fundus lesions

Choroido-retinal lesions are bilateral and start temporal to the macula developing into large, well-defined patches of choroido-retinal degeneration known as the Hissette–Ridley fundus.

Optic neuritis

A post-neuritic optic atrophy may be seen, with sheathing of the retinal vessels near the optic disc. The visual fields are greatly reduced, leaving only tubular vision. Loss of twilight and night vision is a common early diagnostic symptom.

Other manifestations

Extreme wasting, dwarfism with delayed sexual development, epilepsy, and a failure to react immunologically to antigenic stimuli, have all been associated with heavy *O. volvulus* infection.

Diagnosis

Firm diagnosis depends on seeing *O. volvulus* microfilariae in a skin snip or in the eye, or finding a nodule containing adult worms. There is usually some degree of eosinophilia. Skin snips are best taken from over the affected area, or from the iliac crests in Africa, or from the scapula in Latin America. To take a skin snip, the skin is cleaned with spirit, a suitable needle is inserted horizontally into the epidermis to raise up a small cone-shaped fold of skin. The top of this fold is sliced off with a safety razor blade to remove a piece of skin 2–3 mm in diameter and 0.5–1.0 mm deep, which should be bloodless on removal. Alternatively the snip can be taken using a much more expensive scleral punch of the Holth (2 mm) or Walser type. The snip is placed in a drop of normal saline on a slide or in a well-plate and is examined wet at intervals over 24 h (or subsequently, after staining with Giemsa or haemalum), using a 10–50 × magnification, for the presence of motile microfilariae of *O. volvulus*.

In the eye, microfilariae can be seen with a slit-lamp at a magnification of × 20–25. In the cornea, when alive, they are visible in the reflected beam as translucent and slowly motile bodies; when dead, they are seen in the direct beam, straight and opaque, often with cellular reaction around them. In the anterior chamber, they can be seen as shining bodies floating and wriggling in the aqueous humour, and the numbers visible can often be increased by making the patient sit for 1 min with the head inverted between the knees before the examination is carried out. microfilariae can sometimes be found in urine, blood, sputum, cerebrospinal fluid, and hydrocoele fluid, especially in heavily infected patients.

In a suspect case, if microfilariae cannot be found in skin snips or in the eyes, then it is permissible to perform a Mazzotti test without fear of damaging the posterior segment of the eye. Fifty milligrams of diethylcarbamazine citrate (**DEC**) is given by mouth and the test is positive if, within 30 min to 24 h, there develops an acute exacerbation of the itching and the rash, centred on the previously affected parts and due to inflammatory reactions around microfilariae which have been 'unmasked' and are being destroyed in the skin.

Differential diagnosis

The differential diagnosis of early pruritic cutaneous onchocerciasis is from: (1) scabies, which often coexists in Africans; (2) streptocerciasis (q.v.), by identification of the microfilariae of *M. streptocerca*; (3) prickly heat; (4) contact dermatitis; and (5) insect bites, especially those of *Culicoides* or *Simulium*, which may cause great irritation to persons newly arrived in the tropics.

Treatment

Now that ivermectin is freely available (as Mectizan[R]), anyone with onchocerciasis can be provided with safe and effective suppressive therapy, and mass treatment campaigns with this drug are being undertaken in most endemic countries. Nevertheless, there are three groups of sufferers who are in special need of treatment: (1) those with acute pruritic skin eruptions; (2) those under threat of developing severe eye lesions and blindness; and (3) those with disabling skin and lymph node lesions. Those in the last group may require surgical treatment for their conditions in addition to specific therapy for onchocerciasis.

Methods of treatment

Microfilaricides and microfilarial suppressants

The advent of ivermectin (Mectizan[R]) in 1987 has revolutionized the treatment of onchocerciasis for it is the first drug that can be used safely for mass treatment. Ivermectin constitutes a non-toxic, single-dose (150 μg/kg), oral treatment given at least annually, which is both a microfilaricide and a microfilarial suppressant. The drug clears almost all the microfilariae from the skin within 2–3 days and is remarkable in that the clearance is accompanied by little or no Mazzotti reaction. For this reason it should now be used exclusively, instead of DEC, as the microfilaricide for *O. volvulus*. Ivermectin is not directly macrofilaricidal at a single dose so that treatment has to be maintained at least throughout the life-span of the adult worms. However, it does have various deleterious actions on adult *O. volvulus*. The exodus of intrauterine microfilariae from the female is blocked for periods of 3–12 months after a single dose; the numbers of male worms in nodules are reduced and higher proportions of female worms are not inseminated. There is some evidence that repeated doses given over periods of 3 years or more have a slow action of attrition on the adult female worms.

Microfilariae in the eye are not killed directly, probably because the drug does not penetrate into the aqueous or the cornea; but within a few weeks those which were in the eye move out and are not replaced. Thus treatment does not damage either the anterior or the posterior segment of the eye, but it does improve lesions of the anterior segment and prevent their further development. It also prevents the further development of optic neuritis and possibly some other posterior segment lesions.

Ivermectin has now been given to several million persons with onchocerciasis, without serious mishap, in mass distribution programmes. For individual treatment, it should be given at least once a year, but the best clinical results, particularly in those with acute pruritic skin lesions, will probably follow from giving this suppressive treatment every 3 months. Ivermectin should not be given to children under 2 years old, to mothers in the first week of lactation; to persons who are otherwise severely ill; or to those in whom the blood–brain barrier may be deficient, e.g. during outbreaks of cerebrospinal meningitis or African trypanosomiasis. If significant Mazzotti or other adverse reactions occur during the 24–72 h following treatment, palliative symptomatic medication (antipyretics, antihistamines, oral fluids, and possibly corticosteroids) should be given.

The manufacturers (Merck and Co.) have set up a Mectizan Donation Program to provide the drug, free of charge, for treatment of all persons living in areas endemic for onchocerciasis for as long as necessary. Supplies of the drug for compassionate use by physicians may be obtained by writing to Dr Philippe Gaxotte, Directeur Médical, Merck, Sharp and Dohme Interpharma, 106 Avenue Jean-Moulin, 78170 La Celle St. Cloud, France.

Macrofilaricides

The only macrofilaricides currently available to bring about a radical cure of onchocerciasis are suramin, a potentially toxic compound given by weekly intravenous injections over several weeks; and amocarzine, an oral preparation which has proved fairly effective at near-toxic doses in Latin America but not in Africa. As long as ivermectin remains available and effective there will be very few individual patients who are in need of these somewhat heroic radical cures (see OTM3, pp. 916–17).

Nodulectomy

Head nodules, especially common in Mexico and Guatemala, should always be removed as early as possible. Other nodules may be removed if they are a nuisance to the patient. Nodulectomy is done under local anaesthesia (2 per cent lignocaine), preferably without adrenaline, and making sure that all bleeding points are ligated.

Prophylaxis

There is no practically effective chemoprophylactic for *O. volvulus* infection. Personal exposure to *Simulium* can be reduced by wearing clothing that protects those body areas which are most exposed to their bites, i.e. long trousers, stockings and closed footwear help against *S. damnosum* s.l., *S. neavei* s.l., *S. metallicum* and some other South American vectors; long-sleeved shirts, and a hat and veil help against *S. ochraceum*.

Loiasis

Geographical distribution and vectors

Loiasis is caused by *Loa loa*, whose transmission is confined to the West African forest block east of the Dahomey (Benin) gap, and to the Central African equatorial forest block and its fringes. Infections are common in southern Nigeria, Cameroon, Gabon, Equatorial Guinea, Congo, and Zaire; they occur less frequently in southern Chad, Central African Republic, Sudan, Uganda, and Angola. *L. loa* is spread by tabanid flies of the genus *Chrysops*, known as 'red flies'.

Lifecycle of the parasite and pathology

Development of the adult worms takes about 5 months. The males (3–4 cm × 0.35 mm) and females (5–7 cm × 0.5 mm) are freely motile in the subcutaneous tissue and along the fascial planes, and live for up to 15 years. They cause the Calabar swellings that are characteristic of loiasis and occasionally one may traverse the bulbar conjunctiva. The sheathed microfilariae (225–300 μm × 10 μm) show a diurnal periodicity in the blood. They live for about a year and are non-pathogenic except when present in high densities (>10 000 microfilariae/ml) during treatment (see below).

Clinical picture

Infective *Chrysops* bites may cause severe swelling and itching. The L_3 of *L. loa* are 2 mm long and there may be 100–200 in a single fly. Small discrete papules develop in the skin in association with the L_3 or L_4 as they move away from the site of entry over the ensuing 1–4 weeks. Adult worms moving under the skin may cause prickling and itching sensations; those moving deeper in the fascial planes cause shifting aches and pains, and paraesthesiae. Allergic, oedematous, subcutaneous Calabar, or 'fugitive' swellings, 5–10 cm or more in diameter, may develop anywhere but are common on the back of the hand or on the arm. They last from some hours to several days and are often brought on by local muscular activity. The overlying skin is red, hot, and painful, resembling cellulitis; and it may itch.

An adult worm may also cross the conjunctiva (Fig. 6), becoming visible for a matter of 5–30 min, during which it may be removed by prompt surgical intervention under local conjunctival anaesthesia. Its passage is accompanied by allergic swelling of the conjunctiva, eyelids, and periorbital tissues.

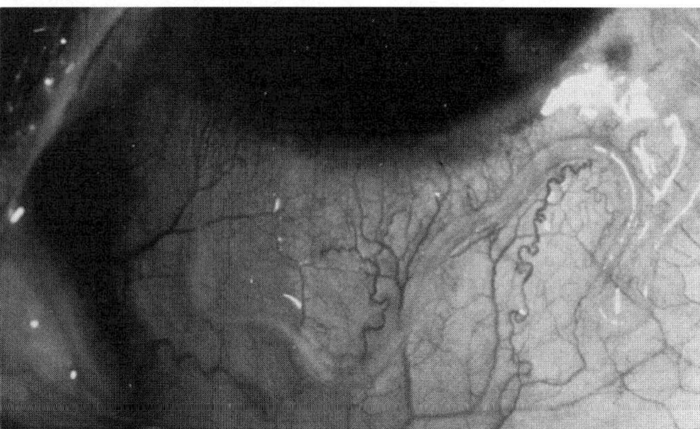

Fig. 6 Adult *L. loa* crossing the bulbar conjunctiva *(photograph by Dr J. Anderson).*

Lightly and recently infected persons may suffer most from Calabar swellings and seek treatment. The swellings may cause a significant loss of working time in labour forces (e.g. on rubber plantations) in endemic areas and this is a good reason for treatment. Persons with infections of long standing who are asymptomatic are probably best left untreated. An association between loiasis and endomyocardial fibrosis has been remarked, possibly attributable to the high eosinophilia.

Diagnosis

The diagnosis is made on the Calabar swellings, which have to be distinguished from insect bites and stings, and septic cellulitis. Eosinophilia (up to 10 000/mm^3) is almost invariable. Finding the microfilariae in day blood, or sight of an adult worm are diagnostic, but in many patients with Calabar swellings no microfilariae can be found.

Treatment

DEC kills the microfilariae, the L_3 and L_4 stages, and a good proportion of the adult worms of *L. loa*. Courses of 7 days duration, at 2 mg/kg three times daily and repeated at intervals of a month, are usually effective, but some adult worms may remain resistant to the drug. Dying adult worms may become visible under the skin.

The dangers of DEC treatment in patients infected with *L. loa* are two. First, many such patients may also harbour infections with *O. volvulus*, which can give rise to severe Mazzotti reactions when DEC is used. Second, especially in patients with a daytime *L. loa* microfilaraemia of >10 000 microfilariae/ml, there is always some risk that the sudden destruction of microfilariae under DEC may, in addition to producing a febrile reaction, give rise to capillary blockage by dead and dying microfilariae in the brain, meninges, and retina (leading to an encephalitic syndrome, which can be fatal). If there is coincident infection with *O. volvulus*, and the *L. loa* microfilaraemia is not dangerously high, the patient should be treated first with ivermectin (150 μg/kg Mectizan[R]) to eliminate the microfilariae of the former species, but it must be remembered that ivermectin itself can induce a *Loa* encephalopathy in a patient with high microfilaraemia. In patients with high *Loa* microfilaraemia (>10 000 microfilariae/ml in peripheral day blood) the risk of capillary blockage in the central nervous system must be taken very seriously, with hospital treatment rapidly accessible. In extreme cases cytophoresis has been used to extract most of the microfilariae from the patient's blood before giving DEC (or possibly ivermectin) at low doses cautiously and under steroid cover. Alternatively, mebendazole (100–500 mg three times a day continued for 4–6 weeks) may gradually reduce the microfilaraemia without complications. Although this drug does not kill adult *Loa*, it may make it safe to use DEC later on for this purpose.

Prophylaxis

DEC has a chemoprophylactic action against *L. loa*. For an adult, a course of 200 mg twice daily for 3 consecutive days once each month will probably kill all infective larvae and immature worms inoculated during the previous month. Prophylaxis may also be achieved by taking 300 mg DEC once a week during periods of exposure. Prevention of *Chrysops* bites depends in large measure on wearing long trousers, fly-screening of houses, and clearance of the forest around dwelling places.

Other filarial infections

Streptocerciasis

Mansonella streptocerca, causing streptocerciasis, occurs in the more humid parts of Ghana, Togo, Nigeria, Cameroon, Gabon, Congo, Equatorial Guinea, and Zaire. Transmission is by *Culicoides* (especially *C. grahamii*), commonly but erroneously known as 'sandflies'.

The adult worms and microfilariae are found in the skin, mainly on the torso. Diagnosis is by finding the characteristic crook-tailed microfilariae in skin snips. Infections are usually asymptomatic but sometimes give rise to a chronic itching rash composed of very small urticarial papules, not unlike that of onchocerciasis. Hypopigmented macules, probably associated with the adult worms which lie very near the surface, may be seen in dark-skinned patients and these may often be taken for early tuberculoid leprosy. The differential diagnosis can only be made by biopsy and it is always possible that both infectious agents may occur together.

DEC at 2 mg/kg three times daily for 7–10 days should suffice to kill both microfilariae and adult worms, without undue reaction.

Mansonella perstans filariasis

Mansonella perstans is common and widespread in tropical Africa south of the Sahara, in parts of South America and in Algeria, Tunisia, and New Guinea. Transmission is by *Culicoides* spp. The adult worms live in serous cavities, in the mesentery and retroperitoneal tissues. The microfilariae are found in the blood and they are non-periodic. High proportions of persons living in endemic areas are infected. *M. perstans* may produce an eosinophilia but is generally considered to be non-pathogenic. Normally no treatment is necessary.

Mansonelliasis *ozzardi*

Mansonella ozzardi is confined to South and Central America and the West Indies. Transmission is by *Simulium* spp. in South America and by *Culicoides* in the Caribbean. The microfilariae occur in the blood and are non-periodic. In the West Indies infections are considered to be non-pathogenic. In the Amazon region, joint pains, fever, lymphadenopathy, and headache have been attributed to this parasite. Treatment with DEC is variously reported as being ineffective against the parasite but effective in reducing the allegedly associated symptoms.

Dirofilariasis

Infections with *Dirofilaria immitis*, the dog heart-worm, with *D. repens* (from dogs or cats), or with *D. tenuis* or *D. ursi* (from the racoon and bear, respectively) are occasionally transmitted by their mosquito vectors to humans. Case reports come from the USA, Japan, Australia, Europe, Africa, Asia, and South America. In humans, *D. immitis* never reaches maturity and the immature worm usually ends up in the lung giving rise to infarction vasculitis and the formation of a granuloma. This may be discovered as a 'silent' coin lesion on chest radiograph, or it may be associated with chest pain, cough, haemoptysis, and fever. There is no certain way to make a prospective diagnosis, for there is never any microfilaraemia and immunological tests cannot be taken as conclusive. Hence the differential diagnosis from bronchial carcinoma, secondary neoplasms, or systemic fungal infections in the lung can only be made with certainty after removal (by lobectomy) and histopathological examination. *D. tenuis*, *D. repens*, and *D. ursi* can give rise to a subcutaneous granuloma anywhere in the body or under the conjunctiva. Surgical removal is the only treatment and subsequent histopathological examination makes the diagnosis.

Further reading

Onchocerciasis

World Health Organization (1974). *Onchocerciasis—symptomatology, pathology, diagnosis* (ed. A.A. Buck), pp. 1–80. WHO, Geneva.

World Health Organization (1995). *Onchocerciasis and its control. Report of a WHO Expert Committee on Onchocerciasis Control*, pp. 1–103. WHO Technical Report Series 852. WHO, Geneva.

Loiasis

Chippaux, J-P., *et al.* (1996). Severe adverse reaction risks during mass treatment with ivermectin in loiasis-endemic areas. *Parasitology Today*, 12, 448–50.

Editorial (1986). *Loa loa*—a pathogenic parasite. *Lancet*, **ii**, 554.

Chapter 16.97

Lymphatic filariasis*

B. O. L. Duke

Global dimensions, geographical distribution, and vectors

Lymphatic filariasis is a chronic disease, widespread in the tropics and subtropics. Over 1.1 billion people live at risk of infection and some 120 million in 73 African, Middle Eastern, South and South-east Asian, Pacific, Latin American, and Caribbean countries are currently infected (107 million with *Wuchereria bancrofti* and 13 million with *Brugia malayi* or *B. timori*). Nearly all suffer variously from lymphoedema or elephantiasis of limbs, genitals or breasts, or

*Contains material from OTM3, pp. 919–24 (B. A. Southgate).

from hydroceles and infections in damaged lymphatics; 43 million have overt chronic physical disabilities as a result.

The vectors of *W. bancrofti* are mosquitoes of the genera *Culex*, *Anopheles* (both night biters), and *Aedes* (day and night biters). The urban or semi-urban *C. quinquefasciatus*, which breeds in sullage water, drains, and cess-pits, etc., accounts for 70 per cent of infections in most regions except the Pacific. In rural surroundings *Anopheles* transmission is more common. *Aedes* mosquitoes, which are small container breeders, are the main vectors in the Pacific and some other islands.

The vectors of nocturnally subperiodic *B. malayi*, originally a rural zoonosis with monkeys and domestic cats as reservoir hosts in Malaysia, Indonesia, and Thailand, are *Mansonia* mosquitoes, whose larvae attach to the roots of water plants. In other areas, notably India (Kerala), this parasite is a nocturnally periodic anthroponosis and the main vectors are *Anopheles*. *B. timori*, localized to a few Indonesian islands, is transmitted by *An. barbirostris*.

Lifecycle of the parasites and pathology

Adult worms are smooth, thread-like, and creamy-white (males, 40 mm × 0.1 mm; females, 80–100 mm × 0.25–0.30 mm). They live in lymphatic vessels and nodes and their life-span is 2–5 years. The microfilariae (mfs), living for up to 12 months, are sheathed (180–290 µm × 7.5–10.0 µm) and blood-dwelling. In stained films they die in graceful curves, and have round nuclei, whose arrangement in the tail is specifically diagnostic. According to the geographical strain, their periodicity may be nocturnal, nocturnally subperiodic, or diurnally subperiodic. The microfilariae develop in the thoracic muscles of compatible mosquito vectors and the infective larvae (L3s) inoculated into humans mature in the lymphatics within 3 or, more usually, 8–24 months.

Pathological damage to the lymphatic vessels results from the effects of the adult worms and their excretory/secretory products, coupled with the immune response of the human host to these antigens and the effects of associated bacterial and fungal superinfections. The microfilariae play no part in lymphatic pathology but are responsible for tropical pulmonary eosinophilia.

Clinical manifestations of lymphatic filariasis

Clinical manifestations vary with the species and strain of parasite, with the area and intensity of transmission, with the age of first exposure (which may be *in utero*), and with the sex and immunological response of the infected person.

'Asymptomatic' amicrofilaraemia and microfilaraemia

Some people living exposed to infection in endemic areas show no microfilaraemia that is detectable by standard methods and they have no obvious clinical disease; yet they can be shown to be infected by means of new, highly-sensitive, diagnostic tests. Other similar people may have patent microfilaraemia but yet appear to be 'asymptomatic'. Although the 'asymptomatic' state may result from a downregulation of their immune–inflammatory response to the parasites, it has recently been recognized that these people have some degree of haematuria and/or proteinuria, reflecting a low-grade renal damage; and lymphoscintography shows dilated lymphatics and abnormal lymph flow. As these changes are reversible by antifilarial chemotherapy, such people are at risk of overt disease and should be treated accordingly.

Acute lymphatic filariasis

In immigrants to endemic areas the clinical incubation period can be as short as 2 months for *B. malayi* and just under 4 months for *W. bancrofti*. In brugian infections, the predominant lesions are lymphadenitis and lymphangitis of the legs; whereas, in bancroftian disease, lesions of the male genitalia predominate.

Filarial fever

This syndrome in known infected persons is well recognized by local inhabitants. It consists of recurrent episodes of fever with chills, rigors, and sweating, accompanied by headache, bone and joint pains, general malaise, anorexia, vomiting, and even delirium. Often typical signs of acute filariasis will supervene during the attack. Some episodes may be due to secondary bacterial (usually streptococcal) infection and respond rapidly to antibiotics, while others are relieved by microfilaricidal therapy. Attacks last 3–7 days, may recur at irregular intervals over many years, and can persist long after the patient has left an endemic area.

Filarial lymphadenitis, lymphangitis, and abscess of the limbs

Attacks may occur from once a year to almost once a week. The onset is abrupt, often precipitated by physical activity and accompanied by filarial fever. The inflammation may affect the inguinal, femoral, popliteal, axillary, or epitrochlear lymph nodes and is sometimes followed by painful retrograde lymphangitis. An abscess in the node may suppurate to form an ulcer. There is oedema in the limb during the attack and, if acute episodes recur, this may pass gradually into chronic lymphatic obstruction.

Filarial funiculitis, epididymitis, and orchitis

Recurrent attacks of retrograde lymphangitis of the spermatic cord, extending from the inguinal ring down the inguinal canal into the scrotum, are known as 'endemic funiculitis' and are characteristic of bancroftian filariasis. There is acute pain and fever, often proceeding to an acute epididymo-orchitis with scrotal oedema and fluid in the tunica vaginalis. The attacks may lead to chronic disease.

Chronic lymphatic filariasis

Chronic disease usually appears 10–20 years after first exposure. It is progressive and cumulative and only rarely resolves without treatment. In tissues whose lymphatic drainage has been compromised by damage from filarial infection, repeated bacterial and fungal superinfections initiate repeated episodes of adenolymphangitis, which further damage the lymph vessels and lead to increasing lymphoedema and later elephantiasis of the affected parts. The features of chronic bancroftian filariasis are hydrocele; lymphoedema and elephantiasis of (in order of decreasing frequency) the legs, scrotum, arms, penis, breasts, and vulva; and chyluria. In brugian filariasis, lymphoedema and elephantiasis are mainly in the legs below the knee, or less commonly in the arm below the elbow. Genital involvement and chyluria do not occur.

Hydrocele

Filarial hydroceles, found exclusively in bancroftian filariasis, are fluid swellings of the tunica vaginalis which may contain microfilariae. Seldom painful, they follow repeated attacks of funiculitis. Unilateral at first, they may soon become bilateral.

Lymphoedema and elephantiasis

The most common site is the leg. The onset is most frequently around the ankles, spreading to the dorsum of the foot, calf, and thigh. Lymphoedema is transient, soft and pitting at first, and responds well to rest and elevation of the leg (grade I). Pitting oedema soon becomes brawny oedema and the swelling is then hard and permanent (grade II) (Plate 1); subcutaneous thickening, hyperkeratosis and fissuring of skin then occur, accompanied by nodular, warty, papillomatous changes (elephantiasis), especially in the feet (grade III).

Chyluria and lymphuria

The rupture of abdominal lymphatic varices into the renal pelvis or bladder gives rise to chyluria when the lymphatic vessel is draining the intestine, or to lymphuria when it is not. Chylous urine is opaque and milky due to suspended fat globules, whereas lymphuria has a normal appearance.

Tropical pulmonary eosinophilia (**TPE**) (see also Chapter 4.24)

TPE is an 'occult' form of lymphatic filariasis, most often seen in South-east Asia. It is rare even in endemic areas and is caused by the rapid destruction of microfilariae as soon as they are produced. There is a persistent, paroxysmal night cough, with wheezing and dyspnoea; hypereosinophilia (absolute counts from 3000 to 50 000/mm^3 of blood); reduction in vital capacity; radiographic signs of diffuse miliary lesions and enhanced bronchovascular markings; high titres of filarial antibodies; and low-grade fever. Untreated, it can progress to chronic pulmonary fibrosis and emphysema.

Diagnosis

Clinical diagnosis depends on careful history taking and a full clinical examination, coupled with the finding of the typical microfilariae in stained blood films (50–100 µl) or on membrane filters (1–5 ml) taken at times of peak periodicity. Recently developed, specific, high-sensitivity tests include a monoclonal antibody assay to detect circulating protein antigens of *W. bancrofti*, and a polymerase chain reaction test to detect parasite DNA of both *W. bancrofti* and *B. malayi*.

Ultrasound techniques allow imaging of the adult worms of *W. bancrofti* to be visualized in the lymphatics, where viability can be confirmed by their movements, known as the 'filarial dance' sign. Using radiolabelled albumin or dextran, lymphoscintigraphy allows monitoring of damaged lymphatics during treatment.

The differential diagnosis in the acute stage is from infective adenolymphangitis; in the chronic stage from mycetoma (Madura foot) and podoconiosis.

Treatment

Chemotherapy

The drugs used against the lymphatic filarial parasites are: diethylcarbamazine citrate (**DEC**), a microfilaricide which also kills a proportion of the adult worms; ivermectin and albendazole, both of which are purely microfilaricidal. The principles of treatment, whether this is mass treatment aimed at controlling transmission in endemic areas or individual treatment, are: to use one or more of these drugs at intervals to eliminate microfilaraemia; to use DEC where possible to kill a proportion of the adult worms; and to control morbidity by measures of simple hygiene, supplemented, where necessary, by more drastic surgical procedures.

DEC can safely be used in patients from all endemic areas except those in sub-Saharan Africa, in whom the possible presence of coincident infections with *Onchocerca volvulus* or *Loa loa* render it liable to cause dangerous reactions. The previously recommended 12-day courses have recently been shown to be no more effective than single doses at 6 mg/kg , which may be repeated at intervals of 3, 6, or (in mass campaigns) 12 months. These regimens have the added advantage that they will kill some, but not all, of the adult worms. Where the domestic salt market can be controlled, DEC-fortified salt (0.2–0.4 per cent w/w) used for cooking and seasoning food over a period of 9–12 months provides a cheap, effective, and safe means of eliminating lymphatic filariasis from a population. DEC is also the correct treatment for TPE.

Ivermectin (Mectizan ®), is an effective microfilaricide that may soon be registered for treatment of lymphatic filariasis. Co-administered with DEC (i.e. 200 µg/kg ivermectin plus 6 mg/kg DEC given annually) it is likely to become the preferred mass treatment in South-east Asia, the Pacific, and the Middle East; whereas in sub-Saharan Africa, it should be replaced by ivermectin co-administered with albendazole (i.e. 200 µg/kg ivermectin plus 400 mg albendazole annually). For individual treatment, these doses may be given at more frequent intervals of 3 or 6 months, if desired, especially where DEC can be used.

Morbidity control

Clinical, immunohistological, and bacteriological evidence has shown that bacterial and fungal superinfections are responsible for most attacks of adenolymphangitis in tissues with compromised lymphatic function, and that these in turn can lead to worsening lymphoedema and eventually elephantiasis. Provided they are kept free of infection, secondary collateral lymph channels can serve to re-establish lymph flow in tissues damaged by repeated filarial infections and, to this end, simple measures of hygiene can have a profound beneficial effect on early lymphoedema. Among them are: twice daily washing of the affected parts with soap and water; raising the limb at night; regularly working the foot up and down to promote lymph flow; keeping the nails clean; wearing shoes; and the use of antiseptic or antibiotic creams to treat small wounds or abrasions. In more advanced or resistant cases, a lymphovenous shunt operation may be necessary, followed by excision of excess tissue. Hydroceles should be drained or treated surgically. Chyluria requires surgical treatment.

Prophylaxis and prevention

The possible prophylactic action of DEC in lymphatic filariasis has never been thoroughly investigated. Biting by infected mosquitoes can be reduced by the use of bed-nets (preferably insecticide impregnated) or protective clothing. Mosquito vector control schemes can be valuable supplements to chemotherapeutic control programmes, but their details vary from species to species and are beyond the scope of this article.

Further reading

Ottesen, E.A., *et al.* (1997). Strategies and tools for the control/elimination of lymphatic filariasis. *Bulletin of the World Health Organization*, 75(6): 491–503.

World Health Organization (1992). *Lymphatic filariasis: the disease and its control. Fifth report of the WHO Expert Committee on Filariasis*, World Health Organization Technical Report Series No. 821, pp. 8–13 and 42–53. WHO, Geneva.

Chapter 16.98

Guinea-worm disease: human dracunculiasis

M. M. Kliks

Dracunculus medinensis, the agent of dracunculiasis, is the largest nematode to infect humans.

Geographical distribution

During 1996, in India, Yemen and the remaining endemic countries (Fig. 1) perhaps 200 000 cases occurred, most of them in Sudan. Elsewhere, the disease is rare, usually occurring in immigrant workers, students, or tourists coming from endemic areas.

Infection occurs only in people who drink from unprotected ground-water sources contaminated with infective larvae contained in the copepod vector. It is not known in casual visitors, tourists, or even long-term expatriate residents of endemic regions who generally live in urban areas with piped water-supply systems. However, 'eco-tourism' may bring outsiders deep into the endemic areas, where some of the most 'primitive' places on earth are to be found.

Life history of the parasite and epidemiology

Copepod crustaceans, 0.5–1.5 mm long, containing infective third-stage larvae of *D. medinensis* are ingested in drinking water.

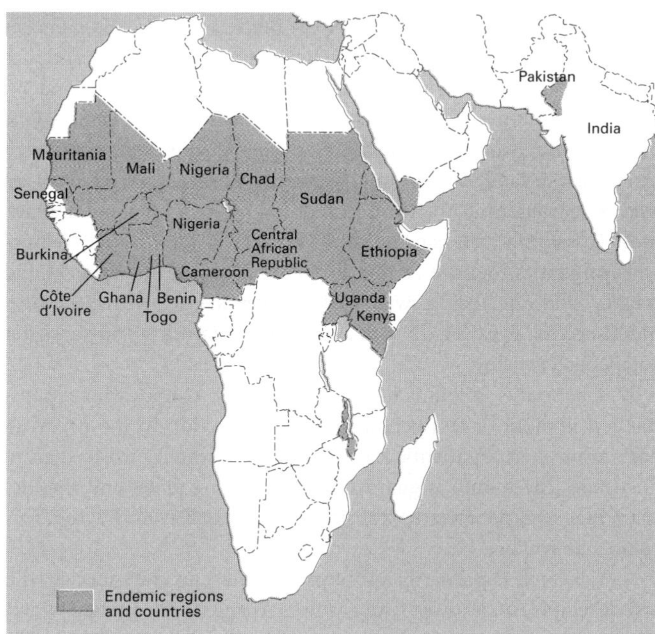

Fig. 1 Geographical distribution of dracunculiasis in 1996.

Immature worms migrate to the body cavities where they mature and mate. Between 9 and 14 months later gravid females, 70–120 cm long, migrate within the subcutaneous connective tissues, usually reaching the extremities. The female releases a chemical that induces the formation of a blister adjacent to her vulva (Fig. 2). The worm protrudes through the ulcer and releases rhabditiform larvae, particularly when stimulated by immersion of the lesion into water, as when the patient enters a pond to fetch drinking water. Larvae are actively ingested by copepods and become infective in about 2 weeks. Acute symptoms develop and the next year's infections are transmitted about the time of the rains and planting. There is evidence of both partial and complete immunity to dracunculiasis (see OTM3, p. 926).

Clinical picture

Gravid worms usually emerge on the extremities (Fig. 2), but also from the scrotum, nipple, sublingual gland, and vulva. Often the worm is not visible, having been broken during extraction and/or having retracted into the lesion, or disintegrated. Ingested larvae may lodge in joints, the orbit, or central or peripheral nervous systems, leading to severe arthritic changes, blindness, or septic subdural abscess. Uncomplicated cases with emergent worms resolve in 2–3 weeks, but most victims are incapacitated for at least 6 weeks. The destruction of worms in host tissues provokes delayed hypersensitivity with massive swelling and exquisite pain. Bacterial infection with cellulitis, abscess formation, and even gangrene and tetanus may occur and chronic inflammation leads to ankylosis and permanent disability. The case fatality rate is approximately 1 per cent.

Diagnosis

Characteristic lesions with or without the female worm in those who have lived or travelled in an endemic country suggests dracunculiasis. Even when adult worms are not visible a saline preparation of the exudate may reveal active larvae. Serodiagnostic methods have been developed to detect prepatent and cryptic infections.

Treatment and patient management

No effective, specific anthelminthic agent has been identified. Clinical management of prepatent, acute, and chronic cases involves surgical and manual extraction, use of appropriate anti-inflammatory, analgesic, and antimicrobial drugs, and supportive nursing care aimed at prevention or elimination of secondary infections, reduction of abscesses, and rehabilitation of effected limbs. However, in the remote, economically deprived villages where guinea worm is a severe social problem, traditional methods of applying poultices made of leaves, charcoal, and mud, and attempts at manual extraction often lead to an exacerbation of symptoms. Under these unhygienic conditions, soaking or applying hot, moist compresses at the affected site and gentle massage toward the opening can promote drainage of the abscess and facilitate removal of worms using light traction. Between treatments the lesions should be carefully bandaged to prevent infection and escape of infective larvae should the patient enter a drinking-water source.

Emerging worms should be removed by making a small incision adjacent to the worm near its mid-point, lifting out a loop of the

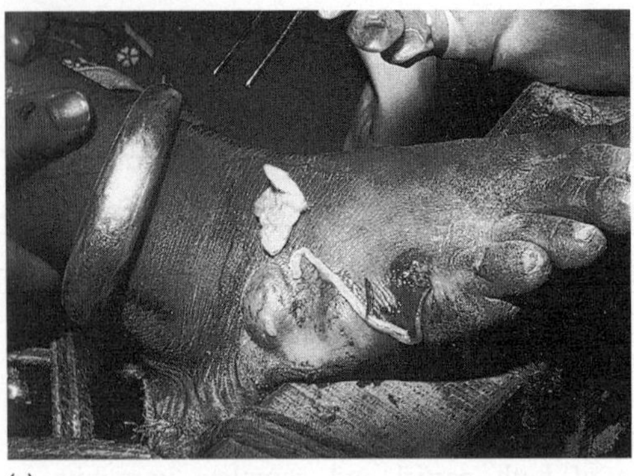
(a)

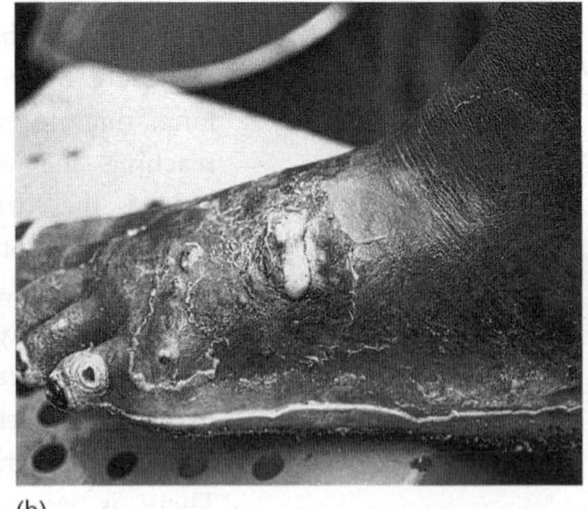
(b)

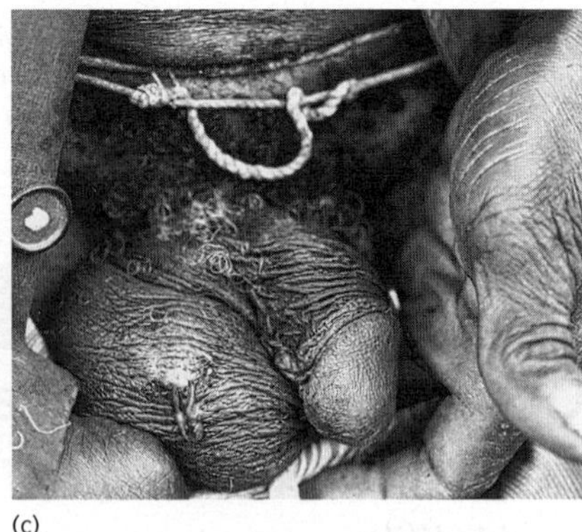
(c)

Fig. 2 Acute inflammation, two blisters; right one opened to reveal intact adult guinea-worm and ulcer beneath; left one spontaneously exuding fluid containing first-stage larvae. After hot water soaking both worms were removed with gentle traction and massage. Rajasthan, India.
(Photograph by M. M. Kliks, CTS Foundation.)

worm using a blunt curved probe, and applying gentle traction to it while firmly massaging the affected limb along the tract of the worm toward the opening. Should the worm rupture, or should it be necessary to ligate it before complete removal, care must be taken to prevent its body fluids from coming into contact with the patient's tissues.

Prophylaxis, prevention, and control

Personal prophylaxis is by avoiding contaminated drinking water or by brief boiling or filtering through cloth to retain copepods (see OTM3, p. 927).

The global eradication effort

Since the mid-1980s, national programmes for the control and eradication of Guinea-worm disease have been developed in almost all endemic countries. The WHO has reported a total of 77 771 cases during 1997, down 49 per cent form the 152 805 cases in 1996: a remarkable reduction from the estimated 5–10 million cases believed to have occurred annually a decade ago. Pakistan and India have both eliminated the disease in humans and significant progress toward control has been made in several of the less heavily affected states of West and East Africa. However, civil disturbances and socio-economic instability have contributed to setbacks in Sudan (43 544), Nigeria (12 590 cases), Ghana (8921 cases): these countries accounted for about 80 per cent of all cases in 1997. For details see OTM3, p. 927.

Further reading

Hopkins, D.R., Ruiz-Tiben, E.T., and Ruebush, T.K. (1997). Dracunculiasis eradication: almost a reality. *American Journal of Tropical Medicine and Hygiene*, 57, 252–9.

Rhode, J.E., Sharma, B.L., Patton, H., Deggan, C., and Sherry, J.M. (1993). Surgical extraction of Guinea worm: disability reduction and contribution to disease control. *American Journal of Tropical Medicine and Hygiene*, **48**, 71–6.

World Health Organization Collaborating Center for Research, Training and Eradication of Dracunculiasis, 1997. (1998). *Guinea worm wrap-up* 78, May 11, 1998. NCID, Centers for Disease Control and Prevention, Atlanta, Georgia, USA.

Chapter 16.99

Ancylostomiasis, strongyloidiasis, and other gut strongyloid nematodes

R. Knight

Ancylostomiasis (hookworm infection)

Biology and epidemiology

Most infections by adult worms are due to *Ancyostoma duodenale* (Plate 1) and *Necator americanus*. Several other carnivore species accidentally infect human beings by the percutaneous route and produce zoonotic cutaneous larva migrans. Adult worms measure 8–13 mm in length; they attach themselves to the wall of the jejunum by drawing mucosa into the buccal cavity (Fig. 1); a vigorous pharyngeal pump enables blood and tissue fluids to be ingested. Females produce 5000–20 000 eggs per day, but output per worm declines as worm load rises. In the soil, development is temperature dependent. Under optimum conditions eggs hatch within 2 days and larvae develop with two moults to the non-feeding infective stage which can persist in sandy soil for up to a month. The first two larval stages feed on bacteria, but the third penetrate host skin after soil contact, most commonly between the toes. After entry into dermal venules and lymphatics they are carried to the lung, ascend the bronchi and trachea, and after being swallowed re-enter the gut where the final moult occurs. Eggs (Fig. 2) can appear in the faeces 50–60 days after cutaneous exposure.

N. americanus is found in the warm, moist tropics where transmission is more or less perennial. Its introduction to the Americas dates from the transatlantic slave trade. It is a smaller worm than *A. duodenale*, the mouth is guarded by two cutting plates and the lifespan may exceed 5 years; transmission is exclusively by the percutaneous route.

A. duodenale is primarily a subtropical and temperate species with soil development at lower temperatures. Formerly it occurred widely in southern Europe; it was responsible for 'miner's anaemia'. The mouth is guarded by two pairs of sharp teeth and the worms live for

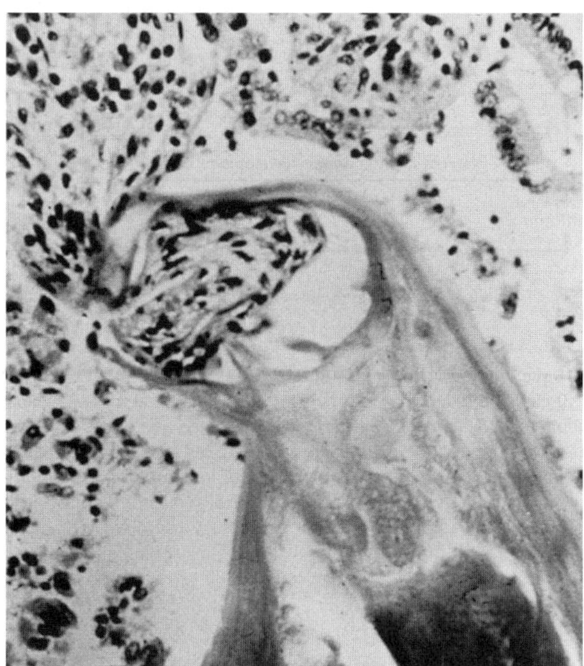

Fig. 1 Adult worm of *N. americanus* showing relationship of its pharynx to a jejunal villus.

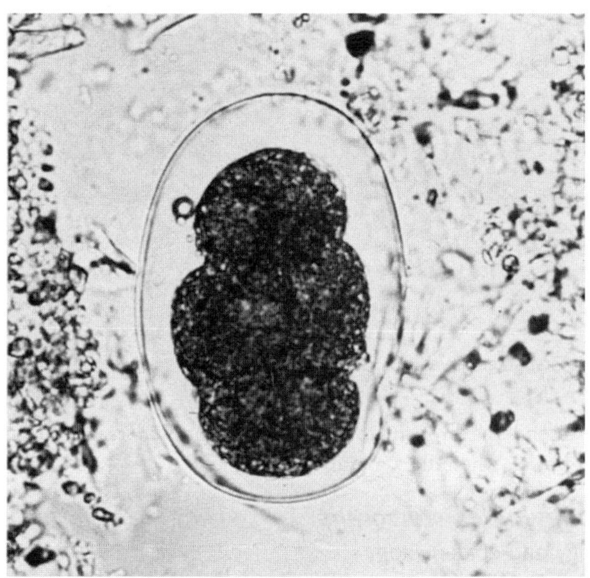

Fig. 2 Egg of *N. americanus*.

about 1 year. Infection is usually by the percutaneous route, but when contaminated vegetables are ingested larvae can penetrate the buccal mucosa or develop directly within the gut mucosa. Infection may also be transplacental; in China severe hookworm disease is reported in very young infants. Another feature of the life cycle is arrested larval development within skeletal muscle or the gut mucosa; this postpones patency and is an adaptive mechanism to irregular or seasonal transmission.

The prevalence of hookworm in the tropics is commonly 20–50 per cent, with higher figures in rural agricultural communities. Aridity and coolness at higher altitudes limit transmission, but irrigation schemes usually favour it by raising the water table. Prevalence of infection and the worm load both rise with age to reach a plateau in adults. Children commonly acquire clinically significant infections between the ages of 5 and 10 years. Within communities, individuals differ greatly in worm load.

Pathology

Hookworms damage the mucosa mechanically and by the inflammatory response they evoke; bleeding continues at former attachment sites. Gut motility is affected, especially in primary infections and in children, and this may affect digestive and absorptive function. *A. duodenale* ingests about 0.15 ml of blood daily, and *N. americanus* 0.05 ml. Because worm loads are commonly above 50, and may reach 500 or more, the cumulative effect can be serious. Children, and pregnant or lactating women, with little reserve iron, can become anaemic in a few months; in a previously healthy adult male it can take 2 years or more. Loss of albumin into the gut may exceed the capacity of the liver to replace it. Hypoalbuminaemia has important haemodynamic consequences because it limits the normal, compensatory expansion of plasma volume that occurs in chronic anaemia. While the risk of pulmonary oedema is less, transition to a state of low cardiac output is made more likely.

Clinical features attributable to adult worms

In acute primary infections and in children, epigastric pain is common and sometimes diarrhoea. Anorexia leads to nutritional deficit. A few patients develop overt gut bleeding, and melaena is reported in transplacentally infected infants in China.

Most patients present with iron-deficiency anaemia; such patients typically have no gut symptoms. Exertional dyspnoea may begin at haemoglobin levels of 8 g/dl, but may not be noted until it falls to 5 g/dl. Palpitations, weakness, and faintness on exertion are common. Some patients have precordial pain, leg claudication or tinnitus, a few are aware of their own jugular vascular bruit. A puffy oedema of the face, arms, and hands is typical, and often unaccompanied by dependent oedema. In severe cases, mental apathy and depression are common, and in adults, amenorrhoea or impotence. Pica is common, especially in pregnancy, and geophagy can lead to acquisition of other soil-transmitted nematodes. Milder degrees of anaemia cause reduced physical work performance in adults. In children, growth and development may be slowed and cognitive impairment can lead to reduced scholastic achievement.

Clinical features attributable to larval worms: cutaneous larval migrans

Wheezy cough due to pneumonitis is more common with *A. duodenale*, especially heavy primary infections; symptoms can continue for many months after one exposure, owing to remobilization of larvae arrested in muscle. Cutaneous lesions take the form of migrating, itchy, red, serpiginous papules, known as creeping eruption or cutaneous larva migrans. They commonly become vesiculated and excoriated, and this leads to bacterial pyoderma. *A. duodenale* or *N. americanus* cause the condition known as 'ground itch'; prominent lesions occur in laboratory infections. Zoonotic infections with the dog hookworms *A. braziliense* and *A. caninum* produce more vigorous lesions that may continue to move for several months, they are most common on the lower legs and buttocks, but also occur on the arms and face. Infections occur on sandy bathing beaches, in children's play areas, and by contact with pet sandboxes.

Diagnosis

Stool microscopy will reveal eggs (Fig. 2), except in patients with prepatent infections; examination of stool concentrates is rarely necessary. It is useful to estimate the faecal egg count as this provides some measure of the intensity of infection; with either species, 1000 eggs per gram is equivalent to 2.2 ml of blood loss per day. Culture to the infective larval stage, using the Harada Mori technique, will differentiate the two major species and the other genera of gut strongyloid nematodes.

Treatment

Safe and effective anthelminthics are now available. A single 400-mg dose of albendazole, or mebendazole, 100 mg twice daily for 3 days, are both very effective. Alternatives are pyrantel, 10 mg/kg daily for three or four doses, or bephenium, 5 g daily for three doses, the latter being less effective for *N. americanus.* Chemotherapy should generally be avoided in pregnancy. To replace iron reserves, oral ferrous sulphate will suffice in most patients, but several weeks of medication may be necessary. When compliance is doubted, consideration should be given to intramuscular iron or total-dose intravenous infusion of iron dextran. Transfusion of red cells may be necessary in pregnancy, and when cardiac output is compromised. Frusemide may be necessary to cover the transfusion, but in other circumstances diuretics should be used with caution. Depletion of plasma volume in hookworm anaemia patients with hypoalbuminaemia can compromise cardiac output.

Cutaneous lesions should be treated with thiabendazole, 25 mg/kg in two divided doses, for 2 days, and, if necessary, after 2 days' rest, a further 5 days at the same dose. A single dose of ivermectin, 200 μg/kg is more effective than a single dose of 400 mg of albendazole. Topical treatment avoids systemic side-effects. One 0.5 g tablet of thiabendazole can be ground up with 5 g of petroleum jelly and applied over the worm tracts daily for 5 days. Alternatively, the thiabendazole can be made up in a dimethylsulphoxide base.

Control

Population-based measures are necessary when endemicity and morbidity are high. Latrines are generally beneficial, but can create foci for transmission when the water table is high. Provision of piped water and protective footwear reduces contact with soil. Where human excreta is used as fertilizer, composting and chemical ovicides are needed. Anthelminthic drugs can be deployed in several ways (see OTM3, p. 932).

Strongyloidiasis

The parasitic female worms of the genus *Strongyloides* are parthenogenic. They measure 2–2.5 mm in length and normally live in tunnels between the enterocytes of the crypts of Lieberkühn in the duodenum and jejunum. In the external environment larvae may develop directly, through two moults, into infective larvae, in a manner similar to that of hookworm (Fig. 3). Or alternatively, by the indirect cycle, into free-living male and female adult worms, about 1 mm in length, that produce a second generation of infective larvae. In either case the cycle is completed when infective larvae penetrate the skin and are carried in the venous circulation to the lungs, whence they ascend the bronchi to be swallowed and so reach the upper small bowel, where they mature.

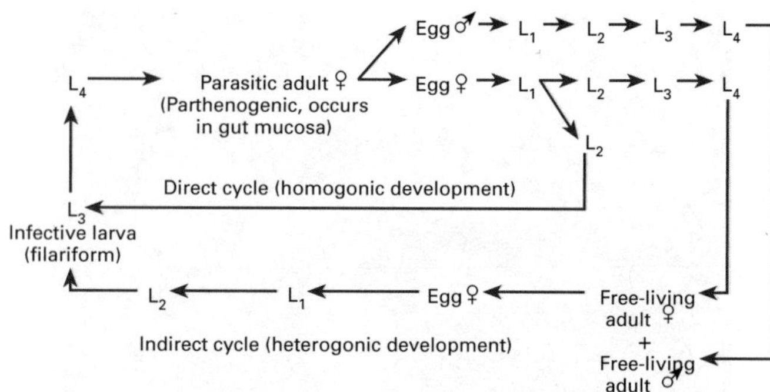

Fig. 3 Basic lifecycle in the genus *Strongyloides*; L_1, L_2, L_3, and L_4 are the larval stages. The indirect cycle occurs in the soil or faecal mass. Eggs of the parasitic female *S. stercoralis* hatch in the gut lumen and direct development may occur not only in the external environment but also on the perianal skin to produce external autoinfection, or in the gut lumen to produce internal autoinfection. The eggs of the parasitic female *S. fuelleborni* appear in the faeces and internal autoinfection is not possible.

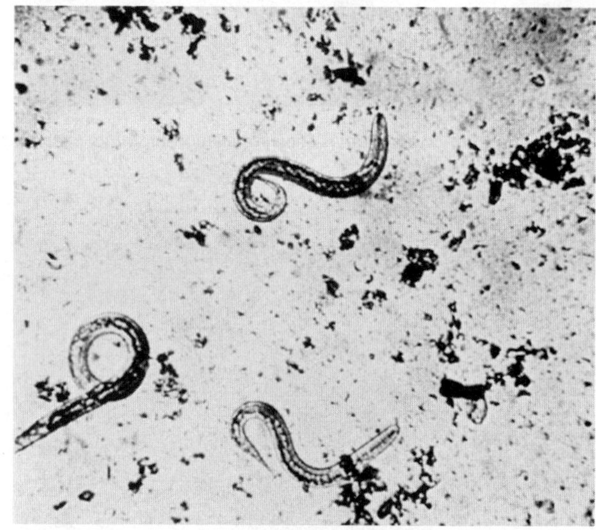

Fig. 4 First-stage larvae of *S. stercoralis* in stool.

Strongyloides stercoralis

Biology and epidemiology

Eggs hatch immediately on reaching the gut lumen, and the first-stage larvae (Fig. 4) then normally pass down the gut without moulting. Direct development in faecally contaminated soil takes 24–48 h; free-living adults mature in 72–96 h, and live for up to 10 days. Infective larvae can persist in the soil for 3 weeks. There is no second generation of free-living adults. Two types of autoinfection enable infection to persist in the host for long periods. In external autoinfection, infective larvae penetrate the perianal skin after rapid direct development on soiled skin. In internal autoinfection, larvae mature to the infective stage within the lumen of the gut and invade the mucosa of the small intestine or colon, and then pass via the gut lymphatics and portal vein to the lungs and back to the gut. In some patients, uncontrolled internal autoinfection leads to hyperinfection with massive worm loads.

S. stercoralis is widely distributed in the tropics, where prevalence may be 5–10 per cent or higher in humid lowlands. It remains endemic in the southern United States, Japan, and in parts of southern Europe, for example, among Swiss and Italian horticulturists. It also occurs in institutions when soil temperatures are high enough. Transmission among male homosexuals is very rare.

Host risk factors are of great importance for internal autoinfection. Steroid and cytotoxic therapy are the most important, but also at risk are those with lymphomas and some other malignancies, hypochlorhydria, diabetic ketosis, hypogammaglobulinaemia, and malnutrition. In the tropics, hyperinfection may occur without evident host factors. Despite co-prevalence with human immunodeficiency virus type 1 over much of its range, it now appears that this viral infection does not predispose significantly to *S. stercoralis* hyperinfection, except in a very few patients with advanced acquired immune deficiency syndrome. Servicemen in the Second World War became infected in Thailand and other parts of South-east Asia, mostly as prisoners of war. Many of these infections still persist and such people are at risk of hyperinfection if given steroids.

Pathology

In most persistent infections the parasite load is very low and evokes little pathological response. In some primary infections and when worm intensities are higher there is villous blunting with oedema and cellular infiltration of the mucosa, leading to malabsorption and protein-losing enteropathy. In more severe infections and in hyperinfection the small gut wall becomes oedematous and thickened with impaired motility, and the mesenteric lymph nodes are enlarged. In massive autoinfection there is patchy mucosal loss and some adult worms are found deep in the mucosa from where larvae may invade directly without entering the gut lumen. Invading infective larvae can produce a diffuse or haemorrhagic colitis; migrating or ectopic larvae may be found in any organ of the body. Peritoneal and pleural effusions occur and the lungs show pneumonitis and terminally alveolar haemorrhages. Rarely, adult female worms develop ectopically in the lungs, and these account for the occasional presence of eggs and rhabditiform larvae in sputum.

Clinical

In light persistent infections symptoms, if any, are usually intermittent, with episodes of upper abdominal pain, wheezy cough, and pruritus ani. Blood eosinophilia is common, and may be the only clinical finding. A pathognomonic sign is a rapidly migrating urticaria known as 'larva currens' that occurs on the buttocks, thighs, and lower trunk; it is a form of cutaneous larva migrans, arising from external autoinfection.

In moderate infections gut symptoms predominate, with diarrhoea and malabsorption. Weight loss and anorexia are prominent and not infrequently there is leg oedema. Pulmonary and skin lesions are not common. In primary infections a Loeffler's pneumonitis can occur, with high eosinophilia.

In hyperinfection diarrhoea is often severe, and sometimes bloody if there is colitis. Vomiting and abdominal distension may progress to pseudo-obstruction. Lung symptoms are common. Patients are often afebrile and without blood eosinophilia; they can deteriorate rapidly and develop Gram-negative septicaemia, shock, or meningitis, especially if they are immunosuppressed. Hypoglycaemia is a feature of autoinfection in malnourished children.

Diagnosis

Rhabditiform larvae should be sought in the stool (Fig. 4). They may be scanty and numbers do not necessarily correlate with symptoms. Live larvae are seen in fresh, wet, microscopical preparations or Baermann concentrates. Using agar-plate co-procultures a result is obtainable in 48 h, earlier than with conventional charcoal cultures. Formol-ether concentrates are also useful but sensitivity can be low. When stool specimens are not fresh, filariform strongyloides larvae may be found, and also rhabditiform hookworm larvae from hatched eggs. Duodenal aspiration is another useful technique. In hyperinfection, larvae may be found in sputum and in pleural, peritoneal, or cerebrospinal fluids.

Serodiagnosis is useful, especially as a screening test in non-endemic areas. In heavy infections, small bowel barium studies show segmental dilatation, narrowing, and abnormal motility; in hyperinfection, plain abdominal films may show fluid levels.

Treatment

Thiabendazole remains the drug of choice; 25 mg/kg is given twice daily (maximum 3 g/day), usually for 3 days. Intolerance is common and drug-induced hepatitis is reported. Treatment may fail in hyperinfection, which continues to have a high mortality. Such patients need supportive care and parenteral antimicrobials. Albendazole is an alternative in non-urgent cases but cure rates are rather low. Ivermectin appears to be effective for this infection, using a single oral dose of 200 μg/kg, repeated after 1 week or 200 μg/kg daily for 3 days, but experience is so far limited. The risks of corticosteroid and cytotoxic therapy are so high in transplant patients, for example, that empirical therapy may be justifiable in those likely to be infected.

Strongyloides fuelleborni

This species differs from *S. stercoralis* in that eggs do not hatch in the gut lumen so there can be no internal autoinfection; in faeces the eggs are thin-walled and contain a larva. In the forests of West and Central Africa, particularly Zaire, this is a zoonotic infection derived from non-human primates. Infections can cause wheezing, upper abdominal pain, and loose stools. In Papua New Guinea a subspecies *S. fuelleborni kellyi* with no known zoonotic reservoir, has a high prevalence in both children and adults in several communities. Infants aged 2 weeks to 6 months may develop 'swollen belly syndrome' with abdominal distension, diarrhoea, breathing difficulties, hypoproteinaemia, and high mortality. External autoinfection of infants occurs when they are nursed in soiled string-bag cradles. Transmammary transmission is suspected but not so far proven.

Other gut strongyloids (see OTM3, p. 932)

Species of *Trichostrongylus*, *Oesophagostomum*, and *Ternidens deminutus* are zoonotic parasites related to hookworm; their eggs are similar and larval culture is needed for reliable identification.

Further reading

Ashford, R.W., Barnish, G., and Viney, M.E. (1992). *Strongyloides fuelleborni kellyi*: infection and disease in Papua New Guinea. *Parasitology Today*, **8**, 314–18.

Grove, D.I. (ed.) (1989). *Strongyloidiasis: a major roundworm infection in man.* Taylor and Francis, London.

Mahmoud, A.A.F. (1996). Strongyloidiasis. *Clinical Infectious Diseases*, **23**, 949–53.

Roche, M. and Layrisse, M. (1966). The nature and causes of hookworm anaemia. *American Journal of Tropical Medicine and Hygiene*, **15**, 1029–102.

Schad, G.A. and Warren, K.S. (ed.) (1990). *Hookworm disease: current status and new directions.* Taylor and Francis, London.

Chapter 16.100

Nematode infections of lesser importance

D. I. Grove

From time to time, a patient may be encountered who harbours an unusual nematode. Some of these organisms are free-living parasites and the patient has a spurious infection, usually as the result of ingestion of the worm or following the *in vitro* contamination of a clinical specimen such as faeces or urine. Other individuals may have true infections with worms being found either in the gastrointestinal tract or in the tissues. Many of these infections are with parasites of animals that are adapted poorly to the human host and are unable to complete their development in humans. Thus, worms in varying stages of development including larvae, adults, and eggs may be found in specimens. Some parasites may be recovered from fluids and are viewed intact whereas others are seen only in histological sections. If there is uncertainty in identifying the worm in the former circumstance, help may often be obtained from a veterinary parasitologist who may be more used to dealing with the species concerned. In the latter instance, definitive diagnosis may be very difficult. Nematode infections of the eye are especially hard to diagnose and sometimes no satisfactory conclusion is reached.

Over 40 unusual species of nematodes have been reported to infect humans. These include species of *Agamomermis, Anatrichosoma, Ancylostoma, Ascaris, Baylisascaris, Bunostomum, Cheilospirura, Contracaecum, Cyclodontostomum, Dioctyphyma, Diploscapter, Eustrongylides, Gongylonema, Haemonchus, Lagochilascaris, Mammomonogamus, Meloidogyne, Meningonema, Mermis, Metastrongylus, Micronema, Necator, Onchocerca, Ostertagia, Parastrongylus, Pelodera, Philometra, Phocanema, Physaloptera, Rhabditis, Rictularia, Spirocerca, Syphacia, Terranova, Tetrameres, Thelazia, Trichuris, Turbatrix*, and *Uncinaria*. Most of these parasites are acquired by ingestion of eggs in contaminated food or infected arthropods such as beetles and cockroaches, while some penetrate the intact skin.

The clinical features are extremely variable depending upon the species of infecting parasite and its location in the patient. Among the more important conditions are cutaneous larva migrans and eosinophilic enteritis caused by the dog hookworm, *Ancylostoma caninum*, which penetrates the intact skin. *Ascaris suum*, the pig roundworm is acquired by ingestion of eggs and may cause pneumonitis (see Section 4) and abdominal discomfort. The mode of infection with *Lagochilascaris minor* is uncertain but it is found in the Americas and may lead to subcutaneous abscesses and nasopharyngeal lesions. Species of *Thelazia* are deposited on the eye by flies and result in conjunctivitis. *Rhabditis* is an example of a spurious infection with environmental worms being found in faeces and urine. *Turbatrix aceti* may contaminate laboratory stains for blood smears and mislead the pathologist.

Nematodes found in the gastrointestinal tract may respond to a benzimidazole agent such as mebendazole (100 mg orally twice daily for up to 3 days). Thiabendazole (25 mg/kg twice daily for several days) has been used traditionally for the treatment of systemic larval infections but its effectiveness is very variable. The related compound, albendazole (10 mg/kg orally daily for up to 1 week), may be more active than thiabendazole and is absorbed better from the gut than mebendazole. If these drugs fail, ivermectin (0.15 mg/kg orally daily for several days) may be tried. Other drugs that have been used in these unusual nematode infections include levamisole and diethylcarbamazine. Unfortunately, some infections are refractory all to anthelmintics. Nevertheless, these worms generally cannot multiply in humans and the parasites will die spontaneously after months or years. In some cases, it is possible to remove the worms surgically.

For further details see OTM3, pp. 933–6.

Further reading

Beaver, P.C., Jung, R.C., and Cupp, W.E. (1984). *Clinical Parasitology*, (9th edn), p. 825. Lea and Febiger, Philadelphia.

Orihel, T.C. and Ash, L.R. (1995). *Parasites in human tissues*, p. 386. American Society of Clinical Parasitologists, Chicago.

Chapter 16.101

Other gut nematodes

V. Zaman

Ascariasis

Adult *Ascaris lumbricoides* (Plate 1) usually live in the small intestine. In unusual circumstances, such as fever, irritation due to drugs, anaesthesia, and bowel manipulation during surgery, the worms may migrate to ectopic sites causing severe disease.

Geographical distribution

The parasite is cosmopolitan but occurs more frequently in moist and warm climates. It is more common in children, who also carry higher worm loads.

Lifecycle (Fig. 1)

The gravid female produces 2 000 000–250 000 eggs daily. These take 3 or 4 weeks to develop into the infective stage. On ingestion, the infective larva hatches out in the small intestine and penetrates the intestinal wall to enter the portal circulation. From the liver it is carried to the heart and via the pulmonary artery to the lungs. In the lungs, it breaks out of the capillaries into the alveoli and moves up to the bronchi and then crawls over the epiglottis to enter the digestive tract. In the intestine, it becomes a sexually mature worm. The lifespan of an adult worm is approximately 1 year, after which it is spontaneously expelled.

Clinical aspects

Most infected individuals remains asymptomatic. However, there is evidence to indicate that *Ascaris* causes nutritional problems and hinders the normal development of children. Occasionally, patients may develop fever, malaise, urticaria, intestinal colic, nausea, vomiting, diarrhoea, and central nervous system disorders.

The migration of larval *Ascaris* through the lungs may produce varying degrees of pneumonitis and bronchospasm. Chest radiographs may show diffuse mottling and increased prominence of peribronchial markings. There is generally high eosinophilia and the condition subsides after 7–10 days unless reinfection occurs. The larva of *A.*

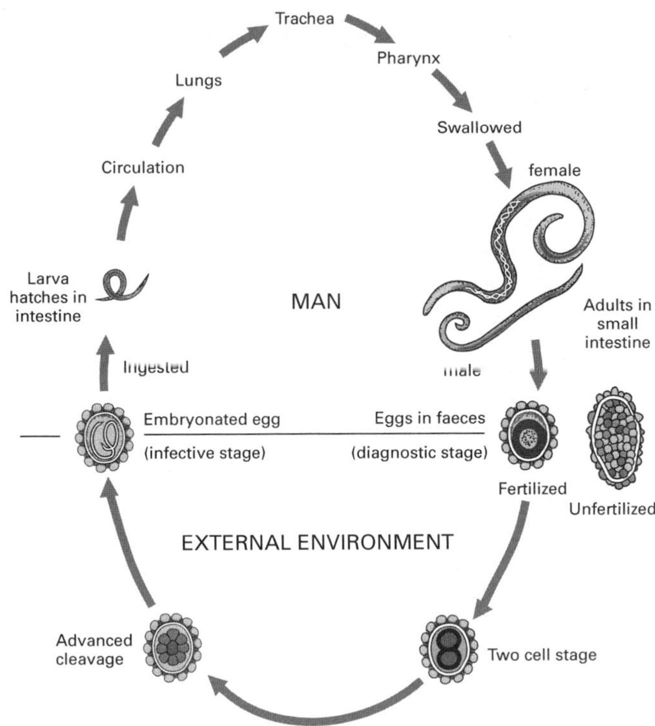

Fig. 1 Lifecycle of *Ascaris lumbricoides* *(adapted from Center for Disease Control, Atlanta, Georgia, USA.*

suum (pig Ascaris) may also produce severe pneumonitis and bronchospasm in areas where pig farming is common. In the following situations, ascariasis can cause severe, life-threatening disease.

1. When large numbers of worms become entangled to form a bolus and block the intestinal lumen producing signs and symptoms of acute intestinal obstruction.
2. When ectopic migration results in the entry of the worm into the appendix, common bile duct, or pancreatic duct. When the biliary tract is invaded, there is severe colic, often followed by suppurative cholangitis and multiple liver abscesses resulting from the disintegration of the trapped worm and secondary bacterial infection.
3. When the worm impacts in the ampulla of Vater causing acute pancreatitis and pancreatic necrosis.

Diagnosis

This is usually made by detecting *Ascaris* eggs in the faeces. Sometimes, the patient brings developing or adult worms that have been passed in the faeces or have emerged from the anus or the nose in a sick child.

Treatment

Whenever possible, all positive cases, irrespective of the worm load, should be treated as even a few worms can undergo ectopic migration with dangerous consequences.

Pyrantel pamoate

A single dose of 10 mg/kg body weight is effective in curing over 90 per cent of cases. Side-effects are mild, if any, and the drug is well tolerated. It has the advantage of also being active against *Enterobius vermicularis* and hookworms. This broad-spectrum activity is useful in endemic areas where multiple nematode infections are common.

Mebendazole

This drug is also a broad-spectrum well tolerated anthelminthic. It is given as 100 mg twice daily for 3 days, irrespective of age. Unfortunately, there are a few reported cases of ectopic migration induced by the drug. The manufacturers now advise against this drug in children under 2 years of age as there is a report of severe neurological toxicity in a young child.

Albendazole

Is effective against infections with *Ascaris*, *Trichuris*, and hookworms. Is taken as a single oral dose of 400 mg by adults and children of more than 2 years. Heavy infections may require therapy for 2–3 days.

Piperazine salts

These are widely used because of their low cost and high degree of efficacy including *E. vermicularis*, but not hookworm. The dose is 75 mg/kg (maximum of 3.5 g) given as a single dose daily for 2 consecutive days. Prior fasting is not required. Occasionally, symptoms involving the central nervous system such as unsteadiness and vertigo have been reported. If signs of intestinal obstruction develop in a child living in an endemic area, ascariasis is a distinct possibility.

In most cases of intestinal obstruction conservative therapy will succeed and the child will rapidly recover. If, however, the signs of obstruction persist and the general condition of the child worsens, laparotomy is required.

Prevention and control

As *Ascaris* eggs can survive in the soil for many years, prevention and control in the endemic areas is difficult. Mass chemotherapy given at intervals of 6 months along with environmental sanitation can break the cycle and has been used in some countries. Prevalence rates of ascariasis and other soil-transmitted helminths are greatly reduced by improvement in housing. Infection is prevented by eating only cooked food and by avoiding green vegetables and salads in countries where human faeces are used as a fertilizer and where this parasite is endemic.

Anisakiasis

Anisakiasis is an infection caused by the larvae of nematodes belonging to the family Anisakidae.

Geographical distribution

The adult worms are commonly found in cetaceans (whales, dolphins, and porpoises) in many parts of the world. Human beings are infected when they eat raw or improperly cooked fish or squid. The incidence is highest in Japan.

Lifecycle

Adults live in the lumen of the intestine of cetaceans, eggs are passed in water, second-stage larvae are ingested by crustaceans, which are then ingested by fish or squid where they enter the muscles; cetaceans and humans get infected by eating fish or squid. In humans, larvae do not develop to maturity but attach themselves to the mucosa of the stomach or intestine.

Clinical aspects

The majority of patients present with gastric symptoms that develop within 4–24 h of eating infected fish. The symptoms are due to ulceration produced by the larvae as they burrow into the mucous membrane. In addition to epigastric pain, nausea, and vomiting, there may be haematemesis during the acute stage of the disease. If there is mild pain and the patient is left untreated, the infection can proceed to a chronic stage with tumour formation.

Diagnosis

Gastroscopy often reveals the lesion and the presence of larvae attached to the mucous membrane. Parasites are usually located in the greater curvature. Radiographs with a barium meal may show the presence of single or multiple ulcers and outline the worm. Serological tests are now available in specialized centres using monoclonal antibodies.

Treatment

In acute infection an attempt should be made to remove all the larvae through a gastroscope. In chronic cases, surgical removal of the ulcerated areas or the tumor may be required. No effective chemotherapy is available. Infection is prevented by avoiding ingestion of raw fish and squid.

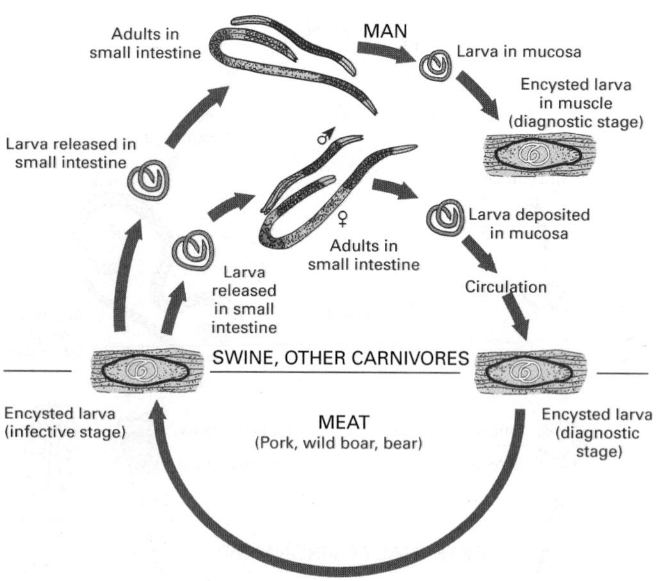

Fig. 2 Lifecycle of *Trichinella spiralis*.
(Adapted from Center for Disease Control, Atlanta, Georgia, USA.)

Capillariasis

Three species of *Capillaria* infect humans: *C. philippinensis*, which produces intestinal capillariasis; *C. hepatica*, which produces hepatic capillariasis; and *C. aerophila*, which produces pulmonary capillariasis.

Geographical distribution

C. philippinensis has been described from the Philippines, Thailand, and some other countries of South-east Asia and Far East.

Lifecycle

The lifecycle of *C. philippinensis* has not been completely worked out, but humans are infected by eating freshwater fish. The main danger with this parasite lies in the possibility of autoinfection, which leads to very heavy worm loads. *C. hepatica* is found in the liver of rodents and other mammals. The eggs are discharged in the liver and remain there until the animal dies. They eventually reach the soil by the decay of the carcass. Human beings are infected by accidentally swallowing embryonated eggs from the soil. *C. aerophila* is a parasite of wild carnivores and humans are rarely infected. Adult worms live under the mucosa of the respiratory tract.

Clinical aspects

C. philippinensis can produce severe and even fatal disease. Patients often present with abdominal pain, diarrhoea, and borborygmi or gurgling stomach. As the worm load increases due to autoinfection, diarrhoea becomes more severe, with anorexia, nausea, and vomiting. In untreated cases, the mortality rate is close to 20 per cent. In *C. hepatica* infection, symptoms of visceral larva migrans may be present. The patient may have an enlarged tender liver with low-grade fever and eosinophilia. In *C. aerophila* infection, dyspnoea, cough, and haemoptysis may be present.

Diagnosis

With *C. philippinensis*, diagnosis is made by finding the typical eggs in the faeces which resemble *Trichuris trichiura* in having polar plugs. Larvae or adult worms may also be present and repeated stool examination may be required in some cases. The parasite may also be found in the jejunal aspirate of the biopsy. With *C. hepatica*, diagnosis is made by identifying the parasite or eggs in the liver biopsy. In *C. aerophila* pulmonary biopsy is required to establish the diagnosis.

Treatment

All cases of *C. philippinesis* should be treated with mebendazole in a dose of 200 mg, twice daily, until the symptoms subside and the eggs completely disappear from the faeces after repeated stool examination. This may take up to 20 days or more. Supportive measures to overcome malnutrition and diarrhoea will be required in severely ill patients. Infection with *C. philippinensis* is prevented by avoiding raw fish in the endemic regions. There is no specific treatment for *C. hepatica* infection and *C. aerophila* infections.

Trichinosis

Geographical distribution

Trichinella spiralis infection is endemic in many parts of the world where pork is consumed.

Lifecycle (Fig. 2)

Humans are infected by eating improperly cooked pork or pork products such as sausages. In some parts of the world, wild boars are heavily infected. After ingestion, the larvae are liberated in the small intestine and mature into adults. The female deposits larvae in the gut wall from where they find their way into the bloodstream and then into the striated muscles. The most heavily parasitized muscles are the diaphragm, tongue, laryngeal, and abdominal muscles. After penetration, the larva undergoes three moults and coils into a spiral, which eventually becomes enclosed in a thick-walled cyst. In this form, the larva may remain viable for many years. Pigs become infected by eating infected scraps and garbage from slaughterhouses or farms, or by eating carcasses of infected rats.

Clinical aspects

Most of those with light infection remain asymptomatic. Heavy infections are manifested in three clinical stages.

The invasion stage

This is seen during the first week of infection and is due to juveniles and adults burrowing into the intestinal tissues. The patient complains of abdominal pain, nausea and vomiting, and diarrhoea of varying intensity. There may be fever, profuse sweating, and tachycardia.

The migration stage

This usually begins after the first week of infection. During this period, the larvae are liberated into the circulation by the gravid female and find their way to skeletal muscles causing generalized myalgia. Symptoms are attributable to toxic effects of the larvae and hypersensitivity reactions triggered by the liberation of parasite antigens. There may be oedema of the face, and periorbital tissues and fever. Complications involving the myocardium, lungs, and the central nervous system may occur due to the migrating larvae.

The encystment stage

This usually begins after the third week of infection. There is usually a gradual recovery from the symptoms. In a few cases with heavy infection, the symptoms may get worse and death may result from myocardiac failure, and respiratory and central nervous involvement.

Diagnosis

This is based on a combination of clinical and epidemiological evidence. In a characteristic case, the patient will give a history of gastrointestinal disturbances (invasion stage) within 48 h of eating pork products, wild boar, or bear meat. If the patient presents at the later stage (migration stage), there is myalgia and irregular fever. Leucocystosis and eosinophilia are usually present. Serum enzymes such as aminotransferases and creatine phosphokinase are elevated. Muscle biopsy is positive in approximately 90 per cent of clinically positive cases.

Treatment

The prognosis is good and most patients recover after the larvae have encysted. The mainstays of treatment are bedrest and salicylates. In myocarditis and severe myalgia, oral prednisone for 3–5 days (0.5–1.0 mg/kg per day) is useful and provides symptomatic relief. In experimental animals, thiabendazole is able to kill encysted larvae. In humans, its efficacy against larvae is doubtful but it provides symptomatic relief. The dosage of 25–50 mg/kg per day for 2–5 days is given and this usually brings down the fever and eosinophilia. Mebendazole appears to be a good alternative to thiabendazole as it has fewer side-effects, and is given at a dosage of 300 mg daily for 7 days. A higher dose of 1000 mg daily for 10–14 days is recommended by some authorities to ensure complete killing of the larvae. Even with this high dosage, side-effects appear not to be serious, consisting of mild Jarisch–Herxheimer type reactions at the start of therapy. The manufacturer does not recommend giving mebendazole to children under 2 years of age.

Control and prevention

Trichonosis in pigs can be greatly reduced or eliminated by hygienic rearing methods. Larvae in pork can be killed by freezing at −18°C for 24 h. Thorough cooking of pork is the best safeguard against infection in all endemic areas.

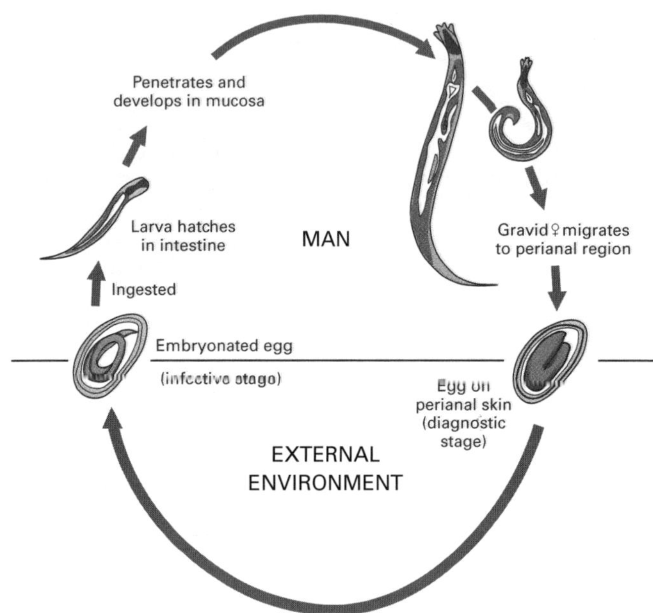

Fig. 3 Lifecycle of *Enterobius vermicularis*. *(Adapted from Center for Disease Control, Atlanta, Georgia, USA.)*

Enterobiasis

Geographical distribution

Enterobius vermicularis (Plate 2) is one of the few parasites that is more prevalent in temperate than tropical regions. Children are more often involved than adults. It occurs in groups such as families living together, inmates of hostels, and in army camps.

Lifecycle (Fig. 3)

Most adult worms live in the caecal region. The female deposits its eggs on the anus and perianal skin. Direct person-to-person infection occurs by inhalation and swallowing of the eggs. In addition, auto-infection occurs by contamination of fingers. *Enterobius* eggs are embryonated when passed, hence there is rapid transmission from person to person.

Clinical aspects

The most common presenting symptom is pruritus ani. Persistent itching may lead to inflammation and secondary bacterial infection of the perianal region. Infected children may suffer from insomnia, emotional disturbance, anorexia, weight loss, and enuresis.

Diagnosis

The eggs are most easily found around the anus, by swabbing or using cellulose adhesive tape. The anal examination for eggs should be done before defecation or bathing. Sometimes intact worms are passed in the faeces and can be easily recognized by their size and shape.

Treatment

Attention to personal hygiene is an important part of treatment and prevention. With simple hygienic measures, infection disappears on its own, due to the short lifespan of the parasite (3–6 weeks). Many drugs are available to treat the infection and it is advisable to treat all the children and adults in the same household at the same time. Piperazine citrate is given in a dose of 65 mg/kg for 7 days. The course

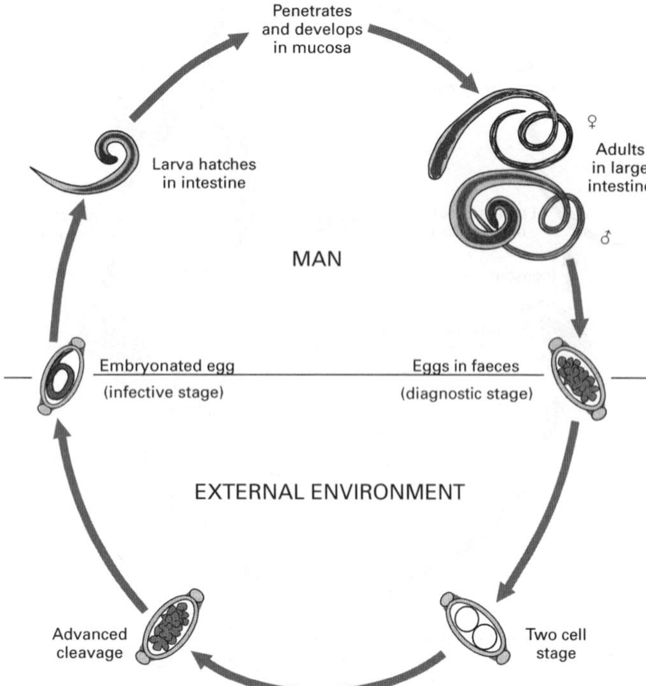

Fig. 4 Lifecycle of *Trichuris trichiura*.
(Adapted from Center for Disease Control, Atlanta, Georgia, USA.)

is repeated after 2 weeks. Piperazine is contraindicated in renal and liver disease and epilepsy. Pyrantel pamoate is equally effective in a single dose of 10 mg/kg (maximum 1 g) and its side-effect profile is better than piperazine. The drug is repeated after 2 weeks. Mebendazole is effective in a single dose of 100 mg, repeated after 2 weeks. This drug is contraindicated in pregnancy.

Trichuriasis

Geographical distribution

Trichuris trichiura (Plate 3) infection is distributed worldwide. It is the most common intestinal nematode in some tropical regions, such as South-east Asia.

Lifecycle (Fig. 4)

Infection results from ingestion of the embryonated egg. The larva does not undergo visceral migration but penetrates the gut for a short period before returning to the lumen to mature into the adult stage. The worms attach themselves to the large intestine by threading their anterior end into the epithelium.

Clinical aspects

Light infections are generally asymptomatic. In heavy infections, there is colitis with the passage of blood and mucus in faeces. The clinical picture is often similar to that of amoebic dysentery. In some cases, prolapse of the rectum occurs, probably due to constant irritation produced by the worms and the weakness of the levator ani muscle.

Diagnosis

This is based on finding characteristic barrel-shaped eggs in the faeces. Eosinophils and Charcot–Leyden crystals are often present.

Treatment

Preventive measures are the same as in ascariasis.

Mebendazole

Dosage is 100 mg, twice daily for 3 days, irrespective of the age of the patient. However, the manufacturers now advise against this drug in children under 2 years of age and it is contraindicated in pregnancy.

Albendazole

Dosage is 4 mg/kg as a single dose.

Further reading

Bratton, R.L. and Nesse, R.E. (1993). Ascariasis. An infection to watch for in immigrants. *Postgraduate Medicine*, **93**, 171–8.

Cross, J.H. (1992). Intestinal capillariasis. *Clinical Microbiology Reviews*, **5**, 120–9.

McAuley, J.B., Michelson, M.K., Hightower, A.W., Engeran, S., Wintermeyer, L.A., and Schantz, P.M. (1992). A trichinoses outbreak among Southeast Asian refugees. *American Journal of Epidemiology*, **135**, 1404–10.

Schantz, P.M. (1989). The dangers of eating raw fish. *New England Journal of Medicine*, **320**, 1143–5.

Walden, J. (1991). Parasitic diseases. Other roundworms. *Trichuris*, hookworm and *Strongyloides*. *Primary Care*, **18**, 53–74.

Chapter 16.102

Toxocariasis and visceral larva migrans

V. Zaman

Visceral larva migrans is characterized by hepatomegaly, fever, respiratory symptoms, and eosinophilia. It is mainly caused by migrating larvae of the dog (*Toxocara canis*) and cat (*T. cati*).

Geographical distribution

Toxocarial infection occurs wherever there is a significant dog and cat population. Many cases have been reported from the United States and other Western countries apparently resulting from close association between these animals and humans.

Lifecycle

The infection of *T. canis* is maintained in the dog population by direct transmission from the soil containing embryonated eggs, from transplacental transmission from bitch to puppies, through the maternal milk to puppies, and by dogs eating infected meat containing larvae. Human beings become infected by ingesting embryonated eggs from the soil. The larvae hatch out in the small intestine and migrate to various organs of the body including the liver, lungs, eye, and brain. They do not mature into adult worms in humans. After some time a granuloma forms around the larvae.

Clinical aspects

Toxocariasis caused mainly two different clinical pictures: classical visceral larva migrans syndrome and ocular toxocariasis. Occasionally, migrating larvae may cause encephalitis, asthma, abdominal distress, and chronic allergy.

Classical visceral larva migrans

This is seen most often in young children because of pica (dirt or soil eating). The majority remain asymptomatic. In a minority symptoms develop consisting of muscular pain, lassitude, anorexia, cough, and urticarial rashes. Physical signs include rhonchi, hepatomegaly, splenomegaly, and lymph-gland enlargement. The acute phase generally lasts for 2–3 weeks after which recovery occurs. Sometimes the resolution of all the signs may take up to 18 months. Rarely the infection may end fatally if a massive dose of parasites has been ingested.

Ocular larva migrans

This is caused by granuloma formation in the eye. If this is near to the macula, impairment of vision or even blindness may occur. The patient may come with the complaint of visual difficulty in one eye, with or without strabismus. As the generalized manifestation of visceral larva migrans may not be present, diagnosis is often difficult. Unlike in visceral larva migrans, eosinophilia may be absent. On fundoscopy a rounded swelling, often near the optic disc, may be detected.

Diagnosis

1. In classical visceral larva migrans there is leucocytosis with marked eosinophilia (20–80 per cent). In ocular larva migrans there may be no peripheral eosinophilia.
2. Serological tests are useful. An enzyme immunoassay is positive in the majority of patients with visceral larva migrans. In ocular larva migrans the vitreous fluid is shown to have antibodies to the parasite.
3. Biopsy of the liver may show larvae with granulomas and eosinophilic infiltration.

Treatment

No anthelminthic drug is completely effective in killing the larvae and most patients recover without specific therapy. Thiabendazole has been tried in a dosage of 25 mg/kg twice daily for 5 days and mebendazole (1 g or 1000 mg three times a day for 21 days). There is a possibility that the use of antihelminthics may sometimes provoke a greater inflammatory response, with worsening of the clinical picture, due to injury of the parasite. In severe cases, corticosteroids have been used with reports of improvement.

In ocular larva migrans, visible larvae can be photocoagulated by laser. Vitrectomy has been used in some cases, and local and intraocular steroids also appear to be of the same value. Recognition of the risk factor for infection is the key to prevention.

Further reading

Glickman, L.T. and Magnaval, J.F. (1993). Zoonotic roundworm infections. *Infectious Diseases Clinics of North America*, 7, 717–32.

Chapter 16.103

Angiostrongyliasis

Sompone Punyagupta

Cerebrospinal angiostrongyliasis ('eosinophilic meningitis')

This is caused by the rat nematode *Angiostrongylus cantonensis*. It is prevalent in many Pacific islands from Hawaii, New Guinea, The Philippines, Indonesia, Southeast Asia, China and Japan, India, and Australia. It has also been reported from Cuba, Egypt, Ivory Coast, and Madagascar. Eosinophilic meningitis is characterized by central nervous system manifestation and eosinophilic pleocytosis.

Epidemiology

Humans are infected by eating uncooked or undercooked snails (e.g. apple snails (*Pila* spp.), giant African snails (*Achatina fulica*)) and possibly shrimps, and even a monitor lizard, fish, and green vegetables contaminated with infective larvae.

Pathogenesis

Adult *A. cantonensis* live in the pulmonary arteries of rats; the first-stage larvae hatch from the eggs lodged in terminal vessels, and migrate along the air passages and intestine. Various slugs, snails, and crustacea serve as intermediate as well as transporting hosts by picking up the larvae from the soil or water. The infective third-stage larvae then develops and infects humans after the animal host is eaten raw or rare. In humans, an accidental host, larvae will migrate from the gastrointestinal tract to the brain and develop into the fifth-stage larvae.

The disease is induced by an immunological reaction to the parasite. Mononuclear and eosinophilic infiltrations are observed along the migration tracks, around the vessels and in the meninges. Tissue reaction around the dead worm is much more severe than around the living one. Scattered areas of minute haemorrhages are evidence of mechanical injury. At autopsy worms may also be found in the spinal cord, eye chambers, and rarely in the lungs.

The disease is usually benign, sometimes subclinical and self-limiting, with complete recovery in most cases. Yet it may be severe, resulting is acute cerebral dysfunction, permanent neurological deficits, or even death. Hundreds of worms may be found in the brain at post mortem. The incubation period varies from 3 to 36 days with an average of 2 weeks but tends to be shorter in severe cases.

Clinical features

Acute, intermittent, unbearable, occipital, and bi-temporal headache persists through the clinical course. There is usually a history of consumption of raw or rare food within 2–4 weeks of the onset of headache. Sometimes there is nausea, vomiting, abdominal discomfort, and urticarial rash soon after ingestion of the suspected food. Fever is usual absent except in patients with severe disease, who may present with deteriorating cerebral symptoms. Meningism can be elicited in only about 15 per cent of mild cases but more in severe cases. Nausea and vomiting are frequent during the first week. Impaired consciousness is uncommon except in severe cases. Some may present with a history of convulsion or psychosis. Mild constitutional symptoms such as malaise, anorexia, and general aching are usual.

Paraesthesia of the trunk and extremities indicating peripheral nerve injury may be observed. Generalized motor weakness and paraplegia due to spinal cord involvement may be noted in some severe cases. Cough, audible rales, and radiographic features of pneumonitis have been recognized in very severe cases. Cranial nerves are sometimes involved, particularly the optic, facial, and abducens nerves. Bilateral or unilateral amblyopia of varying degree, associated with abnormal fundi, is not uncommon. Diplopia, abnormal visual fields, optic atrophy, and periorbital oedema are seldom seen. *A. cantonensis* larvae have been recovered from the eye chambers in many cases. Retinal haemorrhage and detachment are important ocular complications.

Laboratory findings

There is a mild peripheral leucocytosis with 10–50 per cent eosinophilia that persists for about 3 months. Lumbar puncture, the single most useful diagnostic test, must be done in all suspected cases. The opening pressure is usually high, in some cases over 500 mm of cerebrospinal fluid. The fluid may be clear or turbid, colourless or slightly xanthochromic but not purulent. The pleocytosis is usually in the range of 500–2000/mm^3. Red blood cells may be seen occasionally. Eosinophilic pleocytosis varies from 10 per cent to over 90 per cent. The predominant cells may, however, be lymphocytes, and some neutrophils may also be found. Eosinophilic pleocytosis reaches a peak at about the second week after the first symptom and gradually disappears over 3 months. In a few cases, the pleocytosis may recur during the second month with return of some symptoms. The protein concentration is high but the sugar concentration is normal. Spinal fluid should be examined closely under a bright light with the help of a hand lens to detect tiny moving larvae. In Taiwan the recovery rate of worms in the spinal fluid is much higher than elsewhere, ranging from 6.4 to 30 per cent.

Other investigations, including biochemical tests, electroencephalogram, brain scan, and cerebral angiography, are of no diagnostic value. Some abnormalities have been observed in computed axial tomographs of the brain.

Diagnosis

Cerebral angiostrongyliasis should be suspected if a patient who resides in or recently visited the endemic area presents with a history of typical symptoms and eosinophilic pleocytosis within 1 month of eating any of the host species (e.g. snails). A definite diagnosis can only be made by recovering *A. cantonensis* larvae from the spinal fluid or ocular chambers, or at autopsy. Enzyme immune assay, with antigen prepared from fourth-stage larvae, may be used as supporting evidence.

Differential diagnosis

Eosinophilic pleocytosis has been observed rarely in tuberculous meningitis, neurosyphilis, and multiple sclerosis, but for practical purposes it indicates a parasitic infection of the central nervous system: *A. cantonensis*, *Gnathostoma spinigerum*, *Paragonimus westermani*, or schistosomes. Epidemiological information in different geographical areas is most useful. *G. spinigerum* should be suspected if the patient develops paralysis of the extremities following severe radicular pain or impairment of the sensorium with bloody or xanthochromic spinal fluid and eosinophilic pleocytosis.

Treatment and clinical course

Anthelminthics should not be given because the reaction to the dead worms in the brain can be disastrous, leading to clinical deterioration or even death. Headache usually subsides dramatically, but temporarily, after each lumbar puncture. The tap should therefore be repeated at intervals of 3–7 days until there is a definite clinical as well as laboratory improvement. Analgesics and sedatives are helpful. Based on the immunopathological concept, corticosteroids, such as prednisolone, in a dose of 30–60 mg daily, have been advocated in critical cases with cerebral depression, or in those with cranial nerve involvement, but no benefit has been confirmed in milder cases. Although clinical symptoms persist for only 2–4 weeks, the neurological deficit may last longer. In some patients, of acute symptoms may relapse after 2 months of illness, probably representing a reaction to some dead worms in the brain.

Angiostrongylus in the eye should be removed surgically, but complications are inevitable if the posterior chamber is involved.

The overall mortality rate is low: 3.7 per cent in Taiwan, 0.5 per cent in Thailand, and none in Tahiti. However, the fatality among specific groups of patients may be as high as 25 per cent. Patients usually die in coma 2–4 weeks after the onset. Energetic neurological and cardiopulmonary intensive care during the acute stage can be life saving. As there is no specific treatment, preventive measures through public education are necessary.

Abdominal angiostrongyliasis ('eosinophilic enteritis')

This is caused by *Angiostrongylus (Morerastrongylus) costaricensis*. It occurs in Central and South America, from Mexico to Brazil. Eosinophilic gastroenteritis is a clinical syndrome that may be caused by parasites, such as *Eustoma rotundatum*, *Anisakis*, *G. spinigerum*, and *A. costaricensis*.

Pathogenesis

A. costaricensis lives in the mesenteric arteries of various species of rodents. First-stage larvae hatch from eggs in the intestinal capillaries and enter the intestine. Slugs (*Vaginulus plebelus*), which ingest the larvae in rat faeces, serve as intermediate hosts in which second- and third-stage larvae develop. Human beings accidentally ingests vegetable leaves smeared with mucus of slugs containing infective larvae. Humans are not a definitive host, yet the female worms are capable of producing fertile but unhatched eggs. The lesions are confined to the ileocaecal region. Oedema and thickening of the intestinal wall with miliary, yellowish, granulomatous inflammation of the appendix, terminal ileum, caecum, or ascending colon are observed. Regional lymph nodes, liver, omentum, and testicles are occasionally involved. Arteritis or thrombosis of arteries by the 2–4 cm long, filiform, adult worms may be noted. Microscopy of the lesions shows eosinophilic infiltration and characteristic thin-walled eggs or larvae of *A. costaricensis*.

Clinical features

The disease mainly affects children. The incubation period is unknown. Patients experience high fever for 2–4 weeks, anorexia, vomiting, and right-sided, particularly right iliac fossa, abdominal pain resembling that of acute appendicitis. Some present features of partial or complete intestinal obstruction. The worms may migrate to the liver causing hypereosinophilia with hepatomegaly. There is tenderness or a tender mass in the right inferior quadrant and tenderness on rectal examination. Leucocytosis of 10–50 × 10^9/1 with 11–82 per cent eosinophilia is a constant finding. Radiographs may show spasticity, filling defects, and irritability at the caecum and ascending colon. Serodiagnosis may be helpful in chronic as well as acute cases.

Diagnosis and treatment

The diagnosis should be considered in children with features of appendicitis, inflammatory bowel disease, or ileocaecal mass associated with blood eosinophilia. Definitive diagnosis and treatment are best achieved by surgical exploration and resection of affected bowel. Chemotherapy with thiabendazole has achieved inconclusive results.

Further reading

Loria-Cortes, R. and Lobo Sanahuja, J.F. (1980). Clinical abdominal angiostrongylosis. A study of 116 children with intestinal eosinophilic granuloma caused by *Angiostrongylus costaricensis. American Journal of Tropical Medicine and Hygiene*, **29**, 538–44.

Punyagupta, S., Juttijudata, P., and Bunnag, T. (1975). Eosinophilic meningitis in Thailand. Clinical studies of 484 typical cases probably caused by *Angiostrongylus cantonensis. American Journal of Tropical Medicine and Hygiene*, **24**, 921–31.

Yii, C.Y. (1979). Clinical observations on eosinophilic meningitis and meningoencephalitis caused by *Angiostrongylus cantonensis* in Taiwan. *American Journal of Tropical Medicine and Hygiene*, **25**, 233–49.

Chapter 16.104

Gnathostomiasis

Pravan Suntharasamai

Gnathostomiasis is an extraintestinal infection with larval or immature *Gnathostoma spinigerum*, a nematode parasite that lives in the stomachs of cats and dogs. The disease is characterized by intermittent and migratory lesions in the skin and the internal organs, resulting from inflammation or haemorrhage. Occasional deaths are due to the invasion of the central nervous system.

Aetiology

Four species of gnathostomes are known to infect humans. Adult gnathostomes live in the upper gastrointestinal tract of the definitive hosts which for *G. spinigerum*, the most thoroughly studied species, are several carnivores particularly cats and dogs. Cyclops, the first intermediate host, ingests the sheathed, first-stage larvae, which hatch in water from ova shed with the host's faeces. The third-stage larvae are found in the viscera and muscles of second intermediate hosts; such as fish, frog, snake, lizard, chicken, duck, rat, pig, and mongoose; which have ingested the infected cyclops or the infected flesh of another second intermediate host. The lifecycle is shown in Fig. 1.

Consumption of the raw or undercooked flesh of second intermediate and paratenic hosts is the most common mode of transmission. Skin penetration by worms after contamination of the skin of food preparers by infected meat, or the use of such flesh as a poultice, is less important. Prenatal transmission can occur, as larvae have been recovered in neonates as young as 3 days old.

Epidemiology

G. spinigerum infections have been reported frequently in Thailand and Japan, and sporadically in Australia, Bangladesh, Burma, China, Ecuador, India, Indonesia, Laos, Malaysia, Mexico, the Philippines, Sri Lanka, USA, and Vietnam. Prevalence in Bangkok, Thailand, has been estimated to be 4/100. Human infections with the other three species have been reported from Japan. However, it appears that the Japanese acquire *G. hispidum* from infected loaches imported from China; *G. doloresi* and *G. nipponicum* occur naturally in Japan.

Pathogenesis and pathology

After being ingested, the larva penetrates the gut wall and migrates to the liver before wandering, perhaps randomly, through almost any tissue except bone. The migration appears to be facilitated by the architecture of its cuticular spines. As the worm migrates the tissue is destroyed, producing track-like spaces together with varying degrees of haemorrhage and eosinophil-associated acute inflammation that may be the result of an immunological reaction and toxic products of the parasites. Oedema is prominent in some skin lesions, while multiple and sometimes large areas of haematoma are typical of spinal cord and brain involvement.

Clinical features

After consumption of infected material, nausea, vomiting, and abdominal pain may occasionally be noted within 1–2 days, and a syndrome consisting of fever, pain in the right upper quadrant of the abdomen, chest pain, dry cough, and hypereosinophilia may develop within 1–2 weeks. The patients mostly present with only one of the following forms of the infection.

Cutaneous forms

Gnathostomal creeping eruption

This is extremely rare. The serpiginous track is similar to, but bigger and more variable in depth than those caused by dog or cat hookworm larvae. A trail of subcutaneous haemorrhage is sometimes observed.

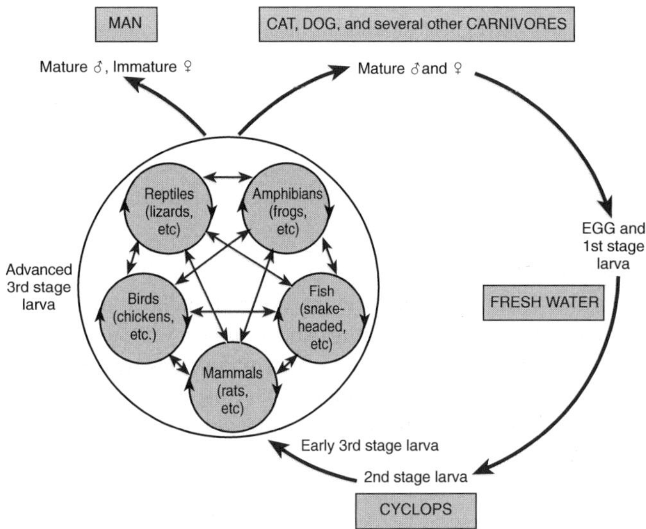

Fig. 1 Lifecycle.

Cutaneous migratory swelling

This is the most common manifestation of human gnathostomiasis. The first swelling may develop 3–4 weeks after ingestion. Swelling can occur any where and may recur close to the original site or at a distance. It develops rapidly and usually lasts for about 1–2 weeks. Frequently it is extensive, involving the whole wrist or hand. Swelling of the digits or plantar surfaces can be very painful and incapacitating. Itching is the main associated symptom. Regional lymphadenitis and fever are usually absent. When swelling involves the eyelid, chemosis and conjunctival haemorrhage may be observed. The worms can escape spontaneously through the skin, or the conjunctiva. The interval between episodes of swelling varies from a few days to a few months and rarely 1–2 years.

Visceral forms

Spinocerebral gnathostomiasis

Involvement of the central nervous system commonly start with intermittent, agonizing, shooting pains with paraesthesia of a limb or a segment of trunk, followed by paraplegia with urinary retention and, rarely, quadriplegia. Sensation is correspondingly impaired and the Brown–Sequard syndrome is sometimes seen. A few patients present with severe headache and vomiting, followed very quickly by coma, cranial nerve palsies, and hemiplegia, resembling a cerebrovascular accident. Physical findings, other than the usual signs of meningeal irritation, depend on the size of the lesions, but a rapidly advancing or changing pattern of neurological deficit is characteristic of the infection. Eosinophilic meningitis without focal neurological deficit or subarachnoid haemorrhage occurs occasionally.

Ocular gnathostomiasis

The gnathostome can be found in the anterior chamber, the vitreous humour, and the retina. Inflammation and destruction markedly impair vision. The parasite usually migrates through the sclera or the cornea, but may die in the vitreous humour.

Intra-abdominal and oral gnathostomiasis

These can result in intestinal obstruction, or cause a painful intra-abdominal mass. The infection may terminate spontaneously when the worm escapes unnoticed into the lumen and is expelled with the faeces.

Pulmonary and respiratory gnathostomiasis

The parasites have been found in the sputum of patients with eosinophilic pneumonitis, or following symptoms indicating irritation of the upper respiratory tract.

Genitourinary gnathostomiasis

The parasites have been found in bloodstained urethral discharge, accompanying haematuria, in the glans penis, or in the uterine cervical mucosa.

Auditory gnathostomiasis

The worms have been found in the external auditory canal in a patient with hearing loss and tinnitus, and in another while penetrating the tympanic membrane. These visceral manifestations are pertaining only to the *G. spinigerum* infection. Cutaneous migratory swelling precedes or follows the episode in only a few of these patients.

Diagnosis

The diagnosis of cutaneous forms is suggested by clinical characteristics, and the geographical and dietary history and by excluding other causes. It is definitive if the worm is obtained and identified. The diagnosis of visceral gnathostomiasis depends mainly on the identification of the worm in surgical specimens and secretions such as sputum, urine, or vaginal discharge.

Laboratory diagnosis

An immunoenzyme test for IgG antibody is indicative of this infection at a titre of 1:400 or above. The Western blot analysis for antibody reacting with 24 000-kDa glycoprotein appears to be more specific. Blood eosinophilia occurs irregularly in about 60 per cent of cases of gnathostomiasis and, therefore, is not necessary in making presumptive diagnosis. With spinocerebral involvement the cerebrospinal fluid can be bloody, xanthochromic, or slightly turbid with a minor increase in protein content. The proportion of eosinophils is higher than expected from haemorrhage *per se.*

Differential diagnosis

The migratory cutaneous swelling should be differentiated from contact dermatitis, angioedema, and urticaria. Calabar swellings (caused by *Lao loa*) occur only in the Central African forest belt and are associated with microfilariae in the blood. Stationary swelling must be differentiated from other infections such as fascioliasis, paragonimiasis, sparganosis, and dirofilariasis, and from non-infectious causes.

Gnathostomal aetiology is highly likely if rapidly advancing myelitis follows radiculitic pain, or if features of cerebral or subarachnoid haemorrhage occur in a person who is otherwise healthy but for a history of cutaneous migratory swelling and blood eosinophilia. Eosinophil pleocytosis is essential for the diagnosis, as is exclusion of non-helminthic encephalomyelitis and Guillain–Barré syndrome. Eosinophilic meningoencephalitis caused by *Angiostrongylus cantonensis* can produce severe headache, meningeal irritation, cranial nerve palsies, and impaired consciousness, but the development is less dramatic. Development of meningoencephalitis after eating poorly cooked, freshwater snails favours the diagnosis of *A. cantonensis* infection. Rarely, *Angiostrongylus* larvae can be identified in the cerebrospinal fluid.

In the case of intraocular infection, the larvae of *A. cantonensis* can be distinguished by being thinner, longer, and folding. They appear in the eyeball 2–3 weeks after the manifestation of eosinophilic meningoencephalitis.

Treatment

Surgical removal of the parasite is curative, but rarely possible. Treatment with albendazole at an adult dosage of 400 mg twice daily for 2 weeks has a unique effect in inducing outward migration of the gnathostome to the skin. The worms have been frequently recovered between days 2 and 14. The recurrence rate of swelling is also markedly diminished after the albendazole treatment. Supportive, symptomatic, and anti-inflammatory treatments are preferable to surgical attempts.

Prognosis

Cerebral gnathostomiasis can be fatal and blindness is usual after intraocular gnathostomiasis. The probability of central nervous or intraocular involvement is less than 1 per cent in patients with cutaneous migratory swelling. Intestinal obstruction may prove fatal if it is complete and prolonged, but more frequently the patient will lose a segment of gut because of a perhaps unnecessary operation.

Prevention

In the endemic area all dishes that contain raw or poorly cooked flesh of animals must be avoided. Food preparers who have had prolonged exposure to potentially infected flesh should use gloves.

Further reading

Miyazaki, I. (1991). *An illustrated book of helminthic zoonoses*, SEAMIC Publication No. 62, pp. 368–409. Southeast Asian Medical Information Centre, International Medical Foundation of Japan, Tokyo.

Rusnak, J.M. and Lucey, D.R. (1993). Clinical gnathostomiasis: case report and review of the English-language literature. *Clinics in Infectious Diseases*, **16**, 33–50.

Suntharasamai, P., Riganti, M., Chittamas, S., and Desakorn, V. (1992). Albendazole stimulates outward migration of *Gnathostoma spinigerum* to the dermis in man. *Southeast Asian Journal of Tropical Medicine and Public Health*, **23**, 716–22.

Cestodes (tapeworms)

Chapter 16.105

Hydatid disease

A. J. Radford

Echinococcosis, hydatidosis, and hydatid disease are synonyms for infection with the dog tapeworm, *Echinococcus granulosus*, which requires another vertebrate host to complete its lifecycle. Less common species which may infect humans include *E. multilocularis* and *E. vogeli*. *E. granulosus* produces cystic hydatid disease and *E. multilocularis* alveolar hydatid disease.

Epidemiology

Overall there is an increasing pandemic. Although decreasing in prevalence in many countries, cystic hydatidosis is widespread throughout the whole Euro-Asian land mass, in northern and eastern Africa, and southern and western South America, much of Canada, and in Australasia (Fig. 1). *E. multilocularis* is found in North America, the former USSR, Japan, parts of central Europe, and in Turkey.

Humans are intruders ('accidental hosts') in the lifecycle and represent a 'dead end' for the parasite whose most usual cycle is between sheep and dogs. Hydatids occur both in domestic and sylvatic (wild) forms. Recently, different strains of *E. granulosus* have been identified and these probably have different levels of pathogenicity in humans. The lifecycle is shown in Fig. 2.

Prevalence rates in animals in excess of 50 per cent have been reported. It is especially prevalent in horses in England, cattle in Italy, some Eskimo dog packs, and dingoes in parts of Australia. A major factor in any recent appearance of hydatidosis is the importation of infected livestock in whom diagnosis is difficult clinically and in which serological cross-reactions occur with closely related tapeworms such as *Taenia ovis* and *T. saginata*.

Familiarity with dogs and ignorance of, or indifference to, the significance and prevalence of the disease are important factors in maintaining human infection rates. Rural rates are almost always higher due to socio-cultural patterns. In the Mediterranean littoral, rates have exceeded 3.5 per cent with micro-endemic areas exceeding 10 per cent.

Lifecycle

The adult cestode worm is bottle-shaped and 3–9 mm long. There may be several thousand adults in the jejunum of an infected animal. The terminal gravid proglottid is shed every 2 weeks, releasing 500 or more eggs which are passed in faeces to the ground where herbivores incidentally ingest them while grazing. Viable in dry conditions, the eggs are sensitive to heat. Humans most commonly ingest them after handling dogs with contaminated hair, or by consuming contaminated vegetables or water. Carnivores acquire the parasite by consuming the infected viscera of intermediate hosts. For *E. granulosus*, this most commonly occurs when dogs devour sheep livers and lungs.

In the intermediate host eggs hatch in the duodenum and the emergent hexacanth embryo passes through the intestinal wall into the portal and lymphatic systems and thence to the liver or lungs, but may pass to any organ. The embryo develops into a simple cyst with an outer elastic laminated layer and more fragile inner germinal layer of epithelial cells from which bud brood capsules may break off forming 'hydatid sand'. Growth is slow taking 5–6 months to become 20 mm in size and infective. The *E. granulosus* cyst is single, filled with clear fluid and sometimes forms daughter cysts, but *E. multilocularis* lesions are honey-combed structures.

Clinical features

There are no specific local or general symptoms and signs of hydatid disease. The diagnosis is usually made in young adults, following incidental findings at radiographic examination or at autopsy. Symptoms and signs are secondary to the progressive expansion of cysts, or due to embolization. Liver and lung involvement are most common, with hepatic lesions being more frequent. In 20–30 per cent there are multiple lesions. Complications are the commonest form of presentation. At diagnosis up to a half of cysts have become secondarily infected.

With the exception of *E. multilocularis*, the parasite has a remarkable capacity to avoid an immunological response by humans who are thus very tolerant to the effects of hydatid infestation walling off the laminated cyst. The growth of most cysts is slow and sometimes arrested. Pulmonary lesions are most common. Symptoms, if present include cough, with or without haemoptysis, and patients cough up pieces of ruptured membrane with a salty taste from cyst fluid. Multiple lesions occur in 40 per cent and are bilateral in 20 per cent of cases.

Similarly, in liver disease most lesions are silent and found incidentally and, when symptomatic, produce pain and discomfort secondary to pressure. Where lesions are near the surface, fluctuation and 'hydatid thrill' may be elicited. The right lobe is involved in 75 per cent of cases and about one-third of cysts are solitary. *E. multilocularis* infections are more invasive, akin to a locally invasive malignancy. Anaphylaxis, which may be fatal, can follow rupture. Bronchopulmonary or hepatobiliary obstruction, and fistulae are

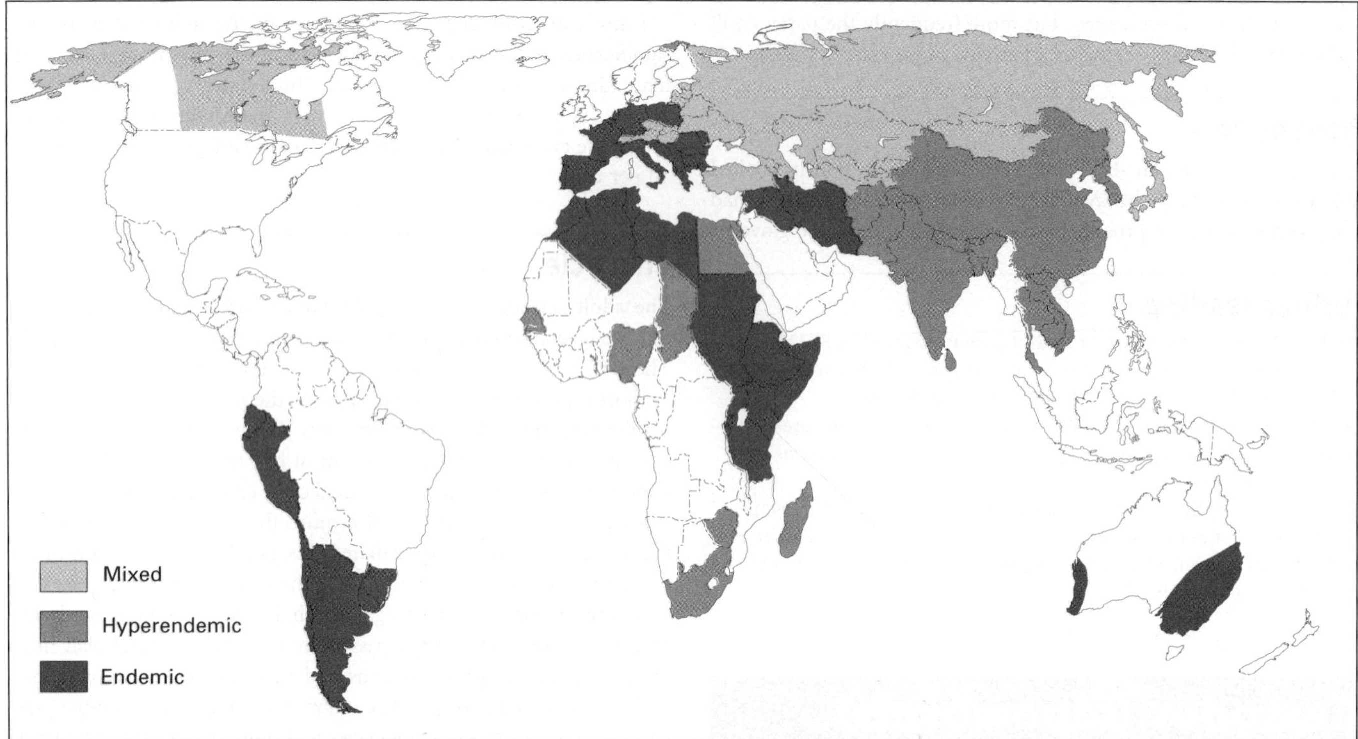

Fig. 1 Distribution of hydatid disease.
(Reproduced from Matossian, R.M., et al. (1977). Hydatosis: a global problem of increasing importance. Bulletin of the World Health Organization, **55***, 449, by permission.)*

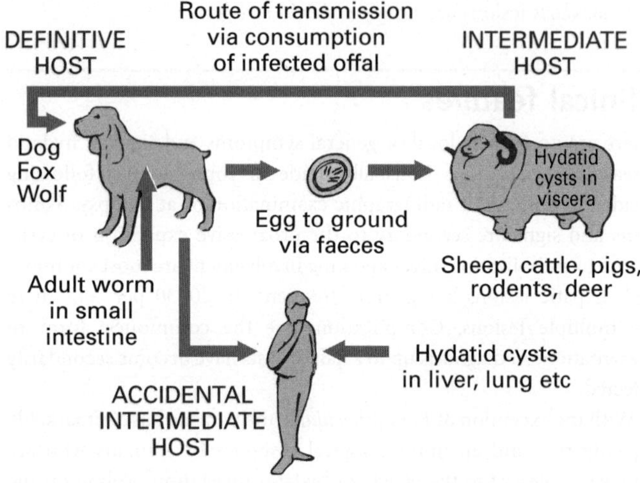

Fig. 2 Lifecycle of *E. granulosus*.

much commoner complications. Less common are spontaneous fractures and hydatiduria. Cerebral lesions give signs and symptoms of a space-occupying lesion.

Diagnosis

The absence of an appropriate geographical history and no contact with dogs makes the diagnosis unlikely.

Over 90 per cent of pulmonary diagnoses can be made radiologically. Lesions are usually round and uniform unless surrounding pneumonitis or atelectasis occurs. Multicystic lesions of *E. multilocularis* infections show notching and budding of cyst walls which vary from 1 to 20 cm in diameter. Various, almost pathognomonic, radiologic appearances may occur. These give rise to 'crescent', 'double arch', or 'water-lily' signs as a result of bronchopulmonary fistulous formation and collapse of the cyst wall. A fluid level may be present after rupture. Cavitation may also occur requiring differentiation from pulmonary abscess. A pleural reaction occurs in about one-third of cases. Sputum microscopy may reveal invaginated or evaginated protoscolices, even when immunodiagnostic tests are negative.

A plain radiograph of the abdomen reveals about a third of cases of hepatic disease, and may reveal 'white line' images for almost the full circumference of the walled cyst. Intralesional gas bubbles may be present if hepatobronchial fistulae have formed. The right hemidiaphragm is deformed and elevated in almost half of liver lesions. In intracranial lesions, radiographs may show signs of increased intracranial pressure with asymmetrical growth or thinning of the underlying bone. Calcification occurs in 3.5 per cent of patients but is more common in hepatic lesions.

Next to plain radiographs, computed tomography and/or magnetic resonance imaging, where available, is the best aid to lesion imaging. Ultrasonography, especially with abdominal locationization, is helpful. The appearances are usually pathognomonic. In the case of liver lesions they usually differentiate hydatid cysts from malignant metastases, hepatomas, angiomas, and abscesses. In intracranial lesions the appearances are cystic, spherical with a sharp border, have a central absorptive value similar to cerebrospinal fluid, and usually show significant ventricular distortion and a shift of mid-line structures.

Immunodiagnosis

An immense array of immunodiagnostic techniques have been developed to confirm diagnosis and to improve species specificity.

The single intact pulmonary cyst gives the fewest positive results. Eosinophilia occurs in only 20 per cent of patients.

The intradermal Casoni test is best known with positivity reported variously to over 90 per cent. At present the immunoelectrophoresis (**IEP**) and polymerase chain reaction (**PCR**) tests are the most specific. Sensitivity of the former is improved by the concentration of serum. False-negative reports of up to 20 per cent of IEP occur, mainly in patients with intact cysts and for the reasons stated above. The Arc 5 band is used as the marker. Whole sheep hydatid cyst fluid is the best source of antigen. Reactions also occur with *E. vogeli* and *E. multilocularis*. Positives occur only if active disease is present or within 12 months after surgery.

Radioimmunoassay, radioallergosorbent test, and enzyme-linked immunosorbent assay (**ELISA**) tests give up to 95 per cent positive results in confirmed cases. Latex agglutination or indirect haemaglutination tests as a screen, and PCR, the IEP test (or complement fixation test or indirect fluorescent antibody test) as a confirmation test appear the best tools for specific diagnosis. Variable cross-reactions occur with paragonimus, cysticercus, a number of the schistosomes and filaria, but some of these results may be due to multiple diagnoses.

Management

Surgery, often using laser techniques, is the main line of treatment and may be technically very demanding. It carries a mortality rate of 1–3 per cent and a recurrence rate of 10 or more per cent when rupture occurs. Rupture on cyst enucleation is reported in up to half of the cases and anaphylactic shock may occur immediately, as may infection in the days or weeks that follow. Several techniques are used to sterilize the contacts of the cysts before enucleation is attempted by a small aspiration followed by the injection of a scolicide. Even simple puncture aspiration of cysts followed by a scolicide injection has had good result where extensive surgery has not been suitable. (For further details, see OTM3, p. 958 and Further reading.)

The benzimidazole derivatives mebendazole, albendazole, fluoromebendazole, and combendazole are undergoing clinical trials. None has consistently demonstrated either its efficiency in humans or its safety at prolonged high dosage. Increasingly both pre- and postoperative courses of either high-dose mebendazole or albendazole are advised, and use of albendazole where lesions are inoperable or where intraperitoneal spillage occurs. Levels above 100 ng/ml are recommended. Repeated courses (up to 60) of albendazole in doses varying from 10 to 20 mg/kg per day for 30 days are showing promising results and some 'cures' have been reported. Praziquantal may have some action on protoscolices and has been used in 'combination' with benzimidazoles.

Control

Hydatid programmes have been some of the world's most successful public health measures. It is significant that the most effective campaigns have been carried out on islands with relatively small populations. Campaigns have one principal objective—'to prevent dogs from getting offal'—thereby interrupting the lifecycle of the parasite (see Fig. 2). Effective control measures include:

1. Prevention of infection of dogs by their exclusion from slaughtering areas and the installation of deep offal pits or incineration systems.
2. Raising the level of public and, especially, farmer awareness and participation in the project with literature, media, and school programmes.
3. On-site farm visits with individual contacts and demonstration of dogs' infection by purgation with arecoline hydrobromide (15–30 mg). Diagnosis by copra antigen detection is now possible.
4. Control of stray dogs in endemic areas.
5. Legislation.
6. Dog immunization is a possibility for the future.

Control or eradication of sylvatic disease is much more difficult.

Other hydatidiform cysts

Other important taeniid larval infections of humans which may cause the development of bladder-like structures in tissue include *Cysticercus cellulosae*, the larvae of *Taeni solium* (see Chapter 16.106); *C. bovis*, the larva of *T. saginata*; *Coenurus cerebralis*, the larval form of *T. (Multiceps) multiceps* in sheep, and *T. brauni*, one of the tape-worms of African dogs. An ELISA test has been developed for *T. solium cysticerci*. For further details see OTM3, p. 959.

Further reading

Beard, T.C. (1969). Hydatid control. A problem in health education. *Medical Journal of Australia*, **2**, 456–9.

Beggs, I. (1983). The radiological appearances of hydatid disease of the liver. *Clinical Radiology*, **34**, 555–63.

Matossian, R.M. (1977). The immunological diagnosis of human hydatid disease. *Transactions of the Royal Society of Tropical Medicine and Hygiene*, **71**, 101–3.

Morris, D.L. and Richards, K.S. (1992). *Hydatid disease: current medical and surgical treatment*. Butterworth-Heinemann, Oxford.

Thompson, R.C.A. (ed.) (1986). *The biology of* Echinococcus *and hydatid disease*. George Allen and Unwin, London.

Chapter 16.106

Gut cestodes

R. Knight

The cyclophyllidean tapeworms maintain anchorage to the host small gut mucosa by means of the scolex, a holdfast structure bearing four adhesive suckers and usually a central evertible rostellum with one or more circlets of hooks (Fig. 1(a,b)). The rest of the body forms the strobila and consists of a chain of flattened proglottids, which bud behind the scolex. Gravid proglottids are lost from the end of the strobila and are replaced by others that have matured as they pass down the strobila. Each proglottid possesses a complete set of hermaphroditic sex organs; eggs accumulate in the uterus of gravid proglottids and only enter the faecal stream when the proglottids are disrupted. In many species the eggs enter the environment within intact proglottids. In either case the eggs are embryonated and contain an onchosphere embryo with three pairs of hooks. After ingestion by the intermediate host, eggs hatch and the released embryo bores its way into the mucosa. The larval stages of the parasite are generally cystic with an invaginated embryonic scolex—the protoscolex. The cycle is completed when the larval stage, within the intermediate host or its tissues, is eaten by the definitive host; the protoscolex evaginates and attaches to the gut mucosa.

In three species, humans are a regular part of the lifecycle (Table 1; Figs 2, 3, and 4); in the rest they are an accidental host. The two *Taenia* spp. are unique among all human infections in that they are zoonoses, that is infections derived from vertebrates, with humans as an obligatory host. For this reason they are described as anthropozoonoses. Symptoms result from local hypersensitivity reactions to the worm and its scolex, and altered gut motility due to the physical mass of the worm. Patients often become aware of proglottids in their faeces.

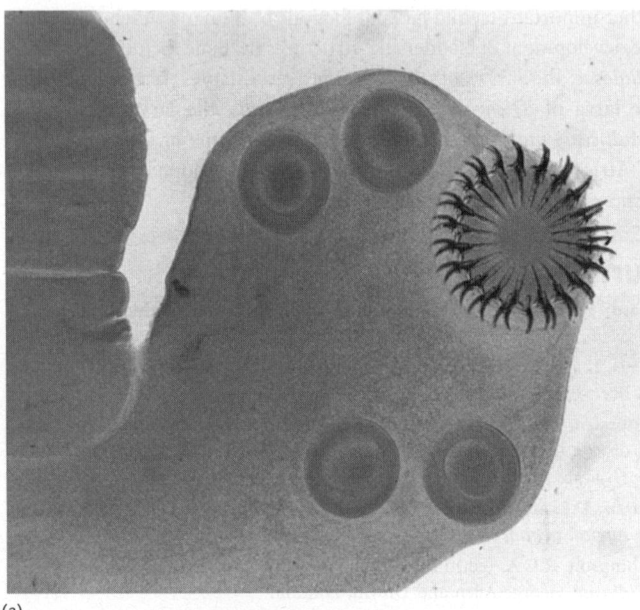

(a)

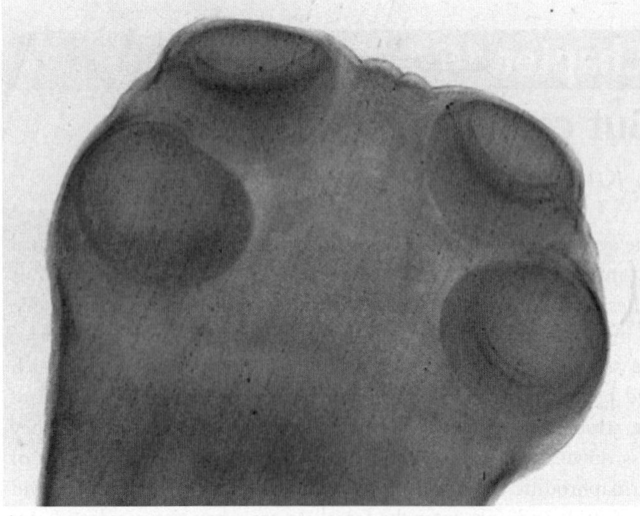

(b)

Fig. 1 (a) *Taenia solium* showing scolex with four suckers and a double row of hooks (×250). (b) *Taenia saginata* showing scolex with four suckers and no hooks (×250).
((a) and (b) by courtesy of Professor V. Zaman.)

Taenia saginata

Epidemiology

The beef tapeworm is prevalent where cattle have access to human faeces and where humans eat undercooked beef. The highest prevalence is in Africa, the Middle East, South America, and South-east Asia. Prevalence is now very low in the United States, Canada, and Australia. It still persists endemically in western Europe; but eastwards prevalence increases progressively.

Gravid proglottids are passed at defecation, often in short chains; free eggs also occur in faeces. The whitish proglottids, approximately 2–3 cm long, are actively motile, elongating, and contracting. Eggs persist on pasture for many months and survive most forms of sewage treatment. Cattle have access to human faeces on farms, at camp sites and recreation areas, and on railway lines. Infected herdsmen can initiate epizootics. Eggs may be dispersed by insects and birds.

In cattle, cysticerci occur in striated muscle; they are whitish, ovoid, and measure 8 × 5 mm; they contain an invaginated protoscolex with no hooks. They become infective within 12 weeks and remain viable in the living host for 2 years; they are viable in stored, chilled meat for several weeks but are killed at −20°C within 1 week. The prepatent period in humans is 3 months and worms may live 30 years. Cattle develop protective immunity to new infection. Prevalence in cattle is best estimated by carcass inspection.

Clinical features

Most worms are solitary; multiple worms are more common in high-transmission areas and probably arise by simultaneous infection. Most patients are first aware of the worm by seeing proglottids on faeces or experiencing active worm migration through the anus. Many have no other symptoms, but others complain of nausea and upper abdominal pains, often relieved by food. A few patients eat to relieve symptoms. In children, impaired appetite can have nutritional consequences. Pruritus ani and anxiety responses are common. The worm may be visible on small bowel barium studies. Proglottids are found in a variety of surgical specimens including resected appendices and the gall bladder; occasionally they obstruct the small intestine, pancreatic duct, or bile duct. After gut perforation they can occur in the peritoneum.

Diagnosis

The typical eggs may be found in faeces, but this is an insensitive method; perianal swabs are also useful. Eggs are indistinguishable from those of *T. solium*; patients should be asked to bring worm specimens. Unless the proglottid is fully gravid the number of uterine branches is an unreliable diagnostic character. In human surveys in endemic areas a 24-h faecal collection after an anthelminthic will give the most reliable prevalence.

Treatment and control

Niclosamide, 2 g, is given to adults and older children as a single morning dose on an empty stomach; the tablets should be chewed. Children of 2–6 years should receive 1 g, and those under 2 only 500 mg. The alternative is praziquantel, 10–20 mg/kg as a single dose after a light breakfast. After either drug the proximal part of the worm disintegrates in the gut and the scolex cannot be found. Failure of proglottids to reappear within 3–4 months indicates cure.

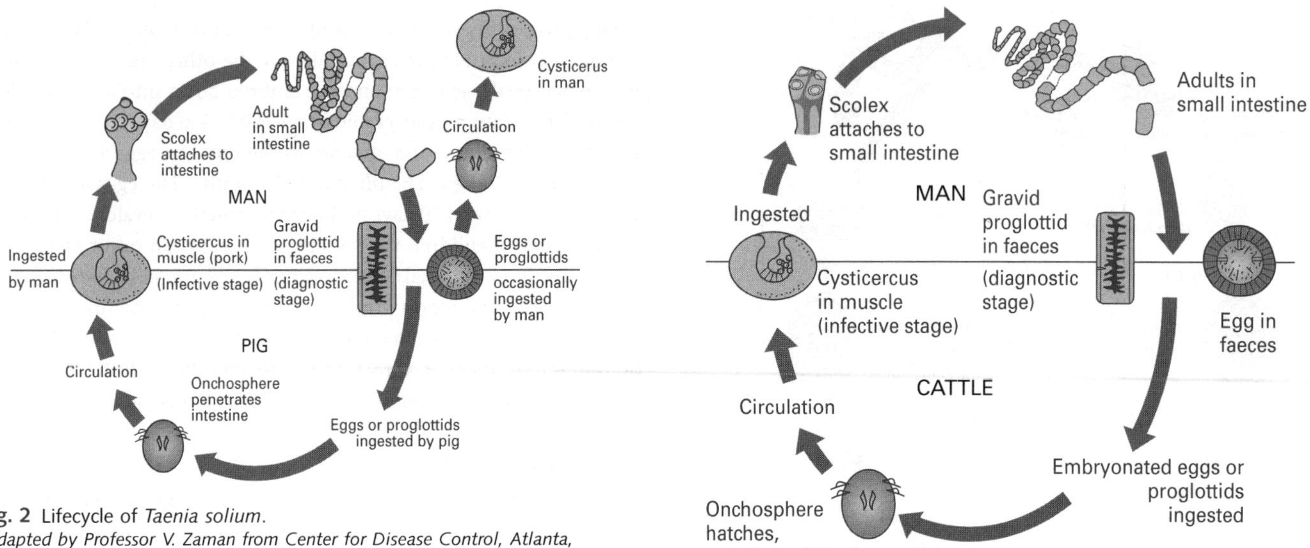

Fig. 2 Lifecycle of *Taenia solium*.
(Adapted by Professor V. Zaman from Center for Disease Control, Atlanta, Georgia, USA.)

Fig. 3 Lifecycle of *Taenia saginata*.
(Adapted by Professor V. Zaman from Center for Disease Control, Atlanta, Georgia, USA.)

Health education concerning raw beef, meat inspection, sanitation and hygiene on cattle farms, and proper sewage treatment and disposal are all effective measures. Mass treatment of herd contacts, or whole adult populations, are the most effective short-term measures when endemicity is high. *T. saginata* causes great economic loss to the beef industry in some developing countries.

Taenia solium

Epidemiology

The pork tapeworm is generally much less common than the beef tapeworm. Its clinical importance relates to cysticercosis (see Chapter 16.107), the occurrence of larval forms in human tissue. This arises when eggs hatch in the upper gut and humans becomes an accidental intermediate host. *T. solium* is now very rare in North America and western Europe, but it remains endemic in sub-Saharan Africa, China, India, and other parts of Asia. High prevalences occur in Mexico and several South American countries. Pig cysticerci are most numerous in the tongue, masseter, heart, and diaphragm, but also occur in the brain. When eaten by humans in undercooked pork the worms mature in 5–12 weeks.

Internal autoinfection from disrupted proglottids is a rare cause of cysticercosis. Conditions favouring this condition include poor personal hygiene, which facilitates external autoinfection and contaminated fingers among food handlers. Faecal pollution of the peridomestic environment, irrigation water or cultivated vegetables are also important. In parts of Africa, tapeworm proglottids are used in traditional medicine. In the absence of these factors, *T. solium* can be endemic with only very sporadic cases of cysticercosis. Cysticercosis is a major health problem in Mexico, some South American countries, and to a lesser extent in Africa and Asia. In 1969, *T. solium* was introduced from Bali into the highlands of

Table 1 Major gut cestodes infecting man

	Taenia saginata (beef tapeworm)	*Taenia solium* (pork tapeworm)	*Hymenolepis nana* (dwarf tapeworm)
Intermediate hosts	Cattle, water buffalo, other bovids, reindeer	Pig, wild boar. Accidentally in man	None
Length	4–12 m	3–5 m	25–40 mm
Number of proglottids	2000 (mean)	700–1000	200 (mean)
Gravid proglottid	Longer than wide 20–30×5–7 mm	Longer than wide 18–25×5–7 mm	Transverse 0.8×0.2 mm
Scolex	No rostellum, no hooks	Rostellum with single circlet of 20–30 minute hooks	Rostellum with double circlet of 22–32 large and small hooks
Gravid uterus	15–20 lateral branches	7–13 lateral branches	Bilobed
Testes	800–1200	394–534	3
Ovary	2-lobed	3-lobed	2-lobed
Egg (contains onchosphere embryo)	Radially striated shell, 31–40 μm in diameter	Radially striated shell, 31–40 μm in diameter	Oval, 30–47 μm long; two membranes; 4–8 filaments arise from each pole of inner membrane

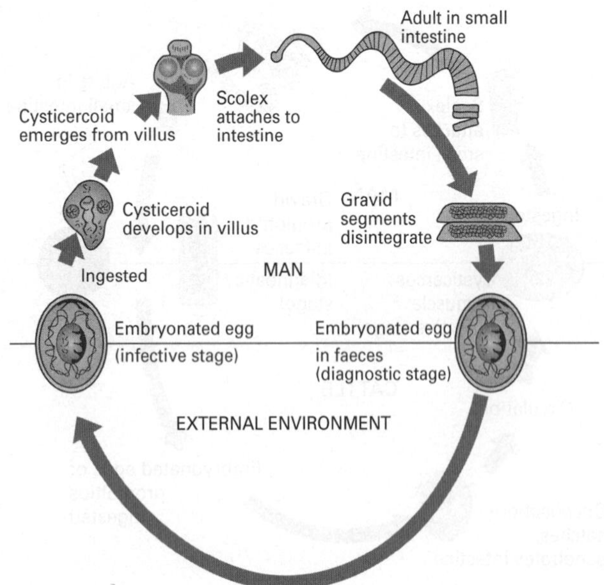

Fig. 4 Lifecycle of *Hymenolepis nana*.
(Adapted by Professor V. Zaman from Center for Disease Control, Atlanta, Georgia, USA.)

Indonesian New Guinea, where the disease is now one of great importance.

Pathology of cysticercosis

Cysts occur especially in striated muscle, subcutaneous tissue, the nervous system, and the eye. Many remain clinically silent until the parasite dies after 3–5 years, when vigorous inflammatory and hypersensitivity reactions may occur; later lesions may calcify. In the brain, particularly in the subarachnoid and the ventricular system, atypical racemose cysts may occur. They appear as irregular or grape-like clusters of cysts that have no protoscolex; they can be mistaken pathologically for non-parasitic cysts.

Clinical features and diagnosis of adult worm infections

Symptoms due to the adult worms are similar to those of *T. saginata* but are often milder and not associated with pruritus ani; proglottids do not actively migrate through the anus. Adult worm infection is detected as for *T. saginata.* Methods for detecting faecal antigen are available and have great potential use in epidemiological studies.

Treatment and control

Adult worms are treated as for *T. saginata.* Drugs causing vomiting must be avoided; it should be remembered that the faeces will be potentially highly infective for several days, both for the patient and attendants. For the treatment of cysticercosis, see Chapter 16.107. Control measures are similar to those of *T. saginata* but local risk factors for human cysticercosis must receive special attention.

Hymenolepis nana

The dwarf tapeworm is the most common cestode in humans; it is also the smallest. When worm loads are high it causes more gut pathology than any other species. It is common in most developing and tropical countries. The lifecycle normally involves only humans (Fig. 4). Fully embryonated infective eggs are passed in the faeces; gravid proglottids normally disintegrate completely in the gut. Infection is commonly direct, but also by the other faecal–oral routes. Eggs hatch in the jejunum and the embryo bores into a villus where it transforms into a cysticercoid larva. After 4–6 days it re-enters the gut, everts the scolex, and attaches to the mucosa; eggs appear in the faeces within 12 days. The lifespan is 3 months. The eggs are delicate and survive less than 10 days in the environment. Prevalence is usually much higher in children than adults; outbreaks can occur in families and institutions. External autoinfection is common in high-risk groups and enables high worm loads to build up. In addition, internal autoinfection occurs when there is gut stasis or retroperistalsis. Because of the importance of direct transmission, this infection may be common in arid environments such as Western Australia.

Clinical features

In heavily infected people, especially children, up to 1000 or more worms may be present. Mucosal damage caused by both larval and adult worms leads to protein loss and sometimes malabsorption. Abdominal pains and anorexia are common. Immunosuppressant or steroid therapy, particularly in lymphoma patients, can lead to the development of bizarre cystic larval forms in the gut wall, mesenteric nodes, liver, and lungs. A similar condition can be produced in immunosuppressed mice.

Diagnosis and treatment

Eggs can be detected in faeces using concentration methods. Proglottids are rarely found in faeces, except after treatment.

Praziquantel in a single dose of 25 mg/kg is the most effective drug. If niclosamide is used, a 7-day course is needed to ensure that larval stages are killed when they re-enter the gut lumen. The dose on the first day is as for *T. saginata*; on the remaining days one-half of this dose is given. Relapses often result from persistence of eggs in the patient's environment.

Accidental gut cestodes (see also OTM3, pp. 962–4)

These have arthropods as intermediate hosts, the larval cysticercoid stage being in the haemocele; the definitive host becomes infected by eating the arthropod intentionally, or accidentally. The means by which humans become infected is sometimes not clear, but fleas, small beetles, and mites are easily overlooked in food. Many species have been recorded in humans, most are rare but three have a worldwide distribution.

Dipylidium caninum infection occurs in children who have groomed their cat or dog and ingested fleas or lice. Worms measure 10–70 cm; proglottids are elongate with a double set of sex organs, they migrate through the anus. *H. nana fraterna* is the murine strain of the human parasite which it resembles; but insects are a necessary intermediate host. The rat tapeworm *H. diminuta,* which measures 20–60 cm in length and has very transverse proglottids is common in rodents but usually rare in humans.

Recognition of accidental gut cestodes is of epidemiological interest and may indicate potential transmission of other zoonotic pathogens. It is certain that these parasites are under-reported. Unusual proglottids or eggs should be preserved in formol saline and sent to a parasitologist.

Further reading

Pawlowski, Z. and Schultz, M.G. (1972). Taeniasis and cysticercosis (*Taenia saginata*). *Advances in Parasitology*, **10**, 269–343.

Chapter 16.107

Cysticercosis

D. Overbosch

Introduction and lifecycle (Fig. 1)

Cysticercosis is caused by the larval stage of the pork tapeworm, *Taenia solium*. The adult tapeworm lives in the human small bowel and each proglottid produces thousands of eggs. For further development, *Taenia* spp. need an intermediate host, which for *T. solium* is the pig. The eggs are ingested by pigs when they feed on human waste contaminated by faeces. When the eggs are digested, the larvae are liberated (onchospheres). They penetrate the intestinal wall and are disseminated throughout the body. They develop in about 2 months into cysts in the muscles (meat!) and brain of the pigs. The cysts, which contain the head (scolex) of the tapeworm, are called cysticercus cellulosae. Humans are infected by eating undercooked pork (barbecued!) containing cysticerci.

People contract cysticercosis after ingestion of *T. solium* eggs, usually in contaminated food or in about 10 per cent of cases by autoinfection (anus–hand–mouth). The onchospheres travel from the gut via the bloodstream through the liver to encyst throughout the body.

The incubation period varies from several months to up to 30 years, average 5 years. Cysticerci may survive for up to 10 years in the body. *T. solium* cysticercosis is associated with poor hygienic conditions and a lack of meat inspection. Central America (Mexico), South America, parts of Africa, India, and South-east Asia are endemic areas. Cysticercosis does not occur in Islamic countries via the intermediate host, as pork is not eaten there. An increasing number of cases of cysticercosis are found in industrialized countries (e.g. USA, Australia, and Europe) due to increased travel into and immigration from the Third World.

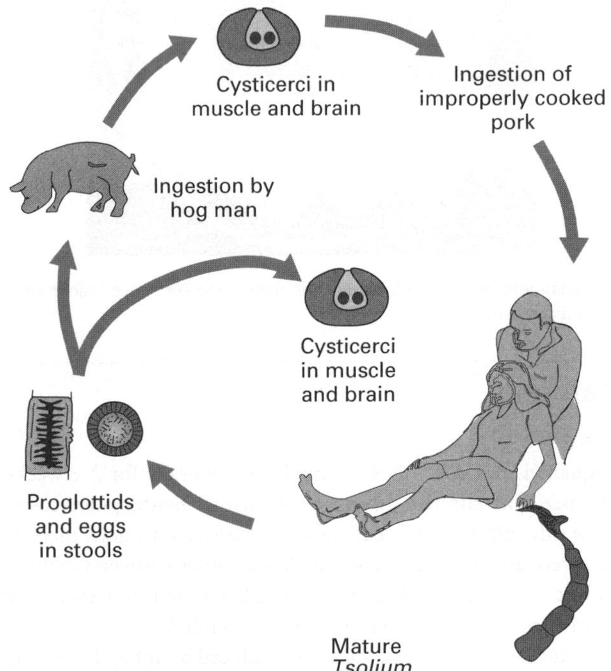

Fig. 1 Lifecycle of Taenia solium (after Overbosch (1992))

Table 1 Classification of neurocysticercosis

Active	Inactive
Arachnoiditis (48.4)	Parenchymal calcifications (57.6)
Meningeal inflammation (25.7)	Meningeal fibrosis (3.8)
Parenchymal cysts (13.2)	
Vasculitis (2.3)	
Mass effect (1.0)	
Intraventricular (0.7)	
Spinal cysts (0.7)	

Occurrence (percentages) in parentheses.

Pathogenesis and clinical pattern

Neurocysticercosis (Table 1)

The clinical picture ranges from asymptomatic infection to severe neurological disease. Cysticerci may lodge in the cortex, ventricles, or basal cisterns.

Neurocysticercosis can be 'active', associated with living and degenerating parasites or 'inactive' arising from the effects of the resulting granulomas, calcifications, or fibrosis.

The most common presenting symptom is epilepsy, especially when cysts are in the cortex. When arachnoiditis blocks the basal cisterns or cysts block the interventricular foramina hydrocephalus develops. Clusters of cysts, like bunches of grapes, in the basal cisterns may cause basal meningitis and cranial nerve dysfunction. Multiple frontal cysts cause dementia, especially in children. Brain infarcts are attributed to vasculitis. Epilepsy and focal neurological deficits occur in both active and inactive disease, depending upon the inflammatory reaction induced within the host or the presence of scar formation or calcification. Subarachnoidal fibrosis, a sequel of arachnoiditis, may result in hydrocephalus and permanent cranial nerve dysfunction. Spinal cysticercosis can cause compression resulting in paresis, radicular symptoms, or cauda equina syndrome.

Muscular and subcutaneous cysticercosis

Cysts frequently go unrecognized, unless they cause discomfort or nerve dysfunction. Firm, round, painless, bean-sized subcutaneous nodules may be palpable. Radiographs reveal multiple calcifications in the muscles (Fig. 2). In India, massive infection results in a syndrome of pseudohypertrophy of the calves and cardiac involvement, together with features of neurocysticercosis including intractable epilepsy, spinal cord lesions, and unilateral blindness.

Ocular cysticercosis

This occurs in about 25 per cent of all patients with cysticercosis. The parasite probably enters the eye via the posterior ciliary artery and lodges in the macular part of the subretinal space. It may reach the vitreous cavity after perforation of the retina. Ocular cysticercosis

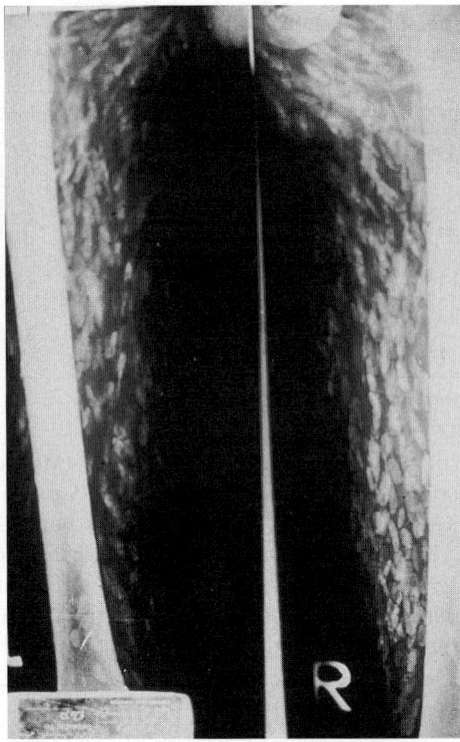

Fig. 2 Calcified cysticercus as seen on a plain radiograph of the thigh.

may lead to severe impairment of vision, blindness, or atrophy of the eye. The patient may experience blurring of vision and may notice slow movements of the parasite, often induced by light.

Computed tomography (CT) and magnetic resonance imaging (MRI), and specific serological reactions against *T. solium* cysticercosis are the mainstay in the diagnosis. CT is especially helpful in detecting cysticerci, which show up as hypodense areas in which the head of the scolex can often be discerned (Fig. 3). Degenerating lesions produce contrasting enhancing ring images. Old, inactive lesions are seen as calcified, hyperdense spots (Fig. 3) and the ventricles may be enlarged. MRI with gadolinium contrasts can detect active neurocysticerci (Fig. 4).

Serological tests are useful. EIA varies in sensitivity and specificity and shows occasional false-positive reactions in patients with cerebral tumours. The enzyme-linked immunoelectrotransfer blot has sensitivity and specificity approaching 100 per cent.

For immunodiagnosis, serum is preferred to cerebrospinal fluid, which may be normal or reveal lymphocytic pleocytosis, sometimes with eosinophilia. An elevated opening pressure, high protein, and low glucose concentration are other non-specific findings.

Differential diagnosis

This includes cerebral tumours or metastases, benign intracranial hypertension, cerebral toxoplasmosis (especially in patients with acquired immune deficiency syndrome) and, if calcification is seen, tuberculoma. Arteriovenous malformations, echinococcosis, syphilitic gumma, bacterial or amoebic cerebral abscesses, paragonimiasis, and cerebral localizations of schistosomiasis (especially *S. japonicum*) may also be considered. Muscular calcifications also occur in trichinosis. Cystic lesions of the eye, other than cysticercosis, may be due to echinococcosis or coenuriasis (caused by larva of *T. multiceps*).

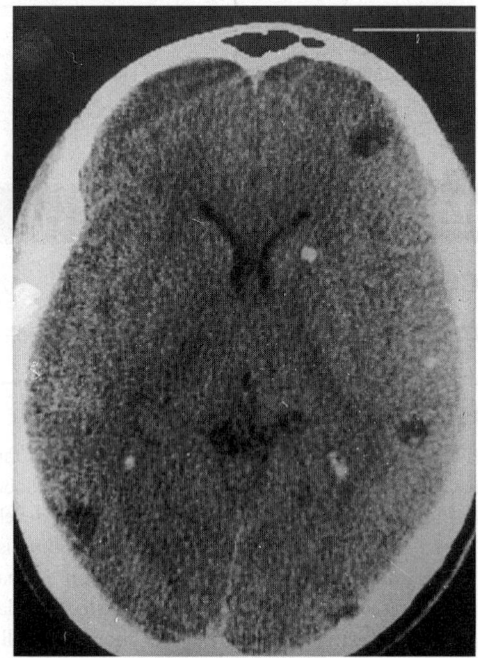

Fig. 3 CT scan of the brain, showing active and calcified lesions simultaneously
(by courtesy of Dr. T. E. Nash, National Institutes of Health, Bethesda, MD, USA).

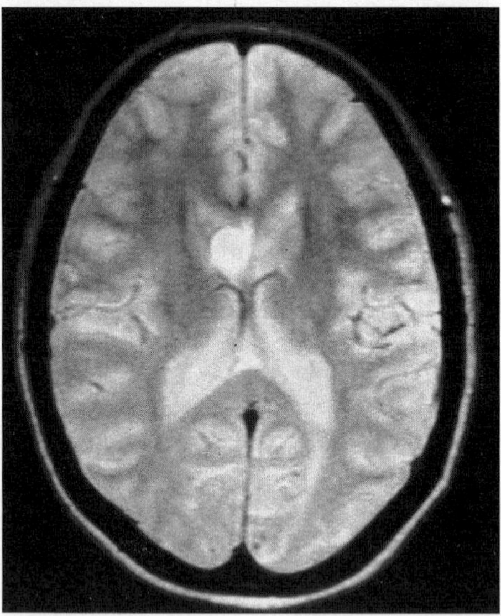

Fig. 4 Magnetic resonance image of the brain showing active lesions of neurocysticercosis.

Treatment

Drug therapy

Praziquantel in a dose of 50–70 mg/kg a day orally for 2–3 weeks is 60–80 per cent effective against parenchymal neurocysticercosis. It has few side-effects, but in patients with massive infections there may be a severe inflammation around degenerating cysticerci. This can aggravate symptoms and lead to cerebral oedema and even death. Glucocorticosteroid prophylaxis is recommended.

The bioavailability of praziquantel is reduced by antiepileptic drugs, which are known to induce its metabolism in the liver. This may be blocked by a P450 cytochrome inhibitor such as cimetidine.

Albendazole is 80–90 per cent effective against parenchymal neurocysticercosis but it has more side-effects than praziquantel on bone marrow and liver and is mutagenic and teratogenic. The generally accepted dose is 15 mg/kg per day orally for 15 days. Praziquantel and albendazole are equally ineffective against intraventricular or meningeal cysticerci. Muscular and subcutaneous cysticercosis can be treated quite successfully with either drug.

Surgical treatment

Drug therapy has largely replaced neurosurgery for neurocysticercosis. However, intraventricular cysts causing obstruction may need surgical removal. Fibreoptic ventriculoscopy is a useful technique. Shunting is sometimes necessary for hydrocephalus. Spinal cord decompression or laminectomy may relieve paresis or radicular symptoms. Surgery remains the treatment of choice for ocular cysticercosis.

Course and prognosis

Mortality of 30–50 per cent in the first 10 years after the onset of symptoms has been greatly reduced by chemotherapy, as has the frequency of seizures.

Further reading

Carpio, A., Santillan, F., Leon, P., Flores, C., and Hauser W. A. (1995). Is the course of neurocysticercosis: modified by treatment with antihelminthic agents? *Archives of Internal Medicine*, **155**, 1982–8.

Martinez, H. R., Rangel-Guerra, R., Arredondo-Estrada, J. H., Marfil, A., and Onofre, J. (1995). Medical and surgical treatment of neurocysticercosis a magnetic resonance study of 161 cases. *Journal of the Neurological Sciences*, **130**, 25–34.

Overbosch, D. (1992). Neurocysticercosis. An introduction with special emphasis on new developments in pharmacotherapy. *Schweizerische Medizinische Wochenschrift*, **122**, 893–8.

Chapter 16.108

Diphyllobothriasis and sparganosis

Seung-Yull Cho

Diphyllobothriasis

The most important intestinal infection with tapeworms of the genus *Diphyllobothrium* is caused by the broad or fish tapeworm, *D. latum*.

Biology and epidemiology

Infection is from consumption of raw freshwater fish (pike, turbot, perch, salmonids) containing plerocercoid larvae (1–1.5 cm long) in their muscles and peritoneal cavity. In the human intestine these larvae develop into adults (usually one per person) 5–6 m long and 0.8–1.5 cm wide. Adults produce a million eggs, 65 × 45 mm in diameter, each day. In fresh water, eggs hatch into swimming coracidia taken up by zooplankters (*Cyclops strenuus, Eudiaptomus gracilis*) and develop into procercoid larvae. These larvae infect fish, which in turn are eaten by larger salmonid fish, in which the plerocercoid develops.

The prevalence of diphyllobothriasis may be as high as 80 per cent in the Baltic, especially Finland, and Siberia. The infection is also reported in Switzerland, Italy, North America, China, Korea, and Japan. Infection can be prevented by freezing fish at −18°C or below for 1 day.

Clinical manifestations

Abdominal discomfort, fatigue, diarrhoea alternating with constipation, dizziness, and urticaria may be the vague presenting symptoms. Rarely, a tapeworm may be vomited up or a mass of worms may cause intestinal obstruction. Strips of gravid segments, 10–80 cm long, may be seen in the stools. Pernicious anaemia associated with *D. latum* infection produces typical haematological and neurological disorders.

Diagnosis and treatment

Racial and geographical origin and predilection for raw fish provide the clue to a diagnosis that can be confirmed by identifying the characteristic eggs in stool. Tapeworm segments are the best material for morphological identification.

Single doses of niclosamide (2 g) or praziquantel (10 mg/kg body weight) are effective. Identification of an expelled scolex confirms a complete cure.

Sparganosis

This is a zoonotic infection in which larval tapeworms of *Spirometra mansoni* or *S. mansonoides* invade a variety of tissues and organs.

Biology

The sparganum is a white, slender, ribbon-shaped, moving plerocercoid larva, 1–100 cm long, with transverse wrinklings and peristaltic waves. It occurs in terrestrial vertebrates. When these animals are eaten by carnivorous mammals, the sparganum matures to an adult in the small intestine. Within 5–6 days adult worms produce operculated eggs. These hatch into swimming coracidia which are taken up by freshwater *Cyclops leuckarti* in which they develop into procercoid larvae. When the procercoid is ingested by terrestrial vertebrates including humans, it becomes a sparganum (Fig. 1).

Epidemiology

Humans are infected by eating the procercoid or the sparganum or swallowing an infected cyclops in unfiltered water. Endemic areas

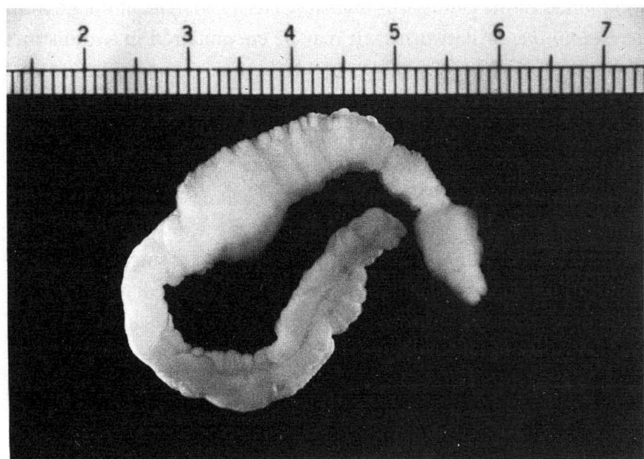

Fig. 1 A sparganum surgically removed from a subcutaneous mass.

include Japan, Korea, China, Vietnam and South-east Asia, where raw poultry, pork, frogs, and snakes are eaten.

Pathology and clinical manifestations

The ingested procercoid larva or sparganum penetrates the intestinal wall to reach the peritoneal cavity and migrates to subcutaneous tissue or muscle in the chest or abdominal walls, limbs, scrotum, or orbit. Migrating worms may cause a lump that appears then spontaneously disappears, only to reappear some weeks or months later at a site remote from the first. There is redness and itching of overlying skin; local bleeding and acute suppurative necrosis may occur. Granulomatous lesions are revealed by imaging in the brain and spinal canal. The sparganum may survive more than 5 years in an infected individual.

Diagnosis and treatment

Usually, the diagnosis is made incidentally by recovering the worm at surgery. Preoperative diagnosis of cerebral sparganosis can be made confidently when computed tomography shows an enhancing nodule that changes shape or position, calcifications, and degeneration of white matter, together with positive specific antibody in serum and cerebrospinal fluid.

Excision is curative but no drugs are known to be effective.

Further reading

von Bonsdorff, B. (1977). *Diphyllobothriasis in man.* Academic Press, London.

Chang, K.H., Chi, J.G., Cho, S.Y., Han, M.H., Han, D.H., and Han, M.C. (1992). Cerebral sparganosis: analysis of 34 cases with emphasis on CT features. *Neuroradiology,* 34, 1–8.

Trematodes (flukes)

Chapter 16.109

Schistosomiasis

A. E. Butterworth and J. E. P. Thomas

Schistosomiasis is the generic term given to disease caused by parasitic blood flukes of the genus *Schistosoma* (Class *Trematoda* of the phylum *Platyhelminthes* or flatworms). It may be encountered in two distinct situations:

- among long-term residents of endemic areas, in whom chronic disease is seen, with damage to the liver and large intestine or to the urinary tract, depending on the species of parasite, and
- among immigrants to endemic areas, or among visitors from non-endemic areas who have been temporarily exposed to infection and who have subsequently returned home. In such individuals, acute schistosomiasis may be seen; this needs immediate treatment, to avoid the possibility of rare but serious sequelae such as transverse myelitis.

Aetiology

Three major species (*Schistosoma mansoni, S. haematobium,* and *S. japonicum*) and two minor species (*S. intercalatum* and *S. mekongi*) affect humans. Many other species affect domestic and wild mammals and birds, but do not infect humans, although their cercariae may penetrate the skin and cause a local itchy reaction (cercarial dermatitis).

All species require two hosts.

- In the *definitive* vertebrate host, sexual maturation and mating of the adult worms occur. In the case of *S. japonicum,* alternative vertebrate hosts can include cattle, water buffalo, pigs, dogs, and various rodents: these serve as important *reservoirs* of infection. Reservoir hosts, including baboons and cane rats, are less important for *S. mansoni*; they are unimportant for *S. haematobium.*
- In the *intermediate* invertebrate host, which is invariably a snail, asexual replication occurs. Different genera of snails serve as intermediate hosts for different schistosome species. The hosts of *S. mansoni* and *S. haematobium* are aquatic snails of the genera *Biomphalaria* and *Bulinus* respectively. These are commonly found in lakes, pools, irrigation canals, or slowly flowing streams or rivers. In contrast, *Oncomelania,* the intermediate host of *S. japonicum,* is an amphibious snail, found not only in open bodies of water but also more widely in rice paddies or damp, marshy ground.

An infected snail releases up to 1000 cercariae each day. These infective larvae, about 200 μm long, can survive in water for up to 24 h before penetrating directly into the skin of the human host, where they transform into young schistosomes or schistosomula. They then migrate via the blood stream, initially to the lungs and eventually to the hepatic portal system, where they mature into adult worms form pairs, and take up their final position in the small venules of the inferior mesenteric vein (*S. mansoni* and *S. japonicum*) or vesical plexus (*S. haematobium*).

Individual worms live for 3–8 years, depending on the species. During this time, the female worm lays eggs at a rate of several hundred to several thousand per day. Some eggs are trapped in the tissues, causing disease, while others pass out into the excreta (urine or faeces, depending on the species). Eggs hatch on contact with fresh water, releasing a free-living larva, the miracidium, which is infective for the appropriate snail intermediate host. Within the snail, the parasite replicates asexually: cercariae are released after about 1 month, and infected snails can remain alive and release cercariae for a further 1–2 months.

Epidemiology

Schistosomiasis has been reported from 74 countries, with *S. mansoni* being found mainly in Africa, South America, and the Caribbean, *S. haematobium* in Africa and the Middle East, and *S. japonicum* in South-east Asia, especially China and the Philippines (Fig. 1). Approximately 500–600 million people throughout the world, mainly living in poor conditions and exposed to numerous other infections, are potentially exposed to schistosomiasis, and it is estimated that 200 million are actually infected.

The adult worms do not replicate within the human host. Each cercaria has the potential to develop into a single worm; infection is acquired cumulatively over a period of years; and each female worm has the capacity to deposit several hundred eggs a day for a period of several years. Because most of the manifestations of disease are attributable to the retention of eggs in the tissues, with ensuing fibrosis, it follows that the severity of disease depends on the actual number of adult worms and the length of time that they are present;

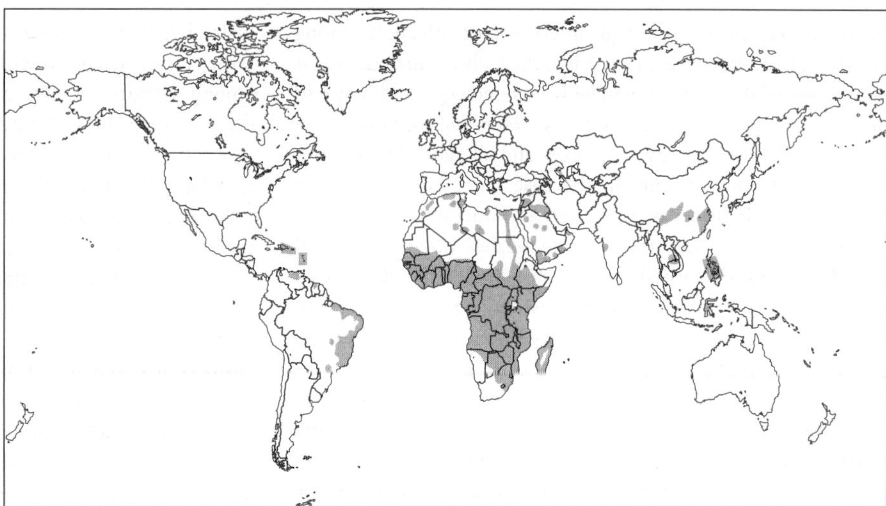

Fig. 1 Global distribution of the schistosomes that affect humans.

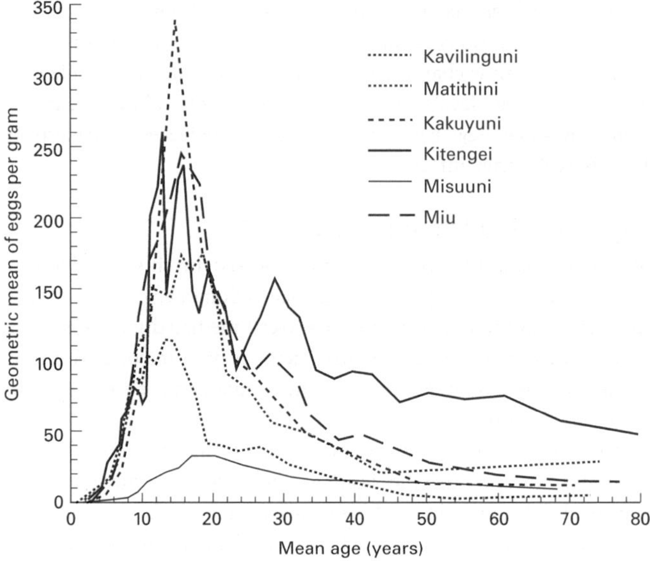

Fig. 2 The characteristically convex age-intensity distribution of *Schistosoma mansoni* infections in six communities in Machakos District, Kenya. *(For source of data see OTM3, p.973.)*

that is, on the *intensity* and *duration* of infection. The distribution of intensities of infection in an endemic community is characteristically overdispersed or aggregated. Even in a community in which the overall prevalence of infection is high, most individuals have only light infections, which cause little or no morbidity, while only a few individuals have very heavy infections that may lead to severe disease.

The shape of the distribution of both prevalence and intensity of infection by age in communities living in endemic areas is characteristically convex (Fig. 2). A typical picture is that young children become infected from about the age of 3–4 years, when they start to have contact with infected water. Both prevalence and mean intensity of infection then rise sharply, reaching a peak during or towards the end of the second decade of life. Thereafter, both prevalence and more markedly intensity of infection decline in the older age groups. There appear to be several reasons for this decline. First, the adult worms from infections acquired early in life, having a limited lifespan of 3–8 years, progressively die. Secondly, in most communities, adults have less contact with infected water than children or teenagers, and are therefore less exposed to new infections. Thirdly, older children and adults progressively develop an immunity to new infections that is mediated particularly by IgE antibodies against adult worm antigens.

One consequence of the relative lack of infection among adults is that, in communities living in endemic areas, schistosomiasis is usually perceived as a disease of children of primary school age. The late sequelae of infection, resulting from fibrosis of egg granulomas, may affect and even kill older children and adults, but these are rare events in comparison with the extensive, although milder, morbidity that is seen in the younger age groups. A typical picture in an area of high transmission is that a majority of young children are infected and have detectable signs or symptoms. In most of these children there is a spontaneous reduction in clinical morbidity as they grow older and lose their worm burden, even without specific treatment. However, in a few, disease progresses to a severe and irreversible state. The introduction into field studies of new techniques, such as large-scale ultrasonography with portable instruments, has revealed that morbidity is greater than was previously thought. Thus, some 20 per cent of those infected with *S. haematobium* may have moderate hydronephrosis, while 10–30 per cent of those with *S. mansoni* or *S. japonicum* may have chronic liver disease. However, the proportion of individuals that go on to develop severe morbidity or to die as a result of their infection cannot be stated with accuracy, as it varies markedly from area to area.

A very different picture is seen in new irrigation schemes or in naïve immigrants or visitors to an endemic area, including foreign tourists and temporary workers. In such individuals, severe acute disease may develop at any age as a consequence of even light infection, which must therefore be taken seriously. This is particularly marked with *S. japonicum* infection, a striking example being reported in 1950 from Jiangsu Province, China, when 'acute schistosomiasis' affected 7000 villagers, of whom 1335 died. However, severe acute schistosomiasis can also occur with *S. mansoni* and *S. haematobium* infections. In 1984, for example, it was reported that 18 touring students swam in an infested lake in Kenya, of whom 15 showed manifestations of acute schistosomiasis, while two developed acute transverse myelitis and paraparesis. There are similar, although less dramatic, accounts of acute disease following bathing in inland lakes from Malawi, Zimbabwe, and Brazil, and the possibility of schistosomiasis should always be born in mind if there is a history of potential exposure.

A further consequence of the high intensities of infection among children living in endemic areas is that it is they who contribute most to contamination of the environment with excreted eggs, and hence to continued transmission. In the case of *S. haematobium*, contamination occurs when urine is voided (by both sexes and all ages) directly into water, especially during bathing. In the case of *S. mansoni* and *S. japonicum*, defecation into water is relatively uncommon. Instead, faeces are deposited, for example, among bushes on the banks of streams, and the eggs are carried into the stream either by rain or by mammals, birds, or flies. Alternatively, eggs may be introduced into the water by the washing of soiled clothes or by washing the anal region following defecation.

In many circumstances, and in particular in communities that have been settled for some generations in an endemic area, the parasite and its human host have reached a state of relative equilibrium: transmission occurs, but at low levels, and severe disease may be uncommon. This has led to the view that schistosomiasis is a disease of minor public health importance. However, this is an overoptimistic attitude. An increasing pressure on land usage throughout much of the tropics leads continuously to attempts to develop new land for agricultural purposes, with the construction of dams and other large or small irrigation schemes. Such projects frequently create conditions that are ideal for the transmission of schistosomiasis and, as immigrants to such schemes or migrant workers employed on a temporary basis may come from non-endemic areas, they rapidly acquire heavy and clinically severe infections. In Africa in particular, schistosomiasis remains a disease of considerable public health, as well as individual, importance.

Pathogenesis and clinical features

The underlying pathology is similar for all species of schistosome, differences in clinical manifestations being attributable to different anatomical locations. Four main stages can be identified, each with distinct pathological and clinical features.

Stage of invasion

Cercarial dermatitis or 'swimmer's itch' occurs with both human and non-human schistosomes. It is therefore encountered in non-endemic areas, such as Western Australia and the Great Lakes of Canada, as well as in endemic areas. The entry of cercariae through the skin in previously exposed individuals provokes a hypersensitivity reaction, with both an immediate element occurring within 15 min, and a delayed element after 12–48 h, with an intense eosinophil infiltrate. An itchy, erythematous, maculopapular rash with varying degrees of oedema occurs on areas of skin that were exposed. A history of recent exposure and the distribution of the rash help to distinguish it from contact dermatitis, scabies, insect bites, and impetigo. It resolves spontaneously.

Stage of maturation: acute schistosomiasis

As the schistosomula migrate through the lungs they may elicit an intense IgE reaction with cough, wheeze, and sometimes an eosinophilic pneumonia. A similar pulmonary response can occur when heavy infestations with hepatosplenic disease are treated and the dead worms are swept into the lungs (the 'lung shift') through anastomotic channels.

People exposed to infection for the first time may also develop an acute illness resembling serum sickness, which in some cases is severe or fatal. Originally described in *S. japonicum* infection, as 'Katayama fever', it can also occur with both *S. mansoni* and, as recently described among visitors to Lake Malawi, *S. haematobium*. Although it can occur as early as 9–14 days after exposure, it is more commonly seen soon after egg laying commences, some 5–9 weeks after infection. It may be associated with immune complex formation and deposition following the release of either worm or egg antigens. Typical features include persistent fever (intermittent or remittent with evening peaks), headache, profound malaise, myalgia, arthralgia, and a dry cough. There may be nausea, vomiting, diarrhoea and weight loss, and the liver and spleen may be enlarged and tender. There is usually an eosinophilia, and sometimes an urticarial rash. Patients may become confused or stuporose, and there may be other major neurological consequences, which are described below.

Acute schistosomiasis should be born in mind in the diagnosis of any febrile illness in a traveller returning from the tropics with a history of potential exposure. The differential diagnosis includes other infections, such as malaria, typhus, typhoid, and hepatitis A, as well as many non-infectious conditions. A leucocytosis with an eosinophilia of 10–75 per cent is characteristic of a helminth infection, while total IgE, IgM, and IgG levels and antischistosome antibodies are elevated at an early stage. Eggs become detectable in the faeces or urine from about 6 weeks after infection.

Stage of established infection

This is the stage that is commonly observed in children living in endemic areas. The key process is the deposition of eggs in the tissues, which leads to the development of a T-cell mediated granulomatous reaction, in which tumour necrosis factor plays a major part and in which there is a marked eosinophilic component. This eventually progresses to fibrosis.

The clinical manifestations of granuloma formation depend on the anatomical location of the lesions, and hence on the species of parasite. In the intestinal schistosomiases due to *S. mansoni* or *S. japonicum* infections, eggs are deposited in the large intestine or liver, and the main clinical consequences are hypogastric pain, bloody diarrhoea, and enlargement of the liver and spleen. In the early stages, the enlarged liver is soft and may be tender. However, this stage is frequently asymptomatic. This is a potential danger, as the condition, which is easily treated in the early stages by antischistosomal chemotherapy, can pass unnoticed until the stage of irreversible complications.

In urinary schistosomiasis due to *S. haematobium* infection, eggs are deposited in the bladder and lower urinary tract, and to a lesser extent the rectum. Haematuria, often terminal, is a common presenting symptom, and there may be suprapubic pain, frequency, and dysuria. The prevalence and severity of the haematuria are related to the intensity of egg output and, in communities in which *S. haematobium* is heavily endemic, haematuria among boys is still considered to be part of the normal process of maturation. In addition, ureteric obstruction may occur as a consequence of granulomatous reactions to eggs in either the ureters or the bladder; in contrast to the later, chronic lesions associated with fibrosis, these acute lesions usually reverse spontaneously after antischistosomal chemotherapy. In adult males there may also be testicular pain and discomfort on ejaculation, with a sensation of gritty semen.

Systemic effects are difficult to assess, but can include a low-grade malaise and fatigue. There is some evidence that children infected with schistosomes have reduced growth and physical and cognitive performance.

Stage of late infection

Two processes occur in untreated individuals. On the one hand, eggs are destroyed, most early granulomas are resolved, and the individual spontaneously loses his or her adult worms. On the other hand, however, some granulomas progress to fibrosis which, like the granulomatous reaction that precedes it, is a T-cell-dependent event attributable to the release of soluble mediators. The fibrosis can be extensive, leading to severe and irreversible chronic tissue damage in a minority of older individuals.

In intestinal schistosomiasis, chronic disease may be restricted to the large intestine, with persistent bloody diarrhoea and pain. The differential diagnosis includes irritable bowel syndrome, amoebiasis, giardiasis, other intestinal helminths, ulcerative colitis, Crohn's disease, and tuberculosis, as well as malignancies. The liver may also be affected, with a characteristic presinusoidal periportal fibrosis, referred to as Symmers' fibrosis, that leads to portal hypertension with hepatosplenomegaly. The liver is usually firm, sharp, non-tender, and nodular, with enlargement especially of the left lobe: the spleen may be massively enlarged, and is firm and non-tender. Liver function is usually retained, and the most important consequence is haematemesis following bleeding from oesophageal varices. With repeated bleeding, especially in the presence of associated hepatitis B infection, liver function is reduced, and there is both anaemia and ascites ('decompensated' hepatosplenic disease). The differential diagnosis includes alcoholic or viral cirrhosis (which may well coexist with schistosomal disease), visceral leishmaniasis, and the tropical splenomegaly syndrome associated with recurrent malaria, as well as malignancies.

In urinary schistosomiasis, there is an obstructive uropathy, often associated with calculus formation and secondary infection. Changes in the bladder include calcification, ulceration, and papilloma formation, leading to nocturia, precipitancy, retention of urine, and severe pain. There is a significant association, which may be causal, between chronic *S. haematobium* infection and carcinoma of the bladder. Changes in the ureters may be unilateral or bilateral, with hydronephrosis that may lead to pyonephrosis or renal failure.

Other manifestations

Central nervous system

There are important, albeit relatively uncommon, complications attributable to ectopic eggs. In *S. japonicum* infection, they present as cerebral lesions, usually focal epilepsy. In *S. mansoni* and *S. haematobium* infection, they occur especially during or after acute infection acquired in adulthood, and are therefore of particular concern in visitors to endemic areas. The spinal cord is affected, especially the cauda equina; there is sacral radiculitis with back pain and sensory changes, that may progress to transverse myelitis.

Pulmonary

In hepatosplenic schistosomiasis mansoni, the opening of portosystemic collaterals allows the passage of eggs from the portal vein to the lungs. Granuloma formation and fibrosis then lead to pulmonary hypertension and cor pulmonale, with fatigue, palpitations, dyspnoea, and occasional haemoptysis.

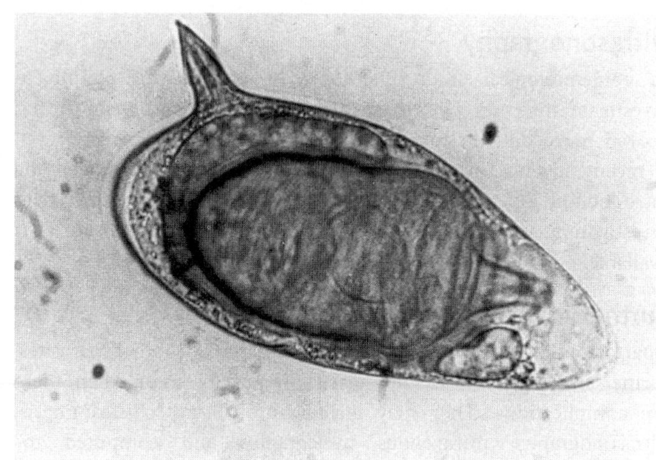

Fig. 3 Egg of *S. mansoni*; note the distinctive lateral spine.

Renal

A chronic glomerulonephritis commonly occurs in chronic *S. mansoni* infections in Brazil. It may present as a nephrotic syndrome, as hypertension, or as simple proteinuria, and may not develop until many years after the onset of hepatosplenic disease.

Miscellaneous

Other late sequelae can include dwarfism and delayed or absent sexual maturation (especially *S. japonicum*, also *S. mansoni*), osteomalacia and lesions of the uterine cervix (*S. haematobium*), chronic dermatitis, and polyarthritis.

Diagnosis and investigations

Diagnosis depends primarily on an appropriate history of exposure and the demonstration of viable eggs, either in the excreta or (for all three species) by rectal biopsy using a Harrison's curette.

Parasitology

Stools can be examined for *S. mansoni* or *S. japonicum* qualitatively in thick smears or by various concentration techniques, and quantitatively by the Kato-Katz method. It is important to examine at least three stools, especially for *S. japonicum*, which tends to produce eggs in clumps. For *S. haematobium* infection, terminal urine specimens collected during the late morning provide the most sensitive indicator; again, three separate samples should be obtained. These are examined for eggs (Fig. 3) following filtration through polycarbonate or polyamide membranes held in an appropriate filter support. Rectal biopsy may prove positive for all three species when stool or urine samples are negative. In *S. haematobium* infections, detection of haematuria or proteinuria by dipstick is a useful additional tool, especially in epidemiological studies.

Immunodiagnosis

An indirect enzyme-linked immunosorbent assay for antibodies against soluble egg antigens (**SEA**) is a useful additional test, especially when rising titres are found. However, it fails to distinguish clearly between present and past infection, and there is extensive cross-reactivity with other helminths. Improved specificity is obtained if a purified fraction (CEF6) of SEA is used. An assay for the detection of circulating schistosome antigens would be much more valuable; such assays have been developed, but are not yet routinely available.

Ultrasonography

In epidemiological studies, although it is relatively simple to investigate infection by systematic stool or urine surveys, it has proved more difficult to assess morbidity at the community level. A recent advance in this area, for all three species, has been the introduction of abdominal ultrasonography as a routine field investigation, using the sensitive portable instruments that are now available.

Further investigations

Apart from a full blood count and a search for other parasites, further investigations are not usually required except when there are complications. They may include, in urinary schistosomiasis, ultrasonography, intravenous pyelography, and computed tomography. In intestinal schistosomiasis, endoscopy, sigmoidoscopy, and ultrasonography may need to be extended to laparoscopy and splenoportography.

Treatment

The drug of choice for all three species is praziquantel, which is both effective and safe, although it is not recommended during the first trimester of pregnancy. There are both species and geographical variations in response, but a single oral dose of 40 mg/kg body weight usually causes at least a 95 per cent reduction in egg output, with complete cure in 70–90 per cent of cases. In heavy *S. japonicum* infections, a total of 60 mg/kg, given in three doses at intervals of 4 h or two doses at intervals of 6–48 h, is preferable. If a complete cure of *S. mansoni* or *S. haematobium* is deemed essential, praziquantel may be given at 20 mg/kg twice daily for 3 days. Side-effects are usually minor, including abdominal pain, which is related to intensity of infection, and urticarial reactions around the lips and eyes. Pulmonary hypersensitivity reactions with bronchospasm and wheezing may occur very occasionally.

Alternative drugs include metrifonate for *S. haematobium*, whose only advantage is its low price (7.5–10 mg/kg body weight, repeated on three occasions at intervals of 14 days), and oxamniquine for *S. mansoni*, although this may cause severe dizziness or epileptiform convulsions (total 15–60 mg/kg according to area, in divided doses at 24 h intervals).

It should be noted that praziquantel is *not* a prophylactic drug, and also that it is not effective against the young migrating schistosomula. A recently infected individual, after an initial treatment, may need to be retreated after 3 months. Effective treatment (i.e. cessation of egg laying) in acute and early schistosomiasis results in complete resolution of disease. Even in chronic schistosomiasis with fibrosis, treatment with praziquantel alone may slowly lead to resolution. In severe late cases, however, additional medical or surgical measures will be required, depending on the organ system involved. In hepatosplenic schistosomiasis mansoni, for example, propranolol has been used to reduce the likelihood of bleeding from oesophageal varices, while endoscopic sclerotherapy or other surgical measures may be required to prevent rebleeding.

The diagnosis and treatment of schistosomiasis in the returning traveller present certain special features. Such travellers should be screened for infection if they are symptomatic, or asymptomatic but potentially exposed. Acute schistosomiasis is common, has potentially dangerous sequelae, and is difficult to diagnose positively: in a majority of cases, neither eggs nor elevated antibody levels can be detected. As praziquantel is safe, it is acceptable to adopt a low threshold for treatment, based on clinical criteria only, once malaria and typhoid have been excluded. If symptoms are severe, patients should be hospitalized and prednisolone (40 mg for 3–5 days) added. The main danger of both acute and established infection is spinal cord disease. If there are suggestive clinical findings, magnetic resonance imaging should be carried out, and treatment started *immediately.* Heavy, chronic infections may occur among individuals returning home from long periods of residence in endemic areas. Apart from specific antischistosomal treatment, such patients may need referral for urological or hepatological investigations.

Prognosis

The prognosis of schistosomiasis depends on the species, the intensity of infection, and the stage at which the infection is detected and treated. In a majority of infected individuals, infection remains asymptomatic or mild, even in the absence of treatment. However, the numbers of individuals who do develop morbidity is sufficiently great, at the level both of the community and of the national health structure, that both treatment of infected individuals and attempts to control transmission (below) are usually warranted.

At the individual level, acute schistosomiasis can be fatal, or can lead to severe residual damage to the central nervous system, but responds well to antischistosomal chemotherapy in conjunction with steroids if started sufficiently early. Early established infections respond extremely well to antischistosomal therapy, leaving little or no residual damage. The main problem about such infections is that, if treatment (especially of young children) is only carried out at the individual level, without attempts to control transmission in the community, then the patient will rapidly become re-exposed and reinfected. Late infections with fibrosis respond less well to specific antischistosomal treatment, although some regression of hepatosplenic disease has been reported. The main purpose of treatment at this stage is to prevent further progression of infection, while the consequences of fibrosis are managed in other ways.

Prevention and control

There are no prophylactic drugs or vaccines available for schistosomiasis, and individual protection against infection depends primarily on avoiding contact with all potentially contaminated fresh water in endemic areas: for example, by avoiding swimming or bathing, and by wearing boots and other waterproof clothing. Water should be boiled before drinking, or left to stand for at least 2 days before use for other purposes such as washing. Should contact with water occur, the skin should be rubbed immediately and vigorously with a towel; the water should not be allowed to evaporate, as this aids cercarial penetration. Soap and alcohol also kill cercariae, and cercaricidal barrier creams can be used.

Thus, prevention of infection in tourists or occasional visitors to an endemic area is relatively straightforward, provided that contact with water is not a necessary part of their work. However, in most endemic areas the local residents do not have the luxury of being able to avoid contact with water. In such areas, the control of schistosomiasis is extremely difficult, and requires a many pronged and integrated attack at the community level.

During recent years, emphasis has switched from control of infection or transmission to control of morbidity. Because morbidity develops primarily in the most heavily infected individuals, the aim is to reduce the mean intensity of infection in a community to levels at which significant morbidity does not occur. Since the introduction of safe and effective drugs, the mainstay of control has been chemotherapy, either of entire communities (mass chemotherapy), or of infected individuals (selective chemotherapy), or of subgroups selectively chosen on the basis of age or intensity of infection (targeted selective chemotherapy). At present, many programmes concentrate on school age children, as they are readily accessible in the primary schools, include the most heavily infected individuals in the community, and contribute most to transmission, but have not yet gone on to develop severe disease. As such children are not immune to reinfection, surveillance and retreatment has to be carried out at intervals of 1–3 years, depending on the area.

An advantage of chemotherapy as a control measure is that, in addition to reducing transmission in the community, it has an immediate impact on infection and illness in individual patients. In addition, other methods of reducing transmission are also valuable. These include snail control through the use of molluscicides, and the use of inexpensive approaches towards the supply of clean water supplies and sanitation. Finally, a key element in any control programme is the close involvement of the community, with extensive health education, especially of children. However, none of the available measures is ideal, and the possible emergence of drug-resistant strains of parasite is a real danger. Alternative measures are being sought, and considerable progress towards a vaccine has been made, although it will be many years before one will be available for routine clinical use.

Further reading

Chen, M.G. and Mott, K.E. (1989). Progress in assessment of morbidity due to *Schistosoma haematobium* infection. A review of the recent literature. *Tropical Diseases Bulletin*, **86**, R1–36.

Hatz, C., Jenkins, J.M., and Tanner, M. (ed.) (1992). Ultrasound in schistosomiasis. *Acta Tropica*, **51**, 1–100.

Jordan, P., Webbe, G., and Sturrock, R.F. (ed.) (1993). *Human schistosomiasis*. CAB International, Wallingford, UK.

World Health Organization (1993). *The control of schistosomiasis: Second Report of the WHO Expert Committee*. WHO Technical Report Series 830. WHO, Geneva

World Health Organization. (1988). *Progress in assessment of morbidity due to* Schistosoma mansoni *infection: a review of recent literature*. WHO/Schisto/88–97, pp. 1–66. WHO, Geneva.

Chapter 16.110

Liver fluke diseases of humans

Swangjai Pungpak and Danai Bunnag

Flukes of the genera *Opisthorchis*, *Clonorchis*, *Fasciola*, and, rarely, *Dicrocoelium* (Table 1) infect the biliary tract of millions of people, especially in eastern Europe and the Far East. Most are asymptomatic.

Opisthorchiasis

Adult *Opisthorchis viverrini* and *O. felineus* flukes live in the distal bile ducts and gallbladder. Fully developed eggs are carried in the bile and passed out in faeces. On reaching water the eggs are eaten by *Bithynia* snails, the first intermediate hosts, in which they hatch. In the snail the miracidia develop further through the stages of sporocyst, redia, and cercaria (Fig. 1). The mature cercariae are released from the snail into the water after 6–8 weeks, and then penetrate the muscle of susceptible freshwater cyprinoid fish or carp to develop into metacercariae. The metacercariae mature and reach an infective stage in 6 weeks. Consumption of infected fish results in infection of the definitive host—humans and other fish-eating mammals, such as cats and dogs. When the metacercariae are liberated by digestion, they enter the duodenum then migrate to the bile ducts where they mature within 4 weeks and begin to produce eggs. The lifespan of these flukes is over 10 years.

Epidemiology (Table 1)

In Thailand, the prevalence of *O. viverrini* is increasing due to the popularity of eating raw fish. In 1991 it was estimated that about 8.7 million Thais harboured the fluke. In some villages, more than 90 per cent of the people are infected, including infants whose diet is supplemented with chopped raw cyprinoid fish (koi pla) from the age of a few weeks. There are about 2.5 million cases of *O. felineus* infection, with a prevalence of up to 8.5 per cent in western Siberia.

Pathology and pathogenesis

In the biliary system, mechanical irritation and toxic substances produced by the flukes and the host's immune response causes epithelial cell hyperplasia, proliferation, and desquamation. In severe infections, there is obstruction of the biliary tract, bile retention,

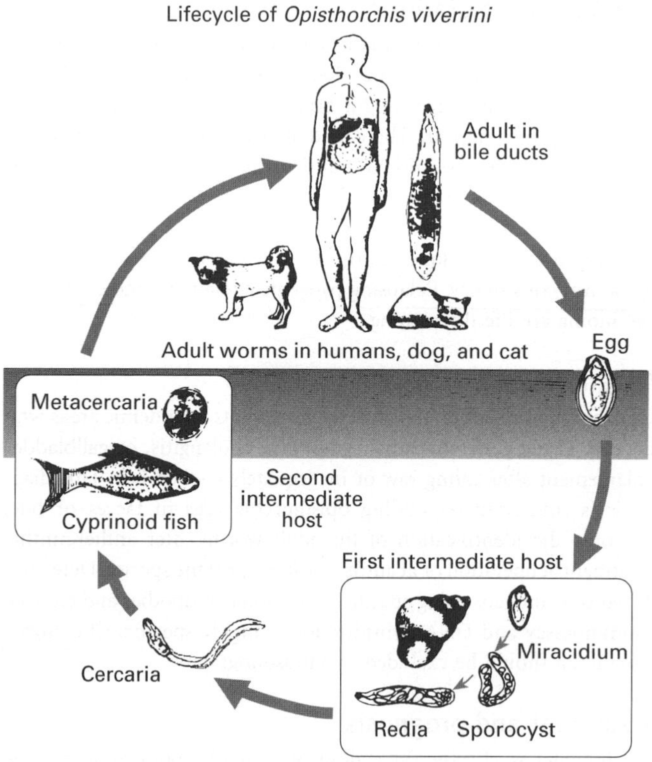

Fig. 1 Lifecycle of *Opisthorchis viverrini*.

Table 1 Human liver flukes

Species	Geographical distribution	Definitive hosts other than man	Source of infection	Size of adults (mm)	Size of ova (μm)
Clonorchis sinensis	Far East	Dog, cat, rat, rabbit	Freshwater fish	10–25 × 3–5	27–35 × 12–19.5
Dicrocoelium dendriticum	Sheep- and cattle-raising areas	Sheep, goat, deer, other herbivorous and omnivorous mammals	Ants (accidentally ingested with food)	6.0–10.0 × 1.5–2.5	36–45 × 22–30
Eurytrema pancreaticum	Japan	Sheep, hare, rabbit	Grasshopper	8–16 × 5.5–8	40–50 × 23–34
Fasciola gigantica	Sheep- and cattle-raising areas	Cattle, water buffalo, herbivorous mammals	Vegetations such as watercress	29–36 × 8	125–157 × 60–100
F. hepatica	Sheep- and cattle-raising areas	Sheep, cattle, herbivorous and omnivorous mammals	Vegetations such as watercress	20–30 × 8–12	130–145 × 70–90
Opisthorchis felineus	Eastern Europe, Vietnam	Dog, cat, rat, pig, beaver, seal, rabbit, and night heron	Freshwater fish	10–18 × 1.25–2.5	26–30 × 10–15
O. viverrini	Thailand, Laos	Dog, cat, piscivorous mammals	Freshwater fish	6.0 × 2.0	26 × 13

papillomatous and adenomatous cholangitis, periductal infiltration with eosinophils and round cells, and fibrosis with necrosis and atrophy of hepatic cells. Intrahepatic bile ducts are uniformly dilated with distal clubbing or cyst formation. The gallbladder is enlarged and contains white bile. Gallstones contain eggs and debris of dead parasites.

At autopsy, cholangitis, cholecystitis, pancreatitis, and cholangiocarcinoma may be found but frank cirrhosis is unusual. As many as 4000 flukes have been found in one patient.

Clinical manifestations

Infection is usually asymptomatic, especially in endemic areas where infection begins early in life. Repeated infections result in accumulation of flukes, reaching a maximum around the fifth decade when symptoms appear. There is dull pain and discomfort in the right hypochondrium, initially transient and later persistent. Other symptoms are lassitude, loss of taste, anorexia, flatulence, diarrhoea, hepatomegaly, weight loss, and mild pedal oedema. The gallbladder is enlarged and functions poorly. The liver is usually enlarged and has a firm consistency. Relapsing pyogenic cholangitis and cholangiocarcinoma are life threatening.

Diagnosis

Opisthorchiasis should be suspected in patients in endemic areas who develop vague gastrointestinal symptoms, cholangitis, or gallbladder enlargement after eating raw or inadequately cooked fish. This diagnosis is supported by finding opisthorchis eggs in faeces or bile, but only the identification of the adult worms after anthelminthic treatment at operation or at autopsy will confirm the species. Detection of parasite antigens using specific monoclonal antibodies and enzyme immunoassay and DNA hybridization is highly specific. Cholangiocarcinoma should be excluded by ultrasonography.

Treatment and prognosis

Praziquantel is effective in a dose of 25 mg/kg body weight three times after meals, or as a single dose of 40–50 mg/kg. Most flukes are expelled dead and damaged with peeling integument; eggs disappear from the stool within 1 week. Symptoms and the enlarged, dysfunctioning gallbladder take a few months to return to normal. To minimize side-effects (headache, dizziness, sleepiness, nausea, and vomiting) the single dose should be given at bed time.

The alternative treatment is mebendazole, 30 mg/kg body weight a day for 3–4 weeks which is more effective than albendazole.

Relapsing pyogenic cholangitis should be treated with antimicrobials. Palliative surgery may be required in complicated cases with obstructive jaundice.

The rare deaths occur in patients with heavy, long-standing infections and result from cholangitis and septic shock or cholangiocarcinoma.

Prevention and control

The practice of eating raw or undercooked fish must be discouraged and sanitation improved. Large-scale chemotherapy with praziquantel reduces transmission in endemic areas.

Clonorchiasis

Clonorchiasis is infection of the biliary tract with the Chinese liver fluke *Clonorchis sinensis* or, more properly, *Opisthorchis sinensis*.

Aetiology

The lifecycle of *Clonorchis* is similar to that of Opisthorchis (see Fig. 1). The first intermediate hosts are hydrobid snails and the second intermediate hosts are cyprinoid fish or carp. Reservoir (definitive) hosts include dogs, cats, mink, rats, and other fish-eating mammals.

Epidemiology

Human clonorchiasis is endemic in Japan, Korea, China, Hong Kong, Taiwan, and Vietnam. It has been reported in the US, Canada, France, Australia, and other countries, because of increased travel and the resettlement of refugees. In the endemic area, fish are kept in ponds fertilized with human and animal faeces. Over 20 million people in China and over 0.5 million in Korea are infected.

Pathology, pathogenesis, clinical manifestations, diagnosis, prognosis, prevention, and control

As for opisthorchiasis. Cholangitis, cholelithiasis, pancreatitis, and cholangiocarcinoma are common potentially fatal complications of chronic infection.

Treatment

The drug of choice is praziquantel, 25 mg/kg body weight after meals three times daily for 1 or 2 days, or as a single does of 40 mg/kg for mass treatment. Albendazole is also effective.

Fascioliasis

This infection is caused by the sheep liver fluke *Fasciola hepatica* or *F. gigantica*. Adult *F. hepatica* live in the large biliary ducts. Eggs, passed in the host's faeces, hatch to release a miracidium which infects a lymnaeid snail, the first intermediate hosts. Cercariae emerge from the snail, encyst on various kinds of aquatic vegetation, swim freely in the water and develop into metacercariae.

A wide range of mammals, the definitive hosts, especially sheep, may become infected when they consume infected vegetation or ingest the encysted metacercariae in water. People are usually infected by eating fresh watercress or drinking contaminated water. Metacercariae excyst in the duodenum and penetrate the intestinal wall to enter the peritoneal cavity. Then they invade the liver capsule and migrate through the parenchyma to the bile ducts.

Epidemiology

Fascioliasis is an important veterinary problem in sheep-raising areas. Human infection is most common where watercress is eaten, including in Britain.

Pathology and pathogenesis

Experimentally excysted metacercariae produce some necrosis of the hepatic parenchyma with fibrosis, cellular infiltration, and abscess formation. Sheep heavily infected with *F. hepatica* develop 'liver rot'. Adult flukes may cause hyperplasia, desquamation, thickening, and dilatation of the bile ducts. A worm load of 600 flukes will kill a sheep.

In humans, exceptionally heavy infection can cause hyperplasia, necrosis, cystic dilation, and leucocytic infiltration of the bile ducts, and subcapsular haematoma. The liver is enlarged, with multiple nodular eosinophilic abscesses. A fluke can block the common bile duct. Wandering flukes in liver parenchyma may result in haemorrhages. Migratory tracks in the liver and other organs are filled with necrotic cellular debris and infiltrated with eosinophils. Outside the liver, flukes calcify or excite granuloma formation.

Each fluke may consume 0.2 ml of blood per day.

Urticaria, granuloma, eosinophilia, and eosinophilic hyperplasia of the bone marrow may be provoked by the fluke's antigens. Various precipitins, haemagglutinins, and other antibodies are detectable in the serum. Serum aminotransferases, alkaline phosphatase, bilirubin, and inflammatory markers may be abnormal.

Clinical manifestations

During the acute migratory period, which may last for several months, patients may experience acute dyspepsia, anorexia, nausea, vomiting, right upper abdominal pain, fever, headache, tender liver enlargement, urticaria, and marked eosinophilia.

During the patent phase, lasting months or years, flukes are lodged in the biliary passage. Usually, there are no symptoms but eggs are detectable in duodenal fluid or stool.

In the obstructive or chronic phase adult flukes inflame and obstruct the bile ducts. Clinical features include right hypochondrial or epigastric pain, dyspepsia, diarrhoea, nausea, vomiting, hepatomegaly, and jaundice. Common findings are eosinophilia, dysproteinaemia, and altered liver function tests. If the extrahepatic bile ducts are occluded the symptoms will be those of cholangitis or cholecystitis. Flukes may cause bleeding into the bile ducts. Prolonged heavy infection can cause sclerosing cholangitis and biliary cirrhosis.

Flukes occasionally migrate to ectopic sites such as the intestinal wall, lungs, heart, brain, and skin, causing pleuritic pain, nodules, or abscesses.

The acute nasopharyngitis known as *halzoun* in Lebanon or *marrara* in Sudan is an allergic response to larval flukes eaten in raw sheep or goat liver. Other causes include the pentastome *Linguatula serrata*, the catfish fluke *Isoparorchis hypselobagri*, and aquatic leeches such as *Limanatis nilotica* and *Dinobdella ferox*.

Diagnosis

In enzootic areas, fascioliasis is suspected in patients suffering from fever, hepatomegaly, and eosinophilia who have eaten freshwater plants. Serological tests are useful early in the illness, before ova appear in the faeces, and in ectopic infections. Chronic fascioliasis is diagnosed by finding the characteristic eggs in stools or material obtained by duodenal or biliary drainage. Cholangiography, ultrasonography, and computed tomography are useful.

Treatment and prognosis

Triclabendazole (single dose 10 mg/kg) is effective but praziquantel is unreliable. Most patients recover completely after the flukes have been evacuated through the intestinal tract.

Prevention and control

Prevention is by avoiding eating fresh aquatic plants especially watercress, by boiling drinking water, and thoroughly cooking sheep and goat liver. Snail intermediate hosts are eliminated by draining sheep pastures and treating with molluscicides (e.g. copper sulphate or Frescon). Sheep and other herbivorous animals are treated.

Dicrocoeliasis

Adult *Dicrocoelium dendriticum* flukes live in the biliary passages of sheep and cattle. Ova excreted in the faeces are ingested by land snails and the resulting cercariae are ingested by ants. Infected ants are eaten inadvertently by grazing herbivores or humans.

Epidemiology

Dicrocoeliasis is enzootic in sheep, goats, deer, and other herbivores in Europe, Turkey, North Africa, and parts of Asia and America.

Pathology, pathogenesis, and clinical manifestations

Symptoms of human dicrocoeliasis are usually mild, but in heavy infections they may include vague biliary and gastrointestinal disturbances including flatulence, biliary colic, vomiting, diarrhoea, or constipation. The liver may be enlarged.

Diagnosis

Ova can be found in faeces, bile, or duodenal fluid.

Treatment

Praziquantel is effective in the same dose that is used for opisthorchiasis.

Prevention and control

Raw vegetables should not be eaten in the endemic area as they may be contaminated by infected snails.

Further reading

Hardman, E.W., Jones, R.L.H., and Davies, A.H. (1970). Fascioliasis a large outbreak. *British Medical Journal*, **iii**, 502–5.

Laird, P.P. and Boray, J.C. (1992). Human fascioliasis successfully treated with triclabendazole. *Australia and New Zealand Journal of Medicine*, **22**, 45–7.

Liu, L.X. and Harinasuta, K.T. (1996). Liver and intestinal flukes. *Gastroenterology Clinics of North America*, **25**(3), 627–36.

Mas-Coma, M.S., Esteban, J.G., and Bargues, M.D. (1999). Epidemiology of human fascioliasis: a review and proposed new classification. *Bulletin of the World Health Organization*, **77**, 340–6.

Pungpak, S., Viravan, C., Radmyos, B., *et al.* (1997). *Opisthorchis viverrini* infection in Thailand: studies on the morbidity of the infection and resolution following praziquantel treatment. *American Journal of Tropical Medicine and Hygiene*, **56**(3), 311–14.

Pungpak, S., Radomyos, P., Radomyos, B., *et al.* (1998). Treatment of *Opisthorchis viverrini* and intestinal fluke infections with praziquantel. *Southeast Asian Journal of Tropical Medicine Public Health*, **29**(2), 246–9.

Chapter 16.111

Lung flukes (paragonimiasis)

Sirivan Vanijanonta

Lung fluke infection is a parasitic infection caused by trematodes of the genus *Paragonimus*. It is estimated that more than 10 million people are infected world wide. The clinical manifestations depend on the duration, intensity, and sites where the parasites lodge in the host's organs.

Aetiology

It is generally agreed that *P. westermani* (see OTM3, p. 971, Fig. 1) the most common and widespread parasite in the Far East. Elsewhere, other species occur including *P. skzjabini*, *P. heterotremus*, *P. ilokstuenensis*, *P. africanus*, *P. uterobilateralis* (central and west Africa), *P. mexicanus*, *P. caliensis*, and *P. peruvianus* (Central and South America). The adults are reddish-brown and plump shaped (8–16 mm in length, 4–8 mm in width). Typically, they are encysted in the lung parenchyma adjacent to the bronchi. The eggs are golden brown and operculated (50–60 μm × 80–120 μm).

Epidemiology

Paragonimiasis is a zoonosis. Human beings enter the cycle accidentally in places where there are suitable reservoir hosts (dog, cat, tiger), first intermediate hosts (certain freshwater snails), and second intermediate hosts (freshwater shrimp, crab), and the intermediate hosts are eaten. Transmission of *Paragonimus* spp. to humans occurs mostly through ingestion of metacercariae in the second intermediate host.

Pathogenesis

In experimental animals the larval flukes penetrate the intestinal wall, the abdominal cavity, then pass through the diaphragm, pleura and finally encyst in the lung parenchyma. Abnormal migration may be found in any internal organ. Migratory larval flukes cause irritation, allergic inflammatory reactions, traumatic tracts, pressure effects, haemorrhage, and necrosis to the affected tissues or organs.

Clinical features

Clinical features are divided into acute and chronic phases. The acute phases is correlated with the invasion and migration of young flukes: these include fever, rashes, urticaria, abdominal pain, or discomfort and a feeling of tightness in the chest. Acute symptoms are usually not serious and patients progress the chronic stage.

Chronic manifestations are classified as pulmonary and extrapulmonary. Pulmonary infection is characterized by chronic productive cough with jam-liked, brownish-red sputum. Breathlessness and chest pain may also occur. Haemoptysis may occur after exertion. Patients with pulmonary paragonimiasis remain relatively well compared with patients with other chronic pulmonary infections. Physical examination shows few abnormality. Chest radiographs show linear infiltrations, exudative pneumonia, nodular or cystic lesions and localized pleural effusion located at the basilar and peripheral regions of both lower lung fields. A thin-walled cyst with a crescentic opacity along one side is the characteristic finding (Fig. 1).

Extrapulmonary paragonimiasis

Extrapulmonary paragonimiasis is caused by aberrant migration of larval and young adult flukes to any organ. Ectopic worms in the liver or spleen may cause clinical manifestations of an abscess. In

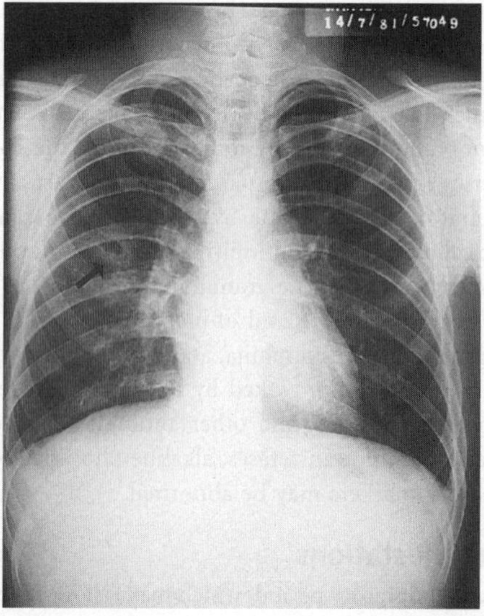

Fig. 1 Pulmonary paragonimiasis; posteroanterior radiograph showing a thick-walled cystic lesion in the right upper lobe with pericystic fibrosis. *(Copyright Dr S. Vanijanonta.)*

the central nervous system it may cause acute meningoencephalitis. Chronic brain abscesses present as paralysis and epilepsy and should be differentiated from cerebral cysticercosis, cryptococcosis, and toxoplasmosis. The cerebrospinal fluid usually shows an eosinophilic leucocytosis with elevated protein in the acute stage and lymphocytic leucocytosis later. *P. skjabini* and *P. ecuadoriensis* can cause migratory subcutaneous swelling and nodules. Spinal cord paragonimiasis produces progressive weakness, back pain, sensory impairment of the lower extremities, and paralysis.

Pathology

Adult worms, larva, and eggs excite inflammation, granulomatous lesions, and abscess formation. Long-term results are fibrosis and calcification.

Laboratory diagnosis

Definitive diagnosis depends upon finding the characteristic operculated ova in the sputum, stool, pleural fluid, or tissue biopsy. Other supportive evidence is obtained by chest radiography. Serology is essential in the diagnosis of extrapulmonary paragonimiasis. Enzyme-linked immunosorbent assay (**ELISA**) and dot ELISA are both highly sensitive and specific. Other less sensitive but more specific tests are complement fixation and indirect haemagglutination tests.

Treatment

Praziquantel is the drug of choice. A total of 75 mg/kg is given in three divided doses for 1–2 days. The cure rate is nearly 100 per cent in multicentre studies. Side-effects are minor and transient, consisting of sleepiness, rashes, headache, and back pain. Alternatively, bithionol may be given as 30–40 mg/kg in divided doses every other day for a total of 10–15 treatment days.

Prognosis

Pulmonary paragonimiasis is rarely fatal. After treatment, the symptoms disappear rapidly, and most of the abnormal lung infiltrations resolve in a few months. Cerebral paragonimiasis may cause chronic morbidity such as epilepsy, mental changes, and neurological sequelae.

Prevention and control

Effective control measures are directed towards interruption of the lifecycle: health education, encouragement of changing the dietary habit of eating raw or inadequately prepared foods, and mass treatment of infected persons in the endemic area (see also OTM3, pp. 988–92).

Further reading

Pozio, E. (1991). Current status of food-borne parasitic zoonoses in Mediterranean and African region. In *Emerging problems in food-borne parasitic zoonosis: impact on agriculture and public health*, (ed. J.H. Cross), pp. 85–7. Thai Watana Panich Press Co. Ltd.

Chapter 16.112

Intestinal trematodiasis

Tranakchit Harinasuta and Prayong Radomyos*

Some 50 million people in the Far East, South-east Asia, the Middle East, and North Africa, harbour hermaphrodite flukes. More than 50 species have been reported in humans but only a few cause disease.

Fasciolopsiasis

The giant intestinal fluke *Fasciolopsis buski* is up to 7.5 × 2 × 0.3 cm in size (Fig. 1). It is found in the small intestine of pigs and humans. The eggs 140 × 85 μm (Fig. 2(e)), are passed with faeces. On reaching the water, miracidia develop in 4–8 weeks, enter *Segmentia*, *Hippeutis*,

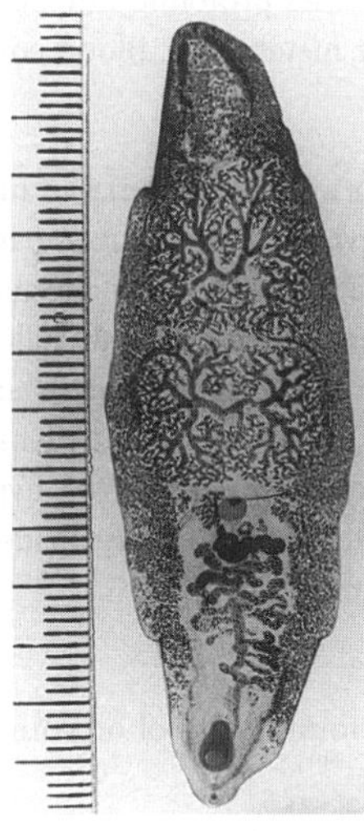

Fig. 1 *Fasciolopsis buski* adult fluke, 5.3 cm long. *(Copyright P. Radomyos.)*

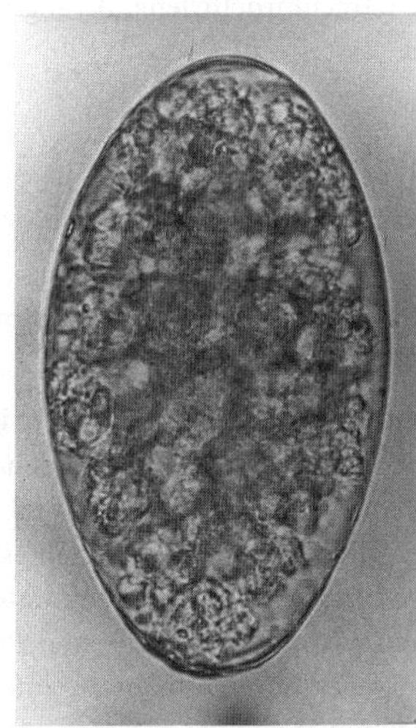

Fig. 2 Ova of *Fasciolopsis buski* 130 μm in diameter (long axis) *(Copyright P. Radomyos.)*

*It is with regret that we report the death of Professor Khunying Tranakchit Harinasuta in 1999.

or *Gyraulus* snails, the first intermediate hosts, forming sporocysts, rediae, and cercariae. The cercariae then swim out and encyst on water plants and develop into metacercariae in approximately 4 weeks. When pigs or humans eat infected water plants such as water caltrop, water morning glory, water chestnut, water bamboo, or watercress, the metacercariae excyst in the duodenum. They attach themselves to the mucosa and in about 90 days develop into mature worms. The life-span of the fluke is only 1 year.

Epidemiology

Over 10 million people in the Far East are thought to be infected with *F. buski* especially in China, Taiwan, Thailand, Laos, Bangladesh, and India. Fasciolopsiasis is restricted to areas where pigs are kept near to the ponds where water plants are grown for human consumption.

Pathology

At their sites of attachment to the duodenal and jejunal mucosa, the flukes cause inflammation followed by ulceration, bleeding, mucous discharge and, in severe cases profound intoxication and sensitization from absorption of their metabolites. Blood eosinophilia is common.

Clinical features

Most infections are light and asymptomatic. In heavy infections, the first symptoms are diarrhoea with hunger pains, simulating peptic ulcer. At first, diarrhoea and constipation alternate, but later diarrhoea becomes persistent. The stool is greenish-yellow and foul smelling, and contains undigested food. Some patients are anorexic and nauseated, and may vomit. In severe cases, oedema of face, trunk, and limbs, and ascites develop, the result of hypoproteinaemia from protein-losing enteropathy. Heavy worm loads may cause intestinal obstruction. Death is rare.

Diagnosis

Flukes and ova may be found in stool or vomitus.

Treatment

Praziquantel in a single dose of 15 mg/kg body weight after supper is effective: flukes will be expelled next day. Niclosamide, 150 mg/kg daily for 1 or 2 days, tetrachloroethylene, 0.1 mg/kg, or albendazole, 200 mg for 2 days, are less effective.

Prevention

Water plants should be cooked or grown in ponds that are not contaminated with human or pig faeces. Molluscicides are used to eradicate snails.

Echinostomiasis

A dozen species of Echinostomatidae are known to infect humans (e.g. *Echinostoma ilocanum, E. lindoense*). These flukes have a characteristic horseshoe-shaped collar of spines around the oral sucker and are up to 15 × 2 mm in size. They live in the small intestine and the eggs, 150 × 95 μm, are passed in faeces. On reaching water, miracidia hatch and enter snails, then develop further and enter Pila snails, fish, and tadpoles, or encyst on vegetation. Humans are infected by eating fish and Pila snails especially in Indonesia and in north-eastern Thailand, where the prevalence is about 50 per cent.

Clinical findings

Heavy infections may produce catarrhal inflammation of the intestinal mucosa. Heavy worm loads may cause vague abdominal complaints of flatulence and loose motions. In children, diarrhoea, abdominal pain, anaemia, and oedema, reminiscent of fasciolopsiasis buski, have been reported. Diagnosis is by finding eggs in faeces or adult worms recovered in faeces after anthelminthics.

Treatment

All drugs recommended for *F. buski* infection are effective. The prognosis is good. Prevention is by thoroughly cooking or avoiding eating Pila snails and other second intermediate hosts.

Heterophyiasis

More than 10 species of minute heterophyid flukes have been found in humans. *Heterophyes heterophyes* is only about 1.7 × 0.7 mm in size. The lifecycle in fresh or brackish-water, involves snails and fish (e.g. mullet and minnows). Human infection is common in parts of the Middle and Far East, Japan, South Korea, Taiwan, China, and the Philippines. People are infected by eating raw fish.

Pathology

Flukes produce ulceration and mild inflammation of the small bowel. Ova deposited in the bowel wall may enter blood vessels and embolize to the heart and central nervous system, damaging the valves and myocardium.

Clinical features

Dyspepsia and gastroenterocolitis with mucous diarrhoea are common. Cardiac involvement may produce chronic congestive cardiac failure or there may be sudden death caused by massive coronary embolization. Diagnosis is by identifying eggs in the faeces. Prevention is by avoiding raw or undercooked fish.

Treatment

Praziquantel at a single dose of 15–25 mg/kg may be effective. Hexylresorcinol, tetrachloroethylene, and bephenium are also effective. The prognosis is good except when brain or heart are involved.

Metagonimiasis

Metagonimus yokogawai is the smallest human fluke (2.5 × 0.7 mm). The lifecycle involves snails and salmonoid and cyprinoid fish.

Epidemiology

M. yokogawai is endemic in China, Japan, Korea, and Taiwan. It has also been reported from Siberia, Manchuria, Israel, the Balkans, and Spain. People are infected by eating raw or undercooked fish.

Pathology

Flukes cause inflammation, granulomatous infiltration, and ulceration of the duodenum and small intestine. Rarely, eggs embolize in the bloodstream to other organs.

Clinical findings

The infection usually causes either mild diarrhoea or no symptoms but egg emboli can result in serious manifestations. Diagnosis is by identifying eggs in stools.

Gastrodisciasis

Gastrodiscoides hominis is about 14 × 8 mm in size with a huge notched acetabulum on its ventral surface. It is a common parasite in parts of India, South-east Asia, and elsewhere. Flukes attach to the mucosa of the caecum and ascending colon. The mucosa is dragged out by the acetabulum, forming a minute papilla in the sharply defined circular imprint made by the discoidal region of the fluke. There is surface desquamation of the mucosa. Both the mucosa and submucosa show infiltration with eosinophils, lymphocytes, and plasma cells.

Clinical findings

The flukes live in the caecum in large numbers, usually producing no symptoms. Mucous diarrhoea has been recorded.

Diagnosis

Diagnosis is by finding ova or adult flukes after anthelminthic treatment.

Treatment

Praziquantel at the same dosage used in fasciolopsiasis may be effective.

For discussion of Alariasis and infection by other minor genera of intestinal flukes see OTM3, pp. 992–9.

Further reading

Cross, J.H. (1969). Fasciolopsiasis in Southeast Asia and the Far East. In *Schistosomiasis and other snail-transmitted helminthiasis, Proceedings of the 4th South-East Asian seminar on parasitology and tropical medicine*, (ed. C. Harinasuta), pp. 177–99. Manila, Philippines.

Liu, L.X. and Harinasuta, K.T. (1996). Liver and intestinal flukes. *Gastroenterology Clinics of North America*, 25(3), 627–36.

Chapter 16.113

Non-venomous arthropods

J. Paul

Of the million or more species in the Phylum Arthropoda, a few hundred, mostly in the Classes Insecta (bugs, flies, fleas, lice, etc.) and Arachnida (mites, ticks), are of special medical importance. Arthropods may bite, feed on secretions, transmit infectious agents, infest or invade the body, be host to stages of human parasites, and stimulate loathing, phobia and delusion. They can be a nuisance by crawling over the skin, invading dwellings or making loud, monotonous noises. (See OTM3, pp. 1000–12 for a detailed account, and for a discussion of venomous arthropods see Chapter 18.2.)

Bites may be important because of the immediate physical discomfort of the bite, sensitization leading to pruritus, excoriation, and secondary infection, other immunological phenomena including anaphylaxis, the transmission of infectious agents and in exceptional circumstances, significant blood loss. Reaction to bites varies with age, past exposure, and other factors which influence immune response. When the patient is able to associate bites with a particular kind of arthropod, management may be directed towards treatment of the bite, if necessary (topical corticosteroids, systemic antihistamines), consideration of the risk of transmitted infection, and prevention of further bites (eradication of ectoparasites, change in behaviour to avoid exposure, repellents, special clothing, insecticide-impregnated bednets). It is often possible to relate bites to infesting ectoparasites, to arthropods which remain attached (ticks), and to predatory bloodsuckers which are highly visible (mosquitoes, midges and black flies, when swarming) and which cause immediately painful bites (tsetse flies, some mosquitoes, tabanid flies). It is harder to ascribe a cause to bites from arthropods which bite at night or when the patient is asleep (some mosquitoes, sand flies, bed bugs, triatomine bugs) or from arthropods which are inconspicuous and which do not cause immediately painful bites (harvest mites, some fleas, some biting flies). Bites of larger arthropods typically have a central punctum and a surrounding area of inflammation and are pruritic. In cases of uncertainty, it may be necessary to obtain a dermatological opinion to exclude other diagnoses, including organic disorders, artefact and delusion.

Blood-sucking flies (Diptera)

Many flies are haematophagous: Suborder Nematocera (mosquitoes, sand flies, black flies, biting midges) and Family Tabanidae of the Suborders Brachycera (horse flies, clegs) and Suborder Cyclorrhapha (tsetse flies, *Glossina* spp.). Bites are often painful and cause sensitization. Biting flies transmit some of the most important human diseases including zoonoses. Among the many species of mosquito (Culicidae) are vectors of filariasis and numerous viral diseases, including yellow fever and dengue. Mosquitoes of the genus *Anopheles* transmit malaria. Sand flies (Phlebotominae) are mainly tropical and subtropical in distribution and transmit leishmaniasis. In South America, sand flies of the genus *Lutzomyia* transmit *Bartonella bacilliformis.* Black flies (Simuliidae) occur worldwide, but in Britain are troublesome only in localities, such as the River Stour, Dorset. In Africa, simuliids transmit onchocerciasis and in South America are associated with the haemorhagic syndrome of Altamira. Black flies pierce the skin and suck blood from the edge of the puncture. The bites, oozing in blood, have a characteristic appearance and may be associated with severe reaction by the host. Biting midges (Ceratopogonidae) are vectors of the filarial worms *Dipetalonema perstans* and *Mansonella ozzardi.* In Africa, tabanid flies transmit *Loa loa.* Tsetse flies, are vectors of African trypanosomiasis.

Bugs (Hemiptera)

Bed bugs (*Cimex* spp.) are cosmopolitan. Triatomines, the vectors of South American trypanosomiasis, occur in the neotropics. Both groups hide during the day in dwellings and painlessly bite the sleeper at night. Control depends on deinfestation of dwellings.

Ticks (Ixodoidea)

Ticks may remain attached to the skin for days. Hard ticks (Ixodidae) and soft ticks (Argasidae) occur worldwide. Stages of the lifecycle are egg, larva (six-legged) and nymph and adult (both eight-legged). Ticks attach and feed with a barbed hypostome and detach when engorged. Smaller stages and ticks in inconspicuous sites, such as the perineum may feed unobserved. Bites are painless but may result in local sensitization, secondary infection, and transmission of infectious agents, including numerous viruses, rickettsias, and Lyme disease. Local reaction to bites may be confused with erythema migrans of Lyme disease (which expands and typically develops a cyanosed centre). Ticks may be removed by gripping with forceps (or in the field, with finger and thumbnail), between the skin and the tick's head and pulling gently. One should avoid squeezing the tick. Careless removal may detach the hypostome, a potential source of secondary infection or inflammation. In Britain, species often found on humans are the sheep tick, *Ixodes ricinus* (a vector of Lyme disease) and the hedgehog tick, *Ixodes hexagonus*, which is doubtfully a vector of borreliosis to humans. In North America and Australia bites by species of hard and soft tick can cause tick paralysis (see OTM3, p. 1149).

Harvest mites (Tromboculidae)

In Britain, larvae of the harvest mite, *Neotrombicula autumnalis* often bite visitors to downland in late Summer. The mites are tiny and seldom noticed. They crawl rapidly on to the body, attach (often under tight-fitting clothes), inject proteolytic enzymes, feed on tissue fluid and detach, causing pruritic, sometimes bullous lesions later. Red bugs or chiggers (also applied to *Tunga penetrans*) are names given to tromboculids in the Americas. In Asia, trombolucids are vectors of scrub typhus. Where tromboculids are troublesome, tucking trousers into boots and application of diethyltoluamide and other repellents may be partially effective.

Accidental bites

Arthropods which do not normally bite humans, but can inflict painful but usually trivial bites when provoked by handling, as by children and entomologists, include: predatory true bugs such as the water boatman (*Notonecta glauca*) and the assassin bug (*Reduvius personatus*) in Britain and wheel bugs (*Arilus* spp.) in the Americas; larger beetles (Coleoptera); dragonflies (Odonata); and bush-crickets (Orthoptera), such as the wartbiter (*Decticus verrucivorus*). Spines used in defence by the great silver diving beetle (*Hydrous piceus*) and larger tropical grasshoppers of the Subfamily Cyrtacanthridinae can cause penetrating injury when handled. Pincers of larger crabs and lobsters (Crustacea) can cause crushing injuries of digits.

Allergy

A wide range of immunological responses to arthropod bites has been described from local pruritus to anaphylaxis. Scabies mites evoke pruritus in immunocompetent patients, but larvae which cause dermal myiasis are poor sensitizing agents. Arthropods, their dead remains, their cast skins (exuviae) or their faeces may act as inhalant allergens. House-dust mites *Dermatophagoides* spp. are a common cause of allergy in Britain and exposure to cockroach allergens in household dust has been associated with asthma in the United States. Following mass emergence, the exuviae of May flies (Ephemeroptera) and caddis flies (Trichoptera) may act as inhalant allergens. Entomologists who collect insects by sucking them into pooters may develop inhalant allergy to their subject of study. Cockroaches wander over sleepers and are attracted to nasal and oral secretions. Herpes blattae is a dermatitis described from Reunion and attributed to cockroach allergy. When the source of an allergy is clear (such as mosquito bites), it may be possible to find a means of avoiding the allergen.

Infestation

Sites of infestation include the hair, body surface, and immediate environment (ectoparasites: lice, fleas), the skin and subdermis (scabies, tungosis, dermal myiasis), wounds, tissues, orifices (myiasis), and the gastrointestinal tract (myiasis, canthariasis). With ectoparasites, the main problems are related to their bites; diagnosis and management may be based on the identification of the ectoparasite. Delusory parasitosis is a condition in which the patient becomes convinced of infestation by parasites despite reassurance by the doctor and absence of clinical or laboratory evidence.

Scabies

This chronic infestation is caused by the human scabies mite *Sarcoptes scabiei* var. *hominis*. Scabies mites adapted to other hosts, such as *Sarcoptes scabiei* var. *canis* cause a self-limiting pruritus in humans. Clinical manifestations of scabies are caused by the adult female mite which burrows through the epidermis. The adult female is oval and about a third of a millimetre long. It lives for about a month, burrowing and ovipositing daily. The burrow may extend to a centimetre in length. Six-legged larvae hatch after a few days and moult to become eight-legged nymphs and later eight-legged adults. Adult males are smaller than females, do not burrow and die after mating on the epidermis. Scabies is cosmopolitan. Prevalence rates are higher in crowded conditions and following social disruption in wartime. Outbreaks sometimes occur in nursing homes and in hospitals. Most cases must be acquired by close contact as the mites do not survive a long away from the body.

The main presenting symptom is pruritus which occurs with sensitization about a month after the onset of infestation. Symptoms may be worse at night and after a hot bath or shower. Burrows commonly occur in web spaces between the fingers and on the wrists, but may be widespread. There is often evidence of excoriation, but the appearance of the skin is variable and may show secondary infection, eczematization, lichenification, and papulovesicles. Careful examination may reveal burrows and mites. Diagnosis may be confirmed by microscopy of scrapings from affected areas, especially interdigital spaces, but many cases are atypical and a dermatological opinion may be required to exclude other causes. Immunsuppressed patients, including transplant recipients, burns victims and patients with acquired immune deficiency syndrome are prone to crusting or so-called 'Norwegian' or hypekeratotic scabies in which crusting lesions of scales and mites accumulate over the hands, feet, and other sites, such as eyebrows, but the patient suffers relatively little discomfort. Such cases and presumably their fomites are highly contagious. Treatment involves topical application of acaricides, including malathion, permethrin, and benzyl benzoate. To prevent reinfection, close contacts should be treated simultaneously. During outbreaks, it may be necessary to treat whole cohorts of patients or health-care teams. Oral ivermectin has been used to treat cases of crusting scabies in immunosuppressed patients.

Louse infestation

Lice are obligate parasites of animals. They bite using piercing mouthparts to feed on blood or tissue fluids. Two cosmopolitan species are associated with humans: *Pthirus pubis*, the pubic louse and *Pediculus humanus* which occurs as two subspecies, *P. humanus* (body louse) and *P. humanus capitis* (head louse). Lice complete their lifecycle on their host. Adult females deposit eggs (nits) on hairshafts (pubic and head lice) or on clothing (body louse). Larvae hatch after about 1 week, begin to feed and over the course of about 2 weeks, undergo several moults before reaching adulthood. Adult females live for about 1 month and may lay about a hundred eggs. Egg cases remain where attached. Most infestations are probably acquired through close contact with an infested case, but some cases may result from contact with clothing, bedclothes, or hairbrushes containing living lice or their eggs which may be attached to shed hairs. As well as the aesthetic and social drawbacks of being able to observe the lice, the medical problems common to all three taxa relate to sensitization of the host to louse antigens from bites and the resulting pruritus which may lead to excoriation and secondary infection. Louse bites have a central punctum and surrounding small red macule. Body lice may transmit a number of agents, including those of endemic typhus (*Rickettsia prowazekii*), trench fever (*Bartonella quintana*), and relapsing fever (*Borrelia recurrentis*). Treatment involves shaving of the head and body hair and topical application of pediculocides, including carbaryl, malathion, and permethrin. Lice may be pediculocide resistant. It may be necessary to treat close contacts, members of institutions or whole populations to prevent reinfestation. Pediculocides should be used with caution in children and asthmatics. Hot washing of clothing or bed clothes will destroy lice and their eggs.

Pubic lice (crab lice)

The lice attach themselves to pubic hairs. Rarely they may be found on eyebrows, eyelashes (phthirus palpebrarum), axillary, head, or chest hair. Eggs are deposited on hair shafts. Most infestations are probably acquired through sexual contact with an infested case. Children may acquire phthirosis at atypical sites through close contact with adults. Lice seldom stray from the body. Transmission is possible, but unlikely without close contact with an infected case. The main symptom is pruritus, sometimes with excoriation and secondary infection. Greyish-blue patches (maculae caeruleae) may occur on the skin. Diagnosis is by observation of the lice, which may be difficult to find, or of eggs or egg cases attached to hairshafts. Adults are 1–2 mm long. The anterior legs are smaller than the other two pairs. The body is squat and crab-like (body length, excluding head, about 1.2 times body width). Infestation may be treated by topical application of carbaryl or malathion to the whole body, repeated a week later to kill newly hatched larvae.

Head lice

Head lice infest the scalp and rarely other body sites. They lay their eggs at the base of hair shafts. Infestation is more common in children than in adults and more common in females than in males. Prevalence rates vary but may be very high in certain communities or institutions, such as schools. Prevalence rates may be high despite good standards of hygiene. Most cases occur probably as a result of close contact. The main symptom is pruritus which may be associated with excoriation, secondary infection, and lymphadenopathy. Diagnosis is by observation of lice, which generally remain close to the scalp, or of eggs or egg cases, attached to hairs. A fine comb (nit comb) may be used to collect material to make the diagnosis. Adults are 3–4 mm long. Infestation may be treated by applications of pediculicide lotion (carbaryl, malathion, or permethrin) to the scalp overnight and repeated a week later to destroy newly hatched larvae. Pediculocide resistance may occur and local expertise should be sought. Regular use of a nit comb may be used to control head lice. In institutions, co-ordinated treatment campaigns may be required to prevent re-infestation.

Body lice

Body lice infest clothing and body hair. They lay their eggs on clothing, often along seams. Body lice are morphologically like head lice, but they are slightly larger. Body louse infestation is associated with poor hygiene and social disruption, as may occur in wartime. Transmission occurs as a result of close contact or through contact with infested clothing. Bites occur on the body, resulting in pruritus which may be associated with excoriation, eczematization, and secondary infection. Diagnosis is confirmed by finding lice, usually on clothing. Infestation may be treated by topical application of carbaryl or malathion to the whole body, repeated a week later to kill newly hatched larvae. Hot washing of clothing will destroy adults and early stages.

Fleas (Siphonaptera)

Fleas are bloodsucking ectoparasites. There are thousands of species, adapted to various host animals. Adults are a few millimetres long, brown, laterally compressed and typically very active. Adults move through the fur or under clothing, but can survive in the environment for long periods without feeding. Eggs are dropped to the ground, where the larvae develop, feeding on organic matter. The pupa may remain in the environment for long periods before the adult emerges. Increasing standards of hygiene in developing countries have made the human flea, *Pulex irritans*, a rarity. Most flea bites in Britain are due to cat and dog flea, *Ctenocephalides felis* and *C.canis*, either through direct exposure to an infested animal or to an environment exposed to an infested animal, possibly months previously. Pigeon fleas may invade homes from pigeon roosts. Flea bites result in intense pruritus at the bite site. There is a central punctum and there may be bulla formation. Flea bites often occur in groups. Although patients may not witness fleas, clues that bites have been caused by fleas include intense pruritus, the appearance of bites in small groups, and a history of exposure to a flea-ridden animal or its domain. Troublesome bites may be treated with topical corticosteroids and systemic antihistamines. Prevention of bites is by good domestic hygiene and treatment of infested animals and environments with insecticides. Certain species of flea are vectors of a number of infectious diseases including plague and murine typhus.

Tungosis

Tungosis is infestation by a flea, *Tunga penetrans*, the jigger, chigger, or chigoe (but popular names are shared with tromboculid mites). The gravid female, about 1 mm long, burrows into exposed skin (usually the foot) or under a toenail and swells to about 1 cm in diameter, causing local discomfort. Local remedies in endemic areas (tropical Africa and the Americas) of shelling out fleas may leave cavities prone to secondary infection and tetanus. Doctors in the developed world seldom have personal experience of the condition and usually opt for surgical enucleation (which provides appropriate treatment) and diagnosis by histology. The wearing of footwear prevents infestation.

Myiasis

Myiasis is the infestation of living animals by the larvae of flies (Diptera). Of many species listed as possible agents of myiasis, most are opportunists whose saprophagous larvae feed on decaying organic matter, which might include necrotic wound tissue. Opportunists usually confine themselves to dead tissue and may even benefit the healing process. There is no dipterous obligate intestinal parasite of humans. Intestinal myiasis may be caused by coprophagous larvae, which invade the rectum or by resilient maggots, such as those of the false stable fly, *Muscina stabulans* and the cheese skipper, *Piophila casei* which survive when swallowed unintentionally among food and may cause intestinal disturbance and scarring. Intestinal myiasis may be spurious following diagnosis based on observation of rapidly-hatching larvae on freshly passed faeces or may be factitious. Flies from several genera, notably *Fannia*, may cause urogential myiasis. Scuttle flies (Phoridae) have been reported to cause pulmonary myiasis, possibly following inhalation of the gravid female fly. A small number of flies are obligate parasites of living tissues and a few species are closely associated but not specific to humans. Many cases of myiasis are benign, self-limiting, and relatively harmless, but aural, nasopharyngeal, and malign wound myiasis are potentially lethal entities that may require removal of the larvae and possibly reconstructive surgery. Myiasis is diagnosed by observing dipterous larvae in a lesion. Identification of larvae may need expert help, but management of the patient, which depending on the type of lesion, may involve the removal of larvae, surgical exploration, debridement or treatment of secondary infection should be based on clinical assessment.

Dermal myiasis

Dermatobia hominis, the human bot fly is a common cause of dermal myiasis in the American tropics. The female fly lays her eggs on biting arthropods, such as mosquitoes. The eggs hatch when in contact with skin into which the larva burrows. The larval stage lasts about 10 weeks, a boil with a small aperture forming as the larva grows. Such boils are not infrequently seen in Europeans returning from the neotropics. The larva may grow to more than a centimetre in length. An early symptom is sporadic pain caused by the spiny larva. Unless in an unusual anatomical site, such as close to the eye, infestation is generally harmless. Secondary infection of the wound is the most common complication. Larvae may be removed through a simple incision. Remedies which include application of raw meat or glue to the lesion may not be successful. Squeezing may rupture the larva to evoke a local granulomatous reaction.

The tumbu fly, *Cordylobia anthropophaga*, is widespread in the Afrotopical region. The female oviposits on sand and also on drying clothes. Ironing destroys eggs. Contact with viable ova on clothing leads to infestation. The larvae pierce the skin and grow rapidly. An uncomfortable boil forms which oozes serosanguinous fluid. Fever and lymphadenopathy may occur. Larvae reach maturity in about 10 days. Larvae may be removed through a simple incision but with care, it may be possible to express larvae following the application of petroleum jelly.

The larvae of warble flies, *Hypoderma* spp. Occasionally cause dermal myiasis in humans. Larvae of horse bot flies, *Gasterophilus* spp. cannot complete their lifecycle in humans, but they can pierce human skin, where they wander for a week or so, causing intense itching (creeping eruption).

Wound myiasis

Many dipterous species are known to cause wound myiasis, but most of them are facultative feeders on necrotic tissue and are rarely destructive to the host, although the presence of maggots in a wound may cause distress. Debridement of necrotic tissue will control such infestation. In contrast, under controlled conditions, clinicians may introduce maggots to debride wounds.

Causes of malign myiasis include the New World screw worm, *Cochliomyia hominivorax*, in the Americas and the Old World screw worm, *Chrysomya bezziana* and Wohlfahrt's wound myiasis fly, *Wohlfahrtia magnifica* in the Old World. Their larvae are obligate parasites of living tissue. Eggs are laid on wounds, in ears, and on mucous membranes. The larvae burrow in groups into health tissue, causing widespread destruction which may be mutilating or fatal. Secondary bacterial infection or secondary wound myiasis may ensue. All species may cause nasopharyngeal, aural, orbital, genital, and malign wound myiasis. Infestation is best avoided by cleaning and dressing wounds as they occur. Treatment involves surgical removal of the larvae, debridement of affected tissue, and treatment of secondary infection. Reconstructive surgery may be required.

Ophthalmic myiasis

Nasal bot flies, *Oestrus* spp., naturally parasitize various herbivorous mammals. They are larviparous and drop their larvae into the nostrils of the host. Dropped into human eyes they cause a self-limiting conjunctivitis. Larvae of warble flies, *hypoderma* spp. are more dangerous: they may burrow into the eye, resulting in pain, nausea, and much damage, and must be surgically removed.

Canthariasis

Infestation of the body by beetles (Coleoptera) or their larvae is called canthariasis. Clinically, it may resemble myiasis but is much rarer. Larvae swallowed with food may dwell temporarily in the intestines, causing discomfort and may be detected in excreta. In Sri Lanka, scarabid dung beetles have been reported to invade the rectum. Rarely, cases of urogenital myiasis have been reported.

Insects and hygiene

Synanthropic insects which feed or wander over faeces, wounds, and food may serve as passive vectors of bacterial and viral diseases. Such insects include pharaoh's ants, *Monomorium pharanois*, which may invade sterile packs and wound dressings in hospitals, flies (especially of the Suborder Cyclorrhapha), and cockroaches (Dictyoptera). Despite many reports of the isolation of pathogenic bacteria and viruses from these insects, there have been few epidemiological studies to define their importance as passive vectors. However, there is evidence that flies may act as passive vectors of shigellosis and that cockroaches acted as passive vectors of hepatitis A, during an outbreak in California and of *Salmonella typhimurium* on a paediatric ward in Belgium. The presence of such insects in hospitals should be monitored and controlled.

Eye-frequenting insects

Flies which feed on eye secretions may act as vectors of trachoma. Some nocturnal moths of the Families Pyralidae, Noctuidae, and Geometridae in Africa and South-east Asia habitually feed on the lacrimal secretions of animals. They may visit human eyes, causing a certain amount of discomfort and may transmit eye infections, including trachoma and viral conjunctivitis. They may also cause mechanical damage to the cornea. The moths stimulate the flow of secretions by vibrating and probing with the probosces. Implicated species include *Lobocraspis griseifulva*, *Arcyophora* spp., and *Filodes fulvidorsalis*. *Calyptra eustrigata* is a skin-piercing, blood sucking noctuid from Malaya. Such Lepidoptera may be avoided by sleeping under a net.

Further reading

Alexander, J., O'D. (1984). *Arthropods and the human skin.* Springer-Verlag, Berlin.

Auerbach, P.S. (ed.) (1995). *Wilderness medicine: management of wilderness and environmental emergencies.* Mosby, St. Louis.

Rosenstreich, D.L., Eggleston, P., Kattan, M., *et al.* (1997). The role of cockroach allergy and exposure to cockroach allergen in causing morbidity among inner-city children with asthma. *New England Journal of Medicine,* **336,** 1356–63.

Roth, L.M. and Willis, E.R. (1957). The medical and veterinary importance of cockroaches. *Smithsonian Miscellaneous Collection,* **134,** 1–147.

Smith, K.G.V. (ed.) (1973). *Insects and arthropods of medical importance.* British Museum (Natural History), London.

Zumpt, F. (1965). *Myiasis in man and animals in the old world.* Butterworths, London.

Chapter 16.114

Pentastomiasis (porocephalosis)

D. A. Warrell

The pentastomida, pentastomes or 'tongue worms' inhabit the respiratory tracts of vertebrates especially snakes, where they feed on blood and other tissues. About 10 species can infect humans. Pentastomida have been classified variously as arthropods, branchiuran crustacea, annelids or in a separate phylum. The most common evidence of *Armillifer armillatus* infection is the discovery of calcified nymphs on radiographs of the abdomen and chest. Visceral pentastomiasis is most often caused by *Linguatula serrata* or *A. armillatus.* Nasopharyngeal pentastomiasis (halzoun or Marrara syndrome) is usually caused by *L. serrata,* although other helminthic parasites have been implicated.

There is no specific treatment for pentastomiasis. Obstruction and compression should be relieved surgically. Hypersensitivity phenomena should be treated with adrenaline, antihistamines, and corticosteroids. Infections could be prevented if all meat were thoroughly cooked or people stopped eating snakes.

More details can be found in OTM3, pp. 1012–14.

Chapter 16.115

Fever of unknown origin

D. T. Durack

Febrile episodes are very common, often transient and often of minor significance. In many cases the cause is obvious, such as an upper respiratory infection in a child. In a few cases, fever is persistent and the cause is not easily diagnosed. Such episodes are termed 'fever of unknown origin' (**FUO**) or 'pyrexia of unknown origin'.

Definitions and terminology

Normal body temperature is 37.0°C or 98.6°F. The normal range is quite wide, being affected by site of measurement, diurnal variation, heavy exercise, hormonal and menstrual status, and individual variation. Patients' body temperature is most often estimated by measurements taken in the mouth or for reasons of convenience, but oral temperatures can be affected by mouth-breathing, by the respiratory rate and by recent drinking of hot or cold liquids. The core body temperature is more closely reflected by rectal measurements, which are usually 0.3–0.6°C higher than oral measurements. Heavy exercise can temporarily raise the core temperature of healthy people by 2°C or more. Another factor is normal circadian variation, which cycles through a range of 0.5°C (0.9°F) daily, with lowest temperatures occurring between 4:00 and 6:00 a.m. and highest between 4:00 and 8:00 p.m. The normal circadian rhythm varies between individuals and is likely to be affected by jet travel between time zones, by work and sleep patterns, and by illnesses. The menstrual cycle affects the baseline temperature of normal women by 0.3–0.5°C, with a small spike at ovulation and higher temperatures from about the 15th to the 25th days of a 28-day cycle. In addition to these factors, there is considerable variation in normal temperature patterns between individuals. Some normal young people, especially women, persistently exhibit slightly 'high' temperatures which are of no pathological significance. This common normal variant, which does not require investigation, may be termed 'habitual hyperthermia'.

Fever and hypothermia may be defined, respectively, as core body temperatures above or below the normal range, allowing for all the factors listed above. For practical clinical purposes, oral or rectal temperatures falling outside the range 35.5–38.0°C (95.9–100.4°F) can be regarded as abnormal. Specific circumstances should be considered; for example, an oral temperature of 37.3°C taken at 6:00 a.m. could represent a clinically significant fever in an elderly patient.

FUO has many possible causes. To help classify these, four distinct types of prolonged fever have been defined: classical FUO, nosocomial FUO, neutropenic FUO, and human immunodeficiency virus (**HIV**) -associated FUO.

Symptoms and signs of FUO

The symptoms and signs of FUO are highly variable. Some patients have mild feverish symptoms, while others may be incapacitated by debilitating chills, rigors, and sweats. The clinical findings may be limited to manifestations of the fever itself, or may reflect the underlying disease as well. The physician should evaluate every symptom or sign, especially new ones, as potential clues to the primary diagnosis.

Certain diseases can produce characteristic patterns of fever, notably malaria, brucellosis, typhoid fever, and some lymphomas, but in practice the shape of the fever curve is seldom of major value in the diagnosis of FUO. Individual host reactions to disease and the common use of antipyretic analgesic drugs confuse the picture. There is a common misconception that drug-induced fevers are usually low-grade, with relatively little variation from peak to trough and a relatively low pulse rate, but in fact the clinical characteristics of drug-induced fevers are highly variable.

Classical FUO

Most of the many causes of classical FUO can be classified into five categories: *infections, malignancies, connective tissue diseases, miscellaneous conditions* including factitious fever and habitual hyperthermia, and *undiagnosed* cases. Within the first three categories,

Table 1 Summary of definitions and major features of four types of FUO

	Classical FUO	Nosocomial FUO	Neutropenic FUO	HIV-related FUO
Definition	>38.0°C, >3 weeks, >2 visits or 3 days in hospital	>38.0°C, >72 h, not present or incubating on admission	>38.0°C, >72 h, <1000PMNs/mm^3, negative cultures after 48 h	>38.0°C, >3 weeks for outpatients, >3 days for inpatients, HIV infection confirmed
Patient location	Community, clinic or hospital	Acute care hospital	Hospital or clinic	Community, clinic, or hospital
Leading aetiologies	Malignancy, infections, inflammatory conditions, undiagnosed, habitual hyperthermia	Nosocomial infections, postoperative complications, drug fevers	Majority due to infections, but aetiology documented in only 40–60%	HIV, typical and atypical mycobacteria, CMV, lymphomas, toxoplasmosis
History emphasis	Travel, contacts, animal and insect exposure, immunizations, family history	Operations and procedures, devices, anatomic considerations, drug treatment	Stage of chemotherapy, drugs administered	Drugs, exposures, risk factors, travel, contacts, staging of HIV infection
Examination emphasis	Abdomen, lymph nodes, spleen, joints, muscles, arteries	Wounds, drains, devices, sinuses, urine	Skin folds, IV sites, lungs, perianal area	Mouth, skin, lymph nodes, eyes, lungs, perianal area
Investigation emphasis	Imaging, biopsies, ESR, PPD	Imaging, bacterial cultures	Chest radiograph, bacterial cultures	Blood and lymphocyte count; serologies; chest radiograph; stool examination; biopsies of lung, bone marrow, liver; cultures and cytologies; brain imaging
Management	Observation, outpatient temperature chart, investigations, avoid empiric drug treatments	Depends on situation	Antimicrobial treatment protocols	AZT, antimicrobial treatment protocols, revision of treatment regimens, nutrition
Time course of disease	Months	Weeks	Days	Weeks to months
Tempo of investigation	Weeks	Days	Hours	Days to weeks
Mortality (attributable to the cause of FUO)	Moderate	Moderate	Low	High

Adapted from Durack and Street (1991).

certain diagnoses predominate (Tables 1 and 2). The leading infectious aetiologies for classical FUO are intra-abdominal infections, complicated urinary tract infections, tuberculosis, and infective endocarditis. The leading malignancies are lymphomas, leukaemias, and some solid tumours, including adenocarcinomas and hypernephromas. Vasculitides including the temporal arteritis-polymyalgia syndromes, Still's disease, systemic lupus erythematosus, and rheumatic fever are important among the connective tissue diseases. Among the miscellaneous conditions that can cause FUO, alcoholic hepatitis and granulomatous conditions such as sarcoidosis or granulomatous hepatitis are important. Self-induced or factitious fever is surprisingly common. Some of the many other miscellaneous, uncommon, or rare diseases that can cause FUO are listed in Table 2. In all published series, a sizeable subgroup of patients with FUO remains undiagnosed.

FUO in children

The proportion of cases of FUO due to infections is higher in children, and the proportion due to malignancy is correspondingly lower. Infections that are particularly common in children are viral syndromes and urinary tract infections. Still's disease and rheumatic fever are more likely to cause FUO in children than in adults, and children are less likely to have factitious fever. The overall mortality of FUO in children is lower than in adults.

FUO in the elderly

In patients over 65 years old, intra-abdominal abscesses including hepatic abscesses, malignancies, and vasculitides cause a higher proportion of cases of FUO. The proportion of FUOs that remain undiagnosed in the elderly is only about half that in children and younger adults. The higher rate of underlying malignancies in any series of elderly patients with FUO means that the long-term prognosis is less favourable than in a younger group. The temporal arteritis/polymyalgia rheumatica syndromes are particularly important because they are common in the elderly, and their many non-specific symptoms may be missed or misdiagnosed. The diagnosis is easily suspected if the erythrocyte sedimentation rate (ESR) is over 100 mm/h, but easily

Table 2 Listing of various causes of FUO.

Leading causes of FUO (by category and approximate frequency)	Uncommon or rare causes of FUO (alphabetical)
Infection (30–50%)	Alcoholic hepatitis
Bacterial abscesses (especially intra-abdominal)	Atrial myxoma
Mycobacterial infections (human and atypical)	Behçet's syndrome
Urinary tract infections	Castleman disease
Infective endocarditis	Chronic meningitis
Viral infections (HIV, CMV,EBV)	Carcinomatous meningitis
Amoebic abscess	Cyclic neutropenia
Leishmaniasis	Drug fever and other hypersensitivities
Brucellosis	Erythema multiforme
Schistosomiasis	Fabry's disease
	Familial Mediterranean fever
Malignancy (15–20%)	Granulomatous hepatitis
Lymphoma	Granulomatous peritonitis
Leukaemia	Haemoglobinopathies
Solid tumours	Haemolytic anaemias
Other haematological malignancies	Histiocytosis X
	Inflammatory bowel disease
Connective tissue diseases (10–20%)	Lymphomatoid granulomatosis
Temporal arteritis/polymyalgia rheumatica	Pancreatitis
Still's disease	Paroxysmal haemoglobinurias
Systemic lupus erythematosus	Pericarditis
Polyarteritis nodosa	Periodic fever
Rheumatic fever (including recurrences)	Phaeochromocytoma
	Pulmonary emboli
Miscellaneous (see right-hand column) (10–15%)	Postpericardiotomy syndrome
	Retroperitoneal fibrosis
Undiagnosed (10–25%)	Sarcoidosis
	Serum sickness
	Sjögren's syndrome
	Thrombotic thrombocytopenic purpura
	Thrombophlebitis
	Thyroiditis and thyrotoxicosis
	Vogt–Koyanaghi–Harada syndrome
	Wegener's granulomatosis
	Whipple's disease

overlooked if an ESR is not obtained. Another hint is a high platelet count. Other connective tissue diseases are less common than in younger patients. Bacterial prostatitis and related urinary tract infections are more common due to prostatic hypertrophy in elderly men. In developed countries, endocarditis has become more common in older patients. Occult pulmonary emboli always should be considered in the differential diagnosis. Factitious fever is rare in the elderly.

Nosocomial FUO

Fever that develops after a patient has been admitted to hospital and then remains undiagnosed is termed nosocomial FUO. These patients usually are being treated for one or more major pre-existing conditions, and have multiple possible reasons for developing fever. Several of these may be contributing simultaneously to the development of fever. After common bacterial infections such as pneumonia, urinary tract infection, and bacteraemia have been excluded, many other conditions remain in the differential diagnosis, for example: local or disseminated candidiasis, *Clostridium difficile* diarrhoea or colitis, cytomegalovirus infection, hepatitis, sinusitis (especially if the patient is intubated), intravascular catheter-related local or bloodstream infections, and infective endocarditis. The possibility that a non-infectious inflammatory condition such as acalculous cholecystitis, gout, or pseudogout has flared during hospitalization for another condition should be considered. Occult pulmonary emboli are an important cause of nosocomial FUO. Drug fever is especially common in this patient group.

Neutropenic FUO

The number of patients with neutropenia caused by cytotoxic chemotherapy for various diseases is increasing, although the duration of neutropenia is now being curtailed by administration of colony-stimulating factors. Fevers in neutropenic patients are very different from the classical FUO defined above. The leading causes of neutropenic FUO are bacteraemias, pneumonias, and skin soft tissue infections. Urinary tract infections are less common than in nosocomial FUOs (above). Focal bacterial infections of intravascular lines and puncture wounds, skin folds, and the perianal area all are common, often associated with bacteraemia. In the early stages of neutropenia, fevers are usually caused by bacteria, but if neutropenia persists, fungal, viral, and other conditions become relatively more common. However, this well-known sequence loses diagnostic value when the patient has received multiple cycles of chemotherapy and antimicrobial drugs.

The natural history of neutropenic FUOs tends to be much shorter than that of classical FUOs. Onset of fever often occurs within days of onset of neutropenia; immediate empiric treatment is usually given, and improvement often is rapid. The aetiology of these FUOs often remains unconfirmed. In the majority of neutropenic FUOs the fever is likely due to infection, but the aetiological organism(s) will be identified in only 40–60 per cent. Recurrent episodes are likely as long as the patient remains neutropenic.

HIV-associated FUO

A self-limited period of fever often occurs during primary HIV infection. After a long asymptomatic interval, fevers and FUOs are extremely common during the later stages of HIV infection. This justifies the introduction of the term 'HIV-associated FUO' in the definitions listed above. The single most common cause of FUO in this setting is mycobacterial infection (tuberculosis in developing countries, *M avium* complex (**MAC**) in the developed world). MAC infection eventually affects up to 40 per cent of acquired immune deficiency syndrome (**AIDS**) patients in developed countries. Many other diagnoses must be considered, especially *Pneumocystis carinii*, cytomegalovirus infection, disseminated cryptococcosis, toxoplasmosis of the central nervous system, lymphomas, and nocardiosis. In the appropriate geographic regions, disseminated leishmaniasis, histoplasmosis and coccidiodomycosis must be considered. Recently, *Bartonella* species, which cause bacillary angiomatosis and peliosis hepatitis, also have been found to cause febrile bacteraemic syndromes and endocarditis in AIDS patients.

Investigation of FUO

At the first encounter, a meticulous history should be taken and a complete physical examination performed. The theme should be attention to detail, for example, careful ophthalmoscopy after dilatation of the pupils could reveal Roth spots or retinal tubercules in classical FUO, retinal candidiasis in nosocomial FUO, or cytomegalovirus retinitis in HIV-associated FUO. Routine test results (chest radiograph, routine blood count, differential cell count, erythrocyte sedimentation rate and serum biochemistry) should be scanned for clues. A raised serum uric acid could signal rapid cell turnover in lymphoma, and alkaline phosphatase can indicate liver involvement. The peripheral blood smear should be carefully examined for abnormalities such as thrombocytosis, leukaemoid reactions, presence of nucleated red blood cells, and other clues that the marrow is reacting to a pathological stimulus. The initial findings should be reviewed in relation to the tempo of disease progression before deciding upon the next round of investigations. What major tests have already been performed elsewhere? Repetition of costly radiographs and scans may be unnecessary. Can further testing be safely postponed? Sometimes more will be learned by waiting, or the FUO may resolve spontaneously.

The next level of investigation usually will involve blood cultures, skin testing for delayed hypersensitivity to tuberculosis, and selected serologic tests for infections and connective tissue diseases. In older patients, tests for prostate-specific antigen and carcinoembryonic antigen should be obtained. If any clues are found that increase the pre-test probability of infective endocarditis (e.g. unexplained heart murmurs, emboli), echocardiography should be performed.

Selection of further investigations requires careful consideration of the likely yield, risks, and costs of each. Because many FUOs are associated with intra-abdominal conditions, computed tomography (**CT**) of the abdomen often is valuable. Sinus radiographs and pulmonary CT can reveal the lesions of Wegener's granulomatosis. Radiographs of the bowel with contrast can reveal abnormalities needing further investigation. Gastrointestinal endoscopy with biopsy is often appropriate if symptoms or imaging studies suggest enteric conditions such as inflammatory bowel disease or cancer. Adjunctive imaging with magnetic resonance imaging scan, ^{67}gallium or ^{111}indium-labelled leucocytes can be helpful, but these tests should be used selectively because they are costly, and of limited sensitivity; the chance that one of these will reveal a diagnosis is quite low if radiographs and CT scans are negative. If the echocardiogram is indeterminate but endocarditis still seems likely, transoesophageal echocardiography should be performed.

Biopsies of bone marrow, lymph nodes, lung tissue, liver, skin, and temporal arteries or other vessels are essential for the diagnosis of many FUOs. Exploratory laparotomy, previously often performed for diagnosis of FUO, is now rarely necessary because of improved imaging techniques. Abnormalities of cytokines occur in over two-thirds of FUO patients, but this finding has not yet proven useful in diagnosis.

Approach to treatment

Treatment of the fever itself is indicated if fever distresses the patient, exacerbates heart failure, or is severe enough to cause a catabolism and wasting. Otherwise, the temperature curve can be observed in the absence of treatment, often yielding useful new information while investigations continue. If the fever must be treated, aspirin, paracetamol, or a non-steroidal anti-inflammatory drug in standard doses usually will suffice. A regular dosage schedule rather than occasional or p.r.n. dosing is recommended.

Classical FUO

If an aetiological diagnosis cannot be made at first, it is usually best to withhold treatment while observing the patient's progress at regular intervals. If he or she is too ill to permit prolonged observation, empirical treatment for FUO may be considered. The most common choice for a therapeutic trial is corticosteroid. The recommended dose for an adult is prednisone 30 mg twice daily initially, or the equivalent dose of another corticosteroid.

Neutropenic FUO

After performing a focused physical examination, obtaining a chest roentgenogram and sending two blood samples and a urine sample for cultures, empiric broad-spectrum antibacterial therapy should be started immediately, before results of laboratory tests are available. Later, antifungal or antiviral therapy may be added according to the patient's progress and the results of investigations.

HIV-associated FUO

For HIV-associated FUO, if the chest radiograph is abnormal or the patient is hypoxic, bronchial washings or biopsy may reveal a pathogen such as *Pneumocystis*, mycobacteria, *Cryptococcus*, or cytomegalovirus. Direct staining of stool may reveal mycobacteria. If the patient is stable, the results of blood cultures for mycobacteria and unusual bacteria such as *Rhodococcus* or *Bartonella* should be awaited before further invasive tests are done. If the fever remains undiagnosed at this stage, bone marrow and liver biopsies are most likely to be informative. Once the cause of HIV-associated FUO has been diagnosed, specific treatment regimens described in Chapter 16.35 can be prescribed.

Prognosis

Classical FUO is a serious condition. Although most of the causes of this type of FUO can be treated, the 1-year mortality remains at 20–30 per cent. Obviously, the prognosis varies depending upon the underlying disease and the age of the patient. If FUO persists undiagnosed for more than 6–12 months, the likelihood that a specific diagnosis will ever be made decreases, and the prognosis improves greatly, to less than 5 per cent mortality. The prognosis for nosocomial FUO depends largely on the underlying diagnoses. The short-term prognosis for neutropenic FUO is excellent, with over 90 per cent response to initial empiric antimicrobial therapy (with appropriate modification as laboratory results return). Again, the long-term prognosis is determined largely by the underlying diagnosis. Most of the causes of HIV-associated FUO can be treated, but these patients have a relatively poor prognosis, with death likely within 2 years because HIV disease is usually advanced by the time the patient has FUO. The prognosis has improved somewhat with the recent introduction of protease inhibitors and combination antiretroviral therapy. Atypical mycobacteria (which are the commonest cause of HIV-associated FUO) can be suppressed but seldom cured, and are likely to develop resistance during therapy.

Further reading

Durack, D.T. and Street, A.C. (1991). Fever of unknown origin—reexamined and redefined. In *Current clinical topics in infectious diseases*, (ed. J.S. Remington and M.N. Swartz), vol. 11, pp. 35–51. Blackwell Scientific Publications, Boston.

Gelfand, J.A. and Wolff, S.M. (1995). Fever of unknown origin. In: *Principles and practice of infectious diseases*, (4th edn), (ed. G.L. Mandell, J.E. Bennett, R. Dolin), pp. 536–49. Churchill Livingstone, New York.

Kazanjian, P.H. (1992). Fever of unknown origin: review of 86 patients treated in community hospitals. *Clinical Infectious Diseases*, **15**, 968–73.

Mackowiak, P. (ed). (1997). *Fever: basic mechanisms and management*, (2nd edn). Raven Press, New York.

Petersdorf, R.G. and Beeson, P.B. (1961). Fever of unexplained origin: report on 100 cases. *Medicine*, **40**, 1–30.

Chapter 16.116

Septicaemia

P. A. Murphy

Septicaemia is the term used for clinical states in which bacteria are present in the bloodstream and cause systemic symptoms such as fever and hypotension. It is the most common cause of the systemic inflammatory response syndrome. However, the manifestations of septicaemia can also be induced by non-bacterial infectious agents, by non-living bacterial or fungal products, or by a variety of non-infectious conditions such as major trauma, burns, or pancreatitis. This reflects the fact that bacteria are only triggers: the host reaction to infection is responsible for all the phenomena observed in septicaemia, and the host reaction can be triggered in other ways.

Table 1 The common causes of community acquired 'primary' septicaemia in adults

Neisseria gonorrhoeae	*Streptococcus faecalis*
Staphylococcus aureus	*Neisseria meningitidis*
Streptococcus pneumoniae	*Listeria monocytogenes*
Streptococcus pyogenes, groups A-T	*Escherichia coli*., Pseudomonas, etc
Non-typhoidal salmonellae	

Perhaps the best evidence that bacteria only start the septic process is provided by the toxic shock syndrome. In this syndrome, toxin-producing staphylococci are located in the vagina, or sometimes in a wound. The toxin is a 'super antigen' which binds to the V β region of the T cell receptors on 15–25 per cent of T cells. Although toxin binding is not actually in the antigen-reactive site, the T cell behaves as if it had bound antigen. A normal antigen activates perhaps one in a million T cells; the response to a super antigen is over 100 000 times as strong. The patient develops all the manifestations of sepsis and may die, even though blood cultures are invariably negative.

Primary and secondary septicaemia

Most septicaemias are 'secondary'. There is a clinically obvious infected focus—a carbuncle, a pneumonia, a urinary tract infection, etc.—and the organisms grow to high levels in that site. Some foci are infected items of hardware such as intravenous lines and intraarterial pressure monitors.

Almost any organism may cause a secondary septicaemia. Some are high-grade pathogens such as the pneumococcus, following its usual path of nasopharyngeal colonization to pneumonia to sepsis. At the other end of the spectrum are organisms such as *Pseudomonas thomasii*, which causes disease only if it is allowed to grow in intravenous fluids, and then is infused into the patient. The essence of secondary septicaemia is that some circumstance allows the generation of a large local population of organisms, which may be virulent, but do not have to be. From the local lesion, organisms are fed into the bloodstream.

'Primary' septicaemias are those without a clinically obvious focus of infection. Of course, there always is a portal of entry, but it may be subtle. Since there is no large local population, the organisms have to be capable of maintaining themselves in the bloodstream. In one kind of primary septicaemia, high-grade capsulated extracellular pathogens infect reasonably well people. In the other kind, organisms of low virulence invade persons whose defences have been abrogated by disease or its treatment.

Primary septicaemia acquired in the community

Most patients in this class are not in the best of health. They are old, alcoholic, malnourished, or suffer from various debilitating diseases such as cirrhosis or diabetes. None the less, they have defences, and a relatively few organisms cause most of the septicaemias (Table 1). This list refers to adults: a paediatric list would be headed by the pneumococcus and *Haemophilus influenzae*, and a neonatal one by Gram-negative rods and Group B streptococci. The list is in approximate order of frequency for times when salmonellae and meningococci are not epidemic. Noteworthy is the position of the Gram-negative rods so common in hospitals: if there is no urinary tract

Table 2 Common sites from which septicaemia arises in relatively normal patients

Site	Likely bacterial causes of sepsis
Urine	Aerobic Gram-negative rods (90%) Aerobic Gram-positive cocci (10%)
Skin	Gram-positive cocci
Respiratory	*Streptococcus pneumoniae*
Abdominal Gallbladder	Aerobic Gram-negative rods, *Str. faecalis*
Bowel perforations	Aerobic Gram-negative rods
Pelvic inflammatory disease	*Neisseria gonorrhoeae* Mixed anaerobes

infection or other local pathology, these are rare causes of sepsis acquired outside hospital.

Since the spleen is a major filter for bacteria in the bloodstream, septicaemias due to organisms such as pneumococci, *H. influenzae*, and *Capnocytophaga canimorsus* are more common in splenectomized persons and may be overwhelming. Septicaemia with shock acquired in the community by a healthy person is a great rarity. If there is no history of splenectomy, then the most likely culprits are *Staphylococcus aureus* and the meningococcus. *S. aureus* sepsis, with or without endocarditis, is particularly common in persons who inject themselves with illegal drugs.

Community-acquired septicaemia with a local focus

Common foci for the origin of sepsis are listed in Table 2, with the classes of organisms most likely to be responsible. Although it is true that septicaemia from a local focus can occur in healthy people, this is rare. Most of the people who develop generalized sepsis from a pneumonia or a urinary tract infection are old, malnourished, or suffer from debilitating disease.

Over half of urinary tract infections are caused by *Escherichia coli*, and most of the rest by other Gram-negative rods. A Gram stain of the spun urinary sediment is a reliable guide to those few cases where enterococci or staphylococci are responsible.

Skin ulcers and areas of cellulitis generally have a Gram-positive flora of streptococci or staphylococci, and those are the organisms recovered from the bloodstream if the patient is septic. This is also true of sepsis related to ischaemic or diabetic feet. The streptococci may be quite diverse: not only Group A, but also B, F, G, and viridans species. Decubitus ulcers may be associated with Gram-positive septicaemia, but anaerobes such as *Bacteroides fragilis* and Clostridia are more common.

Pneumonia with sepsis in a patient who has not been treated with antibiotics is mostly caused by the pneumococcus. In influenza epidemics, some cases are caused by *S. aureus*, haemolytic streptococci, and *H. influenzae*. Gram-negative rods may cause pneumonias in persons previously treated with antibiotics. Persons infected with HIV are most likely to present with pneumococcal pneumonia. However, they may present with pseudomonas pneumonia, which is virtually never seen in normal individuals.

Sometimes the source of sepsis is in the upper respiratory tract. Acute sinusitis and otitis media are highly symptomatic, seldom cause sepsis, and are unlikely to create a diagnostic problem. However, persons with chronic sinusitis or otitis media may be so used to their symptoms that they do not report them. Complications such as cholesteatomas and infective necrosis of bone are usually present, and the sepsis is precipitated by invasion and thrombosis of one of the cerebral veins. A similar condition, occurring in the absence of chronic disease, is Lemierre's septic thrombosis of the internal jugular vein, which is almost always caused by fusiforms.

Abdominal catastrophes usually present as such. However, cholecystitis can be completely silent, especially in an old person, and may give rise to septicaemia with Gram-negative rods or enterococci. Similarly, diverticulitis or appendicitis in an old person may cause few local symptoms. Despite the very large numbers of anaerobes in colonic contents, the organisms in the bloodstream are usually Gram-negative aerobic rods. However, if the patient has an abscess, Bacteroides or other anaerobes may cause septicaemia.

Young women may acquire septicaemia because of pelvic inflammatory disease. Gonorrhoea is probably the most frequent single cause. Infected abortions are now uncommon, but infections of intrauterine devices are quite frequent. Postpartum infections due to retained products of conception are also seen. Most pelvic infections cause septicaemia with *E. coli*, Group B streptococci, or anaerobic cocci. Often several organisms infect the bloodstream simultaneously.

Septicaemia in hospitalized patients

Septicaemia in patients in hospital is no different in principle from sepsis in the community. However, it is vastly more frequent, for a number of reasons. The most important reasons from the diagnostic point of view are the portals of entry for organisms which are provided by surgical wounds, urinary and vascular catheters, and other impedimenta of modern medicine. General factors such as old age, steroid treatment, and diabetes make it more likely that patients will get septicaemia but do not greatly influence the route. However, patients with severe neutropenia are so susceptible to infection that bacteria may invade from trivial local lesions, or from no visible lesion at all.

The most common focus of infection is the urinary tract; it is estimated that 10 per cent of all hospitalized patients have an indwelling urinary catheter, and that even with the best care, 25 per cent of those will be infected by the 14th day. The most common organism is still *E. coli*, but because of the strong selective pressure of antibiotics, it now causes only one-third of cases. Most of the cases are due to other Gram-negative rods with Enterococcus the most common Gram-positive species. In forming an opinion of the likely cause of sepsis in any particular patient, there are two main considerations. First, if the patient's urine is known to be infected with, say, *Enterobacter cloacae*, then that organism is the most likely cause of the sepsis. Second, in most hospitals particular organisms are troublesome on particular wards at particular times. If it is known that three patients on a particular urology ward developed septicaemia with *Serratia marcescens* in the last 10 days, then when a fourth patient on that ward develops sepsis, *Serratia marcescens* is probably the culprit.

The next most common source of sepsis is probably the surgical wound. Included in this category are deep-seated processes such as mediastinitis, leaking intestinal anastomoses, vaginal cuff infections, and infections of the renal transplant bed. In any of these, there may be no evidence of infection in the surface incision. If the patient has recently had an operation, one should be very unwilling to consider any other source of sepsis.

Intravenous line sepsis is rare if the device has been in place less than 24 h, and is uncommon before 72 h. Lines maintained for long periods, such as hyperalimentation lines, inevitably become infected unless cared for by special teams. The most troublesome area for line sepsis in most hospitals is the intensive care unit. It is not uncommon for a patient to have a peripheral line, a central line, a Swan-Ganz catheter, and an arterial line, all inserted in haste under conditions of dubious sterility, and all maintained for several days.

There are several distinct types of intravenous line sepsis. Occasionally the infusion fluid is contaminated, especially if additives have been necessary. Much more often, the fluid is sterile, but there is cellulitis of the puncture wound, infection of the plastic catheter, or septic thrombophlebitis. Over 50 per cent of line sepsis is caused by staphylococci, with *S. epidermidis* more common than *S. aureus* in most series. Viridins streptococci, enterococci, Gram-negative rods and Candida cause most of the other cases.

A very common source of sepsis in patients in hospital is the chest. Some cases have straightforward illnesses such as post-influenzal pneumococcal pneumonia, which are entirely analogous to the same diseases developing in the community. Most cases, however, develop in patients who aspirate pharyngeal contents for one reason or another.

On obstetric and gynaecological wards, sepsis is usually associated with infection of the pregnant or recently pregnant uterine cavity. Attempts to induce abortion by intra-amniotic injections of urea or saline, prolonged labor with ruptured membranes, or the retention of products of conception are the usual predisposing factors. The most dangerous organism is the Group A *Streptococcus pyogenes*, but this has become rare and most cases now are caused by other streptococci.

Burned patients are very susceptible to septicaemia because the dead skin rapidly becomes colonized with bacteria, often in concentrations of 10^8 organisms per gram. The organism causing septicaemia is almost always that most prominent in the burn at the time, and on good burn units this information is available.

A very important patient population is those who do not have normal defences against infection. By far the most important defect is the lack of mature neutrophils; septicaemia becomes progressively more common as the absolute neutrophil count falls below 500/mm^3. Such patients are susceptible to all the usual hospital acquired infections, but in addition are constantly in danger of being overwhelmed by their own flora. They often have several episodes of septicaemia. The initial ones are generally caused by organisms such as *E. coli* and Klebsiella which are normal enteric flora. Antibiotics select out resistant organisms, and subsequent episodes are due to organisms such as Enterobacter or Pseudomonas which are rarely found in the faeces of normal people. Fungaemias due to *Candida* spp. or to *Torulopsis glabrata* also become common. At all stages of the illness, 10–20 per cent of septicaemias are caused by Gram-positive species such as staphylococci and corynebacteria.

The prevention of septicaemia

Septicaemia is a dangerous illness, with a substantial mortality even in fundamentally healthy people. Because of the danger of overwhelming pneumococcal sepsis, most physicians agree that the young person who has lost his/her spleen should receive oral penicillin prophylaxis for perhaps 2 years after the event, in addition to receiving anti-pneumococcal, *H. influenzae*, and meningococcal vaccines. Other than this, we have no control over cases arising in the community, but many of the cases arising in hospital are preventable. Physicians can make a major contribution to infection control by reducing the number of invasive procedures used, and especially by restricting their duration. Surgeons can contribute by following the fundamental principles of surgery in clean procedures, and by the proper use of drains and antibiotics when infection is probable. If it is known that a patient will be aplastic for some time, the incidence of septicaemia can be reduced by selective decontamination of the gut. The aim is to kill the aerobic Gram-negative rods which are the most common causes of septicaemia while leaving the anaerobic population intact. The antibiotic most often used is norfloxacin.

Clinical features

Septicaemia is one of the very few clinical situations in which the patient can give little useful information. He may complain of fever, rigors, or headache, may simply feel very ill, or may be too obtunded to complain of anything. Frequently, septicaemia develops in a patient already gravely ill from some other process, and incapable of communicating with attendants.

Septicaemia should be suspected whenever there is an acute change in the patient's condition. Almost all patients develop some fever, and those in reasonably good condition usually exceed 39°C. Failure to develop a temperature greater than 37.6°C is a bad prognostic sign, and patients whose body temperature stays subnormal virtually all die. Chills and rigors simply mean that the temperature is rising rapidly; they have no independent significance.

If the patient is closely observed, certain signs may be seen even before fever. Unexplained apprehension, lethargy, and clouding of consciousness are commonly noticed by alert relatives or nurses. Tachypnoea and respiratory alkalosis is another early sign.

Hypotension usually follows fever, but if a large number of organisms has been suddenly introduced into the circulation, it may be the initial sign. Hypotension is due to peripheral vasodilation and the cardiac output is high or comparatively high. Cardiac outputs of 20 l/min may be seen in healthy young men; more modest outputs of 7–8 l/min may represent the maximum in a frail elderly patient. By the time most patients come under observation, much fluid has been lost from the circulation through leaky capillaries into the tissues. Cardiac output falls, and the patient appears pale, cold, and clammy.

The pulmonary vascular resistance is persistently elevated, and the arterial oxygen tension becomes subnormal very early. At least some of this pulmonary dysfunction is due to obstruction of pulmonary arterioles with microthrombi: much of the rest appears to be due to leaky pulmonary capillaries. Severe forms of pulmonary dysfunction are associated with gross hypoxaemia, visible infiltrates on chest radiography, and other features of the adult respiratory distress syndrome.

If the patient is already severely ill, septicaemia may present as unexplained deterioration. Bleeding, thrombocytopenia, or leucocytosis may be noticed. Leucopenia may also occur if the patient's marrow reserves of neutrophils become exhausted. Oliguria or anuria, jaundice, or cardiac failure may follow inadequate perfusion of those organs. Organic psychoses of many varieties may occur for the same reason. Some cases present with ecthyma gangrenosum or other skin lesions.

Management

The essentials in the management of septicaemia are to cut off the inflow of organisms to the bloodstream, to kill or inhibit those already there, and to restore the perfusion of vital organs. Bleeding, delirium, and pulmonary and renal failure will generally take care of themselves if the essentials have been achieved. Operationally, the initial steps are the removal or drainage of the source of sepsis (if that is possible), the selection of a suitable antibiotic or antibiotics, and the infusion of large quantities of fluid intravenously.

Clinical assessment

The experienced clinician makes a gestalt assessment of the severity of the patient's state, taking many factors into consideration. The bedside chart shows the height of the fever and the speed of its rise. The pulse rate and blood pressure are measured if not charted. A look at the patient from the foot of the bed may show apathy, clouding of consciousness, or tachypnoea. Other associated findings may include skin rashes or jaundice. A rapid search for the source of the infection should follow. In a patient from outside the hospital, signs of cutaneous ulcers, pneumonia, local or generalized peritonitis, pyelonephritis, and pelvic inflammatory disease are looked for. In a patient already in the hospital, intravascular catheters and monitoring devices, urinary catheters, surgical wounds and deep infections of recent operation sites, pneumonia, and decubitus ulcers should be considered first. This rapid assessment should take no more than 30 minutes. A tentative diagnosis is made, together with a guess at the responsible organism. The most useful diagnostic specimens are taken for culture; these will always include two blood cultures, together with urine, pus, sputum, CSF, etc. as appropriate. Treatment must be got underway immediately. Radiography, sonograms, CT scans, and other time-wasting investigations should be deferred until the patient's condition stabilizes.

Differential diagnosis

There is a very large number of causes of fever, and if there is no evidence of shock it may be reasonable to consider drug reactions, viral infections, and various other non-infectious diagnoses, even to the point of deferring treatment. But the more acute the onset of fever, the higher the value it reaches, and the poorer the appearance of the patient, the more likely it is that bacteria are in the bloodstream. Treatment should not be delayed unless bacterial sepsis is thought to be an improbable explanation of the patient's state. Even then, the patient should be closely observed for evidence of deterioration until the situation clarifies. If the patient is neutropenic, there is no case for delay. It is true that only about half of the febrile episodes occurring in neutropenic patients can be shown to be due to bacterial infection, but untreated sepsis in such patients is generally fatal within 24 hours.

Treatment

Antibiotic selection

It is important not to waste too much time on this. Most organisms are somewhat sensitive to most antibiotics. Even in leukaemic patients, antibiotic regimes which are theoretically unsuitable for the organism which eventually grows out of the bloodstream, often lead to clinical improvement. There is good evidence that the sensitivity or resistance of the organisms in the bloodstream to the antibiotics prescribed during the first 24 hours of the patient's stay in hospital makes little difference to mortality. Therefore, weigh whatever clinical evidence is available, make a guess at the most likely flora, and pick something which covers it. It is better to do anything than to do nothing.

The antibiotics usually selected for treatment of presumed septicaemia are third-generation cephalosporins such as ceftriaxone or an extended spectrum penicillin such as ticarcillin in combination with a β-lactamase inhibitor. Reasonable people differ over whether or not to add an aminoglycoside; personally I only use gentamicin and its relatives if there is a probability of Pseudomonas, if the septicaemia is overwhelming, or if the patient is neutropenic.

A few treatable organisms are completely resistant to cephalosporins and aminoglycosides. Rickettsiae can cause septic shock, and both typhus and Rocky Mountain spotted fever should be thought of in the right parts of the world. Occasionally, psittacosis presents with very high fever and few or no pulmonary signs. Some young women have salpingitis caused by chlamydiae. Chlamydial and rickettsial infections respond to doxycycline. Malaria should be specifically excluded by the examination of blood smears if it is conceivable that the patient might have acquired it by any route including transfusions. *Candida albicans* can cause intravenous line sepsis in normal patients or septicaemia in debilitated ones. Fungal sepsis is seldom immediately lethal, and most oncology units do not treat for it in the first instance, particularly since amphotericin B is so toxic. Viral haemorrhagic fevers are not treatable with antibiotics. However, if the patient has been to Africa, or works with monkeys, they are worth remembering because several pose an infection hazard to the attendants.

Whatever antibiotic regime is chosen, it should be given intravenously in large doses. When the blood cultures are reported, the sensitivities as measured in the laboratory should be checked against the antibiotic regimen being given. If the regimen appears to be inadequate, one should change it, even if the patient appears to be improving. An initial mistake in antibiotic selection is not usually disastrous, but persistence in error commonly is.

Intravenous fluid therapy

A large-bore intravenous line should be inserted as soon as possible. Through it one gives fluid until the haemodynamic parameters become normal, or until there is evidence of fluid overload. There is no evidence that any particular formula of intravenous fluid is better than normal saline. Usually, saline containing some potassium, glucose, and a substrate metabolizable into bicarbonate is given, on the assumption that those additions are harmless and may be useful. Solutions containing albumin or other colloids such as hydroxyethyl starch can be used if available because they may better retain fluid in the bloodstream. If the patient's haematocrit is less than 33 per cent, enough whole blood or packed red cells should be given to raise it above 33 per cent.

A good starting dose of fluid would be 1 litre of Ringers' lactate in the first hour. If marked hypotension is present, it could be given faster and rapidly followed by a second litre. One would then reassess the patient. If the blood pressure has risen to normal, the pulse has slowed somewhat, respiration is no faster, the patient is alert and oriented, and urine flow exceeds 75 ml/h, well and good. One would slow the rate of fluid administration to perhaps 1 litre every 6 hours and await events.

Under most circumstances, when the patient is not desperately ill, this process can be monitored by ordinary clinical methods. The pulse rate, blood pressure, and respiratory rate should be measured and recorded at regular intervals. In most patients it is best to catheterize the urinary bladder to provide accurate information about urine flow. One watches the jugular veins and regularly listens for crepitations at the lung bases.

If the patient remains hypotensive and there is no evidence of fluid overload, one should continue to give fluid, but also look for other correctable problems. The arterial oxygen saturation or pO_2 should be checked; if these are not over 90 per cent or 65 mmHg respectively, the patient should be given oxygen, and intubated if necessary. Obvious electrolyte abnormalities should be corrected. Patients commonly have normal or near normal serum sodium and potassium levels, but very low levels of phosphate or magnesium. Severe hypoglycaemia should also be corrected.

The correction of acidosis is controversial. If the arterial pH is below 7.2, most physicians would cautiously give bicarbonate. However, there is no evidence, in people or in animals, that this is beneficial, and total correction of pH into the normal range is positively harmful. It seems to be true that if the patient's circulatory state can be improved, the acidosis will take care of itself, and that if that cannot be done, bicarbonate will not change the outcome.

If simple management as above appears to be failing, then someone will suggest the use of a Swan-Ganz pulmonary artery catheter. There is no published evidence that the use of these catheters is beneficial for the patient. They certainly are beneficial for the doctor, for they provide accurate left atrial pressures and allow very precise titration of fluid status and haemodynamic values. But what published evidence there is strongly suggests that the use of a pulmonary artery catheter in septic patients is associated with increased mortality, and probably not just because the catheters are used in the sickest patients. It may be more useful to intubate the patient, because that almost certainly will improve oxygenation, and will spare him or her the work of trying to ventilate increasingly oedematous lungs.

Vasoconstrictors and inotropes

If the patient has failed to respond to maximal fluid repletion, and remains hypotensive with now raised atrial pressures, the situation is extremely serious. The expected mortality of such patients is over 50 per cent. The use of inotropes and vasoconstrictors has in the past been controlled by using them to achieve some predetermined mean arterial pressure. The raised blood pressure was often achieved by inducing peripheral vasoconstriction and tissue ischaemia. Death rates for such patients were well over 80 per cent.

We have now retreated from the over-aggressive use of vasoconstrictors. The cardiac blood flow occurs largely during diastole, and a diastolic pressure of 55–60 mmHg is necessary to oxygenate the myocardium adequately. Also, the brain blood flow is autoregulating down to a mean arterial pressure of 70–80 mmHg, but falls if the MAP is below that. These two values are therefore reasonable minimal goals, and it should be noted that both are below normal for most people.

The most useful drugs are those vasoconstrictors which also have positive inotropic action, such as norepinephine and dopamine. Dopamine is especially useful because in doses of 1–5 mg/kg/min it actually increases renal blood flow. In doses above 20 mg/kg/min dopamine is a general vasoconstrictor and probably deleterious.

Although everyone agrees that septic patients who remain hypotensive after maximal fluid repletion should be given vasoconstrictors, there is a remarkable paucity of evidence that such treatment is valuable in terms of improving mortality. Recently, pure inotropes such as dobutamine became fashionable, on the grounds that they improved cardiac output and oxygen delivery to the tissues. It is certainly true that patients who achieve higher oxygen delivery rates do better than these who do not. The question is whether treatment, of any kind, can help achieve this desirable state. A controlled trial failed to show improved mortality, but Shoemaker commented acidly that the trial showed it was 'impossible to prevent organ failure in patients who already have failed organs'.

Removal of septic foci

If a patient in hospital develops septicaemia and no other source is evident, it is advisable to remove all intravascular devices. If they must be replaced, completely new systems should be inserted in vessels far removed from the old sites. If vascular access is limited and a line is precious, a compromise can be achieved by changing the device over a wire, and performing a quantitative culture of the old line. If that culture is negative, the new line can be left in place. However, if culture of the old line is positive then the new line must be removed and a new site selected. If there is evidence of suppurative thrombophlebitis, the affected segment of vein must be removed surgically, or the septicaemia will probably continue.

Localized collections of pus such as empyema or subphrenic abscess should be drained. This is best done by radiologists, using CT or ultrasonic guidance. Foci that are acutely infected but where there is no frank abscess formation are usually left alone in the first instance. Cholecystitis, pneumonia, sinusitis, and pelvic inflammatory disease will all generally respond to antibiotic therapy. If an operation is thought necessary, it can be done later when the patient's condition is stable and the local inflammation has subsided. If the patient has extensive phlegmonous inflammation, but no localized collection, amputation or massive debridement may be lifesaving.

Anticoagulation

Disseminated intravascular coagulation is common in Gram-negative sepsis, and also occurs in Gram-positive infections, but there is no evidence that preventing it by the use of heparin makes any difference to the outcome of sepsis. However, heparin therapy is lifesaving for septic pelvic thrombophlebitis in women, and sometimes for suppurative thrombophlebitis of central veins which cannot be surgically excised. Antibiotic therapy alone does not cure these patients; they continue to have septic pulmonary emboli, abscesses, and empyemas. The addition of heparin generally leads to cure.

Other supportive measures

Septicaemic patients are usually already gravely ill with some other process. They will need all the usual measures for their underlying condition. They may also develop organ failure because of sepsis. It may be necessary to manage postoperative ileus, epileptic fits, and hepatic, renal, or pulmonary failure.

Prognosis

It is important not to be unreasonably optimistic, particularly when talking to relatives. Even with the best care, many patients die. The most important single prognostic factor is the patient's general condition. The mortality also rises with age; most of the excess deaths are attributable to cardiac and pulmonary problems, and to tumours. The species of organism is of some consequence; *Pseudomonas aeruginosa* consistently causes over 50 per cent mortality, probably because of its exotoxin. Mortality of other Gram-negative rods ranges from

25–40 per cent. In most recent series, the mortality of Gram-positive sepsis is also in the 25–40 per cent range.

When death is attributable mainly or entirely to infection, it is often due not so much to the septicaemia as to the consequences of infection in the primary site. Extensive pneumonia, meningitis, or widespread intraperitoneal infection may be impossible to deal with, or may lead to such debilitation that the patient expires of the diseases of the bed-ridden—bedsores, pulmonary emboli, and bronchopneumonia.

The presence of shock suggests a large dose of organisms, and not surprisingly mortality in shocked patients is two or three times that of comparable patients with normal blood pressure. The excess mortality almost all occurs in the first 48 hours, and is directly attributable to septicaemia. A normal or subnormal temperature in the presence of septicaemia is also a very bad prognostic sign.

The effect of antibiotic therapy on prognosis is discernible, but not as great as might be expected. Patients treated with antibiotics to which the organisms are sensitive do survive better than those in whom the treatment was not appropriate. However, the general condition, and the presence or absence of shock, are powerful independent variables.

Septicaemia persisting in the face of therapy

If the patient remains febrile and sick after 48 hours of therapy, a total reassessment should be made. The most important is a complete physical examination looking for infectious foci which might have become apparent since admission. Examination should be detailed, including the fundi, the entire skin surface, and rectal and vaginal examinations. New blood cultures, and cultures of anything else which might be helpful, should be obtained.

If the original blood cultures were positive, and the antibiotic therapy was inappropriate, it should be changed if not already done. If the original blood cultures were positive and the organisms were sensitive to the antibiotics employed, then it is probable that the patient has undrained pus somewhere, and search for that should be made by radiography, sonograms, CT scans, or indium-III scans, as appropriate.

The antibiotic regime should be reviewed to make certain that the route, frequency, and dosage are adequate; subtherapeutic doses are particularly common with aminoglycosides. It is often useful to measure antibiotic levels in blood. Neutropenic patients, and those with large infected tissue foci, respond very slowly, even when the antibiotic regime is adequate. In such patients, it may be right to persist with the same therapy provided one is reasonably certain that there are no other adverse factors.

If the original blood cultures are negative, and the patient remains febrile, the antibiotics should be discontinued, and two new ones substituted. The only exception to this rule is if some acceptable non-infectious cause of the symptoms has declared itself. A search for deep infected foci should be made as outlined above. In neutropenic patients, one should probably add amphotericin B at this stage since Candida and other yeasts may take some days to grow out of the original blood cultures.

Failure to respond to two different antibiotic regimes, with no evidence of local sepsis and no response to antifungal drugs suggests that the diagnosis of septicaemia was wrong. Many fevers in hospitalized patients are caused by drug reactions, tumours, or viral infections of diverse types. High spiking fever may persist for months in alcoholic hepatitis. The best way of managing such situations is to withdraw antibiotics while carefully observing the patient and reculturing as indicated.

Experimental treatment

The mortality for cases of sepsis managed as above averages 30 per cent, and 50 per cent if the patient is still hypotensive after maximal resuscitation. There has been great interest in the idea that mortality could be improved by antagonists of various inflammatory mediators such as IL-1, TNF, arachidonic acid metabolites, platelet activating factor, and nitric oxide. The results of a huge volume of work may be summarized by saying that as yet none of these attempts have led to a significant improvement in mortality.

Further reading

Beal, A.L. and Cerra, F.B. (1994). Multiple organ failure syndrome in the 1990s. *Journal of the American Medical Association*, **271**, 226–33.

Galtinoni, L., Brazzi, L., Pelosi, P., *et al.* (1995). A trial of goal oriented hemodynamic therapy in critically ill patients. *New England Journal of Medicine*, **333**, 1025–32.

Heyland, D.K., Cook, D.J., King, D., *et al.* (1996). Maximizing oxygen delivery in critically ill patients: a methodologic appraisal of the evidence. *Critical Care Medicine*, **24**, 517–24.

Kreger, B.E., Craven, D.E., and McCabe, W. (1980). Gram negative bacteremia. Re-evaluation of clinical features and treatment in 612 patients. *American Jurnal of Medicine*, **68**, 344–55.

Maki, D.G. (1987). Nosocomial bacteremia: an epidemiologic overview. *American Jurnal of Medicine*, **70**, 719–32.

Miller, P.J. and Wenzel, R.P. (1987). Etiologic organisms as independent predictors of death and morbidity associated with bloodstream infections. *Journal of Infectious Diseases*, **156**, 471–7.

Rudio, M.I., Basha, M.A., and Zarowitz, B.J. (1996). Is it time to reposition vasopressors and inotropes in sepsis? *Critical Care Medicine*, **24**, 525–37.

Shoemaker, W.C. and Belzberg, H. (1997). Maximizing oxygen delivery in high risk surgical patients. *Critical Care Medicine*, **25**, 714.

Chapter 16.117

Infection in the immunocompromised host

J. Cohen

The term 'immunocompromised host' implies an impaired response to an infective challenge. The most clear-cut examples are the primary immunodeficiency syndromes (see OTM3, pp. 166–75) and patients with acquired immune deficiency syndrome (**AIDS**) (see Chapter 16.35). This chapter deals with a much broader range of patients who are at increased risk of infection either because of their underlying disease or as a result of therapeutic immunosuppression (Table 1).

Infections in immunosuppressed patients can progress with frightening rapidity; the early physical signs are often muted and the microbiology can be confusing. Patients need to be reviewed frequently and will often need empirical therapy, but this does not need be 'blind'; a structured and informed assessment will generally allow a logical response to what are the most likely pathogens.

Table 1 Conditions associated with impaired immune responses and an increased risk of infection

Organ and bone marrow transplantation	Diabetes mellitus
Neutropenia	Haemochromatosis
• complicating the treatment of haematological malignancy	Uraemia
	Severe liver disease
• as part of aplastic anaemia	Burns
Solid tumours	Cushing's disease
'Vasculitic' diseases	Extremes of life
(Felty's syndrome, rheumatoid	Alcohol abuse
arthritis,etc.)	Malnutrition
Trauma/surgery	Radiation injury
Haemodialysis	Spinal cord injury
Splenectomy	Intravenous drug abuse
Pregnancy	Down's syndrome

Pyrexia of unknown origin (see also Chapter 16.115)

Fever in an immunosuppressed patient should never be ignored. In neutropenic patients, fever is often the first and only sign of bacteraemia, and prompt action is necessary; in non-neutropenic patients there is usually less urgency, but a careful and systematic evaluation should be made.

1 *History.* Note should be made of any past history of infection such as bronchiectasis or tuberculosis, or any recent exposures in the community. A detailed travel history is important; patients who have visited certain parts of the United States may have been exposed to the systemic mycoses such as histoplasmosis or coccidioidomycosis, and travellers to Central America or the Far East, even many years ago, may have acquired an asymptomatic infection with the helminth *Strongyloides stercoralis*; immunosuppression can lead to overt disease (the hyperinfection syndrome), with a high mortality.
2 *Physical examination.* This may be disappointing; immunosuppressed patients often do not mount a good inflammatory response. Nevertheless, careful, and if necessary repeated clinical examination is worthwhile, as signs of inflammation may only become apparent when immune function returns. Particular attention should be paid to the presence of new skin lesions. The perianal area and the insertion sites of indwelling right atrial catheters repay careful examination.
3 *The underlying disease.* Neutropenia is a major risk factor for infection, and renders the patient susceptible to bacteraemias, particularly with Gram-negative organisms. A patient with an obstructing bronchial neoplasm may develop a lung abscess due to inadequate drainage. Corticosteroids are used widely; when given in doses exceeding 15–20 mg daily for long periods they increase susceptibility to infections with viruses, fungi, parasites, and bacteria such as *M. tuberculosis*, which are all organisms normally associated with cellular immune defences.
4 *The duration of the immunosuppression.* This has a marked effect on the risk of infection. For instance, in neutropenia the first 10–14 days are complicated by bacterial infections; fungal and viral infections only occur later.
5 *Speed of progression.* Rapid deterioration over the space of a few hours will suggest a bacterial infection or a non-infectious cause, and will need urgent therapy; a more indolent presentation would point to a fungal or mycobacterial aetiology, and treatment can be delayed for a short period to try and establish the diagnosis.
6 *Investigations.* Aspiration and/or biopsy of any new skin lesion in an immunosuppressed patient is well worthwhile. It is important that the diagnostic laboratories are aware of the clinical problem as handling of specimens—and interpretation of the results—will often differ substantially from routine procedures.

In neutropenic patients, infection is directly related to the severity of the neutropenia; the incidence is greatest at below 1×10^9/litre, and particularly when the count falls to less than 0.1×10^9/litre. The commonest isolates used to be Gram-negative bacteria such as *Escherichia coli*, *Pseudomonas aeruginosa*, and klebsiella, but Gram-positive organisms, notably coagulase negative staphylococci (*S. epidermidis*) and viridans streptococci are now the commonest isolates.

Blood cultures should be drawn before treatment is begun. Ideally two sets should be obtained, at least one of which should be from a peripheral vein (rather than an indwelling catheter). Culturing larger volumes of blood (e.g. 30 ml compared with the more conventional 10 ml) will increase the yield. Appropriate samples must also be taken from other potential foci of infection. Treatment must begin before the results of the cultures are available; delay will lead to unacceptable mortality.

The initial empirical antibiotic regimen for the febrile neutropenic patient should be safe and have good bactericidal activity against all the common pathogens. Choice will depend on the availability (and cost) of antibiotics in a given institution, and on local patterns of antibiotic susceptibility. Two regimens that have been well validated are the combination of an antipseudomonal penicillin plus an aminoglycoside (for example, piperacillin plus gentamicin), or the use of a single extended spectrum cephalosporin, such as ceftazidime. Both regimens are active against all the common Gram-negative organisms, but are relatively ineffective at treating Gram-positive bacteria such as coagulase negative staphylococci, which is nowadays a common problem. Unfortunately, only glycopeptides such as vancomycin are reliably active for these organisms. The disadvantage is the toxicity (and cost) of vancomycin, which may not be justified as, unlike the Gram-negative infections, coagulase negative staphylococci rarely cause death. Clinical trials suggest that vancomycin can usually be withheld until the results of blood cultures are known.

If patients respond to the initial regimen, it should be continued for at least 7 days, and ideally until the neutrophil count has returned to $>0.5 \times 10^9$/litre. When this is not possible, treatment is usually stopped after an arbitrary period such as 14 days; rebound bacteraemias can occur and will need further treatment.

A much more difficult problem is the patient who remains persistently febrile. In cases in which the blood cultures are positive the antibiotics may be modified as necessary, e.g. by the addition of vancomycin. If an indwelling right atrial catheter is incriminated as the possible source (the blood cultures will not necessarily be positive) most clinicians will try to continue treatment without removing the line; however, this is rarely successful in the case of Gram-negative or yeast infections. A common problem is the patient who continues to have high swinging fevers in the absence of any obvious focus or positive microbiology. Sometimes repeated clinical examination or investigations will provide a clue: a new infiltrate on the chest radiograph, for instance. In this situation, deep fungal infection becomes more likely. The few clinical trials that have addressed this problem have concluded that persistent fever for 72 h should be

Table 2 Causes of fever and new pulmonary infiltrates in the immunocompromised host

INFECTIONS
Bacterial
Conventional respiratory pathogens: *S. pneumoniae; H. influenzae; Klebsiella*
Nosocomial pathogens; *E. coli; Pseudomonas* spp; *Legionella* spp.
'Atypical' organisms: *Chlamydia psittaci, C. pneumoniae*; mycoplasmas
Mycobacteria and related organisms: *Mycobacterium tuberculosis*; atypical mycobacteria; Nocardia
Other unusual organisms: *Listeria, Bacillus* spp.
Viral
Herpesviruses; Cytomegalovirus; herpes simplex; Varicella-zoster
Respiratory viruses: Respiratory syncytial virus; (para)influenza; adenovirus; measles
Fungi
Systemic mycoses; Blastomycosis; histoplasmosis; coccidioidomycosis
Opportunistic mycoses: Candida; Aspergillus; Mucor; Cryptococcus
Other rare fungi: Trichosporon; Pseudallescheria
Parasites
Pneumocystis; strongyloides; toxoplasma
NON-INFECTIVE CAUSES
Pulmonary pathology
Pulmonary oedema; pulmonary infarction/emboli; pulmonary haemorrhage
Primary or secondary malignancy
Other causes
Drugs (e.g. busulphan)
Activity of the underlying disease (e.g. systemic lupus)
Radiation pneumonitis

treated by adding amphotericin B. At least 0.3 mg/kg should be given in the first 24 h, followed by 0.5–0.75 mg/kg per day thereafter.

In the non-neutropenic immunosuppressed patient, 'pyrexia of unknown origin' is rarely immediately life-threatening, and because of the wide differential diagnosis, it is generally better to pursue the cause rather than embark on empirical therapy.

Fever and new pulmonary infiltrates

Pneumonia is the commonest infective cause of death in immunocompromised patients. It can progress extremely quickly, and conventional diagnostic procedures may be unhelpful. The list of possible causes is so daunting (Table 2) that clinicians can be tempted to use multiple empirical antimicrobial agents, sometimes to the patient's detriment. It is often impossible to 'guess' the precise cause of the infection and multiple causes may be present simultaneously. However, by considering the available information a 'short list' can be constructed to guide further investigation and treatment.

The initial evaluation should follow the approach outlined above. Factors favouring bacterial aetiology include the presence of neutropenia, a rapid clinical evolution (e.g. deterioration over a period of 12 h), progressive hypoxia, a sputum Gram stain showing a marked predominance of a single bacterial morphology, or a chest radiographic appearance that has worsened over a short period. Non-infective causes such as acute lung haemorrhage or pulmonary oedema can present in an identical fashion. In vasculitis and autoimmune diseases, infection can precipitate a relapse of the underlying disease and treatment must be directed both towards improving oxygenation and the underlying infection.

Certain baseline investigations should be done even if urgent treatment is needed. Blood cultures should always be obtained, and sputum if possible. A chest radiograph and arterial blood gas analysis are essential. The initial treatment will be dictated by the clinical circumstances, but very broad-spectrum cover is best avoided. For community acquired infections, a combination of an extended-spectrum cephalosporin and erythromycin is appropriate. For hospital acquired infections, a cephalosporin (combined with an aminoglycoside if there is strong evidence of pseudomonas infection) is reasonable. Where staphylococcal infection is suspected, flucloxacillin and an aminoglycoside should be used. Unusual ('opportunistic') organisms such as Mycobacteria, Nocardia, or Cytomegalovirus (CMV) rarely cause such a rapid clinical deterioration and are extremely difficult to diagnose on clinical grounds. For these reasons, addition of other drugs is usually not warranted. A possible exception is pneumocystis pneumonia (see below).

Patients not requiring immediate empirical therapy can be investigated further. Tests include serology for atypical organisms, and examination of blood and urine for CMV. Sequential chest radiographs should be obtained, but they are not as sensitive as arterial blood gas measurements, which should be repeated twice daily. The radiographic appearances are rarely sufficiently specific as to suggest a precise diagnosis, although they can provide helpful pointers. Other imaging techniques, such as computed tomography (CT), can often provide useful additional information on the extent of the process, but will rarely allow a more precise identification of the cause. In most cases the investigation of choice is bronchoscopy with broncho-alveolar lavage.

Where a specific cause is identified treatment is straightforward. A more difficult problem is the management of a patient with a non-diagnostic bronchoscopy who continues to deteriorate and in whom the suspicion of occult infection remains. Empirical therapy can never be totally comprehensive, and a judgement must be made of the most probable causes. An extended spectrum cephalosporin plus erythromycin will provide cover against likely bacterial pathogens, and flucloxacillin should be added if *Staph. aureus* is suspected. If tuberculosis is likely three agents should be used (rifampicin, isoniazid and pyrazinamide are suitable). Pneumocystis and CMV are difficult to tell apart on clinical grounds alone and often occur together; high-dose co-trimoxazole and ganciclovir are the drugs of first choice.

Acute neurological syndromes

A large number of conventional and opportunist pathogens can lead to neurological infection in immunocompromised patients. Although there is some degree of overlap, the underlying defect in host defence is a often a good indicator of the likely cause (Table 3).

The clinical features may suggest the diagnosis. Meningitic syndromes are more likely to be associated with conventional bacterial infections, listeriosis and tuberculosis, as well as fungi such as Cryptococcus and Candida. In contrast, infections with Toxoplasma, Aspergillus, or Nocardia more commonly present as space-occupying lesions. Pure encephalitic syndromes are less common, but can occur with herpes simplex (although curiously, herpes simplex encephalitis is remarkably uncommon in immunocompromised patients, despite the frequency of re-activation of cutaneous infection). Rhinocerebral

Table 3 Organisms causing neurological infections in different patient groups

Bacteria	Fungi	Parasites	Virus
Neutropenia			
Enterics	Candida Aspergillus Mucor		
T-cell/monocyte defect			
Listeria	Cryptococcus	Toxoplasma	Varicella-zoster
Legionella	Aspergillus	Strongyloides	Herpes simplex
Nocardia	Mucor		Parvovavirus
Mycobacteria	Coccidioides		
Splenectomy			
Strep. pneumoniae			
Haemophilus influenzae			
Neisseria			

Table 4 Gastrointestinal syndromes in the immunocompromised host

Bacteria	Fungi	Parasites	Virus
Oral infection			
	Candida		Herpes simplex
Diarrhoeal syndromes			
C. difficile	Candida	Giardia	Enterovirus
Mycobacteria		Isospora	Adenovirus
Salmonellae		Cryptosporidia	Cytomegalovirus
Shigellae		Microsporidia	Rotavirus
		Strongyloides	
Hepatic syndromes			
	Candida	Toxoplasma	Cytomegalovirus
			Hepatitis B
			Hepatitis C, D, E
			Herpes simplex
			Varicella-zoster

mucormycosis is a progressive, destructive infection caused by *Mucor* and related moulds, that usually begins in the paranasal sinuses and spreads caudally to involve the orbits or the frontal lobes of the brain. It is seen particularly in patients with uncontrolled diabetes mellitus or as a complication of neutropenia.

The speed of progression can also be helpful: bacterial infections generally proceed rapidly, while fungi and parasites pursue a more indolent course. Examination of the cerebrospinal fluid (**CSF**) is mandatory and should include direct microscopy for (myco)bacteria and fungi, and culture. The cryptococcal latex agglutination test is sensitive and specific; it is better than the India ink test, and should be done on all CSF samples from immunosuppressed patients. Other procedures which can be done include antigen tests for the pneumococcus, serological tests for fungi, and the demonstration of specific antibody production or DNA sequences by the polymerase chain reaction (e.g. for herpes simplex and papovaviruses).

The CSF may reveal only non-specific abnormalities. Certain organisms are notable for their absence on direct microscopy: mycobacteria are seen in less than 10 per cent of cases, Nocardia and Aspergillus only very rarely. A predominance of lymphocytes suggests partially treated bacterial infection, tuberculosis or a viral aetiology but not infection with *Listeria monocytogenes*, despite its name. A low CSF glucose points to tuberculosis but is not specific. Sometimes the only abnormality is a modest elevation of the CSF protein; this should never be ignored. Where appropriate, cytological examination of the CSF should be done to exclude carcinomatous or leukaemic meningitis, which can mimic an acute infective presentation.

A CT scan, which should be contrast enhanced, is valuable. Focal, usually enhancing lesions are particularly associated with pyogenic abscesses and toxoplasmosis. Tuberculomas (and even less often, cryptococcomas) can appear as single lesions. the appearances may suggest herpes simplex encephalitis or progressive multifocal encephalitis (**PML**). Magnetic resonance imaging appears to be better then CT scanning for abnormalities of the brainstem (e.g. the basal meningitis associated with cryptococcal infection), and may reveal lesions in toxoplasmosis which are not seen on CT scans. It may be particularly helpful in avoiding a brain biopsy when a diagnosis of PML is considered.

Any new skin lesions should be biopsied. An electroencephalogram is not helpful, unless herpes simplex encephalitis is suspected. Brain biopsy is done rarely, and it should not be considered unless empirical therapy has failed, and there is a real prospect of therapeutic benefit to the patient.

When the initial examination and investigations reveal the probable diagnosis, treatment is straightforward. If the CSF is non-diagnostic but bacterial infection cannot be excluded, empirical antibiotics should be given immediately. An extended spectrum cephalosporin such as cefotaxime is suitable. Empirical antituberculosis therapy should be with three drugs (see above). A common dilemma is the patient with clinical and radiological features of toxoplasmosis; serological tests for toxoplasmosis are not specific in this setting, and although other infections cannot be excluded with certainty it is better to start empirical therapy with pyrimethamine and sulphadimidine. Cerebral aspergillosis and mucormycosis have a very poor prognosis; treatment should start with high-dose amphotericin B, and surgical debridement considered if possible. There is no effective treatment for PML.

Acute gastrointestinal syndromes

The organisms associated with specific gastrointestinal syndromes in these patients are shown in Table 4.

Severe stomatitis is a common complaint in immunosuppressed patients. Candida, herpes simplex, and chemotherapy induced mucositis are clinically indistinguishable and indeed can coexist. In profoundly immunosuppressed patients such as bone marrow transplant recipients, oral candidiasis is very common, and in patients who are seropositive before transplant, reactivation of herpes simplex almost universal. For these reasons, prophylaxis is usually given. Acylovir is extremely effective for herpes simplex virus (**HSV**), and the new triazole agents such as fluconazole are active against candida. Both HSV and Candida can cause oesophagitis, generally (but not exclusively) as an extension of oral disease. Oesophagoscopy with brush cytology and/or biopsy is the 'gold standard' investigation but is often deferred pending the outcome of a therapeutic trial. Proven oesophageal candidiasis should be regarded as 'invasive' disease and treated with systemic antifungals (amphotericin B or fluconazole).

Table 5 Organisms associated with severe infection as a complication of splenectomy

Streptococcus pneumoniae	*Babesia microti*
Other haemolytic streptococci	*Salmonella* spp.
Haemophilus influenzae	*Plasmodium* spp.
Neisseria meningitidis	*Escherichia coli*
Capnocytophaga canimorsus	

A large number of organisms can cause acute diarrhoeal syndromes; in addition, non-infective conditions such as radiation enteritis, ischaemia, drugs, and graft-versus-host disease must be included in the differential diagnosis. There are no distinguishing clinical features of note, and diagnosis depends on microbiological examination of the faeces.

The diarrhoea caused by *Clostridium difficile* is usually due to a pseudomembranous colitis, but neutropenic patients may develop a fulminating invasive colitis associated with clostridial bacteraemia and a high mortality. *Strongyloides stercoralis* is a helminth that can be carried asymptomatically for many years after exposure, but in immunosuppressed patients a rise in the worm burden results in the hyperinfection syndrome, which may present as pneumonitis or intermittent intestinal obstruction. Treatment is with albendazole or mebendazole (some clinicians add ivermectin), which need to be given for extended periods.

Giardiasis is particularly associated with hypogammaglobulinaemia, and curiously is rarely seen in other groups. *Cryptosporidium, Microsporidia,* and *Isospora* are now well recognized causes of severe and sometimes chronic diarrhoea in AIDS patients, but may also occur in other, less severely immunocompromised patients. Among the viruses, CMV can cause a severe colitis, and in these cases ganciclovir is beneficial. The diagnosis should be confirmed by biopsy, but ultimately may depend on the result of a therapeutic trial as demonstration of the organism does not necessarily indicate that it is causing disease.

Mild abnormalities of liver function tests are a common accompaniment to many systemic infections, but hepatitis is a particular feature of both toxoplasmosis and CMV infection. Immunosuppressed patients frequently need blood transfusions, and for this reason blood-borne *hepatitis viruses* have been a particular problem. Historically, interest has been focused on hepatitis B, but since the advent of effective screening hepatitis C (and latterly, hepatitis D and E) have assumed greater importance. Moreover, not only are immunosuppressed patients more often exposed to these infections, the severity of the acute illness and the long-term consequences can differ markedly from the course in the non-compromised host. Hepatitis B vaccine is safe in immunosuppressed patients; a double-dose regimen is given but the seroconversion rate is not as high as in healthy individuals.

Splenectomy

Patients who have had their spleen removed, or who have functional (or more rarely congenital) asplenia, are at increased risk of certain infections. Approximately 50 per cent of infections are meningitis or bacteraemias, and most of the remainder are pneumonias. The encapsulated bacteria (*S. pneumoniae, H. influenzae, N. meningitidis*) account for about 75 per cent of all infections (Table 5). The degree of risk is related to the underlying cause; overall, 4–12 per cent will suffer a serious infection, but this varies from 1.5 per cent following traumatic splenectomy to as high as 25 per cent in patients with thalassaemia. Serious infections are most common during the first 5 years following splenectomy, and particularly during the first year; recurrent infections occur in about 20 per cent of those affected. The risk of fatal infection is very much higher than in the general population; in the post-traumatic group for instance the risk is up to 200 times higher.

All patients who have had a splenectomy or with a non functioning spleen should receive the pneumococcal vaccine. The 14-valent vaccine which had been available for some years has recently been replaced by a new 23-valent formulation, and patients who received the older vaccine should be revaccinated with the new one. Revaccination should be considered every 6 years. In patients who are to undergo elective splenectomy the vaccine should be given at least 2 weeks preoperatively, but in patients in whom this is not possible (e.g. following trauma) vaccination is still worthwhile. Vaccination will not completely remove the risk of infection, and for those at particularly high risk (e.g. children with sickle cell disease) antibiotic prophylaxis (penicillin or erythromycin) should be given as well. Patient education is also important; they should be advised to wear a warning bracelet, and it may be worthwhile giving the patient a supply of amoxycillin and advising them to start treatment at the earliest signs of infection. It would be logical to give these patients the new *H. influenzae* b vaccine as well, although clinical trials of efficacy in this group have not yet been done.

The clinical features of infection in these patients are characterized by a short prodrome followed by a fulminant illness with high fever and few specific clinical signs. At the onset the focus of infection may not be apparent. Laboratory findings consistent with disseminated intravascular coagulation are common. Empirical treatment is with high-dose intravenous antibiotics (e.g. ampicillin plus gentamicin) and supportive care.

Pregnancy

Cellular immune function is compromised during pregnancy, and there are a number of infections which are more severe when they occur in pregnant women. This increased susceptibility to infection should not be confused with the fact that some infections which occur during pregnancy may be very dangerous to the fetus, even though they have little impact on the mother. These fetal infections (e.g. listeriosis, group B streptococcal infection, and toxoplasmosis) are discussed elsewhere (see Chapters 16.38, 16.70, and 16.86). Table 6 lists those infections which are more severe in pregnancy. Several of these merit further comment.

- *HIV.* Despite some early suggestions that pregnancy accelerated the course of HIV infection the present view is that the effect, if any, is small. There are of course profound implications for the fetus which will need to be addressed.
- *Malaria.* Pregnant women living in endemic areas tend to lose their immunity to malaria. Not only is infection more common, it is also more severe; women in the second trimester of pregnancy are at the greatest risk. The presentation of malaria in pregnant women may be atypical, and the diagnosis should always be considered in the presence of fever or jaundice. The major complications are haemolytic anaemia and hepatorenal syndrome.
- *Hepatitis E (HEV)*: This is found throughout the world and causes an illness very similar to that caused by hepatitis A. However, in

Table 6 Infections which are more common and/or more severe during pregnancy

Viral infections	Bacterial infections
Hepatitis E	Urinary tract infections
Influenza A	Syphilis
Varicella	Chlamydia
Poliomyelitis	Mycoplasma
Measles	(Listeriosis)*
Lassa fever	(Group B streptococcal infection)*
Japanese B encephalitis	**Others**
(HIV)*	Malaria
	Coccidioidomycosis
	Blastomycosis
	(Toxoplasmosis)*

*Infections which occur during pregnancy but are principally a risk to the fetus rather than the mother.

pregnant women (particularly in the third trimester or immediate post-partum) HEV causes a fulminant hepatitis with a case mortality of approximately 20 per cent. The reason for this unusual complication is unknown. No specific therapy is effective.

- *Tuberculosis.* This is worth mentioning mainly to dispel the myth that it presents a problem. Although it has been suggested that the impaired cellular immunity that accompanies pregnancy might be a risk for acquisition of, or reactivation of tuberculosis, the great majority of clinical trials have concluded that if any such risk exists it is negligible.

Further reading

Hibberd, P.L. and Rubin, R.H. (1993). Renal transplantation and related infections. *Seminars in Respiratory Infection*, **8**, 216–24.

Kibbler, C.C. (1997). Infections associated with neutropenia and transplants. In: *Antibiotic and chemotherapy*, (7th edn), (ed. F. O'Grady, H.P. Lambert, R.G. Finch, and D. Greenwood), pp. 614–31. Churchill Livingstone, New York.

Klastersky, J. (ed). 1995. *Infectious complications of cancer.* Kluwer, Boston.

Rubin, R.H. and Young, L.S. (1994). *Clinical approach to infection in the compromised host*, (3rd edn). Plenum, New York.

Warnock, D.W. and Richardson, M.D. (1991). *Fungal infection in the compromised patient*, (2nd edn). Wiley, Chichester.

Chapter 16.118

Chronic fatigue syndrome (postviral fatigue syndrome, neurasthenia, and myalgic encephalomyelitis)

M. Sharpe

Introduction

The terms chronic fatigue syndrome (**CFS**), postviral fatigue syndrome, neurasthenia, and myalgic encephalomyelitis ('**ME**') have all been used to describe an idiopathic syndrome characterized by chronic fatigue and disability, often associated with a history of preceding infection. The nature, pathology and aetiology of this syndrome remain controversial and the purely descriptive term chronic fatigue syndrome is preferred. The current international consensus definition for CFS is shown in Table 1 and its components discussed below.

1. *What is fatigue?* Fatigue is an imprecise term with many meanings. In clinical medicine, concerned with the symptom of fatigue describes a subjective lack of energy and endurance.
2. *When is fatigue abnormal?* Fatigue may be considered abnormal when it is disproportionate to exertion, persistent, and associated with impairment of functioning.
3. *Why 6 months?* Six months is used to define chronicity for purposes of research. Is has the benefit of excluding short lived states of fatigue that can follow any illness.
4. *Which other symptoms?* Patients with CFS commonly complain of symptoms other than fatigue (see clinical features below).
5. *What conditions must be excluded?* Chronic fatigue may be a symptom of most, medical and psychiatric illnesses. The term CFS is reserved for patients in whom the fatigue remains medically unexplained or 'idiopathic' despite careful clinical assessment.

Aetiology

The cause of idiopathic CFS remains controversial. Suggested causes include:

Unidentified organic disease

It is important to consider occult disease (see Table 2) in every case of idiopathic CFS, but follow up studies suggest that it is uncommon.

Depressive and anxiety disorders

Systematic psychiatric assessment has shown that a substantial proportion of patients meeting criteria for CFS also meet criteria for depressive and anxiety disorders. It has consequently been suggested that CFS is a somatically expressed emotional disorder (somatization).

Other aetiological factors

A substantial proportion of cases cannot be readily explained either as occult organic disease or emotional disorder. A number of explanations have been proposed for such cases. These are best considered as predisposing, precipitating, and perpetuating factors. Hence certain individuals may be predisposed to develop CFS by virtue of genetics, personality, or other vulnerability. The condition may be

Table 1 International consensus definition of chronic fatigue syndrome

1. Principal complaint of fatigue
2. At least four of the following additional symptoms: • Subjective memory impairment • Sore throat • Tender lymph nodes • Muscle pain/joint pain • Headache • Unrefreshing sleep • Post-exertional malaise lasting more than 24 h
3. Impairment of functioning
4. Duration at least 6 months
5. Other conditions excluded

Table 2 Conditions to be considered in the differential diagnosis of chronic fatigue syndrome

General	**Respiratory disease**
Occult malignancy	Nocturnal asthma
Autoimmune disease	Obstructive sleep apnoea
Endocrine disease	**Chronic toxicity**
Cardiac, respiratory or renal failure	Alcohol
Neurological	Solvents
Disseminated sclerosis	Heavy metals
Myasthenia gravis	Irradiation
Parkinson's disease	**Psychiatric**
Infectious disease	Major depressive disorder
Chronic active hepatitis (B or C)	Dysthymia
Lyme borreliosis	Anxiety and panic disorder
HIV	Somatization disorder
Tuberculosis	

precipitated in those individuals by factors such as infection or psychological stress (life events). Once established it may be perpetuated by the following:

1 *Chronic infection.* Although an acute infection is often reported at the start of the illness, current evidence suggests that chronic infection is an uncommon perpetuating factor.

2 *Immune dysfunction.* Minor immune abnormalities have been detected in a proportion of patients. However, no consistent abnormality or causal link has been established and the role of immune factors remains unclear.

3 *Inactivity.* Many (but not all) patients with CFS, are profoundly inactive. Inactivity may lead to muscle wasting, changes in the cardiovascular response to exertion, and consequent intolerance of activity.

4 *Central nervous system dysfunction.* Abnormalities have been found in tests of cognitive function, in neuroendocrine tests and neuroimaging. Similar abnormalities have been found in patients with depression and anxiety disorders and their specificity to CFS remains to be established.

5 *Sleep disorder.* Various sleep abnormalities have been found in patients with CFS. These may contribute to daytime fatigue but their role is unclear.

6 *Psychological factors.* There is good evidence that psychological and behavioural factors play a part in perpetuating CFS. These include misconceptions about the nature of the illness. excessive avoidance of any activities, repeated seeking of (ineffective) medical care, and failure to resolve current psychological and social problems.

7 *Social and iatrogenic factors.* Misinformation about CFS or 'ME', whether from doctors, patient groups, or the media; that leads patients to see their illness as mysterious, with a poor prognosis and untreatable other than by rest; is unhelpful and may lead to illness perpetuating behaviour in some individuals.

Epidemiology

Fatigue

As many as one-quarter of the general population complains of persistent fatigue. Fatigue is also a common complaint among patients seen in both primary and secondary medical care. The prevalence of CFS as defined above is much lower. A recent population study in the UK found that less than 1 per cent could be regarded as having CFS.

Chronic fatigue syndrome

Most cases of CFS have arisen sporadically and present individually. Case series from both primary care and hospital outpatient clinics indicate that patients are most commonly aged between 20 and 40 with a predominance of females. The syndrome is also seen in children and adolescents.

Epidemics

Epidemics of a CFS-like syndrome have been described from various parts of the globe. The occurrence of epidemics would appear to favour an infective causation. However, questions have been raised about whether these were true epidemics or the consequence of an artificial linking of cases by doctors, and also whether the clinical picture reported in such apparent epidemics was similar to that of patients presenting sporadically.

Clinical features

The principal symptom of CFS is chronic mental and physical fatigue exacerbated by activity. Patients often report being able to perform for brief periods, but subsequently experiencing severe fatigue for hours or days thereafter. Other symptoms commonly reported include muscular pain, unrefreshing sleep, dizziness and breathlessness, headache, tender lymph glands, and symptoms of irritable bowel syndrome. The patient often describes day to day fluctuations in their symptoms, irrespective of activity. Periods of almost complete recovery may be followed by relapse, often sufficiently severe to make normal daily activity impossible. Depression and anxiety are also common and a proportion of patients suffer panic attacks. Patients and their relatives may hold strong beliefs about the nature and aetiology of their illness (see under Aetiology), and these may be of importance when planning management. Physical examination is typically unremarkable. Complaints of fever and lymphadenopathy are usually found to be within normal variation when assessed. The presence of definite physical signs should not be ascribed to the syndrome and requires an alternative explanation.

Differential diagnosis

Almost any organic disease may present with unexplained fatigue and the differential diagnosis of idiopathic CFS is large (see Table 2). The nature of the fatigue may offer useful clues. Muscular disease should be considered if the patient has no psychological symptoms, and especially if they have a family history. If the patient's complaint of fatigue includes prominent sleepiness, a specific sleep disorder should be considered. In particular prominent night-time snoring and morning headaches in the obese patient raise the possibility of obstructive sleep apnoea.

It is important to assess the patient's mental state. Depression is suggested by fatigue that is worse in the morning and accompanied by loss of motivation, interest, and pleasure. Other symptoms of depression should be sought including sadness, loss of appetite and weight, and feelings of pessimism and failure. If there is evidence of depression it is essential to ask about suicide plans. Chronic anxiety is associated both with fatigue and with many of the symptoms of CFS such as muscle pain, impaired concentration, and poor sleep.

Pathology

There is no established pathology other than changes associated with inactivity.

Laboratory diagnosis

There are no diagnostic tests and no characteristic abnormalities in laboratory investigations which are conducted purely to exclude other diseases. All patients should have a full blood count, erythrocyte sedimentation rate or C-reactive protein, basic biochemistry screen, urine analysis, and possibly thyroid function and antinuclear antibody tests, further investigation depending on the clinical findings and differential diagnosis under consideration.

Treatment

In all cases the doctor should educate the patient about their condition, and correct misconceptions they, and their carers may have about its cause and appropriate treatment. It is especially important to explain that their illness is not progressive or life threatening (see below). A more positive and less sinister explanation may be offered that distinguishes between precipitating causes, such as viral infection and perpetuating factors such as fear of the illness, depression, and the physiological effects of inactivity. The adverse effects of prolonged bed rest should be emphasized and the patient encouraged to adopt a consistent but gradually increasing level of activity, avoiding extremes of both inactivity and exertion.

The prescription of an antidepressant drug may be considered, especially if there is evidence of depression. It is advisable to choose a non-sedating type and to start with as low a dose as possible, as patients with CFS may be particularly sensitive to side-effects. Low doses of antidepressant drugs may reduce anxiety, improve the quality of sleep, and reduce pain. If there is evidence that the patient has a depressive disorder, whatever the cause, it is important to give the antidepressants in an adequate dose for an adequate period. Referral to a psychiatrist should be considered in such cases.

Many patients will have severe continuing difficulties in their work or relationships. These may need to be removed or the patient's ability to cope with them improved before recovery is possible. For some patients long-term follow up may be helpful in encouraging them to persevere with such an approach and in reducing the risk of iatrogenic harm from repeated medical investigation and failed therapy.

Two clinical trials have shown that a rehabilitative psychological therapy (cognitive behaviour therapy) is more effective than conventional medical management. If available a specialist liaison psychiatry or psychology service may be best placed to offer effective treatment in a setting acceptable to the patient.

Many other treatments have been proposed for idiopathic CFS, but none have been adequately evaluated. Patients should be discouraged from pursuing unproven treatments unless they are part of a carefully conducted clinical trial.

Prognosis

The prognosis without treatment for full functional recovery is relatively good for patients seen in general practice, but poor for those severe enough to be referred to hospital clinics. There is no mortality associated with CFS, although there appears to be an increased risk of death by suicide.

Prevention

As the cause is unknown there is no specific primary prevention. It is likely, however, that better initial management would reduce the risk of chronicity.

Further reading

Fukuda, K., *et al.* (1994). Chronic fatigue syndrome: a comprehensive approach to its definition and management. *Annals of Internal Medicine*, **121**, 953–9.

Sharpe, M. (1996). Chronic fatigue syndrome. *Psychiatric Clinics of North America*, **19**, 549–74.

Wessely, S., Sharpe, M., and Hotopf, M. (1998). *Chronic fatigue and its syndromes.* Oxford University Press, Oxford.

Section 17
Sexually transmitted disease

Contents

Chapter 17.1

Sexually-transmitted infections: epidemiology and control

M. W. Adler and A. Meheus

Epidemiology

Introduction

Sexually transmitted diseases are spread by sexual intercourse or, in some cases, by close bodily contact without sexual penetration (e.g. scabies and pediculosis pubis) (Table 1). The range of diseases spread by sexual activity continues to increase. Increased knowledge of the natural history of untreated sexually transmitted diseases has shown that their detrimental effects on pregnancy and the newborn (e.g. miscarriage, prematurity, congenital and neonatal infections, blindness) and their complications in women, such as pelvic inflammatory disease, ectopic pregnancy, infertility, and cervical cancer are more common and severe than had been previously realized.

The incidence, distribution, and development of complications is strongly influenced by behavioural and sociocultural factors, population composition, susceptibility of individuals, changing characteristics of pathogens, society's efforts at primary prevention and disease control, and the complex interaction between these factors.

The HIV/AIDS epidemic has increased attention given to other sexually transmitted diseases; not only are they important causes of morbidity and mortality themselves, but they are also important markers of behaviour associated with a high risk of HIV transmission.

Table 1 Micro-organisms that can be sexually transmitted

Bacteria:	Viruses:
Chlamydia trachomatis	Herpes simplex virus types 1 and 2
Neisseria gonorrhoeae	Wart virus (papillomavirus)
Gardnerella vaginalis	Molluscum contagiosum virus (poxvirus)
Treponema pallidum Group B haemolytic streptococcus	Hepatitis A, B and C virus
Haemophilus ducreyi	Cytomegalovirus
Calymmatobacterium granulomatis	Human immunodeficiency virus types 1 and 2
Shigella spp. Mycoplasmas:	Human T-cell leukaemia virus type 1
Ureaplasma urealyticum *Mycoplasma hominis*	Protozoa:
Parasites:	*Entamoeba histolytica*
Sarcoptes scabei	*Giardia lamblia*
Phthirus pubis	*Trichomonas vaginalis*
	Fungi:
	Candida albicans

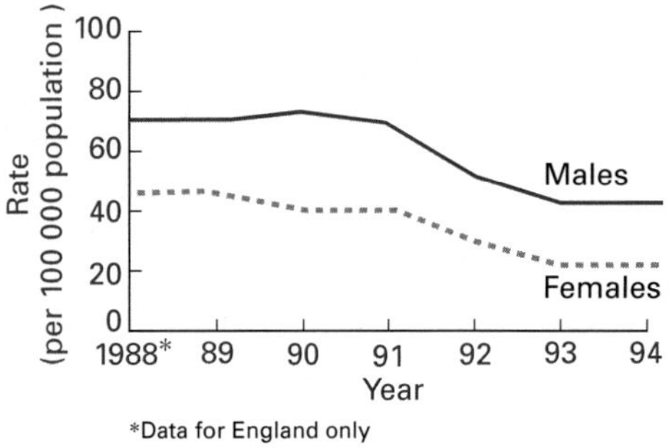

Fig. 1 Attendance rates (per 100 000 population) at genitourinary medicine clinics for gonorrhoea.

Sexually transmitted diseases associated with genital ulcer(s) or genital discharge can enhance both the acquisition and transmission of HIV by increased shedding of the virus within and from the genital tract.

Most countries lack an effective notification system for STDs so it is not possible to estimate accurately the global burden from these diseases. The WHO's 'guesstimate' is of approximately 333 million per annum treatable sexually transmitted infections.

The diseases

In the UK a free and confidential service, for what were called venereal diseases, was started in 1916. The annual number of patients attending specially designated clinics in England is 847 176 (1995, latest figures) compared with 410 711, 14 years ago. Syphilis is no longer a major problem, gonorrhoea still is, but non-specific and chlamydial infections are the most common conditions seen. Other sexually transmitted conditions such as trichomoniasis, pediculosis pubis, and genital warts are increasingly diagnosed. In the last few years the incidence of herpes genitalis has risen, more sexually transmitted hepatitis B and A are being seen, and even more recently, physicians have become aware of the spread of enteric pathogens (*Entamoeba histolytica* and *Giardia lamblia*) by sexual contact. The most recently discovered sexually acquired condition is HIV/AIDS.

Gonorrhoea (see also Chapter 16.42)

Although the rates vary between countries, the trend over the last 30 years has been an increase over most of the period with a flattening out in the mid-1970s and a decrease since. It is difficult to compare rates between countries because of the variation in reporting practices and in the provision of facilities.

In the UK with a network of departments of genitourinary medicine/sexually transmitted disease clinics, and routine notification, figures have been kept. In 1995, there were 12 359 adult cases of gonorrhoea (male 7649, female 4710 in England) (Fig. 1). With the advent of AIDS there has been a marked fall during the 1980s, particularly in men, but this trend has now flattened out. In the US, despite a slow decline in reported cases of gonorrhoea, there are still considerable differences between ethnic groups (Fig. 2). In 1995, cases of gonorrhoea totally 343 010 (179 873 in males and 163 137 in females). The incidence of gonorrhoea in Nordic countries has decreased markedly. In Sweden where the peak incidence of gonorrhoea was approximately 40 000 cases in 1970, the number of gonococcal infections decreased more than 45-fold from 14 097 in 1981 to 307 cases in 1994.

HIV infection and AIDS have brought remarkable changes in behaviour, particularly among homosexual men. Some high risk

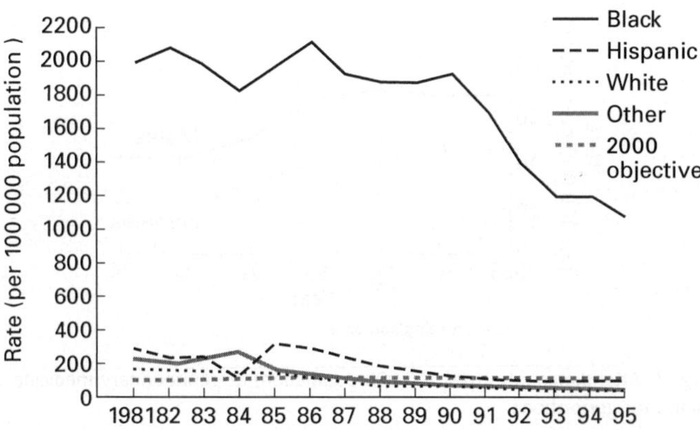

Fig. 2 Gonorrhoea—rates by race and ethnicity: US, 1981–1995 and year 2000 objective.

homosexual men reduced the number of casual partners and adopted safe sex practices. However, measures of syphilis and gonorrhoea incidences suggest that this trend has not been maintained in Europe and the US.

Syphilis (see also Chapter 16.69)

Penicillin made a dramatic impact on the incidence of early infectious syphilis throughout the world in the 1950s. Unfortunately, this effect has not been maintained in all countries. The US has experienced a continuous rise since an initial drop in the 1950s. Since 1956 there has been a seven- to ninefold increase in total cases of primary and secondary syphilis in males and females, respectively. These increases were partly explained by the deployment of resources away from traditional sexually transmitted disease control programmes to AIDS. The lesson from this is that the control of HIV and AIDS will only be effective through integrated sexually transmitted disease/AIDS control programmes. This could be responsible for the ensuing decline in the US to a low of 8122 in 1995.

In the UK the decline in syphilis has been maintained. There had been an increase in all forms of syphilis among males during the 1970s, whereas female rates had continued to fall. This disparity was explained by the fact that the most cases of primary and secondary syphilis (58 per cent) occurred in homosexuals. However, as with gonorrhoea, there has been a decline in cases of syphilis in homosexual men seen in sexually transmitted disease clinics in the UK as a result of changing sexual practices following the HIV epidemic.

Particularly encouraging is the decline in congenital syphilis in developed countries, attributable largely to the control of early acquired infectious syphilis in women and through screening all pregnant women. Unfortunately, congenital syphilis is still a major health problem in many developing countries.

Genital herpes and warts

Genital herpes and warts have shown the greatest increase in England in the 1980s. In 1978, 8406 cases of herpes and 24 136 cases of warts were seen in sexually transmitted disease clinics, rising to 27 065 and 93 317, respectively, by 1995.

There are estimated to be between 200 000 and 500 000 new cases of herpes each year in the US, with a prevalence of approximately 40 million cases.

Pelvic inflammatory disease

Pelvic inflammatory disease is the most serious complication of gonococcal, chlamydial, and non-specific infections. Its incidence and prevalence varies throughout the world but is rapidly increasing in most countries. In Western industrialized countries the annual incidence has been estimated as 10/1000 of women aged 15 to 39 years with a peak incidence of 20/1000 in the age group 15 to 24 years. The factors associated with pelvic inflammatory disease are the sexually transmitted diseases, use of intrauterine devices, abortion, and puerperal infections. The relative importance of these various factors and aetiological agents differs in different parts of the world.

In developed countries, 75 per cent of cases of pelvic inflammatory disease in women below the age of 25 years are due to a sexually transmitted agent. *Chlamydia trachomatis* has replaced gonorrhoea as the commonest cause.

In England and Wales the number of cases of acute pelvic inflammatory disease admitted to hospital has doubled in the last 20 years. The most disastrous consequence of salpingitis is sterility. In Sweden it was found that tubal occlusion occurred in 13 per cent of women with one attack of salpingitis, in 35 per cent after two, rising to 75 per cent with three or more attacks. Even if women with pelvic inflammatory disease are able to conceive, risk of ectopic pregnancy increases 7–10 fold.

Epidemiology of sexually transmitted diseases in developing countries

There are differences in the epidemiology between developed and the developing countries. First, the frequency of sexually transmitted diseases is much higher in developing countries, especially in certain high risk groups such as female prostitutes, their clients, long–distance truck drivers, etc. Prostitutes are blamed by up to 90 per cent of men in developing countries as the source of infection.

Second, among the sexually transmitted diseases, genital ulcers are relatively much more frequent. The so-called tropical sexually transmitted diseases, in particular chancroid, and to a lesser degree lymphogranuloma venereum and granuloma inguinale, are major causes of genital ulcers. The proportion of genital ulcers caused by syphilis is also higher than in industrialized countries; genital herpes accounts for a smaller proportion of ulcerative disease, but has become more important in areas of high AIDS incidence.

Thirdly, the incidence of complications and sequelae of sexually transmitted diseases is much higher, due to lack of resources for adequate diagnosis and treatment. These problems include adverse effects of pregnancy for mothers and babies, neonatal and infant infections, infertility in both sexes, ectopic pregnancy, urethral stricture in males, blindness in infants due to gonococcal ophthalmia neonatorum and in adults due to gonococcal keratoconjunctivitis, and genital cancers, particularly cancer of the cervix uteri and penis.

Fourthly, the epidemiology of AIDS and HIV infection is very different from that in Western countries: frequency rather than orientation of sexual activity is, apparently, the risk factor, and heterosexual transmission of HIV is predominant. There is evidence, however, that genital ulceration, and also other sexually transmitted diseases, facilitate the sexual transmission of HIV infection.

Control

The objectives of control are: (i) to interrupt transmission; (ii) to prevent the development of sexually transmitted diseases, their complications, and sequelae; and (iii) to reduce the risk of sexual transmission of HIV.

Table 2 Structure of a control programme for sexually transmitted diseases (STD)

Intervention strategies
1. Health promotion/counselling; vaccination (HBV) (= primary prevention)
2. Early detection of infection (= secondary prevention)
3. Appropriate management of STD patients: diagnosis and treatment counselling contact tracing (= comprehensive care)
Support components
1. Professional training
2. Laboratory services
3. Research
4. Information system/surveillance

Intervention strategies (Table 2)

Primary prevention is achieved through health promotion (information, education, communication) and counselling activities. The aim is to educate individuals about the advantages of 'discriminative sex' and prophylaxis ('safer sex'). It is necessary to point out the dangers of frequent changes of sexual partner, the importance of using a condom, avoiding partners with symptoms or lesions, and having regular check-ups. Teenagers need to be educated before they become sexually active. The best place for this is at home or school. Since the spread of HIV infection and AIDS, discussion of sexuality is less taboo in many countries. Health workers and educators should take advantage of this new openness. Through campaigns in the mass media targeted at the general public, information, education, and communication have become part of sexually transmitted disease/AIDS control nearly everywhere. A special target group for health promotion and individual counselling are patients with sexually transmitted diseases. Their infection, which is proof of their exposure to sexually transmitted diseases including possibly HIV, may make them more inclined to change risky sexual behaviour.

Secondary prevention aims at early detection of sexually transmitted disease through screening ('check-up') or education about what to do once disease is suspected (health-seeking behaviour). Sexual intercourse should be stopped until medical care has been sought. How and when such advice can be found should be advertised and the importance of adhering to treatment emphasized.

Screening aims to detect asymptomatic or mildly symptomatic infections. Good laboratory support is essential. It is done most often in specific populations where the prevalence of sexually transmitted diseases is high. For instance, in some places pregnant women are screened for syphilis, HIV, or chlamydial infection. Where prostitution is legal or tolerated, prostitutes can be screened for various sexually transmitted diseases. Blood donors are screened for HIV, hepatitis B and viruses, human T-cell leukaemia virus type 1, and syphilis.

Comprehensive patient care aims to: (a) detect or rule out infection; (b) give treatment if necessary; (c) educate and counsel on treatment compliance and on sexually transmitted disease/HIV prevention and condom use; (d) ensure that the sex partner(s) are evaluated and managed (contact tracing); (e) test eventually for other sexually transmitted diseases, including HIV.

Good facilities for accurate diagnosis, rapid treatment, and health education are needed. Such facilities need to be run by doctors who have specialist knowledge and good microbiological back-up. In a developed country it is not appropriate to attempt the management of sexually transmitted diseases without such microbiological facilities. In developing countries, it is more realistic to rely on clinical recognition of sexually transmitted diseases and simple laboratory tests.

To implement the three major intervention strategies, the following support components are needed. These are:

- Training of health workers and health educators, for instance in the use of flow-charts for simplified management of patients with sexually transmitted diseases, or the strengthening of health-education and counselling skills.
- Laboratory services depending on the level of health care provided. A reference laboratory should be developed in each country to allow quality control and analysis of referred specimens.
- Research, including epidemiological and sociobehavioural baseline studies, assessment of antimicrobial sensitivity, and operational research to improve the cost-effectiveness of the programme.
- Information systems, or surveillance, to gather epidemiological data to assess numbers and trends, and to provide information for planning and monitoring the programme. Surveillance methods that can be used are notification by the clinician and laboratory, sentinel-site surveillance (either of syndromes or of aetiological diagnoses), prevalence studies, and aetiological surveys.

Further reading

Adler, M. (1998). *ABC of sexually transmitted diseases*, (4th edn). British Medical Association, London.

De Schryver, A. and Meheus, A. (1990). Epidemiology of sexually transmitted diseases: the global picture. *Bulletin of the World Health Organization*, **68**, 639–54.

World Health Organization. (1995). *An overview of selected curable sexually transmitted diseases.* WHO, Geneva.

World Health Organization. (1990). *WHO features* (December), No. 152. WHO, Geneva.

World Health Organization. (1991). *Management of patients with sexually transmitted diseases.* WHO Technical Report Series No. 810. WHO, Geneva.

Chapter 17.2

Sexual behaviour

A. M. Johnson

Patterns of sexual behaviour vary widely between individuals, within individuals during their lifetime, between societies, and over the course of history. It is important to be able to take a sexual history in clinical practice. Discussion of sexual lifestyle is relevant to the provision of contraceptive advice, the management of common conditions such as vaginal and urethral discharge, counselling following childbirth or pelvic surgery, sexual dysfunction, unwanted pregnancy, infertility, pelvic pain, and a number of rectal and perianal problems.

Resumption of sexual activity may be a concern for patients following major illnesses.

Until recently there had been relatively little systematic study of sexual behaviour in representative population samples, although there are many examples of work carried out in volunteer samples earlier in the century. Kinsey's studies carried out in the US in the 1930s and 1940s were based on volunteer samples, so that the prevalence of different behaviours derived from these studies cannot be regarded as providing valid population estimates. The HIV epidemic has provoked a resurgence of interest in the study of sexual lifestyle and in the late 1980s and early 1990s a number of large-scale surveys have been carried out.

Sexual orientation

Studies in representative population samples show that the majority of men and women are predominantly attracted to, and have experience with, members of the opposite sex throughout their lives. However, sexual orientation is not a simple dichotomy between 'homosexual' and 'heterosexual' but can better be seen as a range of experience from exclusively heterosexual through various shades of attraction and experience with both genders to exclusively homosexual experience. In a large-scale British study of adults aged 16–59, 6.1 per cent of men and 3.4 per cent of women reported sometime having had an experience which they would describe as sexual with someone of the same gender. For some this may be a fleeting experience in adolescence, and many may go on to have exclusively heterosexual partnerships in the future. A smaller proportion of the British population report homosexual partnerships which involve some form of genital contact (3.6 per cent of men and 1.7 per cent of women). Similar findings are reported from French and US surveys. These figures are considerably lower than those reported in the Kinsey studies reflecting the non-representative nature of Kinsey's sample. Most of those with same-gender partners have also had experience of heterosexual intercourse at some time in their lives. Exclusively homosexual experience is thus relatively unusual.

Homosexual experience is more common among men in large metropolitan areas such as London, Amsterdam, New York, and San Francisco. For example, 8.6 per cent of men sampled in Inner London reported having a homosexual partner in the last 5 years. Capital cities typically provide a more tolerant atmosphere and better social facilities for those with a homosexual lifestyle. This is reflected in the high proportion of homosexually-acquired sexually transmitted diseases (STDs) reported from STD clinics in London, and large cities in Europe and the United States.

Age of first heterosexual intercourse

The age of first heterosexual intercourse has been gradually declining over recent decades, while the proportion of men and women reporting experience of sexual intercourse before marriage has rapidly increased so that sex before marriage has become almost universal in Britain. For men born in the years 1930–35, the median age of first intercourse was 20 and for women 21. For men and women born between 1965 and 1975, the median age at first intercourse is 17. Similar trends have been observed in France and the US.

English law gives the age of consent for sexual intercourse as 16 and it is illegal for a man to have sex with a woman under 16 in England. The proportion of men and women reporting first intercourse before the age of 16 has risen rapidly over recent decades to 28 per cent of men and 19 per cent of women aged 16–19 in 1990 in Britain. This has important implications for the provision of sex education in schools. Sexual novices, through lack of knowledge and experience, may be most susceptible to the unwanted consequences of unprotected sexual intercourse. This is reflected in the higher incidence of sexually transmitted diseases and termination of pregnancy in the 16–24 year old age group than in older men and women. HIV is most commonly diagnosed among men and women between 20 and 30.

Heterosexual partners and practice

Most people have few partners, but a small proportion have many. For example, amongst men aged 16–59 in Britain, 65 per cent reported no or one partner(s) in the last 5 years and 5 per cent reported more than 10. A few people are very sexually active and report hundreds or even thousands of partners in the course of their lives. Thus, for example, in the British survey of sexual attitudes and lifestyles, 1 per cent of men with the greatest numbers of partners reported 16 per cent of all partnerships in the last 5 years.

The risk of acquiring an STD increases with the number of partners with whom sexual intercourse occurs. Those with very high numbers of partners are at high risk both of acquiring and transmitting STDs. This subset of the population (which may vary over time) has sometimes been referred to as 'core' groups in STD epidemiology since they may account for a relatively high proportion of STD transmission in a society and for sustaining endemic STD transmission.

Historical data suggest that in the early 20th century a relatively high proportion of STDs could be traced to men who had commercial sexual contacts. This was a particular problem among troops in war time. Prostitutes and their clients remain at high risk of HIV and other STDs in some African urban centres. In Western countries, although prostitutes are at increased risk of STDs, there is evidence of high level of condom use which may protect both them and their clients.

In the British survey, nearly 7 per cent of men reported sometimes paying money for sex with a woman. There is some evidence that the proportion of men seeking commercial partners may have declined over recent decades, possibly in response to the general liberalization of views towards sex outside marriage and multiple partnerships. In other parts of the world such as south-east Asia, initiation by a prostitute remains common.

Multiple heterosexual partnerships are most common among the young, and among those who are not married or cohabiting. For example, close to one in five men aged 16–24 in Britain reported more than 10 partners in the last 5 years, even though this is a group in which a high proportion have not yet become sexually active. Age *per se* is not the only influence on sexual behaviour. Whatever their age, those who are separated, divorced, or widowed are more likely than married people of similar age to have multiple partners.

Heterosexual practices

There is variability in the repertoire and frequency of sexual practices between individuals. In heterosexual relationships, vaginal intercourse is the most common practice, but the majority of couples include other practices in their repertoire, particularly mutual masturbation and orogenital contact.

The frequency of sexual contact varies with age, life stage and the availability of a sexual partner. For married couples, the median frequency of sexual intercourse is in the order of 4 times per month, but is highly variable. Frequency of intercourse appears to decline with age in married and cohabiting couples, although this is partly a function of increasing length of relationship. The excitement of a new relationship may lead to greater frequency of intercourse while the responsibilities and demands, for example of childcare, may lead to decreased frequency.

Among men and women aged 16–59 in Britain, close to 60 per cent reported experience of orogenital contact in the last year and the majority of couples who experience any orogenital contact practise both cunnilingus and fellatio. Orogenital contact may be regarded as a 'safer sexual practice' since in the absence of vaginal intercourse, it protects against unwanted pregnancy and may reduce the risk of transmission of organisms such as HIV. Other organisms such as Herpes simplex virus, gonorrhoea, and syphilis can, however, be transmitted by this route.

Mutual masturbation without intercourse has become a more frequent practice in recent decades. There is little evidence of its being adopted as an alternative to vaginal intercourse in heterosexuals but it may have become a more frequent alternative to anal intercourse among homosexual men since the emergence of the HIV epidemic.

Anal intercourse is a relatively infrequent activity in heterosexual couples. In the British survey, 14 per cent of men and 13 per cent of women had sometime experienced anal intercourse, but only around 6 per cent had experienced it in the last year. Data from France suggest slightly higher rates but in all cultures this appears to be a minority activity. There is little evidence of a major change in the prevalence and practice of anal intercourse over the last decades. Anal intercourse in addition to vaginal intercourse may increase the risk of heterosexual transmission of HIV. However, most heterosexual HIV transmission can be attributed to vaginal intercourse.

Homosexual behaviour

Men with multiple homosexual partnerships are at increased risk of HIV infection as well as other sexually transmitted diseases, including hepatitis B and syphilis. Conversely, women with homosexual partnerships tend to be at low risk of STD and HIV as a result of their different sexual lifestyles and sexual practices such as non-penetrative sex and orogenital contact.

Research in the 1970s of volunteer samples of homosexual men in the US identified a particular lifestyle characterized by multiple casual sexual partners, often encountered at gay meeting places such as bars, clubs, and 'bathhouses'. These men were at high-risk of STDs and were amongst the first to suffer high rates of HIV infection. Research in Britain identified a group of homosexual men with similar lifestyles. However, recent research, suggests greater diversity of lifestyle among men who have sex with men. Volunteer samples recruited outside of STD clinics and gay meeting places show both lower rates of sexual partner change and prevalence of sexually acquired pathogens.

Initial reports of very high numbers (≥ 500) of partners in a high proportion of homosexual men must be revised since many male–male partnerships do not involve penetrative anal intercourse, but are restricted to mutual masturbation or orogenital contact. Anal intercourse, however, is an important mode of transmission of sexually acquired organisms between homosexual men, most of whom practise both anal receptive and insertive intercourse. Receptive anal intercourse is the highest risk behaviour for HIV transmission.

Risk-reduction strategies and sexual health

Preventive activity should take into account the health-promoting qualities of fulfilling sexual relationships which are a key component of adult human lifestyles. Currently, strategies for sexual health are concerned mainly with preventing unplanned pregnancy, STDs, or coercion in sexual relationships.

Young people require education to make informed choices about their sexual expression and to avoid unnecessary risk-taking. This is perhaps best given as part of broader education about human relationships to enable individuals to negotiate adult sexual relationships without fear of disease, coercion, or unwanted pregnancy. Equally important is the provision of services for diagnosis, treatment, and contact tracing for those with STDs.

Individuals can reduce their risk of STD and unwanted pregnancy by reducing the numbers of partners with whom they have unprotected intercourse, by using reliable contraception, by using condoms, and by choosing sexual practices which may reduce transmission risks. Teaching sexual fulfilment is important but more difficult.

Further reading

ACSF investigators. (1992). AIDS and sexual behaviour in France. *Nature,* **360**, 407–9.

Cleland, J. and Ferry, B. (1995). *Sexual behaviour and AIDS in the developing world.* Taylor and Francis, London.

Johnson, A.M., Wadsworth, J., Wellings, K., Bradshaw, S., and Field, J. (1992). Sexual behaviour and HIV risk. *Nature,* **360**, 410–12.

Johnson, A.M., Wadsworth, J., Wellings, K., and Field, J. (1993). *Sexual attitudes and lifestyles.* Blackwell Scientific, Oxford.

Kinsey, A.C., Pomeroy, W.B., and Martin, C.E. (1948). *Sexual behaviour in the human male.* W.B. Saunders, Philadelphia.

Chapter 17.3

Vaginal discharge

J. Schwebke and S. L. Hillier

Vaginal discharge is an extremely common symptom but a poorly understood condition. In the past, it has often been regarded as simply a nuisance. Only recently have accurate diagnosis and treatment of vaginal discharge been recognized as means of preventing future costly morbidity.

The healthy vagina

At puberty the vagina becomes colonized predominantly with lactobacilli, Gram-positive facultative bacilli that metabolize glucose to lactic acid, helping to maintain the normal vaginal pH at less than 4.5. This acidic environment inhibits most pathogens with the exception of *Candida* spp. Women with hydrogen peroxide-producing lactobacilli in the vagina are less likely to have gonorrhoea and have a 50 per cent decreased risk of acquiring bacterial vaginosis.

Factors that predispose the vagina to infection probably include hormonal and immunological factors as well as exogenous influences such as antimicrobial therapy, multiple sexual partners, and the use of vaginal douches.

Vaginitis and vaginosis

There are three main types of vaginal infections: trichomoniasis (see Chapter 6.95), bacterial vaginosis, and vulvovaginal candidiasis (see Chapter 16.81). Trichomoniasis is the only one known to be sexually transmitted, although bacterial vaginosis is most commonly seen in sexually active women and frequently coexists with sexually transmitted infections. Both trichomoniasis and bacterial vaginosis have been associated with preterm delivery and with acquisition of human immunodeficiency virus.

Bacterial vaginosis

Bacterial vaginosis is the most common diagnosis made in women complaining of abnormal vaginal discharge. Complications associated with bacterial vaginosis during pregnancy have been recognized, including an increased incidence of preterm birth, low birth weight, post-abortive endometritis, intra-amniotic infection, and post-partum endometritis. Among non-pregnant women, bacterial vaginosis has been linked to infection of the vaginal cuff following hysterectomy, and possibly pelvic inflammatory disease. Recent studies have also suggested an association between bacterial vaginosis and HIV.

Despite the fact that bacterial vaginosis is most often diagnosed in sexually active women and is frequently seen together with other sexually transmitted infections, it has not been proven to be sexually transmitted. It can occur in monogamous and sexually abstinent women.

Unlike trichomoniasis and candidiasis, bacterial vaginosis does not appear to be caused by a single organism. Instead there is a change in the entire vaginal milieu, resulting in the loss of normal hydrogen peroxide-producing lactobacilli and the appearance of increased numbers of mycoplasmas, *Gardnerella*, and anaerobic bacteria. Included among the anaerobes are the black-pigmented *Bacteroides (Prevotella)* spp., *B. (Prevotella) bivia*, *Peptostreptococcus* spp., and *Mobiluncus* spp. There is no inflammation of the vaginal epithelium, unlike in trichomoniasis and candidiasis, hence the term vaginosis as opposed to vaginitis. However, one-third of women with bacterial vaginosis and without other infections have more than 30 white blood cells per high-power field in the vaginal fluid. The predominant cell type is the squamous epithelial cell, many of which are then covered by adherent bacteria ('clue cells').

The symptoms of bacterial vaginosis are vaginal discharge (90 per cent) and an unpleasant odour (90 per cent). The odour is often first noticed after intercourse as the alkaline semen mixes with the vaginal fluid releasing volatile amines. Pruritus is uncommon, although vaginal irritation may be reported by one-third of women with bacterial vaginosis and without other infections. As with sexually transmitted infections there is a wide range of symptoms and many women with bacterial vaginosis are asymptomatic or unaware of their symptoms. A diagnosis is based upon three of the following four clinical signs:

(1) homogeneous looking, white to grey vaginal discharge;

(2) vaginal pH greater than 4.5;

(3) positive amine odour when vaginal secretions are mixed with 10 per cent potassium hydroxide ('whiff' test);

(4) the presence of 'clue cells'.

It is important to note the type of bacteria present in the vaginal fluid. Careful observation will alert the microscopist to the absence of characteristic lactobacilli and presence of large numbers of coccobacilli and curved, motile rods (*Mobiluncus* spp.). Culture techniques are not helpful in the diagnosis of this infection, as many of the offending organisms are present in the normal vagina but in low numbers. Careful attention should also be paid to the appearance of the cervix because of the frequent coexistence of cervicitis.

Antimicrobial therapy directed at anaerobic organisms is the mainstay of treatment. The most commonly used antibiotic is metronidazole (500 mg orally twice a day for 1 week). Clindamycin is also effective. The introduction of intravaginal therapy in the form of clindamycin 2 per cent cream and metronidazole 0.75 per cent gel is equally effective and has fewer side-effects. Sulpha creams provide symptomatic relief in nearly 80 per cent of women but 50 per cent will have recurrence of symptoms at 1 month. Treatment of the sexual partner(s) of women with bacterial vaginosis does not decrease recurrences.

Although antimicrobial therapy alleviates symptoms in up to 80 per cent of women, recurrences are common. This is probably because therapy is directed towards eliminating organisms rather than re-establishing the normal vaginal flora. Microbiological studies have shown that return to normal is slow, often taking several weeks. During this time the vagina is vulnerable to regrowth of the organisms associated with bacterial vaginosis and to clinical relapse. Future directions in treatment may involve some means of reintroducing healthy lactobacilli into the vaginal ecosystem.

Treatment of women with asymptomatic bacterial vaginosis remains controversial and further studies are needed to define the natural history in these women. However, because of the association of bacterial vaginosis with infectious complications of gynaecological surgery, treatment may be justified in these settings. Although bacterial vaginosis has been associated with complications of pregnancy, routine screening and treatment of low-risk pregnant women with asymptomatic bacterial vaginosis is not yet recommended. Prospective trials of this approach are under way.

Diagnostic approach to the patient with vaginal discharge

As with any problem in medicine, the history is of great importance. This should include a detailed sexual history to help assess the patient's level of risk for sexually transmitted infections. Examination should pay particular attention to the origin of the discharge (i.e. cervical versus vaginal), although this is often difficult to ascertain. Other signs of cervicitis such as oedema and inflammation of the zone of cervical ectopy, and easily induced endocervical bleeding, should also be noted.

During the examination the pH of the vaginal fluid should be determined and a sample of the fluid placed in small amounts of both saline and 10 per cent potassium hydroxide for microscopy. The presence or absence of an amine odour when the potassium hydroxide preparation is made should be noted ('whiff test'). The presence of blood, semen, or exogenous vaginal preparations (douches, creams) will interfere with the determination of pH and with the 'whiff test'. Microscopical examination of the saline preparation should be done at 400 × to look for pseudohyphae, 'clue cells', motile trichomonads,

Table 1 Diagnosis and treatment of vaginal infections

	Bacterial vaginosis	Trichomoniasis	Candidiasis
Symptoms[1]	Odour (fishy), discharge	Pruritus, discharge	Pruritus, discharge
Signs[2]	White-grey, homogeneous discharge	Thick, yellow discharge	Cottage-cheese discharge, erythema, fissures
Laboratory tests			
pH[3]	>4.5	>4.5[5]	<4.5
'Whiff'[3]	Positive	Variable	Negative
Saline wet preparation[6]	'Clue cells', abnormal vaginal flora	Motile trichomonads	Pseudohyphae and budding yeasts
Treatment	Metronidazole (oral or topical), clindamycin (oral or topical)	Metronidazole	Imidazole (oral or creams/ suppositories, triazoles (oral)[4]

[1] Patients may be asymptomatic.

[2] Characteristics of the discharge are quite variable; these are the classical descriptions.

[3] Not reliable during menses or after recent intercourse.

[4] Do not use during pregnancy.

[5] The pH may be <4.5.

[6] Leucocytes may be present in the wet preparation with any of these infections.

and polymorphonuclear leucocytes. The predominant type of bacteria should also be noted.

Vaginal Gram stains may also be used to determine if the bacterial morphotypes suggestive of bacterial vagininosis are present. It is good practice to exclude other diseases such as gonorrhoea and chlamydiae. Table 1 reviews the bedside diagnosis and treatment of vaginal infections.

Further reading

Eschenbach, D.A., Hillier, S., Critchlow, C., Stevens, C., DeRouen, T., and Holmes, K.K. (1988). Diagnosis and clinical manifestations of bacterial vaginosis. *American Journal of Obstetrics and Gynecology*, **158**, 819–28.

Hawes, S.E., Hillier, S.L., Benedetti, J., *et al.* (1996). Hydrogen peroxide-producing lactobacilli and acquisition of vaginal infections. *Journal of Infectious Diseases*, **174**, 1058–63.

Hillier, S.L., Krohn, M.A., Klebanoff, S.J., and Eschenbach, D.A. (1992). The relationship of hydrogen peroxide-producing lactobacilli to bacterial vaginosis and genital microflora in pregnant women. *Obstetrics and Gynecology*, **79**, 369–73.

Lossick, J.G. (1990). Treatment of sexually transmitted vaginosis/vaginitis. *Reviews of Infectious Diseases*, **12**, S665–81.

Nugent, R.P., Krohn, M.A., and Hillier, S.L. (1991). Reliability of diagnosing bacterial vaginosis is improved by a standardized method of Gram stain interpretation. *Journal of Clinical Microbiology*, **29**, 297–301.

Sewankambo, N., Gray, R., Waiver, M.J., *et al.* (1997). HIV-1 infection associated with abnormal vaginal flora morphology and bacterial vaginosis. *Lancet*, **350**: 546–50.

Sobel, J.D. (1997). Vaginitis. *New England Journal of Medicine*, **337**, 1896–903.

Chapter 17.4

Pelvic inflammatory disease

L. Weström

Pelvic inflammatory disease (often used synonymously for acute salpingitis) is defined as 'the acute clinical syndrome associated with ascending spread of micro-organisms (unrelated to pregnancy or surgery) from the vagina/cervix to the endometrium, Fallopian tubes and/or contiguous structures'.

Microbial aetiology and pathogenesis

In young women less than 26 years of age, up to 80 per cent of cases of pelvic inflammatory disease are caused by *Neisseria gonorrhoeae* and/or *Chlamydia trachomatis*. In the remaining cases a variety of facultative and strictly anaerobic bacterial species have been isolated from the upper genital tract, i.e. *Actinomyces israeli*, *Bacteroides* spp., clostridiae, *Escherichia coli*, *Gardnerella vaginalis*, *Peptostreptococcus* spp., staphylococci, streptococci of groups B-D, anaerobic streptococci, mycoplasmas, and others. Many of these species are constituents of the normal vaginal flora as well as of that of bacterial vaginosis (Chapter 17.3).

The factors that determine the ascending spread of causative organisms through the genital tract as well as the host–parasite interactions in the upper genital tract are still poorly understood, but seem to be influenced by sexual activity, hormonal factors, pathogenicity of the organisms, age, behavioural factors, and contraception.

Epidemiology

The cumulative incidence of pelvic inflammatory disease up to the age of 45 years has been estimated as 10 per cent. Three out of four episodes afflict women up to 25 years of age. Therefore, pelvic inflammatory disease in young women should be regarded and dealt with as a sexually transmitted disease. Estimates of pelvic inflammatory disease not associated with sexually transmitted organisms have given age-independent incidences of 2–5 per 1000 women per year.

In the female population, risk-factors include: age under 25, multiple partners, frequent sex, single or divorced, diagnosis of a sexually transmitted disease in patient or partner, no contraception or IUCD-user, urban dweller, low educational status, smoker, and/or drug/alcohol abuser.

Severity ranges from a typical benign infection to severe, life-threatening conditions. Criteria for suspecting pelvic inflammatory

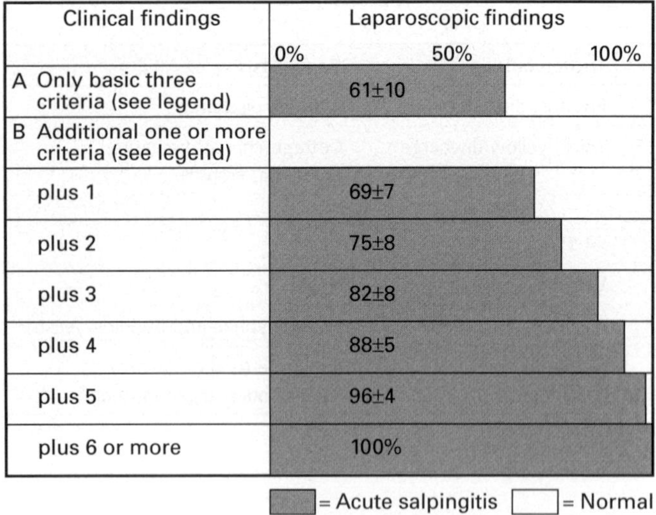

Clinical findings
Laparoscopic findings
0%
50%
100%
A Only basic three criteria (see legend)
61±10
B Additional one or more criteria (see legend)
plus 1
69±7
plus 2
75±8
plus 3
82±8
plus 4
88±5
plus 5
96±4
plus 6 or more
100%
= Acute salpingitis
= Normal

Fig. 1 Distribution of a laparoscopic diagnosis of acute salpingitis and normal intrapelvic findings in 2501 women subjected to laparoscopy on a clinical suspicion of pelvic inflammatory disease. (a) Presenting with the basic clinical criteria for a suspicion of pelvic inflammatory disease: low abdominal pelvic pain, tenderness on moving the cervix, signs of a lower genital tract infection (purulent vaginal secretion or evidence of gonorrhoea or genital chlamydial infection). (b) In addition of one or more of: rectal temperature over 38.0° C or chills, palpable adnexal swelling, erythrocyte sedimentation rate more than 15 mm/h, C-reative protein over 30 mg/l, white cell count in peripheral blood more than 10 000 mm^3, nausea or vomiting, metrorrhagic vaginal bleeding, dysuria.

disease are: low bilateral abdominal or pelvic pain of less than 2 weeks duration, tenderness on moving of the cervix, and signs of an infection of the lower genital tract (Fig. 1).

History

Recent symptoms

The pain is dull, continuous, low abdominal or pelvic, bilateral and has usually lasted for 3 to 9 days before presentation. Often it has started during or shortly after a menstruation. Symptoms of urethritis are common in infections by sexually transmitted organisms. Half of the patients report febrile illness. Chills suggest gonococcal infection. Metrorrhagic, often painful, intermenstrual bleeding is common. Nausea and vomiting are not typical.

Partner symptoms

Infection by sexually transmitted organisms is likely if the patient's sexual partner has urogenital symptoms and signs of urethritis.

Physical examination

General

The patient's general condition is usually good—only 3 per cent are severely ill. Pallor, hollow cheeks, reddening over the cheek-bones, sunken eyeballs, absence of abdominal breathing movements, and abdominal guarding signal an acute 'surgical abdomen' in need of immediate attention.

Pelvic examination

Inspect the external genitals for signs of trauma, haematomas, ulcerations, and warts. For the speculum examination, use tepid sterile saline to ease the insertion instead of antiseptic jellies or creams. Look at the appearances of the mucous surfaces and secretions. Obtain specimens by scraping, cytobrush technique, swabbing, or punch biopsy from any apparently pathological structure as well as from the vaginal and cervical secretions.

On bimanual pelvic examination, tenderness on moving of the cervix indicating an inflammatory reaction of the parametria or pelvic peritoneum and adnexal tenderness are the classical signs. Adnexal tenderness has a high sensitivity (95 per cent), but a low specificity (74 per cent) in predicting pelvic inflammatory disease. Adnexal swelling is often difficult to assess because of pain and abdominal guarding.

Side-room tests

In all women with acute pelvic pain a pregnancy test must be done in order to exclude an ectopic pregnancy. The test should be able to detect β-human chorionic gonadotropin down to 30 i.u./l of urine or blood.

Wet-mounted and air dried specimens of the genital secretions should be spread out on a glass slide, Gram (or methylene blue) stained, and examined under a microscope. In pelvic inflammatory disease, vaginal secretions contain increased numbers of inflammatory cells. In women with pelvic pain, identification of trichomonads or signs of bacterial vaginosis support the presence of an ascending infection. Ten or more polymorphonuclear leucocytes per high power field (× 1000 magnification) in the cervical secretion indicates cervicitis—always present in sexually transmitted disease-associated pelvic infection. Pelvic inflammatory disease is unlikely if the microscopical findings in the vaginal and cervical secretions are perfectly normal.

Laboratory tests

No test result is pathognomonic of pelvic inflammatory disease. In verified pelvic inflammatory disease, an ESR in excess of 15 mm/h is seen in 75 per cent of the patients, a white blood cell count in excess of 10^9/l in 60 per cent, and C-reactive protein over 30 mg/l in 80 per cent. The levels of ESR and C-reactive protein also reflect the severity of the infection. The sensitivity and specificity of these tests have been estimated to 70–93 and 67–90 per cent, respectively, for C-reactive protein, 75 and 56 per cent for ESR and 66 and 33 per cent for the white count. Antichymotrypsin, orosomucoid, or both are elevated in 80 per cent of women with pelvic inflammatory disease, but also in one-quarter of women with pelvic pain and no pelvic infection. The problem with these non-specific tests is that levels are raised in other inflammatory conditions such as appendicitis and inflammatory bowel disease.

Use of the microbiological laboratory

In all women with a suspicion of pelvic inflammatory disease, specimens from the cervix should be examined for gonococci and chlamydia by culture or antigen detection techniques. The results will direct chemotherapy and will be used to inform the partner and to counsel the patient. Unfortunately, the time required for these tests make them less useful for actual diagnosis.

Because of the large number of bacterial species in the normal vaginal flora, unselective bacterial cultures from the lower genital tract are useless. Serology is of little use for the diagnosis of pelvic inflammatory disease.

Table 1 CDC-guidelines for treatment of pelvic inflammatory disease*

Outpatient regimens
Cefoxitin 2 g IM plus probenicid I g orally concurrently or ceftriaxone 250 mg IM, or equivalent cephalosporin. PLUS doxycycline 100 mg 2 times daily for 10–14 days
OR
Ofloxacin 400 mg orally 2 times a day for 14 days, PLUS either clindamycin 450 mg orally 4 times a day, or metronidazole 500 mg orally 2 times a day for 14 days
Inpatient treatment
One of the alternatives A and B below is given for at least 48 h after the patient improves clinically
Regimen A: Cefoxitin IV 2 g every 6 h or cefotetan IV 2 g every 12 h PLUS doxycycline 100 mg every 12 h orally or IV
Regimen B: Clindamycin IV 900 mg every 8 h PLUS gentamicin loading dose IV or IM 2 mg/kg body weight followed by maintenance dose 1.5 mg/kg every 8 h (preferably monitored by determination of serum concentrations)
Continue
after discharge from hospital with doxycycline 100 mg orally 2 times daily for another 10–14 days.

*Management of sex partners:*Sex partners should be empirically treated with regimens effective against *Neisseria gonorrhoeae* and *Chlamydia trachomatis* regardless of the apparent aetiology of pelvic inflammatory disease or pathogens isolated from the infected woman.

**Morbidity and Mortality Weekly Reports* (1993).

Imaging

In advanced pelvic inflammatory disease an ultrasound or computed tomographic examination may help to detect pelvic abscesses.

Invasive diagnostic techniques

Specimens obtained by culdocentesis can be used for microbiological and side-room diagnosis. Frank blood indicates intra-abdominal bleeding and more than 3000 inflammatory cells/mm^3 of fluid an intraperitoneal infection. Entirely normal, clear, cell-free fluid argues against a pelvic infection.

Endometrial biopsy can be done with a Novak curette or other endometrial sampling device. The specimens obtained may be used for microbiological and histopathological analyses. A histopathological diagnosis of endometrial inflammation has a specificity of up to 87 per cent for predicting acute salpingitis.

Laparoscopy is 'the gold standard' for the diagnosis of pelvic inflammatory disease. It should be used freely—especially where delay might endanger the patient.

Treatment

Conservative treatment is the rule. Surgery should be considered only in cases with diffuse peritonitis, large tubo-ovarian abscess, and in somewhat older, parous women who do not plan more pregnancies.

Ambulatory treatment may be used in mild cases in which a 'surgical emergency' or anaerobic soft-tissue infection has been ruled out and in which a close follow-up is possible. Because of the 'polymicrobial' aetiology of pelvic inflammatory disease, multiple-drug regimens are most often necessary. The CDC-guidelines for the antibiotic treatment of pelvic inflammatory disease, given in Table 1 should be followed.

In sexually transmitted disease-associated pelvic inflammatory disease, examination and treatment of the patient's sexual partner is mandatory. It is recommended in all cases of pelvic inflammatory disease in women less than 25 years of age.

One in four women with proven acute salpingitis will suffer from sequelae such as infertility, ectopic pregnancy, and chronic pelvic pain. Antibiotic treatment should therefore be started immediately, and even an apparently uncomplicated genital infection should be treated thoroughly.

Further reading

Berger, G.S. and Weström, L. (ed.). (1992). *Pelvic inflammutory disease.* Raven Press, New York.

Peipert, J.F., Boardman, L., Hogan, J.W., Sung, J., and Mayer, K.H. (1996). Laboratory evaluation of acute upper genital tract infection. *Obstetrics and Gynecology,* **87**, 730–6.

Pelvic inflammatory disease: guidelines for prevention and management. (1993). *Morbidity and Mortality Weekly Report.* **42**, 77–81.

Weström, L. and Wölner-Nahnssen, P. (1993). Pathogenesis of pelvic inflammatory disease. *Genitourinary Medicine,* **69**, 9–17.

Weström, L. and Eschenbach, D.A. (1999). Pelvic inflammatory disease. (*Sexually transmitted diseases,* 3rd edn), pp. 783–810. New York, McGraw Hill Health Professions Division.

Chapter 17.5

Infections and other medical problems in homosexual men

A. McMillan

Many men who have had sexual contact with other men do not regard themselves as homosexual; many are in stable heterosexual relationships.

History

The nature and dates of recent sexual activity should be noted. It is helpful to know if the patient has had contact with someone with a sexually transmitted disease. Many infections, particularly those of the anorectum and pharynx, are symptomless. Some serological tests for syphilis (e.g. *Treponema pallidum* haemagglutination assay) remain positive for years after successful treatment, and so specific enquiry must be made about previous infection. Vaccination against hepatitis B and recent antimicrobial therapy should be noted.

Physical examination and investigations

The skin should be inspected for a rash; a macular rash may indicate primary HIV infection or secondary syphilis. Seborrhoeic dermatitis-like eruptions, extensive pityriasis versicolor, and severe tinea pedis may also occur with HIV.

The mouth and pharynx should be examined. Tender superficial ulceration may be caused by herpes simplex virus infection. Candidiasis, oral hairy leukoplakia, and Kaposi's sarcoma suggest HIV infection. Pharyngeal swabs should always be cultured for *Neisseria gonorrhoeae* even when there are no symptoms.

Generalized lymphadenopathy may be associated with HIV or Epstein-Barr virus infections or secondary syphilis. Tender enlargement of the inguinal or femoral lymph nodes may be found in any inflammatory condition, for example, herpes simplex virus infection of the external genitalia, perianal region, or anal canal.

Hepatic or splenic enlargement may occur in acute viral infections and in secondary syphilis.

The external genitalia should be examined in detail and the anal region should be inspected. Erythema without specific features may be found in patients who have pruritus ani secondary to an anal discharge. Threadworms may be noted at the anus. Multiple tender ulcers in the perianal region are most commonly caused by herpes simplex virus infection. A solitary ulcer at the anal margin may be traumatic in origin, but primary syphilis must always be excluded as a cause. Papillomatous lesions are usually caused by human papillomavirus infection, and, much less commonly, are seen in secondary syphilis.

When there has been receptive anal intercourse and in those with anorectal symptoms, a proctoscope should be passed, and the distal rectum inspected. Table 1 indicates the sexually transmissible causes of proctitis. Ulceration may be noted in herpes simplex virus infection, and, rarely, in primary syphilis, lymphogranuloma venereum, and primary cytomegalovirus infection. At this stage of the examination, material for microbiological examination for *N. gonorrhoeae*, *Chlamydia trachomatis*, and herpes simplex virus should be obtained. As the proctoscope is withdrawn, the anal canal is inspected for ulceration or condylomata.

Sigmoidoscopy is undertaken only if there are persistent symptoms and an infective cause has not been identified. Rectal biopsy is only rarely helpful in the diagnosis of rectal sexually transmitted diseases, but may help to exclude other conditions.

In the diagnosis of a diarrhoeal disease, faecal specimens should be submitted to the microbiology laboratory for culture for bacterial pathogens and for a protozoological examination. Jejunal intubation with biopsy may be necessary for the diagnosis of giardiasis.

The examination of an adhesive cellulose-tape preparation from the perianal skin for ova of *Enterobius vermicularis* should be done in men with a history of pruritus ani.

Serological tests for syphilis and for hepatitis B should be made routinely; in those with jaundice, serological investigations for recent infection with hepatitis A and C, cytomegalovirus, and Epstein-Barr virus should be undertaken. HIV antibody testing can be done after counselling.

Table 1 Organisms that are sexually transmissible amongst homosexual men

Organisms spread by mucosal/skin contact during anal intercourse	Organisms acquired by the faecal-oral route predominantly by oroanal contact)
Bacteria:	Bacteria:
Treponema pallidum ssp. *pallidum*	*Shigella* spp.
Neisseria gonorrhoeae	*Salmonella* spp.
N. meningitidis	*Campylobacter* spp.
Chlamydia trachomatis	
oculogenital serovars (D-K)	Viruses:
lymphogranuloma venereum serovars (L1, 2, 3)	Hepatitis A virus Enteroviruses
Haemophilus ducreyi	
Calymmatobacterium granulomatis	Protozoa:
? *Ureaplasma urealyticum*	*Giardia intestinalis*
? *Mycoplasma* spp.	*Entamoeba histolytica*
? *Brachyspira aalborgi*	*Cryptosporidium parvum*
Viruses:	Nematodes:
Human immunodeficiency virus types 1 and 2	*Enterobius vermicularis* *Strongyloides stercoralis*
Human T-cell leukaemia virus type 1 (rarely)	
Hepatitis B virus	
Hepatitis C virus	
Hepatitis D virus	
Cytomegalovirus	
Human papillomavirus	
Molluscum contagiosum virus	
Anthropods:	
Phthirus pubis	
Sarcoptes scabei	

Homosexually transmissible infections (Table 1) (see also Section 16)

Bacterial infections

Gonorrhoea

In homosexual men, the urethra, rectum, and pharynx may be affected. Pharyngeal gonorrhoea is usually symptomless, but may cause a sore throat.

At least 40 per cent of men with rectal gonorrhoea are symptomless and the rectal mucosa appears normal. Others show distal proctitis. Perianal abscess formation may be a complication.

Neisseria meningitidis infection

About 2 per cent of homosexual men have colonization of the rectum but it is a rare cause of proctitis.

Syphilis

An anal chancre often resembles a traumatic anal fissure—it is often painful, tender, bleeds easily, and lacks induration; there is usually femoral lymph node enlargement. Primary syphilis of the rectum may resemble a carcinoma.

Chlamydial infection

Although non-gonococcal urethritis is common in homosexual men, it is less often caused by *C. trachomatis* than in heterosexual men. Pharyngeal infection is uncommon and usually symptomless. Rectal infection with the oculogenital serovars is generally symptomless and the rectal mucosa appears normal; occasionally there may be a non-specific distal proctitis.

Table 2 Symptoms of sexually transmissible diseases in homosexual men

Symptom	Possible association	Comments
Urethral discharge and dysuria	Urethral gonorrhoea Non-gonococcal urethritis	 Chlamydial infection less common in homosexual men
Sore throat	Pharyngeal gonorrhoea Herpes simplex virus infection Pharyngeal candidiasis	 In HIV infected men
Rash	Primary HIV infection Primary Epstein–Barr virus infection Primary cytomegalovirus infection Acute hepatitis A and B Secondary syphilis Scabies	 More persistent than above
Swollen lymph nodes (generalized)	Primary HIV infection Primary Epstein–Barr virus infection Primary cytomegalovirus infection Acute hepatitis A and B Secondary syphilis	
Swollen inguinal or femoral lymph nodes	Perianal or genital herpes Primary syphilis	
Diarrhoea	*Giardia intestinalis* *Entamoeba histolytica* *Campylobacter* spp. *Shigella* spp. *Salmonella* spp. *Cryptosporidium parvum*	May also be abdominal cramps, nausea and increased flatulence Needs to be differentiated from *E. dispar*
Constipation, anal discharge, anal bleeding, perianal discomfort, pruritus ani	Proctitis associated with *Neisseria gonorrhoeae*, *Chlamydia trachomatis*, herpes simplex virus	
Pruritus ani	*Enterobius vermicularis*	
Perianal pain	Herpes simplex virus Anal fissure Perianal haematoma	
Anorexia, nausea, abdominal discomfort, dark urine, pale stools, jaundice	Acute hepatitis A or B Primary Epstein–Barr virus infection Primary cytomegalovirus infection	

Infection with lymphogranuloma venereum serovars is associated with a severe, distal proctitis with systemic features. Occasionally, the inflammation is more localized, with the formation of an ulcerated mass. Perianal abscess formation, strictures, and fistulae-*in-ano* may complicate untreated disease.

Mycoplasma and ureaplasma infections

Mycoplasmas and ureaplasmas can be cultured from the rectums of homosexual men but there is little evidence that they cause proctitis.

Granuloma inguinale

Perianal granuloma inguinale occurs most commonly in homosexual men. It presents as ulceration. Anal stenosis and basal-cell or squamous cell carcinoma may develop in untreated disease.

Salmonella spp., *Shigella* spp., and *Campylobacter* spp.

These are transmitted by the faecal–oral route, including anilingus, causing diarrhoea.

Viral infections

Human papillomavirus (HPV) infection

Condylomata are found most frequently in the perianal region and anal canal, causing pruritus ani and bleeding during defaecation. Condylomata may be very extensive and persistent in immunocompromised patients, including those with HIV infection.

Non-condylomatous HPV lesions detectable by cytological examination may be associated with anal intraepithelial neoplasia. Lesions are identified by operating microscope after application of dilute acetic acid. They are white, well-demarcated, and punctate. Their natural history is uncertain.

Herpes simplex virus (HSV) infection

In primary perianal herpes caused by either HSV-1 or HSV-2, there is anal pain, constipation, tenesmus, anal discharge, and bleeding on defaecation. Sacral nerve root involvement may result in paraesthesiae in the distribution of the affected nerves, and urinary hesitancy or acute retention and impotence may be features. There are often multiple tender ulcers in the perianal region and within the anal canal. A distal proctitis is common; there may be no specific features but discrete vesicular lesions or ulcers may be seen. Herpetic proctitis can occur in the absence of perianal or anal ulceration.

Recurrences are more likely in HSV-2 than in HSV-1 infection but, generally the symptoms and signs are much less severe and systemic features are not found.

Severe ulceration may be found in the immunocompromised patient, including those with HIV infection.

Cytomegalovirus (CMV)

CMV infection is more prevalent among homosexual men than heterosexual men and women. The virus is present in semen and receptive anal intercourse is the most likely means of acquisition.

Hepatitis A virus (HAV)

Homosexual men are at increased risk of faecal oral infection through oroanal or orogenital contact. HAV vaccine is indicated in homosexually active men.

Hepatitis B virus (HBV)

HBV is more prevalent in homosexual men but this may be declining. Hepatitis B surface antigen is detectable in saliva, seminal fluid, faeces, and the rectal mucosa, and so, particularly when there is superficial ulceration following intercourse, there is a risk of anogenital and oroanal transmission.

Vaccination of sexually active homo- and bisexual men who are antiHBs negative is cost effective. However, the antibody response is frequently impaired in HIV-infected men.

Hepatitis C virus (HCV)

Although there is a risk of infection in homosexual men, the prevalence of infection is low.

Hepatitis D virus (HDV)

Sexual transmission of HDV occurs among homosexual men. Unprotected anal intercourse is the means of spread.

Human immunodeficiency virus

See Chapter 16.35 for further discussion

Human T-cell leukaemia viruses (HTLV) types 1 and 2

Although HTLV-1 and HTLV-2 can be transmitted sexually, their prevalence among homosexual men is low.

Other viral infections

Coronaviruses have been detected in the faeces of homosexual men but their significance remains uncertain.

Protozoal infections

Amoebiasis

In the past, it had been considered that between 10 and 35 per cent of men attending sexually transmitted disease clinics in Europe and the USA were infected with *Entamoeba histolytica*. It is now clear that the majority of these infections were with the non-pathogenic amoeba *Entamoeba dispar* that is morphologically indistinguishable from *E. histolytica*. In tropical and subtropical countries, however, *E. histolytica* may be transmitted sexually and cause dysentery. It is therefore important to take a careful travel history from any homosexual man with diarrhoea.

Giardiasis

The prevalence of *Giardia intestinalis* in homosexual men attending sexually transmitted disease clinics in Western countries is 2–12 per cent. Most have been infected through oroanal sexual contacts. Although most infections are symptomless, a diarrhoeal illness may result.

Cryptosporidiosis

Cryptosporidium parvum is a cause of diarrhoea in some homosexual men. The importance of sexual transmission is uncertain.

Nematode infections

Enterobius vermicularis

Threadworms can be spread amongst homosexual men by oroanal sexual contact.

Strongyloides stercoralis

During oroanal contact ingestion of faeces containing the infective filariform larvae of the nematode can lead to infection in the homosexual man. Penetration of the skin or mucous membrane of the penis by infective larvae may result in infection following or during anal intercourse.

Other medical conditions in homosexual men

Urinary tract infection and epididymitis

Acute epididymitis in homosexual men aged less than 35 years is more likely to be caused by enterobacteria than *N. gonorrhoeae* or *C. trachomatis*, the most common causes of epididymitis in young heterosexual men.

Anorectal trauma

Violent anal intercourse with a penis or dildo can cause anal fissures or the formation of a perianal haematoma. Profuse rectal haemorrhage or rupture of the colon are rare complications of intercourse, but can be the result of the insertion of a hand into the rectum. Extraperitoneal microperforation of the rectum may also result from the latter practice, and is manifest as lower abdominal pain and rectal pain and fever, occurring within a few days. Abdominal examination is often normal, although there may be tenderness in the left iliac fossa; there is marked proctitis and induration of the pararectal tissues.

Anorectal sepsis

This may present as a chronic intersphincteric abscess with or without fistula formation.

Streptococcal infections

Streptococcal infection of the penis may result from fellatio. The lesions are erythematous, exude pus, and crusting may develop. Inguinal lymphadenitis associated with β-haemolytic streptococci may occur in immunocompromised individuals.

Rectal spirochaetosis

In this condition, spirochaetes lie parallel to the microvilli of the epithelial cells of the rectum and superficial portions of the crypts. The condition is indicated by the presence in a haematoxylin-stained section as a haematoxyphil zone, 3 μm wide, on the luminal surface of the cells. At least one species of spirochaete, *Brachyspira aalborgi*, has been associated with this condition.

Rectal spirochaetosis is found in about one-third of homosexual men who attend sexually transmitted disease clinics, a prevalence that is much higher than in patients who attend general medical or surgical clinics. The source of these organisms, and their pathogenicity is uncertain.

Kaposi's sarcoma (HHV8)

Although the incidence of this tumour associated with human herpes virus 8 amongst homosexual men infected with HIV has been declining, it still accounts for considerable morbidity in affected individuals.

Carcinoma of the anorectum

Epidemiological data appear to confirm that receptive anal intercourse may be a risk factor for squamous and transitional cell carcinomas of the anal canal, which are uncommon except in homosexual men. Some tumours are associated with certain types of HPV, particularly type 16, and are being seen with increasing frequency in HIV-infected men.

Further reading

Adler, M. W. (1988). *Diseases in the homosexual male.* Springer-Verlag, London.

Quinn, T.C. and Stamm, W.E. (1990). Proctitis, proctocolitis, enteritis and esophagitis in homosexual men. In: *Sexually transmitted diseases* (ed. K.K. Holmes, P.A. Mardh, P.F. Sparling, and P.J. Wiesner), pp. 663–83. McGraw-Hill, New York.

Chapter 17.6

Cervical cancer and other cancers caused by sexually transmitted infections

V. Beral

Occurrence

Worldwide, cervical cancer is the second most common cancer in women. It is far more frequent in Third World countries than in the West (Fig. 1). About 1 per cent of women in Britain have invasive cervical cancer diagnosed during their lifetime and 0.4 per cent die from it. Mortality rates have been falling throughout the 20th century, except among recent generations of women who became sexually active during the 1960s, a time when exposure to sexually transmitted diseases increased rapidly: 0.2 per cent develop vulval cancer and 0.2 per cent anal cancer.

The role of human papillomaviruses and other factors

There is now overwhelming evidence that the vast majority of cervical, vulval, anal, and penile cancers are caused by specific types of the human papillomavirus (see Chapter 16.32). DNA from human papillomavirus types 16, 18, 31, 33 or 35 (mostly type 16) has been found in cervical and other ano-genital cancers from as many as 90 per cent of those with the malignancy. Fewer than 10 per cent without such cancers have detectable evidence of these types of papillomaviruses in their anogenital cells.

The risk of cervical cancer is increased in women who are poor, have little education, were young when they first had sexual intercourse, had many sexual partners and multiple sexually transmitted infections, had many children, especially when they were young, and who smoked cigarettes and used oral contraceptives. Recent evidence suggests that hormonal and reproductive factors may independently influence the development of cervical cancer in papillomavirus-infected women, whereas cigarette smoking and other sexually transmitted infections may be of no direct aetiological significance.

The natural history of infection with the human papillomavirus and associated changes in the cervical epithelium

Some cervical papillomavirus infections cause no obvious epithelial changes—cervical colposcopy, cytology and biopsy are normal and the only way infection can be identified is by virological study. Other papillomavirus infections cause 'cervical warts', which are asymptomatic but can be seen as white patches at colposcopy after acetic acid has been applied to the cervix. Cervical smears from women with cervical warts may show various degrees of 'dysplasia' or 'dyskaryosis' and cervical biopsy may show various grades of 'cervical intraepithelial neoplasia' (CIN) (or 'squamous intraepithelial lesions' (SIL) according to a new classification known as the 'Bethesda system'). The most extreme change in the epithelium is the development of invasive cervical cancer, which seems to be associated with persistent viral infection and long-standing epithelial abnormalities.

Very little is known about why some lesions progress or regress. Most changes (up to the development of invasive cancer) seem to be reversible and lesions of different severity often coexist in the same woman. The more severe lesions tend to be rarer and found in older women: estimates of the proportion of women in Britain likely to develop various types of lesions are given in Table 1 and the age-specific prevalences of some of these lesions are shown in Fig. 2. At least 1 in 10 women is likely to be infected with human papillomavirus types 16 or 18; 1 in 20 is likely to develop persistent infection or

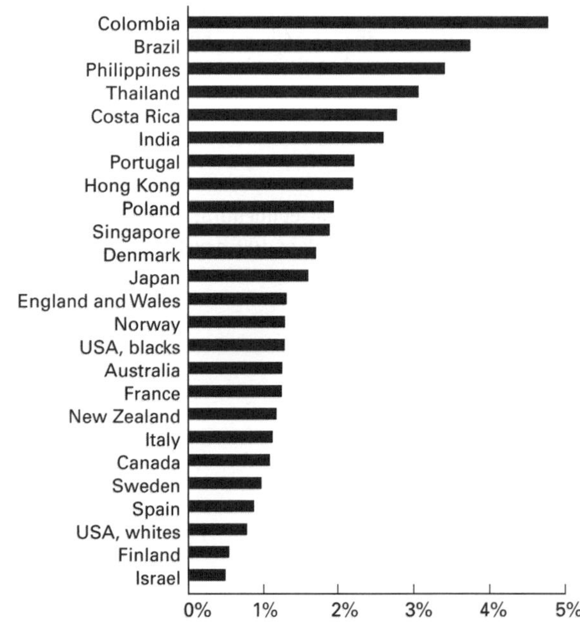

Fig. 1 Percentage of women who develop cervical cancer before age 75, by country.

Table 1 Estimated proportion of women in Britain likely to be infected by the papillomavirus and to develop abnormalities of the cervical epithelium, including cancer.

Outcome	%*
Acquire cervical papillomavirus infection	10–20
Develop persistent infection with papillomavirus	5–10
Develop abnormalities of the cervical epithelium such as 'dyskaryosis' or 'cervical intraepithelial neoplasia' (CIN)	5–10
Have carcinoma *in situ* of the cervix diagnosed	2–5
Have invasive carcinoma of the cervix diagnosed	1.0–1.5
Die from cervical cancer	0.3–0.5

*Ranges are given because exposure to the papillomavirus and the risk of associated abnormalities of the cervical epithelium are not the same for different generations of women; definitions and diagnostic criteria for cervical lesions vary; and screening programmes are leading to a reduction in the incidence of invasive cervical cancer and mortality from it and the magnitude of this reduction cannot be estimated with precision.

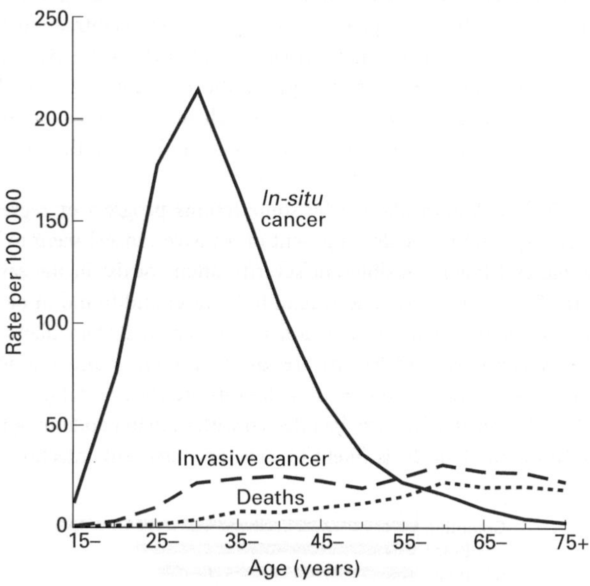

Fig. 2 Age-specific incidence of *in-situ* and invasive cervical cancer and of death from cervical cancer in England and Wales.

some abnormality of her cervical epithelium; 1 in 50 is diagnosed with *in-situ* cervical cancer; and 1 in 100 develops invasive cervical cancer. Papillomavirus infection is most prevalent in women aged in their 20s, corresponding to the age when they acquire other sexually transmitted infections; the peak prevalence of *in-situ* cancer tends to be about 10 years later (in women in their 30s) whereas invasive cancer is rare before 30 years of age.

Clinical implications

Most premalignant cervical changes are caused by papillomaviruses; most infections resolve spontaneously; cervical infection with papillomaviruses is especially common in young women but invasive cervical cancer is rare before the age of 30 years and seems to be associated with persistent infection and long-standing epithelial abnormalities.

We do not know why infection persists in some women and what determines who goes on to develop cervical cancer. Intensity of infection, age at exposure, immune response, genital hygiene, reproductive history, and the use of oral contraceptives could be relevant; future research should clarify. In the meantime it seems sensible not to resort to active treatment in women in their 20s with papillomavirus infection and related mild cervical lesions, but to reassure them that most lesions will resolve spontaneously and encourage them to have regular cervical smears. Only in young women with severe lesions and older women with persistent epithelial abnormalities is there an appreciable risk of progression to invasive cervical cancer, and active treatment is required.

Prevention

Well-organized screening programmes, based on exfoliative cervical cytology, are known to be effective in reducing the incidence and mortality of cervical cancer. Testing for papillomaviruses should not replace cervical cytology as a first-line approach in screening, since this would result in unnecessary treatment in many young women and because not all cervical cancers are associated with papillomavirus infection. Testing for papillomaviruses may be useful, however, in deciding how to manage the large number of women who have equivocal cervical cytology. Its efficacy must be evaluated before it is adopted on a large scale.

Effective vaccines have already been produced for bovine tumours caused by papillomavirus. Vaccines against the human papillomaviruses have been developed in the last few years and are now being tested in clinical trials.

Further reading

Schiffman, M.H. (1992). Recent progress in defining the epidemiology of human papillomavirus infection and cervical neoplasia. *Journal of the National Cancer Institute*, **84**, 394–8.

Section 18

Chemical and physical injuries and environmental factors and diseases

Contents

Poisoning

Environmental factors and disease

Poisoning

Chapter 18.1

Poisoning with drugs and chemicals

J. A. Vale and A. T. Proudfoot

Clinical and metabolic features and general principles of management

Diagnosis

Ideally, diagnosis of acute poisoning requires that the doctor not only establish that exposure to a poison (whether by ingestion, injection, inhalation, or skin contamination) has occurred, but also its chemical composition and magnitude so that the features likely to develop can be anticipated and risk assessed. As in any other branch of medicine, diagnosis of acute poisoning is based on the patient's history and on a combination of circumstantial evidence, the findings on physical examination, and appropriate investigations when a history is not available. However, in acute poisoning, there are many obstacles to establishing the information required. Young children may not be able to give a history, adults are often unreliable, and physical signs are rarely diagnostic. Circumstantial evidence may be only tentative, misleading, or not available, and laboratory diagnosis can never be comprehensive.

History

Since accidental poisoning in childhood is most common between the ages of 9 months and 5 years, an unequivocal history is unlikely to be forthcoming from the victim but may be obtainable from older witnesses. Assessment of amounts must be interpreted with caution since knowledge of the quantities in original containers is frequently inaccurate or unknown.

In contrast, about 90 per cent or more of adults presenting with acute poisoning are conscious or only slightly drowsy and should be able to give a reliable history. A few patients deny having taken poisons, but most admit to it without hesitation although problems arise in trying to establish precisely the nature and quantity of what has been taken. Comparison of patients' statements with poisons detected by laboratory analysis of blood or urine consistently reveals major differences in about half the cases. This is not surprising considering that self-poisoning is commonly an impulsive act. The patient ingests the contents of the first bottle that comes to hand, often when under the influence of alcohol. Although about 60 per cent of episodes involve drugs prescribed for the victims or their relatives, often they do not know their names.

Circumstantial evidence

This becomes important when there is no history.

Circumstances under which found

The mother may return to the kitchen or bathroom to find that her child has hands, face, and clothing covered by some substance, or is surrounded by pills, one of which is being eaten. Adults may be found unconscious with tablet particles around the mouth or on clothing. More often, the presence of empty drug containers close to the patient suggests the diagnosis. Less commonly, they are found unconscious or dead in some remote location. The lack of personal effects to indicate who they are or where they live may suggest a desire not to be identified and should arouse suspicion of drug overdosage. Self-poisoning is a common cause of coma in previously healthy young adults. Protestations by relatives that the patient would never take an overdose are usually wrong.

Table 1 Common feature clusters

Feature cluster	Likely poisons
Coma, hypertonia, hyperreflexia, extensor plantar responses, myoclonus, strabismus, mydriasis, sinus tachycardia	Tricyclic antidepressants—less commonly orphenadrine, thioridazine
Coma, hypotonia, hyporeflexia, plantar responses, either flexor or non-elicitable, hypotension	Barbiturates, benzodiazepines and alcohol combinations, severe tricyclic antidepressant poisoning
Coma, miosis, reduced respiratory rate	Opioid analgesics
Nausea, vomiting, tinnitus, deafness, sweating, hyperventilation, vasodilation, tachycardia	Salicylates
Restlessness, agitation, mydriasis, anxiety, tremor, tachycardia, convulsions, arrhythmias.	Sympathomimetics

Suicide notes

Suicide notes are reliable indicators of drug overdosage in the absence of physical violence as a cause of coma. The note may specify what has been taken in addition to expressing despair, futility, worthlessness, and remorse (Table 1).

Drowsiness, ataxia, dysarthria, and nystagmus are common after ingestion of benzodiazepines. Coma with hypotonia and hyporeflexia may follow, particularly if alcohol has also been taken. Hypotension, hypothermia, and respiratory depression are rare. All these features may occur after overdosage with outmoded drugs such as barbiturates, methaqualone, meprobamate, and ethchlorvynol that are still occasionally prescribed.

At present, tricyclic antidepressants remain among the most common CNS depressants encountered in overdosage. They cause hypertonia, hyperreflexia, extensor plantar responses, and dilated pupils. Sinus tachycardia and prolongation of the ECR QRS interval support the diagnosis. Hypotension and hypothermia are observed. Tricyclic antidepressants and non-steroidal anti-inflammatory agents, particularly mefenamic acid, are the most common causes of seizures after drug overdosage. Coma with pinpoint pupils and a reduced respiratory rate is virtually diagnostic of overdosage with opioid analgesics and is an indication for a therapeutic trial of naloxone. Many patients with opioid poisoning will be habitual drug abusers and have venepuncture marks and evidence of venous tracking in the antecubital fossae. Alcohol may be smelt on the breath as may solvents such as toluene, acetone, or xylene as the result of 'sniffing' glues, cleaning agents, or other preparations. Skin blisters occur in poisoning by many drugs (see below) but rarely in coma due to other causes. Burns around the lips or in the buccal cavity or pharynx indicate ingestion of corrosives, including paraquat.

Lateralizing neurological signs

Since most serious poisonings are associated with impairment of consciousness, neurological signs are particularly important. Lateralizing signs virtually exclude a diagnosis of acute poisoning except in rare cases of barbiturate and phenytoin overdosage. Transient inequality of the pupils has been reported only rarely in acute poisoning but is not an uncommon finding in normal individuals (e.g. due to Holmes-Adie pupils).

Decerebrate and decorticate movements

Unconscious poisoned patients may respond to painful stimuli with flexor and extensor limb movements of the type seen in decorticate and decerebrate states. However, in poisoning, these signs do not indicate irreversible brain damage. Hypoglycaemia must be excluded in these cases.

Strabismus, and internuclear and external ophthalmoplegia

Strabismus has been described in poisoning with phenytoin, carbamazepine, and tricyclic antidepressants. Usually the optic axes diverge in the horizontal plane but in some patients there is additional vertical deviation. It is present transiently and only in patients who are unconscious. Dysconjugate, roving eye movements may also be seen if both eyes are observed for a period of time.

Instillation of ice-cold water into one external auditory meatus should make both eyes turn to that side. Failure of one eye to deviate is evidence of internuclear ophthalmoplegia and a lesion of the medial longitudinal fasciculus. This has been reported in poisoning with a variety of drugs, including tricyclic antidepressants, phenothiazines, benzodiazepines, barbiturates, and ethanol.

In some cases, cold-induced lateral eye movements are followed after an interval of 5–15 seconds by forced downward gaze lasting several min.

In acute poisoning the absence of oculocervical and oculovestibular responses does not indicate irrecoverably severe brainstem damage.

Management

Antidotes and methods of enhancing elimination are available for only a few poisons. The management of the great majority of poisoned patients is supportive.

Emergency treatment

Some poisoned patients arrive at hospital with respiratory obstruction, ventilatory failure, or in cardiorespiratory arrest. In these cases, conventional resuscitation takes precedence over detailed assessment of the patient and attempts to obtain a history. The opioid antagonist, naloxone, can be enormously valuable. It is safe and should be used whenever there is the slightest suspicion that an opioid is involved.

Supportive care

Unconscious patients need scrupulous attention to respiration, hypotension, hypothermia, and other complications if they are to survive. Expert nursing is as important as medical measures.

Airway

The airway may be obstructed by the tongue falling back, dental plates being dislodged, other foreign bodies, buccal secretions, vomitus, and flexion of the neck. Initially, the neck should be extended and the tongue and jaw held forward. Secretions in the oropharynx must be removed and an oropharyngeal airway should be inserted before turning the patient into a semiprone position. If the cough reflex is absent, an endotracheal tube should be inserted to prevent aspiration into the lungs and allow regular aspiration of bronchial secretions. It is then important to ensure that the inspired air is adequately warmed and humidified.

Ventilation

Once a clear airway has been established, the adequacy of spontaneous ventilation should be assessed from the results of arterial blood gas and pH measurements. These should be performed in all comatose patients irrespective of the presence or absence of features suggesting inadequate gas exchange. Unconscious poisoned patients often have a mild, mixed respiratory and metabolic acidosis with carbon dioxide tensions at the upper limit of normal and oxygen tensions which fall with increasing depth of coma. Increasing the oxygen contents of the inspired air is often sufficient to correct hypoxia. Patients in respiratory failure ('carbon dioxide retention') should have an endotracheal tube inserted. If this does not reduce carbon dioxide tensions, assisted ventilation is indicated. High inspired oxygen concentrations are imperative in patients with carbon monoxide and cyanide poisoning and in pulmonary oedema resulting from inhalation of irritant gases.

Hypotension

Hypotension in acute poisoning can be due to a variety of factors including hypovolaemia secondary to increased venous capacitance, metabolic acidosis, arrhythmias, the cardiodepressant effects of some drugs, and blood or fluid loss into the gut. Young patients are generally not at risk of cerebral or renal damage unless the systolic blood pressure falls below 80 mmHg but in those over the age of 40 years it is preferable to keep the systolic blood pressure above 90 mmHg. Hypotension may respond to elevation of the foot of the bed and if this is unsuccessful a venous line should be inserted and the intravascular volume expanded as necessary. Dopamine (2.5–20 μg/kg.min) and dobutamine (5–40 μg/kg.min) are indicated if hypotension is resistant to these measures. The possibility of using techniques to enhance elimination of the poison from the body should then be considered.

Arrhythmias

Although many poisons are potentially cardiotoxic, the incidence of serious cardiac arrhythmias in acute poisoning is very low. Tricyclic antidepressants, (β-adrenoceptor blocking drugs, chloral hydrate, cardiac glycosides, amphetamines, bronchodilators (particularly theophylline and its derivatives), and antimalarial drugs are the most likely causes. Cardiotoxicity usually occurs together with other features of severe poisoning including metabolic acidosis, hypoxia, convulsions, respiratory depression, and abnormalities of electrolyte balance which should be corrected before considering the use of antiarrhythmic drugs. The latter have narrow therapeutic ratios and their use may further impair myocardial function. In general, drug therapy should only be given for persistent, life-threatening arrhythmias associated with peripheral circulatory failure. The drug used must be selected from a knowledge of the pharmacology and toxicology of the poison involved and in such a way that it will not further compromise cardiac function. Lignocaine is probably the drug of choice for serious ventricular tachydysrhythmia since its half-life is short and the dose can be adjusted readily.

Convulsions

Convulsions are potentially life-threatening because they cause hypoxia and metabolic acidosis and may precipitate cardiac arrhythmias and arrest. Short isolated convulsions do not require treatment but those which are recurrent or protracted should be suppressed with intravenous diazepam. This drug is highly effective in adequate doses and alternatives are seldom needed. However, it is important to remember that giving benzodiazepines in this way may potentiate the respiratory depressant effects of other poisons and further complicate management. The combination of convulsions, coma, and vomiting, which may occur with overdosage of theophylline derivatives, is particularly dangerous and in these circumstances it may be preferable to paralyse the patient, insert an endotracheal tube, and start assisted ventilation. However, although this ensures control of the airway and oxygenation, thus avoiding the risk of inhalation of gastric contents, it does not suppress seizure activity; cerebral function must therefore be monitored and parenteral anticonvulsants given as required.

Hypothermia

Any poison that depresses the central nervous system may impair temperature regulation and cause hypothermia, especially when discovery of the patient is delayed and environmental temperatures are low. This important complication may be missed unless temperature is recorded rectally using a low reading thermometer. In severe cases, peripheral and core temperatures should be monitored. Treatment includes nursing the patient in a warm room (27–29°C) and a heat conserving 'space blanket'. Cold intravenous fluids should be avoided and bottles for use should be stored in the room or the lines should pass through a heating device.

Hyperthermia

Rarely, body temperature may increase to potentially fatal levels after overdosage with central nervous system stimulants such as cocaine, amphetamines, phencyclidine, monoamine oxidase inhibitors, and theophylline and its derivatives. In such cases, muscle tone is often grossly increased and convulsions and rhabdomyolysis are common. Cooling measures, including administration of chlorpromazine, are indicated and dantrolene should be considered to reduce muscle tone and temperature.

Acid-base abnormalities

Acid-base disturbances commonly accompany drug-induced coma Some elevation of arterial carbon dioxide tensions towards the upper limit of normal is usual. This, in combination with mild hypoxia in the deeper grades of coma, produces acidaemia. In general, acidosis should be prevented and managed by ensuring adequate ventilation, oxygenation and tissue perfusion, and control of convulsions rather than by giving bicarbonate. However, a number of poisons, particularly methanol and ethylene glycol, cause life-threatening metabolic acidosis which should be corrected by infusion of sodium bicarbonate.

Acute respiratory alkalosis, often in combination with a minor metabolic acidosis, is found commonly in acute salicylate overdosage. The metabolic component may require treatment if it is the dominant feature and is causing overall acidaemia. Respiratory alkalosis should not be treated.

Electrolyte abnormalities

Electrolyte abnormalities may result from acid-base disturbances or the direct effects of poisons. Massive tissue damage, usually rhabdomyolysis, may allow potassium to leak from cells leading to potentially lethal hyperkalaemia. Cardiac glycosides cause hyperkalaemia secondary to loss from cells due to inhibition of the membrane sodium-potassium pump while the reverse occurs with sympathomimetic drugs. Ingestion of potassium salts, even in sustained release formulations, may lead to hyperkalaemia and fatal arrhythmias. Oxalic acid and ethylene glycol (which is metabolized to oxalic acid) may cause hypocalcaemia by leading to the formation of insoluble calcium oxalate which is deposited in tissues. Similarly, ingestion of fluorides is also a possible cause of hypocalcaemia but the amounts children tend to ingest in the form of tablets to prevent dental caries seldom cause serious problems.

Bladder care

Urinary retention is a common complication of acute poisoning, particularly with tricyclic antidepressants and other drugs which have marked anticholinergic actions. Coma *per se* is not an indication for catheterization in poisoned patients, the great majority of whom regain consciousness within 12 hours. The bladder can usually be induced to empty reflexly (provided it is not allowed to become grossly over-distended) by applying gentle suprapubic pressure. Catheterization should be reserved for those patients in whom suprapubic pressure is insufficient to empty the bladder, and in those thought to be developing renal failure.

Skin, muscle, and nerve lesions

Skin blisters may be found after poisoning with a wide variety of drugs, including barbiturates, tricyclic antidepressants and benzodiazepines, and non-drug toxins. They often occur over bony prominences which have been subjected to pressure and less frequently at sites where two skin areas have been in contact, e.g. the inner aspects of the knees. They should be managed as partial thickness burns. Rhabdomyolysis is a further possible result of immobility and may occur in combination with skin lesions or independently. Drug overdosage is the most common non-traumatic cause of this condition and may lead to acute renal failure and, rarely, to ischaemic muscle contractures and long-term disability. Similarly, peripheral nerves such as the radial, ulnar, and common peroneal may be damaged by direct pressure while the patient is unconscious or by being entrapped in fibrosing muscle after rhabdomyolysis.

Antidotes

Naloxone for opioid analgesics, oxygen for carbon monoxide, and, occasionally, flumazenil for benzodiazepines are the only antidotes commonly needed in the management of unconscious poisoned patients. Methionine and *N*-acetylcysteine ('Parvolex') are used frequently for paracetamol overdosage. Other antidotes of proven value are listed in Table 2. They are seldom required. Although potentially life-saving, some are toxic. Further advice should be obtained from a poisons information service.

Prevention of poison absorption

Prevention of absorption of poisons through the lungs obviously requires removal from the toxic atmosphere and occasionally removal of soiled clothing. The latter is also necessary when absorption is thought to have been percutaneous and, in addition, the contaminated skin should be thoroughly washed with soap and water. Measures to limit further absorption of ingested poisons (gut decontamination) include emptying the stomach, either by inducing emesis or by gastric aspiration and lavage, the administration of oral adsorbents, particularly activated charcoal, and the use of whole bowel irrigation.

Table 2 Antidotes of proven value in poisoning and associated complications

Poison or associated complication	Antidote
Anticoagulants (oral)	Vitamin K
Arsenic	Dimercaprol, DMSA, DMPS
Benzodiazepines	Flumazenil
β-Adrenoceptor blockers	Atropine, glucagon
Carbon monoxide	Oxygen
Cyanide	Amyl nitrite, sodium nitrite, dicobalt edetate
Digoxin	Digoxin-specific Fab antibodies
Ethylene glycol	Ethanol, 4-methylpyrazole
Iron salts	Desferrioxamine
Lead (inorganic)	Sodium calciumedetate, DMSA
Methaemoglobinaemia	Methylene blue
Methanol	Ethanol, 4-methylpyrazole
Mercury (inorganic)	DMPS
Opioids	Naloxone
Organophosphate insecticides	Atropine, pralidoxime
Paracetamol	Methionine, *N*-acetylcysteine
Phenothiazine or butyrophenone dystonia	Benztropine, procyclidine

Gastric lavage and syrup of ipecacuanha

Gastric lavage seems logical after ingestion of a poison. However, it is now apparent that gastric lavage (a) retrieves toxicologically significant quantities of drugs in only a small proportion of cases, particularly if carried out later than one hour after ingestion; (b) does not appear to alter the clinical outcome irrespective of the severity of poisoning, and (c) may increase the severity of poisoning by flushing drug from the stomach into the small bowel, thus facilitating rapid absorption.

Induced emesis with syrup of ipecacuanha is no more effective than gastric lavage, and is not without adverse effects. Serious morbidity is rare but protracted vomiting is not uncommon and diarrhoea, abdominal pain, drowsiness, and irritability occur in 10–15 per cent of cases. Aspiration pneumonia occurs in 5 per cent of conscious patients given syrup of ipecacuanha.

Activated charcoal

'Activated' means that the number of pores and channels throughout individual particles is greatly increased, correspondingly enlarging the surface area to which poisons may be adsorbed. *In vitro* studies confirm that charcoal is an effective adsorbent of a wide range of drugs and chemicals. When given within 1 hour of ingestion it can reduce absorption of most drugs commonly taken in overdosage. If given later its efficacy is reduced considerably. Some 50–100 g should be given to adults who have taken a substantial overdose of a toxic substance within the previous hour. If sustained release formulations (e.g. theophylline derivatives) or drugs that delay gastric emptying have been taken (e.g. tricyclic antidepressants and opioid analgesics) the time interval for administration of charcoal can be extended.

Methods of increasing elimination

Once a poison has been absorbed,and providing there is no antidote, it is reasonable to consider the use of treatments that might speed its elimination from the body.

Multiple doses of oral activated charcoal

Multiple doses of activated charcoal aid the elimination of some drugs from the circulation by adsorbing drugs that diffuse into the intestinal juices so interrupting their enterohepatic circulation. The process has been termed 'gut dialysis' since, in effect, the intestinal mucosa is being used as a semipermeable membrane. In poisoned patients repeated doses of oral activated charcoal shorten the plasma half-life of carbamazepine, dapsone, digoxin, phenobarbitone, quinine, and theophylline and, in some cases, are as effective as charcoal haemoperfusion. Recommended adult doses of charcoal for this purpose are 50–100 g initially, followed by 50 g 4-hourly until charcoal appears in the faeces or recovery occurs.

Alkalinization of the urine

Inducing an alkaline urine to enhance elimination is only employed in poisoning by salicylates (see below) and phenoxyacetate herbicides. The urine pH should be maintained between 7.5 and 8.5. As a fall in plasma potassium concentration is likely following bicarbonate administration (due to cellular shift of potassium), hypokalaemia should be corrected before alkalinization and the plasma potassium concentration should therefore be monitored and supplements given as necessary.

Dialysis

In acute poisoning, dialysis is most commonly indicated for the treatment of acute renal failure and only infrequently to increase poisons elimination. It is an inefficient way of trying to remove most poisons. The rate of elimination across the dialysis membrane depends upon the molecular weight of the toxin, the extent to which it is protein bound, the concentration gradient, and pH of blood and dialysate. Haemodialysis is more efficient than peritoneal dialysis and is of value in severe poisoning with salicylates, phenobarbitone, methanol, ethanol, ethylene glycol, lithium, and chlorates. Peritoneal dialysis is useful for the removal of the same toxins when haemodialysis is not available or when renal failure complicates poisoning due to phenobarbitone or salicylates.

Haemoperfusion

Although haemoperfusion was a major advance in the treatment of some of the most serious forms of poisoning 30 years ago, its present day application is extremely limited as a result of the greatly reduced incidence of overdosage with barbiturates, meprobamate, glutethimide, and methaqualone. Unfortunately, it does not remove tricyclic antidepressants. Multiple doses of activated charcoal have been shown to produce similar drug clearances in many cases.

Poisons

Acetone

A clear liquid with a characteristic pungent odour and sweet taste, used widely in industrial and household products.

Metabolism Once absorbed either through the lungs or gut, acetone is exhaled unchanged or metabolized to carbon dioxide.

Clinical features Acetone is highly volatile. Its vapour has an irritating effect on the mucous membranes of the eyes, nose, and throat.

Intoxication results in headache, excitement, restlessness, chest tightness, incoherent speech, nausea, vomiting, occasionally gastrointestinal bleeding, coma, convulsions, and hyperglycaemia.

Treatment If toxicity has followed inhalation, remove from exposure, give supportive treatment, and correct hyperglycaemia. After ingestion gut decontamination is not useful.

Further reading

Gamis, A.S. (1988). Acute acetone intoxication in a pediatric patient. *Pediatric Emergency Care*, **4**, 24–6.

Acids

Acids commonly involved in cases of poisoning include the inorganic acids hydrochloric, hydrofluoric, nitric, phosphoric, and sulphuric acids; and organic acids acetic, formic, lactic, and trichloroacetic acids. Car battery acid typically contains 28 per cent sulphuric acid. Proprietary cleaning agents and antirust compounds often comprise a mixture of hydrochloric and phosphoric acids.

Clinical features On the skin acids behave characteristically as corrosives leading to erythema and burns. In the eyes, intense pain, blepharospasm, and corneal burns may occur. When ingested, acids flow rapidly along the lesser curvature of the stomach to the prepyloric region where they pool because of spasm of the pylorus and antrum to cause almost instantaneous coagulative necrosis of one or more layers of the stomach. In some 80 per cent of cases, acids spare the oesophagus because of rapid transit and resistant squamous epithelium.

There is immediate pain in the mouth, pharynx, and abdomen, intense thirst, vomiting, haematemesis, and diarrhoea. The pain and mucosal oedema cause dysphagia and drooling saliva. Gastric and oesophageal perforation result in chemical peritonitis. Other effects include hoarseness, stridor, respiratory distress, laryngeal and epiglottic oedema, shock, metabolic acidosis, leucocytosis, acute tubular necrosis, renal failure, hypoxaemia , respiratory failure, intravascular coagulation, and haemolysis.

Formic acid ingestion causes systemic acidosis, haematuria, and renal damage. Hydrofluoric acid ingestion causes chelation of calcium, with resultant weakness, paraesthesiae, tetany, convulsions, and disturbed coagulation.

Treatment Acid burns to the skin should be liberally irrigated with water or saline. Dressings are applied as for a thermal burn. Skin grafting may be necessary.

After ocular exposure, the eye should be irrigated, preferably with saline for 15–30 min. Topical local anaesthetic is usually required to relieve pain and to overcome blepharospasm. Ophthalmic advice should be sought.

After ingestion a clear airway should be established. Opioids are often necessary for analgesia.

Dilution and/or neutralization is contraindicated. Urgent panendoscopy is needed. Patients with circumferential ulceration or multiple deep ulcers should be admitted to an intensive care unit. Total parenteral nutrition is often required. Corticosteroids confer no benefit and may mask abdominal signs of perforation; antibiotics should be given for established infection only. Laparotomy with resection of necrotic tissue and surgical repair should be considered.

Acid ingestion may result in antral, pyloric, or jejunal strictures, achlorhydria, protein-losing enteropathy, and gastric carcinoma.

Further reading

Boyce, S.H. and Simpson, K.A. (1996). Hydrochloric acid inhalation: who needs admission? *Journal of Accident and Emergency Medicine*, **13**, 422–4.

Cartotto, R.C., Peters, W.J. Neligan, P.C., Douglas, L.G., and Beeston, J. (1996). Chemical burns. *Canadian Journal of Surgery*, **39**, 205–11.

Alkalis

Those commonly encountered in cases of poisoning include drain, lavatory, and pipe cleaners (sodium hydroxide), dishwashing detergents (sodium carbonate, sodium silicate, sodium tripolyphosphate), denture cleaning tablets (sodium perborate, sodium phosphate, sodium carbonate), urinary glucose testing tablets (sodium hydroxide), water sterilizing tablets (sodium dichloroisocyanurate), alkaline batteries, and sodium hypochlorite (a bleaching agent).

Clinical features The features of eye, skin, and laryngeal contamination with alkalis are similar to those produced by acids (see above). When ingested, alkalis typically damage the oesophagus but usually spare the stomach. There is little immediate oral discomfort but subsequently a burning sensation develops in the mouth and pharynx, together with epigastric pain, vomiting, and diarrhoea. Oesophageal and/or gastric ulceration and their complications may occur.

Treatment The treatment of corrosive injuries caused by alkalis is largely the same as for those produced by acids.

Corticosteroids do not alter the incidence of stricture formation, but may decrease the need for surgical repair of strictures arising from second- or third-degree burns if they are used in conjunction with either anterograde or retrograde oesophageal dilation. Methylprednisolone 40 mg IV 8-hourly in adults or prednisolone 2 mg/kg per day IV can be given, until oral intake is resumed, when an equivalent dosage of prednisolone is given orally and tapered off over a period of 3–6 weeks. A broad-spectrum antibiotic, such as amoxycillin, should be prescribed at the same time.

Alkali ingestion may result in stricture formation and there is a risk of malignancy. The mean latent period for development of carcinoma of the oesophagus following alkali ingestion is more than 40 years.

Further reading

Anderson, K.D., Rouse, T.M., and Randolph, J.G. (1990). A controlled trial of corticosteroids in children with corrosive injury of the esophagus. *New England Journal of Medicine*, **323**, 637–40.

Gaudreault, P., *et al.* (1983). Predictability of esophageal injury from signs and symptoms: a study of caustic ingestion in 378 children. *Pediatrics*, **71**, 767–70.

Ochi, K., Ohashi, T., Sato, S., Watarai, J., Maeda, C., and Takeyama I. (1996). Surgical treatment for caustic ingestion injury of the pharynx, larynx and esophagus. *Acta Oto-laryngologica*, **116**, 116–19.

Aluminium (aluminum)

See Sections 9 and 12 and OTM3, pp. 1105–6.

Ammonia

Ammonia, a colourless gas with a strong irritating odour, is used in aqueous solution in industry and in the home.

Clinical features Ammonia may be absorbed by inhalation, ingestion, or percutaneously. It irritates the eyes, upper respiratory tract, and pharynx. Exposed surfaces may develop chemical burns, blisters, thrombosis of surface vessels, and severe local oedema which may lead to respiratory obstruction and death, if the larynx and glottis are involved. High inhaled concentrations may cause dyspnoea and pulmonary oedema and persistent lung damage.

Treatment The casualty should be removed from the contaminated area. The eyes should be irrigated with water or saline (0.9 per cent) for 15–30 min and an ophthalmic opinion sought as permanent blindness may result. Pulmonary complications should be treated with humidified supplemental oxygen, bronchodilators, and, if necessary, assisted ventilation with positive end-expiratory pressure. There is no conclusive evidence that diuretics and corticosteroids alter the prognosis. Patients who survive for 24 hours are likely to recover fully.

Further reading

Darchy, B., Le Miere, E., Lacour, S., Bavoux, E., and Domart, Y. (1997). Acute ammonia inhalation. *Intensive Care Medicine*, **23**, 597–8.

De La Hoz, R.E., Schlueter, D. P., and Rom, W.N. (1996). Chronic lung disease secondary to ammonia inhalation injury. *American Journal of Industrial Medicine*, **29**, 209–14.

Amphetamines and ecstasy (MDMA)

Clinical features Amphetamine, dexamphetamine, methamphetamine, and 'ecstasy' (3,4-methylenedioxymethamphetamine, MDMA) stimulate the central nervous system causing increased alertness and self-confidence, euphoria, extrovert behaviour, increased talkativeness with rapid speech, lack of desire to eat or sleep, tremor, dilated pupils, tachycardia, and hypertension. More severe intoxication is associated with excitability, agitation, paranoid delusions, hallucinations with violent behaviour, hypertonia, and hyperreflexia. Convulsions, rhabdomyolysis, hyperthermia, and cardiac arrhythmias may develop in the most severe cases. Hyperthyroxinaemia may be found in chronic users. Rarely, intracerebral and subarachnoid haemorrhage, acute cardiomyopathy, and cardiac arrhythmias occur and may be fatal.

Treatment Gastric lavage should be considered if a substantial overdose has been ingested in the preceding hour. Sedation with chlorpromazine, droperidol, or diazepam may be required. The peripheral sympathomimetic actions of amphetamines may be antagonized by β-adrenergic blocking drugs. Acidification of the urine increases the renal elimination of methamphetamine fivefold.

Further reading

Dar, K.J. and McBrien, M.E. (1996). MDMA induced hyperthermia: report of a fatality and review of current therapy. *Intensive Care Medicine*, **22**, 995–6.

Derlet, R.W., Rice, P., Horowitz, B.Z., and Lord, R.V. (1989). Amphetamine toxicity: experience with 127 cases. *Journal of Emergency Medicine*, **7**, 157–61.

Henry, J.A., Jeffreys, D.J., and Dawling, S. (1992). Toxicity and deaths from 3,4-methylenedioxymethamphetamine ('ecstasy'). *Lancet*, **340**, 384–7.

Angiotensin converting enzyme inhibitors

Clinical features Anorexia, nausea, abdominal discomfort, headache, and paraesthesiae have been reported. In addition, hypotension (which may be mediated by the endogenous opioid system), sinus tachycardia, bronchospasm, and hyperkalaemia may develop. Fatalities have been reported.

Treatment Gastric lavage or activated charcoal administration should be considered if the patient presents within 1 hour of a substantial overdose. Supportive therapy should then be employed, including volume expansion with plasma expanders for hypotension. Naloxone in a dose of 0.8–1.2 mg can reverse ACE inhibitor-induced hypotension. Marked hyperkalaemia may require an intravenous infusion of glucose (50 g) and soluble insulin (15 units).

Further reading

Lip, G.Y. and Ferner, R.E. (1995). Poisoning and anti-hypertensive drugs; angiotensin converting enzyme inhibitors. *Journal of Human Hypertension*, **9**, 711–15.

Anticoagulants

Warfarin is the most commonly used oral anticoagulant. Brodifacoum and bromodioline rodenticides are more potent antagonists of vitamin K_1 than warfarin.

Mechanism of toxicity Synthesis of clotting factors II, VII, IX, and X is reduced.

Clinical features Gastrointestinal bleeding, haematuria, and bruising are the commonest features, though the most common site of fatal haemorrhage is intracranial.

Treatment If the International Normalized Ratio (INR) is less than 5, the patient is not bleeding, and continuing anticoagulation is required, no immediate treatment is necessary beyond temporarily stopping warfarin. If continuing anticoagulation is not intended, or the INR is greater than 5, or bleeding has occurred, vitamin K_1 (phytomenadione) 2–5 mg should be given intravenously. The INR will fall within 10 hours. If haemorrhage is severe, fresh-frozen plasma should be given as well.

Further reading

McCarthy, P.T., Cox, A.D., Harrington, *et al.* (1997). Covert poisoning with difenacoum: clinical and toxicological observations. *Human and Experimental Toxicology*, **16**, 166–70.

Parsons, B.J., Day, L.M., Ozanne-Smith, J., and Dobbin, M. (1996). Rodenticide poisoning among children. *Australian and New Zealand Journal of Public Health*, **20**, 488–92.

Antihistamines

First generation antihistamines include brompheniramine, chlorpheniramine, cyclizine, diphenhydramine, mepyramine, methapyrilene, promethazine, and trimeprazine. Second generation drugs include astemizole and terfenadine. The toxicity of the two groups varies.

Clinical features The older antihistamines have anticholinergic actions and their effects are therefore similar to the tricyclic antidepressants (see below) although convulsions, coma, respiratory depression, arrhythmias (other than sinus tachycardia), and death are rare.

Astemizole and terfenadine lack anticholinergic actions but are cardiotoxic, causing QTc interval prolongation and ventricular tachycardia, including the torsade-de-pointes type. Associated giant U waves have been described. Terfenadine in overdose can cause convulsions.

Treatment Gastric lavage may be undertaken or oral activated charcoal may be given if the patient presents less than 1 hour after the ingestion of a substantial overdose of a first generation antihistamine. The patient should be observed for about 12 hours with cardiac monitoring if the QT interval is prolonged. Intravenous magnesium sulphate may abolish serious ventricular arrhythmias.

Further reading

Jumbelic, M.I., Hanzlick, R., and Cohle, S. (1997). Alkylamine antihistamine toxicity and review of Pediatric Toxicology Registry of the National Association of Medical Examiners. *American Journal of Forensic Medicine and Pathology*, **18**, 65–9.

June, R.A. and Nasr, I. (1997). Torsades de pointes and terfenadine ingestion. *American Journal of Emergency Medicine*, **15**, 542–3.

Antimicrobials

Most patients develop no symptoms and require no treatment. Transient nausea, vomiting, and diarrhoea may occur. There have been single case reports of renal failure after overdosage with co-trimoxazole, pancreatitis with erythromycin, and haemorrhagic cystitis with amoxicillin.

Antiparkinsonian drugs

Amantadine, benzhexol, and orphenadrine have anticholinergic effects in overdosage. Orphenadrine is probably the most toxic and has caused deaths.

Clinical features and treatment The features of poisoning are similar to those of the tricyclic antidepressants and should be managed in the same way.

Further reading

Jones, A.L. and Proudfoot, A.T. (1997). The features and management of poisoning with drugs used to treat Parkinson's disease. *Quarterly Journal of Medicine*, **91**, 613–16.

Antiseptics and disinfectants

Once these solutions commonly contained phenol but this has largely been replaced by small quantities of either chlorophenol or chloroxylenol, which although less toxic than phenol can be hazardous if ingested in large quantities. More dangerous are isopropanol and ethanol (see below).

Clinical features Ingestion of a substantial quantity results in a sensation of burning in the mouth and throat, followed by drowsiness, stupor, depression of respiration, and coma.

Treatment Management is supportive (see below for specific advice on ethanol and isopropanol).

Further reading

Chan, T.Y.K. (1996). Poisoning due to Savlon (cetrimide) liquid. *Human and Experimental Toxicology*, **13**, 681–2.

Chan, T.Y.K. and Critchley, J.A.J.H. (1996). Pulmonary aspiration following Dettol poisoning: the scope for prevention. *Human and Experimental Toxicology*, **15**, 843–6.

Arsenic

Arsenic forms both trivalent (e.g. arsenic trioxide, arsenious acid, and arsenites) and pentavalent (e.g. arsenic pentoxide, arsenic acid, and arsenates) derivatives. Inorganic arsenical compounds may generate arsine gas (see below) when in contact with acids and reducing metals (e.g. iron and zinc) or with sodium hydroxide and aluminium. Some 90 per cent of an ingested dose of most inorganic trivalent and pentavalent arsenicals is absorbed, the exception being some insoluble compounds such as arsenic selenide. The half-life is in the range 1–3 days. Excretion is predominantly in the urine, as mono- and dimethyl derivatives. Soluble arsenical compounds can also be absorbed by inhalation but skin absorption is generally poor. In exposed individuals high concentrations of arsenic are present in bone, hair, and nails.

Acute poisoning This can follow accidental, suicidal, or deliberate ingestion, the toxicity being largely dependent on the water solubility of the ingested compound. Within 2 hours of substantial ingestion of a soluble arsenical compound, severe haemorrhagic gastritis or gastroenteritis may ensue with collapse and death, usually within 4 days. A metallic taste, salivation, muscular cramps, facial oedema, difficulty in swallowing, hepatorenal dysfunction, convulsions, and encephalopthy are reported. A peripheral neuropathy (predominantly sensory), striate leukonychia (Mee's lines) and hyperkeratotic, hyperpigmentated skin lesions are common in those surviving a near fatal ingestion. In moderate or severe arsenic poisoning investigations may show anaemia, leucopenia, thrombocytopenia, and disseminated intravascular coagulation. ECG abnormalities have been reported and include QT prolongation and ventricular arrhythmias.

Exposure to arsenic trioxide and trichloride dust causes irritation of the eyes, nose, throat, and lower respiratory tract. Corrosive skin damage may follow skin contact with arsenical compounds such as arsenious acid and arsenic trichloride.

Chronic poisoning The ingestion of arsenic in contaminated drinking water or in 'tonics' containing inorganic trivalent arsenical compounds has led to progressive weakness, anorexia, nausea, vomiting, stomatitis, colitis, increased salivation, epistaxis, bleeding gums, conjunctivitis, weight loss, and low grade fever. Characteristically there is hyperkeratosis of the palms and soles of the feet, 'raindrop' pigmentation of the skin, and 'Mee's lines' on the nails. There is an increased risk of skin cancer (usually squamous cell epithelioma) in affected individuals. A symmetrical peripheral neuropathy is typical. Sensory symptoms predominate but motor involvement is recognized and may cause confusion with the Guillain-Barré syndrome. Central nervous system effects, such as hearing loss, psychological impairment, and EEG changes, have been reported. Other chronic effects include disturbances of liver function and ulceration and perforation of the nasal septum. Chronic exposure to trivalent and pentavalent forms of arsenic has been linked to lung cancer. Lung cancer occurring in lead, tin, and copper smelter workers has been attributed to arsenic.

Treatment Traditionally, dimercaprol (British Anti-Lewisite, BAL) has been the recommended chelator in the treatment of arsenic poisoning. There is now increasing evidence, however, that DMSA (succimer) and DMPS (unithiol) may be preferable. They are more effective in reducing the arsenic content of tissues and, unlike dimercaprol, they do not cause accumulation of arsenic in the brain. DMSA and DMPS may be given orally (in a dose of 30 mg/kg body weight daily), whereas dimercaprol must be given by deep intramuscular injection (2.5–5 mg/kg 4-hourly for 2 days followed by 2.5 mg/kg intramuscularly twice daily for 1–2 weeks).

Further reading

Fielder, R.J., Dale, E.A., and Williams, S.D. (1986). *Toxicity Review 16. Inorganic arsenic compounds.* HMSO, London.

IPCS. (1981). *Environmental Health Criteria 18. Arsenic.* WHO, Geneva.

Kingston, R.L., Hall, S., and Sioris, L. (1993). Clinical observations and medical outcome in 149 cases of arsenate ant killer ingestion. *Clinical Toxicology*, **31**, 581–91.

See also OTM3, p. 1106.

Arsine

See OTM3, p. 1094.

Barbiturates

Amylobarbitone, butobarbitone, cyclobarbitone, heptabarbitone, hexabarbitone, pentobarbitone, and quinalbarbitone are regarded as being short- or medium-acting. The more lipid soluble, shorter-acting preparations are associated commonly with more serious poisoning than phenobarbitone and barbitone, which are much more water soluble.

Clinical features Impairment of consciousness, respiratory depression, hypotension, and hypothermia are typical and are potentiated by alcohol and benzodiazepines. There are no specific neurological signs.

Hypotonia and hyporeflexia are the rule and the plantar responses are either flexor or absent. Hypotension, skin blisters, and rhabdomyolysis may develop. During recovery from coma, with or without hypothermia, it is common to observe a peak of temperature which cannot be explained by infection. Most deaths result from respiratory complications.

Treatment Gastric lavage may be considered if it can be undertaken within one hour of overdose; supportive measures should be used as appropriate. Although charcoal haemoperfusion is very effective for severely poisoned patients, phenobarbitone can be removed efficiently by multiple doses of oral activated charcoal.

Further reading

Bironneu, E., Garrec, F., Kergueris, M.F., Testa, A., and Nicolas, F. (1996). Hemodiafiltration in pentobarbitol poisoning. *Renal Failure*, **18**, 299–303.

Hantson, P., Ziade, D., Evenepoel, M., and Mahieu, P. (1996). Severe hypoxia and hypothermia following barbiturate poisoning. *Intensive Care Medicine*, 22, 998–9.

Benzene

Benzene is a colourless, volatile liquid with a pleasant odour. It is an ingredient in many paints and varnish removers and some petrols.

Mechanisms of toxicity About 10 per cent of inhaled benzene is excreted unchanged in the breath. The remainder is metabolized by mixed function oxidase enzymes predominantly in the liver, but also in the bone marrow, the target organ of benzene toxicity.

Acute exposure Following inhalation or ingestion, euphoria, dizziness, weakness, headache, blurred vision, mucous membrane irritation, tremor, ataxia, chest tightness, respiratory depression, cardiac arrhythmias, coma, and convulsions have been reported. Direct skin contact with liquid benzene may produce marked irritation.

Chronic exposure The toxic effects of chronic poisoning may not become apparent for months or years after initial contact and may develop after all exposure has ceased.

Anorexia, headache, drowsiness, nervousness, and irritability are well described. Anaemia (including aplastic anaemia), leucopenia, thrombocytopenia, pancytopenia, leukaemia, lymphomas, chromosomal abnormalities, and cerebral atrophy have been reported. Patients have recovered after as long as a year of almost complete absence of formation of new blood cells. A dry, scaly dermatitis may develop on prolonged or repeated skin exposure to liquid benzene.

Treatment Following removal from the contaminated atmosphere, treatment should be directed towards symptomatic and supportive measures. Gastric lavage is hazardous as aspiration is likely to occur.

Further reading

Cavender, F. (1994). Benzene. In *Patty's industrial hygiene and toxicology.* (ed. G.D. Clayton and F.E. Clayton), Vol. IIB, 4th edn., pp. 1306–26. John Wiley and Sons, Inc., New York.

Snyder, C.A. (1987). Benzene. In *Ethel Browning's toxicity and metabolism of industrial solvents* (ed. R. Snyder), 2nd ed. pp. 3–37. Elsevier, Amsterdam.

Benzodiazepines

These are widely used as tranquillizers, hypnotics, and sedatives.

Clinical features Although many benzodiazepines have active metabolites which account for their sometimes prolonged sedative effects, they all share a remarkable safety when taken alone in overdosage. As many as 70 or 80 tablets of any of them are unlikely to produce anything more than mild effects in most adults. However, there is individual variation in response; some otherwise healthy elderly people respond to an overdose with prolonged toxicity. Benzodiazepines potentiate the effects of other CNS depressants, particularly alcohol, tricyclic antidepressants, and barbiturates. Dizziness, drowsiness, ataxia, and slurred speech are the usual features while coma, respiratory depression, and hypotension are uncommon and usually mild. Flurazepam is the most likely to cause serious CNS depression.

Treatment Gastric lavage is unnecessary unless the overdose exceeds 30 therapeutic doses in an adult and the patient presents within one hour. In severe poisoning, the specific benzodiazepine antagonist, flumazenil, may be indicated; 0.5 mg is given intravenously over 30 seconds and, if necessary, a further 0.5 mg over 30 s. Most patients will respond to a total dose of between 1 and 3 mg.

Further reading

Hojer, J., Baechrendtz, S., and Gusatfsson, L. (1989). Benzodiazepines poisoning: Experience of 702 admissions to an intensive care unit during a 14-year period. *Journal of Internal Medicine*, **226**, 117–22.

Weinbroum, A., Rudick, V., Sorkine, P., *et al.* (1996). Use of flumazenil in the treatment of drug overdose: a double-blind and open clinical study in 110 patients. *Critical Care Medicine*, **24**, 199–206.

β-Adrenoceptor blocking drugs

β-Adrenoceptor blocking drugs antagonize the effects of endogenous catecholamines on the heart and other tissues by competitive inhibition at β-adrenoceptors. In overdose these drugs exhibit a marked negative inotropic action.

Clinical features Sinus bradycardia may be the only feature following a small overdose, but if a substantial amount has been ingested, coma, convulsions (particularly with propranolol), profound bradycardia, and hypotension may occur. Other effects include drowsiness, delirium, hallucinations, low-output cardiac failure, and cardiorespiratory arrest (asystole or ventricular fibrillation). Bronchospasm and hypoglycaemia occur rarely.

First degree heart block, intraventricular conduction defects, right and left bundle branch block, ST segment elevation, ventricular extrasystoles, and disappearance of the P wave may be noted on the electrocardiogram. Sotalol has been reported to cause QT interval prolongation and ventricular arrhythmias and asystole may follow severe overdose from any β-adrenoceptor blocking drug.

Treatment A delay in treatment may be fatal in patients who are severely poisoned. The blood pressure and cardiac rhythm of the patient should be monitored immediately in an intensive care area and supportive measures implemented. Gastric lavage should be considered in adults who have ingested a substantial overdose less than 1 hour previously; atropine (0.6–1.2 mg intravenously) may prevent vagal-induced cardiovascular collapse during this procedure.

Glucagon is the drug of choice for severe hypotension and should be given in a bolus dose of 50– 150 μg/kg (typically 10 mg in an adult) over 1 min, followed by an infusion of 1–5 mg/h according to response.

Insertion of a temporary transvenous pacemaker wire , atropine, and isoprenaline (5–50 μg/min intravenously) or other inotropic agents, have been recommended but are probably less effective than glucagon. Occasionally, diazepam (5–10 mg intravenously) may be needed for convulsions. If bronchospasm supervenes, salbutamol (albuterol) by nebulizer, or aminophylline by intravenous infusion, should be employed. Hypoglycaemia should be corrected.

Further reading

Critchley, J.A.J.H. and Ungar, A. (1989). The management of acute poisoning due to β-adrenoceptor antagonists. *Medical Toxicology*, **4**, 32–45.

Love, J.N., Litovitz, T.L., Howell, J.M., and Clancy, C. (1997). Characterization of fatal beta blocker ingestion: a review of the American Association of Poison Control Centers data from 1985 to 1995. *Clinical Toxicology*, 35, 353–9.

β_2-Agonists

Poisoning with β_2-agonists, including fenoterol, pirbuterol, reprobuterol, rimiterol, salbutamol, and terbutaline, has followed deliberate and accidental ingestion of these drugs and may also result from confusion over the difference between oral and parenteral doses.

Clinical features These include a feeling of excitement, hallucinations, and agitation, accompanied by palpitations, tachycardia, tremor, and peripheral vasodilation. More serious complications such as hypokalaemia, ventricular tachyarrhythmias, ECG changes of myocardial ischaemia, pulmonary oedema, convulsions, hyperglycaemia, and lactic acidosis are uncommon.

Treatment Gastric lavage may be considered, or activated charcoal administered, if the patient presents within 1 hour of a substantial overdose. Hypokalaemia should be corrected as soon as possible by the administration of an infusion of potassium at a rate of 40–60 mmol/h diluted in 5 per cent dextrose. A non-selective β-blocker, such as propanolol (1–5 mg by slow intravenous injection) will also reverse β_2-agonist-induced hypokalaemia and may be needed. However, its use may exacerbate pre-existing chronic air flow obstruction. Methods to increase elimination have no role.

Further reading

Leikin, J.B., Linowiecki, K.A., Soglin, D.F., and Paloucek, F. (1994). Hypokalemia after pediatric albuterol overdose: a case series. *American Journal of Emergency Medicine*, **12**, 64–6.

Lewis, L.D., Essex, E., Volans, G.N., and Cochrane, G.M. (1993). A study of self-poisoning with oral salbutamol—laboratory and clinical features. *Human and Experimental Toxicology*, **12**, 397–401.

Bismuth chelate (tripotassium dicitratobismuthate)

Mechanism of toxicity Although bismuth absorption from bismuth chelate is low after a therapeutic dose, a significant quantity may be absorbed after overdose. Renal toxicity is dose-dependent in animals and is directed primarily towards the tubular epithelial cells.

Clinical features Self-poisoning with large doses of bismuth chelate has caused reversible renal failure 2 and 10 days after overdose and at least one death. During prolonged (and sometimes high dose) therapy, bismuth-induced encephalopathy has been reported.

Treatment If a patient presents within 1 hour of a substantial overdose, gastric lavage should be considered. Dimercaprol can lower brain bismuth concentrations though there is no evidence that it can prevent nephrotoxicity. DMSA and DMPS may be effective oral alternatives.

Further reading

Akpolat, I., Kahraman, H., Arik, N., Akpolat, T., Kandemir, B., and Cengiz, K. (1996) Acute renal failure due to overdose of colloidal bismuth. *Nephrology, Dialysis, Transplantion*, **11**, 1890–991.

Bleaches and lavatory cleaners

Household bleach is normally a 3–6 per cent solution of sodium hypochlorite, whereas industrial bleaches contain more than 10 per cent. Some bleaches also contain sodium hydroxide. Household bleach may give rise to toxic gases such as chlorine if mixed with other cleaning agents in a lavatory bowl.

Clinical features Ingestion may cause a burning sensation in the mouth, throat, and oesophagus, accompanied by a sensation of thirst, vomiting, and abdominal discomfort. Pharyngeal and laryngeal oedema may develop.

Treatment When small quantities of household bleach have been ingested, liberal fluids by mouth are all that is required. Gastric lavage should only be considered if concentrated bleach has been swallowed less than 1 hour previously.

Inhalation of of gases liberated by mixing bleach with other products may result in severe respiratory irritation and pulmonary oedema. Treat as for inhalation of chlorine.

Further reading

Harley, E.H. and Collins, M.D. (1997). Liquid household bleach ingestion in children: a retrospective review. *Laryngoscope*, **107**, 122–5.

Hilbert, G., Bedry, R., Cardinaud, J., and Benissan, G.G. (1997). Euro bleach:fatal hypernatraemia due to 13.3 per cent sodium hypochlorite. *Clinical Toxicology*, 35, 635–6.

Butyrophenones

Benperidol, haloperidol, and triperidol are used as antipsychotic and neuroleptic agents.

Clinical features Overdosage may result in drowsiness and hypotension, but acute dystonic reactions are the most dramatic consequences.

Treatment Treatment is supportive. Acute dystonic reactions should be treated with benztropine 1–2 mg or procyclidine 5–10 mg intravenously for an adult.

Further reading

Yoshida, I., Sakaguchi, Y., Matsuishi, T., *et al.* (1993). Acute accidental overdosage of haloperidol in children. *Acta Paediatrica Scandinavia*, **82**, 877–80.

Cadmium

Cadmium compounds are poorly absorbed orally but are well absorbed through the lungs (e.g. in tobacco smokers). Cadmium is deposited in the liver and kidneys as a complex with metallothionein and is very slowly excreted in the urine (half-life 10–30 years).

Acute poisoning Inhalation of cadmium oxide fumes produced in welding or cutting can cause severe lung damage and death. Often there are no initial symptoms but after some 4–10 hours there is increasing respiratory distress. Dyspnoea, cough, and chest pain are accompanied by chills and tremor. Severe pulmonary oedema may develop, or chemical pneumonitis in less severe cases. Recovery may be complicated by progressive pulmonary fibrosis.

Ingestion of cadmium salts (>3 mg/kg body weight) can cause gastrointestinal disturbance progressing to circulatory collapse, acute renal failure, pulmonary oedema, and death.

Chronic poisoning Repeated exposure to cadmium leads to renal tubular dysfunction and, at a later stage, emphysema. Glycosuria, aminoaciduria, hypercalciuria, an increased incidence of renal stones, and osteomalacia may result from severe tubular damage. Itai Itai disease was an outbreak of osteomalacia in postmenopausal Japanese women living in areas where the water used for crop irrigation was contaminated with cadmium. Less common features of chronic cadmium exposure include anosmia, anaemia, teeth discoloration, and neuropsychological impairment.

No relationship has been confirmed between cadmium exposure and hypertension. Workers repeatedly exposed to high concentrations of cadmium have developed carcinoma of the prostate or lung.

Treatment There is no specific treatment.

Further reading

IPCS. (1992). Environmental Health Criteria 134. *Cadmium*. WHO, Geneva.

IPCS. (1992). Environmental Health Criteria 135. *Cadmium—environmental aspects*. WHO, Geneva.

See also OTM3, p. 1106–7.

Cannabis

Cannabis is obtained from the plant *Cannabis sativa* which contains many active substances. The most important are the tetrahydrocannabinols.

Smoking is the common route of use of cannabis, but it is occasionally ingested and, rarely, made into a 'tea' and injected intravenously.

Clinical features Euphoria with drowsiness and distorted and heightened images, colours, and sounds are the usual effects of this compound. Tactile sensations may also be altered. A tachycardia is often present and heavy use may lead to conjunctival suffusion, hypotension, and ataxia. Higher doses induce auditory hallucinations, confusion, depersonalization, and panic. Some people find the distortion of perception pleasurable but novice users may panic and seek medical help.

Intravenous injection of cannabis infusions causes serious illness. Within a few minutes, there is nausea, vomiting, and chills followed after an interval of an hour or so by profuse watery diarrhoea, tachycardia, hypotension, and arthralgia. A marked neutrophil leucocytosis is often present and hypoglycaemia has been reported in some cases. There may also be transient renal failure. Long-term use may lead to psychosis.

Treatment Most patients respond to reassurance. Sedation with intravenous diazepam may be required for those whose behaviour is disruptive or who are clearly very distressed. Those who have injected cannabis infusions should be treated supportively.

Further reading

Johnson, B.A. (1990). Psychopharmacological effects of cannabis. *British Journal of Hospital Medicine*, **43**, 114–20.

Carbamate insecticides

Like organophosphorus compounds, carbamate insecticides inhibit acetylcholinesterase. However, the duration of this effect is comparatively short-lived since the carbamate-enzyme complex tends to dissociate spontaneously.

Clinical features See organophosphorus insecticide poisoning.

Treatment Symptomatic cases require atropine, but the use of oximes is usually unnecessary; rapid recovery within 24 hours is the rule.

Further reading

Bardin, P.G., Van Eeden, S.F., Moolman, J.A., Foden, A.P., and Joubert J.R. (1994). Organophosphate and carbamate poisoning. *Archives of Internal Medicine*, **154**, 1433–41.

Saadeh, A.M., Farsakh, N.A., and Al-Ali, M.K. (1997). Cardiac manifestations of acute carbamate and organophosphate poisoning. *Heart*, 77, 461–4.

Carbamazepine

Carbamazepine is structurally related to the tricyclic antidepressants and has similar anticholinergic actions. In overdosage it produces similar clinical features and is treated similarly.

Further reading

Durelli, L., Massazza, U., and Cavallo, R. (1989). Carbamazepine toxicity and poisoning. *Medical Toxicology and Adverse Drug Experience*, **4**, 95–107.

Calcium-channel blockers

Calcium-channel blockers (amlodipine, diltiazem, felodipine, isradipine, nicardipine, nifedipine, nimodipine, verapamil) interfere with the inward transmembrane passage of calcium ions in myocardial cells, the cardiac conducting system, and vascular smooth muscle.

Clinical features In overdose, calcium-channel blockers cause nausea, vomiting, dizziness, slurred speech, confusion, sinus bradycardia and tachycardia, prolonged atrioventricular conduction, atrioventricular dissociation, hypotension, pulmonary oedema, respiratory arrest, convulsions, coma, hyperglycaemia, and metabolic acidosis. Large overdose carries a poor prognosis, particularly in patients with ischaemic heart disease and in those on β-adrenergic blocking agents.

Treatment Gastric lavage should be considered in all patients who present within 1 hour of substantial overdose or, alternatively, 50–100 g of activated charcoal may be administered. Calcium gluconate, (10–20 ml of 10 per cent solution intravenously), may reverse prolonged intracardiac conduction times but inotropic support with dobutamine (5–40 μg/kg/min) or isoprenaline (5–50 μg/kg/min) by intravenous infusion, will also be needed to maintain cardiac output in severe cases.

Further reading

Lip, G.Y. and Ferner, R.E. (1995). Poisoning with anti-hypertensive drugs: calcium antagonists. *Journal of Human Hypertension*, **9**, 155–61.

Carbon dioxide

Carbon dioxide is a colourless gas also used commercially as a solid for refrigeration purposes ('dry ice'). High concentrations may accumulate in wells, silos, manholes, and mines.

Clinical features Dyspnoea, cough, headache, dizziness, sweating, restlessness, paraesthesiae, and sinus tachycardia are features after modest carbon dioxide exposure. Higher concentrations produce psychomotor agitation, myoclonic twitches, eye flickering, coma, and convulsions. Death occurs from acute cardiorespiratory depression.

Skin contact with 'dry ice' may result in frostbite and local blistering.

Treatment The casualty should be removed from the contaminated environment. Thereafter, supportive care should be employed.

Further reading

Baxter, P.J., Kapila, M., and Mfonfu, D. (1989). Lake Nyos disaster, Cameroon, 1986: The medical effects of large scale emission of carbon dioxide? *British Medical Journal*, **298**, 1437–41.

Williams, H.I. (1958). Carbon dioxide poisoning–report of eight cases, with two deaths. *British Medical Journal*, **2**, 1012–4.

Carbon disulphide

Carbon disulphide is used as a fumigant for grain and as a solvent, particularly in the rayon industry. It is a clear, colourless, volatile liquid with an odour like that of decaying cabbage.

Acute exposure Acute poisoning is rare. Absorption occurs through the skin as well as by inhalation. Carbon disulphide, due to its potent defatting activity, causes reddening, cracking, and peeling of the skin and a burn may occur if contact continues for several minutes. Splashes in the eye cause immediate and severe irritation. Acute inhalation may result in irritation of the mucous membranes, blurred vision, nausea and vomiting, headache, delirium, hallucinations, coma, tremor, convulsions, and cardiac and respiratory arrest.

Chronic exposure There is an increased incidence of cardiovascular disease among workers exposed to carbon disulphide. In addition, sleep disturbances, fatigue, anorexia, and weight loss are common complaints among exposed workers. Intellectual decline, depression, stereotyped behaviour, ocular changes, cerebellar and extrapyramidal signs, hepatic damage, and permanent impairment of reproductive performance have been described.

Treatment Treatment involves removal from exposure, washing contaminated skin, irrigation of the eyes with water, and supportive measures. In the majority of cases, however, preventive measures to keep carbon disulphide concentrations in the workplace as low as possible are more important.

Further reading

Fielder, R.J. and Shillaker, R.O. (1981). *Toxicity Review. Carbon disulphide.* HMSO, London.

Spyker, D.A., Gallanosa, A.G., and Suratt, P.M. (1982). Health effects of acute carbon disulfide exposure. *Clinical Toxicology*, **19**, 87–3.

Carbon monoxide

Carbon monoxide is a tasteless, odourless, colourless, non-irritating gas produced by incomplete combustion of organic materials. Normal endogenous carbon monoxide production is sufficient to maintain a resting carboxyhaemoglobin level of 1–3 per cent in urban non-smokers and 5–6 per cent in smokers.

Common sources of carbon monoxide are car exhaust fumes (in the absence of a catalytic converter), improperly maintained and ventilated heating systems, and smoke from all types of fire. Carbon monoxide derived from domestic heating systems is a major cause of accidental death in the developing world. Inhalation of methylene chloride (found in paint strippers) may also lead to carbon monoxide poisoning.

Mechanisms of toxicity Symptoms and signs that follow inhalation of carbon monoxide are the result of tissue hypoxia. The affinity of haemoglobin for carbon monoxide is approximately 240 times greater than that for oxygen. Carbon monoxide combines with haemoglobin to form carboxyhaemoglobin, reducing the total oxygen-carrying capacity of the blood; the oxygen dissociation curve to the left shifts and modifies oxygen-binding sites. As a result, the affinity of the remaining haem groups for oxygen is increased, the oxygen dissociation curve is distorted as well as being shifted, and the resulting tissue hypoxia is thus far greater than that which would result from simple loss of oxygen-carrying capacity.

Carbon monoxide toxicity may also inhibit cellular respiration as a result of reversible binding to cytochrome oxidase a_3. Carbon monoxide mediated brain lipid peroxidation may play a role in the development of delayed neuropsychiatric sequelae.

Clinical features The clinical features of carbon monoxide poisoning are summarized in Table 3.

Table 3 Immediate and delayed clinical features of carbon monoxide poisoning

Agitation, mental confusion, headache (usually frontal and band-like, sometimes occipital)
Nausea and vomiting, incontinence (occasionally), haematemesis, melaena
Hyperventilation, pulmonary oedema, respiratory failure,
Cheyne-Stokes respiration
Metabolic acidosis
Bullous lesions
Hyperpyrexia
Loss of consciousness, hypertonia, hyper-reflexia
Extensor plantar responses, papilloedema, convulsions
Monoplegia or hemiplegia, peripheral neuropathies
Cerebral, cerebellar, and midbrain damage (parkinsonism, akinetic mutism)
Myocardial ischaemia and infarction
Arrhythmias and ECG changes: atrial fibrillation, prolonged PR interval, AV block, bundle-branch block, ventricular extrasystoles, prolonged QT interval, ST depression
Decrease in light sensitivity and dark adaptation, retinal haemorrhages
Hearing loss (central type due to ischaemia of cochlea and brainstem nuclei)
Acute renal failure
Muscle necrosis
Thrombotic thrombocytopenic purpura
Late neuropsychiatric sequelae

Acute exposure The symptoms of moderate exposure to carbon monoxide are mild and may even be mistaken for a viral illness and for this reason it is important that the diagnosis is always borne in mind. Elderly patients and those with pre-existing cardiorespiratory disease are at greater risk. A carboxyhaemoglobin concentration of less than 10 per cent is not normally associated with symptoms and 10–30 per cent carboxyhaemoglobin may cause only headache and mild exertional dyspnoea. It is known that even low concentrations of carbon monoxide produce significant effects on cardiac function during exercise in subjects with coronary artery disease. Coma, convulsions, and cardiorespiratory arrest may be expected to occur with carboxyhaemoglobin concentrations in excess of 60 per cent.

Delayed effects Neuropsychiatric problems after recovery from carbon monoxide intoxication may develop insidiously over a number of weeks. They include intellectual deterioration, memory impairment, cerebral, cerebellar, parkinsonism, akinetic mutism, irritability, verbal aggressiveness, violence, impulsiveness, and moodiness.

Treatment The patient should be removed from exposure and 100 per cent oxygen administered using a tightly-fitting face mask. Endotracheal intubation and mechanical ventilation may be required in those who are unconscious. The administration of oxygen should be continued until the carboxyhaemoglobin concentration is less than 10 per cent.

Controlled studies of hyperbaric oxygen have shown no greater benefit than 100 per cent normobaric oxygen with elective ventilation.

General symptomatic and supportive measures will be required. Diazepam (5–10 mg intravenously) repeated as necessary, is the agent of choice for the management of convulsions. The benefit of corticosteroids for the treatment of cerebral oedema has not been proven but mannitol may be useful.

Further reading

Burney, R.E., Wu, S.C., and Nemiroff, M.J. (1982). Mass carbon monoxide poisoning: clinical effects and results of treatment in 184 victims. *Annals of Emergency Medicine*, **11**, 394–9.

Hardy, K.R. and Thom, S.R. (1994). Pathophysiology and treatment of carbon monoxide poisoning. *Clinical Toxicology*, **32**, 613–29.

Raphael, J.C. *et al.* (1989). Trial of normobaric and hyperbaric oxygen for acute carbon monoxide intoxication. *Lancet*, **ii**, 414–9.

Thom, S.R., Taber, R.L., Mendiguren, I.I., Clark, J.M., Hardy, K.R., and Fisher, A.B. (1995). Delayed neuropsychologic sequelae after carbon monoxide poisoning; prevention by treatment with hyperbaric oxygen. *Annals of Emergency Medicine*, **25**, 474–80.

Carbon tetrachloride (tetrachloromethane)

Carbon tetrachloride was once widely used as a dry-cleaning chemical, degreasing agent, and fire extinguisher but international regulations have now restricted it to laboratory and industrial usage. A complete ban has been proposed by the year 2000.

Acute exposure Immediate effects include nausea, vomiting, abdominal pain, and diarrhoea. High concentrations cause dizziness, confusion, coma, respiratory depression, hypotension, and occasionally convulsions. Death may follow from respiratory failure or ventricular fibrillation due to cardiac sensitization to circulating catecholamines. Hepatorenal damage supervenes after a delay of up to 2 weeks. Hepatic enzyme activities increase before jaundice and a tender swollen liver develop. Maximal liver damage probably occurs within 48 hours of an acute exposure and may progress to fulminant hepatic failure. Acute tubular necrosis is common and may develop in the absence of hepatic dysfunction 1–7 days after exposure. Rarely, cerebellar dysfunction, cerebral haemorrhage, optic atrophy, and parkinsonism may occur.

Alcohol and previous liver damage render the individual more susceptible.

Chronic exposure Repeated exposure to low concentrations of carbon tetrachloride may also cause hepatic and renal damage. Hepatic cirrhosis and hepatoma may develop. Prolonged carbon tetrachloride exposure is associated with polyneuritis, various visual disturbances, anaemia including fatal aplastic anaemia, and mild jaundice.

Treatment After ingestion, gastric emptying is probably best avoided because of the risk of aspiration. If the patient presents within 12 hours of exposure *N*-acetylcysteine should be given as for paracetamol overdose (see below). Renal and liver failure should be managed conventionally.

Further reading

Ruprah, M., Mant, T.G.K., and Flanagan, R.J. (1985). Acute carbon tetrachloride poisoning in 19 patients: Implications for diagnosis and treatment. *Lancet*, **i**, 1027–9.

Torkelson, T.R. and Rowe, V.K. (1981). Carbon tetrachloride. In *Patty's industrial hygiene and toxicology*. (eds. G.D. Clayton and F.E. Clayton), Vol. **2B**. 3rd edn, pp. 3472–8. John Wiley and Sons, New York.

Chloral hydrate

This drug is metabolized by alcohol dehydrogenase to trichlorethanol, the active compound, and further to inactive trichloroacetic acid and trichloroethanol glucuronide.

Clinical features These are similar to barbiturate poisoning, although a retrosternal burning sensation accompanied by vomiting may be prominent in the early stages. Supraventricular tachycardias and ventricular premature beats have occurred. They are often abolished by β-adrenoceptor blocking drugs, provided respiratory depression and hypoxia have been corrected.

Treatment Gastric lavage should be considered if the patient presents within 1 hour of a substantial overdose. Multiple-dose activated charcoal may be of value in severely poisoned patients.

Further reading

Ludwigs, U., Divino Filho, J., Magnusson, A., and Berg, A. (1996). Suicidal chloral hydrate poisoning. *Clinical Toxicology*, **34**, 97–9.

Chlorates

Clinical features Sodium chlorate and potassium chlorate are powerful oxidizing agents and are highly toxic if ingested. The early features include nausea, vomiting, diarrhoea, abdominal pain, and cyanosis secondary to methaemoglobinaemia. Intravascular haemolysis occurs causing hyperkalaemia, jaundice, and oliguric renal failure.

Treatment Gastric lavage should be considered if the patient presents within 1 hour of ingestion. Methaemoglobinaemia can be corrected by slow intravenous injection of methylene blue (2 mg/kg body weight as a 1 per cent solution). Blood transfusion may be required. Plasma potassium concentrations should be monitored and reduced if necessary. Haemodialysis will remove chlorate and may also be required for the management of renal failure and hyperkalaemia. Plasmapheresis has also been employed since it will remove chlorate, circulating free haemoglobin, and red cell stroma and thus help to prevent the development of renal failure.

Chlorine

Chlorine is a greenish-yellow gas, although it is normally transported as a pressurized liquid. Exposure after spillage may be prolonged because gaseous chlorine is heavier than air, causing it to remain near ground level. Chlorine has a pungent odour that can usually be detected by smell at concentrations of less than 0.5 p.p.m. Some workers chronically exposed to the gas become anosmic.

Mechanisms of toxicity Molecular chlorine, a strong oxidizing agent, reacts with many functional groups in cell components, forms chloramines, oxidizes thiol radicals, reacts with tissue water to form hypochlorite and hydrochloric acid, and may generate oxygen free radicals.

Clinical features Symptoms begin within minutes and include irritation of the mucous membranes of the eyes, nose, and throat, followed by cough, breathlessness, expectoration of white sputum (which may be bloodstained), chest pain and tightness, abdominal pain, nausea, headache, dizziness, and palpitation due to ventricular ectopic beats. Laryngeal oedema may cause hoarseness of the voice and stridor, and cardiac arrest may occur secondary to hypoxia.

Restrictive as well as obstructive ventilatory defects arise in those who have inhaled sublethal amounts. Diffusion is impaired, leading to arterial hypoxaemia. In very severe cases, non-cardiogenic pulmonary oedema and respiratory failure may develop. Survival is usually followed by complete resolution of the pulmonary defects.

Treatment The first priority is to remove the casualty from exposure. Skin burns should be treated as for acids (see above). Patients with respiratory symptoms persisting beyond the period of exposure should be admitted to hospital in case they require bronchodilators and humidified oxygen. Some will require mechanical ventilation, particularly if non-cardiogenic pulmonary oedema develops. Frusemide has been reported to be of value. Corticosteroids and prophylactic antibiotics have not been shown to be of value. Correction of serious metabolic acidosis with intravenous sodium bicarbonate may be necessary.

Further reading

Mvros, R., Dean, B.S., and Krenzelok, E.P. (1993). Home exposures to chlorine/chloramine gas: review of 216 cases. *Southern Medical Journal*, **86**, 654–7.

Schonhofer, B., Voshaar, T., and Kohler, D. (1996). Long-term sequelae following accidental chlorine gas exposure. *Respiration*, **63**, 155–9.

Chlormethiazole

Clinical features This hypnotic drug taken in overdose may cause coma, respiratory depression, reduced muscle tone, hypotension, and excessive salivation.The characteristic odour of chlormethiazole is often detected on the breath. Treatment is supportive.

Chlorophenoxyacetate herbicides

These include the widely-used 'hormone' weedkillers. They are often co-formulated with dicamba which is of low toxicity and ioxynil and bromoxynil which uncouple oxidative phosphorylation.

Clinical features Ingestion causes burning in the mouth and throat, nausea, vomiting, and abdominal pain. There is facial flushing, profuse sweating, and fever. Coma, hyperventilation, metabolic acidosis, and pulmonary oedema may develop. ECG abnormalities and skeletal muscle damage leading to proximal myopathy have been reported.

Treatment Gastric lavage should be considered. Alkalinization of the urine is indicated for severe poisoning since it considerably enhances elimination of 2,4-dichlorophenoxy acetic acid (2,4-D) and dichlorprop and, to a lesser extent, mecoprop.

Further reading

Berthelot-Moritz, F., Daudenthun, I., Goulle, J.P., Droy, J.M., Bonmarchand, G., and Leroy, J. (1997). Severe intoxication following ingestion of 2,4-D and MCPP. *Intensive Care Medicine*, **23**, 356–7.

Flanagan, R.J., *et al.* (1990). Alkaline diuresis for acute poisoning with chlorophenoxy herbicides and ioxynil. *Lancet*, **335**, 454–8.

Chloroquine

Chloroquine overdose is probably the most common form of self-poisoning with drugs in Africa, the Far East, and West Pacific and is a growing problem in Europe.

Clinical features Toxicity can result from doses greater than 1 g (about six tablets) in adults. Cardiac arrest is commonly the first clinical manifestation of poisoning, but hypotension usually precedes it and may progress to cardiogenic shock and pulmonary oedema. Electrocardiographic abnormalities, bradyarrhythmias, and tachyarrhythmias are common and are similar to those of quinine (see below). Visual disturbance, agitation, drowsiness, acute psychosis, dystonic reactions, seizures, and coma may ensue. Hypokalaemia is common and is due to potassium channel blockade.

Treatment Gastric lavage or activated charcoal (50–100 g) should be considered if the patient presents within 1 hour. Supportive measures should be employed and hypokalaemia corrected. There is no specific antidote and no means of increasing drug clearance. Mechanical ventilation, epinephrine (0.25 μg/kg. min), and high-doses of diazepam (1 mg/kg as a loading dose and 0.25–0.4 mg/kg.h maintenance) may reduce the mortality to 10 per cent in severe poisoning. Multiple-dose charcoal may enhance chloroquine elimination.

Further reading

Clemessy, J.L., Taboulet, P., Hoffman, J.R., *et al.* (1996). Treatment of acute chloroquine poisoning: a 5-year experience. *Critical Care Medicine*, **24**, 1189–95.

McKenzie, A.G. (1996). Intensive therapy for chloroquine poisoning—a review of 29 cases. *South African Medical Journal*, **86**, 597–9.

Riou, B., Barriot, P., Rimaiho, A., and Baud, F. (1988). Treatment of severe chloroquine poisoning. *New England Journal of Medicine*, **318**, 1–6.

Chromium

See OTM3, pp. 1107–8.

Clonidine

Clonidine exerts its hypotensive action by reduction of sympathetic tone mediated by a central effect on postsynaptic α_2-adrenoceptors in the medulla. Clonidine decreases heart rate, cardiac output, and total peripheral resistance. In the presence of high plasma clonidine concentrations, peripheral α_2-agonist activity predominates and accounts for those instances of vasoconstriction and hypertension reported following clonidine overdose.

Clinical features Poisoning may be severe and life-threatening, particularly in children. Hypertension and severe vasoconstriction are unusual while bradycardia, hypotension, coma, and respiratory depression are common. Toxic effects last about 16 hours, but may extend to several days in severe overdose.

Treatment Gastric lavage should be considered or activated charcoal (50–100 g) administered if a patient presents within 1 hour following a substantial overdose. Bradycardia is usually reversed by atropine (0.6–2.4 mg intravenously). The use of α-adrenergic blocking drugs (tolazoline or phentolamine) has been advocated in severely poisoned patients but their action may be unpredictable. Severe hypotension should first be treated with a plasma expander and then, if necessary, an inotropic agent such as dobutamine, (5–40 μg/kg/min) may be given by intravenous infusion. The use of naloxone has been advocated but its benefit is inconsistent and it may produce hypertension. Sodium nitroprusside (50–400 μg/min) by intravenous infusion is the most effective agent for management of severe hypertension and peripheral vasoconstriction.

Renal elimination is not increased by forced diuresis.

Further reading

Nichols, M.H., King, W.D., and James, L.P. (1997). Clonidine poisoning in Jefferson County, Alabama. *Annals of Emergency Medicine*, **29**, 511–17.

Wiley, J.F., Wiley, C.C., Torrey, S.B., and Henretig, F.M. (1990). Clonidine poisoning in young children. *Journal of Pediatrics*, **116**, 654–8.

Cobalt

See OTM3, p. 1108.

Cocaine

Cocaine is a powerful local anaesthetic and vasoconstrictor and may be abused by smoking, ingestion, injection, or by 'snorting' it intranasally. Users, body packers , and 'stuffers' are at risk of overdose. In the USA, 'street' cocaine is sometimes dissolved in an alkaline solution. and the cocaine extracted into ether which is then evaporated to leave crystals of relatively pure ('freebase') cocaine. 'Crack' (cocaine without the hydrochloride moiety) is also used widely. Other drugs such as ethanol, cannabis, and conventional hypnotics and sedatives are frequently taken with cocaine to reduce the intensity of its less pleasant effects.

Clinical features The features of cocaine overdosage are similar to those of amphetamine. In addition to euphoria, it has sympathomimetic effects including agitation, tachycardia, hypertension, sweating, and hallucinations. Prolonged convulsions with metabolic acidosis, hyperthermia, rhabdomyolysis, ventricular arrhythmias, and cardiorespiratory arrest may follow in the most severe cases. Less common features include dissection of the aorta, myocarditis, myocardial infarction, dilated cardiomyopathy, subarachnoid haemorrhage, cerebral haemorrhage, and cerebral vasculitis.

Rare complications include pulmonary oedema after intravenous injection of freebase cocaine, pneumomediastinum and pneumothorax after sniffing it, and perforation of the nasal septum, CSF rhinorrhoea due to thinning of the cribriform plate, and pulmonary granulomatosis after chronic 'snorting'.

Treatment Diazepam may be needed to control agitation or convulsions. Hypertension and severe tachycardia may be controlled with a β-adrenergic blocking drug but propranolol may cause paradoxical hypertension. Accelerated idioventricular rhythm should not normally require treatment but ventricular fibrillation and asystole should be managed in the usual way.

Further reading

Brown, E., Prager, J., Lee, H-Y., and Ramsey, R.G. (1992). CNS complications of cocaine abuse: prevalence, pathophysiology, and neuroradiology. *American Journal of Roentgenology*, **159**, 137–47.

Kloner, R.A., Hale, S., Alker, K., and Rezkalla, S. (1992). The effects of acute and chronic cocaine use on the heart. *Circulation*, **85**, 407–19.

Marzuk, P.M., Tardiff K., Leon A.C., *et al.* (1995). Fatal injuries after cocaine use as a leading cause of death among young adults in New York city. *New England Journal of Medicine*, **332**, 1753–7.

Sporer, K.A. and Firestone, J. (1997). Clinical course of crack cocaine body stuffers. *Annals of Emergency Medicine*, **29**, 596–601.

Co-phenotrope ('Lomotil')

Co-phenotrope is a mixture of an opioid, diphenoxylate hydrochloride, and atropine.

Clinical features Symptoms may be delayed for up to 12 hours after the overdose. Respiratory depression is the major complication of diphenoxylate poisoning. Vomiting, abdominal pain, drowsiness, and coma also occur. Even the small amount of atropine in co-phenotrope tablets is toxic to children under 5 years and several deaths have been reported. Anticholinergic features are to be expected (see tricyclic antidepressants, below).

Treatment Repeated doses of naloxone may be necessary to reverse respiratory depression because of the long duration of action of diphenoxylate (see opioids and opiates, below). Lavage may be appropriate in an adult presenting within 1 hour of a substantial overdose before toxicity develops; activated charcoal (50–100 g) may also reduce absorption significantly if admitted within 1 hour of overdose.

Further reading

McCarron, M.M., Challoner, K.R., and Thompson, G.A. (1991). Diphenoxylate-atropine (Lomotil) overdose in children: An update (report of eight cases and review of the literature). *Pediatrics*, **87**, 694–700.

Copper

See OTM3, pp. 1109–9 and Chapter 6.10.

Cyanide

Hydrogen cyanide and its derivatives are used widely in industry and are released during the thermal decomposition of polyurethane foams. Cyanide poisoning may also result from the ingestion of the cyanogenic glycoside, amygdalin (vitamin B17) which is found in the kernels of almonds, apples, apricots, cherries, peaches, plums, and other fruits.

Mechanisms of toxicity Cyanide reversibly inhibits cellular enzymes which contain ferric iron, notably cytochrome oxidase a_3, so that electron transfer is blocked, the tricarboxylic acid cycle is paralysed, and cellular respiration ceases.

Acute exposure The ingestion by an adult of 50 ml of (liquid) hydrogen cyanide or 200–300 mg of one of its salts is likely to prove fatal. Inhalation of hydrogen cyanide gas may produce symptoms within seconds and death within minutes.

Acute poisoning is characterized by dizziness, headache, palpitation, anxiety, a feeling of constriction in the chest, dyspnoea, pulmonary oedema, confusion, vertigo, ataxia, coma, and paralysis. Cardiovascular collapse, respiratory arrest, convulsions, and metabolic acidosis are seen in severe cases. Cyanosis may occur, and the classical 'brick-red' colour of the skin is noted occasionally. There is sometimes an odour of bitter almonds on the breath, but the ability to detect it is genetically determined and some 40 per cent of the population are unable to do so.

Chronic exposure Chronic exposure results predominantly in neurological damage including ataxia, peripheral neuropathies, amblyopia, optic atrophy, and nerve deafness..

Treatment Cyanide poisoning is a medical emergency, although specific antidotal treatment may not always be necessary. Where appropriate, the patient should be removed from the source of exposure, contaminated clothing discarded, and the skin washed with soap and water. Gastric lavage should be considered if a cyanide salt has been ingested less than 1 hour previously, but this procedure must not delay treatment if symptoms or signs of toxicity are present. It may be difficult to differentiate between the genuine fear and anxiety of a patient and the early symptoms of cyanide poisoning. However, a patient who has been exposed to hydrogen cyanide gas and who is conscious 30 minutes later is unlikely to require antidotal therapy.

Oxygen The administration of oxygen is of paramount importance in the treatment of cyanide poisoning. It is believed to prevent inhibition of cytochrome oxidase a_3 and to accelerate its reactivation.

Dicobalt edetate Cobalt compounds form stable inert complexes with cyanide. Dicobalt edetate (Kelocyanor), if available, is the treatment of choice for confirmed cyanide poisoning and should be given intravenously in a dose of 300–600 mg over 1 min, with a further 300 mg if recovery does not occur within 1 min. It should be administered only if the diagnosis is certain because, in the absence of cyanide, Kelocyanor may cause serious side-effects including vomiting, tachycardia, hypertension, chest pain, and facial and palpebral oedema.

Sodium thiosulphate Cyanide is detoxified by conversion to thiocyanate. Thiosulphate is required for this reaction. Thiosulphate acts quickly as a cyanide antidote.

Sodium nitrite, 4-dimethylaminophenol Another means of inactivating cyanide is to convert some of the haemoglobin to methaemoglobin which contains ferric iron that binds cyanide. Although the affinity of cyanide for methaemoglobin is less than that of cytochrome oxidase, the presence of a large circulating methaemoglobin pool diminishes cyanide toxicity by binding cyanide ion before tissue penetration occurs. Methaemoglobinaemia may be induced by the administration of either sodium nitrite or 4-dimethylaminophenol (4-DMAP). 4-DMAP may produce unexpectedly high methaemoglobin conentrations and cause acute tubular necrosis and Heinz-body haemolytic anaemia. Nitrites may also mitigate cyanide toxicity by virtue of their vasodilator actions and improvement of tissue perfusion.

Inhalation of amyl nitrite was recommended in the past but it produces only low circulating concentrations of methaemoglobin.

Hydroxocobalamin One mole of hydroxocobalamin inactives one mole of cyanide but on a weight-for-weight basis, 50 times more hydroxocobalamin is needed than cyanide because hydroxocobalamin is a far larger molecule. Concentrated formulations of hydoxocobalamin are not yet available in many countries.

Conclusion If dicobalt edetate or hydroxocobalamin are not available, the treatment of choice for cyanide poisoning is a combination of sodium nitrite (10 ml of a 3 per cent solution (30 mg) IV over 5–20 min) and sodium thiosulphate (50 ml of a 25 per cent solution (12.5 mg) IV over 10 min).

Further reading

Meredith, T.J., Jacobsen, D., Haines, J.A., Berger, J.C., and van Heijst, A.N.P. (1993). IPCS/CEC evaluation of antidotes series. *Antidotes for poisoning by cyanide.* Cambridge University Press, Cambridge.

Rosenow F., Herholz K., Lanfermann H., *et al.* (1995). Neurological sequelae of cyanide intoxication—the patterns of clinical, magnetic resonance imaging and positron emission tomography findings. *Annals of Neurology,* **38**, 825–8.

Dapsone

Dapsone is available formulated alone or in combination with pyrimethamine (as Maloprim for malaria).

Clinical features Dapsone poisoning causes methaemoglobinaemia, haemolysis, hepatitis, drowsiness, coma, seizures, and metabolic acidosis.

Treatment If presentation after overdose is one hour, gastric lavage should be considered or, alternatively, activated charcoal (50–100 g) may be administered. Administration of repeated doses of activated charcoal seems to have comparable efficacy to haemodialysis in increasing dapsone elimination. Methylene blue (2 mg/kg as a 1 per cent solution) should be given intravenously over 5 minutes for severe methaemoglobinaemia.

Further reading

Ferguson A.J. and Lavery G.G. (1997). Deliberate self-poisoning with dapsone—a case report and summary of relevant pharmacology and treatment. *Anaesthesia,* **52**, 359–63.

Jaeger, A., Sauder, P., Kopferschmitt, J., and Flesch, F. (1987). Clinical features and management of poisoning due to antimalarial drugs. *Medical Toxicology,* **2**, 242–73.

Diethylene glycol

Diethylene glycol achieved notoriety in 1985 when it was discovered that for some years it had been added to some wines. Several pharmaceutical errors have also led to fatalities.

Mechanism of toxicity Diethylene glycol is first oxidized by alcohol dehydrogenase to 2-hydroxyethoxyacetaldehyde and then to 2-hydroxyethoxyacetic acid.

Clinical features Nausea, vomiting, and abdominal pain occur frequently and are followed by the development of jaundice and hepatomegaly, pulmonary oedema, metabolic acidosis, coma, and renal failure in most cases.

Treatment This is the same as for ethylene glycol poisoning (see below).

Further reading

Hanif, M., Mobarak, M.R., Ronan, A., Rahman, D., Donovan, J.J.J., and Bennish, M.L. (1995). Fatal renal failure caused by diethylene glycol in paracetamol elixir: the Bangladesh epidemic. *British Medical Journal,* **311**, 88–91.

Scalzo, A.J. (1996). Diethylene glycol revisited: The 1996 Haitian epidemic. *Clinical Toxicology,* **34**, 513–16.

Digoxin and digitoxin

Toxicity occurring during chronic administration of these cardiac glycosides is common. Acute poisoning from digoxin and digitoxin is infrequent but carries a mortality as high as 20 per cent.

Clinical features Nausea, vomiting, dizziness, anorexia, and drowsiness are common. Confusion, diarrhoea, visual disturbances, and hallucinations may also occur. Sinus bradycardia, often marked, is the earliest cardiotoxic effect and may be followed by supraventicular arrhythmias with or without heart block, ventricular premature beats, and ventricular tachycardia. There is hyperkalaemia due to inhibition of the Na+-K+ activated ATPase pump. Diagnosis is confirmed by measuring serum digoxin concentration.

Treatment Gastric lavage should be considered in patients with a history of a substantial overdose less than one hour previously. Alternatively, activated charcoal, (50–100 g) may be administered to reduce absorption; repeated doses will also enhance elimination. Potassium supplements should not be given until the serum potassium concentration is known as severe poisoning is commonly associated with hyperkalaemia which should be treated conventionally.

Sinus bradycardia, ventricular ectopics, atrioventricular block, and sinoatrial standstill or block are often reduced or abolished by atropine, (1.2–2.4 mg). Ventricular ectopics alone should not be treated unless cardiac output is impaired. Ventricular tachydysrhythmias may be treated with intravenous lignocaine, atenolol, phenytoin, or amiodarone. Specific treatment with ovine Fab fragment antidigoxin antibodies ('Digibind', 'DigiTab') (6–8 mg/kg body weight) should be considered. An improvement in the patient's condition should occur within 20–40 minutes. Failure to achieve a satisfactory cardiac output by drug therapy in patients with bradycardia, atrioventricular block, or sinus arrest is an indication for insertion of a right ventricular pacing wire.

Forced diuresis, peritoneal dialysis, haemodialysis, and haemoperfusion do not significantly increase the elimination of the drug.

Further reading

Smith, T.W. (1991). Review of clinical experience with digoxin immune Fab (Ovine). *American Journal of Emergency Medicine*, **9**, 1–6 (supp 1).

Woolf, A.D., Wenger, T., Smith, T.W., and Lovejoy, F.H. (1992). The use of digoxin-specific Fab fragments for severe digitalis intoxication in children. *New England Journal of Medicine*, **326**, 1739–44.

Diphenoxylate ('Lomotil')

See 'Co-phenotrope', above.

Dishwashing liquids

Carpet shampoo, dishwashing rinse aid for dishwashing machines, fabric washing powder and flakes, and scouring liquids, creams, and powders include surfactants that contain both hydrophilic and lipophilic groups to allow dispersal of fat-soluble substances in aqueous media.

Clinical features Anionic detergents irritate the skin by removing natural oils and cause redness, soreness, and even a papular dermatitis. Ingestion may cause mild gastrointestinal irritation, nausea, vomiting, and diarrhoea. Non-ionic surfactants irritate the skin only slightly and appear to be completely harmless when ingested. Cationic surfactants are much more toxic than the others but are rarely found in household cleaning materials.

Treatment After ingestion of non-ionic or anionic surfactants, liberal amounts of water or milk should be swallowed. If a cationic surfactant was ingested, advice should be sought from a poisons information centre.

Further reading

Cornish, L.S., Parsons, B.J., and Dobbin, M.D. (1996). Automatic Dishwasher detergent poisoning: opportunities for prevention. *Australian and New Zealand Journal of Public Health*, **20**, 278–283.

Disulfiram ('Antabuse')

Mechanism of toxicity Disulfiram inhibits the activity of a wide range of enzymes, particularly aldehyde dehydrogenase.

Clinical features Adult cases are likely to be alcoholics who have been taking disulfiram before the overdose and are likely to be malnourished. Sensorimotor neuropathy, flaccid tetraparesis, encephalopathy, vomiting, abdominal pain, and diarrhoea have been described.

In children, drowsiness, pyrexia, hypotonia, ataxia, uncontrollable and inappropriate arm movements, irritability and speech difficulties, hallucinations, coma, and hyperrflexia are the major features.

Disulfiram–ethanol reaction Nausea, vertigo, anxiety, blurred vision, hypotension, chest pain, palpitation, tachycardia, facial flushing, and throbbing headache are the usual features. Symptoms usually last for 3–4 days but may persist for a week. Severe reactions involve respiratory depression, cardiovascular collapse, cardiac arrhythmias, coma, cerebral oedema, hemiplegia, and convulsions: fatalities have been reported.

Further reading

Mahajan, P., Lieh-Lai, M.W., Sarnaik, A., and Kottamasu, S.R. (1997). Basal ganglia infarction in a child with disulfiram poisoning. *Pediatrics*, **99**, 605–8.

Diuretics

When combined diuretic and potassium formulations are ingested, the potassium content is likely to pose the greater risk. More serious consequences are likely if a potassium-sparing diuretic has been ingested.

Clinical features Symptoms and signs of toxicity include anorexia, nausea, vomiting, diarrhoea, profound diuresis, dehydration, hypotension, dizziness, weakness, muscle cramps, tetany, and, occasionally, gastrointestinal bleeding. Hyponatraemia, hypoglycaemia or hyperglycaemia, hyperuricaemia, hypokalaemia, and metabolic alkalosis may develop. Hyperkalaemia may develop following the ingestion of combined diuretic and potassium preparations and potassium-sparing diuretics, such as amiloride, spironolactone, or triamterene. Small-bowel ulceration and stricture formation has followed poisoning from diuretics with an enteric-coated core of potassium chloride.

Treatment Fluid and electrolyte balance should be corrected. Hyperkalaemia is treated by glucose and insulin infusion followed by oral or rectal administration of an ion-exchange resin.

Further reading

Lip, G.Y. and Ferner, R.E. (1995). Poisoning and anti-hypertensive drugs: diuretics and potassium supplements. *Journal of Human Hypertension*, **9**, 295–301.

Ethanol

Alcoholic drink is commonly taken with other substances in overdose. Ethanol is used as a solvent and is found in many cosmetics and antiseptics. It is rapidly absorbed through the gastric and intestinal mucosae. About 95 per cent is oxidized to acetaldehyde and then to acetate. The rest is excreted unchanged in the urine, breath, and through the skin.

Ethanol is a central nervous depressant that exacerbates the effects of other central nervous system depressants, particularly hypnotic

Table 4 Clinical features of ethanol poisoning

Mild intoxication (500–1500 mg/l) Emotional lability, slight impairment of visual acuity, muscular co-ordination and reaction time
Moderate intoxication (1500–3000 mg/l) Visual impairment, sensory loss, muscular inco-ordination, slowed reaction time, slurred speech
Severe intoxication (3000–5000 mg/l) Marked muscular inco-ordination, blurred or double vision, sometimes stupor and hypothermia, and occasionally hypoglycaemia and convulsions
Coma (>5000 mg/l) Depressed reflexes, respiratory depression, hypotension and hypothermia. Death may occur from respiratory or circulatory failure or as the result of aspiration of stomach contents in the absence of a gag reflex

agents. The fatal dose of ethanol alone is between 300 and 500 ml of absolute alcohol, if this is ingested in less than one hour.

Clinical features The clinical features of ethanol intoxication are generally related to blood concentrations (Table 4).

Severe hypoglycaemia results from inhibition of gluconeogenesis. It is more common in children than in adults and typically occurs within 6–36 hours of ingestion of a moderate to large amount of alcohol by either a previously malnourished individual or one who has fasted for the previous 24 hours. The patient is often in coma and hypothermic but flushing, sweating, and tachycardia are frequently absent. Rarely lactic acidosis, ketoacidosis, and acute renal failure have also been described.

Treatment Gastric lavage is not beneficial. Treatment is supportive. Intravenous glucose (50 ml of 50 per cent solution) should be given. Hypoglycaemia is usually unresponsive to glucagon. Haemodialysis should be considered if the blood ethanol concentration exceeds 5000 mg/l and/or if metabolic acidosis is present.

Further reading

Ernst, A.A., Jones, K., Nick, T.G., and Sanchez, J. (1996). Ethanol ingestion and related hypoglycemia in a pediatric and adolescent emergency department population. *Academic Emergency Medicine*, 3, 46–9.

Vogel, C., Caraccio, T., Mofensen, H., and Hart, S. (1995). Alcohol intoxication in young children. *Clinical Toxicology*, 33, 25–33.

Ethylene glycol (1,2-ethanediol)

Ethylene glycol is commonly used as an antifreeze fluid in car radiators. Its sweet taste and ready availability have contributed to its popularity as a suicide agent and as a poor man's substitute for alcohol. The minimum lethal dose is about 100 ml for an adult, although people have recovered after drinking up to 1 litre.

Mechanism of toxicity Ethylene glycol itself is non-toxic but hepatic and renal metabolism leads to accumulation of aldehydes, glycolate, oxalate, and lactic acid.

Clinical features Death may occur during any of the three stages. A serum ethylene glycol concentration in excess of 500 mg/l indicates severe poisoning (Table 5).

Treatment Gastric lavage should be considered when presentation is less than one hour after ingestion. Shock, respiratory distress, hypocalcaemia, and metabolic acidosis must be corrected. Ethanol

Table 5 Clinical features of ethylene glycol poisoning

Stage 1 (30 min–12 hours): gastrointestinal and nervous system involvement Patient appears intoxicated with alcohol (but no ethanol on breath) Nausea, vomiting, haematemesis Coma and convulsions (often focal) Nystagmus, ophthalmoplegias, papilloedema, depressed reflexes, myoclonic jerks, tetanic contractions, V, VII, VIII nerve palsies
Stage 2 (12–24 hours): cardiorespiratory system involvement Tachypnoea Tachycardia Mild hypertension Pulmonary oedema Congestic cardiac failure
Stage 3 (24–72 hours): renal involvement Flank pain Renal angle tenderness Acute tubular necrosis

or 4-methylpyrazole are competitive inhibitors of ethylene glycol metabolism and dialysis increases elimination. A loading dose of 50 g ethanol (conveniently given as approximately 125 ml of gin, whisky, or vodka) should be administered followed by an intravenous infusion of 10–12 g ethanol to provide blood ethanol concentrations of 1 g/l. The infusion should be continued until ethylene glycol is no longer detectable in the blood. If dialysis is also employed, the rate of ethanol administration must be increased (17–22 g/h).

Ethylene glycol, its aldehyde metabolites, and glycolate may be removed by either peritoneal or haemodialysis though the latter is two to three times more efficient. Oxalate, however, is poorly dialysable. Uraemic complications of ethylene glycol poisoning may also required dialysis. Haemodialysis/ultrafiltration may be needed to correct the sodium overload resulting from correction of the metabolic acidosis with sodium bicarbonate. Dialysis should be continued until ethylene glycol is no longer detectable in the blood.

Further reading

Glaser, D.S. (1996). Utility of the serum osmol gap in the diagnosis of methanol or ethylene glycol ingestion. *Annals of Emergency Medicine*, 27, 343–6.

Jacobsen, D. and McMartin, K.E. (1997). Antidotes for methanol and ethylene glycol poisoning. *Clinical Toxicology*, 35, 127–43.

Fluoxetine and fluvoxamine

Clinical features Fluoxetine and fluvoxamine are antidepressants that inhibit serotonin reuptake. Doses of up to 3.6 mg/kg body weight do not appear to cause toxicity and even larger amounts are relatively safe unless potentiated by ethanol. They lack the anticholinergic actions of the tricyclic antidepressants. Drowsiness, nausea, diarrhoea, and sinus tachycardia have been reported. Rarely, junctional bradycardia, seizures, and hypertension have been encountered and influenza-like symptoms may develop after a day or two.

Treatment Activated charcoal may reduce absorption if administered within one hour of substantial overdose.

Further reading

Borys, D.J., Setzer, S.C., Ling, L.J., Reisdorf, J.J., Day, L.C., and Krenzelok, E.P. (1992). Acute fluoxetine overdose: a report of 234 cases. *American Journal of Emergency Medicine*, 10, 115–19.

Formaldehyde

Formaldehyde is a flammable, colourless gas with a pungent odour, most commonly available commercially as a 30–50 per cent w/w aqueous solution. It is used in the synthesis of organic compounds such as plastics and resins.

Metabolism Formaldehyde is oxidized rapidly to formic acid and then converted more slowly to carbon dioxide and water; some formic acid is excreted in the urine.

Acute exposure Severe irritation of the mucous membranes of the eyes, nose, and upper airways occurs after minimal exposure to low (<5 p.p.m.) formaldehyde concentrations, which tends to prevent higher exposure in even the most tolerant subjects. Substantial exposure may result in severe bronchospasm, pulmonary oedema, and death.

Formaldehyde solutions splashed into the eye have caused corneal damage and skin contamination has resulted in dermatitis. Spillage of phenol-formaldehyde resin on to the skin has produced extensive necrotic skin lesions, fever, hypertension, adult respiratory distress syndrome, proteinuria, and renal impairment. Ingestion of formaldehyde solution has resulted in severe corrosive damage to the buccal cavity and tonsils, oesophagus, and stomach with ulceration, necrosis, and subsequent fibrosis and contracture. Shock, metabolic acidosis, respiratory insufficiency, and renal impairment usually ensue. Death may follow ingestion of less than 100 ml in an adult.

Chronic exposure Skin irritation and dermatitis have been observed frequently and allergic sensitization to formaldehyde solutions or resins has been reported.

Treatment Supportive measures including the correction of acid–base disturbance. Haemodialysis is only moderately effective in increasing formate elimination.

Further reading

IPCS. (1989). *Environmental Health Criteria 89. Formaldehyde.* WHO, Geneva.

Glyphosate-containing herbicides

Glyphosate-containing herbicides usually contain the isopropylamine salt together with a surfactant that was probably the main cause of toxicity but has now been changed.

Clinical features There is burning in the mouth and throat, nausea, vomiting, dysphagia, diarrhoea, and sometimes upper gastrointestinal haemorrhage. A polymorph leucocytosis is usual. Hypotension, tachycardia, bradycardia, acute chemical pneumonitis, oliguria, haematuria, and metabolic acidosis occur in severe poisoning.

Treatment Intravenous fluids or blood may be required. Respiratory and renal failure should be managed conventionally.

Further reading

Tominack, R.L., *et al.* (1991). Taiwan National Poison Center survey of glyphosate-surfactant herbicide ingestions. *Clinical Toxicology,* **29**, 91–109.

Hexane

Clinical features Ingestion causes nausea, dizziness, and CNS excitation and then depression, and presents an acute aspiration hazard. Inhalation causes similar symptoms together with progressive sensorimotor neuropathy if exposure is chronic.

Treatment is symptomatic.

Further reading

Low, L.K., Meeks, J.R., and Mackerer, C.R. (1987). The aliphatic hydrocarbons. In Ethel Browning's *toxicity and metabolism of industrial solvents* (ed. R. Snyder), 2nd edn, pp. 253–335. Elsevier, Amsterdam.

Household products

(See antiseptics and disinfectants, dishwashing liquids, fabric conditioners, detergents, bleaches and lavatory cleaners, lavatory sanitizers, and deodorants.)

H_2-receptor antagonists

Clinical features In some patients drowsiness, dryness of the mouth, slurred speech, dizziness, confusion, vomiting, and abdominal discomfort have been reported, Rarely, bradycardia, respiratory depression, and coma may result.

Treatment is symptomatic.

Further reading

Krenzelok, E.P., Litovitz, T., Lippold, K.P., and McNally, C.F. (1987). Cimetidine toxicity: An assessment of 881 cases. *Annals of Emergency Medicine,* **16**, 1217–22.

Hydrogen fluoride

Hydrogen fluoride is a corrosive, fuming, nearly colourless liquid (hydrofluoric acid) at ordinary pressures below 19°C; above 19°C it is gaseous. Aqueous solutions dissolve glass, reacting to form gaseous silicon fluoride.

Mechanisms of toxicity Fluoride inhibits many enzymes (e.g. glycolytic enzymes, cholinesterases, and magnesium and manganese metalloenzymes) and is toxic to nerve and muscle.

Clinical features Inhalation or ingestion of hydrogen fluoride causes severe corrosive damage similar to other acids (see above). Following absorption by whatever route, fluoride chelates calcium and lowers the serum ionized calcium concentration causing weakness, paraesthesiae, tetany, convulsions, hypotension, and cardiac arrhythmias (including ventricular fibrillation). Coma and hepatic and renal failure may develop.

Skin contact with anhydrous hydrogen fluoride produces liquefactive necrosis and severe burns that are felt immediately. Concentrated aqueous solutions are painful but more dilute solutions may give no warning of injury. If the solution is not removed promptly, penetration of the skin by fluoride ion may occur, leading to painful ulcers which heal only slowly.

Treatment Following inhalation of hydrogen fluoride, the casualty should be removed immediately from the contaminated atmosphere. Mechanical ventilation with positive end-expiratory pressure may be needed to treat pulmonary oedema.

If hydrofluoric acid has been ingested soluble calcium tablets (10–20 g) should be given by mouth, followed by an intravenous injection of 10 ml of 10 per cent calcium gluconate solution.

Contaminated skin must be washed with copious quantities of water for 20 minutes, even if there is no apparent burn or pain. Skin burns should be coated repeatedly with 2.5 per cent calcium gluconate gel, or immersed in iced water until the pain subsides. Local subcutaneous injection of 10 per cent calcium gluconate solution (up to 0.5 ml/cm^2) is indicated if pain is persistent.

Further reading

Braun, J., Stob, H., and Zober, A. (1984). Intoxication following the inhalation of hydrogen fluoride. *Archives of Toxicology*, **56**, 50–4.

Dunn, B.J., MacKinnon, M.A., Knowlden, N.F., *et al.* (1996). Topical treatments for hydrofluoric acid dermal burns. *Journal of Occupational and Environmental Medicine*, **38**, 507–14.

Matsuno, K. (1996). The treatment of hydrofluoric acid burns. *Occupational Medicine*, **46**, 313–317.

Hydrogen sulphide

Hydrogen sulphide is a colourless gas which smells of rotten eggs. High concentrations damage the olfactory nerve. The gas is also found in mines and sewers and is liberated from decomposing fish (a hazard in fishing boats if the hold is filled with 'trash' fish used for making fish meal) and liquid manure systems.

Mechanisms of toxicity Hydrogen sulphide is a more potent inhibitor of cytochrome oxidase a_3 than cyanide.

Clinical features Exposure to low concentrations leads to blepharospasm, pain and redness in the eyes, blurred vision, and coloured haloes round lights. Headache, nausea, dizziness, drowsiness, sore throat, and cough may also occur. Higher concentrations cause cyanosis, confusion, pulmonary oedema, coma, and convulsions. Six per cent of cases die.

Treatment The casualty should be moved to fresh air from the contaminated atmosphere by a rescuer wearing breathing apparatus beforehand.

Further reading

Guidotti, T.L. (1996). Hydrogen sulphide. *Occupational Medicine*, **46**, 367–71.

Hypoglycaemic agents

Intentional overdose with insulin and oral hypoglycaemic agents is uncommon. Chlorpropamide, because of its long half-life, may, in overdose, induce hypoglycaemia for a considerable period of time.

Clinical features Drowsiness, coma, twitching, convulsions, depressed limb reflexes, extensor plantar responses, hyperpnoea, pulmonary oedema, tachycardia, and circulatory failure may develop. Hypoglycaemia is to be expected and hypokalaemia, cerebral oedema, and metabolic acidosis may occur.

Treatment Blood glucose must be measured urgently and intravenous glucose given. Glucagon may be ineffective. If the blood sugar is normal, gastric lavage should be considered if the patient has presented within one hour of the ingestion of an oral preparation.

Recurrent hypoglycaemia is highly likely. A continuous infusion of glucose together with carbohydrate-rich meals are required in cases of severe insulin overdosage. In sulphonylurea overdosage, however, further glucose (although its administration may be unavoidable) increases already high circulating insulin concentrations. Diazoxide has therefore been recommended since it increases blood glucose concentrations and raises circulating catecholamine concentrations while blocking insulin release: 1.25 mg/kg body weight is given intravenously over 1 hour, repeated at 6-hourly intervals if necessary.

Further reading

Palatnick, W., Meatherall, R.C., and Tenenbein, M. (1991). Clinical spectrum of sulfonylurea overdose and experience with diazoxide therapy. *Archives of Internal Medicine*, **151**, 1859–62.

Roberge, R.J., Martin, T.G., and Delbridge, T.R. (1993). Intentional massive insulin overdose: recognition and management. *Annals of Emergency Medicine*, **22**, 228–34.

Indomethacin

Clinical features These include headache, nausea, abdominal pain, drowsiness, tinnitus, gastrointestinal bleeding, coma, convulsions, and acute renal failure.

Treatment is symptomatic with haemodialysis/filtration in cases of renal failure.

Iron

Iron overdosage is much more common in preschool children than in adults. Toxic features are unlikely unless more than 60 mg of elemental iron/kg body weight has been ingested.

Mechanism of toxicity Iron salts are corrosive on the upper gastrointestinal tract and affect the circulation; at a cellular level they interfere with intermediary metabolism.

Clinical features Initially there is nausea, vomiting, abdominal pain, and diarrhoea, from direct irritation of the gut. The gastric and upper small bowel mucosae may be stained and impregnated with iron and become ulcerated. The disintegrating tablets may make the vomitus and stools grey or black. Polymorph leucocytosis and hyperglycaemia are common. Iron tablets in the upper gut may be visible in the straight abdominal radiograph, particularly if it is taken within 2 hours of alleged ingestion. A few patients develop haematemesis, hypotension, coma, and shock that may be fatal.

Patients improve permanently or temporarily between about 6–24 hours after ingestion. A few patients deteriorate 12–48 hours after ingestion, often with profound shock, metabolic acidosis, acute renal tubular and hepatocellular necrosis. Some 2–6 weeks after ingestion patients may develop high intestinal obstruction from stricture at the site of corrosive damage to the mucosa. Children are most likely to be affected.

Assessment of the severity of poisoning Shock and coma indicate severe poisoning. Emergency estimation of the serum iron concentration is essential. If concentrations exceed predicted normal iron binding capacity (usually >90 μmol/l) free iron is circulating and treatment is needed. Measurement of the total iron binding capacity in acute iron overdosage is unreliable.

Treatment Gastric lavage without additives should be considered if more than 20 mg of elemental iron/kg body weight has been ingested in the previous one hour. Whole bowel irrigation may have a role if a large amount (particularly of a slow release formulation) has already passed through the pylorus.

Severe poisoning with coma or shock The specific iron chelating agent desferrioxamine, should be given without delay in clinically severe poisoning before the result of the serum iron concentration is available: 15 mg/kg body weight/hour is given intravenously; to a maximum of 80 mg/kg in 24 hours. Clinical improvement can be expected within an hour or two, after which the rate of infusion may be reduced. Desferrioxamine may also be given intramuscularly in a dose of 2 g for adults and 1 g for children.

Hypotension due to desferrioxamine-induced histamine release may develop if the recommended rate of administration is exceeded. Hypersensitivity reactions may occur. Pulmonary oedema and adult respiratory distress syndrome attributed to desferrioxamine have been reported in patients given 15 mg/kg for 65 hours and longer.

Further reading

Chyka P.A., Butler A.Y., and Holley J.E. (1996). Serum iron concentrations and symptoms of acute iron poisoning in children. *Pharmacotherapy*, **16**, 1053–8.

Tenenbein, M. (1996). Benefits of parenteral deferoxamine for acute iron poisoning. *Clinical Toxicology*, **34**, 485–9.

Isoniazid

Poisoning with isoniazid is potentially very serious, but uncommon.
Mechanisms of toxicity Isoniazid depresses brain concentrations of γ-aminobutyric acid (GABA), thus leading to seizures.
Clinical features The ingestion of 80–150 mg isoniazid/kg body weight is likely to cause severe poisoning. Nausea, vomiting, slurred speech, dizziness, and visual hallucinations may develop. Stupor, coma, and convulsions follow rapidly and may be associated with hyperthemia, hyperreflexia, extensor plantar responses, and later, rhabdomyolysis. In addition, dilated pupils, sinus tachycardia, and urinary retention may be observed. In severe cases, hypotension, renal failure, and respiratory failure may ensue. Marked metabolic (lactic) acidosis is common. Less commonly, there is hyperglycaemia, ketoacidosis, glycosuria, and ketonuria.
Treatment Metabolic acidosis must be corrected immediately. Gastric lavage or activated charcoal administration (50 g) should be considered if presentation is less than one hour after overdose. Pyridoxine should be given intravenously in a dose 1 g for 1 g of isoniazid ingested. When the ingested dose of isoniazid is unknown, an initial intravenous dose of 5 g pyridoxine should be given. Diazepam and pyridoxine are synergistic and both should be used in those with convulsions. The 5-g dose of pyridoxine may be repeated if convulsions persist.

Charcoal haemoperfusion is the most effective technique for elimination of isoniazid from the circulation but is rarely needed.

Further reading

Girnani, A., Chawla, R., Kundra, P., and Bhattacharya, A. (1992). Acute izoniazid poisoning. *Anaesthesia*, **47**, 781–3.

Isopropanol (isopropyl alcohol; 2-propanol)

Isopropanol is used as a sterilizing agent and as 'rubbing alcohol'. It is also found in aftershave lotions, disinfectants, and window-cleaning solutions.
Clinical features Ingestion or skin absorption can cause intoxication. Isopropanol is oxidized in the liver to acetone. Coma, respiratory depression, the odour of acetone on the breath, gastritis, haematemesis, hypotension, hypothermia, renal tubular necrosis, acute myopathy, haemolytic anaemia, and cardiac arrest have been described. Hypotension is a poor prognostic feature.
Treatment Gastric lavage should be considered if the patient presents less than one hour after ingestion. Haemodialysis is useful in severely poisoned patients; it removes isopropanol and shortens coma.

Further reading

IPCS. (1990). *Environmental Health Criteria 103. 2-Propanol.* WHO, Geneva.

Lavatory sanitizers and deodorants

Solid lavatory sanitizer or deodorant blocks usually contain paradichlorobenzene. Ingestion may cause nausea, vomiting, diarrhoea, and abdominal pain. If many grams have been ingested and the patient presents within one hour of ingestion, gastric lavage should be considered.

Lead

Exposure to lead occurs in the scrap metal industry, and manufacture of storage batteries and ceramics. Children may chew on lead-painted railings or eat contaminated soil. Drinking from lead-glazed mugs, ingestion of lead-based powders in paints and imported baby tonics, use of lead-containing cosmetics ('surma' in Asian communities), suicidal injections of lead acetate, inhalation or cutaneous absorption of tetraethyl lead (an anti-knock agent in leaded petrol), have all resulted in poisoning.

Lead absorbed into the body is mainly (95 per cent) deposited in the bones and teeth. In blood, 99 per cent is associated with erythrocytes. As the body accumulates lead over many years and releases it into the urine only slowly, even small doses can in time lead to intoxication.
Clinical features Mild intoxication may result in no more than lethargy and occasional abdominal discomfort, whereas diffuse or colicky abdominal pain, vomiting, constipation and encephalopathy develop in more severe cases. Encephalopathy (seizures, mania, delirium, coma) is more common in children than in adults. Foot drop and at a late stage wrist drop are attributable to primary motor peripheral neuropathy. Renal effects include reversible renal tubular dysfunction causing glycosuria, aminoaciduria and phosphaturia, and irreversible interstitial fibrosis with progressive renal insufficiency leading to hypertension. A bluish discoloration of the gum margins from deposition of lead sulphide may be visible.

Lead depresses the enzymes responsible for haem synthesis and shortens erythrocyte lifespan leading to a microcytic or normocytic hypochromic anaemia. In severe intoxication haemolytic anaemia may occur. Basophilic stippling of erythrocytes is due to nuclear remnants. Lead blocks the conversion of δ-aminolaevulinic acid to porphobilinogen, leading to an increase in δ-aminolaevulinic acid in blood and urine. Lead also inhibits ferrochelatase which results in elevated free erythrocyte protoporphyrin (FEP) levels. There is a concomitant increase in urinary coproporphyrins and FEP, commonly assayed as zinc protoporphyrin.

An elevated zinc protoporphyrin concentration (>350 μg/l) reaches a steady state in the blood only after the entire population of circulating erythrocytes has turned over (approximately 120 days). Consequently, it lags behind blood lead concentrations and is an indirect measure of long-term lead exposure. Moreover, zinc protoporphyrin is not a good screening test as it is not sensitive at the lower levels of lead poisoning.
Medical surveillance Workers are recommended to stop exposure to lead when their blood lead concentration exceeds 700 μg/l. In those exposed to organic lead compounds, the urinary lead concentration (>150μg/l) is a good indicator of exposure. In children, blood lead concentrations higher than 100μg/l may be associated with illness.
Treatment The decision to use chelation therapy is based on the blood lead concentration, the symptoms, and, if available, an estimate of the total body burden of lead using X-ray fluorescence. Sodium calcium edetate is more efficient than DMSA (succimer) in increasing lead excretion but it must be given intravenously and may result in increased uptake of lead into the brain. In severe acute lead poisoning sodium calcium edetate (75 mg/kg body weight/day for 5 days) provides rapid relief of symptoms with minimal risk of adverse effect; a second course may be given a week after the first. If hydration is

maintained during chelation proximal tubular damage is not usually observed. Oral DMSA (30 mg/kg body weight).

Further reading

CDC. (1991). *Preventing lead poisoning in young children.* US Department of Health and Human Services, Washington.

Liftshitz, M., Hashkanazi, R., and Phillip, M. (1997). The effect of 2,3-dimercaptosuccinic acid in the treatment of lead poisoning in adults. *Annals of Medicine*, 29, 83–5.

Lignocaine and related drugs

Lignocaine, mexiletine, and tocainide are sodium channel blockers. Intoxication with these agents, particularly lignocaine, occurs most often as a result of therapeutic overdosage in intensive care units. Topical absorption of lignocaine may result in systemic toxicity, particularly in children.

Clinical features There is nausea, vomiting, paraesthesiae, tremor, drowsiness, dizziness, dysarthria, diplopia, nystagmus, ataxia, confusion, convulsions, and coma. Sinus bradycardia, heart block, and hypotension may develop in severe poisoning and cardiac arrest may ensue; mexiletine may also cause atrial fibrillation.

Treatment Gastric lavage should be considered or activated charcoal (50–100 g) administered if an overdose has been ingested less than one hour previously. Diazepam (5–10 mg intravenously) should be given for convulsions. Atropine (1–2 mg intravenously) should be administered for sinus bradycardia. Inotropic support may become necessary if heart block or severe hypotension supervene. Pacing may be attempted but the ventricular response is usually poor. Tocainide elimination is increased significantly with haemodialysis.

Further reading

Denaro, C.P. and Benowitz, N.L. (1989). Poisoning due to class 1B antiarrhythmic drugs: lignocaine, mexilitine and tocainide. *Medical Toxicology*, 4, 412–28.

Lindane

Clinical features There is rapid loss of consciousness with myoclonus, hypertonia, hyperreflexia, convulsions, and rhabdomyolysis. Metabolic acidosis, disseminated intravascular coagulation, renal tubular and hepatocellular necrosis, pancreatitis, and proximal myopathy have been reported.

Treatment Gastric lavage should be considered if lindane has been ingested less than one hour previously, any acid–base abnormality has been corrected, and convulsions have been controlled.

Further reading

IPCS. (1991). *Environmental Health Criteria 124, Lindane.* WHO, Geneva.

Liquefied petroleum gas (LPG 'bottled gas')

Liquefied petroleum gas, (LPG 'bottled gas') contains propane and butane (and sometimes propylene and butylene). Propane and butane may cause vertigo and drowsiness and, at high concentrations, may act as asphyxiants.

Lithium carbonate

The therapeutic index of lithium is low and toxicity is usually the result of therapeutic overdosage rather than deliberate self-poisoning.

Clinical features Thirst, polyuria, diarrhoea, and vomiting, and, in more serious cases, impairment of consciousness, hypertonia, convulsions, and irreversible neurological damage may occur. Serum lithium concentration above 1.5 mmol/l confirms the diagnosis. Acute massive overdosage may produce much higher concentrations without causing toxic features, at least initially.

Treatment Gastric lavage may be considered if the patient presents less than one hour after a substantial overdose. Lithium elimination should be enhanced if symptoms are severe and serum lithium concentration exceeds 3 mmol/l. Forced diuresis is effective but may result in hypernatraemia and increased plasma osmolality. Infusion of low dose dopamine (2.5 μg/kg/min) may be an effective alternative. Haemodialysis may be needed if renal function is impaired and in severe poisoning; peritoneal dialysis is much less effective. Serum lithium concentrations frequently rebound when treatment is stopped.

Further reading

Groleau, G., *et al.* (1987). Lithium intoxication. Manifestation and management. *American Journal of Emergency Medicine*, 5, 527–32.

Scharman, E.J. (1997). Methods used to decrease lithium absorption or enhance elimination. *Clinical Toxicology*, 35, 601–8.

Lysergic acid diethylamide (LSD)

Clinical features Visual hallucinations, distortion of images, agitation, excitement, dilated pupils, tachycardia, hypertension, hyperreflexia, tremor, and hyperthermia are common; auditory hallucinations are rare. Time seems to pass very slowly and behaviour may become disturbed with paranoid delusions. Flashbacks in which the effects of LSD may be re-experienced without further exposure to the drug occur in about 15 per cent of users for several years and are not explained.

Treatment consists of reassurance and sedation.

Manganese

See OTM3, pp. 1110–1.

Mercury

Metallic mercury is very volatile and, when spilt, creates high atmospheric concentrations in an enclosed space when environmental temperature is high.

Non-occupational mercury exposure occurs principally from dietary intake and to a minor extent from dental amalgam. Many foodstuffs contain small amounts of inorganic mercury but organic mercury compounds bioaccumulate in the aquatic food chain so that certain fish (e.g. trout, pike, bass, and tuna) contain significant amounts of methylmercury. The Minamata Bay disaster in 1956 resulted from methylmercury poisoning after eating fish affected by a factory effluent discharged into the Bay. The use of methylmercury as a fungicide led to an outbreak of mercury poisoning in Iraq in the early 1970s, when bread was made with contaminated grain. Creams and soaps containing inorganic mercury have been marketed as skin toners to lighten the complexion; these products are now banned in the European Community and North America.

Acute poisoning Acute mercury vapour inhalation causes headache, nausea, cough, chest pain, bronchitis, and pneumonia. Rarely, renal damage from such acute exposure may produce gross proteinuria or nephrotic syndrome. A fine tremor, neurobehavioural impairment, and peripheral neuropathy may also develop. Kawasaki disease has been reported in exposed children.

Ingestion of metallic mercury, which is poorly absorbed from the gastrointestinal tract, is usually without severe systemic effects. However, mercuric chloride and other inorganic mercuric salts cause an irritant gastroenteritis with corrosive ulceration, bloody diarrhoea, and abdominal cramps and may lead to circulatory collapse and shock. The ingestion of disc batteries containing mercuric oxide may result in potentially toxic mercury levels if the battery opens in transit. Mercurous compounds are less soluble, less corrosive, and less toxic than mercuric salts. Ingestion of mercurous chloride in teething powder has led to 'pink disease' or acrodynia in infants. This condition presents as fever with a pink-coloured rash, irritability, photophobia, painful and swollen extremities, hyperkeratosis, and hypersecretion of sweat glands.

Intravenous or subcutaneous metallic mercury injection may result in pulmonary venous or peripheral arterial embolism, or soft-tissue inflammatory reaction with granuloma formation.

Chronic poisoning Chronic poisoning from inorganic mercury compounds or mercury vapour causes anorexia, insomnia, abnormal sweating, headache, and lassitude. The classical features of chronic mercury poisoning are increased excitability, tremor, gingivitis, and hypersalivation. Other central nervous system effects are extreme shyness, personality changes, and memory and intellectual deterioration. Emotional lability ('mercurial erethism') is thought to be responsible for the phrase 'mad as a hatter' which refers to felt hat makers who were exposed to hot mercuric nitrate used for treating the felt. They also showed a fine tremor ('hatter's shakes') Mercury may be deposited on the lens (mercurialentis). Glomerular and tubular damage and renal tubular acidosis may follow chronic exposure to mercury.

Exposure to organic mercury compounds causes paraesthesiae of the lips, hands, and feet, ataxia, tremor, dysarthria, constriction of visual fields, deafness and emotional and intellectual changes.

Treatment DMPS is effective in improving neurological features. After ingestion of mercuric salts, such as mercuric chloride, gastric lavage is best avoided as significant oesophageal erosions may be present.

Dimercaprol (British Anti-Lewisite, BAL) is used to treat inorganic mercury poisoning. Oral DMPS (unithiol) and DMSA (succimer) (30 mg/kg body weight) enhance mercury elimination, protect against renal damage, and increase survival. DMPS may be more effective than DMSA.

Both DMSA and DMPS are valuable in the treatment of methylmercury poisoning. There is no effective treatment for chronic mercury poisoning.

Further reading

IPCS. (1990). *Environmental Health Criteria 101. Methylmercury.* WHO, Geneva.

IPCS. (1991). *Environmental Health Criteria 118. Inorganic mercury.* WHO, Geneva.

See also Sections 12 and 13 and OTM3, pp. 1111–2.

Metaldehyde

Metaldehyde in the form of pellets is used widely for killing slugs and in some countries as a solid fuel.

Clinical features Nausea, vomiting, abdominal pain, and diarrhoea often occur 1–3 hours after ingestion of any amount while more than 100 mg/kg body weight may cause hypertonia, convulsions, impairment of consciousness, and metabolic acidosis. Hepatic and renal tubular necrosis may become apparent after 2–3 days.

Treatment Gastric lavage should be considered if more than 50 mg/kg has been ingested within 1 hour. Treatment thereafter is supportive.

Methanol (methyl alcohol)

Methanol is used widely as a solvent. It is also found in antifreeze solutions, paints, duplicating fluids, paint removers and varnishes, and shoe polishes. The ingestion of as little as 10 ml of pure methanol has caused permanent blindness and 30 ml is potentially fatal although individual susceptibility varies widely. Toxicity may also occur as a result of inhalation or percutaneous absorption.

Mechanisms of toxicity Methanol is metabolized by alcohol dehydrogenase and catalase enzyme systems to formaldehyde and formic acid (formate) causing metabolic acidosis.

Clinical features Ingested alone, methanol causes mild and transient inebriation and drowsiness. After 8–36 hours, nausea, vomiting, abdominal pain, headaches, dizziness, and coma supervene. Blurred vision, diminished visual acuity, and dilated unreactive pupils presage permanent blindness. A severe metabolic acidosis may develop, accompanied by hyperglycaemia and a raised serum amylase activity. A blood methanol concentration greater than 500 mg/l confirms serious poisoning. Permanent neurological sequelae including blindness, rigidity, hypokinesis, and other parkinsonian-like signs.

Treatment Gastric lavage may be considered in patients who present less than one hour after ingestion. The metabolic acidosis must be corrected. Substantial quantities of bicarbonate (often as much as 2 mol) may be required and since this must be accompanied by sodium, hypernatraemia and hypervolaemia may result. Methanol oxidation must be inhibited and circulating methanol and its toxic metabolites must be removed.

Ethanol inhibits methanol oxidation. If admission plasma concentrations show that most of the methanol has already been metabolized, ethanol administration may not be of benefit and might exacerbate the acidosis. It should therefore be given and monitored as for ethylene glycol (see above). In those undergoing haemodialysis (see below), the dose of ethanol should be increased.

Dialysis is indicated when a patient has ingested more than 30 g methanol, or develops metabolic acidosis, mental, visual, or fundoscopic abnormalities attributable to methanol, or a blood methanol concentration in excess of 500 mg/l. Folinic acid (30 mg IV 6-hourly) may protect against ocular toxicity by accelerating formate metabolism.

Further reading

Burkhart, K. (1997). Methanol and ethylene glycol toxicity. *Clinical Toxicology*, 35, 149–50.

Jacobsen, D. and McMartin, K.E. (1997). Antidotes for methanol and ethylene glycol poisoning. *Clinical Toxicology*, 35, 126–43.

Methyl bromide (bromomethane)

Methyl bromide, increasingly used to fumigate soil, grain, etc., is a colourless, odourless gas at ordinary temperatures. Dangerous concentrations may accumulate without warning. Its high density causes it to settle at floor level.

Mechanism of toxicity Methyl bromide appears to have an affinity for intracellular proteins, particularly those with sulphydryl groups.

Clinical features After a latent period of up to 12 hours dizziness, headache, nausea, vomiting, abdominal pain, malaise, transient blurring of vision, diplopia, and breathlessness may develop. In severe

cases, coma, status epilepticus, tremor, ataxia, hyporeflexia, paraesthesiae, hallucinations, acute psychosis, and polyneuropathy may be found. Proteinuria, oliguria (due to renal tubular and cortical necrosis), and jaundice have been described. Long-term exposure to methyl bromide may lead to a chronic polyneuropathy, lethargy, personality changes, intolerance of alcohol, dysarthria, and epilepsy.
Treatment The casualty should be removed promptly from the contaminated atmosphere and undressed, as methyl bromide can penetrate clothing and rubber gloves. Contaminated skin should be washed with water. Treatment is supportive.

Further reading

De Haro, L., Gastaut, J., Jouglard, J., and Renacco, E. (1997). Central and peripheral neurotoxic effects of chronic methyl bromide intoxication. *Clinical Toxicology*, **35**, 29–34.

Hustinx, W.N.M., van de Laar, R.T.H., van Huffelen, A.C., Verwey J.C., Meulenbelt, J., and Savelkoul, T.J.F. (1993). Systemic effects of inhalational methyl bromide poisoning: a study of nine cases occupationally exposed due to inadvertent spread during fumigation. *British Journal of Industrial Medicine*, **50**, 155–9.

Methyl chloride (chloromethane)

Methyl chloride is a colourless gas used in the production of butyl rubber, tetramethyl lead, and polystyrene foams. Absorption may occur through the skin or by inhalation.
Mechanisms of toxicity Methyl chloride causes marked glutathione depletion.
Clinical features Symptoms may be delayed; they include CNS depression and hepatic, renal, and haematological damage. Following acute poisoning, many patients develop gastrointestinal disturbances, headache, drowsiness, giddiness, ataxia, convulsions, and coma. Chronic exposure may lead to confusion, blurred of vision, slurred speech, staggering gait, and convulsions.
Treatment After evacuation from exposure and removal of contaminated clothing, treatment is symptomatic. Glutathione repletion with *N*-acetylcysteine may be helpful.

Methylene chloride (dichloromethane)

Methylene chloride is used as a paint remover, solvent for plastic films and cements, degreaser, and aerosol propellant.
Mechanism of toxicity Methylene chloride is metabolized to carbon dioxide and carbon monoxide. Carboxyhaemoglobin concentrations of 3–10 per cent (exceptionally 40 per cent) are attained.
Clinical features Skin contact with liquid methylene chloride can be painful. Following inhalation, dizziness, tingling and numbness of the extremities, throbbing headache, nausea, irritability, fatigue, and stupor have been reported. Severe and prolonged exposure may lead to irritative conjunctivitis, lacrimation, respiratory depression, and death. Hepatorenal dysfunction and pulmonary oedema have also been described. Features of acute carbon monoxide poisoning may occur.
Treatment Prompt removal from exposure usually results in complete recovery. Oxygen should be given.

Further reading

Illing, H.P.A. and Shillaker, R.O. (1985). *Toxicity Review. Dichloromethane (methylene chloride)*. HMSO, London.

Metoclopramide

Overdose causes acute dystonic reactions affecting the eyes, tongue, and neck.
Treatment Gastric lavage and activated charcoal may be considered if the patient presents less than one hour after a substantial overdose. Benztropine (1–2 mg in an adult) should be given intravenously if extrapyramidal features are present. Alternatively, diazepam (5–10 mg intravenously) is effective and has the additional advantage of alleviating anxiety and agitation.

Further reading

Miller, L.G. and Jankovic, J. (1989). Metoclopramide-induced movement disorders. *Archives of Internal Medicine*, **149**, 2486–92.

Monoamine-oxidase inhibitors (MAOIs)

Phenalzine, tranylcypromine, and moclobemide are used sometimes to treat depression.
Clinical features Symptoms, due principally to increased sympathetic activity, may be delayed for 12–24 hours after acute overdosage. They include excitement, restlessness (which may be extreme), hyperpyrexia, hyperreflexia, convulsions, opisthotonos, rhabdomyolysis, and coma. Cardiovascular effects include sinus tachycardia and either hypotension or hypertension.
Treatment Gastric lavage and activated charcoal may be considered if the patient presents less than one hour after a substantial overdose. Convulsions and marked excitement are controlled with diazepam. Dantrolene is indicated to minimize the risk of hyperpyrezia and rhabdomyolysis. Hypotension should, in the first instance, be treated by fluid replacement to restore a normal circulating blood volume. Sympathomimetic drugs should be avoided. Hypertension should be treated by the administration of an α-adrenoceptor blocker, such as chlorpromazine.

Natural gas (methane, ethane)

Natural gas contains methane and ethane which are pharmacologically inert and can be tolerated in high concentrations without producing any toxic effects. However, if present in very high concentration (>80 per cent) in poorly ventilated areas, they may produce asphyxia.

Nickel

See OTM3, pp. 1112–3.

Nitrates

Organic nitrates relax smooth muscle cells and undergo extensive 'first pass' metabolism in the liver.
Clinical features Symptoms are attributable to arteriolar and venous dilatation. Headache and vomiting are common, with skin flushing and dizziness. Sinus tachycardia, severe orthostatic hypotension, syncope, convulsions, and coma may develop. Methaemoglobinaemia is rare.
Treatment Mild hypotension may be treated by placing the patient in a head-down position but more severe hypotension will require plasma expanders or a vasopressor agent.

Nitrogen dioxide

Combustion of fossil fuels yields nitrogen dioxide and nitric oxide. Fermentation of silage produces high concentrations within 2 days of filling the silo. It is also a byproduct of many industrial processes.

Clinical features Modest acute exposure (<50 p.p.m.) for a short time often produces no immediate symptoms, although throat irritation, cough, transient choking, tightness in the chest, and sweating have been observed. Massive exposure (e.g. in a silo) can produce severe and immediate hypoxaemia, which may be fatal. In less severe cases, symptoms may be delayed for 3–36 hours; there may be dyspnoea, chest pain (which may be pleuritic), haemoptysis, tachycardia, headache, conjunctivitis, generalized weakness, and dizziness (which may be due to hypotension). Bronchiolitis obliterans may develop within 2–6 weeks.

Treatment Bronchodilator and corticosteroid therapy is sufficient in most cases. Pulmonary oedema responds poorly to diuretics; corticosteroids and mechanical ventilation with positive end-expiratory pressure offer the best hope of reducing the mortality.

Further reading

Berglund, M., Boström, C-E., Bylin, G., *et al.* (1993). Health risk evaluation of nitrogen oxides. *Scandinavian Journal of Work, Environment and Health*, **19** (Suppl.2), 1–72.

Opiates and opioids (see also Section 14)

Acute opioid overdose occurs commonly in 'addicts'. Venipuncture marks and thrombosed veins in the arms and legs suggest the diagnosis.

Clinical features Cardinal signs are pinpoint pupils, reduced respiratory rate (often accompanied by cyanosis), and coma. Depressant effects are increased by alcohol. Hypotension, due to peripheral vasodilation, occurs in less than 10 per cent of cases. Hypothermia and hypoglycaemia may complicate the clinical picture.

Methadone poses particular problems because of its long half-life. As many as 50 per cent of heroin overdose victims develop non-cardiogenic pulmonary oedema, the majority of whom, in turn, develop bacterial pneumonia.

Codeine, dextropropoxyphene, and pethidine cause increased muscle tone, twitching, and convulsions. Rhabdomyolysis and its complications have been reported in diamorphine, dihydrocodeine, dipipanone, methadone, and morphine poisoning.

Management Naloxone reverses respiratory depression and coma due to opioid poisoning. In adults 0.8–1.2 mg is given either intravenously or, less satisfactorily, intramuscularly; the dose in children is 5–10 µg/kg body weight. If the diagnosis of opioid poisoning is correct, the patient should improve within 1 minute with an increase in respiratory rate, an improvement in the level of consciousness, and dilatation of the pupils. In severe opioid poisoning, larger initial doses of naloxone (e.g. 2.4 mg) may be needed. The duration of action of naloxone (1–4 hours) is often less than that of the drug taken in overdose and so careful observation is essential and repeated doses of naloxone may be required. The respiratory-depressant effects of pentazocine and buprenorphine are only partially reversed by naloxone and assisted ventilation may be required.

Gastric lavage and the administration of activated charcoal may be of value if an opioid had been ingested in overdose less than one hour previously.

The development of non-cardiogenic pulmonary oedema may necessitate the use of assisted ventilation. Antibiotics will be required to treat secondary bacterial infection. Hyperkalaemia and renal failure, as a result of rhabdomyolysis, should be treated conventionally.

Organophosphorus insecticides

Organophosphorus compounds are widely used pesticides.

Mechanisms of toxicity They inhibit acetylcholinesterase, causing accumulation of acetylcholine at central and peripheral cholinergic nerve endings, including neuromuscular junctions.

Clinical features Minor exposure may produce subclinical poisoning in which there is reduction of cholinesterase activity but no symptoms or signs. Poisoning is characterized by anxiety, restlessness, insomnia, nightmares, tiredness, dizziness, headache, and muscarinic features such as nausea, vomiting, abdominal colic, diarrhoea, tenesmus, sweating, hypersalivation, and chest tightness. Miosis may be present. Nicotinic effects follow with muscle fasciculation and flaccid paresis of limb muscles, respiratory muscles, and, occasionally, various combinations of extraocular muscle. Respiratory failure is exacerbated by pulmonary oedema and by retention of bronchial secretions. Coma and convulsions may occur. Hyperglycaemia and glycosuria have been reported though ketonuria is absent. Bradycardia occurs in only about 20 per cent of cases. Complete heart block and other arrhythmias are rare.

Diagnosis In the absence of a history of exposure gastroenteritis is a common misdiagnosis. The findings of glycosuria and hyperglycaemia may suggest diabetic pretoma. Miosis is an important diagnostic sign but is not invariable. Reduced plasma, or preferably erythrocyte, cholinesterase activity confirms the diagnosis. In subclinical poisoning cholinesterase activity may be reduced by up to 50 per cent while mild, moderate, and severe poisoning are associated with reduction of cholinesterase activity to approximately 20–50, 10–20, and less than 10 per cent of normal respectively.

Treatment Patients with subclinical poisoning should be kept under observation for about 24 hours to ensure that delayed toxicity does not develop. In patients with symptomatic poisoning soiled clothing should be removed and contaminated skin washed with soap and water to prevent further absorption. Gastric lavage should be considered if the insecticide has been ingested less than one hour previously. A clear airway, effective removal of respiratory secretions, and correction of hypoxia are essential, using endotracheal intubation and assisted ventilation if necessary. The early use of diazepam may reduce morbidity and mortality; 5–10 mg intravenously for an adult reduces anxiety and restlessness but larger doses may be required to control convulsions.

Atropine 2 mg intravenously every 10–30 minutes for an adult, depending on the severity of poisoning, should be given to reduce bronchorrhoea and bronchospasm or until signs of atropinization (flushed dry skin, tachycardia, dilated pupils, and dry mouth) develop. As much as 30 mg and occasionally much more may be required in the first 24 hours. Children should be given 0.02 mg/kg body weight but may require up to 0.05 mg/kg.

Pralidoxime mesylate (P2S) reactivates phosphorylated acetylcholinesterase and should be given together with atropine to every symptomatic patient. The dose is 30 mg/kg body weight by slow intravenous injection. Improvement will usually be apparent within 30 minutes. Further bolus doses of pralidoxime may be required every 4–6 hours. Alternatively, an infusion of pralidoxime 8–10 mg/kg body weight/hour may be administered. Monitoring of erythrocyte (not plasma) cholinesterase activity together with clinical signs guides therapy.

Complications A few patients develop 'intermediate syndrome', comprising cranial nerve and brain-stem lesions and a proximal neuropathy starting 1–4 days after acute intoxication and persisting for

Table 6 Clinical features of paracetamol poisoning

Day 1 Asymptomatic Nausea, vomiting, abdominal pain, anorexia
Day 2 May become asymptomatic Vomiting Hepatic tenderness ± generalized abdominal pain Occasionally, mild jaundice
Day 3 (in severe untreated poisoning) Jaundice → liver failure → hepatic encephalopathy Back pain + renal angle tenderness → renal failure Disseminated intravascular coagulation Cardiac arrhythmias → cardiac arrest Pancreatitis

2–3 weeks. Muscle weakness may cause respiratory failure. Longer-term complications include tiredness, insomnia, inability to concentrate, depression, irritability, and peripheral neuropathy.

Further reading

Ballantyne, B. and Marrs, T.C. (1992). *Organophosphates and carbamates.* Butterworth-Heinemann, Oxford.

Okumura, T., Takasu, N., Ishimatsu, S., *et al.* (1996). Report on 640 victims of the Tokyo subway sarin attack. *Annals of Emergency Medicine*, **28**, 129–35.

Thiermann, H., Mast, U., Klimmek, R., *et al.* (1997). Cholinesterase status, pharmacokinetics and laboratory findings during obidoxime therapy in organophosphate poisoned patients. *Human and Experimental Toxicology*, **16**, 473–80.

Paracetamol (acetaminophen)

Mechanism of toxicity In therapeutic doses, 5–10 per cent of paracetamol is oxidized to a highly reactive compound (*N*-acetyl-*p*-benzoquinoneimine, NAPQI) which is conjugated with glutathione and excreted. In overdose, larger amounts of paracetamol are metabolized by oxidation, liver glutathione stores become depleted, and NAPQI binds to liver cell macromolecules, disrupting cellular architecture and function.

The severity of paracetamol poisoning is dose-related. An absorbed dose of 15 g (200 mg/kg) or more is potentially serious in most patients. There is, however, some variation in individual susceptibility to paracetamol-induced hepatotoxicity and patients with pre-existing liver disease, those with a high alcohol intake, and those receiving enzyme-inducing drugs are at a greater risk. HIV-seropositive people are also vunerable to paracetamol-induced hepatic damage.

Clinical features Patients usually remain asymptomatic or develop anorexia, nausea, and vomiting during the first 24 hours or so (Table 6).

Liver damage is not usually detectable by routine liver function tests until at least 18 hours after ingestion of the drug. Maximum liver damage, as assessed by plasma alanine or aspartate aminotransferase (ALT, AST) activity or prothrombin time, occurs 72–96 hours after ingestion. Hepatic failure, manifest by jaundice and encephalopathy, may then develop between the third and fifth day. More usually there is prolongation of the prothrombin time and a marked rise in aminotransferase activity without the development of

Table 7 Biochemical and haematological abnormalities

AST/ALT ↑↑
Bilirubin ↑
Blood glucose ↓
Creatinine ↑
Lactate ↑
Phosphate ↓
Amylase ↑
PT ↑
Platelets ↓
Clotting factors II ↓ V ↓ VII ↓

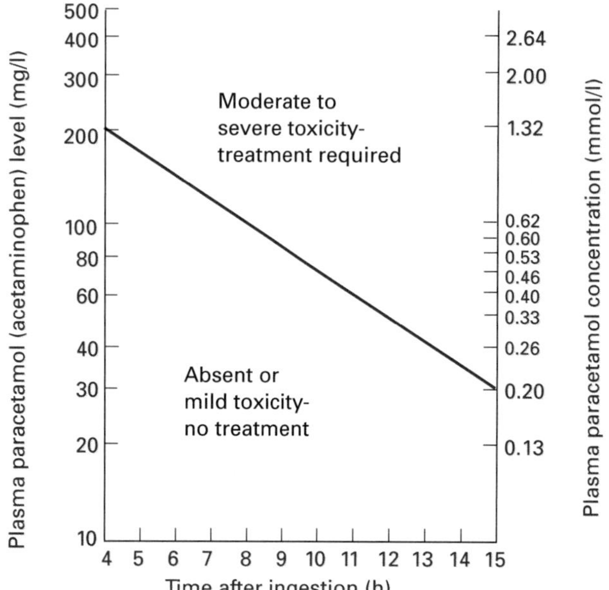

Fig. 1 Graph for use in prediction of liver damage caused by paracetamol and the need for administration of specific protective treatment (see text for further details).

fulminant hepatic failure (Table 7). Acute tubular necrosis develops in about 25 per cent of patients with severe hepatic damage and in a few without serious disturbance of liver function.

In very severe paracetamol poisoning (plasma paracetamol concentration >500 mg/l at 4 hours after ingestion) metabolic acidosis may be associated with coma. Hypophosphataemia, a recognized complication of acute liver failure, may contribute to morbidity and mortality.

Prediction of liver damage The dose ingested is commonly unreliable. However, a single measurement of the plasma paracetamol concentration is an accurate predictor of liver damage provided that it is taken not earlier than 4 hours after ingestion of the overdose. A graph may be used to predict liver damage and to indicate the need for specific treatment with oral methionine or intravenous/ oral *N*-acetylcysteine (Fig. 1). Twelve hours after ingestion, the plasma paracetamol level is still valuable if considered with changes in the prothrombin time (see below).

Prognostic factors The overall untreated mortality of paracetamol poisoning is about 5 per cent. A prothrombin time of more than 20

Table 8 Antidote regimens for paracetamol poisoning

Methionine (orally) 2.5 g initially, then 2.5 g 4-hourly for a further three doses. Total dose 10 g methionine over 12 hours.
N-Acetylcysteine (intravenously) 150 mg/kg over 15 minutes, then 50 mg/kg in 500 ml of 5% dextrose in the next 4 hours and 100 mg/kg in 1000 ml of 5% dextrose over the ensuing 16 hours
Total dose 300 mg/kg over 20 h.
N-Acetylcysteine (orally) 140 mg/kg initially, then 60 mg/kg every 4 hours for 17 additional doses. Total dose 2330 mg/kg over 72 hours

seconds at 24 hours after ingestion indicates that significant hepatic damage has been sustained, and a peak of more than 180 seconds is associated with a chance of survival of less than 8 per cent. Systemic acidosis developing more than 24 hours after overdose, a rise in serum creatinine concentration, and a coagulation Factor VIII/V ratio above 30 indicate a poor prognosis.

Treatment Gastric lavage should be considered if the patient presents less than one hour after a substantial overdose. Alternatively, activated charcoal 50 g may be administered. Parenteral fluid replacement should be given for the first 1 or 2 days after overdose if nausea or vomiting persists.

Methionine and *N*-acetylcysteine ('Parvolex') protect the liver by replenishing cellular glutathione stores. To prevent hepatic damage completely they must be given within 8–10 hours of paracetamol ingestion. Up to 10 per cent of patients treated with intravenous *N*-acetylcysteine develop rashes, angio-oedema, hypotension, and bronchospasm. The infusion should be stopped temporarily and, if the reaction is severe, an antihistamine such as chlorpheniramine given, but these reactions are seldom serious and no fatalities have been reported in patients given the regimen in Table 8.

Only a few patients present more than 12–24 hours after the overdose. In these cases, the morbidity and mortality is greater; 10 per cent glucose is administered to prevent hypoglycaemia and fresh frozen plasma to correct severe coagulation abnormalities. Acute renal failure should be managed conventionally.

If fulminant hepatic failure supervenes, continued intravenous *N*-acetylcysteine may reduce morbidity and mortality even after the onset of encephalopathy and other signs of severe liver damage.

Liver transplantation has been performed successfully in patients with paracetamol-induced fulminant hepatic failure.

Further reading

Jones, A.L. and Prescott, L.F. (1997). Unusual complications of paracetamol poisoning. *Quarterly Journal of Medicine*, **90**, 161–8.

Keayes, P., *et al.* (1991). Intravenous acetylcysteine in paracetamol induced fulminant hepatic failure: a prospective controlled trial. *British Medical Journal*, **303**, 1026–9.

Makin, A.J., Wendon, J., and Williams, R. (1995). A 7-year experience of severe acetaminophen-induced hepatotoxicity (1987–1993). *Gastroenterology*, **109**, 1907–16.

Vale, J.A. and Proudfoot, A.T. (1995). Paracetamol (acetaminophen) poisoning. *Lancet*, **346**, 547–52.

Paraffin oil (kerosene)

Clinical features Repeated local application to the skin results in dryness, dermatitis, and, rarely, epidermal necrolysis. Pulmonary toxicity may occur within one hour of ingestion and aspiration and is characterized by pyrexia, cough, tachypnoea, tachycardia, basal crepitations, and cyanosis. Non-segmental consolidation or collapse is seen radiologically. Pneumatoceles, pneumothorax, pleural effusion, or pulmonary oedema may occur later.

Paraffin ingestion causes respiratory symptoms, a burning sensation in the mouth and throat, vomiting, diarrhoea, abdominal pain and mild hepatomegaly with hepatic dysfunction, and in severe cases atrial fibrillation and ventricular fibrillation.

Treatment Lavage may be considered in adults who have ingested very large quantities of paraffin oil only if the airway can be protected and the procedure can be carried out within the first hour. Corticosteroids and antibiotics have not proved useful. Mechanical ventilation with positive end-expiratory pressure may be necessary in severe cases of aspiration.

Further reading

Baldachin, B.J. and Melmed, R.N. (1964). Clinical and therapeutic aspects of kerosene poisoning : a series of 200 cases. *British Medical Journal*, **2**, 28–30.

Paraquat and related herbicides

The bipyridilium herbicides include diquat, morfamquat, and paraquat.

Clinical features Careless handling has led to reversible changes in the finger nails. Inhalation of spray may cause pain in the throat and epistaxis. Prolonged dermal exposure may cause burns and allow enough paraquat to be absorbed to cause systemic poisoning. Splashes in the eye cause blepharospasm, lacrimation, and corneal ulceration.

Probably no more than 5 per cent of ingested paraquat is absorbed but absorption is rapid, the volume of distribution is high, and there is energy-dependent accumulation particularly in the lungs. Elimination is mainly through the kidneys.

Ingestion of 6 g or more of paraquat ion is likely to be fatal within 24–48 hours while 3–6 g is likely to lead to a more protracted, but still fatal, outcome. Nausea, vomiting, abdominal pain, and diarrhoea, rapidly followed by peripheral circulatory failure, metabolic acidosis, impaired consciousness, convulsions, and increasing breathlessness and cyanosis secondary to acute pneumonitis, are the features of ingestion of large amounts of paraquat. With smaller amounts, the cardiovascular and CNS complications are not seen and the course of poisoning is dominated by alimentary features, particularly painful ulceration of the mouth, tongue, and throat, making it difficult to swallow, speak, and cough. Perforation of the oesophagus causes mediastinitis. Mild jaundice may be seen and renal failure is usually severe. Breathlessness, tachypnoea, widespread crepitations, and central cyanosis may be present by 5–7 days after ingestion and progress relentlessly until the patient dies from hypoxia a few days later.

Ingestion of 1.5–2.0 g of paraquat causes nausea, vomiting and diarrhoea, mild renal tubular necrosis, and pain in the throat. Respiratory involvement may not appear for 10–21 days after ingestion, but may progress till the patient dies of respiratory failure 5–6 weeks later.

Diagnosis The diagnosis can be readily confirmed by a simple qualitative test on urine.

Treatment Administration of activated charcoal is probably more effective than gastric lavage in reducing absorption. Antiemetics, mouth washes, analgesics, and intravenous fluids may be necessary to replace gastrointestinal losses. Skin ulcers should be treated as burns. Currently available techniques are not effective in rapidly removing toxicologically significant quantities of paraquat. There is no evidence that corticosteroids, drugs to prevent free radical formation, free radical scavengers, immunosuppressive agents, radiotherapy to the lungs, or lung transplantation reduce mortality. Early plasma paraquat concentrations help to determine the prognosis. Poisons information services will advise on interpretation.

Further reading

Second European Symposium on Paraquat Poisoning. (1987). *Human Toxicology*, 6, 3–98.

Petrol (gasoline)

Petrol is a complex mixture of hydrocarbons containing a small proportion of non-hydrocarbon additives.

Acute exposure Following the inhalation, dizziness and irritation of the eyes, nose, and throat may occur within 5 minutes followed by euphoria, headache, and blurred vision. If inhalation continues, or significant quantities of petrol are ingested, excitement and depression of the nervous system occurs; inco-ordination, restlessness, excitement, confusion, disorientation, hallucinations, ataxia, nystagmus, tremor, delirium, coma, and convulsions may be seen. Inhalation of high concentrations may cause immediate death, probably from ventricular fibrillation or acute respiratory failure. Chemical pneumonitis may occur as in paraffin oil ingestion (see above) and the clinical features and management are then identical. Intravascular haemolysis, hypofibrinogenaemia, cardiorespiratory arrest, and epiglottitis have been reported.

Chronic exposure Men engaged in cleaning storage tanks and those who habitually sniff may develop both hydrocarbon and lead poisoning.

Treatment Following removal from exposure, supportive measures provide the basis of treatment. Gastric lavage should be considered only if a large amount of petrol has been ingested by an adult within the previous hour and the airway is protected.

Phencyclidine (PCP)

Pseudonyms include PCP, Peace pill, hog, goon, crystal, and angel dust. It is usually smoked with tobacco or marijuana and may also be ingested or injected.

Clinical features There is initial euphoria, a feeling of dissociation, numbness, perceptual distortion, hallucinations, visual nystagmus, hypertension, and tachycardia and hypothermia occurs more frequently than hyperthermia. Severe intoxication may be complicated by hypersalivation, profuse sweating, generalized seizures, prolonged psychotic reactions, dystonias, and hypoglycaemia. Rhabdomyolysis and acute renal failure are common.

Behavioural disturbances include disorientation and confusion with inappropriate affect, a catatonic syndrome with stupor, posturing, catalepsy, mutism, and staring. A minority show bizarre behaviour with excitement, agitation, and a tendency to violence.

Treatment Treatment is supportive and symptomatic. The plasma glucose concentration should be checked and hypoglycaemia treated. Sedation may be necessary.

Phenol ('carbolic acid')

Clinical features If phenol is spilt on the skin, pain is followed promptly by numbness as afferent nerve endings become damaged. The skin becomes blanched, and a dry opaque eschar forms over the burn. When the eschar sloughs off, a brown stain remains. Phenol penetrates intact skin rapidly and is well absorbed through the lungs. After ingestion, vomiting and abdominal pain occur. Systemic toxicity may follow exposure through any route.

Features include coma, loss of vasoconstrictor tone, hypothermia, and cardiac and respiratory depression. Initial central nervous system stimulation, and rarely convulsions, has been observed in children. Grey or black urine, Heinz body haemolytic anaemia, methaemoglobinaemia, and hyperbilirubinaemia are recognized features. Renal complications are common.

Treatment Gastric lavage may be considered if the patient presents less than one hour after ingestion and severe oropharyngeal burns are not suspected. Skin and eye contamination, renal failure, and methaemoglobinaemia are managed appropriately.

Phenothiazines

The phenothiazines block peripheral cholinergic and α-adrenergic receptors, reuptake of amines, and the effects of histamines and 5-hydroxytryptamine.

Clinical features Impairment of consciousness, hypotension, and respiratory depression may develop. Chlorpromazine, perphenazine, and promazine seem more prone to cause hypotension and hypothermia. Anticholinergic effects with tachycardia, ECG changes, and arrhythmias are most common with overdosage of thioridazine and mesoridazine. Acute spasmodic torticollis, oculogyric crises, and orolingual dyskinesias are associated with trifluperazine and prochlorperazine.

Treatment Gastric lavage should be considered if a substantial overdose has been ingested less than one hour previously. Alternatively, activated charcoal (50–100g) should be administered. Acute dystonic reactions should be treated appropriately.

Phenylbutazone

Clinical features See Table 9.

Treatment is supportive and symptomatic.

Phenylpropionic (arylpropionic) acid derivatives

Clinical features Propionic acid derivative poisoning causes nausea, vomiting, abdominal pain, drowsiness, headache, tinnitus, ataxia,

Table 9 Clinical features of poisoning from phenylbutazone

Nausea, vomiting, abdominal pain, gastrointestinal haemorrhage, diarrhoea
Restlessness, agitation, disorientation, hyperthermia, tinnitus, deafness
Respiratory alkalosis (due to hyperventilation, metabolic acidosis, hyperglycaemia, sodium and water retention
Hypotension, sinus tachycardia, cardiorespiratory collapse, sometimes followed by cardiac arrest
Coma, convulsions, nystagmus, hypertonia, hyper-reflexia, extensor plantar responses
Hepatic dysfunction, cholestatic jaundice
Acute renal failure
Hypoprothrombinaemia, thrombocytopenia, leucopenia, leucocytosis, haematuria, red discoloration of urine (due to metabolite)

stupor, and, rarely, coma and convulsions. Hypoventilation, bronchospasm, and hypotension occur more importantly; gastrointestinal haemorrhage and renal failure are rare but reported complications. *Treatment* is supportive.

Phenytoin

Clinical features Acute overdose of phenytoin results in nausea, vomiting, headache, tremor, cerebellar ataxia, nystagmus, and, rarely, loss of consciousness.
Treatment Gastric lavage may be considered if the patient presents within one hour after a substantial overdose. Multiple-dose activated charcoal may increase elimination.

Phosgene

Phosgene is a colourless gas used in the manufacture of isocyanates, polyurethane and polycarbonate resins, dyes, and produced in fires.
Mechanism of toxicity Phosgene reacts with glutathione. When glutathione stores are depleted beyond a critical level binding occurs between phosgene and cell macromolecules causing hepatic and renal necrosis.
Clinical features Exposure causes irritation of the eyes, a dryness or burning sensation in the throat, cough, chest pain, and nausea and vomiting. There is usually a latent period of between 30 minutes and 24 hours followed by the development of pulmonary oedema due to increased capillary permeability; circulatory collapse may follow.
Treatment Administration of *N*-acetylcysteine may confer some protection. Oxygen and bronchodilators should be administered Mechanical ventilation may be life-saving in severe cases.

Further reading

Diller, W.F. and Zante, R. (1985). A literature review: Therapy for phosgene poisoning. *Toxicology and Industrial Health*, 1, 117–28.

Phosphine

Phosphine, a colourless gas with a fish-like odour, is used to fumigate against insects and rodents in stored grain, and in the semiconductor industry.
Clinical features Fatigue, nausea, vomiting, diarrhoea, chest tightness, breathlessness, productive cough, dizziness, and headache are common features of acute exposure. Acute pulmonary oedema, hypertension, cardiac arrhythmias, and convulsions have been described in severe cases. Ataxia, intention tremor, and diplopia may be found on examination.
Treatment The casualty should be removed from exposure as soon as possible. Treatment is symptomatic.

Further reading

IPCS. (1988). *Environmental Health Criteria 73. Phosphine and selected metal phosphides.* WHO, Geneva.

Propylene glycol (1,2-propanediol)

Propylene glycol is used as a preservative, as a vehicle for both oral and intravenous medications, and in preparations used for treating burns.

Mechanism of toxicity

Propylene glycol is oxidized to lactic acid and pyruvate.
Clinical features Ingestion or absorption of large quantities of propylene glycol may cause convulsions, coma, cardiac arrhythmias, hepatorenal damage, intravascular haemolysis, metabolic acidosis, and increased serum osmolality.
Treatment Gastric lavage should be considered if the patient presents within one hour after ingestion. Metabolic acidosis, renal failure, and respiratory depression should be treated conventionally. Haemodialysis removes propylene glycol efficiently.

Pyrethroids

Clinical features Pyrethroids can cause facial paraesthesiae following occupational exposure. After ingestion, percutaneous absorption or inhalational exposure, coma, convulsions, and pulmonary oedema may occur.
Treatment Symptomatic and supportive measures should be employed and reassurance given that facial paraethesiae will not be a long-term problem.

Pyridoxine

High doses (>2–3 g/day) have been used to treat premenstrual syndrome, carpal-tunnel syndrome, schizophrenia, and childhood hyperactivity.
Clinical features Prolonged daily intake of 50–300 mg in women has been reported to cause headaches, irritability, tiredness, shooting pains, circumoral, and limb paraesthesiae, numb extremities, clumsiness, and ataxia, indicating a sensory neuropathy.
Treatment Improvement occurs within 2 months of stopping the drug. There is no specific treatment.

Quinidine and quinine

These are diastereoisomers. Quinine is more oculotoxic and quinidine is more cardiotoxic in overdose. Poisoning may be iatrogenic, suicidal, or from attempted abortion or adulterated heroin (quinine).
Clinical features Doses as low as 2 g can be toxic in adults. Cinchonism (tinnitus, deafness, vertigo, nausea, headache, and diarrhoea) and hypoglycaemia are common at plasma concentrations greater than 5mg/l. In more serious poisoning, collapse with impairment of consciousness (due to ventricular arrhythmias), convulsions, rapid shallow breathing, hypotension, pulmonary oedema and cardiorespiratory arrest may be observed. Ventricular tachycardia and fibrillation and depression of automaticity and intracardiac conduction are potentially lethal. Pulmonary oedema and acute renal failure have been described. About 40 per cent of patients poisoned with quinine develop ocular features, which may be unilateral, including blindness, contracted visual fields, scotomata, dilated pupils, blurred disc margins, macular oedema, arteriolar spasm, and late optic atrophy. Oculotoxicity is likely when plasma concentrations exceed 10 mg/l. Visual loss is permanent in about 50 per cent of cases.
Treatment Gastric lavage is indicated if the patient presents within one hour of ingestion or, alternatively, activated charcoal (50–100 g) may be administered. Multiple doses of activated charcoal increase quinine clearance. Forced diuresis, charcoal haemoperfusion, haemodialysis, stellate ganglion block, and calcium-channel blockers are of no value. Electrolyte and acid–base disturbances and hypoglycaemia should be corrected. Bradyarrhythmias may respond to isoprenaline; overdrive pacing may be required if torsade de pointes occurs. Plasma expanders should be given for hypotension but if the response is poor, an inotrope should be administered.

Further reading

Jaeger, A., Sauder, P., Kopferschmitt, J., and Flesch, F. (1987). Clinical features and management of poisoning due to antimalaria drugs. *Medical Toxicology*, 2, 242–73.

Kim, S.Y. and Benowitz, N.L. (1990). Poisoning due to Class 1A antiarrhythmic drugs: quinidine, procainamide and disopyramide. *Drug Safety*, 5, 393–420.

Rifampicin

Clinical features Poisoning causes 'red man syndrome' which can be fatal. The skin, and subsequently the sclerae, become yellow-orange but the skin discoloration may washed away. This is caused by the intense colour of rifampicin and its metabolites. Nausea, vomiting, abdominal pain , pruritus, a sensation of the skin burning, and convulsions also occur, and less commonly, marked oedema of the forehead, cheeks, chin, and lips with associated eosinophilia. Elevation in serum activities of hepatic enzymes and bilirubin have been noted.
Treatment Gastric lavage may be considered if the patient presents within one hour of a substantial overdose.

Further reading

Holdiness, M.R. (1989). A review of the red man syndrome and rifampicin overdose. *Medical Toxicology and Adverse Drug Experience*, 4, 444–51.

Salicylates

Poisoning is accidental, iatrogenic, or suicidal, and may result from percutaneous absorption of salicylic acid used in keratolytic agents, and ingestion of methyl salicylate ('oil of wintergreen').
Pharmacokinetics and toxicity After overdose, plasma salicylate concentrations may continue to rise for up to 24 hours. Salicyluric acid and salicylphenolic glucuronide formation (Fig. 2) is saturated and renal excretion of salicylate acid becomes increasingly important. This is extremely sensitive to changes in urinary pH.
Mechanisms of toxicity There is direct stimulation of the respiratory centre resulting in hyperventilation and respiratory alkalosis. To compensate, bicarbonate, sodium, and potassium, are excreted in the urine. Dehydration and hypokalaemia result, and the loss of bicarbonate diminishes the buffering capacity allowing acidosis to develop. High brain salicylate concentrations depress the respiratory centre, further increasing acidaemia. Salicylates uncouple oxidative phosphorylation, stimulate nausea and vomiting, and cause hypoglycaemia and hypoprothombinaemia.
Clinical features and assessment of severity of salicylate intoxication The plasma salicylate concentration should be determined on admission

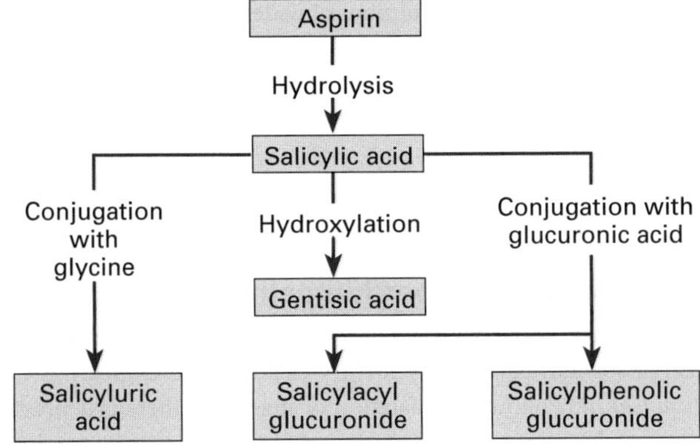

Fig. 2 The principal biotransformation pathways of aspirin.

Table 10 Clinical features of salicylate poisoning

Clinical features
Nausea, vomiting, and epigastric discomfort
Irritability, tremor, tinnitus, deafness, blurring of vision
Hyperpyrexia, sweating, dehydration
Tachypnoea and hyperpnoea
Non-cardiogenic pulmonary oedema
Acute renal failure
Mixed respiratory alkalosis and metabolic acidosis (except in children who usually develop metabolic acidosis alone)
Hypokalaemia, hypernatraemia, or hyponatraemia
Hyperglycaemia or hypoglycaemia
Hypoprothrombinaemia (rare)
Confusion, delirium, stupor, and coma (in severe cases)

Table 11 Management of salicylate poisoning

Management
Gastric lavage or administration of activated charcoal up to one hour after ingestion
Correction of dehydration either orally or parenterally
Correction of hypokalaemia
Correction of hypoglycaemia
Correction of severe metabolic acidosis with intravenous bicarbonate
Tepid sponging for hyperpyrexia
Alkalinization of the urine if blood salicylate concentration >500 mg/l (particularly if metabolic acidosis is present)
Consider haemodialysis if neurological features are present, the serum salicylate concentration is >700 mg/l or if severe acidosis supervenes

and repeated 2 hours later to detect slow absorption, in which case it should be checked again after a further 2 hours. Plasma salicylate concentrations between 300 and 500 mg/l 6 hours after an overdose are associated with only mild toxicity, levels between 500 and 700 mg/l with moderate toxicity; and those in excess of 700 mg/l with severe poisoning.

Salicylate poisoning of any severity is associated with sweating, vomiting, epigastric pain, tinnitus, and deafness (Table 10). Acidaemia allows salicylates to penetrate tissues more readily and leads, in particular, to CNS toxicity. Pulmonary oedema is seen occasionally. It is often due to iatrogenic fluid overload but may be non-cardiac and associated with hypovolaemia. Gastric erosions and gastrointestinal bleeding are rare. Oliguria is usually attributable to dehydration but, rarely, acute renal failure may occur.
Treatment is summarized in Table 11. Sedatives and respiratory depressant drugs should be avoided. In patients with marked salicylism and blood salicylate levels of 500 mg/l alkaline diuresis should be induced. The target urine pH should be above 7.5. Haemodialysis is the treatment of choice for severely poisoned patients, particularly those with features of central nervous system toxicity and metabolic acidosis.

Further reading

Meredith, T.J. and Vale, J.A. (1992). Poisoning due to parcetamol, salicylates, and diflunisal. In: *Therapeutic applications of NSAIDs:*

subpopulations and new formulations. (ed. J.P. Famaey and H.E. Paulus), pp. 67–96. Marcel Dekker, New York.

Smoke

Smoke is a suspension in hot air of small carbon particles coated with organic acids and aldehydes together with gases generated by combustion. Carbon dioxide and carbon monoxide are usually major components. Other toxic compounds commonly contained in the gaseous phase, though not necessarily in high concentration, include acrolein, ammonia, chlorine, hydrogen bromide, hydrogen chloride, hydrogen cyanide, oxides of nitrogen, phosgene, phosphorus pentoxide, and sulphur dioxide.

Clinical features of smoke inhalation The main effects are asphyxia and severe pulmonary irritation and oedema. The release of carbon monoxide, hydrogen cyanide, and carbon dioxide in an enclosed space can cause death from asphyxia. Smaller particles, acids, and aldehydes cause lacrimation, burning of the throat, and nausea and vomiting when swallowed. Highly water soluble gases (e.g. hydrogen chloride, sulphur dioxide) cause immediate upper respiratory tract irritation, whereas gases with low solubility (e.g. chlorine, nitrogen dioxide, phosgene) penetrate further into the lung and cause injury to the distal airways and alveoli. Laryngitis and laryngeal oedema may progress to complete laryngeal obstruction over a period of several hours. Acute hypoxaemia can occur in the absence of notable respiratory symptoms and may cause ventricular ectopics, myocardial ischaemia, and cardiac arrhythmias in subjects with heart disease.

Treatment Casualties should be removed from the smoke and resuscitated. Humidified oxygen should be administered, with a nebulized bronchodilator such as salbutamol if bronchospasm is present. Carboxyhaemoglobin concentration should be obtained and arterial blood gases should be measured.

In case of exposure to burning plastics, the possibility of cyanide poisoning should be considered. Early fibreoptic laryngoscopy or bronchoscopy helps to assess the severity of subglottal injury. Evidence that corticosteroids protect against pulmonary injury is lacking.

Further reading

Hantson, P., Butera, R., Clemessy, J.L., Michel, A., and Baud, F.J. (1997). Early complications and value of initial clinical and paraclinical observations in victims of smoke inhalation without burns. *Chest*, **111**, 671–5.

Demling, R.H. (1993). Smoke inhalation injury. *New Horizons*, **1**, 422–34.

Sodium nitroprusside

This vasodilator is converted *in vivo* to nitric oxide and cyanide. Accumulation of cyanide and thiocyanate occurs if too high an infusion rate of nitroprusside is used.

Clinical features Hypotension may be corrected by reducing infusion rate. Metabolic (lactic) acidosis is usually the first indication of cyanide toxicity (see above). Thiocyanate accumulation may lead to anorexia, nausea, lethargy, fatigue, and psychosis.

Treatment During prolonged infusions the blood cyanide and thiocyanate concentrations should be measured and should not exceed 1 mg/l and 100 mg/l, respectively. The risk of toxicity can be reduced by not exceeding the recommended infusion rates and/or by giving sodium thiosulphate or hydroxocobalamin intravenously. Cyanide toxicity should be treated conventionally (see above).

Further reading

Johanning, R.J., Zaske, D.E., Tschida, S.J., Johnson, S.V., Hoey, L.L., and Vance-Bryan, K.A. (1995). A retrospective study of sodium nitroprusside use and assessment of the potential risk of cyanide poisoning. *Pharmacotherapy*, **15**, 773–7.

Sodium valproate

Clinical features There is impairment of consciousness and respiration and, in severe cases, abnormal liver function tests, hyperammonaemia, increased anion gap acidosis, hypocalcaemia, hypernatraemia, optic nerve atrophy, cerebral oedema, non-cardiogenic pulmonary oedema, renal failure, and pancreatitis.

Treatment Gastric lavage may be considered if the patient presents less than one hour after the ingestion of a substantial overdose, or activated charcoal may be given by mouth.

Further reading

Andersen, G.A. and Ritland, S. (1995). Life threatening intoxication with sodium valproate. *Clinical Toxicology*, **33**, 279–84.

Styrene (vinyl benzene)

Styrene, a yellowish liquid with a pleasant sweet odour is used in the production of plastics.

Mechanism of toxicity Styrene oxide binds covalently to cellular macromolecules when glutathione has been depleted.

Clinical features Exposure is by inhalation and absorption through the skin and gut. It is irritant to the eyes, skin, mucous membranes, and respiratory system accompanied by mucous secretion, a metallic taste, drowsiness, vertigo, and CNS depression.

Treatment The victim should be removed from further exposure, the skin washed, and the eyes irrigated. *N*-Acetylcysteine might protect the liver.

Sulphur dioxide

This colourless gas has a pungent irritating odour. It is the product of burning fuels and is used to manufacture sulphuric acid and may therefore be an occupational problem in paper mills, steel works, and oil refineries.

Clinical features Lacrimation, rhinorrhoea, cough, increased bronchial secretions, bronchoconstriction, and, in severe cases, pulmonary oedema and respiratory arrest occur. Corneal burns can follow eye exposure and liquefied sulphur dioxide can cause skin burns.

Treatment After removal from exposure, victims must be admitted to hospital in case delayed pulmonary oedema develops. The role of corticosteroids is uncertain.

Further reading

IPCS. (1979). *Environmental Health Criteria 8. Sulfur oxides and suspended particulate matter.* WHO, Geneva.

Tetrachloroethylene (perchloroethylene)

This colourless liquid with a chloroform-like odour is used as an industrial solvent, particularly for dry-cleaning and degreasing.

Clinical features Following inhalation or ingestion, there is depression of the central nervous system; nausea and vomiting may be persistent. The eyes, nose, and throat are irritated. Hepatic and renal dysfunction, and also ventricular arrhythmias and non-cardiogenic pulmonary oedema may develop.

Treatment After removal from exposure, treatment is symptomatic.

Further reading

Illing, H.P.A., Mariscotti, S.P., and Smith, A.M. (1987). *Toxicity Review. Tetrachloroethylene. (tetrachloroethene, perchloroethylene).* HMSO, London.

Thallium

See OTM3, pp. 1113–4.

Theophylline

Poisoning may be iatrogenic or suicidal. It is important to establish at an early stage which theophylline product is involved as many are sustained-release formulations that reach peak plasma concentrations 6–12 hours after overdosage with correspondingly delayed symptoms.

Clinical features Most symptomatic patients have concentrations in excess of 25 mg/l. Convulsions are seen more commonly when concentrations are greater than 50 mg/l. Symptoms include nausea, vomiting, hyperventilation, haematemesis, abdominal pain, diarrhoea, sinus tachycardia, supraventricular and ventricular arrhythmias, hypotension, and restlessness, irritability, headache, hyperreflexia, tremors, and convulsions. Hypokalaemia results from $Na+/K+$ ATPase activation. A mixed respiratory alkalosis and metabolic acidosis is common.

Assessment of the severity of poisoning Plasma potassium concentrations of less than 2.6 mmol/l, acidaemia, hypotension, seizures, and arrhythmias are indications for urgent measurement of plasma theophylline concentrations.

Treatment Gastric lavage may be considered in patients who have ingested a lot of theophylline and who present within one hour; administration of activated charcoal 50–100 g (by nasogastric tube, if necessary) is an alternative. Multiple doses of charcoal (e.g. 50 g 4-hourly) enhance systemic elimination. Intractable vomiting may be alleviated by ondansetron, 8 mg intravenously in an adult. Gastrointestinal haemorrhage may require blood transfusion and ranitidine rather than cimetidine which slows the metabolism of theophylline. Tachyarrhythmias may be induced by the rapid flux of potassium across cell membranes and prevented by early correction of hypokalaemia. Potassium supplements will be needed in almost all cases: 60 mmol/h may be required at the outset. Non-selective β-adrenoceptor blocking drugs, such as propranolol, may also be useful in the treatment of tachyarrhythmias secondary to hypokalaemia.

Charcoal haemoperfusion increases theophylline clearance but should be reserved for those in whom intractable vomiting or recurrent seizures make oral charcoal impracticable or hazardous.

Further reading

Sessler, C.N. (1990). Theophylline toxicity: clinical features of 116 consecutive cases. *American Journal of Medicine*, **88**, 567–76.

Thyroxine

Clinical features Few patients who ingest large amounts of thyroid hormones develop toxicity. Symptoms appear within a few hours with tri-iodothyronine (T_3) and after 3–6 days with thyroxine (T_4). Mental confusion, agitation, irritability, and hyperactivity with sinus tachycardia, tachypnoea, pyrexia, and dilated pupils are common while atrial fibrillation, sweating, loose stools, and the ocular features of hyperthyroidism are rare.

Treatment Gastric lavage may be considered if more than 2 mg of thyroxine has been ingested within the preceding one hour; activated charcoal is an alternative. Serum T_4 and T_3 concentrations should be measured 6–12 hours after ingestion. A normal result precludes delayed toxicity. Those with high T_4 concentrations should be reviewed for evidence of toxicity 4–5 days later. Patients who develop toxicity should be given propranolol for 5 days.

Toluene

Toluene, an industrial solvent, is less volatile and toxic than benzene.

Metabolism Following inhalation or ingestion, toluene is oxidized to benzoic acid and then to hippuric acid benzoylglucuronates which are excreted in the urine.

Clinical features Acute poisoning causes euphoria, excitement, dizziness, confusion, increased lacrimation, headache, nervousness, nausea, tinnitus, ataxia, tremor, and coma. Chronic poisoning can cause muscle weakness, abdominal pain and haematemesis, cerebellar abnormalities, optic neuropathy, peripheral neuropathy, altered mental state, dementia, hearing loss, hypokalaemia, and hepatorenal disease, including distal renal tubular acidosis and urinary calculi.

Treatment If poisoning results from inhalation, the patient should be removed from the contaminated environment and given symptomatic treatment.

Further reading

Cavender, F. (1994). Toluene. In *Patty's industrial hygiene and toxicology.* (ed. G.D. Clayton and F.E. Clayton), Vol **IIB**, 4th edn., pp. 1326–32. John Wiley and Sons, Inc., New York.

1,1,1-Trichloroethane (methyl chloroform)

This colourless, volatile liquid is used as a solvent.

Acute exposure Inhalation can cause CNS depression, hepatic and renal dysfunction, and death.

Treatment The casualty should be removed from the contaminated environment. Thereafter treatment is symptomatic and supportive.

Further reading

IPCS. (1992). *Environmental Health Criteria 136. 1,1,1-Trichloroethane.* WHO, Geneva.

Trichloroethylene

This colourless, volatile liquid is an industrial solvent.

Clinical features Following inhalation, ingestion, or dermal absorption, central nervous system depression occurs with nausea and vomiting, hepatic and renal dysfunction, and death. 'Degreaser's flush' (in which the skin on the face and arms becomes markedly reddened) may occur if ethanol is consumed shortly before or after exposure to trichloroethylene. Cranial nerve damage, cerebellar dysfunction, and convulsions have been described.

Treatment Removal from exposure will reduce CNS depression. Thereafter, treatment is symptomatic.

Further reading

Szlatenyi, C.S. and Wang, R.Y. (1996). Encephalopathy and cranial nerve palsies caused by intentional trichloroethylene inhalation. *American Journal of Emergency Medicine*, **14**, 464–7.

Tricyclic antidepressants

These drugs block the reuptake of noradenaline into peripheral and intracerebral neurones (so increasing local concentrations of monoamines) and have anticholinergic and class 1 antiarrhythmic (quinidine-like) activities.

Clinical features Symptoms appear within 30–60 minutes after overdose and usually reach maximum intensity in 4–12 hours. Drowsiness, sinus tachycardia, dry mouth, dilated pupils, urinary retention, increased reflexes, and extensor plantar responses are the usual features of mild poisoning. Severe intoxication leads to coma, often with divergent strabismus, and convulsions. Plantar, oculocephalic, and oculovestibular reflexes may be temporarily abolished. Skin blisters and rhabdomyolysis may be present.

Sinus tachycardia is very common and the dose-related quinidine-like action decreases myocardial contractility and delays conduction producing a bizarre ECG; PR and QRS intervals increase and the P waves diminish in amplitude and may be completely obscured by the preceding T wave. Differentiation between ventricular tachycardia and supraventricular tachycardia with aberrant conduction may be impossible. Serious arrhythmias, particularly ventricular tachycardia, occur in only 4 per cent of cases. The blood pressure and cardiac output fall. Metabolic acidosis and cardiorespiratory depression are the major causes of death.

Treatment Most patients recover with supportive therapy alone. Potentially lethal complications such as convulsions and arrhythmias are most common within 6 hours of overdosage. Coma rarely lasts for more than 24–48 hours. Gastric lavage may be considered in adults when more than 250 mg of the drug has been ingested less than one hour previously. Alternatively, activated charcoal 50–100 g can be administered orally.

Management of cardiotoxicity is difficult. Antiarrhythmic drugs are generally contraindicated. Attention should be given to oxygenation, control of convulsions, and correction of acidosis. Sodium bicarbonate (50 mmol intravenously over 20 minutes) should be given even if there is no acidosis. Lignocaine, (50–100 mg intravenously) may be tried cautiously if ventricular tachycardia is compromising cardiac output.

Physostigmine salicylate, a cholinesterase inhibitor, has no role. When benzodiazepines have been taken in overdose together with tricyclic antidepressants, flumazenil may unmask the tricyclic antidepressant-induced seizure potential and should therefore be used with caution. Forced diuresis and haemodialysis are therefore of no value. Nor is charcoal haemoperfusion effective.

Delirium with auditory and visual hallucinations is a frequent and troublesome complication during the recovery phase. Sedation with oral or intravenous diazepam may be required.

Vanadium

See OTM3, p. 1114.

Vinyl chloride (monochloroethylene, chloroethene)

This colourless, highly flammable, and explosive gas is usually handled as a liquid under pressure.

Mechanisms of toxicity The main route of absorption is through the lungs, although some skin penetration does occur. Metabolism to a reactive metabolite appears to be necessary before toxic effects are seen.

Acute exposure Concentrations in excess of 10 000 p.p.m. cause CNS depression.

Chronic exposure Acro-osteolysis has been described in workers engaged in the handcleaning of autoclaves. The syndrome has three main components: (i) Raynaud's phenomenon, (ii) skin changes resembling scleroderma, and (iii) bony changes of the terminal phalanges of the fingers and sometimes the toes, radial and ulnar styloid processes, sacroiliac joints, and lower poles of the patellae.

Angiosarcoma of the liver, malignances elsewhere, and hepatic fibrosis, often associated with splenomegaly and portal hypertension, have also been reported in vinyl chloride workers.

Volatile substance abuse

Solvent abuse involves the intentional inhalation of volatile organic chemicals such as organic solvents and vapours, hydrocarbon mixtures such as petrol (gasoline), and aerosol propellants.

Volatile substances are either 'bagged' (sprayed into a plastic bag and then inhaled until the subject passes out) or 'huffed' (sprayed on to a cloth held to the mouth). Glue is most often sniffed from a potato crisp bag and repeated abuse in this manner leads to the development of erythematous spots around the mouth and nose ('glue-sniffer's rash'). Most solvent abusers are adolescent males who indulge in the habit as a group activity. Most sniff solvents briefly and on only a few occasions. A few become dependent chronic users, and many of these 'mature out' of the solvent habit.

Clinical features As in alcohol intoxication there is initial CNS stimulation followed by depression. Other symptoms include euphoria, blurring of vision, tinnitus, slurring of speech, ataxia, feelings of omnipotence, headache, abdominal pain, anorexia, nausea, vomiting, jaundice, chest pain, bronchospasm, impaired judgement, irritability, and excitement. Less often a delirious state is seen, with clouding of consciousness and hallucinations. Many chronic users report transient psychotic symptoms which often have an affective component. Convulsions, status epilepticus, and coma may occur. Self-destructive and antisocial acts may be carried out by people under the influence of volatile substances. Psychological dependence and tolerance may develop, but physical dependence is rare. Volatile substance abuse may be associated with the abuse of alcohol and multiple illicit drugs.

Unexplained listlessness, anorexia, and marked moodiness are suggestive of chronic abuse. Poor school adjustment and scholastic performance have been noted in chronic glue sniffers apparently from lack of motivation.

'Glue sniffing' Glues are volatile, semiliquid preparations which usually contain an aromatic hydrocarbon as the vehicle. The physical sequelae of prolonged glue sniffing include aplastic anaemia and acute hepatic and renal damage. Features of renal toxicity include proteinuria, haematuria, distal renal tubular acidosis, and recurrent urinary calculi. Irreversible neurological sequelae such as optic atrophy, encephalopathy, cerebellar degeneration, and equilibrium disorders have been reported in adults who are chronic abusers. Toluene inhalation may cause encephalopathy in children. Neurological damage may occur after 'sniffing' of less than 1 year's duration and symptoms may progress for up to 3 months after the habit has been abandoned. Glues containing *n*-hexane and toluene have been associated with the development of muscle weakness and atrophy and sensory impairment of either the 'glove and stocking' or sensorimotor type, with or without muscle atrophy.

A review of adults who had sniffed toluene indicated three major patterns of presentation: (1) muscle weakness, (2) gastrointestinal complaints (abdominal pain, haematemesis), and (3) neuropsychiatric disorders (altered mental status, cerebellar abnormalities, peripheral neuropathy). In addition, hypokalaemia, hypophosphataemia, and hyperchloraemia were common. Rhabdomyolysis occurred in 40 per cent of cases. Cardiac and haematological toxicity due to toluene appears to be uncommon.

Petrol (gasoline) sniffing Abusers of petrol have reported that 15–20 breaths of the vapours are sufficient to produce intoxication for 3–6 hours. The euphoria of mild intoxication may be accompanied by nausea and vomiting. After prolonged inhalation, or rapid inhalation of highly concentrated vapour, the 'sniffer' may experience a phase of violent excitement followed by loss of consciousness and coma. While unconscious, the subject may suffer convulsions and the pupils may become fixed and dilated or unequal. Nystagmus and conjugate deviation of the eyes may be observed. Death is rare. Cerebral and pulmonary oedema and renal and hepatic damage have been noted at autopsy. The greater danger from petrol 'sniffing' is related to the long-term effects of chronic exposure which include loss of appetite and loss of weight, neurasthenia, muscle weakness and cramps, and permanent neuropsychological damage. Encephalopathy in petrol sniffers may also be due to tetraethyl lead.

Chlorinated hydrocarbon abuse Inhalation of chlorinated hydrocarbons causes a sense of euphoria, and sometimes excitement, associated with headache, dizziness, nausea, vomiting, stupor, coma, and convulsions. Other features may ensue. See under 1,1,1-trichloroethane, trichoroethylene, or dichloropropane as appropriate.

Toxicity due to aerosol inhalation The most commonly abused aerosol propellants are the chlorofluorocarbons (CFCs). Several hundred teenagers have died from this cause. It is likely that the fatalities were due to cardiac arrhythmias.

Diagnosis and management of volatile substance abuse The clinical features described above and the circumstances in which patients are found usually point to the diagnosis, but confirmation may be obtained by detection of solvents in blood or metabolites in the urine.

Acute intoxication from volatile substance abuse is usually brief and self-limiting. If respiratory depression and cardiac arrhythmias supervene they should be treated conventionally and renal and hepatic failure may require further supportive measures and dialysis.

Further reading

Steffee, C.H., Davis, G.J., and Nicol, K.K. (1996). A whiff of death: fatal volatile solvent inhalation abuse. *Southern Medical Journal*, **89**, 879–84.

Xylenes

These are used widely as solvents in paints, lacquers, pesticides, gums, resins, adhesives, and the paper coating industry.

Metabolism Xylene is oxidized and excreted in the urine either free or conjugated with glycine as methylhippuric acid. Ethanol inhibits xylene metabolism.

Clinical features Following inhalation there is dizziness, excitement, flushing of the face, eye irritation, drowsiness, inco-ordination, ataxia, tremor, confusion, coma, respiratory depression, catecholamine-induced ventricular arrhythmias, and hepatorenal damage. Immersion of the hand in liquid xylene may result in erythema and a burning feeling, with some scaling of the skin.

Treatment is supportive.

Zinc

See OTM3, pp. 1114–5.

Chapter 18.2

Injuries, envenoming, poisoning, and allergic reactions caused by animals

D. A. Warrell

Mechanical injuries caused by animals

Lions, tigers, leopards, jaguars, hyenas, wolves, bears, elephants, hippopotamuses, buffaloes, musk ox, moose, wild pigs, and ostriches have mauled or killed humans. About 100 shark attacks are reported each year, mostly between latitudes 30°N and 30°S, 50 of which are fatal. African crocodiles (*Crocodilus niloticus*) and Asian and Australian salt water crocodiles (*C. porosus*) kill several hundreds of people each year (see also OTM3, p. 1125).

Dog bites

Bites by domestic dogs are common. An estimated 6 million dogs live in England and Wales: more than 200 000 patients bitten by dogs attend hospitals each year (4.2 per 1000 population). More than 1 million people are bitten by dogs each year in the USA with 11 deaths in a 2-year period. One hundred thousand Australians are bitten by dogs each year.

Clinical features

Teeth, tusks, claws, and horns tear, crush, and penetrate causing pneumothorax, haemothorax, and penetration of the peritoneal cavity and bowel. Facial and eye injuries are common. Large bovines cause severe crush injuries by trampling and kneeling. Wounds are highly likely to be infected. About one-third of dog and cat bite wounds became infected, commonly by *Pasteurella multocida* or anaerobes (see OTM3, p. 404, Table 2).

Treatment

Urgent thorough cleaning with soap and water is essential; suitable antiseptics are iodine and alcohol solutions. Prophylactic antimicrobials such as co-trimoxazole, penicillins, cephalosporins, or erythromycin have proved effective in dog bite wounds, and are indicated for multiple or severe wounds and bites on the face and hands. Asplenic individuals are at special risk of *Capnocytophaga canimorsus* septicaemia. Fluoroquinolones in combination with penicillins/cephalosporins (e.g. co-amoxiclav) or an aminoglycoside and metronidazole may be required to cover Gram-negative organisms and anaerobes. Blood loss must be replaced. Wounds are irrigated and drained, dead tissue is debrided, and skin suturing is delayed.

Further reading

Cummings, P. (1994). Antibiotics to prevent infection in patients with dog bite wounds: a meta-analysis of randomized trials. *Annals of Emergency Medicine*, **23**, 535–40.

Venomous and poisonous animals

For predation or defence, some animals inject venoms through fangs, stings, spines, hairs, and other specialized venom organs. The flesh of some marine animals is poisonous (see below).

Venomous mammals

See OTM3, p. 1125.

Venomous snakes

Bites by almost 200 species of venomous snake (families Elapidae and Viperidae and rarely Colubridae and Atractaspididae) have caused severe envenoming.

Distribution and classification

Areas free of venomous snakes are the Antarctic, most islands of the western Mediterranean, Atlantic, Caribbean and Eastern Pacific (including Hawaii), Madagascar, New Caledonia, New Zealand, Ireland, Iceland, Chile, and the Atlantic Ocean.

Medically important species have in their upper jaws a pair of enlarged teeth (fangs) that inject venom into the tissues of their victim through grooves or a closed canal (Fig. 1).

Elapidae (cobras (Plate 1), kraits, mambas, coral snakes, Australasian venomous snakes (Plate 2) and sea snakes)

Elapids have short, immobile front fangs. African and Asian 'spitters' (rinkhals and spitting cobras) can eject their venom from the tips of the fangs for a distance of 1–2 m into the eyes of an enemy.

Viperidae (Old World adders and vipers (Plate 3); American rattlesnakes, moccasins, lanceheaded vipers; Asian pit vipers (Plate 4))

The front fangs are long, curved, and erectile. Snakes of the subfamily *Crotalinae* (pit vipers) possess a heat-sensitive pit organ behind the nostril (Plate 4).

Incidence and importance of snake bites

Snake bite is common in some tropical countries. In parts of north-eastern Nigeria, the saw-scaled or carpet viper (*Echis ocellatus*) causes 500 bites per 100 000 population per year with a mortality of 12 per cent. In the Burdwan district of West Bengal almost 30 000 people are bitten each year with 1300 deaths and in Sri Lanka there are 60 000 bites and 900 deaths (6 per 100 000 population) per year. In Burma, Russell's viper bite has been the fifth major cause of death (annual mortality more than 2000, 15 per 100 000 population). In the USA there are approximately 45 000 bites per year, 7000 of which are caused by venomous species, with 9–14 deaths per year. In England, Wales, and Scotland, the adder or viper (*Vipera berus*) is the only venomous species. More than 100 people are admitted to hospital each year but only 14 deaths have been reported since 1876. In Australia there are now about 2–3 deaths per year.

Epidemiology

Snake bite is an occupational disease in rural areas of the tropics. Most bites are inflicted on the lower limbs of farmers, plantation workers, herdsmen, and hunters when they tread on the snake at night or in undergrowth. Asiatic kraits (*Bungarus* sp.) and African spitting cobras (*Naja nigricollis*) enter houses at night and bite people sleeping on the floor. Seasonal peaks of incidence are associated with farming, such as ploughing before the annual rains or harvesting.

Heavy flooding in Colombia, Pakistan, India, Bangladesh, and Vietnam has caused epidemics of snake bite. Snakes are becoming popular pets in Europe and North America and are eaten especially by the Chinese; bites result from their being handled.

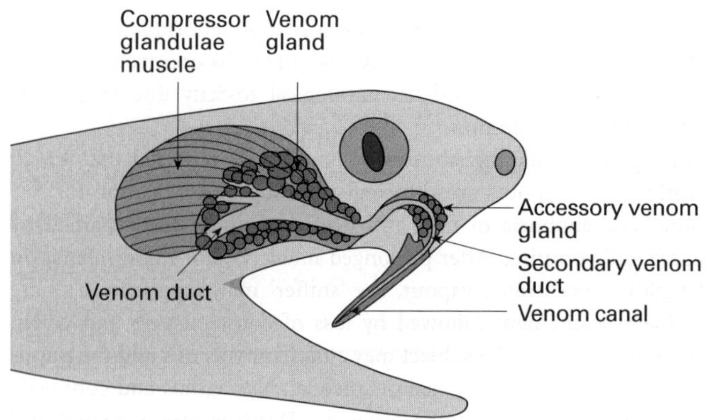

Fig. 1 Venom apparatus of a viper.

Venom apparatus

Venom glands of Elapidae and Viperidae lie behind the eye, surrounded by compressor muscles (Fig. 1). The amount of venom injected into human patients is very variable. Depending on the species 5–70 per cent of those bitten may not be envenomed.

Venom properties

Snake venoms contain more than 20 different compounds. Ninety per cent of the dry weight is protein; enzymes, non-enzymatic polypeptide toxins, and non-toxic proteins. Venom procoagulants include serine proteases (e.g. *Daboia russelii* factor X activator, taipan and tiger snake prothrombin activators), arginine ester-hydrolases (e.g. *D. russelii* factor V activator) and zinc metalloproteinases (e.g. ecarin from *E. carinatus*). Crotaline venoms contain thrombin-like proteases which cleave the fibrinogen molecule, for example, ancrod (*Calloselasma rhodostoma*) and batroxobin (*Bothrops moojeni*). Phospholipase A_2 (lecithinase) is the most widespread venom enzyme; it contributes to myotoxicity, neurotoxicity, cardiotoxicity, haemolysis, and increased vascular permeability.

Polypeptide toxins (neurotoxins)

Postsynaptic (α-) toxins, such as α-bungarotoxin, bind to acetylcholine receptors at peripheral neuromuscular junctions. Toxic phospholipases A_2, such as β-bungarotoxin and taipoxin, paralyse by damaging motor nerve endings and skeletal muscle. Other toxins target other neuronal receptors and ion channels and inhibit acetylcholinesterase.

Pharmacology

Elapid neurotoxins are rapidly absorbed into the bloodstream, whereas the much larger molecules of Viperid venoms are taken up more slowly via lymphatics. Most venoms are concentrated and bound in the kidney and some components are eliminated in the urine. Neurotoxins such as α-bungarotoxin, are tightly bound at neuromuscular junctions. Most venom components do not cross the intact blood–brain barrier.

Pathophysiology

Swelling and bruising of the bitten limb result from increased vascular permeability induced by proteases, phospholipases, membrane-damaging polypeptide cytotoxins, and endogenous autacoids released by the venom, such as histamine, 5-hydroxytryptamine and kinins. Extravasation leads to hypovolaemia, haemoconcentration, hypoalbuminaemia, albuminuria, serous effusions, pulmonary oedema, and conjunctival and facial oedema. Tissue necrosis at the site of the bite is caused by myotoxic and cytolytic factors. Thrombosis, intracompartmental syndrome, or a tight tourniquet may contribute to ischaemia. Hypotension and shock result from hypovolaemia, vasodilatation, and myocardial dysfunction. Some venoms release vasodilating autacoids such as histamine and kinins. Venoms of several pit vipers activate bradykinin and potentiate its hypotensive effect, e.g. by ACE-inhibition. The venom of the Israeli burrowing asp (*Atractaspis engaddensis*) contains four sarafotoxins highly homologous with endothelins with which they share potent effects on the heart and blood vessels. Venom procoagulants activate the clotting cascade at various sites. Fibrinogenases degrade fibrinogen directly. Other toxins activate endogenous plasminogen and induce or inhibit platelet aggregation. Spontaneous systemic bleeding is caused by zinc metalloproteinase haemorrhagins that damage vascular endothelium. The combination of defibrination, thrombocytopenia, and vessel wall damage can result in severe bleeding into the brain or gut, a common cause of death after bites by Viperidae. Acute renal tubular necrosis may be caused by severe hypotension, disseminated intravascular coagulation, direct venom nephrotoxicity, and myoglobinuria resulting from generalized rhabdomyolysis. Neurotoxic polypeptides and phospholipases block neuromuscular transmission, causing death by bulbar or respiratory paralysis.

Clinical features

Fear and effects of first-aid treatment contribute to the symptoms and signs. First there is local pain and bleeding from the fang punctures, followed by pain, tenderness, swelling and bruising extending up the limb, lymphangitis, and tender enlargement of regional lymph nodes.

Anaphylaxis (early syncope, vomiting, colic, diarrhoea, angio-oedema, and wheezing) may occur (e.g. after bites by European vipers). Nausea and vomiting indicate systemic envenoming.

Bites by Elapidae (cobras, kraits, mambas, coral snakes, Australasian snakes, and sea snakes)

Bites by kraits, mambas, coral snakes, some cobras, and most Australasian elapids produce minimal local effects, but the venoms of African spitting cobras and Asian cobras can cause severe local swelling, blistering, and necrosis (Fig. 2). Most elapid venoms are neurotoxic. Before neurological signs appear, there is vomiting, 'heaviness' of the eyelids, blurred vision, paraesthesiae around the mouth, hyperacusis, headache, dizziness, vertigo, hypersalivation, congested conjunctivae, and 'gooseflesh'. Paralysis is first detectable as ptosis and external ophthalmoplegia appearing as early as 15 minutes after the bite, but sometimes delayed for 10 hours or more. Later the face, palate, jaws, tongue, vocal cords, neck muscles, and muscles of deglutition may become paralysed (Fig. 3). Respiratory failure may be precipitated by airway obstruction at this stage, or later after paralysis of intercostal muscles and diaphragm. Neurotoxic effects are reversible, either acutely in response to antivenom or anticholinesterases or spontaneously in 1–7 days.

Envenoming by terrestrial Australasian snakes produces neurotoxicity, haemostatic disturbances, and, rarely, generalized rhabdomyolysis and renal failure. Painful enlarged regional lymph nodes are a useful sign of impending systemic envenoming, but local signs are usually mild. Early symptoms include vomiting, headache, and syncopal attacks.

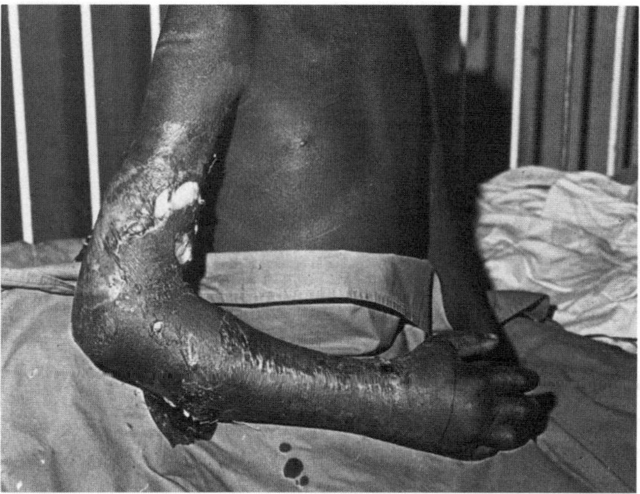

Fig. 2 Extensive necrosis of skin and subcutaneous tissues in a Nigerian girl bitten on the elbow nine days previously by a black-necked or spitting cobra (*Naja nigricollis*)
(copyright D.A. Warrell).

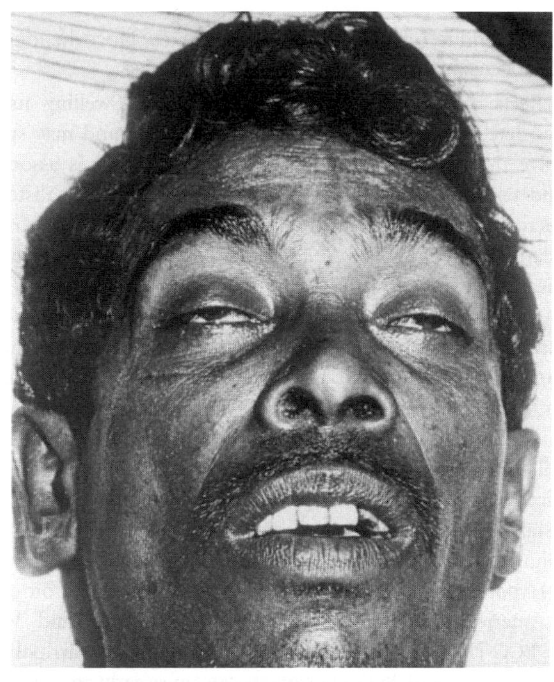

Fig. 3 Neurotoxic envenoming. Ptosis, ophthalmoplegia, and inability to open the mouth and protrude the tongue in a Sri Lankan patient envenomed by the common krait (*Bungarus caeruleus*)
(copyright D.A. Warrell).

Envenoming by sea snakes produces headache, thirst, sweating, and vomiting followed some 30 minutes to 3.5 hours after the bite by generalized aching, stiffness, and tenderness of the muscles.

Trismus is common. Later there is generalized flaccid paralysis. Myoglobinuria appears 3–8 hours after the bite. Myoglobin and potassium released from damaged skeletal muscles can cause renal failure, while hyperkalaemia may precipitate cardiac arrest.

Venom ophthalmia caused by spitting elapids

There is intense pain in the eye, blepharospasm, palpebral oedema, and leucorrhoea (Fig. 4). Secondary infection of corneal erosions may lead to permanent blinding opacities or panophthalmitis.

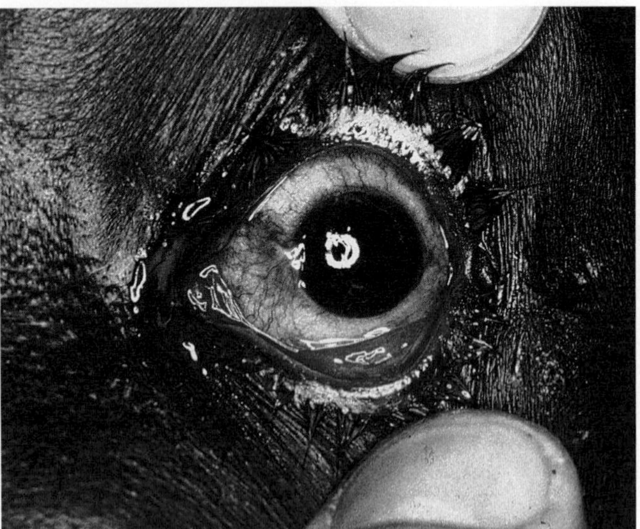

Fig. 4 Acute venom ophthalmia caused by a black-necked or spitting cobra (*Naja nigricollis*)
(copyright D.A. Warrell).

Bites by Viperidae (vipers, adders, rattlesnakes, lance-headed vipers, moccasins, and pit vipers)

Local effects are usually pronounced (Plate 5). Swelling usually becomes detectable within 1–2 hours after the bite and may spread to involve the whole limb and adjacent trunk. There is associated pain and tenderness in regional lymph nodes. Bruising, blistering, and necrosis may appear during the next few days. Necrosis is particularly frequent and severe following bites by some rattlesnakes, lance-headed vipers (genus *Bothrops*), Asian pit vipers, and African vipers (genus *Bitis*). When the envenomed tissue is contained in a tight fascial compartment such as the pulp space of digits or anterior tibial compartment ischaemia may result. Haemostatic abnormalities are common. Persistent bleeding from fang puncture wounds, venepuncture or injection sites, other new and partially healed wounds, and after childbirth, suggests that the blood is incoagulable. Spontaneous systemic haemorrhage is most often detected in the gingival sulci (Plate 6). Epistaxis, haematemesis, cutaneous ecchymoses, haemoptysis, and subconjunctival, retroperitoneal, and intracranial haemorrhages also occur. Hypotension and shock are common in patients bitten by North American rattlesnakes, *Bothrops, Daboia, Bitis,* and *Vipera* species. ECG changes (ST segment, T wave) or cardiac arrhythmias may occur. *Vipera* and *Bothrops* venoms can cause early and recurrent syncopal attacks with anaphylactic symptoms. Renal failure is the major cause of death in patients envenomed by some species of Viperidae. Neurotoxicity, resembling that seen in patients bitten by Elapidae, with rhabdomyolysis (Plate 7) is a feature of envenoming by a few species of Viperidae, but progression to respiratory or generalized paralysis is unusual.

Envenoming by European vipers

Early pain at the site of the bite is usual. Local swelling usually appears within a few minutes but may be delayed. Rarely, blisters containing blood may appear. Swelling and bruising may involve the whole limb within 24 hours and extend on to the trunk. Intracompartmental syndromes and necrosis are rare. Pain, tenderness, and enlargement of local lymph nodes is sometimes noticeable within hours. Marked lymphangitis and bruising of the affected limb appears within a day or two. Dramatic early anaphylactic symptoms may appear within 5 minutes of the bite or later: retching, vomiting, abdominal colic, diarrhoea, incontinence of urine and faeces, sweating, shock, vasoconstriction, tachycardia, and angio-oedema of the face, lips, gums, tongue, throat, and epiglottis, urticaria, and bronchospasm. Hypotension usually develops within 2 hours, may be transient, resolving spontaneously within 2 hours, or persistent, recurrent or progressive, and fatal. ECG changes include flattening or inversion of T waves, ST elevation, second degree heart block and cardiac brady- and tachyarrhythmias, atrial fibrillation, and changes of myocardial infarction. Defibrinogenation (incoagulable blood) or milder degrees of coagulopathy and spontaneous bleeding into the gastrointestinal tract, lungs, or urinary tract are uncommon. Other clinical features include fever, drowsiness and rarely, coma and seizures secondary to hypotension or cerebral oedema, respiratory distress, pulmonary oedema, cerebral oedema, acute renal failure, cardiac arrest, intrauterine death, acute gastric dilatation, and paralytic ileus. Deaths have occurred from 6 to 60 (average 34) hours after the bite.

Laboratory investigations

The peripheral neutrophil count may exceed 20×10^9/l in severely envenomed patients. Initial haemoconcentration, resulting from extravasation of plasma, is followed by anaemia caused by bleeding, dilution as oedema fluid is reabsorbed, or, more rarely, haemolysis. Thrombocytopenia is common following bites by some Viperidae. A useful simple test for venom-induced defibrinogenation or anticoagulation is the 20 minute whole blood clotting test (20WBCT). A few ml of venous blood is placed in a new, clean, dry, glass test tube, left undisturbed for 20 minutes, and then tipped to see if it has clotted. Incoagulable blood indicates systemic envenoming. More sensitive rapid tests of coagulopathy may be used if available. Patients with generalized rhabdomyolysis show a steep rise in serum creatine kinase, myoglobin, and potassium. Black or brown urine suggests generalized rhabdomyolysis or intravascular haemolysis. Concentrations of serum enzymes such as creatine kinase and aspartate aminotransferase are raised in patients with severe local tissue damage. Urine should be examined for blood/haemoglobin, myoglobin, and protein and for microscopic haematuria and red cell casts.

Immunodiagnosis

Snake venom antigens can be detected in wound swabs, aspirates or biopsies, serum, urine, CSF, and other body fluids by enzyme immunoassay (EIA). A commercial test kit for Australian elapids is produced by CSL, Melbourne.

Management of snake bite

First aid

The patient should be reassured and moved to the nearest hospital or dispensary, without exercising any part of the body, especially the bitten limb which should be immobilized with a splint or sling.

Local incisions, suction, potassium permanganate, ice packs, and electric shocks are dangerous and ineffective. Tourniquets and compression bands can cause ischaemia and other complications.

Sutherland's pressure immobilization method (Fig. 5) involves firm but not tight bandaging of the entire bitten limb with a long (4.5 m × 10 cm) crepe bandage, starting over the hand or foot and incorporating a splint. It is recommended for bites by dangerously neurotoxic elapids, but is contraindicated in the case of necrotic venoms.

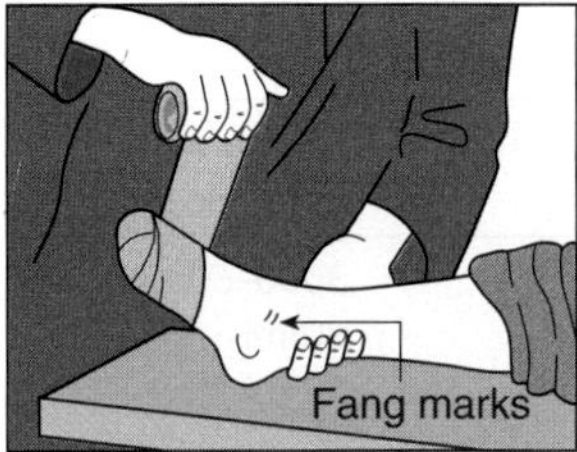

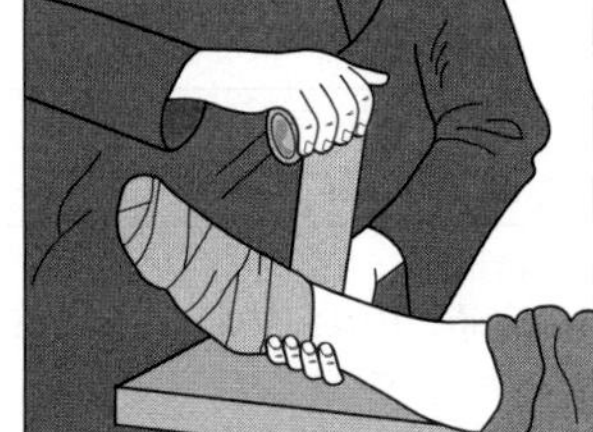
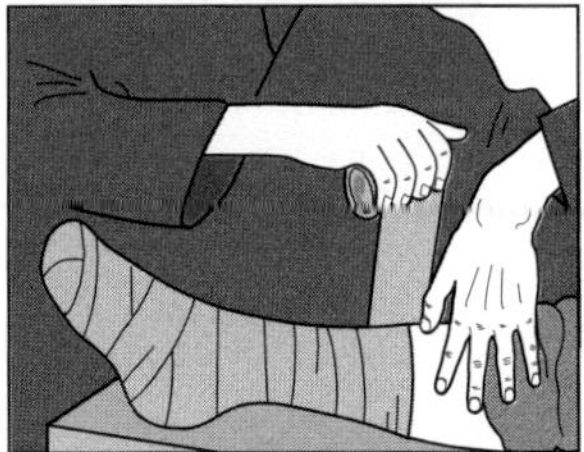
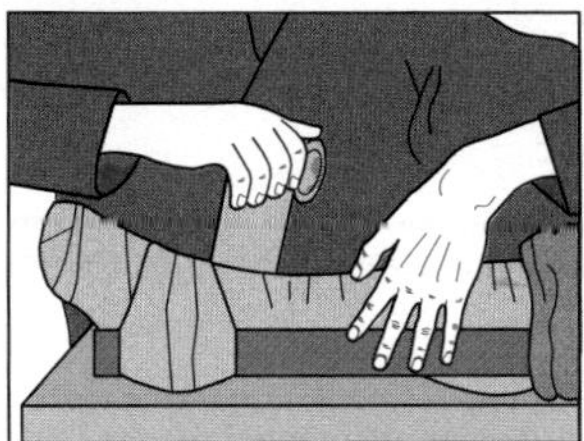
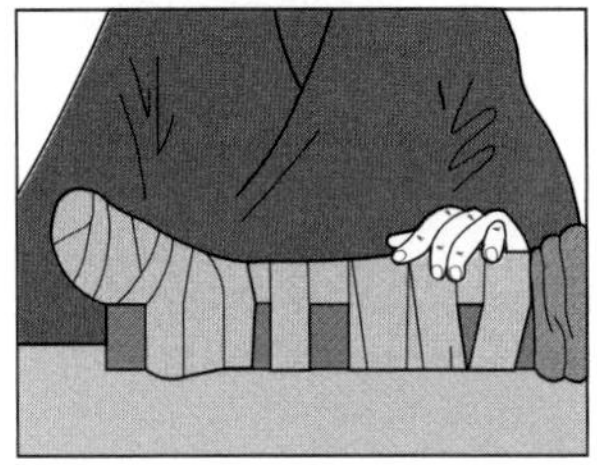
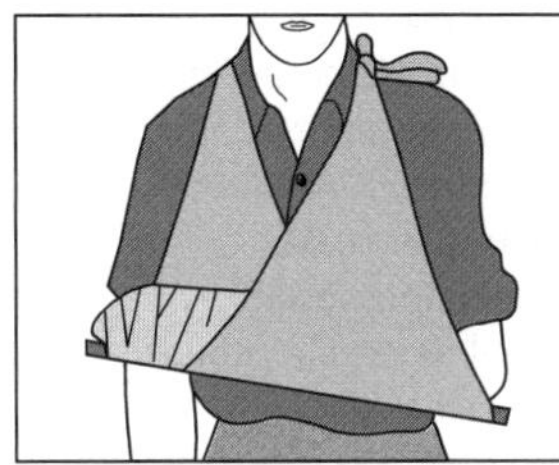

Fig. 5 Pressure immobilization method
(by courtesy of the Australian Venom Research Unit).

If the snake has been killed it should be taken with the patient to hospital but it must not be handled as even a severed head can inject venom.

On the way to hospital patients should lie in the recovery position to prevent aspiration of vomit. Respiratory distress and cyanosis should be treated by clearing the airway, giving oxygen, and, if necessary, assisted ventilation. If the patient is unconscious and no femoral or carotid pulses can be detected, cardiorespiratory resuscitation should be started immediately.

Hospital treatment

Clinical assessment

Uncertainties about the species, quantity, and composition of venom injected can be resolved only by admitting the patient for at least 24 hours of close observation.

Antivenom treatment

Antivenom (heterologous hyperimmune horse or sheep serum) is the only specific treatment. It is indicated for systemic and severe local envenoming (Table 1).

Prediction of antivenom reactions

Skin and conjunctival tests do not predict early (anaphylactic) or late (serum sickness type) antivenom reactions.

Selection and administration of antivenom

Antivenom should be given only if its stated range of specificity includes the species responsible for the bite. Opaque liquid antivenoms should be discarded as precipitation of protein indicates loss of activity and increased risk of reactions. Monospecific (monovalent) antivenom is ideal if the biting species is known. Polyspecific (polyvalent) antivenoms, used in many countries because of the difficulty in identifying the species responsible for bites, may be just as effective but contain less specific activity per unit of immunoglobulin.

Table 1 Antivenom treatment

(a) Indications for antivenom (general)
Systemic envenoming 1. Haemostatic abnormalities such as spontaneous systemic bleeding, incoagulable blood, or thrombocytopenia
2. Neurotoxicity (ptosis, external ophthalmoplegia etc.)
3. Hypotension and shock, abnormal ECG, or other evidence of cardiovascular dysfunction
4. Generalized rhabdomyolysis
Severe local envenoming (venoms known to cause local necrosis)
1. Local swelling involving more than half the bitten limb
2. Extensive blistering or bruising
3. Bites on digits
4. Rapid progression of swelling
(b) Indications for antivenom (adder—*Vipera berus* bites)
1. Sustained fall in blood pressure (systolic to <80 mmHg or by more than 50 mmHg below the normal or admission value confirmed by repeated measurements over 10–15 min) or other signs of shock
2. Other features of systemic envenoming (see above); vomiting, spontaneous bleeding, coagulopathy, pulmonary oedema, or haemorrhage. ECG abnormalities, marked neutrophil leucocytosis, or elevated creatine kinase
3. Severe local envenoming: swelling extending up to or beyond the elbow or knee within 6 hours of the bite and, in adults, swelling beyond the wrist or ankle within 4 hours of the bite

Antivenom should be given as soon as possible but it may be effective as long as signs of systemic envenoming persist. However, local envenoming is probably not affected unless antivenom is given within one or two h of the bite. The intravenous route must be used whenever possible. Infusion of antivenom diluted in approximately 5 ml of isotonic fluid/kg body weight over about 1 h is easier to control than intravenous 'push' injection of undiluted antivenom given at the rate of about 4 ml/min.

Dose of antivenom (Table 2)

Children must be given the same dose as adults

Response to antivenom

Symptomatic improvement may be rapid. In shocked patients, the blood pressure may increase and consciousness return. Neurotoxic signs may improve after several hours. Spontaneous systemic bleeding stops quickly and blood coagulability is restored within 6 hours of a neutralizing dose of antivenom. More antivenom should be given if severe signs of envenoming persist after 1–2 hours, or if blood coagulability is not restored within 6 hours. Systemic envenoming may recur hours or days after an initially good response to antivenom, because of continuing absorption of venom from the injection site after antivenom has been cleared from the bloodstream.

Envenomed patients should be assessed daily for at least 3 or 4 days.

Table 2 Guide to initial dosage of some important antivenoms

Species Latin name	English name	Manufacturer, antivenom	Approximate initial dose
Acanthophis sp.	Death adder	CSL,* monospecific	3000–6000 units
Bitis arietans	Puff adder	SAIMR[d] polyspecific; Pasteur-Mérieux 'IPSER Afrique'	80 ml
Bothrops jararaca	Jararaca	Brazilian manufacturers Bothrops polyspecific	20 ml
Bungarus caeruleus	Common krait	Haffkine polyspecific	100 ml
Calloselasma (Agkistrodon) rhodostoma	Malayan pit viper	Thai Red Cross (Saovabha) Bangkok, monospecific	100 ml
		Thai Government Pharmaceutical Organization, monospecific	50 ml
Crotalus adamanteus	Eastern diamondback rattlesnakes	Wyeth (Crotalidae) polyspecific; Protherics 'CroTab'	30–100 ml
C. atrox	Western diamondback rattlesnakes		
C. viridis subspecies	Western rattlesnakes	Burma Pharmaceutical Industry, monospecific	40 ml
Daboia (Vipera) russelii	Russell's vipers		
		Haffkine polyspecific	100 ml
		Thai manufacturers, monospecific	50 ml
Echis sp.	Saw-scaled or carpet vipers	SAIMR,[d] Echis, monospecific	20 ml
		Pasteur-Mérieux 'IPSER Afrique'	40 ml
Hydrophiidae	Sea snakes	CSL,* sea snake/tiger snake	1000 units
Naja kaouthia	Monocellate Thai cobra	Thai Red Cross, monospecific	100 ml
N. naja	Indian cobra	Haffkine; Central Research Institute, Kasauli; Serum Institute of India, polyspecific	100 ml
N. nigricollis *N. mossambica*	African spitting cobras	SAIMR[d] polyspecific; Pasteur-Mérieux 'IPSER Afrique'	
Notechis scutatus	Tiger snake	CSL,* monospecific	3000–6000 units
Pseudechis textilis	Eastern brown snake		
Oxyuranus scutellatus	Taipan	CSL,* monospecific	12 000 units
Trimeresurus albolabris	Green pit viper	Thai Red Cross, monospecific	100 ml
Vipera berus	European adder	Immunolski Zavod-Zagreb Vipera polyspecific;	10 ml
		Protherics Fab monospecific 'Vipera Tab';	100–200 mg
V. palaestinae	Palestine viper	Rogoff Medical Research Institute, Tel Aviv, Palestine viper monospecific	50–80 ml

* Commonwealth Serum Laboratories, Australia.

[d] South African Institute for Medical Research

Antivenom reactions

Early anaphylactic reactions are common, developing within 10–180 minutes of starting antivenom. They usually result from complement activation by immune complexes or aggregates of IgG fragments and are rarely attributable to lgE mediated Type 1 hypersensitivity. **Pyrogenic reactions** are attributable to endotoxin contamination of the antivenom. Febrile convulsions may be precipitated in children. **Late reactions** of serum sickness, immune complex type may develop 5–24 (mean 7) days after antivenom.

Prevention of antivenom reactions

In adults, 0.5 mg 0.1 per cent epinephrine (adrenaline) given by subcutaneous injection immediately before the start of antivenom treatment reduces the incidence of early antivenom reactions whereas intramuscular promethazine is ineffective.

Treatment of antivenom reactions

Epinephrine is the treatment of first choice for all early reactions; 0.5 ml of 0.1 per cent solution (1 in 1000, 1 mg/ml) is given by intramuscular injection to adults (children 0.01 ml/kg) at the first signs of a reaction, and the dose repeated after 5–10 minutes if the reaction is not controlled. An H_1 blocking antihistamine, such as chlorpheniramine maleate (10 mg for adults, 0.2 mg/kg for children) should be given by intravenous injection to combat the effects of histamine release during the reaction. Pyrogenic reactions are treated by cooling the patient and giving antipyretics. Late reactions respond to an oral antihistamine such as chlorpheniramine (2 mg 6-hourly for adults, 0.25 mg/kg/day in divided doses for children) or to oral prednisolone (5 mg 6-hourly for 5–7 days for adults, 0.7 mg/kg/day in divided doses for children).

Supportive treatment

Neurotoxic envenoming

Bulbar and respiratory paralysis may lead to death from aspiration, airway obstruction, or respiratory failure. The airway must be maintained and, once there is pooling of secretions or respiratory distress, a cuffed endotracheal tube should be inserted or tracheostomy performed.

Provided they are adequately ventilated, patients with neurotoxic envenoming remain fully conscious with intact sensation. Manual ventilation by Ambu bag or anaesthetic bag has proved effective when mechanical ventilation was not available. Anticholinesterases are potentially useful especially when postsynaptic neurotoxins are involved. The 'Tensilon test' should be performed in all cases of severe neurotoxic envenoming as in suspected myasthenia gravis.

Hypotension and shock

If the central venous pressure is low or there is other clinical evidence of hypovolaemia, a plasma expander should be infused. Pressor agents may be needed.

Oliguria and renal failure

Urine output and serum creatinine, urea, and electrolytes should be measured each day in patients with severe envenoming and in those bitten by species known to cause renal failure (Viperidae and sea snakes). If urine output drops below 400 ml in 24 hours and fails to increase after cautious rehydration and diuretics, dopamine (2.5 μg/kg/min by intravenous infusion) should be tried and the patient placed on strict fluid balance. If these measures are ineffective, haemofiltration or peritoneal or haemodialysis is usually required.

Local infection at the site of the bite

Bites by some species (e.g. *Bothrops* sp., *C. rhodostoma*) may be infected by the snake's oral bacteria. Antibiotics (e.g. chloramphenicol) and a tetanus toxoid booster should be given, especially if the wound has been interfered with. An aminoglycoside and metronidazole should be added if there is evidence of tissue necrosis.

Management of local envenoming

Bullae are best left intact. The bitten limb should be elevated. Once definite signs of necrosis have appeared (blackened anaesthetic area with putrid odour or signs of imminent sloughing) surgical debridement, immediate split skin grafting and broad-spectrum antibiotic cover are indicated. Increased pressure within tight fascial compartments such as the digital pulp spaces and anterior tibial compartment may cause ischaemic damage. Fasciotomy may be justified if the intracompartmental pressure exceeds 45 mmHg but this should not be attempted until blood coagulability and a platelet count of more than 50×10^9/l have been restored.

Haemostatic disturbances

Once specific antivenom has been given to neutralize venom procoagulants, restoration of coagulability and platelet function may be accelerated by giving fresh whole blood, fresh frozen plasma, or cryoprecipitates. Heparin should not be used because it may exaggerate haemostatic disturbances and does not neutralize the thrombin generated by most snake venoms.

Other drugs

Corticosteroids, antifibrinolytic agents such as trasylol and ε-aminocaproic acid, and antihistamines have not proved clinically effective and should not be used.

Treatment of snake venom ophthalmia

Irrigate the eyes with water or any other available bland liquid. Unless a corneal abrasion can be excluded by fluorescein staining or slit lamp examination, tetracycline or chloramphenicol should be applied topically. Instillation of antivenom is not recommended. Adrenaline drops 0.5–1.0 per cent relieve pain and inflammation.

Prevention of snake bite

Snakes should never be disturbed, attacked, cornered, or handled even if they are thought to be a harmless species or appear to be dead. Venomous species should not be kept as pets or as performing animals. In snake infested areas, boots, socks, and long trousers should be worn for walks in undergrowth or deep sand and a light should always be carried at night. Unlit paths and roadside gutters are especially dangerous after heavy rains. Various substances toxic to snakes, such as insecticides and methylbromide, have been used to keep human dwellings free of these animals.

Further reading

Gopalakrishnakone, P. (ed.). (1994). *Sea snake toxinology.* National University of Singapore Press, Singapore.

Junghanss, T. and Bodio, M. (1995). *Notfall-Handbuch Gifttiere. Diagnose-Therapie-Biologie.* Georg Thieme Verlag, Stuttgart.

Meier, J. and White, J. (1995). *Clinical toxicology of animal venoms.* CRC Press, Boca Raton.

Warrell, D.A. (ed.). (1999). WHO/SEARO Guidelines for the clinical management of snake bites in the south-east Asian region. *South East Asian Journal of Tropical Medicine and Public Health*, **30**, Suppl. 1, 1–86.

Theakston, R.D.G. and Warrell, D.A. (1991). Antivenoms: a list of hyperimmune sera currently available for the treatment of envenoming by bites and stings. *Toxicon* **29**, 1419–70.

Venomous lizards

The only two venomous species, the gila monster (*Heloderma suspectum*) and Mexican beaded lizard (*H. horridum*) occur in the southwestern USA, western Mexico, and Central America (see OTM3, p. 1140).

Poisonous amphibians

See OTM3, p. 1140.

Poisonous birds

See OTM3, p. 1140.

Marine envenoming and poisoning

Venomous fish

Many species of fish can sting with spines in front of the fins and tail and in the gill covers. The Indo-Pacific region and other tropical waters harbour the largest numbers of venomous species, but sharks, chimaeras, and weevers occur in temperate northern waters. There are freshwater stingrays (*Potamotrygon* sp.) in South America, West Africa, and southeast Asia.

Incidence and epidemiology

Weeverfish are common around the British coast especially in Cornwall. Stings are most frequent in August and September. An estimated 1500 stings by rays and 300 stings by scorpionfish occur in the USA each year. Stings by venomous freshwater rays (*Potamotrygon* sp) are common in the Amazon region. Ornate, but aggressive and venomous members of the genera *Pterois* and *Dendrochirus* (lion, zebra, tiger, turkey, or red fire fish) are popular aquarium pets, that may sting their owners on the fingers. Most fish stings are inflicted on the soles of the feet of people wading near the shore or near coral reefs. Stingrays lash their tails at the intruding limb and usually impale the ankle. Fatalities are rare.

Clinical features

There is immediate sharp, agonizing pain. Hot, erythematous swelling extends up the stung limb. Complications include necrosis and secondary infection, particularly if the spine remains embedded in the wound. Stingray spines up to 30 cm long can lacerate and penetrate the thoracic or abdominal cavities with fatal results.

Systemic effects are uncommon after weever stings (Trachinidae) but patients stung by rays or Scorpaenidae (scorpion- and stonefish) may develop nausea, vomiting, signs of autonomic nervous system stimulation such as diarrhoea, sweating, and hypersalivation, cardiac arrhythmias, hypotension, respiratory distress, neurological signs, and generalized convulsions.

Treatment

Pain is alleviated by immersing the stung limb in water which is uncomfortably hot (less than 45°C) but not scalding. Injection of local anaesthetic is less effective even when applied as a ring block in the case of stung digits but local nerve block with 0.5 per cent plain bupivacaine is effective. The venomous spine, which may be barbed and fragments of membrane should be removed immediately. Cardiopulmonary resuscitation may be needed. Severe hypotension may respond to adrenaline and bradycardia to atropine. Stonefish antivenom (Commonwealth Serum Laboratories, Australia) is effective for envenoming by *Synanceja* sp., North American scorpionfish (*Scorpaena guttata*), and some other Scorpaenidae. One ampoule (2 ml or 2000 units) is given intravenously for each two puncture marks found at the site of the sting. The dose is increased for patients with severe symptoms.

Prevention

Fish stings can be prevented by shuffling the feet when wading, by handling living or dead fish cautiously and by keeping clear of fish in the water especially near tropical reefs. Footwear protects against most species except stingrays.

Poisoning by ingestion of aquatic animals

Acute gastrointestinal symptoms (food poisoning) after eating seafood are usually caused by bacterial or viral infections such as *Vibrio parahaemolyticus* (crustaceans, especially shrimps), *V. cholerae* (crabs and molluscs), non-O group 1 *V. cholerae* (oysters), *V. vulnificus* (oysters), *Aeromonas hydrophila* (frozen oysters), *Plesiomonas shigelloides* (oysters, mussels, mackerel, cuttlefish), *Shigella* sp. (molluscs), *Campylobacter jejuni* (clams), *Salmonella typhi* (molluscs), hepatitis A virus (molluscs, especially clams, and oysters), Norwalk virus (clams and oysters), and astro- and caliciviruses (cockles). Botulism has been caused by eating smoked fish and canned salmon; and in Japan and elsewhere, fish and molluscs became contaminated with methylmercury from industrial waste, causing severe neurological damage and fetal abnormalities (Minamata disease) (see Chapter 18.1).

Toxins in seafood give rise to two main syndromes.

Gastrointestinal/neurotoxic syndrome

Acute nausea, vomiting, abdominal colic, tenesmus, and watery diarrhoea are associated with paraesthesia of the lips, buccal cavity, and extremities; temperature perception is distorted so that cold objects feel burning hot like dry ice; other symptoms include myalgia, progressive flaccid paralysis, ataxia, cardiovascular disturbances, bradycardia, and rashes.

Ciguatera fish poisonings

Symptoms develop 1–6 hours (extreme range, minutes to 30 hours) after eating warm water shore or coral reef fish such as groupers, snappers, parrot fish, mackerel, moray eels, barracudas, and jacks especially in the South Pacific and Caribbean (including Florida) between latitudes 35°N and 34°S. There are more than 50 000 cases each year with an incidence of up to 2 per cent of the population/year and a case fatality of about 0.1 per cent. Ciguatoxin, maitotoxin, and scaritoxin are polyethers ultimately derived through the food chain from bacterial synthesis in benthic dinoflagellates such as *Gambierdiscus toxicus*. They are concentrated in the liver, viscera, and gonads, especially of large old fish. Exotic fish from the Caribbean and elsewhere are imported into Britain, causing cases of ciguatera. Gastrointestinal symptoms resolve within a few hours, but paraesthesiae and myalgias may persist for months.

Tetrodotoxin poisoning

Scaleless porcupine, sun, puffer, and toad fish (order Tetraodontiformes) may contain the aminoperhydroquinazoline, tetrodotoxin, acquired through the food chain. It is one of the most potent non-protein toxins, blocking sodium ion flux through excitable membranes and prolonging nerve conduction. It is concentrated in the ovaries, viscera, and skin of tetraodontiform fish and also occurs in the skin of some frogs, newts, and salamanders, the saliva of octopuses, the digestive glands of several species of gastropod mollusc, in xanthid and horseshoe crabs, flat and ribbon worms, and algae.

The flesh of the puffer fish (fugu) is a delicacy in Japan where, despite stringent regulations, there are still a few cases of tetrodotoxin poisoning each year with four deaths. Neurotoxic symptoms develop within 10–45 minutes and death from respiratory paralysis usually occurs between 2 and 6 hours after eating the fish. There may be no gastrointestinal symptoms. Skin changes include erythema, petechiae, blistering, and desquamation.

Paralytic shellfish poisoning

Bivalve molluscs (mussels, clams, oysters, cockles, and scallops) and some crabs may acquire tetrahydropurine neurotoxins such as saxitoxin from dinoflagellates (*Gonyaulax* sp.). 'Red tides' are caused by blooming of these dinoflagellates. Gastrointestinal symptoms develop within 30 minutes of ingestion. Fatal respiratory paralysis may ensue. In the UK there have been several outbreaks of neurotoxic red whelk (*Neptunea antiqua*) poisoning attributable to tetramine.

Histamine-like syndrome (scrombrotoxic poisoning)

Histidine in the red flesh of scrombroid fish (tuna, mackerel, bonito, and skipjack) and of canned non-scrombroid fish, such as sardines and pilchards, is converted by bacteria (*Morganella morgani* and *Klebsiella pneumoniae*) to saurine, histamine, and other toxins. Histamine absorbed from the gut is normally broken down by *N*-methyltransferase and diamine oxidase (histaminase), but if the histamine concentration is very high, or the patient is taking a diamine oxidase inhibitor such as isoniazid (as antituberculosis chemotherapy) scrombrotoxic poisoning may result. Toxic fish may produce a tingling or smarting sensation in the mouth when eaten. Within minutes or up to a few hours after ingestion, flushing, burning, sweating, urticaria, pruritus, headache, abdominal colic, nausea, vomiting, diarrhoea, bronchial asthma, giddiness, and hypotension may develop. The differential diagnosis includes bacterial and viral food poisoning and allergic reactions.

Treatment

Gastrointestinal contents should be eliminated by emetics and purges. Activated charcoal adsorbs saxitoxin and other shellfish toxins. Mannitol has been advocated for ciguatera poisoning. In adults, 1 g/kg of

10 per cent or 20 per cent mannitol is given by intravenous infusion over 30 minutes as soon as possible after rehydration. Atropine may improve gastrointestinal symptoms and sinus bradycardia. Calcium gluconate relieves mild neuromuscular symptoms. Scrombrotoxic symptoms can be alleviated with antihistamines and bronchodilators.

Prevention

Most toxins are heat stable but some are moderately water soluble and may be leached out by soaking. In tropical areas, the flesh of fish should be separated as soon as possible from the head, skin, intestines, gonads, and other viscera which may contain high concentrations of toxin. Scaleless fish, very large fish, and especially Moray eels should not be eaten. Scrombroid poisoning can be prevented by eating fish fresh or by freezing them as soon as possible after they are caught. Shellfish should not be eaten during red tides and other dangerous seasons.

Poisoning by ingestion of carp's gall bladder

See OTM3, p. 1143.

Venomous marine invertebrates

Cnidarians (jellyfish, cubomedusoids, sea wasps, Portuguese-men-of-war or bluebottles, hydroids, sea anemones etc.)

The tentacles of cnidarian coelenterates are armed with hundreds of thousands of nematocysts which fire stinging hairs into the dermis producing lines of painful irritant weals. Their venoms contain or release vasoactive substances such as histamine and kinins which cause immediate local pain, inflammation, urticaria, and necrosis and, in some cases, severe systemic symptoms.

Epidemiology

The most dangerous species, the box jellyfish, sea wasp, or seastinger (*Chironex fleckeri*) of northern Australia, has caused more than 60 deaths since 1884. Most stings occur in December and January. Fatal stings have also been inflicted by other box jellyfish in the Indo-Pacific region, by the Portuguese man-o-war (*Physalia*) and the Chinese jellyfish *Stomolophus nomurai.* In northern Queensland stings by *Carukia barnesi* (lrukandji stings) are common and potentially dangerous.

Clinical features

The pattern of weals on the skin may be diagnostic. Immediate severe pain is the commonest symptom. Chirodropid box jellyfish (genera *Chironex* and *Chiropsalmus)* cause cough, nausea, vomiting, abdominal colic, diarrhoea, rigors, severe musculoskeletal pains, profuse sweating, respiratory arrest, generalized convulsions, pulmonary oedema, and cardiac arrest which may occur within minutes of the accident. lrukandji syndrome consists of severe musculoskeletal pain, anxiety, trembling, headache, piloerection, sweating, tachycardia, hypertension, and pulmonary oedema starting about 30 minutes after the sting. Stings by *Chrysaora quinquecirrha* (American 'sea nettle'), Cyanea ('Lion's mane'), and Pelagia can be very painful but are rarely; if ever, life-threatening.

Treatment

Stung victims must be removed from the sea as quickly as possible. The aim is to prevent further discharge of nematocysts on fragments of tentacles stuck to the skin. Alcoholic solutions such as methylated spirits, suntan lotion etc., the traditional remedy, cause massive discharge of nematocysts! Commercial vinegar or 3–10 per cent aqueous acetic acid is, however, effective for *Chironex* and *Chiropsalmus* but not for *Physalia* and *Stomolophus*; and baking soda and water (50 per cent w/v) is effective for the widely distributed Atlantic genus, *Chrysaora.* Ice packs can be applied. In patients with extensive stings, firm crepe bandaging of stung limb areas (after inactivation of nematocysts), or the application of tourniquets proximal to the stung areas may delay the absorption of venom. Cardiopulmonary resuscitation on the beach saved the lives of several Australian patients. A specific box jellyfish antivenom for *C. fleckeri* is manufactured in Australia. It is given by intramuscular injection (3 ampoules) on the beach by surf livesavers and, in hospital, by intravenous infusion.

Prevention

Bathers should keep out of the sea when dangerous cnidarians are prevalent, especially when warning notices have been put up, or bathe in stinger-resistant enclosures. Lycra or wet suits and other clothing will protect against nematocyst stings. Divers should look upwards during their ascent to avoid surfacing underneath these animals.

Echinodermata (starfish and sea urchins)

These animals are armed with numerous long, sharp projecting spines and grapples which can envenom when embedded in the skin. Severe pain, local swelling, and, rarely, systemic effects may develop; syncope, numbness, generalized paralysis, aphonia, respiratory distress, cardiac arrhythmias, and even death. Embedded fragments of spines may lead to secondary infection and chronic granulomas or damage to bones and joints.

Treatment

Skin penetrated by the spines, usually the soles of the feet, should be softened with 2 per cent salicylic acid ointment or acetone. The spines can then be squeezed out or removed surgically. No antivenoms are available.

Mollusca (cone shells and octopuses)

Cone shells (genus Conus) are carnivorous marine snails with beautiful shells. They harpoon their prey (fish, polychaete worms, and other molluscs), implanting a radular tooth containing a mixture of peptide neurotoxins. In humans, symptoms include local paraesthesia, numbness,and paralysis which may prove fatal.

Two species of small octopus found in the Australian and West Pacific region (blue ringed octopus *Octopus maculosus and O. lunulatus*) can bite swimmers with their powerful beaks and inject salivary tetrodotoxin. There is pain, local bleeding, swelling, and inflammation. Fatal generalized paralysis may develop within 15 minutes of the bite.

Treatment

No antivenoms are available. Cardiorespiratory resuscitation and mechanical ventilation may be required.

Further reading

Williamson, J.A., *et al.* (ed.). (1996). *Venomous and poisonous marine animals.* University of New South Wales Press, Sydney.

Eastaugh, J. and Shepherd, S. (1989). Infections and toxic syndromes from fish and shellfish consumption. A review. *Archives of Internal Medicine* **149**, 1735–40.

Halstead, B.W. (1988). *Poisonous and venomous marine animals of the world.* 2nd revised edn. Darwin Press, Princeton.

Venomous arthropods

Hymenoptera (bees, wasps, yellowjackets, hornets, and ants)

The commonest and most severe Hymenoptera stings are inflicted by members of the families Apidae (bees), Vespidae (wasps, yellowjackets, and hornets), and Formicidae (fire ants). Allergic reactions to single Hymenoptera stings are common, whereas toxic reactions resulting from many stings are rare. Venom allergens include phospholipases A, hyaluronidase, acid phosphomonoesterases and melittin (bee).

Epidemiology

Less than 10 people die from hymenoptera sting anaphylaxis in Britain each year and in the USA there are between 40 and 50 deaths a year. The prevalence of severe Hymenoptera sting hypersensitivity is about 0.4–0.8 per cent in children and 4 per cent in adults.

Clinical features

Direct toxic effects

In non-sensitized individuals, a sting, which, in the case of Vespidae and Apidae, introduces about 50 μg of venom, will rapidly produce a hot, red, painful swelling and weal a few centimetres in diameter, which persists for a few hours. As few as 30 stings can cause fatal systemic envenoming in children, but children and adults have survived more than 1000 bee stings. In some patients, symptoms suggested histamine toxicity (vasodilatation, hypotension, vomiting, diarrhoea, throbbing headache, coma, and bronchoconstriction). In Latin America, mass attacks by *A. m. scutellata* (Africanized 'killer' bees) have caused generalized rhabdomyolysis, intravascular haemolysis, hypercatecholaminaemia (hypertension, pulmonary oedema, myocardial damage), bleeding, hepatic dysfunction, and acute renal failure.

Allergic effects

Exceptionally, sensitized individuals may die within minutes of the sting. Systemic symptoms include generalized tingling and itching, flushing, dizziness, syncope, shaking, wheezing, abdominal colic, diarrhoea, incontinence of urine and faeces, tachycardia, and visual disturbances, all developing within a few minutes of the sting. Over the next 15–20 minutes, urticaria, angio-oedema, oedema of the glottis, profound hypotension, and coma may develop. Some people develop massive local swelling at the site of the sting; this may be immediate or delayed and can persist for more than a week. A few patients develop serum sickness a week or more after the sting. Many patients with sting allergy have other evidence of an atopic disposition. Reactions are enhanced by β-blockers.

Diagnosis of venom hypersensitivity

Type I hypersensitivity is confirmed by detecting venom specific IgE in the serum using RAST or by prick skin testing. Patients who have suffered a systemic reaction have a 50–60 per cent risk of reacting to the next sting. Children who have generalized urticaria after a sting have only a 10 per cent chance of a systemic reaction when restung. Hypersensitivity to venom may be lost spontaneously especially by children and young adults.

Treatment

Barbed bee stings remain embedded in the skin and continue to inject venom; they should be removed immediately. Wasp stings may become infected. Aspirin and application of ice packs are effective in reducing the pain. Systemic antihistamines can be used for more severe local reactions. Massive local reactions can be treated with a short course of aspirin or corticosteroid. Systemic anaphylaxis must be treated with 0.1 per cent (1:1000) epinephrine (adrenaline) (0.5 ml for adults, 0.01 mg/kg for children) given by intramuscular injection, or, if the patient is unconscious or pulseless or in hospital, by intravenous injection. In rare cases, blood pressure fails to respond even to large doses of epinephrine and plasma expanders. These patients should be given selective bronchodilators such as salbutamol, pressor agents, intravenous histamine H_1 antagonists such as chlorpheniramine maleate (10 mg for adults, 0.2 mg/kg for children) and histamine H_2 antagonists. Corticosteroids are not useful in the treatment of severe systemic anaphylaxis but may prevent relapses. Patients who know they are hypersensitive to venom should wear an identifying tag (such as provided by Medic-Alert in Britain) as they may be discovered unconscious after being stung. They should be trained to give themselves epinephrine intramuscularly and should always carry a preloaded syringe of epinephrine for this purpose (e.g. 'Epipen', 'Anapen', or 'Min-i-Jet'). Epinephrine delivered by a pressurized inhaler can be as effective if at least 20 puffs are taken (10–15 for children) but the effect is more transient than with injected epinephrine. Respiratory tract obstruction and shock are the main causes of death.

Severe envenoming from multiple Hymenoptera stings should be treated with epinephrine, intravenous antihistamines (doses as above), and corticosteroids. Intensive care is essential. Intravenous fluids, with or without mannitol and bicarbonate, may reduce the risk of pigment nephropathy as in crush syndrome. No antivenom is commercially available. Exchange transfusion or plasmapheresis might be considered to remove venom in severe cases. Renal dialysis may be required.

Prevention

Patients over the age of 25 years who have both a history of systemic anaphylaxis following a sting and evidence of Type I hypersensitivity to bee or wasp venoms (venom specific IgE detectable in the serum or a positive skin test) should be considered for desensitization with pure venoms. This treatment has proved to be significantly more effective than placebo or the previously used whole body extracts of Hymenoptera in preventing anaphylactic reactions to sting challenge. Desensitization must be carried out where there are facilities for cardiopulmonary resuscitation, as it is complicated by systemic reactions in 5–15 per cent of patients and by large local reactions in 50 per cent. Patients should be kept under observation for at least 30 minutes after treatment.

Further reading

British Society for Allergy and Clinical Immunology. (1993). Position paper on allergen immunotherapy. Report of a BSACI working party. *Clinical and Experimental Allergy*, **23**, Suppl. 3, 144.

França, F.O.S., *et al.* (1994). Severe and fatal mass attacks by bees (Africanized honey bees- *Apis mellifera scutellata*) in Brazil:

clinicopathological studies with measurement of serum venom concentrations and a review of the literature. *Quarterly Journal of Medicine*, **87**, 269–82.

Mueller, U.R. (1990). *Insect sting allergy. Clinical picture, diagnosis and treatment.* Gustav Fischer, Stuttgart.

Venomous lepidoptera and coleoptera including 'blister beetles'

See OTM3, p. 1146.

Scorpions (Scorpiones: Buthidae, Scorpionidae)

Species capable of inflicting fatal stings occur in North Africa and the Middle East (genus Androctonus, Buthus, and Leiurus), South Africa (Parabuthus), India (*Mesobuthus tamulus*), North, Central, and Southern America and Trinidad (Tityus (Plate 8) and Centruroides).

Epidemiology

In Mexico there are between 1000 and 2000 deaths each year. In Algeria there are an average of 1260 stings and 24 deaths per year. Case fatality is highest among young children (up to 50 per cent in children less than 5 years old).

Clinical features

Intense local pain is the commonest symptom. There may be slight local oedema and tender enlargement of regional lymph nodes. Systemic symptoms may develop within minutes or be delayed for as much as 24 hours. There is some variation in symptoms depending on the species and geographical area. Scorpion venoms stimulate the release of acetylcholine and catecholamines causing initial cholinergic and later adrenergic symptoms. Early symptoms include vomiting, profuse sweating, piloerection, alternating brady- and tachycardia, abdominal colic, diarrhoea, loss of sphincter control, and priapism. Later, severe life-threatening cardiorespiratory effects may appear: hypertension, shock, tachy- and bradyarrhythmias, ECG changes, and pulmonary oedema with or without myocardial dysfunction. Stings by *Androctonus* spp., *Leiurus quinquestriatus, Mesobuthus tamulus,* and *Tityus* spp. can cause severe cardiovascular complications. Stings by North American *Centruroides sculpturatus* produce neurotoxic effects such as fasciculation, spasms, respiratory paralysis, and convulsions. Stings by the Trinidad black scorpion (*Tilyus trinitatis*) cause severe abdominal pain with nausea, vomiting and haematemesis, hyperglycaemia, and biochemical evidence of acute pancreatitis.

Treatment

Pain responds temporarily to local infiltration or ring block with local anaesthetic. In India, local injection of emetine dihydrochloride is preferred but may cause local and systemic toxicity. Strong systemic analgesics may be required.

Specific antivenom should be administered intravenously as soon as possible in patients with systemic envenoming and in young children stung by dangerous species, even before the development of these symptoms. Patients with severe cardiovascular symptoms should be admitted to an intensive care unit. They benefit from vasodilator treatment with α-blockers (e.g. prazosin), calcium channel blockers, or ACE inhibitors. Atropine should not be used except in cases of life-threatening sinus bradycardia. Cardiac glycosides and β-blockers are contraindicated. Anticonvulsants such as phenobarbitone are recommended for neurotoxic symptoms.

Prevention

Scorpions can be kept out of houses by surrounding the base of outside walls with ceramic tiles, making the doorsteps at least 20 cm high, and using residual insecticides, such as 1 per cent lindane or dieldrin powders.

Further reading

Bettini, S. (ed.). (1978). *Arthropod venoms. Handbook of experimental pharmacology,* Vol 48, p. 279. Springer-Verlag, Berlin.

Harvey, A. (ed). (1994). Scorpion envenoming. *Toxicon,* **32**, 1007–44.

Polis, G.A. (ed.). (1990). *The biology of scorpions.* Stanford University Press, Stanford.

Spiders (Araneae)

Spiders bite with a pair of small venom fangs, the chelicerae. There are several important genera of venomous spiders: Loxosceles cause necrotic araneism and Latrodectus, Phoneutria, Atrax, and Hadronyche cause neurotoxic araneism.

Epidemiology

In Chile, the case fatality of *Loxosceles laeta* bites is 1–17 per cent. The brown recluse spider (*L. reclusa*) causes many bites and a few deaths in the USA. Most Loxosceles bites happen in bedrooms while people are asleep or dressing. *Latrodectus tredecemguttatus* ('tarantula') lives in fields in Mediterranean countries and has been responsible for epidemics of bites. In Australia, the redback spider (*Latrodectus hasselti*) causes more than 300 bites each year; 20 deaths have been reported. The black widow spider (*L. mactans*) was responsible for 63 deaths in the USA between 1950 and 1959. *Phoneutria nigriventer*, the Brazilian armed, wandering, or banana spider has been imported to temperate countries on bunches of bananas.

The Sydney funnel web spider (*Atrax robustus*) occurs only within a 160-mile (256 km) radius of Sydney. The aggressive males of this species caused at least 13 deaths between 1927 and 1980. Closely related *Hadronyche* species are potentially as dangerous. In England, mild neurotoxic araneism has been described after bites by *Steatoda nobilis* (Theridiidae) and the woodlouse spider (*Dysdera crocota*).

Necrotic araneism

There is burning at the site of the bite with swelling and development of a characteristic macular lesion which becomes violaceous and then turns into a blackened eschar that sloughs in a few weeks, sometimes leaving a necrotic ulcer. Facial lesions may cause much oedema. Thirteen per cent of cases have systemic symptoms such as fever, scarlatiniform rash, jaundice, and haemoglobinuria resulting from intravascular haemolysis. Renal failure may ensue. The case fatality is about 6 per cent of all reported cases and 30 per cent of those with systemic envenoming.

Neurotoxic araneism

The bite may be painless (*L. hasselti*) or painful (*L. mactans*). Local sweating and piloerection may be the only signs. After about 30 minutes there is painful regional lymphadenopathy, then headache, nausea, vomiting, sweating, goosefiesh, and painful muscle spasms and tremors. Other features include tachycardia, hypertension, restlessness, irritability, psychosis, priapism, and rhabdomyolysis. The 'facies latrodectismica' is a painful grimace caused by facial spasm and trismus associated with swollen eyelids, congested conjunctivae, flushing, and sweating (*L. tredecemguttatus*). Similar effects are seen in patients bitten by Phoneutria and Atrax.

First aid treatment

In the case of bites by spiders with rapidly acting and potent venoms, such as *A. robustus*, firm crepe bandaging and splinting of the bitten limb or a tight tourniquet may delay venom spread until the patient reaches hospital.

Treatment

Antivenoms for Latrodectus, Atrax, Loxosceles, and Phoneutria bites are available.

Further reading

Maretić, Z. and Lebez, D. (1979). *Araneism with special reference to Europe.* Novit, Pula-Ljubjan, Yugoslavia.

Sutherland, S.K. (1983). *Australian animal toxins. The creatures, their toxins and care of the poisoned patient.* Oxford University Press, Melbourne.

Ticks (Acari)

Taxonomy and epidemiology

Some species of hard and soft tick can inject a salivary presynaptic neurotoxin while feeding on human blood. Most cases of tick paralysis have been reported from western North America (*Dermacentor andersoni*), eastern USA (*D. variabilis*), and eastern Australia (*Ixodes holocyclus*). In British Columbia there were 305 cases with 30 deaths between 1900 and 1968 and in New South Wales there were some 20 deaths between 1900 and 1945.

Clinical features

Ticks are picked up in the countryside or from domestic animals, particularly dogs, in the home. The patient, usually a child, develops an ascending flaccid paralysis with paraesthesiae after the tick has been attached for 5–6 days. The child, who may have been irritable for the previous 24 hours, falls on getting out of bed first thing in the morning and is found to be weak or ataxic. Paralysis increases over the next few days: death results from bulbar and respiratory paralysis and aspiration of stomach contents. Vomiting is a feature of the more acute course of *Ixodes holocyclus* envenoming.

Differential diagnosis includes poliomyelitis, Guillain-Barré syndrome, paralytic rabies, Eaton-Lambert syndrome, myasthenia gravis, and botulism. Diagnosis depends on finding the tick, which is likely to be concealed in a crevice, orifice such as the external auditory meatus, scalp, or other hairy area of the body.

Treatment

The tick must be detached without being squeezed. It can be painted with ether, chloroform, paraffin, petrol, or turpentine, or prised out between the partially separated tips of a pair of small curved forceps. Following removal of the tick there is usually rapid and complete recovery, but in Australia, patients have died after the tick has been detached. An antivenom is available in Australia.

Further reading

Murnaghan, M.F. and O'Rourke, F.J. (1978). Tick paralysis. In: *Arthropod venoms. Handbook of experimental pharmacology* ,Vol. 48 (ed S. Bettini), p. 419. Springer-Verlag, Berlin.

Stone, B.F. (1987). Toxicoses induced by ticks and reptiles in domestic animals. In: *Natural toxins: animal, plant and microbial* (ed. J.B. Harris), pp. 56–71.Oxford University Press, Oxford.

Centipedes (Chilopoda) and millipedes (Diplopida)

See OTM3, p. 1149.

Leeches (Phylum Annelida, Class Hirudinea)

Leeches are blood-sucking or carnivorous annelids whose saliva contains a histamine-like vasodilator and anticoagulants, such as hirudin from the medicinal leech (*Hirudo medicinalis*) which inhibits thrombin and factor IXa. Recombinant hirudin is now produced as a therapeutic anticoagulant. The medicinal leech is still used by plastic surgeons to reduce haematomas under skin grafts; the wound may become infected with *Aeromonas hydrophila* which lives symbiotically in the leech's gut.

Land leeches infest the damp, leafy floor and low vegetation of rain forests, especially game trails and watering places. They drop on to the prey or pursue them with a looping or lashing motion. In humans, they usually attach themselves to the lower legs or ankles and are adept at penetrating clothing.

Aquatic leeches may be swallowed by those who drink stagnant water or even mountain stream water or they may attack bathers, entering the mouth, nostrils, eyes, vulva, vagina, urethra, or anus.

Clinical features

The main effect is blood loss, but other symptoms include pain caused by the bite, secondary infection, a residual itching, and phobia. Ingested aquatic leeches usually attach to the nose or pharynx but may penetrate the trachea, bronchi, or oesophagus. The buffalo leech (*Hirudinaria manillensis*) entering through the anus can reach the rectosigmoid junction of the bowel causing perforation and peritonitis. Patients with a leech in the pharynx often have a feeling of movement at the back of the throat with cough, hoarseness, stridor, breathlessness, epistaxis, haemoptysis, haematemesis, and severe anaemia. Fatal upper airway obstruction may result.

Treatment

Leeches will detach if a grain of salt, a lighted match or a cigarette, alcohol, turpentine, or vinegar are applied. Local bleeding can be stopped by applying a styptic, such as silver nitrate or a firm dressing. Aquatic leeches which have penetrated the respiratory, upper gastro-intestinal or genitourinary tracts, or the rectum must be removed by endoscope. Spraying with 30 per cent cocaine, 10 per cent tartaric acid, dilute (1:10 000) adrenaline, or even commercial soda water makes the leech detach in the nasopharynx, larynx, trachea, or oesophagus, while irrigation with concentrated salt solution may be effective in the genitourinary tract and rectum. Leeches should not be pulled off so roughly that the mouth parts are left in the wound as this will lead to a chronic infection. Antimicrobial treatment of secondary bacterial infections (e.g. of *Aeromonas hydrophila* with cefuroxime or a quinolone) may be required.

Prevention is by impregnating clothing, especially the bottoms of trousers and socks, with repellents such as dibutyl phthalate and diethyl toluamide. Children should be discouraged from bathing in leech-infested waters and all drinking water should be boiled or filtered.

Further reading

Sawyer, R.T. (1986). *Leech biology and behaviour.* Oxford University Press, Oxford.

Chapter 18.3

Poisonous plants and fungi

M. R. Cooper and A.W. Johnson

Poisonous plants and fungi are abundant in both urban and rural environments, but only 5–10 per cent of enquiries to poisons centres are about plant poisoning. In most cases there is only mild gastrointestinal irritation. In temperate zones most enquiries involve young children and are concerned with fruits and seeds; some, including those of the cherry laurel (*Prunus laurocerasus*) and *Laburnum*, are toxic, while others are non-toxic or only mildly so: *Cotoneaster* spp., honeysuckle (*Lonicera* spp.), *Pyracantha* spp., Christmas cherry (*Solanum pseudocapsicum*), and *Berberis* spp. A few plants and fungi can cause death; these include deadly nightshade (*Atropa belladonna*), monkshood (*Aconitum napellus*), yew (*Taxus baccata*), oleanders (*Nerium oleander* and *Thevetia* peruviana), castor beans (*Ricinus communis*), jequirity beans (*Abrusprecatorius*), and the death cap fungus (*Amanita phalloides*). As there are no specific antidotes to most plant poisons the general principles of treatment are the same as those for poisoning from any other source (see Chapter 18.1).

Plant poisoning

Clinical effects can be used to classify the different types of plant poisoning:

1. Digestive tract irritation;
2. Cardiovascular disturbances;
3. Central nervous effects;
4. Liver damage;
5. Kidney damage;
6. Skin damage;
7. Nicotine-like effects;
8. Atropine-like effects;
9. Hydrocyanic acid toxicity.

However, poisoning by some plants causes symptoms of more than one type, and the severity may vary according to the sensitivity of the individual.

Digestive tract irritation (Plates 1–5)

Some plants have very irritant sap: that of cuckoo pint (*Arum maculatum*), dumb cane (*Dieffenbachia* spp.), elephant's ear (*Philodendron* spp.) and black bryony (*Tamus communis*) contains calcium oxalate, and that of *Euphorbia* spp. and mezereon and spurge laurel (*Daphne* spp.) diterpene esters. These cause immediate soreness, reddening, and even blistering of the lips and mouth. With most plants, however, the first signs of poisoning are nausea, abdominal pain, and vomiting. In many cases the vomiting eliminates the poisonous substances and prevents the development of further toxic effects; elimination is also promoted by diarrhoea.Toxic agents causing irritation of the stomach and intestines include anthraquinones found in *Aloe* spp., and purging buckthorn (*Rhamnus cathartica*), cytisine in *Laburnum* spp., lectins in *Jatropha*, protoanemonin in *Anemone spp.*, *Helleborus* spp., and *Ranunculus* spp., saponins in horse chestnut (*Aesculus hippocastanum*) and ivy (*Hedera helix*), and viscotoxins in mistletoe (*Viscum album*). Unidentified irritants are present in white bryony (*Bryonia dioica*), holly (*Ilex aquifolium*), *Lantana camara*, privet (*Ligustrum vulgare*), pokeweed (*Phytolacca americana*), and snowberry (*Symphoricarpus alba*). With other plants the start of gastrointestinal symptoms is delayed for several hours (up to 2 days). The toxins responsible include colchicine in autumn crocus (*Colchicum autumnale*) and glory lily (*Gloriosa superba*), lectins in jequirity beans (*Abrusprecatorius*), castor beans (*Ricinus communis*), and false acacia (*Robiniapseudoacacia*), oxalic acid in Virginia creeper (*Parthenocissus* spp.) and some members of the Polygonaceae family, solanine in *Solanum* spp., and unidentified agents, such as that in spindle (*Euonymus europaeus*).

If vomiting has not occurred spontaneously, gastric emptying should be ensured by lavage or use of an emetic, although the value of this type of treatment will depend on the time that has lapsed since ingestion. Fluid and electrolyte balance must be maintained.

Cardiovascular disturbances (Plates 6–9)

In addition to the well-known effects of the cardiac glycosides of the foxglove (*Digitalis purpurea*), there are various other plants that produce the digitalis-like effects seen in digoxin overdosage: lily of the valley (*Convallaria majalis*), bluebell (*Hyacinthoides non-scripta*), oleander (*Nerium oleander*), and yellow oleander (*Thevetia peruviana*). Cardiovascular effects are also induced by aconitine in monkshood (*Aconitum napellus*) and larkspurs (*Delphinium* spp.), andromedotoxins in mountain laurel (*Kalmia latifolia*), *Menziesia* spp., *Pieris* spp., and *Rhododendron* spp., proveratrines in *Veratrum* spp., taxines in yews (*Taxus* spp.), and veratrine in death camas (*Zigadenus* spp.). American mistletoes (*Phoradendron* spp.) cause bradycardia as well as irritating the digestive tract.

Ingested material should be removed, but not with ipecacuanha as this can also have effects on the heart. The Fab fragments of digoxin-specific antibodies (e.g. 'Digibind', 'DigiTAb') are not just specific for digoxin, but can also be used to reverse the toxic effects of some other cardiac glycosides, notably those in *Thevetia peruviana* (Apocynaceae), a common agent of suicide in south Asia. Poisoning by the highly toxic alkaloids in *Aconitum* spp. should always be treated as an emergency.

Central nervous effects (Plate 10)

Some plants contain hallucinogenic compounds, for which they are smoked, chewed, eaten, or infused in water to make teas. Among the plant hallucinogens are tetrahydrocannabinols in cannabis (*Cannabis sativa*, see also Chapter 18.1), alkaloids in khat (*Catha edulis*), lysergic acid and ethylamides in morning glory (*Ipomoea* spp.), mescaline in *peyote* (*Lophophora williamsii*), myristicin in nutmeg (*Myristica fragrans*), and vincristine and vinblastine in periwinkle (*Vinca* spp.).

A number of plants contain convulsants, although actual clinical cases mainly involve Umbelliferae, such as cowbane (*Cicuta virosa*) and hemlock water dropwort (*Oenanthe crocata*) that contain cicutoxin and oenanthetoxin, respectively. Other convulsants include hypoglycin A in akee (*Blighia sapida*), coriariamyrtin in *Coriaria myrtifolia*, anthracenones in Karwinskia humboldtiana, tetranortriterpenes in chinaberry (*Melia azedarach*), alkaloids in moonseed (*Menispermum canadense*), podophylloresin in May apple (*Podophyllum peltatum*), and strychnine and brucine in nux vomica (*Strychnos nia-vomica*).

Patients who have taken hallucinogens require reassurance and supportive treatment. Convulsions must be controlled and respiration supported; gastric lavage may then be possible.

Liver damage (Plate 11)

Various plants in the Compositae (*Senecio* spp.), Leguminosae (*Crotalaria* spp.), and Boraginaceae (*Heliotropium* and *Symphytum* spp.), as well as some in other families contain pyrrolizidine alkaloids, which principally affect the liver. Poisoning has occurred from contamination of cereal crops by these plants and their consequent incorporation into bread, and their use in herbal medicines and bush teas. These alkaloids can cause acute damage to the liver (veno-occlusive disease), which has occurred mainly in Jamaica, India, and Afghanistan. Symptoms, including nausea, abdominal pain and distension, hepatomegaly, and sometimes fever and vomiting, first appear a few days after ingestion. A chronic cirrhosis of the liver can occur in people ingesting small quantities of pyrrolizidine alkaloids over a long period.

Treatment can only be supportive, as once absorbed, there is no specific method of preventing the toxic effects of these alkaloids.

Kidney damage

This can occur after ingestion of plants rich in oxalates, e.g. the leaves of rhubarb (*Rheum rhabarbarum*), and docks and sorrels (*Rumex* spp.).

An emetic should be given, followed by generous fluid replacement to promote renal excretion of the oxalates.

Skin damage (Plates 12–14)

The most common form of skin damage by plants is a non-allergic dermatitis that results from direct contact with various plants that contain irritants, e.g. the stinging hairs of the stinging nettle (*Urtica dioica*), the diterpene-containing latex of *Euphorbia* spp., or the calcium oxalate crystals of *Dieffenbachia* spp. and other members of the Araceae family. There are also allergic forms of dermatitis that result from hypersensitivity to plant allergens. The most common forms of allergic contact dermatitis in the USA are caused by poison ivy (*Toxicodendron radicans*) and western poison oak (*Toxicodendron diversilobum*), and in the UK by primula (*Primula obconica*), but such cutaneous hypersensitivity can occur to a very large number of vascular plants. Some plants contain phototoxic chemicals that increase the reactivity of the skin to ultraviolet light. Exposure to sunlight after eating fat hen (*Chenopodium album*), orache (*Atriplex purpurea*), or other members of the Chenopodiaceae has resulted in severe skin damage. Psoralens (furanocoumarins) are present in various members of the Umbelliferae, including giant hogweed (*Heracleum mantegazzianum*) and parsnips (*Pastinaca sativa*), and also celery (*Apium graveolens*) when infected with the pink rot fungus (*Sclerotinia sclerotiorum*). Other psoralen-containing plants are rue (*Ruta graveolens*) and the gas plant (*Dictamnus album*), both in the Rutaceae family. Typical lesions in dermatitis caused by psoralens are erythema, papules, vesicles, and enormous bullae localized to exposed areas of skin. Psoralens can also induce hyperpigmentation that can last for several months.

Nicotine-like effects (Plate 15)

Nicotine and other alkaloids with similar actions, such as coniine from hemlock (*Conium maculatum*), first stimulate and then paralyse all autonomic ganglia. Centrally, small doses cause respiratory stimulation, while large doses can lead to convulsions and arrest of respiration. Similar effects occur with gelsemine and related alkaloids in yellow jessamine (*Gelsemium sempervirens*), cytisine in *Laburnum* spp., lobeline in *Lobelia* spp., and nicotine in tobacco plants (*Nicotiana tabacum*).

Treatment should be symptomatic. Gastric lavage rather than ipecacuanha-induced emesis is recommended because of the rapid onset of the effects of nicotine.

Atropine-like effects (Plates 16–18)

The tropane alkaloids atropine, hyoscine (scopolamine), and hyoscyamine present in some plants of the Solanaceae competitively inhibit the muscarinic effects of acetylcholine and block the parasympathetic nervous system. They can cause death by depression of the respiratory centre. The plants in this group include deadly nightshade (*Atropa belladonna*), angel's trumpet (*Brugmansia* spp.), thorn apple (*Datura stramonium*), and henbane (*Hyoscyamus rigor*). The clinical signs of poisoning they produce vary with the relative proportions of the different tropane alkaloids they contain. Gardeners who handle these plants and then rub their eyes may develop unilateral or bilateral mydriasis.

Ipecacuanha can be used to induce emesis if given within 30 minutes of ingestion, otherwise gastric lavage should be performed. Physostigmine has been recommended for treatment of the central and peripheral effects, but it is not clear that this is superior to supportive management.

Hydrocyanic acid toxicity

Parts of some plants contain relatively high concentrations of cyanogenic glycosides. The most likely sources are the kernels of fruits of *Prunus* spp. (almonds, apricots, cherries, peaches, etc.) or of loquat (*Eriobotrya japonica*), a large number of apple pips (*Malus* spp.), the berries or leaves of the cherry laurel (*Prunus laurocerasus*), or inadequately prepared cassava (*Manihot esculenta*).

The symptoms and treatment are as for hydrocyanic acid poisoning from any other source (see Chapter 18.1).

Food plant toxicity (Plate 19)

The main toxins present in plants used regularly for food include lectins, cyanogens, alkaloids, oxalates, and polyphenols (mainly tannins).

Lectins

These phytohaemagglutinins are glycoproteins, and beans (Leguminosae) are the main food source. The lectins are not readily digested by pepsin, and have a strong affinity for the intestinal mucosa, where they prevent absorption of carbohydrates. Adequate cooking destroys the lectins, but eating raw or incompletely cooked beans can cause diarrhoea, while long-term exposure can lead to retarded growth and may even be fatal.

Cyanogens

Cyanogenic glycosides are present in some staple foods, such as cassava, sweet potato, and yam, all of which can be made safe to eat by adequate soaking, drying, or fermentation. Chronic poisoning may cause tropical ataxic neuropathy, and spastic paraparesis (konzo).

Alkaloids

Dangerously high quantities of these may develop in some plant foods, e.g. potato tubers that have sprouted or been stored in the light and become green. The green colour is chlorophyll and is harmless, but under conditions where greening occurs the glyco-alkaloid solanine and its derivatives will also have been produced; these exhibit anticholinesterase activity.

Oxalates

These accumulate in some members of the Polygonaceae, notably rhubarb, of which only the red leaf stalks should be eaten, and then only after cooking.

Polyphenols

These are a possible cause of upper digestive tract cancers that may develop after eating sorghum, or taking teas or alcoholic drinks containing high concentrations of tannins.

Some specific diseases attributable to plants are lathyrism, a paralytic disease caused by a neurotoxic amino acid in chick peas (*Lathyrus sativus*), favism that occurs among natives of some Mediterranean and Middle East countries that have a genetic deficiency of glucose 6-phosphate dehydrogenase, and cannot digest broad (fava) beans (*Vicia faba*), and Jamaican vomiting sickness that results from eating the unripe fruits of akee (*Blighia sapida*). Other foods that cause poisoning are the seeds of *Mucuna pruriens*, flour ground from the cones of cycads (e.g. *Zamia* spp.), and young fronds of bracken fern (*Pteridium aquilinum*).

Herbal medicines

It should not be assumed that herbal preparations are safe because they are 'natural', and some may have harmful effects that are not immediately obvious, e.g. carcinogenicity, hepatotoxicity, or teratogenicity. Adulteration of herbal medicines with cheaper ingredients, heavy metals, and orthodox drugs is not uncommon.

Fungal poisoning (Plates 20–23)

Most fungal poisoning results from mistaken identification. The toxicity of fungi may vary with location, season, and in different years, and there is considerable variation in the susceptibility of individuals. Cases of fungal poisoning can be classified into those that develop signs of toxicity:

1. Within 2 hours of ingestion
   - (a) Gastroenteritis;
   - (b) Sweating and vertigo;
   - (c) Mental confusion and sleep;
   - (d) Hallucinations;
   - (e) Alcohol-associated effects.
2. After a delay of 6 hours or more
   - (a) Gastroenteritis;
   - (b) Kidney failure;
   - (c) Gastrointestinal and central nervous effects.

The life-threatening conditions (especially liver and kidney failure) follow apparent recovery from gastrointestinal symptoms that start 6–24 hours after ingestion, or occur after a latent, symptomless period of several days.

Symptoms that develop within 2 hours

Gastroenteritis

Few of the chemical agents responsible for this type of poisoning have been identified. The fungi in this group include *Agaricus placomyces*, yellow-staining mushroom (*Agaricus xanthodermus*), honey fungus (*Armillaria mellea*), the Devil's mushroom (*Boletus satanus*), *Chlorophyllum molybdites*, *Entoloma* spp., *Hebeloma* spp., *Hygrocybe* spp., sulphur tuft (*Hypholoma fasciculare*), *Lactarius* spp., *Macrolepiota rhacodes*, *Megacollybia platyphylla*, *Omphalotus olearius*, *Ramariaformosa*, *Russula* spp., *Scleroderma* spp., and *Tricholoma pardinum*.

Sweating and vertigo

This, associated with nausea, headache, visual disturbances, vertigo, hypotension, and some inco-ordination, results from the parasympathomimetic effects of muscarine, which is present in many *Inocybe* and some *Clitocybe* species. There are only trace amounts of muscarine in *Amanita muscaria*, after which this toxin was named.

Mental confusion and sleep

Fungi that contain ibotenic acid and its derivative muscimol (*Amanita pantherina, A. muscaria, and A. strobiliformis*) affect psychomotor functions and cause gastrointestinal disturbances. Dizziness, delirium, and euphoria are common symptoms, sometimes associated with erratic, or even manic behaviour; deep sleep usually follows. These fungi can have very serious effects on children.

Hallucinations

Psilocybin, a tryptamine derivative with hallucinogenic properties, is found in *Psilocybe* species and several other genera of (usually small) fungi, often called collectively 'magic mushrooms'; among these are some *Conocybe* spp., *Gymnopilus* spp., *Panaeolina foenisecii*, *Panaeolus* spp., *Pluteus* spp., and *Stropharia* spp. These fungi are eaten because of their psychoactive properties. They generally produce a feeling of relaxation, with visual effects, especially heightened perception of colour and shapes. The sensations may, however, be characterized by tension, agitation, and nausea; sometimes frightening flashbacks occur.

Alcohol-associated effects

When alcohol is taken at the same time as some fungi (notably *Coprinus atramentarius* but also *Clitocybe clavipes*) or up to 5 days after they are eaten, a reaction similar to that induced by disulfiram (Antabuse) used for treating alcoholics (see also Chapter 18.1) is produced. The skin becomes flushed, and mydriasis, nausea, and hypotension can occur as a result of the accumulation of acetaldehyde, because the toxin (named coprine in *C. atramentarius*) blocks the liver enzyme aldehyde dehydrogenase.

Symptoms with delayed onset

Gastroenteritis

By far the most common cause of death from the ingestion of fungi is the death cap (*Amanita phalloides*). Specimens vary in size and cap colour (from almost white to yellowish-green). The active toxin in this mushroom and some others including the fool's mushroom

(*Amanita verna*), destroying angel (*Amanita virosa*), *Galerina* spp., and *Lepiota cristata* are cyclopeptides, called amatoxins. Persistent emesis and profuse diarrhoea begin 6–24 hours after ingestion (commonly about 12 hours). A period of apparent recovery often follows, then rapid deterioration. Despite emergency treatment to remove the toxins from the body, and the maintenance of fluid and electrolyte levels, 10–15 per cent of ingestions of half a cap or more result in death from liver and kidney failure.

Kidney failure

Poisoning characterized by oliguria and anuria after a latent period of 3 days to about 2 weeks (sometimes preceded by gastritis) is typical of the group of brownish-orange *Cortinarius* spp. (*C. orellanus*, *C. speciosissimus*, and *C. splendens*) that contain the bipyridyl toxins orelline and orellanin. Death can result from renal failure; kidney transplantation should be considered.

Gastrointestinal and central nervous effects

Gastrointestinal symptoms, associated with headache, cramps, delirium, and sometimes coma, that appear 6–24 hours after ingestion or inhalation of cooking vapour are indicative of poisoning by the false morel (*Gyromitra esculenta*). Monomethylhydrazine is liberated from gyromitrin present in the fungus.

Allergic reactions

The roll-rim cap (*Paxillus involutus*), previously eaten with impunity, may suddenly give rise to an immunohaemolytic anaemia in which decreased haemoglobin levels result in shock and even renal insufficiency. A respiratory allergy, called farmer's lung, results from inhaling spores of the mould *Faenia rectivergula* that is sometimes present on grain or hay. Spores of oyster mushrooms (*Pleurotus ostreatus*) or puffballs (*Lycoperdon* spp.) can also cause respiratory allergies. Skin allergies have been reported with the shiitake mushroom (*Lentinus eludes*).

Ergotism and mycotoxicoses

The ascomycete fungus *Claviceps purpurea* infects cereal crops in which its hard, purplish-black fruiting bodies (ergots) develop in the seed heads. Ergots contain several alkaloids that can cause disease when flour made from contaminated grain is eaten. There are two forms of ergotism: vasoconstriction, sometimes leading to loss of extremities through gangrene (occurring after small quantities of contaminated food have been eaten over a long period); and a less common, acute form characterized by muscular tremors, convulsions, and hallucinations. Other potent toxins (mycotoxins) are produced by some moulds that develop on growing crops, particularly if wet and harvested late, but occur mainly in cereal grains, rice, or nuts stored under damp, inadequately ventilated conditions. Aflatoxins (from *Aspergillus* spp.), ochratoxins (from *Aspergillus* and *Penicillium* spp.), and trichothecenes and zearalenone (from *Fusarium* spp.) have been detected in foods and are suspected of causing hepatitis, hepatocarcinoma, alveolar cell carcinoma, and colonic cancer.

Sources of further information

A directory of about 250 poison information centres is kept for the World Federation of the Association of Clinical Toxicology Centres at the Centre Anti-Poison, Lyon, France. The problem of identifying poisonous plants and fungi in the UK has been addressed by the production of a computerized, image-based system that was developed as a collaborative project by the Royal Botanic Gardens, Kew and the Poisons Unit of Guy's and St Thomas' Hospital Trust, London. The system, called *Poisonous Plants and Fungi in Britain and Ireland*, is available on CD-ROM from Scientific Publication Sales, Sir Joseph Banks Building, Royal Botanic Gardens, Kew, Richmond, TW9 3AE, UK. Similar systems are being developed for other countries.

Further reading

Benjamin, D.R. (1995). *Mushrooms: poisons and panaceas.* W.H. Freeman and Company, New York.

Cooper, M.R. and Johnson, A.W. (1998). *Poisonous plants and fungi in Britain. Animal and human poisoning.* 2nd edn. The Stationery Office, London.

Eddleston, M., *et al.* (2000). Yellow-oleander-induced toxicity treated with anti-digoxin Fab fragments; a randomised controlled trial. *Lancet*, **355**, 967–72.

Everist, S.L. (1981). *Poisonous plants of Australia.* 2nd edn.. Angus and Robertson Publishers, Sydney.

Frohne, D. and Pfander, H.J. (1997). *Giftpflanzen: ein Handbuch für Apotheker, Ärzte, Toxikologen und Biologen.* 4th edn. Wissenschaftliche Verlagsgesellschaft mbH, Stuttgart.

Lovell, C. R. (1993). *Plants and the skin.* Blackwell Scientific Publications, Oxford.

Turner, N.J. and Szczawinski, A.F. (1991, reprinted 1995). *Common poisonous plants and mushrooms of North America.* Timber Press, Portland, Oregon.

Watt, J.M. and Breyer-Brandwijk, M.G. (1962). *The medicinal and poisonous plants of southern and eastern Africa.* 2nd edn. E. and S. Livingstone Ltd., Edinburgh.

Environmental factors and disease

Chapter 18.4

Heat

W. R. Keatinge

Heat stroke

Vasodilatation can dissipate resting heat production in the body in slowly moving air up to about 32°C, but in warmer air, or in cooler air during exercise, the heat produced can only be lost if sweat is formed and can evaporate to cool the skin. Otherwise, progressive rise in body temperature above 38° leads to irritability and confusion, and ultimately to heat stroke with cardiovascular collapse and heat denaturation of proteins. Heat stroke can develop within about 20 minutes in normal people taking severe exercise if heat loss is prevented, for example by external insulation or a hot humid environment. Otherwise, heat stroke is most commonly seen in psychiatric patients receiving drugs such as barbiturates or phenothiazines which depress reflex regulation of body temperature generally, or with anticholinergic drugs which specifically suppress sweating and vasodilatation, or in autonomic hypofunction due to diabetes. Old age without other obvious disability may also be associated with increased liability to heat stroke.

Diagnosis of heat stroke is usually easy, from the history and the presence of irritability, confusion, headache, a hot and often dry skin, and a deep body temperature (oral or rectal) close to or above 41°C. Blood pressure is normal until it falls in the terminal stage of cardiovascular collapse. There is initially respiratory alkalosis due to hyperventilation, often followed by metabolic acidosis due to accumulation of lactic acid as hepatic failure develops. Serum calcium may be low in severe cases due to calcium binding by proteins of damaged cells.

Treatment consists of immediate cooling. Mild cooling by sprinkling or sponging with tepid water which is allowed to evaporate on the skin, is often more effective than very cold water, since it allows high blood flow in the skin to continue. Rapidity of treatment is more important than the method used, since heat stroke can cause sudden death, or lasting cerebellar or cerebral damage.

Postmortem examination may show little abnormality in cases of rapid death from heat stroke. Degeneration of Purkinje cells and other large cells may be present in the cerebellar and cerebral cortex, and oedema and petechial haemorrhages due to microvascular thrombosis occur in the brain, and sometimes in other tissues, in less rapid cases.

Water or salt depletion in hot environments

These often accompany heat stroke, but can occur independently. Water depletion is usually obvious from the history and thirst, sunken face and eyes, and elevated serum sodium and chloride. Haematocrit is normal since the water loss involves cell fluid and extracellular fluid proportionately. Death occurs when weight loss is 15–25 per cent of the body weight, and is due to excess concentration of salts in the body fluids. Drinking of seawater accelerates death in simple water depletion. Treatment consists of giving up to 8 litres of water by mouth during the first 24 hours or up to 5 litres of 5 per cent glucose intravenously if necessary.

Salt depletion usually develops insidiously in people working in hot environments, due to loss of salt in sweat, when water is available but salt intake low. Sodium chloride intake of up to 20 g/day, preferably dissolved, may be needed to prevent it. Classical cases show sunken eyes, fatigue, weakness, headache, nausea, and sometimes vomiting, but with painful muscle cramps (e.g. 'miner's cramp') only if the salt depletion is associated with muscular exercise. It is now rare, but minor salt deficiency contributes to fatigue in exercise, and to mortality among the elderly in warm weather (Chapter 18.6). Haematocrit, plasma proteins, and blood urea are elevated in mild cases. In severe cases, water is retained at the expense of osmotic pressure, and serum sodium and chloride fall. Treatment consists of 25 g sodium chloride in 5 litres of water by mouth, and, in severe cases, intravenous infusion of 500 ml isotonic saline solution.

Further reading

Morbidity and Mortality Weekly Report. (1998). Heat-related mortality–United States, 1997. *Morbidity and Mortality Weekly Report*, 47, 473–6.

Oakley, E.H.N. (1987). Heat exhaustion. *Journal of World Accident, Emergency and Disaster Medicine*, 3, 28–30.

Pandolf, K.B., Sawka, M.N., and Gonzalez, R.R. (ed.). (1988). *Human performance physiology and environmental medicine at terrestrial extremes.* Benchmark, USA.

Chapter 18.5

Drug-induced increases of body temperature

W. I. Cranston

Almost any drug can cause pyrexia. Some drugs can give rise to diseases, of which fever may be a presenting feature, e.g. antibiotic-induced colitis, drug-induced systemic lupus erythematosus, drug-related hepatitis, and infection consequent upon drug-induced agranulocytosis which can be caused by numerous drugs. Injection of drugs can result in local inflammatory changes. Streptokinase commonly causes fever during thrombolysis..

Hypersensitivity may explain febrile reactions to restarting rifampicin. Fever and eosinophilia have been observed following procainamide and methyldopa. Vaccines may contain antibiotics or egg protein to which the patient is sensitive. Fever can follow antineoplastic treatment, particularly with bleomycin and asparaginase. Injection of interferon commonly causes pyrexia.

Direct effects on the central nervous control of body temperatures may explain the pyrexia produced by overdose of sympathomimetics, and monoamine oxidase inhibitors, with or without tricyclic antidepressants. Atropine overdosage commonly causes pyrexia, perhaps by prevention of sweating.

There are two particularly dangerous forms of drug-induced fever, malignant hyperpyrexia and neuroleptic malignant syndrome.

Malignant hyperpyrexia syndrome (MHS)

This is an autosomal dominant condition [17q11.2–24 (MHS2), 7q21–22 (MHS3), or 3q13.1 (MHS4)] affecting the sarcoplasmic reticulum of skeletal muscle in which there is intracellular accumulation of Ca^{2+} in response to inhaled halothane or nitrous oxide, epidural lignocaine or bupivacaine, and suxamethonium, and carries a high mortality. Any suspicious family history should prompt further enquiry. An abnormal resting creatine kinase suggests the likelihood of this condition but a normal level does not exclude it. A similar condition can be provoked by poisoning with 'ecstasy', and it has also been reported after use of its analogue methylenedioxyamphetamine ('eve').

Usually, after induction of anaesthesia, muscle contraction develops and the skin becomes extremely hot; central temperature can rise by 1°C in a few minutes, and thence to fatal levels. If the condition is suspected, anaesthesia should be avoided if possible, but if essential, known inducing agents should be avoided. If time is available, premedication with oral dantrolene (5 mg/kg) should be given in the 24-hour period before anaesthesia. This drug uncouples muscular contraction from excitation by inhibiting release of Ca^{2+} from the sarcoplasmic reticulum. Should unexpected malignant hyperpyrexia develop, the anaesthetic should be stopped, the patient ventilated and cooled, and intravenous dantrolene sodium given in a dose of 1 to 10 mg/kg. This drug is very alkaline and care must be taken not to allow it to extravasate. Metabolic acidosis is common and severe, and should be treated with sodium bicarbonate. Procainamide has been recommended to prevent ventricular fibrillation.

Neuroleptic malignant syndrome (see Chapter 14.6)

Hyperthermia, muscle rigidity, impaired consciousness, and tachycardia develop as an idiosyncratic reaction to therapeutic doses of phenothiazines, thioxanthine, and butyrophenones such as haloperidol, risperidone, and domperidone, all of which interfere with dopaminergic transmission in the central nervous system. Unlike malignant hyperpyrexia, it usually develops more insidiously over 1–3 days, and the recorded temperatures have not usually been as high as those in patients with malignant hyperpyrexia. Mortality of 15–25 per cent is usually associated with respiratory failure or aspiration pneumonia. The increased muscle tone appears to be presynaptically excited: neuromuscular blocking agents will cause paralysis and can be used to treat neuroleptic malignant syndrome. During the illness, creatine kinase levels are elevated and there is one report of elevated resting creatine kinase in the asymptomatic children of a recovered patient.

Treatment is similar to that of MHS, with attention to muscle relaxants, ventilation, and acidosis. Dantrolene is reported as being of value, though there are cases where it was apparently ineffective. Because of the effect of these major tranquillizers on dopaminergic transmission, bromocriptine (a dopamine agonist) has been used to treat some patients.

Further reading

Denborough, M. (1998). Malignant hyperthermia. *Lancet*, **312**, 1131–6

Granto, J.E., *et al.* (1983). Neuroleptic malignant syndrome: successful treatment with dantrolene and bromocriptine. *Annals of Neurology*, **14**, 89–90.

Kellam, A.M.P. (1987). The neuroleptic malignant syndrome, so-called. A survey of the world literature. *British Journal of Psychiatry*, **150**, 752–9.

Pelonero, A.L., Levenson, J.L., and Pandurangi, A.K. (1998). Neuroleptic malignant syndrome: a review. *Psychiatric Service*, **49**, 1163–72.

Chapter 18.6

Cold, drowning, and seasonal mortality

W. R. Keatinge

Effects of cold on the body

Exposure to cold first induces vasoconstriction in the skin and then increase in muscle tone and shivering that increase heat production. These responses enable most healthy and well-fed adults to maintain body temperature for many hours with skin temperatures as low as 12°C if the individual is fat, but only as low as 25–30°C if the individual is thin and has little internal insulation when vasoconstricted. Children are also at a disadvantage because of a high surface area in relation to body mass.

Hypothermia is usually defined by a deep body temperature of less than 35°C. Reliable measurement of this may be made sublingually in air warmer than 24°C, in the external auditory meatus with servocontrolled external heating (zero gradient aural probe) in air warmer than 18°C, rectally in any environment if body temperature is reasonably stable, or oesophageally if the patient is not swallowing cold saliva. Rectal temperature is usually 0.2–0.5°C higher than the others, and lags behind them if deep body temperature is changing rapidly.

If the temperature of the heart and brain fall below 35°C, there is first listlessness and confusion, often with subsequent amnesia for events at the time of low body temperature. Consciousness is lost at a lower but variable temperature of 26–33°C, and at a temperature of 17–26°C cardiac output becomes insufficient to supply even the reduced oxygen requirements of the cold tissues, so that death ultimately ensues unless the patient is rewarmed. Atrial fibrillation may occur at temperatures of 28–35°C and ventricular fibrillation below 33°C. Otherwise, slow cardiac activity can be maintained for a time by a normal or ectopic pacemaker at temperatures as low as 11°C. Respiration is depressed in hypothermia, but generally almost in proportion to metabolic needs. Any metabolic acidosis due to lactic acid is generally mild unless very prolonged hypothermia has resulted in anoxic liver damage. Glucose metabolism is depressed during hypothermia, and blood glucose and serum potassium rise as body temperature falls. If hypothermia develops, inability of renal tubular cells to reabsorb sodium chloride and water at low temperature causes progressive loss of salt and water. Hypotension is therefore common when a victim of hypothermia is warmed and vasodilatation takes place. Gastric erosions and pancreatitis can occur in prolonged, severe hypothermia and may provide postmortem evidence of the cause of death.

Prevention and management of hypothermia and cold injury

Immersion hypothermia

Most people of average fatness, without protection, develop a dangerous degree of hypothermia after several hours of immersion in water at 15–20°C. In colder water they may also suffer cold injury of the limbs.

The most important measures are preventive. Body cooling can be reduced by thick conventional clothing, including gloves and footwear. Body cooling in the water can also, surprisingly, be reduced by advising survivors to float still in lifejackets rather than exercising; exercise in cold water generally increases heat loss more than heat production. Wet suits of foam rubber, or waterproof suits, of course, provide excellent protection if they are available.

After an immersion victim is rescued, it must be determined whether the patient is hypothermic, drowned, or both, and an immediate measure of body temperature is useful. Rectal temperature by a low-reading thermometer is the most reliable, though it must be remembered that it can lag 1–2°C behind cardiac temperature when body temperature is falling very rapidly.

People who have a body core temperature below about 31°C at the time of rescue, and who have not inhaled water, are liable to die suddenly during or shortly after rescue. The probable reason is ventricular fibrillation precipitated by catecholamine drive to the heart during exertion or postural hypotension. People should therefore if possible be rescued from cold water in the horizontal position, and with minimum exertion by the victim.

After rescue, the main principle of treatment in any type of hypothermia is to prevent further heat loss by insulation until the patients can be moved into warm surroundings; to keep them recumbent; and to refrain from any unnecessary action, and particularly intravenous adrenaline, that can precipitate ventricular fibrillation. For those who have developed hypothermia rapidly, for example in cold water, an immediate hot bath (not above 42°C) provides the quickest method of rewarming, but is seldom available within 30 minutes of rescue. After that time victims of immersion hypothermia who are still alive usually recover if left recumbent in warm surroundings with mild heat input such as from hot water bottles not warmer than 42°C. If ventricular fibrillation or cardiac arrest do occur, the patient should be given cardiopulmonary resuscitation and taken straight to hospital for extracorporeal circulation, preferably by femoral bypass. Any active warming must be discontinued as body core temperature rises to 35°C. After initial measures are taken, admission to hospital is always desirable if water is thought to have been inhaled, for chest radiograph and for possible intermittent positive pressure ventilation if late pulmonary oedema develops. Blood glucose, pH, and serum potassium may be measured, once a good flow of blood is restored to the limbs so that a venous sample can give meaningful information. However, attempts to correct apparent abnormalities of pH and potassium should never be made unless the validity of the blood sample itself, and of the assay and any temperature corrections made to it, are known to be dependable.

Non-freezing cold injury

The limbs of people rescued from water below 12°C are initially often anaesthetic and paralysed. If the cooling lasts many hours they will, on warming, develop signs of immersion injury, becoming bright red, hot, oedematous, and painful. They should then be elevated to reduce oedema and analgesics given for the pain. During the next few weeks, muscle and nerve may degenerate, and physiotherapy is needed to prevent contractures. Partial denervation of blood vessels due to degeneration of their motor nerves often leads to vascular instability with excessive vasoconstriction in the cold and dilation in the heat. Some improvement in the disabilities is usual over the course of months as nerves regenerate, but disability may be permanent. Tissues can freeze in sea water, which itself freezes at −1.9°C, but this is much rarer than non-freezing injury during immersion.

Exposure

Hillwalkers, climbers, and skiers who are inadequately clothed are liable to hypothermia even in air above 0°C if they become lost, or immobilized by bad weather or injury. Hypothermia can develop rapidly during even mild exposure to cold if people take ethanol after exercise and without food. When exercise has depleted the body's reserve of carbohydrate, less than 30 ml of ethanol can produce hypoglycaemia. This not only causes mental confusion but suppresses normal responses to cold, so that body temperature falls rapidly.

Apathy and confusion due to exhaustion can be distinguished from mild hypothermia only by temperature measurement. Sublingual readings are affected by local cooling in the cold, and if low, rectal temperature should be measured. In cold air body temperature has usually fallen slowly and so is relatively stable at the time of rescue, and in mild cases is almost invariable if the victim is placed recumbent in a well-insulated sleeping bag while being transported to warm surroundings, preferably breathing through a simple heat exchanger. Loss of plasma volume can be substantial during prolonged exposure. This can usually be controlled with recumbent posture and raising the legs, but 500 ml of saline or dextran intravenously is helpful. Sugary drinks should be given only when body temperature is above 31°C and glucose can be metabolized.

Moderate frostbite

Frostbite, if present, is obvious as hard, white areas of skin on the extremities. As long as it involves only parts of the fingers, toes, hands, or feet and there is no risk of refreezing, it is best treated by sudden thawing in water no hotter than the observer can stand without discomfort. This allows optimal tissue recovery, probably because bloodflow returning is so rapid that it passes through damaged capillaries too rapidly to lose plasma and to block the vessels with sludged red cells. Subsequently, analgesics should be given for pain, the part elevated to reduce oedema, and antibiotics given to prevent infection. The skin may subsequently turn black, but then often sloughs off to leave almost normal tissue beneath. Surgery should be considered only after the necrotic region is fully delineated.

Massive frostbite

People with massive freezing of the limbs, and often with general hypothermia, sometimes survive slow rewarming in warm air without early medical help, but should if possible be transported at once to hospital and rewarmed there under full biochemical control. Such people have extensive tissue damage from freezing, so that rapid thawing otherwise leads to massive release of potassium into the circulation, and to ventricular fibrillation. Haemodialysis, and extracorporeal circulation in cases of persistent ventricular fibrillation, give the best chance of recovery.

Urban hypothermia

Causes

Hypothermia among people indoors in normal homes is rare, and is almost always secondary to disease, alcohol, drugs, or injury. The most common cause is collapse, usually from cardiovascular or respiratory disease, while alone at home and often in heated rooms. People found outdoors with hypothermia in cities also usually suffer from effects of illness or alcohol. Illnesses involved include hypoxia, infection, hypoglycaemia due to alcohol, insulin, or malnutrition, which impair metabolic and vasoconstrictor responses to cold, and hypothyroidism which specifically reduces metabolic rate, and α-adrenergic blocking drugs which impair vasoconstriction. Any central nervous depressant drug in high dosage can impair central thermoregulation and so probably can extreme old age. Such people should be insulated with blankets and taken to hospital for diagnosis and treatment of underlying condition. Hypothermia in the absence of disease or alcohol, though rare, is important. People who die in this way can be mistaken for victims of violence, as confusion and loss of sensation of cold due to hypothermia sometimes cause the patients to shed clothing, damage furniture, and fall and injure themselves.

Seasonal mortality

Mortality in temperate countries increases strikingly in winter and sometimes in summer, mainly in elderly people. About half the excess deaths in the cold are due to coronary and cerebral thrombosis, and about half of the rest to respiratory disease. The thrombosis is due partly to haemoconcentration following the normal vasoconstrictive response to moderate cold, which causes marked increases in red cell count, platelet count, plasma cholesterol, plasma fibrinogen, and blood viscosity, and partly to respiratory infections. Coronary deaths peak a day or two after a cold day, and respiratory deaths about 2 weeks after it. Hypothermia is much rarer, but can be facilitated by undernutrition, and lead to poor co-ordination and falls, causing fractured femurs in the elderly. Angina can be precipitated by cold, and asthma by breathing very cold air.

Even low level heat waves precipitate a variety of premature deaths, but heat waves with daily minima of environmental temperature above 17 to 20°C increase mortality from coronary and cerebral thrombosis, mainly due to haemoconcentration caused by loss of salt in sweat. In temperate countries light clothing, an open window, a fan, and if necessary sprinkling of water on clothing with the fan to provide air movement can prevent serious heat stress in vulnerable people, but in hotter and humid climates air conditioning is desirable. Unacclimatized people are at particular risk.

Further reading

Bull, G.M. and Morton, J. (1978). Environment, temperature and death rates. *Age and Ageing*, 7, 210–24.

Keatinge, W.R., Coleshaw, S.R.K., Easton, J.C., Cotter, F., Mattock, M.B., and Chelliah, R. (1986). Increased platelet and red cell counts, blood viscosity and plasma cholesterol during heat stress, and mortality from coronary and cerebral thrombosis. *American Journal of Medicine*, **81**, 795–800.

Chapter 18.7

Diseases of high terrestrial altitudes

D. Rennie

High altitude terrain and populations

The vast majority of mankind lives below 1000 m, but areas of the world 4000 m or more above sea level have been home to civilizations for thousands of years. Temperature falls some 1°C for every 150-m rise in altitude, so the high altitude climate tends to be an arctic one, with high winds, low humidity, and increased solar radiation.

Hypoxia (see Chapter 18.9)

At the summit of Everest (8848 m), the atmospheric pressure is about 250 torr (33 kPa; one-third that at sea level) and the partial pressure of oxygen is $0.2093 \times 250 = 52.3$ torr (7 kPa). The partial pressure of water, however, reduces the PIO_2 from 52.5 torr to $0.2093 \times (250–47) = 42.5$ torr (5.7 kPa).

Acclimatization

Following a plane's sudden decompression or a rapid balloon ascent, for example, a resting man, just up from sea level, would lose consciousness in a matter of minutes at altitudes between 6400 m and 7300 m (PAO_2 = 24–15 torr; 3.2–2 kPa) and in seconds above 7300 m (PAO_2 below 15 torr; 2 kPa).

The difference between the ineffectual newcomer on arrival at high altitudes and the resident or climber on Everest is the sum of a myriad of physiological adjustments called 'acclimatization'. This seems to depend solely upon the length of exposure and the age when first exposed and has little to do with genetic factors. The time of greatest adjustment is in the hours and days after arrival at a higher altitude, but changes may continue for years.

A few of the principal steps involved may be summarized.

Ventilation

When PAO_2 has fallen to 55 to 60 torr (7.3–7.9 kPa) at an altitude of about 2000–3000 m, the peripheral chemoreceptors are stimulated by hypoxia and ventilation is increased. The PCO_2 falls in a linear manner with altitude, and the resultant respiratory alkalosis is only partly compensated for by a rise in urinary excretion of bicarbonate.

Pulmonary diffusion

In the newcomer to high altitude, exercise is accompanied by a marked fall in arterial oxygen saturation, in contrast to the unchanged values on exercise at sea level, and this may be partly due to a limitation in diffusion.

Circulation

Though there is an abrupt increase in cardiac output on ascent to high altitude, there follows a progressive decrease in stroke volume and maximal cardiac output is reduced at all levels of exercise including maximal exercise. There is no evidence for insufficient myocardial oxygenation and there is argument about whether or not the myocardium is actually depressed by the hypoxia.

The oxygen-carrying ability of the blood is considerably increased by the massive increase in red cell production, in total red cell mass and, more importantly, in tissue capillarity. It is somewhat offset by the higher haematocrit which increases the blood viscosity and decreases the rate of flow.

Tissue adaptations

Apart from the very major role of increased tissue capillarity which reduces the average capillary-mitochondrial distance and so reduces the distance for diffusion, increased myoglobin facilitates oxygen diffusion and there is an increase both in mitochondrial density and in enzymes of the respiratory pathway (e.g. in cytochrome oxidase).

Oxygen uptake

Though the oxygen uptake at rest is not diminished even at very high altitudes, above an altitude of 1500 m the maximal oxygen uptake VO_2max falls about 10 per cent for each gain in altitude of 1000 m between 1500 and 6700 m and though it is improved by administration of pure oxygen, it does not return to normal until several days after descent.

At altitude, as opposed to at sea level, arterial oxygen saturation falls with increasing exertion, but, at moderate altitudes, rises again near maximal exertion. After a few days at high altitude, however, maximal heart rate and particularly maximal cardiac stroke volume are reduced, the cause being unclear, and so the inability of the heart to go on increasing cardiac output seems to be the reason for the fact that VO_2max declines progressively with increases in altitude.

Extreme altitudes

At extreme values, where every increment in height results in a precipitous fall in VO_2max, the oxygen cost of the work of ventilation rises considerably and it assumes an even greater proportion of total oxygen cost when VO_2max is reduced to really low levels. Moreover, the maximal ventilation itself is reduced at such altitudes and in addition there is a diffusion defect within the lungs which becomes very marked on exercise. This, together with the steady decline in maximal cardiac output causes maximal oxygen uptake to fall precipitously when *P*B is below 300 torr, reaching, at around 8000 m altitude, resting or basal levels of oxygen uptake, a figure of about 350 m/kg per min. The state of a climber at 8000 m who is comfortable resting in his tent but whose VO_2max is reached when he puts on his boots, for example, is perilous.

Alveolar gas samples taken on the summit of Everest (8848 m; barometric pressure 253 torr, 33.4 kPa) show an inspired $PO_2 = 43$ torr (5.68 kPa), and alveolar $PO_2 = 35$ torr (4.62 kPa). Estimated arterial gas values are: $PO_2 = 28$ torr (3.7 kPa); $PCO_2 = 7.5$ (0.99 kPa); pH >7.7, oxygen saturation = 70 per cent. A number of reports have suggested mild, possibly permanent defects in cognition in climbers who have ascended to extreme high altitudes.

Illness due to altitude

Acute mountain sickness

When lowland dwellers ascend mountains, some of them become ill. The illness, acute mountain sickness, generally begins after a few hours, and is characterized by non-specific symptoms such as headache and vomiting. In the vast majority of people it is transient and trivial but in a few becomes progressive, severe, and may be fatal. It is to some extent relieved by breathing oxygen and it is cured by descent to sea level. It is thought to be caused by mild oedema of the white matter.

Acute mountain sickness itself is of concern because it may progress to one or both of two very serious conditions, high altitude cerebral oedema and high altitude pulmonary oedema.

Symptoms and signs

Symptoms come on between 8 and 96 hours after ascent and include, after an initial euphoria, lethargy, headache, fitful sleep with arousals, an increasingly severe headache, often occipital, nausea, vomiting, dizziness and loss of balance. The sufferer lies groaning in his sleeping bag, refusing food and dozing. After a day or two of rest, the symptoms disappear and are soon forgotten, yet they may recur on further ascent to a greater altitude.

The signs are few: an irritable, depressed, but usually fit person, often, because he is starved, smelling of ketones and vomit, and holding his aching head. The most useful diagnostic sign is ataxia. Occasionally the patient, especially if vomiting and taking diuretics, may be too dehydrated and hypotensive to stand up. Crackles may be heard in more than a quarter of people examined.

In a few, the symptoms rapidly worsen with the onset of pulmonary oedema. Soon the breathlessness, even at rest, is extreme, with a dry cough. The patient, anxious and sometimes incoherent, becomes progressively more dyspnoeic and sometimes orthopnoeic. He is very cyanosed, with a mild pyrexia (38.3°C) a pronounced tachycardia and sometimes mild hypotension. There are no signs of cardiac failure, but loud crackles can easily be heard all over the chest and frothy sputum, sometimes tinged with blood, wells out of the mouth and nose.

In overt cerebral oedema the patient, having had progressively worsening symptoms of acute mountain sickness for several days, becomes incoherent, hallucinated, and too ataxic and drowsy to stand up or look after himself. He may be unable to get out of his tent, or he may do so and then fall into a snow drift and lie there. Soon he is stuporose and snoring stertorously. His sleeping bag may be wet with urine and in a few hours he is in deepening coma. There are rarely any localizing signs; mild bilateral papilloedema is characteristic.

Predisposing factors

Males and females are equally likely to develop the acute mountain sickness syndrome, and the incidence is inversely related to age. Factors related statistically to the occurrence of acute mountain sickness are severe exertion, starting an ascent at a higher altitude, previous acute mountain sickness, especially pulmonary oedema, and having a low vital capacity and a poor ventilatory response to hypoxia. Healthy high altitude dwellers seem to be at unusually high risk of pulmonary oedema after brief descent to lower altitudes, followed by reascent.

Pathophysiology

Patients with acute mountain sickness, whether this is due to failed or exaggerated physiological adjustments to hypoxia, tend to have ventilation that is inappropriately low for the altitude. They thus have lower blood oxygen and higher PCO_2 levels. Pulmonary oedema causes a vicious cycle of deepening hypoxia.

People with acute mountain sickness also have an antidiuresis and retain fluid. There is movement of fluid into the cells, and considerable hypoxic cerebral vasodilatation. The finding, using MRI, of oedema of the white matter in such people lends support to the concept that in acute mountain sickness there is vasogenic cerebral oedema.

It is known that on ascent to high altitude, there is a shift in blood from the systemic 'capacitance vessels' (veins) to the pulmonary circuit. In addition, there is a greater than normal hypoxic pulmonary arterial vasoconstriction with a rise in pulmonary artery pressure.

The oedema fluid of people suffering from high altitude pulmonary oedema is very high in protein content, which is characteristic of a breakdown in vascular permeability, and not like that of 'high-pressure' cardiogenic pulmonary oedema. Cardiac function is not impaired. Pulmonary wedge pressures are normal, as are atrial pressures.

It is probable that at altitude, there is a patchy closure of some pulmonary vessels and over-perfusion of the rest, which are damaged by the increased pressure and the shear-stress of the resultant large flow and therefore leak.

Incidence

Acute mountain sickness is uncommon below 3000 m. The higher the altitude, the faster the ascent, and the greater the exertion the higher the incidence and the worse the illness.

A bad headache that is not relieved by 600 mg of aspirin, occurs in over half of those lowlanders going to above 4000 m and that over 10 per cent of climbers have more than one severe symptom at that altitude. High altitude pulmonary oedema occurs in about 5 per cent of people at that altitude, but symptomless crackles in the lung in almost a quarter. Cerebral oedema, which takes a few days to develop, is less common, occurring in perhaps 0.5–2 per cent.

Diagnosis

The differential diagnosis is small. For mild acute mountain sickness the non-specific symptoms mean that hypothermia, exhaustion, and dehydration should be considered. The effects of alcohol and marijuana may duplicate those of acute mountain sickness. For pulmonary and cerebral oedema, only infectious diseases (pneumonia, or meningoencephalitis) are likely possibilities, though carbon monoxide poisoning due to poorly ventilated tents occurs. Periodic breathing with apnoeic phases is normal at high altitude and not by itself a cause for alarm. Fever is moderate in high altitude pulmonary oedema, which is accompanied by extreme tachycardia and cyanosis, without purulent sputum. In cerebral oedema there is no meningism and little if any pyrexia, nor evidence of ear infection or of localizing signs. There is a striking absence of any signs of cardiac decompensation (cardiac enlargement, raised neck veins).

All illnesses improve on descent, but the very dramatic recovery on descent in acute mountain sickness, and particularly in pulmonary and cerebral oedema is so striking as to be diagnostic in itself. Numerous cases have been described of people unconscious and worsening at 4000 m who were fully conscious at 3000 m. On descent, the patient recovers fast except in the case of very prolonged cerebral oedema.

Prophylaxis

Acute mountain sickness is the consequence of ascent that for any one individual is too high or too fast, and so it is completely preventable. Everyone going to high altitudes has the responsibility to set a schedule for themselves that includes frequent rests, and that allows them to descend at will. Acute mountain sickness affects the capacity to reason, so everyone must also take responsibility for their fellows, realizing that pulmonary or cerebral oedema can be rapidly fatal and that it is often simple to walk a sufferer down 1000 m, whereas a few hours' delay can endanger the patient's life and scores of rescuers.

Since insensible water loss is increased due to the increased exertion, the extra ventilation and the dry air, every effort must be made to avoid dehydration, by drinking enough to urinate clear, dilute urine. The climber should also eat plenty, especially carbohydrates, and avoid sleeping pills.

Acetazolamide reduces the incidence and severity of acute mountain sickness when taken before and during ascent. Its principal side-effect is tingling in the hands, feet, and around the mouth.

Dexamethasone, a glucocorticoid effective in the management of cerebral oedema, has been shown to prevent acute mountain sickness, while reducing the retinal arterial dilation that follows exposure to hypoxia.

Treatment

Rest, aspirin for headache, and a descent of 500 m or so for a couple of nights usually suffice, though ataxia may require the patient be assisted down further. Acetazolamide increases oxygenation and relieves symptoms. The presence of pulmonary oedema or coma necessitates urgent removal down at least 1000 m, and careful observation. In addition to descent, oxygen should be administered (if necessary through an endotracheal tube at a rate of 5–6 l/min). Immediate descent by even a small amount may save the lives of such critically ill patients, and reliance on air evacuation is dangerous.

In pulmonary oedema, sit the patient up if this makes him comfortable. Give frusemide (20–40 mg orally) and morphine (15 mg intravenously). Both these drugs divert blood from the pulmonary to the systemic circuit. Frusemide causes a diuresis and morphine decreases anxiety and respiration rate.

The calcium blocker nifedipine prevents high altitude pulmonary oedema in susceptible subjects, improves oxygenation, and reduces the excessive rise in pulmonary artery pressure in pulmonary oedema. Its side-effects (hypotension and tachycardia) suggest that its use should be limited to established oedema. Further studies may show that inhaled nitric oxide is useful.

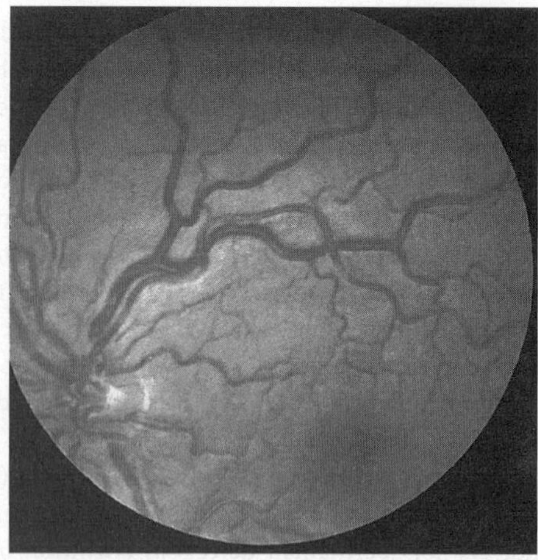

Fig. 1 The left optic fundus of a 26-year-old male climber photographed at 5900 m altitude. Both the veins and arteries are dilated and tortuous and there is hyperaemia of the optic disc as well as mild papilloedema. The climber had severe headache, nausea, and vomiting.

A portable, light-weight hyperbaric bag, made of impermeable nylon, has been developed. The victim lies inside while the air pressure is increased using a foot pump, by 104 torr. For example, at 4200 m, where ambient barometric pressure is 449 torr, the pressure in the bag, 553 torr, would be equivalent to an altitude of 2544 m. This is therefore equivalent to taking the patient down 1656 m. Controlled clinical trials have shown the bag to be effective in acute mountain sickness and mild pulmonary oedema, and expeditions should consider taking such bags with them, though descent is still the safest therapy.

In cerebral oedema, intravenous dexamethasone in large doses (e.g. 16 mg) should be given to reduce the oedema. A cuffed endotracheal tube should be passed, the lungs kept inflated, and the bladder kept empty with a Foley catheter.

Prognosis

This depends not merely on the altitude and terrain but on the speed with which early signs are noticed by the patient's colleagues and their determination and skill in evacuating him to lower altitudes immediately. Once pulmonary oedema and to the rarer but more dangerous cerebral oedema have developed, the patient probably has about a one-third chance of dying. If he lives, full recovery is the rule.

Retinal haemorrhage of high altitude

On ascent, there a considerable increase in cerebral and retinal blood flow. Ophthalmoscopy around 5000–6000 m shows a 20–25 per cent increase in diameter of both arteries and veins, and striking increase in the tortuosity of these vessels (Fig. 1). Suffusion of the the optic disc may simulate papilloedema.

Studies have shown that one-third to one-half of symptomless climbers descending from 7000–8000 m altitude develop flame-shaped retinal haemorrhages which resolve on descent (Fig. 2).

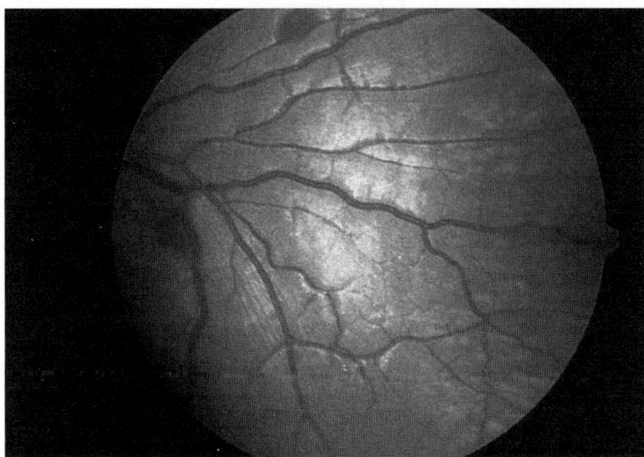

Fig. 2 The left optic fundus of a fit and symptomless 28-year-old male climber photographed at 5900 m altitude. The vessels are dilated, as in Fig. 1, but are less tortuous. Retinal haemorrhages are shown.

Peripheral oedema

Swelling of hands, face, and ankles may occur in climbers on ascent to high altitude, just as on long-continued hiking at sea-level. It is relieved by the diuresis that accompanies descent.

Other illnesses of high altitudes

The normal heart is not limited by heights up to the top of Everest. Unhappily, the doctor has no tests that are sensitive or specific enough to give an accurate prediction, unless the patient has symptoms. On theoretical grounds, people with diseases which limit ventilation, diffusion of oxygen, circulation, and tissue adaptation, will fare badly at high altitudes.

Chronic mountain sickness (Monge's disease)

This disease usually affects middle-aged men and is equivalent to the alveolar hypoventilation syndrome seen at sea level. The symptoms are of headache, dizziness, depression, irritability, and, most strikingly, drowsiness and even episodes of coma. The signs are those of excessive polycythaemia, cyanosis, and clubbing. There is pulmonary hypertension and right ventricular hypertrophy. The disease is cured by descent to sea level.

Myocardial infarction

The physician at sea level is often asked by people whether it is safe for them to go up to 3000 or 4000 m altitude to ski or to climb. People who have poor coronary circulation will be at increased risk when they ascend from sea level and start hard exercise.

Pulmonary emboli

Deep vein thrombosis and embolism occurs because of polycythaemia, dehydration, and enforced inactivity due to storms. Evacuation to lower altitudes and the administration of aspirin as an anticoagulant should be tried.

Sickle-cell anaemia

Cells containing HbS sickle, when hypoxic, become sticky and rigid so homozygous cases of HbS are at danger from high altitude. In Denver, at 1609 m, people who are heterozygotes (sickle-cell trait) apparently lead normal lives, but cases of splenic infarction in people with sickle-cell trait have been described in men at between 3500 and 4500 m. One should be cautious in advising anyone with sickle-cell trait to exercise at altitudes above 2000 m.

Further reading

Hackett, P.H., and Roach, R.C. (1994). High altitude medicine and physiology. In: *Management of wilderness and environmental emergencies* (ed. P.S. Auerbach,) 3rd edn. C.V. Mosby, St Louis.

Reeves, J.T. and Schoene, R.B. (1992). When lungs on mountains leak. *New England Journal of Medicine*, **325**, 1306–7.

Rennie, D. (1986). The great breathlessness mountains. *Journal of the American Medical Association*, **256**, 81–2.

Rennie, D. (1989). Will trekkers have heart attacks? *Journal of the American Medical Association*, **261**, 1045–6.

Chapter 18.8

Aerospace medicine

D. M. Denison

Tthe atmosphere shields the ground below from thermal and other high-energy radiations above. Held to the Earth by gravity and compressed under its own weight, it is denser close to the ground than further away. Long waves of infrared sunlight travel easily through the atmosphere, warming it very little but heating the ground below. The hot ground re-radiates some of this heat at shorter wavelengths, which are absorbed by carbon dioxide and water vapour, making the air close to the ground much warmer than that elsewhere. Short waves of ultraviolet sunlight entering the upper atmosphere create a belt of warm ozone at altitudes of 40 000–140 000 ft which may cause some lung irritation when compressed by aircraft ventilation systems.. Most of the other high-energy rays are also intercepted in the same region but generate secondary rays that extend lower down. Very few of these reach the ground. At sea level, air exerts a pressure of about 1 atm (760 mmHg; approximately 101 kPa), is variably moist, has a temperature in the range –60°C– + 60°C, and usually moves at wind speeds from 0–160 km/h, (the recorded maximum is 496 km/h). With increasing altitude its temperature, pressure, and water content fall and wind speeds increase. In general, on ascent, conditions become more severe and more uniform.

Atmospheric pressure falls with altitude in a regular, almost exponential way, halving every 18 000 ft, (Fig. 1). The oxygen content

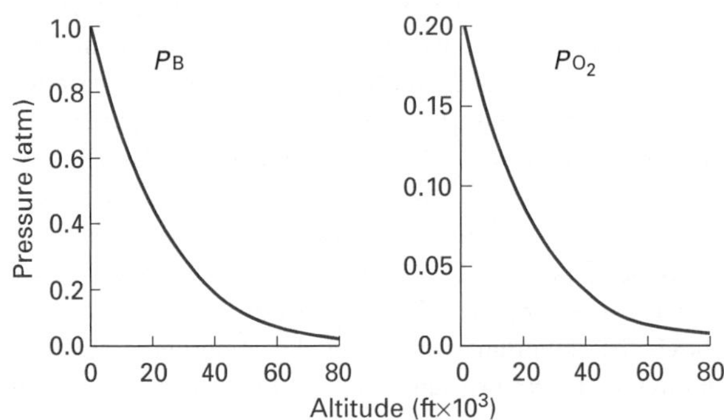

Fig. 1 The variations of barometric pressure and ambient oxygen pressure with altitude.

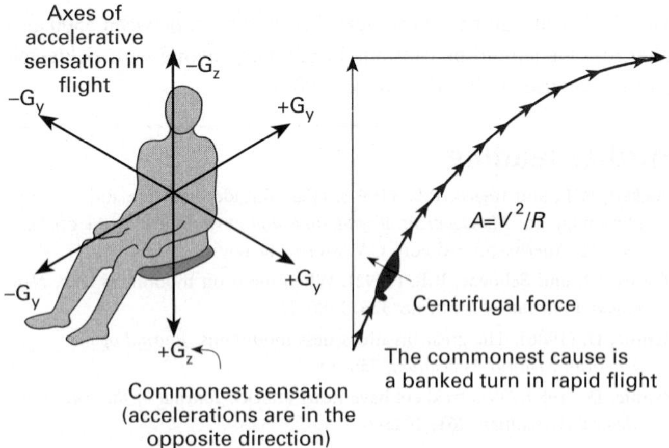

Fig. 2 The axes of acceleration in flight are labelled according to the sensations experienced by the aviator. Thus, when he is accelerated upwards ($+G_z$) he feels his body fluids and tissues sink towards his feet.

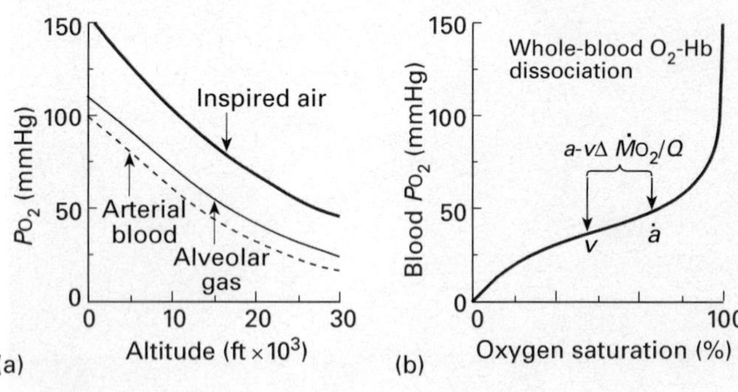

Fig. 3 (a) Variations in moist-inspired, alveolar, and arterial oxygen pressure (Po_2) with altitude in normal men. (b) The conventional oxygen–haemoglobin dissociation curve of whole blood plotted to the same pressure scale as the left-hand graph, so that arterial O_2 content can be read directly (at the same horizontal level as the Po_2 curve. It also emphasizes that the arteriovenous oxygen content difference (a-v ∧) is proportional to the ratio of oxygen uptake (Mo_2) to local blood flow (Q).

of the atmosphere (20.93 per cent) is virtually constant and can be obtained by the same rule (also shown in Fig. 1). The oxygen pressure of physiological importance is that which exists in ambient air when it is warmed and wetted on entering the bronchial tree. This process raises water-vapour pressure to about 47 mmHg. Thus the oxygen pressure in moist inspired gas (PIo_2) fully saturated with water vapour at 37°C is given by the relationship: Equation

$$PIo_2 = Fio_2\ (PB - 47)$$

where Fio_2, the fractional concentration of oxygen in the inspirate, is 0.2093 when air is inspired.

Mechanical aspects

Propeller-driven aircraft need sufficient air to 'bite' on but not enough to slow them down. They fly best at altitudes below 30 000 ft. Jet aircraft are propelled by throwing a stream of hot gas behind them but they need atmospheric oxygen to ignite the fuel that does this. They fly best at altitudes below 65 000 ft. Rockets take an oxygen supply with them, and fly best in a vacuum.

The atmosphere permits vehicles to travel through it at very high speeds. Usually these are achieved and lost so gradually that the changes of pace pass unnoticed, but high-performance aircraft may make continuous high-speed turns that can be sustained for a minute or more. The radial accelerations that such turns produce are proportional to the square of the vehicle's speed and inversely proportional to the radius of its turning circle (as shown in Fig. 2). Because the aircraft turns by applying its broad wing surface to the air, these accelerations are almost perpendicular to that surface and roughly parallel to the long axes of the people within. Usually aircraft make 'head to the middle' turns causing tissue fluids and loosely tethered organs like the liver and the heart to fall footwards (positive 'g' or $+G_z$ accelerations). Occasionally the aircraft makes 'head-out' turns forcing these organs and fluids towards the head.

In brief, the important features of the atmosphere are that its temperature and pressure fall and radiation intensities rise with altitude. In addition there is a poisonous belt of ozone at high altitude. The atmosphere also permits vehicles to travel at high speeds and make sustained severe accelerations.

Physiological aspects

Hypoxia

Enzymes handle virtually all the oxygen uptake measure at the lips but differ in their affinity for oxygen, described by the Michaelis Constant (for oxygen). This constant (KmO_2) is that partial pressure of oxygen which, when all others factors are equal, just allows an oxygen-consuming reaction to proceed at half its maximum velocity. The major oxidase (cytochrome a_3), which is the co-catalyst of oxidative phosphorylation, has a high oxygen affinity and thus a very low KmO_2, of 1 mmHg or less. That means this particular type of oxygen consumption, representing 80–90 per cent of the whole, can proceed full tilt down to very low levels of oxygen supply. By contrast, the other enzymes, which are quantitatively less important but qualitatively critical, have Michaelis constraints for oxygen that vary from 5–250 mmHg. A fall in oxygen supply will influence these processes long before oxidative phosphorylation is affected and at times when overall oxygen consumption is diminished little if at all.

Although Fig. 1 describes how ambient oxygen pressure is related to altitude, it does not convey the measure of oxygen supply critical to man, namely the pressure of oxygen to be found in the lungs. That pressure is determined by two equations. *The alveolar ventilation equation* states that alveolar CO_2 pressure ($Paco_2$) depends only on CO_2 excretion (Mco_2) and alveolar ventilation ($\dot{V}a$), so:

$$Paco_2 = k(\dot{M}co_2/\dot{V}a)$$

The *alveolar air equation* states that since at any one time there is a fixed trading ratio between oxygen uptake and CO_2 excretion ($R = Mco_2/Mo_2$), alveolar oxygen pressure (Pao_2) can be calculated from the moist inspired oxygen pressure (Pio_2*) and alveolar Pco_2 so:

$$Pao_2 = Pio_2^* - (Pco_2/R)$$

Progressive hypoxia leads to a mild hyperventilation i.e. rise in *VA* and fall in $Paco_2$. Knowing that, it is possible to sketch a graph of alveolar oxygen pressure against altitude as in Fig. 3(a).

When arterialized blood leaves a healthy lung it has an oxygen pressure some 10 mmHg less than that in the alveoli, due to uneven matching of ventilation to perfusion, some anatomical shunting, and

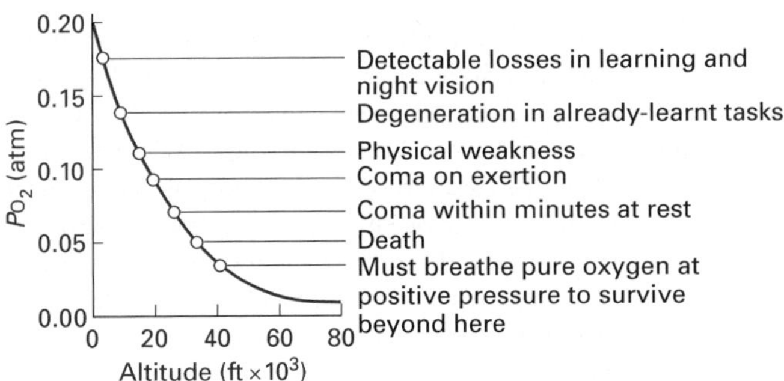

Fig. 4 A Summary of the functional consequences of altitude hypoxia.

an almost nominal obstacle to diffusion. In resting people, the alveolar–arterial oxygen gradient does not change much with altitude, although the relative importance of the factors contributing to it alter considerably; so, subtracting a further 10–15 mmHg describes the relation between arterial oxygen pressure and altitude (also shown in Fig. 3).

People ascending to altitude in a matter of minutes, rather than over several days, make two adaptive responses to hypoxia, an increase in blood flow and modest hyperventilation. These limit but do not abolish the effects of oxygen lack. Consequences (Fig. 4) include loss of night vision, impairment of the ability to learn complex and then simple tasks, a deterioration in the performance of already learnt skills, a progressive loss of muscular power (aerobic capacity), and eventually loss of consciousness, convulsions, and death.

As Fig. 4 shows, people abruptly exposed to altitudes of 10 000 ft and above are mentally unreliable and physically weak. This altitude is taken as the ceiling above which it is mandatory to provide aviators with oxygen. To be safe, the ceiling that is actually used is almost always 8000 ft, at which barometric pressure is 565 mmHg, arterial oxygen pressure is around 55 mmHg (i.e. sitting just at the top of the sloping part of the oxyhaemoglobin dissociation curve), and venous oxygen pressures have only fallen by 1–2 mmHg.

Two physiological features of altitude hypoxia are especially important in aviation. The first is a total lack of awareness that the mind is breaking down. This means that an affected individual cannot be relied on to take corrective action, however well trained. It follows that protective equipment has to be designed to sense the hypoxia and come into operation automatically. The second feature, known as the *time of useful consciousness*, describes how rapidly consciousness is lost and thus dictates how quickly this equipment must respond. Many studies have confirmed the general relation between this time interval and the altitude of sudden exposure. The time of useful consciousness diminishes from about 4 minutes at 25 000 ft to a minimum of roughly 15 seconds, which is reached at 35 000–40 000 ft.

The maximum cabin pressure of 565 mmHg (8000 ft) in commercial passenger aircraft, is sufficiently low to bring a normal person's arterial Pco_2 along the plateau of the oxyhaemoglobin dissociation curve until it is sitting just at the top of the steep part (Fig. 3). Because their blood is still fully saturation with oxygen they will not be cyanosed at this altitude. At ground level, many people with chest diseases have arterial oxygen pressures that are as low as 55–60 mmHg (or even lower, in which case they become cyanosed). As they ascend to 8000 ft their arterial Pco_2 will fall further. If their hypoxaemia at ground level is due to a mismatch of ventilation to perfusion, as is usually the case, the drop in arterial Pco_2 will not be as extensive as in normal people (about 40 mmHg), but if it is due to diffusion defects associated with desaturation on exertion, as in some fibrotic conditions, it may be greater. The fall due to ascent can be reversed by the administration of oxygen (30 per cent oxygen at 8000 ft is equivalent to breathing air at ground level). The medical services of all the major airlines can provide a personal oxygen supply for any passenger if they are given notice beforehand. (It is worth checking the altitudes of the patient's destination and of any stopping point en route at the same time.)

Oxygen equipment and pressure cabins

Aircraft that fly below 10 000 ft need no oxygen equipment. Most of those that fly higher have reinforced cabins capable of holding a higher pressure inside them than out. These are of two sorts, the high-differential type, seen in passenger and transport aircraft generally, and the low-differential variety found in military high-performance aircraft. The former, holding a high transmural pressure, usually prevents pressure falling below 565 mmHg (8000 ft). They provide an environment in which oxygen equipment is not needed routinely and the occupants breathe cabin air. However, it is always possible that the pressure-cabin system can fail, allowing the pressure within to fall to the level of that outside. This fall can be limited by descent to a lower altitude, but it is not always practical to put the aircraft into a very steep dive, for structural reasons. Similarly, it is not always practical to descend below 10 000 ft because, in mid-Atlantic for example, there may not be sufficient fuel for the vehicle to reach the nearest land through the dense air at the lower altitudes. For these reasons, if there is a cabin-pressure failure, people can be exposed to a significant hypoxia for some time.

A high-differential cabin limits the vehicle's range and manoeuvrability. It also increases the risk of catastrophic damage if the fuselage is punctured. For these reasons, military high-performance aircraft are fitted with low-differential cabins. These usually prevent cabin pressure falling below 280 mmHg (equivalent to a pressure altitude of 25 000 ft). That is the level at which decompression sickness becomes a serious hazard (see below). In such aircraft, oxygen equipment is needed routinely.

Sometimes occupants have to escape from aircraft in flight. The faster the aircraft is travelling the more difficult this is to do. All modern fighters are equipped with ejector seats to launch the crew into the high-speed airstream and get them clear of the tail. Usually the people ejected free-fall in their seats until below 10 000 ft. This gets them through the cold hypoxic upper air as quickly as possible. A small seat- or suit-mounted emergency oxygen supply sees them safely through this stage.

Mechanical effects of pressure change

In civilian passenger and transport aircraft the climb from takeoff to cruise altitude takes about 30 minutes and involves a fall of about 200 mmHg in cabin pressure (to 8000 ft). The descent to ground, which involves an equivalent rise in cabin pressure, takes much the same time. Body fluids and tissues generally are virtually incompressible and do not alter shape to any important extent when these pressures are applied (cf. diving), but cavities such as the lungs, gut, middle ear, and facial sinuses, which do contain air, behave differently.

The thoracoabdominal wall is a floppy structure that normally has a transmural pressure of a few millimetres of mercury. Thus, any gas inside the wall must be at a pressure very close to that outside and must also follow Boyle's law. Ascent from ground level (760 mmHg) to 8000 ft (565 mmHg) will expand a given volume of gas in a completely pliable container by about 35 per cent, which is equivalent to a radial increase of 10 per cent if it were in a sphere or 18 per cent in a cylinder of fixed length. In the abdomen this may cause slightly uncomfortable gut distension in healthy people but it is not an important problem.

Evidence from very rapid decompressions in fighter aircraft show healthy people at Functional Residual Capacity can tolerate decompressions of about 200 mmHg (from circa 280 mmHg to 80–120 mmHg) that are complete in as little as 0.1 s. Even very diseased lungs can vent themselves over a minute or so. Most patients with obstructive chest disease are able to fly quite safely and should not be prevented from doing so, but those with very severe asthma, obviously tense cysts, or a pneumothorax should not fly, except in helicopters and aircraft at low altitudes, (1000–2000 ft).

The cavity of the middle ear poses a separate problem since it vents easily but sometimes fails to fill because the lower part of the eustachian tube behaves as a non-return valve, especially when it is inflamed. As a result, the cavity equilibrates quite easily on ascent but does not refill on descent, and the ear-drum bows inwards, causing pain that can be severe. Patients with colds or a history of middle-ear infection should take a decongestant spray with them and use it before descent. In general, people who really cannot move their ear-drums outwards on performing a Valsalva manoeuvre are best advised to delay their flight.

Decompression sickness

One unexpected hazard that passengers in civil aircraft can experience is decompression sickness (see Chapter 18.9). In principle, if the pressure around the person quickly falls to less than half its original value, the gas dissolved in blood and tissue fluids may come out of solution precipitously, forming bubbles and obstructing flow in small blood vessels. Although this cannot develop on simple ascents from ground level to 8000 ft, it may arise if the person has been scuba diving immediately before their flight. It is a particular hazard for holiday-makers on package tours, who often fly back home at night and have all day to swim beforehand. It is customary to advise people not to scuba dive to a depth greater than 30 ft in the 12 hours before take-off. This condition should be kept in mind when looking at anyone who has developed neurological signs or symptoms during or soon after a flight., The correct treatment is immediate descent and ideally transfer to the nearest compression chamber, giving oxygen and other non-specific support meantime.

In aircraft with low-differential pressure cabins, the risk of developing decompression sickness is greater and people flying in them should not dive at all in the preceding 12 hours. The time symptoms take to develop varies widely between individuals and shortens markedly as the altitude of exposure rises.

Medical problems

Because of the very high cost of training pilots, military forces and airlines demand the highest physical and psychological standards on entry, to reduce the chance of crew members having to retire early on medical grounds. The medical standards required for entry into pilot training are usually higher than those for trained pilots. Commercial and private aircrew need a current certificate that they are 'fit to fly' which can only be provided by accredited medical examiners. In Britain, the latter must have a Certificate or Diploma of Aviation Medicine. Courses for these are given jointly by the RAF Centre for Aviation Medicine (Henlow, Beds) and Kings College London. Certificates and Diplomas are awarded by the Faculty of Occupational Medicine of the Royal College of Physicians. Medical standards for commercial aircrew are set by the Joint Aviation Authorities on behalf of the International Civil Aviation Authority. They provide a very readable and reasoned list and manual, (see Further reading). The major English language journal in this field is the *Journal of Aviation, Space and Environmental Medicine* published by the (American) Aerospace Medical Association.

Commercial flying is very safe. Worldwide, the accident rate is 1 in 2 million flying hours with some countries achieving 1 in 5 million flying hours. Medical conditions causing temporary or incomplete incapacitation of passengers are not uncommon in flight. Recent reviews of their nature and incidence are listed under Further reading. The stress of modern travel should not be underestimated. Passengers on international flights are required to check in at least 2 hours before departure, airports often have very long walkways, and it may be difficult to obtain help. Many passengers are elderly with heavy luggage, and flight legs may often take 12 hours or more.

In flight, most commercial airliner cabins are pressurized to 6000–8000 ft. At this altitude the partial pressure of oxygen in the alveoli will have fallen from about 13.5 to about 10 kPa. In healthy people this will lead to a fall of about 3 per cent in the saturation of haemoglobin with oxygen, which is of little functional significance but in patients with cardiorespiratory disease it may be important.

With the decrease in ambient pressure there will be an increase in unrestrained gas volumes of 30 per cent. In the normal individual who is able to clear the ears and has no pockets of gas that cannot be voided, this may cause nothing more than slight discomfort in the ears and abdomen. If, however, the eustachian tube is blocked, otitic and sinus barotrauma may result. Passengers should not fly with sinusitis or otitis media, and those with upper respiratory infections should be treated with decongestants. For similar reasons, patients should not fly after recent ear surgery (particularly stapedectomy), eye surgery, laparotomy, thoracotomy, or spontaneous pneumothorax unless a chest drain is in place. Plaster casts may expand if new and so should be split before travel. Patients who have recently undergone clinical procedures that introduce gas into the body (e.g. arthroscopies, air-encephalograms, pulmonary needle biopsies) should not fly until it is known that the gas has been resorbed.

Patients with severe respiratory or cardiovascular disease should be assessed by appropriate specialists before being allowed to fly. An expectant mother should complete her air travel by the end of the 35th week of her pregnancy. Some neonates may become dangerously hypoxic and suffer 'cot deaths' on long haul flights. Airline medical services are a valuable source of advice and will provide in-flight supplies of oxygen if needed. Specialist organizations can supply medical and nursing support for patients too ill to travel alone. Surprisingly few patients are truly too unfit to fly.

Further reading

DeHart, R.L. (ed.). (1985). *Fundamentals of aerospace medicine.* Lea & Febiger, Philadelphia.

Ernsting, J., Nicholson, A.N., and Rainford, D.J. (1998). *Aviation medicine* (3rd edn). Butterworth Heinemann, London.

Jagoda, A. and Pietrzak, M. (1997). Medical emergencies in commercial air travel. *Emergency Medicine Clinics of North America*, **15**, 251–60.

Joint Aviation Authorities. (1996). *Joint aviation requirements: flight crew medical requirements (JAR/FCL/Part3-Medical)*. Westwood Digital, Cheltenham, Gloucestershire.

Rosenberg, C.A. and Pak, F. (1997). Emergencies in the air: problems, management, and prevention. *Journal of Emergency Medicine*, **15**, 159–64.

Chapter 18.9

Diving medicine

D. M. Denison

In Britain at present there are some 80 000 sports-divers, about 5000 professional divers and around 3000 compressed air workers. On average, one serious incident occurs for each 1000 diver-years. Of these one-fifth are fatal. Adverse events are disproportionately commoner amongst sports than professional divers even though the latter spend much more time underwater, at greater depths, and in more stressful conditions. The low event rate amongst the latter is evidence that most accidents can be prevented by training and discipline. Almost all are due to failures of education, equipment, or communication. Frequently it is too late or impracticable to give effective medical help once they have occurred. Diving medicine is largely concerned with prevention. It depends upon understanding the work divers do and the risks they run completing it.

Figure 1 summarizes the shape of the sea. Diving is confined to the shelves and the uppermost slopes, i.e to a very small fraction of the total volume. At the surface, some tidal currents commonly exceed the speed at which people can swim, so it may only be practical to dive at slack water. Waves are often tall enough to prevent divers being launched or recovered with safety. Dawn arrives late and dusk comes early to the sea. Turbidity surrounding commercial diving sites often limits visibility to a metre or less. Sound localization is poor and auditory thresholds are raised by 30–90 dB. Susceptibility to blast injury is also raised.

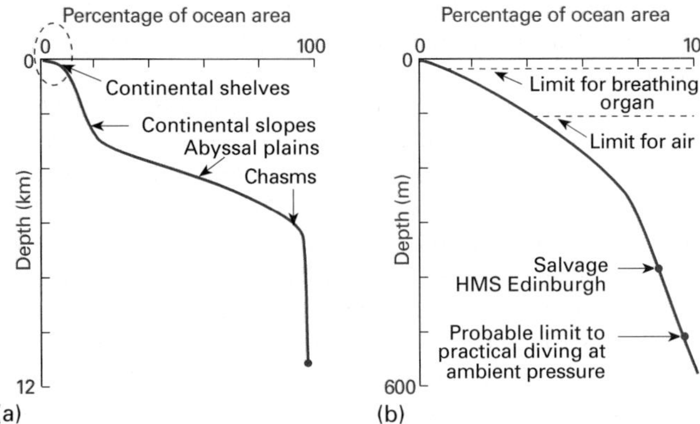

Fig. 1 (a) A cumulative depth versus area of plot of the oceans. (b) A similar plot of the top 600 m including the continental shelves.

Problems of immersion

Except for the surface waters of tropical seas, all of the oceans are too cold for individuals to stay long without insulation. Losses of tactile discrimination and manual dexterity are major problems. Immersion hypovolaemia and weightlessness are two others. Because the immersed body is weightless it can be displaced vertically with ease. Disadvantages are that the diver can no longer use his weight to apply leverage or torque, or to stay in place when a current is running. More important, any vertical movement can quickly become uncontrolled because of the positive feedback between depth and buoyancy. Since the gas in the chest and abdomen is compressible, the deeper a breath-hold diver goes, the denser he becomes and the more rapidly he falls. The higher he rises, the less dense he becomes and the faster he ascends. Such changes should be seen in the context of the person's actual buoyancy and swimming power. The maximum sustained thrust that a swimmer can develop is about 5 kg, which is just enough to propel him at about 1.5 miles an hour. When a normally built man takes a full inspiration he is about 2.5 kg positively buoyant and so requires half of his maximum swim-power to descend. If he breathes out to residual volume he is about 2.5 kg negatively buoyant and needs half his maximum swim-power to ascend. Thermally insulated clothing exaggerates this vertical instability leaving little margin for controlling unexpected ascent or descent.

Gas must be delivered to the diver at the same pressure as the water that surrounds him. This may be sent to him via an umbilical pipe from the surface, in which case it can flush through his helmet or face-mask continuously, which is wasteful of gas, but easily engineered, or it can supply a regulating valve that provides gas on demand only. Alternatively, the diver can take a self-contained underwater breathing apparatus (SCUBA) with him. This always feeds a demand regulator and rarely lasts for more than an hour. Professional divers often use a combination of all three systems, i.e. a surface-demand supply for routine use, with a helmet-flushing capability for occasional comfort or emergency use, and a small, back-mounted gas supply ready in case the surface supply fails.

Problems of descent

Ambient pressure rises linearly with depth by 1 atm for every 10 m descent. The diver may have difficulty in 'clearing his ears' because the mounting pressure on the outside of the drum is not balanced by an equal rise on the inner side, due to the valvular nature of the eustachian tube. This can be very painful, and may lead to drum rupture, but the strain on the drum usually resolves immediately on stopping the descent and ascending slightly. Sometimes the sinuses are affected on ascent or descent, in the same way. Pain on descent is always relieved by ascent.

Pain due to gas trapped in an obstructed space gets worse on ascent. Sometimes blood that has filled a sinus, and partly clotted during descent, is expelled in this manner as the diver returns to the surface. Occasionally, an ethmoid sinus may rupture into the cranial cavity. Usually, no specific treatment is needed for these injuries, but the diver is laid off diving until the cause has been established and he is fit to return.

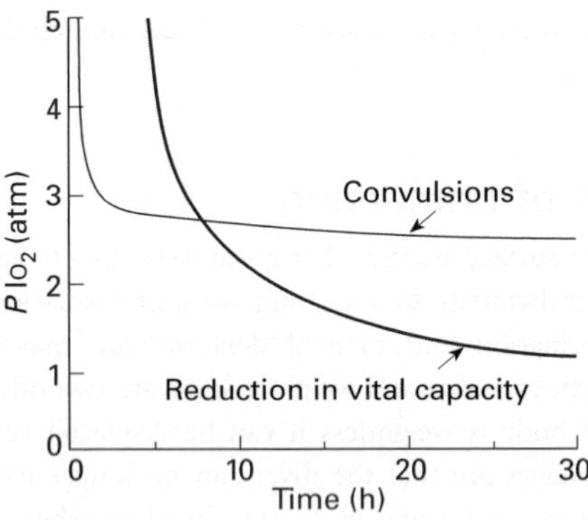

Fig. 2 The pulmonary and central nervous O_2 toxicity versus time curves that are commonly observed
(constructed from the data of many workers).

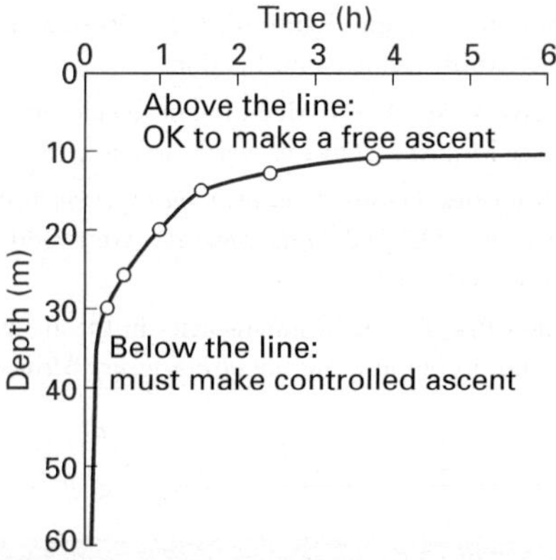

Fig. 3 The 'no-stop' diving curve that determines whether a dive has been shallow and brief enough for the diver to make a free ascent to the surface.

Nowadays, demand regulators and compensated outlet valves are well designed and there are few practical obstacles to providing the diver with gas at the right pressure. The composition of the gas to be breathed is a much more complex decision. Air can be breathed quite safely down to depths of 50 m, although tests of sophisticated cerebral function show there is already some impairment at 20 m. Below 50 m, mental deterioration becomes increasingly obvious, manifested by such actions as the diver offering his mouthpiece to neighbouring fish. If men breathe an oxygen–helium mix, rather than air, they can descend to the lowermost parts of the continental shelves without narcosis but at greater depths show various neurological disturbances due to direct effects of pressure on nerve tissues (the high-pressure nervous syndrome).

Oxygen becomes toxic to the lungs when the alveolar oxygen pressure exceeds half an atmosphere (5 m of sea water) and it becomes toxic to the nervous system when the alveolar, and the arterial, oxygen pressure exceed 2 atm (10 m of sea water). The time taken for symptoms to appear depends upon the dose. It varies from several hours at 0.5 atm to a few hours at 2 atm. Above that pressure the neurological sequelae overshadow the pulmonary damage that still occurs, and appear much earlier (Fig. 2).

Problems of ascent

When a breath-hold diver descends the gas in his lungs is compressed by the surrounding water, according to Boyle's Law. On return to the surface the gas will re-expand to its original volume, with no risk of lung rupture. However, if a diver has access to fresh gas at any time after leaving the surface, he can fill his lungs with enough gas to burst them on ascent, unless they are adequately vented. The lung is a cluster of tubes and balloons with bursting pressure of about 75 mmHg (1 m of sea-water) and time-constants of emptying that are normally close to 0.3 seconds. Divers are taught to exhale continuously when they ascend, and to rise no faster than the bubbles they exhale. Then the alveoli have time to empty and the risk of lung rupture is very low. The mechanics of rupture are not clear (they and other pulmonary aspects of diving are described in detail in Lundgren and Miller (1999), see Further reading). Failure to vent the lungs adequately on ascent is the second commonest cause of death and serious morbidity in diving. Patients with uncomplicated mediastinal and/or subcutaneous emphysema or non-tension pneumothoraces are treated conventionally by the administration of oxygen and aspiration or chest drainage where indicated. They should not be positive-pressure ventilated. Patients with neurological or other serious complications should be recompressed to 18 m depth as soon as possible, and expert diving medicine advice sought immediately.

In most diving accidents there is neither sufficient evidence or equipment to diagnose exactly what has gone on and it is vital to compress the patient in a recompression chamber to a pressure of 2.8 atm or more as quickly as possible. If a chest drain is in place, it must be clamped on compression and be exposed to continuous suction at depth and during decompression.

A separate life-threatening form of decompression illness (*decompression sickness*), occurs because, during any dive, extra inert gas, usually nitrogen or helium, goes into passive solution in the body. On ascent, as the ambient pressure falls, this gas can come out of solution in an uncontrolled way, forming bubbles in the circulation and within tissues. As the ascent continues, these bubbles increase in size and number, blocking blood vessels, and distorting or rupturing cells. On re-descent the bubbles contract and are eventually resorbed. If the first or the subsequent ascent is slow enough, few if any bubbles are formed, the extra gas diffuses into the bloodstream and out of the lungs easily, and the diver reaches the surface unharmed.

A vast amount of experimental work has been done to determine the safe limits to 'no-stop' diving and the depth–time profiles that have to be followed on returning to the surface after any longer dive. The time-limiting curve for 'no-stop' diving is shown in Fig. 3. Knowledge of safe practices is tabulated in a series of lengthy decompression schedules, which vary somewhat from one country to another, and are to be found in any textbook of diving medicine. After long (saturation) dives, the ascent is very slow and can take several days.

About 1 per cent of dives conducted to recommended schedules, and many badly conducted dives, lead to decompression sickness. This can take two forms, skin irritation or limb pain only (type 1 'bends'), or any other serious manifestation (type 2 'bends'). Skin irritation and mottling alone is treated by oxygen inhalation at the surface and does not require recompression. It is the mildest form of decompression sickness. All other cases should be recompressed as soon as possible. This is the only effective treatment. The object is to reduce the size of existing bubbles and prevent the formation of new ones, before irreversible infarction and oedema have occurred. About half of all cases involve the central nervous system, most often the lower cervical, the thoracic, or the upper lumbar segments of the spinal cord. Visual disturbances and then cerebral signs are often seen also. Many others involve limb pain, commonly of the shoulders or elbows in divers and of the knees and hips in tunnel workers. A minority of victims experience sudden chest pain, dyspnoea, and cough, believed to be due to bubbles in the pulmonary circulation. Symptoms appear minutes to hours after the end of a dive. Some of them are due to bubble formation directly—others are believed to be secondary to clumping of red cells. It must be emphasized that the only useful treatment for all of these conditions is immediate recompression, followed by a slow decompression that may take several days. The Duty Diving Officer at the Royal Navy's Institute of Naval Medicine (Alverstoke, Hants) will provide constant and expert advice by telephone (01705 768026).

Problems of assessment

Divers have a physically demanding job and often must work in sites remote from any medical aid. They must have a high exercise tolerance and be free of any active or latent condition that could erupt while they are away from medical help. In Britain, commercial divers have to pass an annual medical examination conducted by a doctor approved by the Health and Safety Executive as competent in diving medicine. If the diver is found to be unfit to dive and disagrees with the decision of the examiner he has the right of appeal to an independent tribunal set up by the Health and Safety Executive. Codes of safe diving practice are given in the Health and Safety Executive's *Diving Operations at Work Regulations 1998* and the *Compressed Air Regulations 1996*, which have been accepted nationally and internationally.

In principle, all divers are expected to be physically fit and mentally stable people, free of conditions such as epilepsy and ill-controlled diabetes or asthma. They should not be addicted to alcohol or any other drug and they should not have a history, or any other evidence, of significant obstructive lung disease, ruptured eardrums, or aural surgery. Divers who are generally fit to dive should not be allowed to do so when they have chest, upper airway or ear infections, or when they are overweight (because obesity predisposes to decompression sickness). Neither should they dive while taking any medication that could impair their ability to think clearly or orientate themselves in space correctly.

Military divers are also obliged to have annual medical examinations for 'fitness to dive', and sports divers are strongly urged to do likewise. The UK Sports Divers Medical Committee provides detailed advice for the latter. The purpose of the medical check is twofold—first to determine whether the candidate is fit to swim in swift currents and rough waters at remote sites, and only second to discover whether there is any bar to him or her also diving. In principle anyone who has more than a 20 per cent reduction in lung function (FEV_1, FVC, or carbon monoxide transfer) or aerobic capacity will not be fit enough to cope with emergencies in water and they should therefore be advised not swim except in calm and supervised sites. Diving is often a relaxed affair, but people normally dive in pairs so that in the case of an emergency one diver can get the other out of trouble. The prime purpose of the medical check is to determine that the candidate has sufficient physical reserves to do that.

Areas of doubt

Currently, four unresolved issues (the significance of a probe-patent foramen ovale, the existence of mild asthma, the role of lung-function tests in annual medical examinations, and possible long-term effects of deep-diving) are causes of concern. They are discussed in detail in the short bibliography listed below.

Conclusion

Diving is a sometimes very vigorous activity that demands a high degree of mental and physical fitness. It exposes people to several physical and chemical challenges that are reasonably well understood. Because it takes place remote from medical help, there is a strong emphasis on prevention of illness by following safe practices, developed empirically on the non-appearance of symptoms in brief trains of dives. There are now indications that these practices may not be quite as safe as first thought, but the cumulative effects are generally slight.

Further reading

Bennett, P.B. and Elliott, D.H. (ed.). (1993). *The physiology and medicine of diving* (4th edn). W.B. Saunders, London.

Bove, A.A. (ed.). (1997). *Diving medicine* (3rd edn). W.B. Saunders, Philadelphia.

Edmonds, C., Lowry, C., and Pennefather, J. (ed.). (1993). *Diving and sub-aquatic medicine* (3rd edn). Butterworth-Heinemann, London.

Hope, H., Lund, T.V., Elliott, D.H., Halsey, M.J., Helge, W. (ed.). (1994). *Long term health effects of diving.* Norwegian Underwater Technology Centre, Bergen.

Lundgren, C. and Miller, J.N. (ed.). (1999). *The lung at depth.* Marcel Dekker. New York.

Paras. (1997). SCUBA diving: A quantitative risk assessment. *Contract Research Report 140/1997.* Health and Safety Executive (Books), Sudbury, Suffolk.

Chapter 18.10

Lightning and electric shock

B. A. Pruitt and A. D. Mason

Between 2 and 8 per cent of all patients admitted to hospital with burns have had an electrical injury, but lightning strikes are very rare.

Pathophysiology of electrical injury

Contact with electric current can produce injury in two ways: electric shock, which may occur at low or high voltage, or thermal injury which occurs principally with higher voltage.

The known determinants of electrical injury include voltage, amperage, type of current, frequency of alternating current, duration of current passage, physical size and configuration of the part involved, and specific points of contact. Unfortunately, the frequencies which are ideal for electric power transmission are within the most dangerous part of the frequency spectrum. A lightning bolt which is a very high voltage and high amperage direct current may cause electric shock and/or severe thermal injury.

Electric shock commonly produces muscular contraction and may cause ventricular fibrillation. Thermal injury may be induced either by electrical arcing outside the body or by power dissipation in tissue. High voltage electric arcs develop very high temperatures that injure

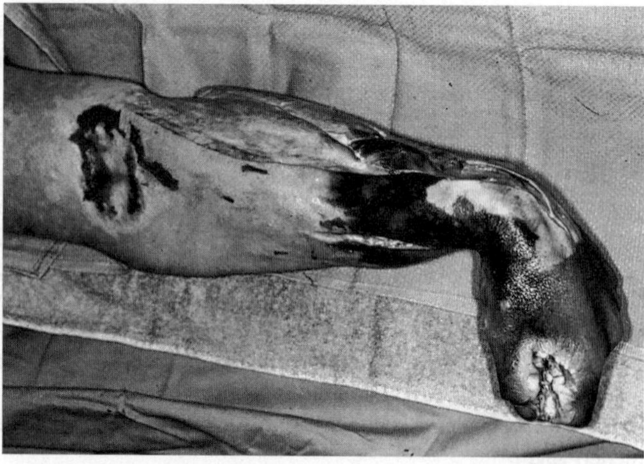

Fig. 1 The left arm and hand of this patient who made contact with a high voltage line show the typical flexion deformities of the digits and wrist, and charring at the contact site in the first web space and at the sites of arcing at the wrist and antecubital space. Note the more severe damage of the tissues of the hand and distal forearm where the cross-sectional area is relatively small, the darkly discoloured oedematous deeper muscle bulging above the more superficial muscles just proximal to the dorsum of the wrist, and the pale oedematous muscle bulging above the incised fascia in the proximal half of the fasciotomy incision.

skin directly and may cause extensive further thermal injury by igniting clothing.

When a part of the body becomes a circuit element, power dissipation within that part produces heat and an increase in temperature. Skin exhibits moderate resistance, especially when dry, but like any insulator, breaks down at sufficient voltage gradient. When this occurs at a contact point, current density and power dissipation reach high levels, producing severe local injury (Fig. 1). In the deeper tissues, current flow is not isotropic, because individual tissues differ in resistance, but except for bone, which has relatively high resistance, these differences are not great. For any specific voltage, power dissipation is greater in tissues of lower resistance and it is a common clinical observation that deep tissues having low resistance are more susceptible to electric injury than those having high resistance. The heat generated within any tissue is not confined to that tissue; it is, instead, distributed within the affected part according to the laws of heat flow. Thus, the low resistance soft tissues, contained between an inner core of high resistance bone and an outer shell of high resistance skin, behave as a nearly isotropic volume electric conductor which is uniformly heated by the passage of current. Soft tissue heating parallels current density, which may be approximated as an inverse function of the square of the radius of the body segment in question; heat production per unit volume and rate of temperature increase are greatest in segments of small diameter.

Thermal injury of tissue is a function of both temperature and duration of exposure. At the threshold for injury, which probably lies between 45 and 50°C, injury occurs when exposure is of the order of 100 s; at higher temperatures, the required time decreases exponentially. A block of tissue heated in such a way as to make its temperature uniform throughout and then exposed to a cooler environment cools more rapidly at its periphery than at its core. This suggests that central segments of body parts are more liable to injury because they sustain longer thermal exposure times. Following such tissue injury, occlusion of small nutrient vessels occurs rapidly and tissue ischaemia ensues. In such areas of injury, the patency of larger vessels is often maintained and the observation of bleeding at the time of early debridement does not necessarily imply vascular integrity.

These pathophysiological characteristics lead to the following predictions:

1. Maximal tissue destruction occurs at contact points and in body segments of small diameter.
2. Injured muscle may underlie intact skin.
3. Injured periosseous muscle may be overlaid by uninjured muscle.
4. The true extent of injury is not correlated with the extent of cutaneous burn.

Cell membrane damage may also be caused by transmembrane potentials of as little as 100–500 mV. This process of electroporation has been implicated as a pathogenic factor in rhabdomyolysis as well as certain otherwise inexplicable neurological signs and symptoms.

Diagnosis and treatment

Cardiopulmonary arrest is common in the immediate post-injury period in patients with high voltage electrical or lightning injury. The arrest may be due to either asystole or fibrillation and must be treated immediately. Cardiac arrhythmias can also occur following resuscitation, and patients with such injuries should undergo ECG monitoring for at least 48 hours following injury even in the absence of arrhythmias and for 48 hours beyond the last ECG evidence of dysrhythmia. Hyperkalaemia may occur and is yet another reason for early post-injury ECG monitoring in patients with high voltage electrical injury. It should be treated as in other patients.

Two factors conspire to increase the incidence of acute renal failure in patients with high voltage electrical injury. Fluid needs may be underestimated because there is little cutaneous injury but extensive deep tissue injury. Accordingly, inadequate volumes of resuscitation fluids may be administered and oliguria results. In addition, myoglobin may be liberated from injured muscle and is more likely to precipitate in the renal tubules in the presence of oliguria. Resuscitation fluids should be infused in sufficient volume to obtain an hourly urinary output of 75–100 ml in patients who exhibit elevated levels of urinary haemochromogens. If oliguria persists or the haemochromogen level does not promptly diminish despite otherwise adequate resuscitation, a diuretic should be administered to prevent the development of acute renal failure. Some advocate the use of a loop diuretic, but we prefer the use of mannitol as an osmotic diuretic, and administer 12.5 g (one ampoule) in each litre of intravenous fluid given until the pigment has cleared from the urine.

If the electric current has caused injury to tissues beneath the investing fascia of a limb, sufficient oedema may be produced in a muscle compartment to impair nutrient blood flow further or to interrupt flow to distal unburned tissue. The clinical signs indicating a need for fasciotomy include stony hardness of muscle compartments upon palpation, cyanosis of distal unburned skin, impaired capillary refilling of distal unburned skin or nail beds, and absent or diminished pulsatile flow in distal vessels as assessed by examination with an ultrasonic flowmeter and a compartment pressure above 40 mmHg as measured with a cannula or wick catheter. When the indications are present, fasciotomy should be performed as an emergency procedure, using general anaesthesia.

Operative exploration should be carried out as soon as the patient is haemodynamically stable and should be performed under general anaesthesia. The involved muscle is thoroughly explored, bearing in mind that non-viable deep periosseous muscle can be present beneath more superficial viable muscle. All necrotic tissue is debrided. Destruction of nerves, tendons, and vessels, or muscle necrosis so extensive as to render a limb useless mandate amputation at a level proximal to the area of tissue necrosis. In a recently treated group of 28 patients with electric injury of the upper limb, 33 amputations, including five shoulder disarticulations, were performed. Oedema of the pectoral muscles in patients with high voltage electrical injuries of the upper limb demands exploration of that area and excision of non-viable muscle if it is present. The amputation or exploration wounds are packed open and the patient scheduled for re-examination of the wounds 24–48 hours later. If, at the time of re-exploration, there is a significant amount of residual necrotic tissue, it is debrided, the wound again packed open, and the patient again scheduled for re-exploration 48–72 hours later. If at the time of initial or subsequent re-exploration, little or no debridement is necessary, an amputation site may be closed by a 'sausage-type' technique and standard delayed primary closure techniques may be applied to other operative wounds.

Bacterial control is best achieved by the use of Sulfamylon® burn cream in those patients in whom electric injury has damaged only skin and subcutaneous tissue or in those patients with burns due to electric ignition of clothing. The active ingredient of this agent (mafenide acetate) can diffuse into the non-viable tissue to limit bacterial proliferation and prevent the development of invasive burn wound sepsis.

Other injuries

Visceral damage is uncommon, but intestinal perforation, focal gall-bladder necrosis, focal pancreatic necrosis, and direct liver injury have been reported. In one series, three-quarters of patients with high voltage electrical injury showed evidence of gastrointestinal dysfunction within 12–18 months of injury and 13 of 45 patients developed cholelithiasis within 2 years

Peripheral nerve or spinal cord injury may be evident immediately following injury, or develop later. Motor nerves are more commonly affected than sensory nerves. If peripheral nerve damage is apparent immediately after injury, recovery is rare. Late appearing peripheral nerve deficits may involve nerves far removed from the points of electrical contact as part of a polyneuritic syndrome with highly variable recovery of function. Immediate post-injury spinal cord deficits reflect direct neuronal injury. Return of function is more common than in the case of spinal cord deficits of delayed onset, which tend to be permanent. Delayed onset abnormalities include localized nerve deficits with signs of ascending paralysis, transverse myelitis, an amyotrophic lateral sclerosis-like syndrome, hemiplegia, and quadriplegia.

Tetanic contractions of the paraspinus muscles induced by electric current may produce compression fractures of one or more vertebral bodies. Vertebral injuries and even long bone fractures may occur in electrical powerline workers who fall from a height following electric shock.

Cataracts may occur in any patient who has sustained high voltage electrical injury (a 6.2 per cent incidence in one series) but this complication is most frequent in those patients in whom the contact point has been on the head or neck. These may develop during the initial hospital period or as late as 3 or more years later.

House current voltage electrical burns of the mouth may occur when a young child bites an electric cord or sucks on the end of a live extension cord. The injury typically has the pearly white appearance of an avascular full-thickness burn and commonly involves the oral commissure. Labial artery bleeding is common (22 per cent in one series) and must be controlled by digital pressure.

Lightning injury

Cardiopulmonary arrest is particularly common in patients who have been struck by lightning. Immediate cardiopulmonary resuscitation is life-saving in such individuals. Recovery has been reported even in patients who were without signs of life for up to 15 or more minutes.

Neurological sequelae are common. They range from coma to isolated nerve deficits and even lower limb paraplegia. These neurological deficits commonly resolve in a matter of hours or, at most, days.

The cutaneous burns caused by lightning are characteristically superficial and often exhibit an arborescent or spidery 'splashed-on' or 'fern leaf' appearance. Myoglobinuria in such patients is surprisingly uncommon in view of the current flow which occurs during lightning injury. Today, two-thirds of patients who have sustained lightning injuries survive as a result of early institution of cardiopulmonary resuscitation and prompt treatment of complications (see also OTM3, pp. 1211–115).

Further reading

Amy, B.W., McManus, W.F., Goodwin, C.W., Jr., and Pruitt, B.A. Jr. (1985). Lightning injury with survival in five patients. *Journal of the American Medical Association*, **253**, 243–5.

Hunt, J.L., Sato, R.M., and Baxter, C.R. (1980). Acute electric burns: current diagnostic and therapeutic approaches to management. *Archives of Surgery*, **115**, 434–8.

Lee, R.C., Gottlieb, L.J., and Krizek, T.J. (1992). Pathophysiology and clinical manifestations of tissue injury in electrical trauma. *Advances in Plastic and Reconstructive Surgery*, **8**, 9–16.

Morbidity and Mortality Weekly Report. (1998). Lightning-associated deaths–United States, 1980–1995. *Morbidity and Mortality Report*, 47, 391–4.

Chapter 18.11

Ionizing radiation

R. J. Berry

Sources of radiation

Natural

Cosmic rays

Throughout their evolution humans have been exposed to cosmic radiation emanating from remote parts of the universe as well as from the sun. Most cosmic rays are very high energy protons and a smaller number of heavier nuclei, mostly helium (alpha-particles). The intensity of exposure of humans to cosmic radiation depends entirely on the altitude at which they are, contributing roughly half of the total external radiation dose from natural sources at sea level but increasing markedly even at high altitudes on land and further still for the crew and passengers of high-flying aircraft.

Secondary radiations

Secondary radiations are generated in the upper atmosphere and consist largely of gamma-rays and high energy electrons (beta-particles), together with other particles with similar biological effects. The contribution from secondary radiations varies with the latitude, being greatest at the poles and lowest at the equator.

Radioactivity

Many of the earth's minerals are naturally radioactive. Atoms are stable only if their nuclei contain an approximately equal number of protons and neutrons and unstable atomic nuclei may undergo spontaneous disintegration. In body fluids the naturally occurring radioactive isotope of potassium ^{40}K makes the largest contribution to the internal radiation background. In the environment, many naturally occurring materials are radioactive and in the UK the primary contribution to radiation dose to people comes from radon in the soil.

Man-made

X-rays used by doctors are the greatest single man-made source of irradiation of the general population. Nuclear reactors are not only sources of direct radiations (usually absorbed in appropriate shielding) but are also copious producers of radioisotopes. Finally, nuclear weapons are intense sources of man-made radiation, although potentially lethal effects of blast and heat can occur at greater distances from the point of detonation than do lethal effects from direct radiation.

For both natural and man-made radioactive substances, the qualities of importance are the type of disintegration, the particles or non-particulate (gamma) radiation produced by the disintegration, the *half-life* (the time for one-half of the initial activity to have disappeared, half of the remaining activity taking the same time to disappear, etc.) and the initial *activity*. This is specified in units of disintegrations per second (becquerels) named after the discoverer of radioactivity. The unit which has been used in the past related the number of radioactive disintegrations to the number of disintegrations taking place in 1 g of pure radium, 3.7×10^{10} per second = 1 curie (1 Ci = 3.7×10^{10} Bq, 1 Bq = 2.7×10^{-11} Ci).

Radiation effects

Ionizing radiations differ in their effects both qualitatively and quantitatively. X-rays and gamma-rays produce their damage by ejecting orbital electrons from atoms of matter with which they interact. These radiations are sparsely ionizing because the ejected particle is of low mass and limited in its capability for producing damage, so that several interactions are needed to cause biological damage. Their effects are dependent upon the rate at which the radiation dose is accumulated, whether protracted in time or fractionated in multiple short bursts.

Protons, neutrons which eject protons from atoms of matter, and other larger particles are more densely ionizing, so that their action is often 'all or none'. Their effects are also less dependent upon dose rate or dose fractionation.

Radiation dose

All effects of radiation depend on the size of the accumulated radiation dose. Absorbed radiation dose is now cited in SI units which have the dimensions of joules (energy) per kilogram (mass of absorbing material). Throughout this chapter these new units will be given, followed by the old units in parentheses. The basic unit of absorbed radiation dose, 1 J/kg, has been given the eponym 1 gray (1 Gy = 100 rad). Conventional SI prefixes are used for multiples and sub-multiples of this unit. To compare the effects of different radiations, the absorbed dose is multiplied by a radiation weighting factor which is selected for the type and energy of the radiation. The value of this factor is determined by the International Commission on Radiological Protection. The product is called *equivalent dose*, and its unit has the special name of sievert (Sv). Table 1 lists a thousand million-fold range of radiation doses, and their effects upon biological systems.

Table 1 Effects of total body irradiation

Equivalent dose (Sv)*	Effect
Sublethal to man	
0.0001	Around 2 weeks' natural background radiation, no detectable effect
0.001 (1 mSv)	Around 6 months' natural background radiation, no detectable effect
0.01	No detectable effect
0.1	Minimal decrease in peripheral lymphocyte count, no clinical effect
1	Mild acute radiation sickness in some individuals (nausea, possible vomiting), no acute deaths, early decrease in peripheral lymphocyte count, decrease in all white blood cells and platelets at 2–3 weeks, increase in late risk of leukaemia, solid tumours
Lethal to man	
10	Severe acute radiation sickness, severe vomiting, diarrhoea, death within 30 days of all exposed individuals Severe depression of blood cell and platelet production, damage to gastrointestinal mucosa
100	Immediate severe vomiting, disorientation, coma, death within hours
1000	Death of some micro-organisms, some insects
10 000	Death of most bacteria, some viruses
100 000	Death of all living organisms, denaturation of proteins

*For X-rays and gamma-radiation equivalent dose in Sv is equal to absorbed dose (gray).

Total body irradiation of man

As seen in Table 1, the major consequence of radiation exposure is life-shortening, either acutely for doses in excess of 5–10 Gy, or due to late effects which may be seen 1–40 years after radiation exposure for smaller doses. Clinically important radiation syndromes are as follows.

Central nervous system syndrome

Above acute exposures of 30–100 Gy (3000–10 000 rad) there is a rapid onset of nausea, vomiting which may be severe and repeated, anxiety, disorientation and, within hours, coma and death due to direct radiation effects on central nervous system conduction and to cerebral oedema.

Gastrointestinal syndrome

People who have received doses in excess of 10 Gy (1000 rad) will also develop nausea and vomiting, usually starting 1–2 hours after radiation exposure, but often resolving by 4–6 hours. However, they are doomed to die within 4–14 days because of radiation damage to the gastrointestinal tract. The convoluted epithelial lining of the small intestine is perhaps the most rapidly renewed tissue in the body; cells born in the intestinal crypts are shed from the tips of villi to the intestinal contents some 7 days later. Radiation inhibition of cell division, followed by the reproductive death of the intestinal stem cells results in, first, a shortening of the intestinal villi until the lining of the intestine is as flat as a garden hose. This drastically reduces the surface area available for nutrient and electrolyte diffusion, and results in intractable diarrhoea. Failure of survival of sufficient intestinal stem cells and their proliferation to replace dying intestinal epithelial cells leads to denudation of areas of the bowel, with consequent free access of bowel contents and infection to the blood and leakage of body fluids into the intestinal contents. Dehydration, overwhelming infection, and death follow.

Haemopoietic syndrome

At doses between 1 and 10 Gy (100–1000 rad) transient nausea and occasional vomiting may be seen in some people, the frequency increasing with increasing dose. These early prodromal symptoms disappear rapidly, followed by a period of relative well-being. Haemopoietic stem cells are damaged by radiation, as are cells of other tissues, primarily by the loss of their ability to divide and by their subsequent death on attempting division. Hence, when the normal division stimuli occur there is an initial abortive repopulation of the peripheral blood achieved by 'short cutting' the normal differentiation steps, which further depletes the already damaged haemopoietic stem cell population. By 2–3 weeks there is no new input of differentiated, functional white cells and platelets, the peripheral blood count falls and the clinical syndrome develops of easy and overwhelming infection due to lack of white cells, and bleeding starting with petechial haemorrhage due to shortage of platelets.

Therapy of acute radiation exposure

If large populations have been irradiated even a crude estimation of the radiation dose received will be of importance. Scarce medical resources will have to be devoted only to those patients who have received doses in the LD_{10}–LD_{50} range; those most ill will have been irretrievably lethally irradiated, and the vast majority of those who have received less than LD_{10} radiation dose will recover spontaneously. Those patients at highest risk of haemopoietic death will have to be identified by the decrease in peripheral blood lymphocytes, which die rapidly over the first 24–48 hours. A better early biological dosimeter, usable when there are only small numbers of exposed individuals, is the number of chromosome aberrations in peripheral blood lymphocytes cultured *in vitro* with phytohaemagglutinin.

Following the nuclear reactor accident at Chernobyl and widespread radioactive contamination of the public from a stolen radioactive source in Goiania, recent experience of management of radiation casualties has been subject to intense scrutiny and an international consensus is beginning to emerge. Successes obtained with therapeutic regimes of fluid and electrolyte replacement and platelet transfusion plus appropriate antibiotics have confirmed that infection and haemorrhage are the primary factors causing death from the haemopoietic syndrome. When the number of casualties is sufficiently small, isolation, antimicrobial decontamination of the intestine, systemic antibiotics, transfusion as required of red cells and platelets and supportive measures for empirical treatment of infection have been shown to be highly effective. The cytokines G-CSF and GM-CSF can accelerate haemopoietic recovery and appear to be of use in treatment of victims of radiation injury who have received a dose large enough to produce sustained neutropenia but not so large that bone marrow recovery will not occur eventually. The role of bone marrow transplantation is limited to the few victims whose marrow is unlikely to recover but who have not received lethal damage to the bowel or lungs. Where there is combined injury due to trauma, conventional injuries require normal medical emergency procedures first, as all but the most severe radiation injury is not immediately life-threatening. In particular, wounds must be treated by early definitive surgery in the narrow window of time before radiation-induced suppression of cellular elements necessary for wound healing occurs.

If a major radiation exposure results not from external irradiation but from contamination by radioactive isotopes as after both the Chernobyl reactor accident and the Goiania lost-source incident, information from Health Physics personnel as to the nature of the hazard expected and determination of the initial amount of radioactivity in and on contaminated casualties is vital—to assess danger to staff as well as to the patients.

First treatment of exposure to radioactive materials by wounding (skin penetration), ingestion, or inhalation may be directed towards removing the radioactive material from the body. Dangerously radioactive material in a wound is treated initially by washing and mechanical scrubbing, and if necessary by adequate surgical excision of the contaminated tissue. Ingestion of radioiodine is treated by giving a single (100–200 mg) dose of stable sodium iodide/iodate so that the amount of the radioisotope which is fixed in the thyroid is minimized. This is most effective if taken before exposure, and only of use within a few hours after exposure. The amount of ^{137}Cs retained in the body can be reduced and its excretion enhanced by treatment with gram quantities of Prussian blue. Ingestion of bone-seeking radionuclides such as ^{90}Sr and actinides such as ^{239}Pu may be treated by administration of chelating agents like diethylenetriamine pentaacetic acid (DTPA) to minimize their deposition in bone. Massive oral doses of stable calcium and parathyroid hormone have also been used with limited success.

Particulate radioactive contamination which has been inhaled may, when the material has particular long-term hazards (e.g. ^{239}Pu), be removed in part by bronchial lavage carried out in centres with appropriate specialist skills.

Late effects of radiation exposure

Leukaemogenesis

Over the period 3–10 years after acute radiation exposure there is increased risk of the development of leukaemia, predominantly myeloid leukaemia. The magnitude of risk is proportional to the total radiation dose received. The dose to double the natural incidence of leukaemia is estimated to lie in the region of a few hundred mGy (a few tens of rads), but as leukaemia represents only around 3 per cent of all new malignancies in the UK, even a relatively large increase in leukaemia incidence may represent a small change in the overall numbers of patients presenting with malignant disease.

Carcinogenesis

Solid tumours are also induced by ionizing radiation exposure, the risk increasing with increasing dose, but over periods up to 40 and more years after radiation exposure. The most common sites of radiation-induced tumours are related to the sites in which cancer is most prevalent in the general population. Skin cancer is inevitably high in incidence; other cancers in which increased incidence following radiation exposure has been demonstrated include breast, lung, thyroid, and bone cancers and lymphomas. A large pool of human experience exists in the early radiation workers, the Hiroshima and Nagasaki survivors, and in specific groups exposed to either inhalation or ingestion of radioactive materials (e.g. uranium miners, radium dial painters) or to the medical use of ionizing radiation for diagnostic or therapeutic purposes (breast cancer in women patients with tuberculosis given a therapeutic artificial pneumothorax, skin and other cancers in patients treated by radiation for ankylosing spondylitis, etc.). Total body exposure of 1 cGy (1 rad) gives at most a risk of about 1 in 2000 of the development of fatal malignant disease in a particular individual. Thus, uniform exposure of a population of 1 million people to 1 cGy may result in the eventual development of about 500 fatal cancers against a background of some 250 000 spontaneous cancer deaths of which some 6000–9000 may have resulted from the unavoidable lifelong exposure to natural background radiation.

Partial body exposure—local radiation effects

When less than the whole body is irradiated, the effect will depend on radiation dose, and upon what parts of the body are irradiated. Radiation therapy, limited to appropriate parts of the body, has been used effectively to treat malignant disease since shortly after Röntgen discovered X-rays in 1895, and there is a considerable literature on the effects of such local irradiation on limiting normal tissues. The radiation effect will also be determined by the fractionation or protraction of the dose in time: the longer the overall time or the larger number of individual radiation exposures, the greater the total dose which can be accumulated before damage is produced. On the skin a single radiation dose in excess of around 8 Gy will cause a transient reddening within a few hours, followed by a more vigorous erythema at 7–10 days, its intensity once again depending on total dose accumulated. With increasing radiation dose to the skin, dry or moist desquamation will result, healing by repopulation of the denuded epithelium from surviving basal epithelial cells. In many organs, although the turnover of parenchymal cells is slow, damage to blood vessels results in focal ischaemia and often leads to fibrosis. Limiting normal tissues for the clinical radiotherapist in the treatment of cancer include lungs, gastrointestinal tract, kidneys, and central nervous system. Modern radiation therapy uses supervoltage (greater than 1 MV) X-rays or the gamma-rays from ^{60}Co which physically spare the skin. The skin is therefore no longer the limiting normal tissue. Normal tissue tolerance is determined by the induction of fibrosis in subcutaneous connective tissues and in limiting organs within the irradiation volume.

Radiation damage to the fetus

The developing fetus is particularly susceptible to damage during the period of organogenesis. In particular, irradiation of the fetus in the period 8–15 weeks after conception during the period of development of the forebrain may lead to severe mental retardation. The fetus, like the adult, is also subject to an increased risk of the development of leukaemia and solid tumours which is related to the total accumulated radiation dose, but this increased risk per unit dose may be several times greater than for an adult.

Genetic damage

Radiation can produce both dominant lethal events, and recessive changes which are not expressed in the first generation. However, with increasing radiation dose, an increased proportion of those cells in which such transformations have taken place are rendered reproductively inert and cannot pass on their genetic misinformation. Hence, somatic rather than genetic damage is the limiting factor in determining permissible radiation exposure to populations.

Controlling human exposure to radiation hazards

ALARA/ALARP

Since the first annual radiation exposure limits, pioneered by the International Congress of Radiology in 1928 and intended for medical radiation workers, progressively more restrictive limits have been imposed for maximum exposure to ionizing radiation, not only for those workers but also for the general public. In 1977 the International Commission on Radiological Protection (ICRP) instituted a new system of radiation protection which was based on three principles.

Justification No practice shall be undertaken involving radiation unless it is likely to bring benefit.

Optimization For any practice involving radiation, the radiation dose used shall be as low as reasonably achievable (ALARA), economic and social considerations being taken into account.

Dose limits No individual shall be exposed to radiation in excess of those limits recommended by the Commission.

In its 1990 recommendations, the Commission developed this system further by identifying *practices*, which increase radiation exposures and *interventions* which reduce them, and by recommending *constraints* on exposure from individual sources, below *dose limits* which are now regarded as the level of dose above which the consequences for the individual would be widely regarded as unacceptable. Current dose limits in the UK are based on the 1977 ICRP recommendations as incorporated into a European Community Directive and given the force of law to keep doses 'As Low as Reasonably Practicable' (ALARP) through regulations made under the Health and Safety at Work, etc. Act, 1974.

Dose limits to the general public

The present average dose to the general public from all sources of radiation is about 2.5 mSv per annum, and the vast majority of this (>85 per cent) is from natural sources of which exposure to radon gas (*circa* 50 per cent) is the largest and most variable part. By far the largest source of man-made exposure to the general public is from medical uses (14 per cent), and of this the largest contribution is from diagnostic X-rays. The current legal dose limit for the general public is 5 mSv, subject to an average dose limit of 1 mSv per year so that the lifetime whole body equivalent dose to any individual member of the public will not normally exceed 70 mSv. This dose limit is designed to keep at an acceptably low level the stochastic harmful effects of radiation exposure (those all-or-none effects which occur with increasing frequency with increasing dose) and to prevent the occurrence of deterministic harmful effects (for which there is a

Table 2 ICRP recommended dose limits (1990)

	Annual dose limit	
	General public	Radiation workers
Total body exposure (effective dose)	1mSv, a higher value allowed in special circumstances provided the average over 5 years does not exceed 1 mSv	20 mSv, averaged over defined periods of 5 years and subject to a maximum 50 mSv in any year
Lens of the eye (equivalent dose)	15 mSv	150 mSv
Skin	50 mSv	500 mSv
Hands, feet	–	500 mSv

dose threshold, above which they increase in severity with increasing dose). If only part of the body is irradiated, proportionately higher doses are allowed. The 1990 ICRP recommended limits are shown in Table 2.

Limits for the inhalation or ingestion of radioactive material depend upon the concentration of those materials in limiting target organs. Thus, the limit for ingestion of radioactive iodine is set by the maximum radiation dose to the thyroid in which it would be concentrated; in fact the limit is set by the concentration in the thyroid of the most susceptible member of the population, a young child.

Dose limits to radiation workers

All occupational exposure is subject to demonstration that it is ALARP, and the National Radiological Protection Board has recommended a dose constraint of 15 mSv per year averaged over 5 years with no more than 20 mSv in a single year. The 1990 ICRP recommendations for occupational dose limits are also shown in Table 2. Present regulations of the European Community require that persons be designated radiation workers if there is a likelihood that their annual radiation exposure will exceed one-third of the current dose limits. Volunteers giving informed consent to participate in medical experiments in which radiation is used may not receive a dose greater than the annual dose limit to radiation workers, except in very special circumstances.

Further reading

MacVittie, T.J., Weiss, J.F., and Browne, D. (ed.). (1996). Advances in the treatment of radiation injuries. *Advances in the Biosciences*, Vol. 94. Pergamon Press, Oxford.

International Commission on Radiological Protection. (1991). Publication 60, 1990. Recommendations of the International Commission on Radiological Protection. *Annals of the ICRP*, Vol. 21, no. 1–3. Pergamon Press, Oxford.

National Radiological Protection Board. (1989). *Living with radiation*, (4th edn). HMSO, London.

National Radiological Protection Board. (1993). Estimates of late radiation risks to the U.K. population. *Documents of the NRPB*, Vol.4, no.4. HMSO, London.

National Radiological Protection Board. (1996). Risk from deterministic effects of ionising radiation. *Documents of the NRPB*, Vol.7, no. 3. HMSO, London.

Chapter 18.12

Noise

R. C. Williams

The most important biological effect of loud noise is hearing loss. Hazardous levels of noise occur most often in the workplace, but the last 40 years have also seen increasing noise exposure in the general community from a variety of sources such as amplified music, motor vehicles, and domestic appliances.

In an otologically normal young adult, the ear can perceive sounds in a frequency range from about 25 Hz to about 20 000 Hz (20 kHz). The human ear is most sensitive in the range 500 Hz to 4 kHz, which corresponds approximately to the speech frequencies. There is a rapid fall off in the sensitivity of the ear in the higher frequencies and a more gradual fall off in the lower frequencies.

The effect of noise on hearing

The level at which sound becomes harmful to hearing remains controversial. Susceptibility to hearing loss is subject to normal biological variation, and in any noise-exposed group there will be individuals who may be at greater risk due to disease, toxic agents, or possibly other environmental factors. Current legislation in the UK, The Noise At Work Regulations 1989, which is based on a European Community Directive, specifies 'a first action level of 85 dB(A)' (decibels in the 'A' scale). This should be sufficient to prevent significant hearing loss in otologically normal persons. Within the UK, the Health and Safety Executive estimated that in 1986 about 1.5 million workers in production industries and construction and around half those in agriculture could be exposed to noise levels above 85 dB(A).

The four main effects on hearing from noise exposure are temporary hearing loss, permanent hearing loss, tinnitus,and recruitment. Initially, exposure to harmful levels of noise causes a temporary loss of hearing, typically in the frequency range 4–6 kHz. Recovery will usually be complete within 2 weeks of ceasing exposure.

Continuing exposure causes permanent threshold shift, i.e. irreversible hearing loss, again typically in the range 4–6 kHz. Initially the lower frequencies are largely unaffected and there is recovery in the higher frequencies. On audiometric testing, this appears as a characteristic notching of the audiogram (Fig. 1). With prolonged exposure, the extent of the loss both increases and extends into the lower frequencies (Fig. 2).

It is now believed that the hearing loss is partly attributable to direct mechanical damage of the cochlea and partly to metabolic overload as a consequence of over-stimulation. The latter raises a future possibility of protecting hearing by the use of pharmacological agents. Tinnitus is subjective , but is associated with noise induced hearing loss. In 5–10 per cent it will cause annoyance and in approximately 1 per cent it will be severe. It may be more common in those exposed to impulse noise.

Recruitment is a distortion of the perception of sound, which occurs in some individuals with severe noise-induced hearing loss. It shows as a characteristic trace on self-recording audiometry.

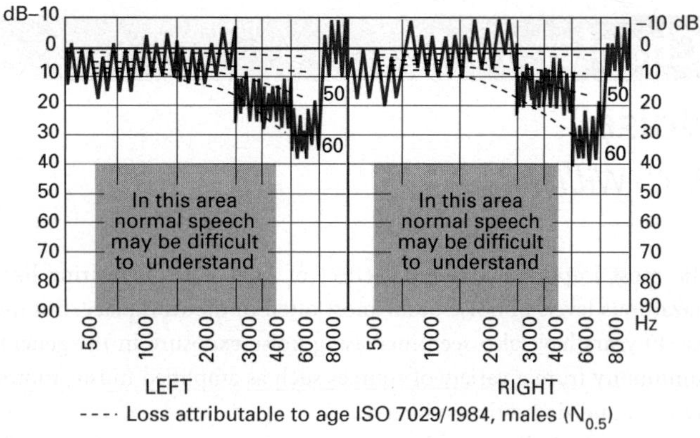

Fig. 1 Hearing loss after continuing noise exposure. Initially the lower frequencies are largely unaffected and there is recovery in the higher frequencies, appearing as a characteristic notching of the audiogram.

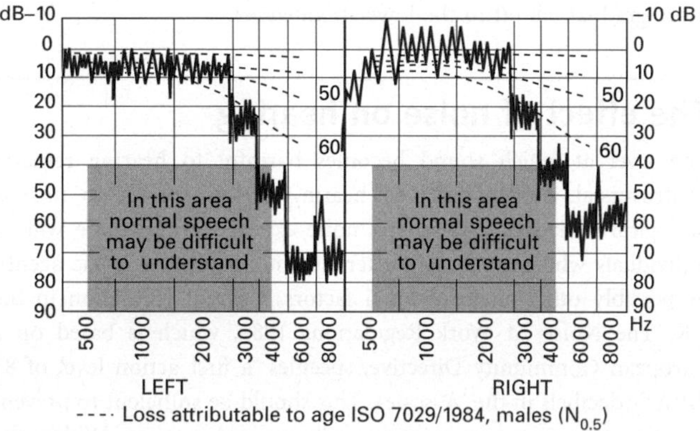

Fig. 2 With prolonged noise exposure the extent of the loss increases and extends into the lower frequencies.

Hearing conservation

In Great Britain the Noise at Work Regulations 1989, which are based on a European Community Directive, require every employer to prevent damage to the hearing of workers from excessive noise at work. Prevention should be by noise reduction at source where reasonably practicable. If not practicable, suitable hearing protection should be issued. Audiometry is not a legal requirement but is recommended as good practice where daily noise exposures exceed 90 dB(A).

Non-auditory effects of noise

Loud noise will obviously interfere with sleep and the perception of speech. The recommended maximum noise level to avoid sleep disturbance is 35 dB(A) averaged over the sleep period. Difficulty with communication may result in hazards to safety.

There is some suggestion that loud noise can affect the cardiovascular system. It may also have psychological and other effects. A recent critical review of the literature suggests that although there are some demonstrable effects of noise on performance and health, the evidence is not conclusive and it is not possible to estimate accurately the impact of the effects or the threshold below which adverse effects will not occur.

Further reading

Alves-Pereira, M. (1999). Noise-induced extra-aural pathology: a review and commentary. *Aviation and Space Environmental Medicine*, **70**, A7–21.

Clarek, W. W. and Bohne, B. A. (1999). Effects of noise on hearing. *Journal of the American Medical Association*, **281**, 1658–9.

King, Coles, Lutman, and Robinson. (1992). *Assessment of hearing disability.* Whurr Publishers, London.

Non-auditory effects of noise. (1999). HSE contract report 241/1999. HSE Books, Sudbury, Suffolk

Chapter 18.13

Vibration

Tar-Ching Aw

The most damaging frequencies of vibration are between 25 and 250 Hz (cycles per second).

Vibration can be transmitted locally usually to the hands and arms of those using hand-held rods such as pneumatic drills, or to the whole body of drivers of tractors, fork-lift trucks, mobile cranes, and helicopters.

Clinical effects

Whole body vibration can cause headache, motion sickness, sleep and visual disturbance, urinary and abdominal complaints, and low back pain. In the case of drivers, low back pain may occur as a result of exposure to whole body vibration and poor posture within the vehicle cab.

Hand transmitted vibration causes secondary Raynaud's phenomenon; 'vibration white-finger'. This manifests as frequent episodic pallor of the digits, usually on exposure to cold. The term refers to vascular changes but there are often accompanying neurological and musculoskeletal effects; 'hand arm vibration syndrome'. The latent period between initial exposure and development of symptoms usually varies from 5–10 years, but may be as little as 1 year.

The vascular effects have been attributed to spasm of the digital vessels. The sequence of colour change in the affected digits include pallor, a bluish hue due to cyanosis, and redness with spontaneous reversal of the vascular spasm. Exposure to cold precipitates attacks of digital pallor, and patients frequently describe pallor in the morning, or following outdoor activity such as fishing or gardening, especially in cold weather. The neurological effects include numbness, reduced temperature perception, loss of manual dexterity, tingling, paraesthesia, and pain. Severe tingling, discomfort, and pain is often described by patients following rapid warming of the hands when the digital blood circulation returns to normal. Inability to distinguish and hold small objects such as coins, and difficulty with manipulating the steering wheel of a car or buttoning up clothes contributes to physical and social disability. Muscle weakness, exostoses and cysts in the carpal bones, carpal tunnel syndrome, osteoarthritis, and Dupuytren's contracture have been associated with exposure to vibration.

Diagnosis

Physical examination may show callosities on the hands, loss of touch, pinprick or temperature sensation in the affected digits, muscle weakness, or may show no obvious abnormalities especially in the early stages of the disease. Phalen's sign (tingling sensation in the fingers following flexion of the wrists) and Tinel's sign (sharp tingling along the path of the median nerve on tapping the wrist over the site of the carpal tunnel) are positive if there is associated carpal tunnel syndrome. In rare severe cases there are trophic changes in the finger tips leading to gangrene.

Compression of the nail bed of affected digits for 10 seconds may show delayed (>5 seconds) return of the digital circulation (Lewis–Prusik test). Finger plethysmography allows measurement of changes in finger systolic blood pressure and finger vascular circulation following local cooling. Digital blood pressure measurements using a Doppler device may demonstrate a fall in pressure after cold provocation. Cold provocation tests are commonly used in an attempt to provoke digital pallor. However, the method of doing these tests has not been standardized, and sensitivity is low. Sensory aesthesiometry may detect early loss of tactile perception. The vibrometer measures thresholds of perception of vibration.

The differential diagnosis should include other causes for Raynaud's phenomenon such as rheumatoid arthritis, lupus erythematosus, scleroderma, other autoimmune disorders, poliomyelitis, syringomyelia, cryoglobulinaemia, occlusive vascular disease, frostbite, and the costoclavicular syndrome. Medications, such as ergot, clonidine, and β-blockers, and heavy cigarette smoking may be contributory factors. Occupational exposure to vinyl chloride monomer, *n*-hexane, carbon disulphide, and methyl *n*-butyl ketone can produce similar effects.

Management, treatment, and prevention

Vibration induced white finger is a prescribed industrial disease in many countries including the UK and may entitle affected workers to financial benefits.

The source of vibration must be reduced or eliminated. Engineering controls may minimize the transmission of vibration from machinery to the body or hands. Specially designed gloves can keep the hands warm and reduce vibration transmission.

Advice to the patient includes avoidance or reduction of further exposure to vibration, use of appropriate gloves, keeping the body and hands warm, especially in cold weather or when working with cold or pneumatic tools, and cessation of cigarette smoking. Vasodilatory drugs have been used in severe cases; tolazoline, inositol, cyclandelate, calcium channel blockers, angiotensin-converting enzyme inhibitors, prostaglandins, and stanazolol have also been tried. Surgical treatment such as sympathectomy is not recommended.

Further reading

Gemne, G. (ed.). (1987). Symptomatology and diagnostic methods in the hand-arm vibration syndrome. *Scandinavian Journal of Work and Environmental Health*, **13**, 271–388.

Tyler, L.E. (ed.). (1993). *FOM Working Party report on hand transmitted vibration.* Royal College of Physicians, London.

Section 19
Geratology

Contents

Chapter 19.1

Medicine in old age

F. I. Caird and J. Grimley Evans

Ageing and medicine

Because of loss of adaptability, illness in old age is often characterized by a cryptic and non-specific presentation. For example, reduced ability to metabolize bacterial toxins and slowness in mounting an inflammatory response may cause pneumonia in an old person to present as acute delirium before there are any physical signs in the chest. A myocardial infarction may be painless in later life and present as mental confusion or as an inexplicable fall. Reduced sensation in the peritoneum may delay the diagnosis of appendicitis or perforated peptic ulcer. The slowness of the aged body in mounting its defences can lead to rapid deterioration unless the diagnosis is made and treatment instituted urgently. Because of this, and of the frequent presence of multiple pathology, older patients require on average more investigations than do younger adults. There is also a much more frequent need for rehabilitation to help an elderly patient recover fully.

Age-associated physiological changes

Alterations in average body composition appear in the fifth decade of life, with a decline in lean body mass and a corresponding fall in oxygen consumption, largely attributable to a decline in muscle bulk. Until extreme old age average body weight remains constant or may increase, owing to an increase in body fat.

The blood volume falls with age, and there is a slight decline in haemoglobin concentration, more evident in women than in men. The white cell count falls slightly, principally the lymphocyte count; some normal ranges for biochemical investigations are also altered.

There is an increase in the amount of fibrous tissue in the myocardium and heart valves, and decrease in the elasticity of the aorta and its main branches. There is also a minor decline of resting heart rate, and in maximum heart rate on exercise. The mean systemic arterial pressure rises in most, but not all populations, and the rise of systolic pressure is greater than that of diastolic; an expression of the reduced elasticity of the aorta. The older heart takes longer to fill during diastole than does the young heart so that the older patient is therefore less tolerant of tachycardia than are the young.

Total lung volume does not alter, but vital capacity falls and residual volume increases, so that over the age of about 60 the critical closing volume exceeds the functional residual volume. Ventilatory capacity falls with age and ventilation-perfusion inequality increases slightly. These changes reflect a decrease in elasticity of the lungs and in respiratory muscular strength, but their overall fractional consequences are minimal.

The glomerular filtration rate falls by approximately 1 per cent per year over the age of 40, as do tubular reabsorptive and secretory capacities, so that serum urea and creatinine concentrations rise slightly. The response to an acid load is impaired, and antidiuretic hormone is reduced. This is accompanied by a delayed response to fluid deprivation, due at least in part to impaired thirst mechanisms, which result in elderly people being at increased risk of dehydration. Some elderly people show an enhanced thirst response to diuretics (perhaps particularly amiloride) with increased water intake and hyponatraemia.

Gastric atrophy becomes increasingly common as age advances, but hydrogen ion secretion is often unaltered. Calcium absorption is reduced because of diminished sensitivity to vitamin D. Reduction in the motility of the large bowel is common and may sometimes reflect diverticular disease or chronic purgative abuse.

There is an age-associated reduction in hepatic mass and blood flow, of approximately 30 per cent. Overall changes in function are minor but reduction in the hepatic metabolism of some drugs is well documented.

The most important manifestation of the decline in bone mass is a reduction in the strength of bone and an increase in the tendency to fracture. The great majority of limb bone fractures in old age are caused by simple falls, and there is an exponential increase in risk of falling after the age of 70 or so. The reasons for the virtually universal occurrence of osteoarthritic changes in many joints are uncertain. There are minor declines in circulating thyroid hormone levels, a reduction in the rate of secretion of insulin in response to raised blood sugar levels, and a decline in insulin sensitivity.

Age changes in the nervous system are important. The numbers of neurones in some parts of the nervous system (for example, the motor neurones of the spinal cord, the Purkinje cells of the cerebellum, the cells of the substantia nigra and the neocortex) fall with age. Anatomical abnormalities of the neurones that remain are also described. The alterations in cortical function may thus be due both to a reduction in number of neurones, and in connections between them. There is a reduction in peripheral nerve conduction velocities, both motor and sensory, and an increase in their variability.

Central autonomic nuclei and first- and second-order autonomic neurones, especially synpathetics, outside the central nervous system show a fall in cell numbers. Changes in autonomic function include alterations in control of heart rate, and abnormalities of temperature regulation. The threshold for appreciation of skin temperature changes may increase by as much as tenfold. There may also be failure of cutaneous vasoconstriction in response to cold, and of vasodilatation and sweating in response to increasing body temperature.

Failure of the blood pressure response to postural change is important. Baroreceptor responses are blunted, and there may be failure of central and perhaps peripheral vasoconstrictor responses to falling blood pressure.

Age changes in the eye include decrease in elasticity of the lens which begins very early in life, but only becomes symptomatic in the fifth decade. High tone deafness is partly an intrinsic age change, but prolonged exposure to industrial and other environmental noise also contributes.

Clinical assessment of the elderly patient

Short standard mental function tests should be part of the routine clinical examination of old people. For patients in hospital the test shown in Table 1 is widely used. Scores of 7 or less imply some form of mental dysfunction such as depression, delirium, dementia, or oligophrenia. The test only detects gross problems and a search for early or mild mental disability requires a more elaborate test such as the Mini-Mental State Examination (MMSE). For physical function

Table 1 Abbreviated mental test score (MTS)

Age (must be correct)
Time (correct to nearest hour without looking at watch or clock)
42 West Street (give this or similar address, ask for it to be repeated to ensure that it has been heard correctly. Ask for it at the end of the test)
Month (exact)
Year (exact, except in January or February when previous year is acceptable)
Name of place (if not in hospital ask for type of place or area of town)
Date of birth (exact)
Start of the Second World War (exact year)
Name of present monarch
Count backwards from 20 to 1 (prompt if necessary, 20, 19, 18 . . ., but no further prompts. Patients can hesitate and self-correct but no other errors allowed)
Score:
8–10 probably normal
7 probably abnormal
0–6 abnormal
Change in score of 3 or more is probably significant

Table 2 The Barthel index of activities of daily living

Bowels		*Transfer*	
Continent	2	Independent	3
Occasional accidents	1	Minor help needed	2
Incontinent	0	Major help (can sit)	1
		Unable	0
Bladder			
Continent	2	*Toilet use*	
Occasional accidents	1	Independent	2
Incontinent	0	Needs some help	1
		Dependent	0
Feeding			
Independent	2	*Walking*	
Needs some help	1	Independent	3
Dependent	0	Walks with one stick	2
		Wheelchair independent	1
Grooming, face/hair/teeth/ shaving		Unable	0
Independent	1	*Stairs*	
Needs help	0	Independent	2
		Needs some help	1
Dressing	2	Dependent	0
Independent			
Can do half	1	*Bathing*	
Dependent	0	Independent	1
		Dependent	0
Total score			

there are many scales available; the Barthel index or one of its modifications (Table 2) is widely used.

A detailed account of the patient's social circumstances is essential, and of the physical and emotional environment at home, often best obtained by a home visit.

Principles of drug therapy in old age

It has been claimed that at least 10 per cent of admissions of elderly patients to hospital in the UK are drug-induced, and likely therefore to be iatrogenic.

Understanding of alterations in pharmacokinetics with age is important. Drug absorption varies little, although a substantial increase in the absorption of levodopa is an important exception. The bioavailability of drugs, which are extensively degraded in the liver, may be greatly increased by a reduction in their first-pass metabolism. Many old people are prescribed several drugs and interactions can be a problem.

The volume of distribution of some drugs is reduced; that of digoxin may be correlated with reduced muscle Na/K ATPase. That of others (for example, diazepam) is increased. Changes in the volume of distribution make it difficult to interpret changes in plasma half-life as a measure of drug elimination; this is most satisfactorily expressed in terms of clearance. The apparent increase in sensitivity of the elderly brain to benzodiazepines, may be due to alterations in the blood–brain barrier, or in the kinetics of drugs in the cerebrospinal fluid, or to a pharmacodynamic effect.

The age-associated fall in glomerular filtration rate is accompanied by a parallel decrease in the elimination of drugs principally excreted by this route (for example, digoxin). Drugs principally eliminated by renal tubular secretion (for example the penicillins and aminoglycosides) share in this reduction in rate of elimination. The situation with regard to drugs eliminated by the liver varies.

There are few examples of age-associated differences in pharmacodynamics but the effect of warfarin is increased in elderly subjects. Some of the cardiac effects of sympathomimetic amines and β-blockers are reduced. In practice this may be cancelled out by the increased bioavailability of some β-blockers.

The chronic administration of thiazide and related diuretics produces little change in whole-body potassium in the middle-aged, but in elderly patients is a prime cause of potassium depletion. The difference lies in the substantially lower average dietary potassium intake of old people.

The compliance of elderly patients with prescribed drug therapy is no more perfect than that of younger ones. Complex drug regimens are inappropriate. Simplicity of prescribing (the use, for instance, of once-daily dosage schedules if possible), clear instruction, reinforced by written indications of what is required, and appropriate packaging and labelling, can do much to improve compliance.

Some common clinical problems

Urinary incontinence

Many patients with dementia become incontinent, but incontinence should never be attributed solely to dementia unless the latter is severe. Incontinence due to inability to reach a toilet in time is unnecessarily prevalent. Overflow incontinence is common in men with prostate difficulties. Urge incontinence is usually mainly due to instability of the detrusor muscle of the bladder, but may also arise through irritation by infected urine. The contractions of an unstable bladder may be inhibited by anticholinergic drugs, but these must be used with care as they may induce glaucoma and constipation, while lipid-soluble anticholinergic drugs may cross the blood–brain barrier and cause delirium.

The certain diagnosis of unstable bladder and associated urethral dysfunctions requires invasive investigation, including cystometry but most cases of urinary incontinence can be dealt with empirically. In many instances urinary incontinence may be a problem only at night, A drug with anticholinergic effects, such as imipramine, may be of value. Another approach is a small dose of a rapidly acting diuretic in the afternoon followed by restriction of fluids until bedtime.

Faecal incontinence

Faecal and double incontinence are associated with a range of anorectal and neurological disorders, including dementia. In later life the commonest cause is faecal impaction readily diagnosed by rectal examination. 'High' impaction can occur at the rectosigmoid junction and above, and may need to be diagnosed by a plain abdominal radiograph. High impaction must always raise the possibility of obstruction by a carcinoma or inflammatory stricture due to diverticulitis. Treatment requires enemas and suppositories, rarely manual evacuation, and then a regular regime of stool-softening medication such as lactulose.

Where faecal incontinence is an intractable problem it can be ameliorated by giving constipating medication such as codeine phosphate or loperamide with bowel lavage once a week.

Falls

One-fifth of people aged 65–69 fall once or more during a year; this proportion doubles by the age of 80. Table 3 lists some of the specific medical causes of falls. If the patients find themselves on the floor and cannot remember falling, this suggests epilepsy or syncope. Full investigation of syncope will include tilt table testing and carotid sinus massage. Postural hypotension (see below) is most commonly due to drugs.

Periods of rest after meals may be effective in treating postprandial hypotension. The unstable knee due to inadequate quadriceps strength is a diagnosis well worth making as it can often be effectively treated by exercises.

Table 3 Some medical causes of falls

Cardiovascular
Hypotension (postural, exertional, postprandial, drug-induced, induced by bed rest)
Cardiac arrhythmia
Syncope (micturition, cough, defaecation, carotid sinus sensitivity)
Neuromuscular
Epilepsy
Transient ischaemic attacks
Menière's disease
Parkinsonism and multisystem disorders
Myopathy
Neuropathy or myelopathy
Unstable knee due to quadriceps weakness
Visual field defect or inattention
Dementia
Intermittent delirium (drugs, alcohol, hypoglycaemia)

Table 4 Some causes of delirium and dementia in old age

Structural damage to the brain e.g. cerebral infarction, Alzheimer's disease, subdural haematoma,
cerebral tumour (primary or secondary)
Disorders of the cerebral circulation e.g. carotid insufficiency, systemic hypotension, congestive cardiac failure
Metabolic brain disorders e.g. hypoxia, uraemia, dehydration, electrolyte disorder, thyroid disease, hypoglycaemia, vitamin deficiency (of vitamin B_1, B_{12}, or folate)
Epilepsy
Drug toxicity e.g. poisoning with barbiturates, phenothiazines, alcohol, digitalis, etc.

Some psychiatric disorders in old age

The recognition of *delirium* should lead to a vigorous search for causes (Table 4). As far as possible, sedative drugs should be avoided and anxiety and disordered behaviour managed by psychological means. Delirious patients have problems with attention, memory, and perception; they are usually also feeling ill and frightened. Patients need to be reassured repeatedly and calmly about where they are and what is happening. The environment should be quiet. It is easier to see what is going on if lighting is adequate for aged eyes. All forms of physical restraint are terrifying; they should not be used.

Assessment of *dementia* requires detailed enquiry from relatives about such manifestations as restlessness, wandering, and aggressive behaviour. The patient's appearance and behaviour during examination provides valuable information; physical examination may show neurological abnormalities. Simple psychometric tests (Table 1) should be a routine part of geriatric clinical examination.

The management of dementia rests on alteration and simplification of the environment so that the sufferer can cope with it. Drug therapy has little place, but disturbed behaviour by day may need to be treated with small doses of thioridazine, with haloperidol as a valuable alternative in more severe cases.

Some patients with dementia may have been living in such a restricted environment and with so much support or that their cognitive impairment has passed unnoticed. When removed suddenly to an unfamiliar environment, they become acutely disorientated and anxious. Unless they are returned rapidly to their familiar environment, this decompensation of dementia may become irreversible.

Depression in old age resembles that at younger ages, except that somatic symptoms are commoner, and differential diagnosis thus wider.There may be uncharacteristic irritability, while poor concentration, and preoccupation with personal worries may lead to lapses in memory, and perhaps to unexpected failure in rehabilitation. Attempts to distinguish endogenous and exogenous forms of depression are unhelpful. Treatment with antidepressants is most useful, and should be persisted in, but relapse and recurrence, sometimes after years of good health, are not uncommon

Some old people whose psychiatric state cannot be called normal defy precise categorization. They have shown persistently odd behaviour throughout their lives, have antagonized and driven away all their relatives and friends, and are in consequence solitary, isolated, and difficult. They may live in self-inflicted squalor which brings them to the attention of neighbours and local authority agencies. They may not be intellectually impaired, and are not paranoid, depressed, nor anxious. The term eccentric is as good as any. Recognition is not difficult, but treatment is, since correction of the squalor and disarray in which they live is only of brief benefit.

When to refer a patient to a psychogeriatrician is a further problem. One indication is undoubtedly difficulty in diagnosis, in particular perhaps in distinguishing between dementia and the pseudodementia of depression, or deciding, when both are present, which is the more important. Interpretation of paranoid states may also constitute an indication for referral. The severely depressed patient should not be denied the benefits of electroconvulsive therapy when the indications exist (for example life-threatening reduction in food or fluid intake). The demented patient whose behaviour is disruptive or aggressive, or manifest by persistent wandering, is best managed in a psychogeriatric ward by appropriately trained nurses.

Cardiovascular disease

The symptoms of heart disease in old age are not infrequently modified. Cardiac pain is often slight; angina may be manifest as a need to stop walking, and the pain of cardiac infarction may be absent. As a symptom of heart failure, breathlessness may be replaced by fatigue, which may reflect reduced cardiac output and changes in muscle metabolism.

Interpretation of cardiovascular signs must also be modified for elderly patients. Reduction in hand blood flow may suppress the signs of increased cardiac output in anaemia or cor pulmonale. Decreased elasticity of the central arterial tree increases pulse pressure, and may mask the peripheral signs of aortic stenosis. Compression of the left innominate vein between an enlarged aorta and the back of the sternum may result in asymmetrical elevation of the venous pressure, that in the left jugular and subclavian veins being higher than that on the right. The true central venous pressure should thus be determined from the right jugular venous system. The cardiac apex may be difficult to feel, and its site may be displaced by thoracic kyphoscoliosis. Basal lung crepitations not cleared by coughing are present in a high proportion of old people without identifiable cause and should not on their own be considered diagnostic of heart failure. A third heart sound is much more suggestive of heart failure than is a fourth sound in later life.

Cardiac failure

Treatable contributory factors, including drugs (sodium-retaining or negatively inotropic), thyrotoxicosis, and ethanol abuse, should be sought for and dealt with. Diuretic therapy is usually the first line of treatment but often causes problems for older patients. Increased urine volumes may precipitate retention in elderly men and may cause incontinence in either sex. Potassium depletion is a common feature and potassium-sparing agents or potassium supplements should be given.

Angiotensin-converting enzyme (ACE) inhibitors are of considerable value in both reducing symptoms and prolonging survival. Treatment needs to be initiated with care because of the possibility of acute hypotension, particularly if the patient is volume-depleted by diuretic therapy. Potassium-sparing diuretics should be discontinued when ACE inhibitors are prescribed on account of a risk of hyperkalaemia.

Where ACE inhibitors are contraindicated vasodilators such as nitrates or hydralazine may help. β–Blockers have also been shown to be beneficial in reducing mortality in cardiac failure but are often contraindicated for older people because of their negative inotropic effects and the danger of inducing bronchospasm in patients with asthma. Digitalization may be required to control the heart rate in patients with fast atrial fibrillation and may have a helpful inotropic effect in other situations.

Paroxysmal cardiac dysrhythmias

Frequent ventricular ectopic beats or left bundle branch block are common findings in routine ECGs of elderly people and are difficult to interpret. If a dysrhythmia has not been demonstrated at the time of a syncopal episode, 24-hour electrocardiogram monitoring is commonly performed, but the relevance of the commonly found brief episodes of dysrhythmia to a patient's symptoms may be difficult to establish. The combination of syncope and complete heart block, bifascicular block, or the sick sinus syndrome, is an indication for cardiac pacing. Elderly patients tolerate cardiac pacing extremely well.

Myocardial infarction

Old age is not a contraindication to thrombolysis and heparin as used in younger patients. Indeed, the evidence suggests that thrombolytic therapy may save more lives when given to older patients than to younger ones. Aspirin and β-blockers where not contraindicated should normally be used in older patients as in younger.

Atrial fibrillation

In the absence of contraindications, patients aged 60 and over with atrial fibrillation should have long-term anticoagulation therapy in order to reduce their three- to fivefold increased risk of stroke. Patients with associated valvular disease or dilated left atrium are at even higher risk of stroke. The risks of oral anticoagulant therapy are greater for older people than younger, but there is evidence that this increased risk of haemorrhagic complications can be overcome by care in prescribing and increased surveillance of therapy. Anticoagulant therapy should only be instituted where good compliance can be expected and adequate surveillance ensured. In atrial fibrillation, an INR of 2–2.5 is an appropriate target. If anticoagulants are contraindicated, aspirin should be considered. Patients aged over 60 with paroxysmal atrial fibillation should be anticoagulated because they are likely to move into established fibrillation.

Deep venous thrombosis

A clot extending above the popliteal vein should be treated in elderly patients along conventional lines with short-term heparin followed by a period of oral anticoagulation. Continuous anticoagulation will need to be considered in a patient with recurrent thrombosis. Anticoagulant therapy is not normally used for elderly patients with venous thrombosis restricted to veins below the knee.

Stroke

Management in elderly patients does not differ significantly from that in younger patients (see Chapter 13.15).

High blood pressure

It is no longer appropriate to consider the rise of blood pressure with age as 'normal ageing' as it clearly carries with it an increased risk of cardiovascular disease, particularly coronary disease and stroke.

Large trials have now established that treatment of high blood pressure in patients at least up to the age of 80 can reduce the risk of stroke. Moreover, the benefits have been shown for the treatment of systolic pressure, regardless of whether diastolic pressure is also raised or not. It is best to regard as in need of treatment a sustained systolic pressure of over 160 mmHg, whether or not the diastolic pressure is over 90 mmHg in a patient under the age of 80. The object of treatment should be to reduce blood pressure to approximately 160/90 mmHg over 2–3 months.

In the absence of contraindications, the first line of treatment in the elderly should be a potassium-sparing thiazide diuretic combination. If this is not effective a second-line drug should be added or substituted. β-Blockers tend not to be very effective in older people and have a fairly high risk of side-effects. Calcium-channel blockers are effective. For diabetic patients and for those with evidence of heart failure, ACE inhibitors may be the best treatment, but the risks of first dose hypotension, functional renal failure due to occult renal artery stenosis, or of a significant increase in plasma potassium levels must be considered.

Orthostatic hypotension

This is a common phenomenon in elderly people. A drop of 20 mmHg or more in systolic pressure on standing is found in 15 per cent of those aged between 65 and 74, and in 25 per cent over that age. The great majority of cases are due to injudicious drug therapy, particularly with thiazides, other antihypertensive drugs, tricyclic antidepressants, phenothiazines, benzodiazepines, levodopa, or combinations of drugs. Orthostatic hypotension may develop if bed rest is prolonged. In the small proportion of cases not due to drugs, primary changes in the autonomic nervous system may be responsible; the complete Shy–Drager syndrome is a rarity. Management begins with reduction or discontinuance of the causal drug therapy. Reduction in levodopa dosage will usually lead to a satisfactory compromise between improvement in parkinsonism and incapacitating orthostatic hypotension. When drug therapy is not implicated, raising the head of the bed at night may be of value, but usually treatment with fludrocortisone, 0.1–0.3 mg/day, should be combined with tight, full-length elastic stockings, and advice on the gradual achievement of the standing position from lying.

Bone disease

Osteoporosis and Paget's disease are common in elderly people but are considered in detail elsewhere (see Section 9). Osteomalacia is now rarely found in the elderly population, in the absence of other specific causative factors such as malabsorption. It may occur in the housebound particularly in the north of the UK. It has also been suggested that minor degrees of vitamin D deficiency may produce osteoporosis. Studies among middle-aged women in the US have shown that in the winter vitamin D levels fall low enough to activate parathyroid hormone, leading to loss of bone that may not be fully made up in the following summer. It may emerge that winter supplements of vitamin D will have a place in the prevention of osteoporosis in older people, but on present knowledge this has to be regarded as speculative.

The manifestations of vitamin D deficiency cover a wide spectrum, from asymptomatic biochemical changes to backache and diffuse bone pain; proximal muscle weakness may lead to immobility and falls; mental changes, especially depression, are common; the combination of muscle weakness and osteomalacic changes in bone may cause fractures, particularly of the proximal femur. The diagnosis should always be considered in elderly patients with these features.

Metabolic and endocrine disorders

Diabetes mellitus

The mean decline in glucose tolerance with age is such that if the standard diagnostic criteria used in middle age are applied to those over the age of 70, over 50 per cent of elderly people would be 'diabetic'. Severe glucose intolerance accompanied by symptoms leaves no doubt that the patient should be treated, but asymptomatic mild impairment of glucose tolerance can scarcely be regarded in the same way. Distinction between criteria for the diagnosis of the diabetes as against impaired glucose tolerance is needed in this context (see Chapter 6.13).

The presentation of diabetes in old age is different from that at younger ages. Many are diagnosed as a result of routine testing, some because of the development of disorders associated with diabetes, and relatively fewer because of classical symptoms. Approximately one case in six of diabetic ketosis occurs in patients over the age of 60. The degree of metabolic decompensation is often greater in the elderly and non-ketotic hyperosmolar coma is virtually confined to elderly patients.

The indications for dietary treatment alone, oral hypoglycaemic agents or insulin in elderly patients are similar to those described in Chapter 6.13 but short acting oral agents (tolbutamide, gliclazide, and glibornuride) are preferred because of the risk of prolonged hypoglycaemia from the longer acting agents. Single rather than multiple injections of insulin are also preferred.

The evidence for the relationship between control of diabetes and the development of complications in old age is not entirely satisfactory. Complications occur more frequently in elderly diabetics. The prognosis of diabetic retinopathy in old age is less favourable than in middle age, but photocoagulation remains effective. Cataract extraction is three or four times more common in elderly diabetics than in non-diabetics. The results of operation are excellent, except when preoperative visual impairment is partly due to pre-existing retinopathy. The neurological complication of diabetes particularly associated with old age is amyotrophy (see Chapter 6.13). Its clinical recognition is important, because of its generally good prognosis, and the need to avoid unnecessary investigation.

Hypothyroidism

Classical clinical presentations probably only occur in a quarter of elderly patients. Cold intolerance, hair loss, and coarsening of the skin, are less common than an insidious decline in general health and mobility, and psychiatric manifestations, in particular depression. Hypothyroid coma, sometimes associated with severe headache and fits, and hypothermia (sometimes precipitated by phenothiazines) are less common but important presentations. The most useful physical signs are change in voice and delayed relaxation of tendon reflexes.

Cautious initial replacement therapy is advisable, beginning with thyroxine 25 μg/day, particularly if overt heart disease coexists. Later doses of 100–150 μg/day are usually adequate. Relapse due to discontinuance of treatment is regrettably frequent. Simplification of treatment by weekly administration of 70 per cent of the total weekly dose of thyroxine or twice-weekly administration of half the dose has its advocates.

Hyperthyroidism

Hyperthyroidism in old age is even more likely to present in an atypical manner. Weight loss, anorexia, gastrointestinal, and cardiovascular symptoms predominate. Cardiac failure, usually with atrial fibrillation resistant to digitalis, is the most important cardiac presentation, and proximal myopathy is not infrequent. The eye signs and goitre are less common in elderly patients, and apathy or depression may be prominent. Treatment is best begun with carbimazole followed by radio-iodine.

Disorders of temperature regulation

Hypothermia

Most elderly patients with hypothermia present after a period of 2 or 3 days of relatively cold weather, but it is entirely possible for hypothermia to develop in midsummer at UK latitudes, especially if disease or drugs play an important part. The fall in temperature occurs over 24–48 hours, and its principal manifestations are progressive ataxia and slowing of cerebration, leading to stupor and finally coma. On examination, the skin feels cold to touch. There may be oedema of the face and eyelids resembling that of myxoedema. The pulse is slow, unless severe physical illness has raised it towards normal, and the blood pressure is difficult to record or low. Cerebration is slow but may be remarkably accurate even in the presence of considerable reduction in body temperature. Tendon reflexes are normal unless there is associated hypothyroidism. The diagnosis is made by recording the rectal temperature; this should be done without delay on all occasions when the oral temperature is recorded at 35°C or less. The principal investigation that may show characteristic but by no means universal features is the electrocardiogram, with bradycardia and J-waves (Fig. 1). In severe hypothermia there is often atrial fibrillation with a slow ventricular response.

Hypothermia in elderly patients has a high fatality, related to its cause in the individual case (those due to drugs usually recover; those due to severe physical illness usually die), its severity, and its complications (particularly pneumonia and pancreatitis). There is no basis for the use of steroids, while intravenous fluids are

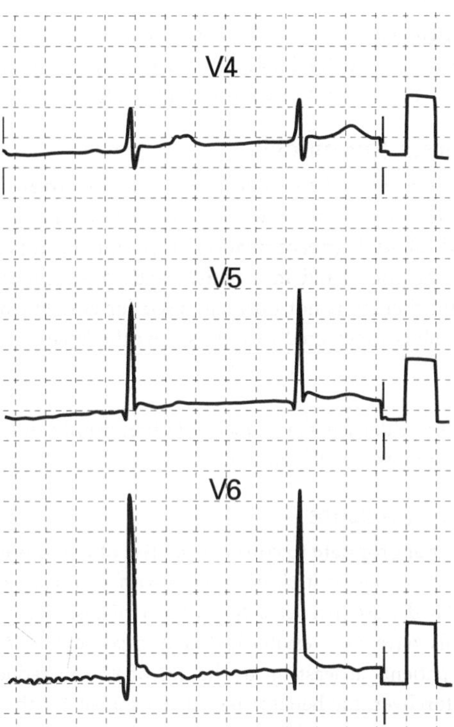

Fig. 1 ECG from a hypothermic patient illustrating the Osborne (J wave) seen in V5 and 6. The characteristic is a deflection lying between the QRS complex and the beginning of the ST segment. The pathophysiology of the J wave is uncertain.

dangerous because they may produce pulmonary oedema; intravenous glucose is not metabolized, since insulin is ineffective in the hypothermic state. A slow rise in body temperature (optimally 0.5°C per hour) should be produced by exposing the patient to a relatively high ambient temperature of 30°C. If hypothyroidism is suspected, liothyronine should be given, but only when the central temperature has risen to normal.

The elderly patient who has recovered from hypothermia should be regarded as at risk from a further episode. The long-term prognosis is better in patients who have survived an episode of known cause.

Hyperthermia

An increase in mortality in continuing care wards and of elderly people at home has been recognized during heat waves. The paramount need is to collect elderly people at risk into environments that can be kept cool. There is little useful guidance about the management of grossly raised body temperatures in elderly patients, except to maintain fluid intake.

Further reading

George, C., Woodhouse, K., MacLennan, W., and Denham, M. (1998). *Drug therapy in old age.* Wiley, Chichester.

Grimley Evans, J., Williams, T.F., Beattie, B.L., Michel, J.-P., and Wilcock, G.K. (2000). *Oxford textbook of geriatric medicine,* (2nd edn). Oxford University Press, Oxford.

O'Mahoney, D. and Martin, U. (1999). *Practical therapeutics for the older patient.* Wiley, Chichester.

Chapter 19.2

Abuse of elderly people

R. Jacoby

Definition

Abuse of elderly people has long been recognized—there are several examples in Dickens' novels—but only in the last 20 years has it been acknowledged as a widespread and serious sociomedical problem. One definition is:

a repeated act against or failure to act for an elderly person which causes distress or damage and so prevents them living a full life.

Five types of abuse are commonly recognized:

1. Psychological—threats, shouting and bullying;
2. Physical—assault of various kinds and varying degrees of severity;
3. Material—theft and undue influence to give money or possessions to the abuser;
4. Sexual;
5. Neglect—when those responsible fail to meet their obligations to provide for dependent old persons who cannot care for themselves.

Prevalence

It is difficult to determine prevalence accurately, because many victims remain silent. Of these, several are incapable of complaining because of dementia. However, epidemiological studies from a variety of countries suggest that the prevalence is approximately 4 per cent of the population over 64. Therefore, a rough calculation for London—assuming a resident population of eight million of which 15 per cent are 65 and over—would yield a figure of some 48 000 elderly victims of abuse.

Clinical features

Psychological, physical, and sexual abuse, and neglect

The typical victim of such abuse has been described as

- female
- aged over 75
- physically disabled
- with cognitive impairment and
- socially isolated

However, this profile, although common, is not invariable, and can be usefully simplified to *the older person who is dependent on others for daily care.*

It is easy to understand that the most likely abusers of such victims are their carers, many of whom have a history of mental disorder or substance abuse themselves. Some are spouses or offspring who are driven beyond their threshold of endurance, because of the physical demands of the victim, such as cleaning up double incontinence, or because of psychological stress. Examples of the latter are where the victim suffers from dementia and might ask the same question dozens of times, or scream repeatedly throughout the 24 hours. Another common situation is where victims are so demented that they perceive intimate care—such as bathing or changing soiled underwear—as an assault, and fight off their carers. In such circumstances, if the carer is himself old and relatively frail, he, too, may be injured. Thus, one person can be both victim and abuser.

Psychological, physical, and even sexual abuse of old people also occurs in institutions such as nursing and residential homes, mainly from staff but occasionally from others, for example male residents sexually harassing or abusing female ones.

Indicators of abuse

Some types of physical injury are characteristic and should immediately arouse suspicion in medical personnel:

- hand slap marks;
- marks appearing to have been made by an implement;
- pinching or grab marks;
- black eyes;
- bruising to the buttocks, lower abdomen, thighs, genital or rectal areas;
- burns (e.g. from cigarettes) or scalds in normally inaccessible areas (mouth, inner surfaces of arms and legs, genitals;
- bites;
- old fractures which have not been medically treated.

Some events or sequences of events should also raise suspicion of abuse:

- several unexplained injuries or falls;
- a prolonged interval between injury and presentation for medical attention;
- deterioration in the level of care—poor personal hygiene, lost dentures, spectacles, and hearing aids;
- malnutrition in someone not living alone.

The behaviour of the victim or the abuser may also be an indicator of abuse:

- the victim is silent and apparently fearful in the presence of the abuser;
- the victim is reluctant to specify how the injuries were sustained;
- the abuser displays an intolerant or dismissive attitude towards the victim;
- the abuser gives implausible reasons for how the injuries came about.

Material abuse

Although only a minority of elderly people have substantial financial assets, the number is increasing. So, too, are the cases of material abuse. This may entail straightforward theft of cash or possessions. Sometimes, workmen carry out house repairs or alterations at grossly inflated prices. The elderly are at particular risk from confidence tricksters who call unannounced at their homes. Much material abuse, however, is committed by carers, often relatives. For example, those with enduring power of attorney donated by someone who has become demented may misuse their authority and spend the donor's money to their own advantage. Pressure may be put on mentally incapacitated old people to change their wills. Sadly, the opportunities to defraud vulnerable old people of their assets have increased with their increasing affluence.

Management

Abuse of older people is such a complex and variable phenomenon that it is not possible to lay down clear-cut procedures to be followed in all cases. Only a few simple points can be made here.

Where abuse is suspected within the victim's own home, the local social services department (SSD), which has statutory responsibilities, and guidelines for action, should be informed. The SSD will investigate the matter and involve the police if necessary. Where abuse is suspected in an independent registered nursing or residential home, it must be reported immediately to the appropriate inspection and registration unit.

Where the victim is thought to be mentally infirm, an urgent psychiatric opinion should be sought. It might then be advisable for the patient to be admitted to a psychiatric facility, informally or under the Mental Health Act, for a period of assessment.

Victims of elder abuse are entitled to the protection of the criminal law in exactly the same way as other citizens. However, the criminal law may be inappropriate in many instances of domestic abuse, say a husband who has cracked under the strain of caring for a wife with advanced dementia. Here, it is clearly better to provide medical and social support that will allow the relationship to resume its normal and more peaceful course.

Case example

A woman in her eighties lived with her 60-year-old son. He was of low intelligence and had a history of minor sexual offences and alcohol abuse. He repeatedly brought his mother to the accident and emergency department of the local hospital in a state of gross neglect and with poorly explained injuries. For example, one of her toenails had been avulsed. He said it had 'come off' when he was trimming her nails. On another occasion she was found to have confluent bruises on the inner aspect of both thighs. At first she said it was where her son had pinched her, but she refused to repeat the allegation. Her son frequently discharged her from the accident and emergency department before further inquiries were made. Eventually, his mother was admitted to a psychiatric ward under the Mental Health Act where she was found to be suffering from dementia. She was not permitted to return home because of her son's repeated physical and sexual abuse, but discharged to a nursing home under a Guardianship order of the Mental Health Act.

Further reading

Fisk, J. (1997). Abuse of the elderly. In: *Psychiatry in the elderly* (ed. R. Jacoby and C. Oppenheimer) (2nd edn), pp. 736–48. Oxford University Press, Oxford.

Tonks, A. and Bennett, G. (1999). Elder abuse (editorial). *British Medical Journal*, 318, 278.

Section 20
Forensic medicine

Contents

Section 20

Forensic medicine (medical jurisprudence: legal medicine)

B. Knight

Here the account is confined to some of the ways in which law impacts on the practice of medicine, bearing in mind that legal systems vary greatly from country to country and even within the same country, as in the UK.

The doctor's duties after a death

Although the procedure to be described is that of England and Wales, most jurisdictions have a broadly similar requirement. First, the doctor must ensure that the fact of death is confirmed. This is a clinical exercise rather than a legal one and consists of the confirmation that cardiorespiratory functions have ceased irreversibly.

In most causes, the marker of the moment of death is cardiac arrest and this must be confirmed by the doctor by auscultation of the heart, as depending upon the radial or even carotid pulse in a moribund patient is often unreliable. Even listening over the apex for heart sounds may be difficult near the point of death and prolonged use of the stethoscope may be required before a decision is made that the heart has finally stopped. Listening for the cessation of respiratory function is less reliable, but attempting to hear air entry over the trachea with a stethoscope may be used. The older traditional tests, such as feathers or mirrors before the mouth or strings tied around the finger, should be relegated to medical history! Rarely, electrocardiograph tracings might be needed. Probably the nearest simulation of death was given by barbituate intoxication, but fortunately this is rarely seen these days, due to the limitation of prescription of these dangerous drugs.

When the fact of death has been confirmed, the time and date should be recorded. The doctor then has to decide whether or not he or she is in a position to issue a death certificate or report the case for medicolegal investigation. In England and Wales, between one-quarter and one-third of deaths are reported to coroners, usually with a withholding of a death certificate, although in strict law, the doctor who has attended the patient in their last illness is statutorily obliged to give a death certificate. However, if the cause of death is thought to be unnatural or is unknown, then it is futile for the doctor to provide such a certificate, this function being taken over by the coroner.

If the doctor was in attendance upon the patient during the 14 days preceding death, is confident of the cause of death and that the cause was natural, then he or she must provide a death certificate on the forms issued by the Registrar General. This must be transmitted to the Registrar of Births and Deaths within 5 days of issue, usually taken personally by the near relatives of the deceased. The book of certificates has a counterfoil for the doctor's own records and a further tear-off strip called 'Notice to Informant', which must be handed to the next-of-kin.

The certificate must avoid undesirable terms that have no aetiological usefulness, such as 'heart failure, syncope, coma'. Useful instructions are given inside the covers of the books of certificates.

Where an autopsy is to be carried out, it is preferable to await the result of the pathologist's findings before completing the death certificate. Many surveys have shown a discrepancy rate of 20–50 per cent between the presumed cause and the cause discovered at autopsy.

Reporting to the coroner

There is no particular duty upon a doctor to report death to the coroner, other than that placed upon every citizen. However, it is conventional that doctors voluntarily report deaths to the coroner wherever the circumstances so indicate. It is better for the doctor, where there is doubt as to whether a death should be reported, to seek the advice of the coroner, the coroner's officer, or a senior pathologist.

The following deaths should be reported:

1. *Where the deceased was not attended in their last illness by a doctor.* Here, if another doctor is called to certify the fact of death or in the mistaken impression that medical treatment or resuscitation can be given, this doctor is in no position to issue a certificate and must report the death to the coroner.
2. *Where the deceased was not seen by a doctor either after death or within the 14 days prior to death.* The alternative of not seeing the body after death should never occur, as only a tiny minority of deceased persons are now not viewed after death by a doctor. In every other country it is mandatory that the body be seen after death, and this may soon be enforced by legislation in the UK. The 14-day rule causes a considerable number of deaths to be reported to the coroner.
3. *Where the cause of death is unknown.*
4. *Where death appears to be due to industrial disease or poisoning.*
5. *Where death may have been unnatural or caused by violence, neglect, or abortion, or attended by suspicious circumstances.*
6. *Where death has occurred during operation or before recovery from an anaesthetic.*

It is a convention with many coroners, although not a legal requirement, that deaths occurring within 24 hours of emergency admission to hospital be reported. Similarly, many coroners will require deaths that occur within 24 hours of surgical operation or other significant medical intervention, and certainly an anaesthetic, to be reported.

Any death that is thought potentially to be related to a medical procedure, either diagnostic or therapeutic, should be reported to the coroner. Whether to do this is the doctor's decision, but it is always preferable to err on the safe side when in doubt.

Once a death is reported to the coroner, no further action should be taken by the doctor. Although a death certificate may be provided if the relatives insist, Box A on the back of the certificate should be signed to indicate that the case has been reported to the coroner and thus the Registrar of Births and Deaths cannot register the death until they hear from the coroner about the final outcome. Similarly, an autopsy cannot be requested and cremation forms cannot be issued in a coroner's case. The donation of organs for transplantation cannot be implemented if the death is reported to the coroner, without the consent of the latter.

Transplantation and Human Tissue Act

In the UK, the donation of cadaver tissue and organs for transplantation together with clinical autopsies is regulated by the Human

Tissue Act (1961). Virtually all cadaver donation must come from patients on artificial ventilation who have been declared brainstem dead (see Chapter 13.14 and OTM3, p. 3317). The consent of the coroner or Procurator Fiscal in Scotland must be obtained before organs are taken from a case that is reportable to the coroner.

The Human Tissue Act (1961) provides that the person lawfully in possession of the body after death (usually the Health Authority or one of their servants, including consultants) may authorize the removal of tissues if the person during their lifetime expressed the wish for this to occur. The display of a signed donor card fulfils this purpose. If no such permission is available, then removal may be authorized if the person lawfully in charge of the body, having made such reasonable enquiry as may be practicable, has no reason to believe that the deceased had ever expressed any objection to donation and that the surviving spouse or any surviving relative has made no such objection. There is usually no specific document for this purpose, but the clinicians must be satisfied that no such objections exist and should record this in the hospital notes.

The use of living donor material is strictly controlled both by the Human Tissue Act and by the Human Organ Transplant Act (1989). The latter Act is to prevent commercial exploitation of live donors and, in summary:

1. Prohibits any payment for donating organs, including any negotiation or advertising for this purpose.
2. Prohibits the removal or transplantation of any organ or tissue from a living person, unless they are genetically related, within certain fixed limits, unless specific consent is obtained. The Act lays down certain serological tests to establish the degree of relationship.
3. Requires that a regulatory authority must give permission to doctors who wish to transplant from live donors who are not within the prescribed limits of genetic relationship. A new registration system has been established.

Medical negligence

Before a patient can succeed in a civil action against a doctor, three criteria must be satisfied:

1. That the doctor had a duty of care to the patient.
2. That there was a breach of this duty either by an act of commission or omission.
3. That the patient suffered physical, financial, or mental damage.

A duty of care depends merely upon the intention of the doctor to act in a healing capacity. Once a doctor assumes a caring role in relation to a patient, the duty of care is established.

The most difficult part of establishing or denying negligent action is in differentiating a true accident or a genuine error of clinical judgement from a failure to discharge a proper duty of care, which is negligent. The only way in which the matter can be resolved is by peer review, in which other knowledgeable doctors of the same seniority and in the same speciality, give their opinion as to whether the actions or omissions of the accused doctor were in line with current medical practice. Such peer opinions need not be unanimous. As long as a substantial body of practice approves the actions of the doctor, that is sufficient to validate the behaviour under dispute.

Finally, the patient must suffer damage, as the whole object of legal actions for negligence is to restore the patient as far as possible to the situation he or she was in before the effects of negligence. Thus, if there are no deleterious effects, no compensation can be claimed.

Risk management in medicine

No admission of negligence should be made to the patient or their relatives at or soon after the event, this being a matter for the medical defence and protection societies and their lawyers. This is certainly not to say that the doctor should not express regret and sympathy for the event, which is quite different from acknowledging blame. One of the major factors in avoiding legal actions for negligence is the maintenance of the doctor–patient relationship. A significant number of negligence actions commence after a breakdown of this relationship and very many patients or their relatives will be forgiving and not initiate complaints where a sympathetic doctor expresses regret (although not admitting culpability).

As protective measures, the most urgent requirement is for every doctor to have the constant support of an expert organization, which will provide specialized medical and legal advice and indemnity against legal costs and damages. Even though, since 1990, doctors in the National Health Service hospitals have financial indemnity provided by the state, this does not extend to general practice or private practice and does not cover any doctor outside their contractual employment with the Health Service. It does not cover issues of professional misconduct, coroners' inquests, disputes with employers, and a whole range of matters other than the strictly limited indemnity within the hospital.

It is vital to keep good clinical records. Many accusations of negligence are sustained not because they were true, but because the doctor's notes failed to contain any indication that some alleged omission was in fact performed. This is particularly true of emergency admissions and general practice visits, where the urgency of a situation overtakes the making of contemporaneous notes. Notes should never be altered. Illegibility, the use of unintelligible abbreviation, and the inclusion of pejorative or even defamatory remarks all contribute to the difficulties of defending a doctor against allegations of malpractice.

Examination of sexual offences

Although in the UK the examination of the victims of alleged sexual offences is largely the province of the police surgeon or 'forensic physician', on some occasions another doctor may be requested to carry out this duty. In other countries the procedure varies. This potentially important subject is fully addressed in OTM3, pp. 4313–14.

Medical confidentiality and consent

There is a firm commitment for all doctors to maintain strict confidentiality concerning the patient's clinical condition. Confidentiality is an essential element of medical practice; without awareness of a doctor's dedication to silence, many patients would be reluctant to provide a full history, to the detriment of their diagnosis and treatment. Confidentiality does not cease with death.

Confidentiality may only be broken in one of the following circumstances:

1. With the consent of the patient or his/her legal representative. Indeed, not only may the doctor release information at the patient's request, but he *must* divulge it.
2. There is no automatic right of relatives to be told medical facts about a patient except in the case of children, although the age at

which this becomes legitimate is rather hazy in English law and depends more upon the maturity of the child than a chronological age. There is very rarely any need to withhold information from spouses, but in the context of sexual matters, venereal disease, pregnancy, or abortion, the patient may not wish the doctor to tell even the closest relative. In such cases the doctor must use judgement and persuasion if necessary. He/she may be required to justify a decision not to accede to the patient's insistence on confidentiality.

3. Many medical conditions have to be notified to some official authority under the law of the land. Examples are various infectious diseases, occupational conditions, drug dependence, and termination of pregnancy.
4. All courts of law have a right to demand that the doctor reveals any medical information whatsoever if the doctor is called as a witness under oath. On rare occasions, the doctor may demur, but if the judge or coroner insists, then further reluctance to divulge is at the risk of being in contempt of court. No legal action can be taken against the doctor who reveals medical information at the behest of a court.
5. Community interest may outweigh the doctor's commitment to confidentiality, for instance in the cases of criminal offence, especially serious assaults, rapes, or even homicide, which may be repeated by a person they know to be dangerous, psychopathic, or mentally disordered.

More often, the danger to the community is less dramatic, but may involve, for example, a public transport driver whom the doctor deems unfit to continue that employment. The patient may be reluctant to alter their employment voluntarily or to undergo further examination at the behest of their employer. If the doctor cannot persuade the employee to do this, the doctor should communicate, preferably with another doctor, such as an industrial medical adviser, but if no such person exists then the managing director of the employing firm should be informed. Where a doctor has a patient who develops epilepsy, there may be need to communicate with the medical officer of the Driving and Vehicle Licence Centre if the patient cannot be persuaded voluntarily to acknowledge their unfitness to drive.

Sometimes infectious diseases may require a breach of confidentiality, but most situations such as this are covered by statutory laws, especially where persons involved in food handling are concerned. A more common situation concerns child abuse, and here the over-riding consideration is the safety of the child. In all these cases, doctors may have to justify their breach of confidentiality to various bodies, including the General Medical Council. Where doubt remains, the protection or defence society can provide expert advice.

Consent

No mentally competent adult (over 16) need seek or accept medical diagnosis and treatment if they do not wish it. Thus all medical intervention must be preceded by consent, otherwise the actions of the doctor may constitute an assault.

Most medical practice is conducted with implied consent, where the very fact of a patient presenting before the doctor implies that he or she is willing to undergo diagnosis and treatment to a certain level. This implied consent covers the usual diagnostic procedures of history-taking, palpation, percussion, auscultation, and general physical examination.

For more invasive techniques of diagnosis or treatment, specific consent has to be obtained for each item of practice. In the taking of a blood sample, for example, the doctor must explain what they wish to do and the reasons for doing it, which the patient is quite entitled to reject. This obtaining of specific consent is known as express consent, and holds good only for one particular action. Express consent is often obtained in writing, almost always where a general anaesthetic or surgical procedure of any significance is contemplated. Written consent is no better in law than oral consent, but is much easier to validate if a dispute arises. Witnessed oral consent can be difficult to prove later if the witness has vanished.

Consent of any type is invalid if it is not informed. This concept has been the subject of many legal actions where patients claim that they did not give proper consent because they did not understand the implications of the procedure due to a failure of the doctor to explain them sufficiently. Explanation given in understandable language, applies not only to surgical operations, anaesthetics, or complex invasive diagnostic procedures, but also to the use of certain drug regimes that carry the risk of side-effects.

The degree to which a patient should have a full explanation varies greatly according to the complexity of the proposed procedure, to the doctor's estimation of the ability of the patient to understand the explanation, and to the relative risks involved. Although in North America it is common for virtually every possible risk to be explained, several legal cases in the UK have been settled on major risks as the criterion for explanation. A balance has to be made between the fullness of information and the possibility of frightening a patient by reciting every risk, including remote ones. Legal cases have established that peer review, i.e. the opinion of practising doctors in the same specialty, should be used to decide what risks should be explained to the patient in relation to any given procedure and, the consensus is that exceptional risks need not be explained.

Where procedures involving marital relations are involved, such as sterilization and termination of pregnancy, the wishes of the spouse are usually sought, although are not legally necessary.

Below the age of 16 years, consent should be sought from the parent or guardian, except in the case of emergencies. However, this does not invalidate consent from some persons below the age of 16 years, if that person is judged to have sufficient maturity of mind to appreciate the significance and risks of the proposed procedure.

Where the parent or guardian of a person below the age of 16 years refuses permission for an urgent procedure, the doctor's position is governed partly by personal ethics and partly by a legal mechanism, usually subservient to the doctor's decision. The situation usually arises from religious objections, notably Jehovah's Witnesses in respect of blood transfusions. Where transfusion is held to be a life-saving matter, the doctor may proceed according to his or her own conscience and trust that the court will uphold his or her view if it should come to litigation. Again the doctor is strongly advised to seek the advice of fellow physicians, especially of more senior level. A formal alternative, now rarely used, is to seek a court order, even in an emergency situation, to transfer the custody of a child to a fit person under the Children Act (1989). The Department of Health in the UK has directed that this procedure be abandoned and, if a doctor acts in good faith in urgent circumstances, they may rest assured that their protection or defence society and employing authority will uphold their decision, even against the parent's objections.

Consent obviously cannot be obtained where a patient is unconscious and, in an emergency situation, the doctor should proceed to act in the patient's best interest.

In the case of mentally impaired persons, if the procedure is not related to the mental defect and the patient is able to understand the nature of the procedure and has given consent, then this is valid. Where the patient is unable to understand the nature of the illness and proposed treatment the legal situation is unclear, as no one, not even the relatives, court, or judge can give consent on behalf of mentally disordered patients. What is usually done is that the doctor seeks approval of his/her actions from the guardian, relative, or responsible medical officer and can even apply to the court for a declaration of approval.

Where the procedure is related to the mental disorder of the patient, then complex rules exist under a variety of legal statutes including the Mental Health Act (1983) and the Mental Health (Hospital Guardianship and Consent to Treatment) Regulations (1983).

Further reading

Cordner, S.M. and Ransom, D.L. (1997). Forensic medicine: grim new role for forensic patholgist. *Lancet*, **350** (supp. III), Siii6.

de Zeeuw, R.A. (1998). Recent developments in analytical toxicology: for better or for worse. *Toxicology Letters*, **102–103**, 103--8.

Peat, M.A. (1998). Advances in forensic toxicology. *Clinics in Laboratory Medicine*, **18**, 263–78.

Index

Page numbers in *italics* refer to pages on which tables are to be found.